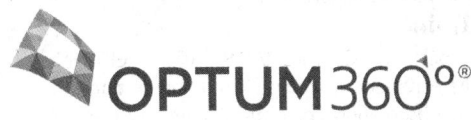

W9-CEF-960

PROFESSIONAL

ICD-10-CM Professional for Hospitals

The complete official code set

Codes valid from October 1, 2021, through September 30, 2022

2022   optum360coding.com

Publisher's Notice

The *ICD-10-CM Professional for Hospitals: The Complete Official Code Set* is designed to be an accurate and authoritative source regarding coding and every reasonable effort has been made to ensure accuracy and completeness of the content. However, Optum360 makes no guarantee, warranty, or representation that this publication is accurate, complete or without errors. It is understood that Optum360 is not rendering any legal or other professional services or advice in this publication and that Optum360 bears no liability for any results or consequences that may arise from the use of this book.

Acknowledgments

Marianne Randall, CPC, *Product Manager*
Anita Schmidt, BS, RHIA, AHIMA-approved ICD-10-CM/PCS Trainer, *Subject Matter Expert*
Karen Krawzik, RHIT, CCS, AHIMA-approved ICD-10-CM/PCS Trainer, *Subject Matter Expert*
Leanne Patterson, CPC, *Subject Matter Expert*
LaJuana Green, RHIA, CCS, *Subject Matter Expert*
Jacqueline R. Petersen, BS, RHIA, CHDA, CPC, *Subject Matter Expert*
Stacy Perry, *Manager, Desktop Publishing*
Tracy Betzler, *Senior Desktop Publishing Specialist*
Hope M. Dunn, *Senior Desktop Publishing Specialist*
Katie Russell, *Desktop Publishing Specialist*
Kate Holden, *Editor*

Our Commitment to Accuracy

Optum360 is committed to producing accurate and reliable materials.

To report corrections, please email accuracy@optum.com. You can also reach customer service by calling 1.800.464.3649, option 1.

Anita Schmidt, BS, RHIA, AHIMA-approved ICD-10-CM/PCS Trainer

Ms. Schmidt has expertise in ICD-10-CM/PCS, DRG, and CPT with more than 15 years' experience in coding in multiple settings, including inpatient, observation, and same-day surgery. Her experience includes analysis of medical record documentation, assignment of ICD-10-CM and PCS codes, and DRG validation. She has conducted training for ICD-10-CM/PCS and electronic health record. She has also collaborated with clinical documentation specialists to identify documentation needs and potential areas for physician education. Most recently she has been developing content for resource and educational products related to ICD-10-CM, ICD-10-PCS, DRG, and CPT. Ms. Schmidt is an AHIMA-approved ICD-10-CM/PCS trainer and is an active member of the American Health Information Management Association (AHIMA) and the Minnesota Health Information Management Association.

Karen Krawzik, RHIT, CCS, AHIMA-approved ICD-10-CM/PCS Trainer

Ms. Krawzik has expertise in ICD-10-CM, ICD-9-CM, CPT/HCPCS, DRG, and data quality and analytics, with more than 30 years' experience coding in multiple settings, including inpatient, observation, ambulatory surgery, ancillary, and emergency room. She has served as a DRG analyst and auditor of commercial and government payer claims, as a contract administrator, and worked on a team providing enterprise-wide conversion of the ICD-9-CM code set to ICD-10. More recently, she has been developing print and electronic content related to ICD-10-CM and ICD-10-PCS coding systems, MS-DRGs, and HCCs. Ms. Krawzik is credentialed by the American Health Information Management Association (AHIMA) as a Registered Health Information Technician (RHIT) and a Certified Coding Specialist (CCS) and is an AHIMA-approved ICD-10-CM/PCS trainer. She is an active member of AHIMA and the Missouri Health Information Management Association.

2022 ICD-10-CM Official Guidelines for Coding and Reporting

Optum360 is pleased to provide you with this 2022 ICD-10-CM code book that INCLUDES the 2022 Official Guidelines for Coding and Reporting.

Welcome to over 25 years of coding expertise.

Every medical organization knows that medical documentation and coding accuracy are vital to the revenue cycle. As a leading health services business, Optum360® has proudly created industry-leading coding, billing and reimbursement solutions for more than 25 years. Serving the broad health market, including physicians, health care organizations, payers and government, we help health systems reduce costs and achieve timely and accurate revenue.

You'll find ICD-10-CM/PCS, CPT®, HCPCS, DRG, specialty and reference content across our full suite of medical coding, billing and reimbursement products. And to ensure you have expert insight and the right information at your fingertips, our subject matter experts have incorporated proprietary features into these resources. These include supplementary edits and notations, coding tips and tools, and appendixes — making each product comprehensive and easy to use. Think of it as coding resources built by coders, for coders like you.

Your coding, billing and reimbursement product team,

Ryan   Nichole   Greg   LaJuana
Ken
Jacqui   Marianne   Denise   Leanne
Anita   Debbie   Elizabeth   Nann
Karen

Put Optum360 medical coding, billing and reimbursement content at your fingertips today. Choose what works for you.

📖 Print books

🖥 Online coding tools

📁 Data files

🖥 Web services

Visit us at **optum360coding.com** to browse our products, or call us at **1-800-464-3649, option 1,** for more information.

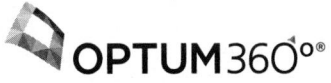

At our core, we're about coding.

Essential medical code sets are just that — essential to your revenue cycle. In our ICD-10-CM/PCS, CPT®, HCPCS and DRG coding tools, we apply our collective coding expertise to present these code set resources in a way that is comprehensive, plus easy to use and apply. Print books are budget-friendly and easily referenced, created with intuitive features and formats, such as visual alerts, color-coding and symbols to identify important coding notes and instructions — plus, great coding tips.

Find the same content, tips and features of our code books in a variety of formats. Choose from print products, online coding tools, data files or web services.

Your coding, billing and reimbursement product team,

Ryan Nichole Greg LaJuana
Ken
Jacqui Marianne Denise Leanne
Anita Debbie Elizabeth Nann
Karen

Put Optum360 medical coding, billing and reimbursement content at your fingertips today. Choose what works for you.

📖 Print books

🛠 Online coding tools

📁 Data files

🖥 Web services

Visit us at **optum360coding.com** to browse our products, or call us at **1-800-464-3649, option 1,** for more information.

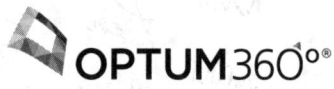

CPT is a registered trademark of the American Medical Association.

Contents

Preface

ICD-10-CM Official Preface

This FY 2022 update of the International Statistical Classification of Diseases and Related Health Problems, 10th revision, Clinical Modification (ICD-10-CM) is being published by the United States government in recognition of its responsibility to promulgate this classification throughout the United States for morbidity coding. The International Statistical Classification of Diseases and Related Health Problems, 10th Revision (ICD-10), published by the World Health Organization (WHO), is the foundation of ICD-10-CM. ICD-10 continues to be the classification used in cause-of-death coding in the United States. The ICD-10-CM is comparable with the ICD-10. The WHO Collaborating Center for the Family of International Classifications in North America, housed at the Centers for Disease Control and Prevention's National Center for Health Statistics (NCHS), has responsibility for the implementation of ICD and other WHO-FIC classifications and serves as a liaison with the WHO, fulfilling international obligations for comparable classifications and the national health data needs of the United States. The historical background of ICD and ICD-10 can be found in the Introduction to the International Classification of Diseases and Related Health Problems (ICD-10), 2010, World Health Organization, Geneva, Switzerland.

ICD-10-CM is the United States' clinical modification of the World Health Organization's ICD-10. The term "clinical" is used to emphasize the modification's intent: to serve as a useful tool in the area of classification of morbidity data for indexing of health records, medical care review, and ambulatory and other health care programs, as well as for basic health statistics. To describe the clinical picture of the patient the codes must be more precise than those needed only for statistical groupings and trend analysis.

Characteristics of ICD-10-CM

ICD-10-CM far exceeds its predecessors in the number of concepts and codes provided. The disease classification has been expanded to include health-related conditions and to provide greater specificity at the sixth and seventh character level. The sixth and seventh characters are not optional and are intended for use in recording the information documented in the clinical record.

ICD-10-CM extensions, interpretations, modifications, addenda, or errata other than those approved by the Centers for Disease Control and Prevention are not to be considered official and should not be utilized. Continuous maintenance of the ICD-10-CM is the responsibility of the aforementioned agencies. However, because the ICD-10-CM represents the best in contemporary thinking of clinicians, nosologists, epidemiologists, and statisticians from both public and private sectors, when future modifications are considered, advice will be sought from all stakeholders.

All official authorized addenda since the last complete update (October 1, 2021) have been included in this revision. For more detailed information please see the complete official authorized addenda to ICD-10-CM, including the "ICD-10-CM Official Guidelines for Coding and Reporting," and a description of the ICD-10-CM updating and maintenance process.

How to Use ICD-10-CM Professional for Hospitals 2022

Introduction

ICD-10-CM Professional for Hospitals: The Complete Official Code Set is your definitive coding resource, combining the work of the National Center for Health Statistics (NCHS), Centers for Medicare and Medicaid Services (CMS), American Hospital Association (AHA), and Optum360 experts to provide the information you need for coding accuracy.

The International Classification of Diseases, 10th Revision, Clinical Modification (ICD-10-CM), is an adaptation of ICD-10, copyrighted by the World Health Organization (WHO). The development and maintenance of this clinical modification (CM) is the responsibility of the NCHS as authorized by WHO. Any new concepts added to ICD-10-CM are based on an established update process through the collaboration of WHO's Update and Revision Committee and the ICD-10-CM Coordination and Maintenance Committee.

In addition to the ICD-10-CM classification, other official government source information has been included in this manual. Depending on the source, updates to information may be annual or quarterly. This manual provides the most current information that was available at the time of publication. For updates to the source documents that may have occurred after this manual was published, please refer to the following:

- **NCHS, International Classification of Diseases, Tenth Revision, Clinical Modification (ICD-10-CM)**

  https://www.cdc.gov/nchs/icd/icd10cm.htm

  https://www.cms.gov/medicare/icd-10/2022-icd-10-cm

- **CMS Inpatient Prospective Payment System Proposed Rule, FY2022**

  https://www.cms.gov/medicare/acute-inpatient-pps/fy-2022-ipps-proposed-rule-home-page

- **CMS Inpatient Prospective Payment System Proposed Rule, FY 2022 — Proposed, version 39, MS-DRG grouper software, Definitions Manual files and Medicare Code Editor (MCE) Files**

  https://www.cms.gov/Medicare/Medicare-Fee-for-Service-Payment/AcuteInpatientPPS/MS-DRG-Classifications-and-Software

- **CMS Risk Adjustment Model, version 24**

  https://www.cms.gov/Medicare/Health-Plans/MedicareAdvtgSpecRateStats/Risk-Adjustors.html

- **CMS Long-term Care Hospital Prospective Payment System Proposed Rule and Data Files, FY 2022**

  https://www.cms.gov/medicaremedicare-fee-service-paymentlong termcarehospitalppsltchpps-regulations-and-notices/cms-1752-p

- **AHA Coding Clinics**

  https://www.codingclinicadvisor.com/

- **Additional specialty-specific resources will also be provided on our product updates page at Optum360coding.com, which can be accessed at the following:**

  https://www.optum360coding.com/ProductUpdates/

  Password: Hospital22

The official NCHS ICD-10-CM classification includes three main sections: the guidelines, the indexes, and the tabular list, all of which make up the bulk of this coding manual. To complement the classification, Optum360's coding experts have incorporated Medicare-related coding edits and proprietary features, such as supplementary notations, coding tools, and appendixes, into a comprehensive and easy-to-use reference. This publication is organized as follows:

What's New for 2022

This section provides a high-level overview of the changes made to the ICD-10-CM official code set for fiscal 2022, identifying codes that have been added and deleted from the classification, codes that had validity changes as a result of these additions and deletions, as well as codes that had revisions to their descriptions. All changes are based on the 2022 official addendum, posted June 23, 2021, by the National Center for Health Statistics (NCHS), the agency charged with maintaining and updating ICD-10-CM. NCHS is part of the Centers for Disease Control and Prevention (CDC).

Conversion Table

The conversion table was developed by National Center for Healthcare Statistics (NCHS) to help facilitate data retrieval as new codes are added to the ICD-10-CM classification. This table provides a crosswalk from each FY 2022 new code to the equivalent code(s) assigned prior to October 1, 2021, for that particular diagnosis or condition. For the full conversion table, including code crosswalks before October 1, 2021 refer to the 2022 Conversion Table zip file at https://www.cms.gov/medicare/icd-10/2022-icd-10-cm.

10 Steps to Correct Coding

This step-by-step tutorial walks the coder through the process of finding the correct code — from locating the code in the official indexes to verifying the code in the tabular section — while following applicable conventions, guidelines, and instructional notes. Specific examples are provided with detailed explanations of each coding step along with advice for proper sequencing.

Official ICD-10-CM Guidelines for Coding and Reporting

This section provides the full official conventions and guidelines regulating the appropriate assignment and reporting of ICD-10-CM codes. These conventions and guidelines are published by the U.S. Department of Health and Human Services (DHHS) and approved by the cooperating parties (American Health Information Management Association [AHIMA], National Center for Health Statistics [NCHS], Centers for Disease Control and Prevention [CDC], and the American Hospital Association [AHA]).

Indexes

Index to Diseases and Injuries

The Index to Diseases and Injuries is arranged in alphabetic order by terms specific to a disease, condition, illness, injury, eponym, or abbreviation as well as terms that describe circumstances other than a disease or injury that may require attention from a health care professional.

Neoplasm Table

The Neoplasm Table is arranged in alphabetic order by anatomical site. Codes are then listed in individual columns based upon the histological behavior (malignant, in situ, benign, uncertain, or unspecified) of the neoplasm.

Table of Drugs and Chemicals

The Table of Drugs and Chemicals is arranged in alphabetic order by the specific drug or chemical name. Codes are listed in individual columns based upon the associated intent (poisoning, adverse effect, or underdosing).

External Causes Index

The External Causes Index is arranged in alphabetic order by main terms that describe the cause, the intent, the place of occurrence, the activity, and the status of the patient at the time the injury occurred or health condition arose.

Index Notations

With

The word "with" or "in" should be interpreted to mean "associated with" or "due to." The classification presumes a causal relationship between the two conditions linked by these terms in the index. These conditions should be coded as related even in the absence of provider documentation explicitly linking them unless the documentation clearly states the conditions are unrelated or when another guideline specifically requires a documented linkage between two conditions (e.g., the sepsis guideline for "acute organ dysfunction that is not clearly associated with the sepsis"). For conditions not specifically linked by these relational terms in the classification or when a guideline requires explicit documentation of a linkage between two conditions, provider documentation must link the conditions to code them as related.

The word "with" in the index is sequenced immediately following the main term, not in alphabetical order.

> **Dermatopolymyositis** M33.90
> with
> myopathy M33.92
> respiratory involvement M33.91
> specified organ involvement NEC M33.99
> in neoplastic disease — *see also* Neoplasm D49.9 *[M36.0]*

See

When the instruction "see" follows a term in the index, it indicates that another term must be referenced to locate the correct code.

> **Hematoperitoneum** — *see* Hemoperitoneum

See Also

The instructional note "see also" simply provides alternative terms the coder may reference that may be useful in determining the correct code but are not necessary to follow if the main term supplies the appropriate code.

> **Hematinuria** — *see also* Hemaglobinuria
> malarial B50.8

Default Codes

In the index, the default code is the code listed next to the main term and represents the condition most commonly associated with that main term. This code may be assigned when documentation does not support reporting a more specific code. Alternatively, it may provide an unspecified code for the condition.

> **Hemiatrophy** R68.89
> cerebellar G31.9
> face, facial, progressive (Romberg) G51.8
> tongue K14.8

Parentheses

Parentheses in the indexes enclose nonessential modifiers, supplementary words that may be present or absent in the statement of a disease without affecting the code.

> **Pseudomeningocele** (cerebral) (infective) (post-traumatic) G96.198
> postprocedural (spinal) G97.82

Brackets

ICD-10-CM has a coding convention addressing code assignment for manifestations that occur as a result of an underlying condition. This convention requires the underlying condition to be sequenced first, followed by the code or codes for the associated manifestation. In the index, italicized codes in brackets identify manifestation codes.

> **Polyneuropathy** (peripheral) G62.9
> alcoholic G62.1
> amyloid (Portuguese) E85.1 *[G63]*
> transthyretin-related (ATTR) familial E85.1 *[G63]*

Shaded Guides

Exclusive vertical shaded guides in the Index to Diseases and Injuries and External Causes Index help the user easily follow the indent levels for the subentries under a main term. Sequencing rules may apply depending on the level of indent for separate subentries.

> **Hemicrania**
> congenital malformation Q00.0
> continua G44.51
> meaning migraine — *see also* Migraine G43.909
> paroxysmal G44.039
> chronic G44.049
> intractable G44.041
> not intractable G44.049
> episodic G44.039
> intractable G44.031
> not intractable G44.039
> intractable G44.031
> not intractable G44.039

Following References

The Index to Diseases and Injuries includes following references to assist in locating out-of-sequence codes in the tabular list. Out-of-sequence codes contain an alphabetic character (letter) in the third- or fourth-character position. These codes are placed according to the classification rules — according to condition — not according to alphabetic or numeric sequencing rules.

> **Carcinoma** (malignant) — *see also* Neoplasm, by site, malignant
> neuroendocrine — *see also* Tumor, neuroendocrine
> high grade, any site C7A.1 (*following* C75)
> poorly differentiated, any site C7A.1 (*following* C75)

Additional Character Required

The Index to Diseases and Injuries, Neoplasm Table, and External Causes Index provide an icon after certain codes to signify to the user that additional characters are required to make the code valid. The tabular list should be consulted for appropriate character selection.

> **Fall, falling** (accidental) W19 ☑
> building W20.1 ☑

Tabular List of Diseases

ICD-10-CM codes and descriptions are arranged numerically within the tabular list of diseases with 19 separate chapters providing codes associated with a particular body system or nature of injury or disease. There is also a chapter providing codes for external causes of an injury or health conditions, a chapter for codes that address encounters with healthcare facilities for circumstances other than a disease or injury, and finally a chapter for codes that capture special circumstances such as new diseases of uncertain etiology or emergency use codes.

Code and Code Descriptions

ICD-10-CM is an alphanumeric classification system that contains categories, subcategories, and valid codes. The first character is always a letter with any additional characters represented by either a letter or number. A three-character category without further subclassification is equivalent to a valid three-character code. Valid codes may be three, four, five, six, or seven characters in length, with each level of subdivision after a three-character category representing a subcategory. The final level of subdivision is a valid code.

Boldface

Boldface type is used for all codes and descriptions in the tabular list.

Italics

Italicized type is used to identify manifestation codes, those codes that should not be reported as first-listed diagnoses.

Deleted Text

~~Strikethrough~~ on a code and code description indicates a deletion from the classification for the current year.

Key Word

Green font is used throughout the Tabular List of Diseases to differentiate the key words that appear in similar code descriptions in a given category or subcategory. The key word convention is used only in those categories in which there are multiple codes with very similar descriptions with only a few words that differentiate them.

For example, refer to the list of codes below from category H55:

☑4ᵗʰ **H55**	**Nystagmus and other** irregular eye movements
☑5ᵗʰ **H55.0**	**Nystagmus**
H55.00	**Unspecified nystagmus**
H55.01	Congenital **nystagmus**
H55.02	Latent **nystagmus**
H55.03	Visual deprivation **nystagmus**
H55.04	Dissociated **nystagmus**
H55.09	**Other forms of nystagmus**

The portion of the code description that appears in green font in the tabular list helps the coder quickly identify the key terms and the correct code. This convention is especially useful when the codes describe laterality, such as the following codes from subcategory H40.22:

☑6ᵗʰ **H40.22**	Chronic **angle-closure glaucoma**
	Chronic primary angle-closure glaucoma
☑7ᵗʰ **H40.221**	**Chronic angle-closure glaucoma,** right **eye**
☑7ᵗʰ **H40.222**	**Chronic angle-closure glaucoma,** left **eye**
☑7ᵗʰ **H40.223**	**Chronic angle-closure glaucoma,** bilateral
☑7ᵗʰ **H40.229**	**Chronic angle-closure glaucoma, unspecified eye**

Tabular Notations

Official parenthetical notes as well as Optum360's supplementary notations are provided at the chapter, code block, category, subcategory, and individual code level to help the user assign proper codes. The information in the notation can apply to one or more codes depending on where the citation is placed.

Official Notations

Includes Notes

The word [INCLUDES] appears immediately under certain categories to further define, clarify, or give examples of the content of a code category.

Inclusion Terms

Lists of inclusion terms are included under certain codes. These terms indicate some of the conditions for which that code number may be used. Inclusion terms may be synonyms with the code title, or, in the case of "other specified" codes, the terms may also provide a list of various conditions included within a classification code. The inclusion terms are not exhaustive. The index may provide additional terms that may also be assigned to a given code.

Excludes Notes

ICD-10-CM has two types of excludes notes. Each note has a different definition for use. However, they are similar in that they both indicate that codes excluded from each other are independent of each other.

Excludes 1

An [EXCLUDES 1] note is a "pure" excludes. It means "NOT CODED HERE!" An Excludes 1 note indicates mutually exclusive codes: two conditions that cannot be reported together. An Excludes1 note indicates that the code excluded should never be used at the same time as the code above the Excludes1 note. An Excludes1 is used when two conditions cannot occur together, such as a congenital form versus an acquired form of the same condition.

An exception to the Excludes 1 definition is when the two conditions are unrelated to each other. If it is not clear whether the two conditions involving an Excludes 1 note are related or not, query the provider. For example, code F45.8 Other somatoform disorders, has an Excludes 1 note for "sleep related teeth grinding (G47.63)" because "teeth grinding" is an inclusion term under F45.8. Only one of these two codes should be assigned for teeth grinding. However, psychogenic dysmenorrhea is also an inclusion term under F45.8, and a patient could have both this condition and sleep-related teeth grinding. In this case, the two conditions are clearly unrelated to each other, so it would be appropriate to report F45.8 and G47.63 together.

Excludes 2

An [EXCLUDES 2] note means "NOT INCLUDED HERE." An Excludes 2 note indicates that although the excluded condition is not part of the condition it is excluded from, a patient may have both conditions at the same time. Therefore, when an Excludes 2 note appears under a code, it may be acceptable to use both the code and the excluded code together if supported by the medical documentation.

Note

The term "NOTE" appears as an icon and precedes the instructional information. These notes function as alerts to highlight coding instructions within the text.

Code First/Use additional code

These instructional notes provide sequencing instruction. They may appear independently of each other or to designate certain etiology/manifestation paired codes. These instructions signal the coder that an additional code should be reported to provide a more complete picture of that diagnosis.

In etiology/manifestation coding, ICD-10-CM requires the underlying condition to be sequenced first, followed by the manifestation. In these situations, codes with "In diseases classified elsewhere" in the code description are never permitted as a first-listed or principal diagnosis code and must be sequenced following the underlying condition code.

Code Also

A "code also" note alerts the coder that more than one code may be required to fully describe the condition. The sequencing depends on the circumstances of the encounter. Factors that may determine sequencing include severity and reason for the encounter.

Revised Text

The revised text ▶◀ "bow ties" alert the user to changes in official notations for the current year. Revised text may include the following:

- A change in a current parenthetical description
- A change in the code(s) associated with a current parenthetical note
- A change in how a current parenthetical note is classified (e.g., an Excludes 1 note that changed to an Excludes 2 note)
- Addition of a new parenthetical note(s) to a code

Deleted Text

~~Strikethrough~~ on official notations indicate a deletion from the classification for the current year.

Optum360 Notations

AHA Coding Clinic Citations

Coding Clinics are official American Hospital Association (AHA) publications that provide coding advice specific to ICD-10-CM and ICD-10-PCS.

Coding Clinic citations included in this manual are current up to the second quarter of 2021.

These citations identify the year, quarter, and page number of one or more *Coding Clinic* publications that may have coding advice relevant to a particular code or group of codes. With the most current citation listed first, these notations are preceded by the symbol **AHA:** and appear in purple type.

I15.1	Hypertension secondary to other renal disorders
	AHA: 2016, 3Q, 22

Definitions

Definitions explain a specific term, condition, or disease process in layman's terms. These notations are preceded by the symbol **DEF:** and appear in purple type.

✓5ᵗʰ M51.4 Schmorl's nodes
DEF: Irregular bone defect in the margin of the vertebral body that causes herniation into the end plate of the vertebral body.

Coding Tips

The tips in the tabular list offer coding advice that is not readily available within the ICD-10-CM classification. It may relate official coding guidelines, indexing nuances, or advice from *AHA's Coding Clinic for ICD-10-CM/PCS*. These notations are preceded by the symbol **TIP:** and appear in brown type.

✓5ᵗʰ B97.2 Coronavirus as the cause of diseases classified elsewhere
TIP: Do not report a code from this subcategory for COVID-19; refer to U07.1.

Icons

Note: The following icons are placed to the left of the code.

● **New Code**
Codes that have been added to the classification system for the current year.

▲ **Revised Code Title**
Codes that have had a change to their description or validity change for the current year. For additional information on codes with validity changes, see the "What's New" section.

☑ **Additional Characters Required**

✓4ᵗʰ This symbol indicates that the code requires a 4th character.

✓5ᵗʰ This symbol indicates that the code requires a 5th character.

✓6ᵗʰ This symbol indicates that the code requires a 6th character.

✓7ᵗʰ This symbol indicates that the code requires a 7th character.

✓5ᵗʰ H60.3 Other infective otitis externa
✓6ᵗʰ H60.31 Diffuse otitis externa
H60.311 Diffuse otitis externa, right ear
H60.312 Diffuse otitis externa, left ear
H60.313 Diffuse otitis externa, bilateral
H60.319 Diffuse otitis externa, unspecified ear

✓x7ᵗʰ **Placeholder Alert**
This symbol indicates that the code requires a 7th character following the placeholder "X". Codes with fewer than six characters that require a 7th character must contain placeholder "X" to fill in the empty character(s).

✓x7ᵗʰ T16.1 Foreign body in right ear

This manual provides the most current information that was available at the time of publication. Except where otherwise noted, the icons and/or color bars reflect edits associated with the inpatient prospective payment system (IPPS). Because the fiscal 2021 IPPS final rule was not available at the time this book was printed, the edits in this manual are based on the proposed, version 39, MS-DRG grouper software, Definitions Manual files, and Medicare Code Editor (MCE) files, published with the fiscal 2022 IPPS proposed rule.

In an effort to provide the most current edit information, Optum360 has provided a searchable data file that includes the final edit designations for all ICD-10-CM codes based on the fiscal 2022 IPPS final rule official files, effective October 1, 2021. The edits included in the data file are as follows:

- Age
- Sex
- Hospital-acquired condition (HAC)
- CC
- MCC
- HIV
- Manifestation code
- Unacceptable principal diagnosis
- Questionable principal diagnosis

This data file can be accessed at the following:

https://www.optum360coding.com/ProductUpdates/
Title: "2022 ICD-10-CM for Hospital IPPS Data File"
Password: Hospital22

Note: The following icons are placed at the end of the code description.

Age Edits

Ⓝ Newborn Age: 0

These diagnoses are intended for newborns and neonates and the patient's age must be 0 years.

N47.0 Adherent prepuce, newborn	Ⓝ♂

Ⓟ Pediatric Age: 0-17

These diagnoses are intended for children and the patient's age must be between 0 and 17 years.

L21.1 Seborrheic infantile dermatitis	Ⓟ

Ⓜ Maternity Age: 9-64

These diagnoses are intended for childbearing patients between the age of 9 and 64 years.

O02.9 Abnormal product of conception, unspecified	Ⓜ♀

Ⓐ Adult Age: 15-124

These diagnoses are intended for patients between the age of 15 and 124 years.

R54 Age-related physical debility	Ⓐ

> Frailty
> Old age
> Senescence
> Senile asthenia
> Senile debility
> **EXCLUDES 1** *age-related cognitive decline (R41.81)*
> *sarcopenia (M62.84)*
> *senile psychosis (F03)*
> *senility NOS (R41.81)*

Sex Edits

♂ Male diagnosis only

Q98.0 Klinefelter syndrome karyotype 47, XXY	♂

♀ Female diagnosis only

N35.12 Postinfective urethral stricture, not elsewhere classified, female	♀

H1 - H14 Hospital Acquired Condition (HAC)

These codes identify conditions that are high cost or high volume or both, are either a complication or comorbidity (CC) or major complication or comorbidity (MCC) that as a secondary diagnosis results in assignment of a case to a higher-paying MS-DRG. These conditions are reasonably preventable through the application of evidence-based guidelines. If the condition is not present on admission (meaning it developed during the hospital admission), the case will not group to the higher-paying MS-DRG based solely upon the reporting of the HAC code. Many of these HACs are conditional, and are based on reporting the specific diagnosis code(s) in combination with certain procedure codes.

Note: Hospital-acquired conditions do not impact MS-LTC-DRG assignment.

N15.1 Renal and perinephric abscess	MCC H6

CC Condition

This symbol designates a complication or comorbidity diagnosis that may affect DRG assignment. A complication or comorbidity diagnosis, CC condition, is defined as a significant acute disease, a significant acute manifestation of a chronic disease, an advanced or end-stage chronic disease, or a chronic disease associated with systemic physiological decompensation and debility that have consistently greater impact on hospital resources.

G90.59 Complex regional pain syndrome I of other specified site	CC

MCC Condition

This symbol designates a major complication or comorbidity diagnosis that may affect DRG assignment. An MCC condition meets the same criteria as a CC condition but is associated with a higher acuity level and hospital resource consumption is expected to be higher than that for a CC condition. There are fewer conditions that meet the criteria as an MCC than those for a CC condition.

✓7ᵗʰ **S35.238 Other injury of inferior mesenteric artery**	MCC

Note: The assignment of an MS-DRG or MS-LTC-DRG often depends on the presence or absence of a secondary diagnosis code that is designated as an MCC or CC. However, in some instances the MCC or CC designation for that secondary diagnosis code is negated due to its relationship with the principal diagnosis; this is referred to as CC exclusion. The ICD-10 MS-DRG Definitions Manual included with the IPPS final rule provides a list of all principal diagnosis codes that would render ineffective the MCC/CC designation for a particular ICD-10-CM code when used as a secondary diagnosis. Optum360 has provided this CC exclusion list in an easily searchable data file, which can be accessed at the following:

https://www.optum360coding.com/ProductUpdates/
Title: "2022 ICD-10-CM for Hospitals CC Excludes Data File"
Password: Hospital22

UPD Unacceptable Principal Diagnosis

This symbol identifies codes that should not be assigned as principal diagnosis for *inpatient* admissions. Codes with an unacceptable principal diagnosis edit are considered supplementary — describing circumstances that influence an individual's health status or an additional code — identifying conditions that are not specific manifestations but may be due to an underlying cause.

✓7ᵗʰ **T48.5X5 Adverse effect** of other anti-common-cold drugs	UPD

HIV HIV-related Condition

This symbol indicates that the condition is considered a major HIV-related diagnosis. When the condition is coded in combination with a diagnosis of human immunodeficiency virus (HIV), code B20, the case will move from MS-DRG/MS-LTC-DRG 977 to MS-DRGs/MS-LTC-DRGs 974-976.

G96.9 Disorder of central nervous system, unspecified	HIV

HCC CMS-HCC Condition

Identify conditions that are considered a CMS-HCC (hierarchical condition category) diagnosis.

The HCC codes represented in this manual have been updated to reflect the 2022 Initial ICD-10-CM Mappings for CMS-HCC Model v24. Midyear final mappings were not available at the time this publication went to print; refer to the following CMS website for final mappings: https://www.cms.gov/Medicare/Health-Plans/MedicareAdvtgSpecRateStats/Risk-Adjustors.html.

Y62.2 Failure of sterile precautions during kidney dialysis and other perfusion	HCC

SW Severe Wound Diagnosis

This symbol indicates that the condition is considered a severe wound diagnosis. Depending on the facility from which the patient is discharged, these conditions may not require that the payment rate for that admission be adjusted.

L89.014 Pressure ulcer of right elbow, stage 4	MCC H4 HCC SW

Color Bars

Manifestation Code

Codes defined as manifestation codes appear in italic type, with a blue color bar over the code description. A manifestation cannot be reported as a first-listed code; it is sequenced as a secondary diagnosis with the underlying disease code listed first.

G32.89	*Other specified degenerative disorders of nervous system in diseases classified elsewhere*
	Degenerative encephalopathy in diseases classified elsewhere

Questionable Admission Diagnoses

Questionable admission diagnoses will appear with a yellow color bar over the code description. These codes, although not unacceptable as a PDx, may be considered a "questionable admission" when used as PDx in an acute care hospital.

E66.09	**Other obesity due to excess calories**

Wrong Procedure Performed Edit

An orange color bar over the code title indicates the Wrong Procedure Performed edit. This edit was created to identify cases in which wrong surgeries occurred. Any claim with a code from Y65.51-Y65.53 will be denied and returned to the provider. A surgical or other invasive procedure is considered to be a wrong procedure if one of the following is true:

- The procedure was performed on the wrong site.

- The procedure was performed on the wrong patient.

- The incorrect procedure was performed on a patient.

Y65.51	**Performance of wrong procedure (operation) on correct patient**
	Wrong device implanted into correct surgical site
	EXCLUDES 1 *performance of correct procedure (operation) on wrong side or body part (Y65.53)*

Unspecified Diagnosis

Codes that appear with a gray color bar over the alphanumeric code identify unspecified diagnoses. These codes should be used in limited circumstances, when neither the diagnostic statement nor the documentation provides enough information to assign a more specific diagnosis code. The abbreviation NOS, "not otherwise specified," in the tabular list may be interpreted as "unspecified."

G03.9	**Meningitis, unspecified**	MCC
	Arachnoiditis (spinal) NOS	

Footnotes

Certain codes in the tabular section have a numerical superscript located to the upper left of the code. This numerical superscript corresponds to a specific footnote description.

For example:

[1] R57.1	Hypovolemic shock	MCC HCC

For convenience, the footnote descriptions are provided on the front cover.

The following list also provides the footnote descriptions of all numerical superscripts found in the Tabular List of Diseases:

1 These codes are considered major complication/comorbidity (MCC) conditions only if the patient is discharged alive.

2 This condition is considered an MCC only when reported as an initial encounter for an open fracture (7th character B or C specific to category).

3 This condition is considered a CC only when reported as an initial encounter for a fracture (7th character A, B, or C specific to category) or a subsequent encounter for nonunion or malunion fracture (7th character K, M, N, P, Q, or R specific to category).

4 This condition is considered a CC only when reported as a subsequent encounter for a nonunion or malunion fracture (7th character K, M, N, P, Q, or R specific to category).

5 This condition is considered a CC only when reported as an initial encounter or subsequent encounter (7th character A or D).

6 This condition is considered an HCC when reported as initial encounter (7th character A, B, or C specific to category).

7 This condition is considered an HCC when reported as initial encounter (7th character A or B specific to category) or as a sequela.

8 This condition is considered an HCC when reported as a sequela.

Chapter-Level Notations

Chapter-Specific Guidelines with Coding Examples

Each chapter begins with the Official Guidelines for Coding and Reporting specific to that chapter, where provided. Coding examples specific to inpatient care settings have been provided to illustrate the coding and/or sequencing guidance in these guidelines.

Muscle and Tendon Table

ICD-10-CM categorizes certain muscles and tendons in the upper and lower extremities by their action (e.g., extension or flexion) as well as their anatomical location. The Muscle/Tendon table is provided at the beginning of chapter 13 and chapter 19 to help users when code selection depends on the action of the muscle and/or tendon.

Note: This table is not all-inclusive, and proper code assignment should be based on the provider's documentation.

Illustrations

This section includes illustrations of normal anatomy with ICD-10-CM-specific terminology.

What's New for 2022

Official Updates

The official ICD-10-CM addendum identifies changes to the ICD-10-CM code set for fiscal 2022, effective October 1, 2021, to September 30, 2022. These changes were made by the agency charged with maintaining and updating the ICD-10-CM code set, the National Center for Health Statistics (NCHS), a section of the Centers for Disease Control and Prevention (CDC). A summary of the changes is provided below.

14 Codes with a Change in Validity

Note: Validity changes are the result of codes being added to or deleted from the classification. Codes that change from valid to invalid allow the creation of a new subcategory to which new codes can be assigned that provide greater detail about the condition. Codes that change from invalid to valid are the result of codes being deleted from a subcategory in the classification, when the detail provided in those codes is no longer required.

Valid to Invalid

D55.2	F78	G92	K22.8	M31.1	M54.5	P09
R05	R35.8	R63.3	Z59.0	Z59.4	Z59.8	Z91.5

Invalid to Valid

No applicable codes

18 Codes Deleted from the Classification

T40.7X1A	Poisoning by cannabis (derivatives), accidental (unintentional), initial encounter
T40.7X1D	Poisoning by cannabis (derivatives), accidental (unintentional), subsequent encounter
T40.7X1S	Poisoning by cannabis (derivatives), accidental (unintentional), sequela
T40.7X2A	Poisoning by cannabis (derivatives), intentional self-harm, initial encounter
T40.7X2D	Poisoning by cannabis (derivatives), intentional self-harm, subsequent encounter
T40.7X2S	Poisoning by cannabis (derivatives), intentional self-harm, sequela
T40.7X3A	Poisoning by cannabis (derivatives), assault, initial encounter
T40.7X3D	Poisoning by cannabis (derivatives), assault, subsequent encounter
T40.7X3S	Poisoning by cannabis (derivatives), assault, sequela
T40.7X4A	Poisoning by cannabis (derivatives), undetermined, initial encounter
T40.7X4D	Poisoning by cannabis (derivatives), undetermined, subsequent encounter
T40.7X4S	Poisoning by cannabis (derivatives), undetermined, sequela
T40.7X5A	Adverse effect of cannabis (derivatives), initial encounter
T40.7X5D	Adverse effect of cannabis (derivatives), subsequent encounter
T40.7X5S	Adverse effect of cannabis (derivatives), sequela
T40.7X6A	Underdosing of cannabis (derivatives), initial encounter
T40.7X6D	Underdosing of cannabis (derivatives), subsequent encounter
T40.7X6S	Underdosing of cannabis (derivatives), sequela

159 New Codes Added to the Classification

A79.82	Anaplasmosis [A. phagocytophilum]
C56.3	Malignant neoplasm of bilateral ovaries
C79.63	Secondary malignant neoplasm of bilateral ovaries
C84.7A	Anaplastic large cell lymphoma, ALK-negative, breast
D55.21	Anemia due to pyruvate kinase deficiency
D55.29	Anemia due to other disorders of glycolytic enzymes
D75.838	Other thrombocytosis
D75.839	Thrombocytosis, unspecified
D89.44	Hereditary alpha tryptasemia
E75.244	Niemann-Pick disease type A/B
F32.A	Depression, unspecified
F78.A1	SYNGAP1-related intellectual disability
F78.A9	Other genetic related intellectual disability
G04.82	Acute flaccid myelitis
G44.86	Cervicogenic headache
G92.00	Immune effector cell-associated neurotoxicity syndrome, grade unspecified
G92.01	Immune effector cell-associated neurotoxicity syndrome, grade 1
G92.02	Immune effector cell-associated neurotoxicity syndrome, grade 2
G92.03	Immune effector cell-associated neurotoxicity syndrome, grade 3
G92.04	Immune effector cell-associated neurotoxicity syndrome, grade 4
G92.05	Immune effector cell-associated neurotoxicity syndrome, grade 5
G92.8	Other toxic encephalopathy
G92.9	Unspecified toxic encephalopathy
I5A	Non-ischemic myocardial injury (non-traumatic)
K22.81	Esophageal polyp
K22.82	Esophagogastric junction polyp
K22.89	Other specified disease of esophagus
K31.A0	Gastric intestinal metaplasia, unspecified
K31.A11	Gastric intestinal metaplasia without dysplasia, involving the antrum
K31.A12	Gastric intestinal metaplasia without dysplasia, involving the body (corpus)
K31.A13	Gastric intestinal metaplasia without dysplasia, involving the fundus
K31.A14	Gastric intestinal metaplasia without dysplasia, involving the cardia
K31.A15	Gastric intestinal metaplasia without dysplasia, involving multiple sites
K31.A19	Gastric intestinal metaplasia without dysplasia, unspecified site
K31.A21	Gastric intestinal metaplasia with low grade dysplasia
K31.A22	Gastric intestinal metaplasia with high grade dysplasia
K31.A29	Gastric intestinal metaplasia with dysplasia, unspecified
L24.A0	Irritant contact dermatitis due to friction or contact with body fluids, unspecified
L24.A1	Irritant contact dermatitis due to saliva
L24.A2	Irritant contact dermatitis due to fecal, urinary or dual incontinence

L24.A9	Irritant contact dermatitis due friction or contact with other specified body fluids	R05.3	Chronic cough
L24.B0	Irritant contact dermatitis related to unspecified stoma or fistula	R05.4	Cough syncope
		R05.8	Other specified cough
L24.B1	Irritant contact dermatitis related to digestive stoma or fistula	R05.9	Cough, unspecified
		R35.81	Nocturnal polyuria
L24.B2	Irritant contact dermatitis related to respiratory stoma or fistula	R35.89	Other polyuria
		R45.88	Nonsuicidal self-harm
L24.B3	Irritant contact dermatitis related to fecal or urinary stoma or fistula	R63.30	Feeding difficulties, unspecified
		R63.31	Pediatric feeding disorder, acute
M31.10	Thrombotic microangiopathy, unspecified	R63.32	Pediatric feeding disorder, chronic
M31.11	Hematopoietic stem cell transplantation-associated thrombotic microangiopathy [HSCT-TMA]	R63.39	Other feeding difficulties
		R79.83	Abnormal findings of blood amino-acid level
M31.19	Other thrombotic microangiopathy	S06.A0XA	Traumatic brain compression without herniation, initial encounter
M35.05	Sjögren syndrome with inflammatory arthritis		
M35.06	Sjögren syndrome with peripheral nervous system involvement	S06.A0XD	Traumatic brain compression without herniation, subsequent encounter
M35.07	Sjögren syndrome with central nervous system involvement	S06.A0XS	Traumatic brain compression without herniation, sequela
		S06.A1XA	Traumatic brain compression with herniation, initial encounter
M35.08	Sjögren syndrome with gastrointestinal involvement		
M35.0A	Sjögren syndrome with glomerular disease	S06.A1XD	Traumatic brain compression with herniation, subsequent encounter
M35.0B	Sjögren syndrome with vasculitis		
M35.0C	Sjögren syndrome with dental involvement	S06.A1XS	Traumatic brain compression with herniation, sequela
M45.A0	Non-radiographic axial spondyloarthritis of unspecified sites in spine	T40.711A	Poisoning by cannabis, accidental (unintentional), initial encounter
M45.A1	Non-radiographic axial spondyloarthritis of occipito-atlanto-axial region	T40.711D	Poisoning by cannabis, accidental (unintentional), subsequent encounter
M45.A2	Non-radiographic axial spondyloarthritis of cervical region	T40.711S	Poisoning by cannabis, accidental (unintentional), sequela
M45.A3	Non-radiographic axial spondyloarthritis of cervicothoracic region	T40.712A	Poisoning by cannabis, intentional self-harm, initial encounter
M45.A4	Non-radiographic axial spondyloarthritis of thoracic region	T40.712D	Poisoning by cannabis, intentional self-harm, subsequent encounter
M45.A5	Non-radiographic axial spondyloarthritis of thoracolumbar region	T40.712S	Poisoning by cannabis, intentional self-harm, sequela
M45.A6	Non-radiographic axial spondyloarthritis of lumbar region	T40.713A	Poisoning by cannabis, assault, initial encounter
M45.A7	Non-radiographic axial spondyloarthritis of lumbosacral region	T40.713D	Poisoning by cannabis, assault, subsequent encounter
		T40.713S	Poisoning by cannabis, assault, sequela
M45.A8	Non-radiographic axial spondyloarthritis of sacral and sacrococcygeal region	T40.714A	Poisoning by cannabis, undetermined, initial encounter
M45.AB	Non-radiographic axial spondyloarthritis of multiple sites in spine	T40.714D	Poisoning by cannabis, undetermined, subsequent encounter
M54.50	Low back pain, unspecified	T40.714S	Poisoning by cannabis, undetermined, sequela
M54.51	Vertebrogenic low back pain	T40.715A	Adverse effect of cannabis, initial encounter
M54.59	Other low back pain	T40.715D	Adverse effect of cannabis, subsequent encounter
P00.82	Newborn affected by (positive) maternal group B streptococcus (GBS) colonization	T40.715S	Adverse effect of cannabis, sequela
		T40.716A	Underdosing of cannabis, initial encounter
P09.1	Abnormal findings on neonatal screening for inborn errors of metabolism	T40.716D	Underdosing of cannabis, subsequent encounter
		T40.716S	Underdosing of cannabis, sequela
P09.2	Abnormal findings on neonatal screening for congenital endocrine disease	T40.721A	Poisoning by synthetic cannabinoids, accidental (unintentional), initial encounter
P09.3	Abnormal findings on neonatal screening for congenital hematologic disorders	T40.721D	Poisoning by synthetic cannabinoids, accidental (unintentional), subsequent encounter
P09.4	Abnormal findings on neonatal screening for cystic fibrosis	T40.721S	Poisoning by synthetic cannabinoids, accidental (unintentional), sequela
P09.5	Abnormal findings on neonatal screening for critical congenital heart disease	T40.722A	Poisoning by synthetic cannabinoids, intentional self-harm, initial encounter
P09.6	Abnormal findings on neonatal screening for neonatal hearing loss	T40.722D	Poisoning by synthetic cannabinoids, intentional self-harm, subsequent encounter
P09.8	Other abnormal findings on neonatal screening	T40.722S	Poisoning by synthetic cannabinoids, intentional self-harm, sequela
P09.9	Abnormal findings on neonatal screening, unspecified		
R05.1	Acute cough	T40.723A	Poisoning by synthetic cannabinoids, assault, initial encounter
R05.2	Subacute cough		

T40.723D	Poisoning by synthetic cannabinoids, assault, subsequent encounter
T40.723S	Poisoning by synthetic cannabinoids, assault, sequela
T40.724A	Poisoning by synthetic cannabinoids, undetermined, initial encounter
T40.724D	Poisoning by synthetic cannabinoids, undetermined, subsequent encounter
T40.724S	Poisoning by synthetic cannabinoids, undetermined, sequela
T40.725A	Adverse effect of synthetic cannabinoids, initial encounter
T40.725D	Adverse effect of synthetic cannabinoids, subsequent encounter
T40.725S	Adverse effect of synthetic cannabinoids, sequela
T40.726A	Underdosing of synthetic cannabinoids, initial encounter
T40.726D	Underdosing of synthetic cannabinoids, subsequent encounter
T40.726S	Underdosing of synthetic cannabinoids, sequela
T80.82XA	Complication of immune effector cellular therapy, initial encounter
T80.82XD	Complication of immune effector cellular therapy, subsequent encounter
T80.82XS	Complication of immune effector cellular therapy, sequela
U09.9	Post COVID-19 condition, unspecified
Y35.899A	Legal intervention involving other specified means, unspecified person injured, initial encounter
Y35.899D	Legal intervention involving other specified means, unspecified person injured, subsequent encounter
Y35.899S	Legal intervention involving other specified means, unspecified person injured, sequela
Z55.5	Less than a high school diploma
Z58.6	Inadequate drinking-water supply
Z59.00	Homelessness unspecified
Z59.01	Sheltered homelessness
Z59.02	Unsheltered homelessness
Z59.41	Food insecurity
Z59.48	Other specified lack of adequate food
Z59.811	Housing instability, housed, with risk of homelessness
Z59.812	Housing instability, housed, homelessness in past 12 months
Z59.819	Housing instability, housed unspecified
Z59.89	Other problems related to housing and economic circumstances
Z71.85	Encounter for immunization safety counseling
Z91.014	Allergy to mammalian meats
Z91.51	Personal history of suicidal behavior
Z91.52	Personal history of nonsuicidal self-harm
Z92.850	Personal history of Chimeric Antigen Receptor T-cell therapy
Z92.858	Personal history of other cellular therapy
Z92.859	Personal history of cellular therapy, unspecified

Z92.86	Personal history of gene therapy

20 Code Descriptions Revised

Note: Each code is listed with its revised description only. Please refer to the full FY 2022 official addenda code files at https://www.cms.gov/medicare/icd-10/2022-icd-10-cm the specific changes made to the codes listed.

G71.20	Congenital myopathy, unspecified
M35.00	Sjögren syndrome, unspecified
M35.01	Sjögren syndrome with keratoconjunctivitis
M35.02	Sjögren syndrome with lung involvement
M35.03	Sjögren syndrome with myopathy
M35.04	Sjögren syndrome with tubulo-interstitial nephropathy
M35.09	Sjögren syndrome with other organ involvement
T63.611A	Toxic effect of contact with Portuguese Man-o-war, accidental (unintentional), initial encounter
T63.611D	Toxic effect of contact with Portuguese Man-o-war, accidental (unintentional), subsequent encounter
T63.611S	Toxic effect of contact with Portuguese Man-o-war, accidental (unintentional), sequela
T63.612A	Toxic effect of contact with Portuguese Man-o-war, intentional self-harm, initial encounter
T63.612D	Toxic effect of contact with Portuguese Man-o-war, intentional self-harm, subsequent encounter
T63.612S	Toxic effect of contact with Portuguese Man-o-war, intentional self-harm, sequela
T63.613A	Toxic effect of contact with Portuguese Man-o-war, assault, initial encounter
T63.613D	Toxic effect of contact with Portuguese Man-o-war, assault, subsequent encounter
T63.613S	Toxic effect of contact with Portuguese Man-o-war, assault, sequela
T63.614A	Toxic effect of contact with Portuguese Man-o-war, undetermined, initial encounter
T63.614D	Toxic effect of contact with Portuguese Man-o-war, undetermined, subsequent encounter
T63.614S	Toxic effect of contact with Portuguese Man-o-war, undetermined, sequela
Z92.25	Personal history of immunosuppression therapy

Proprietary Updates

The following proprietary features have also been added:

- New definitions that describe, in lay terms, a specific condition or disease process

- New coding tips that provide coding advice beyond the code classification

- Updated *AHA Coding Clinic* references through second quarter 2021

Conversion Table of ICD-10-CM Codes

The FY 2022 (October 1, 2021-September 30, 2022) Conversion Table for new ICD-10-CM codes is provided to assist users in data retrieval. For each new code the table shows its previously assigned code equivalent.

Code Assignment Beginning 10/1/2021	Previous Code(s) Assignment	Code Assignment Beginning 10/1/2021	Previous Code(s) Assignment	Code Assignment Beginning 10/1/2021	Previous Code(s) Assignment
A79.82	A77.49	M35.0C	M35.09	T40.715A	T40.7X5A
C56.3	C56.1 and C56.2	M45.A0	M45.9	T40.715D	T40.7X5D
C79.63	C79.61 and C79.62	M45.A1	M45.1	T40.715S	T40.7X5S
C84.7A	C84.79	M45.A2	M45.2	T40.716A	T40.7X6A
D55.21	D55.2	M45.A3	M45.3	T40.716D	T40.7X6D
D55.29	D55.2	M45.A4	M45.4	T40.716S	T40.7X6S
D75.838	D75.83	M45.A5	M45.5	T40.721A	T40.7X1A
D75.839	D75.83	M45.A6	M45.6	T40.721D	T40.7X1D
D89.44	D89.49	M45.A7	M45.7	T40.721S	T40.7X1S
E75.244	E75.240, E75.241, E75.248, E75.249	M45.A8	M45.8	T40.722A	T40.7X2A
		M45.AB	M45.0	T40.722D	T40.7X2D
F32.A	F32.9	M54.50	M54.5	T40.722S	T40.7X2S
F78.A1	F78	M54.51	M54.5	T40.723A	T40.7X3A
F78.A9	F78	M54.59	M54.5	T40.723D	T40.7X3D
G04.82	G04.89	P00.82	P00.89	T40.723S	T40.7X3S
G44.86	G44.89	P09.1	P09	T40.724A	T40.7X4A
G92.00	G92	P09.2	P09	T40.724D	T40.7X4D
G92.01	G92	P09.3	P09	T40.724S	T40.7X4S
G92.02	G92	P09.4	P09	T40.725A	T40.7X5A
G92.03	G92	P09.5	P09	T40.725D	T40.7X5D
G92.04	G92	P09.6	P09	T40.725S	T40.7X5S
G92.05	G92	P09.8	P09	T40.726A	T40.7X6A
G92.8	G92	P09.9	P09	T40.726D	T40.7X6D
G92.9	G92	R05.1	R05	T40.726S	T40.7X6S
I5A	I21.A9	R05.2	R05	T80.82XA	T80.89XA
K22.81	K22.8	R05.3	R05	T80.82XD	T80.89XD
K22.82	K22.8	R05.4	R05	T80.82XS	T80.89XS
K22.89	K22.8	R05.8	R05	U09.9	B94.9
K31.A0	K31.89	R05.9	R05	Y35.899A	Y35.99XA
K31.A11	K31.89	R35.81	R35.8	Y35.899D	Y35.99XD
K31.A12	K31.89	R35.89	R35.8	Y35.899S	Y35.99XS
K31.A13	K31.89	R45.88	R45.89	Z55.5	Z55.8
K31.A14	K31.89	R63.30	R63.3	Z58.6	Z59.4
K31.A15	K31.89	R63.31	R63.3	Z59.00	Z59.0
K31.A19	K31.89	R63.32	R63.3	Z59.01	Z59.0
K31.A21	K31.89	R63.39	R63.3	Z59.02	Z59.0
K31.A22	K31.89	R79.83	R79.89	Z59.41	Z59.4
K31.A29	K31.89	S06.A0XA	S06.890A-S06.899A	Z59.48	Z59.4
L24.A0	L24.89	S06.A0XD	S06.890D-S06.899D	Z59.811	Z59.8
L24.A1	L24.89	S06.A0XS	S06.890D-S06.899S	Z59.812	Z59.8
L24.A2	L24.89	S06.A1XA	S06.890A-S06.899A	Z59.819	Z59.8
L24.A9	L24.89	S06.A1XD	S06.890D-S06.899D	Z59.89	Z59.8
L24.B0	L24.89	S06.A1XS	S06.890D-S06.899S	Z71.85	Z71.89
L24.B1	L24.89	T40.711A	T40.7X1A	Z91.014	Z79.018
L24.B2	L24.89	T40.711D	T40.7X1D	Z91.51	Z91.5
L24.B3	L24.89	T40.711S	T40.7X1S	Z91.52	Z91.5
M31.10	M31.1	T40.712A	T40.7X2A	Z92.850	Z92.89
M31.11	M31.1	T40.712D	T40.7X2D	Z92.858	Z92.89
M31.19	M31.1	T40.712S	T40.7X2S	Z92.859	Z92.89
M35.05	M35.09	T40.713A	T40.7X3A	Z92.86	Z92.89
M35.06	M35.09	T40.713D	T40.7X3D		
M35.07	M35.09	T40.713S	T40.7X3S		
M35.08	M35.09	T40.714A	T40.7X4A		
M35.0A	M35.09	T40.714D	T40.7X4D		
M35.0B	M35.09	T40.714S	T40.7X4S		

10 Steps to Correct Coding

Follow the 10 steps below to correctly code encounters for health care services.

Step 1: Identify the reason for the visit or encounter (i.e., a sign, symptom, diagnosis and/or condition).
The medical record documentation should accurately reflect the patient's condition, using terminology that includes specific diagnoses and symptoms or clearly states the reasons for the encounter.

Choosing the main term that best describes the reason chiefly responsible for the service provided is the most important step in coding. If symptoms are present and documented but a definitive diagnosis has not yet been determined, code the symptoms. *For outpatient cases, do not code conditions that are referred to as "rule out", "suspected," "probable," or "questionable."* Diagnoses often are not established at the time of the initial encounter/visit and may require two or more visits to be established. Code only what is documented in the available outpatient records and only to the highest degree of certainty known at the time of the patient's visit. For inpatient medical records, uncertain diagnoses may be reported if documented at the time of discharge.

Step 2: After selecting the reason for the encounter, consult the alphabetic index.
The most critical rule is to begin code selection in the alphabetic index. Never turn first to the tabular list. The index provides cross-references, essential and nonessential modifiers, and other instructional notations that may not be found in the tabular list.

Step 3: Locate the main term entry.
The alphabetic index lists conditions, which may be expressed as nouns or eponyms, with critical use of adjectives. Some conditions known by several names have multiple main entries. Reasons for encounters may be located under general terms such as admission, encounter, and examination. Other general terms such as history, status (post), or presence (of) can be used to locate other factors influencing health.

Step 4: Scan subterm entries.
Scan the subterm entries, as appropriate, being sure to review continued lines and additional subterms that may appear in the next column or on the next page. Shaded vertical guidelines in the index indicate the indentation level for each subterm in relation to the main terms.

Step 5: Pay close attention to index instructions.
- Parentheses ( ) enclose nonessential modifiers, terms that are supplementary words or explanatory information that may or may not appear in the diagnostic statement and do not affect code selection.
- Brackets [ ] enclose manifestation codes that can be used only as secondary codes to the underlying condition code immediately preceding it. If used, manifestation codes must be reported with the appropriate etiology codes.
- Default codes are listed next to the main term and represent the condition most commonly associated with the main term or the unspecified code for the main term.
- *"See"* cross-references, identified by italicized type and "code by" cross-references indicate that another term *must be referenced* to locate the correct code.
- *"See also"* cross-references, identified by italicized type, provide alternative terms that may be useful to look up but *are not mandatory*.
- "Omit code" cross-references identify instances when a code is not applicable depending on the condition being coded.
- "With" subterms are listed out of alphabetic order and identify a presumed causal relationship between the two conditions they link.

- "Due to" subterms identify a relationship between the two conditions they link.
- "NEC," abbreviation for "not elsewhere classified," follows some main terms or subterms and indicates that there is no specific code for the condition even though the medical documentation may be very specific.
- "NOS," abbreviation for "not otherwise specified," follows some main terms or subterms and is the equivalent of unspecified; NOS signifies that the information in the medical record is insufficient for assigning a more specific code.
- *Following* references help coders locate alphanumeric codes that are out of sequence in the tabular section.
- Check-additional-character symbols flag codes that require additional characters to make the code valid; the characters available to complete the code should be verified in the tabular section.

Step 6: Choose a potential code and locate it in the tabular list.
To prevent coding errors, always use both the alphabetic index (to identify a code) and the tabular list (to verify a code), as the index does not include the important instructional notes found in the tabular list. An added benefit of using the tabular list, which groups like things together, is that while looking at one code in the list, a coder might see a more specific one that would have been missed had the coder relied solely on the alphabetic index. Additionally, many of the codes require a fourth, fifth, sixth, or seventh character to be valid, and many of these characters can be found only in the tabular list.

Step 7: Read all instructional material in the tabular section.
The coder must follow any Includes, Excludes 1 and Excludes 2 notes, and other instructional notes, such as "Code first" and "Use additional code," listed in the tabular list for the chapter, category, subcategory, and subclassification levels of code selection that direct the coder to use a different or additional code. Any codes in the tabular range A00.0- through T88.9- may be used to identify the diagnostic reason for the encounter. The tabular list encompasses many codes describing disease and injury classifications (e.g., infectious and parasitic diseases, neoplasms, symptoms, nervous and circulatory system etc.).

Codes that describe symptoms and signs, as opposed to definitive diagnoses, should be reported when an established diagnosis has not been made (confirmed) by the physician. Chapter 18 of the ICD-10-CM code book, "Symptoms, Signs, and Abnormal Clinical and Laboratory Findings, Not Elsewhere Classified" (codes R00.-–R99), contains many, but not all, codes for symptoms.

ICD-10-CM classifies encounters with health care providers for circumstances other than a disease or injury in chapter 21, "Factors Influencing Health Status and Contact with Health Services" (codes Z00–Z99). Circumstances other than a disease or injury often are recorded as chiefly responsible for the encounter.

A code is invalid if it does not include the full number of characters (greatest level of specificity) required. Codes in ICD-10-CM can contain from three to seven alphanumeric characters. A three-character code is to be used only if the category is not further subdivided into four-, five-, six-, or seven-character codes. Placeholder character X is used as part of an alphanumeric code to allow for future expansion and as a placeholder for empty characters in a code that requires a seventh character but has no fourth, fifth, or sixth character. Note that certain categories require seventh characters that apply to all codes in that category. Always check the category level for applicable seventh characters for that category.

Step 8: Consult the official ICD-10-CM conventions and guidelines.

The *ICD-10-CM Official Guidelines for Coding and Reporting* govern the use of certain codes. These guidelines provide both general and chapter-specific coding guidance.

Step 9: Confirm and assign the code.

Having reviewed all relevant information concerning the possible code choices, assign the code that most completely describes the condition.

Repeat steps 1 through 9 for all additional documented conditions that meet the following criteria:

- They exist at the time of the visit *AND*

- They require or affect patient care, treatment, or management

Step 10: Sequence codes correctly.

Sequencing is the order in which the codes are listed on the claim. List first the ICD-10-CM code for the diagnosis, condition, problem, or other reason for the encounter/visit that is shown in the medical record to be chiefly responsible for the services provided. List additional codes that describe any coexisting conditions. Follow the official coding guidelines (see the guidelines, section II, "Selection of Principal Diagnosis"; section III, "Reporting Additional Diagnoses"; and section IV, "Diagnostic Coding and Reporting Guidelines for Outpatient Services") on proper sequencing of codes.

Coding Examples

Diagnosis: Anorexia

Step 1: The reason for the encounter was the condition, anorexia.

Step 2: Consult the alphabetic index.

Step 3: Locate the main term "Anorexia."

Step 4: Two possible subterms are available, "hysterical" and "nervosa." Neither is documented in this instance, however, so they cannot be used in code selection.

Step 5: The code listed next to the main term is called the default code selection. Because the two subentries (essential modifiers) do not apply in this instance, the default code (R63.0) should be used.

Step 6: Turn to code R63.0 in the tabular list and read all instructional notes.

Step 7: The Excludes 1 note at code R63.0 indicates that anorexia nervosa and loss of appetite determined to be of nonorganic origin should be reported with a code from chapter 5. The diagnostic statement does not describe the condition as anorexia nervosa, however, and does not indicate that the anorexia is of a nonorganic origin. There is no further division of the category past the fourth-character subcategory. Therefore, code R63.0 is at the highest level of specificity.

Step 8: Review of official guideline I.C.18 indicates that a symptom code is appropriate when a more definitive diagnosis is not documented.

Step 9: The default code, R63.0 Anorexia, is the correct code selection.

Repeat steps 1 through 9 for any concomitant diagnoses.

Step 10: Since anorexia is listed as the chief reason for the health care encounter, the first-listed, or principal, diagnosis is R63.0. Note that this is a chapter 18 symptom code but can be assigned for both inpatient and outpatient records since the provider did not establish a more definitive diagnosis, according to sections II.A and IV.D.

Diagnosis: Acute bronchitis

Step 1: The reason for the encounter was the condition, acute bronchitis.

Step 2: Consult the alphabetic index.

Step 3: Locate the main term "Bronchitis."

Step 4: There is a subterm for "acute or subacute." Additional subterms are not included in the diagnostic statement.

Step 5: Review the instructional notes. Nonessential modifiers (with bronchospasm or obstruction) are terms that do not affect code assignment. Since no other subterms indented under "acute" apply here, the code listed next to this subentry—in this case J20.9—should be chosen.

Step 6: Turn to code J20.9 in the tabular list and read all instructional notes.

Step 7: The Includes note under category J20 lists alternative terms for acute bronchitis. Note that the list is not exhaustive but is only a representative selection of diagnoses that are included in the subcategory. The Excludes 1 note refers to category J40 for bronchitis and tracheobronchitis NOS. There are several conditions in the Excludes 2 notes that, if applicable, can be coded in addition to this code.

Note that the codes included in J20 represent acute bronchitis due to various infectious organisms that could be selected if identified in the documentation. In this case, the organism was not identified and there is no further division of the category past the fourth character subcategory. Therefore, code J20.9 is at the highest level of specificity.

Step 8: Review of official guideline I.C.10 provides no additional information affecting the code selected.

Step 9: Assign code J20.9 Acute bronchitis, unspecified.

Repeat steps 1 through 9 for any concomitant diagnoses.

Step 10: In the absence of additional diagnoses that may affect sequencing, code J20.9 should be sequenced as the first-listed, or principal, diagnosis.

Diagnosis: Cerebellar ataxia in myxedema

Step 1: The reason for the encounter was the condition, cerebellar ataxia.

Step 2: Consult the alphabetic index.

Step 3: Locate the main term "Ataxia."

Step 4: Available subterms include "cerebellar (hereditary)," with additional indented subterms for "in" and "myxedema," all essential modifiers that are included in the diagnostic statement. Two codes are provided, E03.9 and G13.2, the latter of which is in brackets.

Step 5: Note the nonessential modifier (in parentheses) after the subterm cerebellar includes the term "hereditary." Because it is in parentheses, this term is not required in the diagnostic statement for this subentry to apply. The brackets around G13.2 identify this code as a manifestation of the condition described by code E03.9 and indicate that the two must be reported together and sequencing rules apply.

Step 6: Locate codes E03.9 and G13.2 in the tabular list, and read all instructional notes.

Step 7: For code E03.9, there are no instructional notes in the tabular list at the category E03 or code level that indicate that this condition should be coded elsewhere in the classification or that additional codes are required. Without further information from the diagnostic statement, myxedema, not otherwise specified (NOS), is appropriately reported with code E03.9 Hypothyroidism, unspecified, according to the inclusion term at this code.

Code G13.2 in the tabular list has an instructional note to "Code first underlying disease," which includes conditions found in category E03.-. Based on this note, codes E03.9 and G13.2 are to be coded together, with G13.2 listed only as a secondary diagnosis. This correlates with what the alphabetic index indicated. As there is no further division of codes in category G13 beyond the fourth character, G13.2 is at the highest level of specificity.

Step 8: Although there are some general conventions, such as how to interpret brackets in the alphabetic index, no chapter-specific guidelines apply to this coding scenario.

Step 9: Assign codes E03.9 Hypothyroidism, unspecified, and G13.2 Systemic atrophy primarily affecting the central nervous system in myxedema.

Repeat steps 1 through 9 for any concomitant diagnoses.

Step 10: Based on the alphabetic index and tabular instructional notations, code E03.9 should be sequenced as the first-listed, or principal, diagnosis followed by G13.2 as a secondary diagnosis.

Diagnosis: Decubitus ulcer of right elbow with skin loss and necrosis of subcutaneous tissue

Step 1: The reason for the encounter was the condition, decubitus ulcer.

Step 2: Consult the alphabetic index.

Step 3: Locate the main term "Ulcer."

Step 4: For the subterm "decubitus," there is no code provided or additional subterms indented, but a cross-reference is listed.

Step 5: The italicized cross-reference instructs the coder to "*see* Ulcer, pressure, by site."

Repeat steps 3 through 5 for the cross-reference.

Step 3: Locate the main term "Ulcer."

Step 4: Review the subentries for the subterm "pressure." The next level of indent lists either the site of the ulcer or the specific stage of the ulcer (stage 1–4, unstageable, and unspecified stages). The diagnostic statement provides the site, right elbow, and the extent of tissue damage (skin loss and necrosis of subcutaneous tissue) but does not specifically state that the ulcer is stage 1, stage 2, etc. Nonessential modifiers (in parentheses) at each stage include a description of the typical extent of damage at each stage. For example, stage 1 describes "pre-ulcer skin changes limited to persistent focal edema." Based on the documentation in the record, the coder can correlate the documentation to the nonessential modifiers and choose the specific stage from the index. The coder can also go directly to the body site, choosing the stage of the ulcer after reviewing the code options and instructional notations in the tabular list.

The diagnostic statement indicates that the extent of the damage to the elbow includes skin loss and necrosis of subcutaneous tissue, coinciding with the nonessential modifier next to the subentry "stage 3." The body site of elbow (L89.0-) is listed as another level of indent with other body sites.

Step 5: Note that code L89.0 is followed by a dash and an additional-character-required icon, which indicate that more characters are needed to complete the code. From here, the tabular listing for L89.0- can be consulted.

Step 6: Locate code L89.0- in the tabular list and read all instructional notes.

Step 7: The tabular listing at category L89 has an Includes note for "decubitus ulcer," which confirms that category L89 is the appropriate category to represent what is documented in the diagnostic statement.

Several Excludes 2 notes are also listed at the category level. Excludes 2 notes represent conditions that can occur concomitantly with the decubitus ulcer and can be coded in addition to code L89, if supported by the documentation.

The subcategory codes under L89.0 indicate that the fifth character describes laterality. Locate the right elbow at subcategory L89.01. See that an additional sixth character to specify the stage of the ulcer is now needed to complete the code. The stage can be determined either by the specific documentation of the stage (e.g., stage 1, stage 2) or, in this case, a description that matches one of the inclusion terms that follow each stage code. For example, the diagnostic description in this case of "skin loss and necrosis of the subcutaneous tissue" matches the inclusion term under L89.013 Pressure ulcer of right elbow, stage 3. No additional characters are required because code L89.013 is at its highest level of specificity.

Step 8: The official guidelines contain quite a bit of information relating to pressure ulcers in chapter-specific guideline I.C.12 as well as information in general guideline I.B.14. These and any other pertinent guidelines should be reviewed to ensure appropriate code assignment.

Step 9: Assign code L89.013 Pressure ulcer of right elbow, stage 3.

Repeat steps 1 through 9 for any concomitant diagnoses.

Step 10: Since the decubitus ulcer is listed as the chief reason for the health care encounter, the first-listed, or principal, diagnosis is L89.013. However, according to the code first instructional note at the L89 category level, gangrene (I96) would be sequenced before the pressure ulcer if it were documented.

Diagnosis: Emergency department visit for bimalleolar fracture of the right ankle due to trauma

Step 1: The reason for the encounter was the condition, bimalleolar fracture.

Step 2: Consult the alphabetic index.

Step 3: Locate the main term "Fracture." Note that many main terms represent fractures: "Fracture, burst,""Fracture, chronic,""Fracture, insufficiency,""Fracture, nontraumatic NEC,""Fracture, pathological," and "Fracture, traumatic." Since the diagnostic statement specifically states that this fracture was the result of trauma, the main term "Fracture, traumatic" should be used.

Step 4: Subterms that should be referenced are "ankle" and "bimalleolar (displaced)," which lists code S82.84-.

Step 5: A nonessential modifier (in parentheses) next to the term bimalleolar for "displaced" indicates that S82.84- is the default category unless the fracture is specifically identified as "nondisplaced."

Note that code S82.84- is followed by a dash and an additional-character icon, both of which indicate that more characters are required. From here, the tabular list can be consulted.

Step 6: Locate code S82.84- in the tabular list and read all instructional notes.

Step: 7 The instructional notes at category S82 indicate that fractures not specified as displaced or nondisplaced default to displaced and that fractures not designated as open or closed default to closed. Additional instructional notes can be found at the category level but none pertain to the current scenario.

Read through the subcategory codes under S82.84, and note that the sixth character specifies displaced or nondisplaced and laterality. Based on the index nonessential modifier (displaced) and the code note at category S82, code selection should identify a displaced fracture of the right side. A displaced bimalleolar fracture of the right lower leg is coded to S82.841.

To complete the code, a seventh character must be assigned to identify the type of encounter (initial, subsequent, or sequela) and whether the fracture is open or closed. Most of the codes in category S82 require a seventh character represented in the list at the category level. However, it is important to note that some subcategories have their own specific set of seventh characters. In this instance, subcategory S82.84- does not have a unique set of seventh characters and the list provided at the category level should be used. Without documentation of the fracture being open, the tabular notation indicates that the default is closed. Character A, representing "initial encounter for closed fracture," listed in the box at the category level is the most appropriate option.

2022 ICD-10-CM Official Guidelines for Coding and Reporting

Narrative changes appear in **bold** text

Items <u>underlined</u> have been moved within the guidelines since the FY 2021 version

Italics are used to indicate revisions to heading changes

The Centers for Medicare and Medicaid Services (CMS) and the National Center for Health Statistics (NCHS), two departments within the U.S. Federal Government's Department of Health and Human Services (DHHS) provide the following guidelines for coding and reporting using the International Classification of Diseases, 10th Revision, Clinical Modification (ICD-10-CM). These guidelines should be used as a companion document to the official version of the ICD-10-CM as published on the NCHS website. The ICD-10-CM is a morbidity classification published by the United States for classifying diagnoses and reason for visits in all health care settings. The ICD-10-CM is based on the ICD-10, the statistical classification of disease published by the World Health Organization (WHO).

These guidelines have been approved by the four organizations that make up the Cooperating Parties for the ICD-10-CM: the American Hospital Association (AHA), the American Health Information Management Association (AHIMA), CMS, and NCHS.

These guidelines are a set of rules that have been developed to accompany and complement the official conventions and instructions provided within the ICD-10-CM itself. The instructions and conventions of the classification take precedence over guidelines. These guidelines are based on the coding and sequencing instructions in the Tabular List and Alphabetic Index of ICD-10-CM, but provide additional instruction. Adherence to these guidelines when assigning ICD-10-CM diagnosis codes is required under the Health Insurance Portability and Accountability Act (HIPAA). The diagnosis codes (Tabular List and Alphabetic Index) have been adopted under HIPAA for all healthcare settings. A joint effort between the healthcare provider and the coder is essential to achieve complete and accurate documentation, code assignment, and reporting of diagnoses and procedures. These guidelines have been developed to assist both the healthcare provider and the coder in identifying those diagnoses that are to be reported. The importance of consistent, complete documentation in the medical record cannot be overemphasized. Without such documentation accurate coding cannot be achieved. The entire record should be reviewed to determine the specific reason for the encounter and the conditions treated.

The term encounter is used for all settings, including hospital admissions. In the context of these guidelines, the term provider is used throughout the guidelines to mean physician or any qualified health care practitioner who is legally accountable for establishing the patient's diagnosis. Only this set of guidelines, approved by the Cooperating Parties, is official.

The guidelines are organized into sections. Section I includes the structure and conventions of the classification and general guidelines that apply to the entire classification, and chapter-specific guidelines that correspond to the chapters as they are arranged in the classification. Section II includes guidelines for selection of principal diagnosis for non-outpatient settings. Section III includes guidelines for reporting additional diagnoses in non-outpatient settings. Section IV is for outpatient coding and reporting. It is necessary to review all sections of the guidelines to fully understand all of the rules and instructions needed to code properly.

Section I. Conventions, general coding guidelines and chapter specific guidelines

The conventions, general guidelines and chapter-specific guidelines are applicable to all health care settings unless otherwise indicated. The conventions and instructions of the classification take precedence over guidelines.

A. Conventions for the ICD-10-CM

The conventions for the ICD-10-CM are the general rules for use of the classification independent of the guidelines. These conventions are incorporated within the Alphabetic Index and Tabular List of the ICD-10-CM as instructional notes.

1. **The Alphabetic Index and Tabular List**

   The ICD-10-CM is divided into the Alphabetic Index, an alphabetical list of terms and their corresponding code, and the Tabular List, a structured list of codes divided into chapters based on body system or condition. The Alphabetic Index consists of the following parts: the Index of Diseases and Injury, the Index of External Causes of Injury, the Table of Neoplasms and the Table of Drugs and Chemicals.

   See Section I.C2. General guidelines

   See Section I.C.19. Adverse effects, poisoning, underdosing and toxic effects

2. **Format and Structure:**

   The ICD-10-CM Tabular List contains categories, subcategories and codes. Characters for categories, subcategories and codes may be either a letter or a number. All categories are 3 characters. A three-character category that has no further subdivision is equivalent to a code. Subcategories are either 4 or 5 characters. Codes may be 3, 4, 5, 6 or 7 characters. That is, each level of subdivision after a category is a subcategory. The final level of subdivision is a code. Codes that have applicable 7th characters are still referred to as codes, not subcategories. A code that has an applicable 7th character is considered invalid without the 7th character.

   The ICD-10-CM uses an indented format for ease in reference.

3. **Use of codes for reporting purposes**

   For reporting purposes only codes are permissible, not categories or subcategories, and any applicable 7th character is required.

4. **Placeholder character**

   The ICD-10-CM utilizes a placeholder character "X". The "X" is used as a placeholder at certain codes to allow for future expansion. An example of this is at the poisoning, adverse effect and underdosing codes, categories T36-T50. Where a placeholder exists, the X must be used in order for the code to be considered a valid code.

5. **7th Characters**

   Certain ICD-10-CM categories have applicable 7th characters. The applicable 7th character is required for all codes within the category, or as the notes in the Tabular List instruct. The 7th character must always be the 7th character in the data field. If a code that requires a 7th character is not 6 characters, a placeholder X must be used to fill in the empty characters.

6. **Abbreviations**

   a. **Alphabetic Index abbreviations**

      NEC "Not elsewhere classifiable"

      This abbreviation in the Alphabetic Index represents "other specified." When a specific code is not available for a condition, the Alphabetic Index directs the coder to the "other specified" code in the Tabular List.

      NOS "Not otherwise specified"

      This abbreviation is the equivalent of unspecified.

   b. **Tabular List abbreviations**

      NEC "Not elsewhere classifiable"

      This abbreviation in the Tabular List represents "other specified". When a specific code is not available for a condition, the Tabular List includes an NEC entry under a code to identify the code as the "other specified" code.

      NOS "Not otherwise specified"

      This abbreviation is the equivalent of unspecified.

7. **Punctuation**

   [ ] Brackets are used in the Tabular List to enclose synonyms, alternative wording or explanatory phrases. Brackets are used in the Alphabetic Index to identify manifestation codes.

   ( ) Parentheses are used in both the Alphabetic Index and Tabular List to enclose supplementary words that may be present or absent in the statement of a disease or procedure without affecting the code

number to which it is assigned. The terms within the parentheses are referred to as nonessential modifiers. The nonessential modifiers in the Alphabetic Index to Diseases apply to subterms following a main term except when a nonessential modifier and a subentry are mutually exclusive, the subentry takes precedence. For example, in the ICD-10-CM Alphabetic Index under the main term Enteritis, "acute" is a nonessential modifier and "chronic" is a subentry. In this case, the nonessential modifier "acute" does not apply to the subentry "chronic".

   : Colons are used in the Tabular List after an incomplete term which needs one or more of the modifiers following the colon to make it assignable to a given category.

8. **Use of "and".**

   See Section I.A.14. Use of the term "And"

9. **Other and Unspecified codes**

   a. **"Other" codes**

      Codes titled "other" or "other specified" are for use when the information in the medical record provides detail for which a specific code does not exist. Alphabetic Index entries with NEC in the line designate "other" codes in the Tabular List. These Alphabetic Index entries represent specific disease entities for which no specific code exists, so the term is included within an "other" code.

   b. **"Unspecified" codes**

      Codes titled "unspecified" are for use when the information in the medical record is insufficient to assign a more specific code. For those categories for which an unspecified code is not provided, the "other specified" code may represent both other and unspecified.

      See Section I.B.18 Use of Signs/Symptom/Unspecified Codes

10. **Includes Notes**

    This note appears immediately under a three-character code title to further define, or give examples of, the content of the category.

11. **Inclusion terms**

    List of terms is included under some codes. These terms are the conditions for which that code is to be used. The terms may be synonyms of the code title, or, in the case of "other specified" codes, the terms are a list of the various conditions assigned to that code. The inclusion terms are not necessarily exhaustive. Additional terms found only in the Alphabetic Index may also be assigned to a code.

12. **Excludes Notes**

    The ICD-10-CM has two types of excludes notes. Each type of note has a different definition for use, but they are all similar in that they indicate that codes excluded from each other are independent of each other.

    a. **Excludes1**

       A type 1 Excludes note is a pure excludes note. It means "NOT CODED HERE!" An Excludes1 note indicates that the code excluded should never be used at the same time as the code above the Excludes1 note. An Excludes1 is used when two conditions cannot occur together, such as a congenital form versus an acquired form of the same condition.

       An exception to the Excludes1 definition is the circumstance when the two conditions are unrelated to each other. If it is not clear whether the two conditions involving an Excludes1 note are related or not, query the provider. For example, code F45.8, Other somatoform disorders, has an Excludes1 note for "sleep related teeth grinding (G47.63)," because "teeth grinding" is an inclusion term under F45.8. Only one of these two codes should be assigned for teeth grinding. However psychogenic dysmenorrhea is also an inclusion term under F45.8, and a patient could have both this condition and sleep related teeth grinding. In this case, the two conditions are clearly unrelated to each other, and so it would be appropriate to report F45.8 and G47.63 together.

    b. **Excludes2**

       A type 2 Excludes note represents "Not included here." An excludes2 note indicates that the condition excluded is not part of the condition represented by the code, but a patient may have both conditions at the same time. When an Excludes2 note appears under a code, it is acceptable to use both the code and the excluded code together, when appropriate.

13. **Etiology/manifestation convention ("code first", "use additional code" and "in diseases classified elsewhere" notes)**

    Certain conditions have both an underlying etiology and multiple body system manifestations due to the underlying etiology. For such conditions, the ICD-10-CM has a coding convention that requires the underlying condition be sequenced first, if applicable, followed by the manifestation. Wherever such a combination exists, there is a "use additional code" note

at the etiology code, and a "code first" note at the manifestation code. These instructional notes indicate the proper sequencing order of the codes, etiology followed by manifestation.

In most cases the manifestation codes will have in the code title, "in diseases classified elsewhere." Codes with this title are a component of the etiology/ manifestation convention. The code title indicates that it is a manifestation code. "In diseases classified elsewhere" codes are never permitted to be used as first listed or principal diagnosis codes. They must be used in conjunction with an underlying condition code and they must be listed following the underlying condition. See category F02, Dementia in other diseases classified elsewhere, for an example of this convention.

There are manifestation codes that do not have "in diseases classified elsewhere" in the title. For such codes, there is a "use additional code" note at the etiology code and a "code first" note at the manifestation code, and the rules for sequencing apply.

In addition to the notes in the Tabular List, these conditions also have a specific Alphabetic Index entry structure. In the Alphabetic Index both conditions are listed together with the etiology code first followed by the manifestation codes in brackets. The code in brackets is always to be sequenced second.

An example of the etiology/manifestation convention is dementia in Parkinson's disease. In the Alphabetic Index, code G20 is listed first, followed by code F02.80 or F02.81 in brackets. Code G20 represents the underlying etiology, Parkinson's disease, and must be sequenced first, whereas code F02.80 and F02.81 represent the manifestation of dementia in diseases classified elsewhere, with or without behavioral disturbance.

"Code first" and "Use additional code" notes are also used as sequencing rules in the classification for certain codes that are not part of an etiology/ manifestation combination.

See Section I.B.7. Multiple coding for a single condition.

14. "And"
The word "and" should be interpreted to mean either "and" or "or" when it appears in a title.

For example, cases of "tuberculosis of bones", "tuberculosis of joints" and "tuberculosis of bones and joints" are classified to subcategory A18.0, Tuberculosis of bones and joints.

15. "With"
The word "with" or "in" should be interpreted to mean "associated with" or "due to" when it appears in a code title, the Alphabetic Index (either under a main term or subterm), or an instructional note in the Tabular List. The classification presumes a causal relationship between the two conditions linked by these terms in the Alphabetic Index or Tabular List. These conditions should be coded as related even in the absence of provider documentation explicitly linking them, unless the documentation clearly states the conditions are unrelated or when another guideline exists that specifically requires a documented linkage between two conditions (e.g., sepsis guideline for "acute organ dysfunction that is not clearly associated with the sepsis").

For conditions not specifically linked by these relational terms in the classification or when a guideline requires that a linkage between two conditions be explicitly documented, provider documentation must link the conditions in order to code them as related.

The word "with" in the Alphabetic Index is sequenced immediately following the main term or subterm, not in alphabetical order.

16. "See" and "See Also"
The "see" instruction following a main term in the Alphabetic Index indicates that another term should be referenced. It is necessary to go to the main term referenced with the "see" note to locate the correct code.

A "see also" instruction following a main term in the Alphabetic Index instructs that there is another main term that may also be referenced that may provide additional Alphabetic Index entries that may be useful. It is not necessary to follow the "see also" note when the original main term provides the necessary code.

17. "Code also" note
A "code also" note instructs that two codes may be required to fully describe a condition, but this note does not provide sequencing direction. The sequencing depends on the circumstances of the encounter.

18. Default codes
A code listed next to a main term in the ICD-10-CM Alphabetic Index is referred to as a default code. The default code represents that condition that is most commonly associated with the main term or is the unspecified code for the condition. If a condition is documented in a medical record (for example, appendicitis) without any additional information, such as acute or chronic, the default code should be assigned.

19. Code assignment and Clinical Criteria
The assignment of a diagnosis code is based on the provider's diagnostic statement that the condition exists. The provider's statement that the patient has a particular condition is sufficient. Code assignment is not based on clinical criteria used by the provider to establish the diagnosis.

B. General Coding Guidelines

1. Locating a code in the ICD-10-CM
To select a code in the classification that corresponds to a diagnosis or reason for visit documented in a medical record, first locate the term in the Alphabetic Index, and then verify the code in the Tabular List. Read and be guided by instructional notations that appear in both the Alphabetic Index and the Tabular List.

It is essential to use both the Alphabetic Index and Tabular List when locating and assigning a code. The Alphabetic Index does not always provide the full code. Selection of the full code, including laterality and any applicable 7th character can only be done in the Tabular List. A dash (-) at the end of an Alphabetic Index entry indicates that additional characters are required. Even if a dash is not included at the Alphabetic Index entry, it is necessary to refer to the Tabular List to verify that no 7th character is required.

2. Level of Detail in Coding
Diagnosis codes are to be used and reported at their highest number of characters available **and to the highest level of specificity documented in the medical record.**

ICD-10-CM diagnosis codes are composed of codes with 3, 4, 5, 6 or 7 characters. Codes with three characters are included in ICD-10-CM as the heading of a category of codes that may be further subdivided by the use of fourth and/or fifth characters and/or sixth characters, which provide greater detail.

A three-character code is to be used only if it is not further subdivided. A code is invalid if it has not been coded to the full number of characters required for that code, including the 7th character, if applicable.

3. Code or codes from A00.0 through T88.9, Z00-Z99.8, U00-U85
The appropriate code or codes from A00.0 through T88.9, Z00-Z99.8, **and U00-U85** must be used to identify diagnoses, symptoms, conditions, problems, complaints or other reason(s) for the encounter/visit.

4. Signs and symptoms
Codes that describe symptoms and signs, as opposed to diagnoses, are acceptable for reporting purposes when a related definitive diagnosis has not been established (confirmed) by the provider. Chapter 18 of ICD-10-CM, Symptoms, Signs, and Abnormal Clinical and Laboratory Findings, Not Elsewhere Classified (codes R00.0-R99) contains many, but not all, codes for symptoms.

See Section I.B.18 Use of Signs/Symptom/Unspecified Codes

5. Conditions that are an integral part of a disease process
Signs and symptoms that are associated routinely with a disease process should not be assigned as additional codes, unless otherwise instructed by the classification.

6. Conditions that are not an integral part of a disease process
Additional signs and symptoms that may not be associated routinely with a disease process should be coded when present.

7. Multiple coding for a single condition
In addition to the etiology/manifestation convention that requires two codes to fully describe a single condition that affects multiple body systems, there are other single conditions that also require more than one code. "Use additional code" notes are found in the Tabular List at codes that are not part of an etiology/manifestation pair where a secondary code is useful to fully describe a condition. The sequencing rule is the same as the etiology/manifestation pair, "use additional code" indicates that a secondary code should be added, if known.

For example, for bacterial infections that are not included in chapter 1, a secondary code from category B95, Streptococcus, Staphylococcus, and Enterococcus, as the cause of diseases classified elsewhere, or B96, Other bacterial agents as the cause of diseases classified elsewhere, may be required to identify the bacterial organism causing the infection. A "use additional code" note will normally be found at the infectious disease code, indicating a need for the organism code to be added as a secondary code.

"Code first" notes are also under certain codes that are not specifically manifestation codes but may be due to an underlying cause. When there is a "code first" note and an underlying condition is present, the underlying condition should be sequenced first, if known.

"Code, if applicable, any causal condition first" notes indicate that this code may be assigned as a principal diagnosis when the causal condition is unknown or not applicable. If a causal condition is known, then the code for that condition should be sequenced as the principal or first-listed diagnosis.

Multiple codes may be needed for sequela, complication codes and obstetric codes to more fully describe a condition. See the specific guidelines for these conditions for further instruction.

8. Acute and Chronic Conditions

If the same condition is described as both acute (subacute) and chronic, and separate subentries exist in the Alphabetic Index at the same indentation level, code both and sequence the acute (subacute) code first.

9. Combination Code

A combination code is a single code used to classify:

   Two diagnoses, or

   A diagnosis with an associated secondary process (manifestation)

   A diagnosis with an associated complication

Combination codes are identified by referring to subterm entries in the Alphabetic Index and by reading the inclusion and exclusion notes in the Tabular List.

Assign only the combination code when that code fully identifies the diagnostic conditions involved or when the Alphabetic Index so directs. Multiple coding should not be used when the classification provides a combination code that clearly identifies all of the elements documented in the diagnosis. When the combination code lacks necessary specificity in describing the manifestation or complication, an additional code should be used as a secondary code.

10. Sequela (Late Effects)

A sequela is the residual effect (condition produced) after the acute phase of an illness or injury has terminated. There is no time limit on when a sequela code can be used. The residual may be apparent early, such as in cerebral infarction, or it may occur months or years later, such as that due to a previous injury. Examples of sequela include: scar formation resulting from a burn, deviated septum due to a nasal fracture, and infertility due to tubal occlusion from old tuberculosis. Coding of sequela generally requires two codes sequenced in the following order: the condition or nature of the sequela is sequenced first. The sequela code is sequenced second.

An exception to the above guidelines are those instances where the code for the sequela is followed by a manifestation code identified in the Tabular List and title, or the sequela code has been expanded (at the fourth, fifth or sixth character levels) to include the manifestation(s). The code for the acute phase of an illness or injury that led to the sequela is never used with a code for the late effect.

See Section I.C.9. Sequelae of cerebrovascular disease

See Section I.C.15. Sequelae of complication of pregnancy, childbirth and the puerperium

See Section I.C.19. Application of 7th characters for Chapter 19

11. Impending or Threatened Condition

Code any condition described at the time of discharge as "impending" or "threatened" as follows:

   If it did occur, code as confirmed diagnosis.

   If it did not occur, reference the Alphabetic Index to determine if the condition has a subentry term for "impending" or "threatened" and also reference main term entries for "Impending" and for "Threatened."

   If the subterms are listed, assign the given code.

   If the subterms are not listed, code the existing underlying condition(s) and not the condition described as impending or threatened.

12. Reporting Same Diagnosis Code More than Once

Each unique ICD-10-CM diagnosis code may be reported only once for an encounter. This applies to bilateral conditions when there are no distinct codes identifying laterality or two different conditions classified to the same ICD-10-CM diagnosis code.

13. Laterality

Some ICD-10-CM codes indicate laterality, specifying whether the condition occurs on the left, right or is bilateral. If no bilateral code is provided and the condition is bilateral, assign separate codes for both the left and right side. If the side is not identified in the medical record, assign the code for the unspecified side.

When a patient has a bilateral condition and each side is treated during separate encounters, assign the "bilateral" code (as the condition still exists on both sides), including for the encounter to treat the first side. For the second encounter for treatment after one side has previously been treated and the condition no longer exists on that side, assign the appropriate unilateral code for the side where the condition still exists (e.g., cataract surgery performed on each eye in separate encounters). The bilateral code would not be assigned for the subsequent encounter, as the patient no longer has the condition in the previously-treated site. If the treatment on the first side did not completely resolve the condition, then the bilateral code would still be appropriate.

When laterality is not documented by the patient's provider, code assignment for the affected side may be based on medical record documentation from other clinicians. If there is conflicting medical record documentation regarding the affected side, the patient's attending provider should be queried for clarification. Codes for "unspecified" side should rarely be used, such as when the documentation in the record is insufficient to determine the affected side and it is not possible to obtain clarification.

14. Documentation by Clinicians Other than the Patient's Provider

Code assignment is based on the documentation by **the** patient's provider (i.e., physician or other qualified healthcare practitioner legally accountable for establishing the patient's diagnosis). There are a few exceptions **when** code assignment may be based on medical record documentation from clinicians who are not the patient's provider (i.e., physician or other qualified healthcare practitioner legally accountable for establishing the patient's diagnosis). **In this context, "clinicians" other than the patient's provider refer to healthcare professionals permitted, based on regulatory or accreditation requirements or internal hospital policies, to document in a patient's official medical record.**

These exceptions include codes for:

- **Body Mass Index (BMI)**
- **Depth of non-pressure chronic ulcers**
- **Pressure ulcer stage**
- **Coma scale**
- **NIH stroke scale (NIHSS)**
- **Social determinants of health (SDOH)**
- **Laterality**
- **Blood alcohol level**

This information is typically**, or may be,** documented by other clinicians involved in the care of the patient (e.g., a dietitian often documents the BMI, a nurse often documents the pressure ulcer stages, and an emergency medical technician often documents the coma scale). However, the associated diagnosis (such as overweight, obesity, acute stroke, pressure ulcer, **or a condition classifiable to category F10, Alcohol related disorders**) must be documented by the patient's provider. If there is conflicting medical record documentation, either from the same clinician or different clinicians, the patient's attending provider should be queried for clarification.

The BMI, coma scale, NIHSS, **blood alcohol level** codes and **codes for social determinants of health** should only be reported as secondary diagnoses.

See Section I.C.21.c.17 for additional information regarding coding social determinants of health.

15. Syndromes

Follow the Alphabetic Index guidance when coding syndromes. In the absence of Alphabetic Index guidance, assign codes for the documented manifestations of the syndrome. Additional codes for manifestations that are not an integral part of the disease process may also be assigned when the condition does not have a unique code.

16. Documentation of Complications of Care

Code assignment is based on the provider's documentation of the relationship between the condition and the care or procedure, unless otherwise instructed by the classification. The guideline extends to any complications of care, regardless of the chapter the code is located in. It is important to note that not all conditions that occur during or following medical care or surgery are classified as complications. There must be a cause-and-effect relationship between the care provided and the condition, and an indication in the documentation that it is a complication. Query the provider for clarification, if the complication is not clearly documented.

17. Borderline Diagnosis

If the provider documents a "borderline" diagnosis at the time of discharge, the diagnosis is coded as confirmed, unless the classification provides a specific entry (e.g., borderline diabetes). If a borderline condition has a specific index entry in ICD-10-CM, it should be coded as such. Since borderline conditions are not uncertain diagnoses, no

distinction is made between the care setting (inpatient versus outpatient). Whenever the documentation is unclear regarding a borderline condition, coders are encouraged to query for clarification.

18. **Use of Sign/Symptom/Unspecified Codes**

Sign/symptom and "unspecified" codes have acceptable, even necessary, uses. While specific diagnosis codes should be reported when they are supported by the available medical record documentation and clinical knowledge of the patient's health condition, there are instances when signs/symptoms or unspecified codes are the best choices for accurately reflecting the healthcare encounter. Each healthcare encounter should be coded to the level of certainty known for that encounter.

As stated in the introductory section of these official coding guidelines, a joint effort between the healthcare provider and the coder is essential to achieve complete and accurate documentation, code assignment, and reporting of diagnoses and procedures. The importance of consistent, complete documentation in the medical record cannot be overemphasized. Without such documentation accurate coding cannot be achieved. The entire record should be reviewed to determine the specific reason for the encounter and the conditions treated.

If a definitive diagnosis has not been established by the end of the encounter, it is appropriate to report codes for sign(s) and/or symptom(s) in lieu of a definitive diagnosis. When sufficient clinical information isn't known or available about a particular health condition to assign a more specific code, it is acceptable to report the appropriate "unspecified" code (e.g., a diagnosis of pneumonia has been determined, but not the specific type). Unspecified codes should be reported when they are the codes that most accurately reflect what is known about the patient's condition at the time of that particular encounter. It would be inappropriate to select a specific code that is not supported by the medical record documentation or conduct medically unnecessary diagnostic testing in order to determine a more specific code.

19. **Coding for Healthcare Encounters in Hurricane Aftermath**
    a. **Use of External Cause of Morbidity Codes**

An external cause of morbidity code should be assigned to identify the cause of the injury(ies) incurred as a result of the hurricane. The use of external cause of morbidity codes is supplemental to the application of ICD-10-CM codes. External cause of morbidity codes are never to be recorded as a principal diagnosis (first-listed in non-inpatient settings). The appropriate injury code should be sequenced before any external cause codes. The external cause of morbidity codes capture how the injury or health condition happened (cause), the intent (unintentional or accidental; or intentional, such as suicide or assault), the place where the event occurred, the activity of the patient at the time of the event, and the person's status (e.g., civilian, military). They should not be assigned for encounters to treat hurricane victims' medical conditions when no injury, adverse effect or poisoning is involved. External cause of morbidity codes should be assigned for each encounter for care and treatment of the injury. External cause of morbidity codes may be assigned in all health care settings. For the purpose of capturing complete and accurate ICD-10-CM data in the aftermath of the hurricane, a healthcare setting should be considered as any location where medical care is provided by licensed healthcare professionals.

    b. **Sequencing of External Causes of Morbidity Codes**

Codes for cataclysmic events, such as a hurricane, take priority over all other external cause codes except child and adult abuse and terrorism and should be sequenced before other external cause of injury codes. Assign as many external cause of morbidity codes as necessary to fully explain each cause. For example, if an injury occurs as a result of a building collapse during the hurricane, external cause codes for both the hurricane and the building collapse should be assigned, with the external causes code for hurricane being sequenced as the first external cause code. For injuries incurred as a direct result of the hurricane, assign the appropriate code(s) for the injuries, followed by the code X37.Ø- Hurricane (with the appropriate 7th character), and any other applicable external cause of injury codes. Code X37.Ø- also should be assigned when an injury is incurred as a result of flooding caused by a levee breaking related to the hurricane. Code X38.-, Flood (with the appropriate 7th character), should be assigned when an injury is from flooding resulting directly from the storm. Code X36.Ø.-, Collapse of dam or man-made structure, should not be assigned when the cause of the collapse is due to the hurricane. Use of code X36.Ø- is limited to collapses of man-made structures due to earth surface movements, not due to storm surges directly from a hurricane.

    c. **Other External Causes of Morbidity Code Issues**

For injuries that are not a direct result of the hurricane, such as an evacuee that has incurred an injury as a result of a motor vehicle accident, assign the appropriate external cause of morbidity code(s) to describe the cause of the injury, but do not assign code X37.Ø-, Hurricane. If it is not clear whether the injury was a direct result of the hurricane, assume the injury is due to the hurricane and assign code X37.Ø-, Hurricane, as well as any other applicable external cause of morbidity codes. In addition to code X37.Ø-, Hurricane, other possible applicable external cause of morbidity codes include:

X30-, Exposure to excessive natural heat

X31-, Exposure to excessive natural cold

X38-, Flood

    d. **Use of Z codes**

Z codes (other reasons for healthcare encounters) may be assigned as appropriate to further explain the reasons for presenting for healthcare services, including transfers between healthcare facilities, **or provide additional information relevant to a patient encounter.** The ICD-10-CM Official Guidelines for Coding and Reporting identify which codes maybe assigned as principal or first-listed diagnosis only, secondary diagnosis only, or principal/first-listed or secondary (depending on the circumstances). Possible applicable Z codes include:

Z59.Ø-,   Homelessness

Z59.1,   Inadequate housing

Z59.5,   Extreme poverty

Z75.1,   Person awaiting admission to adequate facility elsewhere

Z75.3,   Unavailability and inaccessibility of health-care facilities

Z75.4,   Unavailability and inaccessibility of other helping agencies

Z76.2,   Encounter for health supervision and care of other healthy infant and child

Z99.12,   Encounter for respirator [ventilator] dependence during power failure

The external cause of morbidity codes and the Z codes listed above are not an all-inclusive list. Other codes may be applicable to the encounter based upon the documentation. Assign as many codes as necessary to fully explain each healthcare encounter. Since patient history information may be very limited, use any available documentation to assign the appropriate external cause of morbidity and Z codes.

C. Chapter-Specific Coding Guidelines

In addition to general coding guidelines, there are guidelines for specific diagnoses and/or conditions in the classification. Unless otherwise indicated, these guidelines apply to all health care settings. Please refer to Section II for guidelines on the selection of principal diagnosis.

1. **Chapter 1: Certain Infectious and Parasitic Diseases (AØØ-B99), UØ7.1, UØ9.9**
    a. **Human Immunodeficiency Virus (HIV) Infections**
        1) **Code only confirmed cases**

Code only confirmed cases of HIV infection/illness. This is an exception to the hospital inpatient guideline Section II, H.

In this context, "confirmation" does not require documentation of positive serology or culture for HIV; the provider's diagnostic statement that the patient is HIV positive or has an HIV-related illness is sufficient.

        2) **Selection and sequencing of HIV codes**
            (a) **Patient admitted for HIV-related condition**

If a patient is admitted for an HIV-related condition, the principal diagnosis should be B2Ø, Human immunodeficiency virus [HIV] disease followed by additional diagnosis codes for all reported HIV-related conditions.

            (b) **Patient with HIV disease admitted for unrelated condition**

If a patient with HIV disease is admitted for an unrelated condition (such as a traumatic injury), the code for the unrelated condition (e.g., the nature of injury code) should be the principal diagnosis. Other diagnoses would be B2Ø followed by additional diagnosis codes for all reported HIV-related conditions.

(c) **Whether the patient is newly diagnosed**

Whether the patient is newly diagnosed or has had previous admissions/encounters for HIV conditions is irrelevant to the sequencing decision.

(d) **Asymptomatic human immunodeficiency virus**

Z21, Asymptomatic human immunodeficiency virus [HIV] infection status, is to be applied when the patient without any documentation of symptoms is listed as being "HIV positive," "known HIV," "HIV test positive," or similar terminology. Do not use this code if the term "AIDS" **or "HIV disease"** is used or if the patient is treated for any HIV-related illness or is described as having any condition(s) resulting from his/her HIV positive status; use B20 in these cases.

(e) **Patients with inconclusive HIV serology**

Patients with inconclusive HIV serology, but no definitive diagnosis or manifestations of the illness, may be assigned code R75, Inconclusive laboratory evidence of human immunodeficiency virus [HIV].

(f) **Previously diagnosed HIV-related illness**

Patients with any known prior diagnosis of an HIV-related illness should be coded to B20. Once a patient has developed an HIV-related illness, the patient should always be assigned code B20 on every subsequent admission/encounter. Patients previously diagnosed with any HIV illness (B20) should never be assigned to R75 or Z21, Asymptomatic human immunodeficiency virus [HIV] infection status.

(g) **HIV Infection in Pregnancy, Childbirth and the Puerperium**

During pregnancy, childbirth or the puerperium, a patient admitted (or presenting for a health care encounter) because of an HIV-related illness should receive a principal diagnosis code of O98.7-, Human immunodeficiency [HIV] disease complicating pregnancy, childbirth and the puerperium, followed by B20 and the code(s) for the HIV-related illness(es). Codes from Chapter 15 always take sequencing priority.

Patients with asymptomatic HIV infection status admitted (or presenting for a health care encounter) during pregnancy, childbirth, or the puerperium should receive codes of O98.7- and Z21.

(h) **Encounters for testing for HIV**

If a patient is being seen to determine his/her HIV status, use code Z11.4, Encounter for screening for human immunodeficiency virus [HIV]. Use additional codes for any associated high-risk behavior, **if applicable.**

If a patient with signs or symptoms is being seen for HIV testing, code the signs and symptoms. An additional counseling code Z71.7, Human immunodeficiency virus [HIV] counseling, may be used if counseling is provided during the encounter for the test.

When a patient returns to be informed of his/her HIV test results and the test result is negative, use code Z71.7, Human immunodeficiency virus [HIV] counseling.

If the results are positive, see previous guidelines and assign codes as appropriate.

(i) **History of HIV managed by medication**

If a patient with documented history of HIV disease is currently managed on antiretroviral medications, assign code B20, Human immunodeficiency virus [HIV] disease. Code Z79.899, Other long term (current) drug therapy, may be assigned as an additional code to identify the long-term (current) use of antiretroviral medications.

b. **Infectious agents as the cause of diseases classified to other chapters**

Certain infections are classified in chapters other than Chapter 1 and no organism is identified as part of the infection code. In these instances, it is necessary to use an additional code from Chapter 1 to identify the organism. A code from category B95, Streptococcus, Staphylococcus, and Enterococcus as the cause of diseases classified to other chapters, B96, Other bacterial agents as the cause of diseases classified to other chapters, or B97, Viral agents as the cause of diseases classified to other chapters, is to be used as an additional code to identify the organism. An instructional note will be found at the infection code advising that an additional organism code is required.

c. **Infections resistant to antibiotics**

Many bacterial infections are resistant to current antibiotics. It is necessary to identify all infections documented as antibiotic resistant. Assign a code from category Z16, Resistance to antimicrobial drugs, following the infection code only if the infection code does not identify drug resistance.

d. **Sepsis, Severe Sepsis, and Septic Shock Infections resistant to antibiotics**

1) **Coding of Sepsis and Severe Sepsis**

(a) **Sepsis**

For a diagnosis of sepsis, assign the appropriate code for the underlying systemic infection. If the type of infection or causal organism is not further specified, assign code A41.9, Sepsis, unspecified organism.

A code from subcategory R65.2, Severe sepsis, should not be assigned unless severe sepsis or an associated acute organ dysfunction is documented.

(i) **Negative or inconclusive blood cultures and sepsis**

Negative or inconclusive blood cultures do not preclude a diagnosis of sepsis in patients with clinical evidence of the condition; however, the provider should be queried.

(ii) **Urosepsis**

The term urosepsis is a nonspecific term. It is not to be considered synonymous with sepsis. It has no default code in the Alphabetic Index. Should a provider use this term, he/she must be queried for clarification.

(iii) **Sepsis with organ dysfunction**

If a patient has sepsis and associated acute organ dysfunction or multiple organ dysfunction (MOD), follow the instructions for coding severe sepsis.

(iv) **Acute organ dysfunction that is not clearly associated with the sepsis**

If a patient has sepsis and an acute organ dysfunction, but the medical record documentation indicates that the acute organ dysfunction is related to a medical condition other than the sepsis, do not assign a code from subcategory R65.2, Severe sepsis. An acute organ dysfunction must be associated with the sepsis in order to assign the severe sepsis code. If the documentation is not clear as to whether an acute organ dysfunction is related to the sepsis or another medical condition, query the provider.

(b) **Severe sepsis**

The coding of severe sepsis requires a minimum of 2 codes: first a code for the underlying systemic infection, followed by a code from subcategory R65.2, Severe sepsis. If the causal organism is not documented, assign code A41.9, Sepsis, unspecified organism, for the infection. Additional code(s) for the associated acute organ dysfunction are also required.

Due to the complex nature of severe sepsis, some cases may require querying the provider prior to assignment of the codes.

2) **Septic shock**

Septic shock generally refers to circulatory failure associated with severe sepsis, and therefore, it represents a type of acute organ dysfunction.

For cases of septic shock, the code for the systemic infection should be sequenced first, followed by code R65.21, Severe sepsis with septic shock or code T81.12, Postprocedural septic shock. Any additional codes for the other acute organ dysfunctions should also be assigned. As noted in the sequencing instructions in the Tabular List, the code for septic shock cannot be assigned as a principal diagnosis.

3) **Sequencing of severe sepsis**

If severe sepsis is present on admission, and meets the definition of principal diagnosis, the underlying systemic infection should be assigned as principal diagnosis followed by the appropriate code from subcategory R65.2 as required by the sequencing rules in the Tabular List. A code from subcategory R65.2 can never be assigned as a principal diagnosis.

When severe sepsis develops during an encounter (it was not present on admission), the underlying systemic infection and the

appropriate code from subcategory R65.2 should be assigned as secondary diagnoses.

Severe sepsis may be present on admission, but the diagnosis may not be confirmed until sometime after admission. If the documentation is not clear whether severe sepsis was present on admission, the provider should be queried.

4) Sepsis or severe sepsis with a localized infection

If the reason for admission is sepsis or severe sepsis and a localized infection, such as pneumonia or cellulitis, a code(s) for the underlying systemic infection should be assigned first and the code for the localized infection should be assigned as a secondary diagnosis. If the patient has severe sepsis, a code from subcategory R65.2 should also be assigned as a secondary diagnosis. If the patient is admitted with a localized infection, such as pneumonia, and sepsis/severe sepsis doesn't develop until after admission, the localized infection should be assigned first, followed by the appropriate sepsis/severe sepsis codes.

5) Sepsis due to a postprocedural infection

(a) Documentation of causal relationship

As with all postprocedural complications, code assignment is based on the provider's documentation of the relationship between the infection and the procedure.

(b) Sepsis due to a postprocedural infection

For infections following a procedure, a code from T81.40, to T81.43 Infection following a procedure, or a code from O86.00 to O86.03, Infection of obstetric surgical wound, that identifies the site of the infection should be coded first, if known. Assign an additional code for sepsis following a procedure (T81.44) or sepsis following an obstetrical procedure (O86.04). Use an additional code to identify the infectious agent. If the patient has severe sepsis, the appropriate code from subcategory R65.2 should also be assigned with the additional code(s) for any acute organ dysfunction.

For infections following infusion, transfusion, therapeutic injection, or immunization, a code from subcategory T80.2, Infections following infusion, transfusion, and therapeutic injection, or code T88.0-, Infection following immunization, should be coded first, followed by the code for the specific infection. If the patient has severe sepsis, the appropriate code from subcategory R65.2 should also be assigned, with the additional codes(s) for any acute organ dysfunction.

(c) Postprocedural infection and postprocedural septic shock

If a postprocedural infection has resulted in postprocedural septic shock, assign the codes indicated above for sepsis due to a postprocedural infection, followed by code T81.12-, Postprocedural septic shock. Do not assign code R65.21, Severe sepsis with septic shock. Additional code(s) should be assigned for any acute organ dysfunction.

6) Sepsis and severe sepsis associated with a noninfectious process (condition)

In some cases, a noninfectious process (condition) such as trauma, may lead to an infection which can result in sepsis or severe sepsis. If sepsis or severe sepsis is documented as associated with a noninfectious condition, such as a burn or serious injury, and this condition meets the definition for principal diagnosis, the code for the noninfectious condition should be sequenced first, followed by the code for the resulting infection. If severe sepsis is present, a code from subcategory R65.2 should also be assigned with any associated organ dysfunction(s) codes. It is not necessary to assign a code from subcategory R65.1, Systemic inflammatory response syndrome (SIRS) of non-infectious origin, for these cases.

If the infection meets the definition of principal diagnosis, it should be sequenced before the non-infectious condition. When both the associated non-infectious condition and the infection meet the definition of principal diagnosis, either may be assigned as principal diagnosis.

Only one code from category R65, Symptoms and signs specifically associated with systemic inflammation and infection, should be assigned. Therefore, when a non-infectious condition leads to an infection resulting in severe sepsis, assign the appropriate code from subcategory R65.2, Severe sepsis. Do not additionally assign a code from subcategory R65.1, Systemic inflammatory response syndrome (SIRS) of non-infectious origin.

See Section I.C.18. SIRS due to non-infectious process

7) Sepsis and septic shock complicating abortion, pregnancy, childbirth, and the puerperium

See Section I.C.15. Sepsis and septic shock complicating abortion, pregnancy, childbirth and the puerperium

8) Newborn sepsis

See Section I.C.16. f. Bacterial sepsis of Newborn

e. Methicillin Resistant Staphylococcus aureus (MRSA) Conditions

1) Selection and sequencing of MRSA codes

(a) Combination codes for MRSA infection

When a patient is diagnosed with an infection that is due to methicillin resistant *Staphylococcus aureus* (MRSA), and that infection has a combination code that includes the causal organism (e.g., sepsis, pneumonia) assign the appropriate combination code for the condition (e.g., code A41.02, Sepsis due to Methicillin resistant Staphylococcus aureus or code J15.212, Pneumonia due to Methicillin resistant Staphylococcus aureus). Do not assign code B95.62, Methicillin resistant Staphylococcus aureus infection as the cause of diseases classified elsewhere, as an additional code, because the combination code includes the type of infection and the MRSA organism. Do not assign a code from subcategory Z16.11, Resistance to penicillins, as an additional diagnosis.

See Section C.1. for instructions on coding and sequencing of sepsis and severe sepsis.

(b) Other codes for MRSA infection

When there is documentation of a current infection (e.g., wound infection, stitch abscess, urinary tract infection) due to MRSA, and that infection does not have a combination code that includes the causal organism, assign the appropriate code to identify the condition along with code B95.62, Methicillin resistant Staphylococcus aureus infection as the cause of diseases classified elsewhere for the MRSA infection. Do not assign a code from subcategory Z16.11, Resistance to penicillins.

(c) Methicillin susceptible Staphylococcus aureus (MSSA) and MRSA colonization

The condition or state of being colonized or carrying MSSA or MRSA is called colonization or carriage, while an individual person is described as being colonized or being a carrier.

Colonization means that MSSA or MSRA is present on or in the body without necessarily causing illness. A positive MRSA colonization test might be documented by the provider as "MRSA screen positive" or "MRSA nasal swab positive".

Assign code Z22.322, Carrier or suspected carrier of Methicillin resistant Staphylococcus aureus, for patients documented as having MRSA colonization. Assign code Z22.321, Carrier or suspected carrier of Methicillin susceptible Staphylococcus aureus, for patients documented as having MSSA colonization. Colonization is not necessarily indicative of a disease process or as the cause of a specific condition the patient may have unless documented as such by the provider.

(d) MRSA colonization and infection

If a patient is documented as having both MRSA colonization and infection during a hospital admission, code Z22.322, Carrier or suspected carrier of Methicillin resistant Staphylococcus aureus, and a code for the MRSA infection may both be assigned.

f. Zika virus infections

1) Code only confirmed cases

Code only a confirmed diagnosis of Zika virus (A92.5, Zika virus disease) as documented by the provider. This is an exception to the hospital inpatient guideline Section II, H. In this context, "confirmation" does not require documentation of the type of test performed; the provider's diagnostic statement that the condition is confirmed is sufficient. This code should be assigned regardless of the stated mode of transmission.

If the provider documents "suspected", "possible" or "probable" Zika, do not assign code A92.5. Assign a code(s) explaining the reason for encounter (such as fever, rash, or joint pain) or Z20.821, Contact with and (suspected) exposure to Zika virus.

g. **Coronavirus infections**
1) **COVID-19 infection (infection due to SARS-CoV-2)**

(a) **Code only confirmed cases**

Code only a confirmed diagnosis of the 2019 novel coronavirus disease (COVID-19) as documented by the provider, or documentation of a positive COVID-19 test result. For a confirmed diagnosis, assign code U07.1, COVID-19. This is an exception to the hospital inpatient guideline Section II, H. In this context, "confirmation" does not require documentation of a positive test result for COVID-19; the provider's documentation that the individual has COVID-19 is sufficient.

If the provider documents "suspected," "possible," "probable," or "inconclusive" COVID-19, do not assign code U07.1. Instead, code the signs and symptoms reported. See guideline I.C.1.g.1.g.

(b) **Sequencing of codes**

When COVID-19 meets the definition of principal diagnosis, code U07.1, COVID-19, should be sequenced first, followed by the appropriate codes for associated manifestations, except when another guideline requires that certain codes be sequenced first, such as obstetrics, sepsis, or transplant complications.

For a COVID-19 infection that progresses to sepsis, see Section I.C.1.d. Sepsis, Severe Sepsis, and Septic Shock

See Section I.C.15.s. for COVID-19 infection in pregnancy, childbirth, and the puerperium

See Section I.C.16.h. for COVID-19 infection in newborn

For a COVID-19 infection in a lung transplant patient, see Section I.C.19.g.3.a. Transplant complications other than kidney.

(c) **Acute respiratory manifestations of COVID-19**

When the reason for the encounter/admission is a respiratory manifestation of COVID-19, assign code U07.1, COVID-19, as the principal/first-listed diagnosis and assign code(s) for the respiratory manifestation(s) as additional diagnoses.

The following conditions are examples of common respiratory manifestations of COVID-19.

(i) **Pneumonia**

For a patient with pneumonia confirmed as due to COVID-19, assign codes U07.1, COVID-19, and J12.82, Pneumonia due to coronavirus disease 2019.

(ii) **Acute bronchitis**

For a patient with acute bronchitis confirmed as due to COVID-19, assign codes U07.1, and J20.8, Acute bronchitis due to other specified organisms.

Bronchitis not otherwise specified (NOS) due to COVID-19 should be coded using code U07.1 and J40, Bronchitis, not specified as acute or chronic.

(iii) **Lower respiratory infection**

If the COVID-19 is documented as being associated with a lower respiratory infection, not otherwise specified (NOS), or an acute respiratory infection, NOS, codes U07.1 and J22, Unspecified acute lower respiratory infection, should be assigned.

If the COVID-19 is documented as being associated with a respiratory infection, NOS, codes U07.1 and J98.8, Other specified respiratory disorders, should be assigned.

(iv) **Acute respiratory distress syndrome**

For acute respiratory distress syndrome (ARDS) due to COVID-19, assign codes U07.1, and J80, Acute respiratory distress syndrome.

(v) **Acute respiratory failure**

For acute respiratory failure due to COVID-19, assign code U07.1, and code J96.0-, Acute respiratory failure.

(d) **Non-respiratory manifestations of COVID-19**

When the reason for the encounter/admission is a non-respiratory manifestation (e.g., viral enteritis) of COVID-19, assign code U07.1, COVID-19, as the principal/first-listed diagnosis and assign code(s) for the manifestation(s) as additional diagnoses.

(e) **Exposure to COVID-19**

For asymptomatic individuals with actual or suspected exposure to COVID-19, assign code Z20.822, Contact with and (suspected) exposure to COVID-19.

For symptomatic individuals with actual or suspected exposure to COVID-19 and the infection has been ruled out, or test results are inconclusive or unknown, assign code Z20.822, Contact with and (suspected) exposure to COVID-19. See guideline I.C.21.c.1, Contact/Exposure, for additional guidance regarding the use of category Z20 codes.

If COVID-19 is confirmed, see guideline I.C.1.g.1.a.

(f) **Screening for COVID-19**

During the COVID-19 pandemic, a screening code is generally not appropriate. Do not assign code Z11.52, Encounter for screening for COVID-19. For encounters for COVID-19 testing, including preoperative testing, code as exposure to COVID-19 (guideline I.C.1.g.1.e).

Coding guidance will be updated as new information concerning any changes in the pandemic status becomes available.

(g) **Signs and symptoms without definitive diagnosis of COVID-19**

For patients presenting with any signs/symptoms associated with COVID-19 (such as fever, etc.) but a definitive diagnosis has not been established, assign the appropriate code(s) for each of the presenting signs and symptoms such as:

- R05.1, Acute cough, or R05.9, Cough, unspecified
- R06.02 Shortness of breath
- R50.9 Fever, unspecified

If a patient with signs/symptoms associated with COVID-19 also has an actual or suspected contact with or exposure to COVID-19, assign Z20.822, Contact with and (suspected) exposure to COVID-19, as an additional code.

(h) **Asymptomatic individuals who test positive for COVID-19**

For asymptomatic individuals who test positive for COVID-19, see guideline I.C.1.g.1.a. Although the individual is asymptomatic, the individual has tested positive and is considered to have the COVID-19 infection.

(i) **Personal history of COVID-19**

For patients with a history of COVID-19, assign code Z86.16, Personal history of COVID-19.

(j) **Follow-up visits after COVID-19 infection has resolved**

For individuals who previously had COVID-19, **without residual symptom(s) or condition(s),** and are being seen for follow-up evaluation, and COVID-19 test results are negative, assign codes Z09, Encounter for follow-up examination after completed treatment for conditions other than malignant neoplasm, and Z86.16, Personal history of COVID-19.

For follow-up visits for individuals with symptom(s) or condition(s) related to a previous COVID-19 infection, see guideline I.C.1.g.1.m.

See Section I.C.21.c.8, Factors influencing health states and contact with health services, Follow-up

(k) **Encounter for antibody testing**

For an encounter for antibody testing that is not being performed to confirm a current COVID-19 infection, nor is a follow-up test after resolution of COVID-19, assign Z01.84, Encounter for antibody response examination.

Follow the applicable guidelines above if the individual is being tested to confirm a current COVID-19 infection.

For follow-up testing after a COVID-19 infection, see guideline I.C.1.g.1.j.

(l) **Multisystem Inflammatory Syndrome**

For individuals with multisystem inflammatory syndrome (MIS) and COVID-19, assign code U07.1, COVID-19, as the principal/first-listed diagnosis and assign code M35.81, Multisystem inflammatory syndrome, as an additional diagnosis.

If an individual with a history of COVID-19 develops MIS, assign codes M35.81, Multisystem inflammatory syndrome, and **U09.9, Post COVID-19 condition, unspecified**.

If an individual with a known or suspected exposure to COVID-19, and no current COVID-19 infection or history of COVID-19, develops MIS, assign codes M35.81, Multisystem inflammatory syndrome, and Z20.822, Contact with and (suspected) exposure to COVID-19.

Additional codes should be assigned for any associated complications of MIS.

(m) Post COVID-19 Condition

For sequela of COVID-19, or associated symptoms or conditions that develop following a previous COVID-19 infection, assign a code(s) for the specific symptom(s) or condition(s) related to the previous COVID-19 infection, if known, and code U09.9, Post COVID-19 condition, unspecified.

Code U09.9 should not be assigned for manifestations of an active (current) COVID-19 infection.

If a patient has a condition(s) associated with a previous COVID-19 infection and develops a new active (current) COVID-19 infection, code U09.9 may be assigned in conjunction with code U07.1, COVID-19, to identify that the patient also has a condition(s) associated with a previous COVID-19 infection. Code(s) for the specific condition(s) associated with the previous COVID-19 infection and code(s) for manifestation(s) of the new active (current) COVID-19 infection should also be assigned.

2. Chapter 2: Neoplasms (C00-D49)

General Guidelines

Chapter 2 of the ICD-10-CM contains the codes for most benign and all malignant neoplasms. Certain benign neoplasms, such as prostatic adenomas, may be found in the specific body system chapters. To properly code a neoplasm, it is necessary to determine from the record if the neoplasm is benign, in-situ, malignant, or of uncertain histologic behavior. If malignant, any secondary (metastatic) sites should also be determined.

Primary malignant neoplasms overlapping site boundaries

A primary malignant neoplasm that overlaps two or more contiguous (next to each other) sites should be classified to the subcategory/code .8 ('overlapping lesion'), unless the combination is specifically indexed elsewhere. For multiple neoplasms of the same site that are not contiguous such as tumors in different quadrants of the same breast, codes for each site should be assigned.

Malignant neoplasm of ectopic tissue

Malignant neoplasms of ectopic tissue are to be coded to the site of origin mentioned, e.g., ectopic pancreatic malignant neoplasms involving the stomach are coded to malignant neoplasm of pancreas, unspecified (C25.9).

The neoplasm table in the Alphabetic Index should be referenced first. However, if the histological term is documented, that term should be referenced first, rather than going immediately to the Neoplasm Table, in order to determine which column in the Neoplasm Table is appropriate. For example, if the documentation indicates "adenoma," refer to the term in the Alphabetic Index to review the entries under this term and the instructional note to "see also neoplasm, by site, benign." The table provides the proper code based on the type of neoplasm and the site. It is important to select the proper column in the table that corresponds to the type of neoplasm. The Tabular List should then be referenced to verify that the correct code has been selected from the table and that a more specific site code does not exist.

See Section I.C.21. Factors influencing health status and contact with health services, Status, for information regarding Z15.0, codes for genetic susceptibility to cancer.

a. Treatment directed at the malignancy

If the treatment is directed at the malignancy, designate the malignancy as the principal diagnosis.

The only exception to this guideline is if a patient admission/encounter is solely for the administration of chemotherapy, immunotherapy or external beam radiation therapy, assign the appropriate Z51.-- code as the first-listed or principal diagnosis, and the diagnosis or problem for which the service is being performed as a secondary diagnosis.

b. Treatment of secondary site

When a patient is admitted because of a primary neoplasm with metastasis and treatment is directed toward the secondary site only, the secondary neoplasm is designated as the principal diagnosis even though the primary malignancy is still present.

c. Coding and sequencing of complications

Coding and sequencing of complications associated with the malignancies or with the therapy thereof are subject to the following guidelines:

1) Anemia associated with malignancy

When admission/encounter is for management of an anemia associated with the malignancy, and the treatment is only for anemia, the appropriate code for the malignancy is sequenced as the principal or first-listed diagnosis followed by the appropriate code for the anemia (such as code D63.0, Anemia in neoplastic disease).

2) Anemia associated with chemotherapy, immunotherapy and radiation therapy

When the admission/encounter is for management of an anemia associated with an adverse effect of the administration of chemotherapy or immunotherapy and the only treatment is for the anemia, the anemia code is sequenced first followed by the appropriate codes for the neoplasm and the adverse effect (T45.1X5-, Adverse effect of antineoplastic and immunosuppressive drugs).

When the admission/encounter is for management of an anemia associated with an adverse effect of radiotherapy, the anemia code should be sequenced first, followed by the appropriate neoplasm code and code Y84.2, Radiological procedure and radiotherapy as the cause of abnormal reaction of the patient, or of later complication, without mention of misadventure at the time of the procedure.

3) Management of dehydration due to the malignancy

When the admission/encounter is for management of dehydration due to the malignancy and only the dehydration is being treated (intravenous rehydration), the dehydration is sequenced first, followed by the code(s) for the malignancy.

4) Treatment of a complication resulting from a surgical procedure

When the admission/encounter is for treatment of a complication resulting from a surgical procedure, designate the complication as the principal or first-listed diagnosis if treatment is directed at resolving the complication.

d. Primary malignancy previously excised

When a primary malignancy has been previously excised or eradicated from its site and there is no further treatment directed to that site and there is no evidence of any existing primary malignancy at that site, a code from category Z85, Personal history of malignant neoplasm, should be used to indicate the former site of the malignancy. Any mention of extension, invasion, or metastasis to another site is coded as a secondary malignant neoplasm to that site. The secondary site may be the principal or first-listed diagnosis with the Z85 code used as a secondary code.

e. Admissions/Encounters involving chemotherapy, immunotherapy and radiation therapy

1) Episode of care involves surgical removal of neoplasm

When an episode of care involves the surgical removal of a neoplasm, primary or secondary site, followed by adjunct chemotherapy or radiation treatment during the same episode of care, the code for the neoplasm should be assigned as principal or first-listed diagnosis.

2) Patient admission/encounter solely for administration of chemotherapy, immunotherapy and radiation therapy

If a patient admission/encounter is solely for the administration of chemotherapy, immunotherapy or external beam radiation therapy assign code Z51.0, Encounter for antineoplastic radiation therapy, or Z51.11, Encounter for antineoplastic chemotherapy, or Z51.12, Encounter for antineoplastic immunotherapy as the first-listed or principal diagnosis. If a patient receives more than one of these therapies during the same admission more than one of these codes may be assigned, in any sequence.

The malignancy for which the therapy is being administered should be assigned as a secondary diagnosis.

If a patient admission/encounter is for the insertion or implantation of radioactive elements (e.g., brachytherapy) the appropriate code for the malignancy is sequenced as the principal or first-listed diagnosis. Code Z51.0 should not be assigned.

3) **Patient admitted for radiation therapy, chemotherapy or immunotherapy and develops complications**

When a patient is admitted for the purpose of external beam radiotherapy, immunotherapy or chemotherapy and develops complications such as uncontrolled nausea and vomiting or dehydration, the principal or first-listed diagnosis is Z51.0, Encounter for antineoplastic radiation therapy, or Z51.11, Encounter for antineoplastic chemotherapy, or Z51.12, Encounter for antineoplastic immunotherapy followed by any codes for the complications.

When a patient is admitted for the purpose of insertion or implantation of radioactive elements (e.g., brachytherapy) and develops complications such as uncontrolled nausea and vomiting or dehydration, the principal or first-listed diagnosis is the appropriate code for the malignancy followed by any codes for the complications.

f. **Admission/encounter to determine extent of malignancy**

When the reason for admission/encounter is to determine the extent of the malignancy, or for a procedure such as paracentesis or thoracentesis, the primary malignancy or appropriate metastatic site is designated as the principal or first-listed diagnosis, even though chemotherapy or radiotherapy is administered.

g. **Symptoms, signs, and abnormal findings listed in Chapter 18 associated with neoplasms**

Symptoms, signs, and ill-defined conditions listed in Chapter 18 characteristic of, or associated with, an existing primary or secondary site malignancy cannot be used to replace the malignancy as principal or first-listed diagnosis, regardless of the number of admissions or encounters for treatment and care of the neoplasm.

See section I.C.21. Factors influencing health status and contact with health services, Encounter for prophylactic organ removal.

h. **Admission/encounter for pain control/management**

See Section I.C.6. for information on coding admission/encounter for pain control/management.

i. **Malignancy in two or more noncontiguous sites**

A patient may have more than one malignant tumor in the same organ. These tumors may represent different primaries or metastatic disease, depending on the site. Should the documentation be unclear, the provider should be queried as to the status of each tumor so that the correct codes can be assigned.

j. **Disseminated malignant neoplasm, unspecified**

Code C80.0, Disseminated malignant neoplasm, unspecified, is for use only in those cases where the patient has advanced metastatic disease and no known primary or secondary sites are specified. It should not be used in place of assigning codes for the primary site and all known secondary sites.

k. **Malignant neoplasm without specification of site**

Code C80.1, Malignant (primary) neoplasm, unspecified, equates to Cancer, unspecified. This code should only be used when no determination can be made as to the primary site of a malignancy. This code should rarely be used in the inpatient setting.

l. **Sequencing of neoplasm codes**

1) **Encounter for treatment of primary malignancy**

If the reason for the encounter is for treatment of a primary malignancy, assign the malignancy as the principal/first-listed diagnosis. The primary site is to be sequenced first, followed by any metastatic sites.

2) **Encounter for treatment of secondary malignancy**

When an encounter is for a primary malignancy with metastasis and treatment is directed toward the metastatic (secondary) site(s) only, the metastatic site(s) is designated as the principal/first-listed diagnosis. The primary malignancy is coded as an additional code.

3) **Malignant neoplasm in a pregnant patient**

When a pregnant **patient** has a malignant neoplasm, a code from subcategory O9A.1-, Malignant neoplasm complicating pregnancy, childbirth, and the puerperium, should be sequenced first, followed by the appropriate code from Chapter 2 to indicate the type of neoplasm.

4) **Encounter for complication associated with a neoplasm**

When an encounter is for management of a complication associated with a neoplasm, such as dehydration, and the treatment is only for the complication, the complication is coded first, followed by the appropriate code(s) for the neoplasm.

The exception to this guideline is anemia. When the admission/encounter is for management of an anemia associated with the malignancy, and the treatment is only for anemia, the appropriate code for the malignancy is sequenced as the principal or first-listed diagnosis followed by code D63.0, Anemia in neoplastic disease.

5) **Complication from surgical procedure for treatment of a neoplasm**

When an encounter is for treatment of a complication resulting from a surgical procedure performed for the treatment of the neoplasm, designate the complication as the principal/first-listed diagnosis. See the guideline regarding the coding of a current malignancy versus personal history to determine if the code for the neoplasm should also be assigned.

6) **Pathologic fracture due to a neoplasm**

When an encounter is for a pathological fracture due to a neoplasm, and the focus of treatment is the fracture, a code from subcategory M84.5, Pathological fracture in neoplastic disease, should be sequenced first, followed by the code for the neoplasm.

If the focus of treatment is the neoplasm with an associated pathological fracture, the neoplasm code should be sequenced first, followed by a code from M84.5 for the pathological fracture.

m. **Current malignancy versus personal history of malignancy**

When a primary malignancy has been excised but further treatment, such as an additional surgery for the malignancy, radiation therapy or chemotherapy is directed to that site, the primary malignancy code should be used until treatment is completed.

When a primary malignancy has been previously excised or eradicated from its site, there is no further treatment (of the malignancy) directed to that site, and there is no evidence of any existing primary malignancy at that site, a code from category Z85, Personal history of malignant neoplasm, should be used to indicate the former site of the malignancy.

Codes from subcategories Z85.0 – Z85.85 should only be assigned for the former site of a primary malignancy, not the site of a secondary malignancy. Code Z85.89 may be assigned for the former site(s) of either a primary or secondary malignancy.

See Section I.C.21. Factors influencing health status and contact with health services, History (of)

n. **Leukemia, Multiple Myeloma, and Malignant Plasma Cell Neoplasms in remission versus personal history**

The categories for leukemia, and category C90, Multiple myeloma and malignant plasma cell neoplasms, have codes indicating whether or not the leukemia has achieved remission. There are also codes Z85.6, Personal history of leukemia, and Z85.79, Personal history of other malignant neoplasms of lymphoid, hematopoietic and related tissues. If the documentation is unclear as to whether the leukemia has achieved remission, the provider should be queried.

See Section I.C.21. Factors influencing health status and contact with health services, History (of)

o. **Aftercare following surgery for neoplasm**

See Section I.C.21. Factors influencing health status and contact with health services, Aftercare

p. **Follow-up care for completed treatment of a malignancy**

See Section I.C.21. Factors influencing health status and contact with health services, Follow-up

q. **Prophylactic organ removal for prevention of malignancy**

See Section I.C. 21, Factors influencing health status and contact with health services, Prophylactic organ removal

r. **Malignant neoplasm associated with transplanted organ**

A malignant neoplasm of a transplanted organ should be coded as a transplant complication. Assign first the appropriate code from category T86.-, Complications of transplanted organs and tissue, followed by code C80.2, Malignant neoplasm associated with transplanted organ. Use an additional code for the specific malignancy.

s. **Breast Implant Associated Anaplastic Large Cell Lymphoma**

Breast implant associated anaplastic large cell lymphoma (BIA-ALCL) is a type of lymphoma that can develop around breast implants. Assign code C84.7A, Anaplastic large cell lymphoma, ALK-negative, breast, for BIA-ALCL. Do not assign a complication code from chapter 19.

3. **Chapter 3: Disease of the blood and blood-forming organs and certain disorders involving the immune mechanism (D50-D89)**

Reserved for future guideline expansion

4. **Chapter 4: Endocrine, Nutritional, and Metabolic Diseases (E00-E89)**

a. **Diabetes mellitus**

The diabetes mellitus codes are combination codes that include the type of diabetes mellitus, the body system affected, and the complications affecting that body system. As many codes within a particular category as are necessary to describe all of the complications of the disease may be used. They should be sequenced based on the reason for a particular encounter. Assign as many codes from categories E08 – E13 as needed to identify all of the associated conditions that the patient has.

1) **Type of diabetes**

The age of a patient is not the sole determining factor, though most type 1 diabetics develop the condition before reaching puberty. For this reason, type 1 diabetes mellitus is also referred to as juvenile diabetes.

2) **Type of diabetes mellitus not documented**

If the type of diabetes mellitus is not documented in the medical record the default is E11.-, Type 2 diabetes mellitus.

3) **Diabetes mellitus and the use of insulin, oral hypoglycemics, and injectable non-insulin drugs**

If the documentation in a medical record does not indicate the type of diabetes but does indicate that the patient uses insulin, code E11-, Type 2 diabetes mellitus, should be assigned. **Additional** code(s) should be assigned from category Z79 to identify the long-term (current) use of insulin, oral hypoglycemic drugs, **or injectable non-insulin antidiabetic, as follows:**

If the patient is treated with both oral medications and insulin, **both code Z79.4, Long term (current) use of insulin, and code Z79.84, Long term (current) use of oral hypoglycemic drugs,** should be assigned.

If the patient is treated with both insulin and an injectable non-insulin antidiabetic drug, assign codes Z79.4, Long term (current) use of insulin, and Z79.899, Other long term (current) drug therapy.

If the patient is treated with both oral hypoglycemic drugs and an injectable non-insulin antidiabetic drug, assign codes Z79.84, Long term (current) use of oral hypoglycemic drugs, and Z79.899, Other long term (current) drug therapy.

Code Z79.4 should not be assigned if insulin is given temporarily to bring a type 2 patient's blood sugar under control during an encounter.

4) **Diabetes mellitus in pregnancy and gestational diabetes**

See Section I.C.15. Diabetes mellitus in pregnancy.

See Section I.C.15. Gestational (pregnancy induced) diabetes

5) **Complications due to insulin pump malfunction**

(a) **Underdose of insulin due to insulin pump failure**

An underdose of insulin due to an insulin pump failure should be assigned to a code from subcategory T85.6, Mechanical complication of other specified internal and external prosthetic devices, implants and grafts, that specifies the type of pump malfunction, as the principal or first-listed code, followed by code T38.3X6-, Underdosing of insulin and oral hypoglycemic [antidiabetic] drugs. Additional codes for the type of diabetes mellitus and any associated complications due to the underdosing should also be assigned.

(b) **Overdose of insulin due to insulin pump failure**

The principal or first-listed code for an encounter due to an insulin pump malfunction resulting in an overdose of insulin, should also be T85.6-, Mechanical complication of other specified internal and external prosthetic devices, implants and grafts, followed by code T38.3X1-, Poisoning by insulin and oral hypoglycemic [antidiabetic] drugs, accidental (unintentional).

6) **Secondary diabetes mellitus**

Codes under categories E08, Diabetes mellitus due to underlying condition, E09, Drug or chemical induced diabetes mellitus, and E13, Other specified diabetes mellitus, identify complications/manifestations associated with secondary diabetes mellitus. Secondary diabetes is always caused by another condition or event (e.g., cystic fibrosis, malignant neoplasm of pancreas, pancreatectomy, adverse effect of drug, or poisoning).

(a) **Secondary diabetes mellitus and the use of insulin, oral hypoglycemic drugs, or injectable non-insulin drugs**

For patients with secondary diabetes mellitus who routinely use insulin, oral hypoglycemic drugs, **or injectable non-insulin drugs,** additional code(s) from category Z79 should be assigned to identify the long-term (current) use of insulin, oral hypoglycemic drugs, **or non-injectable non-insulin drugs as follows:**

If the patient is treated with both oral medications and insulin, **both code Z79.4, Long term (current) use of insulin, and code Z79.84, Long term (current) use of oral hypoglycemic drugs,** should be assigned.

If the patient is treated with both insulin and an injectable non-insulin antidiabetic drug, assign codes Z79.4, Long-term (current) use of insulin, and Z79.899, Other long term (current) drug therapy.

If the patient is treated with both oral hypoglycemic drugs and an injectable non-insulin antidiabetic drug, assign codes Z79.84, Long-term (current) use of oral hypoglycemic drugs, and Z79.899, Other long-term (current) drug therapy.

Code Z79.4 should not be assigned if insulin is given temporarily to bring a secondary diabetic patient's blood sugar under control during an encounter.

(b) **Assigning and sequencing secondary diabetes codes and its causes**

The sequencing of the secondary diabetes codes in relationship to codes for the cause of the diabetes is based on the Tabular List instructions for categories E08, E09 and E13.

(i) **Secondary diabetes mellitus due to pancreatectomy**

For postpancreatectomy diabetes mellitus (lack of insulin due to the surgical removal of all or part of the pancreas), assign code E89.1, Postprocedural hypoinsulinemia.

Assign a code from category E13 and a code from subcategory Z90.41, Acquired absence of pancreas, as additional codes.

(ii) **Secondary diabetes due to drugs**

Secondary diabetes may be caused by an adverse effect of correctly administered medications, poisoning or sequela of poisoning.

See section I.C.19.e for coding of adverse effects and poisoning, and section I.C.20 for external cause code reporting.

5. **Chapter 5: Mental, Behavioral and Neurodevelopmental disorders (F01-F99)**

a. **Pain disorders related to psychological factors**

Assign code F45.41, for pain that is exclusively related to psychological disorders. As indicated by the Excludes 1 note under category G89, a code from category G89 should not be assigned with code F45.41.

Code F45.42, Pain disorders with related psychological factors, should be used with a code from category G89, Pain, not elsewhere classified, if there is documentation of a psychological component for a patient with acute or chronic pain.

See Section I.C.6. Pain

b. **Mental and behavioral disorders due to psychoactive substance use**

1) **In Remission**

Selection of codes for "in remission" for categories F10-F19, Mental and behavioral disorders due to psychoactive substance use (categories F10-F19 with -.11, -.21) requires the provider's clinical judgment. The appropriate codes for "in remission" are assigned only on the basis of provider documentation (as defined in the Official Guidelines for Coding and Reporting), unless otherwise instructed by the classification.

Mild substance use disorders in early or sustained remission are classified to the appropriate codes for substance abuse in remission, and moderate or severe substance use disorders in

early or sustained remission are classified to the appropriate codes for substance dependence in remission.

2) Psychoactive Substance Use, Abuse and Dependence
When the provider documentation refers to use, abuse and dependence of the same substance (e.g. alcohol, opioid, cannabis, etc.), only one code should be assigned to identify the pattern of use based on the following hierarchy:

- If both use and abuse are documented, assign only the code for abuse
- If both abuse and dependence are documented, assign only the code for dependence
- If use, abuse and dependence are all documented, assign only the code for dependence
- If both use and dependence are documented, assign only the code for dependence.

3) Psychoactive Substance Use, Unspecified
As with all other unspecified diagnoses, the codes for unspecified psychoactive substance use (F10.9-, F11.9-, F12.9-, F13.9-, F14.9-, F15.9-, F16.9-, F18.9-, F19.9-) should only be assigned based on provider documentation and when they meet the definition of a reportable diagnosis (see Section III, Reporting Additional Diagnoses). These codes are to be used only when the psychoactive substance use is associated with a **substance related** disorder (chapter 5 **disorders** such as sexual dysfunction, sleep disorder, or a mental or behavioral disorder) **or medical condition**, and such a relationship is documented by the provider.

4) Medical Conditions Due to Psychoactive Substance Use, Abuse and Dependence
Medical conditions due to substance use, abuse, and dependence are not classified as substance-induced disorders. Assign the diagnosis code for the medical condition as directed by the Alphabetical Index along with the appropriate psychoactive substance use, abuse or dependence code. For example, for alcoholic pancreatitis due to alcohol dependence, assign the appropriate code from subcategory K85.2, Alcohol induced acute pancreatitis, and the appropriate code from subcategory F10.2, such as code F10.20, Alcohol dependence, uncomplicated. It would not be appropriate to assign code F10.288, Alcohol dependence with other alcohol-induced disorder.

5) Blood Alcohol Level
A code from category Y90, Evidence of alcohol involvement determined by blood alcohol level, may be assigned when this information is documented and the patient's provider has documented a condition classifiable to category F10, Alcohol related disorders. The blood alcohol level does not need to be documented by the patient's provider in order for it to be coded.

c. Factitious Disorder
Factitious disorder imposed on self or Munchausen's syndrome is a disorder in which a person falsely reports or causes his or her own physical or psychological signs or symptoms. For patients with documented factitious disorder on self or Munchausen's syndrome, assign the appropriate code from subcategory F68.1-, Factitious disorder imposed on self.

Munchausen's syndrome by proxy (MSBP) is a disorder in which a caregiver (perpetrator) falsely reports or causes an illness or injury in another person (victim) under his or her care, such as a child, an elderly adult, or a person who has a disability. The condition is also referred to as "factitious disorder imposed on another" or "factitious disorder by proxy." The perpetrator, not the victim, receives this diagnosis. Assign code F68.A, Factitious disorder imposed on another, to the perpetrator's record. For the victim of a patient suffering from MSBP, assign the appropriate code from categories T74, Adult and child abuse, neglect and other maltreatment, confirmed, or T76, Adult and child abuse, neglect and other maltreatment, suspected.

See Section I.C.19.f. Adult and child abuse, neglect and other maltreatment

6. Chapter 6: Diseases of the Nervous System (G00-G99)
a. Dominant/nondominant side
Codes from category G81, Hemiplegia and hemiparesis, and subcategories G83.1, Monoplegia of lower limb, G83.2, Monoplegia of upper limb, and G83.3, Monoplegia, unspecified, identify whether the dominant or nondominant side is affected. Should the affected side

be documented, but not specified as dominant or nondominant, and the classification system does not indicate a default, code selection is as follows:

- For ambidextrous patients, the default should be dominant.
- If the left side is affected, the default is non-dominant.
- If the right side is affected, the default is dominant.

b. Pain - Category G89
1) General coding information
Codes in category G89, Pain, not elsewhere classified, may be used in conjunction with codes from other categories and chapters to provide more detail about acute or chronic pain and neoplasm-related pain, unless otherwise indicated below.

If the pain is not specified as acute or chronic, post-thoracotomy, postprocedural, or neoplasm-related, do not assign codes from category G89.

A code from category G89 should not be assigned if the underlying (definitive) diagnosis is known, unless the reason for the encounter is pain control/ management and not management of the underlying condition.

When an admission or encounter is for a procedure aimed at treating the underlying condition (e.g., spinal fusion, kyphoplasty), a code for the underlying condition (e.g., vertebral fracture, spinal stenosis) should be assigned as the principal diagnosis. No code from category G89 should be assigned.

(a) Category G89 Codes as Principal or First-Listed Diagnosis
Category G89 codes are acceptable as principal diagnosis or the first-listed code:

- When pain control or pain management is the reason for the admission/encounter (e.g., a patient with displaced intervertebral disc, nerve impingement and severe back pain presents for injection of steroid into the spinal canal). The underlying cause of the pain should be reported as an additional diagnosis, if known.
- When a patient is admitted for the insertion of a neurostimulator for pain control, assign the appropriate pain code as the principal or first-listed diagnosis. When an admission or encounter is for a procedure aimed at treating the underlying condition and a neurostimulator is inserted for pain control during the same admission/encounter, a code for the underlying condition should be assigned as the principal diagnosis and the appropriate pain code should be assigned as a secondary diagnosis.

(b) Use of Category G89 Codes in Conjunction with Site Specific Pain Codes
(i) Assigning Category G89 and Site-Specific Pain Codes
Codes from category G89 may be used in conjunction with codes that identify the site of pain (including codes from chapter 18) if the category G89 code provides additional information. For example, if the code describes the site of the pain, but does not fully describe whether the pain is acute or chronic, then both codes should be assigned.

(ii) Sequencing of Category G89 Codes with Site-Specific Pain Codes
The sequencing of category G89 codes with site-specific pain codes (including chapter 18 codes), is dependent on the circumstances of the encounter/admission as follows:

- If the encounter is for pain control or pain management, assign the code from category G89 followed by the code identifying the specific site of pain (e.g., encounter for pain management for acute neck pain from trauma is assigned code G89.11, Acute pain due to trauma, followed by code M54.2, Cervicalgia, to identify the site of pain).
- If the encounter is for any other reason except pain control or pain management, and a related definitive diagnosis has not been established (confirmed) by the provider, assign the code for the specific site of

pain first, followed by the appropriate code from category G89.

2) Pain due to devices, implants and grafts
See Section I.C.19. Pain due to medical devices

3) Postoperative Pain
The provider's documentation should be used to guide the coding of postoperative pain, as well as *Section III. Reporting Additional Diagnoses* and *Section IV. Diagnostic Coding and Reporting in the Outpatient Setting.*

The default for post-thoracotomy and other postoperative pain not specified as acute or chronic is the code for the acute form.

Routine or expected postoperative pain immediately after surgery should not be coded.

(a) Postoperative pain not associated with specific postoperative complication
Postoperative pain not associated with a specific postoperative complication is assigned to the appropriate postoperative pain code in category G89.

(b) Postoperative pain associated with specific postoperative complication
Postoperative pain associated with a specific postoperative complication (such as painful wire sutures) is assigned to the appropriate code(s) found in Chapter 19, Injury, poisoning, and certain other consequences of external causes. If appropriate, use additional code(s) from category G89 to identify acute or chronic pain (G89.18 or G89.28).

4) Chronic pain
Chronic pain is classified to subcategory G89.2. There is no time frame defining when pain becomes chronic pain. The provider's documentation should be used to guide use of these codes.

5) Neoplasm Related Pain
Code G89.3 is assigned to pain documented as being related, associated or due to cancer, primary or secondary malignancy, or tumor. This code is assigned regardless of whether the pain is acute or chronic.

This code may be assigned as the principal or first-listed code when the stated reason for the admission/encounter is documented as pain control/pain management. The underlying neoplasm should be reported as an additional diagnosis.

When the reason for the admission/encounter is management of the neoplasm and the pain associated with the neoplasm is also documented, code G89.3 may be assigned as an additional diagnosis. It is not necessary to assign an additional code for the site of the pain.

See Section I.C.2 for instructions on the sequencing of neoplasms for all other stated reasons for the admission/encounter (except for pain control/pain management).

6) Chronic pain syndrome
Central pain syndrome (G89.0) and chronic pain syndrome (G89.4) are different than the term "chronic pain," and therefore codes should only be used when the provider has specifically documented this condition.

See Section I.C.5. Pain disorders related to psychological factors

7. Chapter 7: Diseases of the Eye and Adnexa (H00-H59)
a. Glaucoma
1) Assigning Glaucoma Codes
Assign as many codes from category H40, Glaucoma, as needed to identify the type of glaucoma, the affected eye, and the glaucoma stage.

2) Bilateral glaucoma with same type and stage
When a patient has bilateral glaucoma and both eyes are documented as being the same type and stage, and there is a code for bilateral glaucoma, report only the code for the type of glaucoma, bilateral, with the seventh character for the stage.

When a patient has bilateral glaucoma and both eyes are documented as being the same type and stage, and the classification does not provide a code for bilateral glaucoma (i.e. subcategories H40.10, and H40.20) report only one code for the type of glaucoma with the appropriate seventh character for the stage.

3) Bilateral glaucoma stage with different types or stages
When a patient has bilateral glaucoma and each eye is documented as having a different type or stage, and the classification distinguishes laterality, assign the appropriate code for each eye rather than the code for bilateral glaucoma.

When a patient has bilateral glaucoma and each eye is documented as having a different type, and the classification does not distinguish laterality (i.e., subcategories H40.10, and H40.20), assign one code for each type of glaucoma with the appropriate seventh character for the stage.

When a patient has bilateral glaucoma and each eye is documented as having the same type, but different stage, and the classification does not distinguish laterality (i.e., subcategories H40.10 and H40.20), assign a code for the type of glaucoma for each eye with the seventh character for the specific glaucoma stage documented for each eye.

4) Patient admitted with glaucoma and stage evolves during the admission
If a patient is admitted with glaucoma and the stage progresses during the admission, assign the code for highest stage documented.

5) Indeterminate stage glaucoma
Assignment of the seventh character "4" for "indeterminate stage" should be based on the clinical documentation. The seventh character "4" is used for glaucomas whose stage cannot be clinically determined. This seventh character should not be confused with the seventh character "0", unspecified, which should be assigned when there is no documentation regarding the stage of the glaucoma.

b. Blindness
If "blindness" or "low vision" of both eyes is documented but the visual impairment category is not documented, assign code H54.3, Unqualified visual loss, both eyes. If "blindness" or "low vision" in one eye is documented but the visual impairment category is not documented, assign a code from H54.6-, Unqualified visual loss, one eye. If "blindness" or "visual loss" is documented without any information about whether one or both eyes are affected, assign code H54.7, Unspecified visual loss.

8. Chapter 8: Diseases of the Ear and Mastoid Process (H60-H95)
Reserved for future guideline expansion

9. Chapter 9: Diseases of the Circulatory System (I00-I99)
a. Hypertension
The classification presumes a causal relationship between hypertension and heart involvement and between hypertension and kidney involvement, as the two conditions are linked by the term "with" in the Alphabetic Index. These conditions should be coded as related even in the absence of provider documentation explicitly linking them, unless the documentation clearly states the conditions are unrelated.

For hypertension and conditions not specifically linked by relational terms such as "with," "associated with" or "due to" in the classification, provider documentation must link the conditions in order to code them as related.

1) Hypertension with Heart Disease
Hypertension with heart conditions classified to I50.- or I51.4-I51.7, I51.89, I51.9, are assigned to a code from category I11, Hypertensive heart disease. Use additional code(s) from category I50, Heart failure, to identify the type(s) of heart failure in those patients with heart failure.

The same heart conditions (I50.-, I51.4-I51.7, I51.89, I51.9) with hypertension are coded separately if the provider has documented they are unrelated to the hypertension. Sequence according to the circumstances of the admission/encounter.

2) Hypertensive Chronic Kidney Disease
Assign codes from category I12, Hypertensive chronic kidney disease, when both hypertension and a condition classifiable to category N18, Chronic kidney disease (CKD), are present. CKD should not be coded as hypertensive if the provider indicates the CKD is not related to the hypertension.

The appropriate code from category N18 should be used as a secondary code with a code from category I12 to identify the stage of chronic kidney disease.

See Section I.C.14. Chronic kidney disease.

If a patient has hypertensive chronic kidney disease and acute renal failure, the acute renal failure should also be coded. Sequence according to the circumstances of the admission/encounter.

3) Hypertensive Heart and Chronic Kidney Disease

Assign codes from combination category I13, Hypertensive heart and chronic kidney disease, when there is hypertension with both heart and kidney involvement. If heart failure is present, assign an additional code from category I50 to identify the type of heart failure.

The appropriate code from category N18, Chronic kidney disease, should be used as a secondary code with a code from category I13 to identify the stage of chronic kidney disease.

See Section I.C.14. Chronic kidney disease.

The codes in category I13, Hypertensive heart and chronic kidney disease, are combination codes that include hypertension, heart disease and chronic kidney disease. The Includes note at I13 specifies that the conditions included at I11 and I12 are included together in I13. If a patient has hypertension, heart disease and chronic kidney disease, then a code from I13 should be used, not individual codes for hypertension, heart disease and chronic kidney disease, or codes from I11 or I12.

For patients with both acute renal failure and chronic kidney disease, the acute renal failure should also be coded. Sequence according to the circumstances of the admission/encounter.

4) Hypertensive Cerebrovascular Disease

For hypertensive cerebrovascular disease, first assign the appropriate code from categories I60-I69, followed by the appropriate hypertension code.

5) Hypertensive Retinopathy

Subcategory H35.0, Background retinopathy and retinal vascular changes, should be used **along** with a code from categor**ies** I10-I15, **in the** Hypertensive disease**s section,** to include the systemic hypertension. The sequencing is based on the reason for the encounter.

6) Hypertension, Secondary

Secondary hypertension is due to an underlying condition. Two codes are required: one to identify the underlying etiology and one from category I15 to identify the hypertension. Sequencing of codes is determined by the reason for admission/encounter.

7) Hypertension, Transient

Assign code R03.0, Elevated blood pressure reading without diagnosis of hypertension, unless patient has an established diagnosis of hypertension. Assign code O13.-, Gestational [pregnancy-induced] hypertension without significant proteinuria, or O14.-, Pre-eclampsia, for transient hypertension of pregnancy.

8) Hypertension, Controlled

This diagnostic statement usually refers to an existing state of hypertension under control by therapy. Assign the appropriate code from categories I10-I15, Hypertensive diseases.

9) Hypertension, Uncontrolled

Uncontrolled hypertension may refer to untreated hypertension or hypertension not responding to current therapeutic regimen. In either case, assign the appropriate code from categories I10-I15, Hypertensive diseases.

10) Hypertensive Crisis

Assign a code from category I16, Hypertensive crisis, for documented hypertensive urgency, hypertensive emergency or unspecified hypertensive crisis. Code also any identified hypertensive disease (I10-I15). The sequencing is based on the reason for the encounter.

11) Pulmonary Hypertension

Pulmonary hypertension is classified to category I27, Other pulmonary heart diseases. For secondary pulmonary hypertension (I27.1, I27.2-), code also any associated conditions or adverse effects of drugs or toxins. The sequencing is based on the reason for the encounter, except for adverse effects of drugs (See Section I.C.19.e.).

b. Atherosclerotic Coronary Artery Disease and Angina

ICD-10-CM has combination codes for atherosclerotic heart disease with angina pectoris. The subcategories for these codes are I25.11, Atherosclerotic heart disease of native coronary artery with angina pectoris and I25.7, Atherosclerosis of coronary artery bypass graft(s) and coronary artery of transplanted heart with angina pectoris.

When using one of these combination codes it is not necessary to use an additional code for angina pectoris. A causal relationship can be assumed in a patient with both atherosclerosis and angina pectoris, unless the documentation indicates the angina is due to something other than the atherosclerosis.

If a patient with coronary artery disease is admitted due to an acute myocardial infarction (AMI), the AMI should be sequenced before the coronary artery disease.

See Section I.C.9. Acute myocardial infarction (AMI)

c. Intraoperative and Postprocedural Cerebrovascular Accident

Medical record documentation should clearly specify the cause-and-effect relationship between the medical intervention and the cerebrovascular accident in order to assign a code for intraoperative or postprocedural cerebrovascular accident.

Proper code assignment depends on whether it was an infarction or hemorrhage and whether it occurred intraoperatively or postoperatively. If it was a cerebral hemorrhage, code assignment depends on the type of procedure performed.

d. Sequelae of Cerebrovascular Disease

1) Category I69, Sequelae of Cerebrovascular disease

Category I69 is used to indicate conditions classifiable to categories I60-I67 as the causes of sequela (neurologic deficits), themselves classified elsewhere. These "late effects" include neurologic deficits that persist after initial onset of conditions classifiable to categories I60-I67. The neurologic deficits caused by cerebrovascular disease may be present from the onset or may arise at any time after the onset of the condition classifiable to categories I60-I67.

Codes from category I69, Sequelae of cerebrovascular disease, that specify hemiplegia, hemiparesis and monoplegia identify whether the dominant or nondominant side is affected. Should the affected side be documented, but not specified as dominant or nondominant, and the classification system does not indicate a default, code selection is as follows:

- For ambidextrous patients, the default should be dominant.
- If the left side is affected, the default is non-dominant.
- If the right side is affected, the default is dominant.

2) Codes from category I69 with codes from I60-I67

Codes from category I69 may be assigned on a health care record with codes from I60-I67, if the patient has a current cerebrovascular disease and deficits from an old cerebrovascular disease.

3) Codes from category I69 and Personal history of transient ischemic attack (TIA) and cerebral infarction (Z86.73)

Codes from category I69 should not be assigned if the patient does not have neurologic deficits.

See Section I.C.21. 4. History (of) for use of personal history codes

e. Acute myocardial infarction (AMI)

1) Type 1 ST elevation myocardial infarction (STEMI) and non-ST elevation myocardial infarction (NSTEMI)

The ICD-10-CM codes for type 1 acute myocardial infarction (AMI) identify the site, such as anterolateral wall or true posterior wall. Subcategories I21.0-I21.2 and code I21.3 are used for type 1 ST elevation myocardial infarction (STEMI). Code I21.4, Non-ST elevation (NSTEMI) myocardial infarction, is used for type 1 non-ST elevation myocardial infarction (NSTEMI) and nontransmural MIs.

If a type 1 NSTEMI evolves to STEMI, assign the STEMI code. If a type 1 STEMI converts to NSTEMI due to thrombolytic therapy, it is still coded as STEMI.

For encounters occurring while the myocardial infarction is equal to, or less than, four weeks old, including transfers to another acute setting or a postacute setting, and the myocardial infarction meets the definition for "other diagnoses" (see Section III, Reporting Additional Diagnoses), codes from category I21 may continue to be reported. For encounters after the 4-week time frame and the patient is still receiving care related to the myocardial infarction, the appropriate aftercare code should be assigned, rather than a code from category I21. For old or healed myocardial infarctions not requiring further care, code I25.2, Old myocardial infarction, may be assigned.

2) Acute myocardial infarction, unspecified

Code I21.9, Acute myocardial infarction, unspecified, is the default for unspecified acute myocardial infarction or unspecified type. If only type 1 STEMI or transmural MI without the site is documented, assign code I21.3, ST elevation (STEMI) myocardial infarction of unspecified site.

3) AMI documented as nontransmural or subendocardial but site provided

If an AMI is documented as nontransmural or subendocardial, but the site is provided, it is still coded as a subendocardial AMI.

See Section I.C.21.3 for information on coding status post administration of tPA in a different facility within the last 24 hours.

4) Subsequent acute myocardial infarction

A code from category I22, Subsequent ST elevation (STEMI) and non-ST elevation (NSTEMI) myocardial infarction, is to be used when a patient who has suffered a type 1 or unspecified AMI has a new AMI within the 4 week time frame of the initial AMI. A code from category I22 must be used in conjunction with a code from category I21. The sequencing of the I22 and I21 codes depends on the circumstances of the encounter.

Do not assign code I22 for subsequent myocardial infarctions other than type 1 or unspecified. For subsequent type 2 AMI assign only code I21.A1. For subsequent type 4 or type 5 AMI, assign only code I21.A9.

If a subsequent myocardial infarction of one type occurs within 4 weeks of a myocardial infarction of a different type, assign the appropriate codes from category I21 to identify each type. Do not assign a code from category I22. Codes from category I22 should only be assigned if both the initial and subsequent myocardial infarctions are type 1 or unspecified.

5) Other Types of Myocardial Infarction

The ICD-10-CM provides codes for different types of myocardial infarction. Type 1 myocardial infarctions are assigned to codes I21.0-I21.4.

Type 2 myocardial infarction (myocardial infarction due to demand ischemia or secondary to ischemic imbalance) is assigned to code I21.A1, Myocardial infarction type 2 with the underlying cause coded first. Do not assign code I24.8, Other forms of acute ischemic heart disease, for the demand ischemia. If a type 2 AMI is described as NSTEMI or STEMI, only assign code I21.A1. Codes I21.01-I21.4 should only be assigned for type 1 AMIs.

Acute myocardial infarctions type 3, 4a, 4b, 4c and 5 are assigned to code I21.A9, Other myocardial infarction type.

The "Code also" and "Code first" notes should be followed related to complications, and for coding of postprocedural myocardial infarctions during or following cardiac surgery.

10. Chapter 10: Diseases of the Respiratory System (J00-J99), U07.0

a. Chronic Obstructive Pulmonary Disease [COPD] and Asthma

1) Acute exacerbation of chronic obstructive bronchitis and asthma

The codes in categories J44 and J45 distinguish between uncomplicated cases and those in acute exacerbation. An acute exacerbation is a worsening or a decompensation of a chronic condition. An acute exacerbation is not equivalent to an infection superimposed on a chronic condition, though an exacerbation may be triggered by an infection.

b. Acute Respiratory Failure

1) Acute respiratory failure as principal diagnosis

A code from subcategory J96.0, Acute respiratory failure, or subcategory J96.2, Acute and chronic respiratory failure, may be assigned as a principal diagnosis when it is the condition established after study to be chiefly responsible for occasioning the admission to the hospital, and the selection is supported by the Alphabetic Index and Tabular List. However, chapter-specific coding guidelines (such as obstetrics, poisoning, HIV, newborn) that provide sequencing direction take precedence.

2) Acute respiratory failure as secondary diagnosis

Respiratory failure may be listed as a secondary diagnosis if it occurs after admission, or if it is present on admission, but does not meet the definition of principal diagnosis.

3) Sequencing of acute respiratory failure and another acute condition

When a patient is admitted with respiratory failure and another acute condition, (e.g., myocardial infarction, cerebrovascular accident, aspiration pneumonia), the principal diagnosis will not be the same in every situation. This applies whether the other acute condition is a respiratory or nonrespiratory condition. Selection of the principal diagnosis will be dependent on the circumstances of admission. If both the respiratory failure and the other acute condition are equally responsible for occasioning the admission to the hospital, and there are no chapter-specific sequencing rules, the guideline regarding two or more diagnoses that equally meet the definition for principal diagnosis (Section II, C.) may be applied in these situations.

If the documentation is not clear as to whether acute respiratory failure and another condition are equally responsible for occasioning the admission, query the provider for clarification.

c. Influenza due to certain identified influenza viruses

Code only confirmed cases of influenza due to certain identified influenza viruses (category J09), and due to other identified influenza virus (category J10). This is an exception to the hospital inpatient guideline Section II, H. (Uncertain Diagnosis).

In this context, "confirmation" does not require documentation of positive laboratory testing specific for avian or other novel influenza A or other identified influenza virus. However, coding should be based on the provider's diagnostic statement that the patient has avian influenza, or other novel influenza A, for category J09, or has another particular identified strain of influenza, such as H1N1 or H3N2, but not identified as novel or variant, for category J10.

If the provider records "suspected" or "possible" or "probable" avian influenza, or novel influenza, or other identified influenza, then the appropriate influenza code from category J11, Influenza due to unidentified influenza virus, should be assigned. A code from category J09, Influenza due to certain identified influenza viruses, should not be assigned nor should a code from category J10, Influenza due to other identified influenza virus.

d. Ventilator associated Pneumonia

1) Documentation of Ventilator associated Pneumonia

As with all procedural or postprocedural complications, code assignment is based on the provider's documentation of the relationship between the condition and the procedure.

Code J95.851, Ventilator associated pneumonia, should be assigned only when the provider has documented ventilator associated pneumonia (VAP). An additional code to identify the organism (e.g., Pseudomonas aeruginosa, code B96.5) should also be assigned. Do not assign an additional code from categories J12-J18 to identify the type of pneumonia.

Code J95.851 should not be assigned for cases where the patient has pneumonia and is on a mechanical ventilator and the provider has not specifically stated that the pneumonia is ventilator-associated pneumonia. If the documentation is unclear as to whether the patient has a pneumonia that is a complication attributable to the mechanical ventilator, query the provider.

2) Ventilator associated Pneumonia Develops after Admission

A patient may be admitted with one type of pneumonia (e.g., code J13, Pneumonia due to Streptococcus pneumonia) and subsequently develop VAP. In this instance, the principal diagnosis would be the appropriate code from categories J12-J18 for the pneumonia diagnosed at the time of admission. Code J95.851, Ventilator associated pneumonia, would be assigned as an additional diagnosis when the provider has also documented the presence of ventilator associated pneumonia.

e. Vaping-related disorders

For patients presenting with condition(s) related to vaping, assign code U07.0, Vaping-related disorder, as the principal diagnosis. For lung injury due to vaping, assign only code U07.0. Assign additional codes for other manifestations, such as acute respiratory failure (subcategory J96.0-) or pneumonitis (code J68.0).

Associated respiratory signs and symptoms due to vaping, such as cough, shortness of breath, etc., are not coded separately, when a definitive diagnosis has been established. However, it would be appropriate to code separately any gastrointestinal symptoms, such as diarrhea and abdominal pain.

See Section I.C.1.g.1.c.i. for Pneumonia confirmed as due to COVID-19

11. Chapter 11: Diseases of the Digestive System (K00-K95)

Reserved for future guideline expansion

12. Chapter 12: Diseases of the Skin and Subcutaneous Tissue (L00-L99)

a. Pressure ulcer stage codes

1) Pressure ulcer stages

Codes in category L89, Pressure ulcer, identify the site and stage of the pressure ulcer.

The ICD-10-CM classifies pressure ulcer stages based on severity, which is designated by stages 1-4, deep tissue pressure injury, unspecified stage, and unstageable.

Assign as many codes from category L89 as needed to identify all the pressure ulcers the patient has, if applicable.

See Section I.B.14 for pressure ulcer stage documentation by clinicians other than patient's provider.

2) Unstageable pressure ulcers

Assignment of the code for unstageable pressure ulcer (L89.--0) should be based on the clinical documentation. These codes are used for pressure ulcers whose stage cannot be clinically determined (e.g., the ulcer is covered by eschar or has been treated with a skin or muscle graft). This code should not be confused with the codes for unspecified stage (L89.--9). When there is no documentation regarding the stage of the pressure ulcer, assign the appropriate code for unspecified stage (L89.-- 9).

If during an encounter, the stage of an unstageable pressure ulcer is revealed after debridement, assign only the code for the stage revealed following debridement.

3) Documented pressure ulcer stage

Assignment of the pressure ulcer stage code should be guided by clinical documentation of the stage or documentation of the terms found in the Alphabetic Index. For clinical terms describing the stage that are not found in the Alphabetic Index, and there is no documentation of the stage, the provider should be queried.

4) Patients admitted with pressure ulcers documented as healed

No code is assigned if the documentation states that the pressure ulcer is completely healed at the time of admission.

5) Pressure ulcers documented as healing

Pressure ulcers described as healing should be assigned the appropriate pressure ulcer stage code based on the documentation in the medical record. If the documentation does not provide information about the stage of the healing pressure ulcer, assign the appropriate code for unspecified stage.

If the documentation is unclear as to whether the patient has a current (new) pressure ulcer or if the patient is being treated for a healing pressure ulcer, query the provider.

For ulcers that were present on admission but healed at the time of discharge, assign the code for the site and stage of the pressure ulcer at the time of admission.

6) Patient admitted with pressure ulcer evolving into another stage during the admission

If a patient is admitted to an inpatient hospital with a pressure ulcer at one stage and it progresses to a higher stage, two separate codes should be assigned: one code for the site and stage of the ulcer on admission and a second code for the same ulcer site and the highest stage reported during the stay.

7) Pressure-induced deep tissue damage

For pressure-induced deep tissue damage or deep tissue pressure injury, assign only the appropriate code for pressure-induced deep tissue damage (L89.--6).

b. Non-Pressure Chronic Ulcers

1) Patients admitted with non-pressure ulcers documented as healed

No code is assigned if the documentation states that the non-pressure ulcer is completely healed at the time of admission.

2) Non-pressure ulcers documented as healing

Non-pressure ulcers described as healing should be assigned the appropriate non-pressure ulcer code based on the documentation in the medical record. If the documentation does not provide information about the severity of the healing non-pressure ulcer, assign the appropriate code for unspecified severity.

If the documentation is unclear as to whether the patient has a current (new) non-pressure ulcer or if the patient is being treated for a healing non-pressure ulcer, query the provider.

For ulcers that were present on admission but healed at the time of discharge, assign the code for the site and severity of the non-pressure ulcer at the time of admission.

3) Patient admitted with non-pressure ulcer that progresses to another severity level during the admission

If a patient is admitted to an inpatient hospital with a non-pressure ulcer at one severity level and it progresses to a higher severity level, two separate codes should be assigned: one code for the site and severity level of the ulcer on admission and a second code for the same ulcer site and the highest severity level reported during the stay.

See Section I.B.14 for pressure ulcer stage documentation by clinicians other than patient's provider

13. Chapter 13: Diseases of the Musculoskeletal System and Connective Tissue (M00-M99)

a. Site and laterality

Most of the codes within Chapter 13 have site and laterality designations. The site represents the bone, joint or the muscle involved. For some conditions where more than one bone, joint or muscle is usually involved, such as osteoarthritis, there is a "multiple sites" code available. For categories where no multiple site code is provided and more than one bone, joint or muscle is involved, multiple codes should be used to indicate the different sites involved.

1) Bone versus joint

For certain conditions, the bone may be affected at the upper or lower end, (e.g., avascular necrosis of bone, M87, Osteoporosis, M80, M81). Though the portion of the bone affected may be at the joint, the site designation will be the bone, not the joint.

b. Acute traumatic versus chronic or recurrent musculoskeletal conditions

Many musculoskeletal conditions are a result of previous injury or trauma to a site, or are recurrent conditions. Bone, joint or muscle conditions that are the result of a healed injury are usually found in chapter 13. Recurrent bone, joint or muscle conditions are also usually found in chapter 13. Any current, acute injury should be coded to the appropriate injury code from chapter 19. Chronic or recurrent conditions should generally be coded with a code from chapter 13. If it is difficult to determine from the documentation in the record which code is best to describe a condition, query the provider.

c. Coding of Pathologic Fractures

7th character A is for use as long as the patient is receiving active treatment for the fracture. While the patient may be seen by a new or different provider over the course of treatment for a pathological fracture, assignment of the 7th character is based on whether the patient is undergoing active treatment and not whether the provider is seeing the patient for the first time.

7th character D is to be used for encounters after the patient has completed active treatment for the fracture and is receiving routine care for the fracture during the healing or recovery phase. The other 7th characters, listed under each subcategory in the Tabular List, are to be used for subsequent encounters for treatment of problems associated with the healing, such as malunions, nonunions, and sequelae.

Care for complications of surgical treatment for fracture repairs during the healing or recovery phase should be coded with the appropriate complication codes.

See Section I.C.19. Coding of traumatic fractures.

d. Osteoporosis

Osteoporosis is a systemic condition, meaning that all bones of the musculoskeletal system are affected. Therefore, site is not a component of the codes under category M81, Osteoporosis without current pathological fracture. The site codes under category M80, Osteoporosis with current pathological fracture, identify the site of the fracture, not the osteoporosis.

1) Osteoporosis without pathological fracture

Category M81, Osteoporosis without current pathological fracture, is for use for patients with osteoporosis who do not currently have a pathologic fracture due to the osteoporosis, even if they have had a fracture in the past. For patients with a history of osteoporosis fractures, status code Z87.310, Personal history of (healed) osteoporosis fracture, should follow the code from M81.

2) Osteoporosis with current pathological fracture

Category M80, Osteoporosis with current pathological fracture, is for patients who have a current pathologic fracture at the time of an encounter. The codes under M80 identify the site of the fracture. A code from category M80, not a traumatic fracture code, should be used for any patient with known osteoporosis who suffers a fracture, even if the patient had a minor fall or trauma, if that fall or trauma would not usually break a normal, healthy bone.

e. Multisystem Inflammatory Syndrome

See Section I.C.1.g.1.l for Multisystem Inflammatory Syndrome

14. **Chapter 14: Diseases of Genitourinary System (N00-N99)**
   a. **Chronic kidney disease**
      1) **Stages of chronic kidney disease (CKD)**
         The ICD-10-CM classifies CKD based on severity. The severity of CKD is designated by stages 1-5. Stage 2, code N18.2, equates to mild CKD; stage 3, codes N18.30-N18.32, equate to moderate CKD; and stage 4, code N18.4, equates to severe CKD. Code N18.6, End stage renal disease (ESRD), is assigned when the provider has documented end-stage renal disease (ESRD).

         If both a stage of CKD and ESRD are documented, assign code N18.6 only.

      2) **Chronic kidney disease and kidney transplant status**
         Patients who have undergone kidney transplant may still have some form of chronic kidney disease (CKD) because the kidney transplant may not fully restore kidney function. Therefore, the presence of CKD alone does not constitute a transplant complication. Assign the appropriate N18 code for the patient's stage of CKD and code Z94.0, Kidney transplant status. If a transplant complication such as failure or rejection or other transplant complication is documented, see section I.C.19.g for information on coding complications of a kidney transplant. If the documentation is unclear as to whether the patient has a complication of the transplant, query the provider.

      3) **Chronic kidney disease with other conditions**
         Patients with CKD may also suffer from other serious conditions, most commonly diabetes mellitus and hypertension. The sequencing of the CKD code in relationship to codes for other contributing conditions is based on the conventions in the Tabular List.

         See I.C.9. Hypertensive chronic kidney disease.

         See I.C.19. Chronic kidney disease and kidney transplant complications.

15. **Chapter 15: Pregnancy, Childbirth, and the Puerperium (O00-O9A)**
   a. **General Rules for Obstetric Cases**
      1) **Codes from chapter 15 and sequencing priority**
         Obstetric cases require codes from chapter 15, codes in the range O00-O9A, Pregnancy, Childbirth, and the Puerperium. Chapter 15 codes have sequencing priority over codes from other chapters. Additional codes from other chapters may be used in conjunction with chapter 15 codes to further specify conditions. Should the provider document that the pregnancy is incidental to the encounter, then code Z33.1, Pregnant state, incidental, should be used in place of any chapter 15 codes. It is the provider's responsibility to state that the condition being treated is not affecting the pregnancy.

      2) **Chapter 15 codes used only on the maternal record**
         Chapter 15 codes are to be used only on the maternal record, never on the record of the newborn.

      3) **Final character for trimester**
         The majority of codes in Chapter 15 have a final character indicating the trimester of pregnancy. The timeframes for the trimesters are indicated at the beginning of the chapter. If trimester is not a component of a code, it is because the condition always occurs in a specific trimester, or the concept of trimester of pregnancy is not applicable. Certain codes have characters for only certain trimesters because the condition does not occur in all trimesters, but it may occur in more than just one.

         Assignment of the final character for trimester should be based on the provider's documentation of the trimester (or number of weeks) for the current admission/encounter. This applies to the assignment of trimester for pre-existing conditions as well as those that develop during or are due to the pregnancy. The provider's documentation of the number of weeks may be used to assign the appropriate code identifying the trimester.

         Whenever delivery occurs during the current admission, and there is an "in childbirth" option for the obstetric complication being coded, the "in childbirth" code should be assigned. **When the classification does not provide an obstetric code with an "in childbirth" option, it is appropriate to assign a code describing the current trimester.**

      4) **Selection of trimester for inpatient admissions that encompass more than one trimester**
         In instances when a patient is admitted to a hospital for complications of pregnancy during one trimester and remains in the hospital into a subsequent trimester, the trimester character

for the antepartum complication code should be assigned on the basis of the trimester when the complication developed, not the trimester of the discharge. If the condition developed prior to the current admission/encounter or represents a pre-existing condition, the trimester character for the trimester at the time of the admission/encounter should be assigned.

      5) **Unspecified trimester**
         Each category that includes codes for trimester has a code for "unspecified trimester." The "unspecified trimester" code should rarely be used, such as when the documentation in the record is insufficient to determine the trimester and it is not possible to obtain clarification.

      6) **7th character for Fetus Identification**
         Where applicable, a 7th character is to be assigned for certain categories (O31, O32, O33.3-O33.6, O35, O36, O40, O41, O60.1, O60.2, O64, and O69) to identify the fetus for which the complication code applies.

         Assign 7th character "0":
         • For single gestations
         • When the documentation in the record is insufficient to determine the fetus affected and it is not possible to obtain clarification.
         • When it is not possible to clinically determine which fetus is affected.

   b. **Selection of OB Principal or First-listed Diagnosis**
      1) **Routine outpatient prenatal visits**
         For routine outpatient prenatal visits when no complications are present, a code from category Z34, Encounter for supervision of normal pregnancy, should be used as the first-listed diagnosis. These codes should not be used in conjunction with chapter 15 codes.

      2) **Supervision of High-Risk Pregnancy**
         Codes from category O09, Supervision of high-risk pregnancy, are intended for use only during the prenatal period. For complications during the labor or delivery episode as a result of a high-risk pregnancy, assign the applicable complication codes from Chapter 15. If there are no complications during the labor or delivery episode, assign code O80, Encounter for full-term uncomplicated delivery.

         For routine prenatal outpatient visits for patients with high-risk pregnancies, a code from category O09, Supervision of high-risk pregnancy, should be used as the first-listed diagnosis. Secondary chapter 15 codes may be used in conjunction with these codes if appropriate.

      3) **Episodes when no delivery occurs**
         In episodes when no delivery occurs, the principal diagnosis should correspond to the principal complication of the pregnancy which necessitated the encounter. Should more than one complication exist, all of which are treated or monitored, any of the complication codes may be sequenced first.

      4) **When a delivery occurs**
         When an obstetric patient is admitted and delivers during that admission, the condition that prompted the admission should be sequenced as the principal diagnosis. If multiple conditions prompted the admission, sequence the one most related to the delivery as the principal diagnosis. A code for any complication of the delivery should be assigned as an additional diagnosis. In cases of cesarean delivery, if the patient was admitted with a condition that resulted in the performance of a cesarean procedure, that condition should be selected as the principal diagnosis. If the reason for the admission was unrelated to the condition resulting in the cesarean delivery, the condition related to the reason for the admission should be selected as the principal diagnosis.

      5) **Outcome of delivery**
         A code from category Z37, Outcome of delivery, should be included on every maternal record when a delivery has occurred. These codes are not to be used on subsequent records or on the newborn record.

   c. **Pre-existing conditions versus conditions due to the pregnancy**
      Certain categories in Chapter 15 distinguish between conditions of the mother that existed prior to pregnancy (pre-existing) and those that are a direct result of pregnancy. When assigning codes from Chapter 15, it is important to assess if a condition was pre-existing

prior to pregnancy or developed during or due to the pregnancy in order to assign the correct code.

Categories that do not distinguish between pre-existing and pregnancy-related conditions may be used for either. It is acceptable to use codes specifically for the puerperium with codes complicating pregnancy and childbirth if a condition arises postpartum during the delivery encounter.

d. Pre-existing hypertension in pregnancy

Category O10, Pre-existing hypertension complicating pregnancy, childbirth and the puerperium, includes codes for hypertensive heart and hypertensive chronic kidney disease. When assigning one of the O10 codes that includes hypertensive heart disease or hypertensive chronic kidney disease, it is necessary to add a secondary code from the appropriate hypertension category to specify the type of heart failure or chronic kidney disease.

See Section I.C.9. Hypertension.

e. Fetal Conditions Affecting the Management of the Mother

1) Codes from categories O35 and O36

Codes from categories O35, Maternal care for known or suspected fetal abnormality and damage, and O36, Maternal care for other fetal problems, are assigned only when the fetal condition is actually responsible for modifying the management of the mother, i.e., by requiring diagnostic studies, additional observation, special care, or termination of pregnancy. The fact that the fetal condition exists does not justify assigning a code from this series to the mother's record.

2) In utero surgery

In cases when surgery is performed on the fetus, a diagnosis code from category O35, Maternal care for known or suspected fetal abnormality and damage, should be assigned identifying the fetal condition. Assign the appropriate procedure code for the procedure performed.

No code from Chapter 16, the perinatal codes, should be used on the mother's record to identify fetal conditions. Surgery performed in utero on a fetus is still to be coded as an obstetric encounter.

f. HIV Infection in Pregnancy, Childbirth and the Puerperium

During pregnancy, childbirth or the puerperium, a patient admitted because of an HIV-related illness should receive a principal diagnosis from subcategory O98.7-, Human immunodeficiency [HIV] disease complicating pregnancy, childbirth and the puerperium, followed by the code(s) for the HIV-related illness(es).

Patients with asymptomatic HIV infection status admitted during pregnancy, childbirth, or the puerperium should receive codes of O98.7- and Z21, Asymptomatic human immunodeficiency virus [HIV] infection status.

g. Diabetes mellitus in pregnancy

Diabetes mellitus is a significant complicating factor in pregnancy. Pregnant **patients** who are diabetic should be assigned a code from category O24, Diabetes mellitus in pregnancy, childbirth, and the puerperium, first, followed by the appropriate diabetes code(s) (E08-E13) from Chapter 4.

h. Long term use of insulin and oral hypoglycemics

See section I.C.4.a.3 for information on the long-term use of insulin and oral hypoglycemics.

i. Gestational (pregnancy induced) diabetes

Gestational (pregnancy induced) diabetes can occur during the second and third trimester of pregnancy in **patients** who were not diabetic prior to pregnancy. Gestational diabetes can cause complications in the pregnancy similar to those of pre-existing diabetes mellitus. It also puts the **patient** at greater risk of developing diabetes after the pregnancy.

Codes for gestational diabetes are in subcategory O24.4, Gestational diabetes mellitus. No other code from category O24, Diabetes mellitus in pregnancy, childbirth, and the puerperium, should be used with a code from O24.4.

The codes under subcategory O24.4 include diet controlled, insulin controlled, and controlled by oral hypoglycemic drugs. If a patient with gestational diabetes is treated with both diet and insulin, only the code for insulin-controlled is required. If a patient with gestational diabetes is treated with both diet and oral hypoglycemic medications, only the code for "controlled by oral hypoglycemic drugs" is required. Code Z79.4, Long-term (current) use of insulin or code Z79.84, Long-term (current) use of oral hypoglycemic drugs, should not be assigned with codes from subcategory O24.4.

An abnormal glucose tolerance in pregnancy is assigned a code from subcategory O99.81, Abnormal glucose complicating pregnancy, childbirth, and the puerperium.

j. Sepsis and septic shock complicating abortion, pregnancy, childbirth and the puerperium

When assigning a chapter 15 code for sepsis complicating abortion, pregnancy, childbirth, and the puerperium, a code for the specific type of infection should be assigned as an additional diagnosis. If severe sepsis is present, a code from subcategory R65.2, Severe sepsis, and code(s) for associated organ dysfunction(s) should also be assigned as additional diagnoses.

k. Puerperal sepsis

Code O85, Puerperal sepsis, should be assigned with a secondary code to identify the causal organism (e.g., for a bacterial infection, assign a code from category B95-B96, Bacterial infections in conditions classified elsewhere). A code from category A40, Streptococcal sepsis, or A41, Other sepsis, should not be used for puerperal sepsis. If applicable, use additional codes to identify severe sepsis (R65.2-) and any associated acute organ dysfunction.

Code O85 should not be assigned for sepsis following an obstetrical procedure (See Section I.C.1.d.5.b., Sepsis due to a postprocedural infection).

l. Alcohol, tobacco and drug use during pregnancy, childbirth and the puerperium

1) Alcohol use during pregnancy, childbirth and the puerperium

Codes under subcategory O99.31, Alcohol use complicating pregnancy, childbirth, and the puerperium, should be assigned for any pregnancy case when a **patient** uses alcohol during the pregnancy or postpartum. A secondary code from category F10, Alcohol related disorders, should also be assigned to identify manifestations of the alcohol use.

2) Tobacco use during pregnancy, childbirth and the puerperium

Codes under subcategory O99.33, Smoking (tobacco) complicating pregnancy, childbirth, and the puerperium, should be assigned for any pregnancy case when a **patient** uses any type of tobacco product during the pregnancy or postpartum.

A secondary code from category F17, Nicotine dependence, should also be assigned to identify the type of nicotine dependence.

3) Drug use during pregnancy, childbirth and the puerperium

Codes under subcategory O99.32, Drug use complicating pregnancy, childbirth, and the puerperium, should be assigned for any pregnancy case when a **patient** uses drugs during the pregnancy or postpartum. This can involve illegal drugs, or inappropriate use or abuse of prescription drugs. Secondary code(s) from categories F11-F16 and F18-F19 should also be assigned to identify manifestations of the drug use.

m. Poisoning, toxic effects, adverse effects and underdosing in a pregnant patient

A code from subcategory O9A.2, Injury, poisoning and certain other consequences of external causes complicating pregnancy, childbirth, and the puerperium, should be sequenced first, followed by the appropriate injury, poisoning, toxic effect, adverse effect or underdosing code, and then the additional code(s) that specifies the condition caused by the poisoning, toxic effect, adverse effect or underdosing.

See Section I.C.19. Adverse effects, poisoning, underdosing and toxic effects.

n. Normal Delivery, Code O80

1) Encounter for full term uncomplicated delivery

Code O80 should be assigned when a **patient** is admitted for a full-term normal delivery and delivers a single, healthy infant without any complications antepartum, during the delivery, or postpartum during the delivery episode. Code O80 is always a principal diagnosis. It is not to be used if any other code from chapter 15 is needed to describe a current complication of the antenatal, delivery, or postnatal period. Additional codes from other chapters may be used with code O80 if they are not related to or are in any way complicating the pregnancy.

2) **Uncomplicated delivery with resolved antepartum complication**
Code O80 may be used if the patient had a complication at some point during the pregnancy, but the complication is not present at the time of the admission for delivery.

3) **Outcome of delivery for O80**
Z37.0, Single live birth, is the only outcome of delivery code appropriate for use with O80.

o. **The Peripartum and Postpartum Periods**

1) **Peripartum and Postpartum periods**
The postpartum period begins immediately after delivery and continues for six weeks following delivery. The peripartum period is defined as the last month of pregnancy to five months postpartum.

2) **Peripartum and postpartum complication**
A postpartum complication is any complication occurring within the six-week period.

3) **Pregnancy-related complications after 6-week period**
Chapter 15 codes may also be used to describe pregnancy-related complications after the peripartum or postpartum period if the provider documents that a condition is pregnancy related.

4) **Admission for routine postpartum care following delivery outside hospital**
When the mother delivers outside the hospital prior to admission and is admitted for routine postpartum care and no complications are noted, code Z39.0, Encounter for care and examination of mother immediately after delivery, should be assigned as the principal diagnosis.

5) **Pregnancy associated cardiomyopathy**
Pregnancy associated cardiomyopathy, code O90.3, is unique in that it may be diagnosed in the third trimester of pregnancy but may continue to progress months after delivery. For this reason, it is referred to as peripartum cardiomyopathy. Code O90.3 is only for use when the cardiomyopathy develops as a result of pregnancy in a **patient** who did not have pre-existing heart disease.

p. **Code O94, Sequelae of complication of pregnancy, childbirth, and the puerperium**

1) **Code O94**
Code O94, Sequelae of complication of pregnancy, childbirth, and the puerperium, is for use in those cases when an initial complication of a pregnancy develops a **sequela or** sequelae requiring care or treatment at a future date.

2) **After the initial postpartum period**
This code may be used at any time after the initial postpartum period.

3) **Sequencing of Code O94**
This code, like all sequela codes, is to be sequenced following the code describing the sequelae of the complication.

q. **Termination of Pregnancy and Spontaneous abortions**

1) **Abortion with Liveborn Fetus**
When an attempted termination of pregnancy results in a liveborn fetus, assign code Z33.2, Encounter for elective termination of pregnancy and a code from category Z37, Outcome of Delivery.

2) **Retained Products of Conception following an abortion**
Subsequent encounters for retained products of conception following a spontaneous abortion or elective termination of pregnancy, without complications are assigned O03.4, Incomplete spontaneous abortion without complication, or code O07.4, Failed attempted termination of pregnancy without complication. This advice is appropriate even when the patient was discharged previously with a discharge diagnosis of complete abortion. If the patient has a specific complication associated with the spontaneous abortion or elective termination of pregnancy in addition to retained products of conception, assign the appropriate complication code (e.g., O03.-, O04.-, O07.-) instead of code O03.4 or O07.4.

3) **Complications leading to abortion**
Codes from Chapter 15 may be used as additional codes to identify any documented complications of the pregnancy in conjunction with codes in categories in O04, O07 and O08.

r. **Abuse in a pregnant patient**
For suspected or confirmed cases of abuse of a pregnant patient, a code(s) from subcategories O9A.3, Physical abuse complicating pregnancy, childbirth, and the puerperium, O9A.4, Sexual abuse complicating pregnancy, childbirth, and the puerperium, and O9A.5, Psychological abuse complicating pregnancy, childbirth, and the puerperium, should be sequenced first, followed by the appropriate codes (if applicable) to identify any associated current injury due to physical abuse, sexual abuse, and the perpetrator of abuse.
See Section I.C.19. Adult and child abuse, neglect and other maltreatment.

s. **COVID-19 infection in pregnancy, childbirth, and the puerperium**
During pregnancy, childbirth or the puerperium, when COVID-19 is the reason for admission/encounter , code O98.5-, Other viral diseases complicating pregnancy, childbirth and the puerperium, should be sequenced as the principal/first-listed diagnosis, and code U07.1, COVID-19, and the appropriate codes for associated manifestation(s) should be assigned as additional diagnoses. Codes from Chapter 15 always take sequencing priority.

If the reason for admission/encounter is unrelated to COVID-19 but the patient tests positive for COVID-19 during the admission/encounter, the appropriate code for the reason for admission/encounter should be sequenced as the principal/first-listed diagnosis, and codes O98.5- and U07.1, as well as the appropriate codes for associated COVID-19 manifestations, should be assigned as additional diagnoses.

16. **Chapter 16: Certain Conditions Originating in the Perinatal Period (P00-P96)**
For coding and reporting purposes the perinatal period is defined as before birth through the 28th day following birth. The following guidelines are provided for reporting purposes.

a. **General Perinatal Rules**

1) **Use of Chapter 16 Codes**
Codes in this chapter are <u>never</u> for use on the maternal record. Codes from Chapter 15, the obstetric chapter, are never permitted on the newborn record. Chapter 16 codes may be used throughout the life of the patient if the condition is still present.

2) **Principal Diagnosis for Birth Record**
When coding the birth episode in a newborn record, assign a code from category Z38, Liveborn infants according to place of birth and type of delivery, as the principal diagnosis. A code from category Z38 is assigned only once, to a newborn at the time of birth. If a newborn is transferred to another institution, a code from category Z38 should not be used at the receiving hospital.

A code from category Z38 is used only on the newborn record, not on the mother's record.

3) **Use of Codes from other Chapters with Codes from Chapter 16**
Codes from other chapters may be used with codes from chapter 16 if the codes from the other chapters provide more specific detail. Codes for signs and symptoms may be assigned when a definitive diagnosis has not been established. If the reason for the encounter is a perinatal condition, the code from chapter 16 should be sequenced first.

4) **Use of Chapter 16 Codes after the Perinatal Period**
Should a condition originate in the perinatal period, and continue throughout the life of the patient, the perinatal code should continue to be used regardless of the patient's age.

5) **Birth process or community acquired conditions**
If a newborn has a condition that may be either due to the birth process or community acquired and the documentation does not indicate which it is, the default is due to the birth process and the code from Chapter 16 should be used. If the condition is community-acquired, a code from Chapter 16 should not be assigned.
For COVID-19 infection in a newborn, see guideline I.C.16.h.

6) **Code all clinically significant conditions**
All clinically significant conditions noted on routine newborn examination should be coded. A condition is clinically significant if it requires:

- clinical evaluation; or
- therapeutic treatment; or
- diagnostic procedures; or
- extended length of hospital stay; or

- increased nursing care and/or monitoring; or
- has implications for future health care needs

Note: The perinatal guidelines listed above are the same as the general coding guidelines for "additional diagnoses," except for the final point regarding implications for future health care needs. Codes should be assigned for conditions that have been specified by the provider as having implications for future health care needs.

b. Observation and Evaluation of Newborns for Suspected Conditions not Found

1) Use of Z05 codes

Assign a code from category Z05, Observation and evaluation of newborns and infants for suspected conditions ruled out, to identify those instances when a healthy newborn is evaluated for a suspected condition that is determined after study not to be present. Do not use a code from category Z05 when the patient has identified signs or symptoms of a suspected problem; in such cases code the sign or symptom.

2) Z05 on other than the birth record

A code from category Z05 may also be assigned as a principal or first-listed code for readmissions or encounters when the code from category Z38 code no longer applies. Codes from category Z05 are for use only for healthy newborns and infants for which no condition after study is found to be present.

3) Z05 on a birth record

A code from category Z05 is to be used as a secondary code after the code from category Z38, Liveborn infants according to place of birth and type of delivery.

c. Coding Additional Perinatal Diagnoses

1) Assigning codes for conditions that require treatment

Assign codes for conditions that require treatment or further investigation, prolong the length of stay, or require resource utilization.

2) Codes for conditions specified as having implications for future health care needs

Assign codes for conditions that have been specified by the provider as having implications for future health care needs.

Note: This guideline should not be used for adult patients.

d. Prematurity and Fetal Growth Retardation

Providers utilize different criteria in determining prematurity. A code for prematurity should not be assigned unless it is documented. Assignment of codes in categories P05, Disorders of newborn related to slow fetal growth and fetal malnutrition, and P07, Disorders of newborn related to short gestation and low birth weight, not elsewhere classified, should be based on the recorded birth weight and estimated gestational age.

When both birth weight and gestational age are available, two codes from category P07 should be assigned, with the code for birth weight sequenced before the code for gestational age.

e. Low birth weight and immaturity status

Codes from category P07, Disorders of newborn related to short gestation and low birth weight, not elsewhere classified, are for use for a child or adult who was premature or had a low birth weight as a newborn and this is affecting the patient's current health status.

See Section I.C.21. Factors influencing health status and contact with health services, Status.

f. Bacterial Sepsis of Newborn

Category P36, Bacterial sepsis of newborn, includes congenital sepsis. If a perinate is documented as having sepsis without documentation of congenital or community acquired, the default is congenital and a code from category P36 should be assigned. If the P36 code includes the causal organism, an additional code from category B95, Streptococcus, Staphylococcus, and Enterococcus as the cause of diseases classified elsewhere, or B96, Other bacterial agents as the cause of diseases classified elsewhere, should not be assigned. If the P36 code does not include the causal organism, assign an additional code from category B96. If applicable, use additional codes to identify severe sepsis (R65.2-) and any associated acute organ dysfunction.

g. Stillbirth

Code P95, Stillbirth, is only for use in institutions that maintain separate records for stillbirths. No other code should be used with P95. Code P95 should not be used on the mother's record.

h. COVID-19 Infection in Newborn

For a newborn that tests positive for COVID-19, assign code U07.1, COVID-19, and the appropriate codes for associated manifestation(s)

in neonates/newborns in the absence of documentation indicating a specific type of transmission. For a newborn that tests positive for COVID-19 and the provider documents the condition was contracted in utero or during the birth process, assign codes P35.8, Other congenital viral diseases, and U07.1, COVID-19. When coding the birth episode in a newborn record, the appropriate code from category Z38, Liveborn infants according to place of birth and type of delivery, should be assigned as the principal diagnosis.

17. Chapter 17: Congenital malformations, deformations, and chromosomal abnormalities (Q00-Q99)

Assign an appropriate code(s) from categories Q00-Q99, Congenital malformations, deformations, and chromosomal abnormalities when a malformation/deformation or chromosomal abnormality is documented. A malformation/deformation/or chromosomal abnormality may be the principal/first-listed diagnosis on a record or a secondary diagnosis.

When a malformation/deformation or chromosomal abnormality does not have a unique code assignment, assign additional code(s) for any manifestations that may be present.

When the code assignment specifically identifies the malformation/deformation or chromosomal abnormality, manifestations that are an inherent component of the anomaly should not be coded separately. Additional codes should be assigned for manifestations that are not an inherent component.

Codes from Chapter 17 may be used throughout the life of the patient. If a congenital malformation or deformity has been corrected, a personal history code should be used to identify the history of the malformation or deformity. Although present at birth, a malformation/deformation/or chromosomal abnormality may not be identified until later in life. Whenever the condition is diagnosed by the provider, it is appropriate to assign a code from codes Q00-Q99. For the birth admission, the appropriate code from category Z38, Liveborn infants, according to place of birth and type of delivery, should be sequenced as the principal diagnosis, followed by any congenital anomaly codes, Q00-Q99.

18. Chapter 18: Symptoms, signs, and abnormal clinical and laboratory findings, not elsewhere classified (R00-R99)

Chapter 18 includes symptoms, signs, abnormal results of clinical or other investigative procedures, and ill-defined conditions regarding which no diagnosis classifiable elsewhere is recorded. Signs and symptoms that point to a specific diagnosis have been assigned to a category in other chapters of the classification.

a. Use of symptom codes

Codes that describe symptoms and signs are acceptable for reporting purposes when a related definitive diagnosis has not been established (confirmed) by the provider.

b. Use of a symptom code with a definitive diagnosis code

Codes for signs and symptoms may be reported in addition to a related definitive diagnosis when the sign or symptom is not routinely associated with that diagnosis, such as the various signs and symptoms associated with complex syndromes. The definitive diagnosis code should be sequenced before the symptom code.

Signs or symptoms that are associated routinely with a disease process should not be assigned as additional codes, unless otherwise instructed by the classification.

c. Combination codes that include symptoms

ICD-10-CM contains a number of combination codes that identify both the definitive diagnosis and common symptoms of that diagnosis. When using one of these combination codes, an additional code should not be assigned for the symptom.

d. Repeated falls

Code R29.6, Repeated falls, is for use for encounters when a patient has recently fallen and the reason for the fall is being investigated.

Code Z91.81, History of falling, is for use when a patient has fallen in the past and is at risk for future falls. When appropriate, both codes R29.6 and Z91.81 may be assigned together.

e. Coma

Code R40.20, Unspecified coma, may be assigned in conjunction with codes for any medical condition.

<u>Do not report codes for **unspecified coma**, individual or total Glasgow coma scale scores for a patient with a medically induced coma or a sedated patient.</u>

1) Coma Scale

The coma scale codes (R40.21- to R40.24-) can be used in conjunction with traumatic brain injury codes. These codes are primarily for use by trauma registries, but they may be used in any setting where this information is collected. The coma scale codes should be sequenced after the diagnosis code(s).

These codes, one from each subcategory, are needed to complete the scale. The 7th character indicates when the scale was recorded. The 7th character should match for all three codes.

At a minimum, report the initial score documented on presentation at your facility. This may be a score from the emergency medicine technician (EMT) or in the emergency department. If desired, a facility may choose to capture multiple coma scale scores.

Assign code R40.24-, Glasgow coma scale, total score, when only the total score is documented in the medical record and not the individual score(s).

If multiple coma scores are captured within the first 24 hours after hospital admission, assign only the code for the score at the time of admission. ICD-10-CM does not classify coma scores that are reported after admission but less than 24 hours later.

See Section I.B.14 for coma scale documentation by clinicians other than patient's provider

f. Functional quadriplegia
GUIDELINE HAS BEEN DELETED EFFECTIVE OCTOBER 1, 2017

g. SIRS due to Non-Infectious Process
The systemic inflammatory response syndrome (SIRS) can develop as a result of certain non-infectious disease processes, such as trauma, malignant neoplasm, or pancreatitis. When SIRS is documented with a noninfectious condition, and no subsequent infection is documented, the code for the underlying condition, such as an injury, should be assigned, followed by code R65.10, Systemic inflammatory response syndrome (SIRS) of non-infectious origin without acute organ dysfunction, or code R65.11, Systemic inflammatory response syndrome (SIRS) of non-infectious origin with acute organ dysfunction. If an associated acute organ dysfunction is documented, the appropriate code(s) for the specific type of organ dysfunction(s) should be assigned in addition to code R65.11. If acute organ dysfunction is documented, but it cannot be determined if the acute organ dysfunction is associated with SIRS or due to another condition (e.g., directly due to the trauma), the provider should be queried.

h. Death NOS
Code R99, Ill-defined and unknown cause of mortality, is only for use in the very limited circumstance when a patient who has already died is brought into an emergency department or other healthcare facility and is pronounced dead upon arrival. It does not represent the discharge disposition of death.

i. NIHSS Stroke Scale
The NIH stroke scale (NIHSS) codes (R29.7- -) can be used in conjunction with acute stroke codes (I63) to identify the patient's neurological status and the severity of the stroke. The stroke scale codes should be sequenced after the acute stroke diagnosis code(s).

At a minimum, report the initial score documented. If desired, a facility may choose to capture multiple stroke scale scores.

See Section I.B.14 for NIHSS stroke scale documentation by clinicians other than patient's provider

19. Chapter 19: Injury, poisoning, and certain other consequences of external causes (S00-T88)

a. Application of 7th Characters in Chapter 19
Most categories in chapter 19 have a 7th character requirement for each applicable code. Most categories in this chapter have three 7th character values (with the exception of fractures): A, initial encounter, D, subsequent encounter and S, sequela. Categories for traumatic fractures have additional 7th character values. While the patient may be seen by a new or different provider over the course of treatment for an injury, assignment of the 7th character is based on whether the patient is undergoing active treatment and not whether the provider is seeing the patient for the first time.

For complication codes, active treatment refers to treatment for the condition described by the code, even though it may be related to an earlier precipitating problem. For example, code T84.50XA, Infection and inflammatory reaction due to unspecified internal joint prosthesis, initial encounter, is used when active treatment is provided for the infection, even though the condition relates to the prosthetic device, implant or graft that was placed at a previous encounter.

7th character "A", initial encounter is used for each encounter where the patient is receiving active treatment for the condition.

7th character "D" subsequent encounter is used for encounters after the patient has completed active treatment of the condition and is

receiving routine care for the condition during the healing or recovery phase.

The aftercare Z codes should not be used for aftercare for conditions such as injuries or poisonings, where 7th characters are provided to identify subsequent care. For example, for aftercare of an injury, assign the acute injury code with the 7th character "D" (subsequent encounter).

7th character "S", sequela, is for use for complications or conditions that arise as a direct result of a condition, such as scar formation after a burn. The scars are sequelae of the burn. When using 7th character "S", it is necessary to use both the injury code that precipitated the sequela and the code for the sequela itself. The "S" is added only to the injury code, not the sequela code. The 7th character "S" identifies the injury responsible for the sequela. The specific type of sequela (e.g. scar) is sequenced first, followed by the injury code.

See Section I.B.10 Sequelae, (Late Effects)

b. Coding of Injuries
When coding injuries, assign separate codes for each injury unless a combination code is provided, in which case the combination code is assigned. Codes from category T07, Unspecified multiple injuries should not be assigned in the inpatient setting unless information for a more specific code is not available. Traumatic injury codes (S00-T14.9) are not to be used for normal, healing surgical wounds or to identify complications of surgical wounds.

The code for the most serious injury, as determined by the provider and the focus of treatment, is sequenced first.

1) Superficial injuries
Superficial injuries such as abrasions or contusions are not coded when associated with more severe injuries of the same site.

2) Primary injury with damage to nerves/blood vessels
When a primary injury results in minor damage to peripheral nerves or blood vessels, the primary injury is sequenced first with additional code(s) for injuries to nerves and spinal cord (such as category S04), and/or injury to blood vessels (such as category S15). When the primary injury is to the blood vessels or nerves, that injury should be sequenced first.

3) Iatrogenic injuries
Injury codes from Chapter 19 should not be assigned for injuries that occur during, or as a result of, a medical intervention. Assign the appropriate complication code(s).

c. Coding of Traumatic Fractures
The principles of multiple coding of injuries should be followed in coding fractures. Fractures of specified sites are coded individually by site in accordance with both the provisions within categories S02, S12, S22, S32, S42, S49, S52, S59, S62, S72, S79, S82, S89, S92 and the level of detail furnished by medical record content.

A fracture not indicated as open or closed should be coded to closed. A fracture not indicated whether displaced or not displaced should be coded to displaced.

More specific guidelines are as follows:

1) Initial vs. subsequent encounter for fractures
Traumatic fractures are coded using the appropriate 7th character for initial encounter (A, B, C) for each encounter where the patient is receiving active treatment for the fracture. The appropriate 7th character for initial encounter should also be assigned for a patient who delayed seeking treatment for the fracture or nonunion.

Fractures are coded using the appropriate 7th character for subsequent care for encounters after the patient has completed active treatment of the fracture and is receiving routine care for the fracture during the healing or recovery phase.

Care for complications of surgical treatment for fracture repairs during the healing or recovery phase should be coded with the appropriate complication codes.

Care of complications of fractures, such as malunion and nonunion, should be reported with the appropriate 7th character for subsequent care with nonunion (K, M, N,) or subsequent care with malunion (P, Q, R).

Malunion/nonunion: The appropriate 7th character for initial encounter should also be assigned for a patient who delayed seeking treatment for the fracture or nonunion.

The open fracture designations in the assignment of the 7th character for fractures of the forearm, femur and lower leg, including ankle are based on the Gustilo open fracture

classification. When the Gustilo classification type is not specified for an open fracture, the 7th character for open fracture type I or II should be assigned (B, E, H, M, Q).

A code from category M80, not a traumatic fracture code, should be used for any patient with known osteoporosis who suffers a fracture, even if the patient had a minor fall or trauma, if that fall or trauma would not usually break a normal, healthy bone.

See Section I.C.13. Osteoporosis.

The aftercare Z codes should not be used for aftercare for traumatic fractures. For aftercare of a traumatic fracture, assign the acute fracture code with the appropriate 7th character.

2) **Multiple fractures sequencing**
Multiple fractures are sequenced in accordance with the severity of the fracture.

3) **Physeal fractures**
For physeal fractures, assign only the code identifying the type of physeal fracture. Do not assign a separate code to identify the specific bone that is fractured.

d. **Coding of Burns and Corrosions**
The ICD-10-CM makes a distinction between burns and corrosions. The burn codes are for thermal burns, except sunburns, that come from a heat source, such as a fire or hot appliance. The burn codes are also for burns resulting from electricity and radiation. Corrosions are burns due to chemicals. The guidelines are the same for burns and corrosions.

Current burns (T20-T25) are classified by depth, extent and by agent (X code). Burns are classified by depth as first degree (erythema), second degree (blistering), and third degree (full-thickness involvement). Burns of the eye and internal organs (T26-T28) are classified by site, but not by degree.

1) **Sequencing of burn and related condition codes**
Sequence first the code that reflects the highest degree of burn when more than one burn is present.

   a. When the reason for the admission or encounter is for treatment of external multiple burns, sequence first the code that reflects the burn of the highest degree.

   b. When a patient has both internal and external burns, the circumstances of admission govern the selection of the principal diagnosis or first-listed diagnosis.

   c. When a patient is admitted for burn injuries and other related conditions such as smoke inhalation and/or respiratory failure, the circumstances of admission govern the selection of the principal or first-listed diagnosis.

2) **Burns of the same anatomic site**
Classify burns of the same anatomic site and on the same side but of different degrees to the subcategory identifying the highest degree recorded in the diagnosis (e.g., for second and third degree burns of right thigh, assign only code T24.311-).

3) **Non-healing burns**
Non-healing burns are coded as acute burns.
Necrosis of burned skin should be coded as a non-healed burn.

4) **Infected burn**
For any documented infected burn site, use an additional code for the infection.

5) **Assign separate codes for each burn site**
When coding burns, assign separate codes for each burn site. Category T30, Burn and corrosion, body region unspecified is extremely vague and should rarely be used.

Codes for burns of "multiple sites" should only be assigned when the medical record documentation does not specify the individual sites.

6) **Burns and corrosions classified according to extent of body surface involved**
Assign codes from category T31, Burns classified according to extent of body surface involved, or T32, Corrosions classified according to extent of body surface involved, **for acute burns or corrosions** when the site of the burn **or corrosion** is not specified or when there is a need for additional data. It is advisable to use category T31 as additional coding when needed to provide data for evaluating burn mortality, such as that needed by burn units. It is also advisable to use category T31 as an additional code for reporting purposes when there is mention of a third-degree burn involving 20 percent or more of the body surface. **Codes from categories T31 and T32 should not be used for sequelae of burns or corrosions**.

Categories T31 and T32 are based on the classic "rule of nines" in estimating body surface involved: head and neck are assigned nine percent, each arm nine percent, each leg 18 percent, the anterior trunk 18 percent, posterior trunk 18 percent, and genitalia one percent. Providers may change these percentage assignments where necessary to accommodate infants and children who have proportionately larger heads than adults, and patients who have large buttocks, thighs, or abdomen that involve burns.

7) **Encounters for treatment of sequela of burns**
Encounters for the treatment of the late effects of burns or corrosions (i.e., scars or joint contractures) should be coded with a burn or corrosion code with the 7th character "S" for sequela.

8) **Sequelae with a late effect code and current burn**
When appropriate, both a code for a current burn or corrosion with 7th character "A" or "D" and a burn or corrosion code with 7th character "S" may be assigned on the same record (when both a current burn and sequelae of an old burn exist). Burns and corrosions do not heal at the same rate and a current healing wound may still exist with sequela of a healed burn or corrosion.

See Section I.B.10 Sequela (Late Effects)

9) **Use of an external cause code with burns and corrosions**
An external cause code should be used with burns and corrosions to identify the source and intent of the burn, as well as the place where it occurred.

e. **Adverse Effects, Poisoning, Underdosing and Toxic Effects**
Codes in categories T36-T65 are combination codes that include the substance that was taken as well as the intent. No additional external cause code is required for poisonings, toxic effects, adverse effects and underdosing codes.

1) **Do not code directly from the Table of Drugs**
Do not code directly from the Table of Drugs and Chemicals. Always refer back to the Tabular List.

2) **Use as many codes as necessary to describe**
Use as many codes as necessary to describe completely all drugs, medicinal or biological substances.

3) **If the same code would describe the causative agent**
If the same code would describe the causative agent for more than one adverse reaction, poisoning, toxic effect or underdosing, assign the code only once.

4) **If two or more drugs, medicinal or biological substances**
If two or more drugs, medicinal or biological substances are taken, code each individually unless a combination code is listed in the Table of Drugs and Chemicals.

If multiple unspecified drugs, medicinal or biological substances were taken, assign the appropriate code from subcategory T50.91, Poisoning by, adverse effect of and underdosing of multiple unspecified drugs, medicaments and biological substances.

5) **The occurrence of drug toxicity is classified in ICD-10-CM as follows:**

   (a) Adverse Effect
When coding an adverse effect of a drug that has been correctly prescribed and properly administered, assign the appropriate code for the nature of the adverse effect followed by the appropriate code for the adverse effect of the drug (T36-T50). The code for the drug should have a 5th or 6th character "5" (for example T36.0X5-) Examples of the nature of an adverse effect are tachycardia, delirium, gastrointestinal hemorrhaging, vomiting, hypokalemia, hepatitis, renal failure, or respiratory failure.

   (b) Poisoning
When coding a poisoning or reaction to the improper use of a medication (e.g., overdose, wrong substance given or taken in error, wrong route of administration), first assign the appropriate code from categories T36-T50. The poisoning codes have an associated intent as their 5th or 6th character (accidental, intentional self-harm, assault and undetermined). If the intent of the poisoning is unknown or unspecified, code the intent as accidental intent. The undetermined intent is only for use if the documentation in the record specifies that the intent cannot be determined. Use additional code(s) for all manifestations of poisonings.

If there is also a diagnosis of abuse or dependence of the substance, the abuse or dependence is assigned as an additional code.

Examples of poisoning include:

(i)   Error was made in drug prescription
Errors made in drug prescription or in the administration of the drug by provider, nurse, patient, or other person.

(ii) Overdose of a drug intentionally taken
If an overdose of a drug was intentionally taken or administered and resulted in drug toxicity, it would be coded as a poisoning.

(iii) Nonprescribed drug taken with correctly prescribed and properly administered drug
If a nonprescribed drug or medicinal agent was taken in combination with a correctly prescribed and properly administered drug, any drug toxicity or other reaction resulting from the interaction of the two drugs would be classified as a poisoning.

(iv) Interaction of drug(s) and alcohol
When a reaction results from the interaction of a drug(s) and alcohol, this would be classified as poisoning.

See Section I.C.4. if poisoning is the result of insulin pump malfunctions.

(c)   Underdosing

Underdosing refers to taking less of a medication than is prescribed by a provider or a manufacturer's instruction. Discontinuing the use of a prescribed medication on the patient's own initiative (not directed by the patient's provider) is also classified as an underdosing. For underdosing, assign the code from categories T36-T50 (fifth or sixth character "6").

Codes for underdosing should never be assigned as principal or first-listed codes. If a patient has a relapse or exacerbation of the medical condition for which the drug is prescribed because of the reduction in dose, then the medical condition itself should be coded.

Noncompliance (Z91.12-, Z91.13- and Z91.14-) or complication of care (Y63.6-Y63.9) codes are to be used with an underdosing code to indicate intent, if known.

(d)   Toxic Effects

When a harmful substance is ingested or comes in contact with a person, this is classified as a toxic effect. The toxic effect codes are in categories T51-T65.

Toxic effect codes have an associated intent: accidental, intentional self-harm, assault and undetermined.

f.   Adult and child abuse, neglect and other maltreatment

Sequence first the appropriate code from categories T74, Adult and child abuse, neglect and other maltreatment, confirmed, or T76, Adult and child abuse, neglect and other maltreatment, suspected, for abuse, neglect and other maltreatment, followed by any accompanying mental health or injury code(s).

If the documentation in the medical record states abuse or neglect, it is coded as confirmed (T74.-). It is coded as suspected if it is documented as suspected (T76.-).

For cases of confirmed abuse or neglect an external cause code from the assault section (X92-Y09) should be added to identify the cause of any physical injuries. A perpetrator code (Y07) should be added when the perpetrator of the abuse is known. For suspected cases of abuse or neglect, do not report external cause or perpetrator code.

If a suspected case of abuse, neglect or mistreatment is ruled out during an encounter code Z04.71, Encounter for examination and observation following alleged physical adult abuse, ruled out, or code Z04.72, Encounter for examination and observation following alleged child physical abuse, ruled out, should be used, not a code from T76.

If a suspected case of alleged rape or sexual abuse is ruled out during an encounter code Z04.41, Encounter for examination and observation following alleged adult rape or code Z04.42, Encounter for examination and observation following alleged child rape, should be used, not a code from T76.

If a suspected case of forced sexual exploitation or forced labor exploitation is ruled out during an encounter, code Z04.81, Encounter for examination and observation of victim following forced sexual exploitation, or code Z04.82, Encounter for examination and

observation of victim following forced labor exploitation, should be used, not a code from T76.

See Section I.C.15. Abuse in a pregnant patient.

g.   Complications of care

1)   General guidelines for complications of care

(a)   Documentation of complications of care

See Section I.B.16. for information on documentation of complications of care.

2)   Pain due to medical devices

Pain associated with devices, implants or grafts left in a surgical site (for example painful hip prosthesis) is assigned to the appropriate code(s) found in Chapter 19, Injury, poisoning, and certain other consequences of external causes. Specific codes for pain due to medical devices are found in the T code section of the ICD-10-CM. Use additional code(s) from category G89 to identify acute or chronic pain due to presence of the device, implant or graft (G89.18 or G89.28).

3)   Transplant complications

(a)   Transplant complications other than kidney

Codes under category T86, Complications of transplanted organs and tissues, are for use for both complications and rejection of transplanted organs. A transplant complication code is only assigned if the complication affects the function of the transplanted organ. Two codes are required to fully describe a transplant complication: the appropriate code from category T86 and a secondary code that identifies the complication.

Pre-existing conditions or conditions that develop after the transplant are not coded as complications unless they affect the function of the transplanted organs.

See I.C.21. for transplant organ removal status

See I.C.2. for malignant neoplasm associated with transplanted organ.

(b)   Kidney transplant complications

Patients who have undergone kidney transplant may still have some form of chronic kidney disease (CKD) because the kidney transplant may not fully restore kidney function. Code T86.1- should be assigned for documented complications of a kidney transplant, such as transplant failure or rejection or other transplant complication. Code T86.1- should not be assigned for post kidney transplant patients who have chronic kidney (CKD) unless a transplant complication such as transplant failure or rejection is documented. If the documentation is unclear as to whether the patient has a complication of the transplant, query the provider.

Conditions that affect the function of the transplanted kidney, other than CKD, should be assigned a code from subcategory T86.1, Complications of transplanted organ, Kidney, and a secondary code that identifies the complication.

For patients with CKD following a kidney transplant, but who do not have a complication such as failure or rejection, *see section I.C.14. Chronic kidney disease and kidney transplant status.*

4)   Complication codes that include the external cause

As with certain other T codes, some of the complications of care codes have the external cause included in the code. The code includes the nature of the complication as well as the type of procedure that caused the complication. No external cause code indicating the type of procedure is necessary for these codes.

5)   Complications of care codes within the body system chapters

Intraoperative and postprocedural complication codes are found within the body system chapters with codes specific to the organs and structures of that body system. These codes should be sequenced first, followed by a code(s) for the specific complication, if applicable.

Complication codes from the body system chapters should be assigned for intraoperative and postprocedural complications (e.g., the appropriate complication code from chapter 9 would be assigned for a vascular intraoperative or postprocedural complication) unless the complication is specifically indexed to a T code in chapter 19.

20. **Chapter 20: External Causes of Morbidity (V00-Y99)**

The external causes of morbidity codes should never be sequenced as the first-listed or principal diagnosis.

External cause codes are intended to provide data for injury research and evaluation of injury prevention strategies. These codes capture how the injury or health condition happened (cause), the intent (unintentional or accidental; or intentional, such as suicide or assault), the place where the event occurred the activity of the patient at the time of the event, and the person's status (e.g., civilian, military).

There is no national requirement for mandatory ICD-10-CM external cause code reporting. Unless a provider is subject to a state-based external cause code reporting mandate or these codes are required by a particular payer, reporting of ICD-10-CM codes in Chapter 20, External Causes of Morbidity, is not required. In the absence of a mandatory reporting requirement, providers are encouraged to voluntarily report external cause codes, as they provide valuable data for injury research and evaluation of injury prevention strategies.

a. **General External Cause Coding Guidelines**

1) **Used with any code in the range of A00.0-T88.9, Z00-Z99**
   An external cause code may be used with any code in the range of A00.0-T88.9, Z00-Z99, classification that represents a health condition due to an external cause. Though they are most applicable to injuries, they are also valid for use with such things as infections or diseases due to an external source, and other health conditions, such as a heart attack that occurs during strenuous physical activity.

2) **External cause code used for length of treatment**
   Assign the external cause code, with the appropriate 7th character (initial encounter, subsequent encounter or sequela) for each encounter for which the injury or condition is being treated.

   Most categories in chapter 20 have a 7th character requirement for each applicable code. Most categories in this chapter have three 7th character values: A, initial encounter, D, subsequent encounter and S, sequela. While the patient may be seen by a new or different provider over the course of treatment for an injury or condition, assignment of the 7th character for external cause should match the 7th character of the code assigned for the associated injury or condition for the encounter.

3) **Use the full range of external cause codes**
   Use the full range of external cause codes to completely describe the cause, the intent, the place of occurrence, and if applicable, the activity of the patient at the time of the event, and the patient's status, for all injuries, and other health conditions due to an external cause.

4) **Assign as many external cause codes as necessary**
   Assign as many external cause codes as necessary to fully explain each cause. If only one external code can be recorded, assign the code most related to the principal diagnosis.

5) **The selection of the appropriate external cause code**
   The selection of the appropriate external cause code is guided by the Alphabetic Index of External Causes and by Inclusion and Exclusion notes in the Tabular List.

6) **External cause code can never be a principal diagnosis**
   An external cause code can never be a principal (first-listed) diagnosis.

7) **Combination external cause codes**
   Certain of the external cause codes are combination codes that identify sequential events that result in an injury, such as a fall which results in striking against an object. The injury may be due to either event or both. The combination external cause code used should correspond to the sequence of events regardless of which caused the most serious injury.

8) **No external cause code needed in certain circumstances**
   No external cause code from Chapter 20 is needed if the external cause and intent are included in a code from another chapter (e.g., T36.0X1-, Poisoning by penicillins, accidental (unintentional)).

b. **Place of Occurrence Guideline**
   Codes from category Y92, Place of occurrence of the external cause, are secondary codes for use after other external cause codes to identify the location of the patient at the time of injury or other condition.

   Generally, a place of occurrence code is assigned only once, at the initial encounter for treatment. However, in the rare instance that a new injury occurs during hospitalization, an additional place of occurrence code may be assigned. No 7th characters are used for Y92.

   Do not use place of occurrence code Y92.9 if the place is not stated or is not applicable.

c. **Activity Code**
   Assign a code from category Y93, Activity code, to describe the activity of the patient at the time the injury or other health condition occurred.

   An activity code is used only once, at the initial encounter for treatment. Only one code from Y93 should be recorded on a medical record.

   The activity codes are not applicable to poisonings, adverse effects, misadventures or sequela.

   Do not assign Y93.9, Unspecified activity, if the activity is not stated.

   A code from category Y93 is appropriate for use with external cause and intent codes if identifying the activity provides additional information about the event.

d. **Place of Occurrence, Activity, and Status Codes Used with other External Cause Code**
   When applicable, place of occurrence, activity, and external cause status codes are sequenced after the main external cause code(s). Regardless of the number of external cause codes assigned, generally there should be only one place of occurrence code, one activity code, and one external cause status code assigned to an encounter. However, in the rare instance that a new injury occurs during hospitalization, an additional place of occurrence code may be assigned.

e. **If the Reporting Format Limits the Number of External Cause Codes**
   If the reporting format limits the number of external cause codes that can be used in reporting clinical data, report the code for the cause/intent most related to the principal diagnosis. If the format permits capture of additional external cause codes, the cause/intent, including medical misadventures, of the additional events should be reported rather than the codes for place, activity, or external status.

f. **Multiple External Cause Coding Guidelines**
   More than one external cause code is required to fully describe the external cause of an illness or injury. The assignment of external cause codes should be sequenced in the following priority:

   If two or more events cause separate injuries, an external cause code should be assigned for each cause. The first-listed external cause code will be selected in the following order:

   External codes for child and adult abuse take priority over all other external cause codes.

   See Section I.C.19., Child and Adult abuse guidelines.

   External cause codes for terrorism events take priority over all other external cause codes except child and adult abuse.

   External cause codes for cataclysmic events take priority over all other external cause codes except child and adult abuse and terrorism.

   External cause codes for transport accidents take priority over all other external cause codes except cataclysmic events, child and adult abuse and terrorism.

   Activity and external cause status codes are assigned following all causal (intent) external cause codes.

   The first-listed external cause code should correspond to the cause of the most serious diagnosis due to an assault, accident, or self-harm, following the order of hierarchy listed above.

g. **Child and Adult Abuse Guideline**
   Adult and child abuse, neglect and maltreatment are classified as assault. Any of the assault codes may be used to indicate the external cause of any injury resulting from the confirmed abuse.

   For confirmed cases of abuse, neglect and maltreatment, when the perpetrator is known, a code from Y07, Perpetrator of maltreatment and neglect, should accompany any other assault codes.

   See Section I.C.19. Adult and child abuse, neglect and other maltreatment

h. **Unknown or Undetermined Intent Guideline**
   If the intent (accident, self-harm, assault) of the cause of an injury or other condition is unknown or unspecified, code the intent as accidental intent. All transport accident categories assume accidental intent.

1) **Use of undetermined intent**
   External cause codes for events of undetermined intent are only for use if the documentation in the record specifies that the intent cannot be determined.

i. Sequelae (Late Effects) of External Cause Guidelines

1) Sequelae external cause codes

Sequela are reported using the external cause code with the 7th character "S" for sequela. These codes should be used with any report of a late effect or sequela resulting from a previous injury.

See Section I.B.10 Sequela (Late Effects)

2) Sequela external cause code with a related current injury

A sequela external cause code should never be used with a related current nature of injury code.

3) Use of sequela external cause codes for subsequent visits

Use a late effect external cause code for subsequent visits when a late effect of the initial injury is being treated. Do not use a late effect external cause code for subsequent visits for follow-up care (e.g., to assess healing, to receive rehabilitative therapy) of the injury when no late effect of the injury has been documented.

j. Terrorism Guidelines

1) Cause of injury identified by the Federal Government (FBI) as terrorism

When the cause of an injury is identified by the Federal Government (FBI) as terrorism, the first-listed external cause code should be a code from category Y38, Terrorism. The definition of terrorism employed by the FBI is found at the inclusion note at the beginning of category Y38. Use additional code for place of occurrence (Y92.-). More than one Y38 code may be assigned if the injury is the result of more than one mechanism of terrorism.

2) Cause of an injury is suspected to be the result of terrorism

When the cause of an injury is suspected to be the result of terrorism a code from category Y38 should not be assigned. Suspected cases should be classified as assault.

3) Code Y38.9, Terrorism, secondary effects

Assign code Y38.9, Terrorism, secondary effects, for conditions occurring subsequent to the terrorist event. This code should not be assigned for conditions that are due to the initial terrorist act.

It is acceptable to assign code Y38.9 with another code from Y38 if there is an injury due to the initial terrorist event and an injury that is a subsequent result of the terrorist event.

k. External Cause Status

A code from category Y99, External cause status, should be assigned whenever any other external cause code is assigned for an encounter, including an Activity code, except for the events noted below. Assign a code from category Y99, External cause status, to indicate the work status of the person at the time the event occurred. The status code indicates whether the event occurred during military activity, whether a non-military person was at work, whether an individual including a student or volunteer was involved in a non-work activity at the time of the causal event.

A code from Y99, External cause status, should be assigned, when applicable, with other external cause codes, such as transport accidents and falls. The external cause status codes are not applicable to poisonings, adverse effects, misadventures or late effects.

Do not assign a code from category Y99 if no other external cause codes (cause, activity) are applicable for the encounter.

An external cause status code is used only once, at the initial encounter for treatment. Only one code from Y99 should be recorded on a medical record.

Do not assign code Y99.9, Unspecified external cause status, if the status is not stated.

21. Chapter 21: Factors influencing health status and contact with health services (Z00-Z99)

Note: The chapter specific guidelines provide additional information about the use of Z codes for specified encounters.

a. Use of Z Codes in Any Healthcare Setting

Z codes are for use in any healthcare setting. Z codes may be used as either a first-listed (principal diagnosis code in the inpatient setting) or secondary code, depending on the circumstances of the encounter. Certain Z codes may only be used as first-listed or principal diagnosis.

b. Z Codes Indicate a Reason for an Encounter *or Provide Additional Information about a Patient Encounter*

Z codes are not procedure codes. A corresponding procedure code must accompany a Z code to describe any procedure performed.

c. Categories of Z Codes

1) Contact/Exposure

Category Z20 indicates contact with, and suspected exposure to, communicable diseases. These codes are for patients who are suspected to have been exposed to a disease by close personal contact with an infected individual or are in an area where a disease is epidemic.

Category Z77, Other contact with and (suspected) exposures hazardous to health, indicates contact with and suspected exposures hazardous to health.

Contact/exposure codes may be used as a first-listed code to explain an encounter for testing, or, more commonly, as a secondary code to identify a potential risk.

2) Inoculations and vaccinations

Code Z23 is for encounters for inoculations and vaccinations. It indicates that a patient is being seen to receive a prophylactic inoculation against a disease. Procedure codes are required to identify the actual administration of the injection and the type(s) of immunizations given. Code Z23 may be used as a secondary code if the inoculation is given as a routine part of preventive health care, such as a well-baby visit.

3) Status

Status codes indicate that a patient is either a carrier of a disease or has the sequelae or residual of a past disease or condition. This includes such things as the presence of prosthetic or mechanical devices resulting from past treatment. A status code is informative, because the status may affect the course of treatment and its outcome. A status code is distinct from a history code. The history code indicates that the patient no longer has the condition.

A status code should not be used with a diagnosis code from one of the body system chapters, if the diagnosis code includes the information provided by the status code. For example, code Z94.1, Heart transplant status, should not be used with a code from subcategory T86.2, Complications of heart transplant. The status code does not provide additional information. The complication code indicates that the patient is a heart transplant patient.

For encounters for weaning from a mechanical ventilator, assign a code from subcategory J96.1, Chronic respiratory failure, followed by code Z99.11, Dependence on respirator [ventilator] status.

The status Z codes/categories are:

Z14	Genetic carrier

Genetic carrier status indicates that a person carries a gene, associated with a particular disease, which may be passed to offspring who may develop that disease. The person does not have the disease and is not at risk of developing the disease.

Z15	Genetic susceptibility to disease

Genetic susceptibility indicates that a person has a gene that increases the risk of that person developing the disease.

Codes from category Z15 should not be used as principal or first-listed codes. If the patient has the condition to which he/she is susceptible, and that condition is the reason for the encounter, the code for the current condition should be sequenced first. If the patient is being seen for follow-up after completed treatment for this condition, and the condition no longer exists, a follow-up code should be sequenced first, followed by the appropriate personal history and genetic susceptibility codes. If the purpose of the encounter is genetic counseling associated with procreative management, code Z31.5, Encounter for genetic counseling, should be assigned as the first-listed code, followed by a code from category Z15. Additional codes should be assigned for any applicable family or personal history.

Z16	Resistance to antimicrobial drugs

This code indicates that a patient has a condition that is resistant to antimicrobial drug treatment. Sequence the infection code first.

Z17	Estrogen receptor status
Z18	Retained foreign body fragments
Z19	Hormone sensitivity malignancy status

Z21   Asymptomatic HIV infection status
This code indicates that a patient has tested positive for HIV but has manifested no signs or symptoms of the disease.

Z22   Carrier of infectious disease
Carrier status indicates that a person harbors the specific organisms of a disease without manifest symptoms and is capable of transmitting the infection.

Z28.3   Underimmunization status

Z33.1   Pregnant state, incidental
This code is a secondary code only for use when the pregnancy is in no way complicating the reason for visit. Otherwise, a code from the obstetric chapter is required.

Z66   Do not resuscitate
This code may be used when it is documented by the provider that a patient is on do not resuscitate status at any time during the stay.

Z67   Blood type

Z68   Body mass index (BMI)
BMI codes should only be assigned when there is an associated, reportable diagnosis (such as obesity). Do not assign BMI codes during pregnancy.
See Section I.B.14 for BMI documentation by clinicians other than the patient's provider.

Z74.01 Bed confinement status

Z76.82 Awaiting organ transplant status

Z78   Other specified health status
Code Z78.1, Physical restraint status, may be used when it is documented by the provider that a patient has been put in restraints during the current encounter. Please note that this code should not be reported when it is documented by the provider that a patient is temporarily restrained during a procedure.

Z79   Long-term (current) drug therapy
Codes from this category indicate a patient's continuous use of a prescribed drug (including such things as aspirin therapy) for the long-term treatment of a condition or for prophylactic use. It is not for use for patients who have addictions to drugs. This subcategory is not for use of medications for detoxification or maintenance programs to prevent withdrawal symptoms (e.g., methadone maintenance for opiate dependence). Assign the appropriate code for the drug use, abuse, or dependence instead.

Assign a code from Z79 if the patient is receiving a medication for an extended period as a prophylactic measure (such as for the prevention of deep vein thrombosis) or as treatment of a chronic condition (such as arthritis) or a disease requiring a lengthy course of treatment (such as cancer). Do not assign a code from category Z79 for medication being administered for a brief period of time to treat an acute illness or injury (such as a course of antibiotics to treat acute bronchitis).

Z88   Allergy status to drugs, medicaments and biological substances
Except: Z88.9, Allergy status to unspecified drugs, medicaments and biological substances status

Z89   Acquired absence of limb

Z90   Acquired absence of organs, not elsewhere classified

Z91.0- Allergy status, other than to drugs and biological substances

Z92.82 Status post administration of tPA (rtPA) in a different facility within the last 24 hours prior to admission to a current facility

Assign code Z92.82, Status post administration of tPA (rtPA) in a different facility within the last 24 hours prior to admission to current facility, as a secondary diagnosis when a patient is received by transfer into a facility and documentation indicates they were administered tissue plasminogen activator (tPA) within the last 24 hours prior to admission to the current facility.

This guideline applies even if the patient is still receiving the tPA at the time they are received into the current facility.

The appropriate code for the condition for which the tPA was administered (such as cerebrovascular disease or myocardial infarction) should be assigned first.

Code Z92.82 is only applicable to the receiving facility record and not to the transferring facility record.

Z93   Artificial opening status

Z94   Transplanted organ and tissue status

Z95   Presence of cardiac and vascular implants and grafts Z96 Presence of other functional implants

Z97   Presence of other devices

Z98   Other postprocedural states
Assign code Z98.85, Transplanted organ removal status, to indicate that a transplanted organ has been previously removed. This code should not be assigned for the encounter in which the transplanted organ is removed. The complication necessitating removal of the transplant organ should be assigned for that encounter.
See section I.C19. for information on the coding of organ transplant complications.

Z99   Dependence on enabling machines and devices, not elsewhere classified
Note: Categories Z89-Z90 and Z93-Z99 are for use only if there are no complications or malfunctions of the organ or tissue replaced, the amputation site or the equipment on which the patient is dependent.

4)   **History (of)**
There are two types of history Z codes, personal and family. Personal history codes explain a patient's past medical condition that no longer exists and is not receiving any treatment, but that has the potential for recurrence, and therefore may require continued monitoring.

Family history codes are for use when a patient has a family member(s) who has had a particular disease that causes the patient to be at higher risk of also contracting the disease.

Personal history codes may be used in conjunction with follow-up codes and family history codes may be used in conjunction with screening codes to explain the need for a test or procedure. History codes are also acceptable on any medical record regardless of the reason for visit. A history of an illness, even if no longer present, is important information that may alter the type of treatment ordered.

The reason for the encounter (for example, screening or counseling) should be sequenced first and the appropriate personal and/or family history code(s) should be assigned as additional diagnos(es).

The history Z code categories are:

Z80   Family history of primary malignant neoplasm

Z81   Family history of mental and behavioral disorders

Z82   Family history of certain disabilities and chronic diseases (leading to disablement)

Z83   Family history of other specific disorders

Z84   Family history of other conditions

Z85   Personal history of malignant neoplasm

Z86   Personal history of certain other diseases

Z87   Personal history of other diseases and conditions

Z91.4- Personal history of psychological trauma, not elsewhere classified

Z91.5- Personal history of self-harm

Z91.81 History of falling

Z91.82 Personal history of military deployment

Z92   Personal history of medical treatment
Except: Z92.0, Personal history of contraception
Except: Z92.82, Status post administration of tPA (rtPA) in a different facility within the last 24 hours prior to admission to a current facility

5)   **Screening**
Screening is the testing for disease or disease precursors in seemingly well individuals so that early detection and treatment can be provided for those who test positive for the disease (e.g., screening mammogram).

The testing of a person to rule out or confirm a suspected diagnosis because the patient has some sign or symptom is a diagnostic examination, not a screening. In these cases, the sign or symptom is used to explain the reason for the test.

A screening code may be a first-listed code if the reason for the visit is specifically the screening exam. It may also be used as an additional code if the screening is done during an office visit for other health problems. A screening code is not necessary if the screening is inherent to a routine examination, such as a pap smear done during a routine pelvic examination.

Should a condition be discovered during the screening then the code for the condition may be assigned as an additional diagnosis.

The Z code indicates that a screening exam is planned. A procedure code is required to confirm that the screening was performed.

The screening Z codes/categories:

Z11   Encounter for screening for infectious and parasitic diseases

Z12   Encounter for screening for malignant neoplasms

Z13   Encounter for screening for other diseases and disorders Except: Z13.9, Encounter for screening, unspecified

Z36   Encounter for antenatal screening for mother

6) Observation

There are three observation Z code categories. They are for use in very limited circumstances when a person is being observed for a suspected condition that is ruled out. The observation codes are not for use if an injury or illness or any signs or symptoms related to the suspected condition are present. In such cases the diagnosis/symptom code is used with the corresponding external cause code.

The observation codes are primarily to be used as a principal/first-listed diagnosis. An observation code may be assigned as a secondary diagnosis code when the patient is being observed for a condition that is ruled out and is unrelated to the principal/first-listed diagnosis. Also, when the principal diagnosis is required to be a code from category Z38, Liveborn infants according to place of birth and type of delivery, then a code from category Z05, Encounter for observation and evaluation of newborn for suspected diseases and conditions ruled out, is sequenced after the Z38 code. Additional codes may be used in addition to the observation code, but only if they are unrelated to the suspected condition being observed.

Codes from subcategory Z03.7, Encounter for suspected maternal and fetal conditions ruled out, may either be used as a first-listed or as an additional code assignment depending on the case. They are for use in very limited circumstances on a maternal record when an encounter is for a suspected maternal or fetal condition that is ruled out during that encounter (for example, a maternal or fetal condition may be suspected due to an abnormal test result). These codes should not be used when the condition is confirmed. In those cases, the confirmed condition should be coded. In addition, these codes are not for use if an illness or any signs or symptoms related to the suspected condition or problem are present. In such cases the diagnosis/symptom code is used.

Additional codes may be used in addition to the code from subcategory Z03.7, but only if they are unrelated to the suspected condition being evaluated.

Codes from subcategory Z03.7 may not be used for encounters for antenatal screening of mother. *See Section I.C.21. Screening.*

For encounters for suspected fetal condition that are inconclusive following testing and evaluation, assign the appropriate code from category O35, O36, O40 or O41.

The observation Z code categories:

Z03   Encounter for medical observation for suspected diseases and conditions ruled out

Z04   Encounter for examination and observation for other reasons Except: Z04.9, Encounter for examination and observation for unspecified reason

Z05   Encounter for observation and evaluation of newborn for suspected diseases and conditions ruled out

7) Aftercare

Aftercare visit codes cover situations when the initial treatment of a disease has been performed and the patient requires continued care during the healing or recovery phase, or for the long-term consequences of the disease. The aftercare Z code should not be used if treatment is directed at a current, acute disease. The diagnosis code is to be used in these cases. Exceptions to this rule are codes Z51.0, Encounter for antineoplastic radiation therapy, and codes from subcategory Z51.1, Encounter for antineoplastic chemotherapy and immunotherapy. These codes are to be first listed, followed by the diagnosis code when a patient's encounter is solely to receive radiation therapy, chemotherapy, or immunotherapy for the treatment of a neoplasm. If the reason for the encounter is more than one type of antineoplastic therapy, code Z51.0 and a code from subcategory Z51.1 may be assigned together, in which case one of these codes would be reported as a secondary diagnosis.

The aftercare Z codes should also not be used for aftercare for injuries. For aftercare of an injury, assign the acute injury code with the appropriate 7th character (for subsequent encounter).

The aftercare codes are generally first listed to explain the specific reason for the encounter. An aftercare code may be used as an additional code when some type of aftercare is provided in addition to the reason for admission and no diagnosis code is applicable. An example of this would be the closure of a colostomy during an encounter for treatment of another condition.

Aftercare codes should be used in conjunction with other aftercare codes or diagnosis codes to provide better detail on the specifics of an aftercare encounter visit, unless otherwise directed by the classification. The sequencing of multiple aftercare codes depends on the circumstances of the encounter.

Certain aftercare Z code categories need a secondary diagnosis code to describe the resolving condition or sequelae. For others, the condition is included in the code title.

Additional Z code aftercare category terms include fitting and adjustment, and attention to artificial openings.

Status Z codes may be used with aftercare Z codes to indicate the nature of the aftercare. For example, code Z95.1, Presence of aortocoronary bypass graft, may be used with code Z48.812, Encounter for surgical aftercare following surgery on the circulatory system, to indicate the surgery for which the aftercare is being performed. A status code should not be used when the aftercare code indicates the type of status, such as using Z43.0, Encounter for attention to tracheostomy, with Z93.0, Tracheostomy status.

The aftercare Z category/codes:

Z42   Encounter for plastic and reconstructive surgery following medical procedure or healed injury

Z43   Encounter for attention to artificial openings

Z44   Encounter for fitting and adjustment of external prosthetic device

Z45   Encounter for adjustment and management of implanted device

Z46   Encounter for fitting and adjustment of other devices

Z47   Orthopedic aftercare

Z48   Encounter for other postprocedural aftercare

Z49   Encounter for care involving renal dialysis

Z51   Encounter for other aftercare and medical care

8) Follow-up

The follow-up codes are used to explain continuing surveillance following completed treatment of a disease, condition, or injury. They imply that the condition has been fully treated and no longer exists. They should not be confused with aftercare codes, or injury codes with a 7th character for subsequent encounter, that explain ongoing care of a healing condition or its sequelae. Follow-up codes may be used in conjunction with history codes to provide the full picture of the healed condition and its treatment. The follow-up code is sequenced first, followed by the history code.

A follow-up code may be used to explain multiple visits. Should a condition be found to have recurred on the follow-up visit, then

the diagnosis code for the condition should be assigned in place of the follow-up code.

The follow-up Z code categories:

Z08   Encounter for follow-up examination after completed treatment for malignant neoplasm

Z09   Encounter for follow-up examination after completed treatment for conditions other than malignant neoplasm

Z39   Encounter for maternal postpartum care and examination

9) Donor

Codes in category Z52, Donors of organs and tissues, are used for living individuals who are donating blood or other body tissue. These codes are for individuals donating for others, **as well as** for self-donations. They are not used to identify cadaveric donations.

10) Counseling

Counseling Z codes are used when a patient or family member receives assistance in the aftermath of an illness or injury, or when support is required in coping with family or social problems.

The counseling Z codes/categories:

Z30.0- Encounter for general counseling and advice on contraception

Z31.5   Encounter for procreative genetic counseling

Z31.6- Encounter for general counseling and advice on procreation

Z32.2   Encounter for childbirth instruction

Z32.3   Encounter for childcare instruction

Z69   Encounter for mental health services for victim and perpetrator of abuse

Z70   Counseling related to sexual attitude, behavior and orientation

Z71   Persons encountering health services for other counseling and medical advice, not elsewhere classified
        Note: Code Z71.84, Encounter for health counseling related to travel, is to be used for health risk and safety counseling for future travel purposes.

        Code Z71.85, Encounter for immunization safety counseling, is to be used for counseling of the patient or caregiver regarding the safety of a vaccine. This code should not be used for the provision of general information regarding risks and potential side effects during routine encounters for the administration of vaccines.

Z76.81 Expectant mother prebirth pediatrician visit

11) Encounters for Obstetrical and Reproductive Services

See Section I.C.15. Pregnancy, Childbirth, and the Puerperium, for further instruction on the use of these codes.

Z codes for pregnancy are for use in those circumstances when none of the problems or complications included in the codes from the Obstetrics chapter exist (a routine prenatal visit or postpartum care). Codes in category Z34, Encounter for supervision of normal pregnancy, are always first listed and are not to be used with any other code from the OB chapter.

Codes in category Z3A, Weeks of gestation, may be assigned to provide additional information about the pregnancy. Category Z3A codes should not be assigned for pregnancies with abortive outcomes (categories O00-O08), elective termination of pregnancy (code Z33.2), nor for postpartum conditions, as category Z3A is not applicable to these conditions. The date of the admission should be used to determine weeks of gestation for inpatient admissions that encompass more than one gestational week.

The outcome of delivery, category Z37, should be included on all maternal delivery records. It is always a secondary code.

Codes in category Z37 should not be used on the newborn record.

Z codes for family planning (contraceptive) or procreative management and counseling should be included on an obstetric record either during the pregnancy or the postpartum stage, if applicable.

Z codes/categories for obstetrical and reproductive services:

Z30   Encounter for contraceptive management

Z31   Encounter for procreative management

Z32.2   Encounter for childbirth instruction

Z32.3   Encounter for childcare instruction

Z33   Pregnant state

Z34   Encounter for supervision of normal pregnancy

Z36   Encounter for antenatal screening of mother

Z3A   Weeks of gestation

Z37   Outcome of delivery

Z39   Encounter for maternal postpartum care and examination

Z76.81 Expectant mother prebirth pediatrician visit

12) Newborns and Infants

See Section I.C.16. Newborn (Perinatal) Guidelines, for further instruction on the use of these codes.

Newborn Z codes/categories: ·

Z76.1   Encounter for health supervision and care of foundling

Z00.1- Encounter for routine child health examination

Z38   Liveborn infants according to place of birth and type of delivery

13) Routine and Administrative Examinations

The Z codes allow for the description of encounters for routine examinations, such as, a general check-up, or, examinations for administrative purposes, such as, a pre-employment physical. The codes are not to be used if the examination is for diagnosis of a suspected condition or for treatment purposes. In such cases the diagnosis code is used. During a routine exam, should a diagnosis or condition be discovered, it should be coded as an additional code. Pre-existing and chronic conditions and history codes may also be included as additional codes as long as the examination is for administrative purposes and not focused on any particular condition.

Some of the codes for routine health examinations distinguish between "with" and "without" abnormal findings. Code assignment depends on the information that is known at the time the encounter is being coded. For example, if no abnormal findings were found during the examination, but the encounter is being coded before test results are back, it is acceptable to assign the code for "without abnormal findings." When assigning a code for "with abnormal findings," additional code(s) should be assigned to identify the specific abnormal finding(s).

Pre-operative examination and pre-procedural laboratory examination Z codes are for use only in those situations when a patient is being cleared for a procedure or surgery and no treatment is given.

The Z codes/categories for routine and administrative examinations:

Z00   Encounter for general examination without complaint, suspected or reported diagnosis

Z01   Encounter for other special examination without complaint, suspected or reported diagnosis

Z02   Encounter for administrative examination
        Except: Z02.9, Encounter for administrative examinations, unspecified

Z32.0- Encounter for pregnancy test

14) Miscellaneous Z Codes

The miscellaneous Z codes capture a number of other health care encounters that do not fall into one of the other categories. **Some** of these codes identify the reason for the encounter; others are for use as additional codes that provide useful information on circumstances that may affect a patient's care and treatment.

Prophylactic Organ Removal

For encounters specifically for prophylactic removal of an organ (such as prophylactic removal of breasts due to a genetic susceptibility to cancer or a family history of cancer), the principal or first-listed code should be a code from category Z40, Encounter for prophylactic surgery, followed by the appropriate codes to identify the associated risk factor (such as genetic susceptibility or family history).

If the patient has a malignancy of one site and is having prophylactic removal at another site to prevent either a new primary malignancy or metastatic disease, a code for the malignancy should also be assigned in addition to a code from

subcategory Z40.0, Encounter for prophylactic surgery for risk factors related to malignant neoplasms. A Z40.0 code should not be assigned if the patient is having organ removal for treatment of a malignancy, such as the removal of the testes for the treatment of prostate cancer.

Miscellaneous Z codes/categories:

Z28	Immunization not carried out Except: Z28.3, Underimmunization status
Z29	Encounter for other prophylactic measures
Z40	Encounter for prophylactic surgery
Z41	Encounter for procedures for purposes other than remedying health state Except: Z41.9, Encounter for procedure for purposes other than remedying health state, unspecified
Z53	Persons encountering health services for specific procedures and treatment, not carried out
Z72	Problems related to lifestyle Note: These codes should be assigned only when the documentation specifies that the patient has an associated problem
Z73	Problems related to life management difficulty
Z74	Problems related to care provider dependency Except: Z74.01, Bed confinement status
Z75	Problems related to medical facilities and other health care
Z76.0	Encounter for issue of repeat prescription
Z76.3	Healthy person accompanying sick person
Z76.4	Other boarder to healthcare facility
Z76.5	Malingerer [conscious simulation]
Z91.1-	Patient's noncompliance with medical treatment and regimen
Z91.83	Wandering in diseases classified elsewhere
Z91.84-	Oral health risk factors
Z91.89	Other specified personal risk factors, not elsewhere classified

See Section I.B.14 for Z55-Z65 Persons with potential health hazards related to socioeconomic and psychosocial circumstances, documentation by clinicians other than the patient's provider

15) Nonspecific Z Codes

Certain Z codes are so non-specific, or potentially redundant with other codes in the classification, that there can be little justification for their use in the inpatient setting. Their use in the outpatient setting should be limited to those instances when there is no further documentation to permit more precise coding. Otherwise, any sign or symptom or any other reason for visit that is captured in another code should be used.

Nonspecific Z codes/categories:

Z02.9	Encounter for administrative examinations, unspecified
Z04.9	Encounter for examination and observation for unspecified reason
Z13.9	Encounter for screening, unspecified
Z41.9	Encounter for procedure for purposes other than remedying health state, unspecified
Z52.9	Donor of unspecified organ or tissue
Z86.59	Personal history of other mental and behavioral disorders
Z88.9	Allergy status to unspecified drugs, medicaments and biological substances status
Z92.0	Personal history of contraception

16) Z Codes That May Only be Principal/First-Listed Diagnosis

The following Z codes/categories may only be reported as the principal/first-listed diagnosis, except when there are multiple encounters on the same day and the medical records for the encounters are combined:

Z00	Encounter for general examination without complaint, suspected or reported diagnosis Except: Z00.6
Z01	Encounter for other special examination without complaint, suspected or reported diagnosis
Z02	Encounter for administrative examination
Z04	Encounter for examination and observation for other reasons

Z33.2	Encounter for elective termination of pregnancy
Z31.81	Encounter for male factor infertility in female patient
Z31.83	Encounter for assisted reproductive fertility procedure cycle
Z31.84	Encounter for fertility preservation procedure
Z34	Encounter for supervision of normal pregnancy
Z39	Encounter for maternal postpartum care and examination
Z38	Liveborn infants according to place of birth and type of delivery
Z40	Encounter for prophylactic surgery
Z42	Encounter for plastic and reconstructive surgery following medical procedure or healed injury
Z51.0	Encounter for antineoplastic radiation therapy
Z51.1-	Encounter for antineoplastic chemotherapy and immunotherapy
Z52	Donors of organs and tissues Except: Z52.9, Donor of unspecified organ or tissue
Z76.1	Encounter for health supervision and care of foundling
Z76.2	Encounter for health supervision and care of other healthy infant and child
Z99.12	Encounter for respirator [ventilator] dependence during power failure

17) Social Determinants of Health

Codes describing social determinants of health (SDOH) should be assigned when this information is documented.

For social determinants of health, such as information found in categories Z55-Z65, Persons with potential health hazards related to socioeconomic and psychosocial circumstances, code assignment may be based on medical record documentation from clinicians involved in the care of the patient who are not the patient's provider since this information represents social information, rather than medical diagnoses.

For example, coding professionals may utilize documentation of social information from social workers, community health workers, case managers, or nurses, if their documentation is included in the official medical record.

Patient self-reported documentation may be used to assign codes for social determinants of health, as long as the patient self-reported information is signed-off by and incorporated into the medical record by either a clinician or provider.

Social determinants of health codes are located primarily in these Z code categories:

Z55	**Problems related to education and literacy**
Z56	**Problems related to employment and unemployment**
Z57	**Occupational exposure to risk factors**
Z58	**Problems related to physical environment**
Z59	**Problems related to housing and economic circumstances**
Z60	**Problems related to social environment**
Z62	**Problems related to upbringing**
Z63	**Other problems related to primary support group, including family circumstances**
Z64	**Problems related to certain psychosocial circumstances**
Z65	**Problems related to other psychosocial circumstances**

See Section I.B.14. Documentation by Clinicians Other than the Patient's Provider.

22. Chapter 22: Codes for Special Purposes (U00-U85)

U07.0	Vaping-related disorder (see Section I.C.10.e., Vaping-related disorders)
U07.1	COVID-19 (see Section I.C.1.g.1., COVID-19 infection)
U09.9	**Post COVID-19 condition, unspecified (see Section I.C.1.g.1.m)**

Section II. Selection of Principal Diagnosis

The circumstances of inpatient admission always govern the selection of principal diagnosis. The principal diagnosis is defined in the Uniform Hospital Discharge Data Set (UHDDS) as "that condition established after study to be chiefly responsible for occasioning the admission of the patient to the hospital for care."

The UHDDS definitions are used by hospitals to report inpatient data elements in a standardized manner. These data elements and their definitions can be found in the July 31, 1985, Federal Register (Vol. 50, No, 147), pp. 31038-40.

Since that time, the application of the UHDDS definitions has been expanded to include all non-outpatient settings (acute care, short term, long term care and psychiatric hospitals; home health agencies; rehab facilities; nursing homes, etc.). The UHDDS definitions also apply to hospice services (all levels of care).

In determining principal diagnosis, coding conventions in the ICD-10-CM, the Tabular List and Alphabetic Index take precedence over these official coding guidelines.

(See Section I.A., Conventions for the ICD-10-CM)

The importance of consistent, complete documentation in the medical record cannot be overemphasized. Without such documentation the application of all coding guidelines is a difficult, if not impossible, task.

A. **Codes for symptoms, signs, and ill-defined conditions**
Codes for symptoms, signs, and ill-defined conditions from Chapter 18 are not to be used as principal diagnosis when a related definitive diagnosis has been established.

B. **Two or more interrelated conditions, each potentially meeting the definition for principal diagnosis.**
When there are two or more interrelated conditions (such as diseases in the same ICD-10-CM chapter or manifestations characteristically associated with a certain disease) potentially meeting the definition of principal diagnosis, either condition may be sequenced first, unless the circumstances of the admission, the therapy provided, the Tabular List, or the Alphabetic Index indicate otherwise.

C. **Two or more diagnoses that equally meet the definition for principal diagnosis**
In the unusual instance when two or more diagnoses equally meet the criteria for principal diagnosis as determined by the circumstances of admission, diagnostic workup and/or therapy provided, and the Alphabetic Index, Tabular List, or another coding guidelines does not provide sequencing direction, any one of the diagnoses may be sequenced first.

D. **Two or more comparative or contrasting conditions**
In those rare instances when two or more contrasting or comparative diagnoses are documented as "either/or" (or similar terminology), they are coded as if the diagnoses were confirmed and the diagnoses are sequenced according to the circumstances of the admission. If no further determination can be made as to which diagnosis should be principal, either diagnosis may be sequenced first.

E. **A symptom(s) followed by contrasting/comparative diagnoses**
GUIDELINE HAS BEEN DELETED EFFECTIVE OCTOBER 1, 2014

F. **Original treatment plan not carried out**
Sequence as the principal diagnosis the condition, which after study occasioned the admission to the hospital, even though treatment may not have been carried out due to unforeseen circumstances.

G. **Complications of surgery and other medical care**
When the admission is for treatment of a complication resulting from surgery or other medical care, the complication code is sequenced as the principal diagnosis. If the complication is classified to the T80-T88 series and the code lacks the necessary specificity in describing the complication, an additional code for the specific complication should be assigned.

H. **Uncertain Diagnosis**
If the diagnosis documented at the time of discharge is qualified as "probable," "suspected," "likely," "questionable," "possible," or "still to be ruled out," "compatible with," "consistent with," or other similar terms indicating uncertainty, code the condition as if it existed or was established. The bases for these guidelines are the diagnostic workup, arrangements for further workup or observation, and initial therapeutic approach that correspond most closely with the established diagnosis.
Note: This guideline is applicable only to inpatient admissions to short-term, acute, long-term care and psychiatric hospitals.

I. **Admission from Observation Unit**
1. **Admission Following Medical Observation**
When a patient is admitted to an observation unit for a medical condition, which either worsens or does not improve, and is subsequently admitted as an inpatient of the same hospital for this same medical condition, the principal diagnosis would be the medical condition which led to the hospital admission.

2. **Admission Following Post-Operative Observation**
When a patient is admitted to an observation unit to monitor a condition (or complication) that develops following outpatient surgery, and then is subsequently admitted as an inpatient of the same hospital, hospitals should apply the Uniform Hospital Discharge Data Set (UHDDS) definition of principal diagnosis as "that condition established after study to be chiefly responsible for occasioning the admission of the patient to the hospital for care."

J. **Admission from Outpatient Surgery**
When a patient receives surgery in the hospital's outpatient surgery department and is subsequently admitted for continuing inpatient care at the same hospital, the following guidelines should be followed in selecting the principal diagnosis for the inpatient admission:
- If the reason for the inpatient admission is a complication, assign the complication as the principal diagnosis.
- If no complication, or other condition, is documented as the reason for the inpatient admission, assign the reason for the outpatient surgery as the principal diagnosis.
- If the reason for the inpatient admission is another condition unrelated to the surgery, assign the unrelated condition as the principal diagnosis.

K. **Admissions/Encounters for Rehabilitation**
When the purpose for the admission/encounter is rehabilitation, sequence first the code for the condition for which the service is being performed. For example, for an admission/encounter for rehabilitation for right-sided dominant hemiplegia following a cerebrovascular infarction, report code I69.351, Hemiplegia and hemiparesis following cerebral infarction affecting right dominant side, as the first-listed or principal diagnosis.

If the condition for which the rehabilitation service is being provided is no longer present, report the appropriate aftercare code as the first-listed or principal diagnosis, unless the rehabilitation service is being provided following an injury. For rehabilitation services following active treatment of an injury, assign the injury code with the appropriate seventh character for subsequent encounter as the first-listed or principal diagnosis. For example, if a patient with severe degenerative osteoarthritis of the hip, underwent hip replacement and the current encounter/admission is for rehabilitation, report code Z47.1, Aftercare following joint replacement surgery, as the first-listed or principal diagnosis. If the patient requires rehabilitation post hip replacement for right intertrochanteric femur fracture, report code S72.141D, Displaced intertrochanteric fracture of right femur, subsequent encounter for closed fracture with routine healing, as the first-listed or principal diagnosis.

See Section I.C.21.c.7, Factors influencing health states and contact with health services, Aftercare.

See Section I.C.19.a, for additional information about the use of 7th characters for injury codes.

Section III. Reporting Additional Diagnoses

GENERAL RULES FOR OTHER (ADDITIONAL) DIAGNOSES

For reporting purposes, the definition for "other diagnoses" is interpreted as additional conditions that affect patient care in terms of requiring:

    clinical evaluation; or

    therapeutic treatment; or

    diagnostic procedures; or

    extended length of hospital stay; or

    increased nursing care and/or monitoring.

The UHDDS item #11-b defines Other Diagnoses as "all conditions that coexist at the time of admission, that develop subsequently, or that affect the treatment received and/or the length of stay. Diagnoses that relate to an earlier episode which have no bearing on the current hospital stay are to be excluded." UHDDS definitions apply to inpatients in acute care, short-term, long term care and psychiatric hospital setting. The UHDDS definitions are used by acute care short-term hospitals to report inpatient data elements in a standardized manner. These data elements and their definitions can be found in the July 31, 1985, Federal Register (Vol. 50, No, 147), pp. 31038-40.

Since that time, the application of the UHDDS definitions has been expanded to include all non-outpatient settings (acute care, short term, long term care and psychiatric hospitals; home health agencies; rehab facilities; nursing homes, etc.). The UHDDS definitions also apply to hospice services (all levels of care).

The following guidelines are to be applied in designating "other diagnoses" when neither the Alphabetic Index nor the Tabular List in ICD-10-CM provide direction. The listing of the diagnoses in the patient record is the responsibility of the attending provider.

A. Previous conditions

If the provider has included a diagnosis in the final diagnostic statement, such as the discharge summary or the face sheet, it should ordinarily be coded. Some providers include in the diagnostic statement resolved conditions or diagnoses and status-post procedures from previous admissions that have no bearing on the current stay. Such conditions are not to be reported and are coded only if required by hospital policy.

However, history codes (categories Z80-Z87) may be used as secondary codes if the historical condition or family history has an impact on current care or influences treatment.

B. Abnormal findings

Abnormal findings (laboratory, x-ray, pathologic, and other diagnostic results) are not coded and reported unless the provider indicates their clinical significance. If the findings are outside the normal range and the attending provider has ordered other tests to evaluate the condition or prescribed treatment, it is appropriate to ask the provider whether the abnormal finding should be added.

Please note: This differs from the coding practices in the outpatient setting for coding encounters for diagnostic tests that have been interpreted by a provider.

C. Uncertain Diagnosis

If the diagnosis documented at the time of discharge is qualified as "probable," "suspected," "likely," "questionable," "possible," or "still to be ruled out," "compatible with," "consistent with," or other similar terms indicating uncertainty, code the condition as if it existed or was established. The bases for these guidelines are the diagnostic workup, arrangements for further workup or observation, and initial therapeutic approach that correspond most closely with the established diagnosis.

Note: This guideline is applicable only to inpatient admissions to short-term, acute, long-term care and psychiatric hospitals.

Section IV. Diagnostic Coding and Reporting Guidelines for Outpatient Services

These coding guidelines for outpatient diagnoses have been approved for use by hospitals/ providers in coding and reporting hospital-based outpatient services and provider-based office visits. Guidelines in Section I, Conventions, general coding guidelines and chapter-specific guidelines, should also be applied for outpatient services and office visits.

Information about the use of certain abbreviations, punctuation, symbols, and other conventions used in the ICD-10-CM Tabular List (code numbers and titles), can be found in Section IA of these guidelines, under "Conventions Used in the Tabular List." Section I.B. contains general guidelines that apply to the entire classification. Section I.C. contains chapter-specific guidelines that correspond to the chapters as they are arranged in the classification. Information about the correct sequence to use in finding a code is also described in Section I.

The terms encounter and visit are often used interchangeably in describing outpatient service contacts and, therefore, appear together in these guidelines without distinguishing one from the other.

Though the conventions and general guidelines apply to all settings, coding guidelines for outpatient and provider reporting of diagnoses will vary in a number of instances from those for inpatient diagnoses, recognizing that:

The Uniform Hospital Discharge Data Set (UHDDS) definition of principal diagnosis does not apply to hospital-based outpatient services and provider-based office visits.

Coding guidelines for inconclusive diagnoses (probable, suspected, rule out, etc.) were developed for inpatient reporting and do not apply to outpatients.

A. Selection of first-listed condition

In the outpatient setting, the term first-listed diagnosis is used in lieu of principal diagnosis.

In determining the first-listed diagnosis the coding conventions of ICD-10-CM, as well as the general and disease specific guidelines take precedence over the outpatient guidelines.

Diagnoses often are not established at the time of the initial encounter/visit. It may take two or more visits before the diagnosis is confirmed.

The most critical rule involves beginning the search for the correct code assignment through the Alphabetic Index. Never begin searching initially in the Tabular List as this will lead to coding errors.

1. Outpatient Surgery

When a patient presents for outpatient surgery (same day surgery), code the reason for the surgery as the first-listed diagnosis (reason for the encounter), even if the surgery is not performed due to a contraindication.

2. Observation Stay

When a patient is admitted for observation for a medical condition, assign a code for the medical condition as the first-listed diagnosis.

When a patient presents for outpatient surgery and develops complications requiring admission to observation, code the reason for the surgery as the first reported diagnosis (reason for the encounter), followed by codes for the complications as secondary diagnoses.

B. Codes from A00.0 through T88.9, Z00-Z99, U00-U85

The appropriate code(s) from A00.0 through T88.9, Z00-Z99 **and U00-U85** must be used to identify diagnoses, symptoms, conditions, problems, complaints, or other reason(s) for the encounter/visit.

C. Accurate reporting of ICD-10-CM diagnosis codes

For accurate reporting of ICD-10-CM diagnosis codes, the documentation should describe the patient's condition, using terminology which includes specific diagnoses as well as symptoms, problems, or reasons for the encounter. There are ICD-10-CM codes to describe all of these.

D. Codes that describe symptoms and signs

Codes that describe symptoms and signs, as opposed to diagnoses, are acceptable for reporting purposes when a diagnosis has not been established (confirmed) by the provider. Chapter 18 of ICD-10-CM, Symptoms, Signs, and Abnormal Clinical and Laboratory Findings Not Elsewhere Classified (codes R00-R99) contain many, but not all codes for symptoms.

E. Encounters for circumstances other than a disease or injury

ICD-10-CM provides codes to deal with encounters for circumstances other than a disease or injury. The Factors Influencing Health Status and Contact with Health Services codes (Z00-Z99) are provided to deal with occasions when circumstances other than a disease or injury are recorded as diagnosis or problems.

See Section I.C.21. Factors influencing health status and contact with health services.

F. Level of Detail in Coding

1. ICD-10-CM codes with 3, 4, 5, 6 or 7 characters

ICD-10-CM is composed of codes with 3, 4, 5, 6 or 7 characters. Codes with three characters are included in ICD-10-CM as the heading of a category of codes that may be further subdivided by the use of fourth, fifth, sixth or seventh characters to provide greater specificity.

2. Use of full number of characters required for a code

A three-character code is to be used only if it is not further subdivided. A code is invalid if it has not been coded to the full number of characters required for that code, including the 7th character, if applicable.

3. Highest level of specificity
Code to the highest level of specificity when supported by the medical record documentation.

G. ICD-10-CM code for the diagnosis, condition, problem, or other reason for encounter/visit

List first the ICD-10-CM code for the diagnosis, condition, problem, or other reason for encounter/visit shown in the medical record to be chiefly responsible for the services provided. List additional codes that describe any coexisting conditions. In some cases, the first-listed diagnosis may be a symptom when a diagnosis has not been established (confirmed) by the provider.

H. Uncertain diagnosis

Do not code diagnoses documented as "probable", "suspected," "questionable," "rule out," "compatible with," "consistent with," or "working diagnosis" or other similar terms indicating uncertainty. Rather, code the condition(s) to the highest degree of certainty for that encounter/visit, such as symptoms, signs, abnormal test results, or other reason for the visit.

Please note: This differs from the coding practices used by short-term, acute care, long-term care and psychiatric hospitals.

I. Chronic diseases

Chronic diseases treated on an ongoing basis may be coded and reported as many times as the patient receives treatment and care for the condition(s)

J. Code all documented conditions that coexist

Code all documented conditions that coexist at the time of the encounter/visit and that require or affect patient care, treatment or management. Do not code conditions that were previously treated and no

longer exist. However, history codes (categories Z80-Z87) may be used as secondary codes if the historical condition or family history has an impact on current care or influences treatment.

K. Patients receiving diagnostic services only

For patients receiving diagnostic services only during an encounter/visit, sequence first the diagnosis, condition, problem, or other reason for encounter/visit shown in the medical record to be chiefly responsible for the outpatient services provided during the encounter/visit. Codes for other diagnoses (e.g., chronic conditions) may be sequenced as additional diagnoses.

For encounters for routine laboratory/radiology testing in the absence of any signs, symptoms, or associated diagnosis, assign Z01.89, Encounter for other specified special examinations. If routine testing is performed during the same encounter as a test to evaluate a sign, symptom, or diagnosis, it is appropriate to assign both the Z code and the code describing the reason for the non-routine test.

For outpatient encounters for diagnostic tests that have been interpreted by a physician, and the final report is available at the time of coding, code any confirmed or definitive diagnosis(es) documented in the interpretation. Do not code related signs and symptoms as additional diagnoses.

Please note: This differs from the coding practice in the hospital inpatient setting regarding abnormal findings on test results.

L. Patients receiving therapeutic services only

For patients receiving therapeutic services only during an encounter/visit, sequence first the diagnosis, condition, problem, or other reason for encounter/visit shown in the medical record to be chiefly responsible for the outpatient services provided during the encounter/visit. Codes for other diagnoses (e.g., chronic conditions) may be sequenced as additional diagnoses.

The only exception to this rule is that when the primary reason for the admission/encounter is chemotherapy or radiation therapy, the appropriate Z code for the service is listed first, and the diagnosis or problem for which the service is being performed listed second.

M. Patients receiving preoperative evaluations only

For patients receiving preoperative evaluations only, sequence first a code from subcategory Z01.81, Encounter for pre-procedural examinations, to describe the pre-op consultations. Assign a code for the condition to describe the reason for the surgery as an additional diagnosis. Code also any findings related to the pre-op evaluation.

N. Ambulatory surgery

For ambulatory surgery, code the diagnosis for which the surgery was performed. If the postoperative diagnosis is known to be different from the preoperative diagnosis at the time the diagnosis is confirmed, select the postoperative diagnosis for coding, since it is the most definitive.

O. Routine outpatient prenatal visits

See Section I.C.15. Routine outpatient prenatal visits.

P. Encounters for general medical examinations with abnormal findings

The subcategories for encounters for general medical examinations, Z00.0- and encounter for routine child health examination, Z00.12-, provide codes for with and without abnormal findings. Should a general medical examination result in an abnormal finding, the code for general medical examination with abnormal finding should be assigned as the first-listed diagnosis. An examination with abnormal findings refers to a condition/diagnosis that is newly identified or a change in severity of a chronic condition (such as uncontrolled hypertension, or an acute exacerbation of chronic obstructive pulmonary disease) during a routine physical examination. A secondary code for the abnormal finding should also be coded.

Q. Encounters for routine health screenings

See Section I.C.21. Factors influencing health status and contact with health services, Screening

Appendix I. Present on Admission Reporting Guidelines

Introduction

These guidelines are to be used as a supplement to the *ICD-10-CM Official Guidelines for Coding and Reporting* to facilitate the assignment of the Present on Admission (POA) indicator for each diagnosis and external cause of injury code reported on claim forms (UB-04 and 837 Institutional).

These guidelines are not intended to replace any guidelines in the main body of the *ICD-10-CM Official Guidelines for Coding and Reporting*. The POA guidelines are not intended to provide guidance on when a condition should be coded, but

rather, how to apply the POA indicator to the final set of diagnosis codes that have been assigned in accordance with Sections I, II, and III of the official coding guidelines. Subsequent to the assignment of the ICD-10-CM codes, the POA indicator should then be assigned to those conditions that have been coded.

As stated in the Introduction to the *ICD-10-CM Official Guidelines for Coding and Reporting*, a joint effort between the healthcare provider and the coder is essential to achieve complete and accurate documentation, code assignment, and reporting of diagnoses and procedures. The importance of consistent, complete documentation in the medical record cannot be overemphasized. Medical record documentation from any provider involved in the care and treatment of the patient may be used to support the determination of whether a condition was present on admission or not. In the context of the official coding guidelines, the term "provider" means a physician or any qualified healthcare practitioner who is legally accountable for establishing the patient's diagnosis.

These guidelines are not a substitute for the provider's clinical judgment as to the determination of whether a condition was/was not present on admission. The provider should be queried regarding issues related to the linking of signs/symptoms, timing of test results, and the timing of findings.

Please see the CDC website for the detailed list of ICD-10-CM codes that do not require the use of a POA indicator (https://www.cdc.gov/nchs/icd/icd10cm.htm). The codes and categories on this exempt list are for circumstances regarding the healthcare encounter or factors influencing health status that do not represent a current disease or injury or that describe conditions that are always present on admission.

General Reporting Requirements

All claims involving inpatient admissions to general acute care hospitals or other facilities that are subject to a law or regulation mandating collection of present on admission information.

Present on admission is defined as present at the time the order for inpatient admission occurs -- conditions that develop during an outpatient encounter, including emergency department, observation, or outpatient surgery, are considered as present on admission.

POA indicator is assigned to principal and secondary diagnoses (as defined in Section II of the Official Guidelines for Coding and Reporting) and the external cause of injury codes.

Issues related to inconsistent, missing, conflicting or unclear documentation must still be resolved by the provider.

If a condition would not be coded and reported based on UHDDS definitions and current official coding guidelines, then the POA indicator would not be reported.

> Reporting Options
>> Y – Yes
>> N – No
>> U – Unknown
>> W – Clinically undetermined
>> Unreported/Not used – (Exempt from POA reporting)
> Reporting Definitions
>> Y = present at the time of inpatient admission
>> N = not present at the time of inpatient admission
>> U = documentation is insufficient to determine if condition is present on admission
>> W = provider is unable to clinically determine whether condition was present on admission or not

Timeframe for POA Identification and Documentation

There is no required timeframe as to when a provider (per the definition of "provider" used in these guidelines) must identify or document a condition to be present on admission. In some clinical situations, it may not be possible for a provider to make a definitive diagnosis (or a condition may not be recognized or reported by the patient) for a period of time after admission. In some cases, it may be several days before the provider arrives at a definitive diagnosis. This does not mean that the condition was not present on admission. Determination of whether the condition was present on admission or not will be based on the applicable POA guideline as identified in this document, or on the provider's best clinical judgment.

If at the time of code assignment the documentation is unclear as to whether a condition was present on admission or not, it is appropriate to query the provider for clarification.

Assigning the POA Indicator

Condition is on the "Exempt from Reporting" list

> Leave the "present on admission" field blank if the condition is on the list of ICD-10-CM codes for which this field is not applicable. This is the only circumstance in which the field may be left blank.

POA Explicitly Documented

Assign Y for any condition the provider explicitly documents as being present on admission.

Assign N for any condition the provider explicitly documents as not present at the time of admission.

Conditions diagnosed prior to inpatient admission

Assign "Y" for conditions that were diagnosed prior to admission (example: hypertension, diabetes mellitus, asthma)

Conditions diagnosed during the admission but clearly present before admission

Assign "Y" for conditions diagnosed during the admission that were clearly present but not diagnosed until after admission occurred.

Diagnoses subsequently confirmed after admission are considered present on admission if at the time of admission they are documented as suspected, possible, rule out, differential diagnosis, or constitute an underlying cause of a symptom that is present at the time of admission.

Condition develops during outpatient encounter prior to inpatient admission

Assign Y for any condition that develops during an outpatient encounter prior to a written order for inpatient admission.

Documentation does not indicate whether condition was present on admission

Assign "U" when the medical record documentation is unclear as to whether the condition was present on admission. "U" should not be routinely assigned and used only in very limited circumstances. Coders are encouraged to query the providers when the documentation is unclear.

Documentation states that it cannot be determined whether the condition was or was not present on admission

Assign "W" when the medical record documentation indicates that it cannot be clinically determined whether or not the condition was present on admission.

Chronic condition with acute exacerbation during the admission

If a single code identifies both the chronic condition and the acute exacerbation, see POA guidelines pertaining to codes that contain multiple clinical concepts.

If a single code only identifies the chronic condition and not the acute exacerbation (e.g., acute exacerbation of chronic leukemia), assign "Y."

Conditions documented as possible, probable, suspected, or rule out at the time of discharge

If the final diagnosis contains a possible, probable, suspected, or rule out diagnosis, and this diagnosis was based on signs, symptoms or clinical findings suspected at the time of inpatient admission, assign "Y."

If the final diagnosis contains a possible, probable, suspected, or rule out diagnosis, and this diagnosis was based on signs, symptoms or clinical findings that were not present on admission, assign "N".

Conditions documented as impending or threatened at the time of discharge

If the final diagnosis contains an impending or threatened diagnosis, and this diagnosis is based on symptoms or clinical findings that were present on admission, assign "Y".

If the final diagnosis contains an impending or threatened diagnosis, and this diagnosis is based on symptoms or clinical findings that were not present on admission, assign "N".

Acute and Chronic Conditions

Assign "Y" for acute conditions that are present at time of admission and N for acute conditions that are not present at time of admission.

Assign "Y" for chronic conditions, even though the condition may not be diagnosed until after admission.

If a single code identifies both an acute and chronic condition, see the POA guidelines for codes that contain multiple clinical concepts.

Codes That Contain Multiple Clinical Concepts

Assign "N" if at least one of the clinical concepts included in the code was not present on admission (e.g., COPD with acute exacerbation and the exacerbation was not present on admission; gastric ulcer that does not start bleeding until after admission; asthma patient develops status asthmaticus after admission).

Assign "Y" if all of the clinical concepts included in the code were present on admission (e.g., duodenal ulcer that perforates prior to admission).

For infection codes that include the causal organism, assign "Y" if the infection (or signs of the infection) were present on admission, even though the culture results may not be known until after admission (e.g., patient is admitted with pneumonia and the provider documents Pseudomonas as the causal organism a few days later).

Same Diagnosis Code for Two or More Conditions

When the same ICD-10-CM diagnosis code applies to two or more conditions during the same encounter (e.g. two separate conditions classified to the same ICD-10-CM diagnosis code):

Assign "Y" if all conditions represented by the single ICD-10-CM code were present on admission (e.g. bilateral unspecified age-related cataracts).

Assign "N" if any of the conditions represented by the single ICD-10-CM code was not present on admission (e.g. traumatic secondary and recurrent hemorrhage and seroma is assigned to a single code T79.2, but only one of the conditions was present on admission).

Obstetrical conditions

Whether or not the patient delivers during the current hospitalization does not affect assignment of the POA indicator. The determining factor for POA assignment is whether the pregnancy complication or obstetrical condition described by the code was present at the time of admission or not.

If the pregnancy complication or obstetrical condition was present on admission (e.g., patient admitted in preterm labor), assign "Y".

If the pregnancy complication or obstetrical condition was not present on admission (e.g., 2nd degree laceration during delivery, postpartum hemorrhage that occurred during current hospitalization, fetal distress develops after admission), assign "N".

If the obstetrical code includes more than one diagnosis and any of the diagnoses identified by the code were not present on admission assign "N". (e.g., Category O11, Pre-existing hypertension with pre-eclampsia)

Perinatal conditions

Newborns are not considered to be admitted until after birth. Therefore, any condition present at birth or that developed in utero is considered present at admission and should be assigned "Y". This includes conditions that occur during delivery (e.g., injury during delivery, meconium aspiration, exposure to streptococcus B in the vaginal canal).

Congenital conditions and anomalies

Assign "Y" for congenital conditions and anomalies except for categories Q00-Q99, Congenital anomalies, which are on the exempt list. Congenital conditions are always considered present on admission.

External cause of injury codes

Assign "Y" for any external cause code representing an external cause of morbidity that occurred prior to inpatient admission (e.g., patient fell out of bed at home, patient fell out of bed in emergency room prior to admission)

Assign "N" for any external cause code representing an external cause of morbidity that occurred during inpatient hospitalization (e.g., patient fell out of hospital bed during hospital stay, patient experienced an adverse reaction to a medication administered after inpatient admission).

A

Aarskog's syndrome Q87.19
Abandonment — *see* Maltreatment
Abasia (-astasia) (hysterical) F44.4
Abderhalden-Kaufmann-Lignac syndrome (cystinosis) E72.04
Abdomen, abdominal — *see also* condition
  muscle deficiency syndrome Q79.4
  angina K55.1
    acute R10.0
Abdominalgia — *see* Pain, abdominal
Abduction contracture, hip or other joint — *see* Contraction, joint
Aberrant (congenital) — *see also* Malposition, congenital
  adrenal gland Q89.1
  artery (peripheral) Q27.8
    basilar NEC Q28.1
    cerebral Q28.3
    coronary Q24.5
    digestive system Q27.8
    eye Q15.8
    lower limb Q27.8
    precerebral Q28.1
    pulmonary Q25.79
    renal Q27.2
    retina Q14.1
    specified site NEC Q27.8
    subclavian Q27.8
    upper limb Q27.8
    vertebral Q28.1
  breast Q83.8
  endocrine gland NEC Q89.2
  hepatic duct Q44.5
  pancreas Q45.3
  parathyroid gland Q89.2
  pituitary gland Q89.2
  sebaceous glands, mucous membrane, mouth, congenital Q38.6
  spleen Q89.09
  subclavian artery Q27.8
  thymus (gland) Q89.2
  thyroid gland Q89.2
  vein (peripheral) NEC Q27.8
    cerebral Q28.3
    digestive system Q27.8
    lower limb Q27.8
    precerebral Q28.1
    specified site NEC Q27.8
    upper limb Q27.8
Aberration
  distantial — *see* Disturbance, visual
  mental F99
Abetalipoproteinemia E78.6
Abiotrophy R68.89
Ablatio, ablation
  retinae — *see* Detachment, retina
Ablepharia, ablepharon Q10.3
Abnormal, abnormality, abnormalities — *see also* Anomaly
  acid-base balance (mixed) E87.4
  albumin R77.0
  alphafetoprotein R77.2
  alveolar ridge K08.9
  anatomical relationship Q89.9
  apertures, congenital, diaphragm Q79.1
  auditory perception H93.29- ☑
    diplacusis — *see* Diplacusis
    hyperacusis — *see* Hyperacusis
    recruitment — *see* Recruitment, auditory
    threshold shift — *see* Shift, auditory threshold
  autosomes Q99.9
    fragile site Q95.5
  basal metabolic rate R94.8
  biosynthesis, testicular androgen E29.1
  bleeding time R79.1
  blood amino-acid level R79.83
  blood level (of)
    cobalt R79.0
    copper R79.0
    iron R79.0
    lithium R78.89

Abnormal, abnormality, abnormalities — *continued*
  blood level — *continued*
    magnesium R79.0
    mineral NEC R79.0
    zinc R79.0
  blood pressure
    elevated R03.0
    low reading (nonspecific) R03.1
  blood sugar R73.09
  blood-gas level R79.81
  bowel sounds R19.15
    absent R19.11
    hyperactive R19.12
  brain scan R94.02
  breathing R06.9
  caloric test R94.138
  cerebrospinal fluid R83.9
    cytology R83.6
    drug level R83.2
    enzyme level R83.0
    hormones R83.1
    immunology R83.4
    microbiology R83.5
    nonmedicinal level R83.3
    specified type NEC R83.8
  chemistry, blood R79.9
    C-reactive protein R79.82
    drugs — *see* Findings, abnormal, in blood
    gas level R79.81
    minerals R79.0
    pancytopenia D61.818
    PTT R79.1
    specified NEC R79.89
    toxins — *see* Findings, abnormal, in blood
  chest sounds (friction) (rales) R09.89
  chromosome, chromosomal Q99.9
    with more than three X chromosomes, female Q97.1
    analysis result R89.8
      bronchial washings R84.8
      cerebrospinal fluid R83.8
      cervix uteri NEC R87.89
      nasal secretions R84.8
      nipple discharge R89.8
      peritoneal fluid R85.89
      pleural fluid R84.8
      prostatic secretions R86.8
      saliva R85.89
      seminal fluid R86.8
      sputum R84.8
      synovial fluid R89.8
      throat scrapings R84.8
      vagina R87.89
      vulva R87.89
      wound secretions R89.8
    dicentric replacement Q93.2
    ring replacement Q93.2
    sex Q99.8
      female phenotype Q97.9
        specified NEC Q97.8
      male phenotype Q98.9
        specified NEC Q98.8
      structural male Q98.6
    specified NEC Q99.8
  clinical findings NEC R68.89
  coagulation D68.9
    newborn, transient P61.6
    profile R79.1
    time R79.1
  communication — *see* Fistula
  conjunctiva, vascular H11.41- ☑
  coronary artery Q24.5
  cortisol-binding globulin E27.8
  course, eustachian tube Q17.8
  creatinine clearance R94.4
  cytology
    anus R85.619
      atypical squamous cells cannot exclude high grade squamous intraepithelial lesion (ASC-H) R85.611
      atypical squamous cells of undetermined significance (ASC-US) R85.610
      cytologic evidence of malignancy R85.614

Abnormal, abnormality, abnormalities — *continued*
  cytology — *continued*
    anus — *continued*
      high grade squamous intraepithelial lesion (HGSIL) R85.613
      human papillomavirus (HPV) DNA test
        high risk positive R85.81
        low risk postive R85.82
      inadequate smear R85.615
      low grade squamous intraepithelial lesion (LGSIL) R85.612
      satisfactory anal smear but lacking transformation zone R85.616
      specified NEC R85.618
      unsatisfactory smear R85.615
    female genital organs — *see* Abnormal, Papanicolaou (smear)
  dark adaptation curve H53.61
  dentofacial NEC — *see* Anomaly, dentofacial
  development, developmental Q89.9
    central nervous system Q07.9
  diagnostic imaging
    abdomen, abdominal region NEC R93.5
    biliary tract R93.2
    bladder R93.41
    breast R92.8
    central nervous system NEC R90.89
    cerebrovascular NEC R90.89
    coronary circulation R93.1
    digestive tract NEC R93.3
    gastrointestinal (tract) R93.3
    genitourinary organs R93.89
    head R93.0
    heart R93.1
    intrathoracic organ NEC R93.89
    kidney R93.42- ☑
    limbs R93.6
    liver R93.2
    lung (field) R91.8
    musculoskeletal system NEC R93.7
    renal pelvis R93.41
    retroperitoneum R93.5
    site specified NEC R93.89
    skin and subcutaneous tissue R93.89
    skull R93.0
    testis R93.81- ☑
    ureter R93.41
    urinary organs specified NEC R93.49
  direction, teeth, fully erupted M26.30
  ear ossicles, acquired NEC H74.39- ☑
    ankylosis — *see* Ankylosis, ear ossicles
    discontinuity — *see* Discontinuity, ossicles, ear
    partial loss — *see* Loss, ossicles, ear (partial)
  Ebstein Q22.5
  echocardiogram R93.1
  echoencephalogram R90.81
  echogram — *see* Abnormal, diagnostic imaging
  electrocardiogram [ECG] [EKG] R94.31
  electroencephalogram [EEG] R94.01
  electrolyte — *see* Imbalance, electrolyte
  electromyogram [EMG] R94.131
  electro-oculogram [EOG] R94.110
  electrophysiological intracardiac studies R94.39
  electroretinogram [ERG] R94.111
  erythrocytes
    congenital, with perinatal jaundice D58.9
  feces (color) (contents) (mucus) R19.5
  finding — *see* Findings, abnormal, without diagnosis
  fluid
    amniotic — *see* Abnormal, specimen, specified
    cerebrospinal — *see* Abnormal, cerebrospinal fluid
    peritoneal — *see* Abnormal, specimen, digestive organs
    pleural — *see* Abnormal, specimen, respiratory organs
    synovial — *see* Abnormal, specimen, specified
    thorax (bronchial washings) (pleural fluid) — *see* Abnormal, specimen, respiratory organs
    vaginal — *see* Abnormal, specimen, female genital organs
  form
    teeth K00.2

⬆ Subterms under main terms may continue to next column or page   ☑ Additional Character Required — Refer to the Tabular List for Character Selection   1

Aarskog's syndrome — Abnormal, abnormality, abnormalities

Abnormal, abnormality, abnormalities — *continued*
form — *continued*
    uterus — *see* Anomaly, uterus
function studies
    auditory R94.120
    bladder R94.8
    brain R94.09
    cardiovascular R94.30
    ear R94.128
    endocrine NEC R94.7
    eye NEC R94.118
    kidney R94.4
    liver R94.5
    nervous system
        central NEC R94.09
        peripheral NEC R94.138
    pancreas R94.8
    placenta R94.8
    pulmonary R94.2
    special senses NEC R94.128
    spleen R94.8
    thyroid R94.6
    vestibular R94.121
gait — *see* Gait
    hysterical F44.4
gastrin secretion E16.4
globulin R77.1
    cortisol-binding E27.8
    thyroid-binding E07.89
glomerular, minor — *see also* N00-N07 with fourth character .0 N05.0
glucagon secretion E16.3
glucose tolerance (test) (non-fasting) R73.09
gravitational (G) forces or states (effect of) T75.81 ☑
hair (color) (shaft) L67.9
    specified NEC L67.8
hard tissue formation in pulp (dental) K04.3
head movement R25.0
heart
    rate R00.9
        specified NEC R00.8
    shadow R93.1
    sounds NEC R01.2
hemoglobin (disease) — *see also* Disease, hemoglobin D58.2
    trait — *see* Trait, hemoglobin, abnormal
histology NEC R89.7
immunological findings R89.4
    in serum R76.9
        specified NEC R76.8
increase in appetite R63.2
involuntary movement — *see* Abnormal, movement, involuntary
jaw closure M26.51
karyotype R89.8
kidney function test R94.4
knee jerk R29.2
leukocyte (cell) (differential) NEC D72.9
liver function test — *see also* Elevated, liver function, test R79.89
loss of
    height R29.890
    weight R63.4
mammogram NEC R92.8
    calcification (calculus) R92.1
    microcalcification R92.0
Mantoux test R76.11
movement (disorder) — *see also* Disorder, movement
    head R25.0
    involuntary R25.9
        fasciculation R25.3
        of head R25.0
        spasm R25.2
        specified type NEC R25.8
        tremor R25.1
myoglobin (Aberdeen) (Annapolis) R89.7
neonatal screening P09.9
    for
        congenital adrenal hyperplasia P09.2
        congenital endocrine disease P09.2
        congenital hematologic disorders P09.3
        critical congenital heart disease P09.5
        cystic fibrosis P09.4
        hemoglobinothies P09.3
        hypothyroidism P09.2
        inborn errors of metabolism P09.1
        neonatal hearing loss P09.6

Abnormal, abnormality, abnormalities — *continued*
neonatal screening — *continued*
    for — *continued*
        red cell membrane defects P09.3
        sickle cell P09.3
        specified NEC P09.8
oculomotor study R94.113
palmar creases Q82.8
Papanicolaou (smear)
    anus R85.619
        atypical squamous cells cannot exclude high grade squamous intraepithelial lesion (ASC-H) R85.611
        atypical squamous cells of undetermined significance (ASC-US) R85.610
        cytologic evidence of malignancy R85.614
        high grade squamous intraepithelial lesion (HGSIL) R85.613
        human papillomavirus (HPV) DNA test
            high risk positive R85.81
            low risk postive R85.82
        inadequate smear R85.615
        low grade squamous intraepithelial lesion (LGSIL) R85.612
        satisfactory anal smear but lacking transformation zone R85.616
        specified NEC R85.618
        unsatisfactory smear R85.615
    bronchial washings R84.6
    cerebrospinal fluid R83.6
    cervix R87.619
        atypical squamous cells cannot exclude high grade squamous intraepithelial lesion (ASC-H) R87.611
        atypical squamous cells of undetermined significance (ASC-US) R87.610
        cytologic evidence of malignancy R87.614
        high grade squamous intraepithelial lesion (HGSIL) R87.613
        inadequate smear R87.615
        low grade squamous intraepithelial lesion (LGSIL) R87.612
        non-atypical endometrial cells R87.618
        satisfactory cervical smear but lacking transformation zone R87.616
        specified NEC R87.618
        thin preparaton R87.619
        unsatisfactory smear R87.615
    nasal secretions R84.6
    nipple discharge R89.6
    peritoneal fluid R85.69
    pleural fluid R84.6
    prostatic secretions R86.6
    saliva R85.69
    seminal fluid R86.6
    sites NEC R89.6
    sputum R84.6
    synovial fluid R89.6
    throat scrapings R84.6
    vagina R87.629
        atypical squamous cells cannot exclude high grade squamous intraepithelial lesion (ASC-H) R87.621
        atypical squamous cells of undetermined significance (ASC-US) R87.620
        cytologic evidence of malignancy R87.624
        high grade squamous intraepithelial lesion (HGSIL) R87.623
        inadequate smear R87.625
        low grade squamous intraepithelial lesion (LGSIL) R87.622
        specified NEC R87.628
        thin preparation R87.629
        unsatisfactory smear R87.625
    vulva R87.69
    wound secretions R89.6
partial thromboplastin time (PTT) R79.1
pelvis (bony) — *see* Deformity, pelvis
percussion, chest (tympany) R09.89
periods (grossly) — *see* Menstruation
phonocardiogram R94.39
plantar reflex R29.2
plasma
    protein R77.9
        specified NEC R77.8
    viscosity R70.1
pleural (folds) Q34.0
posture R29.3

Abnormal, abnormality, abnormalities — *continued*
product of conception O02.9
    specified type NEC O02.89
prothrombin time (PT) R79.1
pulmonary
    artery, congenital Q25.79
    function, newborn P28.89
    test results R94.2
pulsations in neck R00.2
pupillary H21.56- ☑
    function (reaction) (reflex) — *see* Anomaly, pupil, function
radiological examination — *see* Abnormal, diagnostic imaging
red blood cell(s) (morphology) (volume) R71.8
reflex — *see* Reflex
renal function test R94.4
response to nerve stimulation R94.130
retinal correspondence H53.31
retinal function study R94.111
rhythm, heart — *see also* Arrhythmia
saliva — *see* Abnormal, specimen, digestive organs
scan
    kidney R94.4
    liver R93.2
    thyroid R94.6
secretion
    gastrin E16.4
    glucagon E16.3
semen, seminal fluid — *see* Abnormal, specimen, male genital organs
serum level (of)
    acid phosphatase R74.8
    alkaline phosphatase R74.8
    amylase R74.8
    enzymes R74.9
        specified NEC R74.8
    lipase R74.8
    triacylglycerol lipase R74.8
shape
    gravid uterus — *see* Anomaly, uterus
sinus venosus Q21.1
size, tooth, teeth K00.2
spacing, tooth, teeth, fully erupted M26.30
specimen
    digestive organs (peritoneal fluid) (saliva) R85.9
        cytology R85.69
        drug level R85.2
        enzyme level R85.0
        histology R85.7
        hormones R85.1
        immunology R85.4
        microbiology R85.5
        nonmedicinal level R85.3
        specified type NEC R85.89
    female genital organs (secretions) (smears) R87.9
        cytology R87.69
            cervix R87.619
                human papillomavirus (HPV) DNA test
                    high risk positive R87.810
                    low risk positive R87.820
                inadequate (unsatisfactory) smear R87.615
                non-atypical endometrial cells R87.618
                specified NEC R87.618
            vagina R87.629
                human papillomavirus (HPV) DNA test
                    high risk positive R87.811
                    low risk positive R87.821
                inadequate (unsatisfactory) smear R87.625
            vulva R87.69
        drug level R87.2
        enzyme level R87.0
        histological R87.7
        hormones R87.1
        immunology R87.4
        microbiology R87.5
        nonmedicinal level R87.3
        specified type NEC R87.89
    male genital organs (prostatic secretions) (semen) R86.9
        cytology R86.6
        drug level R86.2
        enzyme level R86.0
        histological R86.7
        hormones R86.1

- **Abnormal, abnormality, abnormalities** — *continued*
  - specimen — *continued*
    - male genital organs — *continued*
      - immunology R86.4
      - microbiology R86.5
      - nonmedicinal level R86.3
      - specified type NEC R86.8
    - nipple discharge — *see* Abnormal, specimen, specified
    - respiratory organs (bronchial washings) (nasal secretions) (pleural fluid) (sputum) R84.9
      - cytology R84.6
      - drug level R84.2
      - enzyme level R84.Ø
      - histology R84.7
      - hormones R84.1
      - immunology R84.4
      - microbiology R84.5
      - nonmedicinal level R84.3
      - specified type NEC R84.8
    - specified organ, system and tissue NOS R89.9
      - cytology R89.6
      - drug level R89.2
      - enzyme level R89.Ø
      - histology R89.7
      - hormones R89.1
      - immunology R89.4
      - microbiology R89.5
      - nonmedicinal level R89.3
      - specified type NEC R89.8
    - synovial fluid — *see* Abnormal, specimen, specified
    - thorax (bronchial washings) (pleural fluids) — *see* Abnormal, specimen, respiratory organs
    - vagina (secretion) (smear) R87.629
    - vulva (secretion) (smear) R87.69
    - wound secretion — *see* Abnormal, specimen, specified
  - spermatozoa — *see* Abnormal, specimen, male genital organs
  - sputum (amount) (color) (odor) RØ9.3
  - stool (color) (contents) (mucus) R19.5
    - bloody K92.1
    - guaiac positive R19.5
  - synchondrosis Q78.8
  - thermography — *see also* Abnormal, diagnostic imaging R93.89
  - thyroid-binding globulin EØ7.89
  - tooth, teeth (form) (size) KØØ.2
  - toxicology (findings) R78.9
  - transport protein E88.Ø9
  - tumor marker NEC R97.8
  - ultrasound results — *see* Abnormal, diagnostic imaging
  - umbilical cord complicating delivery O69.9 ☑
  - urination NEC R39.198
  - urine (constituents) R82.9Ø
    - bile R82.2
    - cytological examination R82.89
    - drugs R82.5
    - fat R82.Ø
    - glucose R81
    - heavy metals R82.6
    - hemoglobin R82.3
    - histological examination R82.89
    - ketones R82.4
    - microbiological examination (culture) R82.79
    - myoglobin R82.1
    - positive culture R82.79
    - protein — *see* Proteinuria
    - specified substance NEC R82.998
      - chromoabnormality NEC R82.91
    - substances nonmedical R82.6
  - uterine hemorrhage — *see* Hemorrhage, uterus
  - vectorcardiogram R94.39
  - visually evoked potential (VEP) R94.112
  - white blood cells D72.9
    - specified NEC D72.89
  - X-ray examination — *see* Abnormal, diagnostic imaging
- **Abnormity** (any organ or part) — *see* Anomaly
- **Abocclusion** M26.29
  - hemolytic disease (newborn) P55.1
  - incompatibility reaction ABO — *see* Complication(s), transfusion, incompatibility reaction, ABO
- **Abolition, language** R48.8
- **Aborter, habitual or recurrent** — *see* Loss (of), pregnancy, recurrent
- **Abortion** (complete) (spontaneous) OØ3.9
- **Abortion** — *continued*
  - with
    - retained products of conception — *see* Abortion, incomplete
  - attempted (elective) (failed) OØ7.4
    - complicated by OØ7.3Ø
      - afibrinogenemia OØ7.1
      - cardiac arrest OØ7.36
      - chemical damage of pelvic organ(s) OØ7.34
      - circulatory collapse OØ7.31
      - cystitis OØ7.38
      - defibrination syndrome OØ7.1
      - electrolyte imbalance OØ7.33
      - embolism (air) (amniotic fluid) (blood clot) (fat) (pulmonary) (septic) (soap) OØ7.2
      - endometritis OØ7.Ø
      - genital tract and pelvic infection OØ7.Ø
      - hemolysis OØ7.1
      - hemorrhage (delayed) (excessive) OØ7.1
      - infection
        - genital tract or pelvic OØ7.Ø
        - urinary tract tract OØ7.38
      - intravascular coagulation OØ7.1
      - laceration of pelvic organ(s) OØ7.34
      - metabolic disorder OØ7.33
      - oliguria OØ7.32
      - oophoritis OØ7.Ø
      - parametritis OØ7.Ø
      - pelvic peritonitis OØ7.Ø
      - perforation of pelvic organ(s) OØ7.34
      - renal failure or shutdown OØ7.32
      - salpingitis or salpingo-oophoritis OØ7.Ø
      - sepsis OØ7.37
      - shock OØ7.31
      - specified condition NEC OØ7.39
      - tubular necrosis (renal) OØ7.32
      - uremia OØ7.32
      - urinary tract infection OØ7.38
      - venous complication NEC OØ7.35
        - embolism (air) (amniotic fluid) (blood clot) (fat) (pulmonary) (septic) (soap) OØ7.2
  - complicated (by) (following) OØ3.8Ø
    - afibrinogenemia OØ3.6
    - cardiac arrest OØ3.86
    - chemical damage of pelvic organ(s) OØ3.84
    - circulatory collapse OØ3.81
    - cystitis OØ3.88
    - defibrination syndrome OØ3.6
    - electrolyte imbalance OØ3.83
    - embolism (air) (amniotic fluid) (blood clot) (fat) (pulmonary) (septic) (soap) OØ3.7
    - endometritis OØ3.5
    - genital tract and pelvic infection OØ3.5
    - hemolysis OØ3.6
    - hemorrhage (delayed) (excessive) OØ3.6
    - infection
      - genital tract or pelvic OØ3.5
      - urinary tract OØ3.88
    - intravascular coagulation OØ3.6
    - laceration of pelvic organ(s) OØ3.84
    - metabolic disorder OØ3.83
    - oliguria OØ3.82
    - oophoritis OØ3.5
    - parametritis OØ3.5
    - pelvic peritonitis OØ3.5
    - perforation of pelvic organ(s) OØ3.84
    - renal failure or shutdown OØ3.82
    - salpingitis or salpingo-oophoritis OØ3.5
    - sepsis OØ3.87
    - shock OØ3.81
    - specified condition NEC OØ3.89
    - tubular necrosis (renal) OØ3.82
    - uremia OØ3.82
    - urinary tract infection OØ3.88
    - venous complication NEC OØ3.85
      - embolism (air) (amniotic fluid) (blood clot) (fat) (pulmonary) (septic) (soap) OØ3.7
  - failed — *see* Abortion, attempted
  - habitual or recurrent N96
    - with current abortion — *see* categories OØ3-OØ4
    - without current pregnancy N96
    - care in current pregnancy O26.2- ☑
  - incomplete (spontaneous) OØ3.4
    - complicated (by) (following) OØ3.3Ø
      - afibrinogenemia OØ3.1
      - cardiac arrest OØ3.36
      - chemical damage of pelvic organ(s) OØ3.34
      - circulatory collapse OØ3.31
      - cystitis OØ3.38
- **Abortion** — *continued*
  - incomplete — *continued*
    - complicated — *continued*
      - defibrination syndrome OØ3.1
      - electrolyte imbalance OØ3.33
      - embolism (air) (amniotic fluid) (blood clot) (fat) (pulmonary) (septic) (soap) OØ3.2
      - endometritis OØ3.Ø
      - genital tract and pelvic infection OØ3.Ø
      - hemolysis OØ3.1
      - hemorrhage (delayed) (excessive) OØ3.1
      - infection
        - genital tract or pelvic OØ3.Ø
        - urinary tract OØ3.38
      - intravascular coagulation OØ3.1
      - laceration of pelvic organ(s) OØ3.34
      - metabolic disorder OØ3.33
      - oliguria OØ3.32
      - oophoritis OØ3.Ø
      - parametritis OØ3.Ø
      - pelvic peritonitis OØ3.Ø
      - perforation of pelvic organ(s) OØ3.34
      - renal failure or shutdown OØ3.32
      - salpingitis or salpingo-oophoritis OØ3.Ø
      - sepsis OØ3.37
      - shock OØ3.31
      - specified condition NEC OØ3.39
      - tubular necrosis (renal) OØ3.32
      - uremia OØ3.32
      - urinary infection OØ3.38
      - venous complication NEC OØ3.35
        - embolism (air) (amniotic fluid) (blood clot) (fat) (pulmonary) (septic) (soap) OØ3.2
  - induced (encounter for) Z33.2
    - complicated by OØ4.8Ø
      - afibrinogenemia OØ4.6
      - cardiac arrest OØ4.86
      - chemical damage of pelvic organ(s) OØ4.84
      - circulatory collapse OØ4.81
      - cystitis OØ4.88
      - defibrination syndrome OØ4.6
      - electrolyte imbalance OØ4.83
      - embolism (air) (amniotic fluid) (blood clot) (fat) (pulmonary) (septic) (soap) OØ4.7
      - endometritis OØ4.5
      - genital tract and pelvic infection OØ4.5
      - hemolysis OØ4.6
      - hemorrhage (delayed) (excessive) OØ4.6
      - infection
        - genital tract or pelvic OØ4.5
        - urinary tract OØ4.88
      - intravascular coagulation OØ4.6
      - laceration of pelvic organ(s) OØ4.84
      - metabolic disorder OØ4.83
      - oliguria OØ4.82
      - oophoritis OØ4.5
      - parametritis OØ4.5
      - pelvic peritonitis OØ4.5
      - perforation of pelvic organ(s) OØ4.84
      - renal failure or shutdown OØ4.82
      - salpingitis or salpingo-oophoritis OØ4.5
      - sepsis OØ4.87
      - shock OØ4.81
      - specified condition NEC OØ4.89
      - tubular necrosis (renal) OØ4.82
      - uremia OØ4.82
      - urinary tract infection OØ4.88
      - venous complication NEC OØ4.85
        - embolism (air) (amniotic fluid) (blood clot) (fat) (pulmonary) (septic) (soap) OØ4.7
  - inevitable OØ3.4
  - missed OØ2.1
  - spontaneous — *see* Abortion (complete) (spontaneous)
    - threatened O2Ø.Ø
  - threatened (spontaneous) O2Ø.Ø
  - tubal OØØ.1Ø- ☑
    - with intrauterine pregnancy OØØ.11- ☑
- **Abortus fever** A23.1
- **Aboulomania** F6Ø.7
- **Abrami's disease** D59.8
- **Abramov-Fiedler myocarditis** (acute isolated myocarditis) I4Ø.1
- **Abrasion** T14.8 ☑
  - abdomen, abdominal (wall) S3Ø.811 ☑
  - alveolar process SØØ.512 ☑
  - ankle S9Ø.51- ☑
  - antecubital space — *see* Abrasion, elbow
  - anus S3Ø.817 ☑

Abrasion — *continued*
  arm (upper) S40.81- ☑
  auditory canal — *see* Abrasion, ear
  auricle — *see* Abrasion, ear
  axilla — *see* Abrasion, arm
  back, lower S30.810 ☑
  breast S20.11- ☑
  brow S00.81 ☑
  buttock S30.810 ☑
  calf — *see* Abrasion, leg
  canthus — *see* Abrasion, eyelid
  cheek S00.81 ☑
    internal S00.512 ☑
  chest wall — *see* Abrasion, thorax
  chin S00.81 ☑
  clitoris S30.814 ☑
  cornea S05.0- ☑
  costal region — *see* Abrasion, thorax
  dental K03.1
  digit(s)
    foot — *see* Abrasion, toe
    hand — *see* Abrasion, finger
  ear S00.41- ☑
  elbow S50.31- ☑
  epididymis S30.813 ☑
  epigastric region S30.811 ☑
  epiglottis S10.11 ☑
  esophagus (thoracic) S27.818 ☑
    cervical S10.11 ☑
  eyebrow — *see* Abrasion, eyelid
  eyelid S00.21- ☑
  face S00.81 ☑
  finger(s) S60.41- ☑
    index S60.41- ☑
    little S60.41- ☑
    middle S60.41- ☑
    ring S60.41- ☑
  flank S30.811
  foot (except toe(s) alone) S90.81- ☑
    toe — *see* Abrasion, toe
  forearm S50.81- ☑
    elbow only — *see* Abrasion, elbow
  forehead S00.81 ☑
  genital organs, external
    female S30.816 ☑
    male S30.815 ☑
  groin S30.811 ☑
  gum S00.512 ☑
  hand S60.51- ☑
  head S00.91 ☑
    ear — *see* Abrasion, ear
    eyelid — *see* Abrasion, eyelid
    lip S00.511 ☑
    nose S00.31 ☑
    oral cavity S00.512 ☑
    scalp S00.01 ☑
    specified site NEC S00.81 ☑
  heel — *see* Abrasion, foot
  hip S70.21- ☑
  inguinal region S30.811 ☑
  interscapular region S20.419 ☑
  jaw S00.81 ☑
  knee S80.21- ☑
  labium (majus) (minus) S30.814 ☑
  larynx S10.11 ☑
  leg (lower) S80.81- ☑
    knee — *see* Abrasion, knee
    upper — *see* Abrasion, thigh
  lip S00.511 ☑
  lower back S30.810 ☑
  lumbar region S30.810 ☑
  malar region S00.81 ☑
  mammary — *see* Abrasion, breast
  mastoid region S00.81 ☑
  mouth S00.512 ☑
  nail
    finger — *see* Abrasion, finger
    toe — *see* Abrasion, toe
  nape S10.81 ☑
  nasal S00.31 ☑
  neck S10.91 ☑
    specified site NEC S10.81 ☑
    throat S10.11 ☑
  nose S00.31 ☑
  occipital region S00.01 ☑
  oral cavity S00.512 ☑

Abrasion — *continued*
  orbital region — *see* Abrasion, eyelid
  palate S00.512 ☑
  palm — *see* Abrasion, hand
  parietal region S00.01 ☑
  pelvis S30.810 ☑
  penis S30.812 ☑
  perineum
    female S30.814 ☑
    male S30.810 ☑
  periocular area — *see* Abrasion, eyelid
  phalanges
    finger — *see* Abrasion, finger
    toe — *see* Abrasion, toe
  pharynx S10.11 ☑
  pinna — *see* Abrasion, ear
  popliteal space — *see* Abrasion, knee
  prepuce S30.812 ☑
  pubic region S30.810 ☑
  pudendum
    female S30.816 ☑
    male S30.815 ☑
  sacral region S30.810 ☑
  scalp S00.01 ☑
  scapular region — *see* Abrasion, shoulder
  scrotum S30.813 ☑
  shin — *see* Abrasion, leg
  shoulder S40.21- ☑
  skin NEC T14.8 ☑
  sternal region S20.319 ☑
  submaxillary region S00.81 ☑
  submental region S00.81 ☑
  subungual
    finger(s) — *see* Abrasion, finger
    toe(s) — *see* Abrasion, toe
  supraclavicular fossa S10.81 ☑
  supraorbital S00.81 ☑
  temple S00.81 ☑
  temporal region S00.81 ☑
  testis S30.813 ☑
  thigh S70.31- ☑
  thorax, thoracic (wall) S20.91 ☑
    back S20.41- ☑
    front S20.31- ☑
  throat S10.11 ☑
  thumb S60.31- ☑
  toe(s) (lesser) S90.416 ☑
    great S90.41- ☑
  tongue S00.512 ☑
  tooth, teeth (dentifrice) (habitual) (hard tissues) (occupational) (ritual) (traditional) K03.1
  trachea S10.11 ☑
  tunica vaginalis S30.813 ☑
  tympanum, tympanic membrane — *see* Abrasion, ear
  uvula S00.512 ☑
  vagina S30.814 ☑
  vocal cords S10.11 ☑
  vulva S30.814 ☑
  wrist S60.81- ☑
Abrism — *see* Poisoning, food, noxious, plant
Abruptio placentae O45.9- ☑
  with
    afibrinogenemia O45.01- ☑
    coagulation defect O45.00- ☑
      specified NEC O45.09- ☑
    disseminated intravascular coagulation O45.02- ☑
    hypofibrinogenemia O45.01- ☑
  specified NEC O45.8- ☑
Abruption, placenta — *see* Abruptio placentae
Abscess (connective tissue) (embolic) (fistulous) (infective) (metastatic) (multiple) (pernicious) (pyogenic) (septic) L02.91
  with
    diverticular disease (intestine) K57.80
      with bleeding K57.81
      large intestine K57.20
        with
          bleeding K57.21
          small intestine K57.40
            with bleeding K57.41
      small intestine K57.00
        with
          bleeding K57.01
          large intestine K57.40
            with bleeding K57.41

Abscess — *continued*
  with — *continued*
    lymphangitis — *code by* site under Abscess
  abdomen, abdominal
    cavity K65.1
    wall L02.211
  abdominopelvic K65.1
  accessory sinus — *see* Sinusitis
  adrenal (capsule) (gland) E27.8
  alveolar K04.7
    with sinus K04.6
  ambeic A06.4
    brain (and liver or lung abscess) A06.6
    genitourinary tract A06.82
    liver (without mention of brain or lung abscess) A06.4
    lung (and liver) (without mention of brain abscess) A06.5
    specified site NEC A06.89
    spleen A06.89
  anerobic A48.0
  ankle — *see* Abscess, lower limb
  anorectal K61.2
  antecubital space — *see* Abscess, upper limb
  antrum (chronic) (Highmore) — *see* Sinusitis, maxillary
  anus K61.0
  apical (tooth) K04.7
    with sinus (alveolar) K04.6
  appendix K35.33
  areola (acute) (chronic) (nonpuerperal) N61.1
    puerperal, postpartum or gestational — *see* Infection, nipple
  arm (any part) — *see* Abscess, upper limb
  artery (wall) I77.89
  atheromatous I77.2
  auricle, ear — *see* Abscess, ear, external
  axilla (region) L02.41- ☑
    lymph gland or node L04.2
  back (any part, except buttock) L02.212
  Bartholin's gland N75.1
    with
      abortion — *see* Abortion, by type complicated by, sepsis
      ectopic or molar pregnancy O08.0
    following ectopic or molar pregnancy O08.0
  Bezold's — *see* Mastoiditis, acute
  bilharziasis B65.1
  bladder (wall) — *see* Cystitis, specified type NEC
  bone (subperiosteal) — *see also* Osteomyelitis, specified type NEC
    accessory sinus (chronic) — *see* Sinusitis
    chronic or old — *see* Osteomyelitis, chronic
    jaw (lower) (upper) M27.2
    mastoid — *see* Mastoiditis, acute, subperiosteal
    petrous — *see* Petrositis
    spinal (tuberculous) A18.01
      nontuberculous — *see* Osteomyelitis, vertebra
  bowel K63.0
  brain (any part) (cystic) (otogenic) G06.0
    amebic (with abscess of any other site) A06.6
    gonococcal A54.82
    pheomycotic (chromomycotic) B43.1
    tuberculous A17.81
  breast (acute) (chronic) (nonpuerperal) N61.1
    newborn P39.0
    puerperal, postpartum, gestational — *see* Mastitis, obstetric, purulent
  broad ligament N73.2
    acute N73.0
    chronic N73.1
  Brodie's (localized) (chronic) M86.8X- ☑
  bronchi J98.09
  buccal cavity K12.2
  bulbourethral gland N34.0
  bursa M71.00
    ankle M71.07- ☑
    elbow M71.02- ☑
    foot M71.07- ☑
    hand M71.04- ☑
    hip M71.05- ☑
    knee M71.06- ☑
    multiple sites M71.09
    pharyngeal J39.1
    shoulder M71.01- ☑
    specified site NEC M71.08
    wrist M71.03- ☑
  buttock L02.31
  canthus — *see* Blepharoconjunctivitis

☑ **Additional Character Required** — **Refer to the Tabular List for Character Selection**   ▽ **Subterms under main terms may continue to next column or page**

Abscess — *continued*
cartilage — *see* Disorder, cartilage, specified type NEC
cecum K35.33
cerebellum, cerebellar G06.0
    sequelae G09
cerebral (embolic) G06.0
    sequelae G09
cervical (meaning neck) L02.11
    lymph gland or node L04.0
cervix (stump) (uteri) — *see* Cervicitis
cheek (external) L02.01
    inner K12.2
chest J86.9
    with fistula J86.0
    wall L02.213
chin L02.01
choroid — *see* Inflammation, chorioretinal
circumtonsillar J36
cold (lung) (tuberculous) — *see also* Tuberculosis, abscess, lung
    articular — *see* Tuberculosis, joint
colon (wall) K63.0
colostomy K94.02
conjunctiva — *see* Conjunctivitis, acute
cornea H16.31- ☑
corpus
    cavernosum N48.21
    luteum — *see* Oophoritis
Cowper's gland N34.0
cranium G06.0
cul-de-sac (Douglas') (posterior) — *see* Peritonitis, pelvic, female
cutaneous — *see* Abscess, by site
dental K04.7
    with sinus (alveolar) K04.6
dentoalveolar K04.7
    with sinus K04.6
diaphragm, diaphragmatic K65.1
Douglas' cul-de-sac or pouch — *see* Peritonitis, pelvic, female
Dubois A50.59
ear (middle) — *see also* Otitis, media, suppurative
    acute — *see* Otitis, media, suppurative, acute
    external H60- ☑
entamebic — *see* Abscess, amebic
enterostomy K94.12
epididymis N45.4
epidural G06.2
    brain G06.0
    spinal cord G06.1
epiglottis J38.7
epiploon, epiploic K65.1
erysipelatous — *see* Erysipelas
esophagus K20.80
ethmoid (bone) (chronic) (sinus) J32.2
external auditory canal — *see* Abscess, ear, external
extradural G06.2
    brain G06.0
        sequelae G09
    spinal cord G06.1
extraperitoneal K68.19
eye — *see* Endophthalmitis, purulent
eyelid H00.03- ☑
face (any part, except ear, eye and nose) L02.01
fallopian tube — *see* Salpingitis
fascia M72.8
fauces J39.1
fecal K63.0
femoral (region) — *see* Abscess, lower limb
filaria, filarial — *see* Infestation, filarial
finger (any) — *see also* Abscess, hand
    nail — *see* Cellulitis, finger
foot L02.61- ☑
forehead L02.01
frontal sinus (chronic) J32.1
gallbladder K81.0
genital organ or tract
    female (external) N76.4
    male N49.9
        multiple sites N49.8
        specified NEC N49.8
gestational mammary O91.11- ☑
gestational subareolar O91.11- ☑
gingival — *see* Periodontitis, localized
gland, glandular (lymph) (acute) — *see* Lymphadenitis, acute
gluteal (region) L02.31
gonorrheal — *see* Gonococcus

Abscess — *continued*
groin L02.214
gum — *see* Periodontitis, localized
hand L02.51- ☑
head NEC L02.811
    face (any part, except ear, eye and nose) L02.01
heart — *see* Carditis
heel — *see* Abscess, foot
helminthic — *see* Infestation, helminth
hepatic (cholangitic) (hematogenic) (lymphogenic) (pylephlebitic) K75.0
    amebic A06.4
hip (region) — *see* Abscess, lower limb
horseshoe K61.31
ileocecal K35.33
ileostomy (bud) K94.12
iliac (region) L02.214
    fossa K35.33
infraclavicular (fossa) — *see* Abscess, upper limb
inguinal (region) L02.214
    lymph gland or node L04.1
intersphincteric K61.4
intestine, intestinal NEC K63.0
    rectal K61.1
intra-abdominal — *see also* Abscess, peritoneum K65.1
    following procedure T81.43 ☑
        obstetrical O86.03
    postprocedural T81.43 ☑
        retroperitoneal K68.11
intracranial G06.0
intramammary — *see* Abscess, breast
intramuscular, following procedure T81.42 ☑
    obstetrical O86.02
intraorbital — *see* Abscess, orbit
intraperitoneal K65.1
intraspinal G06.1
intrasphincteric (anus) K61.4
intratonsillar J36
ischiorectal (fossa) (specified NEC) K61.39
jaw (bone) (lower) (upper) M27.2
joint — *see* Arthritis, pyogenic or pyemic
    spine (tuberculous) A18.01
        nontuberculous — *see* Spondylopathy, infective
kidney N15.1
    with calculus N20.0
        with hydronephrosis N13.6
    puerperal (postpartum) O86.21
knee — *see also* Abscess, lower limb
    joint M00.9
labium (majus) (minus) N76.4
lacrimal
    caruncle — *see* Inflammation, lacrimal, passages, acute
    gland — *see* Dacryoadenitis
    passages (duct) (sac) — *see* Inflammation, lacrimal, passages, acute
lacunar N34.0
larynx J38.7
lateral (alveolar) K04.7
    with sinus K04.6
leg (any part) — *see* Abscess, lower limb
lens H27.8
lingual K14.0
    tonsil J36
lip K13.0
Littre's gland N34.0
liver (cholangitic) (hematogenic) (lymphogenic) (pylephlebitic) (pyogenic) K75.0
    amebic (due to Entamoeba histolytica) (dysenteric) (tropical) A06.4
        with
            brain abscess (and liver or lung abscess) A06.6
            lung abscess A06.5
loin (region) L02.211
lower limb L02.41- ☑
lumbar (tuberculous) A18.01
    nontuberculous L02.212
lung (miliary) (putrid) J85.2
    with pneumonia J85.1
        due to specified organism (see Pneumonia, in (due to))
    amebic (with liver abscess) A06.5
        with
            brain abscess A06.6
            pneumonia A06.5
lymph, lymphatic, gland or node (acute) — *see also* Lymphadenitis, acute
    mesentery I88.0

Abscess — *continued*
malar M27.2
mammary gland — *see* Abscess, breast
marginal, anus K61.0
mastoid — *see* Mastoiditis, acute
maxilla, maxillary M27.2
    molar (tooth) K04.7
        with sinus K04.6
    premolar K04.7
    sinus (chronic) J32.0
mediastinum J85.3
meibomian gland — *see* Hordeolum
meninges G06.2
mesentery, mesenteric K65.1
mesosalpinx — *see* Salpingitis
mons pubis L02.215
mouth (floor) K12.2
muscle — *see* Myositis, infective
myocardium I40.0
nabothian (follicle) — *see* Cervicitis
nasal J32.9
nasopharyngeal J39.1
navel L02.216
    newborn P38.9
        with mild hemorrhage P38.1
        without hemorrhage P38.9
neck (region) L02.11
    lymph gland or node L04.0
nephritic — *see* Abscess, kidney
nipple N61.1
    associated with
        lactation — *see* Pregnancy, complicated by
        pregnancy — *see* Pregnancy, complicated by
nose (external) (fossa) (septum) J34.0
    sinus (chronic) — *see* Sinusitis
omentum K65.1
operative wound T81.49 ☑
orbit, orbital — *see* Cellulitis, orbit
otogenic G06.0
ovary, ovarian (corpus luteum) — *see* Oophoritis
oviduct — *see* Oophoritis
palate (soft) K12.2
    hard M27.2
palmar (space) — *see* Abscess, hand
pancreas (duct) — *see* Pancreatitis, acute
parafrenal N48.21
parametric, parametrium N73.2
    acute N73.0
    chronic N73.1
paranephric N15.1
parapancreatic — *see* Pancreatitis, acute
parapharyngeal J39.0
pararectal K61.1
parasinus — *see* Sinusitis
parauterine — *see also* Disease, pelvis, inflammatory N73.2
paravaginal — *see* Vaginitis
parietal region (scalp) L02.811
parodontal — *see* Periodontitis, aggressive, localized
parotid (duct) (gland) K11.3
    region K12.2
pectoral (region) L02.213
pelvis, pelvic
    female — *see* Disease, pelvis, inflammatory
    male, peritoneal K65.1
penis N48.21
    gonococcal (accessory gland) (periurethral) A54.1
perianal K61.0
periapical K04.7
    with sinus (alveolar) K04.6
periappendicular K35.33
pericardial I30.1
pericecal K35.33
pericemental — *see* Periodontitis, aggressive, localized
pericholecystic — *see* Cholecystitis, acute
pericoronal — *see* Periodontitis, aggressive, localized
peridental — *see* Periodontitis, aggressive, localized
perimetric — *see also* Disease, pelvis, inflammatory N73.2
perinephric, perinephritic — *see* Abscess, kidney
perineum, perineal (superficial) L02.215
    urethra N34.0
periodontal (parietal) — *see* Periodontitis, aggressive, localized
    apical K04.7
periosteum, periosteal — *see also* Osteomyelitis, specified type NEC

▽ Subterms under main terms may continue to next column or page   ☑ Additional Character Required — Refer to the Tabular List for Character Selection   5

Abscess — Abscess

Abscess — *continued*
periosteum, periosteal — *see also* Osteomyelitis, specified type — *continued*
  with osteomyelitis — *see also* Osteomyelitis, specified type NEC
    acute — *see* Osteomyelitis, acute
    chronic — *see* Osteomyelitis, chronic
peripharyngeal J39.0
peripleuritic J86.9
  with fistula J86.0
periprostatic N41.2
perirectal K61.1
perirenal (tissue) — *see* Abscess, kidney
perisinuous (nose) — *see* Sinusitis
peritoneum, peritoneal (perforated) (ruptured) K65.1
  with appendicitis — *see also* Appendicitis K35.33
  pelvic
    female — *see* Peritonitis, pelvic, female
    male K65.1
  postoperative T81.49 ☑
  puerperal, postpartum, childbirth O85
  tuberculous A18.31
peritonsillar J36
perityphlic K35.33
periureteral N28.89
periurethral N34.0
  gonococcal (accessory gland) (periurethral) A54.1
periuterine — *see also* Disease, pelvis, inflammatory N73.2
perivesical — *see* Cystitis, specified type NEC
petrous bone — *see* Petrositis
phagedenic NOS L02.91
  chancroid A57
pharynx, pharyngeal (lateral) J39.1
pilonidal L05.01
pituitary (gland) E23.6
pleura J86.9
  with fistula J86.0
popliteal — *see* Abscess, lower limb
postcecal K35.33
postlaryngeal J38.7
postnasal J34.0
postoperative (any site) — *see also* Infection, postoperative wound T81.49 ☑
  retroperitoneal K68.11
postpharyngeal J39.0
posttonsillar J36
post-typhoid A01.09
pouch of Douglas — *see* Peritonitis, pelvic, female
premammary — *see* Abscess, breast
prepatellar — *see* Abscess, lower limb
presacral K68.19
prostate N41.2
  gonococcal (acute) (chronic) A54.22
psoas muscle K68.12
puerperal — *code by* site under Puerperal, abscess
pulmonary — *see* Abscess, lung
pulp, pulpal (dental) K04.01
  irreversible K04.02
  reversible K04.01
rectovaginal septum K63.0
rectovesical — *see* Cystitis, specified type NEC
rectum K61.1
renal — *see* Abscess, kidney
retina — *see* Inflammation, chorioretinal
retrobulbar — *see* Abscess, orbit
retrocecal K65.1
retrolaryngeal J38.7
retromammary — *see* Abscess, breast
retroperitoneal NEC K68.19
  postprocedural K68.11
retropharyngeal J39.0
retrouterine — *see* Peritonitis, pelvic, female
retrovesical — *see* Cystitis, specified type NEC
root, tooth K04.7
  with sinus (alveolar) K04.6
round ligament — *see also* Disease, pelvis, inflammatory N73.2
rupture (spontaneous) NOS L02.91
sacrum (tuberculous) A18.01
  nontuberculous M46.28
salivary (duct) (gland) K11.3
scalp (any part) L02.811
scapular — *see* Osteomyelitis, specified type NEC
sclera — *see* Scleritis
scrofulous (tuberculous) A18.2
scrotum N49.2
seminal vesicle N49.0

Abscess — *continued*
septal, dental K04.7
  with sinus (alveolar) K04.6
serous — *see* Periostitis
shoulder (region) — *see* Abscess, upper limb
sigmoid K63.0
sinus (accessory) (chronic) (nasal) — *see also* Sinusitis
  intracranial venous (any) G06.0
Skene's duct or gland N34.1
skin — *see* Abscess, by site
specified site NEC L02.818
spermatic cord N49.1
sphenoidal (sinus) (chronic) J32.3
spinal cord (any part) (staphylococcal) G06.1
  tuberculous A17.81
spine (column) (tuberculous) A18.01
  epidural G06.1
  nontuberculous — *see* Osteomyelitis, vertebra
spleen D73.3
  amebic A06.89
stitch T81.41 ☑
  following an obstetrical procedure O86.01
subarachnoid G06.2
  brain G06.0
  spinal cord G06.1
subareolar — *see* Abscess, breast
subcecal K35.33
subcutaneous — *see also* Abscess, by site
  following procedure T81.41 ☑
    obstetrical O86.01
  pheomycotic (chromomycotic) B43.2
subdiaphragmatic K65.1
subdural G06.2
  brain G06.0
    sequelae G09
  spinal cord G06.1
sub-fascial, following an obstetrical procedure O86.02
subgaleal L02.811
subhepatic K65.1
sublingual K12.2
  gland K11.3
submammary — *see* Abscess, breast
submandibular (region) (space) (triangle) K12.2
  gland K11.3
submaxillary (region) L02.01
  gland K11.3
submental L02.01
  gland K11.3
subperiosteal — *see* Osteomyelitis, specified type NEC
subphrenic K65.1
  following an obstetrical procedure O86.03
  postoperative T81.43 ☑
suburethral N34.0
sudoriparous L75.8
supraclavicular (fossa) — *see* Abscess, upper limb
supralevator K61.5
suprapelvic, acute N73.0
suprarenal (capsule) (gland) E27.8
sweat gland L74.8
tear duct — *see* Inflammation, lacrimal, passages, acute
temple L02.01
temporal region L02.01
temporosphenoidal G06.0
tendon (sheath) M65.00
  ankle M65.07- ☑
  foot M65.07- ☑
  forearm M65.03- ☑
  hand M65.04- ☑
  lower leg M65.06- ☑
  pelvic region M65.05- ☑
  shoulder region M65.01- ☑
  specified site NEC M65.08
  thigh M65.05- ☑
  upper arm M65.02- ☑
testis N45.4
thigh — *see* Abscess, lower limb
thorax J86.9
  with fistula J86.0
throat J39.1
thumb — *see also* Abscess, hand
  nail — *see* Cellulitis, finger
thymus (gland) E32.1
thyroid (gland) E06.0
toe (any) — *see also* Abscess, foot
  nail — *see* Cellulitis, toe
tongue (staphylococcal) K14.0
tonsil(s) (lingual) J36
tonsillopharyngeal J36

Abscess — *continued*
tooth, teeth (root) K04.7
  with sinus (alveolar) K04.6
  supporting structures NEC — *see* Periodontitis, aggressive, localized
trachea J39.8
trunk L02.219
  abdominal wall L02.211
  back L02.212
  chest wall L02.213
  groin L02.214
  perineum L02.215
  umbilicus L02.216
tubal — *see* Salpingitis
tuberculous — *see* Tuberculosis, abscess
tubo-ovarian — *see* Salpingo-oophoritis
tunica vaginalis N49.1
umbilicus L02.216
upper
  limb L02.41- ☑
  respiratory J39.8
urethral (gland) N34.0
urinary N34.0
uterus, uterine (wall) — *see also* Endometritis
  ligament — *see also* Disease, pelvis, inflammatory N73.2
  neck — *see* Cervicitis
uvula K12.2
vagina (wall) — *see* Vaginitis
vaginorectal — *see* Vaginitis
vas deferens N49.1
vermiform appendix K35.33
vertebra (column) (tuberculous) A18.01
  nontuberculous — *see* Osteomyelitis, vertebra
vesical — *see* Cystitis, specified type NEC
vesico-uterine pouch — *see* Peritonitis, pelvic, female
vitreous (humor) — *see* Endophthalmitis, purulent
vocal cord J38.3
von Bezold's — *see* Mastoiditis, acute
vulva N76.4
vulvovaginal gland N75.1
web space — *see* Abscess, hand
wound T81.49 ☑
wrist — *see* Abscess, upper limb
Absence (of) (organ or part) (complete or partial)
adrenal (gland) (congenital) Q89.1
  acquired E89.6
albumin in blood E88.09
alimentary tract (congenital) Q45.8
  upper Q40.8
alveolar process (acquired) — *see* Anomaly, alveolar
ankle (acquired) Z89.44- ☑
anus (congenital) Q42.3
  with fistula Q42.2
aorta (congenital) Q25.41
appendix, congenital Q42.8
arm (acquired) Z89.20- ☑
  above elbow Z89.22- ☑
    congenital (with hand present) — *see* Agenesis, arm, with hand present
    and hand — *see* Agenesis, forearm, and hand
  below elbow Z89.21- ☑
    congenital (with hand present) — *see* Agenesis, arm, with hand present
    and hand — *see* Agenesis, forearm, and hand
  congenital — *see* Defect, reduction, upper limb
  shoulder (following explantation of shoulder joint prosthesis) (joint) (with or without presence of antibiotic-impregnated cement spacer) Z89.23- ☑
    congenital (with hand present) — *see* Agenesis, arm, with hand present
artery (congenital) (peripheral) Q27.8
  brain Q28.3
  coronary Q24.5
  pulmonary Q25.79
  specified NEC Q27.8
  umbilical Q27.0
atrial septum (congenital) Q21.1
auditory canal (congenital) (external) Q16.1
auricle (ear), congenital Q16.0
bile, biliary duct, congenital Q44.5
bladder (acquired) Z90.6
  congenital Q64.5
bowel sounds R19.11
brain Q00.0
  part of Q04.3
breast(s) (and nipple(s)) (acquired) Z90.1- ☑

☑ **Additional Character Required** — Refer to the Tabular List for Character Selection

▽ Subterms under main terms may continue to next column or page

Absence — *continued*
breast(s(s)) — *continued*
congenital Q83.8
broad ligament Q50.6
bronchus (congenital) Q32.4
canaliculus lacrimalis, congenital Q10.4
cerebellum (vermis) Q04.3
cervix (acquired) (with uterus) Z90.710
with remaining uterus Z90.712
congenital Q51.5
chin, congenital Q18.8
cilia (congenital) Q10.3
acquired — *see* Madarosis
clitoris (congenital) Q52.6
coccyx, congenital Q76.49
cold sense R20.8
congenital
lumen — *see* Atresia
organ or site NEC — *see* Agenesis
septum — *see* Imperfect, closure
corpus callosum Q04.0
cricoid cartilage, congenital Q31.8
diaphragm (with hernia), congenital Q79.1
digestive organ(s) or tract, congenital Q45.8
acquired NEC Z90.49
upper Q40.8
ductus arteriosus Q28.8
duodenum (acquired) Z90.49
congenital Q41.0
ear, congenital Q16.9
acquired H93.8- ☑
auricle Q16.0
external Q16.0
inner Q16.5
lobe, lobule Q17.8
middle, except ossicles Q16.4
ossicles Q16.3
ossicles Q16.3
ejaculatory duct (congenital) Q55.4
endocrine gland (congenital) NEC Q89.2
acquired E89.89
epididymis (congenital) Q55.4
acquired Z90.79
epiglottis, congenital Q31.8
esophagus (congenital) Q39.8
acquired (partial) Z90.49
eustachian tube (congenital) Q16.2
extremity (acquired) Z89.9
congenital Q73.0
knee (following explantation of knee joint prosthe-sis) (joint) (with or without presence of antibi-otic-impregnated cement spacer) Z89.52- ☑
lower (above knee) Z89.619
below knee Z89.51- ☑
upper — *see* Absence, arm
eye (acquired) Z90.01
congenital Q11.1
muscle (congenital) Q10.3
eyeball (acquired) Z90.01
eyelid (fold) (congenital) Q10.3
acquired Z90.01
face, specified part NEC Q18.8
fallopian tube(s) (acquired) Z90.79
congenital Q50.6
family member (causing problem in home) NEC — *see also* Disruption, family Z63.32
femur, congenital — *see* Defect, reduction, lower limb, longitudinal, femur
fibrinogen (congenital) D68.2
acquired D65
finger(s) (acquired) Z89.02- ☑
congenital — *see* Agenesis, hand
foot (acquired) Z89.43- ☑
congenital — *see* Agenesis, foot
forearm (acquired) — *see* Absence, arm, below elbow
gallbladder (acquired) Z90.49
congenital Q44.0
gamma globulin in blood D80.1
hereditary D80.0
genital organs
acquired (female) (male) Z90.79
female, congenital Q52.8
external Q52.71
internal NEC Q52.8
male, congenital Q55.8
genitourinary organs, congenital NEC
female Q52.8
male Q55.8

Absence — *continued*
globe (acquired) Z90.01
congenital Q11.1
glottis, congenital Q31.8
hand and wrist (acquired) Z89.11- ☑
congenital — *see* Agenesis, hand
head, part (acquired) NEC Z90.09
heat sense R20.8
hip (following explanation of hip joint prosthesis) (joint) (with or without presence of antibiotic-impregnated cement spacer) Z89.62- ☑
hymen (congenital) Q52.4
ileum (acquired) Z90.49
congenital Q41.2
immunoglobulin, isolated NEC D80.3
IgA D80.2
IgG D80.3
IgM D80.4
incus (acquired) — *see* Loss, ossicles, ear
congenital Q16.3
inner ear, congenital Q16.5
intestine (acquired) (small) Z90.49
congenital Q41.9
specified NEC Q41.8
large Z90.49
congenital Q42.9
specified NEC Q42.8
iris, congenital Q13.1
jejunum (acquired) Z90.49
congenital Q41.1
joint
acquired
hip (following explantation of hip joint prosthe-sis) (with or without presence of antibiotic-impregnated cement spacer) Z89.62- ☑
knee (following explantation of knee joint pros-thesis) (with or without presence of antibi-otic-impregnated cement spacer) Z89.52- ☑
shoulder (following explantation of shoulder joint prosthesis) (with or without presence of antibiotic-impregnated cement spacer) Z89.23- ☑
congenital NEC Q74.8
kidney(s) (acquired) Z90.5
congenital Q60.2
bilateral Q60.1
unilateral Q60.0
knee (following explantation of knee joint prosthesis) (joint) (with or without presence of antibiotic-impregnated cement spacer) Z89.52- ☑
labyrinth, membranous Q16.5
larynx (congenital) Q31.8
acquired Z90.02
leg (acquired) (above knee) Z89.61- ☑
below knee (acquired) Z89.51- ☑
congenital — *see* Defect, reduction, lower limb
lens (acquired) — *see also* Aphakia
congenital Q12.3
post cataract extraction Z98.4- ☑
limb (acquired) — *see* Absence, extremity
lip Q38.6
liver (congenital) Q44.7
lung (fissure) (lobe) (bilateral) (unilateral) (congenital) Q33.3
acquired (any part) Z90.2
menstruation — *see* Amenorrhea
muscle (congenital) (pectoral) Q79.8
ocular Q10.3
neck, part Q18.8
neutrophil — *see* Agranulocytosis
nipple(s) (with breast(s)) (acquired) Z90.1- ☑
congenital Q83.2
nose (congenital) Q30.1
acquired Z90.09
organ
of Corti, congenital Q16.5
or site, congenital NEC Q89.8
acquired NEC Z90.89
osseous meatus (ear) Q16.4
ovary (acquired)
bilateral Z90.722
congenital
bilateral Q50.02
unilateral Q50.01
unilateral Z90.721
oviduct (acquired)
bilateral Z90.722

Absence — *continued*
oviduct — *continued*
congenital Q50.6
unilateral Z90.721
pancreas (congenital) Q45.0
acquired Z90.410
complete Z90.410
partial Z90.411
total Z90.410
parathyroid gland (acquired) E89.2
congenital Q89.2
patella, congenital Q74.1
penis (congenital) Q55.5
acquired Z90.79
pericardium (congenital) Q24.8
pituitary gland (congenital) Q89.2
acquired E89.3
prostate (acquired) Z90.79
congenital Q55.4
pulmonary valve Q22.0
punctum lacrimale (congenital) Q10.4
radius, congenital — *see* Defect, reduction, upper limb, longitudinal, radius
rectum (congenital) Q42.1
with fistula Q42.0
acquired Z90.49
respiratory organ NOS Q34.9
rib (acquired) Z90.89
congenital Q76.6
sacrum, congenital Q76.49
salivary gland(s), congenital Q38.4
scrotum, congenital Q55.29
seminal vesicles (congenital) Q55.4
acquired Z90.79
septum
atrial (congenital) Q21.1
between aorta and pulmonary artery Q21.4
ventricular (congenital) Q20.4
sex chromosome
female phenotype Q97.8
male phenotype Q98.8
skull bone (congenital) Q75.8
with
anencephaly Q00.0
encephalocele — *see* Encephalocele
hydrocephalus Q03.9
with spina bifida — *see* Spina bifida, by site, with hydrocephalus
microcephaly Q02
spermatic cord, congenital Q55.4
spine, congenital Q76.49
spleen (congenital) Q89.01
acquired Z90.81
sternum, congenital Q76.7
stomach (acquired) (partial) Z90.3
congenital Q40.2
superior vena cava, congenital Q26.8
teeth, tooth (congenital) K00.0
acquired (complete) K08.109
class I K08.101
class II K08.102
class III K08.103
class IV K08.104
due to
caries K08.139
class I K08.131
class II K08.132
class III K08.133
class IV K08.134
periodontal disease K08.129
class I K08.121
class II K08.122
class III K08.123
class IV K08.124
specified NEC K08.199
class I K08.191
class II K08.192
class III K08.193
class IV K08.194
trauma K08.119
class I K08.111
class II K08.112
class III K08.113
class IV K08.114
partial K08.409
class I K08.401
class II K08.402
class III K08.403
class IV K08.404

Absence — continued
- teeth, tooth — continued
  - acquired — continued
    - partial — continued
      - due to
        - caries K08.439
          - class I K08.431
          - class II K08.432
          - class III K08.433
          - class IV K08.434
        - periodontal disease K08.429
          - class I K08.421
          - class II K08.422
          - class III K08.423
          - class IV K08.424
        - specified NEC K08.499
          - class I K08.491
          - class II K08.492
          - class III K08.493
          - class IV K08.494
        - trauma K08.419
          - class I K08.411
          - class II K08.412
          - class III K08.413
          - class IV K08.414
- tendon (congenital) Q79.8
- testis (congenital) Q55.0
  - acquired Z90.79
- thumb (acquired) Z89.01- ☑
  - congenital — see Agenesis, hand
- thymus gland Q89.2
- thyroid (gland) (acquired) E89.0
  - cartilage, congenital Q31.8
  - congenital E03.1
- toe(s) (acquired) Z89.42- ☑
  - with foot — see Absence, foot and ankle
  - congenital — see Agenesis, foot
  - great Z89.41- ☑
- tongue, congenital Q38.3
- trachea (cartilage), congenital Q32.1
- transverse aortic arch, congenital Q25.49
- tricuspid valve Q22.4
- umbilical artery, congenital Q27.0
- upper arm and forearm with hand present, congenital — see Agenesis, arm, with hand present
- ureter (congenital) Q62.4
  - acquired Z90.6
- urethra, congenital Q64.5
- uterus (acquired) Z90.710
  - with cervix Z90.710
  - with remaining cervical stump Z90.711
  - congenital Q51.0
- uvula, congenital Q38.5
- vagina, congenital Q52.0
- vas deferens (congenital) Q55.4
  - acquired Z90.79
- vein (peripheral) congenital NEC Q27.8
  - cerebral Q28.3
  - digestive system Q27.8
  - great Q26.8
  - lower limb Q27.8
  - portal Q26.5
  - precerebral Q28.1
  - specified site NEC Q27.8
  - upper limb Q27.8
- vena cava (inferior) (superior), congenital Q26.8
- ventricular septum Q20.4
- vertebra, congenital Q76.49
- vulva, congenital Q52.71
- wrist (acquired) Z89.12- ☑

Absorbent system disease I87.8

Absorption
- carbohydrate, disturbance K90.49
- chemical — see Table of Drugs and Chemicals
  - through placenta (newborn) P04.9
    - environmental substance P04.6
    - nutritional substance P04.5
    - obstetric anesthetic or analgesic drug P04.0
- drug NEC — see Table of Drugs and Chemicals
  - addictive
    - through placenta (newborn) — see also Newborn, affected by, maternal, use of P04.40
      - cocaine P04.41
      - hallucinogens P04.42
      - specified drug NEC P04.49
  - medicinal
    - through placenta (newborn) P04.19
  - through placenta (newborn) P04.19

Absorption — continued
- drug — see Table of Drugs and Chemicals — continued
  - through placenta — continued
    - obstetric anesthetic or analgesic drug P04.0
- fat, disturbance K90.49
  - pancreatic K90.3
- noxious substance — see Table of Drugs and Chemicals
- protein, disturbance K90.49
- starch, disturbance K90.49
- toxic substance — see Table of Drugs and Chemicals
- uremic — see Uremia

Abstinence symptoms, syndrome
- alcohol F10.239
  - with delirium F10.231
- cocaine F14.23
- neonatal P96.1
- nicotine — see Dependence, drug, nicotine, with, withdrawal
- opioid F11.93
  - with dependence F11.23
- psychoactive NEC F19.939
  - with
    - delirium F19.931
    - dependence F19.239
      - with
        - delirium F19.231
        - perceptual disturbance F19.232
        - uncomplicated F19.230
    - perceptual disturbance F19.932
  - uncomplicated F19.930
- sedative F13.939
  - with
    - delirium F13.931
    - dependence F13.239
      - with
        - delirium F13.231
        - perceptual disturbance F13.232
        - uncomplicated F13.230
    - perceptual disturbance F13.932
  - uncomplicated F13.930
- stimulant NEC F15.93
  - with dependence F15.23

Abulia R68.89

Abulomania F60.7

Abuse
- adult — see Maltreatment, adult
  - as reason for
    - couple seeking advice (including offender) Z63.0
- alcohol (non-dependent) F10.10
  - with
    - anxiety disorder F10.180
    - intoxication F10.129
      - with delirium F10.121
      - uncomplicated F10.120
    - mood disorder F10.14
    - other specified disorder F10.188
    - psychosis F10.159
      - delusions F10.150
      - hallucinations F10.151
    - sexual dysfunction F10.181
    - sleep disorder F10.182
    - unspecified disorder F10.19
    - withdrawal F10.139
      - with
        - perceptual disturbance F10.132
      - delirium F10.131
      - uncomplicated F10.130
  - counseling and surveillance Z71.41
  - in remission (early) (sustained) F10.11
- amphetamine (or related substance) — see also Abuse, drug, stimulant NEC
  - stimulant NEC F15.10
    - with
      - anxiety disorder F15.180
      - intoxication F15.129
        - with
          - delirium F15.121
          - perceptual disturbance F15.122
      - withdrawal F15.13
- analgesics (non-prescribed) (over the counter) F55.8
- antacids F55.0
- antidepressants — see Abuse, drug, psychoactive NEC
- anxiolytic — see Abuse, drug, sedative
- barbiturates — see Abuse, drug, sedative
- caffeine — see Abuse, drug, stimulant NEC
- cannabis, cannabinoids — see Abuse, drug, cannabis
- child — see Maltreatment, child

Abuse — continued
- cocaine — see Abuse, drug, cocaine
- drug NEC (non-dependent) F19.10
  - with sleep disorder F19.182
  - amphetamine type — see Abuse, drug, stimulant NEC
  - analgesics (non-prescribed) (over the counter) F55.8
  - antacids F55.0
  - antidepressants — see Abuse, drug, psychoactive NEC
  - anxiolytics — see Abuse, drug, sedative
  - barbiturates — see Abuse, drug, sedative
  - caffeine — see Abuse, drug, stimulant NEC
  - cannabis F12.10
    - with
      - anxiety disorder F12.180
      - intoxication F12.129
        - with
          - delirium F12.121
          - perceptual disturbance F12.122
          - uncomplicated F12.120
      - other specified disorder F12.188
      - psychosis F12.159
        - delusions F12.150
        - hallucinations F12.151
      - unspecified disorder F12.19
      - withdrawal F12.13
    - in remission (early) (sustained) F12.11
  - cocaine F14.10
    - with
      - anxiety disorder F14.180
      - intoxication F14.129
        - with
          - delirium F14.121
          - perceptual disturbance F14.122
          - uncomplicated F14.120
      - mood disorder F14.14
      - other specified disorder F14.188
      - psychosis F14.159
        - delusions F14.150
        - hallucinations F14.151
      - sexual dysfunction F14.181
      - sleep disorder F14.182
      - unspecified disorder F14.19
      - withdrawal F14.13
    - in remission (early) (sustained) F14.11
  - counseling and surveillance Z71.51
  - hallucinogen F16.10
    - with
      - anxiety disorder F16.180
      - flashbacks F16.183
      - intoxication F16.129
        - with
          - delirium F16.121
          - perceptual disturbance F16.122
          - uncomplicated F16.120
      - mood disorder F16.14
      - other specified disorder F16.188
      - perception disorder, persisting F16.183
      - psychosis F16.159
        - delusions F16.150
        - hallucinations F16.151
      - unspecified disorder F16.19
    - in remission (early) (sustained) F16.11
  - hashish — see Abuse, drug, cannabis
  - herbal or folk remedies F55.1
  - hormones F55.3
  - hypnotics — see Abuse, drug, sedative
  - in remission (early) (sustained) F19.11
  - inhalant F18.10
    - with
      - anxiety disorder F18.180
      - dementia, persisting F18.17
      - intoxication F18.129
        - with delirium F18.121
        - uncomplicated F18.120
      - mood disorder F18.14
      - other specified disorder F18.188
      - psychosis F18.159
        - delusions F18.150
        - hallucinations F18.151
      - unspecified disorder F18.19
    - in remission (early) (sustained) F18.11
  - laxatives F55.2
  - LSD — see Abuse, drug, hallucinogen
  - marihuana — see Abuse, drug, cannabis
  - morphine type (opioids) — see Abuse, drug, opioid
  - opioid F11.10

☑ **Additional Character Required — Refer to the Tabular List for Character Selection**   ▼ **Subterms under main terms may continue to next column or page**

Abuse — continued
  drug — continued
    opioid — continued
      with
        intoxication F11.129
          with
            delirium F11.121
            perceptual disturbance F11.122
          uncomplicated F11.120
        mood disorder F11.14
        other specified disorder F11.188
        psychosis F11.159
          delusions F11.150
          hallucinations F11.151
        sexual dysfunction F11.181
        sleep disorder F11.182
        unspecified disorder F11.19
        withdrawal F11.13
      in remission (early) (sustained) F11.11
    PCP (phencyclidine) (or related substance) — see
      Abuse, drug, hallucinogen
    psychoactive NEC F19.10
      with
        amnestic disorder F19.16
        anxiety disorder F19.180
        dementia F19.17
        intoxication F19.129
          with
            delirium F19.121
            perceptual disturbance F19.122
          uncomplicated F19.120
        mood disorder F19.14
        other specified disorder F19.188
        psychosis F19.159
          delusions F19.150
          hallucinations F19.151
        sexual dysfunction F19.181
        sleep disorder F19.182
        unspecified disorder F19.19
        withdrawal F19.139
          with
            perceptual disturbance F19.132
          delirium F19.131
          uncomplicated F19.130
    sedative, hypnotic or anxiolytic F13.10
      with
        anxiety disorder F13.180
        intoxication F13.129
          with delirium F13.121
          uncomplicated F13.120
        mood disorder F13.14
        other specified disorder F13.188
        psychosis F13.159
          delusions F13.150
          hallucinations F13.151
        sexual dysfunction F13.181
        sleep disorder F13.182
        unspecified disorder F13.19
        withdrawal F13.139
          with
            perceptual disturbance F13.132
          delirium F13.131
          uncomplicated F13.130
      in remission (early) (sustained) F13.11
    solvent — see Abuse, drug, inhalant
    steroids F55.3
    stimulant NEC F15.10
      with
        anxiety disorder F15.180
        intoxication F15.129
          with
            delirium F15.121
            perceptual disturbance F15.122
          uncomplicated F15.120
        mood disorder F15.14
        other specified disorder F15.188
        psychosis F15.159
          delusions F15.150
          hallucinations F15.151
        sexual dysfunction F15.181
        sleep disorder F15.182
        unspecified disorder F15.19
        withdrawal F15.13
      in remission (early) (sustained) F15.11
    tranquilizers — see Abuse, drug, sedative
    vitamins F55.4
  hallucinogens — see Abuse, drug, hallucinogen
  hashish — see Abuse, drug, cannabis
  herbal or folk remedies F55.1

Abuse — continued
  hormones F55.3
  hypnotic — see Abuse, drug, sedative
  inhalant — see Abuse, drug, inhalant
  laxatives F55.2
  LSD — see Abuse, drug, hallucinogen
  marihuana — see Abuse, drug, cannabis
  morphine type (opioids) — see Abuse, drug, opioid
  non-psychoactive substance NEC F55.8
    antacids F55.0
    folk remedies F55.1
    herbal remedies F55.1
    hormones F55.3
    laxatives F55.2
    steroids F55.3
    vitamins F55.4
  opioids — see Abuse, drug, opioid
  PCP (phencyclidine) (or related substance) — see
    Abuse, drug, hallucinogen
  physical (adult) (child) — see Maltreatment
  psychoactive substance — see Abuse, drug, psychoac-
    tive NEC
  psychological (adult) (child) — see Maltreatment
  sedative — see Abuse, drug, sedative
  sexual — see Maltreatment
  solvent — see Abuse, drug, inhalant
  steroids F55.3
  vitamins F55.4
Acalculia R48.8
  developmental F81.2
Acanthamebiasis (with) B60.10
  conjunctiva B60.12
  keratoconjunctivitis B60.13
  meningoencephalitis B60.11
  other specified B60.19
Acanthocephaliasis B83.8
Acanthocheilonemiasis B74.4
Acanthocytosis E78.6
Acantholysis L11.9
Acanthosis (acquired) (nigricans) L83
  benign Q82.8
  congenital Q82.8
  seborrheic L82.1
    inflamed L82.0
  tongue K14.3
Acapnia E87.3
Acarbia E87.2
Acardia, acardius Q89.8
Acardiacus amorphus Q89.8
Acardiotrophia I51.4
Acariasis B88.0
  scabies B86
Acarodermatitis (urticarioides) B88.0
Acarophobia F40.218
Acatalasemia, acatalasia E80.3
Acathisia (drug induced) G25.71
Accelerated atrioventricular conduction I45.6
Accentuation of personality traits (type A) Z73.1
Accessory (congenital)
  adrenal gland Q89.1
  anus Q43.4
  appendix Q43.4
  atrioventricular conduction I45.6
  auditory ossicles Q16.3
  auricle (ear) Q17.0
  biliary duct or passage Q44.5
  bladder Q64.79
  blood vessels NEC Q27.9
    coronary Q24.5
  bone NEC Q79.8
  breast tissue, axilla Q83.1
  carpal bones Q74.0
  cecum Q43.4
  chromosome(s) NEC (nonsex) Q92.9
    with complex rearrangements NEC Q92.5
      seen only at prometaphase Q92.8
    13 — see Trisomy, 13
    18 — see Trisomy, 18
    21 — see Trisomy, 21
    partial Q92.9
    sex
      female phenotype Q97.8
  coronary artery Q24.5
  cusp(s), heart valve NEC Q24.8
    pulmonary Q22.3
  cystic duct Q44.5
  digit(s) Q69.9
  ear (auricle) (lobe) Q17.0

Accessory — continued
  endocrine gland NEC Q89.2
  eye muscle Q10.3
  eyelid Q10.3
  face bone(s) Q75.8
  fallopian tube (fimbria) (ostium) Q50.6
  finger(s) Q69.0
  foreskin N47.8
  frontonasal process Q75.8
  gallbladder Q44.1
  genital organ(s)
    female Q52.8
      external Q52.79
      internal NEC Q52.8
    male Q55.8
  genitourinary organs NEC Q89.8
    female Q52.8
    male Q55.8
  hallux Q69.2
  heart Q24.8
    valve NEC Q24.8
      pulmonary Q22.3
  hepatic ducts Q44.5
  hymen Q52.4
  intestine (large) (small) Q43.4
  kidney Q63.0
  lacrimal canal Q10.6
  leaflet, heart valve NEC Q24.8
  ligament, broad Q50.6
  liver Q44.7
    duct Q44.5
  lobule (ear) Q17.0
  lung (lobe) Q33.1
  muscle Q79.8
  navicular of carpus Q74.0
  nervous system, part NEC Q07.8
  nipple Q83.3
  nose Q30.8
  organ or site not listed — see Anomaly, by site
  ovary Q50.31
  oviduct Q50.6
  pancreas Q45.3
  parathyroid gland Q89.2
  parotid gland (and duct) Q38.4
  pituitary gland Q89.2
  preauricular appendage Q17.0
  prepuce N47.8
  renal arteries (multiple) Q27.2
  rib Q76.6
    cervical Q76.5
  roots (teeth) K00.2
  salivary gland Q38.4
  sesamoid bones Q74.8
    foot Q74.2
    hand Q74.0
  skin tags Q82.8
  spleen Q89.09
  sternum Q76.7
  submaxillary gland Q38.4
  tarsal bones Q74.2
  teeth, tooth K00.1
  tendon Q79.8
  thumb Q69.1
  thymus gland Q89.2
  thyroid gland Q89.2
  toes Q69.2
  tongue Q38.3
  tooth, teeth K00.1
  tragus Q17.0
  ureter Q62.5
  urethra Q64.79
  urinary organ or tract NEC Q64.8
  uterus Q51.28
  vagina Q52.10
  valve, heart NEC Q24.8
    pulmonary Q22.3
  vertebra Q76.49
  vocal cords Q31.8
  vulva Q52.79
Accident
  birth — see Birth, injury
  cardiac — see Infarct, myocardium
  cerebral I63.9
  cerebrovascular (embolic) (ischemic) (thrombotic) I63.9
    aborted I63.9
    hemorrhagic — see Hemorrhage, intracranial, intrac-
      erebral
    old (without sequelae) Z86.73

Accident — *continued*
  cerebrovascular — *continued*
    old — *continued*
      with sequelae (of) — *see* Sequelae, infarction, cerebral
    coronary — *see* Infarct, myocardium
    craniovascular I63.9
    vascular, brain I63.9
Accidental — *see* condition
Accommodation (disorder) — *see also* condition
  hysterical paralysis of F44.89
  insufficiency of H52.4
  paresis — *see* Paresis, of accommodation
  spasm — *see* Spasm, of accommodation
Accouchement — *see* Delivery
Accreta placenta O43.21- ☑
Accretio cordis (nonrheumatic) I31.0
Accretions, tooth, teeth K03.6
Acculturation difficulty Z60.3
Accumulation secretion, prostate N42.89
Acephalia, acephalism, acephalus, acephaly Q00.0
Acephalobrachia monster Q89.8
Acephalochirus monster Q89.8
Acephalogaster Q89.8
Acephalostomus monster Q89.8
Acephalothorax Q89.8
Acerophobia F40.298
Acetonemia R79.89
  in Type 1 diabetes E10.10
    with coma E10.11
Acetonuria R82.4
Achalasia (cardia) (esophagus) K22.0
  congenital Q39.5
  pylorus Q40.0
  sphincteral NEC K59.89
Ache(s) — *see* Pain
Acheilia Q38.6
Achillobursitis — *see* Tendinitis, Achilles
Achillodynia — *see* Tendinitis, Achilles
Achlorhydria, achlorhydric (neurogenic) K31.83
  anemia D50.8
  diarrhea K31.83
  psychogenic F45.8
  secondary to vagotomy K91.1
Achluophobia F40.228
Acholia K82.8
Acholuric jaundice (familial) (splenomegalic) — *see also* Spherocytosis
  acquired D59.8
Achondrogenesis Q77.0
Achondroplasia (osteosclerosis congenita) Q77.4
Achroma, cutis L80
Achromat (ism), achromatopsia (acquired) (congenital) H53.51
Achromia, congenital — *see* Albinism
Achromia parasitica B36.0
Achylia gastrica K31.89
  psychogenic F45.8
Acid
  burn — *see* Corrosion
  deficiency
    amide nicotinic E52
    ascorbic E54
    folic E53.8
    nicotinic E52
    pantothenic E53.8
  intoxication E87.2
  peptic disease K30
  phosphatase deficiency E83.39
  stomach K30
    psychogenic F45.8
Acidemia E87.2
  argininosuccinic E72.22
  isovaleric E71.110
  metabolic (newborn) P19.9
    first noted before onset of labor P19.0
    first noted during labor P19.1
    noted at birth P19.2
  methylmalonic E71.120
  pipecolic E72.3
  propionic E71.121
Acidity, gastric (high) K30
  psychogenic F45.8
Acidocytopenia — *see* Agranulocytosis
Acidocytosis D72.10
Acidopenia — *see* Agranulocytosis
Acidosis (lactic) (respiratory) E87.2

Acidosis — *continued*
  in Type 1 diabetes E10.10
    with coma E10.11
  kidney, tubular N25.89
  lactic E87.2
  metabolic NEC E87.2
    with respiratory acidosis E87.4
    hyperchloremic, of newborn P74.421
    late, of newborn P74.0
  mixed metabolic and respiratory, newborn P84
  newborn P84
  renal (hyperchloremic) (tubular) N25.89
  respiratory E87.2
    complicated by
      metabolic
        acidosis E87.4
        alkalosis E87.4
Aciduria
  4-hydroxybutyric E72.81
  argininosuccinic E72.22
  gamma-hydroxybutyric E72.81
  glutaric (type I) E72.3
    type II E71.313
    type III E71.5- ☑
  orotic (congenital) (hereditary) (pyrimidine deficiency) E79.8
    anemia D53.0
Acladiosis (skin) B36.0
Aclasis, diaphyseal Q78.6
Acleistocardia Q21.1
Aclusion — *see* Anomaly, dentofacial, malocclusion
Acne L70.9
  artificialis L70.8
  atrophica L70.2
  cachecticorum (Hebra) L70.8
  conglobata L70.1
  cystic L70.0
  decalvans L66.2
  excoriée (des jeunes filles) L70.5
  frontalis L70.2
  indurata L70.0
  infantile L70.4
  keloid L73.0
  lupoid L70.2
  necrotic, necrotica (miliaris) L70.2
  neonatal L70.4
  nodular L70.0
  occupational L70.8
  picker's L70.5
  pustular L70.0
  rodens L70.2
  rosacea L71.9
  specified NEC L70.8
  tropica L70.3
  varioliformis L70.2
  vulgaris L70.0
Acnitis (primary) A18.4
Acosta's disease T70.29 ☑
Acoustic — *see* condition
Acousticophobia F40.298
ACPO (acute colonic pseudo-obstruction) K59.81
Acquired — *see also* condition
  immunodeficiency syndrome (AIDS) B20
Acrania Q00.0
Acroangiodermatitis I78.9
Acroasphyxia, chronic I73.89
Acrobystitis N47.7
Acrocephalopolysyndactyly Q87.0
Acrocephalosyndactyly Q87.0
Acrocephaly Q75.0
Acrochondrohyperplasia — *see* Syndrome, Marfan's
Acrocyanosis I73.89
  newborn P28.2
    meaning transient blue hands and feet — *omit code*
Acrodermatitis L30.8
  atrophicans (chronica) L90.4
  continua (Hallopeau) L40.2
  enteropathica (hereditary) E83.2
  Hallopeau's L40.2
  infantile papular L44.4
  perstans L40.2
  pustulosa continua L40.2
  recalcitrant pustular L40.2
Acrodynia — *see* Poisoning, mercury
Acromegaly, acromegalia E22.0
Acromelalgia I73.81
Acromicria, acromikria Q79.8
Acronyx L60.0

Acropachy, thyroid — *see* Thyrotoxicosis
Acroparesthesia (simple) (vasomotor) I73.89
Acropathy, thyroid — *see* Thyrotoxicosis
Acrophobia F40.241
Acroposthitis N47.7
Acroscleriasis, acroscleroderma, acrosclerosis — *see* Sclerosis, systemic
Acrosphacelus I96
Acrospiroma, eccrine — *see* Neoplasm, skin, benign
Acrostealgia — *see* Osteochondropathy
Acrotrophodynia — *see* Immersion
ACTH ectopic syndrome E24.3
Actinic — *see* condition
Actinobacillosis, actinobacillus A28.8
  mallei A24.0
  muris A25.1
Actinomyces israelii (infection) — *see* Actinomycosis
Actinomycetoma (foot) B47.1
Actinomycosis, actinomycotic A42.9
  with pneumonia A42.0
  abdominal A42.1
  cervicofacial A42.2
  cutaneous A42.89
  gastrointestinal A42.1
  pulmonary A42.0
  sepsis A42.7
  specified site NEC A42.89
Actinoneuritis G62.82
Action, heart
  disorder I49.9
  irregular I49.9
    psychogenic F45.8
Activated protein C resistance D68.51
Activation
  mast cell (disorder) (syndrome) D89.40
    idiopathic D89.42
    monoclonal D89.41
    secondary D89.43
    specified type NEC D89.49
Active — *see* condition
Acute — *see also* condition
  abdomen R10.0
  gallbladder — *see* Cholecystitis, acute
Acyanotic heart disease (congenital) Q24.9
Acystia Q64.5
Adair-Dighton syndrome (brittle bones and blue sclera, deafness) Q78.0
Adamantinoblastoma — *see* Ameloblastoma
Adamantinoma — *see also* Cyst, calcifying odontogenic
  long bones C40.90
    lower limb C40.2- ☑
    upper limb C40.0- ☑
  malignant C41.1
    jaw (bone) (lower) C41.1
      upper C41.0
  tibial C40.2- ☑
Adamantoblastoma — *see* Ameloblastoma
Adams-Stokes (-Morgagni) disease or syndrome I45.9
Adaption reaction — *see* Disorder, adjustment
Addiction — *see also* Dependence F19.20
  alcohol, alcoholic (ethyl) (methyl) (wood) (without remission) F10.20
    with remission F10.21
  drug — *see* Dependence, drug
  ethyl alcohol (without remission) F10.20
    with remission F10.21
  heroin — *see* Dependence, drug, opioid
  methyl alcohol (without remission) F10.20
    with remission F10.21
  methylated spirit (without remission) F10.20
    with remission F10.21
  morphine (-like substances) — *see* Dependence, drug, opioid
  nicotine — *see* Dependence, drug, nicotine
  opium and opioids — *see* Dependence, drug, opioid
  tobacco — *see* Dependence, drug, nicotine
Addison-Biermer anemia (pernicious) D51.0
Addisonian crisis E27.2
Addison's
  anemia (pernicious) D51.0
  disease (bronze) or syndrome E27.1
    tuberculous A18.7
  keloid L94.0
Addison-Schilder complex E71.528
Additional — *see also* Accessory
  chromosome(s) Q99.8
    21 — *see* Trisomy, 21

Additional — *continued*
　chromosome(s) — *continued*
　　sex — *see* Abnormal, chromosome, sex
Adduction contracture, hip or other joint — *see*
　　Contraction, joint
Adenitis — *see also* Lymphadenitis
　acute, unspecified site L04.9
　axillary I88.9
　　acute L04.2
　　chronic or subacute I88.1
　Bartholin's gland N75.8
　bulbourethral gland — *see* Urethritis
　cervical I88.9
　　acute L04.0
　　chronic or subacute I88.1
　chancroid (Hemophilus ducreyi) A57
　chronic, unspecified site I88.1
　Cowper's gland — *see* Urethritis
　due to Pasteurella multocida (P. septica) A28.0
　epidemic, acute B27.09
　gangrenous L04.9
　gonorrheal NEC A54.89
　groin I88.9
　　acute L04.1
　　chronic or subacute I88.1
　infectious (acute) (epidemic) B27.09
　inguinal I88.9
　　acute L04.1
　　chronic or subacute I88.1
　lymph gland or node, except mesenteric I88.9
　　acute — *see* Lymphadenitis, acute
　　chronic or subacute I88.1
　mesenteric (acute) (chronic) (nonspecific) (subacute)
　　I88.0
　parotid gland (suppurative) — *see* Sialoadenitis
　salivary gland (any) (suppurative) — *see* Sialoadenitis
　scrofulous (tuberculous) A18.2
　Skene's duct or gland — *see* Urethritis
　strumous, tuberculous A18.2
　subacute, unspecified site I88.1
　sublingual gland (suppurative) — *see* Sialoadenitis
　submandibular gland (suppurative) — *see* Sialoadenitis
　submaxillary gland (suppurative) — *see* Sialoadenitis
　tuberculous — *see* Tuberculosis, lymph gland
　urethral gland — *see* Urethritis
　Wharton's duct (suppurative) — *see* Sialoadenitis
Adenoacanthoma — *see* Neoplasm, malignant, by site
Adenoameloblastoma — *see* Cyst, calcifying odonto-
　　genic
Adenocarcinoid (tumor) — *see* Neoplasm, malignant,
　　by site
Adenocarcinoma — *see also* Neoplasm, malignant, by
　　site
　acidophil
　　specified site — *see* Neoplasm, malignant, by site
　　unspecified site C75.1
　adrenal cortical C74.0- ☑
　alveolar — *see* Neoplasm, lung, malignant
　apocrine
　　breast — *see* Neoplasm, breast, malignant
　　in situ
　　　breast D05.8- ☑
　　　specified site NEC — *see* Neoplasm, skin, in situ
　　　unspecified site D04.9
　　specified site NEC — *see* Neoplasm, skin, malignant
　　unspecified site C44.99
　basal cell
　　specified site — *see* Neoplasm, skin, malignant
　　unspecified site C08.9
　basophil
　　specified site — *see* Neoplasm, malignant, by site
　　unspecified site C75.1
　bile duct type C22.1
　　liver C22.1
　　specified site NEC — *see* Neoplasm, malignant, by
　　　site
　　unspecified site C22.1
　bronchiolar — *see* Neoplasm, lung, malignant
　bronchioloalveolar — *see* Neoplasm, lung, malignant
　ceruminous C44.29- ☑
　cervix, in situ — *see also* Carcinoma, cervix uteri, in situ
　　　D06.9
　chromophobe
　　specified site — *see* Neoplasm, malignant, by site
　　unspecified site C75.1
　diffuse type
　　specified site — *see* Neoplasm, malignant, by site
　　unspecified site C16.9

Adenocarcinoma — *continued*
　duct
　　infiltrating
　　　with Paget's disease — *see* Neoplasm, breast,
　　　　malignant
　　　specified site — *see* Neoplasm, malignant, by
　　　　site
　　　unspecified site (female) C50.91- ☑
　　　　male C50.92- ☑
　　specified site — *see* Neoplasm, malignant, by site
　　unspecified site
　　　female C56.9
　　　male C61
　eosinophil
　　specified site — *see* Neoplasm, malignant, by site
　　unspecified site C75.1
　follicular
　　with papillary C73
　　moderately differentiated C73
　　specified site — *see* Neoplasm, malignant, by site
　　trabecular C73
　　unspecified site C73
　　well differentiated C73
　Hurthle cell C73
　in
　　adenomatous
　　　polyposis coli C18.9
　infiltrating duct
　　with Paget's disease — *see* Neoplasm, breast, ma-
　　　lignant
　　specified site — *see* Neoplasm, by site, malignant
　　unspecified site (female) C50.91- ☑
　　　male C50.92- ☑
　inflammatory
　　specified site — *see* Neoplasm, by site, malignant
　　unspecified site (female) C50.91- ☑
　　　male C50.92- ☑
　intestinal type
　　specified site — *see* Neoplasm, by site, malignant
　　unspecified site C16.9
　intracystic papillary
　intraductal
　　breast D05.1- ☑
　　noninfiltrating
　　　breast D05.1- ☑
　　　papillary
　　　　with invasion
　　　　　specified site — *see* Neoplasm, by site,
　　　　　　malignant
　　　　　unspecified site (female) C50.91- ☑
　　　　　　male C50.92- ☑
　　　　breast D05.1- ☑
　　　　specified site NEC — *see* Neoplasm, in situ,
　　　　　by site
　　　　unspecified site D05.1- ☑
　　　specified site NEC — *see* Neoplasm, in situ, by
　　　　site
　　　unspecified site D05.1- ☑
　　papillary
　　　with invasion
　　　　specified site — *see* Neoplasm, malignant, by
　　　　　site
　　　　unspecified site (female) C50.91- ☑
　　　　　male C50.92- ☑
　　　breast D05.1- ☑
　　　specified site — *see* Neoplasm, in situ, by site
　　　unspecified site D05.1- ☑
　　specified site NEC — *see* Neoplasm, in situ, by site
　　unspecified site D05.1- ☑
　islet cell
　　with exocrine, mixed
　　　specified site — *see* Neoplasm, malignant, by
　　　　site
　　　unspecified site C25.9
　　pancreas C25.4
　　specified site NEC — *see* Neoplasm, malignant, by
　　　site
　　unspecified site C25.4
　lobular
　　in situ
　　　breast D05.0- ☑
　　　specified site NEC — *see* Neoplasm, in situ, by
　　　　site
　　　unspecified site D05.0- ☑
　　specified site — *see* Neoplasm, malignant, by site
　　unspecified site (female) C50.91- ☑
　　　male C50.92- ☑

Adenocarcinoma — *continued*
　mucoid — *see also* Neoplasm, malignant, by site
　　cell
　　　specified site — *see* Neoplasm, malignant, by
　　　　site
　　　unspecified site C75.1
　nonencapsulated sclerosing C73
　papillary
　　with follicular C73
　　follicular variant C73
　　intraductal (noninfiltrating)
　　　with invasion
　　　　specified site — *see* Neoplasm, malignant, by
　　　　　site
　　　　unspecified site (female) C50.91- ☑
　　　　　male C50.92- ☑
　　　breast D05.1- ☑
　　　specified site NEC — *see* Neoplasm, in situ, by
　　　　site
　　　unspecified site D05.1- ☑
　　serous
　　　specified site — *see* Neoplasm, malignant, by
　　　　site
　　　unspecified site C56.9
　papillocystic
　　specified site — *see* Neoplasm, malignant, by site
　　unspecified site C56.9
　pseudomucinous
　　specified site — *see* Neoplasm, malignant, by site
　　unspecified site C56.9
　renal cell C64- ☑
　sebaceous — *see* Neoplasm, skin, malignant
　serous — *see also* Neoplasm, malignant, by site
　　papillary
　　　specified site — *see* Neoplasm, malignant, by
　　　　site
　　　unspecified site C56.9
　sweat gland — *see* Neoplasm, skin, malignant
　water-clear cell C75.0
Adenocarcinoma-in-situ — *see also* Neoplasm, in situ,
　　by site
　breast D05.9- ☑
Adenofibroma
　clear cell — *see* Neoplasm, benign, by site
　endometrioid D27.9
　　borderline malignancy D39.10
　　malignant C56- ☑
　mucinous
　　specified site — *see* Neoplasm, benign, by site
　　unspecified site D27.9
　papillary
　　specified site — *see* Neoplasm, benign, by site
　　unspecified site D27.9
　prostate — *see* Enlargement, enlarged, prostate
　serous
　　specified site — *see* Neoplasm, benign, by site
　　unspecified site D27.9
　specified site — *see* Neoplasm, benign, by site
　unspecified site D27.9
Adenofibrosis
　breast — *see* Fibroadenosis, breast
　endometrioid N80.0
Adenoiditis (chronic) J35.02
　with tonsillitis J35.03
　acute J03.90
　　recurrent J03.91
　　specified organism NEC J03.80
　　　recurrent J03.81
　　staphylococcal J03.80
　　　recurrent J03.81
　　streptococcal J03.00
　　　recurrent J03.01
Adenoids — *see* condition
Adenolipoma — *see* Neoplasm, benign, by site
Adenolipomatosis, Launois-Bensaude E88.89
Adenolymphoma
　specified site — *see* Neoplasm, benign, by site
　unspecified site D11.9
Adenoma — *see also* Neoplasm, benign, by site
　acidophil
　　specified site — *see* Neoplasm, benign, by site
　　unspecified site D35.2
　acidophil-basophil, mixed
　　specified site — *see* Neoplasm, benign, by site
　　unspecified site D35.2
　adrenal (cortical) D35.00
　　clear cell D35.00
　　compact cell D35.00

📖 **Subterms under main terms may continue to next column or page**　　　　☑ **Additional Character Required — Refer to the Tabular List for Character Selection**　　　　**11**

Additional — Adenoma

Adenoma — *continued*
adrenal — *continued*
glomerulosa cell D35.ØØ
heavily pigmented variant D35.ØØ
mixed cell D35.ØØ
alpha-cell
pancreas D13.7
specified site NEC — *see* Neoplasm, benign, by site
unspecified site D13.7
alveolar D14.3Ø
apocrine
breast D24- ☑
specified site NEC — *see* Neoplasm, skin, benign, by site
unspecified site D23.9
basal cell D11.9
basophil
specified site — *see* Neoplasm, benign, by site
unspecified site D35.2
basophil-acidophil, mixed
specified site — *see* Neoplasm, benign, by site
unspecified site D35.2
beta-cell
pancreas D13.7
specified site NEC — *see* Neoplasm, benign, by site
unspecified site D13.7
bile duct D13.4
common D13.5
extrahepatic D13.5
intrahepatic D13.4
specified site NEC — *see* Neoplasm, benign, by site
unspecified site D13.4
black D35.ØØ
bronchial D38.1
cylindroid type — *see* Neoplasm, lung, malignant
ceruminous D23.2- ☑
chief cell D35.1
chromophobe
specified site — *see* Neoplasm, benign, by site
unspecified site D35.2
colloid
specified site — *see* Neoplasm, benign, by site
unspecified site D34
eccrine, papillary — *see* Neoplasm, skin, benign
endocrine, multiple
single specified site — *see* Neoplasm, uncertain behavior, by site
two or more specified sites D44- ☑
unspecified site D44.9
endometrioid — *see also* Neoplasm, benign
borderline malignancy — *see* Neoplasm, uncertain behavior, by site
eosinophil
specified site — *see* Neoplasm, benign, by site
unspecified site D35.2
fetal
specified site — *see* Neoplasm, benign, by site
unspecified site D34
follicular
specified site — *see* Neoplasm, benign, by site
unspecified site D34
hepatocellular D13.4
Hurthle cell D34
islet cell
pancreas D13.7
specified site NEC — *see* Neoplasm, benign, by site
unspecified site D13.7
liver cell D13.4
macrofollicular
specified site — *see* Neoplasm, benign, by site
unspecified site D34
malignant, malignum — *see* Neoplasm, malignant, by site
microcystic
pancreas D13.6
specified site NEC — *see* Neoplasm, benign, by site
unspecified site D13.6
microfollicular
specified site — *see* Neoplasm, benign, by site
unspecified site D34
mucoid cell
specified site — *see* Neoplasm, benign, by site
unspecified site D35.2
multiple endocrine
single specified site — *see* Neoplasm, uncertain behavior, by site
two or more specified sites D44- ☑
unspecified site D44.9

Adenoma — *continued*
nipple D24- ☑
papillary — *see also* Neoplasm, benign, by site
eccrine — *see* Neoplasm, skin, benign, by site
Pick's tubular
specified site — *see* Neoplasm, benign, by site
unspecified site
female D27.9
male D29.2Ø
pleomorphic
carcinoma in — *see* Neoplasm, salivary gland, malignant
specified site — *see* Neoplasm, malignant, by site
unspecified site CØ8.9
polypoid — *see also* Neoplasm, benign
adenocarcinoma in — *see* Neoplasm, malignant, by site
adenocarcinoma in situ — *see* Neoplasm, in situ, by site
prostate — *see* Neoplasm, benign, prostate
rete cell D29.2Ø
sebaceous — *see* Neoplasm, skin, benign
Sertoli cell
specified site — *see* Neoplasm, benign, by site
unspecified site
female D27.9
male D29.2Ø
skin appendage — *see* Neoplasm, skin, benign
sudoriferous gland — *see* Neoplasm, skin, benign
sweat gland — *see* Neoplasm, skin, benign
testicular
specified site — *see* Neoplasm, benign, by site
unspecified site
female D27.9
male D29.2Ø
tubular — *see also* Neoplasm, benign, by site
adenocarcinoma in — *see* Neoplasm, malignant, by site
adenocarcinoma in situ — *see* Neoplasm, in situ, by site
Pick's
specified site — *see* Neoplasm, benign, by site
unspecified site
female D27.9
male D29.2Ø
tubulovillous — *see also* Neoplasm, benign, by site
adenocarcinoma in — *see* Neoplasm, malignant, by site
adenocarcinoma in situ — *see* Neoplasm, in situ, by site
villous — *see* Neoplasm, uncertain behavior, by site
adenocarcinoma in — *see* Neoplasm, malignant, by site
adenocarcinoma in situ — *see* Neoplasm, in situ, by site
water-clear cell D35.1

Adenomatosis
endocrine (multiple) E31.2Ø
single specified site — *see* Neoplasm, uncertain behavior, by site
erosive of nipple D24- ☑
pluriendocrine — *see* Adenomatosis, endocrine
pulmonary D38.1
malignant — *see* Neoplasm, lung, malignant
specified site — *see* Neoplasm, benign, by site
unspecified site D12.6

Adenomatous
goiter (nontoxic) EØ4.9
with hyperthyroidism — *see* Hyperthyroidism, with, goiter, nodular
toxic — *see* Hyperthyroidism, with, goiter, nodular

Adenomyoma — *see also* Neoplasm, benign, by site
prostate — *see* Enlarged, prostate

Adenomyometritis N8Ø.Ø

Adenomyosis N8Ø.Ø

Adenopathy (lymph gland) R59.9
generalized R59.1
inguinal R59.Ø
localized R59.Ø
mediastinal R59.Ø
mesentery R59.Ø
syphilitic (secondary) A51.49
tracheobronchial R59.Ø
tuberculous A15.4
primary (progressive) A15.7
tuberculous — *see also* Tuberculosis, lymph gland

Adenopathy — *continued*
tuberculous — *see also* Tuberculosis, lymph gland — *continued*
tracheobronchial A15.4
primary (progressive) A15.7

Adenosalpingitis — *see* Salpingitis

Adenosarcoma — *see* Neoplasm, malignant, by site

Adenosclerosis I88.8

Adenosis (sclerosing) breast — *see* Fibroadenosis, breast

Adenovirus, as cause of disease classified elsewhere B97.Ø

Adentia (complete) (partial) — *see* Absence, teeth

Adherent — *see also* Adhesions
labia (minora) N9Ø.89
pericardium (nonrheumatic) I31.Ø
rheumatic IØ9.2
placenta (with hemorrhage) O72.Ø
without hemorrhage O73.Ø
prepuce, newborn N47.Ø
scar (skin) L9Ø.5
tendon in scar L9Ø.5

Adhesions, adhesive (postinfective) K66.Ø
with intestinal obstruction K56.5Ø
complete K56.52
incomplete K56.51
partial K56.51
abdominal (wall) — *see* Adhesions, peritoneum
appendix K38.8
bile duct (common) (hepatic) K83.8
bladder (sphincter) N32.89
bowel — *see* Adhesions, peritoneum
cardiac I31.Ø
rheumatic IØ9.2
cecum — *see* Adhesions, peritoneum
cervicovaginal N88.1
congenital Q52.8
postpartal O9Ø.89
old N88.1
cervix N88.1
ciliary body NEC — *see* Adhesions, iris
clitoris N9Ø.89
colon — *see* Adhesions, peritoneum
common duct K83.8
congenital — *see also* Anomaly, by site
fingers — *see* Syndactylism, complex, fingers
omental, anomalous Q43.3
peritoneal Q43.3
tongue (to gum or roof of mouth) Q38.3
conjunctiva (acquired) H11.21- ☑
congenital Q15.8
cystic duct K82.8
diaphragm — *see* Adhesions, peritoneum
due to foreign body — *see* Foreign body
duodenum — *see* Adhesions, peritoneum
ear
middle H74.1- ☑
epididymis N5Ø.89
epidural — *see* Adhesions, meninges
epiglottis J38.7
eyelid HØ2.59
female pelvis N73.6
gallbladder K82.8
globe H44.89
heart I31.Ø
rheumatic IØ9.2
ileocecal (coil) — *see* Adhesions, peritoneum
ileum — *see* Adhesions, peritoneum
intestine — *see also* Adhesions, peritoneum
with obstruction K56.5Ø
complete K56.52
incomplete K56.51
partial K56.51
intra-abdominal — *see* Adhesions, peritoneum
iris H21.5Ø- ☑
anterior H21.51- ☑
goniosynechiae H21.52- ☑
posterior H21.54- ☑
to corneal graft T85.898 ☑
joint — *see* Ankylosis
knee M23.8X ☑
temporomandibular M26.61- ☑
labium (majus) (minus), congenital Q52.5
liver — *see* Adhesions, peritoneum
lung J98.4
mediastinum J98.59
meninges (cerebral) (spinal) G96.12
congenital QØ7.8
tuberculous (cerebral) (spinal) A17.Ø

☑ **Additional Character Required — Refer to the Tabular List for Character Selection** ▽ **Subterms under main terms may continue to next column or page**

Adhesions, adhesive — *continued*
mesenteric — *see* Adhesions, peritoneum
nasal (septum) (to turbinates) J34.89
ocular muscle — *see* Strabismus, mechanical
omentum — *see* Adhesions, peritoneum
ovary N73.6
congenital (to cecum, kidney or omentum) Q50.39
paraovarian N73.6
pelvic (peritoneal)
female N73.6
postprocedural N99.4
male — *see* Adhesions, peritoneum
postpartal (old) N73.6
tuberculous A18.17
penis to scrotum (congenital) Q55.8
periappendiceal — *see also* Adhesions, peritoneum
pericardium (nonrheumatic) I31.0
focal I31.8
rheumatic I09.2
tuberculous A18.84
pericholecystic K82.8
perigastric — *see* Adhesions, peritoneum
periovarian N73.6
periprostatic N42.89
perirectal — *see* Adhesions, peritoneum
perirenal N28.89
peritoneum, peritoneal (postinfective) K66.0
with obstruction (intestinal) K56.50
complete K56.52
incomplete K56.51
partial K56.51
congenital Q43.3
pelvic, female N73.6
postprocedural N99.4
postpartal, pelvic N73.6
postprocedural K66.0
to uterus N73.6
peritubal N73.6
periureteral N28.89
periuterine N73.6
perivesical N32.89
perivesicular (seminal vesicle) N50.89
pleura, pleuritic J94.8
tuberculous NEC A15.6
pleuropericardial J94.8
postoperative (gastrointestinal tract) K66.0
with obstruction — *see also* Obstruction, intestine,
postoperative K91.30
due to foreign body accidentally left in wound —
see Foreign body, accidentally left during a
procedure
pelvic peritoneal N99.4
urethra — *see* Stricture, urethra, postprocedural
vagina N99.2
postpartal, old (vulva or perineum) N90.89
preputial, prepuce N47.5
pulmonary J98.4
pylorus — *see* Adhesions, peritoneum
sciatic nerve — *see* Lesion, nerve, sciatic
seminal vesicle N50.89
shoulder (joint) — *see* Capsulitis, adhesive
sigmoid flexure — *see* Adhesions, peritoneum
spermatic cord (acquired) N50.89
congenital Q55.4
spinal canal G96.12
stomach — *see* Adhesions, peritoneum
subscapular — *see* Capsulitis, adhesive
temporomandibular M26.61- ☑
tendinitis (*see also* Tenosynovitis, specified type NEC)
shoulder — *see* Capsulitis, adhesive
testis N44.8
tongue, congenital (to gum or roof of mouth) Q38.3
acquired K14.8
trachea J39.8
tubo-ovarian N73.6
tunica vaginalis N44.8
uterus N73.6
internal N85.6
to abdominal wall N73.6
vagina (chronic) N89.5
postoperative N99.2
vitreomacular H43.82- ☑
vitreous H43.89
vulva N90.89
Adiaspiromycosis B48.8
Adie (-Holmes) **pupil or syndrome** — *see* Anomaly,
pupil, function, tonic pupil
Adiponecrosis neonatorum P83.88

Adiposis — *see also* Obesity
cerebralis E23.6
dolorosa E88.2
Adiposity — *see also* Obesity
heart — *see* Degeneration, myocardial
localized E65
Adiposogenital dystrophy E23.6
Adjustment
disorder — *see* Disorder, adjustment
implanted device — *see* Encounter (for), adjustment
(of)
prosthesis, external — *see* Fitting
reaction — *see* Disorder, adjustment
Administration of tPA (rtPA) in a different facility within
the last 24 hours prior to admission to current facility Z92.82
Admission (for) — *see also* Encounter (for)
adjustment (of)
artificial
arm Z44.00- ☑
complete Z44.01- ☑
partial Z44.02- ☑
eye Z44.2 ☑
leg Z44.10- ☑
complete Z44.11- ☑
partial Z44.12- ☑
brain neuropacemaker Z46.2
implanted Z45.42
breast
implant Z45.81 ☑
prosthesis (external) Z44.3 ☑
colostomy belt Z46.89
contact lenses Z46.0
cystostomy device Z46.6
dental prosthesis Z46.3
device NEC
abdominal Z46.89
implanted Z45.89
cardiac Z45.09
defibrillator (with synchronous cardiac
pacemaker) Z45.02
pacemaker (cardiac resynchronization
therapy (CRT-P) Z45.018
pulse generator Z45.010
resynchronization therapy defibrillator
(CRT-D) Z45.02
hearing device Z45.328
bone conduction Z45.320
cochlear Z45.321
infusion pump Z45.1
nervous system Z45.49
CSF drainage Z45.41
hearing device — *see* Admission, adjustment, device, implanted, hearing
device
neuropacemaker Z45.42
visual substitution Z45.31
specified NEC Z45.89
vascular access Z45.2
visual substitution Z45.31
nervous system Z46.2
implanted — *see* Admission, adjustment,
device, implanted, nervous system
orthodontic Z46.4
prosthetic Z44.9
arm — *see* Admission, adjustment, artificial,
arm
breast Z44.3 ☑
dental Z46.3
eye Z44.2 ☑
leg — *see* Admission, adjustment, artificial,
leg
specified type NEC Z44.8
substitution
auditory Z46.2
implanted — *see* Admission, adjustment,
device, implanted, hearing device
nervous system Z46.2
implanted — *see* Admission, adjustment,
device, implanted, nervous system
visual Z46.2
implanted Z45.31
urinary Z46.6
hearing aid Z46.1
implanted — *see* Admission, adjustment, device,
implanted, hearing device
ileostomy device Z46.89
intestinal appliance or device NEC Z46.89

Admission — *continued*
adjustment — *continued*
neuropacemaker (brain) (peripheral nerve) (spinal
cord) Z46.2
implanted Z45.42
orthodontic device Z46.4
orthopedic (brace) (cast) (device) (shoes) Z46.89
pacemaker (cardiac resynchronization therapy (CRT-
P))
cardiac Z45.018
pulse generator Z45.010
nervous system Z46.2
implanted Z45.42
portacath (port-a-cath) Z45.2
prosthesis Z44.9
arm — *see* Admission, adjustment, artificial, arm
breast Z44.3 ☑
dental Z46.3
eye Z44.2 ☑
leg — *see* Admission, adjustment, artificial, leg
specified NEC Z44.8
spectacles Z46.0
aftercare — *see also* Aftercare Z51.89
postpartum
immediately after delivery Z39.0
routine follow-up Z39.2
radiation therapy (antineoplastic) Z51.0
attention to artificial opening (of) Z43.9
artificial vagina Z43.7
colostomy Z43.3
cystostomy Z43.5
enterostomy Z43.4
gastrostomy Z43.1
ileostomy Z43.2
jejunostomy Z43.4
nephrostomy Z43.6
specified site NEC Z43.8
intestinal tract Z43.4
urinary tract Z43.6
tracheostomy Z43.0
ureterostomy Z43.6
urethrostomy Z43.6
breast augmentation or reduction Z41.1
breast reconstruction following mastectomy Z42.1
change of
dressing (nonsurgical) Z48.00
neuropacemaker device (brain) (peripheral nerve)
(spinal cord) Z46.2
implanted Z45.42
surgical dressing Z48.01
circumcision, ritual or routine (in absence of diagnosis)
Z41.2
clinical research investigation (control) (normal comparison) (participant) Z00.6
contraceptive management Z30.9
cosmetic surgery NEC Z41.1
counseling — *see also* Counseling
dietary Z71.3
gestational carrier Z31.7
HIV Z71.7
human immunodeficiency virus Z71.7
nonattending third party Z71.0
procreative management NEC Z31.69
delivery, full-term, uncomplicated O80
cesarean, without indication O82
desensitization to allergens Z51.6
dietary surveillance and counseling Z71.3
ear piercing Z41.3
examination at health care facility (adult) — *see also*
Examination Z00.00
with abnormal findings Z00.01
clinical research investigation (control) (normal
comparison) (participant) Z00.6
dental Z01.20
with abnormal findings Z01.21
donor (potential) Z00.5
ear Z01.10
with abnormal findings NEC Z01.118
eye Z01.00
with abnormal findings Z01.01
following failed vision screening Z01.020
with abnormal findings Z01.021
general, specified reason NEC Z00.8
hearing Z01.10
with abnormal findings NEC Z01.118
infant or child (over 28 days old) Z00.129
with abnormal findings Z00.121
postpartum checkup Z39.2

Admission — *continued*
  examination at health care facility — *see also* Examination — *continued*
    psychiatric (general) Z00.8
      requested by authority Z04.6
    vision Z01.00
      with abnormal findings Z01.01
      following failed vision screening Z01.020
        with abnormal findings Z01.021
      infant or child (over 28 days old) Z00.129
        with abnormal findings Z00.121
  fitting (of)
    artificial
      arm — *see* Admission, adjustment, artificial, arm
      eye Z44.2 ☑
      leg — *see* Admission, adjustment, artificial, leg
    brain neuropacemaker Z46.2
      implanted Z45.42
    breast prosthesis (external) Z44.3 ☑
    colostomy belt Z46.89
    contact lenses Z46.0
    cystostomy device Z46.6
    dental prosthesis Z46.3
    dentures Z46.3
    device NEC
      abdominal Z46.89
      nervous system Z46.2
        implanted — *see* Admission, adjustment, device, implanted, nervous system
    orthodontic Z46.4
    prosthetic Z44.9
      breast Z44.3 ☑
      dental Z46.3
      eye Z44.2 ☑
    substitution
      auditory Z46.2
        implanted — *see* Admission, adjustment, device, implanted, hearing device
      nervous system Z46.2
        implanted — *see* Admission, adjustment, device, implanted, nervous system
      visual Z46.2
        implanted Z45.31
    hearing aid Z46.1
    ileostomy device Z46.89
    intestinal appliance or device NEC Z46.89
    neuropacemaker (brain) (peripheral nerve) (spinal cord) Z46.2
      implanted Z45.42
    orthodontic device Z46.4
    orthopedic device (brace) (cast) (shoes) Z46.89
    prosthesis Z44.9
      arm — *see* Admission, adjustment, artificial, arm
      breast Z44.3 ☑
      dental Z46.3
      eye Z44.2 ☑
      leg — *see* Admission, adjustment, artificial, leg
      specified type NEC Z44.8
    spectacles Z46.0
  follow-up examination Z09
  intrauterine device management Z30.431
    initial prescription Z30.014
  mental health evaluation Z00.8
    requested by authority Z04.6
  observation — *see* Observation
  Papanicolaou smear, cervix Z12.4
    for suspected malignant neoplasm Z12.4
  plastic and reconstructive surgery following medical procedure or healed injury NEC Z42.8
  plastic surgery, cosmetic NEC Z41.1
  postpartum observation
    immediately after delivery Z39.0
    routine follow-up Z39.2
  poststerilization (for restoration) Z31.0
    aftercare Z31.42
  procreative management Z31.9
  prophylactic (measure) — *see also* Encounter, prophylactic measures
    organ removal Z40.00
      breast Z40.01
      fallopian tube(s) Z40.03
        with ovary(s) Z40.02
      ovary(s) Z40.02
      specified organ NEC Z40.09
      testes Z40.09
    vaccination Z23
  psychiatric examination (general) Z00.8
    requested by authority Z04.6

Admission — *continued*
  radiation therapy (antineoplastic) Z51.0
  reconstructive surgery following medical procedure or healed injury NEC Z42.8
  removal of
    cystostomy catheter Z43.5
    drains Z48.03
    dressing (nonsurgical) Z48.00
    implantable subdermal contraceptive Z30.46
    intrauterine contraceptive device Z30.432
    neuropacemaker (brain) (peripheral nerve) (spinal cord) Z46.2
      implanted Z45.42
    staples Z48.02
    surgical dressing Z48.01
    sutures Z48.02
    ureteral stent Z46.6
  respirator [ventilator] use during power failure Z99.12
  restoration of organ continuity (poststerilization) Z31.0
    aftercare Z31.42
  sensitivity test — *see also* Test, skin
    allergy NEC Z01.82
    Mantoux Z11.1
  tuboplasty following previous sterilization Z31.0
    aftercare Z31.42
  vasoplasty following previous sterilization Z31.0
    aftercare Z31.42
  vision examination Z01.00
    with abnormal findings Z01.01
    following failed vision screening Z01.020
      with abnormal findings Z01.021
    infant or child (over 28 days old) Z00.129
      with abnormal findings Z00.121
  waiting period for admission to other facility Z75.1
Adnexitis (suppurative) — *see* Salpingo-oophoritis
Adolescent X-linked adrenoleukodystrophy E71.521
Adrenal (gland) — *see* condition
Adrenalism, tuberculous A18.7
Adrenalitis, adrenitis E27.8
  autoimmune E27.1
  meningococcal, hemorrhagic A39.1
Adrenarche, premature E27.0
Adrenocortical syndrome — *see* Cushing's, syndrome
Adrenogenital syndrome E25.9
  acquired E25.8
  congenital E25.0
  salt loss E25.0
Adrenogenitalism, congenital E25.0
Adrenoleukodystrophy E71.529
  neonatal E71.511
  X-linked E71.529
    Addison only phenotype E71.528
    Addison-Schilder E71.528
    adolescent E71.521
    adrenomyeloneuropathy E71.522
    childhood cerebral E71.520
    other specified E71.528
Adrenomyeloneuropathy E71.522
Adventitious bursa — *see* Bursopathy, specified type NEC
Adverse effect — *see* Table of Drugs and Chemicals, categories T36-T50, with 6th character 5
Advice — *see* Counseling
Adynamia (episodica) (hereditary) (periodic) G72.3
Aeration lung imperfect, newborn — *see* Atelectasis
Aerobullosis T70.3 ☑
Aerocele — *see* Embolism, air
Aerodermectasia
  subcutaneous (traumatic) T79.7 ☑
Aerodontalgia T70.29 ☑
Aeroembolism T70.3 ☑
Aerogenes capsulatus infection A48.0
Aero-otitis media T70.0 ☑
Aerophagy, aerophagia (psychogenic) F45.8
Aerophobia F40.228
Aerosinusitis T70.1 ☑
Aerotitis T70.0 ☑
Affection — *see* Disease
Afibrinogenemia — *see also* Defect, coagulation D68.8
  acquired D65
  congenital D68.2
  following ectopic or molar pregnancy O08.1
  in abortion — *see* Abortion, by type, complicated by, afibrinogenemia
  puerperal O72.3
African
  sleeping sickness B56.9
  tick fever A68.1

African — *continued*
  trypanosomiasis B56.9
    gambian B56.0
    rhodesian B56.1
Aftercare — *see also* Care Z51.89
  following surgery (for) (on)
    amputation Z47.81
    attention to
      drains Z48.03
      dressings (nonsurgical) Z48.00
        surgical Z48.01
      sutures Z48.02
    circulatory system Z48.812
    delayed (planned) wound closure Z48.1
    digestive system Z48.815
    explantation of joint prosthesis (staged procedure)
      hip Z47.32
      knee Z47.33
      shoulder Z47.31
    genitourinary system Z48.816
    joint replacement Z47.1
    neoplasm Z48.3
    nervous system Z48.811
    oral cavity Z48.814
    organ transplant
      bone marrow Z48.290
      heart Z48.21
      heart-lung Z48.280
      kidney Z48.22
      liver Z48.23
      lung Z48.24
      multiple organs NEC Z48.288
      specified NEC Z48.298
    orthopedic NEC Z47.89
    planned wound closure Z48.1
    removal of internal fixation device Z47.2
    respiratory system Z48.813
    scoliosis Z47.82
    sense organs Z48.810
    skin and subcutaneous tissue Z48.817
    specified body system
      circulatory Z48.812
      digestive Z48.815
      genitourinary Z48.816
      nervous Z48.811
      oral cavity Z48.814
      respiratory Z48.813
      sense organs Z48.810
      skin and subcutaneous tissue Z48.817
      teeth Z48.814
    specified NEC Z48.89
    spinal Z47.89
    teeth Z48.814
  fracture — *code to* fracture with seventh character D
  involving
    removal of
      drains Z48.03
      dressings (nonsurgical) Z48.00
      staples Z48.02
      surgical dressings Z48.01
      sutures Z48.02
  neuropacemaker (brain) (peripheral nerve) (spinal cord) Z46.2
    implanted Z45.42
  orthopedic NEC Z47.89
  postprocedural — *see* Aftercare, following surgery
After-cataract — *see* Cataract, secondary
Agalactia (primary) O92.3
  elective, secondary or therapeutic O92.5
Agammaglobulinemia (acquired (secondary) (nonfamilial) D80.1
  with
    immunoglobulin-bearing B-lymphocytes D80.1
    lymphopenia D81.9
  autosomal recessive (Swiss type) D80.0
  Bruton's X-linked D80.0
  common variable (CVAgamma) D80.1
  congenital sex-linked D80.0
  hereditary D80.0
  lymphopenic D81.9
  Swiss type (autosomal recessive) D80.0
  X-linked (with growth hormone deficiency) (Bruton) D80.0
Aganglionosis (bowel) (colon) Q43.1
Age (old) — *see* Senility
Agenesis
  adrenal (gland) Q89.1
  alimentary tract (complete) (partial) NEC Q45.8

Agenesis — continued
　alimentary tract — continued
　　upper Q40.8
　anus, anal (canal) Q42.3
　　with fistula Q42.2
　aorta Q25.41
　appendix Q42.8
　arm (complete) Q71.0- ☑
　　with hand present Q71.1- ☑
　artery (peripheral) Q27.9
　　brain Q28.3
　　coronary Q24.5
　　pulmonary Q25.79
　　specified NEC Q27.8
　　umbilical Q27.0
　auditory (canal) (external) Q16.1
　auricle (ear) Q16.0
　bile duct or passage Q44.5
　bladder Q64.5
　bone Q79.9
　brain Q00.0
　　part of Q04.3
　breast (with nipple present) Q83.8
　　with absent nipple Q83.0
　bronchus Q32.4
　canaliculus lacrimalis Q10.4
　carpus — see Agenesis, hand
　cartilage Q79.9
　cecum Q42.8
　cerebellum Q04.3
　cervix Q51.5
　chin Q18.8
　cilia Q10.3
　circulatory system, part NOS Q28.9
　clavicle Q74.0
　clitoris Q52.6
　coccyx Q76.49
　colon Q42.9
　　specified NEC Q42.8
　corpus callosum Q04.0
　cricoid cartilage Q31.8
　diaphragm (with hernia) Q79.1
　digestive organ(s) or tract (complete) (partial) NEC Q45.8
　　upper Q40.8
　ductus arteriosus Q28.8
　duodenum Q41.0
　ear Q16.9
　　auricle Q16.0
　　lobe Q17.8
　ejaculatory duct Q55.4
　endocrine (gland) NEC Q89.2
　epiglottis Q31.8
　esophagus Q39.8
　eustachian tube Q16.2
　eye Q11.1
　　adnexa Q15.8
　eyelid (fold) Q10.3
　face
　　bones NEC Q75.8
　　specified part NEC Q18.8
　fallopian tube Q50.6
　femur — see Defect, reduction, lower limb, longitudinal, femur
　fibula — see Defect, reduction, lower limb, longitudinal, fibula
　finger (complete) (partial) — see Agenesis, hand
　foot (and toes) (complete) (partial) Q72.3- ☑
　forearm (with hand present) — see Agenesis, arm, with hand present
　　and hand Q71- ☑
　gallbladder Q44.0
　gastric Q40.2
　genitalia, genital (organ(s))
　　female Q52.8
　　　external Q52.71
　　　internal NEC Q52.8
　　male Q55.8
　glottis Q31.8
　hair Q84.0
　hand (and fingers) (complete) (partial) Q71.3- ☑
　heart Q24.8
　　valve NEC Q24.8
　　　pulmonary Q22.0
　hepatic Q44.7
　humerus — see Defect, reduction, upper limb
　hymen Q52.4
　ileum Q41.2

Agenesis — continued
　incus Q16.3
　intestine (small) Q41.9
　　large Q42.9
　　　specified NEC Q42.8
　iris (dilator fibers) Q13.1
　jaw M26.09
　jejunum Q41.1
　kidney(s) (partial) Q60.2
　　bilateral Q60.1
　　unilateral Q60.0
　labium (majus) (minus) Q52.71
　labyrinth, membranous Q16.5
　lacrimal apparatus Q10.4
　larynx Q31.8
　leg (complete) Q72.0- ☑
　　with foot present Q72.1- ☑
　　lower leg (with foot present) — see Agenesis, leg, with foot present
　　　and foot Q72.2- ☑
　lens Q12.3
　limb (complete) Q73.0
　　lower — see Agenesis, leg
　　upper — see Agenesis, arm
　lip Q38.0
　liver Q44.7
　lung (fissure) (lobe) (bilateral) (unilateral) Q33.3
　mandible, maxilla M26.09
　metacarpus — see Agenesis, hand
　metatarsus — see Agenesis, foot
　muscle Q79.8
　　eyelid Q10.3
　　ocular Q15.8
　musculoskeletal system NEC Q79.8
　nail(s) Q84.3
　neck, part Q18.8
　nerve Q07.8
　nervous system, part NEC Q07.8
　nipple Q83.2
　nose Q30.1
　nuclear Q07.8
　organ
　　of Corti Q16.5
　　or site not listed — see Anomaly, by site
　osseous meatus (ear) Q16.1
　ovary
　　bilateral Q50.02
　　unilateral Q50.01
　oviduct Q50.6
　pancreas Q45.0
　parathyroid (gland) Q89.2
　parotid gland(s) Q38.4
　patella Q74.1
　pelvic girdle (complete) (partial) Q74.2
　penis Q55.5
　pericardium Q24.8
　pituitary (gland) Q89.2
　prostate Q55.4
　punctum lacrimale Q10.4
　radioulnar — see Defect, reduction, upper limb
　radius — see Defect, reduction, upper limb, longitudinal, radius
　rectum Q42.1
　　with fistula Q42.0
　renal Q60.2
　　bilateral Q60.1
　　unilateral Q60.0
　respiratory organ NEC Q34.8
　rib Q76.6
　roof of orbit Q75.8
　round ligament Q52.8
　sacrum Q76.49
　salivary gland Q38.4
　scapula Q74.0
　scrotum Q55.29
　seminal vesicles Q55.4
　septum
　　atrial Q21.1
　　between aorta and pulmonary artery Q21.4
　　ventricular Q20.4
　shoulder girdle (complete) (partial) Q74.0
　skull (bone) Q75.8
　　with
　　　anencephaly Q00.0
　　　encephalocele — see Encephalocele
　　　hydrocephalus Q03.9
　　　　with spina bifida — see Spina bifida, by site, with hydrocephalus

Agenesis — continued
　skull — continued
　　with — continued
　　　microcephaly Q02
　spermatic cord Q55.4
　spinal cord Q06.0
　spine Q76.49
　spleen Q89.01
　sternum Q76.7
　stomach Q40.2
　submaxillary gland(s) (congenital) Q38.4
　tarsus — see Agenesis, foot
　tendon Q79.8
　testicle Q55.0
　thymus (gland) Q89.2
　thyroid (gland) E03.1
　　cartilage Q31.8
　tibia — see Defect, reduction, lower limb, longitudinal, tibia
　tibiofibular — see Defect, reduction, lower limb, specified type NEC
　toe (and foot) (complete) (partial) — see Agenesis, foot
　tongue Q38.3
　trachea (cartilage) Q32.1
　ulna — see Defect, reduction, upper limb, longitudinal, ulna
　upper limb — see Agenesis, arm
　ureter Q62.4
　urethra Q64.5
　urinary tract NEC Q64.8
　uterus Q51.0
　uvula Q38.5
　vagina Q52.0
　vas deferens Q55.4
　vein(s) (peripheral) Q27.9
　　brain Q28.3
　　great NEC Q26.8
　　portal Q26.5
　vena cava (inferior) (superior) Q26.8
　vermis of cerebellum Q04.3
　vertebra Q76.49
　vulva Q52.71
Ageusia R43.2
Agitated — see condition
Agitation R45.1
Aglossia (congenital) Q38.3
Aglossia-adactylia syndrome Q87.0
Aglycogenosis E74.00
Agnosia (body image) (other senses) (tactile) R48.1
　developmental F88
　verbal R48.1
　　auditory R48.1
　　　developmental F80.2
　　developmental F80.2
　visual (object) R48.3
Agoraphobia F40.00
　with panic disorder F40.01
　without panic disorder F40.02
Agrammatism R48.8
Agranulocytopenia — see Agranulocytosis
Agranulocytosis (chronic) (cyclical) (genetic) (infantile) (periodic) (pernicious) — see also Neutropenia D70.9
　congenital D70.0
　cytoreductive cancer chemotherapy sequela D70.1
　drug-induced D70.2
　　due to cytoreductive cancer chemotherapy D70.1
　due to infection D70.3
　secondary D70.4
　　drug-induced D70.2
　　　due to cytoreductive cancer chemotherapy D70.1
Agraphia (absolute) R48.8
　with alexia R48.0
　developmental F81.81
Ague (dumb) — see Malaria
Agyria Q04.3
Ahumada-del Castillo syndrome E23.0
Aichomophobia F40.298
AIDS (related complex) B20
Ailment heart — see Disease, heart
Ailurophobia F40.218
AIN — see Neoplasia, intraepithelial, anal
Ainhum (disease) L94.6
AIPHI (acute idiopathic pulmonary hemorrhage in infants (over 28 days old)) R04.81
Air
　anterior mediastinum J98.2
　compressed, disease T70.3 ☑

Air — *continued*
  conditioner lung or pneumonitis J67.7
  embolism (artery) (cerebral) (any site) T79.0 ☑
    with ectopic or molar pregnancy O08.2
    due to implanted device NEC — *see* Complications, by site and type, specified NEC
    following
      abortion — *see* Abortion by type, complicated by, embolism
      ectopic or molar pregnancy O08.2
      infusion, therapeutic injection or transfusion T80.0 ☑
    in pregnancy, childbirth or puerperium — *see* Embolism, obstetric
    traumatic T79.0 ☑
  hunger, psychogenic F45.8
  rarefied, effects of — *see* Effect, adverse, high altitude
  sickness T75.3 ☑
Airplane sickness T75.3 ☑
Akathisia (drug-induced) (treatment-induced) G25.71
  neuroleptic induced (acute) G25.71
  tardive G25.71
Akinesia R29.898
Akinetic mutism R41.89
Akureyri's disease G93.3
Alactasia, congenital E73.0
Alagille's syndrome Q44.7
Alastrim B03
Albers-Schönberg syndrome Q78.2
Albert's syndrome — *see* Tendinitis, Achilles
Albinism, albino E70.30
  with hematologic abnormality E70.339
    Chédiak-Higashi syndrome E70.330
    Hermansky-Pudlak syndrome E70.331
    other specified E70.338
  I E70.320
  II E70.321
  ocular E70.319
    autosomal recessive E70.311
    other specified E70.318
    X-linked E70.310
  oculocutaneous E70.329
    other specified E70.328
    tyrosinase (ty) negative E70.320
    tyrosinase (ty) positive E70.321
  other specified E70.39
Albinismus E70.30
Albright (-McCune)(-Sternberg) syndrome Q78.1
Albuminous — *see* condition
Albuminuria, albuminuric (acute) (chronic) (subacute)
  — *see also* Proteinuria R80.9
  complicating pregnancy — *see* Proteinuria, gestational
    with
      gestational hypertension — *see* Pre-eclampsia
      pre-existing hypertension — *see* Hypertension, complicating pregnancy, pre-existing, with, pre-eclampsia
  gestational — *see* Proteinuria, gestational
    with
      gestational hypertension — *see* Pre-eclampsia
      pre-existing hypertension — *see* Hypertension, complicating pregnancy, pre-existing, with, pre-eclampsia
  orthostatic R80.2
  postural R80.2
  pre-eclamptic — *see* Pre-eclampsia
  scarlatinal A38.8
Albuminurophobia F40.298
Alcaptonuria E70.29
Alcohol, alcoholic, alcohol-induced
  addiction (without remission) F10.20
    with remission F10.21
  amnestic disorder, persisting F10.96
    with dependence F10.26
  anxiety disorder F10.980
  bipolar and related disorder F10.94
  brain syndrome, chronic F10.97
    with dependence F10.27
  cardiopathy I42.6
  counseling and surveillance Z71.41
    family member Z71.42
  delirium (acute) (tremens) (withdrawal) F10.231
    with intoxication F10.921
      in
        abuse F10.121
        dependence F10.221
  dementia F10.97
    with dependence F10.27

Alcohol, alcoholic, alcohol-induced — *continued*
  depressive disorder F10.94
  deterioration F10.97
    with dependence F10.27
  hallucinosis (acute) F10.951
    in
      abuse F10.151
      dependence F10.251
  insanity F10.959
  intoxication (acute) (without dependence) F10.129
    with
      delirium F10.121
      dependence F10.229
        with delirium F10.221
        uncomplicated F10.220
      uncomplicated F10.120
  jealousy F10.988
  Korsakoff's, Korsakov's, Korsakow's F10.26
  liver K70.9
    acute — *see* Disease, liver, alcoholic, hepatitis
  major neurocognitive disorder, amnestic-confabulatory type F10.96
  major neurocognitive disorder, nonamnestic-confabulatory type F10.97
  mild neurocognitive disorder F10.988
  mania (acute) (chronic) F10.959
  paranoia, paranoid (type) psychosis F10.950
  pellagra E52
  poisoning, accidental (acute) NEC — *see* Table of Drugs and Chemicals, alcohol, poisoning
  psychosis — *see* Psychosis, alcoholic
  psychotic disorder F10.959
  sexual dysfunction F10.981
  sleep disorder F10.982
  withdrawal (without convulsions) F10.239
    with delirium F10.231
Alcoholism (chronic) (without remission) F10.20
  with
    psychosis — *see* Psychosis, alcoholic
    remission F10.21
  Korsakov's F10.96
    with dependence F10.26
Alder (-Reilly) **anomaly or syndrome** (leukocyte granulation) D72.0
Aldosteronism E26.9
  familial (type I) E26.02
  glucocorticoid-remediable E26.02
  primary (due to (bilateral) adrenal hyperplasia) E26.09
  primary NEC E26.09
  secondary E26.1
  specified NEC E26.89
Aldosteronoma D44.10
Aldrich (-Wiskott) **syndrome** (eczema-thrombocytopenia) D82.0
Alektorophobia F40.218
Aleppo boil B55.1
Aleukemic — *see* condition
Aleukia
  congenital D70.0
  hemorrhagica D61.9
    congenital D61.09
  splenica D73.1
Alexia R48.0
  developmental F81.0
  secondary to organic lesion R48.0
Algoneurodystrophy M89.00
  ankle M89.07- ☑
  foot M89.07- ☑
  forearm M89.03- ☑
  hand M89.04- ☑
  lower leg M89.06- ☑
  multiple sites M89.0- ☑
  shoulder M89.01- ☑
  specified site NEC M89.08
  thigh M89.05- ☑
  upper arm M89.02- ☑
Algophobia F40.298
Alienation, mental — *see* Psychosis
Alkalemia E87.3
Alkalosis E87.3
  metabolic E87.3
    with respiratory acidosis E87.4
    of newborn P74.41
  respiratory E87.3
Alkaptonuria E70.29
Allen-Masters syndrome N83.8
Allergy, allergic (reaction) (to) T78.40 ☑
  air-borne substance NEC (rhinitis) J30.89

Allergy, allergic — *continued*
  alveolitis (extrinsic) J67.9
    due to
      Aspergillus clavatus J67.4
      Cryptostroma corticale J67.6
      organisms (fungal, thermophilic actinomycete) growing in ventilation (air conditioning) systems J67.7
    specified type NEC J67.8
  anaphylactic reaction or shock T78.2 ☑
  angioneurotic edema T78.3 ☑
  animal (dander) (epidermal) (hair) (rhinitis) J30.81
  bee sting (anaphylactic shock) — *see* Toxicity, venom, arthropod, bee
  biological — *see* Allergy, drug
  colitis — *see also* Colitis, allergic K52.29
  dander (animal) (rhinitis) J30.81
  dandruff (rhinitis) J30.81
  dental restorative material (existing) K08.55
  dermatitis — *see* Dermatitis, contact, allergic
  diathesis — *see* History, allergy
  drug, medicament & biological (any) (external) (internal) T78.40 ☑
    correct substance properly administered — *see* Table of Drugs and Chemicals, by drug, adverse effect
    wrong substance given or taken NEC (by accident) — *see* Table of Drugs and Chemicals, by drug, poisoning
  due to pollen J30.1
  dust (house) (stock) (rhinitis) J30.89
    with asthma — *see* Asthma, allergic extrinsic
  eczema — *see* Dermatitis, contact, allergic
  epidermal (animal) (rhinitis) J30.81
  feathers (rhinitis) J30.89
  food (any) (ingested) NEC T78.1 ☑
    anaphylactic shock — *see* Shock, anaphylactic, due to food
    dermatitis — *see* Dermatitis, due to, food
    dietary counseling and surveillance Z71.3
    in contact with skin L23.6
    rhinitis J30.5
    status (without reaction) Z91.018
      beef Z91.014
      eggs Z91.012
      lamb Z91.014
      mammalian meats Z91.014
      milk products Z91.011
      peanuts Z91.010
      pork Z91.014
      red meats Z91.014
      seafood Z91.013
      specified NEC Z91.018
  gastrointestinal — *see also* specific type of allergic reaction
    meaning colitis — *see also* Colitis, allergic K52.29
    meaning gastroenteritis — *see also* Gastroenteritis, allergic K52.29
    meaning other adverse food reaction not elsewhere classified T78.1 ☑
  grain J30.1
  grass (hay fever) (pollen) J30.1
    asthma — *see* Asthma, allergic extrinsic
  hair (animal) (rhinitis) J30.81
  history (of) — *see* History, allergy
  horse serum — *see* Allergy, serum
  inhalant (rhinitis) J30.89
    pollen J30.1
  kapok (rhinitis) J30.89
  medicine — *see* Allergy, drug
  milk protein — *see also* Allergy, food Z91.011
    anaphylactic reaction T78.07 ☑
    dermatitis L27.2
    enterocolitis syndrome K52.21
    enteropathy K52.22
    gastroenteritis K52.29
    gastroesophageal reflux — *see also* Reaction, adverse, food K21.9
      with esophagitis (without bleeding) K21.00
        with bleeding K21.01
    proctocolitis K52.29
  nasal, seasonal due to pollen J30.1
  pneumonia J82.89
  pollen (any) (hay fever) J30.1
    asthma — *see* Asthma, allergic extrinsic
  primrose J30.1
  primula J30.1
  proctocolitis K52.29

Allergy, allergic — *continued*
  purpura D69.0
  ragweed (hay fever) (pollen) J30.1
    asthma — *see* Asthma, allergic extrinsic
  rose (pollen) J30.1
  seasonal NEC J30.2
  Senecio jacobae (pollen) J30.1
  serum — *see also* Reaction, serum T80.69 ☑
    anaphylactic shock T80.59 ☑
  shock (anaphylactic) T78.2 ☑
    due to
      administration of blood and blood products T80.51 ☑
      adverse effect of correct medicinal substance properly administered T88.6 ☑
      immunization T80.52 ☑
      serum NEC T80.59 ☑
      vaccination T80.52 ☑
  specific NEC T78.49 ☑
  tree (any) (hay fever) (pollen) J30.1
    asthma — *see* Asthma, allergic extrinsic
  upper respiratory J30.9
  urticaria L50.0
  vaccine — *see* Allergy, serum
  wheat — *see* Allergy, food
Allescheriasis B48.2
Alligator skin disease Q80.9
Allocheiria, allochiria R20.8
Almeida's disease — *see* Paracoccidioidomycosis
Alopecia (hereditaria) (seborrheica) L65.9
  androgenic L64.9
    drug-induced L64.0
    specified NEC L64.8
  areata L63.9
    ophiasis L63.2
    specified NEC L63.8
    totalis L63.0
    universalis L63.1
  cicatricial L66.9
    specified NEC L66.8
  circumscripta L63.9
  congenital, congenitalis Q84.0
  due to cytotoxic drugs NEC L65.8
  mucinosa L65.2
  postinfective NEC L65.8
  postpartum L65.0
  premature L64.8
  specific (syphilitic) A51.32
  specified NEC L65.8
  syphilitic (secondary) A51.32
  totalis (capitis) L63.0
  universalis (entire body) L63.1
  X-ray L58.1
Alpers' disease G31.81
Alpine sickness T70.29 ☑
Alport syndrome Q87.81
ALTE (apparent life threatening event) **in newborn and infant** R68.13
Alteration (of), **Altered**
  awareness
    transient R40.4
    unintended under general anesthesia, during procedure T88.53 ☑
  mental status R41.82
  pattern of family relationships affecting child Z62.898
  sensation
    following
      cerebrovascular disease I69.998
        cerebral infarction I69.398
        intracerebral hemorrhage I69.198
        nontraumatic intracranial hemorrhage NEC I69.298
        specified disease NEC I69.898
        subarachnoid hemorrhage I69.098
Alternating — *see* condition
Altitude, high (effects) — *see* Effect, adverse, high altitude
Aluminosis (of lung) J63.0
Alveolitis
  allergic (extrinsic) — *see* Pneumonitis, hypersensitivity
  due to
    Aspergillus clavatus J67.4
    Cryptostroma corticale J67.6
  fibrosing (cryptogenic) (idiopathic) J84.112
  jaw M27.3
  sicca dolorosa M27.3
Alveolus, alveolar — *see* condition
Alymphocytosis D72.810

Alymphocytosis — *continued*
  thymic (with immunodeficiency) D82.1
Alymphoplasia, thymic D82.1
Alzheimer's disease or sclerosis — *see* Disease, Alzheimer's
Amastia (with nipple present) Q83.8
  with absent nipple Q83.0
Amathophobia F40.228
Amaurosis (acquired) (congenital) — *see also* Blindness
  fugax G45.3
  hysterical F44.6
  Leber's congenital H35.50
  uremic — *see* Uremia
Amaurotic idiocy (infantile) (juvenile) (late) E75.4
Amaxophobia F40.248
Ambiguous genitalia Q56.4
Amblyopia (congenital) (ex anopsia) (partial) (suppression) H53.00- ☑
  anisometropic — *see* Amblyopia, refractive
  deprivation H53.01- ☑
  hysterical F44.6
  nocturnal — *see also* Blindness, night
    vitamin A deficiency E50.5
  refractive H53.02- ☑
  strabismic H53.03- ☑
  suspect H53.04- ☑
  tobacco H53.8
  toxic NEC H53.8
  uremic — *see* Uremia
Ameba, amebic (histolytica) — *see also* Amebiasis
  abscess (liver) A06.4
Amebiasis A06.9
  with abscess — *see* Abscess, amebic
  acute A06.0
  chronic (intestine) A06.1
    with abscess — *see* Abscess, amebic
  cutaneous A06.7
  cutis A06.7
  cystitis A06.81
  genitourinary tract NEC A06.82
  hepatic — *see* Abscess, liver, amebic
  intestine A06.0
  nondysenteric colitis A06.2
  skin A06.7
  specified site NEC A06.89
Ameboma (of intestine) A06.3
Amelia Q73.0
  lower limb — *see* Agenesis, leg
  upper limb — *see* Agenesis, arm
Ameloblastoma — *see also* Cyst, calcifying odontogenic
  long bones C40.9- ☑
    lower limb C40.2- ☑
    upper limb C40.0- ☑
  malignant C41.1
    jaw (bone) (lower) C41.1
      upper C41.0
  tibial C40.2- ☑
Amelogenesis imperfecta K00.5
  nonhereditaria (segmentalis) K00.4
Amenorrhea N91.2
  hyperhormonal E28.8
  primary N91.0
  secondary N91.1
Amentia — *see* Disability, intellectual
  Meynert's (nonalcoholic) F04
American
  leishmaniasis B55.2
  mountain tick fever A93.2
Ametropia — *see* Disorder, refraction
AMH (asymptomatic microscopic hematuria) R31.21
Amianthosis J61
Amimia R48.8
Amino-acid disorder E72.9
  anemia D53.0
Aminoacidopathy E72.9
Aminoaciduria E72.9
Amnesia R41.3
  anterograde R41.1
  auditory R48.8
  dissociative F44.0
    with dissociative fugue F44.1
  hysterical F44.0
  postictal in epilepsy — *see* Epilepsy
  psychogenic F44.0
  retrograde R41.2
  transient global G45.4
Amnes(t)ic syndrome (post-traumatic) F04

Amnes(t)ic syndrome — *continued*
  induced by
    alcohol F10.96
      with dependence F10.26
    psychoactive NEC F19.96
      with
        abuse F19.16
        dependence F19.26
    sedative F13.96
      with dependence F13.26
Amnion, amniotic — *see* condition
Amnionitis — *see* Pregnancy, complicated by
Amok F68.8
Amoral traits F60.89
Amphetamine (or other stimulant) **-induced**
  anxiety disorder F15.980
  bipolar and related disorder F15.94
  delirium F15.921
  depressive disorder F15.94
  obsessive-compulsive and related disorder F15.988
  psychotic disorder F15.959
  sexual dysfunction F15.981
  sleep disorder F15.982
  stimulant withdrawal F15.23
Ampulla
  lower esophagus K22.89
  phrenic K22.89
Amputation — *see also* Absence, by site, acquired
  neuroma (postoperative) (traumatic) — *see* Complications, amputation stump, neuroma
  stump (surgical)
    abnormal, painful, or with complication (late) — *see* Complications, amputation stump
    healed or old NOS Z89.9
  traumatic (complete) (partial)
    arm (upper) (complete) S48.91- ☑
      at
        elbow S58.01- ☑
          partial S58.02- ☑
        shoulder joint (complete) S48.01- ☑
          partial S48.02- ☑
      between
        elbow and wrist (complete) S58.11- ☑
          partial S58.12- ☑
        shoulder and elbow (complete) S48.11- ☑
          partial S48.12- ☑
      partial S48.92- ☑
    breast (complete) S28.21- ☑
      partial S28.22- ☑
    clitoris (complete) S38.211 ☑
      partial S38.212 ☑
    ear (complete) S08.11- ☑
      partial S08.12- ☑
    finger (complete) (metacarpophalangeal) S68.11- ☑
      index S68.11- ☑
      little S68.11- ☑
      middle S68.11- ☑
      partial S68.12- ☑
        index S68.12- ☑
        little S68.12- ☑
        middle S68.12- ☑
        ring S68.12- ☑
      ring S68.11- ☑
      thumb — *see* Amputation, traumatic, thumb
      transphalangeal (complete) S68.61- ☑
        index S68.61- ☑
        little S68.61- ☑
        middle S68.61- ☑
        partial S68.62- ☑
          index S68.62- ☑
          little S68.62- ☑
          middle S68.62- ☑
          ring S68.62- ☑
        ring S68.61- ☑
    foot (complete) S98.91- ☑
      at ankle level S98.01- ☑
        partial S98.02- ☑
      midfoot S98.31- ☑
        partial S98.32- ☑
      partial S98.92- ☑
    forearm (complete) S58.91- ☑
      at elbow level (complete) S58.01- ☑
        partial S58.02- ☑
      between elbow and wrist (complete) S58.11- ☑
        partial S58.12- ☑
      partial S58.92- ☑

▽ **Subterms under main terms may continue to next column or page**   ☑ **Additional Character Required — Refer to the Tabular List for Character Selection**   **17**

Allergy, allergic — Amputation

Amputation — *continued*
  traumatic — *continued*
    genital organ(s) (external)
      female (complete) S38.211 ☑
        partial S38.212 ☑
      male
        penis (complete) S38.221 ☑
          partial S38.222 ☑
        scrotum (complete) S38.231 ☑
          partial S38.232 ☑
        testes (complete) S38.231 ☑
          partial S38.232 ☑
    hand (complete) (wrist level) S68.41- ☑
      finger(s) alone — *see* Amputation, traumatic, finger
      partial S68.42- ☑
      thumb alone — *see* Amputation, traumatic, thumb
      transmetacarpal (complete) S68.71- ☑
        partial S68.72- ☑
    head
      ear — *see* Amputation, traumatic, ear
      nose (partial) S08.812 ☑
        complete S08.811 ☑
      part S08.89 ☑
      scalp S08.0 ☑
    hip (and thigh) (complete) S78.91- ☑
      at hip joint (complete) S78.01- ☑
        partial S78.02- ☑
      between hip and knee (complete) S78.11- ☑
        partial S78.12- ☑
      partial S78.92- ☑
    labium (majus) (minus) (complete) S38.21- ☑
      partial S38.21- ☑
    leg (lower) S88.91- ☑
      at knee level S88.01- ☑
        partial S88.02- ☑
      between knee and ankle S88.11- ☑
        partial S88.12- ☑
      partial S88.92- ☑
    nose (partial) S08.812 ☑
      complete S08.811 ☑
    penis (complete) S38.221 ☑
      partial S38.222 ☑
    scrotum (complete) S38.231 ☑
      partial S38.232 ☑
    shoulder — *see* Amputation, traumatic, arm
      at shoulder joint — *see* Amputation, traumatic, arm, at shoulder joint
    testes (complete) S38.231 ☑
      partial S38.232 ☑
    thigh — *see* Amputation, traumatic, hip
    thorax, part of S28.1 ☑
      breast — *see* Amputation, traumatic, breast
    thumb (complete) (metacarpophalangeal) S68.01- ☑
      partial S68.02- ☑
      transphalangeal (complete) S68.51- ☑
        partial S68.52- ☑
    toe (lesser) S98.13- ☑
      great S98.11- ☑
        partial S98.12- ☑
      more than one S98.21- ☑
        partial S98.22- ☑
      partial S98.14- ☑
    vulva (complete) S38.211 ☑
      partial S38.212 ☑
Amputee (bilateral) (old) Z89.9
Amsterdam dwarfism Q87.19
Amusia R48.8
  developmental F80.89
Amyelencephalus, amyelencephaly Q00.0
Amyelia Q06.0
Amygdalitis — *see* Tonsillitis
Amygdalolith J35.8
Amyloid heart (disease) E85.4 *[I43]*
Amyloidosis (generalized) (primary) E85.9
  with lung involvement E85.4 *[J99]*
  familial E85.2
  genetic E85.2
  heart E85.4 *[I43]*
  hemodialysis-associated E85.3
  light chain (AL) E85.81
  liver E85.4 *[K77]*
  localized E85.4
  neuropathic heredofamilial E85.1

Amyloidosis — *continued*
  non-neuropathic heredofamilial E85.0
  organ limited E85.4
  Portuguese E85.1
  pulmonary E85.4 *[J99]*
  secondary systemic E85.3
  senile systemic (SSA) E85.82
  skin (lichen) (macular) E85.4 *[L99]*
  specified NEC E85.89
  subglottic E85.4 *[J99]*
  wild-type transthyretin-related (ATTR) E85.82
Amylopectinosis (brancher enzyme deficiency) E74.03
Amylophagia — *see* Pica
Amyoplasia congenita Q79.8
Amyotonia M62.89
  congenita G70.2
Amyotrophia, amyotrophy, amyotrophic G71.8
  congenita Q79.8
  diabetic — *see* Diabetes, amyotrophy
  lateral sclerosis G12.21
  neuralgic G54.5
  spinal progressive G12.25
Anacidity, gastric K31.83
  psychogenic F45.8
Anaerosis of newborn P28.89
Analbuminemia E88.09
Analgesia — *see* Anesthesia
Analphalipoproteinemia E78.6
Anaphylactic
  purpura D69.0
  shock or reaction — *see* Shock, anaphylactic
Anaphylactoid shock or reaction — *see* Shock, anaphylactic
Anaphylactoid syndrome of pregnancy O88.01- ☑
Anaphylaxis — *see* Shock, anaphylactic
Anaplasia cervix — *see also* Dysplasia, cervix N87.9
Anaplasmosis [A. phagocytophilum] (transfusion transmitted) A79.82
  human A77.49
Anarthria R47.1
Anasarca R60.1
  cardiac — *see* Failure, heart, congestive
  lung J18.2
  newborn P83.2
  nutritional E43
  pulmonary J18.2
  renal N04.9
Anastomosis
  aneurysmal — *see* Aneurysm
  arteriovenous ruptured brain I60.8
    intracerebral I61.8
    intraparenchymal I61.8
    intraventricular I61.5
    subarachnoid I60.8
  intestinal K63.89
    complicated NEC K91.89
      involving urinary tract N99.89
  retinal and choroidal vessels (congenital) Q14.8
Anatomical narrow angle H40.03- ☑
Ancylostoma, ancylostomiasis (braziliense) (caninum) (ceylanicum) (duodenale) B76.0
  Necator americanus B76.1
Andersen's disease (glycogen storage) E74.09
Anderson-Fabry disease E75.21
Andes disease T70.29 ☑
Andrews' disease (bacterid) L08.89
Androblastoma
  benign
    specified site — *see* Neoplasm, benign, by site
    unspecified site
      female D27.9
      male D29.20
  malignant
    specified site — *see* Neoplasm, malignant, by site
    unspecified site
      female C56.9
      male C62.90
  specified site — *see* Neoplasm, uncertain behavior, by site
  tubular
    with lipid storage
      specified site — *see* Neoplasm, benign, by site
      unspecified site
        female D27.9
        male D29.20
    specified site — *see* Neoplasm, benign, by site

Androblastoma — *continued*
  tubular — *continued*
    unspecified site
      female D27.9
      male D29.20
  unspecified site
    female D39.10
    male D40.10
Androgen insensitivity syndrome — *see also* Syndrome, androgen insensitivity E34.50
Androgen resistance syndrome — *see also* Syndrome, androgen insensitivity E34.50
Android pelvis Q74.2
  with disproportion (fetopelvic) O33.3 ☑
    causing obstructed labor O65.3
Androphobia F40.290
Anectasis, pulmonary (newborn) — *see* Atelectasis
Anemia (essential) (general) (hemoglobin deficiency) (infantile) (primary) (profound) D64.9
  with (due to) (in)
    disorder of
      anaerobic glycolysis D55.29
      pentose phosphate pathway D55.1
    koilonychia D50.9
  achlorhydric D50.8
  achrestic D53.1
  Addison (-Biermer) (pernicious) D51.0
  agranulocytic — *see* Agranulocytosis
  amino-acid-deficiency D53.0
  aplastic D61.9
    congenital D61.09
    drug-induced D61.1
    due to
      drugs D61.1
      external agents NEC D61.2
      infection D61.2
      radiation D61.2
    idiopathic D61.3
    red cell (pure) D60.9
      chronic D60.0
      congenital D61.01
      specified type NEC D60.8
      transient D60.1
    specified type NEC D61.89
    toxic D61.2
  aregenerative
    congenital D61.09
  asiderotic D50.9
  atypical (primary) D64.9
  Baghdad spring D55.0
  Balantidium coli A07.0
  Biermer's (pernicious) D51.0
  blood loss (chronic) D50.0
    acute D62
  bothriocephalus B70.0 *[D63.8]*
  brickmaker's B76.9 *[D63.8]*
  cerebral I67.89
  childhood D58.9
  chlorotic D50.8
  chronic
    blood loss D50.0
    hemolytic D58.9
      idiopathic D59.9
    simple D53.9
  chronica congenita aregenerativa D61.09
  combined system disease NEC D51.0 *[G32.0]*
    due to dietary vitamin B12 deficiency D51.3 *[G32.0]*
  complicating pregnancy, childbirth or puerperium — *see* Pregnancy, complicated by (management affected by), anemia
  congenital P61.4
    aplastic D61.09
    due to isoimmunization NOS P55.9
    dyserythropoietic, dyshematopoietic D64.4
    following fetal blood loss P61.3
    Heinz body D58.2
    hereditary hemolytic NOS D58.9
    pernicious D51.0
    spherocytic D58.0
  Cooley's (erythroblastic) D56.1
  cytogenic D51.0
  deficiency D53.9
    2, 3 diphosphoglycurate mutase D55.29
    2, 3 PG D55.29
    6 phosphogluconate dehydrogenase D55.1
    6-PGD D55.1
    amino-acid D53.0
    combined B12 and folate D53.1

☑ **Additional Character Required** — Refer to the Tabular List for Character Selection   ▽ Subterms under main terms may continue to next column or page

Anemia — *continued*
  deficiency — *continued*
    enzyme D55.9
      drug-induced (hemolytic) D59.2
      glucose-6-phosphate dehydrogenase (G6PD) D55.0
      glycolytic D55.29
      nucleotide metabolism D55.3
      related to hexose monophosphate (HMP) shunt pathway NEC D55.1
      specified type NEC D55.8
    erythrocytic glutathione D55.1
    folate D52.9
      dietary D52.0
      drug-induced D52.1
    folic acid D52.9
      dietary D52.0
      drug-induced D52.1
    G SH D55.1
    G6PD D55.0
    GGS-R D55.1
    glucose-6-phosphate dehydrogenase D55.0
    glutathione reductase D55.1
    glyceraldehyde phosphate dehydrogenase D55.29
    hexokinase D55.29
    iron D50.9
      secondary to blood loss (chronic) D50.0
    nutritional D53.9
      with
        poor iron absorption D50.8
        specified deficiency NEC D53.8
    phosphofructo-aldolase D55.29
    phosphoglycerate kinase D55.29
    PK D55.21
    protein D53.0
    pyruvate kinase D55.21
    transcobalamin II D51.2
    triose-phosphate isomerase D55.29
    vitamin B12 NOS D51.9
      dietary D51.3
      due to
        intrinsic factor deficiency D51.0
        selective vitamin B12 malabsorption with proteinuria D51.1
      pernicious D51.0
      specified type NEC D51.8
  Diamond-Blackfan (congenital hypoplastic) D61.01
  dibothriocephalus B70.0 *[D63.8]*
  dimorphic D53.1
  diphasic D53.1
  Diphyllobothrium (Dibothriocephalus) B70.0 *[D63.8]*
  due to (in) (with)
    antineoplastic chemotherapy D64.81
    blood loss (chronic) D50.0
      acute D62
    chemotherapy, antineoplastic D64.81
    chronic disease classified elsewhere NEC D63.8
    chronic kidney disease D63.1
    deficiency
      amino-acid D53.0
      copper D53.8
      folate (folic acid) D52.9
        dietary D52.0
        drug-induced D52.1
      molybdenum D53.8
      protein D53.0
      zinc D53.8
    dietary vitamin B12 deficiency D51.3
    disorder of
      glutathione metabolism D55.1
      nucleotide metabolism D55.3
    drug — *see* Anemia, by type — *see also* Table of Drugs and Chemicals
    end stage renal disease D63.1
    enzyme disorder D55.9
    fetal blood loss P61.3
    fish tapeworm (D.latum) infestation B70.0 *[D63.8]*
    hemorrhage (chronic) D50.0
      acute D62
    impaired absorption D50.9
    loss of blood (chronic) D50.0
      acute D62
    myxedema E03.9 *[D63.8]*
    Necator americanus B76.1 *[D63.8]*
    prematurity P61.2
    selective vitamin B12 malabsorption with protein-uria D51.1
    transcobalamin II deficiency D51.2
  Dyke-Young type (secondary) (symptomatic) D59.19

Anemia — *continued*
  dyserythropoietic (congenital) D64.4
  dyshematopoietic (congenital) D64.4
  Egyptian B76.9 *[D63.8]*
  elliptocytosis — *see* Elliptocytosis
  enzyme-deficiency, drug-induced D59.2
  epidemic — *see also* Ancylostomiasis B76.9 *[D63.8]*
  erythroblastic
    familial D56.1
    newborn — *see also* Disease, hemolytic P55.9
    of childhood D56.1
  erythrocytic glutathione deficiency D55.1
  erythropoietin-resistant anemia (EPO resistant anemia) D63.1
  Faber's (achlorhydric anemia) D50.9
  factitious (self-induced blood letting) D50.0
  familial erythroblastic D56.1
  Fanconi's (congenital pancytopenia) D61.09
  favism D55.0
  fish tapeworm (D. latum) infestation B70.0 *[D63.8]*
  folate (folic acid) deficiency D52.9
  glucose-6-phosphate dehydrogenase (G6PD) deficiency D55.0
  glutathione-reductase deficiency D55.1
  goat's milk D52.0
  granulocytic — *see* Agranulocytosis
  Heinz body, congenital D58.2
  hemolytic D58.9
    acquired D59.9
      with hemoglobinuria NEC D59.6
      autoimmune NEC D59.19
      infectious D59.4
      specified type NEC D59.8
      toxic D59.4
    acute D59.9
      due to enzyme deficiency specified type NEC D55.8
      Lederer's D59.19
    autoimmune D59.10
      cold D59.12
      drug-induced D59.0
      mixed D59.13
      warm D59.11
    chronic D58.9
      idiopathic D59.9
    cold type (primary) (secondary) (symptomatic) D59.12
    congenital (spherocytic) — *see* Spherocytosis
    due to
      cardiac conditions D59.4
      drugs (nonautoimmune) D59.2
        autoimmune D59.0
      enzyme disorder D55.9
        drug-induced D59.2
      presence of shunt or other internal prosthetic device D59.4
    familial D58.9
    hereditary D58.9
      due to enzyme disorder D55.9
        specified type NEC D55.8
      specified type NEC D58.8
    idiopathic (chronic) D59.9
    mechanical D59.4
    microangiopathic D59.4
    mixed type (primary) (secondary) (symptomatic) D59.13
    nonautoimmune D59.4
      drug-induced D59.2
    nonspherocytic
      congenital or hereditary NEC D55.8
        glucose-6-phosphate dehydrogenase deficien-cy D55.0
        pyruvate kinase deficiency D55.21
        type
          I D55.1
          II D55.29
      type
        I D55.1
        II D55.29
    primary
      autoimmune
        cold type D59.12
        mixed type D59.13
        warm type D59.11
    secondary D59.4
      autoimmune
        cold type D59.12
        mixed type D59.13

Anemia — *continued*
  hemolytic — *continued*
    secondary — *continued*
      autoimmune — *continued*
        warm type D59.11
      specified (hereditary) type NEC D58.8
      Stransky-Regala type — *see also* Hemoglobinopathy D58.8
      symptomatic D59.4
        autoimmune
          cold type D59.12
          mixed type D59.13
          warm type D59.11
      toxic D59.4
      warm type (primary) (secondary) (symptomatic) D59.11
  hemorrhagic (chronic) D50.0
    acute D62
  Herrick's D57.1
  hexokinase deficiency D55.29
  hookworm B76.9 *[D63.8]*
  hypochromic (idiopathic) (microcytic) (normoblastic) D50.9
    due to blood loss (chronic) D50.0
      acute D62
    familial sex-linked D64.0
    pyridoxine-responsive D64.3
    sideroblastic, sex-linked D64.0
  hypoplasia, red blood cells D61.9
    congenital or familial D61.01
  hypoplastic (idiopathic) D61.9
    congenital or familial (of childhood) D61.01
  hypoproliferative (refractive) D61.9
  idiopathic D64.9
    aplastic D61.3
    hemolytic, chronic D59.9
  in (due to) (with)
    chronic kidney disease D63.1
    end stage renal disease D63.1
    failure, kidney (renal) D63.1
    neoplastic disease — *see also* Neoplasm D63.0
  intertropical — *see also* Ancylostomiasis D63.8
  iron deficiency D50.9
    secondary to blood loss (chronic) D50.0
      acute D62
    specified type NEC D50.8
  Joseph-Diamond-Blackfan (congenital hypoplastic) D61.01
  Lederer's (hemolytic) D59.19
  leukoerythroblastic D61.82
  macrocytic D53.9
    nutritional D52.0
    tropical D52.8
  malarial — *see also* Malaria B54 *[D63.8]*
  malignant (progressive) D51.0
  malnutrition D53.9
  marsh — *see also* Malaria B54 *[D63.8]*
  Mediterranean (with other hemoglobinopathy) D56.9
  megaloblastic D53.1
    combined B12 and folate deficiency D53.1
    hereditary D51.1
    nutritional D52.0
    orotic aciduria D53.0
    refractory D53.1
    specified type NEC D53.1
  megalocytic D53.1
  microcytic (hypochromic) D50.9
    due to blood loss (chronic) D50.0
      acute D62
    familial D56.8
  microdrepanocytosis D57.40
  microelliptopoikilocytic (Rietti-Greppi- Micheli) D56.9
  miner's B76.9 *[D63.8]*
  myelodysplastic D46.9
  myelofibrosis D75.81
  myelogenous D64.89
  myelopathic D64.89
  myelophthisic D61.82
  myeloproliferative D47.Z9 *(following D47.4)*
  newborn P61.4
    due to
      ABO (antibodies, isoimmunization, maternal/fetal incompatibility) P55.1
      Rh (antibodies, isoimmunization, maternal/fetal incompatibility) P55.0
    following fetal blood loss P61.3
    posthemorrhagic (fetal) P61.3

Subterms under main terms may continue to next column or page   ☑ **Additional Character Required** — Refer to the Tabular List for Character Selection   **19**

Anemia — Anemia

Anemia — continued

nonspherocytic hemolytic — see Anemia, hemolytic, nonspherocytic

normocytic (infectional) D64.9
    due to blood loss (chronic) D50.0
        acute D62
    myelophthisic D61.82

nutritional (deficiency) D53.9
    with
        poor iron absorption D50.8
        specified deficiency NEC D53.8
    megaloblastic D52.0

of prematurity P61.2

orotaciduric (congenital) (hereditary) D53.0

osteosclerotic D64.89

ovalocytosis (hereditary) — see Elliptocytosis

paludal — see also Malaria B54 *[D63.8]*

pernicious (congenital) (malignant) (progressive) D51.0

pleochromic D64.89
    of sprue D52.8

posthemorrhagic (chronic) D50.0
    acute D62
    newborn P61.3

postoperative (postprocedural)
    due to (acute) blood loss D62
        chronic blood loss D50.0
    specified NEC D64.89

postpartum O90.81

pressure D64.89

progressive D64.9
    malignant D51.0
    pernicious D51.0

protein-deficiency D53.0

pseudoleukemica infantum D64.89

pure red cell D60.9
    congenital D61.01

pyridoxine-responsive D64.3

pyruvate kinase deficiency D55.21

refractory D46.4
    with
        excess of blasts D46.20
            1 (RAEB 1) D46.21
            2 (RAEB 2) D46.22
            in transformation (RAEB T) — see Leukemia, acute myeloblastic
        hemochromatosis D46.1
        sideroblasts (ring) (RARS) D46.1
    megaloblastic D53.1
    sideroblastic D46.1
    sideropenic D50.9
    without ring sideroblasts, so stated D46.0
    without sideroblasts without excess of blasts D46.0

Rietti-Greppi-Micheli D56.9

scorbutic D53.2

secondary to
    blood loss (chronic) D50.0
        acute D62
    hemorrhage (chronic) D50.0
        acute D62

semiplastic D61.89

sickle-cell — see Disease, sickle-cell

sideroblastic D64.3
    hereditary D64.0
    hypochromic, sex-linked D64.0
    pyridoxine-responsive NEC D64.3
    refractory D46.1
    secondary (due to)
        disease D64.1
        drugs and toxins D64.2
    specified type NEC D64.3

sideropenic (refractory) D50.9
    due to blood loss (chronic) D50.0
        acute D62

simple chronic D53.9

specified type NEC D64.89

spherocytic (hereditary) — see Spherocytosis

splenic D64.89

splenomegalic D64.89

stomatocytosis D58.8

syphilitic (acquired) (late) A52.79 *[D63.8]*

target cell D64.89

thalassemia D56.9

thrombocytopenic — see Thrombocytopenia

toxic D61.2

tropical B76.9 *[D63.8]*
    macrocytic D52.8

tuberculous A18.89 *[D63.8]*

vegan D51.3

Anemia — continued

vitamin
    B12 deficiency (dietary) pernicious D51.0
    B6-responsive D64.3
von Jaksch's D64.89
Witts' (achlorhydric anemia) D50.8

Anemophobia F40.228

Anencephalus, anencephaly Q00.0

Anergasia — see Psychosis, organic

Anesthesia, anesthetic R20.0

complication or reaction NEC — see also Complications, anesthesia T88.59 ☑

due to
    correct substance properly administered — see Table of Drugs and Chemicals, by drug, adverse effect
    overdose or wrong substance given — see Table of Drugs and Chemicals, by drug, poisoning

unintended awareness under general anesthesia during procedure T88.53 ☑

personal history of Z92.84

cornea H18.81- ☑

dissociative F44.6

functional (hysterical) F44.6

hyperesthetic, thalamic G89.0

hysterical F44.6

local skin lesion R20.0

sexual (psychogenic) F52.1

shock (due to) T88.2 ☑

skin R20.0

testicular N50.9

Anetoderma (maculosum) (of) L90.8
Jadassohn-Pellizzari L90.2
Schweniger-Buzzi L90.1

Aneurin deficiency E51.9

Aneurysm (anastomotic) (artery) (cirsoid) (diffuse) (false) (fusiform) (multiple) (saccular) I72.9

abdominal (aorta) I71.4
    ruptured I71.3
    syphilitic A52.01

aorta, aortic (nonsyphilitic) I71.9
    abdominal I71.4
        ruptured I71.3
    arch I71.2
        ruptured I71.1
    arteriosclerotic I71.9
        ruptured I71.8
    ascending I71.2
        ruptured I71.1
    congenital Q25.43
    descending I71.9
        abdominal I71.4
            ruptured I71.3
        ruptured I71.8
        thoracic I71.2
            ruptured I71.1
    root Q25.43
    ruptured I71.8
    sinus, congenital Q25.43
    syphilitic A52.01
    thoracic I71.2
        ruptured I71.1
    thoracoabdominal I71.6
        ruptured I71.5
    thorax, thoracic (arch) I71.2
        ruptured I71.1
    transverse I71.2
        ruptured I71.1
    valve (heart) — see also Endocarditis, aortic I35.8

arteriosclerotic I72.9
    cerebral I67.1
        ruptured — see Hemorrhage, intracranial, subarachnoid

arteriovenous (congenital) — see also Malformation, arteriovenous
    acquired I77.0
        brain I67.1
            ruptured — see Aneurysm, arteriovenous, brain, ruptured
        coronary I25.41
        pulmonary I28.0
    brain Q28.2
        ruptured I60.8
            intracerebral I61.8
            intraparenchymal I61.8
            intraventricular I61.5
            subarachnoid I60.8

Aneurysm — continued

arteriovenous — see also Malformation, arteriovenous — continued
    peripheral — see Malformation, arteriovenous, peripheral
    precerebral vessels Q28.0
    specified site NEC — see also Malformation, arteriovenous
    acquired I77.0

basal — see Aneurysm, brain

basilar (trunk) I72.5

berry (congenital) (nonruptured) I67.1
    ruptured I60.7

brain I67.1
    arteriosclerotic I67.1
        ruptured — see Hemorrhage, intracranial, subarachnoid
    arteriovenous (congenital) (nonruptured) Q28.2
        acquired I67.1
            ruptured — see Aneurysm, arteriovenous, brain, ruptured I60.8-
        ruptured — see Aneurysm, arteriovenous, brain, ruptured I60.8-
    berry (congenital) (nonruptured) I67.1
        ruptured — see also Hemorrhage, intracranial, subarachnoid I60.7
    congenital Q28.3
        ruptured I60.7
    meninges I67.1
        ruptured I60.8
    miliary (congenital) (nonruptured) I67.1
        ruptured — see also Hemorrhage, intracranial, subarachnoid I60.7
    mycotic I33.0
    ruptured — see Aneurysm, arteriovenous, brain, ruptured I60.8
    syphilitic (hemorrhage) A52.05

cardiac (false) — see also Aneurysm, heart I25.3

carotid artery (common) (external) I72.0
    internal (intracranial) I67.1
        extracranial portion I72.0
        ruptured into brain I60.0- ☑
    syphilitic A52.09
        intracranial A52.05

cavernous sinus I67.1
    arteriovenous (congenital) (nonruptured) Q28.3
        ruptured I60.8

celiac I72.8

central nervous system, syphilitic A52.05

cerebral — see Aneurysm, brain

chest — see Aneurysm, thorax

circle of Willis I67.1
    congenital Q28.3
        ruptured I60.6
    ruptured I60.6

common iliac artery I72.3

congenital (peripheral) Q27.8
    aorta (root) (sinus) Q25.43
    brain Q28.3
        ruptured I60.7
    coronary Q24.5
    digestive system Q27.8
    lower limb Q27.8
    pulmonary Q25.79
    retina Q14.1
    specified site NEC Q27.8
    upper limb Q27.8

conjunctiva — see Abnormality, conjunctiva, vascular

conus arteriosus — see Aneurysm, heart

coronary (arteriosclerotic) (artery) I25.41
    arteriovenous, congenital Q24.5
    congenital Q24.5
    ruptured — see Infarct, myocardium
    syphilitic A52.06
    vein I25.89

cylindroid (aorta) I71.9
    ruptured I71.8
    syphilitic A52.01

ductus arteriosus Q25.0

endocardial, infective (any valve) I33.0

femoral (artery) (ruptured) I72.4

gastroduodenal I72.8

gastroepiploic I72.8

heart (wall) (chronic or with a stated duration of over 4 weeks) I25.3
    valve — see Endocarditis

hepatic I72.8

iliac (common) (artery) (ruptured) I72.3

Aneurysm — continued
infective I72.9
  endocardial (any valve) I33.0
innominate (nonsyphilitic) I72.8
  syphilitic A52.09
interauricular septum — see Aneurysm, heart
interventricular septum — see Aneurysm, heart
intrathoracic (nonsyphilitic) I71.2
  ruptured I71.1
  syphilitic A52.01
lower limb I72.4
lung (pulmonary artery) I28.1
mediastinal (nonsyphilitic) I72.8
  syphilitic A52.09
miliary (congenital) I67.1
  ruptured — see Hemorrhage, intracerebral, sub-
    arachnoid, intracranial
mitral (heart) (valve) I34.8
mural — see Aneurysm, heart
mycotic I72.9
  endocardial (any valve) I33.0
  ruptured, brain — see Hemorrhage, intracerebral,
    subarachnoid
myocardium — see Aneurysm, heart
neck I72.0
pancreaticoduodenal I72.8
patent ductus arteriosus Q25.0
peripheral NEC I72.8
  congenital Q27.8
    digestive system Q27.8
    lower limb Q27.8
    specified site NEC Q27.8
    upper limb Q27.8
popliteal (artery) (ruptured) I72.4
precerebral
  congenital (nonruptured) Q28.1
  specified site, NEC I72.5
pulmonary I28.1
  arteriovenous Q25.72
    acquired I28.0
  syphilitic A52.09
  valve (heart) — see Endocarditis, pulmonary
racemose (peripheral) I72.9
  congenital — see Aneurysm, congenital
radial I72.1
Rasmussen NEC A15.0
renal (artery) I72.2
retina — see also Disorder, retina, microaneurysms
  congenital Q14.1
  diabetic — see E08-E13 with .3-
sinus of Valsalva Q25.49
specified NEC I72.8
spinal (cord) I72.8
  syphilitic (hemorrhage) A52.09
splenic I72.8
subclavian (artery) (ruptured) I72.8
  syphilitic A52.09
superior mesenteric I72.8
syphilitic (aorta) A52.01
  central nervous system A52.05
  congenital (late) A50.54 [I79.0]
  spine, spinal A52.09
thoracoabdominal (aorta) I71.6
  ruptured I71.5
  syphilitic A52.01
thorax, thoracic (aorta) (arch) (nonsyphilitic) I71.2
  ruptured I71.1
  syphilitic A52.01
traumatic (complication) (early), specified site — see
    Injury, blood vessel
tricuspid (heart) (valve) I07.8
ulnar I72.1
upper limb (ruptured) I72.1
valve, valvular — see Endocarditis
venous — see also Varix I86.8
  congenital Q27.8
    digestive system Q27.8
    lower limb Q27.8
    specified site NEC Q27.8
    upper limb Q27.8
ventricle — see Aneurysm, heart
vertebral artery I72.6
visceral NEC I72.8
Angelman syndrome Q93.51
Anger R45.4
Angiectasis, angiectopia I99.8
Angiitis I77.6
allergic granulomatous M30.1

Angiitis — continued
hypersensitivity M31.0
necrotizing M31.9
  specified NEC M31.8
nervous system, granulomatous I67.7
Angina (attack) (cardiac) (chest) (heart) (pectoris) (syn-
    drome) (vasomotor) I20.9
  with
    atherosclerotic heart disease — see Arteriosclerosis,
      coronary (artery),
    documented spasm I20.1
  abdominal K55.1
  accelerated — see Angina, unstable
  agranulocytic — see Agranulocytosis
  angiospastic — see Angina, with documented spasm
  aphthous B08.5
  crescendo — see Angina, unstable
  croupous J05.0
  cruris I73.9
  de novo effort — see Angina, unstable
  diphtheritic, membranous A36.0
  equivalent I20.8
  exudative, chronic J37.0
  following acute myocardial infarction I23.7
  gangrenous diphtheritic A36.0
  intestinal K55.1
  Ludovici K12.2
  Ludwig's K12.2
  malignant diphtheritic A36.0
  membranous J05.0
    diphtheritic A36.0
    Vincent's A69.1
  mesenteric K55.1
  monocytic — see Mononucleosis, infectious
  of effort — see Angina, specified NEC
  phlegmonous J36
    diphtheritic A36.0
  post-infarctional I23.7
  pre-infarctional — see Angina, unstable
  Prinzmetal — see Angina, with documented spasm
  progressive — see Angina, unstable
  pseudomembranous A69.1
  pultaceous, diphtheritic A36.0
  spasm-induced — see Angina, with documented spasm
  specified NEC I20.8
  stable I20.8
  stenocardia — see Angina, specified NEC
  stridulous, diphtheritic A36.2
  tonsil J36
  trachealis J05.0
  unstable I20.0
  variant — see Angina, with documented spasm
  Vincent's A69.1
  worsening effort — see Angina, unstable
Angioblastoma — see Neoplasm, connective tissue,
    uncertain behavior
Angiocholecystitis — see Cholecystitis, acute
Angiocholitis — see also Cholecystitis, acute K83.09
Angiodysgenesis spinalis G95.19
Angiodysplasia (cecum) (colon) K55.20
  with bleeding K55.21
  duodenum (and stomach) K31.819
    with bleeding K31.811
  stomach (and duodenum) K31.819
    with bleeding K31.811
Angioedema (allergic) (any site) (with urticaria) T78.3 ☑
  episodic, with eosinophilia D72.118
  hereditary D84.1
Angioendothelioma — see Neoplasm, uncertain behav-
    ior, by site
  benign D18.00
    intra-abdominal D18.03
    intracranial D18.02
    skin D18.01
    specified site NEC D18.09
  bone — see Neoplasm, bone, malignant
  Ewing's — see Neoplasm, bone, malignant
Angioendotheliomatosis C85.8- ☑
Angiofibroma — see also Neoplasm, benign, by site
  juvenile
    specified site — see Neoplasm, benign, by site
    unspecified site D10.6
Angiohemophilia (A) (B) D68.0
Angioid streaks (choroid) (macula) (retina) H35.33
Angiokeratoma — see Neoplasm, skin, benign
  corporis diffusum E75.21
Angioleiomyoma — see Neoplasm, connective tissue,
    benign

Angiolipoma — see also Lipoma
  infiltrating — see Lipoma
Angioma — see also Hemangioma, by site
  capillary I78.1
  hemorrhagicum hereditaria I78.0
  intra-abdominal D18.03
  intracranial D18.02
  malignant — see Neoplasm, connective tissue, malig-
    nant
  plexiform D18.00
    intra-abdominal D18.03
    intracranial D18.02
    skin D18.01
    specified site NEC D18.09
  senile I78.1
  serpiginosum L81.7
  skin D18.01
  specified site NEC D18.09
  spider I78.1
  stellate I78.1
  venous Q28.3
Angiomatosis Q82.8
  bacillary A79.89
  encephalotrigeminal Q85.8
  hemorrhagic familial I78.0
  hereditary familial I78.0
  liver K76.4
Angiomyolipoma — see Lipoma
Angiomyoliposarcoma — see Neoplasm, connective
    tissue, malignant
Angiomyoma — see Neoplasm, connective tissue, benign
Angiomyosarcoma — see Neoplasm, connective tissue,
    malignant
Angiomyxoma — see Neoplasm, connective tissue, un-
    certain behavior
Angioneurosis F45.8
Angioneurotic edema (allergic) (any site) (with urticaria)
    T78.3 ☑
  hereditary D84.1
Angiopathia, angiopathy I99.9
  cerebral I67.9
    amyloid E85.4 [I68.0]
  diabetic (peripheral) — see Diabetes, angiopathy
  peripheral I73.9
    diabetic — see Diabetes, angiopathy
    specified type NEC I73.89
  retinae syphilitica A52.05
  retinalis (juvenilis)
    diabetic — see Diabetes, retinopathy
    proliferative — see Retinopathy, proliferative
Angiosarcoma — see also Neoplasm, connective tissue,
    malignant
  liver C22.3
Angiosclerosis — see Arteriosclerosis
Angiospasm (peripheral) (traumatic) (vessel) I73.9
  brachial plexus G54.0
  cerebral G45.9
  cervical plexus G54.2
  nerve
    arm — see Mononeuropathy, upper limb
      axillary G54.0
      median — see Lesion, nerve, median
      ulnar — see Lesion, nerve, ulnar
    axillary G54.0
    leg — see Mononeuropathy, lower limb
    median — see Lesion, nerve, median
    plantar — see Lesion, nerve, plantar
    ulnar — see Lesion, nerve, ulnar
Angiospastic disease or edema I73.9
Angiostrongyliasis
  due to
    Parastrongylus
      cantonensis B83.2
      costaricensis B81.3
  intestinal B81.3
Anguillulosis — see Strongyloidiasis
Angulation
  cecum — see Obstruction, intestine
  coccyx (acquired) — see also subcategory M43.8 ☑
    congenital NEC Q76.49
  femur (acquired) — see also Deformity, limb, specified
    type NEC, thigh
    congenital Q74.2
  intestine (large) (small) — see Obstruction, intestine
  sacrum (acquired) — see also subcategory M43.8 ☑
    congenital NEC Q76.49
  sigmoid (flexure) — see Obstruction, intestine

Angulation — continued
  spine — *see* Dorsopathy, deforming, specified NEC
  tibia (acquired) — *see also* Deformity, limb, specified
    type NEC, lower leg
    congenital Q74.2
  ureter N13.5
    with infection N13.6
  wrist (acquired) — *see also* Deformity, limb, specified
    type NEC, forearm
    congenital Q74.0
Angulus infectiosus (lips) K13.0
Anhedonia R45.84
  sexual F52.0
Anhidrosis L74.4
Anhydration E86.0
Anhydremia E86.0
Anidrosis L74.4
Aniridia (congenital) Q13.1
Anisakiasis (infection) (infestation) B81.0
Anisakis larvae infestation B81.0
Aniseikonia H52.32
Anisocoria (pupil) H57.02
  congenital Q13.2
Anisocytosis R71.8
Anisometropia (congenital) H52.31
Ankle — *see* condition
Ankyloblepharon (eyelid) (acquired) — *see also* Blepharophimosis
  filiforme (adnatum) (congenital) Q10.3
  total Q10.3
Ankyloglossia Q38.1
Ankylosis (fibrous) (osseous) (joint) M24.60
  ankle M24.67- ☑
  arthrodesis status Z98.1
  cricoarytenoid (cartilage) (joint) (larynx) J38.7
  dental K03.5
  ear ossicles H74.31- ☑
  elbow M24.62- ☑
  foot M24.67- ☑
  hand M24.64- ☑
  hip M24.65- ☑
  incostapedial joint (infectional) — *see* Ankylosis, ear
    ossicles
  jaw (temporomandibular) M26.61- ☑
  knee M24.66- ☑
  lumbosacral (joint) M43.27
  postoperative (status) Z98.1
  produced by surgical fusion, status Z98.1
  sacro-iliac (joint) M43.28
  shoulder M24.61- ☑
  specified site NEC M24.69
  spine (joint) — *see also* Fusion, spine
    spondylitic — *see* Spondylitis, ankylosing
  surgical Z98.1
  temporomandibular M26.61- ☑
  tooth, teeth (hard tissues) K03.5
  wrist M24.63- ☑
Ankylostoma — *see* Ancylostoma
Ankylostomiasis — *see* Ancylostomiasis
Ankylurethria — *see* Stricture, urethra
Annular — *see also* condition
  detachment, cervix N88.8
  organ or site, congenital NEC — *see* Distortion
  pancreas (congenital) Q45.1
Anodontia (complete) (partial) (vera) K00.0
  acquired K08.10 ☑
Anomaly, anomalous (congenital) (unspecified type)
  Q89.9
  abdominal wall NEC Q79.59
  acoustic nerve Q07.8
  adrenal (gland) Q89.1
  Alder (-Reilly) (leukocyte granulation) D72.0
  alimentary tract Q45.9
    upper Q40.9
  alveolar M26.70
    hyperplasia M26.79
      mandibular M26.72
      maxillary M26.71
    hypoplasia M26.79
      mandibular M26.74
      maxillary M26.73
    ridge (process) M26.79
    specified NEC M26.79
  ankle (joint) Q74.2
  anus Q43.9
  aorta (arch) NEC Q25.40
    coarctation (preductal) (postductal) Q25.1

Anomaly, anomalous — continued
  aortic cusp or valve Q23.9
  appendix Q43.8
  apple peel syndrome Q41.1
  aqueduct of Sylvius Q03.0
    with spina bifida — *see* Spina bifida, with hydrocephalus
  arm Q74.0
  arteriovenous NEC
    coronary Q24.5
    gastrointestinal Q27.33
      acquired — *see* Angiodysplasia
  artery (peripheral) Q27.9
    basilar NEC Q28.1
    cerebral Q28.3
    coronary Q24.5
    digestive system Q27.8
    eye Q15.8
    great Q25.9
      specified NEC Q25.8
    lower limb Q27.8
    peripheral Q27.9
      specified NEC Q27.8
    pulmonary NEC Q25.79
    renal Q27.2
    retina Q14.1
    specified site NEC Q27.8
    subclavian Q27.8
      origin Q25.48
    umbilical Q27.0
    upper limb Q27.8
    vertebral NEC Q28.1
  aryteno-epiglottic folds Q31.8
  atrial
    bands or folds Q20.8
    septa Q21.1
  atrioventricular
    excitation I45.6
    septum Q21.0
  auditory canal Q17.8
  auricle
    ear Q17.8
      causing impairment of hearing Q16.9
    heart Q20.8
  Axenfeld's Q15.0
  back Q89.9
  band
    atrial Q20.8
    heart Q24.8
    ventricular Q24.8
  Bartholin's duct Q38.4
  biliary duct or passage Q44.5
  bladder Q64.70
    absence Q64.5
    diverticulum Q64.6
    exstrophy Q64.10
      cloacal Q64.12
      extroversion Q64.19
      specified type NEC Q64.19
      supravesical fissure Q64.11
    neck obstruction Q64.31
    specified type NEC Q64.79
  bone Q79.9
    arm Q74.0
    face Q75.9
    leg Q74.2
    pelvic girdle Q74.2
    shoulder girdle Q74.0
    skull Q75.9
      with
        anencephaly Q00.0
        encephalocele — *see* Encephalocele
        hydrocephalus Q03.9
          with spina bifida — *see* Spina bifida, by
            site, with hydrocephalus
        microcephaly Q02
  brain (multiple) Q04.9
    vessel Q28.3
  breast Q83.9
  broad ligament Q50.6
  bronchus Q32.4
  bulbus cordis Q21.9
  bursa Q79.9
  canal of Nuck Q52.4
  canthus Q10.3
  capillary Q27.9
  cardiac Q24.9
    chambers Q20.9
      specified NEC Q20.8

Anomaly, anomalous — continued
  cardiac — continued
    septal closure Q21.9
      specified NEC Q21.8
    valve NEC Q24.8
      pulmonary Q22.3
  cardiovascular system Q28.8
  carpus Q74.0
  caruncle, lacrimal Q10.6
  cascade stomach Q40.2
  cauda equina Q06.3
  cecum Q43.9
  cerebral Q04.9
    vessels Q28.3
  cervix Q51.9
  Chédiak-Higashi (-Steinbrinck) (congenital gigantism
    of peroxidase granules) E70.330
  cheek Q18.9
  chest wall Q67.8
    bones Q76.9
  chin Q18.9
  chordae tendineae Q24.8
  choroid Q14.3
    plexus Q07.8
  chromosomes, chromosomal Q99.9
    D (1) — *see* condition, chromosome 13
    E (3) — *see* condition, chromosome 18
    G — *see* condition, chromosome 21
    sex
      female phenotype Q97.8
      gonadal dysgenesis (pure) Q99.1
      Klinefelter's Q98.4
      male phenotype Q98.9
      Turner's Q96.9
    specified NEC Q99.8
  cilia Q10.3
  circulatory system Q28.9
  clavicle Q74.0
  clitoris Q52.6
  coccyx Q76.49
  colon Q43.9
  common duct Q44.5
  communication
    coronary artery Q24.5
    left ventricle with right atrium Q21.0
  concha (ear) Q17.3
  connection
    portal vein Q26.5
    pulmonary venous Q26.4
      partial Q26.3
      total Q26.2
    renal artery with kidney Q27.2
  cornea (shape) Q13.4
  coronary artery or vein Q24.5
  cranium — *see* Anomaly, skull
  cricoid cartilage Q31.8
  cystic duct Q44.5
  dental
    alveolar — *see* Anomaly, alveolar
    arch relationship M26.20
      specified NEC M26.29
  dentofacial M26.9
    alveolar — *see* Anomaly, alveolar
    dental arch relationship M26.20
      specified NEC M26.29
    functional M26.50
      specified NEC M26.59
    jaw size M26.00
      macrogenia M26.05
      mandibular
        hyperplasia M26.03
        hypoplasia M26.04
      maxillary
        hyperplasia M26.01
        hypoplasia M26.02
      microgenia M26.06
      specified type NEC M26.09
    jaw-cranial base relationship M26.10
      asymmetry M26.12
        maxillary M26.11
      specified type NEC M26.19
    malocclusion M26.4
      dental arch relationship NEC M26.29
      jaw size — *see* Anomaly, dentofacial, jaw size
      jaw-cranial base relationship — *see* Anomaly,
        dentofacial, jaw-cranial base relationship
    specified type NEC M26.89
    temporomandibular joint M26.60- ☑

Anomaly, anomalous — *continued*
dentofacial — *continued*
   temporomandibular joint — *continued*
     adhesions M26.61- ☑
     ankylosis M26.61- ☑
     arthralgia M26.62- ☑
     articular disc M26.63- ☑
     specified type NEC M26.69
   tooth position, fully erupted M26.30
     specified NEC M26.39
dermatoglyphic Q82.8
diaphragm (apertures) NEC Q79.1
digestive organ(s) or tract Q45.9
  lower Q43.9
  upper Q40.9
distance, interarch (excessive) (inadequate) M26.25
distribution, coronary artery Q24.5
ductus
  arteriosus Q25.0
  botalli Q25.0
duodenum Q43.9
dura (brain) Q04.9
  spinal cord Q06.9
ear (external) Q17.9
  causing impairment of hearing Q16.9
  inner Q16.5
  middle (causing impairment of hearing) Q16.4
  ossicles Q16.3
Ebstein's (heart) (tricuspid valve) Q22.5
ectodermal Q82.9
Eisenmenger's (ventricular septal defect) Q21.8
ejaculatory duct Q55.4
elbow Q74.0
endocrine gland NEC Q89.2
epididymis Q55.4
epiglottis Q31.8
esophagus Q39.9
eustachian tube Q17.8
eye Q15.9
  anterior segment Q13.9
    specified NEC Q13.89
  posterior segment Q14.9
    specified NEC Q14.8
  ptosis (eyelid) Q10.0
  specified NEC Q15.8
eyebrow Q18.8
eyelid Q10.3
  ptosis Q10.0
face Q18.9
  bone(s) Q75.9
fallopian tube Q50.6
fascia Q79.9
femur NEC Q74.2
fibula NEC Q74.2
finger Q74.0
fixation, intestine Q43.3
flexion (joint) NOS Q74.9
  hip or thigh Q65.89
foot NEC Q74.2
  varus (congenital) Q66.3- ☑
foramen
  Botalli Q21.1
  ovale Q21.1
forearm Q74.0
forehead Q75.8
form, teeth K00.2
fovea centralis Q14.1
frontal bone — *see* Anomaly, skull
gallbladder (position) (shape) (size) Q44.1
Gartner's duct Q52.4
gastrointestinal tract Q45.9
genitalia, genital organ(s) or system
  female Q52.9
    external Q52.70
    internal NOS Q52.9
  male Q55.9
    hydrocele P83.5
    specified NEC Q55.8
genitourinary NEC
  female Q52.9
  male Q55.9
Gerbode Q21.0
glottis Q31.8
granulation or granulocyte, genetic (constitutional) (leukocyte) D72.0
gum Q38.6
gyri Q07.9
hair Q84.2

Anomaly, anomalous — *continued*
hand Q74.0
hard tissue formation in pulp K04.3
head — *see* Anomaly, skull
heart Q24.9
  auricle Q20.8
  bands or folds Q24.8
  fibroelastosis cordis I42.4
  obstructive NEC Q22.6
  patent ductus arteriosus (Botalli) Q25.0
  septum Q21.9
    auricular Q21.1
    interatrial Q21.1
    interventricular Q21.0
      with pulmonary stenosis or atresia, dextraposition of aorta and hypertrophy of right ventricle Q21.3
    specified NEC Q21.8
    ventricular Q21.0
      with pulmonary stenosis or atresia, dextraposition of aorta and hypertrophy of right ventricle Q21.3
  tetralogy of Fallot Q21.3
  valve NEC Q24.8
    aortic
      bicuspid valve Q23.1
      insufficiency Q23.1
      stenosis Q23.0
        subaortic Q24.4
    mitral
      insufficiency Q23.3
      stenosis Q23.2
    pulmonary Q22.3
      atresia Q22.0
      insufficiency Q22.2
      stenosis Q22.1
        infundibular Q24.3
        subvalvular Q24.3
    tricuspid
      atresia Q22.4
      stenosis Q22.4
  ventricle Q20.8
heel NEC Q74.2
Hegglin's D72.0
hemianencephaly Q00.0
hemicephaly Q00.0
hemicrania Q00.0
hepatic duct Q44.5
hip NEC Q74.2
hourglass stomach Q40.2
humerus Q74.0
hydatid of Morgagni
  female Q50.5
  male (epididymal) Q55.4
    testicular Q55.29
hymen Q52.4
hypersegmentation of neutrophils, hereditary D72.0
hypophyseal Q89.2
ileocecal (coil) (valve) Q43.9
ileum Q43.9
ilium NEC Q74.2
integument Q84.9
  specified NEC Q84.8
interarch distance (excessive) (inadequate) M26.25
intervertebral cartilage or disc Q76.49
intestine (large) (small) Q43.9
  with anomalous adhesions, fixation or malrotation Q43.3
iris Q13.2
ischium NEC Q74.2
jaw — *see* Anomaly, dentofacial
  alveolar — *see* Anomaly, alveolar
jaw-cranial base relationship — *see* Anomaly, dentofacial, jaw-cranial base relationship
jejunum Q43.8
joint Q74.9
  specified NEC Q74.8
Jordan's D72.0
kidney(s) (calyx) (pelvis) Q63.9
  artery Q27.2
  specified NEC Q63.8
Klippel-Feil (brevicollis) Q76.1
knee Q74.1
labium (majus) (minus) Q52.70
labyrinth, membranous Q16.5
lacrimal apparatus or duct Q10.6
larynx, laryngeal (muscle) Q31.9
  web (bed) Q31.0
lens Q12.9

Anomaly, anomalous — *continued*
leukocytes, genetic D72.0
  granulation (constitutional) D72.0
lid (fold) Q10.3
ligament Q79.9
  broad Q50.6
  round Q52.8
limb Q74.9
  lower NEC Q74.2
    reduction deformity — *see* Defect, reduction, lower limb
  upper Q74.0
lip Q38.0
liver Q44.7
  duct Q44.5
lower limb NEC Q74.2
lumbosacral (joint) (region) Q76.49
  kyphosis — *see* Kyphosis, congenital
  lordosis — *see* Lordosis, congenital
lung (fissure) (lobe) Q33.9
mandible — *see* Anomaly, dentofacial
maxilla — *see* Anomaly, dentofacial
May (-Hegglin) D72.0
meatus urinarius NEC Q64.79
meningeal bands or folds Q07.9
  constriction of Q07.8
  spinal Q06.9
meninges Q07.9
  cerebral Q04.8
  spinal Q06.9
meningocele Q05.9
mesentery Q45.9
metacarpus Q74.0
metatarsus NEC Q74.2
middle ear Q16.4
  ossicles Q16.3
mitral (leaflets) (valve) Q23.9
  insufficiency Q23.3
  specified NEC Q23.8
  stenosis Q23.2
mouth Q38.6
Müllerian — *see also* Anomaly, by site
  uterus NEC Q51.818
multiple NEC Q89.7
muscle Q79.9
  eyelid Q10.3
musculoskeletal system, except limbs Q79.9
myocardium Q24.8
nail Q84.6
narrowness, eyelid Q10.3
nasal sinus (wall) Q30.8
neck (any part) Q18.9
nerve Q07.9
  acoustic Q07.8
  optic Q07.8
nervous system (central) Q07.9
nipple Q83.9
nose, nasal (bones) (cartilage) (septum) (sinus) Q30.9
  specified NEC Q30.8
ocular muscle Q15.8
omphalomesenteric duct Q43.0
opening, pulmonary veins Q26.4
optic
  disc Q14.2
  nerve Q07.8
opticociliary vessels Q13.2
orbit (eye) Q10.7
organ Q89.9
  of Corti Q16.5
origin
  artery
    innominate Q25.8
    pulmonary Q25.79
    renal Q27.2
    subclavian Q25.48
osseous meatus (ear) Q16.1
ovary Q50.39
oviduct Q50.6
palate (hard) (soft) NEC Q38.5
pancreas or pancreatic duct Q45.3
papillary muscles Q24.8
parathyroid gland Q89.2
paraurethral ducts Q64.79
parotid (gland) Q38.4
patella Q74.1
Pelger-Huët (hereditary hyposegmentation) D72.0
pelvic girdle NEC Q74.2
pelvis (bony) NEC Q74.2
  rachitic E64.3

Anomaly, anomalous — *continued*
   penis (glans) Q55.69
   pericardium Q24.8
   peripheral vascular system Q27.9
   Peter's Q13.4
   pharynx Q38.8
   pigmentation L81.9
      congenital Q82.8
   pituitary (gland) Q89.2
   pleural (folds) Q34.0
   portal vein Q26.5
      connection Q26.5
   position, tooth, teeth, fully erupted M26.30
      specified NEC M26.39
   precerebral vessel Q28.1
   prepuce Q55.69
   prostate Q55.4
   pulmonary Q33.9
      artery NEC Q25.79
      valve Q22.3
         atresia Q22.0
         insufficiency Q22.2
         specified type NEC Q22.3
         stenosis Q22.1
            infundibular Q24.3
            subvalvular Q24.3
      venous connection Q26.4
         partial Q26.3
         total Q26.2
   pupil Q13.2
      function H57.00
         anisocoria H57.02
         Argyll Robertson pupil H57.01
         miosis H57.03
         mydriasis H57.04
         specified type NEC H57.09
         tonic pupil H57.05- ☑
   pylorus Q40.3
   radius Q74.0
   rectum Q43.9
   reduction (extremity) (limb)
      femur (longitudinal) — *see* Defect, reduction, lower
         limb, longitudinal, femur
      fibula (longitudinal) — *see* Defect, reduction, lower
         limb, longitudinal, fibula
      lower limb — *see* Defect, reduction, lower limb
      radius (longitudinal) — *see* Defect, reduction, upper
         limb, longitudinal, radius
      tibia (longitudinal) — *see* Defect, reduction, lower
         limb, longitudinal, tibia
      ulna (longitudinal) — *see* Defect, reduction, upper
         limb, longitudinal, ulna
      upper limb — *see* Defect, reduction, upper limb
   refraction — *see* Disorder, refraction
   renal Q63.9
      artery Q27.2
      pelvis Q63.9
      specified NEC Q63.8
   respiratory system Q34.9
      specified NEC Q34.8
   retina Q14.1
   rib Q76.6
      cervical Q76.5
   Rieger's Q13.81
   rotation — *see* Malrotation
      hip or thigh Q65.89
   round ligament Q52.8
   sacroiliac (joint) NEC Q74.2
   sacrum NEC Q76.49
      kyphosis — *see* Kyphosis, congenital
      lordosis — *see* Lordosis, congenital
   saddle nose, syphilitic A50.57
   salivary duct or gland Q38.4
   scapula Q74.0
   scrotum — *see* Malformation, testis and scrotum
   sebaceous gland Q82.9
   seminal vesicles Q55.4
   sense organs NEC Q07.8
   sex chromosomes NEC — *see also* Anomaly, chromo-
      somes
      female phenotype Q97.8
      male phenotype Q98.9
   shoulder (girdle) (joint) Q74.0
   sigmoid (flexure) Q43.9
   simian crease Q82.8
   sinus of Valsalva Q25.49
   skeleton generalized Q78.9
   skin (appendage) Q82.9

Anomaly, anomalous — *continued*
   skull Q75.9
      with
         anencephaly Q00.0
         encephalocele — *see* Encephalocele
         hydrocephalus Q03.9
            with spina bifida — *see* Spina bifida, by site,
               with hydrocephalus
         microcephaly Q02
   specified organ or site NEC Q89.8
   spermatic cord Q55.4
   spine, spinal NEC Q76.49
      column NEC Q76.49
         kyphosis — *see* Kyphosis, congenital
         lordosis — *see* Lordosis, congenital
      cord Q06.9
      nerve root Q07.8
   spleen Q89.09
      agenesis Q89.01
   stenonian duct Q38.4
   sternum NEC Q76.7
   stomach Q40.3
   submaxillary gland Q38.4
   tarsus NEC Q74.2
   tendon Q79.9
   testis — *see* Malformation, testis and scrotum
   thigh NEC Q74.2
   thorax (wall) Q67.8
      bony Q76.9
   throat Q38.8
   thumb Q74.0
   thymus gland Q89.2
   thyroid (gland) Q89.2
      cartilage Q31.8
   tibia NEC Q74.2
      saber A50.56
   toe Q74.2
   tongue Q38.3
   tooth, teeth K00.9
      eruption K00.6
      position, fully erupted M26.30
      spacing, fully erupted M26.30
   trachea (cartilage) Q32.1
   tragus Q17.9
   tricuspid (leaflet) (valve) Q22.9
      atresia or stenosis Q22.4
      Ebstein's Q22.5
   Uhl's (hypoplasia of myocardium, right ventricle) Q24.8
   ulna Q74.0
   umbilical artery Q27.0
   union
      cricoid cartilage and thyroid cartilage Q31.8
      thyroid cartilage and hyoid bone Q31.8
      trachea with larynx Q31.8
   upper limb Q74.0
   urachus Q64.4
   ureter Q62.8
      obstructive NEC Q62.39
         cecoureterocele Q62.32
         orthotopic ureterocele Q62.31
   urethra Q64.70
      absence Q64.5
      double Q64.74
      fistula to rectum Q64.73
      obstructive Q64.39
         stricture Q64.32
      prolapse Q64.71
      specified type NEC Q64.79
   urinary tract Q64.9
   uterus Q51.9
      with only one functioning horn Q51.4
   uvula Q38.5
   vagina Q52.4
   valleculae Q31.8
   valve (heart) NEC Q24.8
      coronary sinus Q24.5
      inferior vena cava Q24.8
      pulmonary Q22.3
      sinus coronario Q24.5
      venae cavae inferioris Q24.8
   vas deferens Q55.4
   vascular Q27.9
      brain Q28.3
      ring Q25.45
   vein(s) (peripheral) Q27.9
      brain Q28.3
      cerebral Q28.3
      coronary Q24.5
      developmental Q28.3

Anomaly, anomalous — *continued*
   vein(s) — *continued*
      great Q26.9
         specified NEC Q26.8
   vena cava (inferior) (superior) Q26.9
   venous — *see* Anomaly, vein(s)
   venous return Q26.8
   ventricular
      bands or folds Q24.8
      septa Q21.0
   vertebra Q76.49
      kyphosis — *see* Kyphosis, congenital
      lordosis — *see* Lordosis, congenital
   vesicourethral orifice Q64.79
   vessel(s) Q27.9
      optic papilla Q14.2
      precerebral Q28.1
   vitelline duct Q43.0
   vitreous body or humor Q14.0
   vulva Q52.70
   wrist (joint) Q74.0
Anomia R48.8
Anonychia (congenital) Q84.3
   acquired L60.8
Anophthalmos, anophthalmus (congenital) (globe)
   Q11.1
   acquired Z90.01
Anopia, anopsia H53.46- ☑
   quadrant H53.46- ☑
Anorchia, anorchism, anorchidism Q55.0
Anorexia R63.0
   hysterical F44.89
   nervosa F50.00
      atypical F50.9
      binge-eating type F50.2
         with purging F50.02
      restricting type F50.01
Anorgasmy, psychogenic (female) F52.31
   male F52.32
Anosmia R43.0
   hysterical F44.6
   postinfectional J39.8
Anosognosia R41.89
Anosteoplasia Q78.9
Anovulatory cycle N97.0
Anoxemia R09.02
   newborn P84
Anoxia (pathological) R09.02
   altitude T70.29 ☑
   cerebral G93.1
      complicating
         anesthesia (general) (local) or other sedation
            T88.59 ☑
            in labor and delivery O74.3
            in pregnancy O29.21- ☑
            postpartum, puerperal O89.2
         delivery (cesarean) (instrumental) O75.4
      during a procedure G97.81
      newborn P84
      resulting from a procedure G97.82
   due to
      drowning T75.1 ☑
      high altitude T70.29 ☑
   heart — *see* Insufficiency, coronary
   intrauterine P84
   myocardial — *see* Insufficiency, coronary
   newborn P84
   spinal cord G95.11
   systemic (by suffocation) (low content in atmosphere)
      — *see* Asphyxia, traumatic
Anteflexion — *see* Anteversion
Antenatal
   care (normal pregnancy) Z34.90
   screening (encounter for) of mother — *see also* En-
      counter, antenatal screening Z36.9
Antepartum — *see* condition
Anterior — *see* condition
Antero-occlusion M26.220
Anteversion
   cervix — *see* Anteversion, uterus
   femur (neck), congenital Q65.89
   uterus, uterine (cervix) (postinfectional) (postpartal,
      old) N85.4
      congenital Q51.818
      in pregnancy or childbirth — *see* Pregnancy, com-
         plicated by
Anthophobia F40.228
Anthracosilicosis J60

Anthracosis (lung) (occupational) J60
  lingua K14.3
Anthrax A22.9
  with pneumonia A22.1
  cerebral A22.8
  colitis A22.2
  cutaneous A22.0
  gastrointestinal A22.2
  inhalation A22.1
  intestinal A22.2
  meningitis A22.8
  pulmonary A22.1
  respiratory A22.1
  sepsis A22.7
  specified manifestation NEC A22.8
Anthropoid pelvis Q74.2
  with disproportion (fetopelvic) O33.0
Anthropophobia F40.10
  generalized F40.11
Antibodies, maternal (blood group) — *see* Isoimmunization, affecting management of pregnancy
  anti-D — *see* Isoimmunization, affecting management of pregnancy, Rh
    newborn P55.0
Antibody
  anticardiolipin R76.0
    with
      hemorrhagic disorder D68.312
      hypercoagulable state D68.61
  antiphosphatidylglycerol R76.0
    with
      hemorrhagic disorder D68.312
      hypercoagulable state D68.61
  antiphosphatidylinositol R76.0
    with
      hemorrhagic disorder D68.312
      hypercoagulable state D68.61
  antiphosphatidylserine R76.0
    with
      hemorrhagic disorder D68.312
      hypercoagulable state D68.61
  antiphospholipid R76.0
    with
      hemorrhagic disorder D68.312
      hypercoagulable state D68.61
Anticardiolipin syndrome D68.61
Anticoagulant, circulating (intrinsic) — *see also* Disorder, hemorrhagic D68.318
  drug-induced (extrinsic) — *see also* Disorder, hemorrhagic D68.32
  iatrogenic D68.32
Antidiuretic hormone syndrome E22.2
Antimonial cholera — *see* Poisoning, antimony
Antiphospholipid
  antibody
    with hemorrhagic disorder D68.312
    syndrome D68.61
Antisocial personality F60.2
Antithrombinemia — *see* Circulating anticoagulants
Antithromboplastinemia D68.318
Antithromboplastinogenemia D68.318
Antitoxin complication or reaction — *see* Complications, vaccination
Antlophobia F40.228
Antritis J32.0
  maxilla J32.0
    acute J01.00
      recurrent J01.01
  stomach K29.60
    with bleeding K29.61
Antrum, antral — *see* condition
Anuria R34
  calculous (impacted) (recurrent) — *see also* Calculus, urinary N20.9
  following
    abortion — *see* Abortion by type complicated by, renal failure
    ectopic or molar pregnancy O08.4
  newborn P96.0
  postprocedural N99.0
  postrenal N13.8
  traumatic (following crushing) T79.5 ☑
Anus, anal — *see* condition
Anusitis K62.89
Anxiety F41.9
  depression F41.8
  episodic paroxysmal F41.0
  generalized F41.1

Anxiety — *continued*
  hysteria F41.8
  neurosis F41.1
  panic type F41.0
  reaction F41.1
  separation, abnormal (of childhood) F93.0
  specified NEC F41.8
  state F41.1
Aorta, aortic — *see* condition
Aortectasia — *see* Ectasia, aorta
  with aneurysm — *see* Aneurysm, aorta
Aortitis (nonsyphilitic) (calcific) I77.6
  arteriosclerotic I70.0
  Doehle-Heller A52.02
  luetic A52.02
  rheumatic — *see* Endocarditis, acute, rheumatic
  specific (syphilitic) A52.02
  syphilitic A52.02
    congenital A50.54 *[I79.1]*
Apathetic thyroid storm — *see* Thyrotoxicosis
Apathy R45.3
Apeirophobia F40.228
Apepsia K30
  psychogenic F45.8
Aperistalsis, esophagus K22.0
Apertognathia M26.29
Apert's syndrome Q87.0
Aphagia R13.0
  psychogenic F50.9
Aphakia (acquired) (postoperative) H27.0- ☑
  congenital Q12.3
Aphasia (amnestic) (global) (nominal) (semantic) (syntactic) R47.01
  acquired, with epilepsy (Landau-Kleffner syndrome) — *see* Epilepsy, specified NEC
  auditory (developmental) F80.2
  developmental (receptive type) F80.2
    expressive type F80.1
    Wernicke's F80.2
  following
    cerebrovascular disease I69.920
      cerebral infarction I69.320
      intracerebral hemorrhage I69.120
      nontraumatic intracranial hemorrhage NEC I69.220
      specified disease NEC I69.820
      subarachnoid hemorrhage I69.020
  primary progressive G31.01 *[F02.80]*
    with behavioral disturbance G31.01 *[F02.81]*
  progressive isolated G31.01 *[F02.80]*
    with behavioral disturbance G31.01 *[F02.81]*
  sensory F80.2
  syphilis, tertiary A52.19
  Wernicke's (developmental) F80.2
Aphonia (organic) R49.1
  hysterical F44.4
  psychogenic F44.4
Aphthae, aphthous — *see also* condition
  Bednar's K12.0
  cachectic K14.0
  epizootic B08.8
  fever B08.8
  oral (recurrent) K12.0
  stomatitis (major) (minor) K12.0
  thrush B37.0
  ulcer (oral) (recurrent) K12.0
    genital organ(s) NEC
      female N76.6
      male N50.89
    larynx J38.7
Apical — *see* condition
Apiphobia F40.218
Aplasia — *see also* Agenesis
  abdominal muscle syndrome Q79.4
  alveolar process (acquired) — *see* Anomaly, alveolar
    congenital Q38.6
  aorta (congenital) Q25.41
  axialis extracorticalis (congenita) E75.29
  bone marrow (myeloid) D61.9
    congenital D61.01
  brain Q00.0
    part of Q04.3
  bronchus Q32.4
  cementum K00.4
  cerebellum Q04.3
  cervix (congenital) Q51.5
  congenital pure red cell D61.01
  corpus callosum Q04.0

Aplasia — *continued*
  cutis congenita Q84.8
  erythrocyte congenital D61.01
  extracortical axial E75.29
  eye Q11.1
  fovea centralis (congenital) Q14.1
  gallbladder, congenital Q44.0
  iris Q13.1
  labyrinth, membranous Q16.5
  limb (congenital) Q73.8
    lower — *see* Defect, reduction, lower limb
    upper — *see* Agenesis, arm
  lung, congenital (bilateral) (unilateral) Q33.3
  pancreas Q45.0
  parathyroid-thymic D82.1
  Pelizaeus-Merzbacher E75.29
  penis Q55.5
  prostate Q55.4
  red cell (with thymoma) D60.9
    acquired D60.9
      due to drugs D60.9
    adult D60.9
    chronic D60.0
    congenital D61.01
    constitutional D61.01
    due to drugs D60.9
    hereditary D61.01
    of infants D61.01
    primary D61.01
    pure D61.01
      due to drugs D60.9
    specified type NEC D60.8
    transient D60.1
  round ligament Q52.8
  skin Q84.8
  spermatic cord Q55.4
  spleen Q89.01
  testicle Q55.0
  thymic, with immunodeficiency D82.1
  thyroid (congenital) (with myxedema) E03.1
  uterus Q51.0
  ventral horn cell Q06.1
Apnea, apneic (of) (spells) R06.81
  newborn NEC P28.4
    obstructive P28.4
    sleep (central) (obstructive) (primary) P28.3
  prematurity P28.4
  sleep G47.30
    central (primary) G47.31
      idiopathic G47.31
      in conditions classified elsewhere G47.37
    obstructive (adult) (pediatric) G47.33
      hypopnea G47.33
    primary central G47.31
    specified NEC G47.39
Apneumatosis, newborn P28.0
Apocrine metaplasia (breast) — *see* Dysplasia, mammary, specified type NEC
Apophysitis (bone) — *see also* Osteochondropathy
  calcaneus M92.8
  juvenile M92.9
Apoplectiform convulsions (cerebral ischemia) I67.82
Apoplexia, apoplexy, apoplectic
  adrenal A39.1
  heart (auricle) (ventricle) — *see* Infarct, myocardium
  heat T67.01 ☑
  hemorrhagic (stroke) — *see* Hemorrhage, intracranial
  meninges, hemorrhagic — *see* Hemorrhage, intracranial, subarachnoid
  uremic N18.9 *[I68.8]*
Appearance
  bizarre R46.1
  specified NEC R46.89
  very low level of personal hygiene R46.0
Appendage
  epididymal (organ of Morgagni) Q55.4
  intestine (epiploic) Q43.8
  preauricular Q17.0
  testicular (organ of Morgagni) Q55.29
Appendicitis (pneumococcal) (retrocecal) K37
  with
    gangrene K35.891
    perforation NOS K35.32
    peritoneal abscess K35.33
    peritonitis NEC K35.33
      generalized (with perforation or rupture) K35.20
        with abscess K35.21
      localized K35.30

▽ **Subterms under main terms may continue to next column or page**   ☑ **Additional Character Required** — Refer to the Tabular List for Character Selection   **25**

Anthracosis — Appendicitis

Appendicitis — *continued*
  with — *continued*
    peritonitis — *continued*
      localized — *continued*
        with
          gangrene K35.31
          perforation K35.32
            and abscess K35.33
        rupture (with localized peritonitis) K35.32
  acute (catarrhal) (fulminating) (gangrenous) (obstructive) (retrocecal) (suppurative) K35.80
    with
      gangrene K35.891
      peritoneal abscess K35.33
      peritonitis NEC K35.33
        generalized (with perforation or rupture) K35.20
          with abscess K35.21
        localized K35.30
          with
            gangrene K35.31
            perforation K35.32
              and abscess K35.33
    specified NEC K35.890
      with gangrene K35.891
  amebic A06.89
  chronic (recurrent) K36
  exacerbation — *see* Appendicitis, acute
  gangrenous — *see* Appendicitis, acute
  healed (obliterative) K36
  interval K36
  neurogenic K36
  obstructive K36
  recurrent K36
  relapsing K36
  ruptured NOS (with localized peritonitis) K35.32
  subacute (adhesive) K36
  subsiding K36
  suppurative — *see* Appendicitis, acute
  tuberculous A18.32
Appendicopathia oxyurica B80
Appendix, appendicular — *see also* condition
  epididymis Q55.4
  Morgagni
    female Q50.5
    male (epididymal) Q55.4
      testicular Q55.29
  testis Q55.29
Appetite
  depraved — *see* Pica
  excessive R63.2
  lack or loss — *see also* Anorexia R63.0
    nonorganic origin F50.89
    psychogenic F50.89
  perverted (hysterical) — *see* Pica
Apple peel syndrome Q41.1
Apprehension state F41.1
Apprehensiveness, abnormal F41.9
Approximal wear K03.0
Apraxia (classic) (ideational) (ideokinetic) (ideomotor) (motor) (verbal) R48.2
  following
    cerebrovascular disease I69.990
      cerebral infarction I69.390
      intracerebral hemorrhage I69.190
      nontraumatic intracranial hemorrhage NEC I69.290
      specified disease NEC I69.890
      subarachnoid hemorrhage I69.090
  oculomotor, congenital H51.8
Aptyalism K11.7
Apudoma — *see* Neoplasm, uncertain behavior, by site
Aqueous misdirection H40.83- ☑
Arabicum elephantiasis — *see* Infestation, filarial
Arachnitis — *see* Meningitis
Arachnodactyly — *see* Syndrome, Marfan's
Arachnoiditis (acute) (adhesive) (basal) (brain) (cerebrospinal) — *see* Meningitis
Arachnophobia F40.210
Arboencephalitis, Australian A83.4
Arborization block (heart) I45.5
ARC (AIDS-related complex) B20
Arch
  aortic Q25.49
  bovine Q25.49
Arches — *see* condition
Arcuate uterus Q51.810
Arcuatus uterus Q51.810

Arcus (cornea) senilis — *see* Degeneration, cornea, senile
Arc-welder's lung J63.4
Areflexia R29.2
Areola — *see* condition
Argentaffinoma — *see also* Neoplasm, uncertain behavior, by site
  malignant — *see* Neoplasm, malignant, by site
  syndrome E34.0
Argininemia E72.21
Arginosuccinic aciduria E72.22
Argyll Robertson phenomenon, pupil or syndrome (syphilitic) A52.19
  atypical H57.09
  nonsyphilitic H57.09
Argyria, argyriasis
  conjunctival H11.13- ☑
  from drug or medicament — *see* Table of Drugs and Chemicals, by substance
Argyrosis, conjunctival H11.13- ☑
Arhinencephaly Q04.1
Ariboflavinosis E53.0
Arm — *see* condition
Arnold-Chiari disease, obstruction or syndrome (type II) Q07.00
  with
    hydrocephalus Q07.02
      with spina bifida Q07.03
    spina bifida Q07.01
      with hydrocephalus Q07.03
  type III — *see* Encephalocele
  type IV Q04.8
Aromatic amino-acid metabolism disorder E70.9
  specified NEC E70.89
Arousals, confusional G47.51
Arrest, arrested
  cardiac I46.9
    complicating
      abortion — *see* Abortion, by type, complicated by, cardiac arrest
      anesthesia (general) (local) or other sedation — *see* Table of Drugs and Chemicals, by drug
        in labor and delivery O74.2
        in pregnancy O29.11- ☑
        postpartum, puerperal O89.1
      delivery (cesarean) (instrumental) O75.4
    due to
      cardiac condition I46.2
      specified condition NEC I46.8
    intraoperative I97.71- ☑
    newborn P29.81
    personal history, successfully resuscitated Z86.74
    postprocedural I97.12- ☑
      obstetric procedure O75.4
  cardiorespiratory — *see* Arrest, cardiac
  circulatory — *see* Arrest, cardiac
  deep transverse O64.0 ☑
  development or growth
    bone — *see* Disorder, bone, development or growth
    child R62.50
    tracheal rings Q32.1
  epiphyseal
    complete
      femur M89.15- ☑
      humerus M89.12- ☑
      tibia M89.16- ☑
      ulna M89.13- ☑
      forearm M89.13- ☑
      specified NEC M89.13- ☑
      ulna — *see* Arrest, epiphyseal, by type, ulna
      lower leg M89.16- ☑
        specified NEC M89.168
      tibia — *see* Arrest, epiphyseal, by type, tibia
    partial
      femur M89.15- ☑
      humerus M89.12- ☑
      tibia M89.16- ☑
      ulna M89.13- ☑
      specified NEC M89.18
  granulopoiesis — *see* Agranulocytosis
  growth plate — *see* Arrest, epiphyseal
  heart — *see* Arrest, cardiac
  legal, anxiety concerning Z65.3
  physeal — *see* Arrest, epiphyseal
  respiratory R09.2
    newborn P28.81
  sinus I45.5
  spermatogenesis (complete) — *see* Azoospermia

Arrest, arrested — *continued*
  spermatogenesis — *see* Azoospermia — *continued*
    incomplete — *see* Oligospermia
  transverse (deep) O64.0 ☑
Arrhenoblastoma
  benign
    specified site — *see* Neoplasm, benign, by site
    unspecified site
      female D27.9
      male D29.20
  malignant
    specified site — *see* Neoplasm, malignant, by site
    unspecified site
      female C56.9
      male C62.90
  specified site — *see* Neoplasm, uncertain behavior, by site
  unspecified site
    female D39.10
    male D40.10
Arrhythmia (auricle) (cardiac) (juvenile) (nodal) (reflex) (supraventricular) (transitory) (ventricle) I49.9
  block I45.9
  extrasystolic I49.49
  newborn
    bradycardia P29.12
    occurring before birth P03.819
      before onset of labor P03.810
      during labor P03.811
    tachycardia P29.11
  psychogenic F45.8
  sinus I49.8
  specified NEC I49.8
  vagal R55
  ventricular re-entry I47.0
Arrillaga-Ayerza syndrome (pulmonary sclerosis with pulmonary hypertension) I27.0
Arsenical pigmentation L81.8
  from drug or medicament — *see* Table of Drugs and Chemicals
Arsenism — *see* Poisoning, arsenic
Arterial — *see* condition
Arteriofibrosis — *see* Arteriosclerosis
Arteriolar sclerosis — *see* Arteriosclerosis
Arteriolith — *see* Arteriosclerosis
Arteriolitis I77.6
  necrotizing, kidney I77.5
  renal — *see* Hypertension, kidney
Arteriolosclerosis — *see* Arteriosclerosis
Arterionephrosclerosis — *see* Hypertension, kidney
Arteriopathy I77.9
  cerebral autosomal dominant, with subcortical infarcts and leukoencephalopathy (CADASIL) I67.850
Arteriosclerosis, arteriosclerotic (diffuse) (obliterans) (of) (senile) (with calcification) I70.90
  with
    chronic limb-threatening ischemia — *see* Arteriosclerosis, with critical limb ischemia
    critical limb ischemia
      bypass graft I70.329
        autologous vein graft I70.429
          leg I70.429
            with
              gangrene (and intermittent claudication, rest pain, and ulcer) I70.469
              rest pain (and intermittent claudication) I70.429
          bilateral I70.423
            with
              gangrene (and intermittent claudication, rest pain, and ulcer) I70.463
              rest pain (and intermittent claudication) I70.423
          left I70.422
            with
              gangrene (and intermittent claudication, rest pain, and ulcer) I70.462
              rest pain (and intermittent claudication) I70.422
              ulceration (and intermittent claudication and rest pain) I70.449
                ankle I70.443
                calf I70.442
                foot site NEC I70.445

☑ Additional Character Required — Refer to the Tabular List for Character Selection   ▽ Subterms under main terms may continue to next column or page

Arteriosclerosis, arteriosclerotic — *continued*
  with — *continued*
    critical limb ischemia — *continued*
      bypass graft — *continued*
        autologous vein graft — *continued*
          leg — *continued*
            left — *continued*
              with — *continued*
                ulceration — *continued*
                  heel I70.444
                  lower leg NEC I70.448
                  mid foot I70.444
                  thigh I70.441
            right I70.421
              with
                gangrene (and intermittent clau-dication, rest pain, and ul-cer) I70.461
                rest pain (and intermittent claudi-cation) I70.421
                ulceration (and intermittent claudication and rest pain) I70.439
                  ankle I70.433
                  calf I70.432
                  foot site NEC I70.435
                  heel I70.434
                  lower leg NEC I70.438
                  midfoot I70.434
                  thigh I70.431
        leg I70.329
          with
            gangrene (and intermittent claudica-tion, rest pain, and ulcer) I70.369
            rest pain (and intermittent claudica-tion) I70.329
          bilateral I70.323
            with
              gangrene (and intermittent claudica-tion, rest pain, and ulcer) I70.363
              rest pain (and intermittent claudica-tion) I70.323
          left I70.322
            with
              gangrene (and intermittent claudica-tion, rest pain, and ulcer) I70.362
              rest pain (and intermittent claudica-tion) I70.322
              ulceration (and intermittent claudi-cation and rest pain) I70.349
                ankle I70.343
                calf I70.342
                foot site NEC I70.345
                heel I70.344
                lower leg NEC I70.348
                midfoot I70.344
                thigh I70.341
          right I70.321
            with
              gangrene (and intermittent claudica-tion, rest pain, and ulcer) I70.361
              rest pain (and intermittent claudica-tion) I70.321
              ulceration (and intermittent claudi-cation and rest pain) I70.339
                ankle I70.333
                calf I70.332
                foot site NEC I70.335
                heel I70.334
                lower leg NEC I70.338
                midfoot I70.334
                thigh I70.331
        nonautologous biological graft I70.529
          leg I70.529
            with
              gangrene (and intermittent claudica-tion, rest pain, and ulcer) I70.569
              rest pain (and intermittent claudica-tion) I70.529
            bilateral I70.523
              with
                gangrene (and intermittent clau-dication, rest pain, and ul-cer) I70.563

Arteriosclerosis, arteriosclerotic — *continued*
  with — *continued*
    critical limb ischemia — *continued*
      bypass graft — *continued*
        nonautologous biological graft — *contin-ued*
          leg — *continued*
            bilateral — *continued*
              with — *continued*
                rest pain (and intermittent claudi-cation) I70.523
            left I70.522
              with
                gangrene (and intermittent clau-dication, rest pain, and ul-cer) I70.562
                rest pain (and intermittent claudi-cation) I70.522
                ulceration (and intermittent claudication and rest pain) I70.549
                  ankle I70.543
                  calf I70.542
                  foot site NEC I70.545
                  heel I70.544
                  lower leg NEC I70.548
                  midfoot I70.544
                  thigh I70.541
            right I70.521
              with
                gangrene (and intermittent clau-dication, rest pain, and ul-cer) I70.561
                rest pain (and intermittent claudi-cation) I70.521
                ulceration (and intermittent claudication and rest pain) I70.539
                  ankle I70.533
                  calf I70.532
                  foot site NEC I70.535
                  heel I70.534
                  lower leg NEC I70.538
                  midfoot I70.534
                  thigh I70.531
        nonbiological graft I70.629
          leg I70.629
            with
              gangrene (and intermittent claudica-tion, rest pain, and ulcer) I70.669
              rest pain (and intermittent claudica-tion) I70.629
            bilateral I70.623
              with
                gangrene (and intermittent clau-dication, rest pain, and ul-cer) I70.663
                rest pain (intermittent claudica-tion) I70.623
            left I70.622
              with
                gangrene (and intermittent clau-dication, rest pain, and ul-cer) I70.662
                rest pain (and intermittent claudi-cation) I70.622
                ulceration (and intermittent claudication and rest pain) I70.649
                  ankle I70.643
                  calf I70.642
                  foot site NEC I70.645
                  heel I70.644
                  lower leg NEC I70.648
                  midfoot I70.644
                  thigh I70.641
            right I70.621
              with
                gangrene (and intermittent clau-dication, rest pain, and ul-cer) I70.661
                rest pain (and intermittent claudi-cation) I70.621
                ulceration (and intermittent claudication and rest pain) I70.639
                  ankle I70.633
                  calf I70.632

Arteriosclerosis, arteriosclerotic — *continued*
  with — *continued*
    critical limb ischemia — *continued*
      bypass graft — *continued*
        nonbiological graft — *continued*
          leg — *continued*
            right — *continued*
              with — *continued*
                ulceration — *continued*
                  foot site NEC I70.635
                  heel I70.634
                  lower leg NEC I70.638
                  midfoot I70.634
                  thigh I70.631
        specified graft NEC I70.729
          leg I70.729
            with
              gangrene (and intermittent claudica-tion, rest pain, and ulcer) I70.769
              rest pain (and intermittent claudica-tion) I70.729
            bilateral I70.723
              with
                gangrene (and intermittent clau-dication, rest pain, and ul-cer) I70.763
                rest pain (and intermittent claudi-cation) I70.723
            left I70.722
              with
                gangrene (and intermittent clau-dication, rest pain, and ul-cer) I70.762
                rest pain (and intermittent claudi-cation) I70.722
                ulceration (and intermittent claudication and rest pain) I70.749
                  ankle I70.743
                  calf I70.742
                  foot site NEC I70.745
                  heel I70.744
                  lower leg NEC I70.748
                  midfoot I70.744
                  thigh I70.741
            right I70.721
              with
                gangrene (and intermittent clau-dication, rest pain, and ul-cer) I70.761
                rest pain (and intermittent claudi-cation) I70.721
                ulceration (and intermittent claudication and rest pain) I70.739
                  ankle I70.733
                  calf I70.732
                  foot site NEC I70.735
                  heel I70.734
                  lower leg NEC I70.738
                  midfoot I70.734
                  thigh I70.731
        leg I70.229
          with
            gangrene (and intermittent claudication, rest pain, and ulcer) I70.269
            rest pain (and intermittent claudication) I70.229
          bilateral I70.223
            with
              gangrene (and intermittent claudica-tion, rest pain, and ulcer) I70.263
              rest pain (and intermittent claudica-tion) I70.223
          left I70.222
            with
              gangrene (and intermittent claudica-tion, rest pain, and ulcer) I70.262
              rest pain (and intermittent claudica-tion) I70.222
              ulceration (and intermittent claudica-tion and rest pain) I70.249
                ankle I70.243
                calf I70.242
                foot site NEC I70.245
                heel I70.244

Arteriosclerosis, arteriosclerotic — *continued*
  with — *continued*
    critical limb ischemia — *continued*
      leg — *continued*
        left — *continued*
          with — *continued*
            ulceration — *continued*
              lower leg NEC I70.248
              midfoot I70.244
              thigh I70.241
        right I70.221
          with
            gangrene (and intermittent claudication, rest pain, and ulcer) I70.261
            rest pain (and intermittent claudication) I70.221
            ulceration (and intermittent claudication and rest pain) I70.239
              ankle I70.233
              calf I70.232
              foot site NEC I70.235
              heel I70.234
              lower leg NEC I70.238
              midfoot I70.234
              thigh I70.231
  aorta I70.0
  arteries of extremities — *see* Arteriosclerosis, extremities
    with
      chronic limb-threatening ischemia — *see* Arteriosclerosis, with critical limb ischemia
      critical limb ischemia — *see* Arteriosclerosis, with critical limb ischemia
  brain I67.2
  bypass graft
    with
      chronic limb-threatening ischemia — *see* Arteriosclerosis, with critical limb ischemia
      critical limb ischemia — *see* Arteriosclerosis, with critical limb ischemia
      coronary — *see* Arteriosclerosis, coronary, bypass graft
      extremities — *see* Arteriosclerosis, extremities, bypass graft
  cardiac — *see* Disease, heart, ischemic, atherosclerotic
  cardiopathy — *see* Disease, heart, ischemic, atherosclerotic
  cardiorenal — *see* Hypertension, cardiorenal
  cardiovascular — *see* Disease, heart, ischemic, atherosclerotic
  carotid — *see also* Occlusion, artery, carotid I65.2- ☑
  central nervous system I67.2
  cerebral I67.2
  cerebrovascular I67.2
  coronary (artery) I25.10
    due to
      calcified coronary lesion (severely) I25.84
      lipid rich plaque I25.83
    bypass graft I25.810
      with
        angina pectoris I25.709
          with documented spasm I25.701
          specified type NEC I25.708
          unstable I25.700
        ischemic chest pain I25.709
      autologous artery I25.810
        with
          angina pectoris I25.729
            with documented spasm I25.721
            specified type I25.728
            unstable I25.720
          ischemic chest pain I25.729
      autologous vein I25.810
        with
          angina pectoris I25.719
            with documented spasm I25.711
            specified type I25.718
            unstable I25.710
          ischemic chest pain I25.719
      nonautologous biological I25.810
        with
          angina pectoris I25.739
            with documented spasm I25.731
            specified type I25.738
            unstable I25.730
          ischemic chest pain I25.739
      specified type NEC I25.810

Arteriosclerosis, arteriosclerotic — *continued*
  coronary — *continued*
    bypass graft — *continued*
      specified type — *continued*
        with
          angina pectoris I25.799
            with documented spasm I25.791
            specified type I25.798
            unstable I25.790
          ischemic chest pain I25.799
    native vessel
      with
        angina pectoris I25.119
          with documented spasm I25.111
          specified type NEC I25.118
          unstable I25.110
        ischemic chest pain I25.119
    transplanted heart I25.811
      bypass graft I25.812
        with
          angina pectoris I25.769
            with documented spasm I25.761
            specified type I25.768
            unstable I25.760
          ischemic chest pain I25.769
      native coronary artery I25.811
        with
          angina pectoris I25.759
            with documented spasm I25.751
            specified type I25.758
            unstable I25.750
          ischemic chest pain I25.759
  extremities (native arteries) I70.209
    with
      chronic limb-threatening ischemia — *see* Arteriosclerosis, with critical limb ischemia
      critical limb ischemia — *see* Arteriosclerosis, with critical limb ischemia
    bypass graft I70.309
      with
        chronic limb-threatening ischemia — *see* Arteriosclerosis, with critical limb ischemia
        critical limb ischemia — *see* Arteriosclerosis, with critical limb ischemia
      autologous vein graft I70.409
        leg I70.409
          with
            gangrene (and intermittent claudication, rest pain and ulcer) I70.469
            intermittent claudication I70.419
            rest pain (and intermittent claudication) I70.429
          bilateral I70.403
            with
              gangrene (and intermittent claudication, rest pain and ulcer) I70.463
              intermittent claudication I70.463
              rest pain (and intermittent claudication) I70.423
            specified type NEC I70.493
          left I70.402
            with
              gangrene (and intermittent claudication, rest pain and ulcer) I70.462
              intermittent claudication I70.412
              rest pain (and intermittent claudication) I70.422
              ulceration (and intermittent claudication and rest pain) I70.449
                ankle I70.443
                calf I70.442
                foot site NEC I70.445
                heel I70.444
                lower leg NEC I70.448
                midfoot I70.444
                thigh I70.441
            specified type NEC I70.492
          right I70.401
            with
              gangrene (and intermittent claudication, rest pain and ulcer) I70.461
              intermittent claudication I70.411
              rest pain (and intermittent claudication) I70.421
              ulceration (and intermittent claudication and rest pain) I70.439

Arteriosclerosis, arteriosclerotic — *continued*
  extremities — *continued*
    bypass graft — *continued*
      autologous vein graft — *continued*
        leg — *continued*
          right — *continued*
            with — *continued*
              ulceration — *continued*
                ankle I70.433
                calf I70.432
                foot site NEC I70.435
                heel I70.434
                lower leg NEC I70.438
                midfoot I70.434
                thigh I70.431
            specified type NEC I70.491
          specified type NEC I70.499
        specified NEC I70.408
          with
            gangrene (and intermittent claudication, rest pain and ulcer) I70.468
            intermittent claudication I70.418
            rest pain (and intermittent claudication) I70.428
            ulceration (and intermittent claudication and rest pain) I70.45
          specified type NEC I70.498
      leg I70.309
        with
          gangrene (and intermittent claudication, rest pain and ulcer) I70.369
          intermittent claudication I70.319
          rest pain (and intermittent claudication) I70.329
        bilateral I70.303
          with
            gangrene (and intermittent claudication, rest pain and ulcer) I70.363
            intermittent claudication I70.313
            rest pain (and intermittent claudication) I70.323
          specified type NEC I70.393
        left I70.302
          with
            gangrene (and intermittent claudication, rest pain and ulcer) I70.362
            intermittent claudication I70.312
            rest pain (and intermittent claudication) I70.322
            ulceration (and intermittent claudication and rest pain) I70.349
              ankle I70.343
              calf I70.342
              foot site NEC I70.345
              heel I70.344
              lower leg NEC I70.348
              midfoot I70.344
              thigh I70.341
          specified type NEC I70.392
        right I70.301
          with
            gangrene (and intermittent claudication, rest pain and ulcer) I70.361
            intermittent claudication I70.311
            rest pain (and intermittent claudication) I70.321
            ulceration (and intermittent claudication and rest pain) I70.339
              ankle I70.333
              calf I70.332
              foot site NEC I70.335
              heel I70.334
              lower leg NEC I70.338
              midfoot I70.334
              thigh I70.331
          specified type NEC I70.391
        specified type NEC I70.399
      nonautologous biological graft I70.509
        leg I70.509
          with
            gangrene (and intermittent claudication, rest pain and ulcer) I70.569
            intermittent claudication I70.519
            rest pain (and intermittent claudication) I70.529
          bilateral I70.503

☑ **Additional Character Required** — Refer to the Tabular List for Character Selection   ▽ Subterms under main terms may continue to next column or page

Arteriosclerosis, arteriosclerotic — *continued*
  extremities — *continued*
    bypass graft — *continued*
      nonautologous biological graft — *continued*
        leg — *continued*
          bilateral — *continued*
           with
             gangrene (and intermittent claudication, rest pain and ulcer) I70.563
             intermittent claudication I70.513
             rest pain (and intermittent claudication) I70.523
           specified type NEC I70.593
        left I70.502
          with
           gangrene (and intermittent claudication, rest pain and ulcer) I70.562
           intermittent claudication I70.512
           rest pain (and intermittent claudication) I70.522
           ulceration (and intermittent claudication and rest pain) I70.549
             ankle I70.543
             calf I70.542
             foot site NEC I70.545
             heel I70.544
             lower leg NEC I70.548
             midfoot I70.544
             thigh I70.541
           specified type NEC I70.592
        right I70.501
          with
           gangrene (and intermittent claudication, rest pain and ulcer) I70.561
           intermittent claudication I70.511
           rest pain (and intermittent claudication) I70.521
           ulceration (and intermittent claudication and rest pain) I70.539
             ankle I70.533
             calf I70.532
             foot site NEC I70.535
             heel I70.534
             lower leg NEC I70.538
             midfoot I70.534
             thigh I70.531
           specified type NEC I70.591
        specified type NEC I70.599
        specified NEC I70.508
          with
           gangrene (and intermittent claudication, rest pain and ulcer) I70.568
           intermittent claudication I70.518
           rest pain (and intermittent claudication) I70.528
           ulceration (and intermittent claudication and rest pain) I70.55
          specified type NEC I70.598
      nonbiological graft I70.609
        leg I70.609
          with
           gangrene (and intermittent claudication, rest pain and ulcer) I70.669
           intermittent claudication I70.619
           rest pain (and intermittent claudication) I70.629
         bilateral I70.603
          with
           gangrene (and intermittent claudication, rest pain and ulcer) I70.663
           intermittent claudication I70.613
           rest pain (and intermittent claudication) I70.623
          specified type NEC I70.693
        left I70.602
          with
           gangrene (and intermittent claudication, rest pain and ulcer) I70.662
           intermittent claudication I70.612
           rest pain (and intermittent claudication) I70.622
           ulceration (and intermittent claudication and rest pain) I70.649
             ankle I70.643

Arteriosclerosis, arteriosclerotic — *continued*
  extremities — *continued*
    bypass graft — *continued*
      nonbiological graft — *continued*
        leg — *continued*
          left — *continued*
           with — *continued*
             ulceration — *continued*
               calf I70.642
               foot site NEC I70.645
               heel I70.644
               lower leg NEC I70.648
               midfoot I70.644
               thigh I70.641
           specified type NEC I70.692
          right I70.601
           with
            gangrene (and intermittent claudication, rest pain and ulcer) I70.661
            intermittent claudication I70.611
            rest pain (and intermittent claudication) I70.621
            ulceration (and intermittent claudication and rest pain) I70.639
             ankle I70.633
             calf I70.632
             foot site NEC I70.635
             heel I70.634
             lower leg NEC I70.638
             midfoot I70.634
             thigh I70.631
           specified type NEC I70.691
        specified type NEC I70.699
        specified NEC I70.608
          with
           gangrene (and intermittent claudication, rest pain and ulcer) I70.668
           intermittent claudication I70.618
           rest pain (and intermittent claudication) I70.628
           ulceration (and intermittent claudication and rest pain) I70.65
          specified type NEC I70.698
      specified graft NEC I70.709
        leg I70.709
          with
           gangrene (and intermittent claudication, rest pain and ulcer) I70.769
           intermittent claudication I70.719
           rest pain (and intermittent claudication) I70.729
         bilateral I70.703
          with
           gangrene (and intermittent claudication, rest pain and ulcer) I70.763
           intermittent claudication I70.713
           rest pain (and intermittent claudication) I70.723
          specified type NEC I70.793
        left I70.702
          with
           gangrene (and intermittent claudication, rest pain and ulcer) I70.762
           intermittent claudication I70.712
           rest pain (and intermittent claudication) I70.722
           ulceration (and intermittent claudication and rest pain) I70.749
             ankle I70.743
             calf I70.742
             foot site NEC I70.745
             heel I70.744
             lower leg NEC I70.748
             midfoot I70.744
             thigh I70.741
           specified type NEC I70.792
        right I70.701
          with
           gangrene (and intermittent claudication, rest pain and ulcer) I70.761
           intermittent claudication I70.711
           rest pain (and intermittent claudication) I70.721
           ulceration (and intermittent claudication and rest pain) I70.739

Arteriosclerosis, arteriosclerotic — *continued*
  extremities — *continued*
    bypass graft — *continued*
      specified graft — *continued*
        leg — *continued*
          right — *continued*
           with — *continued*
             ulceration — *continued*
               ankle I70.733
               calf I70.732
               foot site NEC I70.735
               heel I70.734
               lower leg NEC I70.738
               midfoot I70.734
               thigh I70.731
           specified type NEC I70.791
        specified type NEC I70.799
        specified NEC I70.708
          with
           gangrene (and intermittent claudication, rest pain and ulcer) I70.768
           intermittent claudication I70.718
           rest pain (and intermittent claudication) I70.728
           ulceration (and intermittent claudication and rest pain) I70.75
          specified type NEC I70.798
    specified NEC I70.308
      with
        gangrene (and intermittent claudication, rest pain and ulcer) I70.368
        intermittent claudication I70.318
        rest pain (and intermittent claudication) I70.328
        ulceration (and intermittent claudication and rest pain) I70.35
        specifiec type NEC I70.398
    leg I70.209
      with
        gangrene (and intermittent claudication, rest pain and ulcer) I70.269
        intermittent claudication I70.219
        rest pain (and intermittent claudication) I70.229
      bilateral I70.203
        with
          gangrene (and intermittent claudication, rest pain and ulcer) I70.263
          intermittent claudication I70.213
          rest pain (and intermittent claudication) I70.223
          specified type NEC I70.293
      left I70.202
        with
          gangrene (and intermittent claudication, rest pain and ulcer) I70.262
          intermittent claudication I70.212
          rest pain (and intermittent claudication) I70.222
          ulceration (and intermittent claudication and rest pain) I70.249
           ankle I70.243
           calf I70.242
           foot site NEC I70.245
           heel I70.244
           lower leg NEC I70.248
           midfoot I70.244
           thigh I70.241
          specified type NEC I70.292
      right I70.201
        with
          gangrene (and intermittent claudication, rest pain and ulcer) I70.261
          intermittent claudication I70.211
          rest pain (and intermittent claudication) I70.221
          ulceration (and intermittent claudication and rest pain) I70.239
           ankle I70.233
           calf I70.232
           foot site NEC I70.235
           heel I70.234
           lower leg NEC I70.238
           midfoot I70.234
           thigh I70.231
          specified type NEC I70.291
      specified type NEC I70.299
    specified site NEC I70.208

Arteriosclerosis, arteriosclerotic — *continued*
- extremities — *continued*
  - specified site — *continued*
    - with
      - gangrene (and intermittent claudication, rest pain and ulcer) I70.268
      - intermittent claudication I70.218
      - rest pain (and intermittent claudication) I70.228
      - ulceration (and intermittent claudication and rest pain) I70.25
    - specified type NEC I70.298
- generalized I70.91
- heart (disease) — *see* Arteriosclerosis, coronary (artery),
- kidney — *see* Hypertension, kidney
- medial — *see* Arteriosclerosis, extremities
- mesenteric (artery) K55.1
- Mönckeberg's — *see* Arteriosclerosis, extremities
- myocarditis I51.4
- peripheral (of extremities) — *see* Arteriosclerosis, extremities
- pulmonary (idiopathic) I27.0
- renal (arterioles) — *see also* Hypertension, kidney
  - artery I70.1
- retina (vascular) I70.8 [H35.0-] ☑
- specified artery NEC I70.8
- spinal (cord) G95.19
- vertebral (artery) I67.2

Arteriospasm I73.9

Arteriovenous — *see* condition

Arteritis I77.6
- allergic M31.0
- aorta (nonsyphilitic) I77.6
  - syphilitic A52.02
- aortic arch M31.4
- brachiocephalic M31.4
- brain I67.7
  - syphilitic A52.04
- cerebral I67.7
  - in systemic lupus erythematosus M32.19
  - listerial A32.89
  - syphilitic A52.04
  - tuberculous A18.89
- coronary (artery) I25.89
  - rheumatic I01.8
    - chronic I09.89
  - syphilitic A52.06
- cranial (left) (right), giant cell M31.6
- deformans — *see* Arteriosclerosis
- giant cell NEC M31.6
  - with polymyalgia rheumatica M31.5
- necrosing or necrotizing M31.9
  - specified NEC M31.8
- nodosa M30.0
- obliterans — *see* Arteriosclerosis
- pulmonary I28.8
- rheumatic — *see* Fever, rheumatic
- senile — *see* Arteriosclerosis
- suppurative I77.2
- syphilitic (general) A52.09
  - brain A52.04
  - coronary A52.06
  - spinal A52.09
- temporal, giant cell M31.6
- young female aortic arch syndrome M31.4

Artery, arterial — *see also* condition
- abscess I77.89
- single umbilical Q27.0

Arthralgia (allergic) — *see also* Pain, joint
- in caisson disease T70.3 ☑
- temporomandibular M26.62- ☑

Arthritis, arthritic (acute) (chronic) (nonpyogenic) (subacute) M19.90
- allergic — *see* Arthritis, specified form NEC
- ankylosing (crippling) (spine) — *see also* Spondylitis, ankylosing
  - sites other than spine — *see* Arthritis, specified form NEC
- atrophic — *see* Osteoarthritis
  - spine — *see* Spondylitis, ankylosing
- back — *see* Spondylopathy, inflammatory
- blennorrhagic (gonococcal) A54.42
- Charcot's — *see* Arthropathy, neuropathic
  - diabetic — *see* Diabetes, arthropathy, neuropathic
  - syringomyelic G95.0
- chylous (filarial) — *see also* category M01 B74.9
- climacteric (any site) NEC — *see* Arthritis, specified form NEC

Arthritis, arthritic — *continued*
- crystal (-induced) — *see* Arthritis, in, crystals
- deformans — *see* Osteoarthritis
- degenerative — *see* Osteoarthritis
- due to or associated with
  - acromegaly E22.0
  - brucellosis — *see* Brucellosis
  - caisson disease T70.3 ☑
  - diabetes — *see* Diabetes, arthropathy
  - dracontiasis — *see also* category M01 B72
  - enteritis NEC
    - regional — *see* Enteritis, regional
  - erysipelas — *see also* category M01 A46
  - erythema
    - epidemic A25.1
    - nodosum L52
  - filariasis NOS B74.9
  - glanders A24.0
  - helminthiasis — *see also* category M01 B83.9
  - hemophilia D66 [M36.2]
  - Henoch- (Schönlein) purpura D69.0 [M36.4]
  - human parvovirus — *see also* category M01 B97.6
  - infectious disease NEC M01 ☑
  - leprosy (see also category M01) — *see also* Leprosy A30.9
  - Lyme disease A69.23
  - mycobacteria — *see also* category M01 A31.8
  - parasitic disease NEC — *see also* category M01 B89
  - paratyphoid fever (see also category M01) — *see also* Fever, paratyphoid A01.4
  - rat bite fever — *see also* category M01 A25.1
  - regional enteritis — *see* Enteritis, regional
  - respiratory disorder NOS J98.9
  - serum sickness — *see also* Reaction, serum T80.69 ☑
  - syringomyelia G95.0
  - typhoid fever A01.04
- epidemic erythema A25.1
- facet joint — *see also* Spondylosis M47.819
- febrile — *see* Fever, rheumatic
- gonococcal A54.42
- gouty (acute) — *see* Gout
- in (due to)
  - acromegaly — *see also* subcategory M14.8- E22.0
  - amyloidosis — *see also* subcategory M14.8- E85.4
  - bacterial disease — *see also* subcategory M01 A49.9
  - Behçet's syndrome M35.2
  - caisson disease — *see also* subcategory M14.8- T70.3 ☑
  - coliform bacilli (Escherichia coli) — *see* Arthritis, in, pyogenic organism NEC
  - crystals M11.9
    - dicalcium phosphate — *see* Arthritis, in, crystals, specified type NEC
    - hydroxyapatite M11.0- ☑
    - pyrophosphate — *see* Arthritis, in, crystals, specified type NEC
    - specified type NEC M11.80
      - ankle M11.87- ☑
      - elbow M11.82- ☑
      - foot joint M11.87- ☑
      - hand joint M11.84- ☑
      - hip M11.85- ☑
      - knee M11.86- ☑
      - multiple sites M11.8- ☑
      - shoulder M11.81- ☑
      - vertebrae M11.88
      - wrist M11.83- ☑
  - dermatoarthritis, lipoid E78.81
  - dracontiasis (dracunculiasis) — *see also* category M01 B72
  - endocrine disorder NEC — *see also* subcategory M14.8- E34.9
  - enteritis, infectious NEC — *see also* category M01 A09
  - specified organism NEC — *see also* category M01 A08.8
  - erythema
    - multiforme — *see also* subcategory M14.8- L51.9
    - nodosum — *see also* subcategory M14.8- L52
  - gout — *see* Gout
  - helminthiasis NEC — *see also* category M01 B83.9
  - hemochromatosis — *see also* subcategory M14.8- E83.118
  - hemoglobinopathy NEC D58.2 [M36.3]
  - hemophilia NEC D66 [M36.2]
  - Hemophilus influenzae M00.8- ☑ [B96.3]

Arthritis, arthritic — *continued*
- in — *continued*
  - Henoch (-Schönlein) purpura D69.0 [M36.4]
  - hyperparathyroidism NEC — *see also* subcategory M14.8- E21.3
  - hypersensitivity reaction NEC T78.49 ☑ [M36.4]
  - hypogammaglobulinemia — *see also* subcategory M14.8- D80.1
  - hypothyroidism NEC — *see also* subcategory M14.8- E03.9
  - infection — *see* Arthritis, pyogenic or pyemic
    - spine — *see* Spondylopathy, infective
  - infectious disease NEC M01 ☑
  - leprosy — *see also* category M01 A30.9
  - leukemia NEC C95.9- ☑ [M36.1]
  - lipoid dermatoarthritis E78.81
  - Lyme disease A69.23
  - Mediterranean fever, familial — *see also* subcategory M14.8- M04.1
  - Meningococcus A39.83
  - metabolic disorder NEC — *see also* subcategory M14.8- E88.9
  - multiple myelomatosis C90.0- ☑ [M36.1]
  - mumps B26.85
  - mycosis NEC — *see also* category M01 B49
  - myelomatosis (multiple) C90.0- ☑ [M36.1]
  - neurological disorder NEC G98.0
  - ochronosis — *see also* subcategory M14.8- E70.29
  - O'nyong-nyong — *see also* category M01 A92.1
  - parasitic disease NEC — *see also* category M01 B89
  - paratyphoid fever — *see also* category M01 A01.4
  - Pseudomonas — *see* Arthritis, pyogenic, bacterial NEC
  - psoriasis L40.50
  - pyogenic organism NEC — *see* Arthritis, pyogenic, bacterial NEC
  - Reiter's disease — *see* Reiter's disease
  - respiratory disorder NEC — *see also* subcategory M14.8- J98.9
  - reticulosis, malignant — *see also* subcategory M14.8- C86.0
  - rubella B06.82
  - Salmonella (arizonae) (cholerae-suis) (enteritidis) (typhimurium) A02.23
  - sarcoidosis D86.86
  - specified bacteria NEC — *see* Arthritis, pyogenic, bacterial NEC
  - sporotrichosis B42.82
  - syringomyelia G95.0
  - thalassemia NEC D56.9 [M36.3]
  - tuberculosis — *see* Tuberculosis, arthritis
  - typhoid fever A01.04
  - urethritis, Reiter's — *see* Reiter's disease
  - viral disease NEC — *see also* category M01 B34.9
- infectious or infective — *see also* Arthritis, pyogenic or pyemic
  - spine — *see* Spondylopathy, infective
- juvenile M08.90
  - with systemic onset — *see* Still's disease
  - ankle M08.97- ☑
  - elbow M08.92- ☑
  - foot joint M08.97- ☑
  - hand joint M08.94- ☑
  - hip M08.95- ☑
  - knee M08.96- ☑
  - multiple site M08.99
  - pauciarticular M08.40
    - ankle M08.47- ☑
    - elbow M08.42- ☑
    - foot joint M08.47- ☑
    - hand joint M08.44- ☑
    - hip M08.45- ☑
    - knee M08.46- ☑
    - shoulder M08.41- ☑
    - specified site NEC M08.4A
    - vertebrae M08.48
    - wrist M08.43- ☑
  - psoriatic L40.54
  - rheumatoid — *see* Arthritis, rheumatoid, juvenile
  - shoulder M08.91- ☑
  - specified site NEC M08.9A
  - specified type NEC M08.80
    - ankle M08.87- ☑
    - elbow M08.82- ☑
    - foot joint M08.87- ☑
    - hand joint M08.84- ☑
    - hip M08.85- ☑

30

☑ Additional Character Required — Refer to the Tabular List for Character Selection   ▽ Subterms under main terms may continue to next column or page

Arthritis, arthritic — *continued*
  juvenile — *continued*
    specified type — *continued*
      knee M08.86- ☑
      multiple site M08.89
      shoulder M08.81- ☑
      specified joint NEC M08.88
      vertebrae M08.88
      wrist M08.83- ☑
    wrist M08.93- ☑
  meaning osteoarthritis — *see* Osteoarthritis
  meningococcal A39.83
  menopausal (any site) NEC — *see* Arthritis, specified form NEC
  mutilans (psoriatic) L40.52
  mycotic NEC — *see also* category M01 B49
  neuropathic (Charcot) — *see* Arthropathy, neuropathic
    diabetic — *see* Diabetes, arthropathy, neuropathic
    nonsyphilitic NEC G98.0
    syringomyelic G95.0
  ochronotic — *see also* subcategory M14.8- E70.29
  palindromic (any site) — *see* Rheumatism, palindromic
  pneumococcal M00.10
    ankle M00.17- ☑
    elbow M00.12- ☑
    foot joint — *see* Arthritis, pneumococcal, ankle
    hand joint M00.14- ☑
    hip M00.15- ☑
    knee M00.16- ☑
    multiple site M00.19
    shoulder M00.11- ☑
    vertebra M00.18
    wrist M00.13- ☑
  postdysenteric — *see* Arthropathy, postdysenteric
  postmeningococcal A39.84
  postrheumatic, chronic — *see* Arthropathy, postrheumatic, chronic
  primary progressive — *see also* Arthritis, specified form NEC
    spine — *see* Spondylitis, ankylosing
  psoriatic L40.50
  purulent (any site except spine) — *see* Arthritis, pyogenic or pyemic
    spine — *see* Spondylopathy, infective
  pyogenic or pyemic (any site except spine) M00.9
    bacterial NEC M00.80
      ankle M00.87- ☑
      elbow M00.82- ☑
      foot joint — *see* Arthritis, pyogenic, bacterial NEC, ankle
      hand joint M00.84- ☑
      hip M00.85- ☑
      knee M00.86- ☑
      multiple site M00.89
      shoulder M00.81- ☑
      vertebra M00.88
      wrist M00.83- ☑
    pneumococcal — *see* Arthritis, pneumococcal
    spine — *see* Spondylopathy, infective
    staphylococcal — *see* Arthritis, staphylococcal
    streptococcal — *see* Arthritis, streptococcal NEC
      pneumococcal — *see* Arthritis, pneumococcal
  reactive — *see* Reiter's disease
  rheumatic — *see also* Arthritis, rheumatoid
    acute or subacute — *see* Fever, rheumatic
  rheumatoid M06.9
    with
      carditis — *see* Rheumatoid, carditis
      endocarditis — *see* Rheumatoid, carditis
      heart involvement NEC — *see* Rheumatoid, carditis
      lung involvement — *see* Rheumatoid, lung
      myocarditis — *see* Rheumatoid, carditis
      myopathy — *see* Rheumatoid, myopathy
      pericarditis — *see* Rheumatoid, carditis
      polyneuropathy — *see* Rheumatoid, polyneuropathy
      rheumatoid factor — *see* Arthritis, rheumatoid, seropositive
      splenoadenomegaly and leukopenia — *see* Felty's syndrome
      vasculitis — *see* Rheumatoid, vasculitis
      visceral involvement NEC — *see* Rheumatoid, arthritis, with involvement of organs NEC
    juvenile (with or without rheumatoid factor) M08.00
      with systemic onset — *see* Still's disease
      ankle M08.07- ☑

Arthritis, arthritic — *continued*
  rheumatoid — *continued*
    juvenile — *continued*
      elbow M08.02- ☑
      foot joint M08.07- ☑
      hand joint M08.04- ☑
      hip M08.05- ☑
      knee M08.06- ☑
      multiple site M08.09
      shoulder M08.01- ☑
      specified site NEC M08.0A
      vertebra M08.08
      wrist M08.03- ☑
    seronegative M06.00
      ankle M06.07- ☑
      elbow M06.02- ☑
      foot joint M06.07- ☑
      hand joint M06.04- ☑
      hip M06.05- ☑
      knee M06.06- ☑
      multiple site M06.09
      shoulder M06.01- ☑
      specified site NEC M06.0A
      vertebra M06.08
      wrist M06.03- ☑
    seropositive M05.9
      specified NEC M05.80
        ankle M05.87- ☑
        elbow M05.82- ☑
        foot joint M05.87- ☑
        hand joint M05.84- ☑
        hip M05.85- ☑
        knee M05.86- ☑
        multiple sites M05.89
        shoulder M05.81- ☑
        specified site NEC M05.8A
        vertebra — *see* Spondylitis, ankylosing
        wrist M05.83- ☑
      without organ involvement M05.70
        ankle M05.77- ☑
        elbow M05.72- ☑
        foot joint M05.77- ☑
        hand joint M05.74- ☑
        hip M05.75- ☑
        knee M05.76- ☑
        multiple sites M05.79
        shoulder M05.71- ☑
        specified site NEC M05.7A
        vertebra — *see* Spondylitis, ankylosing
        wrist M05.73- ☑
    specified type NEC M06.80
      ankle M06.87- ☑
      elbow M06.82- ☑
      foot joint M06.87- ☑
      hand joint M06.84- ☑
      hip M06.85- ☑
      knee M06.86- ☑
      multiple site M06.89
      shoulder M06.81- ☑
      specified site NEC M06.8A
      vertebra M06.88
      wrist M06.83- ☑
    spine — *see* Spondylitis, ankylosing
  rubella B06.82
  scorbutic — *see also* subcategory M14.8- E54
  senile or senescent — *see* Osteoarthritis
  septic (any site except spine) — *see* Arthritis, pyogenic or pyemic
    spine — *see* Spondylopathy, infective
  serum (nontherapeutic) (therapeutic) — *see* Arthropathy, postimmunization
  specified form NEC M13.80
    ankle M13.87- ☑
    elbow M13.82- ☑
    foot joint M13.87- ☑
    hand joint M13.84- ☑
    hip M13.85- ☑
    knee M13.86- ☑
    multiple site M13.89
    shoulder M13.81- ☑
    specified joint NEC M13.88
    wrist M13.83- ☑
  spine — *see also* Spondylosis
    infectious or infective NEC — *see* Spondylopathy, infective
    Marie-Strümpell — *see* Spondylitis, ankylosing

Arthritis, arthritic — *continued*
  spine — *see also* Spondylosis — *continued*
    pyogenic — *see* Spondylopathy, infective
    rheumatoid — *see* Spondylitis, ankylosing
    traumatic (old) — *see* Spondylopathy, traumatic
    tuberculous A18.01
  staphylococcal M00.00
    ankle M00.07- ☑
    elbow M00.02- ☑
    foot joint — *see* Arthritis, staphylococcal, ankle
    hand joint M00.04- ☑
    hip M00.05- ☑
    knee M00.06- ☑
    multiple site M00.09
    shoulder M00.01- ☑
    vertebra M00.08
    wrist M00.03- ☑
  streptococcal NEC M00.20
    ankle M00.27- ☑
    elbow M00.22- ☑
    foot joint — *see* Arthritis, streptococcal, ankle
    hand joint M00.24- ☑
    hip M00.25- ☑
    knee M00.26- ☑
    multiple site M00.29
    shoulder M00.21- ☑
    vertebra M00.28
    wrist M00.23- ☑
  suppurative — *see* Arthritis, pyogenic or pyemic
  syphilitic (late) A52.16
    congenital A50.55 *[M12.80]*
  syphilitica deformans (Charcot) A52.16
  temporomandibular joint M26.64- ☑
  toxic of menopause (any site) — *see* Arthritis, specified form NEC
  transient — *see* Arthropathy, specified form NEC
  traumatic (chronic) — *see* Arthropathy, traumatic
  tuberculous A18.02
    spine A18.01
  uratic — *see* Gout
  urethritica (Reiter's) — *see* Reiter's disease
  vertebral — *see* Spondylopathy, inflammatory
  villous (any site) — *see* Arthropathy, specified form NEC

Arthrocele — *see* Effusion, joint
Arthrodesis status Z98.1
Arthrodynia — *see also* Pain, joint
Arthrodysplasia Q74.9
Arthrofibrosis, joint — *see* Ankylosis
Arthrogryposis (congenital) Q68.8
  multiplex congenita Q74.3
Arthrokatadysis M24.7
Arthropathy — *see also* Arthritis M12.9
  Charcot's — *see* Arthropathy, neuropathic
    diabetic — *see* Diabetes, arthropathy, neuropathic
    syringomyelic G95.0
  cricoarytenoid J38.7
  crystal (-induced) — *see* Arthritis, in, crystals
  diabetic NEC — *see* Diabetes, arthropathy
  distal interphalangeal, psoriatic L40.51
  enteropathic M07.60
    ankle M07.67- ☑
    elbow M07.62- ☑
    foot joint M07.67- ☑
    hand joint M07.64- ☑
    hip M07.65- ☑
    knee M07.66- ☑
    multiple site M07.69
    shoulder M07.61- ☑
    vertebra M07.68
    wrist M07.63- ☑
  facet joint — *see also* Spondylosis M47.819
  following intestinal bypass M02.00
    ankle M02.07- ☑
    elbow M02.02- ☑
    foot joint M02.07- ☑
    hand joint M02.04- ☑
    hip M02.05- ☑
    knee M02.06- ☑
    multiple site M02.09
    shoulder M02.01- ☑
    vertebra M02.08
    wrist M02.03- ☑
  gouty — *see also* Gout
    in (due to)
      Lesch-Nyhan syndrome E79.1 *[M14.8-]* ☑

▽ **Subterms under main terms may continue to next column or page**   ☑ **Additional Character Required** — Refer to the Tabular List for Character Selection   **31**

Arthritis, arthritic — Arthropathy

Arthropathy — *continued*
  gouty — *see also* Gout — *continued*
    in — *continued*
      sickle-cell disorders D57- ☑ *[M14.8-]* ☑
  hemophilic NEC D66 *[M36.2]*
    in (due to)
      hyperparathyroidism NEC E21.3 *[M14.8-]* ☑
      metabolic disease NOS E88.9 *[M14.8-]* ☑
  in (due to)
    acromegaly E22.0 *[M14.8-]* ☑
    amyloidosis E85.4 *[M14.8-]* ☑
    blood disorder NOS D75.9 *[M36.3]*
    diabetes — *see* Diabetes, arthropathy
    endocrine disease NOS E34.9 *[M14.8-]* ☑
    erythema
      multiforme L51.9 *[M14.8-]* ☑
      nodosum L52 *[M14.8-]* ☑
    hemochromatosis E83.118 *[M14.8-]* ☑
    hemoglobinopathy NEC D58.2 *[M36.3]*
    hemophilia NEC D66 *[M36.2]*
    Henoch-Schönlein purpura D69.0 *[M36.4]*
    hyperthyroidism E05.90 *[M14.8-]* ☑
    hypothyroidism E03.9 *[M14.8-]* ☑
    infective endocarditis I33.0 *[M12.80]*
    leukemia NEC C95.9- ☑ *[M36.1]*
    malignant histiocytosis C96.A *[M36.1]*
    metabolic disease NOS E88.9 *[M14.8-]* ☑
    multiple myeloma C90.0- ☑ *[M36.1]*
    neoplastic disease NOS (*see also* Neoplasm) D49.9 *[M36.1]*
    nutritional deficiency — *see also* subcategory M14.8- E63.9
    psoriasis NOS L40.50
    sarcoidosis D86.86
    syphilis (late) A52.77
      congenital A50.55 *[M12.80]*
    thyrotoxicosis — *see also* subcategory M14.8- E05.90
    ulcerative colitis K51.90 *[M07.60]*
    viral hepatitis (postinfectious) NEC B19.9 *[M12.80]*
    Whipple's disease — *see also* subcategory M14.8- K90.81
  Jaccoud — *see* Arthropathy, postrheumatic, chronic
  juvenile — *see* Arthritis, juvenile
    psoriatic L40.54
  mutilans (psoriatic) L40.52
  neuropathic (Charcot) M14.60
    ankle M14.67- ☑
    diabetic — *see* Diabetes, arthropathy, neuropathic
    elbow M14.62- ☑
    foot joint M14.67- ☑
    hand joint M14.64- ☑
    hip M14.65- ☑
    knee M14.66- ☑
    multiple site M14.69
    nonsyphilitic NEC G98.0
    shoulder M14.61- ☑
    syringomyelic G95.0
    vertebra M14.68
    wrist M14.63- ☑
  osteopulmonary — *see* Osteoarthropathy, hypertrophic, specified NEC
  postdysenteric M02.10
    ankle M02.17- ☑
    elbow M02.12- ☑
    foot joint M02.17- ☑
    hand joint M02.14- ☑
    hip M02.15- ☑
    knee M02.16- ☑
    multiple site M02.19
    shoulder M02.11- ☑
    vertebra M02.18
    wrist M02.13- ☑
  postimmunization M02.20
    ankle M02.27- ☑
    elbow M02.22- ☑
    foot joint M02.27- ☑
    hand joint M02.24- ☑
    hip M02.25- ☑
    knee M02.26- ☑
    multiple site M02.29
    shoulder M02.21- ☑
    vertebra M02.28
    wrist M02.23- ☑
  postinfectious NEC B99 ☑ *[M12.80]*

Arthropathy — *continued*
  postinfectious — *continued*
    in (due to)
      enteritis due to Yersinia enterocolitica A04.6 *[M12.80]*
      syphilis A52.77
      viral hepatitis NEC B19.9 *[M12.80]*
    postrheumatic, chronic (Jaccoud) M12.00
      ankle M12.07- ☑
      elbow M12.02- ☑
      foot joint M12.07- ☑
      hand joint M12.04- ☑
      hip M12.05- ☑
      knee M12.06- ☑
      multiple site M12.09
      shoulder M12.01- ☑
      specified joint NEC M12.08
      vertebrae M12.08
      wrist M12.03- ☑
    psoriatic NEC L40.59
      interphalangeal, distal L40.51
    reactive M02.9
      in (due to)
        infective endocarditis I33.0 *[M02.9]*
      specified type NEC M02.80
        ankle M02.87- ☑
        elbow M02.82- ☑
        foot joint M02.87- ☑
        hand joint M02.84- ☑
        hip M02.85- ☑
        knee M02.86- ☑
        multiple site M02.89
        shoulder M02.81- ☑
        vertebra M02.88
        wrist M02.83- ☑
    specified form NEC M12.80
      ankle M12.87- ☑
      elbow M12.82- ☑
      foot joint M12.87- ☑
      hand joint M12.84- ☑
      hip M12.85- ☑
      knee M12.86- ☑
      multiple site M12.89
      shoulder M12.81- ☑
      specified joint NEC M12.88
      vertebrae M12.88
      wrist M12.83- ☑
    syringomyelic G95.0
    tabes dorsalis A52.16
    tabetic A52.16
    temporomandibular joint M26.65- ☑
    transient — *see* Arthropathy, specified form NEC
    traumatic M12.50
      ankle M12.57- ☑
      elbow M12.52- ☑
      foot joint M12.57- ☑
      hand joint M12.54- ☑
      hip M12.55- ☑
      knee M12.56- ☑
      multiple site M12.59
      shoulder M12.51- ☑
      specified joint NEC M12.58
      vertebrae M12.58
      wrist M12.53- ☑

Arthropyosis — *see* Arthritis, pyogenic or pyemic
Arthrosis (deformans) (degenerative) (localized) — *see also* Osteoarthritis M19.90
  spine — *see* Spondylosis
Arthus' phenomenon or reaction T78.41 ☑
  due to
    drug — *see* Table of Drugs and Chemicals, by drug
Articular — *see* condition
Articulation, reverse (teeth) M26.24
Artificial
  insemination complication — *see* Complications, artificial, fertilization
  opening status (functioning) (without complication) Z93.9
    anus (colostomy) Z93.3
    colostomy Z93.3
    cystostomy Z93.50
      appendico-vesicostomy Z93.52
      cutaneous Z93.51
      specified NEC Z93.59
    enterostomy Z93.4
    gastrostomy Z93.1
    ileostomy Z93.2

Artificial — *continued*
  opening status — *continued*
    intestinal tract NEC Z93.4
    jejunostomy Z93.4
    nephrostomy Z93.6
    specified site NEC Z93.8
    tracheostomy Z93.0
    ureterostomy Z93.6
    urethrostomy Z93.6
    urinary tract NEC Z93.6
    vagina Z93.8
  vagina status Z93.8
Arytenoid — *see* condition
Asbestosis (occupational) J61
Ascariasis B77.9
  with
    complications NEC B77.89
    intestinal complications B77.0
    pneumonia, pneumonitis B77.81
Ascaridosis, ascaridiasis — *see* Ascariasis
Ascaris (infection) (infestation) (lumbricoides) — *see* Ascariasis
Ascending — *see* condition
ASC-H (atypical squamous cells cannot exclude high grade squamous intraepithelial lesion on cytologic smear)
  anus R85.611
  cervix R87.611
  vagina R87.621
Aschoff's bodies — *see* Myocarditis, rheumatic
Ascites (abdominal) R18.8
  cardiac — *see also* Failure, heart, right I50.810
  chylous (nonfilarial) I89.8
    filarial — *see* Infestation, filarial
  due to
    cirrhosis, alcoholic K70.31
    hepatitis
      alcoholic K70.11
      chronic active K71.51
    S. japonicum B65.2
  heart — *see also* Failure, heart, right I50.810
  malignant R18.0
  pseudochylous R18.8
  syphilitic A52.74
  tuberculous A18.31
ASC-US (atypical squamous cells of undetermined significance on cytologic smear)
  anus R85.610
  cervix R87.610
  vagina R87.620
Aseptic — *see* condition
Asherman's syndrome N85.6
Asialia K11.7
Asiatic cholera — *see* Cholera
Asimultagnosia (simultanagnosia) R48.3
Askin's tumor — *see* Neoplasm, connective tissue, malignant
Asocial personality F60.2
Asomatognosia R41.4
Aspartylglucosaminuria E77.1
Asperger's disease or syndrome F84.5
Aspergilloma — *see* Aspergillosis
Aspergillosis (with pneumonia) B44.9
  bronchopulmonary, allergic B44.81
  disseminated B44.7
  generalized B44.7
  pulmonary NEC B44.1
    allergic B44.81
    invasive B44.0
  specified NEC B44.89
  tonsillar B44.2
Aspergillus (flavus) (fumigatus) (infection) (terreus) — *see* Aspergillosis
Aspermatogenesis — *see* Azoospermia
Aspermia (testis) — *see* Azoospermia
Asphyxia, asphyxiation (by) R09.01
  antenatal P84
  birth P84
  bunny bag — *see* Asphyxia, due to, mechanical threat to breathing, trapped in bed clothes
  crushing S28.0 ☑
  drowning T75.1 ☑
  gas, fumes, or vapor — *see* Table of Drugs and Chemicals
  inhalation — *see* Inhalation
  intrauterine P84
  local I73.00
    with gangrene I73.01

☑ **Additional Character Required** — **Refer to the Tabular List for Character Selection**   ▽ Subterms under main terms may continue to next column or page

Asphyxia, asphyxiation — *continued*
　mucus — *see also* Foreign body, respiratory tract, causing asphyxia
　newborn P84
　pathological R09.01
　postnatal P84
　　mechanical — *see* Asphyxia, due to, mechanical threat to breathing
　prenatal P84
　reticularis R23.1
　strangulation — *see* Asphyxia, due to, mechanical threat to breathing
　submersion T75.1 ☑
　traumatic T71.9 ☑
　　due to
　　　crushed chest S28.0 ☑
　　　foreign body (in) — *see* Foreign body, respiratory tract, causing asphyxia
　　　low oxygen content of ambient air T71.20 ☑
　　　　due to
　　　　　being trapped in
　　　　　　low oxygen environment T71.29 ☑
　　　　　　in car trunk T71.221 ☑
　　　　　　　circumstances undetermined T71.224 ☑
　　　　　　　done with intent to harm by
　　　　　　　　another person T71.223 ☑
　　　　　　　　self T71.222 ☑
　　　　　　in refrigerator T71.231 ☑
　　　　　　　circumstances undetermined T71.234 ☑
　　　　　　　done with intent to harm by
　　　　　　　　another person T71.233 ☑
　　　　　　　　self T71.232 ☑
　　　cave-in T71.21 ☑
　　　mechanical threat to breathing (accidental) T71.191 ☑
　　　　circumstances undetermined T71.194 ☑
　　　　done with intent to harm by
　　　　　another person T71.193 ☑
　　　　　self T71.192 ☑
　　　hanging T71.161 ☑
　　　　circumstances undetermined T71.164 ☑
　　　　done with intent to harm by
　　　　　another person T71.163 ☑
　　　　　self T71.162 ☑
　　　plastic bag T71.121 ☑
　　　　circumstances undetermined T71.124 ☑
　　　　done with intent to harm by
　　　　　another person T71.123 ☑
　　　　　self T71.122 ☑
　　　smothering
　　　　in furniture T71.151 ☑
　　　　　circumstances undetermined T71.154 ☑
　　　　　done with intent to harm by
　　　　　　another person T71.153 ☑
　　　　　　self T71.152 ☑
　　　　under
　　　　　another person's body T71.141 ☑
　　　　　　circumstances undetermined T71.144 ☑
　　　　　　done with intent to harm T71.143 ☑
　　　　　pillow T71.111 ☑
　　　　　　circumstances undetermined T71.114 ☑
　　　　　　done with intent to harm by
　　　　　　　another person T71.113 ☑
　　　　　　　self T71.112 ☑
　　　　　trapped in bed clothes T71.131 ☑
　　　　　　circumstances undetermined T71.134 ☑
　　　　　　done with intent to harm by
　　　　　　　another person T71.133 ☑
　　　　　　　self T71.132 ☑
　vomiting, vomitus — *see* Foreign body, respiratory tract, causing asphyxia

Aspiration
　amniotic (clear) fluid (newborn) P24.10
　　with
　　　pneumonia (pneumonitis) P24.11
　　　respiratory symptoms P24.11
　blood
　　newborn (without respiratory symptoms) P24.20
　　　with
　　　　pneumonia (pneumonitis) P24.21
　　　　respiratory symptoms P24.21

Aspiration — *continued*
　blood — *continued*
　　specified age NEC — *see* Foreign body, respiratory tract
　bronchitis J69.0
　food or foreign body — *see* Foreign body, by site
　liquor (amnii) (newborn) P24.10
　　with
　　　pneumonia (pneumonitis) P24.11
　　　respiratory symptoms P24.11
　meconium (newborn) (without respiratory symptoms) P24.00
　　with
　　　pneumonitis (pneumonitis) P24.01
　　　respiratory symptoms P24.01
　milk (newborn) (without respiratory symptoms) P24.30
　　with
　　　pneumonia (pneumonitis) P24.31
　　　respiratory symptoms P24.31
　　specified age NEC — *see* Foreign body, respiratory tract
　mucus — *see also* Foreign body, by site, causing asphyxia
　　newborn P24.10
　　　with
　　　　pneumonia (pneumonitis) P24.11
　　　　respiratory symptoms P24.11
　neonatal P24.9
　　specific NEC (without respiratory symptoms) P24.80
　　　with
　　　　pneumonia (pneumonitis) P24.81
　　　　respiratory symptoms P24.81
　newborn P24.9
　　specific NEC (without respiratory symptoms) P24.80
　　　with
　　　　pneumonia (pneumonitis) P24.81
　　　　respiratory symptoms P24.81
　pneumonia J69.0
　pneumonitis J69.0
　syndrome of newborn — *see* Aspiration, by substance, with pneumonia
　vernix caseosa (newborn) P24.80
　　with
　　　pneumonia (pneumonitis) P24.81
　　　respiratory symptoms P24.81
　vomitus — *see also* Foreign body, respiratory tract
　　newborn (without respiratory symptoms) P24.30
　　　with
　　　　pneumonia (pneumonitis) P24.31
　　　　respiratory symptoms P24.31

Asplenia (congenital) Q89.01
　postsurgical Z90.81
Assam fever B55.0
Assault, sexual — *see* Maltreatment
Assmann's focus NEC A15.0
Astasia (-abasia) (hysterical) F44.4
Asteatosis cutis L85.3
Astereognosia, astereognosis R48.1
Asterixis R27.8
　in liver disease K71.3
Asteroid hyalitis — *see* Deposit, crystalline
Asthenia, asthenic R53.1
　cardiac — *see also* Failure, heart I50.9
　　psychogenic F45.8
　cardiovascular — *see also* Failure, heart I50.9
　　psychogenic F45.8
　heart — *see also* Failure, heart I50.9
　　psychogenic F45.8
　hysterical F44.4
　myocardial — *see also* Failure, heart I50.9
　　psychogenic F45.8
　nervous F48.8
　neurocirculatory F45.8
　neurotic F48.8
　psychogenic F48.8
　psychoneurotic F48.8
　psychophysiologic F48.8
　reaction (psychophysiologic) F48.8
　senile R54
Asthenopia — *see also* Discomfort, visual
　hysterical F44.6
　psychogenic F44.6
Asthenospermia — *see* Abnormal, specimen, male genital organs
Asthma, asthmatic (bronchial) (catarrh) (spasmodic) J45.909
　with
　　chronic obstructive bronchitis J44.9

Asthma, asthmatic — *continued*
　with — *continued*
　　chronic obstructive bronchitis — *continued*
　　　with
　　　　acute lower respiratory infection J44.0
　　　　exacerbation (acute) J44.1
　　chronic obstructive pulmonary disease J44.9
　　　with
　　　　acute lower respiratory infection J44.0
　　　　exacerbation (acute) J44.1
　　exacerbation (acute) J45.901
　　hay fever — *see* Asthma, allergic extrinsic
　　rhinitis, allergic — *see* Asthma, allergic extrinsic
　　status asthmaticus J45.902
　allergic extrinsic J45.909
　　with
　　　exacerbation (acute) J45.901
　　　status asthmaticus J45.902
　atopic — *see* Asthma, allergic extrinsic
　cardiac — *see* Failure, ventricular, left
　cardiobronchial I50.1
　childhood J45.909
　　with
　　　exacerbation (acute) J45.901
　　　status asthmaticus J45.902
　chronic obstructive J44.9
　　with
　　　acute lower respiratory infection J44.0
　　　exacerbation (acute) J44.1
　collier's J60
　cough variant J45.991
　detergent J69.8
　due to
　　detergent J69.8
　　inhalation of fumes J68.3
　eosinophilic J82.83
　extrinsic, allergic — *see* Asthma, allergic extrinsic
　grinder's J62.8
　hay — *see* Asthma, allergic extrinsic
　heart I50.1
　idiosyncratic — *see* Asthma, nonallergic
　intermittent (mild) J45.20
　　with
　　　exacerbation (acute) J45.21
　　　status asthmaticus J45.22
　intrinsic, nonallergic — *see* Asthma, nonallergic
　Kopp's E32.8
　late-onset J45.909
　　with
　　　exacerbation (acute) J45.901
　　　status asthmaticus J45.902
　mild intermittent J45.20
　　with
　　　exacerbation (acute) J45.21
　　　status asthmaticus J45.22
　mild persistent J45.30
　　with
　　　exacerbation (acute) J45.31
　　　status asthmaticus J45.32
　Millar's (laryngismus stridulus) J38.5
　miner's J60
　mixed J45.909
　　with
　　　exacerbation (acute) J45.901
　　　status asthmaticus J45.902
　moderate persistent J45.40
　　with
　　　exacerbation (acute) J45.41
　　　status asthmaticus J45.42
　nervous — *see* Asthma, nonallergic
　nonallergic (intrinsic) J45.909
　　with
　　　exacerbation (acute) J45.901
　　　status asthmaticus J45.902
　persistent
　　mild J45.30
　　　with
　　　　exacerbation (acute) J45.31
　　　　status asthmaticus J45.32
　　moderate J45.40
　　　with
　　　　exacerbation (acute) J45.41
　　　　status asthmaticus J45.42
　　severe J45.50
　　　with
　　　　exacerbation (acute) J45.51
　　　　status asthmaticus J45.52
　platinum J45.998

Asthma, asthmatic — *continued*
  pneumoconiotic NEC J64
  potter's J62.8
  predominantly allergic J45.909
  psychogenic F54
  pulmonary eosinophilic J82.83
  red cedar J67.8
  Rostan's I50.1
  sandblaster's J62.8
  sequoiosis J67.8
  severe persistent J45.50
    with
      exacerbation (acute) J45.51
      status asthmaticus J45.52
  specified NEC J45.998
  stonemason's J62.8
  thymic E32.8
  tuberculous — *see* Tuberculosis, pulmonary
  Wichmann's (laryngismus stridulus) J38.5
  wood J67.8
Astigmatism (compound) (congenital) H52.20- ☑
  irregular H52.21- ☑
  regular H52.22- ☑
Astraphobia F40.220
Astroblastoma
  specified site — *see* Neoplasm, malignant, by site
  unspecified site C71.9
Astrocytoma (cystic)
  anaplastic
    specified site — *see* Neoplasm, malignant, by site
    unspecified site C71.9
  fibrillary
    specified site — *see* Neoplasm, malignant, by site
    unspecified site C71.9
  fibrous
    specified site — *see* Neoplasm, malignant, by site
    unspecified site C71.9
  gemistocytic
    specified site — *see* Neoplasm, malignant, by site
    unspecified site C71.9
  juvenile
    specified site — *see* Neoplasm, malignant, by site
    unspecified site C71.9
  pilocytic
    specified site — *see* Neoplasm, malignant, by site
    unspecified site C71.9
  piloid
    specified site — *see* Neoplasm, malignant, by site
    unspecified site C71.9
  protoplasmic
    specified site — *see* Neoplasm, malignant, by site
    unspecified site C71.9
  specified site NEC — *see* Neoplasm, malignant, by site
  subependymal D43.2
    giant cell
      specified site — *see* Neoplasm, uncertain behavior, by site
      unspecified site D43.2
    specified site — *see* Neoplasm, uncertain behavior, by site
    unspecified site D43.2
  unspecified site C71.9
Astroglioma
  specified site — *see* Neoplasm, malignant, by site
  unspecified site C71.9
Asymbolia R48.8
Asymmetry — *see also* Distortion
  between native and reconstructed breast N65.1
  face Q67.0
  jaw (lower) — *see* Anomaly, dentofacial, jaw-cranial base relationship, asymmetry
Asynergia, asynergy R27.8
  ventricular I51.89
Asystole (heart) — *see* Arrest, cardiac
At risk
  for
    dental caries Z91.849
      high Z91.843
      low Z91.841
      moderate Z91.842
    falling Z91.81
Ataxia, ataxy, ataxic R27.0
  acute R27.8
  autosomal recessive Friedreich G11.11
  brain (hereditary) G11.9
  cerebellar (hereditary) G11.9
    with defective DNA repair G11.3
    alcoholic G31.2

Ataxia, ataxy, ataxic — *continued*
  cerebellar — *continued*
    early-onset G11.10
      with
        essential tremor G11.19
        myoclonus [Hunt's ataxia] G11.19
        retained tendon reflexes G11.19
      in
        alcoholism G31.2
        myxedema E03.9 *[G13.2]*
        neoplastic disease — *see also* Neoplasm D49.9 *[G32.81]*
        specified disease NEC G32.81
    late-onset (Marie's) G11.2
  cerebral (hereditary) G11.9
  congenital nonprogressive G11.0
  family, familial — *see* Ataxia, hereditary
  following
    cerebrovascular disease I69.993
      cerebral infarction I69.393
      intracerebral hemorrhage I69.193
      nontraumatic intracranial hemorrhage NEC I69.293
      specified disease NEC I69.893
      subarachnoid hemorrhage I69.093
  Friedreich's (heredofamilial) (cerebellar) (spinal) (with retained reflexes) G11.11
  gait R26.0
    hysterical F44.4
  general R27.8
  gluten M35.9 *[G32.81]*
    with celiac disease K90.0 *[G32.81]*
  hereditary G11.9
    with neuropathy G60.2
    cerebellar — *see* Ataxia, cerebellar
    spastic G11.4
    specified NEC G11.8
    spinal (Friedreich's) G11.11
  heredofamilial — *see* Ataxia, hereditary
  Hunt's G11.19
  hysterical F44.4
  locomotor (progressive) (syphilitic) (partial) (spastic) A52.11
    diabetic — *see* Diabetes, ataxia
  Marie's (cerebellar) (heredofamilial) (late-onset) G11.2
  nonorganic origin F44.4
  nonprogressive, congenital G11.0
  psychogenic F44.4
  Roussy-Lévy G60.0
  Sanger-Brown's (hereditary) G11.2
  spastic hereditary G11.4
  spinal
    hereditary (Friedreich's) G11.11
    progressive (syphilitic) A52.11
  spinocerebellar, X-linked recessive G11.19
  telangiectasia (Louis-Bar) G11.3
Ataxia-telangiectasia (Louis-Bar) G11.3
Atelectasis (massive) (partial) (pressure) (pulmonary) J98.11
  newborn P28.10
    due to resorption P28.11
    partial P28.19
    primary P28.0
    secondary P28.19
  primary (newborn) P28.0
  tuberculous — *see* Tuberculosis, pulmonary
Atelocardia Q24.9
Atelomyelia Q06.1
Atheroembolism
  of
    extremities
      lower I75.02- ☑
      upper I75.01- ☑
    kidney I75.81
    specified NEC I75.89
Atheroma, atheromatous — *see also* Arteriosclerosis I70.90
  aorta, aortic I70.0
    valve — *see also* Endocarditis, aortic I35.8
  aorto-iliac I70.0
  artery — *see* Arteriosclerosis
  basilar (artery) I67.2
  carotid (artery) (common) (internal) I67.2
  cerebral (arteries) I67.2
  coronary (artery) I25.10
    with angina pectoris — *see* Arteriosclerosis, coronary (artery),
  degeneration — *see* Arteriosclerosis

Atheroma, atheromatous — *continued*
  heart, cardiac — *see* Disease, heart, ischemic, atherosclerotic
  mitral (valve) I34.8
  myocardium, myocardial — *see* Disease, heart, ischemic, atherosclerotic
  pulmonary valve (heart) — *see also* Endocarditis, pulmonary I37.8
  tricuspid (heart) (valve) I36.8
  valve, valvular — *see* Endocarditis
  vertebral (artery) I67.2
Atheromatosis — *see* Arteriosclerosis
Atherosclerosis — *see also* Arteriosclerosis
  coronary
    artery I25.10
      with angina pectoris — *see* Arteriosclerosis, coronary (artery),
      due to
        calcified coronary lesion (severely) I25.84
        lipid rich plaque I25.83
    transplanted heart I25.811
      bypass graft I25.812
        with angina pectoris — *see* Arteriosclerosis, coronary (artery),
      native coronary artery I25.811
        with angina pectoris — *see* Arteriosclerosis, coronary (artery),
Athetosis (acquired) R25.8
  bilateral (congenital) G80.3
  congenital (bilateral) (double) G80.3
  double (congenital) G80.3
  unilateral R25.8
Athlete's
  foot B35.3
  heart I51.7
Athrepsia E41
Athyrea (acquired) — *see also* Hypothyroidism
  congenital E03.1
Atonia, atony, atonic
  bladder (sphincter) (neurogenic) N31.2
  capillary I78.8
  cecum K59.89
    psychogenic F45.8
  colon — *see* Atony, intestine
  congenital P94.2
  esophagus K22.89
  intestine K59.89
    psychogenic F45.8
  stomach K31.89
    neurotic or psychogenic F45.8
  uterus (during labor) O62.2
    with hemorrhage (postpartum) O72.1
    postpartum (with hemorrhage) O72.1
      without hemorrhage O75.89
Atopy — *see* History, allergy
Atransferrinemia, congenital E88.09
Atresia, atretic
  alimentary organ or tract NEC Q45.8
    upper Q40.8
  ani, anus, anal (canal) Q42.3
    with fistula Q42.2
  aorta (ring) Q25.29
  aortic (orifice) (valve) Q23.0
    arch Q25.21
    congenital with hypoplasia of ascending aorta and defective development of left ventricle (with mitral stenosis) Q23.4
    in hypoplastic left heart syndrome Q23.4
  aqueduct of Sylvius Q03.0
    with spina bifida — *see* Spina bifida, with hydrocephalus
  artery NEC Q27.8
    cerebral Q28.3
    coronary Q24.5
    digestive system Q27.8
    eye Q15.8
    lower limb Q27.8
    pulmonary Q25.5
    specified site NEC Q27.8
    umbilical Q27.0
    upper limb Q27.8
  auditory canal (external) Q16.1
  bile duct (common) (congenital) (hepatic) Q44.2
    acquired — *see* Obstruction, bile duct
  bladder (neck) Q64.39
    obstruction Q64.31
  bronchus Q32.4
  cecum Q42.8

☑ **Additional Character Required** — Refer to the Tabular List for Character Selection   ▽ **Subterms under main terms may continue to next column or page**

Atresia, atretic — *continued*
cervix (acquired) N88.2
congenital Q51.828
in pregnancy or childbirth — *see* Anomaly, cervix, in pregnancy or childbirth
causing obstructed labor O65.5
choana Q30.0
colon Q42.9
specified NEC Q42.8
common duct Q44.2
cricoid cartilage Q31.8
cystic duct Q44.2
acquired K82.8
with obstruction K82.0
digestive organs NEC Q45.8
duodenum Q41.0
ear canal Q16.1
ejaculatory duct Q55.4
epiglottis Q31.8
esophagus Q39.0
with tracheoesophageal fistula Q39.1
eustachian tube Q17.8
fallopian tube (congenital) Q50.6
acquired N97.1
follicular cyst N83.0- ☑
foramen of
Luschka Q03.1
with spina bifida — *see* Spina bifida, with hydrocephalus
Magendie Q03.1
with spina bifida — *see* Spina bifida, with hydrocephalus
gallbladder Q44.1
genital organ
external
female Q52.79
male Q55.8
internal
female Q52.8
male Q55.8
glottis Q31.8
gullet Q39.0
with tracheoesophageal fistula Q39.1
heart valve NEC Q24.8
pulmonary Q22.0
tricuspid Q22.4
hymen Q52.3
acquired (postinfective) N89.6
ileum Q41.2
intestine (small) Q41.9
large Q42.9
specified NEC Q42.8
iris, filtration angle Q15.0
jejunum Q41.1
lacrimal apparatus Q10.4
larynx Q31.8
meatus urinarius Q64.33
mitral valve Q23.2
in hypoplastic left heart syndrome Q23.4
nares (anterior) (posterior) Q30.0
nasopharynx Q34.8
nose, nostril Q30.0
acquired J34.89
organ or site NEC Q89.8
osseous meatus (ear) Q16.1
oviduct (congenital) Q50.6
acquired N97.1
parotid duct Q38.4
acquired K11.8
pulmonary (artery) Q25.5
valve Q22.0
pulmonic Q22.0
pupil Q13.2
rectum Q42.1
with fistula Q42.0
salivary duct Q38.4
acquired K11.8
sublingual duct Q38.4
acquired K11.8
submandibular duct Q38.4
acquired K11.8
submaxillary duct Q38.4
acquired K11.8
thyroid cartilage Q31.8
trachea Q32.1
tricuspid valve Q22.4
ureter Q62.10
pelvic junction Q62.11
vesical orifice Q62.12

Atresia, atretic — *continued*
ureteropelvic junction Q62.11
ureterovesical orifice Q62.12
urethra (valvular) Q64.39
stricture Q64.32
urinary tract NEC Q64.8
uterus Q51.818
acquired N85.8
vagina (congenital) Q52.4
acquired (postinfectional) (senile) N89.5
vas deferens Q55.3
vascular NEC Q27.8
cerebral Q28.3
digestive system Q27.8
lower limb Q27.8
specified site NEC Q27.8
upper limb Q27.8
vein NEC Q27.8
digestive system Q27.8
great Q26.8
lower limb Q27.8
portal Q26.5
pulmonary Q26.4
partial Q26.3
total Q26.2
specified site NEC Q27.8
upper limb Q27.8
vena cava (inferior) (superior) Q26.8
vesicourethral orifice Q64.31
vulva Q52.79
acquired N90.5
Atrichia, atrichosis — *see* Alopecia
Atrophia — *see also* Atrophy
cutis senilis L90.8
due to radiation L57.8
gyrata of choroid and retina H31.23
senilis R54
dermatological L90.8
due to radiation (nonionizing) (solar) L57.8
unguium L60.3
congenita Q84.6
Atrophie blanche (en plaque) (de Milian) L95.0
Atrophoderma, atrophodermia (of) L90.9
diffusum (idiopathic) L90.4
maculatum L90.8
et striatum L90.8
due to syphilis A52.79
syphilitic A51.39
neuriticum L90.8
Pasini and Pierini L90.3
pigmentosum Q82.1
reticulatum symmetricum faciei L66.4
senile L90.8
due to radiation (nonionizing) (solar) L57.8
vermiculata (cheeks) L66.4
Atrophy, atrophic (of)
adrenal (capsule) (gland) E27.49
primary (autoimmune) E27.1
alveolar process or ridge (edentulous) K08.20
anal sphincter (disuse) N81.84
appendix K38.8
arteriosclerotic — *see* Arteriosclerosis
bile duct (common) (hepatic) K83.8
bladder N32.89
neurogenic N31.8
blanche (en plaque) (of Milian) L95.0
bone (senile) NEC — *see also* Disorder, bone, specified type NEC
due to
tabes dorsalis (neurogenic) A52.11
brain (cortex) (progressive) G31.9
frontotemporal circumscribed G31.01 *[F02.80]*
with behavioral disturbance G31.01 *[F02.81]*
senile NEC G31.1
breast N64.2
obstetric — *see* Disorder, breast, specified type NEC
buccal cavity K13.79
cardiac — *see* Degeneration, myocardial
cartilage (infectional) (joint) — *see* Disorder, cartilage, specified NEC
cerebellar — *see* Atrophy, brain
cerebral — *see* Atrophy, brain
cervix (mucosa) (senile) (uteri) N88.8
menopausal N95.8
Charcot-Marie-Tooth G60.0
choroid (central) (macular) (myopic) (retina) H31.10- ☑
diffuse secondary H31.12- ☑
gyrate H31.23

Atrophy, atrophic — *continued*
choroid — *continued*
senile H31.11- ☑
ciliary body — *see* Atrophy, iris
conjunctiva (senile) H11.89
corpus cavernosum N48.89
cortical — *see* Atrophy, brain
cystic duct K82.8
Déjérine-Thomas G23.8
disuse NEC — *see* Atrophy, muscle
Duchenne-Aran G12.21
ear H93.8- ☑
edentulous alveolar ridge K08.20
endometrium (senile) N85.8
cervix N88.8
enteric K63.89
epididymis N50.89
eyeball — *see* Disorder, globe, degenerated condition, atrophy
eyelid (senile) — *see* Disorder, eyelid, degenerative
facial (skin) L90.9
fallopian tube (senile) N83.32- ☑
with ovary N83.33- ☑
fascioscapulohumeral (Landouzy- Déjérine) G71.02
fatty, thymus (gland) E32.8
gallbladder K82.8
gastric K29.40
with bleeding K29.41
gastrointestinal K63.89
glandular I89.8
globe H44.52- ☑
gum — *see* Recession, gingival
hair L67.8
heart (brown) — *see* Degeneration, myocardial
hemifacial Q67.4
Romberg G51.8
infantile E41
paralysis, acute — *see* Poliomyelitis, paralytic
intestine K63.89
iris (essential) (progressive) H21.26- ☑
specified NEC H21.29
kidney (senile) (terminal) — *see also* Sclerosis, renal N26.1
congenital or infantile Q60.5
bilateral Q60.4
unilateral Q60.3
hydronephrotic — *see* Hydronephrosis
lacrimal gland (primary) H04.14- ☑
secondary H04.15- ☑
Landouzy-Déjérine G71.02
laryngitis, infective J37.0
larynx J38.7
Leber's optic (hereditary) H47.22
lip K13.0
liver (yellow) K72.90
with coma K72.91
acute, subacute K72.00
with coma K72.01
chronic K72.10
with coma K72.11
lung (senile) J98.4
macular (dermatological) L90.8
syphilitic, skin A51.39
striated A52.79
mandible (edentulous) K08.20
minimal K08.21
moderate K08.22
severe K08.23
maxilla K08.20
minimal K08.24
moderate K08.25
severe K08.26
muscle, muscular (diffuse) (general) (idiopathic) (primary) M62.50
ankle M62.57- ☑
Duchenne-Aran G12.21
foot M62.57- ☑
forearm M62.53- ☑
hand M62.54- ☑
infantile spinal G12.0
lower leg M62.56- ☑
multiple sites M62.59
myelopathic — *see* Atrophy, muscle, spinal
myotonic G71.11
neuritic G58.9
neuropathic (peroneal) (progressive) G60.0
pelvic (disuse) N81.84
peroneal G60.0

Atrophy, atrophic — continued
  muscle, muscular — continued
    progressive (bulbar) G12.21
      adult G12.1
      infantile (spinal) G12.0
      spinal G12.25
        adult G12.1
        infantile G12.0
    pseudohypertrophic G71.02
    shoulder region M62.51- ☑
    specified site NEC M62.58
    spinal G12.9
      adult form G12.1
      Aran-Duchenne G12.21
      childhood form, type II G12.1
      distal G12.1
      hereditary NEC G12.1
      infantile, type I (Werdnig-Hoffmann) G12.0
      juvenile form, type III (Kugelberg- Welander) G12.1
      progressive G12.25
      scapuloperoneal form G12.1
      specified NEC G12.8
    syphilitic A52.78
    thigh M62.55- ☑
    upper arm M62.52- ☑
  myocardium — see Degeneration, myocardial
  myometrium (senile) N85.8
    cervix N88.8
  myopathic NEC — see Atrophy, muscle
  myotonia G71.11
  nail L60.3
  nasopharynx J31.1
  nerve — see also Disorder, nerve
    abducens — see Strabismus, paralytic, sixth nerve
    accessory G52.8
    acoustic or auditory H93.3 ☑
    cranial G52.9
      eighth (auditory) H93.3 ☑
      eleventh (accessory) G52.8
      fifth (trigeminal) G50.8
      first (olfactory) G52.0
      fourth (trochlear) — see Strabismus, paralytic, fourth nerve
      second (optic) H47.20
      sixth (abducens) — see Strabismus, paralytic, sixth nerve
      tenth (pneumogastric) (vagus) G52.2
      third (oculomotor) — see Strabismus, paralytic, third nerve
      twelfth (hypoglossal) G52.3
    hypoglossal G52.3
    oculomotor — see Strabismus, paralytic, third nerve
    olfactory G52.0
    optic (papillomacular bundle)
      syphilitic (late) A52.15
        congenital A50.44
    pneumogastric G52.2
    trigeminal G50.8
    trochlear — see Strabismus, paralytic, fourth nerve
    vagus (pneumogastric) G52.2
  neurogenic, bone, tabetic A52.11
  nutritional E43
    with marasmus E41
  old age R54
  olivopontocerebellar G23.8
  optic (nerve) H47.20
    glaucomatous H47.23- ☑
    hereditary H47.22
    primary H47.21- ☑
    specified type NEC H47.29- ☑
    syphilitic (late) A52.15
      congenital A50.44
  orbit H05.31- ☑
  ovary (senile) N83.31- ☑
    with fallopian tube N83.33- ☑
  oviduct (senile) — see Atrophy, fallopian tube
  palsy, diffuse (progressive) G12.22
  pancreas (duct) (senile) K86.89
  parotid gland K11.0
  pelvic muscle N81.84
  penis N48.89
  pharynx J39.2
  pluriglandular E31.8
    autoimmune E31.0
  polyarthritis M15.9
  prostate N42.89
  pseudohypertrophic (muscle) G71.02

Atrophy, atrophic — continued
  renal — see also Sclerosis, renal N26.1
  retina, retinal (postinfectional) H35.89
  rhinitis J31.0
  salivary gland K11.0
  scar L90.5
  sclerosis, lobar (of brain) G31.09 [F02.80]
    with behavioral disturbance G31.09 [F02.81]
  scrotum N50.89
  seminal vesicle N50.89
  senile R54
    due to radiation (nonionizing) (solar) L57.8
  skin (patches) (spots) L90.9
    degenerative (senile) L90.8
    due to radiation (nonionizing) (solar) L57.8
    senile L90.8
  spermatic cord N50.89
  spinal (acute) (cord) G95.89
    muscular — see Atrophy, muscle, spinal
    paralysis G12.20
      acute — see Poliomyelitis, paralytic
      meaning progressive muscular atrophy G12.25
  spine (column) — see Spondylopathy, specified NEC
  spleen (senile) D73.0
  stomach K29.40
    with bleeding K29.41
  striate (skin) L90.6
    syphilitic A52.79
  subcutaneous L90.9
  sublingual gland K11.0
  submandibular gland K11.0
  submaxillary gland K11.0
  Sudeck's — see Algoneurodystrophy
  suprarenal (capsule) (gland) E27.49
    primary E27.1
  systemic affecting central nervous system in
    myxedema E03.9 [G13.2]
    neoplastic disease — see also Neoplasm D49.9 [G13.1]
    specified disease NEC G13.8
  tarso-orbital fascia, congenital Q10.3
  testis N50.0
  thenar, partial — see Syndrome, carpal tunnel
  thymus (fatty) E32.8
  thyroid (gland) (acquired) E03.4
    with cretinism E03.1
    congenital (with myxedema) E03.1
  tongue (senile) K14.8
    papillae K14.4
  trachea J39.8
  tunica vaginalis N50.89
  turbinate J34.89
  tympanic membrane (nonflaccid) H73.82- ☑
    flaccid H73.81- ☑
  upper respiratory tract J39.8
  uterus, uterine (senile) N85.8
    cervix N88.8
    due to radiation (intended effect) N85.8
      adverse effect or misadventure N99.89
  vagina (senile) N95.2
  vas deferens N50.89
  vascular I99.8
  vertebra (senile) — see Spondylopathy, specified NEC
  vulva (senile) N90.5
  Werdnig-Hoffmann G12.0
  yellow — see Failure, hepatic

Attack, attacks
  with alteration of consciousness (with automatisms) — see Epilepsy, localization-related, symptomatic, with complex partial seizures
  Adams-Stokes I45.9
  akinetic — see Epilepsy, generalized, specified NEC
  angina — see Angina
  atonic — see Epilepsy, generalized, specified NEC
  benign shuddering G25.83
  cataleptic — see Catalepsy
  coronary — see Infarct, myocardium
  cyanotic, newborn P28.2
  drop NEC R55
  epileptic — see Epilepsy
  heart — see Infarct, myocardium
  hysterical F44.9
  jacksonian — see Epilepsy, localization-related, symptomatic, with simple partial seizures
  myocardium, myocardial — see Infarct, myocardium
  myoclonic — see Epilepsy, generalized, specified NEC
  panic F41.0

Attack, attacks — continued
  psychomotor — see Epilepsy, localization-related, symptomatic, with complex partial seizures
  salaam — see Epilepsy, spasms
  schizophreniform, brief F23
  shuddering, benign G25.83
  Stokes-Adams I45.9
  syncope R55
  transient ischemic (TIA) G45.9
    specified NEC G45.8
  unconsciousness R55
    hysterical F44.89
  vasomotor R55
  vasovagal (paroxysmal) (idiopathic) R55
  without alteration of consciousness — see Epilepsy, localization-related, symptomatic, with simple partial seizures
Attention (to)
  artificial
    opening (of) Z43.9
      digestive tract NEC Z43.4
        colon Z43.3
        ilium Z43.2
        stomach Z43.1
      specified NEC Z43.8
      trachea Z43.0
      urinary tract NEC Z43.6
        cystostomy Z43.5
        nephrostomy Z43.6
        ureterostomy Z43.6
        urethrostomy Z43.6
      vagina Z43.7
  colostomy Z43.3
  cystostomy Z43.5
  deficit disorder or syndrome F98.8
    with hyperactivity — see Disorder, attention-deficit hyperactivity
  gastrostomy Z43.1
  ileostomy Z43.2
  jejunostomy Z43.4
  nephrostomy Z43.6
  surgical dressings Z48.01
  sutures Z48.02
  tracheostomy Z43.0
  ureterostomy Z43.6
  urethrostomy Z43.6
Attrition
  gum — see Recession, gingival
  tooth, teeth (excessive) (hard tissues) K03.0
Atypical, atypism — see also condition
  cells (on cytolgocial smear) (endocervical) (endometrial) (glandular)
    cervix R87.619
    vagina R87.629
  cervical N87.9
  endometrium N85.9
    hyperplasia N85.00
  parenting situation Z62.9
Auditory — see condition
Aujeszky's disease B33.8
Aurantiasis, cutis E67.1
Auricle, auricular — see also condition
  cervical Q18.2
Auriculotemporal syndrome G50.8
Austin Flint murmur (aortic insufficiency) I35.1
Australian
  Q fever A78
  X disease A83.4
Autism, autistic (childhood) (infantile) F84.0
  atypical F84.9
  spectrum disorder F84.0
Autodigestion R68.89
Autoerythrocyte sensitization (syndrome) D69.2
Autographism L50.3
Autoimmune
  disease (systemic) M35.9
  inhibitors to clotting factors D68.311
  lymphoproliferative syndrome [ALPS] D89.82
  thyroiditis E06.3
Autointoxication R68.89
Automatism G93.89
  with temporal sclerosis G93.81
  epileptic — see Epilepsy, localization-related, symptomatic, with complex partial seizures
  paroxysmal, idiopathic — see Epilepsy, localization-related, symptomatic, with complex partial seizures

☑ **Additional Character Required** — Refer to the Tabular List for Character Selection   Subterms under main terms may continue to next column or page

Autonomic, autonomous
 bladder (neurogenic) N31.2
 hysteria seizure F44.5
Autosensitivity, erythrocyte D69.2
Autosensitization, cutaneous L30.2
Autosome — *see* condition by chromosome involved
Autotopagnosia R48.1
Autotoxemia R68.89
Autumn — *see* condition
Avellis' syndrome G46.8
Aversion
 oral R63.39
  newborn P92.- ☑
  nonorganic origin F98.2 ☑
 sexual F52.1
Aviator's
 disease or sickness — *see* Effect, adverse, high altitude
 ear T70.0 ☑
Avitaminosis (multiple) — *see also* Deficiency, vitamin
 E56.9
 B E53.9
  with
   beriberi E51.11
   pellagra E52
 B2 E53.0
 B6 E53.1
 B12 E53.8
 D E55.9
  with rickets E55.0
 G E53.0
 K E56.1
 nicotinic acid E52
AVNRT (atrioventricular nodal re-entrant tachycardia)
 I47.1
AVRT (atrioventricular nodal re-entrant tachycardia) I47.1
Avulsion (traumatic)
 blood vessel — *see* Injury, blood vessel
 bone — *see* Fracture, by site
 cartilage — *see also* Dislocation, by site
  symphyseal (inner), complicating delivery O71.6
 external site other than limb — *see* Wound, open, by
  site
 eye S05.7-
 head (intracranial)
  external site NEC S08.89 ☑
  scalp S08.0 ☑
 internal organ or site — *see* Injury, by site
 joint — *see also* Dislocation, by site
  capsule — *see* Sprain, by site
 kidney S37.06- ☑
 ligament — *see* Sprain, by site
 limb — *see also* Amputation, traumatic, by site
  skin and subcutaneous tissue — *see* Wound, open,
   by site
 muscle — *see* Injury, muscle
 nerve (root) — *see* Injury, nerve
 scalp S08.0 ☑
 skin and subcutaneous tissue — *see* Wound, open, by
  site
 spleen S36.032 ☑
 symphyseal cartilage (inner), complicating delivery
  O71.6
 tendon — *see* Injury, muscle
 tooth S03.2 ☑
Awareness of heart beat R00.2
Axenfeld's
 anomaly or syndrome Q15.0
 degeneration (calcareous) Q13.4
Axilla, axillary — *see also* condition
 breast Q83.1
Axonotmesis — *see* Injury, nerve
Ayerza's disease or syndrome (pulmonary artery sclerosis with pulmonary hypertension) I27.0
Azoospermia (organic) N46.01
 due to
  drug therapy N46.021
  efferent duct obstruction N46.023
  infection N46.022
  radiation N46.024
  specified cause NEC N46.029
  systemic disease N46.025
Azotemia R79.89
 meaning uremia N19
Aztec ear Q17.3
Azygos
 continuation inferior vena cava Q26.8
 lobe (lung) Q33.1

B

Baastrup's disease — *see* Kissing spine
Babesiosis B60.00
 due to
  Babesia
   divergens B60.03
   duncani B60.02
   KO-1 B60.09
   microti B60.01
   MO-1 B60.03
   species
    unspecified B60.00
   venatorum B60.09
  specified NEC B60.09
Babington's disease (familial hemorrhagic telangiectasia) I78.0
Babinski's syndrome A52.79
Baby
 crying constantly R68.11
 floppy (syndrome) P94.2
Bacillary — *see* condition
Bacilluria R82.71
Bacillus — *see also* Infection, bacillus
 abortus infection A23.1
 anthracis infection A22.9
 coli infection — *see also* Escherichia coli B96.20
 Flexner's A03.1
 mallei infection A24.0
 Shiga's A03.0
 suipestifer infection — *see* Infection, salmonella
Back — *see* condition
Backache (postural) M54.9
 sacroiliac M53.3
 specified NEC M54.89
Backflow — *see* Reflux
Backward reading (dyslexia) F81.0
Bacteremia R78.81
 with sepsis — *see* Sepsis
Bactericholia — *see* Cholecystitis, acute
Bacterid, bacteride (pustular) L40.3
Bacterium, bacteria, bacterial
 agent NEC, as cause of disease classified elsewhere
  B96.89
 in blood — *see* Bacteremia
 in urine — *see* Bacteriuria
Bacteriuria, bacteruria R82.71
 asymptomatic R82.71
Bacteroides
 fragilis, as cause of disease classified elsewhere B96.6
Bad
 heart — *see* Disease, heart
 trip
  due to drug abuse — *see* Abuse, drug, hallucinogen
  due to drug dependence — *see* Dependence, drug,
   hallucinogen
Baelz's disease (cheilitis glandularis apostematosa) K13.0
Baerensprung's disease (eczema marginatum) B35.6
Bagasse disease or pneumonitis J67.1
Bagassosis J67.1
Baker's cyst — *see* Cyst, Baker's
Bakwin-Krida syndrome (metaphyseal dysplasia) Q78.5
Balancing side interference M26.56
Balanitis (circinata) (erosiva) (gangrenosa) (phagedenic)
 (vulgaris) N48.1
 amebic A06.82
 candidal B37.42
 due to Haemophilus ducreyi A57
 gonococcal (acute) (chronic) A54.23
 xerotica obliterans N48.0
Balanoposthitis N47.6
 gonococcal (acute) (chronic) A54.23
 ulcerative (specific) A63.8
Balanorrhagia — *see* Balanitis
Balantidiasis, balantidiosis A07.0
Bald tongue K14.4
Baldness — *see also* Alopecia
 male-pattern — *see* Alopecia, androgenic
Balkan grippe A78
Balloon disease — *see* Effect, adverse, high altitude
Balo's disease (concentric sclerosis) G37.5
Bamberger-Marie disease — *see* Osteoarthropathy,
 hypertrophic, specified type NEC
Bancroft's filariasis B74.0
Band(s)
 adhesive — *see* Adhesions, peritoneum

Band(s) — *continued*
 anomalous or congenital — *see also* Anomaly, by site
  heart (atrial) (ventricular) Q24.8
  intestine Q43.3
  omentum Q43.3
 cervix N88.1
 constricting, congenital Q79.8
 gallbladder (congenital) Q44.1
 intestinal (adhesive) — *see* Adhesions, peritoneum
 obstructive
  intestine K56.50
   complete K56.52
   incomplete K56.51
   partial K56.51
  peritoneum K56.50
   complete K56.52
   incomplete K56.51
   partial K56.51
 periappendiceal, congenital Q43.3
 peritoneal (adhesive) — *see* Adhesions, peritoneum
 uterus N73.6
  internal N85.6
 vagina N89.5
Bandemia D72.825
Bandl's ring (contraction), complicating delivery O62.4
Bangkok hemorrhagic fever A91
Bang's disease (brucella abortus) A23.1
Bankruptcy, anxiety concerning Z59.89
Bannister's disease T78.3 ☑
 hereditary D84.1
Banti's disease or syndrome (with cirrhosis) (with portal
 hypertension) K76.6
Bar, median, prostate — *see* Enlargement, enlarged,
 prostate
Barcoo disease or rot — *see* Ulcer, skin
Barlow's disease E54
Barodontalgia T70.29 ☑
Baron Münchausen syndrome — *see* Disorder, facti-
 tious
Barosinusitis T70.1 ☑
Barotitis T70.0 ☑
Barotrauma T70.29 ☑
 odontalgia T70.29 ☑
 otitic T70.0 ☑
 sinus T70.1 ☑
Barraquer (-Simons) **disease or syndrome** (progressive
 lipodystrophy) E88.1
Barré-Guillain disease or syndrome G61.0
Barrel chest M95.4
Barré-Liéou syndrome (posterior cervical sympathetic)
 M53.0
Barrett's
 disease — *see* Barrett's, esophagus
 esophagus K22.70
  with dysplasia K22.719
   high grade K22.711
   low grade K22.710
  without dysplasia K22.70
 syndrome — *see* Barrett's, esophagus
 ulcer K22.10
  with bleeding K22.11
  without bleeding K22.10
Bársony (-Polgár) (-Teschendorf) **syndrome** (corkscrew
 esophagus) K22.4
Barth syndrome E78.71
Bartholinitis (suppurating) N75.8
 gonococcal (acute) (chronic) (with abscess) A54.1
Bartonellosis A44.9
 cutaneous A44.1
 mucocutaneous A44.1
 specified NEC A44.8
 systemic A44.0
Barton's fracture S52.56- ☑
Bartter's syndrome E26.81
Basal — *see* condition
Basan's (hidrotic) ectodermal dysplasia Q82.4
Baseball finger — *see* Dislocation, finger
Basedow's disease (exophthalmic goiter) — *see* Hyper-
 thyroidism, with, goiter
Basic — *see* condition
Basilar — *see* condition
Bason's (hidrotic) ectodermal dysplasia Q82.4
Basopenia — *see* Agranulocytosis
Basophilia D72.824
Basophilism (cortico-adrenal) (Cushing's) (pituitary) E24.0
Bassen-Kornzweig disease or syndrome E78.6
Bat ear Q17.5

Bateman's
  disease B08.1
  purpura (senile) D69.2
Bathing cramp T75.1 ☑
Bathophobia F40.248
Batten (-Mayou) **disease** E75.4
  retina E75.4 *[H36]*
Batten-Steinert syndrome G71.11
Battered — *see* Maltreatment
Battey Mycobacterium infection A31.0
Battle exhaustion F43.0
Battledore placenta O43.19- ☑
Baumgarten-Cruveilhier cirrhosis, disease or syndrome K74.69
Bauxite fibrosis (of lung) J63.1
Bayle's disease (general paresis) A52.17
Bazin's disease (primary) (tuberculous) A18.4
Beach ear — *see* Swimmer's, ear
Beaded hair (congenital) Q84.1
Béal conjunctivitis or syndrome B30.2
Beard's disease (neurasthenia) F48.8
Beat(s)
  atrial, premature I49.1
  ectopic I49.49
  elbow — *see* Bursitis, elbow
  escaped, heart I49.49
  hand — *see* Bursitis, hand
  knee — *see* Bursitis, knee
  premature I49.40
    atrial I49.1
    auricular I49.1
    supraventricular I49.1
Beau's
  disease or syndrome — *see* Degeneration, myocardial
  lines (transverse furrows on fingernails) L60.4
Bechterev's syndrome — *see* Spondylitis, ankylosing
Becker's
  cardiomyopathy I42.8
  disease
    idiopathic mural endomyocardial disease I42.3
    myotonia congenita, recessive form G71.12
  dystrophy G71.01
  pigmented hairy nevus D22.5
Beck's syndrome (anterior spinal artery occlusion) I65.8
Beckwith-Wiedemann syndrome Q87.3
Bed confinement status Z74.01
Bed sore — *see* Ulcer, pressure, by site
Bedbug bite(s) — *see* Bite(s), by site, superficial, insect
Bedclothes, asphyxiation or suffocation by — *see* Asphyxia, traumatic, due to, mechanical, trapped
Bednar's
  aphthae K12.0
  tumor — *see* Neoplasm, malignant, by site
Bedridden Z74.01
Bedsore — *see* Ulcer, pressure, by site
Bedwetting — *see* Enuresis
Bee sting (with allergic or anaphylactic shock) — *see* Toxicity, venom, arthropod, bee
Beer drinker's heart (disease) I42.6
Begbie's disease (exophthalmic goiter) — *see* Hyperthyroidism, with, goiter
Behavior
  antisocial
    adult Z72.811
    child or adolescent Z72.810
  disorder, disturbance — *see* Disorder, conduct
  disruptive — *see* Disorder, conduct
  drug seeking Z76.5
  inexplicable R46.2
  marked evasiveness R46.5
  obsessive-compulsive R46.81
  overactivity R46.3
  poor responsiveness R46.4
  self-damaging (life-style) Z72.89
  sleep-incompatible Z72.821
  slowness R46.4
  specified NEC R46.89
  strange (and inexplicable) R46.2
  suspiciousness R46.5
  type A pattern Z73.1
  undue concern or preoccupation with stressful events R46.6
  verbosity and circumstantial detail obscuring reason for contact R46.7
Behçet's disease or syndrome M35.2
Behr's disease — *see* Degeneration, macula
Beigel's disease or morbus (white piedra) B36.2

Bejel A65
Bekhterev's syndrome — *see* Spondylitis, ankylosing
Belching — *see* Eructation
Bell's
  mania F30.8
  palsy, paralysis G51.0
    infant or newborn P11.3
  spasm G51.3- ☑
Bence Jones albuminuria or proteinuria NEC R80.3
Bends T70.3 ☑
Benedikt's paralysis or syndrome G46.3
Benign — *see also* condition
  prostatic hyperplasia — *see* Hyperplasia, prostate
Bennett's fracture (displaced) S62.21- ☑
Benson's disease — *see* Deposit, crystalline
Bent
  back (hysterical) F44.4
  nose M95.0
    congenital Q67.4
Bereavement (uncomplicated) Z63.4
Bergeron's disease (hysterical chorea) F44.4
Berger's disease — *see* Nephropathy, IgA
Beriberi (dry) E51.11
  heart (disease) E51.12
  polyneuropathy E51.11
  wet E51.12
    involving circulatory system E51.11
Berlin's disease or edema (traumatic) S05.8X- ☑
Berlock (berloque) **dermatitis** L56.2
Bernard-Horner syndrome G90.2
Bernard-Soulier disease or thrombopathia D69.1
Bernhardt (-Roth) **disease** — *see* Mononeuropathy, lower limb, meralgia paresthetica
Bernheim's syndrome — *see* Failure, heart, right
Bertielliasis B71.8
Berylliosis (lung) J63.2
Besnier-Boeck (-Schaumann) **disease** — *see* Sarcoidosis
Besnier's
  lupus pernio D86.3
  prurigo L20.0
Bestiality F65.89
Best's disease H35.50
Betalipoproteinemia, broad or floating E78.2
Beta-mercaptolactate-cysteine disulfiduria E72.09
Betting and gambling Z72.6
  pathological (compulsive) F63.0
Bezoar T18.9 ☑
  intestine T18.3 ☑
  stomach T18.2 ☑
Bezold's abscess — *see* Mastoiditis, acute
Bianchi's syndrome R48.8
Bicornate or bicornis uterus Q51.3
  in pregnancy or childbirth O34.00
    causing obstructed labor O65.5
Bicuspid aortic valve Q23.1
Biedl-Bardet syndrome Q87.89
Bielschowsky (-Jansky) disease E75.4
Biermer's (pernicious) anemia or disease D51.0
Biett's disease L93.0
Bifid (congenital)
  apex, heart Q24.8
  clitoris Q52.6
  kidney Q63.8
  nose Q30.2
  patella Q74.1
  scrotum Q55.29
  toe NEC Q74.2
  tongue Q38.3
  ureter Q62.8
  uterus Q51.3
  uvula Q35.7
Biforis uterus (suprasimplex) Q51.3
Bifurcation (congenital)
  gallbladder Q44.1
  kidney pelvis Q63.8
  renal pelvis Q63.8
  rib Q76.6
  tongue, congenital Q38.3
  trachea Q32.1
  ureter Q62.8
  urethra Q64.74
  vertebra Q76.49
Big spleen syndrome D73.1
Bigeminal pulse R00.8
Bilateral — *see* condition
Bile
  duct — *see* condition

Bile — *continued*
  pigments in urine R82.2
Bilharziasis — *see also* Schistosomiasis
  chyluria B65.0
  cutaneous B65.3
  galacturia B65.0
  hematochyluria B65.0
  intestinal B65.1
  lipemia B65.9
  lipuria B65.0
  oriental B65.2
  piarhemia B65.9
  pulmonary NOS B65.9 *[J99]*
    pneumonia B65.9 *[J17]*
  tropical hematuria B65.0
  vesical B65.0
Biliary — *see* condition
Bilirubin metabolism disorder E80.7
  specified NEC E80.6
Bilirubinemia, familial nonhemolytic E80.4
Bilirubinuria R82.2
Biliuria R82.2
Bilocular stomach K31.2
Binswanger's disease I67.3
Biparta, bipartite
  carpal scaphoid Q74.0
  patella Q74.1
  vagina Q52.10
Bird
  face Q75.8
  fancier's disease or lung J67.2
Birth
  complications in mother — *see* Delivery, complicated
  compression during NOS P15.9
  defect — *see* Anomaly
  immature (less than 37 completed weeks) — *see* Preterm, newborn
    extremely (less than 28 completed weeks) — *see* Immaturity, extreme
  inattention, at or after — *see* Maltreatment, child, neglect
  injury NOS P15.9
    basal ganglia P11.1
    brachial plexus NEC P14.3
    brain (compression) (pressure) P11.2
    central nervous system NOS P11.9
    cerebellum P11.1
    cerebral hemorrhage P10.1
    external genitalia P15.5
    eye P15.3
    face P15.4
    fracture
      bone P13.9
        specified NEC P13.8
      clavicle P13.4
      femur P13.2
      humerus P13.3
      long bone, except femur P13.3
      radius and ulna P13.3
      skull P13.0
      spine P11.5
      tibia and fibula P13.3
    intracranial P11.2
      laceration or hemorrhage P10.9
        specified NEC P10.8
    intraventricular hemorrhage P10.2
    laceration
      brain P10.1
      by scalpel P15.8
      peripheral nerve P14.9
    liver P15.0
    meninges
      brain P11.1
      spinal cord P11.5
    nerve
      brachial plexus P14.3
      cranial NEC (except facial) P11.4
      facial P11.3
      peripheral P14.9
      phrenic (paralysis) P14.2
    paralysis
      facial nerve P11.3
      spinal P11.5
    penis P15.5
    rupture
      spinal cord P11.5
    scalp P12.9
    scalpel wound P15.8

☑ **Additional Character Required** — **Refer to the Tabular List for Character Selection**   ⬇ **Subterms under main terms may continue to next column or page**

Birth — *continued*
  injury — *continued*
    scrotum P15.5
    skull NEC P13.1
      fracture P13.0
    specified type NEC P15.8
    spinal cord P11.5
    spine P11.5
    spleen P15.1
    sternomastoid (hematoma) P15.2
    subarachnoid hemorrhage P10.3
    subcutaneous fat necrosis P15.6
    subdural hemorrhage P10.0
    tentorial tear P10.4
    testes P15.5
    vulva P15.5
  lack of care, at or after — *see* Maltreatment, child, neglect
  neglect, at or after — *see* Maltreatment, child, neglect
  palsy or paralysis, newborn, NOS (birth injury) P14.9
  premature (infant) — *see* Preterm, newborn
  shock, newborn P96.89
  trauma — *see* Birth, injury
  weight
    low (2499 grams or less) — *see* Low, birthweight
      extremely (999 grams or less) — *see* Low, birthweight, extreme
    4000 grams to 4499 grams P08.1
    4500 grams or more P08.0
Birthmark Q82.5
Birt-Hogg-Dube syndrome Q87.89
Bisalbuminemia E88.09
Biskra's button B55.1
Bite(s) (animal) (human)
  abdomen, abdominal
    wall S31.159 ☑
      with penetration into peritoneal cavity S31.659 ☑
      epigastric region S31.152 ☑
        with penetration into peritoneal cavity S31.652 ☑
      left
        lower quadrant S31.154 ☑
          with penetration into peritoneal cavity S31.654 ☑
        upper quadrant S31.151 ☑
          with penetration into peritoneal cavity S31.651 ☑
      periumbilic region S31.155 ☑
        with penetration into peritoneal cavity S31.655 ☑
      right
        lower quadrant S31.153 ☑
          with penetration into peritoneal cavity S31.653 ☑
        upper quadrant S31.150 ☑
          with penetration into peritoneal cavity S31.650 ☑
      superficial NEC S30.871 ☑
        insect S30.861 ☑
  alveolar (process) — *see* Bite, oral cavity
  amphibian (venomous) — *see* Venom, bite, amphibian
  animal — *see also* Bite, by site
    venomous — *see* Venom
  ankle S91.05- ☑
    superficial NEC S90.57- ☑
      insect S90.56- ☑
  antecubital space — *see* Bite, elbow
  anus S31.835 ☑
    superficial NEC S30.877 ☑
      insect S30.867 ☑
  arm (upper) S41.15- ☑
    lower — *see* Bite, forearm
    superficial NEC S40.87- ☑
      insect S40.86- ☑
  arthropod NEC — *see* Venom, bite, arthropod
  auditory canal (external) (meatus) — *see* Bite, ear
  auricle, ear — *see* Bite, ear
  axilla — *see* Bite, arm
  back — *see also* Bite, thorax, back
    lower S31.050 ☑
      with penetration into retroperitoneal space S31.051 ☑
      superficial NEC S30.870 ☑
        insect S30.860 ☑
  bedbug — *see* Bite(s), by site, superficial, insect
  breast S21.05- ☑

Bite(s) — *continued*
  breast — *continued*
    superficial NEC S20.17- ☑
      insect S20.16- ☑
  brow — *see* Bite, head, specified site NEC
  buttock S31.805 ☑
    left S31.825 ☑
    right S31.815 ☑
    superficial NEC S30.870 ☑
      insect S30.860 ☑
  calf — *see* Bite, leg
  canaliculus lacrimalis — *see* Bite, eyelid
  canthus, eye — *see* Bite, eyelid
  centipede — *see* Toxicity, venom, arthropod, centipede
  cheek (external) S01.45- ☑
    internal — *see* Bite, oral cavity
    superficial NEC S00.87 ☑
      insect S00.86 ☑
  chest wall — *see* Bite, thorax
  chigger B88.0
  chin — *see* Bite, head, specified site NEC
  clitoris — *see* Bite, vulva
  costal region — *see* Bite, thorax
  digit(s)
    hand — *see* Bite, finger
    toe — *see* Bite, toe
  ear (canal) (external) S01.35- ☑
    superficial NEC S00.47- ☑
      insect S00.46- ☑
  elbow S51.05- ☑
    superficial NEC S50.37- ☑
      insect S50.36- ☑
  epididymis — *see* Bite, testis
  epigastric region — *see* Bite, abdomen
  epiglottis — *see* Bite, neck, specified site NEC
  esophagus, cervical S11.25 ☑
    superficial NEC S10.17 ☑
      insect S10.16 ☑
  eyebrow — *see* Bite, eyelid
  eyelid S01.15- ☑
    superficial NEC S00.27- ☑
      insect S00.26- ☑
  face NEC — *see* Bite, head, specified site NEC
  finger(s) S61.259 ☑
    with
      damage to nail S61.359 ☑
    index S61.258 ☑
      with
        damage to nail S61.358 ☑
      left S61.251 ☑
        with
          damage to nail S61.351 ☑
      right S61.250 ☑
        with
          damage to nail S61.350 ☑
      superficial NEC S60.478 ☑
        insect S60.46- ☑
    little S61.25- ☑
      with
        damage to nail S61.35- ☑
      superficial NEC S60.47- ☑
        insect S60.46- ☑
    middle S61.25- ☑
      with
        damage to nail S61.35- ☑
      superficial NEC S60.47- ☑
        insect S60.46- ☑
    ring S61.25- ☑
      with
        damage to nail S61.35- ☑
      superficial NEC S60.47- ☑
        insect S60.46- ☑
    superficial NEC S60.479 ☑
      insect S60.469 ☑
    thumb — *see* Bite, thumb
  flank — *see* Bite, abdomen, wall
  flea — *see* Bite, by site, superficial, insect
  foot (except toe(s) alone) S91.35- ☑
    superficial NEC S90.87- ☑
      insect S90.86- ☑
    toe — *see* Bite, toe
  forearm S51.85- ☑
    elbow only — *see* Bite, elbow
    superficial NEC S50.87- ☑
      insect S50.86- ☑
  forehead — *see* Bite, head, specified site NEC

Bite(s) — *continued*
  genital organs, external
    female S31.552 ☑
      superficial NEC S30.876 ☑
        insect S30.866 ☑
      vagina and vulva — *see* Bite, vulva
    male S31.551 ☑
      penis — *see* Bite, penis
      scrotum — *see* Bite, scrotum
      superficial NEC S30.875 ☑
        insect S30.865 ☑
      testes — *see* Bite, testis
  groin — *see* Bite, abdomen, wall
  gum — *see* Bite, oral cavity
  hand S61.45- ☑
    finger — *see* Bite, finger
    superficial NEC S60.57- ☑
      insect S60.56- ☑
    thumb — *see* Bite, thumb
  head S01.95 ☑
    cheek — *see* Bite, cheek
    ear — *see* Bite, ear
    eyelid — *see* Bite, eyelid
    lip — *see* Bite, lip
    nose — *see* Bite, nose
    oral cavity — *see* Bite, oral cavity
    scalp — *see* Bite, scalp
    specified site NEC S01.85 ☑
      superficial NEC S00.87 ☑
        insect S00.86 ☑
    superficial NEC S00.97 ☑
      insect S00.96 ☑
    temporomandibular area — *see* Bite, cheek
  heel — *see* Bite, foot
  hip S71.05- ☑
    superficial NEC S70.27- ☑
      insect S70.26- ☑
  hymen S31.45 ☑
  hypochondrium — *see* Bite, abdomen, wall
  hypogastric region — *see* Bite, abdomen, wall
  inguinal region — *see* Bite, abdomen, wall
  insect — *see* Bite, by site, superficial, insect
  instep — *see* Bite, foot
  interscapular region — *see* Bite, thorax, back
  jaw — *see* Bite, head, specified site NEC
  knee S81.05- ☑
    superficial NEC S80.27- ☑
      insect S80.26- ☑
  labium (majus) (minus) — *see* Bite, vulva
  lacrimal duct — *see* Bite, eyelid
  larynx S11.015 ☑
    superficial NEC S10.17 ☑
      insect S10.16 ☑
  leg (lower) S81.85- ☑
    ankle — *see* Bite, ankle
    foot — *see* Bite, foot
    knee — *see* Bite, knee
    superficial NEC S80.87- ☑
      insect S80.86- ☑
    toe — *see* Bite, toe
    upper — *see* Bite, thigh
  lip S01.551 ☑
    superficial NEC S00.571 ☑
      insect S00.561 ☑
  lizard (venomous) — *see* Venom, bite, reptile
  loin — *see* Bite, abdomen, wall
  lower back — *see* Bite, back, lower
  lumbar region — *see* Bite, back, lower
  malar region — *see* Bite, head, specified site NEC
  mammary — *see* Bite, breast
  marine animals (venomous) — *see* Toxicity, venom, marine animal
  mastoid region — *see* Bite, head, specified site NEC
  mouth — *see* Bite, oral cavity
  nail
    finger — *see* Bite, finger
    toe — *see* Bite, toe
  nape — *see* Bite, neck, specified site NEC
  nasal (septum) (sinus) — *see* Bite, nose
  nasopharynx — *see* Bite, head, specified site NEC
  neck S11.95 ☑
    involving
      cervical esophagus — *see* Bite, esophagus, cervical
      larynx — *see* Bite, larynx
      pharynx — *see* Bite, pharynx

Bite(s) — *continued*
  neck — *continued*
    involving — *continued*
      thyroid gland S11.15 ☑
      trachea — *see* Bite, trachea
    specified site NEC S11.85 ☑
      superficial NEC S10.87 ☑
        insect S10.86 ☑
    superficial NEC S10.97 ☑
      insect S10.96 ☑
    throat S11.85 ☑
      superficial NEC S10.17 ☑
        insect S10.16 ☑
  nose (septum) (sinus) S01.25 ☑
    superficial NEC S00.37 ☑
      insect S00.36 ☑
  occipital region — *see* Bite, scalp
  oral cavity S01.552 ☑
    superficial NEC S00.572 ☑
      insect S00.562 ☑
  orbital region — *see* Bite, eyelid
  palate — *see* Bite, oral cavity
  palm — *see* Bite, hand
  parietal region — *see* Bite, scalp
  pelvis S31.050 ☑
    with penetration into retroperitoneal space
      S31.051 ☑
    superficial NEC S30.870 ☑
      insect S30.860 ☑
  penis S31.25 ☑
    superficial NEC S30.872 ☑
      insect S30.862 ☑
  perineum
    female — *see* Bite, vulva
    male — *see* Bite, pelvis
  periocular area (with or without lacrimal passages) —
    see Bite, eyelid
  phalanges
    finger — *see* Bite, finger
    toe — *see* Bite, toe
  pharynx S11.25 ☑
    superficial NEC S10.17 ☑
      insect S10.16 ☑
  pinna — *see* Bite, ear
  poisonous — *see* Venom
  popliteal space — *see* Bite, knee
  prepuce — *see* Bite, penis
  pubic region — *see* Bite, abdomen, wall
  rectovaginal septum — *see* Bite, vulva
  red bug B88.0
  reptile NEC — *see also* Venom, bite, reptile
    nonvenomous — *see* Bite, by site
    snake — *see* Venom, bite, snake
  sacral region — *see* Bite, back, lower
  sacroiliac region — *see* Bite, back, lower
  salivary gland — *see* Bite, oral cavity
  scalp S01.05 ☑
    superficial NEC S00.07 ☑
      insect S00.06 ☑
  scapular region — *see* Bite, shoulder
  scrotum S31.35 ☑
    superficial NEC S30.873 ☑
      insect S30.863 ☑
  sea-snake (venomous) — *see* Toxicity, venom, snake,
    sea snake
  shin — *see* Bite, leg
  shoulder S41.05- ☑
    superficial NEC S40.27- ☑
      insect S40.26- ☑
  snake — *see also* Venom, bite, snake
    nonvenomous — *see* Bite, by site
  spermatic cord — *see* Bite, testis
  spider (venomous) — *see* Toxicity, venom, spider
    nonvenomous — *see* Bite, by site, superficial, insect
  sternal region — *see* Bite, thorax, front
  submaxillary region — *see* Bite, head, specified site
    NEC
  submental region — *see* Bite, head, specified site NEC
  subungual
    finger(s) — *see* Bite, finger
    toe — *see* Bite, toe
  superficial — *see* Bite, by site, superficial
  supraclavicular fossa S11.85 ☑
  supraorbital — *see* Bite, head, specified site NEC
  temple, temporal region — *see* Bite, head, specified
    site NEC

Bite(s) — *continued*
  temporomandibular area — *see* Bite, cheek
  testis S31.35 ☑
    superficial NEC S30.873 ☑
      insect S30.863 ☑
  thigh S71.15- ☑
    superficial NEC S70.37- ☑
      insect S70.36- ☑
  thorax, thoracic (wall) S21.95 ☑
    back S21.25- ☑
      with penetration into thoracic cavity S21.45- ☑
    breast — *see* Bite, breast
    front S21.15- ☑
      with penetration into thoracic cavity S21.35- ☑
    superficial NEC S20.97 ☑
      back S20.47- ☑
      front S20.37- ☑
      insect S20.96 ☑
        back S20.46- ☑
        front S20.36- ☑
  throat — *see* Bite, neck, throat
  thumb S61.05- ☑
    with
      damage to nail S61.15- ☑
    superficial NEC S60.37- ☑
      insect S60.36- ☑
  thyroid S11.15 ☑
    superficial NEC S10.87 ☑
      insect S10.86 ☑
  toe(s) S91.15- ☑
    with
      damage to nail S91.25- ☑
    great S91.15- ☑
      with
        damage to nail S91.25- ☑
    lesser S91.15- ☑
      with
        damage to nail S91.25- ☑
    superficial NEC S90.47- ☑
      great S90.47- ☑
      insect S90.46- ☑
        great S90.46- ☑
  tongue S01.552 ☑
  trachea S11.025 ☑
    superficial NEC S10.17 ☑
      insect S10.16 ☑
  tunica vaginalis — *see* Bite, testis
  tympanum, tympanic membrane — *see* Bite, ear
  umbilical region S31.155 ☑
  uvula — *see* Bite, oral cavity
  vagina — *see* Bite, vulva
  venomous — *see* Venom
  vocal cords S11.035 ☑
    superficial NEC S10.17 ☑
      insect S10.16 ☑
  vulva S31.45 ☑
    superficial NEC S30.874 ☑
      insect S30.864 ☑
  wrist S61.55- ☑
    superficial NEC S60.87- ☑
      insect S60.86- ☑
Biting, cheek or lip K13.1
Biventricular failure (heart) I50.82
Björck (-Thorson) **syndrome** (malignant carcinoid) E34.0
Black
  death A20.9
  eye S00.1- ☑
  hairy tongue K14.3
  heel (foot) S90.3- ☑
  lung (disease) J60
  palm (hand) S60.22- ☑
Blackfan-Diamond anemia or syndrome (congenital
  hypoplastic anemia) D61.01
Blackhead L70.0
Blackout R55
Bladder — *see* condition
Blast (air) (hydraulic) (immersion) (underwater)
  blindness S05.8X- ☑
  injury
    abdomen or thorax — *see* Injury, by site
    ear (acoustic nerve trauma) — *see* Injury, nerve,
      acoustic, specified type NEC
    syndrome NEC T70.8 ☑
Blastoma — *see* Neoplasm, malignant, by site
  pulmonary — *see* Neoplasm, lung, malignant
Blastomycosis, blastomycotic B40.9

Blastomycosis, blastomycotic — *continued*
  Brazilian — *see* Paracoccidioidomycosis
  cutaneous B40.3
  disseminated B40.7
  European — *see* Cryptococcosis
  generalized B40.7
  keloidal B48.0
  North American B40.9
  primary pulmonary B40.0
  pulmonary B40.2
    acute B40.0
    chronic B40.1
  skin B40.3
  South American — *see* Paracoccidioidomycosis
  specified NEC B40.89
Bleb(s) R23.8
  emphysematous (lung) (solitary) J43.9
  endophthalmitis H59.43
  filtering (vitreous), after glaucoma surgery Z98.83
  inflamed (infected), postprocedural H59.40
    stage 1 H59.41
    stage 2 H59.42
    stage 3 H59.43
  lung (ruptured) J43.9
    congenital — *see* Atelectasis
    newborn P25.8
  subpleural (emphysematous) J43.9
Blebitis, postprocedural H59.40
  stage 1 H59.41
  stage 2 H59.42
  stage 3 H59.43
Bleeder (familial) (hereditary) — *see* Hemophilia
Bleeding — *see also* Hemorrhage
  anal K62.5
  anovulatory N97.0
  atonic, following delivery O72.1
  capillary I78.8
    puerperal O72.2
  contact (postcoital) N93.0
  due to uterine subinvolution N85.3
  ear — *see* Otorrhagia
  excessive, associated with menopausal onset N92.4
  familial — *see* Defect, coagulation
  following intercourse N93.0
  gastrointestinal K92.2
  hemorrhoids — *see* Hemorrhoids
  intermenstrual (regular) N92.3
    irregular N92.1
  intraoperative — *see* Complication, intraoperative,
    hemorrhage
  irregular N92.6
  menopausal N92.4
  newborn, intraventricular — *see* Newborn, affected
    by, hemorrhage, intraventricular
  nipple N64.59
  nose R04.0
  ovulation N92.3
  perimenopausal N92.4
  postclimacteric N95.0
  postcoital N93.0
  postmenopausal N95.0
  postoperative — *see* Complication, postprocedural,
    hemorrhage
  preclimacteric N92.4
  pre-pubertal vaginal N93.1
  puberty (excessive, with onset of menstrual periods)
    N92.2
  rectum, rectal K62.5
    newborn P54.2
  tendencies — *see* Defect, coagulation
  throat R04.1
  tooth socket (post-extraction) K91.840
  umbilical stump P51.9
  uterus, uterine NEC N93.9
    climacteric N92.4
    dysfunctional or functional N93.8
    menopausal N92.4
    preclimacteric or premenopausal N92.4
    unrelated to menstrual cycle N93.9
  vagina, vaginal (abnormal) N93.9
    dysfunctional or functional N93.8
    newborn P54.6
    pre-pubertal N93.1
  vicarious N94.89
Blennorrhagia, blennorrhagic — *see* Gonorrhea
Blennorrhea (acute) (chronic) — *see also* Gonorrhea
  inclusion (neonatal) (newborn) P39.1
  lower genitourinary tract (gonococcal) A54.00

☑ **Additional Character Required** — **Refer to the Tabular List for Character Selection** ▽ **Subterms under main terms may continue to next column or page**

Blennorrhea — *continued*
  neonatorum (gonococcal ophthalmia) A54.31
Blepharelosis — *see* Entropion
Blepharitis (angularis) (ciliaris) (eyelid) (marginal)
    (nonulcerative) H01.009
  herpes zoster B02.39
  left H01.006
    lower H01.005
    upper H01.004
    upper and lower H01.00B
  right H01.003
    lower H01.002
    upper H01.001
    upper and lower H01.00A
  squamous H01.029
    left H01.026
      lower H01.025
      upper H01.024
      upper and lower H01.02B
    right H01.023
      lower H01.022
      upper H01.021
      upper and lower H01.02A
  ulcerative H01.019
    left H01.016
      lower H01.015
      upper H01.014
      upper and lower H01.01B
    right H01.013
      lower H01.012
      upper H01.011
      upper and lower H01.01A
Blepharochalasis H02.30
  congenital Q10.0
  left H02.36
    lower H02.35
    upper H02.34
  right H02.33
    lower H02.32
    upper H02.31
Blepharoclonus H02.59
Blepharoconjunctivitis H10.50- ☑
  angular H10.52- ☑
  contact H10.53- ☑
  ligneous H10.51- ☑
Blepharophimosis (eyelid) H02.529
  congenital Q10.3
  left H02.526
    lower H02.525
    upper H02.524
  right H02.523
    lower H02.522
    upper H02.521
Blepharoptosis H02.40- ☑
  congenital Q10.0
  mechanical H02.41- ☑
  myogenic H02.42- ☑
  neurogenic H02.43- ☑
  paralytic H02.43- ☑
Blepharopyorrhea, gonococcal A54.39
Blepharospasm G24.5
  drug induced G24.01
Blighted ovum O02.0
Blind — *see also* Blindness
  bronchus (congenital) Q32.4
  loop syndrome K90.2
    congenital Q43.8
  sac, fallopian tube (congenital) Q50.6
  spot, enlarged — *see* Defect, visual field, localized,
    scotoma, blind spot area
  tract or tube, congenital NEC — *see* Atresia, by site
Blindness (acquired) (congenital) (both eyes) H54.0X- ☑
  blast S05.8X- ☑
  color — *see* Deficiency, color vision
  concussion S05.8X- ☑
  cortical H47.619
    left brain H47.612
    right brain H47.611
  day H53.11
  due to injury (current episode) S05.9- ☑
    sequelae — *code to* injury with seventh character
      S
  eclipse (total) — *see* Retinopathy, solar
  emotional (hysterical) F44.6
  face H53.16
  hysterical F44.6
  legal (both eyes) (USA definition) H54.8
  mind R48.8

Blindness — *continued*
  night H53.60
    abnormal dark adaptation curve H53.61
    acquired H53.62
    congenital H53.63
    specified type NEC H53.69
    vitamin A deficiency E50.5
  one eye (other eye normal) H54.40
    left (normal vision on right) H54.42- ☑
      low vision on right H54.12- ☑
    low vision, other eye H54.10
    right (normal vision on left) H54.41- ☑
      low vision on left H54.11- ☑
  psychic R48.8
  river B73.01
  snow — *see* Photokeratitis
  sun, solar — *see* Retinopathy, solar
  transient — *see* Disturbance, vision, subjective, loss,
    transient
  traumatic (current episode) S05.9- ☑
  word (developmental) F81.0
    acquired R48.0
    secondary to organic lesion R48.0
Blister (nonthermal)
  abdominal wall S30.821 ☑
  alveolar process S00.522 ☑
  ankle S90.52- ☑
  antecubital space — *see* Blister, elbow
  anus S30.827 ☑
  arm (upper) S40.82- ☑
  auditory canal — *see* Blister, ear
  auricle — *see* Blister, ear
  axilla — *see* Blister, arm
  back, lower S30.820 ☑
  beetle dermatitis L24.89
  breast S20.12- ☑
  brow S00.82 ☑
  calf — *see* Blister, leg
  canthus — *see* Blister, eyelid
  cheek S00.82 ☑
    internal S00.522 ☑
  chest wall — *see* Blister, thorax
  chin S00.82 ☑
  costal region — *see* Blister, thorax
  digit(s)
    foot — *see* Blister, toe
    hand — *see* Blister, finger
  due to burn — *see* Burn, by site, second degree
  ear S00.42- ☑
  elbow S50.32- ☑
  epiglottis S10.12 ☑
  esophagus, cervical S10.12 ☑
  eyebrow — *see* Blister, eyelid
  eyelid S00.22- ☑
  face S00.82 ☑
  fever B00.1
  finger(s) S60.429 ☑
    index S60.42- ☑
    little S60.42- ☑
    middle S60.42- ☑
    ring S60.42- ☑
  foot (except toe(s) alone) S90.82- ☑
    toe — *see* Blister, toe
  forearm S50.82- ☑
    elbow only — *see* Blister, elbow
  forehead S00.82 ☑
  fracture — *omit code*
  genital organ
    female S30.826 ☑
    male S30.825 ☑
  gum S00.522 ☑
  hand S60.52- ☑
  head S00.92 ☑
    ear — *see* Blister, ear
    eyelid — *see* Blister, eyelid
    lip S00.521 ☑
    nose S00.32 ☑
    oral cavity S00.522 ☑
    scalp S00.02 ☑
    specified site NEC S00.82 ☑
  heel — *see* Blister, foot
  hip S70.22- ☑
  interscapular region S20.429 ☑
  jaw S00.82 ☑
  knee S80.22- ☑
  larynx S10.12 ☑

Blister — *continued*
  leg (lower) S80.82- ☑
    knee — *see* Blister, knee
    upper — *see* Blister, thigh
  lip S00.521 ☑
  malar region S00.82 ☑
  mammary — *see* Blister, breast
  mastoid region S00.82 ☑
  mouth S00.522 ☑
  multiple, skin, nontraumatic R23.8
  nail
    finger — *see* Blister, finger
    toe — *see* Blister, toe
  nasal S00.32 ☑
  neck S10.92 ☑
    specified site NEC S10.82 ☑
    throat S10.12 ☑
  nose S00.32 ☑
  occipital region S00.02 ☑
  oral cavity S00.522 ☑
  orbital region — *see* Blister, eyelid
  palate S00.522 ☑
  palm — *see* Blister, hand
  parietal region S00.02 ☑
  pelvis S30.820 ☑
  penis S30.822 ☑
  periocular area — *see* Blister, eyelid
  phalanges
    finger — *see* Blister, finger
    toe — *see* Blister, toe
  pharynx S10.12 ☑
  pinna — *see* Blister, ear
  popliteal space — *see* Blister, knee
  scalp S00.02 ☑
  scapular region — *see* Blister, shoulder
  scrotum S30.823 ☑
  shin — *see* Blister, leg
  shoulder S40.22- ☑
  sternal region S20.329 ☑
  submaxillary region S00.82 ☑
  submental region S00.82 ☑
  subungual
    finger(s) — *see* Blister, finger
    toe(s) — *see* Blister, toe
  supraclavicular fossa S10.82 ☑
  supraorbital S00.82 ☑
  temple S00.82 ☑
  temporal region S00.82 ☑
  testis S30.823 ☑
  thermal — *see* Burn, second degree, by site
  thigh S70.32- ☑
  thorax, thoracic (wall) S20.92 ☑
    back S20.42- ☑
    front S20.32- ☑
  throat S10.12 ☑
  thumb S60.32- ☑
  toe(s) S90.42- ☑
    great S90.42- ☑
  tongue S00.522 ☑
  trachea S10.12 ☑
  tympanum, tympanic membrane — *see* Blister, ear
  upper arm — *see* Blister, arm (upper)
  uvula S00.522 ☑
  vagina S30.824 ☑
  vocal cords S10.12 ☑
  vulva S30.824 ☑
  wrist S60.82- ☑
Bloating R14.0
Bloch-Sulzberger disease or syndrome Q82.3
Block, blocked
  alveolocapillary J84.10
  arborization (heart) I45.5
  arrhythmic I45.9
  atrioventricular (incomplete) (partial) I44.30
    with atrioventricular dissociation I44.2
    complete I44.2
      congenital Q24.6
    congenital Q24.6
    first degree I44.0
    second degree (types I and II) I44.1
    specified NEC I44.39
    third degree I44.2
    types I and II I44.1
  auriculoventricular — *see* Block, atrioventricular
  bifascicular (cardiac) I45.2
  bundle-branch (complete) (false) (incomplete) I45.4

Block, blocked — *continued*
  bundle-branch — *continued*
    bilateral I45.2
    left I44.7
      with right bundle branch block I45.2
      hemiblock I44.60
        anterior I44.4
        posterior I44.5
      incomplete I44.7
        with right bundle branch block I45.2
    right I45.10
      with
        left bundle branch block I45.2
        left fascicular block I45.2
      specified NEC I45.19
    Wilson's type I45.19
  cardiac I45.9
  conduction I45.9
    complete I44.2
  fascicular (left) I44.60
    anterior I44.4
    posterior I44.5
    right I45.0
    specified NEC I44.69
  foramen Magendie (acquired) G91.1
    congenital Q03.1
      with spina bifida — *see* Spina bifida, by site, with hydrocephalus
  heart I45.9
    bundle branch I45.4
      bilateral I45.2
    complete (atrioventricular) I44.2
    congenital Q24.6
    first degree (atrioventricular) I44.0
    second degree (atrioventricular) I44.1
    specified type NEC I45.5
    third degree (atrioventricular) I44.2
  hepatic vein I82.0
  intraventricular (nonspecific) I45.4
    bundle branch
      bilateral I45.2
  kidney N28.9
    postcystoscopic or postprocedural N99.0
  Mobitz (types I and II) I44.1
  myocardial — *see* Block, heart
  nodal I45.5
  organ or site, congenital NEC — *see* Atresia, by site
  portal (vein) I81
  second degree (types I and II) I44.1
  sinoatrial I45.5
  sinoauricular I45.5
  third degree I44.2
  trifascicular I45.3
  tubal N97.1
  vein NOS I82.90
  Wenckebach (types I and II) I44.1
Blockage — *see* Obstruction
Blocq's disease F44.4
Blood
  constituents, abnormal R78.9
  disease D75.9
  donor — *see* Donor, blood
  dyscrasia D75.9
    with
      abortion — *see* Abortion, by type, complicated by, hemorrhage
      ectopic pregnancy O08.1
      molar pregnancy O08.1
    following ectopic or molar pregnancy O08.1
    newborn P61.9
    puerperal, postpartum O72.3
  flukes NEC — *see* Schistosomiasis
  in
    feces K92.1
      occult R19.5
    urine — *see* Hematuria
  mole O02.0
  occult in feces R19.5
  pressure
    decreased, due to shock following injury T79.4 ☑
    examination only Z01.30
    fluctuating I99.8
    high — *see* Hypertension
      borderline R03.0
      incidental reading, without diagnosis of hypertension R03.0
    low — *see also* Hypotension

Blood — *continued*
  pressure — *continued*
    low — *see also* Hypotension — *continued*
      incidental reading, without diagnosis of hypotension R03.1
  spitting — *see* Hemoptysis
  staining cornea — *see* Pigmentation, cornea, stromal
  transfusion
    reaction or complication — *see* Complications, transfusion
  type
    A (Rh positive) Z67.10
      Rh negative Z67.11
    AB (Rh positive) Z67.30
      Rh negative Z67.31
    B (Rh positive) Z67.20
      Rh negative Z67.21
    O (Rh positive) Z67.40
      Rh negative Z67.41
    Rh (positive) Z67.90
      negative Z67.91
  vessel rupture — *see* Hemorrhage
  vomiting — *see* Hematemesis
Blood-forming organs, disease D75.9
Bloodgood's disease — *see* Mastopathy, cystic
Bloom (-Machacek)(-Torre) **syndrome** Q82.8
Blount disease or osteochondrosis M92.51- ☑
Blue
  baby Q24.9
  diaper syndrome E72.09
  dome cyst (breast) — *see* Cyst, breast
  dot cataract Q12.0
  nevus D22.9
  sclera Q13.5
    with fragility of bone and deafness Q78.0
  toe syndrome I75.02- ☑
Blueness — *see* Cyanosis
Blues, postpartal O90.6
  baby O90.6
Blurring, visual H53.8
Blushing (abnormal) (excessive) R23.2
BMI — *see* Body, mass index
Boarder, hospital NEC Z76.4
  accompanying sick person Z76.3
  healthy infant or child Z76.2
    foundling Z76.1
Bockhart's impetigo L01.02
Bodechtel-Guttman disease (subacute sclerosing panencephalitis) A81.1
Boder-Sedgwick syndrome (ataxia-telangiectasia) G11.3
Body, bodies
  Aschoff's — *see* Myocarditis, rheumatic
  asteroid, vitreous — *see* Deposit, crystalline
  cytoid (retina) — *see* Occlusion, artery, retina
  drusen (degenerative) (macula) (retinal) — *see also* Degeneration, macula, drusen
    optic disc — *see* Drusen, optic disc
  foreign — *see* Foreign body
  loose
    joint, except knee — *see* Loose, body, joint
      knee M23.4- ☑
    sheath, tendon — *see* Disorder, tendon, specified type NEC
  mass index (BMI)
    adult
      19.9 or less Z68.1
      20.0-20.9 Z68.20
      21.0-21.9 Z68.21
      22.0-22.9 Z68.22
      23.0-23.9 Z68.23
      24.0-24.9 Z68.24
      25.0-25.9 Z68.25
      26.0-26.9 Z68.26
      27.0-27.9 Z68.27
      28.0-28.9 Z68.28
      29.0-29.9 Z68.29
      30.0-30.9 Z68.30
      31.0-31.9 Z68.31
      32.0-32.9 Z68.32
      33.0-33.9 Z68.33
      34.0-34.9 Z68.34
      35.0-35.9 Z68.35
      36.0-36.9 Z68.36
      37.0-37.9 Z68.37
      38.0-38.9 Z68.38
      39.0-39.9 Z68.39
      40.0-44.9 Z68.41
      45.0-49.9 Z68.42

Body, bodies — *continued*
  mass index — *continued*
    adult — *continued*
      50.0-59.9 Z68.43
      60.0-69.9 Z68.44
      70 and over Z68.45
    pediatric
      5th percentile to less than 85th percentile for age Z68.52
      85th percentile to less than 95th percentile for age Z68.53
      greater than or equal to ninety-fifth percentile for age Z68.54
      less than fifth percentile for age Z68.51
  Mooser's A75.2
  rice — *see also* Loose, body, joint
    knee M23.4- ☑
  rocking F98.4
Boeck's
  disease or sarcoid — *see* Sarcoidosis
  lupoid (miliary) D86.3
Boerhaave's syndrome (spontaneous esophageal rupture) K22.3
Boggy
  cervix N88.8
  uterus N85.8
Boil — *see also* Furuncle, by site
  Aleppo B55.1
  Baghdad B55.1
  Delhi B55.1
  lacrimal
    gland — *see* Dacryoadenitis
    passages (duct) (sac) — *see* Inflammation, lacrimal, passages, acute
  Natal B55.1
  orbit, orbital — *see* Abscess, orbit
  tropical B55.1
Bold hives — *see* Urticaria
Bombé, iris — *see* Membrane, pupillary
Bone — *see* condition
Bonnevie-Ullrich syndrome — *see also* Turner's syndrome Q87.19
Bonnier's syndrome H81.8 ☑
Bonvale dam fever T73.3 ☑
Bony block of joint — *see* Ankylosis
BOOP (bronchiolitis obliterans organized pneumonia) J84.89
Borderline
  diabetes mellitus R73.03
  hypertension R03.0
  osteopenia M85.8- ☑
  pelvis, with obstruction during labor O65.1
  personality F60.3
Borna disease A83.9
Bornholm disease B33.0
Boston exanthem A88.0
Botalli, ductus (patent) (persistent) Q25.0
Bothriocephalus latus infestation B70.0
Botulism (foodborne intoxication) A05.1
  infant A48.51
  non-foodborne A48.52
  wound A48.52
Bouba — *see* Yaws
Bouchard's nodes (with arthropathy) M15.2
Bouffée délirante F23
Bouillaud's disease or syndrome (rheumatic heart disease) I01.9
Bourneville's disease Q85.1
Boutonniere deformity (finger) — *see* Deformity, finger, boutonniere
Bouveret (-Hoffmann) **syndrome** (paroxysmal tachycardia) I47.9
Bovine heart — *see* Hypertrophy, cardiac
Bowel — *see* condition
Bowen's
  dermatosis (precancerous) — *see* Neoplasm, skin, in situ
  disease — *see* Neoplasm, skin, in situ
  epithelioma — *see* Neoplasm, skin, in situ
  type
    epidermoid carcinoma-in-situ — *see* Neoplasm, skin, in situ
    intraepidermal squamous cell carcinoma — *see* Neoplasm, skin, in situ
Bowing
  femur — *see also* Deformity, limb, specified type NEC, thigh

Bowing — *continued*
  femur — *see also* Deformity, limb, specified type, thigh
    — *continued*
    congenital Q68.3
  fibula — *see also* Deformity, limb, specified type NEC,
    lower leg
    congenital Q68.4
  forearm — *see* Deformity, limb, specified type NEC,
    forearm
  leg(s), long bones, congenital Q68.5
  radius — *see* Deformity, limb, specified type NEC,
    forearm
  tibia — *see also* Deformity, limb, specified type NEC,
    lower leg
    congenital Q68.4
Bowleg(s) (acquired) M21.16- ☑
  congenital Q68.5
  rachitic E64.3
Boyd's dysentery A03.2
Brachial — *see* condition
Brachycardia R00.1
Brachycephaly Q75.0
Bradley's disease A08.19
Bradyarrhythmia, cardiac I49.8
Bradycardia (sinoatrial) (sinus) (vagal) R00.1
  neonatal P29.12
  reflex G90.09
  tachycardia syndrome I49.5
Bradykinesia R25.8
Bradypnea R06.89
Bradytachycardia I49.5
Brailsford's disease or osteochondrosis — *see* Osteo-
  chondrosis, juvenile, radius
Brain — *see also* condition
  death G93.82
  syndrome — *see* Syndrome, brain
Branched-chain amino-acid disorder E71.2
Branchial — *see* condition
  cartilage, congenital Q18.2
Branchiogenic remnant (in neck) Q18.0
Brandt's syndrome (acrodermatitis enteropathica) E83.2
Brash (water) R12
Bravais-jacksonian epilepsy — *see* Epilepsy, localiza-
  tion-related, symptomatic, with simple partial
  seizures
Braxton Hicks contractions — *see* False, labor
Brazilian leishmaniasis B55.2
BRBPR K62.5
Break, retina (without detachment) H33.30- ☑
  with retinal detachment — *see* Detachment, retina
  horseshoe tear H33.31- ☑
  multiple H33.33- ☑
  round hole H33.32- ☑
Breakdown
  device, graft or implant — *see also* Complications, by
    site and type, mechanical T85.618 ☑
    arterial graft NEC — *see* Complication, cardiovascu-
      lar device, mechanical, vascular
    breast (implant) T85.41 ☑
    catheter NEC T85.618 ☑
      cystostomy T83.010 ☑
      dialysis (renal) T82.41 ☑
        intraperitoneal T85.611 ☑
      Hopkins T83.018 ☑
      ileostomy T83.018 ☑
      infusion NEC T82.514 ☑
        cranial T85.610- ☑
        epidural T85.610 ☑
        intrathecal T85.610 ☑
        spinal T85.610 ☑
        subarachnoid T85.610 ☑
        subdural T85.610 ☑
      nephrostomy T83.012 ☑
      urethral indwelling T83.011 ☑
      urinary NEC T83.018 ☑
      urostomy T83.018 ☑
    electronic (electrode) (pulse generator) (stimulator)
      bone T84.310 ☑
      cardiac T82.119 ☑
        electrode T82.110 ☑
        pulse generator T82.111 ☑
        specified type NEC T82.118 ☑
      nervous system — *see* Complication, prosthetic
        device, mechanical, electronic nervous
        system stimulator
      urinary — *see* Complication, genitourinary, de-
        vice, urinary, mechanical

Breakdown — *continued*
  device, graft or implant — *see also* Complications, by
    site and type, mechanical — *continued*
    fixation, internal (orthopedic) NEC — *see* Complica-
      tion, fixation device, mechanical
    gastrointestinal — *see* Complications, prosthetic
      device, mechanical, gastrointestinal device
    genital NEC T83.418 ☑
      intrauterine contraceptive device T83.31 ☑
      penile prosthesis (cylinder) (implanted) (pump)
        (resevoir) T83.410 ☑
      testicular prosthesis T83.411 ☑
    heart NEC — *see* Complication, cardiovascular de-
      vice, mechanical
    intrathecal infusion pump T85.615 ☑
    joint prosthesis — *see* Complications..., joint pros-
      thesis,internal, mechanical, by site
    nervous system, specified device NEC T85.615 ☑
    ocular NEC — *see* Complications, prosthetic device,
      mechanical, ocular device
    orthopedic NEC — *see* Complication, orthopedic,
      device, mechanical
    specified NEC T85.618 ☑
    subcutaneous device pocket
      nervous system prosthetic device, implant, or
        graft T85.890 ☑
      other internal prosthetic device, implant, or graft
        T85.898 ☑
    sutures, permanent T85.612 ☑
      used in bone repair — *see* Complications, fixation
        device, internal (orthopedic), mechanical
    urinary NEC T83.118 ☑
      graft T83.21 ☑
      sphincter, implanted T83.111 ☑
      stent (ileal conduit) (nephroureteral) T83.113 ☑
      ureteral indwelling T83.112 ☑
    vascular NEC — *see* Complication, cardiovascular
      device, mechanical
    ventricular intracranial shunt T85.01 ☑
  nervous F48.8
  perineum O90.1
  respirator J95.850
    specified NEC J95.859
  ventilator J95.850
    specified NEC J95.859
Breast — *see also* condition
  buds E30.1
    in newborn P96.89
  dense R92.2
  nodule — *see also* Lump, breast N63.0 ☑
Breath
  foul R19.6
  holder, child R06.89
  holding spell R06.89
  shortness R06.02
Breathing
  labored — *see* Hyperventilation
  mouth R06.5
    causing malocclusion M26.5 ☑
  periodic R06.3
    high altitude G47.32
Breathlessness R06.81
Breda's disease — *see* Yaws
Breech presentation (mother) O32.1 ☑
  causing obstructed labor O64.1 ☑
  footling O32.8 ☑
    causing obstructed labor O64.8 ☑
  incomplete O32.8 ☑
    causing obstructed labor O64.8 ☑
Breisky's disease N90.4
Brennemann's syndrome I88.0
Brenner
  tumor (benign) D27.9
    borderline malignancy D39.1- ☑
    malignant C56 ☑
    proliferating D39.1- ☑
Bretonneau's disease or angina A36.0
Breus' mole O02.0
Brevicollis Q76.49
Brickmakers' anemia B76.9 *[D63.8]*
Bridge, myocardial Q24.5
Bright red blood per rectum (BRBPR) K62.5
Bright's disease — *see also* Nephritis
  arteriosclerotic — *see* Hypertension, kidney
Brill (-Zinsser) **disease** (recrudescent typhus) A75.1
Brill-Symmers' disease C82.90
Brion-Kayser disease — *see* Fever, parathyroid

Briquet's disorder or syndrome F45.0
Brissaud's
  infantilism or dwarfism E23.0
  motor-verbal tic F95.2
Brittle
  bones disease Q78.0
  nails L60.3
    congenital Q84.6
Broad — *see also* condition
  beta disease E78.2
  ligament laceration syndrome N83.8
Broad- or floating-betalipoproteinemia E78.2
Brock's syndrome (atelectasis due to enlarged lymph
  nodes) J98.19
Brocq-Duhring disease (dermatitis herpetiformis) L13.0
Brodie's abscess or disease M86.8X- ☑
Broken
  arches — *see also* Deformity, limb, flat foot
  arm (meaning upper limb) — *see* Fracture, arm
  back — *see* Fracture, vertebra
  bone — *see* Fracture
  implant or internal device — *see* Complications, by site
    and type, mechanical
  leg (meaning lower limb) — *see* Fracture, leg
  nose S02.2 ☑
  tooth, teeth — *see* Fracture, tooth
Bromhidrosis, bromidrosis L75.0
Bromidism, bromism G92.8
  due to
    correct substance properly administered — *see* Ta-
      ble of Drugs and Chemicals, by drug, adverse
      effect
    overdose or wrong substance given or taken — *see*
      Table of Drugs and Chemicals, by drug, poi-
      soning
  chronic (dependence) F13.20
Bromidrosiphobia F40.298
Bronchi, bronchial — *see* condition
Bronchiectasis (cylindrical) (diffuse) (fusiform) (localized)
  (saccular) J47.9
  with
    acute
      bronchitis J47.0
      lower respiratory infection J47.0
    exacerbation (acute) J47.1
  congenital Q33.4
  tuberculous NEC — *see* Tuberculosis, pulmonary
Bronchiolectasis — *see* Bronchiectasis
Bronchiolitis (acute) (infective) (subacute) J21.9
  with
    bronchospasm or obstruction J21.9
    influenza, flu or grippe — *see* Influenza, with, respi-
      ratory manifestations NEC
  chemical (chronic) J68.4
    acute J68.0
  chronic (fibrosing) (obliterative) J44.9
  due to
    external agent — *see* Bronchitis, acute, due to
    human metapneumovirus J21.1
    respiratory syncytial virus (RSV) J21.0
    specified organism NEC J21.8
  fibrosa obliterans J44.9
  influenzal — *see* Influenza, with, respiratory manifesta-
    tions NEC
  obliterans J42
    with organizing pneumonia (BOOP) J84.89
  obliterative (chronic) (subacute) J44.9
    due to fumes or vapors J68.4
    due to chemicals, gases, fumes or vapors (inhalation)
      J68.4
  respiratory, interstitial lung disease J84.115
Bronchitis (diffuse) (fibrinous) (hypostatic) (infective)
  (membranous) J40
  with
    influenza, flu or grippe — *see* Influenza, with, respi-
      ratory manifestations NEC
    obstruction (airway) (lung) J44.9
    tracheitis (15 years of age and above) J40
      acute or subacute J20.9
      chronic J42
      under 15 years of age J20.9
  acute or subacute (with bronchospasm or obstruction)
    J20.9
    with
      bronchiectasis J47.0
      chronic obstructive pulmonary disease J44.0
      chemical (due to gases, fumes or vapors) J68.0

Bronchitis — *continued*
  acute or subacute — *continued*
    due to
      fumes or vapors J68.0
      Haemophilus influenzae J20.1
      Mycoplasma pneumoniae J20.0
      radiation J70.0
      specified organism NEC J20.8
      Streptococcus J20.2
      virus
        coxsackie J20.3
        echovirus J20.7
        parainfluenzae J20.4
        respiratory syncytial (RSV) J20.5
        rhinovirus J20.6
      viral NEC J20.8
  allergic (acute) J45.909
    with
      exacerbation (acute) J45.901
      status asthmaticus J45.902
  arachidic T17.528 ☑
  aspiration (due to food and vomit) J69.0
  asthmatic J45.9 ☑
    chronic J44.9
      with
        acute lower respiratory infection J44.0
        exacerbation (acute) J44.1
  capillary — *see* Pneumonia, broncho
  caseous (tuberculous) A15.5
  Castellani's A69.8
  catarrhal (15 years of age and above) J40
    acute — *see* Bronchitis, acute
    chronic J41.0
    under 15 years of age J20.9
  chemical (acute) (subacute) J68.0
    chronic J68.4
    due to fumes or vapors J68.0
      chronic J68.4
  chronic J42
    with
      airways obstruction J44.9
      tracheitis (chronic) J42
    asthmatic (obstructive) J44.9
    catarrhal J41.0
    chemical (due to fumes or vapors) J68.4
    due to
      chemicals, gases, fumes or vapors (inhalation) J68.4
      radiation J70.1
      tobacco smoking J41.0
    emphysematous J44.9
    mucopurulent J41.1
    non-obstructive J41.0
    obliterans J44.9
    obstructive J44.9
    purulent J41.1
    simple J41.0
  croupous — *see* Bronchitis, acute
  due to gases, fumes or vapors (chemical) J68.0
  emphysematous (obstructive) J44.9
  exudative — *see* Bronchitis, acute
  fetid J41.1
  grippal — *see* Influenza, with, respiratory manifestations NEC
  in those under 15 years age — *see* Bronchitis, acute
    chronic — *see* Bronchitis, chronic
  influenzal — *see* Influenza, with, respiratory manifestations NEC
  mixed simple and mucopurulent J41.8
  moulder's J62.8
  mucopurulent (chronic) (recurrent) J41.1
    acute or subacute J20.9
    simple (mixed) J41.8
  obliterans (chronic) J44.9
  obstructive (chronic) (diffuse) J44.9
  pituitous J41.1
  pneumococcal, acute or subacute J20.2
  pseudomembranous, acute or subacute — *see* Bronchitis, acute
  purulent (chronic) (recurrent) J41.1
    acute or subacute — *see* Bronchitis, acute
  putrid J41.1
  senile (chronic) J42
  simple and mucopurulent (mixed) J41.8
  smokers' J41.0
  spirochetal NEC A69.8
  subacute — *see* Bronchitis, acute
  suppurative (chronic) J41.1

Bronchitis — *continued*
  suppurative — *continued*
    acute or subacute — *see* Bronchitis, acute
    tuberculous A15.5
  under 15 years of age — *see* Bronchitis, acute
    chronic — *see* Bronchitis, chronic
  viral NEC, acute or subacute — *see also* Bronchitis, acute J20.8
Bronchoalveolitis J18.0
Bronchoaspergillosis B44.1
Bronchocele meaning goiter E04.0
Broncholithiasis J98.09
  tuberculous NEC A15.5
Bronchomalacia J98.09
  congenital Q32.2
Bronchomycosis NOS B49 *[J99]*
  candidal B37.1
Bronchopleuropneumonia — *see* Pneumonia, broncho
Bronchopneumonia — *see* Pneumonia, broncho
Bronchopneumonitis — *see* Pneumonia, broncho
Bronchopulmonary — *see* condition
Bronchopulmonitis — *see* Pneumonia, broncho
Bronchorrhagia (see Hemoptysis)
Bronchorrhea J98.09
  acute J20.9
  chronic (infective) (purulent) J42
Bronchospasm (acute) J98.01
  with
    bronchiolitis, acute J21.9
    bronchitis, acute (conditions in J20) — *see* Bronchitis, acute
  due to external agent — *see* condition, respiratory, acute, due to
  exercise induced J45.990
Bronchospirochetosis A69.8
  Castellani A69.8
Bronchostenosis J98.09
Bronchus — *see* condition
Brontophobia F40.220
Bronze baby syndrome P83.88
Brooke's tumor — *see* Neoplasm, skin, benign
Brown enamel of teeth (hereditary) K00.5
Brown's sheath syndrome H50.61- ☑
Brown-Séquard disease, paralysis or syndrome G83.81
Bruce sepsis A23.0
Brucellosis (infection) A23.9
  abortus A23.1
  canis A23.3
  dermatitis A23.9
  melitensis A23.0
  mixed A23.8
  sepsis A23.9
    melitensis A23.0
    specified NEC A23.8
  suis A23.2
Bruck-de Lange disease Q87.19
Bruck's disease — *see* Deformity, limb
BRUE (brief resolved unexplained event) R68.13
Brugsch's syndrome Q82.8
Bruise (skin surface intact) — *see also* Contusion
  with
    open wound — *see* Wound, open
  internal organ — *see* Injury, by site
  newborn P54.5
  scalp, due to birth injury, newborn P12.3
  umbilical cord O69.5 ☑
Bruit (arterial) R09.89
  cardiac R01.1
Brush burn — *see* Abrasion, by site
Bruton's X-linked agammaglobulinemia D80.0
Bruxism
  psychogenic F45.8
  sleep related G47.63
Bubbly lung syndrome P27.0
Bubo I88.8
  blennorrhagic (gonococcal) A54.89
  chancroidal A57
  climatic A55
  due to Haemophilus ducreyi A57
  gonococcal A54.89
  indolent (nonspecific) I88.8
  inguinal (nonspecific) I88.8
    chancroidal A57
    climatic A55
    due to H. ducreyi A57
    infective I88.8

Bubo — *continued*
  scrofulous (tuberculous) A18.2
  soft chancre A57
  suppurating — *see* Lymphadenitis, acute
  syphilitic (primary) A51.0
    congenital A50.07
  tropical A55
  virulent (chancroidal) A57
Bubonic plague A20.0
Bubonocele — *see* Hernia, inguinal
Buccal — *see* condition
Buchanan's disease or osteochondrosis M91.0
Buchem's syndrome (hyperostosis corticalis) M85.2
Bucket-handle fracture or tear (semilunar cartilage) — *see* Tear, meniscus
Budd-Chiari syndrome (hepatic vein thrombosis) I82.0
Budgerigar fancier's disease or lung J67.2
Buds
  breast E30.1
    in newborn P96.89
Buerger's disease (thromboangiitis obliterans) I73.1
Bulbar — *see* condition
Bulbus cordis (left ventricle) (persistent) Q21.8
Bulimia (nervosa) F50.2
  atypical F50.9
  normal weight F50.9
Bulky
  stools R19.5
  uterus N85.2
Bulla (e) R23.8
  lung (emphysematous) (solitary) J43.9
    newborn P25.8
Bullet wound — *see also* Wound, open
  fracture — *code as* Fracture, by site
  internal organ — *see* Injury, by site
Bundle
  branch block (complete) (false) (incomplete) — *see* Block, bundle-branch
  of His — *see* condition
Bunion M21.61- ☑
  tailor's M21.62- ☑
Bunionette M21.62- ☑
Buphthalmia, buphthalmos (congenital) Q15.0
Burdwan fever B55.0
Bürger-Grütz disease or syndrome E78.3
Buried
  penis (congenital) Q55.64
    acquired N48.83
  roots K08.3
Burke's syndrome K86.89
Burkitt
  cell leukemia C91.0- ☑
  lymphoma (malignant) C83.7- ☑
    small noncleaved, diffuse C83.7- ☑
    spleen C83.77
    undifferentiated C83.7- ☑
  tumor C83.7- ☑
  type
    acute lymphoblastic leukemia C91.0- ☑
    undifferentiated C83.7- ☑
Burn (electricity) (flame) (hot gas, liquid or hot object) (radiation) (steam) (thermal) T30.0
  abdomen, abdominal (muscle) (wall) T21.02 ☑
    first degree T21.12 ☑
    second degree T21.22 ☑
    third degree T21.32 ☑
  above elbow T22.039 ☑
    first degree T22.139 ☑
    left T22.032 ☑
      first degree T22.132 ☑
      second degree T22.232 ☑
      third degree T22.332 ☑
    right T22.031 ☑
      first degree T22.131 ☑
      second degree T22.231 ☑
      third degree T22.331 ☑
    second degree T22.239 ☑
    third degree T22.339 ☑
  acid (caustic) (external) (internal) — *see* Corrosion, by site
  alimentary tract NEC T28.2 ☑
    esophagus T28.1 ☑
    mouth T28.0 ☑
    pharynx T28.0 ☑
  alkaline (caustic) (external) (internal) — *see* Corrosion, by site

Burn — continued
　ankle T25.019 ☑
　　first degree T25.119 ☑
　　left T25.012 ☑
　　　first degree T25.112 ☑
　　　second degree T25.212 ☑
　　　third degree T25.312 ☑
　　multiple with foot — see Burn, lower, limb, multiple,
　　　　ankle and foot
　　right T25.011 ☑
　　　first degree T25.111 ☑
　　　second degree T25.211 ☑
　　　third degree T25.311 ☑
　　second degree T25.219 ☑
　　third degree T25.319 ☑
　anus — see Burn, buttock
　arm (lower) (upper) — see Burn, upper, limb
　axilla T22.049 ☑
　　first degree T22.149 ☑
　　left T22.042 ☑
　　　first degree T22.142 ☑
　　　second degree T22.242 ☑
　　　third degree T22.342 ☑
　　right T22.041 ☑
　　　first degree T22.141 ☑
　　　second degree T22.241 ☑
　　　third degree T22.341 ☑
　　second degree T22.249 ☑
　　third degree T22.349 ☑
　back (lower) T21.04 ☑
　　first degree T21.14 ☑
　　second degree T21.24 ☑
　　third degree T21.34 ☑
　　upper T21.03 ☑
　　　first degree T21.13 ☑
　　　second degree T21.23 ☑
　　　third degree T21.33 ☑
　blisters — code as Burn, second degree, by site
　breast(s) — see Burn, chest wall
　buttock(s) T21.05 ☑
　　first degree T21.15 ☑
　　second degree T21.25 ☑
　　third degree T21.35 ☑
　calf T24.039 ☑
　　first degree T24.139 ☑
　　left T24.032 ☑
　　　first degree T24.132 ☑
　　　second degree T24.232 ☑
　　　third degree T24.332 ☑
　　right T24.031 ☑
　　　first degree T24.131 ☑
　　　second degree T24.231 ☑
　　　third degree T24.331 ☑
　　second degree T24.239 ☑
　　third degree T24.339 ☑
　canthus (eye) — see Burn, eyelid
　caustic acid or alkaline — see Corrosion, by site
　cervix T28.3 ☑
　cheek T20.06 ☑
　　first degree T20.16 ☑
　　second degree T20.26 ☑
　　third degree T20.36 ☑
　chemical (acids) (alkalines) (caustics) (external) (inter-
　　　nal) — see Corrosion, by site
　chest wall T21.01 ☑
　　first degree T21.11 ☑
　　second degree T21.21 ☑
　　third degree T21.31 ☑
　chin T20.03 ☑
　　first degree T20.13 ☑
　　second degree T20.23 ☑
　　third degree T20.33 ☑
　colon T28.2 ☑
　conjunctiva (and cornea) — see Burn, cornea
　cornea (and conjunctiva) T26.1- ☑
　　chemical — see Corrosion, cornea
　corrosion (external) (internal) — see Corrosion, by site
　deep necrosis of underlying tissue — code as Burn,
　　　third degree, by site
　dorsum of hand T23.069 ☑
　　first degree T23.169 ☑
　　left T23.062 ☑
　　　first degree T23.162 ☑
　　　second degree T23.262 ☑
　　　third degree T23.362 ☑
　　right T23.061 ☑

Burn — continued
　dorsum of hand — continued
　　right — continued
　　　first degree T23.161 ☑
　　　second degree T23.261 ☑
　　　third degree T23.361 ☑
　　second degree T23.269 ☑
　　third degree T23.369 ☑
　due to ingested chemical agent — see Corrosion, by
　　　site
　ear (auricle) (external) (canal) T20.01 ☑
　　first degree T20.11 ☑
　　second degree T20.21 ☑
　　third degree T20.31 ☑
　elbow T22.029 ☑
　　first degree T22.129 ☑
　　left T22.022 ☑
　　　first degree T22.122 ☑
　　　second degree T22.222 ☑
　　　third degree T22.322 ☑
　　right T22.021 ☑
　　　first degree T22.121 ☑
　　　second degree T22.221 ☑
　　　third degree T22.321 ☑
　　second degree T22.229 ☑
　　third degree T22.329 ☑
　epidermal loss — code as Burn, second degree, by site
　erythema, erythematous — code as Burn, first degree,
　　　by site
　esophagus T28.1 ☑
　extent (percentage of body surface)
　　less than 10 percent T31.0
　　10-19 percent T31.10
　　　with 0-9 percent third degree burns T31.10
　　　with 10-19 percent third degree burns T31.11
　　20-29 percent T31.20
　　　with 0-9 percent third degree burns T31.20
　　　with 10-19 percent third degree burns T31.21
　　　with 20-29 percent third degree burns T31.22
　　30-39 percent T31.30
　　　with 0-9 percent third degree burns T31.30
　　　with 10-19 percent third degree burns T31.31
　　　with 20-29 percent third degree burns T31.32
　　　with 30-39 percent third degree burns T31.33
　　40-49 percent T31.40
　　　with 0-9 percent third degree burns T31.40
　　　with 10-19 percent third degree burns T31.41
　　　with 20-29 percent third degree burns T31.42
　　　with 30-39 percent third degree burns T31.43
　　　with 40-49 percent third degree burns T31.44
　　50-59 percent T31.50
　　　with 0-9 percent third degree burns T31.50
　　　with 10-19 percent third degree burns T31.51
　　　with 20-29 percent third degree burns T31.52
　　　with 30-39 percent third degree burns T31.53
　　　with 40-49 percent third degree burns T31.54
　　　with 50-59 percent third degree burns T31.55
　　60-69 percent T31.60
　　　with 0-9 percent third degree burns T31.60
　　　with 10-19 percent third degree burns T31.61
　　　with 20-29 percent third degree burns T31.62
　　　with 30-39 percent third degree burns T31.63
　　　with 40-49 percent third degree burns T31.64
　　　with 50-59 percent third degree burns T31.65
　　　with 60-69 percent third degree burns T31.66
　　70-79 percent T31.70
　　　with 0-9 percent third degree burns T31.70
　　　with 10-19 percent third degree burns T31.71
　　　with 20-29 percent third degree burns T31.72
　　　with 30-39 percent third degree burns T31.73
　　　with 40-49 percent third degree burns T31.74
　　　with 50-59 percent third degree burns T31.75
　　　with 60-69 percent third degree burns T31.76
　　　with 70-79 percent third degree burns T31.77
　　80-89 percent T31.80
　　　with 0-9 percent third degree burns T31.80
　　　with 10-19 percent third degree burns T31.81
　　　with 20-29 percent third degree burns T31.82
　　　with 30-39 percent third degree burns T31.83
　　　with 40-49 percent third degree burns T31.84
　　　with 50-59 percent third degree burns T31.85
　　　with 60-69 percent third degree burns T31.86
　　　with 70-79 percent third degree burns T31.87
　　　with 80-89 percent third degree burns T31.88
　　90 percent or more T31.90
　　　with 0-9 percent third degree burns T31.90
　　　with 10-19 percent third degree burns T31.91
　　　with 20-29 percent third degree burns T31.92

Burn — continued
　extent — continued
　　90 percent or more — continued
　　　with 30-39 percent third degree burns T31.93
　　　with 40-49 percent third degree burns T31.94
　　　with 50-59 percent third degree burns T31.95
　　　with 60-69 percent third degree burns T31.96
　　　with 70-79 percent third degree burns T31.97
　　　with 80-89 percent third degree burns T31.98
　　　with 90 percent or more third degree burns
　　　　T31.99
　extremity — see Burn, limb
　eye(s) and adnexa T26.4- ☑
　　with resulting rupture and destruction of eyeball
　　　T26.2- ☑
　　conjunctival sac — see Burn, cornea
　　cornea — see Burn, cornea
　　lid — see Burn, eyelid
　　periocular area — see Burn, eyelid
　　specified site NEC T26.3- ☑
　eyeball — see Burn, eye
　eyelid(s) T26.0- ☑
　　chemical — see Corrosion, eyelid
　face — see Burn, head
　finger T23.029 ☑
　　first degree T23.129 ☑
　　left T23.022 ☑
　　　first degree T23.122 ☑
　　　second degree T23.222 ☑
　　　third degree T23.322 ☑
　　multiple sites (without thumb) T23.039 ☑
　　　with thumb T23.049 ☑
　　　　first degree T23.149 ☑
　　　　left T23.042 ☑
　　　　　first degree T23.142 ☑
　　　　　second degree T23.242 ☑
　　　　　third degree T23.342 ☑
　　　　right T23.041 ☑
　　　　　first degree T23.141 ☑
　　　　　second degree T23.241 ☑
　　　　　third degree T23.341 ☑
　　　　second degree T23.249 ☑
　　　　third degree T23.349 ☑
　　　first degree T23.139 ☑
　　　left T23.032 ☑
　　　　first degree T23.132 ☑
　　　　second degree T23.232 ☑
　　　　third degree T23.332 ☑
　　　right T23.031 ☑
　　　　first degree T23.131 ☑
　　　　second degree T23.231 ☑
　　　　third degree T23.331 ☑
　　　second degree T23.239 ☑
　　　third degree T23.339 ☑
　　right T23.021 ☑
　　　first degree T23.121 ☑
　　　second degree T23.221 ☑
　　　third degree T23.321 ☑
　　second degree T23.229 ☑
　　third degree T23.329 ☑
　flank — see Burn, abdominal wall
　foot T25.029 ☑
　　first degree T25.129 ☑
　　left T25.022 ☑
　　　first degree T25.122 ☑
　　　second degree T25.222 ☑
　　　third degree T25.322 ☑
　　multiple with ankle — see Burn, lower, limb, multi-
　　　ple, ankle and foot
　　right T25.021 ☑
　　　first degree T25.121 ☑
　　　second degree T25.221 ☑
　　　third degree T25.321 ☑
　　second degree T25.229 ☑
　　third degree T25.329 ☑
　forearm T22.019 ☑
　　first degree T22.119 ☑
　　left T22.012 ☑
　　　first degree T22.112 ☑
　　　second degree T22.212 ☑
　　　third degree T22.312 ☑
　　right T22.011 ☑
　　　first degree T22.111 ☑
　　　second degree T22.211 ☑
　　　third degree T22.311 ☑
　　second degree T22.219 ☑

Burn — *continued*
  forearm — *continued*
    third degree T22.319 ☑
  forehead T20.06 ☑
    first degree T20.16 ☑
    second degree T20.26 ☑
    third degree T20.36 ☑
  fourth degree — *code as* Burn, third degree, by site
  friction — *see* Burn, by site
  from swallowing caustic or corrosive substance NEC
    — *see* Corrosion, by site
  full thickness skin loss — *code as* Burn, third degree,
    by site
  gastrointestinal tract NEC T28.2 ☑
    from swallowing caustic or corrosive substance
      T28.7 ☑
  genital organs
    external
      female T21.07 ☑
        first degree T21.17 ☑
        second degree T21.27 ☑
        third degree T21.37 ☑
      male T21.06 ☑
        first degree T21.16 ☑
        second degree T21.26 ☑
        third degree T21.36 ☑
    internal T28.3 ☑
      from caustic or corrosive substance T28.8 ☑
  groin — *see* Burn, abdominal wall
  hand(s) T23.009 ☑
    back — *see* Burn, dorsum of hand
    finger — *see* Burn, finger
    first degree T23.109 ☑
    left T23.002 ☑
      first degree T23.102 ☑
      second degree T23.202 ☑
      third degree T23.302 ☑
    multiple sites with wrist T23.099 ☑
      first degree T23.199 ☑
      left T23.092 ☑
        first degree T23.192 ☑
        second degree T23.292 ☑
        third degree T23.392 ☑
      right T23.091 ☑
        first degree T23.191 ☑
        second degree T23.291 ☑
        third degree T23.391 ☑
      second degree T23.299 ☑
      third degree T23.399 ☑
    palm — *see* Burn, palm
    right T23.001 ☑
      first degree T23.101 ☑
      second degree T23.201 ☑
      third degree T23.301 ☑
    second degree T23.209 ☑
    third degree T23.309 ☑
    thumb — *see* Burn, thumb
  head (and face) (and neck) T20.00 ☑
    cheek — *see* Burn, cheek
    chin — *see* Burn, chin
    ear — *see* Burn, ear
    eye(s) only — *see* Burn, eye
    first degree T20.10 ☑
    forehead — *see* Burn, forehead
    lip — *see* Burn, lip
    multiple sites T20.09 ☑
      first degree T20.19 ☑
      second degree T20.29 ☑
      third degree T20.39 ☑
    neck — *see* Burn, neck
    nose — *see* Burn, nose
    scalp — *see* Burn, scalp
    second degree T20.20 ☑
    third degree T20.30 ☑
  hip(s) — *see* Burn, thigh
  inhalation — *see* Burn, respiratory tract
    caustic or corrosive substance (fumes) — *see* Corro-
      sion, respiratory tract
  internal organ(s) T28.40 ☑
    alimentary tract T28.2 ☑
      esophagus T28.1 ☑
    eardrum T28.41 ☑
    esophagus T28.1 ☑
    from caustic or corrosive substance (swallowing)
      NEC — *see* Corrosion, by site
    genitourinary T28.3 ☑

Burn — *continued*
  internal organ(s) — *continued*
    mouth T28.0 ☑
    pharynx T28.0 ☑
    respiratory tract — *see* Burn, respiratory tract
    specified organ NEC T28.49 ☑
  interscapular region — *see* Burn, back, upper
  intestine (large) (small) T28.2 ☑
  knee T24.029 ☑
    first degree T24.129 ☑
    left T24.022 ☑
      first degree T24.122 ☑
      second degree T24.222 ☑
      third degree T24.322 ☑
    right T24.021 ☑
      first degree T24.121 ☑
      second degree T24.221 ☑
      third degree T24.321 ☑
    second degree T24.229 ☑
    third degree T24.329 ☑
  labium (majus) (minus) — *see* Burn, genital organs,
    external, female
  lacrimal apparatus, duct, gland or sac — *see* Burn, eye,
    specified site NEC
  larynx T27.0 ☑
    with lung T27.1 ☑
  leg(s) (lower) (upper) — *see* Burn, lower, limb
  lightning — *see* Burn, by site
  limb(s)
    lower (except ankle or foot alone) — *see* Burn,
      lower, limb
    upper — *see* Burn, upper limb
  lip(s) T20.02 ☑
    first degree T20.12 ☑
    second degree T20.22 ☑
    third degree T20.32 ☑
  lower
    back — *see* Burn, back
    limb T24.009 ☑
      ankle — *see* Burn, ankle
      calf — *see* Burn, calf
      first degree T24.109 ☑
      foot — *see* Burn, foot
      hip — *see* Burn, thigh
      knee — *see* Burn, knee
      left T24.002 ☑
        first degree T24.102 ☑
        second degree T24.202 ☑
        third degree T24.302 ☑
      multiple sites, except ankle and foot T24.099 ☑
        ankle and foot T25.099 ☑
          first degree T25.199 ☑
          left T25.092 ☑
            first degree T25.192 ☑
            second degree T25.292 ☑
            third degree T25.392 ☑
          right T25.091 ☑
            first degree T25.191 ☑
            second degree T25.291 ☑
            third degree T25.391 ☑
          second degree T25.299 ☑
          third degree T25.399 ☑
        first degree T24.199 ☑
        left T24.092 ☑
          first degree T24.192 ☑
          second degree T24.292 ☑
          third degree T24.392 ☑
        right T24.091 ☑
          first degree T24.191 ☑
          second degree T24.291 ☑
          third degree T24.391 ☑
        second degree T24.299 ☑
        third degree T24.399 ☑
      right T24.001 ☑
        first degree T24.101 ☑
        second degree T24.201 ☑
        third degree T24.301 ☑
      second degree T24.209 ☑
      thigh — *see* Burn, thigh
      third degree T24.309 ☑
      toe — *see* Burn, toe
  lung (with larynx and trachea) T27.1 ☑
  mouth T28.0 ☑
  neck T20.07 ☑
    first degree T20.17 ☑
    second degree T20.27 ☑

Burn — *continued*
  neck — *continued*
    third degree T20.37 ☑
  nose (septum) T20.04 ☑
    first degree T20.14 ☑
    second degree T20.24 ☑
    third degree T20.34 ☑
  ocular adnexa — *see* Burn, eye
  orbit region — *see* Burn, eyelid
  palm T23.059 ☑
    first degree T23.159 ☑
    left T23.052 ☑
      first degree T23.152 ☑
      second degree T23.252 ☑
      third degree T23.352 ☑
    right T23.051 ☑
      first degree T23.151 ☑
      second degree T23.251 ☑
      third degree T23.351 ☑
    second degree T23.259 ☑
    third degree T23.359 ☑
  partial thickness — *code as* Burn, by site, second degree
  pelvis — *see* Burn, trunk
  penis — *see* Burn, genital organs, external, male
  perineum
    female — *see* Burn, genital organs, external, female
    male — *see* Burn, genital organs, external, male
  periocular area — *see* Burn, eyelid
  pharynx T28.0 ☑
  rectum T28.2 ☑
  respiratory tract T27.3 ☑
    larynx — *see* Burn, larynx
    specified part NEC T27.2 ☑
    trachea — *see* Burn, trachea
  sac, lacrimal — *see* Burn, eye, specified site NEC
  scalp T20.05 ☑
    first degree T20.15 ☑
    second degree T20.25 ☑
    third degree T20.35 ☑
  scapular region T22.069 ☑
    first degree T22.169 ☑
    left T22.062 ☑
      first degree T22.162 ☑
      second degree T22.262 ☑
      third degree T22.362 ☑
    right T22.061 ☑
      first degree T22.161 ☑
      second degree T22.261 ☑
      third degree T22.361 ☑
    second degree T22.269 ☑
    third degree T22.369 ☑
  sclera — *see* Burn, eye, specified site NEC
  scrotum — *see* Burn, genital organs, external, male
  shoulder T22.059 ☑
    first degree T22.159 ☑
    left T22.052 ☑
      first degree T22.152 ☑
      second degree T22.252 ☑
      third degree T22.352 ☑
    right T22.051 ☑
      first degree T22.151 ☑
      second degree T22.251 ☑
      third degree T22.351 ☑
    second degree T22.259 ☑
    third degree T22.359 ☑
  stomach T28.2 ☑
  temple — *see* Burn, head
  testis — *see* Burn, genital organs, external, male
  thigh T24.019 ☑
    first degree T24.119 ☑
    left T24.012 ☑
      first degree T24.112 ☑
      second degree T24.212 ☑
      third degree T24.312 ☑
    right T24.011 ☑
      first degree T24.111 ☑
      second degree T24.211 ☑
      third degree T24.311 ☑
    second degree T24.219 ☑
    third degree T24.319 ☑
  thorax (external) — *see* Burn, trunk
  throat (meaning pharynx) T28.0 ☑
  thumb(s) T23.019 ☑
    first degree T23.119 ☑
    left T23.012 ☑
      first degree T23.112 ☑

☑ **Additional Character Required** — Refer to the Tabular List for Character Selection   ▽ **Subterms under main terms may continue to next column or page**

Burn — *continued*
　thumb(s) — *continued*
　　left — *continued*
　　　　second degree T23.212 ☑
　　　　third degree T23.312 ☑
　　　multiple sites with fingers T23.049 ☑
　　　　first degree T23.149 ☑
　　　　left T23.042 ☑
　　　　　first degree T23.142 ☑
　　　　　second degree T23.242 ☑
　　　　　third degree T23.342 ☑
　　　　right T23.041 ☑
　　　　　first degree T23.141 ☑
　　　　　second degree T23.241 ☑
　　　　　third degree T23.341 ☑
　　　　second degree T23.249 ☑
　　　　third degree T23.349 ☑
　　　right T23.011 ☑
　　　　first degree T23.111 ☑
　　　　second degree T23.211 ☑
　　　　third degree T23.311 ☑
　　　second degree T23.219 ☑
　　　third degree T23.319 ☑
　toe T25.039 ☑
　　first degree T25.139 ☑
　　left T25.032 ☑
　　　first degree T25.132 ☑
　　　second degree T25.232 ☑
　　　third degree T25.332 ☑
　　right T25.031 ☑
　　　first degree T25.131 ☑
　　　second degree T25.231 ☑
　　　third degree T25.331 ☑
　　second degree T25.239 ☑
　　third degree T25.339 ☑
　tongue T28.0 ☑
　tonsil(s) T28.0 ☑
　trachea T27.0 ☑
　　with lung T27.1 ☑
　trunk T21.00 ☑
　　abdominal wall — *see* Burn, abdominal wall
　　anus — *see* Burn, buttock
　　axilla — *see* Burn, upper limb
　　back — *see* Burn, back
　　breast — *see* Burn, chest wall
　　buttock — *see* Burn, buttock
　　chest wall — *see* Burn, chest wall
　　first degree T21.10 ☑
　　flank — *see* Burn, abdominal wall
　　genital
　　　female — *see* Burn, genital organs, external, female
　　　male — *see* Burn, genital organs, external, male
　　groin — *see* Burn, abdominal wall
　　interscapular region — *see* Burn, back, upper
　　labia — *see* Burn, genital organs, external, female
　　lower back — *see* Burn, back
　　penis — *see* Burn, genital organs, external, male
　　perineum
　　　female — *see* Burn, genital organs, external, female
　　　male — *see* Burn, genital organs, external, male
　　scapula region — *see* Burn, scapular region
　　scrotum — *see* Burn, genital organs, external, male
　　second degree T21.20 ☑
　　specified site NEC T21.09 ☑
　　　first degree T21.19 ☑
　　　second degree T21.29 ☑
　　　third degree T21.39 ☑
　　testes — *see* Burn, genital organs, external, male
　　third degree T21.30 ☑
　　upper back — *see* Burn, back, upper
　　vulva — *see* Burn, genital organs, external, female
　unspecified site with extent of body surface involved
　　　specified
　　less than 10 percent T31.0
　　10-19 percent (0-9 percent third degree) T31.10
　　　with 10-19 percent third degree T31.11
　　20-29 percent (0-9 percent third degree) T31.20
　　　with
　　　　10-19 percent third degree T31.21
　　　　20-29 percent third degree T31.22
　　30-39 percent (0-9 percent third degree) T31.30
　　　with
　　　　10-19 percent third degree T31.31
　　　　20-29 percent third degree T31.32

Burn — *continued*
　unspecified site with extent of body surface involved
　　　specified — *continued*
　　30-39 percent — *continued*
　　　with — *continued*
　　　　30-39 percent third degree T31.33
　　40-49 percent (0-9 percent third degree) T31.40
　　　with
　　　　10-19 percent third degree T31.41
　　　　20-29 percent third degree T31.42
　　　　30-39 percent third degree T31.43
　　　　40-49 percent third degree T31.44
　　50-59 percent (0-9 percent third degree) T31.50
　　　with
　　　　10-19 percent third degree T31.51
　　　　20-29 percent third degree T31.52
　　　　30-39 percent third degree T31.53
　　　　40-49 percent third degree T31.54
　　　　50-59 percent third degree T31.55
　　60-69 percent (0-9 percent third degree) T31.60
　　　with
　　　　10-19 percent third degree T31.61
　　　　20-29 percent third degree T31.62
　　　　30-39 percent third degree T31.63
　　　　40-49 percent third degree T31.64
　　　　50-59 percent third degree T31.65
　　　　60-69 percent third degree T31.66
　　70-79 percent (0-9 percent third degree) T31.70
　　　with
　　　　10-19 percent third degree T31.71
　　　　20-29 percent third degree T31.72
　　　　30-39 percent third degree T31.73
　　　　40-49 percent third degree T31.74
　　　　50-59 percent third degree T31.75
　　　　60-69 percent third degree T31.76
　　　　70-79 percent third degree T31.77
　　80-89 percent (0-9 percent third degree) T31.80
　　　with
　　　　10-19 percent third degree T31.81
　　　　20-29 percent third degree T31.82
　　　　30-39 percent third degree T31.83
　　　　40-49 percent third degree T31.84
　　　　50-59 percent third degree T31.85
　　　　60-69 percent third degree T31.86
　　　　70-79 percent third degree T31.87
　　　　80-89 percent third degree T31.88
　　90 percent or more (0-9 percent third degree) T31.90
　　　with
　　　　10-19 percent third degree T31.91
　　　　20-29 percent third degree T31.92
　　　　30-39 percent third degree T31.93
　　　　40-49 percent third degree T31.94
　　　　50-59 percent third degree T31.95
　　　　60-69 percent third degree T31.96
　　　　70-79 percent third degree T31.97
　　　　80-89 percent third degree T31.98
　　　　90-99 percent third degree T31.99
　upper limb T22.00 ☑
　　above elbow — *see* Burn, above elbow
　　axilla — *see* Burn, axilla
　　elbow — *see* Burn, elbow
　　first degree T22.10 ☑
　　forearm — *see* Burn, forearm
　　hand — *see* Burn, hand
　　interscapular region — *see* Burn, back, upper
　　multiple sites T22.099 ☑
　　　first degree T22.199 ☑
　　　left T22.092 ☑
　　　　first degree T22.192 ☑
　　　　second degree T22.292 ☑
　　　　third degree T22.392 ☑
　　　right T22.091 ☑
　　　　first degree T22.191 ☑
　　　　second degree T22.291 ☑
　　　　third degree T22.391 ☑
　　　second degree T22.299 ☑
　　　third degree T22.399 ☑
　　scapular region — *see* Burn, scapular region
　　second degree T22.20 ☑
　　shoulder — *see* Burn, shoulder
　　third degree T22.30 ☑
　　wrist — *see* Burn, wrist
　uterus T28.3 ☑
　vagina T28.3 ☑
　vulva — *see* Burn, genital organs, external, female
　wrist T23.079 ☑
　　first degree T23.179 ☑
　　　left T23.072 ☑

Burn — *continued*
　wrist — *continued*
　　left — *continued*
　　　first degree T23.172 ☑
　　　second degree T23.272 ☑
　　　third degree T23.372 ☑
　　multiple sites with hand T23.099 ☑
　　　first degree T23.199 ☑
　　　left T23.092 ☑
　　　　first degree T23.192 ☑
　　　　second degree T23.292 ☑
　　　　third degree T23.392 ☑
　　　right T23.091 ☑
　　　　first degree T23.191 ☑
　　　　second degree T23.291 ☑
　　　　third degree T23.391 ☑
　　　second degree T23.299 ☑
　　　third degree T23.399 ☑
　　right T23.071 ☑
　　　first degree T23.171 ☑
　　　second degree T23.271 ☑
　　　third degree T23.371 ☑
　　second degree T23.279 ☑
　　third degree T23.379 ☑
Burnett's syndrome E83.52
Burning
　feet syndrome E53.9
　sensation R20.8
　tongue K14.6
Burn-out (state) Z73.0
Burns' disease or osteochondrosis — *see* Osteochondrosis, juvenile, ulna
Bursa — *see* condition
Bursitis M71.9
　Achilles — *see* Tendinitis, Achilles
　adhesive — *see* Bursitis, specified NEC
　ankle — *see* Enthesopathy, lower limb, ankle, specified type NEC
　calcaneal — *see* Enthesopathy, foot, specified type NEC
　collateral ligament, tibial — *see* Bursitis, tibial collateral
　due to use, overuse, pressure — *see also* Disorder, soft tissue, due to use, specified type NEC
　　specified NEC — *see* Disorder, soft tissue, due to use, specified NEC
　Duplay's M75.0 ☑
　elbow NEC M70.3- ☑
　　olecranon M70.2- ☑
　finger — *see* Disorder, soft tissue, due to use, specified type NEC, hand
　foot — *see* Enthesopathy, foot, specified type NEC
　gonococcal A54.49
　gouty — *see* Gout
　hand M70.1- ☑
　hip NEC M70.7- ☑
　　trochanteric M70.6- ☑
　infective NEC M71.10
　　abscess — *see* Abscess, bursa
　　ankle M71.17- ☑
　　elbow M71.12- ☑
　　foot M71.17- ☑
　　hand M71.14- ☑
　　hip M71.15- ☑
　　knee M71.16- ☑
　　multiple sites M71.19
　　shoulder M71.11- ☑
　　specified site NEC M71.18
　　wrist M71.13- ☑
　ischial — *see* Bursitis, hip
　knee NEC M70.5- ☑
　　prepatellar M70.4- ☑
　occupational NEC — *see also* Disorder, soft tissue, due to use
　olecranon — *see* Bursitis, elbow, olecranon
　pharyngeal J39.1
　popliteal — *see* Bursitis, knee
　prepatellar M70.4- ☑
　radiohumeral M70.3- ☑
　rheumatoid M06.20
　　ankle M06.27- ☑
　　elbow M06.22- ☑
　　foot joint M06.27- ☑
　　hand joint M06.24- ☑
　　hip M06.25- ☑
　　knee M06.26- ☑
　　multiple site M06.29
　　shoulder M06.21- ☑

Bursitis — *continued*
  rheumatoid — *continued*
    vertebra M06.28
    wrist M06.23- ☑
  scapulohumeral — *see* Bursitis, shoulder
  semimembranous muscle (knee) — *see* Bursitis, knee
  shoulder M75.5- ☑
    adhesive — *see* Capsulitis, adhesive
  specified NEC M71.50
    ankle M71.57-
    due to use, overuse or pressure — *see* Disorder, soft
      tissue, due to, use
    elbow M71.52- ☑
    foot M71.57- ☑
    hand M71.54- ☑
    hip M71.55- ☑
    knee M71.56- ☑
    shoulder — *see* Bursitis, shoulder
    specified site NEC M71.58
    tibial collateral M76.4- ☑
    wrist M71.53- ☑
  subacromial — *see* Bursitis, shoulder
  subcoracoid — *see* Bursitis, shoulder
  subdeltoid — *see* Bursitis, shoulder
  syphilitic A52.78
  Thornwaldt, Tornwaldt J39.2
  tibial collateral M76.4- ☑
  toe — *see* Enthesopathy, foot, specified type NEC
  trochanteric (area) — *see* Bursitis, hip, trochanteric
  wrist — *see* Bursitis, hand
Bursopathy M71.9
  specified type NEC M71.80
    ankle M71.87- ☑
    elbow M71.82- ☑
    foot M71.87- ☑
    hand M71.84- ☑
    hip M71.85- ☑
    knee M71.86- ☑
    multiple sites M71.89
    shoulder M71.81- ☑
    specified site NEC M71.88
    wrist M71.83- ☑
Burst stitches or sutures (complication of surgery)
  T81.31 ☑
  external operation wound T81.31 ☑
  internal operation wound T81.32 ☑
Buruli ulcer A31.1
Bury's disease L95.1
Buschke's
  disease — *see* Cryptococcosis by site
  scleredema — *see* Sclerosis, systemic
Busse-Buschke disease — *see* Cryptococcosis by site
Buttock — *see* condition
Button
  Biskra B55.1
  Delhi B55.1
  oriental B55.1
Buttonhole deformity (finger) — *see* Deformity, finger,
  boutonniere
Bwamba fever A92.8
Byssinosis J66.0
Bywaters' syndrome T79.5 ☑

C

Cachexia R64
  cancerous R64
  cardiac — *see* Disease, heart
  dehydration E86.0
  due to malnutrition R64
  exophthalmic — *see* Hyperthyroidism
  heart — *see* Disease, heart
  hypophyseal E23.0
  hypopituitary E23.0
  lead — *see* Poisoning, lead
  malignant R64
  marsh — *see* Malaria
  nervous F48.8
  old age R54
  paludal — *see* Malaria
  pituitary E23.0
  pulmonary R64
  renal N28.9
  saturnine — *see* Poisoning, lead
  senile R54
  Simmonds' E23.0
  splenica D73.0

Cachexia — *continued*
  strumipriva E03.4
  tuberculous NEC — *see* Tuberculosis
CADASIL (cerebral autosomal dominant arteriopathy with
  subcortical infarcts and leukoencephalopathy)
  I67.850
Café, au lait spots L81.3
Caffeine-induced
  anxiety disorder F15.980
  sleep disorder F15.982
Caffey's syndrome Q78.8
Caisson disease T70.3 ☑
Cake kidney Q63.1
Caked breast (puerperal, postpartum) O92.79
Calabar swelling B74.3
Calcaneal spur — *see* Spur, bone, calcaneal
Calcaneo-apophysitis M92.8
Calcareous — *see* condition
Calcicosis J62.8
Calciferol (vitamin D) deficiency E55.9
  with rickets E55.0
Calcification
  adrenal (capsule) (gland) E27.49
    tuberculous E35 *[B90.8]*
  aorta I70.0
  artery (annular) — *see* Arteriosclerosis
  auricle (ear) — *see* Disorder, pinna, specified type NEC
  basal ganglia G23.8
  bladder N32.89
    due to Schistosoma hematobium B65.0
  brain (cortex) — *see* Calcification, cerebral
  bronchus J98.09
  bursa M71.40
    ankle M71.47- ☑
    elbow M71.42- ☑
    foot M71.47- ☑
    hand M71.44- ☑
    hip M71.45- ☑
    knee M71.46- ☑
    multiple sites M71.49
    shoulder M75.3- ☑
    specified site NEC M71.48
    wrist M71.43- ☑
  cardiac — *see* Degeneration, myocardial
  cerebral (cortex) G93.89
    artery I67.2
  cervix (uteri) N88.8
  choroid plexus G93.89
  conjunctiva — *see* Concretion, conjunctiva
  corpora cavernosa (penis) N48.89
  cortex (brain) — *see* Calcification, cerebral
  dental pulp (nodular) K04.2
  dentinal papilla K00.4
  fallopian tube N83.8
  falx cerebri G96.198
  gallbladder K82.8
  general E83.59
  heart — *see also* Degeneration, myocardial
    valve — *see* Endocarditis
  idiopathic infantile arterial (IIAC) Q28.8
  intervertebral cartilage or disc (postinfective) — *see*
    Disorder, disc, specified NEC
  intracranial — *see* Calcification, cerebral
  joint — *see* Disorder, joint, specified type NEC
  kidney N28.89
    tuberculous N29 *[B90.1]*
  larynx (senile) J38.7
  lens — *see* Cataract, specified NEC
  lung (active) (postinfectional) J98.4
    tuberculous B90.9
  lymph gland or node (postinfectional) I89.8
    tuberculous — *see also* Tuberculosis, lymph gland
      B90.8
  mammographic R92.1
  massive (paraplegic) — *see* Myositis, ossificans, in,
    quadriplegia
  medial — *see* Arteriosclerosis, extremities
  meninges (cerebral) (spinal) G96.198
  metastatic E83.59
  Mönckeberg's — *see* Arteriosclerosis, extremities
  muscle M61.9
    due to burns — *see* Myositis, ossificans, in, burns
    paralytic — *see* Myositis, ossificans, in, quadriplegia
    specified type NEC M61.40
      ankle M61.47- ☑
      foot M61.47- ☑
      forearm M61.43- ☑

Calcification — *continued*
  muscle — *continued*
    specified type — *continued*
      hand M61.44- ☑
      lower leg M61.46- ☑
      multiple sites M61.49
      pelvic region M61.45- ☑
      shoulder region M61.41- ☑
      specified site NEC M61.48
      thigh M61.45- ☑
      upper arm M61.42- ☑
  myocardium, myocardial — *see* Degeneration, myocar-
    dial
  ovary N83.8
  pancreas K86.89
  penis N48.89
  periarticular — *see* Disorder, joint, specified type NEC
  pericardium — *see also* Pericarditis I31.1
  pineal gland E34.8
  pleura J94.8
    postinfectional J94.8
    tuberculous NEC B90.9
  pulpal (dental) (nodular) K04.2
  sclera H15.89
  spleen D73.89
  subcutaneous L94.2
  suprarenal (capsule) (gland) E27.49
  tendon (sheath) — *see also* Tenosynovitis, specified
    type NEC
    with bursitis, synovitis or tenosynovitis — *see* Ten-
      dinitis, calcific
  trachea J39.8
  ureter N28.89
  uterus N85.8
  vitreous — *see* Deposit, crystalline
Calcified — *see* Calcification
Calcinosis (interstitial) (tumoral) (universalis) E83.59
  with Raynaud's phenomenon, esophageal dysfunction,
    sclerodactyly, telangiectasia (CREST syndrome)
    M34.1
  circumscripta (skin) L94.2
  cutis L94.2
Calciphylaxis — *see also* Calcification, by site E83.59
Calcium
  deposits — *see* Calcification, by site
  metabolism disorder E83.50
  salts or soaps in vitreous — *see* Deposit, crystalline
Calciuria R82.994
Calculi — *see* Calculus
Calculosis, intrahepatic — *see* Calculus, bile duct
Calculus, calculi, calculous
  ampulla of Vater — *see* Calculus, bile duct
  anuria (impacted) (recurrent) — *see also* Calculus, uri-
    nary N20.9
  appendix K38.1
  bile duct (common) (hepatic) K80.50
    with
      calculus of gallbladder — *see* Calculus, gallblad-
        der and bile duct
      cholangitis K80.30
        with
          cholecystitis — *see* Calculus, bile duct,
            with cholecystitis
          obstruction K80.31
        acute K80.32
          with
            chronic cholangitis K80.36
              with obstruction K80.37
            obstruction K80.33
        chronic K80.34
          with
            acute cholangitis K80.36
              with obstruction K80.37
            obstruction K80.35
      cholecystitis (with cholangitis) K80.40
        with obstruction K80.41
        acute K80.42
          with
            chronic cholecystitis K80.46
              with obstruction K80.47
            obstruction K80.43
        chronic K80.44
          with
            acute cholecystitis K80.46
              with obstruction K80.47
            obstruction K80.45
  biliary — *see also* Calculus, gallbladder
    specified NEC K80.80

☑ **Additional Character Required** — Refer to the Tabular List for Character Selection   ⩔ **Subterms under main terms may continue to next column or page**

Calculus, calculi, calculous — *continued*
biliary — *see also* Calculus, gallbladder — *continued*
  specified — *continued*
    with obstruction K80.81
bilirubin, multiple — *see* Calculus, gallbladder
bladder (encysted) (impacted) (urinary) (diverticulum)
  N21.0
bronchus J98.09
calyx (kidney) (renal) — *see* Calculus, kidney
cholesterol (pure) (solitary) — *see* Calculus, gallbladder
common duct (bile) — *see* Calculus, bile duct
conjunctiva — *see* Concretion, conjunctiva
cystic N21.0
  duct — *see* Calculus, gallbladder
dental (subgingival) (supragingival) K03.6
diverticulum
  bladder N21.0
  kidney N20.0
epididymis N50.89
gallbladder K80.20
  with
    bile duct calculus — *see* Calculus, gallbladder
      and bile duct
    cholecystitis K80.10
      with obstruction K80.11
      acute K80.00
        with
          chronic cholecystitis K80.12
            with obstruction K80.13
          obstruction K80.01
      chronic K80.10
        with
          acute cholecystitis K80.12
            with obstruction K80.13
          obstruction K80.11
    specified NEC K80.18
      with obstruction K80.19
    obstruction K80.21
gallbladder and bile duct K80.70
  with
    cholecystitis K80.60
      with obstruction K80.61
      acute K80.62
        with
          chronic cholecystitis K80.66
            with obstruction K80.67
          obstruction K80.63
      chronic K80.64
        with
          acute cholecystitis K80.66
            with obstruction K80.67
          obstruction K80.65
    obstruction K80.71
hepatic (duct) — *see* Calculus, bile duct
ileal conduit N21.8
intestinal (impaction) (obstruction) K56.49
kidney (impacted) (multiple) (pelvis) (recurrent)
  (staghorn) N20.0
  with calculus, ureter N20.2
  congenital Q63.8
lacrimal passages — *see* Dacryolith
liver (impacted) — *see* Calculus, bile duct
lung J98.4
mammographic R92.1
nephritic (impacted) (recurrent) — *see* Calculus, kidney
nose J34.89
pancreas (duct) K86.89
parotid duct or gland K11.5
pelvis, encysted — *see* Calculus, kidney
prostate N42.0
pulmonary J98.4
pyelitis (impacted) (recurrent) N20.0
  with hydronephrosis N13.6
pyelonephritis (impacted) (recurrent) — *see* category
  N20 ☑
  with hydronephrosis N13.6
renal (impacted) (recurrent) — *see* Calculus, kidney
salivary (duct) (gland) K11.5
seminal vesicle N50.89
staghorn — *see* Calculus, kidney
Stensen's duct K11.5
stomach K31.89
sublingual duct or gland K11.5
  congenital Q38.4
submandibular duct, gland or region K11.5
submaxillary duct, gland or region K11.5
suburethral N21.8

Calculus, calculi, calculous — *continued*
tonsil J35.8
tooth, teeth (subgingival) (supragingival) K03.6
tunica vaginalis N50.89
ureter (impacted) (recurrent) N20.1
  with calculus, kidney N20.2
    with hydronephrosis N13.2
      with infection N13.6
ureteropelvic junction N20.1
urethra (impacted) N21.1
urinary (duct) (impacted) (passage) (tract) N20.9
  with hydronephrosis N13.2
    with infection N13.6
  in (due to)
  lower N21.9
    specified NEC N21.8
vagina N89.8
vesical (impacted) N21.0
Wharton's duct K11.5
xanthine E79.8 *[N22]*
Calicectasis N28.89
Caliectasis N28.89
California
disease B38.9
encephalitis A83.5
Caligo cornea — *see* Opacity, cornea, central
Callositas, callosity (infected) L84
Callus (infected) L84
bone — *see* Osteophyte
  excessive, following fracture — *code as* Sequelae
    of fracture
CALME (childhood asymmetric labium majus enlargement) N90.61
Calorie deficiency or malnutrition — *see also* Malnutrition E46
Calvé-Perthes disease — *see* Legg-Calvé-Perthes disease
Calvé's disease — *see* Osteochondrosis, juvenile, spine
Calvities — *see* Alopecia, androgenic
Cameroon fever — *see* Malaria
Camptocormia (hysterical) F44.4
Camurati-Engelmann syndrome Q78.3
Canal — *see also* condition
atrioventricular common Q21.2
Canaliculitis (lacrimal) (acute) (subacute) H04.33- ☑
Actinomyces A42.89
chronic H04.42- ☑
Canavan's disease E75.29
Canceled procedure (surgical) Z53.9
because of
  contraindication Z53.09
    smoking Z53.01
  left against medical advice (AMA) Z53.29
  patient's decision Z53.20
    for reasons of belief or group pressure Z53.1
    specified reason NEC Z53.29
  specified reason NEC Z53.8
Cancer — *see also* Neoplasm, by site, malignant
bile duct type liver C22.1
blood — *see* Leukemia
breast — *see also* Neoplasm, breast, malignant
  C50.91- ☑
hepatocellular C22.0
lung — *see also* Neoplasm, lung, malignant C34.90
ovarian — *see also* Neoplasm ovary, malignant C56.9
unspecified site (primary) C80.1
Cancer (o)phobia F45.29
Cancerous — *see* Neoplasm, malignant, by site
Cancrum oris A69.0
Candidiasis, candidal B37.9
balanitis B37.42
bronchitis B37.1
cheilitis B37.83
congenital P37.5
cystitis B37.41
disseminated B37.7
endocarditis B37.6
enteritis B37.82
esophagitis B37.81
intertrigo B37.2
lung B37.1
meningitis B37.5
mouth B37.0
nails B37.2
neonatal P37.5
onychia B37.2
oral B37.0
osteomyelitis B37.89

Candidiasis, candidal — *continued*
otitis externa B37.84
paronychia B37.2
perionyxis B37.2
pneumonia B37.1
proctitis B37.82
pulmonary B37.1
pyelonephritis B37.49
sepsis B37.7
skin B37.2
specified site NEC B37.89
stomatitis B37.0
systemic B37.7
urethritis B37.41
urogenital site NEC B37.49
vagina B37.3
vulva B37.3
vulvovaginitis B37.3
Candidid L30.2
Candidosis — *see* Candidiasis
Candiru infection or infestation B88.8
Canities (premature) L67.1
congenital Q84.2
Canker (mouth) (sore) K12.0
rash A38.9
Cannabinosis J66.2
Cannabis induced
anxiety disorder F12.980
psychotic disorder F12.959
sleep disorder F12.988
Canton fever A75.9
Cantrell's syndrome Q87.89
Capillariasis (intestinal) B81.1
hepatic B83.8
Capillary — *see* condition
Caplan's syndrome — *see* Rheumatoid, lung
Capsule — *see* condition
Capsulitis (joint) — *see also* Enthesopathy
adhesive (shoulder) M75.0- ☑
hepatic K65.8
labyrinthine — *see* Otosclerosis, specified NEC
thyroid E06.9
Caput
crepitus Q75.8
medusae I86.8
succedaneum P12.81
Car sickness T75.3 ☑
Carapata (disease) A68.0
Carate — *see* Pinta
Carbon lung J60
Carbuncle L02.93
abdominal wall L02.231
anus K61.0
auditory canal, external — *see* Abscess, ear, external
auricle ear — *see* Abscess, ear, external
axilla L02.43- ☑
back (any part) L02.232
breast N61.1
buttock L02.33
cheek (external) L02.03
chest wall L02.233
chin L02.03
corpus cavernosum N48.21
ear (any part) (external) (middle) — *see* Abscess, ear, external
external auditory canal — *see* Abscess, ear, external
eyelid — *see* Abscess, eyelid
face NEC L02.03
femoral (region) — *see* Carbuncle, lower limb
finger — *see* Carbuncle, hand
flank L02.231
foot L02.63- ☑
forehead L02.03
genital — *see* Abscess, genital
gluteal (region) L02.33
groin L02.234
hand L02.53- ☑
head NEC L02.831
heel — *see* Carbuncle, foot
hip — *see* Carbuncle, lower limb
kidney — *see* Abscess, kidney
knee — *see* Carbuncle, lower limb
labium (majus) (minus) N76.4
lacrimal
  gland — *see* Dacryoadenitis
  passages (duct) (sac) — *see* Inflammation, lacrimal, passages, acute

Carbuncle — *continued*
leg — *see* Carbuncle, lower limb
lower limb L02.43- ☑
malignant A22.0
navel L02.236
neck L02.13
nose (external) (septum) J34.0
orbit, orbital — *see* Abscess, orbit
palmar (space) — *see* Carbuncle, hand
partes posteriores L02.33
pectoral region L02.233
penis N48.21
perineum L02.235
pinna — *see* Abscess, ear, external
popliteal — *see* Carbuncle, lower limb
scalp L02.831
seminal vesicle N49.0
shoulder — *see* Carbuncle, upper limb
specified site NEC L02.838
temple (region) L02.03
thumb — *see* Carbuncle, hand
toe — *see* Carbuncle, foot
trunk L02.239
abdominal wall L02.231
back L02.232
chest wall L02.233
groin L02.234
perineum L02.235
umbilicus L02.236
umbilicus L02.236
upper limb L02.43- ☑
urethra N34.0
vulva N76.4
Carbunculus — *see* Carbuncle
Carcinoid (tumor) — *see* Tumor, carcinoid
Carcinoidosis E34.0
Carcinoma (malignant) — *see also* Neoplasm, by site, malignant
acidophil
specified site — *see* Neoplasm, malignant, by site
unspecified site C75.1
acidophil-basophil, mixed
specified site — *see* Neoplasm, malignant, by site
unspecified site C75.1
adnexal (skin) — *see* Neoplasm, skin, malignant
adrenal cortical C74.0- ☑
alveolar — *see* Neoplasm, lung, malignant
cell — *see* Neoplasm, lung, malignant
ameloblastic C41.1
upper jaw (bone) C41.0
apocrine
breast — *see* Neoplasm, breast, malignant
specified site NEC — *see* Neoplasm, skin, malignant
unspecified site C44.99
basal cell (pigmented) (*see also* Neoplasm, skin, malignant) C44.91
fibro-epithelial — *see* Neoplasm, skin, malignant
morphea — *see* Neoplasm, skin, malignant
multicentric — *see* Neoplasm, skin, malignant
basaloid
basal-squamous cell, mixed — *see* Neoplasm, skin, malignant
basophil
specified site — *see* Neoplasm, malignant, by site
unspecified site C75.1
basophil-acidophil, mixed
specified site — *see* Neoplasm, malignant, by site
unspecified site C75.1
basosquamous — *see* Neoplasm, skin, malignant
bile duct
with hepatocellular, mixed C22.0
liver C22.1
specified site NEC — *see* Neoplasm, malignant, by site
unspecified site C22.1
branchial or branchiogenic C10.4
bronchial or bronchogenic — *see* Neoplasm, lung, malignant
bronchiolar — *see* Neoplasm, lung, malignant
bronchioloalveolar — *see* Neoplasm, lung, malignant
C cell
specified site — *see* Neoplasm, malignant, by site
unspecified site C73
ceruminous C44.29- ☑
cervix uteri
in situ D06.9
endocervix D06.0
exocervix D06.1

Carcinoma — *continued*
cervix uteri — *continued*
in situ — *continued*
specified site NEC D06.7
chorionic
specified site — *see* Neoplasm, malignant, by site
unspecified site
female C58
male C62.90
chromophobe
specified site — *see* Neoplasm, malignant, by site
unspecified site C75.1
cloacogenic
specified site — *see* Neoplasm, malignant, by site
unspecified site C21.2
diffuse type
specified site — *see* Neoplasm, malignant, by site
unspecified site C16.9
duct (cell)
with Paget's disease — *see* Neoplasm, breast, malignant
infiltrating
with lobular carcinoma (in situ)
specified site — *see* Neoplasm, malignant, by site
unspecified site (female) C50.91- ☑
male C50.92- ☑
specified site — *see* Neoplasm, malignant, by site
unspecified site (female) C50.91- ☑
male C50.92- ☑
ductal
with lobular
specified site — *see* Neoplasm, malignant, by site
unspecified site (female) C50.91- ☑
male C50.92- ☑
ductular, infiltrating
specified site — *see* Neoplasm, malignant, by site
unspecified site (female) C50.91- ☑
male C50.92- ☑
embryonal
liver C22.7
endometrioid
specified site — *see* Neoplasm, malignant, by site
unspecified site
female C56.9
male C61
eosinophil
specified site — *see* Neoplasm, malignant, by site
unspecified site C75.1
epidermoid — *see also* Neoplasm, skin, malignant
in situ, Bowen's type — *see* Neoplasm, skin, in situ
fibroepithelial, basal cell — *see* Neoplasm, skin, malignant
follicular
with papillary (mixed) C73
moderately differentiated C73
pure follicle C73
specified site — *see* Neoplasm, malignant, by site
trabecular C73
unspecified site C73
well differentiated C73
generalized, with unspecified primary site C80.0
glycogen-rich — *see* Neoplasm, breast, malignant
granulosa cell C56- ☑
hepatic cell C22.0
hepatocellular C22.0
with bile duct, mixed C22.0
fibrolamellar C22.0
hepatocholangiolitic C22.0
Hurthle cell C73
in
adenomatous
polyposis coli C18.9
pleomorphic adenoma — *see* Neoplasm, salivary glands, malignant
situ — *see* Carcinoma-in-situ
infiltrating
duct
with lobular
specified site — *see* Neoplasm, malignant, by site
unspecified site (female) C50.91- ☑
male C50.92- ☑
with Paget's disease — *see* Neoplasm, breast, malignant
specified site — *see* Neoplasm, malignant

Carcinoma — *continued*
infiltrating — *continued*
duct — *continued*
unspecified site (female) C50.91- ☑
male C50.92- ☑
ductular
specified site — *see* Neoplasm, malignant
unspecified site (female) C50.91- ☑
male C50.92- ☑
lobular
specified site — *see* Neoplasm, malignant
unspecified site (female) C50.91- ☑
male C50.92- ☑
inflammatory
specified site — *see* Neoplasm, malignant
unspecified site (female) C50.91- ☑
male C50.92- ☑
intestinal type
specified site — *see* Neoplasm, malignant, by site
unspecified site C16.9
intracystic
noninfiltrating — *see* Neoplasm, in situ, by site
intraductal (noninfiltrating)
with Paget's disease — *see* Neoplasm, breast, malignant
breast D05.1- ☑
papillary
with invasion
specified site — *see* Neoplasm, malignant, by site
unspecified site (female) C50.91- ☑
male C50.92- ☑
breast D05.1- ☑
specified site NEC — *see* Neoplasm, in situ, by site
unspecified site (female) D05.1- ☑
specified site NEC — *see* Neoplasm, in situ, by site
unspecified site (female) D05.1- ☑
intraepidermal — *see* Neoplasm, in situ
squamous cell, Bowen's type — *see* Neoplasm, skin, in situ
intraepithelial — *see* Neoplasm, in situ, by site
squamous cell — *see* Neoplasm, in situ, by site
intraosseous C41.1
upper jaw (bone) C41.0
islet cell
with exocrine, mixed
specified site — *see* Neoplasm, malignant, by site
unspecified site C25.9
pancreas C25.4
specified site NEC — *see* Neoplasm, malignant, by site
unspecified site C25.4
juvenile, breast — *see* Neoplasm, breast, malignant
large cell
small cell
specified site — *see* Neoplasm, malignant, by site
unspecified site C34.90
Leydig cell (testis)
specified site — *see* Neoplasm, malignant, by site
unspecified site
female C56.9
male C62.90
lipid-rich (female) C50.91- ☑
male C50.92- ☑
liver cell C22.0
liver NEC C22.7
lobular (infiltrating)
with intraductal
specified site — *see* Neoplasm, malignant, by site
unspecified site (female) C50.91- ☑
male C50.92- ☑
noninfiltrating
breast D05.0- ☑
specified site NEC — *see* Neoplasm, in situ, by site
unspecified site D05.0- ☑
specified site — *see* Neoplasm, malignant, by site
unspecified site (female) C50.91- ☑
male C50.92- ☑

☑ **Additional Character Required** — Refer to the Tabular List for Character Selection
Ⓥ Subterms under main terms may continue to next column or page

Carcinoma — *continued*
  medullary
    with
      amyloid stroma
        specified site — *see* Neoplasm, malignant, by
          site
        unspecified site C73
      lymphoid stroma
        specified site — *see* Neoplasm, malignant, by
          site
        unspecified site (female) C50.91- ☑
          male C50.92- ☑
  Merkel cell C4A.9 (*following* C43)
    anal margin C4A.51 (*following* C43)
    anal skin C4A.51 (*following* C43)
    canthus C4A.1- ☑ (*following* C43)
    ear and external auricular canal C4A.2- ☑ (*following*
      C43)
    external auricular canal C4A.2- ☑ (*following* C43)
    eyelid, including canthus C4A.1- ☑ (*following* C43)
    face C4A.30 (*following* C43)
      specified NEC C4A.39 (*following* C43)
    hip C4A.7- ☑ (*following* C43)
    lip C4A.0 (*following* C43)
    lower limb, including hip C4A.7- ☑ (*following* C43)
    neck C4A.4 (*following* C43)
    nodal presentation C7B.1 (*following* C75)
    nose C4A.31 (*following* C43)
    overlapping sites C4A.8 (*following* C43)
    perianal skin C4A.51 (*following* C43)
    scalp C4A.4 (*following* C43)
    secondary C7B.1 (*following* C75)
    shoulder C4A.6- ☑ (*following* C43)
    skin of breast C4A.52 (*following* C43)
    trunk NEC C4A.59 (*following* C43)
    upper limb, including shoulder C4A.6- ☑ (*following*
      C43)
    visceral metastatic C7B.1 (*following* C75)
  metastatic — *see* Neoplasm, secondary, by site
  metatypical — *see* Neoplasm, skin, malignant
  morphea, basal cell — *see* Neoplasm, skin, malignant
  mucoid
    cell
      specified site — *see* Neoplasm, malignant, by
        site
      unspecified site C75.1
  neuroendocrine — *see also* Tumor, neuroendocrine
    high grade, any site C7A.1 (*following* C75)
    poorly differentiated, any site C7A.1 (*following* C75)
  nonencapsulated sclerosing C73
  noninfiltrating
    intracystic — *see* Neoplasm, in situ, by site
    intraductal
      breast D05.1- ☑
      papillary
        breast D05.1- ☑
        specified site NEC — *see* Neoplasm, in situ,
          by site
        unspecified site D05.1- ☑
      specified site — *see* Neoplasm, in situ, by site
      unspecified site D05.1- ☑
    lobular
      breast D05.0- ☑
      specified site NEC — *see* Neoplasm, in situ, by
        site
      unspecified site (female) D05.0- ☑
  oat cell
    specified site — *see* Neoplasm, malignant, by site
    unspecified site C34.90
  odontogenic C41.1
    upper jaw (bone) C41.0
  papillary
    with follicular (mixed) C73
    follicular variant C73
    intraductal (noninfiltrating)
      with invasion
        specified site — *see* Neoplasm, malignant, by
          site
        unspecified site (female) C50.91- ☑
          male C50.92- ☑
      breast D05.1- ☑
      specified site NEC — *see* Neoplasm, in situ, by
        site
      unspecified site D05.1- ☑
    serous
      specified site — *see* Neoplasm, malignant, by
        site

Carcinoma — *continued*
  papillary — *continued*
    serous — *continued*
      surface
        specified site — *see* Neoplasm, malignant, by
          site
        unspecified site C56.9
      unspecified site C56.9
  papillocystic
    specified site — *see* Neoplasm, malignant, by site
    unspecified site C56.9
  parafollicular cell
    specified site — *see* Neoplasm, malignant, by site
    unspecified site C73
  pilomatrix — *see* Neoplasm, skin, malignant
  pseudomucinous
    specified site — *see* Neoplasm, malignant, by site
    unspecified site C56.9
  renal cell C64- ☑
  Schmincke — *see* Neoplasm, nasopharynx, malignant
  Schneiderian
    specified site — *see* Neoplasm, malignant, by site
    unspecified site C30.0
  sebaceous — *see* Neoplasm, skin, malignant
  secondary — *see also* Neoplasm, secondary, by site
    Merkel cell C7B.1 (*following* C75)
  secretory, breast — *see* Neoplasm, breast, malignant
  serous
    papillary
      specified site — *see* Neoplasm, malignant, by
        site
      unspecified site C56.9
    surface, papillary
      specified site — *see* Neoplasm, malignant, by
        site
      unspecified site C56.9
  Sertoli cell
    specified site — *see* Neoplasm, malignant, by site
    unspecified site C62.90
      female C56.9
      male C62.90
  skin appendage — *see* Neoplasm, skin, malignant
  small cell
    fusiform cell
      specified site — *see* Neoplasm, malignant, by
        site
      unspecified site C34.90
    intermediate cell
      specified site — *see* Neoplasm, malignant, by
        site
      unspecified site C34.90
    large cell
      specified site — *see* Neoplasm, malignant, by
        site
      unspecified site C34.90
  solid
    with amyloid stroma
      specified site — *see* Neoplasm, malignant, by
        site
      unspecified site C73
    microinvasive
      specified site — *see* Neoplasm, malignant, by
        site
      unspecified site C53.9
  sweat gland — *see* Neoplasm, skin, malignant
  theca cell C56.- ☑
  thymic C37
  unspecified site (primary) C80.1
  water-clear cell C75.0
Carcinoma-in-situ — *see also* Neoplasm, in situ, by site
  breast NOS D05.9- ☑
    specified type NEC D05.8- ☑
  epidermoid — *see also* Neoplasm, in situ, by site
    with questionable stromal invasion
      cervix D06.9
      specified site NEC — *see* Neoplasm, in situ, by
        site
      unspecified site D06.9
    Bowen's type — *see* Neoplasm, skin, in situ
  intraductal
    breast D05.1- ☑
    specified site NEC — *see* Neoplasm, in situ, by site
    unspecified site D05.1- ☑
  lobular
    with
      infiltrating duct
        breast (female) C50.91- ☑
          male C50.92- ☑

Carcinoma-in-situ — *continued*
  lobular — *continued*
    with — *continued*
      infiltrating duct — *continued*
        specified site NEC — *see* Neoplasm, malignant
        unspecified site (female) C50.91- ☑
          male C50.92- ☑
      intraductal
        breast D05.8- ☑
        specified site NEC — *see* Neoplasm, in situ,
          by site
        unspecified site (female) D05.8- ☑
    breast D05.0- ☑
    specified site NEC — *see* Neoplasm, in situ, by site
    unspecified site D05.0- ☑
  squamous cell — *see also* Neoplasm, in situ, by site
    with questionable stromal invasion
      cervix D06.9
      specified site NEC — *see* Neoplasm, in situ, by
        site
      unspecified site D06.9
Carcinomaphobia F45.29
Carcinomatosis C80.0
  peritonei C78.6
  unspecified site (primary) (secondary) C80.0
Carcinosarcoma — *see* Neoplasm, malignant, by site
  embryonal — *see* Neoplasm, malignant, by site
Cardia, cardial — *see* condition
Cardiac — *see also* condition
  death, sudden — *see* Arrest, cardiac
  pacemaker
    in situ Z95.0
    management or adjustment Z45.018
  tamponade I31.4
Cardialgia — *see* Pain, precordial
Cardiectasis — *see* Hypertrophy, cardiac
Cardiochalasia K21.9
Cardiomalacia I51.5
Cardiomegalia glycogenica diffusa E74.02 *[I43]*
Cardiomegaly — *see also* Hypertrophy, cardiac
  congenital Q24.8
  glycogen E74.02 *[I43]*
  idiopathic I51.7
Cardiomyoliposis I51.5
Cardiomyopathy (familial) (idiopathic) I42.9
  alcoholic I42.6
  amyloid E85.4 *[I43]*
    transthyretin-related (ATTR) familial E85.4 *[I43]*
  arteriosclerotic — *see* Disease, heart, ischemic,
    atherosclerotic
  beriberi E51.12
  cobalt-beer I42.6
  congenital I42.4
  congestive I42.0
  constrictive NOS I42.5
  dilated I42.0
  due to
    alcohol I42.6
    beriberi E51.12
    cardiac glycogenosis E74.02 *[I43]*
    drugs I42.7
    external agents NEC I42.7
    Friedreich's ataxia G11.11
    myotonia atrophica G71.11 *[I43]*
    progressive muscular dystrophy G71.09 *[I43]*
  glycogen storage E74.02 *[I43]*
  hypertensive — *see* Hypertension, heart
  hypertrophic (nonobstructive) I42.2
    obstructive I42.1
      congenital Q24.8
  in
    Chagas' disease (chronic) B57.2
      acute B57.0
    sarcoidosis D86.85
  ischemic I25.5
  metabolic E88.9 *[I43]*
    thyrotoxic E05.90 *[I43]*
      with thyroid storm E05.91 *[I43]*
  newborn I42.8
    congenital I42.4
  non-ischemic — *see also* by cause I42.8
  nutritional E63.9 *[I43]*
    beriberi E51.12
  obscure of Africa I42.8
  peripartum O90.3
  postpartum O90.3
  restrictive NEC I42.5

▽ **Subterms under main terms may continue to next column or page**   ☑ **Additional Character Required — Refer to the Tabular List for Character Selection**   **51**

Carcinoma — Cardiomyopathy

Cardiomyopathy — *continued*
　rheumatic I09.0
　secondary I42.9
　specified NEC I42.8
　stress induced I51.81
　takotsubo I51.81
　thyrotoxic E05.90 *[I43]*
　　with thyroid storm E05.91 *[I43]*
　toxic NEC I42.7
　transthyretin-related (ATTR) familial amyloid E85.4
　tuberculous A18.84
　viral B33.24
Cardionephritis — *see* Hypertension, cardiorenal
Cardionephropathy — *see* Hypertension, cardiorenal
Cardionephrosis — *see* Hypertension, cardiorenal
Cardiopathia nigra I27.0
Cardiopathy — *see also* Disease, heart I51.9
　idiopathic I42.9
　mucopolysaccharidosis E76.3 *[I52]*
Cardiopericarditis — *see* Pericarditis
Cardiophobia F45.29
Cardiorenal — *see* condition
Cardiorrhexis — *see* Infarct, myocardium
Cardiosclerosis — *see* Disease, heart, ischemic,
　atherosclerotic
Cardiosis — *see* Disease, heart
Cardiospasm (esophagus) (reflex) (stomach) K22.0
　congenital Q39.5
　　with megaesophagus Q39.5
Cardiostenosis — *see* Disease, heart
Cardiosymphysis I31.0
Cardiovascular — *see* condition
Carditis (acute) (bacterial) (chronic) (subacute) I51.89
　meningococcal A39.50
　rheumatic — *see* Disease, heart, rheumatic
　rheumatoid — *see* Rheumatoid, carditis
　viral B33.20
Care (of) (for) (following)
　child (routine) Z76.2
　family member (handicapped) (sick)
　　creating problem for family Z63.6
　　provided away from home for holiday relief Z75.5
　　unavailable, due to
　　　absence (person rendering care) (sufferer) Z74.2
　　　inability (any reason) of person rendering care
　　　　Z74.2
　foundling Z76.1
　holiday relief Z75.5
　improper — *see* Maltreatment
　lack of (at or after birth) (infant) — *see* Maltreatment,
　　child, neglect
　lactating mother Z39.1
　palliative Z51.5
　postpartum
　　immediately after delivery Z39.0
　　routine follow-up Z39.2
　respite Z75.5
　unavailable, due to
　　absence of person rendering care Z74.2
　　inability (any reason) of person rendering care Z74.2
　well-baby Z76.2
Caries
　bone NEC A18.03
　dental (dentino enamel junction) (early childhood) (of
　　dentine) (pre-eruptive) (recurrent) (to the pulp)
　　K02.9
　　arrested (coronal) (root) K02.3
　　chewing surface
　　　limited to enamel K02.51
　　　penetrating into dentin K02.52
　　　penetrating into pulp K02.53
　　coronal surface
　　　chewing surface
　　　　limited to enamel K02.51
　　　　penetrating into dentin K02.52
　　　　penetrating into pulp K02.53
　　　pit and fissure surface
　　　　limited to enamel K02.51
　　　　penetrating into dentin K02.52
　　　　penetrating into pulp K02.53
　　　smooth surface
　　　　limited to enamel K02.61
　　　　penetrating into dentin K02.62
　　　　penetrating into pulp K02.63
　　pit and fissure surface
　　　limited to enamel K02.51
　　　penetrating into dentin K02.52
　　　penetrating into pulp K02.53

Caries — *continued*
　dental — *continued*
　　primary, cervical origin K02.52
　　root K02.7
　　smooth surface
　　　limited to enamel K02.61
　　　penetrating into dentin K02.62
　　　penetrating into pulp K02.63
　external meatus — *see* Disorder, ear, external, specified
　　type NEC
　hip (tuberculous) A18.02
　initial (tooth)
　　chewing surface K02.51
　　pit and fissure surface K02.51
　　smooth surface K02.61
　knee (tuberculous) A18.02
　labyrinth H83.8 ☑
　limb NEC (tuberculous) A18.03
　mastoid process (chronic) — *see* Mastoiditis, chronic
　　tuberculous A18.03
　middle ear H74.8 ☑
　nose (tuberculous) A18.03
　orbit (tuberculous) A18.03
　ossicles, ear — *see* Abnormal, ear ossicles
　petrous bone — *see* Petrositis
　root (dental) (tooth) K02.7
　sacrum (tuberculous) A18.01
　spine, spinal (column) (tuberculous) A18.01
　syphilitic A52.77
　　congenital (early) A50.02 *[M90.80]*
　tooth, teeth — *see* Caries, dental
　tuberculous A18.03
　vertebra (column) (tuberculous) A18.01
Carious teeth — *see* Caries, dental
Carneous mole O02.0
Carnitine insufficiency E71.40
Carotenemia (dietary) E67.1
Carotenosis (cutis) (skin) E67.1
Carotid body or sinus syndrome G90.01
Carotidynia G90.01
Carpal tunnel syndrome — *see* Syndrome, carpal tunnel
Carpenter's syndrome Q87.0
Carpopedal spasm — *see* Tetany
Carr-Barr-Plunkett syndrome Q97.1
Carrier (suspected) of
　amebiasis Z22.1
　bacterial disease NEC Z22.39
　　diphtheria Z22.2
　　intestinal infectious NEC Z22.1
　　　typhoid Z22.0
　　meningococcal Z22.31
　　sexually transmitted Z22.4
　　specified NEC Z22.39
　　staphylococcal (Methicillin susceptible) Z22.321
　　　Methicillin resistant Z22.322
　　streptococcal Z22.338
　　　group B Z22.330
　　　　complicating pregnancy or delivery
　　　　　O99.82- ☑
　　typhoid Z22.0
　cholera Z22.1
　diphtheria Z22.2
　gastrointestinal pathogens NEC Z22.1
　genetic Z14.8
　　cystic fibrosis Z14.1
　　hemophilia A (asymptomatic) Z14.01
　　　symptomatic Z14.02
　gestational, pregnant Z33.1
　gonorrhea Z22.4
　HAA (hepatitis Australian-antigen) B18.8
　HB (c)(s)-AG B18.1
　hepatitis (viral) B18.9
　　Australia-antigen (HAA) B18.8
　　B surface antigen (HBsAg) B18.1
　　　with acute delta- (super)infection B17.0
　　C B18.2
　　specified NEC B18.8
　human T-cell lymphotropic virus type-1 (HTLV-1) infec-
　　tion Z22.6
　infectious organism Z22.9
　　specified NEC Z22.8
　meningococci Z22.31
　Salmonella typhosa Z22.0
　serum hepatitis — *see* Carrier, hepatitis
　staphylococci (Methicillin susceptible) Z22.321
　　Methicillin resistant Z22.322
　streptococci Z22.338
　　group B Z22.330

Carrier of — *continued*
　streptococci — *continued*
　　group B — *continued*
　　　complicating pregnancy or delivery O99.82- ☑
　syphilis Z22.4
　typhoid Z22.0
　venereal disease NEC Z22.4
Carrion's disease A44.0
Carter's relapsing fever (Asiatic) A68.1
Cartilage — *see* condition
Caruncle (inflamed)
　conjunctiva (acute) — *see* Conjunctivitis, acute
　labium (majus) (minus) N90.89
　lacrimal — *see* Inflammation, lacrimal, passages
　myrtiform N89.8
　urethral (benign) N36.2
Cascade stomach K31.2
Caseation lymphatic gland (tuberculous) A18.2
Cassidy (-Scholte) syndrome (malignant carcinoid) E34.0
Castellani's disease A69.8
Castration, traumatic, male S38.231 ☑
Casts in urine R82.998
Cat
　cry syndrome Q93.4
　ear Q17.3
　eye syndrome Q92.8
Catabolism, senile R54
Catalepsy (hysterical) F44.2
　schizophrenic F20.2
Cataplexy (idiopathic) — *see* Narcolepsy
Cataract (cortical) (immature) (incipient) H26.9
　with
　　neovascularization — *see* Cataract, complicated
　age-related — *see* Cataract, senile
　anterior
　　and posterior axial embryonal Q12.0
　　pyramidal Q12.0
　associated with
　　galactosemia E74.21 *[H28]*
　　myotonic disorders G71.19 *[H28]*
　blue Q12.0
　central Q12.0
　cerulean Q12.0
　complicated H26.20
　　with
　　　neovascularization H26.21- ☑
　　　ocular disorder H26.22- ☑
　　　glaucomatous flecks H26.23- ☑
　congenital Q12.0
　coraliform Q12.0
　coronary Q12.0
　crystalline Q12.0
　diabetic — *see* Diabetes, cataract
　drug-induced H26.3- ☑
　due to
　　ocular disorder — *see* Cataract, complicated
　　radiation H26.8
　electric H26.8
　extraction status Z98.4- ☑
　glass-blower's H26.8
　heat ray H26.8
　heterochromic — *see* Cataract, complicated
　hypermature — *see* Cataract, senile, morgagnian type
　in (due to)
　　chronic iridocyclitis — *see* Cataract, complicated
　　diabetes — *see* Diabetes, cataract
　　endocrine disease E34.9 *[H28]*
　　eye disease — *see* Cataract, complicated
　　hypoparathyroidism E20.9 *[H28]*
　　malnutrition-dehydration E46 *[H28]*
　　metabolic disease E88.9 *[H28]*
　　myotonic disorders G71.19 *[H28]*
　　nutritional disease E63.9 *[H28]*
　infantile — *see* Cataract, presenile
　irradiational — *see* Cataract, specified NEC
　juvenile — *see* Cataract, presenile
　malnutrition-dehydration E46 *[H28]*
　morgagnian — *see* Cataract, senile, morgagnian type
　myotonic G71.19 *[H28]*
　myxedema E03.9 *[H28]*
　nuclear
　　embryonal Q12.0
　　sclerosis — *see* Cataract, senile, nuclear
　presenile H26.00- ☑
　　combined forms H26.06- ☑
　　cortical H26.01- ☑
　　lamellar — *see* Cataract, presenile, cortical

Cataract — *continued*
  presenile — *continued*
    nuclear H26.03-☑
    specified NEC H26.09
    subcapsular polar (anterior) H26.04-☑
      posterior H26.05-☑
    zonular — *see* Cataract, presenile, cortical
  secondary H26.40
    Soemmering's ring H26.41-☑
    specified NEC H26.49-☑
    to eye disease — *see* Cataract, complicated
  senile H25.9
    brunescens — *see* Cataract, senile, nuclear
    combined forms H25.81-☑
    coronary — *see* Cataract, senile, incipient
    cortical H25.01-☑
    hypermature — *see* Cataract, senile, morgagnian
      type
    incipient (mature) (total) H25.09-☑
      cortical — *see* Cataract, senile, cortical
      subcapsular — *see* Cataract, senile, subcapsular
    morgagnian type (hypermature) H25.2-☑
    nuclear (sclerosis) H25.1-☑
    polar subcapsular (anterior) (posterior) — *see*
      Cataract, senile, incipient
    punctate — *see* Cataract, senile, incipient
    specified NEC H25.89
    subcapsular polar (anterior) H25.03-☑
      posterior H25.04-☑
  snowflake — *see* Diabetes, cataract
  specified NEC H26.8
  toxic — *see* Cataract, drug-induced
  traumatic H26.10-☑
    localized H26.11-☑
    partially resolved H26.12-☑
    total H26.13-☑
  zonular (perinuclear) Q12.0
Cataracta — *see also* Cataract
  brunescens — *see* Cataract, senile, nuclear
  centralis pulverulenta Q12.0
  cerulea Q12.0
  complicata — *see* Cataract, complicated
  congenita Q12.0
  coralliformis Q12.0
  coronaria Q12.0
  diabetic — *see* Diabetes, cataract
  membranacea
    accreta — *see* Cataract, secondary
    congenita Q12.0
  nigra — *see* Cataract, senile, nuclear
  sunflower — *see* Cataract, complicated
Catarrh, catarrhal (acute) (febrile) (infectious) (inflammation) — *see also* condition J00
  bronchial — *see* Bronchitis
  chest — *see* Bronchitis
  chronic J31.0
  due to congenital syphilis A50.03
  enteric — *see* Enteritis
  eustachian H68.009
  fauces — *see* Pharyngitis
  gastrointestinal — *see* Enteritis
  gingivitis K05.00
    nonplaque induced K05.01
    plaque induced K05.00
  hay — *see* Fever, hay
  intestinal — *see* Enteritis
  larynx, chronic J37.0
  liver B15.9
    with hepatic coma B15.0
  lung — *see* Bronchitis
  middle ear, chronic — *see* Otitis, media, nonsuppurative, chronic, serous
  mouth K12.1
  nasal (chronic) — *see* Rhinitis
  nasobronchial J31.1
  nasopharyngeal (chronic) J31.1
    acute J00
  pulmonary — *see* Bronchitis
  spring (eye) (vernal) — *see* Conjunctivitis, acute, atopic
  summer (hay) — *see* Fever, hay
  throat J31.2
  tubotympanal — *see also* Otitis, media, nonsuppurative
    chronic — *see* Otitis, media, nonsuppurative, chronic, serous
Catatonia (schizophrenic) F20.2
Catatonic
  disorder due to known physiologic condition F06.1

Catatonic — *continued*
  schizophrenia F20.2
  stupor R40.1
Cat-scratch — *see also* Abrasion
  disease or fever A28.1
Cauda equina — *see* condition
Cauliflower ear M95.1-☑
Causalgia (upper limb) G56.4-☑
  lower limb G57.7-☑
Cause
  external, general effects T75.89 ☑
Caustic burn — *see* Corrosion, by site
Cavare's disease (familial periodic paralysis) G72.3
Cave-in, injury
  crushing (severe) — *see* Crush
  suffocation — *see* Asphyxia, traumatic, due to low
    oxygen, due to cave-in
Cavernitis (penis) N48.29
Cavernositis N48.29
Cavernous — *see* condition
Cavitation of lung — *see also* Tuberculosis, pulmonary
  nontuberculous J98.4
Cavities, dental — *see* Caries, dental
Cavity
  lung — *see* Cavitation of lung
  optic papilla Q14.2
  pulmonary — *see* Cavitation of lung
Cavovarus foot, congenital Q66.1-☑
Cavus foot (congenital) Q66.7-☑
  acquired — *see* Deformity, limb, foot, specified NEC
Cazenave's disease L10.2
CDKL5 (Cyclin-Dependent Kinase-Like 5 Deficiency Disorder) G40.42
Cecitis K52.9
  with perforation, peritonitis, or rupture K65.8
Cecoureterocele Q62.32
Cecum — *see* condition
Celiac
  artery compression syndrome I77.4
  disease (with steatorrhea) K90.0
  infantilism K90.0
Cell(s), **cellular** — *see also* condition
  in urine R82.998
Cellulitis (diffuse) (phlegmonous) (septic) (suppurative)
  L03.90
  abdominal wall L03.311
  anaerobic A48.0
  ankle — *see* Cellulitis, lower limb
  anus K61.0
  arm — *see* Cellulitis, upper limb
  auricle (ear) — *see* Cellulitis, ear
  axilla L03.11-☑
  back (any part) L03.312
  breast (acute) (nonpuerperal) (subacute) N61.0
    nipple N61.0
  broad ligament
    acute N73.0
  buttock L03.317
  cervical (meaning neck) L03.221
  cervix (uteri) — *see* Cervicitis
  cheek (external) L03.211
    internal K12.2
  chest wall L03.313
  chronic L03.90
  clostridial A48.0
  corpus cavernosum N48.22
  digit
    finger — *see* Cellulitis, finger
    toe — *see* Cellulitis, toe
  Douglas' cul-de-sac or pouch
    acute N73.0
  drainage site (following operation) T81.49 ☑
  ear (external) H60.1-☑
  eosinophilic (granulomatous) L98.3
  erysipelatous — *see* Erysipelas
  external auditory canal — *see* Cellulitis, ear
  eyelid — *see* Abscess, eyelid
  face NEC L03.211
  finger (intrathecal) (periosteal) (subcutaneous) (subcuticular) L03.01-☑
  foot — *see* Cellulitis, lower limb
  gangrenous — *see* Gangrene
  genital organ NEC
    female (external) N76.4
    male N49.9
      multiple sites N49.8
      specified NEC N49.8

Cellulitis — *continued*
  gluteal (region) L03.317
  gonococcal A54.89
  groin L03.314
  hand — *see* Cellulitis, upper limb
  head NEC L03.811
    face (any part, except ear, eye and nose) L03.211
  heel — *see* Cellulitis, lower limb
  hip — *see* Cellulitis, lower limb
  jaw (region) L03.211
  knee — *see* Cellulitis, lower limb
  labium (majus) (minus) — *see* Vulvitis
  lacrimal passages — *see* Inflammation, lacrimal, passages
  larynx J38.7
  leg — *see* Cellulitis, lower limb
  lip K13.0
  lower limb L03.11-☑
    toe — *see* Cellulitis, toe
  mouth (floor) K12.2
  multiple sites, so stated L03.90
  nasopharynx J39.1
  navel L03.316
    newborn P38.9
      with mild hemorrhage P38.1
      without hemorrhage P38.9
  neck (region) L03.221
  nipple (acute) (nonpuerperal) (subacute) N61.0
  nose (septum) (external) J34.0
  orbit, orbital H05.01-☑
  palate (soft) K12.2
  pectoral (region) L03.313
  pelvis, pelvic (chronic)
    female — *see also* Disease, pelvis, inflammatory
      N73.2
      acute N73.0
    following ectopic or molar pregnancy O08.0
    male K65.0
  penis N48.22
  perineal, perineum L03.315
  periorbital L03.213
  perirectal K61.1
  peritonsillar J36
  periurethral N34.0
  periuterine — *see also* Disease, pelvis, inflammatory
    N73.2
    acute N73.0
  pharynx J39.1
  preseptal L03.213
  rectum K61.1
  retroperitoneal K68.9
  round ligament
    acute N73.0
  scalp (any part) L03.811
  scrotum N49.2
  seminal vesicle N49.0
  shoulder — *see* Cellulitis, upper limb
  specified site NEC L03.818
  submandibular (region) (space) (triangle) K12.2
    gland K11.3
  submaxillary (region) K12.2
    gland K11.3
  thigh — *see* Cellulitis, lower limb
  thumb (intrathecal) (periosteal) (subcutaneous) (subcuticular) — *see* Cellulitis, finger
  toe (intrathecal) (periosteal) (subcutaneous) (subcuticular) L03.03-☑
  tonsil J36
  trunk L03.319
    abdominal wall L03.311
    back (any part) L03.312
    buttock L03.317
    chest wall L03.313
    groin L03.314
    perineal, perineum L03.315
    umbilicus L03.316
  tuberculous (primary) A18.4
  umbilicus L03.316
  upper limb L03.11-☑
    axilla — *see* Cellulitis, axilla
    finger — *see* Cellulitis, finger
    thumb — *see* Cellulitis, finger
  vaccinal T88.0 ☑
  vocal cord J38.3
  vulva — *see* Vulvitis
  wrist — *see* Cellulitis, upper limb
Cementoblastoma, benign — *see* Cyst, calcifying
  odontogenic

Cementoma — *see* Cyst, calcifying odontogenic
Cementoperiostitis — *see* Periodontitis
Cementosis K03.4
Central auditory processing disorder H93.25
Central pain syndrome G89.0
Cephalematocele, cephal (o)hematocele
　newborn P52.8
　　birth injury P10.8
　traumatic — *see* Hematoma, brain
Cephalematoma, cephalhematoma (calcified)
　newborn (birth injury) P12.0
　traumatic — *see* Hematoma, brain
Cephalgia, cephalalgia — *see also* Headache
　histamine G44.009
　　intractable G44.001
　　not intractable G44.009
　trigeminal autonomic (TAC) NEC G44.099
　　intractable G44.091
　　not intractable G44.099
Cephalic — *see* condition
Cephalitis — *see* Encephalitis
Cephalocele — *see* Encephalocele
Cephalomenia N94.89
Cephalopelvic — *see* condition
Cerclage (with cervical incompetence) in pregnancy —
　　see Incompetence, cervix, in pregnancy
Cerebellitis — *see* Encephalitis
Cerebellum, cerebellar — *see* condition
Cerebral — *see* condition
Cerebritis — *see* Encephalitis
Cerebro-hepato-renal syndrome Q87.89
Cerebromalacia — *see* Softening, brain
　sequelae of cerebrovascular disease I69.398
Cerebroside lipidosis E75.22
Cerebrospasticity (congenital) G80.1
Cerebrospinal — *see* condition
Cerebrum — *see* condition
Ceroid-lipofuscinosis, neuronal E75.4
Cerumen (accumulation) (impacted) H61.2- ☑
Cervical — *see also* condition
　auricle Q18.2
　dysplasia in pregnancy — *see* Abnormal, cervix, in
　　pregnancy or childbirth
　erosion in pregnancy — *see* Abnormal, cervix, in
　　pregnancy or childbirth
　fibrosis in pregnancy — *see* Abnormal, cervix, in preg-
　　nancy or childbirth
　fusion syndrome Q76.1
　rib Q76.5
　shortening (complicating pregnancy) O26.87- ☑
Cervicalgia M54.2
Cervicitis (acute) (chronic) (nonvenereal) (senile (atroph-
　ic)) (subacute) (with ulceration) N72
　with
　　abortion — *see* Abortion, by type complicated by
　　　genital tract and pelvic infection
　　ectopic pregnancy O08.0
　　molar pregnancy O08.0
　chlamydial A56.09
　gonococcal A54.03
　herpesviral A60.03
　puerperal (postpartum) O86.11
　syphilitic A52.76
　trichomonal A59.09
　tuberculous A18.16
Cervicocolpitis (emphysematosa) — *see also* Cervicitis
　N72
Cervix — *see* condition
Cesarean delivery, previous, affecting management
　of pregnancy O34.219
　classical (vertical) scar O34.212
　isthmocele O34.22
　low transverse scar O34.211
　mid-transverse T incision O34.218
　scar
　　defect (isthmocele) O34.22
　　specified type NEC O34.218
Céstan (-Chenais) paralysis or syndrome G46.3
Céstan-Raymond syndrome I65.8
Cestode infestation B71.9
　specified type NEC B71.8
Cestodiasis B71.9
Chabert's disease A22.9
Chacaleh E53.8
Chafing L30.4
Chagas' (-Mazza) disease (chronic) B57.2

Chagas' disease — *continued*
　with
　　cardiovascular involvement NEC B57.2
　　digestive system involvement B57.30
　　　megacolon B57.32
　　　megaesophagus B57.31
　　　other specified B57.39
　　megacolon B57.32
　　megaesophagus B57.31
　　myocarditis B57.2
　　nervous system involvement B57.40
　　　meningitis B57.41
　　　meningoencephalitis B57.42
　　　other specified B57.49
　　specified organ involvement NEC B57.5
　acute (with) B57.1
　　cardiovascular NEC B57.0
　　myocarditis B57.0
Chagres fever B50.9
Chairridden Z74.09
Chalasia (cardiac sphincter) K21.9
Chalazion H00.19
　left H00.16
　　lower H00.15
　　upper H00.14
　right H00.13
　　lower H00.12
　　upper H00.11
Chalcosis — *see also* Disorder, globe, degenerative,
　chalcosis
　cornea — *see* Deposit, cornea
　crystalline lens — *see* Cataract, complicated
　retina H35.89
Chalicosis (pulmonum) J62.8
Chancre (any genital site) (hard) (hunterian) (mixed)
　　(primary) (seronegative) (seropositive) (syphilitic)
　　A51.0
　congenital A50.07
　conjunctiva NEC A51.2
　Ducrey's A57
　extragenital A51.2
　eyelid A51.2
　lip A51.2
　nipple A51.2
　Nisbet's A57
　of
　　carate A67.0
　　pinta A67.0
　　yaws A66.0
　palate, soft A51.2
　phagedenic A57
　simple A57
　soft A57
　　bubo A57
　　palate A51.2
　urethra A51.0
　yaws A66.0
Chancroid (anus) (genital) (penis) (perineum) (rectum)
　　(urethra) (vulva) A57
Chandler's disease (osteochondritis dissecans, hip) —
　　see Osteochondritis, dissecans, hip
Change(s) (in) (of) — *see also* Removal
　arteriosclerotic — *see* Arteriosclerosis
　bone — *see also* Disorder, bone
　　diabetic — *see* Diabetes, bone change
　bowel habit R19.4
　cardiorenal (vascular) — *see* Hypertension, cardiorenal
　cardiovascular — *see* Disease, cardiovascular
　circulatory I99.9
　cognitive (mild) (organic) R41.89
　color, tooth, teeth
　　during formation K00.8
　　posteruptive K03.7
　contraceptive device Z30.433
　corneal membrane H18.30
　　Bowman's membrane fold or rupture H18.31- ☑
　　Descemet's membrane
　　　fold H18.32- ☑
　　　rupture H18.33- ☑
　coronary — *see* Disease, heart, ischemic
　degenerative, spine or vertebra — *see* Spondylosis
　dental pulp, regressive K04.2
　dressing (nonsurgical) Z48.00
　　surgical Z48.01
　heart — *see* Disease, heart
　hip joint — *see* Derangement, joint, hip
　hyperplastic larynx J38.7

Change(s) — *continued*
　hypertrophic
　　nasal sinus J34.89
　　turbinate, nasal J34.3
　　upper respiratory tract J39.8
　indwelling catheter Z46.6
　inflammatory — *see also* Inflammation
　　sacroiliac M46.1
　job, anxiety concerning Z56.1
　joint — *see* Derangement, joint
　life — *see* Menopause
　mental status R41.82
　minimal (glomerular) — *see also* N00-N07 with fourth
　　character .0 N05.0
　myocardium, myocardial — *see* Degeneration, myocar-
　　dial
　of life — *see* Menopause
　pacemaker Z45.018
　　pulse generator Z45.010
　personality (enduring) F68.8
　　due to (secondary to)
　　　general medical condition F07.0
　　secondary (nonspecific) F60.89
　regressive, dental pulp K04.2
　renal — *see* Disease, renal
　retina H35.9
　　myopic — *see also* Myopia, degenerative H44.2- ☑
　sacroiliac joint M53.3
　senile — *see also* condition R54
　sensory R20.8
　skin R23.9
　　acute, due to ultraviolet radiation L56.9
　　　specified NEC L56.8
　　chronic, due to nonionizing radiation L57.9
　　　specified NEC L57.8
　　cyanosis R23.0
　　flushing R23.2
　　pallor R23.1
　　petechiae R23.3
　　specified change NEC R23.8
　　swelling — *see* Mass, localized
　　texture R23.4
　trophic
　　arm — *see* Mononeuropathy, upper limb
　　leg — *see* Mononeuropathy, lower limb
　vascular I99.9
　vasomotor I73.9
　voice R49.9
　　psychogenic F44.4
　　specified NEC R49.8
Changing sleep-work schedule, affecting sleep
　G47.26
Changuinola fever A93.1
Chapping skin T69.8 ☑
Charcot-Marie-Tooth disease, paralysis or syndrome
　G60.0
Charcot's
　arthropathy — *see* Arthropathy, neuropathic
　cirrhosis K74.3
　disease (tabetic arthropathy) A52.16
　joint (disease) (tabetic) A52.16
　　diabetic — *see* Diabetes, with, arthropathy
　　syringomyelic G95.0
　syndrome (intermittent claudication) I73.9
CHARGE association Q89.8
Charley-horse (quadriceps) M62.831
　traumatic (quadriceps) S76.11- ☑
Charlouis' disease — *see* Yaws
Cheadle's disease E54
Checking (of)
　cardiac pacemaker (battery) (electrode(s)) Z45.018
　　pulse generator Z45.010
　implantable subdermal contraceptive Z30.46
　intrauterine contraceptive device Z30.431
　wound Z48.0- ☑
　　due to injury — code to Injury, by site, using appro-
　　　priate seventh character for subsequent en-
　　　counter
Check-up — *see* Examination
Chédiak-Higashi (-Steinbrinck) **syndrome** (congenital
　gigantism of peroxidase granules) E70.330
Cheek — *see* condition
Cheese itch B88.0
Cheese-washer's lung J67.8
Cheese-worker's lung J67.8
Cheilitis (acute) (angular) (catarrhal) (chronic) (exfoliative)
　　(gangrenous) (glandular) (infectional) (suppurative)
　　(ulcerative) (vesicular) K13.0

Cheilitis — *continued*
actinic (due to sun) L56.8
other than from sun L59.8
candidal B37.83
Cheilodynia K13.0
Cheiloschisis — *see* Cleft, lip
Cheilosis (angular) K13.0
with pellagra E52
due to
vitamin B2 (riboflavin) deficiency E53.0
Cheiromegaly M79.89
Cheiropompholyx L30.1
Cheloid — *see* Keloid
Chemical burn — *see* Corrosion, by site
Chemodectoma — *see* Paraganglioma, nonchromaffin
Chemosis, conjunctiva — *see* Edema, conjunctiva
Chemotherapy (session) (for)
cancer Z51.11
neoplasm Z51.11
Cherubism M27.8
Chest — *see* condition
Cheyne-Stokes breathing (respiration) R06.3
Chiari's
disease or syndrome (hepatic vein thrombosis) I82.0
malformation
type I G93.5
type II — *see* Spina bifida
net Q24.8
Chicago disease B40.9
Chickenpox — *see* Varicella
Chiclero ulcer or sore B55.1
Chigger (infestation) B88.0
Chignon (disease) B36.8
newborn (from vacuum extraction) (birth injury) P12.1
Chilaiditi's syndrome (subphrenic displacement, colon) Q43.3
Chilblain(s) (lupus) T69.1 ☑
Child
custody dispute Z65.3
Childbirth — *see* Delivery
Childhood
cerebral X-linked adrenoleukodystrophy E71.520
period of rapid growth Z00.2
Chill(s) R68.83
with fever R50.9
congestive in malarial regions B54
without fever R68.83
Chilomastigiasis A07.8
Chimera 46,XX/46,XY Q99.0
Chin — *see* condition
Chinese dysentery A03.9
Chionophobia F40.228
Chitral fever A93.1
Chlamydia, chlamydial A74.9
cervicitis A56.09
conjunctivitis A74.0
cystitis A56.01
endometritis A56.11
epididymitis A56.19
female
pelvic inflammatory disease A56.11
pelviperitonitis A56.11
orchitis A56.19
peritonitis A74.81
pharyngitis A56.4
proctitis A56.3
psittaci (infection) A70
salpingitis A56.11
sexually-transmitted infection NEC A56.8
specified NEC A74.89
urethritis A56.01
vulvovaginitis A56.02
Chlamydiosis — *see* Chlamydia
Chloasma (skin) (idiopathic) (symptomatic) L81.1
eyelid H02.719
hyperthyroid E05.90 *[H02.719]*
with thyroid storm E05.91 *[H02.719]*
left H02.716
lower H02.715
upper H02.714
right H02.713
lower H02.712
upper H02.711
Chloroma C92.3- ☑
Chlorosis D50.9
Egyptian B76.9 *[D63.8]*
miner's B76.9 *[D63.8]*

Chlorotic anemia D50.8
Chocolate cyst (ovary) N80.1
Choked
disc or disk — *see* Papilledema
on food, phlegm, or vomitus NOS — *see* Foreign body, by site
while vomiting NOS — *see* Foreign body, by site
Chokes (resulting from bends) T70.3 ☑
Choking sensation R09.89
Cholangiectasis K83.8
Cholangiocarcinoma
with hepatocellular carcinoma, combined C22.0
liver C22.1
specified site NEC — *see* Neoplasm, malignant, by site
unspecified site C22.1
Cholangiohepatitis K83.8
due to fluke infestation B66.1
Cholangiohepatoma C22.0
Cholangiolitis (acute) (chronic) (extrahepatic) (gangrenous) (intrahepatic) K83.09
paratyphoidal — *see* Fever, paratyphoid
typhoidal A01.09
Cholangioma D13.4
malignant — *see* Cholangiocarcinoma
Cholangitis (ascending) (recurrent) (secondary) (stenosing) (suppurative) K83.09
with calculus, bile duct — *see* Calculus, bile duct, with cholangitis
chronic nonsuppurative destructive K74.3
primary K83.09
sclerosing K83.01
sclerosing K83.09
Cholecystectasia K82.8
Cholecystitis K81.9
with
calculus, stones in
bile duct (common) (hepatic) — *see* Calculus, bile duct, with cholecystitis
cystic duct — *see* Calculus, gallbladder, with cholecystitis
gallbladder — *see* Calculus, gallbladder, with cholecystitis
choledocholithiasis — *see* Calculus, bile duct, with cholecystitis
cholelithiasis — *see* Calculus, gallbladder, with cholecystitis
gangrene of gallbladder K82.A1
perforation of gallbladder K82.A2
acute (emphysematous) (gangrenous) (suppurative) K81.0
with
calculus, stones in
cystic duct — *see* Calculus, gallbladder, with cholecystitis, acute
gallbladder — *see* Calculus, gallbladder, with cholecystitis, acute
choledocholithiasis — *see* Calculus, bile duct, with cholecystitis, acute
cholelithiasis — *see* Calculus, gallbladder, with cholecystitis, acute
chronic cholecystitis K81.2
with gallbladder calculus K80.12
with obstruction K80.13
chronic K81.1
with acute cholecystitis K81.2
with gallbladder calculus K80.12
with obstruction K80.13
emphysematous (acute) — *see* Cholecystitis, acute
gangrenous — *see* Cholecystitis, acute
paratyphoidal, current A01.4
suppurative — *see* Cholecystitis, acute
typhoidal A01.09
Cholecystolithiasis — *see* Calculus, gallbladder
Cholecystitis (suppurative) K83.09
Choledochith — *see* Calculus, bile duct
Choledocholithiasis (common duct) (hepatic duct) — *see* Calculus, bile duct
cystic — *see* Calculus, gallbladder
typhoidal A01.09
Cholelithiasis (cystic duct) (gallbladder) (impacted) (multiple) — *see* Calculus, gallbladder
bile duct (common) (hepatic) — *see* Calculus, bile duct
hepatic duct — *see* Calculus, bile duct
specified NEC K80.80
with obstruction K80.81
Cholemia — *see also* Jaundice
familial (simple) (congenital) E80.4

Cholemia — *continued*
Gilbert's E80.4
Choleperitoneum, choleperitonitis K65.3
Cholera (Asiatic) (epidemic) (malignant) A00.9
antimonial — *see* Poisoning, antimony
classical A00.0
due to Vibrio cholerae 01 A00.9
biovar cholerae A00.0
biovar eltor A00.1
el tor A00.1
el tor A00.1
Cholerine — *see* Cholera
Cholestasis NEC K83.1
with hepatocyte injury K71.0
due to total parenteral nutrition (TPN) K76.89
pure K71.0
Cholesteatoma (ear) (middle) (with reaction) H71.9- ☑
attic H71.0- ☑
external ear (canal) H60.4- ☑
mastoid H71.2- ☑
postmastoidectomy cavity (recurrent) — *see* Complications, postmastoidectomy, recurrent cholesteatoma
recurrent (postmastoidectomy) — *see* Complications, postmastoidectomy, recurrent cholesteatoma
tympanum H71.1- ☑
Cholesteatosis, diffuse H71.3- ☑
Cholesteremia E78.00
Cholesterin in vitreous — *see* Deposit, crystalline
Cholesterol
deposit
retina H35.89
vitreous — *see* Deposit, crystalline
elevated (high) E78.00
with elevated (high) triglycerides E78.2
screening for Z13.220
imbibition of gallbladder K82.4
Cholesterolemia (essential) (pure) E78.00
familial E78.01
hereditary E78.01
Cholesterolosis, cholesterosis (gallbladder) K82.4
cerebrotendinous E75.5
Cholocolic fistula K82.3
Choluria R82.2
Chondritis M94.8X9
aurical H61.03- ☑
costal (Tietze's) M94.0
external ear H61.03- ☑
patella, posttraumatic — *see* Chondromalacia, patella
pinna H61.03- ☑
purulent M94.8X- ☑
tuberculous NEC A18.02
intervertebral A18.01
Chondroblastoma — *see also* Neoplasm, bone, benign
malignant — *see* Neoplasm, bone, malignant
Chondrocalcinosis M11.20
ankle M11.27- ☑
elbow M11.22- ☑
familial M11.10
ankle M11.17- ☑
elbow M11.12- ☑
foot joint M11.17- ☑
hand joint M11.14- ☑
hip M11.15- ☑
knee M11.16- ☑
multiple site M11.19
shoulder M11.11- ☑
vertebrae M11.18
wrist M11.13- ☑
foot joint M11.27- ☑
hand joint M11.24- ☑
hip M11.25- ☑
knee M11.26- ☑
multiple site M11.29
shoulder M11.21- ☑
specified type NEC M11.20
ankle M11.27- ☑
elbow M11.22- ☑
foot joint M11.27- ☑
hand joint M11.24- ☑
hip M11.25- ☑
knee M11.26- ☑
multiple site M11.29
shoulder M11.21- ☑
vertebrae M11.28
wrist M11.23- ☑
vertebrae M11.28

Chondrocalcinosis — continued
  wrist M11.23- ☑
Chondrodermatitis nodularis helicis or anthelicis —
    see Perichondritis, ear
Chondrodysplasia Q78.9
  with hemangioma Q78.4
  calcificans congenita Q77.3
  fetalis Q77.4
  metaphyseal (Jansen's) (McKusick's) (Schmid's) Q78.8
  punctata Q77.3
Chondrodystrophy, chondrodystrophia (familial) (fetalis) (hypoplastic) Q78.9
  calcificans congenita Q77.3
  myotonic (congenital) G71.13
  punctata Q77.3
Chondroectodermal dysplasia Q77.6
Chondrogenesis imperfecta Q77.4
Chondrolysis M94.35- ☑
Chondroma — see also Neoplasm, cartilage, benign
  juxtacortical — see Neoplasm, bone, benign
  periosteal — see Neoplasm, bone, benign
Chondromalacia (systemic) M94.20
  acromioclavicular joint M94.21- ☑
  ankle M94.27- ☑
  elbow M94.22- ☑
  foot joint M94.27- ☑
  glenohumeral joint M94.21- ☑
  hand joint M94.24- ☑
  hip M94.25- ☑
  knee M94.26- ☑
    patella M22.4- ☑
  multiple sites M94.29
  patella M22.4- ☑
  rib M94.28
  sacroiliac joint M94.259
  shoulder M94.21- ☑
  sternoclavicular joint M94.21- ☑
  vertebral joint M94.28
  wrist M94.23- ☑
Chondromatosis — see also Neoplasm, cartilage, uncertain behavior
  internal Q78.4
Chondromyxosarcoma — see Neoplasm, cartilage, malignant
Chondro-osteodysplasia (Morquio-Brailsford type) E76.219
Chondro-osteodystrophy E76.29
Chondro-osteoma — see Neoplasm, bone, benign
Chondropathia tuberosa M94.0
Chondrosarcoma — see Neoplasm, cartilage, malignant
  juxtacortical — see Neoplasm, bone, malignant
  mesenchymal — see Neoplasm, connective tissue, malignant
  myxoid — see Neoplasm, cartilage, malignant
Chordee (nonvenereal) N48.89
  congenital Q54.4
  gonococcal A54.09
Chorditis (fibrinous) (nodosa) (tuberosa) J38.2
Chordoma — see Neoplasm, vertebral (column), malignant
Chorea (chronic) (gravis) (posthemiplegic) (senile) (spasmodic) G25.5
  with
    heart involvement I02.0
      active or acute (conditions in I01-) I02.0
        rheumatic I02.9
          with valvular disorder I02.0
      rheumatic heart disease (chronic) (inactive)(quiescent) — code to rheumatic heart condition involved
  drug-induced G25.4
  habit F95.8
  hereditary G10
  Huntington's G10
  hysterical F44.4
  minor I02.9
    with heart involvement I02.0
  progressive G25.5
    hereditary G10
  rheumatic (chronic) I02.9
    with heart involvement I02.0
  Sydenham's I02.9
    with heart involvement — see Chorea, with rheumatic heart disease
    nonrheumatic G25.5
Choreoathetosis (paroxysmal) G25.5
Chorioadenoma (destruens) D39.2

Chorioamnionitis O41.12- ☑
Chorioangioma D26.7
Choriocarcinoma — see Neoplasm, malignant, by site
  combined with
    embryonal carcinoma — see Neoplasm, malignant, by site
    other germ cell elements — see Neoplasm, malignant, by site
    teratoma — see Neoplasm, malignant, by site
  specified site — see Neoplasm, malignant, by site
  unspecified site
    female C58
    male C62.90
Chorioencephalitis (acute) (lymphocytic) (serous) A87.2
Chorioepithelioma — see Choriocarcinoma
Choriomeningitis (acute) (lymphocytic) (serous) A87.2
Chorionepithelioma — see Choriocarcinoma
Chorioretinitis — see also Inflammation, chorioretinal
  disseminated — see also Inflammation, chorioretinal, disseminated
    in neurosyphilis A52.19
  Egyptian B76.9 [D63.8]
  focal — see also Inflammation, chorioretinal, focal
  histoplasmic B39.9 [H32]
  in (due to)
    histoplasmosis B39.9 [H32]
    syphilis (secondary) A51.43
      late A52.71
    toxoplasmosis (acquired) B58.01
      congenital (active) P37.1 [H32]
    tuberculosis A18.53
  juxtapapillary, juxtapapillaris — see Inflammation, chorioretinal, focal, juxtapapillary
  leprous A30.9 [H32]
  miner's B76.9 [D63.8]
  progressive myopia (degeneration) — see also Myopia, degenerative H44.2- ☑
  syphilitic (secondary) A51.43
    congenital (early) A50.01 [H32]
      late A50.32
    late A52.71
  tuberculous A18.53
Chorioretinopathy, central serous H35.71- ☑
Choroid — see condition
Choroideremia H31.21
Choroiditis — see Chorioretinitis
Choroidopathy — see Disorder, choroid
Choroidoretinitis — see Chorioretinitis
Choroidoretinopathy, central serous — see Chorioretinopathy, central serous
Christian-Weber disease M35.6
Christmas disease D67
Chromaffinoma — see also Neoplasm, benign, by site
  malignant — see Neoplasm, malignant, by site
Chromatopsia — see Deficiency, color vision
Chromhidrosis, chromidrosis L75.1
Chromoblastomycosis — see Chromomycosis
Chromoconversion R82.91
Chromomycosis B43.9
  brain abscess B43.1
  cerebral B43.1
  cutaneous B43.0
  skin B43.0
  specified NEC B43.8
  subcutaneous abscess or cyst B43.2
Chromophytosis B36.0
Chromosome — see Anomaly, by chromosome involved
  D (1) — see Anomaly, chromosome 13
  E (3) — see Anomaly, chromosome 18
  G — see Anomaly, chromosome 21
Chromotrichomycosis B36.8
Chronic — see condition
  fracture — see Fracture, pathological
Churg-Strauss syndrome M30.1
Chyle cyst, mesentery I89.8
Chylocele (nonfilarial) I89.8
  filarial — see also Infestation, filarial B74.9 [N51]
  tunica vaginalis N50.89
    filarial — see also Infestation, filarial B74.9 [N51]
Chylomicronemia (fasting) (with hyperprebetalipoproteinemia) E78.3
Chylopericardium I31.3
  acute I30.9
Chylothorax (nonfilarial) J94.0
  filarial — see also Infestation, filarial B74.9 [J91.8]
Chylous — see condition
Chyluria (nonfilarial) R82.0

Chyluria — continued
  due to
    bilharziasis B65.0
    Brugia (malayi) B74.1
      timori B74.2
    schistosomiasis (bilharziasis) B65.0
    Wuchereria (bancrofti) B74.0
  filarial — see Infestation, filarial
Cicatricial (deformity) — see Cicatrix
Cicatrix (adherent) (contracted) (painful) (vicious) — see also Scar L90.5
  adenoid (and tonsil) J35.8
  alveolar process M26.79
  anus K62.89
  auricle — see Disorder, pinna, specified type NEC
  bile duct (common) (hepatic) K83.8
  bladder N32.89
  bone — see Disorder, bone, specified type NEC
  brain G93.89
  cervix (postoperative) (postpartal) N88.1
  common duct K83.8
  cornea H17.9
    tuberculous A18.59
  duodenum (bulb), obstructive K31.5
  esophagus K22.2
  eyelid — see Disorder, eyelid function
  hypopharynx J39.2
  lacrimal passages — see Obstruction, lacrimal
  larynx J38.7
  lung J98.4
  middle ear H74.8 ☑
  mouth K13.79
  muscle M62.89
    with contracture — see Contraction, muscle NEC
  nasopharynx J39.2
  palate (soft) K13.79
  penis N48.89
  pharynx J39.2
  prostate N42.89
  rectum K62.89
  retina — see Scar, chorioretinal
  semilunar cartilage — see Derangement, meniscus
  seminal vesicle N50.89
  skin L90.5
    infected L08.89
    postinfective L90.5
    tuberculous B90.8
  specified site NEC L90.5
  throat J39.2
  tongue K14.8
  tonsil (and adenoid) J35.8
  trachea J39.8
  tuberculous NEC B90.9
  urethra N36.8
  uterus N85.8
  vagina N89.8
    postoperative N99.2
  vocal cord J38.3
  wrist, constricting (annular) L90.5
CIDP (chronic inflammatory demyelinating polyneuropathy) G61.81
CIN — see Neoplasia, intraepithelial, cervix
CINCA (chronic infantile neurological, cutaneous and articular syndrome) M04.2
Cinchonism — see Deafness, ototoxic
  correct substance properly administered — see Table of Drugs and Chemicals, by drug, adverse effect
  overdose or wrong substance given or taken — see Table of Drugs and Chemicals, by drug, poisoning
Circle of Willis — see condition
Circular — see condition
Circulating anticoagulants — see also Disorder, hemorrhagic D68.318
  due to drugs — see also Disorder, hemorrhagic D68.32
  following childbirth O72.3
Circulation
  collateral, any site I99.8
  defective (lower extremity) I99.9
    congenital Q28.9
  embryonic Q28.9
  failure (peripheral) R57.9
    newborn P29.89
  fetal, persistent P29.38
  heart, incomplete Q28.9
Circulatory system — see condition
Circulus senilis (cornea) — see Degeneration, cornea, senile

☑ **Additional Character Required** — Refer to the Tabular List for Character Selection   ▽ Subterms under main terms may continue to next column or page

Circumcision (in absence of medical indication) (ritual) (routine) Z41.2
Circumscribed — *see* condition
Circumvallate placenta O43.11- ☑
Cirrhosis, cirrhotic (hepatic) (liver) K74.60
  alcoholic K70.30
    with ascites K70.31
  atrophic — *see* Cirrhosis, liver
  Baumgarten-Cruveilhier K74.69
  biliary (cholangiolitic) (cholangitic) (hypertrophic) (obstructive) (pericholangiolitic) K74.5
    due to
      Clonorchiasis B66.1
      flukes B66.3
    primary K74.3
    secondary K74.4
  cardiac (of liver) K76.1
  Charcot's K74.3
  cholangiolitic, cholangitic, cholostatic (primary) K74.3
  congestive K76.1
  Cruveilhier-Baumgarten K74.69
  cryptogenic (liver) K74.69
  due to
    hepatolenticular degeneration E83.01
    Wilson's disease E83.01
    xanthomatosis E78.2
  fatty K76.0
    alcoholic K70.0
  Hanot's (hypertrophic) K74.3
  hepatic — *see* Cirrhosis, liver
  hypertrophic K74.3
  Indian childhood K74.69
  kidney — *see* Sclerosis, renal
  Laennec's K70.30
    with ascites K70.31
    alcoholic K70.30
      with ascites K70.31
    nonalcoholic K74.69
  liver K74.60
    alcoholic K70.30
      with ascites K70.31
      fatty K70.0
    congenital P78.81
    syphilitic A52.74
  lung (chronic) J84.10
  macronodular K74.69
    alcoholic K70.30
      with ascites K70.31
  micronodular K74.69
    alcoholic K70.30
      with ascites K70.31
  mixed type K74.69
  monolobular K74.3
  nephritis — *see* Sclerosis, renal
  nutritional K74.69
    alcoholic K70.30
      with ascites K70.31
  obstructive — *see* Cirrhosis, biliary
  ovarian N83.8
  pancreas (duct) K86.89
  pigmentary E83.110
  portal K74.69
    alcoholic K70.30
      with ascites K70.31
  postnecrotic K74.69
    alcoholic K70.30
      with ascites K70.31
  pulmonary J84.10
  renal — *see* Sclerosis, renal
  spleen D73.2
  stasis K76.1
  Todd's K74.3
  unilobar K74.3
  xanthomatous (biliary) K74.5
    due to xanthomatosis (familial) (metabolic) (primary) E78.2
Cistern, subarachnoid R93.0
Citrullinemia E72.23
Citrullinuria E72.23
Civatte's disease or poikiloderma L57.3
Clam digger's itch B65.3
Clammy skin R23.1
Clap — *see* Gonorrhea
Clarke-Hadfield syndrome (pancreatic infantilism) K86.89
Clark's paralysis G80.9
Clastothrix L67.8
Claude Bernard-Horner syndrome G90.2

Claude Bernard-Horner syndrome — *continued*
  traumatic — *see* Injury, nerve, cervical sympathetic
Claude's disease or syndrome G46.3
Claudicatio venosa intermittens I87.8
Claudication (intermittent) I73.9
  cerebral (artery) G45.9
  spinal cord (arteriosclerotic) G95.19
    syphilitic A52.09
  venous (axillary) I87.8
Claustrophobia F40.240
Clavus (infected) L84
Clawfoot (congenital) Q66.89
  acquired — *see* Deformity, limb, clawfoot
Clawhand (acquired) — *see also* Deformity, limb, claw-hand
  congenital Q68.1
Clawtoe (congenital) Q66.89
  acquired — *see* Deformity, toe, specified NEC
Clay eating — *see* Pica
Cleansing of artificial opening — *see* Attention to, artificial, opening
Cleft (congenital) — *see also* Imperfect, closure
  alveolar process M26.79
  branchial (persistent) Q18.2
    cyst Q18.0
      fistula Q18.0
      sinus Q18.0
  cricoid cartilage, posterior Q31.8
  cyst Q18.0
    fistula Q18.0
    sinus Q18.0
  foot Q72.7 ☑
  hand Q71.6 ☑
  lip (unilateral) Q36.9
    with cleft palate Q37.9
      hard Q37.1
        with soft Q37.5
      soft Q37.3
        with hard Q37.5
      bilateral Q36.0
        with cleft palate Q37.8
          hard Q37.0
            with soft Q37.4
          soft Q37.2
            with hard Q37.4
      median Q36.1
  nose Q30.2
  palate Q35.9
    with cleft lip (unilateral) Q37.9
      bilateral Q37.8
    hard Q35.1
      with
        cleft lip (unilateral) Q37.1
          bilateral Q37.0
        soft Q35.5
          with cleft lip (unilateral) Q37.5
            bilateral Q37.4
    medial Q35.5
    soft Q35.3
      with
        cleft lip (unilateral) Q37.3
          bilateral Q37.2
        hard Q35.5
          with cleft lip (unilateral) Q37.5
            bilateral Q37.4
  penis Q55.69
  scrotum Q55.29
  thyroid cartilage Q31.8
  uvula Q35.7
Cleidocranial dysostosis Q74.0
Cleptomania F63.2
Clicking hip (newborn) R29.4
Climacteric (female) — *see also* Menopause
  arthritis (any site) NEC — *see* Arthritis, specified form NEC
  depression (single episode) F32.89
    recurrent episode F33.8
  male (symptoms) (syndrome) NEC N50.89
  melancholia (single episode) F32.89
    recurrent episode F33.8
  paranoid state F22
  polyarthritis NEC — *see* Arthritis, specified form NEC
  symptoms (female) N95.1
Clinical research investigation (clinical trial) (control subject) (normal comparison) (participant) Z00.6
Clitoris — *see* condition
Cloaca (persistent) Q43.7
Clonorchiasis, clonorchis infection (liver) B66.1

Clonus R25.8
Closed bite M26.29
Clostridium (C.) **perfringens, as cause of disease classified elsewhere** B96.7
Closure
  congenital, nose Q30.0
  cranial sutures, premature Q75.0
  defective or imperfect NEC — *see* Imperfect, closure
  fistula, delayed — *see* Fistula
  foramen ovale, imperfect Q21.1
  hymen N89.6
  interauricular septum, defective Q21.1
  interventricular septum, defective Q21.0
  lacrimal duct — *see also* Stenosis, lacrimal, duct
    congenital Q10.5
  nose (congenital) Q30.0
    acquired M95.0
  of artificial opening — *see* Attention to, artificial, opening
  vagina N89.5
  valve — *see* Endocarditis
  vulva N90.5
Clot (blood) — *see also* Embolism
  artery (obstruction) (occlusion) — *see* Embolism
  bladder N32.89
  brain (intradural or extradural) — *see* Occlusion, artery, cerebral
  circulation I74.9
  heart — *see also* Infarct, myocardium
    not resulting in infarction I51.3
  vein — *see* Thrombosis
Clouded state R40.1
  epileptic — *see* Epilepsy, specified NEC
  paroxysmal — *see* Epilepsy, specified NEC
Cloudy antrum, antra J32.0
Clouston's (hidrotic) **ectodermal dysplasia** Q82.4
Clubbed nail pachydermoperiostosis M89.40 *[L62]*
Clubbing of finger(s) (nails) R68.3
Clubfinger R68.3
  congenital Q68.1
Clubfoot (congenital) Q66.89
  acquired — *see* Deformity, limb, clubfoot
  equinovarus Q66.0- ☑
  paralytic — *see* Deformity, limb, clubfoot
Clubhand (congenital) (radial) Q71.4- ☑
  acquired — *see* Deformity, limb, clubhand
Clubnail R68.3
  congenital Q84.6
Clump, kidney Q63.1
Clumsiness, clumsy child syndrome F82
Cluttering F80.81
Clutton's joints A50.51 *[M12.80]*
Coagulation, intravascular (diffuse) (disseminated) — *see also* Defibrination syndrome
  complicating abortion — *see* Abortion, by type, complicated by, intravascular coagulation
  following ectopic or molar pregnancy O08.1
Coagulopathy — *see also* Defect, coagulation
  consumption D65
  intravascular D65
    newborn P60
Coalition
  calcaneo-scaphoid Q66.89
  tarsal Q66.89
Coalminer's
  elbow — *see* Bursitis, elbow, olecranon
  lung or pneumoconiosis J60
Coalworker's lung or pneumoconiosis J60
Coarctation
  aorta (preductal) (postductal) Q25.1
  pulmonary artery Q25.71
Coated tongue K14.3
Coats' disease (exudative retinopathy) — *see* Retinopathy, exudative
Cocaine-induced
  anxiety disorder F14.980
  bipolar and related disorder F14.94
  depressive disorder F14.94
  obsessive-compulsive and related disorder F14.988
  psychotic disorder F14.959
  sexual dysfunction F14.981
  sleep disorder F14.982
Cocainism — *see* Disorder, cocaine use
Coccidioidomycosis B38.9
  cutaneous B38.3
  disseminated B38.7
  generalized B38.7

▽ Subterms under main terms may continue to next column or page   ☑ Additional Character Required — Refer to the Tabular List for Character Selection   57

Circumcision — Coccidioidomycosis

Coccidioidomycosis — *continued*
  meninges B38.4
  prostate B38.81
  pulmonary B38.2
    acute B38.0
    chronic B38.1
  skin B38.3
  specified NEC B38.89
Coccidioidosis — *see* Coccidioidomycosis
Coccidiosis (intestinal) A07.3
Coccydynia, coccygodynia M53.3
Coccyx — *see* condition
Cochin-China diarrhea K90.1
Cockayne's syndrome Q87.19
Cocked up toe — *see* Deformity, toe, specified NEC
Cock's peculiar tumor L72.3
Codman's tumor — *see* Neoplasm, bone, benign
Coenurosis B71.8
Coffee-worker's lung J67.8
Cogan's syndrome H16.32- ☑
  oculomotor apraxia H51.8
Coitus, painful (female) N94.10
  male N53.12
  psychogenic F52.6
Cold J00
  with influenza, flu, or grippe — *see* Influenza, with,
    respiratory manifestations NEC
  agglutinin disease or hemoglobinuria (chronic) D59.12
  bronchial — *see* Bronchitis
  chest — *see* Bronchitis
  common (head) J00
  effects of T69.9 ☑
    specified effect NEC T69.8 ☑
  excessive, effects of T69.9 ☑
    specified effect NEC T69.8 ☑
  exhaustion from T69.8 ☑
  exposure to T69.9 ☑
    specified effect NEC T69.8 ☑
  head J00
  injury syndrome (newborn) P80.0
  on lung — *see* Bronchitis
  rose J30.1
  sensitivity, auto-immune D59.12
  symptoms J00
  virus J00
Coldsore B00.1
Colibacillosis A49.8
  as the cause of other disease — *see also* Escherichia
    coli B96.20
  generalized A41.50
Colic (bilious) (infantile) (intestinal) (recurrent) (spasmod-
    ic) R10.83
  abdomen R10.83
    psychogenic F45.8
  appendix, appendicular K38.8
  bile duct — *see* Calculus, bile duct
  biliary — *see* Calculus, bile duct
  common duct — *see* Calculus, bile duct
  cystic duct — *see* Calculus, gallbladder
  Devonshire NEC — *see* Poisoning, lead
  gallbladder — *see* Calculus, gallbladder
  gallstone — *see* Calculus, gallbladder
    gallbladder or cystic duct — *see* Calculus, gallblad-
      der
  hepatic (duct) — *see* Calculus, bile duct
  hysterical F45.8
  kidney N23
  lead NEC — *see* Poisoning, lead
  mucous K58.9
    with diarrhea K58.0
    psychogenic F54
  nephritic N23
  painter's NEC — *see* Poisoning, lead
  pancreas K86.89
  psychogenic F45.8
  renal N23
  saturnine NEC — *see* Poisoning, lead
  ureter N23
  urethral N36.8
    due to calculus N21.1
  uterus NEC N94.89
    menstrual — *see* Dysmenorrhea
  worm NOS B83.9
Colicystitis — *see* Cystitis
Colitis (acute) (catarrhal) (chronic) (noninfective) (hemor-
    rhagic) — *see also* Enteritis K52.9
  allergic K52.29

Colitis — *continued*
  allergic — *continued*
    with
      food protein-induced enterocolitis syndrome
        K52.21
      proctocolitis K52.29
  amebic (acute) — *see also* Amebiasis A06.0
    nondysenteric A06.2
  anthrax A22.2
  bacillary — *see* Infection, Shigella
  balantidial A07.0
  Clostridium difficile
    not specified as recurrent A04.72
    recurrent A04.71
  coccidial A07.3
  collagenous K52.831
  cystica superficialis K52.89
  dietary counseling and surveillance (for) Z71.3
  dietetic — *see also* Colitis, allergic K52.29
  drug-induced K52.1
  due to radiation K52.0
  eosinophilic K52.82
  food hypersensitivity — *see also* Colitis, allergic K52.29
  giardial A07.1
  granulomatous — *see* Enteritis, regional, large intestine
  indeterminate, so stated K52.3
  infectious — *see* Enteritis, infectious
  ischemic K55.9
    acute (subacute) — *see also* Ischemia, intestine,
      acute K55.039
    chronic K55.1
    due to mesenteric artery insufficiency K55.1
    fulminant (acute) — *see also* Ischemia, intestine,
      acute K55.039
  left sided K51.50
    with
      abscess K51.514
      complication K51.519
        specified NEC K51.518
      fistula K51.513
      obstruction K51.512
      rectal bleeding K51.511
  lymphocytic K52.832
  membranous
    psychogenic F54
  microscopic K52.839
    specified NEC K52.838
  mucous — *see* Syndrome, irritable, bowel
    psychogenic F54
  noninfective K52.9
    specified NEC K52.89
  polyposa — *see* Polyp, colon, inflammatory
  protozoal A07.9
  pseudomembranous
    not specified as recurrent A04.72
    recurrent A04.71
  pseudomucinous — *see* Syndrome, irritable, bowel
  regional — *see* Enteritis, regional, large intestine
    infectious A09
  segmental — *see* Enteritis, regional, large intestine
  septic — *see* Enteritis, infectious
  spastic K58.9
    with diarrhea K58.0
    psychogenic F54
  staphylococcal A04.8
    foodborne A05.0
  subacute ischemic — *see also* Ischemia, intestine, acute
    K55.039
  thromboulcerative — *see also* Ischemia, intestine, acute
    K55.039
  toxic NEC K52.1
    due to Clostridium difficile
      not specified as recurrent A04.72
      recurrent A04.71
  transmural — *see* Enteritis, regional, large intestine
  trichomonal A07.8
  tuberculous (ulcerative) A18.32
  ulcerative (chronic) K51.90
    with
      complication K51.919
        abscess K51.914
        fistula K51.913
        obstruction K51.912
        rectal bleeding K51.911
        specified complication NEC K51.918
    enterocolitis — *see* Enterocolitis, ulcerative
    ileocolitis — *see* Ileocolitis, ulcerative
    mucosal proctocolitis — *see* Proctocolitis, mucosal

Colitis — *continued*
  ulcerative — *continued*
    proctitis — *see* Proctitis, ulcerative
    pseudopolyposis — *see* Polyp, colon, inflammatory
    psychogenic F54
    rectosigmoiditis — *see* Rectosigmoiditis, ulcerative
    specified type NEC K51.80
      with
        complication K51.819
          abscess K51.814
          fistula K51.813
          obstruction K51.812
          rectal bleeding K51.811
          specified complication NEC K51.818
Collagenosis, collagen disease (nonvascular) (vascular)
    M35.9
  cardiovascular I42.8
  reactive perforating L87.1
  specified NEC M35.89
Collapse R55
  adrenal E27.2
  cardiorespiratory R57.0
  cardiovascular R57.0
    newborn P29.89
  circulatory (peripheral) R57.9
    during or after labor and delivery O75.1
    following ectopic or molar pregnancy O08.3
    newborn P29.89
  during or
    after labor and delivery O75.1
    resulting from a procedure, not elsewhere classified
      T81.10 ☑
  external ear canal — *see* Stenosis, external ear canal
  general R55
  heart — *see* Disease, heart
  heat T67.1 ☑
  hysterical F44.89
  labyrinth, membranous (congenital) Q16.5
  lung (massive) — *see also* Atelectasis J98.19
    pressure due to anesthesia (general) (local) or other
      sedation T88.2 ☑
      during labor and delivery O74.1
      in pregnancy O29.02- ☑
      postpartum, puerperal O89.09
  myocardial — *see* Disease, heart
  nervous F48.8
  neurocirculatory F45.8
  nose M95.0
  postoperative T81.10 ☑
  pulmonary — *see also* Atelectasis J98.19
    newborn — *see* Atelectasis
  trachea J39.8
  tracheobronchial J98.09
  valvular — *see* Endocarditis
  vascular (peripheral) R57.9
    during or after labor and delivery O75.1
    following ectopic or molar pregnancy O08.3
    newborn P29.89
  vertebra M48.50- ☑
    cervical region M48.52- ☑
    cervicothoracic region M48.53- ☑
    in (due to)
      metastasis — *see* Collapse, vertebra, in, specified
        disease NEC
      osteoporosis — *see also* Osteoporosis M80.88 ☑
        cervical region M80.88 ☑
        cervicothoracic region M80.88 ☑
        lumbar region M80.88 ☑
        lumbosacral region M80.88 ☑
        multiple sites M80.88 ☑
        occipito-atlanto-axial region M80.88 ☑
        sacrococcygeal region M80.88 ☑
        thoracic region M80.88 ☑
        thoracolumbar region M80.88 ☑
      specified disease NEC M48.50- ☑
        cervical region M48.52- ☑
        cervicothoracic region M48.53- ☑
        lumbar region M48.56- ☑
        lumbosacral region M48.57- ☑
        occipito-atlanto-axial region M48.51- ☑
        sacrococcygeal region M48.58- ☑
        thoracic region M48.54- ☑
        thoracolumbar region M48.55- ☑
    lumbar region M48.56- ☑
    lumbosacral region M48.57- ☑
    occipito-atlanto-axial region M48.51- ☑
    sacrococcygeal region M48.58- ☑

Collapse — *continued*
  vertebra — *continued*
    thoracic region M48.54- ☑
    thoracolumbar region M48.55- ☑
Collateral — *see also* condition
  circulation (venous) I87.8
  dilation, veins I87.8
Colles' fracture S52.53- ☑
Collet (-Sicard) syndrome G52.7
Collier's asthma or lung J60
Collodion baby Q80.2
Colloid nodule (of thyroid) (cystic) E04.1
Coloboma (iris) Q13.0
  eyelid Q10.3
  fundus Q14.8
  lens Q12.2
  optic disc (congenital) Q14.2
    acquired H47.31- ☑
Coloenteritis — *see* Enteritis
Colon — *see* condition
Colonization
  MRSA (Methicillin resistant Staphylococcus aureus) Z22.322
  MSSA (Methicillin susceptible Staphylococcus aureus) Z22.321
  status — *see* Carrier (suspected) of
Coloptosis K63.4
Color blindness — *see* Deficiency, color vision
Colostomy
  attention to Z43.3
  fitting or adjustment Z46.89
  malfunctioning K94.03
  status Z93.3
Colpitis (acute) — *see* Vaginitis
Colpocele N81.5
Colpocystitis — *see* Vaginitis
Colpospasm N94.2
Column, spinal, vertebral — *see* condition
Coma R40.20
  with
    motor response (none) R40.231 ☑
      abnormal extensor posturing to pain or noxious stimuli (< 2 years of age) R40.232 ☑
      abnormal flexure posturing to pain or noxious stimuli (0-5 years of age) R40.233 ☑
      extensor posturing to pain or noxious stimuli (2-5 years of age) R40.232 ☑
      flexion/decorticate posturing (< 2 years of age) R40.233 ☑
      localizes pain (2-5 years of age) R40.235 ☑
      normal or spontaneous movement (< 2 years of age) R40.236 ☑
      obeys commands (2-5 years of age) R40.236 ☑
      score of
        1 R40.231 ☑
        2 R40.232 ☑
        3 R40.233 ☑
        4 R40.234 ☑
        5 R40.235 ☑
        6 R40.236 ☑
      withdraws from pain or noxious stimuli (0-5 years of age) R40.234 ☑
      withdraws to touch (< 2 years of age) R40.235 ☑
    opening of eyes (never) R40.211 ☑
      in response to
        pain R40.212 ☑
        sound R40.213 ☑
      score of
        1 R40.211 ☑
        2 R40.212 ☑
        3 R40.213 ☑
        4 R40.214 ☑
      spontaneous R40.214 ☑
    verbal response (none) R40.221 ☑
      confused conversation R40.224 ☑
      cooing or babbling or crying appropriately (<2 years of age) R40.225 ☑
      inappropriate crying or screaming (< 2 years of age) R40.223 ☑
      inappropriate words (2-5 years of age) R40.224 ☑
      inappropriate words R40.223 ☑
      incomprehensible sounds (2-5 years of age) R40.222 ☑
      incomprehensible words R40.222 ☑
      irritable cries (< 2 years of age) R40.224 ☑

Coma — *continued*
  with — *continued*
    verbal response — *continued*
      moans/grunts to pain; restless (< 2 years old) R40.222 ☑
      oriented R40.225 ☑
      score of
        1 R40.221 ☑
        2 R40.222 ☑
        3 R40.223 ☑
        4 R40.224 ☑
        5 R40.225 ☑
      screaming (2-5 years of age) R40.223 ☑
      uses appropriate words (2-5 years of age) R40.225 ☑
  eclamptic — *see* Eclampsia
  epileptic — *see* Epilepsy
  Glasgow, scale score — *see* Glasgow coma scale
  hepatic — *see* Failure, hepatic, by type, with coma
  hyperglycemic (diabetic) — *see* Diabetes, by type, with hyperosmolarity, with coma
  hyperosmolar (diabetic) — *see* Diabetes, by type, with hyperosmolarity, with coma
  hypoglycemic (diabetic) — *see* Diabetes, by type, with hypoglycemia, with coma
    nondiabetic E15
  in diabetes — *see* Diabetes, coma
  insulin-induced — *see* Coma, hypoglycemic
  ketoacidotic (diabetic) — *see* Diabetes, by type, with ketoacidosis, with coma
  myxedematous E03.5
  newborn P91.5
  persistent vegetative state R40.3
  specified NEC, without documented Glasgow coma scale score, or with partial Glasgow coma scale score reported R40.244 ☑
Comatose — *see* Coma
Combat fatigue F43.0
Combined — *see* condition
Comedo, comedones (giant) L70.0
Comedocarcinoma — *see also* Neoplasm, breast, malignant
  noninfiltrating
    breast D05.8- ☑
    specified site — *see* Neoplasm, in situ, by site
    unspecified site D05.8- ☑
Comedomastitis — *see* Ectasia, mammary duct
Comminuted fracture — *code as* Fracture, closed
Common
  arterial trunk Q20.0
  atrioventricular canal Q21.2
  atrium Q21.1
  cold (head) J00
  truncus (arteriosus) Q20.0
  variable immunodeficiency — *see* Immunodeficiency, common variable
  ventricle Q20.4
Commotio, commotion (current)
  brain — *see* Injury, intracranial, concussion
  cerebri — *see* Injury, intracranial, concussion
  retinae S05.8X- ☑
  spinal cord — *see* Injury, spinal cord, by region
  spinalis — *see* Injury, spinal cord, by region
Communication
  between
    base of aorta and pulmonary artery Q21.4
    left ventricle and right atrium Q20.5
    pericardial sac and pleural sac Q34.8
    pulmonary artery and pulmonary vein, congenital Q25.72
    congenital between uterus and digestive or urinary tract Q51.7
Compartment syndrome (deep) (posterior) (traumatic) T79.A0 ☑ (*following* T79.7)
  abdomen T79.A3 ☑ (*following* T79.7)
  lower extremity (hip, buttock, thigh, leg, foot, toes) T79.A2 ☑ (*following* T79.7)
  nontraumatic
    abdomen M79.A3 (*following* M79.7)
    lower extremity (hip, buttock, thigh, leg, foot, toes) M79.A2- ☑ (*following* M79.7)
    specified site NEC M79.A9 (*following* M79.7)
    upper extremity (shoulder, arm, forearm, wrist, hand, fingers) M79.A1- ☑ (*following* M79.7)
  specified site NEC T79.A9 ☑ (*following* T79.7)
  upper extremity (shoulder, arm, forearm, wrist, hand, fingers) T79.A1- ☑ (*following* T79.7)

Compensation
  failure — *see* Disease, heart
  neurosis, psychoneurosis — *see* Disorder, factitious
Complaint — *see also* Disease
  bowel, functional K59.9
    psychogenic F45.8
  intestine, functional K59.9
    psychogenic F45.8
  kidney — *see* Disease, renal
  miners' J60
Complete — *see* condition
Complex
  Addison-Schilder E71.528
  cardiorenal — *see* Hypertension, cardiorenal
  Costen's M26.69
  disseminated mycobacterium avium- intracellulare (DMAC) A31.2
  Eisenmenger's (ventricular septal defect) I27.83
  hypersexual F52.8
  jumped process, spine — *see* Dislocation, vertebra
  primary, tuberculous A15.7
  Schilder-Addison E71.528
  subluxation (vertebral) M99.19
    abdomen M99.19
    acromioclavicular M99.17
    cervical region M99.11
    cervicothoracic M99.11
    costochondral M99.18
    costovertebral M99.18
    head region M99.10
    hip M99.15
    lower extremity M99.16
    lumbar region M99.13
    lumbosacral M99.13
    occipitocervical M99.10
    pelvic region M99.15
    pubic M99.15
    rib cage M99.18
    sacral region M99.14
    sacrococcygeal M99.14
    sacroiliac M99.14
    specified NEC M99.19
    sternochondral M99.18
    sternoclavicular M99.17
    thoracic region M99.12
    thoracolumbar M99.12
    upper extremity M99.17
  Taussig-Bing (transposition, aorta and overriding pulmonary artery) Q20.1
Complication(s) (from) (of)
  accidental puncture or laceration during a procedure (of) — *see* Complications, intraoperative (intraprocedural), puncture or laceration
  amputation stump (surgical) (late) NEC T87.9
    dehiscence T87.81
    infection or inflammation T87.40
      lower limb T87.4- ☑
      upper limb T87.4- ☑
    necrosis T87.50
      lower limb T87.5- ☑
      upper limb T87.5- ☑
    neuroma T87.30
      lower limb T87.3- ☑
      upper limb T87.3- ☑
    specified type NEC T87.89
  anastomosis (and bypass) — *see also* Complications, prosthetic device or implant
    intestinal (internal) NEC K91.89
      involving urinary tract N99.89
    urinary tract (involving intestinal tract) N99.89
    vascular — *see* Complications, cardiovascular device or implant
  anesthesia, anesthetic — *see also* Anesthesia, complication T88.59 ☑
    brain, postpartum, puerperal O89.2
    cardiac
      in
        labor and delivery O74.2
        pregnancy O29.19- ☑
      postpartum, puerperal O89.1
    central nervous system
      in
        labor and delivery O74.3
        pregnancy O29.29- ☑
      postpartum, puerperal O89.2
    difficult or failed intubation T88.4 ☑
      in pregnancy O29.6- ☑

Complication(s) — *continued*
  anesthesia, anesthetic — *see also* Anesthesia, compli-
      cation — *continued*
    failed sedation (conscious) (moderate) during pro-
        cedure T88.52 ☑
    general, unintended awareness during procedure
        T88.53 ☑
    hyperthermia, malignant T88.3 ☑
    hypothermia T88.51 ☑
    intubation failure T88.4 ☑
    malignant hyperthermia T88.3 ☑
    pulmonary
      in
        labor and delivery O74.1
        pregnancy NEC O29.09- ☑
      postpartum, puerperal O89.09
    shock T88.2 ☑
    spinal and epidural
      in
        labor and delivery NEC O74.6
          headache O74.5
        pregnancy NEC O29.5X- ☑
      postpartum, puerperal NEC O89.5
        headache O89.4
    unintended awareness under general anesthesia
        during procedure T88.53 ☑
  anti-reflux device — *see* Complications, esophageal
      anti-reflux device
  aortic (bifurcation) graft — *see* Complications, graft,
      vascular
  aortocoronary (bypass) graft — *see* Complications,
      coronary artery (bypass) graft
  aortofemoral (bypass) graft — *see* Complications, ex-
      tremity artery (bypass) graft
  arteriovenous
    fistula, surgically created T82.9 ☑
      embolism T82.818 ☑
      fibrosis T82.828 ☑
      hemorrhage T82.838 ☑
      infection or inflammation T82.7 ☑
      mechanical
        breakdown T82.510 ☑
        displacement T82.520 ☑
        leakage T82.530 ☑
        malposition T82.520 ☑
        obstruction T82.590 ☑
        perforation T82.590 ☑
        protrusion T82.590 ☑
      pain T82.848 ☑
      specified type NEC T82.898 ☑
      stenosis T82.858 ☑
      thrombosis T82.868 ☑
    shunt, surgically created T82.9 ☑
      embolism T82.818 ☑
      fibrosis T82.828 ☑
      hemorrhage T82.838 ☑
      infection or inflammation T82.7 ☑
      mechanical
        breakdown T82.511 ☑
        displacement T82.521 ☑
        leakage T82.531 ☑
        malposition T82.521 ☑
        obstruction T82.591 ☑
        perforation T82.591 ☑
        protrusion T82.591 ☑
      pain T82.848 ☑
      specified type NEC T82.898 ☑
      stenosis T82.858 ☑
      thrombosis T82.868 ☑
  arthroplasty — *see* Complications, joint prosthesis
  artificial
    fertilization or insemination N98.9
      attempted introduction (of)
        embryo in embryo transfer N98.3
        ovum following in vitro fertilization N98.2
      hyperstimulation of ovaries N98.1
      infection N98.0
      specified NEC N98.8
    heart T82.9 ☑
      embolism T82.817 ☑
      fibrosis T82.827 ☑
      hemorrhage T82.837 ☑
      infection or inflammation T82.7 ☑
      mechanical
        breakdown T82.512 ☑
        displacement T82.522 ☑
        leakage T82.532 ☑

Complication(s) — *continued*
  artificial — *continued*
    heart — *continued*
      mechanical — *continued*
        malposition T82.522 ☑
        obstruction T82.592 ☑
        perforation T82.592 ☑
        protrusion T82.592 ☑
      pain T82.847 ☑
      specified type NEC T82.897 ☑
      stenosis T82.857 ☑
      thrombosis T82.867 ☑
    opening
      cecostomy — *see* Complications, colostomy
      colostomy — *see* Complications, colostomy
      cystostomy — *see* Complications, cystostomy
      enterostomy — *see* Complications, enterostomy
      gastrostomy — *see* Complications, gastrostomy
      ileostomy — *see* Complications, enterostomy
      jejunostomy — *see* Complications, enterostomy
      nephrostomy — *see* Complications, stoma, uri-
          nary tract
      tracheostomy — *see* Complications, tracheosto-
          my
      ureterostomy — *see* Complications, stoma, uri-
          nary tract
      urethrostomy — *see* Complications, stoma, uri-
          nary tract
  balloon implant or device
    gastrointestinal T85.9 ☑
      embolism T85.818 ☑
      fibrosis T85.828 ☑
      hemorrhage T85.838 ☑
      infection and inflammation T85.79 ☑
      pain T85.848 ☑
      specified type NEC T85.898 ·☑
      stenosis T85.858 ☑
      thrombosis T85.868 ☑
    vascular (counterpulsation) T82.9 ☑
      embolism T82.818 ☑
      fibrosis T82.828 ☑
      hemorrhage T82.838 ☑
      infection or inflammation T82.7 ☑
      mechanical
        breakdown T82.513 ☑
        displacement T82.523 ☑
        leakage T82.533 ☑
        malposition T82.523 ☑
        obstruction T82.593 ☑
        perforation T82.593 ☑
        protrusion T82.593 ☑
      pain T82.848 ☑
      specified type NEC T82.898 ☑
      stenosis T82.858 ☑
      thrombosis T82.868 ☑
  bariatric procedure
    gastric band procedure K95.09
      infection K95.01
    specified procedure NEC K95.89
      infection K95.81
  bile duct implant (prosthetic) T85.9 ☑
    embolism T85.818 ☑
    fibrosis T85.828 ☑
    hemorrhage T85.838 ☑
    infection and inflammation T85.79 ☑
    mechanical
      breakdown T85.510 ☑
      displacement T85.520 ☑
      malfunction T85.510 ☑
      malposition T85.520 ☑
      obstruction T85.590 ☑
      perforation T85.590 ☑
      protrusion T85.590 ☑
      specified NEC T85.590 ☑
    pain T85.848 ☑
    specified type NEC T85.898 ☑
    stenosis T85.858 ☑
    thrombosis T85.868 ☑
  bladder device (auxiliary) — *see* Complications, geni-
      tourinary, device or implant, urinary system
  bleeding (postoperative) — *see* Complication, postop-
      erative, hemorrhage
    intraoperative — *see* Complication, intraoperative,
        hemorrhage
  blood vessel graft — *see* Complications, graft, vascular

Complication(s) — *continued*
  bone
    device NEC T84.9 ☑
      embolism T84.81 ☑
      fibrosis T84.82 ☑
      hemorrhage T84.83 ☑
      infection or inflammation T84.7 ☑
      mechanical
        breakdown T84.318 ☑
        displacement T84.328 ☑
        malposition T84.328 ☑
        obstruction T84.398 ☑
        perforation T84.398 ☑
        protrusion T84.398 ☑
      pain T84.84 ☑
      specified type NEC T84.89 ☑
      stenosis T84.85 ☑
      thrombosis T84.86 ☑
    graft — *see* Complications, graft, bone
    growth stimulator (electrode) — *see* Complications,
        electronic stimulator device, bone
    marrow transplant — *see* Complications, transplant,
        bone, marrow
  brain neurostimulator (electrode) — *see* Complications,
      electronic stimulator device, brain
  breast implant (prosthetic) T85.9 ☑
    capsular contracture T85.44 ☑
    embolism T85.818 ☑
    fibrosis T85.828 ☑
    hemorrhage T85.838 ☑
    infection and inflammation T85.79 ☑
    mechanical
      breakdown T85.41 ☑
      displacement T85.42 ☑
      leakage T85.43 ☑
      malposition T85.42 ☑
      obstruction T85.49 ☑
      perforation T85.49 ☑
      protrusion T85.49 ☑
      specified NEC T85.49 ☑
    pain T85.848 ☑
    specified type NEC T85.898 ☑
    stenosis T85.858 ☑
    thrombosis T85.868 ☑
  bypass — *see also* Complications, prosthetic device or
      implant
    aortocoronary — *see* Complications, coronary artery
        (bypass) graft
    arterial — *see also* Complications, graft, vascular
      extremity — *see* Complications, extremity artery
          (bypass) graft
  cardiac — *see also* Disease, heart
    device, implant or graft T82.9 ☑
      embolism T82.817 ☑
      fibrosis T82.827 ☑
      hemorrhage T82.837 ☑
      infection or inflammation T82.7 ☑
        valve prosthesis T82.6 ☑
      mechanical
        breakdown T82.519 ☑
          specified device NEC T82.518 ☑
        displacement T82.529 ☑
          specified device NEC T82.528 ☑
        leakage T82.539 ☑
          specified device NEC T82.538 ☑
        malposition T82.529 ☑
          specified device NEC T82.528 ☑
        obstruction T82.599 ☑
          specified device NEC T82.598 ☑
        perforation T82.599 ☑
          specified device NEC T82.598 ☑
        protrusion T82.599 ☑
          specified device NEC T82.598 ☑
      pain T82.847 ☑
      specified type NEC T82.897 ☑
      stenosis T82.857 ☑
      thrombosis T82.867 ☑
  cardiovascular device, graft or implant T82.9 ☑
    aortic graft — *see* Complications, graft, vascular
    arteriovenous
      fistula, artificial — *see* Complication, arteriove-
          nous, fistula, surgically created
      shunt — *see* Complication, arteriovenous, shunt,
          surgically created
    artificial heart — *see* Complication, artificial, heart

☑ **Additional Character Required — Refer to the Tabular List for Character Selection**   ▽ **Subterms under main terms may continue to next column or page**

Complication(s) — *continued*
  cardiovascular device, graft or implant — *continued*
    balloon (counterpulsation) device — *see* Complication, balloon implant, vascular
    carotid artery graft — *see* Complications, graft, vascular
    coronary bypass graft — *see* Complication, coronary artery (bypass) graft
    dialysis catheter (vascular) — *see* Complication, catheter, dialysis
    electronic T82.9 ☑
      electrode T82.9 ☑
        embolism T82.817 ☑
        fibrosis T82.827 ☑
        hemorrhage T82.837 ☑
        infection T82.7 ☑
        mechanical
          breakdown T82.110 ☑
          displacement T82.120 ☑
          leakage T82.190 ☑
          obstruction T82.190 ☑
          perforation T82.190 ☑
          protrusion T82.190 ☑
          specified type NEC T82.190 ☑
        pain T82.847 ☑
        specified NEC T82.897 ☑
        stenosis T82.857 ☑
        thrombosis T82.867 ☑
      embolism T82.817 ☑
      fibrosis T82.827 ☑
      hemorrhage T82.837 ☑
      infection T82.7 ☑
      mechanical
        breakdown T82.119 ☑
        displacement T82.129 ☑
        leakage T82.199 ☑
        obstruction T82.199 ☑
        perforation T82.199 ☑
        protrusion T82.199 ☑
        specified type NEC T82.199 ☑
      pain T82.847 ☑
      pulse generator T82.9 ☑
        embolism T82.817 ☑
        fibrosis T82.827 ☑
        hemorrhage T82.837 ☑
        infection T82.7 ☑
        mechanical
          breakdown T82.111 ☑
          displacement T82.121 ☑
          leakage T82.191 ☑
          obstruction T82.191 ☑
          perforation T82.191 ☑
          protrusion T82.191 ☑
          specified type NEC T82.191 ☑
        pain T82.847 ☑
        specified NEC T82.897 ☑
        stenosis T82.857 ☑
        thrombosis T82.867 ☑
      specified condition NEC T82.897 ☑
      specified device NEC T82.9 ☑
        embolism T82.817 ☑
        fibrosis T82.827 ☑
        hemorrhage T82.837 ☑
        infection T82.7 ☑
        mechanical
          breakdown T82.118 ☑
          displacement T82.128 ☑
          leakage T82.198 ☑
          obstruction T82.198 ☑
          perforation T82.198 ☑
          protrusion T82.198 ☑
          specified type NEC T82.198 ☑
        pain T82.847 ☑
        specified NEC T82.897 ☑
        stenosis T82.857 ☑
        thrombosis T82.867 ☑
      stenosis T82.857 ☑
      thrombosis T82.867 ☑
    extremity artery graft — *see* Complication, extremity artery (bypass) graft
    femoral artery graft — *see* Complication, extremity artery (bypass) graft
    heart
      transplant — *see* Complication, transplant, heart
      valve — *see* Complication, prosthetic device, heart valve

Complication(s) — *continued*
  cardiovascular device, graft or implant — *continued*
    heart — *continued*
      valve — *see* Complication, prosthetic device, heart valve — *continued*
        graft — *see* Complication, heart, valve, graft
    heart-lung transplant — *see* Complication, transplant, heart, with lung
    infection or inflammation T82.7 ☑
    umbrella device — *see* Complication, umbrella device, vascular
    vascular graft (or anastosis) — *see* Complication, graft, vascular
  carotid artery (bypass) graft — *see* Complications, graft, vascular
  catheter (device) NEC — *see also* Complications, prosthetic device or implant
    cranial infusion
      infection and inflammation T85.735 ☑
      mechanical
        breakdown T85.610 ☑
        displacement T85.620 ☑
        leakage T85.630 ☑
        malfunction T85.690 ☑
        malposition T85.620 ☑
        obstruction T85.690 ☑
        perforation T85.690 ☑
        protrusion T85.690 ☑
        specified NEC T85.690 ☑
    cystostomy T83.9 ☑
      embolism T83.81 ☑
      fibrosis T83.82 ☑
      hemorrhage T83.83 ☑
      infection and inflammation T83.510 ☑
      mechanical
        breakdown T83.010 ☑
        displacement T83.020 ☑
        leakage T83.030 ☑
        malposition T83.020 ☑
        obstruction T83.090 ☑
        perforation T83.090 ☑
        protrusion T83.090 ☑
        specified NEC T83.090 ☑
      pain T83.84 ☑
      specified type NEC T83.89 ☑
      stenosis T83.85 ☑
      thrombosis T83.86 ☑
    dialysis (vascular) T82.9 ☑
      embolism T82.818 ☑
      fibrosis T82.828 ☑
      hemorrhage T82.838 ☑
      infection and inflammation T82.7 ☑
      intraperitoneal — *see* Complications, catheter, intraperitoneal
      mechanical
        breakdown T82.41 ☑
        displacement T82.42 ☑
        leakage T82.43 ☑
        malposition T82.42 ☑
        obstruction T82.49 ☑
        perforation T82.49 ☑
        protrusion T82.49 ☑
      pain T82.848 ☑
      specified type NEC T82.898 ☑
      stenosis T82.858 ☑
      thrombosis T82.868 ☑
    epidural infusion T85.9 ☑
      embolism T85.810 ☑
      fibrosis T85.820 ☑
      hemorrhage T85.830 ☑
      infection and inflammation T85.735 ☑
      mechanical
        breakdown T85.610 ☑
        displacement T85.620 ☑
        leakage T85.630 ☑
        malfunction T85.610 ☑
        malposition T85.620 ☑
        obstruction T85.690 ☑
        perforation T85.690 ☑
        protrusion T85.690 ☑
        specified NEC T85.690 ☑
      pain T85.840 ☑
      specified type NEC T85.890 ☑
      stenosis T85.850 ☑
      thrombosis T85.860 ☑
    intraperitoneal dialysis T85.9 ☑

Complication(s) — *continued*
  catheter — *see also* Complications, prosthetic device or implant — *continued*
    intraperitoneal dialysis — *continued*
      embolism T85.818 ☑
      fibrosis T85.828 ☑
      hemorrhage T85.838 ☑
      infection and inflammation T85.71 ☑
      mechanical
        breakdown T85.611 ☑
        displacement T85.621 ☑
        leakage T85.631 ☑
        malfunction T85.611 ☑
        malposition T85.621 ☑
        obstruction T85.691 ☑
        perforation T85.691 ☑
        protrusion T85.691 ☑
        specified NEC T85.691 ☑
      pain T85.848 ☑
      specified type NEC T85.898 ☑
      stenosis T85.858 ☑
      thrombosis T85.868 ☑
    intrathecal infusion
      infection and inflammation T85.735 ☑
      mechanical
        breakdown T85.610 ☑
        displacement T85.620 ☑
        leakage T85.630 ☑
        malfunction T85.690 ☑
        malposition T85.620 ☑
        obstruction T85.690 ☑
        perforation T85.690 ☑
        protrusion T85.690 ☑
        specified NEC T85.690 ☑
    intravenous infusion T82.9 ☑
      embolism T82.818 ☑
      fibrosis T82.828 ☑
      hemorrhage T82.838 ☑
      infection or inflammation T82.7 ☑
      mechanical
        breakdown T82.514 ☑
        displacement T82.524 ☑
        leakage T82.534 ☑
        malposition T82.524 ☑
        obstruction T82.594 ☑
        perforation T82.594 ☑
        protrusion T82.594 ☑
      pain T82.848 ☑
      specified type NEC T82.898 ☑
      stenosis T82.858 ☑
      thrombosis T82.868 ☑
    spinal infusion
      infection and inflammation T85.735 ☑
      mechanical
        breakdown T85.610 ☑
        displacement T85.620 ☑
        leakage T85.630 ☑
        malfunction T85.690 ☑
        malposition T85.620 ☑
        obstruction T85.690 ☑
        perforation T85.690 ☑
        protrusion T85.690 ☑
        specified NEC T85.690 ☑
    subarachnoid infusion
      infection and inflammation T85.735 ☑
      mechanical
        breakdown T85.610 ☑
        displacement T85.620 ☑
        leakage T85.630 ☑
        malfunction T85.690 ☑
        malposition T85.620 ☑
        obstruction T85.690 ☑
        perforation T85.690 ☑
        protrusion T85.690 ☑
        specified NEC T85.690 ☑
    subdural infusion T85.9 ☑
      embolism T85.810 ☑
      fibrosis T85.820 ☑
      hemorrhage T85.830 ☑
      infection and inflammation T85.735 ☑
      mechanical
        breakdown T85.610 ☑
        displacement T85.620 ☑
        leakage T85.630 ☑
        malfunction T85.610 ☑
        malposition T85.620 ☑

▽ Subterms under main terms may continue to next column or page   ☑ Additional Character Required — Refer to the Tabular List for Character Selection   61

Complication — Complication

Complication(s) — *continued*
catheter — *see also* Complications, prosthetic device or implant — *continued*
  subdural infusion — *continued*
    mechanical — *continued*
      obstruction T85.690 ☑
      perforation T85.690 ☑
      protrusion T85.690 ☑
      specified NEC T85.690 ☑
    pain T85.840 ☑
    specified type NEC T85.890 ☑
    stenosis T85.850 ☑
    thrombosis T85.860 ☑
  urethral T83.9
    displacement T83.028 ☑
    embolism T83.81 ☑
    fibrosis T83.82 ☑
    hemorrhage T83.83 ☑
    indwelling
      breakdown T83.011 ☑
      displacement T83.021 ☑
      infection and inflammation T83.511 ☑
      leakage T83.031 ☑
      specified complication NEC T83.091 ☑
    infection and inflammation T83.511 ☑
    leakage T83.038 ☑
    malposition T83.028 ☑
    mechanical
      breakdown T83.011 ☑
    obstruction (mechanical) T83.091 ☑
    pain T83.84 ☑
    perforation T83.091 ☑
    protrusion T83.091 ☑
    specified type NEC T83.091 ☑
    stenosis T83.85 ☑
    thrombosis T83.86 ☑
  urinary NEC
    breakdown T83.018 ☑
    displacement T83.028 ☑
    infection and inflammation T83.518 ☑
    leakage T83.038 ☑
    specified complication NEC T83.098 ☑
cecostomy (stoma) — *see* Complications, colostomy
cesarean delivery wound NEC O90.89
  disruption O90.0
  hematoma O90.2
  infection (following delivery) O86.00
chemotherapy (antineoplastic) NEC T88.7 ☑
chimeric antigen receptor (CAR-T) cell therapy T80.82 ☑
chin implant (prosthetic) — *see* Complication, prosthetic device or implant, specified NEC
circulatory system I99.8
  intraoperative I97.88
  postprocedural I97.89
    following cardiac surgery — *see also* Infarct, myocardium, associated with revascularization procedure I97.19- ☑
      postcardiotomy syndrome I97.0
    hypertension I97.3
    lymphedema after mastectomy I97.2
    postcardiotomy syndrome I97.0
    specified NEC I97.89
colostomy (stoma) K94.00
  hemorrhage K94.01
  infection K94.02
  malfunction K94.03
  mechanical K94.03
  specified complication NEC K94.09
contraceptive device, intrauterine — *see* Complications, intrauterine, contraceptive device
cord (umbilical) — *see* Complications, umbilical cord
corneal graft — *see* Complications, graft, cornea
coronary artery (bypass) graft T82.9 ☑
  atherosclerosis — *see* Arteriosclerosis, coronary (artery),
  embolism T82.818 ☑
  fibrosis T82.828 ☑
  hemorrhage T82.838 ☑
  infection and inflammation T82.7 ☑
  mechanical
    breakdown T82.211 ☑
    displacement T82.212 ☑
    leakage T82.213 ☑
    malposition T82.212 ☑
    obstruction T82.218 ☑
    perforation T82.218 ☑

Complication(s) — *continued*
coronary artery graft — *continued*
  mechanical — *continued*
    protrusion T82.218 ☑
    specified NEC T82.218 ☑
  pain T82.848 ☑
  specified type NEC T82.898 ☑
  stenosis T82.858 ☑
  thrombosis T82.868 ☑
counterpulsation device (balloon), intra-aortic — *see* Complications, balloon implant, vascular
cystostomy (stoma) N99.518
  catheter — *see* Complications, catheter, cystostomy
  hemorrhage N99.510
  infection N99.511
  malfunction N99.512
  specified type NEC N99.518
delivery — *see also* Complications, obstetric O75.9
  procedure (instrumental) (manual) (surgical) O75.4
  specified NEC O75.89
dialysis (peritoneal) (renal) — *see also* Complications, infusion
  catheter (vascular) — *see* Complication, catheter, dialysis
    peritoneal, intraperitoneal — *see* Complications, catheter, intraperitoneal
dorsal column (spinal) neurostimulator — *see* Complications, electronic stimulator device, spinal cord
drug NEC T88.7 ☑
ear procedure — *see also* Disorder, ear
  intraoperative H95.88
    hematoma — *see* Complications, intraoperative, hemorrhage (hematoma) (of), ear
    hemorrhage — *see* Complications, intraoperative, hemorrhage (hematoma) (of), ear
    laceration — *see* Complications, intraoperative, puncture or laceration..., ear
    specified NEC H95.88
  postoperative H95.89
    external ear canal stenosis H95.81- ☑
    hematoma — *see* Complications, postprocedural, hematoma (of), ear
    hemorrhage — *see* Complications, postprocedural, hemorrhage (of), ear
    postmastoidectomy — *see* Complications, postmastoidectomy
    seroma — *see* Complications, postprocedural, seroma (of), mastoid process
    specified NEC H95.89
ectopic pregnancy O08.9
  damage to pelvic organs O08.6
  embolism O08.2
  genital infection O08.0
  hemorrhage (delayed) (excessive) O08.1
  metabolic disorder O08.5
  renal failure O08.4
  shock O08.3
  specified type NEC O08.0
  venous complication NEC O08.7
electronic stimulator device
  bladder (urinary) — *see* Complications, electronic stimulator device, urinary
  bone T84.9 ☑
    breakdown T84.310 ☑
    displacement T84.320 ☑
    embolism T84.81 ☑
    fibrosis T84.82 ☑
    hemorrhage T84.83 ☑
    infection or inflammation T84.7 ☑
    malfunction T84.310 ☑
    malposition T84.320 ☑
    mechanical NEC T84.390 ☑
    obstruction T84.390 ☑
    pain T84.84 ☑
    perforation T84.390 ☑
    protrusion T84.390 ☑
    specified type NEC T84.89 ☑
    stenosis T84.85 ☑
    thrombosis T84.86 ☑
  brain T85.9 ☑
    embolism T85.810 ☑
    fibrosis T85.820 ☑
    hemorrhage T85.830 ☑
    infection and inflammation T85.731 ☑
    mechanical
      breakdown T85.110 ☑
      displacement T85.120 ☑

Complication(s) — *continued*
electronic stimulator device — *continued*
  brain — *continued*
    mechanical — *continued*
      leakage T85.190 ☑
      malposition T85.120 ☑
      obstruction T85.190 ☑
      perforation T85.190 ☑
      protrusion T85.190 ☑
      specified NEC T85.190 ☑
    pain T85.840 ☑
    specified type NEC T85.890 ☑
    stenosis T85.850 ☑
    thrombosis T85.860 ☑
  cardiac (defibrillator) (pacemaker) — *see* Complications, cardiovascular device or implant, electronic
  generator (brain) (gastric) (peripheral) (sacral) (spinal)
    breakdown T85.113 ☑
    displacement T85.123 ☑
    leakage T85.193 ☑
    malposition T85.123 ☑
    obstruction T85.193 ☑
    perforation T85.193 ☑
    protrusion T85.193 ☑
    specified type NEC T85.193 ☑
  muscle T84.9 ☑
    breakdown T84.418 ☑
    displacement T84.428 ☑
    embolism T84.81 ☑
    fibrosis T84.82 ☑
    hemorrhage T84.83 ☑
    infection or inflammation T84.7 ☑
    mechanical NEC T84.498 ☑
    pain T84.84 ☑
    specified type NEC T84.89 ☑
    stenosis T84.85 ☑
    thrombosis T84.86 ☑
  nervous system T85.9 ☑
    brain — *see* Complications, electronic stimulator device, brain
    cranial nerve — *see* Complications, electronic stimulator device, peripheral nerve
    embolism T85.810 ☑
    fibrosis T85.820 ☑
    gastric nerve — *see* Complications, electronic stimulator device, peripheral nerve
    hemorrhage T85.830 ☑
    infection and inflammation T85.738 ☑
    mechanical
      breakdown T85.118 ☑
      displacement T85.128 ☑
      leakage T85.199 ☑
      malposition T85.128 ☑
      obstruction T85.199 ☑
      perforation T85.199 ☑
      protrusion T85.199 ☑
      specified NEC T85.199 ☑
    pain T85.840 ☑
    peripheral nerve — *see* Complications, electronic stimulator device, peripheral nerve
    sacral nerve — *see* Complications, electronic stimulator device, peripheral nerve
    specified type NEC T85.890 ☑
    spinal cord — *see* Complications, electronic stimulator device, spinal cord
    stenosis T85.850 ☑
    thrombosis T85.860 ☑
    vagal nerve — *see* Complications, electronic stimulator device, peripheral nerve
  peripheral nerve T85.9 ☑
    embolism T85.810 ☑
    fibrosis T85.820 ☑
    hemorrhage T85.830 ☑
    infection and inflammation T85.732 ☑
    mechanical
      breakdown T85.111 ☑
      displacement T85.121 ☑
      leakage T85.191 ☑
      malposition T85.121 ☑
      obstruction T85.191 ☑
      perforation T85.191 ☑
      protrusion T85.191 ☑
      specified NEC T85.191 ☑
    pain T85.840 ☑

☑ Additional Character Required — Refer to the Tabular List for Character Selection   ▽ Subterms under main terms may continue to next column or page

Complication(s) — *continued*
electronic stimulator device — *continued*
  peripheral nerve — *continued*
    specified type NEC T85.890 ☑
    stenosis T85.850 ☑
    thrombosis T85.860 ☑
  spinal cord T85.9 ☑
    embolism T85.810 ☑
    fibrosis T85.820 ☑
    hemorrhage T85.830 ☑
    infection and inflammation T85.733 ☑
    mechanical
      breakdown T85.112 ☑
      displacement T85.122 ☑
      leakage T85.192 ☑
      malposition T85.122 ☑
      obstruction T85.192 ☑
      perforation T85.192 ☑
      protrusion T85.192 ☑
      specified NEC T85.192 ☑
    pain T85.840 ☑
    specified type NEC T85.890 ☑
    stenosis T85.850 ☑
    thrombosis T85.860 ☑
  urinary T83.9 ☑
    embolism T83.81 ☑
    fibrosis T83.82 ☑
    hemorrhage T83.83 ☑
    infection and inflammation T83.598 ☑
    mechanical
      breakdown T83.110 ☑
      displacement T83.120 ☑
      malposition T83.120 ☑
      perforation T83.190 ☑
      protrusion T83.190 ☑
      specified NEC T83.190 ☑
    pain T83.84 ☑
    specified type NEC T83.89 ☑
    stenosis T83.85 ☑
    thrombosis T83.86 ☑
electroshock therapy T88.9 ☑
  specified NEC T88.8 ☑
endocrine E34.9
  postprocedural
    adrenal hypofunction E89.6
    hypoinsulinemia E89.1
    hypoparathyroidism E89.2
    hypopituitarism E89.3
    hypothyroidism E89.0
    ovarian failure E89.40
      asymptomatic E89.40
      symptomatic E89.41
    specified NEC E89.89
    testicular hypofunction E89.5
endodontic treatment NEC M27.59
enterostomy (stoma) K94.10
  hemorrhage K94.11
  infection K94.12
  malfunction K94.13
  mechanical K94.13
  specified complication NEC K94.19
episiotomy, disruption O90.1
esophageal anti-reflux device T85.9 ☑
  embolism T85.818 ☑
  fibrosis T85.828 ☑
  hemorrhage T85.838 ☑
  infection and inflammation T85.79 ☑
  mechanical
    breakdown T85.511 ☑
    displacement T85.521 ☑
    malfunction T85.511 ☑
    malposition T85.521 ☑
    obstruction T85.591 ☑
    perforation T85.591 ☑
    protrusion T85.591 ☑
    specified NEC T85.591 ☑
  pain T85.848 ☑
  specified type NEC T85.898 ☑
  stenosis T85.858 ☑
  thrombosis T85.868 ☑
esophagostomy K94.30
  hemorrhage K94.31
  infection K94.32
  malfunction K94.33
  mechanical K94.33
  specified complication NEC K94.39
extracorporeal circulation T80.90 ☑

Complication(s) — *continued*
extremity artery (bypass) graft T82.9 ☑
  arteriosclerosis — *see* Arteriosclerosis, extremities, bypass graft
  embolism T82.818 ☑
  fibrosis T82.828 ☑
  hemorrhage T82.838 ☑
  infection and inflammation T82.7 ☑
  mechanical
    breakdown T82.318 ☑
      femoral artery T82.312 ☑
    displacement T82.328 ☑
      femoral artery T82.322 ☑
    leakage T82.338 ☑
      femoral artery T82.332 ☑
    malposition T82.328 ☑
      femoral artery T82.322 ☑
    obstruction T82.398 ☑
      femoral artery T82.392 ☑
    perforation T82.398 ☑
      femoral artery T82.392 ☑
    protrusion T82.398 ☑
      femoral artery T82.392 ☑
  pain T82.848 ☑
  specified type NEC T82.898 ☑
  stenosis T82.858 ☑
  thrombosis T82.868 ☑
eye H57.9
  corneal graft — *see* Complications, graft, cornea
  implant (prosthetic) T85.9 ☑
    embolism T85.818 ☑
    fibrosis T85.828 ☑
    hemorrhage T85.838 ☑
    infection and inflammation T85.79 ☑
    mechanical
      breakdown T85.318 ☑
      displacement T85.328 ☑
      leakage T85.398 ☑
      malposition T85.328 ☑
      obstruction T85.398 ☑
      perforation T85.398 ☑
      protrusion T85.398 ☑
      specified NEC T85.398 ☑
    pain T85.848 ☑
    specified type NEC T85.898 ☑
    stenosis T85.858 ☑
    thrombosis T85.868 ☑
  intraocular lens — *see* Complications, intraocular lens
  orbital prosthesis — *see* Complications, orbital prosthesis
female genital N94.9
  device, implant or graft NEC — *see* Complications, genitourinary, device or implant, genital tract
femoral artery (bypass) graft — *see* Complication, extremity artery (bypass) graft
fixation device, internal (orthopedic) T84.9 ☑
  infection and inflammation T84.60 ☑
    arm T84.61- ☑
      humerus T84.61- ☑
      radius T84.61- ☑
      ulna T84.61- ☑
    leg T84.629 ☑
      femur T84.62- ☑
      fibula T84.62- ☑
      tibia T84.62- ☑
    specified site NEC T84.89 ☑
    spine T84.63 ☑
  mechanical
    breakdown
      limb T84.119 ☑
        carpal T84.210 ☑
        femur T84.11- ☑
        fibula T84.11- ☑
        humerus T84.11- ☑
        metacarpal T84.210 ☑
        metatarsal T84.213 ☑
        phalanx
          foot T84.213 ☑
          hand T84.210 ☑
        radius T84.11- ☑
        tarsal T84.213 ☑
        tibia T84.11- ☑
        ulna T84.11- ☑
      specified bone NEC T84.218 ☑
      spine T84.216 ☑

Complication(s) — *continued*
fixation device, internal — *continued*
  mechanical — *continued*
    displacement
      limb T84.129 ☑
        carpal T84.220 ☑
        femur T84.12- ☑
        fibula T84.12- ☑
        humerus T84.12- ☑
        metacarpal T84.220 ☑
        metatarsal T84.223 ☑
        phalanx
          foot T84.223 ☑
          hand T84.220 ☑
        radius T84.12- ☑
        tarsal T84.223 ☑
        tibia T84.12- ☑
        ulna T84.12- ☑ .
      specified bone NEC T84.228 ☑
      spine T84.226 ☑
    malposition — *see* Complications, fixation device, internal, mechanical, displacement
    obstruction — *see* Complications, fixation device, internal, mechanical, specified type NEC
    perforation — *see* Complications, fixation device, internal, mechanical, specified type NEC
    protrusion — *see* Complications, fixation device, internal, mechanical, specified type NEC
    specified type NEC
      limb T84.199 ☑
        carpal T84.290 ☑
        femur T84.19- ☑
        fibula T84.19- ☑
        humerus T84.19- ☑
        metacarpal T84.290 ☑
        metatarsal T84.293 ☑
        phalanx
          foot T84.293 ☑
          hand T84.290 ☑
        radius T84.19- ☑
        tarsal T84.293 ☑
        tibia T84.19- ☑
        ulna T84.19- ☑
      specified bone NEC T84.298 ☑
      vertebra T84.296 ☑
  specified type NEC T84.89 ☑
    embolism T84.81 ☑
    fibrosis T84.82 ☑
    hemorrhage T84.83 ☑
    pain T84.84 ☑
    specified complication NEC T84.89 ☑
    stenosis T84.85 ☑
    thrombosis T84.86 ☑
following
  acute myocardial infarction NEC I23.8
    aneurysm (false) (of cardiac wall) (of heart wall) (ruptured) I23.3
    angina I23.7
    atrial
      septal defect I23.1
      thrombosis I23.6
    cardiac wall rupture I23.3
    chordae tendinae rupture I23.4
    defect
      septal
        atrial (heart) I23.1
        ventricular (heart) I23.2
    hemopericardium I23.0
    papillary muscle rupture I23.5
    rupture
      cardiac wall I23.3
        with hemopericardium I23.0
      chordae tendineae I23.4
      papillary muscle I23.5
    specified NEC I23.8
    thrombosis
      atrium I23.6
      auricular appendage I23.6
      ventricle (heart) I23.6
    ventricular
      septal defect I23.2
      thrombosis I23.6
  ectopic or molar pregnancy O08.9
    cardiac arrest O08.81
    sepsis O08.82
    specified type NEC O08.89
    urinary tract infection O08.83

Index

Complication(s) — *continued*
  following — *continued*
    termination of pregnancy — *see* Abortion
  gastrointestinal K92.9
    bile duct prosthesis — *see* Complications, bile duct implant
    esophageal anti-reflux device — *see* Complications, esophageal anti-reflux device
    postoperative
      colostomy — *see* Complications, colostomy
      dumping syndrome K91.1
      enterostomy — *see* Complications, enterostomy
      gastrostomy — *see* Complications, gastrostomy
      malabsorption NEC K91.2
      obstruction — *see also* Obstruction, intestine, postoperative K91.30
      postcholecystectomy syndrome K91.5
      specified NEC K91.89
      vomiting after GI surgery K91.0
    prosthetic device or implant
      bile duct prosthesis — *see* Complications, bile duct implant
      esophageal anti-reflux device — *see* Complications, esophageal anti-reflux device
      specified type NEC
        embolism T85.818 ☑
        fibrosis T85.828 ☑
        hemorrhage T85.838 ☑
        mechanical
          breakdown T85.518 ☑
          displacement T85.528 ☑
          malfunction T85.518 ☑
          malposition T85.528 ☑
          obstruction T85.598 ☑
          perforation T85.598 ☑
          protrusion T85.598 ☑
          specified NEC T85.598 ☑
        pain T85.848 ☑
        specified complication NEC T85.898 ☑
        stenosis T85.858 ☑
        thrombosis T85.868 ☑
  gastrostomy (stoma) K94.20
    hemorrhage K94.21
    infection K94.22
    malfunction K94.23
    mechanical K94.23
    specified complication NEC K94.29
  genitourinary
    device or implant T83.9 ☑
      genital tract T83.9 ☑
        infection or inflammation T83.69 ☑
        intrauterine contraceptive device — *see* Complications, intrauterine, contraceptive device
        mechanical — *see* Complications, by device, mechanical
        mesh — *see* Complications, prosthetic device or implant, mesh
        penile prosthesis — *see* Complications, prosthetic device, penile
        specified type NEC T83.89 ☑
          embolism T83.81 ☑
          fibrosis T83.82 ☑
          hemorrhage T83.83 ☑
          pain T83.84 ☑
          specified complication NEC T83.89 ☑
          stenosis T83.85 ☑
          thrombosis T83.86 ☑
        vaginal mesh — *see* Complications, prosthetic device or implant, mesh
      urinary system T83.9 ☑
        cystostomy catheter — *see* Complication, catheter, cystostomy
        electronic stimulator — *see* Complications, electronic stimulator device, urinary
        indwelling urethral catheter — *see* Complications, catheter, urethral, indwelling
        infection or inflammation T83.598 ☑
          indwelling urethral catheter T83.511 ☑
        kidney transplant — *see* Complication, transplant, kidney
        organ graft — *see* Complication, graft, urinary organ
        specified type NEC T83.89 ☑
          embolism T83.81 ☑
          fibrosis T83.82 ☑
          hemorrhage T83.83 ☑

Complication(s) — *continued*
  genitourinary — *continued*
    device or implant — *continued*
      urinary system — *continued*
        specified type — *continued*
          mechanical T83.198 ☑
            breakdown T83.118 ☑
            displacement T83.128 ☑
            malfunction T83.118 ☑
            malposition T83.128 ☑
            obstruction T83.198 ☑
            perforation T83.198 ☑
            protrusion T83.198 ☑
            specified NEC T83.198 ☑
        sphincter implant — *see* Complications, implant, urinary sphincter
        sphincter, implanted T83.191 ☑
        stent (ileal conduit) (nephroureteral) T83.193 ☑
          pain T83.84 ☑
          specified complication NEC T83.89 ☑
          stenosis T83.85 ☑
          thrombosis T83.86 ☑
          ureteral indwelling T83.192 ☑
    postprocedural
      pelvic peritoneal adhesions N99.4
      renal failure N99.0
      specified NEC N99.89
      stoma — *see* Complications, stoma, urinary tract
      urethral stricture — *see* Stricture, urethra, postprocedural
      vaginal
        adhesions N99.2
        vault prolapse N99.3
  graft (bypass) (patch) — *see also* Complications, prosthetic device or implant
    aorta — *see* Complications, graft, vascular
    arterial — *see* Complication, graft, vascular
    bone T86.839
      failure T86.831
      infection T86.832
      mechanical T84.318 ☑
        breakdown T84.318 ☑
        displacement T84.328 ☑
        protrusion T84.398 ☑
        specified type NEC T84.398 ☑
      rejection T86.830
      specified type NEC T86.838
    carotid artery — *see* Complications, graft, vascular
    cornea T86.849-
      failure T86.841- ☑
      infection T86.842- ☑
      mechanical T85.398 ☑
        breakdown T85.318 ☑
        displacement T85.328 ☑
        protrusion T85.398 ☑
        specified type NEC T85.398 ☑
      rejection T86.840- ☑
      retroprosthetic membrane T85.398 ☑
      specified type NEC T86.848- ☑
    femoral artery (bypass) — *see* Complication, extremity artery (bypass) graft
    genital organ or tract — *see* Complications, genitourinary, device or implant, genital tract
    muscle T84.9 ☑
      breakdown T84.410 ☑
      displacement T84.420 ☑
      embolism T84.81 ☑
      fibrosis T84.82 ☑
      hemorrhage T84.83 ☑
      infection and inflammation T84.7 ☑
      mechanical NEC T84.490 ☑
      pain T84.84 ☑
      specified type NEC T84.89 ☑
      stenosis T84.85 ☑
      thrombosis T84.86 ☑
    nerve — *see* Complication, prosthetic device or implant, specified NEC
    skin — *see* Complications, prosthetic device or implant, skin graft
    tendon T84.9 ☑
      breakdown T84.410 ☑
      displacement T84.420 ☑
      embolism T84.81 ☑
      fibrosis T84.82 ☑
      hemorrhage T84.83 ☑

Complication(s) — *continued*
  graft — *see also* Complications, prosthetic device or implant — *continued*
    tendon — *continued*
      infection and inflammation T84.7 ☑
      mechanical NEC T84.490 ☑
      pain T84.84 ☑
      specified type NEC T84.89 ☑
      stenosis T84.85 ☑
      thrombosis T84.86 ☑
    urinary organ T83.9 ☑
      embolism T83.81 ☑
      fibrosis T83.82 ☑
      hemorrhage T83.83 ☑
      infection and inflammation T83.598 ☑
        indwelling urethral catheter T83.511 ☑
      mechanical
        breakdown T83.21 ☑
        displacement T83.22 ☑
        erosion T83.24 ☑
        exposure T83.25 ☑
        leakage T83.23 ☑
        malposition T83.22 ☑
        obstruction T83.29 ☑
        perforation T83.29 ☑
        protrusion T83.29 ☑
        specified NEC T83.29 ☑
      pain T83.84 ☑
      specified type NEC T83.89 ☑
      stenosis T83.85 ☑
      thrombosis T83.86 ☑
    vascular T82.9 ☑
      embolism T82.818 ☑
      femoral artery — *see* Complication, extremity artery (bypass) graft
      fibrosis T82.828 ☑
      hemorrhage T82.838 ☑
      mechanical
        breakdown T82.319 ☑
          aorta (bifurcation) T82.310 ☑
          carotid artery T82.311 ☑
          specified vessel NEC T82.318 ☑
        displacement T82.329 ☑
          aorta (bifurcation) T82.320 ☑
          carotid artery T82.321 ☑
          specified vessel NEC T82.328 ☑
        leakage T82.339 ☑
          aorta (bifurcation) T82.330 ☑
          carotid artery T82.331 ☑
          specified vessel NEC T82.338 ☑
        malposition T82.329 ☑
          aorta (bifurcation) T82.320 ☑
          carotid artery T82.321 ☑
          specified vessel NEC T82.328 ☑
        obstruction T82.399 ☑
          aorta (bifurcation) T82.390 ☑
          carotid artery T82.391 ☑
          specified vessel NEC T82.398 ☑
        perforation T82.399 ☑
          aorta (bifurcation) T82.390 ☑
          carotid artery T82.391 ☑
          specified vessel NEC T82.398 ☑
        protrusion T82.399 ☑
          aorta (bifurcation) T82.390 ☑
          carotid artery T82.391 ☑
          specified vessel NEC T82.398 ☑
      pain T82.848 ☑
      specified complication NEC T82.898 ☑
      stenosis T82.858 ☑
      thrombosis T82.868 ☑
  heart I51.9
    assist device
      infection and inflammation T82.7 ☑
    following acute myocardial infarction — *see* Complications, following, acute myocardial infarction
    postoperative — *see* Complications, circulatory system
    transplant — *see* Complication, transplant, heart and lung(s) — *see* Complications, transplant, heart, with lung
    valve
      graft (biological) T82.9 ☑
        embolism T82.817 ☑
        fibrosis T82.827 ☑
        hemorrhage T82.837 ☑

☑ Additional Character Required — Refer to the Tabular List for Character Selection   Subterms under main terms may continue to next column or page

Complication(s) — *continued*
　heart — *continued*
　　valve — *continued*
　　　graft — *continued*
　　　　infection and inflammation T82.7 ☑
　　　　mechanical T82.228 ☑
　　　　　breakdown T82.221 ☑
　　　　　displacement T82.222 ☑
　　　　　leakage T82.223 ☑
　　　　　malposition T82.222 ☑
　　　　　obstruction T82.228 ☑
　　　　　perforation T82.228 ☑
　　　　　protrusion T82.228 ☑
　　　　pain T82.847 ☑
　　　　specified type NEC T82.897 ☑
　　　　stenosis T82.857 ☑
　　　　thrombosis T82.867 ☑
　　　prosthesis T82.9
　　　　embolism T82.817 ☑
　　　　fibrosis T82.827 ☑
　　　　hemorrhage T82.837 ☑
　　　　infection or inflammation T82.6 ☑
　　　　mechanical T82.09
　　　　　breakdown T82.01 ☑
　　　　　displacement T82.02 ☑
　　　　　leakage T82.03 ☑
　　　　　malposition T82.02 ☑
　　　　　obstruction T82.09 ☑
　　　　　perforation T82.09 ☑
　　　　　protrusion T82.09 ☑
　　　　pain T82.847 ☑
　　　　specified type NEC T82.897 ☑
　　　　　mechanical T82.09
　　　　stenosis T82.857 ☑
　　　　thrombosis T82.867 ☑
　hematoma
　　intraoperative — *see* Complication, intraoperative, hemorrhage
　　postprocedural — *see* Complication, postprocedural, hematoma
　hemodialysis — *see* Complications, dialysis
　hemorrhage
　　intraoperative — *see* Complication, intraoperative, hemorrhage
　　postprocedural — *see* Complication, postprocedural, hemorrhage
　IEC (immune effector cellular) therapy T80.82 ☑
　ileostomy (stoma) — *see* Complications, enterostomy
　immune effector cellular (IEC) therapy T80.82 ☑
　immunization (procedure) — *see* Complications, vaccination
　implant — *see also* Complications, by site and type
　　urinary sphincter T83.9 ☑
　　　embolism T83.81 ☑
　　　fibrosis T83.82 ☑
　　　hemorrhage T83.83 ☑
　　　infection and inflammation T83.591 ☑
　　　mechanical
　　　　breakdown T83.111 ☑
　　　　displacement T83.121 ☑
　　　　leakage T83.191 ☑
　　　　malposition T83.121 ☑
　　　　obstruction T83.191 ☑
　　　　perforation T83.191 ☑
　　　　protrusion T83.191 ☑
　　　　specified NEC T83.191 ☑
　　　pain T83.84 ☑
　　　specified type NEC T83.89 ☑
　　　stenosis T83.85 ☑
　　　thrombosis T83.86 ☑
　infusion (procedure) T80.90 ☑
　　air embolism T80.0 ☑
　　blood — *see* Complications, transfusion
　　catheter — *see* Complications, catheter
　　infection T80.29 ☑
　　pump — *see* Complications, cardiovascular, device or implant
　　sepsis T80.29 ☑
　　serum reaction — *see also* Reaction, serum T80.69 ☑
　　　anaphylactic shock — *see also* Shock, anaphylactic T80.59 ☑
　　specified type NEC T80.89 ☑
　inhalation therapy NEC T81.81 ☑
　injection (procedure) T80.90 ☑
　　drug reaction — *see* Reaction, drug

Complication(s) — *continued*
　injection — *continued*
　　infection T80.29 ☑
　　sepsis T80.29 ☑
　　serum (prophylactic) (therapeutic) — *see* Complications, vaccination
　　specified type NEC T80.89 ☑
　　vaccine (any) — *see* Complications, vaccination
　inoculation (any) — *see* Complications, vaccination
　insulin pump
　　infection and inflammation T85.72 ☑
　　mechanical
　　　breakdown T85.614 ☑
　　　displacement T85.624 ☑
　　　leakage T85.633 ☑
　　　malposition T85.624 ☑
　　　obstruction T85.694 ☑
　　　perforation T85.694 ☑
　　　protrusion T85.694 ☑
　　　specified NEC T85.694 ☑
　intestinal pouch NEC K91.858 ☑
　intraocular lens (prosthetic) T85.9 ☑
　　embolism T85.818 ☑
　　fibrosis T85.828 ☑
　　hemorrhage T85.838 ☑
　　infection and inflammation T85.79 ☑
　　mechanical
　　　breakdown T85.21 ☑
　　　displacement T85.22 ☑
　　　malposition T85.22 ☑
　　　obstruction T85.29 ☑
　　　perforation T85.29 ☑
　　　protrusion T85.29 ☑
　　　specified NEC T85.29 ☑
　　pain T85.848 ☑
　　specified type NEC T85.898 ☑
　　stenosis T85.858 ☑
　　thrombosis T85.868 ☑
　intraoperative (intraprocedural)
　　cardiac arrest — *see also* Infarct, myocardium, associated with revascularization procedure
　　　during cardiac surgery I97.710
　　　during other surgery I97.711
　　cardiac functional disturbance NEC — *see also* Infarct, myocardium, associated with revascularization procedure
　　　during cardiac surgery I97.790
　　　during other surgery I97.791
　　hemorrhage (hematoma) (of)
　　　circulatory system organ or structure
　　　　during cardiac bypass I97.411
　　　　during cardiac catheterization I97.410
　　　　during other circulatory system procedure I97.418
　　　　during other procedure I97.42
　　　digestive system organ
　　　　during procedure on digestive system K91.61
　　　　during procedure on other organ K91.62
　　　ear
　　　　during procedure on ear and mastoid process H95.21
　　　　during procedure on other organ H95.22
　　　endocrine system organ or structure
　　　　during procedure on endocrine system organ or structure E36.01
　　　　during procedure on other organ E36.02
　　　eye and adnexa
　　　　during ophthalmic procedure H59.11- ☑
　　　　during other procedure H59.12- ☑
　　　genitourinary organ or structure
　　　　during procedure on genitourinary organ or structure N99.61
　　　　during procedure on other organ N99.62
　　　mastoid process
　　　　during procedure on ear and mastoid process H95.21
　　　　during procedure on other organ H95.22
　　　musculoskeletal structure
　　　　during musculoskeletal surgery M96.810
　　　　during non-orthopedic surgery M96.811
　　　　during orthopedic surgery M96.810
　　　nervous system
　　　　during a nervous system procedure G97.31
　　　　during other procedure G97.32
　　　respiratory system
　　　　during other procedure J95.62

Complication(s) — *continued*
　intraoperative — *continued*
　　hemorrhage — *continued*
　　　respiratory system — *continued*
　　　　during procedure on respiratory system organ or structure J95.61
　　　skin and subcutaneous tissue
　　　　during a dermatologic procedure L76.01
　　　　during a procedure on other organ L76.02
　　　spleen
　　　　during a procedure on other organ D78.02
　　　　during a procedure on the spleen D78.01
　　puncture or laceration (accidental) (unintentional) (of)
　　　brain
　　　　during a nervous system procedure G97.48
　　　　during other procedure G97.49
　　　circulatory system organ or structure
　　　　during circulatory system procedure I97.51
　　　　during other procedure I97.52
　　　digestive system
　　　　during procedure on digestive system K91.71
　　　　during procedure on other organ K91.72
　　　ear
　　　　during procedure on ear and mastoid process H95.31
　　　　during procedure on other organ H95.32
　　　endocrine system organ or structure
　　　　during procedure on endocrine system organ or structure E36.11
　　　　during procedure on other organ E36.12
　　　eye and adnexa
　　　　during ophthalmic procedure H59.21- ☑
　　　　during other procedure H59.22- ☑
　　　genitourinary organ or structure
　　　　during procedure on genitourinary organ or structure N99.71
　　　　during procedure on other organ N99.72
　　　mastoid process
　　　　during procedure on ear and mastoid process H95.31
　　　　during procedure on other organ H95.32
　　　musculoskeletal structure
　　　　during musculoskeletal surgery M96.820
　　　　during non-orthopedic surgery M96.821
　　　　during orthopedic surgery M96.820
　　　nervous system
　　　　during a nervous system procedure G97.48
　　　　during other procedure G97.49
　　　respiratory system
　　　　during other procedure J95.72
　　　　during procedure on respiratory system organ or structure J95.71
　　　skin and subcutaneous tissue
　　　　during a dermatologic procedure L76.11
　　　　during a procedure on other organ L76.12
　　　spleen
　　　　during a procedure on other organ D78.12
　　　　during a procedure on the spleen D78.11
　　specified NEC
　　　circulatory system I97.88
　　　digestive system K91.81
　　　ear H95.88
　　　endocrine system E36.8
　　　eye and adnexa H59.88
　　　genitourinary system N99.81
　　　mastoid process H95.88
　　　musculoskeletal structure M96.89
　　　nervous system G97.81
　　　respiratory system J95.88
　　　skin and subcutaneous tissue L76.81
　　　spleen D78.81
　intraperitoneal catheter (dialysis) (infusion) — *see* Complication(s), catheter, intraperitoneal dialysis
　intrathecal infusion pump
　　infection and inflammation T85.738 ☑
　　mechanical
　　　breakdown T85.615 ☑
　　　displacement T85.625 ☑
　　　leakage T85.635 ☑
　　　malfunction T85.695 ☑
　　　malposition T85.625 ☑
　　　obstruction T85.695 ☑
　　　perforation T85.695 ☑
　　　protrusion T85.695 ☑
　　　specified NEC T85.695 ☑

Complication(s) — *continued*
  intrauterine
    contraceptive device
      embolism T83.81 ☑
      fibrosis T83.82 ☑
      hemorrhage T83.83 ☑
      infection and inflammation T83.69 ☑
      mechanical
        breakdown T83.31 ☑
        displacement T83.32 ☑
        malposition T83.32 ☑
        obstruction T83.39 ☑
        perforation T83.39 ☑
        protrusion T83.39 ☑
        specified NEC T83.39 ☑
      pain T83.84 ☑
      specified type NEC T83.89 ☑
      stenosis T83.85 ☑
      thrombosis T83.86 ☑
    procedure (fetal), to newborn P96.5
  jejunostomy (stoma) — *see* Complications, enterostomy
  joint prosthesis, internal T84.9 ☑
    breakage (fracture) T84.01- ☑
    dislocation T84.02- ☑
    fracture T84.01- ☑
    infection or inflammation T84.50 ☑
      hip T84.5- ☑
      knee T84.5- ☑
      specified joint NEC T84.59 ☑
    instability T84.02- ☑
    malposition — *see* Complications, joint prosthesis, mechanical, displacement
    mechanical
      breakage, broken T84.01- ☑
      dislocation T84.02- ☑
      fracture T84.01- ☑
      instability T84.02- ☑
      leakage — *see* Complications, joint prosthesis, mechanical, specified NEC
      loosening T84.039 ☑
        hip T84.03- ☑
        knee T84.03- ☑
        specified joint NEC T84.038 ☑
      obstruction — *see* Complications, joint prosthesis, mechanical, specified NEC
      perforation — *see* Complications, joint prosthesis, mechanical, specified NEC
        osteolysis T84.059 ☑
          hip T84.05- ☑
          knee T84.05- ☑
          other specified joint T84.058 ☑
      periprosthetic osteolysis T84.059 ☑
      protrusion — *see* Complications, joint prosthesis, mechanical, specified NEC
      specified complication NEC T84.099 ☑
        hip T84.09- ☑
        knee T84.09- ☑
        other specified joint T84.098 ☑
      subluxation T84.02- ☑
      wear of articular bearing surface T84.069 ☑
        hip T84.06- ☑
        knee T84.06- ☑
        other specified joint T84.068 ☑
    specified joint NEC T84.89 ☑
      embolism T84.81 ☑
      fibrosis T84.82 ☑
      hemorrhage T84.83 ☑
      pain T84.84 ☑
      specified complication NEC T84.89 ☑
      stenosis T84.85 ☑
      thrombosis T84.86 ☑
    subluxation T84.02- ☑
  kidney transplant — *see* Complications, transplant, kidney
  labor O75.9
    specified NEC O75.89
  liver transplant (immune or nonimmune) — *see* Complications, transplant, liver
  lumbar puncture G97.1
    cerebrospinal fluid leak G97.0
    headache or reaction G97.1
  lung transplant — *see* Complications, transplant, lung and heart — *see* Complications, transplant, lung, with heart
  male genital N50.9

Complication(s) — *continued*
  male genital — *continued*
    device, implant or graft — *see* Complications, genitourinary, device or implant, genital tract
    postprocedural or postoperative — *see* Complications, genitourinary, postprocedural
    specified NEC N99.89
  mastoid (process) procedure
    intraoperative H95.88
      hematoma — *see* Complications, intraoperative, hemorrhage (hematoma) (of), mastoid process
      hemorrhage — *see* Complications, intraoperative, hemorrhage (hematoma) (of), mastoid process
      laceration — *see* Complications, intraoperative, puncture or laceration, mastoid process
      specified NEC H95.88
    postmastoidectomy — *see* Complications, postmastoidectomy
    postoperative H95.89
      external ear canal stenosis H95.81 ☑
      hematoma — *see* Complications, postprocedural, hematoma (of), mastoid process
      hemorrhage — *see* Complications, postprocedural, hemorrhage (of), mastoid process
      postmastoidectomy — *see* Complications, postmastoidectomy
      seroma — *see* Complications, postprocedural, seroma (of), mastoid process
      specified NEC H95.89
  mastoidectomy cavity — *see* Complications, postmastoidectomy
  mechanical — *see* Complications, by site and type, mechanical
  medical procedures — *see also* Complication(s), intraoperative T88.9 ☑
  metabolic E88.9
    postoperative E89.89
    specified NEC E89.89
  molar pregnancy NOS O08.9
    damage to pelvic organs O08.6
    embolism O08.2
    genital infection O08.0
    hemorrhage (delayed) (excessive) O08.1
    metabolic disorder O08.5
    renal failure O08.4
    shock O08.3
    specified type NEC O08.0
    venous complication NEC O08.7
  musculoskeletal system — *see also* Complication, intraoperative (intraprocedural), by site
    device, implant or graft NEC — *see* Complications, orthopedic, device or implant
    internal fixation (nail) (plate) (rod) — *see* Complications, fixation device, internal
    joint prosthesis — *see* Complications, joint prosthesis
    post radiation M96.89
      kyphosis M96.2
      scoliosis M96.5
      specified complication NEC M96.89
    postoperative (postprocedural) M96.89
      with osteoporosis — *see* Osteoporosis
      fracture following insertion of device — *see* Fracture, following insertion of orthopedic implant, joint prosthesis or bone plate
      joint instability after prosthesis removal M96.89
      lordosis M96.4
      postlaminectomy syndrome NEC M96.1
        kyphosis M96.3
      pseudarthrosis M96.0
      specified complication NEC M96.89
  nephrostomy (stoma) — *see* Complications, stoma, urinary tract, external NEC
  nervous system G98.8
    central G96.9
    device, implant or graft — *see also* Complication, prosthetic device or implant, specified NEC
    electronic stimulator (electrode(s)) — *see* Complications, electronic stimulator device
    specified NEC
      infection and inflammation T85.738 ☑
      mechanical T85.695 ☑
        breakdown T85.615 ☑
        displacement T85.625 ☑
        leakage T85.635 ☑
        malfunction T85.695 ☑

Complication(s) — *continued*
  nervous system — *continued*
    device, implant or graft — *see also* Complication, prosthetic device or implant, specified — *continued*
      specified — *continued*
        mechanical — *continued*
          malposition T85.625 ☑
          obstruction T85.695 ☑
          perforation T85.695 ☑
          protrusion T85.695 ☑
          specified NEC T85.695 ☑
      ventricular shunt — *see* Complications, ventricular shunt
    electronic stimulator (electrode(s)) — *see* Complications, electronic stimulator device
    postprocedural G97.82
      intracranial hypotension G97.2
      specified NEC G97.82
      spinal fluid leak G97.0
  newborn, due to intrauterine (fetal) procedure P96.5
  nonabsorbable (permanent) sutures — *see* Complication, sutures, permanent
  obstetric O75.9
    procedure (instrumental) (manual) (surgical) specified NEC O75.4
    specified NEC O75.89
    surgical wound NEC O90.89
      hematoma O90.2
      infection O86.00
  ocular lens implant — *see* Complications, intraocular lens
  ophthalmologic
    postprocedural bleb — *see* Blebitis
  orbital prosthesis T85.9 ☑
    embolism T85.818 ☑
    fibrosis T85.828 ☑
    hemorrhage T85.838 ☑
    infection and inflammation T85.79 ☑
    mechanical
      breakdown T85.31- ☑
      displacement T85.32- ☑
      malposition T85.32- ☑
      obstruction T85.39- ☑
      perforation T85.39- ☑
      protrusion T85.39- ☑
      specified NEC T85.39- ☑
    pain T85.848 ☑
    specified type NEC T85.898 ☑
    stenosis T85.858 ☑
    thrombosis T85.868 ☑
  organ or tissue transplant (partial) (total) — *see* Complications, transplant
  orthopedic — *see also* Disorder, soft tissue
    device or implant T84.9 ☑
      bone
        device or implant — *see* Complication, bone, device NEC
        graft — *see* Complication, graft, bone
      breakdown T84.418 ☑
      displacement T84.428 ☑
      electronic bone stimulator — *see* Complications, electronic stimulator device, bone
      embolism T84.81 ☑
      fibrosis T84.82 ☑
      fixation device — *see* Complication, fixation device, internal
      hemorrhage T84.83 ☑
      infection or inflammation T84.7 ☑
      joint prosthesis — *see* Complication, joint prosthesis, internal
      malfunction T84.418 ☑
      malposition T84.428 ☑
      mechanical NEC T84.498 ☑
      muscle graft — *see* Complications, graft, muscle
      obstruction T84.498 ☑
      pain T84.84 ☑
      perforation T84.498 ☑
      protrusion T84.498 ☑
      specified complication NEC T84.89 ☑
      stenosis T84.85 ☑
      tendon graft — *see* Complications, graft, tendon
      thrombosis T84.86 ☑
    fracture (following insertion of device) — *see* Fracture, following insertion of orthopedic implant, joint prosthesis or bone plate
    postprocedural M96.89

Complication(s) — *continued*
  orthopedic — *see also* Disorder, soft tissue — *continued*
    postprocedural — *continued*
      fracture — *see* Fracture, following insertion of orthopedic implant, joint prosthesis or bone plate
      postlaminectomy syndrome NEC M96.1
        kyphosis M96.3
        lordosis M96.4
      postradiation
        kyphosis M96.2
        scoliosis M96.5
      pseudarthrosis post-fusion M96.0
      specified type NEC M96.89
  pacemaker (cardiac) — *see* Complications, cardiovascular device or implant, electronic
  pancreas transplant — *see* Complications, transplant, pancreas
  penile prosthesis (implant) — *see* Complications, prosthetic device, penile
  perfusion NEC T80.90 ☑
  perineal repair (obstetrical) NEC O90.89
    disruption O90.1
    hematoma O90.2
    infection (following delivery) O86.09
  phototherapy T88.9 ☑
    specified NEC T88.8 ☑
  postmastoidectomy NEC H95.19- ☑
    cyst, mucosal H95.13- ☑
    granulation H95.12- ☑
    inflammation, chronic H95.11- ☑
    recurrent cholesteatoma H95.0- ☑
  postoperative — *see* Complications, postprocedural
    circulatory — *see* Complications, circulatory system
    ear — *see* Complications, ear
    endocrine — *see* Complications, endocrine
    eye — *see* Complications, eye
    lumbar puncture G97.1
      cerebrospinal fluid leak G97.0
    nervous system (central) (peripheral) — *see* Complications, nervous system
    respiratory system — *see* Complications, respiratory system
  postprocedural — *see also* Complications, surgical procedure
    cardiac arrest — *see also* Infarct, myocardium, associated with revascularization procedure
      following cardiac surgery I97.120
      following other surgery I97.121
    cardiac functional disturbance NEC — *see also* Infarct, myocardium, associated with revascularization procedure
      following cardiac surgery I97.190
      following other surgery I97.191
    cardiac insufficiency
      following cardiac surgery I97.110
      following other surgery I97.111
    chorioretinal scars following retinal surgery H59.81- ☑
    following cataract surgery
      cataract (lens) fragments H59.02- ☑
      cystoid macular edema H59.03- ☑
      specified NEC H59.09- ☑
      vitreous (touch) syndrome H59.01- ☑
    heart failure
      following cardiac surgery I97.130
      following other surgery I97.131
    hematoma (of)
      circulatory system organ or structure
        following cardiac bypass I97.631
        following cardiac catheterization I97.630
        following other circulatory system procedure I97.638
        following other procedure I97.621
      digestive system
        following procedure on digestive system K91.870
        following procedure on other organ K91.871
      ear
        following other procedure H95.52
        following procedure on ear and mastoid process H95.51
      endocrine system
        following endocrine system procedure E89.820
        following other procedure E89.821

Complication(s) — *continued*
  postprocedural — *see also* Complications, surgical procedure — *continued*
    hematoma — *continued*
      eye and adnexa
        following ophthalmic procedure H59.33- ☑
        following other procedure H59.34- ☑
      genitourinary organ or structure
        following procedure on genitourinary organ or structure N99.840
        following procedure on other organ N99.841
      mastoid process
        following other procedure H95.52
        following procedure on ear and mastoid process H95.51
      musculoskeletal structure
        following musculoskeletal surgery M96.840
        following non-orthopedic surgery M96.841
        following orthopedic surgery M96.840
      nervous system
        following nervous system procedure G97.61
        following other procedure G97.62
      respiratory system
        following other procedure J95.861
        following procedure on respiratory system organ or structure J95.860
      skin and subcutaneous tissue
        following dermatologic procedure L76.31
        following procedure on other organ L76.32
      spleen
        following procedure on other organ D78.32
        following procedure on the spleen D78.31
    hemorrhage (of)
      circulatory system organ or structure
        following cardiac bypass I97.611
        following cardiac catheterization I97.610
        following other circulatory system procedure I97.618
        following other procedure I97.620
      digestive system
        following procedure on digestive system K91.840
        following procedure on other organ K91.841
      ear
        following other procedure H95.42
        following procedure on ear and mastoid process H95.41
      endocrine system
        following endocrine system procedure E89.810
        following other procedure E89.811
      eye and adnexa
        following ophthalmic procedure H59.31- ☑
        following other procedure H59.32- ☑
      genitourinary organ or structure
        following procedure on genitourinary organ or structure N99.820
        following procedure on other organ N99.821
      mastoid process
        following other procedure H95.42
        following procedure on ear and mastoid process H95.41
      musculoskeletal structure
        following musculoskeletal surgery M96.830
        following non-orthopedic surgery M96.831
        following orthopedic surgery M96.830
      nervous system
        following nervous system procedure G97.51
        following other procedure G97.52
      respiratory system
        following a respiratory system procedure J95.830
        following other procedure J95.831
      skin and subcutaneous tissue
        following a procedure on other organ L76.22
        following dermatologic procedure L76.21
      spleen
        following procedure on other organ D78.22
        following procedure on the spleen D78.21
    seroma (of)
      circulatory system organ or structure
        following cardiac bypass I97.641
        following cardiac catheterization I97.640
        following other circulatory system procedure I97.648
        following other procedure I97.622
      digestive system
        following procedure on digestive system K91.872

Complication(s) — *continued*
  postprocedural — *see also* Complications, surgical procedure — *continued*
    seroma — *continued*
      digestive system — *continued*
        following procedure on other organ K91.873
      ear
        following other procedure H95.54
        following procedure on ear and mastoid process H95.53
      endocrine system
        following endocrine system procedure E89.822
        following other procedure E89.823
      eye and adnexa
        following ophthalmic procedure H59.35- ☑
        following other procedure H59.36- ☑
      genitourinary organ or structure
        following procedure on genitourinary organ or structure N99.842
        following procedure on other organ N99.843
      mastoid process
        following other procedure H95.54
        following procedure on ear and mastoid process H95.53
      musculoskeletal structure
        following musculoskeletal surgery M96.842
        following non-orthopedic surgery M96.843
        following orthopedic surgery M96.842
      nervous system
        following nervous system procedure G97.63
        following other procedure G97.64
      respiratory system
        following other procedure J95.863
        following procedure on respiratory system organ or structure J95.862
      skin and subcutaneous tissue
        following dermatologic procedure L76.33
        following procedure on other organ L76.34
      spleen
        following procedure on other organ D78.34
        following procedure on the spleen D78.33
    specified NEC
      circulatory system I97.89
      digestive K91.89
      ear H95.89
      endocrine E89.89
      eye and adnexa H59.89
      genitourinary N99.89
      mastoid process H95.89
      metabolic E89.89
      musculoskeletal structure M96.89
      nervous system G97.82
      respiratory system J95.89
      skin and subcutaneous tissue L76.82
      spleen D78.89
  pregnancy NEC — *see* Pregnancy, complicated by
  prosthetic device or implant T85.9 ☑
    bile duct — *see* Complications, bile duct implant
    breast — *see* Complications, breast implant
    bulking agent
      ureteral
        erosion T83.714 ☑
        exposure T83.724 ☑
      urethral
        erosion T83.713 ☑
        exposure T83.723 ☑
    cardiac and vascular NEC — *see* Complications, cardiovascular device or implant
    corneal transplant — *see* Complications, graft, cornea
    electronic nervous system stimulator — *see* Complications, electronic stimulator device
    epidural infusion catheter — *see* Complications, catheter, epidural
    esophageal anti-reflux device — *see* Complications, esophageal anti-reflux device
    genital organ or tract — *see* Complications, genitourinary, device or implant, genital tract
      specified NEC T83.79- ☑
    heart valve — *see* Complications, heart, valve, prosthesis
    infection or inflammation T85.79 ☑
      intestine transplant T86.892
      liver transplant T86.43
      lung transplant T86.812
      pancreas transplant T86.892
      skin graft T86.822

▽ Subterms under main terms may continue to next column or page   ☑ Additional Character Required — Refer to the Tabular List for Character Selection   **67**

Complication — Complication

Complication(s) — *continued*
  prosthetic device or implant — *continued*
    intraocular lens — *see* Complications, intraocular lens
    intraperitoneal (dialysis) catheter — *see* Complication(s), catheter, intraperitoneal dialysis
    joint — *see* Complications, joint prosthesis, internal
    mechanical NEC T85.698 ☑
      dialysis catheter (vascular) — *see also* Complication, catheter, dialysis, mechanical
      peritoneal — *see* Complication(s), catheter, intraperitoneal dialysis
      gastrointestinal device T85.598 ☑
      ocular device T85.398 ☑
      subdural (infusion) catheter T85.690 ☑
      suture, permanent T85.692 ☑
        that for bone repair — *see* Complications, fixation device, internal (orthopedic), mechanical
      ventricular shunt
        breakdown T85.01 ☑
        displacement T85.02 ☑
        leakage T85.03 ☑
        malposition T85.02 ☑
        obstruction T85.09 ☑
        perforation T85.09 ☑
        protrusion T85.09 ☑
        specified NEC T85.09 ☑
    mesh
      erosion (to surrounding organ or tissue) T83.718 ☑
        urethral (into pelvic floor muscles) T83.712 ☑
        vaginal (into pelvic floor muscles) T83.711 ☑
      exposure (into surrounding organ or tissue) T83.728 ☑
        urethral (through urethral wall) T83.722 ☑
        vaginal (into vagina) (through vaginal wall) T83.721 ☑
    orbital — *see* Complications, orbital prosthesis
    penile T83.9 ☑
      embolism T83.81 ☑
      fibrosis T83.82 ☑
      hemorrhage T83.83 ☑
      infection and inflammation T83.61 ☑
      mechanical
        breakdown T83.410 ☑
        displacement T83.420 ☑
        leakage T83.490 ☑
        malposition T83.420 ☑
        obstruction T83.490 ☑
        perforation T83.490 ☑
        protrusion T83.490 ☑
        specified NEC T83.490 ☑
      pain T83.84 ☑
      specified type NEC T83.89 ☑
      stenosis T83.85 ☑
      thrombosis T83.86 ☑
    prosthetic materials NEC
      erosion (to surrounding organ or tissue) T83.718 ☑
      exposure (into surrounding organ or tissue) T83.728 ☑
    skin graft T86.829
      artificial skin or decellularized allodermis
        embolism T85.818 ☑
        fibrosis T85.828 ☑
        hemorrhage T85.838 ☑
        infection and inflammation T85.79 ☑
        mechanical
          breakdown T85.613 ☑
          displacement T85.623 ☑
          malfunction T85.613 ☑
          malposition T85.623 ☑
          obstruction T85.693 ☑
          perforation T85.693 ☑
          protrusion T85.693 ☑
          specified NEC T85.693 ☑
        pain T85.848 ☑
        specified type NEC T85.898 ☑
        stenosis T85.858 ☑
        thrombosis T85.868 ☑
      failure T86.821
      infection T86.822
      rejection T86.820
      specified NEC T86.828

Complication(s) — *continued*
  prosthetic device or implant — *continued*
    sling
      urethral (female) (male)
        erosion T83.712 ☑
        exposure T83.722 ☑
    specified NEC T85.9 ☑
      embolism T85.818 ☑
      fibrosis T85.828 ☑
      hemorrhage T85.838 ☑
      infection and inflammation T85.79 ☑
      mechanical
        breakdown T85.618 ☑
        displacement T85.628 ☑
        leakage T85.638 ☑
        malfunction T85.618 ☑
        malposition T85.628 ☑
        obstruction T85.698 ☑
        perforation T85.698 ☑
        protrusion T85.698 ☑
        specified NEC T85.698 ☑
      pain T85.848 ☑
      specified type NEC T85.898 ☑
      stenosis T85.858 ☑
      thrombosis T85.868 ☑
    subdural infusion catheter — *see* Complications, catheter, subdural
    sutures — *see* Complications, sutures
    urinary organ or tract NEC — *see* Complications, genitourinary, device or implant, urinary system
    vascular — *see* Complications, cardiovascular device or implant
    ventricular shunt — *see* Complications, ventricular shunt (device)
  puerperium — *see* Puerperal
  puncture, spinal G97.1
    cerebrospinal fluid leak G97.0
    headache or reaction G97.1
  pyelogram N99.89
  radiation
    kyphosis M96.2
    scoliosis M96.5
  reattached
    extremity (infection) (rejection)
      lower T87.1X- ☑
      upper T87.0X- ☑
    specified body part NEC T87.2
  reconstructed breast
    asymmetry between native and reconstructed breast N65.1
    deformity N65.0
    disproportion between native and reconstructed breast N65.1
    excess tissue N65.0
    misshappen N65.0
  reimplant NEC — *see also* Complications, prosthetic device or implant
    limb (infection) (rejection) — *see* Complications, reattached, extremity
    organ (partial) (total) — *see* Complications, transplant
    prosthetic device NEC — *see* Complications, prosthetic device
  renal N28.9
    allograft — *see* Complications, transplant, kidney
    dialysis — *see* Complications, dialysis
  respirator
    mechanical J95.850
      specified NEC J95.859
  respiratory system J98.9
    device, implant or graft — *see* Complication, prosthetic device or implant, specified NEC
    lung transplant — *see* Complications, prosthetic device or implant, lung transplant
    postoperative J95.89
      air leak J95.812
      Mendelson's syndrome (chemical pneumonitis) J95.4
      pneumothorax J95.811
      pulmonary insufficiency (acute) (after nonthoracic surgery) J95.2
        chronic J95.3
        following thoracic surgery J95.1
      respiratory failure (acute) J95.821
        acute and chronic J95.822
      specified NEC J95.89

Complication(s) — *continued*
  respiratory system — *continued*
    postoperative — *continued*
      subglottic stenosis J95.5
      tracheostomy complication — *see* Complications, tracheostomy
    therapy T81.89 ☑
  sedation during labor and delivery O74.9
    cardiac O74.2
    central nervous system O74.3
    pulmonary NEC O74.1
  shunt — *see also* Complications, prosthetic device or implant
    arteriovenous — *see* Complications, arteriovenous, shunt
    ventricular (communicating) — *see* Complications, ventricular shunt
  skin
    graft T86.829
      failure T86.821
      infection T86.822
      rejection T86.820
      specified type NEC T86.828
  spinal
    anesthesia — *see* Complications, anesthesia, spinal
    catheter (epidural) (subdural) — *see* Complications, catheter
    puncture or tap G97.1
      cerebrospinal fluid leak G97.0
      headache or reaction G97.1
  stent
    bile duct — *see* Complications, bile duct prosthesis
    ureteral indwelling
      breakdown T83.112 ☑
      displacement T83.122 ☑
      leakage T83.192 ☑
      malposition T83.122 ☑
      obstruction T83.192 ☑
      perforation T83.192 ☑
      protrusion T83.192 ☑
      specified NEC T83.192 ☑
    urinary NEC (ileal conduit) (nephroureteral) T83.193 ☑
      embolism T83.81 ☑
      fibrosis T83.82 ☑
      hemorrhage T83.83 ☑
      infection and inflammation T83.593 ☑
      mechanical
        breakdown T83.113 ☑
        displacement T83.123 ☑
        leakage T83.193 ☑
        malposition T83.123 ☑
        obstruction T83.193 ☑
        perforation T83.193 ☑
        protrusion T83.193 ☑
        specified NEC T83.193 ☑
      pain T83.84 ☑
      specified type NEC T83.89 ☑
      stenosis T83.85 ☑
      thrombosis T83.86 ☑
    vascular
      end stent stenosis — *see* Restenosis, stent
      in stent stenosis — *see* Restenosis, stent
  stoma
    digestive tract
      colostomy — *see* Complications, colostomy
      enterostomy — *see* Complications, enterostomy
      esophagostomy — *see* Complications, esophagostomy
      gastrostomy — *see* Complications, gastrostomy
    urinary tract N99.528
      continent N99.538
        hemorrhage N99.530
        herniation N99.533
        infection N99.531
        malfunction N99.532
        specified type NEC N99.538
        stenosis N99.534
      cystostomy — *see* Complications, cystostomy
      external NOS N99.528
      hemorrhage N99.520
      herniation N99.523
      incontinent N99.528
        hemorrhage N99.520
        herniation N99.523
        infection N99.521
        malfunction N99.522

☑ **Additional Character Required — Refer to the Tabular List for Character Selection** ☞ Subterms under main terms may continue to next column or page

Complication(s) — *continued*
  stoma — *continued*
    urinary tract — *continued*
      incontinent — *continued*
        specified type NEC N99.528
        stenosis N99.524
      infection N99.521
      malfunction N99.522
      specified type NEC N99.528
      stenosis N99.524
  stomach banding — *see* Complication(s), bariatric procedure
  stomach stapling — *see* Complication(s), bariatric procedure
  surgical material, nonabsorbable — *see* Complication, suture, permanent
  surgical procedure (on) T81.9 ☑
    amputation stump (late) — *see* Complications, amputation stump
    cardiac — *see* Complications, circulatory system
    cholesteatoma, recurrent — *see* Complications, postmastoidectomy, recurrent cholesteatoma
    circulatory (early) — *see* Complications, circulatory system
    digestive system — *see* Complications, gastrointestinal
    dumping syndrome (postgastrectomy) K91.1
    ear — *see* Complications, ear
    elephantiasis or lymphedema I97.89
      postmastectomy I97.2
    emphysema (surgical) T81.82 ☑
    endocrine — *see* Complications, endocrine
    eye — *see* Complications, eye
    fistula (persistent postoperative) T81.83 ☑
    foreign body inadvertently left in wound (sponge) (suture) (swab) — *see* Foreign body, accidentally left during a procedure
    gastrointestinal — *see* Complications, gastrointestinal
    genitourinary NEC N99.89
    hematoma
      intraoperative — *see* Complication, intraoperative, hemorrhage
      postprocedural — *see* Complication, postprocedural, hematoma
    hemorrhage
      intraoperative — *see* Complication, intraoperative, hemorrhage
      postprocedural — *see* Complication, postprocedural, hemorrhage
    hepatic failure K91.82
    hyperglycemia (postpancreatectomy) E89.1
    hypoinsulinemia (postpancreatectomy) E89.1
    hypoparathyroidism (postparathyroidectomy) E89.2
    hypopituitarism (posthypophysectomy) E89.3
    hypothyroidism (post-thyroidectomy) E89.0
    intestinal obstruction — *see also* Obstruction, intestine, postoperative K91.30
    intracranial hypotension following ventricular shunting (ventriculostomy) G97.2
    lymphedema I97.89
      postmastectomy I97.2
    malabsorption (postsurgical) NEC K91.2
      osteoporosis — *see* Osteoporosis, postsurgical malabsorption
    mastoidectomy cavity NEC — *see* Complications, postmastoidectomy
    metabolic E89.89
      specified NEC E89.89
    musculoskeletal — *see* Complications, musculoskeletal system
    nervous system (central) (peripheral) — *see* Complications, nervous system
    ovarian failure E89.40
      asymptomatic E89.40
      symptomatic E89.41
    peripheral vascular — *see* Complications, surgical procedure, vascular
    postcardiotomy syndrome I97.0
    postcholecystectomy syndrome K91.5
    postcommissurotomy syndrome I97.0
    postgastrectomy dumping syndrome K91.1
    postlaminectomy syndrome NEC M96.1
      kyphosis M96.3
    postmastectomy lymphedema syndrome I97.2
    postmastoidectomy cholesteatoma — *see* Complications, postmastoidectomy, recurrent cholesteatoma

Complication(s) — *continued*
  surgical procedure — *continued*
    postvagotomy syndrome K91.1
    postvalvulotomy syndrome I97.0
    pulmonary insufficiency (acute) J95.2
      chronic J95.3
      following thoracic surgery J95.1
    reattached body part — *see* Complications, reattached
    respiratory — *see* Complications, respiratory system
    shock (hypovolemic) T81.19 ☑
    spleen (postoperative) D78.89
      intraoperative D78.81
    stitch abscess T81.41 ☑
    subglottic stenosis (postsurgical) J95.5
    testicular hypofunction E89.5
    transplant — *see* Complications, organ or tissue transplant
    urinary NEC N99.89
    vaginal vault prolapse (posthysterectomy) N99.3
    vascular (peripheral)
      artery T81.719 ☑
        mesenteric T81.710 ☑
        renal T81.711 ☑
        specified NEC T81.718 ☑
      vein T81.72 ☑
    wound infection T81.49 ☑
  suture, permanent (wire) NEC T85.9 ☑
    with repair of bone — *see* Complications, fixation device, internal
    embolism T85.818 ☑
    fibrosis T85.828 ☑
    hemorrhage T85.838 ☑
    infection and inflammation T85.79 ☑
    mechanical
      breakdown T85.612 ☑
      displacement T85.622 ☑
      malfunction T85.612 ☑
      malposition T85.622 ☑
      obstruction T85.692 ☑
      perforation T85.692 ☑
      protrusion T85.692 ☑
      specified NEC T85.692 ☑
    pain T85.848 ☑
    specified type NEC T85.898 ☑
    stenosis T85.858 ☑
    thrombosis T85.868 ☑
  tracheostomy J95.00
    granuloma J95.09
    hemorrhage J95.01
    infection J95.02
    malfunction J95.03
    mechanical J95.03
    obstruction J95.03
    specified type NEC J95.09
    tracheo-esophageal fistula J95.04
  transfusion (blood) (lymphocytes) (plasma) T80.92 ☑
    air emblism T80.0 ☑
    circulatory overload E87.71
    febrile nonhemolytic transfusion reaction R50.84
    hemochromatosis E83.111
    hemolysis T80.89 ☑
    hemolytic reaction (antigen unspecified) T80.919 ☑
    incompatibility reaction (antigen unspecified) T80.919 ☑
      ABO T80.30 ☑
        delayed serologic (DSTR) T80.39 ☑
        hemolytic transfusion reaction (HTR) (unspecified time after transfusion) T80.319 ☑
        acute (AHTR) (less than 24 hours after transfusion) T80.310 ☑
        delayed (DHTR) (24 hours or more after transfusion) T80.311 ☑
        specified NEC T80.39 ☑
      acute (antigen unspecified) T80.910 ☑
      delayed (antigen unspecified) T80.911 ☑
      delayed serologic (DSTR) T80.89 ☑
      non-ABO (minor antigens (Duffy) (K) (Kell) (Kidd) (Lewis) (M) (N) (P) (S)) T80.A0 ☑ (*following* T80.4)
        delayed serologic (DSTR) T80.A9 ☑ (*following* T80.4)
        hemolytic transfusion reaction (HTR) (unspecified time after transfusion) T80.A19 ☑ (*following* T80.4)

Complication(s) — *continued*
  transfusion — *continued*
    incompatibility reaction — *continued*
      non-ABO (S) — *continued*
        hemolytic transfusion reaction — *continued*
          acute (AHTR) (less than 24 hours after transfusion) T80.A10 ☑ (*following* T80.4)
          delayed (DHTR) (24 hours or more after transfusion) T80.A11 ☑ (*following* T80.4)
          specified NEC T80.A9 ☑ (*following* T80.4)
      Rh (antigens (C) (c) (D) (E) (e)) (factor) T80.40 ☑
        delayed serologic (DSTR) T80.49 ☑
        hemolytic transfusion reaction (HTR) (unspecified time after transfusion) T80.419 ☑
        acute (AHTR) (less than 24 hours after transfusion) T80.410 ☑
        delayed (DHTR) (24 hours or more after transfusion) T80.411 ☑
        specified NEC T80.49 ☑
    infection T80.29 ☑
      acute T80.22- ☑
    reaction NEC T80.89 ☑
    sepsis T80.29 ☑
    shock T80.89 ☑
  transplant T86.90
    bone T86.839
      failure T86.831
      infection T86.832
      rejection T86.830
      specified type NEC T86.838
    bone marrow T86.00
      failure T86.02
      infection T86.03
      rejection T86.01
      specified type NEC T86.09
    cornea T86.849-
      failure T86.841- ☑
      infection T86.842- ☑
      rejection T86.840- ☑
      specified type NEC T86.848- ☑
    failure T86.92
    heart T86.20
      with lung T86.30
      cardiac allograft vasculopathy T86.290
        failure T86.32
        infection T86.33
        rejection T86.31
        specified type NEC T86.39
      failure T86.22
      infection T86.23
      rejection T86.21
      specified type NEC T86.298
    infection T86.93
    intestine T86.859
      failure T86.851
      infection T86.852
      rejection T86.850
      specified type NEC T86.858
    kidney T86.10
      failure T86.12
      infection T86.13
      rejection T86.11
      specified type NEC T86.19
    liver T86.40
      failure T86.42
      infection T86.43
      rejection T86.41
      specified type NEC T86.49
    lung T86.819
      with heart T86.30
        failure T86.32
        infection T86.33
        rejection T86.31
        specified type NEC T86.39
      failure T86.811
      infection T86.812
      rejection T86.810
      specified type NEC T86.818
    malignant neoplasm C80.2
    pancreas T86.899
      failure T86.891
      infection T86.892
      rejection T86.890
      specified type NEC T86.898
    peripheral blood stem cells T86.5

Index

Complication — Complication

Complication(s) — *continued*
  transplant — *continued*
    post-transplant lymphoproliferative disorder (PTLD) D47.Z1 (*following* D47.4)
    rejection T86.91
    skin T86.829
      failure T86.821
      infection T86.822
      rejection T86.820
      specified type NEC T86.828
    specified
      tissue T86.899
        failure T86.891
        infection T86.892
        rejection T86.890
        specified type NEC T86.898
      type NEC T86.99
    stem cell (from peripheral blood) (from umbilical cord) T86.5
    umbilical cord stem cells T86.5
  trauma (early) T79.9 ☑
    specified NEC T79.8 ☑
  ultrasound therapy NEC T88.9 ☑
  umbilical cord NEC
    complicating delivery O69.9 ☑
    specified NEC O69.89 ☑
  umbrella device, vascular T82.9 ☑
    embolism T82.818 ☑
    fibrosis T82.828 ☑
    hemorrhage T82.838 ☑
    infection or inflammation T82.7 ☑
    mechanical
      breakdown T82.515 ☑
      displacement T82.525 ☑
      leakage T82.535 ☑
      malposition T82.525 ☑
      obstruction T82.595 ☑
      perforation T82.595 ☑
      protrusion T82.595 ☑
    pain T82.848 ☑
    specified type NEC T82.898 ☑
    stenosis T82.858 ☑
    thrombosis T82.868 ☑
  urethral catheter — *see* Complications, catheter, urethral, indwelling
  vaccination T88.1 ☑
    anaphylaxis NEC T80.52 ☑
    arthropathy — *see* Arthropathy, postimmunization
    cellulitis T88.0 ☑
    encephalitis or encephalomyelitis G04.02
    infection (general) (local) NEC T88.0 ☑
    meningitis G03.8
    myelitis G04.02
    protein sickness T80.62 ☑
    rash T88.1 ☑
    reaction (allergic) T88.1 ☑
      serum T80.62 ☑
    sepsis T88.0 ☑
    serum intoxication, sickness, rash, or other serum reaction NEC T80.62 ☑
      anaphylactic shock T80.52 ☑
    shock (allergic) (anaphylactic) T80.52 ☑
    vaccinia (generalized) (localized) T88.1 ☑
  vas deferens device or implant — *see* Complications, genitourinary, device or implant, genital tract
  vascular I99.9
    device or implant T82.9 ☑
      embolism T82.818 ☑
      fibrosis T82.828 ☑
      hemorrhage T82.838 ☑
      infection or inflammation T82.7 ☑
      mechanical
        breakdown T82.519 ☑
          specified device NEC T82.518 ☑
        displacement T82.529 ☑
          specified device NEC T82.528 ☑
        leakage T82.539 ☑
          specified device NEC T82.538 ☑
        malposition T82.529 ☑
          specified device NEC T82.528 ☑
        obstruction T82.599 ☑
          specified device NEC T82.598 ☑
        perforation T82.599 ☑
          specified device NEC T82.598 ☑
        protrusion T82.599 ☑
          specified device NEC T82.598 ☑
      pain T82.848 ☑

Complication(s) — *continued*
  vascular — *continued*
    device or implant — *continued*
      specified type NEC T82.898 ☑
      stenosis T82.858 ☑
      thrombosis T82.868 ☑
    dialysis catheter — *see* Complication, catheter, dialysis
    following infusion, therapeutic injection or transfusion T80.1 ☑
    graft T82.9 ☑
      embolism T82.818 ☑
      fibrosis T82.828 ☑
      hemorrhage T82.838 ☑
      mechanical
        breakdown T82.319 ☑
          aorta (bifurcation) T82.310 ☑
          carotid artery T82.311 ☑
          specified vessel NEC T82.318 ☑
        displacement T82.329 ☑
          aorta (bifurcation) T82.320 ☑
          carotid artery T82.321 ☑
          specified vessel NEC T82.328 ☑
        leakage T82.339 ☑
          aorta (bifurcation) T82.330 ☑
          carotid artery T82.331 ☑
          specified vessel NEC T82.338 ☑
        malposition T82.329 ☑
          aorta (bifurcation) T82.320 ☑
          carotid artery T82.321 ☑
          specified vessel NEC T82.328 ☑
        obstruction T82.399 ☑
          aorta (bifurcation) T82.390 ☑
          carotid artery T82.391 ☑
          specified vessel NEC T82.398 ☑
        perforation T82.399 ☑
          aorta (bifurcation) T82.390 ☑
          carotid artery T82.391 ☑
          specified vessel NEC T82.398 ☑
        protrusion T82.399 ☑
          aorta (bifurcation) T82.390 ☑
          carotid artery T82.391 ☑
          specified vessel NEC T82.398 ☑
      pain T82.848 ☑
      specified complication NEC T82.898 ☑
      stenosis T82.858 ☑
      thrombosis T82.868 ☑
    postoperative — *see* Complications, postoperative, circulatory
    vena cava device (filter) (sieve) (umbrella) — *see* Complications, umbrella device, vascular
  ventilation therapy NEC T81.81 ☑
  ventilator
    mechanical J95.850
      specified NEC J95.859
  ventricular (communicating) shunt (device) T85.9 ☑
    embolism T85.810 ☑
    fibrosis T85.820 ☑
    hemorrhage T85.830 ☑
    infection and inflammation T85.730 ☑
    mechanical
      breakdown T85.01 ☑
      displacement T85.02 ☑
      leakage T85.03 ☑
      malposition T85.02 ☑
      obstruction T85.09 ☑
      perforation T85.09 ☑
      protrusion T85.09 ☑
      specified NEC T85.09 ☑
    pain T85.840 ☑
    specified type NEC T85.890 ☑
    stenosis T85.850 ☑
    thrombosis T85.860 ☑
  wire suture, permanent (implanted) — *see* Complications, suture, permanent

Compressed air disease T70.3 ☑
Compression
  with injury — *code by* Nature of injury
  artery I77.1
    celiac, syndrome I77.4
  brachial plexus G54.0
  brain (stem) G93.5
    due to
      contusion (diffuse) — *see also* Injury, intracranial, diffuse S06.A0 ☑
        with herniation S06.A1 ☑

Compression — *continued*
  brain — *continued*
    due to — *continued*
      contusion — *see also* Injury, intracranial, diffuse — *continued*
        focal — *see also* Injury, intracranial, focal S06.A0 ☑
          with herniation S06.A1 ☑
      injury NEC — *see also* Injury, intracranial, diffuse S06.A0 ☑
      nontraumatic G93.5
      traumatic — *see also* Injury, intracranial, diffuse S06.A0 ☑
        with herniation S06.A1 ☑
  bronchus J98.09
  cauda equina G83.4
  celiac (artery) (axis) I77.4
  cerebral — *see* Compression, brain
  cervical plexus G54.2
  cord
    spinal — *see* Compression, spinal
    umbilical — *see* Compression, umbilical cord
  cranial nerve G52.9
    eighth H93.3 ☑
    eleventh G52.8
    fifth G50.8
    first G52.0
    fourth — *see* Strabismus, paralytic, fourth nerve
    ninth G52.1
    second — *see* Disorder, nerve, optic
    seventh G51.8
    sixth — *see* Strabismus, paralytic, sixth nerve
    tenth G52.2
    third — *see* Strabismus, paralytic, third nerve
    twelfth G52.3
  diver's squeeze T70.3 ☑
  during birth (newborn) P15.9
  esophagus K22.2
  eustachian tube — *see* Obstruction, eustachian tube, cartilaginous
  facies Q67.1
  fracture
    nontraumatic NOS — *see* Collapse, vertebra
    pathological — *see* Fracture, pathological
    traumatic — *see* Fracture, traumatic
  heart — *see* Disease, heart
  intestine — *see* Obstruction, intestine
  laryngeal nerve, recurrent G52.2
    with paralysis of vocal cords and larynx J38.00
      bilateral J38.02
      unilateral J38.01
  lumbosacral plexus G54.1
  lung J98.4
  lymphatic vessel I89.0
  medulla — *see* Compression, brain
  nerve — *see also* Disorder, nerve G58.9
    arm NEC — *see* Mononeuropathy, upper limb
    axillary G54.0
    cranial — *see* Compression, cranial nerve
    leg NEC — *see* Mononeuropathy, lower limb
    median (in carpal tunnel) — *see* Syndrome, carpal tunnel
    optic — *see* Disorder, nerve, optic
    plantar — *see* Lesion, nerve, plantar
    posterior tibial (in tarsal tunnel) — *see* Syndrome, tarsal tunnel
    root or plexus NOS (in) G54.9
      intervertebral disc disorder NEC — *see* Disorder, disc, with, radiculopathy
        with myelopathy — *see* Disorder, disc, with, myelopathy
      neoplastic disease — *see also* Neoplasm D49.9 *[G55]*
      spondylosis — *see* Spondylosis, with radiculopathy
    sciatic (acute) — *see* Lesion, nerve, sciatic
    sympathetic G90.8
    traumatic — *see* Injury, nerve
    ulnar — *see* Lesion, nerve, ulnar
    upper extremity NEC — *see* Mononeuropathy, upper limb
  spinal (cord) G95.20
    by displacement of intervertebral disc NEC — *see also* Disorder, disc, with, myelopathy
    nerve root NOS G54.9
      due to displacement of intervertebral disc NEC — *see* Disorder, disc, with, radiculopathy

☑ Additional Character Required — Refer to the Tabular List for Character Selection   ▽ Subterms under main terms may continue to next column or page

Compression — *continued*
  spinal — *continued*
    nerve root — *continued*
      due to displacement of intervertebral disc — *see*
        Disorder, disc, with, radiculopathy — *continued*
        with myelopathy — *see* Disorder, disc, with,
          myelopathy
    specified NEC G95.29
    spondylogenic (cervical) (lumbar, lumbosacral)
      (thoracic) — *see* Spondylosis, with myelopathy NEC
    anterior — *see* Syndrome, anterior, spinal artery,
      compression
    traumatic — *see* Injury, spinal cord, by region
  subcostal nerve (syndrome) — *see* Mononeuropathy,
    upper limb, specified NEC
  sympathetic nerve NEC G90.8
  syndrome T79.5 ☑
  trachea J39.8
  ulnar nerve (by scar tissue) — *see* Lesion, nerve, ulnar
  umbilical cord
    complicating delivery O69.2 ☑
      cord around neck O69.1 ☑
      prolapse O69.0 ☑
      specified NEC O69.2 ☑
  ureter N13.5
  vein I87.1
  vena cava (inferior) (superior) I87.1
Compulsion, compulsive
  gambling F63.0
  neurosis F42.8
  personality F60.5
  states F42.8
  swearing F42.8
    in Gilles de la Tourette's syndrome F95.2
  tics and spasms F95.9
Concato's disease (pericardial polyserositis) A19.9
  nontubercular I31.1
  pleural — *see* Pleurisy, with effusion
Concavity chest wall M95.4
Concealed penis Q55.64
Concern (normal) **about sick person in family** Z63.6
Concrescence (teeth) K00.2
Concretio cordis I31.1
  rheumatic I09.2
Concretion — *see also* Calculus
  appendicular K38.1
  canaliculus — *see* Dacryolith
  clitoris N90.89
  conjunctiva H11.12- ☑
  eyelid — *see* Disorder, eyelid, specified type NEC
  lacrimal passages — *see* Dacryolith
  prepuce (male) N47.8
  salivary gland (any) K11.5
  seminal vesicle N50.89
  tonsil J35.8
Concussion (brain) (cerebral) (current) S06.0X9 ☑
  with
    loss of consciousness of 30 minutes or less
      S06.0X1 ☑
    loss of consciousness of unspecified duration
      S06.0X9 ☑
  blast (air) (hydraulic) (immersion) (underwater)
    abdomen or thorax — *see* Injury, blast, by site
    ear with acoustic nerve injury — *see* Injury, nerve,
      acoustic, specified type NEC
  cauda equina S34.3 ☑
  conus medullaris S34.02 ☑
  ocular S05.8X- ☑
  spinal (cord)
    cervical S14.0 ☑
    lumbar S34.01 ☑
    sacral S34.02 ☑
    thoracic S24.0 ☑
  syndrome F07.81
  without loss of consciousness S06.0X0 ☑
Condition — *see also* Disease
  post COVID-19 U09.9
Conditions arising in the perinatal period — *see*
  Newborn, affected by
Conduct disorder — *see* Disorder, conduct
Condyloma A63.0
  acuminatum A63.0
  gonorrheal A54.09
  latum A51.31
  syphilitic A51.31

Condyloma — *continued*
  syphilitic — *continued*
    congenital A50.07
  venereal, syphilitic A51.31
Conflagration — *see also* Burn
  asphyxia (by inhalation of gases, fumes or vapors) —
    see also Table of Drugs and Chemicals T59.9- ☑
Conflict (with) — *see also* Discord
  family Z73.9
  marital Z63.0
    involving divorce or estrangement Z63.5
  parent-child Z62.820
    parent-adopted child Z62.821
    parent-biological child Z62.820
    parent-foster child Z62.822
  social role NEC Z73.5
Confluent — *see* condition
Confusion, confused R41.0
  epileptic F05
  mental state (psychogenic) F44.89
  psychogenic F44.89
  reactive (from emotional stress, psychological trauma)
    F44.89
Confusional arousals G47.51
Congelation T69.9 ☑
Congenital — *see also* condition
  aortic septum Q25.49
  intrinsic factor deficiency D51.0
  malformation — *see* Anomaly
Congestion, congestive
  bladder N32.89
  bowel K63.89
  brain G93.89
  breast N64.59
  bronchial J98.09
  catarrhal J31.0
  chest R09.89
  chill, malarial — *see* Malaria
  circulatory NEC I99.8
  duodenum K31.89
  eye — *see* Hyperemia, conjunctiva
  facial, due to birth injury P15.4
  general R68.89
  glottis J37.0
  heart — *see* Failure, heart, congestive
  hepatic K76.1
  hypostatic (lung) — *see* Edema, lung
  intestine K63.89
  kidney N28.89
  labyrinth H83.8 ☑
  larynx J37.0
  liver K76.1
  lung R09.89
    active or acute — *see* Pneumonia
  malaria, malarial — *see* Malaria
  nasal R09.81
  nose R09.81
  orbit, orbital — *see also* Exophthalmos
    inflammatory (chronic) — *see* Inflammation, orbit
  ovary N83.8
  pancreas K86.89
  pelvic, female N94.89
  pleural J94.8
  prostate (active) N42.1
  pulmonary — *see* Congestion, lung
  renal N28.89
  retina H35.81
  seminal vesicle N50.1
  spinal cord G95.19
  spleen (chronic) D73.2
  stomach K31.89
  trachea — *see* Tracheitis
  urethra N36.8
  uterus N85.8
    with subinvolution N85.3
  venous (passive) I87.8
  viscera R68.89
Congestive — *see* Congestion
Conical
  cervix (hypertrophic elongation) N88.4
  cornea — *see* Keratoconus
  teeth K00.2
Conjoined twins Q89.4
Conjugal maladjustment Z63.0
  involving divorce or estrangement Z63.5
Conjunctiva — *see* condition
Conjunctivitis (staphylococcal) (streptococcal) NOS H10.9
  Acanthamoeba B60.12

Conjunctivitis — *continued*
  acute H10.3- ☑
    atopic H10.1- ☑
    chemical — *see also* Corrosion, cornea H10.21- ☑
    mucopurulent H10.02- ☑
      follicular H10.01- ☑
    pseudomembranous H10.22- ☑
    serous except viral H10.23- ☑
    viral — *see* Conjunctivitis, viral
    toxic H10.21- ☑
  adenoviral (acute) (follicular) B30.1
  allergic (acute) — *see* Conjunctivitis, acute, atopic
    chronic H10.45
    vernal H10.44
  anaphylactic — *see* Conjunctivitis, acute, atopic
  Apollo B30.3
  atopic (acute) — *see* Conjunctivitis, acute, atopic
  Béal's B30.2
  blennorrhagic (gonococcal) (neonatorum) A54.31
  chemical (acute) — *see also* Corrosion, cornea
    H10.21- ☑
  chlamydial A74.0
    due to trachoma A71.1
    neonatal P39.1
  chronic (nodosa) (petrificans) (phlyctenular) H10.40- ☑
    allergic H10.45
      vernal H10.44
    follicular H10.43- ☑
    giant papillary H10.41- ☑
    simple H10.42- ☑
    vernal H10.44
  coxsackievirus 24 B30.3
  diphtheritic A36.86
  due to
    dust — *see* Conjunctivitis, acute, atopic
    filariasis B74.9
    mucocutaneous leishmaniasis B55.2
  enterovirus type 70 (hemorrhagic) B30.3
  epidemic (viral) B30.9
    hemorrhagic B30.3
  gonococcal (neonatorum) A54.31
  granular (trachomatous) A71.1
    sequelae (late effect) B94.0
  hemorrhagic (acute) (epidemic) B30.3
  herpes zoster B02.31
  in (due to)
    Acanthamoeba B60.12
    adenovirus (acute) (follicular) B30.1
    Chlamydia A74.0
    coxsackievirus 24 B30.3
    diphtheria A36.86
    enterovirus type 70 (hemorrhagic) B30.3
    filariasis B74.9
    gonococci A54.31
    herpes (simplex) virus B00.53
      zoster B02.31
    infectious disease NEC B99 ☑
    meningococci A39.89
    mucocutaneous leishmaniasis B55.2
    rosacea H10.82- ☑
    syphilis (late) A52.71
    zoster B02.31
  inclusion A74.0
  infantile P39.1
    gonococcal A54.31
  Koch-Weeks' — *see* Conjunctivitis, acute, mucopurulent
  light — *see* Conjunctivitis, acute, atopic
  ligneous — *see* Blepharoconjunctivitis, ligneous
  meningococcal A39.89
  mucopurulent — *see* Conjunctivitis, acute, mucopurulent
  neonatal P39.1
    gonococcal A54.31
  Newcastle B30.8
  of Béal B30.2
  parasitic
    filariasis B74.9
    mucocutaneous leishmaniasis B55.2
  Parinaud's H10.89
  petrificans H10.89
  rosacea H10.82- ☑
  specified NEC H10.89
  swimming-pool B30.1
  trachomatous A71.1
    acute A71.0
    sequelae (late effect) B94.0
  traumatic NEC H10.89
  tuberculous A18.59

Conjunctivitis — continued
tularemic A21.1
tularensis A21.1
viral B30.9
due to
adenovirus B30.1
enterovirus B30.3
specified NEC B30.8
Conjunctivochalasis H11.82- ☑
Connective tissue — see condition
Conn's syndrome E26.01
Conradi (-Hunermann) **disease** Q77.3
Consanguinity Z84.3
counseling Z71.89
Conscious simulation (of illness) Z76.5
Consecutive — see condition
Consolidation lung (base) — see Pneumonia, lobar
Constipation (atonic) (neurogenic) (simple) (spastic) K59.00
chronic K59.09
idiopathic K59.04
drug-induced K59.03
functional K59.04
outlet dysfunction K59.02
psychogenic F45.8
slow transit K59.01
specified NEC K59.09
Constitutional — see also condition
substandard F60.7
Constitutionally substandard F60.7
Constriction — see also Stricture
auditory canal — see Stenosis, external ear canal
bronchial J98.09
duodenum K31.5
esophagus K22.2
external
abdomen, abdominal (wall) S30.841 ☑
alveolar process S00.542 ☑
ankle S90.54- ☑
antecubital space — see Constriction, external, forearm
arm (upper) S40.84- ☑
auricle — see Constriction, external, ear
axilla — see Constriction, external, arm
back, lower S30.840 ☑
breast S20.14- ☑
brow S00.84 ☑
buttock S30.840 ☑
calf — see Constriction, external, leg
canthus — see Constriction, external, eyelid
cheek S00.84 ☑
internal S00.542 ☑
chest wall — see Constriction, external, thorax
chin S00.84 ☑
clitoris S30.844 ☑
costal region — see Constriction, external, thorax
digit(s)
foot — see Constriction, external, toe
hand — see Constriction, external, finger
ear S00.44- ☑
elbow S50.34- ☑
epididymis S30.843 ☑
epigastric region S30.841 ☑
esophagus, cervical S10.14 ☑
eyebrow — see Constriction, external, eyelid
eyelid S00.24- ☑
face S00.84 ☑
finger(s) S60.44- ☑
index S60.44- ☑
little S60.44- ☑
middle S60.44- ☑
ring S60.44- ☑
flank S30.841 ☑
foot (except toe(s) alone) S90.84- ☑
toe — see Constriction, external, toe
forearm S50.84- ☑
elbow only — see Constriction, external, elbow
forehead S00.84 ☑
genital organs, external
female S30.846 ☑
male S30.845 ☑
groin S30.841 ☑
gum S00.542 ☑
hand S60.54- ☑
head S00.94 ☑
ear — see Constriction, external, ear
eyelid — see Constriction, external, eyelid

Constriction — continued
external — continued
head — continued
lip S00.541 ☑
nose S00.34 ☑
oral cavity S00.542 ☑
scalp S00.04 ☑
specified site NEC S00.84 ☑
heel — see Constriction, external, foot
hip S70.24- ☑
inguinal region S30.841 ☑
interscapular region S20.449 ☑
jaw S00.84 ☑
knee S80.24- ☑
labium (majus) (minus) S30.844 ☑
larynx S10.14 ☑
leg (lower) S80.84- ☑
knee — see Constriction, external, knee
upper — see Constriction, external, thigh
lip S00.541 ☑
lower back S30.840 ☑
lumbar region S30.840 ☑
malar region S00.84 ☑
mammary — see Constriction, external, breast
mastoid region S00.84 ☑
mouth S00.542 ☑
nail
finger — see Constriction, external, finger
toe — see Constriction, external, toe
nasal S00.34 ☑
neck S10.94 ☑
specified site NEC S10.84 ☑
throat S10.14 ☑
nose S00.34 ☑
occipital region S00.04 ☑
oral cavity S00.542 ☑
orbital region — see Constriction, external, eyelid
palate S00.542 ☑
palm — see Constriction, external, hand
parietal region S00.04 ☑
pelvis S30.840 ☑
penis S30.842 ☑
perineum
female S30.844 ☑
male S30.840 ☑
periocular area — see Constriction, external, eyelid
phalanges
finger — see Constriction, external, finger
toe — see Constriction, external, toe
pharynx S10.14 ☑
pinna — see Constriction, external, ear
popliteal space — see Constriction, external, knee
prepuce S30.842 ☑
pubic region S30.840 ☑
pudendum
female S30.846 ☑
male S30.845 ☑
sacral region S30.840 ☑
scalp S00.04 ☑
scapular region — see Constriction, external, shoulder
scrotum S30.843 ☑
shin — see Constriction, external, leg
shoulder S40.24- ☑
sternal region S20.349 ☑
submaxillary region S00.84 ☑
submental region S00.84 ☑
subungual
finger(s) — see Constriction, external, finger
toe(s) — see Constriction, external, toe
supraclavicular fossa S10.84 ☑
supraorbital S00.84 ☑
temple S00.84 ☑
temporal region S00.84 ☑
testis S30.843 ☑
thigh S70.34- ☑
thorax, thoracic (wall) S20.94 ☑
back S20.44- ☑
front S20.34- ☑
throat S10.14 ☑
thumb S60.34- ☑
toe(s) (lesser) S90.44- ☑
great S90.44- ☑
tongue S00.542 ☑
trachea S10.14 ☑
tunica vaginalis S30.843 ☑

Constriction — continued
external — continued
uvula S00.542 ☑
vagina S30.844 ☑
vulva S30.844 ☑
wrist S60.84- ☑
gallbladder — see Obstruction, gallbladder
intestine — see Obstruction, intestine
larynx J38.6
congenital Q31.8
specified NEC Q31.8
subglottic Q31.1
organ or site, congenital NEC — see Atresia, by site
prepuce (acquired) (congenital) N47.1
pylorus (adult hypertrophic) K31.1
congenital or infantile Q40.0
newborn Q40.0
ring dystocia (uterus) O62.4
spastic — see also Spasm
ureter N13.5
ureter N13.5
with infection N13.6
urethra — see Stricture, urethra
visual field (peripheral) (functional) — see Defect, visual field
Constrictive — see condition
Consultation
medical — see Counseling, medical
religious Z71.81
specified reason NEC Z71.89
spiritual Z71.81
without complaint or sickness Z71.9
feared complaint unfounded Z71.1
specified reason NEC Z71.89
Consumption — see Tuberculosis
Contact (with) — see also Exposure (to)
acariasis Z20.7
AIDS virus Z20.6
air pollution Z77.110
algae and algae toxins Z77.121
algae bloom Z77.121
anthrax Z20.810
aromatic amines Z77.020
aromatic (hazardous) compounds NEC Z77.028
aromatic dyes NOS Z77.028
arsenic Z77.010
asbestos Z77.090
bacterial disease NEC Z20.818
benzene Z77.021
blue-green algae bloom Z77.121
body fluids (potentially hazardous) Z77.21
brown tide Z77.121
chemicals (chiefly nonmedicinal) (hazardous) NEC Z77.098
cholera Z20.09
chromium compounds Z77.018
communicable disease Z20.9
bacterial NEC Z20.818
specified NEC Z20.89
viral NEC Z20.828
Zika virus Z20.821
coronavirus (disease) (novel) 2019 Z20.822
COVID-19 Z20.822
cyanobacteria bloom Z77.121
dyes Z77.098
Escherichia coli (E. coli) Z20.01
fiberglass — see Table of Drugs and Chemicals, fiberglass
German measles Z20.4
gonorrhea Z20.2
hazardous metals NEC Z77.018
hazardous substances NEC Z77.29
hazards in the physical environment NEC Z77.128
hazards to health NEC Z77.9
HIV Z20.6
HTLV-III/LAV Z20.6
human immunodeficiency virus (HIV) Z20.6
infection Z20.9
specified NEC Z20.89
infestation (parasitic) NEC Z20.7
intestinal infectious disease NEC Z20.09
Escherichia coli (E. coli) Z20.01
lead Z77.011
meningococcus Z20.811
mold (toxic) Z77.120
nickel dust Z77.018
noise Z77.122
parasitic disease Z20.7

☑ Additional Character Required — Refer to the Tabular List for Character Selection   ▼ Subterms under main terms may continue to next column or page

Contact — *continued*
 pediculosis Z20.7
 pfiesteria piscicida Z77.121
 poliomyelitis Z20.89
 pollution
  air Z77.110
  environmental NEC Z77.118
  soil Z77.112
  water Z77.111
 polycyclic aromatic hydrocarbons Z77.028
 positive maternal group B streptococcus P00.82
 rabies Z20.3
 radiation, naturally occurring NEC Z77.123
 radon Z77.123
 red tide (Florida) Z77.121
 rubella Z20.4
 SARS-CoV-2 Z20.822
 sexually-transmitted disease Z20.2
 smallpox (laboratory) Z20.89
 syphilis Z20.2
 tuberculosis Z20.1
 uranium Z77.012
 varicella Z20.820
 venereal disease Z20.2
 viral disease NEC Z20.828
 viral hepatitis Z20.5
 water pollution Z77.111
 Zika virus Z20.821
Contamination, food — *see* Intoxication, foodborne
Contraception, contraceptive
 advice Z30.09
 counseling Z30.09
 device (intrauterine) (in situ) Z97.5
  causing menorrhagia T83.83 ☑
  checking Z30.431
  complications — *see* Complications, intrauterine, contraceptive device
  in place Z97.5
  initial prescription Z30.014
  reinsertion Z30.433
  removal Z30.432
  replacement Z30.433
 emergency (postcoital) Z30.012
 initial prescription Z30.019
  barrier Z30.018
  diaphragm Z30.018
  injectable Z30.013
  intrauterine device Z30.014
  pills Z30.011
  postcoital (emergency) Z30.012
  specified type NEC Z30.018
  subdermal implantable Z30.017
  transdermal patch hormonal Z30.016
  vaginal ring hormonal Z30.015
 maintenance Z30.40
  barrier Z30.49
  diaphragm Z30.49
  examination Z30.8
  injectable Z30.42
  intrauterine device Z30.431
  pills Z30.41
  specified type NEC Z30.49
  subdermal implantable Z30.46
  transdermal patch hormonal Z30.45
  vaginal ring hormonal Z30.44
 management Z30.9
  specified NEC Z30.8
 postcoital (emergency) Z30.012
 prescription Z30.019
  repeat Z30.40
 sterilization Z30.2
 surveillance (drug) — *see* Contraception, maintenance
Contraction(s), contracture, contracted
 Achilles tendon — *see also* Short, tendon, Achilles
  congenital Q66.89
 amputation stump (surgical) (flexion) (late) (next proximal joint) T87.89
 anus K59.89
 bile duct (common) (hepatic) K83.8
 bladder N32.89
  neck or sphincter N32.0
 bowel, cecum, colon or intestine, any part — *see* Obstruction, intestine
 Braxton Hicks — *see* False, labor
 breast implant, capsular T85.44 ☑
 bronchial J98.09
 burn (old) — *see* Cicatrix
 cervix — *see* Stricture, cervix

Contraction(s), contracture, contracted — *continued*
 cicatricial — *see* Cicatrix
 conjunctiva, trachomatous, active A71.1
  sequelae (late effect) B94.0
 Dupuytren's M72.0
 eyelid — *see* Disorder, eyelid function
 fascia (lata) (postural) M72.8
  Dupuytren's M72.0
  palmar M72.0
  plantar M72.2
 finger NEC — *see also* Deformity, finger
  congenital Q68.1
  joint — *see* Contraction, joint, hand
 flaccid — *see* Contraction, paralytic
 gallbladder K82.0
 heart valve — *see* Endocarditis
 hip — *see* Contraction, joint, hip
 hourglass
  bladder N32.89
   congenital Q64.79
  gallbladder K82.0
   congenital Q44.1
  stomach K31.89
   congenital Q40.2
   psychogenic F45.8
  uterus (complicating delivery) O62.4
 hysterical F44.4
 internal os — *see* Stricture, cervix
 joint (abduction) (acquired) (adduction) (flexion) (rotation) M24.50
  ankle M24.57- ☑
  congenital NEC Q68.8
   hip Q65.89
  elbow M24.52- ☑
  foot joint M24.57- ☑
  hand joint M24.54- ☑
  hip M24.55- ☑
   congenital Q65.89
  hysterical F44.4
  knee M24.56- ☑
  shoulder M24.51- ☑
  specified site NEC M24.59
  wrist M24.53- ☑
 kidney (granular) (secondary) N26.9
  congenital Q63.8
  hydronephritic — *see* Hydronephrosis Page N26.2
  pyelonephritic — *see* Pyelitis, chronic
  tuberculous A18.11
 ligament — *see also* Disorder, ligament
  congenital Q79.8
 muscle (postinfective) (postural) NEC M62.40
  with contracture of joint — *see* Contraction, joint
  ankle M62.47- ☑
  congenital Q79.8
   sternocleidomastoid Q68.0
  extraocular — *see* Strabismus
  eye (extrinsic) — *see* Strabismus
  foot M62.47- ☑
  forearm M62.43- ☑
  hand M62.44- ☑
  hysterical F44.4
  ischemic (Volkmann's) T79.6 ☑
  lower leg M62.46- ☑
  multiple sites M62.49
  pelvic region M62.45- ☑
  posttraumatic — *see* Strabismus, paralytic
  psychogenic F45.8
   conversion reaction F44.4
  shoulder region M62.41- ☑
  specified site NEC M62.48
  thigh M62.45- ☑
  upper arm M62.42- ☑
 neck — *see* Torticollis
 ocular muscle — *see* Strabismus
 organ or site, congenital NEC — *see* Atresia, by site
 outlet (pelvis) — *see* Contraction, pelvis
 palmar fascia M72.0
 paralytic
  joint — *see* Contraction, joint
  muscle — *see also* Contraction, muscle NEC
   ocular — *see* Strabismus, paralytic
 pelvis (acquired) (general) M95.5
  with disproportion (fetopelvic) O33.1
   causing obstructed labor O65.1
   inlet O33.2

Contraction(s), contracture, contracted — *continued*
 pelvis — *continued*
  with disproportion — *continued*
   mid-cavity O33.3 ☑
   outlet O33.3 ☑
 plantar fascia M72.2
 premature
  atrium I49.1
  auriculoventricular I49.49
  heart I49.49
  junctional I49.2
  supraventricular I49.1
  ventricular I49.3
 prostate N42.89
 pylorus NEC — *see also* Pylorospasm
  psychogenic F45.8
 rectum, rectal (sphincter) K59.89
 ring (Bandl's) (complicating delivery) O62.4
 scar — *see* Cicatrix
 spine — *see* Dorsopathy, deforming
 sternocleidomastoid (muscle), congenital Q68.0
 stomach K31.89
  hourglass K31.89
   congenital Q40.2
   psychogenic F45.8
  psychogenic F45.8
 tendon (sheath) M62.40
  with contracture of joint — *see* Contraction, joint
  Achilles — *see* Short, tendon, Achilles
  ankle M62.47- ☑
   Achilles — *see* Short, tendon, Achilles
  foot M62.47- ☑
  forearm M62.43- ☑
  hand M62.44- ☑
  lower leg M62.46- ☑
  multiple sites M62.49
  neck M62.48
  pelvic region M62.45- ☑
  shoulder region M62.41- ☑
  specified site NEC M62.48
  thigh M62.45- ☑
  thorax M62.48
  trunk M62.48
  upper arm M62.42- ☑
 toe — *see* Deformity, toe, specified NEC
 ureterovesical orifice (postinfectional) N13.5
  with infection N13.6
 urethra — *see also* Stricture, urethra
  orifice N32.0
 uterus N85.8
  abnormal NEC O62.9
  clonic (complicating delivery) O62.4
  dyscoordinate (complicating delivery) O62.4
  hourglass (complicating delivery) O62.4
  hypertonic O62.4
  hypotonic NEC O62.2
  inadequate
   primary O62.0
   secondary O62.1
  incoordinate (complicating delivery) O62.4
  poor O62.2
  tetanic (complicating delivery) O62.4
 vagina (outlet) N89.5
 vesical N32.89
  neck or urethral orifice N32.0
 visual field — *see* Defect, visual field, generalized
 Volkmann's (ischemic) T79.6 ☑
Contusion (skin surface intact) T14.8 ☑
 abdomen, abdominal (muscle) (wall) S30.1 ☑
 adnexa, eye NEC S05.8X- ☑
 adrenal gland S37.812 ☑
 alveolar process S00.532 ☑
 ankle S90.0- ☑
 antecubital space — *see* Contusion, forearm
 anus S30.3 ☑
 arm (upper) S40.02- ☑
  lower (with elbow) — *see* Contusion, forearm
 auditory canal — *see* Contusion, ear
 auricle — *see* Contusion, ear
 axilla — *see* Contusion, arm, upper
 back — *see also* Contusion, thorax, back
  lower S30.0 ☑
 bile duct S36.13 ☑
 bladder S37.22 ☑
 bone NEC T14.8 ☑
 brain (diffuse) — *see* Injury, intracranial, diffuse

⬇ **Subterms under main terms may continue to next column or page**   ☑ **Additional Character Required — Refer to the Tabular List for Character Selection**   **73**

Contact — Contusion

Contusion — *continued*

brain — *see* Injury, intracranial, diffuse — *continued*
   focal — *see* Injury, intracranial, focal
brainstem S06.38- ☑
breast S20.0- ☑
broad ligament S37.892 ☑
brow S00.83 ☑
buttock S30.0 ☑
canthus, eye S00.1- ☑
cauda equina S34.3 ☑
cerebellar, traumatic S06.37- ☑
cerebral S06.33- ☑
   left side S06.32- ☑
   right side S06.31- ☑
cheek S00.83 ☑
   internal S00.532 ☑
chest (wall) — *see* Contusion, thorax
chin S00.83 ☑
clitoris S30.23 ☑
colon — *see* Injury, intestine, large, contusion
common bile duct S36.13 ☑
conjunctiva S05.1- ☑
   with foreign body (in conjunctival sac) — *see* Foreign body, conjunctival sac
conus medullaris (spine) S34.139 ☑
cornea — *see* Contusion, eyeball
   with foreign body — *see* Foreign body, cornea
corpus cavernosum S30.21 ☑
cortex (brain) (cerebral) — *see* Injury, intracranial, diffuse
   focal — *see* Injury, intracranial, focal
costal region — *see* Contusion, thorax
cystic duct S36.13 ☑
diaphragm S27.802 ☑
duodenum S36.420 ☑
ear S00.43- ☑
elbow S50.0- ☑
   with forearm — *see* Contusion, forearm
epididymis S30.22 ☑
epigastric region S30.1 ☑
epiglottis S10.0 ☑
esophagus (thoracic) S27.812 ☑
   cervical S10.0 ☑
eyeball S05.1- ☑
eyebrow S00.1- ☑
eyelid (and periocular area) S00.1- ☑
face NEC S00.83 ☑
fallopian tube S37.529 ☑
   bilateral S37.522 ☑
   unilateral S37.521 ☑
femoral triangle S30.1 ☑
finger(s) S60.00 ☑
   with damage to nail (matrix) S60.10 ☑
   index S60.02- ☑
     with damage to nail S60.12- ☑
   little S60.05- ☑
     with damage to nail S60.15- ☑
   middle S60.03- ☑
     with damage to nail S60.13- ☑
   ring S60.04- ☑
     with damage to nail S60.14- ☑
   thumb — *see* Contusion, thumb
flank S30.1 ☑
foot (except toe(s) alone) S90.3- ☑
   toe — *see* Contusion, toe
forearm S50.1- ☑
   elbow only — *see* Contusion, elbow
forehead S00.83 ☑
gallbladder S36.122 ☑
genital organs, external
   female S30.202 ☑
   male S30.201 ☑
globe (eye) — *see* Contusion, eyeball
groin S30.1 ☑
gum S00.532 ☑
hand S60.22- ☑
   finger(s) — *see* Contusion, finger
   wrist — *see* Contusion, wrist
head S00.93 ☑
   ear — *see* Contusion, ear
   eyelid — *see* Contusion, eyelid
   lip S00.531 ☑
   nose S00.33 ☑
   oral cavity S00.532 ☑
   scalp S00.03 ☑
   specified part NEC S00.83 ☑

Contusion — *continued*

heart — *see also* Injury, heart S26.91 ☑
heel — *see* Contusion, foot
hepatic duct S36.13 ☑
hip S70.0- ☑
ileum S36.428 ☑
iliac region S30.1 ☑
inguinal region S30.1 ☑
interscapular region S20.229 ☑
intra-abdominal organ S36.92 ☑
   colon — *see* Injury, intestine, large, contusion
   liver S36.112 ☑
   pancreas — *see* Contusion, pancreas
   rectum S36.62 ☑
   small intestine — *see* Injury, intestine, small, contusion
   specified organ NEC S36.892 ☑
   spleen — *see* Contusion, spleen
   stomach S36.32 ☑
iris (eye) — *see* Contusion, eyeball
jaw S00.83 ☑
jejunum S36.428 ☑
kidney S37.01- ☑
   major (greater than 2 cm) S37.02- ☑
   minor (less than 2 cm) S37.01- ☑
knee S80.0- ☑
labium (majus) (minus) S30.23 ☑
lacrimal apparatus, gland or sac S05.8X- ☑
larynx S10.0 ☑
leg (lower) S80.1- ☑
   knee — *see* Contusion, knee
lens — *see* Contusion, eyeball
lip S00.531 ☑
liver S36.112 ☑
lower back S30.0 ☑
lumbar region S30.0 ☑
lung S27.329 ☑
   bilateral S27.322 ☑
   unilateral S27.321 ☑
malar region S00.83 ☑
mastoid region S00.83 ☑
membrane, brain — *see* Injury, intracranial, diffuse
   focal — *see* Injury, intracranial, focal
mesentery S36.892 ☑
mesosalpinx S37.892 ☑
mouth S00.532 ☑
muscle — *see* Contusion, by site
nail
   finger — *see* Contusion, finger, with damage to nail
   toe — *see* Contusion, toe, with damage to nail
nasal S00.33 ☑
neck S10.93 ☑
   specified site NEC S10.83 ☑
   throat S10.0 ☑
nerve — *see* Injury, nerve
newborn P54.5
nose S00.33 ☑
occipital
   lobe (brain) — *see* Injury, intracranial, diffuse
     focal — *see* Injury, intracranial, focal
   region (scalp) S00.03 ☑
orbit (region) (tissues) S05.1- ☑
ovary S37.429 ☑
   bilateral S37.422 ☑
   unilateral S37.421 ☑
palate S00.532 ☑
pancreas S36.229 ☑
   body S36.221 ☑
   head S36.220 ☑
   tail S36.222 ☑
parietal
   lobe (brain) — *see* Injury, intracranial, diffuse
     focal — *see* Injury, intracranial, focal
   region (scalp) S00.03 ☑
pelvic organ S37.92 ☑
   adrenal gland S37.812 ☑
   bladder S37.22 ☑
   fallopian tube — *see* Contusion, fallopian tube
   kidney — *see* Contusion, kidney
   ovary — *see* Contusion, ovary
   prostate S37.822 ☑
   specified organ NEC S37.892 ☑
   ureter S37.12 ☑
   urethra S37.32 ☑
   uterus S37.62 ☑
pelvis S30.0 ☑

Contusion — *continued*

penis S30.21 ☑
perineum
   female S30.23 ☑
   male S30.0 ☑
periocular area S00.1- ☑
peritoneum S36.81 ☑
periurethral tissue — *see* Contusion, urethra
pharynx S10.0 ☑
pinna — *see* Contusion, ear
popliteal space — *see* Contusion, knee
prepuce S30.21 ☑
prostate S37.822 ☑
pubic region S30.1 ☑
pudendum
   female S30.202 ☑
   male S30.201 ☑
quadriceps femoris — *see* Contusion, thigh
rectum S36.62 ☑
retroperitoneum S36.892 ☑
round ligament S37.892 ☑
sacral region S30.0 ☑
scalp S00.03 ☑
   due to birth injury P12.3
scapular region — *see* Contusion, shoulder
sclera — *see* Contusion, eyeball
scrotum S30.22 ☑
seminal vesicle S37.892 ☑
shoulder S40.01- ☑
skin NEC T14.8 ☑
small intestine — *see* Injury, intestine, small, contusion
spermatic cord S30.22 ☑
spinal cord — *see* Injury, spinal cord, by region
   cauda equina S34.3 ☑
   conus medullaris S34.139 ☑
spleen S36.029 ☑
   major S36.021 ☑
   minor S36.020 ☑
sternal region S20.219 ☑
stomach S36.32 ☑
subconjunctival S05.1- ☑
subcutaneous NEC T14.8 ☑
submaxillary region S00.83 ☑
submental region S00.83 ☑
subperiosteal NEC T14.8 ☑
subungual
   finger — *see* Contusion, finger, with damage to nail
   toe — *see* Contusion, toe, with damage to nail
supraclavicular fossa S10.83 ☑
supraorbital S00.83 ☑
suprarenal gland S37.812 ☑
temple (region) S00.83 ☑
temporal
   lobe (brain) — *see* Injury, intracranial, diffuse
     focal — *see* Injury, intracranial, focal
   region S00.83 ☑
testis S30.22 ☑
thigh S70.1- ☑
thorax (wall) S20.20 ☑
   back S20.22- ☑
   front S20.21- ☑
throat S10.0 ☑
thumb S60.01- ☑
   with damage to nail S60.11- ☑
toe(s) (lesser) S90.12- ☑
   with damage to nail S90.22- ☑
   great S90.11- ☑
     with damage to nail S90.21- ☑
tongue S00.532 ☑
trachea (cervical) S10.0 ☑
   thoracic S27.52 ☑
tunica vaginalis S30.22 ☑
tympanum, tympanic membrane — *see* Contusion, ear
ureter S37.12 ☑
urethra S37.32 ☑
urinary organ NEC S37.892 ☑
uterus S37.62 ☑
uvula S00.532 ☑
vagina S30.23 ☑
vas deferens S37.892 ☑
vesical S37.22 ☑
vocal cord(s) S10.0 ☑
vulva S30.23 ☑
wrist S60.21- ☑

Conus (congenital) (any type) Q14.8

Conus — *continued*
  cornea — *see* Keratoconus
  medullaris syndrome G95.81
Conversion hysteria, neurosis or reaction F44.9
Converter, tuberculosis (test reaction) R76.11
Conviction (legal), **anxiety concerning** Z65.0
  with imprisonment Z65.1
Convulsions (idiopathic) — *see also* Seizure(s) R56.9
  apoplectiform (cerebral ischemia) I67.82
  dissociative F44.5
  epileptic — *see* Epilepsy
  epileptiform, epileptoid — *see* Seizure, epileptiform
  ether (anesthetic) — *see* Table of Drugs and Chemicals,
    by drug
  febrile R56.00
    with status epilepticus G40.901
      complex R56.01
        with status epilepticus G40.901
      simple R56.00
  hysterical F44.5
  infantile P90
    epilepsy — *see* Epilepsy
  jacksonian — *see* Epilepsy, localization-related, symp-
    tomatic, with simple partial seizures
  myoclonic G25.3
  newborn P90
  obstetrical (nephritic) (uremic) — *see* Eclampsia
  paretic A52.17
  post traumatic R56.1
  psychomotor — *see* Epilepsy, localization-related,
    symptomatic, with complex partial seizures
  recurrent R56.9
  reflex R25.8
  scarlatinal A38.8
  tetanus, tetanic — *see* Tetanus
  thymic E32.8
Convulsive — *see also* Convulsions
Cooley's anemia D56.1
Coolie itch B76.9
Cooper's
  disease — *see* Mastopathy, cystic
  hernia — *see* Hernia, abdomen, specified site NEC
Copra itch B88.0
Coprophagy F50.89
Coprophobia F40.298
Coproporphyria, hereditary E80.29
Cor
  biloculare Q20.8
  bovis, bovinum — *see* Hypertrophy, cardiac
  pulmonale (chronic) I27.81
    acute I26.09
  triatriatum, triatrium Q24.2
  triloculare Q20.8
    biatrium Q20.4
    biventriculare Q21.1
Corbus' disease (gangrenous balanitis) N48.1
Cord — *see also* condition
  around neck
    complicating delivery O69.81
      with compression O69.1 ☑
  bladder G95.89
    tabetic A52.19
Cordis ectopia Q24.8
Corditis (spermatic) N49.1
Corectopia Q13.2
Cori's disease (glycogen storage) E74.03
Corkhandler's disease or lung J67.3
Corkscrew esophagus K22.4
Corkworker's disease or lung J67.3
Corn (infected) L84
Cornea — *see also* condition
  donor Z52.5
  plana Q13.4
Cornelia de Lange syndrome Q87.19
Cornu cutaneum L85.8
Cornual gestation or pregnancy O00.80
  with intrauterine pregnancy O00.81
Coronary (artery) — *see* condition
Coronavirus (infection)
  2019 — *see also* COVID-19 U07.1
  as cause of diseases classified elsewhere B97.29
  coronavirus-19 — *see also* COVID-19 U07.1
  COVID-19 — *see also* COVID-19 U07.1
  SARS-associated B97.21
Corpora — *see also* condition
  amylacea, prostate N42.89
  cavernosa — *see* condition

Corpulence — *see* Obesity
Corpus — *see* condition
Corrected transposition Q20.5
Corrosion (injury) (acid) (caustic) (chemical) (lime) (external) (internal) T30.4
  abdomen, abdominal (muscle) (wall) T21.42 ☑
    first degree T21.52 ☑
    second degree T21.62 ☑
    third degree T21.72 ☑
  above elbow T22.439 ☑
    first degree T22.539 ☑
    left T22.432 ☑
      first degree T22.532 ☑
      second degree T22.632 ☑
      third degree T22.732 ☑
    right T22.431 ☑
      first degree T22.531 ☑
      second degree T22.631 ☑
      third degree T22.731 ☑
    second degree T22.639 ☑
    third degree T22.739 ☑
  alimentary tract NEC T28.7 ☑
  ankle T25.419 ☑
    first degree T25.519 ☑
    left T25.412 ☑
      first degree T25.512 ☑
      second degree T25.612 ☑
      third degree T25.712 ☑
    multiple with foot — *see* Corrosion, lower, limb,
      multiple, ankle and foot
    right T25.411 ☑
      first degree T25.511 ☑
      second degree T25.611 ☑
      third degree T25.711 ☑
    second degree T25.619 ☑
    third degree T25.719 ☑
  anus — *see* Corrosion, buttock
  arm(s) (meaning upper limb(s)) — *see* Corrosion, upper
    limb
  axilla T22.449 ☑
    first degree T22.549 ☑
    left T22.442 ☑
      first degree T22.542 ☑
      second degree T22.642 ☑
      third degree T22.742 ☑
    right T22.441 ☑
      first degree T22.541 ☑
      second degree T22.641 ☑
      third degree T22.741 ☑
    second degree T22.649 ☑
    third degree T22.749 ☑
  back (lower) T21.44 ☑
    first degree T21.54 ☑
    second degree T21.64 ☑
    third degree T21.74 ☑
    upper T21.43 ☑
      first degree T21.53 ☑
      second degree T21.63 ☑
      third degree T21.73 ☑
  blisters — *code as* Corrosion, second degree, by site
  breast(s) — *see* Corrosion, chest wall
  buttock(s) T21.45 ☑
    first degree T21.55 ☑
    second degree T21.65 ☑
    third degree T21.75 ☑
  calf T24.439 ☑
    first degree T24.539 ☑
    left T24.432 ☑
      first degree T24.532 ☑
      second degree T24.632 ☑
      third degree T24.732 ☑
    right T24.431 ☑
      first degree T24.531 ☑
      second degree T24.631 ☑
      third degree T24.731 ☑
    second degree T24.639 ☑
    third degree T24.739 ☑
  canthus (eye) — *see* Corrosion, eyelid
  cervix T28.8 ☑
  cheek T20.46 ☑
    first degree T20.56 ☑
    second degree T20.66 ☑
    third degree T20.76 ☑
  chest wall T21.41 ☑
    first degree T21.51 ☑
    second degree T21.61 ☑

Corrosion — *continued*
  chest wall — *continued*
    third degree T21.71 ☑
  chin T20.43 ☑
    first degree T20.53 ☑
    second degree T20.63 ☑
    third degree T20.73 ☑
  colon T28.7 ☑
  conjunctiva (and cornea) — *see* Corrosion, cornea
  cornea (and conjunctiva) T26.6- ☑
  deep necrosis of underlying tissue — *code as* Corrosion,
    third degree, by site
  dorsum of hand T23.469 ☑
    first degree T23.569 ☑
    left T23.462 ☑
      first degree T23.562 ☑
      second degree T23.662 ☑
      third degree T23.762 ☑
    right T23.461 ☑
      first degree T23.561 ☑
      second degree T23.661 ☑
      third degree T23.761 ☑
    second degree T23.669 ☑
    third degree T23.769 ☑
  ear (auricle) (external) (canal) T20.41 ☑
    drum T28.91 ☑
    first degree T20.51 ☑
    second degree T20.61 ☑
    third degree T20.71 ☑
  elbow T22.429 ☑
    first degree T22.529 ☑
    left T22.422 ☑
      first degree T22.522 ☑
      second degree T22.622 ☑
      third degree T22.722 ☑
    right T22.421 ☑
      first degree T22.521 ☑
      second degree T22.621 ☑
      third degree T22.721 ☑
    second degree T22.629 ☑
    third degree T22.729 ☑
  entire body — *see* Corrosion, multiple body regions
  epidermal loss — *code as* Corrosion, second degree,
    by site
  epiglottis T27.4 ☑
  erythema, erythematous — *code as* Corrosion, first
    degree, by site
  esophagus T28.6 ☑
  extent (percentage of body surface)
    less than 10 percent T32.0
    10-19 percent (0-9 percent third degree) T32.10
      with 10-19 percent third degree T32.11
    20-29 percent (0-9 percent third degree) T32.20
      with
        10-19 percent third degree T32.21
        20-29 percent third degree T32.22
    30-39 percent (0-9 percent third degree) T32.30
      with
        10-19 percent third degree T32.31
        20-29 percent third degree T32.32
        30-39 percent third degree T32.33
    40-49 percent (0-9 percent third degree) T32.40
      with
        10-19 percent third degree T32.41
        20-29 percent third degree T32.42
        30-39 percent third degree T32.43
        40-49 percent third degree T32.44
    50-59 percent (0-9 percent third degree) T32.50
      with
        10-19 percent third degree T32.51
        20-29 percent third degree T32.52
        30-39 percent third degree T32.53
        40-49 percent third degree T32.54
        50-59 percent third degree T32.55
    60-69 percent (0-9 percent third degree) T32.60
      with
        10-19 percent third degree T32.61
        20-29 percent third degree T32.62
        30-39 percent third degree T32.63
        40-49 percent third degree T32.64
        50-59 percent third degree T32.65
        60-69 percent third degree T32.66
    70-79 percent (0-9 percent third degree) T32.70
      with
        10-19 percent third degree T32.71
        20-29 percent third degree T32.72
        30-39 percent third degree T32.73

Corrosion — *continued*
extent — *continued*
70-79 percent — *continued*
with — *continued*
40-49 percent third degree T32.74
50-59 percent third degree T32.75
60-69 percent third degree T32.76
70-79 percent third degree T32.77
80-89 percent (0-9 percent third degree) T32.80
with
10-19 percent third degree T32.81
20-29 percent third degree T32.82
30-39 percent third degree T32.83
40-49 percent third degree T32.84
50-59 percent third degree T32.85
60-69 percent third degree T32.86
70-79 percent third degree T32.87
80-89 percent third degree T32.88
90 percent or more (0-9 percent third degree) T32.90
with
10-19 percent third degree T32.91
20-29 percent third degree T32.92
30-39 percent third degree T32.93
40-49 percent third degree T32.94
50-59 percent third degree T32.95
60-69 percent third degree T32.96
70-79 percent third degree T32.97
80-89 percent third degree T32.98
90-99 percent third degree T32.99
extremity — *see* Corrosion, limb
eye(s) and adnexa T26.9- ☑
with resulting rupture and destruction of eyeball T26.7- ☑
conjunctival sac — *see* Corrosion, cornea
cornea — *see* Corrosion, cornea
lid — *see* Corrosion, eyelid
periocular area — *see* Corrosion eyelid
specified site NEC T26.8- ☑
eyeball — *see* Corrosion, eye
eyelid(s) T26.5- ☑
face — *see* Corrosion, head
finger T23.429 ☑
first degree T23.529 ☑
left T23.422 ☑
first degree T23.522 ☑
second degree T23.622 ☑
third degree T23.722 ☑
multiple sites (without thumb) T23.439 ☑
with thumb T23.449 ☑
first degree T23.549 ☑
left T23.442 ☑
first degree T23.542 ☑
second degree T23.642 ☑
third degree T23.742 ☑
right T23.441 ☑
first degree T23.541 ☑
second degree T23.641 ☑
third degree T23.741 ☑
second degree T23.649 ☑
third degree T23.749 ☑
first degree T23.539 ☑
left T23.432 ☑
first degree T23.532 ☑
second degree T23.632 ☑
third degree T23.732 ☑
right T23.431 ☑
first degree T23.531 ☑
second degree T23.631 ☑
third degree T23.731 ☑
second degree T23.639 ☑
third degree T23.739 ☑
right T23.421 ☑
first degree T23.521 ☑
second degree T23.621 ☑
third degree T23.721 ☑
second degree T23.629 ☑
third degree T23.729 ☑
flank — *see* Corrosion, abdomen
foot T25.429 ☑
first degree T25.529 ☑
left T25.422 ☑
first degree T25.522 ☑
second degree T25.622 ☑
third degree T25.722 ☑
multiple with ankle — *see* Corrosion, lower, limb, multiple, ankle and foot
right T25.421 ☑

Corrosion — *continued*
foot — *continued*
right — *continued*
first degree T25.521 ☑
second degree T25.621 ☑
third degree T25.721 ☑
second degree T25.629 ☑
third degree T25.729 ☑
forearm T22.419 ☑
first degree T22.519 ☑
left T22.412 ☑
first degree T22.512 ☑
second degree T22.612 ☑
third degree T22.712 ☑
right T22.411 ☑
first degree T22.511 ☑
second degree T22.611 ☑
third degree T22.711 ☑
second degree T22.619 ☑
third degree T22.719 ☑
forehead T20.46 ☑
first degree T20.56 ☑
second degree T20.66 ☑
third degree T20.76 ☑
fourth degree — *code as* Corrosion, third degree, by site
full thickness skin loss — *code as* Corrosion, third degree, by site
gastrointestinal tract NEC T28.7 ☑
genital organs
external
female T21.47 ☑
first degree T21.57 ☑
second degree T21.67 ☑
third degree T21.77 ☑
male T21.46 ☑
first degree T21.56 ☑
second degree T21.66 ☑
third degree T21.76 ☑
internal T28.8 ☑
groin — *see* Corrosion, abdominal wall
hand(s) T23.409 ☑
back — *see* Corrosion, dorsum of hand
finger — *see* Corrosion, finger
first degree T23.509 ☑
left T23.402 ☑
first degree T23.502 ☑
second degree T23.602 ☑
third degree T23.702 ☑
multiple sites with wrist T23.499 ☑
first degree T23.599 ☑
left T23.492 ☑
first degree T23.592 ☑
second degree T23.692 ☑
third degree T23.792 ☑
right T23.491 ☑
first degree T23.591 ☑
second degree T23.691 ☑
third degree T23.791 ☑
second degree T23.699 ☑
third degree T23.799 ☑
palm — *see* Corrosion, palm
right T23.401 ☑
first degree T23.501 ☑
second degree T23.601 ☑
third degree T23.701 ☑
second degree T23.609 ☑
third degree T23.709 ☑
thumb — *see* Corrosion, thumb
head (and face) (and neck) T20.40 ☑
cheek — *see* Corrosion, cheek
chin — *see* Corrosion, chin
ear — *see* Corrosion, ear
eye(s) only — *see* Corrosion, eye
first degree T20.50 ☑
forehead — *see* Corrosion, forehead
lip — *see* Corrosion, lip
multiple sites T20.49 ☑
first degree T20.59 ☑
second degree T20.69 ☑
third degree T20.79 ☑
neck — *see* Corrosion, neck
nose — *see* Corrosion, nose
scalp — *see* Corrosion, scalp
second degree T20.60 ☑
third degree T20.70 ☑

Corrosion — *continued*
hip(s) — *see* Corrosion, lower, limb
inhalation — *see* Corrosion, respiratory tract
internal organ(s) — *see also* Corrosion, by site
T28.90 ☑
alimentary tract T28.7 ☑
esophagus T28.6 ☑
esophagus T28.6 ☑
genitourinary T28.8 ☑
mouth T28.5 ☑
pharynx T28.5 ☑
specified organ NEC T28.99 ☑
interscapular region — *see* Corrosion, back, upper
intestine (large) (small) T28.7 ☑
knee T24.429 ☑
first degree T24.529 ☑
left T24.422 ☑
first degree T24.522 ☑
second degree T24.622 ☑
third degree T24.722 ☑
right T24.421 ☑
first degree T24.521 ☑
second degree T24.621 ☑
third degree T24.721 ☑
second degree T24.629 ☑
third degree T24.729 ☑
labium (majus) (minus) — *see* Corrosion, genital organs, external, female
lacrimal apparatus, duct, gland or sac — *see* Corrosion, eye, specified site NEC
larynx T27.4 ☑
with lung T27.5 ☑
leg(s) (meaning lower limb(s)) — *see* Corrosion, lower, limb
limb(s)
lower — *see* Corrosion, lower, limb
upper — *see* Corrosion, upper limb
lip(s) T20.42 ☑
first degree T20.52 ☑
second degree T20.62 ☑
third degree T20.72 ☑
lower
back — *see* Corrosion, back
limb T24.409 ☑
ankle — *see* Corrosion, ankle
calf — *see* Corrosion, calf
first degree T24.509 ☑
foot — *see* Corrosion, foot
knee — *see* Corrosion, knee
left T24.402 ☑
first degree T24.502 ☑
second degree T24.602 ☑
third degree T24.702 ☑
multiple sites, except ankle and foot T24.499 ☑
ankle and foot T25.499 ☑
first degree T25.599 ☑
left T25.492 ☑
first degree T25.592 ☑
second degree T25.692 ☑
third degree T25.792 ☑
right T25.491 ☑
first degree T25.591 ☑
second degree T25.691 ☑
third degree T25.791 ☑
second degree T25.699 ☑
third degree T25.799 ☑
first degree T24.599 ☑
left T24.492 ☑
first degree T24.592 ☑
second degree T24.692 ☑
third degree T24.792 ☑
right T24.491 ☑
first degree T24.591 ☑
second degree T24.691 ☑
third degree T24.791 ☑
second degree T24.699 ☑
third degree T24.799 ☑
right T24.401 ☑
first degree T24.501 ☑
second degree T24.601 ☑
third degree T24.701 ☑
second degree T24.609 ☑
thigh — *see* Corrosion, thigh
third degree T24.709 ☑
lung (with larynx and trachea) T27.5 ☑
mouth T28.5 ☑

Corrosion — *continued*
- neck T20.47 ☑
  - first degree T20.57 ☑
  - second degree T20.67 ☑
  - third degree T20.77 ☑
- nose (septum) T20.44 ☑
  - first degree T20.54 ☑
  - second degree T20.64 ☑
  - third degree T20.74 ☑
- ocular adnexa — *see* Corrosion, eye
- orbit region — *see* Corrosion, eyelid
- palm T23.459 ☑
  - first degree T23.559 ☑
  - left T23.452 ☑
    - first degree T23.552 ☑
    - second degree T23.652 ☑
    - third degree T23.752 ☑
  - right T23.451 ☑
    - first degree T23.551 ☑
    - second degree T23.651 ☑
    - third degree T23.751 ☑
  - second degree T23.659 ☑
  - third degree T23.759 ☑
- partial thickness — *code as* Corrosion, unspecified degree, by site
- pelvis — *see* Corrosion, trunk
- penis — *see* Corrosion, genital organs, external, male
- perineum
  - female — *see* Corrosion, genital organs, external, female
  - male — *see* Corrosion, genital organs, external, male
- periocular area — *see* Corrosion, eyelid
- pharynx T28.5 ☑
- rectum T28.7 ☑
- respiratory tract T27.7 ☑
  - larynx — *see* Corrosion, larynx
  - specified part NEC T27.6 ☑
  - trachea — *see* Corrosion, larynx
- sac, lacrimal — *see* Corrosion, eye, specified site NEC
- scalp T20.45 ☑
  - first degree T20.55 ☑
  - second degree T20.65 ☑
  - third degree T20.75 ☑
- scapular region T22.469 ☑
  - first degree T22.569 ☑
  - left T22.462 ☑
    - first degree T22.562 ☑
    - second degree T22.662 ☑
    - third degree T22.762 ☑
  - right T22.461 ☑
    - first degree T22.561 ☑
    - second degree T22.661 ☑
    - third degree T22.761 ☑
  - second degree T22.669 ☑
  - third degree T22.769 ☑
- sclera — *see* Corrosion, eye, specified site NEC
- scrotum — *see* Corrosion, genital organs, external, male
- shoulder T22.459 ☑
  - first degree T22.559 ☑
  - left T22.452 ☑
    - first degree T22.552 ☑
    - second degree T22.652 ☑
    - third degree T22.752 ☑
  - right T22.451 ☑
    - first degree T22.551 ☑
    - second degree T22.651 ☑
    - third degree T22.751 ☑
  - second degree T22.659 ☑
  - third degree T22.759 ☑
- stomach T28.7 ☑
- temple — *see* Corrosion, head
- testis — *see* Corrosion, genital organs, external, male
- thigh T24.419 ☑
  - first degree T24.519 ☑
  - left T24.412 ☑
    - first degree T24.512 ☑
    - second degree T24.612 ☑
    - third degree T24.712 ☑
  - right T24.411 ☑
    - first degree T24.511 ☑
    - second degree T24.611 ☑
    - third degree T24.711 ☑
  - second degree T24.619 ☑
  - third degree T24.719 ☑
- thorax (external) — *see* Corrosion, trunk

- throat (meaning pharynx) T28.5 ☑
- thumb(s) T23.419 ☑
  - first degree T23.519 ☑
  - left T23.412 ☑
    - first degree T23.512 ☑
    - second degree T23.612 ☑
    - third degree T23.712 ☑
  - multiple sites with fingers T23.449 ☑
    - first degree T23.549 ☑
    - left T23.442 ☑
      - first degree T23.542 ☑
      - second degree T23.642 ☑
      - third degree T23.742 ☑
    - right T23.441 ☑
      - first degree T23.541 ☑
      - second degree T23.641 ☑
      - third degree T23.741 ☑
    - second degree T23.649 ☑
    - third degree T23.749 ☑
  - right T23.411 ☑
    - first degree T23.511 ☑
    - second degree T23.611 ☑
    - third degree T23.711 ☑
  - second degree T23.619 ☑
  - third degree T23.719 ☑
- toe T25.439 ☑
  - first degree T25.539 ☑
  - left T25.432 ☑
    - first degree T25.532 ☑
    - second degree T25.632 ☑
    - third degree T25.732 ☑
  - right T25.431 ☑
    - first degree T25.531 ☑
    - second degree T25.631 ☑
    - third degree T25.731 ☑
  - second degree T25.639 ☑
  - third degree T25.739 ☑
- tongue T28.5 ☑
- tonsil(s) T28.5 ☑
- total body — *see* Corrosion, multiple body regions
- trachea T27.4 ☑
  - with lung T27.5 ☑
- trunk T21.40 ☑
  - abdominal wall — *see* Corrosion, abdominal wall
  - anus — *see* Corrosion, buttock
  - axilla — *see* Corrosion, upper limb
  - back — *see* Corrosion, back
  - breast — *see* Corrosion, chest wall
  - buttock — *see* Corrosion, buttock
  - chest wall — *see* Corrosion, chest wall
  - first degree T21.50 ☑
  - flank — *see* Corrosion, abdominal wall
  - genital
    - female — *see* Corrosion, genital organs, external, female
    - male — *see* Corrosion, genital organs, external, male
  - groin — *see* Corrosion, abdominal wall
  - interscapular region — *see* Corrosion, back, upper
  - labia — *see* Corrosion, genital organs, external, female
  - lower back — *see* Corrosion, back
  - penis — *see* Corrosion, genital organs, external, male
  - perineum
    - female — *see* Corrosion, genital organs, external, female
    - male — *see* Corrosion, genital organs, external, male
  - scapular region — *see* Corrosion, upper limb
  - scrotum — *see* Corrosion, genital organs, external, male
  - second degree T21.60 ☑
  - shoulder — *see* Corrosion, upper limb
  - specified site NEC T21.49 ☑
    - first degree T21.59 ☑
    - second degree T21.69 ☑
    - third degree T21.79 ☑
  - testes — *see* Corrosion, genital organs, external, male
  - third degree T21.70 ☑
  - upper back — *see* Corrosion, back, upper
- vagina T28.8 ☑
- vulva — *see* Corrosion, genital organs, external, female

- unspecified site with extent of body surface involved specified
  - less than 10 percent T32.0
  - 10-19 percent (0-9 percent third degree) T32.10
    - with 10-19 percent third degree T32.11
  - 20-29 percent (0-9 percent third degree) T32.20
    - with
      - 10-19 percent third degree T32.21
      - 20-29 percent third degree T32.22
  - 30-39 percent (0-9 percent third degree) T32.30
    - with
      - 10-19 percent third degree T32.31
      - 20-29 percent third degree T32.32
      - 30-39 percent third degree T32.33
  - 40-49 percent (0-9 percent third degree) T32.40
    - with
      - 10-19 percent third degree T32.41
      - 20-29 percent third degree T32.42
      - 30-39 percent third degree T32.43
      - 40-49 percent third degree T32.44
  - 50-59 percent (0-9 percent third degree) T32.50
    - with
      - 10-19 percent third degree T32.51
      - 20-29 percent third degree T32.52
      - 30-39 percent third degree T32.53
      - 40-49 percent third degree T32.54
      - 50-59 percent third degree T32.55
  - 60-69 percent (0-9 percent third degree) T32.60
    - with
      - 10-19 percent third degree T32.61
      - 20-29 percent third degree T32.62
      - 30-39 percent third degree T32.63
      - 40-49 percent third degree T32.64
      - 50-59 percent third degree T32.65
      - 60-69 percent third degree T32.66
  - 70-79 percent (0-9 percent third degree) T32.70
    - with
      - 10-19 percent third degree T32.71
      - 20-29 percent third degree T32.72
      - 30-39 percent third degree T32.73
      - 40-49 percent third degree T32.74
      - 50-59 percent third degree T32.75
      - 60-69 percent third degree T32.76
      - 70-79 percent third degree T32.77
  - 80-89 percent (0-9 percent third degree) T32.80
    - with
      - 10-19 percent third degree T32.81
      - 20-29 percent third degree T32.82
      - 30-39 percent third degree T32.83
      - 40-49 percent third degree T32.84
      - 50-59 percent third degree T32.85
      - 60-69 percent third degree T32.86
      - 70-79 percent third degree T32.87
      - 80-89 percent third degree T32.88
  - 90 percent or more (0-9 percent third degree) T32.90
    - with
      - 10-19 percent third degree T32.91
      - 20-29 percent third degree T32.92
      - 30-39 percent third degree T32.93
      - 40-49 percent third degree T32.94
      - 50-59 percent third degree T32.95
      - 60-69 percent third degree T32.96
      - 70-79 percent third degree T32.97
      - 80-89 percent third degree T32.98
      - 90-99 percent third degree T32.99
- upper limb (axilla) (scapular region) T22.40 ☑
  - above elbow — *see* Corrosion, above elbow
  - axilla — *see* Corrosion, axilla
  - elbow — *see* Corrosion, elbow
  - first degree T22.50 ☑
  - forearm — *see* Corrosion, forearm
  - hand — *see* Corrosion, hand
  - interscapular region — *see* Corrosion, back, upper
  - multiple sites T22.499 ☑
    - first degree T22.599 ☑
    - left T22.492 ☑
      - first degree T22.592 ☑
      - second degree T22.692 ☑
      - third degree T22.792 ☑
    - right T22.491 ☑
      - first degree T22.591 ☑
      - second degree T22.691 ☑
      - third degree T22.791 ☑
    - second degree T22.699 ☑
    - third degree T22.799 ☑
  - scapular region — *see* Corrosion, scapular region
  - second degree T22.60 ☑

▽ **Subterms under main terms may continue to next column or page**   ☑ **Additional Character Required — Refer to the Tabular List for Character Selection**   **77**

Corrosion — Corrosion

Corrosion — continued
  upper limb — continued
    shoulder — see Corrosion, shoulder
    third degree T22.70 ☑
    wrist — see Corrosion, hand
  uterus T28.8 ☑
  vagina T28.8 ☑
  vulva — see Corrosion, genital organs, external, female
  wrist T23.479 ☑
    first degree T23.579 ☑
    left T23.472 ☑
      first degree T23.572 ☑
      second degree T23.672 ☑
      third degree T23.772 ☑
    multiple sites with hand T23.499 ☑
      first degree T23.599 ☑
      left T23.492 ☑
        first degree T23.592 ☑
        second degree T23.692 ☑
        third degree T23.792 ☑
      right T23.491 ☑
        first degree T23.591 ☑
        second degree T23.691 ☑
        third degree T23.791 ☑
      second degree T23.699 ☑
      third degree T23.799 ☑
    right T23.471 ☑
      first degree T23.571 ☑
      second degree T23.671 ☑
      third degree T23.771 ☑
    second degree T23.679 ☑
    third degree T23.779 ☑
Corrosive burn — see Corrosion
Corsican fever — see Malaria
Cortical — see condition
Cortico-adrenal — see condition
Coryza (acute) J00
  with grippe or influenza — see Influenza, with, respiratory manifestations NEC
  syphilitic
    congenital (chronic) A50.05
Costen's syndrome or complex M26.69
Costiveness — see Constipation
Costochondritis M94.0
Cot death R99
Cotard's syndrome F22
Cotia virus B08.8
Cotton wool spots (retinal) H35.81
Cotungo's disease — see Sciatica
Cough (affected) (epidemic) (nervous) R05.9
  with hemorrhage — see Hemoptysis
  acute R05.1
  bronchial R05.8
    with grippe or influenza — see Influenza, with, respiratory manifestations NEC
  chronic R05.3
  functional F45.8
  hysterical F45.8
  laryngeal, spasmodic R05.8
  paroxysmal, due to Bordetella pertussis (without pneumonia) A37.00
    with pneumonia A37.01
  persistent R05.3
  psychogenic F45.8
  refractory R05.3
  smokers' J41.0
  specified NEC R05.8
  subacute R05.2
  syncope R05.4
  tea taster's B49
  unexplained R05.3
Counseling (for) Z71.9
  abuse NEC
    perpetrator Z69.82
    victim Z69.81
  alcohol abuser Z71.41
    family Z71.42
  child abuse
    nonparental
      perpetrator Z69.021
      victim Z69.020
    parental
      perpetrator Z69.011
      victim Z69.010
  consanguinity Z71.89
  contraceptive Z30.09
  dietary Z71.3

Counseling — continued
  drug abuser Z71.51
    family member Z71.52
  exercise Z71.82
  family Z71.89
  fertility preservation (prior to cancer therapy) (prior to removal of gonads) Z31.62
  for non-attending third party Z71.0
    related to sexual behavior or orientation Z70.2
  genetic
    nonprocreative Z71.83
    procreative NEC Z31.5
  gestational carrier Z31.7
  health (advice) (education) (instruction) — see Counseling, medical
    risk for travel (international) Z71.84
  human immunodeficiency virus (HIV) Z71.7
  immunization safety Z71.85
  impotence Z70.1
  insulin pump use Z46.81
  medical (for) Z71.9
    boarding school resident Z59.3
    consanguinity Z71.89
    feared complaint and no disease found Z71.1
    human immunodeficiency virus (HIV) Z71.7
    institutional resident Z59.3
    on behalf of another Z71.0
      related to sexual behavior or orientation Z70.2
    person living alone Z60.2
    specified reason NEC Z71.89
  natural family planning
    procreative Z31.61
    to avoid pregnancy Z30.02
  perpetrator (of)
    abuse NEC Z69.82
    child abuse
      non-parental Z69.021
      parental Z69.011
    rape NEC Z69.82
    spousal abuse Z69.12
  procreative NEC Z31.69
    fertility preservation (prior to cancer therapy) (prior to removal of gonads) Z31.62
    using natural family planning Z31.61
  promiscuity Z70.1
  rape victim Z69.81
  religious Z71.81
  safety for travel (international) Z71.84
  sex, sexual (related to) Z70.9
    attitude(s) Z70.0
    behavior or orientation Z70.1
    combined concerns Z70.3
    non-responsiveness Z70.1
    on behalf of third party Z70.2
    specified reason NEC Z70.8
  specified reason NEC Z71.89
  spiritual Z71.81
  spousal abuse (perpetrator) Z69.12
    victim Z69.11
  substance abuse Z71.89
    alcohol Z71.41
    drug Z71.51
    tobacco Z71.6
  tobacco use Z71.6
  travel (international) Z71.84
  use (of)
    insulin pump Z46.81
  vaccine product safety Z71.85
  victim (of)
    abuse Z69.81
    child abuse
      by parent Z69.010
      non-parental Z69.020
    rape NEC Z69.81
Coupled rhythm R00.8
Couvelaire syndrome or uterus (complicating delivery) O45.8X- ☑
COVID-19 U07.1
  condition post U09.9
  contact (with) Z20.822
  exposure (to) Z20.822
  history of (personal) Z86.16
  long (haul) U09.9
  pneumonia J12.82
  screening Z11.52
  sequelae (post acute) U09.9
Cowperitis — see Urethritis
Cowper's gland — see condition

Cowpox B08.010
  due to vaccination T88.1 ☑
Coxa
  magna M91.4- ☑
  plana M91.2- ☑
  valga (acquired) — see also Deformity, limb, specified type NEC, thigh
    congenital Q65.81
    sequelae (late effect) of rickets E64.3
  vara (acquired) — see also Deformity, limb, specified type NEC, thigh
    congenital Q65.82
    sequelae (late effect) of rickets E64.3
Coxalgia, coxalgic (nontuberculous) — see also Pain, joint, hip
  tuberculous A18.02
Coxitis — see Monoarthritis, hip
Coxsackie (virus) (infection) B34.1
  as cause of disease classified elsewhere B97.11
  carditis B33.20
  central nervous system NEC A88.8
  endocarditis B33.21
  enteritis A08.39
  meningitis (aseptic) A87.0
  myocarditis B33.22
  pericarditis B33.23
  pharyngitis B08.5
  pleurodynia B33.0
  specific disease NEC B33.8
Crabs, meaning pubic lice B85.3
Crack baby P04.41
Cracked nipple N64.0
  associated with
    lactation O92.13
    pregnancy O92.11- ☑
    puerperium O92.12
Cracked tooth K03.81
Cradle cap L21.0
Craft neurosis F48.8
Cramp(s) R25.2
  abdominal — see Pain, abdominal
  bathing T75.1 ☑
  colic R10.83
    psychogenic F45.8
  due to immersion T75.1 ☑
  fireman T67.2 ☑
  heat T67.2 ☑
  immersion T75.1 ☑
  intestinal — see Pain, abdominal
    psychogenic F45.8
  leg, sleep related G47.62
  limb (lower) (upper) NEC R25.2
    sleep related G47.62
  linotypist's F48.8
    organic G25.89
  muscle (limb) (general) R25.2
    due to immersion T75.1 ☑
    psychogenic F45.8
  occupational (hand) F48.8
    organic G25.89
  salt-depletion E87.1
  sleep related, leg G47.62
  stoker's T67.2 ☑
  swimmer's T75.1 ☑
  telegrapher's F48.8
    organic G25.89
  typist's F48.8
    organic G25.89
  uterus N94.89
    menstrual — see Dysmenorrhea
  writer's F48.8
    organic G25.89
Cranial — see condition
Craniocleidodysostosis Q74.0
Craniofenestria (skull) Q75.8
Craniolacunia (skull) Q75.8
Craniopagus Q89.4
Craniopathy, metabolic M85.2
Craniopharyngeal — see condition
Craniopharyngioma D44.4
Craniorachischisis (totalis) Q00.1
Cranioschisis Q75.8
Craniostenosis Q75.0
Craniosynostosis Q75.0
Craniotabes (cause unknown) M83.8
  neonatal P96.3
  rachitic E64.3

☑ Additional Character Required — Refer to the Tabular List for Character Selection   ▽ Subterms under main terms may continue to next column or page

Craniotabes — *continued*
  syphilitic A50.56
Cranium — *see* condition
Craw-craw — *see* Onchocerciasis
Creaking joint — *see* Derangement, joint, specified type
  NEC
Creeping
  eruption B76.9
  palsy or paralysis G12.22
Crenated tongue K14.8
Creotoxism A05.9
Crepitus
  caput Q75.8
  joint — *see* Derangement, joint, specified type NEC
Crescent or conus choroid, congenital Q14.3
CREST syndrome M34.1
Cretin, cretinism (congenital) (endemic) (nongoitrous)
  (sporadic) E00.9
  pelvis
    with disproportion (fetopelvic) O33.0
      causing obstructed labor O65.0
  type
    hypothyroid E00.1
    mixed E00.2
    myxedematous E00.1
    neurological E00.0
Creutzfeldt-Jakob disease or syndrome (with dementia) A81.00
  familial A81.09
  iatrogenic A81.09
  specified NEC A81.09
  sporadic A81.09
  variant (vCJD) A81.01
Crib death R99
Cribriform hymen Q52.3
Cri-du-chat syndrome Q93.4
Crigler-Najjar disease or syndrome E80.5
Crime, victim of Z65.4
Crimean hemorrhagic fever A98.0
Criminalism F60.2
Crisis
  abdomen R10.0
  acute reaction F43.0
  addisonian E27.2
  adrenal (cortical) E27.2
  celiac K90.0
  Dietl's N13.8
  emotional — *see also* Disorder, adjustment
    acute reaction to stress F43.0
    specific to childhood and adolescence F93.8
  glaucomatocyclitic — *see* Glaucoma, secondary, inflam-
    mation
  heart — *see* Failure, heart
  nitritoid I95.2
    correct substance properly administered — *see* Ta-
      ble of Drugs and Chemicals, by drug, adverse
      effect
    overdose or wrong substance given or taken — *see*
      Table of Drugs and Chemicals, by drug, poi-
      soning
  oculogyric H51.8
    psychogenic F45.8
  Pel's (tabetic) A52.11
  psychosexual identity F64.2
  renal N28.0
  sickle-cell D57.00
    with
      acute chest syndrome D57.01
      cerebral vascular involvement D57.03
      crisis (painful) D57.00
        with complication specified NEC D57.09
      splenic sequestration D57.02
      vasoocclusive pain D57.00
  state (acute reaction) F43.0
  tabetic A52.11
  thyroid — *see* Thyrotoxicosis with thyroid storm
  thyrotoxic — *see* Thyrotoxicosis with thyroid storm
Crocq's disease (acrocyanosis) I73.89
Crohn's disease — *see* Enteritis, regional
Crooked septum, nasal J34.2
Cross syndrome E70.328
Crossbite (anterior) (posterior) M26.24
Cross-eye — *see* Strabismus, convergent concomitant
Croup, croupous (catarrhal) (infectious) (inflammatory)
  (nondiphtheritic) J05.0
  bronchial J20.9
  diphtheritic A36.2
  false J38.5

Croup, croupous — *continued*
  spasmodic J38.5
    diphtheritic A36.2
  stridulous J38.5
    diphtheritic A36.2
Crouzon's disease Q75.1
Crowding, tooth, teeth, fully erupted M26.31
CRST syndrome M34.1
Cruchet's disease A85.8
Cruelty in children — *see also* Disorder, conduct
Crural ulcer — *see* Ulcer, lower limb
Crush, crushed, crushing T14.8 ☑
  abdomen S38.1 ☑
  ankle S97.0- ☑
  arm (upper) (and shoulder) S47.- ☑
  axilla — *see* Crush, arm
  back, lower S38.1 ☑
  buttock S38.1 ☑
  cheek S07.0 ☑
  chest S28.0 ☑
  cranium S07.1 ☑
  ear S07.0 ☑
  elbow S57.0- ☑
  extremity
    lower
      ankle — *see* Crush, ankle
      below knee — *see* Crush, leg
      foot — *see* Crush, foot
      hip — *see* Crush, hip
      knee — *see* Crush, knee
      thigh — *see* Crush, thigh
      toe — *see* Crush, toe
    upper
      below elbow S67.9- ☑
      elbow — *see* Crush, elbow
      finger — *see* Crush, finger
      forearm — *see* Crush, forearm
      hand — *see* Crush, hand
      thumb — *see* Crush, thumb
      upper arm — *see* Crush, arm
      wrist — *see* Crush, wrist
  face S07.0 ☑
  finger(s) S67.1- ☑
    with hand (and wrist) — *see* Crush, hand, specified
      site NEC
    index S67.19- ☑
    little S67.19- ☑
    middle S67.19- ☑
    ring S67.19- ☑
    thumb — *see* Crush, thumb
  foot S97.8- ☑
    toe — *see* Crush, toe
  forearm S57.8- ☑
  genitalia, external
    female S38.002 ☑
      vagina S38.03 ☑
      vulva S38.03 ☑
    male S38.001 ☑
      penis S38.01 ☑
      scrotum S38.02 ☑
      testis S38.02 ☑
  hand (except fingers alone) S67.2- ☑
    with wrist S67.4- ☑
  head S07.9 ☑
    specified NEC S07.8 ☑
  heel — *see* Crush, foot
  hip S77.0- ☑
    with thigh S77.2- ☑
  internal organ (abdomen, chest, or pelvis) NEC T14.8 ☑
  knee S87.0- ☑
  labium (majus) (minus) S38.03 ☑
  larynx S17.0 ☑
  leg (lower) S87.8- ☑
    knee — *see* Crush, knee
  lip S07.0 ☑
  lower
    back S38.1 ☑
    leg — *see* Crush, leg
  neck S17.9 ☑
  nerve — *see* Injury, nerve
  nose S07.0 ☑
  pelvis S38.1 ☑
  penis S38.01 ☑
  scalp S07.8 ☑
  scapular region — *see* Crush, arm
  scrotum S38.02 ☑

Crush, crushed, crushing — *continued*
  severe, unspecified site T14.8 ☑
  shoulder (and upper arm) — *see* Crush, arm
  skull S07.1 ☑
  syndrome (complication of trauma) T79.5 ☑
  testis S38.02 ☑
  thigh S77.1- ☑
    with hip S77.2- ☑
  throat S17.8 ☑
  thumb S67.0- ☑
    with hand (and wrist) — *see* Crush, hand, specified
      site NEC
  toe(s) S97.10- ☑
    great S97.11- ☑
    lesser S97.12- ☑
  trachea S17.0 ☑
  vagina S38.03 ☑
  vulva S38.03 ☑
  wrist S67.3- ☑
    with hand S67.4- ☑
Crusta lactea L21.0
Crusts R23.4
Crutch paralysis — *see* Injury, brachial plexus
**Cruveilhier-Baumgarten cirrhosis, disease or syn-
  drome** K74.69
Cruveilhier's atrophy or disease G12.8
Crying (constant) (continuous) (excessive)
  child, adolescent, or adult R45.83
  infant (baby) (newborn) R68.11
Cryofibrinogenemia D89.2
Cryoglobulinemia (essential) (idiopathic) (mixed) (primary) (purpura) (secondary) (vasculitis) D89.1
  with lung involvement D89.1 *[J99]*
Cryptitis (anal) (rectal) K62.89
Cryptococcosis, cryptococcus (infection) (neoformans)
  B45.9
  bone B45.3
  cerebral B45.1
  cutaneous B45.2
  disseminated B45.7
  generalized B45.7
  meningitis B45.1
  meningocerebralis B45.1
  osseous B45.3
  pulmonary B45.0
  skin B45.2
  specified NEC B45.8
Cryptopapillitis (anus) K62.89
Cryptophthalmos Q11.2
  syndrome Q87.0
Cryptorchid, cryptorchism, cryptorchidism Q53.9
  bilateral Q53.20
    abdominal Q53.211
    perineal Q53.22
  unilateral Q53.10
    abdominal Q53.111
    perineal Q53.12
Cryptosporidiosis A07.2
  hepatobiliary B88.8
  respiratory B88.8
Cryptostromosis J67.6
Crystalluria R82.998
Cubitus
  congenital Q68.8
  valgus (acquired) M21.0- ☑
    congenital Q68.8
    sequelae (late effect) of rickets E64.3
  varus (acquired) M21.1- ☑
    congenital Q68.8
    sequelae (late effect) of rickets E64.3
Cultural deprivation or shock Z60.3
Curling esophagus K22.4
Curling's ulcer — *see* Ulcer, peptic, acute
Curschmann (-Batten) (-Steinert) **disease or syndrome**
  G71.11
Curse, Ondine's — *see* Apnea, sleep
Curvature
  organ or site, congenital NEC — *See* Distortion
  penis (lateral) Q55.61
  Pott's (spinal) A18.01
  radius, idiopathic, progressive (congenital) Q74.0
  spine (acquired) (angular) (idiopathic) (incorrect)
    (postural) — *see* Dorsopathy, deforming
    congenital Q67.5
    due to or associated with
      Charcot-Marie-Tooth disease — *see also* subcat-
        egory M49.8 G60.0

Curvature — *continued*
  spine — *see* Dorsopathy, deforming — *continued*
    due to or associated with — *continued*
      osteitis
        deformans M88.88
        fibrosa cystica — *see also* subcategory M49.8
          E21.0
      tuberculosis (Pott's curvature) A18.01
      sequelae (late effect) of rickets E64.3
      tuberculous A18.01
Cushingoid due to steroid therapy E24.2
  correct substance properly administered — *see* Table of Drugs and Chemicals, by drug, adverse effect
  overdose or wrong substance given or taken — *see* Table of Drugs and Chemicals, by drug, poisoning
Cushing's
  syndrome or disease E24.9
    drug-induced E24.2
    iatrogenic E24.2
    pituitary-dependent E24.0
    specified NEC E24.8
  ulcer — *see* Ulcer, peptic, acute
Cusp, Carabelli — *omit code*
Cut (external) — *see also* Laceration
  muscle — *see* Injury, muscle
Cutaneous — *see also* condition
  hemorrhage R23.3
  larva migrans B76.9
Cutis — *see also* condition
  hyperelastica Q82.8
    acquired L57.4
  laxa (hyperelastica) — *see* Dermatolysis
  marmorata R23.8
  osteosis L94.2
  pendula — *see* Dermatolysis
  rhomboidalis nuchae L57.2
  verticis gyrata Q82.8
    acquired L91.8
Cyanosis R23.0
  due to
    patent foramen botalli Q21.1
    persistent foramen ovale Q21.1
  enterogenous D74.8
  paroxysmal digital — *see* Raynaud's disease
    with gangrene I73.01
  retina, retinal H35.89
Cyanotic heart disease I24.9
  congenital Q24.9
Cycle
  anovulatory N97.0
  menstrual, irregular N92.6
Cyclencephaly Q04.9
Cyclical vomiting, in migraine — *see also* Vomiting, cyclical G43.A0 (*following* G43.7)
  psychogenic F50.89
Cyclitis — *see also* Iridocyclitis H20.9
  chronic — *see* Iridocyclitis, chronic
  Fuchs' heterochromic H20.81- ☑
  granulomatous — *see* Iridocyclitis, chronic
  lens-induced — *see* Iridocyclitis, lens-induced
  posterior H30.2- ☑
Cycloid personality F34.0
Cyclophoria H50.54
Cyclopia, cyclops Q87.0
Cyclopism Q87.0
Cyclosporiasis A07.4
Cyclothymia F34.0
Cyclothymic personality F34.0
Cyclotropia H50.41- ☑
Cylindroma — *see also* Neoplasm, malignant, by site
  eccrine dermal — *see* Neoplasm, skin, benign
  skin — *see* Neoplasm, skin, benign
Cylindruria R82.998
Cynanche
  diphtheritic A36.2
  tonsillaris J36
Cynophobia F40.218
Cynorexia R63.2
Cyphosis — *see* Kyphosis
Cyprus fever — *see* Brucellosis
Cyst (colloid) (mucous) (simple) (retention)
  adenoid (infected) J35.8
  adrenal gland E27.8
    congenital Q89.1
  air, lung J98.4
  allantoic Q64.4
  alveolar process (jaw bone) M27.40

Cyst — *continued*
  amnion, amniotic O41.8X- ☑
  aneurysmal M27.49
  anterior
    chamber (eye) — *see* Cyst, iris
    nasopalatine K09.1
  antrum J34.1
  anus K62.89
  apical (tooth) (periodontal) K04.8
  appendix K38.8
  arachnoid, brain (acquired) G93.0
    congenital Q04.6
  arytenoid J38.7
  Baker's M71.2- ☑
    ruptured M66.0
    tuberculous A18.02
  Bartholin's gland N75.0
  bile duct (common) (hepatic) K83.5
  bladder (multiple) (trigone) N32.89
  blue dome (breast) — *see* Cyst, breast
  bone (local) NEC M85.60
    aneurysmal M85.50
      ankle M85.57- ☑
      foot M85.57- ☑
      forearm M85.53- ☑
      hand M85.54- ☑
      jaw M27.49
      lower leg M85.56- ☑
      multiple site M85.59
      neck M85.58
      rib M85.58
      shoulder M85.51- ☑
      skull M85.58
      specified site NEC M85.58
      thigh M85.55- ☑
      toe M85.57- ☑
      upper arm M85.52- ☑
      vertebra M85.58
    solitary M85.40
      ankle M85.47- ☑
      fibula M85.46- ☑
      foot M85.47- ☑
      hand M85.44- ☑
      humerus M85.42- ☑
      jaw M27.49
      neck M85.48
      pelvis M85.45- ☑
      radius M85.43- ☑
      rib M85.48
      shoulder M85.41- ☑
      skull M85.48
      specified site NEC M85.48
      tibia M85.46- ☑
      toe M85.47- ☑
      ulna M85.43- ☑
      vertebra M85.48
    specified type NEC M85.60
      ankle M85.67- ☑
      foot M85.67- ☑
      forearm M85.63- ☑
      hand M85.64- ☑
      jaw M27.40
        developmental (nonodontogenic) K09.1
        odontogenic K09.0
        latent M27.0
      lower leg M85.66- ☑
      multiple site M85.69
      neck M85.68
      rib M85.68
      shoulder M85.61- ☑
      skull M85.68
      specified site NEC M85.68
      thigh M85.65- ☑
      toe M85.67- ☑
      upper arm M85.62- ☑
      vertebra M85.68
  brain (acquired) G93.0
    congenital Q04.6
    hydatid B67.99 *[G94]*
    third ventricle (colloid), congenital Q04.6
  branchial (cleft) Q18.0
  branchiogenic Q18.0
  breast (benign) (blue dome) (pedunculated) (solitary) N60.0- ☑
    involution — *see* Dysplasia, mammary, specified type NEC

Cyst — *continued*
  breast — *continued*
    sebaceous — *see* Dysplasia, mammary, specified type NEC
  broad ligament (benign) N83.8
  bronchogenic (mediastinal) (sequestration) J98.4
    congenital Q33.0
  buccal K09.8
  bulbourethral gland N36.8
  bursa, bursal NEC M71.30
    with rupture — *see* Rupture, synovium
    ankle M71.37- ☑
    elbow M71.32- ☑
    foot M71.37- ☑
    hand M71.34- ☑
    hip M71.35- ☑
    multiple sites M71.39
    pharyngeal J39.2
    popliteal space — *see* Cyst, Baker's
    shoulder M71.31- ☑
    specified site NEC M71.38
    wrist M71.33- ☑
  calcifying odontogenic D16.5
    upper jaw (bone) (maxilla) D16.4
  canal of Nuck (female) N94.89
    congenital Q52.4
  canthus — *see* Cyst, conjunctiva
  carcinomatous — *see* Neoplasm, malignant, by site
  cauda equina G95.89
  cavum septi pellucidi — *see* Cyst, brain
  celomic (pericardium) Q24.8
  cerebellopontine (angle) — *see* Cyst, brain
  cerebellum — *see* Cyst, brain
  cerebral — *see* Cyst, brain
  cervical lateral Q18.0
  cervix NEC N88.8
    embryonic Q51.6
    nabothian N88.8
  chiasmal optic NEC — *see* Disorder, optic, chiasm
  chocolate (ovary) N80.1
  choledochus, congenital Q44.4
  chorion O41.8X- ☑
  choroid plexus G93.0
    congenital Q04.6
  ciliary body — *see* Cyst, iris
  clitoris N90.7
  colon K63.89
  common (bile) duct K83.5
  congenital NEC Q89.8
    adrenal gland Q89.1
    epiglottis Q31.8
    esophagus Q39.8
    fallopian tube Q50.4
    kidney Q61.00
      more than one (multiple) Q61.02
        specified as polycystic Q61.3
          adult type Q61.2
          infantile type NEC Q61.19
            collecting duct dilation Q61.11
      solitary Q61.01
    larynx Q31.8
    liver Q44.6
    lung Q33.0
    mediastinum Q34.1
    ovary Q50.1
    oviduct Q50.4
    periurethral (tissue) Q64.79
    prepuce Q55.69
    salivary gland (any) Q38.4
    sublingual Q38.6
    submaxillary gland Q38.6
    thymus (gland) Q89.2
    tongue Q38.3
    ureterovesical orifice Q62.8
    vulva Q52.79
  conjunctiva H11.44- ☑
  cornea H18.89- ☑
  corpora quadrigemina G93.0
  corpus
    albicans N83.29- ☑
    luteum (hemorrhagic) (ruptured) N83.1- ☑
  Cowper's gland (benign) (infected) N36.8
  cranial meninges G93.0
  craniobuccal pouch E23.6
  craniopharyngeal pouch E23.6
  cystic duct K82.8
  Cysticercus — *see* Cysticercosis
  Dandy-Walker Q03.1

☑ **Additional Character Required** — Refer to the Tabular List for Character Selection   ▽ **Subterms under main terms may continue to next column or page**

Cyst — continued
 Dandy-Walker — continued
  with spina bifida — see Spina bifida
 dental (root) K04.8
  developmental K09.0
  eruption K09.0
  primordial K09.0
 dentigerous (mandible) (maxilla) K09.0
 dermoid — see Neoplasm, benign, by site
  with malignant transformation C56.- ☑
  implantation
   external area or site (skin) NEC L72.0
   iris — see Cyst, iris, implantation
   vagina N89.8
   vulva N90.7
  mouth K09.8
  oral soft tissue K09.8
  sacrococcygeal — see Cyst, pilonidal
 developmental K09.1
  odontogenic K09.0
  oral region (nonodontogenic) K09.1
  ovary, ovarian Q50.1
 dura (cerebral) G93.0
  spinal G96.198
 ear (external) Q18.1
 echinococcal — see Echinococcus
 embryonic
  cervix uteri Q51.6
  fallopian tube Q50.4
  vagina Q52.4
 endometrium, endometrial (uterus) N85.8
  ectopic — see Endometriosis
 enterogenous Q43.8
 epidermal, epidermoid (inclusion) (see also Cyst, skin)
   L72.0
  mouth K09.8
  oral soft tissue K09.8
 epididymis N50.3
 epiglottis J38.7
 epiphysis cerebri E34.8
 epithelial (inclusion) L72.0
 epoophoron Q50.5
 eruption K09.0
 esophagus K22.89
 ethmoid sinus J34.1
 external female genital organs NEC N90.7
 eyelid (sebaceous) H02.829
  infected — see Hordeolum
  left H02.826
   lower H02.825
   upper H02.824
  right H02.823
   lower H02.822
   upper H02.821
 eye NEC H57.89
  congenital Q15.8
 fallopian tube N83.8
  congenital Q50.4
 fimbrial (twisted) Q50.4
 fissural (oral region) K09.1
 follicle (graafian) (hemorrhagic) N83.0- ☑
  nabothian N88.8
 follicular (atretic) (hemorrhagic) (ovarian) N83.0- ☑
  dentigerous K09.0
  odontogenic K09.0
  skin L72.9
   specified NEC L72.8
 frontal sinus J34.1
 gallbladder K82.8
 ganglion — see Ganglion
 Gartner's duct Q52.4
 gingiva K09.0
 gland of Moll — see Cyst, eyelid
 globulomaxillary K09.1
 graafian follicle (hemorrhagic) N83.0- ☑
 granulosal lutein (hemorrhagic) N83.1- ☑
 hemangiomatous D18.00
  intra-abdominal D18.03
  intracranial D18.02
  skin D18.01
  specified site NEC D18.09
 hemorrhagic M27.49
 hydatid — see also Echinococcus B67.90
  brain B67.99 [G94]
  liver — see also Cyst, liver, hydatid B67.8
  lung NEC B67.99 [J99]
  Morgagni
   female Q50.5

Cyst — continued
 hydatid — see also Echinococcus — continued
  Morgagni — continued
   male (epididymal) Q55.4
    testicular Q55.29
  specified site NEC B67.99
 hymen N89.8
  embryonic Q52.4
 hypopharynx J39.2
 hypophysis, hypophyseal (duct) (recurrent) E23.6
  cerebri E23.6
 implantation (dermoid)
  external area or site (skin) NEC L72.0
  iris — see Cyst, iris, implantation
  vagina N89.8
  vulva N90.7
 incisive canal K09.1
 inclusion (epidermal) (epithelial) (epidermoid) (squamous) L72.0
  not of skin — code under Cyst, by site
 intestine (large) (small) K63.89
 intracranial — see Cyst, brain
 intraligamentous — see also Disorder, ligament
  knee — see Derangement, knee
 intrasellar E23.6
 iris H21.309
  exudative H21.31- ☑
  idiopathic H21.30- ☑
  implantation H21.32- ☑
  parasitic H21.33- ☑
  pars plana (primary) H21.34- ☑
   exudative H21.35- ☑
 jaw (bone) M27.40
  aneurysmal M27.49
  developmental (odontogenic) K09.0
  fissural K09.1
  hemorrhagic M27.49
  traumatic M27.49
 joint NEC — see Disorder, joint, specified type NEC
 kidney (acquired) N28.1
  calyceal — see Hydronephrosis
  congenital Q61.00
   more than one (multiple) Q61.02
    specified as polycystic Q61.3
     adult type (autosomal dominant) Q61.2
     infantile type (autosomal recessive) NEC
      Q61.19
     collecting duct dilation Q61.11
  pyelogenic — see Hydronephrosis
  simple N28.1
  solitary (single) Q61.01
   acquired N28.1
 labium (majus) (minus) N90.7
  sebaceous N90.7
 lacrimal — see also Disorder, lacrimal system, specified
   NEC
  gland H04.13- ☑
  passages or sac — see Disorder, lacrimal system,
    specified NEC
 larynx J38.7
 lateral periodontal K09.0
 lens H27.8
  congenital Q12.8
 lip (gland) K13.0
 liver (idiopathic) (simple) K76.89
  congenital Q44.6
  hydatid B67.8
   granulosus B67.0
   multilocularis B67.5
 lung J98.4
  congenital Q33.0
  giant bullous J43.9
 lutein N83.1- ☑
 lymphangiomatous D18.1
 lymphoepithelial, oral soft tissue K09.8
 macula — see Degeneration, macula, hole
 malignant — see Neoplasm, malignant, by site
 mammary gland — see Cyst, breast
 mandible M27.40
  dentigerous K09.0
  radicular K04.8
 maxilla M27.40
  dentigerous K09.0
  radicular K04.8
 medial, face and neck Q18.8
 median
  anterior maxillary K09.1
  palatal K09.1

Cyst — continued
 mediastinum, congenital Q34.1
 meibomian (gland) — see Chalazion
  infected — see Hordeolum
 membrane, brain G93.0
 meninges (cerebral) G93.0
  spinal G96.198
 meniscus, knee — see Derangement, knee, meniscus,
   cystic
 mesentery, mesenteric K66.8
  chyle I89.8
 mesonephric duct
  female Q50.5
  male Q55.4
 milk N64.89
 Morgagni (hydatid)
  female Q50.5
  male (epididymal) Q55.4
   testicular Q55.29
 mouth K09.8
 Müllerian duct Q50.4
  appendix testis Q55.29
  cervix Q51.6
  fallopian tube Q50.4
  female Q50.4
  male Q55.29
  prostatic utricle Q55.4
  vagina (embryonal) Q52.4
 multilocular (ovary) D39.10
  benign — see Neoplasm, benign, by site
 myometrium N85.8
 nabothian (follicle) (ruptured) N88.8
 nasoalveolar K09.1
 nasolabial K09.1
 nasopalatine (anterior) (duct) K09.1
 nasopharynx J39.2
 neoplastic — see Neoplasm, uncertain behavior, by
   site
  benign — see Neoplasm, benign, by site
 nerve root
  cervical G96.191
  lumbar G96.191
  sacral G96.191
  thoracic G96.191
 nervous system NEC G96.89
 neuroenteric (congenital) Q06.8
 nipple — see Cyst, breast
 nose (turbinates) J34.1
  sinus J34.1
 odontogenic, developmental K09.0
 omentum (lesser) K66.8
  congenital Q45.8
 ora serrata — see Cyst, retina, ora serrata
 oral
  region K09.9
   developmental (nonodontogenic) K09.1
   specified NEC K09.8
  soft tissue K09.9
   specified NEC K09.8
 orbit H05.81- ☑
 ovary, ovarian (twisted) N83.20- ☑
  adherent N83.20- ☑
  chocolate N80.1
  corpus
   albicans N83.29- ☑
   luteum (hemorrhagic) N83.1- ☑
  dermoid D27.9
  developmental Q50.1
  due to failure of involution NEC N83.20- ☑
  endometrial N80.1
  follicular (graafian) (hemorrhagic) N83.0- ☑
  hemorrhagic N83.20- ☑
  in pregnancy or childbirth O34.8- ☑
   with obstructed labor O65.5
  multilocular D39.10
  pseudomucinous D27.9
  retention N83.29- ☑
  serous N83.20- ☑
  specified NEC N83.29- ☑
  theca lutein (hemorrhagic) N83.1- ☑
  tuberculous A18.18
 oviduct N83.8
 palate (median) (fissural) K09.1
 palatine papilla (jaw) K09.1
 pancreas, pancreatic (hemorrhagic) (true) K86.2
  congenital Q45.2
  false K86.3

Cyst — *continued*
paralabral
  hip M24.85- ☑
  shoulder S43.43- ☑
paramesonephric duct Q50.4
  female Q50.4
  male Q55.29
paranephric N28.1
paraphysis, cerebri, congenital Q04.6
parasitic B89
parathyroid (gland) E21.4
paratubal N83.8
paraurethral duct N36.8
paroophoron Q50.5
parotid gland K11.6
parovarian Q50.5
pelvis, female N94.89
  in pregnancy or childbirth O34.8- ☑
    causing obstructed labor O65.5
penis (sebaceous) N48.89
periapical K04.8
pericardial (congenital) Q24.8
  acquired (secondary) I31.8
pericoronal K09.0
perineural G96.191
periodontal K04.8
  lateral K09.0
peripelvic (lymphatic) N28.1
peritoneum K66.8
  chylous I89.8
periventricular, acquired, newborn P91.1
pharynx (wall) J39.2
pilar L72.11
pilonidal (infected) (rectum) L05.91
  with abscess L05.01
  malignant C44.59- ☑
pituitary (duct) (gland) E23.6
placenta O43.19- ☑
pleura J94.8
popliteal — *see* Cyst, Baker's
porencephalic Q04.6
  acquired G93.0
postanal (infected) — *see* Cyst, pilonidal
postmastoidectomy cavity (mucosal) — *see* Complications, postmastoidectomy, cyst
preauricular Q18.1
prepuce N47.4
  congenital Q55.69
primordial (jaw) K09.0
prostate N42.83
pseudomucinous (ovary) D27.9
pupillary, miotic H21.27- ☑
radicular (residual) K04.8
radiculodental K04.8
ranular K11.8
Rathke's pouch E23.6
rectum (epithelium) (mucous) K62.89
renal — *see* Cyst, kidney
residual (radicular) K04.8
retention (ovary) N83.29- ☑
  salivary gland K11.6
retina H33.19- ☑
  ora serrata H33.11- ☑
  parasitic H33.12- ☑
retroperitoneal K68.9
sacrococcygeal (dermoid) — *see* Cyst, pilonidal
salivary gland or duct (mucous extravasation or retention) K11.6
Sampson's N80.1
sclera H15.89
scrotum L72.9
  sebaceous L72.3
sebaceous (duct) (gland) L72.3
  breast — *see* Dysplasia, mammary, specified type NEC
  eyelid — *see* Cyst, eyelid
  genital organ NEC
    female N94.89
    male N50.89
  scrotum L72.3
semilunar cartilage (knee) (multiple) — *see* Derangement, knee, meniscus, cystic
seminal vesicle N50.89
serous (ovary) N83.20- ☑
sinus (accessory) (nasal) J34.1
Skene's gland N36.8
skin L72.9

Cyst — *continued*
skin — *continued*
  breast — *see* Dysplasia, mammary, specified type NEC
  epidermal, epidermoid L72.0
  epithelial L72.0
  eyelid — *see* Cyst, eyelid
  genital organ NEC
    female N90.7
    male N50.89
  inclusion L72.0
  scrotum L72.9
  sebaceous L72.3
  sweat gland or duct L74.8
solitary
  bone — *see* Cyst, bone, solitary
  jaw M27.40
  kidney N28.1
spermatic cord N50.89
sphenoid sinus J34.1
spinal meninges G96.198
spleen NEC D73.4
  congenital Q89.09
  hydatid — *see also* Echinococcus B67.99 [D77]
Stafne's M27.0
subarachnoid intrasellar R93.0
subcutaneous, pheomycotic (chromomycotic) B43.2
subdural (cerebral) G93.0
  spinal cord G96.198
sublingual gland K11.6
submandibular gland K11.6
submaxillary gland K11.6
suburethral N36.8
suprarenal gland E27.8
suprasellar — *see* Cyst, brain
sweat gland or duct L74.8
synovial — *see also* Cyst, bursa
  ruptured — *see* Rupture, synovium
Tarlov G96.191
tarsal — *see* Chalazion
tendon (sheath) — *see* Disorder, tendon, specified type NEC
testis N44.2
  tunica albuginea N44.1
theca lutein (ovary) N83.1- ☑
Thornwaldt's J39.2
thymus (gland) E32.8
thyroglossal duct (infected) (persistent) Q89.2
thyroid (gland) E04.1
thyrolingual duct (infected) (persistent) Q89.2
tongue K14.8
tonsil J35.8
tooth — *see* Cyst, dental
Tornwaldt's J39.2
trichilemmal (proliferating) L72.12
trichodermal L72.12
tubal (fallopian) N83.8
  inflammatory — *see* Salpingitis, chronic
tubo-ovarian N83.8
  inflammatory N70.13
tunica
  albuginea testis N44.1
  vaginalis N50.89
turbinate (nose) J34.1
Tyson's gland N48.89
urachus, congenital Q64.4
ureter N28.89
ureterovesical orifice N28.89
urethra, urethral (gland) N36.8
uterine ligament N83.8
uterus (body) (corpus) (recurrent) N85.8
  embryonic Q51.818
    cervix Q51.6
vagina, vaginal (implantation) (inclusion) (squamous cell) (wall) N89.8
  embryonic Q52.4
vallecula, vallecular (epiglottis) J38.7
vesical (orifice) N32.89
vitreous body H43.89
vulva (implantation) (inclusion) N90.7
  congenital Q52.79
  sebaceous gland N90.7
vulvovaginal gland N90.7
wolffian
  female Q50.5
  male Q55.4

Cystadenocarcinoma — *see* Neoplasm, malignant, by site

Cystadenocarcinoma — *continued*
bile duct C22.1
endometrioid — *see* Neoplasm, malignant, by site
  specified site — *see* Neoplasm, malignant, by site
  unspecified site
    female C56.9
    male C61
mucinous
  papillary
    specified site — *see* Neoplasm, malignant, by site
    unspecified site C56.9
  specified site — *see* Neoplasm, malignant, by site
  unspecified site C56.9
papillary
  mucinous
    specified site — *see* Neoplasm, malignant, by site
    unspecified site C56.9
  pseudomucinous
    specified site — *see* Neoplasm, malignant, by site
    unspecified site C56.9
  serous
    specified site — *see* Neoplasm, malignant, by site
    unspecified site C56.9
  specified site — *see* Neoplasm, malignant, by site
  unspecified site C56.9
pseudomucinous
  papillary
    specified site — *see* Neoplasm, malignant, by site
    unspecified site C56.9
  specified site — *see* Neoplasm, malignant, by site
  unspecified site C56.9
serous
  papillary
    specified site — *see* Neoplasm, malignant, by site
    unspecified site C56.9
  specified site — *see* Neoplasm, malignant, by site
  unspecified site C56.9

Cystadenofibroma
clear cell — *see* Neoplasm, benign, by site
endometrioid D27.9
  borderline malignancy D39.1- ☑
  malignant C56.- ☑
mucinous
  specified site — *see* Neoplasm, benign, by site
  unspecified site D27.9
serous
  specified site — *see* Neoplasm, benign, by site
  unspecified site D27.9
specified site — *see* Neoplasm, benign, by site
unspecified site D27.9

Cystadenoma — *see also* Neoplasm, benign, by site
bile duct D13.4
endometrioid — *see* Neoplasm, benign, by site
  borderline malignancy — *see* Neoplasm, uncertain behavior, by site
malignant — *see* Neoplasm, malignant, by site
mucinous
  borderline malignancy
    ovary C56.- ☑
    specified site NEC — *see* Neoplasm, uncertain behavior, by site
    unspecified site C56.9
  papillary
    borderline malignancy
      ovary C56.- ☑
      specified site NEC — *see* Neoplasm, uncertain behavior, by site
      unspecified site C56.9
    specified site — *see* Neoplasm, benign, by site
    unspecified site D27.9
  specified site — *see* Neoplasm, benign, by site
  unspecified site D27.9
papillary
  borderline malignancy
    ovary C56.- ☑
    specified site NEC — *see* Neoplasm, uncertain behavior, by site
    unspecified site C56.9
  lymphomatosum
    specified site — *see* Neoplasm, benign, by site
    unspecified site D11.9

☑ **Additional Character Required** — Refer to the Tabular List for Character Selection   ▽ **Subterms under main terms may continue to next column or page**

Cystadenoma — continued
  papillary — continued
    mucinous
      borderline malignancy
        ovary C56.- ☑
        specified site NEC — see Neoplasm, uncertain
          behavior, by site
        unspecified site C56.9
      specified site — see Neoplasm, benign, by site
      unspecified site D27.9
    pseudomucinous
      borderline malignancy
        ovary C56.- ☑
        specified site NEC — see Neoplasm, uncertain
          behavior, by site
        unspecified site C56.9
      specified site — see Neoplasm, benign, by site
      unspecified site D27.9
    serous
      borderline malignancy
        ovary C56.- ☑
        specified site NEC — see Neoplasm, uncertain
          behavior, by site
        unspecified site C56.9
      specified site — see Neoplasm, benign, by site
      unspecified site D27.9
    specified site — see Neoplasm, benign, by site
    unspecified site D27.9
  pseudomucinous
    borderline malignancy
      ovary C56.- ☑
      specified site NEC — see Neoplasm, uncertain
        behavior, by site
      unspecified site C56.9
    papillary
      borderline malignancy
        ovary C56.- ☑
        specified site NEC — see Neoplasm, uncertain
          behavior, by site
        unspecified site C56.9
      specified site — see Neoplasm, benign, by site
      unspecified site D27.9
    specified site — see Neoplasm, benign, by site
    unspecified site D27.9
  serous
    borderline malignancy
      ovary C56.- ☑
      specified site NEC — see Neoplasm, uncertain
        behavior, by site
      unspecified site C56.9
    papillary
      borderline malignancy
        ovary C56.- ☑
        specified site NEC — see Neoplasm, uncertain
          behavior, by site
        unspecified site C56.9
      specified site — see Neoplasm, benign, by site
      unspecified site D27.9
    specified site — see Neoplasm, benign, by site
    unspecified site D27.9

Cystathionine synthase deficiency E72.11
Cystathioninemia E72.19
Cystathioninuria E72.19
Cystic — see also condition
  breast (chronic) — see Mastopathy, cystic
  corpora lutea (hemorrhagic) N83.1- ☑
  duct — see condition
  eyeball (congenital) Q11.0
  fibrosis — see Fibrosis, cystic
  kidney (congenital) Q61.9

Cystic — continued
  kidney — continued
    adult type Q61.2
    infantile type NEC Q61.19
      collecting duct dilatation Q61.11
    medullary Q61.5
  liver, congenital Q44.6
  lung disease J98.4
    congenital Q33.0
  mastitis, chronic — see Mastopathy, cystic
  medullary, kidney Q61.5
  meniscus — see Derangement, knee, meniscus, cystic
  ovary N83.20- ☑
Cysticercosis, cysticerciasis B69.9
  with
    epileptiform fits B69.0
    myositis B69.81
  brain B69.0
  central nervous system B69.0
  cerebral B69.0
  ocular B69.1
  specified NEC B69.89
Cysticercus cellulose infestation — see Cysticercosis
Cystinosis (malignant) E72.04
Cystinuria E72.01
Cystitis (exudative) (hemorrhagic) (septic) (suppurative)
  N30.90
  with
    fibrosis — see Cystitis, chronic, interstitial
    hematuria N30.91
    leukoplakia — see Cystitis, chronic, interstitial
    malakoplakia — see Cystitis, chronic, interstitial
    metaplasia — see Cystitis, chronic, interstitial
    prostatitis N41.3
  acute N30.00
    with hematuria N30.01
    of trigone N30.30
      with hematuria N30.31
  allergic — see Cystitis, specified type NEC
  amebic A06.81
  bilharzial B65.9 [N33]
  blennorrhagic (gonococcal) A54.01
  bullous — see Cystitis, specified type NEC
  calculous N21.0
  chlamydial A56.01
  chronic N30.20
    with hematuria N30.21
    interstitial N30.10
      with hematuria N30.11
    of trigone N30.30
      with hematuria N30.31
    specified NEC N30.20
      with hematuria N30.21
  cystic (a) — see Cystitis, specified type NEC
  diphtheritic A36.85
  echinococcal
    granulosus B67.39
    multilocularis B67.69
  emphysematous — see Cystitis, specified type NEC
  encysted — see Cystitis, specified type NEC
  eosinophilic — see Cystitis, specified type NEC
  follicular — see Cystitis, of trigone
  gangrenous — see Cystitis, specified type NEC
  glandularis — see Cystitis, specified type NEC
  gonococcal A54.01
  incrusted — see Cystitis, specified type NEC
  interstitial (chronic) — see Cystitis, chronic, interstitial
  irradiation N30.40
    with hematuria N30.41
  irritation — see Cystitis, specified type NEC

Cystitis — continued
  malignant — see Cystitis, specified type NEC
  of trigone N30.30
    with hematuria N30.31
  panmural — see Cystitis, chronic, interstitial
  polyposa — see Cystitis, specified type NEC
  prostatic N41.3
  puerperal (postpartum) O86.22
  radiation — see Cystitis, irradiation
  specified type NEC N30.80
    with hematuria N30.81
  subacute — see Cystitis, chronic
  submucous — see Cystitis, chronic, interstitial
  syphilitic (late) A52.76
  trichomonal A59.03
  tuberculous A18.12
  ulcerative — see Cystitis, chronic, interstitial
Cystocele (-urethrocele)
  female N81.10
    with prolapse of uterus — see Prolapse, uterus
    lateral N81.12
    midline N81.11
    paravaginal N81.12
  in pregnancy or childbirth O34.8- ☑
    causing obstructed labor O65.5
  male N32.89
Cystolithiasis N21.0
Cystoma — see also Neoplasm, benign, by site
  endometrial, ovary N80.1
  mucinous
    specified site — see Neoplasm, benign, by site
    unspecified site D27.9
  serous
    specified site — see Neoplasm, benign, by site
    unspecified site D27.9
  simple (ovary) N83.29- ☑
Cystoplegia N31.2
Cystoptosis N32.89
Cystopyelitis — see Pyelonephritis
Cystorrhagia N32.89
Cystosarcoma phyllodes D48.6- ☑
  benign D24- ☑
  malignant — see Neoplasm, breast, malignant
Cystostomy
  attention to Z43.5
  complication — see Complications, cystostomy
  status Z93.50
    appendico-vesicostomy Z93.52
    cutaneous Z93.51
    specified NEC Z93.59
Cystourethritis — see Urethritis
Cystourethrocele — see also Cystocele
  female N81.10
    with uterine prolapse — see Prolapse, uterus
    lateral N81.12
    midline N81.11
    paravaginal N81.12
  male N32.89
Cytomegalic inclusion disease
  congenital P35.1
Cytomegalovirus infection B25.9
Cytomycosis (reticuloendothelial) B39.4
Cytopenia D75.9
  refractory
    with multilineage dysplasia D46.A (following D46.2)
    and ring sideroblasts (RCMD RS) D46.B (following
      D46.2)
Czerny's disease (periodic hydrarthrosis of the knee) —
  see Effusion, joint, knee

D

Da Costa's syndrome F45.8
Daae (-Finsen) **disease** (epidemic pleurodynia) B33.0
Dabney's grip B33.0
Dacryoadenitis, dacryadenitis H04.00- ☑
  acute H04.01- ☑
  chronic H04.02- ☑
Dacryocystitis H04.30- ☑
  acute H04.32- ☑
  chronic H04.41- ☑
  neonatal P39.1
  phlegmonous H04.31- ☑
  syphilitic A52.71
    congenital (early) A50.01
  trachomatous, active A71.1
    sequelae (late effect) B94.0
Dacryocystoblenorrhea — see Inflammation, lacrimal, passages, chronic
Dacryocystocele — see Disorder, lacrimal system, changes
Dacryolith, dacryolithiasis H04.51- ☑
Dacryoma — see Disorder, lacrimal system, changes
Dacryopericystitis — see Dacryocystitis
Dacryops H04.11- ☑
Dacryostenosis — see also Stenosis, lacrimal
  congenital Q10.5
Dactylitis
  bone — see Osteomyelitis
  sickle-cell D57.00
    Hb C D57.219
    Hb SS D57.00
    specified NEC D57.819
  skin L08.9
  syphilitic A52.77
  tuberculous A18.03
Dactylolysis spontanea (ainhum) L94.6
Dactylosymphysis Q70.9
  fingers — see Syndactylism, complex, fingers
  toes — see Syndactylism, complex, toes
Damage
  arteriosclerotic — see Arteriosclerosis
  brain (nontraumatic) G93.9
    anoxic, hypoxic G93.1
      resulting from a procedure G97.82
    child NEC G80.9
    due to birth injury P11.2
  cardiorenal (vascular) — see Hypertension, cardiorenal
  cerebral NEC — see Damage, brain
  coccyx, complicating delivery O71.6
  coronary — see Disease, heart, ischemic
  deep tissue, pressure-induced — see also L89 with final character .6
  eye, birth injury P15.3
  liver (nontraumatic) K76.9
    alcoholic K70.9
    due to drugs — see Disease, liver, toxic
    toxic — see Disease, liver, toxic
  lung
    dabbing (related) U07.0
    electronic cigarette (related) U07.0
    vaping (associated) (device) (product) (use) U07.0
  medication T88.7 ☑
  organ
    dabbing (related) U07.0
    electronic cigarette (related) U07.0
    vaping (associated) (device) (product) (use) U07.0
  pelvic
    joint or ligament, during delivery O71.6
    organ NEC
      during delivery O71.5
      following ectopic or molar pregnancy O08.6
  renal — see Disease, renal
  subendocardium, subendocardial — see Degeneration, myocardial
  vascular I99.9
Dana-Putnam syndrome (subacute combined sclerosis with pernicious anemia) — see Degeneration, combined
Danbolt (-Cross) **syndrome** (acrodermatitis enteropathica) E83.2
Dandruff L21.0
Dandy-Walker syndrome Q03.1
  with spina bifida — see Spina bifida
Danlos' syndrome — see also Syndrome, Ehlers-Danlos Q79.60

Darier (-White) **disease** (congenital) Q82.8
  meaning erythema annulare centrifugum L53.1
Darier-Roussy sarcoid D86.3
Darling's disease or histoplasmosis B39.4
Darwin's tubercle Q17.8
Dawson's (inclusion body) **encephalitis** A81.1
De Beurmann (-Gougerot) **disease** B42.1
De la Tourette's syndrome F95.2
De Lange's syndrome Q87.19
De Morgan's spots (senile angiomas) I78.1
De Quervain's
  disease (tendon sheath) M65.4
  syndrome E34.51
  thyroiditis (subacute granulomatous thyroiditis) E06.1
De Toni-Fanconi (-Debré) **syndrome** E72.09
  with cystinosis E72.04
Dead
  fetus, retained (mother) O36.4 ☑
    early pregnancy O02.1
  labyrinth H83.2 ☑
  ovum, retained O02.0
Deaf nonspeaking NEC H91.3
Deafmutism (acquired) (congenital) NEC H91.3
  hysterical F44.6
  syphilitic, congenital — see also subcategory H94.8 A50.09
Deafness (acquired) (complete) (hereditary) (partial) H91.9- ☑
  with blue sclera and fragility of bone Q78.0
  auditory fatigue — see Deafness, specified type NEC
  aviation T70.0 ☑
    nerve injury — see Injury, nerve, acoustic, specified type NEC
  boilermaker's H83.3 ☑
  central — see Deafness, sensorineural
  conductive H90.2
    and sensorineural
      mixed H90.8
        bilateral H90.6
    bilateral H90.0
    unilateral H90.1- ☑
      with restricted hearing on the contralateral side H90.A- ☑
  congenital H90.5
    with blue sclera and fragility of bone Q78.0
  due to toxic agents — see Deafness, ototoxic
  emotional (hysterical) F44.6
  functional (hysterical) F44.6
  high frequency H91.9- ☑
  hysterical F44.6
  low frequency H91.9- ☑
  mental R48.8
  mixed conductive and sensorineural H90.8
    bilateral H90.6
    unilateral H90.7- ☑
  nerve — see Deafness, sensorineural
  neural — see Deafness, sensorineural
  noise-induced — see also subcategory H83.3 ☑
    nerve injury — see Injury, nerve, acoustic, specified type NEC
  nonspeaking H91.3
  ototoxic H91.0 ☑
  perceptive — see Deafness, sensorineural
  psychogenic (hysterical) F44.6
  sensorineural H90.5
    and conductive
      bilateral H90.6
      mixed H90.8
        bilateral H90.6
    bilateral H90.3
    unilateral H90.4- ☑
      with restricted hearing on the contralateral side H90.A- ☑
  sensory — see Deafness, sensorineural
  specified type NEC H91.8 ☑
  sudden (idiopathic) H91.2- ☑
  syphilitic A52.15
  transient ischemic H93.01- ☑
  traumatic — see Injury, nerve, acoustic, specified type NEC
  word (developmental) H93.25
Death (cause unknown) (of) (unexplained) (unspecified cause) R99
  brain G93.82
  cardiac (sudden) (with successful resuscitation) — code to underlying disease
    family history of Z82.41

Death — continued
  cardiac — code to underlying disease — continued
    personal history of Z86.74
    family member (assumed) Z63.4
Debility (chronic) (general) (nervous) R53.81
  congenital or neonatal NOS P96.9
  nervous R53.81
  old age R54
  senile R54
Débove's disease (splenomegaly) R16.1
Decalcification
  bone — see Osteoporosis
  teeth K03.89
Decapsulation, kidney N28.89
Decay
  dental — see Caries, dental
  senile R54
  tooth, teeth — see Caries, dental
Deciduitis (acute)
  following ectopic or molar pregnancy O08.0
Decline (general) — see Debility
  cognitive, age-associated R41.81
Decompensation
  cardiac (acute) (chronic) — see Disease, heart
  cardiovascular — see Disease, cardiovascular
  heart — see Disease, heart
  hepatic — see Failure, hepatic
  myocardial (acute) (chronic) — see Disease, heart
  respiratory J98.8
Decompression sickness T70.3 ☑
Decrease (d)
  absolute neutrophil count — see Neutropenia
  blood
    platelets — see Thrombocytopenia
    pressure R03.1
      due to shock following
        injury T79.4 ☑
        operation T81.19 ☑
  estrogen E28.39
    postablative E89.40
      asymptomatic E89.40
      symptomatic E89.41
  fragility of erythrocytes D58.8
  function
    lipase (pancreatic) K90.3
    ovary in hypopituitarism E23.0
    parenchyma of pancreas K86.89
    pituitary (gland) (anterior) (lobe) E23.0
    posterior (lobe) E23.0
  functional activity R68.89
  glucose R73.09
  hematocrit R71.0
  hemoglobin R71.0
  leukocytes D72.819
    specified NEC D72.818
  libido R68.82
  lymphocytes D72.810
  platelets D69.6
  respiration, due to shock following injury T79.4 ☑
  sexual desire R68.82
  tear secretion NEC — see Syndrome, dry eye
  tolerance
    fat K90.49
    glucose R73.09
    pancreatic K90.3
    salt and water E87.8
  vision NEC H54.7
  white blood cell count D72.819
    specified NEC D72.818
Decubitus (ulcer) — see Ulcer, pressure, by site
  cervix N86
Deepening acetabulum — see Derangement, joint, specified type NEC, hip
Defect, defective Q89.9
  3-beta-hydroxysteroid dehydrogenase E25.0
  11-hydroxylase E25.0
  21-hydroxylase E25.0
  abdominal wall, congenital Q79.59
  antibody immunodeficiency D80.9
  aorticopulmonary septum Q21.4
  atrial septal (ostium secundum type) Q21.1
    following acute myocardial infarction (current complication) I23.1
    ostium primum type Q21.2
  atrioventricular
    canal Q21.2
    septum Q21.2
  auricular septal Q21.1

☑ Additional Character Required — Refer to the Tabular List for Character Selection   Subterms under main terms may continue to next column or page

Defect, defective — *continued*
  bilirubin excretion NEC E80.6
  biosynthesis, androgen (testicular) E29.1
  bulbar septum Q21.0
  catalase E80.3
  cell membrane receptor complex (CR3) D71
  circulation I99.9
    congenital Q28.9
    newborn Q28.9
  coagulation (factor) — *see also* Deficiency, factor D68.9
    with
      ectopic pregnancy O08.1
      molar pregnancy O08.1
    acquired D68.4
    antepartum with hemorrhage — *see* Hemorrhage, antepartum, with coagulation defect
    due to
      liver disease D68.4
      vitamin K deficiency D68.4
    hereditary NEC D68.2
    intrapartum O67.0
    newborn, transient P61.6
    postpartum O99.13
      with hemorrhage O72.3
    specified type NEC D68.8
  complement system D84.1
  conduction (heart) I45.9
    bone — *see* Deafness, conductive
  congenital, organ or site not listed — *see* Anomaly, by site
  coronary sinus Q21.1
  cushion, endocardial Q21.2
  degradation, glycoprotein E77.1
  dental bridge, crown, fillings — *see* Defect, dental restoration
  dental restoration K08.50
    specified NEC K08.59
  dentin (hereditary) K00.5
  Descemet's membrane, congenital Q13.89
  developmental — *see also* Anomaly
    cauda equina Q06.3
  diaphragm
    with elevation, eventration or hernia — *see* Hernia, diaphragm
    congenital Q79.1
      with hernia Q79.0
      gross (with hernia) Q79.0
  ectodermal, congenital Q82.9
  Eisenmenger's Q21.8
  enzyme
    catalase E80.3
    peroxidase E80.3
  esophagus, congenital Q39.9
  extensor retinaculum M62.89
  fibrin polymerization D68.2
  filling
    bladder R93.41
    kidney R93.42- ☑
    renal pelvis R93.41
    stomach R93.3
    ureter R93.41
    urinary organs, specified NEC R93.49
  GABA (gamma aminobutyric acid) metabolic E72.81
  Gerbode Q21.0
  glucose transport, blood-brain barrier E74.810
  glycoprotein degradation E77.1
  Hageman (factor) D68.2
  hearing — *see* Deafness
  high grade F70
  interatrial septal Q21.1
  interauricular septal Q21.1
  interventricular septal Q21.0
    with dextroposition of aorta, pulmonary stenosis and hypertrophy of right ventricle Q21.3
    in tetralogy of Fallot Q21.3
  learning (specific) — *see* Disorder, learning
  lymphocyte function antigen-1 (LFA-1) D84.0
  lysosomal enzyme, post-translational modification E77.0
  major osseous M89.70
    ankle M89.77- ☑
    carpus M89.74- ☑
    clavicle M89.71- ☑
    femur M89.75- ☑
    fibula M89.76- ☑
    fingers M89.74- ☑
    foot M89.77- ☑
    forearm M89.73- ☑

Defect, defective — *continued*
  major osseous — *continued*
    hand M89.74- ☑
    humerus M89.72- ☑
    lower leg M89.76- ☑
    metacarpus M89.74- ☑
    metatarsus M89.77- ☑
    multiple sites M89.79
    pelvic region M89.75- ☑
    pelvis M89.75- ☑
    radius M89.73- ☑
    scapula M89.71- ☑
    shoulder region M89.71- ☑
    specified NEC M89.78
    tarsus M89.77- ☑
    thigh M89.75- ☑
    tibia M89.76- ☑
    toes M89.77- ☑
    ulna M89.73- ☑
  mental — *see* Disability, intellectual
  modification, lysosomal enzymes, post-translational E77.0
  obstructive, congenital
    renal pelvis Q62.39
    ureter Q62.39
      atresia — *see* Atresia, ureter
      cecoureterocele Q62.32
      megaureter Q62.2
      orthotopic ureterocele Q62.31
  osseous, major M89.70
    ankle M89.77- ☑
    carpus M89.74- ☑
    clavicle M89.71- ☑
    femur M89.75- ☑
    fibula M89.76- ☑
    fingers M89.74- ☑
    foot M89.77- ☑
    forearm M89.73- ☑
    hand M89.74- ☑
    humerus M89.72- ☑
    lower leg M89.76- ☑
    metacarpus M89.74- ☑
    metatarsus M89.77- ☑
    multiple sites M89.9
    pelvic region M89.75- ☑
    pelvis M89.75- ☑
    radius M89.73- ☑
    scapula M89.71- ☑
    shoulder region M89.71- ☑
    specified NEC M89.78
    tarsus M89.77- ☑
    thigh M89.75- ☑
    tibia M89.76- ☑
    toes M89.77- ☑
    ulna M89.73- ☑
  osteochondral NEC — *see also* Deformity M95.8
  ostium
    primum Q21.2
    secundum Q21.1
  peroxidase E80.3
  placental blood supply — *see* Insufficiency, placental
  platelets, qualitative D69.1
    constitutional D68.0
  postural NEC, spine — *see* Dorsopathy, deforming
  reduction
    limb Q73.8
      lower Q72.9- ☑
        absence — *see* Agenesis, leg
          foot — *see* Agenesis, foot
        longitudinal
          femur Q72.4- ☑
          fibula Q72.6- ☑
          tibia Q72.5- ☑
        specified type NEC Q72.89- ☑
        split foot Q72.7- ☑
      specified type NEC Q73.8
      upper Q71.9- ☑
        absence — *see* Agenesis, arm
          forearm — *see* Agenesis, forearm
          hand — *see* Agenesis, hand
        lobster-claw hand Q71.6- ☑
        longitudinal
          radius Q71.4- ☑
          ulna Q71.5- ☑
        specified type NEC Q71.89- ☑
  renal pelvis Q63.8

Defect, defective — *continued*
  renal pelvis — *continued*
    obstructive Q62.39
  respiratory system, congenital Q34.9
  restoration, dental K08.50
    specified NEC K08.59
  retinal nerve bundle fibers H35.89
  septal (heart) NOS Q21.9
    acquired (atrial) (auricular) (ventricular) (old) I51.0
    atrial Q21.1
      concurrent with acute myocardial infarction — *see* Infarct, myocardium
      following acute myocardial infarction (current complication) I23.1
    ventricular — *see also* Defect, ventricular septal Q21.0
  sinus venosus Q21.1
  speech — *see* Disorder, speech
    developmental F80.9
    specified NEC R47.89
  Taussig-Bing (aortic transposition and overriding pulmonary artery) Q20.1
  teeth, wedge K03.1
  vascular (local) I99.9
    congenital Q27.9
  ventricular septal Q21.0
    concurrent with acute myocardial infarction — *see* Infarct, myocardium
    following acute myocardial infarction (current complication) I23.2
    in tetralogy of Fallot Q21.3
  vision NEC H54.7
  visual field H53.40
    bilateral
      heteronymous H53.47
      homonymous H53.46- ☑
    generalized contraction H53.48- ☑
    localized
      arcuate H53.43- ☑
      scotoma (central area) H53.41- ☑
        blind spot area H53.42- ☑
      sector H53.43- ☑
      specified type NEC H53.45- ☑
  voice R49.9
    specified NEC R49.8
  wedge, tooth, teeth (abrasion) K03.1
Deferentitis N49.1
  gonorrheal (acute) (chronic) A54.23
Defibrination (syndrome) D65
  antepartum — *see* Hemorrhage, antepartum, with coagulation defect, disseminated intravascular coagulation
  following ectopic or molar pregnancy O08.1
  intrapartum O67.0
  newborn P60
  postpartum O72.3
Deficiency, deficient
  3-beta hydroxysteroid dehydrogenase E25.0
  5-alpha reductase (with male pseudohermaphroditism) E29.1
  11-hydroxylase E25.0
  21-hydroxylase E25.0
  AADC (aromatic L-amino acid decarboxylase) E70.81
  abdominal muscle syndrome Q79.4
  AC globulin (congenital) (hereditary) D68.2
    acquired D68.4
  accelerator globulin (Ac G) (blood) D68.2
  acid phosphatase E83.39
  acid sphingomyelinase (ASMD) E75.249
    type
      A E75.240
      A/B E75.244
      B E75.241
  activating factor (blood) D68.2
  ADA2 (adenosine deaminase 2) D81.32
  adenosine deaminase (ADA) D81.30
    with severe combined immunodeficiency (SCID) D81.31
    partial (type 1) D81.39
    specified NEC D81.39
    type 1 (without SCID) (without severe combined immunodeficiency) D81.39
    type 2 D81.32
  aldolase (hereditary) E74.19
  alpha-1-antitrypsin E88.01
  amino-acids E72.9
  anemia — *see* Anemia
  aneurin E51.9

Deficiency, deficient — *continued*
- antibody with
  - hyperimmunoglobulinemia D80.6
  - near-normal immunoglobins D80.6
- antidiuretic hormone E23.2
- anti-hemophilic
  - factor (A) D66
    - B D67
    - C D68.1
  - globulin (AHG) NEC D66
- antithrombin (antithrombin III) D68.59
- aromatic L-amino acid decarboxylase (AADC) E70.81
- ascorbic acid E54
- attention (disorder) (syndrome) F98.8
  - with hyperactivity — *see* Disorder, attention-deficit hyperactivity
- autoprothrombin
  - I D68.2
  - II D67
  - C D68.2
- beta-glucuronidase E76.29
- biotin E53.8
- biotin-dependent carboxylase D81.819
- biotinidase D81.810
- brancher enzyme (amylopectinosis) E74.03
- C1 esterase inhibitor (C1-INH) D84.1
- calciferol E55.9
  - with
    - adult osteomalacia M83.8
    - rickets — *see* Rickets
- calcium (dietary) E58
- calorie, severe E43
  - with marasmus E41
    - and kwashiorkor E42
- cardiac — *see* Insufficiency, myocardial
- carnitine E71.40
  - due to
    - hemodialysis E71.43
    - inborn errors of metabolism E71.42
    - Valproic acid therapy E71.43
  - iatrogenic E71.43
  - muscle palmityltransferase E71.314
  - primary E71.41
  - secondary E71.448
- carotene E50.9
- central nervous system G96.89
- ceruloplasmin (Wilson) E83.01
- choline E53.8
- Christmas factor D67
- chromium E61.4
- chronic neurovisceral acid sphingomyelinase E75.244
- chronic visceral acid sphingomyelinase E75.241
- clotting (blood) — *see also* Deficiency, coagulation factor D68.9
- clotting factor NEC (hereditary) — *see also* Deficiency, factor D68.2
- coagulation NOS D68.9
  - with
    - ectopic pregnancy O08.1
    - molar pregnancy O08.1
  - acquired (any) D68.4
  - antepartum hemorrhage — *see* Hemorrhage, antepartum, with coagulation defect
  - clotting factor NEC — *see also* Deficiency, factor D68.2
  - due to
    - hyperprothrombinemia D68.4
    - liver disease D68.4
    - vitamin K deficiency D68.4
  - newborn, transient P61.6
  - postpartum O72.3
  - specified NEC D68.8
- cognitive F09
- color vision H53.50
  - achromatopsia H53.51
  - acquired H53.52
  - deuteranomaly H53.53
  - protanomaly H53.54
  - specified type NEC H53.59
  - tritanomaly H53.55
- combined glucocorticoid and mineralocorticoid E27.49
- contact factor D68.2
- copper (nutritional) E61.0
- corticoadrenal E27.40
  - primary E27.1
- craniofacial axis Q75.0
- cyanocobalamin E53.8
- debrancher enzyme (limit dextrinosis) E74.03

Deficiency, deficient — *continued*
- dehydrogenase
  - long chain/very long chain acyl CoA E71.310
  - medium chain acyl CoA E71.311
  - short chain acyl CoA E71.312
- diet E63.9
- dihydropyrimidine dehydrogenase (DPD) E88.89
- disaccharidase E73.9
- edema — *see* Malnutrition, severe
- endocrine E34.9
- energy-supply — *see* Malnutrition
- enzymes, circulating NEC E88.09
- ergosterol E55.9
  - with
    - adult osteomalacia M83.8
    - rickets — *see* Rickets
- essential fatty acid (EFA) E63.0
- eye movements
  - saccadic H55.81
  - smooth pursuit H55.82
- factor — *see also* Deficiency, coagulation
  - Hageman D68.2
  - I (congenital) (hereditary) D68.2
  - II (congenital) (hereditary) D68.2
  - IX (congenital) (functional) (hereditary) (with functional defect) D67
  - multiple (congenital) D68.8
    - acquired D68.4
  - V (congenital) (hereditary) D68.2
  - VII (congenital) (hereditary) D68.2
  - VIII (congenital) (functional) (hereditary) (with functional defect) D66
    - with vascular defect D68.0
  - X (congenital) (hereditary) D68.2
  - XI (congenital) (hereditary) D68.1
  - XII (congenital) (hereditary) D68.2
  - XIII (congenital) (hereditary) D68.2
- femoral, proximal focal (congenital) — *see* Defect, reduction, lower limb, longitudinal, femur
- fibrinase D68.2
- fibrinogen (congenital) (hereditary) D68.2
  - acquired D65
- fibrin-stabilizing factor (congenital) (hereditary) D68.2
  - acquired D68.4
- folate E53.8
- folic acid E53.8
- foreskin N47.3
- fructokinase E74.11
- fructose 1,6-diphosphatase E74.19
- fructose-1-phosphate aldolase E74.19
- GABA (gamma aminobutyric acid) transaminase E72.81
- GABA-T (gamma aminobutyric acid transaminase) E72.81
- galactokinase E74.29
- galactose-1-phosphate uridyl transferase E74.29
- gammaglobulin in blood D80.1
  - hereditary D80.0
- glass factor D68.2
- glucocorticoid E27.49
  - mineralocorticoid E27.49
- glucose transporter protein type 1 E74.810
- glucose-6-phosphatase E74.01
- glucose-6-phosphate dehydrogenase
  - anemia D55.0
  - without anemia D75.A
- glucuronyl transferase E80.5
- Glut1 E74.810
- glycogen synthetase E74.09
- gonadotropin (isolated) E23.0
- growth hormone (idiopathic) (isolated) E23.0
- Hageman factor D68.2
- hemoglobin D64.9
- hepatophosphorylase E74.09
- homogentisate 1,2-dioxygenase E70.29
- hormone
  - anterior pituitary (partial) NEC E23.0
    - growth E23.0
  - growth (isolated) E23.0
  - pituitary E23.0
  - testicular E29.1
- hypoxanthine- (guanine)-phosphoribosyltransferase (HG- PRT) (total H-PRT) E79.1
- immunity D84.9
  - cell-mediated D84.89
    - with thrombocytopenia and eczema D82.0
  - combined D81.9
  - humoral D80.9
  - IgA (secretory) D80.2
  - IgG D80.3

Deficiency, deficient — *continued*
- immunity — *continued*
  - IgM D80.4
- immuno — *see* Immunodeficiency
- immunoglobulin, selective
  - A (IgA) D80.2
  - G (IgG) (subclasses) D80.3
  - M (IgM) D80.4
- infantile neurovisceral acid sphingomyelinase E75.240
- inositol (B complex) E53.8
- intrinsic
  - factor (congenital) D51.0
  - sphincter N36.42
    - with urethral hypermobility N36.43
- iodine E61.8
  - congenital syndrome — *see* Syndrome, iodine-deficiency, congenital
- iron E61.1
  - anemia D50.9
- kalium E87.6
- kappa-light chain D80.8
- labile factor (congenital) (hereditary) D68.2
  - acquired D68.4
- lacrimal fluid (acquired) — *see also* Syndrome, dry eye
  - congenital Q10.6
- lactase
  - congenital E73.0
  - secondary E73.1
- Laki-Lorand factor D68.2
- lecithin cholesterol acyltransferase E78.6
- lipocaic K86.89
- lipoprotein (familial) (high density) E78.6
- liver phosphorylase E74.09
- lysosomal alpha-1, 4 glucosidase E74.02
- magnesium E61.2
- major histocompatibility complex
  - class I D81.6
  - class II D81.7
- manganese E61.3
- menadione (vitamin K) E56.1
  - newborn P53
- mental (familial) (hereditary) — *see* Disability, intellectual
- methylenetetrahydrofolate reductase (MTHFR) E72.12
- mevalonate kinase M04.1
- mineralocorticoid E27.49
  - with glucocorticoid E27.49
- mineral NEC E61.8
- molybdenum (nutritional) E61.5
- moral F60.2
- multiple nutrient elements E61.7
- multiple sulfatase (MSD) E75.26
- muscle
  - carnitine (palmityltransferase) E71.314
  - phosphofructokinase E74.09
- myoadenylate deaminase E79.2
- myocardial — *see* Insufficiency, myocardial
- myophosphorylase E74.04
- NADH diaphorase or reductase (congenital) D74.0
- NADH-methemoglobin reductase (congenital) D74.0
- natrium E87.1
- niacin (amide) (-tryptophan) E52
- nicotinamide E52
- nicotinic acid E52
- number of teeth — *see* Anodontia
- nutrient element E61.9
  - multiple E61.7
  - specified NEC E61.8
- nutrition, nutritional E63.9
  - sequelae — *see* Sequelae, nutritional deficiency
  - specified NEC E63.8
- of interleukin 1 receptor antagonist [DIRA] M04.8
- ornithine transcarbamylase E72.4
- ovarian E28.39
- oxygen — *see* Anoxia
- pantothenic acid E53.8
- parathyroid (gland) E20.9
- perineum (female) N81.89
- phenylalanine hydroxylase E70.1
- phosphoenolpyruvate carboxykinase E74.4
- phosphofructokinase E74.19
- phosphomannomutuse E74.818
- phosphomannose isomerase E74.818
- phosphomannosyl mutase E74.818
- phosphorylase kinase, liver E74.09
- pituitary hormone (isolated) E23.0
- plasma thromboplastin
  - antecedent (PTA) D68.1

Deficiency, deficient — *continued*
  plasma thromboplastin — *continued*
    component (PTC) D67
  plasminogen (type 1) (type 2) E88.02
  platelet NEC D69.1
    constitutional D68.0
  polyglandular E31.8
    autoimmune E31.0
  potassium (K) E87.6
  prepuce N47.3
  proaccelerin (congenital) (hereditary) D68.2
    acquired D68.4
  proconvertin factor (congenital) (hereditary) D68.2
    acquired D68.4
  protein — *see also* Malnutrition E46
    anemia D53.0
    C D68.59
    S D68.59
  prothrombin (congenital) (hereditary) D68.2
    acquired D68.4
  Prower factor D68.2
  pseudocholinesterase E88.09
  PTA (plasma thromboplastin antecedent) D68.1
  PTC (plasma thromboplastin component) D67
  purine nucleoside phosphorylase (PNP) D81.5
  pyracin (alpha) (beta) E53.1
  pyridoxal E53.1
  pyridoxamine E53.1
  pyridoxine (derivatives) E53.1
  pyruvate
    carboxylase E74.4
    dehydrogenase E74.4
  riboflavin (vitamin B2) E53.0
  salt E87.1
  secretion
    ovary E28.39
    salivary gland (any) K11.7
    urine R34
  selenium (dietary) E59
  serum antitrypsin, familial E88.01
  short stature homeobox gene (SHOX)
    with
      dyschondrosteosis Q78.8
      short stature (idiopathic) E34.3
      Turner's syndrome Q96.9
  sodium (Na) E87.1
  SPCA (factor VII) D68.2
  sphincter, intrinsic N36.42
    with urethral hypermobility N36.43
  stable factor (congenital) (hereditary) D68.2
    acquired D68.4
  Stuart-Prower (factor X) D68.2
  succinic semialdehyde dehydrogenase E72.81
  sucrase E74.39
  sulfatase E75.26
  sulfite oxidase E72.19
  thiamin, thiaminic (chloride) E51.9
    beriberi (dry) E51.11
      wet E51.12
  thrombokinase D68.2
    newborn P53
  thyroid (gland) — *see* Hypothyroidism
  tocopherol E56.0
  tooth bud K00.0
  transcobalamine II (anemia) D51.2
  vanadium E61.6
  vascular I99.9
  vasopressin E23.2
  vertical ridge K06.8
  viosterol — *see* Deficiency, calciferol
  vitamin (multiple) NOS E56.9
    A E50.9
      with
        Bitot's spot (corneal) E50.1
        follicular keratosis E50.8
        keratomalacia E50.4
        manifestations NEC E50.8
        night blindness E50.5
        scar of cornea, xerophthalmic E50.6
        xeroderma E50.8
        xerophthalmia E50.7
        xerosis
          conjunctival E50.0
            and Bitot's spot E50.1
          cornea E50.2
            and ulceration E50.3
      sequelae E64.1
    B (complex) NOS E53.9

Deficiency, deficient — *continued*
  vitamin — *continued*
    B — *continued*
      with
        beriberi (dry) E51.11
          wet E51.12
        pellagra E52
      B1 NOS E51.9
        beriberi (dry) E51.11
          with circulatory system manifestations E51.11
          wet E51.12
      B12 E53.8
      B2 (riboflavin) E53.0
      B6 E53.1
      C E54
        sequelae E64.2
      D E55.9
        with
          adult osteomalacia M83.8
          rickets — *see* Rickets
        25-hydroxylase E83.32
      E E56.0
      folic acid E53.8
      G E53.0
      group B E53.9
        specified NEC E53.8
      H (biotin) E53.8
      K E56.1
        of newborn P53
      nicotinic E52
      P E56.8
      PP (pellagra-preventing) E52
      specified NEC E56.8
      thiamin E51.9
        beriberi — *see* Beriberi
  zinc, dietary E60
Deficit — *see also* Deficiency
  attention and concentration R41.840
    disorder — *see* Attention, deficit
    following
      cerebral infarction I69.310
      cerebrovascular disease I69.910
        specified disease NEC I69.810
      nontraumatic
        intracerebral hemorrhage I69.110
        specified intracranial hemorrhage NEC I69.210
        subarachnoid hemorrhage I69.010
  cognitive
    communication R41.841
    emotional
      following
        cerebral infarction I69.315
        cerebrovascular disease I69.915
          specified disease NEC I69.815
        nontraumatic
          intracerebral hemorrhage I69.115
          specified intracranial hemorrhage NEC I69.215
          subarachnoid hemorrhage I69.015
    following
      cerebral infarction I69.319
      cerebrovascular disease I69.919
        specified disease NEC I69.819
      nontraumatic
        intracerebral hemorrhage I69.119
        specified intracranial hemorrhage NEC I69.219
        subarachnoid hemorrhage I69.019
    social
      following
        cerebral infarction I69.315
        cerebrovascular disease I69.915
          specified disease NEC I69.815
        nontraumatic
          intracerebral hemorrhage I69.115
          specified intracranial hemorrhage NEC I69.215
          subarachnoid hemorrhage I69.015
  cognitive NEC R41.89
    following
      cerebral infarction I69.318
      cerebrovascular disease I69.918
        specified disease NEC I69.818
      nontraumatic
        intracerebral hemorrhage I69.118
        specified intracranial hemorrhage NEC I69.218
        subarachnoid hemorrhage I69.018
  concentration R41.840
  executive function R41.844

Deficit — *continued*
  executive function — *continued*
    following
      cerebral infarction I69.314
      cerebrovascular disease I69.914
        specified disease NEC I69.814
      nontraumatic
        intracerebral hemorrhage I69.114
        specified intracranial hemorrhage NEC I69.214
        subarachnoid hemorrhage I69.014
  frontal lobe R41.844
    following
      cerebral infarction I69.314
      cerebrovascular disease I69.914
        specified disease NEC I69.814
      nontraumatic
        intracerebral hemorrhage I69.114
        specified intracranial hemorrhage NEC I69.214
        subarachnoid hemorrhage I69.014
  memory
    following
      cerebral infarction I69.311
      cerebrovascular disease I69.911
        specified disease NEC I69.811
      nontraumatic
        intracerebral hemorrhage I69.111
        specified intracranial hemorrhage NEC I69.211
        subarachnoid hemorrhage I69.011
  neurologic NEC R29.818
    ischemic
      reversible (RIND) I63.9
        prolonged (PRIND) I63.9
  oxygen R09.02
  prolonged reversible ischemic neurologic (PRIND) I63.9
  psychomotor R41.843
    following
      cerebral infarction I69.313
      cerebrovascular disease I69.913
        specified disease NEC I69.813
      nontraumatic
        intracerebral hemorrhage I69.113
        specified intracranial hemorrhage NEC I69.213
        subarachnoid hemorrhage I69.013
  visuospatial R41.842
    following
      cerebral infarction I69.312
      cerebrovascular disease I69.912
        specified disease NEC I69.812
      nontraumatic
        intracerebral hemorrhage I69.112
        specified intracranial hemorrhage NEC I69.212
        subarachnoid hemorrhage I69.012
Deflection
  radius — *see* Deformity, limb, specified type NEC, forearm
  septum (acquired) (nasal) (nose) J34.2
  spine — *see* Curvature, spine
  turbinate (nose) J34.2
Defluvium
  capillorum — *see* Alopecia
  ciliorum — *see* Madarosis
  unguium L60.8
Deformity Q89.9
  abdomen, congenital Q89.9
  abdominal wall
    acquired M95.8
    congenital Q79.59
  acquired (unspecified site) M95.9
  adrenal gland Q89.1
  alimentary tract, congenital Q45.9
    upper Q40.9
  ankle (joint) (acquired) — *see also* Deformity, limb, lower leg
    abduction — *see* Contraction, joint, ankle
    congenital Q68.8
    contraction — *see* Contraction, joint, ankle
    specified type NEC — *see* Deformity, limb, foot, specified NEC
  anus (acquired) K62.89
    congenital Q43.9
  aorta (arch) (congenital) Q25.40
    acquired I77.89
  aortic
    arch, acquired I77.89
    cusp or valve (congenital) Q23.8
      acquired — *see also* Endocarditis, aortic I35.8
  arm (acquired) (upper) — *see also* Deformity, limb, upper arm

Deformity — *continued*
  arm — *see also* Deformity, limb, upper arm — *continued*
    congenital Q68.8
    forearm — *see* Deformity, limb, forearm
  artery (congenital) (peripheral) NOS Q27.9
    acquired I77.89
    coronary (acquired) I25.9
      congenital Q24.5
    umbilical Q27.0
  atrial septal Q21.1
  auditory canal (external) (congenital) — *see also* Malformation, ear, external
    acquired — *see* Disorder, ear, external, specified type NEC
  auricle
    ear (congenital) — *see also* Malformation, ear, external
      acquired — *see* Disorder, pinna, deformity
  back — *see* Dorsopathy, deforming
  bile duct (common) (congenital) (hepatic) Q44.5
    acquired K83.8
  biliary duct or passage (congenital) Q44.5
    acquired K83.8
  bladder (neck) (trigone) (sphincter) (acquired) N32.89
    congenital Q64.79
  bone (acquired) NOS M95.9
    congenital Q79.9
    turbinate M95.0
  brain (congenital) Q04.9
    acquired G93.89
    reduction Q04.3
  breast (acquired) N64.89
    congenital Q83.9
    reconstructed N65.0
  bronchus (congenital) Q32.4
    acquired NEC J98.09
  bursa, congenital Q79.9
  canaliculi (lacrimalis) (acquired) — *see also* Disorder, lacrimal system, changes
    congenital Q10.6
  canthus, acquired — *see* Disorder, eyelid, specified type NEC
  capillary (acquired) I78.8
  cardiovascular system, congenital Q28.9
  caruncle, lacrimal (acquired) — *see also* Disorder, lacrimal system, changes
    congenital Q10.6
  cascade, stomach K31.2
  cecum (congenital) Q43.9
    acquired K63.89
  cerebral, acquired G93.89
    congenital Q04.9
  cervix (uterus) (acquired) NEC N88.8
    congenital Q51.9
  cheek (acquired) M95.2
    congenital Q18.9
  chest (acquired) (wall) M95.4
    congenital Q67.8
    sequelae (late effect) of rickets E64.3
  chin (acquired) M95.2
    congenital Q18.9
  choroid (congenital) Q14.3
    acquired H31.8
    plexus Q07.8
      acquired G96.198
  cicatricial — *see* Cicatrix
  cilia, acquired — *see* Disorder, eyelid, specified type NEC
  clavicle (acquired) M95.8
    congenital Q68.8
  clitoris (congenital) Q52.6
    acquired N90.89
  clubfoot — *see* Clubfoot
  coccyx (acquired) — *see* subcategory M43.8 ☑
  colon (congenital) Q43.9
    acquired K63.89
  concha (ear), congenital — *see also* Malformation, ear, external
    acquired — *see* Disorder, pinna, deformity
  cornea (acquired) H18.70
    congenital Q13.4
    descemetocele — *see* Descemetocele
    ectasia — *see* Ectasia, cornea
    specified NEC H18.79- ☑
    staphyloma — *see* Staphyloma, cornea
  coronary artery (acquired) I25.9
    congenital Q24.5

Deformity — *continued*
  cranium (acquired) — *see* Deformity, skull
  cricoid cartilage (congenital) Q31.8
    acquired J38.7
  cystic duct (congenital) Q44.5
    acquired K82.8
  Dandy-Walker Q03.1
    with spina bifida — *see* Spina bifida
  diaphragm (congenital) Q79.1
    acquired J98.6
  digestive organ NOS Q45.9
  ductus arteriosus Q25.0
  duodenal bulb K31.89
  duodenum (congenital) Q43.9
    acquired K31.89
  dura — *see* Deformity, meninges
  ear (acquired) — *see also* Disorder, pinna, deformity
    congenital (external) Q17.9
      internal Q16.5
      middle Q16.4
        ossicles Q16.3
      ossicles Q16.3
  ectodermal (congenital) NEC Q84.9
  ejaculatory duct (congenital) Q55.4
    acquired N50.89
  elbow (joint) (acquired) — *see also* Deformity, limb, upper arm
    congenital Q68.8
    contraction — *see* Contraction, joint, elbow
  endocrine gland NEC Q89.2
  epididymis (congenital) Q55.4
    acquired N50.89
  epiglottis (congenital) Q31.8
    acquired J38.7
  esophagus (congenital) Q39.9
    acquired K22.89
  eustachian tube (congenital) NEC Q17.8
  eye, congenital Q15.9
  eyebrow (congenital) Q18.8
  eyelid (acquired) — *see also* Disorder, eyelid, specified type NEC
    congenital Q10.3
  face (acquired) M95.2
    congenital Q18.9
  fallopian tube, acquired N83.8
  femur (acquired) — *see* Deformity, limb, specified type NEC, thigh
  fetal
    with fetopelvic disproportion O33.7 ☑
    causing obstructed labor O66.3
  finger (acquired) M20.00- ☑
    boutonniere M20.02- ☑
    congenital Q68.1
    flexion contracture — *see* Contraction, joint, hand
    mallet finger M20.01- ☑
    specified NEC M20.09- ☑
    swan-neck M20.03- ☑
  flexion (joint) (acquired) — *see also* Deformity, limb, flexion M21.20
    congenital NOS Q74.9
      hip Q65.89
  foot (acquired) — *see also* Deformity, limb, lower leg
    cavovarus (congenital) Q66.1- ☑
    congenital NOS Q66.9- ☑
      specified type NEC Q66.89
    specified type NEC — *see* Deformity, limb, foot, specified NEC
    valgus (congenital) Q66.6
      acquired — *see* Deformity, valgus, ankle
    varus (congenital) NEC Q66.3- ☑
      acquired — *see* Deformity, varus, ankle
  forearm (acquired) — *see also* Deformity, limb, forearm
    congenital Q68.8
  forehead (acquired) M95.2
    congenital Q75.8
  frontal bone (acquired) M95.2
    congenital Q75.8
  gallbladder (congenital) Q44.1
    acquired K82.8
  gastrointestinal tract (congenital) NOS Q45.9
    acquired K63.89
  genitalia, genital organ(s) or system NEC
    female (congenital) Q52.9
      acquired N94.89
      external Q52.70
    male (congenital) Q55.9
      acquired N50.89
  globe (eye) (congenital) Q15.8

Deformity — *continued*
  globe — *continued*
    acquired H44.89
  gum, acquired NEC K06.8
  hand (acquired) — *see* Deformity, limb, hand
    congenital Q68.1
  head (acquired) M95.2
    congenital Q75.8
  heart (congenital) Q24.9
    septum Q21.9
      auricular Q21.1
      ventricular Q21.0
    valve (congenital) NEC Q24.8
      acquired — *see* Endocarditis
  heel (acquired) — *see* Deformity, foot
  hepatic duct (congenital) Q44.5
    acquired K83.8
  hip (joint) (acquired) (*see also* Deformity, limb, thigh)
    congenital Q65.9
    due to (previous) juvenile osteochondrosis — *see* Coxa, plana
    flexion — *see* Contraction, joint, hip
  hourglass — *see* Contraction, hourglass
  humerus (acquired) M21.82- ☑
    congenital Q74.0
  hypophyseal (congenital) Q89.2
  ileocecal (coil) (valve) (acquired) K63.89
    congenital Q43.9
  ileum (congenital) Q43.9
    acquired K63.89
  ilium (acquired) M95.5
    congenital Q74.2
  integument (congenital) Q84.9
  intervertebral cartilage or disc (acquired) — *see* Disorder, disc, specified NEC
  intestine (large) (small) (congenital) NOS Q43.9
    acquired K63.89
  intrinsic minus or plus (hand) — *see* Deformity, limb, specified type NEC, forearm
  iris (acquired) H21.89
    congenital Q13.2
  ischium (acquired) M95.5
    congenital Q74.2
  jaw (acquired) (congenital) M26.9
  joint (acquired) NEC M21.90
    congenital Q68.8
    elbow M21.92- ☑
    hand M21.94- ☑
    hip M21.95- ☑
    knee M21.96- ☑
    shoulder M21.92- ☑
    wrist M21.93- ☑
  kidney(s) (calyx) (pelvis) (congenital) Q63.9
    acquired N28.89
    artery (congenital) Q27.2
      acquired I77.89
  Klippel-Feil (brevicollis) Q76.1
  knee (acquired) NEC — *see also* Deformity, limb, lower leg
    congenital Q68.2
  labium (majus) (minus) (congenital) Q52.79
    acquired N90.89
  lacrimal passages or duct (congenital) NEC Q10.6
    acquired — *see* Disorder, lacrimal system, changes
  larynx (muscle) (congenital) Q31.8
    acquired J38.7
    web (glottic) Q31.0
  leg (upper) (acquired) NEC — *see also* Deformity, limb, thigh
    congenital Q68.8
    lower leg — *see* Deformity, limb, lower leg
  lens (acquired) H27.8
    congenital Q12.9
  lid (fold) (acquired) — *see also* Disorder, eyelid, specified type NEC
    congenital Q10.3
  ligament (acquired) — *see* Disorder, ligament
    congenital Q79.9
  limb (acquired) M21.90
    clawfoot M21.53- ☑
    clawhand M21.51- ☑
    clubfoot M21.54- ☑
    clubhand M21.52- ☑
    congenital, except reduction deformity Q74.9
    flat foot M21.4- ☑
    flexion M21.20
      ankle M21.27- ☑
      elbow M21.22- ☑

☑ **Additional Character Required** — Refer to the Tabular List for Character Selection   ▽ **Subterms under main terms may continue to next column or page**

Deformity — *continued*
limb — *continued*
  flexion — *continued*
    finger M21.24- ☑
    hip M21.25- ☑
    knee M21.26- ☑
    shoulder M21.21- ☑
    toe M21.27- ☑
    wrist M21.23- ☑
  foot
    claw — *see* Deformity, limb, clawfoot
    club — *see* Deformity, limb, clubfoot
    drop M21.37- ☑
    flat — *see* Deformity, limb, flat foot
    specified NEC M21.6X- ☑
  forearm M21.93- ☑
  hand M21.94- ☑
  lower leg M21.96- ☑
  specified type NEC M21.80
    forearm M21.83- ☑
    lower leg M21.86- ☑
    thigh M21.85- ☑
    upper arm M21.82- ☑
  thigh M21.95- ☑
  unequal length M21.70
    short site is
      femur M21.75- ☑
      fibula M21.76- ☑
      humerus M21.72- ☑
      radius M21.73- ☑
      tibia M21.76- ☑
      ulna M21.73- ☑
    upper arm M21.92- ☑
  valgus — *see* Deformity, valgus
  varus — *see* Deformity, varus
  wrist drop M21.33- ☑
lip (acquired) NEC K13.0
  congenital Q38.0
liver (congenital) Q44.7
  acquired K76.89
lumbosacral (congenital) (joint) (region) Q76.49
  acquired — *see* subcategory M43.8 ☑
  kyphosis — *see* Kyphosis, congenital
  lordosis — *see* Lordosis, congenital
lung (congenital) Q33.9
  acquired J98.4
lymphatic system, congenital Q89.9
Madelung's (radius) Q74.0
mandible (acquired) (congenital) M26.9
maxilla (acquired) (congenital) M26.9
meninges or membrane (congenital) Q07.9
  cerebral Q04.8
    acquired G96.198
  spinal cord (congenital) Q06.- ☑
    acquired G96.198
metacarpus (acquired) — *see* Deformity, limb, forearm
  congenital Q74.0
metatarsus (acquired) — *see* Deformity, foot
  congenital Q66.9- ☑
middle ear (congenital) Q16.4
  ossicles Q16.3
mitral (leaflets) (valve) I05.8
  parachute Q23.2
  stenosis, congenital Q23.2
mouth (acquired) K13.79
  congenital Q38.6
multiple, congenital NEC Q89.7
muscle (acquired) M62.89
  congenital Q79.9
    sternocleidomastoid Q68.0
musculoskeletal system (acquired) M95.9
  congenital Q79.9
  specified NEC M95.8
nail (acquired) L60.8
  congenital Q84.6
nasal — *see* Deformity, nose
neck (acquired) M95.3
  congenital Q18.9
    sternocleidomastoid Q68.0
nervous system (congenital) Q07.9
nipple (congenital) Q83.9
  acquired N64.89
nose (acquired) (cartilage) M95.0
  bone (turbinate) M95.0
  congenital Q30.9
    bent or squashed Q67.4
  saddle M95.0

Deformity — *continued*
nose — *continued*
  saddle — *continued*
    syphilitic A50.57
  septum (acquired) J34.2
    congenital Q30.8
  sinus (wall) (congenital) Q30.8
    acquired M95.0
  syphilitic (congenital) A50.57
    late A52.73
ocular muscle (congenital) Q10.3
  acquired — *see* Strabismus, mechanical
opticociliary vessels (congenital) Q13.2
orbit (eye) (acquired) H05.30
  atrophy — *see* Atrophy, orbit
  congenital Q10.7
  due to
    bone disease NEC H05.32- ☑
    trauma or surgery H05.33- ☑
  enlargement — *see* Enlargement, orbit
  exostosis — *see* Exostosis, orbit
organ of Corti (congenital) Q16.5
ovary (congenital) Q50.39
  acquired N83.8
oviduct, acquired N83.8
palate (congenital) Q38.5
  acquired M27.8
  cleft (congenital) — *see* Cleft, palate
pancreas (congenital) Q45.3
  acquired K86.89
parathyroid (gland) Q89.2
parotid (gland) (congenital) Q38.4
  acquired K11.8
patella (acquired) — *see* Disorder, patella, specified NEC
pelvis, pelvic (acquired) (bony) M95.5
  with disproportion (fetopelvic) O33.0
    causing obstructed labor O65.0
  congenital Q74.2
  rachitic sequelae (late effect) E64.3
penis (glans) (congenital) Q55.69
  acquired N48.89
pericardium (congenital) Q24.8
  acquired — *see* Pericarditis
pharynx (congenital) Q38.8
  acquired J39.2
pinna, acquired — *see also* Disorder, pinna, deformity
  congenital Q17.9
pituitary (congenital) Q89.2
posture — *see* Dorsopathy, deforming
prepuce (congenital) Q55.69
  acquired N47.8
prostate (congenital) Q55.4
  acquired N42.89
pupil (congenital) Q13.2
  acquired — *see* Abnormality, pupillary
pylorus (congenital) Q40.3
  acquired K31.89
rachitic (acquired), old or healed E64.3
radius (acquired) — *see also* Deformity, limb, forearm
  congenital Q68.8
rectum (congenital) Q43.9
  acquired K62.89
reduction (extremity) (limb), congenital — *see also* condition and site Q73.8
  brain Q04.3
  lower — *see* Defect, reduction, lower limb
  upper — *see* Defect, reduction, upper limb
renal — *see* Deformity, kidney
respiratory system (congenital) Q34.9
rib (acquired) M95.4
  congenital Q76.6
  cervical Q76.5
rotation (joint) (acquired) — *see* Deformity, limb, specified site NEC
  congenital Q74.9
  hip — *see* Deformity, limb, specified type NEC, thigh
    congenital Q65.89
sacroiliac joint (congenital) — *see* subcategory Q74.2
  acquired — *see* subcategory M43.8 ☑
sacrum (acquired) — *see* subcategory M43.8 ☑
saddle
  back — *see* Lordosis
  nose M95.0
    syphilitic A50.57
salivary gland or duct (congenital) Q38.4
  acquired K11.8
scapula (acquired) M95.8

Deformity — *continued*
scapula — *continued*
  congenital Q68.8
scrotum (congenital) — *see also* Malformation, testis and scrotum
  acquired N50.89
seminal vesicles (congenital) Q55.4
  acquired N50.89
septum, nasal (acquired) J34.2
shoulder (joint) (acquired) — *see* Deformity, limb, upper arm
  congenital Q74.0
  contraction — *see* Contraction, joint, shoulder
sigmoid (flexure) (congenital) Q43.9
  acquired K63.89
skin (congenital) Q82.9
skull (acquired) M95.2
  congenital Q75.8
    with
      anencephaly Q00.0
      encephalocele — *see* Encephalocele
      hydrocephalus Q03.9
        with spina bifida — *see* Spina bifida, by site, with hydrocephalus
      microcephaly Q02
soft parts, organs or tissues (of pelvis)
  in pregnancy or childbirth NEC O34.8- ☑
    causing obstructed labor O65.5
spermatic cord (congenital) Q55.4
  acquired N50.89
  torsion — *see* Torsion, spermatic cord
spinal — *see* Dorsopathy, deforming
  column (acquired) — *see* Dorsopathy, deforming
    congenital Q67.5
  cord (congenital) Q06.9
    acquired G95.89
  nerve root (congenital) Q07.9
spine (acquired) — *see also* Dorsopathy, deforming
  congenital Q67.5
  rachitic E64.3
  specified NEC — *see* Dorsopathy, deforming, specified NEC
spleen
  acquired D73.89
  congenital Q89.09
Sprengel's (congenital) Q74.0
sternocleidomastoid (muscle), congenital Q68.0
sternum (acquired) M95.4
  congenital NEC Q76.7
stomach (congenital) Q40.3
  acquired K31.89
submandibular gland (congenital) Q38.4
submaxillary gland (congenital) Q38.4
  acquired K11.8
talipes — *see* Talipes
testis (congenital) — *see also* Malformation, testis and scrotum
  acquired N44.8
  torsion — *see* Torsion, testis
thigh (acquired) — *see also* Deformity, limb, thigh
  congenital NEC Q68.8
thorax (acquired) (wall) M95.4
  congenital Q67.8
  sequelae of rickets E64.3
thumb (acquired) — *see also* Deformity, finger
  congenital NEC Q68.1
thymus (tissue) (congenital) Q89.2
thyroid (gland) (congenital) Q89.2
  cartilage Q31.8
    acquired J38.7
tibia (acquired) — *see also* Deformity, limb, specified type NEC, lower leg
  congenital NEC Q68.8
  saber (syphilitic) A50.56
toe (acquired) M20.6- ☑
  congenital Q66.9- ☑
  hallux rigidus M20.2- ☑
  hallux valgus M20.1- ☑
  hallux varus M20.3- ☑
  hammer toe M20.4- ☑
  specified NEC M20.5X- ☑
tongue (congenital) Q38.3
  acquired K14.8
tooth, teeth K00.2
trachea (rings) (congenital) Q32.1
  acquired J39.8
transverse aortic arch (congenital) Q25.49
tricuspid (leaflets) (valve) I07.8

Deformity — *continued*
  tricuspid — *continued*
    atresia or stenosis Q22.4
    Ebstein's Q22.5
  trunk (acquired) M95.8
    congenital Q89.9
  ulna (acquired) — *see also* Deformity, limb, forearm
    congenital NEC Q68.8
  urachus, congenital Q64.4
  ureter (opening) (congenital) Q62.8
    acquired N28.89
  urethra (congenital) Q64.79
    acquired N36.8
  urinary tract (congenital) Q64.9
    urachus Q64.4
  uterus (congenital) Q51.9
    acquired N85.8
  uvula (congenital) Q38.5
  vagina (acquired) N89.8
    congenital Q52.4
  valgus NEC M21.00
    ankle M21.07- ☑
    elbow M21.02- ☑
    hip M21.05- ☑
    knee M21.06- ☑
  valve, valvular (congenital) (heart) Q24.8
    acquired — *see* Endocarditis
  varus NEC M21.10
    ankle M21.17- ☑
    elbow M21.12- ☑
    hip M21.15 ☑
    knee M21.16- ☑
  tibia — *see* Osteochondrosis, juvenile, tibia
  vas deferens (congenital) Q55.4
    acquired N50.89
  vein (congenital) Q27.9
    great Q26.9
  vertebra — *see* Dorsopathy, deforming
  vertical talus (congenital) Q66.80
    left foot Q66.82
    right foot Q66.81
  vesicourethral orifice (acquired) N32.89
    congenital NEC Q64.79
  vessels of optic papilla (congenital) Q14.2
  visual field (contraction) — *see* Defect, visual field
  vitreous body, acquired H43.89
  vulva (congenital) Q52.79
    acquired N90.89
  wrist (joint) (acquired) — *see also* Deformity, limb, forearm
    congenital Q68.8
    contraction — *see* Contraction, joint, wrist

Degeneration, degenerative
  adrenal (capsule) (fatty) (gland) (hyaline) (infectional) E27.8
  amyloid — *see also* Amyloidosis E85.9
  anterior cornua, spinal cord G12.29
  anterior labral S43.49- ☑
  aorta, aortic I70.0
    fatty I77.89
  aortic valve (heart) — *see* Endocarditis, aortic
  arteriovascular — *see* Arteriosclerosis
  artery, arterial (atheromatous) (calcareous) — *see also* Arteriosclerosis
    cerebral, amyloid E85.4 [I68.0]
    medial — *see* Arteriosclerosis, extremities
  articular cartilage NEC — *see* Derangement, joint, articular cartilage, by site
  atheromatous — *see* Arteriosclerosis
  basal nuclei or ganglia G23.9
    specified NEC G23.8
  bone NEC — *see* Disorder, bone, specified type NEC
  brachial plexus G54.0
  brain (cortical) (progressive) G31.9
    alcoholic G31.2
    arteriosclerotic I67.2
    childhood G31.9
      specified NEC G31.89
    cystic G31.89
      congenital Q04.6
    in
      alcoholism G31.2
      beriberi E51.2
      cerebrovascular disease I67.9
      congenital hydrocephalus Q03.9
        with spina bifida — *see also* Spina bifida
      Fabry-Anderson disease E75.21
      Gaucher's disease E75.22

Degeneration, degenerative — *continued*
  brain — *continued*
    in — *continued*
      Hunter's syndrome E76.1
      lipidosis
        cerebral E75.4
        generalized E75.6
      mucopolysaccharidosis — *see* Mucopolysaccharidosis
      myxedema E03.9 [G32.89]
      neoplastic disease — *see also* Neoplasm D49.6 [G32.89]
      Niemann-Pick disease E75.249 [G32.89]
      sphingolipidosis E75.3 [G32.89]
      vitamin B12 deficiency E53.8 [G32.89]
    senile NEC G31.1
  breast N64.89
  Bruch's membrane — *see* Degeneration, choroid
  capillaries (fatty) I78.8
    amyloid E85.89 [I79.8]
  cardiac — *see also* Degeneration, myocardial
    valve, valvular — *see* Endocarditis
  cardiorenal — *see* Hypertension, cardiorenal
  cardiovascular — *see also* Disease, cardiovascular
    renal — *see* Hypertension, cardiorenal
  cerebellar NOS G31.9
    alcoholic G31.2
    primary (hereditary) (sporadic) G11.9
  cerebral — *see* Degeneration, brain
  cerebrovascular I67.9
    due to hypertension I67.4
  cervical plexus G54.2
  cervix N88.8
    due to radiation (intended effect) N88.8
      adverse effect or misadventure N99.89
  chamber angle H21.21- ☑
  changes, spine or vertebra — *see* Spondylosis
  chorioretinal — *see also* Degeneration, choroid
    hereditary H31.20
  choroid (colloid) (drusen) H31.10- ☑
    atrophy — *see* Atrophy, choroidal
    hereditary — *see* Dystrophy, choroidal, hereditary
  ciliary body H21.22- ☑
  cochlear — *see* subcategory H83.8 ☑
  combined (spinal cord) (subacute) E53.8 [G32.0]
    with anemia (pernicious) D51.0 [G32.0]
      due to dietary vitamin B12 deficiency D51.3 [G32.0]
    in (due to)
      vitamin B12 deficiency E53.8 [G32.0]
      anemia D51.9 [G32.0]
  conjunctiva H11.10
    concretions — *see* Concretion, conjunctiva
    deposits — *see* Deposit, conjunctiva
    pigmentations — *see* Pigmentation, conjunctiva
    pinguecula — *see* Pinguecula
    xerosis — *see* Xerosis, conjunctiva
  cornea H18.40
    calcerous H18.43
      band keratopathy H18.42- ☑
    familial, hereditary — *see* Dystrophy, cornea
    hyaline (of old scars) H18.49
    keratomalacia — *see* Keratomalacia
    nodular H18.45- ☑
    peripheral H18.46- ☑
    senile H18.41- ☑
    specified type NEC H18.49
  cortical (cerebellar) (parenchymatous) G31.89
    alcoholic G31.2
    diffuse, due to arteriopathy I67.2
  corticobasal G31.85
  cutis L98.8
    amyloid E85.4 [L99]
  dental pulp K04.2
  disc disease — *see* Degeneration, intervertebral disc NEC
  dorsolateral (spinal cord) — *see* Degeneration, combined
  extrapyramidal G25.9
  eye, macular — *see also* Degeneration, macula
    congenital or hereditary — *see* Dystrophy, retina
  facet joints — *see* Spondylosis
  fatty
    liver NEC K76.0
      alcoholic K70.0
  grey matter (brain) (Alpers') G31.81
  heart — *see also* Degeneration, myocardial

Degeneration, degenerative — *continued*
  heart — *see also* Degeneration, myocardial — *continued*
    amyloid E85.4 [I43]
    atheromatous — *see* Disease, heart, ischemic, atherosclerotic
    ischemic — *see* Disease, heart, ischemic
  hepatolenticular (Wilson's) E83.01
  hepatorenal K76.7
  hyaline (diffuse) (generalized)
    localized — *see* Degeneration, by site
  infrapatellar fat pad M79.4
  intervertebral disc NOS
    with
      myelopathy — *see* Disorder, disc, with, myelopathy
      radiculitis or radiculopathy — *see* Disorder, disc, with, radiculopathy
    cervical, cervicothoracic — *see* Disorder, disc, cervical, degeneration
    with
      myelopathy — *see* Disorder, disc, cervical, with myelopathy
      neuritis, radiculitis or radiculopathy — *see* Disorder, disc, cervical, with neuritis
    lumbar region M51.36
    with
      myelopathy M51.06
      neuritis, radiculitis, radiculopathy or sciatica M51.16
    lumbosacral region M51.37
    with
      neuritis, radiculitis, radiculopathy or sciatica M51.17
    sacrococcygeal region M53.3
    thoracic region M51.34
    with
      myelopathy M51.04
      neuritis, radiculitis, radiculopathy M51.14
    thoracolumbar region M51.35
    with
      myelopathy M51.05
      neuritis, radiculitis, radiculopathy M51.15
  intestine, amyloid E85.4
  iris (pigmentary) H21.23- ☑
  ischemic — *see* Ischemia
  joint disease — *see* Osteoarthritis
  kidney N28.89
    amyloid E85.4 [N29]
    cystic, congenital Q61.9
    fatty N28.89
    polycystic Q61.3
      adult type (autosomal dominant) Q61.2
      infantile type (autosomal recessive) NEC Q61.19
        collecting duct dilatation Q61.11
  Kuhnt-Junius — *see also* Degeneration, macula H35.32- ☑
  lens — *see* Cataract
  lenticular (familial) (progressive) (Wilson's) (with cirrhosis of liver) E83.01
  liver (diffuse) NEC K76.89
    amyloid E85.4 [K77]
    cystic K76.89
      congenital Q44.6
    fatty NEC K76.0
      alcoholic K70.0
    hypertrophic K76.89
    parenchymatous, acute or subacute K72.00
      with coma K72.01
    pigmentary K76.89
    toxic (acute) K71.9
  lung J98.4
  lymph gland I89.8
    hyaline I89.8
  macula, macular (acquired) (age-related) (senile) H35.30
    angioid streaks H35.33
    atrophic age-related H35.31- ☑
    congenital or hereditary — *see* Dystrophy, retina
    cystoid H35.35- ☑
    drusen H35.36- ☑
    dry age-related H35.31- ☑
    exudative H35.32- ☑
    hole H35.34- ☑
    nonexudative H35.31- ☑
    puckering H35.37- ☑
    toxic H35.38- ☑
    wet age-related H35.32- ☑

Degeneration, degenerative — *continued*
  membranous labyrinth, congenital (causing impairment of hearing) Q16.5
  meniscus — *see* Derangement, meniscus
  mitral — *see* Insufficiency, mitral
  Mönckeberg's — *see* Arteriosclerosis, extremities
  motor centers, senile G31.1
  multi-system G90.3
  mural — *see* Degeneration, myocardial
  muscle (fatty) (fibrous) (hyaline) (progressive) M62.89
    heart — *see* Degeneration, myocardial
  myelin, central nervous system G37.9
  myocardial, myocardium (fatty) (hyaline) (senile) I51.5
    with rheumatic fever (conditions in I00) I09.0
      active, acute or subacute I01.2
        with chorea I02.0
      inactive or quiescent (with chorea) I09.0
    hypertensive — *see* Hypertension, heart
    rheumatic — *see* Degeneration, myocardial, with rheumatic fever
    syphilitic A52.06
  nasal sinus (mucosa) J32.9
    frontal J32.1
    maxillary J32.0
  nerve — *see* Disorder, nerve
  nervous system G31.9
    alcoholic G31.2
    amyloid E85.4 *[G99.8]*
    autonomic G90.9
    fatty G31.89
    specified NEC G31.89
  nipple N64.89
  olivopontocerebellar (hereditary) (familial) G23.8
  osseous labyrinth — *see* subcategory H83.8 ☑
  ovary N83.8
    cystic N83.20- ☑
    microcystic N83.20- ☑
  pallidal pigmentary (progressive) G23.0
  pancreas K86.89
    tuberculous A18.83
  penis N48.89
  pigmentary (diffuse) (general)
    localized — *see* Degeneration, by site
    pallidal (progressive) G23.0
  pineal gland E34.8
  pituitary (gland) E23.6
  popliteal fat pad M79.4
  posterolateral (spinal cord) — *see* Degeneration, combined
  pulmonary valve (heart) I37.8
  pulp (tooth) K04.2
  pupillary margin H21.24- ☑
  renal — *see* Degeneration, kidney
  retina H35.9
    hereditary (cerebroretinal) (congenital) (juvenile) (macula) (peripheral) (pigmentary) — *see* Dystrophy, retina
    Kuhnt-Junius — *see also* Degeneration, macula H35.32- ☑
    macula (cystic) (exudative) (hole) (nonexudative) (pseudohole) (senile) (toxic) — *see* Degeneration, macula
    peripheral H35.40
      lattice H35.41- ☑
      microcystoid H35.42- ☑
      paving stone H35.43- ☑
      secondary
        pigmentary H35.45- ☑
        vitreoretinal H35.46- ☑
      senile reticular H35.44- ☑
    pigmentary (primary) — *see also* Dystrophy, retina
      secondary — *see* Degeneration, retina, peripheral, secondary
    posterior pole — *see* Degeneration, macula
  saccule, congenital (causing impairment of hearing) Q16.5
  senile R54
    brain G31.1
    cardiac, heart or myocardium — *see* Degeneration, myocardial
    motor centers G31.1
    vascular — *see* Arteriosclerosis
  sinus (cystic) — *see also* Sinusitis
    polypoid J33.1
  skin L98.8
    amyloid E85.4 *[L99]*
    colloid L98.8
  spinal (cord) G31.89

Degeneration, degenerative — *continued*
  spinal — *continued*
    amyloid E85.4 *[G32.89]*
    combined (subacute) — *see* Degeneration, combined
    dorsolateral — *see* Degeneration, combined
    familial NEC G31.89
    fatty G31.89
    funicular — *see* Degeneration, combined
    posterolateral — *see* Degeneration, combined
    subacute combined — *see* Degeneration, combined
    tuberculous A17.81
  spleen D73.0
    amyloid E85.4 *[D77]*
  stomach K31.89
  striatonigral G23.2
  suprarenal (capsule) (gland) E27.8
  synovial membrane (pulpy) — *see* Disorder, synovium, specified type NEC
  tapetoretinal — *see* Dystrophy, retina
  thymus (gland) E32.8
    fatty E32.8
  thyroid (gland) E07.89
  tricuspid (heart) (valve) I07.9
  tuberculous NEC — *see* Tuberculosis
  turbinate J34.89
  uterus (cystic) N85.8
  vascular (senile) — *see* Arteriosclerosis
    hypertensive — *see* Hypertension
  vitreoretinal, secondary — *see* Degeneration, retina, peripheral, secondary, vitreoretinal
  vitreous (body) H43.81- ☑
  Wallerian — *see* Disorder, nerve
  Wilson's hepatolenticular E83.01

Deglutition
  paralysis R13.0
    hysterical F44.4
  pneumonia J69.0

Degos' disease I77.89

Dehiscence (of)
  amputation stump T87.81
  cesarean wound O90.0
  closure of
    cornea T81.31 ☑
    craniotomy T81.32 ☑
    fascia (muscular) (superficial) T81.32 ☑
    internal organ or tissue T81.32 ☑
    laceration (external) (internal) T81.33 ☑
    ligament T81.32 ☑
    mucosa T81.31 ☑
    muscle or muscle flap T81.32 ☑
    ribs or rib cage T81.32 ☑
    skin and subcutaneous tissue (full-thickness) (superficial) T81.31 ☑
    skull T81.32 ☑
    sternum (sternotomy) T81.32 ☑
    tendon T81.32 ☑
    traumatic laceration (external) (internal) T81.33 ☑
  episiotomy O90.1
  operation wound NEC T81.31 ☑
    external operation wound (superficial) T81.31 ☑
    internal operation wound (deep) T81.32 ☑
  perineal wound (postpartum) O90.1
  traumatic injury wound repair T81.33 ☑
  wound T81.30 ☑
    traumatic repair T81.33 ☑

Dehydration E86.0
  newborn P74.1

Déjérine-Roussy syndrome G89.0

Déjérine-Sottas disease or neuropathy (hypertrophic) G60.0

Déjérine-Thomas atrophy G23.8

Delay, delayed
  any plane in pelvis
    complicating delivery O66.9
  birth or delivery NOS O63.9
  closure, ductus arteriosus (Botalli) P29.38
  coagulation — *see* Defect, coagulation
  conduction (cardiac) (ventricular) I45.9
  delivery, second twin, triplet, etc O63.2
  development R62.50
    global F88
    intellectual (specific) F81.9
    language F80.9
      due to hearing loss F80.4
    learning F81.9
    pervasive F84.9

Delay, delayed — *continued*
  development — *continued*
    physiological R62.50
      specified stage NEC R62.0
    reading F81.0
    sexual E30.0
    speech F80.9
      due to hearing loss F80.4
    spelling F81.81
  ejaculation F52.32
  gastric emptying K30
  menarche E30.0
  menstruation (cause unknown) N91.0
  milestone R62.0
  passage of meconium (newborn) P76.0
  primary respiration P28.9
  puberty (constitutional) E30.0
  separation of umbilical cord P96.82
  sexual maturation, female E30.0
  sleep phase syndrome G47.21
  union, fracture — *see* Fracture, by site
  vaccination Z28.9

Deletion(s)
  autosome Q93.9
    identified by fluorescence in situ hybridization (FISH) Q93.89
    identified by in situ hybridization (ISH) Q93.89
  chromosome
    with complex rearrangements NEC Q93.7
    part of NEC Q93.59
    seen only at prometaphase Q93.89
    short arm
      22q11.2 Q93.81
      4 Q93.3
      5p Q93.4
    specified NEC Q93.89
  long arm chromosome 18 or 21 Q93.89
    with complex rearrangements NEC Q93.7
  microdeletions NEC Q93.88

Delhi boil or button B55.1

Delinquency (juvenile) (neurotic) F91.8
  group Z72.810

Delinquent immunization status Z28.3

Delirium, delirious (acute or subacute) (not alcohol- or drug-induced) (with dementia) R41.0
  alcoholic (acute) (tremens) (withdrawal) F10.921
    with intoxication F10.921
      in
        abuse F10.121
        dependence F10.221
  due to (secondary to)
    alcohol
      intoxication F10.921
        in
          abuse F10.121
          dependence F10.221
      withdrawal F10.231
    amphetamine intoxication F15.921
      in
        abuse F15.121
        dependence F15.221
    anxiolytic
      intoxication F13.921
        in
          abuse F13.121
          dependence F13.221
      withdrawal F13.231
    cannabis intoxication (acute) F12.921
      in
        abuse F12.121
        dependence F12.221
    cocaine intoxication (acute) F14.921
      in
        abuse F14.121
        dependence F14.221
    general medical condition F05
    hallucinogen intoxication F16.921
      in
        abuse F16.121
        dependence F16.221
    hypnotic
      intoxication F13.921
        in
          abuse F13.121
          dependence F13.221
      withdrawal F13.231
    inhalant intoxication (acute) F18.921
      in
        abuse F18.121

Delirium, delirious — *continued*
  due to — *continued*
    inhalant intoxication — *continued*
      in — *continued*
        dependence F18.221
    multiple etiologies F05
    opioid intoxication (acute) F11.921
      in
        abuse F11.121
        dependence F11.221
    other (or unknown) substance F19.921
    phencyclidine intoxication (acute) F16.921
      in
        abuse F16.121
        dependence F16.221
    psychoactive substance NEC intoxication (acute) F19.921
      in
        abuse F19.121
        dependence F19.221
    sedative
      intoxication F13.921
        in
          abuse F13.121
          dependence F13.221
      withdrawal F13.231
    unknown etiology R41.0
  exhaustion F43.0
  hysterical F44.89
  postprocedural (postoperative) F05
  puerperal F05
  thyroid — *see* Thyrotoxicosis with thyroid storm
  traumatic — *see* Injury, intracranial
  tremens (alcohol-induced) F10.231
    sedative-induced F13.231
Delivery (childbirth) (labor)
  arrested active phase O62.1
  cesarean (for)
    abnormal
      pelvis (bony) (deformity) (major) NEC with disproportion (fetopelvic) O33.0
        with obstructed labor O65.0
      presentation or position O32.9 ☑
    abruptio placentae — *see also* Abruptio placentae O45.9- ☑
    acromion presentation O32.2 ☑
    atony, uterus O62.2
    breech presentation O32.1 ☑
      incomplete O32.8 ☑
    brow presentation O32.3 ☑
    cephalopelvic disproportion O33.9
    cerclage O34.3- ☑
    chin presentation O32.3 ☑
    cicatrix of cervix O34.4- ☑
    contracted pelvis (general)
      inlet O33.2
      outlet O33.3 ☑
    cord presentation or prolapse O69.0 ☑
    cystocele O34.8- ☑
    deformity (acquired) (congenital)
      pelvic organs or tissues NEC O34.8- ☑
      pelvis (bony) NEC O33.0
    disproportion NOS O33.9
    eclampsia — *see* Eclampsia
    face presentation O32.3 ☑
    failed
      forceps O66.5
      induction of labor O61.9
        instrumental O61.1
        mechanical O61.1
        medical O61.0
        specified NEC O61.8
        surgical O61.1
      trial of labor NOS O66.40
        following previous cesarean delivery O66.41
      vacuum extraction O66.5
      ventouse O66.5
    fetal-maternal hemorrhage O43.01- ☑
    hemorrhage (intrapartum) O67.9
      with coagulation defect O67.0
      specified cause NEC O67.8
    high head at term O32.4 ☑
    hydrocephalic fetus O33.6 ☑
    incarceration of uterus O34.51- ☑
    incoordinate uterine action O62.4
    increased size, fetus O33.5 ☑
    inertia, uterus O62.2
      primary O62.0

Delivery — *continued*
  cesarean — *continued*
    inertia, uterus — *continued*
      secondary O62.1
    isthmocele O34.22
    lateroversion, uterus O34.59- ☑
    mal lie O32.9 ☑
    malposition
      fetus O32.9 ☑
      pelvic organs or tissues NEC O34.8- ☑
      uterus NEC O34.59- ☑
    malpresentation NOS O32.9 ☑
    oblique presentation O32.2 ☑
    occurring after 37 completed weeks of gestation but before 39 completed weeks gestation due to (spontaneous) onset of labor O75.82
    oversize fetus O33.5 ☑
    pelvic tumor NEC O34.8- ☑
    placenta previa O44.0- ☑
      complete O44.0- ☑
        with hemorrhage O44.1- ☑
    placental insufficiency O36.51- ☑
    planned, occurring after 37 completed weeks of gestation but before 39 completed weeks gestation due to (spontaneous) onset of labor O75.82
    polyp, cervix O34.4- ☑
      causing obstructed labor O65.5
    poor dilatation, cervix O62.0
    pre-eclampsia O14.94
      mild O14.04
      moderate O14.04
      severe O14.14
        with hemolysis, elevated liver enzymes and low platelet count (HELLP) O14.24
    previous
      cesarean delivery O34.219
        classical (vertical) scar O34.212
        isthmocele O34.22
        low transverse scar O34.211
        mid-transverse T incision O34.218
        scar
          defect (isthmocele) O34.22
          specified type NEC O34.218
      surgery (to)
        cervix O34.4- ☑
        gynecological NEC O34.8- ☑
        rectum O34.7- ☑
        uterus O34.29
        vagina O34.6- ☑
    prolapse
      arm or hand O32.2 ☑
      uterus O34.52- ☑
    prolonged labor NOS O63.9
    rectocele O34.8- ☑
    retroversion
      uterus O34.53- ☑
    rigid
      cervix O34.4- ☑
      pelvic floor O34.8- ☑
      perineum O34.7- ☑
      vagina O34.6- ☑
      vulva O34.7- ☑
    sacculation, pregnant uterus O34.59- ☑
    scar(s)
      cervix O34.4- ☑
      cesarean delivery O34.219
        classical (vertical) O34.212
        isthmocele O34.22
        low transverse O34.211
        mid-transverse T incision O34.218
        scar
          defect (isthmocele) O34.22
          specified type NEC O34.218
      defect (isthmocele) O34.22
      transmural uterine O34.29
      uterus O34.29
    Shirodkar suture in situ O34.3- ☑
    shoulder presentation O32.2 ☑
    stenosis or stricture, cervix O34.4- ☑
    streptococcus group B (GBS) carrier state O99.824
    transmural uterine scar O34.29
    transverse presentation or lie O32.2 ☑
    tumor, pelvic organs or tissues NEC O34.8- ☑
      cervix O34.4- ☑
    umbilical cord presentation or prolapse O69.0 ☑
  without indication O82

Delivery — *continued*
  completely normal case O80
  complicated O75.9
    by
      abnormal, abnormality (of)
        forces of labor O62.9
          specified type NEC O62.8
        glucose O99.814
        uterine contractions NOS O62.9
      abruptio placentae — *see also* Abruptio placentae O45.9- ☑
      abuse
        physical O9A.32 (*following* O99)
        psychological O9A.52 (*following* O99)
        sexual O9A.42 (*following* O99)
      adherent placenta O72.0
        without hemorrhage O73.0
      alcohol use O99.314
      anemia (pre-existing) O99.02
      anesthetic death O74.8
      annular detachment of cervix O71.3
      atony, uterus O62.2
      attempted vacuum extraction and forceps O66.5
      Bandl's ring O62.4
      bariatric surgery status O99.844
      biliary tract disorder O26.62
      bleeding — *see* Delivery, complicated by, hemorrhage
      blood disorder NEC O99.12
      cervical dystocia (hypotonic) O62.2
        primary O62.0
        secondary O62.1
      circulatory system disorder O99.42
      compression of cord (umbilical) NEC O69.2 ☑
      condition NEC O99.892
      contraction, contracted ring O62.4
      cord (umbilical)
        around neck
          with compression O69.1 ☑
          without compression O69.81 ☑
        bruising O69.5 ☑
        complication O69.9 ☑
          specified NEC O69.89 ☑
        compression NEC O69.2 ☑
        entanglement O69.2 ☑
          without compression O69.82 ☑
        hematoma O69.5 ☑
        presentation O69.0 ☑
        prolapse O69.0 ☑
        short O69.3 ☑
        thrombosis (vessels) O69.5 ☑
        vascular lesion O69.5 ☑
      Couvelaire uterus O45.8X- ☑
      damage to (injury to) NEC
        perineum O71.82
        periurethral tissue O71.82
        vulva O71.82
      delay following rupture of membranes (spontaneous) — *see* Pregnancy, complicated by, premature rupture of membranes
      depressed fetal heart tones O76
      diabetes O24.92
        gestational O24.429
          diet controlled O24.420
          insulin controlled O24.424
          oral drug controlled (antidiabetic) (hypoglycemic) O24.425
        pre-existing O24.32
          specified NEC O24.82
          type 1 O24.02
          type 2 O24.12
      diastasis recti (abdominis) O71.89
      dilatation
        bladder O66.8
        cervix incomplete, poor or slow O62.0
      disease NEC O99.892
      disruptio uteri — *see* Delivery, complicated by, rupture, uterus
      drug use O99.324
      dysfunction, uterus NOS O62.9
        hypertonic O62.4
        hypotonic O62.2
          primary O62.0
          secondary O62.1
        incoordinate O62.4
      eclampsia O15.1
      embolism (pulmonary) — *see* Embolism, obstetric

Delivery — *continued*
  complicated — *continued*
    by — *continued*
      endocrine, nutritional or metabolic disease NEC
        O99.284
      failed
        attempted vaginal birth after previous cesarean delivery O66.41
        induction of labor O61.9
          instrumental O61.1
          mechanical O61.1
          medical O61.0
          specified NEC O61.8
          surgical O61.1
        trial of labor O66.40
      female genital mutilation O65.5
      fetal
        abnormal acid-base balance O68
        acidemia O68
        acidosis O68
        alkalosis O68
        death, early O02.1
        deformity O66.3
        heart rate or rhythm (abnormal) (non-reassuring) O76
        hypoxia O77.8
        stress O77.9
          due to drug administration O77.1
          electrocardiographic evidence of O77.8
          specified NEC O77.8
          ultrasound evidence of O77.8
      fever during labor O75.2
      gastric banding status O99.844
      gastric bypass status O99.844
      gastrointestinal disease NEC O99.62
      gestational
        diabetes O24.429
          diet controlled O24.420
          insulin (and diet) controlled O24.424
          oral drug controlled (antidiabetic) (hypoglycemic) O24.425
        edema O12.04
          with proteinuria O12.24
        proteinuria O12.14
      gonorrhea O98.22
      hematoma O71.7
        ischial spine O71.7
        pelvic O71.7
        vagina O71.7
        vulva or perineum O71.7
      hemorrhage (uterine) O67.9
        associated with
          afibrinogenemia O67.0
          coagulation defect O67.0
          hyperfibrinolysis O67.0
          hypofibrinogenemia O67.0
        due to
          low implantation of placenta O44.5- ☑
          low-lying placenta O44.5- ☑
          placenta previa O44.1- ☑
            marginal O44.3- ☑
            partial O44.3- ☑
          premature separation of placenta (normally implanted) — *see also* Abruptio placentae O45.9- ☑
          retained placenta O72.0
          uterine leiomyoma O67.8
        placenta NEC O67.8
        postpartum NEC (atonic) (immediate) O72.1
          with retained or trapped placenta O72.0
          delayed O72.2
          secondary O72.2
          third stage O72.0
      hourglass contraction, uterus O62.4
      hypertension, hypertensive (pre-existing) — *see* Hypertension, complicated by, childbirth (labor)
      hypotension O26.5- ☑
      incomplete dilatation (cervix) O62.0
      incoordinate uterus contractions O62.4
      inertia, uterus O62.2
        during latent phase of labor O62.0
        primary O62.0
        secondary O62.1
      infection (maternal) O98.92
        carrier state NEC O99.834
        gonorrhea O98.22
        human immunodeficiency virus (HIV) O98.72

Delivery — *continued*
  complicated — *continued*
    by — *continued*
      infection — *continued*
        sexually transmitted NEC O98.32
        specified NEC O98.82
        syphilis O98.12
        tuberculosis O98.02
        viral hepatitis O98.42
        viral NEC O98.52
      injury (to mother) — *see also* Delivery, complicated, by, damage to O71.9
        nonobstetric O9A.22 (*following* O99)
        caused by abuse — *see* Delivery, complicated by, abuse
      intrauterine fetal death, early O02.1
      inversion, uterus O71.2
      laceration (perineal) O70.9
        anus (sphincter) O70.4
          with third degree laceration — *see also* Delivery, complicated, by, laceration, perineum, third degree O70.20
            with mucosa O70.3
          without third degree laceration O70.2 ☑
        bladder (urinary) O71.5
        bowel O71.5
        cervix (uteri) O71.3
        fourchette O70.0
        hymen O70.0
        labia O70.0
        pelvic
          floor O70.1
          organ NEC O71.5
        perineum, perineal O70.9
          first degree O70.0
          fourth degree O70.3
          muscles O70.1
          second degree O70.1
          skin O70.0
          slight O70.0
          third degree O70.20
            with
              both external anal sphincter (EAS) and internal anal sphincter (IAS) torn (IIIc) O70.23
              less than 50% of external anal sphincter (EAS) thickness torn (IIIa) O70.21
              more than 50% external anal sphincter (EAS) thickness torn (IIIb) O70.22
            IIIa O70.21
            IIIb O70.22
            IIIc O70.23
        peritoneum (pelvic) O71.5
        rectovaginal (septum) (without perineal laceration) O71.4
          with perineum — *see also* Delivery, complicated, by, laceration, perineum, third degree O70.20
            with anal or rectal mucosa O70.3
        specified NEC O71.89
        sphincter ani — *see* Delivery, complicated, by, laceration, anus (sphincter)
        urethra O71.5
        uterus O71.81
          before labor O71.81
        vagina, vaginal (deep) (high) (without perineal laceration) O71.4
          with perineum O70.0
          muscles, with perineum O70.1
        vulva O70.0
      liver disorder O26.62
      malignancy O9A.12 (*following* O99)
      malnutrition O25.2
      malposition, malpresentation
        uterus or cervix O65.5
        placenta O44.0- ☑
          with hemorrhage O44.1- ☑
        without obstruction — *see also* Delivery, complicated by, obstruction O32.9 ☑
          breech O32.1 ☑
          compound O32.6 ☑
          face (brow) (chin) O32.3 ☑
          footling O32.8 ☑
          high head O32.4 ☑
          oblique O32.2 ☑

Delivery — *continued*
  complicated — *continued*
    by — *continued*
      malposition, malpresentation — *continued*
        without obstruction — *see also* Delivery, complicated by, obstruction — *continued*
          specified NEC O32.8 ☑
          transverse O32.2 ☑
          unstable lie O32.0 ☑
      meconium in amniotic fluid O77.0
      mental disorder NEC O99.344
      metrorrhexis — *see* Delivery, complicated by, rupture, uterus
      nervous system disorder O99.354
      obesity (pre-existing) O99.214
      obesity surgery status O99.844
      obstetric trauma O71.9
        specified NEC O71.89
      obstructed labor
        due to
          breech (complete) (frank) presentation O64.1 ☑
            incomplete O64.8 ☑
          brow presentation O64.3 ☑
          buttock presentation O64.1 ☑
          chin presentation O64.2 ☑
          compound presentation O64.5 ☑
          contracted pelvis O65.1
          deep transverse arrest O64.0 ☑
          deformed pelvis O65.0
          dystocia (fetal) O66.9
            due to
              conjoined twins O66.3
              fetal
                abnormality NEC O66.3
                ascites O66.3
                hydrops O66.3
                meningomyelocele O66.3
                sacral teratoma O66.3
                tumor O66.3
              hydrocephalic fetus O66.3
              shoulder O66.0
          face presentation O64.2 ☑
          fetopelvic disproportion O65.4
          footling presentation O64.8 ☑
          impacted shoulders O66.0
          incomplete rotation of fetal head O64.0 ☑
          large fetus O66.2
          locked twins O66.1
          malposition O64.9 ☑
            specified NEC O64.8 ☑
          malpresentation O64.9 ☑
            specified NEC O64.8 ☑
          multiple fetuses NEC O66.6
          pelvic
            abnormality (maternal) O65.9
              organ O65.5
              specified NEC O65.8
            contraction
              inlet O65.2
              mid-cavity O65.3
              outlet O65.3
          persistent (position)
            occipitoiliac O64.0 ☑
            occipitoposterior O64.0 ☑
            occipitosacral O64.0 ☑
            occipitotransverse O64.0 ☑
          prolapsed arm O64.4 ☑
          shoulder presentation O64.4 ☑
        specified NEC O66.8
      pathological retraction ring, uterus O62.4
      penetration, pregnant uterus by instrument O71.1
      perforation — *see* Delivery, complicated by, laceration
      placenta, placental
        ablatio — *see also* Abruptio placentae O45.9- ☑
        abnormality O43.9- ☑
          specified NEC O43.89- ☑
        abruptio — *see also* Abruptio placentae O45.9- ☑
        accreta O43.21- ☑
        adherent (with hemorrhage) O72.0
          without hemorrhage O73.0

Delivery — *continued*
  complicated — *continued*
    by — *continued*
      placenta, placental — *continued*
        detachment (premature) — *see also* Abruptio
            placentae O45.9- ☑
        disorder O43.9- ☑
          specified NEC O43.89- ☑
        hemorrhage NEC O67.8
        increta O43.22- ☑
        low (implantation) (lying) O44.4- ☑
          with hemorrhage O44.5- ☑
        malformation O43.10- ☑
        malposition O44.0- ☑
          without hemorrhage O44.1- ☑
        percreta O43.23- ☑
        previa (central) (complete) (lateral) (total)
            O44.0- ☑
          with hemorrhage O44.1- ☑
          marginal O44.2- ☑
            with hemorrhage O44.3- ☑
          partial O44.2- ☑
            with hemorrhage O44.3- ☑
        retained (with hemorrhage) O72.0
          without hemorrhage O73.0
        separation (premature) O45.9- ☑
          specified NEC O45.8X- ☑
        vicious insertion O44.1- ☑
    precipitate labor O62.3
    premature rupture, membranes — *see also*
        Pregnancy, complicated by, premature
        rupture of membranes O42.90
    prolapse
      arm or hand O32.2 ☑
      cord (umbilical) O69.0 ☑
      foot or leg O32.8 ☑
      uterus O34.52- ☑
    prolonged labor O63.9
      first stage O63.0
      second stage O63.1
    protozoal disease (maternal) O98.62
    respiratory disease NEC O99.52
    retained membranes or portions of placenta
        O72.2
      without hemorrhage O73.1
    retarded birth O63.9
    retention of secundines (with hemorrhage) O72.0
      without hemorrhage O73.0
      partial O72.2
        without hemorrhage O73.1
    rupture
      bladder (urinary) O71.5
      cervix O71.3
      pelvic organ NEC O71.5
      urethra O71.5
      uterus (during or after labor) O71.1
        before labor O71.0- ☑
    separation, pubic bone (symphysis pubis) O71.6
    shock O75.1
    shoulder presentation O64.4 ☑
    skin disorder NEC O99.72
    spasm, cervix O62.4
    stenosis or stricture, cervix O65.5
    streptococcus group B (GBS) carrier state O99.824
    subluxation of symphysis (pubis) O26.72
    syphilis (maternal) O98.12
    tear — *see* Delivery, complicated by, laceration
    tetanic uterus O62.4
    trauma (obstetrical) — *see also* Delivery, compli-
        cated, by, damage to O71.9
      non-obstetric O9A.22 (*following* O99)
      periurethral O71.82
      specified NEC O71.89
    tuberculosis (maternal) O98.02
    tumor, pelvic organs or tissues NEC O65.5
    umbilical cord around neck
      with compression O69.1 ☑
      without compression O69.81 ☑
    uterine inertia O62.2
      during latent phase of labor O62.0
      primary O62.0
      secondary O62.1
    vasa previa O69.4 ☑
    velamentous insertion of cord O43.12- ☑
  specified complication NEC O75.89
  delayed NOS O63.9

Delivery — *continued*
  delayed — *continued*
    following rupture of membranes
      artificial O75.5
    second twin, triplet, etc. O63.2
  forceps, low following failed vacuum extraction O66.5
  missed (at or near term) O36.4 ☑
  normal O80
  obstructed — *see* Delivery, complicated by, obstructed
      labor
  precipitate O62.3
  preterm — *see also* Pregnancy, complicated by,
      preterm labor O60.10 ☑
  spontaneous O80
  term pregnancy NOS O80
  uncomplicated O80
  vaginal, following previous cesarean delivery O34.219
    classical (vertical) scar O34.212
    low transverse scar O34.211
    mid-transverse T incision O34.218
    scar
      defect (isthmocele) O34.22
      specified type NEC O34.218
Delusions (paranoid) — *see* Disorder, delusional
Dementia (degenerative (primary)) (old age) (persisting)
    F03.90
  with
    aggressive behavior F03.91
    behavioral disturbance F03.91
    combative behavior F03.91
    Lewy bodies G31.83 *[F02.80]*
      with behavioral disturbance G31.83 *[F02.81]*
    Parkinsonism G31.83 *[F02.80]*
      with behavioral disturbance G31.83 *[F02.81]*
    Parkinson's disease G20 *[F02.80]*
      with behavioral disturbance G20 *[F02.81]*
    violent behavior F03.91
  alcoholic F10.97
    with dependence F10.27
  Alzheimer's type — *see* Disease, Alzheimer's
  arteriosclerotic — *see* Dementia, vascular
  atypical, Alzheimer's type — *see* Disease, Alzheimer's,
      specified NEC
  congenital — *see* Disability, intellectual
  frontal (lobe) G31.09 *[F02.80]*
    with behavioral disturbance G31.09 *[F02.81]*
  frontotemporal G31.09 *[F02.80]*
    with behavioral disturbance G31.09 *[F02.81]*
    specified NEC G31.09 *[F02.80]*
      with behavioral disturbance G31.09 *[F02.81]*
  in (due to)
    alcohol F10.97
      with dependence F10.27
    Alzheimer's disease — *see* Disease, Alzheimer's
    arteriosclerotic brain disease — *see* Dementia, vas-
        cular
    cerebral lipidoses E75.- ☑ *[F02.80]*
      with behavioral disturbance E75.- ☑ *[F02.81]*
    Creutzfeldt-Jakob disease — *see also* Creutzfeldt-
        Jakob disease or syndrome (with dementia)
        A81.00
    epilepsy G40.- ☑ *[F02.80]*
      with behavioral disturbance G40.- ☑ *[F02.81]*
    hepatolenticular degeneration E83.01 *[F02.80]*
      with behavioral disturbance E83.01 *[F02.81]*
    human immunodeficiency virus (HIV) disease
        B20 *[F02.80]*
      with behavioral disturbance B20 *[F02.81]*
    Huntington's disease or chorea G10 *[F02.80]*
      with behavioral disturbance G10 *[F02.81]*
    hypercalcemia E83.52 *[F02.80]*
      with behavioral disturbance E83.52 *[F02.81]*
    hypothyroidism, acquired E03.9 *[F02.80]*
      with behavioral disturbance E03.9 *[F02.81]*
      due to iodine deficiency E01.8 *[F02.80]*
        with behavioral disturbance E01.8 *[F02.81]*
    inhalants F18.97
      with dependence F18.27
    multiple
      etiologies F03 ☑
      sclerosis G35 *[F02.80]*
        with behavioral disturbance G35 *[F02.81]*
    neurosyphilis A52.17 *[F02.80]*
      with behavioral disturbance A52.17 *[F02.81]*
      juvenile A50.49 *[F02.80]*
        with behavioral disturbance A50.49 *[F02.81]*
    niacin deficiency E52 *[F02.80]*

Dementia — *continued*
  in — *continued*
    niacin deficiency — *continued*
      with behavioral disturbance E52 *[F02.81]*
    paralysis agitans G20 *[F02.80]*
      with behavioral disturbance G20 *[F02.81]*
    Parkinson's disease G20 *[F02.80]*
    pellagra E52 *[F02.80]*
      with behavioral disturbance E52 *[F02.81]*
    Pick's G31.01 *[F02.80]*
      with behavioral disturbance G31.01 *[F02.81]*
    polyarteritis nodosa M30.0 *[F02.80]*
      with behavioral disturbance M30.0 *[F02.81]*
    psychoactive drug F19.97
      with dependence F19.27
      inhalants F18.97
        with dependence F18.27
      sedatives, hypnotics or anxiolytics F13.97
        with dependence F13.27
    sedatives, hypnotics or anxiolytics F13.97
      with dependence F13.27
    systemic lupus erythematosus M32.- ☑ *[F02.80]*
      with behavioral disturbance M32.- ☑ *[F02.81]*
    trypanosomiasis
      African B56.9 *[F02.80]*
        with behavioral disturbance B56.9 *[F02.81]*
    unknown etiology F03
    vitamin B12 deficiency E53.8 *[F02.80]*
      with behavioral disturbance E53.8 *[F02.81]*
    volatile solvents F18.97
      with dependence F18.27
    with behavioral disturbance G31.83 *[F02.81]*
  infantile, infantilis F84.3
  Lewy body G31.83 *[F02.80]*
    with behavioral disturbance G31.83 *[F02.81]*
  multi-infarct — *see* Dementia, vascular
  paralytica, paralytic (syphilitic) A52.17 *[F02.80]*
    with behavioral disturbance A52.17 *[F02.81]*
    juvenilis A50.45
  paretic A52.17
  praecox — *see* Schizophrenia
  presenile F03 ☑
    Alzheimer's type — *see* Disease, Alzheimer's, early
        onset
  primary degenerative F03 ☑
  progressive, syphilitic A52.17
  senile F03 ☑
    with acute confusional state F05
    Alzheimer's type — *see* Disease, Alzheimer's, late
        onset
    depressed or paranoid type F03 ☑
  vascular (acute onset) (mixed) (multi-infarct) (subcorti-
      cal) F01.50
    with behavioral disturbance F01.51
Demineralization, bone — *see* Osteoporosis
Demodex folliculorum (infestation) B88.0
Demophobia F40.248
Demoralization R45.3
Demyelination, demyelinization
  central nervous system G37.9
    specified NEC G37.8
  corpus callosum (central) G37.1
  disseminated, acute G36.9
    specified NEC G36.8
  global G35
  in optic neuritis G36.0
Dengue (classical) (fever) A90
  hemorrhagic A91
  sandfly A93.1
Dennie-Marfan syphilitic syndrome A50.45
Dens evaginatus, in dente or invaginatus K00.2
Dense breasts R92.2
Density
  increased, bone (disseminated) (generalized) (spotted)
      — *see* Disorder, bone, density and structure,
        specified type NEC
  lung (nodular) J98.4
Dental — *see also* condition
  examination Z01.20
    with abnormal findings Z01.21
  restoration
    aesthetically inadequate or displeasing K08.56
    defective K08.50
      specified NEC K08.59
    failure of marginal integrity K08.51
    failure of periodontal anatomical integrity K08.54
Dentia praecox K00.6

Index

Delivery — Dentia praecox

Denticles (pulp) K04.2
Dentigerous cyst K09.0
Dentin
  irregular (in pulp) K04.3
  opalescent K00.5
  secondary (in pulp) K04.3
  sensitive K03.89
Dentinogenesis imperfecta K00.5
Dentinoma — *see* Cyst, calcifying odontogenic
Dentition (syndrome) K00.7
  delayed K00.6
  difficult K00.7
  precocious K00.6
  premature K00.6
  retarded K00.6
Dependence (on) (syndrome) F19.20
  with remission F19.21
  alcohol (ethyl) (methyl) (without remission) F10.20
    with
      amnestic disorder, persisting F10.26
      anxiety disorder F10.280
      dementia, persisting F10.27
      intoxication F10.229
        with delirium F10.221
        uncomplicated F10.220
      mood disorder F10.24
      psychotic disorder F10.259
        with
          delusions F10.250
          hallucinations F10.251
      remission F10.21
      sexual dysfunction F10.281
      sleep disorder F10.282
      specified disorder NEC F10.288
      withdrawal F10.239
        with
          delirium F10.231
          perceptual disturbance F10.232
        uncomplicated F10.230
    counseling and surveillance Z71.41
    in remission F10.21
  amobarbital — *see* Dependence, drug, sedative
  amphetamine(s) (type) — *see* Dependence, drug, stimulant NEC
  amytal (sodium) — *see* Dependence, drug, sedative
  analgesic NEC F55.8
  anesthetic (agent) (gas) (general) (local) NEC — *see* Dependence, drug, psychoactive NEC
  anxiolytic NEC — *see* Dependence, drug, sedative
  barbital(s) — *see* Dependence, drug, sedative
  barbiturate(s) (compounds) (drugs classifiable to T42) — *see* Dependence, drug, sedative
  benzedrine — *see* Dependence, drug, stimulant NEC
  bhang — *see* Dependence, drug, cannabis
  bromide(s) NEC — *see* Dependence, drug, sedative
  caffeine — *see* Dependence, drug, stimulant NEC
  cannabis (sativa) (indica) (resin) (derivatives) (type) — *see* Dependence, drug, cannabis
  chloral (betaine) (hydrate) — *see* Dependence, drug, sedative
  chlordiazepoxide — *see* Dependence, drug, sedative
  coca (leaf) (derivatives) — *see* Dependence, drug, cocaine
  cocaine — *see* Dependence, drug, cocaine
  codeine — *see* Dependence, drug, opioid
  combinations of drugs F19.20
  dagga — *see* Dependence, drug, cannabis
  demerol — *see* Dependence, drug, opioid
  dexamphetamine — *see* Dependence, drug, stimulant NEC
  dexedrine — *see* Dependence, drug, stimulant NEC
  dextromethorphan — *see* Dependence, drug, opioid
  dextromoramide — *see* Dependence, drug, opioid
  dextro-nor-pseudo-ephedrine — *see* Dependence, drug, stimulant NEC
  dextrorphan — *see* Dependence, drug, opioid
  diazepam — *see* Dependence, drug, sedative
  dilaudid — *see* Dependence, drug, opioid
  D-lysergic acid diethylamide — *see* Dependence, drug, hallucinogen
  drug NEC F19.20
    with sleep disorder F19.282
    cannabis F12.20
      with
        anxiety disorder F12.280
        intoxication F12.229
          with
            delirium F12.221

Dependence — *continued*
  drug — *continued*
    cannabis — *continued*
      with — *continued*
        intoxication — *continued*
          with — *continued*
            perceptual disturbance F12.222
          uncomplicated F12.220
        other specified disorder F12.288
        psychosis F12.259
          delusions F12.250
          hallucinations F12.251
        unspecified disorder F12.29
        withdrawal F12.23
      in remission F12.21
    cocaine F14.20
      with
        anxiety disorder F14.280
        intoxication F14.229
          with
            delirium F14.221
            perceptual disturbance F14.222
          uncomplicated F14.220
        mood disorder F14.24
        other specified disorder F14.288
        psychosis F14.259
          delusions F14.250
          hallucinations F14.251
        sexual dysfunction F14.281
        sleep disorder F14.282
        unspecified disorder F14.29
        withdrawal F14.23
      in remission F14.21
      withdrawal symptoms in newborn P96.1
    counseling and surveillance Z71.51
    hallucinogen F16.20
      with
        anxiety disorder F16.280
        flashbacks F16.283
        intoxication F16.229
          with delirium F16.221
          uncomplicated F16.220
        mood disorder F16.24
        other specified disorder F16.288
        perception disorder, persisting F16.283
        psychosis F16.259
          delusions F16.250
          hallucinations F16.251
        unspecified disorder F16.29
      in remission F16.21
    in remission F19.21
    inhalant F18.20
      with
        anxiety disorder F18.280
        dementia, persisting F18.27
        intoxication F18.229
          with delirium F18.221
          uncomplicated F18.220
        mood disorder F18.24
        other specified disorder F18.288
        psychosis F18.259
          delusions F18.250
          hallucinations F18.251
        unspecified disorder F18.29
      in remission F18.21
    nicotine F17.200
      with disorder F17.209
        in remission F17.201
        specified disorder NEC F17.208
        withdrawal F17.203
      chewing tobacco F17.220
        with disorder F17.229
          in remission F17.221
          specified disorder NEC F17.228
          withdrawal F17.223
      cigarettes F17.210
        with disorder F17.219
          in remission F17.211
          specified disorder NEC F17.218
          withdrawal F17.213
      specified product NEC F17.290
        with disorder F17.299
          remission F17.291
          specified disorder NEC F17.298
          withdrawal F17.293
    opioid F11.20
      with
        intoxication F11.229

Dependence — *continued*
  drug — *continued*
    opioid — *continued*
      with — *continued*
        intoxication — *continued*
          with
            delirium F11.221
            perceptual disturbance F11.222
          uncomplicated F11.220
        mood disorder F11.24
        other specified disorder F11.288
        psychosis F11.259
          delusions F11.250
          hallucinations F11.251
        sexual dysfunction F11.281
        sleep disorder F11.282
        unspecified disorder F11.29
        withdrawal F11.23
      in remission F11.21
    psychoactive NEC F19.20
      with
        amnestic disorder F19.26
        anxiety disorder F19.280
        dementia F19.27
        intoxication F19.229
          with
            delirium F19.221
            perceptual disturbance F19.222
          uncomplicated F19.220
        mood disorder F19.24
        other specified disorder F19.288
        psychosis F19.259
          delusions F19.250
          hallucinations F19.251
        sexual dysfunction F19.281
        sleep disorder F19.282
        unspecified disorder F19.29
        withdrawal F19.239
          with
            delirium F19.231
            perceptual disturbance F19.232
          uncomplicated F19.230
    sedative, hypnotic or anxiolytic F13.20
      with
        amnestic disorder F13.26
        anxiety disorder F13.280
        dementia, persisting F13.27
        intoxication F13.229
          with delirium F13.221
          uncomplicated F13.220
        mood disorder F13.24
        other specified disorder F13.288
        psychosis F13.259
          delusions F13.250
          hallucinations F13.251
        sexual dysfunction F13.281
        sleep disorder F13.282
        unspecified disorder F13.29
        withdrawal F13.239
          with
            delirium F13.231
            perceptual disturbance F13.232
          uncomplicated F13.230
      in remission F13.21
    stimulant NEC F15.20
      with
        anxiety disorder F15.280
        intoxication F15.229
          with
            delirium F15.221
            perceptual disturbance F15.222
          uncomplicated F15.220
        mood disorder F15.24
        other specified disorder F15.288
        psychosis F15.259
          delusions F15.250
          hallucinations F15.251
        sexual dysfunction F15.281
        sleep disorder F15.282
        unspecified disorder F15.29
        withdrawal F15.23
      in remission F15.21
  ethyl
    alcohol (without remission) F10.20
      with remission F10.21
  bromide — *see* Dependence, drug, sedative
  carbamate F19.20
  chloride F19.20
  morphine — *see* Dependence, drug, opioid

Dependence — *continued*

ganja — *see* Dependence, drug, cannabis
glue (airplane) (sniffing) — *see* Dependence, drug, inhalant
glutethimide — *see* Dependence, drug, sedative
hallucinogenics — *see* Dependence, drug, hallucinogen
hashish — *see* Dependence, drug, cannabis
hemp — *see* Dependence, drug, cannabis
heroin (salt) (any) — *see* Dependence, drug, opioid
hypnotic NEC — *see* Dependence, drug, sedative
Indian hemp — *see* Dependence, drug, cannabis
inhalants — *see* Dependence, drug, inhalant
khat — *see* Dependence, drug, stimulant NEC
laudanum — *see* Dependence, drug, opioid
LSD (-25) (derivatives) — *see* Dependence, drug, hallucinogen
luminal — *see* Dependence, drug, sedative
lysergic acid — *see* Dependence, drug, hallucinogen
maconha — *see* Dependence, drug, cannabis
marihuana — *see* Dependence, drug, cannabis
meprobamate — *see* Dependence, drug, sedative
mescaline — *see* Dependence, drug, hallucinogen
methadone — *see* Dependence, drug, opioid
methamphetamine(s) — *see* Dependence, drug, stimulant NEC
methaqualone — *see* Dependence, drug, sedative
methyl
    alcohol (without remission) F10.20
        with remission F10.21
    bromide — *see* Dependence, drug, sedative
    morphine — *see* Dependence, drug, opioid
    phenidate — *see* Dependence, drug, stimulant NEC
    sulfonal — *see* Dependence, drug, sedative
morphine (sulfate) (sulfite) (type) — *see* Dependence, drug, opioid
narcotic (drug) NEC — *see* Dependence, drug, opioid
nembutal — *see* Dependence, drug, sedative
neraval — *see* Dependence, drug, sedative
neravan — *see* Dependence, drug, sedative
neurobarb — *see* Dependence, drug, sedative
nicotine — *see* Dependence, drug, nicotine
nitrous oxide F19.20
nonbarbiturate sedatives and tranquilizers with similar effect — *see* Dependence, drug, sedative
on
    artificial heart (fully implantable) (mechanical) Z95.812
    aspirator Z99.0
    care provider (because of) Z74.9
        impaired mobility Z74.09
        need for
            assistance with personal care Z74.1
            continuous supervision Z74.3
            no other household member able to render care Z74.2
        specified reason NEC Z74.8
    machine Z99.89
        enabling NEC Z99.89
        specified type NEC Z99.89
    renal dialysis (hemodialysis) (peritoneal) Z99.2
    respirator Z99.11
    ventilator Z99.11
    wheelchair Z99.3
opiate — *see* Dependence, drug, opioid
opioids — *see* Dependence, drug, opioid
opium (alkaloids) (derivatives) (tincture) — *see* Dependence, drug, opioid
oxygen (long-term) (supplemental) Z99.81
paraldehyde — *see* Dependence, drug, sedative
paregoric — *see* Dependence, drug, opioid
PCP (phencyclidine) (or related substance) — *see* Dependence, drug, hallucinogen
pentobarbital — *see* Dependence, drug, sedative
pentobarbitone (sodium) — *see* Dependence, drug, sedative
pentothal — *see* Dependence, drug, sedative
peyote — *see* Dependence, drug, hallucinogen
phencyclidine (PCP) (or related substance) — *see* Dependence, drug, hallucinogen
phenmetrazine — *see* Dependence, drug, stimulant NEC
phenobarbital — *see* Dependence, drug, sedative
polysubstance F19.20
psilocibin, psilocin, psilocyn, psilocyline — *see* Dependence, drug, hallucinogen
psychostimulant NEC — *see* Dependence, drug, stimulant NEC

Dependence — *continued*

secobarbital — *see* Dependence, drug, sedative
seconal — *see* Dependence, drug, sedative
sedative NEC — *see* Dependence, drug, sedative
specified drug NEC — *see* Dependence, drug, sedative
stimulant NEC — *see* Dependence, drug, stimulant NEC
substance NEC — *see* Dependence, drug
supplemental oxygen Z99.81
tobacco — *see* Dependence, drug, nicotine
    counseling and surveillance Z71.6
tranquilizer NEC — *see* Dependence, drug, sedative
vitamin B6 E53.1
volatile solvents — *see* Dependence, drug, inhalant

Dependency
care-provider Z74.9
passive F60.7
reactions (persistent) F60.7

Depersonalization (in neurotic state) (neurotic) (syndrome) F48.1

Depletion
extracellular fluid E86.9
plasma E86.1
potassium E87.6
    nephropathy N25.89
salt or sodium E87.1
    causing heat exhaustion or prostration T67.4 ☑
    nephropathy N28.9
volume NOS E86.9

Deployment (current) (military) status Z56.82
in theater or in support of military war, peacekeeping and humanitarian operations Z56.82
personal history of Z91.82
    military war, peacekeeping and humanitarian deployment (current or past conflict) Z91.82
returned from Z91.82

Depolarization, premature I49.40
atrial I49.1
junctional I49.2
specified NEC I49.49
ventricular I49.3

Deposit
bone in Boeck's sarcoid D86.89
calcareous, calcium — *see* Calcification
cholesterol
    retina H35.89
    vitreous (body) (humor) — *see* Deposit, crystalline
conjunctiva H11.11- ☑
cornea H18.00- ☑
    argentous H18.02- ☑
    due to metabolic disorder H18.03- ☑
    Kayser-Fleischer ring H18.04- ☑
    pigmentation — *see* Pigmentation, cornea
crystalline, vitreous (body) (humor) H43.2- ☑
hemosiderin in old scars of cornea — *see* Pigmentation, cornea, stromal
metallic in lens — *see* Cataract, specified NEC
skin R23.8
tooth, teeth (betel) (black) (green) (materia alba) (orange) (tobacco) K03.6
urate, kidney — *see* Calculus, kidney

Depraved appetite — *see* Pica

Depressed
HDL cholesterol E78.6

Depression (acute) (mental) F32.A
agitated (single episode) F32.2
anaclitic — *see* Disorder, adjustment
anxiety F41.8
    persistent F34.1
arches — *see also* Deformity, limb, flat foot
atypical (single episode) F32.89
    recurrent episode F33.8
basal metabolic rate R94.8
bone marrow D75.89
central nervous system R09.2
cerebral R29.818
    newborn P91.4
cerebrovascular I67.9
chest wall M95.4
climacteric (single episode) F32.89
    recurrent episode F33.8
endogenous (without psychotic symptoms) F33.2
    with psychotic symptoms F33.3
functional activity R68.89
hysterical F44.89
involutional (single episode) F32.89
    recurrent episode F33.8
major F32.9
    with psychotic symptoms F32.3

Depression — *continued*

major — *continued*
    recurrent — *see* Disorder, depressive, recurrent
manic-depressive — *see* Disorder, depressive, recurrent
masked (single episode) F32.89
medullary G93.89
menopausal (single episode) F32.89
    recurrent episode F33.8
metatarsus — *see* Depression, arches
monopolar F33.9
nervous F34.1
neurotic F34.1
nose M95.0
postnatal (NOS) F53.0
postpartum (NOS) F53.0
post-psychotic of schizophrenia F32.89
post-schizophrenic F32.89
psychogenic (reactive) (single episode) F32.9
psychoneurotic F34.1
psychotic (single episode) F32.3
    recurrent F33.3
reactive (psychogenic) (single episode) F32.9
    psychotic (single episode) F32.3
recurrent — *see* Disorder, depressive, recurrent
respiratory center G93.89
seasonal — *see* Disorder, depressive, recurrent
senile F03 ☑
severe, single episode F32.2
situational F43.21
skull Q67.4
specified NEC (single episode) F32.89
sternum M95.4
visual field — *see* Defect, visual field
vital (recurrent) (without psychotic symptoms) F33.2
    with psychotic symptoms F33.3
    single episode F32.2

Deprivation
cultural Z60.3
effects NOS T73.9 ☑
    specified NEC T73.8 ☑
emotional NEC Z65.8
    affecting infant or child — *see* Maltreatment, child, psychological
food T73.0 ☑
protein — *see* Malnutrition
sleep Z72.820
social Z60.4
    affecting infant or child — *see* Maltreatment, child, psychological
specified NEC T73.8 ☑
vitamins — *see* Deficiency, vitamin
water T73.1 ☑

Derangement
ankle (internal) — *see* Derangement, joint, ankle
cartilage (articular) NEC — *see* Derangement, joint, articular cartilage, by site
    recurrent — *see* Dislocation, recurrent
cruciate ligament, anterior, current injury — *see* Sprain, knee, cruciate, anterior
elbow (internal) — *see* Derangement, joint, elbow
hip (joint) (internal) (old) — *see* Derangement, joint, hip
joint (internal) M24.9
    ankylosis — *see* Ankylosis
    articular cartilage M24.10
        ankle M24.17- ☑
        elbow M24.12- ☑
        foot M24.17- ☑
        hand M24.14- ☑
        hip M24.15- ☑
        knee NEC M23.9- ☑
        loose body — *see* Loose, body
        shoulder M24.11- ☑
        specified site NEC M24.19
        wrist M24.13- ☑
    contracture — *see* Contraction, joint
    current injury — *see also* Dislocation
        knee, meniscus or cartilage — *see* Tear, meniscus
    dislocation
        pathological — *see* Dislocation, pathological
        recurrent — *see* Dislocation, recurrent
    knee — *see* Derangement, knee
    ligament — *see* Disorder, ligament
    loose body — *see* Loose, body
    recurrent — *see* Dislocation, recurrent
    specified type NEC M24.80
        ankle M24.87- ☑

☑ **Additional Character Required** — Refer to the Tabular List for Character Selection   ▽ **Subterms under main terms may continue to next column or page**

Derangement — *continued*
  joint — *continued*
    specified type — *continued*
      elbow M24.82- ☑
      foot joint M24.87- ☑
      hand joint M24.84- ☑
      hip M24.85- ☑
      shoulder M24.81- ☑
      specified site NEC M24.89
      wrist M24.83- ☑
    temporomandibular M26.69
  knee (recurrent) M23.9- ☑
    ligament disruption, spontaneous M23.60- ☑
      anterior cruciate M23.61- ☑
      capsular M23.67- ☑
      instability, chronic M23.5- ☑
      lateral collateral M23.64- ☑
      medial collateral M23.63- ☑
      posterior cruciate M23.62- ☑
    loose body M23.4- ☑
    meniscus M23.30- ☑
      cystic M23.00- ☑
        lateral M23.002
          anterior horn M23.04- ☑
          posterior horn M23.05- ☑
          specified NEC M23.06- ☑
        medial M23.005
          anterior horn M23.01- ☑
          posterior horn M23.02- ☑
          specified NEC M23.03- ☑
      degenerate — *see* Derangement, knee, meniscus, specified NEC
      detached — *see* Derangement, knee, meniscus, specified NEC
      due to old tear or injury M23.20- ☑
        lateral M23.20- ☑
          anterior horn M23.24- ☑
          posterior horn M23.25- ☑
          specified NEC M23.26- ☑
        medial M23.20- ☑
          anterior horn M23.21- ☑
          posterior horn M23.22- ☑
          specified NEC M23.23- ☑
      retained — *see* Derangement, knee, meniscus, specified NEC
      specified NEC M23.30- ☑
        lateral M23.30- ☑
          anterior horn M23.34- ☑
          posterior horn M23.35- ☑
          specified NEC M23.36- ☑
        medial M23.30- ☑
          anterior horn M23.31- ☑
          posterior horn M23.32- ☑
          specified NEC M23.33- ☑
    old M23.8X- ☑
    specified NEC — *see* subcategory M23.8 ☑
  low back NEC — *see* Dorsopathy, specified NEC
  meniscus — *see* Derangement, knee, meniscus
  mental — *see* Psychosis
  patella, specified NEC — *see* Disorder, patella, derangement NEC
  semilunar cartilage (knee) — *see* Derangement, knee, meniscus, specified NEC
  shoulder (internal) — *see* Derangement, joint, shoulder

Dercum's disease E88.2
Derealization (neurotic) F48.1
Dermal — *see* condition
Dermaphytid — *see* Dermatophytosis
Dermatitis (eczematous) L30.9
  ab igne L59.0
  acarine B88.0
  actinic (due to sun) L57.8
    other than from sun L59.8
  allergic — *see* Dermatitis, contact, allergic
  ambustionis, due to burn or scald — *see* Burn
  amebic A06.7
  ammonia L22
  arsenical (ingested) L27.8
  artefacta L98.1
    psychogenic F54
  atopic L20.9
    psychogenic F54
    specified NEC L20.89
  autoimmune progesterone L30.8
  berlock, berloque L56.2
  blastomycotic B40.3
  blister beetle L24.89

Dermatitis — *continued*
  bullous, bullosa L13.9
    mucosynechial, atrophic L12.1
    seasonal L30.8
    specified NEC L13.8
  calorica L59.0
    due to burn or scald — *see* Burn
  caterpillar L24.89
  cercarial B65.3
  combustionis L59.0
    due to burn or scald — *see* Burn
  congelationis T69.1 ☑
  contact (occupational) L25.9
    allergic L23.9
      due to
        adhesives L23.1
        cement L23.5
        chemical products NEC L23.5
        chromium L23.0
        cosmetics L23.2
        dander (cat) (dog) L23.81
        drugs in contact with skin L23.3
        dyes L23.4
        food in contact with skin L23.6
        hair (cat) (dog) L23.81
        insecticide L23.5
        metals L23.0
        nickel L23.0
        plants, non-food L23.7
        plastic L23.5
        rubber L23.5
        specified agent NEC L23.89
    due to
      cement L25.3
      chemical products NEC L25.3
      cosmetics L25.0
      dander (cat) (dog) L23.81
      drugs in contact with skin L25.1
      dyes L25.2
      food in contact with skin L25.4
      hair (cat) (dog) L23.81
      plants, non-food L25.5
      specified agent NEC L25.8
    irritant L24.9
      due to
        body fluids L24.A0
          incontinence (dual) (fecal) (urinary) L24.A2
          saliva L24.A1
          specified NEC L24.A9
        cement L24.5
        chemical products NEC L24.5
        cosmetics L24.3
        detergents L24.0
        drugs in contact with skin L24.4
        food in contact with skin L24.6
        oils and greases L24.1
        plants, non-food L24.7
        solvents L24.2
        specified agent NEC L24.89
      related to
        colostomy L24.B3
        endotracheal tube L24.A9
        enterocutaneous fistula L24.B3
        gastrostomy L24.B1
        ileostomy L24.B3
        jejunostomy L24.B1
        saliva or spit fistula L24.B1
        stoma or fistula L24.B0
          digestive L24.B1
          fecal or urinary L24.B3
          respiratory L24.B2
        tracheostomy L24.B2
  contusiformis L52
  desquamative L30.8
  diabetic — *see* E08-E13 with .620
  diaper L22
  diphtheritica A36.3
  dry skin L85.3
  due to
    acetone (contact) (irritant) L24.2
    acids (contact) (irritant) L24.5
    adhesive(s) (allergic) (contact) (plaster) L23.1
      irritant L24.5
    alcohol (irritant) (skin contact) (substances in category T51) L24.2
      taken internally L27.8
    alkalis (contact) (irritant) L24.5
    arsenic (ingested) L27.8

Dermatitis — *continued*
  due to — *continued*
    carbon disulfide (contact) (irritant) L24.2
    caustics (contact) (irritant) L24.5
    cement (contact) L25.3
    cereal (ingested) L27.2
    chemical(s) NEC L25.3
      taken internally L27.8
    chlorocompounds L24.2
    chromium (contact) (irritant) L24.81
    coffee (ingested) L27.2
    cold weather L30.8
    cosmetics (contact) L25.0
      allergic L23.2
      irritant L24.3
    cyclohexanes L24.2
    dander (cat) (dog) L23.81
    Demodex species B88.0
    Dermanyssus gallinae B88.0
    detergents (contact) (irritant) L24.0
    dichromate L24.81
    drugs and medicaments (generalized) (internal use) L27.0
      external — *see* Dermatitis, due to, drugs, in contact with skin
      in contact with skin L25.1
        allergic L23.3
        irritant L24.4
      localized skin eruption L27.1
      specified substance — *see* Table of Drugs and Chemicals
    dyes (contact) L25.2
      allergic L23.4
      irritant L24.89
    epidermophytosis — *see* Dermatophytosis
    esters L24.2
    external irritant NEC L24.9
    fish (ingested) L27.2
    flour (ingested) L27.2
    food (ingested) L27.2
      in contact with skin L25.4
    fruit (ingested) L27.2
    furs (allergic) (contact) L23.81
    glues — *see* Dermatitis, due to, adhesives
    glycols L24.2
    greases NEC (contact) (irritant) L24.1
    hair (cat) (dog) L23.81
    hot
      objects and materials — *see* Burn
      weather or places L59.0
    hydrocarbons L24.2
    infrared rays L59.8
    ingestion, ingested substance L27.9
      chemical NEC L27.8
      drugs and medicaments — *see* Dermatitis, due to, drugs
      food L27.2
      specified NEC L27.8
    insecticide in contact with skin L24.5
    internal agent L27.9
      drugs and medicaments (generalized) — *see* Dermatitis, due to, drugs
      food L27.2
    irradiation — *see* Dermatitis, due to, radioactive substance
    ketones L24.2
    lacquer tree (allergic) (contact) L23.7
    light (sun) NEC L57.8
      acute L56.8
      other L59.8
    Liponyssoides sanguineus B88.0
    low temperature L30.8
    meat (ingested) L27.2
    metals, metal salts (contact) (irritant) L24.81
    milk (ingested) L27.2
    nickel (contact) (irritant) L24.81
    nylon (contact) (irritant) L24.5
    oils NEC (contact) (irritant) L24.1
    paint solvent (contact) (irritant) L24.2
    petroleum products (contact) (irritant) (substances in T52.0) L24.2
    plants NEC (contact) L25.5
      allergic L23.7
      irritant L24.7
    plasters (adhesive) (any) (allergic) (contact) L23.1
      irritant L24.5
    plastic (contact) L25.3

▽ **Subterms under main terms may continue to next column or page**   ☑ **Additional Character Required** — Refer to the Tabular List for Character Selection   **97**

Derangement — Dermatitis

Dermatitis — *continued*
  due to — *continued*
    preservatives (contact) — *see* Dermatitis, due to, chemical, in contact with skin
    primrose (allergic) (contact) L23.7
    primula (allergic) (contact) L23.7
    radiation L59.8
      nonionizing (chronic exposure) L57.8
      sun NEC L57.8
        acute L56.8
    radioactive substance L58.9
      acute L58.0
      chronic L58.1
    radium L58.9
      acute L58.0
      chronic L58.1
    ragweed (allergic) (contact) L23.7
    Rhus (allergic) (contact) (diversiloba) (radicans) (toxicodendron) (venenata) (verniciflua) L23.7
    rubber (contact) L24.5
    Senecio jacobaea (allergic) (contact) L23.7
    solvents (contact) (irritant) (substances in category T52) L24.2
    specified agent NEC (contact) L25.8
      allergic L23.89
      irritant L24.89
    sunshine NEC L57.8
      acute L56.8
    tetrachlorethylene (contact) (irritant) L24.2
    toluene (contact) (irritant) L24.2
    turpentine (contact) L24.2
    ultraviolet rays (sun NEC) (chronic exposure) L57.8
      acute L56.8
    vaccine or vaccination L27.0
      specified substance — *see* Table of Drugs and Chemicals
    varicose veins — *see* Varix, leg, with, inflammation
    X-rays L58.9
      acute L58.0
      chronic L58.1
  dyshydrotic L30.1
  dysmenorrheica N94.6
  escharotica — *see* Burn
  exfoliative, exfoliativa (generalized) L26
    neonatorum L00
  eyelid — *see also* Dermatosis, eyelid H01.9
    allergic H01.119
      left H01.116
        lower H01.115
        upper H01.114
      right H01.113
        lower H01.112
        upper H01.111
    contact — *see* Dermatitis, eyelid, allergic
    due to
      Demodex species B88.0
      herpes (zoster) B02.39
        simplex B00.59
    eczematous H01.139
      left H01.136
        lower H01.135
        upper H01.134
      right H01.133
        lower H01.132
        upper H01.131
    specified NEC H01.8
  facta, factitia, factitial L98.1
    psychogenic F54
  flexural NEC L20.82
  friction L30.4
  fungus B36.9
    specified type NEC B36.8
  gangrenosa, gangrenous infantum L08.0
  harvest mite B88.0
  heat L59.0
  herpesviral, vesicular (ear) (lip) B00.1
  herpetiformis (bullous) (erythematous) (pustular) (vesicular) L13.0
    juvenile L12.2
    senile L12.0
  hiemalis L30.8
  hypostatic, hypostatica — *see* Varix, leg, with, inflammation
  infectious eczematoid L30.3
  infective L30.3
  irritant — *see* Dermatitis, contact, irritant
  Jacquet's (diaper dermatitis) L22
  Leptus B88.0

Dermatitis — *continued*
  lichenified NEC L28.0
  medicamentosa (generalized) (internal use) — *see* Dermatitis, due to drugs
  mite B88.0
  multiformis L13.0
    juvenile L12.2
  napkin L22
  neurotica L13.0
  nummular L30.0
  papillaris capillitii L73.0
  pellagrous E52
  perioral L71.0
  photocontact L56.2
  polymorpha dolorosa L13.0
  pruriginosa L13.0
  pruritic NEC L30.8
  psychogenic F54
  purulent L08.0
  pustular
    contagious B08.02
    subcorneal L13.1
  pyococcal L08.0
  pyogenica L08.0
  repens L40.2
  Ritter's (exfoliativa) L00
  Schamberg's L81.7
  schistosome B65.3
  seasonal bullous L30.8
  seborrheic L21.9
    infantile L21.1
    specified NEC L21.8
  sensitization NOS L23.9
  septic L08.0
  solare L57.8
  specified NEC L30.8
  stasis I87.2
    with
      varicose ulcer — *see* Varix, leg, with ulcer, with inflammation
      varicose veins — *see* Varix, leg, with, inflammation
    due to postthrombotic syndrome — *see* Syndrome, postthrombotic
  suppurative L08.0
  traumatic NEC L30.4
  trophoneurotica L13.0
  ultraviolet (sun) (chronic exposure) L57.8
    acute L56.8
  varicose — *see* Varix, leg, with, inflammation
  vegetans L10.1
  verrucosa B43.0
  vesicular, herpesviral B00.1

Dermatoarthritis, lipoid E78.81
Dermatochalasis, eyelid H02.839
  left H02.836
    lower H02.835
    upper H02.834
  right H02.833
    lower H02.832
    upper H02.831
Dermatofibroma (lenticulare) — *see* Neoplasm, skin, benign
  protuberans — *see* Neoplasm, skin, uncertain behavior
Dermatofibrosarcoma (pigmented) (protuberans) — *see* Neoplasm, skin, malignant
Dermatographia L50.3
Dermatolysis (exfoliativa) (congenital) Q82.8
  acquired L57.4
  eyelids — *see* Blepharochalasis
  palpebrarum — *see* Blepharochalasis
  senile L57.4
Dermatomegaly NEC Q82.8
Dermatomucosomyositis M33.10
  with
    myopathy M33.12
    respiratory involvement M33.11
    specified organ involvement NEC M33.19
Dermatomycosis B36.9
  furfuracea B36.0
  specified type NEC B36.8
Dermatomyositis (acute) (chronic) — *see also* Dermatopolymyositis
  adult — *see also* Dermatomyositis, specified NEC M33.10
  in (due to) neoplastic disease — *see also* Neoplasm D49.9 [M36.0]
  juvenile M33.00

Dermatomyositis — *continued*
  juvenile — *continued*
    with
      myopathy M33.02
      respiratory involvement M33.01
      specified organ involvement NEC M33.09
    without myopathy M33.03
  specified NEC M33.10
    with
      myopathy M33.12
      respiratory involvement M33.11
      specified organ involvement NEC M33.19
    without myopathy M33.13
Dermatoneuritis of children — *see* Poisoning, mercury
Dermatophilosis A48.8
Dermatophytid L30.2
Dermatophytide — *see* Dermatophytosis
Dermatophytosis (epidermophyton) (infection) (Microsporum) (tinea) (Trichophyton) B35.9
  beard B35.0
  body B35.4
  capitis B35.0
  corporis B35.4
  deep-seated B35.8
  disseminated B35.8
  foot B35.3
  granulomatous B35.8
  groin B35.6
  hand B35.2
  nail B35.1
  perianal (area) B35.6
  scalp B35.0
  specified NEC B35.8
Dermatopolymyositis M33.90
  with
    myopathy M33.92
    respiratory involvement M33.91
    specified organ involvement NEC M33.99
  in neoplastic disease — *see also* Neoplasm D49.9 [M36.0]
  juvenile M33.00
    with
      myopathy M33.02
      respiratory involvement M33.01
      specified organ involvement NEC M33.09
  specified NEC M33.10
    myopathy M33.12
    respiratory involvement M33.11
    specified organ involvement NEC M33.19
  without myopathy M33.93
Dermatopolyneuritis — *see* Poisoning, mercury
Dermatorrhexis — *see also* Syndrome, Ehlers-Danlos Q79.60
  acquired L57.4
Dermatosclerosis — *see also* Scleroderma
  localized L94.0
Dermatosis L98.9
  Andrews' L08.89
  Bowen's — *see* Neoplasm, skin, in situ
  bullous L13.9
    specified NEC L13.8
  exfoliativa L26
  eyelid (noninfectious) — *see also* Dermatitis, eyelid H01.9
    discoid lupus erythematosus — *see* Lupus, erythematosus, eyelid
    xeroderma — *see* Xeroderma, acquired, eyelid
  factitial L98.1
  febrile neutrophilic L98.2
  gonococcal A54.89
  herpetiformis L13.0
    juvenile L12.2
  linear IgA L13.8
  menstrual NEC L98.8
  neutrophilic, febrile L98.2
  occupational — *see* Dermatitis, contact
  papulosa nigra L82.1
  pigmentary L81.9
    progressive L81.7
    Schamberg's L81.7
  psychogenic F54
  purpuric, pigmented L81.7
  pustular, subcorneal L13.1
  transient acantholytic L11.1
Dermographia, dermographism L50.3
Dermoid (cyst) — *see also* Neoplasm, benign, by site
  with malignant transformation C56- ☑
  due to radiation (nonionizing) L57.8

☑ **Additional Character Required** — Refer to the Tabular List for Character Selection   ▽ **Subterms under main terms may continue to next column or page**

Dermopathy
infiltrative with thyrotoxicosis — *see* Thyrotoxicosis
nephrogenic fibrosing L90.8
Dermophytosis — *see* Dermatophytosis
Descemetocele H18.73- ☑
Descemet's membrane — *see* condition
Descending — *see* condition
Descensus uteri — *see* Prolapse, uterus
Desert
rheumatism B38.0
sore — *see* Ulcer, skin
Desertion (newborn) — *see* Maltreatment
Desmoid (extra-abdominal) (tumor) — *see* Neoplasm, connective tissue, uncertain behavior
abdominal D48.1
Despondency F32.A
Desquamation, skin R23.4
Destruction, destructive — *see also* Damage
articular facet — *see also* Derangement, joint, specified type NEC
knee M23.8X- ☑
vertebra — *see* Spondylosis
bone — *see also* Disorder, bone, specified type NEC
syphilitic A52.77
joint — *see also* Derangement, joint, specified type NEC
sacroiliac M53.3
rectal sphincter K62.89
septum (nasal) J34.89
tuberculous NEC — *see* Tuberculosis
tympanum, tympanic membrane (nontraumatic) — *see* Disorder, tympanic membrane, specified NEC
vertebral disc — *see* Degeneration, intervertebral disc
Destructiveness — *see also* Disorder, conduct
adjustment reaction — *see* Disorder, adjustment
Desultory labor O62.2
Detachment
cartilage — *see* Sprain
cervix, annular N88.8
complicating delivery O71.3
choroid (old) (postinfectional) (simple) (spontaneous) H31.40- ☑
hemorrhagic H31.41- ☑
serous H31.42- ☑
ligament — *see* Sprain
meniscus (knee) — *see also* Derangement, knee, meniscus, specified NEC
current injury — *see* Tear, meniscus
due to old tear or injury — *see* Derangement, knee, meniscus, due to old tear
retina (without retinal break) (serous) H33.2- ☑
with retinal:
break H33.00- ☑
giant H33.03- ☑
multiple H33.02- ☑
single H33.01- ☑
dialysis H33.04- ☑
pigment epithelium — *see* Degeneration, retina, separation of layers, pigment epithelium detachment
rhegmatogenous — *see* Detachment, retina, with retinal, break
specified NEC H33.8
total H33.05- ☑
traction H33.4- ☑
vitreous (body) H43.81 ☑
Detergent asthma J69.8
Deterioration
epileptic F06.8
general physical R53.81
heart, cardiac — *see* Degeneration, myocardial
mental — *see* Psychosis
myocardial, myocardium — *see* Degeneration, myocardial
senile (simple) R54
Deuteranomaly (anomalous trichromat) H53.53
Deuteranopia (complete) (incomplete) H53.53
Development
abnormal, bone Q79.9
arrested R62.50
bone — *see* Arrest, development or growth, bone
child R62.50
due to malnutrition E45
defective, congenital — *see also* Anomaly, by site
cauda equina Q06.3
left ventricle Q24.8
in hypoplastic left heart syndrome Q23.4

Development — *continued*
defective, congenital — *see also* Anomaly, by site — *continued*
valve Q24.8
pulmonary Q22.3
delayed — *see also* Delay, development R62.50
arithmetical skills F81.2
language (skills) (expressive) F80.1
learning skill F81.9
mixed skills F88
motor coordination F82
reading F81.0
specified learning skill NEC F81.89
speech F80.9
spelling F81.81
written expression F81.81
imperfect, congenital — *see also* Anomaly, by site
heart Q24.9
lungs Q33.6
incomplete
bronchial tree Q32.4
organ or site not listed — *see* Hypoplasia, by site
respiratory system Q34.9
sexual, precocious NEC E30.1
tardy, mental — *see also* Disability, intellectual F79
Developmental — *see* condition
testing, infant or child — *see* Examination, child
Devergie's disease (pityriasis rubra pilaris) L44.0
Deviation (in)
conjugate palsy (eye) (spastic) H51.0
esophagus (acquired) K22.89
eye, skew H51.8
midline (jaw) (teeth) (dental arch) M26.29
specified site NEC — *see* Malposition
nasal septum J34.2
congenital Q67.4
opening and closing of the mandible M26.53
organ or site, congenital NEC — *see* Malposition, congenital
septum (nasal) (acquired) J34.2
congenital Q67.4
sexual F65.9
bestiality F65.89
erotomania F52.8
exhibitionism F65.2
fetishism, fetishistic F65.0
transvestism F65.1
frotteurism F65.81
masochism F65.51
multiple F65.89
necrophilia F65.89
nymphomania F52.8
pederosis F65.4
pedophilia F65.4
sadism, sadomasochism F65.52
satyriasis F52.8
specified type NEC F65.89
transvestism F64.1
voyeurism F65.3
teeth, midline M26.29
trachea J39.8
ureter, congenital Q62.61
Device
cerebral ventricle (communicating) in situ Z98.2
contraceptive — *see* Contraceptive, device
drainage, cerebrospinal fluid, in situ Z98.2
Devic's disease G36.0
Devil's
grip B33.0
pinches (purpura simplex) D69.2
Devitalized tooth K04.99
Devonshire colic — *see* Poisoning, lead
Dextraposition, aorta Q20.3
in tetralogy of Fallot Q21.3
Dextrinosis, limit (debrancher enzyme deficiency) E74.03
Dextrocardia (true) Q24.0
with
complete transposition of viscera Q89.3
situs inversus Q89.3
Dextrotransposition, aorta Q20.3
d-glyceric acidemia E72.59
Dhat syndrome F48.8
Dhobi itch B35.6
Di George's syndrome D82.1
Di Guglielmo's disease C94.0- ☑
Diabetes, diabetic (mellitus) (sugar) E11.9
with
amyotrophy E11.44

Diabetes, diabetic — *continued*
with — *continued*
arthropathy NEC E11.618
autonomic (poly)neuropathy E11.43
cataract E11.36
Charcot's joints E11.610
chronic kidney disease E11.22
circulatory complication NEC E11.59
coma due to
hyperosmolarity E11.01
hypoglycemia E11.641
ketoacidosis E11.11
complication E11.8
specified NEC E11.69
dermatitis E11.620
foot ulcer E11.621
gangrene E11.52
gastroparalysis E11.43
gastroparesis E11.43
glomerulonephrosis, intracapillary E11.21
glomerulosclerosis, intercapillary E11.21
hyperglycemia E11.65
hyperosmolarity E11.00
with coma E11.01
hypoglycemia E11.649
with coma E11.641
ketoacidosis E11.10
with coma E11.11
kidney complications NEC E11.29
Kimmelstiel-Wilson disease E11.21
loss of protective sensation (LOPS) — *see* Diabetes, by type, with neuropathy
mononeuropathy E11.41
myasthenia E11.44
necrobiosis lipoidica E11.620
nephropathy E11.21
neuralgia E11.42
neurologic complication NEC E11.49
neuropathic arthropathy E11.610
neuropathy E11.40
ophthalmic complication NEC E11.39
oral complication NEC E11.638
osteomyelitis E11.69
periodontal disease E11.630
peripheral angiopathy E11.51
with gangrene E11.52
polyneuropathy E11.42
renal complication NEC E11.29
renal tubular degeneration E11.29
retinopathy E11.319
with macular edema E11.311
resolved following treatment E11.37- ☑
nonproliferative E11.329 ☑
with macular edema E11.321 ☑
mild E11.329 ☑
with macular edema E11.321 ☑
moderate E11.339 ☑
with macular edema E11.331 ☑
severe E11.349 ☑
with macular edema E11.341 ☑
proliferative E11.359 ☑
with
combined traction retinal detachment and rhegmatogenous retinal detachment E11.354 ☑
macular edema E11.351 ☑
stable proliferative diabetic retinopathy E11.355 ☑
traction retinal detachment involving the macula E11.352 ☑
traction retinal detachment not involving the macula E11.353 ☑
resolved following treatment E09.37 ☑
skin complication NEC E11.628
skin ulcer NEC E11.622
brittle — *see* Diabetes, type 1
bronzed E83.110
complicating pregnancy — *see* Pregnancy, complicated by, diabetes
dietary counseling and surveillance Z71.3
due to
autoimmune process — *see* Diabetes, type 1
immune mediated pancreatic islet beta-cell destruction — *see* Diabetes, type 1
due to drug or chemical E09.9
with
amyotrophy E09.44
arthropathy NEC E09.618

Diabetes, diabetic — *continued*
  due to drug or chemical — *continued*
    with — *continued*
      autonomic (poly)neuropathy E09.43
      cataract E09.36
      Charcot's joints E09.610
      chronic kidney disease E09.22
      circulatory complication NEC E09.59
      complication E09.8
        specified NEC E09.69
      dermatitis E09.620
      foot ulcer E09.621
      gangrene E09.52
      gastroparalysis E09.43
      gastroparesis E09.43
      glomerulonephrosis, intracapillary E09.21
      glomerulosclerosis, intercapillary E09.21
      hyperglycemia E09.65
      hyperosmolarity E09.00
        with coma E09.01
      hypoglycemia E09.649
        with coma E09.641
      ketoacidosis E09.10
        with coma E09.11
      kidney complications NEC E09.29
      Kimmelstein-Wilson disease E09.21
      mononeuropathy E09.41
      myasthenia E09.44
      necrobiosis lipoidica E09.620
      nephropathy E09.21
      neuralgia E09.42
      neurologic complication NEC E09.49
      neuropathic arthropathy E09.610
      neuropathy E09.40
      ophthalmic complication NEC E09.39
      oral complication NEC E09.638
      periodontal disease E09.630
      peripheral angiopathy E09.51
        with gangrene E09.52
      polyneuropathy E09.42
      renal complication NEC E09.29
      renal tubular degeneration E09.29
      retinopathy E09.319
        with macular edema E09.311
        resolved following treatment E09.37 ☑
        nonproliferative E09.329 ☑
          with macular edema E09.321 ☑
          mild E09.329 ☑
            with macular edema E09.321 ☑
          moderate E09.339 ☑
            with macular edema E09.331 ☑
          severe E09.349 ☑
            with macular edema E09.341 ☑
        proliferative E09.359 ☑
          with
            combined traction retinal detachment
              and rhegmatogenous retinal
              detachment E09.354 ☑
            macular edema E09.351 ☑
            stable proliferative diabetic retinopa-
              thy E09.355 ☑
            traction retinal detachment involving
              the macula E09.352 ☑
            traction retinal detachment not involv-
              ing the macula E09.353 ☑
      skin complication NEC E09.628
      skin ulcer NEC E09.622
  due to underlying condition E08.9
    with
      amyotrophy E08.44
      arthropathy NEC E08.618
      autonomic (poly)neuropathy E08.43
      cataract E08.36
      Charcot's joints E08.610
      chronic kidney disease E08.22
      circulatory complication NEC E08.59
      complication E08.8
        specified NEC E08.69
      dermatitis E08.620
      foot ulcer E08.621
      gangrene E08.52
      gastroparalysis E08.43
      gastroparesis E08.43
      glomerulonephrosis, intracapillary E08.21
      glomerulosclerosis, intercapillary E08.21
      hyperglycemia E08.65
      hyperosmolarity E08.00
        with coma E08.01

Diabetes, diabetic — *continued*
  due to underlying condition — *continued*
    with — *continued*
      hypoglycemia E08.649
        with coma E08.641
      ketoacidosis E08.10
        with coma E08.11
      kidney complications NEC E08.29
      Kimmelsteil-Wilson disease E08.21
      mononeuropathy E08.41
      myasthenia E08.44
      necrobiosis lipoidica E08.620
      nephropathy E08.21
      neuralgia E08.42
      neurologic complication NEC E08.49
      neuropathic arthropathy E08.610
      neuropathy E08.40
      ophthalmic complication NEC E08.39
      oral complication NEC E08.638
      periodontal disease E08.630
      peripheral angiopathy E08.51
        with gangrene E08.52
      polyneuropathy E08.42
      renal complication NEC E08.29
      renal tubular degeneration E08.29
      retinopathy E08.319
        with macular edema E08.311
        resolved following treatment E08.37 ☑
        nonproliferative E08.329 ☑
          with macular edema E08.321 ☑
          mild E08.329 ☑
            with macular edema E08.321 ☑
          moderate E08.339 ☑
            with macular edema E08.331 ☑
          severe E08.349 ☑
            with macular edema E08.341 ☑
        proliferative E08.359 ☑
          with
            combined traction retinal detachment
              and rhegmatogenous retinal
              detachment E08.354 ☑
            macular edema E08.351 ☑
            stable proliferative diabetic retinopa-
              thy E08.355 ☑
            traction retinal detachment involving
              the macula E08.352 ☑
            traction retinal detachment not involv-
              ing the macula E08.353 ☑
      skin complication NEC E08.628
      skin ulcer NEC E08.622
  gestational (in pregnancy) O24.419
    affecting newborn P70.0
    diet controlled O24.410
    in childbirth O24.429
      diet controlled O24.420
      insulin (and diet) controlled O24.424
      oral drug controlled (antidiabetic) (hypo-
        glycemic) O24.425
    insulin (and diet) controlled O24.414
    oral drug controlled (antidiabetic) (hypoglycemic)
      O24.415
    puerperal O24.439
      diet controlled O24.430
      insulin (and diet) controlled O24.434
      oral drug controlled (antidiabetic) (hypo-
        glycemic) O24.435
  hepatogenous E13.9
  idiopathic — *see* Diabetes, type 1
  inadequately controlled — *code to* Diabetes, by type,
    with hyperglycemia
  insipidus E23.2
    nephrogenic N25.1
    pituitary E23.2
    vasopressin resistant N25.1
  insulin dependent — *code to* type of diabetes
  juvenile-onset — *see* Diabetes, type 1
  ketosis-prone — *see* Diabetes, type 1
  latent R73.03
  neonatal (transient) P70.2
  non-insulin dependent — *code to* type of diabetes
  out of control — *code to* Diabetes, by type, with hyper-
    glycemia
  phosphate E83.39
  poorly controlled — *code to* Diabetes, by type, with
    hyperglycemia
  postpancreatectomy — *see* Diabetes, specified type
    NEC
  postprocedural — *see* Diabetes, specified type NEC

Diabetes, diabetic — *continued*
  secondary diabetes mellitus NEC — *see* Diabetes,
    specified type NEC
  specified type NEC E13.9
    with
      amyotrophy E13.44
      arthropathy NEC E13.618
      autonomic (poly)neuropathy E13.43
      cataract E13.36
      Charcot's joints E13.610
      chronic kidney disease E13.22
      circulatory complication NEC E13.59
      complication E13.8
        specified NEC E13.69
      dermatitis E13.620
      foot ulcer E13.621
      gangrene E13.52
      gastroparalysis E13.43
      gastroparesis E13.43
      glomerulonephrosis, intracapillary E13.21
      glomerulosclerosis, intercapillary E13.21
      hyperglycemia E13.65
      hyperosmolarity E13.00
        with coma E13.01
      hypoglycemia E13.649
        with coma E13.641
      ketoacidosis E13.10
        with coma E13.11
      kidney complications NEC E13.29
      Kimmelsteil-Wilson disease E13.21
      mononeuropathy E13.41
      myasthenia E13.44
      necrobiosis lipoidica E13.620
      nephropathy E13.21
      neuralgia E13.42
      neurologic complication NEC E13.49
      neuropathic arthropathy E13.610
      neuropathy E13.40
      ophthalmic complication NEC E13.39
      oral complication NEC E13.638
      periodontal disease E13.630
      peripheral angiopathy E13.51
        with gangrene E13.52
      polyneuropathy E13.42
      renal complication NEC E13.29
      renal tubular degeneration E13.29
      retinopathy E13.319
        with macular edema E13.311
        resolved following treatment E13.37 ☑
        nonproliferative E13.329 ☑
          with macular edema E13.321 ☑
          mild E13.329 ☑
            with macular edema E13.321 ☑
          moderate E13.339 ☑
            with macular edema E13.331 ☑
          severe E13.349 ☑
            with macular edema E13.341 ☑
        proliferative E13.359 ☑
          with
            combined traction retinal detachment
              and rhegmatogenous retinal
              detachment E13.354 ☑
            macular edema E13.351 ☑
            stable proliferative diabetic retinopa-
              thy E13.355 ☑
            traction retinal detachment involving
              the macula E13.352 ☑
            traction retinal detachment not involv-
              ing the macula E13.353 ☑
    skin complication NEC E13.628
    skin ulcer NEC E13.622
  steroid-induced — *see* Diabetes, due to, drug or
    chemical
  type 1 E10.9
    with
      amyotrophy E10.44
      arthropathy NEC E10.618
      autonomic (poly)neuropathy E10.43
      cataract E10.36
      Charcot's joints E10.610
      chronic kidney disease E10.22
      circulatory complication NEC E10.59
      coma due to
        hyperosmolarity E11.01
        hypoglycemia E11.641
        ketoacidosis E10.11
      complication E10.8
        specified NEC E10.69

☑ **Additional Character Required** — **Refer to the Tabular List for Character Selection**   ▽ Subterms under main terms may continue to next column or page

Diabetes, diabetic — continued
  type 1 — continued
    with — continued
      dermatitis E10.620
      foot ulcer E10.621
      gangrene E10.52
      gastroparalysis E10.43
      gastroparesis E10.43
      glomerulonephrosis, intracapillary E10.21
      glomerulosclerosis, intercapillary E10.21
      hyperglycemia E10.65
      hypoglycemia E10.649
        with coma E10.641
      ketoacidosis E10.10
        with coma E10.11
      kidney complications NEC E10.29
      Kimmelsteil-Wilson disease E10.21
      mononeuropathy E10.41
      myasthenia E10.44
      necrobiosis lipoidica E10.620
      nephropathy E10.21
      neuralgia E10.42
      neurologic complication NEC E10.49
      neuropathic arthropathy E10.610
      neuropathy E10.40
      ophthalmic complication NEC E10.39
      oral complication NEC E10.638
      osteomyelitis E10.69
      periodontal disease E10.630
      peripheral angiopathy E10.51
        with gangrene E10.52
      polyneuropathy E10.42
      renal complication NEC E10.29
      renal tubular degeneration E10.29
      retinopathy E10.319
        with macular edema E10.311
        resolved following treatment E10.37 ☑
        nonproliferative E10.329 ☑
          with macular edema E10.321 ☑
          mild E10.329 ☑
            with macular edema E10.321 ☑
          moderate E10.339 ☑
            with macular edema E10.331 ☑
          severe E10.349 ☑
            with macular edema E10.341 ☑
        proliferative E10.359 ☑
          with
            combined traction retinal detachment and rhegmatogenous retinal detachment E10.354 ☑
            macular edema E10.351 ☑
            stable proliferative diabetic retinopathy E10.355 ☑
            traction retinal detachment involving the macula E10.352 ☑
            traction retinal detachment not involving the macula E10.353 ☑
      skin complication NEC E10.628
      skin ulcer NEC E10.622
  type 2 E11.9
    with
      amyotrophy E11.44
      arthropathy NEC E11.618
      autonomic (poly)neuropathy E11.43
      cataract E11.36
      Charcot's joints E11.610
      chronic kidney disease E11.22
      circulatory complication NEC E11.59
      coma due to
        hyperosmolarity E11.01
        hypoglycemia E11.641
        ketoacidosis
      complication E11.8
        specified NEC E11.69
      dermatitis E11.620
      foot ulcer E11.621
      gangrene E11.52
      gastroparalysis E11.43
      gastroparesis E11.43
      glomerulonephrosis, intracapillary E11.21
      glomerulosclerosis, intercapillary E11.21
      hyperglycemia E11.65
      hyperosmolarity E11.00
        with coma E11.01
      hypoglycemia E11.649
        with coma E11.641
      ketoacidosis E11.10
        with coma E11.11

Diabetes, diabetic — continued
  type 2 — continued
    with — continued
      kidney complications NEC E11.29
      Kimmelsteil-Wilson disease E11.21
      mononeuropathy E11.41
      myasthenia E11.44
      necrobiosis lipoidica E11.620
      nephropathy E11.21
      neuralgia E11.42
      neurologic complication NEC E11.49
      neuropathic arthropathy E11.610
      neuropathy E11.42
      ophthalmic complication NEC E11.39
      oral complication NEC E11.638
      osteomyelitis E11.69
      periodontal disease E11.630
      peripheral angiopathy E11.51
        with gangrene E11.52
      polyneuropathy E11.42
      renal complication NEC E11.29
      renal tubular degeneration E11.29
      retinopathy E11.319
        with macular edema E11.311
        resolved following treatment E11.37 ☑
        nonproliferative E11.329 ☑
          with macular edema E11.321 ☑
          mild E11.329 ☑
            with macular edema E11.321 ☑
          moderate E11.339 ☑
            with macular edema E11.331 ☑
          severe E11.349 ☑
            with macular edema E11.341 ☑
        proliferative E11.359 ☑
          with
            combined traction retinal detachment and rhegmatogenous retinal detachment E11.354 ☑
            macular edema E11.351 ☑
            stable proliferative diabetic retinopathy E11.355 ☑
            traction retinal detachment involving the macula E11.352 ☑
            traction retinal detachment not involving the macula E11.353 ☑
      skin complication NEC E11.628
      skin ulcer NEC E11.622
  uncontrolled
    meaning
      hyperglycemia — see Diabetes, by type, with, hyperglycemia
      hypoglycemia — see Diabetes, by type, with, hypoglycemia
Diacyclothrombopathia D69.1
Diagnosis deferred R69
Dialysis (intermittent) (treatment)
  noncompliance (with) Z91.15
  renal (hemodialysis) (peritoneal), status Z99.2
  retina, retinal — see Detachment, retina, with retinal, dialysis
Diamond-Blackfan anemia (congenital hypoplastic) D61.01
Diamond-Gardener syndrome (autoerythrocyte sensitization) D69.2
Diaper rash L22
Diaphoresis (excessive) R61
Diaphragm — see condition
Diaphragmalgia R07.1
Diaphragmatitis, diaphragmitis J98.6
Diaphysial aclasis Q78.6
Diaphysitis — see Osteomyelitis, specified type NEC
Diarrhea, diarrheal (disease) (infantile) (inflammatory) R19.7
  achlorhydric K31.83
  allergic K52.29
    due to
      colitis — see Colitis, allergic
      enteritis — see Enteritis, allergic
  amebic — see also Amebiasis A06.0
    with abscess — see Abscess, amebic
    acute A06.0
    chronic A06.1
    nondysenteric A06.2
  bacillary — see Dysentery, bacillary
  balantidial A07.0
  cachectic NEC K52.89
  Chilomastix A07.8

Diarrhea, diarrheal — continued
  choleriformis A00.1
  chronic (noninfectious) K52.9
  coccidial A07.3
  Cochin-China K90.1
    strongyloidiasis B78.0
  Dientamoeba A07.8
  dietetic — see also Diarrhea, allergic K52.29
  drug-induced K52.1
  due to
    bacteria A04.9
      specified NEC A04.8
    Campylobacter A04.5
    Capillaria philippinensis B81.1
    Clostridium difficile
      not specified as recurrent A04.72
      recurrent A04.71
    Clostridium perfringens (C) (F) A04.8
    Cryptosporidium A07.2
    drugs K52.1
    Escherichia coli A04.4
      enteroaggregative A04.4
      enterohemorrhagic A04.3
      enteroinvasive A04.2
      enteropathogenic A04.0
      enterotoxigenic A04.1
      specified NEC A04.4
    food hypersensitivity — see also Diarrhea, allergic K52.29
    Necator americanus B76.1
    S. japonicum B65.2
    specified organism NEC A08.8
      bacterial A04.8
      viral A08.39
    Staphylococcus A04.8
    Trichuris trichiura B79
    virus — see Enteritis, viral
    Yersinia enterocolitica A04.6
  dysenteric A09
  endemic A09
  epidemic A09
  flagellate A07.9
  Flexner's (ulcerative) A03.1
  functional K59.1
    following gastrointestinal surgery K91.89
    psychogenic F45.8
  Giardia lamblia A07.1
  giardial A07.1
  hill K90.1
  infectious A09
  malarial — see Malaria
  mite B88.0
  mycotic NEC B49
  neonatal (noninfectious) P78.3
  nervous F45.8
  neurogenic K59.1
  noninfectious K52.9
  postgastrectomy K91.1
  postvagotomy K91.1
  protozoal A07.9
    specified NEC A07.8
  psychogenic F45.8
  specified
    bacterium NEC A04.8
    virus NEC A08.39
  strongyloidiasis B78.0
  toxic K52.1
  trichomonal A07.8
  tropical K90.1
  tuberculous A18.32
  viral — see Enteritis, viral
Diastasis
  cranial bones M84.88
    congenital NEC Q75.8
  joint (traumatic) — see Dislocation
  muscle M62.00
    ankle M62.07- ☑
    congenital Q79.8
    foot M62.07- ☑
    forearm M62.03- ☑
    hand M62.04- ☑
    lower leg M62.06- ☑
    pelvic region M62.05- ☑
    shoulder region M62.01- ☑
    specified site NEC M62.08
    thigh M62.05- ☑
    upper arm M62.02- ☑

ⱲⱲⱲ Subterms under main terms may continue to next column or page   ☑ Additional Character Required — Refer to the Tabular List for Character Selection   101

Diabetes, diabetic — Diastasis

Diastasis — continued
recti (abdomen)
complicating delivery O71.89
congenital Q79.59
Diastema, tooth, teeth, fully erupted M26.32
Diastematomyelia Q06.2
Diataxia, cerebral G80.4
Diathesis
allergic — see History, allergy
bleeding (familial) D69.9
cystine (familial) E72.00
gouty — see Gout
hemorrhagic (familial) D69.9
newborn NEC P53
spasmophilic R29.0
Diaz's disease or osteochondrosis (juvenile) (talus) —
see Osteochondrosis, juvenile, tarsus
Dibothriocephalus, dibothriocephaliasis (latus) (infection) (infestation) B70.0
larval B70.1
Dicephalus, dicephaly Q89.4
Dichotomy, teeth K00.2
Dichromat, dichromatopsia (congenital) — see Deficiency, color vision
Dichuchwa A65
Dicroceliasis B66.2
Didelphia, didelphys — see Double uterus
Didymytis N45.1
with orchitis N45.3
Dietary
inadequacy or deficiency E63.9
surveillance and counseling Z71.3
Dietl's crisis N13.8
Dieulafoy lesion (hemorrhagic)
duodenum K31.82
esophagus K22.89
intestine (colon) K63.81
stomach K31.82
Difficult, difficulty (in)
acculturation Z60.3
feeding R63.30
newborn P92.9
breast P92.5
specified NEC P92.8
nonorganic (infant or child) F98.29
specified NEC R63.39
intubation, in anesthesia T88.4 ☑
mechanical, gastroduodenal stoma K91.89
causing obstruction — see also Obstruction, intestine, postoperative K91.30
micturition
need to immediately re-void R39.191
position dependent R39.192
specified NEC R39.198
reading (developmental) F81.0
secondary to emotional disorders F93.9
spelling (specific) F81.81
with reading disorder F81.89
due to inadequate teaching Z55.8
swallowing — see Dysphagia
walking R26.2
work
conditions NEC Z56.5
schedule Z56.3
Diffuse — see condition
Digestive — see condition
Dihydropyrimidine dehydrogenase disease (DPD)
E88.89
Diktyoma — see Neoplasm, malignant, by site
Dilaceration, tooth K00.4
Dilatation
anus K59.89
venule — see Hemorrhoids
aorta (focal) (general) — see Ectasia, aorta
with aneuysm — see Aneurysm, aorta
congenital Q25.44
artery — see Aneurysm
bladder (sphincter) N32.89
congenital Q64.79
blood vessel I99.8
bronchial J47.9
with
exacerbation (acute) J47.1
lower respiratory infection J47.0
calyx N28.89
due to obstruction — see Hydronephrosis
capillaries I78.8

Dilatation — continued
cardiac (acute) (chronic) — see also Hypertrophy, cardiac
congenital Q24.8
valve NEC Q24.8
pulmonary Q22.3
valve — see Endocarditis
cavum septi pellucidi Q06.8
cervix (uteri) — see also Incompetency, cervix
incomplete, poor, slow complicating delivery O62.0
colon K59.39
congenital Q43.1
psychogenic F45.8
toxic K59.31
common duct (acquired) K83.8
congenital Q44.5
cystic duct (acquired) K82.8
congenital Q44.5
duct, mammary — see Ectasia, mammary duct
duodenum K59.89
esophagus K22.89
congenital Q39.5
due to achalasia K22.0
eustachian tube, congenital Q17.8
gallbladder K82.8
gastric — see Dilatation, stomach
heart (acute) (chronic) — see also Hypertrophy, cardiac
congenital Q24.8
valve — see Endocarditis
ileum K59.89
psychogenic F45.8
jejunum K59.89
psychogenic F45.8
kidney (calyx) (collecting structures) (cystic)
(parenchyma) (pelvis) (idiopathic) N28.89
due to obstruction — see Hydronephrosis
lacrimal passages or duct — see Disorder, lacrimal system, changes
lymphatic vessel I89.0
mammary duct — see Ectasia, mammary duct
Meckel's diverticulum (congenital) Q43.0
malignant — see Table of Neoplasms, small intestine, malignant
myocardium (acute) (chronic) — see Hypertrophy, cardiac
organ or site, congenital NEC — see Distortion
pancreatic duct K86.89
pericardium — see Pericarditis
pharynx J39.2
prostate N42.89
pulmonary
artery (idiopathic) I28.8
valve, congenital Q22.3
pupil H57.04
rectum K59.39
saccule, congenital Q16.5
salivary gland (duct) K11.8
sphincter ani K62.89
stomach K31.89
acute K31.0
psychogenic F45.8
submaxillary duct K11.8
trachea, congenital Q32.1
ureter (idiopathic) N28.82
congenital Q62.2
due to obstruction N13.4
urethra (acquired) N36.8
vasomotor I73.9
vein I86.8
ventricular, ventricle (acute) (chronic) — see also Hypertrophy, cardiac
cerebral, congenital Q04.8
venule NEC I86.8
vesical orifice N32.89
Dilated, dilation — see Dilatation
Diminished, diminution
hearing (acuity) — see Deafness
sense or sensation (cold) (heat) (tactile) (vibratory)
R20.8
vision NEC H54.7
vital capacity R94.2
Diminuta taenia B71.0
Dimitri-Sturge-Weber disease Q85.8
Dimple
congenital sacral Q82.6
parasacral Q82.6
pilonidal or postanal — see Cyst, pilonidal
Dioctophyme renalis (infection) (infestation) B83.8

Dipetalonemiasis B74.4
Diphallus Q55.69
Diphtheria, diphtheritic (gangrenous) (hemorrhagic)
A36.9
carrier (suspected) Z22.2
cutaneous A36.3
faucial A36.0
infection of wound A36.3
laryngeal A36.2
myocarditis A36.81
nasal, anterior A36.89
nasopharyngeal A36.1
neurological complication A36.89
pharyngeal A36.0
specified site NEC A36.89
tonsillar A36.0
Diphyllobothriasis (intestine) B70.0
larval B70.1
Diplacusis H93.22- ☑
Diplegia (upper limbs) G83.0
congenital (cerebral) G80.8
facial G51.0
lower limbs G82.20
spastic G80.1
Diplococcus, diplococcal — see condition
Diplopia H53.2
Dipsomania F10.20
with
psychosis — see Psychosis, alcoholic
remission F10.21
Dipylidiasis B71.1
DIRA (deficiency of interleukin 1 receptor antagonist)
M04.8
Direction, teeth, abnormal, fully erupted M26.30
Dirofilariasis B74.8
Dirt-eating child F98.3
Disability, disabilities
heart — see Disease, heart
intellectual F79
with
autistic features F84.9
pathogenic CHAMP1 (genetic) (variant) F78.A9
pathogenic HNRNPH2 (genetic) (variant) F78.A9
pathogenic SATB2 (genetic) (variant) F78.A9
pathogenic SETBP1 (genetic) (variant) F78.A9
pathogenic STXBP1 (genetic) (variant) F78.A9
pathogenic SYNGAP1 (genetic) (variant) F78.A1
autosomal dominant F78.A9
autosomal recessive F78.A9
genetic related F78.A9
with
pathogenic CHAMP1 (variant) F78.A9
pathogenic HNRNPH2 (variant) F78.A9
pathogenic SATB2 (variant) F78.A9
pathogenic SETBP1 (variant) F78.A9
pathogenic STXBP1 (variant) F78.A9
pathogenic SYNGAP1 (variant) F78.A1
specified NEC F78.A9
SYNGAP1-related F78.A1
in
autosomal dominant mental retardation F78.A9
autosomal recessive mental retardation F78.A9
SATB2-associated syndrome F78.A9
SETBP1 disorder F78.A9
STXBP1 encephalopathy with epilepsy — see
also Encephalopathy; and — see also
Epilepsy
X-linked mental retardation (syndromic) (Bain
type) F78.A9
mild (I.Q. 50-69) F70
moderate (I.Q. 35-49) F71
profound (I.Q. under 20) F73
severe (I.Q. 20-34) F72
specified level NEC F78.A9
SYNGAP1-related F78.A1
X-linked (syndromic) (Bain type) F78.A9
knowledge acquisition F81.9
learning F81.9
limiting activities Z73.6
spelling, specific F81.81
Disappearance of family member Z63.4
Disarticulation — see Amputation
meaning traumatic amputation — see Amputation,
traumatic
Discharge (from)
abnormal finding in — see Abnormal, specimen
breast (female) (male) N64.52

Discharge — *continued*
  diencephalic autonomic idiopathic — *see* Epilepsy,
      specified NEC
  ear — *see also* Otorrhea
    blood — *see* Otorrhagia
  excessive urine R35.89
  nipple N64.52
  penile R36.9
  postnasal R09.82
  prison, anxiety concerning Z65.2
  urethral R36.9
    without blood R36.0
    hematospermia R36.1
  vaginal N89.8

Discitis, diskitis M46.40
  cervical region M46.42
  cervicothoracic region M46.43
  lumbar region M46.46
  lumbosacral region M46.47
  multiple sites M46.49
  occipito-atlanto-axial region M46.41
  pyogenic — *see* Infection, intervertebral disc, pyogenic
  sacrococcygeal region M46.48
  thoracic region M46.44
  thoracolumbar region M46.45

Discoid
  meniscus (congenital) Q68.6
  semilunar cartilage (congenital) — *see* Derangement,
    knee, meniscus, specified NEC

Discoloration
  nails L60.8
  teeth (posteruptive) K03.7
    during formation K00.8

Discomfort
  chest R07.89
  visual H53.14- ☑

Discontinuity, ossicles, ear H74.2- ☑

Discord (with)
  boss Z56.4
  classmates Z55.4
  counselor Z64.4
  employer Z56.4
  family Z63.8
  fellow employees Z56.4
  in-laws Z63.1
  landlord Z59.2
  lodgers Z59.2
  neighbors Z59.2
  probation officer Z64.4
  social worker Z64.4
  teachers Z55.4
  workmates Z56.4

Discordant connection
  atrioventricular (congenital) Q20.5
  ventriculoarterial Q20.3

Discrepancy
  centric occlusion maximum intercuspation M26.55
  leg length (acquired) — *see* Deformity, limb, unequal
    length
    congenital — *see* Defect, reduction, lower limb
  uterine size date O26.84- ☑

Discrimination
  ethnic Z60.5
  political Z60.5
  racial Z60.5
  religious Z60.5
  sex Z60.5

Disease, diseased — *see also* Syndrome
  absorbent system I87.8
  acid-peptic K30
  Acosta's T70.29 ☑
  Adams-Stokes (-Morgagni) (syncope with heart block)
    I45.9
  Addison's anemia (pernicious) D51.0
  adenoids (and tonsils) J35.9
  adrenal (capsule) (cortex) (gland) (medullary) E27.9
    hyperfunction E27.0
    specified NEC E27.8
  ainhum L94.6
  airway
    obstructive, chronic J44.9
      due to
        cotton dust J66.0
        specific organic dusts NEC J66.8
    reactive — *see* Asthma
  akamushi (scrub typhus) A75.3
  Albers-Schönberg (marble bones) Q78.2
  Albert's — *see* Tendinitis, Achilles

Disease, diseased — *continued*
  alimentary canal K63.9
  alligator-skin Q80.9
    acquired L85.0
  alpha heavy chain C88.3
  alpine T70.29 ☑
  altitude T70.20 ☑
  alveolar ridge
    edentulous K06.9
      specified NEC K06.8
  alveoli, teeth K08.9
  Alzheimer's G30.9 *[F02.80]*
    with behavioral disturbance G30.9 *[F02.81]*
    early onset G30.0 *[F02.80]*
      with behavioral disturbance G30.0 *[F02.81]*
    late onset G30.1 *[F02.80]*
      with behavioral disturbance G30.1 *[F02.81]*
    specified NEC G30.8 *[F02.80]*
      with behavioral disturbance G30.8 *[F02.81]*
  amyloid — *see* Amyloidosis
  Andersen's (glycogenosis IV) E74.09
  Andes T70.29 ☑
  Andrews' (bacterid) L08.89
  angiospastic I73.9
    cerebral G45.9
    vein I87.8
  anterior
    chamber H21.9
    horn cell G12.29
  antiglomerular basement membrane (anti- GBM) anti-
    body M31.0
    tubulo-interstitial nephritis N12
  antral — *see* Sinusitis, maxillary
  anus K62.9
    specified NEC K62.89
  aorta (nonsyphilitic) I77.9
    syphilitic NEC A52.02
  aortic (heart) (valve) I35.9
    rheumatic I06.9
  Apollo B30.3
  aponeuroses — *see* Enthesopathy
  appendix K38.9
    specified NEC K38.8
  aqueous (chamber) H21.9
  Arnold-Chiari — *see* Arnold-Chiari disease
  arterial I77.9
    occlusive — *see* Occlusion, by site
      due to stricture or stenosis I77.1
    peripheral I73.9
  arteriocardiorenal — *see* Hypertension, cardiorenal
  arteriolar (generalized) (obliterative) I77.9
  arteriorenal — *see* Hypertension, kidney
  arteriosclerotic — *see also* Arteriosclerosis
    cardiovascular — *see* Disease, heart, ischemic,
      atherosclerotic
    coronary (artery) — *see* Disease, heart, ischemic,
      atherosclerotic
    heart — *see* Disease, heart, ischemic, atherosclerotic
  artery I77.9
    cerebral I67.9
    coronary I25.10
      with angina pectoris — *see* Arteriosclerosis,
        coronary (artery)
    peripheral I73.9
  arthropod-borne NOS (viral) A94
    specified type NEC A93.8
  atticoantral, chronic H66.20
    left H66.22
      with right H66.23
    right H66.21
      with left H66.23
  auditory canal — *see* Disorder, ear, external
  auricle, ear NEC — *see* Disorder, pinna
  Australian X A83.4
  autoimmune (systemic) NOS M35.9
    hemolytic D59.10
      cold type (primary) (secondary) (symptomatic)
        D59.12
      drug-induced D59.0
      mixed type (primary) (secondary) (symptomatic)
        D59.13
      warm type (primary) (secondary) (symptomatic)
        D59.11
    thyroid E06.3
  autoinflammatory M04.9
    NOD2-associated M04.8
    specified type NEC M04.8
  aviator's — *see* Effect, adverse, high altitude

Disease, diseased — *continued*
  Ayerza's (pulmonary artery sclerosis with pulmonary
    hypertension) I27.0
  Babington's (familial hemorrhagic telangiectasia) I78.0
  bacterial A49.9
    specified NEC A48.8
    zoonotic A28.9
      specified type NEC A28.8
  Baelz's (cheilitis glandularis apostematosa) K13.0
  bagasse J67.1
  balloon — *see* Effect, adverse, high altitude
  Bang's (brucella abortus) A23.1
  Bannister's T78.3 ☑
  barometer makers' — *see* Poisoning, mercury
  Barraquer (-Simons') (progressive lipodystrophy) E88.1
  Barrett's — *see* Barrett's, esophagus
  Bartholin's gland N75.9
  basal ganglia G25.9
    degenerative G23.9
      specified NEC G23.8
    specified NEC G25.89
  Basedow's (exophthalmic goiter) — *see* Hyperthy-
    roidism, with, goiter (diffuse)
  Bateman's B08.1
  Batten-Steinert G71.11
  Battey A31.0
  Beard's (neurasthenia) F48.8
  Becker
    idiopathic mural endomyocardial I42.3
    myotonia congenita G71.12
  Begbie's (exophthalmic goiter) — *see* Hyperthyroidism,
    with, goiter (diffuse)
  behavioral, organic F07.9
  Beigel's (white piedra) B36.2
  Benson's — *see* Deposit, crystalline
  Bernard-Soulier (thrombopathy) D69.1
  Bernhardt (-Roth) — *see* Mononeuropathy, lower limb,
    meralgia paresthetica
  Biermer's (pernicious anemia) D51.0
  bile duct (common) (hepatic) K83.9
    with calculus, stones — *see* Calculus, bile duct
    specified NEC K83.8
  biliary (tract) K83.9
    specified NEC K83.8
  Billroth's — *see* Spina bifida
  bird fancier's J67.2
  black lung J60
  bladder N32.9
    in (due to)
      schistosomiasis (bilharziasis) B65.0 *[N33]*
    specified NEC N32.89
  bleeder's D66
  blood D75.9
    forming organs D75.9
    vessel I99.9
  Bloodgood's — *see* Mastopathy, cystic
  Blount M92.51- ☑
  Bodechtel-Guttmann (subacute sclerosing panen-
    cephalitis) A81.1
  bone — *see also* Disorder, bone
    aluminum M83.4
    fibrocystic NEC
      jaw M27.49
  bone-marrow D75.9
  Borna A83.9
  Bornholm (epidemic pleurodynia) B33.0
  Bouchard's (myopathic dilatation of the stomach) K31.0
  Bouillaud's (rheumatic heart disease) I01.9
  Bourneville (-Brissaud) (tuberous sclerosis) Q85.1
  Bouveret (-Hoffmann) (paroxysmal tachycardia) I47.9
  bowel K63.9
    functional K59.9
      psychogenic F45.8
  brain G93.9
    arterial, artery I67.9
    arteriosclerotic I67.2
    congenital Q04.9
    degenerative — *see* Degeneration, brain
    inflammatory — *see* Encephalitis
    organic G93.9
      arteriosclerotic I67.2
    parasitic NEC B71.9 *[G94]*
    senile NEC G31.1
    specified NEC G93.89
  breast — *see also* Disorder, breast N64.9
    cystic (chronic) — *see* Mastopathy, cystic
    fibrocystic — *see* Mastopathy, cystic

Disease, diseased — *continued*
- breast — *see also* Disorder, breast — *continued*
    - Paget's
        - female, unspecified side C50.91- ✓
        - male, unspecified side C50.92- ✓
        - specified NEC N64.89
- Breda's — *see* Yaws
- Bretonneau's (diphtheritic malignant angina) A36.0
- Bright's — *see* Nephritis
    - arteriosclerotic — *see* Hypertension, kidney
- Brill's (recrudescent typhus) A75.1
- Brill-Zinsser (recrudescent typhus) A75.1
- Brion-Kayser — *see* Fever, paratyphoid
- broad
    - beta E78.2
    - ligament (noninflammatory) N83.9
        - inflammatory — *see* Disease, pelvis, inflammatory
        - specified NEC N83.8
- Brocq-Duhring (dermatitis herpetiformis) L13.0
- Brocq's
    - meaning
        - dermatitis herpetiformis L13.0
        - prurigo L28.2
- bronchopulmonary J98.4
- bronchus NEC J98.09
- bronze Addison's E27.1
    - tuberculous A18.7
- budgerigar fancier's J67.2
- Buerger's (thromboangiitis obliterans) I73.1
- bullous L13.9
    - chronic of childhood L12.2
    - specified NEC L13.8
- Bürger-Grütz (essential familial hyperlipemia) E78.3
- bursa — *see* Bursopathy
- caisson T70.3 ✓
- California — *see* Coccidioidomycosis
- capillaries I78.9
    - specified NEC I78.8
- Carapata A68.0
- cardiac — *see* Disease, heart
- cardiopulmonary, chronic I27.9
- cardiorenal (hepatic) (hypertensive) (vascular) — *see* Hypertension, cardiorenal
- cardiovascular (atherosclerotic) I25.10
    - with angina pectoris — *see* Arteriosclerosis, coronary (artery),
    - congenital Q28.9
    - hypertensive — *see* Hypertension, heart
    - newborn P29.9
        - specified NEC P29.89
    - renal (hypertensive) — *see* Hypertension, cardiorenal
    - syphilitic (asymptomatic) A52.00
- cartilage — *see* Disorder, cartilage
- Castellani's A69.8
- Castleman (unicentric) (multicentric) D47.Z2
    - HHV-8-associated — *see also* Herpesvirus, human, 8 D47.Z2
- cat-scratch A28.1
- Cavare's (familial periodic paralysis) G72.3
- cecum K63.9
- celiac (adult) (infantile) (with steatorrhea) K90.0
- cellular tissue L98.9
- central core G71.29
- cerebellar, cerebellum — *see* Disease, brain
- cerebral — *see also* Disease, brain
    - degenerative — *see* Degeneration, brain
- cerebrospinal G96.9
- cerebrovascular I67.9
    - acute I67.89
        - embolic I63.4- ✓
        - thrombotic I63.3- ✓
    - arteriosclerotic I67.2
    - hereditary NEC I67.858
    - specified NEC I67.89
- cervix (uteri) (noninflammatory) N88.9
    - inflammatory — *see* Cervicitis
    - specified NEC N88.8
- Chabert's A22.9
- Chandler's (osteochondritis dissecans, hip) — *see* Osteochondritis, dissecans, hip
- Charlouis — *see* Yaws
- Chédiak-Steinbrinck (-Higashi) (congenital gigantism of peroxidase granules) E70.330
- chest J98.9
- Chiari's (hepatic vein thrombosis) I82.0
- Chicago B40.9

Disease, diseased — *continued*
- Chignon B36.8
- chigo, chigoe B88.1
- childhood granulomatous D71
- Chinese liver fluke B66.1
- chlamydial A74.9
    - specified NEC A74.89
- cholecystic K82.9
- choroid H31.9
    - specified NEC H31.8
- Christmas D67
- chronic bullous of childhood L12.2
- chylomicron retention E78.3
- ciliary body H21.9
    - specified NEC H21.89
- circulatory (system) NEC I99.8
    - newborn P29.9
    - syphilitic A52.00
        - congenital A50.54
- coagulation factor deficiency (congenital) — *see* Defect, coagulation
- coccidioidal — *see* Coccidioidomycosis
- cold
    - agglutinin or hemoglobinuria D59.12
        - paroxysmal D59.6
    - hemagglutinin (chronic) D59.12
- collagen NOS (nonvascular) (vascular) M35.9
    - specified NEC M35.89
- colon K63.9
    - functional K59.9
        - congenital Q43.2
    - ischemic — *see also* Ischemia, intestine, acute K55.039
- colonic inflammatory bowel, unclassified (IBDU) K52.3
- combined system — *see* Degeneration, combined
- compressed air T70.3 ✓
- Concato's (pericardial polyserositis) A19.9
    - nontubercular I31.1
    - pleural — *see* Pleurisy, with effusion
- conjunctiva H11.9
    - chlamydial A74.0
    - specified NEC H11.89
    - viral B30.9
        - specified NEC B30.8
- connective tissue, systemic (diffuse) M35.9
    - in (due to)
        - hypogammaglobulinemia D80.1 *[M36.8]*
        - ochronosis E70.29 *[M36.8]*
    - specified NEC M35.89
- Conor and Bruch's (boutonneuse fever) A77.1
- Cooper's — *see* Mastopathy, cystic
- Cori's (glycogenosis III) E74.03
- corkhandler's or corkworker's J67.3
- cornea H18.9
    - specified NEC H18.89- ✓
- coronary (artery) — *see* Disease, heart, ischemic, atherosclerotic
    - congenital Q24.5
    - ostial, syphilitic (aortic) (mitral) (pulmonary) A52.03
- corpus cavernosum N48.9
    - specified NEC N48.89
- Cotugno's — *see* Sciatica
- COVID-19 U07.1
- coxsackie (virus) NEC B34.1
- cranial nerve NOS G52.9
- Creutzfeldt-Jakob — *see* Creutzfeldt-Jakob disease or syndrome
- Crocq's (acrocyanosis) I73.89
- Crohn's — *see* Enteritis, regional
- Curschmann G71.11
- cystic
    - breast (chronic) — *see* Mastopathy, cystic
    - kidney, congenital Q61.9
    - liver, congenital Q44.6
    - lung J98.4
        - congenital Q33.0
- cytomegalic inclusion (generalized) B25.9
    - with pneumonia B25.0
    - congenital P35.1
- cytomegaloviral B25.9
    - specified NEC B25.8
- Czerny's (periodic hydrarthrosis of the knee) — *see* Effusion, joint, knee
- Daae (-Finsen) (epidemic pleurodynia) B33.0
- Darling's — *see* Histoplasmosis capsulati
- de Quervain's (tendon sheath) M65.4
    - thyroid (subacute granulomatous thyroiditis) E06.1
- Débove's (splenomegaly) R16.1

Disease, diseased — *continued*
- deer fly — *see* Tularemia
- Degos' I77.89
- demyelinating, demyelinizating (nervous system) G37.9
    - multiple sclerosis G35
    - specified NEC G37.8
- dense deposit — *see also* N00-N07 with fourth character .6 N05.6
- deposition, hydroxyapatite — *see* Disease, hydroxyapatite deposition
- Devergie's (pityriasis rubra pilaris) L44.0
- Devic's G36.0
- diaphorase deficiency D74.0
- diaphragm J98.6
- diarrheal, infectious NEC A09
- digestive system K92.9
    - specified NEC K92.89
- disc, degenerative — *see* Degeneration, intervertebral disc
- discogenic — *see also* Displacement, intervertebral disc NEC
    - with myelopathy — *see* Disorder, disc, with, myelopathy
- diverticular — *see* Diverticula
- Dubois (thymus) A50.59 *[E35]*
- Duchenne-Griesinger G71.01
- Duchenne's
    - muscular dystrophy G71.01
    - pseudohypertrophy, muscles G71.01
- ductless glands E34.9
- Duhring's (dermatitis herpetiformis) L13.0
- duodenum K31.9
    - specified NEC K31.89
- Dupré's (meningism) R29.1
- Dupuytren's (muscle contracture) M72.0
- Durand-Nicholas-Favre (climatic bubo) A55
- Duroziez's (congenital mitral stenosis) Q23.2
- ear — *see* Disorder, ear
- Eberth's — *see* Fever, typhoid
- Ebola (virus) A98.4
- Ebstein's heart Q22.5
- Echinococcus — *see* Echinococcus
- echovirus NEC B34.1
- Eddowes' (brittle bones and blue sclera) Q78.0
- edentulous (alveolar) ridge K06.9
    - specified NEC K06.8
- Edsall's T67.2 ✓
- Eichstedt's (pityriasis versicolor) B36.0
- Eisenmenger's (irreversible) I27.83
- Ellis-van Creveld (chondroectodermal dysplasia) Q77.6
- end stage renal (ESRD) N18.6
    - due to hypertension I12.0
- endocrine glands or system NEC E34.9
- endomyocardial (eosinophilic) I42.3
- English (rickets) E55.0
- enteroviral, enterovirus NEC B34.1
    - central nervous system NEC A88.8
- epidemic B99.9
    - specified NEC B99.8
- epididymis N50.9
- Erb (-Landouzy) G71.02
- Erdheim-Chester (ECD) E88.89
- esophagus K22.9
    - functional K22.4
    - psychogenic F45.8
    - specified NEC K22.89
- Eulenburg's (congenital paramyotonia) G71.19
- eustachian tube — *see* Disorder, eustachian tube
- external
    - auditory canal — *see* Disorder, ear, external
    - ear — *see* Disorder, ear, external
- extrapyramidal G25.9
    - specified NEC G25.89
- eye H57.9
    - anterior chamber H21.9
    - inflammatory NEC H57.89
    - muscle (external) — *see* Strabismus
    - specified NEC H57.89
    - syphilitic — *see* Oculopathy, syphilitic
- eyeball H44.9
    - specified NEC H44.89
- eyelid — *see* Disorder, eyelid
    - specified NEC — *see* Disorder, eyelid, specified type NEC
- eyeworm of Africa B74.3
- facial nerve (seventh) G51.9
    - newborn (birth injury) P11.3
- Fahr (of brain) G23.8

✓ **Additional Character Required** — **Refer to the Tabular List for Character Selection**   ▽ **Subterms under main terms may continue to next column or page**

Index

Disease, diseased — Disease, diseased

Disease, diseased — *continued*
Fahr Volhard (of kidney) I12.- ☑
fallopian tube (noninflammatory) N83.9
  inflammatory — *see* Salpingo-oophoritis
  specified NEC N83.8
familial periodic paralysis G72.3
Fanconi's (congenital pancytopenia) D61.09
fascia NEC — *see also* Disorder, muscle
  inflammatory — *see* Myositis
  specified NEC M62.89
Fauchard's (periodontitis) — *see* Periodontitis
Favre-Durand-Nicolas (climatic bubo) A55
Fede's K14.0
Feer's — *see* Poisoning, mercury
female pelvic inflammatory — *see also* Disease, pelvis,
  inflammatory N73.9
  syphilitic (secondary) A51.42
  tuberculous A18.17
Fernels' (aortic aneurysm) I71.9
fibrocaseous of lung — *see* Tuberculosis, pulmonary
fibrocystic — *see* Fibrocystic disease
Fiedler's (leptospiral jaundice) A27.0
fifth B08.3
file-cutter's — *see* Poisoning, lead
fish-skin Q80.9
  acquired L85.0
Flajani (-Basedow) (exophthalmic goiter) — *see* Hyperthyroidism, with, goiter (diffuse)
flax-dresser's J66.1
fluke — *see* Infestation, fluke
foot and mouth B08.8
foot process N04.9
Forbes' (glycogenosis III) E74.03
Fordyce-Fox (apocrine miliaria) L75.2
Fordyce's (ectopic sebaceous glands) (mouth) Q38.6
Forestier's (rhizomelic pseudopolyarthritis) M35.3
  meaning ankylosing hyperostosis — *see* Hyperosto-
    sis, ankylosing
Fothergill's
  neuralgia — *see* Neuralgia, trigeminal
  scarlatina anginosa A38.9
Fournier (gangrene) N49.3
  female N76.89
fourth B08.8
Fox (-Fordyce) (apocrine miliaria) L75.2
Francis' — *see* Tularemia
Franklin C88.2
Frei's (climatic bubo) A55
Friedreich's
  combined systemic or ataxia G11.11
  myoclonia G25.3
frontal sinus — *see* Sinusitis, frontal
fungus NEC B49
Gaisböck's (polycythemia hypertonica) D75.1
gallbladder K82.9
  calculus — *see* Calculus, gallbladder
  cholecystitis — *see* Cholecystitis
  cholesterolosis K82.4
  fistula — *see* Fistula, gallbladder
  hydrops K82.1
  obstruction — *see* Obstruction, gallbladder
  perforation K82.2
  specified NEC K82.8
gamma heavy chain C88.2
Gamna's (sideritic splenomegaly) D73.2
Gamstorp's (adynamia episodica hereditaria) G72.3
Gandy-Nanta (sideritic splenomegaly) D73.2
ganister J62.8
gastric — *see* Disease, stomach
gastroesophageal reflux (GERD) K21.9
  with esophagitis (without bleeding) K21.00
    with bleeding K21.01
gastrointestinal (tract) K92.9
  amyloid E85.4
  functional K59.9
    psychogenic F45.8
  specified NEC K92.89
Gee (-Herter) (-Heubner) (-Thaysen) (nontropical sprue)
  K90.0
genital organs
  female N94.9
  male N50.9
Gerhardt's (erythromelalgia) I73.81
Gibert's (pityriasis rosea) L42
Gierke's (glycogenosis I) E74.01
Gilles de la Tourette's (motor-verbal tic) F95.2
gingiva K06.9
  plaque induced K05.00

Disease, diseased — *continued*
gingiva — *continued*
  specified NEC K06.8
gland (lymph) I89.9
Glanzmann's (hereditary hemorrhagic thrombasthenia)
  D69.1
glass-blower's (cataract) — *see* Cataract, specified NEC
  salivary gland hypertrophy K11.1
Glisson's — *see* Rickets
globe H44.9
  specified NEC H44.89
glomerular — *see also* Glomerulonephritis
  with edema — *see* Nephrosis
  acute — *see* Nephritis, acute
  chronic — *see* Nephritis, chronic
  minimal change N05.0
  rapidly progressive N01.9
glycogen storage E74.00
  Andersen's E74.09
  Cori's E74.03
  Forbes' E74.03
  generalized E74.00
  glucose-6-phosphatase deficiency E74.01
  heart E74.02 *[I43]*
  hepatorenal E74.09
  Hers' E74.09
  liver and kidney E74.09
  McArdle's E74.04
  muscle phosphofructokinase E74.09
  myocardium E74.02 *[I43]*
  Pompe's E74.02
  Tauri's E74.09
  type 0 E74.09
  type I E74.01
  type II E74.02
  type III E74.03
  type IV E74.09
  type V E74.04
  type VI-XI E74.09
  Von Gierke's E74.01
Goldstein's (familial hemorrhagic telangiectasia) I78.0
gonococcal NOS A54.9
graft-versus-host (GVH) D89.813
  acute D89.810
  acute on chronic D89.812
  chronic D89.811
grainhandler's J67.8
granulomatous (childhood) (chronic) D71
Graves' (exophthalmic goiter) — *see* Hyperthyroidism,
  with, goiter (diffuse)
Griesinger's — *see* Ancylostomiasis
Grisel's M43.6
Gruby's (tinea tonsurans) B35.0
Guillain-Barré G61.0
Guinon's (motor-verbal tic) F95.2
gum K06.9
gynecological N94.9
H (Hartnup's) E72.02
Haff — *see* Poisoning, mercury
Hageman (congenital factor XII deficiency) D68.2
hair (color) (shaft) L67.9
  follicles L73.9
    specified NEC L73.8
Hamman's (spontaneous mediastinal emphysema)
  J98.2
hand, foot and mouth B08.4
Hansen's — *see* Leprosy
Hantavirus, with pulmonary manifestations B33.4
  with renal manifestations A98.5
Harada's H30.81- ☑
Hartnup (pellagra-cerebellar ataxia-renal
  aminoaciduria) E72.02
Hart's (pellagra-cerebellar ataxia-renal aminoaciduria)
  E72.02
Hashimoto's (struma lymphomatosa) E06.3
Hb — *see* Disease, hemoglobin
heart (organic) I51.9
  with
    pulmonary edema (acute) — *see also* Failure,
      ventricular, left I50.1
    rheumatic fever (conditions in I00)
      active I01.9
        with chorea I02.0
        specified NEC I01.8
      inactive or quiescent (with chorea) I09.9
        specified NEC I09.89
  amyloid E85.4 *[I43]*
  aortic (valve) I35.9

Disease, diseased — *continued*
heart — *continued*
  arteriosclerotic or sclerotic (senile) — *see* Disease,
    heart, ischemic, atherosclerotic
  artery, arterial — *see* Disease, heart, ischemic,
    atherosclerotic
  beer drinkers' I42.6
  beriberi (wet) E51.12
  black I27.0
  congenital Q24.9
    cyanotic Q24.9
    specified NEC Q24.8
  coronary — *see* Disease, heart, ischemic
  cryptogenic I51.9
  fibroid — *see* Myocarditis
  functional I51.89
    psychogenic F45.8
  glycogen storage E74.02 *[I43]*
  gonococcal A54.83
  hypertensive — *see* Hypertension, heart
  hyperthyroid — *see also* Hyperthyroidism
    E05.90 *[I43]*
    with thyroid storm E05.91 *[I43]*
  ischemic (chronic or with a stated duration of over
    4 weeks) I25.9
    atherosclerotic (of) I25.10
      with angina pectoris — *see* Arteriosclerosis,
        coronary (artery)
      coronary artery bypass graft — *see* Arterioscle-
        rosis, coronary (artery),
      cardiomyopathy I25.5
    diagnosed on ECG or other special investigation,
      but currently presenting no symptoms
      I25.6
    silent I25.6
    specified form NEC I25.89
  kyphoscoliotic I27.1
  meningococcal A39.50
    endocarditis A39.51
    myocarditis A39.52
    pericarditis A39.53
  mitral I05.9
    specified NEC I05.8
  muscular — *see* Degeneration, myocardial
  psychogenic (functional) F45.8
  pulmonary (chronic) I27.9
    in schistosomiasis B65.9 *[I52]*
    specified NEC I27.89
  rheumatic (chronic) (inactive) (old) (quiescent) (with
    chorea) I09.9
    active or acute I01.9
      with chorea (acute) (rheumatic) (Sydenham's)
        I02.0
    specified NEC I09.89
  senile — *see* Myocarditis
  syphilitic A52.06
    aortic A52.03
      aneurysm A52.01
    congenital A50.54 *[I52]*
  thyrotoxic — *see also* Thyrotoxicosis E05.90 *[I43]*
    with thyroid storm E05.91 *[I43]*
  valve, valvular (obstructive) (regurgitant) — *see also*
    Endocarditis
    congenital NEC Q24.8
    pulmonary Q22.3
  vascular — *see* Disease, cardiovascular
heavy chain NEC C88.2
  alpha C88.3
  gamma C88.2
  mu C88.2
Hebra's
  pityriasis
    maculata et circinata L42
    rubra pilaris L44.0
  prurigo L28.2
hematopoietic organs D75.9
hemoglobin or Hb
  abnormal (mixed) NEC D58.2
    with thalassemia D56.9
  AS genotype D57.3
  Bart's D56.0
  C (Hb-C) D58.2
    with other abnormal hemoglobin NEC D58.2
    elliptocytosis D58.1
    Hb-S D57.2- ☑
    sickle-cell D57.2- ☑
    thalassemia D56.8
  Constant Spring D58.2

Disease, diseased — *continued*
 hemoglobin or Hb — *continued*
  D (Hb-D) D58.2
  E (Hb-E) D58.2
  E-beta thalassemia D56.5
  elliptocytosis D58.1
  H (Hb-H) (thalassemia) D56.0
   with other abnormal hemoglobin NEC D56.9
   Constant Spring D56.0
  I thalassemia D56.9
  M D74.0
  S or SS D57.1
   with
    acute chest syndrome D57.01
    cerebral vascular involvement D57.03
    crisis (painful) D57.00
     with complication specified NEC D57.09
    splenic sequestration D57.02
    vasoocclusive pain D57.00
   beta plus D57.44
    with
     acute chest syndrome D57.451
     cerebral vascular involvement D57.453
     crisis D57.459
      with specified complication NEC D57.458
     splenic sequestration D57.452
     vasoocclusive pain D57.459
    without crisis D57.44
   beta zero D57.42
    with
     acute chest syndrome D57.431
     cerebral vascular involvement D57.433
     crisis D57.439
      with specified complication NEC D57.438
     splenic sequestration D57.432
     vasoocclusive pain
    without crisis D57.42
  SC D57.2- ☑
  SD D57.8- ☑
  SE D57.8- ☑
  spherocytosis D58.0
  unstable, hemolytic D58.2
 hemolytic (newborn) P55.9
  autoimmune D59.10
   cold type (primary) (secondary) (symptomatic) D59.12
   mixed type (primary) (secondary) (symptomatic) D59.13
   warm type (primary) (secondary) (symptomatic) D59.11
  drug-induced D59.0
  due to or with
   incompatibility
    ABO (blood group) P55.1
    blood (group) (Duffy) (K) (Kell) (Kidd) (Lewis) (M) (S) NEC P55.8
    Rh (blood group) (factor) P55.0
   Rh negative mother P55.0
  specified type NEC P55.8
  unstable hemoglobin D58.2
 hemorrhagic D69.9
  newborn P53
 Henoch (-Schönlein) (purpura nervosa) D69.0
 hepatic — *see* Disease, liver
 hepatolenticular E83.01
 heredodegenerative NEC
  spinal cord G95.89
 herpesviral, disseminated B00.7
 Hers' (glycogenosis VI) E74.09
 Herter (-Gee) (-Heubner) (nontropical sprue) K90.0
 Heubner-Herter (nontropical sprue) K90.0
 high fetal gene or hemoglobin thalassemia D56.9
 Hildenbrand's — *see* Typhus
 hip (joint) M25.9
  congenital Q65.89
  suppurative M00.9
  tuberculous A18.02
 His (-Werner) (trench fever) A79.0
 Hodgson's I71.2
  ruptured I71.1
 Holla — *see* Spherocytosis
 hookworm B76.9
  specified NEC B76.8
 host-versus-graft D89.813
  acute D89.810
  acute on chronic D89.812
  chronic D89.811

 human immunodeficiency virus (HIV) B20
 Huntington's G10
  with dementia G10 *[F02.80]*
 Hutchinson's (cheiropompholyx) — *see* Hutchinson's disease
 hyaline (diffuse) (generalized)
  membrane (lung) (newborn) P22.0
   adult J80
 hydatid — *see* Echinococcus
 hydroxyapatite deposition M11.00
  ankle M11.07- ☑
  elbow M11.02- ☑
  foot joint M11.07- ☑
  hand joint M11.04- ☑
  hip M11.05- ☑
  knee M11.06- ☑
  multiple site M11.09
  shoulder M11.01- ☑
  vertebra M11.08
  wrist M11.03- ☑
 hyperkinetic — *see* Hyperkinesia
 hypertensive — *see* Hypertension
 hypophysis E23.7
 Iceland G93.3
 I-cell E77.0
 immune D89.9
 immunoproliferative (malignant) C88.9
  small intestinal C88.3
  specified NEC C88.8
 inclusion B25.9
  salivary gland B25.9
 infectious, infective B99.9
  congenital P37.9
   specified NEC P37.8
   viral P35.9
    specified type NEC P35.8
  specified NEC B99.8
 inflammatory
  penis N48.29
   abscess N48.21
   cellulitis N48.22
  prepuce N47.7
   balanoposthitis N47.6
  tubo-ovarian — *see* Salpingo-oophoritis
 intervertebral disc — *see also* Disorder, disc
  with myelopathy — *see* Disorder, disc, with, myelopathy
  cervical, cervicothoracic — *see* Disorder, disc, cervical
   with
    myelopathy — *see* Disorder, disc, cervical, with myelopathy
    neuritis, radiculitis or radiculopathy — *see* Disorder, disc, cervical, with neuritis
   specified NEC — *see* Disorder, disc, cervical, specified type NEC
  lumbar (with)
   myelopathy M51.06
   neuritis, radiculitis, radiculopathy or sciatica M51.16
   specified NEC M51.86
  lumbosacral (with)
   neuritis, radiculitis, radiculopathy or sciatica M51.17
   specified NEC M51.87
  specified NEC — *see* Disorder, disc, specified NEC
  thoracic (with)
   myelopathy M51.04
   neuritis, radiculitis or radiculopathy M51.14
   specified NEC M51.84
  thoracolumbar (with)
   myelopathy M51.05
   neuritis, radiculitis or radiculopathy M51.15
   specified NEC M51.85
 intestine K63.9
  functional K59.9
   psychogenic F45.8
   specified NEC K59.89
  organic K63.9
  protozoal A07.9
  specified NEC K63.89
 iris H21.9
  specified NEC H21.89
 iron metabolism or storage E83.10
 island (scrub typhus) A75.3
 itai-itai — *see* Poisoning, cadmium

 Jakob-Creutzfeldt — *see* Creutzfeldt-Jakob disease or syndrome
 jaw M27.9
  fibrocystic M27.49
  specified NEC M27.8
 jigger B88.1
 joint — *see also* Disorder, joint
  Charcot's — *see* Arthropathy, neuropathic (Charcot)
  degenerative — *see* Osteoarthritis
   multiple M15.9
   spine — *see* Spondylosis
  facet joint — *see also* Spondylosis M47.819
  hypertrophic — *see* Osteoarthritis
  sacroiliac M53.3
  specified NEC — *see* Disorder, joint, specified type NEC
  spine NEC — *see* Dorsopathy
  suppurative — *see* Arthritis, pyogenic or pyemic
 Jourdain's (acute gingivitis) K05.00
  nonplaque induced K05.01
  plaque induced K05.00
 Kaschin-Beck (endemic polyarthritis) M12.10
  ankle M12.17- ☑
  elbow M12.12- ☑
  foot joint M12.17- ☑
  hand joint M12.14- ☑
  hip M12.15- ☑
  knee M12.16- ☑
  multiple site M12.19
  shoulder M12.11- ☑
  vertebra M12.18
  wrist M12.13- ☑
 Katayama B65.2
 Kedani (scrub typhus) A75.3
 Keshan E59
 kidney (functional) (pelvis) N28.9
  chronic N18.9
   hypertensive — *see* Hypertension, kidney
   stage 1 N18.1
   stage 2 (mild) N18.2
   stage 3 (moderate) N18.30
   stage 3a N18.31
   stage 3b N18.32
   stage 4 (severe) N18.4
   stage 5 N18.5
  complicating pregnancy — *see* Pregnancy, complicated by, renal disease
  cystic (congenital) Q61.9
  fibrocystic (congenital) Q61.8
  hypertensive — *see* Hypertension, kidney
  in (due to)
   schistosomiasis (bilharziasis) B65.9 *[N29]*
  multicystic Q61.4
  polycystic Q61.3
   adult type Q61.2
   childhood type NEC Q61.19
    collecting duct dilatation Q61.11
 Kimmelstiel (-Wilson) (intercapillary polycystic (congenital) glomerulosclerosis) — *see* E08-E13 with .21
 Kinnier Wilson's (hepatolenticular degeneration) E83.01
 kissing — *see* Mononucleosis, infectious
 Klebs' — *see also* Glomerulonephritis N05- ☑
 Klippel-Feil (brevicollis) Q76.1
 Köhler-Pellegrini-Stieda (calcification, knee joint) — *see* Bursitis, tibial collateral
 Kok Q89.8
 König's (osteochondritis dissecans) — *see* Osteochondritis, dissecans
 Korsakoff's (nonalcoholic) F04
  alcoholic F10.96
   with dependence F10.26
 Kostmann's (infantile genetic agranulocytosis) D70.0
 kuru A81.81
 Kyasanur Forest A98.2
 labyrinth, ear — *see* Disorder, ear, inner
 lacrimal system — *see* Disorder, lacrimal system
 Lafora's — *see* Epilepsy, generalized, idiopathic
 Lancereaux-Mathieu (leptospiral jaundice) A27.0
 Landry's G61.0
 Larrey-Weil (leptospiral jaundice) A27.0
 larynx J38.7
 legionnaires' A48.1
  nonpneumonic A48.2
 Lenegre's I44.2
 lens H27.9
  specified NEC H27.8
 Lev's (acquired complete heart block) I44.2

  ☑ **Additional Character Required — Refer to the Tabular List for Character Selection**   ▽ Subterms under main terms may continue to next column or page

Disease, diseased — *continued*
- Lewy body (dementia) G31.83 *[F02.80]*
  - with behavioral disturbance G31.83 *[F02.81]*
- Lichtheim's (subacute combined sclerosis with pernicious anemia) D51.0
- Lightwood's (renal tubular acidosis) N25.89
- Lignac's (cystinosis) E72.04
- lip K13.0
- lipid-storage E75.6
  - specified NEC E75.5
- Lipschütz's N76.6
- liver (chronic) (organic) K76.9
  - alcoholic (chronic) K70.9
    - acute — *see* Disease, liver, alcoholic, hepatitis
    - cirrhosis K70.30
      - with ascites K70.31
    - failure K70.40
      - with coma K70.41
    - fatty liver K70.0
    - fibrosis K70.2
    - hepatitis K70.10
      - with ascites K70.11
    - sclerosis K70.2
  - cystic, congenital Q44.6
  - drug-induced (idiosyncratic) (toxic) (predictable) (unpredictable) — *see* Disease, liver, toxic
  - end stage K72.10
    - due to hepatitis — *see* Hepatitis
    - with coma K72.11
  - fatty, nonalcoholic (NAFLD) K76.0
    - alcoholic K70.0
  - fibrocystic (congenital) Q44.6
  - fluke
    - Chinese B66.1
    - oriental B66.1
    - sheep B66.3
  - gestational alloimmune (GALD) P78.84
  - glycogen storage E74.09 *[K77]*
  - in (due to)
    - schistosomiasis (bilharziasis) B65.9 *[K77]*
  - inflammatory K75.9
    - alcoholic K70.1 ☑
    - specified NEC K75.89
  - polycystic (congenital) Q44.6
  - toxic K71.9
    - with
      - cholestasis K71.0
      - cirrhosis (liver) K71.7
      - fibrosis (liver) K71.7
      - focal nodular hyperplasia K71.8
      - hepatic granuloma K71.8
      - hepatic necrosis K71.10
        - with coma K71.11
      - hepatitis NEC K71.6
        - acute K71.2
        - chronic
          - active K71.50
            - with ascites K71.51
          - lobular K71.4
          - persistent K71.3
        - lupoid K71.50
          - with ascites K71.51
      - peliosis hepatis K71.8
      - veno-occlusive disease (VOD) of liver K71.8
  - veno-occlusive K76.5
- Lobo's (keloid blastomycosis) B48.0
- Lobstein's (brittle bones and blue sclera) Q78.0
- Ludwig's (submaxillary cellulitis) K12.2
- lumbosacral region M53.87
- lung J98.4
  - black J60
  - congenital Q33.9
  - cystic J98.4
    - congenital Q33.0
  - dabbing (related) U07.0
  - electronic cigarette (related) U07.0
  - fibroid (chronic) — *see* Fibrosis, lung
  - fluke B66.4
    - oriental B66.4
  - in
    - amyloidosis E85.4 *[J99]*
    - sarcoidosis D86.0
    - Sjögren's syndrome M35.02
    - systemic
      - lupus erythematosus M32.13
      - sclerosis M34.81
  - interstitial J84.9
    - of childhood, specified NEC J84.848

Disease, diseased — *continued*
- lung — *continued*
  - interstitial — *continued*
    - respiratory bronchiolitis J84.115
    - specified NEC J84.89
    - with progressive fibrotic phenotype, in diseases classified elsewhere J84.170
  - obstructive (chronic) J44.9
    - with
      - acute
        - bronchitis J44.0
          - exacerbation NEC J44.1
          - lower respiratory infection J44.0
      - alveolitis, allergic J67.9
      - asthma J44.9
      - bronchiectasis J47.9
        - with
          - exacerbation (acute) J47.1
          - lower respiratory infection J47.0
      - bronchitis J44.9
        - with
          - exacerbation (acute) J44.1
          - lower respiratory infection J44.0
      - emphysema J43.9
      - hypersensitivity pneumonitis J67.9
    - decompensated J44.1
      - with
        - exacerbation (acute) J44.1
  - polycystic J98.4
    - congenital Q33.0
  - rheumatoid (diffuse) (interstitial) — *see* Rheumatoid, lung
  - vaping (associated) (device) (product) (use) U07.0
- Lutembacher's (atrial septal defect with mitral stenosis) Q21.1
- Lyme A69.20
- lymphatic (gland) (system) (channel) (vessel) I89.9
- lymphoproliferative D47.9
  - specified NEC D47.Z9 *(following* D47.4)
  - T-gamma D47.Z9 *(following* D47.4)
  - X-linked D82.3
- Magitot's M27.2
- malarial — *see* Malaria
- malignant — *see also* Neoplasm, malignant, by site
- Manson's B65.1
- maple bark J67.6
- maple-syrup-urine E71.0
- Marburg (virus) A98.3
- Marion's (bladder neck obstruction) N32.0
- Marsh's (exophthalmic goiter) — *see* Hyperthyroidism, with goiter (diffuse)
- mastoid (process) — *see* Disorder, ear, middle
- Mathieu's (leptospiral jaundice) A27.0
- Maxcy's A75.2
- McArdle (-Schmid-Pearson) (glycogenosis V) E74.04
- mediastinum J98.59
- medullary center (idiopathic) (respiratory) G93.89
- Meige's (chronic hereditary edema) Q82.0
- meningococcal — *see* Infection, meningococcal
- mental F99
  - organic F09
- mesenchymal M35.9
- mesenteric embolic — *see also* Ischemia, intestine, acute K55.039
- metabolic, metabolism E88.9
  - bilirubin E80.7
- metal-polisher's J62.8
- metastatic — *see also* Neoplasm, secondary, by site C79.9
- microvascular - code to condition
- microvillus
  - atrophy Q43.8
  - inclusion (MVD) Q43.8
- middle ear — *see* Disorder, ear, middle
- Mikulicz' (dryness of mouth, absent or decreased lacrimation) K11.8
- Milroy's (chronic hereditary edema) Q82.0
- Minamata — *see* Poisoning, mercury
- minicore G71.29
- Minor's G95.19
- Minot's (hemorrhagic disease, newborn) P53
- Minot-von Willebrand-Jürgens (angiohemophilia) D68.0
- Mitchell's (erythromelalgia) I73.81
- mitral (valve) I05.9
  - nonrheumatic I34.9
- mixed connective tissue M35.1
- moldy hay J67.0
- Monge's T70.29 ☑

Disease, diseased — *continued*
- Morgagni-Adams-Stokes (syncope with heart block) I45.9
- Morgagni's (syndrome) (hyperostosis frontalis interna) M85.2
- Morton's (with metatarsalgia) — *see* Lesion, nerve, plantar
- Morvan's G60.8
- motor neuron (bulbar) (mixed type) (spinal) G12.20
  - amyotrophic lateral sclerosis G12.21
  - familial G12.24
  - progressive bulbar palsy G12.22
  - specified NEC G12.29
- moyamoya I67.5
- mu heavy chain disease C88.2
- multicore G71.29
- multiminicore G71.29
- muscle — *see also* Disorder, muscle
  - inflammatory — *see* Myositis
  - ocular (external) — *see* Strabismus
- musculoskeletal system, soft tissue — *see also* Disorder, soft tissue
  - specified NEC — *see* Disorder, soft tissue, specified type NEC
- mushroom workers' J67.5
- mycotic B49
- myelodysplastic, not classified — *see also* Syndrome, myelodysplasia C94.6
- myeloproliferative, not classified C94.6
  - chronic D47.1
- myocardium, myocardial — *see also* Degeneration, myocardial I51.5
  - primary (idiopathic) I42.9
- myoneural G70.9
- Naegeli's D69.1
- nails L60.9
  - specified NEC L60.8
- Nairobi (sheep virus) A93.8
- nasal J34.9
- nemaline body G71.21
- nerve — *see* Disorder, nerve
- nervous system G98.8
  - autonomic G90.9
  - central G96.9
    - specified NEC G96.89
  - congenital Q07.9
  - parasympathetic G90.9
  - specified NEC G98.8
  - sympathetic G90.9
  - vegetative G90.9
- neuromuscular system G70.9
- Newcastle B30.8
- Nicolas (-Durand)-Favre (climatic bubo) A55
- nipple N64.9
  - Paget's C50.01- ☑
    - female C50.01- ☑
    - male C50.02- ☑
- Nishimoto (-Takeuchi) I67.5
- nonarthropod-borne NOS (viral) B34.9
  - enterovirus NEC B34.1
- nonautoimmune hemolytic D59.4
  - drug-induced D59.2
- Nonne-Milroy-Meige (chronic hereditary edema) Q82.0
- nose J34.9
- nucleus pulposus — *see* Disorder, disc
- nutritional E63.9
- oast-house-urine E72.19
  - ocular
    - herpesviral B00.50
    - zoster B02.30
- obliterative vascular I77.1
- Ohara's — *see* Tularemia
- Opitz's (congestive splenomegaly) D73.2
- Oppenheim-Urbach (necrobiosis lipoidica diabeticorum) — *see* E08-E13 with .620
- optic nerve NEC — *see* Disorder, nerve, optic
- orbit — *see* Disorder, orbit
- organ
  - dabbing (related) U07.0
  - electronic cigarette (related) U07.0
  - vaping (associated) (device) (product) (use) U07.0
- Oriental liver fluke B66.1
- Oriental lung fluke B66.4
- Ormond's N13.5
- Osler-Rendu (familial hemorrhagic telangiectasia) I78.0
- osteofibrocystic E21.0
- Otto's M24.7

Disease, diseased — *continued*

outer ear — *see* Disorder, ear, external
ovary (noninflammatory) N83.9
  cystic N83.20- ☑
  inflammatory — *see* Salpingo-oophoritis
  polycystic E28.2
  specified NEC N83.8
Owren's (congenital) — *see* Defect, coagulation
pancreas K86.9
  cystic K86.2
  fibrocystic E84.9
  specified NEC K86.89
panvalvular I08.9
  specified NEC I08.8
parametrium (noninflammatory) N83.9
parasitic B89
  cerebral NEC B71.9 [*G94*]
  intestinal NOS B82.9
  mouth B37.0
  skin NOS B88.9
  specified type — *see* Infestation
  tongue B37.0
parathyroid (gland) E21.5
  specified NEC E21.4
Parkinson's G20
parodontal K05.6
Parrot's (syphilitic osteochondritis) A50.02
Parry's (exophthalmic goiter) — *see* Hyperthyroidism, with, goiter (diffuse)
Parson's (exophthalmic goiter) — *see* Hyperthyroidism, with, goiter (diffuse)
Paxton's (white piedra) B36.2
pearl-worker's — *see* Osteomyelitis, specified type NEC
Pellegrini-Stieda (calcification, knee joint) — *see* Bursitis, tibial collateral
pelvis, pelvic
  female NOS N94.9
    specified NEC N94.89
  gonococcal (acute) (chronic) A54.24
  inflammatory (female) N73.9
    acute N73.0
    chlamydial A56.11
    chronic N73.1
    specified NEC N73.8
    syphilitic (secondary) A51.42
      late A52.76
    tuberculous A18.17
  organ, female N94.9
  peritoneum, female NEC N94.89
penis N48.9
  inflammatory N48.29
    abscess N48.21
    cellulitis N48.22
  specified NEC N48.89
periapical tissues NOS K04.90
periodontal K05.6
  specified NEC K05.5
periosteum — *see* Disorder, bone, specified type NEC
peripheral
  arterial I73.9
  autonomic nervous system G90.9
  nerves — *see* Polyneuropathy
  vascular NOS I73.9
peritoneum K66.9
  pelvic, female NEC N94.89
  specified NEC K66.8
persistent mucosal (middle ear) H66.20
  left H66.22
    with right H66.23
  right H66.21
    with left H66.23
Petit's — *see* Hernia, abdomen, specified site NEC
pharynx J39.2
  specified NEC J39.2
Phocas' — *see* Mastopathy, cystic
photochromogenic (acid-fast bacilli) (pulmonary) A31.0
  nonpulmonary A31.9
Pick's G31.01 [*F02.80*]
  with behavioral disturbance G31.01 [*F02.81*]
  brain G31.01 [*F02.80*]
    with behavioral disturbance G31.01 [*F02.81*]
  of pericardium (pericardial pseudocirrhosis of liver) I31.1
pigeon fancier's J67.2
pineal gland E34.8
pink — *see* Poisoning, mercury
Pinkus' (lichen nitidus) L44.1
pinworm B80

Disease, diseased — *continued*

Piry virus A93.8
pituitary (gland) E23.7
pituitary-snuff-taker's J67.8
pleura (cavity) J94.9
  specified NEC J94.8
pneumatic drill (hammer) T75.21 ☑
Pollitzer's (hidradenitis suppurativa) L73.2
polycystic
  kidney or renal Q61.3
    adult type Q61.2
    childhood type NEC Q61.19
      collecting duct dilatation Q61.11
  liver or hepatic Q44.6
  lung or pulmonary J98.4
    congenital Q33.0
  ovary, ovaries E28.2
  spleen Q89.09
polyethylene T84.05- ☑
Pompe's (glycogenosis II) E74.02
Posadas-Wernicke B38.9
Potain's (pulmonary edema) — *see* Edema, lung
prepuce N47.8
  inflammatory N47.7
    balanoposthitis N47.6
Pringle's (tuberous sclerosis) Q85.1
prion, central nervous system A81.9
  specified NEC A81.89
prostate N42.9
  specified NEC N42.89
protozoal B64
  acanthamebiasis — *see* Acanthamebiasis
  African trypanosomiasis — *see* African trypanosomiasis
  babesiosis — *see also* Babesiosis B60.00
  Chagas disease — *see* Chagas disease
  intestine, intestinal A07.9
  leishmaniasis — *see* Leishmaniasis
  malaria — *see* Malaria
  naegleriasis B60.2
  pneumocystosis B59
  specified organism NEC B60.8
  toxoplasmosis — *see* Toxoplasmosis
pseudo-Hurler's E77.0
psychiatric F99
psychotic — *see* Psychosis
Puente's (simple glandular cheilitis) K13.0
puerperal — *see also* Puerperal O90.89
pulmonary — *see also* Disease, lung
  artery I28.9
  chronic obstructive J44.9
    with
      acute bronchitis J44.0
      exacerbation (acute) J44.1
      lower respiratory infection (acute) J44.0
    decompensated J44.1
      with
        exacerbation (acute) J44.1
  heart I27.9
    specified NEC I27.89
  hypertensive (vascular) — *see also* Hypertension, pulmonary I27.20
  NEC I27.2 ☑
    primary (idiopathic) I27.0
  valve I37.9
    rheumatic I09.89
pulp (dental) NOS K04.90
pulseless M31.4
Putnam's (subacute combined sclerosis with pernicious anemia) D51.0
Pyle (-Cohn) (metaphyseal dysplasia) Q78.5
ragpicker's or ragsorter's A22.1
Raynaud's — *see* Raynaud's disease
reactive airway — *see* Asthma
Reclus' (cystic) — *see* Mastopathy, cystic
rectum K62.9
  specified NEC K62.89
Refsum's (heredopathia atactica polyneuritiformis) G60.1
renal (functional) (pelvis) — *see also* Disease, kidney N28.9
  with
    edema — *see* Nephrosis
    glomerular lesion — *see* Glomerulonephritis
      with edema — *see* Nephrosis
    interstitial nephritis N12
  acute N28.9
  chronic — *see also* Disease, kidney, chronic N18.9

Disease, diseased — *continued*

renal — *see also* Disease, kidney — *continued*
  cystic, congenital Q61.9
  diabetic — *see* E08-E13 with .22
  end-stage (failure) N18.6
    due to hypertension I12.0
  fibrocystic (congenital) Q61.8
  hypertensive — *see* Hypertension, kidney
  lupus M32.14
  phosphate-losing (tubular) N25.0
  polycystic (congenital) Q61.3
    adult type Q61.2
    childhood type NEC Q61.19
      collecting duct dilatation Q61.11
  rapidly progressive N01.9
  subacute N01.9
Rendu-Osler-Weber (familial hemorrhagic telangiectasia) I78.0
renovascular (arteriosclerotic) — *see* Hypertension, kidney
respiratory (tract) J98.9
  acute or subacute NOS J06.9
    due to
      chemicals, gases, fumes or vapors (inhalation) J68.3
      external agent J70.9
        specified NEC J70.8
      radiation J70.0
      smoke inhalation J70.5
    noninfectious J39.8
  chronic NOS J98.9
    due to
      chemicals, gases, fumes or vapors J68.4
      external agent J70.9
        specified NEC J70.8
      radiation J70.1
  newborn P27.9
    specified NEC P27.8
  due to
    chemicals, gases, fumes or vapors J68.9
      acute or subacute NEC J68.3
      chronic J68.4
    external agent J70.9
      specified NEC J70.8
  newborn P28.9
    specified type NEC P28.89
  upper J39.9
    acute or subacute J06.9
    noninfectious NEC J39.8
    specified NEC J39.8
    streptococcal J06.9
retina, retinal H35.9
  Batten's or Batten-Mayou E75.4 [*H36*]
  specified NEC H35.89
rheumatoid — *see* Arthritis, rheumatoid
rickettsial NOS A79.9
  specified type NEC A79.89
Riga (-Fede) (cachectic aphthae) K14.0
Riggs' (compound periodontitis) — *see* Periodontitis
Ritter's L00
Rivalta's (cervicofacial actinomycosis) A42.2
Robles' (onchocerciasis) B73.01
rod body G71.21
Roger's (congenital interventricular septal defect) Q21.0
Rosenthal's (factor XI deficiency) D68.1
Ross River B33.1
Rossbach's (hyperchlorhydria) K31.89
  psychogenic F45.8
Rotes Quérol — *see* Hyperostosis, ankylosing
Roth (-Bernhardt) — *see* Mononeuropathy, lower limb, meralgia paresthetica
Runeberg's (progressive pernicious anemia) D51.0
sacroiliac NEC M53.3
salivary gland or duct K11.9
  inclusion B25.9
  specified NEC K11.8
  virus B25.9
sandworm B76.9
Schimmelbusch's — *see* Mastopathy, cystic
Schmorl's — *see* Schmorl's disease or nodes
Schönlein (-Henoch) (purpura rheumatica) D69.0
Schottmüller's — *see* Fever, paratyphoid
Schultz's (agranulocytosis) — *see* Agranulocytosis
Schwalbe-Ziehen-Oppenheim G24.1
Schwartz-Jampel G71.13
sclera H15.9
  specified NEC H15.89
scrofulous (tuberculous) A18.2

☑ Additional Character Required — Refer to the Tabular List for Character Selection   ▽ Subterms under main terms may continue to next column or page

Disease, diseased — *continued*
  scrotum N50.9
  sebaceous glands L73.9
  semilunar cartilage, cystic — *see also* Derangement,
    knee, meniscus, cystic
  seminal vesicle N50.9
  serum NEC — *see also* Reaction, serum T80.69 ☑
  sexually transmitted A64
    anogenital
      herpesviral infection — *see* Herpes, anogenital
      warts A63.0
    chancroid A57
    chlamydial infection — *see* Chlamydia
    gonorrhea — *see* Gonorrhea
    granuloma inguinale A58
    specified organism NEC A63.8
    syphilis — *see* Syphilis
    trichomoniasis — *see* Trichomoniasis
  Sézary C84.1- ☑
  shimamushi (scrub typhus) A75.3
  shipyard B30.0
  sickle-cell D57.1
    with
      acute chest syndrome D57.01
      cerebral vascular involvement D57.03
      crisis (painful) D57.00
        with complication specified NEC D57.09
      splenic sequestration D57.02
      vasoocclusive pain D57.00
    elliptocytosis D57.8- ☑
    Hb-C D57.20
      with
        acute chest syndrome D57.211
        cerebral vascular involvement D57.213
        crisis D57.219
          with specified complication NEC D57.218
        splenic sequestration D57.212
        vasoocclusive pain D57.219
      without crisis D57.20
    Hb-SD D57.80
      with
        acute chest syndrome D57.811
        cerebral vascular involvement D57.813
        crisis D57.819
          with complication specified NEC D57.818
        splenic sequestration D57.812
        vasoocclusive pain D57.819
      without crisis D57.80
    Hb-SE D57.80
      with
        acute chest syndrome D57.811
        cerebral vascular involvement D57.813
        crisis D57.819
          with complication specified NEC D57.818
        splenic sequestration D57.812
        vasoocclusive pain D57.819
      without crisis D57.80
    specified NEC D57.80
      with
        acute chest syndrome D57.811
        cerebral vascular involvement D57.813
        crisis D57.819
          with complication specified NEC D57.818
        splenic sequestration D57.812
        vasoocclusive pain D57.819
      without crisis D57.80
    spherocytosis D57.80
      with
        acute chest syndrome D57.811
        cerebral vascular involvement D57.813
        crisis D57.819
          with complication specified NEC D57.818
        splenic sequestration D57.812
        vasoocclusive pain D57.819
      without crisis D57.80
    thalassemia D57.40
      with
        acute chest syndrome D57.411
        cerebral vascular involvement D57.413
        crisis (painful) D57.419
          with specified complication NEC D57.418
        splenic sequestration D57.412
        vasoocclusive pain D57.419
      beta plus D57.44
        with
          acute chest syndrome D57.451
          cerebral vascular involvement D57.453
          crisis D57.459

Disease, diseased — *continued*
  sickle-cell — *continued*
    thalassemia — *continued*
      beta plus — *continued*
        with — *continued*
          crisis — *continued*
            with specified complication NEC
              D57.458
          splenic sequestration D57.452
          vasoocclusive pain D57.459
        without crisis D57.44
      beta zero D57.42
        with
          acute chest syndrome D57.431
          cerebral vascular involvement D57.433
          crisis D57.439
            with specified complication NEC
              D57.438
          splenic sequestration D57.432
          vasoocclusive pain D57.439
        without crisis D57.42
  silo-filler's J68.8
    bronchitis J68.0
    pneumonitis J68.0
    pulmonary edema J68.1
  simian B B00.4
  Simons' (progressive lipodystrophy) E88.1
  sin nombre virus B33.4
  sinus — *see* Sinusitis
  Sirkari's B55.0
  sixth B08.20
    due to human herpesvirus 6 B08.21
    due to human herpesvirus 7 B08.22
  skin L98.9
    due to metabolic disorder NEC E88.9 *[L99]*
    specified NEC L98.8
  slim (HIV) B20
  small vessel I73.9
  Sneddon-Wilkinson (subcorneal pustular dermatosis)
    L13.1
  South African creeping B88.0
  spinal (cord) G95.9
    congenital Q06.9
    specified NEC G95.89
  spine — *see also* Spondylopathy
    joint — *see* Dorsopathy
    tuberculous A18.01
  spinocerebellar (hereditary) G11.9
    specified NEC G11.8
  spleen D73.9
    amyloid E85.4 *[D77]*
    organic D73.9
    polycystic Q89.09
    postinfectional D73.89
  sponge-diver's — *see* Toxicity, venom, marine animal,
    sea anemone
  Startle Q89.8
  Steinert's G71.11
  Sticker's (erythema infectiosum) B08.3
  Stieda's (calcification, knee joint) — *see* Bursitis, tibial
    collateral
  Stokes' (exophthalmic goiter) — *see* Hyperthyroidism,
    with, goiter (diffuse)
  Stokes-Adams (syncope with heart block) I45.9
  stomach K31.9
    functional, psychogenic F45.8
    specified NEC K31.89
  stonemason's J62.8
  storage
    glycogen — *see* Disease, glycogen storage
    mucopolysaccharide — *see* Mucopolysaccharidosis
  striatopallidal system NEC G25.89
  Stuart-Prower (congenital factor X deficiency) D68.2
  Stuart's (congenital factor X deficiency) D68.2
  subcutaneous tissue — *see* Disease, skin
  supporting structures of teeth K08.9
    specified NEC K08.89
  suprarenal (capsule) (gland) E27.9
    hyperfunction E27.0
    specified NEC E27.8
  sweat glands L74.9
    specified NEC L74.8
  Sweeley-Klionsky E75.21
  Swift (-Feer) — *see* Poisoning, mercury
  swimming-pool granuloma A31.1
  Sylvest's (epidemic pleurodynia) B33.0
  sympathetic nervous system G90.9
  synovium — *see* Disorder, synovium

Disease, diseased — *continued*
  syphilitic — *see* Syphilis
  systemic tissue mast cell D47.02
  tanapox (virus) B08.71
  Tangier E78.6
  Tarral-Besnier (pityriasis rubra pilaris) L44.0
  Tauri's E74.09
  tear duct — *see* Disorder, lacrimal system
  tendon, tendinous — *see also* Disorder, tendon
    nodular — *see* Trigger finger
  terminal vessel I73.9
  testis N50.9
  thalassemia Hb-S — *see* Disease, sickle-cell, thalassemia
  Thaysen-Gee (nontropical sprue) K90.0
  Thomsen G71.12
  throat J39.2
    septic J02.0
  thromboembolic — *see* Embolism
  thymus (gland) E32.9
    specified NEC E32.8
  thyroid (gland) E07.9
    heart — *see also* Hyperthyroidism E05.90 *[I43]*
      with thyroid storm E05.91 *[I43]*
    specified NEC E07.89
  Tietze's M94.0
  tongue K14.9
    specified NEC K14.8
  tonsils, tonsillar (and adenoids) J35.9
  tooth, teeth K08.9
    hard tissues K03.9
      specified NEC K03.89
    pulp NEC K04.99
    specified NEC K08.89
  Tourette's F95.2
  trachea NEC J39.8
  tricuspid I07.9
    nonrheumatic I36.9
  triglyceride-storage E75.5
  trophoblastic — *see* Mole, hydatidiform
  tsutsugamushi A75.3
  tube (fallopian) (noninflammatory) N83.9
    inflammatory — *see* Salpingitis
    specified NEC N83.8
  tuberculous NEC — *see* Tuberculosis
  tubo-ovarian (noninflammatory) N83.9
    inflammatory — *see* Salpingo-oophoritis
    specified NEC N83.8
  tubotympanic, chronic — *see* Otitis, media, suppura-
    tive, chronic, tubotympanic
  tubulo-interstitial N15.9
    specified NEC N15.8
  tympanum — *see* Disorder, tympanic membrane
  Uhl's Q24.8
  Underwood's (sclerema neonatorum) P83.0
  Unverricht (-Lundborg) — *see* Epilepsy, generalized,
    idiopathic
  Urbach-Oppenheim (necrobiosis lipoidica diabetico-
    rum) — *see* E08-E13 with .620
  ureter N28.9
    in (due to)
      schistosomiasis (bilharziasis) B65.0 *[N29]*
  urethra N36.9
    specified NEC N36.8
  urinary (tract) N39.9
    bladder N32.9
      specified NEC N32.89
    specified NEC N39.8
  uterus (noninflammatory) N85.9
    infective — *see* Endometritis
    inflammatory — *see* Endometritis
    specified NEC N85.8
  uveal tract (anterior) H21.9
    posterior H31.9
  vagabond's B85.1
  vagina, vaginal (noninflammatory) N89.9
    inflammatory NEC N76.89
    specified NEC N89.8
  valve, valvular I38
    multiple I08.9
      specified NEC I08.8
  van Creveld-von Gierke (glycogenosis I) E74.01
  vas deferens N50.9
  vascular I99.9
    arteriosclerotic — *see* Arteriosclerosis
    ciliary body NEC — *see* Disorder, iris, vascular
    hypertensive — *see* Hypertension
    iris NEC — *see* Disorder, iris, vascular
    obliterative I77.1

Disease, diseased — *continued*
  vascular — *continued*
    obliterative — *continued*
      peripheral I73.9
    occlusive I99.8
    peripheral (occlusive) I73.9
      in diabetes mellitus — *see* E08-E13 with .51
    vasomotor I73.9
    vasospastic I73.9
    vein I87.9
  venereal — *see also* Disease, sexually transmitted A64
    chlamydial NEC A56.8
      anus A56.3
      genitourinary NOS A56.2
      pharynx A56.4
      rectum A56.3
    fifth A55
    sixth A55
    specified nature or type NEC A63.8
  vertebra, vertebral — *see also* Spondylopathy
    disc — *see* Disorder, disc
  vibration — *see* Vibration, adverse effects
  viral, virus — *see also* Disease, by type of virus B34.9
    arbovirus NOS A94
    arthropod-borne NOS A94
    congenital P35.9
      specified NEC P35.8
    Hanta (with renal manifestations) (Dobrava) (Pu-
      umala) (Seoul) A98.5
      with pulmonary manifestations (Andes) (Bayou)
        (Bermejo) (Black Creek Canal) (Choclo)
        (Juquitiba) (Laguna negra) (Lechiguanas)
        (New York) (Oran) (Sin nombre) B33.4
    Hantaan (Korean hemorrhagic fever) A98.5
    human immunodeficiency (HIV) B20
    Kunjin A83.4
    nonarthropod-borne NOS B34.9
    Powassan A84.81
    Rocio (encephalitis) A83.6
    Sin nombre (Hantavirus) (cardio)-pulmonary syn-
      drome) B33.4
    Tahyna B33.8
    vesicular stomatitis A93.8
  vitreous H43.9
    specified NEC H43.89
  vocal cord J38.3
  Volkmann's, acquired T79.6 ☑
  von Eulenburg's (congenital paramyotonia) G71.19
  von Gierke's (glycogenosis I) E74.01
  von Graefe's — *see* Strabismus, paralytic, ophthalmo-
    plegia, progressive
  von Willebrand (-Jürgens) (angiohemophilia) D68.0
  Vrolik's (osteogenesis imperfecta) Q78.0
  vulva (noninflammatory) N90.9
    inflammatory NEC N76.89
    specified NEC N90.89
  Wallgren's (obstruction of splenic vein with collateral
    circulation) I87.8
  Wassilieff's (leptospiral jaundice) A27.0
  wasting NEC R64
    due to malnutrition E43
      with marasmus E41
  Waterhouse-Friderichsen A39.1
  Wegner's (syphilitic osteochondritis) A50.02
  Weil's (leptospiral jaundice of lung) A27.0
  Weir Mitchell's (erythromelalgia) I73.81
  Werdnig-Hoffmann G12.0
  Wermer's E31.21
  Werner-His (trench fever) A79.0
  Werner-Schultz (neutropenic splenomegaly) D73.81
  Wernicke-Posadas B38.9
  whipworm B79
  white blood cells D72.9
    specified NEC D72.89
  white matter R90.82
  white-spot, meaning lichen sclerosus et atrophicus
    L90.0
    penis N48.0
    vulva N90.4
  Wilkie's K55.1
  Wilkinson-Sneddon (subcorneal pustular dermatosis)
    L13.1
  Willis' — *see* Diabetes
  Wilson's (hepatolenticular degeneration) E83.01
  woolsorter's A22.1
  yaba monkey tumor B08.72
  yaba pox (virus) B08.72
  Zika virus A92.5

Disease, diseased — *continued*
  Zika virus — *continued*
    congenital P35.4
  zoonotic, bacterial A28.9
    specified type NEC A28.8
Disfigurement (due to scar) L90.5
Disgerminoma — *see* Dysgerminoma
DISH (diffuse idiopathic skeletal hyperostosis) — *see* Hyperostosis, ankylosing
Disinsertion, retina — *see* Detachment, retina
Dislocatable hip, congenital Q65.6
Dislocation (articular)
  with fracture — *see* Fracture
  acromioclavicular (joint) S43.10- ☑
    with displacement
      100%-200% S43.12- ☑
      more than 200% S43.13- ☑
    inferior S43.14- ☑
    posterior S43.15- ☑
  ankle S93.0- ☑
  astragalus — *see* Dislocation, ankle
  atlantoaxial S13.121 ☑
  atlantooccipital S13.111 ☑
  atloidooccipital S13.111 ☑
  breast bone S23.29 ☑
  capsule, joint — *code by* site under Dislocation
  carpal (bone) — *see* Dislocation, wrist
  carpometacarpal (joint) NEC S63.05- ☑
    thumb S63.04- ☑
  cartilage (joint) — *code by* site under Dislocation
  cervical spine (vertebra) — *see* Dislocation, vertebra,
    cervical
  chronic — *see* Dislocation, recurrent
  clavicle — *see* Dislocation, acromioclavicular joint
  coccyx S33.2 ☑
  congenital NEC Q68.8
  coracoid — *see* Dislocation, shoulder
  costal cartilage S23.29 ☑
  costochondral S23.29 ☑
  cricoarytenoid articulation S13.29 ☑
  cricothyroid articulation S13.29 ☑
  dorsal vertebra — *see* Dislocation, vertebra, thoracic
  ear ossicle — *see* Discontinuity, ossicles, ear
  elbow S53.10- ☑
    congenital Q68.8
    pathological — *see* Dislocation, pathological NEC,
      elbow
    radial head alone — *see* Dislocation, radial head
    recurrent — *see* Dislocation, recurrent, elbow
    traumatic S53.10- ☑
      anterior S53.11- ☑
      lateral S53.14- ☑
      medial S53.13- ☑
      posterior S53.12- ☑
      specified type NEC S53.19- ☑
  eye, nontraumatic — *see* Luxation, globe
  eyeball, nontraumatic — *see* Luxation, globe
  femur
    distal end — *see* Dislocation, knee
    proximal end — *see* Dislocation, hip
  fibula
    distal end — *see* Dislocation, ankle
    proximal end — *see* Dislocation, knee
  finger S63.25- ☑
    index S63.25- ☑
    interphalangeal S63.27- ☑
      distal S63.29- ☑
        index S63.29- ☑
        little S63.29- ☑
        middle S63.29- ☑
        ring S63.29- ☑
      index S63.27- ☑
      little S63.27- ☑
      middle S63.27- ☑
      proximal S63.28- ☑
        index S63.28- ☑
        little S63.28- ☑
        middle S63.28- ☑
        ring S63.28- ☑
      ring S63.27- ☑
    little S63.25- ☑
    metacarpophalangeal S63.26- ☑
      index S63.26- ☑
      little S63.26- ☑
      middle S63.26- ☑
      ring S63.26- ☑

Dislocation — *continued*
  finger — *continued*
    middle S63.25- ☑
    recurrent — *see* Dislocation, recurrent, finger
    ring S63.25- ☑
    thumb — *see* Dislocation, thumb
  foot S93.30- ☑
    recurrent — *see* Dislocation, recurrent, foot
    specified site NEC S93.33- ☑
    tarsal joint S93.31- ☑
    tarsometatarsal joint S93.32- ☑
    toe — *see* Dislocation, toe
  fracture — *see* Fracture
  glenohumeral (joint) — *see* Dislocation, shoulder
  glenoid — *see* Dislocation, shoulder
  habitual — *see* Dislocation, recurrent
  hip S73.00- ☑
    anterior S73.03- ☑
      obturator S73.02- ☑
    central S73.04- ☑
    congenital (total) Q65.2
      bilateral Q65.1
      partial Q65.5
        bilateral Q65.4
        unilateral Q65.3- ☑
      unilateral Q65.0- ☑
    developmental M24.85- ☑
    pathological — *see* Dislocation, pathological NEC,
      hip
    posterior S73.01- ☑
    recurrent — *see* Dislocation, recurrent, hip
  humerus, proximal end — *see* Dislocation, shoulder
  incomplete — *see* Subluxation, by site
  incus — *see* Discontinuity, ossicles, ear
  infracoracoid — *see* Dislocation, shoulder
  innominate (pubic junction) (sacral junction) S33.39 ☑
    acetabulum — *see* Dislocation, hip
  interphalangeal (joint(s))
    finger S63.279 ☑
      distal S63.29- ☑
        index S63.29- ☑
        little S63.29- ☑
        middle S63.29- ☑
        ring S63.29- ☑
      index S63.27- ☑
      little S63.27- ☑
      middle S63.27- ☑
      proximal S63.28- ☑
        index S63.28- ☑
        little S63.28- ☑
        middle S63.28- ☑
        ring S63.28- ☑
      ring S63.27- ☑
    foot or toe — *see* Dislocation, toe
    thumb S63.12- ☑
  jaw (cartilage) (meniscus) S03.0- ☑
  joint prosthesis — *see* Complications, joint prosthesis,
    mechanical, displacement, by site
  knee S83.106 ☑
    cap — *see* Dislocation, patella
    congenital Q68.2
    old M23.8X- ☑
    patella — *see* Dislocation, patella
    pathological — *see* Dislocation, pathological NEC,
      knee
    proximal tibia
      anteriorly S83.11- ☑
      laterally S83.14- ☑
      medially S83.13- ☑
      posteriorly S83.12- ☑
    recurrent — *see also* Derangement, knee, specified
      NEC
    specified type NEC S83.19- ☑
  lacrimal gland H04.16- ☑
  lens (complete) H27.10
    anterior H27.12- ☑
    congenital Q12.1
    ocular implant — *see* Complications, intraocular
      lens
    partial H27.11- ☑
    posterior H27.13- ☑
    traumatic S05.8X- ☑
  ligament — *code by* site under Dislocation
  lumbar (vertebra) — *see* Dislocation, vertebra, lumbar
  lumbosacral (vertebra) — *see also* Dislocation, vertebra,
    lumbar

Dislocation — continued
    lumbosacral — see also Dislocation, vertebra, lumbar
        — continued
        congenital Q76.49
    mandible S03.0- ☑
    meniscus (knee) — see Tear, meniscus
        other sites - code by site under Dislocation
    metacarpal (bone)
        distal end — see Dislocation, finger
        proximal end S63.06- ☑
    metacarpophalangeal (joint)
        finger S63.26- ☑
            index S63.26- ☑
            little S63.26- ☑
            middle S63.26- ☑
            ring S63.26- ☑
            thumb S63.11- ☑
    metatarsal (bone) — see Dislocation, foot
    metatarsophalangeal (joint(s)) — see Dislocation, toe
    midcarpal (joint) S63.03- ☑
    midtarsal (joint) — see Dislocation, foot
    neck S13.20 ☑
        specified site NEC S13.29 ☑
        vertebra — see Dislocation, vertebra, cervical
    nose (septal cartilage) S03.1 ☑
    occipitoatloid S13.111 ☑
    old — see Derangement, joint, specified type NEC
    ossicles, ear — see Discontinuity, ossicles, ear
    partial — see Subluxation, by site
    patella S83.006 ☑
        congenital Q74.1
        lateral S83.01- ☑
        recurrent (nontraumatic) M22.0- ☑
            incomplete M22.1- ☑
        specified type NEC S83.09- ☑
    pathological NEC M24.30
        ankle M24.37- ☑
        elbow M24.32- ☑
        foot joint M24.37- ☑
        hand joint M24.34- ☑
        hip M24.35- ☑
        knee M24.36- ☑
        lumbosacral joint — see subcategory M53.2 ☑
        pelvic region — see Dislocation, pathological, hip
        sacroiliac — see subcategory M53.2 ☑
        shoulder M24.31- ☑
        specified site NEC M24.39
        wrist M24.33- ☑
    pelvis NEC S33.30 ☑
        specified NEC S33.39 ☑
    phalanx
        finger or hand — see Dislocation, finger
        foot or toe — see Dislocation, toe
    prosthesis, internal — see Complications, prosthetic
        device, by site, mechanical
    radial head S53.006 ☑
        anterior S53.01- ☑
        posterior S53.02- ☑
        specified type NEC S53.09- ☑
    radiocarpal (joint) S63.02- ☑
    radiohumeral (joint) — see Dislocation, radial head
    radioulnar (joint)
        distal S63.01- ☑
        proximal — see Dislocation, elbow
    radius
        distal end — see Dislocation, wrist
        proximal end — see Dislocation, radial head
    recurrent M24.40
        ankle M24.47- ☑
        elbow M24.42- ☑
        finger M24.44- ☑
        foot joint M24.47- ☑
        hand joint M24.44- ☑
        hip M24.45- ☑
        knee M24.46- ☑
            patella — see Dislocation, patella, recurrent
        patella — see Dislocation, patella, recurrent
        sacroiliac — see subcategory M53.2 ☑
        shoulder M24.41- ☑
        specified site NEC M24.49
        toe M24.47- ☑
        vertebra — see also subcategory M43.5 ☑
            atlantoaxial M43.4
                with myelopathy M43.3
        wrist M24.43- ☑
    rib (cartilage) S23.29 ☑

Dislocation — continued
    sacrococcygeal S33.2 ☑
    sacroiliac (joint) (ligament) S33.2 ☑
        congenital Q74.2
        recurrent — see subcategory M53.2 ☑
    sacrum S33.2 ☑
    scaphoid (bone) (hand) (wrist) — see Dislocation, wrist
        foot — see Dislocation, foot
    scapula — see Dislocation, shoulder, girdle, scapula
    semilunar cartilage, knee — see Tear, meniscus
    septal cartilage (nose) S03.1 ☑
    septum (nasal) (old) J34.2
    sesamoid bone — code by site under Dislocation
    shoulder (blade) (ligament) (joint) (traumatic)
        S43.006 ☑
        acromioclavicular — see Dislocation, acromioclavic-
            ular
        chronic — see Dislocation, recurrent, shoulder
        congenital Q68.8
        girdle S43.30- ☑
            scapula S43.31- ☑
            specified site NEC S43.39- ☑
        humerus S43.00- ☑
            anterior S43.01- ☑
            inferior S43.03- ☑
            posterior S43.02- ☑
        pathological — see Dislocation, pathological NEC,
            shoulder
        recurrent — see Dislocation, recurrent, shoulder
        specified type NEC S43.08- ☑
    spine
        cervical — see Dislocation, vertebra, cervical
        congenital Q76.49
        due to birth trauma P11.5
        lumbar — see Dislocation, vertebra, lumbar
        thoracic — see Dislocation, vertebra, thoracic
    spontaneous — see Dislocation, pathological
    sternoclavicular (joint) S43.206 ☑
        anterior S43.21- ☑
        posterior S43.22- ☑
    sternum S23.29 ☑
    subglenoid — see Dislocation, shoulder
    symphysis pubis S33.4 ☑
    talus — see Dislocation, ankle
    tarsal (bone(s)) (joint(s)) — see Dislocation, foot
    tarsometatarsal (joint(s)) — see Dislocation, foot
    temporomandibular (joint) S03.0- ☑
    thigh, proximal end — see Dislocation, hip
    thorax S23.20 ☑
        specified site NEC S23.29 ☑
        vertebra — see Dislocation, vertebra
    thumb S63.10- ☑
        interphalangeal joint — see Dislocation, interpha-
            langeal (joint), thumb
        metacarpophalangeal joint — see Dislocation,
            metacarpophalangeal (joint), thumb
    thyroid cartilage S13.29 ☑
    tibia
        distal end — see Dislocation, ankle
        proximal end — see Dislocation, knee
    tibiofibular (joint)
        distal — see Dislocation, ankle
        superior — see Dislocation, knee
    toe(s) S93.106 ☑
        great S93.10- ☑
            interphalangeal joint S93.11- ☑
            metatarsophalangeal joint S93.12- ☑
        interphalangeal joint S93.119 ☑
        lesser S93.106 ☑
            interphalangeal joint S93.11- ☑
            metatarsophalangeal joint S93.12- ☑
        metatarsophalangeal joint S93.12- ☑
    tooth S03.2 ☑
    trachea S23.29 ☑
    ulna
        distal end S63.07- ☑
        proximal end — see Dislocation, elbow
    ulnohumeral (joint) — see Dislocation, elbow
    vertebra (articular process) (body) (traumatic)
        cervical S13.101 ☑
            atlantoaxial joint S13.121 ☑
            atlantooccipital joint S13.111 ☑
            atloidooccipital joint S13.111 ☑
            joint between
                C0 and C1 S13.111 ☑
                C1 and C2 S13.121 ☑

Dislocation — continued
    vertebra — continued
        cervical — continued
            joint between — continued
                C2 and C3 S13.131 ☑
                C3 and C4 S13.141 ☑
                C4 and C5 S13.151 ☑
                C5 and C6 S13.161 ☑
                C6 and C7 S13.171 ☑
                C7 and T1 S13.181 ☑
            occipitoatloid joint S13.111 ☑
        congenital Q76.49
        lumbar S33.101 ☑
            joint between
                L1 and L2 S33.111 ☑
                L2 and L3 S33.121 ☑
                L3 and L4 S33.131 ☑
                L4 and L5 S33.141 ☑
        nontraumatic — see Displacement, intervertebral
            disc
        partial — see Subluxation, by site
        recurrent NEC — see subcategory M43.5 ☑
        thoracic S23.101 ☑
            joint between
                T1 and T2 S23.111 ☑
                T2 and T3 S23.121 ☑
                T3 and T4 S23.123 ☑
                T4 and T5 S23.131 ☑
                T5 and T6 S23.133 ☑
                T6 and T7 S23.141 ☑
                T7 and T8 S23.143 ☑
                T8 and T9 S23.151 ☑
                T9 and T10 S23.153 ☑
                T10 and T11 S23.161 ☑
                T11 and T12 S23.163 ☑
                T12 and L1 S23.171 ☑
    wrist (carpal bone) S63.006 ☑
        carpometacarpal joint — see Dislocation, car-
            pometacarpal (joint)
        distal radioulnar joint — see Dislocation, radioulnar
            (joint), distal
        metacarpal bone, proximal — see Dislocation,
            metacarpal (bone), proximal end
        midcarpal — see Dislocation, midcarpal (joint)
        radiocarpal joint — see Dislocation, radiocarpal
            (joint)
        recurrent — see Dislocation, recurrent, wrist
        specified site NEC S63.09- ☑
        ulna — see Dislocation, ulna, distal end
    xiphoid cartilage S23.29 ☑
Disorder (of) — see also Disease
    acantholytic L11.9
        specified NEC L11.8
    acute
        psychotic — see Psychosis, acute
        stress F43.0
    adjustment (grief) F43.20
        with
            anxiety F43.22
                with depressed mood F43.23
            conduct disturbance F43.24
                with emotional disturbance F43.25
            depressed mood F43.21
                with anxiety F43.23
            other specified symptom F43.29
    adrenal (capsule) (gland) (medullary) E27.9
        specified NEC E27.8
    adrenogenital E25.9
        drug-induced E25.8
        iatrogenic E25.8
        idiopathic E25.8
    adult personality (and behavior) F69
        specified NEC F68.8
    affective (mood) — see Disorder, mood
    aggressive, unsocialized F91.1
    alcohol use
        mild F10.10
            with
                alcohol intoxication F10.129
                    delirium F10.121
                alcohol-induced
                    anxiety disorder F10.180
                    bipolar and related disorder F10.14
                    depressive disorder F10.14
                    psychotic disorder F10.159
                    sexual dysfunction F10.181
                    sleep disorder F10.182

▽ Subterms under main terms may continue to next column or page   ☑ **Additional Character Required** — Refer to the Tabular List for Character Selection   **111**

Dislocation — Disorder

Disorder — *continued*
 alcohol use — *continued*
  mild — *continued*
   in remission (early) (sustained) F10.11
  moderate or severe F10.20
   with
    alcohol intoxication F10.229
     delirium F10.221
    alcohol-induced
     anxiety disorder F10.280
     bipolar and related disorder F10.24
     depressive disorder F10.24
     major neurocognitive disorder, amnestic-confabulatory type F10.26
     major neurocognitive disorder, non-amnestic-confabulatory type F10.27
     mild neurocognitive disorder F10.288
     psychotic disorder F10.259
     sexual dysfunction F10.281
     sleep disorder F10.282
   in remission (early) (sustained) F10.21
 alcohol-related F10.99
  with
   amnestic disorder, persisting F10.96
   anxiety disorder F10.980
   dementia, persisting F10.97
   intoxication F10.929
    with delirium F10.921
    uncomplicated F10.920
   mood disorder F10.94
   other specified F10.988
   psychotic disorder F10.959
    with
     delusions F10.950
     hallucinations F10.951
   sexual dysfunction F10.981
   sleep disorder F10.982
 allergic — *see* Allergy
 alveolar NEC J84.09
 amino-acid
  cystathioninuria E72.19
  cystinosis E72.04
  cystinuria E72.01
  glycinuria E72.09
  homocystinuria E72.11
  metabolism — *see* Disturbance, metabolism, amino-acid
   specified NEC E72.89
  neonatal, transitory P74.8
  renal transport NEC E72.09
  transport NEC E72.09
 amnesic, amnestic
  alcohol-induced F10.96
   with dependence F10.26
  due to (secondary to) general medical condition F04
  psychoactive NEC-induced F19.96
   with
    abuse F19.16
    dependence F19.26
  sedative, hypnotic or anxiolytic-induced F13.96
   with dependence F13.26
 amphetamine (or other stimulant) use
  mild
   with
    amphetamine, cocaine, or other stimulant intoxication
     with perceptual disturbances F15.122
     without perceptual disturbances F15.129
    amphetamine (or other stimulant)-induced
     anxiety disorder F15.180
     bipolar and related disorder F15.14
     depressive disorder F15.14
     obsessive-compulsive and related disorder F15.188
     psychotic disorder F15.159
     sexual dysfunction F15.181
    intoxication delirium F15.121
  moderate or severe
   with
    amphetamine, cocaine, or other stimulant intoxication
     with perceptual disturbances F15.222
     without perceptual disturbances F15.229
    amphetamine (or other stimulant)-induced
     anxiety disorder F15.280
     bipolar and related disorder F15.24
     depressive disorder F15.24

Disorder — *continued*
 amphetamine use — *continued*
  moderate or severe — *continued*
   with — *continued*
    amphetamine-induced — *continued*
     obsessive-compulsive and related disorder F15.288
     psychotic disorder F15.259
     sexual dysfunction F15.281
    intoxication delirium F15.221
 amphetamine-type substance use
  mild F15.10
   in remission (early) (sustained) F15.11
  moderate F15.20
   in remission (early) (sustained) F15.21
  severe F15.20
   in remission (early) (sustained) F15.21
 anaerobic glycolysis with anemia D55.29
 anxiety F41.9
  due to (secondary to)
   alcohol F10.980
    in
     abuse F10.180
     dependence F10.280
   amphetamine F15.980
    in
     abuse F15.180
     dependence F15.280
   anxiolytic F13.980
    in
     abuse F13.180
     dependence F13.280
   caffeine F15.980
    in
     abuse F15.180
     dependence F15.280
   cannabis F12.980
    in
     abuse F12.180
     dependence F12.280
   cocaine F14.980
    in
     abuse F14.180
     dependence F14.180
   general medical condition F06.4
   hallucinogen F16.980
    in
     abuse F16.180
     dependence F16.280
   hypnotic F13.980
    in
     abuse F13.180
     dependence F13.280
   inhalant F18.980
    in
     abuse F18.180
     dependence F18.280
   phencyclidine F16.980
    in
     abuse F16.180
     dependence F16.280
   psychoactive substance NEC F19.980
    in
     abuse F19.180
     dependence F19.280
   sedative F13.980
    in
     abuse F13.180
     dependence F13.280
   volatile solvents F18.980
    in
     abuse F18.180
     dependence F18.280
  generalized F41.1
  illness F45.21
  mixed
   with depression (mild) F41.8
   specified NEC F41.3
  organic F06.4
  phobic F40.9
   of childhood F40.8
  specified NEC F41.8
 aortic valve — *see* Endocarditis, aortic
 aromatic amino-acid metabolism E70.9
  specified NEC E70.89
 arteriole NEC I77.89
 artery NEC I77.89
 articulation — *see* Disorder, joint

Disorder — *continued*
 attachment (childhood)
  disinhibited F94.2
  reactive F94.1
 attention-deficit hyperactivity (adolescent) (adult) (child) F90.9
  combined
   presentation F90.2
   type F90.2
  hyperactive
   impulsive presentation F90.1
   type F90.1
  inattentive
   presentation F90.0
   type F90.0
  specified type NEC F90.8
 attention-deficit without hyperactivity (adolescent) (adult) (child) F98.8
 auditory processing (central) H93.25
 autism spectrum F84.0
 autistic F84.0
 autoimmune D89.89
 autonomic nervous system G90.9
  specified NEC G90.8
 avoidant
  child or adolescent F40.10
  restrictive food intake F50.82
 balance
  acid-base E87.8
   mixed E87.4
  electrolyte E87.8
  fluid NEC E87.8
 behavioral (disruptive) — *see* Disorder, conduct
 beta-amino-acid metabolism E72.89
 bile acid and cholesterol metabolism E78.70
  Barth syndrome E78.71
  other specified E78.79
  Smith-Lemli-Opitz syndrome E78.72
 bilirubin excretion E80.6
 binge eating F50.81
 binocular
  movement H51.9
   convergence
    excess H51.12
    insufficiency H51.11
   internuclear ophthalmoplegia — *see* Ophthalmoplegia, internuclear
   palsy of conjugate gaze H51.0
   specified type NEC H51.8
  vision NEC — *see* Disorder, vision, binocular
 bipolar (I) (type I) F31.9
  and related due to a known physiological condition
   with
    manic features F06.33
    manic- or hypomanic-like episodes F06.33
    mixed features F06.34
  current (or most recent) episode
   depressed F31.9
    with psychotic features F31.5
    without psychotic features F31.30
     mild F31.31
     moderate F31.32
     severe (without psychotic features) F31.4
      with psychotic features F31.5
   hypomanic F31.0
   manic F31.9
    with psychotic features F31.2
    without psychotic features F31.10
     mild F31.11
     moderate F31.12
     severe (without psychotic features) F31.13
      with psychotic features F31.2
   mixed F31.60
    mild F31.61
    moderate F31.62
    severe (without psychotic features) F31.63
     with psychotic features F31.64
    severe depression (without psychotic features) F31.4
     with psychotic features F31.5
  in remission (currently) F31.70
   in full remission
    most recent episode
     depressed F31.76
     hypomanic F31.72
     manic F31.74
     mixed F31.78

Disorder — *continued*
  bipolar — *continued*
    in remission — *continued*
      in partial remission
        most recent episode
          depressed F31.75
          hypomanic F31.71
          manic F31.73
          mixed F31.77
    organic F06.30
    single manic episode F30.9
      mild F30.11
      moderate F30.12
      severe (without psychotic symptoms) F30.13
        with psychotic symptoms F30.2
    specified NEC F31.89
  bipolar II (type 2) F31.81
  bladder N32.9
    functional NEC N31.9
    in schistosomiasis B65.0 *[N33]*
    specified NEC N32.89
  bleeding D68.9
  blood D75.9
    in congenital early syphilis A50.09 *[D77]*
  body dysmorphic F45.22
  bone M89.9
    continuity M84.9
      specified type NEC M84.80
        ankle M84.87- ☑
        fibula M84.86- ☑
        foot M84.87- ☑
        hand M84.84- ☑
        humerus M84.82- ☑
        neck M84.88
        pelvis M84.859
        radius M84.83- ☑
        rib M84.88
        shoulder M84.81- ☑
        skull M84.88
        thigh M84.85- ☑
        tibia M84.86- ☑
        ulna M84.83- ☑
        vertebra M84.88
    density and structure M85.9
      cyst — *see also* Cyst, bone, specified type NEC
        aneurysmal — *see* Cyst, bone, aneurysmal
        solitary — *see* Cyst, bone, solitary
      diffuse idiopathic skeletal hyperostosis — *see* Hyperostosis, ankylosing
      fibrous dysplasia (monostotic) — *see* Dysplasia, fibrous, bone
      fluorosis — *see* Fluorosis, skeletal
      hyperostosis of skull M85.2
      osteitis condensans — *see* Osteitis, condensans
      specified type NEC M85.8- ☑
        ankle M85.87- ☑
        foot M85.87- ☑
        forearm M85.83- ☑
        hand M85.84- ☑
        lower leg M85.86- ☑
        multiple sites M85.89
        neck M85.88
        rib M85.88
        shoulder M85.81- ☑
        skull M85.88
        thigh M85.85- ☑
        upper arm M85.82- ☑
        vertebra M85.88
    development and growth NEC M89.20
      carpus M89.24- ☑
      clavicle M89.21- ☑
      femur M89.25- ☑
      fibula M89.26- ☑
      finger M89.24- ☑
      humerus M89.22- ☑
      ilium M89.259
      ischium M89.259
      metacarpus M89.24- ☑
      metatarsus M89.27- ☑
      multiple sites M89.29
      neck M89.28
      radius M89.23- ☑
      rib M89.28
      scapula M89.21- ☑
      skull M89.28
      tarsus M89.27- ☑
      tibia M89.26- ☑

Disorder — *continued*
  bone — *continued*
    development and growth — *continued*
      toe M89.27- ☑
      ulna M89.23- ☑
      vertebra M89.28
    specified type NEC M89.8X- ☑
  brachial plexus G54.0
  branched-chain amino-acid metabolism E71.2
    specified NEC E71.19
  breast N64.9
    agalactia — *see* Agalactia
    associated with
      lactation O92.70
        specified NEC O92.79
      pregnancy O92.20
        specified NEC O92.29
      puerperium O92.20
        specified NEC O92.29
    cracked nipple — *see* Cracked nipple
    galactorrhea — *see* Galactorrhea
    hypogalactia O92.4
    lactation disorder NEC O92.79
    mastitis — *see* Mastitis
    nipple infection — *see* Infection, nipple
    retracted nipple — *see* Retraction, nipple
    specified type NEC N64.89
  Briquet's F45.0
  bullous, in diseases classified elsewhere L14
  caffeine use
    mild
      with
        caffeine-induced
          anxiety disorder F15.180
          sleep disorder F15.182
    moderate or severe
      with
        caffeine-induced
          anxiety disorder F15.280
          sleep disorder F15.282
  cannabis use
    mild F12.10
      with
        cannabis intoxication delirium F12.121
          with perceptual disturbances F12.122
          without perceptual disturbances F12.129
        cannabis-induced
          anxiety disorder F12.180
          psychotic disorder F12.159
          sleep disorder F12.188
      in remission (early) (sustained) F12.11
    moderate or severe F12.20
      with
        cannabis intoxication
          with perceptual disturbances F12.222
          without perceptual disturbances F12.229
        cannabis-induced
          anxiety disorder F12.280
          psychotic disorder F12.259
          sleep disorder F12.288
        delirium F12.221
      in remission (early) (sustained) F12.21
  carbohydrate
    absorption, intestinal NEC E74.39
    metabolism (congenital) E74.9
      specified NEC E74.89
  cardiac, functional I51.89
  carnitine metabolism E71.40
  cartilage M94.9
    articular NEC — *see* Derangement, joint, articular cartilage
    chondrocalcinosis — *see* Chondrocalcinosis
    specified type NEC M94.8X- ☑
      articular — *see* Derangement, joint, articular cartilage
      multiple sites M94.8X0
  catatonia (due to known physiological condition) (with another mental disorder) F06.1
  catatonic
    due to (secondary to) known physiological condition F06.1
    organic F06.1
  central auditory processing H93.25
  cervical
    region NEC M53.82
    root (nerve) NEC G54.2
  character NOS F60.9
  childhood disintegrative NEC F84.3

Disorder — *continued*
  cholesterol and bile acid metabolism E78.70
    Barth syndrome E78.71
    other specified E78.79
    Smith-Lemli-Opitz syndrome E78.72
  choroid H31.9
    atrophy — *see* Atrophy, choroid
    degeneration — *see* Degeneration, choroid
    detachment — *see* Detachment, choroid
    dystrophy — *see* Dystrophy, choroid
    hemorrhage — *see* Hemorrhage, choroid
    rupture — *see* Rupture, choroid
    scar — *see* Scar, chorioretinal
    solar retinopathy — *see* Retinopathy, solar
    specified type NEC H31.8
  ciliary body — *see* Disorder, iris
    degeneration — *see* Degeneration, ciliary body
  coagulation (factor) — *see also* Defect, coagulation D68.9
    newborn, transient P61.6
  cocaine use
    mild F14.10
      with
        amphetamine, cocaine, or other stimulant intoxication
          with perceptual disturbances F14.122
          without perceptual disturbances F14.129
        cocaine intoxication delirium F14.121
        cocaine-induced
          anxiety disorder F14.180
          bipolar and related disorder F14.14
          depressive disorder F14.14
          obsessive-compulsive and related disorder F14.188
          psychotic disorder F14.159
          sexual dysfunction F14.181
          sleep disorder F14.182
      in remission (early) (sustained) F14.11
    moderate or severe F14.20
      with
        amphetamine, cocaine, or other stimulant intoxication
          with perceptual disturbances F14.222
          without perceptual disturbances F14.229
        cocaine intoxication delirium F14.221
        cocaine-induced
          anxiety disorder F14.280
          bipolar and related disorder F14.24
          depressive disorder F14.24
          obsessive-compulsive and related disorder F14.288
          psychotic disorder F14.259
          sexual dysfunction F14.281
          sleep disorder F14.282
      in remission (early) (sustained) F14.21
  coccyx NEC M53.3
  cognitive F09
    due to (secondary to) general medical condition F09
    persisting R41.89
      due to
        alcohol F10.97
          with dependence F10.27
        anxiolytics F13.97
          with dependence F13.27
        hypnotics F13.97
          with dependence F13.27
        sedatives F13.97
          with dependence F13.27
        specified substance NEC F19.97
          with
            abuse F19.17
            dependence F19.27
  communication F80.9
    social pragmatic F80.82
  conduct (childhood) F91.9
    adjustment reaction — *see* Disorder, adjustment
    adolescent onset type F91.2
    childhood onset type F91.1
    compulsive F63.9
    confined to family context F91.0
    depressive F91.8
    group type F91.2
    hyperkinetic — *see* Disorder, attention-deficit hyperactivity
    oppositional defiance F91.3
    socialized F91.2
    solitary aggressive type F91.1
    specified NEC F91.8

Index

Disorder — *continued*
- conduct — *continued*
  - unsocialized (aggressive) F91.1
- conduction, heart I45.9
- congenital glycosylation (CDG) E74.89
- conjunctiva H11.9
  - infection — *see* Conjunctivitis
- connective tissue, localized L94.9
  - specified NEC L94.8
- conversion (functional neurological symptom disorder)
  - with
    - abnormal movement F44.4
    - anesthesia or sensory loss F44.6
    - attacks or seizures F44.5
    - mixed symptoms F44.7
    - special sensory symptoms F44.6
    - speech symptoms F44.4
    - swallowing symptoms F44.4
    - weakness or paralysis F44.4
- convulsive (secondary) — *see* Convulsions
- cornea H18.9
  - deformity — *see* Deformity, cornea
  - degeneration — *see* Degeneration, cornea
  - deposits — *see* Deposit, cornea
  - due to contact lens H18.82- ☑
    - specified as edema — *see* Edema, cornea
  - edema — *see* Edema, cornea
  - keratitis — *see* Keratitis
  - keratoconjunctivitis — *see* Keratoconjunctivitis
  - membrane change — *see* Change, corneal membrane
  - neovascularization — *see* Neovascularization, cornea
  - scar — *see* Opacity, cornea
  - specified type NEC H18.89- ☑
  - ulcer — *see* Ulcer, cornea
- corpus cavernosum N48.9
- cranial nerve — *see* Disorder, nerve, cranial
- Cyclin-Dependent Kinase-Like 5 Deficiency (CDKL5) G40.42
- cyclothymic F34.0
- defiant oppositional F91.3
- delusional (persistent) (systematized) F22
  - induced F24
- depersonalization F48.1
- depressive F32.A
  - due to known physiological condition
    - with
      - depressive features F06.31
      - major depressive-like episode F06.32
      - mixed features F06.34
  - major F32.9
    - with psychotic symptoms F32.3
    - in remission (full) F32.5
      - partial F32.4
    - recurrent F33.9
      - with psychotic features F33.3
    - single episode F32.9
      - mild F32.0
      - moderate F32.1
      - severe (without psychotic symptoms) F32.2
        - with psychotic symptoms F32.3
  - organic F06.31
  - persistent F34.1
  - recurrent F33.9
    - current episode
      - mild F33.0
      - moderate F33.1
      - severe (without psychotic symptoms) F33.2
        - with psychotic symptoms F33.3
    - in remission F33.40
      - full F33.42
      - partial F33.41
    - specified NEC F33.8
  - single episode — *see* Episode, depressive
  - specified NEC F32.89
- developmental F89
  - arithmetical skills F81.2
  - coordination (motor) F82
  - expressive writing F81.81
  - language F80.9
    - expressive F80.1
    - mixed receptive and expressive F80.2
    - receptive type F80.2
    - specified NEC F80.89
  - learning F81.9
    - arithmetical F81.2
    - reading F81.0

Disorder — *continued*
- developmental — *continued*
  - mixed F88
  - motor coordination or function F82
  - pervasive F84.9
    - specified NEC F84.8
  - phonological F80.0
  - reading F81.0
  - scholastic skills — *see also* Disorder, learning
    - mixed F81.89
  - specified NEC F88
  - speech F80.9
    - articulation F80.0
    - specified NEC F80.89
  - written expression F81.81
- diaphragm J98.6
- digestive (system) K92.9
  - newborn P78.9
    - specified NEC P78.89
  - postprocedural — *see* Complication, gastrointestinal
  - psychogenic F45.8
- disc (intervertebral) M51.9
  - with
    - myelopathy
      - cervical region M50.00
      - cervicothoracic region M50.03
      - high cervical region M50.01
      - lumbar region M51.06
      - mid-cervical region M50.020
      - sacrococcygeal region M53.3
      - thoracic region M51.04
      - thoracolumbar region M51.05
    - radiculopathy
      - cervical region M50.10
      - cervicothoracic region M50.13
      - high cervical region M50.11
      - lumbar region M51.16
      - lumbosacral region M51.17
      - mid-cervical region M50.120
      - sacrococcygeal region M53.3
      - thoracic region M51.14
      - thoracolumbar region M51.15
  - cervical M50.90
    - with
      - myelopathy M50.00
        - C2-C3 M50.01
        - C3-C4 M50.01
        - C4-C5 M50.021
        - C5-C6 M50.022
        - C6-C7 M50.023
        - C7-T1 M50.03
        - cervicothoracic region M50.03
        - high cervical region M50.01
        - mid-cervical region M50.020
      - neuritis, radiculitis or radiculopathy M50.10
        - C2-C3 M50.11
        - C3-C4 M50.11
        - C4-C5 M50.121
        - C5-C6 M50.122
        - C6-C7 M50.123
        - C7-T1 M50.13
        - cervicothoracic region M50.13
        - high cervical region M50.11
        - mid-cervical region M50.120
    - C2-C3 M50.91
    - C3-C4 M50.91
    - C4-C5 M50.921
    - C5-C6 M50.922
    - C6-C7 M50.923
    - C7-T1 M50.93
    - cervicothoracic region M50.93
    - degeneration M50.30
      - C2-C3 M50.31
      - C3-C4 M50.31
      - C4-C5 M50.321
      - C5-C6 M50.322
      - C6-C7 M50.323
      - C7-T1 M50.33
      - cervicothoracic region M50.33
      - high cervical region M50.31
      - mid-cervical region M50.320
    - displacement M50.20
      - C2-C3 M50.21
      - C3-C4 M50.21
      - C4-C5 M50.221
      - C5-C6 M50.222
      - C6-C7 M50.223
      - C7-T1 M50.23
      - cervicothoracic region M50.23

Disorder — *continued*
- disc — *continued*
  - cervical — *continued*
    - displacement — *continued*
      - high cervical region M50.21
      - mid-cervical region M50.220
    - high cervical region M50.91
    - mid-cervical region M50.920
    - specified type NEC M50.80
      - C2-C3 M50.81
      - C3-C4 M50.81
      - C4-C5 M50.821
      - C5-C6 M50.822
      - C6-C7 M50.823
      - C7-T1 M50.83
      - cervicothoracic region M50.83
      - high cervical region M50.81
      - mid-cervical region M50.820
  - specified NEC
    - lumbar region M51.86
    - lumbosacral region M51.87
    - sacrococcygeal region M53.3
    - thoracic region M51.84
    - thoracolumbar region M51.85
- disinhibited attachment (childhood) F94.2
- disintegrative, childhood NEC F84.3
- disruptive F91.9
  - mood dysregulation F34.81
  - specified NEC F91.8
- disruptive behavior — *see* Disorder, conduct
- dissocial personality F60.2
- dissociative F44.9
  - affecting
    - motor function F44.4
      - and sensation F44.7
    - sensation F44.6
      - and motor function F44.7
  - brief reactive F43.0
  - due to (secondary to) general medical condition F06.8
  - mixed F44.7
  - organic F06.8
  - other specified NEC F44.89
- double heterozygous sickling — *see* Disease, sickle-cell
- dream anxiety F51.5
- drug induced hemorrhagic D68.32
- drug related F19.99
  - abuse — *see* Abuse, drug
  - dependence — *see* Dependence, drug
- dysmorphic body F45.22
- dysthymic F34.1
- ear H93.9- ☑
  - bleeding — *see* Otorrhagia
  - deafness — *see* Deafness
  - degenerative H93.09- ☑
  - discharge — *see* Otorrhea
  - external H61.9- ☑
    - auditory canal stenosis — *see* Stenosis, external ear canal
    - exostosis — *see* Exostosis, external ear canal
    - impacted cerumen — *see* Impaction, cerumen
    - otitis — *see* Otitis, externa
    - perichondritis — *see* Perichondritis, ear
    - pinna — *see* Disorder, pinna
    - specified type NEC H61.89- ☑
  - inner H83.9- ☑
    - vestibular dysfunction — *see* Disorder, vestibular function
  - middle H74.9- ☑
    - adhesive H74.1- ☑
    - ossicle — *see* Abnormal, ear ossicles
    - polyp — *see* Polyp, ear (middle)
    - specified NEC, in diseases classified elsewhere H75.8- ☑
  - postprocedural — *see* Complications, ear, procedure
  - specified NEC, in diseases classified elsewhere H94.8- ☑
- eating (adult) (psychogenic) F50.9
  - anorexia — *see* Anorexia
  - binge F50.81
  - bulimia F50.2
  - child F98.29
    - pica F98.3
    - rumination disorder F98.21
  - pica F50.89
    - childhood F98.3
- electrolyte (balance) NEC E87.8

☑ Additional Character Required — Refer to the Tabular List for Character Selection   ▽ Subterms under main terms may continue to next column or page

Disorder — Disorder

Disorder — continued
  electrolyte — continued
    with
      abortion — see Abortion by type complicated
        by specified condition NEC
      ectopic pregnancy O08.5
      molar pregnancy O08.5
    acidosis (metabolic) (respiratory) E87.2
    alkalosis (metabolic) (respiratory) E87.3
  elimination, transepidermal L87.9
    specified NEC L87.8
  emotional (persistent) F34.9
    of childhood F93.9
      specified NEC F93.8
  endocrine E34.9
    postprocedural E89.89
      specified NEC E89.89
  erectile (male) (organic) — see also Dysfunction, sexual, male, erectile N52.9
    nonorganic F52.21
  erythematous — see Erythema
  esophagus K22.9
    functional K22.4
    psychogenic F45.8
  eustachian tube H69.9- ☑
    infection — see Salpingitis, eustachian
    obstruction — see Obstruction, eustachian tube
    patulous — see Patulous, eustachian tube
    specified NEC H69.8- ☑
  exhibitionistic F65.2
  extrapyramidal G25.9
    in deseases classified elsewhere — see category G26
    specified type NEC G25.89
  eye H57.9
    postprocedural — see Complication, postprocedural, eye
  eyelid H02.9
    cyst — see Cyst, eyelid
    degenerative H02.70
      chloasma — see Chloasma, eyelid
      madarosis — see Madarosis
      specified type NEC H02.79
      vitiligo — see Vitiligo, eyelid
      xanthelasma — see Xanthelasma
    dermatochalasis — see Dermatochalasis
    edema — see Edema, eyelid
    elephantiasis — see Elephantiasis, eyelid
    foreign body, retained — see Foreign body, retained, eyelid
    function H02.59
      abnormal innervation syndrome — see Syndrome, abnormal innervation
      blepharochalasis — see Blepharochalasis
      blepharoclonus — see Blepharoclonus
      blepharophimosis — see Blepharophimosis
      blepharoptosis — see Blepharoptosis
      lagophthalmos — see Lagophthalmos
      lid retraction — see Retraction, lid
    hypertrichosis — see Hypertrichosis, eyelid
    specified type NEC H02.89
    vascular H02.879
      left H02.876
        lower H02.875
        upper H02.874
      right H02.873
        lower H02.872
        upper H02.871
  factitious
    by proxy F68.A
    imposed on another F68.A
    imposed on self F68.10
      with predominantly
        psychological symptoms F68.11
          with physical symptoms F68.13
        physical symptoms F68.12
          with psychological symptoms F68.13
  factor, coagulation — see Defect, coagulation
  fatty acid
    metabolism E71.30
      specified NEC E71.39
    oxidation
      LCAD E71.310
      MCAD E71.311
      SCAD E71.312
      specified deficiency NEC E71.318
  feeding (infant or child) — see also Disorder, eating R63.30

Disorder — continued
  feeding — see also Disorder, eating — continued
    or eating disorder F50.9
    pediatric
      acute R63.31
      chronic R63.32
      specified NEC F50.9
  feigned (with obvious motivation) Z76.5
    without obvious motivation — see Disorder, factitious
  female
    hypoactive sexual desire F52.0
    orgasmic F52.31
    sexual interest/arousal F52.22
  fetishistic F65.0
  fibroblastic M72.9
    specified NEC M72.8
  fluency
    adult onset F98.5
    childhood onset F80.81
    following
      cerebral infarction I69.323
      cerebrovascular disease I69.923
        specified disease NEC I69.823
      intracerebral hemorrhage I69.123
      nontraumatic intracranial hemorrhage NEC I69.223
      subarachnoid hemorrhage I69.023
    in conditions classified elsewhere R47.82
  fluid balance E87.8
  follicular (skin) L73.9
    specified NEC L73.8
  frotteuristic F65.81
  fructose metabolism E74.10
    essential fructosuria E74.11
    fructokinase deficiency E74.11
    fructose-1, 6-diphosphatase deficiency E74.19
    hereditary fructose intolerance E74.12
    other specified E74.19
  functional polymorphonuclear neutrophils D71
  gallbladder, biliary tract and pancreas in diseases classified elsewhere K87
  gambling F63.0
  gamma aminobutyric acid (GABA) metabolism E72.81
  gamma-glutamyl cycle E72.89
  gastric (functional) K31.9
    motility K30
    psychogenic F45.8
    secretion K30
  gastrointestinal (functional) NOS K92.9
    newborn P78.9
    psychogenic F45.8
  gender-identity or -role F64.9
    childhood F64.2
    effect on relationship F66
    of adolescence or adulthood F64.0
      nontranssexual F64.8
    specified NEC F64.8
    uncertainty F66
  genito-pelvic pain penetration F52.6
  genitourinary system
    female N94.9
    male N50.9
    psychogenic F45.8
  globe H44.9
    degenerated condition H44.50
      absolute glaucoma H44.51- ☑
      atrophy H44.52- ☑
      leucocoria H44.53- ☑
    degenerative H44.30
      chalcosis H44.31- ☑
      myopia — see also Myopia, degenerative H44.2- ☑
      siderosis H44.32- ☑
      specified type NEC H44.39- ☑
    endophthalmitis — see Endophthalmitis
    foreign body, retained — see Foreign body, intraocular, old, retained
    hemophthalmos — see Hemophthalmos
    hypotony H44.40
      due to
        ocular fistula H44.42- ☑
        specified disorder NEC H44.43- ☑
      flat anterior chamber H44.41- ☑
      primary H44.44- ☑
    luxation — see Luxation, globe
    specified type NEC H44.89
  glomerular (in) N05.9

Disorder — continued
  glomerular — continued
    amyloidosis E85.4 [N08]
    cryoglobulinemia D89.1 [N08]
    disseminated intravascular coagulation D65 [N08]
    Fabry's disease E75.21 [N08]
    familial lecithin cholesterol acyltransferase deficiency E78.6 [N08]
    Goodpasture's syndrome M31.0
    hemolytic-uremic syndrome D59.3
    Henoch (-Schönlein) purpura D69.0 [N08]
    malariae malaria B52.0
    microscopic polyangiitis M31.7 [N08]
    multiple myeloma C90.0- ☑ [N08]
    mumps B26.83
    schistosomiasis B65.9 [N08]
    sepsis NEC A41.- ☑ [N08]
      streptococcal A40.- ☑ [N08]
    sickle-cell disorders D57.- ☑ [N08]
    strongyloidiasis B78.9 [N08]
    subacute bacterial endocarditis I33.0 [N08]
    syphilis A52.75
    systemic lupus erythematosus M32.14
    thrombotic thrombocytopenic purpura M31.19 [N08]
    Waldenström macroglobulinemia C88.0 [N08]
    Wegener's granulomatosis M31.31
  gluconeogenesis E74.4
  glucosaminoglycan metabolism — see Disorder, metabolism, glucosaminoglycan
  glucose transport E74.819
    specified NEC E74.818
  glycine metabolism E72.50
    d-glycericacidemia E72.59
    hyperhydroxyprolinemia E72.59
    hyperoxaluria R82.992
      primary E72.53
    hyperprolinemia E72.59
    non-ketotic hyperglycinemia E72.51
    oxalosis E72.53
    oxaluria E72.53
    sarcosinemia E72.59
    trimethylaminuria E72.52
  glycoprotein metabolism E77.9
    specified NEC E77.8
  habit (and impulse) F63.9
    involving sexual behavior NEC F65.9
    specified NEC F63.89
  hallucinogen use
    mild F16.10
      with
        hallucinogen intoxication delirium F16.121
        hallucinogen-induced
          anxiety disorder F16.180
          bipolar and related disorder F16.14
          depressive disorder F16.14
          psychotic disorder F16.159
        other hallucinogen intoxication F16.129
      in remission (early) (sustained) F16.11
    moderate or severe F16.20
      with
        hallucinogen intoxication delirium F16.221
        hallucinogen-induced
          anxiety disorder F16.280
          bipolar and related disorder F16.24
          depressive disorder F16.24
          psychotic disorder F16.259
        other hallucinogen intoxication F16.229
      in remission (early) (sustained) F16.21
  heart action I49.9
  hematological D75.9
    newborn (transient) P61.9
      specified NEC P61.8
  hematopoietic organs D75.9
  hemorrhagic NEC D69.9
    drug-induced D68.32
    due to
      extrinsic circulating anticoagulants D68.32
      increase in
        anti-IIa D68.32
        anti-Xa D68.32
      intrinsic
        circulating anticoagulants D68.318
        increase in
          anti-IXa D68.318
          antithrombin D68.318
          anti-VIIIa D68.318
          anti-XIa D68.318

▽ Subterms under main terms may continue to next column or page   ☑ Additional Character Required — Refer to the Tabular List for Character Selection   115

Disorder — Disorder

Disorder — *continued*
hemorrhagic — *continued*
following childbirth O72.3
hemostasis — *see* Defect, coagulation
histidine metabolism E70.40
histidinemia E70.41
other specified E70.49
hoarding F42.3
hyperkinetic — *see* Disorder, attention-deficit hyperactivity
hyperleucine-isoleucinemia E71.19
hypervalinemia E71.19
hypoactive sexual desire F52.0
hypochondriacal F45.20
body dysmorphic F45.22
neurosis F45.21
other specified F45.29
identity
dissociative F44.81
illness anxiety F45.21
of childhood F93.8
immune mechanism (immunity) D89.9
specified type NEC D89.89
impaired renal tubular function N25.9
specified NEC N25.89
impulse (control) F63.9
inflammatory
pelvic, in diseases classified elsewhere — *see* category N74
penis N48.29
abscess N48.21
cellulitis N48.22
inhalant use
mild F18.10
with
inhalant intoxication F18.129
inhalant intoxication delirium F18.121
inhalant-induced
anxiety disorder F18.180
depressive disorder F18.14
major neurocognitive disorder F18.17
mild neurocognitive disorder F18.188
psychotic disorder F18.159
in remission (early) (sustained) F18.11
moderate or severe F18.20
with
inhalant intoxication F18.229
inhalant intoxication delirium F18.221
inhalant-induced
anxiety disorder F18.280
depressive disorder F18.24
major neurocognitive disorder F18.27
mild neurocognitive disorder F18.288
psychotic disorder F18.259
in remission (early) (sustained) F18.21
integument, newborn P83.9
specified NEC P83.88
intermittent explosive F63.81
internal secretion pancreas — *see* Increased, secretion, pancreas, endocrine
intestine, intestinal
carbohydrate absorption NEC E74.39
postoperative K91.2
functional NEC K59.9
postoperative K91.89
psychogenic F45.8
vascular K55.9
chronic K55.1
specified NEC K55.8
intraoperative (intraprocedural) — *see* Complications, intraoperative
involuntary emotional expression (IEED) F07.89
iris H21.9
adhesions — *see* Adhesions, iris
atrophy — *see* Atrophy, iris
chamber angle recession — *see* Recession, chamber angle
cyst — *see* Cyst, iris
degeneration — *see* Degeneration, iris
in diseases classified elsewhere H22
iridodialysis — *see* Iridodialysis
iridoschisis — *see* Iridoschisis
miotic pupillary cyst — *see* Cyst, pupillary
pupillary
abnormality — *see* Abnormality, pupillary
membrane — *see* Membrane, pupillary
specified type NEC H21.89
vascular NEC H21.1X- ☑

Disorder — *continued*
iron metabolism E83.10
specified NEC E83.19
isovaleric acidemia E71.110
jaw, developmental M27.0
temporomandibular — *see also* Anomaly, dentofacial, temporomandibular joint M26.60- ☑
joint M25.9
derangement — *see* Derangement, joint
effusion — *see* Effusion, joint
fistula — *see* Fistula, joint
hemarthrosis — *see* Hemarthrosis
instability — *see* Instability, joint
osteophyte — *see* Osteophyte
pain — *see* Pain, joint
psychogenic F45.8
specified type NEC M25.80
ankle M25.87- ☑
elbow M25.82- ☑
foot joint M25.87- ☑
hand joint M25.84- ☑
hip M25.85- ☑
knee M25.86- ☑
shoulder M25.81- ☑
wrist M25.83- ☑
stiffness — *see* Stiffness, joint
ketone metabolism E71.32
kidney N28.9
functional (tubular) N25.9
in
schistosomiasis B65.9 [N29]
tubular function N25.9
specified NEC N25.89
lacrimal system H04.9
changes H04.69
fistula — *see* Fistula, lacrimal
gland H04.19
atrophy — *see* Atrophy, lacrimal gland
cyst — *see* Cyst, lacrimal, gland
dacryops — *see* Dacryops
dislocation — *see* Dislocation, lacrimal gland
dry eye syndrome — *see* Syndrome, dry eye
infection — *see* Dacryoadenitis
granuloma — *see* Granuloma, lacrimal
inflammation — *see* Inflammation, lacrimal
obstruction — *see* Obstruction, lacrimal
specified NEC H04.89
lactation NEC O92.79
language (developmental) F80.9
expressive F80.1
mixed receptive and expressive F80.2
receptive F80.2
late luteal phase dysphoric N94.89
learning (specific) F81.9
acalculia R48.8
alexia R48.0
mathematics F81.2
reading F81.0
specified
with impairment in
mathematics F81.2
reading F81.0
written expression F81.81
specified NEC F81.89
spelling F81.81
written expression F81.81
lens H27.9
aphakia — *see* Aphakia
cataract — *see* Cataract
dislocation — *see* Dislocation, lens
specified type NEC H27.8
ligament M24.20
ankle M24.27- ☑
attachment, spine — *see* Enthesopathy, spinal
elbow M24.22- ☑
foot joint M24.27- ☑
hand joint M24.24- ☑
hip M24.25- ☑
knee — *see* Derangement, knee, specified NEC
shoulder M24.21- ☑
specified site NEC M24.29
vertebra M24.28
wrist M24.23- ☑
ligamentous attachments — *see also* Enthesopathy
spine — *see* Enthesopathy, spinal
lipid
metabolism, congenital E78.9

Disorder — *continued*
lipid — *continued*
storage E75.6
specified NEC E75.5
lipoprotein
deficiency (familial) E78.6
metabolism E78.9
specified NEC E78.89
liver K76.9
malarial B54 [K77]
low back — *see also* Dorsopathy, specified NEC
lumbosacral
plexus G54.1
root (nerve) NEC G54.4
lung, interstitial, drug-induced J70.4
acute J70.2
chronic J70.3
dabbing (related) U07.0
e-cigarette (related) U07.0
electronic cigarette (related) U07.0
vaping (associated) (device) (product) (related) (use) U07.0
lymphoproliferative, post-transplant (PTLD) D47.Z1 (*following* D47.4)
lysine and hydroxylysine metabolism E72.3
major neurocognitive — *see* Dementia, in (due to)
male
erectile (organic) — *see also* Dysfunction, sexual, male, erectile N52.9
nonorganic F52.21
hypoactive sexual desire F52.0
orgasmic F52.32
manic F30.9
organic F06.33
mast cell activation — *see* Activation, mast cell
mastoid — *see also* Disorder, ear, middle
postprocedural — *see* Complications, ear, procedure
meninges, specified type NEC G96.198
meniscus — *see* Derangement, knee, meniscus
menopausal N95.9
specified NEC N95.8
menstrual N92.6
psychogenic F45.8
specified NEC N92.5
mental (or behavioral) (nonpsychotic) F99
due to (secondary to)
amphetamine
due to drug abuse — *see* Abuse, drug, stimulant
due to drug dependence — *see* Dependence, drug, stimulant
brain disease, damage and dysfunction F09
caffeine use
due to drug abuse — *see* Abuse, drug, stimulant
due to drug dependence — *see* Dependence, drug, stimulant
cannabis use
due to drug abuse — *see* Abuse, drug, cannabis
due to drug dependence — *see* Dependence, drug, cannabis
general medical condition F09
sedative or hypnotic use
due to drug abuse — *see* Abuse, drug, sedative
due to drug dependence — *see* Dependence, drug, sedative
tobacco (nicotine) use — *see* Dependence, drug, nicotine
following organic brain damage F07.9
frontal lobe syndrome F07.0
personality change F07.0
postconcussional syndrome F07.81
specified NEC F07.89
infancy, childhood or adolescence F98.9
neurotic — *see* Neurosis
organic or symptomatic F09
presenile, psychotic F03 ☑
problem NEC
psychoneurotic — *see* Neurosis
psychotic — *see* Psychosis
puerperal F53.0
senile, psychotic NEC F03 ☑
metabolic, amino acid, transitory, newborn P74.8
metabolism NOS E88.9
amino-acid E72.9
aromatic E70.9

☑ **Additional Character Required** — Refer to the Tabular List for Character Selection   ▽ **Subterms under main terms may continue to next column or page**

Disorder — *continued*
  metabolism — *continued*
    amino-acid — *continued*
      aromatic — *continued*
        albinism — *see* Albinism
        histidine E70.40
          histidinemia E70.41
          other specified E70.49
        hyperphenylalaninemia E70.1
          classical phenylketonuria E70.0
        other specified E70.89
        tryptophan E70.5
        tyrosine E70.20
          hypertyrosinemia E70.21
          other specified E70.29
      branched chain E71.2
        3-methylglutaconic aciduria E71.111
        hyperleucine-isoleucinemia E71.19
        hypervalinemia E71.19
        isovaleric acidemia E71.110
        maple syrup urine disease E71.0
        methylmalonic acidemia E71.120
        organic aciduria NEC E71.118
        other specified E71.19
        proprionate NEC E71.128
        proprionic acidemia E71.121
      glycine E72.50
        d-glycericacidemia E72.59
        hyperhydroxyprolinemia E72.59
        hyperoxaluria R82.992
          primary E72.53
        hyperprolinemia E72.59
        non-ketotic hyperglycinemia E72.51
        other specified E72.59
        sarcosinemia E72.59
        trimethylaminuria E72.52
      hydroxylysine E72.3
      lysine E72.3
      ornithine E72.4
      other specified E72.89
        beta-amino acid E72.89
        gamma-glutamyl cycle E72.89
      straight-chain E72.89
      sulfur-bearing E72.10
        homocystinuria E72.11
        methylenetetrahydrofolate reductase deficiency E72.12
        other specified E72.19
    bile acid and cholesterol metabolism E78.70
    bilirubin E80.7
      specified NEC E80.6
    calcium E83.50
      hypercalcemia E83.52
      hypocalcemia E83.51
      other specified E83.59
    carbohydrate E74.9
      specified NEC E74.89
    cholesterol and bile acid metabolism E78.70
    congenital E88.9
    copper E83.00
      specified type NEC E83.09
      Wilson's disease E83.01
    cystinuria E72.01
    fructose E74.10
    galactose E74.20
    glucosaminoglycan E76.9
      mucopolysaccharidosis — *see* Mucopolysaccharidosis
      specified NEC E76.8
    glutamine E72.89
    glycine E72.50
    glycogen storage (hepatorenal) E74.09
    glycoprotein E77.9
      specified NEC E77.8
    glycosaminoglycan E76.9
      specified NEC E76.8
    in labor and delivery O75.89
    iron E83.10
    isoleucine E71.19
    leucine E71.19
    lipoid E78.9
    lipoprotein E78.9
      specified NEC E78.89
    magnesium E83.40
      hypermagnesemia E83.41
      hypomagnesemia E83.42
      other specified E83.49
    mineral E83.9
      specified NEC E83.89

Disorder — *continued*
  metabolism — *continued*
    mitochondrial E88.40
      MELAS syndrome E88.41
      MERRF syndrome (myoclonic epilepsy associated with ragged-red fibers) E88.42
      other specified E88.49
    ornithine E72.4
    phosphatases E83.30
    phosphorus E83.30
      acid phosphatase deficiency E83.39
      hypophosphatasia E83.39
      hypophosphatemia E83.39
        familial E83.31
      other specified E83.39
      pseudovitamin D deficiency E83.32
    plasma protein NEC E88.09
    porphyrin — *see* Porphyria
    postprocedural E89.89
      specified NEC E89.89
    purine E79.9
      specified NEC E79.8
    pyrimidine E79.9
      specified NEC E79.8
    pyruvate E74.4
    serine E72.89
    sodium E87.8
    specified NEC E88.89
    threonine E72.89
    valine E71.19
    zinc E83.2
  methylmalonic acidemia E71.120
  micturition NEC — *see also* Difficulty, micturition R39.198
    feeling of incomplete emptying R39.14
    hesitancy R39.11
    poor stream R39.12
    psychogenic F45.8
    split stream R39.13
    straining R39.16
    urgency R39.15
  mild neurocognitive G31.84
  mitochondrial metabolism E88.40
  mitral (valve) — *see* Endocarditis, mitral
  mixed
    anxiety and depressive F41.8
    of scholastic skills (developmental) F81.89
    receptive expressive language F80.2
  mood F39
    bipolar — *see* Disorder, bipolar
    depressive — *see* Disorder, depressive
    due to (secondary to)
      alcohol F10.94
      amphetamine F15.94
        in
          abuse F15.14
          dependence F15.24
      anxiolytic F13.94
        in
          abuse F13.14
          dependence F13.24
      cocaine F14.94
        in
          abuse F14.14
          dependence F14.24
      general medical condition F06.30
      hallucinogen F16.94
        in
          abuse F16.14
          dependence F16.24
      hypnotic F13.94
        in
          abuse F13.14
          dependence F13.24
      inhalant F18.94
        in
          abuse F18.14
          dependence F18.24
      opioid F11.94
        in
          abuse F11.14
          dependence F11.24
      phencyclidine (PCP) F16.94
        in
          abuse F16.14
          dependence F16.24
      physiological condition F06.30
        with
          depressive features F06.31

Disorder — *continued*
  mood — *continued*
    due to — *continued*
      physiological condition — *continued*
        with — *continued*
          major depressive-like episode F06.32
          manic features F06.33
          mixed features F06.34
      psychoactive substance NEC F19.94
        in
          abuse F19.14
          dependence F19.24
      sedative F13.94
        in
          abuse F13.14
          dependence F13.24
      volatile solvents F18.94
        in
          abuse F18.14
          dependence F18.24
    manic episode F30.9
      with psychotic symptoms F30.2
      in remission (full) F30.4
        partial F30.3
      specified type NEC F30.8
      without psychotic symptoms F30.10
        mild F30.11
        moderate F30.12
        severe F30.13
    organic F06.30
      right hemisphere F07.89
    persistent F34.9
      cyclothymia F34.0
      dysthymia F34.1
      specified type NEC F34.89
    recurrent F39
    right hemisphere organic F07.89
  movement G25.9
    drug-induced G25.70
      akathisia G25.71
      specified NEC G25.79
    hysterical F44.4
    in diseases classified elsewhere — *see* category G26
    periodic limb G47.61
      sleep related G47.61
    sleep related NEC G47.69
    specified NEC G25.89
    stereotyped F98.4
    treatment-induced G25.9
  multiple personality F44.81
  muscle M62.9
    attachment, spine — *see* Enthesopathy, spinal
    in trichinellosis — *see* Trichinellosis, with muscle disorder
    psychogenic F45.8
    specified type NEC M62.89
    tone, newborn P94.9
      specified NEC P94.8
  muscular
    attachments — *see also* Enthesopathy
      spine — *see* Enthesopathy, spinal
    urethra N36.44
  musculoskeletal system, soft tissue — *see* Disorder, soft tissue
    postprocedural M96.89
    psychogenic F45.8
  myoneural G70.9
    due to lead G70.1
    specified NEC G70.89
    toxic G70.1
  myotonic NEC G71.19
  nail, in diseases classified elsewhere L62
  neck region NEC — *see* Dorsopathy, specified NEC
  neonatal onset multisystemic inflammatory (NOMID) M04.2
  nerve G58.9
    abducent NEC — *see* Strabismus, paralytic, sixth nerve
    accessory G52.8
    acoustic — *see* subcategory H93.3 ☑
    auditory — *see* subcategory H93.3 ☑
    auriculotemporal G50.8
    axillary G54.0
    cerebral — *see* Disorder, nerve, cranial
    cranial G52.9
      eighth — *see* subcategory H93.3 ☑
      eleventh G52.8
      fifth G50.9

Disorder — *continued*
  nerve — *continued*
    cranial — *continued*
      first G52.0
      fourth NEC — *see* Strabismus, paralytic, fourth
        nerve
      multiple G52.7
      ninth G52.1
      second NEC — *see* Disorder, nerve, optic
      seventh NEC G51.8
      sixth NEC — *see* Strabismus, paralytic, sixth nerve
      specified NEC G52.8
      tenth G52.2
      third NEC — *see* Strabismus, paralytic, third nerve
      twelfth G52.3
    entrapment — *see* Neuropathy, entrapment
    facial G51.9
      specified NEC G51.8
    femoral — *see* Lesion, nerve, femoral
    glossopharyngeal NEC G52.1
    hypoglossal G52.3
    intercostal G58.0
    lateral
      cutaneous of thigh — *see* Mononeuropathy,
        lower limb, meralgia paresthetica
      popliteal — *see* Lesion, nerve, popliteal
    lower limb — *see* Mononeuropathy, lower limb
    medial popliteal — *see* Lesion, nerve, popliteal,
      medial
    median NEC — *see* Lesion, nerve, median
    multiple G58.7
    oculomotor NEC — *see* Strabismus, paralytic, third
      nerve
    olfactory G52.0
    optic NEC H47.09- ☑
      hemorrhage into sheath — *see* Hemorrhage,
        optic nerve
      ischemic H47.01- ☑
    peroneal — *see* Lesion, nerve, popliteal
    phrenic G58.8
    plantar — *see* Lesion, nerve, plantar
    pneumogastric G52.2
    posterior tibial — *see* Syndrome, tarsal tunnel
    radial — *see* Lesion, nerve, radial
    recurrent laryngeal G52.2
    root G54.9
      cervical G54.2
      lumbosacral G54.1
      specified NEC G54.8
      thoracic G54.3
    sciatic NEC — *see* Lesion, nerve, sciatic
    specified NEC G58.8
      lower limb — *see* Mononeuropathy, lower limb,
        specified NEC
      upper limb — *see* Mononeuropathy, upper limb,
        specified NEC
    sympathetic G90.9
    tibial — *see* Lesion, nerve, popliteal, medial
    trigeminal G50.9
      specified NEC G50.8
    trochlear NEC — *see* Strabismus, paralytic, fourth
      nerve
    ulnar — *see* Lesion, nerve, ulnar
    upper limb — *see* Mononeuropathy, upper limb
    vagus G52.2
  nervous system G98.8
    autonomic (peripheral) G90.9
      specified NEC G90.8
    central G96.9
      specified NEC G96.89
    parasympathetic G90.9
    specified NEC G98.8
    sympathetic G90.9
    vegetative G90.9
  neurocognitive R41.9
    major
      with
        aggressive behavior F01.51
        combative behavior F01.51
        violent behavior F01.51
      due to vascular disease, with behavioral distur-
        bance F01.51
      in (due to) (other diseases classified elsewhere)
        — *see also* Dementia, in (due to) F02.80
        with
          aggressive behavior F02.81
          combative behavior F02.81
          violent behavior F02.81

Disorder — *continued*
  neurocognitive — *continued*
    major — *continued*
      without behavioral disturbance F01.50
    mild G31.84
  neurodevelopmental F89
    specified NEC F88
  neurohypophysis NEC E23.3
  neurological NEC R29.818
  neuromuscular G70.9
    hereditary NEC G71.9
    specified NEC G70.89
    toxic G70.1
  neurotic F48.9
    specified NEC F48.8
  neutrophil, polymorphonuclear D71
  nicotine use — *see* Dependence, drug, nicotine
  nightmare F51.5
  non-rapid eye movement sleep arousal
    sleep terror type F51.4
    sleepwalking type F51.3
  nose J34.9
    specified NEC J34.89
  obsessive-compulsive F42.9
    and related disorder due to a known physiological
      condition F06.8
  odontogenesis NOS K00.9
  opioid use
    with
      opioid-induced psychotic disorder F11.959
        with
          delusions F11.950
          hallucinations F11.951
      due to drug abuse — *see* Abuse, drug, opioid
      due to drug dependence — *see* Dependence, drug,
        opioid
    mild F11.10
      with
        opioid-induced
          anxiety disorder F11.188
          depressive disorder F11.14
          sexual dysfunction F11.181
        opioid intoxication
          with perceptual disturbances F11.122
          delirium F11.121
          without perceptual disturbances F11.129
      in remission (early) (sustained) F11.11
    moderate or severe F11.20
      with
        opioid-induced
          anxiety disorder F11.288
          anxiety disorder F11.988
          depressive disorder F11.24
          depressive disorder F11.94
          sexual dysfunction F11.281
          sexual dysfunction F11.981
        opioid intoxication
          with perceptual disturbances F11.222
          delirium F11.221
          without perceptual disturbances F11.229
      in remission (early) (sustained) F11.21
  oppositional defiant F91.3
  optic
    chiasm H47.49
      due to
        inflammatory disorder H47.41
        neoplasm H47.42
        vascular disorder H47.43
    disc H47.39- ☑
      coloboma — *see* Coloboma, optic disc
      drusen — *see* Drusen, optic disc
      pseudopapilledema — *see* Pseudopapilledema
    radiations — *see* Disorder, visual, pathway
    tracts — *see* Disorder, visual, pathway
  orbit H05.9
    cyst — *see* Cyst, orbit
    deformity — *see* Deformity, orbit
    edema — *see* Edema, orbit
    enophthalmos — *see* Enophthalmos
    exophthalmos — *see* Exophthalmos
    hemorrhage — *see* Hemorrhage, orbit
    inflammation — *see* Inflammation, orbit
    myopathy — *see* Myopathy, extraocular muscles
    retained foreign body — *see* Foreign body, orbit,
      old
    specified type NEC H05.89
  organic
    anxiety F06.4

Disorder — *continued*
  organic — *continued*
    catatonic F06.1
    delusional F06.2
    dissociative F06.8
    emotionally labile (asthenic) F06.8
    mood (affective) F06.30
    schizophrenia-like F06.2
  orgasmic (female) F52.31
    male F52.32
  ornithine metabolism E72.4
  overanxious F41.1
    of childhood F93.8
  pain
    with related psychological factors F45.42
    exclusively related to psychological factors F45.41
    genito-pelvic penetration disorder F52.6
  pancreatic internal secretion E16.9
    specified NEC E16.8
  panic F41.0
    with agoraphobia F40.01
  papulosquamous L44.9
    in diseases classified elsewhere L45
    specified NEC L44.8
  paranoid F22
    induced F24
    shared F24
  paraphilic F65.9
    specified NEC F65.89
  parathyroid (gland) E21.5
    specified NEC E21.4
  parietoalveolar NEC J84.09
  paroxysmal, mixed R56.9
  patella M22.9- ☑
    chondromalacia — *see* Chondromalacia, patella
    derangement NEC M22.3X- ☑
    recurrent
      dislocation — *see* Dislocation, patella, recurrent
      subluxation — *see* Dislocation, patella, recurrent,
        incomplete
    specified NEC M22.8X- ☑
  patellofemoral M22.2X- ☑
  pedophilic F65.4
  pentose phosphate pathway with anemia D55.1
  perception, due to hallucinogens F16.983
    in
      abuse F16.183
      dependence F16.283
  peripheral nervous system NEC G64
  peroxisomal E71.50
    biogenesis
      neonatal adrenoleukodystrophy E71.511
      specified disorder NEC E71.518
      Zellweger syndrome E71.510
    rhizomelic chondrodysplasia punctata E71.540
    specified form NEC E71.548
      group 1 E71.518
      group 2 E71.53
      group 3 E71.542
    X-linked adrenoleukodystrophy E71.529
      adolescent E71.521
      adrenomyeloneuropathy E71.522
      childhood E71.520
      specified form NEC E71.528
    Zellweger-like syndrome E71.541
  persistent
    (somatoform) pain F45.41
    affective (mood) F34.9
  personality — *see also* Personality F60.9
    affective F34.0
    aggressive F60.3
    amoral F60.2
    anankastic F60.5
    antisocial F60.2
    anxious F60.6
    asocial F60.2
    asthenic F60.7
    avoidant F60.6
    borderline F60.3
    change (secondary) due to general medical condi-
      tion F07.0
    compulsive F60.5
    cyclothymic F34.0
    dependent (passive) F60.7
    depressive F34.1
    dissocial F60.2
    emotional instability F60.3
    expansive paranoid F60.0

☑ Additional Character Required — Refer to the Tabular List for Character Selection   ▽ Subterms under main terms may continue to next column or page

Disorder — continued
- personality — see also Personality — continued
  - explosive F60.3
  - following organic brain damage F07.9
  - histrionic F60.4
  - hyperthymic F34.0
  - hypothymic F34.1
  - hysterical F60.4
  - immature F60.89
  - inadequate F60.7
  - labile F60.3
  - mixed (nonspecific) F60.89
  - moral deficiency F60.2
  - narcissistic F60.81
  - negativistic F60.89
  - obsessional F60.5
  - obsessive (-compulsive) F60.5
  - organic F07.9
  - overconscientious F60.5
  - paranoid F60.0
  - passive (-dependent) F60.7
  - passive-aggressive F60.89
  - pathological NEC F60.9
  - pseudosocial F60.2
  - psychopathic F60.2
  - schizoid F60.1
  - schizotypal F21
  - self-defeating F60.7
  - specified NEC F60.89
  - type A F60.5
  - unstable (emotional) F60.3
- pervasive, developmental F84.9
- phencyclidine use
  - mild F16.10
    - with
      - phencyclidine intoxication F16.129
      - phencyclidine intoxication delirium F16.121
      - phencyclidine-induced
        - anxiety disorder F16.180
        - bipolar and related disorder F16.14
        - depressive disorder F16.14
        - psychotic disorder F16.159
      - in remission (early) (sustained) F16.11
  - moderate or severe F16.20
    - with
      - phencyclidine intoxication F16.229
      - phencyclidine intoxication delirium F16.221
      - phencyclidine-induced
        - anxiety disorder F16.280
        - bipolar and related disorder F16.14
        - depressive disorder F16.24
        - psychotic disorder F16.259
      - in remission (early) (sustained) F16.21
- phobic anxiety, childhood F40.8
- phosphate-losing tubular N25.0
- pigmentation L81.9
  - choroid, congenital Q14.3
  - diminished melanin formation L81.6
  - iron L81.8
  - specified NEC L81.8
- pinna (noninfective) H61.10- ✓
  - deformity, acquired H61.11- ✓
  - hematoma H61.12- ✓
  - perichondritis — see Perichondritis, ear
  - specified type NEC H61.19- ✓
- pituitary gland E23.7
  - iatrogenic (postprocedural) E89.3
  - specified NEC E23.6
- platelets D69.1
- plexus G54.9
  - specified NEC G54.8
- polymorphonuclear neutrophils D71
- porphyrin metabolism — see Porphyria
- postconcussional F07.81
- posthallucinogen perception F16.983
  - in
    - abuse F16.183
    - dependence F16.283
- postmenopausal N95.9
  - specified NEC N95.8
- postprocedural (postoperative) — see Complications, postprocedural
- post-transplant lymphoproliferative D47.Z1 (following D47.4)
- post-traumatic stress (PTSD) F43.10
  - acute F43.11
  - chronic F43.12
- premenstrual dysphoric (PMDD) F32.81

Disorder — continued
- prepuce N47.8
- propionic acidemia E71.121
- prostate N42.9
  - specified NEC N42.89
- psychogenic NOS — see also condition F45.9
  - anxiety F41.8
  - appetite F50.9
  - asthenic F48.8
  - cardiovascular (system) F45.8
  - compulsive F42.8
  - cutaneous F54
  - depressive F32.9
  - digestive (system) F45.8
  - dysmenorrheic F45.8
  - dyspneic F45.8
  - endocrine (system) F54
  - eye NEC F45.8
  - feeding — see Disorder, eating
  - functional NEC F45.8
  - gastric F45.8
  - gastrointestinal (system) F45.8
  - genitourinary (system) F45.8
  - heart (function) (rhythm) F45.8
  - hyperventilatory F45.8
  - hypochondriacal — see Disorder, hypochondriacal
  - intestinal F45.8
  - joint F45.8
  - learning F81.9
  - limb F45.8
  - lymphatic (system) F45.8
  - menstrual F45.8
  - micturition F45.8
  - monoplegic NEC F44.4
  - motor F44.4
  - muscle F45.8
  - musculoskeletal F45.8
  - neurocirculatory F45.8
  - obsessive F42.8
  - occupational F48.8
  - organ or part of body NEC F45.8
  - paralytic NEC F44.4
  - phobic F40.9
  - physical NEC F45.8
  - rectal F45.8
  - respiratory (system) F45.8
  - rheumatic F45.8
  - sexual (function) F52.9
  - skin (allergic) (eczematous) F54
  - sleep F51.9
  - specified part of body NEC F45.8
  - stomach F45.8
- psychological F99
  - associated with
    - disease classified elsewhere F54
    - sexual
      - development F66
      - relationship F66
      - uncertainty about gender identity F64.9
- psychomotor NEC F44.4
  - hysterical F44.4
- psychoneurotic — see also Neurosis
  - mixed NEC F48.8
- psychophysiologic — see Disorder, somatoform
- psychosexual F65.9
  - development F66
  - identity of childhood F64.2
- psychosomatic NOS — see Disorder, somatoform
  - multiple F45.0
  - undifferentiated F45.1
- psychotic — see Psychosis
  - transient (acute) F23
- puberty E30.9
  - specified NEC E30.8
- pulmonary (valve) — see Endocarditis, pulmonary
- purine metabolism E79.9
- pyrimidine metabolism E79.9
- pyruvate metabolism E74.4
- reactive attachment (childhood) F94.1
- reading R48.0
  - developmental (specific) F81.0
- receptive language F80.2
- receptor, hormonal, peripheral — see also Syndrome, androgen insensitivity E34.50
- recurrent brief depressive F33.8
- reflex R29.2
- refraction H52.7
  - aniseikonia H52.32

Disorder — continued
- refraction — continued
  - anisometropia H52.31
  - astigmatism — see Astigmatism
  - hypermetropia — see Hypermetropia
  - myopia — see Myopia
  - presbyopia H52.4
  - specified NEC H52.6
- relationship F68.8
  - due to sexual orientation F66
- REM sleep behavior G47.52
- renal function, impaired (tubular) N25.9
- resonance R49.9
  - specified NEC R49.8
- respiratory function, impaired — see also Failure, respiration
  - postprocedural — see Complication, postoperative, respiratory system
  - psychogenic F45.8
- retina H35.9
  - angioid streaks H35.33
  - changes in vascular appearance H35.01- ✓
  - degeneration — see Degeneration, retina
  - dystrophy (hereditary) — see Dystrophy, retina
  - edema H35.81
  - hemorrhage — see Hemorrhage, retina
  - ischemia H35.82
  - macular degeneration — see Degeneration, macula
  - microaneurysms H35.04- ✓
  - microvascular abnormality NEC H35.09
  - neovascularization — see Neovascularization, retina
  - retinopathy — see Retinopathy
  - separation of layers H35.70
    - central serous chorioretinopathy H35.71- ✓
    - pigment epithelium detachment (serous) H35.72- ✓
      - hemorrhagic H35.73- ✓
  - specified type NEC H35.89
  - telangiectasis — see Telangiectasis, retina
  - vasculitis — see Vasculitis, retina
- retroperitoneal K68.9
- right hemisphere organic affective F07.89
- rumination (infant or child) F98.21
- sacrum, sacrococcygeal NEC M53.3
- schizoaffective F25.9
  - bipolar type F25.0
  - depressive type F25.1
  - manic type F25.0
  - mixed type F25.0
  - specified NEC F25.8
- schizoid of childhood F84.5
- schizophrenia spectrum and other psychotic disorder F29
  - specified NEC F28
- schizophreniform F20.81
  - brief F23
- schizotypal (personality) F21
- secretion, thyrocalcitonin E07.0
- sedative, hypnotic, or anxiolytic use
  - mild F13.10
    - with
      - sedative, hypnotic, or anxiolytic intoxication F13.129
      - sedative, hypnotic, or anxiolytic intoxication delirium F13.121
      - sedative, hypnotic, or anxiolytic-induced
        - anxiety disorder F13.180
        - bipolar and related disorder F13.14
        - depressive disorder F13.14
        - psychotic disorder F13.159
        - sexual dysfunction F13.181
      - in remission (early) (sustained) F13.11
  - moderate or severe F13.20
    - with
      - sedative, hypnotic, or anxiolytic intoxication F13.229
      - sedative, hypnotic, or anxiolytic intoxication delirium F13.221
      - sedative, hypnotic, or anxiolytic-induced
        - anxiety disorder F13.280
        - bipolar and related disorder F13.24
        - depressive disorder F13.24
        - major neurocognitive disorder F13.27
        - mild neurocognitive disorder F13.288
        - psychotic disorder F13.259
        - sexual dysfunction F13.281
      - in remission (early) (sustained) F13.21
- seizure — see also Epilepsy G40.909

✎ Subterms under main terms may continue to next column or page   ✓ Additional Character Required — Refer to the Tabular List for Character Selection   **119**

Disorder — Disorder

Disorder — *continued*
 seizure — *see also* Epilepsy — *continued*
  intractable G40.919
   with status epilepticus G40.911
 semantic pragmatic F80.89
  with autism F84.0
 sense of smell R43.1
  psychogenic F45.8
 separation anxiety, of childhood F93.0
 sexual
  aversion F52.1
  function, psychogenic F52.9
  interest/arousal, female F52.22
  masochism F65.51
  maturation F66
  nonorganic F52.9
  preference — *see also* Deviation, sexual F65.9
   fetishistic transvestism F65.1
  relationship F66
  sadism F65.52
 shyness, of childhood and adolescence F40.10
 sibling rivalry F93.8
 sickle-cell (sickling) (homozygous) — *see* Disease, sickle-cell
  heterozygous D57.3
  specified type NEC D57.8- ☑
  trait D57.3
 sinus (nasal) J34.9
  specified NEC J34.89
 skin L98.9
  atrophic L90.9
   specified NEC L90.8
  granulomatous L92.9
   specified NEC L92.8
  hypertrophic L91.9
   specified NEC L91.8
  infiltrative NEC L98.6
  newborn P83.9
   specified NEC P83.88
  picking F42.4
  psychogenic (allergic) (eczematous) F54
 sleep G47.9
  breathing-related — *see* Apnea, sleep
  circadian rhythm G47.20
   advance sleep phase type G47.22
   delayed sleep phase type G47.21
   due to
    alcohol
     abuse F10.182
     dependence F10.282
     use F10.982
    amphetamines
     abuse F15.182
     dependence F15.282
     use F15.982
    caffeine
     abuse F15.182
     dependence F15.282
     use F15.982
    cocaine
     abuse F14.182
     dependence F14.282
     use F14.982
    drug NEC
     abuse F19.182
     dependence F19.282
     use F19.982
    opioid
     abuse F11.182
     dependence F11.282
     use F11.982
    psychoactive substance NEC
     abuse F19.182
     dependence F19.282
     use F19.982
    sedative, hypnotic, or anxiolytic
     abuse F13.182
     dependence F13.282
     use F13.982
    stimulant NEC
     abuse F15.182
     dependence F15.282
     use F15.982
   free running type G47.24
   in conditions classified elsewhere G47.27
   irregular sleep wake type G47.23
   jet lag type G47.25
   non-24-hour sleep-wake type G47.24
   shift work type G47.26

Disorder — *continued*
 sleep — *continued*
  circadian rhythm — *continued*
   specified NEC G47.29
   due to
    alcohol
     abuse F10.182
     dependence F10.282
     use F10.982
    amphetamine
     abuse F15.182
     dependence F15.282
     use F15.982
    anxiolytic
     abuse F13.182
     dependence F13.282
     use F13.982
    caffeine
     abuse F15.182
     dependence F15.282
     use F15.982
    cocaine
     abuse F14.182
     dependence F14.282
     use F14.982
    drug NEC
     abuse F19.182
     dependence F19.282
     use F19.982
    hypnotic
     abuse F13.182
     dependence F13.282
     use F13.982
    opioid
     abuse F11.182
     dependence F11.282
     use F11.982
    psychoactive substance NEC
     abuse F19.182
     dependence F19.282
     use F19.982
    sedative
     abuse F13.182
     dependence F13.282
     use F13.982
    stimulant NEC
     abuse F15.182
     dependence F15.282
     use F15.982
  emotional F51.9
  excessive somnolence — *see* Hypersomnia
  hypersomnia type — *see* Hypersomnia
  initiating or maintaining — *see* Insomnia
  nightmares F51.5
  nonorganic F51.9
   specified NEC F51.8
  parasomnia type G47.50
  specified NEC G47.8
  terrors F51.4
  walking F51.3
 sleep-wake pattern or schedule — *see also* Disorder, sleep, circadian rhythm G47.9
  specified NEC G47.8
 social
  anxiety (of childhood) F40.10
   generalized F40.11
  functioning in childhood F94.9
   specified NEC F94.8
  pragmatic F80.82
 soft tissue M79.9
  ankle M79.9
  due to use, overuse and pressure M70.90
   ankle M70.97- ☑
   bursitis — *see* Bursitis
   foot M70.97- ☑
   forearm M70.93- ☑
   hand M70.94- ☑
   lower leg M70.96- ☑
   multiple sites M70.99
   pelvic region M70.95- ☑
   shoulder region M70.91- ☑
   specified site NEC M70.98
   specified type NEC M70.80
    ankle M70.87- ☑
    foot M70.87- ☑
    forearm M70.83- ☑
    hand M70.84- ☑
    lower leg M70.86- ☑

Disorder — *continued*
 soft tissue — *continued*
  due to use, overuse and pressure — *continued*
   specified type — *continued*
    multiple sites M70.89
    pelvic region M70.85- ☑
    shoulder region M70.81- ☑
    specified site NEC M70.88
    thigh M70.85- ☑
    upper arm M70.82- ☑
   thigh M70.95- ☑
   upper arm M70.92- ☑
  foot M79.9
  forearm M79.9
  hand M79.9
  lower leg M79.9
  multiple sites M79.9
  occupational — *see* Disorder, soft tissue, due to use, overuse and pressure
  pelvic region M79.9
  shoulder region M79.9
  specified type NEC M79.89
  thigh M79.9
  upper arm M79.9
 somatic symptom F45.1
 somatization F45.0
 somatoform F45.9
  pain (persistent) F45.41
  somatization (multiple) (long-lasting) F45.0
  specified NEC F45.8
  undifferentiated F45.1
 somnolence, excessive — *see* Hypersomnia
 specific
  arithmetical F81.2
  developmental, of motor F82
  reading F81.0
  speech and language F80.9
  spelling F81.81
  written expression F81.81
 speech R47.9
  articulation (functional) (specific) F80.0
  developmental F80.9
  specified NEC R47.89
 speech-sound F80.0
 spelling (specific) F81.81
 spine — *see also* Dorsopathy
  ligamentous or muscular attachments, peripheral — *see* Enthesopathy, spinal
  specified NEC — *see* Dorsopathy, specified NEC
 stereotyped, habit or movement F98.4
 stimulant use (other) (unspecified)
  mild F15.10
   in remission (early) (sustained) F15.11
  moderate or severe F15.20
   in remission (early) (sustained) F15.21
 stomach (functional) — *see* Disorder, gastric
 stress F43.9
  acute F43.0
  post-traumatic F43.10
   acute F43.11
   chronic F43.12
 substance use (other) (unknown)
  mild F19.10
   with substance-induced
    anxiety disorder F19.180
    bipolar and related disorder F19.14
    depressive disorder F19.14
    major neurocognitive disorder F19.17
    mild neurocognitive disorder F19.188
    obsessive-compulsive and related disorder F19.188
    sexual dysfunction F19.181
   substance intoxication F19.129
   substance intoxication delirium F19.121
  moderate or severe F19.20
   with substance-induced
    anxiety disorder F19.280
    bipolar and related disorder F19.24
    depressive disorder F19.24
    major neurocognitive disorder F19.27
    mild neurocognitive disorder F19.288
    obsessive-compulsive and related disorder F19.288
    sexual dysfunction F19.281
   in remission (early) (sustained) F19.21
   substance intoxication F19.229
   substance intoxication delirium F19.221
 sulfur-bearing amino-acid metabolism E72.10

120

☑ **Additional Character Required** — Refer to the Tabular List for Character Selection   ▽ **Subterms under main terms may continue to next column or page**

Disorder — *continued*
　sweat gland (eccrine) L74.9
　　apocrine L75.9
　　　specified NEC L75.8
　　specified NEC L74.8
　synovium M67.9Ø
　　acromioclavicular M67.91- ☑
　　ankle M67.97- ☑
　　elbow M67.92- ☑
　　foot M67.97- ☑
　　forearm M67.93- ☑
　　hand M67.94- ☑
　　hip M67.95- ☑
　　knee M67.96- ☑
　　multiple sites M67.99
　　rupture — *see* Rupture, synovium
　　shoulder M67.91- ☑
　　specified type NEC M67.8Ø
　　　acromioclavicular M67.81- ☑
　　　ankle M67.87- ☑
　　　elbow M67.82- ☑
　　　foot M67.87- ☑
　　　hand M67.84- ☑
　　　hip M67.85- ☑
　　　knee M67.86- ☑
　　　multiple sites M67.89
　　　wrist M67.83- ☑
　　synovitis — *see* Synovitis
　　upper arm M67.92- ☑
　　wrist M67.93- ☑
　temperature regulation, newborn P81.9
　　specified NEC P81.8
　temporomandibular joint M26.6Ø- ☑
　tendon M67.9Ø
　　acromioclavicular M67.91- ☑
　　ankle M67.97- ☑
　　contracture — *see* Contracture, tendon
　　elbow M67.92- ☑
　　foot M67.97- ☑
　　forearm M67.93- ☑
　　hand M67.94- ☑
　　hip M67.95- ☑
　　knee M67.96- ☑
　　multiple sites M67.99
　　rupture — *see* Rupture, tendon
　　shoulder M67.91- ☑
　　specified type NEC M67.8Ø
　　　acromioclavicular M67.81- ☑
　　　ankle M67.87- ☑
　　　elbow M67.82- ☑
　　　foot M67.87- ☑
　　　hand M67.84- ☑
　　　hip M67.85- ☑
　　　knee M67.86- ☑
　　　multiple sites M67.89
　　　trunk M67.88
　　　wrist M67.83- ☑
　　synovitis — *see* Synovitis
　　tendinitis — *see* Tendinitis
　　tenosynovitis — *see* Tenosynovitis
　　trunk M67.98
　　upper arm M67.92- ☑
　　wrist M67.93- ☑
　thoracic root (nerve) NEC G54.3
　thyrocalcitonin hypersecretion EØ7.Ø
　thyroid (gland) EØ7.9
　　function NEC, neonatal, transitory P72.2
　　iodine-deficiency related EØ1.8
　　specified NEC EØ7.89
　tic — *see* Tic
　tobacco use
　　chewing tobacco (mild) (moderate) (severe)
　　　in remission (early) (sustained) F17.221
　　cigarettes (mild) (moderate) (severe)
　　　in remission (early) (sustained) F17.211
　　mild F17.2ØØ
　　　in remission (early) (sustained) F17.2Ø1
　　moderate F17.2ØØ
　　　in remission (early) (sustained) F17.2Ø1
　　severe F17.2ØØ
　　　in remission (early) (sustained) F17.2Ø1
　　specified product NEC (mild) (moderate) (severe)
　　　in remission (early) (sustained) F17.291
　tooth KØ8.9
　　development KØØ.9
　　　specified NEC KØØ.8
　　eruption KØØ.6

Disorder — *continued*
　Tourette's F95.2
　trance and possession F44.89
　transvestic F65.1
　trauma and stressor-related F43.9
　　other specified F43.8
　tricuspid (valve) — *see* Endocarditis, tricuspid
　tryptophan metabolism E7Ø.5
　tubular, phosphate-losing N25.Ø
　tubulo-interstitial (in)
　　brucellosis A23.9 *[N16]*
　　cystinosis E72.Ø4
　　diphtheria A36.84
　　glycogen storage disease E74.ØØ *[N16]*
　　leukemia NEC C95.9- ☑ *[N16]*
　　lymphoma NEC C85.9- ☑ *[N16]*
　　mixed cryoglobulinemia D89.1 *[N16]*
　　multiple myeloma C9Ø.Ø- ☑ *[N16]*
　　Salmonella infection AØ2.25
　　sarcoidosis D86.84
　　sepsis A41.9 *[N16]*
　　　streptococcal A4Ø.9 *[N16]*
　　systemic lupus erythematosus M32.15
　　toxoplasmosis B58.83
　　transplant rejection T86.91 *[N16]*
　　Wilson's disease E83.Ø1 *[N16]*
　tubulo-renal function, impaired N25.9
　　specified NEC N25.89
　tympanic membrane H73.9- ☑
　　atrophy — *see* Atrophy, tympanic membrane
　　infection — *see* Myringitis
　　perforation — *see* Perforation, tympanum
　　specified NEC H73.89- ☑
　unsocialized aggressive F91.1
　urea cycle metabolism E72.2Ø
　　argininemia E72.21
　　arginosuccinic aciduria E72.22
　　citrullinemia E72.23
　　ornithine transcarbamylase deficiency E72.4
　　other specified E72.29
　ureter (in) N28.9
　　schistosomiasis B65.Ø *[N29]*
　　tuberculosis A18.11
　urethra N36.9
　　specified NEC N36.8
　urinary system N39.9
　　specified NEC N39.8
　valve, heart
　　aortic — *see* Endocarditis, aortic
　　mitral — *see* Endocarditis, mitral
　　pulmonary — *see* Endocarditis, pulmonary
　　rheumatic
　　　aortic — *see* Endocarditis, aortic, rheumatic
　　　mitral — *see* Endocarditis, mitral
　　　pulmonary — *see* Endocarditis, pulmonary,
　　　　rheumatic
　　　tricuspid — *see* Endocarditis, tricuspid
　　tricuspid — *see* Endocarditis, tricuspid
　vestibular function H81.9- ☑
　　specified NEC — *see* subcategory H81.8 ☑
　　in diseases classified elsewhere H82.- ☑
　　vertigo — *see* Vertigo
　vision, binocular H53.3Ø
　　abnormal retinal correspondence H53.31
　　diplopia H53.2
　　fusion with defective stereopsis H53.32
　　simultaneous perception H53.33
　　suppression H53.34
　visual
　　cortex
　　　blindness H47.619
　　　　left brain H47.612
　　　　right brain H47.611
　　　due to
　　　　inflammatory disorder H47.629
　　　　　left brain H47.622
　　　　　right brain H47.621
　　　　neoplasm H47.639
　　　　　left brain H47.632
　　　　　right brain H47.631
　　　　vascular disorder H47.649
　　　　　left brain H47.642
　　　　　right brain H47.641
　　pathway H47.9
　　　due to
　　　　inflammatory disorder H47.51- ☑
　　　　neoplasm H47.52- ☑
　　　　vascular disorder H47.53- ☑

Disorder — *continued*
　visual — *continued*
　　pathway — *continued*
　　　optic chiasm — *see* Disorder, optic, chiasm
　　vitreous body H43.9
　　　crystalline deposits — *see* Deposit, crystalline
　　　degeneration — *see* Degeneration, vitreous
　　　hemorrhage — *see* Hemorrhage, vitreous
　　　opacities — *see* Opacity, vitreous
　　　prolapse — *see* Prolapse, vitreous
　　　specified type NEC H43.89
　　voice R49.9
　　　specified type NEC R49.8
　　volatile solvent use
　　　due to drug abuse — *see* Abuse, drug, inhalant
　　　due to drug dependence — *see* Dependence, drug,
　　　　inhalant
　　voyeuristic F65.3
　　white blood cells D72.9
　　　specified NEC D72.89
　　withdrawing, child or adolescent F4Ø.1Ø
Disorientation R41.Ø
Displacement, displaced
　acquired traumatic of bone, cartilage, joint, tendon
　　NEC — *see* Dislocation
　adrenal gland (congenital) Q89.1
　appendix, retrocecal (congenital) Q43.8
　auricle (congenital) Q17.4
　bladder (acquired) N32.89
　　congenital Q64.19
　brachial plexus (congenital) QØ7.8
　brain stem, caudal (congenital) QØ4.8
　canaliculus (lacrimalis), congenital Q1Ø.6
　cardia through esophageal hiatus (congenital) Q4Ø.1
　cerebellum, caudal (congenital) QØ4.8
　cervix — *see* Malposition, uterus
　colon (congenital) Q43.3
　device, implant or graft — *see also* Complications, by
　　site and type, mechanical T85.628 ☑
　　arterial graft NEC — *see* Complication, cardiovascu-
　　　lar device, mechanical, vascular
　　breast (implant) T85.42 ☑
　　catheter NEC T85.628 ☑
　　　dialysis (renal) T82.42 ☑
　　　　intraperitoneal T85.621 ☑
　　　infusion NEC T82.524 ☑
　　　　spinal (epidural) (subdural) T85.62Ø ☑
　　　urinary
　　　　cystostomy T83.Ø2Ø ☑
　　　　Hopkins T83.Ø28 ☑
　　　　ileostomy T83.Ø28 ☑
　　　　indwelling T83.Ø21 ☑
　　　　nephrostomy T83.Ø22 ☑
　　　　specified NEC T83.Ø28 ☑
　　　　urostomy T83.Ø28 ☑
　　electronic (electrode) (pulse generator) (stimulator)
　　　— *see* Complication, electronic stimulator
　　fixation, internal (orthopedic) NEC — *see* Complica-
　　　tion, fixation device, mechanical
　　gastrointestinal — *see* Complications, prosthetic
　　　device, mechanical, gastrointestinal device
　　genital NEC T83.428 ☑
　　　intrauterine contraceptive device (string)
　　　　T83.32 ☑
　　　penile prosthesis (cylinder) (implanted) (pump)
　　　　(reservoir) T83.42Ø ☑
　　　testicular prosthesis T83.421 ☑
　　heart NEC — *see* Complication, cardiovascular de-
　　　vice, mechanical
　　joint prosthesis — *see* Complications, joint prosthe-
　　　sis, mechanical
　　ocular — *see* Complications, prosthetic device,
　　　mechanical, ocular device
　　orthopedic NEC — *see* Complication, orthopedic,
　　　device or graft, mechanical
　　specified NEC T85.628 ☑
　　urinary NEC T83.128 ☑
　　　graft T83.22 ☑
　　　sphincter, implanted T83.121 ☑
　　　stent (ileal conduit) (nephroureteral) T83.123 ☑
　　　　ureteral indwelling T83.122 ☑
　　vascular NEC — *see* Complication, cardiovascular
　　　device, mechanical
　　ventricular intracranial shunt T85.Ø2 ☑
　electronic stimulator
　　bone T84.32Ø ☑

Displacement, displaced — *continued*
  electronic stimulator — *continued*
    cardiac — *see* Complications, cardiac device, electronic
    nervous system — *see* Complication, prosthetic device, mechanical, electronic nervous system stimulator
    urinary — *see* Complications, electronic stimulator, urinary
  esophageal mucosa into cardia of stomach, congenital Q39.8
  esophagus (acquired) K22.89
    congenital Q39.8
  eyeball (acquired) (lateral) (old) — *see* Displacement, globe
    congenital Q15.8
    current — *see* Avulsion, eye
  fallopian tube (acquired) N83.4- ☑
    congenital Q50.6
    opening (congenital) Q50.6
  gallbladder (congenital) Q44.1
  gastric mucosa (congenital) Q40.2
  globe (acquired) (old) (lateral) H05.21- ☑
    current — *see* Avulsion, eye
  heart (congenital) Q24.8
    acquired I51.89
  hymen (upward) (congenital) Q52.4
  intervertebral disc NEC
    with myelopathy — *see* Disorder, disc, with, myelopathy
    cervical, cervicothoracic (with) M50.20
      myelopathy — *see* Disorder, disc, cervical, with myelopathy
      neuritis, radiculitis or radiculopathy — *see* Disorder, disc, cervical, with neuritis
    due to trauma — *see* Dislocation, vertebra
    lumbar region M51.26
      with
        myelopathy M51.06
        neuritis, radiculitis, radiculopathy or sciatica M51.16
    lumbosacral region M51.27
      with
        neuritis, radiculitis, radiculopathy or sciatica M51.17
    sacrococcygeal region M53.3
    thoracic region M51.24
      with
        myelopathy M51.04
        neuritis, radiculitis, radiculopathy M51.14
    thoracolumbar region M51.25
      with
        myelopathy M51.05
        neuritis, radiculitis, radiculopathy M51.15
  intrauterine device (string) T83.32 ☑
  kidney (acquired) N28.83
    congenital Q63.2
  lachrymal, lacrimal apparatus or duct (congenital) Q10.6
  lens, congenital Q12.1
  macula (congenital) Q14.1
  Meckel's diverticulum Q43.0
    malignant — *see* Table of Neoplasms, small intestine, malignant
  nail (congenital) Q84.6
    acquired L60.8
  opening of Wharton's duct in mouth Q38.4
  organ or site, congenital NEC — *see* Malposition, congenital
  ovary (acquired) N83.4- ☑
    congenital Q50.39
    free in peritoneal cavity (congenital) Q50.39
    into hernial sac N83.4- ☑
  oviduct (acquired) N83.4- ☑
    congenital Q50.6
  parathyroid (gland) E21.4
  parotid gland (congenital) Q38.4
  punctum lacrimale (congenital) Q10.6
  sacro-iliac (joint) (congenital) Q74.2
    current injury S33.2 ☑
    old — *see* subcategory M53.2 ☑
  salivary gland (any) (congenital) Q38.4
  spleen (congenital) Q89.09
  stomach, congenital Q40.2
  sublingual duct Q38.4
  tongue (downward) (congenital) Q38.3
  tooth, teeth, fully erupted M26.30
    horizontal M26.33
    vertical M26.34

Displacement, displaced — *continued*
  trachea (congenital) Q32.1
  ureter or ureteric opening or orifice (congenital) Q62.62
  uterine opening of oviducts or fallopian tubes Q50.6
  uterus, uterine — *see* Malposition, uterus
  ventricular septum Q21.0
    with rudimentary ventricle Q20.4
Disproportion
  between native and reconstructed breast N65.1
  fiber-type G71.20
    congenital G71.29
Disruptio uteri — *see* Rupture, uterus
Disruption (of)
  ciliary body NEC H21.89
  closure of
    cornea T81.31 ☑
    craniotomy T81.32 ☑
    fascia (muscular) (superficial) T81.32 ☑
    internal organ or tissue T81.32 ☑
    laceration (external) (internal) T81.33 ☑
    ligament T81.32 ☑
    mucosa T81.31 ☑
    muscle or muscle flap T81.32 ☑
    ribs or rib cage T81.32 ☑
    skin and subcutaneous tissue (full-thickness) (superficial) T81.31 ☑
    skull T81.32 ☑
    sternum (sternotomy) T81.32 ☑
    tendon T81.32 ☑
    traumatic laceration (external) (internal) T81.33 ☑
  family Z63.8
    due to
      absence of family member due to military deployment Z63.31
      absence of family member NEC Z63.32
      alcoholism and drug addiction in family Z63.72
      bereavement Z63.4
      death (assumed) or disappearance of family member Z63.4
      divorce or separation Z63.5
      drug addiction in family Z63.72
      return of family member from military deployment (current or past conflict) Z63.71
      stressful life events NEC Z63.79
  iris NEC H21.89
  ligament(s) — *see also* Sprain
    knee
      current injury — *see* Dislocation, knee
      old (chronic) — *see* Derangement, knee, instability
      spontaneous NEC — *see* Derangement, knee, disruption ligament
  ossicular chain — *see* Discontinuity, ossicles, ear
  pelvic ring (stable) S32.810 ☑
    unstable S32.811 ☑
  traumatic injury wound repair T81.33 ☑
  wound T81.30 ☑
    episiotomy O90.1
    operation T81.31 ☑
      cesarean O90.0
      external operation wound (superficial) T81.31 ☑
      internal operation wound (deep) T81.32 ☑
    perineal (obstetric) O90.1
    traumatic injury repair T81.33 ☑
Dissatisfaction with
  employment Z56.9
  school environment Z55.4
Dissecting — *see* condition
Dissection
  aorta I71.00
    abdominal I71.02
    thoracic I71.01
    thoracoabdominal I71.03
  artery I77.70
    basilar (trunk) I77.75
    carotid I77.71
    cerebral (nonruptured) I67.0
      ruptured — *see* Hemorrhage, intracranial, subarachnoid
    coronary I25.42
    extremity
      lower I77.77
      upper I77.76
    iliac I77.72
    precerebral
      congenital (nonruptured) Q28.1
      specified site NEC I77.75

Dissection — *continued*
  artery — *continued*
    renal I77.73
    specified NEC I77.79
    vertebral I77.74
  precerebral artery, congenital (nonruptured) Q28.1
    Heartland A93.8
  traumatic — *see* Wound, open, by site
  vascular I99.8
  wound — *see* Wound, open
Disseminated — *see* condition
Dissociation
  auriculoventricular or atrioventricular (AV) (any degree) (isorhythmic) I45.89
    with heart block I44.2
  interference I45.89
Dissociative reaction, state F44.9
Dissolution, vertebra — *see* Osteoporosis
Distension, distention
  abdomen R14.0
  bladder N32.89
  cecum K63.89
  colon K63.89
  gallbladder K82.8
  intestine K63.89
  kidney N28.89
  liver K76.89
  seminal vesicle N50.89
  stomach K31.89
    acute K31.0
    psychogenic F45.8
  ureter — *see* Dilatation, ureter
  uterus N85.8
Distoma hepaticum infestation B66.3
Distomiasis B66.9
  bile passages B66.3
  hemic B65.9
  hepatic B66.3
    due to Clonorchis sinensis B66.1
  intestinal B66.5
  liver B66.3
    due to Clonorchis sinensis B66.1
  lung B66.4
  pulmonary B66.4
Distomolar (fourth molar) K00.1
Disto-occlusion (Division I) (Division II) M26.212
Distortion(s) (congenital)
  adrenal (gland) Q89.1
  arm NEC Q68.8
  bile duct or passage Q44.5
  bladder Q64.79
  brain Q04.9
  cervix (uteri) Q51.9
  chest (wall) Q67.8
    bones Q76.8
  clavicle Q74.0
  clitoris Q52.6
  coccyx Q76.49
  common duct Q44.5
  coronary Q24.5
  cystic duct Q44.5
  ear (auricle) (external) Q17.3
    inner Q16.5
    middle Q16.4
      ossicles Q16.3
  endocrine NEC Q89.2
  eustachian tube Q17.8
  eye (adnexa) Q15.8
  face bone(s) NEC Q75.8
  fallopian tube Q50.6
  femur NEC Q68.8
  fibula NEC Q68.8
  finger(s) Q68.1
  foot Q66.9- ☑
  genitalia, genital organ(s)
    female Q52.8
      external Q52.79
      internal NEC Q52.8
  gyri Q04.8
  hand bone(s) Q68.1
  heart (auricle) (ventricle) Q24.8
    valve (cusp) Q24.8
  hepatic duct Q44.5
  humerus NEC Q68.8
  hymen Q52.4
  intrafamilial communications Z63.8
  jaw NEC M26.89
  labium (majus) (minus) Q52.79

☑ **Additional Character Required** — Refer to the Tabular List for Character Selection   ▽ **Subterms under main terms may continue to next column or page**

Distortion(s) — continued
- leg NEC Q68.8
- lens Q12.8
- liver Q44.7
- lumbar spine Q76.49
  - with disproportion O33.8
    - causing obstructed labor O65.0
- lumbosacral (joint) (region) Q76.49
  - kyphosis — see Kyphosis, congenital
  - lordosis — see Lordosis, congenital
- nerve Q07.8
- nose Q30.8
- organ
  - of Corti Q16.5
  - or site not listed — see Anomaly, by site
- ossicles, ear Q16.3
- oviduct Q50.6
- pancreas Q45.3
- parathyroid (gland) Q89.2
- pituitary (gland) Q89.2
- radius NEC Q68.8
- sacroiliac joint Q74.2
- sacrum Q76.49
- scapula Q74.0
- shoulder girdle Q74.0
- skull bone(s) NEC Q75.8
  - with
    - anencephalus Q00.0
    - encephalocele — see Encephalocele
    - hydrocephalus Q03.9
      - with spina bifida — see Spina bifida, with hydrocephalus
    - microcephaly Q02
- spinal cord Q06.8
- spine Q76.49
  - kyphosis — see Kyphosis, congenital
  - lordosis — see Lordosis, congenital
- spleen Q89.09
- sternum NEC Q76.7
- thorax (wall) Q67.8
  - bony Q76.8
- thymus (gland) Q89.2
- thyroid (gland) Q89.2
- tibia NEC Q68.8
- toe(s) Q66.9- ☑
- tongue Q38.3
- trachea (cartilage) Q32.1
- ulna NEC Q68.8
- ureter Q62.8
- urethra Q64.79
  - causing obstruction Q64.39
- uterus Q51.9
- vagina Q52.4
- vertebra Q76.49
  - kyphosis — see Kyphosis, congenital
  - lordosis — see Lordosis, congenital
- visual — see also Disturbance, vision
  - shape and size H53.15
- vulva Q52.79
- wrist (bones) (joint) Q68.8

Distress
- abdomen — see Pain, abdominal
- acute respiratory R06.03
  - syndrome (adult) (child) J80
- epigastric R10.13
- fetal P84
  - complicating pregnancy — see Stress, fetal
- gastrointestinal (functional) K30
  - psychogenic F45.8
- intestinal (functional) NOS K59.9
  - psychogenic F45.8
- maternal, during labor and delivery O75.0
- relationship, with spouse or intimate partner Z63.0
- respiratory (adult) (child) R06.03
  - newborn P22.9
    - specified NEC P22.8
  - orthopnea R06.01
  - psychogenic F45.8
  - shortness of breath R06.02
  - specified type NEC R06.09

Distribution vessel, atypical Q27.9
- coronary artery Q24.5
- precerebral Q28.1

Districhiasis L68.8

Disturbance(s) — see also Disease
- absorption K90.9
  - calcium E58
  - carbohydrate K90.49

Disturbance(s) — continued
- absorption — continued
  - fat K90.49
    - pancreatic K90.3
  - protein K90.49
  - starch K90.49
  - vitamin — see Deficiency, vitamin
- acid-base equilibrium E87.8
  - mixed E87.4
- activity and attention (with hyperkinesis) — see Disorder, attention-deficit hyperactivity
- amino acid transport E72.00
- assimilation, food K90.9
- auditory nerve, except deafness — see subcategory H93.3 ☑
- behavior — see Disorder, conduct
- blood clotting (mechanism) — see also Defect, coagulation D68.9
- cerebral
  - nerve — see Disorder, nerve, cranial
  - status, newborn P91.9
    - specified NEC P91.88
- circulatory I99.9
- conduct — see also Disorder, conduct F91.9
  - adjustment reaction — see Disorder, adjustment
  - compulsive F63.9
  - disruptive F91.9
  - hyperkinetic — see Disorder, attention-deficit hyperactivity
  - socialized F91.2
  - specified NEC F91.8
  - unsocialized F91.1
- coordination R27.8
- cranial nerve — see Disorder, nerve, cranial
- deep sensibility — see Disturbance, sensation
- digestive K30
  - psychogenic F45.8
- electrolyte — see also Imbalance, electrolyte
  - newborn, transitory P74.49
    - hyperammonemia P74.6
    - hyperchloremia P74.421
    - hyperchloremic metabolic acidosis P74.421
    - hypochloremia P74.422
    - potassium balance
      - hyperkalemia P74.31
      - hypokalemia P74.32
    - sodium balance
      - hypernatremia P74.21
      - hyponatremia P74.22
    - specified type NEC P74.49
- emotions specific to childhood and adolescence F93.9
  - with
    - anxiety and fearfulness NEC F93.8
    - elective mutism F94.0
    - oppositional disorder F91.3
    - sensitivity (withdrawal) F40.10
    - shyness F40.10
    - social withdrawal F40.10
  - involving relationship problems F93.8
  - mixed F93.8
  - specified NEC F93.8
- endocrine (gland) E34.9
  - neonatal, transitory P72.9
    - specified NEC P72.8
- equilibrium R42
- fructose metabolism E74.10
- gait — see Gait
  - hysterical F44.4
  - psychogenic F44.4
- gastrointestinal (functional) K30
  - psychogenic F45.8
- habit, child F98.9
- hearing, except deafness and tinnitus — see Abnormal, auditory perception
- heart, functional (conditions in I44-I50)
  - due to presence of (cardiac) prosthesis I97.19- ☑
  - postoperative I97.89
    - cardiac surgery — see also Infarct, myocardium, associated with revascularization procedure I97.19- ☑
- hormones E34.9
- innervation uterus (parasympathetic) (sympathetic) N85.8
- keratinization NEC
  - gingiva K05.10
    - nonplaque induced K05.11
    - plaque induced K05.10
  - lip K13.0

Disturbance(s) — continued
- keratinization — continued
  - oral (mucosa) (soft tissue) K13.29
  - tongue K13.29
- learning (specific) — see Disorder, learning
- memory — see Amnesia
  - mild, following organic brain damage F06.8
- mental F99
  - associated with diseases classified elsewhere F54
- metabolism E88.9
  - with
    - abortion — see Abortion, by type with other specified complication
    - ectopic pregnancy O08.5
    - molar pregnancy O08.5
  - amino-acid E72.9
    - aromatic E70.9
    - branched-chain E71.2
    - straight-chain E72.89
    - sulfur-bearing E72.10
  - ammonia E72.20
  - arginine E72.21
  - arginosuccinic acid E72.22
  - carbohydrate E74.9
  - cholesterol E78.9
  - citrulline E72.23
  - cystathionine E72.19
  - general E88.9
  - glutamine E72.89
  - histidine E70.40
  - homocystine E72.19
  - hydroxylysine E72.3
  - in labor or delivery O75.89
  - iron E83.10
  - lipoid E78.9
  - lysine E72.3
  - methionine E72.19
  - neonatal, transitory P74.9
    - calcium and magnesium P71.9
      - specified type NEC P71.8
    - carbohydrate metabolism P70.9
      - specified type NEC P70.8
    - specified NEC P74.8
  - ornithine E72.4
  - phosphate E83.39
  - sodium NEC E87.8
  - threonine E72.89
  - tryptophan E70.5
  - tyrosine E70.20
  - urea cycle E72.20
- motor R29.2
- nervous, functional R45.0
- neuromuscular mechanism (eye), due to syphilis A52.15
- nutritional E63.9
  - nail L60.3
- ocular motion H51.9
  - psychogenic F45.8
- oculogyric H51.8
  - psychogenic F45.8
- oculomotor H51.9
  - psychogenic F45.8
- olfactory nerve R43.1
- optic nerve NEC — see Disorder, nerve, optic
- oral epithelium, including tongue NEC K13.29
- perceptual due to
  - alcohol withdrawal F10.232
  - amphetamine intoxication F15.922
    - in
      - abuse F15.122
      - dependence F15.222
  - anxiolytic withdrawal F13.232
  - cannabis intoxication (acute) F12.922
    - in
      - abuse F12.122
      - dependence F12.222
  - cocaine intoxication (acute) F14.922
    - in
      - abuse F14.122
      - dependence F14.222
  - hypnotic withdrawal F13.232
  - opioid intoxication (acute) F11.922
    - in
      - abuse F11.122
      - dependence F11.222
  - phencyclidine intoxication (acute) F16.122
  - sedative withdrawal F13.232
- personality (pattern) (trait) — see also Disorder, personality F60.9
  - following organic brain damage F07.9

⚐ Subterms under main terms may continue to next column or page   ☑ Additional Character Required — Refer to the Tabular List for Character Selection   123

Distortion — Disturbance(s)

Disturbance(s) — *continued*
  polyglandular E31.9
    specified NEC E31.8
  potassium balance, newborn
    hyperkalemia P74.31
    hypokalemia P74.32
  psychogenic F45.9
  psychomotor F44.4
  psychophysical visual H53.16
  pupillary — *see* Anomaly, pupil, function
  reflex R29.2
  rhythm, heart I49.9
  salivary secretion K11.7
  sensation (cold) (heat) (localization) (tactile discrimination) (texture) (vibratory) NEC R20.9
    hysterical F44.6
    skin R20.9
      anesthesia R20.0
      hyperesthesia R20.3
      hypoesthesia R20.1
      paresthesia R20.2
      specified type NEC R20.8
    smell R43.9
      and taste (mixed) R43.8
      anosmia R43.0
      parosmia R43.1
      specified NEC R43.8
    taste R43.9
      and smell (mixed) R43.8
      parageusia R43.2
      specified NEC R43.8
  sensory — *see* Disturbance, sensation
  situational (transient) — *see also* Disorder, adjustment
    acute F43.0
  sleep G47.9
    nonorganic origin F51.9
  smell — *see* Disturbance, sensation, smell
  sociopathic F60.2
  sodium balance, newborn
    hypernatremia P74.21
    hyponatremia P74.22
  speech R47.9
    developmental F80.9
    specified NEC R47.89
  stomach (functional) K31.9
  sympathetic (nerve) G90.9
  taste — *see* Disturbance, sensation, taste
  temperature
    regulation, newborn P81.9
      specified NEC P81.8
    sense R20.8
      hysterical F44.6
  tooth
    eruption K00.6
    formation K00.4
    structure, hereditary NEC K00.5
  touch — *see* Disturbance, sensation
  vascular I99.9
    arteriosclerotic — *see* Arteriosclerosis
  vasomotor I73.9
  vasospastic I73.9
  vision, visual H53.9
    following
      cerebral infarction I69.398
      cerebrovascular disease I69.998
        specified NEC I69.898
      intracerebral hemorrhage I69.198
      nontraumatic intracranial hemorrhage NEC I69.298
      specified disease NEC I69.898
      subarachnoid hemorrhage I69.098
    psychophysical H53.16
    specified NEC H53.8
    subjective H53.10
      day blindness H53.11
      discomfort H53.14- ☑
      distortions of shape and size H53.15
      loss
        sudden H53.13- ☑
        transient H53.12- ☑
      specified type NEC H53.19
  voice R49.9
    psychogenic F44.4
    specified NEC R49.8
Diuresis R35.89
Diver's palsy, paralysis or squeeze T70.3 ☑
Diverticulitis (acute) K57.92
  bladder — *see* Cystitis

Diverticulitis — *continued*
  ileum — *see* Diverticulitis, intestine, small
  intestine K57.92
    with
      abscess, perforation K57.80
        with bleeding K57.81
      bleeding K57.93
    congenital Q43.8
    large K57.32
      with
        abscess, perforation K57.20
          with bleeding K57.21
        bleeding K57.33
        small intestine K57.52
          with
            abscess, perforation K57.40
              with bleeding K57.41
            bleeding K57.53
    small K57.12
      with
        abscess, perforation K57.00
          with bleeding K57.01
        bleeding K57.13
        large intestine K57.52
          with
            abscess, perforation K57.40
              with bleeding K57.41
            bleeding K57.53
Diverticulosis K57.90
  with bleeding K57.91
  large intestine K57.30
    with
      bleeding K57.31
      small intestine K57.50
        with bleeding K57.51
  small intestine K57.10
    with
      bleeding K57.11
      large intestine K57.50
        with bleeding K57.51
Diverticulum, diverticula (multiple) K57.90
  appendix (noninflammatory) K38.2
  bladder (sphincter) N32.3
    congenital Q64.6
  bronchus (congenital) Q32.4
    acquired J98.09
  calyx, calyceal (kidney) N28.89
  cardia (stomach) K31.4
  cecum — *see* Diverticulosis, intestine, large
    congenital Q43.8
  colon — *see* Diverticulosis, intestine, large
    congenital Q43.8
  duodenum — *see* Diverticulosis, intestine, small
    congenital Q43.8
  epiphrenic (esophagus) K22.5
  esophagus (congenital) Q39.6
    acquired (epiphrenic) (pulsion) (traction) K22.5
  eustachian tube — *see* Disorder, eustachian tube, specified NEC
  fallopian tube N83.8
  gastric K31.4
  heart (congenital) Q24.8
  ileum — *see* Diverticulosis, intestine, small
  jejunum — *see* Diverticulosis, intestine, small
  kidney (pelvis) (calyces) N28.89
    with calculus — *see* Calculus, kidney
  Meckel's (displaced) (hypertrophic) Q43.0
    malignant — *see* Table of Neoplasms, small intestine, malignant
  midthoracic K22.5
  organ or site, congenital NEC — *see* Distortion
  pericardium (congenital) (cyst) Q24.8
    acquired I31.8
  pharyngoesophageal (congenital) Q39.6
    acquired K22.5
  pharynx (congenital) Q38.7
  rectosigmoid — *see* Diverticulosis, intestine, large
    congenital Q43.8
  rectum — *see* Diverticulosis, intestine, large
  Rokitansky's K22.5
  seminal vesicle N50.89
  sigmoid — *see* Diverticulosis, intestine, large
    congenital Q43.8
  stomach (acquired) K31.4
    congenital Q40.2
  trachea (acquired) J39.8
  ureter (acquired) N28.89
    congenital Q62.8

Diverticulum, diverticula — *continued*
  ureterovesical orifice N28.89
  urethra (acquired) N36.1
    congenital Q64.79
  ventricle, left (congenital) Q24.8
  vesical N32.3
    congenital Q64.6
  Zenker's (esophagus) K22.5
Division
  cervix uteri (acquired) N88.8
  glans penis Q55.69
  labia minora (congenital) Q52.79
  ligament (partial or complete) (current) — *see also* Sprain
    with open wound — *see* Wound, open
  muscle (partial or complete) (current) — *see also* Injury, muscle
    with open wound — *see* Wound, open
  nerve (traumatic) — *see* Injury, nerve
  spinal cord — *see* Injury, spinal cord, by region
  vein I87.8
Divorce, causing family disruption Z63.5
Dix-Hallpike neurolabyrinthitis — *see* Neuronitis, vestibular
Dizziness R42
  hysterical F44.89
  psychogenic F45.8
DMAC (disseminated mycobacterium avium- intracellulare complex) A31.2
DNR (do not resuscitate) Z66
Doan-Wiseman syndrome (primary splenic neutropenia) — *see* Agranulocytosis
Doehle-Heller aortitis A52.02
Dog bite — *see* Bite
Dohle body panmyelopathic syndrome D72.0
Dolichocephaly Q67.2
Dolichocolon Q43.8
Dolichostenomelia — *see* Syndrome, Marfan's
Donohue's syndrome E34.8
Donor (organ or tissue) Z52.9
  blood (whole) Z52.000
    autologous Z52.010
    specified component (lymphocytes) (platelets) NEC Z52.008
      autologous Z52.018
      specified donor NEC Z52.098
    specified donor NEC Z52.090
    stem cells Z52.001
      autologous Z52.011
      specified donor NEC Z52.091
  bone Z52.20
    autologous Z52.21
    marrow Z52.3
    specified type NEC Z52.29
  cornea Z52.5
  egg (Oocyte) Z52.819
    age 35 and over Z52.812
      anonymous recipient Z52.812
      designated recipient Z52.813
    under age 35 Z52.810
      anonymous recipient Z52.810
      designated recipient Z52.811
  kidney Z52.4
  liver Z52.6
  lung Z52.89
  lymphocyte — *see* Donor, blood, specified components NEC
  Oocyte — *see* Donor, egg
  platelets Z52.008
  potential, examination of Z00.5
  semen Z52.89
  skin Z52.10
    autologous Z52.11
    specified type NEC Z52.19
  specified organ or tissue NEC Z52.89
  sperm Z52.89
Donovanosis A58
Dorsalgia M54.9
  psychogenic F45.41
  specified NEC M54.89
Dorsopathy M53.9
  deforming M43.9
    specified NEC — *see* subcategory M43.8 ☑
  specified NEC M53.80
    cervical region M53.82
    cervicothoracic region M53.83
    lumbar region M53.86
    lumbosacral region M53.87

Dorsopathy — *continued*
    specified — *continued*
        occipito-atlanto-axial region M53.81
        sacrococcygeal region M53.88
        thoracic region M53.84
        thoracolumbar region M53.85
Double
    albumin E88.09
    aortic arch Q25.45
    auditory canal Q17.8
    auricle (heart) Q20.8
    bladder Q64.79
    cervix Q51.820
        with doubling of uterus (and vagina) Q51.10
            with obstruction Q51.11
    inlet ventricle Q20.4
    kidney with double pelvis (renal) Q63.0
    meatus urinarius Q64.75
    monster Q89.4
    outlet
        left ventricle Q20.2
        right ventricle Q20.1
    pelvis (renal) with double ureter Q62.5
    tongue Q38.3
    ureter (one or both sides) Q62.5
        with double pelvis (renal) Q62.5
    urethra Q64.74
    urinary meatus Q64.75
    uterus Q51.28
        with
            doubling of cervix (and vagina) Q51.10
                with obstruction Q51.11
            complete Q51.21
        in pregnancy or childbirth O34.0- ☑
            causing obstructed labor O65.5
        partial Q51.22
        specified NEC Q51.28
    vagina Q52.10
        with doubling of uterus (and cervix) Q51.10
            with obstruction Q51.11
    vision H53.2
    vulva Q52.79
Doubled up Z59.01
Douglas' pouch, cul-de-sac — *see* condition
Down syndrome Q90.9
    meiotic nondisjunction Q90.0
    mitotic nondisjunction Q90.1
    mosaicism Q90.1
    translocation Q90.2
DPD (dihydropyrimidine dehydrogenase deficiency)
    E88.89
Dracontiasis B72
Dracunculiasis, dracunculosis B72
Dream state, hysterical F44.89
Drepanocytic anemia — *see* Disease, sickle-cell
Dresbach's syndrome (elliptocytosis) D58.1
Dreschlera (hawaiiensis) (infection) B43.8
Dressler's syndrome I24.1
Drift, ulnar — *see* Deformity, limb, specified type NEC,
    forearm
Drinking (alcohol)
    excessive, to excess NEC (without dependence) F10.10
        habitual (continual) (without remission) F10.20
            with remission F10.21
Drip, postnasal (chronic) R09.82
    due to
        allergic rhinitis — *see* Rhinitis, allergic
        common cold J00
        gastroesophageal reflux — *see* Reflux, gastroe-
            sophageal
        nasopharyngitis — *see* Nasopharyngitis
        other known condition — *code to* condition
        sinusitis — *see* Sinusitis
Droop
    facial R29.810
        cerebrovascular disease I69.992
            cerebral infarction I69.392
            intracerebral hemorrhage I69.192
            nontraumatic intracranial hemorrhage NEC
                I69.292
            specified disease NEC I69.892
            subarachnoid hemorrhage I69.092
Drop (in)
    attack NEC R55
    finger — *see* Deformity, finger
    foot — *see* Deformity, limb, foot, drop
    hematocrit (precipitous) R71.0
    hemoglobin R71.0

Drop — *continued*
    toe — *see* Deformity, toe, specified NEC
    wrist — *see* Deformity, limb, wrist drop
Dropped heart beats I45.9
Dropsy, dropsical — *see also* Hydrops
    abdomen R18.8
    brain — *see* Hydrocephalus
    cardiac, heart — *see* Failure, heart, congestive
    gangrenous — *see* Gangrene
    heart — *see* Failure, heart, congestive
    kidney — *see* Nephrosis
    lung — *see* Edema, lung
    newborn due to isoimmunization P56.0
    pericardium — *see* Pericarditis
Drowned, drowning (near) T75.1 ☑
Drowsiness R40.0
Drug
    abuse counseling and surveillance Z71.51
    addiction — *see* Dependence
    dependence — *see* Dependence
    habit — *see* Dependence
    harmful use — *see* Abuse, drug
    induced fever R50.2
    overdose — *see* Table of Drugs and Chemicals, by drug,
        poisoning
    poisoning — *see* Table of Drugs and Chemicals, by
        drug, poisoning
    resistant organism infection — *see also* Resistant, or-
        ganism, to, drug Z16.30
    therapy
        long term (current) (prophylactic) — *see* Therapy,
            drug long-term (current) (prophylactic)
        short term — *omit code*
    wrong substance given or taken in error — *see* Table
        of Drugs and Chemicals, by drug, poisoning
Drunkenness (without dependence) F10.129
    acute in alcoholism F10.229
    chronic (without remission) F10.20
        with remission F10.21
    pathological (without dependence) F10.129
        with dependence F10.229
    sleep F51.9
Drusen
    macula (degenerative) (retina) — *see* Degeneration,
        macula, drusen
    optic disc H47.32- ☑
Dry, dryness — *see also* condition
    larynx J38.7
    mouth R68.2
        due to dehydration E86.0
    nose J34.89
    socket (teeth) M27.3
    throat J39.2
DSAP L56.5
Duane's syndrome H50.81- ☑
Dubin-Johnson disease or syndrome E80.6
Dubois' disease (thymus gland) A50.59 *[E35]*
Dubowitz' syndrome Q87.19
Duchenne-Aran muscular atrophy G12.21
Duchenne-Griesinger disease G71.01
Duchenne's
    disease or syndrome
        motor neuron disease G12.22
        muscular dystrophy G71.01
    locomotor ataxia (syphilitic) A52.11
    paralysis
        birth injury P14.0
        due to or associated with
            motor neuron disease G12.22
            muscular dystrophy G71.01
Ducrey's chancre A57
Duct, ductus — *see* condition
Duhring's disease (dermatitis herpetiformis) L13.0
Dullness, cardiac (decreased) (increased) R01.2
Dumb ague — *see* Malaria
Dumbness — *see* Aphasia
Dumdum fever B55.0
Dumping syndrome (postgastrectomy) K91.1
Duodenitis (nonspecific) (peptic) K29.80
    with bleeding K29.81
Duodenocholangitis — *see* Cholangitis
Duodenum, duodenal — *see* condition
Duplay's bursitis or periarthritis M75.0 ☑
Duplication, duplex — *see also* Accessory
    alimentary tract Q45.8
    anus Q43.4
    appendix (and cecum) Q43.4

Duplication, duplex — *continued*
    biliary duct (any) Q44.5
    bladder Q64.79
    cecum (and appendix) Q43.4
    cervix Q51.820
    chromosome NEC
        with complex rearrangements NEC Q92.5
        seen only at prometaphase Q92.8
    cystic duct Q44.5
    digestive organs Q45.8
    esophagus Q39.8
    frontonasal process Q75.8
    intestine (large) (small) Q43.4
    kidney Q63.0
    liver Q44.7
    pancreas Q45.3
    penis Q55.69
    respiratory organs NEC Q34.8
    salivary duct Q38.4
    spinal cord (incomplete) Q06.2
    stomach Q40.2
Dupré's disease (meningism) R29.1
Dupuytren's contraction or disease M72.0
Durand-Nicolas-Favre disease A55
Durotomy (inadvertent) (incidental) G97.41
Duroziez's disease (congenital mitral stenosis) Q23.2
Dutton's relapsing fever (West African) A68.1
Dwarfism E34.3
    achondroplastic Q77.4
    congenital E34.3
    constitutional E34.3
    hypochondroplastic Q77.4
    hypophyseal E23.0
    infantile E34.3
    Laron-type E34.3
    Lorain (-Levi) type E23.0
    metatropic Q77.8
    nephrotic-glycosuric (with hypophosphatemic rickets)
        E72.09
    nutritional E45
    pancreatic K86.89
    pituitary E23.0
    renal N25.0
    thanatophoric Q77.1
Dyke-Young anemia (secondary) (symptomatic) D59.19
Dysacusis — *see* Abnormal, auditory perception
Dysadrenocortism E27.9
    hyperfunction E27.0
Dysarthria R47.1
    following
        cerebral infarction I69.322
        cerebrovascular disease I69.922
            specified disease NEC I69.822
        intracerebral hemorrhage I69.122
        nontraumatic intracranial hemorrhage NEC I69.222
        subarachnoid hemorrhage I69.022
Dysautonomia (familial) G90.1
Dysbarism T70.3 ☑
Dysbasia R26.2
    angiosclerotica intermittens I73.9
    hysterical F44.4
    lordotica (progressiva) G24.1
    nonorganic origin F44.4
    psychogenic F44.4
Dysbetalipoproteinemia (familial) E78.2
Dyscalculia R48.8
    developmental F81.2
Dyschezia K59.00
Dyschondroplasia (with hemangiomata) Q78.4
Dyschromia (skin) L81.9
Dyscollagenosis M35.9
Dyscranio-pygo-phalangy Q87.0
Dyscrasia
    blood (with) D75.9
        antepartum hemorrhage — *see* Hemorrhage, an-
            tepartum, with coagulation defect
        intrapartum hemorrhage O67.0
        newborn P61.9
            specified type NEC P61.8
        puerperal, postpartum O72.3
    polyglandular, pluriglandular E31.9
Dysendocrinism E34.9
Dysentery, dysenteric (catarrhal) (diarrhea) (epidemic)
    (hemorrhagic) (infectious) (sporadic) (tropical) A09
    abscess, liver A06.4
    amebic — *see also* Amebiasis A06.0
        with abscess — *see* Abscess, amebic
        acute A06.0

Dysentery, dysenteric — *continued*
- amebic — *see also* Amebiasis — *continued*
  - chronic A06.1
  - arthritis — *see also* category M01 A09
    - bacillary (*see also* category M01) A03.9
  - bacillary A03.9
    - arthritis — *see also* category M01 A03.9
    - Boyd A03.2
    - Flexner A03.1
    - Schmitz (-Stutzer) A03.0
    - Shiga (-Kruse) A03.0
    - Shigella A03.9
      - boydii A03.2
      - dysenteriae A03.0
      - flexneri A03.1
      - group A A03.0
      - group B A03.1
      - group C A03.2
      - group D A03.3
      - sonnei A03.3
      - specified type NEC A03.8
    - Sonne A03.3
    - specified type NEC A03.8
  - balantidial A07.0
  - Balantidium coli A07.0
  - Boyd's A03.2
  - candidal B37.82
  - Chilomastix A07.8
  - Chinese A03.9
  - coccidial A07.3
  - Dientamoeba (fragilis) A07.8
  - Embadomonas A07.8
  - Entamoeba, entamebic — *see* Dysentery, amebic
  - Flexner-Boyd A03.2
  - Flexner's A03.1
  - Giardia lamblia A07.1
  - Hiss-Russell A03.1
  - Lamblia A07.1
  - leishmanial B55.0
  - malarial — *see* Malaria
  - metazoal B82.0
  - monilial B37.82
  - protozoal A07.9
  - Salmonella A02.0
  - schistosomal B65.1
  - Schmitz (-Stutzer) A03.0
  - Shiga (-Kruse) A03.0
  - Shigella NOS — *see* Dysentery, bacillary
  - Sonne A03.3
  - strongyloidiasis B78.0
  - trichomonal A07.8
  - viral — *see also* Enteritis, viral A08.4

Dysequilibrium R42
Dysesthesia R20.8
- hysterical F44.6
Dysfibrinogenemia (congenital) D68.2
Dysfunction
- adrenal E27.9
  - hyperfunction E27.0
- autonomic
  - due to alcohol G31.2
  - somatoform F45.8
- bladder N31.9
  - neurogenic NOS — *see* Dysfunction, bladder, neuromuscular
  - neuromuscular NOS N31.9
    - atonic (motor) (sensory) N31.2
    - autonomous N31.2
    - flaccid N31.2
    - nonreflex N31.2
    - reflex N31.1
    - specified NEC N31.8
    - uninhibited N31.0
- bleeding, uterus N93.8
- cerebral G93.89
- colon K59.9
  - psychogenic F45.8
- colostomy K94.03
- cystic duct K82.8
- cystostomy (stoma) — *see* Complications, cystostomy
- ejaculatory N53.19
  - anejaculatory orgasm N53.13
  - painful N53.12
  - premature F52.4
  - retarded N53.11
- endocrine NOS E34.9
- endometrium N85.8
- enterostomy K94.13

Dysfunction — *continued*
- erectile — *see* Dysfunction, sexual, male, erectile
- feeding, pediatric
  - acute R63.31
  - chronic R63.32
- gallbladder K82.8
- gastrostomy (stoma) K94.23
- gland, glandular NOS E34.9
  - meibomian, of eyelid — *see* Dysfunction, meibomian gland
- heart I51.89
- hemoglobin D75.89
- hepatic K76.89
- hypophysis E23.7
- hypothalamic NEC E23.3
- ileostomy (stoma) K94.13
- jejunostomy (stoma) K94.13
- kidney — *see* Disease, renal
- labyrinthine — *see* subcategory H83.2 ☑
- left ventricular, following sudden emotional stress I51.81
- liver K76.89
- male — *see* Dysfunction, sexual, male
- meibomian gland, of eyelid H02.889
  - left H02.886
    - lower H02.885
    - upper H02.884
    - upper and lower eyelids H02.88B
  - right H02.883
    - lower H02.882
    - upper H02.881
    - upper and lower eyelids H02.88A
- orgasmic (female) F52.31
  - male F52.32
- ovary E28.9
  - specified NEC E28.8
- papillary muscle I51.89
- parathyroid E21.4
- physiological NEC R68.89
  - psychogenic F59
- pineal gland E34.8
- pituitary (gland) E23.3
- platelets D69.1
- polyglandular E31.9
  - specified NEC E31.8
- psychophysiologic F59
- psychosexual F52.9
  - with
    - dyspareunia F52.6
    - premature ejaculation F52.4
    - vaginismus F52.5
- pylorus K31.9
- rectum K59.9
  - psychogenic F45.8
- reflex (sympathetic) — *see* Syndrome, pain, complex regional I
- segmental — *see* Dysfunction, somatic
- senile R54
- sexual (due to) R37
  - alcohol F10.981
  - amphetamine F15.981
    - in
      - abuse F15.181
      - dependence F15.281
  - anxiolytic F13.981
    - in
      - abuse F13.181
      - dependence F13.281
  - cocaine F14.981
    - in
      - abuse F14.181
      - dependence F14.281
  - excessive sexual drive F52.8
  - failure of genital response (male) F52.21
    - female F52.22
  - female N94.9
    - aversion F52.1
    - dyspareunia N94.10
      - psychogenic F52.6
    - frigidity F52.22
    - nymphomania F52.8
    - orgasmic F52.31
    - psychogenic F52.9
      - aversion F52.1
      - dyspareunia F52.6
      - frigidity F52.22
      - nymphomania F52.8
      - orgasmic F52.31

Dysfunction — *continued*
- sexual — *continued*
  - female — *continued*
    - psychogenic — *continued*
      - vaginismus F52.5
    - vaginismus N94.2
      - psychogenic F52.5
  - hypnotic F13.981
    - in
      - abuse F13.181
      - dependence F13.281
  - inhibited orgasm (female) F52.31
    - male F52.32
  - lack
    - of sexual enjoyment F52.1
    - or loss of sexual desire F52.0
  - male N53.9
    - anejaculatory orgasm N53.13
    - ejaculatory N53.19
      - painful N53.12
      - premature F52.4
      - retarded N53.11
    - erectile N52.9
      - drug induced N52.2
      - due to
        - disease classified elsewhere N52.1
        - drug N52.2
      - postoperative (postprocedural) N52.39
        - following
          - cryotherapy N52.37
          - interstitial seed therapy N52.36
          - prostate ablative therapy N52.37
          - prostatectomy N52.34
            - radical N52.31
          - radiation therapy N52.35
          - radical cystectomy N52.32
          - ultrasound ablative therapy N52.37
          - urethral surgery N52.33
      - psychogenic F52.21
      - specified cause NEC N52.8
      - vasculogenic
        - arterial insufficiency N52.01
          - with corporo-venous occlusive N52.03
        - corporo-venous occlusive N52.02
          - with arterial insufficiency N52.03
    - impotence — *see* Dysfunction, sexual, male, erectile
    - psychogenic F52.9
      - aversion F52.1
      - erectile F52.21
      - orgasmic F52.32
      - premature ejaculation F52.4
      - satyriasis F52.8
      - specified type NEC F52.8
    - specified type NEC N53.8
  - nonorganic F52.9
    - specified NEC F52.8
  - opioid F11.981
    - in
      - abuse F11.181
      - dependence F11.281
  - orgasmic dysfunction (female) F52.31
    - male F52.32
  - premature ejaculation F52.4
  - psychoactive substances NEC F19.981
    - in
      - abuse F19.181
      - dependence F19.281
  - psychogenic F52.9
  - sedative F13.981
    - in
      - abuse F13.181
      - dependence F13.281
  - sexual aversion F52.1
  - vaginismus (nonorganic) (psychogenic) F52.5
- sinoatrial node I49.5
- somatic M99.09
  - abdomen M99.09
  - acromioclavicular M99.07
  - cervical region M99.01
  - cervicothoracic M99.01
  - costochondral M99.08
  - costovertebral M99.08
  - head region M99.00
  - hip M99.05
  - lower extremity M99.06
  - lumbar region M99.03
  - lumbosacral M99.03
  - occipitocervical M99.00

☑ **Additional Character Required — Refer to the Tabular List for Character Selection** ▽ **Subterms under main terms may continue to next column or page**

Dysfunction — *continued*
  somatic — *continued*
    pelvic region M99.05
    pubic M99.05
    rib cage M99.08
    sacral region M99.04
    sacrococcygeal M99.04
    sacroiliac M99.04
    specified NEC M99.09
    sternochondral M99.08
    sternoclavicular M99.07
    thoracic region M99.02
    thoracolumbar M99.02
    upper extremity M99.07
  somatoform autonomic F45.8
  stomach K31.89
    psychogenic F45.8
  suprarenal E27.9
    hyperfunction E27.0
  symbolic R48.9
    specified type NEC R48.8
  temporomandibular (joint) M26.69
    joint-pain syndrome M26.62- ☑
  testicular (endocrine) E29.9
    specified NEC E29.8
  thymus E32.9
  thyroid E07.9
  ureterostomy (stoma) — *see* Complications, stoma,
    urinary tract
  urethrostomy (stoma) — *see* Complications, stoma,
    urinary tract
  uterus, complicating delivery O62.9
    hypertonic O62.4
    hypotonic O62.2
      primary O62.0
      secondary O62.1
  ventricular I51.9
    with congestive heart failure — *see also* Failure,
      heart I50.9
    left, reversible, following sudden emotional stress
      I51.81
Dysgenesis
  gonadal (due to chromosomal anomaly) Q96.9
    pure Q99.1
  renal Q60.5
    bilateral Q60.4
    unilateral Q60.3
  reticular D72.0
  tidal platelet D69.3
Dysgerminoma
  specified site — *see* Neoplasm, malignant, by site
  unspecified site
    female C56.9
    male C62.90
Dysgeusia R43.2
Dysgraphia R27.8
Dyshidrosis, dysidrosis L30.1
Dyskaryotic cervical smear R87.619
Dyskeratosis L85.8
  cervix — *see* Dysplasia, cervix
  congenital Q82.8
  uterus NEC N85.8
Dyskinesia G24.9
  biliary (cystic duct or gallbladder) K82.8
  drug induced
    orofacial G24.01
  esophagus K22.4
  hysterical F44.4
  intestinal K59.89
  nonorganic origin F44.4
  orofacial (idiopathic) G24.4
    drug induced G24.01
  psychogenic F44.4
  subacute, drug induced G24.01
  tardive G24.01
    neuroleptic induced G24.01
  trachea J39.8
  tracheobronchial J98.09
Dyslalia (developmental) F80.0
Dyslexia R48.0
  developmental F81.0
Dyslipidemia E78.5
  depressed HDL cholesterol E78.6
  elevated fasting triglycerides E78.1
Dysmaturity — *see also* Light for dates
  pulmonary (newborn) (Wilson-Mikity) P27.0
Dysmenorrhea (essential) (exfoliative) N94.6
  congestive (syndrome) N94.6

Dysmenorrhea — *continued*
  primary N94.4
  psychogenic F45.8
  secondary N94.5
Dysmetabolic syndrome X E88.81
Dysmetria R27.8
Dysmorphism (due to)
  alcohol Q86.0
  exogenous cause NEC Q86.8
  hydantoin Q86.1
  warfarin Q86.2
Dysmorphophobia (nondelusional) F45.22
  delusional F22
Dysnomia R47.01
Dysorexia R63.0
  psychogenic F50.89
Dysostosis
  cleidocranial, cleidocranialis Q74.0
  craniofacial Q75.1
  Fairbank's (idiopathic familial generalized osteophyto-
    sis) Q78.9
  mandibulofacial (incomplete) Q75.4
  multiplex E76.01
  oculomandibular Q75.5
Dyspareunia (female) N94.10
  deep N94.12
  male N53.12
  nonorganic F52.6
  psychogenic F52.6
  secondary N94.19
  specified NEC N94.19
  superficial (introital) N94.11
Dyspepsia R10.13
  atonic K30
  functional (allergic) (congenital) (gastrointestinal) (oc-
    cupational) (reflex) K30
  intestinal K59.89
  nervous F45.8
  neurotic F45.8
  psychogenic F45.8
Dysphagia R13.10
  cervical R13.19
  following
    cerebral infarction I69.391
    cerebrovascular disease I69.991
      specified NEC I69.891
    intracerebral hemorrhage I69.191
    nontraumatic intracranial hemorrhage NEC I69.291
    specified disease NEC I69.891
    subarachnoid hemorrhage I69.091
  functional (hysterical) F45.8
  hysterical F45.8
  nervous (hysterical) F45.8
  neurogenic R13.19
  oral phase R13.11
  oropharyngeal phase R13.12
  pharyngeal phase R13.13
  pharyngoesophageal phase R13.14
  psychogenic F45.8
  sideropenic D50.1
  spastica K22.4
  specified NEC R13.19
Dysphagocytosis, congenital D71
Dysphasia R47.02
  developmental
    expressive type F80.1
    receptive type F80.2
  following
    cerebrovascular disease I69.921
      cerebral infarction I69.321
      intracerebral hemorrhage I69.121
      nontraumatic intracranial hemorrhage NEC
        I69.221
      specified disease NEC I69.821
      subarachnoid hemorrhage I69.021
Dysphonia R49.0
  functional F44.4
  hysterical F44.4
  psychogenic F44.4
  spastica J38.3
Dysphoria
  gender F64.9
    in
      adolescence and adulthood F64.0
      children F64.2
    specified NEC F64.8
  postpartal O90.6
Dyspituitarism E23.3

Dysplasia — *see also* Anomaly
  acetabular, congenital Q65.89
  alveolar capillary, with vein misalignment J84.843
  anus (histologically confirmed) (mild) (moderate)
    K62.82
    severe D01.3
  arrhythmogenic right ventricular I42.8
  arterial, fibromuscular I77.3
  asphyxiating thoracic (congenital) Q77.2
  brain Q07.9
  bronchopulmonary, perinatal P27.1
  cervix (uteri) N87.9
    mild N87.0
    moderate N87.1
    severe D06.9
  chondroectodermal Q77.6
  colon D12.6
  craniometaphyseal Q78.8
  dentinal K00.5
  diaphyseal, progressive Q78.3
  dystrophic Q77.5
  ectodermal (anhidrotic) (congenital) (hereditary) Q82.4
    hydrotic Q82.8
  epithelial, uterine cervix — *see* Dysplasia, cervix
  eye (congenital) Q11.2
  fibrous
    bone NEC (monostotic) M85.00
      ankle M85.07- ☑
      foot M85.07- ☑
      forearm M85.03- ☑
      hand M85.04- ☑
      lower leg M85.06- ☑
      multiple site M85.09
      neck M85.08
      rib M85.08
      shoulder M85.01- ☑
      skull M85.08
      specified site NEC M85.08
      thigh M85.05- ☑
      toe M85.07- ☑
      upper arm M85.02- ☑
      vertebra M85.08
  diaphyseal, progressive Q78.3
  jaw M27.8
  polyostotic Q78.1
  florid osseous — *see also* Cyst, calcifying odontogenic
  high grade, focal D12.6
  hip, congenital Q65.89
  joint, congenital Q74.8
  kidney Q61.4
    multicystic Q61.4
  leg Q74.2
  lung, congenital (not associated with short gestation)
    Q33.6
  mammary (gland) (benign) N60.9- ☑
    cyst (solitary) — *see* Cyst, breast
    cystic — *see* Mastopathy, cystic
    duct ectasia — *see* Ectasia, mammary duct
    fibroadenosis — *see* Fibroadenosis, breast
    fibrosclerosis — *see* Fibrosclerosis, breast
    specified type NEC N60.8- ☑
  metaphyseal Q78.5
  muscle Q79.8
  oculodentodigital Q87.0
  periapical (cemental) (cemento-osseous) — *see* Cyst,
    calcifying odontogenic
  periosteum — *see* Disorder, bone, specified type NEC
  polyostotic fibrous Q78.1
  prostate — *see also* Neoplasia, intraepithelial, prostate
    N42.30
    severe D07.5
    specified NEC N42.39
  renal Q61.4
    multicystic Q61.4
  retinal, congenital Q14.1
  right ventricular, arrhythmogenic I42.8
  septo-optic Q04.4
  skin L98.8
  spinal cord Q06.1
  spondyloepiphyseal Q77.7
  thymic, with immunodeficiency D82.1
  vagina N89.3
    mild N89.0
    moderate N89.1
    severe NEC D07.2
  vulva N90.3
    mild N90.0
    moderate N90.1

Dysplasia — *continued*
  vulva — *continued*
    severe NEC D07.1
Dysplasminogenemia E88.02
Dyspnea (nocturnal) (paroxysmal) R06.00
  asthmatic (bronchial) J45.909
    with
      bronchitis J45.909
        with
          exacerbation (acute) J45.901
          status asthmaticus J45.902
      chronic J44.9
      exacerbation (acute) J45.901
      status asthmaticus J45.902
  cardiac — *see* Failure, ventricular, left
  cardiac — *see* Failure, ventricular, left
  functional F45.8
  hyperventilation R06.4
  hysterical F45.8
  newborn P28.89
  orthopnea R06.01
  psychogenic F45.8
  shortness of breath R06.02
  specified type NEC R06.09
Dyspraxia R27.8
  developmental (syndrome) F82
Dysproteinemia E88.09
Dysreflexia, autonomic G90.4
Dysrhythmia
  cardiac I49.9
    newborn
      bradycardia P29.12
        occurring before birth P03.819
          before onset of labor P03.810
          during labor P03.811
      tachycardia P29.11
  postoperative I97.89
  cerebral or cortical — *see* Epilepsy
Dyssomnia — *see* Disorder, sleep
Dyssynergia
  biliary K83.8
  bladder sphincter N36.44
  cerebellaris myoclonica (Hunt's ataxia) G11.19
Dysthymia F34.1
Dysthyroidism E07.9
Dystocia O66.9
  affecting newborn P03.1
  cervical (hypotonic) O62.2
    affecting newborn P03.6
    primary O62.0
    secondary O62.1
  contraction ring O62.4
  fetal O66.9
    abnormality NEC O66.3
    conjoined twins O66.3
    oversize O66.2
  maternal O66.9
  positional O64.9 ☑
  shoulder (girdle) O66.0
    causing obstructed labor O66.0
  uterine NEC O62.4
Dystonia G24.9
  cervical G24.3
  deformans progressiva G24.1
  drug induced NEC G24.09
    acute G24.02
    specified NEC G24.09
  familial G24.1
  idiopathic G24.1
    familial G24.1
    nonfamilial G24.2
    orofacial G24.4
  lenticularis G24.8
  musculorum deformans G24.1
  neuroleptic induced (acute) G24.02
  orofacial (idiopathic) G24.4
  oromandibular G24.4
    due to drug G24.01
  specified NEC G24.8
  torsion (familial) (idiopathic) G24.1
    acquired G24.8
    genetic G24.1
    symptomatic (nonfamilial) G24.2
Dystonic movements R25.8
Dystrophy, dystrophia
  adiposogenital E23.6
  autosomal recessive, childhood type, muscular dystrophy resembling Duchenne or Becker G71.01

Dystrophy, dystrophia — *continued*
  Becker's type G71.01
  cervical sympathetic G90.2
  choroid (hereditary) H31.20
    central areolar H31.22
    choroideremia H31.21
    gyrate atrophy H31.23
    specified type NEC H31.29
  cornea (hereditary) H18.50- ☑
    endothelial H18.51- ☑
    epithelial H18.52- ☑
    granular H18.53- ☑
    lattice H18.54- ☑
    macular H18.55- ☑
    specified type NEC H18.59- ☑
  Duchenne's type G71.01
  due to malnutrition E45
  Erb's G71.02
  Fuchs' H18.51- ☑
  Gower's muscular G71.01
  hair L67.8
  infantile neuraxonal G31.89
  Landouzy-Déjérine G71.02
  Leyden-Möbius G71.09
  muscular G71.00
    autosomal recessive, childhood type, muscular dystrophy resembling Duchenne or Becker G71.01
    benign (Becker type) G71.01
      scapuloperoneal with early contractures [Emery-Dreifuss] G71.09
    congenital (hereditary) (progressive) (with specific morphological abnormalities of the muscle fiber) G71.09
      myotonic G71.11
    distal G71.09
    Duchenne type G71.01
    Emery-Dreifuss G71.09
    Erb type G71.02
    facioscapulohumeral G71.02
    Gower's G71.01
    hereditary (progressive) G71.09
    Landouzy-Déjérine type G71.02
    limb-girdle G71.09
    myotonic G71.11
    progressive (hereditary) G71.09
      Charcot-Marie (-Tooth) type G60.0
    pseudohypertrophic (infantile) G71.01
    scapulohumeral G71.02
    scapuloperoneal G71.09
    severe (Duchenne type) G71.01
    specified type NEC G71.09
  myocardium, myocardial — *see* Degeneration, myocardial
  nail L60.3
    congenital Q84.6
  nutritional E45
  ocular G71.09
  oculocerebrorenal E72.03
  oculopharyngeal G71.09
  ovarian N83.8
  polyglandular E31.8
  reflex (neuromuscular) (sympathetic) — *see* Syndrome, pain, complex regional I
  retinal (hereditary) H35.50
    in
      lipid storage disorders E75.6 *[H36]*
      systemic lipidoses E75.6 *[H36]*
    involving
      pigment epithelium H35.54
      sensory area H35.53
    pigmentary H35.52
    vitreoretinal H35.51
  Salzmann's nodular — *see* Degeneration, cornea, nodular
  scapuloperoneal G71.09
  skin NEC L98.8
  sympathetic (reflex) — *see* Syndrome, pain, complex regional I
    cervical G90.2
  tapetoretinal H35.54
  thoracic, asphyxiating Q77.2
  unguium L60.3
    congenital Q84.6
  vitreoretinal H35.51
  vulva N90.4
  yellow (liver) — *see* Failure, hepatic
Dysuria R30.0

Dysuria — *continued*
  psychogenic F45.8

E

Eales' disease H35.06- ☑
Ear — *see also* condition
  piercing Z41.3
  tropical NEC B36.9 *[H62.40]*
    in
      aspergillosis B44.89
      candidiasis B37.84
      moniliasis B37.84
  wax (impacted) H61.20
    left H61.22
      with right H61.23
    right H61.21
      with left H61.23
Earache — *see* subcategory H92.0 ☑
Early satiety R68.81
Eaton-Lambert syndrome — *see* Syndrome, Lambert-Eaton
Eberth's disease (typhoid fever) A01.00
Ebola virus disease A98.4
Ebstein's anomaly or syndrome (heart) Q22.5
Eccentro-osteochondrodysplasia E76.29
Ecchondroma — *see* Neoplasm, bone, benign
Ecchondrosis D48.0
Ecchymosis R58
  conjunctiva — *see* Hemorrhage, conjunctiva
  eye (traumatic) — *see* Contusion, eyeball
  eyelid (traumatic) — *see* Contusion, eyelid
  newborn P54.5
  spontaneous R23.3
  traumatic — *see* Contusion
Echinococciasis — *see* Echinococcus
Echinococcosis — *see* Echinococcus
Echinococcus (infection) B67.90
  granulosus B67.4
    bone B67.2
    liver B67.0
    lung B67.1
    multiple sites B67.32
    specified site NEC B67.39
    thyroid B67.31
  liver NOS B67.8
    granulosus B67.0
    multilocularis B67.5
  lung NEC B67.99
    granulosus B67.1
    multilocularis B67.69
  multilocularis B67.7
    liver B67.5
    multiple sites B67.61
    specified site NEC B67.69
  specified site NEC B67.99
    granulosus B67.39
    multilocularis B67.69
  thyroid NEC B67.99
    granulosus B67.31
    multilocularis B67.69 *[E35]*
Echinorhynchiasis B83.8
Echinostomiasis B66.8
Echolalia R48.8
Echovirus, as cause of disease classified elsewhere B97.12
Eclampsia, eclamptic (coma) (convulsions) (delirium) (with hypertension) NEC O15.9
  complicating
    labor and delivery O15.1
    postpartum O15.2
    pregnancy O15.0- ☑
    puerperium O15.2
Economic circumstances affecting care Z59.9
Economo's disease A85.8
Ectasia, ectasis
  annuloaortic I35.8
  aorta I77.819
    with aneurysm — *see* Aneurysm, aorta
    abdominal I77.811
    thoracic I77.810
    thoracoabdominal I77.812
  breast — *see* Ectasia, mammary duct
  capillary I78.8
  cornea H18.71- ☑
  gastric antral vascular (GAVE) K31.819
    with hemorrhage K31.811

Ectasia, ectasis — *continued*
  gastric antral vascular — *continued*
    without hemorrhage K31.819
  mammary duct N60.4- ☑
  salivary gland (duct) K11.8
  sclera — *see* Sclerectasia
Ecthyma L08.0
  contagiosum B08.02
  gangrenosum L08.0
  infectiosum B08.02
Ectocardia Q24.8
Ectodermal dysplasia (anhidrotic) Q82.4
Ectodermosis erosiva pluriorificialis L51.1
Ectopic, ectopia (congenital)
  abdominal viscera Q45.8
    due to defect in anterior abdominal wall Q79.59
  ACTH syndrome E24.3
  adrenal gland Q89.1
  anus Q43.5
  atrial beats I49.1
  beats I49.49
    atrial I49.1
    ventricular I49.3
  bladder Q64.10
  bone and cartilage in lung Q33.5
  brain Q04.8
  breast tissue Q83.8
  cardiac Q24.8
  cerebral Q04.8
  cordis Q24.8
  endometrium — *see* Endometriosis
  gastric mucosa Q40.2
  gestation — *see* Pregnancy, by site
  heart Q24.8
  hormone secretion NEC E34.2
  kidney (crossed) (pelvis) Q63.2
  lens, lentis Q12.1
  mole — *see* Pregnancy, by site
  organ or site NEC — *see* Malposition, congenital
  pancreas Q45.3
  pregnancy — *see* Pregnancy, ectopic
  pupil — *see* Abnormality, pupillary
  renal Q63.2
  sebaceous glands of mouth Q38.6
  spleen Q89.09
  testis Q53.00
    bilateral Q53.02
    unilateral Q53.01
  thyroid Q89.2
  tissue in lung Q33.5
  ureter Q62.63
  ventricular beats I49.3
  vesicae Q64.10
Ectromelia Q73.8
  lower limb — *see* Defect, reduction, limb, lower, specified type NEC
  upper limb — *see* Defect, reduction, limb, upper, specified type NEC
Ectropion H02.109
  cervix N86
    with cervicitis N72
  congenital Q10.1
  eyelid H02.109
    cicatricial H02.119
      left H02.116
        lower H02.115
        upper H02.114
      right H02.113
        lower H02.112
        upper H02.111
    congenital Q10.1
    left H02.106
      lower H02.105
      upper H02.104
    mechanical H02.129
      left H02.126
        lower H02.125
        upper H02.124
      right H02.123
        lower H02.122
        upper H02.121
    paralytic H02.159
      left H02.156
        lower H02.155
        upper H02.154
      right H02.153
        lower H02.152
        upper H02.151

Ectropion — *continued*
  eyelid — *continued*
    right H02.103
      lower H02.102
      upper H02.101
    senile H02.139
      left H02.136
        lower H02.135
        upper H02.134
      right H02.133
        lower H02.132
        upper H02.131
    spastic H02.149
      left H02.146
        lower H02.145
        upper H02.144
      right H02.143
        lower H02.142
        upper H02.141
  iris H21.89
  lip (acquired) K13.0
    congenital Q38.0
  urethra N36.8
  uvea H21.89
Eczema (acute) (chronic) (erythematous) (fissum) (rubrum) (squamous) — *see also* Dermatitis L30.9
  contact — *see* Dermatitis, contact
  dyshydrotic L30.1
  external ear — *see* Otitis, externa, acute, eczematoid
  flexural L20.82
  herpeticum B00.0
  hypertrophicum L28.0
  hypostatic — *see* Varix, leg, with, inflammation
  impetiginous L01.1
  infantile (due to any substance) L20.83
    intertriginous L21.1
    seborrheic L21.1
  intertriginous NEC L30.4
    infantile L21.1
  intrinsic (allergic) L20.84
  lichenified NEC L28.0
  marginatum (hebrae) B35.6
  pustular L30.3
  stasis I87.2
    with varicose veins — *see* Varix, leg, with, inflammation
  vaccination, vaccinatum T88.1 ☑
  varicose — *see* Varix, leg, with, inflammation
Eczematid L30.2
Eddowes (-Spurway) **syndrome** Q78.0
Edema, edematous (infectious) (pitting) (toxic) R60.9
  with nephritis — *see* Nephrosis
  allergic T78.3 ☑
  amputation stump (surgical) (sequelae (late effect)) T87.89
  angioneurotic (allergic) (any site) (with urticaria) T78.3 ☑
    hereditary D84.1
  angiospastic I73.9
  Berlin's (traumatic) S05.8X- ☑
  brain (cytotoxic) (vasogenic) G93.6
    due to birth injury P11.0
    newborn (anoxia or hypoxia) P52.4
      birth injury P11.0
    traumatic — *see* Injury, intracranial, cerebral edema
  cardiac — *see* Failure, heart, congestive
  cardiovascular — *see* Failure, heart, congestive
  cerebral — *see* Edema, brain
  cerebrospinal — *see* Edema, brain
  cervix (uteri) (acute) N88.8
    puerperal, postpartum O90.89
  chronic hereditary Q82.0
  circumscribed, acute T78.3 ☑
    hereditary D84.1
  conjunctiva H11.42- ☑
  cornea H18.2- ☑
    idiopathic H18.22- ☑
    secondary H18.23- ☑
      due to contact lens H18.21- ☑
  due to
    lymphatic obstruction I89.0
    salt retention E87.0
  epiglottis — *see* Edema, glottis
  essential, acute T78.3 ☑
    hereditary D84.1
  extremities, lower — *see* Edema, legs
  eyelid NEC H02.849
    left H02.846

Edema, edematous — *continued*
  eyelid — *continued*
    left — *continued*
      lower H02.845
      upper H02.844
    right H02.843
      lower H02.842
      upper H02.841
  familial, hereditary Q82.0
  famine — *see* Malnutrition, severe
  generalized R60.1
  glottis, glottic, glottidis (obstructive) (passive) J38.4
    allergic T78.3 ☑
      hereditary D84.1
  heart — *see* Failure, heart, congestive
  heat T67.7 ☑
  hereditary Q82.0
  inanition — *see* Malnutrition, severe
  intracranial G93.6
  iris H21.89
  joint — *see* Effusion, joint
  larynx — *see* Edema, glottis
  legs R60.0
    due to venous obstruction I87.1
    hereditary Q82.0
  localized R60.0
    due to venous obstruction I87.1
  lower limbs — *see* Edema, legs
  lung J81.1
    with heart condition or failure — *see* Failure, ventricular, left
    acute J81.0
      chemical (acute) J68.1
        chronic J68.1
      chronic J81.1
        due to
          chemicals, gases, fumes or vapors (inhalation) J68.1
          external agent J70.9
            specified NEC J70.8
          radiation J70.1
    due to
      chemicals, fumes or vapors (inhalation) J68.1
      external agent J70.9
        specified NEC J70.8
      high altitude T70.29 ☑
      near drowning T75.1 ☑
      radiation J70.0
    meaning failure, left ventricle I50.1
  lymphatic I89.0
    due to mastectomy I97.2
  macula H35.81
    cystoid, following cataract surgery — *see* Complications, postprocedural, following cataract surgery
    diabetic — *see* Diabetes, by type, with, retinopathy, with macular edema
  malignant — *see* Gangrene, gas
  Milroy's Q82.0
  nasopharynx J39.2
  newborn P83.30
    hydrops fetalis — *see* Hydrops, fetalis
    specified NEC P83.39
  nutritional — *see also* Malnutrition, severe
    with dyspigmentation, skin and hair E40
  optic disc or nerve — *see* Papilledema
  orbit H05.22- ☑
  pancreas K86.89
  papilla, optic — *see* Papilledema
  penis N48.89
  periodic T78.3 ☑
    hereditary D84.1
  pharynx J39.2
  pulmonary — *see* Edema, lung
  Quincke's T78.3 ☑
    hereditary D84.1
  renal — *see* Nephrosis
  retina H35.81
    diabetic — *see* Diabetes, by type, with, retinopathy, with macular edema
  salt E87.0
  scrotum N50.89
  seminal vesicle N50.89
  spermatic cord N50.89
  spinal (cord) (vascular) (nontraumatic) G95.19
  starvation — *see* Malnutrition, severe
  stasis — *see* Hypertension, venous, (chronic)
  subglottic — *see* Edema, glottis

Edema, edematous — *continued*
  supraglottic — *see* Edema, glottis
  testis N44.8
  tunica vaginalis N50.89
  vas deferens N50.89
  vulva (acute) N90.89
Edentulism — *see* Absence, teeth, acquired
Edsall's disease T67.2 ☑
Educational handicap Z55.9
  less than a high school diploma Z55.5
  no general equivalence degree (GED) Z55.5
  specified NEC Z55.8
Edward's syndrome — *see* Trisomy, 18
Effect(s) (of) (from) — *see* Effect, adverse NEC
Effect, adverse
  abnormal gravitational (G) forces or states T75.81 ☑
  abuse — *see* Maltreatment
  air pressure T70.9 ☑
    specified NEC T70.8 ☑
  altitude (high) — *see* Effect, adverse, high altitude
  anesthesia — *see also* Anesthesia T88.59 ☑
    in labor and delivery O74.9
    local, toxic
      in labor and delivery O74.4
      in pregnancy NEC O29.3-
      postpartum, puerperal O89.3
    postpartum, puerperal O89.9
    specified NEC T88.59 ☑
      in labor and delivery O74.8
      postpartum, puerperal O89.8
    spinal and epidural T88.59 ☑
      headache T88.59 ☑
        in labor and delivery O74.5
        postpartum, puerperal O89.4
      specified NEC
        in labor and delivery O74.6
        postpartum, puerperal O89.5
  antitoxin — *see* Complications, vaccination
  atmospheric pressure T70.9 ☑
    due to explosion T70.8 ☑
    high T70.3 ☑
    low — *see* Effect, adverse, high altitude
    specified effect NEC T70.8 ☑
  biological, correct substance properly administered — *see* Effect, adverse, drug
  blood (derivatives) (serum) (transfusion) — *see* Complications, transfusion
  chemical substance — *see* Table of Drugs and Chemicals
  cold (temperature) (weather) T69.9 ☑
    chilblains T69.1 ☑
    frostbite — *see* Frostbite
    specified effect NEC T69.8 ☑
  drugs and medicaments T88.7 ☑
    specified drug — *see* Table of Drugs and Chemicals, by drug, adverse effect
    specified effect — *code to* condition
  electric current, electricity (shock) T75.4 ☑
    burn — *see* Burn
  exertion (excessive) T73.3 ☑
  exposure — *see* Exposure
  external cause NEC T75.89 ☑
  foodstuffs T78.1 ☑
    allergic reaction — *see* Allergy, food
      causing anaphylaxis — *see* Shock, anaphylactic, due to food
    noxious — *see* Poisoning, food, noxious
  gases, fumes, or vapors T59.9- ☑
    specified agent — *see* Table of Drugs and Chemicals
  glue (airplane) sniffing
    due to drug abuse — *see* Abuse, drug, inhalant
    due to drug dependence — *see* Dependence, drug, inhalant
  heat — *see* Heat
  high altitude NEC T70.29 ☑
    anoxia T70.29 ☑
    on
      ears T70.0 ☑
      sinuses T70.1 ☑
    polycythemia D75.1
  high pressure fluids T70.4 ☑
  hot weather — *see* Heat
  hunger T73.0 ☑
  immersion, foot — *see* Immersion
  immunization — *see* Complications, vaccination
  immunological agents — *see* Complications, vaccination

Effect, adverse — *continued*
  infrared (radiation) (rays) NOS T66 ☑
    dermatitis or eczema L59.8
  infusion — *see* Complications, infusion
  lack of care of infants — *see* Maltreatment, child
  lightning — *see* Lightning
  medical care T88.9 ☑
    specified NEC T88.8 ☑
  medicinal substance, correct, properly administered — *see* Effect, adverse, drug
  motion T75.3 ☑
  noise, on inner ear — *see* subcategory H83.3 ☑
  overheated places — *see* Heat
  psychosocial, of work environment Z56.5
  radiation (diagnostic) (infrared) (natural source) (therapeutic) (ultraviolet) (X-ray) NOS T66 ☑
    dermatitis or eczema — *see* Dermatitis, due to, radiation
    fibrosis of lung J70.1
    pneumonitis J70.0
    pulmonary manifestations
      acute J70.0
      chronic J70.1
    skin L59.9
  radioactive substance NOS
    dermatitis or eczema — *see* Radiodermatitis
  reduced temperature T69.9 ☑
    immersion foot or hand — *see* Immersion
    specified effect NEC T69.8 ☑
  serum NEC — *see also* Reaction, serum T80.69 ☑
  specified NEC T78.8 ☑
    external cause NEC T75.89 ☑
  strangulation — *see* Asphyxia, traumatic
  submersion T75.1 ☑
  thirst T73.1 ☑
  toxic — *see* Toxicity
  transfusion — *see* Complications, transfusion
  ultraviolet (radiation) (rays) NOS T66 ☑
    burn — *see* Burn
    dermatitis or eczema — *see* Dermatitis, due to, ultraviolet rays
      acute L56.8
  vaccine (any) — *see* Complications, vaccination
  vibration — *see* Vibration, adverse effects
  water pressure NEC T70.9 ☑
    specified NEC T70.8 ☑
  weightlessness T75.82 ☑
  whole blood — *see* Complications, transfusion
  work environment Z56.5
Effects, late — *see* Sequelae
Effluvium
  anagen L65.1
  telogen L65.0
Effort syndrome (psychogenic) F45.8
Effusion
  amniotic fluid — *see* Pregnancy, complicated by, premature rupture of membranes
  brain (serous) G93.6
  bronchial — *see* Bronchitis
  cerebral G93.6
  cerebrospinal — *see also* Meningitis
    vessel G93.6
  chest — *see* Effusion, pleura
  chylous, chyliform (pleura) J94.0
  intracranial G93.6
  joint M25.40
    ankle M25.47- ☑
    elbow M25.42- ☑
    foot joint M25.47- ☑
    hand joint M25.44- ☑
    hip M25.45- ☑
    knee M25.46- ☑
    shoulder M25.41- ☑
    specified joint NEC M25.48
    wrist M25.43- ☑
  malignant pleural J91.0
  meninges — *see* Meningitis
  pericardium, pericardial (noninflammatory) I31.3
    acute — *see* Pericarditis, acute
  peritoneal (chronic) R18.8
  pleura, pleurisy, pleuritic, pleuropericardial J90
    chylous, chyliform J94.0
    due to systemic lupus erythematosis M32.13
    in conditions classified elsewhere J91.8
    influenzal — *see* Influenza, with, respiratory manifestations NEC
    malignant J91.0

Effusion — *continued*
  pleura, pleurisy, pleuritic, pleuropericardial — *continued*
    newborn P28.89
    tuberculous NEC A15.6
      primary (progressive) A15.7
  spinal — *see* Meningitis
  thorax, thoracic — *see* Effusion, pleura
Egg shell nails L60.3
  congenital Q84.6
EGPA (eosinophilic granulomatosis with polyangiitis) M30.1
Egyptian splenomegaly B65.1
Ehlers-Danlos syndrome — *see also* Syndrome, Ehlers-Danlos Q79.60
Ehrlichiosis A77.40
  due to
    E. chafeensis A77.41
    E. ewingii A77.49
    E. muris euclairensis A77.49
    E. sennetsu A79.81
    specified organism NEC A77.49
Eichstedt's disease B36.0
Eisenmenger's
  complex or syndrome I27.83
  defect Q21.8
Ejaculation
  delayed F52.32
  painful N53.12
  premature F52.4
  retarded N53.11
  retrograde N53.14
  semen, painful N53.12
    psychogenic F52.6
Ekbom's syndrome (restless legs) G25.81
Ekman's syndrome (brittle bones and blue sclera) Q78.0
Elastic skin Q82.8
  acquired L57.4
Elastofibroma — *see* Neoplasm, connective tissue, benign
Elastoma (juvenile) Q82.8
  Miescher's L87.2
Elastomyofibrosis I42.4
Elastosis
  actinic, solar L57.8
  atrophicans (senile) L57.4
  perforans serpiginosa L87.2
  senilis L57.4
Elbow — *see* condition
Electric current, electricity, effects (concussion) (fatal) (nonfatal) (shock) T75.4 ☑
  burn — *see* Burn
Electric feet syndrome E53.8
Electrocution T75.4 ☑
  from electroshock gun (taser) T75.4 ☑
Electrolyte imbalance E87.8
  with
    abortion — *see* Abortion by type, complicated by, electrolyte imbalance
    ectopic pregnancy O08.5
    molar pregnancy O08.5
Elephantiasis (nonfilarial) I89.0
  arabicum — *see* Infestation, filarial
  bancroftian B74.0
  congenital (any site) (hereditary) Q82.0
  due to
    Brugia (malayi) B74.1
      timori B74.2
    mastectomy I97.2
    Wuchereria (bancrofti) B74.0
  eyelid H02.859
    left H02.856
      lower H02.855
      upper H02.854
    right H02.853
      lower H02.852
      upper H02.851
  filarial, filariensis — *see* Infestation, filarial
  glandular I89.0
  graecorum A30.9
  lymphangiectatic I89.0
  lymphatic vessel I89.0
    due to mastectomy I97.2
  scrotum (nonfilarial) I89.0
  streptococcal I89.0
  surgical I97.89
    postmastectomy I97.2
  telangiectodes I89.0

130

☑ **Additional Character Required** — Refer to the Tabular List for Character Selection
▽ **Subterms under main terms may continue to next column or page**

Elephantiasis — *continued*
  vulva (nonfilarial) N90.89
Elevated, elevation
  alanine transaminase (ALT) R74.01
  ALT (alanine transaminase) R74.01
  antibody titer R76.0
  aspartate transaminase (AST) R74.01
  AST (aspartate transaminase) R74.01
  basal metabolic rate R94.8
  blood pressure — *see also* Hypertension
    reading (incidental) (isolated) (nonspecific), no diag-
      nosis of hypertension R03.0
  blood sugar R73.9
  body temperature (of unknown origin) R50.9
  cancer antigen 125 [CA 125] R97.1
  carcinoembryonic antigen [CEA] R97.0
  cholesterol E78.00
    with high triglycerides E78.2
  conjugate, eye H51.0
  C-reactive protein (CRP) R79.82
  diaphragm, congenital Q79.1
  erythrocyte sedimentation rate R70.0
  fasting glucose R73.01
  fasting triglycerides E78.1
  finding on laboratory examination — *see* Findings,
    abnormal, inconclusive, without diagnosis, by
    type of exam
  GFR (glomerular filtration rate) — *see* Findings, abnor-
    mal, inconclusive, without diagnosis, by type of
    exam
  glucose tolerance (oral) R73.02
  immunoglobulin level R76.8
  indoleacetic acid R82.5
  lactic acid dehydrogenase (LDH) level R74.02
  leukocytes D72.829
  lipoprotein a (Lp(a)) level E78.41
  liver function
    study R94.5
    test R79.89
      alkaline phosphatase R74.8
      aminotransferase R74.01
      bilirubin R17
      hepatic enzyme R74.8
      lactate dehydrogenase R74.02
  Lp(a) (lipoprotein(a)) E78.41
  lymphocytes D72.820
  prostate specific antigen [PSA] R97.20
  Rh titer — *see* Complication(s), transfusion, incompat-
    ibility reaction, Rh (factor)
  scapula, congenital Q74.0
  sedimentation rate R70.0
  SGOT R74.01
  SGPT R74.01
  transaminase level R74.01
  triglycerides E78.1
    with high cholesterol E78.2
  troponin R77.8
  tumor associated antigens [TAA] NEC R97.8
  tumor specific antigens [TSA] NEC R97.8
  urine level of
    17-ketosteroids R82.5
    catecholamine R82.5
    indoleacetic acid R82.5
    steroids R82.5
    vanillylmandelic acid (VMA) R82.5
  venous pressure I87.8
  white blood cell count D72.829
    specified NEC D72.828
Elliptocytosis (congenital) (hereditary) D58.1
  Hb C (disease) D58.1
  hemoglobin disease D58.1
  sickle-cell (disease) D57.8- ☑
    trait D57.3
Ellison-Zollinger syndrome E16.4
Ellis-van Creveld syndrome (chondroectodermal dysplasia) Q77.6
Elongated, elongation (congenital) — *see also* Distortion
  bone Q79.9
  cervix (uteri) Q51.828
    acquired N88.4
    hypertrophic N88.4
  colon Q43.8
  common bile duct Q44.5
  cystic duct Q44.5
  frenulum, penis Q55.69
  labia minora (acquired) N90.69
  ligamentum patellae Q74.1

Elongated, elongation — *continued*
  petiolus (epiglottidis) Q31.8
  tooth, teeth K00.2
  uvula Q38.6
Eltor cholera A00.1
Emaciation R64
  due to malnutrition E43
Embadomoniasis A07.8
Embedded tooth, teeth K01.0
  root only K08.3
Embolic — *see* condition
Embolism (multiple) (paradoxical) I74.9
  air (any site) (traumatic) T79.0 ☑
    following
      abortion — *see* Abortion by type complicated
        by embolism
      ectopic pregnancy O08.2
      infusion, therapeutic injection or transfusion
        T80.0 ☑
      molar pregnancy O08.2
      procedure NEC
        artery T81.719 ☑
          mesenteric T81.710 ☑
          renal T81.711 ☑
          specified NEC T81.718 ☑
        vein T81.72 ☑
    in pregnancy, childbirth or puerperium — *see* Em-
      bolism, obstetric
  amniotic fluid (pulmonary) — *see also* Embolism, ob-
    stetric
    following
      abortion — *see* Abortion by type complicated
        by embolism
      ectopic pregnancy O08.2
      molar pregnancy O08.2
  aorta, aortic I74.10
    abdominal I74.09
      saddle I74.01
    bifurcation I74.09
    saddle I74.01
    thoracic I74.11
  artery I74.9
    auditory, internal I65.8
    basilar — *see* Occlusion, artery, basilar
    carotid (common) (internal) — *see* Occlusion, artery,
      carotid
    cerebellar (anterior inferior) (posterior inferior) (su-
      perior) I66.3
    cerebral — *see* Occlusion, artery, cerebral
    choroidal (anterior) I65.8
    communicating posterior I65.8
    coronary — *see also* Infarct, myocardium
      not resulting in infarction I24.0
    extremity I74.4
      lower I74.3
      upper I74.2
    hypophyseal I65.8
    iliac I74.5
    limb I74.4
      lower I74.3
      upper I74.2
    mesenteric (with gangrene) — *see also* Ischemia,
      intestine, acute K55.059
    ophthalmic — *see* Occlusion, artery, retina
    peripheral I74.4
    pontine I65.8
    precerebral — *see* Occlusion, artery, precerebral
    pulmonary — *see* Embolism, pulmonary
    renal N28.0
    retinal — *see* Occlusion, artery, retina
    septic I76
    specified NEC I74.8
    vertebral — *see* Occlusion, artery, vertebral
  basilar (artery) I65.1
  blood clot
    following
      abortion — *see* Abortion by type complicated
        by embolism
      ectopic or molar pregnancy O08.2
    in pregnancy, childbirth or puerperium — *see* Em-
      bolism, obstetric
  brain — *see also* Occlusion, artery, cerebral
    following
      abortion — *see* Abortion by type complicated
        by embolism
      ectopic or molar pregnancy O08.2
    puerperal, postpartum, childbirth — *see* Embolism,
      obstetric

Embolism — *continued*
  capillary I78.8
  cardiac — *see also* Infarct, myocardium
    not resulting in infarction I51.3
  carotid (artery) (common) (internal) — *see* Occlusion,
    artery, carotid
  cavernous sinus (venous) — *see* Embolism, intracranial,
    venous sinus
  cerebral — *see* Occlusion, artery, cerebral
  cholesterol — *see* Atheroembolism
  coronary (artery or vein) (systemic) — *see* Occlusion,
    coronary
  due to device, implant or graft — *see also* Complica-
    tions, by site and type, specified NEC
    arterial graft NEC T82.818 ☑
    breast (implant) T85.818 ☑
    catheter NEC T85.818 ☑
      dialysis (renal) T82.818 ☑
        intraperitoneal T85.818 ☑
      infusion NEC T82.818 ☑
        spinal (epidural) (subdural) T85.810 ☑
      urinary (indwelling) T83.81 ☑
    electronic (electrode) (pulse generator) (stimulator)
      bone T84.81 ☑
      cardiac T82.817 ☑
      nervous system (brain) (peripheral nerve) (spinal)
        T85.810 ☑
      urinary T83.81 ☑
    fixation, internal (orthopedic) NEC T84.81 ☑
    gastrointestinal (bile duct) (esophagus) T85.818 ☑
    genital NEC T83.81 ☑
    heart (graft) (valve) T82.817 ☑
    joint prosthesis T84.81 ☑
    ocular (corneal graft) (orbital implant) T85.818 ☑
    orthopedic (bone graft) NEC T86.838
    specified NEC T85.818 ☑
    urinary (graft) NEC T83.81 ☑
    vascular NEC T82.818 ☑
    ventricular intracranial shunt T85.810 ☑
  extremities
    lower — *see* Embolism, vein, lower extremity
      arterial I74.3
    upper I74.2
  eye H34.9
  fat (cerebral) (pulmonary) (systemic) T79.1 ☑
    complicating delivery — *see* Embolism, obstetric
    following
      abortion — *see* Abortion by type complicated
        by embolism
      ectopic or molar pregnancy O08.2
  following
    abortion — *see* Abortion by type complicated by
      embolism
    ectopic or molar pregnancy O08.2
    infusion, therapeutic injection or transfusion
      air T80.0 ☑
  heart (fatty) — *see also* Infarct, myocardium
    not resulting in infarction I51.3
  hepatic (vein) I82.0
  in pregnancy, childbirth or puerperium — *see* Em-
    bolism, obstetric
  intestine (artery) (vein) (with gangrene) — *see also* Is-
    chemia, intestine, acute K55.039
  intracranial — *see also* Occlusion, artery, cerebral
    venous sinus (any) G08
      nonpyogenic I67.6
  intraspinal venous sinuses or veins G08
    nonpyogenic G95.19
  kidney (artery) N28.0
  lateral sinus (venous) — *see* Embolism, intracranial,
    venous sinus
  leg — *see* Embolism, vein, lower extremity
    arterial I74.3
  longitudinal sinus (venous) — *see* Embolism, intracra-
    nial, venous sinus
  lung (massive) — *see* Embolism, pulmonary
  meninges I66.8
  mesenteric (artery) (vein) (with gangrene) — *see also*
    Ischemia, intestine, acute K55.059
  obstetric (in) (pulmonary)
    childbirth O88.22
      air O88.02
      amniotic fluid O88.12
      blood clot O88.22
      fat O88.82
      pyemic O88.32
      septic O88.32

▽ Subterms under main terms may continue to next column or page   ☑ **Additional Character Required** — **Refer to the Tabular List for Character Selection**   **131**

Elephantiasis — Embolism

Embolism — *continued*
  obstetric — *continued*
    childbirth — *continued*
      specified type NEC O88.82
      pregnancy O88.21- ☑
        air O88.01- ☑
        amniotic fluid O88.11- ☑
        blood clot O88.21- ☑
        fat O88.81- ☑
        pyemic O88.31- ☑
        septic O88.31- ☑
        specified type NEC O88.81- ☑
      puerperal O88.23
        air O88.03
        amniotic fluid O88.13
        blood clot O88.23
        fat O88.83
        pyemic O88.33
        septic O88.33
        specified type NEC O88.83
  ophthalmic — *see* Occlusion, artery, retina
  penis N48.81
  peripheral artery NOS I74.4
  pituitary E23.6
  popliteal (artery) I74.3
  portal (vein) I81
  postoperative, postprocedural
    artery T81.719
      mesenteric T81.710 ☑
      renal T81.711 ☑
      specified NEC T81.718 ☑
    vein T81.72 ☑
  precerebral artery — *see* Occlusion, artery, precerebral
  puerperal — *see* Embolism, obstetric
  pulmonary (acute) (artery) (vein) I26.99
    with acute cor pulmonale I26.09
    chronic I27.82
    following
      abortion — *see* Abortion by type complicated
        by embolism
      ectopic or molar pregnancy O08.2
    healed or old Z86.711
    in pregnancy, childbirth or puerperium — *see* Embolism, obstetric
    multiple subsegmental without acute cor pulmonale
      I26.94
    personal history of Z86.711
    saddle I26.92
      with acute cor pulmonale I26.02
    septic I26.90
      with acute cor pulmonale I26.01
    single subsegmental without acute cor pulmonale
      I26.93
    subsegmental NOS I26.93
  pyemic (multiple) I76
    following
      abortion — *see* Abortion by type complicated
        by embolism
      ectopic or molar pregnancy O08.2
    Hemophilus influenzae A41.3
    pneumococcal A40.3
      with pneumonia J13
    puerperal, postpartum, childbirth (any organism)
      — *see* Embolism, obstetric
    specified organism NEC A41.89
    staphylococcal A41.2
    streptococcal A40.9
  renal (artery) N28.0
    vein I82.3
  retina, retinal — *see* Occlusion, artery, retina
  saddle
    abdominal aorta I74.01
    pulmonary artery I26.92
      with acute cor pulmonale I26.02
  septic (arterial) I76
    complicating abortion — *see* Abortion, by type,
      complicated by, embolism
  sinus — *see* Embolism, intracranial, venous sinus
  soap complicating abortion — *see* Abortion, by type,
    complicated by, embolism
  spinal cord G95.19
    pyogenic origin G06.1
  spleen, splenic (artery) I74.8
  upper extremity I74.2
  vein (acute) I82.90
    antecubital I82.61- ☑
      chronic I82.71- ☑
    axillary I82.A1- ☑ (*following* I82.7)

Embolism — *continued*
  vein — *continued*
    axillary — *continued*
      chronic I82.A2- ☑ (*following* I82.7)
    basilic I82.61- ☑
      chronic I82.71- ☑
    brachial I82.62- ☑
      chronic I82.72- ☑
    brachiocephalic (innominate) I82.290
      chronic I82.291
    cephalic I82.61- ☑
      chronic I82.71- ☑
    chronic I82.91
    deep (DVT) I82.40- ☑
      calf I82.4Z- ☑
        chronic I82.5Z- ☑
      lower leg I82.4Z- ☑
        chronic I82.5Z- ☑
      thigh I82.4Y- ☑
        chronic I82.5Y- ☑
      upper leg I82.4Y
        chronic I82.5Y-
    femoral I82.41- ☑
      chronic I82.51- ☑
    iliac (iliofemoral) I82.42- ☑
      chronic I82.52- ☑
    innominate I82.290
      chronic I82.291
    internal jugular I82.C1- ☑ (*following* I82.7)
      chronic I82.C2- ☑ (*following* I82.7)
    lower extremity
      deep I82.40- ☑
        chronic I82.50- ☑
        specified NEC I82.49- ☑
          chronic NEC I82.59- ☑
      distal
        deep I82.4Z- ☑
      proximal
        deep I82.4Y- ☑
          chronic I82.5Y- ☑
      superficial I82.81- ☑
    popliteal I82.43- ☑
      chronic I82.53- ☑
    radial I82.62- ☑
      chronic I82.72- ☑
    renal I82.3
    saphenous (greater) (lesser) I82.81- ☑
    specified NEC I82.890
      chronic NEC I82.891
    subclavian I82.B1- ☑ (*following* I82.7)
      chronic I82.B2- ☑ (*following* I82.7)
    thoracic NEC I82.290
      chronic I82.291
    tibial I82.44- ☑
      chronic I82.54- ☑
    ulnar I82.62- ☑
      chronic I82.72- ☑
    upper extremity I82.60- ☑
      chronic I82.70- ☑
      deep I82.62- ☑
        chronic I82.72- ☑
      superficial I82.61- ☑
        chronic I82.71- ☑
    vena cava
      inferior (acute) I82.220
        chronic I82.221
      superior (acute) I82.210
        chronic I82.211
    venous sinus G08
    vessels of brain — *see* Occlusion, artery, cerebral
Embolus — *see* Embolism
Embryoma — *see also* Neoplasm, uncertain behavior,
  by site
  benign — *see* Neoplasm, benign, by site
  kidney C64.- ☑
  liver C22.0
  malignant — *see also* Neoplasm, malignant, by site
    kidney C64.- ☑
    liver C22.0
    testis C62.9- ☑
      descended (scrotal) C62.1- ☑
      undescended C62.0- ☑
  testis C62.9- ☑
    descended (scrotal) C62.1- ☑
    undescended C62.0- ☑

Embryonic
  circulation Q28.9
  heart Q28.9
  vas deferens Q55.4
Embryopathia NOS Q89.9
Embryotoxon Q13.4
Emesis — *see* Vomiting
Emotional lability R45.86
Emotionality, pathological F60.3
Emotogenic disease — *see* Disorder, psychogenic
Emphysema (atrophic) (bullous) (chronic) (interlobular)
  (lung) (obstructive) (pulmonary) (senile) (vesicular)
  J43.9
  cellular tissue (traumatic) T79.7 ☑
    surgical T81.82 ☑
  centrilobular J43.2
  compensatory J98.3
  congenital (interstitial) P25.0
  conjunctiva H11.89
  connective tissue (traumatic) T79.7 ☑
    surgical T81.82 ☑
  due to chemicals, gases, fumes or vapors J68.4
  eyelid(s) — *see* Disorder, eyelid, specified type NEC
    surgical T81.82 ☑
    traumatic T79.7 ☑
  interstitial J98.2
    congenital P25.0
    perinatal period P25.0
  laminated tissue T79.7 ☑
    surgical T81.82 ☑
  mediastinal J98.2
    newborn P25.2
  orbit, orbital — *see* Disorder, orbit, specified type NEC
  panacinar J43.1
  panlobular J43.1
  specified NEC J43.8
  subcutaneous (traumatic) T79.7 ☑
    nontraumatic J98.2
    postprocedural T81.82 ☑
    surgical T81.82 ☑
  surgical T81.82 ☑
  thymus (gland) (congenital) E32.8
  traumatic (subcutaneous) T79.7 ☑
  unilateral J43.0
Empty nest syndrome Z60.0
Empyema (acute) (chest) (double) (pleura) (supradiaphragmatic) (thorax) J86.9
  with fistula J86.0
  accessory sinus (chronic) — *see* Sinusitis
  antrum (chronic) — *see* Sinusitis, maxillary
  brain (any part) — *see* Abscess, brain
  ethmoidal (chronic) (sinus) — *see* Sinusitis, ethmoidal
  extradural — *see* Abscess, extradural
  frontal (chronic) (sinus) — *see* Sinusitis, frontal
  gallbladder K81.0
  mastoid (process) (acute) — *see* Mastoiditis, acute
  maxilla, maxillary M27.2
    sinus (chronic) — *see* Sinusitis, maxillary
  nasal sinus (chronic) — *see* Sinusitis
  sinus (accessory) (chronic) (nasal) — *see* Sinusitis
  sphenoidal (sinus) (chronic) — *see* Sinusitis, sphenoidal
  subarachnoid — *see* Abscess, extradural
  subdural — *see* Abscess, subdural
  tuberculous A15.6
  ureter — *see* Ureteritis
  ventricular — *see* Abscess, brain
En coup de sabre lesion L94.1
Enamel pearls K00.2
Enameloma K00.2
Enanthema, viral B09
Encephalitis (chronic) (hemorrhagic) (idiopathic)
  (nonepidemic) (spurious) (subacute) G04.90
  acute — *see also* Encephalitis, viral A86
    disseminated G04.00
      infectious G04.01
      noninfectious G04.81
      postimmunization (postvaccination) G04.02
      postinfectious G04.01
    inclusion body A85.8
    necrotizing hemorrhagic G04.30
      postimmunization G04.32
      postinfectious G04.31
      specified NEC G04.39
  arboviral, arbovirus NEC A85.2
  arthropod-borne NEC (viral) A85.2
  Australian A83.4
  California (virus) A83.5

☑ **Additional Character Required** — Refer to the Tabular List for Character Selection   ▼ Subterms under main terms may continue to next column or page

Encephalitis — *continued*
    Central European (tick-borne) A84.1
    Czechoslovakian A84.1
    Dawson's (inclusion body) A81.1
    diffuse sclerosing A81.1
    disseminated, acute G04.00
    due to
        cat scratch disease A28.1
        human immunodeficiency virus (HIV) disease
            B20 *[G05.3]*
        malaria — *see* Malaria
        rickettsiosis — *see* Rickettsiosis
        smallpox inoculation G04.02
        typhus — *see* Typhus
    Eastern equine A83.2
    endemic (viral) A86
    epidemic NEC (viral) A86
    equine (acute) (infectious) (viral) A83.9
        Eastern A83.2
        Venezuelan A92.2
        Western A83.1
    Far Eastern (tick-borne) A84.0
    following vaccination or other immunization procedure
        G04.02
    herpes zoster B02.0
    herpesviral B00.4
        due to herpesvirus 6 B10.01
        due to herpesvirus 7 B10.09
        specified NEC B10.09
    Ilheus (virus) A83.8
    in (due to)
        actinomycosis A42.82
        adenovirus A85.1
        African trypanosomiasis B56.9 *[G05.3]*
        Chagas' disease (chronic) B57.42
        cytomegalovirus B25.8
        enterovirus A85.0
        herpes (simplex) virus B00.4
            due to herpesvirus 6 B10.01
            due to herpesvirus 7 B10.09
            specified NEC B10.09
        infectious disease NEC B99 ☑ *[G05.3]*
        influenza — *see* Influenza, with, encephalopathy
        listeriosis A32.12
        measles B05.0
        mumps B26.2
        naegleriasis B60.2
        parasitic disease NEC B89 *[G05.3]*
        poliovirus A80.9 *[G05.3]*
        rubella B06.01
        syphilis
            congenital A50.42
            late A52.14
        systemic lupus erythematosus M32.19
        toxoplasmosis (acquired) B58.2
            congenital P37.1
        tuberculosis A17.82
        zoster B02.0
    inclusion body A81.1
    infectious (acute) (virus) NEC A86
    Japanese (B type) A83.0
    La Crosse A83.5
    lead — *see* Poisoning, lead
    lethargica (acute) (infectious) A85.8
    louping ill A84.89
    lupus erythematosus, systemic M32.19
    lymphatica A87.2
    Mengo A85.8
    meningococcal A39.81
    Murray Valley A83.4
    otitic NEC H66.40 *[G05.3]*
    parasitic NOS B71.9
    periaxial G37.0
    periaxialis (concentrica) (diffuse) G37.5
    postchickenpox B01.11
    postexanthematous NEC B09
    postimmunization G04.02
    postinfectious NEC G04.01
    postmeasles B05.0
    postvaccinal G04.02
    postvaricella B01.11
    postviral NEC A86
    Powassan A84.81
    Rasmussen G04.81
    Rio Bravo A85.8
    Russian
        autumnal A83.0
        spring-summer (taiga) A84.0

Encephalitis — *continued*
    saturnine — *see* Poisoning, lead
    specified NEC G04.81
    St. Louis A83.3
    subacute sclerosing A81.1
    summer A83.0
    suppurative G04.81
    tick-borne A84.9
    Torula, torular (cryptococcal) B45.1
    toxic NEC G92.8
    trichinosis B75 *[G05.3]*
    type
        B A83.0
        C A83.3
    van Bogaert's A81.1
    Venezuelan equine A92.2
    Vienna A85.8
    viral, virus A86
        arthropod-borne NEC A85.2
            mosquito-borne A83.9
                Australian X disease A83.4
                California virus A83.5
                Eastern equine A83.2
                Japanese (B type) A83.0
                Murray Valley A83.4
                specified NEC A83.8
                St. Louis A83.3
                type B A83.0
                type C A83.3
                Western equine A83.1
            tick-borne A84.9
                biundulant A84.1
                central European A84.1
                Czechoslovakian A84.1
                diphasic meningoencephalitis A84.1
                Far Eastern A84.0
                Russian spring-summer (taiga) A84.0
                specified NEC A84.89
        specified type NEC A85.8
        tick-borne, specified NEC A84.89
    Western equine A83.1
Encephalocele Q01.9
    frontal Q01.0
    nasofrontal Q01.1
    occipital Q01.2
    specified NEC Q01.8
Encephalocystocele — *see* Encephalocele
Encephaloduroarteriomyosynangiosis (EDAMS) I67.5
Encephalomalacia (brain) (cerebellar) (cerebral) — *see*
    Softening, brain
Encephalomeningitis — *see* Meningoencephalitis
Encephalomeningocele — *see* Encephalocele
Encephalomeningomyelitis — *see* Meningoencephalitis
Encephalomyelitis — *see also* Encephalitis G04.90
    acute disseminated G04.00
        infectious G04.01
        noninfectious G04.81
        postimmunization G04.02
        postinfectious G04.01
    acute necrotizing hemorrhagic G04.30
        postimmunization G04.32
        postinfectious G04.31
        specified NEC G04.39
    benign myalgic G93.3
    equine A83.9
        Eastern A83.2
        Venezuelan A92.2
        Western A83.1
    in diseases classified elsewhere G05.3
    myalgic, benign G93.3
    postchickenpox B01.11
    postinfectious NEC G04.01
    postmeasles B05.0
    postvaccinal G04.02
    postvaricella B01.11
    rubella B06.01
    specified NEC G04.81
    Venezuelan equine A92.2
Encephalomyelocele — *see* Encephalocele
Encephalomyelomeningitis — *see* Meningoencephalitis
Encephalomyelopathy G96.9
Encephalomyeloradiculitis (acute) G61.0
Encephalomyeloradiculoneuritis (acute) (Guillain-
    Barré) G61.0
Encephalomyeloradiculopathy G96.9
Encephalopathia hyperbilirubinemica, newborn
    P57.9
    due to isoimmunization (conditions in P55) P57.0

Encephalopathy (acute) G93.40
    acute necrotizing hemorrhagic G04.30
        postimmunization G04.32
        postinfectious G04.31
        specified NEC G04.39
    alcoholic G31.2
    anoxic — *see* Damage, brain, anoxic
    arteriosclerotic I67.2
    centrolobar progressive (Schilder) G37.0
    congenital Q07.9
    degenerative, in specified disease NEC G32.89
    demyelinating callosal G37.1
    due to
        drugs — *see also* Table of Drugs and Chemicals
            G92.8
    hepatic — *see* Failure, hepatic
    hyperbilirubinemic, newborn P57.9
        due to isoimmunization (conditions in P55) P57.0
    hypertensive I67.4
    hypoglycemic E16.2
    hypoxic — *see* Damage, brain, anoxic
    hypoxic ischemic P91.60
        mild P91.61
        moderate P91.62
        severe P91.63
    in (due to) (with)
        birth injury P11.1
        hyperinsulinism E16.1 *[G94]*
        influenza — *see* Influenza, with, encephalopathy
        lack of vitamin — *see also* Deficiency, vitamin
            E56.9 *[G32.89]*
        neoplastic disease — *see also* Neoplasm
            D49.9 *[G13.1]*
        serum — *see also* Reaction, serum T80.69 ☑
        syphilis A52.17
        trauma (postconcussional) F07.81
            current injury — *see* Injury, intracranial
        vaccination G04.02
    lead — *see* Poisoning, lead
    metabolic G93.41
        drug induced G92.8
        toxic G92.8
    myoclonic, early, symptomatic — *see* Epilepsy, gener-
        alized, specified NEC
    necrotizing, subacute (Leigh) G31.82
    neonatal P91.819
        in diseases classified elsewhere P91.811
    pellagrous E52 *[G32.89]*
    portosystemic — *see* Failure, hepatic
    postcontusional F07.81
        current injury — *see* Injury, intracranial, diffuse
    posthypoglycemic (coma) E16.1 *[G94]*
    postradiation G93.89
    saturnine — *see* Poisoning, lead
    septic G93.41
    specified NEC G93.49
    spongiform, subacute (viral) A81.09
    toxic G92.9
        metabolic G92.8
    traumatic (postconcussional) F07.81
        current injury — *see* Injury, intracranial
    vitamin B deficiency NEC E53.9 *[G32.89]*
        vitamin B1 E51.2
    Wernicke's E51.2
Encephalorrhagia — *see* Hemorrhage, intracranial, in-
    tracerebral
Encephalosis, posttraumatic F07.81
Enchondroma — *see also* Neoplasm, bone, benign
Enchondromatosis (cartilaginous) (multiple) Q78.4
Encopresis R15.9
    functional F98.1
    nonorganic origin F98.1
    psychogenic F98.1
Encounter (with health service) (for) Z76.89
    adjustment and management (of)
        breast implant Z45.81 ☑
        implanted device NEC Z45.89
        myringotomy device (stent) (tube) Z45.82
        neurostimulator (brain) (gastric) (peripheral nerve)
            (sacral nerve) (spinal cord) (vagus nerve)
            Z45.42
    administrative purpose only Z02.9
        examination for
            adoption Z02.82
            armed forces Z02.3
            disability determination Z02.71
            driving license Z02.4
            employment Z02.1

Encounter — *continued*
administrative purpose only — *continued*
examination for — *continued*
insurance Z02.6
medical certificate NEC Z02.79
paternity testing Z02.81
residential institution admission Z02.2
school admission Z02.0
sports Z02.5
specified reason NEC Z02.89
aftercare — *see* Aftercare
antenatal screening Z36.9
cervical length Z36.86
chromosomal anomalies Z36.0
congenital cardiac abnormalities Z36.83
elevated maternal serum alphafetoprotein Z36.1
fetal growth retardation Z36.4
fetal lung maturity Z36.84
fetal macrosomia Z36.88
hydrops fetalis Z36.81
intrauterine growth restriction (IUGR) /small-for-dates Z36.4
isoimmunization Z36.5
large-for-dates Z36.88
malformations Z36.3
non-visualized anatomy on a previous scan Z36.2
nuchal translucency Z36.82
raised alphafetoprotein level Z36.1
risk of pre-term labor Z36.86
specified follow-up NEC Z36.2
specified genetic defects NEC Z36.8A
specified type NEC Z36.89
Streptococcus B Z36.85
suspected anomaly Z36.3
uncertain dates Z36.87
assisted reproductive fertility procedure cycle Z31.83
blood typing Z01.83
Rh typing Z01.83
breast augmentation or reduction Z41.1
breast implant exchange (different material) (different size) Z45.81 ☑
breast reconstruction following mastectomy Z42.1
check-up — *see* Examination
chemotherapy for neoplasm Z51.11
colonoscopy, screening Z12.11
counseling — *see* Counseling
delivery, full-term, uncomplicated O80
cesarean, without indication O82
desensitization to allergens Z51.6
ear piercing Z41.3
examination — *see* Examination
expectant parent(s) (adoptive) pre-birth pediatrician visit Z76.81
fertility preservation procedure (prior to cancer therapy) (prior to removal of gonads) Z31.84
fitting (of) — *see* Fitting (and adjustment) (of)
genetic
counseling
nonprocreative Z71.83
procreative Z31.5
testing — *see* Test, genetic
hearing conservation and treatment Z01.12
immunotherapy for neoplasm Z51.12
in vitro fertilization cycle Z31.83
instruction (in)
child care (postpartal) (prenatal) Z32.3
childbirth Z32.2
natural family planning
procreative Z31.61
to avoid pregnancy Z30.02
insulin pump titration Z46.81
joint prosthesis insertion following prior explantation of joint prosthesis (staged procedure)
hip Z47.32
knee Z47.33
shoulder Z47.31
laboratory (as part of a general medical examination) Z00.00
with abnormal findings Z00.01
mental health services (for)
abuse NEC
perpetrator Z69.82
victim Z69.81
child abuse
nonparental
perpetrator Z69.021
victim Z69.020

Encounter — *continued*
mental health services — *continued*
child abuse — *continued*
parental
perpetrator Z69.011
victim Z69.010
child neglect
nonparental
perpetrator Z69.021
victim Z69.020
parental
perpetrator Z69.011
victim Z69.010
child psychological abuse
nonparental
perpetrator Z69.021
victim Z69.020
parental
perpetrator Z69.011
victim Z69.010
child sexual abuse
nonparental
perpetrator Z69.021
victim Z69.020
parental
perpetrator Z69.011
victim Z69.010
non-spousal adult abuse
perpetrator Z69.82
victim Z69.81
spousal or partner
abuse
perpetrator Z69.12
victim Z69.11
neglect
perpetrator Z69.12
victim Z69.11
psychological abuse
perpetrator Z69.12
victim Z69.11
violence
perpetrator (physical) (sexual) Z69.12
victim (physical) Z69.11
sexual Z69.81
observation (for) (ruled out)
exposure to (suspected)
anthrax Z03.810
biological agent NEC Z03.818
pediatrician visit, by expectant parent(s) (adoptive) Z76.81
placental sample (taken vaginally) — *see also* Encounter, antenatal screening Z36.9
plastic and reconstructive surgery following medical procedure or healed injury NEC Z42.8
pregnancy
supervision of — *see* Pregnancy, supervision of
test Z32.00
result negative Z32.02
result positive Z32.01
procreative management and counseling for gestational carrier Z31.7
prophylactic measures Z29.9
antivenin Z29.12
fluoride administration Z29.3
immunotherapy for respiratory syncytial virus (RSV) Z29.11
rabies immune globin Z29.14
Rho (D) immune globulin Z29.13
specified NEC Z29.8
radiation therapy (antineoplastic) Z51.0
radiological (as part of a general medical examination) Z00.00
with abnormal findings Z00.01
reconstructive surgery following medical procedure or healed injury NEC Z42.8
removal (of) — *see also* Removal
artificial
arm Z44.00- ☑
complete Z44.01- ☑
partial Z44.02- ☑
eye Z44.2- ☑
leg Z44.10- ☑
complete Z44.11- ☑
partial Z44.12- ☑
breast implant Z45.81 ☑
tissue expander (with or without synchronous insertion of permanent implant) Z45.81 ☑
device Z46.9

Encounter — *continued*
removal — *see also* Removal — *continued*
device — *continued*
specified NEC Z46.89
external
fixation device — *code to* fracture with seventh character D
prosthesis, prosthetic device Z44.9
breast Z44.3- ☑
specified NEC Z44.8
implanted device NEC Z45.89
insulin pump Z46.81
internal fixation device Z47.2
myringotomy device (stent) (tube) Z45.82
nervous system device NEC Z46.2
brain neuropacemaker Z46.2
visual substitution device Z46.2
implanted Z45.31
non-vascular catheter Z46.82
orthodontic device Z46.4
stent
ureteral Z46.6
urinary device Z46.6
repeat cervical smear to confirm findings of recent normal smear following initial abnormal smear Z01.42
respirator [ventilator] use during power failure Z99.12
Rh typing Z01.83
screening — *see* Screening
specified NEC Z76.89
sterilization Z30.2
suspected condition, ruled out
amniotic cavity and membrane Z03.71
cervical shortening Z03.75
fetal anomaly Z03.73
fetal growth Z03.74
maternal and fetal conditions NEC Z03.79
oligohydramnios Z03.71
placental problem Z03.72
polyhydramnios Z03.71
suspected exposure (to), ruled out
anthrax Z03.810
biological agents NEC Z03.818
termination of pregnancy, elective Z33.2
testing — *see* Test
therapeutic drug level monitoring Z51.81
titration, insulin pump Z46.81
to determine fetal viability of pregnancy O36.80 ☑
training
insulin pump Z46.81
X-ray of chest (as part of a general medical examination) Z00.00
with abnormal findings Z00.01
Encystment — *see* Cyst
Endarteritis (bacterial, subacute) (infective) I77.6
brain I67.7
cerebral or cerebrospinal I67.7
deformans — *see* Arteriosclerosis
embolic — *see* Embolism
obliterans — *see also* Arteriosclerosis
pulmonary I28.8
pulmonary I28.8
retina — *see* Vasculitis, retina
senile — *see* Arteriosclerosis
syphilitic A52.09
brain or cerebral A52.04
congenital A50.54 [I79.8]
tuberculous A18.89
Endemic — *see* condition
Endocarditis (chronic) (marantic) (nonbacterial) (thrombotic) (valvular) I38
with rheumatic fever (conditions in I00)
active — *see* Endocarditis, acute, rheumatic
inactive or quiescent (with chorea) I09.1
acute or subacute I33.9
infective I33.0
rheumatic (aortic) (mitral) (pulmonary) (tricuspid) I01.1
with chorea (acute) (rheumatic) (Sydenham's) I02.0
aortic (heart) (nonrheumatic) (valve) I35.8
with
mitral disease I08.0
with tricuspid (valve) disease I08.3
active or acute I01.1
with chorea (acute) (rheumatic) (Sydenham's) I02.0

Endocarditis — *continued*
  aortic — *continued*
    with — *continued*
      rheumatic fever (conditions in I00)
        active — *see* Endocarditis, acute, rheumatic
        inactive or quiescent (with chorea) I06.9
      tricuspid (valve) disease I08.2
        with mitral (valve) disease I08.3
    acute or subacute I33.9
    arteriosclerotic I35.8
    rheumatic I06.9
      with mitral disease I08.0
        with tricuspid (valve) disease I08.3
          active or acute I01.1
            with chorea (acute) (rheumatic) (Sydenham's) I02.0
        active or acute I01.1
          with chorea (acute) (rheumatic) (Sydenham's) I02.0
      specified NEC I06.8
    specified cause NEC I35.8
    syphilitic A52.03
  arteriosclerotic I38
  atypical verrucous (Libman-Sacks) M32.11
  bacterial (acute) (any valve) (subacute) I33.0
  candidal B37.6
  congenital Q24.8
  constrictive I33.0
  Coxiella burnetii A78 *[I39]*
  Coxsackie B33.21
  due to
    prosthetic cardiac valve T82.6 ☑
    Q fever A78 *[I39]*
    Serratia marcescens I33.0
    typhoid (fever) A01.02
  gonococcal A54.83
  infectious or infective (acute) (any valve) (subacute) I33.0
  lenta (acute) (any valve) (subacute) I33.0
  Libman-Sacks M32.11
  listerial A32.82
  Löffler's I42.3
  malignant (acute) (any valve) (subacute) I33.0
  meningococcal A39.51
  mitral (chronic) (double) (fibroid) (heart) (inactive) (valve) (with chorea) I05.9
    with
      aortic (valve) disease I08.0
        with tricuspid (valve) disease I08.3
          active or acute I01.1
            with chorea (acute) (rheumatic) (Sydenham's) I02.0
      rheumatic fever (conditions in I00)
        active — *see* Endocarditis, acute, rheumatic
        inactive or quiescent (with chorea) I05.9
      tricuspid (valve) disease I08.1
        with aortic (valve) disease I08.3
    active or acute I01.1
      with chorea (acute) (rheumatic) (Sydenham's) I02.0
    bacterial I33.0
    arteriosclerotic I34.8
    nonrheumatic I34.8
      acute or subacute I33.9
    specified NEC I05.8
  monilial B37.6
  multiple valves I08.9
    specified disorders I08.8
  mycotic (acute) (any valve) (subacute) I33.0
  pneumococcal (acute) (any valve) (subacute) I33.0
  pulmonary (chronic) (heart) (valve) I37.8
    with rheumatic fever (conditions in I00)
      active — *see* Endocarditis, acute, rheumatic
      inactive or quiescent (with chorea) I09.89
        with aortic, mitral or tricuspid disease I08.8
    acute or subacute I33.9
      rheumatic I01.1
        with chorea (acute) (rheumatic) (Sydenham's) I02.0
    arteriosclerotic I37.8
    congenital Q22.2
    rheumatic (chronic) (inactive) (with chorea) I09.89
      active or acute I01.1
        with chorea (acute) (rheumatic) (Sydenham's) I02.0
    syphilitic A52.03
  purulent (acute) (any valve) (subacute) I33.0
  Q fever A78 *[I39]*

Endocarditis — *continued*
  rheumatic (chronic) (inactive) (with chorea) I09.1
    active or acute (aortic) (mitral) (pulmonary) (tricuspid) I01.1
      with chorea (acute) (rheumatic) (Sydenham's) I02.0
  rheumatoid — *see* Rheumatoid, carditis
  septic (acute) (any valve) (subacute) I33.0
  streptococcal (acute) (any valve) (subacute) I33.0
  subacute — *see* Endocarditis, acute
  suppurative (acute) (any valve) (subacute) I33.0
  syphilitic A52.03
  toxic I33.9
  tricuspid (chronic) (heart) (inactive) (rheumatic) (valve) (with chorea) I07.9
    with
      aortic (valve) disease I08.2
        mitral (valve) disease I08.3
      mitral (valve) disease I08.1
        aortic (valve) disease I08.3
      rheumatic fever (conditions in I00)
        active — *see* Endocarditis, acute, rheumatic
        inactive or quiescent (with chorea) I07.8
    active or acute I01.1
      with chorea (acute) (rheumatic) (Sydenham's) I02.0
    arteriosclerotic I36.8
    nonrheumatic I36.8
      acute or subacute I33.9
    specified cause, except rheumatic I36.8
  tuberculous — *see* Tuberculosis, endocarditis
  typhoid A01.02
  ulcerative (acute) (any valve) (subacute) I33.0
  vegetative (acute) (any valve) (subacute) I33.0
  verrucous (atypical) (nonbacterial) (nonrheumatic) M32.11
Endocardium, endocardial — *see also* condition
  cushion defect Q21.2
Endocervicitis — *see also* Cervicitis
  due to intrauterine (contraceptive) device T83.69 ☑
  hyperplastic N72
Endocrine — *see* condition
Endocrinopathy, pluriglandular E31.9
Endodontic
  overfill M27.52
  underfill M27.53
Endodontitis K04.01
  irreversible K04.02
  reversible K04.01
Endomastoiditis — *see* Mastoiditis
Endometrioma N80.9
Endometriosis N80.9
  appendix N80.5
  bladder N80.8
  bowel N80.5
  broad ligament N80.3
  cervix N80.0
  colon N80.5
  cul-de-sac (Douglas') N80.3
  exocervix N80.0
  fallopian tube N80.2
  female genital organ NEC N80.8
  gallbladder N80.8
  in scar of skin N80.6
  internal N80.0
  intestine N80.5
  lung N80.8
  myometrium N80.0
  ovary N80.1
  parametrium N80.3
  pelvic peritoneum N80.3
  peritoneal (pelvic) N80.3
  rectovaginal septum N80.4
  rectum N80.5
  round ligament N80.3
  skin (scar) N80.6
  specified site NEC N80.8
  stromal D39.0
  thorax N80.8
  umbilicus N80.8
  uterus (internal) N80.0
  vagina N80.4
  vulva N80.8
Endometritis (decidual) (nonspecific) (purulent) (senile) (atrophic) (suppurative) N71.9
  with ectopic pregnancy O08.0
  acute N71.0
  blenorrhagic (gonococcal) (acute) (chronic) A54.24

Endometritis — *continued*
  cervix, cervical (with erosion or ectropion) — *see also* Cervicitis
    hyperplastic N72
  chlamydial A56.11
  chronic N71.1
  following
    abortion — *see* Abortion by type complicated by genital infection
    ectopic or molar pregnancy O08.0
  gonococcal, gonorrheal (acute) (chronic) A54.24
  hyperplastic — *see also* Hyperplasia, endometrial N85.00
    cervix N72
  puerperal, postpartum, childbirth O86.12
  subacute N71.0
  tuberculous A18.17
Endometrium — *see* condition
Endomyocardiopathy, South African I42.3
Endomyocarditis — *see* Endocarditis
Endomyofibrosis I42.3
Endomyometritis — *see* Endometritis
Endopericarditis — *see* Endocarditis
Endoperineuritis — *see* Disorder, nerve
Endophlebitis — *see* Phlebitis
Endophthalmia — *see* Endophthalmitis, purulent
Endophthalmitis (acute) (infective) (metastatic) (subacute) H44.009
  bleb associated — *see also* Bleb, inflamed (infected), postprocedural H59.4 ☑
  gonorrheal A54.39
  in (due to)
    cysticercosis B69.1
    onchocerciasis B73.01
    toxocariasis B83.0
  panuveitis — *see* Panuveitis
  parasitic H44.12- ☑
  purulent H44.00- ☑
    panophthalmitis — *see* Panophthalmitis
    vitreous abscess H44.02- ☑
  specified NEC H44.19
  sympathetic — *see* Uveitis, sympathetic
Endosalpingioma D28.2
Endosalpingiosis N94.89
Endosteitis — *see* Osteomyelitis
Endothelioma, bone — *see* Neoplasm, bone, malignant
Endotheliosis (hemorrhagic infectional) D69.8
Endotoxemia — code to condition
Endotrachelitis — *see* Cervicitis
Engelmann (-Camurati) **syndrome** Q78.3
English disease — *see* Rickets
Engman's disease L30.3
Engorgement
  breast N64.59
    newborn P83.4
    puerperal, postpartum O92.79
  lung (passive) — *see* Edema, lung
  pulmonary (passive) — *see* Edema, lung
  stomach K31.89
  venous, retina — *see* Occlusion, retina, vein, engorgement
Enlargement, enlarged — *see also* Hypertrophy
  adenoids J35.2
    with tonsils J35.3
  alveolar ridge K08.89
    congenital — *see* Anomaly, alveolar
  apertures of diaphragm (congenital) Q79.1
  gingival K06.1
  heart, cardiac — *see* Hypertrophy, cardiac
  labium majus, childhood asymmetric (CALME) N90.61
  lacrimal gland, chronic H04.03- ☑
  liver — *see* Hypertrophy, liver
  lymph gland or node R59.9
    generalized R59.1
    localized R59.0
  orbit H05.34- ☑
  organ or site, congenital NEC — *see* Anomaly, by site
  parathyroid (gland) E21.0
  pituitary fossa R93.0
  prostate N40.0
    with lower urinary tract symptoms (LUTS) N40.1
    without lower urinary tract symtpoms (LUTS) N40.0
  sella turcica R93.0
  spleen — *see* Splenomegaly
  thymus (gland) (congenital) E32.0
  thyroid (gland) — *see* Goiter
  tongue K14.8

Enlargement, enlarged — continued
  tonsils J35.1
    with adenoids J35.3
  uterus N85.2
  vestibular aqueduct Q16.5
Enophthalmos H05.40- ☑
  due to
    orbital tissue atrophy H05.41- ☑
    trauma or surgery H05.42- ☑
Enostosis M27.8
Entamebic, entamebiasis — see Amebiasis
Entanglement
  umbilical cord(s) O69.82 ☑
    with compression O69.2 ☑
      around neck (with compression) O69.81 ☑
        with compression O69.1 ☑
        without compression O69.81 ☑
      of twins in monoamniotic sac O69.2 ☑
    without compression O69.82 ☑
Enteralgia — see Pain, abdominal
Enteric — see condition
Enteritis (acute) (diarrheal) (hemorrhagic) (noninfective)
    K52.9
  adenovirus A08.2
  aertrycke infection A02.0
  allergic K52.29
    with
      eosinophilic gastritis or gastroenteritis K52.81
      food protein-induced enterocolitis syndrome
          K52.21
      food protein-induced enteropathy K52.22
      FPIES K52.21
  amebic (acute) A06.0
    with abscess — see Abscess, amebic
    chronic A06.1
      with abscess — see Abscess, amebic
      nondysenteric A06.2
    nondysenteric A06.2
  astrovirus A08.32
  bacillary NOS A03.9
  bacterial A04.9
    specified NEC A04.8
  calicivirus A08.31
  candidal B37.82
  Chilomastix A07.8
  choleriformis A00.1
  chronic (noninfectious) K52.9
    ulcerative — see Colitis, ulcerative
  cicatrizing (chronic) — see Enteritis, regional, small in-
      testine
  Clostridium
    botulinum (food poisoning) A05.1
    difficile
      not specified as recurrent A04.72
      recurrent A04.71
  coccidial A07.3
  coxsackie virus A08.39
  dietetic — see also Enteritis, allergic K52.29
  drug-induced K52.1
  due to
    astrovirus A08.32
    calicivirus A08.31
    coxsackie virus A08.39
    drugs K52.1
    echovirus A08.39
    enterovirus NEC A08.39
    food hypersensitivity — see also Enteritis, allergic
        K52.29
    infectious organism (bacterial) (viral) — see Enteritis,
        infectious
    torovirus A08.39
    Yersinia enterocolitica A04.6
  echovirus A08.39
  eltor A00.1
  enterovirus NEC A08.39
  eosinophilic K52.81
  epidemic (infectious) A09
  fulminant — see also Ischemia, intestine, acute K55.019
  gangrenous — see Enteritis, infectious
  giardial A07.1
  infectious NOS A09
    due to
      adenovirus A08.2
      Aerobacter aerogenes A04.8
      Arizona (bacillus) A02.0
      bacteria NOS A04.9
        specified NEC A04.8
      Campylobacter A04.5

Enteritis — continued
  infectious — continued
    due to — continued
      Clostridium difficile
        not specified as recurrent A04.72
        recurrent A04.71
      Clostridium perfringens A04.8
      Enterobacter aerogenes A04.8
      enterovirus A08.39
      Escherichia coli A04.4
        enteroaggregative A04.4
        enterohemorrhagic A04.3
        enteroinvasive A04.2
        enteropathogenic A04.0
        enterotoxigenic A04.1
        specified NEC A04.4
      specified
        bacteria NEC A04.8
        virus NEC A08.39
      Staphylococcus A04.8
      virus NEC A08.4
        specified type NEC A08.39
      Yersinia enterocolitica A04.6
    specified organism NEC A08.8
  influenzal — see Influenza, with, digestive manifesta-
      tions
  ischemic K55.9
    acute — see also Ischemia, intestine, acute K55.019
    chronic K55.1
  microsporidial A07.8
  mucomembranous, myxomembranous — see Syn-
      drome, irritable bowel
  mucous — see Syndrome, irritable bowel
  necroticans A05.2
  necrotizing of newborn — see Enterocolitis, necrotiz-
      ing, in newborn
  neurogenic — see Syndrome, irritable bowel
  newborn necrotizing — see Enterocolitis, necrotizing,
      in newborn
  noninfectious K52.9
  norovirus A08.11
  parasitic NEC B82.9
  paratyphoid (fever) — see Fever, paratyphoid
  protozoal A07.9
    specified NEC A07.8
  radiation K52.0
  regional (of) K50.90
    with
      complication K50.919
        abscess K50.914
        fistula K50.913
        intestinal obstruction K50.912
        rectal bleeding K50.911
        specified complication NEC K50.918
    colon — see Enteritis, regional, large intestine
    duodenum — see Enteritis, regional, small intestine
    ileum — see Enteritis, regional, small intestine
    jejunum — see Enteritis, regional, small intestine
    large bowel — see Enteritis, regional, large intestine
    large intestine (colon) (rectum) K50.10
      with
        complication K50.119
          abscess K50.114
          fistula K50.113
          intestinal obstruction K50.112
          rectal bleeding K50.111
          small intestine (duodenum) (ileum) (je-
              junum) involvement K50.80
            with
              complication K50.819
                abscess K50.814
                fistula K50.813
                intestinal obstruction K50.812
                rectal bleeding K50.811
                specified complication NEC
                    K50.818
          specified complication NEC K50.118
    rectum — see Enteritis, regional, large intestine
    small intestine (duodenum) (ileum) (jejunum)
        K50.00
      with
        complication K50.019
          abscess K50.014
          fistula K50.013
          intestinal obstruction K50.012
          large intestine (colon) (rectum) involve-
              ment K50.80

Enteritis — continued
  regional — continued
    small intestine — continued
      with — continued
        complication — continued
          large intestine involvement — contin-
              ued
            with
              complication K50.819
                abscess K50.814
                fistula K50.813
                intestinal obstruction K50.812
                rectal bleeding K50.811
                specified complication NEC
                    K50.818
        rectal bleeding K50.011
        specified complication NEC K50.018
  rotaviral A08.0
  Salmonella, salmonellosis (arizonae) (cholerae-suis)
      (enteritidis) (typhimurium) A02.0
  segmental — see Enteritis, regional
  septic A09
  Shigella — see Infection, Shigella
  small round structured NEC A08.19
  spasmodic, spastic — see Syndrome, irritable bowel
  staphylococcal A04.8
    due to food A05.0
  torovirus A08.39
  toxic NEC K52.1
    due to Clostridium difficile
      not specified as recurrent A04.72
      recurrent A04.71
  trichomonal A07.8
  tuberculous A18.32
  typhosa A01.00
  ulcerative (chronic) — see Colitis, ulcerative
  viral A08.4
    adenovirus A08.2
    enterovirus A08.39
    Rotavirus A08.0
    small round structured NEC A08.19
    specified NEC A08.39
    virus specified NEC A08.39
Enterobiasis B80
Enterobius vermicularis (infection) (infestation) B80
Enterocele — see also Hernia, abdomen
  pelvic, pelvis (acquired) (congenital) N81.5
  vagina, vaginal (acquired) (congenital) NEC N81.5
Enterocolitis — see also Enteritis K52.9
  due to Clostridium difficile
    not specified as recurrent A04.72
    recurrent A04.71
  fulminant ischemic — see also Ischemia, intestine,
      acute K55.059
  granulomatous — see Enteritis, regional
  hemorrhagic (acute) — see also Ischemia, intestine,
      acute K55.059
    chronic K55.1
  infectious NEC A09
  ischemic K55.9
  necrotizing K55.30
    with
      perforation K55.33
      pneumatosis K55.32
        and perforation K55.33
    due to Clostridium difficile
      not specified as recurrent A04.72
      recurrent A04.71
    in non-newborn K55.30
      stage 1 (without pneumatosis, without perfora-
          tion) K55.31
      stage 2 (with pneumatosis, without perforation)
          K55.32
      stage 3 (with pneumatosis, with perforation)
          K55.33
    in newborn P77.9
      stage 1 (without pneumatosis, without perfora-
          tion) P77.1
      stage 2 (with pneumatosis, without perforation)
          P77.2
      stage 3 (with pneumatosis, with perforation)
          P77.3
    without pneumatosis or perforation K55.31
  noninfectious K52.9
  newborn — see Enterocolitis, necrotizing, in new-
      born
  pseudomembranous (newborn)
    not specified as recurrent A04.72

Enterocolitis — *continued*
pseudomembranous — *continued*
recurrent A04.71
radiation K52.0
newborn — *see* Enterocolitis, necrotizing, in new-born
ulcerative (chronic) — *see* Pancolitis, ulcerative (chronic)
Enterogastritis — *see* Enteritis
Enteropathy K63.9
celiac-gluten-sensitive K90.0
non-celiac K90.41
food protein-induced K52.22
hemorrhagic, terminal — *see also* Ischemia, intestine, acute K55.059
protein-losing K90.49
Enteroperitonitis — *see* Peritonitis
Enteroptosis K63.4
Enterorrhagia K92.2
Enterospasm — *see also* Syndrome, irritable, bowel
psychogenic F45.8
Enterostenosis — *see also* Obstruction, intestine, specified NEC K56.699
Enterostomy
complication — *see* Complication, enterostomy
status Z93.4
Enterovirus, as cause of disease classified elsewhere B97.10
coxsackievirus B97.11
echovirus B97.12
other specified B97.19
Enthesopathy (peripheral) M77.9
Achilles tendinitis — *see* Tendinitis, Achilles
ankle and tarsus M77.5- ☑
specified type NEC — *see* Enthesopathy, foot, specified type NEC
anterior tibial syndrome M76.81- ☑
calcaneal spur — *see* Spur, bone, calcaneal
elbow region M77.8
lateral epicondylitis — *see* Epicondylitis, lateral
medial epicondylitis — *see* Epicondylitis, medial
foot NEC M77.8
metatarsalgia — *see* Metatarsalgia
specified type NEC M77.5- ☑
forearm M77.8
gluteal tendinitis — *see* Tendinitis, gluteal
hand M77.8
hip — *see* Enthesopathy, lower limb, specified type NEC
iliac crest spur — *see* Spur, bone, iliac crest
iliotibial band syndrome — *see* Syndrome, iliotibial band
knee — *see* Enthesopathy, lower limb, lower leg, specified type NEC
lateral epicondylitis — *see* Epicondylitis, lateral
lower limb (excluding foot) M76.9
Achilles tendinitis — *see* Tendinitis, Achilles
ankle and tarsus M77.5- ☑
specified type NEC — *see* Enthesopathy, foot, specified type NEC
anterior tibial syndrome M76.81- ☑
gluteal tendinitis — *see* Tendinitis, gluteal
iliac crest spur — *see* Spur, bone, iliac crest
iliotibial band syndrome — *see* Syndrome, iliotibial band
patellar tendinitis — *see* Tendinitis, patellar
pelvic region — *see* Enthesopathy, lower limb, specified type NEC
peroneal tendinitis — *see* Tendinitis, peroneal
posterior tibial syndrome M76.82- ☑
psoas tendinitis — *see* Tendinitis, psoas
specified type NEC M76.89- ☑
tibial collateral bursitis — *see* Bursitis, tibial collateral
medial epicondylitis — *see* Epicondylitis, medial
metatarsalgia — *see* Metatarsalgia
multiple sites M77.8
patellar tendinitis — *see* Tendinitis, patellar
pelvis M77.8
periarthritis of wrist — *see* Periarthritis, wrist
peroneal tendinitis — *see* Tendinitis, peroneal
posterior tibial syndrome M76.82- ☑
psoas tendinitis — *see* Tendinitis, psoas
shoulder M77.8
shoulder region — *see* Lesion, shoulder
specified type NEC M77.8
spinal M46.00

Enthesopathy — *continued*
spinal — *continued*
cervical region M46.02
cervicothoracic region M46.03
lumbar region M46.06
lumbosacral region M46.07
multiple sites M46.09
occipito-atlanto-axial region M46.01
sacrococcygeal region M46.08
thoracic region M46.04
thoracolumbar region M46.05
tibial collateral bursitis — *see* Bursitis, tibial collateral
upper arm M77.8
wrist and carpus NEC M77.8
calcaneal spur — *see* Spur, bone, calcaneal
periarthritis of wrist — *see* Periarthritis, wrist
Entomophobia F40.218
Entomophthoromycosis B46.8
Entrance, air into vein — *see* Embolism, air
Entrapment, nerve — *see* Neuropathy, entrapment
Entropion (eyelid) (paralytic) H02.009
cicatricial H02.019
left H02.016
lower H02.015
upper H02.014
right H02.013
lower H02.012
upper H02.011
congenital Q10.2
left H02.006
lower H02.005
upper H02.004
mechanical H02.029
left H02.026
lower H02.025
upper H02.024
right H02.023
lower H02.022
upper H02.021
right H02.003
lower H02.002
upper H02.001
senile H02.039
left H02.036
lower H02.035
upper H02.034
right H02.033
lower H02.032
upper H02.031
spastic H02.049
left H02.046
lower H02.045
upper H02.044
right H02.043
lower H02.042
upper H02.041
Enucleated eye (traumatic, current) S05.7- ☑
Enuresis R32
functional F98.0
habit disturbance F98.0
nocturnal N39.44
psychogenic F98.0
nonorganic origin F98.0
psychogenic F98.0
Eosinopenia — *see* Agranulocytosis
Eosinophilia (allergic) (idiopathic) (secondary) D72.10
with
angiolymphoid hyperplasia (ALHE) D18.01
familial D72.19
hereditary D72.19
in disease classified elsewhere D72.18
infiltrative — *see* Eosinophilia, pulmonary
Löffler's J82.89
peritoneal — *see* Peritonitis, eosinophilic
pulmonary NEC J82.89
acute J82.82
asthmatic J82.83
chronic J82.81
specified NEC D72.19
tropical (pulmonary) J82.89
Eosinophilia-myalgia syndrome M35.89
Ependymitis (acute) (cerebral) (chronic) (granular) — *see* Encephalomyelitis
Ependymoblastoma
specified site — *see* Neoplasm, malignant, by site
unspecified site C71.9

Ependymoma (epithelial) (malignant)
anaplastic
specified site — *see* Neoplasm, malignant, by site
unspecified site C71.9
benign
specified site — *see* Neoplasm, benign, by site
unspecified site D33.2
myxopapillary D43.2
specified site — *see* Neoplasm, uncertain behavior, by site
unspecified site D43.2
papillary D43.2
specified site — *see* Neoplasm, uncertain behavior, by site
unspecified site D43.2
specified site — *see* Neoplasm, malignant, by site
unspecified site C71.9
Ependymopathy G93.89
Ephelis, ephelides L81.2
Epiblepharon (congenital) Q10.3
Epicanthus, epicanthic fold (eyelid) (congenital) Q10.3
Epicondylitis (elbow)
lateral M77.1- ☑
medial M77.0- ☑
Epicystitis — *see* Cystitis
Epidemic — *see* condition
Epidermidalization, cervix — *see* Dysplasia, cervix
Epidermis, epidermal — *see* condition
Epidermodysplasia verruciformis B07.8
Epidermolysis
bullosa (congenital) Q81.9
acquired L12.30
drug-induced L12.31
specified cause NEC L12.35
dystrophica Q81.2
letalis Q81.1
simplex Q81.0
specified NEC Q81.8
necroticans combustiformis L51.2
due to drug — *see* Table of Drugs and Chemicals, by drug
Epidermophytid — *see* Dermatophytosis
Epidermophytosis (infected) — *see* Dermatophytosis
Epididymis — *see* condition
Epididymitis (acute) (nonvenereal) (recurrent) (residual) N45.1
with orchitis N45.3
blennorrhagic (gonococcal) A54.23
caseous (tuberculous) A18.15
chlamydial A56.19
filarial — *see also* Infestation, filarial B74.9 *[N51]*
gonococcal A54.23
syphilitic A52.76
tuberculous A18.15
Epididymo-orchitis — *see also* Epididymitis N45.3
Epidural — *see* condition
Epigastrium, epigastric — *see* condition
Epigastrocele — *see* Hernia, ventral
Epiglottis — *see* condition
Epiglottitis, epiglottiditis (acute) J05.10
with obstruction J05.11
chronic J37.0
Epignathus Q89.4
Epilepsia partialis continua — *see also* Kozhevnikof's epilepsy G40.1- ☑
Epilepsy, epileptic, epilepsia (attack) (cerebral) (convulsion) (fit) (seizure) G40.909

Note: the following terms are to be considered equivalent to intractable: pharmacoresistant (pharmacologically resistant), treatment resistant, refractory (medically) and poorly controlled

with
complex partial seizures — *see* Epilepsy, localization-related, symptomatic, with complex partial seizures
grand mal seizures on awakening — *see* Epilepsy, generalized, specified NEC
myoclonic absences — *see* Epilepsy, generalized, specified NEC
myoclonic-astatic seizures — *see* Epilepsy, generalized, specified NEC
simple partial seizures — *see* Epilepsy, localization-related, symptomatic, with simple partial seizures
akinetic — *see* Epilepsy, generalized, specified NEC

Epilepsy, epileptic, epilepsia — *continued*
benign childhood with centrotemporal EEG spikes — *see* Epilepsy, localization-related, idiopathic
benign myoclonic in infancy G40.80- ☑
Bravais-jacksonian — *see* Epilepsy, localization-related, symptomatic, with simple partial seizures
childhood
with occipital EEG paroxysms — *see* Epilepsy, localization-related, idiopathic
absence G40.A09 (*following* G40.3)
intractable G40.A19 (*following* G40.3)
with status epilepticus G40.A11 (*following* G40.3)
without status epilepticus G40.A19 (*following* G40.3)
not intractable G40.A09 (*following* G40.3)
with status epilepticus G40.A01 (*following* G40.3)
without status epilepticus G40.A09 (*following* G40.3)
climacteric — *see* Epilepsy, specified NEC
cysticercosis B69.0
deterioration (mental) F06.8
due to syphilis A52.19
focal — *see* Epilepsy, localization-related, symptomatic, with simple partial seizures
generalized
idiopathic G40.309
intractable G40.319
with status epilepticus G40.311
without status epilepticus G40.319
not intractable G40.309
with status epilepticus G40.301
without status epilepticus G40.309
specified NEC G40.409
intractable G40.419
with status epilepticus G40.411
without status epilepticus G40.419
not intractable G40.409
with status epilepticus G40.401
without status epilepticus G40.409
impulsive petit mal — *see* Epilepsy, juvenile myoclonic
intractable G40.919
with status epilepticus G40.911
without status epilepticus G40.919
juvenile absence G40.A09 (*following* G40.3)
intractable G40.A19 (*following* G40.3)
with status epilepticus G40.A11 (*following* G40.3)
without status epilepticus G40.A19 (*following* G40.3)
not intractable G40.A09 (*following* G40.3)
with status epilepticus G40.A01 (*following* G40.3)
without status epilepticus G40.A09 (*following* G40.3)
juvenile myoclonic G40.B09 (*following* G40.3)
intractable G40.B19 (*following* G40.3)
with status epilepticus G40.B11 (*following* G40.3)
without status epilepticus G40.B19 (*following* G40.3)
not intractable G40.B09 (*following* G40.3)
with status epilepticus G40.B01 (*following* G40.3)
without status epilepticus G40.B09 (*following* G40.3)
localization-related (focal) (partial)
idiopathic G40.009
with seizures of localized onset G40.009
intractable G40.019
with status epilepticus G40.011
without status epilepticus G40.019
not intractable G40.009
with status epilepticus G40.001
without status epilepticus G40.009
symptomatic
with complex partial seizures G40.209
intractable G40.219
with status epilepticus G40.211
without status epilepticus G40.219
not intractable G40.209
with status epilepticus G40.201
without status epilepticus G40.209
with simple partial seizures G40.109
intractable G40.119
with status epilepticus G40.111
without status epilepticus G40.119
not intractable G40.109
with status epilepticus G40.101
without status epilepticus G40.109

Epilepsy, epileptic, epilepsia — *continued*
myoclonus, myoclonic — *see also* Epilepsy, generalized, specified NEC
progressive — *see* Epilepsy, generalized, idiopathic
severe, in infancy (SMEI) G40.83- ☑
not intractable G40.909
with status epilepticus G40.901
without status epilepticus G40.909
on awakening — *see* Epilepsy, generalized, specified NEC
parasitic NOS B71.9 [G94]
partialis continua — *see also* Kozhevnikof's epilepsy G40.1- ☑
peripheral — *see* Epilepsy, specified NEC
polymorphic, in infancy (PMEI) G40.83- ☑
procursiva — *see* Epilepsy, localization-related, symptomatic, with simple partial seizures
progressive (familial) myoclonic — *see* Epilepsy, generalized, idiopathic
reflex — *see* Epilepsy, specified NEC
related to
alcohol G40.509
not intractable G40.509
with status epilepticus G40.501
without status epilepticus G40.509
drugs G40.509
not intractable G40.509
with status epilepticus G40.501
without status epilepticus G40.509
external causes G40.509
not intractable G40.509
with status epilepticus G40.501
without status epilepticus G40.509
hormonal changes G40.509
not intractable G40.509
with status epilepticus G40.501
without status epilepticus G40.509
sleep deprivation G40.509
not intractable G40.509
with status epilepticus G40.501
without status epilepticus G40.509
stress G40.509
not intractable G40.509
with status epilepticus G40.501
without status epilepticus G40.509
somatomotor — *see* Epilepsy, localization-related, symptomatic, with simple partial seizures
somatosensory — *see* Epilepsy, localization-related, symptomatic, with simple partial seizures
spasms G40.822
intractable G40.824
with status epilepticus G40.823
without status epilepticus G40.824
not intractable G40.822
with status epilepticus G40.821
without status epilepticus G40.822
specified NEC G40.802
intractable G40.804
with status epilepticus G40.803
without status epilepticus G40.804
not intractable G40.802
with status epilepticus G40.801
without status epilepticus G40.802
syndromes
generalized
idiopathic G40.309
intractable G40.319
with status epilepticus G40.311
without status epilepticus G40.319
not intractable G40.309
with status epilepticus G40.301
without status epilepticus G40.309
specified NEC G40.409
intractable G40.419
with status epilepticus G40.411
without status epilepticus G40.419
not intractable G40.409
with status epilepticus G40.401
without status epilepticus G40.409
localization-related (focal) (partial)
idiopathic G40.009
with seizures of localized onset G40.009
intractable G40.019
with status epilepticus G40.011
without status epilepticus G40.019
not intractable G40.009
with status epilepticus G40.001
without status epilepticus G40.009

Epilepsy, epileptic, epilepsia — *continued*
syndromes — *continued*
localization-related — *continued*
symptomatic
with complex partial seizures G40.209
intractable G40.219
with status epilepticus G40.211
without status epilepticus G40.219
not intractable G40.209
with status epilepticus G40.201
without status epilepticus G40.209
with simple partial seizures G40.109
intractable G40.119
with status epilepticus G40.111
without status epilepticus G40.119
not intractable G40.109
with status epilepticus G40.101
without status epilepticus G40.109
specified NEC G40.802
intractable G40.804
with status epilepticus G40.803
without status epilepticus G40.804
not intractable G40.802
with status epilepticus G40.801
without status epilepticus G40.802
tonic (-clonic) — *see* Epilepsy, generalized, specified NEC
twilight F05
uncinate (gyrus) — *see* Epilepsy, localization-related, symptomatic, with complex partial seizures
Unverricht (-Lundborg) (familial myoclonic) — *see* Epilepsy, generalized, idiopathic
visceral — *see* Epilepsy, specified NEC
visual — *see* Epilepsy, specified NEC
Epiloia Q85.1
Epimenorrhea N92.0
Epipharyngitis — *see* Nasopharyngitis
Epiphora H04.20- ☑
due to
excess lacrimation H04.21- ☑
insufficient drainage H04.22- ☑
Epiphyseal arrest — *see* Arrest, epiphyseal
Epiphyseolysis, epiphysiolysis — *see* Osteochondropathy
Epiphysitis — *see also* Osteochondropathy
juvenile M92.9
syphilitic (congenital) A50.02
Epiplocele — *see* Hernia, abdomen
Epiploitis — *see* Peritonitis
Epiplosarcomphalocele — *see* Hernia, umbilicus
Episcleritis (suppurative) H15.10- ☑
in (due to)
syphilis A52.71
tuberculosis A18.51
nodular H15.12- ☑
periodica fugax H15.11- ☑
angioneurotic — *see* Edema, angioneurotic
syphilitic (late) A52.71
tuberculous A18.51
Episode
affective, mixed F39
depersonalization (in neurotic state) F48.1
depressive F32.A
major F32.9
mild F32.0
moderate F32.1
severe (without psychotic symptoms) F32.2
with psychotic symptoms F32.3
recurrent F33.9
brief F33.8
specified NEC F32.89
hypomanic F30.8
manic F30.9
with
psychotic symptoms F30.2
remission (full) F30.4
partial F30.3
other specified F30.8
recurrent F31.89
without psychotic symptoms F30.10
mild F30.11
moderate F30.12
severe (without psychotic symptoms) F30.13
with psychotic symptoms F30.2
psychotic F23
organic F06.8
schizophrenic (acute) NEC, brief F23
Epispadias (female) (male) Q64.0

▽ Subterms under main terms may continue to next column or page   ☑ Additional Character Required — Refer to the Tabular List for Character Selection   139

Episplenitis — Esophagus

Esophoria H50.51
  convergence, excess H51.12
  divergence, insufficiency H51.8
Esotropia — *see* Strabismus, convergent concomitant
Espundia B55.2
Essential — *see* condition
Esthesioneuroblastoma C30.0
Esthesioneurocytoma C30.0
Esthesioneuroepithelioma C30.0
Esthiomene A55
Estivo-autumnal malaria (fever) B50.9
Estrangement (marital) Z63.5
  parent-child NEC Z62.890
Estriasis — *see* Myiasis
Ethanolism — *see* Alcoholism
Etherism — *see* Dependence, drug, inhalant
Ethmoid, ethmoidal — *see* condition
Ethmoiditis (chronic) (nonpurulent) (purulent) — *see also* Sinusitis, ethmoidal
  influenzal — *see* Influenza, with, respiratory manifestations NEC
  Woakes' J33.1
Ethylism — *see* Alcoholism
Eulenburg's disease (congenital paramyotonia) G71.19
Eumycetoma B47.0
Eunuchoidism E29.1
  hypogonadotropic E23.0
European blastomycosis — *see* Cryptococcosis
Eustachian — *see* condition
Evaluation (for) (of)
  development state
    adolescent Z00.3
    period of
      delayed growth in childhood Z00.70
        with abnormal findings Z00.71
      rapid growth in childhood Z00.2
    puberty Z00.3
  growth and developmental state (period of rapid growth) Z00.2
    delayed growth Z00.70
      with abnormal findings Z00.71
  mental health (status) Z00.8
    requested by authority Z04.6
  period of
    delayed growth in childhood Z00.70
      with abnormal findings Z00.71
    rapid growth in childhood Z00.2
  suspected condition — *see* Observation
Evans syndrome D69.41
Event
  apparent life threatening in newborn and infant (ALTE) R68.13
  brief resolved unexplained event (BRUE) R68.13
Eventration — *see also* Hernia, ventral
  colon into chest — *see* Hernia, diaphragm
  diaphragm (congenital) Q79.1
Eversion
  bladder N32.89
  cervix (uteri) N86
    with cervicitis N72
  foot NEC — *see also* Deformity, valgus, ankle
    congenital Q66.6
  punctum lacrimale (postinfectional) (senile) H04.52- ☑
  ureter (meatus) N28.89
  urethra (meatus) N36.8
  uterus N81.4
Evidence
  cytologic
    of malignancy on anal smear R85.614
    of malignancy on cervical smear R87.614
    of malignancy on vaginal smear R87.624
Evisceration
  birth injury P15.8
  traumatic NEC
    eye — *see* Enucleated eye
Evulsion — *see* Avulsion
Ewing's sarcoma or tumor — *see* Neoplasm, bone, malignant
Examination (for) (following) (general) (of) (routine) Z00.00
  with abnormal findings Z00.01
  abuse, physical (alleged), ruled out
    adult Z04.71
    child Z04.72
  adolescent (development state) Z00.3
  alleged rape or sexual assault (victim), ruled out
    adult Z04.41
    child Z04.42

Examination — *continued*
  allergy Z01.82
  annual (adult) (periodic) (physical) Z00.00
    with abnormal findings Z00.01
    gynecological Z01.419
      with abnormal findings Z01.411
  antibody response Z01.84
  blood — *see* Examination, laboratory
  blood pressure Z01.30
    with abnormal findings Z01.31
  cancer staging — *see* Neoplasm, malignant, by site
  cervical Papanicolaou smear Z12.4
    as part of routine gynecological examination Z01.419
      with abnormal findings Z01.411
  child (over 28 days old) Z00.129
    with abnormal findings Z00.121
    under 28 days old — *see* Newborn, examination
  clinical research control or normal comparison (control) (participant) Z00.6
  contraceptive (drug) maintenance (routine) Z30.8
    device (intrauterine) Z30.431
  dental Z01.20
    with abnormal findings Z01.21
  developmental — *see* Examination, child
  donor (potential) Z00.5
  ear Z01.10
    with abnormal findings NEC Z01.118
  eye Z01.00
    with abnormal findings Z01.01
    following failed vision screening Z01.020
      with abnormal findings Z01.021
  follow-up (routine) (following) Z09
    chemotherapy NEC Z09
      malignant neoplasm Z08
    fracture Z09
    malignant neoplasm Z08
    postpartum Z39.2
    psychotherapy Z09
    radiotherapy NEC Z09
      malignant neoplasm Z08
    surgery NEC Z09
      malignant neoplasm Z08
  following
    accident NEC Z04.3
      transport Z04.1
      work Z04.2
    assault, alleged, ruled out
      adult Z04.71
      child Z04.72
    motor vehicle accident Z04.1
    treatment (for) Z09
      combined NEC Z09
        fracture Z09
        malignant neoplasm Z08
      malignant neoplasm Z08
      mental disorder Z09
      specified condition NEC Z09
  forced sexual exploitation Z04.81
  forced labor exploitation Z04.82
  gynecological Z01.419
    with abnormal findings Z01.411
    for contraceptive maintenance Z30.8
  health — *see* Examination, medical
  hearing Z01.10
    with abnormal findings NEC Z01.118
    following failed hearing screening Z01.110
    infant or child (over 28 days old) Z00.129
      with abnormal findings Z00.121
  immunity status testing Z01.84
  laboratory (as part of a general medical examination) Z00.00
    with abnormal findings Z00.01
    preprocedural Z01.812
  lactating mother Z39.1
  medical (adult) (for) (of) Z00.00
    with abnormal findings Z00.01
    administrative purpose only Z02.9
      specified NEC Z02.89
    admission to
      armed forces Z02.3
      old age home Z02.2
      prison Z02.89
      residential institution Z02.2
      school Z02.0
        following illness or medical treatment Z02.0
      summer camp Z02.89
    adoption Z02.82
    blood alcohol or drug level Z02.83

Examination — *continued*
  medical — *continued*
    camp (summer) Z02.89
    clinical research, normal subject (control) (participant) Z00.6
    control subject in clinical research (normal comparison) (participant) Z00.6
    donor (potential) Z00.5
    driving license Z02.4
    general (adult) Z00.00
      with abnormal findings Z00.01
    immigration Z02.89
    insurance purposes Z02.6
    marriage Z02.89
    medicolegal reasons NEC Z04.89
    naturalization Z02.89
    participation in sport Z02.5
    paternity testing Z02.81
    population survey Z00.8
    pre-employment Z02.1
    pre-operative — *see* Examination, pre-procedural
    pre-procedural
      cardiovascular Z01.810
      respiratory Z01.811
      specified NEC Z01.818
    preschool children
      for admission to school Z02.0
    prisoners
      for entrance into prison Z02.89
    recruitment for armed forces Z02.3
    specified NEC Z00.8
    sport competition Z02.5
  medicolegal reason NEC Z04.89
    following
      forced sexual exploitation Z04.81
      forced labor exploitation Z04.82
  newborn — *see* Newborn, examination
  pelvic (annual) (periodic) Z01.419
    with abnormal findings Z01.411
  period of rapid growth in childhood Z00.2
  periodic (adult) (annual) (routine) Z00.00
    with abnormal findings Z00.01
  physical (adult) — *see also* Examination, medical Z00.00
    sports Z02.5
  postpartum
    immediately after delivery Z39.0
    routine follow-up Z39.2
  pre-chemotherapy (antineoplastic) Z01.818
  prenatal (normal pregnancy) — *see also* Pregnancy, normal Z34.9- ☑
  pre-procedural (pre-operative)
    cardiovascular Z01.810
    laboratory Z01.812
    respiratory Z01.811
    specified NEC Z01.818
  prior to chemotherapy (antineoplastic) Z01.818
  psychiatric NEC Z00.8
    follow-up not needing further care Z09
    requested by authority Z04.6
  radiological (as part of a general medical examination) Z00.00
    with abnormal findings Z00.01
  repeat cervical smear to confirm findings of recent normal smear following initial abnormal smear Z01.42
  skin (hypersensitivity) Z01.82
  special — *see also* Examination, by type Z01.89
    specified type NEC Z01.89
  specified type or reason NEC Z04.89
  teeth Z01.20
    with abnormal findings Z01.21
  urine — *see* Examination, laboratory
  vision Z01.00
    with abnormal findings Z01.01
    following failed vision screening Z01.020
      with abnormal findings Z01.021
    infant or child (over 28 days old) Z00.129
      with abnormal findings Z00.121
Exanthem, exanthema — *see also* Rash
  with enteroviral vesicular stomatitis B08.4
  Boston A88.0
  epidemic with meningitis A88.0 *[G02]*
  subitum B08.20
    due to human herpesvirus 6 B08.21
    due to human herpesvirus 7 B08.22
  viral, virus B09
    specified type NEC B08.8

☑ **Additional Character Required** — Refer to the Tabular List for Character Selection   ▽ **Subterms under main terms may continue to next column or page**

Excess, excessive, excessively

alcohol level in blood R78.0
androgen (ovarian) E28.1
attrition, tooth, teeth K03.0
carotene, carotin (dietary) E67.1
cold, effects of T69.9 ☑
  specified effect NEC T69.8 ☑
convergence H51.12
crying
  in child, adolescent, or adult R45.83
  in infant R68.11
development, breast N62
divergence H51.8
drinking (alcohol) NEC (without dependence) F10.10
  habitual (continual) (without remission) F10.20
eating R63.2
estrogen E28.0
fat — see also Obesity
  in heart — see Degeneration, myocardial
  localized E65
foreskin N47.8
gas R14.0
glucagon E16.3
heat — see Heat
intermaxillary vertical dimension of fully erupted teeth M26.37
interocclusal distance of fully erupted teeth M26.37
kalium E87.5
large
  colon K59.39
    congenital Q43.8
  infant P08.0
  organ or site, congenital NEC — see Anomaly, by site
long
  organ or site, congenital NEC — see Anomaly, by site
menstruation (with regular cycle) N92.0
  with irregular cycle N92.1
napping Z72.821
natrium E87.0
number of teeth K00.1
nutrient (dietary) NEC R63.2
potassium (K) E87.5
salivation K11.7
secretion — see also Hypersecretion
  milk O92.6
  sputum R09.3
  sweat R61
sexual drive F52.8
short
  organ or site, congenital NEC — see Anomaly, by site
  umbilical cord in labor or delivery O69.3 ☑
skin L98.7
  and subcutaneous tissue L98.7
  eyelid (acquired) — see Blepharochalasis
    congenital Q10.3
sodium (Na) E87.0
spacing of fully erupted teeth M26.32
sputum R09.3
sweating R61
thirst R63.1
  due to deprivation of water T73.1 ☑
tuberosity of jaw M26.07
vitamin
  A (dietary) E67.0
    administered as drug (prolonged intake) — see Table of Drugs and Chemicals, vitamins, adverse effect
    overdose or wrong substance given or taken — see Table of Drugs and Chemicals, vitamins, poisoning
  D (dietary) E67.3
    administered as drug (prolonged intake) — see Table of Drugs and Chemicals, vitamins, adverse effect
    overdose or wrong substance given or taken — see Table of Drugs and Chemicals, vitamins, poisoning
weight
  gain R63.5
  loss R63.4

Excitability, abnormal, under minor stress (personality disorder) F60.3

Excitation

anomalous atrioventricular I45.6
psychogenic F30.8

Excitation — continued

reactive (from emotional stress, psychological trauma) F30.8

Excitement

hypomanic F30.8
manic F30.9
mental, reactive (from emotional stress, psychological trauma) F30.8
state, reactive (from emotional stress, psychological trauma) F30.8

Excoriation (traumatic) — see also Abrasion

neurotic L98.1
skin picking disorder F42.4

Exfoliation

due to erythematous conditions according to extent of body surface involved L49.0
  10-19 percent of body surface L49.1
  20-29 percent of body surface L49.2
  30-39 percent of body surface L49.3
  40-49 percent of body surface L49.4
  50-59 percent of body surface L49.5
  60-69 percent of body surface L49.6
  70-79 percent of body surface L49.7
  80-89 percent of body surface L49.8
  90-99 percent of body surface L49.9
  less than 10 percent of body surface L49.0
teeth, due to systemic causes K08.0

Exfoliative — see condition

Exhaustion, exhaustive (physical NEC) R53.83

battle F43.0
cardiac — see Failure, heart
delirium F43.0
due to
  cold T69.8 ☑
  excessive exertion T73.3 ☑
  exposure T73.2 ☑
  neurasthenia F48.8
heart — see Failure, heart
heat — see also Heat, exhaustion T67.5 ☑
  due to
    salt depletion T67.4 ☑
    water depletion T67.3 ☑
maternal, complicating delivery O75.81
mental F48.8
myocardium, myocardial — see Failure, heart
nervous F48.8
old age R54
psychogenic F48.8
psychosis F43.0
senile R54
vital NEC Z73.0

Exhibitionism F65.2

Exocervicitis — see Cervicitis

Exomphalos Q79.2

meaning hernia — see Hernia, umbilicus

Exophoria H50.52

convergence, insufficiency H51.11
divergence, excess H51.8

Exophthalmos H05.2- ☑

congenital Q15.8
constant NEC H05.24- ☑
displacement, globe — see Displacement, globe
due to thyrotoxicosis (hyperthyroidism) — see Hyperthyroidism, with, goiter (diffuse)
dysthyroid — see Hyperthyroidism, with, goiter (diffuse)
goiter — see Hyperthyroidism, with, goiter (diffuse)
intermittent NEC H05.25- ☑
malignant — see Hyperthyroidism, with, goiter (diffuse)
orbital
  edema — see Edema, orbit
  hemorrhage — see Hemorrhage, orbit
pulsating NEC H05.26- ☑
thyrotoxic, thyrotropic — see Hyperthyroidism, with, goiter (diffuse)

Exostosis — see also Disorder, bone

cartilaginous — see Neoplasm, bone, benign
congenital (multiple) Q78.6
external ear canal H61.81- ☑
gonococcal A54.49
jaw (bone) M27.8
multiple, congenital Q78.6
orbit H05.35- ☑
osteocartilaginous — see Neoplasm, bone, benign
syphilitic A52.77

Exotropia — see Strabismus, divergent concomitant

Explanation of

investigation finding Z71.2
medication Z71.89

Exploitation

labor
  confirmed
    adult forced T74.61 ☑
    child forced T74.62 ☑
  suspected
    adult forced T76.61 ☑
    child forced T76.62 ☑
sexual
  confirmed
    adult forced T74.51 ☑
    child T74.52 ☑
  suspected
    adult forced T76.51 ☑
    child T76.52 ☑

Exposure (to) — see also Contact, with T75.89 ☑

acariasis Z20.7
AIDS virus Z20.6
air pollution Z77.110
algae and algae toxins Z77.121
algae bloom Z77.121
anthrax Z20.810
aromatic amines Z77.020
aromatic (hazardous) compounds NEC Z77.028
aromatic dyes NOS Z77.028
arsenic Z77.010
asbestos Z77.090
bacterial disease NEC Z20.818
benzene Z77.021
blue-green algae bloom Z77.121
body fluids (potentially hazardous) Z77.21
brown tide Z77.121
chemicals (chiefly nonmedicinal) (hazardous) NEC Z77.098
cholera Z20.09
chromium compounds Z77.018
cold, effects of T69.9 ☑
  specified effect NEC T69.8 ☑
communicable disease Z20.9
  bacterial NEC Z20.818
  specified NEC Z20.89
  viral NEC Z20.828
  Zika virus Z20.821
coronavirus (disease) (novel) 2019 Z20.822
COVID-19 Z20.822
cyanobacteria bloom Z77.121
disaster Z65.5
discrimination Z60.5
dyes Z77.098
effects of T73.9 ☑
environmental tobacco smoke (acute) (chronic) Z77.22
Escherichia coli (E. coli) Z20.01
exhaustion due to T73.2 ☑
fiberglass — see Table of Drugs and Chemicals, fiberglass
German measles Z20.4
gonorrhea Z20.2
hazardous metals NEC Z77.018
hazardous substances NEC Z77.29
hazards in the physical environment NEC Z77.128
hazards to health NEC Z77.9
human immunodeficiency virus (HIV) Z20.6
human T-lymphotropic virus type-1 (HTLV-1) Z20.89
implanted
  mesh — see Complications, prosthetic device or implant, mesh
  prosthetic materials NEC — see Complications, prosthetic materials NEC
infestation (parasitic) NEC Z20.7
intestinal infectious disease NEC Z20.09
  Escherichia coli (E. coli) Z20.01
lead Z77.011
meningococcus Z20.811
mold (toxic) Z77.120
nickel dust Z77.018
noise Z77.122
occupational
  air contaminants NEC Z57.39
  dust Z57.2
  environmental tobacco smoke Z57.31
  extreme temperature Z57.6
  noise Z57.0
  radiation Z57.1
  risk factors Z57.9
    specified NEC Z57.8

Exposure — *continued*
  occupational — *continued*
    toxic agents (gases) (liquids) (solids) (vapors) in agriculture Z57.4
    toxic agents (gases) (liquids) (solids) (vapors) in industry NEC Z57.5
    vibration Z57.7
  parasitic disease NEC Z20.7
  pediculosis Z20.7
  persecution Z60.5
  pfiesteria piscicida Z77.121
  poliomyelitis Z20.89
  pollution
    air Z77.110
    environmental NEC Z77.118
    soil Z77.112
    water Z77.111
  polycyclic aromatic hydrocarbons Z77.028
  prenatal (drugs) (toxic chemicals) — *see* Newborn, affected by, noxious substances transmitted via placenta or breast milk
  rabies Z20.3
  radiation, naturally occurring NEC Z77.123
  radon Z77.123
  red tide (Florida) Z77.121
  rubella Z20.4
  SARS-CoV-2 Z20.822
  second hand tobacco smoke (acute) (chronic) Z77.22
    in the perinatal period P96.81
  sexually-transmitted disease Z20.2
  smallpox (laboratory) Z20.89
  syphilis Z20.2
  terrorism Z65.4
  torture Z65.4
  tuberculosis Z20.1
  uranium Z77.012
  varicella Z20.820
  venereal disease Z20.2
  viral disease NEC Z20.828
  war Z65.5
  water pollution Z77.111
  Zika virus Z20.821
Exsanguination — *see* Hemorrhage
Exstrophy
  abdominal contents Q45.8
  bladder Q64.10
    cloacal Q64.12
    specified type NEC Q64.19
    supravesical fissure Q64.11
Extensive — *see* condition
Extra — *see also* Accessory
  marker chromosomes (normal individual) Q92.61
    in abnormal individual Q92.62
  rib Q76.6
    cervical Q76.5
Extrasystoles (supraventricular) I49.49
  atrial I49.1
  auricular I49.1
  junctional I49.2
  ventricular I49.3
Extrauterine gestation or pregnancy — *see* Pregnancy, by site
Extravasation
  blood R58
  chyle into mesentery I89.8
  pelvicalyceal N13.8
  pyelosinus N13.8
  urine (from ureter) R39.0
  vesicant agent
    antineoplastic chemotherapy T80.810 ☑
    other agent NEC T80.818 ☑
Extremity — *see* condition, limb
Extrophy — *see* Exstrophy
Extroversion
  bladder Q64.19
  uterus N81.4
    complicating delivery O71.2
    postpartal (old) N81.4
Extruded tooth (teeth) M26.34
Extrusion
  breast implant (prosthetic) T85.42 ☑
  eye implant (globe) (ball) T85.328 ☑
  intervertebral disc — *see* Displacement, intervertebral disc
  ocular lens implant (prosthetic) — *see* Complications, intraocular lens
  vitreous — *see* Prolapse, vitreous

Exudate
  pleural — *see* Effusion, pleura
  retina H35.89
  wound fluids L24.A9
Exudative — *see* condition
Eye, eyeball, eyelid — *see* condition
Eyestrain — *see* Disturbance, vision, subjective
Eyeworm disease of Africa B74.3

F

Faber's syndrome (achlorhydric anemia) D50.9
Fabry (-Anderson) **disease** E75.21
Facet syndrome M47.89- ☑
Faciocephalalgia, autonomic — *see also* Neuropathy, peripheral, autonomic G90.09
Factor(s)
  psychic, associated with diseases classified elsewhere F54
  psychological
    affecting physical conditions F54
    or behavioral
      affecting general medical condition F54
      associated with disorders or diseases classified elsewhere F54
Fahr disease (of brain) G23.8
Fahr Volhard disease (of kidney) I12.- ☑
Failure, failed
  abortion — *see* Abortion, attempted
  aortic (valve) I35.8
    rheumatic I06.8
  attempted abortion — *see* Abortion, attempted
  biventricular I50.82
    due to left heart failure I50.814
  bone marrow — *see* Anemia, aplastic
  cardiac — *see* Failure, heart
  cardiorenal (chronic) — *see also* Failure, renal, and Failure, heart I50.9
    hypertensive I13.2
  cardiorespiratory — *see also* Failure, heart R09.2
  cardiovascular (chronic) — *see* Failure, heart
  cerebrovascular I67.9
  cervical dilatation in labor O62.0
  circulation, circulatory (peripheral) R57.9
    newborn P29.89
  compensation — *see* Disease, heart
  compliance with medical treatment or regimen — *see* Noncompliance
  congestive — *see* Failure, heart, congestive
  dental implant (endosseous) M27.69
    due to
      failure of dental prosthesis M27.63
      lack of attached gingiva M27.62
      occlusal trauma (poor prosthetic design) M27.62
      parafunctional habits M27.62
      periodontal infection (peri-implantitis) M27.62
      poor oral hygiene M27.62
    osseointegration M27.61
      due to
        complications of systemic disease M27.61
        poor bone quality M27.61
      iatrogenic M27.61
    post-osseointegration
      biological M27.62
      due to complications of systemic disease M27.62
      iatrogenic M27.62
      mechanical M27.63
    pre-integration M27.61
    pre-osseointegration M27.61
    specified NEC M27.69
  descent of head (at term) of pregnancy (mother) O32.4 ☑
  endosseous dental implant — *see* Failure, dental implant
  engagement of head (term of pregnancy) (mother) O32.4 ☑
  erection (penile) — *see also* Dysfunction, sexual, male, erectile N52.9
    nonorganic F52.21
  examination(s), anxiety concerning Z55.2
  expansion terminal respiratory units (newborn) (primary) P28.0
  forceps NOS (with subsequent cesarean delivery) O66.5
  gain weight (child over 28 days old) R62.51
    adult R62.7
    newborn P92.6
  genital response (male) F52.21
    female F52.22

Failure, failed — *continued*
  heart (acute) (senile) (sudden) I50.9
    with
      acute pulmonary edema — *see* Failure, ventricular, left
      decompensation I50.9
        with
          normal ejection fraction I50.33
          preserved ejection fraction I50.33
          reduced ejection fraction I50.23
            with diastolic dysfunction I50.43
          combined systolic and diastolic I50.43
          diastolic I50.33
          right I50.813
          systolic I50.23
    dilatation — *see* Disease, heart
    hypertension — *see* Hypertension, heart
    normal ejection fraction — *see* Failure, heart, diastolic
    preserved ejection fraction — *see* Failure, heart, diastolic
    reduced ejection fraction — *see* Failure, heart, systolic
    arteriosclerotic I70.90
    biventricular I50.82
      due to left heart failure I50.814
    combined left-right sided I50.82
      due to left heart failure I50.814
    compensated — *see also* Failure, heart, by type as diastolic or systolic, chronic I50.9
    complicating
      anesthesia (general) (local) or other sedation in labor and delivery O74.2
        in pregnancy O29.12- ☑
        postpartum, puerperal O89.1
      delivery (cesarean) (instrumental) O75.4
    congestive I50.9
      with rheumatic fever (conditions in I00)
        active I01.8
        inactive or quiescent (with chorea) I09.81
      newborn P29.0
      rheumatic (chronic) (inactive) (with chorea) I09.81
        active or acute I01.8
          with chorea I02.0
    decompensated — *see also* Failure, heart, by type as diastolic or systolic, acute and chronic I50.9
    degenerative — *see* Degeneration, myocardial
    diastolic (congestive) (left ventricular) I50.30
      acute (congestive) I50.31
        and (on) chronic (congestive) I50.33
      chronic (congestive) I50.32
        and (on) acute (congestive) I50.33
      combined with systolic (congestive) I50.40
        acute (congestive) I50.41
          and (on) chronic (congestive) I50.43
        chronic (congestive) I50.42
          and (on) acute (congestive) I50.43
    due to presence of cardiac prosthesis I97.13- ☑
    end stage — *see also* Failure, heart, by type as diastolic or systolic, chronic I50.84
    following cardiac surgery I97.13- ☑
    high output NOS I50.83
    hypertensive — *see* Hypertension, heart
    left (ventricular) — *see also* Failure, ventricular, left
      combined diastolic and systolic — *see* Failure, heart, diastolic, combined with systolic
      diastolic — *see* Failure, heart, diastolic
      systolic — *see* Failure, heart, systolic
    low output (syndrome) NOS I50.9
    newborn P29.0
    organic — *see* Disease, heart
    peripartum O90.3
    postprocedural I97.13- ☑
    rheumatic (chronic) (inactive) I09.9
    right (isolated) (ventricular) I50.810
      acute I50.811
        and (on) chronic I50.813
      chronic I50.812
        and acute I50.813
      secondary to left heart failure I50.814
    specified NEC I50.89

> *Note: heart failure stages A, B, C, and D are based on the American College of Cardiology and American Heart Association stages of heart failure, which complement and should not be confused with the New York Heart Association Classification of Heart Failure, into Class I, Class II, Class III, and Class IV*

☑ **Additional Character Required** — Refer to the Tabular List for Character Selection   ⚐ **Subterms under main terms may continue to next column or page**

Failure, failed — *continued*
- heart — *continued*
  - stage A Z91.89
  - stage B — *see also* Failure, heart, by type as diastolic or systolic I50.9
  - stage C — *see also* Failure, heart, by type as diastolic or systolic I50.9
  - stage D — *see also* Failure, heart, by type as diastolic or systolic, chronic I50.84
  - systolic (congestive) (left ventricular) I50.20
    - acute (congestive) I50.21
      - and (on) chronic (congestive) I50.23
    - chronic (congestive) I50.22
      - and (on) acute (congestive) I50.23
    - combined with diastolic (congestive) I50.40
      - acute (congestive) I50.41
        - and (on) chronic (congestive) I50.43
      - chronic (congestive) I50.42
        - and (on) acute (congestive) I50.43
  - thyrotoxic — *see also* Thyrotoxicosis E05.90 *[I43]*
    - with
      - high output — *see also* Thyrotoxicosis I50.83
      - thyroid storm E05.91 *[I43]*
        - high output — *see also* Thyrotoxicosis I50.83
  - valvular — *see* Endocarditis
- hepatic K72.90
  - with coma K72.91
  - acute or subacute K72.00
    - with coma K72.01
    - due to drugs K71.10
      - with coma K71.11
  - alcoholic (acute) (chronic) (subacute) K70.40
    - with coma K70.41
  - chronic K72.10
    - with coma K72.11
    - due to drugs (acute) (subacute) (chronic) K71.10
      - with coma K71.11
  - due to drugs (acute) (subacute) (chronic) K71.10
    - with coma K71.11
  - postprocedural K91.82
- hepatorenal K76.7
- induction (of labor) O61.9
  - abortion — *see* Abortion, attempted
  - by
    - oxytocic drugs O61.0
    - prostaglandins O61.0
  - instrumental O61.1
  - mechanical O61.1
  - medical O61.0
  - specified NEC O61.8
  - surgical O61.1
- intubation during anesthesia T88.4 ☑
  - in pregnancy O29.6- ☑
  - labor and delivery O74.7
  - postpartum, puerperal O89.6
- involution, thymus (gland) E32.0
- kidney — *see also* Disease, kidney, chronic N19
  - acute — *see also* Failure, renal, acute N17.9
- lactation (complete) O92.3
  - partial O92.4
- Leydig's cell, adult E29.1
- liver — *see* Failure, hepatic
- menstruation at puberty N91.0
- mitral I05.8
- myocardial, myocardium — *see also* Failure, heart I50.9
  - chronic — *see also* Failure, heart, congestive I50.9
  - congestive — *see also* Failure, heart, congestive I50.9
- newborn screening — *see* Abnormal, neonatal screening
  - neonatal congenital heart disease P09.5
- orgasm (female) (psychogenic) F52.31
  - male F52.32
- ovarian (primary) E28.39
  - iatrogenic E89.40
    - asymptomatic E89.40
    - symptomatic E89.41
  - postprocedural (postablative) (postirradiation) (postsurgical) E89.40
    - asymptomatic E89.40
    - symptomatic E89.41
- ovulation causing infertility N97.0
- polyglandular, autoimmune E31.0
- prosthetic joint implant — *see* Complications, joint prosthesis, mechanical, breakdown, by site
- renal N19

Failure, failed — *continued*
- renal — *continued*
  - with
    - tubular necrosis (acute) N17.0
  - acute N17.9
    - with
      - cortical necrosis N17.1
      - medullary necrosis N17.2
      - tubular necrosis N17.0
    - specified NEC N17.8
  - chronic N18.9
    - hypertensive — *see* Hypertension, kidney
  - congenital P96.0
  - end stage (chronic) N18.6
    - due to hypertension I12.0
  - following
    - abortion — *see* Abortion by type complicated by specified condition NEC
    - crushing T79.5 ☑
    - ectopic or molar pregnancy O08.4
    - labor and delivery (acute) O90.4
  - hypertensive — *see* Hypertension, kidney
  - postprocedural N99.0
- respiration, respiratory J96.90
  - with
    - hypercapnia J96.92
    - hypercarbia J96.92
    - hypoxia J96.91
  - acute J96.00
    - with
      - hypercapnia J96.02
      - hypercarbia J96.02
      - hypoxia J96.01
  - center G93.89
  - acute and (on) chronic J96.20
    - with
      - hypercapnia J96.22
      - hypercarbia J96.22
      - hypoxia J96.21
  - chronic J96.10
    - with
      - hypercapnia J96.12
      - hypercarbia J96.12
      - hypoxia J96.11
  - newborn P28.5
  - postprocedural (acute) J95.821
    - acute and chronic J95.822
- rotation
  - cecum Q43.3
  - colon Q43.3
  - intestine Q43.3
  - kidney Q63.2
- sedation (conscious) (moderate) during procedure T88.52 ☑
  - history of Z92.83
- segmentation — *see also* Fusion
  - fingers — *see* Syndactylism, complex, fingers
  - vertebra Q76.49
    - with scoliosis Q76.3
- seminiferous tubule, adult E29.1
- senile (general) R54
- sexual arousal (male) F52.21
  - female F52.22
- testicular endocrine function E29.1
- to thrive (child over 28 days old) R62.51
  - adult R62.7
  - newborn P92.6
- transplant T86.92
  - bone T86.831
    - marrow T86.02
  - cornea T86.841- ☑
  - heart T86.22
    - with lung(s) T86.32
  - intestine T86.851
  - kidney T86.12
  - liver T86.42
  - lung(s) T86.811
    - with heart T86.32
  - pancreas T86.891
  - skin (allograft) (autograft) T86.821
  - specified organ or tissue NEC T86.891
  - stem cell (peripheral blood) (umbilical cord) T86.5
- trial of labor (with subsequent cesarean delivery) O66.40
  - following previous cesarean delivery O66.41
- tubal ligation N99.89
- urinary — *see* Disease, kidney, chronic

Failure, failed — *continued*
- vacuum extraction NOS (with subsequent cesarean delivery) O66.5
- vasectomy N99.89
- ventouse NOS (with subsequent cesarean delivery) O66.5
- ventricular — *see also* Failure, heart I50.9
  - left — *see also* Failure, heart, left I50.1
    - with rheumatic fever (conditions in I00)
      - active I01.8
        - with chorea I02.0
      - inactive or quiescent (with chorea) I09.81
      - rheumatic (chronic) (inactive) (with chorea) I09.81
        - active or acute I01.8
          - with chorea I02.0
  - right — *see* Failure, heart, right
- vital centers, newborn P91.88

Fainting (fit) R55

Fallen arches — *see* Deformity, limb, flat foot

Falling, falls (repeated) R29.6
- any organ or part — *see* Prolapse

Fallopian
- insufflation Z31.41
- tube — *see* condition

Fallot's
- pentalogy Q21.8
- tetrad or tetralogy Q21.3
- triad or trilogy Q22.3

False — *see also* condition
- croup J38.5
- joint — *see* Nonunion, fracture
- labor (pains) O47.9
  - at or after 37 completed weeks of gestation O47.1
  - before 37 completed weeks of gestation O47.0- ☑
- passage, urethra (prostatic) N36.5
- pregnancy F45.8

Family, familial — *see also* condition
- disruption Z63.8
  - involving divorce or separation Z63.5
- Li-Fraumeni (syndrome) Z15.01
- planning advice Z30.09
- problem Z63.9
  - specified NEC Z63.8
- retinoblastoma C69.2- ☑

Famine (effects of) T73.0 ☑
- edema — *see* Malnutrition, severe

Fanconi (-de Toni)(-Debré) **syndrome** E72.09
- with cystinosis E72.04

Fanconi's anemia (congenital pancytopenia) D61.09

Farber's disease or syndrome E75.29

Farcy A24.0

Farmer's
- lung J67.0
- skin L57.8

Farsightedness — *see* Hypermetropia

Fascia — *see* condition

Fasciculation R25.3

Fasciitis M72.9
- diffuse (eosinophilic) M35.4
- infective M72.8
  - necrotizing M72.6
- necrotizing M72.6
- nodular M72.4
- perirenal (with ureteral obstruction) N13.5
  - with infection N13.6
- plantar M72.2
- specified NEC M72.8
- traumatic (old) M72.8
  - current — *code by* site under Sprain

Fascioliasis B66.3

Fasciolopsis, fasciolopsiasis (intestinal) B66.5

Fascioscapulohumeral myopathy G71.02

Fast pulse R00.0

Fat
- embolism — *see* Embolism, fat
- excessive — *see also* Obesity
  - in heart — *see* Degeneration, myocardial
- in stool R19.5
- localized (pad) E65
  - heart — *see* Degeneration, myocardial
  - knee M79.4
  - retropatellar M79.4
- necrosis
  - breast N64.1
  - mesentery K65.4
  - omentum K65.4
- pad E65

Fat — *continued*
  pad — *continued*
    knee M79.4
Fatigue R53.83
  auditory deafness — *see* Deafness
  chronic R53.82
  combat F43.0
  general R53.83
    psychogenic F48.8
  heat (transient) T67.6 ☑
  muscle M62.89
  myocardium — *see* Failure, heart
  neoplasm-related R53.0
  nervous, neurosis F48.8
  operational F48.8
  psychogenic (general) F48.8
  senile R54
  voice R49.8
Fatness — *see* Obesity
Fatty — *see also* condition
  apron E65
  degeneration — *see* Degeneration, fatty
  heart (enlarged) — *see* Degeneration, myocardial
  liver NEC K76.0
    alcoholic K70.0
    nonalcoholic K76.0
  necrosis — *see* Degeneration, fatty
Fauces — *see* condition
Fauchard's disease (periodontitis) — *see* Periodontitis
Faucitis J02.9
Favism (anemia) D55.0
Favus — *see* Dermatophytosis
Fazio-Londe disease or syndrome G12.1
Fear complex or reaction F40.9
Fear of — *see* Phobia
Feared complaint unfounded Z71.1
Febris, febrile — *see also* Fever
  flava — *see also* Fever, yellow A95.9
  melitensis A23.0
  pestis — *see* Plague
  recurrens — *see* Fever, relapsing
  rubra A38.9
Fecal
  incontinence R15.9
  smearing R15.1
  soiling R15.1
  urgency R15.2
Fecalith (impaction) K56.41
  appendix K38.1
  congenital P76.8
Fede's disease K14.0
Feeble rapid pulse due to shock following injury T79.4 ☑
Feeble-minded F70
Feeding
  difficulties R63.30
  problem (elderly) (infant) R63.39
    newborn P92.9
      specified NEC P92.8
    nonorganic (adult) — *see* Disorder, eating
Feeling (of)
  foreign body in throat R09.89
Feer's disease — *see* Poisoning, mercury
Feet — *see* condition
Feigned illness Z76.5
Feil-Klippel syndrome (brevicollis) Q76.1
Feinmesser's (hidrotic) **ectodermal dysplasia** Q82.4
Felinophobia F40.218
Felon — *see also* Cellulitis, digit
  with lymphangitis — *see* Lymphangitis, acute, digit
Felty's syndrome M05.00
  ankle M05.07- ☑
  elbow M05.02- ☑
  foot joint M05.07- ☑
  hand joint M05.04- ☑
  hip M05.05- ☑
  knee M05.06- ☑
  multiple site M05.09
  shoulder M05.01- ☑
  vertebra — *see* Spondylitis, ankylosing
  wrist M05.03- ☑
Female genital cutting status — *see* Female genital mutilation status (FGM)
Female genital mutilation status (FGM) N90.810
  specified NEC N90.818
  type I (clitorectomy status) N90.811

Female genital mutilation status — *continued*
  type II (clitorectomy with excision of labia minora status) N90.812
  type III (infibulation status) N90.813
  type IV N90.818
Femur, femoral — *see* condition
Fenestration, fenestrated — *see also* Imperfect, closure
  aortico-pulmonary Q21.4
  cusps, heart valve NEC Q24.8
    pulmonary Q22.3
  pulmonic cusps Q22.3
Fernell's disease (aortic aneurysm) I71.9
Fertile eunuch syndrome E23.0
Fetid
  breath R19.6
  sweat L75.0
Fetishism F65.0
  transvestic F65.1
Fetus, fetal — *see also* condition
  alcohol syndrome (dysmorphic) Q86.0
  compressus O31.0- ☑
  hydantoin syndrome Q86.1
  lung tissue P28.0
  papyraceous O31.0- ☑
Fever (inanition) (of unknown origin) (persistent) (with chills) (with rigor) R50.9
  abortus A23.1
  Aden (dengue) A90
  African tick bite A77.8
  African tick-borne A68.1
  American
    mountain (tick) A93.2
    spotted A77.0
  aphthous B08.8
  arbovirus, arboviral A94
    hemorrhagic A94
    specified NEC A93.8
  Argentinian hemorrhagic A96.0
  Assam B55.0
  Australian Q A78
  Bangkok hemorrhagic A91
  Barmah forest A92.8
  Bartonella A44.0
  bilious, hemoglobinuric B50.8
  blackwater B50.8
  blister B00.1
  Bolivian hemorrhagic A96.1
  Bonvale dam T73.3 ☑
  boutonneuse A77.1
  brain — *see* Encephalitis
  Brazilian purpuric A48.4
  breakbone A90
  Bullis A77.0
  Bunyamwera A92.8
  Burdwan B55.0
  Bwamba A92.8
  Cameroon — *see* Malaria
  Canton A75.9
  catarrhal (acute) J00
    chronic J31.0
  cat-scratch A28.1
  Central Asian hemorrhagic A98.0
  cerebral — *see* Encephalitis
  cerebrospinal meningococcal A39.0
  Chagres B50.9
  Chandipura A92.8
  Changuinola A93.1
  Charcot's (biliary) (hepatic) (intermittent) — *see* Calculus, bile duct
  Chikungunya (viral) (hemorrhagic) A92.0
  Chitral A93.1
  Colombo — *see* Fever, paratyphoid
  Colorado tick (virus) A93.2
  congestive (remittent) — *see* Malaria
  Congo virus A98.0
  continued malarial B50.9
  Corsican — *see* Malaria
  Crimean-Congo hemorrhagic A98.0
  Cyprus — *see* Brucellosis
  dandy A90
  deer fly — *see* Tularemia
  dengue (virus) A90
    hemorrhagic A91
    sandfly A93.1
  desert B38.0
  drug induced R50.2
  due to
    conditions classified elsewhere R50.81

Fever — *continued*
  due to — *continued*
    heat T67.01 ☑
  enteric A01.00
  enteroviral exanthematous (Boston exanthem) A88.0
  ephemeral (of unknown origin) R50.9
  epidemic hemorrhagic A98.5
  erysipelatous — *see* Erysipelas
  estivo-autumnal (malarial) B50.9
  famine A75.0
  five day A79.0
  following delivery O86.4
  Fort Bragg A27.89
  gastroenteric A01.00
  gastromalarial — *see* Malaria
  Gibraltar — *see* Brucellosis
  glandular — *see* Mononucleosis, infectious
  Guama (viral) A92.8
  Haverhill A25.1
  hay (allergic) J30.1
    with asthma (bronchial) J45.909
      with
        exacerbation (acute) J45.901
        status asthmaticus J45.902
    due to
      allergen other than pollen J30.89
      pollen, any plant or tree J30.1
  heat (effects) T67.01 ☑
  hematuric, bilious B50.8
  hemoglobinuric (malarial) (bilious) B50.8
  hemorrhagic (arthropod-borne) NOS A94
    with renal syndrome A98.5
    arenaviral A96.9
      specified NEC A96.8
    Argentinian A96.0
    Bangkok A91
    Bolivian A96.1
    Central Asian A98.0
    Chikungunya A92.0
    Crimean-Congo A98.0
    dengue (virus) A91
    epidemic A98.5
    Junin (virus) A96.0
    Korean A98.5
    Kyasanur forest A98.2
    Machupo (virus) A96.1
    mite-borne A93.8
    mosquito-borne A92.8
    Omsk A98.1
    Philippine A91
    Russian A98.5
    Singapore A91
    Southeast Asia A91
    Thailand A91
    tick-borne NEC A93.8
    viral A99
      specified NEC A98.8
  hepatic — *see* Cholecystitis
  herpetic — *see* Herpes
  icterohemorrhagic A27.0
  Indiana A93.8
  infective B99.9
    specified NEC B99.8
  intermittent (bilious) — *see also* Malaria
    of unknown origin R50.9
    pernicious B50.9
  iodide R50.2
  Japanese river A75.3
  jungle — *see also* Malaria
    yellow A95.0
  Junin (virus) hemorrhagic A96.0
  Katayama B65.2
  kedani A75.3
  Kenya (tick) A77.1
  Kew Garden A79.1
  Korean hemorrhagic A98.5
  Lassa A96.2
  Lone Star A77.0
  Machupo (virus) hemorrhagic A96.1
  malaria, malarial — *see* Malaria
  Malta A23.9
  Marseilles A77.1
  marsh — *see* Malaria
  Mayaro (viral) A92.8
  Mediterranean — *see also* Brucellosis A23.9
    familial M04.1
    tick A77.1
  meningeal — *see* Meningitis

☑ **Additional Character Required** — Refer to the Tabular List for Character Selection
  Subterms under main terms may continue to next column or page

Fever — *continued*
Meuse A79.0
Mexican A75.2
mianeh A68.1
miasmatic — *see* Malaria
mosquito-borne (viral) A92.9
  hemorrhagic A92.8
mountain — *see also* Brucellosis
  meaning Rocky Mountain spotted fever A77.0
  tick (American) (Colorado) (viral) A93.2
Mucambo (viral) A92.8
mud A27.9
Neapolitan — *see* Brucellosis
neutropenic D70.9
newborn P81.9
  environmental P81.0
Nine-Mile A78
non-exanthematous tick A93.2
North Asian tick-borne A77.2
Omsk hemorrhagic A98.1
O'nyong-nyong (viral) A92.1
Oropouche (viral) A93.0
Oroya A44.0
pacific coast tick A77.8
paludal — *see* Malaria
Panama (malarial) B50.9
Pappataci A93.1
paratyphoid A01.4
  A A01.1
  B A01.2
  C A01.3
parrot A70
periodic (Mediterranean) M04.1
persistent (of unknown origin) R50.9
petechial A39.0
pharyngoconjunctival B30.2
Philippine hemorrhagic A91
phlebotomus A93.1
Piry (virus) A93.8
Pixuna (viral) A92.8
Plasmodium ovale B53.0
polioviral (nonparalytic) A80.4
Pontiac A48.2
postimmunization R50.83
postoperative R50.82
  due to infection T81.40 ☑
posttransfusion R50.84
postvaccination R50.83
presenting with conditions classified elsewhere R50.81
pretibial A27.89
puerperal O86.4
Q A78
quadrilateral A78
quartan (malaria) B52.9
Queensland (coastal) (tick) A77.3
quintan A79.0
rabbit — *see* Tularemia
rat-bite A25.9
  due to
    Spirillum A25.0
    Streptobacillus moniliformis A25.1
recurrent — *see* Fever, relapsing
relapsing (Borrelia) A68.9
  Carter's (Asiatic) A68.1
  Dutton's (West African) A68.1
  Koch's A68.9
  louse-borne A68.0
  Novy's
    louse-borne A68.0
    tick-borne A68.1
  Obermeyer's (European) A68.0
  tick-borne A68.1
remittent (bilious) (congestive) (gastric) — *see* Malaria
rheumatic (active) (acute) (chronic) (subacute) I00
  with central nervous system involvement I02.9
  active with heart involvement — *see* category I01 ☑
  inactive or quiescent with
    cardiac hypertrophy I09.89
    carditis I09.9
    endocarditis I09.1
      aortic (valve) I06.9
        with mitral (valve) disease I08.0
      mitral (valve) I05.9
        with aortic (valve) disease I08.0
      pulmonary (valve) I09.89
      tricuspid (valve) I07.8
    heart disease NEC I09.89

Fever — *continued*
rheumatic — *continued*
  inactive or quiescent with — *continued*
    heart failure (congestive) (conditions in category I50.) I09.81
    left ventricular failure (conditions in I50.1-I50.4-) I09.81
    myocarditis, myocardial degeneration (conditions in I51.4) I09.0
    pancarditis I09.9
    pericarditis I09.2
Rift Valley (viral) A92.4
Rocky Mountain spotted A77.0
rose J30.1
Ross River B33.1
Russian hemorrhagic A98.5
San Joaquin (Valley) B38.0
sandfly A93.1
Sao Paulo A77.0
scarlet A38.9
seven day (leptospirosis) (autumnal) (Japanese) A27.89
  dengue A90
shin-bone A79.0
Singapore hemorrhagic A91
solar A90
Songo A98.5
sore B00.1
South African tick-bite A68.1
Southeast Asia hemorrhagic A91
spinal — *see* Meningitis
spirillary A25.0
splenic — *see* Anthrax
spotted A77.9
  American A77.0
  Brazilian A77.0
  cerebrospinal meningitis A39.0
  Colombian A77.0
  due to Rickettsia
    africae (African tick bite fever) A77.8
    australis A77.3
    conorii A77.1
    parkeri A77.8
    rickettsii A77.0
    sibirica A77.2
    specified type NEC A77.8
  Ehrlichiosis A77.40
    due to
      E. chaffeensis A77.41
      specified organism NEC A77.49
  Rocky Mountain A77.0
steroid R50.2
streptobacillary A25.1
subtertian B50.9
Sumatran mite A75.3
sun A90
swamp A27.9
swine A02.8
sylvatic, yellow A95.0
Tahyna B33.8
tertian — *see* Malaria, tertian
Thailand hemorrhagic A91
thermic T67.01 ☑
three-day A93.1
tick
  American mountain A93.2
  Colorado A93.2
  Kemerovo A93.8
  Mediterranean A77.1
  mountain A93.2
  nonexanthematous A93.2
  Quaranfil A93.8
tick-bite NEC A93.8
tick-borne (hemorrhagic) NEC A93.8
trench A79.0
tsutsugamushi A75.3
typhogastric A01.00
typhoid (abortive) (hemorrhagic) (intermittent) (malignant) A01.00
  complicated by
    arthritis A01.04
    heart involvement A01.02
    meningitis A01.01
    osteomyelitis A01.05
    pneumonia A01.03
    specified NEC A01.09
typhomalarial — *see* Malaria
typhus — *see* Typhus (fever)
undulant — *see* Brucellosis

Fever — *continued*
unknown origin R50.9
uveoparotid D86.89
valley B38.0
Venezuelan equine A92.2
vesicular stomatitis A93.8
viral hemorrhagic — *see* Fever, hemorrhagic, by type of virus
Volhynian A79.0
Wesselsbron (viral) A92.8
West
  African B50.8
  Nile (viral) A92.30
    with
      complications NEC A92.39
      cranial nerve disorders A92.32
      encephalitis A92.31
      encephalomyelitis A92.31
      neurologic manifestation NEC A92.32
      optic neuritis A92.32
      polyradiculitis A92.32
Whitmore's — *see* Melioidosis
Wolhynian A79.0
worm B83.9
yellow A95.9
  jungle A95.0
  sylvatic A95.0
  urban A95.1
Zika virus A92.5
Fibrillation
atrial or auricular (established) I48.91
  chronic I48.20
    persistent I48.19
  paroxysmal I48.0
  permanent I48.21
  persistent (chronic) (NOS) (other) I48.19
    longstanding I48.11
cardiac I49.8
heart I49.8
muscular M62.89
ventricular I49.01
Fibrin
ball or bodies, pleural (sac) J94.1
chamber, anterior (eye) (gelatinous exudate) — *see* Iridocyclitis, acute
Fibrinogenolysis — *see* Fibrinolysis
Fibrinogenopenia D68.8
acquired D65
congenital D68.2
Fibrinolysis (hemorrhagic) (acquired) D65
antepartum hemorrhage — *see* Hemorrhage, antepartum, with coagulation defect
following
  abortion — *see* Abortion by type complicated by hemorrhage
  ectopic or molar pregnancy O08.1
intrapartum O67.0
newborn, transient P60
postpartum O72.3
Fibrinopenia (hereditary) D68.2
acquired D68.4
Fibrinopurulent — *see* condition
Fibrinous — *see* condition
Fibroadenoma
cellular intracanalicular D24- ☑
giant D24- ☑
intracanalicular
  cellular D24- ☑
  giant D24- ☑
  specified site — *see* Neoplasm, benign, by site
  unspecified site D24- ☑
juvenile D24- ☑
pericanalicular
  specified site — *see* Neoplasm, benign, by site
  unspecified site D24- ☑
phyllodes D24- ☑
prostate D29.1
specified site NEC — *see* Neoplasm, benign, by site
unspecified site D24- ☑
Fibroadenosis, breast (chronic) (cystic) (diffuse) (periodic) (segmental) N60.2- ☑
Fibroangioma — *see also* Neoplasm, benign, by site
juvenile
  specified site — *see* Neoplasm, benign, by site
  unspecified site D10.6
Fibrochondrosarcoma — *see* Neoplasm, cartilage, malignant

Fibrocystic — Fiedler's

Fibrocystic
disease — *see also* Fibrosis, cystic
  breast — *see* Mastopathy, cystic
  jaw M27.49
  kidney (congenital) Q61.8
  liver Q44.6
  pancreas E84.9
kidney (congenital) Q61.8
Fibrodysplasia ossificans progressiva — *see* Myositis, ossificans, progressiva
Fibroelastosis (cordis) (endocardial) (endomyocardial) I42.4
Fibroid (tumor) — *see also* Neoplasm, connective tissue, benign
disease, lung (chronic) — *see* Fibrosis, lung
heart (disease) — *see* Myocarditis
in pregnancy or childbirth O34.1- ☑
  causing obstructed labor O65.5
induration, lung (chronic) — *see* Fibrosis, lung
lung — *see* Fibrosis, lung
pneumonia (chronic) — *see* Fibrosis, lung
uterus — *see also* Leiomyoma, uterus D25.9
Fibrolipoma — *see* Lipoma
Fibroliposarcoma — *see* Neoplasm, connective tissue, malignant
Fibroma — *see also* Neoplasm, connective tissue, benign
ameloblastic — *see* Cyst, calcifying odontogenic
bone (nonossifying) — *see* Disorder, bone, specified type NEC
  ossifying — *see* Neoplasm, bone, benign
cementifying — *see* Neoplasm, bone, benign
chondromyxoid — *see* Neoplasm, bone, benign
desmoplastic — *see* Neoplasm, connective tissue, uncertain behavior
durum — *see* Neoplasm, connective tissue, benign
fascial — *see* Neoplasm, connective tissue, benign
invasive — *see* Neoplasm, connective tissue, uncertain behavior
molle — *see* Lipoma
myxoid — *see* Neoplasm, connective tissue, benign
nasopharynx, nasopharyngeal (juvenile) D10.6
nonosteogenic (nonossifying) — *see* Dysplasia, fibrous
odontogenic (central) — *see* Cyst, calcifying odontogenic
ossifying — *see* Neoplasm, bone, benign
periosteal — *see* Neoplasm, bone, benign
soft — *see* Lipoma
Fibromatosis M72.9
abdominal — *see* Neoplasm, connective tissue, uncertain behavior
aggressive — *see* Neoplasm, connective tissue, uncertain behavior
congenital generalized — *see* Neoplasm, connective tissue, uncertain behavior
Dupuytren's M72.0
gingival K06.1
palmar (fascial) M72.0
plantar (fascial) M72.2
pseudosarcomatous (proliferative) (subcutaneous) M72.4
retroperitoneal D48.3
specified NEC M72.8
Fibromyalgia M79.7
Fibromyoma — *see also* Neoplasm, connective tissue, benign
uterus (corpus) — *see also* Leiomyoma, uterus
  in pregnancy or childbirth — *see* Fibroid, in pregnancy or childbirth
    causing obstructed labor O65.5
Fibromyositis M79.7
Fibromyxolipoma D17.9
Fibromyxoma — *see* Neoplasm, connective tissue, benign
Fibromyxosarcoma — *see* Neoplasm, connective tissue, malignant
Fibro-odontoma, ameloblastic — *see* Cyst, calcifying odontogenic
Fibro-osteoma — *see* Neoplasm, bone, benign
Fibroplasia, retrolental H35.17- ☑
Fibropurulent — *see* condition
Fibrosarcoma — *see also* Neoplasm, connective tissue, malignant
ameloblastic C41.1
  upper jaw (bone) C41.0
congenital — *see* Neoplasm, connective tissue, malignant
fascial — *see* Neoplasm, connective tissue, malignant

Fibrosarcoma — *continued*
infantile — *see* Neoplasm, connective tissue, malignant
odontogenic C41.1
  upper jaw (bone) C41.0
periosteal — *see* Neoplasm, bone, malignant
Fibrosclerosis
breast N60.3- ☑
multifocal M35.5
penis (corpora cavernosa) N48.6
Fibrosis, fibrotic
adrenal (gland) E27.8
amnion O41.8X- ☑
anal papillae K62.89
arteriocapillary — *see* Arteriosclerosis
bladder N32.89
  interstitial — *see* Cystitis, chronic, interstitial
  localized submucosal — *see* Cystitis, chronic, interstitial
  panmural — *see* Cystitis, chronic, interstitial
breast — *see* Fibrosclerosis, breast
capillary — *see also* Arteriosclerosis I70.90
  lung (chronic) — *see* Fibrosis, lung
cardiac — *see* Myocarditis
cervix N88.8
chorion O41.8X- ☑
corpus cavernosum (sclerosing) N48.6
cystic (of pancreas) E84.9
  with
    distal intestinal obstruction syndrome E84.19
    fecal impaction E84.19
    intestinal manifestations NEC E84.19
    pulmonary manifestations E84.0
    specified manifestations NEC E84.8
due to device, implant or graft — *see also* Complications, by site and type, specified NEC T85.828 ☑
  arterial graft NEC T82.828 ☑
  breast (implant) T85.828 ☑
  catheter NEC T85.828 ☑
    dialysis (renal) T82.828 ☑
      intraperitoneal T85.828 ☑
    infusion NEC T82.828 ☑
      spinal (epidural) (subdural) T85.820 ☑
    urinary (indwelling) T83.82 ☑
  electronic (electrode) (pulse generator) (stimulator)
    bone T84.82 ☑
    cardiac T82.827 ☑
    nervous system (brain) (peripheral nerve) (spinal) T85.820 ☑
    urinary T83.82 ☑
  fixation, internal (orthopedic) NEC T84.82 ☑
  gastrointestinal (bile duct) (esophagus) T85.828 ☑
  genital NEC T83.82 ☑
  heart NEC T82.827 ☑
  joint prosthesis T84.82 ☑
  ocular (corneal graft) (orbital implant) NEC T85.828 ☑
  orthopedic NEC T84.82 ☑
  specified NEC T85.828 ☑
  urinary NEC T83.82 ☑
  vascular NEC T82.828 ☑
  ventricular intracranial shunt T85.820 ☑
ejaculatory duct N50.89
endocardium — *see* Endocarditis
endomyocardial (tropical) I42.3
epididymis N50.89
eye muscle — *see* Strabismus, mechanical
heart — *see* Myocarditis
hepatic — *see* Fibrosis, liver
hepatolienal (portal hypertension) K76.6
hepatosplenic (portal hypertension) K76.6
infrapatellar fat pad M79.4
intrascrotal N50.89
kidney N26.9
liver K74.00
  with sclerosis K74.2
  advanced K74.02
  alcoholic K70.2
  early K74.01
  stage
    F1 or F2 K74.01
    F3 K74.02
lung (atrophic) (chronic) (confluent) (massive) (perialveolar) (peribronchial) J84.10
  with
    anthracosilicosis J60
    anthracosis J60
    asbestosis J61

Fibrosis, fibrotic — *continued*
lung — *continued*
  with — *continued*
    bagassosis J67.1
    bauxite J63.1
    berylliosis J63.2
    byssinosis J66.0
    calcicosis J62.8
    chalicosis J62.8
    dust reticulation J64
    farmer's lung J67.0
    ganister disease J62.8
    graphite J63.3
    pneumoconiosis NOS J64
    siderosis J63.4
    silicosis J62.8
  capillary J84.10
  congenital P27.8
  diffuse (idiopathic) J84.10
    chemicals, gases, fumes or vapors (inhalation) J68.4
    interstitial J84.10
      acute J84.114
    talc J62.0
  following radiation J70.1
  idiopathic J84.112
  postinflammatory J84.10
  silicotic J62.8
  tuberculous — *see* Tuberculosis, pulmonary
lymphatic gland I89.8
median bar — *see* Hyperplasia, prostate
mediastinum (idiopathic) J98.59
meninges G96.198
myocardium, myocardial — *see* Myocarditis
ovary N83.8
oviduct N83.8
pancreas K86.89
penis NEC N48.6
pericardium I31.0
perineum, in pregnancy or childbirth O34.7- ☑
  causing obstructed labor O65.5
pleura J94.1
popliteal fat pad M79.4
prostate (chronic) — *see* Hyperplasia, prostate
pulmonary — *see also* Fibrosis, lung J84.10
  congenital P27.8
  idiopathic J84.112
rectal sphincter K62.89
retroperitoneal, idiopathic (with ureteral obstruction) N13.5
  with infection N13.6
sclerosing mesenteric (idiopathic) K65.4
scrotum N50.89
seminal vesicle N50.89
senile R54
skin L90.5
spermatic cord N50.89
spleen D73.89
  in schistosomiasis (bilharziasis) B65.9 [D77]
subepidermal nodular — *see* Neoplasm, skin, benign
submucous (oral) (tongue) K13.5
testis N44.8
  chronic, due to syphilis A52.76
thymus (gland) E32.8
tongue, submucous K13.5
tunica vaginalis N50.89
uterus (non-neoplastic) N85.8
vagina N89.8
valve, heart — *see* Endocarditis
vas deferens N50.89
vein I87.8
Fibrositis (periarticular) M79.7
nodular, chronic (Jaccoud's) (rheumatoid) — *see* Arthropathy, postrheumatic, chronic
Fibrothorax J94.1
Fibrotic — *see* Fibrosis
Fibrous — *see* condition
Fibroxanthoma — *see also* Neoplasm, connective tissue, benign
atypical — *see* Neoplasm, connective tissue, uncertain behavior
malignant — *see* Neoplasm, connective tissue, malignant
Fibroxanthosarcoma — *see* Neoplasm, connective tissue, malignant
Fiedler's
disease (icterohemorrhagic leptospirosis) A27.0
myocarditis (acute) I40.1

Fifth disease B08.3
    venereal A55
Filaria, filarial, filariasis — *see* Infestation, filarial
Filatov's disease — *see* Mononucleosis, infectious
File-cutter's disease — *see* Poisoning, lead
Filling defect
    biliary tract R93.2
    bladder R93.41
    duodenum R93.3
    gallbladder R93.2
    gastrointestinal tract R93.3
    intestine R93.3
    kidney R93.42- ☑
    stomach R93.3
    ureter R93.41
    urinary organs, specified NEC R93.49
Fimbrial cyst Q50.4
Financial problem affecting care NOS Z59.9
    bankruptcy Z59.89
    foreclosure on loan Z59.89
    home loan Z59.81- ☑
Findings, abnormal, inconclusive, without diagnosis
    — *see also* Abnormal
    17-ketosteroids, elevated R82.5
    acetonuria R82.4
    alcohol in blood R78.0
    anisocytosis R71.8
    antenatal screening of mother O28.9
        biochemical O28.1
        chromosomal O28.5
        cytological O28.2
        genetic O28.5
        hematological O28.0
        radiological O28.4
        specified NEC O28.8
        ultrasonic O28.3
    antibody titer, elevated R76.0
    anticardiolipin antibody R76.0
    antiphosphatidylglycerol antibody R76.0
    antiphosphatidylinositol antibody R76.0
    antiphosphatidylserine antibody R76.0
    antiphospholipid antibody R76.0
    bacteriuria R82.71
    bicarbonate E87.8
    bile in urine R82.2
    blood sugar R73.09
        high R73.9
        low (transient) E16.2
    body fluid or substance, specified NEC R88.8
    casts, urine R82.998
    catecholamines R82.5
    cells, urine R82.998
    chloride E87.8
    cholesterol E78.9
        high E78.00
            with high triglycerides E78.2
    chyluria R82.0
    cloudy
        dialysis effluent R88.0
        urine R82.90
    creatinine clearance R94.4
    crystals, urine R82.998
    culture
        blood R78.81
        positive — *see* Positive, culture
    echocardiogram R93.1
    electrolyte level, urinary R82.998
    function study NEC R94.8
        bladder R94.8
        endocrine NEC R94.7
            thyroid R94.6
        kidney R94.4
        liver R94.5
        pancreas R94.8
        placenta R94.8
        pulmonary R94.2
        spleen R94.8
    gallbladder, nonvisualization R93.2
    glucose (tolerance test) (non-fasting) R73.09
    glycosuria R81
    heart
        shadow R93.1
        sounds R01.2
    hematinuria R82.3
    hematocrit drop (precipitous) R71.0
    hemoglobinuria R82.3

Findings, abnormal, inconclusive, without diagnosis
    — *continued*
    human papillomavirus (HPV) DNA test positive
        cervix
            high risk R87.810
            low risk R87.820
        vagina
            high risk R87.811
            low risk R87.821
    in blood (of substance not normally found in blood)
        R78.9
        addictive drug NEC R78.4
        alcohol (excessive level) R78.0
        cocaine R78.2
        hallucinogen R78.3
        heavy metals (abnormal level) R78.79
        lead R78.71
        lithium (abnormal level) R78.89
        opiate drug R78.1
        psychotropic drug R78.5
        specified substance NEC R78.89
        steroid agent R78.6
    indoleacetic acid, elevated R82.5
    ketonuria R82.4
    lactic acid dehydrogenase (LDH) R74.02
    liver function test — *see also* Elevated, liver function,
        test R79.89
    mammogram NEC R92.8
        calcification (calculus) R92.1
        inconclusive result (due to dense breasts) R92.2
        microcalcification R92.0
    mediastinal shift R93.89
    melanin, urine R82.998
    myoglobinuria R82.1
    neonatal screening — *see* Abnormal, neonatal
        screening
    newborn screens, state mandated — *see* Abnormal,
        neonatal screening
    nonvisualization of gallbladder R93.2
    odor of urine NOS R82.90
    Papanicolaou cervix R87.619
        non-atypical endometrial cells R87.618
    pneumoencephalogram R93.0
    poikilocytosis R71.8
    potassium (deficiency) E87.6
        excess E87.5
    PPD R76.11
    radiologic (X-ray) R93.89
        abdomen R93.5
        biliary tract R93.2
        breast R92.8
        gastrointestinal tract R93.3
        genitourinary organs R93.89
        head R93.0
        inconclusive due to excess body fat of patient R93.9
        intrathoracic organs NEC R93.1
        musculoskeletal
            limbs R93.6
            other than limb R93.7
        placenta R93.89
        retroperitoneum R93.5
        skin R93.89
        skull R93.0
        subcutaneous tissue R93.89
        testis R93.81- ☑
    red blood cell (count) (morphology) (sickling) (volume)
        R71.8
    scan NEC R94.8
        bladder R94.8
        bone R94.8
        kidney R94.4
        liver R93.2
        lung R94.2
        pancreas R94.8
        placental R94.8
        spleen R94.8
        thyroid R94.6
    sedimentation rate, elevated R70.0
    SGOT R74.01
    SGPT R74.01
    sodium (deficiency) E87.1
        excess E87.0
    specified body fluid NEC R88.8
    stress test R94.39
    testis R93.81- ☑
    thyroid (function) (metabolic rate) (scan) (uptake) R94.6
    transaminase (level) R74.01
    triglycerides E78.9
        high E78.1

Findings, abnormal, inconclusive, without diagnosis
    — *continued*
    triglycerides — *continued*
        high — *continued*
            with high cholesterol E78.2
    tuberculin skin test (without active tuberculosis) R76.11
    urine R82.90
        acetone R82.4
        bacteria R82.71
        bile R82.2
        casts or cells R82.998
        chyle R82.0
        culture positive R82.79
        glucose R81
        hemoglobin R82.3
        ketone R82.4
        sugar R81
    vanillylmandelic acid (VMA), elevated R82.5
    vectorcardiogram (VCG) R94.39
    ventriculogram R93.0
    white blood cell (count) (differential) (morphology)
        D72.9
    xerography R92.8
Finger — *see* condition
Fire, Saint Anthony's — *see* Erysipelas
Fire-setting
    pathological (compulsive) F63.1
Fish hook stomach K31.89
Fishmeal-worker's lung J67.8
Fissure, fissured
    anus, anal K60.2
        acute K60.0
        chronic K60.1
        congenital Q43.8
    ear, lobule, congenital Q17.8
    epiglottis (congenital) Q31.8
    larynx J38.7
        congenital Q31.8
    lip K13.0
        congenital — *see* Cleft, lip
    nipple N64.0
        associated with
            lactation O92.13
            pregnancy O92.11- ☑
            puerperium O92.12
    nose Q30.2
    palate (congenital) — *see* Cleft, palate
    skin R23.4
    spine (congenital) — *see also* Spina bifida
        with hydrocephalus — *see* Spina bifida, by site, with
            hydrocephalus
    tongue (acquired) K14.5
        congenital Q38.3
Fistula (cutaneous) L98.8
    abdomen (wall) K63.2
        bladder N32.2
        intestine NEC K63.2
        ureter N28.89
        uterus N82.5
    abdominorectal K63.2
    abdominosigmoidal K63.2
    abdominothoracic J86.0
    abdominouterine N82.5
        congenital Q51.7
    abdominovesical N32.2
    accessory sinuses — *see* Sinusitis
    actinomycotic — *see* Actinomycosis
    alveolar antrum — *see* Sinusitis, maxillary
    alveolar process K04.6
    anorectal K60.5
    antrobuccal — *see* Sinusitis, maxillary
    antrum — *see* Sinusitis, maxillary
    anus, anal (recurrent) (infectional) K60.3
        congenital Q43.6
            with absence, atresia and stenosis Q42.2
        tuberculous A18.32
    aorta-duodenal I77.2
    appendix, appendicular K38.3
    arteriovenous (acquired) (nonruptured) I77.0
        brain I67.1
            congenital Q28.2
                ruptured — *see* Fistula, arteriovenous, brain,
                    ruptured
                ruptured I60.8
                    intracerebral I61.8
                    intraparenchymal I61.8
                    intraventricular I61.5
                    subarachnoid I60.8

▽ **Subterms under main terms may continue to next column or page**   ☑ **Additional Character Required** — **Refer to the Tabular List for Character Selection**   **147**

Fifth disease — Fistula

Fistula — *continued*
  arteriovenous — *continued*
    cerebral — *see* Fistula, arteriovenous, brain
    congenital (peripheral) — *see also* Malformation, arteriovenous
      brain Q28.2
        ruptured — *see* Fistula, arteriovenous, brain, ruptured
      coronary Q24.5
      pulmonary Q25.72
    coronary I25.41
      congenital Q24.5
    pulmonary I28.0
      congenital Q25.72
    surgically created (for dialysis) Z99.2
      complication — *see* Complication, arteriovenous, fistula, surgically created
    traumatic — *see* Injury, blood vessel
  artery I77.2
  aural (mastoid) — *see* Mastoiditis, chronic
  auricle — *see also* Disorder, pinna, specified type NEC
    congenital Q18.1
  Bartholin's gland N82.8
  bile duct (common) (hepatic) K83.3
    with calculus, stones — *see also* Calculus, bile duct K83.3
  biliary (tract) — *see* Fistula, bile duct
  bladder (sphincter) NEC — *see also* Fistula, vesico- N32.2
    into seminal vesicle N32.2
  bone — *see also* Disorder, bone, specified type NEC
    with osteomyelitis, chronic — *see* Osteomyelitis, chronic, with draining sinus
  brain G93.89
    arteriovenous (acquired) — *see also* Fistula, arteriovenous, brain I67.1
      congenital Q28.2
  branchial (cleft) Q18.0
  branchiogenous Q18.0
  breast N61.0
    puerperal, postpartum or gestational, due to mastitis (purulent) — *see* Mastitis, obstetric, purulent
  bronchial J86.0
  bronchocutaneous, bronchomediastinal, bronchopleural, bronchopleuromediastinal (infective) J86.0
    tuberculous NEC A15.5
  bronchoesophageal J86.0
    congenital Q39.2
      with atresia of esophagus Q39.1
  bronchovisceral J86.0
  buccal cavity (infective) K12.2
  cecosigmoidal K63.2
  cecum K63.2
  cerebrospinal (fluid) G96.08
  cervical, lateral Q18.1
  cervicoaural Q18.1
  cervicosigmoidal N82.4
  cervicovesical N82.1
  cervix N82.8
  chest (wall) J86.0
  cholecystenteric — *see* Fistula, gallbladder
  cholecystocolic — *see* Fistula, gallbladder
  cholecystocolonic — *see* Fistula, gallbladder
  cholecystoduodenal — *see* Fistula, gallbladder
  cholecystogastric — *see* Fistula, gallbladder
  cholecystointestinal — *see* Fistula, gallbladder
  choledochoduodenal — *see* Fistula, bile duct
  cholocolic K82.3
  coccyx — *see* Sinus, pilonidal
  colon K63.2
  colostomy K94.09
  colovesical N32.1
  common duct — *see* Fistula, bile duct
  congenital, site not listed — *see* Anomaly, by site
  coronary, arteriovenous I25.41
    congenital Q24.5
  costal region J86.0
  cul-de-sac, Douglas' N82.8
  cystic duct — *see also* Fistula, gallbladder
    congenital Q44.5
  dental K04.6
  diaphragm J86.0
  duodenum K31.6
  ear (external) (canal) — *see* Disorder, ear, external, specified type NEC
  enterocolic K63.2
  enterocutaneous K63.2
  enterouterine N82.4

Fistula — *continued*
  enterouterine — *continued*
    congenital Q51.7
  enterovaginal N82.4
    congenital Q52.2
    large intestine N82.3
    small intestine N82.2
  enterovesical N32.1
  epididymis N50.89
    tuberculous A18.15
  esophagobronchial J86.0
    congenital Q39.2
      with atresia of esophagus Q39.1
  esophagocutaneous K22.89
  esophagopleural-cutaneous J86.0
  esophagotracheal J86.0
    congenital Q39.2
      with atresia of esophagus Q39.1
  esophagus K22.89
    congenital Q39.2
      with atresia of esophagus Q39.1
  ethmoid — *see* Sinusitis, ethmoidal
  eyeball (cornea) (sclera) — *see* Disorder, globe, hypotony
  eyelid H01.8
  fallopian tube, external N82.5
  fecal K63.2
    congenital Q43.6
  from periapical abscess K04.6
  frontal sinus — *see* Sinusitis, frontal
  gallbladder K82.3
    with calculus, cholelithiasis, stones — *see* Calculus, gallbladder
  gastric K31.6
  gastrocolic K31.6
    congenital Q40.2
    tuberculous A18.32
  gastroenterocolic K31.6
  gastroesophageal K31.6
  gastrojejunal K31.6
  gastrojejunocolic K31.6
  genital tract (female) N82.9
    specified NEC N82.8
    to intestine NEC N82.4
    to skin N82.5
  hepatic artery-portal vein, congenital Q26.6
  hepatopleural J86.0
  hepatopulmonary J86.0
  ileorectal or ileosigmoidal K63.2
  ileovaginal N82.2
  ileovesical N32.1
  ileum K63.2
  in ano K60.3
    tuberculous A18.32
  inner ear (labyrinth) — *see* subcategory H83.1 ☑
  intestine NEC K63.2
  intestinocolonic (abdominal) K63.2
  intestinoureteral N28.89
  intestinouterine N82.4
  intestinovaginal N82.4
    large intestine N82.3
    small intestine N82.2
  intestinovesical N32.1
  ischiorectal (fossa) K61.39
  jejunum K63.2
  joint M25.10
    ankle M25.17- ☑
    elbow M25.12- ☑
    foot joint M25.17- ☑
    hand joint M25.14- ☑
    hip M25.15- ☑
    knee M25.16- ☑
    shoulder M25.11- ☑
    specified joint NEC M25.18
    tuberculous — *see* Tuberculosis, joint
    vertebrae M25.18
    wrist M25.13- ☑
  kidney N28.89
  labium (majus) (minus) N82.8
  labyrinth — *see* subcategory H83.1 ☑
  lacrimal (gland) (sac) H04.61- ☑
  lacrimonasal duct — *see* Fistula, lacrimal
  laryngotracheal, congenital Q34.8
  larynx J38.7
  lip K13.0
    congenital Q38.0
  lumbar, tuberculous A18.01
  lung J86.0

Fistula — *continued*
  lymphatic I89.8
  mammary (gland) N61.0
  mastoid (process) (region) — *see* Mastoiditis, chronic
  maxillary J32.0
  medial, face and neck Q18.8
  mediastinal J86.0
  mediastinobronchial J86.0
  mediastinocutaneous J86.0
  middle ear — *see* subcategory H74.8 ☑
  mouth K12.2
  nasal J34.89
    sinus — *see* Sinusitis
  nasopharynx J39.2
  nipple N64.0
  nose J34.89
  oral (cutaneous) K12.2
    maxillary J32.0
    nasal (with cleft palate) — *see* Cleft, palate
  orbit, orbital — *see* Disorder, orbit, specified type NEC
  oroantral J32.0
  oviduct, external N82.5
  palate (hard) M27.8
  pancreatic K86.89
  pancreaticoduodenal K86.89
  parotid (gland) K11.4
    region K12.2
  penis N48.89
  perianal K60.3
  pericardium (pleura) (sac) — *see* Pericarditis
  pericecal K63.2
  perineorectal K60.4
  perineosigmoidal K63.2
  perineum, perineal (with urethral involvement) NEC N36.0
    tuberculous A18.13
    ureter N28.89
  perirectal K60.4
    tuberculous A18.32
  peritoneum K65.9
  pharyngoesophageal J39.2
  pharynx J39.2
    branchial cleft (congenital) Q18.0
  pilonidal (infected) (rectum) — *see* Sinus, pilonidal
  pleura, pleural, pleurocutaneous, pleuroperitoneal J86.0
    tuberculous NEC A15.6
  pleuropericardial I31.8
  portal vein-hepatic artery, congenital Q26.6
  postauricular H70.81- ☑
  postoperative, persistent T81.83 ☑
    specified site — *see* Fistula, by site
  preauricular (congenital) Q18.1
  prostate N42.89
  pulmonary J86.0
    arteriovenous I28.0
      congenital Q25.72
    tuberculous — *see* Tuberculosis, pulmonary
  pulmonoperitoneal J86.0
  rectolabial N82.4
  rectosigmoid (intercommunicating) K63.2
  rectoureteral N28.89
  rectourethral N36.0
    congenital Q64.73
  rectouterine N82.4
    congenital Q51.7
  rectovaginal N82.3
    congenital Q52.2
    tuberculous A18.18
  rectovesical N32.1
    congenital Q64.79
  rectovesicovaginal N82.3
  rectovulval N82.4
    congenital Q52.79
  rectum (to skin) K60.4
    congenital Q43.6
      with absence, atresia and stenosis Q42.0
    tuberculous A18.32
  renal N28.89
  retroauricular — *see* Fistula, postauricular
  salivary duct or gland (any) K11.4
    congenital Q38.4
  scrotum (urinary) N50.89
    tuberculous A18.15
  semicircular canals — *see* subcategory H83.1 ☑
  sigmoid K63.2
    to bladder N32.1
  sinus — *see* Sinusitis

☑ **Additional Character Required** — Refer to the Tabular List for Character Selection   ▽ Subterms under main terms may continue to next column or page

Fistula — *continued*
  skin L98.8
    to genital tract (female) N82.5
  splenocolic D73.89
  stercoral K63.2
  stomach K31.6
  sublingual gland K11.4
  submandibular gland K11.4
  submaxillary (gland) K11.4
    region K12.2
  thoracic J86.0
    duct I89.8
  thoracoabdominal J86.0
  thoracogastric J86.0
  thoracointestinal J86.0
  thorax J86.0
  thyroglossal duct Q89.2
  thyroid E07.89
  trachea, congenital (external) (internal) Q32.1
  tracheoesophageal J86.0
    congenital Q39.2
      with atresia of esophagus Q39.1
    following tracheostomy J95.04
  traumatic arteriovenous — *see* Injury, blood vessel, by site
  tuberculous — *code by* site under Tuberculosis
  typhoid A01.09
  umbilicourinary Q64.8
  urachus, congenital Q64.4
  ureter (persistent) N28.89
  ureteroabdominal N28.89
  ureterorectal N28.89
  ureterosigmoido-abdominal N28.89
  ureterovaginal N82.1
  ureterovesical N32.2
  urethra N36.0
    congenital Q64.79
    tuberculous A18.13
  urethroperineal N36.0
  urethroperineovesical N32.2
  urethrorectal N36.0
    congenital Q64.73
  urethroscrotal N50.89
  urethrovaginal N82.1
  urethrovesical N32.2
  urinary (tract) (persistent) (recurrent) N36.0
  uteroabdominal N82.5
    congenital Q51.7
  uteroenteric, uterointestinal N82.4
    congenital Q51.7
  uterorectal N82.4
    congenital Q51.7
  uteroureteric N82.1
  uterourethral Q51.7
  uterovaginal N82.8
  uterovesical N82.1
    congenital Q51.7
  uterus N82.8
  vagina (postpartal) (wall) N82.8
  vaginocutaneous (postpartal) N82.5
  vaginointestinal NEC N82.4
    large intestine N82.3
    small intestine N82.2
  vaginoperineal N82.5
  vasocutaneous, congenital Q55.7
  vesical NEC N32.2
  vesicoabdominal N32.2
  vesicocervicovaginal N82.1
  vesicocolic N32.1
  vesicocutaneous N32.2
  vesicoenteric N32.1
  vesicointestinal N32.1
  vesicometrorectal N82.4
  vesicoperineal N32.2
  vesicorectal N32.1
    congenital Q64.79
  vesicosigmoidal N32.1
  vesicosigmoidovaginal N82.3
  vesicoureteral N32.2
  vesicoureterovaginal N82.1
  vesicourethral N32.2
  vesicourethrorectal N32.1
  vesicouterine N82.1
    congenital Q51.7
  vesicovaginal N82.0
  vulvorectal N82.4
    congenital Q52.79
Fit R56.9
  epileptic — *see* Epilepsy

Fit — *continued*
  fainting R55
  hysterical F44.5
  newborn P90
Fitting (and adjustment) (of)
  artificial
    arm — *see* Admission, adjustment, artificial, arm
    breast Z44.3 ☑
    eye Z44.2 ☑
    leg — *see* Admission, adjustment, artificial, leg
  automatic implantable cardiac defibrillator (with synchronous cardiac pacemaker) Z45.02
  brain neuropacemaker Z46.2
    implanted Z45.42
  cardiac defibrillator — *see* Fitting (and adjustment) (of), automatic implantable cardiac defibrillator
  catheter, non-vascular Z46.82
  colostomy belt Z46.89
  contact lenses Z46.0
  CRT-D (resynchronization therapy defibrillator) Z45.02
  CRT-P (cardiac resynchronization therapy pacemaker) Z45.018
    pulse generator Z45.010
  cystostomy device Z46.6
  defibrillator, cardiac — *see* Fitting (and adjustment) (of), automatic implantable cardiac defibrillator
  dentures Z46.3
  device NOS Z46.9
    abdominal Z46.89
    gastrointestinal NEC Z46.59
    implanted NEC Z45.89
    nervous system Z46.2
      implanted — *see* Admission, adjustment, device, implanted, nervous system
    orthodontic Z46.4
    orthoptic Z46.0
    orthotic Z46.89
    prosthetic (external) Z44.9
      breast Z44.3 ☑
      dental Z46.3
      eye Z44.2 ☑
      specified NEC Z44.8
    specified NEC Z46.89
    substitution
      auditory Z46.2
        implanted — *see* Admission, adjustment, device, implanted, hearing device
      nervous system Z46.2
        implanted — *see* Admission, adjustment, device, implanted, nervous system
      visual Z46.2
        implanted Z45.31
    urinary Z46.6
  gastric lap band Z46.51
  gastrointestinal appliance NEC Z46.59
  glasses (reading) Z46.0
  hearing aid Z46.1
  ileostomy device Z46.89
  insulin pump Z46.81
  intestinal appliance NEC Z46.89
  myringotomy device (stent) (tube) Z45.82
  neuropacemaker Z46.2
    implanted Z45.42
  non-vascular catheter Z46.82
  orthodontic device Z46.4
  orthopedic device (brace) (cast) (corset) (shoes) Z46.89
  pacemaker (cardiac) (cardiac resynchronization therapy (CRT-P)) Z45.018
    nervous system (brain) (peripheral nerve) (spinal cord) Z46.2
      implanted Z45.42
    pulse generator Z45.010
  portacath (port-a-cath) Z45.2
  prosthesis (external) Z44.9
    arm — *see* Admission, adjustment, artificial, arm
    breast Z44.3 ☑
    dental Z46.3
    eye Z44.2 ☑
    leg — *see* Admission, adjustment, artificial, leg
    specified NEC Z44.8
  spectacles Z46.0
  wheelchair Z46.89
Fitzhugh-Curtis syndrome
  due to
    Chlamydia trachomatis A74.81
    Neisseria gonorrhorea (gonococcal peritonitis) A54.85

Fitz's syndrome (acute hemorrhagic pancreatitis) — *see also* Pancreatitis, acute K85.80
Fixation
  joint — *see* Ankylosis
  larynx J38.7
  stapes — *see* Ankylosis, ear ossicles
    deafness — *see* Deafness, conductive
  uterus (acquired) — *see* Malposition, uterus
  vocal cord J38.3
Flabby ridge K06.8
Flaccid — *see also* condition
  palate, congenital Q38.5
Flail
  chest S22.5 ☑
    newborn (birth injury) P13.8
  joint (paralytic) M25.20
    ankle M25.27- ☑
    elbow M25.22- ☑
    foot joint M25.27- ☑
    hand joint M25.24- ☑
    hip M25.25- ☑
    knee M25.26- ☑
    shoulder M25.21- ☑
    specified joint NEC M25.28
    wrist M25.23- ☑
Flajani's disease — *see* Hyperthyroidism, with, goiter (diffuse)
Flap, liver K71.3
Flashbacks (residual to hallucinogen use) F16.283
Flat
  chamber (eye) — *see* Disorder, globe, hypotony, flat anterior chamber
  chest, congenital Q67.8
  foot (acquired) (fixed type) (painful) (postural) — *see also* Deformity, limb, flat foot
    congenital (rigid) (spastic (everted)) Q66.5- ☑
    rachitic sequelae (late effect) E64.3
  organ or site, congenital NEC — *see* Anomaly, by site
  pelvis M95.5
    with disproportion (fetopelvic) O33.0
      causing obstructed labor O65.0
    congenital Q74.2
Flatau-Schilder disease G37.0
Flatback syndrome M40.30
  lumbar region M40.36
  lumbosacral region M40.37
  thoracolumbar region M40.35
Flattening
  head, femur M89.8X5
  hip — *see* Coxa, plana
  lip (congenital) Q18.8
  nose (congenital) Q67.4
    acquired M95.0
Flatulence R14.3
  psychogenic F45.8
Flatus R14.3
  vaginalis N89.8
Flax-dresser's disease J66.1
Flea bite — *see* Injury, bite, by site, superficial, insect
Flecks, glaucomatous (subcapsular) — *see* Cataract, complicated
Fleischer (-Kayser) **ring** (cornea) H18.04- ☑
Fleshy mole O02.0
Flexibilitas cerea — *see* Catalepsy
Flexion
  amputation stump (surgical) T87.89
  cervix — *see* Malposition, uterus
  contracture, joint — *see* Contraction, joint
  deformity, joint — *see also* Deformity, limb, flexion M21.20
    hip, congenital Q65.89
  uterus — *see also* Malposition, uterus
    lateral — *see* Lateroversion, uterus
Flexner-Boyd dysentery A03.2
Flexner's dysentery A03.1
Flexure — *see* Flexion
Flint murmur (aortic insufficiency) I35.1
Floater, vitreous — *see* Opacity, vitreous
Floating
  cartilage (joint) — *see also* Loose, body, joint
    knee — *see* Derangement, knee, loose body
  gallbladder, congenital Q44.1
  kidney N28.89
    congenital Q63.8
  spleen D73.89
Flooding N92.0
Floor — *see* condition

▽ **Subterms under main terms may continue to next column or page**   ☑ **Additional Character Required** — Refer to the Tabular List for Character Selection   **149**

Fistula — Floor

Floppy
 baby syndrome (nonspecific) P94.2
 iris syndrome (intraoperative) (IFIS) H21.81
 nonrheumatic mitral valve syndrome I34.1
Flu — see also Influenza
 avian — see also Influenza, due to, identified novel influenza A virus J09.X2
 bird — see also Influenza, due to, identified novel influenza A virus J09.X2
 intestinal NEC A08.4
 swine (viruses that normally cause infections in pigs) — see also Influenza, due to, identified novel influenza A virus J09.X2
Fluctuating blood pressure I99.8
Fluid
 abdomen R18.8
 chest J94.8
 heart — see Failure, heart, congestive
 joint — see Effusion, joint
 loss (acute) E86.9
 lung — see Edema, lung
 overload E87.70
  specified NEC E87.79
 peritoneal cavity R18.8
 pleural cavity J94.8
 retention R60.9
Flukes NEC — see also Infestation, fluke
 blood NEC — see Schistosomiasis
 liver B66.3
Fluor (vaginalis) N89.8
 trichomonal or due to Trichomonas (vaginalis) A59.00
Fluorosis
 dental K00.3
 skeletal M85.10
  ankle M85.17- ☑
  foot M85.17- ☑
  forearm M85.13- ☑
  hand M85.14- ☑
  lower leg M85.16- ☑
  multiple site M85.19
  neck M85.18
  rib M85.18
  shoulder M85.11- ☑
  skull M85.18
  specified site NEC M85.18
  thigh M85.15- ☑
  toe M85.17- ☑
  upper arm M85.12- ☑
  vertebra M85.18
Flush syndrome E34.0
Flushing R23.2
 menopausal N95.1
Flutter
 atrial or auricular I48.92
  atypical I48.4
  type I I48.3
  type II I48.4
  typical I48.3
 heart I49.8
  atrial or auricular I48.92
   atypical I48.4
   type I I48.3
   type II I48.4
   typical I48.3
  ventricular I49.02
 ventricular I49.02
FNHTR (febrile nonhemolytic transfusion reaction) R50.84
Fochier's abscess — code by site under Abscess
Focus, Assmann's — see Tuberculosis, pulmonary
Fogo selvagem L10.3
Foix-Alajouanine syndrome G95.19
Fold, folds (anomalous) — see also Anomaly, by site
 Descemet's membrane — see Change, corneal membrane, Descemet's, fold
 epicanthic Q10.3
 heart Q24.8
Folie à deux F24
Follicle
 cervix (nabothian) (ruptured) N88.8
 graafian, ruptured, with hemorrhage N83.0- ☑
 nabothian N88.8
Follicular — see condition
Folliculitis (superficial) L73.9
 abscedens et suffodiens L66.3
 cyst N83.0- ☑
 decalvans L66.2
 deep — see Furuncle, by site

Folliculitis — continued
 gonococcal (acute) (chronic) A54.01
 keloid, keloidalis L73.0
 pustular L01.02
 ulerythematosa reticulata L66.4
Folliculome lipidique
 specified site — see Neoplasm, benign, by site
 unspecified site
  female D27.9
  male D29.20
Følling's disease E70.0
Follow-up — see Examination, follow-up
Fong's syndrome (hereditary osteo-onychodysplasia) Q87.2
Food
 allergy L27.2
 asphyxia (from aspiration or inhalation) — see Foreign body, by site
 choked on — see Foreign body, by site
 deprivation T73.0 ☑
  specified kind of food NEC E63.8
 insecurity Z59.41
 intoxication — see Poisoning, food
 lack of T73.0 ☑
 poisoning — see Poisoning, food
 rejection NEC — see Disorder, eating
 strangulation or suffocation — see Foreign body, by site
 toxemia — see Poisoning, food
Foot — see condition
Foramen ovale (nonclosure) (patent) (persistent) Q21.1
Forbes' glycogen storage disease E74.03
Fordyce-Fox disease L75.2
Fordyce's disease (mouth) Q38.6
Forearm — see condition
Foreclosure on loan Z59.89
Foreign body
 with
  laceration — see Laceration, by site, with foreign body
  puncture wound — see Puncture, by site, with foreign body
 accidentally left following a procedure T81.509 ☑
  aspiration T81.506 ☑
   resulting in
    adhesions T81.516 ☑
    obstruction T81.526 ☑
    perforation T81.536 ☑
    specified complication NEC T81.596 ☑
  cardiac catheterization T81.505 ☑
   resulting in
    acute reaction T81.60 ☑
     aseptic peritonitis T81.61 ☑
     specified NEC T81.69 ☑
    adhesions T81.515 ☑
    obstruction T81.525 ☑
    perforation T81.535 ☑
    specified complication NEC T81.595 ☑
   causing
    acute reaction T81.60 ☑
     aseptic peritonitis T81.61 ☑
     specified complication NEC T81.69 ☑
    adhesions T81.519 ☑
    aseptic peritonitis T81.61 ☑
    obstruction T81.529 ☑
    perforation T81.539 ☑
    specified complication NEC T81.599 ☑
  endoscopy T81.504 ☑
   resulting in
    adhesions T81.514 ☑
    obstruction T81.524 ☑
    perforation T81.534 ☑
    specified complication NEC T81.594 ☑
  immunization T81.503 ☑
   resulting in
    adhesions T81.513 ☑
    obstruction T81.523 ☑
    perforation T81.533 ☑
    specified complication NEC T81.593 ☑
  infusion T81.501 ☑
   resulting in
    adhesions T81.511 ☑
    obstruction T81.521 ☑
    perforation T81.531 ☑
    specified complication NEC T81.591 ☑
  injection T81.503 ☑

Foreign body — continued
 accidentally left following a procedure — continued
  injection — continued
   resulting in
    adhesions T81.513 ☑
    obstruction T81.523 ☑
    perforation T81.533 ☑
    specified complication NEC T81.593 ☑
  kidney dialysis T81.502 ☑
   resulting in
    adhesions T81.512 ☑
    obstruction T81.522 ☑
    perforation T81.532 ☑
    specified complication NEC T81.592 ☑
  packing removal T81.507 ☑
   resulting in
    acute reaction T81.60 ☑
     aseptic peritonitis T81.61 ☑
     specified NEC T81.69 ☑
    adhesions T81.517 ☑
    obstruction T81.527 ☑
    perforation T81.537 ☑
    specified complication NEC T81.597 ☑
  puncture T81.506 ☑
   resulting in
    adhesions T81.516 ☑
    obstruction T81.526 ☑
    perforation T81.536 ☑
    specified complication NEC T81.596 ☑
  specified procedure NEC T81.508 ☑
   resulting in
    acute reaction T81.60 ☑
     aseptic peritonitis T81.61 ☑
     specified NEC T81.69 ☑
    adhesions T81.518 ☑
    obstruction T81.528 ☑
    perforation T81.538 ☑
    specified complication NEC T81.598 ☑
  surgical operation T81.500 ☑
   resulting in
    acute reaction T81.60 ☑
     aseptic peritonitis T81.61 ☑
     specified NEC T81.69 ☑
    adhesions T81.510 ☑
    obstruction T81.520 ☑
    perforation T81.530 ☑
    specified complication NEC T81.590 ☑
  transfusion T81.501 ☑
   resulting in
    adhesions T81.511 ☑
    obstruction T81.521 ☑
    perforation T81.531 ☑
    specified complication NEC T81.591 ☑
 alimentary tract T18.9 ☑
  anus T18.5 ☑
  colon T18.4 ☑
  esophagus — see Foreign body, esophagus
  mouth T18.0 ☑
  multiple sites T18.8 ☑
  rectosigmoid (junction) T18.5 ☑
  rectum T18.5 ☑
  small intestine T18.3 ☑
  specified site NEC T18.8 ☑
  stomach T18.2 ☑
 anterior chamber (eye) S05.5- ☑
 auditory canal — see Foreign body, entering through orifice, ear
 bronchus T17.508 ☑
  causing
   asphyxiation T17.500 ☑
    food (bone) (seed) T17.520 ☑
    gastric contents (vomitus) T17.510 ☑
    specified type NEC T17.590 ☑
   injury NEC T17.508 ☑
    food (bone) (seed) T17.528 ☑
    gastric contents (vomitus) T17.518 ☑
    specified type NEC T17.598 ☑
 canthus — see Foreign body, conjunctival sac
 ciliary body (eye) S05.5- ☑
 conjunctival sac T15.1- ☑
 cornea T15.0- ☑
 entering through orifice
  accessory sinus T17.0 ☑
  alimentary canal T18.9 ☑
   multiple parts T18.8 ☑
   specified part NEC T18.8 ☑

☑ Additional Character Required — Refer to the Tabular List for Character Selection ▽ Subterms under main terms may continue to next column or page

Foreign body — *continued*
  entering through orifice — *continued*
    alveolar process T18.0 ☑
    antrum (Highmore's) T17.0 ☑
    anus T18.5 ☑
    appendix T18.4 ☑
    auditory canal — *see* Foreign body, entering through orifice, ear
    auricle — *see* Foreign body, entering through orifice, ear
    bladder T19.1 ☑
    bronchioles — *see* Foreign body, respiratory tract, specified site NEC
    bronchus (main) — *see* Foreign body, bronchus
    buccal cavity T18.0 ☑
    canthus (inner) — *see* Foreign body, conjunctival sac
    cecum T18.4 ☑
    cervix (canal) (uteri) T19.3 ☑
    colon T18.4 ☑
    conjunctival sac — *see* Foreign body, conjunctival sac
    cornea — *see* Foreign body, cornea
    digestive organ or tract NOS T18.9 ☑
      multiple parts T18.8 ☑
      specified part NEC T18.8 ☑
    duodenum T18.3 ☑
    ear (external) T16.- ☑
    esophagus — *see* Foreign body, esophagus
    eye (external) NOS T15.9- ☑
      conjunctival sac — *see* Foreign body, conjunctival sac
      cornea — *see* Foreign body, cornea
      specified part NEC T15.8- ☑
    eyeball — *see also* Foreign body, entering through orifice, eye, specified part NEC
      with penetrating wound — *see* Puncture, eyeball
    eyelid — *see also* Foreign body, conjunctival sac
      with
        laceration — *see* Laceration, eyelid, with foreign body
        puncture — *see* Puncture, eyelid, with foreign body
        superficial injury — *see* Foreign body, superficial, eyelid
    gastrointestinal tract T18.9 ☑
      multiple parts T18.8 ☑
      specified part NEC T18.8 ☑
    genitourinary tract T19.9 ☑
      multiple parts T19.8 ☑
      specified part NEC T19.8 ☑
    globe — *see* Foreign body, entering through orifice, eyeball
    gum T18.0 ☑
    Highmore's antrum T17.0 ☑
    hypopharynx — *see* Foreign body, pharynx
    ileum T18.3 ☑
    intestine (small) T18.3 ☑
      large T18.4 ☑
    lacrimal apparatus (punctum) — *see* Foreign body, entering through orifice, eye, specified part NEC
    large intestine T18.4 ☑
    larynx — *see* Foreign body, larynx
    lung — *see* Foreign body, respiratory tract, specified site NEC
    maxillary sinus T17.0 ☑
    mouth T18.0 ☑
    nasal sinus T17.0 ☑
    nasopharynx — *see* Foreign body, pharynx
    nose (passage) T17.1 ☑
    nostril T17.1 ☑
    oral cavity T18.0 ☑
    palate T18.0 ☑
    penis T19.4 ☑
    pharynx — *see* Foreign body, pharynx
    piriform sinus — *see* Foreign body, pharynx
    rectosigmoid (junction) T18.5 ☑
    rectum T18.5 ☑
    respiratory tract — *see* Foreign body, respiratory tract
    sinus (accessory) (frontal) (maxillary) (nasal) T17.0 ☑
      piriform — *see* Foreign body, pharynx
    small intestine T18.3 ☑
    stomach T18.2 ☑
    suffocation by — *see* Foreign body, by site

Foreign body — *continued*
  entering through orifice — *continued*
    tear ducts or glands — *see* Foreign body, entering through orifice, eye, specified part NEC
    throat — *see* Foreign body, pharynx
    tongue T18.0 ☑
    tonsil, tonsillar (fossa) — *see* Foreign body, pharynx
    trachea — *see* Foreign body, trachea
    ureter T19.8 ☑
    urethra T19.0 ☑
    uterus (any part) T19.3 ☑
    vagina T19.2 ☑
    vulva T19.2 ☑
  esophagus T18.108 ☑
    causing
      injury NEC T18.108 ☑
        food (bone) (seed) T18.128 ☑
        gastric contents (vomitus) T18.118 ☑
        specified type NEC T18.198 ☑
      tracheal compression T18.100 ☑
        food (bone) (seed) T18.120 ☑
        gastric contents (vomitus) T18.110 ☑
        specified type NEC T18.190 ☑
  feeling of, in throat R09.89
  fragment — *see* Retained, foreign body fragments (type of)
  genitourinary tract T19.9 ☑
    bladder T19.1 ☑
    multiple parts T19.8 ☑
    penis T19.4 ☑
    specified site NEC T19.8 ☑
    urethra T19.0 ☑
    uterus T19.3 ☑
      IUD Z97.5
    vagina T19.2 ☑
      contraceptive device Z97.5
    vulva T19.2 ☑
  granuloma (old) (soft tissue) — *see also* Granuloma, foreign body
    skin L92.3
  in
    laceration — *see* Laceration, by site, with foreign body
    puncture wound — *see* Puncture, by site, with foreign body
    soft tissue (residual) M79.5
  inadvertently left in operation wound — *see* Foreign body, accidentally left during a procedure
  ingestion, ingested NOS T18.9 ☑
  inhalation or inspiration — *see* Foreign body, by site
  internal organ, not entering through a natural orifice — code as specific injury with foreign body
  intraocular S05.5- ☑
    old, retained (nonmagnetic) H44.70- ☑
      anterior chamber H44.71- ☑
      ciliary body H44.72- ☑
      iris H44.72- ☑
      lens H44.73- ☑
      magnetic H44.60- ☑
        anterior chamber H44.61- ☑
        ciliary body H44.62- ☑
        iris H44.62- ☑
        lens H44.63- ☑
        posterior wall H44.64- ☑
        specified site NEC H44.69- ☑
        vitreous body H44.65- ☑
      posterior wall H44.74- ☑
      specified site NEC H44.79- ☑
      vitreous body H44.75- ☑
    iris — *see* Foreign body, intraocular
  lacrimal punctum — *see* Foreign body, entering through orifice, eye, specified part NEC
  larynx T17.308 ☑
    causing
      asphyxiation T17.300 ☑
        food (bone) (seed) T17.320 ☑
        gastric contents (vomitus) T17.310 ☑
        specified type NEC T17.390 ☑
      injury NEC T17.308 ☑
        food (bone) (seed) T17.328 ☑
        gastric contents (vomitus) T17.318 ☑
        specified type NEC T17.398 ☑
  lens — *see* Foreign body, intraocular
  ocular muscle S05.4- ☑
    old, retained — *see* Foreign body, orbit, old

Foreign body — *continued*
  old or residual
    soft tissue (residual) M79.5
  operation wound, left accidentally — *see* Foreign body, accidentally left during a procedure
  orbit S05.4- ☑
    old, retained H05.5- ☑
  pharynx T17.208 ☑
    causing
      asphyxiation T17.200 ☑
        food (bone) (seed) T17.220 ☑
        gastric contents (vomitus) T17.210 ☑
        specified type NEC T17.290 ☑
      injury NEC T17.208 ☑
        food (bone) (seed) T17.228 ☑
        gastric contents (vomitus) T17.218 ☑
        specified type NEC T17.298 ☑
  respiratory tract T17.908 ☑
    bronchioles — *see* Foreign body, respiratory tract, specified site NEC
    bronchus — *see* Foreign body, bronchus
    causing
      asphyxiation T17.900 ☑
        food (bone) (seed) T17.920 ☑
        gastric contents (vomitus) T17.910 ☑
        specified type NEC T17.990 ☑
      injury NEC T17.908 ☑
        food (bone) (seed) T17.928 ☑
        gastric contents (vomitus) T17.918 ☑
        specified type NEC T17.998 ☑
    larynx — *see* Foreign body, larynx
    lung — *see* Foreign body, respiratory tract, specified site NEC
    multiple parts — *see* Foreign body, respiratory tract, specified site NEC
    nasal sinus T17.0 ☑
    nasopharynx — *see* Foreign body, pharynx
    nose T17.1 ☑
    nostril T17.1 ☑
    pharynx — *see* Foreign body, pharynx
    specified site NEC T17.808 ☑
      causing
        asphyxiation T17.800 ☑
          food (bone) (seed) T17.820 ☑
          gastric contents (vomitus) T17.810 ☑
          specified type NEC T17.890 ☑
        injury NEC T17.808 ☑
          food (bone) (seed) T17.828 ☑
          gastric contents (vomitus) T17.818 ☑
          specified type NEC T17.898 ☑
    throat — *see* Foreign body, pharynx
    trachea — *see* Foreign body, trachea
  retained (old) (nonmagnetic) (in)
    anterior chamber (eye) — *see* Foreign body, intraocular, old, retained, anterior chamber
      magnetic — *see* Foreign body, intraocular, old, retained, magnetic, anterior chamber
    ciliary body — *see* Foreign body, intraocular, old, retained, ciliary body
      magnetic — *see* Foreign body, intraocular, old, retained, magnetic, ciliary body
    eyelid H02.819
      left H02.816
        lower H02.815
        upper H02.814
      right H02.813
        lower H02.812
        upper H02.811
    fragments — *see* Retained, foreign body fragments (type of)
    globe — *see* Foreign body, intraocular, old, retained
      magnetic — *see* Foreign body, intraocular, old, retained, magnetic
    intraocular — *see* Foreign body, intraocular, old, retained
      magnetic — *see* Foreign body, intraocular, old, retained, magnetic
    iris — *see* Foreign body, intraocular, old, retained, iris
      magnetic — *see* Foreign body, intraocular, old, retained, magnetic, iris
    lens — *see* Foreign body, intraocular, old, retained, lens
      magnetic — *see* Foreign body, intraocular, old, retained, magnetic, lens
    muscle — *see* Foreign body, retained, soft tissue
    orbit — *see* Foreign body, orbit, old

▽ Subterms under main terms may continue to next column or page   ☑ Additional Character Required — Refer to the Tabular List for Character Selection   **151**

Foreign body — Foreign body

Foreign body — *continued*
  retained — *continued*
    posterior wall of globe — *see* Foreign body, intraocular, old, retained, posterior wall
      magnetic — *see* Foreign body, intraocular, old, retained, magnetic, posterior wall
    retrobulbar — *see* Foreign body, orbit, old, retrobulbar
    soft tissue M79.5
    vitreous — *see* Foreign body, intraocular, old, retained, vitreous body
      magnetic — *see* Foreign body, intraocular, old, retained, magnetic, vitreous body
  retina S05.5- ☑
  superficial, without open wound
    abdomen, abdominal (wall) S30.851 ☑
    alveolar process S00.552 ☑
    ankle S90.55- ☑
    antecubital space — *see* Foreign body, superficial, forearm
    anus S30.857 ☑
    arm (upper) S40.85- ☑
    auditory canal — *see* Foreign body, superficial, ear
    auricle — *see* Foreign body, superficial, ear
    axilla — *see* Foreign body, superficial, arm
    back, lower S30.850 ☑
    breast S20.15- ☑
    brow S00.85 ☑
    buttock S30.850 ☑
    calf — *see* Foreign body, superficial, leg
    canthus — *see* Foreign body, superficial, eyelid
    cheek S00.85 ☑
      internal S00.552 ☑
    chest wall — *see* Foreign body, superficial, thorax
    chin S00.85 ☑
    clitoris S30.854 ☑
    costal region — *see* Foreign body, superficial, thorax
    digit(s)
      foot — *see* Foreign body, superficial, toe
      hand — *see* Foreign body, superficial, finger
    ear S00.45- ☑
    elbow S50.35- ☑
    epididymis S30.853 ☑
    epigastric region S30.851 ☑
    epiglottis S10.15 ☑
    esophagus, cervical S10.15 ☑
    eyebrow — *see* Foreign body, superficial, eyelid
    eyelid S00.25- ☑
    face S00.85 ☑
    finger(s) S60.459 ☑
      index S60.45- ☑
      little S60.45- ☑
      middle S60.45- ☑
      ring S60.45- ☑
    flank S30.851 ☑
    foot (except toe(s) alone) S90.85- ☑
      toe — *see* Foreign body, superficial, toe
    forearm S50.85- ☑
      elbow only — *see* Foreign body, superficial, elbow
    forehead S00.85 ☑
    genital organs, external
      female S30.856 ☑
      male S30.855 ☑
    groin S30.851 ☑
    gum S00.552 ☑
    hand S60.55- ☑
    head S00.95 ☑
      ear — *see* Foreign body, superficial, ear
      eyelid — *see* Foreign body, superficial, eyelid
      lip S00.551 ☑
      nose S00.35 ☑
      oral cavity S00.552 ☑
      scalp S00.05 ☑
      specified site NEC S00.85 ☑
    heel — *see* Foreign body, superficial, foot
    hip S70.25- ☑
    inguinal region S30.851 ☑
    interscapular region S20.459 ☑
    jaw S00.85 ☑
    knee S80.25- ☑
    labium (majus) (minus) S30.854 ☑
    larynx S10.15 ☑
    leg (lower) S80.85- ☑
      knee — *see* Foreign body, superficial, knee
      upper — *see* Foreign body, superficial, thigh

Foreign body — *continued*
  superficial, without open wound — *continued*
    lip S00.551 ☑
    lower back S30.850 ☑
    lumbar region S30.850 ☑
    malar region S00.85 ☑
    mammary — *see* Foreign body, superficial, breast
    mastoid region S00.85 ☑
    mouth S00.552 ☑
    nail
      finger — *see* Foreign body, superficial, finger
      toe — *see* Foreign body, superficial, toe
    nape S10.85 ☑
    nasal S00.35 ☑
    neck S10.95 ☑
      specified site NEC S10.85 ☑
      throat S10.15 ☑
    nose S00.35 ☑
    occipital region S00.05 ☑
    oral cavity S00.552 ☑
    orbital region — *see* Foreign body, superficial, eyelid
    palate S00.552 ☑
    palm — *see* Foreign body, superficial, hand
    parietal region S00.05 ☑
    pelvis S30.850 ☑
    penis S30.852 ☑
    perineum
      female S30.854 ☑
      male S30.850 ☑
    periocular area — *see* Foreign body, superficial, eyelid
    phalanges
      finger — *see* Foreign body, superficial, finger
      toe — *see* Foreign body, superficial, toe
    pharynx S10.15 ☑
    pinna — *see* Foreign body, superficial, ear
    popliteal space — *see* Foreign body, superficial, knee
    prepuce S30.852 ☑
    pubic region S30.850 ☑
    pudendum
      female S30.856 ☑
      male S30.855 ☑
    sacral region S30.850 ☑
    scalp S00.05 ☑
    scapular region — *see* Foreign body, superficial, shoulder
    scrotum S30.853 ☑
    shin — *see* Foreign body, superficial, leg
    shoulder S40.25- ☑
    sternal region S20.359 ☑
    submaxillary region S00.85 ☑
    submental region S00.85 ☑
    subungual
      finger(s) — *see* Foreign body, superficial, finger
      toe(s) — *see* Foreign body, superficial, toe
    supraclavicular fossa S10.85 ☑
    supraorbital S00.85 ☑
    temple S00.85 ☑
    temporal region S00.85 ☑
    testis S30.853 ☑
    thigh S70.35- ☑
    thorax, thoracic (wall) S20.95 ☑
      back S20.45- ☑
      front S20.35- ☑
    throat S10.15 ☑
    thumb S60.35- ☑
    toe(s) (lesser) S90.456 ☑
      great S90.45- ☑
    tongue S00.552 ☑
    trachea S10.15 ☑
    tunica vaginalis S30.853 ☑
    tympanum, tympanic membrane — *see* Foreign body, superficial, ear
    uvula S00.552 ☑
    vagina S30.854 ☑
    vocal cords S10.15 ☑
    vulva S30.854 ☑
    wrist S60.85- ☑
  swallowed T18.9 ☑
  trachea T17.408 ☑
    causing
      asphyxiation T17.400 ☑
        food (bone) (seed) T17.420 ☑
        gastric contents (vomitus) T17.410 ☑
        specified type NEC T17.490 ☑

Foreign body — *continued*
  trachea — *continued*
    causing — *continued*
      injury NEC T17.408 ☑
        food (bone) (seed) T17.428 ☑
        gastric contents (vomitus) T17.418 ☑
        specified type NEC T17.498 ☑
    type of fragment — *see* Retained, foreign body fragments (type of)
  vitreous (humor) S05.5- ☑
Forestier's disease (rhizomelic pseudopolyarthritis) M35.3
  meaning ankylosing hyperostosis — *see* Hyperostosis, ankylosing
Formation
  hyalin in cornea — *see* Degeneration, cornea
  sequestrum in bone (due to infection) — *see* Osteomyelitis, chronic
  valve
    colon, congenital Q43.8
    ureter (congenital) Q62.39
Formication R20.2
Fort Bragg fever A27.89
Fossa — *see also* condition
  pyriform — *see* condition
Foster-Kennedy syndrome H47.14- ☑
Fothergill's
  disease (trigeminal neuralgia) — *see also* Neuralgia, trigeminal
    scarlatina anginosa A38.9
Foul breath R19.6
Foundling Z76.1
Fournier disease or gangrene N49.3
  female N76.89
Fourth
  cranial nerve — *see* condition
  molar K00.1
Foville's (peduncular) **disease or syndrome** G46.3
Fox (-Fordyce) disease (apocrine miliaria) L75.2
FPIES (food protein-induced enterocolitis syndrome) K52.21
Fracture, burst — *see* Fracture, traumatic, by site
Fracture, chronic — *see* Fracture, pathological, by site
Fracture, insufficiency — *see* Fracture, pathological, by site
Fracture, nontraumatic, NEC
  atypical
    femur M84.750- ☑
      complete
        oblique M84.759 ☑
          left side M84.758 ☑
          right side M84.757 ☑
        transverse M84.756 ☑
          left side M84.755 ☑
          right side M84.754 ☑
      incomplete M84.753 ☑
        left side M84.752 ☑
        right side M84.751 ☑
Fracture, pathological (pathologic) — *see also* Fracture, traumatic M84.40 ☑
  ankle M84.47- ☑
  carpus M84.44- ☑
  clavicle M84.41- ☑
  compression (not due to trauma) — *see also* Collapse, vertebra M48.50- ☑
  dental implant M27.63
  dental restorative material K08.539
    with loss of material K08.531
    without loss of material K08.530
  due to
    neoplastic disease NEC — *see also* Neoplasm M84.50 ☑
      ankle M84.57- ☑
      carpus M84.54- ☑
      clavicle M84.51- ☑
      femur M84.55- ☑
      fibula M84.56- ☑
      finger M84.54- ☑
      hip M84.559 ☑
      humerus M84.52- ☑
      ilium M84.550 ☑
      ischium M84.550 ☑
      metacarpus M84.54- ☑
      metatarsus M84.57- ☑
      neck M84.58 ☑
      pelvis M84.550 ☑

Fracture, pathological — *continued*
- due to — *continued*
  - neoplastic disease — *see also* Neoplasm — *continued*
    - radius M84.53- ☑
    - rib M84.58 ☑
    - scapula M84.51- ☑
    - skull M84.58 ☑
    - specified site NEC M84.58 ☑
    - tarsus M84.57- ☑
    - tibia M84.56- ☑
    - toe M84.57- ☑
    - ulna M84.53- ☑
    - vertebra M84.58 ☑
  - osteoporosis M80.00 ☑
    - disuse — *see* Osteoporosis, specified type NEC, with pathological fracture
    - drug-induced — *see* Osteoporosis, drug induced, with pathological fracture
    - idiopathic — *see* Osteoporosis, specified type NEC, with pathological fracture
    - postmenopausal — *see* Osteoporosis, postmenopausal, with pathological fracture
    - postoophorectomy — *see* Osteoporosis, postoophorectomy, with pathological fracture
    - postsurgical malabsorption — *see* Osteoporosis, specified type NEC, with pathological fracture
    - specified cause NEC — *see* Osteoporosis, specified type NEC, with pathological fracture
  - specified disease NEC M84.60 ☑
    - ankle M84.67- ☑
    - carpus M84.64- ☑
    - clavicle M84.61- ☑
    - femur M84.65- ☑
    - fibula M84.66- ☑
    - finger M84.64- ☑
    - hip M84.65- ☑
    - humerus M84.62- ☑
    - ilium M84.650 ☑
    - ischium M84.650 ☑
    - metacarpus M84.64- ☑
    - metatarsus M84.67- ☑
    - neck M84.68 ☑
    - radius M84.63- ☑
    - rib M84.68 ☑
    - scapula M84.61- ☑
    - skull M84.68 ☑
    - tarsus M84.67- ☑
    - tibia M84.66- ☑
    - toe M84.67- ☑
    - ulna M84.63- ☑
    - vertebra M84.68 ☑
- femur M84.45- ☑
- fibula M84.46- ☑
- finger M84.44- ☑
- hip M84.459 ☑
- humerus M84.42- ☑
- ilium M84.454 ☑
- ischium M84.454 ☑
- joint prosthesis — *see* Complications, joint prosthesis, mechanical, breakdown, by site
  - periprosthetic — *see* Fracture, pathological, periprosthetic
- metacarpus M84.44- ☑
- metatarsus M84.47- ☑
- neck M84.48 ☑
- pelvis M84.454 ☑
- periprosthetic M97.9 ☑
  - ankle M97.2- ☑
  - elbow M97.4- ☑
  - finger M97.8 ☑
  - hip M97.0- ☑
  - knee M97.1- ☑
  - other specified joint M97.8 ☑
  - shoulder M97.3- ☑
  - spinal joint M97.8 ☑
  - toe joint M97.8 ☑
  - wrist joint M97.8 ☑
- radius M84.43- ☑
- restorative material (dental) K08.539
  - with loss of material K08.531
  - without loss of material K08.530
- rib M84.48 ☑
- scapula M84.41- ☑
- skull M84.48 ☑

Fracture, pathological — *continued*
- tarsus M84.47- ☑
- tibia M84.46- ☑
- toe M84.47- ☑
- ulna M84.43- ☑
- vertebra M84.48 ☑

Fracture, traumatic (abduction) (adduction) (separation) — *see also* Fracture, pathological T14.8 ☑
- acetabulum S32.40- ☑
  - column
    - anterior (displaced) (iliopubic) S32.43- ☑
      - nondisplaced S32.436 ☑
    - posterior (displaced) (ilioischial) S32.443 ☑
      - nondisplaced S32.44- ☑
  - dome (displaced) S32.48- ☑
    - nondisplaced S32.48 ☑
  - specified NEC S32.49- ☑
  - transverse (displaced) S32.45- ☑
    - with associated posterior wall fracture (displaced) S32.46- ☑
      - nondisplaced S32.46- ☑
    - nondisplaced S32.45- ☑
  - wall
    - anterior (displaced) S32.41- ☑
      - nondisplaced S32.41- ☑
    - medial (displaced) S32.47- ☑
      - nondisplaced S32.47- ☑
    - posterior (displaced) S32.42- ☑
      - with associated transverse fracture (displaced) S32.46- ☑
        - nondisplaced S32.46- ☑
      - nondisplaced S32.42- ☑
- acromion — *see* Fracture, scapula, acromial process
- ankle S82.899 ☑
  - bimalleolar (displaced) S82.84- ☑
    - nondisplaced S82.84- ☑
  - lateral malleolus only (displaced) S82.6- ☑
    - nondisplaced S82.6- ☑
  - medial malleolus (displaced) S82.5- ☑
    - associated with Maisonneuve's fracture — *see* Fracture, Maisonneuve's
    - nondisplaced S82.5- ☑
  - talus — *see* Fracture, tarsal, talus
  - trimalleolar (displaced) S82.85- ☑
    - nondisplaced S82.85- ☑
- arm (upper) — *see also* Fracture, humerus, shaft
  - humerus — *see* Fracture, humerus
  - radius — *see* Fracture, radius
  - ulna — *see* Fracture, ulna
- astragalus — *see* Fracture, tarsal, talus
- atlas — *see* Fracture, neck, cervical vertebra, first
- axis — *see* Fracture, neck, cervical vertebra, second
- back — *see* Fracture, vertebra
- Barton's — *see* Barton's fracture
- base of skull — *see* Fracture, skull, base
- basicervical (basal) (femoral) S72.0 ☑
- Bennett's — *see* Bennett's fracture
- bimalleolar — *see* Fracture, ankle, bimalleolar
- blow-out S02.3- ☑
- bone NEC T14.8 ☑
  - birth injury P13.9
  - following insertion of orthopedic implant, joint prosthesis or bone plate — *see* Fracture, following insertion of orthopedic implant, joint prosthesis or bone plate
  - in (due to) neoplastic disease NEC — *see* Fracture, pathological, due to, neoplastic disease
  - pathological (cause unknown) — *see* Fracture, pathological
- breast bone — *see* Fracture, sternum
- bucket handle (semilunar cartilage) — *see* Tear, meniscus
- buckle — *see* Fracture, by site, torus
- burst — *see* Fracture, traumatic, by site
- calcaneus — *see* Fracture, tarsal, calcaneus
- carpal bone(s) S62.10- ☑
  - capitate (displaced) S62.13- ☑
    - nondisplaced S62.13- ☑
  - cuneiform — *see* Fracture, carpal bone, triquetrum
  - hamate (body) (displaced) S62.143 ☑
    - hook process (displaced) S62.15- ☑
      - nondisplaced S62.15- ☑
    - nondisplaced S62.14- ☑
  - larger multangular — *see* Fracture, carpal bones, trapezium
  - lunate (displaced) S62.12- ☑

Fracture, traumatic — *continued*
- carpal bone(s) — *continued*
  - lunate — *continued*
    - nondisplaced S62.12- ☑
  - navicular S62.00- ☑
    - distal pole (displaced) S62.01- ☑
      - nondisplaced S62.01- ☑
    - middle third (displaced) S62.02- ☑
      - nondisplaced S62.02- ☑
    - proximal third (displaced) S62.03- ☑
      - nondisplaced S62.03- ☑
    - volar tuberosity — *see* Fracture, carpal bones, navicular, distal pole
  - os magnum — *see* Fracture, carpal bones, capitate
  - pisiform (displaced) S62.16- ☑
    - nondisplaced S62.16- ☑
  - semilunar — *see* Fracture, carpal bones, lunate
  - smaller multangular — *see* Fracture, carpal bones, trapezoid
  - trapezium (displaced) S62.17- ☑
    - nondisplaced S62.17- ☑
  - trapezoid (displaced) S62.18- ☑
    - nondisplaced S62.18- ☑
  - triquetrum (displaced) S62.11- ☑
    - nondisplaced S62.11- ☑
  - unciform — *see* Fracture, carpal bones, hamate
- cervical — *see* Fracture, vertebra, cervical
- clavicle S42.00- ☑
  - acromial end (displaced) S42.03- ☑
    - nondisplaced S42.03- ☑
  - birth injury P13.4
  - lateral end — *see* Fracture, clavicle, acromial end
  - shaft (displaced) S42.02- ☑
    - nondisplaced S42.02- ☑
  - sternal end (anterior) (displaced) S42.01- ☑
    - nondisplaced S42.01- ☑
    - posterior S42.01- ☑
- coccyx S32.2
- collapsed — *see* Collapse, vertebra
- collar bone — *see* Fracture, clavicle
- Colles' — *see* Colles' fracture
- coronoid process — *see* Fracture, ulna, upper end, coronoid process
- corpus cavernosum penis S39.840 ☑
- costochondral cartilage S23.41 ☑
- costochondral, costosternal junction — *see* Fracture, rib
- cranium — *see* Fracture, skull
- cricoid cartilage S12.8 ☑
- cuboid (ankle) — *see* Fracture, tarsal, cuboid
- cuneiform
  - foot — *see* Fracture, tarsal, cuneiform
  - wrist — *see* Fracture, carpal, triquetrum
- delayed union — *see* Delay, union, fracture
- dental restorative material K08.539
  - with loss of material K08.531
  - without loss of material K08.530
- due to
  - birth injury — *see* Birth, injury, fracture
  - osteoporosis — *see* Osteoporosis, with fracture
- Dupuytren's — *see* Fracture, ankle, lateral malleolus
- elbow S42.40- ☑
- ethmoid (bone) (sinus) — *see* Fracture, skull, base
- face bone S02.92 ☑
- fatigue — *see also* Fracture, stress
  - vertebra M48.40 ☑
    - cervical region M48.42 ☑
    - cervicothoracic region M48.43 ☑
    - lumbar region M48.46 ☑
    - lumbosacral region M48.47 ☑
    - occipito-atlanto-axial region M48.41 ☑
    - sacrococcygeal region M48.48 ☑
    - thoracic region M48.44 ☑
    - thoracolumbar region M48.45 ☑
- femur, femoral S72.9- ☑
  - basicervical (basal) S72.0 ☑
  - birth injury P13.2
  - capital epiphyseal S79.01- ☑
  - condyles, epicondyles — *see* Fracture, femur, lower end
  - distal end — *see* Fracture, femur, lower end
  - epiphysis
    - head — *see* Fracture, femur, upper end, epiphysis
    - lower — *see* Fracture, femur, lower end, epiphysis

Fracture, traumatic — *continued*
  femur, femoral — *continued*
    epiphysis — *continued*
      upper — *see* Fracture, femur, upper end, epiphysis
    following insertion of implant, prosthesis or plate M96.66- ☑
    head — *see* Fracture, femur, upper end, head
    intertrochanteric — *see* Fracture, femur, trochanteric
    intratrochanteric — *see* Fracture, femur, trochanteric
    lower end S72.40- ☑
      condyle (displaced) S72.41- ☑
        lateral (displaced) S72.42- ☑
          nondisplaced S72.42- ☑
        medial (displaced) S72.43- ☑
          nondisplaced S72.43- ☑
        nondisplaced S72.41- ☑
      epiphysis (displaced) S72.44- ☑
        nondisplaced S72.44- ☑
      physeal S79.10- ☑
        Salter-Harris
          Type I S79.11- ☑
          Type II S79.12- ☑
          Type III S79.13- ☑
          Type IV S79.14- ☑
        specified NEC S79.19- ☑
      specified NEC S72.49- ☑
      supracondylar (displaced) S72.45- ☑
        with intracondylar extension (displaced) S72.46- ☑
          nondisplaced S72.46- ☑
        nondisplaced S72.45- ☑
      torus S72.47- ☑
    neck — *see* Fracture, femur, upper end, neck
    pertrochanteric — *see* Fracture, femur, trochanteric
    shaft (lower third) (middle third) (upper third) S72.30- ☑
      comminuted (displaced) S72.35- ☑
        nondisplaced S72.35- ☑
      oblique (displaced) S72.33- ☑
        nondisplaced S72.33- ☑
      segmental (displaced) S72.36- ☑
        nondisplaced S72.36- ☑
      specified NEC S72.39- ☑
      spiral (displaced) S72.34- ☑
        nondisplaced S72.34- ☑
      transverse (displaced) S72.32- ☑
        nondisplaced S72.32- ☑
    specified site NEC — *see* subcategory S72.8 ☑
    subcapital (displaced) S72.01- ☑
    subtrochanteric (region) (section) (displaced) S72.2- ☑
      nondisplaced S72.2- ☑
    transcervical — *see* Fracture, femur, midcervical
    transtrochanteric — *see* Fracture, femur, trochanteric
    trochanteric S72.10- ☑
      apophyseal (displaced) S72.13- ☑
        nondisplaced S72.13- ☑
      greater trochanter (displaced) S72.11- ☑
        nondisplaced S72.11- ☑
      intertrochanteric (displaced) S72.14- ☑
        nondisplaced S72.14- ☑
      lesser trochanter (displaced) S72.12- ☑
        nondisplaced S72.12- ☑
    upper end S72.00- ☑
      apophyseal (displaced) S72.13- ☑
        nondisplaced S72.13- ☑
      cervicotrochanteric — *see* Fracture, femur, upper end, neck, base
      epiphysis (displaced) S72.02- ☑
        nondisplaced S72.02- ☑
      head S72.05- ☑
        articular (displaced) S72.06- ☑
          nondisplaced S72.06- ☑
        specified NEC S72.09- ☑
      intertrochanteric (displaced) S72.14- ☑
        nondisplaced S72.14- ☑
      intracapsular S72.01- ☑
      midcervical (displaced) S72.03- ☑
        nondisplaced S72.03- ☑
      neck S72.00- ☑
        base (displaced) S72.04- ☑
          nondisplaced S72.04- ☑

Fracture, traumatic — *continued*
  femur, femoral — *continued*
    upper end — *continued*
      neck — *continued*
        specified NEC S72.09- ☑
      pertrochanteric — *see* Fracture, femur, upper end, trochanteric
      physeal S79.00- ☑
        Salter-Harris type I S79.01- ☑
        specified NEC S79.09- ☑
      subcapital (displaced) S72.01- ☑
      subtrochanteric (displaced) S72.2- ☑
        nondisplaced S72.2- ☑
      transcervical — *see* Fracture, femur, upper end, midcervical
      trochanteric S72.10- ☑
        greater (displaced) S72.11- ☑
          nondisplaced S72.11- ☑
        lesser (displaced) S72.12- ☑
          nondisplaced S72.12- ☑
  fibula (shaft) (styloid) S82.40- ☑
    comminuted (displaced) S82.45- ☑
      nondisplaced S82.45- ☑
    following insertion of implant, prosthesis or plate M96.67- ☑
    involving ankle or malleolus — *see* Fracture, fibula, lateral malleolus
    lateral malleolus (displaced) S82.6- ☑
      nondisplaced S82.6- ☑
    lower end
      physeal S89.30- ☑
        Salter-Harris
          Type I S89.31- ☑
          Type II S89.32- ☑
        specified NEC S89.39- ☑
      specified NEC S82.83- ☑
      torus S82.82- ☑
    oblique (displaced) S82.43- ☑
      nondisplaced S82.43- ☑
    segmental (displaced) S82.46- ☑
      nondisplaced S82.46- ☑
    specified NEC S82.49- ☑
    spiral (displaced) S82.44- ☑
      nondisplaced S82.44- ☑
    transverse (displaced) S82.42- ☑
      nondisplaced S82.42- ☑
    upper end
      physeal S89.20- ☑
        Salter-Harris
          Type I S89.21- ☑
          Type II S89.22- ☑
        specified NEC S89.29- ☑
      specified NEC S82.83- ☑
      torus S82.81- ☑
  finger (except thumb) S62.60- ☑
    distal phalanx (displaced) S62.63- ☑
      nondisplaced S62.66- ☑
    index S62.60- ☑
      distal phalanx (displaced) S62.63- ☑
        nondisplaced S62.66- ☑
      middle phalanx (displaced) S62.62- ☑
        nondisplaced S62.65- ☑
      proximal phalanx (displaced) S62.61- ☑
        nondisplaced S62.64- ☑
    little S62.60- ☑
      distal phalanx (displaced) S62.63- ☑
        nondisplaced S62.66- ☑
      middle phalanx (displaced) S62.62- ☑
        nondisplaced S62.65- ☑
      proximal phalanx (displaced) S62.61- ☑
        nondisplaced S62.64- ☑
    middle S62.60- ☑
      distal phalanx (displaced) S62.63- ☑
        nondisplaced S62.66- ☑
      middle phalanx (displaced) S62.62- ☑
        nondisplaced S62.65- ☑
      proximal phalanx (displaced) S62.61- ☑
        nondisplaced S62.64- ☑
    middle phalanx (displaced) S62.62- ☑
      nondisplaced S62.65- ☑
    proximal phalanx (displaced) S62.61- ☑
      nondisplaced S62.64- ☑
    ring S62.60- ☑
      distal phalanx (displaced) S62.63- ☑
        nondisplaced S62.66- ☑
      middle phalanx (displaced) S62.62- ☑

Fracture, traumatic — *continued*
  finger — *continued*
    ring — *continued*
      middle phalanx — *continued*
        nondisplaced S62.65- ☑
      proximal phalanx (displaced) S62.61- ☑
        nondisplaced S62.64- ☑
    thumb — *see* Fracture, thumb
    following insertion (intraoperative) (postoperative) of orthopedic implant, joint prosthesis or bone plate M96.69
    femur M96.66- ☑
    fibula M96.67- ☑
    humerus M96.62- ☑
    pelvis M96.65
    radius M96.63- ☑
    specified bone NEC M96.69
    tibia M96.67- ☑
    ulna M96.63- ☑
  foot S92.90- ☑
    astragalus — *see* Fracture, tarsal, talus
    calcaneus — *see* Fracture, tarsal, calcaneus
    cuboid — *see* Fracture, tarsal, cuboid
    cuneiform — *see* Fracture, tarsal, cuneiform
    metatarsal — *see* Fracture, metatarsal
    navicular — *see* Fracture, tarsal, navicular
    sesamoid S92.81- ☑
    specified NEC S92.81- ☑
    talus — *see* Fracture, tarsal, talus
    tarsal — *see* Fracture, tarsal
    toe — *see* Fracture, toe
  forearm S52.9- ☑
    radius — *see* Fracture, radius
    ulna — *see* Fracture, ulna
  fossa (anterior) (middle) (posterior) S02.19 ☑
  fragility — *see* Fracture, pathological, due to osteoporosis
  frontal (bone) (skull) S02.0 ☑
    sinus S02.19 ☑
  glenoid (cavity) (scapula) — *see* Fracture, scapula, glenoid cavity
  greenstick — *see* Fracture, by site
  hallux — *see* Fracture, toe, great
  hand S62.9- ☑
    carpal — *see* Fracture, carpal bone
    finger (except thumb) — *see* Fracture, finger
    metacarpal — *see* Fracture, metacarpal
    navicular (scaphoid) (hand) — *see* Fracture, carpal bone, navicular
    thumb — *see* Fracture, thumb
  healed or old
    with complications — *code by* Nature of the complication
  heel bone — *see* Fracture, tarsal, calcaneus
  Hill-Sachs S42.29- ☑
  hip — *see* Fracture, femur, neck
  humerus S42.30- ☑
    anatomical neck — *see* Fracture, humerus, upper end
    articular process — *see* Fracture, humerus, lower end
    capitellum — *see* Fracture, humerus, lower end, condyle, lateral
    distal end — *see* Fracture, humerus, lower end
    epiphysis
      lower — *see* Fracture, humerus, lower end, physeal
      upper — *see* Fracture, humerus, upper end, physeal
    external condyle — *see* Fracture, humerus, lower end, condyle, lateral
    following insertion of implant, prosthesis or plate M96.62- ☑
    great tuberosity — *see* Fracture, humerus, upper end, greater tuberosity
    intercondylar — *see* Fracture, humerus, lower end
    internal epicondyle — *see* Fracture, humerus, lower end, epicondyle, medial
    lesser tuberosity — *see* Fracture, humerus, upper end, lesser tuberosity
    lower end S42.40- ☑
      condyle
        lateral (displaced) S42.45- ☑
          nondisplaced S42.45- ☑
        medial (displaced) S42.46- ☑
          nondisplaced S42.46- ☑

☑ Additional Character Required — Refer to the Tabular List for Character Selection   ▽ Subterms under main terms may continue to next column or page

Fracture, traumatic — *continued*
  humerus — *continued*
    lower end — *continued*
      epicondyle
        lateral (displaced) S42.43- ☑
          nondisplaced S42.43- ☑
        medial (displaced) S42.44- ☑
          incarcerated S42.44- ☑
          nondisplaced S42.44- ☑
      physeal S49.10- ☑
        Salter-Harris
          Type I S49.11- ☑
          Type II S49.12- ☑
          Type III S49.13- ☑
          Type IV S49.14- ☑
        specified NEC S49.19- ☑
      specified NEC (displaced) S42.49- ☑
        nondisplaced S42.49- ☑
      supracondylar (simple) (displaced) S42.41- ☑
        with intercondylar fracture — *see* Fracture,
          humerus, lower end
        comminuted (displaced) S42.42- ☑
          nondisplaced S42.42- ☑
        nondisplaced S42.41- ☑
      torus S42.48- ☑
      transcondylar (displaced) S42.47- ☑
        nondisplaced S42.47- ☑
    proximal end — *see* Fracture, humerus, upper end
    shaft S42.30- ☑
      comminuted (displaced) S42.35- ☑
        nondisplaced S42.35- ☑
      greenstick S42.31- ☑
      oblique (displaced) S42.33- ☑
        nondisplaced S42.33- ☑
      segmental (displaced) S42.36- ☑
        nondisplaced S42.36- ☑
      specified NEC S42.39- ☑
      spiral (displaced) S42.34- ☑
        nondisplaced S42.34- ☑
      transverse (displaced) S42.32- ☑
        nondisplaced S42.32- ☑
    supracondylar — *see* Fracture, humerus, lower end
    surgical neck — *see* Fracture, humerus, upper end,
      surgical neck
    trochlea — *see* Fracture, humerus, lower end,
      condyle, medial
    tuberosity — *see* Fracture, humerus, upper end
    upper end S42.20- ☑
      anatomical neck — *see* Fracture, humerus, upper
        end, specified NEC
      articular head — *see* Fracture, humerus, upper
        end, specified NEC
      epiphysis — *see* Fracture, humerus, upper end,
        physeal
      greater tuberosity (displaced) S42.25- ☑
        nondisplaced S42.25- ☑
      lesser tuberosity (displaced) S42.26- ☑
        nondisplaced S42.26- ☑
      physeal S49.00- ☑
        Salter-Harris
          Type I S49.01- ☑
          Type II S49.02- ☑
          Type III S49.03- ☑
          Type IV S49.04- ☑
        specified NEC S49.09- ☑
      specified NEC (displaced) S42.29- ☑
        nondisplaced S42.29- ☑
      surgical neck (displaced) S42.21- ☑
        four-part S42.24- ☑
        nondisplaced S42.21- ☑
        three-part S42.23- ☑
        two-part (displaced) S42.22- ☑
          nondisplaced S42.22- ☑
      torus S42.27- ☑
      transepiphyseal — *see* Fracture, humerus, upper
        end, physeal
  hyoid bone S12.8 ☑
  ilium S32.30- ☑
    with disruption of pelvic ring — *see* Disruption,
      pelvic ring
    avulsion (displaced) S32.31- ☑
      nondisplaced S32.31- ☑
    specified NEC S32.39- ☑
  impaction, impacted — *code as* Fracture, by site
  innominate bone — *see* Fracture, ilium
  instep — *see* Fracture, foot

Fracture, traumatic — *continued*
  ischium S32.60- ☑
    with disruption of pelvic ring — *see* Disruption,
      pelvic ring
    avulsion (displaced) S32.61- ☑
      nondisplaced S32.61- ☑
    specified NEC S32.69- ☑
  jaw (bone) (lower) — *see* Fracture, mandible
    upper — *see* Fracture, maxilla
  joint prosthesis — *see* Complications, joint prosthesis,
    mechanical, breakdown, by site
    periprosthetic — *see* Fracture, traumatic, peripros-
      thetic
  knee cap — *see* Fracture, patella
  larynx S12.8 ☑
  late effects — *see* Sequelae, fracture
  leg (lower) S82.9- ☑
    ankle — *see* Fracture, ankle
    femur — *see* Fracture, femur
    fibula — *see* Fracture, fibula
    malleolus — *see* Fracture, ankle
    patella — *see* Fracture, patella
    specified site NEC S82.89- ☑
    tibia — *see* Fracture, tibia
  lumbar spine — *see* Fracture, vertebra, lumbar
  lumbosacral spine S32.9 ☑
  Maisonneuve's (displaced) S82.86- ☑
    nondisplaced S82.86- ☑
  malar bone — *see also* Fracture, maxilla S02.400 ☑
    left side S02.40B ☑
    right side S02.40A ☑
  malleolus — *see* Fracture, ankle
  malunion — *see* Fracture, by site
  mandible (lower jaw (bone)) S02.609 ☑
    alveolus S02.67- ☑
    angle (of jaw) S02.65- ☑
    body, unspecified S02.600 ☑
      left side S02.602 ☑
      right side S02.601 ☑
    condylar process S02.61- ☑
    coronoid process S02.63- ☑
    ramus, unspecified S02.64- ☑
    specified site NEC S02.69 ☑
    subcondylar process S02.62- ☑
    symphysis S02.66 ☑
  manubrium (sterni) S22.21 ☑
    dissociation from sternum S22.23 ☑
  march — *see* Fracture, traumatic, stress, by site
  maxilla, maxillary (bone) (sinus) (superior) (upper jaw)
    S02.401 ☑
    alveolus S02.42 ☑
    inferior — *see* Fracture, mandible
    LeFort I S02.411 ☑
    LeFort II S02.412 ☑
    LeFort III S02.413 ☑
    left side S02.40D ☑
    right side S02.40C ☑
  metacarpal S62.309 ☑
    base (displaced) S62.319 ☑
      nondisplaced S62.349 ☑
    fifth S62.30- ☑
      base (displaced) S62.31- ☑
        nondisplaced S62.34- ☑
      neck (displaced) S62.33- ☑
        nondisplaced S62.36- ☑
      shaft (displaced) S62.32- ☑
        nondisplaced S62.35- ☑
      specified NEC S62.398 ☑
    first S62.20- ☑
      base NEC (displaced) S62.23- ☑
        nondisplaced S62.23- ☑
      Bennett's — *see* Bennett's fracture
      neck (displaced) S62.25- ☑
        nondisplaced S62.25- ☑
      shaft (displaced) S62.24- ☑
        nondisplaced S62.24- ☑
      specified NEC S62.29- ☑
    fourth S62.30- ☑
      base (displaced) S62.31- ☑
        nondisplaced S62.34- ☑
      neck (displaced) S62.33- ☑
        nondisplaced S62.36- ☑
      shaft (displaced) S62.32- ☑
        nondisplaced S62.35- ☑
      specified NEC S62.39- ☑
    neck (displaced) S62.33- ☑

Fracture, traumatic — *continued*
  metacarpal — *continued*
    neck — *continued*
      nondisplaced S62.36- ☑
    Rolando's — *see* Rolando's fracture
    second S62.30- ☑
      base (displaced) S62.31- ☑
        nondisplaced S62.34- ☑
      neck (displaced) S62.33- ☑
        nondisplaced S62.36- ☑
      shaft (displaced) S62.32- ☑
        nondisplaced S62.35- ☑
      specified NEC S62.39- ☑
    shaft (displaced) S62.32- ☑
      nondisplaced S62.35- ☑
    specified NEC S62.399 ☑
    third S62.30- ☑
      base (displaced) S62.31- ☑
        nondisplaced S62.34- ☑
      neck (displaced) S62.33- ☑
        nondisplaced S62.36- ☑
      shaft (displaced) S62.32- ☑
        nondisplaced S62.35- ☑
      specified NEC S62.39- ☑
  metaphyseal — *see* Fracture, traumatic, by site, shaft
  metastatic — *see* Fracture, pathological, due to, neo-
    plastic disease — *see also* Neoplasm
  metatarsal bone S92.30- ☑
    fifth (displaced) S92.35- ☑
      nondisplaced S92.35- ☑
    first (displaced) S92.31- ☑
      nondisplaced S92.31- ☑
    fourth (displaced) S92.34- ☑
      nondisplaced S92.34- ☑
    physeal S99.10- ☑
      Salter-Harris
        Type I S99.11- ☑
        Type II S99.12- ☑
        Type III S99.13- ☑
        Type IV S99.14- ☑
      specified NEC S99.19- ☑
    second (displaced) S92.32- ☑
      nondisplaced S92.32- ☑
    third (displaced) S92.33- ☑
      nondisplaced S92.33- ☑
  Monteggia's — *see* Monteggia's fracture
  multiple
    hand (and wrist) NEC — *see* Fracture, by site
    ribs — *see* Fracture, rib, multiple
  nasal (bone(s)) S02.2 ☑
  navicular (scaphoid) (foot) — *see also* Fracture, tarsal,
    navicular
    hand — *see* Fracture, carpal, navicular
  neck S12.9 ☑
    cervical vertebra S12.9 ☑
      fifth (displaced) S12.400 ☑
        nondisplaced S12.401 ☑
        specified type NEC (displaced) S12.490 ☑
          nondisplaced S12.491 ☑
      first (displaced) S12.000 ☑
        burst (stable) S12.01 ☑
          unstable S12.02 ☑
        lateral mass (displaced) S12.040 ☑
          nondisplaced S12.041 ☑
        nondisplaced S12.001 ☑
        posterior arch (displaced) S12.030 ☑
          nondisplaced S12.031 ☑
        specified type NEC (displaced) S12.090 ☑
          nondisplaced S12.091 ☑
      fourth (displaced) S12.300 ☑
        nondisplaced S12.301 ☑
        specified type NEC (displaced) S12.390 ☑
          nondisplaced S12.391 ☑
      second (displaced) S12.100 ☑
        dens (anterior) (displaced) (type II) S12.110 ☑
          nondisplaced S12.112 ☑
          posterior S12.111 ☑
        specified type NEC (displaced) S12.120 ☑
          nondisplaced S12.121 ☑
        nondisplaced S12.101 ☑
        specified type NEC (displaced) S12.190 ☑
          nondisplaced S12.191 ☑
      seventh (displaced) S12.600 ☑
        nondisplaced S12.601 ☑
        specified type NEC (displaced) S12.690 ☑
          nondisplaced S12.691 ☑

Fracture, traumatic — *continued*
  neck — *continued*
    cervical vertebra — *continued*
      sixth (displaced) S12.500 ☑
        nondisplaced S12.501 ☑
        specified type NEC (displaced) S12.590 ☑
          nondisplaced S12.591 ☑
      third (displaced) S12.200 ☑
        nondisplaced S12.201 ☑
        specified type NEC (displaced) S12.290 ☑
          nondisplaced S12.291 ☑
    hyoid bone S12.8 ☑
    larynx S12.8 ☑
    specified site NEC S12.8 ☑
    thyroid cartilage S12.8 ☑
    trachea S12.8 ☑
  neoplastic NEC — *see* Fracture, pathological, due to,
    neoplastic disease
  neural arch — *see* Fracture, vertebra
  newborn — *see* Birth, injury, fracture
  nontraumatic — *see* Fracture, pathological
  nonunion — *see* Nonunion, fracture
  nose, nasal (bone) (septum) S02.2 ☑
  occiput — *see* Fracture, skull, base, occiput
  odontoid process — *see* Fracture, neck, cervical verte-
    bra, second
  olecranon (process) (ulna) — *see* Fracture, ulna, upper
    end, olecranon process
  orbit, orbital (bone) (region) S02.85 ☑
    floor (blow-out) S02.3- ☑
    roof S02.12- ☑
    wall S02.85 ☑
      lateral S02.84- ☑
      medial S02.83- ☑
  os
    calcis — *see* Fracture, tarsal, calcaneus
    magnum — *see* Fracture, carpal, capitate
    pubis — *see* Fracture, pubis
  palate S02.8- ☑
  parietal bone (skull) S02.0 ☑
  patella S82.00- ☑
    comminuted (displaced) S82.04- ☑
      nondisplaced S82.04- ☑
    longitudinal (displaced) S82.02- ☑
      nondisplaced S82.02- ☑
    osteochondral (displaced) S82.01- ☑
      nondisplaced S82.01- ☑
    specified NEC S82.09- ☑
    transverse (displaced) S82.03- ☑
      nondisplaced S82.03- ☑
  pedicle (of vertebral arch) — *see* Fracture, vertebra
  pelvis, pelvic (bone) S32.9 ☑
    acetabulum — *see* Fracture, acetabulum
    circle — *see* Disruption, pelvic ring
    following insertion of implant, prosthesis or plate
      M96.65
    ilium — *see* Fracture, ilium
    ischium — *see* Fracture, ischium
    multiple
      with disruption of pelvic ring (circle) — *see* Dis-
        ruption, pelvic ring
      without disruption of pelvic ring (circle)
        S32.82 ☑
    pubis — *see* Fracture, pubis
    sacrum — *see* Fracture, sacrum
    specified site NEC S32.89 ☑
  periprosthetic, around internal prosthetic joint
    M97.9 ☑
    ankle M97.2- ☑
    elbow M97.4- ☑
    finger M97.8 ☑
    hip M97.0- ☑
    knee M97.1- ☑
    shoulder M97.3- ☑
    specified joint NEC M97.8 ☑
    spine M97.8 ☑
    toe M97.8 ☑
    wrist M97.8 ☑
  phalanx
    foot — *see* Fracture, toe
    hand — *see* Fracture, finger
  pisiform — *see* Fracture, carpal, pisiform
  pond — *see* Fracture, skull
  prosthetic device, internal — *see* Complications, pros-
    thetic device, by site, mechanical
  pubis S32.50- ☑

Fracture, traumatic — *continued*
  pubis — *continued*
    with disruption of pelvic ring — *see* Disruption,
      pelvic ring
    specified site NEC S32.59- ☑
    superior rim S32.51- ☑
  radius S52.9- ☑
    distal end — *see* Fracture, radius, lower end
    following insertion of implant, prosthesis or plate
      M96.63- ☑
    head — *see* Fracture, radius, upper end, head
    lower end S52.50- ☑
      Barton's — *see* Barton's fracture
      Colles' — *see* Colles' fracture
      extraarticular NEC S52.55- ☑
      intraarticular NEC S52.57- ☑
      physeal S59.20- ☑
        Salter-Harris
          Type I S59.21- ☑
          Type II S59.22- ☑
          Type III S59.23- ☑
          Type IV S59.24- ☑
        specified NEC S59.29- ☑
      Smith's — *see* Smith's fracture
      specified NEC S52.59- ☑
      styloid process (displaced) S52.51- ☑
        nondisplaced S52.51- ☑
      torus S52.52- ☑
    neck — *see* Fracture, radius, upper end
    proximal end — *see* Fracture, radius, upper end
    shaft S52.30- ☑
      bent bone S52.38- ☑
      comminuted (displaced) S52.35- ☑
        nondisplaced S52.35- ☑
      Galeazzi's — *see* Galeazzi's fracture
      greenstick S52.31- ☑
      oblique (displaced) S52.33- ☑
        nondisplaced S52.33- ☑
      segmental (displaced) S52.36- ☑
        nondisplaced S52.36- ☑
      specified NEC S52.39- ☑
      spiral (displaced) S52.34- ☑
        nondisplaced S52.34- ☑
      transverse (displaced) S52.32- ☑
        nondisplaced S52.32- ☑
    upper end S52.10- ☑
      head (displaced) S52.12- ☑
        nondisplaced S52.12- ☑
      neck (displaced) S52.13- ☑
        nondisplaced S52.13- ☑
      physeal S59.10- ☑
        Salter-Harris
          Type I S59.11- ☑
          Type II S59.12- ☑
          Type III S59.13- ☑
          Type IV S59.14- ☑
        specified NEC S59.19- ☑
      specified NEC S52.18- ☑
      torus S52.11- ☑
  ramus
    inferior or superior, pubis — *see* Fracture, pubis
    mandible — *see* Fracture, mandible
  restorative material (dental) K08.539
    with loss of material K08.531
    without loss of material K08.530
  rib S22.3- ☑
    with flail chest — *see* Flail, chest
    multiple S22.4- ☑
      with flail chest — *see* Flail, chest
  root, tooth — *see* Fracture, tooth
  sacrum S32.10 ☑
    specified NEC S32.19 ☑
    Type
      1 S32.14 ☑
      2 S32.15 ☑
      3 S32.16 ☑
      4 S32.17 ☑
    Zone
      I S32.119 ☑
        displaced (minimally) S32.111 ☑
          severely S32.112 ☑
        nondisplaced S32.110 ☑
      II S32.129 ☑
        displaced (minimally) S32.121 ☑
          severely S32.122 ☑
        nondisplaced S32.120 ☑

Fracture, traumatic — *continued*
  sacrum — *continued*
    Zone — *continued*
      III S32.139 ☑
        displaced (minimally) S32.131 ☑
          severely S32.132 ☑
        nondisplaced S32.130 ☑
  scaphoid (hand) — *see also* Fracture, carpal, navicular
    foot — *see* Fracture, tarsal, navicular
  scapula S42.10- ☑
    acromial process (displaced) S42.12- ☑
      nondisplaced S42.12- ☑
    body (displaced) S42.11- ☑
      nondisplaced S42.11- ☑
    coracoid process (displaced) S42.13- ☑
      nondisplaced S42.13- ☑
    glenoid cavity (displaced) S42.14- ☑
      nondisplaced S42.14- ☑
    neck (displaced) S42.15- ☑
      nondisplaced S42.15- ☑
    specified NEC S42.19- ☑
  semilunar bone, wrist — *see* Fracture, carpal, lunate
  sequelae — *see* Sequelae, fracture
  sesamoid bone
    foot S92.81- ☑
    hand — *see* Fracture, carpal
    other — *see* Fracture, traumatic, by site
  shepherd's — *see* Fracture, tarsal, talus
  shoulder (girdle) S42.9- ☑
    blade — *see* Fracture, scapula
  sinus (ethmoid) (frontal) S02.19 ☑
  skull S02.91 ☑
    base S02.10- ☑
      occiput S02.119 ☑
        condyle S02.113 ☑
          specified NEC S02.118 ☑
            left side S02.11H ☑
            right side S02.11G ☑
          type I S02.110 ☑
            left side S02.11B ☑
            right side S02.11A ☑
          type II S02.111 ☑
            left side S02.11D ☑
            right side S02.11C ☑
          type III S02.112 ☑
            left side S02.11F ☑
            right side S02.11E ☑
      specified NEC S02.19 ☑
    birth injury P13.0
    frontal bone S02.0 ☑
    parietal bone S02.0 ☑
    specified site NEC S02.8- ☑
    temporal bone S02.19 ☑
    vault S02.0 ☑
  Smith's — *see* Smith's fracture
  sphenoid (bone) (sinus) S02.19 ☑
  spine — *see* Fracture, vertebra
  spinous process — *see* Fracture, vertebra
  spontaneous (cause unknown) — *see* Fracture, patho-
    logical
  stave (of thumb) — *see* Fracture, metacarpal, first
  sternum S22.20 ☑
    with flail chest — *see* Flail, chest
    body S22.22 ☑
    manubrium S22.21 ☑
    xiphoid (process) S22.24 ☑
  stress M84.30 ☑
    ankle M84.37- ☑
    carpus M84.34- ☑
    clavicle M84.31- ☑
    femoral neck M84.359 ☑
    femur M84.35- ☑
    fibula M84.36- ☑
    finger M84.34- ☑
    hip M84.359 ☑
    humerus M84.32- ☑
    ilium M84.350 ☑
    ischium M84.350 ☑
    metacarpus M84.34- ☑
    metatarsus M84.37- ☑
    neck — *see* Fracture, fatigue, vertebra
    pelvis M84.350 ☑
    radius M84.33- ☑
    rib M84.38 ☑
    scapula M84.31- ☑
    skull M84.38 ☑

☑ Additional Character Required — Refer to the Tabular List for Character Selection   ▽ Subterms under main terms may continue to next column or page

Fracture, traumatic — *continued*
  stress — *continued*
    tarsus M84.37- ☑
    tibia M84.36- ☑
    toe M84.37- ☑
    ulna M84.33- ☑
    vertebra — *see* Fracture, fatigue, vertebra
  supracondylar, elbow — *see* Fracture, humerus, lower
      end, supracondylar
  symphysis pubis — *see* Fracture, pubis
  talus (ankle bone) — *see* Fracture, tarsal, talus
  tarsal bone(s) S92.20- ☑
    astragalus — *see* Fracture, tarsal, talus
    calcaneus S92.00- ☑
      anterior process (displaced) S92.02- ☑
        nondisplaced S92.02- ☑
      body (displaced) S92.01- ☑
        nondisplaced S92.01- ☑
      extraarticular NEC (displaced) S92.05- ☑
        nondisplaced S92.05- ☑
      intraarticular (displaced) S92.06- ☑
        nondisplaced S92.06- ☑
      physeal S99.00- ☑
        Salter-Harris
          Type I S99.01- ☑
          Type II S99.02- ☑
          Type III S99.03- ☑
          Type IV S99.04- ☑
        specified NEC S99.09- ☑
      tuberosity (displaced) S92.04- ☑
        avulsion (displaced) S92.03- ☑
          nondisplaced S92.03- ☑
        nondisplaced S92.04- ☑
    cuboid (displaced) S92.21- ☑
      nondisplaced S92.21- ☑
    cuneiform
      intermediate (displaced) S92.23- ☑
        nondisplaced S92.23- ☑
      lateral (displaced) S92.22- ☑
        nondisplaced S92.22- ☑
      medial (displaced) S92.24- ☑
        nondisplaced S92.24- ☑
    navicular (displaced) S92.25- ☑
      nondisplaced S92.25- ☑
    scaphoid — *see* Fracture, tarsal, navicular
    talus S92.10- ☑
      avulsion (displaced) S92.15- ☑
        nondisplaced S92.15- ☑
      body (displaced) S92.12- ☑
        nondisplaced S92.12- ☑
      dome (displaced) S92.14- ☑
        nondisplaced S92.14- ☑
      head (displaced) S92.12- ☑
        nondisplaced S92.12- ☑
      lateral process (displaced) S92.14- ☑
        nondisplaced S92.14- ☑
      neck (displaced) S92.11- ☑
        nondisplaced S92.11- ☑
      posterior process (displaced) S92.13- ☑
        nondisplaced S92.13- ☑
      specified NEC S92.19- ☑
  temporal bone (styloid) S02.19 ☑
  thorax (bony) S22.9 ☑
    with flail chest — *see* Flail, chest
    rib S22.3- ☑
      multiple S22.4- ☑
        with flail chest — *see* Flail, chest
    sternum S22.20 ☑
      body S22.22 ☑
      manubrium S22.21 ☑
      xiphoid process S22.24 ☑
    vertebra (displaced) S22.009 ☑
      burst (stable) S22.001 ☑
        unstable S22.002 ☑
      eighth S22.069 ☑
        burst (stable) S22.061 ☑
          unstable S22.062 ☑
        specified type NEC S22.068 ☑
        wedge compression S22.060 ☑
      eleventh S22.089 ☑
        burst (stable) S22.081 ☑
          unstable S22.082 ☑
        specified type NEC S22.088 ☑
        wedge compression S22.080 ☑
      fifth S22.059 ☑
        burst (stable) S22.051

Fracture, traumatic — *continued*
  thorax — *continued*
    vertebra — *continued*
      fifth — *continued*
        burst — *continued*
          unstable S22.052 ☑
        specified type NEC S22.058 ☑
        wedge compression S22.050 ☑
      first S22.019 ☑
        burst (stable) S22.011 ☑
          unstable S22.012 ☑
        specified type NEC S22.018 ☑
        wedge compression S22.010 ☑
      fourth S22.049 ☑
        burst (stable) S22.041 ☑
          unstable S22.042 ☑
        specified type NEC S22.048 ☑
        wedge compression S22.040 ☑
      ninth S22.079 ☑
        burst (stable) S22.071 ☑
          unstable S22.072 ☑
        specified type NEC S22.078 ☑
        wedge compression S22.070 ☑
      nondisplaced S22.001 ☑
      second S22.029 ☑
        burst (stable) S22.021 ☑
          unstable S22.022 ☑
        specified type NEC S22.028 ☑
        wedge compression S22.020 ☑
      seventh S22.069 ☑
        burst (stable) S22.061 ☑
          unstable S22.062 ☑
        specified type NEC S22.068 ☑
        wedge compression S22.060 ☑
      sixth S22.059 ☑
        burst (stable) S22.051 ☑
          unstable S22.052 ☑
        specified type NEC S22.058 ☑
        wedge compression S22.050 ☑
      specified type NEC S22.008 ☑
      tenth S22.079 ☑
        burst (stable) S22.071 ☑
          unstable S22.072 ☑
        specified type NEC S22.078 ☑
        wedge compression S22.070 ☑
      third S22.039 ☑
        burst (stable) S22.031 ☑
          unstable S22.032 ☑
        specified type NEC S22.038 ☑
        wedge compression S22.030 ☑
      twelfth S22.089 ☑
        burst (stable) S22.081 ☑
          unstable S22.082 ☑
        specified type NEC S22.088 ☑
        wedge compression S22.080 ☑
      wedge compression S22.000 ☑
  thumb S62.50- ☑
    distal phalanx (displaced) S62.52- ☑
      nondisplaced S62.52- ☑
    proximal phalanx (displaced) S62.51- ☑
      nondisplaced S62.51- ☑
  thyroid cartilage S12.8 ☑
  tibia (shaft) S82.20- ☑
    comminuted (displaced) S82.25- ☑
      nondisplaced S82.25- ☑
    condyles — *see* Fracture, tibia, upper end
    distal end — *see* Fracture, tibia, lower end
    epiphysis
      lower — *see* Fracture, tibia, lower end
      upper — *see* Fracture, tibia, upper end
    following insertion of implant, prosthesis or plate
        M96.67- ☑
    head (involving knee joint) — *see* Fracture, tibia,
        upper end
    intercondyloid eminence — *see* Fracture, tibia, up-
        per end
    involving ankle or malleolus — *see* Fracture, ankle,
        medial malleolus
    lower end S82.30- ☑
      physeal S89.10- ☑
        Salter-Harris
          Type I S89.11- ☑
          Type II S89.12- ☑
          Type III S89.13- ☑
          Type IV S89.14- ☑
        specified NEC S89.19- ☑

Fracture, traumatic — *continued*
  tibia — *continued*
    lower end — *continued*
      pilon (displaced) S82.87- ☑
        nondisplaced S82.87- ☑
      specified NEC S82.39- ☑
      torus S82.31- ☑
    malleolus — *see* Fracture, ankle, medial malleolus
    oblique (displaced) S82.23- ☑
      nondisplaced S82.23- ☑
    pilon — *see* Fracture, tibia, lower end, pilon
    proximal end — *see* Fracture, tibia, upper end
    segmental (displaced) S82.26- ☑
      nondisplaced S82.26- ☑
    specified NEC S82.29- ☑
    spine — *see* Fracture, tibia, upper end, spine
    spiral (displaced) S82.24- ☑
      nondisplaced S82.24- ☑
    transverse (displaced) S82.22- ☑
      nondisplaced S82.22- ☑
    tuberosity — *see* Fracture, tibia, upper end,
        tuberosity
    upper end S82.10- ☑
      bicondylar (displaced) S82.14- ☑
        nondisplaced S82.14- ☑
      lateral condyle (displaced) S82.12- ☑
        nondisplaced S82.12- ☑
      medial condyle (displaced) S82.13- ☑
        nondisplaced S82.13- ☑
      physeal S89.00- ☑
        Salter-Harris
          Type I S89.01- ☑
          Type II S89.02- ☑
          Type III S89.03- ☑
          Type IV S89.04- ☑
        specified NEC S89.09- ☑
      plateau — *see* Fracture, tibia, upper end, bicondy-
          lar
      specified NEC S82.19- ☑
      spine (displaced) S82.11- ☑
        nondisplaced S82.11- ☑
      torus S82.16- ☑
      tuberosity (displaced) S82.15- ☑
        nondisplaced S82.15- ☑
  toe S92.91- ☑
    great (displaced) S92.40- ☑
      distal phalanx (displaced) S92.42- ☑
        nondisplaced S92.42- ☑
      nondisplaced S92.40- ☑
      proximal phalanx (displaced) S92.41- ☑
        nondisplaced S92.41- ☑
      specified NEC S92.49- ☑
    lesser (displaced) S92.50- ☑
      distal phalanx (displaced) S92.53- ☑
        nondisplaced S92.53- ☑
      middle phalanx (displaced) S92.52- ☑
        nondisplaced S92.52- ☑
      nondisplaced S92.50- ☑
      proximal phalanx (displaced) S92.51- ☑
        nondisplaced S92.51- ☑
      specified NEC S92.59- ☑
    physeal
      phalanx S99.20- ☑
        Salter-Harris
          Type I S99.21- ☑
          Type II S99.22- ☑
          Type III S99.23- ☑
          Type IV S99.24- ☑
        specified NEC S99.29- ☑
  tooth (root) S02.5 ☑
  trachea (cartilage) S12.8 ☑
  transverse process — *see* Fracture, vertebra
  trapezium or trapezoid bone — *see* Fracture, carpal
  trimalleolar — *see* Fracture, ankle, trimalleolar
  triquetrum (cuneiform of carpus) — *see* Fracture,
      carpal, triquetrum
  trochanter — *see* Fracture, femur, trochanteric
  tuberosity (external) — *see* Fracture, traumatic, by site
  ulna (shaft) S52.20- ☑
    bent bone S52.28- ☑
    coronoid process — *see* Fracture, ulna, upper end,
        coronoid process
    distal end — *see* Fracture, ulna, lower end
    following insertion of implant, prosthesis or plate
        M96.63- ☑
    head S52.60- ☑

Fructokinase deficiency E74.11
Fructose 1,6 diphosphatase deficiency E74.19
Fructosemia (benign) (essential) E74.12
Fructosuria (benign) (essential) E74.11
Fuchs'
    black spot (myopic) — see also Myopia, degenerative
        H44.2- ☑
    dystrophy (corneal endothelium) H18.51- ☑
    heterochromic cyclitis — see Cyclitis, Fuchs' hete-
        rochromic
Fucosidosis E77.1
Fugue R68.89
    dissociative F44.1
    hysterical (dissociative) F44.1
    postictal in epilepsy — see Epilepsy
    reaction to exceptional stress (transient) F43.0
Fulminant, fulminating — see condition
Functional — see also condition
    bleeding (uterus) N93.8
Functioning, intellectual, borderline R41.83
Fundus — see condition
Fungemia NOS B49
Fungus, fungous
    cerebral G93.89
    disease NOS B49
    infection — see Infection, fungus
Funiculitis (acute) (chronic) (endemic) N49.1
    gonococcal (acute) (chronic) A54.23
    tuberculous A18.15
Funnel
    breast (acquired) M95.4
        congenital Q67.6
        sequelae (late effect) of rickets E64.3
    chest (acquired) M95.4
        congenital Q67.6
        sequelae (late effect) of rickets E64.3
    pelvis (acquired) M95.5
        with disproportion (fetopelvic) O33.3 ☑
            causing obstructed labor O65.3
        congenital Q74.2
FUO (fever of unknown origin) R50.9
Furfur L21.0
    microsporon B36.0
Furrier's lung J67.8
Furrowed K14.5
    nail(s) (transverse) L60.4
        congenital Q84.6
    tongue K14.5
        congenital Q38.3
Furuncle L02.92
    abdominal wall L02.221
    ankle — see Furuncle, lower limb
    antecubital space — see Furuncle, upper limb
    anus K61.0
    arm — see Furuncle, upper limb
    auditory canal, external — see Abscess, ear, external
    auricle (ear) — see Abscess, ear, external
    axilla (region) L02.42- ☑
    back (any part) L02.222
    breast N61.1
    buttock L02.32
    cheek (external) L02.02
    chest wall L02.223

Furuncle — continued
    chin L02.02
    corpus cavernosum N48.21
    ear, external — see Abscess, ear, external
    external auditory canal — see Abscess, ear, external
    eyelid — see Abscess, eyelid
    face L02.02
    femoral (region) — see Furuncle, lower limb
    finger — see Furuncle, hand
    flank L02.221
    foot L02.62- ☑
    forehead L02.02
    gluteal (region) L02.32
    groin L02.224
    hand L02.52- ☑
    head L02.821
        face L02.02
    hip — see Furuncle, lower limb
    kidney — see Abscess, kidney
    knee — see Furuncle, lower limb
    labium (majus) (minus) N76.4
    lacrimal
        gland — see Dacryoadenitis
        passages (duct) (sac) — see Inflammation, lacrimal,
            passages, acute
    leg (any part) — see Furuncle, lower limb
    lower limb L02.42- ☑
    malignant A22.0
    mouth K12.2
    navel L02.226
    neck L02.12
    nose J34.0
    orbit, orbital — see Abscess, orbit
    palmar (space) — see Furuncle, hand
    partes posteriores L02.32
    pectoral region L02.223
    penis N48.21
    perineum L02.225
    pinna — see Abscess, ear, external
    popliteal — see Furuncle, lower limb
    prepatellar — see Furuncle, lower limb
    scalp L02.821
    seminal vesicle N49.0
    shoulder — see Furuncle, upper limb
    specified site NEC L02.828
    submandibular K12.2
    temple (region) L02.02
    thumb — see Furuncle, hand
    toe — see Furuncle, foot
    trunk L02.229
        abdominal wall L02.221
        back L02.222
        chest wall L02.223
        groin L02.224
        perineum L02.225
        umbilicus L02.226
    umbilicus L02.226
    upper limb L02.42- ☑
    vulva N76.4
Furunculosis — see Furuncle
Fused — see Fusion, fused
Fusion, fused (congenital)
    astragaloscaphoid Q74.2

Fusion, fused — continued
    atria Q21.1
    auditory canal Q16.1
    auricles, heart Q21.1
    binocular with defective stereopsis H53.32
    bone Q79.8
    cervical spine M43.22
    choanal Q30.0
    commissure, mitral valve Q23.2
    cusps, heart valve NEC Q24.8
        mitral Q23.2
        pulmonary Q22.1
        tricuspid Q22.4
    ear ossicles Q16.3
    fingers Q70.0 ☑
    hymen Q52.3
    joint (acquired) — see also Ankylosis
        congenital Q74.8
    kidneys (incomplete) Q63.1
    labium (majus) (minus) Q52.5
    larynx and trachea Q34.8
    limb, congenital Q74.8
        lower Q74.2
        upper Q74.0
    lobes, lung Q33.8
    lumbosacral (acquired) M43.27
        arthrodesis status Z98.1
        congenital Q76.49
        postprocedural status Z98.1
    nares, nose, nasal, nostril(s) Q30.0
    organ or site not listed — see Anomaly, by site
    ossicles Q79.9
        auditory Q16.3
    pulmonic cusps Q22.1
    ribs Q76.6
    sacroiliac (joint) (acquired) M43.28
        arthrodesis status Z98.1
        congenital Q74.2
        postprocedural status Z98.1
    spine (acquired) NEC M43.20
        arthrodesis status Z98.1
        cervical region M43.22
        cervicothoracic region M43.23
        congenital Q76.49
        lumbar M43.26
        lumbosacral region M43.27
        occipito-atlanto-axial region M43.21
        postoperative status Z98.1
        sacrococcygeal region M43.28
        thoracic region M43.24
        thoracolumbar region M43.25
    sublingual duct with submaxillary duct at opening in
        mouth Q38.4
    testes Q55.1
    toes Q70.2- ☑
    tooth, teeth K00.2
    trachea and esophagus Q39.8
    twins Q89.4
    vagina Q52.4
    ventricles, heart Q21.0
    vertebra (arch) — see Fusion, spine
    vulva Q52.5
Fusospirillosis (mouth) (tongue) (tonsil) A69.1
Fussy baby R68.12

G

Gain in weight (abnormal) (excessive) — *see also* Weight, gain
Gaisböck's disease (polycythemia hypertonica) D75.1
Gait abnormality R26.9
  ataxic R26.0
  falling R29.6
  hysterical (ataxic) (staggering) F44.4
  paralytic R26.1
  spastic R26.1
  specified type NEC R26.89
  staggering R26.0
  unsteadiness R26.81
  walking difficulty NEC R26.2
Galactocele (breast) N64.89
  puerperal, postpartum O92.79
Galactokinase deficiency E74.29
Galactophoritis N61.0
  gestational, puerperal, postpartum O91.2- ☑
Galactorrhea O92.6
  not associated with childbirth N64.3
Galactosemia (classic) (congenital) E74.21
Galactosuria E74.29
Galacturia R82.0
  schistosomiasis (bilharziasis) B65.0
GALD (gestational alloimmune liver disease) P78.84
Galeazzi's fracture S52.37- ☑
Galen's vein — *see* condition
Galeophobia F40.218
Gall duct — *see* condition
Gallbladder — *see also* condition
  acute K81.0
Gallop rhythm R00.8
Gallstone (colic) (cystic duct) (gallbladder) (impacted) (multiple) — *see also* Calculus, gallbladder
  with
    cholecystitis — *see* Calculus, gallbladder, with cholecystitis
    bile duct (common) (hepatic) — *see* Calculus, bile duct
  causing intestinal obstruction K56.3
  specified NEC K80.80
    with obstruction K80.81
Gambling Z72.6
  pathological (compulsive) F63.0
Gammopathy (of undetermined significance [MGUS]) D47.2
  associated with lymphoplasmacytic dyscrasia D47.2
  monoclonal D47.2
  polyclonal D89.0
Gamna's disease (siderotic splenomegaly) D73.1
Gamophobia F40.298
Gampsodactylia (congenital) Q66.7- ☑
Gamstorp's disease (adynamia episodica hereditaria) G72.3
Gandy-Nanta disease (siderotic splenomegaly) D73.1
Gang
  membership offenses Z72.810
Gangliocytoma D36.10
Ganglioglioma — *see* Neoplasm, uncertain behavior, by site
Ganglion (compound) (diffuse) (joint) (tendon (sheath)) M67.40
  ankle M67.47- ☑
  foot M67.47- ☑
  forearm M67.43- ☑
  hand M67.44- ☑
  lower leg M67.46- ☑
  multiple sites M67.49
  of yaws (early) (late) A66.6
  pelvic region M67.45- ☑
  periosteal — *see* Periostitis
  shoulder region M67.41- ☑
  specified site NEC M67.48
  thigh region M67.45- ☑
  tuberculous A18.09
  upper arm M67.42- ☑
  wrist M67.43- ☑
Ganglioneuroblastoma — *see* Neoplasm, nerve, malignant
Ganglioneuroma D36.10
  malignant — *see* Neoplasm, nerve, malignant
Ganglioneuromatosis D36.10
Ganglionitis
  fifth nerve — *see* Neuralgia, trigeminal
  gasserian (postherpetic) (postzoster) B02.21

Ganglionitis — *continued*
  geniculate G51.1
    newborn (birth injury) P11.3
    postherpetic, postzoster B02.21
  herpes zoster B02.21
  postherpetic geniculate B02.21
Gangliosidosis E75.10
  GM1 E75.19
  GM2 E75.00
    other specified E75.09
    Sandhoff disease E75.01
    Tay-Sachs disease E75.02
  GM3 E75.19
  mucolipidosis IV E75.11
Gangosa A66.5
Gangrene, gangrenous (connective tissue) (dropsical) (dry) (moist) (skin) (ulcer) — *see also* Necrosis I96
  with diabetes (mellitus) — *see* Diabetes, with, gangrene
  abdomen (wall) I96
  alveolar M27.3
  appendix K35.80
    with
      peritonitis, localized — *see also* Appendicitis K35.31
  arteriosclerotic (general) (senile) — *see* Arteriosclerosis, extremities, with, gangrene
  auricle I96
  Bacillus welchii A48.0
  bladder (infectious) — *see* Cystitis, specified type NEC
  bowel, cecum, or colon — *see* Gangrene, intestine
  Clostridium perfringens or welchii A48.0
  cornea H18.89- ☑
  corpora cavernosa N48.29
    noninfective N48.89
  cutaneous, spreading I96
  decubital — *see* Ulcer, pressure, by site
  diabetic (any site) — *see* Diabetes, with, gangrene
  emphysematous — *see* Gangrene, gas
  epidemic — *see* Poisoning, food, noxious, plant
  epididymis (infectional) N45.1
  erysipelas — *see* Erysipelas
  extremity (lower) (upper) I96
  Fournier N49.3
    female N76.89
  fusospirochetal A69.0
  gallbladder — *see* Cholecystitis, acute
  gas (bacillus) A48.0
    following
      abortion — *see* Abortion by type complicated by infection
      ectopic or molar pregnancy O08.0
  glossitis K14.0
  hernia — *see* Hernia, by site, with gangrene
  intestine, intestinal (hemorrhagic) (massive) — *see also* Infarct, intestine K55.069
    with
      mesenteric embolism — *see also* Infarct, intestine K55.069
      obstruction — *see* Obstruction, intestine
  laryngitis J04.0
  limb (lower) (upper) I96
  lung J85.0
    spirochetal A69.8
  lymphangitis I89.1
  Meleney's (synergistic) — *see* Ulcer, skin
  mesentery — *see also* Infarct, intestine K55.069
    with
      embolism — *see also* Infarct, intestine K55.069
      intestinal obstruction — *see* Obstruction, intestine
  mouth A69.0
  ovary — *see* Oophoritis
  pancreas — *see* Pancreatitis, acute
  penis N48.29
    noninfective N48.89
  perineum I96
  pharynx — *see also* Pharyngitis
    Vincent's A69.1
  presenile I73.1
  progressive synergistic — *see* Ulcer, skin
  pulmonary J85.0
  pulpal (dental) K04.1
  quinsy J36
  Raynaud's (symmetric gangrene) I73.01
  retropharyngeal J39.2
  scrotum N49.3
    noninfective N50.89

Gangrene, gangrenous — *continued*
  senile (atherosclerotic) — *see* Arteriosclerosis, extremities, with, gangrene
  spermatic cord N49.1
    noninfective N50.89
  spine I96
  spirochetal NEC A69.8
  spreading cutaneous I96
  stomatitis A69.0
  symmetrical I73.01
  testis (infectional) N45.2
    noninfective N44.8
  throat — *see also* Pharyngitis
    diphtheritic A36.0
    Vincent's A69.1
  thyroid (gland) E07.89
  tooth (pulp) K04.1
  tuberculous NEC — *see* Tuberculosis
  tunica vaginalis N49.1
    noninfective N50.89
  umbilicus I96
  uterus — *see* Endometritis
  uvulitis K12.2
  vas deferens N49.1
    noninfective N50.89
  vulva N76.89
Ganister disease J62.8
Ganser's syndrome (hysterical) F44.89
Gardner-Diamond syndrome (autoerythrocyte sensitization) D69.2
Gargoylism E76.01
Garré's disease, osteitis (sclerosing), osteomyelitis — *see* Osteomyelitis, specified type NEC
Garrod's pad, knuckle M72.1
Gartner's duct
  cyst Q52.4
  persistent Q50.6
Gas R14.3
  asphyxiation, inhalation, poisoning, suffocation NEC — *see* Table of Drugs and Chemicals
  excessive R14.0
  gangrene A48.0
    following
      abortion — *see* Abortion by type complicated by infection
      ectopic or molar pregnancy O08.0
  on stomach R14.0
  pains R14.1
Gastralgia — *see also* Pain, abdominal
Gastrectasis K31.0
  psychogenic F45.8
Gastric — *see* condition
Gastrinoma
  malignant
    pancreas C25.4
    specified site NEC — *see* Neoplasm, malignant, by site
    unspecified site C25.4
  specified site — *see* Neoplasm, uncertain behavior
  unspecified site D37.9
Gastritis (simple) K29.70
  with bleeding K29.71
  acute (erosive) K29.00
    with bleeding K29.01
  alcoholic K29.20
    with bleeding K29.21
  allergic K29.60
    with bleeding K29.61
  atrophic (chronic) K29.40
    with bleeding K29.41
  chronic (antral) (fundal) K29.50
    with bleeding K29.51
    atrophic K29.40
      with bleeding K29.41
    superficial K29.30
      with bleeding K29.31
  dietary counseling and surveillance Z71.3
  due to diet deficiency E63.9
  eosinophilic K52.81
  giant hypertrophic K29.60
    with bleeding K29.61
  granulomatous K29.60
    with bleeding K29.61
  hypertrophic (mucosa) K29.60
    with bleeding K29.61
  nervous F54
  spastic K29.60
    with bleeding K29.61

Gastritis — *continued*
  specified NEC K29.60
    with bleeding K29.61
  superficial chronic K29.30
    with bleeding K29.31
  tuberculous A18.83
  viral NEC A08.4
Gastrocarcinoma — *see* Neoplasm, malignant, stomach
Gastrocolic — *see* condition
Gastrodisciasis, gastrodiscoidiasis B66.8
Gastroduodenitis K29.90
  with bleeding K29.91
  virus, viral A08.4
    specified type NEC A08.39
Gastrodynia — *see* Pain, abdominal
Gastroenteritis (acute) (chronic) (noninfectious) — *see also* Enteritis K52.9
  allergic K52.29
    with
      eosinophilic gastritis or gastroenteritis K52.81
      food protein-induced enterocolitis syndrome K52.21
      food protein-induced enteropathy K52.22
  dietetic — *see also* Gastroenteritis, allergic K52.29
  drug-induced K52.1
  due to
    Cryptosporidium A07.2
    drugs K52.1
    food poisoning — *see* Intoxication, foodborne
    radiation K52.0
  eosinophilic K52.81
  epidemic (infectious) A09
  food hypersensitivity — *see also* Gastroenteritis, allergic K52.29
  infectious — *see* Enteritis, infectious
  influenzal — *see* Influenza, with gastroenteritis
  noninfectious K52.9
    specified NEC K52.89
  rotaviral A08.0
  Salmonella A02.0
  toxic K52.1
  viral NEC A08.4
    acute infectious A08.39
      type Norwalk A08.11
    infantile (acute) A08.39
    Norwalk agent A08.11
    rotaviral A08.0
    severe of infants A08.39
    specified type NEC A08.39
Gastroenteropathy — *see also* Gastroenteritis K52.9
  acute, due to Norovirus A08.11
  acute, due to Norwalk agent A08.11
  infectious A09
Gastroenteroptosis K63.4
Gastroesophageal laceration- hemorrhage syndrome K22.6
Gastrointestinal — *see* condition
Gastrojejunal — *see* condition
Gastrojejunitis — *see also* Enteritis K52.9
Gastrojejunocolic — *see* condition
Gastroliths K31.89
Gastromalacia K31.89
Gastroparalysis K31.84
  diabetic — *see* Diabetes, gastroparalysis
Gastroparesis K31.84
  diabetic — *see* Diabetes, by type, with gastroparesis
Gastropathy K31.9
  congestive portal — *see also* Hypertension, portal K31.89
  erythematous K29.70
  exudative K90.89
  portal hypertensive — *see also* Hypertension, portal K31.89
Gastroptosis K31.89
Gastrorrhagia K92.2
  psychogenic F45.8
Gastroschisis (congenital) Q79.3
Gastrospasm (neurogenic) (reflex) K31.89
  neurotic F45.8
  psychogenic F45.8
Gastrostaxis — *see* Gastritis, with bleeding
Gastrostenosis K31.89
Gastrostomy
  attention to Z43.1
  status Z93.1
Gastrosuccorrhea (continuous) (intermittent) K31.89
  neurotic F45.8
  psychogenic F45.8

Gatophobia F40.218
Gaucher's disease or splenomegaly (adult) (infantile) E75.22
Gee (-Herter)(-Thaysen) **disease** (nontropical sprue) K90.0
Gélineau's syndrome G47.419
  with cataplexy G47.411
Gemination, tooth, teeth K00.2
Gemistocytoma
  specified site — *see* Neoplasm, malignant, by site
  unspecified site C71.9
General, generalized — *see* condition
Genetic
  carrier (status)
    cystic fibrosis Z14.1
    hemophilia A (asymptomatic) Z14.01
      symptomatic Z14.02
    specified NEC Z14.8
  susceptibility to disease NEC Z15.89
    malignant neoplasm Z15.09
      breast Z15.01
      endometrium Z15.04
      ovary Z15.02
      prostate Z15.03
      specified NEC Z15.09
    multiple endocrine neoplasia Z15.81
Genital — *see* condition
Genito-anorectal syndrome A55
Genitourinary system — *see* condition
Genu
  congenital Q74.1
  extrorsum (acquired) — *see also* Deformity, varus, knee
    congenital Q74.1
    sequelae (late effect) of rickets E64.3
  introrsum (acquired) — *see also* Deformity, valgus, knee
    congenital Q74.1
    sequelae (late effect) of rickets E64.3
  rachitic (old) E64.3
  recurvatum (acquired) — *see also* Deformity, limb, specified type NEC, lower leg
    congenital Q68.2
    sequelae (late effect) of rickets E64.3
  valgum (acquired) (knock-knee) M21.06- ☑
    congenital Q74.1
    sequelae (late effect) of rickets E64.3
  varum (acquired) (bowleg) M21.16- ☑
    congenital Q74.1
    sequelae (late effect) of rickets E64.3
Geographic tongue K14.1
Geophagia — *see* Pica
Geotrichosis B48.3
  stomatitis B48.3
Gephyrophobia F40.242
Gerbode defect Q21.0
GERD (gastroesophageal reflux disease) K21.9
Gerhardt's
  disease (erythromelalgia) I73.81
  syndrome (vocal cord paralysis) J38.00
    bilateral J38.02
    unilateral J38.01
German measles — *see also* Rubella
  exposure to Z20.4
Germinoblastoma (diffuse) C85.9- ☑
  follicular C82.9- ☑
Germinoma — *see* Neoplasm, malignant, by site
Gerontoxon — *see* Degeneration, cornea, senile
Gerstmann's syndrome R48.8
  developmental F81.2
Gerstmann-Sträussler-Scheinker syndrome (GSS) A81.82
Gestation (period) — *see also* Pregnancy
  ectopic — *see* Pregnancy, by site
  multiple O30.9- ☑
    greater than quadruplets — *see* Pregnancy, multiple (gestation), specified NEC
    specified NEC — *see* Pregnancy, multiple (gestation), specified NEC
Gestational
  mammary abscess O91.11- ☑
  purulent mastitis O91.11- ☑
  subareolar abscess O91.11- ☑
Ghon tubercle, primary infection A15.7
Ghost
  teeth K00.4
  vessels (cornea) H16.41- ☑
Ghoul hand A66.3
Gianotti-Crosti disease L44.4

Giant
  cell
    epulis K06.8
    peripheral granuloma K06.8
  esophagus, congenital Q39.5
  kidney, congenital Q63.3
  urticaria T78.3 ☑
    hereditary D84.1
Giardiasis A07.1
Gibert's disease or pityriasis L42
Giddiness R42
  hysterical F44.89
  psychogenic F45.8
Gierke's disease (glycogenosis I) E74.01
Gigantism (cerebral) (hypophyseal) (pituitary) E22.0
  constitutional E34.4
Gilbert's disease or syndrome E80.4
Gilchrist's disease B40.9
Gilford-Hutchinson disease E34.8
Gilles de la Tourette's disease or syndrome (motor-verbal tic) F95.2
Gingivitis K05.10
  acute (catarrhal) K05.00
    necrotizing A69.1
    nonplaque induced K05.01
    plaque induced K05.00
  chronic (desquamative) (hyperplastic) (simple marginal) (pregnancy associated) (ulcerative) K05.10
    nonplaque induced K05.11
    plaque induced K05.10
  expulsiva — *see* Periodontitis
  necrotizing ulcerative (acute) A69.1
  pellagrous E52
    acute necrotizing A69.1
  Vincent's A69.1
Gingivoglossitis K14.0
Gingivopericementitis — *see* Periodontitis
Gingivosis — *see* Gingivitis, chronic
Gingivostomatitis K05.10
  herpesviral B00.2
  necrotizing ulcerative (acute) A69.1
Gland, glandular — *see* condition
Glanders A24.0
Glanzmann (-Naegeli) **disease or thrombasthenia** D69.1
Glasgow coma scale
  total score
    3-8 R40.243 ☑
    9-12 R40.242 ☑
    13-15 R40.241 ☑
Glass-blower's disease (cataract) — *see* Cataract, specified NEC
Glaucoma H40.9
  with
    increased episcleral venous pressure H40.81- ☑
    pseudoexfoliation of lens — *see* Glaucoma, open angle, primary, capsular
  absolute H44.51- ☑
  angle-closure (primary) H40.20- ☑
    acute (attack) (crisis) H40.21- ☑
    chronic H40.22- ☑
    intermittent H40.23- ☑
    residual stage H40.24- ☑
  borderline H40.00- ☑
  capsular (with pseudoexfoliation of lens) — *see* Glaucoma, open angle, primary, capsular
  childhood Q15.0
  closed angle — *see* Glaucoma, angle-closure
  congenital Q15.0
  corticosteroid-induced — *see* Glaucoma, secondary, drugs
  hypersecretion H40.82- ☑
  in (due to)
    amyloidosis E85.4 [H42]
    aniridia Q13.1 [H42]
    concussion of globe — *see* Glaucoma, secondary, trauma
    dislocation of lens — *see* Glaucoma, secondary
    disorder of lens NEC — *see* Glaucoma, secondary
    drugs — *see* Glaucoma, secondary, drugs
    endocrine disease NOS E34.9 [H42]
    eye
      inflammation — *see* Glaucoma, secondary, inflammation
      trauma — *see* Glaucoma, secondary, trauma
    hypermature cataract — *see* Glaucoma, secondary

Glaucoma — continued
  in — continued
    iridocyclitis — see Glaucoma, secondary, inflammation
    lens disorder — see Glaucoma, secondary
    Lowe's syndrome E72.03 [H42]
    metabolic disease NOS E88.9 [H42]
    ocular disorders NEC — see Glaucoma, secondary
    onchocerciasis B73.02
    pupillary block — see Glaucoma, secondary
    retinal vein occlusion — see Glaucoma, secondary
    Rieger's anomaly Q13.81 [H42]
    rubeosis of iris — see Glaucoma, secondary
    tumor of globe — see Glaucoma, secondary
  infantile Q15.0
  low tension — see Glaucoma, open angle, primary, low-tension
  malignant H40.83- ☑
  narrow angle — see Glaucoma, angle-closure
  newborn Q15.0
  noncongestive (chronic) — see Glaucoma, open angle
  nonobstructive — see Glaucoma, open angle
  obstructive — see also Glaucoma, angle-closure
    due to lens changes — see Glaucoma, secondary
  open angle H40.10- ☑
    primary H40.11- ☑
      capsular (with pseudoexfoliation of lens) H40.14- ☑
      low-tension H40.12- ☑
      pigmentary H40.13- ☑
      residual stage H40.15- ☑
  phacolytic — see Glaucoma, secondary
  pigmentary — see Glaucoma, open angle, primary, pigmentary
  postinfectious — see Glaucoma, secondary, inflammation
  secondary (to) H40.5- ☑
    drugs H40.6- ☑
    inflammation H40.4- ☑
    trauma H40.3- ☑
  simple (chronic) H40.11- ☑
  simplex H40.11- ☑
  specified type NEC H40.89
  suspect H40.00- ☑
  syphilitic A52.71
  traumatic — see also Glaucoma, secondary, trauma
    newborn (birth injury) P15.3
  tuberculous A18.59
Glaucomatous flecks (subcapsular) — see Cataract, complicated
Glazed tongue K14.4
Gleet (gonococcal) A54.01
Glénard's disease K63.4
Glioblastoma (multiforme)
  with sarcomatous component
    specified site — see Neoplasm, malignant, by site
    unspecified site C71.9
  giant cell
    specified site — see Neoplasm, malignant, by site
    unspecified site C71.9
  specified site — see Neoplasm, malignant, by site
  unspecified site C71.9
Glioma (malignant)
  astrocytic
    specified site — see Neoplasm, malignant, by site
    unspecified site C71.9
  mixed
    specified site — see Neoplasm, malignant, by site
    unspecified site C71.9
  nose Q30.8
  specified site NEC — see Neoplasm, malignant, by site
  subependymal D43.2
    specified site — see Neoplasm, uncertain behavior, by site
    unspecified site D43.2
  unspecified site C71.9
Gliomatosis cerebri C71.0
Glioneuroma — see Neoplasm, uncertain behavior, by site
Gliosarcoma
  specified site — see Neoplasm, malignant, by site
  unspecified site C71.9
Gliosis (cerebral) G93.89
  spinal G95.89
Glisson's disease — see Rickets
Globinuria R82.3
Globus (hystericus) F45.8

Glomangioma D18.00
  intra-abdominal D18.03
  intracranial D18.02
  skin D18.01
  specified site NEC D18.09
Glomangiomyoma D18.00
  intra-abdominal D18.03
  intracranial D18.02
  skin D18.01
  specified site NEC D18.09
Glomangiosarcoma — see Neoplasm, connective tissue, malignant
Glomerular
  disease in syphilis A52.75
  nephritis — see Glomerulonephritis
Glomerulitis — see Glomerulonephritis
Glomerulonephritis — see also Nephritis N05.9
  with
    C3
      glomerulonephritis N05.A
      glomerulopathy N05.A
        with dense deposit disease N05.6
    edema — see Nephrosis
    minimal change N05.0
    minor glomerular abnormality N05.0
  acute N00.9
  chronic N03.9
  crescentic (diffuse) NEC — see also N00-N07 with fourth character .7 N05.7
  dense deposit — see also N00-N07 with fourth character .6 N05.6
  diffuse
    crescentic — see also N00-N07 with fourth character .7 N05.7
    endocapillary proliferative — see also N00-N07 with fourth character .4 N05.4
    membranous — see also N00-N07 with fourth character .2 N05.2
    mesangial proliferative — see also N00-N07 with fourth character .3 N05.3
    mesangiocapillary — see also N00-N07 with fourth character .5 N05.5
    sclerosing N18.9
  endocapillary proliferative (diffuse) NEC — see also N00-N07 with fourth character .4 N05.4
  extracapillary NEC — see also N00-N07 with fourth character .7 N05.7
  focal (and segmental) — see also N00-N07 with fourth character .1 N05.1
  hypocomplementemic — see Glomerulonephritis, membranoproliferative
  IgA — see Nephropathy, IgA
  immune complex (circulating) NEC N05.8
  in (due to)
    amyloidosis E85.4 [N08]
    bilharziasis B65.9 [N08]
    cryoglobulinemia D89.1 [N08]
    defibrination syndrome D65 [N08]
    diabetes mellitus — see Diabetes, glomerulosclerosis
    disseminated intravascular coagulation D65 [N08]
    Fabry (-Anderson) disease E75.21 [N08]
    Goodpasture's syndrome M31.0
    hemolytic-uremic syndrome D59.3
    Henoch (-Schönlein) purpura D69.0 [N08]
    lecithin cholesterol acyltransferase deficiency E78.6 [N08]
    microscopic polyangiitis M31.7 [N08]
    multiple myeloma C90.0- ☑ [N08]
    Plasmodium malariae B52.0
    schistosomiasis B65.9 [N08]
    sepsis A41.9 [N08]
      streptococcal A40- ☑ [N08]
    sickle-cell disorders D57.- ☑ [N08]
    strongyloidiasis B78.9 [N08]
    subacute bacterial endocarditis I33.0 [N08]
    syphilis (late) congenital A50.59 [N08]
    systemic lupus erythematosus M32.14
    thrombotic thrombocytopenic purpura M31.19 [N08]
    typhoid fever A01.09
    Waldenström macroglobulinemia C88.0 [N08]
    Wegener's granulomatosis M31.31
  latent or quiescent N03.9
  lobular, lobulonodular — see Glomerulonephritis, membranoproliferative

Glomerulonephritis — continued
  membranoproliferative (diffuse)(type 1 or 3) — see also N00-N07 with fourth character .5 N05.5
    dense deposit (type 2) NEC — see also N00-N07 with fourth character .6 N05.6
  membranous (diffuse) NEC — see also N00-N07 with fourth character .2 N05.2
  mesangial
    IgA/IgG — see Nephropathy, IgA
    proliferative (diffuse) NEC — see also N00-N07 with fourth character .3 N05.3
  mesangiocapillary (diffuse) NEC — see also N00-N07 with fourth character .5 N05.5
  necrotic, necrotizing NEC — see also N00-N07 with fourth character .8 N05.8
  nodular — see Glomerulonephritis, membranoproliferative
  poststreptococcal NEC N05.9
    acute N00.9
    chronic N03.9
    rapidly progressive N01.9
  proliferative NEC — see also N00-N07 with fourth character .8 N05.8
    diffuse (lupus) M32.14
    rapidly progressive N01.9
  sclerosing, diffuse N18.9
  specified pathology NEC — see also N00-N07 with fourth character .8 N05.8
  subacute N01.9
Glomerulopathy — see Glomerulonephritis
Glomerulosclerosis — see also Sclerosis, renal
  intercapillary (nodular) (with diabetes) — see Diabetes, glomerulosclerosis
  intracapillary — see Diabetes, glomerulosclerosis
Glossagra K14.6
Glossalgia K14.6
Glossitis (chronic superficial) (gangrenous) (Moeller's) K14.0
  areata exfoliativa K14.1
  atrophic K14.4
  benign migratory K14.1
  cortical superficial, sclerotic K14.0
  Hunter's D51.0
  interstitial, sclerous K14.0
  median rhomboid K14.2
  pellagrous E52
  superficial, chronic K14.0
Glossocele K14.8
Glossodynia K14.6
  exfoliativa K14.4
Glossoncus K14.8
Glossopathy K14.9
Glossophytia K14.3
Glossoplegia K14.8
Glossoptosis K14.8
Glossopyrosis K14.6
Glossotrichia K14.3
Glossy skin L90.8
Glottis — see condition
Glottitis — see also Laryngitis J04.0
Glucagonoma
  pancreas
    benign D13.7
    malignant C25.4
    uncertain behavior D37.8
  specified site NEC
    benign — see Neoplasm, benign, by site
    malignant — see Neoplasm, malignant, by site
    uncertain behavior — see Neoplasm, uncertain behavior, by site
  unspecified site
    benign D13.7
    malignant C25.4
    uncertain behavior D37.8
Glucoglycinuria E72.51
Glucose-galactose malabsorption E74.39
Glue
  ear — see Otitis, media, nonsuppurative, chronic, mucoid
  sniffing (airplane) — see Abuse, drug, inhalant
    dependence — see Dependence, drug, inhalant
GLUT1 deficiency syndrome 1, infantile onset E74.810
GLUT1 deficiency syndrome 2, childhood onset E74.810
Glutaric aciduria E72.3
Glycinemia E72.51
Glycinuria (renal) (with ketosis) E72.09

☑ Additional Character Required — Refer to the Tabular List for Character Selection   ▼ Subterms under main terms may continue to next column or page

Glycogen
  infiltration — see Disease, glycogen storage
  storage disease — see Disease, glycogen storage
Glycogenosis (diffuse) (generalized) — see also Disease, glycogen storage
  cardiac E74.02 [I43]
  diabetic, secondary — see Diabetes, glycogenosis, secondary
  pulmonary interstitial J84.842
Glycopenia E16.2
Glycosuria R81
  renal E74.818
Gnathostoma spinigerum (infection) (infestation), **gnathostomiasis** (wandering swelling) B83.1
Goiter (plunging) (substernal) E04.9
  with
    hyperthyroidism (recurrent) — see Hyperthyroidism, with, goiter
    thyrotoxicosis — see Hyperthyroidism, with, goiter
  adenomatous — see Goiter, nodular
  cancerous C73
  congenital (nontoxic) E03.0
    diffuse E03.0
    parenchymatous E03.0
    transitory, with normal functioning P72.0
  cystic E04.2
    due to iodine-deficiency E01.1
  due to
    enzyme defect in synthesis of thyroid hormone E07.1
    iodine-deficiency (endemic) E01.2
  dyshormonogenetic (familial) E07.1
  endemic (iodine-deficiency) E01.2
    diffuse E01.0
    multinodular E01.1
  exophthalmic — see Hyperthyroidism, with, goiter
  iodine-deficiency (endemic) E01.2
    diffuse E01.0
    multinodular E01.1
    nodular E01.1
  lingual Q89.2
  lymphadenoid E06.3
  malignant C73
  multinodular (cystic) (nontoxic) E04.2
    toxic or with hyperthyroidism E05.20
      with thyroid storm E05.21
  neonatal NEC P72.0
  nodular (nontoxic) (due to) E04.9
    with
      hyperthyroidism E05.20
        with thyroid storm E05.21
      thyrotoxicosis E05.20
        with thyroid storm E05.21
    endemic E01.1
    iodine-deficiency E01.1
    sporadic E04.9
    toxic E05.20
      with thyroid storm E05.21
  nontoxic E04.9
    diffuse (colloid) E04.0
    multinodular E04.2
    simple E04.0
    specified NEC E04.8
    uninodular E04.1
  simple E04.0
  toxic — see Hyperthyroidism, with, goiter
  uninodular (nontoxic) E04.1
    toxic or with hyperthyroidism E05.10
      with thyroid storm E05.11
Goiter-deafness syndrome E07.1
Goldberg syndrome Q89.8
Goldberg-Maxwell syndrome E34.51
Goldblatt's hypertension or kidney I70.1
Goldenhar (-Gorlin) **syndrome** Q87.0
Goldflam-Erb disease or syndrome G70.00
  with exacerbation (acute) G70.01
  in crisis G70.01
Goldscheider's disease Q81.8
Goldstein's disease (familial hemorrhagic telangiectasia) I78.0
Golfer's elbow — see Epicondylitis, medial
Gonadoblastoma
  specified site — see Neoplasm, uncertain behavior, by site
  unspecified site
    female D39.10
    male D40.10
Gonecystitis — see Vesiculitis

Gongylonemiasis B83.8
Goniosynechiae — see Adhesions, iris, goniosynechiae
Gonococcemia A54.86
Gonococcus, gonococcal (disease) (infection) — see also condition A54.9
  anus A54.6
  bursa, bursitis A54.49
  conjunctiva, conjunctivitis (neonatorum) A54.31
  endocardium A54.83
  eye A54.30
    conjunctivitis A54.31
    iridocyclitis A54.32
    keratitis A54.33
    newborn A54.31
    other specified A54.39
  fallopian tubes (acute) (chronic) A54.24
  genitourinary (organ) (system) (tract) (acute)
    lower A54.00
      with abscess (accessory gland) (periurethral) A54.1
    upper — see also condition A54.29
  heart A54.83
  iridocyclitis A54.32
  joint A54.42
  lymphatic (gland) (node) A54.89
  meninges, meningitis A54.81
  musculoskeletal A54.40
    arthritis A54.42
    osteomyelitis A54.43
    other specified A54.49
    spondylopathy A54.41
  pelviperitonitis A54.24
  pelvis (acute) (chronic) A54.24
  pharynx A54.5
  proctitis A54.6
  pyosalpinx (acute) (chronic) A54.24
  rectum A54.6
  skin A54.89
  specified site NEC A54.89
  tendon sheath A54.49
  throat A54.5
  urethra (acute) (chronic) A54.01
    with abscess (accessory gland) (periurethral) A54.1
  vulva (acute) (chronic) A54.02
Gonocytoma
  specified site — see Neoplasm, uncertain behavior, by site
  unspecified site
    female D39.10
    male D40.10
Gonorrhea (acute) (chronic) A54.9
  Bartholin's gland (acute) (chronic) (purulent) A54.02
    with abscess (accessory gland) (periurethral) A54.1
  bladder A54.01
  cervix A54.03
  conjunctiva, conjunctivitis (neonatorum) A54.31
  contact Z20.2
  Cowper's gland (with abscess) A54.1
  exposure to Z20.2
  fallopian tube (acute) (chronic) A54.24
  kidney (acute) (chronic) A54.21
  lower genitourinary tract A54.00
    with abscess (accessory gland) (periurethral) A54.1
  ovary (acute) (chronic) A54.24
  pelvis (acute) (chronic) A54.24
    female pelvic inflammatory disease A54.24
  penis A54.09
  prostate (acute) (chronic) A54.22
  seminal vesicle (acute) (chronic) A54.23
  specified site not listed — see also Gonococcus A54.89
  spermatic cord (acute) (chronic) A54.23
  urethra A54.01
    with abscess (accessory gland) (periurethral) A54.1
  vagina A54.02
  vas deferens (acute) (chronic) A54.23
  vulva A54.02
Goodall's disease A08.19
Goodpasture's syndrome M31.0
Gopalan's syndrome (burning feet) E53.0
Gorlin-Chaudry-Moss syndrome Q87.0
Gottron's papules L94.4
Gougerot-Blum syndrome (pigmented purpuric lichenoid dermatitis) L81.7
Gougerot-Carteaud disease or syndrome (confluent reticulate papillomatosis) L83
Gougerot's syndrome (trisymptomatic) L81.7
Gouley's syndrome (constrictive pericarditis) I31.1
Goundou A66.6

Gout, chronic — see also Gout, gouty M1A.9 ☑ (following M08)
  drug-induced M1A.20 ☑ (following M08)
    ankle M1A.27- ☑ (following M08)
    elbow M1A.22- ☑ (following M08)
    foot joint M1A.27- ☑ (following M08)
    hand joint M1A.24- ☑ (following M08)
    hip M1A.25- ☑ (following M08)
    knee M1A.26- ☑ (following M08)
    multiple site M1A.29- ☑ (following M08)
    shoulder M1A.21- ☑ (following M08)
    vertebrae M1A.28 ☑ (following M08)
    wrist M1A.23- ☑ (following M08)
  idiopathic M1A.00 ☑ (following M08)
    ankle M1A.07- ☑ (following M08)
    elbow M1A.02- ☑ (following M08)
    foot joint M1A.07- ☑ (following M08)
    hand joint M1A.04- ☑ (following M08)
    hip M1A.05- ☑ (following M08)
    knee M1A.06- ☑ (following M08)
    multiple site M1A.09 ☑ (following M08)
    shoulder M1A.01- ☑ (following M08)
    vertebrae M1A.08 ☑ (following M08)
    wrist M1A.03- ☑ (following M08)
  in (due to) renal impairment M1A.30 ☑ (following M08)
    ankle M1A.37- ☑ (following M08)
    elbow M1A.32- ☑ (following M08)
    foot joint M1A.37- ☑ (following M08)
    hand joint M1A.34- ☑ (following M08)
    hip M1A.35- ☑ (following M08)
    knee M1A.36- ☑ (following M08)
    multiple site M1A.39 ☑ (following M08)
    shoulder M1A.31- ☑ (following M08)
    vertebrae M1A.38 ☑ (following M08)
    wrist M1A.33- ☑ (following M08)
  lead-induced M1A.10 ☑ (following M08)
    ankle M1A.17- ☑ (following M08)
    elbow M1A.12- ☑ (following M08)
    foot joint M1A.17- ☑ (following M08)
    hand joint M1A.14- ☑ (following M08)
    hip M1A.15- ☑ (following M08)
    knee M1A.16- ☑ (following M08)
    multiple site M1A.19 ☑ (following M08)
    shoulder M1A.11- ☑ (following M08)
    vertebrae M1A.18 ☑ (following M08)
    wrist M1A.13- ☑ (following M08)
  primary — see Gout, chronic, idiopathic
  saturnine — see Gout, chronic, lead-induced
  secondary NEC M1A.40 ☑ (following M08)
    ankle M1A.47- ☑ (following M08)
    elbow M1A.42- ☑ (following M08)
    foot joint M1A.47- ☑ (following M08)
    hand joint M1A.44- ☑ (following M08)
    hip M1A.45- ☑ (following M08)
    knee M1A.46- ☑ (following M08)
    multiple site M1A.49 ☑ (following M08)
    shoulder M1A.41- ☑ (following M08)
    vertebrae M1A.48 ☑ (following M08)
    wrist M1A.43- ☑ (following M08)
  syphilitic — see also subcategory M14.8- A52.77
  tophi M1A.9 ☑ (following M08)
Gout, gouty (acute) (attack) (flare) — see also Gout, chronic M10.9
  drug-induced M10.20
    ankle M10.27- ☑
    elbow M10.22- ☑
    foot joint M10.27- ☑
    hand joint M10.24- ☑
    hip M10.25- ☑
    knee M10.26- ☑
    multiple site M10.29
    shoulder M10.21- ☑
    vertebrae M10.28
    wrist M10.23- ☑
  idiopathic M10.00
    ankle M10.07- ☑
    elbow M10.02- ☑
    foot joint M10.07- ☑
    hand joint M10.04- ☑
    hip M10.05- ☑
    knee M10.06- ☑
    multiple site M10.09
    shoulder M10.01- ☑
    vertebrae M10.08
    wrist M10.03- ☑
  in (due to) renal impairment M10.30

Gout, gouty — *continued*
  in renal impairment — *continued*
    ankle M10.37- ☑
    elbow M10.32- ☑
    foot joint M10.37- ☑
    hand joint M10.34- ☑
    hip M10.35- ☑
    knee M10.36- ☑
    multiple site M10.39
    shoulder M10.31- ☑
    vertebrae M10.38
    wrist M10.33- ☑
  lead-induced M10.10
    ankle M10.17- ☑
    elbow M10.12- ☑
    foot joint M10.17- ☑
    hand joint M10.14- ☑
    hip M10.15- ☑
    knee M10.16- ☑
    multiple site M10.19
    shoulder M10.11- ☑
    vertebrae M10.18
    wrist M10.13- ☑
  primary — *see* Gout, idiopathic
  saturnine — *see* Gout, lead-induced
  secondary NEC M10.40
    ankle M10.47- ☑
    elbow M10.42- ☑
    foot joint M10.47- ☑
    hand joint M10.44- ☑
    hip M10.45- ☑
    knee M10.46- ☑
    multiple site M10.49
    shoulder M10.41- ☑
    vertebrae M10.48
    wrist M10.43- ☑
  syphilitic — *see also* subcategory M14.8- A52.77
  tophi — *see* Gout, chronic
Gower's
  muscular dystrophy G71.01
  syndrome (vasovagal attack) R55
Gradenigo's syndrome — *see* Otitis, media, suppurative, acute
Graefe's disease — *see* Strabismus, paralytic, ophthalmoplegia, progressive
Graft-versus-host disease D89.813
  acute D89.810
  acute on chronic D89.812
  chronic D89.811
Grain mite (itch) B88.0
Grainhandler's disease or lung J67.8
Grand mal — *see* Epilepsy, generalized, specified NEC
Grand multipara status only (not pregnant) Z64.1
  pregnant — *see* Pregnancy, complicated by, grand multiparity
Granite worker's lung J62.8
Granular — *see also* condition
  inflammation, pharynx J31.2
  kidney (contracting) — *see* Sclerosis, renal
  liver K74.69
Granulation tissue (abnormal) (excessive) L92.9
  postmastoidectomy cavity — *see* Complications, postmastoidectomy, granulation
Granulocytopenia (primary) (malignant) — *see* Agranulocytosis
Granuloma L92.9
  abdomen K66.8
    from residual foreign body L92.3
    pyogenicum L98.0
  actinic L57.5
  annulare (perforating) L92.0
  apical K04.5
  aural — *see* Otitis, externa, specified NEC
  beryllium (skin) L92.3
  bone
    eosinophilic C96.6
    from residual foreign body — *see* Osteomyelitis, specified type NEC
    lung C96.6
  brain (any site) G06.0
    schistosomiasis B65.9 [G07]
  canaliculus lacrimalis — *see* Granuloma, lacrimal
  candidal (cutaneous) B37.2
  cerebral (any site) G06.0
  coccidioidal (primary) (progressive) B38.7
    lung B38.1
    meninges B38.4

Granuloma — *continued*
  colon K63.89
  conjunctiva H11.22- ☑
  dental K04.5
  ear, middle — *see* Cholesteatoma
  eosinophilic C96.6
    bone C96.6
    lung C96.6
    oral mucosa K13.4
    skin L92.2
  eyelid H01.8
  facial (e) L92.2
  foreign body (in soft tissue) NEC M60.20
    ankle M60.27- ☑
    foot M60.27- ☑
    forearm M60.23- ☑
    hand M60.24- ☑
    in operation wound — *see* Foreign body, accidentally left during a procedure
    lower leg M60.26- ☑
    pelvic region M60.25- ☑
    shoulder region M60.21- ☑
    skin L92.3
    specified site NEC M60.28
    subcutaneous tissue L92.3
    thigh M60.25- ☑
    upper arm M60.22- ☑
  gangraenescens M31.2
  genito-inguinale A58
  giant cell (central) (reparative) (jaw) M27.1
    gingiva (peripheral) K06.8
  gland (lymph) I88.8
  hepatic NEC K75.3
    in (due to)
      berylliosis J63.2 [K77]
      sarcoidosis D86.89
  Hodgkin C81.9 ☑
  ileum K63.89
  infectious B99.9
    specified NEC B99.8
  inguinale (Donovan) (venereal) A58
  intestine NEC K63.89
  intracranial (any site) G06.0
  intraspinal (any part) G06.1
  iridocyclitis — *see* Iridocyclitis, chronic
  jaw (bone) (central) M27.1
    reparative giant cell M27.1
  kidney — *see also* Infection, kidney N15.8
  lacrimal H04.81- ☑
  larynx J38.7
  lethal midline (faciale(e)) M31.2
  liver NEC — *see* Granuloma, hepatic
  lung (infectious) — *see also* Fibrosis, lung
    coccidioidal B38.1
    eosinophilic C96.6
  Majocchi's B35.8
  malignant (facial(e)) M31.2
  mandible (central) M27.1
  midline (lethal) M31.2
  monilial (cutaneous) B37.2
  nasal sinus — *see* Sinusitis
  operation wound T81.89 ☑
    foreign body — *see* Foreign body, accidentally left during a procedure
    stitch T81.89 ☑
    talc — *see* Foreign body, accidentally left during a procedure
  oral mucosa K13.4
  orbit, orbital H05.11- ☑
  paracoccidioidal B41.8
  penis, venereal A58
  periapical K04.5
  peritoneum K66.8
    due to ova of helminths NOS — *see also* Helminthiasis B83.9 [K67]
  postmastoidectomy cavity — *see* Complications, postmastoidectomy, recurrent cholesteatoma
  prostate N42.89
  pudendi (ulcerating) A58
  pulp, internal (tooth) K03.3
  pyogenic, pyogenicum (of) (skin) L98.0
    gingiva K06.8
    maxillary alveolar ridge K04.5
    oral mucosa K13.4
  rectum K62.89
  reticulohistiocytic D76.3
  rubrum nasi L74.8
  Schistosoma — *see* Schistosomiasis

Granuloma — *continued*
  septic (skin) L98.0
  silica (skin) L92.3
  sinus (accessory) (infective) (nasal) — *see* Sinusitis
  skin L92.9
    from residual foreign body L92.3
    pyogenicum L98.0
  spine
    syphilitic (epidural) A52.19
    tuberculous A18.01
  stitch (postoperative) T81.89 ☑
  suppurative (skin) L98.0
  swimming pool A31.1
  talc — *see also* Granuloma, foreign body
    in operation wound — *see* Foreign body, accidentally left during a procedure
  telangiectaticum (skin) L98.0
  tracheostomy J95.09
  trichophyticum B35.8
  tropicum A66.4
  umbilical P83.81
  umbilicus P83.81
  urethra N36.8
  uveitis — *see* Iridocyclitis, chronic
  vagina A58
  venereum A58
  vocal cord J38.3
Granulomatosis L92.9
  with polyangiitis M31.3 ☑
  eosinophilic, with polyangiitis [EGPA] M30.1
  lymphoid C83.8- ☑
  miliary (listerial) A32.89
  necrotizing, respiratory M31.30
  progressive septic D71
  specified NEC L92.8
  Wegener's M31.30
    with renal involvement M31.31
Granulomatous tissue (abnormal) (excessive) L92.9
Granulosis rubra nasi L74.8
Graphite fibrosis (of lung) J63.3
Graphospasm F48.8
  organic G25.89
Grating scapula M89.8X1
Gravel (urinary) — *see* Calculus, urinary
Graves' disease — *see* Hyperthyroidism, with, goiter
Gravis — *see* condition
Grawitz tumor C64.- ☑
Gray syndrome (newborn) P93.0
Grayness, hair (premature) L67.1
  congenital Q84.2
Green sickness D50.8
Greenfield's disease
  meaning
    concentric sclerosis (encephalitis periaxialis concentrica) G37.5
    metachromatic leukodystrophy E75.25
Greenstick fracture — *code as* Fracture, by site
Grey syndrome (newborn) P93.0
Grief F43.21
  prolonged F43.29
  reaction — *see also* Disorder, adjustment F43.20
Griesinger's disease B76.0
Grinder's lung or pneumoconiosis J62.8
Grinding, teeth
  psychogenic F45.8
  sleep related G47.63
Grip
  Dabney's B33.0
  devil's B33.0
Grippe, grippal — *see also* Influenza
  Balkan A78
  summer, of Italy A93.1
Grisel's disease M43.6
Groin — *see* condition
Grooved tongue K14.5
Ground itch B76.9
Grover's disease or syndrome L11.1
Growing pains, children R29.898
Growth (fungoid) (neoplastic) (new) — *see also* Neoplasm
  adenoid (vegetative) J35.8
  benign — *see* Neoplasm, benign, by site
  malignant — *see* Neoplasm, malignant, by site
  rapid, childhood Z00.2
  secondary — *see* Neoplasm, secondary, by site
Gruby's disease B35.0
Gubler-Millard paralysis or syndrome G46.3
Guerin-Stern syndrome Q74.3

☑ Additional Character Required — Refer to the Tabular List for Character Selection

▽ Subterms under main terms may continue to next column or page

Guidance, insufficient anterior (occlusal) M26.54
Guillain-Barré disease or syndrome G61.0
  sequelae G65.0
Guinea worms (infection) (infestation) B72
Guinon's disease (motor-verbal tic) F95.2
Gull's disease E03.4
Gum — see condition
Gumboil K04.7
  with sinus K04.6
Gumma (syphilitic) A52.79
  artery A52.09
    cerebral A52.04
  bone A52.77
    of yaws (late) A66.6
  brain A52.19
  cauda equina A52.19
  central nervous system A52.3
  ciliary body A52.71
  congenital A50.59
  eyelid A52.71
  heart A52.06
  intracranial A52.19
  iris A52.71
  kidney A52.75
  larynx A52.73
  leptomeninges A52.19
  liver A52.74
  meninges A52.19
  myocardium A52.06
  nasopharynx A52.73
  neurosyphilitic A52.3
  nose A52.73
  orbit A52.71
  palate (soft) A52.79
  penis A52.76
  pericardium A52.06
  pharynx A52.73
  pituitary A52.79
  scrofulous (tuberculous) A18.4
  skin A52.79
  specified site NEC A52.79
  spinal cord A52.19
  tongue A52.79
  tonsil A52.73
  trachea A52.73
  tuberculous A18.4
  ulcerative due to yaws A66.4
  ureter A52.75
  yaws A66.4
    bone A66.6
Gunn's syndrome Q07.8
Gunshot wound — see also Puncture, open
  fracture — code as Fracture, by site
  internal organs — see Injury, by site
Gynandrism Q56.0
Gynandroblastoma
  specified site — see Neoplasm, uncertain behavior, by site
  unspecified site
    female D39.10
    male D40.10
Gynecological examination (periodic) (routine) Z01.419
  with abnormal findings Z01.411
Gynecomastia N62
Gynephobia F40.291
Gyrate scalp Q82.8

H

H (Hartnup's) **disease** E72.02
Haas' disease or osteochondrosis (juvenile) (head of humerus) — see Osteochondrosis, juvenile, humerus
Habit, habituation
  bad sleep Z72.821
  chorea F95.8
  disturbance, child F98.9
  drug — see Dependence, drug
  irregular sleep Z72.821
  laxative F55.2
  spasm — see Tic
  tic — see Tic
Haemophilus (H.) **influenzae, as cause of disease classified elsewhere** B96.3
Haff disease — see Poisoning, mercury
Hageman's factor defect, deficiency or disease D68.2
Haglund's disease or osteochondrosis (juvenile) (os tibiale externum) — see Osteochondrosis, juvenile, tarsus

Hailey-Hailey disease Q82.8
Hair — see also condition
  plucking F63.3
    in stereotyped movement disorder F98.4
  tourniquet syndrome — see also Constriction, external, by site
    finger S60.44- ☑
    penis S30.842 ☑
    thumb S60.34- ☑
    toe S90.44- ☑
Hairball in stomach T18.2 ☑
Hair-pulling, pathological (compulsive) F63.3
Hairy black tongue K14.3
Half vertebra Q76.49
Halitosis R19.6
Hallerman-Streiff syndrome Q87.0
Hallervorden-Spatz disease G23.0
Hallopeau's acrodermatitis or disease L40.2
Hallucination R44.3
  auditory R44.0
  gustatory R44.2
  olfactory R44.2
  specified NEC R44.2
  tactile R44.2
  visual R44.1
Hallucinosis (chronic) F28
  alcoholic (acute) F10.951
    in
      abuse F10.151
      dependence F10.251
  drug-induced F19.951
    cannabis F12.951
    cocaine F14.951
    hallucinogen F16.151
      in
        abuse F19.151
          cannabis F12.151
          cocaine F14.151
          hallucinogen F16.151
          inhalant F18.151
          opioid F11.151
          sedative, anxiolytic or hypnotic F13.151
          stimulant NEC F15.151
        dependence F19.251
          cannabis F12.251
          cocaine F14.251
          hallucinogen F16.251
          inhalant F18.251
          opioid F11.251
          sedative, anxiolytic or hypnotic F13.251
          stimulant NEC F15.251
    inhalant F18.951
    opioid F11.951
    sedative, anxiolytic or hypnotic F13.951
    stimulant NEC F15.951
  organic F06.0
Hallux
  deformity (acquired) NEC M20.5X- ☑
  limitus M20.5X- ☑
  malleus (acquired) NEC M20.3- ☑
  rigidus (acquired) M20.2- ☑
    congenital Q74.2
    sequelae (late effect) of rickets E64.3
  valgus (acquired) M20.1- ☑
    congenital Q66.6
  varus (acquired) M20.3- ☑
    congenital Q66.3- ☑
Halo, visual H53.19
Hamartoma, hamartoblastoma Q85.9
  epithelial (gingival), odontogenic, central or peripheral — see Cyst, calcifying odontogenic
Hamartosis Q85.9
Hamman-Rich syndrome J84.114
Hammer toe (acquired) NEC — see also Deformity, toe, hammer toe
  congenital Q66.89
  sequelae (late effect) of rickets E64.3
Hand — see condition
Hand-foot syndrome L27.1
Handicap, handicapped
  educational Z55.9
    specified NEC Z55.8
Hand-Schüller-Christian disease or syndrome C96.5
Hanging (asphyxia) (strangulation) (suffocation) — see Asphyxia, traumatic, due to mechanical threat
Hangnail — see also Cellulitis, digit
  with lymphangitis — see Lymphangitis, acute, digit

Hangover (alcohol) F10.129
Hanhart's syndrome Q87.0
Hanot-Chauffard (-Troisier) **syndrome** E83.19
Hanot's cirrhosis or disease K74.3
Hansen's disease — see Leprosy
Hantaan virus disease (Korean hemorrhagic fever) A98.5
Hantavirus disease (with renal manifestations) (Dobrava) (Puumala) (Seoul) A98.5
  with pulmonary manifestations (Andes) (Bayou) (Bermejo) (Black Creek Canal) (Choclo) (Juquitiba) (Laguna negra) (Lechiguanas) (New York) (Oran) (Sin nombre) B33.4
Happy puppet syndrome Q93.51
Harada's disease or syndrome H30.81- ☑
Hardening
  artery — see Arteriosclerosis
  brain G93.89
Harelip (complete) (incomplete) — see Cleft, lip
Harlequin (newborn) Q80.4
Harley's disease D59.6
Harmful use (of)
  alcohol F10.10
  anxiolytics — see Abuse, drug, sedative
  cannabinoids — see Abuse, drug, cannabis
  cocaine — see Abuse, drug, cocaine
  drug — see Abuse, drug
  hallucinogens — see Abuse, drug, hallucinogen
  hypnotics — see Abuse, drug, sedative
  opioids — see Abuse, drug, opioid
  PCP (phencyclidine) — see Abuse, drug, hallucinogen
  sedatives — see Abuse, drug, sedative
  stimulants NEC — see Abuse, drug, stimulant
Harris' lines — see Arrest, epiphyseal
Hartnup's disease E72.02
Harvester's lung J67.0
Harvesting ovum for in vitro fertilization Z31.83
Hashimoto's disease or thyroiditis E06.3
Hashitoxicosis (transient) E06.3
Hassal-Henle bodies or warts (cornea) H18.49
Haut mal — see Epilepsy, generalized, specified NEC
Haverhill fever A25.1
Hay fever — see also Fever, hay J30.1
Hayem-Widal syndrome D59.8
Haygarth's nodes M15.8
Haymaker's lung J67.0
Hb (abnormal)
  Bart's disease D56.0
  disease — see Disease, hemoglobin
  trait — see Trait
Head — see condition
Headache R51.9
  with
    orthostatic component NEC R51.0
    positional component NEC R51.0
  allergic NEC G44.89
  associated with sexual activity G44.82
  cervicogenic G44.86
  chronic daily R51.9
  cluster G44.009
    chronic G44.029
      intractable G44.021
      not intractable G44.029
    episodic G44.019
      intractable G44.011
      not intractable G44.019
    intractable G44.001
    not intractable G44.009
  cough (primary) G44.83
  daily chronic R51.9
  drug-induced NEC G44.40
    intractable G44.41
    not intractable G44.40
  exertional (primary) G44.84
  histamine G44.009
    intractable G44.001
    not intractable G44.009
  hypnic G44.81
  lumbar puncture G97.1
  medication overuse G44.40
    intractable G44.41
    not intractable G44.40
  menstrual — see Migraine, menstrual
  migraine (type) — see also Migraine G43.909
  nasal septum R51.9
  neuralgiform, short lasting unilateral, with conjunctival injection and tearing (SUNCT) G44.059
    intractable G44.051

Headache — *continued*
　neuralgiform, short lasting unilateral, with conjunctival injection and tearing — *continued*
　　not intractable G44.059
　new daily persistent (NDPH) G44.52
　orgasmic G44.82
　periodic syndromes in adults and children G43.C0 (*following* G43.7)
　　with refractory migraine G43.C1 (*following* G43.7)
　　intractable G43.C1 (*following* G43.7)
　　not intractable G43.C0 (*following* G43.7)
　　without refractory migraine G43.C0 (*following* G43.7)
　postspinal puncture G97.1
　post-traumatic G44.309
　　acute G44.319
　　　intractable G44.311
　　　not intractable G44.319
　　chronic G44.329
　　　intractable G44.321
　　　not intractable G44.329
　　intractable G44.301
　　not intractable G44.309
　pre-menstrual — *see* Migraine, menstrual
　preorgasmic G44.82
　primary
　　cough G44.83
　　exertional G44.84
　　stabbing G44.85
　　thunderclap G44.53
　rebound G44.40
　　intractable G44.41
　　not intractable G44.40
　short lasting unilateral neuralgiform, with conjunctival injection and tearing (SUNCT) G44.059
　　intractable G44.051
　　not intractable G44.059
　specified syndrome NEC G44.89
　spinal and epidural anesthesia - induced T88.59 ☑
　　in labor and delivery O74.5
　　in pregnancy O29.4- ☑
　　postpartum, puerperal O89.4
　spinal fluid loss (from puncture) G97.1
　stabbing (primary) G44.85
　tension (-type) G44.209
　　chronic G44.229
　　　intractable G44.221
　　　not intractable G44.229
　　episodic G44.219
　　　intractable G44.211
　　　not intractable G44.219
　　intractable G44.201
　　not intractable G44.209
　thunderclap (primary) G44.53
　vascular NEC G44.1
Healthy
　infant
　　accompanying sick mother Z76.3
　　receiving care Z76.2
　person accompanying sick person Z76.3
Hearing examination Z01.10
　with abnormal findings NEC Z01.118
　following failed hearing screening Z01.110
　for hearing conservation and treatment Z01.12
　infant or child (over 28 days old) Z00.129
　　with abnormal findings Z00.121
Heart — *see* condition
Heart beat
　abnormality R00.9
　　specified NEC R00.8
　awareness R00.2
　rapid R00.0
　slow R00.1
Heartburn R12
　psychogenic F45.8
Heartland virus disease A93.8
Heat (effects) T67.9 ☑
　apoplexy T67.01 ☑
　burn — *see also* Burn L55.9
　collapse T67.1 ☑
　cramps T67.2 ☑
　dermatitis or eczema L59.0
　edema T67.7 ☑
　erythema — *code by site under* Burn, first degree
　excessive T67.9 ☑
　　specified effect NEC T67.8 ☑
　exhaustion T67.5 ☑
　　anhydrotic T67.3 ☑

Heat — *continued*
　exhaustion — *continued*
　　due to
　　　salt (and water) depletion T67.4 ☑
　　　water depletion T67.3 ☑
　　　　with salt depletion T67.4 ☑
　fatigue (transient) T67.6 ☑
　fever T67.01 ☑
　hyperpyrexia T67.01 ☑
　prickly L74.0
　prostration — *see* Heat, exhaustion
　pyrexia T67.01 ☑
　rash L74.0
　specified effect NEC T67.8 ☑
　stroke T67.01 ☑
　　exertional T67.02 ☑
　　specified NEC T67.09 ☑
　sunburn — *see* Sunburn
　syncope T67.1 ☑
Heavy-for-dates NEC (infant) (4000g to 4499g) P08.1
　exceptionally (4500g or more) P08.0
Hebephrenia, hebephrenic (schizophrenia) F20.1
Heberden's disease or nodes (with arthropathy) M15.1
Hebra's
　pityriasis L26
　prurigo L28.2
Heel — *see* condition
Heerfordt's disease D86.89
Hegglin's anomaly or syndrome D72.0
Heilmeyer-Schoner disease D45
Heine-Medin disease A80.9
Heinz body anemia, congenital D58.2
Heliophobia F40.228
Heller's disease or syndrome F84.3
HELLP syndrome (hemolysis, elevated liver enzymes and low platelet count) O14.2- ☑
　complicating
　　childbirth O14.24
　　puerperium O14.25
Helminthiasis — *see also* Infestation, helminth
　Ancylostoma B76.0
　intestinal B82.0
　　mixed types (types classifiable to more than one of the titles B65.0-B81.3 and B81.8) B81.4
　　specified type NEC B81.8
　mixed types (intestinal) (types classifiable to more than one of the titles B65.0-B81.3 and B81.8) B81.4
　Necator (americanus) B76.1
　specified type NEC B83.8
Heloma L84
Hemangioblastoma — *see* Neoplasm, connective tissue, uncertain behavior
　malignant — *see* Neoplasm, connective tissue, malignant
Hemangioendothelioma — *see also* Neoplasm, uncertain behavior, by site
　benign D18.00
　　intra-abdominal D18.03
　　intracranial D18.02
　　skin D18.01
　　specified site NEC D18.09
　bone (diffuse) — *see* Neoplasm, bone, malignant
　epithelioid — *see also* Neoplasm, uncertain behavior, by site
　　malignant — *see* Neoplasm, malignant, by site
　malignant — *see* Neoplasm, connective tissue, malignant
Hemangiofibroma — *see* Neoplasm, benign, by site
Hemangiolipoma — *see* Lipoma
Hemangioma D18.00
　arteriovenous D18.00
　　intra-abdominal D18.03
　　intracranial D18.02
　　skin D18.01
　　specified site NEC D18.09
　capillary I78.1
　　intra-abdominal D18.03
　　intracranial D18.02
　　skin D18.01
　　specified site NEC D18.09
　cavernous D18.00
　　intra-abdominal D18.03
　　intracranial D18.02
　　skin D18.01
　　specified site NEC D18.09
　epithelioid D18.00
　　intra-abdominal D18.03

Hemangioma — *continued*
　epithelioid — *continued*
　　intracranial D18.02
　　skin D18.01
　　specified site NEC D18.09
　histiocytoid D18.00
　　intra-abdominal D18.03
　　intracranial D18.02
　　skin D18.01
　　specified site NEC D18.09
　infantile D18.00
　　intra-abdominal D18.03
　　intracranial D18.02
　　skin D18.01
　　specified site NEC D18.09
　intra-abdominal D18.03
　intracranial D18.02
　intramuscular D18.00
　　intra-abdominal D18.03
　　intracranial D18.02
　　skin D18.01
　　specified site NEC D18.09
　intrathoracic structures D18.09
　juvenile D18.00
　malignant — *see* Neoplasm, connective tissue, malignant
　plexiform D18.00
　　intra-abdominal D18.03
　　intracranial D18.02
　　skin D18.01
　　specified site NEC D18.09
　racemose D18.00
　　intra-abdominal D18.03
　　intracranial D18.02
　　skin D18.01
　　specified site NEC D18.09
　sclerosing — *see* Neoplasm, skin, benign
　simplex D18.00
　　intra-abdominal D18.03
　　intracranial D18.02
　　skin D18.01
　　specified site NEC D18.09
　skin D18.01
　specified site NEC D18.09
　venous D18.00
　　intra-abdominal D18.03
　　intracranial D18.02
　　skin D18.01
　　specified site NEC D18.09
　verrucous keratotic D18.00
　　intra-abdominal D18.03
　　intracranial D18.02
　　skin D18.01
　　specified site NEC D18.09
Hemangiomatosis (systemic) I78.8
　involving single site — *see* Hemangioma
Hemangiopericytoma — *see also* Neoplasm, connective tissue, uncertain behavior
　benign — *see* Neoplasm, connective tissue, benign
　malignant — *see* Neoplasm, connective tissue, malignant
Hemangiosarcoma — *see* Neoplasm, connective tissue, malignant
Hemarthrosis (nontraumatic) M25.00
　ankle M25.07- ☑
　elbow M25.02- ☑
　foot joint M25.07- ☑
　hand joint M25.04- ☑
　hip M25.05- ☑
　in hemophilic arthropathy — *see* Arthropathy, hemophilic
　knee M25.06- ☑
　shoulder M25.01- ☑
　specified joint NEC M25.08
　traumatic — *see* Sprain, by site
　vertebrae M25.08
　wrist M25.03- ☑
Hematemesis K92.0
　with ulcer — *code by site under* Ulcer, with hemorrhage K27.4
　newborn, neonatal P54.0
　　due to swallowed maternal blood P78.2
Hematidrosis L74.8
Hematinuria — *see also* Hemoglobinuria
　malarial B50.8
Hematobilia K83.8
Hematocele
　female NEC N94.89

☑ **Additional Character Required** — **Refer to the Tabular List for Character Selection**
▽ **Subterms under main terms may continue to next column or page**

Hematocele — *continued*
  female — *continued*
    with ectopic pregnancy O00.90
      with intrauterine pregnancy O00.91
    ovary N83.8
  male N50.1
Hematochezia — *see also* Melena K92.1
Hematochyluria — *see also* Infestation, filarial
  schistosomiasis (bilharziasis) B65.0
Hematocolpos (with hematometra or hematosalpinx)
  N89.7
Hematocornea — *see* Pigmentation, cornea, stromal
Hematogenous — *see* condition
Hematoma (traumatic) (skin surface intact) — *see also*
  Contusion
  with
    injury of internal organs — *see* Injury, by site
    open wound — *see* Wound, open
  amputation stump (surgical) (late) T87.89
  aorta, dissecting I71.00
    abdominal I71.02
    thoracic I71.01
    thoracoabdominal I71.03
  aortic intramural — *see* Dissection, aorta
  arterial (complicating trauma) — *see* Injury, blood
    vessel, by site
  auricle — *see* Contusion, ear
    nontraumatic — *see* Disorder, pinna, hematoma
  birth injury NEC P15.8
  brain (traumatic)
    with
      cerebral laceration or contusion (diffuse) — *see*
        Injury, intracranial, diffuse
        focal — *see* Injury, intracranial, focal
    cerebellar, traumatic S06.37- ☑
    intracerebral, traumatic — *see* Injury, intracranial,
      intracerebral hemorrhage
    newborn NEC P52.4
      birth injury P10.1
    nontraumatic — *see* Hemorrhage, intracranial
    subarachnoid, arachnoid, traumatic — *see* Injury,
      intracranial, subarachnoid hemorrhage
    subdural, traumatic — *see* Injury, intracranial, sub-
      dural hemorrhage
  breast (nontraumatic) N64.89
  broad ligament (nontraumatic) N83.7
    traumatic S37.892 ☑
  cerebellar, traumatic S06.37- ☑
  cerebral — *see* Hematoma, brain
  cerebrum S06.36- ☑
    left S06.35- ☑
    right S06.34- ☑
  cesarean delivery wound O90.2
  complicating delivery (perineal) (pelvic) (vagina) (vulva)
    O71.7
  corpus cavernosum (nontraumatic) N48.89
  epididymis (nontraumatic) N50.1
  epidural (traumatic) — *see* Injury, intracranial, epidural
    hemorrhage
    spinal — *see* Injury, spinal cord, by region
  episiotomy O90.2
  face, birth injury P15.4
  genital organ NEC (nontraumatic)
    female (nonobstetric) N94.89
      traumatic S30.202 ☑
    male N50.1
      traumatic S30.201 ☑
  internal organs — *see* Injury, by site
  intracerebral, traumatic — *see* Injury, intracranial, in-
    tracerebral hemorrhage
  intraoperative — *see* Complications, intraoperative,
    hemorrhage
  labia (nontraumatic) (nonobstetric) N90.89
  liver (subcapsular) (nontraumatic) K76.89
    birth injury P15.0
  mediastinum — *see* Injury, intrathoracic
  mesosalpinx (nontraumatic) N83.7
    traumatic S37.898 ☑
  muscle — code by site under Contusion
  nontraumatic
    muscle M79.81
    soft tissue M79.81
  obstetrical surgical wound O90.2
  orbit, orbital (nontraumatic) — *see also* Hemorrhage,
    orbit
    traumatic — *see* Contusion, orbit
  pelvis (female) (nontraumatic) (nonobstetric) N94.89
    obstetric O71.7

Hematoma — *continued*
  pelvis — *continued*
    traumatic — *see* Injury, by site
  penis (nontraumatic) N48.89
    birth injury P15.5
  perianal (nontraumatic) K64.5
  perineal S30.23 ☑
    complicating delivery O71.7
  perirenal — *see* Injury, kidney
  pinna — *see* Contusion, ear
    nontraumatic — *see* Disorder, pinna, hematoma
  placenta O43.89- ☑
  postoperative (postprocedural) — *see* Complication,
    postprocedural, hematoma
  retroperitoneal (nontraumatic) K66.1
    traumatic S36.892 ☑
  scrotum, superficial S30.22 ☑
    birth injury P15.5
  seminal vesicle (nontraumatic) N50.1
    traumatic S37.892 ☑
  spermatic cord (traumatic) S37.892 ☑
    nontraumatic N50.1
  spinal (cord) (meninges) — *see also* Injury, spinal cord,
    by region
    newborn (birth injury) P11.5
  spleen D73.5
    intraoperative — *see* Complications, intraoperative,
      hemorrhage, spleen
    postprocedural (postoperative) — *see* Complica-
      tions, postprocedural, hemorrhage, spleen
  sternocleidomastoid, birth injury P15.2
  sternomastoid, birth injury P15.2
  subarachnoid (traumatic) — *see* Injury, intracranial,
    subarachnoid hemorrhage
    newborn (nontraumatic) P52.5
      due to birth injury P10.3
    nontraumatic — *see* Hemorrhage, intracranial,
      subarachnoid
  subdural (traumatic) — *see* Injury, intracranial, subdural
    hemorrhage
    newborn (localized) P52.8
      birth injury P10.0
    nontraumatic — *see* Hemorrhage, intracranial,
      subdural
  superficial, newborn P54.5
  testis (nontraumatic) N50.1
    birth injury P15.5
  tunica vaginalis (nontraumatic) N50.1
  umbilical cord, complicating delivery O69.5 ☑
  uterine ligament (broad) (nontraumatic) N83.7
    traumatic S37.892 ☑
  vagina (ruptured) (nontraumatic) N89.8
    complicating delivery O71.7
  vas deferens (nontraumatic) N50.1
    traumatic S37.892 ☑
  vitreous — *see* Hemorrhage, vitreous
  vulva (nontraumatic) (nonobstetric) N90.89
    complicating delivery O71.7
    newborn (birth injury) P15.5
Hematometra N85.7
  with hematocolpos N89.7
Hematomyelia (central) G95.19
  newborn (birth injury) P11.5
  traumatic T14.8 ☑
Hematomyelitis G04.90
Hematoperitoneum — *see* Hemoperitoneum
Hematophobia F40.230
Hematopneumothorax (see Hemothorax)
Hematopoiesis, cyclic D70.4
Hematoporphyria — *see* Porphyria
Hematorachis, hematorrhachis G95.19
  newborn (birth injury) P11.5
Hematosalpinx N83.6
  with
    hematocolpos N89.7
    hematometra N85.7
      with hematocolpos N89.7
  infectional — *see* Salpingitis
Hematospermia R36.1
Hematothorax (see Hemothorax)
Hematuria R31.9
  benign (familial) (of childhood) — *see also* Hematuria,
    idiopathic
    essential microscopic R31.1
  due to sulphonamide, sulfonamide — *see* Table of
    Drugs and Chemicals, by drug
  endemic — *see also* Schistosomiasis B65.0

Hematuria — *continued*
  gross R31.0
  idiopathic N02.9
    with glomerular lesion
      C3
        glomerulonephritis N02.A
        glomerulopathy N02.A
          with dense deposit disease N02.6
      crescentic (diffuse) glomerulonephritis N02.7
      dense deposit disease N02.6
      endocapillary proliferative glomerulonephritis
        N02.4
      focal and segmental hyalinosis or sclerosis N02.1
      membranoproliferative (diffuse) N02.5
      membranous (diffuse) N02.2
      mesangial proliferative (diffuse) N02.3
      mesangiocapillary (diffuse) N02.5
      minor abnormality N02.0
      proliferative NEC N02.8
      specified pathology NEC N02.8
  intermittent — *see* Hematuria, idiopathic
  malarial B50.8
  microscopic NEC (with symptoms) R31.29
    asymptomatic R31.21
    benign essential R31.1
  paroxysmal — *see also* Hematuria, idiopathic
    nocturnal D59.5
  persistent — *see* Hematuria, idiopathic
  recurrent — *see* Hematuria, idiopathic
  tropical — *see also* Schistosomiasis B65.0
  tuberculous A18.13
Hemeralopia (day blindness) H53.11
  vitamin A deficiency E50.5
Hemi-akinesia R41.4
Hemianalgesia R20.0
Hemianencephaly Q00.0
Hemianesthesia R20.0
Hemianopia, hemianopsia (heteronymous) H53.47
  homonymous H53.46- ☑
  syphilitic A52.71
Hemiathetosis R25.8
Hemiatrophy R68.89
  cerebellar G31.9
  face, facial, progressive (Romberg) G51.8
  tongue K14.8
Hemiballism (us) G25.5
Hemicardia Q24.8
Hemicephalus, hemicephaly Q00.0
Hemichorea G25.5
Hemicolitis, left — *see* Colitis, left sided
Hemicrania
  congenital malformation Q00.0
  continua G44.51
  meaning migraine — *see also* Migraine G43.909
  paroxysmal G44.039
    chronic G44.049
      intractable G44.041
      not intractable G44.049
    episodic G44.039
      intractable G44.031
      not intractable G44.039
    intractable G44.031
    not intractable G44.039
Hemidystrophy — *see* Hemiatrophy
Hemiectromelia Q73.8
Hemihypalgesia R20.8
Hemihypesthesia R20.1
Hemi-inattention R41.4
Hemimelia Q73.8
  lower limb — *see* Defect, reduction, lower limb, speci-
    fied type NEC
  upper limb — *see* Defect, reduction, upper limb, spec-
    ified type NEC
Hemiparalysis — *see* Hemiplegia
Hemiparesis — *see* Hemiplegia
Hemiparesthesia R20.2
Hemiparkinsonism G20
Hemiplegia G81.9- ☑
  alternans facialis G83.89
  ascending NEC G81.90
    spinal G95.89
  congenital (cerebral) G80.8
    spastic G80.2
  embolic (current episode) I63.4- ☑
  flaccid G81.0- ☑
  following
    cerebrovascular disease I69.959

Hemiplegia — *continued*
  following — *continued*
    cerebrovascular disease — *continued*
      cerebral infarction I69.35- ☑
      intracerebral hemorrhage I69.15- ☑
      nontraumatic intracranial hemorrhage NEC I69.25- ☑
      specified disease NEC I69.85- ☑
      stroke NOS I69.35- ☑
      subarachnoid hemorrhage I69.05- ☑
  hysterical F44.4
  newborn NEC P91.88
    birth injury P11.9
  spastic G81.1- ☑
    congenital G80.2
  thrombotic (current episode) I63.3- ☑
Hemisection, spinal cord — *see* Injury, spinal cord, by region
Hemispasm (facial) R25.2
Hemisporosis B48.8
Hemitremor R25.1
Hemivertebra Q76.49
  failure of segmentation with scoliosis Q76.3
  fusion with scoliosis Q76.3
Hemochromatosis E83.119
  with refractory anemia D46.1
  due to repeated red blood cell transfusion E83.111
  hereditary (primary) E83.110
  neonatal P78.84
  primary E83.110
  specified NEC E83.118
Hemoglobin — *see also* condition
  abnormal (disease) — *see* Disease, hemoglobin
  AS genotype D57.3
  Constant Spring D58.2
  E-beta thalassemia D56.5
  fetal, hereditary persistence (HPFH) D56.4
  H Constant Spring D56.0
  low NOS D64.9
  S (Hb S), heterozygous D57.3
Hemoglobinemia D59.9
  due to blood transfusion T80.89 ☑
  paroxysmal D59.6
    nocturnal D59.5
Hemoglobinopathy (mixed) D58.2
  with thalassemia D56.8
  sickle-cell D57.1
    with thalassemia D57.40
      with
        acute chest syndrome D57.411
        cerebral vascular involvement D57.413
        crisis (painful) D57.419
          with specified complication NEC D57.418
        splenic sequestration D57.412
        vasoocclusive pain D57.419
      without crisis D57.40
Hemoglobinuria R82.3
  with anemia, hemolytic, acquired (chronic) NEC D59.6
  cold (paroxysmal) (with Raynaud's syndrome) D59.6
    agglutinin D59.12
  due to exertion or hemolysis NEC D59.6
  intermittent D59.6
  malarial B50.8
  march D59.6
  nocturnal (paroxysmal) D59.5
  paroxysmal (cold) D59.6
    nocturnal D59.5
Hemolymphangioma D18.1
Hemolysis
  intravascular
    with
      abortion — *see* Abortion, by type, complicated by, hemorrhage
      ectopic or molar pregnancy O08.1
      hemorrhage
        antepartum — *see* Hemorrhage, antepartum, with coagulation defect
        intrapartum — *see also* Hemorrhage, complicating, delivery O67.0
      postpartum O72.3
  neonatal (excessive) P58.9
    specified NEC P58.8
Hemolytic — *see* condition
Hemopericardium I31.2
  following acute myocardial infarction (current complication) I23.0
  newborn P54.8
  traumatic — *see* Injury, heart, with hemopericardium

Hemoperitoneum K66.1
  infectional K65.9
  traumatic S36.899 ☑
    with open wound — *see* Wound, open, with penetration into peritoneal cavity
Hemophilia (classical) (familial) (hereditary) D66
  A D66
  acquired D68.311
  autoimmune D68.311
  B D67
  C D68.1
  calcipriva — *see also* Defect, coagulation D68.4
  nonfamilial — *see also* Defect, coagulation D68.4
  secondary D68.311
  vascular D68.0
Hemophthalmos H44.81- ☑
Hemopneumothorax — *see also* Hemothorax
  traumatic S27.2 ☑
Hemoptysis R04.2
  newborn P26.9
  tuberculous — *see* Tuberculosis, pulmonary
Hemorrhage, hemorrhagic (concealed) R58
  abdomen R58
  accidental antepartum — *see* Hemorrhage, antepartum
  acute idiopathic pulmonary, in infants R04.81
  adenoid J35.8
  adrenal (capsule) (gland) E27.49
    medulla E27.8
    newborn P54.4
  after delivery — *see* Hemorrhage, postpartum
  alveolar
    lung, newborn P26.8
    process K08.89
  alveolus K08.89
  amputation stump (surgical) T87.89
  anemia (chronic) D50.0
    acute D62
  antepartum (with) O46.90
    with coagulation defect O46.00- ☑
      afibrinogenemia O46.01- ☑
      disseminated intravascular coagulation O46.02- ☑
      hypofibrinogenemia O46.01- ☑
      specified defect NEC O46.09- ☑
    before 20 weeks gestation O20.9
      specified type NEC O20.8
      threatened abortion O20.0
    due to
      abruptio placenta — *see also* Abruptio placentae O45.9- ☑
      leiomyoma, uterus — *see* Hemorrhage, antepartum, specified cause NEC
      placenta previa O44.1- ☑
    specified cause NEC — *see* subcategory O46.8X- ☑
  anus (sphincter) K62.5
  apoplexy (stroke) — *see* Hemorrhage, intracranial, intracerebral
  arachnoid — *see* Hemorrhage, intracranial, subarachnoid
  artery R58
    brain — *see* Hemorrhage, intracranial, intracerebral
  basilar (ganglion) I61.0
  bladder N32.89
  bowel K92.2
    newborn P54.3
  brain (miliary) (nontraumatic) — *see* Hemorrhage, intracranial, intracerebral
    due to
      birth injury P10.1
      syphilis A52.05
    epidural or extradural (traumatic) — *see* Injury, intracranial, epidural hemorrhage
    newborn P52.4
      birth injury P10.1
    subarachnoid — *see* Hemorrhage, intracranial, subarachnoid
    subdural — *see* Hemorrhage, intracranial, subdural
  brainstem (nontraumatic) I61.3
    traumatic S06.38- ☑
  breast N64.59
  bronchial tube — *see* Hemorrhage, lung
  bronchopulmonary — *see* Hemorrhage, lung
  bronchus — *see* Hemorrhage, lung
  bulbar I61.5
  capillary I78.8
    primary D69.8
  cecum K92.2
  cerebellar, cerebellum (nontraumatic) I61.4

Hemorrhage, hemorrhagic — *continued*
  cerebellar, cerebellum — *continued*
    newborn P52.6
    traumatic S06.37- ☑
  cerebral, cerebrum — *see also* Hemorrhage, intracranial, intracerebral
    lobe I61.1
    newborn (anoxic) P52.4
      birth injury P10.1
  cerebromeningeal I61.8
  cerebrospinal — *see* Hemorrhage, intracranial, intracerebral
  cervix (uteri) (stump) NEC N88.8
  chamber, anterior (eye) — *see* Hyphema
  childbirth — *see* Hemorrhage, complicating, delivery
  choroid H31.30- ☑
    expulsive H31.31- ☑
  ciliary body — *see* Hyphema
  cochlea — *see* subcategory H83.8 ☑
  colon K92.2
  complicating
    abortion — *see* Abortion, by type, complicated by, hemorrhage
    delivery O67.9
      associated with coagulation defect (afibrinogenemia) (DIC) (hyperfibrinolysis) O67.0
      specified cause NEC O67.8
    surgical procedure — *see* Hemorrhage, intraoperative
  conjunctiva H11.3- ☑
    newborn P54.8
  cord, newborn (stump) P51.9
  corpus luteum (ruptured) cyst N83.1- ☑
  cortical (brain) I61.1
  cranial — *see* Hemorrhage, intracranial
  cutaneous R23.3
    due to autosensitivity, erythrocyte D69.2
    newborn P54.5
  delayed
    following ectopic or molar pregnancy O08.1
    postpartum O72.2
  diathesis (familial) D69.9
  disease D69.9
    newborn P53
    specified type NEC D69.8
  due to or associated with
    afibrinogenemia or other coagulation defect (conditions in categories D65- D69)
      antepartum — *see* Hemorrhage, antepartum, with coagulation defect
      intrapartum O67.0
  dental implant M27.61
  device, implant or graft — *see also* Complications, by site and type, specified NEC T85.838 ☑
    arterial graft NEC T82.838 ☑
    breast T85.838 ☑
    catheter NEC T85.838 ☑
      dialysis (renal) T82.838 ☑
        intraperitoneal T85.838 ☑
      infusion NEC T82.838 ☑
        spinal (epidural) (subdural) T85.830 ☑
      urinary (indwelling) T83.83 ☑
    electronic (electrode) (pulse generator) (stimulator)
      bone T84.83 ☑
      cardiac T82.837 ☑
      nervous system (brain) (peripheral nerve) (spinal) T85.830 ☑
      urinary T83.83 ☑
    fixation, internal (orthopedic) NEC T84.83 ☑
    gastrointestinal (bile duct) (esophagus) T85.838 ☑
    genital NEC T83.83 ☑
    heart NEC T82.837 ☑
    joint prosthesis T84.83 ☑
    ocular (corneal graft) (orbital implant) NEC T85.838 ☑
    orthopedic NEC T84.83 ☑
      bone graft T86.838
    specified NEC T85.838 ☑
    urinary NEC T83.83 ☑
    vascular NEC T82.838 ☑
    ventricular intracranial shunt T85.830 ☑
  duodenum, duodenal K92.2
    ulcer — *see* Ulcer, duodenum, with hemorrhage
  dura mater — *see* Hemorrhage, intracranial, subdural
  endotracheal — *see* Hemorrhage, lung

Hemorrhage, hemorrhagic — *continued*
- epicranial subaponeurotic (massive), birth injury P12.2
- epidural (traumatic) — *see also* Injury, intracranial, epidural hemorrhage
  - nontraumatic I62.1
- esophagus K22.89
  - varix I85.01
    - secondary I85.11
- excessive, following ectopic gestation (subsequent episode) O08.1
- extradural (traumatic) — *see* Injury, intracranial, epidural hemorrhage
  - birth injury P10.8
  - newborn (anoxic) (nontraumatic) P52.8
  - nontraumatic I62.1
- eye NEC H57.89
  - fundus — *see* Hemorrhage, retina
  - lid — *see* Disorder, eyelid, specified type NEC
- fallopian tube N83.6
- fibrinogenolysis — *see* Fibrinolysis
- fibrinolytic (acquired) — *see* Fibrinolysis
- from
  - ear (nontraumatic) — *see* Otorrhagia
  - tracheostomy stoma J95.01
- fundus, eye — *see* Hemorrhage, retina
- funis — *see* Hemorrhage, umbilicus, cord
- gastric — *see* Hemorrhage, stomach
- gastroenteric K92.2
  - newborn P54.3
- gastrointestinal (tract) K92.2
  - newborn P54.3
- genital organ, male N50.1
- genitourinary (tract) NOS R31.9
- gingiva K06.8
- globe (eye) — *see* Hemophthalmos
- graafian follicle cyst (ruptured) N83.0- ☑
- gum K06.8
- heart I51.89
- hypopharyngeal (throat) R04.1
- intermenstrual (regular) N92.3
  - irregular N92.1
- internal (organs) NEC R58
  - capsule I61.0
  - ear — *see* subcategory H83.8 ☑
  - newborn P54.8
- intestine K92.2
  - newborn P54.3
- intra-abdominal R58
- intra-alveolar (lung), newborn P26.8
- intracerebral (nontraumatic) — *see* Hemorrhage, intracranial, intracerebral
- intracranial (nontraumatic) I62.9
  - birth injury P10.9
  - epidural, nontraumatic I62.1
  - extradural, nontraumatic I62.1
  - intracerebral (nontraumatic) (in) I61.9
    - brain stem I61.3
    - cerebellum I61.4
    - hemisphere I61.2
      - cortical (superficial) I61.1
      - subcortical (deep) I61.0
    - intraoperative
      - during a nervous system procedure G97.31
      - during other procedure G97.32
    - intraventricular I61.5
    - multiple localized I61.6
    - newborn P52.4
      - birth injury P10.1
    - postprocedural
      - following a nervous system procedure G97.51
      - following other procedure G97.52
    - specified NEC I61.8
    - superficial I61.1
    - traumatic (diffuse) — *see* Injury, intracranial, diffuse
      - focal — *see* Injury, intracranial, focal
  - newborn P52.9
    - specified NEC P52.8
  - subarachnoid (nontraumatic) (from) I60.9
    - intracranial (cerebral) artery I60.7
      - anterior communicating I60.2
      - basilar I60.4
      - carotid siphon and bifurcation I60.0- ☑
      - communicating I60.7
        - anterior I60.2
        - posterior I60.3- ☑
      - middle cerebral I60.1- ☑
      - posterior communicating I60.3- ☑

Hemorrhage, hemorrhagic — *continued*
- intracranial — *continued*
  - subarachnoid — *continued*
    - intracranial artery — *continued*
      - specified artery NEC I60.6
      - vertebral I60.5- ☑
    - newborn P52.5
      - birth injury P10.3
    - specified NEC I60.8
    - traumatic S06.6X- ☑
  - subdural (nontraumatic) I62.00
    - acute I62.01
    - birth injury P10.0
    - chronic I62.03
    - newborn (anoxic) (hypoxic) P52.8
      - birth injury P10.0
    - spinal G95.19
    - subacute I62.02
    - traumatic — *see* Injury, intracranial, subdural hemorrhage
  - traumatic — *see* Injury, intracranial, focal brain injury
- intramedullary NEC G95.19
- intraocular — *see* Hemophthalmos
- intraoperative, intraprocedural — *see* Complication, hemorrhage (hematoma), intraoperative (intraprocedural), by site
- intrapartum — *see* Hemorrhage, complicating, delivery
- intrapelvic
  - female N94.89
  - male K66.1
- intraperitoneal K66.1
- intrapontine I61.3
- intraprocedural — *see* Complication, hemorrhage (hematoma), intraoperative (intraprocedural), by site
- intrauterine N85.7
  - complicating delivery — *see also* Hemorrhage, complicating, delivery O67.9
  - postpartum — *see* Hemorrhage, postpartum
- intraventricular I61.5
  - newborn (nontraumatic) — *see also* Newborn, affected by, hemorrhage P52.3
    - due to birth injury P10.2
    - grade
      - 1 P52.0
      - 2 P52.1
      - 3 P52.21
      - 4 P52.22
- intravesical N32.89
- iris (postinfectional) (postinflammatory) (toxic) — *see* Hyphema
- joint (nontraumatic) — *see* Hemarthrosis
- kidney N28.89
- knee (joint) (nontraumatic) — *see* Hemarthrosis, knee
- labyrinth — *see* subcategory H83.8 ☑
- lenticular striate artery I61.0
- ligature, vessel — *see* Hemorrhage, postoperative
- liver K76.89
- lung R04.89
  - newborn P26.9
    - massive P26.1
    - specified NEC P26.8
  - tuberculous — *see* Tuberculosis, pulmonary
- massive umbilical, newborn P51.0
- mediastinum — *see* Hemorrhage, lung
- medulla I61.3
- membrane (brain) I60.8
  - spinal cord — *see* Hemorrhage, spinal cord
- meninges, meningeal (brain) (middle) I60.8
  - spinal cord — *see* Hemorrhage, spinal cord
- mesentery K66.1
- metritis — *see* Endometritis
- mouth K13.79
- mucous membrane NEC R58
  - newborn P54.8
- muscle M62.89
- nail (subungual) L60.8
- nasal turbinate R04.0
  - newborn P54.8
- navel, newborn P51.9
- newborn P54.9
  - specified NEC P54.8
- nipple N64.59
- nose R04.0
  - newborn P54.8
- omentum K66.1
- optic nerve (sheath) H47.02- ☑

Hemorrhage, hemorrhagic — *continued*
- orbit, orbital H05.23- ☑
- ovary NEC N83.8
- oviduct N83.6
- pancreas K86.89
- parathyroid (gland) (spontaneous) E21.4
- parturition — *see* Hemorrhage, complicating, delivery
- penis N48.89
- pericardium, pericarditis I31.2
- peritoneum, peritoneal K66.1
- peritonsillar tissue J35.8
  - due to infection J36
- petechial R23.3
  - due to autosensitivity, erythrocyte D69.2
- pituitary (gland) E23.6
- pleura — *see* Hemorrhage, lung
- polioencephalitis, superior E51.2
- polymyositis — *see* Polymyositis
- pons, pontine I61.3
- posterior fossa (nontraumatic) I61.8
  - newborn P52.6
- postmenopausal N95.0
- postnasal R04.0
- postoperative — *see* Complications, postprocedural, hemorrhage, by site
- postpartum NEC (following delivery of placenta) O72.1
  - delayed or secondary O72.2
  - retained placenta O72.0
  - third stage O72.0
- pregnancy — *see* Hemorrhage, antepartum
- preretinal — *see* Hemorrhage, retina
- prostate N42.1
- puerperal — *see* Hemorrhage, postpartum
  - delayed or secondary O72.2
- pulmonary R04.89
  - newborn P26.9
    - massive P26.1
    - specified NEC P26.8
  - tuberculous — *see* Tuberculosis, pulmonary
- purpura (primary) D69.3
- rectum (sphincter) K62.5
  - newborn P54.2
- recurring, following initial hemorrhage at time of injury T79.2 ☑
- renal N28.89
- respiratory passage or tract R04.9
  - specified NEC R04.89
- retina, retinal (vessels) H35.6- ☑
  - diabetic — *see* Diabetes, retinal, hemorrhage
- retroperitoneal R58
- scalp R58
- scrotum N50.1
- secondary (nontraumatic) R58
  - following initial hemorrhage at time of injury T79.2 ☑
- seminal vesicle N50.1
- skin R23.3
  - newborn P54.5
- slipped umbilical ligature P51.8
- spermatic cord N50.1
- spinal (cord) G95.19
  - newborn (birth injury) P11.5
- spleen D73.5
  - intraoperative — *see* Complications, intraoperative, hemorrhage, spleen
  - postprocedural — *see* Complications, postprocedural, hemorrhage, spleen
- stomach K92.2
  - newborn P54.3
  - ulcer — *see* Ulcer, stomach, with hemorrhage
- subarachnoid (nontraumatic) — *see* Hemorrhage, intracranial, subarachnoid
- subconjunctival — *see also* Hemorrhage, conjunctiva
  - birth injury P15.3
- subcortical (brain) I61.0
- subcutaneous R23.3
- subdiaphragmatic R58
- subdural (acute) (nontraumatic) — *see* Hemorrhage, intracranial, subdural
- subependymal
  - newborn P52.0
    - with intraventricular extension P52.1
      - and intracerebral extension P52.22
- subgaleal P12.2
- subhyaloid — *see* Hemorrhage, retina
- subperiosteal — *see* Disorder, bone, specified type NEC
- subretinal — *see* Hemorrhage, retina
- subtentorial — *see* Hemorrhage, intracranial, subdural

Hemorrhage, hemorrhagic — Hemorrhage, hemorrhagic

⬇ Subterms under main terms may continue to next column or page   ☑ Additional Character Required — Refer to the Tabular List for Character Selection   169

Hemorrhage, hemorrhagic — *continued*
  subungual L60.8
  suprarenal (capsule) (gland) E27.49
    newborn P54.4
  tentorium (traumatic) NEC — *see* Hemorrhage, brain
    newborn (birth injury) P10.4
  testis N50.1
  third stage (postpartum) O72.0
  thorax — *see* Hemorrhage, lung
  throat R04.1
  thymus (gland) E32.8
  thyroid (cyst) (gland) E07.89
  tongue K14.8
  tonsil J35.8
  trachea — *see* Hemorrhage, lung
  tracheobronchial R04.89
    newborn P26.0
  traumatic — *code to* specific injury
    cerebellar — *see* Hemorrhage, brain
    intracranial — *see* Hemorrhage, brain
    recurring or secondary (following initial hemorrhage
      at time of injury) T79.2 ☑
  tuberculous NEC — *see also* Tuberculosis, pulmonary
    A15.0
  tunica vaginalis N50.1
  ulcer — *code by* site under Ulcer, with hemorrhage
    K27.4
  umbilicus, umbilical
    cord
      after birth, newborn P51.9
      complicating delivery O69.5 ☑
    newborn P51.9
      massive P51.0
      slipped ligature P51.8
    stump P51.9
  urethra (idiopathic) N36.8
  uterus, uterine (abnormal) N93.9
    climacteric N92.4
    complicating delivery — *see* Hemorrhage, compli-
      cating, delivery
    dysfunctional or functional N93.8
    intermenstrual (regular) N92.3
      irregular N92.1
    postmenopausal N95.0
    postpartum — *see* Hemorrhage, postpartum
    preclimacteric or premenopausal N92.4
    prepubertal N93.8
    pubertal N92.2
  vagina (abnormal) N93.9
    newborn P54.6
  vas deferens N50.1
  vasa previa O69.4 ☑
  ventricular I61.5
  vesical N32.89
  viscera NEC R58
    newborn P54.8
  vitreous (humor) (intraocular) H43.1- ☑
  vulva N90.89
Hemorrhoids (bleeding) (without mention of degree)
  K64.9
  1st degree (grade/stage I) (without prolapse outside
    of anal canal) K64.0
  2nd degree (grade/stage II) (that prolapse with strain-
    ing but retract spontaneously) K64.1
  3rd degree (grade/stage III) (that prolapse with strain-
    ing and require manual replacement back inside
    anal canal) K64.2
  4th degree (grade/stage IV) (with prolapsed tissue that
    cannot be manually replaced) K64.3
  complicating
    pregnancy O22.4 ☑
    puerperium O87.2
  external K64.4
    with
      thrombosis K64.5
  internal (without mention of degree) K64.8
  prolapsed K64.8
  skin tags
    anus K64.4
    residual K64.4
  specified NEC K64.8
  strangulated — *see also* Hemorrhoids, by degree K64.8
  thrombosed — *see also* Hemorrhoids, by degree K64.5
  ulcerated — *see also* Hemorrhoids, by degree K64.8
Hemosalpinx N83.6
  with
    hematocolpos N89.7
    hematometra N85.7

Hemosalpinx — *continued*
  with — *continued*
    hematometra — *continued*
      with hematocolpos N89.7
Hemosiderosis (dietary) E83.19
  pulmonary, idiopathic E83.1- ☑ *[J84.03]*
  transfusion T80.89 ☑
Hemothorax (bacterial) (nontuberculous) J94.2
  newborn P54.8
  traumatic S27.1 ☑
    with pneumothorax S27.2 ☑
  tuberculous NEC A15.6
Henoch (-Schönlein) **disease or syndrome** (purpura)
  D69.0
Henpue, henpuye A66.6
Hepar lobatum (syphilitic) A52.74
Hepatalgia K76.89
Hepatitis K75.9
  acute B17.9
    with coma K72.01
    with hepatic failure — *see* Failure, hepatic
    alcoholic — *see* Hepatitis, alcoholic
    infectious B17.9
    non-viral K72.0 ☑
    viral B17.9
  alcoholic (acute) (chronic) K70.10
    with ascites K70.11
  amebic — *see* Abscess, liver, amebic
  anicteric, (viral) — *see* Hepatitis, viral
  antigen-associated (HAA) — *see* Hepatitis, B
  Australia-antigen (positive) — *see* Hepatitis, B
  autoimmune K75.4
  B B19.10
    with hepatic coma B19.11
    acute B16.9
      with
        delta-agent (coinfection) (without hepatic
          coma) B16.1
          with hepatic coma B16.0
        hepatic coma (without delta-agent coinfec-
          tion) B16.2
    chronic B18.1
      with delta-agent B18.0
  bacterial NEC K75.89
  C (viral) B19.20
    with hepatic coma B19.21
    acute B17.10
      with hepatic coma B17.11
    chronic B18.2
  catarrhal (acute) B15.9
    with hepatic coma B15.0
  cholangiolitic K75.89
  cholestatic K75.89
  chronic K73.9
    active NEC K73.2
    lobular NEC K73.1
    persistent NEC K73.0
    specified NEC K73.8
  cytomegaloviral B25.1
  due to ethanol (acute) (chronic) — *see* Hepatitis, alco-
    holic
  epidemic B15.9
    with hepatic coma B15.0
  fulminant NEC (viral) — *see* Hepatitis, viral
  granulomatous NEC K75.3
  herpesviral B00.81
  history of
    B Z86.19
    C Z86.19
  homologous serum — *see* Hepatitis, viral, type B
  in (due to)
    mumps B26.81
    toxoplasmosis (acquired) B58.1
      congenital (active) P37.1 *[K77]*
  infectious, infective B15.9
    acute (subacute) B17.9
    chronic B18.9
  inoculation — *see* Hepatitis, viral, type B
  interstitial (chronic) K74.69
  ischemia, ischemic K72.00
  lupoid NEC K75.4
  malignant NEC (with hepatic failure) K72.90
    with coma K72.91
  neonatal (idiopathic) (toxic) P59.29
  neonatal giant cell P59.29
  newborn P59.29
  non-viral K72.0 ☑
  postimmunization — *see* Hepatitis, viral, type B

Hepatitis — *continued*
  post-transfusion — *see* Hepatitis, viral, type B
  reactive, nonspecific K75.2
  serum — *see* Hepatitis, viral, type B
  shock K72.00
  specified type NEC
    with hepatic failure — *see* Failure, hepatic
  syphilitic (late) A52.74
    congenital (early) A50.08 *[K77]*
      late A50.59 *[K77]*
    secondary A51.45
  toxic — *see also* Disease, liver, toxic K71.6
  tuberculous A18.83
  viral, virus B19.9
    with hepatic coma B19.0
    acute B17.9
    chronic B18.9
      specified NEC B18.8
      type
        B B18.1
          with delta-agent B18.0
        C B18.2
    congenital P35.3
    coxsackie B33.8 *[K77]*
    cytomegalic inclusion B25.1
    in remission, any type — *code to* Hepatitis, chronic,
      by type
    non-A, non-B B17.8
    specified type NEC (with or without coma) B17.8
    type
      A B15.9
        with hepatic coma B15.0
      B B19.10
        with hepatic coma B19.11
        acute B16.9
          with
            delta-agent (coinfection) (without
              hepatic coma) B16.1
              with hepatic coma B16.0
            hepatic coma (without delta-agent
              coinfection) B16.2
        chronic B18.1
          with delta-agent B18.0
      C B19.20
        with hepatic coma B19.21
        acute B17.10
          with hepatic coma B17.11
        chronic B18.2
      E B17.2
      non-A, non-B B17.8
Hepatization lung (acute) — *see* Pneumonia, lobar
Hepatoblastoma C22.2
Hepatocarcinoma C22.0
Hepatocholangiocarcinoma C22.0
Hepatocholangioma, benign D13.4
Hepatocholangitis K75.89
Hepatolenticular degeneration E83.01
Hepatoma (malignant) C22.0
  benign D13.4
  embryonal C22.0
Hepatomegaly — *see also* Hypertrophy, liver
  with splenomegaly R16.2
  congenital Q44.7
  in mononucleosis
    gammaherpesviral B27.09
    infectious specified NEC B27.89
Hepatoptosis K76.89
Hepatorenal syndrome following labor and delivery
  O90.4
Hepatosis K76.89
Hepatosplenomegaly R16.2
  hyperlipemic (Bürger-Grütz type) E78.3 *[K77]*
Hereditary — *see* condition
Hereditary alpha tryptasemia (syndrome) D89.44
Heredodegeneration, macular — *see* Dystrophy, retina
Heredopathia atactica polyneuritiformis G60.1
Heredosyphilis — *see* Syphilis, congenital
Herlitz' syndrome Q81.1
Hermansky-Pudlak syndrome E70.331
Hermaphrodite, hermaphroditism (true) Q56.0
  46,XX with streak gonads Q99.1
  46,XX/46,XY Q99.0
  46,XY with streak gonads Q99.1
  chimera 46,XX/46,XY Q99.0
Hernia, hernial (acquired) (recurrent) K46.9
  with
    gangrene — *see* Hernia, by site, with, gangrene
    incarceration — *see* Hernia, by site, with, obstruction

Hernia, hernial — *continued*
  with — *continued*
    irreducible — *see* Hernia, by site, with, obstruction
    obstruction — *see* Hernia, by site, with, obstruction
    strangulation — *see* Hernia, by site, with, obstruction
  abdomen, abdominal K46.9
    with
      gangrene (and obstruction) K46.1
      obstruction K46.0
    femoral — *see* Hernia, femoral
    incisional — *see* Hernia, incisional
    inguinal — *see* Hernia, inguinal
    specified site NEC K45.8
      with
        gangrene (and obstruction) K45.1
        obstruction K45.0
    umbilical — *see* Hernia, umbilical
    wall — *see* Hernia, ventral
  appendix — *see* Hernia, abdomen
  bladder (mucosa) (sphincter)
    congenital (female) (male) Q79.51
    female — *see* Cystocele
    male N32.89
  brain, congenital — *see* Encephalocele
  cartilage, vertebra — *see* Displacement, intervertebral disc
  cerebral, congenital — *see also* Encephalocele
    endaural Q01.8
  ciliary body (traumatic) S05.2- ☑
  colon — *see* Hernia, abdomen
  Cooper's — *see* Hernia, abdomen, specified site NEC
  crural — *see* Hernia, femoral
  diaphragm, diaphragmatic K44.9
    with
      gangrene (and obstruction) K44.1
      obstruction K44.0
    congenital Q79.0
  direct (inguinal) — *see* Hernia, inguinal
  diverticulum, intestine — *see* Hernia, abdomen
  double (inguinal) — *see* Hernia, inguinal, bilateral
  due to adhesions (with obstruction) K56.50
  epigastric — *see also* Hernia, ventral K43.9
  esophageal hiatus — *see* Hernia, hiatal
  external (inguinal) — *see* Hernia, inguinal
  fallopian tube N83.4- ☑
  fascia M62.89
  femoral K41.90
    with
      gangrene (and obstruction) K41.40
        not specified as recurrent K41.40
        recurrent K41.41
      obstruction K41.30
        not specified as recurrent K41.30
        recurrent K41.31
    not specified as recurrent K41.90
    recurrent K41.91
    bilateral K41.20
      with
        gangrene (and obstruction) K41.10
          not specified as recurrent K41.10
          recurrent K41.11
        obstruction K41.00
          not specified as recurrent K41.00
          recurrent K41.01
      not specified as recurrent K41.20
      recurrent K41.21
    unilateral K41.90
      with
        gangrene (and obstruction) K41.40
          not specified as recurrent K41.40
          recurrent K41.41
        obstruction K41.30
          not specified as recurrent K41.30
          recurrent K41.31
      not specified as recurrent K41.90
      recurrent K41.91
  foramen magnum G93.5
    congenital Q01.8
  funicular (umbilical) — *see also* Hernia, umbilicus
    spermatic (cord) — *see* Hernia, inguinal
  gastrointestinal tract — *see* Hernia, abdomen
  Hesselbach's — *see* Hernia, femoral, specified site NEC
  hiatal (esophageal) (sliding) K44.9
    with
      gangrene (and obstruction) K44.1
      obstruction K44.0
    congenital Q40.1

Hernia, hernial — *continued*
  hypogastric — *see* Hernia, ventral
  incarcerated — *see also* Hernia, by site, with obstruction
    with gangrene — *see* Hernia, by site, with gangrene
  incisional K43.2
    with
      gangrene (and obstruction) K43.1
      obstruction K43.0
  indirect (inguinal) — *see* Hernia, inguinal
  inguinal (direct) (external) (funicular) (indirect) (internal) (oblique) (scrotal) (sliding) K40.90
    with
      gangrene (and obstruction) K40.40
        not specified as recurrent K40.40
        recurrent K40.41
      obstruction K40.30
        not specified as recurrent K40.30
        recurrent K40.31
    not specified as recurrent K40.90
    recurrent K40.91
    bilateral K40.20
      with
        gangrene (and obstruction) K40.10
          not specified as recurrent K40.10
          recurrent K40.11
        obstruction K40.00
          not specified as recurrent K40.00
          recurrent K40.01
      not specified as recurrent K40.20
      recurrent K40.21
    unilateral K40.90
      with
        gangrene (and obstruction) K40.40
          not specified as recurrent K40.40
          recurrent K40.41
        obstruction K40.30
          not specified as recurrent K40.30
          recurrent K40.31
      not specified as recurrent K40.90
      recurrent K40.91
  internal — *see also* Hernia, abdomen
    inguinal — *see* Hernia, inguinal
  interstitial — *see* Hernia, abdomen
  intervertebral cartilage or disc — *see* Displacement, intervertebral disc
  intestine, intestinal — *see* Hernia, by site
  intra-abdominal — *see* Hernia, abdomen
  iris (traumatic) S05.2- ☑
  irreducible — *see also* Hernia, by site, with obstruction
    with gangrene — *see* Hernia, by site, with gangrene
  ischiatic — *see* Hernia, abdomen, specified site NEC
  ischiorectal — *see* Hernia, abdomen, specified site NEC
  lens (traumatic) S05.2- ☑
  linea (alba) (semilunaris) — *see* Hernia, ventral
  Littre's — *see* Hernia, abdomen
  lumbar — *see* Hernia, abdomen, specified site NEC
  lung (subcutaneous) J98.4
  mediastinum J98.59
  mesenteric (internal) — *see* Hernia, abdomen
  midline — *see* Hernia, ventral
  muscle (sheath) M62.89
  nucleus pulposus — *see* Displacement, intervertebral disc
  oblique (inguinal) — *see* Hernia, inguinal
  obstructive — *see also* Hernia, by site, with obstruction
    with gangrene — *see* Hernia, by site, with gangrene
  obturator — *see* Hernia, abdomen, specified site NEC
  omental — *see* Hernia, abdomen
  ovary N83.4- ☑
  oviduct N83.4- ☑
  paraesophageal — *see also* Hernia, diaphragm
    congenital Q40.1
  parastomal K43.5
    with
      gangrene (and obstruction) K43.4
      obstruction K43.3
  paraumbilical — *see* Hernia, umbilicus
  perineal — *see* Hernia, abdomen, specified site NEC
  Petit's — *see* Hernia, abdomen, specified site NEC
  postoperative — *see* Hernia, incisional
  pregnant uterus — *see* Abnormal, uterus in pregnancy or childbirth
  prevesical N32.89
  properitoneal — *see* Hernia, abdomen, specified site NEC
  pudendal — *see* Hernia, abdomen, specified site NEC
  rectovaginal N81.6

Hernia, hernial — *continued*
  retroperitoneal — *see* Hernia, abdomen, specified site NEC
  Richter's — *see* Hernia, abdomen, with obstruction
  Rieux's, Riex's — *see* Hernia, abdomen, specified site NEC
  sac condition (adhesion) (dropsy) (inflammation) (laceration) (suppuration) — *code by site under* Hernia
  sciatic — *see* Hernia, abdomen, specified site NEC
  scrotum, scrotal — *see* Hernia, inguinal
  sliding (inguinal) — *see also* Hernia, inguinal
    hiatus — *see* Hernia, hiatal
  spigelian — *see* Hernia, ventral
  spinal — *see* Spina bifida
  strangulated — *see also* Hernia, by site, with obstruction
    with gangrene — *see* Hernia, by site, with gangrene
  subxiphoid — *see* Hernia, ventral
  supra-umbilicus — *see* Hernia, ventral
  tendon — *see* Disorder, tendon, specified type NEC
  Treitz's (fossa) — *see* Hernia, abdomen, specified site NEC
  tunica vaginalis Q55.29
  umbilicus, umbilical K42.9
    with
      gangrene (and obstruction) K42.1
      obstruction K42.0
  ureter N28.89
  urethra, congenital Q64.79
  urinary meatus, congenital Q64.79
  uterus N81.4
    pregnant — *see* Abnormal, uterus in pregnancy or childbirth
  vaginal (anterior) (wall) — *see* Cystocele
  Velpeau's — *see* Hernia, femoral
  ventral K43.9
    with
      gangrene (and obstruction) K43.7
      obstruction K43.6
    incisional K43.2
      with
        gangrene (and obstruction) K43.1
        obstruction K43.0
      recurrent — *see* Hernia, incisional
    specified NEC K43.9
      with
        gangrene (and obstruction) K43.7
        obstruction K43.6
  vesical
    congenital (female) (male) Q79.51
    female — *see* Cystocele
    male N32.89
  vitreous (into wound) S05.2- ☑
    into anterior chamber — *see* Prolapse, vitreous
Herniation — *see also* Hernia
  brain (stem) G93.5
    nontraumatic G93.5
    traumatic S06.A1 ☑
      cerebellar S06.A1 ☑
      subfalcine (cingulate) S06.A1 ☑
      tonsillar S06.A1 ☑
      transtentorial (central) (upward cerebellar) S06.A1 ☑
      uncal S06.A1 ☑
  cerebral G93.5
    nontraumatic G93.5
    traumatic S06.A1 ☑
  mediastinum J98.59
  nucleus pulposus — *see* Displacement, intervertebral disc
Herpangina B08.5
Herpes, herpesvirus, herpetic B00.9
  anogenital A60.9
    perianal skin A60.1
    rectum A60.1
    urogenital tract A60.00
      cervix A60.03
      male genital organ NEC A60.02
      penis A60.01
      specified site NEC A60.09
      vagina A60.04
      vulva A60.04
  blepharitis (zoster) B02.39
    simplex B00.59
  circinatus B35.4
    bullosus L12.0
  conjunctivitis (simplex) B00.53

Herpes, herpesvirus, herpetic — *continued*
  conjunctivitis — *continued*
    zoster B02.31
  cornea B02.33
  encephalitis B00.4
    due to herpesvirus 6 B10.01
    due to herpesvirus 7 B10.09
    specified NEC B10.09
  eye (zoster) B02.30
    simplex B00.50
  eyelid (zoster) B02.39
    simplex B00.59
  facialis B00.1
  febrilis B00.1
  geniculate ganglionitis B02.21
  genital, genitalis A60.00
    female A60.09
    male A60.02
  gestational, gestationis O26.4- ☑
  gingivostomatitis B00.2
  human B00.9
    1 — *see* Herpes, simplex
    2 — *see* Herpes, simplex
    3 — *see* Varicella
    4 — *see* Mononucleosis, Epstein-Barr (virus)
    5 — *see* Disease, cytomegalic inclusion (generalized)
    6
      encephalitis B10.01
      specified NEC B10.81
    7
      encephalitis B10.09
      specified NEC B10.82
    8 B10.89
  infection NEC B10.89
    Kaposi's sarcoma associated B10.89
  iridocyclitis (simplex) B00.51
    zoster B02.32
  iris (vesicular erythema multiforme) L51.9
  iritis (simplex) B00.51
  Kaposi's sarcoma associated B10.89
  keratitis (simplex) (dendritic) (disciform) (interstitial)
      B00.52
    zoster (interstitial) B02.33
  keratoconjunctivitis (simplex) B00.52
    zoster B02.33
  labialis B00.1
  lip B00.1
  meningitis (simplex) B00.3
    zoster B02.1
  ophthalmicus (zoster) NEC B02.30
    simplex B00.50
  penis A60.01
  perianal skin A60.1
  pharyngitis, pharyngotonsillitis B00.2
  rectum A60.1
  scrotum A60.02
  sepsis B00.7
  simplex B00.9
    complicated NEC B00.89
    congenital P35.2
    conjunctivitis B00.53
    external ear B00.1
    eyelid B00.59
    hepatitis B00.81
    keratitis (interstitial) B00.52
    myleitis B00.82
    specified complication NEC B00.89
    visceral B00.89
  stomatitis B00.2
  tonsurans B35.0
  visceral B00.89
  vulva A60.04
  whitlow B00.89
  zoster — *see also* condition B02.9
    auricularis B02.21
    complicated NEC B02.8
    conjunctivitis B02.31
    disseminated B02.7
    encephalitis B02.0
    eye (lid) B02.39
    geniculate ganglionitis B02.21
    keratitis (interstitial) B02.33
    meningitis B02.1
    myelitis B02.24
    neuritis, neuralgia B02.29
    ophthalmicus NEC B02.30
    oticus B02.21
    polyneuropathy B02.23

Herpes, herpesvirus, herpetic — *continued*
  zoster — *see also* condition — *continued*
    specified complication NEC B02.8
    trigeminal neuralgia B02.22
Herpesvirus (human) — *see* Herpes
Herpetophobia F40.218
Herrick's anemia — *see* Disease, sickle-cell
Hers' disease E74.09
Herter-Gee syndrome K90.0
Herxheimer's reaction R68.89
Hesitancy
  of micturition R39.11
  urinary R39.11
Hesselbach's hernia — *see* Hernia, femoral, specified
    site NEC
Heterochromia (congenital) Q13.2
  cataract — *see* Cataract, complicated
  cyclitis (Fuchs) — *see* Cyclitis, Fuchs' heterochromic
  hair L67.1
  iritis — *see* Cyclitis, Fuchs' heterochromic
  retained metallic foreign body (nonmagnetic) — *see*
      Foreign body, intraocular, old, retained
    magnetic — *see* Foreign body, intraocular, old, retained, magnetic
  uveitis — *see* Cyclitis, Fuchs' heterochromic
Heterophoria — *see* Strabismus, heterophoria
Heterophyes, heterophyiasis (small intestine) B66.8
Heterotopia, heterotopic — *see also* Malposition,
    congenital
  cerebralis Q04.8
Heterotropia — *see* Strabismus
Heubner-Herter disease K90.0
Hexadactylism Q69.9
HGSIL (cytology finding) (high grade squamous intraep-
    ithelial lesion on cytologic smear) (Pap smear find-
    ing)
  anus R85.613
  cervix R87.613
    biopsy (histology) finding — *see* Neoplasia, intraep-
        ithelial, cervix, grade II or grade III
  vagina R87.623
    biopsy (histology) finding — *see* Neoplasia, intraep-
        ithelial, cervix, grade II or grade III
Hibernoma — *see* Lipoma
Hiccup, hiccough R06.6
  epidemic B33.0
  psychogenic F45.8
Hidden penis (congenital) Q55.64
  acquired N48.83
Hidradenitis (axillaris) (suppurative) L73.2
Hidradenoma (nodular) — *see also* Neoplasm, skin, be-
    nign
  clear cell — *see* Neoplasm, skin, benign
  papillary — *see* Neoplasm, skin, benign
Hidrocystoma — *see* Neoplasm, skin, benign
High
  altitude effects T70.20 ☑
    anoxia T70.29 ☑
    on
      ears T70.0 ☑
      sinuses T70.1 ☑
    polycythemia D75.1
  arch
    foot Q66.7- ☑
    palate, congenital Q38.5
  arterial tension — *see* Hypertension
  basal metabolic rate R94.8
  blood pressure — *see also* Hypertension
    borderline R03.0
    reading (incidental) (isolated) (nonspecific), without
        diagnosis of hypertension R03.0
  cholesterol E78.00
    with high triglycerides E78.2
  diaphragm (congenital) Q79.1
  expressed emotional level within family Z63.8
  head at term O32.4 ☑
  palate, congenital Q38.5
  risk
    infant NEC Z76.2
    sexual behavior (heterosexual) Z72.51
      bisexual Z72.53
      homosexual Z72.52
  scrotal testis, testes
    bilateral Q53.23
    unilateral Q53.13
  temperature (of unknown origin) R50.9
  thoracic rib Q76.6

High — *continued*
  triglycerides E78.1
    with high cholesterol E78.2
Hildenbrand's disease A75.0
Hilum — *see* condition
Hip — *see* condition
Hippel's disease Q85.8
Hippophobia F40.218
Hippus H57.09
Hirschsprung's disease or megacolon Q43.1
Hirsutism, hirsuties L68.0
Hirudiniasis
  external B88.3
  internal B83.4
Hiss-Russell dysentery A03.1
Histidinemia, histidinuria E70.41
Histiocytoma — *see also* Neoplasm, skin, benign
  fibrous — *see also* Neoplasm, skin, benign
    atypical — *see* Neoplasm, connective tissue, uncer-
        tain behavior
    malignant — *see* Neoplasm, connective tissue, ma-
        lignant
Histiocytosis D76.3
  acute differentiated progressive C96.0
  Langerhans' cell NEC C96.6
    multifocal X
      multisystemic (disseminated) C96.0
      unisystemic C96.5
    pulmonary, adult (adult PLCH) J84.82
    unifocal (X) C96.6
  lipid, lipoid D76.3
    essential E75.29
  malignant C96.A (*following* C96.6)
  mononuclear phagocytes NEC D76.1
    Langerhans' cells C96.6
  non-Langerhans cell D76.3
  polyostotic sclerosing D76.3
  sinus, with massive lymphadenopathy D76.3
  syndrome NEC D76.3
  X NEC C96.6
    acute (progressive) C96.0
    chronic C96.6
    multifocal C96.5
    multisystemic C96.0
    unifocal C96.6
Histoplasmosis B39.9
  with pneumonia NEC B39.2
  African B39.5
  American — *see* Histoplasmosis, capsulati
  capsulati B39.4
    disseminated B39.3
    generalized B39.3
    pulmonary B39.2
      acute B39.0
      chronic B39.1
  Darling's B39.4
  duboisii B39.5
  lung NEC B39.2
History
  family (of) — *see also* History, personal (of)
    alcohol abuse Z81.1
    allergy NEC Z84.89
    anemia Z83.2
    arthritis Z82.61
    asthma Z82.5
    blindness Z82.1
    cardiac death (sudden) Z82.41
    carrier of genetic disease Z84.81
    chromosomal anomaly Z82.79
    chronic
      disabling disease NEC Z82.8
      lower respiratory disease Z82.5
    colonic polyps Z83.71
    congenital malformations and deformations Z82.79
      polycystic kidney Z82.71
    consanguinity Z84.3
    deafness Z82.2
    diabetes mellitus Z83.3
    disability NEC Z82.8
    disease or disorder (of)
      allergic NEC Z84.89
      behavioral NEC Z81.8
      blood and blood-forming organs Z83.2
      cardiovascular NEC Z82.49
      chronic disabling NEC Z82.8
      digestive Z83.79
      ear NEC Z83.52
      elevated lipoprotein (a) (Lp(a)) Z83.430

☑ **Additional Character Required** — **Refer to the Tabular List for Character Selection**   Subterms under main terms may continue to next column or page

History — *continued*
  family — *see also* History, personal — *continued*
    disease or disorder — *continued*
      endocrine NEC Z83.49
      eye NEC Z83.518
        glaucoma Z83.511
      familial hypercholesterolemia Z83.42
      genitourinary NEC Z84.2
      glaucoma Z83.511
      hematological Z83.2
      immune mechanism Z83.2
      infectious NEC Z83.1
      ischemic heart Z82.49
      kidney Z84.1
      lipoprotein metabolism Z83.438
      mental NEC Z81.8
      metabolic Z83.49
      musculoskeletal NEC Z82.69
      neurological NEC Z82.0
      nutritional Z83.49
      parasitic NEC Z83.1
      psychiatric NEC Z81.8
      respiratory NEC Z83.6
      skin and subcutaneous tissue NEC Z84.0
      specified NEC Z84.89
    drug abuse NEC Z81.3
    elevated lipoprotein (a) (Lp(a)) Z83.430
    epilepsy Z82.0
    familial hypercholesterolemia Z83.42
    genetic disease carrier Z84.81
    glaucoma Z83.511
    hearing loss Z82.2
    human immunodeficiency virus (HIV) infection Z83.0
    Huntington's chorea Z82.0
    hyperlipidemia, familial combined Z83.438
    intellectual disability Z81.0
    leukemia Z80.6
    lipidemia NEC Z83.438
    malignant neoplasm (of) NOS Z80.9
      bladder Z80.52
      breast Z80.3
      bronchus Z80.1
      digestive organ Z80.0
      gastrointestinal tract Z80.0
      genital organ Z80.49
        ovary Z80.41
        prostate Z80.42
        specified organ NEC Z80.49
        testis Z80.43
      hematopoietic NEC Z80.7
      intrathoracic organ NEC Z80.2
      kidney Z80.51
      lung Z80.1
      lymphatic NEC Z80.7
      ovary Z80.41
      prostate Z80.42
      respiratory organ NEC Z80.2
      specified site NEC Z80.8
      testis Z80.43
      trachea Z80.1
      urinary organ or tract Z80.59
        bladder Z80.52
        kidney Z80.51
    mental
      disorder NEC Z81.8
    multiple endocrine neoplasia (MEN) syndrome Z83.41
    osteoporosis Z82.62
    polycystic kidney Z82.71
    polyps (colon) Z83.71
    psychiatric disorder Z81.8
    psychoactive substance abuse NEC Z81.3
    respiratory condition NEC Z83.6
      asthma and other lower respiratory conditions Z82.5
    self-harmful behavior Z81.8
    SIDS (sudden infant death syndrome) Z84.82
    skin condition Z84.0
    specified condition NEC Z84.89
    stroke (cerebrovascular) Z82.3
    substance abuse NEC Z81.4
      alcohol Z81.1
      drug NEC Z81.3
      psychoactive NEC Z81.3
      tobacco Z81.2
    sudden
      cardiac death Z82.41
      infant death syndrome (SIDS) Z84.82
    tobacco abuse Z81.2

History — *continued*
  family — *see also* History, personal — *continued*
    violence, violent behavior Z81.8
    visual loss Z82.1
  personal (of) — *see also* History, family (of)
    abuse
      adult Z91.419
        forced labor or sexual exploitation Z91.42
        physical and sexual Z91.410
        psychological Z91.411
      childhood Z62.819
        forced labor or sexual exploitation in childhood Z62.813
        physical Z62.810
        psychological Z62.811
        sexual Z62.810
    alcohol dependence F10.21
    allergy (to) Z88.9
      analgesic agent NEC Z88.6
      anesthetic Z88.4
      antibiotic agent NEC Z88.1
      anti-infective agent NEC Z88.3
      contrast media Z91.041
      drugs, medicaments and biological substances Z88.9
        specified NEC Z88.8
      food Z91.018
        additives Z91.02
        beef Z91.014
        eggs Z91.012
        lamb Z91.014
        mammalian meats Z91.014
        milk products Z91.011
        peanuts Z91.010
        pork Z91.014
        red meats Z91.014
        seafood Z91.013
        specified food NEC Z91.018
      insect Z91.038
        bee Z91.030
      latex Z91.040
      medicinal agents Z88.9
        specified NEC Z88.8
      narcotic agent NEC Z88.5
      nonmedicinal agents Z91.048
      penicillin Z88.0
      serum Z88.7
      specified NEC Z91.09
      sulfonamides Z88.2
      vaccine Z88.7
    anaphylactic shock Z87.892
    anaphylaxis Z87.892
    behavioral disorders Z86.59
    benign carcinoid tumor Z86.012
    benign neoplasm Z86.018
      brain Z86.011
      carcinoid Z86.012
      colonic polyps Z86.010
    brain injury (traumatic) Z87.820
    breast implant removal Z98.86
    calculi, renal Z87.442
    cancer — *see* History, personal (of), malignant neoplasm (of)
    cardiac arrest (death), successfully resuscitated Z86.74
    CAR-T (Chimeric Antigen Receptor T-cell) therapy Z92.850
    cellular therapy Z92.859
      specified NEC Z92.858
    cerebral infarction without residual deficit Z86.73
    cervical dysplasia Z87.410
    chemotherapy for neoplastic condition Z92.21
    childhood abuse — *see* History, personal (of), abuse
    Chimeric Antigen Receptor T-cell (CAR-T) therapy Z92.850
    cleft lip (corrected) Z87.730
    cleft palate (corrected) Z87.730
    collapsed vertebra (healed) Z87.311
      due to osteoporosis Z87.310
    combat and operational stress reaction Z86.51
    congenital malformation (corrected) Z87.798
      circulatory system (corrected) Z87.74
      digestive system (corrected) NEC Z87.738
      ear (corrected) Z87.721
      eye (corrected) Z87.720
      face and neck (corrected) Z87.790
      genitourinary system (corrected) NEC Z87.718
      heart (corrected) Z87.74
      integument (corrected) Z87.76

History — *continued*
  personal — *see also* History, family — *continued*
    congenital malformation — *continued*
      limb(s) (corrected) Z87.76
      musculoskeletal system (corrected) Z87.76
      neck (corrected) Z87.790
      nervous system (corrected) NEC Z87.728
      respiratory system (corrected) Z87.75
      sense organs (corrected) NEC Z87.728
      specified NEC Z87.798
    contraception Z92.0
    coronavirus (disease) (novel) 2019 Z86.16
    COVID-19 Z86.16
    deployment (military) Z91.82
    diabetic foot ulcer Z86.31
    disease or disorder (of) Z87.898
      anaphylaxis Z87.892
      blood and blood-forming organs Z86.2
      circulatory system Z86.79
        specified condition NEC Z86.79
      connective tissue Z87.39
      digestive system Z87.19
        colonic polyp Z86.010
        peptic ulcer disease Z87.11
        specified condition NEC Z87.19
      ear Z86.69
      endocrine Z86.39
        diabetic foot ulcer Z86.31
        gestational diabetes Z86.32
        specified type NEC Z86.39
      eye Z86.69
      genital (track) system NEC
        female Z87.42
        male Z87.438
      hematological Z86.2
      Hodgkin Z85.71
      immune mechanism Z86.2
      infectious Z86.19
        coronavirus (disease) (novel) 2019 Z86.16
        COVID-19 Z86.16
        malaria Z86.13
        Methicillin resistant Staphylococcus aureus (MRSA) Z86.14
        poliomyelitis Z86.12
        SARS-CoV-2 Z86.16
        specified NEC Z86.19
        tuberculosis Z86.11
      mental NEC Z86.59
      metabolic Z86.39
        diabetic foot ulcer Z86.31
        gestational diabetes Z86.32
        specified type NEC Z86.39
      musculoskeletal NEC Z87.39
      nervous system Z86.69
      nutritional Z86.39
      parasitic Z86.19
      respiratory system NEC Z87.09
      sense organs Z86.69
      skin Z87.2
      specified site or type NEC Z87.898
      subcutaneous tissue Z87.2
      trophoblastic Z87.59
      urinary system NEC Z87.448
    drug dependence — *see* Dependence, drug, by type, in remission
    drug therapy
      antineoplastic chemotherapy Z92.21
      estrogen Z92.23
      immunosuppression Z92.25
      inhaled steroids Z92.240
      monoclonal drug Z92.22
      specified NEC Z92.29
      steroid Z92.241
      systemic steroids Z92.241
    dysplasia
      cervical (mild) (moderate) Z87.410
        severe (grade III) Z86.001
      prostatic Z87.430
      vaginal (mild) (moderate) Z87.411
        severe (grade III) Z86.002
      vulvar (mild) (moderate) Z87.412
        severe (grade III) Z86.002
    embolism (venous) Z86.718
      pulmonary Z86.711
    encephalitis Z86.61
    estrogen therapy Z92.23
    extracorporeal membrane oxygenation (ECMO) Z92.81
    failed conscious sedation Z92.83

History — continued
  personal — *see also* History, family — *continued*
    failed moderate sedation Z92.83
    fall, falling Z91.81
    forced labor or sexual exploitation Z91.42
      in childhood Z62.813
    fracture (healed)
      fatigue Z87.312
      fragility Z87.310
      osteoporosis Z87.310
      pathological NEC Z87.311
      stress Z87.312
      traumatic Z87.81
    gene therapy Z92.86
    gestational diabetes Z86.32
    hepatitis
      B Z86.19
      C Z86.19
    Hodgkin disease Z85.71
    hyperthermia, malignant Z88.4
    hypospadias (corrected) Z87.710
    hysterectomy Z90.710
    immunosuppression therapy Z92.25
    in situ neoplasm
      breast Z86.000
      cervix uteri Z86.001
      digestive organs, specified NEC Z86.004
      esophagus Z86.003
      genital organs, specified NEC Z86.002
      melanoma Z86.006
      middle ear Z86.005
      oral cavity Z86.003
      respiratory system Z86.005
      skin Z86.007
      specified NEC Z86.008
      stomach Z86.003
    in utero procedure during pregnancy Z98.870
    in utero procedure while a fetus Z98.871
    infection NEC Z86.19
      central nervous system Z86.61
      coronavirus (disease) (novel) 2019 Z86.16
      COVID-19 Z86.16
      latent tuberculosis Z86.15
      Methicillin resistant Staphylococcus aureus
        (MRSA) Z86.14
      SARS-CoV-2 Z86.16
      urinary (recurrent) (tract) Z87.440
    injury NEC Z87.828
    irradiation Z92.3
    kidney stones Z87.442
    latent tuberculosis infection Z86.15
    leukemia Z85.6
    lymphoma (non-Hodgkin) Z85.72
    malignant melanoma (skin) Z85.820
    malignant neoplasm (of) Z85.9
      accessory sinuses Z85.22
      anus NEC Z85.048
        carcinoid Z85.040
      bladder Z85.51
      bone Z85.830
      brain Z85.841
      breast Z85.3
      bronchus NEC Z85.118
        carcinoid Z85.110
      carcinoid — *see* History, personal (of), malignant
        neoplasm, by site, carcinioid
      cervix Z85.41
      colon NEC Z85.038
        carcinoid Z85.030
      digestive organ Z85.00
        specified NEC Z85.09
      endocrine gland NEC Z85.858
      epididymis Z85.48
      esophagus Z85.01
      eye Z85.840
      gastrointestinal tract — *see* History, malignant
        neoplasm, digestive organ
      genital organ
        female Z85.40
          specified NEC Z85.44
        male Z85.45
          specified NEC Z85.49
      hematopoietic NEC Z85.79
      intrathoracic organ Z85.20
      kidney NEC Z85.528
        carcinoid Z85.520
      large intestine NEC Z85.038
        carcinoid Z85.030
      larynx Z85.21

History — continued
  personal — *see also* History, family — *continued*
    malignant neoplasm — *continued*
      liver Z85.05
      lung NEC Z85.118
        carcinoid Z85.110
      mediastinum Z85.29
      Merkel cell Z85.821
      middle ear Z85.22
      nasal cavities Z85.22
      nervous system NEC Z85.848
      oral cavity Z85.819
        specified site NEC Z85.818
      ovary Z85.43
      pancreas Z85.07
      pelvis Z85.53
      pharynx Z85.819
        specified site NEC Z85.818
      pleura Z85.29
      prostate Z85.46
      rectosigmoid junction NEC Z85.048
        carcinoid Z85.040
      rectum NEC Z85.048
        carcinoid Z85.040
      respiratory organ Z85.20
      sinuses, accessory Z85.22
      skin NEC Z85.828
        melanoma Z85.820
        Merkel cell Z85.821
      small intestine NEC Z85.068
        carcinoid Z85.060
      soft tissue Z85.831
      specified site NEC Z85.89
      stomach NEC Z85.028
        carcinoid Z85.020
      testis Z85.47
      thymus NEC Z85.238
        carcinoid Z85.230
      thyroid Z85.850
      tongue Z85.810
      trachea Z85.12
      urinary organ or tract Z85.50
        specified NEC Z85.59
      uterus Z85.42
    maltreatment Z91.89
    medical treatment NEC Z92.89
    melanoma Z85.820
      in situ Z86.006
      malignant (skin) Z85.820
    meningitis Z86.61
    mental disorder Z86.59
    Merkel cell carcinoma (skin) Z85.821
    Methicillin resistant Staphylococcus aureus (MRSA)
      Z86.14
    military deployment Z91.82
    military war, peacekeeping and humanitarian de-
      ployment (current or past conflict) Z91.82
    myocardial infarction (old) I25.2
    neglect (in)
      adult Z91.412
      childhood Z62.812
    neoplasia
      anal intraepithelial, III [AIN III] Z86.004
      high-grade prostatic intraepithelial, III [HGPIN
        III] Z86.002
      vaginal intraepithelial, III [VAIN III] Z86.002
      vulvar intraepithelial, III [VIN III] Z86.002
    neoplasm
      benign Z86.018
        brain Z86.011
        colon polyp Z86.010
      in situ
        breast Z86.000
        cervix uteri Z86.001
        digestive organs, specified NEC Z86.004
        esophagus Z86.003
        genital organs, specified NEC Z86.002
        melanoma Z86.006
        middle ear Z86.005
        oral cavity Z86.003
        respiratory system Z86.005
        skin Z86.007
        specified NEC Z86.008
        stomach Z86.003
      malignant — *see* History of, malignant neoplasm
      uncertain behavior Z86.03
    nephrotic syndrome Z87.441
    nicotine dependence Z87.891

History — continued
  personal — *see also* History, family — *continued*
    noncompliance with medical treatment or regimen
      — *see* Noncompliance
    nutritional deficiency Z86.39
    obstetric complications Z87.59
      childbirth Z87.59
      pregnancy Z87.59
      pre-term labor Z87.51
      puerperium Z87.59
    osteoporosis fractures Z87.31 ☑
    parasuicide (attempt) Z91.51
    physical trauma NEC Z87.828
      self-harm or suicide attempt Z91.51
    pneumonia (recurrent) Z87.01
    poisoning NEC Z91.89
      self-harm or suicide attempt Z91.51
    poor personal hygiene Z91.89
    preterm labor Z87.51
    procedure during pregnancy Z98.870
    procedure while a fetus Z98.871
    prolonged reversible ischemic neurologic deficit
      (PRIND) Z86.73
    prostatic dysplasia Z87.430
    psychological
      abuse
        adult Z91.411
        child Z62.811
      trauma, specified NEC Z91.49
    radiation therapy Z92.3
    removal
      implant
        breast Z98.86
    renal calculi Z87.442
    respiratory condition NEC Z87.09
    retained foreign body fully removed Z87.821
    risk factors NEC Z91.89
    SARS-CoV-2 infection Z86.16
    self-harm
      nonsuicidal Z91.52
      suicidal Z91.51
    self-inflicted injury without suicidal intent Z91.52
    self-injury
      nonsuicidal Z91.52
    self-mutilation Z91.52
    self-poisoning attempt Z91.51
    sex reassignment Z87.890
    sleep-wake cycle problem Z72.821
    specified NEC Z87.898
    steroid therapy (systemic) Z92.241
      inhaled Z92.240
    stroke without residual deficits Z86.73
    substance abuse NEC F10-F19
    sudden cardiac arrest Z86.74
    sudden cardiac death successfully resuscitated
      Z86.74
    suicidal behavior Z91.51
    suicide attempt Z91.51
    surgery NEC Z98.890
      with uterine scar Z98.891
      sex reassignment Z87.890
      transplant — *see* Transplant
    thrombophlebitis Z86.72
    thrombosis (venous) Z86.718
      pulmonary Z86.711
    tobacco dependence Z87.891
    transient ischemic attack (TIA) without residual
      deficits Z86.73
    trauma (physical) NEC Z87.828
      psychological NEC Z91.49
      self-harm Z91.51
    traumatic brain injury Z87.820
    tuberculosis, latent infection Z86.15
    unhealthy sleep-wake cycle Z72.821
    unintended awareness under general anesthesia
      Z92.84
    urinary calculi Z87.442
    urinary (recurrent) (tract) infection(s) Z87.440
    uterine scar from previous surgery Z98.891
    vaginal dysplasia Z87.411
    venous thrombosis or embolism Z86.718
      pulmonary Z86.711
    vulvar dysplasia Z87.412
His-Werner disease A79.0
HIV — *see also* Human, immunodeficiency virus B20
  laboratory evidence (nonconclusive) R75
  nonconclusive test (in infants) R75
  positive, seropositive Z21

☑ **Additional Character Required — Refer to the Tabular List for Character Selection**   ⬇ **Subterms under main terms may continue to next column or page**

Hives (bold) — *see* Urticaria
Hoarseness R49.0
Hobo Z59.00
Hodgkin disease — *see* Lymphoma, Hodgkin
Hodgson's disease I71.2
  ruptured I71.1
Hoffa-Kastert disease E88.89
Hoffa's disease E88.89
Hoffmann-Bouveret syndrome I47.9
Hoffmann's syndrome E03.9 *[G73.7]*
Hole (round)
  macula H35.34- ☑
  retina (without detachment) — *see* Break, retina, round hole
    with detachment — *see* Detachment, retina, with retinal, break
Holiday relief care Z75.5
Hollenhorst's plaque — *see* Occlusion, artery, retina
Hollow foot (congenital) Q66.7- ☑
  acquired — *see* Deformity, limb, foot, specified NEC
Holoprosencephaly Q04.2
Holt-Oram syndrome Q87.2
Homelessness Z59.00
  sheltered Z59.01
  unsheltered Z59.02
Homesickness — *see* Disorder, adjustment
Homocysteinemia R79.83
Homocystinemia, homocystinuria E72.11
Homogentisate 1,2-dioxygenase deficiency E70.29
Homologous serum hepatitis (prophylactic) (therapeutic) — *see* Hepatitis, viral, type B
Honeycomb lung J98.4
  congenital Q33.0
Hooded
  clitoris Q52.6
  penis Q55.69
Hookworm (disease) (infection) (infestation) B76.9
  with anemia B76.9 *[D63.8]*
  specified NEC B76.8
Hordeolum (eyelid) (externum) (recurrent) H00.019
  internum H00.029
    left H00.026
      lower H00.025
      upper H00.024
    right H00.023
      lower H00.022
      upper H00.021
  left H00.016
    lower H00.015
    upper H00.014
  right H00.013
    lower H00.012
    upper H00.011
Horn
  cutaneous L85.8
  nail L60.2
    congenital Q84.6
Horner (-Claude Bernard) **syndrome** G90.2
  traumatic — *see* Injury, nerve, cervical sympathetic
Horseshoe kidney (congenital) Q63.1
Horton's headache or neuralgia G44.099
  intractable G44.091
  not intractable G44.099
Hospital hopper syndrome — *see* Disorder, factitious
Hospitalism in children — *see* Disorder, adjustment
Hostility R45.5
  towards child Z62.3
Hot flashes
  menopausal N95.1
Hourglass (contracture) — *see also* Contraction, hourglass
  stomach K31.89
    congenital Q40.2
    stricture K31.2
Household, housing circumstance affecting care Z59.9
  specified NEC Z59.89
Housemaid's knee — *see* Bursitis, prepatellar
HSCT-TMA (hematopoietic stem cell transplantation-associated thrombotic microangiopathy) M31.11
Hudson (-Stähli) **line** (cornea) — *see* Pigmentation, cornea, anterior
Human
  bite (open wound) — *see also* Bite
    intact skin surface — *see* Bite, superficial
  herpesvirus — *see* Herpes
  immunodeficiency virus (HIV) disease (infection) B20

Human — *continued*
  immunodeficiency virus disease — *continued*
    asymptomatic status Z21
    contact Z20.6
    counseling Z71.7
    dementia B20 *[F02.80]*
      with behavioral disturbance B20 *[F02.81]*
    exposure to Z20.6
    laboratory evidence R75
    type-2 (HIV 2) as cause of disease classified elsewhere B97.35
  papillomavirus (HPV)
    DNA test positive
      high risk
        cervix R87.810
        vagina R87.811
      low risk
        cervix R87.820
        vagina R87.821
    screening for Z11.51
  T-cell lymphotropic virus
    type-1 (HTLV-I) infection B33.3
      as cause of disease classified elsewhere B97.33
      carrier Z22.6
    type-2 (HTLV-II) as cause of disease classified elsewhere B97.34
Humidifier lung or pneumonitis J67.7
Humiliation (experience) **in childhood** Z62.898
Humpback (acquired) — *see* Kyphosis
Hunchback (acquired) — *see* Kyphosis
Hunger T73.0 ☑
  air, psychogenic F45.8
Hungry bone syndrome E83.81
Hunner's ulcer — *see* Cystitis, chronic, interstitial
Hunter's
  glossitis D51.0
  syndrome E76.1
Huntington's disease or chorea G10
  with dementia G10 *[F02.80]*
    with behavioral disturbance G10 *[F02.81]*
Hunt's
  disease or syndrome (herpetic geniculate ganglionitis) B02.21
    dyssynergia cerebellaris myoclonica G11.19
  neuralgia B02.21
Hurler (-Scheie) **disease or syndrome** E76.02
Hurst's disease G36.1
Hurthle cell
  adenocarcinoma C73
  adenoma D34
  carcinoma C73
  tumor D34
Hutchinson-Boeck disease or syndrome — *see* Sarcoidosis
Hutchinson-Gilford disease or syndrome E34.8
Hutchinson's
  disease, meaning
    angioma serpiginosum L81.7
    pompholyx (cheiropompholyx) L30.1
    prurigo estivalis L56.4
    summer eruption or summer prurigo L56.4
  melanotic freckle — *see* Melanoma, in situ
    malignant melanoma in — *see* Melanoma
  teeth or incisors (congenital syphilis) A50.52
  triad (congenital syphilis) A50.53
Hyalin plaque, sclera, senile H15.89
Hyaline membrane (disease) (lung) (pulmonary) (newborn) P22.0
Hyalinosis
  cutis (et mucosae) E78.89
  focal and segmental (glomerular) — *see also* N00-N07
    with fourth character .1 N05.1
Hyalitis, hyalosis, asteroid — *see also* Deposit, crystalline
  syphilitic (late) A52.71
Hydatid
  cyst or tumor — *see* Echinococcus
  mole — *see* Hydatidiform mole
  Morgagni
    female Q50.5
    male (epididymal) Q55.4
      testicular Q55.29
Hydatidiform mole (benign) (complicating pregnancy) (delivered) (undelivered) O01.9
  classical O01.0
  complete O01.0
  incomplete O01.1
  invasive D39.2

Hydatidiform mole — *continued*
  malignant D39.2
  partial O01.1
Hydatidosis — *see* Echinococcus
Hydradenitis (axillaris) (suppurative) L73.2
Hydradenoma — *see* Hidradenoma
Hydramnios O40.-
Hydrancephaly, hydranencephaly Q04.3
  with spina bifida — *see* Spina bifida, with hydrocephalus
Hydrargyrism NEC — *see* Poisoning, mercury
Hydrarthrosis — *see also* Effusion, joint
  gonococcal A54.42
  intermittent M12.40
    ankle M12.47- ☑
    elbow M12.42- ☑
    foot joint M12.47- ☑
    hand joint M12.44- ☑
    hip M12.45- ☑
    knee M12.46- ☑
    multiple site M12.49
    shoulder M12.41- ☑
    specified joint NEC M12.48
    wrist M12.43- ☑
  of yaws (early) (late) — *see also* subcategory M14.8-A66.6
  syphilitic (late) A52.77
    congenital A50.55 *[M12.80]*
Hydremia D64.89
Hydrencephalocele (congenital) — *see* Encephalocele
Hydrencephalomeningocele (congenital) — *see* Encephalocele
Hydroa R23.8
  aestivale L56.4
  vacciniforme L56.4
Hydroadenitis (axillaris) (suppurative) L73.2
Hydrocalycosis — *see* Hydronephrosis
Hydrocele (spermatic cord) (testis) (tunica vaginalis) N43.3
  canal of Nuck N94.89
  communicating N43.2
    congenital P83.5
  congenital P83.5
  encysted N43.0
  female NEC N94.89
  infected N43.1
  newborn P83.5
  round ligament N94.89
  specified NEC N43.2
  spinalis — *see* Spina bifida
  vulva N90.89
Hydrocephalus (acquired) (external) (internal) (malignant) (recurrent) G91.9
  aqueduct Sylvius stricture Q03.0
  causing disproportion O33.6 ☑
    with obstructed labor O66.3
  communicating G91.0
  congenital (external) (internal) Q03.9
    with spina bifida Q05.4
      cervical Q05.0
      dorsal Q05.1
      lumbar Q05.2
      lumbosacral Q05.2
      sacral Q05.3
      thoracic Q05.1
      thoracolumbar Q05.1
    specified NEC Q03.8
  due to toxoplasmosis (congenital) P37.1
  foramen Magendie block (acquired) G91.1
    congenital — *see also* Hydrocephalus, congenital Q03.1
  in (due to)
    infectious disease NEC B89 *[G91.4]*
    neoplastic disease NEC — *see also* Neoplasm G91.4
    parasitic disease B89 *[G91.4]*
  newborn Q03.9
    with spina bifida — *see* Spina bifida, with hydrocephalus
  noncommunicating G91.1
  normal pressure G91.2
    secondary G91.0
  obstructive G91.1
  otitic G93.2
  post-traumatic NEC G91.3
  secondary G91.4
    post-traumatic G91.3
  specified NEC G91.8
  syphilitic, congenital A50.49

Hydrocolpos (congenital) N89.8
Hydrocystoma — see Neoplasm, skin, benign
Hydroencephalocele (congenital) — see Encephalocele
Hydroencephalomeningocele (congenital) — see Encephalocele
Hydrohematopneumothorax — see Hemothorax
Hydromeningitis — see Meningitis
Hydromeningocele (spinal) — see also Spina bifida
   cranial — see Encephalocele
Hydrometra N85.8
Hydrometrocolpos N89.8
Hydromicrocephaly Q02
Hydromphalos (since birth) Q45.8
Hydromyelia Q06.4
Hydromyelocele — see Spina bifida
Hydronephrosis (atrophic) (early) (functionless) (intermittent) (primary) (secondary) NEC N13.30
  with
    infection N13.6
    obstruction (by) (of)
      renal calculus N13.2
        with infection N13.6
      ureteral NEC N13.1
        with infection N13.6
        calculus N13.2
          with infection N13.6
      ureteropelvic junction (congenital) Q62.11
        acquired N13.0
          with infection N13.6
      ureteral stricture NEC N13.1
        with infection N13.6
  congenital Q62.0
  due to acquired occlusion of ureteropelvic junction N13.0
  specified type NEC N13.39
  tuberculous A18.11
Hydropericarditis — see Pericarditis
Hydropericardium — see Pericarditis
Hydroperitoneum R18.8
Hydrophobia — see Rabies
Hydrophthalmos Q15.0
Hydropneumohemothorax — see Hemothorax
Hydropneumopericarditis — see Pericarditis
Hydropneumopericardium — see Pericarditis
Hydropneumothorax J94.8
  traumatic — see Injury, intrathoracic, lung
  tuberculous NEC A15.6
Hydrops R60.9
  abdominis R18.8
  articulorum intermittens — see Hydrarthrosis, intermittent
  cardiac — see Failure, heart, congestive
  causing obstructed labor (mother) O66.3
  endolymphatic H81.0- ☑
  fetal — see Pregnancy, complicated by, hydrops, fetalis
  fetalis P83.2
    due to
      ABO isoimmunization P56.0
      alpha thalassemia D56.0
      hemolytic disease P56.90
        specified NEC P56.99
      isoimmunization (ABO) (Rh) P56.0
      other specified nonhemolytic disease NEC P83.2
      Rh incompatibility P56.0
    during pregnancy — see Pregnancy, complicated by, hydrops, fetalis
  gallbladder K82.1
  joint — see Effusion, joint
  labyrinth H81.0- ☑
  newborn (idiopathic) P83.2
    due to
      ABO isoimmunization P56.0
      alpha thalassemia D56.0
      hemolytic disease P56.90
        specified NEC P56.99
      isoimmunization (ABO) (Rh) P56.0
      Rh incompatibility P56.0
  nutritional — see Malnutrition, severe
  pericardium — see Pericarditis
  pleura — see Hydrothorax
  spermatic cord — see Hydrocele
Hydropyonephrosis N13.6
Hydrorachis Q06.4
Hydrorrhea (nasal) J34.89
  pregnancy — see Rupture, membranes, premature
Hydrosadenitis (axillaris) (suppurative) L73.2
Hydrosalpinx (fallopian tube) (follicularis) N70.11

Hydrothorax (double) (pleura) J94.8
  chylous (nonfilarial) I89.8
    filarial — see also Infestation, filarial B74.9 [J91.8]
  traumatic — see Injury, intrathoracic
  tuberculous NEC (non primary) A15.6
Hydroureter — see also Hydronephrosis N13.4
  with infection N13.6
  congenital Q62.39
Hydroureteronephrosis — see Hydronephrosis
Hydrourethra N36.8
Hydroxykynureninuria E70.89
Hydroxylysinemia E72.3
Hydroxyprolinemia E72.59
Hygiene, sleep
  abuse Z72.821
  inadequate Z72.821
  poor Z72.821
Hygroma (congenital) (cystic) D18.1
  praepatellare, prepatellar — see Bursitis, prepatellar
Hymen — see condition
Hymenolepis, hymenolepiasis (diminuta) (infection) (infestation) (nana) B71.0
Hypalgesia R20.8
Hyperacidity (gastric) K31.89
  psychogenic F45.8
Hyperactive, hyperactivity F90.9
  basal cell, uterine cervix — see Dysplasia, cervix
  bowel sounds R19.12
  cervix epithelial (basal) — see Dysplasia, cervix
  child F90.9
    attention deficit — see Disorder, attention-deficit hyperactivity
  detrusor muscle N32.81
  gastrointestinal K31.89
    psychogenic F45.8
  nasal mucous membrane J34.3
  stomach K31.89
  thyroid (gland) — see Hyperthyroidism
Hyperacusis H93.23- ☑
Hyperadrenalism E27.5
Hyperadrenocorticism E24.9
  congenital E25.0
  iatrogenic E24.2
    correct substance properly administered — see Table of Drugs and Chemicals, by drug, adverse effect
    overdose or wrong substance given or taken — see Table of Drugs and Chemicals, by drug, poisoning
  not associated with Cushing's syndrome E27.0
  pituitary-dependent E24.0
Hyperaldosteronism E26.9
  familial (type I) E26.02
  glucocorticoid-remediable E26.02
  primary (due to (bilateral) adrenal hyperplasia) E26.09
  primary NEC E26.09
  secondary E26.1
  specified NEC E26.89
Hyperalgesia R20.8
Hyperalimentation R63.2
  carotene, carotin E67.1
  specified NEC E67.8
  vitamin
    A E67.0
    D E67.3
Hyperaminoaciduria
  arginine E72.21
  cystine E72.01
  lysine E72.3
  ornithine E72.4
Hyperammonemia (congenital) E72.20
Hyperazotemia — see Uremia
Hyperbetalipoproteinemia (familial) E78.00
  with prebetalipoproteinemia E78.2
Hyperbicarbonatemia P74.41
Hyperbilirubinemia
  constitutional E80.6
  familial conjugated E80.6
  neonatal (transient) — see Jaundice, newborn
Hypercalcemia, hypocalciuric, familial E83.52
Hypercalciuria, idiopathic R82.994
Hypercapnia R06.89
  newborn P84
Hypercarotenemia (dietary) E67.1
Hypercementosis K03.4
Hyperchloremia E87.8
Hyperchlorhydria K31.89

Hyperchlorhydria — continued
  neurotic F45.8
  psychogenic F45.8
Hypercholesterinemia — see Hypercholesterolemia
Hypercholesterolemia (essential) (primary) (pure) E78.00
  with hyperglyceridemia, endogenous E78.2
  dietary counseling and surveillance Z71.3
  familial E78.01
  hereditary E78.01
Hyperchylia gastrica, psychogenic F45.8
Hyperchylomicronemia (familial) (primary) E78.3
  with hyperbetalipoproteinemia E78.3
Hypercoagulable (state) D68.59
  activated protein C resistance D68.51
  antithrombin (III) deficiency D68.59
  factor V Leiden mutation D68.51
  primary NEC D68.59
  protein C deficiency D68.59
  protein S deficiency D68.59
  prothrombin gene mutation D68.52
  secondary D68.69
  specified NEC D68.69
Hypercoagulation (state) D68.59
Hypercorticalism, pituitary-dependent E24.0
Hypercorticosolism — see Cushing's, syndrome
Hypercorticosteronism E24.2
  correct substance properly administered — see Table of Drugs and Chemicals, by drug, adverse effect
  overdose or wrong substance given or taken — see Table of Drugs and Chemicals, by drug, poisoning
Hypercortisonism E24.2
  correct substance properly administered — see Table of Drugs and Chemicals, by drug, adverse effect
  overdose or wrong substance given or taken — see Table of Drugs and Chemicals, by drug, poisoning
Hyperekplexia Q89.8
Hyperelectrolytemia E87.8
Hyperemesis R11.10
  with nausea R11.2
  gravidarum (mild) O21.0
    with
      carbohydrate depletion O21.1
      dehydration O21.1
      electrolyte imbalance O21.1
      metabolic disturbance O21.1
      severe (with metabolic disturbance) O21.1
  projectile R11.12
  psychogenic F45.8
Hyperemia (acute) (passive) R68.89
  anal mucosa K62.89
  bladder N32.89
  cerebral I67.89
  conjunctiva H11.43- ☑
  ear internal, acute — see subcategory H83.0 ☑
  enteric K59.89
  eye — see Hyperemia, conjunctiva
  eyelid (active) (passive) — see Disorder, eyelid, specified type NEC
  intestine K59.89
  iris — see Disorder, iris, vascular
  kidney N28.89
  labyrinth — see subcategory H83.0 ☑
  liver (active) K76.89
  lung (passive) — see Edema, lung
  pulmonary (passive) — see Edema, lung
  renal N28.89
  retina H35.89
  stomach K31.89
Hyperesthesia (body surface) R20.3
  larynx (reflex) J38.7
    hysterical F44.89
  pharynx (reflex) J39.2
    hysterical F44.89
Hyperestrogenism (drug-induced) (iatrogenic) E28.0
Hyperexplexia Q89.8
Hyperfibrinolysis — see Fibrinolysis
Hyperfructosemia E74.19
Hyperfunction
  adrenal cortex, not associated with Cushing's syndrome E27.0
    medulla E27.5
      adrenomedullary E27.5
    virilism E25.9
      congenital E25.0
  ovarian E28.8
  pancreas K86.89
  parathyroid (gland) E21.3
  pituitary (gland) (anterior) E22.9

Hyperfunction — continued
  pituitary — continued
    specified NEC E22.8
  polyglandular E31.1
  testicular E29.0
Hypergammaglobulinemia D89.2
  polyclonal D89.0
  Waldenström D89.0
Hypergastrinemia E16.4
Hyperglobulinemia R77.1
Hyperglycemia, hyperglycemic (transient) R73.9
  coma — see Diabetes, by type, with coma
  postpancreatectomy E89.1
Hyperglyceridemia (endogenous) (essential) (familial) (hereditary) (pure) E78.1
  mixed E78.3
Hyperglycinemia (non-ketotic) E72.51
Hypergonadism
  ovarian E28.8
  testicular (primary) (infantile) E29.0
Hyperheparinemia D68.32
Hyperhidrosis, hyperidrosis R61
  focal
    primary L74.519
      axilla L74.510
      face L74.511
      palms L74.512
      soles L74.513
    secondary L74.52
  generalized R61
  localized
    primary L74.519
      axilla L74.510
      face L74.511
      palms L74.512
      soles L74.513
    secondary L74.52
  psychogenic F45.8
  secondary R61
    focal L74.52
Hyperhistidinemia E70.41
Hyperhomocysteinemia E72.11
Hyperhydroxyprolinemia E72.59
Hyperinsulinism (functional) E16.1
  with
    coma (hypoglycemic) E15
    encephalopathy E16.1 [G94]
  ectopic E16.1
  therapeutic misadventure (from administration of insulin) — see subcategory T38.3 ☑
Hyperkalemia E87.5
Hyperkeratosis — see also Keratosis L85.9
  cervix N88.0
  due to yaws (early) (late) (palmar or plantar) A66.3
  follicularis Q82.8
    penetrans (in cutem) L87.0
  palmoplantaris climacterica L85.1
  pinta A67.1
  senile (with pruritus) L57.0
  universalis congenita Q80.8
  vocal cord J38.3
  vulva N90.4
Hyperkinesia, hyperkinetic (disease) (reaction) (syndrome) (childhood) (adolescence) — see also Disorder, attention-deficit hyperactivity
  heart I51.89
Hyperleucine-isoleucinemia E71.19
Hyperlipemia, hyperlipidemia E78.5
  combined E78.2
    familial E78.49
  group
    A E78.00
    B E78.1
    C E78.2
    D E78.3
  mixed E78.2
  specified NEC E78.49
Hyperlipidosis E75.6
  hereditary NEC E75.5
Hyperlipoproteinemia E78.5
  Fredrickson's type
    I E78.3
    IIa E78.00
    IIb E78.2
    III E78.2
    IV E78.1
    V E78.3
  low-density-lipoprotein-type (LDL) E78.00

Hyperlipoproteinemia — continued
  very-low-density-lipoprotein-type (VLDL) E78.1
Hyperlucent lung, unilateral J43.0
Hyperlysinemia E72.3
Hypermagnesemia E83.41
  neonatal P71.8
Hypermenorrhea N92.0
Hypermethioninemia E72.19
Hypermetropia (congenital) H52.0- ☑
Hypermobility, hypermotility
  cecum — see Syndrome, irritable bowel
  coccyx — see subcategory M53.2 ☑
  colon — see Syndrome, irritable bowel
    psychogenic F45.8
  ileum K58.9
  intestine — see also Syndrome, irritable bowel K58.9
    psychogenic F45.8
  meniscus (knee) — see Derangement, knee, meniscus
  scapula — see Instability, joint, shoulder
  stomach K31.89
    psychogenic F45.8
  syndrome M35.7
  urethra N36.41
    with intrinsic sphincter deficiency N36.43
Hypernasality R49.21
Hypernatremia E87.0
Hypernephroma C64.- ☑
Hyperopia — see Hypermetropia
Hyperorexia nervosa F50.2
Hyperornithinemia E72.4
Hyperosmia R43.1
Hyperosmolality E87.0
Hyperostosis (monomeric) — see also Disorder, bone, density and structure, specified NEC
  ankylosing (spine) M48.10
    cervical region M48.12
    cervicothoracic region M48.13
    lumbar region M48.16
    lumbosacral region M48.17
    multiple sites M48.19
    occipito-atlanto-axial region M48.11
    sacrococcygeal region M48.18
    thoracic region M48.14
    thoracolumbar region M48.15
  cortical (skull) M85.2
    infantile M89.8X- ☑
  frontal, internal of skull M85.2
  interna frontalis M85.2
  skeletal, diffuse idiopathic — see Hyperostosis, ankylosing
  skull M85.2
    congenital Q75.8
  vertebral, ankylosing — see Hyperostosis, ankylosing
Hyperovarism E28.8
Hyperoxaluria R82.992
  primary E72.53
Hyperparathyroidism E21.3
  primary E21.0
  secondary (renal) N25.81
    non-renal E21.1
  specified NEC E21.2
  tertiary E21.2
Hyperpathia R20.8
Hyperperistalsis R19.2
  psychogenic F45.8
Hyperpermeability, capillary I78.8
Hyperphagia R63.2
Hyperphenylalaninemia NEC E70.1
Hyperphoria (alternating) H50.53
Hyperphosphatemia E83.39
Hyperpiesis, hyperpiesia — see Hypertension
Hyperpigmentation — see also Pigmentation
  melanin NEC L81.4
  postinflammatory L81.0
Hyperpinealism E34.8
Hyperpituitarism E22.9
Hyperplasia, hyperplastic
  adenoids J35.2
  adrenal (capsule) (cortex) (gland) E27.8
    with
      sexual precocity (male) E25.9
        congenital E25.0
      virilism, adrenal E25.9
        congenital E25.0
      virilization (female) E25.9
        congenital E25.0
    congenital E25.0

Hyperplasia, hyperplastic — continued
  adrenal — continued
    congenital — continued
      salt-losing E25.0
  adrenomedullary E27.5
  angiolymphoid, eosinophilia (ALHE) D18.01
  appendix (lymphoid) K38.0
  artery, fibromuscular I77.3
  bone — see also Hypertrophy, bone
    marrow D75.89
  breast — see also Hypertrophy, breast
    atypical, atypia N60.9- ☑
      ductal N60.9- ☑
      lobular N60.9- ☑
  C-cell, thyroid E07.0
  cementation (tooth) (teeth) K03.4
  cervical gland R59.0
  cervix (uteri) (basal cell) (endometrium) (polypoid) — see also Dysplasia, cervix
    congenital Q51.828
  clitoris, congenital Q52.6
  denture K06.2
  endocervicitis N72
  endometrium, endometrial (adenomatous) (cystic) (glandular) (glandular-cystic) (polypoid) N85.00
    with atypia N85.02
    benign N85.01
    cervix — see Dysplasia, cervix
    complex (without atypia) N85.01
    simple (without atypia) N85.01
  epithelial L85.9
    focal, oral, including tongue K13.29
    nipple N62
    skin L85.9
    tongue K13.29
    vaginal wall N89.3
  erythroid D75.89
  fibromuscular of artery (carotid) (renal) I77.3
  genital
    female NEC N94.89
    male N50.89
  gingiva K06.1
  glandularis cystica uteri (interstitialis) — see also Hyperplasia, endometrial N85.00
  gum K06.1
  hymen, congenital Q52.4
  irritative, edentulous (alveolar) K06.2
  jaw M26.09
    alveolar M26.79
      lower M26.03
        alveolar M26.72
      upper M26.01
        alveolar M26.71
  kidney (congenital) Q63.3
  labia N90.69
    epithelial N90.3
  liver (congenital) Q44.7
    nodular, focal K76.89
  lymph gland or node R59.9
  mandible, mandibular M26.03
    alveolar M26.72
    unilateral condylar M27.8
  maxilla, maxillary M26.01
    alveolar M26.71
  myometrium, myometrial N85.2
  neuroendocrine cell, of infancy J84.841
  nose
    lymphoid J34.89
    polypoid J33.9
  oral mucosa (irritative) K13.6
  organ or site, congenital NEC — see Anomaly, by site
  ovary N83.8
  palate, papillary (irritative) K13.6
  pancreatic islet cells E16.9
    alpha E16.8
      with excess
        gastrin E16.4
        glucagon E16.3
    beta E16.1
  parathyroid (gland) E21.0
  pharynx (lymphoid) J39.2
  prostate (adenofibromatous) (nodular) N40.0
    with lower urinary tract symptoms (LUTS) N40.1
    without lower urinary tract symtpoms (LUTS) N40.0
  renal artery I77.89
  reticulo-endothelial (cell) D75.89
  salivary gland (any) K11.1
  Schimmelbusch's — see Mastopathy, cystic

☞ Subterms under main terms may continue to next column or page   ☑ Additional Character Required — Refer to the Tabular List for Character Selection   177

Hyperfunction — Hyperplasia, hyperplastic

Hyperplasia, hyperplastic — *continued*
- suprarenal capsule (gland) E27.8
- thymus (gland) (persistent) E32.0
- thyroid (gland) — *see* Goiter
- tonsils (faucial) (infective) (lingual) (lymphoid) J35.1
  - with adenoids J35.3
- unilateral condylar M27.8
- uterus, uterine N85.2
  - endometrium (glandular) — *see also* Hyperplasia, endometrial N85.00
- vulva N90.69
  - epithelial N90.3

Hyperpnea — *see* Hyperventilation
Hyperpotassemia E87.5
Hyperprebetalipoproteinemia (familial) E78.1
Hyperprolactinemia E22.1
Hyperprolinemia (type I) (type II) E72.59
Hyperproteinemia E88.09
Hyperprothrombinemia, causing coagulation factor deficiency D68.4
Hyperpyrexia R50.9
- heat (effects) T67.01 ☑
- malignant, due to anesthetic T88.3 ☑
- rheumatic — *see* Fever, rheumatic
- unknown origin R50.9

Hyper-reflexia R29.2
Hypersalivation K11.7
Hypersecretion
- ACTH (not associated with Cushing's syndrome) E27.0
  - pituitary E24.0
- adrenaline E27.5
- adrenomedullary E27.5
- androgen (testicular) E29.0
  - ovarian (drug-induced) (iatrogenic) E28.1
- calcitonin E07.0
- catecholamine E27.5
- corticoadrenal E24.9
- cortisol E24.9
- epinephrine E27.5
- estrogen E28.0
- gastric K31.89
  - psychogenic F45.8
- gastrin E16.4
- glucagon E16.3
- hormone(s)
  - ACTH (not associated with Cushing's syndrome) E27.0
    - pituitary E24.0
  - antidiuretic E22.2
  - growth E22.0
  - intestinal NEC E34.1
  - ovarian androgen E28.1
  - pituitary E22.9
  - testicular E29.0
  - thyroid stimulating E05.80
    - with thyroid storm E05.81
- insulin — *see* Hyperinsulinism
- lacrimal glands — *see* Epiphora
- medulloadrenal E27.5
- milk O92.6
- ovarian androgens E28.1
- salivary gland (any) K11.7
- thyrocalcitonin E07.0
- upper respiratory J38.8

Hypersegmentation, leukocytic, hereditary D72.0
Hypersensitive, hypersensitiveness, hypersensitivity
— *see also* Allergy
- carotid sinus G90.01
- colon — *see* Irritable, colon
- drug T88.7 ☑
- gastrointestinal K52.29
  - immediate K52.29
  - psychogenic F45.8
- labyrinth — *see* subcategory H83.2 ☑
- pain R20.8
- pneumonitis — *see* Pneumonitis, allergic
- reaction T78.40 ☑
  - upper respiratory tract NEC J39.3

Hypersomnia (organic) G47.10
- due to
  - alcohol
    - abuse F10.182
    - dependence F10.282
    - use F10.982
  - amphetamines
    - abuse F15.182
    - dependence F15.282
    - use F15.982

Hypersomnia — *continued*
- due to — *continued*
  - caffeine
    - abuse F15.182
    - dependence F15.282
    - use F15.982
  - cocaine
    - abuse F14.182
    - dependence F14.282
    - use F14.982
  - drug NEC
    - abuse F19.182
    - dependence F19.282
    - use F19.982
  - medical condition G47.14
  - mental disorder F51.13
  - opioid
    - abuse F11.182
    - dependence F11.282
    - use F11.982
  - psychoactive substance NEC
    - abuse F19.182
    - dependence F19.282
    - use F19.982
  - sedative, hypnotic, or anxiolytic
    - abuse F13.182
    - dependence F13.282
    - use F13.982
  - stimulant NEC
    - abuse F15.182
    - dependence F15.282
    - use F15.982
- idiopathic G47.11
  - with long sleep time G47.11
  - without long sleep time G47.12
- menstrual related G47.13
- nonorganic origin F51.11
  - specified NEC F51.19
- not due to a substance or known physiological condition F51.11
  - specified NEC F51.19
- primary F51.11
- recurrent G47.13
- specified NEC G47.19

Hypersplenia, hypersplenism D73.1
Hyperstimulation, ovaries (associated with induced ovulation) N98.1
Hypersusceptibility — *see* Allergy
Hypertelorism (ocular) (orbital) Q75.2
Hypertension, hypertensive (accelerated) (benign) (essential) (idiopathic) (malignant) (systemic) I10
- with
  - heart failure (congestive) I11.0
  - heart involvement (conditions in I50.- or I51.4-I51.7, I51.89, I51.9, due to hypertension) — *see* Hypertension, heart
  - kidney involvement — *see* Hypertension, kidney
- benign, intracranial G93.2
- borderline R03.0
- cardiorenal (disease) I13.10
  - with heart failure I13.0
    - with stage 1 through stage 4 chronic kidney disease I13.0
    - with stage 5 or end stage renal disease I13.2
  - without heart failure I13.10
    - with stage 1 through stage 4 chronic kidney disease I13.10
    - with stage 5 or end stage renal disease I13.11
- cardiovascular
  - disease (arteriosclerotic) (sclerotic) — *see* Hypertension, heart
  - renal (disease) — *see* Hypertension, cardiorenal
- chronic venous — *see* Hypertension, venous (chronic)
- complicating
  - childbirth (labor) O16.4
    - pre-existing O10.92
      - with
        - heart disease O10.12
          - with renal disease O10.32
        - pre-eclampsia O11.4
        - renal disease O10.22
          - with heart disease O10.32
        - essential O10.02
      - secondary O10.42
  - pregnancy O16.- ☑
    - with edema — *see also* Pre-eclampsia O14.9- ☑
    - gestational (pregnancy induced) (without proteinuria) O13.- ☑

Hypertension, hypertensive — *continued*
- complicating — *continued*
  - pregnancy — *continued*
    - gestational — *continued*
      - with proteinuria O14.9- ☑
        - mild pre-eclampsia O14.0- ☑
        - moderate pre-eclampsia O14.0- ☑
        - severe pre-eclampsia O14.1- ☑
          - with hemolysis, elevated liver enzymes and low platelet count (HELLP) O14.2- ☑
    - pre-existing O10.91- ☑
      - with
        - heart disease O10.11- ☑
          - with renal disease O10.31- ☑
        - pre-eclampsia — *see* category O11
        - renal disease O10.21- ☑
          - with heart disease O10.31- ☑
        - essential O10.01- ☑
      - secondary O10.41- ☑
    - transient O13- ☑
  - puerperium, pre-existing O16.5
    - pre-existing
      - with
        - heart disease O10.13
          - with renal disease O10.33
        - pre-eclampsia O11.5
        - renal disease O10.23
          - with heart disease O10.33
        - essential O10.03
      - pregnancy-induced O13.9
      - secondary O10.43
- crisis I16.9
- due to
  - endocrine disorders I15.2
  - pheochromocytoma I15.2
  - renal disorders NEC I15.1
    - arterial I15.0
  - renovascular disorders I15.0
  - specified disease NEC I15.8
- emergency I16.1
- encephalopathy I67.4
- gestational (without significant proteinuria) (pregnancy-induced) (transient) O13.- ☑
  - with significant proteinuria — *see* Pre-eclampsia
  - complicating
    - delivery O13.4
    - puerperium O13.5
- Goldblatt's I70.1
- heart (disease) (conditions in I51.4-I51.9 due to hypertension) I11.9
  - with
    - heart failure (congestive) I11.0
    - kidney disease (chronic) — *see* Hypertension, cardiorenal
- intracranial, benign G93.2
- kidney I12.9
  - with
    - heart disease — *see* Hypertension, cardiorenal
    - stage 1 through stage 4 chronic kidney disease I12.9
    - stage 5 chronic kidney disease (CKD) or end stage renal disease (ESRD) I12.0
- lesser circulation I27.0
- maternal O16- ☑
- newborn P29.2
  - pulmonary (persistent) P29.30
- ocular H40.05- ☑
- pancreatic duct — *code to* underlying condition
  - with chronic pancreatitis K86.1
- portal (due to chronic liver disease) (idiopathic) K76.6
  - gastropathy K31.89
  - in (due to) schistosomiasis (bilharziasis) B65.9 *[K77]*
- postoperative I97.3
- psychogenic F45.8
- pulmonary I27.20
  - with
    - cor pulmonale (chronic) I27.29
      - acute I26.09
    - right heart ventricular strain/failure I27.29
      - acute I26.09
    - right to left shunt related to congenital heart disease I27.83
    - unclear multifactorial mechanisms I27.29
  - arterial (associated) (drug-induced) (toxin-induced) I27.21
  - chronic thromboembolic I27.24

Hypertension, hypertensive — *continued*
  pulmonary — *continued*
    due to
      hematologic disorders I27.29
      kyphoscoliotic heart disease I27.1
      left heart disease I27.22
      lung diseases and hypoxia I27.23
      metabolic disorders I27.29
      specified systemic disorders I27.29
    group 1 (associated) (drug-induced) (toxin-induced)
      I27.21
    group 2 I27.22
    group 3 I27.23
    group 4 I27.24
    group 5 I27.29
    of newborn (persistent) P29.30
    primary (idiopathic) I27.0
    secondary
      arterial I27.21
      specified NEC I27.29
  renal — *see* Hypertension, kidney
  renovascular I15.0
  secondary NEC I15.9
    due to
      endocrine disorders I15.2
      pheochromocytoma I15.2
      renal disorders NEC I15.1
        arterial I15.0
      renovascular disorders I15.0
    specified NEC I15.8
  transient R03.0
    of pregnancy O13.- ☑
  urgency I16.0
  venous (chronic)
    due to
      deep vein thrombosis — *see* Syndrome, post-
        thrombotic
      idiopathic I87.309
        with
          inflammation I87.32- ☑
            with ulcer I87.33- ☑
          specified complication NEC I87.39- ☑
          ulcer I87.31- ☑
            with inflammation I87.33- ☑
          asymptomatic I87.30- ☑
Hypertensive urgency — *see* Hypertension
Hyperthecosis ovary E28.8
Hyperthermia (of unknown origin) — *see also* Hyper-
    pyrexia
  malignant, due to anesthesia T88.3 ☑
  newborn P81.9
    environmental P81.0
Hyperthyroid (recurrent) — *see* Hyperthyroidism
Hyperthyroidism (latent) (pre-adult) (recurrent) E05.90
  with
    goiter (diffuse) E05.00
      with thyroid storm E05.01
    nodular (multinodular) E05.20
      with thyroid storm E05.21
      uninodular E05.10
        with thyroid storm E05.11
    storm E05.91
  due to ectopic thyroid tissue E05.30
    with thyroid storm E05.31
  neonatal, transitory P72.1
  specified NEC E05.80
    with thyroid storm E05.81
Hypertony, hypertonia, hypertonicity
  bladder N31.8
  congenital P94.1
  stomach K31.89
    psychogenic F45.8
  uterus, uterine (contractions) (complicating delivery)
    O62.4
Hypertrichosis L68.9
  congenital Q84.2
  eyelid H02.869
    left H02.866
      lower H02.865
      upper H02.864
    right H02.863
      lower H02.862
      upper H02.861
  lanuginosa Q84.2
    acquired L68.1
  localized L68.2
  specified NEC L68.8
Hypertriglyceridemia, essential E78.1

Hypertrophy, hypertrophic
  adenofibromatous, prostate — *see* Enlargement, en-
    larged, prostate
  adenoids (infective) J35.2
    with tonsils J35.3
  adrenal cortex E27.8
  alveolar process or ridge — *see* Anomaly, alveolar
  anal papillae K62.89
  artery I77.89
    congenital NEC Q27.8
      digestive system Q27.8
      lower limb Q27.8
      specified site NEC Q27.8
      upper limb Q27.8
  auricular — *see* Hypertrophy, cardiac
  Bartholin's gland N75.8
  bile duct (common) (hepatic) K83.8
  bladder (sphincter) (trigone) N32.89
  bone M89.30
    carpus M89.34- ☑
    clavicle M89.31- ☑
    femur M89.35- ☑
    fibula M89.36- ☑
    finger M89.34- ☑
    humerus M89.32- ☑
    ilium M89.359
    ischium M89.359
    metacarpus M89.34- ☑
    metatarsus M89.37- ☑
    multiple sites M89.39
    neck M89.38
    radius M89.33- ☑
    rib M89.38
    scapula M89.31- ☑
    skull M89.38
    tarsus M89.37- ☑
    tibia M89.36- ☑
    toe M89.37- ☑
    ulna M89.33- ☑
    vertebra M89.38
  brain G93.89
  breast N62
    cystic — *see* Mastopathy, cystic
    newborn P83.4
    pubertal, massive N62
    puerperal, postpartum — *see* Disorder, breast,
      specified type NEC
    senile (parenchymatous) N62
  cardiac (chronic) (idiopathic) I51.7
    with rheumatic fever (conditions in I00)
      active I01.8
      inactive or quiescent (with chorea) I09.89
    congenital NEC Q24.8
    fatty — *see* Degeneration, myocardial
    hypertensive — *see* Hypertension, heart
    rheumatic (with chorea) I09.89
      active or acute I01.8
        with chorea I02.0
    valve — *see* Endocarditis
  cartilage — *see* Disorder, cartilage, specified type NEC
  cecum — *see* Megacolon
  cervix (uteri) N88.8
    congenital Q51.828
    elongation N88.4
  clitoris (cirrhotic) N90.89
    congenital Q52.6
  colon — *see also* Megacolon
    congenital Q43.2
  conjunctiva, lymphoid H11.89
  corpora cavernosa N48.89
  cystic duct K82.8
  duodenum K31.89
  endometrium (glandular) — *see also* Hyperplasia, en-
    dometrial N85.00
    cervix N88.8
  epididymis N50.89
  esophageal hiatus (congenital) Q79.1
    with hernia — *see* Hernia, hiatal
  eyelid — *see* Disorder, eyelid, specified type NEC
  facet joint — *see also* Spondylosis M47.819
  fat pad E65
    knee (infrapatellar) (popliteal) (prepatellar)
      (retropatellar) M79.4
  foot (congenital) Q74.2
  frenulum, frenum (tongue) K14.8
    lip K13.0
  gallbladder K82.8
  gastric mucosa K29.60

Hypertrophy, hypertrophic — *continued*
  gastric mucosa — *continued*
    with bleeding K29.61
  gland, glandular R59.9
    generalized R59.1
    localized R59.0
  gum (mucous membrane) K06.1
  heart (idiopathic) — *see also* Hypertrophy, cardiac
    valve — *see also* Endocarditis I38
  hemifacial Q67.4
  hepatic — *see* Hypertrophy, liver
  hiatus (esophageal) Q79.1
  hilus gland R59.0
  hymen, congenital Q52.4
  ileum K63.89
  intestine NEC K63.89
  jejunum K63.89
  kidney (compensatory) N28.81
    congenital Q63.3
  labium (majus) (minus) N90.60
  ligament — *see* Disorder, ligament
  lingual tonsil (infective) J35.1
    with adenoids J35.3
  lip K13.0
    congenital Q18.6
  liver R16.0
    acute K76.89
    cirrhotic — *see* Cirrhosis, liver
    congenital Q44.7
    fatty — *see* Fatty, liver
  lymph, lymphatic gland R59.9
    generalized R59.1
    localized R59.0
    tuberculous — *see* Tuberculosis, lymph gland
  mammary gland — *see* Hypertrophy, breast
  Meckel's diverticulum (congenital) Q43.0
    malignant — *see* Table of Neoplasms, small intes-
      tine, malignant
  median bar — *see* Hyperplasia, prostate
  meibomian gland — *see* Chalazion
  meniscus, knee, congenital Q74.1
  metatarsal head — *see* Hypertrophy, bone, metatarsus
  metatarsus — *see* Hypertrophy, bone, metatarsus
  mucous membrane
    alveolar ridge K06.2
    gum K06.1
    nose (turbinate) J34.3
  muscle M62.89
  muscular coat, artery I77.89
  myocardium — *see also* Hypertrophy, cardiac
    idiopathic I42.2
  myometrium N85.2
  nail L60.2
    congenital Q84.5
  nasal J34.89
    alae J34.89
    bone J34.89
    cartilage J34.89
    mucous membrane (septum) J34.3
    sinus J34.89
    turbinate J34.3
  nasopharynx, lymphoid (infectional) (tissue) (wall) J35.2
  nipple N62
  organ or site, congenital NEC — *see* Anomaly, by site
  ovary N83.8
  palate (hard) M27.8
    soft K13.79
  pancreas, congenital Q45.3
  parathyroid (gland) E21.0
  parotid gland K11.1
  penis N48.89
  pharyngeal tonsil J35.2
  pharynx J39.2
    lymphoid (infectional) (tissue) (wall) J35.2
  pituitary (anterior) (fossa) (gland) E23.6
  prepuce (congenital) N47.8
    female N90.89
  prostate — *see* Enlargement, enlarged, prostate
    congenital Q55.4
  pseudomuscular G71.09
  pylorus (adult) (muscle) (sphincter) K31.1
    congenital or infantile Q40.0
  rectal, rectum (sphincter) K62.89
  rhinitis (turbinate) J31.0
  salivary gland (any) K11.1
    congenital Q38.4
  scaphoid (tarsal) — *see* Hypertrophy, bone, tarsus
  scar L91.0

Hypertrophy, hypertrophic — *continued*
  scrotum N50.89
  seminal vesicle N50.89
  sigmoid — *see* Megacolon
  skin L91.9
    specified NEC L91.8
  spermatic cord N50.89
  spleen — *see* Splenomegaly
  spondylitis — *see* Spondylosis
  stomach K31.89
  sublingual gland K11.1
  submandibular gland K11.1
  suprarenal cortex (gland) E27.8
  synovial NEC M67.20
    acromioclavicular M67.21- ☑
    ankle M67.27- ☑
    elbow M67.22- ☑
    foot M67.27- ☑
    hand M67.24- ☑
    hip M67.25- ☑
    knee M67.26- ☑
    multiple sites M67.29
    specified site NEC M67.28
    wrist M67.23- ☑
  tendon — *see* Disorder, tendon, specified type NEC
  testis N44.8
    congenital Q55.29
  thymic, thymus (gland) (congenital) E32.0
  thyroid (gland) — *see* Goiter
  toe (congenital) Q74.2
    acquired — *see also* Deformity, toe, specified NEC
  tongue K14.8
    congenital Q38.2
    papillae (foliate) K14.3
  tonsils (faucial) (infective) (lingual) (lymphoid) J35.1
    with adenoids J35.3
  tunica vaginalis N50.89
  ureter N28.89
  urethra N36.8
  uterus N85.2
    neck (with elongation) N88.4
    puerperal O90.89
  uvula K13.79
  vagina N89.8
  vas deferens N50.89
  vein I87.8
  ventricle, ventricular (heart) — *see also* Hypertrophy, cardiac
    congenital Q24.8
    in tetralogy of Fallot Q21.3
  verumontanum N36.8
  vocal cord J38.3
  vulva N90.60
    stasis (nonfilarial) N90.69
Hypertropia H50.2- ☑
Hypertyrosinemia E70.21
Hyperuricemia (asymptomatic) E79.0
Hyperuricosuria R82.993
Hypervalinemia E71.19
Hyperventilation (tetany) R06.4
  hysterical F45.8
  psychogenic F45.8
  syndrome F45.8
Hypervitaminosis (dietary) NEC E67.8
  A E67.0
    administered as drug (prolonged intake) — *see* Table of Drugs and Chemicals, vitamins, adverse effect
    overdose or wrong substance given or taken — *see* Table of Drugs and Chemicals, vitamins, poisoning
  B6 E67.2
  D E67.3
    administered as drug (prolonged intake) — *see* Table of Drugs and Chemicals, vitamins, adverse effect
    overdose or wrong substance given or taken — *see* Table of Drugs and Chemicals, vitamins, poisoning
  K E67.8
    administered as drug (prolonged intake) — *see* Table of Drugs and Chemicals, vitamins, adverse effect
    overdose or wrong substance given or taken — *see* Table of Drugs and Chemicals, vitamins, poisoning
Hypervolemia E87.70
  specified NEC E87.79

Hypesthesia R20.1
  cornea — *see* Anesthesia, cornea
Hyphema H21.0- ☑
  traumatic S05.1- ☑
Hypoacidity, gastric K31.89
  psychogenic F45.8
Hypoadrenalism, hypoadrenia E27.40
  primary E27.1
  tuberculous A18.7
Hypoadrenocorticism E27.40
  pituitary E23.0
  primary E27.1
Hypoalbuminemia E88.09
Hypoaldosteronism E27.40
Hypoalphalipoproteinemia E78.6
Hypobarism T70.29 ☑
Hypobaropathy T70.29 ☑
Hypobetalipoproteinemia (familial) E78.6
Hypocalcemia E83.51
  dietary E58
  neonatal P71.1
    due to cow's milk P71.0
    phosphate-loading (newborn) P71.1
Hypochloremia E87.8
Hypochlorhydria K31.89
  neurotic F45.8
  psychogenic F45.8
Hypochondria, hypochondriac, hypochondriasis (reaction) F45.21
  sleep F51.03
Hypochondrogenesis Q77.0
Hypochondroplasia Q77.4
Hypochromasia, blood cells D50.8
Hypocitraturia R82.991
Hypodontia — *see* Anodontia
Hypoeosinophilia D72.89
Hypoesthesia R20.1
Hypofibrinogenemia D68.8
  acquired D65
  congenital (hereditary) D68.2
Hypofunction
  adrenocortical E27.40
    drug-induced E27.3
    postprocedural E89.6
    primary E27.1
  adrenomedullary, postprocedural E89.6
  cerebral R29.818
  corticoadrenal NEC E27.40
  intestinal K59.89
  labyrinth — *see* subcategory H83.2 ☑
  ovary E28.39
  pituitary (gland) (anterior) E23.0
  testicular E29.1
    postprocedural (postsurgical) (postirradiation) (iatrogenic) E89.5
Hypogalactia O92.4
Hypogammaglobulinemia — *see also* Agammaglobulinemia D80.1
  hereditary D80.0
  nonfamilial D80.1
  transient, of infancy D80.7
Hypogenitalism (congenital) — *see* Hypogonadism
Hypoglossia Q38.3
Hypoglycemia (spontaneous) E16.2
  coma E15
    diabetic — *see* Diabetes, by type, with hypoglycemia, with coma
  diabetic — *see* Diabetes, hypoglycemia
  dietary counseling and surveillance Z71.3
  drug-induced E16.0
    with coma (nondiabetic) E15
  due to insulin E16.0
    with coma (nondiabetic) E15
    therapeutic misadventure — *see* subcategory T38.3 ☑
  functional, nonhyperinsulinemic E16.1
  iatrogenic E16.0
    with coma (nondiabetic) E15
  in infant of diabetic mother P70.1
    gestational diabetes P70.0
  infantile E16.1
  leucine-induced E71.19
  neonatal (transitory) P70.4
    iatrogenic P70.3
  reactive (not drug-induced) E16.1
  transitory neonatal P70.4

Hypogonadism
  female E28.39
  hypogonadotropic E23.0
  male E29.1
  ovarian (primary) E28.39
  pituitary E23.0
  testicular (primary) E29.1
Hypohidrosis, hypoidrosis L74.4
Hypoinsulinemia, postprocedural E89.1
Hypokalemia E87.6
Hypoleukocytosis — *see* Agranulocytosis
Hypolipoproteinemia (alpha) (beta) E78.6
Hypomagnesemia E83.42
  neonatal P71.2
Hypomania, hypomanic reaction F30.8
Hypomenorrhea — *see* Oligomenorrhea
Hypometabolism R63.8
Hypomotility
  gastrointestinal (tract) K31.89
    psychogenic F45.8
  intestine K59.89
    psychogenic F45.8
  stomach K31.89
    psychogenic F45.8
Hyponasality R49.22
Hyponatremia E87.1
Hypo-osmolality E87.1
Hypo-ovarianism, hypo-ovarism E28.39
Hypoparathyroidism E20.9
  familial E20.8
  idiopathic E20.0
  neonatal, transitory P71.4
  postprocedural E89.2
  specified NEC E20.8
Hypoperfusion (in)
  newborn P96.89
Hypopharyngitis — *see* Laryngopharyngitis
Hypophoria H50.53
Hypophosphatemia, hypophosphatasia (acquired) (congenital) (renal) E83.39
  familial E83.31
Hypophyseal, hypophysis — *see also* condition
  dwarfism E23.0
  gigantism E22.0
Hypopiesis — *see* Hypotension
Hypopinealism E34.8
Hypopituitarism (juvenile) E23.0
  drug-induced E23.1
  due to
    hypophysectomy E89.3
    radiotherapy E89.3
  iatrogenic NEC E23.1
  postirradiation E89.3
  postpartum O99.285
  postprocedural E89.3
Hypoplasia, hypoplastic
  adrenal (gland), congenital Q89.1
  alimentary tract, congenital Q45.8
    upper Q40.8
  anus, anal (canal) Q42.3
    with fistula Q42.2
  aorta, aortic Q25.42
    ascending, in hypoplastic left heart syndrome Q23.4
    valve Q23.1
      in hypoplastic left heart syndrome Q23.4
  areola, congenital Q83.8
  arm (congenital) — *see* Defect, reduction, upper limb
  artery (peripheral) Q27.8
    brain (congenital) Q28.3
    coronary Q24.5
    digestive system Q27.8
    lower limb Q27.8
    pulmonary Q25.79
      functional, unilateral J43.0
    retinal (congenital) Q14.1
    specified site NEC Q27.8
    umbilical Q27.0
    upper limb Q27.8
  auditory canal Q17.8
    causing impairment of hearing Q16.9
  biliary duct or passage Q44.5
  bone NOS Q79.9
    face Q75.8
    marrow D61.9
      megakaryocytic D69.49
    skull — *see* Hypoplasia, skull
  brain Q02
    gyri Q04.3

☑ **Additional Character Required** — Refer to the Tabular List for Character Selection

▽ **Subterms under main terms may continue to next column or page**

Hypoplasia, hypoplastic — continued
  brain — continued
    part of Q04.3
  breast (areola) N64.82
  bronchus Q32.4
  cardiac Q24.8
  carpus — see Defect, reduction, upper limb, specified type NEC
  cartilage hair Q78.8
  cecum Q42.8
  cementum K00.4
  cephalic Q02
  cerebellum Q04.3
  cervix (uteri), congenital Q51.821
  clavicle (congenital) Q74.0
  coccyx Q76.49
  colon Q42.9
    specified NEC Q42.8
  corpus callosum Q04.0
  cricoid cartilage Q31.2
  digestive organ(s) or tract NEC Q45.8
    upper (congenital) Q40.8
  ear (auricle) (lobe) Q17.2
    middle Q16.4
  enamel of teeth (neonatal) (postnatal) (prenatal) K00.4
  endocrine (gland) NEC Q89.2
  endometrium N85.8
  epididymis (congenital) Q55.4
  epiglottis Q31.2
  erythroid, congenital D61.01
  esophagus (congenital) Q39.8
  eustachian tube Q17.8
  eye Q11.2
  eyelid (congenital) Q10.3
  face Q18.8
    bone(s) Q75.8
  femur (congenital) — see Defect, reduction, lower limb, specified type NEC
  fibula (congenital) — see Defect, reduction, lower limb, specified type NEC
  finger (congenital) — see Defect, reduction, upper limb, specified type NEC
  focal dermal Q82.8
  foot — see Defect, reduction, lower limb, specified type NEC
  gallbladder Q44.0
  genitalia, genital organ(s)
    female, congenital Q52.8
      external Q52.79
      internal NEC Q52.8
    in adiposogenital dystrophy E23.6
  glottis Q31.2
  hair Q84.2
  hand (congenital) — see Defect, reduction, upper limb, specified type NEC
  heart Q24.8
  humerus (congenital) — see Defect, reduction, upper limb, specified type NEC
  intestine (small) Q41.9
    large Q42.9
      specified NEC Q42.8
  jaw M26.09
    alveolar M26.79
    lower M26.04
      alveolar M26.74
    upper M26.02
      alveolar M26.73
  kidney(s) Q60.5
    bilateral Q60.4
    unilateral Q60.3
  labium (majus) (minus), congenital Q52.79
  larynx Q31.2
  left heart syndrome Q23.4
  leg (congenital) — see Defect, reduction, lower limb
  limb Q73.8
    lower (congenital) — see Defect, reduction, lower limb
    upper (congenital) — see Defect, reduction, upper limb
  liver Q44.7
  lung (lobe) (not associated with short gestation) Q33.6
    associated with immaturity, low birth weight, prematurity, or short gestation P28.0
  mammary (areola), congenital Q83.8
  mandible, mandibular M26.04
    alveolar M26.74
    unilateral condylar M27.8
  maxillary M26.02

Hypoplasia, hypoplastic — continued
  maxillary — continued
    alveolar M26.73
  medullary D61.9
  megakaryocytic D69.49
  metacarpus — see Defect, reduction, upper limb, specified type NEC
  metatarsus — see Defect, reduction, lower limb, specified type NEC
  muscle Q79.8
  nail(s) Q84.6
  nose, nasal Q30.1
  optic nerve H47.03- ☑
  osseous meatus (ear) Q17.8
  ovary, congenital Q50.39
  pancreas Q45.0
  parathyroid (gland) Q89.2
  parotid gland Q38.4
  patella Q74.1
  pelvis, pelvic girdle Q74.2
  penis (congenital) Q55.62
  peripheral vascular system Q27.8
    digestive system Q27.8
    lower limb Q27.8
    specified site NEC Q27.8
    upper limb Q27.8
  pituitary (gland) (congenital) Q89.2
  pulmonary (not associated with short gestation) Q33.6
    artery, functional J43.0
    associated with short gestation P28.0
  radioulnar — see Defect, reduction, upper limb, specified type NEC
  radius — see Defect, reduction, upper limb
  rectum Q42.1
    with fistula Q42.0
  respiratory system NEC Q34.8
  rib Q76.6
  right heart syndrome Q22.6
  sacrum Q76.49
  scapula Q74.0
  scrotum Q55.1
  shoulder girdle Q74.0
  skin Q82.8
  skull (bone) Q75.8
    with
      anencephaly Q00.0
      encephalocele — see Encephalocele
      hydrocephalus Q03.9
        with spina bifida — see Spina bifida, by site, with hydrocephalus
      microcephaly Q02
  spinal (cord) (ventral horn cell) Q06.1
  spine Q76.49
  sternum Q76.7
  tarsus — see Defect, reduction, lower limb, specified type NEC
  testis Q55.1
  thymic, with immunodeficiency D82.1
  thymus (gland) Q89.2
    with immunodeficiency D82.1
  thyroid (gland) E03.1
    cartilage Q31.2
  tibiofibular (congenital) — see Defect, reduction, lower limb, specified type NEC
  toe — see Defect, reduction, lower limb, specified type NEC
  tongue Q38.3
  Turner's K00.4
  ulna (congenital) — see Defect, reduction, upper limb
  umbilical artery Q27.0
  unilateral condylar M27.8
  ureter Q62.8
  uterus, congenital Q51.811
  vagina Q52.4
  vascular NEC peripheral Q27.8
    brain Q28.3
    digestive system Q27.8
    lower limb Q27.8
    specified site NEC Q27.8
    upper limb Q27.8
  vein(s) (peripheral) Q27.8
    brain Q28.3
    digestive system Q27.8
    great Q26.8
    lower limb Q27.8
    specified site NEC Q27.8
    upper limb Q27.8
  vena cava (inferior) (superior) Q26.8

Hypoplasia, hypoplastic — continued
  vertebra Q76.49
  vulva, congenital Q52.79
  zonule (ciliary) Q12.8
Hypoplasminogenemia E88.02
Hypopnea, obstructive sleep apnea G47.33
Hypopotassemia E87.6
Hypoproconvertinemia, congenital (hereditary) D68.2
Hypoproteinemia E77.8
Hypoprothrombinemia (congenital) (hereditary) (idiopathic) D68.2
  acquired D68.4
  newborn, transient P61.6
Hypoptyalism K11.7
Hypopyon (eye) (anterior chamber) — see Iridocyclitis, acute, hypopyon
Hypopyrexia R68.0
Hyporeflexia R29.2
Hyposecretion
  ACTH E23.0
  antidiuretic hormone E23.2
  ovary E28.39
  salivary gland (any) K11.7
  vasopressin E23.2
Hyposegmentation, leukocytic, hereditary D72.0
Hyposiderinemia D50.9
Hypospadias Q54.9
  balanic Q54.0
  coronal Q54.0
  glandular Q54.0
  penile Q54.1
  penoscrotal Q54.2
  perineal Q54.3
  specified NEC Q54.8
Hypospermatogenesis — see Oligospermia
Hyposplenism D73.0
Hypostasis pulmonary, passive — see Edema, lung
Hypostatic — see condition
Hyposthenuria N28.89
Hypotension (arterial) (constitutional) I95.9
  chronic I95.89
  due to (of) hemodialysis I95.3
  drug-induced I95.2
  iatrogenic I95.89
  idiopathic (permanent) I95.0
  intracranial G96.810
    following
      lumbar cerebrospinal fluid shunting G97.83
      specified procedure NEC G97.84
      ventricular shunting (ventriculostomy) G97.2
    specified NEC G96.819
    spontaneous G96.811
  intra-dialytic I95.3
  maternal, syndrome (following labor and delivery) O26.5- ☑
  neurogenic, orthostatic G90.3
  orthostatic (chronic) I95.1
    due to drugs I95.2
    neurogenic G90.3
  postoperative I95.81
  postural I95.1
  specified NEC I95.89
Hypothermia (accidental) T68 ☑
  due to anesthesia, anesthetic T88.51 ☑
  low environmental temperature T68 ☑
  neonatal P80.9
    environmental (mild) NEC P80.8
    mild P80.8
    severe (chronic) (cold injury syndrome) P80.0
    specified NEC P80.8
  not associated with low environmental temperature R68.0
Hypothyroidism (acquired) E03.9
  autoimmune — see Thyroiditis, autoimmune
  congenital (without goiter) E03.1
    with goiter (diffuse) E03.0
  due to
    exogenous substance NEC E03.2
    iodine-deficiency, acquired E01.8
      subclinical E02
    irradiation therapy E89.0
    medicament NEC E03.2
    P-aminosalicylic acid (PAS) E03.2
    phenylbutazone E03.2
    resorcinol E03.2
    sulfonamide E03.2
    surgery E89.0
    thiourea group drugs E03.2

Hypothyroidism — *continued*
iatrogenic NEC E03.2
iodine-deficiency (acquired) E01.8
congenital — *see* Syndrome, iodine- deficiency, congenital
subclinical E02
neonatal, transitory P72.2
postinfectious E03.3
postirradiation E89.0
postprocedural E89.0
postsurgical E89.0
specified NEC E03.8
subclinical, iodine-deficiency related E02
Hypotonia, hypotonicity, hypotony
bladder N31.2
congenital (benign) P94.2
eye — *see* Disorder, globe, hypotony
Hypotrichosis — *see* Alopecia
Hypotropia H50.2- ☑
Hypoventilation R06.89
congenital central alveolar G47.35
sleep related
idiopathic nonobstructive alveolar G47.34
in conditions classified elsewhere G47.36
Hypovitaminosis — *see* Deficiency, vitamin
Hypovolemia E86.1
surgical shock T81.19 ☑
traumatic (shock) T79.4 ☑
Hypoxemia R09.02
newborn P84
sleep related, in conditions classified elsewhere G47.36
Hypoxia — *see also* Anoxia R09.02
cerebral, during a procedure NEC G97.81
postprocedural NEC G97.82
intrauterine P84
myocardial — *see* Insufficiency, coronary
newborn P84
sleep-related G47.34
Hypsarhythmia — *see* Epilepsy, generalized, specified NEC
Hysteralgia, pregnant uterus O26.89- ☑
Hysteria, hysterical (conversion) (dissociative state) F44.9
anxiety F41.8
convulsions F44.5
psychosis, acute F44.9
Hysteroepilepsy F44.5

I

IBDU (colonic inflammatory bowel dissease unclassified) K52.3
ICANS (immune effector cell-associated neurotoxicity syndrome) — *see* Syndrome, immune effector cell-associated neurotoxicity
Ichthyoparasitism due to Vandellia cirrhosa B88.8
Ichthyosis (congenital) Q80.9
acquired L85.0
fetalis Q80.4
hystrix Q80.8
lamellar Q80.2
lingual K13.29
palmaris and plantaris Q82.8
simplex Q80.0
vera Q80.8
vulgaris Q80.0
X-linked Q80.1
Ichthyotoxism — *see* Poisoning, fish
bacterial — *see* Intoxication, foodborne
Icteroanemia, hemolytic (acquired) D59.9
congenital — *see* Spherocytosis
Icterus — *see also* Jaundice
conjunctiva R17
gravis, newborn P55.0
hematogenous (acquired) D59.9
hemolytic (acquired) D59.9
congenital — *see* Spherocytosis
hemorrhagic (acute) (leptospiral) (spirochetal) A27.0
newborn P53
infectious B15.9
with hepatic coma B15.0
leptospiral A27.0
spirochetal A27.0
neonatorum — *see* Jaundice, newborn
newborn P59.9
spirochetal A27.0
Ictus solaris, solis T67.01 ☑

Id reaction (due to bacteria) L30.2
Ideation
homicidal R45.850
suicidal R45.851
Identity disorder (child) F64.9
gender role F64.2
psychosexual F64.2
Idioglossia F80.0
Idiopathic — *see* condition
Idiot, idiocy (congenital) F73
amaurotic (Bielschowsky(-Jansky)) (family) (infantile (late)) (juvenile (late)) (Vogt-Spielmeyer) E75.4
microcephalic Q02
IgE asthma J45.909
IIAC (idiopathic infantile arterial calcification) Q28.8
Ileitis (chronic) (noninfectious) — *see also* Enteritis K52.9
backwash — *see* Pancolitis, ulcerative (chronic)
infectious A09
regional (ulcerative) — *see* Enteritis, regional, small intestine
segmental — *see* Enteritis, regional
terminal (ulcerative) — *see* Enteritis, regional, small intestine
Ileocolitis — *see also* Enteritis K52.9
infectious A09
regional — *see* Enteritis, regional
ulcerative K51.0- ☑
Ileostomy
attention to Z43.2
malfunctioning K94.13
status Z93.2
with complication — *see* Complications, enterostomy
Ileotyphus — *see* Typhoid
Ileum — *see* condition
Ileus (bowel) (colon) (inhibitory) (intestine) K56.7
adynamic K56.0
due to gallstone (in intestine) K56.3
duodenal (chronic) K31.5
gallstone K56.3
mechanical NEC — *see also* Obstruction, intestine, specified NEC K56.699
meconium P76.0
in cystic fibrosis E84.11
meaning meconium plug (without cystic fibrosis) P76.0
myxedema K59.89
neurogenic K56.0
Hirschsprung's disease or megacolon Q43.1
newborn
due to meconium P76.0
in cystic fibrosis E84.11
meaning meconium plug (without cystic fibrosis) P76.0
transitory P76.1
obstructive — *see also* Obstruction, intestine, specified NEC K56.699
paralytic K56.0
postoperative K91.89
Iliac — *see* condition
Iliotibial band syndrome M76.3- ☑
Illiteracy Z55.0
Illness — *see also* Disease R69
manic-depressive — *see* Disorder, bipolar
Imbalance R26.89
autonomic G90.8
constituents of food intake E63.1
electrolyte E87.8
with
abortion — *see* Abortion by type, complicated by, electrolyte imbalance
molar pregnancy O08.5
due to hyperemesis gravidarum O21.1
following ectopic or molar pregnancy O08.5
neonatal, transitory NEC P74.49
potassium
hyperkalemia P74.31
hypokalemia P74.32
sodium
hypernatremia P74.21
hyponatremia P74.22
endocrine E34.9
eye muscle NOS H50.9
hormone E34.9
hysterical F44.4
labyrinth — *see* subcategory H83.2 ☑
posture R29.3
protein-energy — *see* Malnutrition

Imbalance — *continued*
sympathetic G90.8
Imbecile, imbecility (I.Q. 35-49) F71
Imbedding, intrauterine device T83.39 ☑
Imbibition, cholesterol (gallbladder) K82.4
Imbrication, teeth,, fully erupted M26.30
Imerslund (-Gräsbeck) **syndrome** D51.1
Immature — *see also* Immaturity
birth (less than 37 completed weeks) — *see* Preterm, newborn
extremely (less than 28 completed weeks) — *see* Immaturity, extreme
personality F60.89
Immaturity (less than 37 completed weeks) — *see also* Preterm, newborn
extreme of newborn (less than 28 completed weeks of gestation) (less than 196 completed days of gestation) (unspecified weeks of gestation) P07.20
gestational age
23 completed weeks (23 weeks, 0 days through 23 weeks, 6 days) P07.22
24 completed weeks (24 weeks, 0 days through 24 weeks, 6 days) P07.23
25 completed weeks (25 weeks, 0 days through 25 weeks, 6 days) P07.24
26 completed weeks (26 weeks, 0 days through 26 weeks, 6 days) P07.25
27 completed weeks (27 weeks, 0 days through 27 weeks, 6 days) P07.26
less than 23 completed weeks P07.21
fetus or infant light-for-dates — *see* Light-for-dates
lung, newborn P28.0
organ or site NEC — *see* Hypoplasia
pulmonary, newborn P28.0
reaction F60.89
sexual (female) (male), after puberty E30.0
Immersion T75.1 ☑
foot T69.02- ☑
hand T69.01- ☑
Immobile, immobility
complete, due to severe physical disability or frailty R53.2
intestine K59.89
syndrome (paraplegic) M62.3
Immune reconstitution (inflammatory) syndrome [IRIS] D89.3
Immunization — *see also* Vaccination
ABO — *see* Incompatibility, ABO
in newborn P55.1
appropriate for age
child (over 28 days old) Z00.129
with abnormal findings Z00.121
complication — *see* Complications, vaccination
encounter for Z23
not done (not carried out) Z28.9
because (of)
acute illness of patient Z28.01
allergy to vaccine (or component) Z28.04
caregiver refusal Z28.82
chronic illness of patient Z28.02
contraindication NEC Z28.09
delay in delivery of vaccine Z28.83
group pressure Z28.1
guardian refusal Z28.82
immune compromised state of patient Z28.03
lack of availability of vaccine Z28.83
manufacturer delay of vaccine Z28.83
parent refusal Z28.82
patient had disease being vaccinated against Z28.81
patient refusal Z28.21
patient's belief Z28.1
religious beliefs of patient Z28.1
specified reason NEC Z28.89
of patient Z28.29
unavailability of vaccine Z28.83
unspecified patient reason Z28.20
Rh factor
affecting management of pregnancy NEC O36.09- ☑
anti-D antibody O36.01- ☑
from transfusion — *see* Complication(s), transfusion, incompatibility reaction, Rh (factor)
Immunocompromised NOS D84.9
Immunocytoma C83.0- ☑
Immunodeficiency D84.9

☑ Additional Character Required — Refer to the Tabular List for Character Selection   ▽ Subterms under main terms may continue to next column or page

Immunodeficiency — *continued*
  with
    adenosine-deaminase deficiency — *see also* Deficiency, adenosine deaminase D81.30
    antibody defects D80.9
      specified type NEC D80.8
    hyperimmunoglobulinemia D80.6
    increased immunoglobulin M (IgM) D80.5
    major defect D82.9
      specified type NEC D82.8
    partial albinism D82.8
    short-limbed stature D82.2
    thrombocytopenia and eczema D82.0
  antibody with
    hyperimmunoglobulinemia D80.6
    near-normal immunoglobulins D80.6
  autosomal recessive, Swiss type D80.0
  combined D81.9
    biotin-dependent carboxylase D81.819
      biotinidase D81.810
      holocarboxylase synthetase D81.818
      specified type NEC D81.818
    severe (SCID) D81.9
      with
        low or normal B-cell numbers D81.2
        low T- and B-cell numbers D81.1
        reticular dysgenesis D81.0
    specified type NEC D81.89
  common variable D83.9
    with
      abnormalities of B-cell numbers and function D83.0
      autoantibodies to B- or T-cells D83.2
      immunoregulatory T-cell disorders D83.1
    specified type NEC D83.8
  due to
    conditions classified elsewhere D84.81
    drugs D84.821
    external causes D84.822
    medication (current or past) D84.821
  following hereditary defective response to Epstein-Barr virus (EBV) D82.3
  selective, immunoglobulin
    A (IgA) D80.2
    G (IgG) (subclasses) D80.3
    M (IgM) D80.4
  severe combined (SCID) D81.9
    due to adenosine deaminase deficiency D81.31
  specified type NEC D84.89
  X-linked, with increased IgM D80.5
Immunodeficient NOS D84.9
Immunosuppressed NOS D84.9
Immunotherapy (encounter for)
  antineoplastic Z51.12
Impaction, impacted
  bowel, colon, rectum — *see also* Impaction, fecal K56.49
    by gallstone K56.3
  calculus — *see* Calculus
  cerumen (ear) (external) H61.2- ☑
  cuspid — *see* Impaction, tooth
  dental (same or adjacent tooth) K01.1
  fecal, feces K56.41
  fracture — *see* Fracture, by site
  gallbladder — *see* Calculus, gallbladder
  gallstone(s) — *see* Calculus, gallbladder
    bile duct (common) (hepatic) — *see* Calculus, bile duct
    cystic duct — *see* Calculus, gallbladder
    in intestine, with obstruction (any part) K56.3
  intestine (calculous) NEC — *see also* Impaction, fecal K56.49
    gallstone, with ileus K56.3
  intrauterine device (IUD) T83.39 ☑
  molar — *see* Impaction, tooth
  shoulder, causing obstructed labor O66.0
  tooth, teeth K01.1
  turbinate J34.89
Impaired, impairment (function)
  auditory discrimination — *see* Abnormal, auditory perception
  cognitive, mild, so stated G31.84
  dual sensory Z73.82
  fasting glucose R73.01
  glucose tolerance (oral) R73.02
  hearing — *see* Deafness
  heart — *see* Disease, heart
  kidney N28.9

Impaired, impairment — *continued*
  kidney — *continued*
    disorder resulting from N25.9
      specified NEC N25.89
    liver K72.90
      with coma K72.91
    mastication K08.89
    mild cognitive, so stated G31.84
    mobility
      ear ossicles — *see* Ankylosis, ear ossicles
      requiring care provider Z74.09
    myocardium, myocardial — *see* Insufficiency, myocardial
    rectal sphincter R19.8
    renal (acute) (chronic) N28.9
      disorder resulting from N25.9
        specified NEC N25.89
    vision NEC H54.7
      both eyes H54.3
Impediment, speech — *see also* Disorder, speech R47.9
  psychogenic (childhood) F98.8
  slurring R47.81
  specified NEC R47.89
Impending
  coronary syndrome I20.0
  delirium tremens F10.239
  myocardial infarction I20.0
Imperception auditory (acquired) — *see also* Deafness
  congenital H93.25
Imperfect
  aeration, lung (newborn) NEC — *see* Atelectasis
  closure (congenital)
    alimentary tract NEC Q45.8
      lower Q43.8
      upper Q40.8
    atrioventricular ostium Q21.2
    atrium (secundum) Q21.1
    branchial cleft NOS Q18.2
      cyst Q18.0
      fistula Q18.0
      sinus Q18.0
    choroid Q14.3
    cricoid cartilage Q31.8
    cusps, heart valve NEC Q24.8
      pulmonary Q22.3
    ductus
      arteriosus Q25.0
      Botalli Q25.0
    ear drum (causing impairment of hearing) Q16.4
    esophagus with communication to bronchus or trachea Q39.1
    eyelid Q10.3
    foramen
      botalli Q21.1
      ovale Q21.1
    genitalia, genital organ(s) or system
      female Q52.8
        external Q52.79
        internal NEC Q52.8
      male Q55.8
    glottis Q31.8
    interatrial ostium or septum Q21.1
    interauricular ostium or septum Q21.1
    interventricular ostium or septum Q21.0
    larynx Q31.8
    lip — *see* Cleft, lip
    nasal septum Q30.3
    nose Q30.2
    omphalomesenteric duct Q43.0
    optic nerve entry Q14.2
    organ or site not listed — *see* Anomaly, by site
    ostium
      interatrial Q21.1
      interauricular Q21.1
      interventricular Q21.0
    palate — *see* Cleft, palate
    preauricular sinus Q18.1
    retina Q14.1
    roof of orbit Q75.8
    sclera Q13.5
    septum
      aorticopulmonary Q21.4
      atrial (secundum) Q21.1
      between aorta and pulmonary artery Q21.4
      heart Q21.9
      interatrial (secundum) Q21.1
      interauricular (secundum) Q21.1
      interventricular Q21.0

Imperfect — *continued*
  closure — *continued*
    septum — *continued*
      interventricular — *continued*
        in tetralogy of Fallot Q21.3
      nasal Q30.3
      ventricular Q21.0
        with pulmonary stenosis or atresia, dextraposition of aorta, and hypertrophy of right ventricle Q21.3
        in tetralogy of Fallot Q21.3
    skull Q75.0
      with
        anencephaly Q00.0
        encephalocele — *see* Encephalocele
        hydrocephalus Q03.9
          with spina bifida — *see* Spina bifida, by site, with hydrocephalus
        microcephaly Q02
    spine (with meningocele) — *see* Spina bifida
    trachea Q32.1
    tympanic membrane (causing impairment of hearing) Q16.4
    uterus Q51.818
    vitelline duct Q43.0
  erection — *see* Dysfunction, sexual, male, erectile
  fusion — *see* Imperfect, closure
  inflation, lung (newborn) — *see* Atelectasis
  posture R29.3
  rotation, intestine Q43.3
  septum, ventricular Q21.0
Imperfectly descended testis — *see* Cryptorchid
Imperforate (congenital) — *see also* Atresia
  anus Q42.3
    with fistula Q42.2
  cervix (uteri) Q51.828
  esophagus Q39.0
    with tracheoesophageal fistula Q39.1
  hymen Q52.3
  jejunum Q41.1
  pharynx Q38.8
  rectum Q42.1
    with fistula Q42.0
  urethra Q64.39
  vagina Q52.4
Impervious (congenital) — *see also* Atresia
  anus Q42.3
    with fistula Q42.2
  bile duct Q44.2
  esophagus Q39.0
    with tracheoesophageal fistula Q39.1
  intestine (small) Q41.9
    large Q42.9
      specified NEC Q42.8
  rectum Q42.1
    with fistula Q42.0
  ureter — *see* Atresia, ureter
  urethra Q64.39
Impetiginization of dermatoses L01.1
Impetigo (any organism) (any site) (circinate) (contagiosa) (simplex) (vulgaris) L01.00
  Bockhart's L01.02
  bullous, bullosa L01.03
  external ear L01.00 [H62.40]
  follicularis L01.02
  furfuracea L30.5
  herpetiformis L40.1
    nonobstetrical L40.1
  neonatorum L01.03
  nonbullous L01.01
  specified type NEC L01.09
  ulcerative L01.09
Impingement (on teeth)
  joint — *see* Disorder, joint, specified type NEC
  soft tissue
    anterior M26.81
    posterior M26.82
Implant, endometrial N80.9
Implantation
  anomalous — *see* Anomaly, by site
    ureter Q62.63
  cyst
    external area or site (skin) NEC L72.0
    iris — *see* Cyst, iris, implantation
    vagina N89.8
    vulva N90.7
  dermoid (cyst) — *see* Implantation, cyst
Impotence (sexual) N52.9

Impotence — *continued*
  counseling Z70.1
  organic origin — *see also* Dysfunction, sexual, male, erectile N52.9
  psychogenic F52.21
Impression, basilar Q75.8
Imprisonment, anxiety concerning Z65.1
Improper care (child) (newborn) — *see* Maltreatment
Improperly tied umbilical cord (causing hemorrhage) P51.8
Impulsiveness (impulsive) R45.87
Inability to swallow — *see* Aphagia
Inaccessible, inaccessibility
  health care NEC Z75.3
    due to
      waiting period Z75.2
        for admission to facility elsewhere Z75.1
      other helping agencies Z75.4
Inactive — *see* condition
Inadequate, inadequacy
  aesthetics of dental restoration K08.56
  biologic, constitutional, functional, or social F60.7
  development
    child R62.50
    genitalia
      after puberty NEC E30.0
      congenital
        female Q52.8
          external Q52.79
          internal Q52.8
        male Q55.8
    lungs Q33.6
      associated with short gestation P28.0
    organ or site not listed — *see* Anomaly, by site
  diet (causing nutritional deficiency) E63.9
  drinking-water supply Z58.6
  eating habits Z72.4
  environment, household Z59.1
  family support Z63.8
  food (supply) NEC Z59.48
    hunger effects T73.0 ☑
  functional F60.7
  household care, due to
    family member
      handicapped or ill Z74.2
      on vacation Z75.5
      temporarily away from home Z74.2
    technical defects in home Z59.1
    temporary absence from home of person rendering care Z74.2
  housing (heating) (space) Z59.1
  income (financial) Z59.6
  intrafamilial communication Z63.8
  material resources Z59.9
  mental — *see* Disability, intellectual
  parental supervision or control of child Z62.0
  personality F60.7
  pulmonary
    function R06.89
      newborn P28.5
    ventilation, newborn P28.5
  sample of cytologic smear
    anus R85.615
    cervix R87.615
    vagina R87.625
  social F60.7
    insurance Z59.7
    skills NEC Z73.4
  supervision of child by parent Z62.0
  teaching affecting education Z55.8
  welfare support Z59.7
Inanition R64
  with edema — *see* Malnutrition, severe
  due to
    deprivation of food T73.0 ☑
    malnutrition — *see* Malnutrition
  fever R50.9
Inappropriate
  change in quantitative human chorionic gonadotropin (hCG) in early pregnancy O02.81
  diet or eating habits Z72.4
  level of quantitative human chorionic gonadotropin (hCG) for gestational age in early pregnancy O02.81
  secretion
    antidiuretic hormone (ADH) (excessive) E22.2
      deficiency E23.2
    pituitary (posterior) E22.2

Inattention at or after birth — *see* Neglect
Incarceration, incarcerated
  enterocele K46.0
    gangrenous K46.1
  epiplocele K46.0
    gangrenous K46.1
  exomphalos K42.0
    gangrenous K42.1
  hernia — *see also* Hernia, by site, with obstruction
    with gangrene — *see* Hernia, by site, with gangrene
  iris, in wound — *see* Injury, eye, laceration, with prolapse
  lens, in wound — *see* Injury, eye, laceration, with prolapse
  omphalocele K42.0
  prison, anxiety concerning Z65.1
  rupture — *see* Hernia, by site
  sarcoepiplocele K46.0
    gangrenous K46.1
  sarcoepiplomphalocele K42.0
    with gangrene K42.1
  uterus N85.8
    gravid O34.51- ☑
      causing obstructed labor O65.5
Incised wound
  external — *see* Laceration
  internal organs — *see* Injury, by site
Incision, incisional
  hernia K43.2
    with
      gangrene (and obstruction) K43.1
      obstruction K43.0
  surgical, complication — *see* Complications, surgical procedure
  traumatic
    external — *see* Laceration
    internal organs — *see* Injury, by site
Inclusion
  azurophilic leukocytic D72.0
  blennorrhea (neonatal) (newborn) P39.1
  gallbladder in liver (congenital) Q44.1
Incompatibility
  ABO
    affecting management of pregnancy O36.11- ☑
      anti-A sensitization O36.11- ☑
      anti-B sensitization O36.19- ☑
      specified NEC O36.19- ☑
    infusion or transfusion reaction — *see* Complication(s), transfusion, incompatibility reaction, ABO
    newborn P55.1
  blood (group) (Duffy) (K) (Kell) (Kidd) (Lewis) (M) (S) NEC
    affecting management of pregnancy O36.11- ☑
      anti-A sensitization O36.11- ☑
      anti-B sensitization O36.19- ☑
    infusion or transfusion reaction T80.89 ☑
    newborn P55.8
  divorce or estrangement Z63.5
  Rh (blood group) (factor) Z31.82
    affecting management of pregnancy NEC O36.09- ☑
      anti-D antibody O36.01- ☑
    infusion or transfusion reaction — *see* Complication(s), transfusion, incompatibility reaction, Rh (factor)
    newborn P55.0
  rhesus — *see* Incompatibility, Rh
Incompetency, incompetent, incompetence
  annular
    aortic (valve) — *see* Insufficiency, aortic
    mitral (valve) I34.0
    pulmonary valve (heart) I37.1
  aortic (valve) — *see* Insufficiency, aortic
  cardiac valve — *see* Endocarditis
  cervix, cervical (os) N88.3
    in pregnancy O34.3- ☑
  chronotropic I45.89
    with
      autonomic dysfunction G90.8
      ischemic heart disease I25.89
      left ventricular dysfunction I51.89
      sinus node dysfunction I49.8
  esophagogastric (junction) (sphincter) K22.0
  mitral (valve) — *see* Insufficiency, mitral
  pelvic fundus N81.89
  pubocervical tissue N81.82
  pulmonary valve (heart) I37.1
    congenital Q22.3

Incompetency, incompetent, incompetence — *continued*
  rectovaginal tissue N81.83
  tricuspid (annular) (valve) — *see* Insufficiency, tricuspid
  valvular — *see* Endocarditis
    congenital Q24.8
  vein, venous (saphenous) (varicose) — *see* Varix, leg
Incomplete — *see also* condition
  bladder, emptying R33.9
  defecation R15.0
  expansion lungs (newborn) NEC — *see* Atelectasis
  rotation, intestine Q43.3
Inconclusive
  diagnostic imaging due to excess body fat of patient R93.9
  findings on diagnostic imaging of breast NEC R92.8
  mammogram (due to dense breasts) R92.2
Incontinence R32
  anal sphincter R15.9
  coital N39.491
  feces R15.9
    nonorganic origin F98.1
  insensible (urinary) N39.42
  overflow N39.490
  postural (urinary) N39.492
  psychogenic F45.8
  rectal R15.9
  reflex N39.498
  stress (female) (male) N39.3
    and urge N39.46
  urethral sphincter R32
  urge N39.41
    and stress (female) (male) N39.46
  urine (urinary) R32
    continuous N39.45
    due to cognitive impairment, or severe physical disability or immobility R39.81
    functional R39.81
    insensible N39.42
    mixed (stress and urge) N39.46
    nocturnal N39.44
    nonorganic origin F98.0
    overflow N39.490
    post dribbling N39.43
    postural N39.492
    reflex N39.498
    specified NEC N39.498
    stress (female) (male) N39.3
      and urge N39.46
    total N39.498
    unaware N39.42
    urge N39.41
      and stress (female) (male) N39.46
Incontinentia pigmenti Q82.3
Incoordinate, incoordination
  esophageal-pharyngeal (newborn) — *see* Dysphagia
  muscular R27.8
  uterus (action) (contractions) (complicating delivery) O62.4
Increase, increased
  abnormal, in development R63.8
  androgens (ovarian) E28.1
  anticoagulants (antithrombin) (anti-VIIIa) (anti-IXa) (anti-Xa) (anti-XIa) — *see* Circulating anticoagulants
  cold sense R20.8
  estrogen E28.0
  function
    adrenal
      cortex — *see* Cushing's, syndrome
      medulla E27.5
    pituitary (gland) (anterior) (lobe) E22.9
      posterior E22.2
  heat sense R20.8
  intracranial pressure (benign) G93.2
  permeability, capillaries I78.8
  pressure, intracranial G93.2
  secretion
    gastrin E16.4
    glucagon E16.3
    pancreas, endocrine E16.9
      growth hormone-releasing hormone E16.8
      pancreatic polypeptide E16.8
      somatostatin E16.8
      vasoactive-intestinal polypeptide E16.8
  sphericity, lens Q12.4
  splenic activity D73.1
  venous pressure I87.8

☑ **Additional Character Required** — **Refer to the Tabular List for Character Selection**   ▽ **Subterms under main terms may continue to next column or page**

Increase, increased — *continued*
  venous pressure — *continued*
    portal K76.6
Increta placenta O43.22- ☑
Incrustation, cornea, foreign body (lead)(zinc) — *see* Foreign body, cornea
Incyclophoria H50.54
Incyclotropia — *see* Cyclotropia
Indeterminate sex Q56.4
India rubber skin Q82.8
Indigestion (acid) (bilious) (functional) K30
  catarrhal K31.89
  due to decomposed food NOS A05.9
  nervous F45.8
  psychogenic F45.8
Indirect — *see* condition
Induratio penis plastica N48.6
Induration, indurated
  brain G93.89
  breast (fibrous) N64.51
    puerperal, postpartum O92.29
  broad ligament N83.8
  chancre
    anus A51.1
    congenital A50.07
    extragenital NEC A51.2
  corpora cavernosa (penis) (plastic) N48.6
  liver (chronic) K76.89
  lung (black) (chronic) (fibroid) — *see also* Fibrosis, lung J84.10
    essential brown J84.03
  penile (plastic) N48.6
  phlebitic — *see* Phlebitis
  skin R23.4
Inebriety (without dependence) — *see* Alcohol, intoxication
Inefficiency, kidney N28.9
Inelasticity, skin R23.4
Inequality, leg (length) (acquired) — *see also* Deformity, limb, unequal length
  congenital — *see* Defect, reduction, lower limb
  lower leg — *see* Deformity, limb, unequal length
Inertia
  bladder (neurogenic) N31.2
  stomach K31.89
    psychogenic F45.8
  uterus, uterine during labor O62.2
    during latent phase of labor O62.0
    primary O62.0
    secondary O62.1
  vesical (neurogenic) N31.2
Infancy, infantile, infantilism — *see also* condition
  celiac K90.0
  genitalia, genitals (after puberty) E30.0
  Herter's (nontropical sprue) K90.0
  intestinal K90.0
  Lorain E23.0
  pancreatic K86.89
  pelvis M95.5
    with disproportion (fetopelvic) O33.1
      causing obstructed labor O65.1
  pituitary E23.0
  renal N25.0
  uterus — *see* Infantile, genitalia
Infant(s) — *see also* Infancy
  excessive crying R68.11
  irritable child R68.12
  lack of care — *see* Neglect
  liveborn (singleton) Z38.2
    born in hospital Z38.00
      by cesarean Z38.01
    born outside hospital Z38.1
    multiple NEC Z38.8
      born in hospital Z38.68
        by cesarean Z38.69
      born outside hospital Z38.7
    quadruplet Z38.8
      born in hospital Z38.63
        by cesarean Z38.64
      born outside hospital Z38.7
    quintuplet Z38.8
      born in hospital Z38.65
        by cesarean Z38.66
      born outside hospital Z38.7
    triplet Z38.8
      born in hospital Z38.61
        by cesarean Z38.62
      born outside hospital Z38.7

Infant(s) — *continued*
  liveborn — *continued*
    twin Z38.5
      born in hospital Z38.30
        by cesarean Z38.31
      born outside hospital Z38.4
    of diabetic mother (syndrome of) P70.1
      gestational diabetes P70.0
Infantile — *see also* condition
  genitalia, genitals E30.0
  os, uterine E30.0
  penis E30.0
  testis E29.1
  uterus E30.0
Infantilism — *see* Infancy
Infarct, infarction
  adrenal (capsule) (gland) E27.49
  appendices epiploicae — *see also* Infarct, intestine K55.069
  bowel — *see also* Infarct, intestine K55.069
  brain (stem) — *see* Infarct, cerebral
  breast N64.89
  brewer's (kidney) N28.0
  cardiac — *see* Infarct, myocardium
  cerebellar — *see* Infarct, cerebral
  cerebral (acute) (chronic) — *see also* Occlusion, artery cerebral or precerebral, with infarction I63.9-
    aborted I63.9
    cortical I63.9
    due to
      cerebral venous thrombosis, nonpyogenic I63.6
      embolism
        cerebral arteries I63.4- ☑
        precerebral arteries I63.1- ☑
      occlusion NEC
        cerebral arteries I63.5- ☑
        precerebral arteries I63.2- ☑
        small artery I63.81
      stenosis NEC
        cerebral arteries I63.5- ☑
        precerebral arteries I63.2- ☑
        small artery I63.81
      thrombosis
        cerebral artery I63.3- ☑
        precerebral artery I63.0- ☑
    intraoperative
      during cardiac surgery I97.810
      during other surgery I97.811
    neonatal P91.82- ☑
    perinatal (arterial ischemic) P91.82- ☑
    postprocedural
      following cardiac surgery I97.820
      following other surgery I97.821
    specified NEC I63.89
  colon (acute) (agnogenic) (embolic) (hemorrhagic) (nonocclusive) (nonthrombotic) (occlusive) (segmental) (thrombotic) (with gangrene) — *see also* Infarct, intestine K55.049
  coronary artery — *see* Infarct, myocardium
  embolic — *see* Embolism
  fallopian tube N83.8
  gallbladder K82.8
  heart — *see* Infarct, myocardium
  hepatic K76.3
  hypophysis (anterior lobe) E23.6
  impending (myocardium) I20.0
  intestine (acute) (agnogenic) (embolic) (hemorrhagic) (nonocclusive) (nonthrombotic) (occlusive) (thrombotic) (with gangrene) K55.069
    diffuse K55.062
    focal K55.061
    large K55.049
      diffuse K55.042
      focal K55.041
    small K55.029
      diffuse K55.022
      focal K55.021
  kidney N28.0
  lacunar I63.81
  liver K76.3
  lung (embolic) (thrombotic) — *see* Embolism, pulmonary
  lymph node I89.8
  mesentery, mesenteric (embolic) (thrombotic) (with gangrene) — *see also* Infarct, intestine K55.069
  muscle (ischemic) M62.20
    ankle M62.27- ☑
    foot M62.27- ☑

Infarct, infarction — *continued*
  muscle — *continued*
    forearm M62.23- ☑
    hand M62.24- ☑
    lower leg M62.26- ☑
    pelvic region M62.25- ☑
    shoulder region M62.21- ☑
    specified site NEC M62.28
    thigh M62.25- ☑
    upper arm M62.22- ☑
  myocardium, myocardial (acute) (with stated duration of 4 weeks or less) I21.9
    associated with revascularization procedure I21.A9
    diagnosed on ECG, but presenting no symptoms I25.2
    due to
      demand ischemia I21.A1
      ischemic imbalance I21.A1
    healed or old I25.2
    intraoperative — *see also* Infarct, myocardium, associated with revascularization procedure
      during cardiac surgery I97.790
      during other surgery I97.791
    non-Q wave I21.4
    non-ST elevation (NSTEMI) I21.4
      subsequent I22.2
    nontransmural I21.4
    past (diagnosed on ECG or other investigation, but currently presenting no symptoms) I25.2
    postprocedural — *see also* Infarct, myocardium, associated with revascularization procedure
      following cardiac surgery — *see also* Infarct, myocardium, type 4 or type 5 I97.190
      following other surgery I97.191
    Q wave (*see also* Infarct, myocardium, by site) I21.3
    secondary to
      demand ischemia I21.A1
      ischemic imbalance I21.A1
    ST elevation (STEMI) I21.3
      anterior (anteroapical) (anterolateral) (anteroseptal) (Q wave) (wall) I21.09
        subsequent I22.0
      inferior (diaphragmatic) (inferolateral) (inferoposterior) (wall) NEC I21.19
        subsequent I22.1
      inferoposterior transmural (Q wave) I21.11
      involving
        coronary artery of anterior wall NEC I21.09
        coronary artery of inferior wall NEC I21.19
        diagonal coronary artery I21.02
        left anterior descending coronary artery I21.02
        left circumflex coronary artery I21.21
        left main coronary artery I21.01
        oblique marginal coronary artery I21.21
        right coronary artery I21.11
      lateral (apical-lateral) (basal-lateral) (high) I21.29
        subsequent I22.8
      posterior (posterobasal) (posterolateral) (posteroseptal) (true) I21.29
        subsequent I22.8
      septal I21.29
        subsequent I22.8
      specified site NEC I21.29
        subsequent I22.8
    subsequent I22.9
    subsequent (recurrent) (reinfarction) I22.9
      anterior (anteroapical) (anterolateral) (anteroseptal) (wall) I22.0
      diaphragmatic (wall) I22.1
      inferior (diaphragmatic) (inferolateral) (inferoposterior) (wall) I22.1
      lateral (apical-lateral) (basal-lateral) (high) I22.8
      non-ST elevation (NSTEMI) I22.2
      posterior (posterobasal) (posterolateral) (posteroseptal) (true) I22.8
      septal I22.8
      specified NEC I22.8
      ST elevation I22.9
        anterior (anteroapical) (anterolateral) (anteroseptal) (wall) I22.0
        inferior (diaphragmatic) (inferolateral) (inferoposterior) (wall) I22.1
        specified NEC I22.8
      subendocardial I22.2
      transmural I21.3
        anterior (anteroapical) (anterolateral) (anteroseptal) (wall) I22.0
        diaphragmatic (wall) I22.1

Infarct, infarction — *continued*
  myocardium, myocardial — *continued*
    subsequent — *continued*
      transmural — *continued*
        inferior (diaphragmatic) (inferolateral) (infer-oposterior) (wall) I22.1
        lateral (apical-lateral) (basal-lateral) (high) I22.8
        posterior (posterobasal) (posterolateral) (posteroseptal) (true) I22.8
        specified NEC I22.8
        type 1 — *see also* Infarction, myocardial, subsequent, by site, or by ST elevation or non-ST elevation I22.9
        type 2 I21.A1
        type 3 I21.A9
        type 4 I21.A9
        type 5 I21.A9
      syphilitic A52.06
      transmural I21.9
        anterior (anteroapical) (anterolateral) (anteroseptal) (Q wave) (wall) NEC I21.09
        inferior (diaphragmatic) (inferolateral) (inferoposterior) (Q wave) (wall) NEC I21.19
        inferoposterior (Q wave) I21.11
        lateral (apical-lateral) (basal-lateral) (high) NEC I21.29
        posterior (posterobasal) (posterolateral) (posteroseptal) (true) NEC I21.29
        septal NEC I21.29
        specified NEC I21.29
        type 1 — *see also* Infarction, myocardial, by site, or by ST elevation or non-ST elevation I21.9
        type 2 I21.A1
        type 3 I21.A9
        type 4 (a) (b) (c) I21.A9
        type 5 I21.A9
  nontransmural I21.4
  omentum — *see also* Infarct, intestine K55.069
  ovary N83.8
  pancreas K86.89
  papillary muscle — *see* Infarct, myocardium
  parathyroid gland E21.4
  pituitary (gland) E23.6
  placenta O43.81- ☑
  prostate N42.89
  pulmonary (artery) (vein) (hemorrhagic) — *see* Embolism, pulmonary
  renal (embolic) (thrombotic) N28.0
  retina, retinal (artery) — *see* Occlusion, artery, retina
  spinal (cord) (acute) (embolic) (nonembolic) G95.11
  spleen D73.5
    embolic or thrombotic I74.8
  subendocardial (acute) (nontransmural) I21.4
  suprarenal (capsule) (gland) E27.49
  testis N50.1
  thrombotic — *see also* Thrombosis
    artery, arterial — *see* Embolism
  thyroid (gland) E07.89
  ventricle (heart) — *see* Infarct, myocardium
Infecting — *see* condition
Infection, infected, infective (opportunistic) B99.9
  with
    drug resistant organism — *see* Resistance (to), drug
      — *see also* specific organism
    lymphangitis — *see* Lymphangitis
    organ dysfunction (acute) R65.20
      with septic shock R65.21
  abscess (skin) — *code by* site under Abscess
  Absidia — *see* Mucormycosis
  Acanthamoeba — *see* Acanthamebiasis
  Acanthocheilonema (perstans) (streptocerca) B74.4
  accessory sinus (chronic) — *see* Sinusitis
  achorion — *see* Dermatophytosis
  Acremonium falciforme B47.0
  acromioclavicular M00.9
  Actinobacillus (actinomycetem-comitans) A28.8
    mallei A24.0
    muris A25.1
  Actinomadura B47.1
  Actinomyces (israelii) — *see also* Actinomycosis A42.9
  Actinomycetales — *see* Actinomycosis
  actinomycotic NOS — *see* Actinomycosis
  adenoid (and tonsil) J03.90
    chronic J35.02
  adenovirus NEC
    as cause of disease classified elsewhere B97.0
    unspecified nature or site B34.0

Infection, infected, infective — *continued*
  aerogenes capsulatus A48.0
  aertrycke — *see* Infection, salmonella
  alimentary canal NOS — *see* Enteritis, infectious
  Allescheria boydii B48.2
  Alternaria B48.8
  alveolus, alveolar (process) K04.7
  Ameba, amebic (histolytica) — *see* Amebiasis
  amniotic fluid, sac or cavity O41.10- ☑
    chorioamnionitis O41.12- ☑
    placentitis O41.14- ☑
  amputation stump (surgical) — *see* Complication, amputation stump, infection
  Ancylostoma (duodenalis) B76.0
  Anisakiasis, Anisakis larvae B81.0
  anthrax — *see* Anthrax
  antrum (chronic) — *see* Sinusitis, maxillary
  anus, anal (papillae) (sphincter) K62.89
  arbovirus (arbor virus) A94
    specified type NEC A93.8
  artificial insemination N98.0
  Ascaris lumbricoides — *see* Ascariasis
  Ascomycetes B47.0
  Aspergillus (flavus) (fumigatus) (terreus) — *see* Aspergillosis
  atypical
    acid-fast (bacilli) — *see* Mycobacterium, atypical
    mycobacteria — *see* Mycobacterium, atypical
    virus A81.9
      specified type NEC A81.89
  auditory meatus (external) — *see* Otitis, externa, infective
  auricle (ear) — *see* Otitis, externa, infective
  axillary gland (lymph) L04.2
  Bacillus A49.9
    abortus A23.1
    anthracis — *see* Anthrax
    Ducrey's (any location) A57
    Flexner's A03.1
    Friedländer's NEC A49.8
    gas (gangrene) A48.0
    mallei A24.0
    melitensis A23.0
    paratyphoid, paratyphosus A01.4
      A A01.1
      B A01.2
      C A01.3
    Shiga (-Kruse) A03.0
    suipestifer — *see* Infection, salmonella
    swimming pool A31.1
    typhosa A01.00
    welchii — *see* Gangrene, gas
  bacterial NOS A49.9
    as cause of disease classified elsewhere B96.89
      Bacteroides fragilis [B. fragilis] B96.6
      Clostridium perfringens [C. perfringens] B96.7
      Enterobacter sakazakii B96.89
      Enterococcus B95.2
      Escherichia coli [E. coli] — *see also* Escherichia coli B96.20
      Helicobacter pylori [H.pylori] B96.81
      Hemophilus influenzae [H. influenzae] B96.3
      Klebsiella pneumoniae [K. pneumoniae] B96.1
      Mycoplasma pneumoniae [M. pneumoniae] B96.0
      Proteus (mirabilis) (morganii) B96.4
      Pseudomonas (aeruginosa) (mallei) (pseudomallei) B96.5
      Staphylococcus B95.8
        aureus (methicillin susceptible) (MSSA) B95.61
          methicillin resistant (MRSA) B95.62
        specified NEC B95.7
      Streptococcus B95.5
        group A B95.0
        group B B95.1
        pneumoniae B95.3
        specified NEC B95.4
      Vibrio vulnificus B96.82
    specified NEC A48.8
  Bacterium
    paratyphosum A01.4
      A A01.1
      B A01.2
      C A01.3
    typhosum A01.00
  Bacteroides NEC A49.8
    fragilis, as cause of disease classified elsewhere B96.6

Infection, infected, infective — *continued*
  Balantidium coli A07.0
  Bartholin's gland N75.8
  Basidiobolus B46.8
  bile duct (common) (hepatic) — *see* Cholangitis
  bladder — *see* Cystitis
  Blastomyces, blastomycotic — *see also* Blastomycosis
    brasiliensis — *see* Paracoccidioidomycosis
    dermatitidis — *see* Blastomycosis
    European — *see* Cryptococcosis
    Loboi B48.0
    North American B40.9
    South American — *see* Paracoccidioidomycosis
  bleb, postprocedure — *see* Blebitis
  bone — *see* Osteomyelitis
  Bordetella — *see* Whooping cough
  Borrelia bergdorfi A69.20
  brain — *see also* Encephalitis G04.90
    membranes — *see* Meningitis
    septic G06.0
      meninges — *see* Meningitis, bacterial
  branchial cyst Q18.0
  breast — *see* Mastitis
  bronchus — *see* Bronchitis
  Brucella A23.9
    abortus A23.1
    canis A23.3
    melitensis A23.0
    mixed A23.8
    specified NEC A23.8
    suis A23.2
  Brugia (malayi) B74.1
    timori B74.2
  bursa — *see* Bursitis, infective
  buttocks (skin) L08.9
  Campylobacter, intestinal A04.5
    as cause of disease classified elsewhere B96.81
  Candida (albicans) (tropicalis) — *see* Candidiasis
  candiru B88.8
  Capillaria (intestinal) B81.1
    hepatica B83.8
    philippinensis B81.1
  cartilage — *see* Disorder, cartilage, specified type NEC
  cat liver fluke B66.0
  catheter-related bloodstream (CRBSI) T80.211 ☑
  cellulitis — *code by* site under Cellulitis
  central line-associated T80.219 ☑
    bloodstream (CLABSI) T80.211 ☑
    specified NEC T80.218 ☑
  Cephalosporium falciforme B47.0
  cerebrospinal — *see* Meningitis
  cervical gland (lymph) L04.0
  cervix — *see* Cervicitis
  cesarean delivery wound (puerperal) O86.00
  cestodes — *see* Infestation, cestodes
  chest J22
  Chilomastix (intestinal) A07.8
  Chlamydia, chlamydial A74.9
    anus A56.3
    genitourinary tract A56.2
      lower A56.00
      specified NEC A56.19
    lymphogranuloma A55
    pharynx A56.4
    psittaci A70
    rectum A56.3
    sexually transmitted NEC A56.8
  cholera — *see* Cholera
  Cladosporium
    bantianum (brain abscess) B43.1
    carrionii B43.0
    castellanii B36.1
    trichoides (brain abscess) B43.1
    werneckii B36.1
  Clonorchis (sinensis) (liver) B66.1
  Clostridium NEC
    bifermentans A48.0
    botulinum (food poisoning) A05.1
      infant A48.51
      wound A48.52
    difficile
      as cause of disease classified elsewhere B96.89
      foodborne (disease)
        not specified as recurrent A04.72
        recurrent A04.71
      gas gangrene A48.0
      necrotizing enterocolitis
        not specified as recurrent A04.72

☑ **Additional Character Required** — Refer to the Tabular List for Character Selection   ▽ **Subterms under main terms may continue to next column or page**

Infection, infected, infective — *continued*
Clostridium — *continued*
  difficile — *continued*
    necrotizing enterocolitis — *continued*
      recurrent A04.71
    sepsis A41.4
  gas-forming NEC A48.0
  histolyticum A48.0
  novyi, causing gas gangrene A48.0
  oedematiens A48.0
  perfringens
    as cause of disease classified elsewhere B96.7
    due to food A05.2
    foodborne (disease) A05.2
    gas gangrene A48.0
    sepsis A41.4
  septicum, causing gas gangrene A48.0
  sordellii, causing gas gangrene A48.0
  welchii
    as cause of disease classified elsewhere B96.7
    foodborne (disease) A05.2
    gas gangrene A48.0
    necrotizing enteritis A05.2
    sepsis A41.4
Coccidioides (immitis) — *see* Coccidioidomycosis
colon — *see* Enteritis, infectious
colostomy K94.02
common duct — *see* Cholangitis
congenital P39.9
  Candida (albicans) P37.5
  cytomegalovirus P35.1
  hepatitis, viral P35.3
  herpes simplex P35.2
  infectious or parasitic disease P37.9
    specified NEC P37.8
  listeriosis (disseminated) P37.2
  malaria NEC P37.4
    falciparum P37.3
  Plasmodium falciparum P37.3
  poliomyelitis P35.8
  rubella P35.0
  skin P39.4
  toxoplasmosis (acute) (subacute) (chronic) P37.1
  tuberculosis P37.0
  urinary (tract) P39.3
  vaccinia P35.8
  virus P35.9
    specified type NEC P35.8
Conidiobolus B46.8
coronavirus-2019 U07.1
coronavirus NEC B34.2
  as cause of disease classified elsewhere B97.29
  severe acute respiratory syndrome (SARS associated) B97.21
corpus luteum — *see* Salpingo-oophoritis
Corynebacterium diphtheriae — *see* Diphtheria
cotia virus B08.8
COVID-19 — *see also* COVID-19 U07.1
Coxiella burnetii A78
coxsackie — *see* Coxsackie
Cryptococcus neoformans — *see* Cryptococcosis
Cryptosporidium A07.2
Cunninghamella — *see* Mucormycosis
cyst — *see* Cyst
cystic duct — *see also* Cholecystitis K81.9
Cysticercus cellulosae — *see* Cysticercosis
cytomegalovirus, cytomegaloviral B25.9
  congenital P35.1
  maternal, maternal care for (suspected) damage to fetus O35.3
  mononucleosis B27.10
    with
      complication NEC B27.19
      meningitis B27.12
      polyneuropathy B27.11
delta-agent (acute), in hepatitis B carrier B17.0
dental (pulpal origin) K04.7
Deuteromycetes B47.0
Dicrocoelium dendriticum B66.2
Dipetalonema (perstans) (streptocerca) B74.4
diphtherial — *see* Diphtheria
Diphyllobothrium (adult) (latum) (pacificum) B70.0
  larval B70.1
Diplogonoporus (grandis) B71.8
Dipylidium caninum B67.4
Dirofilaria B74.8
Dracunculus medinensis B72
Drechslera (hawaiiensis) B43.8

Infection, infected, infective — *continued*
Ducrey Haemophilus (any location) A57
due to or resulting from
  artificial insemination N98.0
  Babesia
    divergens (-like) strain B60.03
    duncani (-type) species B60.02
    microti B60.01
    species
      specified NEC B60.09
  central venous catheter T80.219 ☑
    bloodstream T80.211 ☑
    exit or insertion site T80.212 ☑
    localized T80.212 ☑
    port or reservoir T80.212 ☑
    specified NEC T80.218 ☑
    tunnel T80.212 ☑
  device, implant or graft — *see also* Complications, by site and type, infection or inflammation T85.79 ☑
    arterial graft NEC T82.7 ☑
    breast (implant) T85.79 ☑
    catheter NEC T85.79 ☑
      dialysis (renal) T82.7 ☑
        central line T80.211 ☑
        intraperitoneal T85.71 ☑
      infusion NEC T82.7 ☑
        cranial T85.735 ☑
        intrathecal T85.735 ☑
        spinal (epidural) (subdural) T85.735 ☑
        subarachnoid T85.735 ☑
      urinary T83.518 ☑
        cystostomy T83.510 ☑
        Hopkins T83.518 ☑
        ileostomy T83.518 ☑
        nephrostomy T83.512 ☑
        specified NEC T83.518 ☑
        urethral indwelling T83.511 ☑
        urostomy T83.518 ☑
    electronic (electrode) (pulse generator) (stimulator)
      bone T84.7 ☑
      cardiac T82.7 ☑
      nervous system T85.738 ☑
        brain T85.731 ☑
        cranial nerve T85.732 ☑
        gastric nerve T85.732 ☑
        generator pocket T85.734 ☑
        neurostimulator generator T85.734 ☑
        peripheral nerve T85.732 ☑
        sacral nerve T85.732 ☑
        spinal cord T85.733 ☑
        vagal nerve T85.732 ☑
    urinary (indwelling) T83.51 ☑
    fixation, internal (orthopedic) NEC — *see* Complication, fixation device, infection
    gastrointestinal (bile duct) (esophagus) T85.79 ☑
      neurostimulator electrode (lead) T85.732 ☑
    genital NEC T83.69 ☑
    heart NEC T82.7 ☑
      valve (prosthesis) T82.6 ☑
      graft T82.7 ☑
    joint prosthesis — *see* Complication, joint prosthesis, infection
    ocular (corneal graft) (orbital implant) NEC T85.79 ☑
    orthopedic NEC T84.7 ☑
    penile (cylinder) (pump) (resevoir) T83.61 ☑
    specified NEC T85.79 ☑
    testicular T83.62 ☑
    urinary NEC T83.598 ☑
      ileal conduit stent T83.593 ☑
      implanted neurostimulation T83.590 ☑
      implanted sphincter T83.591 ☑
      indwelling ureteral stent T83.592 ☑
      nephroureteral stent T83.593 ☑
      specified stent NEC T83.593 ☑
    vascular NEC T82.7 ☑
    ventricular intracranial (communicating) shunt T85.730 ☑
  Hickman catheter T80.219 ☑
    bloodstream T80.211 ☑
    localized T80.212 ☑
    specified NEC T80.218 ☑
  immunization or vaccination T88.0 ☑
  infusion, injection or transfusion NEC T80.29 ☑

Infection, infected, infective — *continued*
due to or resulting from — *continued*
  injury NEC — *code by* site under Wound, open
  peripherally inserted central catheter (PICC) T80.219 ☑
    bloodstream T80.211 ☑
    localized T80.212 ☑
    specified NEC T80.218 ☑
  portacath (port-a-cath) T80.219 ☑
    bloodstream T80.211 ☑
    localized T80.212 ☑
    specified NEC T80.218 ☑
  protozoa of the order Piroplasmida NEC B60.09
  pulmonary artery catheter — *see* Infection, due to or resulting from, central venous catheter
  surgery T81.40 ☑
  Swan Ganz catheter — *see* Infection, due to or resulting from, central venous catheter
  triple lumen catheter T80.219 ☑
    bloodstream T80.211 ☑
    localized T80.212 ☑
    specified NEC T80.218 ☑
  umbilical venous catheter T80.219 ☑
    bloodstream T80.211 ☑
    localized T80.212 ☑
    specified NEC T80.218 ☑
during labor NEC O75.3
ear (middle) — *see also* Otitis media
  external — *see* Otitis, externa, infective
  inner — *see* subcategory H83.0 ☑
Eberthella typhosa A01.00
Echinococcus — *see* Echinococcus
echovirus
  as cause of disease classified elsewhere B97.12
  unspecified nature or site B34.1
endocardium I33.0
endocervix — *see* Cervicitis
Entamoeba — *see* Amebiasis
enteric — *see* Enteritis, infectious
Enterobacter sakazakii B96.89
Enterobius vermicularis B80
enterostomy K94.12
enterovirus B34.1
  as cause of disease classified elsewhere B97.10
    coxsackievirus B97.11
    echovirus B97.12
    specified NEC B97.19
Entomophthora B46.8
Epidermophyton — *see* Dermatophytosis
epididymis — *see* Epididymitis
episiotomy (puerperal) O86.09
Erysipelothrix (insidiosa) (rhusiopathiae) — *see* Erysipeloid
erythema infectiosum B08.3
Escherichia (E.) coli NEC A49.8
  as cause of disease classified elsewhere — *see also* Escherichia coli B96.20
  congenital P39.8
    sepsis P36.4
  generalized A41.51
  intestinal — *see* Enteritis, infectious, due to, Escherichia coli
ethmoidal (chronic) (sinus) — *see* Sinusitis, ethmoidal
eustachian tube (ear) — *see* Salpingitis, eustachian
external auditory canal (meatus) NEC — *see* Otitis, externa, infective
eye (purulent) — *see* Endophthalmitis, purulent
eyelid — *see* Inflammation, eyelid
fallopian tube — *see* Salpingo-oophoritis
Fasciola (gigantica) (hepatica) (indica) B66.3
Fasciolopsis (buski) B66.5
filarial — *see* Infestation, filarial
finger (skin) L08.9
  nail L03.01- ☑
    fungus B35.1
fish tapeworm B70.0
  larval B70.1
flagellate, intestinal A07.9
fluke — *see* Infestation, fluke
focal
  teeth (pulpal origin) K04.7
  tonsils J35.01
Fonsecaea (compactum) (pedrosoi) B43.0
food — *see* Intoxication, foodborne
foot (skin) L08.9
  dermatophytic fungus B35.3
Francisella tularensis — *see* Tularemia

Infection, infected, infective — *continued*
  frontal (sinus) (chronic) — *see* Sinusitis, frontal
  fungus NOS B49
    beard B35.0
    dermatophytic — *see* Dermatophytosis
    foot B35.3
    groin B35.6
    hand B35.2
    nail B35.1
    pathogenic to compromised host only B48.8
    perianal (area) B35.6
    scalp B35.0
    skin B36.9
      foot B35.3
      hand B35.2
      toenails B35.1
  Fusarium B48.8
  gallbladder — *see* Cholecystitis
  gas bacillus — *see* Gangrene, gas
  gastrointestinal — *see* Enteritis, infectious
  generalized NEC — *see* Sepsis
  generator pocket, implanted electronic neurostimulator T85.734 ☑
  genital organ or tract
    female — *see* Disease, pelvis, inflammatory
    male N49.9
      multiple sites N49.8
      specified NEC N49.8
  Ghon tubercle, primary A15.7
  Giardia lamblia A07.1
  gingiva (chronic) K05.10
    acute K05.00
      nonplaque induced K05.01
      plaque induced K05.00
    nonplaque induced K05.11
    plaque induced K05.10
  glanders A24.0
  glenosporopsis B48.0
  Gnathostoma (spinigerum) B83.1
  Gongylonema B83.8
  gonococcal — *see* Gonococcus
  gram-negative bacilli NOS A49.9
  guinea worm B72
  gum (chronic) K05.10
    acute K05.00
      nonplaque induced K05.01
      plaque induced K05.00
    nonplaque induced K05.11
    plaque induced K05.10
  Haemophilus — *see* Infection, Hemophilus
  heart — *see* Carditis
  Helicobacter pylori A04.8
    as cause of disease classified elsewhere B96.81
  helminths B83.9
    intestinal B82.0
      mixed (types classifiable to more than one of the titles B65.0-B81.3 and B81.8) B81.4
      specified type NEC B81.8
    specified type NEC B83.8
  Hemophilus
    aegyptius, systemic A48.4
    ducrey (any location) A57
    generalized A41.3
    influenzae NEC A49.2
      as cause of disease classified elsewhere B96.3
  herpes (simplex) — *see also* Herpes
    congenital P35.2
    disseminated B00.7
    zoster B02.9
  herpesvirus, herpesviral — *see* Herpes
  Heterophyes (heterophyes) B66.8
  hip (joint) NEC M00.9
    due to internal joint prosthesis
      left T84.52 ☑
      right T84.51 ☑
    skin NEC L08.9
  Histoplasma — *see* Histoplasmosis
    American B39.4
    capsulatum B39.4
  hookworm B76.9
  human
    papilloma virus A63.0
    T-cell lymphotropic virus type-1 (HTLV-1) B33.3
  hydrocele N43.0
  Hymenolepis B71.0
  hypopharynx — *see* Pharyngitis
  inguinal (lymph) glands L04.1
    due to soft chancre A57

Infection, infected, infective — *continued*
  intervertebral disc, pyogenic M46.30
    cervical region M46.32
    cervicothoracic region M46.33
    lumbar region M46.36
    lumbosacral region M46.37
    multiple sites M46.39
    occipito-atlanto-axial region M46.31
    sacrococcygeal region M46.38
    thoracic region M46.34
    thoracolumbar region M46.35
  intestine, intestinal — *see* Enteritis, infectious
    specified NEC A08.8
  intra-amniotic affecting newborn NEC P39.2
  intrauterine inflammation O41.12- ☑
  Isospora belli or hominis A07.3
  Japanese B encephalitis A83.0
  jaw (bone) (lower) (upper) M27.2
  joint NEC M00.9
    due to internal joint prosthesis T84.50 ☑
  kidney (cortex) (hematogenous) N15.9
    with calculus N20.0
      with hydronephrosis N13.6
    following ectopic gestation O08.83
    pelvis and ureter (cystic) N28.85
    puerperal (postpartum) O86.21
    specified NEC N15.8
  Klebsiella (K.) pneumoniae NEC A49.8
    as cause of disease classified elsewhere B96.1
  knee (joint) NEC M00.9
    joint M00.9
    due to internal joint prosthesis
      left T84.54 ☑
      right T84.53 ☑
    skin L08.9
  Koch's — *see* Tuberculosis
  labia (majora) (minora) (acute) — *see* Vulvitis
  lacrimal
    gland — *see* Dacryoadenitis
    passages (duct) (sac) — *see* Inflammation, lacrimal, passages
  lancet fluke B66.2
  larynx NEC J38.7
  leg (skin) NOS L08.9
  Legionella pneumophila A48.1
    nonpneumonic A48.2
  Leishmania — *see also* Leishmaniasis
    aethiopica B55.1
    braziliensis B55.2
    chagasi B55.0
    donovani B55.0
    infantum B55.0
    major B55.1
    mexicana B55.1
    tropica B55.1
  lentivirus, as cause of disease classified elsewhere B97.31
  Leptosphaeria senegalensis B47.0
  Leptospira interrogans A27.9
    autumnalis A27.89
    canicola A27.89
    hebdomadis A27.89
    icterohaemorrhagiae A27.0
    pomona A27.89
    specified type NEC A27.89
  leptospirochetal NEC — *see* Leptospirosis
  Listeria monocytogenes — *see also* Listeriosis
    congenital P37.2
  Loa loa B74.3
    with conjunctival infestation B74.3
    eyelid B74.3
  Loboa loboi B48.0
  local, skin (staphylococcal) (streptococcal) L08.9
    abscess — *code by* site under Abscess
    cellulitis — *code by* site under Cellulitis
    specified NEC L08.89
    ulcer — *see* Ulcer, skin
  Loefflerella mallei A24.0
  lung — *see also* Pneumonia J18.9
    atypical Mycobacterium A31.0
    spirochetal A69.8
    tuberculous — *see* Tuberculosis, pulmonary
    virus — *see* Pneumonia, viral
  lymph gland — *see also* Lymphadenitis, acute
    mesenteric I88.0
  lymphoid tissue, base of tongue or posterior pharynx, NEC (chronic) J35.03
  Madurella (grisea) (mycetomii) B47.0

Infection, infected, infective — *continued*
  major
    following ectopic or molar pregnancy O08.0
    puerperal, postpartum, childbirth O85
  Malassezia furfur B36.0
  Malleomyces
    mallei A24.0
    pseudomallei (whitmori) — *see* Melioidosis
  mammary gland N61.0
  Mansonella (ozzardi) (perstans) (streptocerca) B74.4
  mastoid — *see* Mastoiditis
  maxilla, maxillary M27.2
    sinus (chronic) — *see* Sinusitis, maxillary
  mediastinum J98.51
  Medina (worm) B72
  meibomian cyst or gland — *see* Hordeolum
  meninges — *see* Meningitis, bacterial
  meningococcal — *see also* condition A39.9
    adrenals A39.1
    brain A39.81
    cerebrospinal A39.0
    conjunctiva A39.89
    endocardium A39.51
    heart A39.50
      endocardium A39.51
      myocardium A39.52
      pericardium A39.53
    joint A39.83
    meninges A39.0
    meningococcemia A39.4
      acute A39.2
      chronic A39.3
    myocardium A39.52
    pericardium A39.53
    retrobulbar neuritis A39.82
    specified site NEC A39.89
  mesenteric lymph nodes or glands NEC I88.0
  Metagonimus B66.8
  metatarsophalangeal M00.9
  methicillin
    resistant Staphylococcus aureus (MRSA) A49.02
    susceptible Staphylococcus aureus (MSSA) A49.01
  Microsporum, microsporic — *see* Dermatophytosis
  mixed flora (bacterial) NEC A49.8
  Monilia — *see* Candidiasis
  Monosporium apiospermum B48.2
  mouth, parasitic B37.0
  Mucor — *see* Mucormycosis
  muscle NEC — *see* Myositis, infective
  mycelium NOS B49
  mycetoma B47.9
    actinomycotic NEC B47.1
    mycotic NEC B47.0
  Mycobacterium, mycobacterial — *see* Mycobacterium
  Mycoplasma NEC A49.3
    pneumoniae, as cause of disease classified elsewhere B96.0
  mycotic NOS B49
    pathogenic to compromised host only B48.8
    skin NOS B36.9
  myocardium NEC I40.0
  nail (chronic)
    with lymphangitis — *see* Lymphangitis, acute, digit
    finger L03.01- ☑
      fungus B35.1
    ingrowing L60.0
    toe L03.03- ☑
      fungus B35.1
  nasal sinus (chronic) — *see* Sinusitis
  nasopharynx — *see* Nasopharyngitis
  navel L08.82
  Necator americanus B76.1
  Neisseria — *see* Gonococcus
  Neotestudina rosatii B47.0
  newborn P39.9
    intra-amniotic NEC P39.2
    skin P39.4
    specified type NEC P39.8
  nipple N61.0
    associated with
      lactation O91.03
      pregnancy O91.01- ☑
      puerperium O91.02
  Nocardia — *see* Nocardiosis
  obstetrical surgical wound (puerperal) O86.00
    incisional site
      deep O86.02
      superficial O86.01

☑ **Additional Character Required** — Refer to the Tabular List for Character Selection   ▽ **Subterms under main terms may continue to next column or page**

Infection, infected, infective — *continued*
obstetrical surgical wound — *continued*
  organ and space site O86.03
  surgical site specified NEC O86.09
Oesophagostomum (apiostomum) B81.8
Oestrus ovis — *see* Myiasis
Oidium albicans B37.9
Onchocerca (volvulus) — *see* Onchocerciasis
oncovirus, as cause of disease classified elsewhere
  B97.32
operation wound T81.49 ☑
Opisthorchis (felineus) (viverrini) B66.0
orbit, orbital — *see* Inflammation, orbit
orthopoxvirus NEC B08.09
ovary — *see* Salpingo-oophoritis
Oxyuris vermicularis B80
pancreas (acute) — *see* Pancreatitis, acute
  abscess — *see* Pancreatitis, acute
  specified NEC — *see also* Pancreatitis, acute K85.80
papillomavirus, as cause of disease classified elsewhere
  B97.7
papovavirus NEC B34.4
Paracoccidioides brasiliensis — *see* Paracoccidioidomycosis
Paragonimus (westermani) B66.4
parainfluenza virus B34.8
parameningococcus NOS A39.9
parapoxvirus B08.60
  specified NEC B08.69
parasitic B89
Parastrongylus
  cantonensis B83.2
  costaricensis B81.3
  paratyphoid A01.4
    Type A A01.1
    Type B A01.2
    Type C A01.3
paraurethral ducts N34.2
parotid gland — *see* Sialoadenitis
parvovirus NEC B34.3
  as cause of disease classified elsewhere B97.6
Pasteurella NEC A28.0
  multocida A28.0
  pestis — *see* Plague
  pseudotuberculosis A28.0
  septica (cat bite) (dog bite) A28.0
  tularensis — *see* Tularemia
pelvic, female — *see* Disease, pelvis, inflammatory
Penicillium (marneffei) B48.4
penis (glans) (retention) NEC N48.29
periapical K04.5
peridental, periodontal K05.20
  generalized — *see* Periodontitis, aggressive, gener-
    alized
  localized — *see* Periodontitis, aggressive, localized
perinatal period P39.9
  specified type NEC P39.8
perineal repair (puerperal) O86.09
periorbital — *see* Inflammation, orbit
perirectal K62.89
perirenal — *see* Infection, kidney
peritoneal — *see* Peritonitis
periureteral N28.89
Petriellidium boydii B48.2
pharynx — *see also* Pharyngitis
  coxsackievirus B08.5
  posterior, lymphoid (chronic) J35.03
Phialophora
  gougerotii (subcutaneous abscess or cyst) B43.2
  jeanselmei (subcutaneous abscess or cyst) B43.2
  verrucosa (skin) B43.0
Piedraia hortae B36.3
pinta A67.9
  intermediate A67.1
  late A67.2
  mixed A67.3
  primary A67.0
pinworm B80
pityrosporum furfur B36.0
pleuro-pneumonia-like organism (PPLO) NEC A49.3
  as cause of disease classified elsewhere B96.0
pneumococcus, pneumococcal NEC A49.1
  as cause of disease classified elsewhere B95.3
  generalized (purulent) A40.3
    with pneumonia J13
Pneumocystis carinii (pneumonia) B59
Pneumocystis jiroveci (pneumonia) B59
port or reservoir T80.212 ☑

Infection, infected, infective — *continued*
postoperative T81.40 ☑
postoperative wound T81.49 ☑
  surgical site
    deep incisional T81.42 ☑
    organ and space T81.43 ☑
    specified NEC T81.49 ☑
    superficial incisional T81.41 ☑
postprocedural T81.40 ☑
postvaccinal T88.0 ☑ ·
prepuce NEC N47.7
  with penile inflammation N47.6
prion — *see* Disease, prion, central nervous system
prostate (capsule) — *see* Prostatitis
Proteus (mirabilis) (morganii) (vulgaris) NEC A49.8
  as cause of disease classified elsewhere B96.4
protozoal NEC B64
  intestinal A07.9
    specified NEC A07.8
  specified NEC B60.8
Pseudoallescheria boydii B48.2
Pseudomonas NEC A49.8
  as cause of disease classified elsewhere B96.5
  mallei A24.0
  pneumonia J15.1
  pseudomallei — *see* Melioidosis
puerperal O86.4
  genitourinary tract NEC O86.89
  major or generalized O85
  minor O86.4
  specified NEC O86.89
pulmonary — *see* Infection, lung
purulent — *see* Abscess
Pyrenochaeta romeroi B47.0
Q fever A78
rectum (sphincter) K62.89
renal — *see also* Infection, kidney
  pelvis and ureter (cystic) N28.85
reovirus, as cause of disease classified elsewhere B97.5
respiratory (tract) NEC J98.8
  acute J22
  chronic J98.8
  influenzal (upper) (acute) — *see* Influenza, with,
    respiratory manifestations NEC
  lower (acute) J22
    chronic — *see* Bronchitis, chronic
  rhinovirus J00
  syncytial virus (RSV) — *see* Infection, virus, respira-
    tory syncytial (RSV)
  upper (acute) NOS J06.9
    chronic J39.8
    streptococcal J06.9
    viral NOS J06.9
      due to respiratory syncytial virus (RSV)
      J06.9 [B97.4]
resulting from
  presence of internal prosthesis, implant, graft —
    see Complications, by site and type, infection
retortamoniasis A07.8
retroperitoneal NEC K68.9
retrovirus B33.3
  as cause of disease classified elsewhere B97.30
  human
    immunodeficiency, type 2 (HIV 2) B97.35
    T-cell lymphotropic
      type I (HTLV-I) B97.33
      type II (HTLV-II) B97.34
  lentivirus B97.31
  oncovirus B97.32
  specified NEC B97.39
Rhinosporidium (seeberi) B48.1
rhinovirus
  as cause of disease classified elsewhere B97.89
  unspecified nature or site B34.8
Rhizopus — *see* Mucormycosis
rickettsial NOS A79.9
roundworm (large) NEC B82.0
  Ascariasis — *see also* Ascariasis B77.9
  rubella — *see* Rubella
Saccharomyces — *see* Candidiasis
salivary duct or gland (any) — *see* Sialoadenitis
Salmonella (aertrycke) (arizonae) (callinarum) (cholerae-
  suis) (enteritidis) (suipestifer) (typhimurium)
  A02.9
  with
    (gastro)enteritis A02.0
    sepsis A02.1
    specified manifestation NEC A02.8

Infection, infected, infective — *continued*
Salmonella — *continued*
  due to food (poisoning) A02.9
  hirschfeldii A01.3
  localized A02.20
    arthritis A02.23
    meningitis A02.21
    osteomyelitis A02.24
    pneumonia A02.22
    pyelonephritis A02.25
    specified NEC A02.29
  paratyphi A01.4
    A A01.1
    B A01.2
    C A01.3
  schottmuelleri A01.2
  typhi, typhosa — *see* Typhoid
Sarcocystis A07.8
SARS-CoV-2 — *see* Infection, COVID-19
scabies B86
Schistosoma — *see* Infestation, Schistosoma
scrotum (acute) NEC N49.2
seminal vesicle — *see* Vesiculitis
septic
  localized, skin — *see* Abscess
sheep liver fluke B66.3
Shigella A03.9
  boydii A03.2
  dysenteriae A03.0
  flexneri A03.1
  group
    A A03.0
    B A03.1
    C A03.2
    D A03.3
  Schmitz (-Stutzer) A03.0
  schmitzii A03.0
  shigae A03.0
  sonnei A03.3
  specified NEC A03.8
shoulder (joint) NEC M00.9
  due to internal joint prosthesis T84.59 ☑
  skin NEC L08.9
sinus (accessory) (chronic) (nasal) — *see also* Sinusitis
  pilonidal — *see* Sinus, pilonidal
  skin NEC L08.89
Skene's duct or gland — *see* Urethritis
skin (local) (staphylococcal) (streptococcal) L08.9
  abscess — *code by* site under Abscess
  cellulitis — *code by* site under Cellulitis
  due to fungus B36.9
    specified type NEC B36.8
  mycotic B36.9
    specified type NEC B36.8
  newborn P39.4
  ulcer — *see* Ulcer, skin
slow virus A81.9
  specified NEC A81.89
Sparganum (mansoni) (proliferum) (baxteri) B70.1
specific — *see also* Syphilis
  to perinatal period — *see* Infection, congenital
specified NEC B99.8
spermatic cord NEC N49.1
sphenoidal (sinus) — *see* Sinusitis, sphenoidal
spinal cord NOS — *see also* Myelitis G04.91
  abscess G06.1
  meninges — *see* Meningitis
  streptococcal G04.89
Spirillum A25.0
spirochetal NOS A69.9
  lung A69.8
  specified NEC A69.8
Spirometra larvae B70.1
spleen D73.89
Sporotrichum, Sporothrix (schenckii) — *see* Sporotrichosis
staphylococcal, unspecified site
  as cause of disease classified elsewhere B95.8
    aureus (methicillin susceptible) (MSSA) B95.61
      methicillin resistant (MRSA) B95.62
    specified NEC B95.7
  aureus (methicillin susceptible) (MSSA) A49.01
    methicillin resistant (MRSA) A49.02
  food poisoning A05.0
  generalized (purulent) A41.2
  pneumonia — *see* Pneumonia, staphylococcal
Stellantchasmus falcatus B66.8
streptobacillus moniliformis A25.1

Infection, infected, infective — *continued*
streptococcal NEC A49.1
  as cause of disease classified elsewhere B95.5
  B genitourinary complicating
    childbirth O98.82
    pregnancy O98.81- ☑
    puerperium O98.83
  congenital
    sepsis P36.10
      group B P36.0
      specified NEC P36.19
  generalized (purulent) A40.9
Streptomyces B47.1
Strongyloides (stercoralis) — *see* Strongyloidiasis
stump (amputation) (surgical) — *see* Complication, amputation stump, infection
subcutaneous tissue, local L08.9
suipestifer — *see* Infection, salmonella
swimming pool bacillus A31.1
Taenia — *see* Infestation, Taenia
Taeniarhynchus saginatus B68.1
tapeworm — *see* Infestation, tapeworm
tendon (sheath) — *see* Tenosynovitis, infective NEC
Ternidens diminutus B81.8
testis — *see* Orchitis
threadworm B80
throat — *see* Pharyngitis
thyroglossal duct K14.8
toe (skin) L08.9
  cellulitis L03.03- ☑
    fungus B35.1
  nail L03.03- ☑
    fungus B35.1
tongue NEC K14.0
  parasitic B37.0
tonsil (and adenoid) (faucial) (lingual) (pharyngeal) — *see* Tonsillitis
tooth, teeth K04.7
  periapical K04.7
  peridental, periodontal K05.20
    generalized — *see* Periodontitis, aggressive, generalized
    localized — *see* Periodontitis, aggressive, localized
  pulp K04.01
    irreversible K04.02
    reversible K04.01
  socket M27.3
TORCH — *see* Infection, congenital
  without active infection P00.2
Torula histolytica — *see* Cryptococcosis
Toxocara (canis) (cati) (felis) B83.0
Toxoplasma gondii — *see* Toxoplasma
trachea, chronic J42
trematode NEC — *see* Infestation, fluke
trench fever A79.0
Treponema pallidum — *see* Syphilis
Trichinella (spiralis) B75
Trichomonas A59.9
  cervix A59.09
  intestine A07.8
  prostate A59.02
  specified site NEC A59.8
  urethra A59.03
  urogenitalis A59.00
  vagina A59.01
  vulva A59.01
Trichophyton, trichophytic — *see* Dermatophytosis
Trichosporon (beigelii) cutaneum B36.2
Trichostrongylus B81.2
Trichuris (trichiura) B79
Trombicula (irritans) B88.0
Trypanosoma
  brucei
    gambiense B56.0
    rhodesiense B56.1
  cruzi — *see* Chagas' disease
tubal — *see* Salpingo-oophoritis
tuberculous
  latent (LTBI) Z22.7
  NEC — *see* Tuberculosis
tubo-ovarian — *see* Salpingo-oophoritis
tunica vaginalis N49.1
tunnel T80.212 ☑
tympanic membrane NEC — *see* Myringitis
typhoid (abortive) (ambulant) (bacillus) — *see* Typhoid
typhus A75.9
  flea-borne A75.2

Infection, infected, infective — *continued*
typhus — *continued*
  mite-borne A75.3
  recrudescent A75.1
  tick-borne A77.9
    African A77.1
    North Asian A77.2
umbilicus L08.82
ureter — *see* Ureteritis
urethra — *see* Urethritis
urinary (tract) N39.0
  bladder — *see* Cystitis
  complicating
    pregnancy O23.4- ☑
      specified type NEC O23.3- ☑
  kidney — *see* Infection, kidney
  newborn P39.3
  puerperal (postpartum) O86.20
  tuberculous A18.13
  urethra — *see* Urethritis
uterus, uterine — *see* Endometritis
vaccination T88.0 ☑
vaccinia not from vaccination B08.011
vagina (acute) — *see* Vaginitis
varicella B01.9
varicose veins — *see* Varix
vas deferens NEC N49.1
vesical — *see* Cystitis
Vibrio
  cholerae A00.0
    El Tor A00.1
  parahaemolyticus (food poisoning) A05.3
  vulnificus
    as cause of disease classified elsewhere B96.82
    foodborne intoxication A05.5
Vincent's (gum) (mouth) (tonsil) A69.1
virus, viral NOS B34.9
  adenovirus
    as cause of disease classified elsewhere B97.0
    unspecified nature or site B34.0
  arbovirus, arbovirus arthropod-borne A94
  as cause of disease classified elsewhere B97.89
    adenovirus B97.0
    coronavirus B97.29
      SARS-associated B97.21
    coxsackievirus B97.11
    echovirus B97.12
    enterovirus B97.10
      coxsackievirus B97.11
      echovirus B97.12
      specified NEC B97.19
    human
      immunodeficiency, type 2 (HIV 2) B97.35
      metapneumovirus B97.81
      T-cell lymphotropic,
        type I (HTLV-I) B97.33
        type II (HTLV-II) B97.34
    papillomavirus B97.7
    parvovirus B97.6
    reovirus B97.5
    respiratory syncytial (RSV) — *see* Infection, virus, respiratory syncytial (RSV)
    retrovirus B97.30
      human
        immunodeficiency, type 2 (HIV 2) B97.35
        T-cell lymphotropic,
          type I (HTLV-I) B97.33
          type II (HTLV-II) B97.34
      lentivirus B97.31
      oncovirus B97.32
      specified NEC B97.39
    specified NEC B97.89
  central nervous system A89
    atypical A81.9
      specified NEC A81.89
    enterovirus NEC A88.8
      meningitis A87.0
    slow virus A81.9
      specified NEC A81.89
    specified NEC A88.8
  chest J98.8
  cotia B08.8
  COVID-19 U07.1
  coxsackie — *see also* Infection, coxsackie B34.1
    as cause of disease classified elsewhere B97.11
  ECHO
    as cause of disease classified elsewhere B97.12
    unspecified nature or site B34.1

Infection, infected, infective — *continued*
virus, viral — *continued*
  encephalitis, tick-borne A84.9
  enterovirus, as cause of disease classified elsewhere B97.10
    coxsackievirus B97.11
    echovirus B97.12
    specified NEC B97.19
  exanthem NOS B09
  human metapneumovirus as cause of disease classified elsewhere B97.81
  human papilloma as cause of disease classified elsewhere B97.7
  intestine — *see* Enteritis, viral
  respiratory syncytial (RSV)
    as cause of disease classified elsewhere B97.4
    bronchiolitis J21.0
    bronchitis J20.5
    bronchopneumonia J12.1
    otitis media H65- ☑ *[B97.4]*
    pneumonia J12.1
    upper respiratory infection J06.9 *[B97.4]*
  rhinovirus
    as cause of disease classified elsewhere B97.89
    unspecified nature or site B34.8
  slow A81.9
    specified NEC A81.89
  specified type NEC B33.8
    as cause of disease classified elsewhere B97.89
    unspecified nature or site B34.8
  unspecified nature or site B34.9
  West Nile — *see* Virus, West Nile
  vulva (acute) — *see* Vulvitis
  West Nile — *see* Virus, West Nile
  whipworm B79
  worms B83.9
    specified type NEC B83.8
  Wuchereria (bancrofti) B74.0
    malayi B74.1
  yatapoxvirus B08.70
    specified NEC B08.79
  yeast — *see also* Candidiasis B37.9
  yellow fever — *see* Fever, yellow
  Yersinia
    enterocolitica (intestinal) A04.6
    pestis — *see* Plague
    pseudotuberculosis A28.2
  Zeis' gland — *see* Hordeolum
  Zika virus A92.5
    congenital P35.4
  zoonotic bacterial NOS A28.9
  Zopfia senegalensis B47.0
Infective, infectious — *see* condition
Infertility
  female N97.9
    age-related N97.8
    associated with
      anovulation N97.0
      cervical (mucus) disease or anomaly N88.3
      congenital anomaly
        cervix N88.3
        fallopian tube N97.1
        uterus N97.2
        vagina N97.8
      dysmucorrhea N88.3
      fallopian tube disease or anomaly N97.1
      pituitary-hypothalamic origin E23.0
      specified origin NEC N97.8
      Stein-Leventhal syndrome E28.2
      uterine disease or anomaly N97.2
      vaginal disease or anomaly N97.8
    due to
      cervical anomaly N88.3
      fallopian tube anomaly N97.1
      ovarian failure E28.39
      Stein-Leventhal syndrome E28.2
      uterine anomaly N97.2
      vaginal anomaly N97.8
    nonimplantation N97.2
    origin
      cervical N88.3
      tubal (block) (occlusion) (stenosis) N97.1
      uterine N97.2
      vaginal N97.8
  male N46.9
    azoospermia N46.01
      extratesticular cause N46.029
        drug therapy N46.021

☑ **Additional Character Required** — **Refer to the Tabular List for Character Selection**   ▽ **Subterms under main terms may continue to next column or page**

Infertility — *continued*
  male — *continued*
    azoospermia — *continued*
      extratesticular cause — *continued*
        efferent duct obstruction N46.023
        infection N46.022
        radiation N46.024
        specified cause NEC N46.029
        systemic disease N46.025
    oligospermia N46.11
      extratesticular cause N46.129
        drug therapy N46.121
        efferent duct obstruction N46.123
        infection N46.122
        radiation N46.124
        specified cause NEC N46.129
        systemic disease N46.125
    specified type NEC N46.8
Infestation B88.9
  Acanthocheilonema (perstans) (streptocerca) B74.4
  Acariasis B88.0
    demodex folliculorum B88.0
    sarcoptes scabiei B86
    trombiculae B88.0
  Agamofilaria streptocerca B74.4
  Ancylostoma, ankylostoma (braziliense) (caninum) (ceylanicum) (duodenale) B76.0
    americanum B76.1
    new world B76.1
  Anisakis larvae, anisakiasis B81.0
  arthropod NEC B88.2
  Ascaris lumbricoides — *see* Ascariasis
  Balantidium coli A07.0
  beef tapeworm B68.1
  Bothriocephalus (latus) B70.0
    larval B70.1
  broad tapeworm B70.0
    larval B70.1
  Brugia (malayi) B74.1
    timori B74.2
  candiru B88.8
  Capillaria
    hepatica B83.8
    philippinensis B81.1
  cat liver fluke B66.0
  cestodes B71.9
    diphyllobothrium — *see* Infestation, diphyllobothrium
    dipylidiasis B71.1
    hymenolepiasis B71.0
    specified type NEC B71.8
  chigger B88.0
  chigo, chigoe B88.1
  Clonorchis (sinensis) (liver) B66.1
  coccidial A07.3
  crab-lice B85.3
  Cysticercus cellulosae — *see* Cysticercosis
  Demodex (folliculorum) B88.0
  Dermanyssus gallinae B88.0
  Dermatobia (hominis) — *see* Myiasis
  Dibothriocephalus (latus) B70.0
    larval B70.1
  Dicrocoelium dendriticum B66.2
  Diphyllobothrium (adult) (latum) (intestinal) (pacificum) B70.0
    larval B70.1
  Diplogonoporus (grandis) B71.8
  Dipylidium caninum B67.4
  Distoma hepaticum B66.3
  dog tapeworm B67.4
  Dracunculus medinensis B72
  dragon worm B72
  dwarf tapeworm B71.0
  Echinococcus — *see* Echinococcus
  Echinostomum ilocanum B66.8
  Entamoeba (histolytica) — *see* Infection, Ameba
  Enterobius vermicularis B80
  eyelid
    in (due to)
      leishmaniasis B55.1
      loiasis B74.3
      onchocerciasis B73.09
      phthiriasis B85.3
    parasitic NOS B89
  eyeworm B74.3
  Fasciola (gigantica) (hepatica) (indica) B66.3
  Fasciolopsis (buski) (intestine) B66.5
  filarial B74.9

Infestation
  filarial — *continued*
    bancroftian B74.0
    conjunctiva B74.9
    due to
      Acanthocheilonema (perstans) (streptocerca) B74.4
      Brugia (malayi) B74.1
        timori B74.2
      Dracunculus medinensis B72
      guinea worm B72
      loa loa B74.3
      Mansonella (ozzardi) (perstans) (streptocerca) B74.4
      Onchocerca volvulus B73.00
        eye B73.00
        eyelid B73.09
      Wuchereria (bancrofti) B74.0
    Malayan B74.1
    ozzardi B74.4
    specified type NEC B74.8
  fish tapeworm B70.0
    larval B70.1
  fluke B66.9
    blood NOS — *see* Schistosomiasis
    cat liver B66.0
    intestinal B66.5
    lancet B66.2
    liver (sheep) B66.3
      cat B66.0
      Chinese B66.1
      due to clonorchiasis B66.1
      oriental B66.1
    lung (oriental) B66.4
    sheep liver B66.3
    specified type NEC B66.8
  fly larvae — *see* Myiasis
  Gasterophilus (intestinalis) — *see* Myiasis
  Gastrodiscoides hominis B66.8
  Giardia lamblia A07.1
  Gnathostoma (spinigerum) B83.1
  Gongylonema B83.8
  guinea worm B72
  helminth B83.9
    angiostrongyliasis B83.2
      intestinal B81.3
    gnathostomiasis B83.1
    hirudiniasis, internal B83.4
    intestinal B82.0
      angiostrongyliasis B81.3
      anisakiasis B81.0
      ascariasis — *see* Ascariasis
      capillariasis B81.1
      cysticercosis — *see* Cysticercosis
      diphyllobothriasis — *see* Infestation, diphyllobothriasis
      dracunculiasis B72
      echinococcus — *see* Echinococcosis
      enterobiasis B80
      filariasis — *see* Infestation, filarial
      fluke — *see* Infestation, fluke
      hookworm — *see* Infestation, hookworm
      mixed (types classifiable to more than one of the titles B65.0-B81.3 and B81.8) B81.4
      onchocerciasis — *see* Onchocerciasis
      schistosomiasis — *see* Infestation, schistosoma
      specified
        cestode NEC — *see* Infestation, cestode
        type NEC B81.8
      strongyloidiasis — *see* Strongyloidiasis
      taenia — *see* Infestation, taenia
      trichinellosis B75
      trichostrongyliasis B81.2
      trichuriasis B79
    specified type NEC B83.8
    syngamiasis B83.3
    visceral larva migrans B83.0
  Heterophyes (heterophyes) B66.8
  hookworm B76.9
    ancylostomiasis B76.0
    necatoriasis B76.1
    specified type NEC B76.8
  Hymenolepis (diminuta) (nana) B71.0
  intestinal NEC B82.9
  leeches (aquatic) (land) — *see* Hirudiniasis
  Leishmania — *see* Leishmaniasis
  lice, louse — *see* Infestation, Pediculus
  Linguatula B88.8

Infestation — *continued*
  Liponyssoides sanguineus B88.0
  Loa loa B74.3
    conjunctival B74.3
    eyelid B74.3
  louse — *see* Infestation, Pediculus
  maggots — *see* Myiasis
  Mansonella (ozzardi) (perstans) (streptocerca) B74.4
  Medina (worm) B72
  Metagonimus (yokogawai) B66.8
  microfilaria streptocerca — *see* Onchocerciasis
    eye B73.00
    eyelid B73.09
  mites B88.9
    scabic B86
  Monilia (albicans) — *see* Candidiasis
  mouth B37.0
  Necator americanus B76.1
  nematode NEC (intestinal) B82.0
    Ancylostoma B76.0
    conjunctiva NEC B83.9
    Enterobius vermicularis B80
    Gnathostoma spinigerum B83.1
    physaloptera B80
    specified NEC B81.8
    trichostrongylus B81.2
    trichuris (trichuria) B79
  Oesophagostomum (apiostomum) B81.8
  Oestrus ovis — *see also* Myiasis B87.9
  Onchocerca (volvulus) — *see* Onchocerciasis
  Opisthorchis (felineus) (viverrini) B66.0
  orbit, parasitic NOS B89
  Oxyuris vermicularis B80
  Paragonimus (westermani) B66.4
  parasite, parasitic B89
    eyelid B89
    intestinal NOS B82.9
    mouth B37.0
    skin B88.9
    tongue B37.0
  Parastrongylus
    cantonensis B83.2
    costaricensis B81.3
  Pediculus B85.2
    body B85.1
    capitis (humanus) (any site) B85.0
    corporis (humanus) (any site) B85.1
    head B85.0
    mixed (classifiable to more than one of the titles B85.0 - B85.3) B85.4
    pubis (any site) B85.3
  Pentastoma B88.8
  Phthirus (pubis) (any site) B85.3
    with any infestation classifiable to B85.0 - B85.2 B85.4
  pinworm B80
  pork tapeworm (adult) B68.0
  protozoal NEC B64
    intestinal A07.9
      specified NEC A07.8
    specified NEC B60.8
  pubic, louse B85.3
  rat tapeworm B71.0
  red bug B88.0
  roundworm (large) NEC B82.0
    Ascariasis — *see also* Ascariasis B77.9
  sandflea B88.1
  Sarcoptes scabiei B86
  scabies B86
  Schistosoma B65.9
    bovis B65.8
    cercariae B65.3
    haematobium B65.0
    intercalatum B65.8
    japonicum B65.2
    mansoni B65.1
    mattheei B65.8
    mekongi B65.8
    specified type NEC B65.8
    spindale B65.8
  screw worms — *see* Myiasis
  skin NOS B88.9
  Sparganum (mansoni) (proliferum) (baxteri) B70.1
    larval B70.1
  specified type NEC B88.8
  Spirometra larvae B70.1
  Stellantchasmus falcatus B66.8
  Strongyloides stercoralis — *see* Strongyloidiasis

Infestation — *continued*
    Taenia B68.9
        diminuta B71.0
        echinococcus — *see* Echinococcus
        mediocanellata B68.1
        nana B71.0
        saginata B68.1
        solium (intestinal form) B68.0
            larval form — *see* Cysticercosis
    Taeniarhynchus saginatus B68.1
    tapeworm B71.9
        beef B68.1
        broad B70.0
            larval B70.1
        dog B67.4
        dwarf B71.0
        fish B70.0
            larval B70.1
        pork B68.0
        rat B71.0
    Ternidens diminutus B81.8
    Tetranychus molestissimus B88.0
    threadworm B80
    tongue B37.0
    Toxocara (canis) (cati) (felis) B83.0
    trematode(s) NEC — *see* Infestation, fluke
    Trichinella (spiralis) B75
    Trichocephalus B79
    Trichomonas — *see* Trichomoniasis
    Trichostrongylus B81.2
    Trichuris (trichiura) B79
    Trombicula (irritans) B88.0
    Tunga penetrans B88.1
    Uncinaria americana B76.1
    Vandellia cirrhosa B88.8
    whipworm B79
    worms B83.9
        intestinal B82.0
    Wuchereria (bancrofti) B74.0
Infiltrate, infiltration
    amyloid (generalized) (localized) — *see* Amyloidosis
    calcareous NEC R89.7
        localized — *see* Degeneration, by site
    calcium salt R89.7
    cardiac
        fatty — *see* Degeneration, myocardial
        glycogenic E74.02 *[I43]*
    corneal — *see* Edema, cornea
    eyelid — *see* Inflammation, eyelid
    glycogen, glycogenic — *see* Disease, glycogen storage
    heart, cardiac
        fatty — *see* Degeneration, myocardial
        glycogenic E74.02 *[I43]*
    inflammatory in vitreous H43.89
    kidney N28.89
    leukemic — *see* Leukemia
    liver K76.89
        fatty — *see* Fatty, liver NEC
        glycogen — *see also* Disease, glycogen storage
            E74.03 *[K77]*
    lung R91.8
        eosinophilic — *see* Eosinophilia, pulmonary
    lymphatic — *see also* Leukemia, lymphatic C91.9- ☑
        gland I88.9
    muscle, fatty M62.89
    myocardium, myocardial
        fatty — *see* Degeneration, myocardial
        glycogenic E74.02 *[I43]*
    on chest x-ray R91.8
    pulmonary R91.8
        with eosinophilia — *see* Eosinophilia, pulmonary
    skin (lymphocytic) L98.6
    thymus (gland) (fatty) E32.8
    urine R39.0
    vesicant agent
        antineoplastic chemotherapy T80.810 ☑
        other agent NEC T80.818 ☑
    vitreous body H43.89
Infirmity R68.89
    senile R54
Inflammation, inflamed, inflammatory (with exudation)
    abducent (nerve) — *see* Strabismus, paralytic, sixth nerve
    accessory sinus (chronic) — *see* Sinusitis
    adrenal (gland) E27.8
    alveoli, teeth M27.3
        scorbutic E54

Inflammation, inflamed, inflammatory — *continued*
    anal canal, anus K62.89
    antrum (chronic) — *see* Sinusitis, maxillary
    appendix — *see* Appendicitis
    arachnoid — *see* Meningitis
    areola N61.0
        puerperal, postpartum or gestational — *see* Infection, nipple
    areolar tissue NOS L08.9
    artery — *see* Arteritis
    auditory meatus (external) — *see* Otitis, externa
    Bartholin's gland N75.8
    bile duct (common) (hepatic) or passage — *see* Cholangitis
    bladder — *see* Cystitis
    bone — *see* Osteomyelitis
    brain — *see also* Encephalitis
        membrane — *see* Meningitis
    breast N61.0
        puerperal, postpartum, gestational — *see* Mastitis, obstetric
    broad ligament — *see* Disease, pelvis, inflammatory
    bronchi — *see* Bronchitis
    catarrhal J00
    cecum — *see* Appendicitis
    cerebral — *see also* Encephalitis
        membrane — *see* Meningitis
    cerebrospinal
        meningococcal A39.0
    cervix (uteri) — *see* Cervicitis
    chest J98.8
    chorioretinal H30.9- ☑
        cyclitis — *see* Cyclitis
        disseminated H30.10- ☑
            generalized H30.13- ☑
            peripheral H30.12- ☑
            posterior pole H30.11- ☑
        epitheliopathy — *see* Epitheliopathy
        focal H30.00- ☑
            juxtapapillary H30.01- ☑
            macular H30.04- ☑
            paramacular — *see* Inflammation, chorioretinal, focal, macular
            peripheral H30.03- ☑
            posterior pole H30.02- ☑
        specified type NEC H30.89- ☑
    choroid — *see* Inflammation, chorioretinal
    chronic, postmastoidectomy cavity — *see* Complications, postmastoidectomy, inflammation
    colon — *see* Enteritis
    connective tissue (diffuse) NEC — *see* Disorder, soft tissue, specified type NEC
    cornea — *see* Keratitis
    corpora cavernosa N48.29
    cranial nerve — *see* Disorder, nerve, cranial
    Douglas' cul-de-sac or pouch (chronic) N73.0
    due to device, implant or graft — *see also* Complications, by site and type, infection or inflammation
        arterial graft T82.7 ☑
        breast (implant) T85.79 ☑
        catheter T85.79 ☑
            dialysis (renal) T82.7 ☑
                intraperitoneal T85.71 ☑
            infusion T82.7 ☑
                cranial T85.735 ☑
                intrathecal T85.735 ☑
                spinal (epidural) (subdural) T85.735 ☑
                subarachnoid T85.735 ☑
            urinary T83.518 ☑
                cystostomy T83.510 ☑
                Hopkins T83.518 ☑
                ileostomy T83.518 ☑
                nephrostomy T83.512 ☑
                specified NEC T83.518 ☑
                urethral indwelling T83.511 ☑
                urostomy T83.518 ☑
        electronic (electrode) (pulse generator) (stimulator)
            bone T84.7 ☑
            cardiac T82.7 ☑
            nervous system T85.738 ☑
                brain T85.731 ☑
                cranial nerve T85.732 ☑
                gastric nerve T85.732 ☑
                neurostimulator generator T85.734 ☑
                peripheral nerve T85.732 ☑

Inflammation, inflamed, inflammatory — *continued*
    due to device, implant or graft — *see also* Complications, by site and type, infection or inflammation — *continued*
        electronic — *continued*
            nervous system — *continued*
                sacral nerve T85.732 ☑
                spinal cord T85.733 ☑
                vagal nerve T85.732 ☑
            urinary T83.590 ☑
        fixation, internal (orthopedic) NEC — *see* Complication, fixation device, infection
        gastrointestinal (bile duct) (esophagus) T85.79 ☑
            neurostimulator electrode (lead) T85.732 ☑
        genital NEC T83.69 ☑
        heart NEC T82.7 ☑
            valve (prosthesis) T82.6 ☑
                graft T82.7 ☑
        joint prosthesis — *see* Complication, joint prosthesis, infection
        ocular (corneal graft) (orbital implant) NEC T85.79 ☑
        orthopedic NEC T84.7 ☑
        penile (cylinder) (pump) (resevoir) T83.61 ☑
        specified NEC T85.79 ☑
        testicular T83.62 ☑
        urinary NEC T83.598 ☑
            ileal conduit stent T83.593 ☑
            implanted neurostimulation T83.590 ☑
            implanted sphincter T83.591 ☑
            indwelling ureteral stent T83.592 ☑
            nephroureteral stent T83.593 ☑
            specified stent NEC T83.593 ☑
        vascular NEC T82.7 ☑
        ventricular intracranial (communicating) shunt T85.730 ☑
    duodenum K29.80
        with bleeding K29.81
    dura mater — *see* Meningitis
    ear (middle) — *see also* Otitis, media
        external — *see* Otitis, externa
        inner — *see* subcategory H83.0 ☑
    epididymis — *see* Epididymitis
    esophagus — *see* Esophagitis
    ethmoidal (sinus) (chronic) — *see* Sinusitis, ethmoidal
    eustachian tube (catarrhal) — *see* Salpingitis, eustachian
    eyelid H01.9
        abscess — *see* Abscess, eyelid
        blepharitis — *see* Blepharitis
        chalazion — *see* Chalazion
        dermatosis (noninfectious) — *see* Dermatosis, eyelid
        hordeolum — *see* Hordeolum
        specified NEC H01.8
    fallopian tube — *see* Salpingo-oophoritis
    fascia — *see* Myositis
    follicular, pharynx J31.2
    frontal (sinus) (chronic) — *see* Sinusitis, frontal
    gallbladder — *see* Cholecystitis
    gastric — *see* Gastritis
    gastrointestinal — *see* Enteritis
    genital organ (internal) (diffuse)
        female — *see* Disease, pelvis, inflammatory
        male N49.9
            multiple sites N49.8
            specified NEC N49.8
    gland (lymph) — *see* Lymphadenitis
    glottis — *see* Laryngitis
    granular, pharynx J31.2
    gum K05.10
        nonplaque induced K05.11
        plaque induced K05.10
    heart — *see* Carditis
    hepatic duct — *see* Cholangitis
    ileoanal (internal) pouch K91.850
    ileum — *see also* Enteritis
        regional or terminal — *see* Enteritis, regional
    intestinal pouch K91.850
    intestine (any part) — *see* Enteritis
    jaw (acute) (bone) (chronic) (lower) (suppurative) (upper) M27.2
    joint NEC — *see* Arthritis
        sacroiliac M46.1
    kidney — *see* Nephritis
    knee (joint) M13.169
        tuberculous A18.02
    labium (majus) (minus) — *see* Vulvitis

☑ **Additional Character Required** — Refer to the Tabular List for Character Selection   ▽ **Subterms under main terms may continue to next column or page**

Inflammation, inflamed, inflammatory — *continued*
- lacrimal
  - gland — *see* Dacryoadenitis
  - passages (duct) (sac) — *see also* Dacryocystitis
    - canaliculitis — *see* Canaliculitis, lacrimal
- larynx — *see* Laryngitis
- leg NOS L08.9
- lip K13.0
- liver (capsule) — *see also* Hepatitis
  - chronic K73.9
  - suppurative K75.0
- lung (acute) — *see also* Pneumonia
  - chronic J98.4
- lymph gland or node — *see* Lymphadenitis
- lymphatic vessel — *see* Lymphangitis
- maxilla, maxillary M27.2
  - sinus (chronic) — *see* Sinusitis, maxillary
- membranes of brain or spinal cord — *see* Meningitis
- meninges — *see* Meningitis
- mouth K12.1
- muscle — *see* Myositis
- myocardium — *see* Myocarditis
- nasal sinus (chronic) — *see* Sinusitis
- nasopharynx — *see* Nasopharyngitis
- navel L08.82
- nerve NEC — *see* Neuritis
- nipple N61.0
  - puerperal, postpartum or gestational — *see* Infection, nipple
- nose — *see* Rhinitis
- oculomotor (nerve) — *see* Strabismus, paralytic, third nerve
- optic nerve — *see* Neuritis, optic
- orbit (chronic) H05.10
  - acute H05.00
    - abscess — *see* Abscess, orbit
    - cellulitis — *see* Cellulitis, orbit
    - osteomyelitis — *see* Osteomyelitis, orbit
    - periostitis — *see* Periostitis, orbital
    - tenonitis — *see* Tenonitis, eye
  - granuloma — *see* Granuloma, orbit
  - myositis — *see* Myositis, orbital
- ovary — *see* Salpingo-oophoritis
- oviduct — *see* Salpingo-oophoritis
- pancreas (acute) — *see* Pancreatitis
- parametrium N73.0
- parotid region L08.9
- pelvis, female — *see* Disease, pelvis, inflammatory
- penis (corpora cavernosa) N48.29
- perianal K62.89
- pericardium — *see* Pericarditis
- perineum (female) (male) L08.9
- perirectal K62.89
- peritoneum — *see* Peritonitis
- periuterine — *see* Disease, pelvis, inflammatory
- perivesical — *see* Cystitis
- petrous bone (acute) (chronic) — *see* Petrositis
- pharynx (acute) — *see* Pharyngitis
- pia mater — *see* Meningitis
- pleura — *see* Pleurisy
- polyp, colon — *see also* Polyp, colon, inflammatory K51.40
- prostate — *see also* Prostatitis
  - specified type NEC N41.8
- rectosigmoid — *see* Rectosigmoiditis
- rectum — *see also* Proctitis K62.89
- respiratory, upper — *see also* Infection, respiratory, upper J06.9
  - acute, due to radiation J70.0
  - chronic, due to external agent — *see* condition, respiratory, chronic, due to
  - due to
    - chemicals, gases, fumes or vapors (inhalation) J68.2
    - radiation J70.1
- retina — *see* Chorioretinitis
- retrocecal — *see* Appendicitis
- retroperitoneal — *see* Peritonitis
- salivary duct or gland (any) (suppurative) — *see* Sialoadenitis
- scorbutic, alveoli, teeth E54
- scrotum N49.2
- seminal vesicle — *see* Vesiculitis
- sigmoid — *see* Enteritis
- sinus — *see* Sinusitis
- Skene's duct or gland — *see* Urethritis

Inflammation, inflamed, inflammatory — *continued*
- skin L08.9
- spermatic cord N49.1
- sphenoidal (sinus) — *see* Sinusitis, sphenoidal
- spinal
  - cord — *see* Encephalitis
  - membrane — *see* Meningitis
  - nerve — *see* Disorder, nerve
- spine — *see* Spondylopathy, inflammatory
- spleen (capsule) D73.89
- stomach — *see* Gastritis
- subcutaneous tissue L08.9
- suprarenal (gland) E27.8
- synovial — *see* Tenosynovitis
- tendon (sheath) NEC — *see* Tenosynovitis
- testis — *see* Orchitis
- throat (acute) — *see* Pharyngitis
- thymus (gland) E32.8
- thyroid (gland) — *see* Thyroiditis
- tongue K14.0
- tonsil — *see* Tonsillitis
- trachea — *see* Tracheitis
- trochlear (nerve) — *see* Strabismus, paralytic, fourth nerve
- tubal — *see* Salpingo-oophoritis
- tuberculous NEC — *see* Tuberculosis
- tubo-ovarian — *see* Salpingo-oophoritis
- tunica vaginalis N49.1
- tympanic membrane — *see* Tympanitis
- umbilicus, umbilical L08.82
- uterine ligament — *see* Disease, pelvis, inflammatory
- uterus (catarrhal) — *see* Endometritis
- uveal tract (anterior) NOS — *see also* Iridocyclitis
  - posterior — *see* Chorioretinitis
- vagina — *see* Vaginitis
- vas deferens N49.1
- vein — *see also* Phlebitis
  - intracranial or intraspinal (septic) G08
  - thrombotic I80.9
    - leg — *see* Phlebitis, leg
    - lower extremity — *see* Phlebitis, leg
- vocal cord J38.3
- vulva — *see* Vulvitis
- Wharton's duct (suppurative) — *see* Sialoadenitis

Inflation, lung, imperfect (newborn) — *see* Atelectasis

Influenza (bronchial) (epidemic) (respiratory (upper)) (unidentified influenza virus) J11.1
- with
  - digestive manifestations J11.2
  - encephalopathy J11.81
  - enteritis J11.2
  - gastroenteritis J11.2
  - gastrointestinal manifestations J11.2
  - laryngitis J11.1
  - myocarditis J11.82
  - otitis media J11.83
  - pharyngitis J11.1
  - pneumonia J11.00
    - specified type J11.08
  - respiratory manifestations NEC J11.1
  - specified manifestation NEC J11.89
- A (non-novel) J10- ☑
- A/H5N1 — *see also* Influenza, due to, identified novel influenza A virus J09.X2
- avian — *see also* Influenza, due to, identified novel influenza A virus J09.X2
- B J10- ☑
- bird — *see also* Influenza, due to, identified novel influenza A virus J09.X2
- C J10- ☑
- due to
  - avian — *see also* Influenza, due to, identified novel influenza A virus J09.X2
  - identified influenza virus NEC J10.1
    - with
      - digestive manifestations J10.2
      - encephalopathy J10.81
      - enteritis J10.2
      - gastroenteritis J10.2
      - gastrointestinal manifestations J10.2
      - laryngitis J10.1
      - myocarditis J10.82
      - otitis media J10.83
      - pharyngitis J10.1
      - pneumonia (unspecified type) J10.00
        - with same identified influenza virus J10.01

Influenza — *continued*
- due to — *continued*
  - identified influenza virus — *continued*
    - with — *continued*
      - pneumonia — *continued*
        - specified type NEC J10.08
      - respiratory manifestations NEC J10.1
      - specified manifestation NEC J10.89
    - identified novel influenza A virus J09.X2
      - with
        - digestive manifestations J09.X3
        - encephalopathy J09.X9
        - enteritis J09.X3
        - gastroenteritis J09.X3
        - gastrointestinal manifestations J09.X3
        - laryngitis J09.X2
        - myocarditis J09.X9
        - otitis media J09.X9
        - pharyngitis J09.X2
        - pneumonia J09.X1
        - respiratory manifestations NEC J09.X2
        - specified manifestation NEC J09.X9
        - upper respiratory symptoms J09.X2
  - novel (2009) H1N1 influenza — *see also* Influenza, due to, identified influenza virus NEC J10.1
  - novel influenza A/H1N1 — *see also* Influenza, due to, identified influenza virus NEC J10.1
  - of other animal origin, not bird or swine — *see also* Influenza, due to, identified novel influenza A virus J09.X2
  - swine (viruses that normally cause infections in pigs) — *see also* Influenza, due to, identified novel influenza A virus J09.X2

Influenzal — *see* Influenza

Influenza-like disease — *see* Influenza

Infraction, Freiberg's (metatarsal head) — *see* Osteochondrosis, juvenile, metatarsus

Infraeruption of tooth (teeth) M26.34

Infusion complication, misadventure, or reaction — *see* Complications, infusion

Ingestion
- chemical — *see* Table of Drugs and Chemicals, by substance, poisoning
- drug or medicament
  - correct substance properly administered — *see* Table of Drugs and Chemicals, by drug, adverse effect
  - overdose or wrong substance given or taken — *see* Table of Drugs and Chemicals, by drug, poisoning
- foreign body — *see* Foreign body, alimentary tract
- multiple drug — *see* Table of Drugs and Chemicals, multiple
- tularemia A21.3

Ingrowing
- hair (beard) L73.1
- nail (finger) (toe) L60.0

Inguinal — *see also* condition
- testicle Q53.9
  - bilateral Q53.212
  - unilateral Q53.112

Inhalant-induced
- anxiety disorder F18.980
- depressive disorder F18.94
- major neurocognitive disorder F18.97
- mild neurocognitive disorder F18.988
- psychotic disorder F18.959

Inhalation
- anthrax A22.1
- flame T27.3 ☑
- food or foreign body — *see* Foreign body, by site
- gases, fumes, or vapors T59.9- ☑
  - specified agent NEC — *see* Table of Drugs and Chemicals, by substance T59.89- ☑
- liquid or vomitus — *see* Asphyxia
- meconium (newborn) P24.00
  - with
    - with respiratory symptoms P24.01
    - pneumonia (pneumonitis) P24.01
- mucus — *see* Asphyxia, mucus
- oil or gasoline (causing suffocation) — *see* Foreign body, by site
- smoke T59.81- ☑
  - with respiratory conditions J70.5
    - due to chemicals, gases, fumes and vapors J68.9
- steam — *see also* Burn, respiratory tract T59.9- ☑
- stomach contents or secretions — *see* Foreign body, by site

Inhalation — continued
- stomach contents or secretions — see Foreign body, by site — continued
  - due to anesthesia (general) (local) or other sedation T88.59 ☑
  - in labor and delivery O74.0
  - in pregnancy O29.01- ☑
  - postpartum, puerperal O89.01

Inhibition, orgasm
- female F52.31
- male F52.32

Inhibitor, systemic lupus erythematosus (presence of) D68.62

Iniencephalus, iniencephaly Q00.2

Injection, traumatic jet (air) (industrial) (water) (paint or dye) T70.4 ☑

Injury — see also specified injury type T14.90 ☑
- abdomen, abdominal S39.91 ☑
  - blood vessel — see Injury, blood vessel, abdomen
  - cavity — see Injury, intra-abdominal
  - contusion S30.1
  - internal — see Injury, intra-abdominal
  - intra-abdominal organ — see Injury, intra-abdominal
  - nerve — see Injury, nerve, abdomen
  - open — see Wound, open, abdomen
  - specified NEC S39.81 ☑
  - superficial — see Injury, superficial, abdomen
- Achilles tendon S86.00- ☑
  - laceration S86.02- ☑
  - specified type NEC S86.09- ☑
  - strain S86.01- ☑
- acoustic, resulting in deafness — see Injury, nerve, acoustic
- adrenal (gland) S37.819 ☑
  - contusion S37.812 ☑
  - laceration S37.813 ☑
  - specified type NEC S37.818 ☑
- alveolar (process) S09.93 ☑
- ankle S99.91- ☑
  - contusion — see Contusion, ankle
  - dislocation — see Dislocation, ankle
  - fracture — see Fracture, ankle
  - nerve — see Injury, nerve, ankle
  - open — see Wound, open, ankle
  - specified type NEC S99.81- ☑
  - sprain — see Sprain, ankle
  - superficial — see Injury, superficial, ankle
- anterior chamber, eye — see Injury, eye, specified site NEC
- anus — see Injury, abdomen
- aorta (thoracic) S25.00 ☑
  - abdominal S35.00 ☑
    - laceration (minor) (superficial) S35.01 ☑
      - major S35.02 ☑
    - specified type NEC S35.09 ☑
  - laceration (minor) (superficial) S25.01 ☑
    - major S25.02 ☑
  - specified type NEC S25.09 ☑
- arm (upper) S49.9- ☑
  - blood vessel — see Injury, blood vessel, arm
  - contusion — see Contusion, arm, upper
  - fracture — see Fracture, humerus
  - lower — see Injury, forearm
  - muscle — see Injury, muscle, shoulder
  - nerve — see Injury, nerve, arm
  - open — see Wound, open, arm
  - specified type NEC S49.8- ☑
  - superficial — see Injury, superficial, arm
- artery (complicating trauma) — see also Injury, blood vessel, by site
  - cerebral or meningeal — see Injury, intracranial
- auditory canal (external) (meatus) S09.91 ☑
- auricle, auris, ear S09.91 ☑
- axilla — see Injury, shoulder
- back — see Injury, back, lower
- bile duct S36.13 ☑
- birth — see also Birth, injury P15.9
- bladder (sphincter) S37.20 ☑
  - at delivery O71.5
  - contusion S37.22 ☑
  - laceration S37.23 ☑
  - obstetrical trauma O71.5
  - specified type NEC S37.29 ☑
- blast (air) (hydraulic) (immersion) (underwater) NEC T14.8 ☑

Injury — continued
- blast — continued
  - acoustic nerve trauma — see Injury, nerve, acoustic
  - bladder — see Injury, bladder
  - brain — see Concussion
  - colon — see Injury, intestine, large
  - ear (primary) S09.31- ☑
    - secondary S09.39- ☑
  - generalized T70.8 ☑
  - lung — see Injury, intrathoracic, lung
  - multiple body organs T70.8 ☑
  - peritoneum S36.81 ☑
  - rectum S36.61 ☑
  - retroperitoneum S36.898 ☑
  - small intestine S36.419 ☑
    - duodenum S36.410 ☑
    - specified site NEC S36.418 ☑
  - specified
    - intra-abdominal organ NEC S36.898 ☑
    - pelvic organ NEC S37.899 ☑
- blood vessel NEC T14.8 ☑
  - abdomen S35.9 ☑
    - aorta — see Injury, aorta, abdominal
    - celiac artery — see Injury, blood vessel, celiac artery
    - iliac vessel — see Injury, blood vessel, iliac
    - laceration S35.91 ☑
    - mesenteric vessel — see Injury, mesenteric
    - portal vein — see Injury, blood vessel, portal vein
    - renal vessel — see Injury, blood vessel, renal
    - specified vessel NEC S35.8X- ☑
    - splenic vessel — see Injury, blood vessel, splenic
    - vena cava — see Injury, vena cava, inferior
  - ankle — see Injury, blood vessel, foot
  - aorta (abdominal) (thoracic) — see Injury, aorta
  - arm (upper) NEC S45.90- ☑
    - forearm — see Injury, blood vessel, forearm
    - laceration S45.91- ☑
    - specified
      - site NEC S45.80- ☑
        - laceration S45.81- ☑
        - specified type NEC S45.89- ☑
      - type NEC S45.99- ☑
    - superficial vein S45.30- ☑
      - laceration S45.31- ☑
      - specified type NEC S45.39- ☑
  - axillary
    - artery S45.00- ☑
      - laceration S45.01- ☑
      - specified type NEC S45.09- ☑
    - vein S45.20- ☑
      - laceration S45.21- ☑
      - specified type NEC S45.29- ☑
  - azygos vein — see Injury, blood vessel, thoracic, specified site NEC
  - brachial
    - artery S45.10- ☑
      - laceration S45.11- ☑
      - specified type NEC S45.19- ☑
    - vein S45.20- ☑
      - laceration S45.219 ☑
      - specified type NEC S45.29- ☑
  - carotid artery (common) (external) (internal, extracranial) S15.00- ☑
    - internal, intracranial S06.8- ☑
    - laceration (minor) (superficial) S15.01- ☑
      - major S15.02- ☑
    - specified type NEC S15.09- ☑
  - celiac artery S35.219 ☑
    - branch S35.299 ☑
      - laceration (minor) (superficial) S35.291
        - major S35.292 ☑
      - specified NEC S35.298 ☑
    - laceration (minor) (superficial) S35.211 ☑
      - major S35.212 ☑
    - specified type NEC S35.218 ☑
  - cerebral — see Injury, intracranial
  - deep plantar — see Injury, blood vessel, plantar artery
  - digital (hand) — see Injury, blood vessel, finger
  - dorsal
    - artery (foot) S95.00- ☑
      - laceration S95.01- ☑
      - specified type NEC S95.09- ☑
    - vein (foot) S95.20- ☑
      - laceration S95.21- ☑

Injury — continued
- blood vessel — continued
  - dorsal — continued
    - vein — continued
      - specified type NEC S95.29- ☑
  - due to accidental laceration during procedure — see Laceration, accidental complicating surgery
  - extremity — see Injury, blood vessel, limb
  - femoral
    - artery (common) (superficial) S75.00- ☑
      - laceration (minor) (superficial) S75.01- ☑
        - major S75.02- ☑
      - specified type NEC S75.09- ☑
    - vein (hip level) (thigh level) S75.10- ☑
      - laceration (minor) (superficial) S75.11- ☑
        - major S75.12- ☑
      - specified type NEC S75.19- ☑
  - finger S65.50- ☑
    - index S65.50- ☑
      - laceration S65.51- ☑
      - specified type NEC S65.59- ☑
    - laceration S65.51- ☑
    - little S65.50- ☑
      - laceration S65.51- ☑
      - specified type NEC S65.59- ☑
    - middle S65.50- ☑
      - laceration S65.51- ☑
      - specified type NEC S65.59- ☑
    - specified type NEC S65.59- ☑
    - thumb — see Injury, blood vessel, thumb
  - foot S95.90- ☑
    - dorsal
      - artery — see Injury, blood vessel, dorsal, artery
      - vein — see Injury, blood vessel, dorsal, vein
    - laceration S95.91- ☑
    - plantar artery — see Injury, blood vessel, plantar artery
    - specified
      - site NEC S95.80- ☑
        - laceration S95.81- ☑
        - specified type NEC S95.89- ☑
      - specified type NEC S95.99- ☑
  - forearm S55.90- ☑
    - laceration S55.91- ☑
    - radial artery — see Injury, blood vessel, radial artery
    - specified
      - site NEC S55.80- ☑
        - laceration S55.81- ☑
        - specified type NEC S55.89- ☑
      - type NEC S55.99- ☑
    - ulnar artery — see Injury, blood vessel, ulnar artery
    - vein S55.20- ☑
      - laceration S55.21- ☑
      - specified type NEC S55.29- ☑
  - gastric
    - artery — see Injury, mesenteric, artery, branch
    - vein — see Injury, blood vessel, abdomen
  - gastroduodenal artery — see Injury, mesenteric, artery, branch
  - greater saphenous vein (lower leg level) S85.30- ☑
    - hip (and thigh) level S75.20- ☑
      - laceration (minor) (superficial) S75.21- ☑
        - major S75.22- ☑
      - specified type NEC S75.29- ☑
    - laceration S85.31- ☑
    - specified type NEC S85.39- ☑
  - hand (level) S65.90- ☑
    - finger — see Injury, blood vessel, finger
    - laceration S65.91- ☑
    - palmar arch — see Injury, blood vessel, palmar arch
    - radial artery — see Injury, blood vessel, radial artery, hand
    - specified
      - site NEC S65.80- ☑
        - laceration S65.81- ☑
        - specified type NEC S65.89- ☑
      - type NEC S65.99- ☑
    - thumb — see Injury, blood vessel, thumb
    - ulnar artery — see Injury, blood vessel, ulnar artery, hand
  - head S09.0 ☑

☑ **Additional Character Required** — Refer to the Tabular List for Character Selection

☒ Subterms under main terms may continue to next column or page

Injury — continued
  blood vessel — continued
    head — continued
      intracranial — see Injury, intracranial
      multiple S09.0 ☑
    hepatic
      artery — see Injury, mesenteric, artery
      vein — see Injury, vena cava, inferior
    hip S75.90- ☑
      femoral artery — see Injury, blood vessel,
        femoral, artery
      femoral vein — see Injury, blood vessel, femoral,
        vein
      greater saphenous vein — see Injury, blood ves-
        sel, greater saphenous, hip level
      laceration S75.91- ☑
      specified
        site NEC S75.80- ☑
          laceration S75.81- ☑
          specified type NEC S75.89- ☑
        type NEC S75.99- ☑
    hypogastric (artery) (vein) — see Injury, blood ves-
      sel, iliac
    iliac S35.5- ☑
      artery S35.51- ☑
      specified vessel NEC S35.5- ☑
      uterine vessel — see Injury, blood vessel, uterine
      vein S35.51- ☑
    innominate — see Injury, blood vessel, thoracic, in-
      nominate
    intercostal (artery) (vein) — see Injury, blood vessel,
      thoracic, intercostal
    jugular vein (external) S15.20- ☑
      internal S15.30- ☑
        laceration (minor) (superficial) S15.31- ☑
          major S15.32- ☑
        specified type NEC S15.39- ☑
      laceration (minor) (superficial) S15.21- ☑
        major S15.22- ☑
      specified type NEC S15.29- ☑
    leg (level) (lower) S85.90- ☑
      greater saphenous — see Injury, blood vessel,
        greater saphenous
      laceration S85.91- ☑
      lesser saphenous — see Injury, blood vessel,
        lesser saphenous
      peroneal artery — see Injury, blood vessel, per-
        oneal artery
      popliteal
        artery — see Injury, blood vessel, popliteal,
          artery
        vein — see Injury, blood vessel, popliteal, vein
      specified
        site NEC S85.80- ☑
          laceration S85.81- ☑
          specified type NEC S85.89- ☑
        type NEC S85.99- ☑
      thigh — see Injury, blood vessel, hip
      tibial artery — see Injury, blood vessel, tibial
        artery
    lesser saphenous vein (lower leg level) S85.40- ☑
      laceration S85.41- ☑
      specified type NEC S85.49- ☑
    limb
      lower — see Injury, blood vessel, leg
      upper — see Injury, blood vessel, arm
    lower back — see Injury, blood vessel, abdomen
      specified NEC — see Injury, blood vessel, ab-
        domen, specified, site NEC
    mammary (artery) (vein) — see Injury, blood vessel,
      thoracic, specified site NEC
    mesenteric (inferior) (superior)
      artery — see Injury, mesenteric, artery
      vein — see Injury, blood vessel, mesenteric, vein
    neck S15.9 ☑
      specified site NEC S15.8 ☑
    ovarian (artery) (vein) — see subcategory S35.8 ☑
    palmar arch (superficial) S65.20- ☑
      deep S65.30- ☑
        laceration S65.31- ☑
        specified type NEC S65.39- ☑
      laceration S65.21- ☑
      specified type NEC S65.29- ☑
    pelvis — see Injury, blood vessel, abdomen
      specified NEC — see Injury, blood vessel, ab-
        domen, specified, site NEC

Injury — continued
  blood vessel — continued
    peroneal artery S85.20- ☑
      laceration S85.21- ☑
      specified type NEC S85.29- ☑
    plantar artery (deep) (foot) S95.10- ☑
      laceration S95.11- ☑
      specified type NEC S95.19- ☑
    popliteal
      artery S85.00- ☑
        laceration S85.01- ☑
        specified type NEC S85.09- ☑
      vein S85.50- ☑
        laceration S85.51- ☑
        specified type NEC S85.59- ☑
    portal vein S35.319 ☑
      laceration S35.311 ☑
      specified type NEC S35.318 ☑
    precerebral — see Injury, blood vessel, neck
    pulmonary (artery) (vein) — see Injury, blood vessel,
      thoracic, pulmonary
    radial artery (forearm level) S55.10- ☑
      hand and wrist (level) S65.10- ☑
        laceration S65.11- ☑
        specified type NEC S65.19- ☑
      laceration S55.11- ☑
      specified type NEC S55.19- ☑
    renal
      artery S35.40- ☑
        laceration S35.41- ☑
        specified type NEC S35.49- ☑
      vein S35.40- ☑
        laceration S35.41- ☑
        specified NEC S35.49- ☑
    saphenous vein (greater) (lower leg level) — see
      Injury, blood vessel, greater saphenous
      hip and thigh level — see Injury, blood vessel,
        greater saphenous, hip level
      lesser — see Injury, blood vessel, lesser saphe-
        nous
    shoulder
      specified NEC — see Injury, blood vessel, arm,
        specified site NEC
      superficial vein — see Injury, blood vessel, arm,
        superficial vein
    specified NEC T14.8 ☑
    splenic
      artery — see Injury, blood vessel, celiac artery,
        branch
      vein S35.329 ☑
        laceration S35.321 ☑
        specified NEC S35.328 ☑
    subclavian — see Injury, blood vessel, thoracic, in-
      nominate
    thigh — see Injury, blood vessel, hip
    thoracic S25.90 ☑
      aorta S25.00 ☑
        laceration (minor) (superficial) S25.01 ☑
          major S25.02 ☑
        specified type NEC S25.09 ☑
      azygos vein — see Injury, blood vessel, thoracic,
        specified, site NEC
      innominate
        artery S25.10- ☑
          laceration (minor) (superficial) S25.11- ☑
            major S25.12- ☑
          specified type NEC S25.19- ☑
        vein S25.30- ☑
          laceration (minor) (superficial) S25.31- ☑
            major S25.32- ☑
          specified type NEC S25.39- ☑
      intercostal S25.50- ☑
        laceration S25.51- ☑
        specified type NEC S25.59- ☑
      laceration S25.91 ☑
      mammary vessel — see Injury, blood vessel,
        thoracic, specified, site NEC
      pulmonary S25.40- ☑
        laceration (minor) (superficial) S25.41- ☑
          major S25.42- ☑
        specified type NEC S25.49- ☑
      specified
        site NEC S25.80- ☑
          laceration S25.81 ☑
          specified type NEC S25.89 ☑
        type NEC S25.99 ☑

Injury — continued
  blood vessel — continued
    thoracic — continued
      subclavian — see Injury, blood vessel, thoracic,
        innominate
      vena cava (superior) S25.20 ☑
        laceration (minor) (superficial) S25.21 ☑
          major S25.22 ☑
        specified type NEC S25.29 ☑
    thumb S65.40- ☑
      laceration S65.41- ☑
      specified type NEC S65.49- ☑
    tibial artery S85.10- ☑
      anterior S85.13- ☑
        laceration S85.14- ☑
        specified injury NEC S85.15- ☑
      laceration S85.11- ☑
      posterior S85.16- ☑
        laceration S85.17- ☑
        specified injury NEC S85.18- ☑
      specified injury NEC S85.12- ☑
    ulnar artery (forearm level) S55.00- ☑
      hand and wrist (level) S65.00- ☑
        laceration S65.01- ☑
        specified type NEC S65.09- ☑
      laceration S55.01- ☑
      specified type NEC S55.09- ☑
    upper arm (level) — see Injury, blood vessel, arm
      superficial vein — see Injury, blood vessel, arm,
        superficial vein
    uterine S35.5- ☑
      artery S35.53- ☑
      vein S35.53- ☑
    vena cava — see Injury, vena cava
    vertebral artery S15.10- ☑
      laceration (minor) (superficial) S15.11- ☑
        major S15.12- ☑
      specified type NEC S15.19- ☑
    wrist (level) — see Injury, blood vessel, hand
  brachial plexus S14.3 ☑
    newborn P14.3
  brain (traumatic) S06.9- ☑
    diffuse (axonal) S06.2X- ☑
    focal S06.30- ☑
  brainstem S06.38- ☑
  breast NOS S29.9 ☑
  broad ligament — see Injury, pelvic organ, specified
    site NEC
  bronchus, bronchi — see Injury, intrathoracic, bronchus
  brow S09.90 ☑
  buttock S39.92 ☑
  canthus, eye S05.90 ☑
  cardiac plexus — see Injury, nerve, thorax, sympathetic
  cauda equina S34.3 ☑
  cavernous sinus — see Injury, intracranial
  cecum — see Injury, colon
  celiac ganglion or plexus — see Injury, nerve, lum-
    bosacral, sympathetic
  cerebellum — see Injury, intracranial
  cerebral — see Injury, intracranial
  cervix (uteri) — see Injury, uterus
  cheek (wall) S09.93 ☑
  chest — see Injury, thorax
  childbirth (newborn) — see also Birth, injury
    maternal NEC O71.9
  chin S09.93 ☑
  choroid (eye) — see Injury, eye, specified site NEC
  clitoris S39.94 ☑
  coccyx — see also Injury, back, lower
    complicating delivery O71.6
  colon — see Injury, intestine, large
  common bile duct — see Injury, liver
  conjunctiva (superficial) — see Injury, eye, conjunctiva
  conus medullaris — see Injury, spinal, sacral
  cord
    spermatic (pelvic region) S37.898 ☑
      scrotal region S39.848 ☑
    spinal — see Injury, spinal cord, by region
  cornea — see Injury, eye, specified site NEC
    abrasion — see Injury, eye, cornea, abrasion
  cortex (cerebral) — see also Injury, intracranial
    visual — see Injury, nerve, optic
  costal region NEC S29.9 ☑
  costochondral NEC S29.9 ☑
  cranial
    cavity — see Injury, intracranial

Injury — *continued*
cranial — *continued*
   nerve — *see* Injury, nerve, cranial
  crushing — *see* Crush
  cutaneous sensory nerve
  cystic duct — *see* Injury, liver
  deep tissue — *see* Contusion, by site
   meaning pressure ulcer — *see* Ulcer, pressure L89
    with final character .6
  delivery (newborn) P15.9
   maternal NEC O71.9
  Descemet's membrane — *see* Injury, eyeball, penetrating
  diaphragm — *see* Injury, intrathoracic, diaphragm
  duodenum — *see* Injury, intestine, small, duodenum
  ear (auricle) (external) (canal) S09.91 ☑
   abrasion — *see* Abrasion, ear
   bite — *see* Bite, ear
   blister — *see* Blister, ear
   bruise — *see* Contusion, ear
   contusion — *see* Contusion, ear
   external constriction — *see* Constriction, external, ear
   hematoma — *see* Hematoma, ear
   inner — *see* Injury, ear, middle
   laceration — *see* Laceration, ear
   middle S09.30- ☑
    blast — *see* Injury, blast, ear
    specified NEC S09.39- ☑
   puncture — *see* Puncture, ear
   superficial — *see* Injury, superficial, ear
  eighth cranial nerve (acoustic or auditory) — *see* Injury, nerve, acoustic
  elbow S59.90- ☑
   contusion — *see* Contusion, elbow
   dislocation — *see* Dislocation, elbow
   fracture — *see* Fracture, ulna, upper end
   open — *see* Wound, open, elbow
   specified NEC S59.80- ☑
   sprain — *see* Sprain, elbow
   superficial — *see* Injury, superficial, elbow
  eleventh cranial nerve (accessory) — *see* Injury, nerve, accessory
  epididymis S39.94 ☑
  epigastric region S39.91 ☑
  epiglottis NEC S19.89 ☑
  esophageal plexus — *see* Injury, nerve, thorax, sympathetic
  esophagus (thoracic part) — *see also* Injury, intrathoracic, esophagus
   cervical NEC S19.85 ☑
  eustachian tube S09.30 ☑
  eye S05.9- ☑
   avulsion S05.7- ☑
   ball — *see* Injury, eyeball
   conjunctiva S05.0- ☑
   cornea
    abrasion S05.0- ☑
   laceration S05.3- ☑
    with prolapse S05.2- ☑
   lacrimal apparatus S05.8X- ☑
   orbit penetration S05.4- ☑
   specified site NEC S05.8X- ☑
  eyeball S05.8X- ☑
   contusion S05.1- ☑
   penetrating S05.6- ☑
    with
     foreign body S05.5- ☑
     prolapse or loss of intraocular tissue S05.2- ☑
     without prolapse or loss of intraocular tissue S05.3- ☑
   specified type NEC S05.8- ☑
  eyebrow S09.93 ☑
  eyelid S09.93 ☑
   abrasion — *see* Abrasion, eyelid
   contusion — *see* Contusion, eyelid
   open — *see* Wound, open, eyelid
  face S09.93 ☑
  fallopian tube S37.509 ☑
   bilateral S37.502 ☑
    blast injury S37.512 ☑
    contusion S37.522 ☑
    laceration S37.532 ☑
    specified type NEC S37.592 ☑
   blast injury (primary) S37.519 ☑
    bilateral S37.512 ☑

Injury — *continued*
fallopian tube — *continued*
  blast injury — *continued*
   secondary — *see* Injury, fallopian tube, specified type NEC
   unilateral S37.511 ☑
  contusion S37.529 ☑
   bilateral S37.522 ☑
   unilateral S37.521 ☑
  laceration S37.539 ☑
   bilateral S37.532 ☑
   unilateral S37.531 ☑
  specified type NEC S37.599 ☑
   bilateral S37.592 ☑
   unilateral S37.591 ☑
  unilateral S37.501 ☑
   blast injury S37.511 ☑
   contusion S37.521 ☑
   laceration S37.531 ☑
   specified type NEC S37.591 ☑
  fascia — *see* Injury, muscle
  fifth cranial nerve (trigeminal) — *see* Injury, nerve, trigeminal
  finger (nail) S69.9- ☑
   blood vessel — *see* Injury, blood vessel, finger
   contusion — *see* Contusion, finger
   dislocation — *see* Dislocation, finger
   fracture — *see* Fracture, finger
   muscle — *see* Injury, muscle, finger
   nerve — *see* Injury, nerve, digital, finger
   open — *see* Wound, open, finger
   specified NEC S69.8- ☑
   sprain — *see* Sprain, finger
   superficial — *see* Injury, superficial, finger
  first cranial nerve (olfactory) — *see* Injury, nerve, olfactory
  flank — *see* Injury, abdomen
  foot S99.92- ☑
   blood vessel — *see* Injury, blood vessel, foot
   contusion — *see* Contusion, foot
   dislocation — *see* Dislocation, foot
   fracture — *see* Fracture, foot
   muscle — *see* Injury, muscle, foot
   open — *see* Wound, open, foot
   specified type NEC S99.82- ☑
   sprain — *see* Sprain, foot
   superficial — *see* Injury, superficial, foot
  forceps NOS P15.9
  forearm S59.91- ☑
   blood vessel — *see* Injury, blood vessel, forearm
   contusion — *see* Contusion, forearm
   fracture — *see* Fracture, forearm
   muscle — *see* Injury, muscle, forearm
   nerve — *see* Injury, nerve, forearm
   open — *see* Wound, open, forearm
   specified NEC S59.81- ☑
   superficial — *see* Injury, superficial, forearm
  forehead S09.90 ☑
  fourth cranial nerve (trochlear) — *see* Injury, nerve, trochlear
  gallbladder S36.129 ☑
   contusion S36.122 ☑
   laceration S36.123 ☑
   specified NEC S36.128 ☑
  ganglion
   celiac, coeliac — *see* Injury, nerve, lumbosacral, sympathetic
   gasserian — *see* Injury, nerve, trigeminal
   stellate — *see* Injury, nerve, thorax, sympathetic
   thoracic sympathetic — *see* Injury, nerve, thorax, sympathetic
  gasserian ganglion — *see* Injury, nerve, trigeminal
  gastric artery — *see* Injury, blood vessel, celiac artery, branch
  gastroduodenal artery — *see* Injury, blood vessel, celiac artery, branch
  gastrointestinal tract — *see* Injury, intra-abdominal
   with open wound into abdominal cavity — *see* Wound, open, with penetration into peritoneal cavity
   colon — *see* Injury, intestine, large
   rectum — *see* Injury, intestine, large, rectum
    with open wound into abdominal cavity S36.61 ☑
   small intestine — *see* Injury, intestine, small

Injury — *continued*
gastrointestinal tract — *see* Injury, intra-abdominal — *continued*
  specified site NEC — *see* Injury, intra-abdominal, specified, site NEC
  stomach — *see* Injury, stomach
  genital organ(s)
   external S39.94 ☑
    specified NEC S39.848 ☑
   internal S37.90 ☑
    fallopian tube — *see* Injury, fallopian tube
    ovary — *see* Injury, ovary
    prostate — *see* Injury, prostate
    seminal vesicle — *see* Injury, pelvis, organ, specified site NEC
    uterus — *see* Injury, uterus
    vas deferens — *see* Injury, pelvis, organ, specified site NEC
   obstetrical trauma O71.9
  gland
   lacrimal laceration — *see* Injury, eye, specified site NEC
   salivary S09.93 ☑
   thyroid NEC S19.84 ☑
  globe (eye) S05.90 ☑
   specified NEC S05.8X- ☑
  groin — *see* Injury, abdomen
  gum S09.90 ☑
  hand S69.9- ☑
   blood vessel — *see* Injury, blood vessel, hand
   contusion — *see* Contusion, hand
   fracture — *see* Fracture, hand
   muscle — *see* Injury, muscle, hand
   nerve — *see* Injury, nerve, hand
   open — *see* Wound, open, hand
   specified NEC S69.8- ☑
   sprain — *see* Sprain, hand
   superficial — *see* Injury, superficial, hand
  head S09.90 ☑
   with loss of consciousness S06.9- ☑
   specified NEC S09.8 ☑
  heart (traumatic) S26.90 ☑
   with hemopericardium S26.00 ☑
    contusion S26.01 ☑
    laceration (mild) S26.020 ☑
     major S26.022 ☑
     moderate S26.021 ☑
    specified type NEC S26.09 ☑
   contusion S26.91 ☑
   laceration S26.92 ☑
   non-traumatic (acute) (chronic) (non-ischemic) I5A
   specified type NEC S26.99 ☑
   without hemopericardium S26.10 ☑
    contusion S26.11 ☑
    laceration S26.12 ☑
    specified type NEC S26.19 ☑
  heel — *see* Injury, foot
  hepatic
   artery — *see* Injury, blood vessel, celiac artery, branch
   duct — *see* Injury, liver
   vein — *see* Injury, vena cava, inferior
  hip S79.91- ☑
   blood vessel — *see* Injury, blood vessel, hip
   contusion — *see* Contusion, hip
   dislocation — *see* Dislocation, hip
   fracture — *see* Fracture, femur, neck
   muscle — *see* Injury, muscle, hip
   nerve — *see* Injury, nerve, hip
   open — *see* Wound, open, hip
   specified NEC S79.81- ☑
   sprain — *see* Sprain, hip
   superficial — *see* Injury, superficial, hip
  hymen S39.94 ☑
  hypogastric
   blood vessel — *see* Injury, blood vessel, iliac
   plexus — *see* Injury, nerve, lumbosacral, sympathetic
  ileum — *see* Injury, intestine, small
  iliac region S39.91 ☑
  instrumental (during surgery) — *see* Laceration, accidental complicating surgery
   birth injury — *see* Birth, injury
   nonsurgical — *see* Injury, by site
   obstetrical O71.9
    bladder O71.5

☑ **Additional Character Required** — **Refer to the Tabular List for Character Selection**   ▽ **Subterms under main terms may continue to next column or page**

Injury — *continued*
- instrumental — *see* Laceration, accidental complicating
  - surgery — *continued*
  - obstetrical — *continued*
    - cervix O71.3
    - high vaginal O71.4
    - perineal NOS O70.9
    - urethra O71.5
    - uterus O71.5
      - with rupture or perforation O71.1
- internal T14.8 ☑
  - aorta — *see* Injury, aorta
  - bladder (sphincter) — *see* Injury, bladder
    - with
      - ectopic or molar pregnancy O08.6
      - following ectopic or molar pregnancy O08.6
      - obstetrical trauma O71.5
  - bronchus, bronchi — *see* Injury, intrathoracic, bronchus
  - cecum — *see* Injury, intestine, large
  - cervix (uteri) — *see also* Injury, uterus
    - with ectopic or molar pregnancy O08.6
    - following ectopic or molar pregnancy O08.6
    - obstetrical trauma O71.3
  - chest — *see* Injury, intrathoracic
  - gastrointestinal tract — *see* Injury, intra-abdominal
  - heart — *see* Injury, heart
  - intestine NEC — *see* Injury, intestine
  - intrauterine — *see* Injury, uterus
  - mesentery — *see* Injury, intra-abdominal, specified, site NEC
  - pelvis, pelvic (organ) S37.90 ☑
    - following ectopic or molar pregnancy (subsequent episode) O08.6
    - obstetrical trauma NEC O71.5
    - rupture or perforation O71.1
    - specified NEC S39.83 ☑
  - rectum — *see* Injury, intestine, large, rectum
  - stomach — *see* Injury, stomach
  - ureter — *see* Injury, ureter
  - urethra (sphincter) following ectopic or molar pregnancy O08.6
  - uterus — *see* Injury, uterus
- interscapular area — *see* Injury, thorax
- intestine
  - large S36.509 ☑
    - ascending (right) S36.500 ☑
      - blast injury (primary) S36.510 ☑
        - secondary S36.590 ☑
      - contusion S36.520 ☑
      - laceration S36.530 ☑
      - specified type NEC S36.590 ☑
    - blast injury (primary) S36.519 ☑
      - ascending (right) S36.510 ☑
      - descending (left) S36.512 ☑
      - rectum S36.61 ☑
      - sigmoid S36.513 ☑
      - specified site NEC S36.518 ☑
      - transverse S36.511 ☑
    - contusion S36.529 ☑
      - ascending (right) S36.520 ☑
      - descending (left) S36.522 ☑
      - rectum S36.62 ☑
      - sigmoid S36.523 ☑
      - specified site NEC S36.528 ☑
      - transverse S36.521 ☑
    - descending (left) S36.502 ☑
      - blast injury (primary) S36.512 ☑
        - secondary S36.592 ☑
      - contusion S36.522 ☑
      - laceration S36.532 ☑
      - specified type NEC S36.592 ☑
    - laceration S36.539 ☑
      - ascending (right) S36.530 ☑
      - descending (left) S36.532 ☑
      - rectum S36.63 ☑
      - sigmoid S36.533 ☑
      - specified site NEC S36.538 ☑
      - transverse S36.531 ☑
    - rectum S36.60 ☑
      - blast injury (primary) S36.61 ☑
        - secondary S36.69 ☑
      - contusion S36.62 ☑
      - laceration S36.63 ☑
      - specified type NEC S36.69 ☑
    - sigmoid S36.503 ☑

Injury — *continued*
- intestine — *continued*
  - large — *continued*
    - sigmoid — *continued*
      - blast injury (primary) S36.513 ☑
        - secondary S36.593 ☑
      - contusion S36.523 ☑
      - laceration S36.533 ☑
      - specified type NEC S36.593 ☑
    - specified
      - site NEC S36.508 ☑
        - blast injury (primary) S36.518 ☑
          - secondary S36.598 ☑
        - contusion S36.528 ☑
        - laceration S36.538 ☑
        - specified type NEC S36.598 ☑
      - type NEC S36.599 ☑
        - ascending (right) S36.590 ☑
        - descending (left) S36.592 ☑
        - rectum S36.69 ☑
        - sigmoid S36.593 ☑
        - specified site NEC S36.598 ☑
        - transverse S36.591 ☑
    - transverse S36.501 ☑
      - blast injury (primary) S36.511 ☑
        - secondary S36.591 ☑
      - contusion S36.521 ☑
      - laceration S36.531 ☑
      - specified type NEC S36.591 ☑
  - small S36.409 ☑
    - blast injury (primary) S36.419 ☑
      - duodenum S36.410 ☑
      - secondary S36.499 ☑
        - duodenum S36.490 ☑
        - specified site NEC S36.498 ☑
      - specified site NEC S36.418 ☑
    - contusion S36.429 ☑
      - duodenum S36.420 ☑
      - specified site NEC S36.428 ☑
    - duodenum S36.400 ☑
      - blast injury (primary) S36.410 ☑
        - secondary S36.490 ☑
      - contusion S36.420 ☑
      - laceration S36.430 ☑
      - specified NEC S36.490 ☑
    - laceration S36.439 ☑
      - duodenum S36.430 ☑
      - specified site NEC S36.438 ☑
    - specified
      - site NEC S36.408 ☑
      - type NEC S36.499 ☑
        - duodenum S36.490 ☑
        - specified site NEC S36.498 ☑
  - intra-abdominal S36.90 ☑
    - adrenal gland — *see* Injury, adrenal gland
    - bladder — *see* Injury, bladder
    - colon — *see* Injury, intestine, large
    - contusion S36.92 ☑
    - fallopian tube — *see* Injury, fallopian tube
    - gallbladder — *see* Injury, gallbladder
    - intestine — *see* Injury, intestine
    - kidney — *see* Injury, kidney
    - laceration S36.93 ☑
    - liver — *see* Injury, liver
    - ovary — *see* Injury, ovary
    - pancreas — *see* Injury, pancreas
    - pelvic NOS S37.90 ☑
    - peritoneum — *see* Injury, intra-abdominal, specified, site NEC
    - prostate — *see* Injury, prostate
    - rectum — *see* Injury, intestine, large, rectum
    - retroperitoneum — *see* Injury, intra-abdominal, specified, site NEC
    - seminal vesicle — *see* Injury, pelvis, organ, specified site NEC
    - small intestine — *see* Injury, intestine, small
    - specified
      - pelvic S37.90 ☑
        - specified
          - site NEC S37.899 ☑
            - specified type NEC S37.898 ☑
          - type NEC S37.99 ☑
      - site NEC S36.899 ☑
        - contusion S36.892 ☑
        - laceration S36.893 ☑
        - specified type NEC S36.898 ☑

Injury — *continued*
- intra-abdominal — *continued*
  - specified — *continued*
    - type NEC S36.99 ☑
  - spleen — *see* Injury, spleen
  - stomach — *see* Injury, stomach
  - ureter — *see* Injury, ureter
  - urethra — *see* Injury, urethra
  - uterus — *see* Injury, uterus
  - vas deferens — *see* Injury, pelvis, organ, specified site NEC
- intracranial (traumatic) — *see also* if applicable, Compression, brain, traumatic S06.9- ☑
  - cerebellar hemorrhage, traumatic — *see* Injury, intracranial, focal
  - cerebral edema, traumatic S06.1X- ☑
    - diffuse S06.1X- ☑
    - focal S06.1X- ☑
  - diffuse (axonal) S06.2X- ☑
  - epidural hemorrhage (traumatic) S06.4X- ☑
  - focal brain injury S06.30- ☑
    - contusion — *see* Contusion, cerebral
    - laceration — *see* Laceration, cerebral
    - intracerebral hemorrhage, traumatic S06.36- ☑
      - left side S06.35- ☑
      - right side S06.34- ☑
    - subarachnoid hemorrhage, traumatic S06.6X- ☑
    - subdural hemorrhage, traumatic S06.5X- ☑
- intraocular — *see* Injury, eyeball, penetrating
- intrathoracic S27.9 ☑
  - bronchus S27.409 ☑
    - bilateral S27.402 ☑
    - blast injury (primary) S27.419 ☑
      - bilateral S27.412 ☑
      - secondary — *see* Injury, intrathoracic, bronchus, specified type NEC
      - unilateral S27.411 ☑
    - contusion S27.429 ☑
      - bilateral S27.422 ☑
      - unilateral S27.421 ☑
    - laceration S27.439 ☑
      - bilateral S27.432 ☑
      - unilateral S27.431 ☑
    - specified type NEC S27.499 ☑
      - bilateral S27.492 ☑
      - unilateral S27.491 ☑
    - unilateral S27.401 ☑
  - diaphragm S27.809 ☑
    - contusion S27.802 ☑
    - laceration S27.803 ☑
    - specified type NEC S27.808 ☑
  - esophagus (thoracic) S27.819 ☑
    - contusion S27.812 ☑
    - laceration S27.813 ☑
    - specified type NEC S27.818 ☑
  - heart — *see* Injury, heart
  - hemopneumothorax S27.2 ☑
  - hemothorax S27.1 ☑
  - lung S27.309 ☑
    - aspiration J69.0
    - bilateral S27.302 ☑
    - blast injury (primary) S27.319 ☑
      - bilateral S27.312 ☑
      - secondary — *see* Injury, intrathoracic, lung, specified type NEC
      - unilateral S27.311 ☑
    - contusion S27.329 ☑
      - bilateral S27.322 ☑
      - unilateral S27.321 ☑
    - laceration S27.339 ☑
      - bilateral S27.332 ☑
      - unilateral S27.331 ☑
    - specified type NEC S27.399 ☑
      - bilateral S27.392 ☑
      - unilateral S27.391 ☑
    - unilateral S27.301 ☑
  - pleura S27.60 ☑
    - laceration S27.63 ☑
    - specified type NEC S27.69 ☑
  - pneumothorax S27.0 ☑
  - specified organ NEC S27.899 ☑
    - contusion S27.892 ☑
    - laceration S27.893 ☑
    - specified type NEC S27.898 ☑
  - thoracic duct — *see* Injury, intrathoracic, specified organ NEC

Injury — *continued*
  intrathoracic — *continued*
    thymus gland — *see* Injury, intrathoracic, specified organ NEC
    trachea, thoracic S27.50 ☑
      blast (primary) S27.51 ☑
      contusion S27.52 ☑
      laceration S27.53 ☑
      specified type NEC S27.59 ☑
  iris — *see* Injury, eye, specified site NEC
    penetrating — *see* Injury, eyeball, penetrating
  jaw S09.93 ☑
  jejunum — *see* Injury, intestine, small
  joint NOS T14.8 ☑
    old or residual — *see* Disorder, joint, specified type NEC
  kidney S37.00- ☑
    acute (nontraumatic) N17.9
    contusion — *see* Contusion, kidney
    laceration — *see* Laceration, kidney
    specified NEC S37.09- ☑
  knee S89.9- ☑
    contusion — *see* Contusion, knee
    dislocation — *see* Dislocation, knee
    meniscus (lateral) (medial) — *see* Sprain, knee, specified site NEC
      old injury or tear — *see* Derangement, knee, meniscus, due to old injury
    open — *see* Wound, open, knee
    specified NEC S89.8- ☑
    sprain — *see* Sprain, knee
    superficial — *see* Injury, superficial, knee
  labium (majus) (minus) S39.94 ☑
  labyrinth, ear S09.30- ☑
  lacrimal apparatus, duct, gland, or sac — *see* Injury, eye, specified site NEC
  larynx NEC S19.81 ☑
  leg (lower) S89.9- ☑
    blood vessel — *see* Injury, blood vessel, leg
    contusion — *see* Contusion, leg
    fracture — *see* Fracture, leg
    muscle — *see* Injury, muscle, leg
    nerve — *see* Injury, nerve, leg
    open — *see* Wound, open, leg
    specified NEC S89.8- ☑
    superficial — *see* Injury, superficial, leg
  lens, eye — *see* Injury, eye, specified site NEC
    penetrating — *see* Injury, eyeball, penetrating
  limb NEC T14.8 ☑
  lip S09.93 ☑
  liver S36.119 ☑
    contusion S36.112 ☑
    laceration S36.113 ☑
      major (stellate) S36.116 ☑
      minor S36.114 ☑
      moderate S36.115 ☑
    specified NEC S36.118 ☑
  lower back S39.92 ☑
    specified NEC S39.82 ☑
  lumbar, lumbosacral (region) S39.92 ☑
    plexus — *see* Injury, lumbosacral plexus
  lumbosacral plexus S34.4 ☑
  lung — *see also* Injury, intrathoracic, lung
    aspiration J69.0
    dabbing (related) U07.0
    electronic cigarette (related) U07.0
    EVALI - [e-cigarette, or vaping, product use associated] U07.0
    transfusion-related (TRALI) J95.84
    vaping (associated) (device) (product) (use) U07.0
  lymphatic thoracic duct — *see* Injury, intrathoracic, specified organ NEC
  malar region S09.93 ☑
  mastoid region S09.90 ☑
  maxilla S09.93 ☑
  mediastinum — *see* Injury, intrathoracic, specified organ NEC
  membrane, brain — *see* Injury, intracranial
  meningeal artery — *see* Injury, intracranial, subdural hemorrhage
  meninges (cerebral) — *see* Injury, intracranial
  mesenteric
    artery
      branch S35.299 ☑
        laceration (minor) (superficial) S35.291 ☑
          major S35.292 ☑

Injury — *continued*
  mesenteric — *continued*
    artery — *continued*
      branch — *continued*
        specified NEC S35.298 ☑
      inferior S35.239 ☑
        laceration (minor) (superficial) S35.231 ☑
          major S35.232 ☑
        specified NEC S35.238 ☑
      superior S35.229 ☑
        laceration (minor) (superficial) S35.221 ☑
          major S35.222 ☑
        specified NEC S35.228 ☑
    plexus (inferior) (superior) — *see* Injury, nerve, lumbosacral, sympathetic
    vein
      inferior S35.349 ☑
        laceration S35.341 ☑
        specified NEC S35.348 ☑
      superior S35.339 ☑
        laceration S35.331 ☑
        specified NEC S35.338 ☑
  mesentery — *see* Injury, intra-abdominal, specified site NEC
  mesosalpinx — *see* Injury, pelvic organ, specified site NEC
  middle ear S09.30- ☑
  midthoracic region NOS S29.9 ☑
  mouth S09.93 ☑
  multiple NOS T07 ☑
  muscle (and fascia) (and tendon)
    abdomen S39.001 ☑
      laceration S39.021 ☑
      specified type NEC S39.091 ☑
      strain S39.011 ☑
    abductor
      thumb, forearm level — *see* Injury, muscle, thumb, abductor
    adductor
      thigh S76.20- ☑
        laceration S76.22- ☑
        specified type NEC S76.29- ☑
        strain S76.21- ☑
    ankle — *see* Injury, muscle, foot
    anterior muscle group, at leg level (lower) S86.20- ☑
      laceration S86.22- ☑
      specified type NEC S86.29- ☑
      strain S86.21- ☑
    arm (upper) — *see* Injury, muscle, shoulder
    biceps (parts NEC) S46.20- ☑
      laceration S46.22- ☑
      long head S46.10- ☑
        laceration S46.12- ☑
        specified type NEC S46.19- ☑
        strain S46.11- ☑
      specified type NEC S46.29- ☑
      strain S46.21- ☑
    extensor
      finger(s) (other than thumb) — *see* Injury, muscle, finger by site, extensor
      forearm level, specified NEC — *see* Injury, muscle, forearm, extensor
      thumb — *see* Injury, muscle, thumb, extensor
      toe (large) (ankle level) (foot level) — *see* Injury, muscle, toe, extensor
    finger
      extensor (forearm level) S56.40- ☑
        hand level S66.309 ☑
          laceration S66.329 ☑
          specified type NEC S66.399 ☑
          strain S66.319 ☑
        laceration S56.429 ☑
        specified type NEC S56.499 ☑
        strain S56.419 ☑
      flexor (forearm level) S56.10- ☑
        hand level S66.109 ☑
          laceration S66.129 ☑
          specified type NEC S66.199 ☑
          strain S66.119 ☑
        laceration S56.129 ☑
        specified type NEC S56.199 ☑
        strain S56.119 ☑
      index
        extensor (forearm level)
          hand level S66.308 ☑
            laceration S66.32- ☑

Injury — *continued*
  muscle — *continued*
    finger — *continued*
      index — *continued*
        extensor — *continued*
          hand level — *continued*
            specified type NEC S66.39- ☑
            strain S66.31- ☑
          specified type NEC S56.492- ☑
        flexor (forearm level)
          hand level S66.108 ☑
            laceration S66.12- ☑
            specified type NEC S66.19- ☑
            strain S66.11- ☑
          specified type NEC S56.19- ☑
          strain S56.11- ☑
        intrinsic S66.50- ☑
          laceration S66.52- ☑
          specified type NEC S66.59- ☑
          strain S66.51- ☑
      intrinsic S66.509 ☑
        laceration S66.529 ☑
        specified type NEC S66.599 ☑
        strain S66.519 ☑
      little
        extensor (forearm level)
          hand level S66.30- ☑
            laceration S66.32- ☑
            specified type NEC S66.39- ☑
            strain S66.31- ☑
          laceration S56.42- ☑
          specified type NEC S56.49- ☑
          strain S56.41- ☑
        flexor (forearm level)
          hand level S66.10- ☑
            laceration S66.12- ☑
            specified type NEC S66.19- ☑
            strain S66.11- ☑
          laceration S56.12- ☑
          specified type NEC S56.19- ☑
          strain S56.11- ☑
        intrinsic S66.50- ☑
          laceration S66.52- ☑
          specified type NEC S66.59- ☑
          strain S66.51- ☑
      middle
        extensor (forearm level)
          hand level S66.30- ☑
            laceration S66.32- ☑
            specified type NEC S66.39- ☑
            strain S66.31- ☑
          laceration S56.42- ☑
          specified type NEC S56.49- ☑
          strain S56.41- ☑
        flexor (forearm level)
          hand level S66.10- ☑
            laceration S66.12- ☑
            specified type NEC S66.19- ☑
            strain S66.11- ☑
          laceration S56.12- ☑
          specified type NEC S56.19- ☑
          strain S56.11- ☑
        intrinsic S66.50- ☑
          laceration S66.52- ☑
          specified type NEC S66.59- ☑
          strain S66.51- ☑
      ring
        extensor (forearm level)
          hand level S66.30- ☑
            laceration S66.32- ☑
            specified type NEC S66.39- ☑
            strain S66.31- ☑
          laceration S56.42- ☑
          specified type NEC S56.49- ☑
          strain S56.41- ☑
        flexor (forearm level)
          hand level S66.10- ☑
            laceration S66.12- ☑
            specified type NEC S66.19- ☑
            strain S66.11- ☑
          laceration S56.12- ☑
          specified type NEC S56.19- ☑
          strain S56.11- ☑
        intrinsic S66.50- ☑
          laceration S66.52- ☑
          specified type NEC S66.59- ☑

☑ **Additional Character Required** — Refer to the Tabular List for Character Selection   ▽ **Subterms under main terms may continue to next column or page**

Injury — *continued*
  muscle — *continued*
    finger — *continued*
      ring — *continued*
        intrinsic — *continued*
          strain S66.51- ☑
      flexor
        finger(s) (other than thumb) — *see* Injury, muscle, finger
        forearm level, specified NEC — *see* Injury, muscle, forearm, flexor
        thumb — *see* Injury, muscle, thumb, flexor
        toe (long) (ankle level) (foot level) — *see* Injury, muscle, toe, flexor
    foot S96.90- ☑
      intrinsic S96.20- ☑
        laceration S96.22- ☑
        specified type NEC S96.29- ☑
        strain S96.21- ☑
      laceration S96.92- ☑
      long extensor, toe — *see* Injury, muscle, toe, extensor
      long flexor, toe — *see* Injury, muscle, toe, flexor
      specified
        site NEC S96.80- ☑
          laceration S96.82- ☑
          specified type NEC S96.89- ☑
          strain S96.81- ☑
          type S96.99- ☑
        strain S96.91- ☑
    forearm (level) S56.90- ☑
      extensor S56.50- ☑
        laceration S56.52- ☑
        specified type NEC S56.59- ☑
        strain S56.51- ☑
      flexor S56.20- ☑
        laceration S56.22- ☑
        specified type NEC S56.29- ☑
        strain S56.21- ☑
      laceration S56.92- ☑
      specified S56.99- ☑
        site NEC S56.80- ☑
          laceration S56.82- ☑
          strain S56.81- ☑
          type NEC S56.89- ☑
        strain S56.91- ☑
    hand (level) S66.90- ☑
      laceration S66.92- ☑
      specified
        site NEC S66.80- ☑
          laceration S66.82- ☑
          specified type NEC S66.89- ☑
          strain S66.81- ☑
          type NEC S66.99- ☑
        strain S66.91- ☑
    head S09.10 ☑
      laceration S09.12 ☑
      specified type NEC S09.19 ☑
      strain S09.11 ☑
    hip NEC S76.00- ☑
      laceration S76.02- ☑
      specified type NEC S76.09- ☑
      strain S76.01- ☑
    intrinsic
      ankle and foot level — *see* Injury, muscle, foot, intrinsic
      finger (other than thumb) — *see* Injury, muscle, finger by site, intrinsic
      foot (level) — *see* Injury, muscle, foot, intrinsic
      thumb — *see* Injury, muscle, thumb, intrinsic
    leg (level) (lower) S86.90- ☑
      Achilles tendon — *see* Injury, Achilles tendon
      anterior muscle group — *see* Injury, muscle, anterior muscle group
      laceration S86.92- ☑
      peroneal muscle group — *see* Injury, muscle, peroneal muscle group
      posterior muscle group — *see* Injury, muscle, posterior muscle group, leg level
      specified
        site NEC S86.80- ☑
          laceration S86.82- ☑
          specified type NEC S86.89- ☑
          strain S86.81- ☑
          type NEC S86.99- ☑
        strain S86.91- ☑

Injury — *continued*
  muscle — *continued*
    long
      extensor toe, at ankle and foot level — *see* Injury, muscle, toe, extensor
      flexor, toe, at ankle and foot level — *see* Injury, muscle, toe, flexor
      head, biceps — *see* Injury, muscle, biceps, long head
    lower back S39.002 ☑
      laceration S39.022 ☑
      specified type NEC S39.092 ☑
      strain S39.012 ☑
    neck (level) S16.9 ☑
      laceration S16.2 ☑
      specified type NEC S16.8 ☑
      strain S16.1 ☑
    pelvis S39.003 ☑
      laceration S39.023 ☑
      specified type NEC S39.093 ☑
      strain S39.013 ☑
    peroneal muscle group, at leg level (lower) S86.30- ☑
      laceration S86.32- ☑
      specified type NEC S86.39- ☑
      strain S86.31- ☑
    posterior muscle (group)
      leg level (lower) S86.10- ☑
        laceration S86.12- ☑
        specified type NEC S86.19- ☑
        strain S86.11- ☑
      thigh level S76.30- ☑
        laceration S76.32- ☑
        specified type NEC S76.39- ☑
        strain S76.31- ☑
    quadriceps (thigh) S76.10- ☑
      laceration S76.12- ☑
      specified type NEC S76.19- ☑
      strain S76.11- ☑
    shoulder S46.90- ☑
      laceration S46.92- ☑
      rotator cuff — *see* Injury, rotator cuff
      specified site NEC S46.80- ☑
        laceration S46.82- ☑
        specified type NEC S46.89- ☑
        strain S46.81- ☑
      specified type NEC S46.99- ☑
      strain S46.91- ☑
    thigh NEC (level) S76.90- ☑
      adductor — *see* Injury, muscle, adductor, thigh
      laceration S76.92- ☑
      posterior muscle (group) — *see* Injury, muscle, posterior muscle, thigh level
      quadriceps — *see* Injury, muscle, quadriceps
      specified
        site NEC S76.80- ☑
          laceration S76.82- ☑
          specified type NEC S76.89- ☑
          strain S76.81- ☑
          type NEC S76.99- ☑
        strain S76.91- ☑
    thorax (level) S29.009 ☑
      back wall S29.002 ☑
      front wall S29.001 ☑
      laceration S29.029 ☑
        back wall S29.022 ☑
        front wall S29.021 ☑
      specified type NEC S29.099 ☑
        back wall S29.092 ☑
        front wall S29.091 ☑
      strain S29.019 ☑
        back wall S29.012 ☑
        front wall S29.011 ☑
    thumb
      abductor (forearm level) S56.30- ☑
        laceration S56.32- ☑
        specified type NEC S56.39- ☑
        strain S56.31- ☑
      extensor (forearm level) S56.30- ☑
        hand level S66.20- ☑
          laceration S66.22- ☑
          specified type NEC S66.29- ☑
          strain S66.21- ☑
        laceration S56.32- ☑
        specified type NEC S56.39- ☑
        strain S56.31- ☑

Injury — *continued*
  muscle — *continued*
    thumb — *continued*
      flexor (forearm level) S56.00- ☑
        hand level S66.00- ☑
          laceration S66.02- ☑
          specified type NEC S66.09- ☑
          strain S66.01- ☑
        laceration S56.02- ☑
        specified type NEC S56.09- ☑
        strain S56.01- ☑
        wrist level — *see* Injury, muscle, thumb, flexor, hand level
      intrinsic S66.40- ☑
        laceration S66.42- ☑
        specified type NEC S66.49- ☑
        strain S66.41- ☑
    toe — *see also* Injury, muscle, foot
      extensor, long S96.10- ☑
        laceration S96.12- ☑
        specified type NEC S96.19- ☑
        strain S96.11- ☑
      flexor, long S96.00- ☑
        laceration S96.02- ☑
        specified type NEC S96.09- ☑
        strain S96.01- ☑
    triceps S46.30- ☑
      laceration S46.32- ☑
      specified type NEC S46.39- ☑
      strain S46.31- ☑
    wrist (and hand) level — *see* Injury, muscle, hand
  musculocutaneous nerve — *see* Injury, nerve, musculocutaneous
  myocardial (acute) (chronic) (non-ischemic) (non-traumatic) I5A
    traumatic — *see* Injury, heart
  myocardium — *see also* Injury, heart
    non-traumatic — *see* Injury, myocardial
  nape — *see* Injury, neck
  nasal (septum) (sinus) S09.92 ☑
  nasopharynx S09.92 ☑
  neck S19.9 ☑
    specified NEC S19.80 ☑
      specified site NEC S19.89 ☑
  nerve NEC T14.8 ☑
    abdomen S34.9 ☑
      peripheral S34.6 ☑
      specified site NEC S34.8 ☑
    abducens S04.4- ☑
      contusion S04.4- ☑
      laceration S04.4- ☑
      specified type NEC S04.4- ☑
    abducent — *see* Injury, nerve, abducens
    accessory S04.7- ☑
      contusion S04.7- ☑
      laceration S04.7- ☑
      specified type NEC S04.7- ☑
    acoustic S04.6- ☑
      contusion S04.6- ☑
      laceration S04.6- ☑
      specified type NEC S04.6- ☑
    ankle S94.9- ☑
      cutaneous sensory S94.3- ☑
      specified site NEC — *see* subcategory S94.8 ☑
    anterior crural, femoral — *see* Injury, nerve, femoral
    arm (upper) S44.9- ☑
      axillary — *see* Injury, nerve, axillary
      cutaneous — *see* Injury, nerve, cutaneous, arm
      median — *see* Injury, nerve, median, upper arm
      musculocutaneous — *see* Injury, nerve, musculocutaneous
      radial — *see* Injury, nerve, radial, upper arm
      specified site NEC — *see* subcategory S44.8 ☑
      ulnar — *see* Injury, nerve, ulnar, arm
    auditory — *see* Injury, nerve, acoustic
    axillary S44.3- ☑
    brachial plexus — *see* Injury, brachial plexus
    cervical sympathetic S14.5 ☑
    cranial S04.9 ☑
      contusion S04.9 ☑
      eighth (acoustic or auditory) — *see* Injury, nerve, acoustic
      eleventh (accessory) — *see* Injury, nerve, accessory
      fifth (trigeminal) — *see* Injury, nerve, trigeminal
      first (olfactory) — *see* Injury, nerve, olfactory

Injury — continued
  nerve — continued
    cranial — continued
      fourth (trochlear) — see Injury, nerve, trochlear
      laceration S04.9 ☑
      ninth (glossopharyngeal) — see Injury, nerve, glossopharyngeal
      second (optic) — see Injury, nerve, optic
      seventh (facial) — see Injury, nerve, facial
      sixth (abducent) — see Injury, nerve, abducens
      specified
        nerve NEC S04.89- ☑
          contusion S04.89- ☑
          laceration S04.89- ☑
          specified type NEC S04.89- ☑
        type NEC S04.9 ☑
      tenth (pneumogastric or vagus) — see Injury, nerve, vagus
      third (oculomotor) — see Injury, nerve, oculomotor
      twelfth (hypoglossal) — see Injury, nerve, hypoglossal
    cutaneous sensory
      ankle (level) S94.3- ☑
      arm (upper) (level) S44.5- ☑
      foot (level) — see Injury, nerve, cutaneous sensory, ankle
      forearm (level) S54.3- ☑
      hip (level) S74.2- ☑
      leg (lower level) S84.2- ☑
      shoulder (level) — see Injury, nerve, cutaneous sensory, arm
      thigh (level) — see Injury, nerve, cutaneous sensory, hip
    deep peroneal — see Injury, nerve, peroneal, foot
    digital
      finger S64.4- ☑
        index S64.49- ☑
        little S64.49- ☑
        middle S64.49- ☑
        ring S64.49- ☑
      thumb S64.3- ☑
      toe — see Injury, nerve, ankle, specified site NEC
    eighth cranial (acoustic or auditory) — see Injury, nerve, acoustic
    eleventh cranial (accessory) — see Injury, nerve, accessory
    facial S04.5- ☑
      contusion S04.5- ☑
      laceration S04.5- ☑
      newborn P11.3
      specified type NEC S04.5- ☑
    femoral (hip level) (thigh level) S74.1- ☑
    fifth cranial (trigeminal) — see Injury, nerve, trigeminal
    finger (digital) — see Injury, nerve, digital, finger
    first cranial (olfactory) — see Injury, nerve, olfactory
    foot S94.9- ☑
      cutaneous sensory S94.3- ☑
      deep peroneal S94.2- ☑
      lateral plantar S94.0- ☑
      medial plantar S94.1- ☑
      specified site NEC — see subcategory S94.8 ☑
    forearm (level) S54.9- ☑
      cutaneous sensory — see Injury, nerve, cutaneous sensory, forearm
      median — see Injury, nerve, median
      radial — see Injury, nerve, radial
      specified site NEC — see subcategory S54.8 ☑
      ulnar — see Injury, nerve, ulnar
    fourth cranial (trochlear) — see Injury, nerve, trochlear
    glossopharyngeal S04.89- ☑
      specified type NEC S04.89- ☑
    hand S64.9- ☑
      median — see Injury, nerve, median, hand
      radial — see Injury, nerve, radial, hand
      specified NEC — see subcategory S64.8 ☑
      ulnar — see Injury, nerve, ulnar, hand
    hip (level) S74.9- ☑
      cutaneous sensory — see Injury, nerve, cutaneous sensory, hip
      femoral — see Injury, nerve, femoral
      sciatic — see Injury, nerve, sciatic
      specified site NEC — see subcategory S74.8 ☑
    hypoglossal S04.89- ☑

Injury — continued
  nerve — continued
    hypoglossal — continued
      specified type NEC S04.89- ☑
    lateral plantar S94.0- ☑
    leg (lower) S84.9- ☑
      cutaneous sensory — see Injury, nerve, cutaneous sensory, leg
      peroneal — see Injury, nerve, peroneal
      specified site NEC — see subcategory S84.8 ☑
      tibial — see Injury, nerve, tibial
      upper — see Injury, nerve, thigh
    lower
      back — see Injury, nerve, abdomen, specified site NEC
        peripheral — see Injury, nerve, abdomen, peripheral
      limb — see Injury, nerve, leg
    lumbar plexus — see Injury, nerve, lumbosacral, sympathetic
    lumbar spinal
      peripheral S34.6 ☑
      root S34.21 ☑
      sympathetic S34.5 ☑
    lumbosacral
      plexus — see Injury, nerve, lumbosacral, sympathetic
      sympathetic S34.5 ☑
    medial plantar S94.1- ☑
    median (forearm level) S54.1- ☑
      hand (level) S64.1- ☑
      upper arm (level) S44.1- ☑
      wrist (level) — see Injury, nerve, median, hand
    musculocutaneous S44.4- ☑
    musculospiral (upper arm level) — see Injury, nerve, radial, upper arm
    neck S14.9 ☑
      peripheral S14.4 ☑
      specified site NEC S14.8 ☑
      sympathetic S14.5 ☑
    ninth cranial (glossopharyngeal) — see Injury, nerve, glossopharyngeal
    oculomotor S04.1- ☑
      contusion S04.1- ☑
      laceration S04.1- ☑
      specified type NEC S04.1- ☑
    olfactory S04.81- ☑
      specified type NEC S04.81- ☑
    optic S04.01- ☑
      contusion S04.01- ☑
      laceration S04.01- ☑
      specified type NEC S04.01- ☑
    pelvic girdle — see Injury, nerve, hip
    pelvis — see Injury, nerve, abdomen, specified site NEC
      peripheral — see Injury, nerve, abdomen, peripheral
    peripheral NEC T14.8 ☑
      abdomen — see Injury, nerve, abdomen, peripheral
      lower back — see Injury, nerve, abdomen, peripheral
      neck — see Injury, nerve, neck, peripheral
      pelvis — see Injury, nerve, abdomen, peripheral
      specified NEC T14.8 ☑
    peroneal (lower leg level) S84.1- ☑
      foot S94.2- ☑
    plexus
      brachial — see Injury, brachial plexus
      celiac, coeliac — see Injury, nerve, lumbosacral, sympathetic
      mesenteric, inferior — see Injury, nerve, lumbosacral, sympathetic
      sacral — see Injury, lumbosacral plexus
      spinal
        brachial — see Injury, brachial plexus
        lumbosacral — see Injury, lumbosacral plexus
    pneumogastric — see Injury, nerve, vagus
    radial (forearm level) S54.2- ☑
      hand (level) S64.2- ☑
      upper arm (level) S44.2- ☑
      wrist (level) — see Injury, nerve, radial, hand
    root — see Injury, nerve, spinal, root
    sacral plexus — see Injury, lumbosacral plexus
    sacral spinal
      peripheral S34.6 ☑

Injury — continued
  nerve — continued
    sacral spinal — continued
      root S34.22 ☑
      sympathetic S34.5 ☑
    sciatic (hip level) (thigh level) S74.0- ☑
    second cranial (optic) — see Injury, nerve, optic
    seventh cranial (facial) — see Injury, nerve, facial
    shoulder — see Injury, nerve, arm
    sixth cranial (abducent) — see Injury, nerve, abducens
    spinal
      plexus — see Injury, nerve, plexus, spinal
      root
        cervical S14.2 ☑
        dorsal S24.2 ☑
        lumbar S34.21 ☑
        sacral S34.22 ☑
        thoracic — see Injury, nerve, spinal, root, dorsal
    splanchnic — see Injury, nerve, lumbosacral, sympathetic
    sympathetic NEC — see Injury, nerve, lumbosacral, sympathetic
      cervical — see Injury, nerve, cervical sympathetic
    tenth cranial (pneumogastric or vagus) — see Injury, nerve, vagus
    thigh (level) — see Injury, nerve, hip
      cutaneous sensory — see Injury, nerve, cutaneous sensory, hip
      femoral — see Injury, nerve, femoral
      sciatic — see Injury, nerve, sciatic
      specified NEC — see Injury, nerve, hip
    third cranial (oculomotor) — see Injury, nerve, oculomotor
    thorax S24.9 ☑
      peripheral S24.3 ☑
      specified site NEC S24.8 ☑
      sympathetic S24.4 ☑
    thumb, digital — see Injury, nerve, digital, thumb
    tibial (lower leg level) (posterior) S84.0- ☑
    toe — see Injury, nerve, ankle
    trigeminal S04.3- ☑
      contusion S04.3- ☑
      laceration S04.3- ☑
      specified type NEC S04.3- ☑
    trochlear S04.2- ☑
      contusion S04.2- ☑
      laceration S04.2- ☑
      specified type NEC S04.2- ☑
    twelfth cranial (hypoglossal) — see Injury, nerve, hypoglossal
    ulnar (forearm level) S54.0- ☑
      arm (upper) (level) S44.0- ☑
      hand (level) S64.0- ☑
      wrist (level) — see Injury, nerve, ulnar, hand
    vagus S04.89- ☑
      specified type NEC S04.89- ☑
    wrist (level) — see Injury, nerve, hand
  ninth cranial nerve (glossopharyngeal) — see Injury, nerve, glossopharyngeal
  nose (septum) S09.92 ☑
  obstetrical O71.9
    specified NEC O71.89
  occipital (region) (scalp) S09.90 ☑
    lobe — see Injury, intracranial
  optic chiasm S04.02 ☑
  optic radiation S04.03- ☑
  optic tract and pathways S04.03- ☑
  orbit, orbital (region) — see Injury, eye
    penetrating (with foreign body) — see Injury, eye, orbit, penetrating
    specified NEC — see Injury, eye, specified site NEC
  ovary, ovarian S37.409 ☑
    bilateral S37.402 ☑
      contusion S37.422 ☑
      laceration S37.432 ☑
      specified type NEC S37.492 ☑
    blood vessel — see Injury, blood vessel, ovarian
    contusion S37.429 ☑
      bilateral S37.422 ☑
      unilateral S37.421 ☑
    laceration S37.439 ☑
      bilateral S37.432 ☑
      unilateral S37.431 ☑
    specified type NEC S37.499 ☑

☑ Additional Character Required — Refer to the Tabular List for Character Selection   🔺 Subterms under main terms may continue to next column or page

Injury — *continued*

ovary, ovarian — *continued*
  specified type — *continued*
    bilateral S37.492 ☑
    unilateral S37.491 ☑
  unilateral S37.401 ☑
    contusion S37.421 ☑
    laceration S37.431 ☑
    specified type NEC S37.491 ☑
palate (hard) (soft) S09.93 ☑
pancreas S36.209 ☑
  body S36.201 ☑
    contusion S36.221 ☑
    laceration S36.231 ☑
      major S36.261 ☑
      minor S36.241 ☑
      moderate S36.251 ☑
    specified type NEC S36.291 ☑
  contusion S36.229 ☑
  head S36.200 ☑
    contusion S36.220 ☑
    laceration S36.230 ☑
      major S36.260 ☑
      minor S36.240 ☑
      moderate S36.250 ☑
    specified type NEC S36.290 ☑
  laceration S36.239 ☑
    major S36.269 ☑
    minor S36.249 ☑
    moderate S36.259 ☑
  specified type NEC S36.299 ☑
  tail S36.202 ☑
    contusion S36.222 ☑
    laceration S36.232 ☑
      major S36.262 ☑
      minor S36.242 ☑
      moderate S36.252 ☑
    specified type NEC S36.292 ☑
parietal (region) (scalp) S09.90 ☑
  lobe — *see* Injury, intracranial
patellar ligament (tendon) S76.10- ☑
  laceration S76.12- ☑
  specified NEC S76.19- ☑
  strain S76.11- ☑
pelvis, pelvic (floor) S39.93 ☑
  complicating delivery O70.1
  joint or ligament, complicating delivery O71.6
  organ S37.90 ☑
    with ectopic or molar pregnancy O08.6
    complication of abortion — *see* Abortion
    contusion S37.92 ☑
    following ectopic or molar pregnancy O08.6
    laceration S37.93 ☑
    obstetrical trauma NEC O71.5
    specified
      site NEC S37.899 ☑
        contusion S37.892 ☑
        laceration S37.893 ☑
        specified type NEC S37.898 ☑
      type NEC S37.99 ☑
  specified NEC S39.83 ☑
penis S39.94 ☑
perineum S39.94 ☑
peritoneum S36.81 ☑
  laceration S36.893 ☑
periurethral tissue — *see* Injury, urethra
  complicating delivery O71.82
phalanges
  foot — *see* Injury, foot
  hand — *see* Injury, hand
pharynx NEC S19.85 ☑
pleura — *see* Injury, intrathoracic, pleura
plexus
  brachial — *see* Injury, brachial plexus
  cardiac — *see* Injury, nerve, thorax, sympathetic
  celiac, coeliac — *see* Injury, nerve, lumbosacral, sympathetic
  esophageal — *see* Injury, nerve, thorax, sympathetic
  hypogastric — *see* Injury, nerve, lumbosacral, sympathetic
  lumbar, lumbosacral — *see* Injury, lumbosacral plexus
  mesenteric — *see* Injury, nerve, lumbosacral, sympathetic
  pulmonary — *see* Injury, nerve, thorax, sympathetic
postcardiac surgery (syndrome) I97.0

Injury — *continued*

prepuce S39.94 ☑
pressure
  injury — *see* Ulcer, pressure, by site
prostate S37.829 ☑
  contusion S37.822 ☑
  laceration S37.823 ☑
  specified type NEC S37.828 ☑
pubic region S39.94 ☑
pudendum S39.94 ☑
pulmonary plexus — *see* Injury, nerve, thorax, sympathetic
rectovaginal septum NEC S39.83 ☑
rectum — *see* Injury, intestine, large, rectum
retina — *see* Injury, eye, specified site NEC
  penetrating — *see* Injury, eyeball, penetrating
retroperitoneal — *see* Injury, intra-abdominal, specified site NEC
rotator cuff (muscle(s)) (tendon(s)) S46.00- ☑
  laceration S46.02- ☑
  specified type NEC S46.09- ☑
  strain S46.01- ☑
round ligament — *see* Injury, pelvic organ, specified site NEC
sacral plexus — *see* Injury, lumbosacral plexus
salivary duct or gland S09.93 ☑
scalp S09.90 ☑
  newborn (birth injury) P12.9
    due to monitoring (electrode) (sampling incision) P12.4
    specified NEC P12.89
      caput succedaneum P12.81
scapular region — *see* Injury, shoulder
sclera — *see* Injury, eye, specified site NEC
  penetrating — *see* Injury, eyeball, penetrating
scrotum S39.94 ☑
second cranial nerve (optic) — *see* Injury, nerve, optic
self-inflicted, without suicidal intent R45.88
seminal vesicle — *see* Injury, pelvic organ, specified site NEC
seventh cranial nerve (facial) — *see* Injury, nerve, facial
shoulder S49.9- ☑
  blood vessel — *see* Injury, blood vessel, arm
  contusion — *see* Contusion, shoulder
  dislocation — *see* Dislocation, shoulder
  fracture — *see* Fracture, shoulder
  muscle — *see* Injury, muscle, shoulder
  nerve — *see* Injury, nerve, shoulder
  open — *see* Wound, open, shoulder
  specified type NEC S49.8- ☑
  sprain — *see* Sprain, shoulder girdle
  superficial — *see* Injury, superficial, shoulder
sinus
  cavernous — *see* Injury, intracranial
  nasal S09.92 ☑
sixth cranial nerve (abducent) — *see* Injury, nerve, abducens
skeleton, birth injury P13.9
  specified part NEC P13.8
skin NEC T14.8 ☑
  surface intact — *see* Injury, superficial
skull NEC S09.90 ☑
  specified NEC T14.8 ☑
spermatic cord (pelvic region) S37.898 ☑
  scrotal region S39.848 ☑
spinal (cord)
  cervical (neck) S14.109 ☑
    anterior cord syndrome S14.139 ☑
      C1 level S14.131 ☑
      C2 level S14.132 ☑
      C3 level S14.133 ☑
      C4 level S14.134 ☑
      C5 level S14.135 ☑
      C6 level S14.136 ☑
      C7 level S14.137 ☑
      C8 level S14.138 ☑
    Brown-Séquard syndrome S14.149 ☑
      C1 level S14.141 ☑
      C2 level S14.142 ☑
      C3 level S14.143 ☑
      C4 level S14.144 ☑
      C5 level S14.145 ☑
      C6 level S14.146 ☑
      C7 level S14.147 ☑
      C8 level S14.148 ☑
    C1 level S14.101 ☑

Injury — *continued*

spinal — *continued*
  cervical — *continued*
    C2 level S14.102 ☑
    C3 level S14.103 ☑
    C4 level S14.104 ☑
    C5 level S14.105 ☑
    C6 level S14.106 ☑
    C7 level S14.107 ☑
    C8 level S14.108 ☑
    central cord syndrome S14.129 ☑
      C1 level S14.121 ☑
      C2 level S14.122 ☑
      C3 level S14.123 ☑
      C4 level S14.124 ☑
      C5 level S14.125 ☑
      C6 level S14.126 ☑
      C7 level S14.127 ☑
      C8 level S14.128 ☑
    complete lesion S14.119 ☑
      C1 level S14.111 ☑
      C2 level S14.112 ☑
      C3 level S14.113 ☑
      C4 level S14.114 ☑
      C5 level S14.115 ☑
      C6 level S14.116 ☑
      C7 level S14.117 ☑
      C8 level S14.118 ☑
    concussion S14.0 ☑
    edema S14.0 ☑
    incomplete lesion specified NEC S14.159 ☑
      C1 level S14.151 ☑
      C2 level S14.152 ☑
      C3 level S14.153 ☑
      C4 level S14.154 ☑
      C5 level S14.155 ☑
      C6 level S14.156 ☑
      C7 level S14.157 ☑
      C8 level S14.158 ☑
    posterior cord syndrome S14.159 ☑
      C1 level S14.151 ☑
      C2 level S14.152 ☑
      C3 level S14.153 ☑
      C4 level S14.154 ☑
      C5 level S14.155 ☑
      C6 level S14.156 ☑
      C7 level S14.157 ☑
      C8 level S14.158 ☑
  dorsal — *see* Injury, spinal, thoracic
  lumbar S34.109 ☑
    complete lesion S34.119 ☑
      L1 level S34.111 ☑
      L2 level S34.112 ☑
      L3 level S34.113 ☑
      L4 level S34.114 ☑
      L5 level S34.115 ☑
    concussion S34.01 ☑
    edema S34.01 ☑
    incomplete lesion S34.129 ☑
      L1 level S34.121 ☑
      L2 level S34.122 ☑
      L3 level S34.123 ☑
      L4 level S34.124 ☑
      L5 level S34.125 ☑
    L1 level S34.101 ☑
    L2 level S34.102 ☑
    L3 level S34.103 ☑
    L4 level S34.104 ☑
    L5 level S34.105 ☑
  nerve root NEC
    cervical — *see* Injury, nerve, spinal, root, cervical
    dorsal — *see* Injury, nerve, spinal, root, dorsal
    lumbar S34.21 ☑
    sacral S34.22 ☑
    thoracic — *see* Injury, nerve, spinal, root, dorsal
  plexus
    brachial — *see* Injury, brachial plexus
    lumbosacral — *see* Injury, lumbosacral plexus
  sacral S34.139 ☑
    complete lesion S34.131 ☑
    incomplete lesion S34.132 ☑
  thoracic S24.109 ☑
    anterior cord syndrome S24.139 ☑
      T1 level S24.131 ☑
      T2-T6 level S24.132 ☑
      T7-T10 level S24.133 ☑

Injury — *continued*
  spinal — *continued*
    thoracic — *continued*
      anterior cord syndrome — *continued*
        T11-T12 level S24.134 ☑
      Brown-Séquard syndrome S24.149 ☑
        T1 level S24.141 ☑
        T2-T6 level S24.142 ☑
        T7-T10 level S24.143 ☑
        T11-T12 level S24.144 ☑
      complete lesion S24.119 ☑
        T1 level S24.111 ☑
        T2-T6 level S24.112 ☑
        T7-T10 level S24.113 ☑
        T11-T12 level S24.114 ☑
      concussion S24.0 ☑
      edema S24.0 ☑
      incomplete lesion specified NEC S24.159 ☑
        T1 level S24.151 ☑
        T2-T6 level S24.152 ☑
        T7-T10 level S24.153 ☑
        T11-T12 level S24.154 ☑
      posterior cord syndrome S24.159 ☑
        T1 level S24.151 ☑
        T2-T6 level S24.152 ☑
        T7-T10 level S24.153 ☑
        T11-T12 level S24.154 ☑
      T1 level S24.101 ☑
      T2-T6 level S24.102 ☑
      T7-T10 level S24.103 ☑
      T11-T12 level S24.104 ☑
  splanchnic nerve — *see* Injury, nerve, lumbosacral, sympathetic
  spleen S36.00 ☑
    contusion S36.029 ☑
      major S36.021 ☑
      minor S36.020 ☑
    laceration S36.039 ☑
      major (massive) (stellate) S36.032 ☑
      moderate S36.031 ☑
      superficial (capsular) (minor) S36.030 ☑
    specified type NEC S36.09 ☑
  splenic artery — *see* Injury, blood vessel, celiac artery, branch
  stellate ganglion — *see* Injury, nerve, thorax, sympathetic
  sternal region S29.9 ☑
  stomach S36.30 ☑
    contusion S36.32 ☑
    laceration S36.33 ☑
    specified type NEC S36.39 ☑
  subconjunctival — *see* Injury, eye, conjunctiva
  subcutaneous NEC T14.8 ☑
  submaxillary region S09.93 ☑
  submental region S09.93 ☑
  subungual
    fingers — *see* Injury, hand
    toes — *see* Injury, foot
  superficial NEC T14.8 ☑
    abdomen, abdominal (wall) S30.92 ☑
      abrasion S30.811 ☑
      bite S30.871 ☑
        insect S30.861 ☑
      contusion S30.1 ☑
      external constriction S30.841 ☑
      foreign body S30.851 ☑
    abrasion — *see* Abrasion, by site
    adnexa, eye NEC — *see* Injury, eye, specified site NEC
    alveolar process — *see* Injury, superficial, oral cavity
    ankle S90.91- ☑
      abrasion — *see* Abrasion, ankle
      bite — *see* Bite, ankle
      blister — *see* Blister, ankle
      contusion — *see* Contusion, ankle
      external constriction — *see* Constriction, external, ankle
      foreign body — *see* Foreign body, superficial, ankle
    anus S30.98 ☑
    arm (upper) S40.92- ☑
      abrasion — *see* Abrasion, arm
      bite — *see* Bite, superficial, arm
      blister — *see* Blister, arm (upper)
      contusion — *see* Contusion, arm

Injury — *continued*
  superficial — *continued*
    arm — *continued*
      external constriction — *see* Constriction, external, arm
      foreign body — *see* Foreign body, superficial, arm
    auditory canal (external) (meatus) — *see* Injury, superficial, ear
    auricle — *see* Injury, superficial, ear
    axilla — *see* Injury, superficial, arm
    back — *see also* Injury, superficial, thorax, back
      lower S30.91 ☑
        abrasion S30.810 ☑
        contusion S30.0 ☑
        external constriction S30.840 ☑
        superficial
          bite NEC S30.870 ☑
            insect S30.860 ☑
          foreign body S30.850 ☑
    bite NEC — *see* Bite, superficial NEC, by site
    blister — *see* Blister, by site
    breast S20.10- ☑
      abrasion — *see* Abrasion, breast
      bite — *see* Bite, superficial, breast
      contusion — *see* Contusion, breast
      external constriction — *see* Constriction, external, breast
      foreign body — *see* Foreign body, superficial, breast
    brow — *see* Injury, superficial, head, specified NEC
    buttock S30.91 ☑
    calf — *see* Injury, superficial, leg
    canthus, eye — *see* Injury, superficial, periocular area
    cheek (external) — *see* Injury, superficial, head, specified NEC
      internal — *see* Injury, superficial, oral cavity
    chest wall — *see* Injury, superficial, thorax
    chin — *see* Injury, superficial, head NEC
    clitoris S30.95 ☑
    conjunctiva — *see* Injury, eye, conjunctiva
      with foreign body (in conjunctival sac) — *see* Foreign body, conjunctival sac
    contusion — *see* Contusion, by site
    costal region — *see* Injury, superficial, thorax
    digit(s)
      hand — *see* Injury, superficial, finger
    ear (auricle) (canal) (external) S00.40- ☑
      abrasion — *see* Abrasion, ear
      bite — *see* Bite, superficial, ear
      contusion — *see* Contusion, ear
      external constriction — *see* Constriction, external, ear
      foreign body — *see* Foreign body, superficial, ear
    elbow S50.90- ☑
      abrasion — *see* Abrasion, elbow
      bite — *see* Bite, superficial, elbow
      blister — *see* Blister, elbow
      contusion — *see* Contusion, elbow
      external constriction — *see* Constriction, external, elbow
      foreign body — *see* Foreign body, superficial, elbow
    epididymis S30.94 ☑
    epigastric region S30.92 ☑
    epiglottis — *see* Injury, superficial, throat
    esophagus
      cervical — *see* Injury, superficial, throat
    external constriction — *see* Constriction, external, by site
    extremity NEC T14.8 ☑
    eyeball NEC — *see* Injury, eye, specified site NEC
    eyebrow — *see* Injury, superficial, periocular area
    eyelid S00.20- ☑
      abrasion — *see* Abrasion, eyelid
      bite — *see* Bite, superficial, eyelid
      contusion — *see* Contusion, eyelid
      external constriction — *see* Constriction, external, eyelid
      foreign body — *see* Foreign body, superficial, eyelid
    face NEC — *see* Injury, superficial, head, specified NEC
    finger(s) S60.949 ☑
      abrasion — *see* Abrasion, finger

Injury — *continued*
  superficial — *continued*
    finger(s) — *continued*
      bite — *see* Bite, superficial, finger
      blister — *see* Blister, finger
      contusion — *see* Contusion, finger
      external constriction — *see* Constriction, external, finger
      foreign body — *see* Foreign body, superficial, finger
      index S60.94- ☑
      insect bite — *see* Bite, by site, superficial, insect
      little S60.94- ☑
      middle S60.94- ☑
      ring S60.94- ☑
    flank S30.92 ☑
    foot S90.92- ☑
      abrasion — *see* Abrasion, foot
      bite — *see* Bite, foot
      blister — *see* Blister, foot
      contusion — *see* Contusion, foot
      external constriction — *see* Constriction, external, foot
      foreign body — *see* Foreign body, superficial, foot
    forearm S50.91- ☑
      abrasion — *see* Abrasion, forearm
      bite — *see* Bite, forearm, superficial
      blister — *see* Blister, forearm
      contusion — *see* Contusion, forearm
      elbow only — *see* Injury, superficial, elbow
      external constriction — *see* Constriction, external, forearm
      foreign body — *see* Foreign body, superficial, forearm
    forehead — *see* Injury, superficial, head NEC
    foreign body — *see* Foreign body, superficial
    genital organs, external
      female S30.97 ☑
      male S30.96 ☑
    globe (eye) — *see* Injury, eye, specified site NEC
    groin S30.92 ☑
    gum — *see* Injury, superficial, oral cavity
    hand S60.92- ☑
      abrasion — *see* Abrasion, hand
      bite — *see* Bite, superficial, hand
      contusion — *see* Contusion, hand
      external constriction — *see* Constriction, external, hand
      foreign body — *see* Foreign body, superficial, hand
    head S00.90 ☑
      ear — *see* Injury, superficial, ear
      eyelid — *see* Injury, superficial, eyelid
      nose S00.30 ☑
      oral cavity S00.502 ☑
      scalp S00.00 ☑
      specified site NEC S00.80 ☑
    heel — *see* Injury, superficial, foot
    hip S70.91- ☑
      abrasion — *see* Abrasion, hip
      bite — *see* Bite, superficial, hip
      blister — *see* Blister, hip
      contusion — *see* Contusion, hip
      external constriction — *see* Constriction, external, hip
      foreign body — *see* Foreign body, superficial, hip
    iliac region — *see* Injury, superficial, abdomen
    inguinal region — *see* Injury, superficial, abdomen
    insect bite — *see* Bite, by site, superficial, insect
    interscapular region — *see* Injury, superficial, thorax, back
    jaw — *see* Injury, superficial, head, specified NEC
    knee S80.91- ☑
      abrasion — *see* Abrasion, knee
      bite — *see* Bite, superficial, knee
      blister — *see* Blister, knee
      contusion — *see* Contusion, knee
      external constriction — *see* Constriction, external, knee
      foreign body — *see* Foreign body, superficial, knee
    labium (majus) (minus) S30.95 ☑
    lacrimal (apparatus) (gland) (sac) — *see* Injury, eye, specified site NEC

☑ **Additional Character Required** — **Refer to the Tabular List for Character Selection**   ▽ Subterms under main terms may continue to next column or page

Injury — continued
　superficial — continued
　　larynx — see Injury, superficial, throat
　　leg (lower) S80.92- ☑
　　　abrasion — see Abrasion, leg
　　　bite — see Bite, superficial, leg
　　　contusion — see Contusion, leg
　　　external constriction — see Constriction, external, leg
　　　foreign body — see Foreign body, superficial, leg
　　　knee — see Injury, superficial, knee
　　limb NEC T14.8 ☑
　　lip S00.501 ☑
　　lower back S30.91 ☑
　　lumbar region S30.91 ☑
　　malar region — see Injury, superficial, head, specified NEC
　　mammary — see Injury, superficial, breast
　　mastoid region — see Injury, superficial, head, specified NEC
　　mouth — see Injury, superficial, oral cavity
　　muscle NEC T14.8 ☑
　　nail NEC T14.8 ☑
　　　finger — see Injury, superficial, finger
　　　toe — see Injury, superficial, toe
　　nasal (septum) — see Injury, superficial, nose
　　neck S10.90 ☑
　　　specified site NEC S10.80 ☑
　　nose (septum) S00.30 ☑
　　occipital region — see Injury, superficial, scalp
　　oral cavity S00.502 ☑
　　orbital region — see Injury, superficial, periocular area
　　palate — see Injury, superficial, oral cavity
　　palm — see Injury, superficial, hand
　　parietal region — see Injury, superficial, scalp
　　pelvis S30.91 ☑
　　　girdle — see Injury, superficial, hip
　　penis S30.93 ☑
　　perineum
　　　female S30.95 ☑
　　　male S30.91 ☑
　　periocular area S00.20- ☑
　　　abrasion — see Abrasion, eyelid
　　　bite — see Bite, superficial, eyelid
　　　contusion — see Contusion, eyelid
　　　external constriction — see Constriction, external, eyelid
　　　foreign body — see Foreign body, superficial, eyelid
　　phalanges
　　　finger — see Injury, superficial, finger
　　　toe — see Injury, superficial, toe
　　pharynx — see Injury, superficial, throat
　　pinna — see Injury, superficial, ear
　　popliteal space — see Injury, superficial, knee
　　prepuce S30.93 ☑
　　pubic region S30.91 ☑
　　pudendum
　　　female S30.97 ☑
　　　male S30.96 ☑
　　sacral region S30.91 ☑
　　scalp S00.00 ☑
　　scapular region — see Injury, superficial, shoulder
　　sclera — see Injury, eye, specified site NEC
　　scrotum S30.94 ☑
　　shin — see Injury, superficial, leg
　　shoulder S40.91- ☑
　　　abrasion — see Abrasion, shoulder
　　　bite — see Bite, superficial, shoulder
　　　blister — see Blister, shoulder
　　　contusion — see Contusion, shoulder
　　　external constriction — see Constriction, external, shoulder
　　　foreign body — see Foreign body, superficial, shoulder
　　skin NEC T14.8 ☑
　　sternal region — see Injury, superficial, thorax, front
　　subconjunctival — see Injury, eye, specified site NEC
　　subcutaneous NEC T14.8 ☑
　　submaxillary region — see Injury, superficial, head, specified NEC
　　submental region — see Injury, superficial, head, specified NEC

Injury — continued
　superficial — continued
　　subungual
　　　finger(s) — see Injury, superficial, finger
　　　toe(s) — see Injury, superficial, toe
　　supraclavicular fossa — see Injury, superficial, neck
　　supraorbital — see Injury, superficial, head, specified NEC
　　temple — see Injury, superficial, head, specified NEC
　　temporal region — see Injury, superficial, head, specified NEC
　　testis S30.94 ☑
　　thigh S70.92- ☑
　　　abrasion — see Abrasion, thigh
　　　bite — see Bite, superficial, thigh
　　　blister — see Blister, thigh
　　　contusion — see Contusion, thigh
　　　external constriction — see Constriction, external, thigh
　　　foreign body — see Foreign body, superficial, thigh
　　thorax, thoracic (wall) S20.90 ☑
　　　abrasion — see Abrasion, thorax
　　　back S20.40- ☑
　　　bite — see Bite, thorax, superficial
　　　blister — see Blister, thorax
　　　contusion — see Contusion, thorax
　　　external constriction — see Constriction, external, thorax
　　　foreign body — see Foreign body, superficial, thorax
　　　front S20.30- ☑
　　throat S10.10 ☑
　　　abrasion S10.11 ☑
　　　bite S10.17 ☑
　　　　insect S10.16 ☑
　　　blister S10.12 ☑
　　　contusion S10.0 ☑
　　　external constriction S10.14 ☑
　　　foreign body S10.15 ☑
　　thumb S60.93- ☑
　　　abrasion — see Abrasion, thumb
　　　bite — see Bite, superficial, thumb
　　　blister — see Blister, thumb
　　　contusion — see Contusion, thumb
　　　external constriction — see Constriction, external, thumb
　　　foreign body — see Foreign body, superficial, thumb
　　　insect bite — see Bite, by site, superficial, insect
　　　specified type NEC S60.39 ☑
　　toe(s) S90.93- ☑
　　　abrasion — see Abrasion, toe
　　　bite — see Bite, toe
　　　blister — see Blister, toe
　　　contusion — see Contusion, toe
　　　external constriction — see Constriction, external, toe
　　　foreign body — see Foreign body, superficial, toe
　　　great S90.93- ☑
　　tongue — see Injury, superficial, oral cavity
　　tooth, teeth — see Injury, superficial, oral cavity
　　trachea S10.10 ☑
　　tunica vaginalis S30.94 ☑
　　tympanum, tympanic membrane — see Injury, superficial, ear
　　uvula — see Injury, superficial, oral cavity
　　vagina S30.95 ☑
　　vocal cords — see Injury, superficial, throat
　　vulva S30.95 ☑
　　wrist S60.91- ☑
　supraclavicular region — see Injury, neck
　supraorbital S09.93 ☑
　suprarenal gland (multiple) — see Injury, adrenal
　surgical complication (external or internal site) — see Laceration, accidental complicating surgery
　temple S09.90 ☑
　temporal region S09.90 ☑
　tendon — see also Injury, muscle, by site
　　abdomen — see Injury, muscle, abdomen
　　Achilles — see Injury, Achilles tendon
　　lower back — see Injury, muscle, lower back
　　pelvic organs — see Injury, muscle, pelvis
　tenth cranial nerve (pneumogastric or vagus) — see Injury, nerve, vagus

Injury — continued
　testis S39.94 ☑
　thigh S79.92- ☑
　　blood vessel — see Injury, blood vessel, hip
　　contusion — see Contusion, thigh
　　fracture — see Fracture, femur
　　muscle — see Injury, muscle, thigh
　　nerve — see Injury, nerve, thigh
　　open — see Wound, open, thigh
　　specified NEC S79.82- ☑
　　superficial — see Injury, superficial, thigh
　third cranial nerve (oculomotor) — see Injury, nerve, oculomotor
　thorax, thoracic S29.9 ☑
　　blood vessel — see Injury, blood vessel, thorax
　　cavity — see Injury, intrathoracic
　　dislocation — see Dislocation, thorax
　　external (wall) S29.9 ☑
　　　contusion — see Contusion, thorax
　　　nerve — see Injury, nerve, thorax
　　　open — see Wound, open, thorax
　　　specified NEC S29.8 ☑
　　　sprain — see Sprain, thorax
　　　superficial — see Injury, superficial, thorax
　　fracture — see Fracture, thorax
　　internal — see Injury, intrathoracic
　　intrathoracic organ — see Injury, intrathoracic
　　sympathetic ganglion — see Injury, nerve, thorax, sympathetic
　throat — see also Injury, neck S19.9 ☑
　thumb S69.9- ☑
　　blood vessel — see Injury, blood vessel, thumb
　　contusion — see Contusion, thumb
　　dislocation — see Dislocation, thumb
　　fracture — see Fracture, thumb
　　muscle — see Injury, muscle, thumb
　　nerve — see Injury, nerve, digital, thumb
　　open — see Wound, open, thumb
　　specified NEC S69.8- ☑
　　sprain — see Sprain, thumb
　　superficial — see Injury, superficial, thumb
　thymus (gland) — see Injury, intrathoracic, specified organ NEC
　thyroid (gland) NEC S19.84 ☑
　toe S99.92- ☑
　　contusion — see Contusion, toe
　　dislocation — see Dislocation, toe
　　fracture — see Fracture, toe
　　muscle — see Injury, muscle, toe
　　open — see Wound, open, toe
　　specified type NEC S99.82- ☑
　　sprain — see Sprain, toe
　　superficial — see Injury, superficial, toe
　tongue S09.93 ☑
　tonsil S09.93 ☑
　tooth S09.93 ☑
　trachea (cervical) NEC S19.82 ☑
　　thoracic — see Injury, intrathoracic, trachea, thoracic
　transfusion-related acute lung (TRALI) J95.84
　tunica vaginalis S39.94 ☑
　twelfth cranial nerve (hypoglossal) — see Injury, nerve, hypoglossal
　ureter S37.10 ☑
　　contusion S37.12 ☑
　　laceration S37.13 ☑
　　specified type NEC S37.19 ☑
　urethra (sphincter) S37.30 ☑
　　at delivery O71.5
　　contusion S37.32 ☑
　　laceration S37.33 ☑
　　specified type NEC S37.39 ☑
　urinary organ S37.90 ☑
　　contusion S37.92 ☑
　　laceration S37.93 ☑
　　specified
　　　site NEC S37.899 ☑
　　　　contusion S37.892 ☑
　　　　laceration S37.893 ☑
　　　　specified type NEC S37.898 ☑
　　　type NEC S37.99 ☑
　uterus, uterine S37.60 ☑
　　with ectopic or molar pregnancy O08.6
　　blood vessel — see Injury, blood vessel, iliac
　　contusion S37.62 ☑
　　laceration S37.63 ☑
　　　cervix at delivery O71.3

�ураSubterms under main terms may continue to next column or page　　☑ Additional Character Required — Refer to the Tabular List for Character Selection　　**203**

Injury — Injury

Injury — *continued*
  uterus, uterine — *continued*
    rupture associated with obstetrics — *see* Rupture, uterus
    specified type NEC S37.69 ☑
  uvula S09.93 ☑
  vagina S39.93 ☑
    abrasion S30.814 ☑
    bite S31.45 ☑
      insect S30.864 ☑
      superficial NEC S30.874 ☑
    contusion S30.23 ☑
    crush S38.03 ☑
    during delivery — *see* Laceration, vagina, during delivery
    external constriction S30.844 ☑
    insect bite S30.864 ☑
    laceration S31.41 ☑
      with foreign body S31.42 ☑
    open wound S31.40 ☑
    puncture S31.43 ☑
      with foreign body S31.44 ☑
    superficial S30.95 ☑
      foreign body S30.854 ☑
  vas deferens — *see* Injury, pelvic organ, specified site NEC
  vascular NEC T14.8 ☑
  vein — *see* Injury, blood vessel
  vena cava (superior) S25.20 ☑
    inferior S35.10 ☑
      laceration (minor) (superficial) S35.11 ☑
        major S35.12 ☑
      specified type NEC S35.19 ☑
    laceration (minor) (superficial) S25.21 ☑
      major S25.22 ☑
    specified type NEC S25.29 ☑
  vesical (sphincter) — *see* Injury, bladder
  visual cortex S04.04- ☑
  vitreous (humor) S05.90 ☑
    specified NEC S05.8X- ☑
  vocal cord NEC S19.83 ☑
  vulva S39.94 ☑
    abrasion S30.814 ☑
    bite S31.45 ☑
      insect S30.864 ☑
      superficial NEC S30.874 ☑
    contusion S30.23 ☑
    crush S38.03 ☑
    during delivery — *see* Laceration, perineum, female, during delivery
    external constriction S30.844 ☑
    insect bite S30.864 ☑
    laceration S31.41 ☑
      with foreign body S31.42 ☑
    open wound S31.40 ☑
    puncture S31.43 ☑
      with foreign body S31.44 ☑
    superficial S30.95 ☑
      foreign body S30.854 ☑
  whiplash (cervical spine) S13.4 ☑
  wrist S69.9- ☑
    blood vessel — *see* Injury, blood vessel, hand
    contusion — *see* Contusion, wrist
    dislocation — *see* Dislocation, wrist
    fracture — *see* Fracture, wrist
    muscle — *see* Injury, muscle, hand
    nerve — *see* Injury, nerve, hand
    open — *see* Wound, open, wrist
    specified NEC S69.8- ☑
    sprain — *see* Sprain, wrist
    superficial — *see* Injury, superficial, wrist
Inoculation — *see also* Vaccination
  complication or reaction — *see* Complications, vaccination
Insanity, insane — *see also* Psychosis
  adolescent — *see* Schizophrenia
  confusional F28
    acute or subacute F05
  delusional F22
  senile F03 ☑
Insect
  bite — *see* Bite, by site, superficial, insect
  venomous, poisoning NEC (by) — *see* Venom, arthropod
Insecurity, food Z59.41

Insensitivity
  adrenocorticotropin hormone (ACTH) E27.49
  androgen E34.50
    complete E34.51
    partial E34.52
Insertion
  cord (umbilical) lateral or velamentous O43.12- ☑
  intrauterine contraceptive device (encounter for) — *see* Intrauterine contraceptive device
Insolation (sunstroke) T67.01 ☑
Insomnia (organic) G47.00
  adjustment F51.02
  adjustment disorder F51.02
  behavioral, of childhood Z73.819
    combined type Z73.812
    limit setting type Z73.811
    sleep-onset association type Z73.810
  childhood Z73.819
  chronic F51.04
    somatized tension F51.04
  conditioned F51.04
  due to
    alcohol
      abuse F10.182
      dependence F10.282
      use F10.982
    amphetamines
      abuse F15.182
      dependence F15.282
      use F15.982
    anxiety disorder F51.05
    caffeine
      abuse F15.182
      dependence F15.282
      use F15.982
    cocaine
      abuse F14.182
      dependence F14.282
      use F14.982
    depression F51.05
    drug NEC
      abuse F19.182
      dependence F19.282
      use F19.982
    medical condition G47.01
    mental disorder NEC F51.05
    opioid
      abuse F11.182
      dependence F11.282
      use F11.982
    psychoactive substance NEC
      abuse F19.182
      dependence F19.182
      use F19.982
    sedative, hypnotic, or anxiolytic
      abuse F13.182
      dependence F13.282
      use F13.982
    stimulant NEC
      abuse F15.182
      dependence F15.282
      use F15.982
  fatal familial (FFI) A81.83
  idiopathic F51.01
  learned F51.3
  nonorganic origin F51.01
  not due to a substance or known physiological condition F51.01
    specified NEC F51.09
  paradoxical F51.03
  primary F51.01
  psychiatric F51.05
  psychophysiologic F51.04
  related to psychopathology F51.05
  short-term F51.02
  specified NEC G47.09
  stress-related F51.02
  transient F51.02
  without objective findings F51.02
Inspiration
  food or foreign body — *see* Foreign body, by site
  mucus — *see* Asphyxia, mucus
Inspissated bile syndrome (newborn) P59.1
Instability
  emotional (excessive) F60.3
  housing
    housed Z59.819
      with risk of homelessness Z59.811

Instability — *continued*
  housing — *continued*
    housed — *continued*
      homelessness in past 12 months Z59.812
  joint (post-traumatic) M25.30
    ankle M25.37- ☑
    due to old ligament injury — *see* Disorder, ligament
    elbow M25.32- ☑
    flail — *see* Flail, joint
    foot M25.37- ☑
    hand M25.34- ☑
    hip M25.35- ☑
    knee M25.36- ☑
    lumbosacral — *see* subcategory M53.2 ☑
    prosthesis — *see* Complications, joint prosthesis, mechanical, displacement, by site
    sacroiliac — *see* subcategory M53.2 ☑
    secondary to
      old ligament injury — *see* Disorder, ligament
      removal of joint prosthesis M96.89
    shoulder (region) M25.31- ☑
    specified site NEC M25.39
    spine — *see* subcategory M53.2 ☑
    wrist M25.33- ☑
  knee (chronic) M23.5- ☑
  lumbosacral — *see* subcategory M53.2 ☑
  nervous F48.8
  personality (emotional) F60.3
  spine — *see* Instability, joint, spine
  vasomotor R55
Institutional syndrome (childhood) F94.2
Institutionalization, affecting child Z62.22
  disinhibited attachment F94.2
Insufficiency, insufficient
  accommodation, old age H52.4
  adrenal (gland) E27.40
    primary E27.1
  adrenocortical E27.40
    drug-induced E27.3
    iatrogenic E27.3
    primary E27.1
  anatomic crown height K08.89
  anterior (occlusal) guidance M26.54
  anus K62.89
  aortic (valve) I35.1
    with
      mitral (valve) disease I08.0
        with tricuspid (valve) disease I08.3
      stenosis I35.2
      tricuspid (valve) disease I08.2
        with mitral (valve) disease I08.3
    congenital Q23.1
    rheumatic I06.1
      with
        mitral (valve) disease I08.0
          with tricuspid (valve) disease I08.3
        stenosis I06.2
          with mitral (valve) disease I08.0
            with tricuspid (valve) disease I08.3
        tricuspid (valve) disease I08.2
          with mitral (valve) disease I08.3
    specified cause NEC I35.1
    syphilitic A52.03
  arterial I77.1
    basilar G45.0
    carotid (hemispheric) G45.1
    cerebral I67.81
    coronary (acute or subacute) I24.8
    mesenteric K55.1
    peripheral I73.9
    precerebral (multiple) (bilateral) G45.2
    vertebral G45.0
  arteriovenous I99.8
  biliary K83.8
  cardiac — *see also* Insufficiency, myocardial
    due to presence of (cardiac) prosthesis I97.11- ☑
    postprocedural I97.11- ☑
  cardiorenal, hypertensive I13.2
  cardiovascular — *see* Disease, cardiovascular
  cerebrovascular (acute) I67.81
    with transient focal neurological signs and symptoms G45.8
  circulatory NEC I99.8
    newborn P29.89
  clinical crown length K08.89
  convergence H51.11
  coronary (acute or subacute) I24.8

Insufficiency, insufficient — *continued*
  coronary — *continued*
    chronic or with a stated duration of over 4 weeks
      I25.89
  corticoadrenal E27.40
    primary E27.1
  dietary E63.9
  divergence H51.8
  food T73.0 ☑
  gastroesophageal K22.89
  gonadal
    ovary E28.39
    testis E29.1
  heart — *see also* Insufficiency, myocardial
    newborn P29.0
    valve — *see* Endocarditis
  hepatic — *see* Failure, hepatic
  idiopathic autonomic G90.09
  interocclusal distance of fully erupted teeth (ridge)
    M26.36
  kidney N28.9
    acute N28.9
    chronic N18.9
  lacrimal (secretion) H04.12- ☑
    passages — *see* Stenosis, lacrimal
  liver — *see* Failure, hepatic
  lung — *see* Insufficiency, pulmonary
  mental (congenital) — *see* Disability, intellectual
  mesenteric K55.1
  mitral (valve) I34.0
    with
      aortic valve disease I08.0
        with tricuspid (valve) disease I08.3
      obstruction or stenosis I05.2
        with aortic valve disease I08.0
      tricuspid (valve) disease I08.1
        with aortic (valve) disease I08.3
    congenital Q23.3
    rheumatic I05.1
      with
        aortic valve disease I08.0
          with tricuspid (valve) disease I08.3
        obstruction or stenosis I05.2
          with aortic valve disease I08.0
            with tricuspid (valve) disease I08.3
        tricuspid (valve) disease I08.1
          with aortic (valve) disease I08.3
    active or acute I01.1
      with chorea, rheumatic (Sydenham's) I02.0
    specified cause, except rheumatic I34.0
  muscle — *see also* Disease, muscle
    heart — *see* Insufficiency, myocardial
    ocular NEC H50.9
  myocardial, myocardium (with arteriosclerosis) — *see*
    also Failure, heart I50.9
    with
      rheumatic fever (conditions in I00) I09.0
        active, acute or subacute I01.2
          with chorea I02.0
        inactive or quiescent (with chorea) I09.0
    congenital Q24.8
    hypertensive — *see* Hypertension, heart
    newborn P29.0
    rheumatic I09.0
      active, acute, or subacute I01.2
    syphilitic A52.06
  nourishment T73.0 ☑
  pancreatic K86.89
    exocrine K86.81
  parathyroid (gland) E20.9
  peripheral vascular (arterial) I73.9
  pituitary E23.0
  placental (mother) O36.51- ☑
  platelets D69.6
  prenatal care affecting management of pregnancy
    O09.3- ☑
  progressive pluriglandular E31.0
  pulmonary J98.4
    acute, following surgery (nonthoracic) J95.2
      thoracic J95.1
    chronic, following surgery J95.3
    following
      shock J98.4
      trauma J98.4
    newborn P28.89
    valve I37.1
      with stenosis I37.2
      congenital Q22.2

Insufficiency, insufficient — *continued*
  pulmonary — *continued*
    valve — *continued*
      rheumatic I09.89
        with aortic, mitral or tricuspid (valve) disease
          I08.8
  pyloric K31.89
  renal (acute) N28.9
    chronic N18.9
  respiratory R06.89
    newborn P28.5
  rotation — *see* Malrotation
  sleep syndrome F51.12
  social insurance Z59.7
  suprarenal E27.40
    primary E27.1
  tarso-orbital fascia, congenital Q10.3
  testis E29.1
  thyroid (gland) (acquired) E03.9
    congenital E03.1
  tricuspid (valve) (rheumatic) I07.1
    with
      aortic (valve) disease I08.2
        with mitral (valve) disease I08.3
      mitral (valve) disease I08.1
        with aortic (valve) disease I08.3
      obstruction or stenosis I07.2
        with aortic (valve) disease I08.2
          with mitral (valve) disease I08.3
    congenital Q22.8
    nonrheumatic I36.1
      with stenosis I36.2
  urethral sphincter R32
  valve, valvular (heart) I38
    aortic — *see* Insufficiency, aortic (valve)
    congenital Q24.8
    mitral — *see* Insufficiency, mitral (valve)
    pulmonary — *see* Insufficiency, pulmonary, valve
    tricuspid — *see* Insufficiency, tricuspid (valve)
  vascular I99.8
    intestine K55.9
      acute — *see also* Ischemia, intestine, acute
        K55.059
    mesenteric K55.1
    peripheral I73.9
    renal — *see* Hypertension, kidney
  venous (chronic) (peripheral) I87.2
  velopharyngeal
    acquired K13.79
    congenital Q38.8
  ventricular — *see* Insufficiency, myocardial
  welfare support Z59.7
Insufflation, fallopian Z31.41
Insular — *see* condition
Insulinoma
  pancreas
    benign D13.7
    malignant C25.4
    uncertain behavior D37.8
  specified site
    benign — *see* Neoplasm, by site, benign
    malignant — *see* Neoplasm, by site, malignant
    uncertain behavior — *see* Neoplasm, by site, uncer-
      tain behavior
  unspecified site
    benign D13.7
    malignant C25.4
    uncertain behavior D37.8
Insuloma — *see* Insulinoma
Interference
  balancing side M26.56
  non-working side M26.56
Intermenstrual — *see* condition
Intermittent — *see* condition
Internal — *see* condition
Interrogation
  cardiac defibrillator (automatic) (implantable) Z45.02
  cardiac pacemaker Z45.018
  cardiac (event) (loop) recorder Z45.09
  infusion pump (implanted) (intrathecal) Z45.1
  neurostimulator Z46.2
Interruption
  aortic arch Q25.21
  bundle of His I44.30
  phase-shift, sleep cycle — *see* Disorder, sleep, circadian
    rhythm
  sleep phase-shift, or 24 hour sleep-wake cycle — *see*
    Disorder, sleep, circadian rhythm

Interstitial — *see* condition
Intertrigo L30.4
  labialis K13.0
Intervertebral disc — *see* condition
Intestine, intestinal — *see* condition
Intolerance
  carbohydrate K90.49
  disaccharide, hereditary E73.0
  fat NEC K90.49
    pancreatic K90.3
  food K90.49
    dietary counseling and surveillance Z71.3
  fructose E74.10
    hereditary E74.12
  glucose (-galactose) E74.39
  gluten K90.41
  lactose E73.9
    specified NEC E73.8
  lysine E72.3
  milk NEC K90.49
    lactose E73.9
  protein K90.49
  starch NEC K90.49
  sucrose (-isomaltose) E74.31
Intoxicated NEC (without dependence) — *see* Alcohol,
  intoxication
Intoxication
  acid E87.2
  alcoholic (acute) (without dependence) — *see* Alcohol,
    intoxication
  alimentary canal K52.1
  amphetamine (without dependence) — *see also* Abuse,
    drug, stimulant, with intoxication
    with dependence — *see* Dependence, drug, stimu-
      lant, with intoxication
    stimulant NEC F15.10
      with
        anxiety disorder F15.180
        intoxication F15.129
          with
            delirium F15.121
            perceptual disturbance F15.122
  anxiolytic (acute) (without dependence) — *see* Abuse,
    drug, sedative, with intoxication
    with dependence — *see* Dependence, drug, seda-
      tive, with intoxication
  caffeine F15.929
    with dependence — *see* Dependence, drug, stimu-
      lant, with intoxication
  cannabinoids (acute) (without dependence) — *see*
    Use, cannabis, with intoxication
    with
      abuse — *see* Abuse, drug, cannabis, with intoxi-
        cation
      dependence — *see* Dependence, drug, cannabis,
        with intoxication
  chemical — *see* Table of Drugs and Chemicals
    via placenta or breast milk — *see* - Absorption,
      chemical, through placenta
  cocaine (acute) (without dependence) — *see* Abuse,
    drug, cocaine, with intoxication
    with dependence — *see* Dependence, drug, cocaine,
      with intoxication
  drug
    acute (without dependence) — *see* Abuse, drug, by
      type with intoxication
      with dependence — *see* Dependence, drug, by
        type with intoxication
    addictive
      via placenta or breast milk — *see* Absorption,
        drug, addictive, through placenta
    newborn P93.8
      gray baby syndrome P93.0
    overdose or wrong substance given or taken — *see*
      Table of Drugs and Chemicals, by drug, poi-
      soning
  enteric K52.1
  foodborne A05.9
    bacterial A05.9
    classical (Clostridium botulinum) A05.1
    due to
      Bacillus cereus A05.4
      bacterium A05.9
        specified NEC A05.8
      Clostridium
        botulinum A05.1
        perfringens A05.2
        welchii A05.2

Intoxication — continued
  foodborne — continued
    due to — continued
      Salmonella A02.9
        with
          (gastro)enteritis A02.0
          localized infection(s) A02.20
            arthritis A02.23
            meningitis A02.21
            osteomyelitis A02.24
            pneumonia A02.22
            pyelonephritis A02.25
            specified NEC A02.29
        sepsis A02.1
        specified manifestation NEC A02.8
      Staphylococcus A05.0
      Vibrio
        parahaemolyticus A05.3
        vulnificus A05.5
    enterotoxin, staphylococcal A05.0
    noxious — see Poisoning, food, noxious
  gastrointestinal K52.1
  hallucinogenic (without dependence) — see Abuse, drug, hallucinogen, with intoxication
    with dependence — see Dependence, drug, hallucinogen, with intoxication
  hypnotic (acute) (without dependence) — see Abuse, drug, sedative, with intoxication
    with dependence — see Dependence, drug, sedative, with intoxication
  inhalant (acute) (without dependence) — see Abuse, drug, inhalant, with intoxication
    with dependence — see Dependence, drug, inhalant, with intoxication
  meaning
    inebriation — see category F10 ☑
    poisoning — see Table of Drugs and Chemicals
  methyl alcohol (acute) (without dependence) — see Alcohol, intoxication
  opioid (acute) (without dependence) — see Abuse, drug, opioid, with intoxication
    with dependence — see Dependence, drug, opioid, with intoxication
  pathologic NEC (without dependence) — see Alcohol, intoxication
  phencyclidine (without dependence) — see Abuse, drug, hallucinogen, with intoxication
    with dependence — see Dependence, drug, hallucinogen, with intoxication
  potassium (K) E87.5
  psychoactive substance NEC (without dependence) — see Abuse, drug, psychoactive NEC, with intoxication
    with dependence — see Dependence, drug, psychoactive NEC, with intoxication
  sedative (acute) (without dependence) — see Abuse, drug, sedative, with intoxication
    with dependence — see Dependence, drug, sedative, with intoxication
  serum — see also Reaction, serum T80.69 ☑
  uremic — see Uremia
  volatile solvents (acute) (without dependence) — see Abuse, drug, inhalant, with intoxication
    with dependence — see Dependence, drug, inhalant, with intoxication
  water E87.79
Intraabdominal testis, testes
  bilateral Q53.211
  unilateral Q53.111
Intracranial — see condition
Intrahepatic gallbladder Q44.1
Intraligamentous — see condition
Intrathoracic — see also condition
  kidney Q63.2
Intrauterine contraceptive device
  checking Z30.431
  in situ Z97.5
  insertion Z30.430
    immediately following removal Z30.433
  management Z30.431
  reinsertion Z30.433
  removal Z30.432
  replacement Z30.433
  retention in pregnancy O26.3- ☑
Intraventricular — see condition
Intrinsic deformity — see Deformity
Intubation, difficult or failed T88.4 ☑
Intumescence, lens (eye) (cataract) — see Cataract

Intussusception (bowel) (colon) (enteric) (ileocecal) (ileocolic) (intestine) (rectum) K56.1
  appendix K38.8
  congenital Q43.8
  ureter (with obstruction) N13.5
Invagination (bowel, colon, intestine or rectum) K56.1
Inversion
  albumin-globulin (A-G) ratio E88.09
  bladder N32.89
  cecum — see Intussusception
  cervix N88.8
  chromosome in normal individual Q95.1
  circadian rhythm — see Disorder, sleep, circadian rhythm
  nipple N64.59
    congenital Q83.8
    gestational — see Retraction, nipple
    puerperal, postpartum — see Retraction, nipple
  nyctohemeral rhythm — see Disorder, sleep, circadian rhythm
  optic papilla Q14.2
  organ or site, congenital NEC — see Anomaly, by site
  sleep rhythm — see Disorder, sleep, circadian rhythm
  testis (congenital) Q55.29
  uterus (chronic) (postinfectional) (postpartal, old) N85.5
    postpartum O71.2
  vagina (posthysterectomy) N99.3
  ventricular Q20.5
Investigation — see also Examination Z04.9
  clinical research subject (control) (normal comparison) (participant) Z00.6
Involuntary movement, abnormal R25.9
Involution, involutional — see also condition
  breast, cystic — see Dysplasia, mammary, specified type NEC
  depression (single episode) F32.89
    recurrent episode F33.9
  melancholia (single episode) F32.89
    recurrent episode F33.8
  ovary, senile — see Atrophy, ovary
  thymus failure E32.8
I.Q.
  20-34 F72
  35-49 F71
  50-69 F70
  under 20 F73
IRDS (type I) P22.0
  type II P22.1
Irideremia Q13.1
Iridis rubeosis — see Disorder, iris, vascular
Iridochoroiditis (panuveitis) — see Panuveitis
Iridocyclitis H20.9
  acute H20.0- ☑
    hypopyon H20.05- ☑
    primary H20.01- ☑
    recurrent H20.02- ☑
    secondary (noninfectious) H20.04- ☑
      infectious H20.03- ☑
  chronic H20.1- ☑
  due to allergy — see Iridocyclitis, acute, secondary
  endogenous — see Iridocyclitis, acute, primary
  Fuchs' — see Cyclitis, Fuchs' heterochromic
  gonococcal A54.32
  granulomatous — see Iridocyclitis, chronic
  herpes, herpetic (simplex) B00.51
    zoster B02.32
  hypopyon — see Iridocyclitis, acute, hypopyon
  in (due to)
    ankylosing spondylitis M45.9
    gonococcal infection A54.32
    herpes (simplex) virus B00.51
      zoster B02.32
    infectious disease NOS B99 ☑
    parasitic disease NOS B89 [H22]
    sarcoidosis D86.83
    syphilis A51.43
    tuberculosis A18.54
    zoster B02.32
  lens-induced H20.2- ☑
  nongranulomatous — see Iridocyclitis, acute
  recurrent — see Iridocyclitis, acute, recurrent
  rheumatic — see Iridocyclitis, chronic
  subacute — see Iridocyclitis, acute
  sympathetic — see Uveitis, sympathetic
  syphilitic (secondary) A51.43
  tuberculous (chronic) A18.54
  Vogt-Koyanagi H20.82- ☑

Iridocyclochoroiditis (panuveitis) — see Panuveitis
Iridodialysis H21.53- ☑
Iridodonesis H21.89
Iridoplegia (complete) (partial) (reflex) H57.09
Iridoschisis H21.25- ☑
Iris — see also condition
  bombé — see Membrane, pupillary
Iritis — see also Iridocyclitis
  chronic — see Iridocyclitis, chronic
  diabetic — see E08-E13 with .39
  due to
    herpes simplex B00.51
    leprosy A30.9 [H22]
  gonococcal A54.32
  gouty — see also Gout, by type M10.9 [H22]
  granulomatous — see Iridocyclitis, chronic
  lens induced — see Iridocyclitis, lens-induced
  papulosa (syphilitic) A52.71
  rheumatic — see Iridocyclitis, chronic
  syphilitic (secondary) A51.43
    congenital (early) A50.01
    late A52.71
  tuberculous A18.54
Iron — see condition
Iron-miner's lung J63.4
Irradiated enamel (tooth, teeth) K03.89
Irradiation effects, adverse T66 ☑
Irreducible, irreducibility — see condition
Irregular, irregularity
  action, heart I49.9
  alveolar process K08.89
  bleeding N92.6
  breathing R06.89
  contour of cornea (acquired) — see Deformity, cornea
    congenital Q13.4
  contour, reconstructed breast N65.0
  dentin (in pulp) K04.3
  eye movements H55.89
    deficient
      saccadic H55.81
      smooth H55.82
    nystagmus — see Nystagmus
  labor O62.2
  menstruation (cause unknown) N92.6
  periods N92.6
  prostate N42.9
  pupil — see Abnormality, pupillary
  reconstructed breast N65.0
  respiratory R06.89
  septum (nasal) J34.2
  shape, organ or site, congenital NEC — see Distortion
  sleep-wake pattern (rhythm) G47.23
Irritable, irritability R45.4
  bladder N32.89
  bowel (syndrome) K58.9
    with
      constipation K58.1
      diarrhea K58.0
      mixed K58.2
      psychogenic F45.8
      specified NEC K58.8
  bronchial — see Bronchitis
  cerebral, in newborn P91.3
  colon — see also Irritable, bowel K58.9
    with diarrhea K58.0
    psychogenic F45.8
  duodenum K59.89
  heart (psychogenic) F45.8
  hip — see Derangement, joint, specified type NEC, hip
  ileum K59.89
  infant R68.12
  jejunum K59.89
  rectum K59.89
  stomach K31.89
    psychogenic F45.8
  sympathetic G90.8
  urethra N36.8
Irritation
  anus K62.89
  axillary nerve G54.0
  bladder N32.89
  brachial plexus G54.0
  bronchial — see Bronchitis
  cervical plexus G54.2
  cervix — see Cervicitis
  choroid, sympathetic — see Endophthalmitis
  cranial nerve — see Disorder, nerve, cranial
  gastric K31.89

☑ **Additional Character Required** — Refer to the Tabular List for Character Selection   Subterms under main terms may continue to next column or page

Irritation — *continued*
　gastric — *continued*
　　psychogenic F45.8
　globe, sympathetic — *see* Uveitis, sympathetic
　labyrinth — *see* subcategory H83.2 ☑
　lumbosacral plexus G54.1
　meninges (traumatic) — *see* Injury, intracranial
　　nontraumatic — *see* Meningismus
　nerve — *see* Disorder, nerve
　nervous R45.0
　penis N48.89
　perineum NEC L29.3
　peripheral autonomic nervous system G90.8
　peritoneum — *see* Peritonitis
　pharynx J39.2
　plantar nerve — *see* Lesion, nerve, plantar
　spinal (cord) (traumatic) — *see also* Injury, spinal cord, by region
　　nerve G58.9
　　　root NEC — *see* Radiculopathy
　　nontraumatic — *see* Myelopathy
　stomach K31.89
　　psychogenic F45.8
　sympathetic nerve NEC G90.8
　ulnar nerve — *see* Lesion, nerve, ulnar
　vagina N89.8
Ischemia, ischemic I99.8
　bowel (transient)
　　acute — *see also* Ischemia, intestine, acute K55.059
　　chronic K55.1
　　due to mesenteric artery insufficiency K55.1
　brain — *see* Ischemia, cerebral
　cardiac (see Disease, heart, ischemic)
　cardiomyopathy I25.5
　cerebral (chronic) (generalized) I67.82
　　arteriosclerotic I67.2
　　intermittent G45.9
　　newborn P91.0
　　recurrent focal G45.8
　　transient G45.9
　colon chronic (due to mesenteric artery insufficiency) K55.1
　coronary — *see* Disease, heart, ischemic
　demand (coronary) — *see also* Angina I24.8
　　with myocardial infarction I21.A1
　　resulting in myocardial infarction I21.A1
　heart (chronic or with a stated duration of over 4 weeks) I25.9
　　acute or with a stated duration of 4 weeks or less I24.9
　　subacute I24.9
　infarction, muscle — *see* Infarct, muscle
　intestine (large) (small) (transient) K55.9
　　acute K55.059
　　　diffuse K55.052
　　　focal K55.051
　　　large K55.039
　　　　diffuse K55.032
　　　　focal K55.031
　　　small K55.019
　　　　diffuse K55.012
　　　　focal K55.011
　　chronic K55.1
　　due to mesenteric artery insufficiency K55.1
　kidney N28.0
　limb, critical — *see* Arteriosclerosis, with critical limb ischemia
　limb-threatening, chronic — *see* Arteriosclerosis, with critical limb ischemia
　mesenteric, acute — *see also* Ischemia, intestine, acute K55.059
　muscle, traumatic T79.6 ☑
　myocardium, myocardial (chronic or with a stated duration of over 4 weeks) I25.9
　　acute, without myocardial infarction I51.3
　　silent (asymptomatic) I25.6
　　transient of newborn P29.4
　renal N28.0
　retina, retinal — *see* Occlusion, artery, retina
　small bowel
　　acute K55.019
　　　diffuse K55.012
　　　focal K55.011
　　chronic K55.1
　　due to mesenteric artery insufficiency K55.1
　spinal cord G95.11
　subendocardial — *see* Insufficiency, coronary
　supply (coronary) — *see also* Angina I25.9

Ischemia, ischemic — *continued*
　supply — *see also* Angina — *continued*
　　due to vasospasm I20.1
Ischial spine — *see* condition
Ischialgia — *see* Sciatica
Ischiopagus Q89.4
Ischium, ischial — *see* condition
Ischuria R34
Iselin's disease or osteochondrosis — *see* Osteochondrosis, juvenile, metatarsus
Islands of
　parotid tissue in
　　lymph nodes Q38.6
　　neck structures Q38.6
　submaxillary glands in
　　fascia Q38.6
　　lymph nodes Q38.6
　　neck muscles Q38.6
Islet cell tumor, pancreas D13.7
Isoimmunization NEC — *see also* Incompatibility
　affecting management of pregnancy (ABO) (with hydrops fetalis) O36.11- ☑
　　anti-A sensitization O36.11- ☑
　　anti-B sensitization O36.19- ☑
　　anti-c sensitization O36.09- ☑
　　anti-C sensitization O36.09- ☑
　　anti-e sensitization O36.09- ☑
　　anti-E sensitization O36.09- ☑
　　Rh NEC O36.09- ☑
　　　anti-D antibody O36.01- ☑
　　specified NEC O36.19- ☑
　newborn P55.9
　　with
　　　hydrops fetalis P56.0
　　　kernicterus P57.0
　　　ABO (blood groups) P55.1
　　　Rhesus (Rh) factor P55.0
　　　specified type NEC P55.8
Isolation, isolated
　dwelling Z59.89
　family Z63.79
　social Z60.4
Isoleucinosis E71.19
Isomerism atrial appendages (with asplenia or polysplenia) Q20.6
Isosporiasis, isosporosis A07.3
Isovaleric acidemia E71.110
Issue of
　medical certificate Z02.79
　　for disability determination Z02.71
　repeat prescription (appliance) (glasses) (medicinal substance, medicament, medicine) Z76.0
　　contraception — *see* Contraception
Itch, itching — *see also* Pruritus
　baker's L23.6
　barber's B35.0
　bricklayer's L24.5
　cheese B88.0
　clam digger's B65.3
　coolie B76.9
　copra B88.0
　dew B76.9
　dhobi B35.6
　filarial — *see* Infestation, filarial
　grain B88.0
　grocer's B88.0
　ground B76.9
　harvest B88.0
　jock B35.6
　Malabar B35.5
　　beard B35.0
　　foot B35.3
　　scalp B35.0
　meaning scabies B86
　Norwegian B86
　perianal L29.0
　poultrymen's B88.0
　sarcoptic B86
　scabies B86
　scrub B88.0
　straw B88.0
　swimmer's B65.3
　water B76.9
　winter L29.8
Ivemark's syndrome (asplenia with congenital heart disease) Q89.01
Ivory bones Q78.2
Ixodiasis NEC B88.8

J

Jaccoud's syndrome — *see* Arthropathy, postrheumatic, chronic
Jackson's
　membrane Q43.3
　paralysis or syndrome G83.89
　veil Q43.3
Jacquet's dermatitis (diaper dermatitis) L22
Jadassohn-Pellizari's disease or anetoderma L90.2
Jadassohn's
　blue nevus — *see* Nevus
　intraepidermal epithelioma — *see* Neoplasm, skin, benign
Jaffe-Lichtenstein (-Uehlinger) **syndrome** — *see* Dysplasia, fibrous, bone NEC
Jakob-Creutzfeldt disease or syndrome — *see* Creutzfeldt-Jakob disease or syndrome
Jaksch-Luzet disease D64.89
Jamaican
　neuropathy G92.8
　paraplegic tropical ataxic-spastic syndrome G92.8
Janet's disease F48.8
Janiceps Q89.4
Jansky-Bielschowsky amaurotic idiocy E75.4
Japanese
　B-type encephalitis A83.0
　river fever A75.3
Jaundice (yellow) R17
　acholuric (familial) (splenomegalic) — *see also* Spherocytosis
　　acquired D59.8
　breast-milk (inhibitor) P59.3
　catarrhal (acute) B15.9
　　with hepatic coma B15.0
　cholestatic (benign) R17
　due to or associated with
　　delayed conjugation P59.8
　　　associated with (due to) preterm delivery P59.0
　　preterm delivery P59.0
　epidemic (catarrhal) B15.9
　　with hepatic coma B15.0
　　leptospiral A27.0
　　spirochetal A27.0
　familial nonhemolytic (congenital) (Gilbert) E80.4
　　Crigler-Najjar E80.5
　febrile (acute) B15.9
　　with hepatic coma B15.0
　　leptospiral A27.0
　　spirochetal A27.0
　hematogenous D59.9
　hemolytic (acquired) D59.9
　　congenital — *see* Spherocytosis
　hemorrhagic (acute) (leptospiral) (spirochetal) A27.0
　infectious (acute) (subacute) B15.9
　　with hepatic coma B15.0
　　leptospiral A27.0
　　spirochetal A27.0
　leptospiral (hemorrhagic) A27.0
　malignant (without coma) K72.90
　　with coma K72.91
　neonatal — *see* Jaundice, newborn
　newborn P59.9
　　due to or associated with
　　　ABO
　　　　antibodies P55.1
　　　　incompatibility, maternal/fetal P55.1
　　　　isoimmunization P55.1
　　　absence or deficiency of enzyme system for bilirubin conjugation (congenital) P59.8
　　　bleeding P58.1
　　　breast milk inhibitors to conjugation P59.3
　　　　associated with preterm delivery P59.0
　　　bruising P58.0
　　　Crigler-Najjar syndrome E80.5
　　　delayed conjugation P59.8
　　　　associated with preterm delivery P59.0
　　　drugs or toxins
　　　　given to newborn P58.42
　　　　transmitted from mother P58.41
　　　excessive hemolysis P58.9
　　　　due to
　　　　　bleeding P58.1
　　　　　bruising P58.0
　　　　　drugs or toxins
　　　　　　given to newborn P58.42
　　　　　　transmitted from mother P58.41

▽ **Subterms under main terms may continue to next column or page**　　☑ **Additional Character Required** — **Refer to the Tabular List for Character Selection**　　　**207**

Irritation — Jaundice

Jaundice — *continued*
  newborn — *continued*
    due to or associated with — *continued*
      excessive hemolysis — *continued*
        due to — *continued*
          infection P58.2
          polycythemia P58.3
          swallowed maternal blood P58.5
        specified type NEC P58.8
      galactosemia E74.21
      Gilbert syndrome E80.4
      hemolytic disease P55.9
        ABO isoimmunization P55.1
        Rh isoimmunization P55.0
        specified NEC P55.8
      hepatocellular damage P59.20
        specified NEC P59.29
      hereditary hemolytic anemia P58.8
      hypothyroidism, congenital E03.1
      incompatibility, maternal/fetal NOS P55.9
      infection P58.2
      inspissated bile syndrome P59.1
      isoimmunization NOS P55.9
      mucoviscidosis E84.9
      polycythemia P58.3
      preterm delivery P59.0
      Rh
        antibodies P55.0
        incompatibility, maternal/fetal P55.0
        isoimmunization P55.0
      specified cause NEC P59.8
      swallowed maternal blood P58.5
    spherocytosis (congenital) D58.0
    nonhemolytic congenital familial (Gilbert) E80.4
    nuclear, newborn — *see also* Kernicterus of newborn P57.9
    obstructive — *see also* Obstruction, bile duct K83.1
    post-immunization — *see* Hepatitis, viral, type, B
    post-transfusion — *see* Hepatitis, viral, type, B
    regurgitation — *see also* Obstruction, bile duct K83.1
    serum (homologous) (prophylactic) (therapeutic) — *see* Hepatitis, viral, type, B
    spirochetal (hemorrhagic) A27.0
    symptomatic R17
      newborn P59.9
Jaw — *see* condition
Jaw-winking phenomenon or syndrome Q07.8
Jealousy
  alcoholic F10.988
  childhood F93.8
  sibling F93.8
Jejunitis — *see* Enteritis
Jejunostomy status Z93.4
Jejunum, jejunal — *see* condition
Jensen's disease — *see* Inflammation, chorioretinal, focal, juxtapapillary
Jerks, myoclonic G25.3
Jervell-Lange-Nielsen syndrome I45.81
Jeune's disease Q77.2
Jigger disease B88.1
Job's syndrome (chronic granulomatous disease) D71
Joint — *see also* condition
  mice — *see* Loose, body, joint
    knee M23.4-
Jordan's anomaly or syndrome D72.0
Joseph-Diamond-Blackfan anemia (congenital hypoplastic) D61.01
Jungle yellow fever A95.0
Jüngling's disease — *see* Sarcoidosis
Juvenile — *see* condition

K

Kahler's disease C90.0- ☑
Kakke E51.11
Kala-azar B55.0
Kallmann's syndrome E23.0
Kanner's syndrome (autism) — *see* Psychosis, childhood
Kaposi's
  dermatosis (xeroderma pigmentosum) Q82.1
  lichen ruber L44.0
    acuminatus L44.0
  sarcoma
    colon C46.4
    connective tissue C46.1
    gastrointestinal organ C46.4
    lung C46.5- ☑

Kaposi's — *continued*
  sarcoma — *continued*
    lymph node (multiple) C46.3
    palate (hard) (soft) C46.2
    rectum C46.4
    skin (multiple sites) C46.0
    specified site NEC C46.7
    stomach C46.4
    unspecified site C46.9
  varicelliform eruption B00.0
    vaccinia T88.1 ☑
Kartagener's syndrome or triad (sinusitis, bronchiectasis, situs inversus) Q89.3
Karyotype
  with abnormality except iso (Xq) Q96.2
  45,X Q96.0
  46,X
    iso (Xq) Q96.1
  46,XX Q98.3
    with streak gonads Q50.32
    hermaphrodite (true) Q99.1
    male Q98.3
  46,XY
    with streak gonads Q56.1
    female Q97.3
    hermaphrodite (true) Q99.1
  47,XXX Q97.0
  47,XXY Q98.0
  47,XYY Q98.5
Kaschin-Beck disease — *see* Disease, Kaschin-Beck
Katayama's disease or fever B65.2
Kawasaki's syndrome M30.3
Kayser-Fleischer ring (cornea) (pseudosclerosis) H18.04- ☑
Kaznelson's syndrome (congenital hypoplastic anemia) D61.01
Kearns-Sayre syndrome H49.81- ☑
Kedani fever A75.3
Kelis L91.0
Kelly (-Patterson) **syndrome** (sideropenic dysphagia) D50.1
Keloid, cheloid L91.0
  acne L73.0
  Addison's L94.0
  cornea — *see* Opacity, cornea
  Hawkin's L91.0
  scar L91.0
Keloma L91.0
Kenya fever A77.1
Keratectasia — *see also* Ectasia, cornea
  congenital Q13.4
Keratinization of alveolar ridge mucosa
  excessive K13.23
  minimal K13.22
Keratinized residual ridge mucosa
  excessive K13.23
  minimal K13.22
Keratitis (nodular) (nonulcerative) (simple) (zonular) H16.9
  with ulceration (central) (marginal) (perforated) (ring) — *see* Ulcer, cornea
  actinic — *see* Photokeratitis
  arborescens (herpes simplex) B00.52
  areolar H16.11- ☑
  bullosa H16.8
  deep H16.309
    specified type NEC H16.399
  dendritic (a) (herpes simplex) B00.52
  disciform (is) (herpes simplex) B00.52
    varicella B01.81
  filamentary H16.12- ☑
  gonococcal (congenital or prenatal) A54.33
  herpes, herpetic (simplex) B00.52
    zoster B02.33
  in (due to)
    acanthamebiasis B60.13
    adenovirus B30.0
    exanthema — *see also* Exanthem B09
    herpes (simplex) virus B00.52
    measles B05.81
    syphilis A50.31
    tuberculosis A18.52
    zoster B02.33
  interstitial (nonsyphilitic) H16.30- ☑
    diffuse H16.32- ☑
    herpes, herpetic (simplex) B00.52
      zoster B02.33
    sclerosing H16.33- ☑

Keratitis — *continued*
  interstitial — *continued*
    specified type NEC H16.39- ☑
    syphilitic (congenital) (late) A50.31
    tuberculous A18.52
  macular H16.11- ☑
  nummular H16.11- ☑
  oyster shuckers' H16.8
  parenchymatous — *see* Keratitis, interstitial
  petrificans H16.8
  postmeasles B05.81
  punctata
    leprosa A30.9 [H16.14-] ☑
    syphilitic (profunda) A50.31
  punctate H16.14- ☑
  purulent H16.8
  rosacea L71.8
  sclerosing H16.33- ☑
  specified type NEC H16.8
  stellate H16.11- ☑
  striate H16.11- ☑
  superficial H16.10- ☑
    with conjunctivitis — *see* Keratoconjunctivitis
    due to light — *see* Photokeratitis
  suppurative H16.8
  syphilitic (congenital) (prenatal) A50.31
  trachomatous A71.1
    sequelae B94.0
  tuberculous A18.52
  vesicular H16.8
  xerotic — *see also* Keratomalacia H16.8
    vitamin A deficiency E50.4
Keratoacanthoma L85.8
Keratocele — *see* Descemetocele
Keratoconjunctivitis H16.20- ☑
  Acanthamoeba B60.13
  adenoviral B30.0
  epidemic B30.0
  exposure H16.21- ☑
  herpes, herpetic (simplex) B00.52
    zoster B02.33
  in exanthema — *see also* Exanthem B09
  infectious B30.0
  lagophthalmic — *see* Keratoconjunctivitis, specified type NEC
  neurotrophic H16.23- ☑
  phlyctenular H16.25- ☑
  postmeasles B05.81
  shipyard B30.0
  sicca (Sjogren's) M35.0- ☑
    not Sjogren's H16.22- ☑
  specified type NEC H16.29- ☑
  tuberculous (phlyctenular) A18.52
  vernal H16.26- ☑
Keratoconus H18.60- ☑
  congenital Q13.4
  stable H18.61- ☑
  unstable H18.62- ☑
Keratocyst (dental) (odontogenic) — *see* Cyst, calcifying odontogenic
Keratoderma, keratodermia (congenital) (palmaris et plantaris) (symmetrical) Q82.8
  acquired L85.1
    in diseases classified elsewhere L86
  climactericum L85.1
  gonococcal A54.89
  gonorrheal A54.89
  punctata L85.2
  Reiter's — *see* Reiter's disease
Keratodermatocele — *see* Descemetocele
Keratoglobus H18.79 ☑
  congenital Q15.8
    with glaucoma Q15.0
Keratohemia — *see* Pigmentation, cornea, stromal
Keratoiritis — *see also* Iridocyclitis
  syphilitic A50.39
  tuberculous A18.54
Keratoma L57.0
  palmaris and plantaris hereditarium Q82.8
  senile L57.0
Keratomalacia H18.44- ☑
  vitamin A deficiency E50.4
Keratomegaly Q13.4
Keratomycosis B49
  nigrans, nigricans (palmaris) B36.1
Keratopathy H18.9
  band H18.42- ☑

Keratopathy — *continued*
  bullous (aphakic), following cataract surgery H59.Ø1- ☑
  bullous H18.1- ☑
Keratoscleritis, tuberculous A18.52
Keratosis L57.Ø
  actinic L57.Ø
  arsenical L85.8
  congenital, specified NEC Q8Ø.8
  female genital NEC N94.89
  follicularis Q82.8
    acquired L11.Ø
    congenita Q82.8
    et parafollicularis in cutem penetrans L87.Ø
    spinulosa (decalvans) Q82.8
    vitamin A deficiency E5Ø.8
  gonococcal A54.89
  male genital (external) N5Ø.89
  nigricans L83
  obturans, external ear (canal) — *see* Cholesteatoma,
    external ear
  palmaris et plantaris (inherited) (symmetrical) Q82.8
    acquired L85.1
  penile N48.89
  pharynx J39.2
  pilaris, acquired L85.8
  punctata (palmaris et plantaris) L85.2
  scrotal N5Ø.89
  seborrheic L82.1
    inflamed L82.Ø
  senile L57.Ø
  solar L57.Ø
  tonsillaris J35.8
  vagina N89.4
  vegetans Q82.8
  vitamin A deficiency E5Ø.8
  vocal cord J38.3
Kerato-uveitis — *see* Iridocyclitis
Kerion (celsi) B35.Ø
Kernicterus of newborn (not due to isoimmunization)
    P57.9
  due to isoimmunization (conditions in P55.Ø-P55.9)
    P57.Ø
  specified type NEC P57.8
Kerunoparalysis T75.Ø9 ☑
Keshan disease E59
Ketoacidosis E87.2
  diabetic — *see* Diabetes, by type, with ketoacidosis
Ketonuria R82.4
Ketosis NEC E88.89
  diabetic — *see* Diabetes, by type, with ketoacidosis
Kew Garden fever A79.1
Kidney — *see* condition
Kienböck's disease — *see also* Osteochondrosis, juvenile,
    hand, carpal lunate
  adult M93.1
Kimmelstiel (-Wilson) **disease** — *see* Diabetes, Kimmel-
    stiel (-Wilson) disease
Kink, kinking
  artery I77.1
  hair (acquired) L67.8
  ileum or intestine — *see* Obstruction, intestine
  Lane's — *see* Obstruction, intestine
  organ or site, congenital NEC — *see* Anomaly, by site
  ureter (pelvic junction) N13.5
    with
      hydronephrosis N13.1
        with infection N13.6
      pyelonephritis (chronic) N11.1
    congenital Q62.39
  vein(s) I87.8
    caval I87.1
    peripheral I87.1
Kinnier Wilson's disease (hepatolenticular degenera-
    tion) E83.Ø1
Kissing spine M48.2Ø
  cervical region M48.22
  cervicothoracic region M48.23
  lumbar region M48.26
  lumbosacral region M48.27
  occipito-atlanto-axial region M48.21
  thoracic region M48.24
  thoracolumbar region M48.25
Klatskin's tumor C22.1
Klauder's disease A26.8
Klebs' disease — *see also* Glomerulonephritis NØ5- ☑
Klebsiella (K.) **pneumoniae, as cause of disease clas-
    sified elsewhere** B96.1
Klein (e)-**Levin syndrome** G47.13

Kleptomania F63.2
Klinefelter's syndrome Q98.4
  karyotype 47,XXY Q98.Ø
  male with more than two X chromosomes Q98.1
Klippel-Feil deficiency, disease, or syndrome (brevi-
    collis) Q76.1
Klippel's disease I67.2
Klippel-Trenaunay (-Weber) **syndrome** Q87.2
Klumpke (-Déjerine) **palsy, paralysis** (birth) (newborn)
    P14.1
Knee — *see* condition
Knock knee (acquired) M21.Ø6- ☑
  congenital Q74.1
Knot(s)
  intestinal, syndrome (volvulus) K56.2
  surfer S89.8- ☑
  umbilical cord (true) O69.2 ☑
Knotting (of)
  hair L67.8
  intestine K56.2
Knuckle pad (Garrod's) M72.1
Koch's
  infection — *see* Tuberculosis
  relapsing fever A68.9
Koch-Weeks' conjunctivitis — *see* Conjunctivitis, acute,
    mucopurulent
Köebner's syndrome Q81.8
Köenig's disease (osteochondritis dissecans) — *see* Os-
    teochondritis, dissecans
Köhler-Pellegrini-Steida disease or syndrome (calci-
    fication, knee joint) — *see* Bursitis, tibial collateral
Köhler's disease
  patellar — *see* Osteochondrosis, juvenile, patella
  tarsal navicular — *see* Osteochondrosis, juvenile, tarsus
Koilonychia L6Ø.3
  congenital Q84.6
Kojevnikov's, epilepsy — *see* Kozhevnikof's epilepsy
Koplik's spots BØ5.9
Kopp's asthma E32.8
Korsakoff's (Wernicke) **disease, psychosis or syn-
    drome** (alcoholic) F1Ø.96
  with dependence F1Ø.26
  drug-induced
    due to drug abuse — *see* Abuse, drug, by type, with
      amnestic disorder
    due to drug dependence — *see* Dependence, drug,
      by type, with amnestic disorder
  nonalcoholic FØ4
Korsakov's disease, psychosis or syndrome — *see*
    Korsakoff's disease
Korsakow's disease, psychosis or syndrome — *see*
    Korsakoff's disease
Kostmann's disease or syndrome (infantile genetic
    agranulocytosis) — *see* Agranulocytosis
Kozhevnikof's epilepsy G4Ø.1Ø9
  intractable G4Ø.119
    with status epilepticus G4Ø.111
    without status epilepticus G4Ø.119
  not intractable G4Ø.1Ø9
    with status epilepticus G4Ø.1Ø1
    without status epilepticus G4Ø.1Ø9
Krabbe's
  disease E75.23
  syndrome, congenital muscle hypoplasia Q79.8
Kraepelin-Morel disease — *see* Schizophrenia
Kraft-Weber-Dimitri disease Q85.8
Kraurosis
  ani K62.89
  penis N48.Ø
  vagina N89.8
  vulva N9Ø.4
Kreotoxism AØ5.9
Krukenberg's
  spindle — *see* Pigmentation, cornea, posterior
  tumor C79.6- ☑
Kufs' disease E75.4
Kugelberg-Welander disease G12.1
Kuhnt-Junius degeneration — *see also* Degeneration,
    macula H35.32- ☑
Kümmell's disease or spondylitis — *see* Spondylopa-
    thy, traumatic
Kupffer cell sarcoma C22.3
Kuru A81.81
Kussmaul's
  disease M3Ø.Ø
  respiration E87.2

Kussmaul's — *continued*
  respiration — *continued*
    in diabetic acidosis — *see* Diabetes, by type, with
      ketoacidosis
Kwashiorkor E4Ø
  marasmic, marasmus type E42
Kyasanur Forest disease A98.2
Kyphoscoliosis, kyphoscoliotic (acquired) — *see also*
    Scoliosis M41.9
  congenital Q67.5
  heart (disease) I27.1
  sequelae of rickets E64.3
  tuberculous A18.Ø1
Kyphosis, kyphotic (acquired) M4Ø.2Ø9
  cervical region M4Ø.2Ø2
  cervicothoracic region M4Ø.2Ø3
  congenital Q76.419
    cervical region Q76.412
    cervicothoracic region Q76.413
    occipito-atlanto-axial region Q76.411
    thoracic region Q76.414
    thoracolumbar region Q76.415
  Morquio-Brailsford type (spinal) — *see also* subcatego-
    ry M49.8 E76.219
  postlaminectomy M96.3
  postradiation therapy M96.2
  postural (adolescent) M4Ø.ØØ
    cervicothoracic region M4Ø.Ø3
    thoracic region M4Ø.Ø4
    thoracolumbar region M4Ø.Ø5
  secondary NEC M4Ø.1Ø
    cervical region M4Ø.12
    cervicothoracic region M4Ø.13
    thoracic region M4Ø.14
    thoracolumbar region M4Ø.15
  sequelae of rickets E64.3
  specified type NEC M4Ø.299
    cervical region M4Ø.292
    cervicothoracic region M4Ø.293
    thoracic region M4Ø.294
    thoracolumbar region M4Ø.295
  syphilitic, congenital A5Ø.56
  thoracic region M4Ø.2Ø4
  thoracolumbar region M4Ø.2Ø5
  tuberculous A18.Ø1
Kyrle disease L87.Ø

L

Labia, labium — *see* condition
Labile
  blood pressure RØ9.89
  vasomotor system I73.9
Labioglossal paralysis G12.29
Labium leporinum — *see* Cleft, lip
Labor — *see* Delivery
Labored breathing — *see* Hyperventilation
Labyrinthitis (circumscribed) (destructive) (diffuse) (inner
    ear) (latent) (purulent) (suppurative) — *see also*
    subcategory H83.Ø ☑
  syphilitic A52.79
Laceration
  with abortion — *see* Abortion, by type, complicated
    by laceration of pelvic organs
  abdomen, abdominal
    wall S31.119 ☑
      with
        foreign body S31.129 ☑
        penetration into peritoneal cavity S31.619 ☑
          with foreign body S31.629 ☑
        epigastric region S31.112 ☑
          with
            foreign body S31.122 ☑
            penetration into peritoneal cavity
              S31.612 ☑
              with foreign body S31.622 ☑
        left
          lower quadrant S31.114 ☑
            with
              foreign body S31.124 ☑
              penetration into peritoneal cavity
                S31.614 ☑
                with foreign body S31.624 ☑
          upper quadrant S31.111 ☑
            with
              foreign body S31.121 ☑

Laceration — *continued*
abdomen, abdominal — *continued*
    wall — *continued*
        left — *continued*
            upper quadrant — *continued*
                with — *continued*
                    penetration into peritoneal cavity
                        S31.611 ☑
                        with foreign body S31.621 ☑
        periumbilic region S31.115 ☑
            with
                foreign body S31.125 ☑
                penetration into peritoneal cavity
                    S31.615 ☑
                    with foreign body S31.625 ☑
        right
            lower quadrant S31.113 ☑
                with
                    foreign body S31.123 ☑
                    penetration into peritoneal cavity
                        S31.613 ☑
                        with foreign body S31.623 ☑
            upper quadrant S31.110 ☑
                with
                    foreign body S31.120 ☑
                    penetration into peritoneal cavity
                        S31.610 ☑
                        with foreign body S31.620 ☑
accidental, complicating surgery — *see* Complications,
    surgical, accidental puncture or laceration
Achilles tendon S86.02- ☑
adrenal gland S37.813 ☑
alveolar (process) — *see* Laceration, oral cavity
ankle S91.01- ☑
    with
        foreign body S91.02- ☑
antecubital space — *see* Laceration, elbow
anus (sphincter) S31.831 ☑
    with
        ectopic or molar pregnancy O08.6
        foreign body S31.832 ☑
    complicating delivery — *see* Delivery, complicated,
        by, laceration, anus (sphincter)
    following ectopic or molar pregnancy O08.6
    nontraumatic, nonpuerperal — *see* Fissure, anus
arm (upper) S41.11- ☑
    with foreign body S41.12- ☑
    lower — *see* Laceration, forearm
auditory canal (external) (meatus) — *see* Laceration,
    ear
auricle, ear — *see* Laceration, ear
axilla — *see* Laceration, arm
back — *see also* Laceration, thorax, back
    lower S31.010 ☑
        with
            foreign body S31.020 ☑
                with penetration into retroperitoneal
                    space S31.021 ☑
            penetration into retroperitoneal space
                S31.011 ☑
bile duct S36.13 ☑
bladder S37.23 ☑
    with ectopic or molar pregnancy O08.6
    following ectopic or molar pregnancy O08.6
    obstetrical trauma O71.5
blood vessel — *see* Injury, blood vessel
bowel — *see also* Laceration, intestine
    with ectopic or molar pregnancy O08.6
    complicating abortion — *see* Abortion, by type,
        complicated by, specified condition NEC
    following ectopic or molar pregnancy O08.6
    obstetrical trauma O71.5
brain (any part) (cortex) (diffuse) (membrane) — *see
    also* Injury, intracranial, diffuse
    during birth P10.8
        with hemorrhage P10.1
    focal — *see* Injury, intracranial, focal brain injury
brainstem S06.38- ☑
breast S21.01- ☑
    with foreign body S21.02- ☑
broad ligament S37.893 ☑
    with ectopic or molar pregnancy O08.6
    following ectopic or molar pregnancy O08.6
    laceration syndrome N83.8
    obstetrical trauma O71.6
    syndrome (laceration) N83.8
buttock S31.801 ☑

Laceration — *continued*
buttock — *continued*
    with foreign body S31.802 ☑
        left S31.821 ☑
            with foreign body S31.822 ☑
        right S31.811 ☑
            with foreign body S31.812 ☑
calf — *see* Laceration, leg
canaliculus lacrimalis — *see* Laceration, eyelid
canthus, eye — *see* Laceration, eyelid
capsule, joint — *see* Sprain
causing eversion of cervix uteri (old) N86
central (perineal), complicating delivery O70.9
cerebellum, traumatic S06.37-
cerebral S06.33- ☑
    during birth P10.8
        with hemorrhage P10.1
    left side S06.32-
    right side S06.31- ☑
cervix (uteri)
    with ectopic or molar pregnancy O08.6
    following ectopic or molar pregnancy O08.6
    nonpuerperal, nontraumatic N88.1
    obstetrical trauma (current) O71.3
    old (postpartal) N88.1
    traumatic S37.63 ☑
cheek (external) S01.41- ☑
    with foreign body S01.42-
    internal — *see* Laceration, oral cavity
chest wall — *see* Laceration, thorax
chin — *see* Laceration, head, specified site NEC
chordae tendinae NEC I51.1
    concurrent with acute myocardial infarction — *see*
        Infarct, myocardium
    following acute myocardial infarction (current
        complication) I23.4
clitoris — *see* Laceration, vulva
colon — *see* Laceration, intestine, large, colon
common bile duct S36.13 ☑
cortex (cerebral) — *see* Injury, intracranial, diffuse
costal region — *see* Laceration, thorax
cystic duct S36.13 ☑
diaphragm S27.803 ☑
digit(s)
    foot — *see* Laceration, toe
    hand — *see* Laceration, finger
duodenum S36.430 ☑
ear (canal) (external) S01.31- ☑
    with foreign body S01.32- ☑
    drum S09.2- ☑
elbow S51.01- ☑
    with
        foreign body S51.02- ☑
epididymis — *see* Laceration, testis
epigastric region — *see* Laceration, abdomen, wall,
    epigastric region
esophagus K22.89
    traumatic
        cervical S11.21 ☑
            with foreign body S11.22 ☑
        thoracic S27.813 ☑
eye (ball) S05.3- ☑
    with prolapse or loss of intraocular tissue S05.2- ☑
    penetrating S05.6- ☑
eyebrow — *see* Laceration, eyelid
eyelid S01.11- ☑
    with foreign body S01.12- ☑
face NEC — *see* Laceration, head, specified site NEC
fallopian tube S37.539 ☑
    bilateral S37.532 ☑
    unilateral S37.531 ☑
finger(s) S61.219 ☑
    with
        damage to nail S61.319 ☑
            with
                foreign body S61.329 ☑
        foreign body S61.229 ☑
    index S61.218 ☑
        with
            damage to nail S61.318 ☑
                with
                    foreign body S61.328 ☑
            foreign body S61.228 ☑
        left S61.211 ☑
            with
                damage to nail S61.311 ☑

Laceration — *continued*
finger(s) — *continued*
    index — *continued*
        left — *continued*
            with — *continued*
                damage to nail — *continued*
                    with
                        foreign body S61.321 ☑
                    foreign body S61.221 ☑
            right S61.210 ☑
                with
                    damage to nail S61.310 ☑
                        with
                            foreign body S61.320 ☑
                    foreign body S61.220 ☑
    little S61.218 ☑
        with
            damage to nail S61.318 ☑
                with
                    foreign body S61.328 ☑
            foreign body S61.228 ☑
        left S61.217 ☑
            with
                damage to nail S61.317 ☑
                    with
                        foreign body S61.327 ☑
                foreign body S61.227 ☑
        right S61.216 ☑
            with
                damage to nail S61.316 ☑
                    with
                        foreign body S61.326 ☑
                foreign body S61.226 ☑
    middle S61.218 ☑
        with
            damage to nail S61.318 ☑
                with
                    foreign body S61.328 ☑
            foreign body S61.228 ☑
        left S61.213 ☑
            with
                damage to nail S61.313 ☑
                    with
                        foreign body S61.323 ☑
                foreign body S61.223 ☑
        right S61.212 ☑
            with
                damage to nail S61.312 ☑
                    with
                        foreign body S61.322 ☑
                foreign body S61.222 ☑
    ring S61.218 ☑
        with
            damage to nail S61.318 ☑
                with
                    foreign body S61.328 ☑
            foreign body S61.228 ☑
        left S61.215 ☑
            with
                damage to nail S61.315 ☑
                    with
                        foreign body S61.325 ☑
                foreign body S61.225 ☑
        right S61.214 ☑
            with
                damage to nail S61.314 ☑
                    with
                        foreign body S61.324 ☑
                foreign body S61.224 ☑
flank S31.119 ☑
    with foreign body S31.129 ☑
foot (except toe(s) alone) S91.319 ☑
    with foreign body S91.329 ☑
    left S91.312 ☑
        with foreign body S91.322 ☑
    right S91.311 ☑
        with foreign body S91.321 ☑
    toe — *see* Laceration, toe
forearm S51.819 ☑
    with
        foreign body S51.829 ☑
    elbow only — *see* Laceration, elbow
    left S51.812 ☑
        with
            foreign body S51.822 ☑
    right S51.811 ☑

☑ **Additional Character Required** — Refer to the Tabular List for Character Selection   ▽ **Subterms under main terms may continue to next column or page**

Laceration — continued
  forearm — continued
    right — continued
      with
        foreign body S51.821 ☑
  forehead S01.81 ☑
    with foreign body S01.82 ☑
  fourchette O70.0
    with ectopic or molar pregnancy O08.6
    complicating delivery O70.0
    following ectopic or molar pregnancy O08.6
  gallbladder S36.123 ☑
  genital organs, external
    female S31.512 ☑
      with foreign body S31.522 ☑
      vagina — see Laceration, vagina
      vulva — see Laceration, vulva
    male S31.511 ☑
      with foreign body S31.521 ☑
      penis — see Laceration, penis
      scrotum — see Laceration, scrotum
      testis — see Laceration, testis
  groin — see Laceration, abdomen, wall
  gum — see Laceration, oral cavity
  hand S61.419 ☑
    with
      foreign body S61.429 ☑
      finger — see Laceration, finger
    left S61.412 ☑
      with
        foreign body S61.422 ☑
    right S61.411 ☑
      with
        foreign body S61.421 ☑
    thumb — see Laceration, thumb
  head S01.91 ☑
    with foreign body S01.92 ☑
    cheek — see Laceration, cheek
    ear — see Laceration, ear
    eyelid — see Laceration, eyelid
    lip — see Laceration, lip
    nose — see Laceration, nose
    oral cavity — see Laceration, oral cavity
    scalp S01.01 ☑
      with foreign body S01.02 ☑
    specified site NEC S01.81 ☑
      with foreign body S01.82 ☑
    temporomandibular area — see Laceration, cheek
  heart — see Injury, heart, laceration
  heel — see Laceration, foot
  hepatic duct S36.13 ☑
  hip S71.019 ☑
    with foreign body S71.029 ☑
    left S71.012 ☑
      with foreign body S71.022 ☑
    right S71.011 ☑
      with foreign body S71.021 ☑
  hymen — see Laceration, vagina
  hypochondrium — see Laceration, abdomen, wall
  hypogastric region — see Laceration, abdomen, wall
  ileum S36.438 ☑
  inguinal region — see Laceration, abdomen, wall
  instep — see Laceration, foot
  internal organ — see Injury, by site
  interscapular region — see Laceration, thorax, back
  intestine
    large
      colon S36.539 ☑
        ascending S36.530 ☑
        descending S36.532 ☑
        sigmoid S36.533 ☑
        specified site NEC S36.538 ☑
      rectum S36.63 ☑
      transverse S36.531 ☑
    small S36.439 ☑
      duodenum S36.430 ☑
      specified site NEC S36.438 ☑
  intra-abdominal organ S36.93 ☑
    intestine — see Laceration, intestine
    liver — see Laceration, liver
    pancreas — see Laceration, pancreas
    peritoneum S36.81 ☑
    specified site NEC S36.893 ☑
    spleen — see Laceration, spleen
    stomach — see Laceration, stomach
  intracranial NEC — see also Injury, intracranial, diffuse

Laceration — continued
  intracranial — see also Injury, intracranial, diffuse —
    continued
    birth injury P10.9
  jaw — see Laceration, head, specified site NEC
  jejunum S36.438 ☑
  joint capsule — see Sprain, by site
  kidney S37.03-
    major (greater than 3 cm) (massive) (stellate)
      S37.06-
    minor (less than 1 cm) S37.04- ☑
    moderate (1 to 3 cm) S37.05- ☑
    multiple S37.06- ☑
  knee S81.01- ☑
    with foreign body S81.02- ☑
  labium (majus) (minus) — see Laceration, vulva
  lacrimal duct — see Laceration, eyelid
  large intestine — see Laceration, intestine, large
  larynx S11.011 ☑
    with foreign body S11.012 ☑
  leg (lower) S81.819 ☑
    with foreign body S81.829 ☑
    foot — see Laceration, foot
    knee — see Laceration, knee
    left S81.812 ☑
      with foreign body S81.822 ☑
    right S81.811 ☑
      with foreign body S81.821 ☑
    upper — see Laceration, thigh
  ligament — see Sprain
  lip S01.511 ☑
    with foreign body S01.521 ☑
  liver S36.113 ☑
    major (stellate) S36.116 ☑
    minor S36.114 ☑
    moderate S36.115 ☑
  loin — see Laceration, abdomen, wall
  lower back — see Laceration, back, lower
  lumbar region — see Laceration, back, lower
  lung S27.339 ☑
    bilateral S27.332 ☑
    unilateral S27.331 ☑
  malar region — see Laceration, head, specified site NEC
  mammary — see Laceration, breast
  mastoid region — see Laceration, head, specified site
    NEC
  meninges — see Injury, intracranial, diffuse
  meniscus — see Tear, meniscus
  mesentery S36.893 ☑
  mesosalpinx S37.893 ☑
  mouth — see Laceration, oral cavity
  muscle — see Injury, muscle, by site, laceration
  nail
    finger — see Laceration, finger, with damage to nail
    toe — see Laceration, toe, with damage to nail
  nasal (septum) (sinus) — see Laceration, nose
  nasopharynx — see Laceration, head, specified site
    NEC
  neck S11.91 ☑
    with foreign body S11.92 ☑
    involving
      cervical esophagus S11.21 ☑
        with foreign body S11.22 ☑
      larynx — see Laceration, larynx
      pharynx — see Laceration, pharynx
      thyroid gland — see Laceration, thyroid gland
      trachea — see Laceration, trachea
      specified site NEC S11.81 ☑
        with foreign body S11.82 ☑
  nerve — see Injury, nerve
  nose (septum) (sinus) S01.21 ☑
    with foreign body S01.22 ☑
  ocular NOS S05.3- ☑
    adnexa NOS S01.11- ☑
  oral cavity S01.512 ☑
    with foreign body S01.522 ☑
  orbit (eye) — see Wound, open, ocular, orbit
  ovary S37.439 ☑
    bilateral S37.432 ☑
    unilateral S37.431 ☑
  palate — see Laceration, oral cavity
  palm — see Laceration, hand
  pancreas S36.239 ☑
  pelvic S31.010 ☑
    with
      foreign body S31.020 ☑

Laceration — continued
  pelvic — continued
    with — continued
      foreign body — continued
        penetration into retroperitoneal cavity
          S31.021 ☑
      penetration into retroperitoneal cavity
        S31.011 ☑
    floor — see also Laceration, back, lower
      with ectopic or molar pregnancy O08.6
      complicating delivery O70.1
      following ectopic or molar pregnancy O08.6
      old (postpartal) N81.89
    organ S37.93 ☑
  penis S31.21 ☑
    with foreign body S31.22 ☑
  perineum
    female S31.41 ☑
      with
        ectopic or molar pregnancy O08.6
        foreign body S31.42 ☑
      during delivery O70.9
        first degree O70.0
        fourth degree O70.3
        second degree O70.1
        third degree — see also Delivery, complicat-
          ed, by, laceration, perineum, third de-
          gree O70.20
      old (postpartal) N81.89
      postpartal N81.89
      secondary (postpartal) O90.1
    male S31.119 ☑
      with foreign body S31.129 ☑
  periocular area (with or without lacrimal passages) —
    see Laceration, eyelid
  peritoneum S36.893 ☑
  periumbilic region — see Laceration, abdomen, wall,
    periumbilic
  periurethral tissue — see Laceration, urethra
  phalanges
    finger — see Laceration, finger
    toe — see Laceration, toe
  pharynx S11.21 ☑
    with foreign body S11.22 ☑
  pinna — see Laceration, ear
  popliteal space — see Laceration, knee
  prepuce — see Laceration, penis
  prostate S37.823 ☑
  pubic region S31.119 ☑
    with foreign body S31.129 ☑
  pudendum — see Laceration, genital organs, external
  rectovaginal septum — see Laceration, vagina
  rectum S36.63 ☑
  retroperitoneum S36.893 ☑
  round ligament S37.893 ☑
  sacral region — see Laceration, back, lower
  sacroiliac region — see Laceration, back, lower
  salivary gland — see Laceration, oral cavity
  scalp S01.01 ☑
    with foreign body S01.02 ☑
  scapular region — see Laceration, shoulder
  scrotum S31.31 ☑
    with foreign body S31.32 ☑
  seminal vesicle S37.893 ☑
  shin — see Laceration, leg
  shoulder S41.019 ☑
    with foreign body S41.029 ☑
    left S41.012 ☑
      with foreign body S41.022 ☑
    right S41.011 ☑
      with foreign body S41.021 ☑
  small intestine — see Laceration, intestine, small
  spermatic cord — see Laceration, testis
  spinal cord (meninges) — see also Injury, spinal cord,
    by region
    due to injury at birth P11.5
    newborn (birth injury) P11.5
  spleen S36.039 ☑
    major (massive) (stellate) S36.032 ☑
    moderate S36.031 ☑
    superficial (minor) S36.030 ☑
  sternal region — see Laceration, thorax, front
  stomach S36.33 ☑
  submaxillary region — see Laceration, head, specified
    site NEC
  submental region — see Laceration, head, specified
    site NEC

Laceration — continued
   subungual
      finger(s) — see Laceration, finger, with damage to nail
      toe(s) — see Laceration, toe, with damage to nail
   suprarenal gland — see Laceration, adrenal gland
   temple, temporal region — see Laceration, head, specified site NEC
   temporomandibular area — see Laceration, cheek
   tendon — see Injury, muscle, by site, laceration
      Achilles S86.02- ☑
   tentorium cerebelli — see Injury, intracranial, diffuse
   testis S31.31 ☑
      with foreign body S31.32 ☑
   thigh S71.11- ☑
      with foreign body S71.12- ☑
   thorax, thoracic (wall) S21.91 ☑
      with foreign body S21.92 ☑
         back S21.22- ☑
            with penetration into thoracic cavity S21.42- ☑
         front S21.12- ☑
            with penetration into thoracic cavity S21.32- ☑
      back S21.21- ☑
         with
            foreign body S21.22- ☑
               with penetration into thoracic cavity S21.42- ☑
            penetration into thoracic cavity S21.41- ☑
      breast — see Laceration, breast
      front S21.11- ☑
         with
            foreign body S21.12- ☑
               with penetration into thoracic cavity S21.32- ☑
            penetration into thoracic cavity S21.31- ☑
   thumb S61.019 ☑
      with
         damage to nail S61.119 ☑
            with
               foreign body S61.129 ☑
         foreign body S61.029 ☑
      left S61.012 ☑
         with
            damage to nail S61.112 ☑
               with
                  foreign body S61.122 ☑
            foreign body S61.022 ☑
      right S61.011 ☑
         with
            damage to nail S61.111 ☑
               with
                  foreign body S61.121 ☑
            foreign body S61.021 ☑
   thyroid gland S11.11 ☑
      with foreign body S11.12 ☑
   toe(s) S91.119 ☑
      with
         damage to nail S91.219 ☑
            with
               foreign body S91.229 ☑
         foreign body S91.129 ☑
      great S91.113 ☑
         with
            damage to nail S91.213 ☑
               with
                  foreign body S91.223 ☑
            foreign body S91.123 ☑
         left S91.112 ☑
            with
               damage to nail S91.212 ☑
                  with
                     foreign body S91.222 ☑
               foreign body S91.122 ☑
         right S91.111 ☑
            with
               damage to nail S91.211 ☑
                  with
                     foreign body S91.221 ☑
               foreign body S91.121 ☑
      lesser S91.116 ☑
         with
            damage to nail S91.216 ☑
               with
                  foreign body S91.226 ☑

Laceration — continued
   toe(s) — continued
      lesser — continued
         with — continued
               foreign body S91.126 ☑
            left S91.115 ☑
               with
                  damage to nail S91.215 ☑
                     with
                        foreign body S91.225 ☑
                  foreign body S91.125 ☑
            right S91.114 ☑
               with
                  damage to nail S91.214 ☑
                     with
                        foreign body S91.224 ☑
                  foreign body S91.124 ☑
   tongue — see Laceration, oral cavity
   trachea S11.021 ☑
      with foreign body S11.022 ☑
   tunica vaginalis — see Laceration, testis
   tympanum, tympanic membrane — see Laceration, ear, drum
   umbilical region S31.115 ☑
      with foreign body S31.125 ☑
   ureter S37.13 ☑
   urethra S37.33 ☑
      with or following ectopic or molar pregnancy O08.6
      obstetrical trauma O71.5
   urinary organ NEC S37.893 ☑
   uterus S37.63 ☑
      with ectopic or molar pregnancy O08.6
      following ectopic or molar pregnancy O08.6
      nonpuerperal, nontraumatic N85.8
      obstetrical trauma NEC O71.81
      old (postpartal) N85.8
   uvula — see Laceration, oral cavity
   vagina S31.41 ☑
      with
         ectopic or molar pregnancy O08.6
         foreign body S31.42 ☑
      during delivery O71.4
         with perineal laceration — see Laceration, perineum, female, during delivery
      following ectopic or molar pregnancy O08.6
      nonpuerperal, nontraumatic N89.8
      old (postpartal) N89.8
   vas deferens S37.893 ☑
   vesical — see Laceration, bladder
   vocal cords S11.031 ☑
      with foreign body S11.032 ☑
   vulva S31.41 ☑
      with
         ectopic or molar pregnancy O08.6
         foreign body S31.42 ☑
      complicating delivery O70.0
      following ectopic or molar pregnancy O08.6
      nonpuerperal, nontraumatic N90.89
      old (postpartal) N90.89
   wrist S61.519 ☑
      with
         foreign body S61.529 ☑
      left S61.512 ☑
         with
            foreign body S61.522 ☑
      right S61.511 ☑
         with
            foreign body S61.521 ☑

Lack of
   achievement in school Z55.3
   adequate
      food Z59.48
      intermaxillary vertical dimension of fully erupted teeth M26.36
      sleep Z72.820
   appetite (see Anorexia) R63.0
   awareness R41.9
   care
      in home Z74.2
      of infant (at or after birth) T76.02 ☑
         confirmed T74.02 ☑
   cognitive functions R41.9
   coordination R27.9
      ataxia R27.0
      specified type NEC R27.8
   development (physiological) R62.50
      failure to thrive (child over 28 days old) R62.51

Lack of — continued
   development — continued
      failure to thrive — continued
         adult R62.7
         newborn P92.6
      short stature R62.52
      specified type NEC R62.59
   energy R53.83
   financial resources Z59.6
   food Z59.48
   growth R62.52
   heating Z59.1
   housing (permanent) (temporary) Z59.00
      adequate Z59.1
   learning experiences in childhood Z62.898
   leisure time (affecting life-style) Z73.2
   material resources Z59.9
   memory — see also Amnesia
      mild, following organic brain damage F06.8
   ovulation N97.0
   parental supervision or control of child Z62.0
   person able to render necessary care Z74.2
   physical exercise Z72.3
   play experience in childhood Z62.898
   posterior occlusal support M26.57
   relaxation (affecting life-style) Z73.2
   safe drinking water Z58.6
   sexual
      desire F52.0
      enjoyment F52.1
   shelter Z59.02
   sleep (adequate) Z72.820
   supervision of child by parent Z62.0
   support, posterior occlusal M26.57
   water T73.1
      safe drinking Z58.6
Lacrimal — see condition
Lacrimation, abnormal — see Epiphora
Lacrimonasal duct — see condition
Lactation, lactating (breast) (puerperal, postpartum)
   associated
      cracked nipple O92.13
      retracted nipple O92.03
   defective O92.4
   disorder NEC O92.79
   excessive O92.6
   failed (complete) O92.3
      partial O92.4
   mastitis NEC — see Mastitis, obstetric
   mother (care and/or examination) Z39.1
   nonpuerperal N64.3
Lacticemia, excessive E87.2
Lacunar skull Q75.8
Laennec's cirrhosis K70.30
   with ascites K70.31
   nonalcoholic K74.69
Lafora's disease — see Epilepsy, generalized, idiopathic
Lag, lid (nervous) — see Retraction, lid
Lagophthalmos (eyelid) (nervous) H02.209
   bilateral, upper and lower eyelids H02.20C
   cicatricial H02.219
      bilateral, upper and lower eyelids H02.21C
      left H02.216
         lower H02.215
         upper H02.214
         upper and lower eyelids H02.21B
      right H02.213
         lower H02.212
         upper H02.211
         upper and lower eyelids H02.21A
   keratoconjunctivitis — see Keratoconjunctivitis
   left H02.206
      lower H02.205
      upper H02.204
      upper and lower eyelids H02.20B
   mechanical H02.229
      bilateral, upper and lower eyelids H02.22C
      left H02.226
         lower H02.225
         upper H02.224
         upper and lower eyelids H02.22B
      right H02.223
         lower H02.222
         upper H02.221
         upper and lower eyelids H02.22A
   paralytic H02.239
      bilateral, upper and lower eyelids H02.23C
      left H02.236

☑ **Additional Character Required** — Refer to the Tabular List for Character Selection   ▽ **Subterms under main terms may continue to next column or page**

Lagophthalmos — *continued*
  paralytic — *continued*
    left — *continued*
      lower H02.235
      upper H02.234
      upper and lower eyelids H02.23B
      right H02.233
        lower H02.232
        upper H02.231
        upper and lower eyelids H02.23A
    right H02.203
      lower H02.202
      upper H02.201
      upper and lower eyelids H02.20A
Laki-Lorand factor deficiency — *see* Defect, coagulation, specified type NEC
Lalling F80.0
Lambert-Eaton syndrome — *see* Syndrome, Lambert-Eaton
Lambliasis, lambliosis A07.1
Landau-Kleffner syndrome — *see* Epilepsy, specified NEC
Landouzy-Déjérine dystrophy or facioscapulohumeral atrophy G71.02
Landouzy's disease (icterohemorrhagic leptospirosis) A27.0
Landry-Guillain-Barré, syndrome or paralysis G61.0
Landry's disease or paralysis G61.0
Lane's
  band Q43.3
  kink — *see* Obstruction, intestine
  syndrome K90.2
Langdon Down syndrome — *see* Trisomy, 21
Lapsed immunization schedule status Z28.3
Large
  baby (regardless of gestational age) (4000g to 4499g) P08.1
  ear, congenital Q17.1
  physiological cup Q14.2
  stature R68.89
Large-for-dates NEC (infant) (4000g to 4499g) P08.1
  affecting management of pregnancy O36.6- ☑
  exceptionally (4500g or more) P08.0
Larsen-Johansson disease orosteochondrosis — *see* Osteochondrosis, juvenile, patella
Larsen's syndrome (flattened facies and multiple congenital dislocations) Q74.8
Larva migrans
  cutaneous B76.9
    Ancylostoma B76.0
  visceral B83.0
Laryngeal — *see* condition
Laryngismus (stridulus) J38.5
  congenital P28.89
  diphtheritic A36.2
Laryngitis (acute) (edematous) (fibrinous) (infective) (infiltrative) (malignant) (membranous) (phlegmonous) (pneumococcal) (pseudomembranous) (septic) (subglottic) (suppurative) (ulcerative) J04.0
  with
    influenza, flu, or grippe — *see* Influenza, with, laryngitis
    tracheitis (acute) — *see* Laryngotracheitis
  atrophic J37.0
  catarrhal J37.0
  chronic J37.0
    with tracheitis (chronic) J37.1
  diphtheritic A36.2
  due to external agent — *see* Inflammation, respiratory, upper, due to
  H. influenzae J04.0
  Hemophilus influenzae J04.0
  hypertrophic J37.0
  influenzal — *see* Influenza, with, respiratory manifestations NEC
  obstructive J05.0
  sicca J37.0
  spasmodic J05.0
    acute J04.0
  streptococcal J04.0
  stridulous J05.0
  syphilitic (late) A52.73
    congenital A50.59 *[J99]*
    early A50.03 *[J99]*
  tuberculous A15.5
  Vincent's A69.1
Laryngocele (congenital) (ventricular) Q31.3
Laryngofissure J38.7

Laryngofissure — *continued*
  congenital Q31.8
Laryngomalacia (congenital) Q31.5
Laryngopharyngitis (acute) J06.0
  chronic J37.0
  due to external agent — *see* Inflammation, respiratory, upper, due to
Laryngoplegia J38.00
  bilateral J38.02
  unilateral J38.01
Laryngoptosis J38.7
Laryngospasm J38.5
Laryngostenosis J38.6
Laryngotracheitis (acute) (Infectional) (infective) (viral) J04.2
  atrophic J37.1
  catarrhal J37.1
  chronic J37.1
  diphtheritic A36.2
  due to external agent — *see* Inflammation, respiratory, upper, due to
  Hemophilus influenzae J04.2
  hypertrophic J37.1
  influenzal — *see* Influenza, with, respiratory manifestations NEC
  pachydermic J38.7
  sicca J37.1
  spasmodic J38.5
    acute J05.0
  streptococcal J04.2
  stridulous J38.5
  syphilitic (late) A52.73
    congenital A50.59 *[J99]*
    early A50.03 *[J99]*
  tuberculous A15.5
  Vincent's A69.1
Laryngotracheobronchitis — *see* Bronchitis
Larynx, laryngeal — *see* condition
Lassa fever A96.2
Lassitude — *see* Weakness
Late
  talker R62.0
  walker R62.0
Late effect(s) — *see* Sequelae
Latent — *see* condition
Laterocession — *see* Lateroversion
Lateroflexion — *see* Lateroversion
Lateroversion
  cervix — *see* Lateroversion, uterus
  uterus, uterine (cervix) (postinfectional) (postpartal, old) N85.4
    congenital Q51.818
    in pregnancy or childbirth O34.59- ☑
Lathyrism — *see* Poisoning, food, noxious, plant
Launois' syndrome (pituitary gigantism) E22.0
Launois-Bensaude adenolipomatosis E88.89
Laurence-Moon (-Bardet)-**Biedl syndrome** Q87.89
Lax, laxity — *see also* Relaxation
  ligament (ous) — *see also* Disorder, ligament
    familial M35.7
    knee — *see* Derangement, knee
  skin (acquired) L57.4
    congenital Q82.8
Laxative habit F55.2
Lazy leukocyte syndrome D70.8
Lead miner's lung J63.6
Leak, leakage
  air NEC J93.82
    postprocedural J95.812
  amniotic fluid — *see* Rupture, membranes, premature
  blood (microscopic), fetal, into maternal circulation
    affecting management of pregnancy — *see* Pregnancy, complicated by
  cerebrospinal fluid G96.00
    cranial
      postoperative G96.08
      specified NEC G96.08
      spontaneous G96.01
      traumatic G96.08
    from spinal (lumbar) puncture G97.0
    spinal
      postoperative G96.09
      post-traumatic G96.09
      specified NEC G96.09
      spontaneous G96.02
    spontaneous
      from
        skull base G96.01

Leak, leakage — *continued*
  cerebrospinal fluid — *continued*
    spontaneous — *continued*
      from — *continued*
        spine G96.02
  CSF — *see* Leak, cerebrospinal fluid
  device, implant or graft — *see also* Complications, by site and type, mechanical
    arterial graft NEC — *see* Complication, cardiovascular device, mechanical, vascular
    breast (implant) T85.43 ☑
    catheter NEC T85.638 ☑
      dialysis (renal) T82.43 ☑
        intraperitoneal T85.631 ☑
      infusion NEC T82.534 ☑
        spinal (epidural) (subdural) T85.630 ☑
      urinary T83.038 ☑
        cystostomy T83.030 ☑
        Hopkins T83.038 ☑
        ileostomy T83.038 ☑
        indwelling T83.031 ☑
        nephrostomy T83.032 ☑
        specified T83.038 ☑
        urostomy T83.038 ☑
    gastrointestinal — *see* Complications, prosthetic device, mechanical, gastrointestinal device
    genital NEC T83.498 ☑
      penile prosthesis (cylinder) (implanted) (pump) (reservoir) T83.490 ☑
      testicular prosthesis T83.491 ☑
    heart NEC — *see* Complication, cardiovascular device, mechanical
    joint prosthesis — *see* Complications, joint prosthesis, mechanical, specified NEC, by site
    ocular NEC — *see* Complications, prosthetic device, mechanical, ocular device
    orthopedic NEC — *see* Complication, orthopedic, device, mechanical
    persistent air J93.82
    specified NEC T85.638 ☑
    urinary NEC — *see also* Complication, genitourinary, device, urinary, mechanical
      graft T83.23 ☑
    vascular NEC — *see* Complication, cardiovascular device, mechanical
    ventricular intracranial shunt T85.03 ☑
  urine — *see* Incontinence
Leaky heart — *see* Endocarditis
Learning defect (specific) F81.9
Leather bottle stomach C16.9
Leber's
  congenital amaurosis H35.50
  optic atrophy (hereditary) H47.22
Lederer's anemia D59.19
Leeches (external) — *see* Hirudiniasis
Leg — *see* condition
Legg (-Calvé)-**Perthes disease, syndrome or osteochondrosis** M91.1- ☑
Legionellosis A48.1
  nonpneumonic A48.2
Legionnaires'
  disease A48.1
    nonpneumonic A48.2
  pneumonia A48.1
Leigh's disease G31.82
Leiner's disease L21.1
Leiofibromyoma — *see* Leiomyoma
Leiomyoblastoma — *see* Neoplasm, connective tissue, benign
Leiomyofibroma — *see also* Neoplasm, connective tissue, benign
  uterus (cervix) (corpus) D25.9
Leiomyoma — *see also* Neoplasm, connective tissue, benign
  bizarre — *see* Neoplasm, connective tissue, benign
  cellular — *see* Neoplasm, connective tissue, benign
  epithelioid — *see* Neoplasm, connective tissue, benign
  uterus (cervix) (corpus) D25.9
    intramural D25.1
    submucous D25.0
    subserosal D25.2
  vascular — *see* Neoplasm, connective tissue, benign
Leiomyoma, leiomyomatosis (intravascular) — *see* Neoplasm, connective tissue, uncertain behavior
Leiomyosarcoma — *see also* Neoplasm, connective tissue, malignant

Index

Leiomyosarcoma — *continued*
  epithelioid — *see* Neoplasm, connective tissue, malignant
  myxoid — *see* Neoplasm, connective tissue, malignant
Leishmaniasis B55.9
  American (mucocutaneous) B55.2
    cutaneous B55.1
  Asian Desert B55.1
  Brazilian B55.2
  cutaneous (any type) B55.1
  dermal — *see also* Leishmaniasis, cutaneous
    post-kala-azar B55.0
  eyelid B55.1
  infantile B55.0
  Mediterranean B55.0
  mucocutaneous (American) (New World) B55.2
  naso-oral B55.2
  nasopharyngeal B55.2
  old world B55.1
  tegumentaria diffusa B55.1
  visceral B55.0
Leishmanoid, dermal — *see also* Leishmaniasis, cutaneous
  post-kala-azar B55.0
Lenegre's disease I44.2
Lengthening, leg — *see* Deformity, limb, unequal length
Lennert's lymphoma — *see* Lymphoma, Lennert's
Lennox-Gastaut syndrome G40.812
  intractable G40.814
    with status epilepticus G40.813
    without status epilepticus G40.814
  not intractable G40.812
    with status epilepticus G40.811
    without status epilepticus G40.812
Lens — *see* condition
Lenticonus (anterior) (posterior) (congenital) Q12.8
Lenticular degeneration, progressive E83.01
Lentiglobus (posterior) (congenital) Q12.8
Lentigo (congenital) L81.4
  maligna — *see also* Melanoma, in situ
    melanoma — *see* Melanoma
Lentivirus, as cause of disease classified elsewhere B97.31
Leontiasis
  ossium M85.2
  syphilitic (late) A52.78
    congenital A50.59
Lepothrix A48.8
Lepra — *see* Leprosy
Leprechaunism E34.8
Leprosy A30.- ☑
  with muscle disorder A30.9 *[M63.80]*
    ankle A30.9 *[M63.87-]* ☑
    foot A30.9 *[M63.87-]* ☑
    forearm A30.9 *[M63.83-]* ☑
    hand A30.9 *[M63.84-]* ☑
    lower leg A30.9 *[M63.86-]* ☑
    multiple sites A30.9 *[M63.89]*
    pelvic region A30.9 *[M63.85-]* ☑
    shoulder region A30.9 *[M63.81-]* ☑
    specified site NEC A30.9 *[M63.88]*
    thigh A30.9 *[M63.85-]* ☑
    upper arm A30.9 *[M63.82-]* ☑
  anesthetic A30.9
  BB A30.3
  BL A30.4
  borderline (infiltrated) (neuritic) A30.3
    lepromatous A30.4
    tuberculoid A30.2
  BT A30.2
  dimorphous (infiltrated) (neuritic) A30.3
  I A30.0
  indeterminate (macular) (neuritic) A30.0
  lepromatous (diffuse) (infiltrated) (macular) (neuritic) (nodular) A30.5
  LL A30.5
  macular (early) (neuritic) (simple) A30.9
  maculoanesthetic A30.9
  mixed A30.3
  neural A30.9
  nodular A30.5
  primary neuritic A30.3
  specified type NEC A30.8
  TT A30.1
  tuberculoid (major) (minor) A30.1
Leptocytosis, hereditary D56.9

Leptomeningitis (chronic) (circumscribed) (hemorrhagic) (nonsuppurative) — *see* Meningitis
Leptomeningopathy G96.198
Leptospiral — *see* condition
Leptospirochetal — *see* condition
Leptospirosis A27.9
  canicola A27.89
  due to Leptospira interrogans serovar icterohaemorrhagiae A27.0
  icterohemorrhagica A27.0
  pomona A27.89
  Weil's disease A27.0
Leptus dermatitis B88.0
Leriche's syndrome (aortic bifurcation occlusion) I74.09
Leri's pleonosteosis Q78.8
Leri-Weill syndrome Q77.8
Lermoyez' syndrome — *see* Vertigo, peripheral NEC
Lesch-Nyhan syndrome E79.1
Leser-Trélat disease L82.1
  inflamed L82.0
Lesion(s) (nontraumatic)
  abducens nerve — *see* Strabismus, paralytic, sixth nerve
  alveolar process K08.9
  angiocentric immunoproliferative D47.Z9 (*following* D47.4)
  anorectal K62.9
  aortic (valve) I35.9
  auditory nerve — *see* subcategory H93.3 ☑
  basal ganglion G25.9
  bile duct — *see* Disease, bile duct
  biomechanical M99.9
    specified type NEC M99.89
      abdomen M99.89
      acromioclavicular M99.87
      cervical region M99.81
      cervicothoracic M99.81
      costochondral M99.88
      costovertebral M99.88
      head region M99.80
      hip M99.85
      lower extremity M99.86
      lumbar region M99.83
      lumbosacral M99.83
      occipitocervical M99.80
      pelvic region M99.85
      pubic M99.85
      rib cage M99.88
      sacral region M99.84
      sacrococcygeal M99.84
      sacroiliac M99.84
      specified NEC M99.89
      sternochondral M99.88
      sternoclavicular M99.87
      thoracic region M99.82
      thoracolumbar M99.82
      upper extremity M99.87
  bladder N32.9
  bone — *see* Disorder, bone
  brachial plexus G54.0
  brain G93.9
    congenital Q04.9
    vascular I67.9
      degenerative I67.9
      hypertensive I67.4
  buccal cavity K13.79
  calcified — *see* Calcification
  canthus — *see* Disorder, eyelid
  carate — *see* Pinta, lesions
  cardia K31.9
  cardiac — *see also* Disease, heart I51.9
    congenital Q24.9
    valvular — *see* Endocarditis
  cauda equina G83.4
  cecum K63.9
  cerebral — *see* Lesion, brain
  cerebrovascular I67.9
    degenerative I67.9
    hypertensive I67.4
  cervical (nerve) root NEC G54.2
  chiasmal — *see* Disorder, optic, chiasm
  chorda tympani G51.8
  coin, lung R91.1
  colon K63.9
  combined periodontic - endodontic K05.5
  congenital — *see* Anomaly, by site
  conjunctiva H11.9
  conus medullaris — *see* Injury, conus medullaris
  coronary artery — *see* Ischemia, heart

Lesion(s) — *continued*
  cranial nerve G52.9
    eighth — *see* Disorder, ear
    eleventh G52.9
    fifth G50.9
    first G52.0
    fourth — *see* Strabismus, paralytic, fourth nerve
    seventh G51.9
    sixth — *see* Strabismus, paralytic, sixth nerve
    tenth G52.2
    twelfth G52.3
  cystic — *see* Cyst
  degenerative — *see* Degeneration
  duodenum K31.9
  edentulous (alveolar) ridge, associated with trauma, due to traumatic occlusion K06.2
  en coup de sabre L94.1
  eyelid — *see* Disorder, eyelid
  gasserian ganglion G50.8
  gastric K31.9
  gastroduodenal K31.9
  gastrointestinal K63.9
  gingiva, associated with trauma K06.2
  glomerular
    focal and segmental — *see also* N00-N07 with fourth character .1 N05.1
    minimal change — *see also* N00-N07 with fourth character .0 N05.0
  heart (organic) — *see* Disease, heart
  hyperchromic, due to pinta (carate) A67.1
  hyperkeratotic — *see* Hyperkeratosis
  hypothalamic E23.7
  ileocecal K63.9
  ileum K63.9
  iliohypogastric nerve G57.8- ☑
  inflammatory — *see* Inflammation
  intestine K63.9
  intracerebral — *see* Lesion, brain
  intrachiasmal (optic) — *see* Disorder, optic, chiasm
  intracranial, space-occupying R90.0
  joint — *see* Disorder, joint
    sacroiliac (old) M53.3
  keratotic — *see* Keratosis
  kidney — *see* Disease, renal
  laryngeal nerve (recurrent) G52.2
  lip K13.0
  liver K76.9
  lumbosacral
    plexus G54.1
    root (nerve) NEC G54.4
  lung (coin) R91.1
  maxillary sinus J32.0
  mitral I05.9
  Morel-Lavallée — *see* Hematoma, by site
  motor cortex NEC G93.89
  mouth K13.79
  nerve G58.9
    femoral G57.2- ☑
    median G56.1- ☑
      carpal tunnel syndrome — *see* Syndrome, carpal tunnel
    plantar G57.6- ☑
    popliteal (lateral) G57.3- ☑
      medial G57.4- ☑
    radial G56.3- ☑
    sciatic G57.0- ☑
    spinal — *see* Injury, nerve, spinal
    ulnar G56.2- ☑
  nervous system, congenital Q07.9
  nonallopathic — *see* Lesion, biomechanical
  nose (internal) J34.89
  obstructive — *see* Obstruction
  obturator nerve G57.8- ☑
  oral mucosa K13.70
  organ or site NEC — *see* Disease, by site
  osteolytic — *see* Osteolysis
  peptic K27.9
  periodontal, due to traumatic occlusion K05.5
  pharynx J39.2
  pigment, pigmented (skin) L81.9
  pinta — *see* Pinta, lesions
  polypoid — *see* Polyp
  prechiasmal (optic) — *see* Disorder, optic, chiasm
  primary — *see also* Syphilis, primary A51.0
    carate A67.0
    pinta A67.0
    yaws A66.0

☑ **Additional Character Required** — Refer to the Tabular List for Character Selection   ▽ **Subterms under main terms may continue to next column or page**

Leiomyosarcoma — Lesion

Lesion(s) — *continued*
pulmonary J98.4
   valve I37.9
pylorus K31.9
rectosigmoid K63.9
retina, retinal H35.9
sacroiliac (joint) (old) M53.3
salivary gland K11.9
   benign lymphoepithelial K11.8
saphenous nerve G57.8- ☑
sciatic nerve G57.0- ☑
secondary — *see* Syphilis, secondary
shoulder (region) M75.9- ☑
   specified NEC M75.8- ☑
sigmoid K63.9
sinus (accessory) (nasal) J34.89
skin L98.9
   suppurative L08.0
SLAP S43.43- ☑
spinal cord G95.9
   congenital Q06.9
spleen D73.89
stomach K31.9
superior glenoid labrum S43.43- ☑
syphilitic — *see* Syphilis
tertiary — *see* Syphilis, tertiary
thoracic root (nerve) NEC G54.3
tonsillar fossa J35.9
tooth, teeth K08.9
   white spot
      chewing surface K02.51
      pit and fissure surface K02.51
      smooth surface K02.61
traumatic — *see* specific type of injury by site
tricuspid (valve) I07.9
   nonrheumatic I36.9
trigeminal nerve G50.9
ulcerated or ulcerative — *see* Ulcer, skin
uterus N85.9
vagina N89.8
vagus nerve G52.2
valvular — *see* Endocarditis
vascular I99.9
   affecting central nervous system I67.9
   following trauma NEC T14.8 ☑
   umbilical cord, complicating delivery O69.5 ☑
vulva N90.89
warty — *see* Verruca
white spot (tooth)
   chewing surface K02.51
   pit and fissure surface K02.51
   smooth surface K02.61
Less than a high school diploma Z55.5
Lethargic — *see* condition
Lethargy R53.83
Letterer-Siwe's disease C96.0
Leukemia, leukemic C95.9- ☑
acute basophilic C94.8- ☑
acute bilineal C95.0- ☑
acute erythroid C94.0- ☑
acute lymphoblastic C91.0- ☑
acute megakaryoblastic C94.2- ☑
acute megakaryocytic C94.2- ☑
acute mixed lineage C95.0- ☑
acute monoblastic (monoblastic/monocytic) C93.0- ☑
acute monocytic (monoblastic/monocytic) C93.0- ☑
acute myeloblastic (minimal differentiation) (with maturation) C92.0- ☑
acute myeloid, NOS C92.0- ☑
   with
      11q23-abnormality C92.6- ☑
      dysplasia of remaining hematopoesis and/or myelodysplastic disease in its history C92.A- ☑ (*following* C92.6)
      multilineage dysplasia C92.A- ☑ (*following* C92.6)
      variation of MLL-gene C92.6- ☑
   M6 (a)(b) C94.0- ☑
   M7 C94.2- ☑
acute myelomonocytic C92.5- ☑
acute promyelocytic C92.4- ☑
adult T-cell (HTLV-1-associated) (acute variant) (chronic variant) (lymphomatoid variant) (smouldering variant) C91.5- ☑
aggressive NK-cell C94.8- ☑
AML (1/ETO) (M0) (M1) (M2) (without a FAB classification) C92.0- ☑

Leukemia, leukemic — *continued*
AML M3 C92.4- ☑
AML M4 (Eo with inv(16) or t(16;16)) C92.5- ☑
AML M5 C93.0- ☑
AML M5a C93.0- ☑
AML M5b C93.0- ☑
AML Me with t (15;17) and variants C92.4- ☑
atypical chronic myeloid, BCR/ABL-negative C92.2- ☑
biphenotypic acute C95.0- ☑
blast cell C95.0- ☑
Burkitt-type, mature B-cell C91.A- ☑ (*following* C91.6)
chronic eosinophilic — *see also* Syndrome, hypereosinophilic, myeloid C94.8- ☑
chronic lymphocytic, of B-cell type C91.1- ☑
chronic monocytic C93.1- ☑
chronic myelogenous (Philadelphia chromosome (Ph1) positive) (t(9;22)) (q34;q11) (with crisis of blast cells) C92.1- ☑
chronic myeloid, BCR/ABL-positive C92.1- ☑
   atypical, BCR/ABL-negative C92.2- ☑
chronic myelomonocytic C93.1- ☑
chronic neutrophilic D47.1
CMML (-1) (-2) (with eosinophilia) C93.1- ☑
granulocytic — *see also* Category C92 C92.9- ☑
hairy cell C91.4- ☑
juvenile myelomonocytic C93.3- ☑
lymphoid C91.9- ☑
   specified NEC C91.Z- ☑ (*following* C91.6)
mast cell C94.3- ☑
mature B-cell, Burkitt-type C91.A- ☑ (*following* C91.6)
monocytic (subacute) C93.9- ☑
   specified NEC C93.Z- ☑ (*following* C93.3)
myelogenous — *see also* Category C92 C92.9- ☑
myeloid C92.9- ☑
   specified NEC C92.Z- ☑ (*following* C92.6)
plasma cell C90.1- ☑
plasmacytic C90.1- ☑
prolymphocytic
   of B-cell type C91.3- ☑
   of T-cell type C91.6- ☑
specified NEC C94.8- ☑
stem cell, of unclear lineage C95.0- ☑
subacute lymphocytic C91.9- ☑
T-cell large granular lymphocytic C91.Z- ☑ (*following* C91.6)
unspecified cell type C95.9- ☑
   acute C95.0- ☑
   chronic C95.1- ☑
Leukemoid reaction — *see also* Reaction, leukemoid D72.823
Leukoaraiosis (hypertensive) I67.81
Leukoariosis — *see* Leukoaraiosis
Leukocoria — *see* Disorder, globe, degenerated condition, leucocoria
Leukocytopenia D72.819
Leukocytosis D72.829
eosinophilic D72.19
Leukoderma, leukodermia NEC L81.5
syphilitic A51.39
   late A52.79
Leukodystrophy E75.29
Leukoedema, oral epithelium K13.29
Leukoencephalitis G04.81
acute (subacute) hemorrhagic G36.1
   postimmunization or postvaccinal G04.02
postinfectious G04.01
subacute sclerosing A81.1
van Bogaert's (sclerosing) A81.1
Leukoencephalopathy — *see also* Encephalopathy G93.49
Binswanger's I67.3
heroin vapor G92.8
metachromatic E75.25
multifocal (progressive) A81.2
postimmunization and postvaccinal G04.02
progressive multifocal A81.2
reversible, posterior G93.6
van Bogaert's (sclerosing) A81.1
vascular, progressive I67.3
Leukoerythroblastosis D75.9
Leukokeratosis — *see also* Leukoplakia
mouth K13.21
nicotina palati K13.24
oral mucosa K13.21
tongue K13.21
vocal cord J38.3
Leukokraurosis vulva (e) N90.4

Leukoma (cornea) — *see also* Opacity, cornea
adherent H17.0- ☑
interfering with central vision — *see* Opacity, cornea, central
Leukomalacia, cerebral, newborn P91.2
periventricular P91.2
Leukomelanopathy, hereditary D72.0
Leukonychia (punctata) (striata) L60.8
congenital Q84.4
Leukopathia unguium L60.8
congenital Q84.4
Leukopenia D72.819
basophilic D72.818
chemotherapy (cancer) induced D70.1
congenital D70.0
cyclic D70.0
drug induced NEC D70.2
   due to cytoreductive cancer chemotherapy D70.1
eosinophilic D72.818
familial D70.0
infantile genetic D70.0
malignant D70.9
periodic D70.0
transitory neonatal P61.5
Leukopenic — *see* condition
Leukoplakia
anus K62.89
bladder (postinfectional) N32.89
buccal K13.21
cervix (uteri) N88.0
esophagus K22.89
gingiva K13.21
hairy (oral mucosa) (tongue) K13.3
kidney (pelvis) N28.89
larynx J38.7
lip K13.21
mouth K13.21
oral epithelium, including tongue (mucosa) K13.21
palate K13.21
pelvis (kidney) N28.89
penis (infectional) N48.0
rectum K62.89
syphilitic (late) A52.79
tongue K13.21
ureter (postinfectional) N28.89
urethra (postinfectional) N36.8
uterus N85.8
vagina N89.4
vocal cord J38.3
vulva N90.4
Leukorrhea N89.8
due to Trichomonas (vaginalis) A59.00
trichomonal A59.00
Leukosarcoma C85.9- ☑
Levocardia (isolated) Q24.1
with situs inversus Q89.3
Levotransposition Q20.5
Lev's disease or syndrome (acquired complete heart block) I44.2
Levulosuria — *see* Fructosuria
Levurid L30.2
Lewy body (ies) (dementia) (disease) G31.83
Leyden-Moebius dystrophy G71.09
Leydig cell
carcinoma
   specified site — *see* Neoplasm, malignant, by site
   unspecified site
      female C56.9
      male C62.9- ☑
tumor
   benign
      specified site — *see* Neoplasm, benign, by site
      unspecified site
         female D27.- ☑
         male D29.2- ☑
   malignant
      specified site — *see* Neoplasm, malignant, by site
      unspecified site
         female C56.- ☑
         male C62.9- ☑
   specified site — *see* Neoplasm, uncertain behavior, by site
   unspecified site
      female D39.1- ☑
      male D40.1- ☑
Leydig-Sertoli cell tumor
specified site — *see* Neoplasm, benign, by site

Leydig-Sertoli cell tumor — *continued*
  unspecified site
    female D27.- ☑
    male D29.2- ☑
LGSIL (Low grade squamous intraepithelial lesion on cytologic smear of)
  anus R85.612
  cervix R87.612
  vagina R87.622
Liar, pathologic F60.2
Libido
  decreased R68.82
Libman-Sacks disease M32.11
Lice (infestation) B85.2
  body (Pediculus corporis) B85.1
  crab B85.3
  head (Pediculus capitis) B85.0
  mixed (classifiable to more than one of the titles B85.0-B85.3) B85.4
  pubic (Phthirus pubis) B85.3
Lichen L28.0
  albus L90.0
    penis N48.0
    vulva N90.4
  amyloidosis E85.4 [L99]
  atrophicus L90.0
    penis N48.0
    vulva N90.4
  congenital Q82.8
  myxedematosus L98.5
  nitidus L44.1
  pilaris Q82.8
    acquired L85.8
  planopilaris L66.1
  planus (chronicus) L43.9
    annularis L43.8
    bullous L43.1
    follicular L66.1
    hypertrophic L43.0
    moniliformis L44.3
    of Wilson L43.9
    specified NEC L43.8
    subacute (active) L43.3
    tropicus L43.3
  ruber
    acuminatus L44.0
    moniliformis L44.3
    planus L43.9
  sclerosus (et atrophicus) L90.0
    penis N48.0
    vulva N90.4
  scrofulosus (primary) (tuberculous) A18.4
  simplex (chronicus) (circumscriptus) L28.0
  striatus L44.2
  urticatus L28.2
Lichenification L28.0
Lichenoides tuberculosis (primary) A18.4
Lichtheim's disease or syndrome D51.0
Lien migrans D73.89
Ligament — *see* condition
Light
  for gestational age — *see* Light for dates
  headedness R42
Light-for-dates (infant) P05.00
  with weight of
    499 grams or less P05.01
    500-749 grams P05.02
    750-999 grams P05.03
    1000-1249 grams P05.04
    1250-1499 grams P05.05
    1500-1749 grams P05.06
    1750-1999 grams P05.07
    2000-2499 grams P05.08
    2500 grams and over P05.09
  affecting management of pregnancy O36.59- ☑
  and small-for-dates — *see* Small for dates
  specified NEC P05.09
Lightning (effects) (stroke) (struck by) T75.00 ☑
  burn — *see* Burn
  foot E53.8
  shock T75.01 ☑
  specified effect NEC T75.09 ☑
Lightwood-Albright syndrome N25.89
Lightwood's disease or syndrome (renal tubular acidosis) N25.89
Lignac (-de Toni) (-Fanconi) (-Debré) **disease or syndrome** E72.09
  with cystinosis E72.04

Ligneous thyroiditis E06.5
Likoff's syndrome I20.8
Limb — *see* condition
Limbic epilepsy personality syndrome F07.0
Limitation, limited
  activities due to disability Z73.6
  cardiac reserve — *see* Disease, heart
  eye muscle duction, traumatic — *see* Strabismus, mechanical
  mandibular range of motion M26.52
Lindau (-von Hippel) **disease** Q85.8
Line(s)
  Beau's L60.4
  Harris' — *see* Arrest, epiphyseal
  Hudson's (cornea) — *see* Pigmentation, cornea, anterior
  Stähli's (cornea) — *see* Pigmentation, cornea, anterior
Linea corneae senilis — *see* Change, cornea, senile
Lingua
  geographica K14.1
  nigra (villosa) K14.3
  plicata K14.5
  tylosis K13.29
Lingual — *see* condition
Linguatulosis B88.8
Linitis (gastric) **plastica** C16.9
Lip — *see* condition
Lipedema — *see* Edema
Lipemia — *see also* Hyperlipidemia
  retina, retinalis E78.3
Lipidosis E75.6
  cerebral (infantile) (juvenile) (late) E75.4
  cerebroretinal E75.4
  cerebroside E75.22
  cholesterol (cerebral) E75.5
  glycolipid E75.21
  hepatosplenomegalic E78.3
  sphingomyelin — *see* Niemann-Pick disease or syndrome
  sulfatide E75.29
Lipoadenoma — *see* Neoplasm, benign, by site
Lipoblastoma — *see* Lipoma
Lipoblastomatosis — *see* Lipoma
Lipochondrodystrophy E76.01
Lipochrome histiocytosis (familial) D71
Lipodermatosclerosis — *see* Varix, leg, with, inflammation
  ulcerated — *see* Varix, leg, with, ulcer, with inflammation by site
Lipodystrophia progressiva E88.1
Lipodystrophy (progressive) E88.1
  insulin E88.1
  intestinal K90.81
  mesenteric K65.4
Lipofibroma — *see* Lipoma
Lipofuscinosis, neuronal (with ceroidosis) E75.4
Lipogranuloma, sclerosing L92.8
Lipogranulomatosis E78.89
Lipoid — *see also* condition
  histiocytosis D76.3
    essential E75.29
  nephrosis N04.9
  proteinosis of Urbach E78.89
Lipoidemia — *see* Hyperlipidemia
Lipoidosis — *see* Lipidosis
Lipoma D17.9
  fetal D17.9
    fat cell D17.9
  infiltrating D17.9
  intramuscular D17.9
  pleomorphic D17.9
  site classification
    arms (skin) (subcutaneous) D17.2- ☑
    connective tissue D17.30
      intra-abdominal D17.5
      intrathoracic D17.4
      peritoneum D17.79
      retroperitoneum D17.79
      specified site NEC D17.39
      spermatic cord D17.6
    face (skin) (subcutaneous) D17.0
    genitourinary organ NEC D17.72
    head (skin) (subcutaneous) D17.0
    intra-abdominal D17.5
    intrathoracic D17.4
    kidney D17.71
    legs (skin) (subcutaneous) D17.2- ☑
    neck (skin) (subcutaneous) D17.0

Lipoma — *continued*
  site classification — *continued*
    peritoneum D17.79
    retroperitoneum D17.79
    skin D17.30
      specified site NEC D17.39
    specified site NEC D17.79
    spermatic cord D17.6
    subcutaneous D17.30
      specified site NEC D17.39
    trunk (skin) (subcutaneous) D17.1
    unspecified D17.9
  spindle cell D17.9
Lipomatosis E88.2
  dolorosa (Dercum) E88.2
  fetal — *see* Lipoma
  Launois-Bensaude E88.89
Lipomyoma — *see* Lipoma
Lipomyxoma — *see* Lipoma
Lipomyxosarcoma — *see* Neoplasm, connective tissue, malignant
Lipoprotein metabolism disorder E78.9
Lipoproteinemia E78.5
  broad-beta E78.2
  floating-beta E78.2
  hyper-pre-beta E78.1
Liposarcoma — *see also* Neoplasm, connective tissue, malignant
  dedifferentiated — *see* Neoplasm, connective tissue, malignant
  differentiated type — *see* Neoplasm, connective tissue, malignant
  embryonal — *see* Neoplasm, connective tissue, malignant
  mixed type — *see* Neoplasm, connective tissue, malignant
  myxoid — *see* Neoplasm, connective tissue, malignant
  pleomorphic — *see* Neoplasm, connective tissue, malignant
  round cell — *see* Neoplasm, connective tissue, malignant
  well differentiated type — *see* Neoplasm, connective tissue, malignant
Liposynovitis prepatellaris E88.89
Lipping, cervix N86
Lipschütz disease or ulcer N76.6
Lipuria R82.0
  schistosomiasis (bilharziasis) B65.0
Lisping F80.0
Lissauer's paralysis A52.17
Lissencephalia, lissencephaly Q04.3
Listeriosis, listerellosis A32.9
  congenital (disseminated) P37.2
  cutaneous A32.0
  neonatal, newborn (disseminated) P37.2
  oculoglandular A32.81
  specified NEC A32.89
Lithemia E79.0
Lithiasis — *see* Calculus
Lithosis J62.8
Lithuria R82.998
Litigation, anxiety concerning Z65.3
Little leaguer's elbow — *see* Epicondylitis, medial
Little's disease G80.9
Littre's
  gland — *see* condition
  hernia — *see* Hernia, abdomen
Littritis — *see* Urethritis
Livedo (annularis) (racemosa) (reticularis) R23.1
Liver — *see* condition
Living alone (problems with) Z60.2
  with handicapped person Z74.2
Living in a shelter (motel) (scattered site housing) (temporary or transitional living situation) Z59.01
Lloyd's syndrome — *see* Adenomatosis, endocrine
Loa loa, loaiasis, loasis B74.3
Lobar — *see* condition
Lobomycosis B48.0
Lobo's disease B48.0
Lobotomy syndrome F07.0
Lobstein (-Ekman) **disease or syndrome** Q78.0
Lobster-claw hand Q71.6- ☑
Lobulation (congenital) — *see also* Anomaly, by site
  kidney, Q63.1
  liver, abnormal Q44.7
  spleen Q89.09
Lobule, lobular — *see* condition

Local, localized — *see* condition
Locked twins causing obstructed labor O66.1
Locked-in state G83.5
Locking
  joint — *see* Derangement, joint, specified type NEC
    knee — *see* Derangement, knee
Lockjaw — *see* Tetanus
Löffler's
  endocarditis I42.3
  eosinophilia J82.89
  pneumonia J82.89
  syndrome (eosinophilic pneumonitis) J82.89
Loiasis (with conjunctival infestation) (eyelid) B74.3
Lone Star fever A77.0
Long
  COVID (-19) — *see also* COVID-19 U09.9
  labor O63.9
    first stage O63.0
    second stage O63.1
  QT syndrome I45.81
Longitudinal stripes or grooves, nails L60.8
  congenital Q84.6
Long-term (current) (prophylactic) **drug therapy** (use of)
  agents affecting estrogen receptors and estrogen levels NEC Z79.818
  anastrozole (Arimidex) Z79.811
  antibiotics Z79.2
    short-term use — *omit code*
  anticoagulants Z79.01
  anti-inflammatory, non-steroidal (NSAID) Z79.1
  antiplatelet Z79.02
  antithrombotics Z79.02
  aromatase inhibitors Z79.811
  aspirin Z79.82
  birth control pill or patch Z79.3
  bisphosphonates Z79.83
  contraceptive, oral Z79.3
  drug, specified NEC Z79.899
  estrogen receptor downregulators Z79.818
  Evista Z79.810
  exemestane (Aromasin) Z79.811
  Fareston Z79.810
  fulvestrant (Faslodex) Z79.818
  gonadotropin-releasing hormone (GnRH) agonist Z79.818
  goserelin acetate (Zoladex) Z79.818
  hormone replacement Z79.890
  insulin Z79.4
  letrozole (Femara) Z79.811
  leuprolide acetate (leuprorelin) (Lupron) Z79.818
  megestrol acetate (Megace) Z79.818
  methadone for pain management Z79.891
  Nolvadex Z79.810
  non-insulin antidiabetic drug, injectable Z79.899
  non-steroidal anti-inflammatories (NSAID) Z79.1
  opiate analgesic Z79.891
  oral
    antidiabetic Z79.84
    contraceptive Z79.3
    hypoglycemic Z79.84
  raloxifene (Evista) Z79.810
  selective estrogen receptor modulators (SERMs) Z79.810
  steroids
    inhaled Z79.51
    systemic Z79.52
  tamoxifen (Nolvadex) Z79.810
  toremifene (Fareston) Z79.810
Loop
  intestine — *see* Volvulus
  vascular on papilla (optic) Q14.2
Loose — *see also* condition
  body
    joint M24.00
      ankle M24.07- ☑
      elbow M24.02- ☑
      hand M24.04- ☑
      hip M24.05- ☑
      knee M23.4- ☑
      shoulder (region) M24.01- ☑
      specified site NEC M24.08
      toe M24.07- ☑
      vertebra M24.08
      wrist M24.03- ☑
    knee M23.4- ☑
    sheath, tendon — *see* Disorder, tendon, specified type NEC

Loose — *continued*
  cartilage — *see* Loose, body, joint
  skin and subcutaneous tissue (following bariatric surgery weight loss) (following dietary weight loss) L98.7
  tooth, teeth K08.89
Loosening
  aseptic
    joint prosthesis — *see* Complications, joint prosthesis, mechanical, loosening, by site
    epiphysis — *see* Osteochondropathy
  mechanical
    joint prosthesis — *see* Complications, joint prosthesis, mechanical, loosening, by site
Looser-Milkman (-Debray) **syndrome** M83.8
Lop ear (deformity) Q17.3
Lorain (-Levi) **short stature syndrome** E23.0
Lordosis M40.50
  acquired — *see* Lordosis, specified type NEC
  congenital Q76.429
    lumbar region Q76.426
    lumbosacral region Q76.427
    sacral region Q76.428
    sacrococcygeal region Q76.428
    thoracolumbar region Q76.425
  lumbar region M40.56
  lumbosacral region M40.57
  postsurgical M96.4
  postural — *see* Lordosis, specified type NEC
  rachitic (late effect) (sequelae) E64.3
  sequelae of rickets E64.3
  specified type NEC M40.40
    lumbar region M40.46
    lumbosacral region M40.47
    thoracolumbar region M40.45
  thoracolumbar region M40.55
  tuberculous A18.01
Loss (of)
  appetite — *see also* Anorexia R63.0
    hysterical F50.89
    nonorganic origin F50.89
    psychogenic F50.89
  blood — *see* Hemorrhage
  bone —*see* Loss, substance of, bone
  consciousness, transient R55
    traumatic — *see* Injury, intracranial
  control, sphincter, rectum R15.9
    nonorganic origin F98.1
  elasticity, skin R23.4
  family (member) in childhood Z62.898
  fluid (acute) E86.9
  function of labyrinth — *see* subcategory H83.2 ☑
  hair, nonscarring — *see* Alopecia
  hearing — *see also* Deafness
    central NOS H90.5
    conductive H90.2
      bilateral H90.0
      unilateral
        with
          restricted hearing on the contralateral side H90.A1- ☑
          unrestricted hearing on the contralateral side H90.1- ☑
    mixed conductive and sensorineural hearing loss H90.8
      bilateral H90.6
      unilateral
        with
          restricted hearing on the contralateral side H90.A3- ☑
          unrestricted hearing on the contralateral side H90.7- ☑
    neural NOS H90.5
    perceptive NOS H90.5
    sensorineural NOS H90.5
      bilateral H90.3
      unilateral
        with
          restricted hearing onthe contralateral side H90.A2- ☑
          unrestricted hearing on the contralateral side H90.4- ☑
    sensory NOS H90.5
  height R29.890
  limb or member, traumatic, current — *see* Amputation, traumatic
  love relationship in childhood Z62.898
  memory — *see also* Amnesia

Loss — *continued*
  memory — *see also* Amnesia — *continued*
    mild, following organic brain damage F06.8
    mind — *see* Psychosis
  occlusal vertical dimension of fully erupted teeth M26.37
  organ or part — *see* Absence, by site, acquired
  ossicles, ear (partial) H74.32- ☑
  parent in childhood Z63.4
  pregnancy, recurrent N96
    care in current pregnancy O26.2- ☑
    without current pregnancy N96
  recurrent pregnancy — *see* Loss, pregnancy, recurrent
  self-esteem, in childhood Z62.898
  sense of
    smell — *see* Disturbance, sensation, smell
    taste — *see* Disturbance, sensation, taste
    touch R20.8
  sensory R44.9
    dissociative F44.6
  sexual desire F52.0
  sight (acquired) (complete) (congenital) — *see* Blindness
  substance of
    bone — *see* Disorder, bone, density and structure, specified NEC
      horizontal alveolar K06.3
    cartilage — *see* Disorder, cartilage, specified type NEC
      auricle (ear) — *see* Disorder, pinna, specified type NEC
    vitreous (humor) H15.89
  tooth, teeth — *see* Absence, teeth, acquired
  vision, visual H54.7
    both eyes H54.3
    one eye H54.60
      left (normal vision on right) H54.62
      right (normal vision on left) H54.61
    specified as blindness — *see* Blindness
    subjective
      sudden H53.13- ☑
      transient H53.12- ☑
  vitreous — *see* Prolapse, vitreous
  voice — *see* Aphonia
  weight (abnormal) (cause unknown) R63.4
Louis-Bar syndrome (ataxia-telangiectasia) G11.3
Louping ill (encephalitis) A84.89
Louse, lousiness — *see* Lice
Low
  achiever, school Z55.3
  back syndrome M54.50
  basal metabolic rate R94.8
  birthweight (2499 grams or less) P07.10
    with weight of
      1000-1249 grams P07.14
      1250-1499 grams P07.15
      1500-1749 grams P07.16
      1750-1999 grams P07.17
      2000-2499 grams P07.18
    extreme (999 grams or less) P07.00
      with weight of
        499 grams or less P07.01
        500-749 grams P07.02
        750-999 grams P07.03
    for gestational age — *see* Light for dates
  blood pressure — *see also* Hypotension
    reading (incidental) (isolated) (nonspecific) R03.1
  cardiac reserve — *see* Disease, heart
  function — *see also* Hypofunction
    kidney N28.9
  hematocrit D64.9
  hemoglobin D64.9
  income Z59.6
  level of literacy Z55.0
  lying
    kidney N28.89
    organ or site, congenital — *see* Malposition, congenital
  output syndrome (cardiac) — *see* Failure, heart
  platelets (blood) — *see* Thrombocytopenia
  reserve, kidney N28.89
  salt syndrome E87.1
  self esteem R45.81
  set ears Q17.4
  vision H54.2X- ☑
    one eye (other eye normal) H54.50
      left (normal vision on right) H54.52A- ☑
      other eye blind — *see* Blindness

Low — continued
  vision — continued
    one eye — continued
      right (normal vision on left) H54.511- ☑
Low-density-lipoprotein-type (LDL) **hyperlipopro-
    teinemia** E78.00
Lowe's syndrome E72.03
Lown-Ganong-Levine syndrome I45.6
LSD reaction (acute) (without dependence) F16.90
    with dependence F16.20
L-shaped kidney Q63.8
LTBI (latent tuberculosis infection) Z22.7
Ludwig's angina or disease K12.2
Lues (venerea), **luetic** — see Syphilis
Luetscher's syndrome (dehydration) E86.0
Lumbago, lumbalgia M54.50
    with sciatica M54.4- ☑
      due to intervertebral disc disorder M51.17
    due to displacement, intervertebral disc M51.27
      with sciatica M51.17
Lumbar — see condition
Lumbarization, vertebra, congenital Q76.49
Lumbermen's itch B88.0
Lump — see also Mass
  breast N63.0
    axillary tail
      left N63.32
      right N63.31
    left
      lower inner quadrant N63.24
      lower outer quadrant N63.23
      overlapping quadrants N63.25
      unspecified quadrant N63.20
      upper inner quadrant N63.22
      upper outer quadrant N63.21
    right
      lower inner quadrant N63.14
      lower outer quadrant N63.13
      overlapping quadrants N63.15
      unspecified quadrant N63.10
      upper inner quadrant N63.12
      upper outer quadrant N63.11
    subareolar
      left N63.42
      right N63.41
Lunacy — see Psychosis
Lung — see condition
Lupoid (miliary) **of Boeck** D86.3
Lupus
  anticoagulant D68.62
    with
      hemorrhagic disorder D68.312
      hypercoagulable state D68.62
    finding without diagnosis R76.0
  discoid (local) L93.0
  erythematosus (discoid) (local) L93.0
    disseminated — see Lupus, erythematosus, systemic
    eyelid H01.129
      left H01.126
        lower H01.125
        upper H01.124
      right H01.123
        lower H01.122
        upper H01.121
    profundus L93.2
    specified NEC L93.2
    subacute cutaneous L93.1
    systemic M32.9
      with organ or system involvement M32.10
        endocarditis M32.11
        lung M32.13
        pericarditis M32.12
        renal (glomerular) M32.14
          tubulo-interstitial M32.15
        specified organ or system NEC M32.19
      drug-induced M32.0
      inhibitor (presence of) D68.62
        with
          hemorrhagic disorder D68.312
          hypercoagulable state D68.62
        finding without diagnosis R76.0
      specified NEC M32.8
  exedens A18.4
  hydralazine M32.0
    correct substance properly administered — see Ta-
      ble of Drugs and Chemicals, by drug, adverse
      effect

Lupus — continued
  hydralazine — continued
    overdose or wrong substance given or taken — see
      Table of Drugs and Chemicals, by drug, poi-
      soning
  nephritis (chronic) M32.14
  nontuberculous, not disseminated L93.0
  panniculitis L93.2
  pernio (Besnier) D86.3
  systemic — see Lupus, erythematosus, systemic
  tuberculous A18.4
    eyelid A18.4
  vulgaris A18.4
    eyelid A18.4
Luteinoma D27.- ☑
Lutembacher's disease or syndrome (atrial septal de-
    fect with mitral stenosis) Q21.1
Luteoma D27.- ☑
Lutz (-Splendore-de Almeida) **disease** — see Paracoccid-
    ioidomycosis
Luxation — see also Dislocation
  eyeball (nontraumatic) — see Luxation, globe
    birth injury P15.3
  globe, nontraumatic H44.82- ☑
  lacrimal gland — see Dislocation, lacrimal gland
  lens (old) (partial) (spontaneous)
    congenital Q12.1
    syphilitic A50.39
Lycanthropy F22
Lyell's syndrome L51.2
  due to drug L51.2
    correct substance properly administered — see Ta-
      ble of Drugs and Chemicals, by drug, adverse
      effect
    overdose or wrong substance given or taken — see
      Table of Drugs and Chemicals, by drug, poi-
      soning
Lyme disease A69.20
Lymph
  gland or node — see condition
  scrotum — see Infestation, filarial
Lymphadenitis I88.9
  with ectopic or molar pregnancy O08.0
  acute L04.9
    axilla L04.2
    face L04.0
    head L04.0
    hip L04.3
    limb
      lower L04.3
      upper L04.2
    neck L04.0
    shoulder L04.2
    specified site NEC L04.8
    trunk L04.1
  anthracosis (occupational) J60
  any site, except mesenteric I88.9
    chronic I88.1
    subacute I88.1
  breast
    gestational — see Mastitis, obstetric
    puerperal, postpartum (nonpurulent) O91.22
  chancroidal (congenital) A57
  chronic I88.1
    mesenteric I88.0
  due to
    Brugia (malayi) B74.1
      timori B74.2
    chlamydial lymphogranuloma A55
    diphtheria (toxin) A36.89
    lymphogranuloma venereum A55
    Wuchereria bancrofti B74.0
  following ectopic or molar pregnancy O08.0
  gonorrheal A54.89
  infective — see Lymphadenitis, acute
  mesenteric (acute) (chronic) (nonspecific) (subacute)
    I88.0
    due to Salmonella typhi A01.09
    tuberculous A18.39
  mycobacterial A31.8
  purulent — see Lymphadenitis, acute
  pyogenic — see Lymphadenitis, acute
  regional, nonbacterial I88.8
  septic — see Lymphadenitis, acute
  subacute, unspecified site I88.1
  suppurative — see Lymphadenitis, acute
  syphilitic (early) (secondary) A51.49
    late A52.79

Lymphadenitis — continued
  tuberculous — see Tuberculosis, lymph gland
  venereal (chlamydial) A55
Lymphadenoid goiter E06.3
Lymphadenopathy (generalized) R59.1
  angioimmunoblastic, with dysproteinemia (AILD) C86.5
  due to toxoplasmosis (acquired) B58.89
    congenital (acute) (subacute) (chronic) P37.1
  localized R59.0
  syphilitic (early) (secondary) A51.49
Lymphadenosis R59.1
Lymphangiectasis I89.0
  conjunctiva H11.89
  postinfectional I89.0
  scrotum I89.0
Lymphangiectatic elephantiasis, nonfilarial I89.0
Lymphangioendothelioma D18.1
  malignant — see Neoplasm, connective tissue, malig-
    nant
Lymphangioleiomyomatosis J84.81
Lymphangioma D18.1
  capillary D18.1
  cavernous D18.1
  cystic D18.1
  malignant — see Neoplasm, connective tissue, malig-
    nant
Lymphangiomyoma D18.1
Lymphangiomyomatosis J84.81
Lymphangiosarcoma — see Neoplasm, connective tis-
    sue, malignant
Lymphangitis I89.1
  with
    abscess — code by site under Abscess
    cellulitis — code by site under Cellulitis
  ectopic or molar pregnancy O08.0
  acute L03.91
    abdominal wall L03.321
    ankle — see Lymphangitis, acute, lower limb
    arm — see Lymphangitis, acute, upper limb
    auricle (ear) — see Lymphangitis, acute, ear
    axilla L03.12- ☑
    back (any part) L03.322
    buttock L03.327
    cervical (meaning neck) L03.222
    cheek (external) L03.212
    chest wall L03.323
    digit
      finger — see Lymphangitis, acute, finger
      toe — see Lymphangitis, acute, toe
    ear (external) H60.1- ☑
    external auditory canal — see Lymphangitis, acute,
      ear
    eyelid — see Abscess, eyelid
    face NEC L03.212
    finger (intrathecal) (periosteal) (subcutaneous)
      (subcuticular) L03.02- ☑
    foot — see Lymphangitis, acute, lower limb
    gluteal (region) L03.327
    groin L03.324
    hand — see Lymphangitis, acute, upper limb
    head NEC L03.891
      face (any part, except ear, eye and nose) L03.212
    heel — see Lymphangitis, acute, lower limb
    hip — see Lymphangitis, acute, lower limb
    jaw (region) L03.212
    knee — see Lymphangitis, acute, lower limb
    leg — see Lymphangitis, acute, lower limb
    lower limb L03.12- ☑
      toe — see Lymphangitis, acute, toe
    navel L03.326
    neck (region) L03.222
    orbit, orbital — see Cellulitis, orbit
    pectoral (region) L03.323
    perineal, perineum L03.325
    scalp (any part) L03.891
    shoulder — see Lymphangitis, acute, upper limb
    specified site NEC L03.898
    thigh — see Lymphangitis, acute, lower limb
    thumb (intrathecal) (periosteal) (subcutaneous)
      (subcuticular) — see Lymphangitis, acute,
      finger
    toe (intrathecal) (periosteal) (subcutaneous) (subcu-
      ticular) L03.04- ☑
    trunk L03.329
      abdominal wall L03.321
      back (any part) L03.322
      buttock L03.327

Lymphangitis — *continued*
  acute — *continued*
    trunk — *continued*
      chest wall L03.323
      groin L03.324
      perineal, perineum L03.325
      umbilicus L03.326
      umbilicus L03.326
      upper limb L03.12- ☑
        axilla — *see* Lymphangitis, acute, axilla
        finger — *see* Lymphangitis, acute, finger
        thumb — *see* Lymphangitis, acute, finger
        wrist — *see* Lymphangitis, acute, upper limb
  breast
    gestational — *see* Mastitis, obstetric
  chancroidal A57
  chronic (any site) I89.1
  due to
    Brugia (malayi) B74.1
      timori B74.2
    Wuchereria bancrofti B74.0
  following ectopic or molar pregnancy O08.89
  penis
    acute N48.29
    gonococcal (acute) (chronic) A54.09
  puerperal, postpartum, childbirth O86.89
  strumous, tuberculous A18.2
  subacute (any site) I89.1
  tuberculous — *see* Tuberculosis, lymph gland
Lymphatic (vessel) — *see* condition
Lymphatism E32.8
Lymphectasia I89.0
Lymphedema (acquired) — *see also* Elephantiasis
  congenital Q82.0
  hereditary (chronic) (idiopathic) Q82.0
  postmastectomy I97.2
  praecox I89.0
  secondary I89.0
  surgical NEC I97.89
    postmastectomy (syndrome) I97.2
Lymphoblastic — *see* condition
Lymphoblastoma (diffuse) — *see* Lymphoma, lymphoblastic (diffuse)
  giant follicular — *see* Lymphoma, lymphoblastic (diffuse)
  macrofollicular — *see* Lymphoma, lymphoblastic (diffuse)
Lymphocele I89.8
Lymphocytic
  chorioencephalitis (acute) (serous) A87.2
  choriomeningitis (acute) (serous) A87.2
  meningoencephalitis A87.2
Lymphocytoma, benign cutis L98.8
Lymphocytopenia D72.810
Lymphocytosis (symptomatic) D72.820
  infectious (acute) B33.8
Lymphoepithelioma — *see* Neoplasm, malignant, by site
Lymphogranuloma (malignant) — *see also* Lymphoma, Hodgkin
  chlamydial A55
  inguinale A55
  venereum (any site) (chlamydial) (with stricture of rectum) A55
Lymphogranulomatosis (malignant) — *see also* Lymphoma, Hodgkin
  benign (Boeck's sarcoid) (Schaumann's) D86.1
Lymphohistiocytosis, hemophagocytic (familial) D76.1
Lymphoid — *see* condition
Lymphoma (of) (malignant) C85.90
  adult T-cell (HTLV-1-associated) (acute variant) (chronic variant) (lymphomatoid variant) (smouldering variant) C91.5- ☑
  anaplastic large cell
    ALK-negative C84.7- ☑
    ALK-positive C84.6- ☑
    breast implant associated (BIA-ALCL) C84.7A
    CD30-positive C84.6- ☑
    primary cutaneous C86.6
  angioimmunoblastic T-cell C86.5
  BALT C88.4
  B-cell C85.1- ☑
  blastic NK-cell C86.4
  blastic plasmacytoid dendritic cell neoplasm (BPDCN) C86.4
  B-precursor C83.5- ☑
  bronchial-associated lymphoid tissue [BALT-lymphoma] C88.4

Lymphoma — *continued*
  Burkitt (atypical) C83.7- ☑
  Burkitt-like C83.7- ☑
  centrocytic C82.6- ☑
  cutaneous follicle center C82.6- ☑
  cutaneous T-cell C84.A- ☑ (*following* C84.7)
  diffuse follicle center C82.5- ☑
  diffuse large cell C83.3- ☑
    anaplastic C83.3- ☑
    B-cell C83.3- ☑
    CD30-positive C83.3- ☑
    centroblastic C83.3- ☑
    immunoblastic C83.3- ☑
    plasmablastic C83.3- ☑
    subtype not specified C83.3- ☑
    T-cell rich C83.3- ☑
  enteropathy-type (associated) (intestinal) T-cell C86.2
  extranodal marginal zone B-cell lymphoma of mucosa-associated lymphoid tissue [MALT-lymphoma] C88.4
  extranodal NK/T-cell, nasal type C86.0
  follicular C82.9- ☑
    grade
      I C82.0- ☑
      II C82.1- ☑
      III C82.2- ☑
      IIIa C82.3- ☑
      IIIb C82.4- ☑
    specified NEC C82.8- ☑
  hepatosplenic T-cell (alpha-beta) (gamma-delta) C86.1
  histiocytic C85.9- ☑
    true C96.A (*following* C96.6)
  Hodgkin C81.9
    lymphocyte depleted (classical) C81.3- ☑
    lymphocyte-rich (classical) C81.4- ☑
    mixed cellularity (classical) C81.2- ☑
    nodular
      lymphocyte predominant C81.0- ☑
      sclerosis (classical) C81.1- ☑
    nodular sclerosis (classical) C81.1- ☑
    specified NEC (classical) C81.7- ☑
  intravascular large B-cell C83.8- ☑
  Lennert's C84.4- ☑
  lymphoblastic (diffuse) C83.5- ☑
  lymphoblastic B-cell C83.5- ☑
  lymphoblastic T-cell C83.5- ☑
  lymphoepithelioid C84.4- ☑
  lymphoplasmacytic C83.0- ☑
    with IgM-production C88.0
  MALT C88.4
  mantle cell C83.1- ☑
  mature T-cell NEC C84.4- ☑
  mature T/NK-cell C84.9- ☑
    specified NEC C84.Z- ☑ (*following* C84.7)
  mediastinal (thymic) large B-cell C85.2- ☑
  Mediterranean C88.3
  mucosa-associated lymphoid tissue [MALT-lymphoma] C88.4
  NK/T cell C84.9- ☑
  nodal marginal zone C83.0- ☑
  non-follicular (diffuse) C83.9- ☑
    specified NEC C83.8- ☑
  non-Hodgkin — *see also* Lymphoma, by type C85.9- ☑
    specified NEC C85.8- ☑
  non-leukemic variant of B-CLL C83.0- ☑
  peripheral T-cell, not classified C84.4- ☑
  primary cutaneous
    anaplastic large cell C86.6
    CD30-positive large T-cell C86.6
  primary effusion B-cell C83.8- ☑
  SALT C88.4
  skin-associated lymphoid tissue [SALT-lymphoma] C88.4
  small cell B-cell C83.0- ☑
  splenic marginal zone C83.0- ☑
  subcutaneous panniculitis-like T-cell C86.3
  T-precursor C83.5- ☑
  true histiocytic C96.A (*following* C96.6)
Lymphomatosis — *see* Lymphoma
Lymphopathia venereum, veneris A55
Lymphopenia D72.810
Lymphoplasmacytic leukemia — *see* Leukemia, chronic lymphocytic, B-cell type
Lymphoproliferation, X-linked disease D82.3
Lymphoreticulosis, benign (of inoculation) A28.1
Lymphorrhea I89.8

Lymphosarcoma (diffuse) — *see also* Lymphoma C85.9- ☑
Lymphostasis I89.8
Lypemania — *see* Melancholia
Lysine and hydroxylysine metabolism disorder E72.3
Lyssa — *see* Rabies

M

Macacus ear Q17.3
Maceration, wet feet, tropical (syndrome) T69.02- ☑
MacLeod's syndrome J43.0
Macrocephalia, macrocephaly Q75.3
Macrocheilia, macrochilia (congenital) Q18.6
Macrocolon — *see also* Megacolon Q43.1
Macrocornea Q15.8
  with glaucoma Q15.0
Macrocytic — *see* condition
Macrocytosis D75.89
Macrodactylia, macrodactylism (fingers) (thumbs) Q74.0
  toes Q74.2
Macrodontia K00.2
Macrogenia M26.05
Macrogenitosomia (adrenal) (male) (praecox) E25.9
  congenital E25.0
Macroglobulinemia (idiopathic) (primary) C88.0
  monoclonal (essential) D47.2
  Waldenström C88.0
Macroglossia (congenital) Q38.2
  acquired K14.8
Macrognathia, macrognathism (congenital) (mandibular) (maxillary) M26.09
Macrogyria (congenital) Q04.8
Macrohydrocephalus — *see* Hydrocephalus
Macromastia — *see* Hypertrophy, breast
Macrophthalmos Q11.3
  in congenital glaucoma Q15.0
Macropsia H53.15
Macrosigmoid K59.39
  congenital Q43.2
Macrospondylitis , acromegalic E22.0
Macrostomia (congenital) Q18.4
Macrotia (external ear) (congenital) Q17.1
Macula
  cornea, corneal — *see* Opacity, cornea
  degeneration (atrophic) (exudative) (senile) — *see also* Degeneration, macula
  hereditary — *see* Dystrophy, retina
Maculae ceruleae B85.1
Maculopathy, toxic — *see* Degeneration, macula, toxic
Madarosis (eyelid) H02.729
  left H02.726
    lower H02.725
    upper H02.724
  right H02.723
    lower H02.722
    upper H02.721
Madelung's
  deformity (radius) Q74.0
  disease
    radial deformity Q74.0
    symmetrical lipomas, neck E88.89
Madness — *see* Psychosis
Madura
  foot B47.9
    actinomycotic B47.1
    mycotic B47.0
Maduromycosis B47.0
Maffucci's syndrome Q78.4
Magnesium metabolism disorder — *see* Disorder, metabolism, magnesium
Main en griffe (acquired) — *see also* Deformity, limb, clawhand
  congenital Q74.0
Maintenance (encounter for)
  antineoplastic chemotherapy Z51.11
  antineoplastic radiation therapy Z51.0
  methadone F11.20
Majocchi's
  disease L81.7
  granuloma B35.8
Major — *see* condition
Mal de los pintos — *see* Pinta
Mal de mer T75.3
Malabar itch (any site) B35.5
Malabsorption K90.9

▽ Subterms under main terms may continue to next column or page   ☑ Additional Character Required — Refer to the Tabular List for Character Selection   **219**

Lymphangitis — Malabsorption

Malabsorption — *continued*
  calcium K90.89
  carbohydrate K90.49
  disaccharide E73.9
  fat K90.49
  galactose E74.20
  glucose (-galactose) E74.39
  intestinal K90.9
    specified NEC K90.89
  isomaltose E74.31
  lactose E73.9
  methionine E72.19
  monosaccharide E74.39
  postgastrectomy K91.2
  postsurgical K91.2
  protein K90.49
  starch K90.49
  sucrose E74.39
  syndrome K90.9
    postsurgical K91.2
Malacia, bone (adult) M83.9
  juvenile — *see* Rickets
Malacoplakia
  bladder N32.89
  pelvis (kidney) N28.89
  ureter N28.89
  urethra N36.8
Malacosteon, juvenile — *see* Rickets
Maladaptation — *see* Maladjustment
Maladie de Roger Q21.0
Maladjustment
  conjugal Z63.0
    involving divorce or estrangement Z63.5
  educational Z55.4
  family Z63.9
  marital Z63.0
    involving divorce or estrangement Z63.5
  occupational NEC Z56.89
  simple, adult — *see* Disorder, adjustment
  situational — *see* Disorder, adjustment
  social Z60.9
    due to
      acculturation difficulty Z60.3
      discrimination and persecution (perceived) Z60.5
      exclusion and isolation Z60.4
      life-cycle (phase of life) transition Z60.0
      rejection Z60.4
      specified reason NEC Z60.8
Malaise R53.81
Malakoplakia — *see* Malacoplakia
Malaria, malarial (fever) B54
  with
    blackwater fever B50.8
      hemoglobinuric (bilious) B50.8
    hemoglobinuria B50.8
  accidentally induced (therapeutically) — *code by* type
    under Malaria
  algid B50.9
  cerebral B50.0 *[G94]*
  clinically diagnosed (without parasitological confirmation) B54
  congenital NEC P37.4
    falciparum P37.3
  congestion, congestive B54
  continued (fever) B50.9
  estivo-autumnal B50.9
  falciparum B50.9
    with complications NEC B50.8
      cerebral B50.0 *[G94]*
    severe B50.8
  hemorrhagic B54
  malariae B52.9
    with
      complications NEC B52.8
      glomerular disorder B52.0
  malignant (tertian) — *see* Malaria, falciparum
  mixed infections — *code to* first listed type in B50-B53
  ovale B53.0
  parasitologically confirmed NEC B53.8
  pernicious, acute — *see* Malaria, falciparum
  Plasmodium (P.)
    falciparum NEC — *see* Malaria, falciparum
    malariae NEC B52.9
      with Plasmodium
        falciparum (and or vivax) — *see* Malaria, falciparum
        vivax — *see also* Malaria, vivax
          and falciparum — *see* Malaria, falciparum

Malaria, malarial — *continued*
  Plasmodium — *continued*
    ovale B53.0
      with Plasmodium malariae — *see also* Malaria, malariae
        and vivax — *see also* Malaria, vivax
          and falciparum — *see* Malaria, falciparum
    simian B53.1
      with Plasmodium malariae — *see also* Malaria, malariae
        and vivax — *see also* Malaria, vivax
          and falciparum — *see* Malaria, falciparum
    vivax NEC B51.9
      with Plasmodium falciparum — *see* Malaria, falciparum
  quartan — *see* Malaria, malariae
  quotidian — *see* Malaria, falciparum
  recurrent B54
  remittent B54
  specified type NEC (parasitologically confirmed) B53.8
  spleen B54
  subtertian (fever) — *see* Malaria, falciparum
  tertian (benign) — *see also* Malaria, vivax
    malignant B50.9
  tropical B50.9
  typhoid B54
  vivax B51.9
    with
      complications NEC B51.8
      ruptured spleen B51.0
Malassez's disease (cystic) N50.89
Malassimilation K90.9
Maldescent, testis Q53.9
  bilateral Q53.20
    abdominal Q53.211
    perineal Q53.22
  unilateral Q53.10
    abdominal Q53.111
    perineal Q53.12
Maldevelopment — *see also* Anomaly
  brain Q07.9
  colon Q43.9
  hip Q74.2
    congenital dislocation Q65.2
      bilateral Q65.1
      unilateral Q65.0- ☑
  mastoid process Q75.8
  middle ear Q16.4
    except ossicles Q16.4
    ossicles Q16.3
  ossicles Q16.3
  spine Q76.49
  toe Q74.2
Male type pelvis Q74.2
  with disproportion (fetopelvic) O33.3 ☑
    causing obstructed labor O65.3
Malformation (congenital) — *see also* Anomaly
  adrenal gland Q89.1
  affecting multiple systems with skeletal changes NEC Q87.5
  alimentary tract Q45.9
    specified type NEC Q45.8
    upper Q40.9
      specified type NEC Q40.8
  aorta Q25.40
    absence Q25.41
    aneurysm, congenital Q25.43
    aplasia Q25.41
    atresia Q25.29
      aortic arch Q25.21
    coarctation (preductal) (postductal) Q25.1
    dilatation, congenital Q25.44
    hypoplasia Q25.42
    patent ductus arteriosus Q25.0
    specified type NEC Q25.49
    stenosis Q25.1
      supravalvular Q25.3
  aortic valve Q23.9
    specified NEC Q23.8
  arteriovenous, aneurysmatic (congenital) Q27.30
    brain Q28.2
      ruptured I60.8
        intracerebral I61.8
        intraparenchymal I61.8
        intraventricular I61.5
        subarachnoid I60.8
    cerebral — *see also* Malformation, arteriovenous, brain Q28.2

Malformation — *continued*
  arteriovenous, aneurysmatic — *continued*
    peripheral Q27.30
      digestive system — *see* Angiodysplasia
        congenital Q27.33
      lower limb Q27.32
      other specified site Q27.39
      renal vessel Q27.34
      upper limb Q27.31
    precerebral vessels (nonruptured) Q28.0
  auricle
    ear (congenital) Q17.3
      acquired H61.119
        left H61.112
          with right H61.113
        right H61.111
          with left H61.113
  bile duct Q44.5
  bladder Q64.79
    aplasia Q64.5
    diverticulum Q64.6
    exstrophy — *see* Exstrophy, bladder
    neck obstruction Q64.31
  bone Q79.9
    face Q75.9
      specified type NEC Q75.8
    skull Q75.9
      specified type NEC Q75.8
  brain (multiple) Q04.9
    arteriovenous Q28.2
    specified type NEC Q04.8
  branchial cleft Q18.2
  breast Q83.9
    specified type NEC Q83.8
  broad ligament Q50.6
  bronchus Q32.4
  bursa Q79.9
  cardiac
    chambers Q20.9
      specified type NEC Q20.8
    septum Q21.9
      specified type NEC Q21.8
  cerebral Q04.9
    vessels Q28.3
  cervix uteri Q51.9
    specified type NEC Q51.828
  Chiari
    Type I G93.5
    Type II Q07.01
  choroid (congenital) Q14.3
    plexus Q07.8
  circulatory system Q28.9
  cochlea Q16.5
  cornea Q13.4
  coronary vessels Q24.5
  corpus callosum (congenital) Q04.0
  diaphragm Q79.1
  digestive system NEC, specified type NEC Q45.8
  dura Q07.9
    brain Q04.9
    spinal Q06.9
  ear Q17.9
    causing impairment of hearing Q16.9
    external Q17.9
      accessory auricle Q17.0
      causing impairment of hearing Q16.9
        absence of
          auditory canal Q16.1
          auricle Q16.0
      macrotia Q17.1
      microtia Q17.2
      misplacement Q17.4
      misshapen NEC Q17.3
      prominence Q17.5
      specified type NEC Q17.8
    inner Q16.5
    middle Q16.4
      absence of eustachian tube Q16.2
      ossicles (fusion) Q16.3
    ossicles Q16.3
    specified type NEC Q17.8
  epididymis Q55.4
  esophagus Q39.9
    specified type NEC Q39.8
  eye Q15.9
    lid Q10.3
    specified NEC Q15.8
  fallopian tube Q50.6
  genital organ — *see* Anomaly, genitalia

☑ **Additional Character Required** — Refer to the Tabular List for Character Selection   ⬇ **Subterms under main terms may continue to next column or page**

Malformation — continued
great
  artery Q25.9
    aorta — see Malformation, aorta
    pulmonary artery — see Malformation, pulmonary, artery
    specified type NEC Q25.8
  vein Q26.9
    anomalous
      portal venous connection Q26.5
      pulmonary venous connection Q26.4
        partial Q26.3
        total Q26.2
    persistent left superior vena cava Q26.1
    portal vein-hepatic artery fistula Q26.6
    specified type NEC Q26.8
    vena cava stenosis, congenital Q26.0
gum Q38.6
hair Q84.2
heart Q24.9
  specified type NEC Q24.8
integument Q84.9
  specified type NEC Q84.8
internal ear Q16.5
intestine Q43.9
  specified type NEC Q43.8
iris Q13.2
joint Q74.9
  ankle Q74.2
  lumbosacral Q76.49
  sacroiliac Q74.2
  specified type NEC Q74.8
kidney Q63.9
  accessory Q63.0
  giant Q63.3
  horseshoe Q63.1
  hydronephrosis Q62.0
  malposition Q63.2
  specified type NEC Q63.8
lacrimal apparatus Q10.6
lingual Q38.3
lip Q38.0
liver Q44.7
lung Q33.9
meninges or membrane (congenital) Q07.9
  cerebral Q04.8
  spinal (cord) Q06.9
middle ear Q16.4
  ossicles Q16.3
mitral valve Q23.9
  specified type NEC Q23.8
Mondini's (congenital) (malformation, cochlea) Q16.5
mouth (congenital) Q38.6
multiple types NEC Q89.7
musculoskeletal system Q79.9
myocardium Q24.8
nail Q84.6
nervous system (central) Q07.9
nose Q30.9
  specified type NEC Q30.8
optic disc Q14.2
orbit Q10.7
ovary Q50.39
palate Q38.5
parathyroid gland Q89.2
pelvic organs or tissues NEC
  in pregnancy or childbirth O34.8- ☑
    causing obstructed labor O65.5
penis Q55.69
  aplasia Q55.5
  curvature (lateral) Q55.61
  hypoplasia Q55.62
pericardium Q24.8
peripheral vascular system Q27.9
  specified type NEC Q27.8
pharynx Q38.8
precerebral vessels Q28.1
prostate Q55.4
pulmonary
  arteriovenous Q25.72
  artery Q25.9
    atresia Q25.5
    specified type NEC Q25.79
    stenosis Q25.6
  valve Q22.3
renal artery Q27.2
respiratory system Q34.9
retina Q14.1
scrotum — see Malformation, testis and scrotum

Malformation — continued
seminal vesicles Q55.4
sense organs NEC Q07.9
skin Q82.9
specified NEC Q89.8
spinal
  cord Q06.9
  nerve root Q07.8
spine Q76.49
  kyphosis — see Kyphosis, congenital
  lordosis — see Lordosis, congenital
spleen Q89.09
stomach Q40.3
  specified type NEC Q40.2
teeth, tooth K00.9
tendon Q79.9
testis and scrotum Q55.20
  aplasia Q55.0
  hypoplasia Q55.1
  polyorchism Q55.21
  retractile testis Q55.22
  scrotal transposition Q55.23
  specified NEC Q55.29
thorax, bony Q76.9
throat Q38.8
thyroid gland Q89.2
tongue (congenital) Q38.3
  hypertrophy Q38.2
  tie Q38.1
trachea Q32.1
tricuspid valve Q22.9
  specified type NEC Q22.8
umbilical cord NEC (complicating delivery) O69.89 ☑
umbilicus Q89.9
ureter Q62.8
  agenesis Q62.4
  duplication Q62.5
  malposition — see Malposition, congenital, ureter
  obstructive defect — see Defect, obstructive, ureter
  vesico-uretero-renal reflux Q62.7
urethra Q64.79
  aplasia Q64.5
  duplication Q64.74
  posterior valves Q64.2
  prolapse Q64.71
  stricture Q64.32
urinary system Q64.9
uterus Q51.9
  specified type NEC Q51.818
vagina Q52.4
vas deferens Q55.4
  atresia Q55.3
vascular system, peripheral Q27.9
venous — see Anomaly, vein(s)
vulva Q52.70
Malfunction — see also Dysfunction
cardiac electronic device T82.119 ☑
  electrode T82.110 ☑
  pulse generator T82.111 ☑
  specified type NEC T82.118 ☑
catheter device NEC T85.618 ☑
  cystostomy T83.010 ☑
  dialysis (renal) (vascular) T82.41 ☑
    intraperitoneal T85.611 ☑
  infusion NEC T82.514 ☑
    cranial T85.610 ☑
    epidural T85.610 ☑
    intrathecal T85.610 ☑
    spinal T85.610 ☑
    subarachnoid T85.610 ☑
    subdural T85.610 ☑
  urinary — see also Breakdown, device, catheter
    T83.018 ☑
colostomy K94.03
  valve K94.03
cystostomy (stoma) N99.512
  catheter T83.010 ☑
enteric stoma K94.13
enterostomy K94.13
esophagostomy K94.33
gastroenteric K31.89
gastrostomy K94.23
ileostomy K94.13
  valve K94.13
intrathecal infusion pump T85.615 ☑
jejunostomy K94.13
nervous system device, implant or graft, specified NEC
    T85.615 ☑

Malfunction — continued
pacemaker — see Malfunction, cardiac electronic device
prosthetic device, internal — see Complications, prosthetic device, by site, mechanical
tracheostomy J95.03
urinary device NEC — see Complication, genitourinary, device, urinary, mechanical
valve
  colostomy K94.03
  heart T82.09 ☑
  ileostomy K94.13
vascular graft or shunt NEC — see Complication, cardiovascular device, mechanical, vascular
ventricular (communicating shunt) T85.01 ☑
Malherbe's tumor — see Neoplasm, skin, benign
Malibu disease L98.8
Malignancy — see also Neoplasm, malignant, by site
  unspecified site (primary) C80.1
Malignant — see condition
Malingerer, malingering Z76.5
Mallet finger (acquired) — see Deformity, finger, mallet
  finger
  congenital Q74.0
  sequelae of rickets E64.3
Malleus A24.0
Mallory's bodies R89.7
Mallory-Weiss syndrome K22.6
Malnutrition E46
degree
  first E44.1
    mild (protein) E44.1
    moderate (protein) E44.0
  second E44.0
  severe (protein-energy) E43
    intermediate form E42
      with
        kwashiorkor (and marasmus) E42
        marasmus E41
  third E43
following gastrointestinal surgery K91.2
intrauterine
  light-for-dates — see Light for dates
  small-for-dates — see Small for dates
lack of care, or neglect (child) (infant) T76.02 ☑
  confirmed T74.02 ☑
malignant E40
protein E46
  calorie E46
    mild E44.1
    moderate E44.0
    severe E43
      intermediate form E42
        with
          kwashiorkor (and marasmus) E42
          marasmus E41
  energy E46
    mild E44.1
    moderate E44.0
    severe E43
      intermediate form E42
        with
          kwashiorkor (and marasmus) E42
          marasmus E41
severe (protein-energy) E43
  with
    kwashiorkor (and marasmus) E42
    marasmus E41
Malocclusion (teeth) M26.4
Angle's M26.219
  class I M26.211
  class II M26.212
  class III M26.213
due to
  abnormal swallowing M26.59
  mouth breathing M26.59
  tongue, lip or finger habits M26.59
temporomandibular (joint) M26.69
Malposition
cervix — see Malposition, uterus
congenital
  adrenal (gland) Q89.1
  alimentary tract Q45.8
    lower Q43.8
    upper Q40.8
  aorta Q25.49
  appendix Q43.8
  arterial trunk Q20.0

Malposition — *continued*
congenital — *continued*
 artery (peripheral) Q27.8
  coronary Q24.5
  digestive system Q27.8
  lower limb Q27.8
  pulmonary Q25.79
  specified site NEC Q27.8
  upper limb Q27.8
 auditory canal Q17.8
  causing impairment of hearing Q16.9
 auricle (ear) Q17.4
  causing impairment of hearing Q16.9
  cervical Q18.2
 biliary duct or passage Q44.5
 bladder (mucosa) — *see* Exstrophy, bladder
 brachial plexus Q07.8
 brain tissue Q04.8
 breast Q83.8
 bronchus Q32.4
 cecum Q43.8
 clavicle Q74.0
 colon Q43.8
 digestive organ or tract NEC Q45.8
  lower Q43.8
  upper Q40.8
 ear (auricle) (external) Q17.4
  ossicles Q16.3
 endocrine (gland) NEC Q89.2
 epiglottis Q31.89
 eustachian tube Q17.8
 eye Q15.8
 facial features Q18.8
 fallopian tube Q50.6
 finger(s) Q68.1
  supernumerary Q69.0
 foot Q66.9- ☑
 gallbladder Q44.1
 gastrointestinal tract Q45.8
 genitalia, genital organ(s) or tract
  female Q52.8
   external Q52.79
   internal NEC Q52.8
  male Q55.8
 glottis Q31.8
 hand Q68.1
 heart Q24.8
  dextrocardia Q24.0
   with complete transposition of viscera Q89.3
 hepatic duct Q44.5
 hip (joint) Q65.89
 intestine (large) (small) Q43.8
  with anomalous adhesions, fixation or malrotation Q43.3
 joint NEC Q68.8
 kidney Q63.2
 larynx Q31.8
 limb Q68.8
  lower Q68.8
  upper Q68.8
 liver Q44.7
 lung (lobe) Q33.8
 nail(s) Q84.6
 nerve Q07.8
 nervous system NEC Q07.8
 nose, nasal (septum) Q30.8
 organ or site not listed — *see* Anomaly, by site
 ovary Q50.39
 pancreas Q45.3
 parathyroid (gland) Q89.2
 patella Q74.1
 peripheral vascular system Q27.8
 pituitary (gland) Q89.2
 respiratory organ or system NEC Q34.8
 rib (cage) Q76.6
  supernumerary in cervical region Q76.5
 scapula Q74.0
 shoulder Q74.0
 spinal cord Q06.8
 spleen Q89.09
 sternum NEC Q76.7
 stomach Q40.2
 symphysis pubis Q74.2
 thymus (gland) Q89.2
 thyroid (gland) (tissue) Q89.2
  cartilage Q31.8
 toe(s) Q66.9- ☑
  supernumerary Q69.2
 tongue Q38.3

Malposition — *continued*
congenital — *continued*
 trachea Q32.1
 ureter Q62.60
  deviation Q62.61
  displacement Q62.62
  ectopia Q62.63
  specified type NEC Q62.69
 uterus Q51.818
 vein(s) (peripheral) Q27.8
  great Q26.8
 vena cava (inferior) (superior) Q26.8
device, implant or graft — *see also* Complications, by site and type, mechanical T85.628 ☑
 arterial graft NEC — *see* Complication, cardiovascular device, mechanical, vascular
 breast (implant) T85.42 ☑
 catheter NEC T85.628 ☑
  cystostomy T83.020 ☑
  dialysis (renal) T82.42 ☑
   intraperitoneal T85.621 ☑
  infusion NEC T82.524 ☑
   spinal (epidural) (subdural) T85.620 ☑
  urinary — *see also* Displacement, device, catheter, urinary T83.028 ☑
 electronic (electrode) (pulse generator) (stimulator)
  bone T84.320 ☑
  cardiac T82.129 ☑
   electrode T82.120 ☑
   pulse generator T82.121 ☑
   specified type NEC T82.128 ☑
  nervous system — *see* Complication, prosthetic device, mechanical, electronic nervous system stimulator
  urinary — *see* Complication, genitourinary, device, urinary, mechanical
 fixation, internal (orthopedic) NEC — *see* Complication, fixation device, mechanical
 gastrointestinal — *see* Complications, prosthetic device, mechanical, gastrointestinal device
 genital NEC T83.428 ☑
  intrauterine contraceptive device (string) T83.32 ☑
  penile prosthesis (cylinder) (implanted) (pump) (reservoir) T83.420 ☑
  testicular prosthesis T83.421 ☑
 heart NEC — *see* Complication, cardiovascular device, mechanical
 joint prosthesis — *see* Complication, joint prosthesis, mechanical
 ocular NEC — *see* Complications, prosthetic device, mechanical, ocular device
 orthopedic NEC — *see* Complication, orthopedic, device, mechanical
 specified NEC T85.628 ☑
 urinary NEC — *see also* Complication, genitourinary, device, urinary, mechanical
  graft T83.22 ☑
 vascular NEC — *see* Complication, cardiovascular device, mechanical
 ventricular intracranial shunt T85.02 ☑
fetus — *see* Pregnancy, complicated by (management affected by), presentation, fetal
gallbladder K82.8
gastrointestinal tract, congenital Q45.8
heart, congenital NEC Q24.8
joint prosthesis — *see* Complications, joint prosthesis, mechanical, displacement, by site
stomach K31.89
 congenital Q40.2
tooth, teeth, fully erupted M26.30
uterus (acute) (acquired) (adherent) (asymptomatic) (postinfectional) (postpartal) (old) N85.4
 anteflexion or anteversion N85.4
  congenital Q51.818
 flexion N85.4
  lateral — *see* Lateroversion, uterus
 inversion N85.5
 lateral (flexion) (version) — *see* Lateroversion, uterus
  in pregnancy or childbirth — *see* subcategory O34.5 ☑
 retroflexion or retroversion — *see* Retroversion, uterus
Malposture R29.3
Malrotation
cecum Q43.3
colon Q43.3

Malrotation — *continued*
intestine Q43.3
kidney Q63.2
Malta fever — *see* Brucellosis
Maltreatment
adult
 abandonment
  confirmed T74.01 ☑
  suspected T76.01 ☑
 bullying
  confirmed T74.31 ☑
  suspected T76.31 ☑
 confirmed T74.91 ☑
 history of Z91.419
 intimidation (through social media)
  confirmed T74.31 ☑
  suspected T76.31 ☑
 neglect
  confirmed T74.01 ☑
  suspected T76.01 ☑
 physical abuse
  confirmed T74.11 ☑
  suspected T76.11 ☑
 psychological abuse
  confirmed T74.31 ☑
  history of Z91.411
  suspected T76.31 ☑
 sexual abuse
  confirmed T74.21 ☑
  suspected T76.21 ☑
 suspected T76.91 ☑
child
 abandonment
  confirmed T74.02 ☑
  suspected T76.02 ☑
 bullying
  confirmed T74.32 ☑
  suspected T76.32 ☑
 confirmed T74.92 ☑
 history of — *see* History, personal (of), abuse
 intimidation (through social media)
  confirmed T74.32 ☑
  suspected T76.32 ☑
 neglect
  confirmed T74.02 ☑
  history of — *see* History, personal (of), abuse
  suspected T76.02 ☑
 physical abuse
  confirmed T74.12 ☑
  history of — *see* History, personal (of), abuse
  suspected T76.12 ☑
 psychological abuse
  confirmed T74.32 ☑
  history of — *see* History, personal (of), abuse
  suspected T76.32 ☑
 sexual abuse
  confirmed T74.22 ☑
  history of — *see* History, personal (of), abuse
  suspected T76.22 ☑
 suspected T76.92 ☑
personal history of Z91.89
Maltworker's lung J67.4
Malunion, fracture — *see* Fracture, by site
Mammillitis N61.0
 puerperal, postpartum O91.02
Mammitis — *see* Mastitis
Mammogram (examination) Z12.39
 routine Z12.31
Mammoplasia N62
Management (of)
 bone conduction hearing device (implanted) Z45.320
 cardiac pacemaker NEC Z45.018
 cerebrospinal fluid drainage device Z45.41
 cochlear device (implanted) Z45.321
 contraceptive Z30.9
  specified NEC Z30.8
 implanted device Z45.9
  specified NEC Z45.89
 infusion pump Z45.1
 procreative Z31.9
  male factor infertility in female Z31.81
  specified NEC Z31.89
 prosthesis (external) — *see also* Fitting Z44.9
  implanted Z45.9
   specified NEC Z45.89
 renal dialysis catheter Z49.01
 vascular access device Z45.2

222

☑ **Additional Character Required** — **Refer to the Tabular List for Character Selection**   ▽ **Subterms under main terms may continue to next column or page**

Malposition — Management

Mangled — *see* specified injury by site
Mania (monopolar) — *see also* Disorder, mood, manic
    episode
    with psychotic symptoms F30.2
    without psychotic symptoms F30.10
        mild F30.11
        moderate F30.12
        severe F30.13
    Bell's F30.8
    chronic (recurrent) F31.89
    hysterical F44.89
    puerperal F30.8
    recurrent F31.89
Manic depression F31.9
Manic-depressive insanity, psychosis, or syndrome
    — *see* Disorder, bipolar
Mannosidosis E77.1
Mansonelliasis, mansonellosis B74.4
Manson's
    disease B65.1
    schistosomiasis B65.1
Manual — *see* condition
Maple-bark-stripper's lung (disease) J67.6
Maple-syrup-urine disease E71.0
Marable's syndrome (celiac artery compression) I77.4
Marasmus E41
    due to malnutrition E41
    intestinal E41
    nutritional E41
    senile R54
    tuberculous NEC — *see* Tuberculosis
Marble
    bones Q78.2
    skin R23.8
Marburg virus disease A98.3
March
    fracture — *see* Fracture, traumatic, stress, by site
    hemoglobinuria D59.6
Marchesani (-Weill) **syndrome** Q87.0
Marchiafava (-Bignami) **syndrome or disease** G37.1
Marchiafava-Micheli syndrome D59.5
Marcus Gunn's syndrome Q07.8
Marfan's syndrome — *see* Syndrome, Marfan's
Marie-Bamberger disease — *see* Osteoarthropathy,
    hypertrophic, specified NEC
Marie-Charcot-Tooth neuropathic muscular atrophy
    G60.0
Marie's
    cerebellar ataxia (late-onset) G11.2
    disease or syndrome (acromegaly) E22.0
Marie-Strümpell arthritis, disease or spondylitis —
    see Spondylitis, ankylosing
Marion's disease (bladder neck obstruction) N32.0
Marital conflict Z63.0
Mark
    port wine Q82.5
    raspberry Q82.5
    strawberry Q82.5
    stretch L90.6
    tattoo L81.8
Marker heterochromatin — *see* Extra, marker chromo-
    somes
Maroteaux-Lamy syndrome (mild) (severe) E76.29
Marrow (bone)
    arrest D61.9
    poor function D75.89
Marseilles fever A77.1
Marsh fever — *see* Malaria
Marshall's (hidrotic) **ectodermal dysplasia** Q82.4
Marsh's disease (exophthalmic goiter) E05.00
    with storm E05.01
Masculinization (female) **with adrenal hyperplasia**
    E25.9
    congenital E25.0
Masculinovoblastoma D27.- ☑
Masochism (sexual) F65.51
Mason's lung J62.8
Mass
    abdominal R19.00
        epigastric R19.06
        generalized R19.07
        left lower quadrant R19.04
        left upper quadrant R19.02
        periumbilic R19.05
        right lower quadrant R19.03
        right upper quadrant R19.01
        specified site NEC R19.09

Mass — *continued*
    breast — *see also* Lump, breast N63.0
    chest R22.2
    cystic — *see* Cyst
    ear H93.8- ☑
    head R22.0
    intra-abdominal (diffuse) (generalized) — *see* Mass,
        abdominal
    kidney N28.89
    liver R16.0
    localized (skin) R22.9
        chest R22.2
        head R22.0
        limb
            lower R22.4- ☑
            upper R22.3- ☑
        neck R22.1
        trunk R22.2
    lung R91.8
    malignant — *see* Neoplasm, malignant, by site
    neck R22.1
    pelvic (diffuse) (generalized) — *see* Mass, abdominal
    specified organ NEC — *see* Disease, by site
    splenic R16.1
    substernal thyroid — *see* Goiter
    superficial (localized) R22.9
    umbilical (diffuse) (generalized) R19.09
Massive — *see* condition
Mast cell
    disease, systemic tissue D47.02
    leukemia C94.3- ☑
    neoplasm
        malignant C96.20
            specified type NEC C96.29
        of uncertain behavior NEC D47.09
    sarcoma C96.22
    tumor D47.09
Mastalgia N64.4
Masters-Allen syndrome N83.8
Mastitis (acute) (diffuse) (nonpuerperal) (subacute) N61.0
    with abscess N61.1
    chronic (cystic) — *see* Mastopathy, cystic
    cystic (Schimmelbusch's type) — *see* Mastopathy, cystic
    fibrocystic — *see* Mastopathy, cystic
    granulomatous N61.2- ☑
    infective N61.0
        newborn P39.0
    interstitial, gestational or puerperal — *see* Mastitis,
        obstetric
    neonatal (noninfective) P83.4
        infective P39.0
    obstetric (interstitial) (nonpurulent)
        associated with
            lactation O91.23
            pregnancy O91.21- ☑
            puerperium O91.22
        purulent
            associated with
                lactation O91.13
                pregnancy O91.11- ☑
                puerperium O91.12
    periductal — *see* Ectasia, mammary duct
    phlegmonous — *see* Mastopathy, cystic
    plasma cell — *see* Ectasia, mammary duct
    without abscess N61.0
Mastocytoma (extracutaneous) D47.09
    malignant C96.29
    solitary D47.01
Mastocytosis D47.09
    aggressive systemic C96.21
    cutaneous (diffuse) (maculopapular) D47.01
        congenital Q82.2
        of neonatal onset Q82.2
        of newborn onset Q82.2
    indolent systemic D47.02
    isolated bone marrow D47.02
    malignant C96.29
    systemic (indolent) (smoldering)
        with an associated hematological non-mast cell
            lineage disease (SM-AHNMD) D47.02
Mastodynia N64.4
Mastoid — *see* condition
Mastoidalgia — *see* subcategory H92.0 ☑
Mastoiditis (coalescent) (hemorrhagic) (suppurative)
    H70.9- ☑
    acute, subacute H70.00- ☑
        complicated NEC H70.09- ☑

Mastoiditis — *continued*
    acute, subacute — *continued*
        subperiosteal H70.01- ☑
    chronic (necrotic) (recurrent) H70.1- ☑
    in (due to)
        infectious disease NEC B99 ☑ *[H75.0-]* ☑
        parasitic disease NEC B89 *[H75.0-]* ☑
        tuberculosis A18.03
    petrositis — *see* Petrositis
    postauricular fistula — *see* Fistula, postauricular
    specified NEC H70.89- ☑
    tuberculous A18.03
Mastopathy, mastopathia N64.9
    chronica cystica — *see* Mastopathy, cystic
    cystic (chronic) (diffuse) N60.1- ☑
        with epithelial proliferation N60.3- ☑
    diffuse cystic — *see* Mastopathy, cystic
    estrogenic, oestrogenica N64.89
    ovarian origin N64.89
Mastoplasia, mastoplastia N62
Masturbation (excessive) F98.8
Maternal care (for) — *see* Pregnancy (complicated by)
    (management affected by)
Matheiu's disease (leptospiral jaundice) A27.0
Mauclaire's disease or osteochondrosis — *see* Osteo-
    chondrosis, juvenile, hand, metacarpal
Maxcy's disease A75.2
Maxilla, maxillary — *see* condition
May (-Hegglin) **anomaly or syndrome** D72.0
McArdle (-Schmid)(-Pearson) **disease** (glycogen storage)
    E74.04
McCune-Albright syndrome Q78.1
McQuarrie's syndrome (idiopathic familial hypo-
    glycemia) E16.2
Meadow's syndrome Q86.1
Measles (black) (hemorrhagic) (suppressed) B05.9
    with
        complications NEC B05.89
        encephalitis B05.0
        intestinal complications B05.4
        keratitis (keratoconjunctivitis) B05.81
        meningitis B05.1
        otitis media B05.3
        pneumonia B05.2
    French — *see* Rubella
    German — *see* Rubella
    Liberty — *see* Rubella
Meatitis, urethral — *see* Urethritis
Meatus, meatal — *see* condition
Meat-wrappers' asthma J68.9
Meckel-Gruber syndrome Q61.9
Meckel's diverticulitis, diverticulum (displaced) (hy-
    pertrophic) Q43.0
    malignant — *see* Table of Neoplasms, small intestine,
        malignant
Meconium
    ileus, newborn P76.0
        in cystic fibrosis E84.11
        meaning meconium plug (without cystic fibrosis)
            P76.0
    obstruction, newborn P76.0
        due to fecaliths P76.0
        in mucoviscidosis E84.11
    peritonitis P78.0
    plug syndrome (newborn) NEC P76.0
Median — *see also* condition
    arcuate ligament syndrome I77.4
    bar (prostate) (vesical orifice) — *see* Hyperplasia,
        prostate
    rhomboid glossitis K14.2
Mediastinal shift R93.89
Mediastinitis (acute) (chronic) J98.51
    syphilitic A52.73
    tuberculous A15.8
Mediastinopericarditis — *see also* Pericarditis
    acute I30.9
    adhesive I31.0
    chronic I31.8
        rheumatic I09.2
Mediastinum, mediastinal — *see* condition
Medicine poisoning — *see* Table of Drugs and Chemi-
    cals, by drug, poisoning
Mediterranean
    fever — *see* Brucellosis
        familial M04.1
        tick A77.1
    kala-azar B55.0

Mediterranean — *continued*
  leishmaniasis B55.0
  tick fever A77.1
Medulla — *see* condition
Medullary cystic kidney Q61.5
Medullated fibers
  optic (nerve) Q14.8
  retina Q14.1
Medulloblastoma
  desmoplastic C71.6
  specified site — *see* Neoplasm, malignant, by site
  unspecified site C71.6
Medulloepithelioma — *see also* Neoplasm, malignant, by site
  teratoid — *see* Neoplasm, malignant, by site
Medullomyoblastoma
  specified site — *see* Neoplasm, malignant, by site
  unspecified site C71.6
Meekeren-Ehlers-Danlos syndrome — *see also* Syndrome, Ehlers-Danlos Q79.69
Megacolon (acquired) (functional) (not Hirschsprung's disease) (in) K59.39
  Chagas' disease B57.32
  congenital, congenitum (aganglionic) Q43.1
  Hirschsprung's (disease) Q43.1
  toxic NEC K59.31
    due to Clostridium difficile
      not specified as recurrent A04.72
      recurrent A04.71
Megaesophagus (functional) K22.0
  congenital Q39.5
  in (due to) Chagas' disease B57.31
Megalencephaly Q04.5
Megalerythema (epidemic) B08.3
Megaloappendix Q43.8
Megalocephalus, megalocephaly NEC Q75.3
Megalocornea Q15.8
  with glaucoma Q15.0
Megalocytic anemia D53.1
Megalodactylia (fingers) (thumbs) (congenital) Q74.0
  toes Q74.2
Megaloduodenum Q43.8
Megaloesophagus (functional) K22.0
  congenital Q39.5
Megalogastria (acquired) K31.89
  congenital Q40.2
Megalophthalmos Q11.3
Megalopsia H53.15
Megalosplenia — *see* Splenomegaly
Megaloureter N28.82
  congenital Q62.2
Megarectum K62.89
Megasigmoid K59.39
  congenital Q43.2
Megaureter N28.82
  congenital Q62.2
Megavitamin-B6 syndrome E67.2
Megrim — *see* Migraine
Meibomian
  cyst, infected — *see* Hordeolum
  gland — *see* condition
  sty, stye — *see* Hordeolum
Meibomitis — *see* Hordeolum
Meige-Milroy disease (chronic hereditary edema) Q82.0
Meige's syndrome Q82.0
Melalgia, nutritional E53.8
Melancholia F32.A
  climacteric (single episode) F32.89
    recurrent episode F33.8
  hypochondriac F45.29
  intermittent (single episode) F32.89
    recurrent episode F33.8
  involutional (single episode) F32.89
    recurrent episode F33.8
  menopausal (single episode) F32.89
    recurrent episode F33.8
  puerperal F32.89
  reactive (emotional stress or trauma) F32.3
  recurrent F33.9
  senile F03 ☑
  stuporous (single episode) F32.89
    recurrent episode F33.8
Melanemia R79.89
Melanoameloblastoma — *see* Neoplasm, bone, benign
Melanoblastoma — *see* Melanoma
Melanocarcinoma — *see* Melanoma
Melanocytoma, eyeball D31.9- ☑

Melanocytosis, neurocutaneous Q82.8
Melanoderma, melanodermia L81.4
Melanodontia, infantile K03.89
Melanodontoclasia K03.89
Melanoepithelioma — *see* Melanoma
Melanoma (malignant) C43.9
  acral lentiginous, malignant — *see* Melanoma, skin, by site
  amelanotic — *see* Melanoma, skin, by site
  balloon cell — *see* Melanoma, skin, by site
  benign — *see* Nevus
  desmoplastic, malignant — *see* Melanoma, skin, by site
  epithelioid cell — *see* Melanoma, skin, by site
    with spindle cell, mixed — *see* Melanoma, skin, by site
  in
    giant pigmented nevus — *see* Melanoma, skin, by site
    Hutchinson's melanotic freckle — *see* Melanoma, skin, by site
    junctional nevus — *see* Melanoma, skin, by site
    precancerous melanosis — *see* Melanoma, skin, by site
  in situ D03.9
    abdominal wall D03.59
    ala nasi D03.39
    ankle D03.7- ☑
    anus, anal (margin) (skin) D03.51
    arm D03.6- ☑
    auditory canal D03.2- ☑
    auricle (ear) D03.2- ☑
    auricular canal (external) D03.2- ☑
    axilla, axillary fold D03.59
    back D03.59
    breast D03.52
    brow D03.39
    buttock D03.59
    canthus (eye) D03.1- ☑
    cheek (external) D03.39
    chest wall D03.59
    chin D03.39
    choroid D03.8
    conjunctiva D03.8
    ear (external) D03.2- ☑
    external meatus (ear) D03.2- ☑
    eye D03.8
    eyebrow D03.39
    eyelid (lower) (upper) D03.1- ☑
    face D03.30
      specified NEC D03.39
    female genital organ (external) NEC D03.8
    finger D03.6- ☑
    flank D03.59
    foot D03.7- ☑
    forearm D03.6- ☑
    forehead D03.39
    foreskin D03.8
    gluteal region D03.59
    groin D03.59
    hand D03.6- ☑
    heel D03.7- ☑
    helix D03.2- ☑
    hip D03.7- ☑
    interscapular region D03.59
    iris D03.8
    jaw D03.39
    knee D03.7- ☑
    labium (majus) (minus) D03.8
    lacrimal gland D03.8
    leg D03.7- ☑
    lip (lower) (upper) D03.0
    lower limb NEC D03.7- ☑
    male genital organ (external) NEC D03.8
    nail D03.9
      finger D03.6- ☑
      toe D03.7- ☑
    neck D03.4
    nose (external) D03.39
    orbit D03.8
    penis D03.8
    perianal skin D03.51
    perineum D03.51
    pinna D03.2- ☑
    popliteal fossa or space D03.7- ☑
    prepuce D03.8
    pudendum D03.8

Melanoma — *continued*
  in situ — *continued*
    retina D03.8
    retrobulbar D03.8
    scalp D03.4
    scrotum D03.8
    shoulder D03.6- ☑
    specified site NEC D03.8
    submammary fold D03.52
    temple D03.39
    thigh D03.7- ☑
    toe D03.7- ☑
    trunk NEC D03.59
    umbilicus D03.59
    upper limb NEC D03.6- ☑
    vulva D03.8
  juvenile — *see* Nevus
  malignant, of soft parts except skin — *see* Neoplasm, connective tissue, malignant
  metastatic
    breast C79.81
    genital organ C79.82
    specified site NEC C79.89
  neurotropic, malignant — *see* Melanoma, skin, by site
  nodular — *see* Melanoma, skin, by site
  regressing, malignant — *see* Melanoma, skin, by site
  skin C43.9
    abdominal wall C43.59
    ala nasi C43.31
    ankle C43.7- ☑
    anus, anal (skin) C43.51
    arm C43.6- ☑
    auditory canal (external) C43.2- ☑
    auricle (ear) C43.2- ☑
    auricular canal (external) C43.2- ☑
    axilla, axillary fold C43.59
    back C43.59
    breast (female) (male) C43.52
    brow C43.39
    buttock C43.59
    canthus (eye) C43.1- ☑
    cheek (external) C43.39
    chest wall C43.59
    chin C43.39
    ear (external) C43.2- ☑
    elbow C43.6- ☑
    external meatus (ear) C43.2- ☑
    eyebrow C43.39
    eyelid (lower) (upper) C43.1- ☑
    face C43.30
      specified NEC C43.39
    female genital organ (external) NEC C51.9
    finger C43.6- ☑
    flank C43.59
    foot C43.7- ☑
    forearm C43.6- ☑
    forehead C43.39
    foreskin C60.0
    glabella C43.39
    gluteal region C43.59
    groin C43.59
    hand C43.6- ☑
    heel C43.7- ☑
    helix C43.2- ☑
    hip C43.7- ☑
    interscapular region C43.59
    jaw (external) C43.39
    knee C43.7- ☑
    labium C51.9
      majus C51.0
      minus C51.1
    leg C43.7- ☑
    lip (lower) (upper) C43.0
    lower limb NEC C43.7- ☑
    male genital organ (external) NEC C63.9
    nail
      finger C43.6- ☑
      toe C43.7- ☑
    nasolabial groove C43.39
    nates C43.59
    neck C43.4
    nose (external) C43.31
    overlapping site C43.8
    palpebra C43.1- ☑
    penis C60.9
    perianal skin C43.51
    perineum C43.51

☑ **Additional Character Required** — **Refer to the Tabular List for Character Selection**   **Subterms under main terms may continue to next column or page**

Melanoma — *continued*
  skin — *continued*
    pinna C43.2- ☑
    popliteal fossa or space C43.7- ☑
    prepuce C60.0
    pudendum C51.9
    scalp C43.4
    scrotum C63.2
    shoulder C43.6- ☑
    skin NEC C43.9
    submammary fold C43.52
    temple C43.39
    thigh C43.7- ☑
    toe C43.7- ☑
    trunk NEC C43.59
    umbilicus C43.59
    upper limb NEC C43.6- ☑
    vulva C51.9
      overlapping sites C51.8
  spindle cell
    with epithelioid, mixed — *see* Melanoma, skin, by site
    type A C69.4- ☑
    type B C69.4- ☑
  superficial spreading — *see* Melanoma, skin, by site
Melanosarcoma — *see also* Melanoma
  epithelioid cell — *see* Melanoma
Melanosis L81.4
  addisonian E27.1
    tuberculous A18.7
  adrenal E27.1
  colon K63.89
  conjunctiva — *see* Pigmentation, conjunctiva
    congenital Q13.89
  cornea (presenile) (senile) — *see also* Pigmentation, cornea
    congenital Q13.4
  eye NEC H57.89
    congenital Q15.8
  lenticularis progressiva Q82.1
  liver K76.89
  precancerous — *see also* Melanoma, in situ
    malignant melanoma in — *see* Melanoma
  Riehl's L81.4
  sclera H15.89
    congenital Q13.89
  suprarenal E27.1
  tar L81.4
  toxic L81.4
Melanuria R82.998
MELAS syndrome E88.41
Melasma L81.1
  adrenal (gland) E27.1
  suprarenal (gland) E27.1
Melena K92.1
  with ulcer — *code by* site under Ulcer, with hemorrhage K27.4
  due to swallowed maternal blood P78.2
  newborn, neonatal P54.1
    due to swallowed maternal blood P78.2
Meleney's
  gangrene (cutaneous) — *see* Ulcer, skin
  ulcer (chronic undermining) — *see* Ulcer, skin
Melioidosis A24.9
  acute A24.1
  chronic A24.2
  fulminating A24.1
  pneumonia A24.1
  pulmonary (chronic) A24.2
    acute A24.1
    subacute A24.2
  sepsis A24.1
  specified NEC A24.3
  subacute A24.2
Melitensis, febris A23.0
Melkersson (-Rosenthal) **syndrome** G51.2
Mellitus, diabetes — *see* Diabetes
Melorheostosis (bone) — *see* Disorder, bone, density and structure, specified NEC
Meloschisis Q18.4
Melotia Q17.4
Membrana
  capsularis lentis posterior Q13.89
  epipapillaris Q14.2
Membranacea placenta O43.19- ☑
Membranaceous uterus N85.8
Membrane(s), membranous — *see also* condition

Membrane(s), membranous — *continued*
  cyclitic — *see* Membrane, pupillary
  folds, congenital — *see* Web
  Jackson's Q43.3
  over face of newborn P28.9
  premature rupture — *see* Rupture, membranes, premature
  pupillary H21.4- ☑
    persistent Q13.89
  retained (with hemorrhage) (complicating delivery) O72.2
    without hemorrhage O73.1
  secondary cataract — *see* Cataract, secondary
  unruptured (causing asphyxia) — *see* Asphyxia, newborn
  vitreous — *see* Opacity, vitreous, membranes and strands
Membranitis — *see* Chorioamnionitis
Memory disturbance, lack or loss — *see also* Amnesia
  mild, following organic brain damage F06.8
Menadione deficiency E56.1
Menarche
  delayed E30.0
  precocious E30.1
Mendacity, pathologic F60.2
Mendelson's syndrome (due to anesthesia) J95.4
  in labor and delivery O74.0
  in pregnancy O29.01- ☑
  obstetric O74.0
  postpartum, puerperal O89.01
Ménétrier's disease or syndrome K29.60
  with bleeding K29.61
Ménière's disease, syndrome or vertigo H81.0- ☑
Meninges, meningeal — *see* condition
Meningioma — *see also* Neoplasm, meninges, benign
  angioblastic — *see* Neoplasm, meninges, benign
  angiomatous — *see* Neoplasm, meninges, benign
  atypical — *see* Neoplasm, meninges, uncertain behavior
  endotheliomatous — *see* Neoplasm, meninges, benign
  fibroblastic — *see* Neoplasm, meninges, benign
  fibrous — *see* Neoplasm, meninges, benign
  hemangioblastic — *see* Neoplasm, meninges, benign
  hemangiopericytic — *see* Neoplasm, meninges, benign
  malignant — *see* Neoplasm, meninges, malignant
  meningiothelial — *see* Neoplasm, meninges, benign
  meningotheliomatous — *see* Neoplasm, meninges, benign
  mixed — *see* Neoplasm, meninges, benign
  multiple — *see* Neoplasm, meninges, uncertain behavior
  papillary — *see* Neoplasm, meninges, uncertain behavior
  psammomatous — *see* Neoplasm, meninges, benign
  syncytial — *see* Neoplasm, meninges, benign
  transitional — *see* Neoplasm, meninges, benign
Meningiomatosis (diffuse) — *see* Neoplasm, meninges, uncertain behavior
Meningism — *see* Meningismus
Meningismus (infectional) (pneumococcal) R29.1
  due to serum or vaccine R29.1
  influenzal — *see* Influenza, with, manifestations NEC
Meningitis (basal) (basic) (brain) (cerebral) (cervical) (congestive) (diffuse) (hemorrhagic) (infantile) (membranous) (metastatic) (nonspecific) (pontine) (progressive) (simple) (spinal) (subacute) (sympathetic) (toxic) G03.9
  abacterial G03.0
  actinomycotic A42.81
  adenoviral A87.1
  arbovirus A87.8
  aseptic (acute) G03.0
  bacterial G00.9
    Escherichia coli (E. coli) G00.8
    Friedländer (bacillus) G00.8
    gram-negative G00.9
    H. influenzae G00.0
    Klebsiella G00.8
    pneumococcal G00.1
    specified organism NEC G00.8
    staphylococcal G00.3
    streptococcal (acute) G00.2
  benign recurrent (Mollaret) G03.2
  candidal B37.5
  caseous (tuberculous) A17.0
  cerebrospinal A39.0
  chronic NEC G03.1

Meningitis — *continued*
  clear cerebrospinal fluid NEC G03.0
  coxsackievirus A87.0
  cryptococcal B45.1
  diplococcal (gram positive) A39.0
  echovirus A87.0
  enteroviral A87.0
  eosinophilic B83.2
  epidemic NEC A39.0
  Escherichia coli (E. coli) G00.8
  fibrinopurulent G00.9
    specified organism NEC G00.8
  Friedländer (bacillus) G00.8
  gonococcal A54.81
  gram-negative cocci G00.9
  gram-positive cocci G00.9
  H. influenzae G00.0
  Haemophilus (influenzae) G00.0
  in (due to)
    adenovirus A87.1
    African trypanosomiasis B56.9 *[G02]*
    anthrax A22.8
    bacterial disease NEC A48.8 *[G01]*
    Chagas' disease (chronic) B57.41
    chickenpox B01.0
    coccidioidomycosis B38.4
    Diplococcus pneumoniae G00.1
    enterovirus A87.0
    herpes (simplex) virus B00.3
      zoster B02.1
    infectious mononucleosis B27.92
    leptospirosis A27.81
    Listeria monocytogenes A32.11
    Lyme disease A69.21
    measles B05.1
    mumps (virus) B26.1
    neurosyphilis (late) A52.13
    parasitic disease NEC B89 *[G02]*
    poliovirus A80.9 *[G02]*
    preventive immunization, inoculation or vaccination G03.8
    rubella B06.02
    Salmonella infection A02.21
    specified cause NEC G03.8
    Streptococcal pneumoniae G00.1
    typhoid fever A01.01
    varicella B01.0
    viral disease NEC A87.8
    whooping cough A37.90
    zoster B02.1
  infectious G00.9
  influenzal (H. influenzae) G00.0
  Klebsiella G00.8
  leptospiral (aseptic) A27.81
  lymphocytic (acute) (benign) (serous) A87.2
  meningococcal A39.0
  Mima polymorpha G00.8
  Mollaret (benign recurrent) G03.2
  monilial B37.5
  mycotic NEC B49 *[G02]*
  Neisseria A39.0
  nonbacterial G03.0
  nonpyogenic NEC G03.0
  ossificans G96.198
  pneumococcal streptococcus pneumoniae G00.1
  poliovirus A80.9 *[G02]*
  postmeasles B05.1
  purulent G00.9
    specified organism NEC G00.8
  pyogenic G00.9
    specified organism NEC G00.8
  Salmonella (arizonae) (Cholerae-Suis) (enteritidis) (typhimurium) A02.21
  septic G00.9
    specified organism NEC G00.8
  serosa circumscripta NEC G03.0
  serous NEC G93.2
  specified organism NEC G00.8
  sporotrichosis B42.81
  staphylococcal G00.3
  sterile G03.0
  Streptococcal (acute) G00.2
    pneumoniae G00.1
  suppurative G00.9
    specified organism NEC G00.8
  syphilitic (late) (tertiary) A52.13
    acute A51.41
    congenital A50.41
    secondary A51.41

Melanoma — Meningitis

Subterms under main terms may continue to next column or page   ☑ Additional Character Required — Refer to the Tabular List for Character Selection   **225**

Meningitis — continued
  Torula histolytica (cryptococcal) B45.1
  traumatic (complication of injury) T79.8 ☑
  tuberculous A17.0
  typhoid A01.01
  viral NEC A87.9
  Yersinia pestis A20.3
Meningocele (spinal) — see also Spina bifida
  with hydrocephalus — see Spina bifida, by site, with
    hydrocephalus
  acquired (traumatic) G96.198
  cerebral — see Encephalocele
Meningocerebritis — see Meningoencephalitis
Meningococcemia A39.4
  acute A39.2
  chronic A39.3
Meningococcus, meningococcal — see also condition
  A39.9
  adrenalitis, hemorrhagic A39.1
  carrier (suspected) of Z22.31
  meningitis (cerebrospinal) A39.0
Meningoencephalitis — see also Encephalitis G04.90
  acute NEC — see also Encephalitis, viral A86
  bacterial NEC G04.2
  California A83.5
  diphasic A84.1
  eosinophilic B83.2
  epidemic A39.81
  herpesviral, herpetic B00.4
    due to herpesvirus 6 B10.01
    due to herpesvirus 7 B10.09
    specified NEC B10.09
  in (due to)
    blastomycosis NEC B40.81
    diseases classified elsewhere G05.3
    free-living amebae B60.2
    H. influenzae G00.0
    Hemophilus influenzae (H .influenzae) G00.0
    herpes B00.4
      due to herpesvirus 6 B10.01
      due to herpesvirus 7 B10.09
      specified NEC B10.09
    Lyme disease A69.22
    mercury — see subcategory T56.1 ☑
    mumps B26.2
    Naegleria (amebae) (organisms) (fowleri) B60.2
    Parastrongylus cantonensis B83.2
    toxoplasmosis (acquired) B58.2
      congenital P37.1
  infectious (acute) (viral) A86
  influenzal (H. influenzae) G00.0
  Listeria monocytogenes A32.12
  lymphocytic (serous) A87.2
  mumps B26.2
  parasitic NEC B89 [G05.3]
  pneumococcal G04.2
  primary amebic B60.2
  specific (syphilitic) A52.14
  specified organism NEC G04.81
  staphylococcal G04.2
  streptococcal G04.2
  syphilitic A52.14
  toxic NEC G92.8
    due to mercury — see subcategory T56.1 ☑
  tuberculous A17.82
  virus NEC A86
Meningoencephalocele — see also Encephalocele
  syphilitic A52.19
    congenital A50.49
Meningoencephalomyelitis — see also Meningoencephalitis
  acute NEC (viral) A86
    disseminated G04.00
      postimmunization or postvaccination G04.02
      postinfectious G04.01
  due to
    actinomycosis A42.82
    Torula B45.1
    Toxoplasma or toxoplasmosis (acquired) B58.2
      congenital P37.1
  postimmunization or postvaccination G04.02
Meningoencephalomyelopathy G96.9
Meningoencephalopathy G96.9
Meningomyelitis — see also Meningoencephalitis
  bacterial NEC G04.2
  blastomycotic NEC B40.81
  cryptococcal B45.1
  in diseases classified elsewhere G05.4

Meningomyelitis — continued
  meningococcal A39.81
  syphilitic A52.14
  tuberculous A17.82
Meningomyelocele — see also Spina bifida
  syphilitic A52.19
Meningomyeloneuritis — see Meningoencephalitis
Meningoradiculitis — see Meningitis
Meningovascular — see condition
Menkes' disease or syndrome E83.09
  meaning maple-syrup-urine disease E71.0
Menometrorrhagia N92.1
Menopause, menopausal (asymptomatic) (state) Z78.0
  arthritis (any site) NEC — see Arthritis, specified form
    NEC
  bleeding N92.4
  depression (single episode) F32.89
    agitated (single episode) F32.2
      recurrent episode F33.9
    psychotic (single episode) F32.89
      recurrent episode F33.9
    recurrent episode F33.8
    melancholia (single episode) F32.89
      recurrent episode F33.8
  paranoid state F22
  premature E28.319
    asymptomatic E28.319
      postirradiation E89.40
      postsurgical E89.40
    symptomatic E28.310
      postirradiation E89.41
      postsurgical E89.41
  psychosis NEC F28
  symptomatic N95.1
  toxic polyarthritis NEC — see Arthritis, specified form
    NEC
Menorrhagia (primary) N92.0
  climacteric N92.4
    menopausal N92.4
  menopausal N92.4
  perimenopausal N92.4
  postclimacteric N95.0
  postmenopausal N95.0
  preclimacteric or premenopausal N92.4
  pubertal (menses retained) N92.2
Menostaxis N92.0
Menses, retention N94.89
Menstrual — see Menstruation
Menstruation
  absent — see Amenorrhea
  anovulatory N97.0
  cycle, irregular N92.6
  delayed N91.0
  disorder N93.9
    psychogenic F45.8
  during pregnancy O20.8
  excessive (with regular cycle) N92.0
    with irregular cycle N92.1
    at puberty N92.2
  frequent N92.0
  infrequent — see Oligomenorrhea
  irregular N92.6
    specified NEC N92.5
  latent N92.5
  membranous N92.5
  painful — see also Dysmenorrhea N94.6
    primary N94.4
    psychogenic F45.8
    secondary N94.5
  passage of clots N92.0
  precocious E30.1
  protracted N92.5
  rare — see Oligomenorrhea
  retained N94.89
  retrograde N92.5
  scanty — see Oligomenorrhea
  suppression N94.89
  vicarious (nasal) N94.89
Mental — see also condition
  deficiency — see Disability, intellectual
  deterioration — see Psychosis
  disorder — see Disorder, mental
  exhaustion F48.8
  insufficiency (congenital) — see Disability, intellectual
  observation without need for further medical care
    Z03.89
  retardation — see Disability, intellectual
  subnormality — see Disability, intellectual

Mental — continued
  upset — see Disorder, mental
Meralgia paresthetica G57.1- ☑
Mercurial — see condition
Mercurialism — see subcategory T56.1 ☑
Merkel cell tumor — see Carcinoma, Merkel cell
Merocele — see Hernia, femoral
Meromelia
  lower limb — see Defect, reduction, lower limb
    intercalary
      femur — see Defect, reduction, lower limb,
        specified type NEC
      tibiofibular (complete) (incomplete) — see
        Defect, reduction, lower limb
  upper limb — see Defect, reduction, upper limb
    intercalary, humeral, radioulnar — see Agenesis,
      arm, with hand present
MERRF syndrome (myoclonic epilepsy associated with
  ragged-red fiber) E88.42
Merzbacher-Pelizaeus disease E75.29
Mesaortitis — see Aortitis
Mesarteritis — see Arteritis
Mesencephalitis — see Encephalitis
Mesenchymoma — see also Neoplasm, connective tis-
  sue, uncertain behavior
  benign — see Neoplasm, connective tissue, benign
  malignant — see Neoplasm, connective tissue, malig-
    nant
Mesenteritis
  retractile K65.4
  sclerosing K65.4
Mesentery, mesenteric — see condition
Mesiodens, mesiodentes K00.1
Mesio-occlusion M26.213
Mesocolon — see condition
Mesonephroma (malignant) — see Neoplasm, malig-
  nant, by site
  benign — see Neoplasm, benign, by site
Mesophlebitis — see Phlebitis
Mesostromal dysgenesis Q13.89
Mesothelioma (malignant) C45.9
  benign
    mesentery D19.1
    mesocolon D19.1
    omentum D19.1
    peritoneum D19.1
    pleura D19.0
    specified site NEC D19.7
    unspecified site D19.9
  biphasic C45.9
    benign
      mesentery D19.1
      mesocolon D19.1
      omentum D19.1
      peritoneum D19.1
      pleura D19.0
      specified site NEC D19.7
      unspecified site D19.9
  cystic D48.4
  epithelioid C45.9
    benign
      mesentery D19.1
      mesocolon D19.1
      omentum D19.1
      peritoneum D19.1
      pleura D19.0
      specified site NEC D19.7
      unspecified site D19.9
  fibrous C45.9
    benign
      mesentery D19.1
      mesocolon D19.1
      omentum D19.1
      peritoneum D19.1
      pleura D19.0
      specified site NEC D19.7
      unspecified site D19.9
  site classification
    liver C45.7
    lung C45.7
    mediastinum C45.7
    mesentery C45.1
    mesocolon C45.1
    omentum C45.1
    pericardium C45.2
    peritoneum C45.1
    pleura C45.0
      parietal C45.0

Mesothelioma — *continued*
  site classification — *continued*
    retroperitoneum C45.7
    specified site NEC C45.7
    unspecified C45.9
Metabolic syndrome E88.81
Metagonimiasis B66.8
Metagonimus infestation (intestine) B66.8
Metal
  pigmentation L81.8
  polisher's disease J62.8
Metamorphopsia H53.15
Metaplasia
  apocrine (breast) — *see* Dysplasia, mammary, specified type NEC
  cervix (squamous) — *see* Dysplasia, cervix
  endometrium (squamous) (uterus) N85.8
  esophagus K22.7- ☑
  gastric intestinal K31.A0
    with dysplasia K31.A29
      high grade K31.A22
      low grade K31.A21
    indefinite for dysplasia K31.A0
    without dysplasia K31.A19
      involving
        antrum K31.A11
        body (corpus) K31.A12
        cardia K31.A14
        fundus K31.A13
        multiple sites K31.A15
  kidney (pelvis) (squamous) N28.89
  myelogenous D73.1
  myeloid (agnogenic) (megakaryocytic) D73.1
  spleen D73.1
  squamous cell, bladder N32.89
Metastasis, metastatic
  abscess — *see* Abscess
  calcification E83.59
  cancer
    from specified site — *see* Neoplasm, malignant, by site
    to specified site — *see* Neoplasm, secondary, by site
  deposits (in) — *see* Neoplasm, secondary, by site
  disease — *see also* Neoplasm, secondary, by site C79.9
  spread (to) — *see* Neoplasm, secondary, by site
Metastrongyliasis B83.8
Metatarsalgia M77.4- ☑
  anterior G57.6- ☑
  Morton's G57.6- ☑
Metatarsus, metatarsal — *see also* condition
  adductus, congenital Q66.22- ☑
  valgus (abductus), congenital Q66.6
  varus (congenital) Q66.22- ☑
    primus Q66.21- ☑
Methadone use — *see* Use, opioid
Methemoglobinemia D74.9
  acquired (with sulfhemoglobinemia) D74.8
  congenital D74.0
  enzymatic (congenital) D74.0
  Hb M disease D74.0
  hereditary D74.0
  toxic D74.8
Methemoglobinuria — *see* Hemoglobinuria
Methioninemia E72.19
Methylmalonic acidemia E71.120
Metritis (catarrhal) (hemorrhagic) (septic) (suppurative) — *see also* Endometritis
  cervical — *see* Cervicitis
Metropathia hemorrhagica N93.8
Metroperitonitis — *see* Peritonitis, pelvic, female
Metrorrhagia N92.1
  climacteric N92.4
  menopausal N92.4
  perimenopausal N92.4
  postpartum NEC (atonic) (following delivery of placenta) O72.1
    delayed or secondary O72.2
  preclimacteric or premenopausal N92.4
  psychogenic F45.8
Metrorrhexis — *see* Rupture, uterus
Metrosalpingitis N70.91
Metrostaxis N93.8
Metrovaginitis — *see* Endometritis
Meyer-Schwickerath and Weyers syndrome Q87.0
Meynert's amentia (nonalcoholic) F04
  alcoholic F10.96
    with dependence F10.26

Mibelli's disease (porokeratosis) Q82.8
Mice, joint — *see* Loose, body, joint
  knee M23.4- ☑
Micrencephalon, micrencephaly Q02
Microalbuminuria R80.9
Microaneurysm, retinal — *see also* Disorder, retina, microaneurysms
  diabetic — *see* E08-E13 with .31
Microangiopathy (peripheral) I73.9
  thrombotic M31.10
    hematopoietic stem cell transplantation-associated [HSCT-TMA] M31.10
Microcalcifications, breast R92.0
Microcephalus, microcephalic, microcephaly Q02
  due to toxoplasmosis (congenital) P37.1
Microcheilia Q18.7
Microcolon (congenital) Q43.8
Microcornea (congenital) Q13.4
Microcytic — *see* condition
Microdeletions NEC Q93.88
Microdontia K00.2
Microdrepanocytosis D57.40
  with
    acute chest syndrome D57.411
    cerebral vascular involvement D57.413
    crisis (painful) D57.419
      with specified complication NEC D57.418
    splenic sequestration D57.412
    vasoocclusive pain D57.419
Microembolism
  atherothrombotic — *see* Atheroembolism
  retinal — *see* Occlusion, artery, retina
Microencephalon Q02
Microfilaria streptocerca infestation — *see* Onchocerciasis
Microgastria (congenital) Q40.2
Microgenia M26.06
Microgenitalia, congenital
  female Q52.8
  male Q55.8
Microglioma — *see* Lymphoma, non-Hodgkin, specified NEC
Microglossia (congenital) Q38.3
Micrognathia, micrognathism (congenital) (mandibular) (maxillary) M26.09
Microgyria (congenital) Q04.3
Microinfarct of heart — *see* Insufficiency, coronary
Microlentia (congenital) Q12.8
Microlithiasis, alveolar, pulmonary J84.02
Micromastia N64.82
Micromyelia (congenital) Q06.8
Micropenis Q55.62
Microphakia (congenital) Q12.8
Microphthalmos, microphthalmia (congenital) Q11.2
  due to toxoplasmosis P37.1
Micropsia H53.15
Microscopic polyangiitis (polyarteritis) M31.7
Microsporidiosis B60.8
  intestinal A07.8
Microsporon furfur infestation B36.0
Microsporosis — *see also* Dermatophytosis
  nigra B36.1
Microstomia (congenital) Q18.5
Microtia (congenital) (external ear) Q17.2
Microtropia H50.40
Microvillus inclusion disease (MVD) (MVID) Q43.8
Micturition
  disorder NEC — *see also* Difficulty, micturition R39.198
    psychogenic F45.8
  frequency R35.0
    psychogenic F45.8
  hesitancy R39.11
  incomplete emptying R39.14
  nocturnal R35.1
  painful R30.9
    dysuria R30.0
    psychogenic F45.8
    tenesmus R30.1
  poor stream R39.12
  position dependent R39.192
  split stream R39.13
  straining R39.16
  urgency R39.15
Mid plane — *see* condition
Middle
  ear — *see* condition
  lobe (right) syndrome J98.19

Miescher's elastoma L87.2
Mietens' syndrome Q87.2
Migraine (idiopathic) G43.909
  with refractory migraine G43.919
    with status migrainosus G43.911
    without status migrainosus G43.919
  with aura (acute-onset) (prolonged) (typical) (without headache) G43.109
    with refractory migraine G43.119
      with status migrainosus G43.111
      without status migrainosus G43.119
    intractable G43.119
      with status migrainosus G43.111
      without status migrainosus G43.119
    not intractable G43.109
      with status migrainosus G43.101
      without status migrainosus G43.109
    persistent G43.509
      with cerebral infarction G43.609
        with refractory migraine G43.619
          with status migrainosus G43.611
          without status migrainosus G43.619
        intractable G43.619
          with status migrainosus G43.611
          without status migrainosus G43.619
        not intractable G43.609
          with status migrainosus G43.601
          without status migrainosus G43.609
        without refractory migraine G43.609
          with status migrainosus G43.601
          without status migrainosus G43.609
      without cerebral infarction G43.509
        with refractory migraine G43.519
          with status migrainosus G43.511
          without status migrainosus G43.519
        intractable G43.519
          with status migrainosus G43.511
          without status migrainosus G43.519
        not intractable G43.509
          with status migrainosus G43.501
          without status migrainosus G43.509
        without refractory migraine G43.509
          with status migrainosus G43.501
          without status migrainosus G43.509
    without mention of refractory migraine G43.109
      with status migrainosus G43.101
      without status migrainosus G43.109
  abdominal G43.D0 (*following* G43.7)
    with refractory migraine G43.D1 (*following* G43.7)
    intractable G43.D1 (*following* G43.7)
    not intractable G43.D0 (*following* G43.7)
    without refractory migraine G43.D0 (*following* G43.7)
  basilar — *see* Migraine, with aura
  classical — *see* Migraine, with aura
  common — *see* Migraine, without aura
  complicated G43.109
  equivalents — *see* Migraine, with aura
  familiar — *see* Migraine, hemiplegic
  hemiplegic G43.409
    with refractory migraine G43.419
      with status migrainosus G43.411
      without status migrainosus G43.419
    intractable G43.419
      with status migrainosus G43.411
      without status migrainosus G43.419
    not intractable G43.409
      with status migrainosus G43.401
      without status migrainosus G43.409
    without refractory migraine G43.409
      with status migrainosus G43.401
      without status migrainosus G43.409
  intractable G43.919
    with status migrainosus G43.911
    without status migrainosus G43.919
  menstrual G43.829
    with refractory migraine G43.839
      with status migrainosus G43.831
      without status migrainosus G43.839
    intractable G43.839
      with status migrainosus G43.831
      without status migrainosus G43.839
    not intractable G43.829
      with status migrainosus G43.821
      without status migrainosus G43.829
    without refractory migraine G43.829
      with status migrainosus G43.821
      without status migrainosus G43.829
  menstrually related — *see* Migraine, menstrual

Migraine — *continued*
  not intractable G43.909
    with status migrainosus G43.901
    without status migrainosus G43.919
  ophthalmoplegic G43.B0 (*following* G43.7)
    with refractory migraine G43.B1 (*following* G43.7)
    intractable G43.B1 (*following* G43.7)
    not intractable G43.B0 (*following* G43.7)
    without refractory migraine G43.B0 (*following* G43.7)
  persistent aura (with, without) cerebral infarction —
    see Migraine, with aura
  preceded or accompanied by transient focal neurolog-
    ical phenomena — *see* Migraine, with aura
  pre-menstrual — *see* Migraine, menstrual
  pure menstrual — *see* Migraine, menstrual
  retinal — *see* Migraine, with aura
  specified NEC G43.809
    intractable G43.819
      with status migrainosus G43.811
      without status migrainosus G43.819
    not intractable G43.809
      with status migrainosus G43.801
      without status migrainosus G43.809
  sporadic — *see* Migraine, hemiplegic
  transformed — *see* Migraine, without aura, chronic
  triggered seizures — *see* Migraine, with aura
  without aura G43.009
    with refractory migraine G43.019
      with status migrainosus G43.011
      without status migrainosus G43.019
    chronic G43.709
      with refractory migraine G43.719
        with status migrainosus G43.711
        without status migrainosus G43.719
      intractable
        with status migrainosus G43.711
        without status migrainosus G43.719
      not intractable
        with status migrainosus G43.701
        without status migrainosus G43.709
      without refractory migraine G43.709
        with status migrainosus G43.701
        without status migrainosus G43.709
    intractable
      with status migrainosus G43.011
      without status migrainosus G43.019
    not intractable
      with status migrainosus G43.001
      without status migrainosus G43.009
    without mention of refractory migraine G43.009
      with status migrainosus G43.001
      without status migrainosus G43.009
  without refractory migraine G43.909
    with status migrainosus G43.901
    without status migrainosus G43.919
Migrant, social Z59.00
Migration, anxiety concerning Z60.3
Migratory, migrating — *see also* condition
  person Z59.00
  testis Q55.29
Mikity-Wilson disease or syndrome P27.0
Mikulicz' disease or syndrome K11.8
Miliaria L74.3
  alba L74.1
  apocrine L75.2
  crystallina L74.1
  profunda L74.2
  rubra L74.0
  tropicalis L74.2
Miliary — *see* condition
Milium L72.0
  colloid L57.8
Milk
  crust L21.0
  excessive secretion O92.6
  poisoning — *see* Poisoning, food, noxious
  retention O92.79
  sickness — *see* Poisoning, food, noxious
  spots I31.0
Milk-alkali disease or syndrome E83.52
Milk-leg (deep vessels) (nonpuerperal) — *see* Embolism,
    vein, lower extremity
  complicating pregnancy O22.3- ☑
  puerperal, postpartum, childbirth O87.1
Milkman's disease or syndrome M83.8
Milky urine — *see* Chyluria
Millard-Gubler (-Foville) **paralysis or syndrome** G46.3
Millar's asthma J38.5

Miller Fisher syndrome G61.0
Mills' disease — *see* Hemiplegia
Millstone maker's pneumoconiosis J62.8
Milroy's disease (chronic hereditary edema) Q82.0
Minamata disease T56.1 ☑
Miners' asthma or lung J60
Minkowski-Chauffard syndrome — *see* Spherocytosis
Minor — *see* condition
Minor's disease (hematomyelia) G95.19
Minot's disease (hemorrhagic disease), newborn P53
Minot-von Willebrand-Jurgens disease or syndrome
    (angiohemophilia) D68.0
Minus (and plus) **hand** (intrinsic) — *see* Deformity, limb,
    specified type NEC, forearm
Miosis (pupil) H57.03
Mirizzi's syndrome (hepatic duct stenosis) K83.1
Mirror writing F81.0
MIS-A M35.81
Misadventure (of) (prophylactic) (therapeutic) — *see*
    also Complications T88.9 ☑
  administration of insulin (by accident) — *see* subcate-
    gory T38.3 ☑
  infusion — *see* Complications, infusion
  local applications (of fomentations, plasters, etc.)
    T88.9 ☑
    burn or scald — *see* Burn
    specified NEC T88.8 ☑
  medical care (early) (late) T88.9 ☑
    adverse effect of drugs or chemicals — *see* Table of
      Drugs and Chemicals
    burn or scald — *see* Burn
    specified NEC T88.8 ☑
  specified NEC T88.8 ☑
  surgical procedure (early) (late) — *see* Complications,
    surgical procedure
  transfusion — *see* Complications, transfusion
  vaccination or other immunological procedure — *see*
    Complications, vaccination
MIS-C M35.81
Miscarriage O03.9
Misdirection, aqueous H40.83- ☑
Misperception, sleep state F51.02
Misplaced, misplacement
  ear Q17.4
  kidney (acquired) N28.89
    congenital Q63.2
  organ or site, congenital NEC — *see* Malposition, con-
    genital
Missed
  abortion O02.1
  delivery O36.4 ☑
Missing — *see also* Absence
  string of intrauterine contraceptive device T83.32- ☑
Misuse of drugs F19.99
Mitchell's disease (erythromelalgia) I73.81
Mite(s) (infestation) B88.9
  diarrhea B88.0
  grain (itch) B88.0
  hair follicle (itch) B88.0
  in sputum B88.0
Mitral — *see* condition
Mittelschmerz N94.0
Mixed — *see* condition
MMN (multifocal motor neuropathy) G61.82
MNGIE (Mitochondrial Neurogastrointestinal Encephalopa-
    thy) **syndrome** E88.49
Mobile, mobility
  cecum Q43.3
  excessive — *see* Hypermobility
  gallbladder, congenital Q44.1
  kidney N28.89
  organ or site, congenital NEC — *see* Malposition, con-
    genital
Mobitz heart block (atrioventricular) I44.1
Moebius, Möbius
  disease (ophthalmoplegic migraine) — *see* Migraine,
    ophthalmoplegic
  syndrome Q87.0
    congenital oculofacial paralysis (with other anoma-
      lies) Q87.0
    ophthalmoplegic migraine — *see* Migraine, ophthal-
      moplegic
Moeller's glossitis K14.0
Mohr's syndrome (Types I and II) Q87.0
Mola destruens D39.2
Molar pregnancy O02.0
Molarization of premolars K00.2

Molding, head (during birth) — *omit code*
Mole (pigmented) — *see also* Nevus
  blood O02.0
  Breus' O02.0
  cancerous — *see* Melanoma
  carneous O02.0
  destructive D39.2
  fleshy O02.0
  hydatid, hydatidiform (benign) (complicating pregnan-
      cy) (delivered) (undelivered) O01.9
    classical O01.0
    complete O01.0
    incomplete O01.1
    invasive D39.2
    malignant D39.2
    partial O01.1
  intrauterine O02.0
  invasive (hydatidiform) D39.2
  malignant
    meaning
      malignant hydatidiform mole D39.2
      melanoma — *see* Melanoma
  nonhydatidiform O02.0
  nonpigmented — *see* Nevus
  pregnancy NEC O02.0
  skin — *see* Nevus
  tubal O00.10- ☑
    with intrauterine pregnancy O00.11- ☑
  vesicular — *see* Mole, hydatidiform
Molimen, molimina (menstrual) N94.3
Molluscum contagiosum (epitheliale) B08.1
Mönckeberg's arteriosclerosis, disease, or sclerosis
    — *see* Arteriosclerosis, extremities
Mondini's malformation (cochlea) Q16.5
Mondor's disease I80.8
Monge's disease T70.29 ☑
Monilethrix (congenital) Q84.1
Moniliasis — *see also* Candidiasis B37.9
  neonatal P37.5
Monitoring (encounter for)
  therapeutic drug level Z51.81
Monkey malaria B53.1
Monkeypox B04
Monoarthritis M13.10
  ankle M13.17- ☑
  elbow M13.12- ☑
  foot joint M13.17- ☑
  hand joint M13.14- ☑
  hip M13.15- ☑
  knee M13.16- ☑
  shoulder M13.11- ☑
  wrist M13.13- ☑
Monoblastic — *see* condition
Monochromat (ism), monochromatopsia (acquired)
    (congenital) H53.51
Monocytic — *see* condition
Monocytopenia D72.818
Monocytosis (symptomatic) D72.821
Monomania — *see* Psychosis
Mononeuritis G58.9
  cranial nerve — *see* Disorder, nerve, cranial
  femoral nerve G57.2- ☑
  lateral
    cutaneous nerve of thigh G57.1- ☑
    popliteal nerve G57.3- ☑
  lower limb G57.9- ☑
    specified nerve NEC G57.8- ☑
  medial popliteal nerve G57.4- ☑
  median nerve G56.1- ☑
  multiplex G58.7
  plantar nerve G57.6- ☑
  posterior tibial nerve G57.5- ☑
  radial nerve G56.3- ☑
  sciatic nerve G57.0- ☑
  specified NEC G58.8
  tibial nerve G57.4- ☑
  ulnar nerve G56.2- ☑
  upper limb G56.9- ☑
    specified nerve NEC G56.8- ☑
  vestibular — *see* subcategory H93.3 ☑
Mononeuropathy G58.9
  carpal tunnel syndrome — *see* Syndrome, carpal tunnel
  diabetic NEC — *see* E08-E13 with .41
  femoral nerve — *see* Lesion, nerve, femoral
  ilioinguinal nerve G57.8- ☑
  in diseases classified elsewhere — *see* category G59
  intercostal G58.0

Mononeuropathy — *continued*
lower limb G57.9- ☑
  causalgia — *see* Causalgia, lower limb
  femoral nerve — *see* Lesion, nerve, femoral
  meralgia paresthetica G57.1- ☑
  plantar nerve — *see* Lesion, nerve, plantar
  popliteal nerve — *see* Lesion, nerve, popliteal
  sciatic nerve — *see* Lesion, nerve, sciatic
  specified NEC G57.8- ☑
  tarsal tunnel syndrome — *see* Syndrome, tarsal tunnel
median nerve — *see* Lesion, nerve, median
multiplex G58.7
obturator nerve G57.8- ☑
popliteal nerve — *see* Lesion, nerve, popliteal
radial nerve — *see* Lesion, nerve, radial
saphenous nerve G57.8- ☑
specified NEC G58.8
tarsal tunnel syndrome — *see* Syndrome, tarsal tunnel
tuberculous A17.83
ulnar nerve — *see* Lesion, nerve, ulnar
upper limb G56.9- ☑
  carpal tunnel syndrome — *see* Syndrome, carpal tunnel
  causalgia — *see* Causalgia
  median nerve — *see* Lesion, nerve, median
  radial nerve — *see* Lesion, nerve, radial
  specified site NEC G56.8- ☑
  ulnar nerve — *see* Lesion, nerve, ulnar
Mononucleosis, infectious B27.90
with
  complication NEC B27.99
  meningitis B27.92
  polyneuropathy B27.91
cytomegaloviral B27.10
  with
    complication NEC B27.19
    meningitis B27.12
    polyneuropathy B27.11
Epstein-Barr (virus) B27.00
  with
    complication NEC B27.09
    meningitis B27.02
    polyneuropathy B27.01
gammaherpesviral B27.00
  with
    complication NEC B27.09
    meningitis B27.02
    polyneuropathy B27.01
specified NEC B27.80
  with
    complication NEC B27.89
    meningitis B27.82
    polyneuropathy B27.81
Monoplegia G83.3- ☑
congenital (cerebral) G80.8
  spastic G80.1
embolic (current episode) I63.4- ☑
following
  cerebrovascular disease
    cerebral infarction
      lower limb I69.34- ☑
      upper limb I69.33- ☑
    intracerebral hemorrhage
      lower limb I69.14- ☑
      upper limb I69.13- ☑
    lower limb I69.94- ☑
    nontraumatic intracranial hemorrhage NEC
      lower limb I69.24- ☑
      upper limb I69.23- ☑
    specified disease NEC
      lower limb I69.84- ☑
      upper limb I69.83- ☑
    stroke NOS
      lower limb I69.34- ☑
      upper limb I69.33- ☑
    subarachnoid hemorrhage
      lower limb I69.04- ☑
      upper limb I69.03- ☑
    upper limb I69.93- ☑
hysterical (transient) F44.4
lower limb G83.1- ☑
psychogenic (conversion reaction) F44.4
thrombotic (current episode) I63.3- ☑
transient R29.818
upper limb G83.2- ☑
Monorchism, monorchidism Q55.0

Monosomy — *see also* Deletion, chromosome Q93.9
specified NEC Q93.89
whole chromosome
  meiotic nondisjunction Q93.0
  mitotic nondisjunction Q93.1
  mosaicism Q93.1
X Q96.9
Monster, monstrosity (single) Q89.7
acephalic Q00.0
twin Q89.4
Monteggia's fracture (-dislocation) S52.27- ☑
Mooren's ulcer (cornea) — *see* Ulcer, cornea, Mooren's
Moore's syndrome — *see* Epilepsy, specified NEC
Mooser-Neill reaction A75.2
Mooser's bodies A75.2
Morbidity not stated or unknown R69
Morbilli — *see* Measles
Morbus — *see also* Disease
angelicus, anglorum E55.0
Beigel B36.2
caducus — *see* Epilepsy
celiacus K90.0
comitialis — *see* Epilepsy
cordis — *see also* Disease, heart I51.9
  valvulorum — *see* Endocarditis
coxae senilis M16.9
  tuberculous A18.02
hemorrhagicus neonatorum P53
maculosus neonatorum P54.5
Morel (-Stewart)(-Morgagni) **syndrome** M85.2
Morel-Kraepelin disease — *see* Schizophrenia
Morel-Moore syndrome M85.2
Morgagni's
cyst, organ, hydatid, or appendage
  female Q50.5
  male (epididymal) Q55.4
    testicular Q55.29
syndrome M85.2
Morgagni-Stewart-Morel syndrome M85.2
Morgagni-Stokes-Adams syndrome I45.9
Morgagni-Turner (-Albright) **syndrome** Q96.9
Moria F07.0
Moron (I.Q. 50-69) F70
Morphea L94.0
Morphinism (without remission) F11.20
with remission F11.21
Morphinomania (without remission) F11.20
with remission F11.21
Morquio (-Ullrich)(-Brailsford) **disease or syndrome** — *see* Mucopolysaccharidosis
Mortification (dry) (moist) — *see* Gangrene
Morton's metatarsalgia (neuralgia)(neuroma) (syndrome) G57.6- ☑
Morvan's disease or syndrome G60.8
Mosaicism, mosaic (autosomal) (chromosomal)
45,X/46,XX Q96.3
45,X/other cell lines NEC with abnormal sex chromosome Q96.4
sex chromosome
  female Q97.8
    lines with various numbers of X chromosomes Q97.2
  male Q98.7
XY Q96.3
Moschowitz' disease M31.19
Mother yaw A66.0
Motion sickness (from travel, any vehicle) (from roundabouts or swings) T75.3 ☑
Mottled, mottling, teeth (enamel) (endemic) (nonendemic) K00.3
Mounier-Kuhn syndrome Q32.4
with bronchiectasis J47.9
  exacerbation (acute) J47.1
  lower respiratory infection J47.0
acquired J98.09
  with bronchiectasis J47.9
    with
      exacerbation (acute) J47.1
      lower respiratory infection J47.0
Mountain
sickness T70.29 ☑
  with polycythemia , acquired (acute) D75.1
tick fever A93.2
Mouse, joint — *see* Loose, body, joint
knee M23.4- ☑
Mouth — *see* condition
Movable
coccyx — *see* subcategory M53.2 ☑

Movable — *continued*
kidney N28.89
  congenital Q63.8
spleen D73.89
Movements, dystonic R25.8
Moyamoya disease I67.5
MRSA (Methicillin resistant Staphylococcus aureus)
infection A49.02
  as the cause of diseases classified elsewhere B95.62
sepsis A41.02
MSD (multiple sulfatase deficiency) E75.26
MSSA (Methicillin susceptible Staphylococcus aureus)
infection A49.01
  as the cause of diseases classified elsewhere B95.61
sepsis A41.01
Mucha-Habermann disease L41.0
Mucinosis (cutaneous) (focal) (papular) (skin) L98.5
oral K13.79
Mucocele
appendix K38.8
buccal cavity K13.79
gallbladder K82.1
lacrimal sac, chronic H04.43- ☑
nasal sinus J34.1
nose J34.1
salivary gland (any) K11.6
sinus (accessory) (nasal) J34.1
turbinate (bone) (middle) (nasal) J34.1
uterus N85.8
Mucolipidosis
I E77.1
II, III E77.0
IV E75.11
Mucopolysaccharidosis E76.3
beta-gluduronidase deficiency E76.29
cardiopathy E76.3 *[I52]*
Hunter's syndrome E76.1
Hurler's syndrome E76.01
Hurler-Scheie syndrome E76.02
Maroteaux-Lamy syndrome E76.29
Morquio syndrome E76.219
  A E76.210
  B E76.211
  classic E76.210
Sanfilippo syndrome E76.22
Scheie's syndrome E76.03
specified NEC E76.29
type
  I
    Hurler's syndrome E76.01
    Hurler-Scheie syndrome E76.02
    Scheie's syndrome E76.03
  II E76.1
  III E76.22
  IV E76.219
  IVA E76.210
  IVB E76.211
  VI E76.29
  VII E76.29
Mucormycosis B46.5
cutaneous B46.3
disseminated B46.4
gastrointestinal B46.2
generalized B46.4
pulmonary B46.0
rhinocerebral B46.1
skin B46.3
subcutaneous B46.3
Mucositis (ulcerative) K12.30
due to drugs NEC K12.32
gastrointestinal K92.81
mouth (oral) (oropharyngeal) K12.30
  due to antineoplastic therapy K12.31
  due to drugs NEC K12.32
  due to radiation K12.33
  specified NEC K12.39
  viral K12.39
nasal J34.81
oral cavity — *see* Mucositis, mouth
oral soft tissues — *see* Mucositis, mouth
vagina and vulva N76.81
Mucositis necroticans agranulocytica — *see* Agranulocytosis
Mucous — *see also* condition
patches (syphilitic) A51.39
  congenital A50.07
Mucoviscidosis E84.9
with meconium obstruction E84.11

▽ Subterms under main terms may continue to next column or page   ☑ Additional Character Required — Refer to the Tabular List for Character Selection   **229**

Mononeuropathy — Mucoviscidosis

Mucus
- asphyxia or suffocation — *see* Asphyxia, mucus
- in stool R19.5
- plug — *see* Asphyxia, mucus

Muguet B37.0

Mulberry molars (congenital syphilis) A50.52

Müllerian mixed tumor
- specified site — *see* Neoplasm, malignant, by site
- unspecified site C54.9

Multicystic kidney (development) Q61.4

Multiparity (grand) Z64.1
- affecting management of pregnancy, labor and delivery (supervision only) O09.4- ☑
- requiring contraceptive management — *see* Contraception

Multipartita placenta O43.19- ☑

Multiple, multiplex — *see also* condition
- digits (congenital) Q69.9
- endocrine neoplasia — *see* Neoplasia, endocrine, multiple (MEN)
- personality F44.81

Multisystem inflammatory syndrome (in adult) (in children) M35.81

Mumps B26.9
- arthritis B26.85
- complication NEC B26.89
- encephalitis B26.2
- hepatitis B26.81
- meningitis (aseptic) B26.1
- meningoencephalitis B26.2
- myocarditis B26.82
- oophoritis B26.89
- orchitis B26.0
- pancreatitis B26.3
- polyneuropathy B26.84

Mumu — *see also* Infestation, filarial B74.9 [N51]

Münchhausen's syndrome — *see* Disorder, factitious

Münchmeyer's syndrome — *see* Myositis, ossificans, progressiva

Mural — *see* condition

Murmur (cardiac) (heart) (organic) R01.1
- abdominal R19.15
- aortic (valve) — *see* Endocarditis, aortic
- benign R01.0
- diastolic — *see* Endocarditis
- Flint I35.1
- functional R01.0
- Graham Steell I37.1
- innocent R01.0
- mitral (valve) — *see* Insufficiency, mitral
- nonorganic R01.0
- presystolic, mitral — *see* Insufficiency, mitral
- pulmonic (valve) I37.8
- systolic R01.1
- tricuspid (valve) I07.9
- valvular — *see* Endocarditis

Murri's disease (intermittent hemoglobinuria) D59.6

Muscle, muscular — *see also* condition
- carnitine (palmityltransferase) deficiency E71.314

Musculoneuralgia — *see* Neuralgia

Mushrooming hip — *see* Derangement, joint, specified NEC, hip

Mushroom-workers' (pickers') **disease or lung** J67.5

Mutation(s)
- factor V Leiden D68.51
- prothrombin gene D68.52
- surfactant, of lung J84.83

Mutism — *see also* Aphasia
- deaf (acquired) (congenital) NEC H91.3
- elective (adjustment reaction) (childhood) F94.0
- hysterical F44.4
- selective (childhood) F94.0

MVD (microvillus inclusion disease) Q43.8

MVID (microvillus inclusion disease) Q43.8

Myalgia M79.10
- auxiliary muscles, head and neck M79.12
- epidemic (cervical) B33.0
- mastication muscle M79.11
- site specified NEC M79.18
- traumatic NEC T14.8 ☑

Myasthenia G70.9
- congenital G70.2
- cordis — *see* Failure, heart
- developmental G70.2
- gravis G70.00
  - with exacerbation (acute) G70.01
  - in crisis G70.01

Myasthenia — *continued*
- gravis — *continued*
  - neonatal, transient P94.0
  - pseudoparalytica G70.00
    - with exacerbation (acute) G70.01
    - in crisis G70.01
  - stomach, psychogenic F45.8
  - syndrome
    - in
      - diabetes mellitus — *see* E08-E13 with .44
      - neoplastic disease — *see also* Neoplasm D49.9 [G73.3]
      - pernicious anemia D51.0 [G73.3]
      - thyrotoxicosis E05.90 [G73.3]
        - with thyroid storm E05.91 [G73.3]

Myasthenic M62.81

Mycelium infection B49

Mycetismus — *see* Poisoning, food, noxious, mushroom

Mycetoma B47.9
- actinomycotic B47.1
- bone (mycotic) B47.9 [M90.80]
- eumycotic B47.0
- foot B47.9
  - actinomycotic B47.1
  - mycotic B47.0
- madurae NEC B47.9
  - mycotic B47.0
- maduromycotic B47.0
- mycotic B47.0
- nocardial B47.1

Mycobacteriosis — *see* Mycobacterium

Mycobacterium, mycobacterial (infection) A31.9
- anonymous A31.9
- atypical A31.9
  - cutaneous A31.1
  - pulmonary A31.0
    - tuberculous — *see* Tuberculosis, pulmonary
  - specified site NEC A31.8
- avium (intracellulare complex) A31.0
- balnei A31.1
- Battey A31.0
- chelonei A31.8
- cutaneous A31.1
- extrapulmonary systemic A31.8
- fortuitum A31.8
- intracellulare (Battey bacillus) A31.0
- kakaferifu A31.8
- kansasii (yellow bacillus) A31.0
- kasongo A31.8
- leprae — *see also* Leprosy A30.9
- luciflavum A31.1
- marinum (M. balnei) A31.1
- nonspecific — *see* Mycobacterium, atypical
- pulmonary (atypical) A31.0
  - tuberculous — *see* Tuberculosis, pulmonary
- scrofulaceum A31.8
- simiae A31.8
- systemic, extrapulmonary A31.8
- szulgai A31.8
- terrae A31.8
- triviale A31.8
- tuberculosis (human, bovine) — *see* Tuberculosis
- ulcerans A31.1
- xenopi A31.8

Mycoplasma (M.) **pneumoniae, as cause of disease classified elsewhere** B96.0

Mycosis, mycotic B49
- cutaneous NEC B36.9
- ear B36.9
  - in
    - aspergillosis B44.89
    - candidiasis B37.84
    - moniliasis B37.84
- fungoides (extranodal) (solid organ) C84.0- ☑
- mouth B37.0
- nails B35.1
- opportunistic B48.8
- skin NEC B36.9
- specified NEC B48.8
- stomatitis B37.0
- vagina, vaginitis (candidal) B37.3

Mydriasis (pupil) H57.04

Myelatelia Q06.1

Myelinolysis, pontine, central G37.2

Myelitis (acute) (ascending) (childhood) (chronic) (descending) (diffuse) (disseminated) (idiopathic) (pressure) (progressive) (spinal cord) (subacute) — *see also* Encephalitis G04.91

Myelitis — *continued*
- flaccid G04.82
- herpes simplex B00.82
- herpes zoster B02.24
- in diseases classified elsewhere G05.4
- necrotizing, subacute G37.4
- optic neuritis in G36.0
- postchickenpox B01.12
- postherpetic B02.24
- postimmunization G04.02
- postinfectious NEC G04.89
- postvaccinal G04.02
- specified NEC G04.89
- syphilitic (transverse) A52.14
- toxic G92.9
- transverse (in demyelinating diseases of central nervous system) G37.3
- tuberculous A17.82
- varicella B01.12

Myeloblastic — *see* condition

Myeloblastoma
- granular cell — *see also* Neoplasm, connective tissue
  - malignant — *see* Neoplasm, connective tissue, malignant
- tongue D10.1

Myelocele — *see* Spina bifida

Myelocystocele — *see* Spina bifida

Myelocytic — *see* condition

Myelodysplasia D46.9
- specified NEC D46.Z (following D46.4)
- spinal cord (congenital) Q06.1

Myelodysplastic syndrome — *see also* Syndrome, myelodysplastic D46.9
- with
  - 5q deletion D46.C (following D46.2)
  - isolated del (5q) chromosomal abnormality D46.C (following D46.2)
- specified NEC D46.Z (following D46.4)

Myeloencephalitis — *see* Encephalitis

Myelofibrosis D75.81
- with myeloid metaplasia D47.4
- acute C94.4- ☑
- idiopathic (chronic) D47.4
- primary D47.1
- secondary D75.81
  - in myeloproliferative disease D47.4

Myelogenous — *see* condition

Myeloid — *see* condition

Myelokathexis D70.9

Myeloleukodystrophy E75.29

Myelolipoma — *see* Lipoma

Myeloma (multiple) C90.0- ☑
- monostotic C90.3 ☑
  - plasma cell C90.0- ☑
- plasma cell C90.0- ☑
- solitary — *see also* Plasmacytoma, solitary C90.3- ☑

Myelomalacia G95.89

Myelomatosis C90.0- ☑

Myelomeningitis — *see* Meningoencephalitis

Myelomeningocele (spinal cord) — *see* Spina bifida

Myelo-osteo-musculodysplasia hereditaria Q79.8

Myelopathic
- anemia D64.89
- muscle atrophy — *see* Atrophy, muscle, spinal
- pain syndrome G89.0

Myelopathy (spinal cord) G95.9
- drug-induced G95.89
- in (due to)
  - degeneration or displacement, intervertebral disc NEC — *see* Disorder, disc, with, myelopathy
  - infection — *see* Encephalitis
  - intervertebral disc disorder — *see also* Disorder, disc, with, myelopathy
  - mercury — *see* subcategory T56.1 ☑
  - neoplastic disease — *see also* Neoplasm D49.9 [G99.2]
  - pernicious anemia D51.0 [G99.2]
  - spondylosis — *see* Spondylosis, with myelopathy NEC
- necrotic (subacute) (vascular) G95.19
- radiation-induced G95.89
- spondylogenic NEC — *see* Spondylosis, with myelopathy NEC
- toxic G95.89
- transverse, acute G37.3
- vascular G95.19
- vitamin B12 E53.8 [G32.0]

☑ **Additional Character Required** — Refer to the Tabular List for Character Selection   ▽ **Subterms under main terms may continue to next column or page**

Myelophthisis D61.82
Myeloradiculitis G04.91
Myeloradiculodysplasia (spinal) Q06.1
Myelosarcoma C92.3-
Myelosclerosis D75.89
  with myeloid metaplasia D47.4
  disseminated, of nervous system G35
  megakaryocytic D47.4
    with myeloid metaplasia D47.4
Myelosis
  acute C92.0-
  aleukemic C92.9-
  chronic D47.1
  erythremic (acute) C94.0-
  megakaryocytic C94.2-
  nonleukemic D72.828
  subacute C92.9-
Myiasis (cavernous) B87.9
  aural B87.4
  creeping B87.0
  cutaneous B87.0
  dermal B87.0
  ear (external) (middle) B87.4
  eye B87.2
  genitourinary B87.81
  intestinal B87.82
  laryngeal B87.3
  nasopharyngeal B87.3
  ocular B87.2
  orbit B87.2
  skin B87.0
  specified site NEC B87.89
  traumatic B87.1
  wound B87.1
Myoadenoma, prostate — see Hyperplasia, prostate
Myoblastoma
  granular cell — see also Neoplasm, connective tissue, benign
    malignant — see Neoplasm, connective tissue, malignant
  tongue D10.1
Myocardial — see condition
Myocardiopathy (congestive) (constrictive) (familial) (hypertrophic nonobstructive) (idiopathic) (infiltrative) (obstructive) (primary) (restrictive) (sporadic) — see also Cardiomyopathy I42.9
  alcoholic I42.6
  cobalt-beer I42.6
  glycogen storage E74.02 [I43]
  hypertrophic obstructive I42.1
  in (due to)
    beriberi E51.12
    cardiac glycogenosis E74.02 [I43]
    Friedreich's ataxia G11.11 [I43]
    myotonia atrophica G71.11 [I43]
    progressive muscular dystrophy G71.09 [I43]
  obscure (African) I42.8
  secondary I42.9
  thyrotoxic E05.90 [I43]
    with storm E05.91 [I43]
  toxic NEC I42.7
Myocarditis (with arteriosclerosis)(chronic)(fibroid) (interstitial) (old) (progressive) (senile) I51.4
  with
    rheumatic fever (conditions in I00) I09.0
      active — see Myocarditis, acute, rheumatic
      inactive or quiescent (with chorea) I09.0
  active I40.9
    rheumatic I01.2
      with chorea (acute) (rheumatic) (Sydenham's) I02.0
  acute or subacute (interstitial) I40.9
    due to
      streptococcus (beta-hemolytic) I01.2
    idiopathic I40.1
    rheumatic I01.2
      with chorea (acute) (rheumatic) (Sydenham's) I02.0
    specified NEC I40.8
  aseptic of newborn B33.22
  bacterial (acute) I40.0
  Coxsackie (virus) B33.22
  diphtheritic A36.81
  eosinophilic I40.1
  epidemic of newborn (Coxsackie) B33.22
  Fiedler's (acute) (isolated) I40.1
  giant cell (acute) (subacute) I40.1
  gonococcal A54.83

Myocarditis — continued
  granulomatous (idiopathic) (isolated) (nonspecific) I40.1
  hypertensive — see Hypertension, heart
  idiopathic (granulomatous) I40.1
  in (due to)
    diphtheria A36.81
    epidemic louse-borne typhus A75.0 [I41]
    Lyme disease A69.29
    sarcoidosis D86.85
    scarlet fever A38.1
    toxoplasmosis (acquired) B58.81
    typhoid A01.02
    typhus NEC A75.9 [I41]
  infective I40.0
  influenzal — see Influenza, with, myocarditis
  isolated (acute) I40.1
  meningococcal A39.52
  mumps B26.82
  nonrheumatic, active I40.9
  parenchymatous I40.9
  pneumococcal I40.0
  rheumatic (chronic) (inactive) (with chorea) I09.0
    active or acute I01.2
      with chorea (acute) (rheumatic) (Sydenham's) I02.0
  rheumatoid — see Rheumatoid, carditis
  septic I40.0
  staphylococcal I40.0
  suppurative I40.0
  syphilitic (chronic) A52.06
  toxic I40.8
    rheumatic — see Myocarditis, acute, rheumatic
  tuberculous A18.84
  typhoid A01.02
  valvular — see Endocarditis
  virus, viral I40.0
    of newborn (Coxsackie) B33.22
Myocardium, myocardial — see condition
Myocardosis — see Cardiomyopathy
Myoclonus, myoclonic, myoclonia (familial) (essential) (multifocal) (simplex) G25.3
  drug-induced G25.3
  epilepsy — see also Epilepsy, generalized, specified NEC G40.4-
    familial (progressive) G25.3
  epileptica G40.409
    with status epilepticus G40.401
  facial G51.3-
  familial progressive G25.3
  Friedreich's G25.3
  jerks G25.3
  massive G25.3
  palatal G25.3
  pharyngeal G25.3
Myocytolysis I51.5
Myodiastasis — see Diastasis, muscle
Myoendocarditis — see Endocarditis
Myoepithelioma — see Neoplasm, benign, by site
Myofasciitis (acute) — see Myositis
Myofibroma — see also Neoplasm, connective tissue, benign
  uterus (cervix) (corpus) — see Leiomyoma
Myofibromatosis D48.1
  infantile Q89.8
Myofibrosis M62.89
  heart — see Myocarditis
  scapulohumeral — see Lesion, shoulder, specified NEC
Myofibrositis M79.7
  scapulohumeral — see Lesion, shoulder, specified NEC
Myoglobulinuria, myoglobinuria (primary) R82.1
Myokymia, facial G51.4
Myolipoma — see Lipoma
Myoma — see also Neoplasm, connective tissue, benign
  malignant — see Neoplasm, connective tissue, malignant
  prostate D29.1
  uterus (cervix) (corpus) — see Leiomyoma
Myomalacia M62.89
Myometritis — see Endometritis
Myometrium — see condition
Myonecrosis, clostridial A48.0
Myopathy G72.9
  acute
    necrotizing G72.81
      quadriplegic G72.81
  alcoholic G72.1
  benign congenital G71.20
  central core G71.29

Myopathy — continued
  centronuclear G71.228
    autosomal (dominant) (recessive) G71.228
    other specified NEC G71.228
  congenital (benign) G71.20
  critical illness G72.81
  distal G71.09
  drug-induced G72.0
  endocrine NEC E34.9 [G73.7]
  extraocular muscles H05.82-
  facioscapulohumeral G71.02
  hereditary G71.9
    specified NEC G71.8
  hyaline body G71.29
  immune NEC G72.49
  in (due to)
    Addison's disease E27.1 [G73.7]
    alcohol G72.1
    amyloidosis E85.0 [G73.7]
    cretinism E00.9 [G73.7]
    Cushing's syndrome E24.9 [G73.7]
    drugs G72.0
    endocrine disease NEC E34.9 [G73.7]
    giant cell arteritis M31.6 [G73.7]
    glycogen storage disease E74.00 [G73.7]
    hyperadrenocorticism E24.9 [G73.7]
    hyperparathyroidism NEC E21.3 [G73.7]
    hypoparathyroidism E20.9 [G73.7]
    hypopituitarism E23.0 [G73.7]
    hypothyroidism E03.9 [G73.7]
    infectious disease NEC B99 [G73.7]
    lipid storage disease E75.6 [G73.7]
    metabolic disease NEC E88.9 [G73.7]
    myxedema E03.9 [G73.7]
    parasitic disease NEC B89 [G73.7]
    polyarteritis nodosa M30.0 [G73.7]
    rheumatoid arthritis — see Rheumatoid, myopathy
    sarcoidosis D86.87
    scleroderma M34.82
    sicca syndrome M35.03
    Sjögren's syndrome M35.03
    systemic lupus erythematosus M32.19
    thyrotoxicosis (hyperthyroidism) E05.90 [G73.7]
      with thyroid storm E05.91 [G73.7]
    toxic agent NEC G72.2
  inflammatory NEC G72.49
  intensive care (ICU) G72.81
  limb-girdle G71.09
  mitochondrial NEC G71.3
  myosin storage G71.29
  myotubular (centronuclear) G71.220
    X-linked G71.220
  mytonic, proximal (PROMM) G71.11
  nemaline G71.21
  ocular G71.09
  oculopharyngeal G71.09
  of critical illness G72.81
  primary G71.9
    specified NEC G71.8
  progressive NEC G72.89
  proximal myotonic (PROMM) G71.11
  rod (body) G71.21
  scapulohumeral G71.02
  specified NEC G72.89
  toxic G72.2
Myopericarditis — see also Pericarditis
  chronic rheumatic I09.2
Myopia (axial) (congenital) H52.1-
  degenerative (malignant) H44.20
    with
      choroidal neovascularization H44.2A-
      foveoschisis H44.2D-
      macular hole H44.2B-
      retinal detachment H44.2C-
      specified maculopathy NEC H44.2E-
    bilateral H44.23
    left eye H44.22
    right eye H44.21
  malignant — see also Myopia, degenerative H44.2-
  pernicious — see also Myopia, degenerative H44.2-
  progressive high (degenerative) — see also Myopia, degenerative H44.2-
Myosarcoma — see Neoplasm, connective tissue, malignant
Myosis (pupil) H57.03
  stromal (endolymphatic) D39.0
Myositis M60.9

▼ Subterms under main terms may continue to next column or page   ☑ **Additional Character Required** — Refer to the Tabular List for Character Selection   **231**

Myelophthisis — Myositis

Myositis — *continued*
clostridial A48.0
due to posture — *see* Myositis, specified type NEC
epidemic B33.0
fibrosa or fibrous (chronic), Volkmann's T79.6 ☑
foreign body granuloma — *see* Granuloma, foreign
    body
in (due to)
    bilharziasis B65.9 *[M63.8-]* ☑
    cysticercosis B69.81
    leprosy A30.9 *[M63.8-]* ☑
    mycosis B49 *[M63.8-]* ☑
    sarcoidosis D86.87
    schistosomiasis B65.9 *[M63.8-]* ☑
    syphilis
      late A52.78
      secondary A51.49
    toxoplasmosis (acquired) B58.82
    trichinellosis B75 *[M63.8-]* ☑
    tuberculosis A18.09
inclusion body [IBM] G72.41
infective M60.009
  arm M60.002
    left M60.001
    right M60.000
  leg M60.005
    left M60.004
    right M60.003
  lower limb M60.005
    ankle M60.07- ☑
    foot M60.07- ☑
    lower leg M60.06- ☑
    thigh M60.05- ☑
    toe M60.07- ☑
  multiple sites M60.09
  specified site NEC M60.08
  upper limb M60.002
    finger M60.04- ☑
    forearm M60.03- ☑
    hand M60.04- ☑
    shoulder region M60.01- ☑
    upper arm M60.02- ☑
interstitial M60.10
  ankle M60.17- ☑
  foot M60.17- ☑
  forearm M60.13- ☑
  hand M60.14- ☑
  lower leg M60.16- ☑
  multiple sites M60.19
  shoulder region M60.11- ☑
  specified site NEC M60.18
  thigh M60.15- ☑
  upper arm M60.12- ☑
mycotic B49 *[M63.8-]* ☑
orbital, chronic H05.12- ☑
ossificans or ossifying (circumscripta) — *see also* Ossi-
    fication, muscle, specified NEC
  in (due to)
    burns M61.30
      ankle M61.37- ☑

Myositis — *continued*
ossificans or ossifying — *see also* Ossification, muscle,
    specified — *continued*
  in — *continued*
    burns — *continued*
      foot M61.37- ☑
      forearm M61.33- ☑
      hand M61.34- ☑
      lower leg M61.36- ☑
      multiple sites M61.39
      pelvic region M61.35- ☑
      shoulder region M61.31- ☑
      specified site NEC M61.38
      thigh M61.35- ☑
      upper arm M61.32- ☑
    quadriplegia or paraplegia M61.20
      ankle M61.27- ☑
      foot M61.27- ☑
      forearm M61.23- ☑
      hand M61.24- ☑
      lower leg M61.26- ☑
      multiple sites M61.29
      pelvic region M61.25- ☑
      shoulder region M61.21- ☑
      specified site NEC M61.28
      thigh M61.25- ☑
      upper arm M61.22- ☑
  progressiva M61.10
    ankle M61.17- ☑
    finger M61.14- ☑
    foot M61.17- ☑
    forearm M61.13- ☑
    hand M61.14- ☑
    lower leg M61.16- ☑
    multiple sites M61.19
    pelvic region M61.15- ☑
    shoulder region M61.11- ☑
    specified site NEC M61.18
    thigh M61.15- ☑
    toe M61.17- ☑
    upper arm M61.12- ☑
  traumatica M61.00
    ankle M61.07- ☑
    foot M61.07- ☑
    forearm M61.03- ☑
    hand M61.04- ☑
    lower leg M61.06- ☑
    multiple sites M61.09
    pelvic region M61.05- ☑
    shoulder region M61.01- ☑
    specified site NEC M61.08
    thigh M61.05- ☑
    upper arm M61.02- ☑
purulent — *see* Myositis, infective
specified type NEC M60.80
  ankle M60.87- ☑
  foot M60.87- ☑
  forearm M60.83- ☑
  hand M60.84- ☑
  lower leg M60.86- ☑

Myositis — *continued*
specified type — *continued*
  multiple sites M60.89
  pelvic region M60.85- ☑
  shoulder region M60.81- ☑
  specified site NEC M60.88
  thigh M60.85- ☑
  upper arm M60.82- ☑
suppurative — *see* Myositis, infective
traumatic (old) — *see* Myositis, specified type NEC
Myospasia impulsiva F95.2
Myotonia (acquisita) (intermittens) M62.89
atrophica G71.11
chondrodystrophic G71.13
congenita (acetazolamide responsive) (dominant) (re-
    cessive) G71.12
drug-induced G71.14
dystrophica G71.11
fluctuans G71.19
levior G71.12
permanens G71.19
symptomatic G71.19
Myotonic pupil — *see* Anomaly, pupil, function, tonic
    pupil
Myriapodiasis B88.2
Myringitis H73.2- ☑
with otitis media — *see* Otitis, media
acute H73.00- ☑
  bullous H73.01- ☑
  specified NEC H73.09- ☑
bullous — *see* Myringitis, acute, bullous
chronic H73.1-
Mysophobia F40.228
Mytilotoxism — *see* Poisoning, fish
Myxadenitis labialis K13.0
Myxedema (adult) (idiocy) (infantile) (juvenile) — *see
    also* Hypothyroidism E03.9
circumscribed E05.90
  with storm E05.91
coma E03.5
congenital E00.1
cutis L98.5
localized (pretibial) E05.90
  with storm E05.91
papular L98.5
Myxochondrosarcoma — *see* Neoplasm, cartilage, ma-
    lignant
Myxofibroma — *see* Neoplasm, connective tissue, benign
odontogenic — *see* Cyst, calcifying odontogenic
Myxofibrosarcoma — *see* Neoplasm, connective tissue,
    malignant
Myxolipoma D17.9
Myxoliposarcoma — *see* Neoplasm, connective tissue,
    malignant
Myxoma — *see also* Neoplasm, connective tissue, benign
nerve sheath — *see* Neoplasm, nerve, benign
odontogenic — *see* Cyst, calcifying odontogenic
Myxosarcoma — *see* Neoplasm, connective tissue, ma-
    lignant

☑ **Additional Character Required** — Refer to the Tabular List for Character Selection   ▽ **Subterms under main terms may continue to next column or page**

N

Naegeli's
disease Q82.8
leukemia, monocytic C93.1- ☑
Nageleriasis (with meningoencephalitis) B60.2
Naffziger's syndrome G54.0
Naga sore — *see* Ulcer, skin
Nägele's pelvis M95.5
with disproportion (fetopelvic) O33.0
causing obstructed labor O65.0
Nail — *see also* condition
biting F98.8
patella syndrome Q87.2
Nanism, nanosomia — *see* Dwarfism
Nanophyetiasis B66.8
Nanukayami A27.89
Napkin rash L22
Narcolepsy G47.419
with cataplexy G47.411
in conditions classified elsewhere G47.429
with cataplexy G47.421
Narcosis R06.89
Narcotism — *see* Dependence
NARP (Neuropathy, Ataxia and Retinitis pigmentosa)
syndrome E88.49
Narrow
anterior chamber angle H40.03- ☑
gingival width (of periodontal soft tissue) K05.5
pelvis — *see* Contraction, pelvis
Narrowing — *see also* Stenosis
artery I77.1
auditory, internal I65.8
basilar — *see* Occlusion, artery, basilar
carotid — *see* Occlusion, artery, carotid
cerebellar — *see* Occlusion, artery, cerebellar
cerebral — *see* Occlusion artery, cerebral
choroidal — *see* Occlusion, artery, precerebral,
specified NEC
communicating posterior — *see* Occlusion, artery,
precerebral, specified NEC
coronary — *see also* Disease, heart, ischemic,
atherosclerotic
congenital Q24.5
syphilitic A50.54 [I52]
due to syphilis NEC A52.06
hypophyseal — *see* Occlusion, artery, precerebral,
specified NEC
pontine — *see* Occlusion, artery, precerebral, specified NEC
precerebral — *see* Occlusion, artery, precerebral
vertebral — *see* Occlusion, artery, vertebral
auditory canal (external) — *see* Stenosis, external ear
canal
eustachian tube — *see* Obstruction, eustachian tube
eyelid — *see* Disorder, eyelid function
larynx J38.6
mesenteric artery — *see also* Ischemia, intestine, acute
K55.059
palate M26.89
palpebral fissure — *see* Disorder, eyelid function
ureter N13.5
with infection N13.6
urethra — *see* Stricture, urethra
Narrowness, abnormal, eyelid Q10.3
Nasal — *see* condition
Nasolachrymal, nasolacrimal — *see* condition
Nasopharyngeal — *see also* condition
pituitary gland Q89.2
torticollis M43.6
Nasopharyngitis (acute) (infective) (streptococcal)
(subacute) J00
chronic (suppurative) (ulcerative) J31.1
Nasopharynx, nasopharyngeal — *see* condition
Natal tooth, teeth K00.6
Nausea (without vomiting) R11.0
with vomiting R11.2
gravidarum — *see* Hyperemesis, gravidarum
marina T75.3 ☑
navalis T75.3 ☑
Navel — *see* condition
Neapolitan fever — *see* Brucellosis
Near drowning T75.1 ☑
Nearsightedness — *see* Myopia
Near-syncope R55
Nebula, cornea — *see* Opacity, cornea

Necator americanus infestation B76.1
Necatoriasis B76.1
Neck — *see* condition
Necrobiosis R68.89
lipoidica NEC L92.1
with diabetes — *see* E08-E13 with .620
Necrolysis, toxic epidermal L51.2
due to drug
correct substance properly administered — *see* Table of Drugs and Chemicals, by drug, adverse
effect
overdose or wrong substance given or taken — *see*
Table of Drugs and Chemicals, by drug, poisoning
Necrophilia F65.89
Necrosis, necrotic (ischemic) — *see also* Gangrene
adrenal (capsule) (gland) E27.49
amputation stump (surgical) (late) T87.50
arm T87.5- ☑
leg T87.5- ☑
antrum J32.0
aorta (hyaline) — *see also* Aneurysm, aorta
cystic medial — *see* Dissection, aorta
artery I77.5
bladder (aseptic) (sphincter) N32.89
bone — *see also* Osteonecrosis M87.9
aseptic or avascular — *see* Osteonecrosis
idiopathic M87.00
ethmoid J32.2
jaw M27.2
tuberculous — *see* Tuberculosis, bone
brain I67.89
breast (aseptic) (fat) (segmental) N64.1
bronchus J98.09
central nervous system NEC I67.89
cerebellar I67.89
cerebral I67.89
colon — *see also* Infarct, intestine K55.049
cornea H18.89- ☑
cortical (acute) (renal) N17.1
cystic medial (aorta) — *see* Dissection, aorta
dental pulp K04.1
esophagus K22.89
ethmoid (bone) J32.2
eyelid — *see* Disorder, eyelid, degenerative
fat, fatty (generalized) — *see also* Disorder, soft tissue,
specified type NEC)
abdominal wall K65.4
breast (aseptic) (segmental) N64.1
localized — *see* Degeneration, by site, fatty
mesentery K65.4
omentum K65.4
pancreas K86.89
peritoneum K65.4
skin (subcutaneous), newborn P83.0
subcutaneous, due to birth injury P15.6
gallbladder — *see* Cholecystitis, acute
heart — *see* Infarct, myocardium
hip, aseptic or avascular — *see* Osteonecrosis, by type,
femur
intestine (acute) (hemorrhagic) (massive) — *see also*
Infarct, intestine K55.069
jaw M27.2
kidney (bilateral) N28.0
acute N17.9
cortical (acute) (bilateral) N17.1
with ectopic or molar pregnancy O08.4
medullary (bilateral) (in acute renal failure) (papillary) N17.2
papillary (bilateral) (in acute renal failure) N17.2
tubular N17.0
with ectopic or molar pregnancy O08.4
complicating
abortion — *see* Abortion, by type, complicated by, tubular necrosis
ectopic or molar pregnancy O08.4
pregnancy — *see* Pregnancy, complicated by,
diseases of, specified type or system
NEC
following ectopic or molar pregnancy O08.4
traumatic T79.5 ☑
larynx J38.7
liver (with hepatic failure) (cell) — *see* Failure, hepatic
hemorrhagic, central K76.2
lung J85.0
lymphatic gland — *see* Lymphadenitis, acute
mammary gland (fat) (segmental) N64.1
mastoid (chronic) — *see* Mastoiditis, chronic

Necrosis, necrotic — *continued*
medullary (acute) (renal) N17.2
mesentery — *see also* Infarct, intestine K55.069
fat K65.4
mitral valve — *see* Insufficiency, mitral
myocardium, myocardial — *see* Infarct, myocardium
nose J34.0
omentum (with mesenteric infarction) — *see also* Infarct, intestine K55.069
fat K65.4
orbit, orbital — *see* Osteomyelitis, orbit
ossicles, ear — *see* Abnormal, ear ossicles
ovary N70.92
pancreas (aseptic) (duct) (fat) K86.89
acute (infective) — *see* Pancreatitis, acute
infective — *see* Pancreatitis, acute
papillary (acute) (renal) N17.2
perineum N90.89
peritoneum (with mesenteric infarction) — *see also*
Infarct, intestine K55.069
fat K65.4
pharynx J02.9
in granulocytopenia — *see* Neutropenia
Vincent's A69.1
phosphorus — *see* subcategory T54.2 ☑
pituitary (gland) E23.0
postpartum O99.285
Sheehan O99.285
pressure — *see* Ulcer, pressure, by site
pulmonary J85.0
pulp (dental) K04.1
radiation — *see* Necrosis, by site
radium — *see* Necrosis, by site
renal — *see* Necrosis, kidney
sclera H15.89
scrotum N50.89
skin or subcutaneous tissue NEC I96
spine, spinal (column) — *see* Osteonecrosis, by
type, vertebra
cord G95.19
spleen D73.5
stomach K31.89
stomatitis (ulcerative) A69.0
subcutaneous fat, newborn P83.88
subendocardial (acute) I21.4
chronic I25.89
suprarenal (capsule) (gland) E27.49
testis N50.89
thymus (gland) E32.8
tonsil J35.8
trachea J39.8
tuberculous NEC — *see* Tuberculosis
tubular (acute) (anoxic) (renal) (toxic) N17.0
postprocedural N99.0
vagina N89.8
vertebra — *see also* Osteonecrosis, by type, vertebra
tuberculous A18.01
vulva N90.89
X-ray — *see* Necrosis, by site
Necrospermia — *see* Infertility, male
Need (for)
care provider because (of)
assistance with personal care Z74.1
continuous supervision required Z74.3
impaired mobility Z74.09
no other household member able to render care
Z74.2
specified reason NEC Z74.8
immunization — *see* Vaccination
vaccination — *see* Vaccination
Neglect
adult
confirmed T74.01 ☑
history of Z91.412
suspected T76.01 ☑
child (childhood)
confirmed T74.02 ☑
history of Z62.812
suspected T76.02 ☑
emotional, in childhood Z62.898
hemispatial R41.4
left-sided R41.4
sensory R41.4
visuospatial R41.4
Neisserian infection NEC — *see* Gonococcus
Nelaton's syndrome G60.8
Nelson's syndrome E24.1
Nematodiasis (intestinal) B82.0

Nematodiasis — *continued*
Ancylostoma B76.0
Neonatal — *see also* Newborn
acne L70.4
bradycardia P29.12
screening, abnormal findings on — *see* Abnormal,
neonatal screening
tachycardia P29.11
tooth, teeth K00.6
Neonatorum — *see* condition
Neoplasia
endocrine, multiple (MEN) E31.20
type I E31.21
type IIA E31.22
type IIB E31.23
intraepithelial (histologically confirmed)
anal (AIN) (histologically confirmed) K62.82
grade I K62.82
grade II K62.82
severe D01.3
cervical glandular (histologically confirmed) D06.9
cervix (uteri) (CIN) (histologically confirmed) N87.9
glandular D06.9
grade I N87.0
grade II N87.1
grade III (severe dysplasia) — *see also* Carcinoma,
cervix uteri, in situ D06.9
prostate (histologically confirmed) (PIN) N42.31
grade I N42.31
grade II N42.31
grade III (severe dysplasia) D07.5
vagina (histologically confirmed) (VAIN) N89.3
grade I N89.0
grade II N89.1
grade III (severe dysplasia) D07.2
vulva (histologically confirmed) (VIN) N90.3
grade I N90.0
grade II N90.1
grade III (severe dysplasia) D07.1
Neoplasm, neoplastic — *see also* Table of Neoplasms
lipomatous, benign — *see* Lipoma
malignant mast cell C96.20
specified type NEC C96.29
mast cell, of uncertain behavior NEC D47.09
Neovascularization
ciliary body — *see* Disorder, iris, vascular
cornea H16.40- ☑
deep H16.44- ☑
ghost vessels — *see* Ghost, vessels
localized H16.43- ☑
pannus — *see* Pannus
iris — *see* Disorder, iris, vascular
retina H35.05- ☑
Nephralgia N23
Nephritis, nephritic (albuminuric) (azotemic) (congenital) (disseminated) (epithelial) (familial) (focal)
(granulomatous) (hemorrhagic) (infantile) (nonsuppurative, excretory) (uremic) N05.9
with
C3
glomerulonephritis N05.A
glomerulopathy N05.A
with dense deposit disease N05.6
dense deposit disease N05.6
diffuse
crescentic glomerulonephritis N05.7
endocapillary proliferative glomerulonephritis
N05.4
membranous glomerulonephritis N05.2
mesangial proliferative glomerulonephritis N05.3
mesangiocapillary glomerulonephritis N05.5
edema — *see* Nephrosis
focal and segmental glomerular lesions N05.1
foot process disease N04.9
glomerular lesion
diffuse sclerosing N05.8
hypocomplementemic — *see* Nephritis, membranoproliferative
IgA — *see* Nephropathy, IgA
lobular, lobulonodular — *see* Nephritis, membranoproliferative
nodular — *see* Nephritis, membranoproliferative
lesion of
glomerulonephritis, proliferative N05.8
renal necrosis N05.9
minor glomerular abnormality N05.0
specified morphological changes NEC N05.8
acute N00.9

Nephritis, nephritic — *continued*
acute — *continued*
with
C3
glomerulonephritis N00.A
glomerulopathy N00.A
with dense deposit disease N00.6
dense deposit disease N00.6
diffuse
crescentic glomerulonephritis N00.7
endocapillary proliferative glomerulonephritis
N00.4
membranous glomerulonephritis N00.2
mesangial proliferative glomerulonephritis
N00.3
mesangiocapillary glomerulonephritis N00.5
focal and segmental glomerular lesions N00.1
minor glomerular abnormality N00.0
specified morphological changes NEC N00.8
amyloid E85.4 *[N08]*
antiglomerular basement membrane (anti-GBM) antibody NEC
in Goodpasture's syndrome M31.0
antitubular basement membrane (tubulo-interstitial)
NEC N12
toxic — *see* Nephropathy, toxic
arteriolar — *see* Hypertension, kidney
arteriosclerotic — *see* Hypertension, kidney
ascending — *see* Nephritis, tubulo-interstitial
atrophic N03.9
Balkan (endemic) N15.0
calculous, calculus — *see* Calculus, kidney
cardiac — *see* Hypertension, kidney
cardiovascular — *see* Hypertension, kidney
chronic N03.9
with
C3
glomerulonephritis N03.A
glomerulopathy N03.A
with dense deposit disease N03.6
dense deposit disease N03.6
diffuse
crescentic glomerulonephritis N03.7
endocapillary proliferative glomerulonephritis
N03.4
membranous glomerulonephritis N03.2
mesangial proliferative glomerulonephritis
N03.3
mesangiocapillary glomerulonephritis N03.5
focal and segmental glomerular lesions N03.1
minor glomerular abnormality N03.0
specified morphological changes NEC N03.8
arteriosclerotic — *see* Hypertension, kidney
cirrhotic N26.9
complicating pregnancy O26.83- ☑
croupous N00.9
degenerative — *see* Nephrosis
diffuse sclerosing N05.8
due to
diabetes mellitus — *see* E08-E13 with .21
subacute bacterial endocarditis I33.0
systemic lupus erythematosus (chronic) M32.14
typhoid fever A01.09
gonococcal (acute) (chronic) A54.21
hypocomplementemic — *see* Nephritis, membranoproliferative
IgA — *see* Nephropathy, IgA
immune complex (circulating) NEC N05.8
infective — *see* Nephritis, tubulo-interstitial
interstitial — *see* Nephritis, tubulo-interstitial
lead N14.3
membranoproliferative (diffuse) (type 1 or 3) — *see
also* N00-N07 with fourth character .5 N05.5
type 2 — *see also* N00-N07 with fourth character .6
N05.6
minimal change N05.8
necrotic, necrotizing NEC — *see also* N00-N07 with
fourth character .8 N05.8
nephrotic — *see* Nephrosis
nodular — *see* Nephritis, membranoproliferative
polycystic Q61.3
adult type Q61.2
autosomal
dominant Q61.2
recessive NEC Q61.19
childhood type NEC Q61.19
infantile type NEC Q61.19
poststreptococcal N05.9

Nephritis, nephritic — *continued*
poststreptococcal — *continued*
acute N00.9
chronic N03.9
rapidly progressive N01.9
proliferative NEC — *see also* N00-N07 with fourth
character .8 N05.8
purulent — *see* Nephritis, tubulo-interstitial
rapidly progressive N01.9
with
C3
glomerulonephritis N01.A
glomerulopathy N01.A
with dense deposit disease N01.6
dense deposit disease N01.6
diffuse
crescentic glomerulonephritis N01.7
endocapillary proliferative glomerulonephritis
N01.4
membranous glomerulonephritis N01.2
mesangial proliferative glomerulonephritis
N01.3
mesangiocapillary glomerulonephritis N01.5
focal and segmental glomerular lesions N01.1
minor glomerular abnormality N01.0
specified morphological changes NEC N01.8
salt losing or wasting NEC N28.89
saturnine N14.3
sclerosing, diffuse N05.8
septic — *see* Nephritis, tubulo-interstitial
specified pathology NEC — *see also* N00-N07 with
fourth character .8 N05.8
subacute N01.9
suppurative — *see* Nephritis, tubulo-interstitial
syphilitic (late) A52.75
congenital A50.59 *[N08]*
early (secondary) A51.44
toxic — *see* Nephropathy, toxic
tubal, tubular — *see* Nephritis, tubulo-interstitial
tuberculous A18.11
tubulo-interstitial (in) N12
acute (infectious) N10
chronic (infectious) N11.9
nonobstructive N11.8
reflux-associated N11.0
obstructive N11.1
specified NEC N11.8
due to
brucellosis A23.9 *[N16]*
cryoglobulinemia D89.1 *[N16]*
glycogen storage disease E74.00 *[N16]*
Sjögren's syndrome M35.04
vascular — *see* Hypertension, kidney
war N00.9
Nephroblastoma (epithelial) (mesenchymal) C64- ☑
Nephrocalcinosis E83.59 *[N29]*
Nephrocystitis, pustular — *see* Nephritis, tubulo-interstitial
Nephrolithiasis (congenital) (pelvis) (recurrent) — *see
also* Calculus, kidney
Nephroma C64- ☑
mesoblastic D41.0- ☑
Nephronephritis — *see* Nephrosis
Nephronophthisis Q61.5
Nephropathia epidemica A98.5
Nephropathy — *see also* Nephritis N28.9
with
edema — *see* Nephrosis
glomerular lesion — *see* Glomerulonephritis
amyloid, hereditary E85.0
analgesic N14.0
with medullary necrosis, acute N17.2
Balkan (endemic) N15.0
chemical — *see* Nephropathy, toxic
diabetic — *see* E08-E13 with .21
drug-induced N14.2
specified NEC N14.1
focal and segmental hyalinosis or sclerosis N02.1
heavy metal-induced N14.3
hereditary NEC N07.9
with
C3
glomerulonephritis N07.A
glomerulopathy N07.A
with dense deposit disease N07.6
dense deposit disease N07.6
diffuse
crescentic glomerulonephritis N07.7

☑ **Additional Character Required** — Refer to the Tabular List for Character Selection   ▽ **Subterms under main terms may continue to next column or page**

Nephropathy — *continued*
  hereditary — *continued*
    with — *continued*
      diffuse — *continued*
        endocapillary proliferative glomerulonephritis N07.4
        membranous glomerulonephritis N07.2
        mesangial proliferative glomerulonephritis N07.3
        mesangiocapillary glomerulonephritis N07.5
      focal and segmental glomerular lesions N07.1
      minor glomerular abnormality N07.0
      specified morphological changes NEC N07.8
  hypercalcemic N25.89
  hypertensive — *see* Hypertension, kidney
  hypokalemic (vacuolar) N25.89
  IgA N02.8
    with glomerular lesion N02.9
      focal and segmental hyalinosis or sclerosis N02.1
      membranoproliferative (diffuse) N02.5
      membranous (diffuse) N02.2
      mesangial proliferative (diffuse) N02.3
      mesangiocapillary (diffuse) N02.5
      proliferative NEC N02.8
      specified pathology NEC N02.8
  lead N14.3
  membranoproliferative (diffuse) N02.5
  membranous (diffuse) N02.2
  mesangial (IgA/IgG) — *see* Nephropathy, IgA
    proliferative (diffuse) N02.3
  mesangiocapillary (diffuse) N02.5
  obstructive N13.8
  phenacetin N17.2
  phosphate-losing N25.0
  potassium depletion N25.89
  pregnancy-related O26.83- ☑
  proliferative NEC — *see also* N00-N07 with fourth character .8 N05.8
  protein-losing N25.89
  saturnine N14.3
  sickle-cell D57.- ☑ *[N08]*
  toxic NEC N14.4
    due to
      drugs N14.2
        analgesic N14.0
        specified NEC N14.1
      heavy metals N14.3
  vasomotor N17.0
  water-losing N25.89
Nephroptosis N28.83
Nephropyosis — *see* Abscess, kidney
Nephrorrhagia N28.89
Nephrosclerosis (arteriolar)(arteriosclerotic) (chronic) (hyaline) — *see also* Hypertension, kidney
  hyperplastic — *see* Hypertension, kidney
  senile N26.9
Nephrosis, nephrotic (Epstein's) (syndrome) (congenital) N04.9
  with
    foot process disease N04.9
    glomerular lesion N04.1
    hypocomplementemic N04.5
  acute N04.9
  anoxic — *see* Nephrosis, tubular
  chemical — *see* Nephrosis, tubular
  cholemic K76.7
  diabetic — *see* E08-E13 with .21
  Finnish type (congenital) Q89.8
  hemoglobin N10
  hemoglobinuric — *see* Nephrosis, tubular
  in
    amyloidosis E85.4 *[N08]*
    diabetes mellitus — *see* E08-E13 with .21
    epidemic hemorrhagic fever A98.5
    malaria (malariae) B52.0
  ischemic — *see* Nephrosis, tubular
  lipoid N04.9
  lower nephron — *see* Nephrosis, tubular
  malarial (malariae) B52.0
  minimal change N04.0
  myoglobin N10
  necrotizing — *see* Nephrosis, tubular
  osmotic (sucrose) N25.89
  radiation N04.9
  syphilitic (late) A52.75
  toxic — *see* Nephrosis, tubular
  tubular (acute) N17.0
    postprocedural N99.0

Nephrosis, nephrotic — *continued*
  tubular — *continued*
    radiation N04.9
Nephrosonephritis, hemorrhagic (endemic) A98.5
Nephrostomy
  attention to Z43.6
  status Z93.6
Nerve — *see also* condition
  injury — *see* Injury, nerve, by body site
Nerves R45.0
Nervous — *see also* condition R45.0
  heart F45.8
  stomach F45.8
  tension R45.0
Nervousness R45.0
Nesidioblastoma
  pancreas D13.7
  specified site NEC — *see* Neoplasm, benign, by site
  unspecified site D13.7
Nettleship's syndrome — *see* Urticaria pigmentosa
Neumann's disease or syndrome L10.1
Neuralgia, neuralgic (acute) M79.2
  accessory (nerve) G52.8
  acoustic (nerve) — *see* subcategory H93.3 ☑
  auditory (nerve) — *see* subcategory H93.3 ☑
  ciliary G44.009
    intractable G44.001
    not intractable G44.009
  cranial
    nerve — *see also* Disorder, nerve, cranial
      fifth or trigeminal — *see* Neuralgia, trigeminal
    postherpetic, postzoster B02.29
  ear — *see* subcategory H92.0 ☑
  facialis vera G51.1
  Fothergill's — *see* Neuralgia, trigeminal
  glossopharyngeal (nerve) G52.1
  Horton's G44.099
    intractable G44.091
    not intractable G44.099
  Hunt's B02.21
  hypoglossal (nerve) G52.3
  infraorbital — *see* Neuralgia, trigeminal
  malarial — *see* Malaria
  migrainous G44.009
    intractable G44.001
    not intractable G44.009
  Morton's G57.6- ☑
  nerve, cranial — *see* Disorder, nerve, cranial
  nose G52.0
  occipital M54.81
  olfactory G52.0
  penis N48.9
  perineum R10.2
  postherpetic NEC B02.29
    trigeminal B02.22
  pubic region R10.2
  scrotum R10.2
  Sluder's G44.89
  specified nerve NEC G58.8
  spermatic cord R10.2
  sphenopalatine (ganglion) G90.09
  trifacial — *see* Neuralgia, trigeminal
  trigeminal G50.0
    postherpetic, postzoster B02.22
  vagus (nerve) G52.2
  writer's F48.8
    organic G25.89
Neurapraxia — *see* Injury, nerve
Neurasthenia F48.8
  cardiac F45.8
  gastric F45.8
  heart F45.8
Neurilemmoma — *see also* Neoplasm, nerve, benign
  acoustic (nerve) D33.3
  malignant — *see also* Neoplasm, nerve, malignant
    acoustic (nerve) C72.4- ☑
Neurilemmosarcoma — *see* Neoplasm, nerve, malignant
Neurinoma — *see* Neoplasm, nerve, benign
Neurinomatosis — *see* Neoplasm, nerve, uncertain behavior
Neuritis (rheumatoid) M79.2
  abducens (nerve) — *see* Strabismus, paralytic, sixth nerve
  accessory (nerve) G52.8
  acoustic (nerve) — *see also* subcategory H93.3 ☑
    in (due to)
      infectious disease NEC B99 ☑ *[H94.0-]* ☑

Neuritis — *continued*
  acoustic — *see also* subcategory — *continued*
    in — *continued*
      parasitic disease NEC B89 *[H94.0-]* ☑
      syphilitic A52.15
  alcoholic G62.1
    with psychosis — *see* Psychosis, alcoholic
  amyloid, any site E85.4 *[G63]*
  auditory (nerve) — *see* subcategory H93.3 ☑
  brachial — *see* Radiculopathy
    due to displacement, intervertebral disc — *see* Disorder, disc, cervical, with neuritis
  cranial nerve
    due to Lyme disease A69.22
    eighth or acoustic or auditory — *see* subcategory H93.3 ☑
    eleventh or accessory G52.8
    fifth or trigeminal G51.0
    first or olfactory G52.0
    fourth or trochlear — *see* Strabismus, paralytic, fourth nerve
    second or optic — *see* Neuritis, optic
    seventh or facial G51.8
      newborn (birth injury) P11.3
    sixth or abducent — *see* Strabismus, paralytic, sixth nerve
    tenth or vagus G52.2
    third or oculomotor — *see* Strabismus, paralytic, third nerve
    twelfth or hypoglossal G52.3
  Déjérine-Sottas G60.0
  diabetic (mononeuropathy) — *see* E08-E13 with .41
    polyneuropathy — *see* E08-E13 with .42
  due to
    beriberi E51.11
    displacement, prolapse or rupture, intervertebral disc — *see* Disorder, disc, with, radiculopathy
    herniation, nucleus pulposus M51.9 *[G55]*
  endemic E51.11
  facial G51.8
    newborn (birth injury) P11.3
  general — *see* Polyneuropathy
  geniculate ganglion G51.1
    due to herpes (zoster) B02.21
  gouty — *see also* Gout, by type M10.9 *[G63]*
  hypoglossal (nerve) G52.3
  ilioinguinal (nerve) G57.9- ☑
  infectious (multiple) NEC G61.0
  interstitial hypertrophic progressive G60.0
  lumbar M54.16
  lumbosacral M54.17
  multiple — *see also* Polyneuropathy
    endemic E51.11
    infective, acute G61.0
  multiplex endemica E51.11
  nerve root — *see* Radiculopathy
  oculomotor (nerve) — *see* Strabismus, paralytic, third nerve
  olfactory nerve G52.0
  optic (nerve) (hereditary) (sympathetic) H46.9
    with demyelination G36.0
      in myelitis G36.0
    nutritional H46.2
    papillitis — *see* Papillitis, optic
    retrobulbar H46.1- ☑
    specified type NEC H46.8
    toxic H46.3
  peripheral (nerve) G62.9
    multiple — *see* Polyneuropathy
    single — *see* Mononeuritis
  pneumogastric (nerve) G52.2
  postherpetic, postzoster B02.29
  progressive hypertrophic interstitial G60.0
  retrobulbar — *see also* Neuritis, optic, retrobulbar
    in (due to)
      late syphilis A52.15
      meningococcal infection A39.82
    meningococcal A39.82
    syphilitic A52.15
  sciatic (nerve) — *see also* Sciatica
    due to displacement of intervertebral disc — *see* Disorder, disc, with, radiculopathy
  serum — *see also* Reaction, serum T80.69 ☑
  shoulder-girdle G54.5
  specified nerve NEC G58.8
  spinal root — *see* Radiculopathy
  syphilitic A52.15
  thenar (median) G56.1- ☑

Neuritis — continued
- thoracic M54.14
- toxic NEC G62.2
- trochlear (nerve) — see Strabismus, paralytic, fourth nerve
- vagus (nerve) G52.2

Neuroastrocytoma — see Neoplasm, uncertain behavior, by site

Neuroavitaminosis E56.9 [G99.8]

Neuroblastoma
- olfactory C30.0
- specified site — see Neoplasm, malignant, by site
- unspecified site C74.90

Neurochorioretinitis — see Chorioretinitis

Neurocirculatory asthenia F45.8

Neurocysticercosis B69.0

Neurocytoma — see Neoplasm, benign, by site

Neurodermatitis (circumscribed) (circumscripta) (local) L28.0
- atopic L20.81
- diffuse (Brocq) L20.81
- disseminated L20.81

Neuroencephalomyelopathy, optic G36.0

Neuroepithelioma — see also Neoplasm, malignant, by site
- olfactory C30.0

Neurofibroma — see also Neoplasm, nerve, benign
- melanotic — see Neoplasm, nerve, benign
- multiple — see Neurofibromatosis
- plexiform — see Neoplasm, nerve, benign

Neurofibromatosis (multiple) (nonmalignant) Q85.00
- acoustic Q85.02
- malignant — see Neoplasm, nerve, malignant
- specified NEC Q85.09
- type 1 (von Recklinghausen) Q85.01
- type 2 Q85.02

Neurofibrosarcoma — see Neoplasm, nerve, malignant

Neurogenic — see also condition
- bladder — see also Dysfunction, bladder, neuromuscular N31.9
  - cauda equina syndrome G83.4
- bowel NEC K59.2
- heart F45.8

Neuroglioma — see Neoplasm, uncertain behavior, by site

Neurolabyrinthitis (of Dix and Hallpike) — see Neuronitis, vestibular

Neurolathyrism — see Poisoning, food, noxious, plant

Neuroleprosy A30.9

Neuroma — see also Neoplasm, nerve, benign
- acoustic (nerve) D33.3
- amputation (stump) (traumatic) (surgical complication) (late) T87.3- ☑
  - arm T87.3- ☑
  - leg T87.3- ☑
- digital (toe) G57.6- ☑
- interdigital G58.8
  - lower limb (toe) G57.8- ☑
  - upper limb G56.8- ☑
- intermetatarsal G57.8- ☑
- Morton's G57.6- ☑
- nonneoplastic
  - arm G56.9- ☑
  - leg G57.9- ☑
  - lower extremity G57.9- ☑
  - upper extremity G56.9- ☑
- optic (nerve) D33.3
- plantar G57.6- ☑
- plexiform — see Neoplasm, nerve, benign
- surgical (nonneoplastic)
  - arm G56.9- ☑
  - leg G57.9- ☑
  - lower extremity G57.9- ☑
  - upper extremity G56.9- ☑

Neuromyalgia — see Neuralgia

Neuromyasthenia (epidemic) (postinfectious) G93.3

Neuromyelitis G36.9
- ascending G61.0
- optica G36.0

Neuromyopathy G70.9
- paraneoplastic D49.9 [G13.0]

Neuromyotonia (Isaacs) G71.19

Neuronevus — see Nevus

Neuronitis G58.9
- ascending (acute) G57.2- ☑
- vestibular H81.2- ☑

Neuroparalytic — see condition

Neuropathy, neuropathic G62.9
- acute motor G62.81
- alcoholic G62.1
  - with psychosis — see Psychosis, alcoholic
- arm G56.9- ☑
- autonomic, peripheral — see Neuropathy, peripheral, autonomic
- axillary G56.9- ☑
- bladder N31.9
  - atonic (motor) (sensory) N31.2
  - autonomous N31.2
  - flaccid N31.2
  - nonreflex N31.2
  - reflex N31.1
  - uninhibited N31.0
- brachial plexus G54.0
- cervical plexus G54.2
- chronic
  - progressive segmentally demyelinating G62.89
  - relapsing demyelinating G62.89
- Déjérine-Sottas G60.0
- diabetic — see E08-E13 with .40
  - mononeuropathy — see E08-E13 with .41
  - polyneuropathy — see E08-E13 with .42
- entrapment G58.9
  - iliohypogastric nerve G57.8- ☑
  - ilioinguinal nerve G57.8- ☑
  - lateral cutaneous nerve of thigh G57.1- ☑
  - median nerve G56.0- ☑
  - obturator nerve G57.8- ☑
  - peroneal nerve G57.3- ☑
  - posterior tibial nerve G57.5- ☑
  - saphenous nerve G57.8- ☑
  - ulnar nerve G56.2- ☑
- facial nerve G51.9
- hereditary G60.9
  - motor and sensory (types I-IV) G60.0
  - sensory G60.8
  - specified NEC G60.8
- hypertrophic G60.0
  - Charcot-Marie-Tooth G60.0
  - Déjérine-Sottas G60.0
  - interstitial progressive G60.0
  - of infancy G60.0
  - Refsum G60.1
- idiopathic G60.9
  - progressive G60.3
  - specified NEC G60.8
- in association with hereditary ataxia G60.2
- intercostal G58.0
- ischemic — see Disorder, nerve
- Jamaica (ginger) G62.2
- leg NEC G57.9- ☑
- lower extremity G57.9- ☑
- lumbar plexus G54.1
- median nerve G56.1- ☑
- motor and sensory — see also Polyneuropathy
  - hereditary (types I-IV) G60.0
- multifocal motor (MMN) G61.82
- multiple (acute) (chronic) — see Polyneuropathy
- optic (nerve) — see also Neuritis, optic
  - ischemic H47.01- ☑
- paraneoplastic (sensorial) (Denny Brown) D49.9 [G13.0]
- peripheral (nerve) — see also Polyneuropathy G62.9
  - autonomic G90.9
    - idiopathic G90.09
    - in (due to)
      - amyloidosis E85.4 [G99.0]
      - diabetes mellitus — see E08-E13 with .43
      - endocrine disease NEC E34.9 [G99.0]
      - gout M10.00 [G99.0]
      - hyperthyroidism E05.90 [G99.0]
        - with thyroid storm E05.91 [G99.0]
      - metabolic disease NEC E88.9 [G99.0]
  - idiopathic G60.9
    - progressive G60.3
  - in (due to)
    - antitetanus serum G62.0
    - arsenic G62.2
    - drugs NEC G62.0
    - lead G62.2
    - organophosphate compounds G62.2
    - toxic agent NEC G62.2
- plantar nerves G57.6- ☑
- progressive
  - hypertrophic interstitial G60.0
  - inflammatory G62.81

Neuropathy, neuropathic — continued
- radicular NEC — see Radiculopathy
- sacral plexus G54.1
- sciatic G57.0- ☑
- serum G61.1
- toxic NEC G62.2
- trigeminal sensory G50.8
- ulnar nerve G56.2- ☑
- uremic N18.9 [G63]
- vitamin B12 E53.8 [G63]
  - with anemia (pernicious) D51.0 [G63]
    - due to dietary deficiency D51.3 [G63]

Neurophthisis — see also Disorder, nerve
- peripheral, diabetic — see E08-E13 with .42

Neuroretinitis — see Chorioretinitis

Neuroretinopathy, hereditary optic H47.22

Neurosarcoma — see Neoplasm, nerve, malignant

Neurosclerosis — see Disorder, nerve

Neurosis, neurotic F48.9
- anankastic F42.8
- anxiety (state) F41.1
  - panic type F41.0
- asthenic F48.8
- bladder F45.8
- cardiac (reflex) F45.8
- cardiovascular F45.8
- character F60.9
- colon F45.8
- compensation F68.10
- compulsive, compulsion F42.8
- conversion F44.9
- craft F48.8
- cutaneous F45.8
- depersonalization F48.1
- depressive (reaction) (type) F34.1
- environmental F48.8
- excoriation L98.1
- fatigue F48.8
- functional — see Disorder, somatoform
- gastric F45.8
- gastrointestinal F45.8
- heart F45.8
- hypochondriacal F45.21
- hysterical F44.9
- incoordination F45.8
  - larynx F45.8
  - vocal cord F45.8
- intestine F45.8
- larynx (sensory) F45.8
  - hysterical F44.4
- mixed NEC F48.8
- musculoskeletal F45.8
- obsessional F42.8
- obsessive-compulsive F42.8
- occupational F48.8
- ocular NEC F45.8
- organ — see Disorder, somatoform
- pharynx F45.8
- phobic F40.9
- posttraumatic (situational) F43.10
  - acute F43.11
  - chronic F43.12
- psychasthenic (type) F48.8
- railroad F48.8
- rectum F45.8
- respiratory F45.8
- rumination F45.8
- sexual F65.9
- situational F48.8
- social F40.10
  - generalized F40.11
- specified type NEC F48.8
- state F48.9
  - with depersonalization episode F48.1
- stomach F45.8
- traumatic F43.10
  - acute F43.11
  - chronic F43.12
- vasomotor F45.8
- visceral F45.8
- war F48.8

Neurospongioblastosis diffusa Q85.1

Neurosyphilis (arrested) (early) (gumma) (late) (latent) (recurrent) (relapse) A52.3
- with ataxia (cerebellar) (locomotor) (spastic) (spinal) A52.19
- aneurysm (cerebral) A52.05
- arachnoid (adhesive) A52.13

☑ Additional Character Required — Refer to the Tabular List for Character Selection　　　▽ Subterms under main terms may continue to next column or page

Neurosyphilis — *continued*
 arteritis (any artery) (cerebral) A52.04
 asymptomatic A52.2
 congenital A50.40
 dura (mater) A52.13
 general paresis A52.17
 hemorrhagic A52.05
 juvenile (asymptomatic) (meningeal) A50.40
 leptomeninges (aseptic) A52.13
 meningeal, meninges (adhesive) A52.13
 meningitis A52.13
 meningovascular (diffuse) A52.13
 optic atrophy A52.15
 parenchymatous (degenerative) A52.19
 paresis, paretic A52.17
  juvenile A50.45
 remission in (sustained) A52.3
 serological (without symptoms) A52.2
 specified nature or site NEC A52.19
 tabes, tabetic (dorsalis) A52.11
  juvenile A50.45
 taboparesis A52.17
  juvenile A50.45
 thrombosis (cerebral) A52.05
 vascular (cerebral) NEC A52.05
Neurothekeoma — *see* Neoplasm, nerve, benign
Neurotic — *see* Neurosis
Neurotoxemia — *see* Toxemia
Neutroclusion M26.211
Neutropenia, neutropenic (chronic) (genetic) (idiopathic) (immune) (infantile) (malignant) (pernicious) (splenic) D70.9
 congenital (primary) D70.0
 cyclic D70.4
 cytoreductive cancer chemotherapy sequela D70.1
 drug-induced D70.2
  due to cytoreductive cancer chemotherapy D70.1
 due to infection D70.3
 fever D70.9
 neonatal, transitory (isoimmune) (maternal transfer) P61.5
 periodic D70.4
 secondary (cyclic) (periodic) (splenic) D70.4
  drug-induced D70.2
   due to cytoreductive cancer chemotherapy D70.1
 toxic D70.8
Neutrophilia, hereditary giant D72.0
Nevocarcinoma — *see* Melanoma
Nevus D22.9
 achromic — *see* Neoplasm, skin, benign
 amelanotic — *see* Neoplasm, skin, benign
 angiomatous D18.00
  intra-abdominal D18.03
  intracranial D18.02
  skin D18.01
  specified site NEC D18.09
 araneus I78.1
 balloon cell — *see* Neoplasm, skin, benign
 bathing trunk D48.5
 blue — *see* Neoplasm, skin, benign
  cellular — *see* Neoplasm, skin, benign
  giant — *see* Neoplasm, skin, benign
  Jadassohn's — *see* Neoplasm, skin, benign
  malignant — *see* Melanoma
 capillary D18.00
  intra-abdominal D18.03
  intracranial D18.02
  skin D18.01
  specified site NEC D18.09
 cavernous D18.00
  intra-abdominal D18.03
  intracranial D18.02
  skin D18.01
  specified site NEC D18.09
 cellular — *see* Neoplasm, skin, benign
  blue — *see* Neoplasm, skin, benign
 choroid D31.3- ☑
 comedonicus Q82.0-
 conjunctiva D31.0- ☑
 dermal — *see* Neoplasm, skin, benign
  with epidermal nevus — *see* Neoplasm, skin, benign
 dysplastic — *see* Neoplasm, skin, benign
 eye D31.9- ☑
 flammeus Q82.5
 hemangiomatous D18.00
  intra-abdominal D18.03
  intracranial D18.02
  skin D18.01

Nevus — *continued*
 hemangiomatous — *continued*
  specified site NEC D18.09
 iris D31.4- ☑
 lacrimal gland D31.5- ☑
 lymphatic D18.1
 magnocellular
  specified site — *see* Neoplasm, benign, by site
  unspecified site D31.40
 malignant — *see* Melanoma
 meaning hemangioma D18.00
  intra-abdominal D18.03
  intracranial D18.02
  skin D18.01
  specified site NEC D18.09
 mouth (mucosa) D10.30
  specified site NEC D10.39
  white sponge Q38.6
 multiplex Q85.1
 non-neoplastic I78.1
 oral mucosa D10.30
  specified site NEC D10.39
  white sponge Q38.6
 orbit D31.6- ☑
 pigmented
  giant — *see also* Neoplasm, skin, uncertain behavior D48.5
   malignant melanoma in — *see* Melanoma
 portwine Q82.5
 retina D31.2- ☑
 retrobulbar D31.6- ☑
 sanguineous Q82.5
 senile I78.1
 skin D22.9
  abdominal wall D22.5
  ala nasi D22.39
  ankle D22.7- ☑
  anus, anal D22.5
  arm D22.6- ☑
  auditory canal (external) D22.2- ☑
  auricle (ear) D22.2- ☑
  auricular canal (external) D22.2- ☑
  axilla, axillary fold D22.5
  back D22.5
  breast D22.5
  brow D22.39
  buttock D22.5
  canthus (eye) D22.1- ☑
  cheek (external) D22.39
  chest wall D22.5
  chin D22.39
  ear (external) D22.2- ☑
  external meatus (ear) D22.2- ☑
  eyebrow D22.39
  eyelid (lower) (upper) D22.1- ☑
  face D22.30
   specified NEC D22.39
  female genital organ (external) NEC D28.0
  finger D22.6- ☑
  flank D22.5
  foot D22.7- ☑
  forearm D22.6- ☑
  forehead D22.39
  foreskin D29.0
  genital organ (external) NEC
   female D28.0
   male D29.9
  gluteal region D22.5
  groin D22.5
  hand D22.6- ☑
  heel D22.7- ☑
  helix D22.2- ☑
  hip D22.7- ☑
  interscapular region D22.5
  jaw D22.39
  knee D22.7- ☑
  labium (majus) (minus) D28.0
  leg D22.7- ☑
  lip (lower) (upper) D22.0
  lower limb D22.7- ☑
  male genital organ (external) D29.9
  nail D22.9
   finger D22.6- ☑
   toe D22.7- ☑
  nasolabial groove D22.39
  nates D22.5
  neck D22.4
  nose (external) D22.39

Nevus — *continued*
 skin — *continued*
  palpebra D22.1- ☑
  penis D29.0
  perianal skin D22.5
  perineum D22.5
  pinna D22.2- ☑
  popliteal fossa or space D22.7- ☑
  prepuce D29.0
  pudendum D28.0
  scalp D22.4
  scrotum D29.4
  shoulder D22.6- ☑
  submammary fold D22.5
  temple D22.39
  thigh D22.7- ☑
  toe D22.7- ☑
  trunk NEC D22.5
  umbilicus D22.5
  upper limb D22.6- ☑
  vulva D28.0
 specified site NEC — *see* Neoplasm, by site, benign
 spider I78.1
 stellar I78.1
 strawberry Q82.5
 Sutton's benign D22.9
 unius lateris Q82.5
 Unna's Q82.5
 vascular Q82.5
 verrucous Q82.5
Newborn (infant) (liveborn) (singleton) Z38.2
 abstinence syndrome P96.1
 acne L70.4
 affected by
  abnormalities of membranes P02.9
   specified NEC P02.8
  abruptio placenta P02.1
  amino-acid metabolic disorder, transitory P74.8
  amniocentesis (while in utero) P00.6
  amnionitis P02.78
  apparent life threatening event (ALTE) R68.13
  bleeding (into)
   cerebral cortex P52.22
   germinal matrix P52.0
   ventricles P52.1
  breech delivery P03.0
  cardiac arrest P29.81
  cardiomyopathy I42.8
   congenital I42.4
  cerebral ischemia P91.0
  Cesarean delivery P03.4
  chemotherapy agents P04.11
  chorioamnionitis P02.78
  cocaine (crack) P04.41
  complications of labor and delivery P03.9
   specified NEC P03.89
  compression of umbilical cord NEC P02.5
  contracted pelvis P03.1
  cyanosis P28.2
  delivery P03.9
   Cesarean P03.4
   forceps P03.2
   vacuum extractor P03.3
  drugs of addiction P04.40
   cocaine P04.41
   hallucinogens P04.42
   specified drug NEC P04.49
  entanglement (knot) in umbilical cord P02.5
  environmental chemicals P04.6
  fetal (intrauterine)
   growth retardation P05.9
   inflammatory response syndrome (FIRS) P02.70
   malnutrition not light or small for gestational age P05.2
  FIRS (fetal inflammatory response syndrome) P02.70
  forceps delivery P03.2
  heart rate abnormalities
   bradycardia P29.12
   intrauterine P03.819
    before onset of labor P03.810
    during labor P03.811
   tachycardia P29.11
  hemorrhage (antepartum) P02.1
   cerebellar (nontraumatic) P52.6
   intracerebral (nontraumatic) P52.4
   intracranial (nontraumatic) P52.9
    specified NEC P52.8
   intraventricular (nontraumatic) P52.3

Neurosyphilis — Newborn

▼ Subterms under main terms may continue to next column or page   ☑ Additional Character Required — Refer to the Tabular List for Character Selection   237

Newborn — *continued*
  affected by — *continued*
    hemorrhage — *continued*
      intraventricular — *continued*
        grade 1 P52.0
        grade 2 P52.1
        grade 3 P52.21
        grade 4 P52.22
      posterior fossa (nontraumatic) P52.6
      subarachnoid (nontraumatic) P52.5
      subependymal P52.0
        with intracerebral extension P52.22
        with intraventricular extension P52.1
          with enlargment of ventricles P52.21
        without intraventricular extension P52.0
    hypoxic ischemic encephalopathy [HIE] P91.60
      mild P91.61
      moderate P91.62
      severe P91.63
    induction of labor P03.89
    intestinal perforation P78.0
    intrauterine (fetal) blood loss P50.9
      due to (from)
        cut end of co-twin cord P50.5
        hemorrhage into
          co-twin P50.3
          maternal circulation P50.4
        placenta P50.2
        ruptured cord blood P50.1
        vasa previa P50.0
      specified NEC P50.8
    intrauterine (fetal) hemorrhage P50.9
    intrauterine (in utero) procedure P96.5
    malpresentation (malposition) NEC P03.1
    maternal (complication of) (use of)
      alcohol P04.3
      amphetamines P04.16
      analgesia (maternal) P04.0
      anesthesia (maternal) P04.0
      anticonvulsants P04.13
      antidepressants P04.15
      antineoplastic chemotherapy P04.11
      anxiolytics P04.1A
      blood loss P02.1
      cannabis P04.81
      circulatory disease P00.3
      condition P00.9
        specified NEC P00.89
      cytotoxic drugs P04.12
      delivery P03.9
        Cesarean P03.4
        forceps P03.2
        vacuum extractor P03.3
      diabetes mellitus (pre-existing) P70.1
      disorder P00.9
        specified NEC P00.89
      drugs (addictive) (illegal) NEC P04.49
      ectopic pregnancy P01.4
      gestational diabetes P70.0
      group B streptococcus (GBS) colonization (posi-
        tive) P00.82
      hemorrhage P02.1
      hypertensive disorder P00.0
      incompetent cervix P01.0
      infectious disease P00.2
      injury P00.5
      labor and delivery P03.9
      malpresentation before labor P01.7
      maternal death P01.6
      medical procedure P00.7
      medication P04.19
        specified type NEC P04.18
      multiple pregnancy P01.5
      nutritional disorder P00.4
      oligohydramnios P01.2
      opiates P04.14
        administered for procedures during pregnan-
          cy or labor and delivery P04.0
      parasitic disease P00.2
      periodontal disease P00.81
      placenta previa P02.0
      polyhydramnios P01.3
      precipitate delivery P03.5
      pregnancy P01.9
        specified P01.8
      premature rupture of membranes P01.1
      renal disease P00.1
      respiratory disease P00.3
      sedative-hypnotics P04.17
      surgical procedure P00.6
      tranquilizers administered for procedures during
        pregnancy or labor and delivery P04.0
      urinary tract disease P00.1
      uterine contraction (abnormal) P03.6
    meconium peritonitis P78.0
    medication (legal) (maternal use) (prescribed)
      P04.19
    membrane abnormalities P02.9
      specified NEC P02.8
    membranitis P02.78
    methamphetamine(s) P04.49
    mixed metabolic and respiratory acidosis P84
    neonatal abstinence syndrome P96.1
    noxious substances transmitted via placenta or
      breast milk P04.9
      cannabis P04.81
      specified NEC P04.89
    nutritional supplements P04.5
    placenta previa P02.0
    placental
      abnormality (functional) (morphological) P02.20
        specified NEC P02.29
      dysfunction P02.29
      infarction P02.29
      insufficiency P02.29
      separation NEC P02.1
      transfusion syndromes P02.3
    placentitis P02.78
    precipitate delivery P03.5
    prolapsed cord P02.4
    respiratory arrest P28.81
    slow intrauterine growth P05.9
    tobacco P04.2
    twin to twin transplacental transfusion P02.3
    umbilical cord (tightly) around neck P02.5
    umbilical cord condition P02.60
      short cord P02.69
      specified NEC P02.69
    uterine contractions (abnormal) P03.6
    vasa previa P02.69
      from intrauterine blood loss P50.0
  apnea P28.4
    obstructive P28.4
    primary P28.3
    sleep (central) (obstructive) (primary) P28.3
  born in hospital Z38.00
    by cesarean Z38.01
  born outside hospital Z38.1
  breast buds P96.89
  breast engorgement P83.4
  check-up — *see* Newborn, examination
  convulsion P90
  dehydration P74.1
  examination
    8 to 28 days old Z00.111
    under 8 days old Z00.110
  fever P81.9
    environmentally-induced P81.0
  hyperbilirubinemia P59.9
    of prematurity P59.0
  hypernatremia P74.21
  hyponatremia P74.22
  infection P39.9
    candidal P37.5
    specified NEC P39.8
    urinary tract P39.3
  jaundice P59.9
    due to
      breast milk inhibitor P59.3
      hepatocellular damage P59.20
        specified NEC P59.29
      preterm delivery P59.0
    of prematurity P59.0
    specified NEC P59.8
  late metabolic acidosis P74.0
  mastitis P39.0
    infective P39.0
    noninfective P83.4
  multiple born NEC Z38.8
    born in hospital Z38.68
      by cesarean Z38.69
    born outside hospital Z38.7
  omphalitis P38.9
    with mild hemorrhage P38.1
    without hemorrhage P38.9

Newborn — *continued*
  post-term P08.21
  prolonged gestation (over 42 completed weeks) P08.22
  quadruplet Z38.8
    born in hospital Z38.63
      by cesarean Z38.64
    born outside hospital Z38.7
  quintuplet Z38.8
    born in hospital Z38.65
      by cesarean Z38.66
    born outside hospital Z38.7
  seizure P90
  sepsis (congenital) P36.9
    due to
      anaerobes NEC P36.5
      Escherichia coli P36.4
      Staphylococcus P36.30
        aureus P36.2
        specified NEC P36.39
      Streptococcus P36.10
        group B P36.0
        specified NEC P36.19
      specified NEC P36.8
  triplet Z38.8
    born in hospital Z38.61
      by cesarean Z38.62
    born outside hospital Z38.7
  twin Z38.5
    born in hospital Z38.30
      by cesarean Z38.31
    born outside hospital Z38.4
  vomiting P92.09
    bilious P92.01
  weight check Z00.111
Newcastle conjunctivitis or disease B30.8
Nezelof's syndrome (pure alymphocytosis) D81.4
Niacin (amide) **deficiency** E52
Nicolas (-Durand)-**Favre disease** A55
Nicotine — *see* Tobacco
Nicotinic acid deficiency E52
Niemann-Pick disease or syndrome E75.249
  specified NEC E75.248
  type
    A E75.240
    A/B E75.244
    B E75.241
    C E75.242
    D E75.243
Night
  blindness — *see* Blindness, night
  sweats R61
  terrors (child) F51.4
Nightmares (REM sleep type) F51.5
NIHSS (National Institutes of Health Stroke Scale) **score**
  R29.7- ☑
Nipple — *see* condition
Nisbet's chancre A57
Nishimoto (-Takeuchi) **disease** I67.5
Nitritoid crisis or reaction — *see* Crisis, nitritoid
Nitrosohemoglobinemia D74.8
Njovera A65
No general equivalence degree (GED) Z55.5
Nocardiosis, nocardiasis A43.9
  cutaneous A43.1
  lung A43.0
  pneumonia A43.0
  pulmonary A43.0
  specified site NEC A43.8
Nocturia R35.1
  psychogenic F45.8
Nocturnal — *see* condition
Nodal rhythm I49.8
Node(s) — *see also* Nodule
  Bouchard's (with arthropathy) M15.2
  Haygarth's M15.8
  Heberden's (with arthropathy) M15.1
  larynx J38.7
  lymph — *see* condition
  milker's B08.03
  Osler's I33.0
  Schmorl's — *see* Schmorl's disease
  singer's J38.2
  teacher's J38.2
  tuberculous — *see* Tuberculosis, lymph gland
  vocal cord J38.2
Nodule(s), **nodular**
  actinomycotic — *see* Actinomycosis
  breast NEC — *see also* Lump, breast N63.0

☑ **Additional Character Required** — Refer to the Tabular List for Character Selection   ▽ **Subterms under main terms may continue to next column or page**

Nodule(s), **nodular** — *continued*
  colloid (cystic), thyroid E04.1
  cutaneous — *see* Swelling, localized
  endometrial (stromal) D26.1
  Haygarth's M15.8
  inflammatory — *see* Inflammation
  juxta-articular
    syphilitic A52.77
    yaws A66.7
  larynx J38.7
  lung, solitary (subsegmental branch of the bronchial
    tree) R91.1
    multiple R91.8
  milker's B08.03
  prostate N40.2
    with lower urinary tract symptoms (LUTS) N40.3
    without lower urinary tract symptoms (LUTS) N40.2
  pulmonary, solitary (subsegmental branch of the
    bronchial tree) R91.1
  retrocardiac R09.89
  rheumatoid M06.30
    ankle M06.37- ☑
    elbow M06.32- ☑
    foot joint M06.37- ☑
    hand joint M06.34- ☑
    hip M06.35- ☑
    knee M06.36- ☑
    multiple site M06.39
    shoulder M06.31- ☑
    vertebra M06.38
    wrist M06.33- ☑
  scrotum (inflammatory) N49.2
  singer's J38.2
  solitary, lung (subsegmental branch of the bronchial
    tree) R91.1
    multiple R91.8
  subcutaneous — *see* Swelling, localized
  teacher's J38.2
  thyroid (cold) (gland) (nontoxic) E04.1
    with thyrotoxicosis E05.20
      with thyroid storm E05.21
    toxic or with hyperthyroidism E05.20
      with thyroid storm E05.21
  vocal cord J38.2
Noma (gangrenous) (hospital) (infective) A69.0
  auricle I96
  mouth A69.0
  pudendi N76.89
  vulvae N76.89
Nomad, nomadism Z59.00
NOMID (neonatal onset multisystemic inflammatory disorder) M04.2
Nonadherence to medical treatment Z91.19
Nonautoimmune hemolytic anemia D59.4
  drug-induced D59.2
Nonclosure — *see also* Imperfect, closure
  ductus arteriosus (Botallo's) Q25.0
  foramen
    botalli Q21.1
    ovale Q21.1
Noncompliance Z91.19
  with
    dialysis Z91.15
    dietary regimen Z91.11
    medical treatment Z91.19
    medication regimen NEC Z91.14
      underdosing — *see also* Table of Drugs and
        Chemicals, categories T36-T50, with final
        character 6 Z91.14
        intentional NEC Z91.128
          due to financial hardship of patient
            Z91.120
        unintentional NEC Z91.138
          due to patient's age related debility
            Z91.130
    renal dialysis Z91.15
Nondescent (congenital) — *see also* Malposition, congenital
  cecum Q43.3
  colon Q43.3
  testicle Q53.9
    bilateral Q53.20
      abdominal Q53.211
      perineal Q53.22
    unilateral Q53.10
      abdominal Q53.111
      perineal Q53.12

Nondevelopment
  brain Q02
    part of Q04.3
  heart Q24.8
  organ or site, congenital NEC — *see* Hypoplasia
Nonengagement
  head NEC O32.4 ☑
    in labor, causing obstructed labor O64.8 ☑
Nonexanthematous tick fever A93.2
Nonexpansion, lung (newborn) P28.0
Nonfunctioning
  cystic duct — *see also* Disease, gallbladder K82.8
  gallbladder — *see also* Disease, gallbladder K82.8
  kidney N28.9
  labyrinth — *see* subcategory H83.2 ☑
Non-Hodgkin lymphoma NEC — *see* Lymphoma, non-
  Hodgkin
Nonimplantation, ovum N97.2
Noninsufflation, fallopian tube N97.1
Non-ketotic hyperglycinemia E72.51
Nonne-Milroy syndrome Q82.0
Nonovulation N97.0
Non-palpable testicle(s)
  bilateral R39.84
  unilateral R39.83
Nonpatent fallopian tube N97.1
Nonpneumatization, lung NEC P28.0
Nonrotation — *see* Malrotation
Nonsecretion, urine — *see* Anuria
Nonunion
  fracture — *see* Fracture, by site
  joint, following fusion or arthrodesis M96.0
  organ or site, congenital NEC — *see* Imperfect, closure
  symphysis pubis, congenital Q74.2
Nonvisualization, gallbladder R93.2
Nonvital, nonvitalized tooth K04.99
Non-working side interference M26.56
Noonan's syndrome Q87.19
Normocytic anemia (infectional) due to blood loss
  (chronic) D50.0
  acute D62
Norrie's disease (congenital) Q15.8
North American blastomycosis B40.9
Norwegian itch B86
Nose, nasal — *see* condition
Nosebleed R04.0
Nose-picking F98.8
Nosomania F45.21
Nosophobia F45.22
Nostalgia F43.20
Notch of iris Q13.2
Notching nose, congenital (tip) Q30.2
Nothnagel's
  syndrome — *see* Strabismus, paralytic, third nerve
  vasomotor acroparesthesia I73.89
Novy's relapsing fever A68.9
  louse-borne A68.0
  tick-borne A68.1
Noxious
  foodstuffs, poisoning by — *see* Poisoning, food, nox-
    ious, plant
  substances transmitted through placenta or breast milk
    P04.9
Nucleus pulposus — *see* condition
Numbness R20.0
Nuns' knee — *see* Bursitis, prepatellar
Nursemaid's elbow S53.03- ☑
Nutcracker esophagus K22.4
Nutmeg liver K76.1
Nutrient element deficiency E61.9
  specified NEC E61.8
Nutrition deficient or insufficient — *see also* Malnutri-
  tion E46
  due to
    insufficient food T73.0 ☑
    lack of
      care (child) T76.02 ☑
        adult T76.01 ☑
      food T73.0 ☑
Nutritional stunting E45
Nyctalopia (night blindness) — *see* Blindness, night
Nycturia R35.1
  psychogenic F45.8
Nymphomania F52.8
Nystagmus H55.00
  benign paroxysmal — *see* Vertigo, benign paroxysmal
  central positional H81.4

Nystagmus — *continued*
  congenital H55.01
  dissociated H55.04
  latent H55.02
  miners' H55.09
  positional
    benign paroxysmal H81.4
    central H81.4
  specified form NEC H55.09
  visual deprivation H55.03

O

Obermeyer's relapsing fever (European) A68.0
Obesity E66.9
  with alveolar hypoventilation E66.2
  adrenal E27.8
  complicating
    childbirth O99.214
    pregnancy O99.21- ☑
    puerperium O99.215
  constitutional E66.8
  dietary counseling and surveillance Z71.3
  drug-induced E66.1
  due to
    drug E66.1
    excess calories E66.09
      morbid E66.01
      severe E66.01
  endocrine E66.8
  endogenous E66.8
  exogenous E66.09
  familial E66.8
  glandular E66.8
  hypothyroid — *see* Hypothyroidism
  hypoventilation syndrome (OHS) E66.2
  morbid E66.01
    with
      alveolar hypoventilation E66.2
      obesity hypoventilation syndrome (OHS) E66.2
    due to excess calories E66.01
  nutritional E66.09
  pituitary E23.6
  severe E66.01
  specified type NEC E66.8
Oblique — *see* condition
Obliteration
  appendix (lumen) K38.8
  artery I77.1
  bile duct (noncalculous) K83.1
  common duct (noncalculous) K83.1
  cystic duct — *see* Obstruction, gallbladder
  disease, arteriolar I77.1
  endometrium N85.8
  eye, anterior chamber — *see* Disorder, globe, hypotony
  fallopian tube N97.1
  lymphatic vessel I89.0
    due to mastectomy I97.2
  organ or site, congenital NEC — *see* Atresia, by site
  ureter N13.5
    with infection N13.6
  urethra — *see* Stricture, urethra
  vein I87.8
  vestibule (oral) K08.89
Observation (following) (for) (without need for further
  medical care) Z04.9
  accident NEC Z04.3
    at work Z04.2
    transport Z04.1
  adverse effect of drug Z03.6
  alleged rape or sexual assault (victim), ruled out
    adult Z04.41
    child Z04.42
  criminal assault Z04.89
  development state
    adolescent Z00.3
    period of rapid growth in childhood Z00.2
    puberty Z00.3
  disease, specified NEC Z03.89
  following work accident Z04.2
  forced sexual exploitation Z04.81
  forced labor exploitation Z04.82
  growth and development state — *see* Observation,
    development state
  injuries (accidental) NEC — *see also* Observation, acci-
    dent

Observation — *continued*
  newborn (for)
    suspected condition, related to exposure from the mother or birth process — *see* Newborn, affected by, maternal
    ruled out Z05.9
      cardiac Z05.0
      connective tissue Z05.73
      gastrointestinal Z05.5
      genetic Z05.41
      genitourinary Z05.6
      immunologic Z05.43
      infectious Z05.1
      metabolic Z05.42
      musculoskeletal Z05.72
      neurological Z05.2
      respiratory Z05.3
      skin and subcutaneous tissue Z05.71
      specified condition NEC Z05.8
  postpartum
    immediately after delivery Z39.0
    routine follow-up Z39.2
  pregnancy (normal) (without complication) Z34.9- ☑
    high risk O09.9- ☑
  suicide attempt, alleged NEC Z03.89
    self-poisoning Z03.6
  suspected, ruled out — *see also* Suspected condition, ruled out
    abuse, physical
      adult Z04.71
      child Z04.72
    accident at work Z04.2
    adult battering victim Z04.71
    child battering victim Z04.72
    condition NEC Z03.89
      newborn — *see also* Observation, newborn (for), suspected condition, ruled out Z05.9
    drug poisoning or adverse effect Z03.6
    exposure (to)
      anthrax Z03.810
      biological agent NEC Z03.818
    foreign body
      aspirated (inhaled) Z03.822
      ingested Z03.821
      inserted (injected), in (eye) (orifice) (skin) Z03.823
    inflicted injury NEC Z04.89
    suicide attempt, alleged Z03.89
      self-poisoning Z03.6
    toxic effects from ingested substance (drug) (poison) Z03.6
  toxic effects from ingested substance (drug) (poison) Z03.6
Obsession, obsessional state F42.8
  mixed thoughts and acts F42.2
Obsessive-compulsive neurosis or reaction F42.8
Obstetric embolism, septic — *see* Embolism, obstetric, septic
Obstetrical trauma (complicating delivery) O71.9
  with or following ectopic or molar pregnancy O08.6
  specified type NEC O71.89
Obstipation — *see* Constipation
Obstruction, obstructed, obstructive
  airway J98.8
    with
      allergic alveolitis J67.9
      asthma J45.909
        with
          exacerbation (acute) J45.901
          status asthmaticus J45.902
      bronchiectasis J47.9
        with
          exacerbation (acute) J47.1
          lower respiratory infection J47.0
      bronchitis (chronic) J44.9
      emphysema J43.9
    chronic J44.9
      with
        allergic alveolitis — *see* Pneumonitis, hypersensitivity
        bronchiectasis J47.9
          with
            exacerbation (acute) J47.1
            lower respiratory infection J47.0
    due to
      foreign body — *see* Foreign body, by site, causing asphyxia
      inhalation of fumes or vapors J68.9
      laryngospasm J38.5

Obstruction, obstructed, obstructive — *continued*
  ampulla of Vater K83.1
  aortic (heart) (valve) — *see* Stenosis, aortic
  aortoiliac I74.09
  aqueduct of Sylvius G91.1
    congenital Q03.0
      with spina bifida — *see* Spina bifida, by site, with hydrocephalus
  Arnold-Chiari — *see* Arnold-Chiari disease
  artery — *see also* Atherosclerosis, artery I70.9 ☑
    basilar (complete) (partial) — *see* Occlusion, artery, basilar
    carotid (complete) (partial) — *see* Occlusion, artery, carotid
    cerebellar — *see* Occlusion, artery, cerebellar
    cerebral (anterior) (middle) (posterior) — *see* Occlusion, artery, cerebral
    precerebral — *see* Occlusion, artery, precerebral
    renal N28.0
    retinal NEC — *see* Occlusion, artery, retina
    stent — *see* Restenosis, stent
    vertebral (complete) (partial) — *see* Occlusion, artery, vertebral
  band (intestinal) — *see also* Obstruction, intestine, specified NEC K56.699
  bile duct or passage (common) (hepatic) (noncalculous) K83.1
    with calculus K80.51
    congenital (causing jaundice) Q44.3
  biliary (duct) (tract) K83.1
    gallbladder K82.0
  bladder-neck (acquired) N32.0
    congenital Q64.31
    due to hyperplasia (hypertrophy) of prostate — *see* Hyperplasia, prostate
  bowel — *see* Obstruction, intestine
  bronchus J98.09
  canal, ear — *see* Stenosis, external ear canal
  cardia K22.2
  caval veins (inferior) (superior) I87.1
  cecum — *see* Obstruction, intestine
  circulatory I99.8
  colon — *see* Obstruction, intestine
  common duct (noncalculous) K83.1
  coronary (artery) — *see* Occlusion, coronary
  cystic duct — *see also* Obstruction, gallbladder
    with calculus K80.21
  device, implant or graft — *see also* Complications, by site and type, mechanical T85.698 ☑
    arterial graft NEC — *see* Complication, cardiovascular device, mechanical, vascular
    catheter NEC T85.628 ☑
      cystostomy T83.090 ☑
      dialysis (renal) T82.49 ☑
        intraperitoneal T85.691 ☑
      Hopkins T83.098 ☑
      ileostomy T83.098 ☑
      infusion NEC T82.594 ☑
        spinal (epidural) (subdural) T85.690 ☑
      nephrostomy T83.092 ☑
      urethral indwelling T83.091 ☑
      urinary T83.098 ☑
      urostomy T83.098 ☑
    due to infection T85.79 ☑
    gastrointestinal — *see* Complications, prosthetic device, mechanical, gastrointestinal device
    genital NEC T83.498 ☑
      intrauterine contraceptive device T83.39 ☑
      penile prosthesis (cylinder) (implanted) (pump) (resevoir) T83.490 ☑
      testicular prosthesis T83.491 ☑
    heart NEC — *see* Complication, cardiovascular device, mechanical
    joint prosthesis — *see* Complications, joint prosthesis, mechanical, specified NEC, by site
    orthopedic NEC — *see* Complication, orthopedic, device, mechanical
    specified NEC T85.628 ☑
    urinary NEC — *see also* Complication, genitourinary, device, urinary, mechanical
      graft T83.29 ☑
    vascular NEC — *see* Complication, cardiovascular device, mechanical
    ventricular intracranial shunt T85.09 ☑
  due to foreign body accidentally left in operative wound T81.529 ☑
  duodenum K31.5

Obstruction, obstructed, obstructive — *continued*
  ejaculatory duct N50.89
  esophagus K22.2
  eustachian tube (complete) (partial) H68.10- ☑
    cartilagenous (extrinsic) H68.13- ☑
      intrinsic H68.12- ☑
    osseous H68.11- ☑
  fallopian tube (bilateral) N97.1
  fecal K56.41
    with hernia — *see* Hernia, by site, with obstruction
  foramen of Monro (congenital) Q03.8
    with spina bifida — *see* Spina bifida, by site, with hydrocephalus
  foreign body — *see* Foreign body
  gallbladder K82.0
    with calculus, stones K80.21
    congenital Q44.1
  gastric outlet K31.1
  gastrointestinal — *see* Obstruction, intestine
  hepatic K76.89
    duct (noncalculous) K83.1
  ileum — *see* Obstruction, intestine
  iliofemoral (artery) I74.5
  intestine K56.609
    with
      adhesions (intestinal) (peritoneal) K56.50
        complete K56.52
        incomplete K56.51
        partial K56.51
    adynamic K56.0
    by gallstone K56.3
    complete K56.601
    congenital (small) Q41.9
      large Q42.9
        specified part NEC Q42.8
    incomplete K56.600
    neurogenic K56.0
      Hirschsprung's disease or megacolon Q43.1
    newborn P76.9
      due to
        fecaliths P76.8
        inspissated milk P76.2
        meconium (plug) P76.0
          in mucoviscidosis E84.11
      specified NEC P76.8
    partial K56.600
    postoperative K91.30
      complete K91.32
      incomplete K91.31
      partial K91.31
    reflex K56.0
    specified NEC K56.699
      complete K56.691
      incomplete K56.690
      partial K56.690
    volvulus K56.2
  intracardiac ball valve prosthesis T82.09 ☑
  jejunum — *see* Obstruction, intestine
  joint prosthesis — *see* Complications, joint prosthesis, mechanical, specified NEC, by site
  kidney (calices) — *see also* Hydronephrosis N28.89
  labor — *see* Delivery
  lacrimal (passages) (duct)
    by
      dacryolith — *see* Dacryolith
      stenosis — *see* Stenosis, lacrimal
    congenital Q10.5
    neonatal H04.53- ☑
  lacrimonasal duct — *see* Obstruction, lacrimal
  lacteal, with steatorrhea K90.2
  laryngitis — *see* Laryngitis
  larynx NEC J38.6
    congenital Q31.8
  lung J98.4
    disease, chronic J44.9
  lymphatic I89.0
  meconium (plug)
    newborn P76.0
      due to fecaliths P76.0
      in mucoviscidosis E84.11
  mitral — *see* Stenosis, mitral
  nasal J34.89
  nasolacrimal duct — *see also* Obstruction, lacrimal
    congenital Q10.5
  nasopharynx J39.2
  nose J34.89
  organ or site, congenital NEC — *see* Atresia, by site
  pancreatic duct K86.89

☑ **Additional Character Required** — **Refer to the Tabular List for Character Selection**   ▽ **Subterms under main terms may continue to next column or page**

Obstruction, obstructed, obstructive — *continued*
  parotid duct or gland K11.8
  pelviureteral junction N13.5
    with hydronephrosis N13.0
      congenital Q62.39
  pharynx J39.2
  portal (circulation) (vein) I81
  prostate — *see also* Hyperplasia, prostate
    valve (urinary) N32.0
  pulmonary valve (heart) I37.0
  pyelonephritis (chronic) N11.1
  pylorus
    adult K31.1
    congenital or infantile Q40.0
  rectosigmoid — *see* Obstruction, intestine
  rectum K62.4
  renal — *see also* Hydronephrosis N28.89
    outflow N13.8
    pelvis, congenital Q62.39
  respiratory J98.8
    chronic J44.9
  retinal (vessels) H34.9
  salivary duct (any) K11.8
    with calculus K11.5
  sigmoid — *see* Obstruction, intestine
  sinus (accessory) (nasal) J34.89
  Stensen's duct K11.8
  stomach NEC K31.89
    acute K31.0
    congenital Q40.2
    due to pylorospasm K31.3
  submandibular duct K11.8
  submaxillary gland K11.8
    with calculus K11.5
  thoracic duct I89.0
  thrombotic — *see* Thrombosis
  trachea J39.8
  tracheostomy airway J95.03
  tricuspid (valve) — *see* Stenosis, tricuspid
  upper respiratory, congenital Q34.8
  ureter (functional) (pelvic junction) NEC N13.5
    with
      hydronephrosis N13.1
        with infection N13.6
        congenital Q62.39
      pyelonephritis (chronic) N11.1
    congenital Q62.39
    due to calculus — *see* Calculus, ureter
  urethra NEC N36.8
    congenital Q64.39
  urinary (moderate) N13.9
    due to hyperplasia (hypertrophy) of prostate — *see* Hyperplasia, prostate
    organ or tract (lower) N13.9
    prostatic valve N32.0
    specified NEC N13.8
  uropathy N13.9
  uterus N85.8
  vagina N89.5
  valvular — *see* Endocarditis
  vein, venous I87.1
    caval (inferior) (superior) I87.1
    thrombotic — *see* Thrombosis
  vena cava (inferior) (superior) I87.1
  vesical NEC N32.0
  vesicourethral orifice N32.0
    congenital Q64.31
  vessel NEC I99.8
  stent — *see* Restenosis, stent
Obturator — *see* condition
Occlusal wear, teeth K03.0
Occlusio pupillae — *see* Membrane, pupillary
Occlusion, occluded
  anus K62.4
    congenital Q42.3
      with fistula Q42.2
  aortoiliac (chronic) I74.09
  aqueduct of Sylvius G91.1
    congenital Q03.0
      with spina bifida — *see* Spina bifida, by site, with hydrocephalus
  artery — *see also* Atherosclerosis, artery I70.9 ☑
    auditory, internal I65.8
    basilar I65.1
      with
        infarction I63.22
          due to
            embolism I63.12

Occlusion, occluded — *continued*
  artery — *see also* Atherosclerosis, artery — *continued*
    basilar — *continued*
      with — *continued*
        infarction — *continued*
          due to — *continued*
            thrombosis I63.02
    brain or cerebral I66.9
      with infarction (due to) I63.5- ☑
        embolism I63.4- ☑
        thrombosis I63.3- ☑
    carotid I65.2- ☑
      with
        infarction I63.23- ☑
          due to
            embolism I63.13- ☑
            thrombosis I63.03- ☑
    cerebellar (anterior inferior) (posterior inferior) (superior) I66.3
      with infarction I63.54- ☑
        due to
          embolism I63.44- ☑
          thrombosis I63.34- ☑
    cerebral I66.9
      with infarction I63.50
        due to
          embolism I63.40
            specified NEC I63.49
          thrombosis I63.30
            specified NEC I63.39
      anterior I66.1- ☑
        with infarction I63.52- ☑
          due to
            embolism I63.42- ☑
            thrombosis I63.32- ☑
      middle I66.0- ☑
        with infarction I63.51- ☑
          due to
            embolism I63.41- ☑
            thrombosis I63.31- ☑
      posterior I66.2- ☑
        with infarction I63.53- ☑
          due to
            embolism I63.43- ☑
            thrombosis I63.33- ☑
      specified NEC I66.8
        with infarction I63.59
          due to
            embolism I63.4- ☑
            thrombosis I63.3- ☑
    choroidal (anterior) — *see* Occlusion, artery, precerebral, specified NEC
    communicating posterior — *see* Occlusion, artery, precerebral, specified NEC
    complete
      coronary I25.82
      extremities I70.92
    coronary (acute) (thrombotic) (without myocardial infarction) I24.0
      with myocardial infarction — *see* Infarction, myocardium
      chronic total I25.82
      complete I25.82
      healed or old I25.2
      total (chronic) I25.82
    hypophyseal — *see* Occlusion, artery, precerebral, specified NEC
    iliac I74.5
    lower extremities due to stenosis or stricture I77.1
    mesenteric (embolic) (thrombotic) — *see also* Infarct, intestine K55.069
    perforating — *see* Occlusion, artery, cerebral, specified NEC
    peripheral I77.9
      thrombotic or embolic I74.4
    pontine — *see* Occlusion, artery, precerebral, specified NEC
    precerebral I65.9
      with infarction I63.20
        specified NEC I63.29
        due to
          embolism I63.10
            specified NEC I63.19
          thrombosis I63.00
            specified NEC I63.09
    basilar — *see* Occlusion, artery, basilar

Occlusion, occluded — *continued*
  artery — *see also* Atherosclerosis, artery — *continued*
    precerebral — *continued*
      carotid — *see* Occlusion, artery, carotid
      puerperal O88.23
      specified NEC I65.8
        with infarction I63.29
          due to
            embolism I63.19
            thrombosis I63.09
      vertebral — *see* Occlusion, artery, vertebral
    renal N28.0
    retinal
      branch H34.23- ☑
      central H34.1- ☑
      partial H34.21- ☑
      transient H34.0- ☑
    spinal — *see* Occlusion, artery, precerebral, vertebral
    total (chronic)
      coronary I25.82
      extremities I70.92
    vertebral I65.0- ☑
      with
        infarction I63.21- ☑
          due to
            embolism I63.11- ☑
            thrombosis I63.01- ☑
  basilar artery — *see* Occlusion, artery, basilar
  bile duct (common) (hepatic) (noncalculous) K83.1
  bowel — *see* Obstruction, intestine
  carotid (artery) (common) (internal) — *see* Occlusion, artery, carotid
  centric (of teeth) M26.59
    maximum intercuspation discrepancy M26.55
  cerebellar (artery) — *see* Occlusion, artery, cerebellar
  cerebral (artery) — *see* Occlusion, artery, cerebral
  cerebrovascular — *see also* Occlusion, artery, cerebral
    with infarction I63.5- ☑
  cervical canal — *see* Stricture, cervix
  cervix (uteri) — *see* Stricture, cervix
  choanal Q30.0
  choroidal (artery) — *see* Occlusion, artery, precerebral, specified NEC
  colon — *see* Obstruction, intestine
  communicating posterior artery — *see* Occlusion, artery, precerebral, specified NEC
  coronary (artery) (vein) (thrombotic) — *see also* Infarct, myocardium
    chronic total I25.82
    healed or old I25.2
    not resulting in infarction I24.0
    total (chronic) I25.82
  cystic duct — *see* Obstruction, gallbladder
  embolic — *see* Embolism
  fallopian tube N97.1
    congenital Q50.6
  gallbladder — *see also* Obstruction, gallbladder
    congenital (causing jaundice) Q44.1
  gingiva, traumatic K06.2
  hymen N89.6
    congenital Q52.3
  hypophyseal (artery) — *see* Occlusion, artery, precerebral, specified NEC
  iliac artery I74.5
  intestine — *see* Obstruction, intestine
  lacrimal passages — *see* Obstruction, lacrimal
  lung J98.4
  lymph or lymphatic channel I89.0
  mammary duct N64.89
  mesenteric artery (embolic) (thrombotic) — *see also* Infarct, intestine K55.069
  nose J34.89
    congenital Q30.0
  organ or site, congenital NEC — *see* Atresia, by site
  oviduct N97.1
    congenital Q50.6
  peripheral arteries
    due to stricture or stenosis I77.1
    upper extremity I74.2
  pontine (artery) — *see* Occlusion, artery, precerebral, specified NEC
  posterior lingual, of mandibular teeth M26.29
  precerebral artery — *see* Occlusion, artery, precerebral
  punctum lacrimale — *see* Obstruction, lacrimal
  pupil — *see* Membrane, pupillary
  pylorus, adult — *see also* Stricture, pylorus K31.1

Occlusion, occluded — *continued*
　renal artery N28.0
　retina, retinal
　　artery — *see* Occlusion, artery, retinal
　　vein (central) H34.81- ☑
　　　engorgement H34.82- ☑
　　　tributary H34.83- ☑
　　vessels H34.9
　spinal artery — *see* Occlusion, artery, precerebral, vertebral
　teeth (mandibular) (posterior lingual) M26.29
　thoracic duct I89.0
　thrombotic — *see* Thrombosis, artery
　traumatic
　　edentulous (alveolar) ridge K06.2
　　gingiva K06.2
　　periodontal K05.5
　tubal N97.1
　ureter (complete) (partial) N13.5
　　congenital Q62.10
　ureteropelvic junction N13.5
　　congenital Q62.11
　ureterovesical orifice N13.5
　　congenital Q62.12
　urethra — *see* Stricture, urethra
　uterus N85.8
　vagina N89.5
　vascular NEC I99.8
　vein — *see* Thrombosis
　　retinal — *see* Occlusion, retinal, vein
　vena cava (inferior) (superior) — *see* Embolism, vena cava
　ventricle (brain) NEC G91.1
　vertebral (artery) — *see* Occlusion, artery, vertebral
　vessel (blood) I99.8
　vulva N90.5
Occult
　blood in feces (stools) R19.5
Occupational
　problems NEC Z56.89
Ochlophobia — *see* Agoraphobia
Ochronosis (endogenous) E70.29
Ocular muscle — *see* condition
Oculogyric crisis or disturbance H51.8
　psychogenic F45.8
Oculomotor syndrome H51.9
Oculopathy
　syphilitic NEC A52.71
　　congenital
　　　early A50.01
　　　late A50.30
　　early (secondary) A51.43
　　late A52.71
Oddi's sphincter spasm K83.4
Odontalgia K08.89
Odontoameloblastoma — *see* Cyst, calcifying odontogenic
Odontoclasia K03.89
Odontodysplasia, regional K00.4
Odontogenesis imperfecta K00.5
Odontoma (ameloblastic) (complex) (compound) (fibroameloblastic) — *see* Cyst, calcifying odontogenic
Odontomyelitis (closed) (open) K04.01
　irreversible K04.02
　reversible K04.01
Odontorrhagia K08.89
Odontosarcoma, ameloblastic C41.1
　upper jaw (bone) C41.0
Oestriasis — *see* Myiasis
Oguchi's disease H53.63
Ohara's disease — *see* Tularemia
OHS (obesity hypoventilation syndrome) E66.2
Oidiomycosis — *see* Candidiasis
Oidium albicans infection — *see* Candidiasis
Old age (without mention of debility) R54
　dementia F03 ☑
Old (previous) **myocardial infarction** I25.2
Olfactory — *see* condition
Oligemia — *see* Anemia
Oligoastrocytoma
　specified site — *see* Neoplasm, malignant, by site
　unspecified site C71.9
Oligocythemia D64.9
Oligodendroblastoma
　specified site — *see* Neoplasm, malignant
　unspecified site C71.9

Oligodendroglioma
　anaplastic type
　　specified site — *see* Neoplasm, malignant, by site
　　unspecified site C71.9
　specified site — *see* Neoplasm, malignant, by site
　unspecified site C71.9
Oligodontia — *see* Anodontia
Oligoencephalon Q02
Oligohidrosis L74.4
Oligohydramnios O41.0- ☑
Oligohydrosis L74.4
Oligomenorrhea N91.5
　primary N91.3
　secondary N91.4
Oligophrenia — *see also* Disability, intellectual
　phenylpyruvic E70.0
Oligospermia N46.11
　due to
　　drug therapy N46.121
　　efferent duct obstruction N46.123
　　infection N46.122
　　radiation N46.124
　　specified cause NEC N46.129
　　systemic disease N46.125
Oligotrichia — *see* Alopecia
Oliguria R34
　with, complicating or following ectopic or molar pregnancy O08.4
　postprocedural N99.0
Ollier's disease Q78.4
Omenotocele — *see* Hernia, abdomen, specified site NEC
Omentitis — *see* Peritonitis
Omentum, omental — *see* condition
Omphalitis (congenital) (newborn) P38.9
　with mild hemorrhage P38.1
　without hemorrhage P38.9
　not of newborn L08.82
　tetanus A33
Omphalocele Q79.2
Omphalomesenteric duct, persistent Q43.0
Omphalorrhagia, newborn P51.9
Omsk hemorrhagic fever A98.1
Onanism (excessive) F98.8
Onchocerciasis, onchocercosis B73.1
　with
　　eye disease B73.00
　　　endophthalmitis B73.01
　　　eyelid B73.09
　　　glaucoma B73.02
　　　specified NEC B73.09
　　eyelid B73.09
　　eye NEC B73.00
Oncocytoma — *see* Neoplasm, benign, by site
Oncovirus, as cause of disease classified elsewhere B97.32
Ondine's curse — *see* Apnea, sleep
Oneirophrenia F23
Onychauxis L60.2
　congenital Q84.5
Onychia — *see also* Cellulitis, digit
　with lymphangitis — *see* Lymphangitis, acute, digit
　candidal B37.2
　dermatophytic B35.1
Onychitis — *see also* Cellulitis, digit
　with lymphangitis — *see* Lymphangitis, acute, digit
Onychocryptosis L60.0
Onychodystrophy L60.3
　congenital Q84.6
Onychogryphosis, onychogryposis L60.2
Onycholysis L60.1
Onychomadesis L60.8
Onychomalacia L60.3
Onychomycosis (finger) (toe) B35.1
Onycho-osteodysplasia Q87.2
Onychophagia F98.8
Onychophosis L60.8
Onychoptosis L60.8
Onychorrhexis L60.3
　congenital Q84.6
Onychoschizia L60.3
Onyxis (finger) (toe) L60.0
Onyxitis — *see also* Cellulitis, digit
　with lymphangitis — *see* Lymphangitis, acute, digit
Oophoritis (cystic) (infectional) (interstitial) N70.92
　with salpingitis N70.93
　acute N70.02
　　with salpingitis N70.03

Oophoritis — *continued*
　chronic N70.12
　　with salpingitis N70.13
　complicating abortion — *see* Abortion, by type, complicated by, oophoritis
Oophorocele N83.4- ☑
Opacity, opacities
　cornea H17.- ☑
　　central H17.1- ☑
　　congenital Q13.3
　　degenerative — *see* Degeneration, cornea
　　hereditary — *see* Dystrophy, cornea
　　inflammatory — *see* Keratitis
　　minor H17.81- ☑
　　peripheral H17.82- ☑
　　sequelae of trachoma (healed) B94.0
　　specified NEC H17.89
　enamel (teeth) (fluoride) (nonfluoride) K00.3
　lens — *see* Cataract
　snowball — *see* Deposit, crystalline
　vitreous (humor) NEC H43.39- ☑
　　congenital Q14.0
　　membranes and strands H43.31- ☑
Opalescent dentin (hereditary) K00.5
Open, opening
　abnormal, organ or site, congenital — *see* Imperfect, closure
　angle with
　　borderline
　　　findings
　　　　high risk H40.02- ☑
　　　　low risk H40.01- ☑
　　　　intraocular pressure H40.00- ☑
　　cupping of discs H40.01- ☑
　　glaucoma (primary) — *see* Glaucoma, open angle
　bite
　　anterior M26.220
　　posterior M26.221
　false — *see* Imperfect, closure
　margin on tooth restoration K08.51
　restoration margins of tooth K08.51
　wound — *see* Wound, open
Operational fatigue F48.8
Operative — *see* condition
Operculitis — *see* Periodontitis
Operculum — *see* Break, retina
Ophiasis L63.2
Ophthalmia — *see also* Conjunctivitis H10.9
　actinic rays — *see* Photokeratitis
　allergic (acute) — *see* Conjunctivitis, acute, atopic
　blennorrhagic (gonococcal) (neonatorum) A54.31
　diphtheritic A36.86
　Egyptian A71.1
　electrica — *see* Photokeratitis
　gonococcal (neonatorum) A54.31
　metastatic — *see* Endophthalmitis, purulent
　migraine — *see* Migraine, ophthalmoplegic
　neonatorum, newborn P39.1
　　gonococcal A54.31
　nodosa H16.24- ☑
　purulent — *see* Conjunctivitis, acute, mucopurulent
　spring — *see* Conjunctivitis, acute, atopic
　sympathetic — *see* Uveitis, sympathetic
Ophthalmitis — *see* Ophthalmia
Ophthalmocele (congenital) Q15.8
Ophthalmoneuromyelitis G36.0
Ophthalmoplegia — *see also* Strabismus, paralytic
　anterior internuclear — *see* Ophthalmoplegia, internuclear
　ataxia-areflexia G61.0
　diabetic — *see* E08-E13 with .39
　exophthalmic E05.00
　　with thyroid storm E05.01
　external H49.88- ☑
　　progressive H49.4- ☑
　　　with pigmentary retinopathy — *see* Kearns-Sayre syndrome
　　total H49.3- ☑
　internal (complete) (total) H52.51- ☑
　internuclear H51.2- ☑
　migraine — *see* Migraine, ophthalmoplegic
　Parinaud's H49.88- ☑
　progressive external — *see* Ophthalmoplegia, external, progressive
　supranuclear, progressive G23.1
　total (external) — *see* Ophthalmoplegia, external, total

Opioid(s)
  abuse — *see* Abuse, drug, opioids
  dependence — *see* Dependence, drug, opioids
  induced, without use disorder
    anxiety disorder F11.988
    delirium F11.921
    depressive disorder F11.94
    sexual dysfunction F11.981
    sleep disorder F11.982
Opisthognathism M26.09
Opisthorchiasis (felineus) (viverrini) B66.0
Opitz' disease D73.2
Opiumism — *see* Dependence, drug, opioid
Oppenheim's disease G70.2
Oppenheim-Urbach disease (necrobiosis lipoidica diabeticorum) — *see* E08-E13 with .620
Optic nerve — *see* condition
Orbit — *see* condition
Orchioblastoma C62.9- ☑
Orchitis (gangrenous) (nonspecific) (septic) (suppurative) N45.2
  blennorrhagic (gonococcal) (acute) (chronic) A54.23
  chlamydial A56.19
  filarial — *see also* Infestation, filarial B74.9 *[N51]*
  gonococcal (acute) (chronic) A54.23
  mumps B26.0
  syphilitic A52.76
  tuberculous A18.15
Orf (virus disease) B08.02
Organic — *see also* condition
  brain syndrome F09
  heart — *see* Disease, heart
  mental disorder F09
  psychosis F09
Orgasm
  anejaculatory N53.13
Oriental
  bilharziasis B65.2
  schistosomiasis B65.2
Orifice — *see* condition
Origin of both great vessels from right ventricle Q20.1
Ormond's disease (with ureteral obstruction) N13.5
  with infection N13.6
Ornithine metabolism disorder E72.4
Ornithinemia (Type I) (Type II) E72.4
Ornithosis A70
Orotaciduria, oroticaciduria (congenital) (hereditary) (pyrimidine deficiency) E79.8
  anemia D53.0
Orthodontics
  adjustment Z46.4
  fitting Z46.4
Orthopnea R06.01
Orthopoxvirus B08.09
Os, uterus — *see* condition
Osgood-Schlatter disease or osteochondrosis M92.52- ☑
Osler (-Weber)-**Rendu disease** I78.0
Osler's nodes I33.0
Osmidrosis L75.0
Osseous — *see* condition
Ossification
  artery — *see* Arteriosclerosis
  auricle (ear) — *see* Disorder, pinna, specified type NEC
  bronchial J98.09
  cardiac — *see* Degeneration, myocardial
  cartilage (senile) — *see* Disorder, cartilage, specified type NEC
  coronary (artery) — *see* Disease, heart, ischemic, atherosclerotic
  diaphragm J98.6
  ear, middle — *see* Otosclerosis
  falx cerebri G96.198
  fontanel, premature Q75.0
  heart — *see also* Degeneration, myocardial
    valve — *see* Endocarditis
  larynx J38.7
  ligament — *see* Disorder, tendon, specified type NEC
    posterior longitudinal — *see* Spondylopathy, specified NEC
  meninges (cerebral) (spinal) G96.198
  multiple, eccentric centers — *see* Disorder, bone, development or growth
  muscle — *see also* Calcification, muscle
    due to burns — *see* Myositis, ossificans, in, burns
    paralytic — *see* Myositis, ossificans, in, quadriplegia

Ossification — *continued*
  muscle — *see also* Calcification, muscle — *continued*
    progressive — *see* Myositis, ossificans, progressiva
    specified NEC M61.50
      ankle M61.57- ☑
      foot M61.57- ☑
      forearm M61.53- ☑
      hand M61.54- ☑
      lower leg M61.56- ☑
      multiple sites M61.59
      pelvic region M61.55- ☑
      shoulder region M61.51- ☑
      specified site NEC M61.58
      thigh M61.55- ☑
      upper arm M61.52- ☑
    traumatic — *see* Myositis, ossificans, traumatica
  myocardium, myocardial — *see* Degeneration, myocardial
  penis N48.89
  periarticular — *see* Disorder, joint, specified type NEC
  pinna — *see* Disorder, pinna, specified type NEC
  rider's bone — *see* Ossification, muscle, specified NEC
  sclera H15.89
  subperiosteal, post-traumatic M89.8X- ☑
  tendon — *see* Disorder, tendon, specified type NEC
  trachea J39.8
  tympanic membrane — *see* Disorder, tympanic membrane, specified NEC
  vitreous (humor) — *see* Deposit, crystalline
Osteitis — *see also* Osteomyelitis
  alveolar M27.3
  condensans M85.30
    ankle M85.37- ☑
    foot M85.37- ☑
    forearm M85.33- ☑
    hand M85.34- ☑
    lower leg M85.36- ☑
    multiple site M85.39
    neck M85.38
    rib M85.38
    shoulder M85.31- ☑
    skull M85.38
    specified site NEC M85.38
    thigh M85.35- ☑
    toe M85.37- ☑
    upper arm M85.32- ☑
    vertebra M85.38
  deformans M88.9
    in (due to)
      malignant neoplasm of bone C41.9 *[M90.60]*
      neoplastic disease — *see also* Neoplasm D49.9 *[M90.60]*
        carpus D49.9 *[M90.64-]* ☑
        clavicle D49.9 *[M90.61-]* ☑
        femur D49.9 *[M90.65-]* ☑
        fibula D49.9 *[M90.66-]* ☑
        finger D49.9 *[M90.64-]* ☑
        humerus D49.9 *[M90.62-]* ☑
        ilium D49.9 *[M90.65-]* ☑
        ischium D49.9 *[M90.65-]* ☑
        metacarpus D49.9 *[M90.64-]* ☑
        metatarsus D49.9 *[M90.67-]* ☑
        multiple sites D49.9 *[M90.69]*
        neck D49.9 *[M90.68]*
        radius D49.9 *[M90.63-]* ☑
        rib D49.9 *[M90.68]*
        scapula D49.9 *[M90.61-]* ☑
        skull D49.9 *[M90.68]*
        tarsus D49.9 *[M90.67-]* ☑
        tibia D49.9 *[M90.66-]* ☑
        toe D49.9 *[M90.67-]* ☑
        ulna D49.9 *[M90.63-]* ☑
        vertebra D49.9 *[M90.68]*
    skull M88.0
    specified NEC — *see* Paget's disease, bone, by site
    vertebra M88.1
  due to yaws A66.6
  fibrosa NEC — *see* Cyst, bone, by site
    circumscripta — *see* Dysplasia, fibrous, bone NEC
    cystica (generalisata) E21.0
    disseminata Q78.1
    osteoplastica E21.0
  fragilitans Q78.0
  Garr's (sclerosing) — *see* Osteomyelitis, specified type NEC

Osteitis — *continued*
  jaw (acute) (chronic) (lower) (suppurative) (upper) M27.2
  parathyroid E21.0
  petrous bone (acute) (chronic) — *see* Petrositis
  sclerotic, nonsuppurative — *see* Osteomyelitis, specified type NEC
  tuberculosa A18.09
    cystica D86.89
    multiplex cystoides D86.89
Osteoarthritis M19.90
  ankle M19.07- ☑
  elbow M19.02- ☑
  foot joint M19.07- ☑
  generalized (multiple joints) M15.9
    erosive M15.4
    primary M15.0
    specified NEC M15.8
  hand joint M19.04- ☑
    first carpometacarpal joint M18.9
  hip M16.1- ☑
    bilateral M16.0
    due to hip dysplasia (unilateral) M16.3- ☑
      bilateral M16.2
  interphalangeal
    distal (Heberden) M15.1
    proximal (Bouchard) M15.2
  knee M17.1- ☑
    bilateral M17.0
  post-traumatic NEC M19.92
    ankle M19.17- ☑
    elbow M19.12- ☑
    foot joint M19.17- ☑
    hand joint M19.14- ☑
      first carpometacarpal joint M18.3- ☑
        bilateral M18.2
    hip M16.5- ☑
      bilateral M16.4
    knee M17.3- ☑
      bilateral M17.2
    shoulder M19.11- ☑
    specified site NEC M19.19
    wrist M19.13- ☑
  primary M19.91
    ankle M19.07- ☑
    elbow M19.02- ☑
    foot joint M19.07- ☑
    hand joint M19.04- ☑
      first carpometacarpal joint M18.1- ☑
        bilateral M18.0
    hip M16.1- ☑
      bilateral M16.0
    knee M17.1- ☑
      bilateral M17.0
    multiple sites M15.9
    shoulder M19.01- ☑
    spine — *see* Spondylosis
    wrist M19.03- ☑
  secondary M19.93
    ankle M19.27- ☑
    elbow M19.22- ☑
    foot joint M19.27- ☑
    hand joint M19.24- ☑
      first carpometacarpal joint M18.5- ☑
        bilateral M18.4
    hip M16.7
      bilateral M16.6
    knee M17.5
      bilateral M17.4
    multiple M15.3
    shoulder M19.21- ☑
    specified site NEC M19.29
    spine — *see* Spondylosis
    wrist M19.23- ☑
  shoulder M19.01- ☑
  specified site NEC M19.09
  spine — *see* Spondylosis
  wrist M19.03- ☑
Osteoarthropathy (hypertrophic) M19.90
  ankle — *see* Osteoarthritis, primary, ankle
  elbow — *see* Osteoarthritis, primary, elbow
  foot joint — *see* Osteoarthritis, primary, foot
  hand joint — *see* Osteoarthritis, primary, hand joint
  knee joint — *see* Osteoarthritis, primary, knee
  multiple site — *see* Osteoarthritis, primary, multiple joint

Osteoarthropathy — *continued*
  pulmonary — *see also* Osteoarthropathy, specified
      type NEC
    hypertrophic — *see* Osteoarthropathy, hypertrophic,
        specified type NEC
  secondary — *see* Osteoarthropathy, specified type NEC
  secondary hypertrophic — *see* Osteoarthropathy,
      specified type NEC
  shoulder — *see* Osteoarthritis, primary, shoulder
  specified joint NEC — *see* Osteoarthritis, primary,
      specified joint NEC
  specified type NEC M89.40
    carpus M89.44- ☑
    clavicle M89.41- ☑
    femur M89.45- ☑
    fibula M89.46- ☑
    finger M89.44- ☑
    humerus M89.42- ☑
    ilium M89.459
    ischium M89.459
    metacarpus M89.44- ☑
    metatarsus M89.47- ☑
    multiple sites M89.49
    neck M89.48
    radius M89.43- ☑
    rib M89.48
    scapula M89.41- ☑
    skull M89.48
    tarsus M89.47- ☑
    tibia M89.46- ☑
    toe M89.47- ☑
    ulna M89.43- ☑
    vertebra M89.48
  spine — *see* Spondylosis
  wrist — *see* Osteoarthritis, primary, wrist
Osteoarthrosis (degenerative) (hypertrophic) (joint) —
    see also Osteoarthritis
  deformans alkaptonurica E70.29 *[M36.8]*
  erosive M15.4
  generalized M15.9
    primary M15.0
  polyarticular M15.9
  spine — *see* Spondylosis
Osteoblastoma — *see* Neoplasm, bone, benign
  aggressive — *see* Neoplasm, bone, uncertain behavior
Osteochondritis — *see also* Osteochondropathy, by site
  Brailsford's — *see* Osteochondrosis, juvenile, radius
  dissecans M93.20
    ankle M93.27- ☑
    elbow M93.22- ☑
    foot M93.27- ☑
    hand M93.24- ☑
    hip M93.25- ☑
    knee M93.26- ☑
    multiple sites M93.29
    shoulder joint M93.21- ☑
    specified site NEC M93.28
    wrist M93.23- ☑
  juvenile M92.9
  patellar — *see* Osteochondrosis, juvenile, patella
  syphilitic (congenital) (early) A50.02 *[M90.80]*
    ankle A50.02 *[M90.87-]* ☑
    elbow A50.02 *[M90.82-]* ☑
    foot A50.02 *[M90.87-]* ☑
    forearm A50.02 *[M90.83-]* ☑
    hand A50.02 *[M90.84-]* ☑
    hip A50.02 *[M90.85-]* ☑
    knee A50.02 *[M90.86-]* ☑
    multiple sites A50.02 *[M90.89]*
    shoulder joint A50.02 *[M90.81-]* ☑
    specified site NEC A50.02 *[M90.88]*
Osteochondroarthrosis deformans endemica — *see*
    Disease, Kaschin-Beck
Osteochondrodysplasia Q78.9
  with defects of growth of tubular bones and spine
      Q77.9
    specified NEC Q77.8
  specified NEC Q78.8
Osteochondrodystrophy E78.9
Osteochondrolysis — *see* Osteochondritis, dissecans
Osteochondroma — *see* Neoplasm, bone, benign
Osteochondromatosis D48.0
  syndrome Q78.4
Osteochondromyxosarcoma — *see* Neoplasm, bone,
    malignant
Osteochondropathy M93.90
  ankle M93.97- ☑

Osteochondropathy — *continued*
  elbow M93.92- ☑
  foot M93.97- ☑
  hand M93.94- ☑
  hip M93.95- ☑
  Kienböck's disease of adults M93.1
  knee M93.96- ☑
  multiple joints M93.99
  osteochondritis dissecans — *see* Osteochondritis, dis-
      secans
  osteochondrosis — *see* Osteochondrosis
  shoulder region M93.91- ☑
  slipped upper femoral epiphysis — *see* Slipped, epiph-
      ysis, upper femoral
  specified joint NEC M93.98
  specified type NEC M93.80
    ankle M93.87- ☑
    elbow M93.82- ☑
    foot M93.87- ☑
    hand M93.84- ☑
    hip M93.85- ☑
    knee M93.86- ☑
    multiple joints M93.89
    shoulder region M93.81- ☑
    specified joint NEC M93.88
    wrist M93.83- ☑
  syphilitic, congenital
    early A50.02 *[M90.80]*
    late A50.56 *[M90.80]*
  wrist M93.93- ☑
Osteochondrosarcoma — *see* Neoplasm, bone, malig-
    nant
Osteochondrosis — *see also* Osteochondropathy, by
    site
  acetabulum (juvenile) M91.0
  adult — *see* Osteochondropathy, specified type NEC,
      by site
  astragalus (juvenile) — *see* Osteochondrosis, juvenile,
      tarsus
  Blount M92.51- ☑
  Buchanan's M91.0
  Burns' — *see* Osteochondrosis, juvenile, ulna
  calcaneus (juvenile) — *see* Osteochondrosis, juvenile,
      tarsus
  capitular epiphysis (femur) (juvenile) — *see* Legg-Calvé-
      Perthes disease
  carpal (juvenile) (lunate) (scaphoid) — *see* Osteochon-
      drosis, juvenile, hand, carpal lunate
    adult M93.1
  coxa juvenilis — *see* Legg-Calvé-Perthes disease
  deformans juvenilis, coxae — *see* Legg-Calvé-Perthes
      disease
  Diaz's — *see* Osteochondrosis, juvenile, tarsus
  dissecans (knee) (shoulder) — *see* Osteochondritis,
      dissecans
  femoral capital epiphysis (juvenile) — *see* Legg-Calvé-
      Perthes disease
  femur (head), juvenile — *see* Legg-Calvé-Perthes dis-
      ease
  fibula (juvenile) — *see* Osteochondrosis, juvenile,
      fibula
  foot NEC (juvenile) M92.8
  Freiberg's — *see* Osteochondrosis, juvenile, metatarsus
  Haas' (juvenile) — *see* Osteochondrosis, juvenile,
      humerus
  Haglund's — *see* Osteochondrosis, juvenile, tarsus
  hip (juvenile) — *see* Legg-Calvé-Perthes disease
  humerus (capitulum) (head) (juvenile) — *see* Osteo-
      chondrosis, juvenile, humerus
  ilium, iliac crest (juvenile) M91.0
  ischiopubic synchondrosis M91.0
  Iselin's — *see* Osteochondrosis, juvenile, metatarsus
  juvenile, juvenilis M92.9
    after congenital dislocation of hip reduction — *see*
        Osteochondrosis, juvenile, hip, specified NEC
    arm — *see* Osteochondrosis, juvenile, upper limb
        NEC
    capitular epiphysis (femur) — *see* Legg-Calvé-
        Perthes disease
    clavicle, sternal epiphysis — *see* Osteochondrosis,
        juvenile, upper limb NEC
    coxae — *see* Legg-Calvé-Perthes disease
    deformans M92.9
    fibula M92.50- ☑
    foot NEC M92.8
    hand M92.20- ☑
      carpal lunate M92.21- ☑

Osteochondrosis — *continued*
  juvenile, juvenilis — *continued*
    hand — *continued*
      metacarpal head M92.22- ☑
      specified site NEC M92.29- ☑
    head of femur — *see* Legg-Calvé-Perthes disease
    hip and pelvis M91.9- ☑
      coxa plana — *see* Coxa, plana
      femoral head — *see* Legg-Calvé-Perthes disease
      pelvis M91.0
      pseudocoxalgia — *see* Pseudocoxalgia
      specified NEC M91.8- ☑
    humerus M92.0- ☑
    limb
      lower NEC M92.8
      upper NEC — *see* Osteochondrosis, juvenile,
          upper limb NEC
    medial cuneiform bone — *see* Osteochondrosis,
        juvenile, tarsus
    metatarsus M92.7- ☑
    patella M92.4- ☑
    radius M92.1- ☑
    specified
      site NEC M92.8
      type NEC M92.8
        tibia and fibula M92.59- ☑
    spine M42.00
      cervical region M42.02
      cervicothoracic region M42.03
      lumbar region M42.06
      lumbosacral region M42.07
      multiple sites M42.09
      occipito-atlanto-axial region M42.01
      sacrococcygeal region M42.08
      thoracic region M42.04
      thoracolumbar region M42.05
    tarsus M92.6- ☑
    tibia M92.50- ☑
      proximal M92.51- ☑
      tubercle M92.52- ☑
    ulna M92.1- ☑
    upper limb NEC M92.3- ☑
    vertebra (body) (epiphyseal plates) (Calvé's)
        (Scheuermann's) — *see* Osteochondrosis, ju-
        venile, spine
  Kienböck's — *see* Osteochondrosis, juvenile, hand,
      carpal lunate
    adult M93.1
  Köhler's
    patellar — *see* Osteochondrosis, juvenile, patella
    tarsal navicular — *see* Osteochondrosis, juvenile,
        tarsus
  Legg-Perthes (-Calvé)(-Waldenström) — *see* Legg-
      Calvé-Perthes disease
  limb
    lower NEC (juvenile) M92.8
      tibia and fibula M92.59- ☑
    upper NEC (juvenile) — *see* Osteochondrosis, juve-
        nile, upper limb NEC
  lunate bone (carpal) (juvenile) — *see also* Osteochon-
      drosis, juvenile, hand, carpal lunate
    adult M93.1
  Mauclaire's — *see* Osteochondrosis, juvenile, hand,
      metacarpal
  metacarpal (head) (juvenile) — *see* Osteochondrosis,
      juvenile, hand, metacarpal
  metatarsus (fifth) (head) (juvenile) (second) — *see* Os-
      teochondrosis, juvenile, metatarsus
  navicular (juvenile) — *see* Osteochondrosis, juvenile,
      tarsus
  os
    calcis (juvenile) — *see* Osteochondrosis, juvenile,
        tarsus
    tibiale externum (juvenile) — *see* Osteochondrosis,
        juvenile, tarsus
  Osgood-Schlatter M92.52- ☑
  Panner's — *see* Osteochondrosis, juvenile, humerus
  patellar center (juvenile) (primary) (secondary) — *see*
      Osteochondrosis, juvenile, patella
  pelvis (juvenile) M91.0
  Pierson's M91.0
  radius (head) (juvenile) — *see* Osteochondrosis, juve-
      nile, radius
  Scheuermann's — *see* Osteochondrosis, juvenile, spine
  Sever's — *see* Osteochondrosis, juvenile, tarsus
  Sinding-Larsen — *see* Osteochondrosis, juvenile,
      patella

☑ **Additional Character Required** — Refer to the Tabular List for Character Selection   ▽ **Subterms under main terms may continue to next column or page**

Osteochondrosis — continued
  spine M42.9
    adult M42.10
      cervical region M42.12
      cervicothoracic region M42.13
      lumbar region M42.16
      lumbosacral region M42.17
      multiple sites M42.19
      occipito-atlanto-axial region M42.11
      sacrococcygeal region M42.18
      thoracic region M42.14
      thoracolumbar region M42.15
    juvenile — see Osteochondrosis, juvenile, spine
  symphysis pubis (juvenile) M91.0
  syphilitic (congenital) A50.02
  talus (juvenile) — see Osteochondrosis, juvenile, tarsus
  tarsus (navicular) (juvenile) — see Osteochondrosis, juvenile, tarsus
  tibia (proximal) (tubercle) (juvenile) — see Osteochondrosis, juvenile, tibia
  tuberculous — see Tuberculosis, bone
  ulna (lower) (juvenile) — see Osteochondrosis, juvenile, ulna
  van Neck's M91.0
  vertebral — see Osteochondrosis, spine
Osteoclastoma D48.0
  malignant — see Neoplasm, bone, malignant
Osteodynia — see Disorder, bone, specified type NEC
Osteodystrophy Q78.9
  azotemic N25.0
  congenital Q78.9
  parathyroid, secondary E21.1
  renal N25.0
Osteofibroma — see Neoplasm, bone, benign
Osteofibrosarcoma — see Neoplasm, bone, malignant
Osteogenesis imperfecta Q78.0
Osteogenic — see condition
Osteolysis M89.50
  carpus M89.54-
  clavicle M89.51-
  femur M89.55-
  fibula M89.56-
  finger M89.54-
  humerus M89.52-
  ilium M89.559
  ischium M89.559
  joint prosthesis (periprosthetic) — see Complications, joint prosthesis, mechanical, periprosthetic, osteolysis, by site
  metacarpus M89.54-
  metatarsus M89.57-
  multiple sites M89.59
  neck M89.58
  periprosthetic — see Complications, joint prosthesis, mechanical, periprosthetic, osteolysis, by site
  radius M89.53-
  rib M89.58
  scapula M89.51-
  skull M89.58
  tarsus M89.57-
  tibia M89.56-
  toe M89.57-
  ulna M89.53-
  vertebra M89.58
Osteoma — see also Neoplasm, bone, benign
  osteoid — see also Neoplasm, bone, benign
    giant — see Neoplasm, bone, benign
Osteomalacia M83.9
  adult M83.9
    drug-induced NEC M83.5
    due to
      malabsorption (postsurgical) M83.2
      malnutrition M83.3
    specified NEC M83.8
  aluminium-induced M83.4
  infantile — see Rickets
  juvenile — see Rickets
  oncogenic E83.89
  pelvis M83.8
  puerperal M83.0
  senile M83.1
  vitamin-D-resistant in adults E83.31 [M90.8-]
    carpus E83.31 [M90.84-]
    clavicle E83.31 [M90.81-]
    femur E83.31 [M90.85-]
    fibula E83.31 [M90.86-]
    finger E83.31 [M90.84-]

Osteomalacia — continued
  vitamin-D-resistant in adults — continued
    humerus E83.31 [M90.82-]
    ilium E83.31 [M90.859]
    ischium E83.31 [M90.859]
    metacarpus E83.31 [M90.84-]
    metatarsus E83.31 [M90.87-]
    multiple sites E83.31 [M90.89]
    neck E83.31 [M90.88]
    radius E83.31 [M90.83-]
    rib E83.31 [M90.88]
    scapula E83.31 [M90.819]
    skull E83.31 [M90.88]
    tarsus E83.31 [M90.879]
    tibia E83.31 [M90.869]
    toe E83.31 [M90.879]
    ulna E83.31 [M90.839]
    vertebra E83.31 [M90.88]
Osteomyelitis (general) (infective) (localized) (neonatal) (purulent) (septic) (staphylococcal) (streptococcal) (suppurative) (with periostitis) M86.9
  acute M86.10
    carpus M86.14-
    clavicle M86.11-
    femur M86.15-
    fibula M86.16-
    finger M86.14-
    hematogenous M86.00
      carpus M86.04-
      clavicle M86.01-
      femur M86.05-
      fibula M86.06-
      finger M86.04-
      humerus M86.02-
      ilium M86.08
      ischium M86.08
      mandible M27.2
      metacarpus M86.04-
      metatarsus M86.07-
      multiple sites M86.09
      neck M86.08
      orbit H05.02-
      petrous bone — see Petrositis
      radius M86.03-
      rib M86.08
      scapula M86.01-
      skull M86.08
      tarsus M86.07-
      tibia M86.06-
      toe M86.07-
      ulna M86.03-
      vertebra — see Osteomyelitis, vertebra
    humerus M86.12-
    ilium M86.18
    ischium M86.18
    mandible M27.2
    metacarpus M86.14-
    metatarsus M86.17-
    multiple sites M86.19
    neck M86.18
    orbit H05.02-
    petrous bone — see Petrositis
    radius M86.13-
    rib M86.18
    scapula M86.11-
    skull M86.18
    tarsus M86.17-
    tibia M86.16-
    toe M86.17-
    ulna M86.13-
    vertebra — see Osteomyelitis, vertebra
  chronic (or old) M86.60
    with draining sinus M86.40
      carpus M86.44-
      clavicle M86.41-
      femur M86.45-
      fibula M86.46-
      finger M86.44-
      humerus M86.42-
      ilium M86.459
      ischium M86.459
      mandible M27.2
      metacarpus M86.44-
      metatarsus M86.47-
      multiple sites M86.49
      neck M86.48

Osteomyelitis — continued
  chronic — continued
    with draining sinus — continued
      orbit H05.02-
      petrous bone — see Petrositis
      radius M86.43-
      rib M86.48
      scapula M86.41-
      skull M86.48
      tarsus M86.47-
      tibia M86.46-
      toe M86.47-
      ulna M86.43-
      vertebra — see Osteomyelitis, vertebra
    carpus M86.64-
    clavicle M86.61-
    femur M86.65-
    fibula M86.66-
    finger M86.64-
    hematogenous NEC M86.50
      carpus M86.54-
      clavicle M86.51-
      femur M86.55-
      fibula M86.56-
      finger M86.54-
      humerus M86.52-
      ilium M86.559
      ischium M86.559
      mandible M27.2
      metacarpus M86.54-
      metatarsus M86.57-
      multifocal M86.30
        carpus M86.34-
        clavicle M86.31-
        femur M86.35-
        fibula M86.36-
        finger M86.34-
        humerus M86.32-
        ilium M86.359
        ischium M86.359
        metacarpus M86.34-
        metatarsus M86.37-
        multiple sites M86.39
        neck M86.38
        radius M86.33-
        rib M86.38
        scapula M86.31-
        skull M86.38
        tarsus M86.37-
        tibia M86.36-
        toe M86.37-
        ulna M86.33-
        vertebra — see Osteomyelitis, vertebra
      multiple sites M86.59
      neck M86.58
      orbit H05.02-
      petrous bone — see Petrositis
      radius M86.53-
      rib M86.58
      scapula M86.51-
      skull M86.58
      tarsus M86.57-
      tibia M86.56-
      toe M86.57-
      ulna M86.53-
      vertebra — see Osteomyelitis, vertebra
    humerus M86.62-
    ilium M86.659
    ischium M86.659
    mandible M27.2
    metacarpus M86.64-
    metatarsus M86.67-
    multifocal — see Osteomyelitis, chronic, hematogenous, multifocal
    multiple sites M86.69
    neck M86.68
    orbit H05.02-
    petrous bone — see Petrositis
    radius M86.63-
    rib M86.68
    scapula M86.61-
    skull M86.68
    tarsus M86.67-
    tibia M86.66-
    toe M86.67-
    ulna M86.63-

Osteomyelitis — continued
  chronic — continued
    vertebra — see Osteomyelitis, vertebra
  echinococcal B67.2
  Garr's — see Osteomyelitis, specified type NEC
  in diabetes mellitus — see E08-E13 with .69
  jaw (acute) (chronic) (lower) (neonatal) (suppurative) (upper) M27.2
  nonsuppurating — see Osteomyelitis, specified type NEC
  orbit H05.02- ☑
  petrous bone — see Petrositis
  Salmonella (arizonae) (cholerae-suis) (enteritidis) (typhimurium) A02.24
  sclerosing, nonsuppurative — see Osteomyelitis, specified type NEC
  specified type NEC — see also subcategory M86.8X- ☑
    mandible M27.2
    orbit H05.02- ☑
    petrous bone — see Petrositis
    vertebra — see Osteomyelitis, vertebra
  subacute M86.20
    carpus M86.24- ☑
    clavicle M86.21- ☑
    femur M86.25- ☑
    fibula M86.26- ☑
    finger M86.24- ☑
    humerus M86.22- ☑
    mandible M27.2
    metacarpus M86.24- ☑
    metatarsus M86.27- ☑
    multiple sites M86.29
    neck M86.28
    orbit H05.02- ☑
    petrous bone — see Petrositis
    radius M86.23- ☑
    rib M86.28
    scapula M86.21- ☑
    skull M86.28
    tarsus M86.27- ☑
    tibia M86.26- ☑
    toe M86.27- ☑
    ulna M86.23- ☑
    vertebra — see Osteomyelitis, vertebra
  syphilitic A52.77
    congenital (early) A50.02 [M90.80]
  tuberculous — see Tuberculosis, bone
  typhoid A01.05
  vertebra M46.20
    cervical region M46.22
    cervicothoracic region M46.23
    lumbar region M46.26
    lumbosacral region M46.27
    occipito-atlanto-axial region M46.21
    sacrococcygeal region M46.28
    thoracic region M46.24
    thoracolumbar region M46.25
Osteomyelofibrosis D47.4
Osteomyelosclerosis D75.89
Osteonecrosis M87.9
  due to
    drugs — see Osteonecrosis, secondary, due to, drugs
    trauma — see Osteonecrosis, secondary, due to, trauma
  idiopathic aseptic M87.00
    ankle M87.07- ☑
    carpus M87.03- ☑
    clavicle M87.01- ☑
    femur M87.05- ☑
    fibula M87.06- ☑
    finger M87.04- ☑
    humerus M87.02- ☑
    ilium M87.050
    ischium M87.050
    metacarpus M87.04- ☑
    metatarsus M87.07- ☑
    multiple sites M87.09
    neck M87.08
    pelvis M87.050
    radius M87.03- ☑
    rib M87.08
    scapula M87.01- ☑
    skull M87.08
    tarsus M87.07- ☑
    tibia M87.06- ☑
    toe M87.07- ☑
    ulna M87.03- ☑

Osteonecrosis — continued
  idiopathic aseptic — continued
    vertebra M87.08
  secondary NEC M87.30
    carpus M87.33- ☑
    clavicle M87.31- ☑
    due to
      drugs M87.10
        carpus M87.13- ☑
        clavicle M87.11- ☑
        femur M87.15- ☑
        fibula M87.16- ☑
        finger M87.14- ☑
        humerus M87.12- ☑
        ilium M87.159
        ischium M87.159
        jaw M87.180
        metacarpus M87.14- ☑
        metatarsus M87.17- ☑
        multiple sites M87.19
        neck M87.18 ☑
        radius M87.13- ☑
        rib M87.18 ☑
        scapula M87.11- ☑
        skull M87.18 ☑
        tarsus M87.17- ☑
        tibia M87.16- ☑
        toe M87.17- ☑
        ulna M87.13- ☑
        vertebra M87.18 ☑
      hemoglobinopathy NEC D58.2 [M90.50]
        carpus D58.2 [M90.54-] ☑
        clavicle D58.2 [M90.51-] ☑
        femur D58.2 [M90.55-] ☑
        fibula D58.2 [M90.56-] ☑
        finger D58.2 [M90.54-] ☑
        humerus D58.2 [M90.52-] ☑
        ilium D58.2 [M90.55-] ☑
        ischium D58.2 [M90.55-] ☑
        metacarpus D58.2 [M90.54-] ☑
        metatarsus D58.2 [M90.57-] ☑
        multiple sites D58.2 [M90.58]
        neck D58.2 [M90.58]
        radius D58.2 [M90.53-] ☑
        rib D58.2 [M90.58]
        scapula D58.2 [M90.51-] ☑
        skull D58.2 [M90.58]
        tarsus D58.2 [M90.57-] ☑
        tibia D58.2 [M90.56-] ☑
        toe D58.2 [M90.57-] ☑
        ulna D58.2 [M90.53-] ☑
        vertebra D58.2 [M90.58]
      trauma (previous) M87.20
        carpus M87.23- ☑
        clavicle M87.21- ☑
        femur M87.25- ☑
        fibula M87.26- ☑
        finger M87.24- ☑
        humerus M87.22- ☑
        ilium M87.25- ☑
        ischium M87.25- ☑
        metacarpus M87.24- ☑
        metatarsus M87.27- ☑
        multiple sites M87.29
        neck M87.28
        radius M87.23- ☑
        rib M87.28
        scapula M87.21- ☑
        skull M87.28
        tarsus M87.27- ☑
        tibia M87.26- ☑
        toe M87.27- ☑
        ulna M87.23- ☑
        vertebra M87.28
    femur M87.35- ☑
    fibula M87.36- ☑
    finger M87.34- ☑
    humerus M87.32- ☑
    ilium M87.350
    in
      caisson disease T70.3 ☑ [M90.50]
        carpus T70.3 ☑ [M90.54-] ☑
        clavicle T70.3 ☑ [M90.51-] ☑
        femur T70.3 ☑ [M90.55-] ☑
        fibula T70.3 ☑ [M90.56-] ☑
        finger T70.3 ☑ [M90.54-] ☑

Osteonecrosis — continued
  secondary — continued
    in — continued
      caisson disease — continued
        humerus T70.3 ☑ [M90.52-] ☑
        ilium T70.3 ☑ [M90.55-]
        ischium T70.3 ☑ [M90.55-]
        metacarpus T70.3 ☑ [M90.54-] ☑
        metatarsus T70.3 ☑ [M90.57-] ☑
        multiple sites T70.3 ☑ [M90.59]
        neck T70.3 ☑ [M90.58]
        radius T70.3 ☑ [M90.53-] ☑
        rib T70.3 ☑ [M90.58]
        scapula T70.3 ☑ [M90.51-] ☑
        skull T70.3 ☑ [M90.58]
        tarsus T70.3 ☑ [M90.57-] ☑
        tibia T70.3 ☑ [M90.56-] ☑
        toe T70.3 ☑ [M90.57-] ☑
        ulna T70.3 ☑ [M90.53-] ☑
        vertebra T70.3 ☑ [M90.58]
    ischium M87.350
    metacarpus M87.34- ☑
    metatarsus M87.37- ☑
    multiple site M87.39
    neck M87.38
    radius M87.33- ☑
    rib M87.38
    scapula M87.319
    skull M87.38
    tarsus M87.379
    tibia M87.366
    toe M87.379
    ulna M87.33- ☑
    vertebra M87.38
  specified type NEC M87.80
    carpus M87.83- ☑
    clavicle M87.81- ☑
    femur M87.85- ☑
    fibula M87.86- ☑
    finger M87.84- ☑
    humerus M87.82- ☑
    ilium M87.85- ☑
    ischium M87.85- ☑
    metacarpus M87.84- ☑
    metatarsus M87.87- ☑
    multiple sites M87.89
    neck M87.88
    radius M87.83- ☑
    rib M87.88
    scapula M87.81- ☑
    skull M87.88
    tarsus M87.87- ☑
    tibia M87.86- ☑
    toe M87.87- ☑
    ulna M87.83- ☑
    vertebra M87.88
Osteo-onycho-arthro-dysplasia Q87.2
Osteo-onychodysplasia, hereditary Q87.2
Osteopathia condensans disseminata Q78.8
Osteopathy — see also Osteomyelitis, Osteonecrosis, Osteoporosis
  after poliomyelitis M89.60
    carpus M89.64- ☑
    clavicle M89.61- ☑
    femur M89.65- ☑
    fibula M89.66- ☑
    finger M89.64- ☑
    humerus M89.62- ☑
    ilium M89.659
    ischium M89.659
    metacarpus M89.64- ☑
    metatarsus M89.67- ☑
    multiple sites M89.69
    neck M89.68
    radius M89.63- ☑
    rib M89.68
    scapula M89.61- ☑
    skull M89.68
    tarsus M89.67- ☑
    tibia M89.66- ☑
    toe M89.67- ☑
    ulna M89.63- ☑
    vertebra M89.68
  in (due to)
    renal osteodystrophy N25.0

☑ **Additional Character Required** — Refer to the Tabular List for Character Selection   ▽ Subterms under main terms may continue to next column or page

Osteopathy — *continued*
  in — *continued*
    specified diseases classified elsewhere — *see* sub-
      category M90.8 ☑
Osteopenia M85.8- ☑
  borderline M85.8- ☑
Osteoperiostitis — *see* Osteomyelitis, specified type
  NEC
Osteopetrosis (familial) Q78.2
Osteophyte M25.70
  ankle M25.77- ☑
  elbow M25.72- ☑
  foot joint M25.77- ☑
  hand joint M25.74- ☑
  hip M25.75- ☑
  knee M25.76- ☑
  shoulder M25.71- ☑
  spine M25.78
  vertebrae M25.78
  wrist M25.73- ☑
Osteopoikilosis Q78.8
Osteoporosis (female) (male) M81.0
  with current pathological fracture M80.00 ☑
  age-related M81.0
    with current pathologic fracture M80.00 ☑
      carpus M80.04- ☑
      clavicle M80.01- ☑
      fibula M80.06- ☑
      finger M80.04- ☑
      humerus M80.02- ☑
      ilium M80.05- ☑
      ischium M80.05- ☑
      metacarpus M80.04- ☑
      metatarsus M80.07- ☑
      pelvis M80.05- ☑
      radius M80.03- ☑
      scapula M80.01- ☑
      site specified NEC M80.0A ☑
      tarsus M80.07- ☑
      tibia M80.06- ☑
      toe M80.07- ☑
      ulna M80.03- ☑
      vertebra M80.08 ☑
  disuse M81.8
    with current pathological fracture M80.80 ☑
      carpus M80.84- ☑
      clavicle M80.81- ☑
      fibula M80.86- ☑
      finger M80.84- ☑
      humerus M80.82- ☑
      ilium M80.85- ☑
      ischium M80.85- ☑
      metacarpus M80.84- ☑
      metatarsus M80.87- ☑
      pelvis M80.85- ☑
      radius M80.83- ☑
      scapula M80.81- ☑
      site specified NEC M80.8A ☑
      tarsus M80.87- ☑
      tibia M80.86- ☑
      toe M80.87- ☑
      ulna M80.83- ☑
      vertebra M80.88 ☑
  drug-induced — *see* Osteoporosis, specified type NEC
  idiopathic — *see* Osteoporosis, specified type NEC
  involutional — *see* Osteoporosis, age-related
  Lequesne M81.6
  localized M81.6
  postmenopausal M81.0
    with pathological fracture M80.00 ☑
      carpus M80.04- ☑
      clavicle M80.01- ☑
      fibula M80.06- ☑
      finger M80.04- ☑
      humerus M80.02- ☑
      ilium M80.05- ☑
      ischium M80.05- ☑
      metacarpus M80.04- ☑
      metatarsus M80.07- ☑
      pelvis M80.05- ☑
      radius M80.03- ☑
      scapula M80.01- ☑
      site specified NEC M80.0A ☑
      tarsus M80.07- ☑
      tibia M80.06- ☑
      toe M80.07- ☑

Osteoporosis — *continued*
  postmenopausal — *continued*
    with pathological fracture — *continued*
      ulna M80.03- ☑
      vertebra M80.08 ☑
  postoophorectomy — *see* Osteoporosis, specified type
    NEC
  postsurgical malabsorption — *see* Osteoporosis,
    specified type NEC
  post-traumatic — *see* Osteoporosis, specified type NEC
  senile — *see* Osteoporosis, age-related
  specified type NEC M81.8
    with pathological fracture M80.80 ☑
      carpus M80.84- ☑
      clavicle M80.81- ☑
      fibula M80.86- ☑
      finger M80.84- ☑
      humerus M80.82- ☑
      ilium M80.85- ☑
      ischium M80.85- ☑
      metacarpus M80.84- ☑
      metatarsus M80.87- ☑
      pelvis M80.85- ☑
      radius M80.83- ☑
      scapula M80.81- ☑
      site specified NEC M80.8A ☑
      tarsus M80.87- ☑
      tibia M80.86- ☑
      toe M80.87- ☑
      ulna M80.83- ☑
      vertebra M80.88 ☑
Osteopsathyrosis (idiopathica) Q78.0
Osteoradionecrosis, jaw (acute) (chronic) (lower) (suppurative) (upper) M27.2
Osteosarcoma (any form) — *see* Neoplasm, bone, malignant
Osteosclerosis Q78.2
  acquired M85.8- ☑
  congenita Q77.4
  fragilitas (generalisata) Q78.2
  myelofibrosis D75.81
Osteosclerotic anemia D64.89
Osteosis
  cutis L94.2
  renal fibrocystic N25.0
Österreicher-Turner syndrome Q87.2
Ostium
  atrioventriculare commune Q21.2
  primum (arteriosum) (defect) (persistent) Q21.2
  secundum (arteriosum) (defect) (patent) (persistent)
    Q21.1
Ostrum-Furst syndrome Q75.8
Otalgia H92.0 ☑
Otitis (acute) H66.90
  with effusion — *see also* Otitis, media, nonsuppurative
    purulent — *see* Otitis, media, suppurative
  adhesive — *see* subcategory H74.1 ☑
  chronic — *see also* Otitis, media, chronic
    with effusion — *see also* Otitis, media, nonsuppura-
      tive, chronic
  externa H60.9- ☑
    abscess — *see* Abscess, ear, external
    acute (noninfective) H60.50- ☑
      actinic H60.51- ☑
      chemical H60.52- ☑
      contact H60.53- ☑
      eczematoid H60.54- ☑
      infective — *see* Otitis, externa, infective
      reactive H60.55- ☑
      specified NEC H60.59- ☑
    cellulitis — *see* Cellulitis, ear
    chronic H60.6- ☑
    diffuse — *see* Otitis, externa, infective, diffuse
    hemorrhagic — *see* Otitis, externa, infective, hem-
      orrhagic
    in (due to)
      aspergillosis B44.89
      candidiasis B37.84
      erysipelas A46 *[H62.40]*
      herpes (simplex) virus infection B00.1
        zoster B02.8
      impetigo L01.00 *[H62.40]*
      infectious disease NEC B99 ☑ *[H62.4-]* ☑
      mycosis NEC B36.9 *[H62.40]*
      parasitic disease NEC B89 *[H62.40]*
      viral disease NEC B34.9 *[H62.40]*

Otitis — *continued*
  externa — *continued*
    in — *continued*
      zoster B02.8
    infective NEC H60.39- ☑
      abscess — *see* Abscess, ear, external
      cellulitis — *see* Cellulitis, ear
      diffuse H60.31- ☑
      hemorrhagic H60.32- ☑
      swimmer's ear — *see* Swimmer's, ear
    malignant H60.2- ☑
    mycotic NEC B36.9 *[H62.40]*
      in
        aspergillosis B44.89
        candidiasis B37.84
        moniliasis B37.84
    necrotizing — *see* Otitis, externa, malignant
    Pseudomonas aeruginosa — *see* Otitis, externa,
      malignant
    reactive — *see* Otitis, externa, acute, reactive
    specified NEC — *see* subcategory H60.8 ☑
    tropical NEC B36.9 *[H62.40]*
      in
        aspergillosis B44.89
        candidiasis B37.84
        moniliasis B37.84
  insidiosa — *see* Otosclerosis
  interna H83.0 ☑
  media (hemorrhagic) (staphylococcal) (streptococcal)
    H66.9- ☑
    with effusion (nonpurulent) — *see* Otitis, media,
      nonsuppurative
    acute, subacute H66.90
      allergic — *see* Otitis, media, nonsuppurative,
        acute, allergic
      exudative — *see* Otitis, media, suppurative, acute
      mucoid — *see* Otitis, media, nonsuppurative,
        acute
      necrotizing — *see also* Otitis, media, suppurative,
        acute
        in
          measles B05.3
          scarlet fever A38.0
      nonsuppurative NEC — *see* Otitis, media, non-
        suppurative, acute
      purulent — *see* Otitis, media, suppurative, acute
      sanguinous — *see* Otitis, media, nonsuppurative,
        acute
      secretory — *see* Otitis, media, nonsuppurative,
        acute, serous
      seromucinous — *see* Otitis, media, nonsuppura-
        tive, acute
      serous — *see* Otitis, media, nonsuppurative,
        acute, serous
      suppurative — *see* Otitis, media, suppurative,
        acute
    allergic — *see* Otitis, media, nonsuppurative
    catarrhal — *see* Otitis, media, nonsuppurative
    chronic H66.90
      with effusion (nonpurulent) — *see* Otitis, media,
        nonsuppurative, chronic
      allergic — *see* Otitis, media, nonsuppurative,
        chronic, allergic
      benign suppurative — *see* Otitis, media, suppu-
        rative, chronic, tubotympanic
      catarrhal — *see* Otitis, media, nonsuppurative,
        chronic, serous
      exudative — *see* Otitis, media, nonsuppurative,
        chronic
      mucinous — *see* Otitis, media, nonsuppurative,
        chronic, mucoid
      mucoid — *see* Otitis, media, nonsuppurative,
        chronic, mucoid
      nonsuppurative NEC — *see* Otitis, media, non-
        suppurative, chronic
      purulent — *see* Otitis, media, suppurative,
        chronic
      secretory — *see* Otitis, media, nonsuppurative,
        chronic, mucoid
      seromucinous — *see* Otitis, media, nonsuppura-
        tive, chronic
      serous — *see* Otitis, media, nonsuppurative,
        chronic, serous
      suppurative — *see* Otitis, media, suppurative,
        chronic
      transudative — *see* Otitis, media, nonsuppura-
        tive, chronic, mucoid

Otitis — *continued*
  media — *continued*
    exudative — *see* Otitis, media, suppurative
    in (due to) (with)
      influenza — *see* Influenza, with, otitis media
      measles B05.3
      scarlet fever A38.0
      tuberculosis A18.6
      viral disease NEC B34.- ☑ *[H67.-]* ☑
    mucoid — *see* Otitis, media, nonsuppurative
    nonsuppurative H65.9- ☑
      acute or subacute NEC H65.19- ☑
        allergic H65.11- ☑
          recurrent H65.11- ☑
        recurrent H65.19- ☑
        secretory — *see* Otitis, media, nonsuppurative, serous
        serous H65.0- ☑
          recurrent H65.0- ☑
      chronic H65.49- ☑
        allergic H65.41- ☑
        mucoid H65.3- ☑
        serous H65.2- ☑
    postmeasles B05.3
    purulent — *see* Otitis, media, suppurative
    secretory — *see* Otitis, media, nonsuppurative
    seromucinous — *see* Otitis, media, nonsuppurative
    serous — *see* Otitis, media, nonsuppurative
    suppurative H66.4- ☑
      acute H66.00- ☑
        with rupture of ear drum H66.01- ☑
        recurrent H66.00- ☑
          with rupture of ear drum H66.01- ☑
      chronic — *see also* subcategory H66.3 ☑
        atticoantral H66.2- ☑
        benign — *see* Otitis, media, suppurative, chronic, tubotympanic
        tubotympanic H66.1- ☑
    transudative — *see* Otitis, media, nonsuppurative
    tuberculous A18.6
Otocephaly Q18.2
Otolith syndrome — *see* subcategory H81.8 ☑
Otomycosis (diffuse) **NEC** B36.9 *[H62.40]*
  in
    aspergillosis B44.89
    candidiasis B37.84
    moniliasis B37.84
Otoporosis — *see* Otosclerosis
Otorrhagia (nontraumatic) H92.2- ☑
  traumatic — *code by* Type of injury
Otorrhea H92.1- ☑
  cerebrospinal (fluid) G96.01
    postoperative G96.08
    specified NEC G96.08
    spontaneous G96.01
    traumatic G96.08
Otosclerosis (general) H80.9- ☑
  cochlear (endosteal) H80.2- ☑
  involving
    otic capsule — *see* Otosclerosis, cochlear
    oval window
      nonobliterative H80.0- ☑
      obliterative H80.1- ☑
    round window — *see* Otosclerosis, cochlear
  nonobliterative — *see* Otosclerosis, involving, oval window, nonobliterative
  obliterative — *see* Otosclerosis, involving, oval window, obliterative
  specified NEC H80.8- ☑
Otospongiosis — *see* Otosclerosis
Otto's disease or pelvis M24.7
Outcome of delivery Z37.9
  multiple births Z37.9
    all liveborn Z37.50
      quadruplets Z37.52
      quintuplets Z37.53
      sextuplets Z37.54
      specified number NEC Z37.59
      triplets Z37.51
    all stillborn Z37.7
    some liveborn Z37.60
      quadruplets Z37.62
      quintuplets Z37.63
      sextuplets Z37.64
      specified number NEC Z37.69
      triplets Z37.61
  single NEC Z37.9

Outcome of delivery — *continued*
  single — *continued*
    liveborn Z37.0
    stillborn Z37.1
  twins NEC Z37.9
    both liveborn Z37.2
    both stillborn Z37.4
    one liveborn, one stillborn Z37.3
Outlet — *see* condition
Ovalocytosis (congenital) (hereditary) — *see* Elliptocytosis
Ovarian — *see* Condition
Ovariocele N83.4-
Ovaritis (cystic) — *see* Oophoritis
Ovary, ovarian — *see also* condition
  resistant syndrome E28.39
  vein syndrome N13.8
Overactive — *see also* Hyperfunction
  adrenal cortex NEC E27.0
  bladder N32.81
  hypothalamus E23.3
  thyroid — *see* Hyperthyroidism
Overactivity R46.3
  child — *see* Disorder, attention-deficit hyperactivity
Overbite (deep) (excessive) (horizontal) (vertical) M26.29
Overbreathing — *see* Hyperventilation
Overconscientious personality F60.5
Overdevelopment — *see* Hypertrophy
Overdistension — *see* Distension
Overdose, overdosage (drug) — *see* Table of Drugs and Chemicals, by drug, poisoning
Overeating R63.2
  nonorganic origin F50.89
  psychogenic F50.89
Overexertion (effects) (exhaustion) T73.3 ☑
Overexposure (effects) T73.9 ☑
  exhaustion T73.2 ☑
Overfeeding — *see* Overeating
  newborn P92.4
Overfill, endodontic M27.52
Overgrowth, bone — *see* Hypertrophy, bone
Overhanging of dental restorative material (unrepairable) K08.52
Overheated (places) (effects) — *see* Heat
Overjet (excessive horizontal) M26.23
Overlaid, overlying (suffocation) — *see* Asphyxia, traumatic, due to mechanical threat
Overlap, excessive horizontal (teeth) M26.23
Overlapping toe (acquired) — *see also* Deformity, toe, specified NEC
  congenital (fifth toe) Q66.89
Overload
  circulatory, due to transfusion (blood) (blood components) (TACO) E87.71
  fluid E87.70
    due to transfusion (blood) (blood components) E87.71
    specified NEC E87.79
  iron, due to repeated red blood cell transfusions E83.111
  potassium (K) E87.5
  sodium (Na) E87.0
Overnutrition — *see* Hyperalimentation
Overproduction — *see also* Hypersecretion
  ACTH E27.0
  catecholamine E27.5
  growth hormone E22.0
Overprotection, child by parent Z62.1
Overriding
  aorta Q25.49
  finger (acquired) — *see* Deformity, finger
    congenital Q68.1
  toe (acquired) — *see also* Deformity, toe, specified NEC
    congenital Q66.89
Overstrained R53.83
  heart — *see* Hypertrophy, cardiac
Overuse, muscle NEC M70.8- ☑
Overweight E66.3
Overworked R53.83
Oviduct — *see* condition
Ovotestis Q56.0
Ovulation (cycle)
  failure or lack of N97.0
  pain N94.0
Ovum — *see* condition
Owren's disease or syndrome (parahemophilia) D68.2
Ox heart — *see* Hypertrophy, cardiac

Oxalosis E72.53
Oxaluria E72.53
Oxycephaly, oxycephalic Q75.0
  syphilitic, congenital A50.02
Oxyuriasis B80
Oxyuris vermicularis (infestation) B80
Ozena J31.0

P

Pachyderma, pachydermia L85.9
  larynx (verrucosa) J38.7
Pachydermatocele (congenital) Q82.8
Pachydermoperiostosis — *see also* Osteoarthropathy, hypertrophic, specified type NEC
  clubbed nail M89.40 *[L62]*
Pachygyria Q04.3
Pachymeningitis (adhesive) (basal) (brain) (cervical) (chronic)(circumscribed) (external) (fibrous) (hemorrhagic) (hypertrophic) (internal) (purulent) (spinal) (suppurative) — *see* Meningitis
Pachyonychia (congenital) Q84.5
Pacinian tumor — *see* Neoplasm, skin, benign
Pad, knuckle or Garrod's M72.1
Paget's disease
  with infiltrating duct carcinoma — *see* Neoplasm, breast, malignant
  bone M88.9
    carpus M88.84- ☑
    clavicle M88.81- ☑
    femur M88.85- ☑
    fibula M88.86- ☑
    finger M88.84- ☑
    humerus M88.82- ☑
    ilium M88.85- ☑
    in neoplastic disease — *see* Osteitis, deformans, in neoplastic disease
    ischium M88.85- ☑
    metacarpus M88.84- ☑
    metatarsus M88.87- ☑
    multiple sites M88.89
    neck M88.88
    radius M88.83- ☑
    rib M88.88
    scapula M88.81- ☑
    skull M88.0
    specified NEC M88.88
    tarsus M88.87- ☑
    tibia M88.86- ☑
    toe M88.87- ☑
    ulna M88.83- ☑
    vertebra M88.1
  breast (female) C50.01- ☑
    male C50.02- ☑
  extramammary — *see also* Neoplasm, skin, malignant
    anus C21.0
      margin C44.590
      skin C44.590
  intraductal carcinoma — *see* Neoplasm, breast, malignant
  malignant — *see* Neoplasm, skin, malignant
    breast (female) C50.01- ☑
      male C50.02- ☑
    unspecified site (female) C50.01- ☑
      male C50.02- ☑
  mammary — *see* Paget's disease, breast
  nipple — *see* Paget's disease, breast
  osteitis deformans — *see* Paget's disease, bone
Paget-Schroetter syndrome I82.890
Pain(s) — *see also* Painful R52
  abdominal R10.9
    colic R10.83
    generalized R10.84
      with acute abdomen R10.0
    lower R10.30
      left quadrant R10.32
      pelvic or perineal R10.2
      periumbilical R10.33
      right quadrant R10.31
    rebound — *see* Tenderness, abdominal, rebound
    severe with abdominal rigidity R10.0
    tenderness — *see* Tenderness, abdominal
    upper R10.10
      epigastric R10.13
      left quadrant R10.12
      right quadrant R10.11
  acute R52

Pain(s) — *continued*
　acute — *continued*
　　due to trauma G89.11
　　neoplasm related G89.3
　　postprocedural NEC G89.18
　　post-thoracotomy G89.12
　　specified by site — *code to* Pain, by site
　adnexa (uteri) R10.2
　anginoid — *see* Pain, precordial
　anus K62.89
　arm — *see* Pain, limb, upper
　axillary (axilla) M79.62- ☑
　back (postural) M54.9
　bladder R39.89
　　associated with micturition — *see* Micturition,
　　　painful
　　chronic R39.82
　bone — *see* Disorder, bone, specified type NEC
　breast N64.4
　broad ligament R10.2
　cancer associated (acute) (chronic) G89.3
　cecum — *see* Pain, abdominal
　cervicobrachial M53.1
　chest (central) R07.9
　　anterior wall R07.89
　　atypical R07.89
　　ischemic I20.9
　　musculoskeletal R07.89
　　non-cardiac R07.89
　　on breathing R07.1
　　pleurodynia R07.81
　　precordial R07.2
　　wall (anterior) R07.89
　chronic G89.29
　　associated with significant psychosocial dysfunction
　　　G89.4
　　due to trauma G89.21
　　neoplasm related G89.3
　　postoperative NEC G89.28
　　postprocedural NEC G89.28
　　post-thoracotomy G89.22
　　specified NEC G89.29
　coccyx M53.3
　colon — *see* Pain, abdominal
　coronary — *see* Angina
　costochondral R07.1
　diaphragm R07.1
　due to cancer G89.3
　due to device, implant or graft — *see also* Complica-
　　tions, by site and type, specified NEC T85.848 ☑
　　arterial graft NEC T82.848 ☑
　　breast (implant) T85.848 ☑
　　catheter NEC T85.848 ☑
　　　dialysis (renal) T82.848 ☑
　　　　intraperitoneal T85.848 ☑
　　　infusion NEC T82.848 ☑
　　　　spinal (epidural) (subdural) T85.840 ☑
　　　urinary (indwelling) T83.84 ☑
　　electronic (electrode) (pulse generator) (stimulator)
　　　bone T85.840 ☑
　　　cardiac T82.847 ☑
　　　nervous system (brain) (peripheral nerve) (spinal)
　　　　T85.84 ☑
　　　urinary T83.84 ☑
　　fixation, internal (orthopedic) NEC T84.84 ☑
　　gastrointestinal (bile duct) (esophagus) T85.848 ☑
　　genital NEC T83.84 ☑
　　heart NEC T82.847 ☑
　　infusion NEC T85.848 ☑
　　joint prosthesis T84.84 ☑
　　ocular (corneal graft) (orbital implant) NEC
　　　T85.848 ☑
　　orthopedic NEC T84.84 ☑
　　specified NEC T85.848 ☑
　　urinary NEC T83.84 ☑
　　vascular NEC T82.848 ☑
　　ventricular intracranial shunt T85.840 ☑
　due to malignancy (primary) (secondary) G89.3
　ear — *see* subcategory H92.0 ☑
　epigastric, epigastrium R10.13
　eye — *see* Pain, ocular
　face, facial R51.9
　　atypical G50.1
　female genital organs NEC N94.89
　finger — *see* Pain, limb, upper
　flank — *see* Pain, abdominal
　foot — *see* Pain, limb, lower

Pain(s) — *continued*
　gallbladder K82.9
　gas (intestinal) R14.1
　gastric — *see* Pain, abdominal
　generalized NOS R52
　genital organ
　　female N94.89
　　male N50.89
　groin — *see* Pain, abdominal, lower
　hand — *see* Pain, limb, upper
　head — *see* Headache
　heart — *see* Pain, precordial
　infra-orbital — *see* Neuralgia, trigeminal
　intercostal R07.82
　intermenstrual N94.0
　jaw R68.84
　joint M25.50
　　ankle M25.57- ☑
　　elbow M25.52- ☑
　　finger M25.54- ☑
　　foot M25.57- ☑
　　hand M25.54- ☑
　　hip M25.55- ☑
　　knee M25.56- ☑
　　shoulder M25.51- ☑
　　specified site NEC M25.59
　　toe M25.57- ☑
　　wrist M25.53- ☑
　kidney N23
　laryngeal R07.0
　leg — *see* Pain, limb, lower
　limb M79.609
　　lower M79.60- ☑
　　　foot M79.67- ☑
　　　lower leg M79.66- ☑
　　　thigh M79.65- ☑
　　　toe M79.67- ☑
　　upper M79.60- ☑
　　　axilla M79.62- ☑
　　　finger M79.64- ☑
　　　forearm M79.63- ☑
　　　hand M79.64- ☑
　　　upper arm M79.62- ☑
　loin M54.50
　low back M54.50
　　specified NEC M54.59
　　vertebral end plate M54.51
　　vertebrogenic M54.51
　lumbar region M54.50
　　vertebral end plate M54.51
　　vertebrogenic M54.51
　mandibular R68.84
　mastoid — *see* subcategory H92.0 ☑
　maxilla R68.84
　menstrual — *see also* Dysmenorrhea N94.6
　metacarpophalangeal (joint) — *see* Pain, joint, hand
　metatarsophalangeal (joint) — *see* Pain, joint, foot
　mouth K13.79
　muscle — *see* Myalgia
　musculoskeletal — *see also* Pain, by site M79.18
　myofascial M79.18
　nasal J34.89
　nasopharynx J39.2
　neck NEC M54.2
　nerve NEC — *see* Neuralgia
　neuromuscular — *see* Neuralgia
　nose J34.89
　ocular H57.1- ☑
　ophthalmic — *see* Pain, ocular
　orbital region — *see* Pain, ocular
　ovary N94.89
　over heart — *see* Pain, precordial
　ovulation N94.0
　pelvic (female) R10.2
　penis N48.89
　pericardial — *see* Pain, precordial
　perineal, perineum R10.2
　pharynx J39.2
　pleura, pleural, pleuritic R07.81
　postoperative NOS G89.18
　postprocedural NOS G89.18
　post-thoracotomy G89.12
　precordial (region) R07.2
　premenstrual N94.3
　psychogenic (persistent) (any site) F45.41
　radicular (spinal) — *see* Radiculopathy
　rectum K62.89

Pain(s) — *continued*
　respiration R07.1
　retrosternal R07.2
　rheumatoid, muscular — *see* Myalgia
　rib R07.81
　root (spinal) — *see* Radiculopathy
　round ligament (stretch) R10.2
　sacroiliac M53.3
　sciatic — *see* Sciatica
　scrotum N50.82
　seminal vesicle N50.89
　shoulder M25.51- ☑
　spermatic cord N50.89
　spinal root — *see* Radiculopathy
　spine M54.9
　　cervical M54.2
　　low back M54.50
　　　with sciatica M54.4- ☑
　　thoracic M54.6
　stomach — *see* Pain, abdominal
　substernal R07.2
　temporomandibular (joint) M26.62- ☑
　testis N50.81- ☑
　thoracic spine M54.6
　　with radicular and visceral pain M54.14
　throat R07.0
　tibia — *see* Pain, limb, lower
　toe — *see* Pain, limb, lower
　tongue K14.6
　tooth K08.89
　trigeminal — *see* Neuralgia, trigeminal
　tumor associated G89.3
　ureter N23
　urinary (organ) (system) N23
　uterus NEC N94.89
　vagina R10.2
　vertebral end plate — *see* Pain, vertebrogenic
　vertebrogenic M54.89
　　low back M54.51
　　lumbar M54.51
　　syndrome M54.89
　vesical R39.89
　　associated with micturition — *see* Micturition,
　　　painful
　vulva R10.2
Painful — *see also* Pain
　coitus
　　female N94.10
　　male N53.12
　　psychogenic F52.6
　ejaculation (semen) N53.12
　　psychogenic F52.6
　erection — *see* Priapism
　feet syndrome E53.8
　joint replacement (hip) (knee) T84.84 ☑
　menstruation — *see also* Dysmenorrhea
　　psychogenic F45.8
　micturition — *see* Micturition, painful
　respiration R07.1
　scar NEC L90.5
　wire sutures T81.89 ☑
Painter's colic — *see* subcategory T56.0 ☑
Palate — *see* condition
Palatoplegia K13.79
Palatoschisis — *see* Cleft, palate
Palilalia R48.8
Palliative care Z51.5
Pallor R23.1
　optic disc, temporal — *see* Atrophy, optic
Palmar — *see also* condition
　fascia — *see* condition
Palpable
　cecum K63.89
　kidney N28.89
　ovary N83.8
　prostate N42.9
　spleen — *see* Splenomegaly
Palpitations (heart) R00.2
　psychogenic F45.8
Palsy — *see also* Paralysis G83.9
　atrophic diffuse (progressive) G12.22
　Bell's — *see also* Palsy, facial
　　newborn P11.3
　brachial plexus NEC G54.0
　　newborn (birth injury) P14.3
　brain — *see* Palsy, cerebral
　bulbar (progressive) (chronic) G12.22
　　of childhood (Fazio-Londe) G12.1

▽ **Subterms under main terms may continue to next column or page**　　　☑ **Additional Character Required** — **Refer to the Tabular List for Character Selection**　　　**249**

Pain — Palsy

Palsy — *continued*
  bulbar — *continued*
    pseudo NEC G12.29
    supranuclear (progressive) G23.1
  cerebral (congenital) G80.9
    ataxic G80.4
    athetoid G80.3
    choreathetoid G80.3
    diplegic G80.8
      spastic G80.1
    dyskinetic G80.3
      athetoid G80.3
      choreathetoid G80.3
      distonic G80.3
    dystonic G80.3
    hemiplegic G80.8
      spastic G80.2
    mixed G80.8
    monoplegic G80.8
      spastic G80.1
    paraplegic G80.8
      spastic G80.1
    quadriplegic G80.8
      spastic G80.0
    spastic G80.1
      diplegic G80.1
      hemiplegic G80.2
      monoplegic G80.1
      quadriplegic G80.0
      specified NEC G80.1
      tetrapelgic G80.0
    specified NEC G80.8
    syphilitic A52.12
      congenital A50.49
    tetraplegic G80.8
      spastic G80.0
  cranial nerve — *see also* Disorder, nerve, cranial
    multiple G52.7
      in
        infectious disease B99 ☑ *[G53]*
        neoplastic disease — *see also* Neoplasm
          D49.9 *[G53]*
        parasitic disease B89 *[G53]*
        sarcoidosis D86.82
  creeping G12.22
  diver's T70.3 ☑
  Erb's P14.0
  facial G51.0
    newborn (birth injury) P11.3
  glossopharyngeal G52.1
  Klumpke (-Déjérine) P14.1
  lead — *see* subcategory T56.0 ☑
  median nerve (tardy) G56.1- ☑
  nerve G58.9
    specified NEC G58.8
  peroneal nerve (acute) (tardy) G57.3- ☑
  progressive supranuclear G23.1
  pseudobulbar NEC G12.29
  radial nerve (acute) G56.3- ☑
  seventh nerve — *see also* Palsy, facial
    newborn P11.3
  shaking — *see* Parkinsonism
  spastic (cerebral) (spinal) G80.1
  ulnar nerve (tardy) G56.2- ☑
  wasting G12.29
Paludism — *see* Malaria
Panangiitis M30.0
Panaris, panaritium — *see also* Cellulitis, digit
  with lymphangitis — *see* Lymphangitis, acute, digit
Panarteritis nodosa M30.0
  brain or cerebral I67.7
Pancake heart R93.1
  with cor pulmonale (chronic) I27.81
Pancarditis (acute) (chronic) I51.89
  rheumatic I09.89
    active or acute I01.8
Pancoast's syndrome or tumor C34.1- ☑
Pancolitis, ulcerative (chronic) K51.00
  with
    abscess K51.014
    complication K51.019
    fistula K51.013
    obstruction K51.012
    rectal bleeding K51.011
    specified complication NEC K51.018
Pancreas, pancreatic — *see* condition

Pancreatitis (annular) (apoplectic) (calcareous) (edematous) (hemorrhagic) (malignant) (subacute) (suppurative) K85.90
  with necrosis (uninfected) K85.91
    infected K85.92
  acute (without necrosis or infection) K85.90
    with necrosis (uninfected) K85.91
      infected K85.92
    alcohol induced (without necrosis or infection) K85.20
      with necrosis (uninfected) K85.21
        infected K85.22
    biliary (without necrosis or infection) K85.10
      with necrosis (uninfected) K85.11
        infected K85.12
    drug induced (without necrosis or infection) K85.30
      with necrosis (uninfected) K85.31
        infected K85.32
    gallstone (without necrosis or infection) K85.10
      with necrosis (uninfected) K85.11
        infected K85.12
    idiopathic (without necrosis or infection) K85.00
      with necrosis (uninfected) K85.01
        infected K85.02
    specified NEC (without necrosis or infection) K85.80
      with necrosis (uninfected) K85.81
        infected K85.82
  chronic (infectious) K86.1
    alcohol-induced K86.0
    recurrent K86.1
    relapsing K86.1
  cystic (chronic) K86.1
  cytomegaloviral B25.2
  fibrous (chronic) K86.1
  gallstone (without necrosis or infection) K85.10
    with necrosis (uninfected) K85.11
      infected K85.12
  gangrenous — *see* Pancreatitis, acute
  interstitial (chronic) K86.1
    acute — *see also* Pancreatitis, acute K85.80
  mumps B26.3
  recurrent
    acute — *see* Pancreatitis, acute by type
    chronic K86.1
  relapsing, chronic K86.1
  syphilitic A52.74
Pancreatoblastoma — *see* Neoplasm, pancreas, malignant
Pancreolithiasis K86.89
Pancytolysis D75.89
Pancytopenia (acquired) D61.818
  with
    malformations D61.09
    myelodysplastic syndrome — *see* Syndrome, myelodysplastic
  antineoplastic chemotherapy induced D61.810
  congenital D61.09
  drug-induced NEC D61.811
PANDAS (pediatric autoimmune neuropsychiatric disorders associated with streptococcal infections syndrome) D89.89
Panencephalitis, subacute, sclerosing A81.1
Panhematopenia D61.9
  congenital D61.09
  constitutional D61.09
  splenic, primary D73.1
Panhemocytopenia D61.9
  congenital D61.09
  constitutional D61.09
Panhypogonadism E29.1
Panhypopituitarism E23.0
  prepubertal E23.0
Panic (attack) (state) F41.0
  reaction to exceptional stress (transient) F43.0
Panmyelopathy, familial, constitutional D61.09
Panmyelophthisis D61.82
  congenital D61.09
Panmyeiosis (acute) (with myelofibrosis) C94.4- ☑
Panner's disease — *see* Osteochondrosis, juvenile, humerus
Panneuritis endemica E51.11
Panniculitis (nodular) (nonsuppurative) M79.3
  back M54.00
    cervical region M54.02
    cervicothoracic region M54.03
    lumbar region M54.06
    lumbosacral region M54.07
    multiple sites M54.09

Panniculitis — *continued*
  back — *continued*
    occipito-atlanto-axial region M54.01
    sacrococcygeal region M54.08
    thoracic region M54.04
    thoracolumbar region M54.05
  lupus L93.2
  mesenteric K65.4
  neck M54.02
    cervicothoracic region M54.03
    occipito-atlanto-axial region M54.01
  relapsing M35.6
Panniculus adiposus (abdominal) E65
Pannus (allergic) (cornea) (degenerativus) (keratic) H16.42- ☑
  abdominal (symptomatic) E65
  trachomatosus, trachomatous (active) A71.1
Panophthalmitis H44.01- ☑
Pansinusitis (chronic) (hyperplastic) (nonpurulent) (purulent) J32.4
  acute J01.40
    recurrent J01.41
  tuberculous A15.8
Panuveitis (sympathetic) H44.11- ☑
Panvalvular disease I08.9
  specified NEC I08.8
PAPA (pyogenic arthritis, pyoderma gangrenosum, and acne syndrome) M04.8
Papanicolaou smear, cervix Z12.4
  as part of routine gynecological examination Z01.419
    with abnormal findings Z01.411
  for suspected neoplasm Z12.4
  nonspecific abnormal finding R87.619
  routine Z01.419
    with abnormal findings Z01.411
Papilledema (choked disc) H47.10
  associated with
    decreased ocular pressure H47.12
    increased intracranial pressure H47.11
    retinal disorder H47.13
  Foster-Kennedy syndrome H47.14- ☑
Papillitis H46.00
  anus K62.89
  chronic lingual K14.4
  necrotizing, kidney N17.2
  optic H46.0- ☑
  rectum K62.89
  renal, necrotizing N17.2
  tongue K14.0
Papilloma — *see also* Neoplasm, benign, by site
  acuminatum (female) (male) (anogenital) A63.0
  basal cell L82.1
    inflamed L82.0
  benign pinta (primary) A67.0
  bladder (urinary) (transitional cell) D41.4
  choroid plexus (lateral ventricle) (third ventricle) D33.0
    anaplastic C71.5
    fourth ventricle D33.1
    malignant C71.5
  renal pelvis (transitional cell) D41.1- ☑
    benign D30.1- ☑
  Schneiderian
    specified site — *see* Neoplasm, benign, by site
    unspecified site D14.0
  serous surface
    borderline malignancy
      specified site — *see* Neoplasm, uncertain behavior, by site
      unspecified site D39.10
    specified site — *see* Neoplasm, benign, by site
    unspecified site D27.9
  transitional (cell)
    bladder (urinary) D41.4
    inverted type — *see* Neoplasm, uncertain behavior, by site
    renal pelvis D41.1- ☑
    ureter D41.2- ☑
  ureter (transitional cell) D41.2- ☑
    benign D30.2- ☑
  urothelial — *see* Neoplasm, uncertain behavior, by site
  villous — *see* Neoplasm, uncertain behavior, by site
    adenocarcinoma in — *see* Neoplasm, malignant, by site
    in situ — *see* Neoplasm, in situ
  yaws, plantar or palmar A66.1
Papillomata, multiple, of yaws A66.1
Papillomatosis — *see also* Neoplasm, benign, by site
  confluent and reticulated L83

☑ **Additional Character Required** — Refer to the Tabular List for Character Selection   ▽ Subterms under main terms may continue to next column or page

Papillomatosis — *continued*
  cystic, breast — *see* Mastopathy, cystic
  ductal, breast — *see* Mastopathy, cystic
  intraductal (diffuse) — *see* Neoplasm, benign, by site
  subareolar duct D24- ☑
Papillomavirus, as cause of disease classified elsewhere B97.7
Papillon-Léage and Psaume syndrome Q87.0
Papule(s) R23.8
  carate (primary) A67.0
  fibrous, of nose D22.39
  Gottron's L94.4
  pinta (primary) A67.0
Papulosis
  lymphomatoid C86.6
  malignant I77.89
Papyraceous fetus O31.0- ☑
Para-albuminemia E88.09
Paracephalus Q89.7
Parachute mitral valve Q23.2
Paracoccidioidomycosis B41.9
  disseminated B41.7
  generalized B41.7
  mucocutaneous-lymphangitic B41.8
  pulmonary B41.0
  specified NEC B41.8
  visceral B41.8
Paradentosis K05.4
Paraffinoma T88.8 ☑
Paraganglioma D44.7
  adrenal D35.0- ☑
    malignant C74.1- ☑
  aortic body D44.7
    malignant C75.5
  carotid body D44.6
    malignant C75.4
  chromaffin — *see also* Neoplasm, benign, by site
    malignant — *see* Neoplasm, malignant, by site
  extra-adrenal D44.7
    malignant C75.5
      specified site — *see* Neoplasm, malignant, by site
      unspecified site C75.5
    specified site — *see* Neoplasm, uncertain behavior, by site
    unspecified site D44.7
  gangliocytic D13.2
    specified site — *see* Neoplasm, benign, by site
    unspecified site D13.2
  glomus jugulare D44.7
    malignant C75.5
  jugular D44.7
  malignant C75.5
    specified site — *see* Neoplasm, malignant, by site
    unspecified site C75.5
  nonchromaffin D44.7
    malignant C75.5
      specified site — *see* Neoplasm, malignant, by site
      unspecified site C75.5
    specified site — *see* Neoplasm, uncertain behavior, by site
    unspecified site D44.7
  parasympathetic D44.7
    specified site — *see* Neoplasm, uncertain behavior, by site
    unspecified site D44.7
  specified site — *see* Neoplasm, uncertain behavior, by site
  sympathetic D44.7
    specified site — *see* Neoplasm, uncertain behavior, by site
    unspecified site D44.7
  unspecified site D44.7
Parageusia R43.2
  psychogenic F45.8
Paragonimiasis B66.4
Paragranuloma, Hodgkin — *see* Lymphoma, Hodgkin, specified NEC
Parahemophilia — *see also* Defect, coagulation D68.2
Parakeratosis R23.4
  variegata L41.0
Paralysis, paralytic (complete) (incomplete) G83.9
  with
    syphilis A52.17
  abducens, abducent (nerve) — *see* Strabismus, paralytic, sixth nerve

Paralysis, paralytic — *continued*
  abductor, lower extremity G57.9- ☑
  accessory nerve G52.8
  accommodation — *see also* Paresis, of accommodation
    hysterical F44.89
  acoustic nerve (except Deafness) H93.3 ☑
  agitans — *see also* Parkinsonism G20
    arteriosclerotic G21.4
  alternating (oculomotor) G83.89
  amyotrophic G12.21
  ankle G57.9- ☑
  anus (sphincter) K62.89
  arm — *see* Monoplegia, upper limb
  ascending (spinal), acute G61.0
  association G12.29
  asthenic bulbar G70.00
    with exacerbation (acute) G70.01
    in crisis G70.01
  ataxic (hereditary) G11.9
    general (syphilitic) A52.17
  atrophic G58.9
    infantile, acute — *see* Poliomyelitis, paralytic
    progressive G12.22
    spinal (acute) — *see* Poliomyelitis, paralytic
  axillary G54.0
  Babinski-Nageotte's G83.89
  Bell's G51.0
    newborn P11.3
  Benedikt's G46.3
  birth injury P14.9
    spinal cord P11.5
  bladder (neurogenic) (sphincter) N31.2
  bowel, colon or intestine K56.0
  brachial plexus G54.0
    birth injury P14.3
    newborn (birth injury) P14.3
  brain G83.9
    diplegia G83.0
    triplegia G83.89
  bronchial J98.09
  Brown-Séquard G83.81
  bulbar (chronic) (progressive) G12.22
    infantile — *see* Poliomyelitis, paralytic
    poliomyelitic — *see* Poliomyelitis, paralytic
    pseudo G12.29
  bulbospinal G70.00
    with exacerbation (acute) G70.01
    in crisis G70.01
  cardiac — *see also* Failure, heart I50.9
  cerebrocerebellar, diplegic G80.1
  cervical
    plexus G54.2
    sympathetic G90.09
  Céstan-Chenais G46.3
  Charcot-Marie-Tooth type G60.0
  Clark's G80.9
  colon K56.0
  compressed air T70.3 ☑
  compression
    arm G56.9- ☑
    leg G57.9- ☑
    lower extremity G57.9- ☑
    upper extremity G56.9- ☑
  congenital (cerebral) — *see* Palsy, cerebral
  conjugate movement (gaze) (of eye) H51.0
    cortical (nuclear) (supranuclear) H51.0
  cordis — *see* Failure, heart
  cranial or cerebral nerve G52.9
  creeping G12.22
  crossed leg G83.89
  crutch — *see* Injury, brachial plexus
  deglutition R13.0
    hysterical F44.4
  dementia A52.17
  descending (spinal) NEC G12.29
  diaphragm (flaccid) J98.6
    due to accidental dissection of phrenic nerve during procedure — *see* Puncture, accidental complicating surgery
  digestive organs NEC K59.89
  diplegic — *see* Diplegia
  divergence (nuclear) H51.8
  diver's T70.3 ☑
  Duchenne's
    birth injury P14.0
    due to or associated with
      motor neuron disease G12.22
      muscular dystrophy G71.01

Paralysis, paralytic — *continued*
  due to intracranial or spinal birth injury — *see* Palsy, cerebral
  embolic (current episode) I63.4- ☑
  Erb (-Duchenne) (birth) (newborn) P14.0
  Erb's syphilitic spastic spinal A52.17
  esophagus K22.89
  eye muscle (extrinsic) H49.9
    intrinsic — *see also* Paresis, of accommodation
  facial (nerve) G51.0
    birth injury P11.3
    congenital P11.3
    following operation NEC — *see* Puncture, accidental complicating surgery
    newborn (birth injury) P11.3
  familial (recurrent) (periodic) G72.3
    spastic G11.4
  fauces J39.2
  finger G56.9- ☑
  gait R26.1
  gastric nerve (nondiabetic) G52.2
  gaze, conjugate H51.0
  general (progressive) (syphilitic) A52.17
    juvenile A50.45
  glottis J38.00
    bilateral J38.02
    unilateral J38.01
  gluteal G54.1
  Gubler (-Millard) G46.3
  hand — *see* Monoplegia, upper limb
  heart — *see* Arrest, cardiac
  hemiplegic — *see* Hemiplegia
  hyperkalemic periodic (familial) G72.3
  hypoglossal (nerve) G52.3
  hypokalemic periodic G72.3
  hysterical F44.4
  ileus K56.0
  infantile — *see also* Poliomyelitis, paralytic A80.30
    bulbar — *see* Poliomyelitis, paralytic
    cerebral — *see* Palsy, cerebral
    spastic — *see* Palsy, cerebral, spastic
  infective — *see* Poliomyelitis, paralytic
  inferior nuclear G83.9
  internuclear — *see* Ophthalmoplegia, internuclear
  intestine K56.0
  iris H57.09
    due to diphtheria (toxin) A36.89
  ischemic, Volkmann's (complicating trauma) T79.6 ☑
  Jackson's G83.89
  jake — *see* Poisoning, food, noxious, plant
  Jamaica ginger (jake) G62.2
  juvenile general A50.45
  Klumpke (-Déjérine) (birth) (newborn) P14.1
  labioglossal (laryngeal) (pharyngeal) G12.29
  Landry's G61.0
  laryngeal nerve (recurrent) (superior) (unilateral) J38.00
    bilateral J38.02
    unilateral J38.01
  larynx J38.00
    bilateral J38.02
    due to diphtheria (toxin) A36.2
    unilateral J38.01
  lateral G12.23
  lead T56.0 ☑
  left side — *see* Hemiplegia
  leg G83.1- ☑
    both — *see* Paraplegia
    crossed G83.89
    hysterical F44.4
    psychogenic F44.4
    transient or transitory R29.818
      traumatic NEC — *see* Injury, nerve, leg
  levator palpebrae superioris — *see* Blepharoptosis, paralytic
  limb — *see* Monoplegia
  lip K13.0
  Lissauer's A52.17
  lower limb — *see* Monoplegia, lower limb
    both — *see* Paraplegia
  lung J98.4
  median nerve G56.1- ☑
  medullary (tegmental) G83.89
  mesencephalic NEC G83.89
    tegmental G83.89
  middle alternating G83.89
  Millard-Gubler-Foville G46.3
  monoplegic — *see* Monoplegia
  motor G83.9

Paralysis, paralytic — *continued*
  muscle, muscular NEC G72.89
    due to nerve lesion G58.9
    eye (extrinsic) H49.9
      intrinsic — *see* Paresis, of accommodation
      oblique — *see* Strabismus, paralytic, fourth nerve
    iris sphincter H21.9
    ischemic (Volkmann's) (complicating trauma) T79.6 ☑
    progressive G12.21
    progressive, spinal G12.25
    pseudohypertrophic G71.02
    spinal progressive G12.25
  musculocutaneous nerve G56.9- ☑
  musculospiral G56.9- ☑
  nerve — *see also* Disorder, nerve
    abducent — *see* Strabismus, paralytic, sixth nerve
    accessory G52.8
    auditory (except Deafness) H93.3 ☑
    birth injury P14.9
    cranial or cerebral G52.9
    facial G51.0
      birth injury P11.3
      congenital P11.3
      newborn (birth injury) P11.3
    fourth or trochlear — *see* Strabismus, paralytic, fourth nerve
    newborn (birth injury) P14.9
    oculomotor — *see* Strabismus, paralytic, third nerve
    phrenic (birth injury) P14.2
    radial G56.3- ☑
    seventh or facial G51.0
      newborn (birth injury) P11.3
    sixth or abducent — *see* Strabismus, paralytic, sixth nerve
    syphilitic A52.15
    third or oculomotor — *see* Strabismus, paralytic, third nerve
    trigeminal G50.9
    trochlear — *see* Strabismus, paralytic, fourth nerve
    ulnar G56.2- ☑
  normokalemic periodic G72.3
  ocular H49.9
    alternating G83.89
  oculofacial, congenital (Moebius) Q87.0
  oculomotor (external bilateral) (nerve) — *see* Strabismus, paralytic, third nerve
  palate (soft) K13.79
  paratrigeminal G50.9
  periodic (familial) (hyperkalemic) (hypokalemic) (myotonic) (normokalemic) (potassium sensitive) (secondary) G72.3
  peripheral autonomic nervous system — *see* Neuropathy, peripheral, autonomic
  peroneal (nerve) G57.3- ☑
  pharynx J39.2
  phrenic nerve G56.8- ☑
  plantar nerve(s) G57.6- ☑
  pneumogastric nerve G52.2
  poliomyelitis (current) — *see* Poliomyelitis, paralytic
  popliteal nerve G57.3- ☑
  postepileptic transitory G83.84
  progressive (atrophic) (bulbar) (spinal) G12.22
    general A52.17
    infantile acute — *see* Poliomyelitis, paralytic
    supranuclear G23.1
  pseudobulbar G12.29
  pseudohypertrophic (muscle) G71.09
  psychogenic F44.4
  quadriceps G57.9- ☑
  quadriplegic — *see* Tetraplegia
  radial nerve G56.3- ☑
  rectus muscle (eye) H49.9
  recurrent isolated sleep G47.53
  respiratory (muscle) (system) (tract) R06.81
    center NEC G93.89
    congenital P28.89
    newborn P28.89
  right side — *see* Hemiplegia
  saturnine T56.0 ☑
  sciatic nerve G57.0- ☑
  senile G83.9
  shaking — *see* Parkinsonism
  shoulder G56.9- ☑
  sleep, recurrent isolated G47.53
  spastic G83.9
    cerebral — *see* Palsy, cerebral, spastic
    congenital (cerebral) — *see* Palsy, cerebral, spastic

Paralysis, paralytic — *continued*
  spastic — *continued*
    familial G11.4
    hereditary G11.4
    quadriplegic G80.0
    syphilitic (spinal) A52.17
  sphincter, bladder — *see* Paralysis, bladder
  spinal (cord) G83.9
    accessory nerve G52.8
    acute — *see* Poliomyelitis, paralytic
    ascending acute G61.0
    atrophic (acute) — *see also* Poliomyelitis, paralytic
      spastic, syphilitic A52.17
    congenital NEC — *see* Palsy, cerebral
    hereditary G95.89
    infantile — *see* Poliomyelitis, paralytic
    progressive G12.21
      muscle G12.25
    sequelae NEC G83.89
  sternomastoid G52.8
  stomach K31.84
    diabetic — *see* Diabetes, by type, with gastroparesis
    nerve G52.2
      diabetic — *see* Diabetes, by type, with gastroparesis
  stroke — *see* Infarct, brain
  subcapsularis G56.8- ☑
  supranuclear (progressive) G23.1
  sympathetic G90.8
    cervical G90.09
    nervous system — *see* Neuropathy, peripheral, autonomic
  syndrome G83.9
    specified NEC G83.89
  syphilitic spastic spinal (Erb's) A52.17
  thigh G57.9- ☑
  throat J39.2
    diphtheritic A36.0
    muscle J39.2
  thrombotic (current episode) I63.3- ☑
  thumb G56.9- ☑
  tick — *see* Toxicity, venom, arthropod, specified NEC
  Todd's (postepileptic transitory paralysis) G83.84
  toe G57.6- ☑
  tongue K14.8
  transient R29.5
    arm or leg NEC R29.818
    traumatic NEC — *see* Injury, nerve
  trapezius G52.8
  traumatic, transient NEC — *see* Injury, nerve
  trembling — *see* Parkinsonism
  triceps brachii G56.9- ☑
  trigeminal nerve G50.9
  trochlear (nerve) — *see* Strabismus, paralytic, fourth nerve
  ulnar nerve G56.2- ☑
  upper limb — *see* Monoplegia, upper limb
  uremic N18.9 [G99.8]
  uveoparotitic D86.89
  uvula K13.79
    postdiphtheritic A36.0
  vagus nerve G52.2
  vasomotor NEC G90.8
  velum palati K13.79
  vesical — *see* Paralysis, bladder
  vestibular nerve (except Vertigo) H93.3 ☑
  vocal cords J38.00
    bilateral J38.02
    unilateral J38.01
  Volkmann's (complicating trauma) T79.6 ☑
  wasting G12.29
  Weber's G46.3
  wrist G56.9- ☑
Paramedial urethrovesical orifice Q64.79
Paramenia N92.6
Parametritis — *see also* Disease, pelvis, inflammatory N73.2
  acute N73.0
  complicating abortion — *see* Abortion, by type, complicated by, parametritis
Parametrium, parametric — *see* condition
Paramnesia — *see* Amnesia
Paramolar K00.1
Paramyloidosis E85.89
Paramyoclonus multiplex G25.3
Paramyotonia (congenita) G71.19
Parangi — *see* Yaws

Paranoia (querulans) F22
  senile F03 ☑
Paranoid
  dementia (senile) F03 ☑
    praecox — *see* Schizophrenia
  personality F60.0
  psychosis (climacteric) (involutional) (menopausal) F22
    psychogenic (acute) F23
    senile F03 ☑
  reaction (acute) F23
    chronic F22
  schizophrenia F20.0
  state (climacteric) (involutional) (menopausal) (simple) F22
    senile F03 ☑
  tendencies F60.0
  traits F60.0
  trends F60.0
  type, psychopathic personality F60.0
Paraparesis — *see* Paraplegia
Paraphasia R47.02
Paraphilia F65.9
Paraphimosis (congenital) N47.2
  chancroidal A57
Paraphrenia, paraphrenic (late) F22
  schizophrenia F20.0
Paraplegia (lower) G82.20
  ataxic — *see* Degeneration, combined, spinal cord
  complete G82.21
  congenital (cerebral) G80.8
    spastic G80.1
  familial spastic G11.4
  functional (hysterical) F44.4
  hereditary, spastic G11.4
  hysterical F44.4
  incomplete G82.22
  Pott's A18.01
  psychogenic F44.4
  spastic
    Erb's spinal, syphilitic A52.17
    hereditary G11.4
    tropical G04.1
  syphilitic (spastic) A52.17
  traumatic
    current injury — code to injury with seventh character A
    sequela of previous injury — code to injury with seventh character S
  tropical spastic G04.1
Parapoxvirus B08.60
  specified NEC B08.69
Paraproteinemia D89.2
  benign (familial) D89.2
  monoclonal D47.2
  secondary to malignant disease D47.2
Parapsoriasis L41.9
  en plaques L41.4
  guttata L41.1
  large plaque L41.4
  retiform, retiformis L41.5
  small plaque L41.3
  specified NEC L41.8
  varioliformis (acuta) L41.0
Parasitic — *see also* condition
  disease NEC B89
  stomatitis B37.0
  sycosis (beard) (scalp) B35.0
  twin Q89.4
Parasitism B89
  intestinal B82.9
  skin B88.9
  specified — *see* Infestation
Parasitophobia F40.218
Parasomnia G47.50
  due to
    alcohol
      abuse F10.182
      dependence F10.282
      use F10.982
    amphetamines
      abuse F15.182
      dependence F15.282
      use F15.982
    caffeine
      abuse F15.182
      dependence F15.282
      use F15.982

Parasomnia — *continued*
  due to — *continued*
    cocaine
      abuse F14.182
      dependence F14.282
      use F14.982
    drug NEC
      abuse F19.182
      dependence F19.282
      use F19.982
    opioid
      abuse F11.182
      dependence F11.282
      use F11.982
    psychoactive substance NEC
      abuse F19.182
      dependence F19.282
      use F19.982
    sedative, hypnotic, or anxiolytic
      abuse F13.182
      dependence F13.282
      use F13.982
    stimulant NEC
      abuse F15.182
      dependence F15.282
      use F15.982
  in conditions classified elsewhere G47.54
  nonorganic origin F51.8
  organic G47.50
  specified NEC G47.59
Paraspadias Q54.9
Paraspasmus facialis G51.8
Parasuicide (attempt)
  history of (personal) Z91.51
    in family Z81.8
Parathyroid gland — *see* condition
Parathyroid tetany E20.9
Paratrachoma A74.0
Paratyphilitis — *see* Appendicitis
Paratyphoid (fever) — *see* Fever, paratyphoid
Paratyphus — *see* Fever, paratyphoid
Paraurethral duct Q64.79
Paraurethritis — *see also* Urethritis
  gonococcal (acute) (chronic) (with abscess) A54.1
Paravaccinia NEC B08.04
Paravaginitis — *see* Vaginitis
Parencephalitis — *see also* Encephalitis
  sequelae G09
Parent-child conflict — *see* Conflict, parent-child
  estrangement NEC Z62.890
Paresis — *see also* Paralysis
  accommodation — *see* Paresis, of accommodation
  Bernhardt's G57.1- ☑
  bladder (sphincter) — *see also* Paralysis, bladder
    tabetic A52.17
  bowel, colon or intestine K56.0
  extrinsic muscle, eye H49.9
  general (progressive) (syphilitic) A52.17
    juvenile A50.45
  heart — *see* Failure, heart
  insane (syphilitic) A52.17
  juvenile (general) A50.45
  of accommodation H52.52- ☑
  peripheral progressive (idiopathic) G60.3
  pseudohypertrophic G71.09
  senile G83.9
  syphilitic (general) A52.17
    congenital A50.45
  vesical NEC N31.2
Paresthesia — *see also* Disturbance, sensation, skin R20.2
  Bernhardt G57.1- ☑
Paretic — *see* condition
Parinaud's
  conjunctivitis H10.89
  oculoglandular syndrome H10.89
  ophthalmoplegia H49.88- ☑
Parkinsonism (idiopathic) (primary) G20
  with neurogenic orthostatic hypotension (symptomatic) G90.3
  arteriosclerotic G21.4
  dementia G31.83 *[F02.80]*
    with behavioral disturbance G31.83 *[F02.81]*
  due to
    drugs NEC G21.19
      neuroleptic G21.11
  medication-induced NEC G21.19
  neuroleptic induced G21.11
  postencephalitic G21.3

Parkinsonism — *continued*
  secondary G21.9
    due to
      arteriosclerosis G21.4
      drugs NEC G21.19
        neuroleptic G21.11
      encephalitis G21.3
      external agents NEC G21.2
      syphilis A52.19
    specified NEC G21.8
  syphilitic A52.19
  treatment-induced NEC G21.19
  vascular G21.4
Parkinson's disease, syndrome or tremor — *see* Parkinsonism
Parodontitis — *see* Periodontitis
Parodontosis K05.4
Paronychia — *see also* Cellulitis, digit
  with lymphangitis — *see* Lymphangitis, acute, digit
  candidal (chronic) B37.2
  tuberculous (primary) A18.4
Parorexia (psychogenic) F50.89
Parosmia R43.1
  psychogenic F45.8
Parotid gland — *see* condition
Parotitis, parotiditis (allergic)(nonspecific toxic) (purulent) (septic) (suppurative) — *see also* Sialoadenitis
  epidemic — *see* Mumps
  infectious — *see* Mumps
  postoperative K91.89
  surgical K91.89
Parrot fever A70
Parrot's disease (early congenital syphilitic pseudoparalysis) A50.02
Parry-Romberg syndrome G51.8
Parry's disease or syndrome E05.00
  with thyroid storm E05.01
Pars planitis — *see* Cyclitis
Parsonage (-Aldren)-**Turner syndrome** G54.5
Parson's disease (exophthalmic goiter) E05.00
  with thyroid storm E05.01
Particolored infant Q82.8
Parturition — *see* Delivery
Parulis K04.7
  with sinus K04.6
Parvovirus, as cause of disease classified elsewhere B97.6
Pasini and Pierini's atrophoderma L90.3
Passage
  false, urethra N36.5
  meconium (newborn) during delivery P03.82
  of sounds or bougies — *see* Attention to, artificial, opening
Passive — *see* condition
  smoking Z77.22
Past due on rent or mortgage Z59.81- ☑
Pasteurella septica A28.0
Pasteurellosis — *see* Infection, Pasteurella
PAT (paroxysmal atrial tachycardia) I47.1
Patau's syndrome — *see* Trisomy, 13
Patches
  mucous (syphilitic) A51.39
    congenital A50.07
  smokers' (mouth) K13.24
Patellar — *see* condition
Patent — *see also* Imperfect, closure
  canal of Nuck Q52.4
  cervix N88.3
  ductus arteriosus or Botallo's Q25.0
  foramen
    botalli Q21.1
    ovale Q21.1
  interauricular septum Q21.1
  interventricular septum Q21.0
  omphalomesenteric duct Q43.0
  os (uteri) — *see* Patent, cervix
  ostium secundum Q21.1
  urachus Q64.4
  vitelline duct Q43.0
Paterson (-Brown)(-Kelly) **syndrome or web** D50.1
Pathologic, pathological — *see also* condition
  asphyxia R09.01
  fire-setting F63.1
  gambling F63.0
  ovum O02.0
  resorption, tooth K03.3
  stealing F63.2

Pathology (of) — *see* Disease
  periradicular, associated with previous endodontic treatment NEC M27.59
Pattern, sleep-wake, irregular G47.23
Patulous — *see also* Imperfect, closure (congenital)
  alimentary tract Q45.8
    lower Q43.8
    upper Q40.8
  eustachian tube H69.0- ☑
Pause, sinoatrial I49.5
Paxton's disease B36.2
Pearl(s)
  enamel K00.2
  Epstein's K09.8
Pearl-worker's disease — *see* Osteomyelitis, specified type NEC
Pectenosis K62.4
Pectoral — *see* condition
Pectus
  carinatum (congenital) Q67.7
    acquired M95.4
      rachitic sequelae (late effect) E64.3
  excavatum (congenital) Q67.6
    acquired M95.4
      rachitic sequelae (late effect) E64.3
  recurvatum (congenital) Q67.6
Pedatrophia E41
Pederosis F65.4
Pediatric inflammatory multisystem syndrome M35.81
Pediculosis (infestation) B85.2
  capitis (head-louse) (any site) B85.0
  corporis (body-louse) (any site) B85.1
  eyelid B85.0
  mixed (classifiable to more than one of the titles B85.0-B85.3) B85.4
  pubis (pubic louse) (any site) B85.3
  vestimenti B85.1
  vulvae B85.3
Pediculus (infestation) — *see* Pediculosis
Pedophilia F65.4
Peg-shaped teeth K00.2
Pelade — *see* Alopecia, areata
Pelger-Huët anomaly or syndrome D72.0
Peliosis (rheumatica) D69.0
  hepatis K76.4
    with toxic liver disease K71.8
Pelizaeus-Merzbacher disease E75.29
Pellagra (alcoholic) (with polyneuropathy) E52
Pellagra-cerebellar-ataxia-renal aminoaciduria syndrome E72.02
Pellegrini (-Stieda) **disease or syndrome** — *see* Bursitis, tibial collateral
Pellizzi's syndrome E34.8
Pel's crisis A52.11
Pelvic — *see also* condition
  examination (periodic) (routine) Z01.419
    with abnormal findings Z01.411
  kidney, congenital Q63.2
Pelviolithiasis — *see* Calculus, kidney
Pelviperitonitis — *see also* Peritonitis, pelvic
  gonococcal A54.24
  puerperal O85
Pelvis — *see* condition or type
Pemphigoid L12.9
  benign, mucous membrane L12.1
  bullous L12.0
  cicatricial L12.1
  juvenile L12.2
  ocular L12.1
  specified NEC L12.8
Pemphigus L10.9
  benign familial (chronic) Q82.8
  Brazilian L10.3
  circinatus L13.0
  conjunctiva L12.1
  drug-induced L10.5
  erythematosus L10.4
  foliaceous L10.2
  gangrenous — *see* Gangrene
  neonatorum L01.03
  ocular L12.1
  paraneoplastic L10.81
  specified NEC L10.89
  syphilitic (congenital) A50.06
  vegetans L10.1
  vulgaris L10.0
  wildfire L10.3

Pendred's syndrome E07.1
Pendulous
  abdomen, in pregnancy — *see* Pregnancy, complicated
    by, abnormal, pelvic organs or tissues NEC
  breast N64.89
Penetrating wound — *see also* Puncture
  with internal injury — *see* Injury, by site
  eyeball — *see* Puncture, eyeball
  orbit (with or without foreign body) — *see* Puncture,
    orbit
  uterus by instrument with or following ectopic or molar
    pregnancy O08.6
Penicillosis B48.4
Penis — *see* condition
Penitis N48.29
Pentalogy of Fallot Q21.8
Pentasomy X syndrome Q97.1
Pentosuria (essential) E74.89
Percreta placenta - O43.23 ☑
Peregrinating patient — *see* Disorder, factitious
Perforation, perforated (nontraumatic) (of)
  accidental during procedure (blood vessel) (nerve)
    (organ) — *see* Complication, accidental puncture
    or laceration
  antrum — *see* Sinusitis, maxillary
  appendix K35.32
    with localized peritonitis K35.32
  atrial septum, multiple Q21.1
  attic, ear — *see* Perforation, tympanum, attic
  bile duct (common) (hepatic) K83.2
    cystic K82.2
  bladder (urinary)
    with or following ectopic or molar pregnancy O08.6
    obstetrical trauma O71.5
    traumatic S37.29 ☑
      at delivery O71.5
  bowel K63.1
    with or following ectopic or molar pregnancy O08.6
    newborn P78.0
    obstetrical trauma O71.5
    traumatic — *see* Laceration, intestine
  broad ligament N83.8
    with or following ectopic or molar pregnancy O08.6
    obstetrical trauma O71.6
  by
    device, implant or graft — *see also* Complications,
      by site and type, mechanical T85.628 ☑
      arterial graft NEC — *see* Complication, cardiovas-
        cular device, mechanical, vascular
      breast (implant) T85.49 ☑
      catheter NEC T85.698 ☑
        cystostomy T83.090 ☑
        dialysis (renal) T82.49 ☑
          intraperitoneal T85.691 ☑
        infusion NEC T82.594 ☑
          spinal (epidural) (subdural) T85.690 ☑
        urinary — *see also* Complications, catheter,
          urinary T83.098 ☑
      electronic (electrode) (pulse generator) (stimula-
        tor)
        bone T84.390 ☑
        cardiac T82.199 ☑
          electrode T82.190 ☑
          pulse generator T82.191 ☑
          specified type NEC T82.198 ☑
        nervous system — *see* Complication, prosthet-
          ic device, mechanical, electronic ner-
          vous system stimulator
        urinary — *see* Complication, genitourinary,
          device, urinary, mechanical
      fixation, internal (orthopedic) NEC — *see* Compli-
        cation, fixation device, mechanical
      gastrointestinal — *see* Complications, prosthetic
        device, mechanical, gastrointestinal device
      genital NEC T83.498 ☑
        intrauterine contraceptive device T83.39 ☑
        penile prosthesis T83.490 ☑
      heart NEC — *see* Complication, cardiovascular
        device, mechanical
      joint prosthesis — *see* Complications, joint
        prosthesis, mechanical, specified NEC, by
        site
      ocular NEC — *see* Complications, prosthetic de-
        vice, mechanical, ocular device
      orthopedic NEC — *see* Complication, orthopedic,
        device, mechanical
      specified NEC T85.628 ☑

Perforation, perforated — *continued*
  by — *continued*
    device, implant or graft — *see also* Complications,
      by site and type, mechanical — *continued*
      urinary NEC — *see also* Complication, genitouri-
        nary, device, urinary, mechanical
        graft T83.29 ☑
      vascular NEC — *see* Complication, cardiovascular
        device, mechanical
      ventricular intracranial shunt T85.09 ☑
    foreign body left accidentally in operative wound
      T81.539 ☑
    instrument (any) during a procedure, accidental —
      see Puncture, accidental complicating surgery
  cecum K35.32
    with localized peritonitis K35.32
  cervix (uteri) N88.8
    with or following ectopic or molar pregnancy O08.6
    obstetrical trauma O71.3
  colon K63.1
    newborn P78.0
    obstetrical trauma O71.5
    traumatic — *see* Laceration, intestine, large
  common duct (bile) K83.2
  cornea (due to ulceration) — *see* Ulcer, cornea, perfo-
    rated
  cystic duct K82.2
  diverticulum (intestine) K57.80
    with bleeding K57.81
    large intestine K57.20
      with
        bleeding K57.21
        small intestine K57.40
          with bleeding K57.41
    small intestine K57.00
      with
        bleeding K57.01
        large intestine K57.40
          with bleeding K57.41
  ear drum — *see* Perforation, tympanum
  esophagus K22.3
  ethmoidal sinus — *see* Sinusitis, ethmoidal
  frontal sinus — *see* Sinusitis, frontal
  gallbladder K82.2
  heart valve — *see* Endocarditis
  ileum K63.1
    newborn P78.0
    obstetrical trauma O71.5
    traumatic — *see* Laceration, intestine, small
  instrumental, surgical (accidental) (blood vessel) (nerve)
    (organ) — *see* Puncture, accidental complicating
    surgery
  intestine NEC K63.1
    with ectopic or molar pregnancy O08.6
    newborn P78.0
    obstetrical trauma O71.5
    traumatic — *see* Laceration, intestine
    ulcerative NEC K63.1
      newborn P78.0
  jejunum, jejunal K63.1
    obstetrical trauma O71.5
    traumatic — *see* Laceration, intestine, small
    ulcer — *see* Ulcer, gastrojejunal, with perforation
  joint prosthesis — *see* Complications, joint prosthesis,
    mechanical, specified NEC, by site
  mastoid (antrum) (cell) — *see* Disorder, mastoid,
    specified NEC
  maxillary sinus — *see* Sinusitis, maxillary
  membrana tympani — *see* Perforation, tympanum
  nasal
    septum J34.89
      congenital Q30.3
      syphilitic A52.73
    sinus J34.89
      congenital Q30.8
      due to sinusitis — *see* Sinusitis
  palate — *see also* Cleft, palate Q35.9
    syphilitic A52.79
  palatine vault — *see also* Cleft, palate, hard Q35.1
    syphilitic A52.79
      congenital A50.59
  pars flaccida (ear drum) — *see* Perforation, tympanum,
    attic
  pelvic
    floor S31.030 ☑
      with
        ectopic or molar pregnancy O08.6

Perforation, perforated — *continued*
  pelvic — *continued*
    floor — *continued*
      with — *continued*
        penetration into retroperitoneal space
          S31.031 ☑
        retained foreign body S31.040 ☑
          with penetration into retroperitoneal
            space S31.041 ☑
      following ectopic or molar pregnancy O08.6
      obstetrical trauma O70.1
    organ S37.99 ☑
      adrenal gland S37.818 ☑
      bladder — *see* Perforation, bladder
      fallopian tube S37.599 ☑
        bilateral S37.592 ☑
        unilateral S37.591 ☑
      kidney S37.09- ☑
      obstetrical trauma O71.5
      ovary S37.499 ☑
        bilateral S37.492 ☑
        unilateral S37.491 ☑
      prostate S37.828 ☑
      specified organ NEC S37.898 ☑
      ureter — *see* Perforation, ureter
      urethra — *see* Perforation, urethra
      uterus — *see* Perforation, uterus
  perineum — *see* Laceration, perineum
  pharynx J39.2
  rectum K63.1
    newborn P78.0
    obstetrical trauma O71.5
    traumatic S36.63 ☑
  root canal space due to endodontic treatment M27.51
  sigmoid K63.1
    newborn P78.0
    obstetrical trauma O71.5
    traumatic S36.533 ☑
  sinus (accessory) (chronic) (nasal) J34.89
  sphenoidal sinus — *see* Sinusitis, sphenoidal
  surgical (accidental) (by instrument) (blood vessel)
    (nerve) (organ) — *see* Puncture, accidental
    complicating surgery
  traumatic
    external — *see* Puncture
    eye — *see* Puncture, eyeball
    internal organ — *see* Injury, by site
  tympanum, tympanic (membrane) (persistent post-
    traumatic) (postinflammatory) H72.9- ☑
    attic H72.1- ☑
      multiple — *see* Perforation, tympanum, multiple
      total — *see* Perforation, tympanum, total
    central H72.0- ☑
      multiple — *see* Perforation, tympanum, multiple
      total — *see* Perforation, tympanum, total
    marginal NEC — *see* subcategory H72.2 ☑
    multiple H72.81- ☑
    pars flaccida — *see* Perforation, tympanum, attic
    total H72.82- ☑
    traumatic, current episode S09.2- ☑
  typhoid, gastrointestinal — *see* Typhoid
  ulcer — *see* Ulcer, by site, with perforation
  ureter N28.89
    traumatic S37.19 ☑
  urethra N36.8
    with ectopic or molar pregnancy O08.6
    following ectopic or molar pregnancy O08.6
    obstetrical trauma O71.5
    traumatic S37.39 ☑
      at delivery O71.5
  uterus
    with ectopic or molar pregnancy O08.6
    by intrauterine contraceptive device T83.39 ☑
    following ectopic or molar pregnancy O08.6
    obstetrical trauma O71.1
    traumatic S37.69 ☑
      obstetric O71.1
  uvula K13.79
    syphilitic A52.79
  vagina K57.4
    obstetrical trauma O71.4
    other trauma — *see* Puncture, vagina
Periadenitis mucosa necrotica recurrens K12.0
Periappendicitis (acute) — *see* Appendicitis
Periarteritis nodosa (disseminated) (infectious) (necro-
  tizing) M30.0
Periarthritis (joint) — *see also* Enthesopathy

☑ **Additional Character Required** — **Refer to the Tabular List for Character Selection**   ▽ **Subterms under main terms may continue to next column or page**

Periarthritis — *continued*
  Duplay's M75.0- ☑
  gonococcal A54.42
  humeroscapularis — *see* Capsulitis, adhesive
  scapulohumeral — *see* Capsulitis, adhesive
  shoulder — *see* Capsulitis, adhesive
  wrist M77.2- ☑
Periarthrosis (angioneural) — *see* Enthesopathy
Pericapsulitis, adhesive (shoulder) — *see* Capsulitis, adhesive
Pericarditis (with decompensation) (with effusion) I31.9
  with rheumatic fever (conditions in I00)
    active — *see* Pericarditis, rheumatic
    inactive or quiescent I09.2
  acute (hemorrhagic) (nonrheumatic) (Sicca) I30.9
    with chorea (acute) (rheumatic) (Sydenham's) I02.0
    benign I30.8
    nonspecific I30.0
    rheumatic I01.0
      with chorea (acute) (Sydenham's) I02.0
  adhesive or adherent (chronic) (external) (internal) I31.0
    acute — *see* Pericarditis, acute
    rheumatic I09.2
  bacterial (acute) (subacute) (with serous or seropurulent effusion) I30.1
  calcareous I31.1
  cholesterol (chronic) I31.8
    acute I30.9
  chronic (nonrheumatic) I31.9
    rheumatic I09.2
  constrictive (chronic) I31.1
  coxsackie B33.23
  fibrinocaseous (tuberculous) A18.84
  fibrinopurulent I30.1
  fibrinous I30.8
  fibrous I31.0
  gonococcal A54.83
  idiopathic I30.0
  in systemic lupus erythematosus M32.12
  infective I30.1
  meningococcal A39.53
  neoplastic (chronic) I31.8
    acute I30.9
  obliterans, obliterating I31.0
  plastic I31.0
  pneumococcal I30.1
  postinfarction I24.1
  purulent I30.1
  rheumatic (active) (acute) (with effusion) (with pneumonia) I01.0
    with chorea (acute) (rheumatic) (Sydenham's) I02.0
    chronic or inactive (with chorea) I09.2
  rheumatoid — *see* Rheumatoid, carditis
  septic I30.1
  serofibrinous I30.8
  staphylococcal I30.1
  streptococcal I30.1
  suppurative I30.1
  syphilitic A52.06
  tuberculous A18.84
  uremic N18.9 [I32]
  viral I30.1
Pericardium, pericardial — *see* condition
Pericellulitis — *see* Cellulitis
Pericementitis (chronic) (suppurative) — *see also* Periodontitis
  acute K05.20
    generalized — *see* Periodontitis, aggressive, generalized
    localized — *see* Periodontitis, aggressive, localized
Perichondritis
  auricle — *see* Perichondritis, ear
  bronchus J98.09
  ear (external) H61.00- ☑
    acute H61.01- ☑
    chronic H61.02- ☑
  external auditory canal — *see* Perichondritis, ear
  larynx J38.7
    syphilitic A52.73
    typhoid A01.09
  nose J34.89
  pinna — *see* Perichondritis, ear
  trachea J39.8
Periclasia K05.4
Pericoronitis — *see* Periodontitis
Pericystitis N30.90
  with hematuria N30.91
Peridiverticulitis (intestine) K57.92

Peridiverticulitis — *continued*
  cecum — *see* Diverticulitis, intestine, large
  colon — *see* Diverticulitis, intestine, large
  duodenum — *see* Diverticulitis, intestine, small
  intestine — *see* Diverticulitis, intestine
  jejunum — *see* Diverticulitis, intestine, small
  rectosigmoid — *see* Diverticulitis, intestine, large
  rectum — *see* Diverticulitis, intestine, large
  sigmoid — *see* Diverticulitis, intestine, large
Periendocarditis — *see* Endocarditis
Periepididymitis N45.1
Perifolliculitis L01.02
  abscedens, caput, scalp L66.3
  capitis, abscedens (et suffodiens) L66.3
  superficial pustular L01.02
Perihepatitis K65.8
Perilabyrinthitis (acute) — *see* subcategory H83.0 ☑
Perimeningitis — *see* Meningitis
Perimetritis — *see* Endometritis
Perimetrosalpingitis — *see* Salpingo-oophoritis
Perineocele N81.81
Perinephric, perinephritic — *see* condition
Perinephritis — *see also* Infection, kidney
  purulent — *see* Abscess, kidney
Perineum, perineal — *see* condition
Perineuritis NEC — *see* Neuralgia
Periodic — *see* condition
Periodontitis (chronic) (complex) (compound) (local) (simplex) K05.30
  acute K05.20
    generalized K05.229
      moderate K05.222
      severe K05.223
      slight K05.221
    localized K05.219
      moderate K05.212
      severe K05.213
      slight K05.211
  apical K04.5
    acute (pulpal origin) K04.4
  generalized K05.329
    moderate K05.322
    severe K05.323
    slight K05.321
  localized K05.319
    moderate K05.312
    severe K05.313
    slight K05.311
Periodontoclasia K05.4
Periodontosis (juvenile) K05.4
Periods — *see also* Menstruation
  heavy N92.0
  irregular N92.6
  shortened intervals (irregular) N92.1
Perionychia — *see also* Cellulitis, digit
  with lymphangitis — *see* Lymphangitis, acute, digit
Perioophoritis — *see* Salpingo-oophoritis
Periorchitis N45.2
Periosteum, periosteal — *see* condition
Periostitis (albuminosa) (circumscribed) (diffuse) (infective) (monomelic) — *see also* Osteomyelitis
  alveolar M27.3
  alveolodental M27.3
  dental M27.3
  gonorrheal A54.43
  jaw (lower) (upper) M27.2
  orbit H05.03- ☑
  syphilitic A52.77
    congenital (early) A50.02 [M90.80]
    secondary A51.46
  tuberculous — *see* Tuberculosis, bone
  yaws (hypertrophic) (early) (late) A66.6 [M90.80]
Periostosis (hyperplastic) — *see also* Disorder, bone, specified type NEC
  with osteomyelitis — *see* Osteomyelitis, specified type NEC
Peripartum
  cardiomyopathy O90.3
Periphlebitis — *see* Phlebitis
Periproctitis K62.89
Periprostatitis — *see* Prostatitis
Perirectal — *see* condition
Perirenal — *see* condition
Perisalpingitis — *see* Salpingo-oophoritis
Perisplenitis (infectional) D73.89
Peristalsis, visible or reversed R19.2
Peritendinitis — *see* Enthesopathy

Peritoneum, peritoneal — *see* condition
Peritonitis (adhesive) (bacterial) (fibrinous) (hemorrhagic) (idiopathic) (localized) (perforative) (primary) (with adhesions) (with effusion) K65.9
  with or following
    abscess K65.1
    appendicitis
      with perforation or rupture K35.32
      generalized — *see also* Appendicitis K35.20
      localized — *see also* Appendicitis K35.30
    diverticular disease (intestine) K57.80
      with bleeding K57.81
      ectopic or molar pregnancy O08.0
      large intestine K57.20
        with
          bleeding K57.21
          small intestine K57.40
            with bleeding K57.41
      small intestine K57.00
        with
          bleeding K57.01
          large intestine K57.40
            with bleeding K57.41
  acute (generalized) K65.0
  aseptic T81.61 ☑
  bile, biliary K65.3
  chemical T81.61 ☑
  chlamydial A74.81
  chronic proliferative K65.8
  complicating abortion — *see* Abortion, by type, complicated by, pelvic peritonitis
  congenital P78.1
  diaphragmatic K65.0
  diffuse K65.0
  diphtheritic A36.89
  disseminated K65.0
  due to
    bile K65.3
    foreign
      body or object accidentally left during a procedure (instrument) (sponge) (swab) T81.599 ☑
      substance accidentally left during a procedure (chemical) (powder) (talc) T81.61 ☑
    talc T81.61 ☑
    urine K65.8
  eosinophilic K65.8
    acute K65.0
  fibrocaseous (tuberculous) A18.31
  fibropurulent K65.0
  following ectopic or molar pregnancy O08.0
  general (ized) K65.0
  gonococcal A54.85
  meconium (newborn) P78.0
  neonatal P78.1
    meconium P78.0
  pancreatic K65.0
  paroxysmal, familial E85.0
    benign E85.0
  pelvic
    female N73.5
      acute N73.3
      chronic N73.4
        with adhesions N73.6
    male K65.0
  periodic, familial E85.0
  proliferative, chronic K65.8
  puerperal, postpartum, childbirth O85
  purulent K65.0
  septic K65.0
  specified NEC K65.8
  spontaneous bacterial K65.2
  subdiaphragmatic K65.0
  subphrenic K65.0
  suppurative K65.0
  syphilitic A52.74
    congenital (early) A50.08 [K67]
  talc T81.61 ☑
  tuberculous A18.31
  urine K65.8
Peritonsillar — *see* condition
Peritonsillitis J36
Perityphlitis K37
Periureteritis N28.89
Periurethral — *see* condition
Periurethritis (gangrenous) — *see* Urethritis
Periuterine — *see* condition
Perivaginitis — *see* Vaginitis

Perivasculitis, retinal H35.06- ☑
Perivasitis (chronic) N49.1
Perivesiculitis (seminal) — see Vesiculitis
Perlèche NEC K13.0
  due to
    candidiasis B37.83
    moniliasis B37.83
    riboflavin deficiency E53.0
    vitamin B2 (riboflavin) deficiency E53.0
Pernicious — see condition
Pernio, perniosis T69.1 ☑
Perpetrator (of abuse) — see Index to External Causes of Injury, Perpetrator
Persecution
  delusion F22
  social Z60.5
Perseveration (tonic) R48.8
Persistence, persistent (congenital)
  anal membrane Q42.3
    with fistula Q42.2
  arteria stapedia Q16.3
  atrioventricular canal Q21.2
  branchial cleft NOS Q18.2
    cyst Q18.0
    fistula Q18.0
    sinus Q18.0
  bulbus cordis in left ventricle Q21.8
  canal of Cloquet Q14.0
  capsule (opaque) Q12.8
  cilioretinal artery or vein Q14.8
  cloaca Q43.7
  communication — see Fistula, congenital
  convolutions
    aortic arch Q25.46
    fallopian tube Q50.6
    oviduct Q50.6
    uterine tube Q50.6
  double aortic arch Q25.45
  ductus arteriosus (Botalli) Q25.0
  fetal
    circulation P29.38
    form of cervix (uteri) Q51.828
    hemoglobin, hereditary (HPFH) D56.4
  foramen
    Botalli Q21.1
    ovale Q21.1
  Gartner's duct Q52.4
  hemoglobin, fetal (hereditary) (HPFH) D56.4
  hyaloid
    artery (generally incomplete) Q14.0
    system Q14.8
  hymen, in pregnancy or childbirth — see Pregnancy, complicated by, abnormal, vulva
  lanugo Q84.2
  left
    posterior cardinal vein Q26.8
    root with right arch of aorta Q25.49
    superior vena cava Q26.1
  Meckel's diverticulum Q43.0
    malignant — see Table of Neoplasms, small intestine, malignant
  mucosal disease (middle ear) — see Otitis, media, suppurative, chronic, tubotympanic
  nail(s), anomalous Q84.6
  omphalomesenteric duct Q43.0
  organ or site not listed — see Anomaly, by site
  ostium
    atrioventriculare commune Q21.2
    primum Q21.2
    secundum Q21.1
  ovarian rests in fallopian tube Q50.6
  pancreatic tissue in intestinal tract Q43.8
  primary (deciduous)
    teeth K00.6
    vitreous hyperplasia Q14.0
  pupillary membrane Q13.89
  rhesus (Rh) titer — see Complication(s), transfusion, incompatibility reaction, Rh (factor)
  right aortic arch Q25.47
  sinus
    urogenitalis
      female Q52.8
      male Q55.8
    venosus with imperfect incorporation in right auricle Q26.8
  thymus (gland) (hyperplasia) E32.0
  thyroglossal duct Q89.2
  thyrolingual duct Q89.2

Persistence, persistent — continued
  truncus arteriosus or communis Q20.0
  tunica vasculosa lentis Q12.2
  umbilical sinus Q64.4
  urachus Q64.4
  vitelline duct Q43.0
Person (with)
  admitted for clinical research, as a control subject (normal comparison) (participant) Z00.6
  awaiting admission to adequate facility elsewhere Z75.1
  concern (normal) about sick person in family Z63.6
  consulting on behalf of another Z71.0
  feigning illness Z76.5
  living (in)
    alone Z60.2
    boarding school Z59.3
    residential institution Z59.3
    without
      adequate housing (heating) (space) Z59.1
      housing (permanent) (temporary) Z59.00
      person able to render necessary care Z74.2
      shelter Z59.02
  on waiting list Z75.1
  sick or handicapped in family Z63.6
Personality (disorder) F60.9
  accentuation of traits (type A pattern) Z73.1
  affective F34.0
  aggressive F60.3
  amoral F60.2
  anacastic, anankastic F60.5
  antisocial F60.2
  anxious F60.6
  asocial F60.2
  asthenic F60.7
  avoidant F60.6
  borderline F60.3
  change due to organic condition (enduring) F07.0
  compulsive F60.5
  cycloid F34.0
  cyclothymic F34.0
  dependent F60.7
  depressive F34.1
  dissocial F60.2
  dual F44.81
  eccentric F60.89
  emotionally unstable F60.3
  expansive paranoid F60.0
  explosive F60.3
  fanatic F60.0
  haltose type F60.89
  histrionic F60.4
  hyperthymic F34.0
  hypothymic F34.1
  hysterical F60.4
  immature F60.89
  inadequate F60.7
  labile (emotional) F60.3
  mixed (nonspecific) F60.89
  morally defective F60.2
  multiple F44.81
  narcissistic F60.81
  obsessional F60.5
  obsessive (-compulsive) F60.5
  organic F07.0
  overconscientious F60.5
  paranoid F60.0
  passive (-dependent) F60.7
  passive-aggressive F60.89
  pathologic F60.9
  pattern defect or disturbance F60.9
  pseudopsychopathic (organic) F07.0
  pseudoretarded (organic) F07.0
  psychoinfantile F60.4
  psychoneurotic NEC F60.89
  psychopathic F60.2
  querulant F60.0
  sadistic F60.89
  schizoid F60.1
  self-defeating F60.89
  sensitive paranoid F60.0
  sociopathic (amoral) (antisocial) (asocial) (dissocial) F60.2
  specified NEC F60.89
  type A Z73.1
  unstable (emotional) F60.3
Perthes' disease — see Legg-Calvé-Perthes disease
Pertussis — see also Whooping cough A37.90

Perversion, perverted
  appetite F50.89
    psychogenic F50.89
  function
    pituitary gland E23.2
      posterior lobe E22.2
  sense of smell and taste R43.8
    psychogenic F45.8
  sexual — see Deviation, sexual
Pervious, congenital — see also Imperfect, closure
  ductus arteriosus Q25.0
Pes (congenital) — see also Talipes
  acquired — see also Deformity, limb, foot, specified NEC
    planus — see Deformity, limb, flat foot
  adductus Q66.89
  cavus Q66.7- ☑
  deformity NEC, acquired — see Deformity, limb, foot, specified NEC
  planus (acquired) (any degree) — see also Deformity, limb, flat foot
    rachitic sequelae (late effect) E64.3
  valgus Q66.6
Pest, pestis — see Plague
Petechia, petechiae R23.3
  newborn P54.5
Petechial typhus A75.9
Peter's anomaly Q13.4
Petit mal seizure — see Epilepsy, childhood, absence
Petit's hernia — see Hernia, abdomen, specified site NEC
Petrellidosis B48.2
Petrositis H70.20- ☑
  acute H70.21- ☑
  chronic H70.22- ☑
Peutz-Jeghers disease or syndrome Q85.8
Peyronie's disease N48.6
PFAPA (periodic fever, aphthous stomatitis, pharyngitis, and adenopathy syndrome) M04.8
Pfeiffer's disease — see Mononucleosis, infectious
Phagedena (dry) (moist) (sloughing) — see also Gangrene
  geometric L88
  penis N48.29
  tropical — see Ulcer, skin
  vulva N76.6
Phagedenic — see condition
Phakoma H35.89
Phakomatosis — see also specific eponymous syndromes Q85.9
  Bourneville's Q85.1
  specified NEC Q85.8
Phantom limb syndrome (without pain) G54.7
  with pain G54.6
Pharyngeal pouch syndrome D82.1
Pharyngitis (acute) (catarrhal)(gangrenous) (infective) (malignant) (membranous) (phlegmonous) (pseudomembranous) (simple) (subacute) (suppurative) (ulcerative) (viral) J02.9
  with influenza, flu, or grippe — see Influenza, with, pharyngitis
  aphthous B08.5
  atrophic J31.2
  chlamydial A56.4
  chronic (atrophic) (granular) (hypertrophic) J31.2
  coxsackievirus B08.5
  diphtheritic A36.0
  enteroviral vesicular B08.5
  follicular (chronic) J31.2
  fusospirochetal A69.1
  gonococcal A54.5
  granular (chronic) J31.2
  herpesviral B00.2
  hypertrophic J31.2
  infectional, chronic J31.2
  influenzal — see Influenza, with, respiratory manifestations NEC
  lymphonodular, acute (enteroviral) B08.8
  pneumococcal J02.8
  purulent J02.9
  putrid J02.9
  septic J02.0
  sicca J31.2
  specified organism NEC J02.8
  staphylococcal J02.8
  streptococcal J02.0
  syphilitic, congenital (early) A50.03
  tuberculous A15.8
  vesicular, enteroviral B08.5

☑ Additional Character Required — Refer to the Tabular List for Character Selection   ▽ Subterms under main terms may continue to next column or page

Pharyngitis — *continued*
  viral NEC J02.8
Pharyngoconjunctivitis, viral B30.2
Pharyngolaryngitis (acute) J06.0
  chronic J37.0
Pharyngoplegia J39.2
Pharyngotonsillitis, herpesviral B00.2
Pharyngotracheitis, chronic J42
Pharynx, pharyngeal — *see* condition
Phencyclidine-induced
  anxiety disorder F16.980
  bipolar and related disorder F16.94
  depressive disorder F16.94
  psychotic disorder F16.959
Phenomenon
  Arthus' — *see* Arthus' phenomenon
  jaw-winking Q07.8
  lupus erythematosus (LE) cell M32.9
  Raynaud's (secondary) I73.00
    with gangrene I73.01
  vasomotor R55
  vasospastic I73.9
  vasovagal R55
  Wenckebach's I44.1
Phenylketonuria E70.1
  classical E70.0
  maternal E70.1
Pheochromoblastoma
  specified site — *see* Neoplasm, malignant, by site
  unspecified site C74.10
Pheochromocytoma
  malignant
    specified site — *see* Neoplasm, malignant, by site
    unspecified site C74.10
  specified site — *see* Neoplasm, benign, by site
  unspecified site D35.00
Pheohyphomycosis — *see* Chromomycosis
Pheomycosis — *see* Chromomycosis
Phimosis (congenital) (due to infection) N47.1
  chancroidal A57
Phlebectasia — *see also* Varix
  congenital Q27.4
Phlebitis (infective) (pyemic) (septic) (suppurative) I80.9
  antepartum — *see* Thrombophlebitis, antepartum
  blue — *see* Phlebitis, leg, deep
  breast, superficial I80.8
  calf muscular vein (NOS) I80.25- ☑
  cavernous (venous) sinus — *see* Phlebitis, intracranial
    (venous) sinus
  cerebral (venous) sinus — *see* Phlebitis, intracranial
    (venous) sinus
  chest wall, superficial I80.8
  cranial (venous) sinus — *see* Phlebitis, intracranial
    (venous) sinus
  deep (vessels) — *see* Phlebitis, leg, deep
  due to implanted device — *see* Complications, by site
    and type, specified NEC
  during or resulting from a procedure T81.72 ☑
  femoral vein (superficial) I80.1- ☑
  femoropopliteal vein I80.0- ☑
  gastrocnemial vein I80.25- ☑
  gestational — *see* Phlebopathy, gestational
  hepatic veins I80.8
  iliac vein (common) (external) (internal) I80.21- ☑
  iliofemoral — *see* Phlebitis, femoral vein
  intracranial (venous) sinus (any) G08
    nonpyogenic I67.6
  intraspinal venous sinuses and veins G08
    nonpyogenic G95.19
  lateral (venous) sinus — *see* Phlebitis, intracranial (ve-
    nous) sinus
  leg I80.3
    antepartum — *see* Thrombophlebitis, antepartum
    deep (vessels) NEC I80.20- ☑
      iliac I80.21- ☑
      popliteal vein I80.22- ☑
      specified vessel NEC I80.29- ☑
      tibial vein (anterior) (posterior) I80.23- ☑
    femoral vein (superficial) I80.1- ☑
    superficial (vessels) I80.0- ☑
  longitudinal sinus — *see* Phlebitis, intracranial (venous)
    sinus
  lower limb — *see* Phlebitis, leg
  migrans, migrating (superficial) I82.1
  pelvic
    with ectopic or molar pregnancy O08.0
    following ectopic or molar pregnancy O08.0

Phlebitis — *continued*
  pelvic — *continued*
    puerperal, postpartum O87.1
  peroneal vein I80.24- ☑
  popliteal vein — *see* Phlebitis, leg, deep, popliteal
  portal (vein) K75.1
  postoperative T81.72 ☑
  pregnancy — *see* Thrombophlebitis, antepartum
  puerperal, postpartum, childbirth O87.0
    deep O87.1
    pelvic O87.1
    superficial O87.0
  retina — *see* Vasculitis, retina
  saphenous (accessory) (great) (long) (small) — *see*
    Phlebitis, leg, superficial
  sinus (meninges) — *see* Phlebitis, intracranial (venous)
    sinus
  soleal vein I80.25- ☑
  specified site NEC I80.8
  syphilitic A52.09
  tibial vein — *see* Phlebitis, leg, deep, tibial
  ulcerative I80.9
    leg — *see* Phlebitis, leg
  umbilicus I80.8
  uterus (septic) — *see* Endometritis
  varicose (leg) (lower limb) — *see* Varix, leg, with, inflam-
    mation
Phlebofibrosis I87.8
Phleboliths I87.8
Phlebopathy,
  gestational O22.9- ☑
  puerperal O87.9
Phlebosclerosis I87.8
Phlebothrombosis — *see also* Thrombosis
  antepartum — *see* Thrombophlebitis, antepartum
  pregnancy — *see* Thrombophlebitis, antepartum
  puerperal — *see* Thrombophlebitis, puerperal
Phlebotomus fever A93.1
Phlegmasia
  alba dolens O87.1
    nonpuerperal — *see* Phlebitis, femoral vein
  cerulea dolens — *see* Phlebitis, leg, deep
Phlegmon — *see* Abscess
Phlegmonous — *see* condition
Phlyctenulosis (allergic) (keratoconjunctivitis) (nontuberculous) — *see also* Keratoconjunctivitis
  cornea — *see* Keratoconjunctivitis
  tuberculous A18.52
Phobia, phobic F40.9
  animal F40.218
    spiders F40.210
  examination F40.298
  reaction F40.9
  simple F40.298
  social F40.10
    generalized F40.11
  specific (isolated) F40.298
    animal F40.218
      spiders F40.210
    blood F40.230
    injection F40.231
    injury F40.233
    men F40.290
    natural environment F40.228
      thunderstorms F40.220
    situational F40.248
      bridges F40.242
      closed in spaces F40.240
      flying F40.243
      heights F40.241
    specified focus NEC F40.298
    transfusion F40.231
    women F40.291
  specified NEC F40.8
    medical care NEC F40.232
  state F40.9
Phocas' disease — *see* Mastopathy, cystic
Phocomelia Q73.1
  lower limb — *see* Agenesis, leg, with foot present
  upper limb — *see* Agenesis, arm, with hand present
Phoria H50.50
Phosphate-losing tubular disorder N25.0
Phosphatemia E83.39
Phosphaturia E83.39
Photodermatitis (sun) L56.8
  chronic L57.8
  due to drug L56.8

Photodermatitis — *continued*
  light other than sun L59.8
Photokeratitis H16.13- ☑
Photophobia H53.14- ☑
Photophthalmia — *see* Photokeratitis
Photopsia H53.19
Photoretinitis — *see* Retinopathy, solar
Photosensitivity, photosensitization (sun) skin L56.8
  light other than sun L59.8
Phrenitis — *see* Encephalitis
Phrynoderma (vitamin A deficiency) E50.8
Phthiriasis (pubis) B85.3
  with any infestation classifiable to B85.0-B85.2 B85.4
Phthirus infestation — *see* Phthiriasis
Phthisis — *see also* Tuberculosis
  bulbi (infectional) — *see* Disorder, globe, degenerated
    condition, atrophy
  eyeball (due to infection) — *see* Disorder, globe, degen-
    erated condition, atrophy
Phycomycosis — *see* Zygomycosis
Physalopteriasis B81.8
Physical restraint status Z78.1
Phytobezoar T18.9 ☑
  intestine T18.3 ☑
  stomach T18.2 ☑
Pian — *see* Yaws
Pianoma A66.1
Pica F50.89
  in adults F50.89
  infant or child F98.3
Picking, nose F98.8
Pick-Niemann disease — *see* Niemann-Pick disease or
  syndrome
Pick's
  cerebral atrophy G31.01 *[F02.80]*
    with behavioral disturbance G31.01 *[F02.81]*
  disease or syndrome (brain) G31.01 *[F02.80]*
    with behavioral disturbance G31.01 *[F02.81]*
      brain G31.01 *[F02.80]*
        with behavioral disturbance G31.01 *[F02.81]*
    pericardium (pericardial pseudocirrhosis of liver)
      I31.1
  syndrome
    brain G31.01 *[F02.80]*
      with behavioral disturbance G31.01 *[F02.81]*
    of heart (pericardial pseudocirrhosis of liver) I31.1
Pickwickian syndrome E66.2
Piebaldism E70.39
Piedra (beard) (scalp) B36.8
  black B36.3
  white B36.2
Pierre Robin deformity or syndrome Q87.0
Pierson's disease or osteochondrosis M91.0
Pig-bel A05.2
Pigeon
  breast or chest (acquired) M95.4
    congenital Q67.7
    rachitic sequelae (late effect) E64.3
  breeder's disease or lung J67.2
  fancier's disease or lung J67.2
  toe — *see* Deformity, toe, specified NEC
Pigmentation (abnormal) (anomaly) L81.9
  conjunctiva H11.13- ☑
  cornea (anterior) H18.01- ☑
    posterior H18.05- ☑
    stromal H18.06- ☑
  diminished melanin formation NEC L81.6
  iron L81.8
  lids, congenital Q82.8
  limbus corneae — *see* Pigmentation, cornea
  metals L81.8
  optic papilla, congenital Q14.2
  retina, congenital (grouped) (nevoid) Q14.1
  scrotum, congenital Q82.8
  tattoo L81.8
Piles — *see also* Hemorrhoids K64.9
Pili
  annulati or torti (congenital) Q84.1
  incarnati L73.1
Pill roller hand (intrinsic) — *see* Parkinsonism
Pilomatrixoma — *see* Neoplasm, skin, benign
  malignant — *see* Neoplasm, skin, malignant
Pilonidal — *see* condition
Pimple R23.8
PIMS M35.81
PIN — *see* Neoplasia, intraepithelial, prostate
Pinched nerve — *see* Neuropathy, entrapment

Pindborg tumor — see Cyst, calcifying odontogenic
Pineal body or gland — see condition
Pinealoblastoma C75.3
Pinealoma D44.5
  malignant C75.3
Pineoblastoma C75.3
Pineocytoma D44.5
Pinguecula H11.15- ☑
Pingueculitis H10.81- ☑
Pinhole meatus — see also Stricture, urethra N35.919
Pink
  disease — see subcategory T56.1 ☑
  eye — see Conjunctivitis, acute, mucopurulent
Pinkus' disease (lichen nitidus) L44.1
Pinpoint
  meatus — see Stricture, urethra
  os (uteri) — see Stricture, cervix
Pins and needles R20.2
Pinta A67.9
  cardiovascular lesions A67.2
  chancre (primary) A67.0
  erythematous plaques A67.1
  hyperchromic lesions A67.1
  hyperkeratosis A67.1
  lesions A67.9
    cardiovascular A67.2
    hyperchromic A67.1
    intermediate A67.1
    late A67.2
    mixed A67.3
    primary A67.0
    skin (achromic) (cicatricial) (dyschromic) A67.2
      hyperchromic A67.1
      mixed (achromic and hyperchromic) A67.3
    papule (primary) A67.0
  skin lesions (achromic) (cicatricial) (dyschromic) A67.2
    hyperchromic A67.1
    mixed (achromic and hyperchromic) A67.3
  vitiligo A67.2
Pintids A67.1
Pinworm (disease) (infection) (infestation) B80
Piroplasmosis — see also Babesiosis B60.00
  specified NEC B60.09
Pistol wound — see Gunshot wound
Pitchers' elbow — see Derangement, joint, specified type NEC, elbow
Pithecoid pelvis Q74.2
  with disproportion (fetopelvic) O33.0
    causing obstructed labor O65.0
Pithiatism F48.8
Pitted — see Pitting
Pitting — see also Edema R60.9
  lip R60.0
  nail L60.8
  teeth K00.4
Pituitary gland — see condition
Pituitary-snuff-taker's disease J67.8
Pityriasis (capitis) L21.0
  alba L30.5
  circinata (et maculata) L42
  furfuracea L21.0
  Hebra's L26
  lichenoides L41.0
    chronica L41.1
    et varioliformis (acuta) L41.0
  maculata (et circinata) L30.5
  nigra B36.1
  pilaris, Hebra's L44.0
  rosea L42
  rotunda L44.8
  rubra (Hebra) pilaris L44.0
  simplex L30.5
  specified type NEC L30.5
  streptogenes L30.5
  versicolor (scrotal) B36.0
Placenta, placental — see Pregnancy, complicated by (care of) (management affected by), specified condition
Placentitis O41.14- ☑
Plagiocephaly Q67.3
Plague A20.9
  abortive A20.8
  ambulatory A20.8
  asymptomatic A20.8
  bubonic A20.0
  cellulocutaneous A20.1
  cutaneobubonic A20.1
  lymphatic gland A20.0

Plague — continued
  meningitis A20.3
  pharyngeal A20.8
  pneumonic (primary) (secondary) A20.2
  pulmonary, pulmonic A20.2
  septicemic A20.7
  tonsillar A20.8
    septicemic A20.7
Planning, family
  contraception Z30.9
  procreation Z31.69
Plaque(s)
  artery, arterial — see Arteriosclerosis
  calcareous — see Calcification
  coronary, lipid rich I25.83
  epicardial I31.8
  erythematous, of pinta A67.1
  Hollenhorst's — see Occlusion, artery, retina
  lipid rich, coronary I25.83
  pleural (without asbestos) J92.9
    with asbestos J92.0
  tongue K13.29
Plasmacytoma C90.3- ☑
  extramedullary C90.2- ☑
  medullary C90.0- ☑
  solitary C90.3- ☑
Plasmacytopenia D72.818
Plasmacytosis D72.822
Plaster ulcer — see Ulcer, pressure, by site
Plateau iris syndrome (post-iridectomy) (postprocedural) (without glaucoma) H21.82
  with glaucoma H40.22- ☑
Platybasia Q75.8
Platyonychia (congenital) Q84.6
  acquired L60.8
Platypelloid pelvis M95.5
  with disproportion (fetopelvic) O33.0
    causing obstructed labor O65.0
  congenital Q74.2
Platyspondylisis Q76.49
Plaut (-Vincent) **disease** — see also Vincent's A69.1
Plethora R23.2
  newborn P61.1
Pleura, pleural — see condition
Pleuralgia R07.81
Pleurisy (acute) (adhesive) (chronic) (costal) (diaphragmatic) (double) (dry) (fibrinous) (fibrous) (interlobar) (latent) (plastic) (primary) (residual) (sicca) (sterile) (subacute) (unresolved) R09.1
  with
    adherent pleura J86.0
    effusion J90
      chylous, chyliform J94.0
      tuberculous (non primary) A15.6
        primary (progressive) A15.7
    tuberculosis — see Pleurisy, tuberculous (non primary)
  encysted — see Pleurisy, with effusion
  exudative — see Pleurisy, with effusion
  fibrinopurulent, fibropurulent — see Pyothorax
  hemorrhagic — see Hemothorax
  pneumococcal J90
  purulent — see Pyothorax
  septic — see Pyothorax
  serofibrinous — see Pleurisy, with effusion
  seropurulent — see Pyothorax
  serous — see Pleurisy, with effusion
  staphylococcal J86.9
  streptococcal J90
  suppurative — see Pyothorax
  traumatic (post) (current) — see Injury, intrathoracic, pleura
  tuberculous (with effusion) (non primary) A15.6
    primary (progressive) A15.7
Pleuritis sicca — see Pleurisy
Pleurobronchopneumonia — see Pneumonia, broncho-
Pleurodynia R07.81
  epidemic B33.0
  viral B33.0
Pleuropericarditis — see also Pericarditis
  acute I30.9
Pleuropneumonia (acute) (bilateral) (double) (septic) — see also Pneumonia J18.8
  chronic — see Fibrosis, lung
Pleuro-pneumonia-like-organism (PPLO), as cause of disease classified elsewhere B96.0
Pleurorrhea — see Pleurisy, with effusion

Plexitis, brachial G54.0
Plica
  polonica B85.0
  syndrome, knee M67.5- ☑
  tonsil J35.8
Plicated tongue K14.5
Plug
  bronchus NEC J98.09
  meconium (newborn) NEC syndrome P76.0
  mucus — see Asphyxia, mucus
Plumbism — see subcategory T56.0 ☑
Plummer's disease E05.20
  with thyroid storm E05.21
Plummer-Vinson syndrome D50.1
Pluricarential syndrome of infancy E40
Plus (and minus) **hand** (intrinsic) — see Deformity, limb, specified type NEC, forearm
PMEI (polymorphic epilepsy in infancy) G40.83- ☑
Pneumathemia — see Air, embolism
Pneumatic hammer (drill) syndrome T75.21 ☑
Pneumatocele (lung) J98.4
  intracranial G93.89
  tension J44.9
Pneumatosis
  cystoides intestinalis K63.89
  intestinalis K63.89
  peritonei K66.8
Pneumaturia R39.89
Pneumoblastoma — see Neoplasm, lung, malignant
Pneumocephalus G93.89
Pneumococcemia A40.3
Pneumococcus, pneumococcal — see condition
Pneumoconiosis (due to) (inhalation of) J64
  with tuberculosis (any type in A15) J65
  aluminum J63.0
  asbestos J61
  bagasse, bagassosis J67.1
  bauxite J63.1
  beryllium J63.2
  coal miners' (simple) J60
  coalworkers' (simple) J60
  collier's J60
  cotton dust J66.0
  diatomite (diatomaceous earth) J62.8
  dust
    inorganic NEC J63.6
    lime J62.8
    marble J62.8
    organic NEC J66.8
  fumes or vapors (from silo) J68.9
  graphite J63.3
  grinder's J62.8
  kaolin J62.8
  mica J62.8
  millstone maker's J62.8
  mineral fibers NEC J61
  miner's J60
  moldy hay J67.0
  potter's J62.8
  rheumatoid — see Rheumatoid, lung
  sandblaster's J62.8
  silica, silicate NEC J62.8
    with carbon J60
  stonemason's J62.8
  talc (dust) J62.0
Pneumocystis carinii pneumonia B59
Pneumocystis jiroveci (pneumonia) B59
Pneumocystosis (with pneumonia) B59
Pneumohemopericardium I31.2
Pneumohemothorax J94.2
  traumatic S27.2 ☑
Pneumohydropericardium — see Pericarditis
Pneumohydrothorax — see Hydrothorax
Pneumomediastinum J98.2
  congenital or perinatal P25.2
Pneumomycosis B49 [J99]
Pneumonia (acute) (double) (migratory) (purulent) (septic) (unresolved) J18.9
  with
    influenza — see Influenza, with, pneumonia
    lung abscess J85.1
      due to specified organism — see Pneumonia, in (due to)
  2019 (novel) coronavirus J12.82
  adenoviral J12.0
  adynamic J18.2
  alba A50.04
  allergic — see also Pneumonitis, hypersensitivity J82.89

Pneumonia — *continued*
  alveolar — *see* Pneumonia, lobar
  anaerobes J15.8
  anthrax A22.1
  apex, apical — *see* Pneumonia, lobar
  Ascaris B77.81
  aspiration J69.0
    due to
      aspiration of microorganisms
        bacterial J15.9
        viral J12.9
      food (regurgitated) J69.0
      gastric secretions J69.0
      milk (regurgitated) J69.0
      oils, essences J69.1
      solids, liquids NEC J69.8
      vomitus J69.0
    newborn P24.81
      amniotic fluid (clear) P24.11
      blood P24.21
      food (regurgitated) P24.31
      liquor (amnii) P24.11
      meconium P24.01
      milk P24.31
      mucus P24.11
      specified NEC P24.81
      stomach contents P24.31
    postprocedural J95.4
  atypical NEC J18.9
  bacillus J15.9
    specified NEC J15.8
  bacterial J15.9
    specified NEC J15.8
  Bacteroides (fragilis) (oralis) (melaninogenicus) J15.8
  basal, basic, basilar — *see* Pneumonia, by type
  bronchiolitis obliterans organized (BOOP) J84.89
  broncho-, bronchial (confluent) (croupous) (diffuse)
    (disseminated) (hemorrhagic) (involving lobes)
    (lobar) (terminal) J18.0
    allergic — *see also* Pneumonitis, hypersensitivity
      J82.89
    aspiration — *see* Pneumonia, aspiration
    bacterial J15.9
      specified NEC J15.8
    chronic — *see* Fibrosis, lung
    diplococcal J13
    Eaton's agent J15.7
    Escherichia coli (E. coli) J15.5
    Friedländer's bacillus J15.0
    Hemophilus influenzae J14
    hypostatic J18.2
    inhalation — *see also* Pneumonia, aspiration
      due to fumes or vapors (chemical) J68.0
      of oils or essences J69.1
    Klebsiella (pneumoniae) J15.0
    lipid, lipoid J69.1
      endogenous J84.89
    Mycoplasma (pneumoniae) J15.7
    pleuro-pneumonia-like-organisms (PPLO) J15.7
    pneumococcal J13
    Proteus J15.6
    Pseudomonas J15.1
    Serratia marcescens J15.6
    specified organism NEC J16.8
    staphylococcal — *see* Pneumonia, staphylococcal
    streptococcal NEC J15.4
      group B J15.3
      pneumoniae J13
    viral, virus — *see* Pneumonia, viral
  Butyrivibrio (fibriosolvens) J15.8
  Candida B37.1
  caseous — *see* Tuberculosis, pulmonary
  catarrhal — *see* Pneumonia, broncho
  chlamydial J16.0
    congenital P23.1
  cholesterol J84.89
  cirrhotic (chronic) — *see* Fibrosis, lung
  Clostridium (haemolyticum) (novyi) J15.8
  confluent — *see* Pneumonia, broncho
  congenital (infective) P23.9
    due to
      bacterium NEC P23.6
      Chlamydia P23.1
      Escherichia coli P23.4
      Haemophilus influenzae P23.6
      infective organism NEC P23.8
      Klebsiella pneumoniae P23.6
      Mycoplasma P23.6

Pneumonia — *continued*
  congenital — *continued*
    due to — *continued*
      Pseudomonas P23.5
      Staphylococcus P23.2
      Streptococcus (except group B) P23.6
        group B P23.3
      viral agent P23.0
    specified NEC P23.8
  coronavirus (novel) (disease) 2019 J12.82
  COVID-19 J12.82
  croupous — *see* Pneumonia, lobar
  cryptogenic organizing J84.116
  cytomegalic inclusion B25.0
  cytomegaloviral B25.0
  deglutition — *see* Pneumonia, aspiration
  desquamative interstitial J84.117
  diffuse — *see* Pneumonia, broncho
  diplococcal, diplococcus (broncho-) (lobar) J13
  disseminated (focal) — *see* Pneumonia, broncho
  Eaton's agent J15.7
  embolic, embolism — *see* Embolism, pulmonary
  Enterobacter J15.6
  eosinophilic J82.81
    acute J82.82
    chronic J82.81
  Escherichia coli (E. coli) J15.5
  Eubacterium J15.8
  fibrinous — *see* Pneumonia, lobar
  fibroid, fibrous (chronic) — *see* Fibrosis, lung
  Friedländer's bacillus J15.0
  Fusobacterium (nucleatum) J15.8
  gangrenous J85.0
  giant cell (measles) B05.2
  gonococcal A54.84
  gram-negative bacteria NEC J15.6
    anaerobic J15.8
  Hemophilus influenzae (broncho) (lobar) J14
  human metapneumovirus J12.3
  hypostatic (broncho) (lobar) J18.2
  in (due to)
    actinomycosis A42.0
    adenovirus J12.0
    anthrax A22.1
    ascariasis B77.81
    aspergillosis B44.9
    Bacillus anthracis A22.1
    Bacterium anitratum J15.6
    candidiasis B37.1
    chickenpox B01.2
    Chlamydia J16.0
      neonatal P23.1
    coccidioidomycosis B38.2
      acute B38.0
      chronic B38.1
    cytomegalovirus disease B25.0
    Diplococcus (pneumoniae) J13
    Eaton's agent J15.7
    Enterobacter J15.6
    Escherichia coli (E. coli) J15.5
    Friedländer's bacillus J15.0
    fumes and vapors (chemical) (inhalation) J68.0
    gonorrhea A54.84
    Hemophilus influenzae (H. influenzae) J14
    Herellea J15.6
    histoplasmosis B39.2
      acute B39.0
      chronic B39.1
    human metapneumovirus J12.3
    Klebsiella (pneumoniae) J15.0
    measles B05.2
    Mycoplasma (pneumoniae) J15.7
    nocardiosis, nocardiasis A43.0
    ornithosis A70
    parainfluenza virus J12.2
    pleuro-pneumonia-like-organism (PPLO) J15.7
    pneumococcus J13
    pneumocystosis (Pneumocystis carinii) (Pneumocystis jiroveci) B59
    Proteus J15.6
    Pseudomonas NEC J15.1
      pseudomallei A24.1
    psittacosis A70
    Q fever A78
    respiratory syncytial virus (RSV) J12.1
    rheumatic fever I00 [J17]
    rubella B06.81
    Salmonella (infection) A02.22

Pneumonia — *continued*
  in — *continued*
    Salmonella — *continued*
      typhi A01.03
    schistosomiasis B65.9 [J17]
    Serratia marcescens J15.6
    specified
      bacterium NEC J15.8
      organism NEC J16.8
    spirochetal NEC A69.8
    Staphylococcus J15.20
      aureus (methicillin susceptible) (MSSA) J15.211
        methicillin resistant (MRSA) J15.212
      specified NEC J15.29
    Streptococcus J15.4
      group B J15.3
      pneumoniae J13
      specified NEC J15.4
    toxoplasmosis B58.3
    tularemia A21.2
    typhoid (fever) A01.03
    varicella B01.2
    virus — *see* Pneumonia, viral
    whooping cough A37.91
      due to
        Bordetella parapertussis A37.11
        Bordetella pertussis A37.01
        specified NEC A37.81
    Yersinia pestis A20.2
  inhalation of food or vomit — *see* Pneumonia, aspiration
  interstitial J84.9
    chronic J84.111
    desquamative J84.117
    due to
      collagen vascular disease J84.178
      known underlying cause J84.178
    idiopathic NOS J84.111
    in disease classified elsewhere J84.178
    lymphocytic (due to collagen vascular disease) (in diseases classified elsewhere) J84.178
    lymphoid J84.2
    non-specific J84.89
      due to
        collagen vascular disease J84.178
        known underlying cause J84.178
      idiopathic J84.113
      in diseases classified elsewhere J84.178
    plasma cell B59
    pseudomonas J15.1
    usual J84.112
      due to collagen vascular disease J84.178
      idiopathic J84.112
      in diseases classified elsewhere J84.178
  Klebsiella (pneumoniae) J15.0
  lipid, lipoid (exogenous) J69.1
    endogenous J84.89
  lobar (disseminated) (double) (interstitial) J18.1
    bacterial J15.9
      specified NEC J15.8
    chronic — *see* Fibrosis, lung
    Escherichia coli (E. coli) J15.5
    Friedländer's bacillus J15.0
    Hemophilus influenzae J14
    hypostatic J18.2
    Klebsiella (pneumoniae) J15.0
    pneumococcal J13
    Proteus J15.6
    Pseudomonas J15.1
    specified organism NEC J16.8
    staphylococcal — *see* Pneumonia, staphylococcal
    streptococcal NEC J15.4
    Streptococcus pneumoniae J13
    viral, virus — *see* Pneumonia, viral
  lobular — *see* Pneumonia, broncho
  Löffler's J82.89
  lymphoid interstitial J84.2
  massive — *see* Pneumonia, lobar
  meconium P24.01
  MRSA (methicillin resistant Staphylococcus aureus) J15.212
  MSSA (methicillin susceptible Staphylococcus aureus) J15.211
  multilobar — *see* Pneumonia, by type
  Mycoplasma (pneumoniae) J15.7
  necrotic J85.0
  neonatal P23.9

Pneumonia — continued
- neonatal — continued
  - aspiration — see Aspiration, by substance, with pneumonia
- nitrogen dioxide J68.0
- organizing J84.89
  - due to
    - collagen vascular disease J84.178
    - known underlying cause J84.178
  - in diseases classified elsewhere J84.178
- orthostatic J18.2
- parainfluenza virus J12.2
- parenchymatous — see Fibrosis, lung
- passive J18.2
- patchy — see Pneumonia, broncho
- Peptococcus J15.8
- Peptostreptococcus J15.8
- plasma cell (of infants) B59
- pleurolobar — see Pneumonia, lobar
- pleuro-pneumonia-like organism (PPLO) J15.7
- pneumococcal (broncho) (lobar) J13
- Pneumocystis (carinii) (jiroveci) B59
- postinfectional NEC B99 ☑ [J17]
- postmeasles B05.2
- Proteus J15.6
- Pseudomonas J15.1
- psittacosis A70
- radiation J70.0
- respiratory syncytial virus (RSV) J12.1
- resulting from a procedure J95.89
- rheumatic I00 [J17]
- Salmonella (arizonae) (cholerae-suis) (enteritidis) (typhimurium) A02.22
  - typhi A01.03
  - typhoid fever A01.03
- SARS-associated coronavirus J12.81
- SARS-CoV-2 J12.82
- segmented, segmental — see Pneumonia, broncho-
- Serratia marcescens J15.6
- specified NEC J18.8
  - bacterium NEC J15.8
  - organism NEC J16.8
  - virus NEC J12.89
- spirochetal NEC A69.8
- staphylococcal (broncho) (lobar) J15.20
  - aureus (methicillin susceptible) (MSSA) J15.211
    - methicillin resistant (MRSA) J15.212
  - specified NEC J15.29
- static, stasis J18.2
- streptococcal NEC (broncho) (lobar) J15.4
  - group
    - A J15.4
    - B J15.3
    - specified NEC J15.4
- Streptococcus pneumoniae J13
- syphilitic, congenital (early) A50.04
- traumatic (complication) (early) (secondary) T79.8 ☑
- tuberculous (any) — see Tuberculosis, pulmonary
- tularemic A21.2
- varicella B01.2
- Veillonella J15.8
- ventilator associated J95.851
- viral, virus (broncho) (interstitial) (lobar) J12.9
  - adenoviral J12.0
  - congenital P23.0
  - human metapneumovirus J12.3
  - parainfluenza J12.2
  - respiratory syncytial (RSV) J12.1
  - SARS-associated coronavirus J12.81
  - specified NEC J12.89
- white (congenital) A50.04

Pneumonic — see condition

Pneumonitis (acute) (primary) — see also Pneumonia
- air-conditioner J67.7
- allergic (due to) J67.9
  - organic dust NEC J67.8
  - red cedar dust J67.8
  - sequoiosis J67.8
  - wood dust J67.8
- aspiration J69.0
  - due to
    - anesthesia J95.4
      - during
        - labor and delivery O74.0
        - pregnancy O29.01- ☑
        - puerperium O89.01
    - fumes or gases J68.0
  - obstetric O74.0

Pneumonitis — continued
- chemical (due to gases, fumes or vapors) (inhalation) J68.0
  - due to anesthesia J95.4
- cholesterol J84.89
- chronic — see Fibrosis, lung
- congenital rubella P35.0
- crack (cocaine) J68.0
- due to
  - beryllium J68.0
  - cadmium J68.0
  - crack (cocaine) J68.0
  - detergent J69.8
  - fluorocarbon-polymer J68.0
  - food, vomit (aspiration) J69.0
  - fumes or vapors J68.0
  - gases, fumes or vapors (inhalation) J68.0
  - inhalation
    - blood J69.8
    - essences J69.1
    - food (regurgitated), milk, vomit J69.0
    - oils, essences J69.1
    - saliva J69.0
    - solids, liquids NEC J69.8
  - manganese J68.0
  - nitrogen dioxide J68.0
  - oils, essences J69.1
  - solids, liquids NEC J69.8
  - toxoplasmosis (acquired) B58.3
    - congenital P37.1
  - vanadium J68.0
  - ventilator J95.851
- eosinophilic J82.81
  - acute J82.82
  - chronic J82.81
- hypersensitivity J67.9
  - air conditioner lung J67.7
  - bagassosis J67.1
  - bird fancier's lung J67.2
  - farmer's lung J67.0
  - maltworker's lung J67.4
  - maple bark-stripper's lung J67.6
  - mushroom worker's lung J67.5
  - specified organic dust NEC J67.8
  - suberosis J67.3
- interstitial (chronic) J84.89
  - acute J84.114
  - lymphoid J84.2
  - non-specific J84.89
    - idiopathic J84.113
- lymphoid, interstitial J84.2
- meconium P24.01
- postanesthetic J95.4
  - correct substance properly administered — see Table of Drugs and Chemicals, by drug, adverse effect
  - in labor and delivery O74.0
  - in pregnancy O29.01- ☑
  - obstetric O74.0
  - overdose or wrong substance given or taken (by accident) — see Table of Drugs and Chemicals, by drug, poisoning
  - postpartum, puerperal O89.01
- postoperative J95.4
  - obstetric O74.0
- radiation J70.0
- rubella, congenital P35.0
- ventilation (air-conditioning) J67.7
- ventilator associated J95.851
- wood-dust J67.8

Pneumonoconiosis — see Pneumoconiosis
Pneumoparotid K11.8
Pneumopathy NEC J98.4
- alveolar J84.09
- due to organic dust NEC J66.8
- parietoalveolar J84.09
Pneumopericarditis — see also Pericarditis
- acute I30.9
Pneumopericardium — see also Pericarditis
- congenital P25.3
- newborn P25.3
- traumatic (post) — see Injury, heart
Pneumophagia (psychogenic) F45.8
Pneumopleurisy, pneumopleuritis — see also Pneumonia J18.8
Pneumopyopericardium I30.1
Pneumopyothorax — see Pyopneumothorax
- with fistula J86.0

Pneumorrhagia — see also Hemorrhage, lung
- tuberculous — see Tuberculosis, pulmonary
Pneumothorax NOS J93.9
- acute J93.83
- chronic J93.81
- congenital P25.1
- perinatal period P25.1
- postprocedural J95.811
- specified NEC J93.83
- spontaneous NOS J93.83
  - newborn P25.1
  - primary J93.11
  - secondary J93.12
  - tension J93.0
- tense valvular, infectional J93.0
- tension (spontaneous) J93.0
- traumatic S27.0 ☑
  - with hemothorax S27.2 ☑
- tuberculous — see Tuberculosis, pulmonary
Podagra — see also Gout M10.9
Podencephalus Q01.9
Poikilocytosis R71.8
Poikiloderma L81.6
- Civatte's L57.3
- congenital Q82.8
- vasculare atrophicans L94.5
Poikilodermatomyositis M33.10
- with
  - myopathy M33.12
  - respiratory involvement M33.11
  - specified organ involvement NEC M33.19
Pointed ear (congenital) Q17.3
Poison ivy, oak, sumac or other plant dermatitis (allergic) (contact) L23.7
Poisoning (acute) — see also Table of Drugs and Chemicals
- algae and toxins T65.82- ☑
- Bacillus B (aertrycke) (cholerae (suis)) (paratyphosus) (suipestifer) A02.9
  - botulinus A05.1
- bacterial toxins A05.9
- berries, noxious — see Poisoning, food, noxious, berries
- botulism A05.1
- ciguatera fish T61.0- ☑
- Clostridium botulinum A05.1
- death-cap (Amanita phalloides) (Amanita verna) — see Poisoning, food, noxious, mushrooms
- drug — see Table of Drugs and Chemicals, by drug, poisoning
- epidemic, fish (noxious) — see Poisoning, seafood bacterial A05.9
- fava bean D55.0
- fish (noxious) T61.9- ☑
  - bacterial — see Intoxication, foodborne, by agent
  - ciguatera fish — see Poisoning, ciguatera fish
  - scombroid fish — see Poisoning, scombroid fish
  - specified type NEC T61.77- ☑
- food NEC A05.9
  - bacterial — see Intoxication, foodborne, by agent
  - due to
    - Bacillus (aertrycke) (choleraesuis) (paratyphosus) (suipestifer) A02.9
      - botulinus A05.1
    - Clostridium (perfringens) (Welchii) A05.2
    - salmonella (aertrycke) (callinarum) (choleraesuis) (enteritidis) (paratyphi) (suipestifer) A02.9
      - with
        - gastroenteritis A02.0
        - sepsis A02.1
    - staphylococcus A05.0
    - Vibrio
      - parahaemolyticus A05.3
      - vulnificus A05.5
  - noxious or naturally toxic T62.9- ☑
    - berries — see subcategory T62.1 ☑
    - fish — see Poisoning, seafood
    - mushrooms — see subcategory T62.0X ☑
    - plants NEC — see subcategory T62.2X ☑
    - seafood — see Poisoning, seafood
    - specified NEC — see subcategory T62.8X ☑
- ichthyotoxism — see Poisoning, seafood
- kreotoxism, food A05.9
- latex T65.81- ☑
- lead T56.0- ☑
- mushroom — see Poisoning, food, noxious, mushroom
- mussels — see also Poisoning, shellfish
  - bacterial — see Intoxication, foodborne, by agent

☑ Additional Character Required — Refer to the Tabular List for Character Selection   ▽ Subterms under main terms may continue to next column or page

Poisoning — *continued*
  nicotine (tobacco) T65.2- ☑
  noxious foodstuffs — *see* Poisoning, food, noxious
  plants, noxious — *see* Poisoning, food, noxious, plants NEC
  ptomaine — *see* Poisoning, food
  radiation J70.0
  Salmonella (arizonae) (cholerae-suis) (enteritidis) (typhimurium) A02.9
  scombroid fish T61.1- ☑
  seafood (noxious) T61.9- ☑
    bacterial — *see* Intoxication, foodborne, by agent
    fish — *see* Poisoning, fish
    shellfish — *see* Poisoning, shellfish
    specified NEC — *see* subcategory T61.8X ☑
  shellfish (amnesic) (azaspiracid) (diarrheic) (neurotoxic) (noxious) (paralytic) T61.78- ☑
    bacterial — *see* Intoxication, foodborne, by agent
    ciguatera mollusk — *see* Poisoning, ciguatera fish
  specified substance NEC T65.891 ☑
  Staphylococcus, food A05.0
  tobacco (nicotine) T65.2- ☑
  water E87.79
Poker spine — *see* Spondylitis, ankylosing
Poland syndrome Q79.8
Polioencephalitis (acute) (bulbar) A80.9
  inferior G12.22
  influenzal — *see* Influenza, with, encephalopathy
  superior hemorrhagic (acute) (Wernicke's) E51.2
  Wernicke's E51.2
Polioencephalomyelitis (acute) (anterior) A80.9
  with beriberi E51.2
Polioencephalopathy, superior hemorrhagic E51.2
  with
    beriberi E51.11
    pellagra E52
Poliomeningoencephalitis — *see* Meningoencephalitis
Poliomyelitis (acute) (anterior) (epidemic) A80.9
  with paralysis (bulbar) — *see* Poliomyelitis, paralytic
  abortive A80.4
  ascending (progressive) — *see* Poliomyelitis, paralytic
  bulbar (paralytic) — *see* Poliomyelitis, paralytic
  congenital P35.8
  nonepidemic A80.9
  nonparalytic A80.4
  paralytic A80.30
    specified NEC A80.39
    vaccine-associated A80.0
    wild virus
      imported A80.1
      indigenous A80.2
  spinal, acute A80.9
Poliosis (eyebrow) (eyelashes) L67.1
  circumscripta, acquired L67.1
Pollakiuria R35.0
  psychogenic F45.8
Pollinosis J30.1
Pollitzer's disease L73.2
Polyadenitis — *see also* Lymphadenitis
  malignant A20.0
Polyalgia M79.89
Polyangiitis M30.0
  microscopic M31.7
  overlap syndrome M30.8
Polyarteritis
  microscopic M31.7
  nodosa M30.0
    with lung involvement M30.1
    juvenile M30.2
    related condition NEC M30.8
Polyarthralgia — *see* Pain, joint
Polyarthritis, polyarthropathy — *see also* Arthritis M13.0
  due to or associated with other specified conditions — *see* Arthritis
  epidemic (Australian) (with exanthema) B33.1
  infective — *see* Arthritis, pyogenic or pyemic
  inflammatory M06.4
  juvenile (chronic) (seronegative) M08.3
  migratory M13.8- ☑
  rheumatic, acute — *see* Fever, rheumatic
Polyarthrosis M15.9
  post-traumatic M15.3
  primary M15.0
  specified NEC M15.8
Polycarential syndrome of infancy E40

Polychondritis (atrophic) (chronic) — *see also* Disorder, cartilage, specified type NEC
  relapsing M94.1
Polycoria Q13.2
Polycystic (disease)
  degeneration, kidney Q61.3
    autosomal dominant (adult type) Q61.2
    autosomal recessive (infantile type) NEC Q61.19
  kidney Q61.3
    autosomal
      dominant Q61.2
      recessive NEC Q61.19
    autosomal dominant (adult type) Q61.2
    autosomal recessive (childhood type) NEC Q61.19
    infantile type NEC Q61.19
  liver Q44.6
  lung J98.4
    congenital Q33.0
  ovary, ovaries E28.2
  spleen Q89.09
Polycythemia (secondary) D75.1
  acquired D75.1
  benign (familial) D75.0
  due to
    donor twin P61.1
    erythropoietin D75.1
    fall in plasma volume D75.1
    high altitude D75.1
    maternal-fetal transfusion P61.1
    stress D75.1
  emotional D75.1
  erythropoietin D75.1
  familial (benign) D75.0
  Gaisböck's (hypertonica) D75.1
  high altitude D75.1
  hypertonica D75.1
  hypoxemic D75.1
  neonatorum P61.1
  nephrogenous D75.1
  relative D75.1
  secondary D75.1
  spurious D75.1
  stress D75.1
  vera D45
Polycytosis cryptogenica D75.1
Polydactylism, polydactyly Q69.9
  toes Q69.2
Polydipsia R63.1
Polydystrophy, pseudo-Hurler E77.0
Polyembryoma — *see* Neoplasm, malignant, by site
Polyglandular
  deficiency E31.0
  dyscrasia E31.9
  dysfunction E31.9
  syndrome E31.8
Polyhydramnios O40.- ☑
Polymastia Q83.1
Polymenorrhea N92.0
Polymyalgia M35.3
  arteritica, giant cell M31.5
  rheumatica M35.3
    with giant cell arteritis M31.5
Polymyositis (acute) (chronic) (hemorrhagic) M33.20
  with
    myopathy M33.22
    respiratory involvement M33.21
    skin involvement — *see* Dermatopolymyositis
    specified organ involvement NEC M33.29
  ossificans (generalisata) (progressiva) — *see* Myositis, ossificans, progressiva
Polyneuritis, polyneuritic — *see also* Polyneuropathy
  acute (post-)infective G61.0
  alcoholic G62.1
  cranialis G52.7
  demyelinating, chronic inflammatory (CIDP) G61.81
  diabetic — *see* Diabetes, polyneuropathy
  diphtheritic A36.83
  due to lack of vitamin NEC E56.9 *[G63]*
  endemic E51.11
  erythredema — *see* subcategory T56.1 ☑
  febrile, acute G61.0
  hereditary ataxic G60.1
  idiopathic, acute G61.0
  infective (acute) G61.0
  inflammatory, chronic demyelinating (CIDP) G61.81
  nutritional E63.9 *[G63]*
  postinfective (acute) G61.0
  specified NEC G62.89

Polyneuropathy (peripheral) G62.9
  alcoholic G62.1
  amyloid (Portuguese) E85.1 *[G63]*
    transthyretin-related (ATTR) familial E85.1 *[G63]*
  arsenical G62.2
  critical illness G62.81
  demyelinating, chronic inflammatory (CIDP) G61.81
  diabetic — *see* Diabetes, polyneuropathy
  drug-induced G62.0
  hereditary G60.9
    specified NEC G60.8
  idiopathic G60.9
    progressive G60.3
  in (due to)
    alcohol G62.1
      sequelae G65.2
    amyloidosis, familial (Portuguese) E85.1 *[G63]*
    antitetanus serum G61.1
    arsenic G62.2
      sequelae G65.2
    avitaminosis NEC E56.9 *[G63]*
    beriberi E51.11
    collagen vascular disease NEC M35.9 *[G63]*
    deficiency (of)
      B (-complex) vitamins E53.9 *[G63]*
      vitamin B6 E53.1 *[G63]*
    diabetes — *see* Diabetes, polyneuropathy
    diphtheria A36.83
    drug or medicament G62.0
      correct substance properly administered — *see* Table of Drugs and Chemicals, by drug, adverse effect
      overdose or wrong substance given or taken — *see* Table of Drugs and Chemicals, by drug, poisoning
    endocrine disease NEC E34.9 *[G63]*
    herpes zoster B02.23
    hypoglycemia E16.2 *[G63]*
    infectious
      disease NEC B99 ☑ *[G63]*
      mononucleosis B27.91
    lack of vitamin NEC E56.9 *[G63]*
    lead G62.2
      sequelae G65.2
    leprosy A30.9 *[G63]*
    Lyme disease A69.22
    metabolic disease NEC E88.9 *[G63]*
    microscopic polyangiitis M31.7 *[G63]*
    mumps B26.84
    neoplastic disease — *see also* Neoplasm D49.9 *[G63]*
    nutritional deficiency NEC E63.9 *[G63]*
    organophosphate compounds G62.2
      sequelae G65.2
    parasitic disease NEC B89 *[G63]*
    pellagra E52 *[G63]*
    polyarteritis nodosa M30.0
    porphyria E80.20 *[G63]*
    radiation G62.82
    rheumatoid arthritis — *see* Rheumatoid, polyneuropathy
    sarcoidosis D86.89
    serum G61.1
    syphilis (late) A52.15
      congenital A50.43
    systemic
      connective tissue disorder M35.9 *[G63]*
      lupus erythematosus M32.19
    toxic agent NEC G62.2
      sequelae G65.2
    transthyretin-related (ATTR) familial amyloid E85.1
    triorthocresyl phosphate G62.2
      sequelae G65.2
    tuberculosis A17.89
    uremia N18.9 *[G63]*
    vitamin B12 deficiency E53.8 *[G63]*
      with anemia (pernicious) D51.0 *[G63]*
        due to dietary deficiency D51.3, G63
    zoster B02.23
  inflammatory G61.9
    chronic demyelinating (CIDP) G61.81
    sequelae G65.1
    specified NEC G61.89
  lead G62.2
    sequelae G65.2
  nutritional NEC E63.9 *[G63]*
  postherpetic (zoster) B02.23
  progressive G60.3
  radiation-induced G62.82

Polyneuropathy — *continued*
  sensory (hereditary) (idiopathic) G60.8
  specified NEC G62.89
  syphilitic (late) A52.15
    congenital A50.43
Polyopia H53.8
Polyorchism, polyorchidism Q55.21
Polyosteoarthritis — *see also* Osteoarthritis, generalized M15.9
  post-traumatic M15.3
  specified NEC M15.8
Polyostotic fibrous dysplasia Q78.1
Polyotia Q17.0
Polyp, polypus
  accessory sinus J33.8
  adenocarcinoma in — *see* Neoplasm, malignant, by site
  adenocarcinoma in situ in — *see* Neoplasm, in situ, by site
  adenoid tissue J33.0
  adenomatous — *see also* Neoplasm, benign, by site
    adenocarcinoma in — *see* Neoplasm, malignant, by site
    adenocarcinoma in situ in — *see* Neoplasm, in situ, by site
    carcinoma in — *see* Neoplasm, malignant, by site
    carcinoma in situ in — *see* Neoplasm, in situ, by site
    multiple — *see* Neoplasm, benign
      adenocarcinoma in — *see* Neoplasm, malignant, by site
      adenocarcinoma in situ in — *see* Neoplasm, in situ, by site
  antrum J33.8
  anus, anal (canal) K62.0
  Bartholin's gland N84.3
  bladder D41.4
  carcinoma in — *see* Neoplasm, malignant, by site
  carcinoma in situ in — *see* Neoplasm, in situ, by site
  cecum D12.0
  cervix (uteri) N84.1
    in pregnancy or childbirth — *see* Pregnancy, complicated by, abnormal, cervix
    mucous N84.1
    nonneoplastic N84.1
  choanal J33.0
  cholesterol K82.4
  clitoris N84.3
  colon K63.5
    adenomatous D12.6
      ascending D12.2
      cecum D12.0
      descending D12.4
      sigmoid D12.5
      transverse D12.3
    ascending K63.5
    cecum K63.5
    descending K63.5
    hyperplastic, (any site) K63.5
    inflammatory K51.40
      with
        abscess K51.414
        complication K51.419
          specified NEC K51.418
        fistula K51.413
        intestinal obstruction K51.412
        rectal bleeding K51.411
    sigmoid K63.5
    transverse K63.5
  corpus uteri N84.0
  dental K04.01
    irreversible K04.02
    reversible K04.01
  duodenum K31.7
  ear (middle) H74.4- ☑
  endometrium N84.0
  esophageal K22.81
  esophagogastric junction K22.82
  ethmoidal (sinus) J33.8
  fallopian tube N84.8
  female genital tract N84.9
    specified NEC N84.8
  frontal (sinus) J33.8
  gallbladder K82.4
  gingiva, gum K06.8
  labia, labium (majus) (minus) N84.3
  larynx (mucous) J38.1
    adenomatous D14.1
  malignant — *see* Neoplasm, malignant, by site

Polyp, polypus — *continued*
  maxillary (sinus) J33.8
  middle ear — *see* Polyp, ear (middle)
  myometrium N84.0
  nares
    anterior J33.9
    posterior J33.0
  nasal (mucous) J33.9
    cavity J33.0
    septum J33.0
  nasopharyngeal J33.0
  nose (mucous) J33.9
  oviduct N84.8
  pharynx J39.2
  placenta O90.89
  prostate — *see* Enlargement, enlarged, prostate
  pudenda, pudendum N84.3
  pulpal (dental) K04.01
    irreversible K04.02
    reversible K04.01
  rectum (nonadenomatous) K62.1
    adenomatous — *see* Polyp, adenomatous
  septum (nasal) J33.0
  sinus (accessory) (ethmoidal) (frontal) (maxillary) (sphenoidal) J33.8
  sphenoidal (sinus) J33.8
  stomach K31.7
    adenomatous D13.1
  tube, fallopian N84.8
  turbinate, mucous membrane J33.8
  umbilical, newborn P83.6
  ureter N28.89
  urethra N36.2
  uterus (body) (corpus) (mucous) N84.0
    cervix N84.1
    in pregnancy or childbirth — *see* Pregnancy, complicated by, tumor, uterus
  vagina N84.2
  vocal cord (mucous) J38.1
  vulva N84.3
Polyphagia R63.2
Polyploidy Q92.7
Polypoid — *see* condition
Polyposis — *see also* Polyp
  coli (adenomatous) D12.6
    adenocarcinoma in C18.9
    adenocarcinoma in situ in — *see* Neoplasm, in situ, by site
    carcinoma in C18.9
  colon (adenomatous) D12.6
  familial D12.6
    adenocarcinoma in situ in — *see* Neoplasm, in situ, by site
  intestinal (adenomatous) D12.6
  malignant lymphomatous C83.1- ☑
  multiple, adenomatous — *see also* Neoplasm, benign D36.9
Polyradiculitis — *see* Polyneuropathy
Polyradiculoneuropathy (acute) (postinfective) (segmentally demyelinating) G61.0
Polyserositis
  due to pericarditis I31.1
  pericardial I31.1
  periodic, familial E85.0
  tuberculous A19.9
    acute A19.1
    chronic A19.8
Polysplenia syndrome Q89.09
Polysyndactyly — *see also* Syndactylism, syndactyly Q70.4
Polytrichia L68.3
Polyunguia Q84.6
Polyuria R35.89
  nocturnal R35.81
  psychogenic F45.8
  specified NEC R35.89
Pompe's disease (glycogen storage) E74.02
Pompholyx L30.1
Poncet's disease (tuberculous rheumatism) A18.09
Pond fracture — *see* Fracture, skull
Ponos B55.0
Pons, pontine — *see* condition
Poor
  aesthetic of existing restoration of tooth K08.56
  contractions, labor O62.2
  gingival margin to tooth restoration K08.51
  personal hygiene R46.0

Poor — *continued*
  prenatal care, affecting management of pregnancy — *see* Pregnancy, complicated by, insufficient, prenatal care
  sucking reflex (newborn) R29.2
  urinary stream R39.12
  vision NEC H54.7
Poradenitis, nostras inguinalis or venerea A55
Porencephaly (congenital) (developmental) (true) Q04.6
  acquired G93.0
  nondevelopmental G93.0
  traumatic (post) F07.89
Porocephaliasis B88.8
Porokeratosis Q82.8
Poroma, eccrine — *see* Neoplasm, skin, benign
Porphyria (South African) E80.20
  acquired E80.20
  acute intermittent (hepatic) (Swedish) E80.21
  cutanea tarda (hereditary) (symptomatic) E80.1
  due to drugs E80.20
    correct substance properly administered — *see* Table of Drugs and Chemicals, by drug, adverse effect
    overdose or wrong substance given or taken — *see* Table of Drugs and Chemicals, by drug, poisoning
  erythropoietic (congenital) (hereditary) E80.0
  hepatocutaneous type E80.1
  secondary E80.20
  toxic NEC E80.20
  variegata E80.20
Porphyrinuria — *see* Porphyria
Porphyruria — *see* Porphyria
Port wine nevus, mark, or stain Q82.5
Portal — *see* condition
Posadas-Wernicke disease B38.9
Positive
  culture (nonspecific)
    blood R78.81
    bronchial washings R84.5
    cerebrospinal fluid R83.5
    cervix uteri R87.5
    nasal secretions R84.5
    nipple discharge R89.5
    nose R84.5
      staphylococcus (Methicillin susceptible) Z22.321
      Methicillin resistant Z22.322
    peritoneal fluid R85.5
    pleural fluid R84.5
    prostatic secretions R86.5
    saliva R85.5
    seminal fluid R86.5
    sputum R84.5
    synovial fluid R89.5
    throat scrapings R84.5
    urine R82.79
    vagina R87.5
    vulva R87.5
    wound secretions R89.5
  PPD (skin test) R76.11
  serology for syphilis A53.0
    false R76.8
    with signs or symptoms — *code as* Syphilis, by site and stage
  skin test, tuberculin (without active tuberculosis) R76.11
  test, human immunodeficiency virus (HIV) R75
  VDRL A53.0
    with signs or symptoms — *code by* site and stage under Syphilis A53.9
  Wassermann reaction A53.0
Post COVID-19 condition, unspecified U09.9
Postcardiotomy syndrome I97.0
Postcaval ureter Q62.62
Postcholecystectomy syndrome K91.5
Postclimacteric bleeding N95.0
Postcommissurotomy syndrome I97.0
Postconcussional syndrome F07.81
Postcontusional syndrome F07.81
Postcricoid region — *see* condition
Post-dates (40-42 weeks) (pregnancy) (mother) O48.0
  more than 42 weeks gestation O48.1
Postencephalitic syndrome F07.89
Posterior — *see* condition
Posterolateral sclerosis (spinal cord) — *see* Degeneration, combined
Postexanthematous — *see* condition
Postfebrile — *see* condition
Postgastrectomy dumping syndrome K91.1

☑ **Additional Character Required** — Refer to the Tabular List for Character Selection   🔻 **Subterms under main terms may continue to next column or page**

Posthemiplegic chorea — *see* Monoplegia
Posthemorrhagic anemia (chronic) D50.0
　acute D62
　newborn P61.3
Postherpetic neuralgia (zoster) B02.29
　trigeminal B02.22
Posthitis N47.7
Postimmunization complication or reaction — *see*
　Complications, vaccination
Postinfectious — *see* condition
Postlaminectomy syndrome NEC M96.1
Postleukotomy syndrome F07.0
Postmastectomy lymphedema (syndrome) I97.2
Postmaturity, postmature (over 42 weeks)
　maternal (over 42 weeks gestation) O48.1
　newborn P08.22
Postmeasles complication NEC — *see also* condition
　B05.89
Postmenopausal
　endometrium (atrophic) N95.8
　　suppurative — *see also* Endometritis N71.9
　osteoporosis — *see* Osteoporosis, postmenopausal
Postnasal drip R09.82
　due to
　　allergic rhinitis — *see* Rhinitis, allergic
　　common cold J00
　　gastroesophageal reflux — *see* Reflux, gastroe-
　　　sophageal
　　nasopharyngitis — *see* Nasopharyngitis
　　other known condition — *code to* condition
　　sinusitis — *see* Sinusitis
Postnatal — *see* condition
Postoperative (postprocedural) — *see* Complication,
　postoperative
　pneumothorax, therapeutic Z98.3
　state NEC Z98.890
Postpancreatectomy hyperglycemia E89.1
Postpartum — *see* Puerperal
Postphlebitic syndrome — *see* Syndrome, postthrom-
　botic
Postpolio (myelitic) **syndrome** G14
Postpoliomyelitic — *see also* condition
　osteopathy — *see* Osteopathy, after poliomyelitis
Postprocedural — *see also* Postoperative
　hypoinsulinemia E89.1
Postschizophrenic depression F32.89
Postsurgery status — *see also* Status (post)
　pneumothorax, therapeutic Z98.3
Post-term (40-42 weeks) (pregnancy) (mother) O48.0
　infant P08.21
　more than 42 weeks gestation (mother) O48.1
Post-traumatic brain syndrome, nonpsychotic F07.81
Post-typhoid abscess A01.09
Postures, hysterical F44.2
Postvaccinal reaction or complication — *see* Compli-
　cations, vaccination
Postvalvulotomy syndrome I97.0
Potain's
　disease (pulmonary edema) — *see* Edema, lung
　syndrome (gastrectasis with dyspepsia) K31.0
Potter's
　asthma J62.8
　facies Q60.6
　lung J62.8
　syndrome (with renal agenesis) Q60.6
Pott's
　curvature (spinal) A18.01
　disease or paraplegia A18.01
　spinal curvature A18.01
　tumor, puffy — *see* Osteomyelitis, specified type NEC
Pouch
　bronchus Q32.4
　Douglas' — *see* condition
　esophagus, esophageal, congenital Q39.6
　　acquired K22.5
　gastric K31.4
　Hartmann's K82.8
　pharynx, pharyngeal (congenital) Q38.7
Pouchitis K91.850
Poultrymen's itch B88.0
Poverty NEC Z59.6
　extreme Z59.5
Poxvirus NEC B08.8
Prader-Willi syndrome Q87.11
Prader-Willi-like syndrome Q87.19
Preauricular appendage or tag Q17.0

Prebetalipoproteinemia (acquired) (essential) (familial)
　(hereditary) (primary) (secondary) E78.1
　with chylomicronemia E78.3
Precipitate labor or delivery O62.3
Preclimacteric bleeding (menorrhagia) N92.4
Precocious
　adrenarche E30.1
　menarche E30.1
　menstruation E30.1
　pubarche E30.1
　puberty E30.1
　　central E22.8
　sexual development NEC E30.1
　thelarche E30.8
Precocity, sexual (constitutional) (cryptogenic) (female)
　(idiopathic) (male) E30.1
　with adrenal hyperplasia E25.9
　　congenital E25.0
Precordial pain R07.2
Predeciduous teeth K00.2
Prediabetes, prediabetic R73.03
　complicating
　　pregnancy — *see* Pregnancy, complicated by, dis-
　　　eases of, specified type or system NEC
　　puerperium O99.893
Predislocation status of hip at birth Q65.6
Pre-eclampsia O14.9- ☑
　with pre-existing hypertension — *see* Hypertension,
　　complicating pregnancy, pre-existing, with, pre-
　　eclampsia
　complicating
　　childbirth O14.94
　　puerperium O14.95
　mild O14.0- ☑
　　complicating
　　　childbirth O14.04
　　　puerperium O14.05
　moderate O14.0- ☑
　　complicating
　　　childbirth O14.04
　　　puerperium O14.05
　severe O14.1- ☑
　　with hemolysis, elevated liver enzymes and low
　　　platelet count (HELLP) O14.2- ☑
　　complicating
　　　childbirth O14.24
　　　puerperium O14.25
　　complicating
　　　childbirth O14.14
　　　puerperium O14.15
Pre-eruptive color change, teeth, tooth K00.8
Pre-excitation atrioventricular conduction I45.6
Preglaucoma H40.00- ☑
Pregnancy (single) (uterine) — *see also* Delivery and
　Puerperal Z33.1

---
*Note: The Tabular must be reviewed for assign-
ment of appropriate seventh character for multiple gestation codes in Chapter 15*

---
*Note: The Tabular must be reviewed for assign-
ment of the appropriate character indicating the
trimester of the pregnancy*

---
　abdominal (ectopic) O00.00
　　with intrauterine pregnancy O00.01
　　with viable fetus O36.7-
　ampullar O00.10- ☑
　　with intrauterine pregnancy O00.11- ☑
　biochemical O02.81
　broad ligament O00.80
　　with intrauterine pregnancy O00.81
　cervical O00.8
　　with intrauterine pregnancy O00.81
　chemical O02.81
　complicated by (care of) (management affected by)
　　abnormal, abnormality
　　　cervix O34.4- ☑
　　　　causing obstructed labor O65.5
　　　cord (umbilical) O69.9 ☑
　　　fetal heart rate or rhythm O36.83- ☑
　　　findings on antenatal screening of mother O28.9
　　　　biochemical O28.1
　　　　chromosomal O28.5
　　　　cytological O28.2
　　　　genetic O28.5
　　　　hematological O28.0
　　　　radiological O28.4
　　　　specified NEC O28.8

Pregnancy — *continued*
　complicated by — *continued*
　　abnormal, abnormality — *continued*
　　　findings on antenatal screening of mother —
　　　　continued
　　　　ultrasonic O28.3
　　　glucose (tolerance) NEC O99.810
　　　pelvic organs O34.9- ☑
　　　　specified NEC O34.8- ☑
　　　　　causing obstructed labor O65.5
　　　pelvis (bony) (major) NEC O33.0
　　　perineum O34.7- ☑
　　　position
　　　　placenta O44.0- ☑
　　　　　with hemorrhage O44.1- ☑
　　　　uterus O34.59- ☑
　　　uterus O34.59- ☑
　　　　causing obstructed labor O65.5
　　　　congenital O34.0- ☑
　　　vagina O34.6- ☑
　　　　causing obstructed labor O65.5
　　　vulva O34.7- ☑
　　　　causing obstructed labor O65.5
　　abruptio placentae — *see* Abruptio placentae
　　abscess or cellulitis
　　　bladder O23.1- ☑
　　　breast O91.11- ☑
　　　genital organ or tract O23.9- ☑
　　abuse
　　　physical O9A.31 ☑ (*following* O99)
　　　psychological O9A.51 ☑ (*following* O99)
　　　sexual O9A.41 ☑ (*following* O99)
　　adverse effect anesthesia O29.9- ☑
　　　aspiration pneumonitis O29.01- ☑
　　　cardiac arrest O29.11- ☑
　　　cardiac complication NEC O29.19- ☑
　　　cardiac failure O29.12- ☑
　　　central nervous system complication NEC
　　　　O29.29- ☑
　　　cerebral anoxia O29.21- ☑
　　　failed or difficult intubation O29.6- ☑
　　　inhalation of stomach contents or secretions NOS
　　　　O29.01- ☑
　　　local, toxic reaction O29.3X ☑
　　　Mendelson's syndrome O29.01- ☑
　　　pressure collapse of lung O29.02- ☑
　　　pulmonary complications NEC O29.09- ☑
　　　specified NEC O29.8X- ☑
　　　spinal and epidural type NEC O29.5X ☑
　　　　induced headache O29.4- ☑
　　albuminuria — *see also* Proteinuria, gestational
　　　O12.1- ☑
　　alcohol use O99.31- ☑
　　amnionitis O41.12- ☑
　　anaphylactoid syndrome of pregnancy O88.01- ☑
　　anemia (conditions in D50-D64) (pre-existing)
　　　O99.01- ☑
　　　complicating the puerperium O99.03
　　antepartum hemorrhage O46.9- ☑
　　　with coagulation defect — *see* Hemorrhage,
　　　　antepartum, with coagulation defect
　　　specified NEC O46.8X- ☑
　　appendicitis O99.61- ☑
　　atrophy (yellow) (acute) liver (subacute) O26.61- ☑
　　bariatric surgery status O99.84- ☑
　　bicornis or bicornuate uterus O34.0- ☑
　　biliary tract problems O26.61- ☑
　　breech presentation O32.1
　　cardiovascular diseases (conditions in I00-I09, I20-
　　　I52, I70-I99) O99.41- ☑
　　cerebrovascular disorders (conditions in I60-I69)
　　　O99.41- ☑
　　cervical shortening O26.87- ☑
　　cervicitis O23.51- ☑
　　cesarean scar defect (isthmocele) O34.22
　　chloasma (gravidarum) O26.89- ☑
　　cholecystitis O99.61- ☑
　　cholestasis (intrahepatic) O26.61- ☑
　　chorioamnionitis O41.12- ☑
　　circulatory system disorder (conditions in I00-I09,
　　　I20-I99, O99.41-)
　　compound presentation O32.6
　　conjoined twins O30.02- ☑
　　connective system disorders (conditions in M00-
　　　M99) O99.891
　　contracted pelvis (general) O33.1

☒ **Subterms under main terms may continue to next column or page**　　　☑ **Additional Character Required** — Refer to the Tabular List for Character Selection　　　**263**

Posthemiplegic chorea — Pregnancy

Pregnancy — *continued*
  complicated by — *continued*
    contracted pelvis — *continued*
      inlet O33.2
      outlet O33.3 ☑
    convulsions (eclamptic) (uremic) — *see also*
        Eclampsia O15.9
    cracked nipple O92.11- ☑
    cystitis O23.1- ☑
    cystocele O34.8- ☑
    death of fetus (near term) O36.4 ☑
      early pregnancy O02.1
      of one fetus or more in multiple gestation
          O31.2- ☑
    deciduitis O41.14- ☑
    decreased fetal movement O36.81- ☑
    dental problems O99.61- ☑
    diabetes (mellitus) O24.91- ☑
      gestational (pregnancy induced) — *see* Diabetes,
          gestational
      pre-existing O24.31- ☑
        specified NEC O24.81- ☑
        type 1 O24.01- ☑
        type 2 O24.11- ☑
    digestive system disorders (conditions in K00-K93)
        O99.61- ☑
    diseases of — *see* Pregnancy, complicated by,
        specified body system disease
      biliary tract O26.61- ☑
      blood NEC (conditions in D65-D77) O99.11- ☑
      liver O26.61- ☑
      specified NEC O99.891
    disorders of — *see* Pregnancy, complicated by,
        specified body system disorder
      amniotic fluid and membranes O41.9- ☑
        specified NEC O41.8X- ☑
      biliary tract O26.61- ☑
      ear and mastoid process (conditions in H60-H95)
          O99.891
      eye and adnexa (conditions in H00-H59) O99.891
      liver O26.61- ☑
      skin (conditions in L00-L99) O99.71- ☑
      specified NEC O99.891
    displacement, uterus NEC O34.59- ☑
      causing obstructed labor O65.5
    disproportion (due to) O33.9
      fetal (ascites) (hydrops) (meningomyelocele)
          (sacral teratoma) (tumor) deformities NEC
          O33.7 ☑
      generally contracted pelvis O33.1
      hydrocephalic fetus O33.6 ☑
      inlet contraction of pelvis O33.2
      mixed maternal and fetal origin O33.4 ☑
      specified NEC O33.8
    double uterus O34.0- ☑
      causing obstructed labor O65.5
    drug use (conditions in F11-F19) O99.32- ☑
    eclampsia, eclamptic (coma) (convulsions) (delirium)
        (nephritis) (uremia) — *see also* Eclampsia
        O15.- ☑
    ectopic pregnancy — *see* Pregnancy, ectopic
    edema O12.0- ☑
      with
        gestational hypertension, mild — *see also*
            Pre-eclampsia O14.0- ☑
        proteinuria O12.2- ☑
    effusion, amniotic fluid — *see* Pregnancy, compli-
        cated by, premature rupture of membranes
    elderly
      multigravida O09.52- ☑
      primigravida O09.51- ☑
    embolism — *see also* Embolism, obstetric, pregnan-
        cy O88.- ☑
    endocrine diseases NEC O99.28- ☑
    endometritis O86.12
    excessive weight gain O26.0- ☑
    exhaustion O26.81- ☑
      during labor and delivery O75.81
    face presentation O32.3 ☑
    failed induction of labor O61.9
      instrumental O61.1
      mechanical O61.1
      medical O61.0
      specified NEC O61.8
      surgical O61.1
    failed or difficult intubation for anesthesia O29.6- ☑
    false labor (pains) O47.9

Pregnancy — *continued*
  complicated by — *continued*
    false labor — *continued*
      at or after 37 completed weeks of pregnancy
          O47.1
      before 37 completed weeks of pregnancy
          O47.0- ☑
    fatigue O26.81- ☑
      during labor and delivery O75.81
    fatty metamorphosis of liver O26.61- ☑
    female genital mutilation O34.8- ☑ [N90.81-] ☑
    fetal (maternal care for)
      abnormality or damage O35.9 ☑
        acid-base balance O68
        specified type NEC O35.8 ☑
      acidemia O68
      acidosis O68
      alkalosis O68
      anemia and thrombocytopenia O36.82- ☑
      anencephaly O35.0 ☑
      bradycardia O36.83- ☑
      chromosomal abnormality (conditions in Q90-
          Q99) O35.1 ☑
      conjoined twins O30.02- ☑
      damage from
        amniocentesis O35.7 ☑
        biopsy procedures O35.7 ☑
        drug addiction O35.5 ☑
        hematological investigation O35.7 ☑
        intrauterine contraceptive device O35.7 ☑
        maternal
          alcohol addiction O35.4 ☑
          cytomegalovirus infection O35.3 ☑
          disease NEC O35.8 ☑
          drug addiction O35.5 ☑
          listeriosis O35.8 ☑
          rubella O35.3 ☑
          toxoplasmosis O35.8 ☑
          viral infection O35.3 ☑
        medical procedure NEC O35.7 ☑
        radiation O35.6 ☑
      death (near term) O36.4 ☑
        early pregnancy O02.1
      decreased movement O36.81- ☑
      depressed heart rate tones O36.83- ☑
      disproportion due to deformity (fetal) O33.7 ☑
      excessive growth (large for dates) O36.6- ☑
      growth retardation O36.59- ☑
        light for dates O36.59- ☑
        small for dates O36.59- ☑
      heart rate irregularity (abnormal variability)
          (bradycardia) (decelerations) (tachycardia)
          O36.83- ☑
      hereditary disease O35.2 ☑
      hydrocephalus O35.0 ☑
      intrauterine death O36.4 ☑
      non-reassuring heart rate or rhythm O36.83- ☑
      poor growth O36.59- ☑
        light for dates O36.59- ☑
        small for dates O36.59- ☑
      problem O36.9- ☑
        specified NEC O36.89- ☑
      reduction (elective) O31.3- ☑
      selective termination O31.3- ☑
      spina bifida O35.0 ☑
      thrombocytopenia O36.82- ☑
    fibroid (tumor) (uterus) O34.1- ☑
    fissure of nipple O92.11- ☑
    gallstones O99.61- ☑
    gastric banding status O99.84- ☑
    gastric bypass status O99.84- ☑
    genital herpes (asymptomatic) (history of) (inactive)
        O98.3- ☑
    genital tract infection O23.9- ☑
    glomerular diseases (conditions in N00-N07)
        O26.83- ☑
      with hypertension, pre-existing — *see* Hyperten-
          sion, complicating, pregnancy, pre-exist-
          ing, with, renal disease
    gonorrhea O98.21- ☑
    grand multiparity O09.4 ☑
    habitual aborter — *see* Pregnancy, complicated by,
        recurrent pregnancy loss
    HELLP syndrome (hemolysis, elevated liver enzymes
        and low platelet count) O14.2- ☑

Pregnancy — *continued*
  complicated by — *continued*
    hemorrhage
      antepartum — *see* Hemorrhage, antepartum
      before 20 completed weeks gestation O20.9
        specified NEC O20.8
        due to premature separation, placenta — *see
            also* Abruptio placentae O45.9- ☑
      early O20.9
        specified NEC O20.8
      threatened abortion O20.0
    hemorrhoids O22.4- ☑
    hepatitis (viral) O98.41- ☑
    herniation of uterus O34.59- ☑
    high
      head at term O32.4 ☑
      risk — *see* Supervision (of) (for), high-risk
    history of in utero procedure during previous preg-
        nancy O09.82- ☑
    HIV O98.71- ☑
    human immunodeficiency virus (HIV) disease
        O98.71- ☑
    hydatidiform mole — *see also* Mole, hydatidiform
        O01.9
    hydramnios O40.- ☑
    hydrocephalic fetus (disproportion) O33.6 ☑
    hydrops
      amnii O40.- ☑
      fetalis O36.2- ☑
        associated with isoimmunization — *see also*
            Pregnancy, complicated by, isoimmu-
            nization O36.11- ☑
    hydrorrhea O42.90
    hyperemesis (gravidarum) (mild) — *see also* Hyper-
        emesis, gravidarum O21.0
    hypertension — *see* Hypertension, complicating
        pregnancy
    hypertensive
      heart and renal disease, pre-existing — *see* Hy-
          pertension, complicating, pregnancy, pre-
          existing, with, heart disease, with renal
          disease
      heart disease, pre-existing — *see* Hypertension,
          complicating, pregnancy, pre-existing,
          with, heart disease
      renal disease, pre-existing — *see* Hypertension,
          complicating, pregnancy, pre-existing,
          with, renal disease
    hypotension O26.5- ☑
    immune disorders NEC (conditions in D80-D89)
        O99.11- ☑
    incarceration, uterus O34.51- ☑
    incompetent cervix O34.3- ☑
    inconclusive fetal viability O36.80 ☑
    infection(s) O98.91- ☑
      amniotic fluid or sac O41.10- ☑
      bladder O23.1- ☑
      carrier state NEC O99.830
        streptococcus B O99.820
      genital organ or tract O23.9- ☑
        specified NEC O23.59- ☑
      genitourinary tract O23.9- ☑
      gonorrhea O98.21- ☑
      hepatitis (viral) O98.41- ☑
      HIV O98.71- ☑
      human immunodeficiency virus (HIV) O98.71- ☑
      intrauterine O41.12 ☑
      kidney O23.0- ☑
      nipple O91.01- ☑
      parasitic disease O98.91- ☑
        specified NEC O98.81- ☑
      protozoal disease O98.61- ☑
      sexually transmitted NEC O98.31- ☑
      specified type NEC O98.81- ☑
      syphilis O98.11- ☑
      tuberculosis O98.01- ☑
      urethra O23.2- ☑
      urinary (tract) O23.4- ☑
        specified NEC O23.3- ☑
      viral disease O98.51- ☑
    inflammation
      intrauterine O41.12 ☑
    injury or poisoning (conditions in S00-T88)
        O9A.21- ☑ (*following* O99)
      due to abuse
        physical O9A.31- ☑ (*following* O99)
        psychological O9A.51- ☑ (*following* O99)

☑ **Additional Character Required — Refer to the Tabular List for Character Selection**   ▽ **Subterms under main terms may continue to next column or page**

Pregnancy — *continued*
  complicated by — *continued*
    injury or poisoning — *continued*
      due to abuse — *continued*
        sexual O9A.41- ☑ *(following O99)*
    insufficient
      prenatal care O09.3- ☑
      weight gain O26.1- ☑
    insulin resistance O26.89 ☑
    intrauterine fetal death (near term) O36.4 ☑
      early pregnancy O02.1
      multiple gestation (one fetus or more) O31.2- ☑
    isoimmunization O36.11- ☑
      anti-A sensitization O36.11- ☑
      anti-B sensitization O36.19- ☑
      Rh O36.09- ☑
        anti-D antibody O36.01- ☑
      specified NEC O36.19- ☑
    laceration of uterus NEC O71.81
    malformation
      placenta, placental (vessel) O43.10- ☑
        specified NEC O43.19- ☑
      uterus (congenital) O34.0- ☑
    malnutrition (conditions in E40-E46) O25.1- ☑
    maternal hypotension syndrome O26.5- ☑
    mental disorders (conditions in F01-F09, F20-F52
        and F54-F99) O99.34- ☑
      alcohol use O99.31- ☑
      drug use O99.32- ☑
      smoking O99.33- ☑
    mentum presentation O32.3 ☑
    metabolic disorders O99.28- ☑
    missed
      abortion O02.1
      delivery O36.4 ☑
    multiple gestations O30.9- ☑
      conjoined twins O30.02- ☑
      quadruplet — *see* Pregnancy, quadruplet
      specified complication NEC O31.8X- ☑
      specified number of multiples NEC — *see* Pregnancy, multiple (gestation), specified NEC
      triplet — *see* Pregnancy, triplet
      twin — *see* Pregnancy, twin
    musculoskeletal condition (conditions is M00-M99)
        O99.891
    necrosis, liver (conditions in K72) O26.61- ☑
    neoplasm
      benign
        cervix O34.4- ☑
        corpus uteri O34.1- ☑
        uterus O34.1- ☑
      malignant O9A.11- ☑ *(following O99)*
    nephropathy NEC O26.83- ☑
    nervous system condition (conditions in G00-G99)
        O99.35- ☑
    nutritional diseases NEC O99.28- ☑
    obesity (pre-existing) O99.21- ☑
    obesity surgery status O99.84- ☑
    oblique lie or presentation O32.2 ☑
    older mother — *see* Pregnancy, complicated by, elderly
    oligohydramnios O41.0- ☑
      with premature rupture of membranes — *see also* Pregnancy, complicated by, premature rupture of membranes O42.- ☑
    onset (spontaneous) of labor after 37 completed weeks of gestation but before 39 completed weeks gestation, with delivery by (planned) cesarean section O75.82
    oophoritis O23.52- ☑
    overdose, drug — *see also* Table of Drugs and Chemicals, by drug, poisoning O9A.21- ☑ *(following O99)*
    oversize fetus O33.5 ☑
    papyraceous fetus O31.0- ☑
    pelvic inflammatory disease O99.891
    periodontal disease O99.61- ☑
    peripheral neuritis O26.82- ☑
    peritoneal (pelvic) adhesions O99.891
    phlebitis O22.9- ☑
    phlebopathy O22.9- ☑
    phlebothrombosis (superficial) O22.2- ☑
      deep O22.3- ☑
    placenta accreta O43.21- ☑
    placenta increta O43.22- ☑
    placenta percreta O43.23- ☑

Pregnancy — *continued*
  complicated by — *continued*
    placenta previa O44.0- ☑
      complete O44.0- ☑
        with hemorrhage O44.1- ☑
      marginal O44.2- ☑
        with hemorrhage O44.3- ☑
      partial O44.2- ☑
        with hemorrhage O44.3- ☑
    placental disorder O43.9- ☑
      specified NEC O43.89- ☑
    placental dysfunction O43.89- ☑
    placental infarction O43.81- ☑
    placental insufficiency O36.51- ☑
    placental transfusion syndromes
      fetomaternal O43.01- ☑
      fetus to fetus O43.02- ☑
      maternofetal O43.01- ☑
    placentitis O41.14- ☑
    pneumonia O99.51- ☑
    poisoning — *see also* Table of Drugs and Chemicals O9A.21 ☑ *(following O99)*
    polyhydramnios O40- ☑
    polymorphic eruption of pregnancy O26.86
    poor obstetric history NEC O09.29- ☑
    postmaturity (post-term) (40 to 42 weeks) O48.0
      more than 42 completed weeks gestation (prolonged) O48.1
    pre-eclampsia O14.9- ☑
      mild O14.0- ☑
      moderate O14.0- ☑
      severe O14.1- ☑
        with hemolysis, elevated liver enzymes and low platelet count (HELLP) O14.2- ☑
    premature labor — *see* Pregnancy, complicated by, preterm labor
    premature rupture of membranes O42.90
      with onset of labor
        within 24 hours O42.00
          at or after 37 weeks gestation, onset of labor within 24 hours of rupture O42.02
          pre-term (before 37 completed weeks of gestation) O42.01- ☑
        after 24 hours O42.10
          at or after 37 weeks gestation, onset of labor more than 24 hours following rupture O42.12
          pre-term (before 37 completed weeks of gestation) O42.11- ☑
      at or after 37 weeks gestation, unspecified as to length of time between rupture and onset of labor O42.92
      full-term, unspecified as to length of time between rupture and onset of labor O42.92
      pre-term (before 37 completed weeks of gestation) O42.91- ☑
    premature separation of placenta — *see also* Abruptio placentae O45.9- ☑
    presentation, fetal — *see* Delivery, complicated by, malposition
    preterm delivery O60.10 ☑
    preterm labor
      with delivery O60.10 ☑
        preterm O60.10 ☑
        term O60.20 ☑
      second trimester
        with term delivery O60.22 ☑
        without delivery O60.02
        with preterm delivery
          second trimester O60.12 ☑
          third trimester O60.13 ☑
      third trimester
        with term delivery O60.23 ☑
        without delivery O60.03
        with third trimester preterm delivery O60.14 ☑
      without delivery O60.00
        second trimester O60.02
        third trimester O60.03
    previous history of — *see* Pregnancy, supervision of, high-risk
    prolapse, uterus O34.52- ☑
    proteinuria (gestational) — *see also* Proteinuria, gestational O12.1- ☑
      with edema O12.2- ☑

Pregnancy — *continued*
  complicated by — *continued*
    pruritic urticarial papules and plaques of pregnancy (PUPPP) O26.86
    pruritus (neurogenic) O26.89- ☑
    psychosis or psychoneurosis (puerperal) F53.1
    ptyalism O26.89- ☑
    PUPPP (pruritic urticarial papules and plaques of pregnancy) O26.86
    pyelitis O23.0- ☑
    recurrent pregnancy loss O26.2- ☑
    renal disease or failure NEC O26.83- ☑
      with secondary hypertension, pre-existing — *see* Hypertension, complicating, pregnancy, pre-existing, secondary
      hypertensive, pre-existing — *see* Hypertension, complicating, pregnancy, pre-existing, with, renal disease
    respiratory condition (conditions in J00-J99) O99.51- ☑
    retained, retention
      dead ovum O02.0
      intrauterine contraceptive device O26.3- ☑
    retroversion, uterus O34.53- ☑
    Rh immunization, incompatibility or sensitization NEC O36.09- ☑
      anti-D antibody O36.01- ☑
    rupture
      amnion (premature) — *see also* Pregnancy, complicated by, premature rupture of membranes O42- ☑
      membranes (premature) — *see also* Pregnancy, complicated by, premature rupture of membranes O42- ☑
      uterus (during labor) O71.1
        before onset of labor O71.0- ☑
    salivation (excessive) O26.89- ☑
    salpingitis O23.52- ☑
    salpingo-oophoritis O23.52- ☑
    sepsis (conditions in A40, A41) O98.81- ☑
    size date discrepancy (uterine) O26.84- ☑
    skin condition (conditions in L00-L99) O99.71- ☑
    smoking (tobacco) O99.33- ☑
    social problem O09.7- ☑
    specified condition NEC O26.89- ☑
    spotting O26.85- ☑
    streptococcus group B (GBS) carrier state O99.820
    subluxation of symphysis (pubis) O26.71- ☑
    syphilis (conditions in A50-A53) O98.11- ☑
    threatened
      abortion O20.0
      labor O47.9
        at or after 37 completed weeks of gestation O47.1
        before 37 completed weeks of gestation O47.0- ☑
    thrombophlebitis (superficial) O22.2- ☑
    thrombosis O22.9- ☑
      cerebral venous O22.5- ☑
      cerebrovenous sinus O22.5- ☑
      deep O22.3- ☑
    tobacco use disorder (smoking) O99.33- ☑
    torsion of uterus O34.59- ☑
    toxemia O14.9- ☑
    transverse lie or presentation O32.2 ☑
    tuberculosis (conditions in A15-A19) O98.01- ☑
    tumor (benign)
      cervix O34.4- ☑
      malignant O9A.11- ☑ *(following O99)*
      uterus O34.1- ☑
    unstable lie O32.0 ☑
    upper respiratory infection O99.51- ☑
    urethritis O23.2- ☑
    uterine size date discrepancy O26.84- ☑
    vaginitis or vulvitis O23.59- ☑
    varicose veins (lower extremities) O22.0- ☑
      genitals O22.1- ☑
      legs O22.0- ☑
      perineal O22.1- ☑
      vaginal or vulval O22.1- ☑
    venereal disease NEC (conditions in A63.8) O98.31- ☑
    venous disorders O22.9- ☑
      specified NEC O22.8X- ☑
    very young mother — *see* Pregnancy, complicated by, young mother

☟ Subterms under main terms may continue to next column or page   ☑ Additional Character Required — Refer to the Tabular List for Character Selection   265

Pregnancy — Pregnancy

Pregnancy — *continued*
  complicated by — *continued*
    viral diseases (conditions in A80-B09, B25-B34) O98.51- ☑
    vomiting O21.9
      due to diseases classified elsewhere O21.8
      hyperemesis gravidarum (mild) — *see also* Hyperemesis, gravidarum O21.0
      late (occurring after 20 weeks of gestation) O21.2
    young mother
      multigravida O09.62- ☑
      primigravida O09.61- ☑
  complicated NOS O26.9- ☑
  concealed O09.3- ☑
  continuing following
    elective fetal reduction of one or more fetus O31.3- ☑
    intrauterine death of one or more fetus O31.2- ☑
    spontaneous abortion of one or more fetus O31.1- ☑
  cornual O00.80
    with intrauterine pregnancy O00.81
  ectopic (ruptured) O00.90
    with intrauterine pregnancy O00.91
    abdominal O00.00
      with
        intrauterine pregnancy O00.01
        viable fetus O36.7- ☑
    cervical O00.80
      with intrauterine pregnancy O00.81
    complicated (by) O08.9
      afibrinogenemia O08.1
      cardiac arrest O08.81
      chemical damage of pelvic organ(s) O08.6
      circulatory collapse O08.3
      defibrination syndrome O08.1
      electrolyte imbalance O08.5
      embolism (amniotic fluid) (blood clot) (pulmonary) (septic) O08.2
      endometritis O08.0
      genital tract and pelvic infection O08.0
      hemorrhage (delayed) (excessive) O08.1
      infection
        genital tract or pelvic O08.0
        kidney O08.83
        urinary tract O08.3
      intravascular coagulation O08.1
      laceration of pelvic organ(s) O08.6
      metabolic disorder O08.5
      oliguria O08.4
      oophoritis O08.0
      parametritis O08.0
      pelvic peritonitis O08.0
      perforation of pelvic organ(s) O08.6
      renal failure or shutdown O08.4
      salpingitis or salpingo-oophoritis O08.0
      sepsis O08.82
      shock O08.83
        septic O08.82
      specified condition NEC O08.89
      tubular necrosis (renal) O08.4
      uremia O08.4
      urinary infection O08.83
      venous complication NEC O08.7
        embolism O08.2
    cornual O00.80
      with intrauterine pregnancy O00.81
    intraligamentous O00.80
      with intrauterine pregnancy O00.81
    mural O00.80
      with intrauterine pregnancy O00.81
    ovarian O00.20- ☑
      with intrauterine pregnancy O00.21- ☑
    specified site NEC O00.80
      with intrauterine pregnancy O00.81
    tubal (ruptured) O00.10- ☑
      with intrauterine pregnancy O00.11- ☑
  examination (normal) Z34.9- ☑
    first Z34.0- ☑
    high-risk — *see* Pregnancy, supervision of, high-risk
    specified Z34.8- ☑
  extrauterine — *see* Pregnancy, ectopic
  fallopian O00.10- ☑
    with intrauterine pregnancy O00.11- ☑
  false F45.8
  gestational carrier Z33.3
  heptachorionic, hepta-amniotic (septuplets) O30.83- ☑
  hexachorionic, hexa-amniotic (sextuplets) O30.83- ☑

Pregnancy — *continued*
  hidden O09.3- ☑
  high-risk — *see* Pregnancy, supervision of, high-risk
  incidental finding Z33.1
  interstitial O00.80
    with intrauterine pregnancy O00.81
  intraligamentous O00.80
    with intrauterine pregnancy O00.81
  intramural O00.80
    with intrauterine pregnancy O00.81
  intraperitoneal O00.00
    with intrauterine pregnancy O00.01
  isthmian O00.10- ☑
    with intrauterine pregnancy O00.11- ☑
  mesometric (mural) O00.80
    with intrauterine pregnancy O00.81
  molar NEC O02.0
    complicated (by) O08.9
      afibrinogenemia O08.1
      cardiac arrest O08.81
      chemical damage of pelvic organ(s) O08.6
      circulatory collapse O08.3
      defibrination syndrome O08.1
      electrolyte imbalance O08.5
      embolism (amniotic fluid) (blood clot) (pulmonary) (septic) O08.2
      endometritis O08.0
      genital tract and pelvic infection O08.0
      hemorrhage (delayed) (excessive) O08.1
      infection
        genital tract or pelvic O08.0
        kidney O08.83
        urinary tract O08.83
      intravascular coagulation O08.1
      laceration of pelvic organ(s) O08.6
      metabolic disorder O08.5
      oliguria O08.4
      oophoritis O08.0
      parametritis O08.0
      pelvic peritonitis O08.0
      perforation of pelvic organ(s) O08.6
      renal failure or shutdown O08.4
      salpingitis or salpingo-oophoritis O08.0
      sepsis O08.82
      shock O08.3
        septic O08.82
      specified condition NEC O08.89
      tubular necrosis (renal) O08.4
      uremia O08.4
      urinary infection O08.83
      venous complication NEC O08.7
        embolism O08.2
    hydatidiform — *see also* Mole, hydatidiform O01.9
  multiple (gestation) O30.9- ☑
    greater than quadruplets — *see* Pregnancy, multiple (gestation), specified NEC
    specified NEC O30.80- ☑
      with
        two or more monoamniotic fetuses O30.82- ☑
        two or more monochorionic fetuses O30.81- ☑
        number of chorions and amnions are both equal to the number of fetuses O30.83- ☑
      two or more monoamniotic fetuses O30.82- ☑
      two or more monochorionic fetuses O30.81- ☑
      unable to determine number of placenta and number of amniotic sacs O30.89- ☑
      unspecified number of placenta and unspecified number of amniotic sacs O30.80- ☑
  mural O00.80
    with intrauterine pregnancy O00.81
  normal (supervision of) Z34.9- ☑
    first Z34.0- ☑
    high-risk — *see* Pregnancy, supervision of, high-risk
    specified Z34.8- ☑
  ovarian O00.20- ☑
    with intrauterine pregnancy O00.21- ☑
  pentachorionic, penta-amniotic (quintuplets) O30.83- ☑
  postmature (40 to 42 weeks) O48.0
    more than 42 weeks gestation O48.1
  post-term (40 to 42 weeks) O48.0
  prenatal care only Z34.9- ☑
    first Z34.0- ☑
    high-risk — *see* Pregnancy, supervision of, high-risk
    specified Z34.8- ☑
  prolonged (more than 42 weeks gestation) O48.1

Pregnancy — *continued*
  quadruplet O30.20- ☑
    with
      two or more monoamniotic fetuses O30.22- ☑
      two or more monochorionic fetuses O30.21- ☑
    quadrachorionic/quadra-amniotic O30.23- ☑
    two or more monoamniotic fetuses O30.22- ☑
    two or more monochorionic fetuses O30.21- ☑
    unable to determine number of placenta and number of amniotic sacs O30.29- ☑
    unspecified number of placenta and unspecified number of amniotic sacs O30.20- ☑
  quintuplet — *see* Pregnancy, multiple (gestation), specified NEC
  sextuplet — *see* Pregnancy, multiple (gestation), specified NEC
  supervision of
    concealed pregnancy O09.3- ☑
    elderly mother
      multigravida O09.52- ☑
      primigravida O09.51- ☑
    hidden pregnancy O09.3- ☑
    high-risk O09.9- ☑
      due to (history of)
        ectopic pregnancy O09.1- ☑
        elderly — *see* Pregnancy, supervision, elderly mother
        grand multiparity O09.4 ☑
        in utero procedure during previous pregnancy O09.82- ☑
        in vitro fertilization O09.81- ☑
        infertility O09.0- ☑
        insufficient prenatal care O09.3- ☑
        molar pregnancy O09.A- ☑
        multiple previous pregnancies O09.4- ☑
        older mother — *see* Pregnancy, supervision of, elderly mother
        poor reproductive or obstetric history NEC O09.29- ☑
        pre-term labor O09.21- ☑
        previous
          neonatal death O09.29- ☑
        social problems O09.7- ☑
        specified NEC O09.89- ☑
        very young mother — *see* Pregnancy, supervision, young mother
      resulting from in vitro fertilization O09.81- ☑
    normal Z34.9- ☑
      first Z34.0- ☑
      specified NEC Z34.8- ☑
    young mother
      multigravida O09.62- ☑
      primigravida O09.61- ☑
  triplet O30.10- ☑
    with
      two or more monoamniotic fetuses O30.12- ☑
      two or more monochorionic fetuses O30.11- ☑
    trichorionic/triamniotic O30.13- ☑
    two or more monoamniotic fetuses O30.12- ☑
    two or more monochorionic fetuses O30.11- ☑
    unable to determine number of placenta and number of amniotic sacs O30.19- ☑
    unspecified number of placenta and unspecified number of amniotic sacs O30.10- ☑
  tubal (with abortion) (with rupture) O00.10- ☑
    with intrauterine pregnancy O00.11- ☑
  twin O30.00- ☑
    conjoined O30.02- ☑
    dichorionic/diamniotic (two placenta, two amniotic sacs) O30.04- ☑
    monochorionic/diamniotic (one placenta, two amniotic sacs) O30.03- ☑
    monochorionic/monoamniotic (one placenta, one amniotic sac) O30.01- ☑
    unable to determine number of placenta and number of amniotic sacs O30.09- ☑
    unspecified number of placenta and unspecified number of amniotic sacs O30.00- ☑
  unwanted Z64.0
  weeks of gestation
    8 weeks Z3A.08 (*following* Z36)
    9 weeks Z3A.09 (*following* Z36)
    10 weeks Z3A.10 (*following* Z36)
    11 weeks Z3A.11 (*following* Z36)
    12 weeks Z3A.12 (*following* Z36)
    13 weeks Z3A.13 (*following* Z36)
    14 weeks Z3A.14 (*following* Z36)

☑ **Additional Character Required — Refer to the Tabular List for Character Selection**   ▽ **Subterms under main terms may continue to next column or page**

Pregnancy — continued
  weeks of gestation — continued
    15 weeks Z3A.15 (following Z36)
    16 weeks Z3A.16 (following Z36)
    17 weeks Z3A.17 (following Z36)
    18 weeks Z3A.18 (following Z36)
    19 weeks Z3A.19 (following Z36)
    20 weeks Z3A.20 (following Z36)
    21 weeks Z3A.21 (following Z36)
    22 weeks Z3A.22 (following Z36)
    23 weeks Z3A.23 (following Z36)
    24 weeks Z3A.24 (following Z36)
    25 weeks Z3A.25 (following Z36)
    26 weeks Z3A.26 (following Z36)
    27 weeks Z3A.27 (following Z36)
    28 weeks Z3A.28 (following Z36)
    29 weeks Z3A.29 (following Z36)
    30 weeks Z3A.30 (following Z36)
    31 weeks Z3A.31 (following Z36)
    32 weeks Z3A.32 (following Z36)
    33 weeks Z3A.33 (following Z36)
    34 weeks Z3A.34 (following Z36)
    35 weeks Z3A.35 (following Z36)
    36 weeks Z3A.36 (following Z36)
    37 weeks Z3A.37 (following Z36)
    38 weeks Z3A.38 (following Z36)
    39 weeks Z3A.39 (following Z36)
    40 weeks Z3A.40 (following Z36)
    41 weeks Z3A.41 (following Z36)
    42 weeks Z3A.42 (following Z36)
    greater than 42 weeks Z3A.49 (following Z36)
    less than 8 weeks Z3A.01 (following Z36)
    not specified Z3A.00 (following Z36)
Preiser's disease — see Osteonecrosis, secondary, due to, trauma, metacarpus
Pre-kwashiorkor — see Malnutrition, severe
Preleukemia (syndrome) D46.9
Preluxation, hip, congenital Q65.6
Premature — see also condition
  adrenarche E27.0
  aging E34.8
  beats I49.40
    atrial I49.1
    auricular I49.1
    supraventricular I49.1
  birth NEC — see Preterm, newborn
  closure, foramen ovale Q21.8
  contraction
    atrial I49.1
    atrioventricular I49.2
    auricular I49.1
    auriculoventricular I49.49
    heart (extrasystole) I49.49
    junctional I49.2
    ventricular I49.3
  delivery — see also Pregnancy, complicated by, preterm labor O60.10 ☑
  ejaculation F52.4
  infant NEC — see Preterm, newborn
    light-for-dates — see Light for dates
  labor — see Pregnancy, complicated by, preterm labor
  lungs P28.0
  menopause E28.319
    asymptomatic E28.319
    symptomatic E28.310
  newborn
    extreme (less than 28 completed weeks) — see Immaturity, extreme
    less than 37 completed weeks — see Preterm, newborn
  puberty E30.1
  rupture membranes or amnion — see Pregnancy, complicated by, premature rupture of membranes
  senility E34.8
  thelarche E30.8
  ventricular systole I49.3
Prematurity NEC (less than 37 completed weeks) — see Preterm, newborn
  extreme (less than 28 completed weeks) — see Immaturity, extreme
Premenstrual
  dysphoric disorder (PMDD) F32.81
  tension (syndrome) N94.3
Premolarization, cuspids K00.2
Prenatal
  care, normal pregnancy — see Pregnancy, normal

Prenatal — continued
  screening of mother — see also Encounter, antenatal screening Z36.9
  teeth K00.6
Preparatory care for subsequent treatment NEC
  for dialysis Z49.01
    peritoneal Z49.02
Prepartum — see condition
Preponderance, left or right ventricular I51.7
Prepuce — see condition
PRES (posterior reversible encephalopathy syndrome) I67.83
Presbycardia R54
Presbycusis, presbyacusia H91.1- ☑
Presbyesophagus K22.89
Presbyophrenia F03 ☑
Presbyopia H52.4
Prescription of contraceptives (initial) Z30.019
  barrier Z30.018
  diaphragm Z30.018
  emergency (postcoital) Z30.012
  implantable subdermal Z30.017
  injectable Z30.013
  intrauterine contraceptive device Z30.014
  pills Z30.011
  postcoital (emergency) Z30.012
  repeat Z30.40
    barrier Z30.49
    diaphragm Z30.49
    implantable subdermal Z30.46
    injectable Z30.42
    pills Z30.41
    specified type NEC Z30.49
    transdermal patch hormonal Z30.45
    vaginal ring hormonal Z30.44
  specified type NEC Z30.018
    transdermal patch hormonal Z30.016
    vaginal ring hormonal Z30.015
Presence (of)
  ankle-joint implant (functional) (prosthesis) Z96.66- ☑
  aortocoronary (bypass) graft Z95.1
  arterial-venous shunt (dialysis) Z99.2
  artificial
    eye (globe) Z97.0
    heart (fully implantable) (mechanical) Z95.812
      valve Z95.2
    larynx Z96.3
    lens (intraocular) Z96.1
    limb (complete) (partial) Z97.1- ☑
      arm Z97.1- ☑
        bilateral Z97.15
      leg Z97.1- ☑
        bilateral Z97.16
  audiological implant (functional) Z96.29
  bladder implant (functional) Z96.0
  bone
    conduction hearing device Z96.29
    implant (functional) NEC Z96.7
    joint (prosthesis) — see Presence, joint implant
  cardiac
    defibrillator (functional) (with synchronous cardiac pacemaker) Z95.810
    implant or graft Z95.9
      specified type NEC Z95.818
    pacemaker Z95.0
    resynchronization therapy
      defibrillator Z95.810
      pacemaker Z95.0
  cardioverter-defibrillator (ICD) Z95.810
  cerebrospinal fluid drainage device Z98.2
  cochlear implant (functional) Z96.21
  contact lens (es) Z97.3
  coronary artery graft or prosthesis Z95.5
  CRT-D (cardiac resynchronization therapy defibrillator) Z95.810
  CRT-P (cardiac resynchronization therapy pacemaker) Z95.0
  CSF shunt Z98.2
  dental prosthesis device Z97.2
  dentures Z97.2
  device (external) NEC Z97.8
    cardiac NEC Z95.818
    heart assist Z95.811
    implanted (functional) Z96.9
      specified NEC Z96.89
    prosthetic Z97.8
  ear implant Z96.20
    cochlear implant Z96.21

Presence — continued
  ear implant — continued
    myringotomy tube Z96.22
    specified type NEC Z96.29
  elbow-joint implant (functional) (prosthesis) Z96.62- ☑
  endocrine implant (functional) NEC Z96.49
  eustachian tube stent or device (functional) Z96.29
  external hearing-aid or device Z97.4
  finger-joint implant (functional) (prosthetic) Z96.69- ☑
  functional implant Z96.9
    specified NEC Z96.89
  graft
    cardiac NEC Z95.818
    vascular NEC Z95.828
  hearing-aid or device (external) Z97.4
    implant (bone) (cochlear) (functional) Z96.21
  heart assist device Z95.811
  heart valve implant (functional) Z95.2
    prosthetic Z95.2
    specified type NEC Z95.4
    xenogenic Z95.3
  hip-joint implant (functional) (prosthesis) Z96.64- ☑
  ICD (cardioverter-defibrillator) Z95.810
  implanted device (artificial) (functional) (prosthetic) Z96.9
    automatic cardiac defibrillator (with synchronous cardiac pacemaker) Z95.810
    cardiac pacemaker Z95.0
    cochlear Z96.21
    dental Z96.5
    heart Z95.812
    heart valve Z95.2
      prosthetic Z95.2
      specified NEC Z95.4
      xenogenic Z95.3
    insulin pump Z96.41
    intraocular lens Z96.1
    joint Z96.60
      ankle Z96.66- ☑
      elbow Z96.62- ☑
      finger Z96.69- ☑
      hip Z96.64- ☑
      knee Z96.65- ☑
      shoulder Z96.61- ☑
      specified NEC Z96.698
      wrist Z96.63- ☑
    larynx Z96.3
    myringotomy tube Z96.22
    otological Z96.20
      cochlear Z96.21
      eustachian stent Z96.29
      myringotomy Z96.22
      specified NEC Z96.29
      stapes Z96.29
    skin Z96.81
    skull plate Z96.7
    specified NEC Z96.89
    urogenital Z96.0
  insulin pump (functional) Z96.41
  intestinal bypass or anastomosis Z98.0
  intraocular lens (functional) Z96.1
  intrauterine contraceptive device (IUD) Z97.5
  intravascular implant (functional) (prosthetic) NEC Z95.9
    coronary artery Z95.5
    defibrillator (with synchronous cardiac pacemaker) Z95.810
    peripheral vessel (with angioplasty) Z95.820
  joint implant (prosthetic) (any) Z96.60
    ankle — see Presence, ankle joint implant
    elbow — see Presence, elbow joint implant
    finger — see Presence, finger joint implant
    hip — see Presence, hip joint implant
    knee — see Presence, knee joint implant
    shoulder — see Presence, shoulder joint implant
    specified joint NEC Z96.698
    wrist — see Presence, wrist joint implant
  knee-joint implant (functional) (prosthesis) Z96.65- ☑
  laryngeal implant (functional) Z96.3
  mandibular implant (dental) Z96.5
  myringotomy tube(s) Z96.22
  neurostimulator (brain) (gastric) (peripheral nerve) (sacral nerve) (spinal cord) (vagus nerve) Z96.82
  orthopedic-joint implant (prosthetic) (any) — see Presence, joint implant
  otological implant (functional) Z96.29
  shoulder-joint implant (functional) (prosthesis) Z96.61- ☑

▽ Subterms under main terms may continue to next column or page   ☑ Additional Character Required — Refer to the Tabular List for Character Selection   267

Pregnancy — Presence

Presence — *continued*
  skull-plate implant Z96.7
  spectacles Z97.3
  stapes implant (functional) Z96.29
  systemic lupus erythematosus [SLE] inhibitor D68.62
  tendon implant (functional) (graft) Z96.7
  tooth root(s) implant Z96.5
  ureteral stent Z96.0
  urethral stent Z96.0
  urogenital implant (functional) Z96.0
  vascular implant or device Z95.9
    access port device Z95.828
    specified type NEC Z95.828
  wrist-joint implant (functional) (prosthesis) Z96.63- ☑
Presenile — *see also* condition
  dementia F03 ☑
  premature aging E34.8
Presentation, fetal — *see* Delivery, complicated by, malposition
Prespondylolisthesis (congenital) Q76.2
Pressure
  area, skin — *see* Ulcer, pressure, by site
  brachial plexus G54.0
  brain G93.5
    injury at birth NEC P11.1
  cerebral — *see* Pressure, brain
  chest R07.89
  cone, tentorial G93.5
  hyposystolic — *see also* Hypotension
    incidental reading, without diagnosis of hypotension R03.1
  increased
    intracranial benign G93.2
      injury at birth P11.0
    intraocular H40.05- ☑
  injury — *see* Ulcer, pressure, by site
  lumbosacral plexus G54.1
  mediastinum J98.59
  necrosis (chronic) — *see* Ulcer, pressure, by site
  parental, inappropriate (excessive) Z62.6
  sore (chronic) — *see* Ulcer, pressure, by site
  spinal cord G95.20
  ulcer (chronic) — *see* Ulcer, pressure, by site
  venous, increased I87.8
Pre-syncope R55
Preterm
  delivery — *see also* Pregnancy, complicated by, preterm labor O60.10 ☑
  labor — *see* Pregnancy, complicated by, preterm labor
  newborn (infant) P07.30
    gestational age
      28 completed weeks (28 weeks, 0 days through 28 weeks, 6 days) P07.31
      29 completed weeks (29 weeks, 0 days through 29 weeks, 6 days) P07.32
      30 completed weeks (30 weeks, 0 days through 30 weeks, 6 days) P07.33
      31 completed weeks (31 weeks, 0 days through 31 weeks, 6 days) P07.34
      32 completed weeks (32 weeks, 0 days through 32 weeks, 6 days) P07.35
      33 completed weeks (33 weeks, 0 days through 33 weeks, 6 days) P07.36
      34 completed weeks (34 weeks, 0 days through 34 weeks, 6 days) P07.37
      35 completed weeks (35 weeks, 0 days through 35 weeks, 6 days) P07.38
      36 completed weeks (36 weeks, 0 days through 36 weeks, 6 days) P07.39
Previa
  placenta (total) (without hemorrhage) O44.0- ☑
    with hemorrhage O44.1- ☑
    complete O44.0- ☑
      with hemorrhage O44.1- ☑
    low — *see also* Delivery, complicated, by, placenta, low O44.4- ☑
      with hemorrhage O44.5- ☑
    marginal O44.2- ☑
      with hemorrhage O44.3- ☑
    partial O44.2- ☑
      with hemorrhage O44.3- ☑
  vasa O69.4 ☑
Priapism N48.30
  due to
    disease classified elsewhere N48.32
    drug N48.33
    specified cause NEC N48.39
    trauma N48.31

Prickling sensation (skin) R20.2
Prickly heat L74.0
Primary — *see* condition
Primigravida
  elderly, affecting management of pregnancy, labor and delivery (supervision only) — *see* Pregnancy, complicated by, elderly, primigravida
  older, affecting management of pregnancy, labor and delivery (supervision only) — *see* Pregnancy, complicated by, elderly, primigravida
  very young, affecting management of pregnancy, labor and delivery (supervision only) — *see* Pregnancy, complicated by, young mother, primigravida
Primipara
  elderly, affecting management of pregnancy, labor and delivery (supervision only) — *see* Pregnancy, complicated by, elderly, primigravida
  older, affecting management of pregnancy, labor and delivery (supervision only) — *see* Pregnancy, complicated by, elderly, primigravida
  very young, affecting management of pregnancy, labor and delivery (supervision only) — *see* Pregnancy, complicated by, young mother, primigravida
Primus varus Q66.21- ☑
PRIND (Prolonged reversible ischemic neurologic deficit) I63.9
Pringle's disease (tuberous sclerosis) Q85.1
Prinzmetal angina I20.1
Prizefighter ear — *see* Cauliflower ear
Problem (with) (related to)
  academic Z55.8
  acculturation Z60.3
  adjustment (to)
    change of job Z56.1
    life-cycle transition Z60.0
    pension Z60.0
    retirement Z60.0
  adopted child Z62.821
  alcoholism in family Z63.72
  atypical parenting situation Z62.9
  bankruptcy Z59.89
  behavioral (adult) F69
    drug seeking Z76.5
  birth of sibling affecting child Z62.898
  care (of)
    provider dependency Z74.9
      specified NEC Z74.8
    sick or handicapped person in family or household Z63.6
  child
    abuse (affecting the child) — *see* Maltreatment, child
    custody or support proceedings Z65.3
    in care of non-parental family member Z62.21
    in foster care Z62.21
    in welfare custody Z62.21
    living in orphanage or group home Z62.22
  child-rearing Z62.9
    specified NEC Z62.898
  communication (developmental) F80.9
  conflict or discord (with)
    boss Z56.4
    classmates Z55.4
    counselor Z64.4
    employer Z56.4
    family Z63.9
      specified NEC Z63.8
    probation officer Z64.4
    social worker Z64.4
    teachers Z55.4
    workmates Z56.4
  conviction in legal proceedings Z65.0
    with imprisonment Z65.1
  counselor Z64.4
  creditors Z59.89
  digestive K92.9
  drug addict in family Z63.72
  ear — *see* Disorder, ear
  economic Z59.9
    affecting care Z59.9
    specified NEC Z59.89
  education Z55.9
    specified NEC Z55.8
  employment Z56.9
    change of job Z56.1
    discord Z56.4
    environment Z56.5
    sexual harassment Z56.81

Problem — *continued*
  employment — *continued*
    specified NEC Z56.89
    stressful schedule Z56.3
    stress NEC Z56.6
    threat of job loss Z56.2
    unemployment Z56.0
  enuresis, child F98.0
  eye H57.9
  failed examinations (school) Z55.2
  falling Z91.81
  family — *see also* Disruption, family Z63.9
    specified NEC Z63.8
  feeding (elderly) (infant) R63.39
    newborn P92.9
      breast P92.5
      overfeeding P92.4
      slow P92.2
      specified NEC P92.8
      underfeeding P92.3
    nonorganic F50.89
  finance Z59.9
    specified NEC Z59.89
  foreclosure on loan Z59.89
  foster child Z62.822
  frightening experience(s) in childhood Z62.898
  genital NEC
    female N94.9
    male N50.9
  health care Z75.9
    specified NEC Z75.8
  hearing — *see* Deafness
  homelessness Z59.00
  housing Z59.9
    inadequate Z59.1
    isolated Z59.89
    specified NEC Z59.89
  identity (of childhood) F93.8
  illegitimate pregnancy (unwanted) Z64.0
  illiteracy Z55.0
  impaired mobility Z74.09
  imprisonment or incarceration Z65.1
  inadequate teaching affecting education Z55.8
  inappropriate (excessive) parental pressure Z62.6
  influencing health status NEC Z78.9
  in-law Z63.1
  institutionalization, affecting child Z62.22
  intrafamilial communication Z63.8
  jealousy, child F93.8
  landlord Z59.2
  language (developmental) F80.9
  learning (developmental) F81.9
  legal Z65.3
    conviction without imprisonment Z65.0
    imprisonment Z65.1
    release from prison Z65.2
  life-management Z73.9
    specified NEC Z73.89
  life-style Z72.9
    gambling Z72.6
    high-risk sexual behavior (heterosexual) Z72.51
      bisexual Z72.53
      homosexual Z72.52
    inappropriate eating habits Z72.4
    self-damaging behavior NEC Z72.89
    specified NEC Z72.89
    tobacco use Z72.0
  literacy Z55.9
    low level Z55.0
    specified NEC Z55.8
  living alone Z60.2
  lodgers Z59.2
  loss of love relationship in childhood Z62.898
  marital Z63.0
    involving
      divorce Z63.5
      estrangement Z63.5
      gender identity F66
  mastication K08.89
  medical
    care, within family Z63.6
    facilities Z75.9
      specified NEC Z75.8
  mental F48.9
  multiparity Z64.1
  negative life events in childhood Z62.9
    altered pattern of family relationships Z62.898
    frightening experience Z62.898

Problem — *continued*
  negative life events in childhood — *continued*
    loss of
      love relationship Z62.898
      self-esteem Z62.898
    physical abuse (alleged) — *see* Maltreatment, child
    removal from home Z62.29
    specified event NEC Z62.898
  neighbor Z59.2
  neurological NEC R29.818
  new step-parent affecting child Z62.898
  none (feared complaint unfounded) Z71.1
  occupational NEC Z56.89
  parent-child — *see* Conflict, parent-child
  personal hygiene Z91.89
  personality F69
  phase-of-life transition, adjustment Z60.0
  presence of sick or disabled person in family or house-
      hold Z63.79
    needing care Z63.6
  primary support group (family) Z63.9
    specified NEC Z63.8
  probation officer Z64.4
  psychiatric F99
  psychosexual (development) F66
  psychosocial Z65.9
    religious or spiritual Z65.8
    specified NEC Z65.8
  relationship Z63.9
    childhood F93.8
  release from prison Z65.2
    religious or spiritual Z65.8
  removal from home affecting child Z62.29
  seeking and accepting known hazardous and harmful
    behavioral or psychological interventions Z65.8
    chemical, nutritional or physical interventions Z65.8
  sexual function (nonorganic) F52.9
  sight H54.7
  sleep disorder, child F51.9
  smell — *see* Disturbance, sensation, smell
  social
    environment Z60.9
      specified NEC Z60.8
    exclusion and rejection Z60.4
    worker Z64.4
  speech R47.9
    developmental F80.9
    specified NEC R47.89
  swallowing — *see* Dysphagia
  taste — *see* Disturbance, sensation, taste
  tic, child F95.0
  underachievement in school Z55.3
  unemployment Z56.0
    threatened Z56.2
  unwanted pregnancy Z64.0
  upbringing Z62.9
    specified NEC Z62.898
  urinary N39.9
  voice production R47.89
  work schedule (stressful) Z56.3
Procedure (surgical)
  converted
    arthroscopic to open Z53.33
    laparoscopic to open Z53.31
    specified procedure NEC to open Z53.39
    thoracoscopic to open Z53.32
  for purpose other than remedying health state Z41.9
    specified NEC Z41.8
  not done Z53.9
    because of
      administrative reasons Z53.8
      contraindication Z53.09
        smoking Z53.01
      patient's decision Z53.20
        for reasons of belief or group pressure Z53.1
        left against medical advice (AMA) Z53.29
        left without being seen Z53.21
        specified reason NEC Z53.29
      specified reason NEC Z53.8
Procidentia (uteri) N81.3
Proctalgia K62.89
  fugax K59.4
  spasmodic K59.4
Proctitis K62.89
  amebic (acute) A06.0
  chlamydial A56.3
  gonococcal A54.6
  granulomatous — *see* Enteritis, regional, large intestine

Proctitis — *continued*
  herpetic A60.1
  radiation K62.7
  tuberculous A18.32
  ulcerative (chronic) K51.20
    with
      complication K51.219
        abscess K51.214
        fistula K51.213
        obstruction K51.212
        rectal bleeding K51.211
        specified NEC K51.218
Proctocele
  female (without uterine prolapse) N81.6
    with uterine prolapse N81.2
      complete N81.3
  male K62.3
Proctocolitis
  allergic K52.29
  food protein-induced K52.29
  food-induced eosinophilic K52.29
  milk protein-induced K52.29
  mucosal — *see* Rectosigmoiditis, ulcerative
Proctoptosis K62.3
Proctorrhagia K62.5
Proctosigmoiditis K63.89
  ulcerative (chronic) — *see* Rectosigmoiditis, ulcerative
Proctospasm K59.4
  psychogenic F45.8
Profichet's disease — *see* Disorder, soft tissue, specified
    type NEC
Progeria E34.8
Prognathism (mandibular) (maxillary) M26.19
Progonoma (melanotic) — *see* Neoplasm, benign, by
    site
Progressive — *see* condition
Prolactinoma
  specified site — *see* Neoplasm, benign, by site
  unspecified site D35.2
Prolapse, prolapsed
  anus, anal (canal) (sphincter) K62.2
  arm or hand O32.2 ☑
    causing obstructed labor O64.4 ☑
  bladder (mucosa) (sphincter) (acquired)
    congenital Q79.4
    female — *see* Cystocele
    male N32.89
  breast implant (prosthetic) T85.49 ☑
  cecostomy K94.09
  cecum K63.4
  cervix, cervical (hypertrophied) N81.2
    anterior lip, obstructing labor O65.5
    congenital Q51.828
    postpartal, old N81.2
    stump N81.85
  ciliary body (traumatic) — *see* Laceration, eye(ball),
    with prolapse or loss of interocular tissue
  colon (pedunculated) K63.4
  colostomy K94.09
  disc (intervertebral) — *see* Displacement, intervertebral
    disc
  eye implant (orbital) T85.398 ☑
    lens (ocular) — *see* Complications, intraocular lens
  fallopian tube N83.4- ☑
  gastric (mucosa) K31.89
  genital, female N81.9
    specified NEC N81.89
  globe, nontraumatic — *see* Luxation, globe
  ileostomy bud K94.19
  intervertebral disc — *see* Displacement, intervertebral
    disc
  intestine (small) K63.4
  iris (traumatic) — *see* Laceration, eye(ball), with pro-
    lapse or loss of interocular tissue
    nontraumatic H21.89
  kidney N28.83
    congenital Q63.2
  laryngeal muscles or ventricle J38.7
  liver K76.89
  meatus urinarius N36.8
  mitral (valve) I34.1
  ocular lens implant — *see* Complications, intraocular
    lens
  organ or site, congenital NEC — *see* Malposition, con-
    genital
  ovary N83.4- ☑
  pelvic floor, female N81.89
  perineum, female N81.89

Prolapse, prolapsed — *continued*
  rectum (mucosa) (sphincter) K62.3
    due to trichuris trichuria B79
  spleen D73.89
  stomach K31.89
  umbilical cord
    complicating delivery O69.0 ☑
  urachus, congenital Q64.4
  ureter N28.89
    with obstruction N13.5
      with infection N13.6
  ureterovesical orifice N28.89
  urethra (acquired) (infected) (mucosa) N36.8
    congenital Q64.71
  urinary meatus N36.8
    congenital Q64.72
  uterovaginal N81.4
    complete N81.3
    incomplete N81.2
  uterus (with prolapse of vagina) N81.4
    complete N81.3
    congenital Q51.818
    first degree N81.2
    in pregnancy or childbirth — *see* Pregnancy, com-
      plicated by, abnormal, uterus
    incomplete N81.2
    postpartal (old) N81.4
    second degree N81.2
    third degree N81.3
  uveal (traumatic) — *see* Laceration, eye(ball), with
    prolapse or loss of interocular tissue
  vagina (anterior) (wall) — *see* Cystocele
    with prolapse of uterus N81.4
      complete N81.3
      incomplete N81.2
    posterior wall N81.6
    posthysterectomy N99.3
  vitreous (humor) H43.0- ☑
    in wound — *see* Laceration, eye(ball), with prolapse
      or loss of interocular tissue
  womb — *see* Prolapse, uterus
Prolapsus, female N81.9
  specified NEC N81.89
Proliferation(s)
  primary cutaneous CD30-positive large T-cell C86.6
  prostate, atypical small acinar N42.32
Proliferative — *see* condition
Prolonged, prolongation (of)
  bleeding (time) (idiopathic) R79.1
  coagulation (time) R79.1
  gestation (over 42 completed weeks)
    mother O48.1
    newborn P08.22
  interval I44.0
  labor O63.9
    first stage O63.0
    second stage O63.1
  partial thromboplastin time (PTT) R79.1
  pregnancy (more than 42 weeks gestation) O48.1
  prothrombin time R79.1
  QT interval R94.31
  uterine contractions in labor O62.4
Prominence, prominent
  auricle (congenital) (ear) Q17.5
  ischial spine or sacral promontory with disproportion
    (fetopelvic) O33.0
    causing obstructed labor O65.0
  nose (congenital) acquired M95.0
Promiscuity — *see* High, risk, sexual behavior
Pronation
  ankle — *see* Deformity, limb, foot, specified NEC
  foot — *see also* Deformity, limb, foot, specified NEC
    congenital Q74.2
Prophylactic
  administration of
    antibiotics, long-term Z79.2
      short-term use — *omit code*
    drug — *see also* Long-term (current) drug therapy
      (use of) Z79.899
    medication Z79.899
    organ removal (for neoplasia management) Z40.00
      breast Z40.01
      fallopian tube(s) Z40.03
        with ovary(s) Z40.02
      ovary(s) Z40.02
      specified site NEC Z40.09
    surgery Z40.9

▽ **Subterms under main terms may continue to next column or page**   ☑ **Additional Character Required — Refer to the Tabular List for Character Selection**   **269**

Problem — Prophylactic

Prophylactic — *continued*
  surgery — *continued*
    for risk factors related to malignant neoplasm —
      see Prophylactic, organ removal
    specified NEC Z40.8
  vaccination Z23
Propionic acidemia E71.121
Proptosis (ocular) — *see also* Exophthalmos
  thyroid — *see* Hyperthyroidism, with goiter
Prosecution, anxiety concerning Z65.3
Prosopagnosia R48.3
Prostadynia N42.81
Prostate, prostatic — *see* condition
Prostatism — *see* Hyperplasia, prostate
Prostatitis (congestive) (suppurative) (with cystitis) N41.9
  acute N41.0
  cavitary N41.8
  chronic N41.1
  diverticular N41.8
  due to Trichomonas (vaginalis) A59.02
  fibrous N41.1
  gonococcal (acute) (chronic) A54.22
  granulomatous N41.4
  hypertrophic N41.1
  subacute N41.1
  trichomonal A59.02
  tuberculous A18.14
Prostatocystitis N41.3
Prostatorrhea N42.89
Prostatosis N42.82
Prostration R53.83
  heat — *see also* Heat, exhaustion
    anhydrotic T67.3 ☑
    due to
      salt (and water) depletion T67.4 ☑
      water depletion T67.3 ☑
  nervous F48.8
  senile R54
Protanomaly (anomalous trichromat) H53.54
Protanopia (complete) (incomplete) H53.54
Protection (against) (from) — *see* Prophylactic
Protein
  deficiency NEC — *see* Malnutrition
  malnutrition — *see* Malnutrition
  sickness — *see also* Reaction, serum T80.69 ☑
Proteinemia R77.9
Proteinosis
  alveolar (pulmonary) J84.01
  lipid or lipoid (of Urbach) E78.89
Proteinuria R80.9
  Bence Jones R80.3
  complicating pregnancy — *see* Proteinuria, gestational
  gestational
    complicating
      childbirth O12.14
      pregnancy O12.1- ☑
        with edema O12.2- ☑
      puerperium O12.15
  idiopathic R80.0
  isolated R80.0
    with glomerular lesion N06.9
      C3
        glomerulonephritis N06.A
        glomerulopathy N06.A
          with dense deposit disease N06.6
        dense deposit disease N06.6
        diffuse
          crescentic glomerulonephritis N06.7
          endocapillary proliferative glomerulonephritis N06.4
          mesangiocapillary glomerulonephritis N06.5
          focal and segmental hyalinosis or sclerosis N06.1
          membranous (diffuse) N06.2
          mesangial proliferative (diffuse) N06.3
          minimal change N06.0
          specified pathology NEC N06.8
  orthostatic R80.2
    with glomerular lesion — *see* Proteinuria, isolated, with glomerular lesion
  persistent R80.1
    with glomerular lesion — *see* Proteinuria, isolated, with glomerular lesion
  postural R80.2
    with glomerular lesion — *see* Proteinuria, isolated, with glomerular lesion
  pre-eclamptic — *see* Pre-eclampsia
  puerperal O12.15
  specified type NEC R80.8

Proteolysis, pathologic D65
Proteus (mirabilis) (morganii), **as cause of disease classified elsewhere** B96.4
Prothrombin gene mutation D68.52
Protoporphyria, erythropoietic E80.0
Protozoal — *see also* condition
  disease B64
    specified NEC B60.8
Protrusion, protrusio
  acetabuli M24.7
  acetabulum (into pelvis) M24.7
  device, implant or graft — *see also* Complications, by site and type, mechanical T85.698 ☑
    arterial graft NEC — *see* Complication, cardiovascular device, mechanical, vascular
    breast (implant) T85.49 ☑
    catheter NEC T85.698 ☑
      cystostomy T83.090 ☑
      dialysis (renal) T82.49 ☑
        intraperitoneal T85.691 ☑
      infusion NEC T82.594 ☑
        spinal (epidural) (subdural) T85.690 ☑
      urinary — *see also* Complications, catheter, urinary T83.098 ☑
    electronic (electrode) (pulse generator) (stimulator) bone T84.390 ☑
    nervous system — *see* Complication, prosthetic device, mechanical, electronic nervous system stimulator
    fixation, internal (orthopedic) NEC — *see* Complication, fixation device, mechanical
    gastrointestinal — *see* Complications, prosthetic device, mechanical, gastrointestinal device
    genital NEC T83.498 ☑
      intrauterine contraceptive device T83.39 ☑
      penile prosthesis (cylinder) (implanted) (pump) (resevoir) T83.490 ☑
      testicular prosthesis T83.491 ☑
    heart NEC — *see* Complication, cardiovascular device, mechanical
    joint prosthesis — *see* Complications, joint prosthesis, mechanical, specified NEC, by site
    ocular NEC — *see* Complications, prosthetic device, mechanical, ocular device
    orthopedic NEC — *see* Complication, orthopedic, device, mechanical
    specified NEC T85.628 ☑
    urinary NEC — *see also* Complication, genitourinary, device, urinary, mechanical
      graft T83.29 ☑
    vascular NEC — *see* Complication, cardiovascular device, mechanical
    ventricular intracranial shunt T85.09 ☑
  intervertebral disc — *see* Displacement, intervertebral disc
  joint prosthesis — *see* Complications, joint prosthesis, mechanical, specified NEC, by site
  nucleus pulposus — *see* Displacement, intervertebral disc
Prune belly (syndrome) Q79.4
Prurigo (ferox) (gravis) (Hebrae) (Hebra's) (mitis) (simplex) L28.2
  Besnier's L20.0
  estivalis L56.4
  nodularis L28.1
  psychogenic F45.8
Pruritus, pruritic (essential) L29.9
  ani, anus L29.0
    psychogenic F45.8
  anogenital L29.3
    psychogenic F45.8
  due to onchocerca volvulus B73.1
  gravidarum — *see* Pregnancy, complicated by, specified pregnancy-related condition NEC
  hiemalis L29.8
  neurogenic (any site) F45.8
  perianal L29.0
  psychogenic (any site) F45.8
  scroti, scrotum L29.1
    psychogenic F45.8
  senile, senilis L29.8
  specified NEC L29.8
    psychogenic F45.8
  Trichomonas A59.9
  vulva, vulvae L29.2
    psychogenic F45.8

Pseudarthrosis, pseudoarthrosis (bone) — *see* Nonunion, fracture
  clavicle, congenital Q74.0
  joint, following fusion or arthrodesis M96.0
Pseudoaneurysm — *see* Aneurysm
Pseudoangina (pectoris) — *see* Angina
Pseudoangioma I81
Pseudoarteriosus Q28.8
Pseudoarthrosis — *see* Pseudarthrosis
Pseudobulbar affect (PBA) F48.2
Pseudochromhidrosis L67.8
Pseudocirrhosis, liver, pericardial I31.1
Pseudocowpox B08.03
Pseudocoxalgia M91.3- ☑
Pseudocroup J38.5
Pseudo-Cushing's syndrome, alcohol-induced E24.4
Pseudocyesis F45.8
Pseudocyst
  lung J98.4
  pancreas K86.3
  retina — *see* Cyst, retina
Pseudoelephantiasis neuroarthritica Q82.0
Pseudoexfoliation, capsule (lens) — *see* Cataract, specified NEC
Pseudofolliculitis barbae L73.1
Pseudoglioma H44.89
Pseudohemophilia (Bernuth's) (hereditary) (type B) D68.0
  Type A D69.8
  vascular D69.8
Pseudohermaphroditism Q56.3
  adrenal E25.8
  female Q56.2
    with adrenocortical disorder E25.8
    without adrenocortical disorder Q56.2
    adrenal (congenital) E25.0
    unspecified E25.9
  male Q56.1
    with
      5-alpha-reductase deficiency E29.1
      adrenocortical disorder E25.8
      androgen resistance E34.51
      cleft scrotum Q56.1
      feminizing testis E34.51
    without gonadal disorder Q56.1
    adrenal E25.8
    unspecified E25.9
Pseudo-Hurler's polydystrophy E77.0
Pseudohydrocephalus G93.2
Pseudohypertrophic muscular dystrophy (Erb's) G71.02
Pseudohypertrophy, muscle G71.09
Pseudohypoparathyroidism E20.1
Pseudoinsomnia F51.03
Pseudoleukemia, infantile D64.89
Pseudomembranous — *see* condition
Pseudomeningocele (cerebral) (infective) (post-traumatic) G96.198
  postprocedural (spinal) G97.82
Pseudomenses (newborn) P54.6
Pseudomenstruation (newborn) P54.6
Pseudomonas
  aeruginosa, as cause of disease classified elsewhere B96.5
  mallei infection A24.0
    as cause of disease classified elsewhere B96.5
  pseudomallei, as cause of disease classified elsewhere B96.5
Pseudomyotonia G71.19
Pseudomyxoma peritonei C78.6
Pseudoneuritis, optic (nerve) (disc) (papilla), **congenital** Q14.2
Pseudo-obstruction intestine (acute) (chronic) (idiopathic) (intermittent secondary) (primary) K59.89
  colonic K59.81
Pseudopapilledema H47.33- ☑
  congenital Q14.2
Pseudoparalysis
  arm or leg R29.818
  atonic, congenital P94.2
Pseudopelade L66.0
Pseudophakia Z96.1
Pseudopolyarthritis, rhizomelic M35.3
Pseudopolycythemia D75.1
Pseudopseudohypoparathyroidism E20.1
Pseudopterygium H11.81- ☑
Pseudoptosis (eyelid) — *see* Blepharochalasis

270

☑ Additional Character Required — Refer to the Tabular List for Character Selection   Subterms under main terms may continue to next column or page

Pseudopuberty, precocious
  female heterosexual E25.8
  male isosexual E25.8
Pseudorickets (renal) N25.0
Pseudorubella B08.20
Pseudosclerema, newborn P83.88
Pseudosclerosis (brain)
  Jakob's — see Creutzfeldt-Jakob disease or syndrome
    of Westphal (Strümpell) E83.01
  spastic — see Creutzfeldt-Jakob disease or syndrome
Pseudotetanus — see Convulsions
Pseudotetany R29.0
  hysterical F44.5
Pseudotruncus arteriosus Q25.49
Pseudotuberculosis A28.2
  enterocolitis A04.8
  pasteurella (infection) A28.0
Pseudotumor G93.2
  cerebri G93.2
  orbital H05.11 ☑
Pseudoxanthoma elasticum Q82.8
Psilosis (sprue) (tropical) K90.1
  nontropical K90.0
Psittacosis A70
Psoitis M60.88
Psoriasis L40.9
  arthropathic L40.50
    arthritis mutilans L40.52
    distal interphalangeal L40.51
    juvenile L40.54
    other specified L40.59
    spondylitis L40.53
  buccal K13.29
  flexural L40.8
  guttate L40.4
  mouth K13.29
  nummular L40.0
  plaque L40.0
  psychogenic F54
  pustular (generalized) L40.1
    palmaris et plantaris L40.3
  specified NEC L40.8
  vulgaris L40.0
Psychasthenia F48.8
Psychiatric disorder or problem F99
Psychogenic — see also condition
  factors associated with physical conditions F54
Psychological and behavioral factors affecting medical condition F59
Psychoneurosis, psychoneurotic — see also Neurosis
  anxiety (state) F41.1
  depersonalization F48.1
  hypochondriacal F45.21
  hysteria F44.9
  neurasthenic F48.8
  personality NEC F60.89
Psychopathy, psychopathic
  affectionless F94.2
  autistic F84.5
  constitution, post-traumatic F07.81
  personality — see Disorder, personality
  sexual — see Deviation, sexual
  state F60.2
Psychosexual identity disorder of childhood F64.2
Psychosis, psychotic F29
  acute (transient) F23
    hysterical F44.9
  affective — see Disorder, mood
  alcoholic F10.959
    with
      abuse F10.159
      anxiety disorder F10.980
        with
          abuse F10.180
          dependence F10.280
      delirium tremens F10.231
      delusions F10.950
        with
          abuse F10.150
          dependence F10.250
      dementia F10.97
        with dependence F10.27
      dependence F10.259
      hallucinosis F10.951
        with
          abuse F10.151
          dependence F10.251
      mood disorder F10.94

Psychosis, psychotic — continued
  alcoholic — continued
    with — continued
      mood disorder — continued
        with
          abuse F10.14
          dependence F10.24
      paranoia F10.950
        with
          abuse F10.150
          dependence F10.250
      persisting amnesia F10.96
        with dependence F10.26
    amnestic confabulatory F10.96
      with dependence F10.26
    delirium tremens F10.231
    Korsakoff's, Korsakov's, Korsakow's F10.26
    paranoid type F10.950
      with
        abuse F10.150
        dependence F10.250
  anergastic — see Psychosis, organic
  arteriosclerotic (simple type) (uncomplicated) F01.50
    with behavioral disturbance F01.51
  childhood F84.0
    atypical F84.8
  climacteric — see Psychosis, involutional
  confusional F29
    acute or subacute F05
    reactive F23
  cycloid F23
  depressive — see Disorder, depressive
  disintegrative (childhood) F84.3
  drug-induced — see F11-F19 with .X59
    paranoid and hallucinatory states — see F11-F19 with .X50 or .X51
  due to or associated with
    addiction, drug — see F11-F19 with .X59
    dependence
      alcohol F10.259
      drug — see F11-F19 with .X59
    epilepsy F06.8
    Huntington's chorea F06.8
    ischemia, cerebrovascular (generalized) F06.8
    multiple sclerosis F06.8
    physical disease F06.8
    presenile dementia F03 ☑
    senile dementia F03 ☑
    vascular disease (arteriosclerotic) (cerebral) F01.50
      with behavioral disturbance F01.51
  epileptic F06.8
  episode F23
    due to or associated with physical condition F06.8
  exhaustive F43.0
  hallucinatory, chronic F28
  hypomanic F30.8
  hysterical (acute) F44.9
  induced F24
  infantile F84.0
    atypical F84.8
  infective (acute) (subacute) F05
  involutional F28
    depressive — see Disorder, depressive
    melancholic — see Disorder, depressive
    paranoid (state) F22
  Korsakoff's, Korsakov's, Korsakow's (nonalcoholic) F04
    alcoholic F10.96
      in dependence F10.26
    induced by other psychoactive substance — see categories F11-F19 with .X5X
  mania, manic (single episode) F30.2
    recurrent type F31.89
  manic-depressive — see Disorder, bipolar
  menopausal — see Psychosis, involutional
  mixed schizophrenic and affective F25.8
  multi-infarct (cerebrovascular) F01.50
    with behavioral disturbance F01.51
  nonorganic F29
    specified NEC F28
  organic F09
    due to or associated with
      arteriosclerosis (cerebral) — see Psychosis, arteriosclerotic
      cerebrovascular disease, arteriosclerotic — see Psychosis, arteriosclerotic
      childbirth — see Psychosis, puerperal
      Creutzfeldt-Jakob disease or syndrome — see Creutzfeldt-Jakob disease or syndrome

Psychosis, psychotic — continued
  organic — continued
    due to or associated with — continued
      dependence, alcohol F10.259
      disease
        alcoholic liver F10.259
        brain, arteriosclerotic — see Psychosis, arteriosclerotic
        cerebrovascular F01.50
          with behavioral disturbance F01.51
        Creutzfeldt-Jakob — see Creutzfeldt-Jakob disease or syndrome
        endocrine or metabolic F06.8
          acute or subacute F05
        liver, alcoholic F10.259
      epilepsy transient (acute) F05
      infection
        brain (intracranial) F06.8
          acute or subacute F05
      intoxication
        alcoholic (acute) F10.259
        drug F11-F19 with .x59
      ischemia, cerebrovascular (generalized) — see Psychosis, arteriosclerotic
      puerperium — see Psychosis, puerperal
      trauma, brain (birth) (from electric current) (surgical) F06.8
        acute or subacute F05
    infective F06.8
      acute or subacute F05
    post-traumatic F06.8
      acute or subacute F05
  paranoiac F22
  paranoid (climacteric) (involutional) (menopausal) F22
    psychogenic (acute) F23
    schizophrenic F20.0
    senile F03 ☑
  postpartum (NOS) F53.1
  presbyophrenic (type) F03 ☑
  presenile F03 ☑
  psychogenic (paranoid) F23
    depressive F32.3
  puerperal (NOS) F53.1
    specified type — see Psychosis, by type
  reactive (brief) (transient) (emotional stress) (psychological trauma) F23
    depressive F32.3
      recurrent F33.3
    excitative type F30.8
  schizoaffective F25.9
    depressive type F25.1
    manic type F25.0
  schizophrenia, schizophrenic — see Schizophrenia
  schizophrenia-like, in epilepsy F06.2
  schizophreniform F20.81
    affective type F25.9
    brief F23
    confusional type F23
    mixed type F25.0
  senile NEC F03 ☑
    depressed or paranoid type F03 ☑
    simple deterioration F03 ☑
    specified type — code to condition
  shared F24
  situational (reactive) F23
  symbiotic (childhood) F84.3
  symptomatic F09
Psychosomatic — see Disorder, psychosomatic
Psychosyndrome, organic F07.9
Psychotic episode due to or associated with physical condition F06.8
Pterygium (eye) H11.00- ☑
  amyloid H11.01- ☑
  central H11.02- ☑
  colli Q18.3
  double H11.03- ☑
  peripheral
    progressive H11.05- ☑
    stationary H11.04- ☑
  recurrent H11.06- ☑
Ptilosis (eyelid) — see Madarosis
Ptomaine (poisoning) — see Poisoning, food
Ptosis — see also Blepharoptosis
  adiposa (false) — see Blepharoptosis
  breast N64.81-
  brow H57.81- ☑
  cecum K63.4
  colon K63.4

Ptosis — *continued*
  congenital (eyelid) Q10.0
    specified site NEC — *see* Anomaly, by site
  eyebrow H57.81- ☑
  eyelid — *see* Blepharoptosis
    congenital Q10.0
  gastric K31.89
  intestine K63.4
  kidney N28.83
  liver K76.89
  renal N28.83
  splanchnic K63.4
  spleen D73.89
  stomach K31.89
  viscera K63.4
PTP D69.51
Ptyalism (periodic) K11.7
  hysterical F45.8
  pregnancy — *see* Pregnancy, complicated by, specified
    pregnancy-related condition NEC
  psychogenic F45.8
Ptyalolithiasis K11.5
Pubarche, precocious E30.1
Pubertas praecox E30.1
Puberty (development state) Z00.3
  bleeding (excessive) N92.2
  delayed E30.0
  precocious (constitutional) (cryptogenic) (idiopathic)
    E30.1
    central E22.8
    due to
      ovarian hyperfunction E28.1
        estrogen E28.0
      testicular hyperfunction E29.0
  premature E30.1
    due to
      adrenal cortical hyperfunction E25.8
      pineal tumor E34.8
      pituitary (anterior) hyperfunction E22.8
Puckering, macula — *see* Degeneration, macula, puckering
Pudenda, pudendum — *see* condition
Puente's disease (simple glandular cheilitis) K13.0
Puerperal, puerperium (complicated by, complications)
  abnormal glucose (tolerance test) O99.815
  abscess
    areola O91.02
      associated with lactation O91.03
    Bartholin's gland O86.19
    breast O91.12
      associated with lactation O91.13
    cervix (uteri) O86.11
    genital organ NEC O86.19
    kidney O86.21
    mammary O91.12
      associated with lactation O91.13
    nipple O91.02
      associated with lactation O91.03
    peritoneum O85
    subareolar O91.12
      associated with lactation O91.13
    urinary tract — *see* Puerperal, infection, urinary
    uterus O86.12
    vagina (wall) O86.13
    vaginorectal O86.13
    vulvovaginal gland O86.13
  adnexitis O86.19
  afibrinogenemia, or other coagulation defect O72.3
  albuminuria (acute) (subacute) — *see* Proteinuria, gestational
  alcohol use O99.315
  anemia O90.81
    pre-existing (pre-pregnancy) O99.03
  anesthetic death O89.8
  apoplexy O99.43
  bariatric surgery status O99.845
  blood disorder NEC O99.13
  blood dyscrasia O72.3
  cardiomyopathy O90.3
  cerebrovascular disorder (conditions in I60-I69) O99.43
  cervicitis O86.11
  circulatory system disorder O99.43
  coagulopathy (any) O99.13
    with hemorrhage O72.3
  complications O90.9
    specified NEC O90.89
  convulsions — *see* Eclampsia
  cystitis O86.22

Puerperal, puerperium — *continued*
  cystopyelitis O86.29
  delirium NEC F05
  diabetes O24.93
    gestational — *see* Puerperal, gestational diabetes
    pre-existing O24.33
      specified NEC O24.83
      type 1 O24.03
      type 2 O24.13
  digestive system disorder O99.63
  disease O90.9
    breast O92.29
    cerebrovascular (acute) O99.43
    nonobstetric NEC O99.893
    tubo-ovarian O86.19
    Valsuani's O99.03
  disorder O90.9
    biliary tract O26.63
    lactation O92.70
    liver O26.63
    nonobstetric NEC O99.893
  disruption
    cesarean wound O90.0
    episiotomy wound O90.1
    perineal laceration wound O90.1
  drug use O99.325
  eclampsia (with pre-existing hypertension) O15.2
  embolism (pulmonary) (blood clot) — *see* Embolism, obstetric, puerperal
  endocrine, nutritional or metabolic disease NEC
    O99.285
  endophlebitis — *see* Puerperal, phlebitis
  endotrachelitis O86.11
  failure
    lactation (complete) O92.3
      partial O92.4
    renal, acute O90.4
  fever (of unknown origin) O86.4
    septic O85
  fissure, nipple O92.12
    associated with lactation O92.13
  fistula
    breast (due to mastitis) O91.12
      associated with lactation O91.13
    nipple O91.02
      associated with lactation O91.03
  galactophoritis O91.22
    associated with lactation O91.23
  galactorrhea O92.6
  gastric banding status O99.845
  gastric bypass status O99.845
  gastrointestinal disease NEC O99.63
  gestational
    diabetes O24.439
      diet controlled O24.430
      insulin (and diet) controlled O24.434
      oral drug controlled (antidiabetic) (hypoglycemic) O24.435
    edema O12.05
      with proteinuria O12.25
    proteinuria O12.15
  gonorrhea O98.23
  hematoma, subdural O99.43
  hemiplegia, cerebral O99.355
    due to cerbrovascular disorder O99.43
  hemorrhage O72.1
    brain O99.43
    bulbar O99.43
    cerebellar O99.43
    cerebral O99.43
    cortical O99.43
    delayed or secondary O72.2
    extradural O99.43
    internal capsule O99.43
    intracranial O99.43
    intrapontine O99.43
    meningeal O99.43
    pontine O99.43
    retained placenta O72.0
    subarachnoid O99.43
    subcortical O99.43
    subdural O99.43
    third stage O72.0
    uterine, delayed O72.2
    ventricular O99.43
  hemorrhoids O87.2
  hepatorenal syndrome O90.4
  hypertension — *see* Hypertension, complicating, puerperium

Puerperal, puerperium — *continued*
  hypertrophy, breast O92.29
  induration breast (fibrous) O92.29
  infection O86.4
    cervix O86.11
    generalized O85
    genital tract NEC O86.19
      obstetric surgical wound O86.09
    kidney (bacillus coli) O86.21
    maternal O98.93
      carrier state NEC O99.835
      gonorrhea O98.23
      human immunodeficiency virus (HIV) O98.73
      protozoal O98.63
      sexually transmitted NEC O98.33
      specified NEC O98.83
      streptococcus group B (GBS) carrier state O99.825
      syphilis O98.13
      tuberculosis O98.03
      viral hepatitis O98.43
      viral NEC O98.53
    nipple O91.02
      associated with lactation O91.03
    peritoneum O85
    renal O86.21
    specified NEC O86.89
    urinary (asymptomatic) (tract) NEC O86.20
      bladder O86.22
      kidney O86.21
      specified site NEC O86.29
      urethra O86.22
    vagina O86.13
    vein — *see* Puerperal, phlebitis
  ischemia, cerebral O99.43
  lymphangitis O86.89
    breast O91.22
      associated with lactation O91.23
  malignancy O9A.13 (*following* O99)
  malnutrition O25.3
  mammillitis O91.02
    associated with lactation O91.03
  mammitis O91.22
    associated with lactation O91.23
  mania F30.8
  mastitis O91.22
    associated with lactation O91.23
    purulent O91.12
      associated with lactation O91.13
  melancholia — *see* Disorder, depressive
  mental disorder NEC O99.345
  metroperitonitis O85
  metrorrhagia — *see* Hemorrhage, postpartum
  metrosalpingitis O86.19
  metrovaginitis O86.13
  milk leg O87.1
  monoplegia, cerebral O99.43
  mood disturbance O90.6
  necrosis, liver (acute) (subacute) (conditions in subcategory K72.0) O26.63
    with renal failure O90.4
  nervous system disorder O99.355
  obesity (pre-existing prior to pregnancy) O99.215
  obesity surgery status O99.845
  occlusion, precerebral artery O99.43
  paralysis
    bladder (sphincter) O90.89
    cerebral O99.43
  paralytic stroke O99.43
  parametritis O85
  paravaginitis O86.13
  pelviperitonitis O85
  perimetritis O86.12
  perimetrosalpingitis O86.19
  perinephritis O86.21
  periphlebitis — *see* Puerperal phlebitis
  peritoneal infection O85
  peritonitis (pelvic) O85
  perivaginitis O86.13
  phlebitis O87.0
    deep O87.1
    pelvic O87.1
    superficial O87.0
  phlebothrombosis, deep O87.1
  phlegmasia alba dolens O87.1
  placental polyp O90.89
  pneumonia, embolic — *see* Embolism, obstetric, puerperal
  pre-eclampsia — *see* Pre-eclampsia
  psychosis (NOS) F53.1

☑ Additional Character Required — Refer to the Tabular List for Character Selection   ▽ Subterms under main terms may continue to next column or page

Puerperal, puerperium — *continued*
pyelitis O86.21
pyelocystitis O86.29
pyelonephritis O86.21
pyelonephrosis O86.21
pyemia O85
pyocystitis O86.29
pyohemia O85
pyometra O86.12
pyonephritis O86.21
pyosalpingitis O86.19
pyrexia (of unknown origin) O86.4
renal
   disease NEC O90.89
   failure O90.4
respiratory disease NEC O99.53
retention
   decidua — *see* Retention, decidua
   placenta O72.0
   secundines — *see* Retention, secundines
retrated nipple O92.02
salpingo-ovaritis O86.19
salpingoperitonitis O85
secondary perineal tear O90.1
sepsis (pelvic) O85
sepsis O85
septic thrombophlebitis O86.81
skin disorder NEC O99.73
specified condition NEC O99.893
stroke O99.43
subinvolution (uterus) O90.89
subluxation of symphysis (pubis) O26.73
suppuration — *see* Puerperal, abscess
tetanus A34
thelitis O91.02
   associated with lactation O91.03
thrombocytopenia O72.3
thrombophlebitis (superficial) O87.0
   deep O87.1
   pelvic O87.1
   septic O86.81
thrombosis (venous) — *see* Thrombosis, puerperal
thyroiditis O90.5
toxemia (eclamptic) (pre-eclamptic) (with convulsions) O15.2
trauma, non-obstetric O9A.23 (*following* O99)
   caused by abuse (physical) (suspected) O9A.33 (*following* O99)
      confirmed O9A.33 (*following* O99)
   psychological (suspected) O9A.53 (*following* O99)
      confirmed O9A.53 (*following* O99)
   sexual (suspected) O9A.43 (*following* O99)
      confirmed O9A.43 (*following* O99)
uremia (due to renal failure) O90.4
urethritis O86.22
vaginitis O86.13
varicose veins (legs) O87.4
   vulva or perineum O87.8
venous O87.9
vulvitis O86.19
vulvovaginitis O86.13
white leg O87.1
Puerperium — *see* Puerperal
Pulmolithiasis J98.4
Pulmonary — *see* condition
Pulpitis (acute) (anachoretic) (chronic) (hyperplastic) (putrescent) (suppurative) (ulcerative) K04.01
   irreversible K04.02
   reversible K04.01
Pulpless tooth K04.99
Pulse
   alternating R00.8
   bigeminal R00.8
   fast R00.0
   feeble, rapid due to shock following injury T79.4 ☑
   rapid R00.0
   weak R09.89
Pulsus alternans or trigeminus R00.8
Punch drunk F07.81
Punctum lacrimale occlusion — *see* Obstruction, lacrimal
Puncture
   abdomen, abdominal
      wall S31.139 ☑
         with
            foreign body S31.149 ☑
               penetration into peritoneal cavity S31.639 ☑
                  with foreign body S31.649 ☑

Puncture — *continued*
   abdomen, abdominal — *continued*
      wall — *continued*
         epigastric region S31.132 ☑
            with
               foreign body S31.142 ☑
                  penetration into peritoneal cavity S31.632 ☑
                     with foreign body S31.642 ☑
         left
            lower quadrant S31.134 ☑
               with
                  foreign body S31.144 ☑
                     penetration into peritoneal cavity S31.634 ☑
                        with foreign body S31.644 ☑
            upper quadrant S31.131 ☑
               with
                  foreign body S31.141 ☑
                     penetration into peritoneal cavity S31.631 ☑
                        with foreign body S31.641 ☑
         periumbilic region S31.135 ☑
            with
               foreign body S31.145 ☑
                  penetration into peritoneal cavity S31.635 ☑
                     with foreign body S31.645 ☑
         right
            lower quadrant S31.133 ☑
               with
                  foreign body S31.143 ☑
                     penetration into peritoneal cavity S31.633 ☑
                        with foreign body S31.643 ☑
            upper quadrant S31.130 ☑
               with
                  foreign body S31.140 ☑
                     penetration into peritoneal cavity S31.630 ☑
                        with foreign body S31.640 ☑
   accidental, complicating surgery — *see* Complication, accidental puncture or laceration
   alveolar (process) — *see* Puncture, oral cavity
   ankle S91.039 ☑
      with
         foreign body S91.049 ☑
      left S91.032 ☑
         with
            foreign body S91.042 ☑
      right S91.031 ☑
         with
            foreign body S91.041 ☑
   anus S31.833 ☑
      with foreign body S31.834 ☑
   arm (upper) S41.139 ☑
      with foreign body S41.149 ☑
      left S41.132 ☑
         with foreign body S41.142 ☑
      lower — *see* Puncture, forearm
      right S41.131 ☑
         with foreign body S41.141 ☑
   auditory canal (external) (meatus) — *see* Puncture, ear
   auricle, ear — *see* Puncture, ear
   axilla — *see* Puncture, arm
   back — *see also* Puncture, thorax, back
      lower S31.030 ☑
         with
            foreign body S31.040 ☑
               with penetration into retroperitoneal space S31.041 ☑
            penetration into retroperitoneal space S31.031 ☑
   bladder (traumatic) S37.29 ☑
      nontraumatic N32.89
   breast S21.039 ☑
      with foreign body S21.049 ☑
      left S21.032 ☑
         with foreign body S21.042 ☑
      right S21.031 ☑
         with foreign body S21.041 ☑
   buttock S31.803 ☑
      with foreign body S31.804 ☑
      left S31.823 ☑
         with foreign body S31.824 ☑
      right S31.813 ☑

Puncture — *continued*
   buttock — *continued*
      right — *continued*
         with foreign body S31.814 ☑
   by
      device, implant or graft — *see* Complications, by site and type, mechanical
      foreign body left accidentally in operative wound T81.539 ☑
      instrument (any) during a procedure, accidental — *see* Puncture, accidental complicating surgery
   calf — *see* Puncture, leg
   canaliculus lacrimalis — *see* Puncture, eyelid
   canthus, eye — *see* Puncture, eyelid
   cervical esophagus S11.23 ☑
      with foreign body S11.24 ☑
   cheek (external) S01.439 ☑
      with foreign body S01.449 ☑
      internal — *see* Puncture, oral cavity
      left S01.432 ☑
         with foreign body S01.442 ☑
      right S01.431 ☑
         with foreign body S01.441 ☑
   chest wall — *see* Puncture, thorax
   chin — *see* Puncture, head, specified site NEC
   clitoris — *see* Puncture, vulva
   costal region — *see* Puncture, thorax
   digit(s)
      foot — *see* Puncture, toe
      hand — *see* Puncture, finger
   ear (canal) (external) S01.339 ☑
      with foreign body S01.349 ☑
      drum S09.2- ☑
      left S01.332 ☑
         with foreign body S01.342 ☑
      right S01.331 ☑
         with foreign body S01.341 ☑
   elbow S51.039 ☑
      with
         foreign body S51.049 ☑
      left S51.032 ☑
         with
            foreign body S51.042 ☑
      right S51.031 ☑
         with
            foreign body S51.041 ☑
   epididymis — *see* Puncture, testis
   epigastric region — *see* Puncture, abdomen, wall, epigastric
   epiglottis S11.83 ☑
      with foreign body S11.84 ☑
   esophagus
      cervical S11.23 ☑
         with foreign body S11.24 ☑
      thoracic S27.818 ☑
   eyeball S05.6- ☑
      with foreign body S05.5- ☑
   eyebrow — *see* Puncture, eyelid
   eyelid S01.13- ☑
      with foreign body S01.14- ☑
      left S01.132 ☑
         with foreign body S01.142 ☑
      right S01.131 ☑
         with foreign body S01.141 ☑
   face NEC — *see* Puncture, head, specified site NEC
   finger(s) S61.239 ☑
      with
         damage to nail S61.339 ☑
            with
               foreign body S61.349 ☑
         foreign body S61.249 ☑
      index S61.238 ☑
         with
            damage to nail S61.338 ☑
               with
                  foreign body S61.348 ☑
            foreign body S61.248 ☑
         left S61.231 ☑
            with
               damage to nail S61.331 ☑
                  with
                     foreign body S61.341 ☑
               foreign body S61.241 ☑
         right S61.230 ☑
            with
               damage to nail S61.330 ☑

Puncture — *continued*
finger(s) — *continued*
    index — *continued*
        right — *continued*
            with — *continued*
                damage to nail — *continued*
                    with
                        foreign body S61.340 ✓
                    foreign body S61.240 ✓
        little S61.238 ✓
            with
                damage to nail S61.338 ✓
                    with
                        foreign body S61.348 ✓
                foreign body S61.248 ✓
            left S61.237 ✓
                with
                    damage to nail S61.337 ✓
                        with
                            foreign body S61.347 ✓
                    foreign body S61.247 ✓
            right S61.236 ✓
                with
                    damage to nail S61.336 ✓
                        with
                            foreign body S61.346 ✓
                    foreign body S61.246 ✓
        middle S61.238 ✓
            with
                damage to nail S61.338 ✓
                    with
                        foreign body S61.348 ✓
                foreign body S61.248 ✓
            left S61.233 ✓
                with
                    damage to nail S61.333 ✓
                        with
                            foreign body S61.343 ✓
                    foreign body S61.243 ✓
            right S61.232 ✓
                with
                    damage to nail S61.332 ✓
                        with
                            foreign body S61.342 ✓
                    foreign body S61.242 ✓
        ring S61.238 ✓
            with
                damage to nail S61.338 ✓
                    with
                        foreign body S61.348 ✓
                foreign body S61.248 ✓
            left S61.235 ✓
                with
                    damage to nail S61.335 ✓
                        with
                            foreign body S61.345 ✓
                    foreign body S61.245 ✓
            right S61.234 ✓
                with
                    damage to nail S61.334 ✓
                        with
                            foreign body S61.344 ✓
                    foreign body S61.244 ✓
flank S31.139 ✓
    with foreign body S31.149 ✓
foot (except toe(s) alone) S91.339 ✓
    with foreign body S91.349 ✓
    left S91.332 ✓
        with foreign body S91.342 ✓
    right S91.331 ✓
        with foreign body S91.341 ✓
    toe — *see* Puncture, toe
forearm S51.839 ✓
    with
        foreign body S51.849 ✓
    elbow only — *see* Puncture, elbow
    left S51.832 ✓
        with
            foreign body S51.842 ✓
    right S51.831 ✓
        with
            foreign body S51.841 ✓
forehead — *see* Puncture, head, specified site NEC
genital organs, external
    female S31.532 ✓
        with foreign body S31.542 ✓

Puncture — *continued*
    genital organs, external — *continued*
        female — *continued*
            vagina — *see* Puncture, vagina
            vulva — *see* Puncture, vulva
        male S31.531 ✓
            with foreign body S31.541 ✓
            penis — *see* Puncture, penis
            scrotum — *see* Puncture, scrotum
            testis — *see* Puncture, testis
    groin — *see* Puncture, abdomen, wall
    gum — *see* Puncture, oral cavity
    hand S61.439 ✓
        with
            foreign body S61.449 ✓
        finger — *see* Puncture, finger
        left S61.432 ✓
            with
                foreign body S61.442 ✓
        right S61.431 ✓
            with
                foreign body S61.441 ✓
        thumb — *see* Puncture, thumb
    head S01.93 ✓
        with foreign body S01.94 ✓
        cheek — *see* Puncture, cheek
        ear — *see* Puncture, ear
        eyelid — *see* Puncture, eyelid
        lip — *see* Puncture, oral cavity
        nose — *see* Puncture, nose
        oral cavity — *see* Puncture, oral cavity
        scalp S01.03 ✓
            with foreign body S01.04 ✓
        specified site NEC S01.83 ✓
            with foreign body S01.84 ✓
        temporomandibular area — *see* Puncture, cheek
    heart S26.99 ✓
        with hemopericardium S26.09 ✓
        without hemopericardium S26.19 ✓
    heel — *see* Puncture, foot
    hip S71.039 ✓
        with foreign body S71.049 ✓
        left S71.032 ✓
            with foreign body S71.042 ✓
        right S71.031 ✓
            with foreign body S71.041 ✓
    hymen — *see* Puncture, vagina
    hypochondrium — *see* Puncture, abdomen, wall
    hypogastric region — *see* Puncture, abdomen, wall
    inguinal region — *see* Puncture, abdomen, wall
    instep — *see* Puncture, foot
    internal organs — *see* Injury, by site
    interscapular region — *see* Puncture, thorax, back
    intestine
        large
            colon S36.599 ✓
                ascending S36.590 ✓
                descending S36.592 ✓
                sigmoid S36.593 ✓
                specified site NEC S36.598 ✓
                transverse S36.591 ✓
            rectum S36.69 ✓
        small S36.499 ✓
            duodenum S36.490 ✓
            specified site NEC S36.498 ✓
    intra-abdominal organ S36.99 ✓
        gallbladder S36.128 ✓
        intestine — *see* Puncture, intestine
        liver S36.118 ✓
        pancreas — *see* Puncture, pancreas
        peritoneum S36.81 ✓
        specified site NEC S36.898 ✓
        spleen S36.09 ✓
        stomach S36.39 ✓
    jaw — *see* Puncture, head, specified site NEC
    knee S81.039 ✓
        with foreign body S81.049 ✓
        left S81.032 ✓
            with foreign body S81.042 ✓
        right S81.031 ✓
            with foreign body S81.041 ✓
    labium (majus) (minus) — *see* Puncture, vulva
    lacrimal duct — *see* Puncture, eyelid
    larynx S11.013 ✓
        with foreign body S11.014 ✓
    leg (lower) S81.839 ✓

Puncture — *continued*
    leg — *continued*
        with foreign body S81.849 ✓
        foot — *see* Puncture, foot
        knee — *see* Puncture, knee
        left S81.832 ✓
            with foreign body S81.842 ✓
        right S81.831 ✓
            with foreign body S81.841 ✓
        upper — *see* Puncture, thigh
    lip S01.531 ✓
        with foreign body S01.541 ✓
    loin — *see* Puncture, abdomen, wall
    lower back — *see* Puncture, back, lower
    lumbar region — *see* Puncture, back, lower
    malar region — *see* Puncture, head, specified site NEC
    mammary — *see* Puncture, breast
    mastoid region — *see* Puncture, head, specified site NEC
    mouth — *see* Puncture, oral cavity
    nail
        finger — *see* Puncture, finger, with damage to nail
        toe — *see* Puncture, toe, with damage to nail
    nasal (septum) (sinus) — *see* Puncture, nose
    nasopharynx — *see* Puncture, head, specified site NEC
    neck S11.93 ✓
        with foreign body S11.94 ✓
        involving
            cervical esophagus — *see* Puncture, cervical esophagus
            larynx — *see* Puncture, larynx
            pharynx — *see* Puncture, pharynx
            thyroid gland — *see* Puncture, thyroid gland
            trachea — *see* Puncture, trachea
        specified site NEC S11.83 ✓
            with foreign body S11.84 ✓
    nose (septum) (sinus) S01.23 ✓
        with foreign body S01.24 ✓
    ocular — *see* Puncture, eyeball
    oral cavity S01.532 ✓
        with foreign body S01.542 ✓
    orbit S05.4-
    palate — *see* Puncture, oral cavity
    palm — *see* Puncture, hand
    pancreas S36.299 ✓
        body S36.291 ✓
        head S36.290 ✓
        tail S36.292 ✓
    pelvis — *see* Puncture, back, lower
    penis S31.23 ✓
        with foreign body S31.24 ✓
    perineum
        female S31.43 ✓
            with foreign body S31.44 ✓
        male S31.139 ✓
            with foreign body S31.149 ✓
    periocular area (with or without lacrimal passages) — *see* Puncture, eyelid
    phalanges
        finger — *see* Puncture, finger
        toe — *see* Puncture, toe
    pharynx S11.23 ✓
        with foreign body S11.24 ✓
    pinna — *see* Puncture, ear
    popliteal space — *see* Puncture, knee
    prepuce — *see* Puncture, penis
    pubic region S31.139 ✓
        with foreign body S31.149 ✓
    pudendum — *see* Puncture, genital organs, external
    rectovaginal septum — *see* Puncture, vagina
    sacral region — *see* Puncture, back, lower
    sacroiliac region — *see* Puncture, back, lower
    salivary gland — *see* Puncture, oral cavity
    scalp S01.03 ✓
        with foreign body S01.04 ✓
    scapular region — *see* Puncture, shoulder
    scrotum S31.33 ✓
        with foreign body S31.34 ✓
    shin — *see* Puncture, leg
    shoulder S41.039 ✓
        with foreign body S41.049 ✓
        left S41.032 ✓
            with foreign body S41.042 ✓
        right S41.031 ✓
            with foreign body S41.041 ✓
    spermatic cord — *see* Puncture, testis

✓ **Additional Character Required** — Refer to the Tabular List for Character Selection   ▽ Subterms under main terms may continue to next column or page

Puncture — *continued*
- sternal region — *see* Puncture, thorax, front
- submaxillary region — *see* Puncture, head, specified site NEC
- submental region — *see* Puncture, head, specified site NEC
- subungual
  - finger(s) — *see* Puncture, finger, with damage to nail
  - toe — *see* Puncture, toe, with damage to nail
- supraclavicular fossa — *see* Puncture, neck, specified site NEC
- temple, temporal region — *see* Puncture, head, specified site NEC
- temporomandibular area — *see* Puncture, cheek
- testis S31.33 ☑
  - with foreign body S31.34 ☑
- thigh S71.139 ☑
  - with foreign body S71.149 ☑
  - left S71.132 ☑
    - with foreign body S71.142 ☑
  - right S71.131 ☑
    - with foreign body S71.141 ☑
- thorax, thoracic (wall) S21.93 ☑
  - with foreign body S21.94 ☑
  - back S21.23- ☑
    - with
      - foreign body S21.24- ☑
        - with penetration S21.44 ☑
      - penetration S21.43 ☑
  - breast — *see* Puncture, breast
  - front S21.13- ☑
    - with
      - foreign body S21.14- ☑
        - with penetration S21.34 ☑
      - penetration S21.33 ☑
- throat — *see* Puncture, neck
- thumb S61.039 ☑
  - with
    - damage to nail S61.139 ☑
      - with
        - foreign body S61.149 ☑
    - foreign body S61.049 ☑
  - left S61.032 ☑
    - with
      - damage to nail S61.132 ☑
        - with
          - foreign body S61.142 ☑
      - foreign body S61.042 ☑
  - right S61.031 ☑
    - with
      - damage to nail S61.131 ☑
        - with
          - foreign body S61.141 ☑
      - foreign body S61.041 ☑
- thyroid gland S11.13 ☑
  - with foreign body S11.14 ☑
- toe(s) S91.139 ☑
  - with
    - damage to nail S91.239 ☑
      - with
        - foreign body S91.249 ☑
    - foreign body S91.149 ☑
  - great S91.133 ☑
    - with
      - damage to nail S91.233 ☑
        - with
          - foreign body S91.243 ☑
      - foreign body S91.143 ☑
    - left S91.132 ☑
      - with
        - damage to nail S91.232 ☑
          - with
            - foreign body S91.242 ☑
        - foreign body S91.142 ☑
    - right S91.131 ☑
      - with
        - damage to nail S91.231 ☑
          - with
            - foreign body S91.241 ☑
        - foreign body S91.141 ☑
  - lesser S91.136 ☑
    - with
      - damage to nail S91.236 ☑
        - with
          - foreign body S91.246 ☑

Puncture — *continued*
- toe(s) — *continued*
  - lesser — *continued*
    - with — *continued*
      - foreign body S91.146 ☑
    - left S91.135 ☑
      - with
        - damage to nail S91.235 ☑
          - with
            - foreign body S91.245 ☑
        - foreign body S91.145 ☑
    - right S91.134 ☑
      - with
        - damage to nail S91.234 ☑
          - with
            - foreign body S91.244 ☑
        - foreign body S91.144 ☑
- tongue — *see* Puncture, oral cavity
- trachea S11.023 ☑
  - with foreign body S11.024 ☑
- tunica vaginalis — *see* Puncture, testis
- tympanum, tympanic membrane S09.2- ☑
- umbilical region S31.135 ☑
  - with foreign body S31.145 ☑
- uvula — *see* Puncture, oral cavity
- vagina S31.43 ☑
  - with foreign body S31.44 ☑
- vocal cords S11.033 ☑
  - with foreign body S11.034 ☑
- vulva S31.43 ☑
  - with foreign body S31.44 ☑
- wrist S61.539 ☑
  - with
    - foreign body S61.549 ☑
  - left S61.532 ☑
    - with
      - foreign body S61.542 ☑
  - right S61.531 ☑
    - with
      - foreign body S61.541 ☑

PUO (pyrexia of unknown origin) R50.9
Pupillary membrane (persistent) Q13.89
Pupillotonia — *see* Anomaly, pupil, function, tonic pupil
Purpura D69.2
- abdominal D69.0
- allergic D69.0
- anaphylactoid D69.0
- annularis telangiectodes L81.7
- arthritic D69.0
- autoerythrocyte sensitization D69.2
- autoimmune D69.0
- bacterial D69.0
- Bateman's (senile) D69.2
- capillary fragility (hereditary) (idiopathic) D69.8
- cryoglobulinemic D89.1
- Devil's pinches D69.2
- fibrinolytic — *see* Fibrinolysis
- fulminans, fulminous D65
- gangrenous D65
- hemorrhagic, hemorrhagica D69.3
  - not due to thrombocytopenia D69.0
- Henoch (-Schönlein) (allergic) D69.0
- hypergammaglobulinemic (benign) (Waldenström) D89.0
- idiopathic (thrombocytopenic) D69.3
  - nonthrombocytopenic D69.0
- immune thrombocytopenic D69.3
- infectious D69.0
- malignant D69.0
- neonatorum P54.5
- nervosa D69.0
- newborn P54.5
- nonthrombocytopenic D69.2
  - hemorrhagic D69.0
  - idiopathic D69.0
- nonthrombopenic D69.2
- peliosis rheumatica D69.0
- posttransfusion (post-transfusion) (from (fresh) whole blood or blood products) D69.51
- primary D69.49
- red cell membrane sensitivity D69.2
- rheumatica D69.0
- Schönlein (-Henoch) (allergic) D69.0
- scorbutic E54 [D77]
- senile D69.2
- simplex D69.2
- symptomatica D69.0

Purpura — *continued*
- telangiectasia annularis L81.7
- thrombocytopenic D69.49
  - congenital D69.42
  - hemorrhagic D69.3
  - hereditary D69.42
  - idiopathic D69.3
  - immune D69.3
  - neonatal, transitory P61.0
  - thrombotic M31.19
- thrombohemolytic — *see* Fibrinolysis
- thrombolytic — *see* Fibrinolysis
- thrombopenic D69.49
- thrombotic, thrombocytopenic M31.19
- toxic D69.0
- vascular D69.0
- visceral symptoms D69.0
Purpuric spots R23.3
Purulent — *see* condition
Pus
- in
  - stool R19.5
  - urine N39.0
- tube (rupture) — *see* Salpingo-oophoritis
Pustular rash L08.0
Pustule (nonmalignant) L08.9
- malignant A22.0
Pustulosis palmaris et plantaris L40.3
Putnam (-Dana) **disease or syndrome** — *see* Degeneration, combined
Putrescent pulp (dental) K04.1
Pyarthritis, pyarthrosis — *see* Arthritis, pyogenic or pyemic
- tuberculous — *see* Tuberculosis, joint
Pyelectasis — *see* Hydronephrosis
Pyelitis (congenital) (uremic) — *see also* Pyelonephritis
- with
  - calculus — *see* category N20 ☑
    - with hydronephrosis N13.6
  - contracted kidney N11.9
- acute N10
- chronic N11.9
  - with calculus — *see* category N20 ☑
    - with hydronephrosis N13.6
- cystica N28.84
- puerperal (postpartum) O86.21
- tuberculous A18.11
Pyelocystitis — *see* Pyelonephritis
Pyelonephritis — *see also* Nephritis, tubulo-interstitial
- with
  - calculus — *see* category N20 ☑
    - with hydronephrosis N13.6
  - contracted kidney N11.9
- acute N10
- calculous — *see* category N20 ☑
  - with hydronephrosis N13.6
- chronic N11.9
  - with calculus — *see* category N20 ☑
    - with hydronephrosis N13.6
  - associated with ureteral obstruction or stricture N11.1
  - nonobstructive N11.8
    - with reflux (vesicoureteral) N11.0
  - obstructive N11.1
  - specified NEC N11.8
- in (due to)
  - brucellosis A23.9 [N16]
  - cryoglobulinemia (mixed) D89.1 [N16]
  - cystinosis E72.04
  - diphtheria A36.84
  - glycogen storage disease E74.09 [N16]
  - leukemia NEC C95.9- ☑ [N16]
  - lymphoma NEC C85.90 [N16]
  - multiple myeloma C90.0- ☑ [N16]
  - obstruction N11.1
  - Salmonella infection A02.25
  - sarcoidosis D86.84
  - sepsis A41.9 [N16]
  - Sjögren's disease M35.04
  - toxoplasmosis B58.83
  - transplant rejection T86.91 [N16]
  - Wilson's disease E83.01 [N16]
- nonobstructive N12
  - with reflux (vesicoureteral) N11.0
  - chronic N11.8
- syphilitic A52.75
Pyelonephrosis (obstructive) N11.1
- chronic N11.9

Pyelophlebitis I80.8
Pyeloureteritis cystica N28.85
Pyemia, pyemic (fever) (infection) (purulent) — *see also*
    Sepsis
  joint — *see* Arthritis, pyogenic or pyemic
  liver K75.1
  pneumococcal A40.3
  portal K75.1
  postvaccinal T88.0 ☑
  puerperal, postpartum, childbirth O85
  specified organism NEC A41.89
  tuberculous — *see* Tuberculosis, miliary
Pygopagus Q89.4
Pyknoepilepsy (idiopathic) — *see* Pyknolepsy
Pyknolepsy G40.A09 (*following* G40.3)
  intractable G40.A19 (*following* G40.3)
    with status epilepticus G40.A11 (*following* G40.3)
    without status epilepticus G40.A19 (*following* G40.3)
  not intractable G40.A09 (*following* G40.3)
    with status epilepticus G40.A01 (*following* G40.3)
    without status epilepticus G40.A09 (*following* G40.3)
Pylephlebitis K75.1
Pyle's syndrome Q78.5
Pylethrombophlebitis K75.1
Pylethrombosis K75.1
Pyloritis K29.90
  with bleeding K29.91
Pylorospasm (reflex) **NEC** K31.3
  congenital or infantile Q40.0
  neurotic F45.8
  newborn Q40.0
  psychogenic F45.8
Pylorus, pyloric — *see* condition
Pyoarthrosis — *see* Arthritis, pyogenic or pyemic
Pyocele
  mastoid — *see* Mastoiditis, acute
  sinus (accessory) — *see* Sinusitis
  turbinate (bone) J32.9
  urethra — *see also* Urethritis N34.0
Pyocolpos — *see* Vaginitis
Pyocystitis N30.80
  with hematuria N30.81
Pyoderma, pyodermia L08.0
  gangrenosum L88
  newborn P39.4
  phagedenic L88
  vegetans L08.81
Pyodermatitis L08.0
  vegetans L08.81
Pyogenic — *see* condition
Pyohydronephrosis N13.6
Pyometra, pyometrium, pyometritis — *see* Endometri-
  tis
Pyomyositis (tropical) — *see* Myositis, infective
Pyonephritis N12
Pyonephrosis N13.6
  tuberculous A18.11
Pyo-oophoritis — *see* Salpingo-oophoritis
Pyo-ovarium — *see* Salpingo-oophoritis
Pyopericarditis, pyopericardium I30.1
Pyophlebitis — *see* Phlebitis
Pyopneumopericardium I30.1
Pyopneumothorax (infective) J86.9
  with fistula J86.0
  tuberculous NEC A15.6
Pyosalpinx, pyosalpingitis — *see also* Salpingo-
  oophoritis
Pyothorax J86.9
  with fistula J86.0
  tuberculous NEC A15.6
Pyoureter N28.89
  tuberculous A18.11
Pyramidopallidonigral syndrome G20
Pyrexia (of unknown origin) R50.9
  atmospheric T67.01 ☑
  during labor NEC O75.2
  heat T67.01 ☑
  newborn P81.9
    environmentally-induced P81.0
  persistent R50.9
  puerperal O86.4
Pyroglobulinemia NEC E88.09
Pyromania F63.1
Pyrosis R12
Pyuria (bacterial) (sterile) R82.81

Q

Q fever A78
  with pneumonia A78
Quadricuspid aortic valve Q23.8
Quadrilateral fever A78
Quadriparesis — *see* Quadriplegia
  meaning muscle weakness M62.81
Quadriplegia G82.50
  complete
    C1-C4 level G82.51
    C5-C7 level G82.53
  congenital (cerebral) (spinal) G80.8
    spastic G80.0
  embolic (current episode) I63.4- ☑
  functional R53.2
  incomplete
    C1-C4 level G82.52
    C5-C7 level G82.54
  thrombotic (current episode) I63.3- ☑
  traumatic — *code to* injury with seventh character S
    current episode — *see* Injury, spinal (cord), cervical
Quadruplet, pregnancy — *see* Pregnancy, quadruplet
Quarrelsomeness F60.3
Queensland fever A77.3
Quervain's disease M65.4
  thyroid E06.1
Queyrat's erythroplasia D07.4
  penis D07.4
  specified site — *see* Neoplasm, skin, in situ
  unspecified site D07.4
Quincke's disease or edema T78.3 ☑
  hereditary D84.1
Quinsy (gangrenous) J36
Quintan fever A79.0
Quintuplet, pregnancy — *see* Pregnancy, quintuplet

R

Rabbit fever — *see* Tularemia
Rabies A82.9
  contact Z20.3
  exposure to Z20.3
  inoculation reaction — *see* Complications, vaccination
  sylvatic A82.0
  urban A82.1
Rachischisis — *see* Spina bifida
Rachitic — *see also* condition
  deformities of spine (late effect) (sequelae) E64.3
  pelvis (late effect) (sequelae) E64.3
    with disproportion (fetopelvic) O33.0
      causing obstructed labor O65.0
Rachitis, rachitism (acute) (tarda) — *see also* Rickets
  renalis N25.0
  sequelae E64.3
Radial nerve — *see* condition
Radiation
  burn — *see* Burn
  effects NOS T66 ☑
  sickness NOS T66 ☑
  therapy, encounter for Z51.0
Radiculitis (pressure) (vertebrogenic) — *see* Radiculopathy
Radiculomyelitis — *see also* Encephalitis
  toxic, due to
    Clostridium tetani A35
    Corynebacterium diphtheriae A36.82
Radiculopathy M54.10
  cervical region M54.12
  cervicothoracic region M54.13
  due to
    disc disorder
      C3 M50.11
      C4 M50.11
      C5 M50.121
      C6 M50.122
      C7 M50.123
    displacement of intervertebral disc — *see* Disorder,
      disc, with, radiculopathy
  leg M54.1- ☑
  lumbar region M54.16
  lumbosacral region M54.17
  occipito-atlanto-axial region M54.11
  postherpetic B02.29
  sacrococcygeal region M54.18
  syphilitic A52.11

Radiculopathy — *continued*
  thoracic region (with visceral pain) M54.14
  thoracolumbar region M54.15
Radiodermal burns (acute, chronic, or occupational) —
  see Burn
Radiodermatitis L58.9
  acute L58.0
  chronic L58.1
Radiotherapy session Z51.0
RAEB (refractory anemia with excess blasts) D46.2- ☑
Rage, meaning rabies — *see* Rabies
Ragpicker's disease A22.1
Ragsorter's disease A22.1
Raillietiniasis B71.8
Railroad neurosis F48.8
Railway spine F48.8
Raised — *see also* Elevated
  antibody titer R76.0
Rake teeth, tooth M26.39
Rales R09.89
Ramifying renal pelvis Q63.8
Ramsay-Hunt disease or syndrome — *see also* Hunt's
  disease B02.21
  meaning dyssynergia cerebellaris myoclonica G11.19
Ranula K11.6
  congenital Q38.4
Rape
  adult
    confirmed T74.21 ☑
    suspected T76.21 ☑
  alleged, observation or examination, ruled out
    adult Z04.41
    child Z04.42
  child
    confirmed T74.22 ☑
    suspected T76.22 ☑
Rapid
  feeble pulse, due to shock, following injury T79.4 ☑
  heart (beat) R00.0
    psychogenic F45.8
  second stage (delivery) O62.3
  time-zone change syndrome G47.25
Rarefaction, bone — *see* Disorder, bone, density and
  structure, specified NEC
Rash (toxic) R21
  canker A38.9
  diaper L22
  drug (internal use) L27.0
    contact — *see also* Dermatitis, due to, drugs, exter-
      nal L25.1
  following immunization T88.1 ☑
  food — *see* Dermatitis, due to, food
  heat L74.0
  napkin (psoriasiform) L22
  nettle — *see* Urticaria
  pustular L08.0
  rose R21
    epidemic B06.9
  scarlet A38.9
  serum — *see also* Reaction, serum T80.69 ☑
  wandering tongue K14.1
Rasmussen aneurysm — *see* Tuberculosis, pulmonary
Rasmussen encephalitis G04.81
Rat-bite fever A25.9
  due to Streptobacillus moniliformis A25.1
  spirochetal (morsus muris) A25.0
Rathke's pouch tumor D44.3
Raymond (-Céstan) **syndrome** I65.8
Raynaud's disease, phenomenon or syndrome (secondary) I73.00
  with gangrene (symmetric) I73.01
RDS (newborn) (type I) P22.0
  type II P22.1
Reaction — *see also* Disorder
  withdrawing, child or adolescent F93.8
  adaptation — *see* Disorder, adjustment
  adjustment (anxiety) (conduct disorder) (depressive-
    ness) (distress) — *see* Disorder, adjustment
    with
      mutism, elective (child) (adolescent) F94.0
  adverse
    food (any) (ingested) NEC T78.1 ☑
      anaphylactic — *see* Shock, anaphylactic, due to
        food
  affective — *see* Disorder, mood
  allergic — *see* Allergy
  anaphylactic — *see* Shock, anaphylactic

Reaction — *continued*
　anaphylactoid — *see* Shock, anaphylactic
　anesthesia — *see* Anesthesia, complication
　antitoxin (prophylactic) (therapeutic) — *see* Complications, vaccination
　anxiety F41.1
　Arthus — *see* Arthus' phenomenon
　asthenic F48.8
　combat and operational stress F43.0
　compulsive F42.8
　conversion F44.9
　crisis, acute F43.0
　deoxyribonuclease (DNA) (DNase) hypersensitivity D69.2
　depressive (single episode) F32.9
　　affective (single episode) F31.4
　　　recurrent episode F33.9
　　neurotic F34.1
　　psychoneurotic F34.1
　　psychotic F32.3
　　recurrent — *see* Disorder, depressive, recurrent
　dissociative F44.9
　drug NEC T88.7 ☑
　　addictive — *see* Dependence, drug
　　　transmitted via placenta or breast milk — *see* Absorption, drug, addictive, through placenta
　　allergic — *see* Allergy, drug
　　lichenoid L43.2
　　newborn P93.8
　　　gray baby syndrome P93.0
　　overdose or poisoning (by accident) — *see* Table of Drugs and Chemicals, by drug, poisoning
　　photoallergic L56.1
　　phototoxic L56.0
　　withdrawal — *see* Dependence, by drug, with, withdrawal
　　　infant of dependent mother P96.1
　　　newborn P96.1
　　wrong substance given or taken (by accident) — *see* Table of Drugs and Chemicals, by drug, poisoning
　fear F40.9
　　child (abnormal) F93.8
　febrile nonhemolytic transfusion (FNHTR) R50.84
　fluid loss, cerebrospinal G97.1
　foreign
　　body NEC — *see* Granuloma, foreign body
　　　in operative wound (inadvertently left) — *see* Foreign body, accidentally left during a procedure
　　substance accidentally left during a procedure (chemical) (powder) (talc) T81.60 ☑
　　　aseptic peritonitis T81.61 ☑
　　　body or object (instrument) (sponge) (swab) — *see* Foreign body, accidentally left during a procedure
　　　specified reaction NEC T81.69 ☑
　grief — *see* Disorder, adjustment
　Herxheimer's R68.89
　hyperkinetic — *see* Hyperkinesia
　hypochondriacal F45.20
　hypoglycemic, due to insulin E16.0
　　with coma (diabetic) — *see* Diabetes, coma
　　nondiabetic E15
　　therapeutic misadventure — *see* subcategory T38.3 ☑
　hypomanic F30.8
　hysterical F44.9
　immunization — *see* Complications, vaccination
　incompatibility
　　ABO blood group (infusion) (transfusion) — *see* Complication(s), transfusion, incompatibility reaction, ABO
　　　delayed serologic T80.39 ☑
　　　minor blood group (Duffy) (E) (K) (Kell) (Kidd) (Lewis) (M) (N) (P) (S) T80.89 ☑
　　　Rh (factor) (infusion) (transfusion) — *see* Complication(s), transfusion, incompatibility reaction, Rh (factor)
　inflammatory — *see* Infection
　infusion — *see* Complications, infusion
　inoculation (immune serum) — *see* Complications, vaccination
　insulin T38.3- ☑
　involutional psychotic — *see* Disorder, depressive
　leukemoid D72.823
　　basophilic D72.823

Reaction — *continued*
　leukemoid — *continued*
　　lymphocytic D72.823
　　monocytic D72.823
　　myelocytic D72.823
　　neutrophilic D72.823
　LSD (acute)
　　due to drug abuse — *see* Abuse, drug, hallucinogen
　　due to drug dependence — *see* Dependence, drug, hallucinogen
　lumbar puncture G97.1
　manic-depressive — *see* Disorder, bipolar
　neurasthenic F48.8
　neurogenic — *see* Neurosis
　neurotic F48.9
　neurotic-depressive F34.1
　nitritoid — *see* Crisis, nitritoid
　nonspecific
　　to
　　　cell mediated immunity measurement of gamma interferon antigen response without active tuberculosis R76.12
　　　QuantiFERON-TB test (QFT) without active tuberculosis R76.12
　　　tuberculin test — *see also* Reaction, tuberculin skin test R76.11
　obsessive-compulsive F42.8
　organic, acute or subacute — *see* Delirium
　paranoid (acute) F23
　　chronic F22
　　senile F03 ☑
　passive dependency F60.7
　phobic F40.9
　post-traumatic stress, uncomplicated Z73.3
　psychogenic F99
　psychoneurotic — *see also* Neurosis
　　compulsive F42.8
　　depersonalization F48.1
　　depressive F34.1
　　hypochondriacal F45.20
　　neurasthenic F48.8
　　obsessive F42.8
　psychophysiologic — *see* Disorder, somatoform
　psychosomatic — *see* Disorder, somatoform
　psychotic — *see* Psychosis
　scarlet fever toxin — *see* Complications, vaccination
　schizophrenic F23
　　acute (brief) (undifferentiated) F23
　　latent F21
　　undifferentiated (acute) (brief) F23
　serological for syphilis — *see* Serology for syphilis
　serum T80.69 ☑
　　anaphylactic (immediate) — *see also* Shock, anaphylactic T80.59 ☑
　　specified reaction NEC
　　　due to
　　　　administration of blood and blood products T80.61 ☑
　　　　immunization T80.62 ☑
　　　　serum specified NEC T80.69 ☑
　　　　vaccination T80.62 ☑
　situational — *see* Disorder, adjustment
　somatization — *see* Disorder, somatoform
　spinal puncture G97.1
　　dural G97.1
　stress (severe) F43.9
　　acute (agitation) ("daze") (disorientation) (disturbance of consciousness) (flight reaction) (fugue) F43.0
　　specified NEC F43.8
　surgical procedure — *see* Complications, surgical procedure
　tetanus antitoxin — *see* Complications, vaccination
　toxic, to local anesthesia T88.59 ☑
　　in labor and delivery O74.4
　　in pregnancy O29.3X- ☑
　　postpartum, puerperal O89.3
　toxin-antitoxin — *see* Complications, vaccination
　transfusion (blood) (bone marrow) (lymphocytes) (allergic) — *see* Complications, transfusion
　tuberculin skin test, abnormal R76.11
　vaccination (any) — *see* Complications, vaccination
Reactive airway disease — *see* Asthma
Reactive depression — *see* Reaction, depressive
Rearrangement
　chromosomal
　　balanced (in) Q95.9
　　　abnormal individual (autosomal) Q95.2

Rearrangement — *continued*
　chromosomal — *continued*
　　balanced — *continued*
　　　abnormal individual — *continued*
　　　　non-sex (autosomal) chromosomes Q95.2
　　　　sex/non-sex chromosomes Q95.3
　　　　specified NEC Q95.8
Recalcitrant patient — *see* Noncompliance
Recanalization, thrombus — *see* Thrombosis
Recession, receding
　chamber angle (eye) H21.55- ☑
　chin M26.09
　gingival (postinfective) (postoperative)
　　generalized K06.020
　　　minimal K06.021
　　　moderate K06.022
　　　severe K06.023
　　localized K06.010
　　　minimal K06.011
　　　moderate K06.012
　　　severe K06.013
Recklinghausen disease Q85.01
　bones E21.0
Reclus' disease (cystic) — *see* Mastopathy, cystic
Recrudescent typhus (fever) A75.1
Recruitment, auditory H93.21- ☑
Rectalgia K62.89
Rectitis K62.89
Rectocele
　female (without uterine prolapse) N81.6
　　with uterine prolapse N81.4
　　　incomplete N81.2
　in pregnancy — *see* Pregnancy, complicated by, abnormal, pelvic organs or tissues NEC
　male K62.3
Rectosigmoid junction — *see* condition
Rectosigmoiditis K63.89
　ulcerative (chronic) K51.30
　　with
　　　complication K51.319
　　　　abscess K51.314
　　　　fistula K51.313
　　　　obstruction K51.312
　　　　rectal bleeding K51.311
　　　　specified NEC K51.318
Rectourethral — *see* condition
Rectovaginal — *see* condition
Rectovesical — *see* condition
Rectum, rectal — *see* condition
Recurrent — *see* condition
　pregnancy loss — *see* Loss (of), pregnancy, recurrent
Red bugs B88.0
Red tide — *see also* Table of Drugs and Chemicals T65.82- ☑
Red-cedar lung or pneumonitis J67.8
Reduced
　mobility Z74.09
　ventilatory or vital capacity R94.2
Redundant, redundancy
　anus (congenital) Q43.8
　clitoris N90.89
　colon (congenital) Q43.8
　foreskin (congenital) N47.8
　intestine (congenital) Q43.8
　labia N90.69
　organ or site, congenital NEC — *see* Accessory
　panniculus (abdominal) E65
　prepuce (congenital) N47.8
　pylorus K31.89
　rectum (congenital) Q43.8
　scrotum N50.89
　sigmoid (congenital) Q43.8
　skin L98.7
　　and subcutaneous tissue L98.7
　　of face L57.4
　　　eyelids — *see* Blepharochalasis
　stomach K31.89
Reduplication — *see* Duplication
Reflex R29.2
　hyperactive gag J39.2
　pupillary, abnormal — *see* Anomaly, pupil, function
　vasoconstriction I73.9
　vasovagal R55
Reflux K21.9
　acid K21.9
　esophageal K21.9
　　with esophagitis (without bleeding) K21.00
　　　with bleeding K21.01

Reflux — continued
  esophageal — continued
    newborn P78.83
  gastroesophageal K21.9
    with esophagitis (without bleeding) K21.00
      with bleeding K21.01
  mitral — see Insufficiency, mitral
  ureteral — see Reflux, vesicoureteral
  vesicoureteral (with scarring) N13.70
    with
      nephropathy N13.729
        with hydroureter N13.739
          bilateral N13.732
          unilateral N13.731
        bilateral N13.722
        unilateral N13.721
        without hydroureter N13.729
          bilateral N13.722
          unilateral N13.721
      pyelonephritis (chronic) N11.0
    congenital Q62.7
    without nephropathy N13.71
Reforming, artificial openings — see Attention to, artificial, opening
Refractive error — see Disorder, refraction
Refsum's disease or syndrome G60.1
Refusal of
  food, psychogenic F50.89
  treatment (because of) Z53.20
    left against medical advice (AMA) Z53.29
    left without being seen Z53.21
    patient's decision NEC Z53.29
    reasons of belief or group pressure Z53.1
Regional — see condition
Regurgitation R11.10
  aortic (valve) — see Insufficiency, aortic
  food — see also Vomiting
    with reswallowing — see Rumination
    newborn P92.1
  gastric contents — see Vomiting
  heart — see Endocarditis
  mitral (valve) — see Insufficiency, mitral
    congenital Q23.3
  myocardial — see Endocarditis
  pulmonary (valve) (heart) I37.1
    congenital Q22.2
    syphilitic A52.03
  tricuspid — see Insufficiency, tricuspid
  valve, valvular — see Endocarditis
    congenital Q24.8
  vesicoureteral — see Reflux, vesicoureteral
Reichmann's disease or syndrome K31.89
Reifenstein syndrome E34.52
Reinsertion
  implantable subdermal contraceptive Z30.46
  intrauterine contraceptive device Z30.433
Reiter's disease, syndrome, or urethritis M02.30
  ankle M02.37- ☑
  elbow M02.32- ☑
  foot joint M02.37- ☑
  hand joint M02.34- ☑
  hip M02.35- ☑
  knee M02.36- ☑
  multiple site M02.39
  shoulder M02.31- ☑
  vertebra M02.38
  wrist M02.33- ☑
Rejection
  food, psychogenic F50.89
  transplant T86.91
    bone T86.830
      marrow T86.01
    cornea T86.840- ☑
    heart T86.21
      with lung(s) T86.31
    intestine T86.850
    kidney T86.11
    liver T86.41
    lung(s) T86.810
      with heart T86.31
    organ (immune or nonimmune cause) T86.91
    pancreas T86.890
    skin (allograft) (autograft) T86.820
    specified NEC T86.890
    stem cell (peripheral blood) (umbilical cord) T86.5
Relapsing fever A68.9
  Carter's (Asiatic) A68.1
  Dutton's (West African) A68.1

Relapsing fever — continued
  Koch's A68.9
  louse-borne (epidemic) A68.0
  Novy's (American) A68.1
  Obermeyers's (European) A68.0
  Spirillum A68.9
  tick-borne (endemic) A68.1
Relationship
  occlusal
    open anterior M26.220
    open posterior M26.221
Relaxation
  anus (sphincter) K62.89
    psychogenic F45.8
  arch (foot) — see also Deformity, limb, flat foot
  back ligaments — see Instability, joint, spine
  bladder (sphincter) N31.2
  cardioesophageal K21.9
  cervix — see Incompetency, cervix
  diaphragm J98.6
  joint (capsule) (ligament) (paralytic) — see Flail, joint
    congenital NEC Q74.8
  lumbosacral (joint) — see subcategory M53.2 ☑
  pelvic floor N81.89
  perineum N81.89
  posture R29.3
  rectum (sphincter) K62.89
  sacroiliac (joint) — see subcategory M53.2 ☑
  scrotum N50.89
  urethra (sphincter) N36.44
  vesical N31.2
Release from prison, anxiety concerning Z65.2
Remains
  canal of Cloquet Q14.0
  capsule (opaque) Q14.8
Remittent fever (malarial) B54
Remnant
  canal of Cloquet Q14.0
  capsule (opaque) Q14.8
  cervix, cervical stump (acquired) (postoperative) N88.8
  cystic duct, postcholecystectomy K91.5
  fingernail L60.8
    congenital Q84.6
  meniscus, knee — see Derangement, knee, meniscus, specified NEC
  thyroglossal duct Q89.2
  tonsil J35.8
    infected (chronic) J35.01
  urachus Q64.4
Removal (from) (of)
  artificial
    arm Z44.00- ☑
      complete Z44.01- ☑
      partial Z44.02- ☑
    eye Z44.2- ☑
    leg Z44.10- ☑
      complete Z44.11- ☑
      partial Z44.12- ☑
  breast implant Z45.81 ☑
  cardiac pulse generator (battery) (end-of-life) Z45.010
  catheter (urinary) (indwelling) Z46.6
    from artificial opening — see Attention to, artificial, opening
    non-vascular Z46.82
    vascular NEC Z45.2
  device Z46.9
    contraceptive Z30.432
      implantable subdermal Z30.46
    implanted NEC Z45.89
    specified NEC Z46.89
  drains Z48.03
  dressing (nonsurgical) Z48.00
    surgical Z48.01
  external
    fixation device — code to fracture with seventh character D
    prosthesis, prosthetic device Z44.9
      breast Z44.3- ☑
      specified NEC Z44.8
  home in childhood (to foster home or institution) Z62.29
  ileostomy Z43.2
  insulin pump Z46.81
  myringotomy device (stent) (tube) Z45.82
  nervous system device NEC Z46.2
    brain neuropacemaker Z46.2
    visual substitution device Z46.2
      implanted Z45.31

Removal — continued
  non-vascular catheter Z46.82
  organ, prophylactic (for neoplasia management) — see Prophylactic, organ removal
  orthodontic device Z46.4
  staples Z48.02
  stent
    ureteral Z46.6
  suture Z48.02
  urinary device Z46.6
  vascular access device or catheter Z45.2
Ren
  arcuatus Q63.1
  mobile, mobilis N28.89
    congenital Q63.8
  unguliformis Q63.1
Renal — see condition
Rendu-Osler-Weber disease or syndrome I78.0
Reninoma D41.0- ☑
Renon-Delille syndrome E23.3
Reovirus, as cause of disease classified elsewhere B97.5
Repeated falls NEC R29.6
Replaced chromosome by dicentric ring Q93.2
Replacement by artificial or mechanical device or prosthesis of
  bladder Z96.0
  blood vessel NEC Z95.828
  bone NEC Z96.7
  cochlea Z96.21
  coronary artery Z95.5
  eustachian tube Z96.29
  eye globe Z97.0
  heart Z95.812
    valve Z95.2
      prosthetic Z95.2
      specified NEC Z95.4
      xenogenic Z95.3
  intestine Z96.89
  joint Z96.60
    hip — see Presence, hip joint implant
    knee — see Presence, knee joint implant
    specified site NEC Z96.698
  larynx Z96.3
  lens Z96.1
  limb(s) — see Presence, artificial, limb
  mandible NEC (for tooth root implant(s)) Z96.5
  organ NEC Z96.89
  peripheral vessel NEC Z95.828
  stapes Z96.29
  teeth Z97.2
  tendon Z96.7
  tissue NEC Z96.89
  tooth root(s) Z96.5
  vessel NEC Z95.828
    coronary (artery) Z95.5
Request for expert evidence Z04.89
Reserve, decreased or low
  cardiac — see Disease, heart
  kidney N28.89
Residing
  in place not meant for human habitation (abandoned building) (car) (park) (sidewalk) Z59.02
  on the street Z59.02
Residual — see also condition
  ovary syndrome N99.83
  state, schizophrenic F20.5
  urine R39.198
Resistance, resistant (to)
  activated protein C D68.51
  complicating pregnancy O26.89 ☑
  insulin E88.81
  organism(s)
    to
      drug Z16.30
        aminoglycosides Z16.29
        amoxicillin Z16.11
        ampicillin Z16.11
        antibiotic(s) Z16.20
          multiple Z16.24
          specified NEC Z16.29
        antifungal Z16.32
        antimicrobial (single) Z16.30
          multiple Z16.35
          specified NEC Z16.39
        antimycobacterial (single) Z16.341
          multiple Z16.342
        antiparasitic Z16.31

☑ Additional Character Required — Refer to the Tabular List for Character Selection   ▽ Subterms under main terms may continue to next column or page

Resistance, resistant — continued
  organism(s) — continued
    to — continued
      drug — continued
        antiviral Z16.33
        beta lactam antibiotics Z16.10
          specified NEC Z16.19
        cephalosporins Z16.19
        extended beta lactamase (ESBL) Z16.12
        fluoroquinolones Z16.23
        macrolides Z16.29
        methicillin — see MRSA
        multiple drugs (MDRO)
          antibiotics Z16.24
          antimicrobial Z16.35
          antimycobacterials Z16.342
        penicillins Z16.11
        quinine (and related compounds) Z16.31
        quinolones Z16.23
        sulfonamides Z16.29
        tetracyclines Z16.29
        tuberculostatics (single) Z16.341
          multiple Z16.342
        vancomycin Z16.21
          related antibiotics Z16.22
    thyroid hormone E07.89
Resorption
  dental (roots) K03.3
    alveoli M26.79
  teeth (external) (internal) (pathological) (roots) K03.3
Respiration
  Cheyne-Stokes R06.3
  decreased due to shock, following injury T79.4 ☑
  disorder of, psychogenic F45.8
  insufficient, or poor R06.89
    newborn P28.5
  painful R07.1
  sighing, psychogenic F45.8
Respiratory — see also condition
  distress syndrome (newborn) (type I) P22.0
    type II P22.1
  syncytial virus, as cause of disease classified elsewhere
    — see also Virus, respiratory syncytial (RSV) B97.4
Respite care Z75.5
Response (drug)
  photoallergic L56.1
  phototoxic L56.0
Restenosis
  stent
    vascular
      end stent
        adjacent to stent — see Arteriosclerosis
        within the stent
          coronary T82.855 ☑
          peripheral T82.856 ☑
      in stent
        coronary vessel T82.855 ☑
        peripheral vessel T82.856 ☑
Restless legs (syndrome) G25.81
Restlessness R45.1
Restoration (of)
  dental
    aesthetically inadequate or displeasing K08.56
    defective K08.50
      specified NEC K08.59
    failure of marginal integrity K08.51
    failure of periodontal anatomical intergrity K08.54
    organ continuity from previous sterilization (tuboplasty) (vasoplasty) Z31.0
      aftercare Z31.42
    tooth (existing)
      contours biologically incompatible with oral health K08.54
      open margins K08.51
      overhanging K08.52
      poor aesthetic K08.56
      poor gingival margins K08.51
    unsatisfactory, of tooth K08.50
      specified NEC K08.59
Restorative material (dental)
  allergy to K08.55
  fractured K08.539
    with loss of material K08.531
    without loss of material K08.530
  unrepairable overhanging of K08.52
Restriction of housing space Z59.1
Rests, ovarian, in fallopian tube Q50.6
Restzustand (schizophrenic) F20.5

Retained — see also Retention
  cholelithiasis following cholecystectomy K91.86
  foreign body fragments (type of) Z18.9
    acrylics Z18.2
    animal quill(s) or spines Z18.31
    cement Z18.83
    concrete Z18.83
    crystalline Z18.83
    depleted isotope Z18.09
    depleted uranium Z18.01
    diethylhexyl phthalates Z18.2
    glass Z18.81
    isocyanate Z18.2
    magnetic metal Z18.11
    metal Z18.10
    nonmagnectic metal Z18.12
    nontherapeutic radioactive Z18.09
    organic NEC Z18.39
    plastic Z18.2
    quill(s) (animal) Z18.31
    radioactive (nontherapeutic) NEC Z18.09
    specified NEC Z18.89
    spine(s) (animal) Z18.31
    stone Z18.83
    tooth (teeth) Z18.32
    wood Z18.33
  fragments (type of) Z18.9
    acrylics Z18.2
    animal quill(s) or spines Z18.31
    cement Z18.83
    concrete Z18.83
    crystalline Z18.83
    depleted isotope Z18.09
    depleted uranium Z18.01
    diethylhexyl phthalates Z18.2
    glass Z18.81
    isocyanate Z18.2
    magnetic metal Z18.11
    metal Z18.10
    nonmagnectic metal Z18.12
    nontherapeutic radioactive Z18.09
    organic NEC Z18.39
    plastic Z18.2
    quill(s) (animal) Z18.31
    radioactive (nontherapeutic) NEC Z18.09
    specified NEC Z18.89
    spine(s) (animal) Z18.31
    stone Z18.83
    tooth (teeth) Z18.32
    wood Z18.33
  gallstones, following cholecystectomy K91.86
Retardation
  development, developmental, specific — see Disorder, developmental
  endochondral bone growth — see Disorder, bone, development or growth
  growth R62.50
    due to malnutrition E45
  mental — see Disability, intellectual
  motor function, specific F82
  physical (child) R62.52
    due to malnutrition E45
  reading (specific) F81.0
  spelling (specific) (without reading disorder) F81.81
Retching — see Vomiting
Retention — see also Retained
  bladder — see Retention, urine
  carbon dioxide E87.2
  cholelithiasis following cholecystectomy K91.86
  cyst — see Cyst
  dead
    fetus (at or near term) (mother) O36.4 ☑
      early fetal death O02.1
    ovum O02.0
  decidua (fragments) (following delivery) (with hemorrhage) O72.2
    without hemorrhage O73.1
  deciduous tooth K00.6
  dental root K08.3
  fecal — see Constipation
  fetus
    dead O36.4 ☑
      early O02.1
  fluid R60.9
  foreign body — see also Foreign body, retained
    current trauma — code as Foreign body, by site or type
  gallstones, following cholecystectomy K91.86

Retention — continued
  gastric K31.89
  intrauterine contraceptive device, in pregnancy — see Pregnancy, complicated by, retention, intrauterine device
  membranes (complicating delivery) (with hemorrhage) O72.2
    with abortion — see Abortion, by type
    without hemorrhage O73.1
  meniscus — see Derangement, meniscus
  menses N94.89
  milk (puerperal, postpartum) O92.79
  nitrogen, extrarenal R39.2
  ovary syndrome N99.83
  placenta (total) (with hemorrhage) O72.0
    without hemorrhage O73.0
    portions or fragments (with hemorrhage) O72.2
      without hemorrhage O73.1
  products of conception
    early pregnancy (dead fetus) O02.1
    following
      delivery (with hemorrhage) O72.2
        without hemorrhage O73.1
  secundines (following delivery) (with hemorrhage) O72.0
    without hemorrhage O73.0
    complicating puerperium (delayed hemorrhage) O72.2
    partial O72.2
      without hemorrhage O73.1
  smegma, clitoris N90.89
  urine R33.9
    due to hyperplasia (hypertrophy) of prostate — see Hyperplasia, prostate
    drug-induced R33.0
    organic R33.8
      drug-induced R33.0
    psychogenic F45.8
    specified NEC R33.8
  water (in tissues) — see Edema
Reticulation, dust — see Pneumoconiosis
Reticulocytosis R70.1
Reticuloendotheliosis
  acute infantile C96.0
  leukemic C91.4- ☑
  nonlipid C96.0
Reticulohistiocytoma (giant-cell) D76.3
Reticuloid, actinic L57.1
Reticulosis (skin)
  acute of infancy C96.0
  hemophagocytic, familial D76.1
  histiocytic medullary C96.A (following C96.6)
  lipomelanotic I89.8
  malignant (midline) C86.0
  polymorphic C83.8- ☑
  Sézary — see Sézary disease
Retina, retinal — see also condition
  dark area D49.81
Retinitis — see also Inflammation, chorioretinal
  albuminurica N18.9 [H32]
  diabetic — see Diabetes, retinitis
  disciformis — see Degeneration, macula
  focal — see Inflammation, chorioretinal, focal
  gravidarum — see Pregnancy, complicated by, specified pregnancy-related condition NEC
  juxtapapillaris — see Inflammation, chorioretinal, focal, juxtapapillary
  luetic — see Retinitis, syphilitic
  pigmentosa H35.52
  proliferans — see Disorder, globe, degenerative, specified type NEC
  proliferating — see Disorder, globe, degenerative, specified type NEC
  renal N18.9 [H32]
  syphilitic (early) (secondary) A51.43
    central, recurrent A52.71
    congenital (early) A50.01 [H32]
    late A52.71
  tuberculous A18.53
Retinoblastoma C69.2- ☑
  differentiated C69.2- ☑
  undifferentiated C69.2- ☑
Retinochoroiditis — see also Inflammation, chorioretinal
  disseminated — see Inflammation, chorioretinal, disseminated
  syphilitic A52.71
  focal — see Inflammation, chorioretinal

Retinochoroiditis — *continued*
- juxtapapillaris — *see* Inflammation, chorioretinal, focal, juxtapapillary

Retinopathy (background) H35.00
- arteriosclerotic I70.8 [H35.0-] ☑
- atherosclerotic I70.8 [H35.0-] ☑
- central serous — *see* Chorioretinopathy, central serous
- Coats H35.02- ☑
- diabetic — *see* Diabetes, retinopathy
- exudative H35.02- ☑
- hypertensive H35.03- ☑
- in (due to)
  - diabetes — *see* Diabetes, retinopathy
  - sickle-cell disorders D57.- ☑ [H36]
- of prematurity H35.10- ☑
  - stage 0 H35.11- ☑
  - stage 1 H35.12- ☑
  - stage 2 H35.13- ☑
  - stage 3 H35.14- ☑
  - stage 4 H35.15- ☑
  - stage 5 H35.16- ☑
- pigmentary, congenital — *see* Dystrophy, retina
- proliferative NEC H35.2- ☑
  - diabetic — *see* Diabetes, retinopathy, proliferative
  - sickle-cell D57.- ☑ [H36]
- solar H31.02- ☑

Retinoschisis H33.10- ☑
- congenital Q14.1
- specified type NEC H33.19- ☑

Retortamoniasis A07.8

Retractile testis Q55.22

Retraction
- cervix — *see* Retroversion, uterus
- drum (membrane) — *see* Disorder, tympanic membrane, specified NEC
- finger — *see* Deformity, finger
- lid H02.539
  - left H02.536
    - lower H02.535
    - upper H02.534
  - right H02.533
    - lower H02.532
    - upper H02.531
- lung J98.4
- mediastinum J98.59
- nipple N64.53
  - associated with
    - lactation O92.03
    - pregnancy O92.01- ☑
    - puerperium O92.02
  - congenital Q83.8
- palmar fascia M72.0
- pleura — *see* Pleurisy
- ring, uterus (Bandl's) (pathological) O62.4
- sternum (congenital) Q76.7
  - acquired M95.4
- uterus — *see* Retroversion, uterus
- valve (heart) — *see* Endocarditis

Retrobulbar — *see* condition

Retrocecal — *see* condition

Retrocession — *see* Retroversion

Retrodisplacement — *see* Retroversion

Retroflection, retroflexion — *see* Retroversion

Retrognathia, retrognathism (mandibular) (maxillary) M26.19

Retrograde menstruation N92.5

Retroperineal — *see* condition

Retroperitoneal — *see* condition

Retroperitonitis K68.9

Retropharyngeal — *see* condition

Retroplacental — *see* condition

Retroposition — *see* Retroversion

Retroprosthetic membrane T85.398 ☑

Retrosternal thyroid (congenital) Q89.2

Retroversion, retroverted
- cervix — *see* Retroversion, uterus
- female NEC — *see* Retroversion, uterus
- iris H21.89
- testis (congenital) Q55.29
- uterus (acquired) (acute) (any degree) (asymptomatic) (cervix) (postinfectional) (postpartal, old) N85.4
  - congenital Q51.818
  - in pregnancy O34.53- ☑

Retrovirus, as cause of disease classified elsewhere B97.30
- human
  - immunodeficiency, type 2 (HIV 2) B97.35

Retrovirus, as cause of disease classified elsewhere — *continued*
- human — *continued*
  - T-cell lymphotropic
    - type I (HTLV-I) B97.33
    - type II (HTLV-II) B97.34
  - lentivirus B97.31
  - oncovirus B97.32
  - specified NEC B97.39

Retrusion, premaxilla (developmental) M26.09

Rett's disease or syndrome F84.2

Reverse peristalsis R19.2

Reye's syndrome G93.7

Rh (factor)
- hemolytic disease (newborn) P55.0
- incompatibility, immunization or sensitization
  - affecting management of pregnancy NEC O36.09- ☑
    - anti-D antibody O36.01- ☑
  - newborn P55.0
  - transfusion reaction — *see* Complication(s), transfusion, incompatibility reaction, Rh (factor)
- negative mother affecting newborn P55.0
- titer elevated — *see* Complication(s), transfusion, incompatibility reaction, Rh (factor)
- transfusion reaction — *see* Complication(s), transfusion, incompatibility reaction, Rh (factor)

Rhabdomyolysis (idiopathic) NEC M62.82
- traumatic T79.6 ☑

Rhabdomyoma — *see also* Neoplasm, connective tissue, benign
- adult — *see* Neoplasm, connective tissue, benign
- fetal — *see* Neoplasm, connective tissue, benign
- glycogenic — *see* Neoplasm, connective tissue, benign

Rhabdomyosarcoma (any type) — *see* Neoplasm, connective tissue, malignant

Rhabdosarcoma — *see* Rhabdomyosarcoma

Rhesus (factor) **incompatibility** — *see* Rh, incompatibility

Rheumatic (acute) (subacute)
- adherent pericardium I09.2
- chronic I09.89
- coronary arteritis I01.8
- degeneration, myocardium I09.0
- fever (acute) — *see* Fever, rheumatic
- heart — *see* Disease, heart, rheumatic
- myocardial degeneration — *see* Degeneration, myocardium
- myocarditis (chronic) (inactive) (with chorea) I09.0
  - active or acute I01.2
  - with chorea (acute) (rheumatic) (Sydenham's) I02.0
- pancarditis, acute I01.8
  - with chorea (acute) (rheumatic) Sydenham's) I02.0
- pericarditis (active) (acute) (with effusion) (with pneumonia) I01.0
  - with chorea (acute) (rheumatic) (Sydenham's) I02.0
  - chronic or inactive I09.2
- pneumonia I00 [J17]
- torticollis M43.6
- typhoid fever A01.09

Rheumatism (articular) (neuralgic) (nonarticular) M79.0
- gout — *see* Arthritis, rheumatoid
- intercostal, meaning Tietze's disease M94.0
- palindromic (any site) M12.30
  - ankle M12.37- ☑
  - elbow M12.32- ☑
  - foot joint M12.37- ☑
  - hand joint M12.34- ☑
  - hip M12.35- ☑
  - knee M12.36- ☑
  - multiple site M12.39
  - shoulder M12.31- ☑
  - specified joint NEC M12.38
  - vertebrae M12.38
  - wrist M12.33- ☑
- sciatic M54.4- ☑

Rheumatoid — *see also* condition
- arthritis — *see also* Arthritis, rheumatoid
  - with involvement of organs NEC M05.60
    - ankle M05.67- ☑
    - elbow M05.62- ☑
    - foot joint M05.67- ☑
    - hand joint M05.64- ☑
    - hip M05.65- ☑
    - knee M05.66- ☑
    - multiple site M05.69
    - shoulder M05.61- ☑
    - vertebra — *see* Spondylitis, ankylosing

Rheumatoid — *continued*
- arthritis — *see also* Arthritis, rheumatoid — *continued*
  - with involvement of organs — *continued*
    - wrist M05.63- ☑
  - seronegative — *see* Arthritis, rheumatoid, seronegative
  - seropositive — *see* Arthritis, rheumatoid, seropositive
- carditis M05.30
  - ankle M05.37- ☑
  - elbow M05.32- ☑
  - foot joint M05.37- ☑
  - hand joint M05.34- ☑
  - hip M05.35- ☑
  - knee M05.36- ☑
  - multiple site M05.39
  - shoulder M05.31- ☑
  - vertebra — *see* Spondylitis, ankylosing
  - wrist M05.33- ☑
- endocarditis — *see* Rheumatoid, carditis
- lung (disease) M05.10
  - ankle M05.17- ☑
  - elbow M05.12- ☑
  - foot joint M05.17- ☑
  - hand joint M05.14- ☑
  - hip M05.15- ☑
  - knee M05.16- ☑
  - multiple site M05.19
  - shoulder M05.11- ☑
  - vertebra — *see* Spondylitis, ankylosing
  - wrist M05.13- ☑
- myocarditis — *see* Rheumatoid, carditis
- myopathy M05.40
  - ankle M05.47- ☑
  - elbow M05.42- ☑
  - foot joint M05.47- ☑
  - hand joint M05.44- ☑
  - hip M05.45- ☑
  - knee M05.46- ☑
  - multiple site M05.49
  - shoulder M05.41- ☑
  - vertebra — *see* Spondylitis, ankylosing
  - wrist M05.43- ☑
- pericarditis — *see* Rheumatoid, carditis
- polyarthritis — *see* Arthritis, rheumatoid
- polyneuropathy M05.50
  - ankle M05.57- ☑
  - elbow M05.52- ☑
  - foot joint M05.57- ☑
  - hand joint M05.54- ☑
  - hip M05.55- ☑
  - knee M05.56- ☑
  - multiple site M05.59
  - shoulder M05.51- ☑
  - vertebra — *see* Spondylitis, ankylosing
  - wrist M05.53- ☑
- vasculitis M05.20
  - ankle M05.27- ☑
  - elbow M05.22- ☑
  - foot joint M05.27- ☑
  - hand joint M05.24- ☑
  - hip M05.25- ☑
  - knee M05.26- ☑
  - multiple site M05.29
  - shoulder M05.21- ☑
  - vertebra — *see* Spondylitis, ankylosing
  - wrist M05.23- ☑

Rhinitis (atrophic) (catarrhal) (chronic) (croupous) (fibrinous) (granulomatous) (hyperplastic) (hypertrophic) (membranous) (obstructive) (purulent) (suppurative) (ulcerative) J31.0
- with
  - sore throat — *see* Nasopharyngitis
- acute J00
- allergic J30.9
  - with asthma J45.909
    - with
      - exacerbation (acute) J45.901
      - status asthmaticus J45.902
  - due to
    - food J30.5
    - pollen J30.1
  - nonseasonal J30.89
  - perennial J30.89
  - seasonal NEC J30.2
  - specified NEC J30.89

☑ **Additional Character Required** — Refer to the Tabular List for Character Selection ▽ **Subterms under main terms may continue to next column or page**

Rhinitis — *continued*
  infective J00
  pneumococcal J00
  syphilitic A52.73
    congenital A50.05 *[J99]*
  tuberculous A15.8
  vasomotor J30.0
Rhinoantritis (chronic) — *see* Sinusitis, maxillary
Rhinodacryolith — *see* Dacryolith
Rhinolith (nasal sinus) J34.89
Rhinomegaly J34.89
Rhinopharyngitis (acute) (subacute) — *see also* Nasopharyngitis
  chronic J31.1
  destructive ulcerating A66.5
  mutilans A66.5
Rhinophyma L71.1
Rhinorrhea J34.89
  cerebrospinal (fluid) G96.01
    postoperative G96.08
    specified NEC G96.08
    spontaneous G96.01
    traumatic G96.08
  paroxysmal — *see* Rhinitis, allergic
  spasmodic — *see* Rhinitis, allergic
Rhinosalpingitis — *see* Salpingitis, eustachian
Rhinoscleroma A48.8
Rhinosporidiosis B48.1
Rhinovirus infection NEC B34.8
Rhizomelic chondrodysplasia punctata E71.540
Rhythm
  atrioventricular nodal I49.8
  disorder I49.9
    coronary sinus I49.8
    ectopic I49.8
    nodal I49.8
  escape I49.9
  heart, abnormal I49.9
  idioventricular I44.2
  nodal I49.8
  sleep, inversion G47.2- ☑
    nonorganic origin — *see* Disorder, sleep, circadian
      rhythm, psychogenic
Rhytidosis facialis L98.8
Rib — *see also* condition
  cervical Q76.5
Riboflavin deficiency E53.0
Rice bodies — *see also* Loose, body, joint
  knee M23.4- ☑
Richter syndrome — *see* Leukemia, chronic lymphocytic,
  B-cell type
Richter's hernia — *see* Hernia, abdomen, with obstruction
Ricinism — *see* Poisoning, food, noxious, plant
Rickets (active) (acute) (adolescent) (chest wall) (congenital) (current) (infantile) (intestinal) E55.0
  adult — *see* Osteomalacia
  celiac K90.0
  hypophosphatemic with nephrotic-glycosuric dwarfism
    E72.09
  inactive E64.3
  kidney N25.0
  renal N25.0
  sequelae, any E64.3
  vitamin-D-resistant E83.31 *[M90.80]*
Rickettsia 364D/R. philipii (Pacific Coast tick fever)
  A77.8
Rickettsial disease A79.9
  specified type NEC A79.89
Rickettsialpox (Rickettsia akari) A79.1
Rickettsiosis A79.9
  due to
    Ehrlichia sennetsu A79.81
    Neorickettsia sennetsu A79.81
    Rickettsia akari (rickettsialpox) A79.1
  specified type NEC A79.89
  tick-borne A77.9
  vesicular A79.1
Rider's bone — *see* Ossification, muscle, specified NEC
Ridge, alveolus — *see also* condition
  flabby K06.8
Ridged ear, congenital Q17.3
Riedel's
  lobe, liver Q44.7
  struma, thyroiditis or disease E06.5
Rieger's anomaly or syndrome Q13.81
Riehl's melanosis L81.4

Rietti-Greppi-Micheli anemia D56.9
Rieux's hernia — *see* Hernia, abdomen, specified site
  NEC
Riga (-Fede) **disease** K14.0
Riggs' disease — *see* Periodontitis
Right aortic arch Q25.47
Right middle lobe syndrome J98.11
Rigid, rigidity — *see also* condition
  abdominal R19.30
    with severe abdominal pain R10.0
    epigastric R19.36
    generalized R19.37
    left lower quadrant R19.34
    left upper quadrant R19.32
    periumbilic R19.35
    right lower quadrant R19.33
    right upper quadrant R19.31
  articular, multiple, congenital Q68.8
  cervix (uteri) in pregnancy — *see* Pregnancy, complicated by, abnormal, cervix
  hymen (acquired) (congenital) N89.6
  nuchal R29.1
  pelvic floor in pregnancy — *see* Pregnancy, complicated by, abnormal, pelvic organs or tissues NEC
  perineum or vulva in pregnancy — *see* Pregnancy, complicated by, abnormal, vulva
  spine — *see* Dorsopathy, specified NEC
  vagina in pregnancy — *see* Pregnancy, complicated by, abnormal, vagina
Rigors R68.89
  with fever R50.9
Riley-Day syndrome G90.1
RIND (reversible ischemic neurologic deficit) I63.9
Ring(s)
  aorta (vascular) Q25.45
  Bandl's O62.4
  contraction, complicating delivery O62.4
  esophageal, lower (muscular) K22.2
  Fleischer's (cornea) H18.04- ☑
  hymenal, tight (acquired) (congenital) N89.6
  Kayser-Fleischer (cornea) H18.04- ☑
  retraction, uterus, pathological O62.4
  Schatzki's (esophagus) (lower) K22.2
    congenital Q39.3
  Soemmerring's — *see* Cataract, secondary
  vascular (congenital) Q25.8
    aorta Q25.45
Ringed hair (congenital) Q84.1
Ringworm B35.9
  beard B35.0
  black dot B35.0
  body B35.4
  Burmese B35.5
  corporeal B35.4
  foot B35.3
  groin B35.6
  hand B35.2
  honeycomb B35.0
  nails B35.1
  perianal (area) B35.6
  scalp B35.0
  specified NEC B35.8
  Tokelau B35.5
Rise, venous pressure I87.8
Rising, PSA following treatment for malignant neoplasm of prostate R97.21
Risk
  for
    dental caries Z91.849
      high Z91.843
      low Z91.841
      moderate Z91.842
    homelessness, imminent Z59.811
  suicidal
    meaning personal history of attempted suicide
      Z91.51
    meaning suicidal ideation — *see* Ideation, suicidal
Ritter's disease L00
Rivalry, sibling Z62.891
Rivalta's disease A42.2
River blindness B73.01
Robert's pelvis Q74.2
  with disproportion (fetopelvic) O33.0
    causing obstructed labor O65.0
Robin (-Pierre) **syndrome** Q87.0
Robinow-Silvermann-Smith syndrome Q87.19
Robinson's (hidrotic) **ectodermal dysplasia or syndrome** Q82.4

Robles' disease B73.01
Rocky Mountain (spotted) **fever** A77.0
Roetheln — *see* Rubella
Roger's disease Q21.0
Rokitansky-Aschoff sinuses (gallbladder) K82.8
Rolando's fracture (displaced) S62.22- ☑
  nondisplaced S62.22- ☑
Romano-Ward (prolonged QT interval) **syndrome** I45.81
Romberg's disease or syndrome G51.8
Roof, mouth — *see* condition
Rosacea L71.9
  acne L71.9
  keratitis L71.8
  specified NEC L71.8
Rosary, rachitic E55.0
Rose
  cold J30.1
  fever J30.1
  rash R21
    epidemic B06.9
Rosenbach's erysipeloid A26.0
Rosenthal's disease or syndrome D68.1
Roseola B09
  infantum B08.20
    due to human herpesvirus 6 B08.21
    due to human herpesvirus 7 B08.22
Ross River disease or fever B33.1
Rossbach's disease K31.89
  psychogenic F45.8
Rostan's asthma (cardiac) — *see* Failure, ventricular, left
Rotation
  anomalous, incomplete or insufficient, intestine Q43.3
  cecum (congenital) Q43.3
  colon (congenital) Q43.3
  spine, incomplete or insufficient — *see* Dorsopathy,
    deforming, specified NEC
  tooth, teeth, fully erupted M26.35
  vertebra, incomplete or insufficient — *see* Dorsopathy,
    deforming, specified NEC
Rotes Quérol disease or syndrome — *see* Hyperostosis,
  ankylosing
Roth (-Bernhardt) **disease or syndrome** — *see* Meralgia
  paraesthetica
Rothmund (-Thomson) **syndrome** Q82.8
Rotor's disease or syndrome E80.6
Round
  back (with wedging of vertebrae) — *see* Kyphosis
    sequelae (late effect) of rickets E64.3
  worms (large) (infestation) NEC B82.0
    Ascariasis — *see also* Ascariasis B77.9
Roussy-Lévy syndrome G60.0
Rubella (German measles) B06.9
  complication NEC B06.09
    neurological B06.00
  congenital P35.0
  contact Z20.4
  exposure to Z20.4
  maternal
    care for (suspected) damage to fetus O35.3 ☑
      manifest rubella in infant P35.0
    suspected damage to fetus affecting management
      of pregnancy O35.3 ☑
  specified complications NEC B06.89
Rubeola (meaning measles) — *see* Measles
  meaning rubella — *see* Rubella
Rubeosis, iris — *see* Disorder, iris, vascular
Rubinstein-Taybi syndrome Q87.2
Rudimentary (congenital) — *see also* Agenesis
  arm — *see* Defect, reduction, upper limb
  bone Q79.9
  cervix uteri Q51.828
  eye Q11.2
  lobule of ear Q17.3
  patella Q74.1
  respiratory organs in thoracopagus Q89.4
  tracheal bronchus Q32.4
  uterus Q51.818
    in male Q56.1
  vagina Q52.0
Ruled out condition — *see* Observation, suspected
Rumination R11.10
  with nausea R11.2
  disorder of infancy F98.21
  neurotic F42.8
  newborn P92.1
  obsessional F42.8
  psychogenic F42.8

△ **Subterms under main terms may continue to next column or page**   ☑ **Additional Character Required — Refer to the Tabular List for Character Selection**

Runeberg's disease D51.0
Runny nose R09.89
Rupia (syphilitic) A51.39
  congenital A50.06
  tertiary A52.79
Rupture, ruptured
  abscess (spontaneous) — *code by* site under Abscess
  aneurysm — *see* Aneurysm
  anus (sphincter) — *see* Laceration, anus
  aorta, aortic I71.8
    abdominal I71.3
    arch I71.1
    ascending I71.1
    descending I71.8
      abdominal I71.3
      thoracic I71.1
    syphilitic A52.01
    thoracoabdominal I71.5
    thorax, thoracic I71.1
    transverse I71.1
    traumatic — *see* Injury, aorta, laceration, major
    valve or cusp — *see also* Endocarditis, aortic I35.8
  appendix (with peritonitis) — *see also* Appendicitis K35.32
    with localized peritonitis — *see also* Appendicitis K35.32
  arteriovenous fistula, brain — *see* Fistula, arteriovenous, brain, ruptured
  artery I77.2
    brain — *see* Hemorrhage, intracranial, intracerebral
    coronary — *see* Infarct, myocardium
    heart — *see* Infarct, myocardium
    pulmonary I28.8
    traumatic (complication) — *see* Injury, blood vessel
  bile duct (common) (hepatic) K83.2
    cystic K82.2
  bladder (sphincter) (nontraumatic) (spontaneous) N32.89
    following ectopic or molar pregnancy O08.6
    obstetrical trauma O71.5
    traumatic S37.29 ☑
  blood vessel — *see also* Hemorrhage
    brain — *see* Hemorrhage, intracranial, intracerebral
    heart — *see* Infarct, myocardium
    traumatic (complication) — *see* Injury, blood vessel, laceration, major, by site
  bone — *see* Fracture
  bowel (nontraumatic) K63.1
  brain
    aneurysm (congenital) — *see also* Hemorrhage, intracranial, subarachnoid
      syphilitic A52.05
    hemorrhagic — *see* Hemorrhage, intracranial, intracerebral
  capillaries I78.8
  cardiac (auricle) (ventricle) (wall) I23.3
    with hemopericardium I23.0
    infectional I40.9
    traumatic — *see* Injury, heart
  cartilage (articular) (current) — *see also* Sprain
    knee S83.3- ☑
    semilunar — *see* Tear, meniscus
  cecum (with peritonitis) K65.0
    with peritoneal abscess K35.33
    traumatic S36.598 ☑
  celiac artery, traumatic — *see* Injury, blood vessel, celiac artery, laceration, major
  cerebral aneurysm (congenital) (see Hemorrhage, intracranial, subarachnoid)
  cervix (uteri)
    with ectopic or molar pregnancy O08.6
    following ectopic or molar pregnancy O08.6
    obstetrical trauma O71.3
    traumatic S37.69 ☑
  chordae tendineae NEC I51.1
    concurrent with acute myocardial infarction — *see* Infarct, myocardium
    following acute myocardial infarction (current complication) I23.4
  choroid (direct) (indirect) (traumatic) H31.32- ☑
  circle of Willis I60.6
  colon (nontraumatic) K63.1
    traumatic — *see* Injury, intestine, large
  cornea (traumatic) — *see* Injury, eye, laceration
  coronary (artery) (thrombotic) — *see* Infarct, myocardium
  corpus luteum (infected) (ovary) N83.1- ☑

Rupture, ruptured — *continued*
  cyst — *see* Cyst
  cystic duct K82.2
  Descemet's membrane — *see* Change, corneal membrane, Descemet's, rupture
    traumatic — *see* Injury, eye, laceration
  diaphragm, traumatic — *see* Injury, intrathoracic, diaphragm
  disc — *see* Rupture, intervertebral disc
  diverticulum (intestine) K57.80
    with bleeding K57.81
    bladder N32.3
    large intestine K57.20
      with
        bleeding K57.21
        small intestine K57.40
          with bleeding K57.41
      small intestine K57.00
        with
          bleeding K57.01
          large intestine K57.40
            with bleeding K57.41
  duodenal stump K31.89
  ear drum (nontraumatic) — *see also* Perforation, tympanum
    traumatic S09.2- ☑
      due to blast injury — *see* Injury, blast, ear
  esophagus K22.3
  eye (without prolapse or loss of intraocular tissue) — *see* Injury, eye, laceration
  fallopian tube NEC (nonobstetric) (nontraumatic) N83.8
    due to pregnancy O00.10- ☑
      with intrauterine pregnancy O00.11- ☑
  fontanel P13.1
  gallbladder K82.2
    traumatic S36.128 ☑
  gastric — *see also* Rupture, stomach
    vessel K92.2
  globe (eye) (traumatic) — *see* Injury, eye, laceration
  graafian follicle (hematoma) N83.0- ☑
  heart — *see* Rupture, cardiac
  hymen (nontraumatic) (nonintentional) N89.8
  internal organ, traumatic — *see* Injury, by site
  intervertebral disc — *see* Displacement, intervertebral disc
    traumatic — *see* Rupture, traumatic, intervertebral disc
  intestine NEC (nontraumatic) K63.1
    traumatic — *see* Injury, intestine
  iris — *see also* Abnormality, pupillary
    traumatic — *see* Injury, eye, laceration
  joint capsule, traumatic — *see* Sprain
  kidney (traumatic) S37.06- ☑
    birth injury P15.8
    nontraumatic N28.89
  lacrimal duct (traumatic) — *see* Injury, eye, specified site NEC
  lens (cataract) (traumatic) — *see* Cataract, traumatic
  ligament, traumatic — *see* Rupture, traumatic, ligament, by site
  liver S36.116 ☑
    birth injury P15.0
  lymphatic vessel I89.8
  marginal sinus (placental) (with hemorrhage) — *see* Hemorrhage, antepartum, specified cause NEC
  membrana tympani (nontraumatic) — *see* Perforation, tympanum
  membranes (spontaneous)
    artificial
      delayed delivery following O75.5
    delayed delivery following — *see* Pregnancy, complicated by, premature rupture of membranes
  meningeal artery I60.8
  meniscus (knee) — *see also* Tear, meniscus
    old — *see* Derangement, meniscus
    site other than knee — *code as* Sprain
  mesenteric artery, traumatic — *see* Injury, mesenteric, artery, laceration, major
  mesentery (nontraumatic) K66.8
    traumatic — *see* Injury, intra-abdominal, specified, site NEC
  mitral (valve) I34.8
  muscle (traumatic) — *see also* Strain
    diastasis — *see* Diastasis, muscle
    nontraumatic M62.10
      ankle M62.17- ☑
      foot M62.17- ☑

Rupture, ruptured — *continued*
  muscle — *see also* Strain — *continued*
    nontraumatic — *continued*
      forearm M62.13- ☑
      hand M62.14- ☑
      lower leg M62.16- ☑
      pelvic region M62.15- ☑
      shoulder region M62.11- ☑
      specified site NEC M62.18
      thigh M62.15- ☑
      upper arm M62.12- ☑
    traumatic — *see* Strain, by site
  musculotendinous junction NEC, nontraumatic — *see* Rupture, tendon, spontaneous
  mycotic aneurysm causing cerebral hemorrhage — *see* Hemorrhage, intracranial, subarachnoid
  myocardium, myocardial — *see* Rupture, cardiac
    traumatic — *see* Injury, heart
  nontraumatic, meaning hernia — *see* Hernia
  obstructed — *see* Hernia, by site, obstructed
  operation wound — *see* Disruption, wound, operation
  ovary, ovarian N83.8
    corpus luteum cyst N83.1- ☑
    follicle (graafian) N83.0- ☑
  oviduct (nonobstetric) (nontraumatic) N83.8
    due to pregnancy O00.10- ☑
      with intrauterine pregnancy O00.11- ☑
  pancreas (nontraumatic) K86.89
    traumatic S36.299 ☑
  papillary muscle NEC I51.2
    following acute myocardial infarction (current complication) I23.5
  pelvic
    floor, complicating delivery O70.1
    organ NEC, obstetrical trauma O71.5
  perineum (nonobstetric) (nontraumatic) N90.89
    complicating delivery — *see* Delivery, complicated, by, laceration, anus (sphincter)
  postoperative wound — *see* Disruption, wound, operation
  prostate (traumatic) S37.828 ☑
  pulmonary
    artery I28.8
    valve (heart) I37.8
    vein I28.8
    vessel I28.8
  pus tube — *see* Salpingitis
  pyosalpinx — *see* Salpingitis
  rectum (nontraumatic) K63.1
    traumatic S36.69 ☑
  retina, retinal (traumatic) (without detachment) — *see also* Break, retina
    with detachment — *see* Detachment, retina, with retinal, break
  rotator cuff (nontraumatic) M75.10- ☑
    complete M75.12- ☑
    incomplete M75.11- ☑
  sclera — *see* Injury, eye, laceration
  sigmoid (nontraumatic) K63.1
    traumatic S36.593 ☑
  spinal cord — *see also* Injury, spinal cord, by region
    due to injury at birth P11.5
    newborn (birth injury) P11.5
  spleen (traumatic) S36.09 ☑
    birth injury P15.1
    congenital (birth injury) P15.1
    due to P. vivax malaria B51.0
    nontraumatic D73.5
    spontaneous D73.5
  splenic vein R58
    traumatic — *see* Injury, blood vessel, splenic vein
  stomach (nontraumatic) (spontaneous) K31.89
    traumatic S36.39 ☑
  supraspinatus (complete) (incomplete) (nontraumatic) — *see* Tear, rotator cuff
  symphysis pubis
    obstetric O71.6
    traumatic S33.4 ☑
  synovium (cyst) M66.10
    ankle M66.17- ☑
    elbow M66.12- ☑
    finger M66.14- ☑
    foot M66.17- ☑
    forearm M66.13- ☑
    hand M66.14- ☑
    pelvic region M66.15- ☑
    shoulder region M66.11- ☑

Rupture, ruptured — *continued*
  synovium — *continued*
    specified site NEC M66.18
    thigh M66.15- ☑
    toe M66.17- ☑
    upper arm M66.12- ☑
    wrist M66.13- ☑
  tendon (traumatic) — *see* Strain
    nontraumatic (spontaneous) M66.9
      ankle M66.87- ☑
      extensor M66.20
        ankle M66.27- ☑
        foot M66.27- ☑
        forearm M66.23- ☑
        hand M66.24- ☑
        lower leg M66.26- ☑
        multiple sites M66.29
        pelvic region M66.25- ☑
        shoulder region M66.21- ☑
        specified site NEC M66.28
        thigh M66.25- ☑
        upper arm M66.22- ☑
      flexor M66.30
        ankle M66.37- ☑
        foot M66.37- ☑
        forearm M66.33- ☑
        hand M66.34- ☑
        lower leg M66.36- ☑
        multiple sites M66.39
        pelvic region M66.35- ☑
        shoulder region M66.31- ☑
        specified site NEC M66.38
        thigh M66.35- ☑
        upper arm M66.32- ☑
      foot M66.87- ☑
      forearm M66.83- ☑
      hand M66.84- ☑
      lower leg M66.86- ☑
      multiple sites M66.89
      pelvic region M66.85- ☑
      shoulder region M66.81- ☑
      specified
        site NEC M66.88
        tendon M66.80
      thigh M66.85- ☑
      upper arm M66.82- ☑
  thoracic duct I89.8
  tonsil J35.8
  traumatic
    aorta — *see* Injury, aorta, laceration, major
    diaphragm — *see* Injury, intrathoracic, diaphragm
    external site — *see* Wound, open, by site
    eye — *see* Injury, eye, laceration
    internal organ — *see* Injury, by site
    intervertebral disc
      cervical S13.0 ☑
      lumbar S33.0 ☑
      thoracic S23.0 ☑
    kidney S37.06- ☑
    ligament — *see also* Sprain
      ankle — *see* Sprain, ankle
      carpus — *see* Rupture, traumatic, ligament, wrist
      collateral (hand) — *see* Rupture, traumatic, ligament, finger, collateral
      finger (metacarpophalangeal) (interphalangeal) S63.40- ☑
        collateral S63.41- ☑
          index S63.41- ☑
          little S63.41- ☑
          middle S63.41- ☑
          ring S63.41- ☑
        index S63.40- ☑
        little S63.40- ☑
        middle S63.40- ☑
        palmar S63.42- ☑
          index S63.42- ☑
          little S63.42- ☑
          middle S63.42- ☑
          ring S63.42- ☑
        ring S63.40- ☑
        specified site NEC S63.499 ☑
          index S63.49- ☑
          little S63.49- ☑
          middle S63.49- ☑
          ring S63.49- ☑
        volar plate S63.43- ☑

Rupture, ruptured — *continued*
  traumatic — *continued*
    ligament — *see also* Sprain — *continued*
      finger — *continued*
        volar plate — *continued*
          index S63.43- ☑
          little S63.43- ☑
          middle S63.43- ☑
          ring S63.43- ☑
      foot — *see* Sprain, foot
      radial collateral S53.2- ☑
      radiocarpal — *see* Rupture, traumatic, ligament, wrist, radiocarpal
      ulnar collateral S53.3- ☑
      ulnocarpal — *see* Rupture, traumatic, ligament, wrist, ulnocarpal
      wrist S63.30- ☑
        collateral S63.31- ☑
        radiocarpal S63.32- ☑
        specified site NEC S63.39- ☑
        ulnocarpal (palmar) S63.33- ☑
    liver S36.116 ☑
    membrana tympani — *see* Rupture, ear drum, traumatic
    muscle or tendon — *see* Strain
    myocardium — *see* Injury, heart
    pancreas S36.299 ☑
    rectum S36.69 ☑
    sigmoid S36.593 ☑
    spleen S36.09 ☑
    stomach S36.39 ☑
    symphysis pubis S33.4 ☑
    tympanum, tympanic (membrane) — *see* Rupture, ear drum, traumatic
    ureter S37.19 ☑
    uterus S37.69 ☑
    vagina — *see* Injury, vagina
    vena cava — *see* Injury, vena cava, laceration, major
  tricuspid (heart) (valve) I07.8
  tube, tubal (nonobstetric) (nontraumatic) N83.8
    abscess — *see* Salpingitis
    due to pregnancy O00.10- ☑
      with intrauterine pregnancy O00.11- ☑
  tympanum, tympanic (membrane) (nontraumatic) — *see also* Perforation, tympanic membrane H72.9- ☑
    traumatic — *see* Rupture, ear drum, traumatic
  umbilical cord, complicating delivery O69.89 ☑
  ureter (traumatic) S37.19 ☑
    nontraumatic N28.89
  urethra (nontraumatic) N36.8
    with ectopic or molar pregnancy O08.6
    following ectopic or molar pregnancy O08.6
    obstetrical trauma O71.5
    traumatic S37.39 ☑
  uterosacral ligament (nonobstetric) (nontraumatic) N83.8
  uterus (traumatic) S37.69 ☑
    before labor O71.0- ☑
    during or after labor O71.1
    nonpuerperal, nontraumatic N85.8
    pregnant (during labor) O71.1
      before labor O71.0- ☑
  vagina — *see* Injury, vagina
  valve, valvular (heart) — *see* Endocarditis
  varicose vein — *see* Varix
  varix — *see* Varix
  vena cava R58
    traumatic — *see* Injury, vena cava, laceration, major
  vesical (urinary) N32.89
  vessel (blood) R58
    pulmonary I28.8
    traumatic — *see* Injury, blood vessel
  viscus R19.8
  vulva complicating delivery O70.0
Russell-Silver syndrome Q87.19
Russian spring-summer type encephalitis A84.0
Rust's disease (tuberculous cervical spondylitis) A18.01
Ruvalcaba-Myhre-Smith syndrome E71.440
Rytand-Lipsitch syndrome I44.2

S

Saber, sabre shin or tibia (syphilitic) A50.56 [M90.8-] ☑
Sac lacrimal — *see* condition
Saccharomyces infection B37.9

Saccharopinuria E72.3
Saccular — *see* condition
Sacculation
  aorta (nonsyphilitic) — *see* Aneurysm, aorta
  bladder N32.3
  intralaryngeal (congenital) (ventricular) Q31.3
  larynx (congenital) (ventricular) Q31.3
  organ or site, congenital — *see* Distortion
  pregnant uterus — *see* Pregnancy, complicated by, abnormal, uterus
  ureter N28.89
  urethra N36.1
  vesical N32.3
Sachs' amaurotic familial idiocy or disease E75.02
Sachs-Tay disease E75.02
Sacks-Libman disease M32.11
Sacralgia M53.3
Sacralization Q76.49
Sacrodynia M53.3
Sacroiliac joint — *see* condition
Sacroiliitis NEC M46.1
Sacrum — *see* condition
Saddle
  back — *see* Lordosis
  embolus
    abdominal aorta I74.01
    pulmonary artery I26.92
      with acute cor pulmonale I26.02
  injury — *code to* condition
  nose M95.0
    due to syphilis A50.57
Sadism (sexual) F65.52
Sadness, postpartal O90.6
Sadomasochism F65.50
Saemisch's ulcer (cornea) — *see* Ulcer, cornea, central
Sagging
  skin and subcutaneous tissue (following bariatric surgery weight loss) (following dietary weight loss) L98.7
Sahib disease B55.0
Sailors' skin L57.8
Saint
  Anthony's fire — *see* Erysipelas
  triad — *see* Hernia, diaphragm
  Vitus' dance — *see* Chorea, Sydenham's
Salaam
  attack(s) — *see* Epilepsy, spasms
  tic R25.8
Salicylism
  abuse F55.8
  overdose or wrong substance given — *see* Table of Drugs and Chemicals, by drug, poisoning
Salivary duct or gland — *see* condition
Salivation, excessive K11.7
Salmonella — *see* Infection, Salmonella
Salmonellosis A02.0
Salpingitis (catarrhal) (fallopian tube) (nodular) (pseudofollicular) (purulent) (septic) N70.91
  with oophoritis N70.93
  acute N70.01
    with oophoritis N70.03
  chlamydial A56.11
  chronic N70.11
    with oophoritis N70.13
  complicating abortion — *see* Abortion, by type, complicated by, salpingitis
  ear — *see* Salpingitis, eustachian
  eustachian (tube) H68.00- ☑
    acute H68.01- ☑
    chronic H68.02- ☑
  follicularis N70.11
    with oophoritis N70.13
  gonococcal (acute) (chronic) A54.24
  interstitial, chronic N70.11
    with oophoritis N70.13
  isthmica nodosa N70.11
    with oophoritis N70.13
  specific (gonococcal) (acute) (chronic) A54.24
  tuberculous (acute) (chronic) A18.17
  venereal (gonococcal) (acute) (chronic) A54.24
Salpingocele N83.4- ☑
Salpingo-oophoritis (catarrhal) (purulent) (ruptured) (septic) (suppurative) N70.93
  acute N70.03
    with ectopic or molar pregnancy O08.0
    following ectopic or molar pregnancy O08.0
    gonococcal A54.24

Salpingo-oophoritis — *continued*
- chronic N70.13
- following ectopic or molar pregnancy O08.0
- gonococcal (acute) (chronic) A54.24
- puerperal O86.19
- specific (gonococcal) (acute) (chronic) A54.24
- subacute N70.03
- tuberculous (acute) (chronic) A18.17
- venereal (gonococcal) (acute) (chronic) A54.24

Salpingo-ovaritis — *see* Salpingo-oophoritis

Salpingoperitonitis — *see* Salpingo-oophoritis

Salzmann's nodular dystrophy — *see* Degeneration, cornea, nodular

Sampson's cyst or tumor N80.1

San Joaquin (Valley) **fever** B38.0

Sandblaster's asthma, lung or pneumoconiosis J62.8

Sander's disease (paranoia) F22

Sandfly fever A93.1

Sandhoff's disease E75.01

Sanfilippo (Type B) (Type C) (Type D) **syndrome** E76.22

Sanger-Brown ataxia G11.2

Sao Paulo fever or typhus A77.0

Saponification, mesenteric K65.8

Sarcocele (benign)
- syphilitic A52.76
- congenital A50.59

Sarcocystosis A07.8

Sarcoepiplocele — *see* Hernia

Sarcoepiplomphalocele Q79.2

Sarcoid — *see also* Sarcoidosis
- arthropathy D86.86
- Boeck's D86.9
- Darier-Roussy D86.3
- iridocyclitis D86.83
- meningitis D86.81
- myocarditis D86.85
- myositis D86.87
- pyelonephritis D86.84
- Spiegler-Fendt L08.89

Sarcoidosis D86.9
- with
  - cranial nerve palsies D86.82
  - hepatic granuloma D86.89
  - polyarthritis D86.86
  - tubulo-interstitial nephropathy D86.84
- combined sites NEC D86.89
- lung D86.0
  - and lymph nodes D86.2
- lymph nodes D86.1
  - and lung D86.2
- meninges D86.81
- skin D86.3
- specified type NEC D86.89

Sarcoma (of) — *see also* Neoplasm, connective tissue, malignant
- alveolar soft part — *see* Neoplasm, connective tissue, malignant
- ameloblastic C41.1
  - upper jaw (bone) C41.0
- botryoid — *see* Neoplasm, connective tissue, malignant
- botryoides — *see* Neoplasm, connective tissue, malignant
- cerebellar C71.6
  - circumscribed (arachnoidal) C71.6
- circumscribed (arachnoidal) cerebellar C71.6
- clear cell — *see also* Neoplasm, connective tissue, malignant
  - kidney C64.- ☑
- dendritic cells (accessory cells) C96.4
- embryonal — *see* Neoplasm, connective tissue, malignant
- endometrial (stromal) C54.1
  - isthmus C54.0
- epithelioid (cell) — *see* Neoplasm, connective tissue, malignant
- Ewing's — *see* Neoplasm, bone, malignant
- follicular dendritic cell C96.4
- germinoblastic (diffuse) — *see* Lymphoma, diffuse large cell
  - follicular — *see* Lymphoma, follicular, specified NEC
- giant cell (except of bone) — *see also* Neoplasm, connective tissue, malignant
  - bone — *see* Neoplasm, bone, malignant
- glomoid — *see* Neoplasm, connective tissue, malignant
- granulocytic C92.3- ☑
- hemangioendothelial — *see* Neoplasm, connective tissue, malignant
- hemorrhagic, multiple — *see* Sarcoma, Kaposi's

Sarcoma — *continued*
- histiocytic C96.A (*following* C96.6)
- Hodgkin — *see* Lymphoma, Hodgkin
- immunoblastic (diffuse) — *see* Lymphoma, diffuse large cell
- interdigitating dendritic cell C96.4
- Kaposi's
  - colon C46.4
  - connective tissue C46.1
  - gastrointestinal organ C46.4
  - lung C46.5- ☑
  - lymph node(s) C46.3
  - palate (hard) (soft) C46.2
  - rectum C46.4
  - skin C46.0
  - specified site NEC C46.7
  - stomach C46.4
  - unspecified site C46.9
- Kupffer cell C22.3
- Langerhans cell C96.4
- leptomeningeal — *see* Neoplasm, meninges, malignant
- liver NEC C22.4
- lymphangioendothelial — *see* Neoplasm, connective tissue, malignant
- lymphoblastic — *see* Lymphoma, lymphoblastic (diffuse)
- lymphocytic — *see* Lymphoma, small cell B-cell
- mast cell C96.22
- melanotic — *see* Melanoma
- meningeal — *see* Neoplasm, meninges, malignant
- meningothelial — *see* Neoplasm, meninges, malignant
- mesenchymal — *see also* Neoplasm, connective tissue, malignant
  - mixed — *see* Neoplasm, connective tissue, malignant
- mesothelial — *see* Mesothelioma
- monstrocellular
  - specified site — *see* Neoplasm, malignant, by site
  - unspecified site C71.9
- myeloid C92.3- ☑
- neurogenic — *see* Neoplasm, nerve, malignant
- odontogenic C41.1
  - upper jaw (bone) C41.0
- osteoblastic — *see* Neoplasm, bone, malignant
- osteogenic — *see also* Neoplasm, bone, malignant
  - juxtacortical — *see* Neoplasm, bone, malignant
  - periosteal — *see* Neoplasm, bone, malignant
- periosteal — *see also* Neoplasm, bone, malignant
  - osteogenic — *see* Neoplasm, bone, malignant
- pleomorphic cell — *see* Neoplasm, connective tissue, malignant
- reticulum cell (diffuse) — *see* Lymphoma, diffuse large cell
  - nodular — *see* Lymphoma, follicular
  - pleomorphic cell type — *see* Lymphoma, diffuse large cell
- rhabdoid — *see* Neoplasm, malignant, by site
- round cell — *see* Neoplasm, connective tissue, malignant
- small cell — *see* Neoplasm, connective tissue, malignant
- soft tissue — *see* Neoplasm, connective tissue, malignant
- spindle cell — *see* Neoplasm, connective tissue, malignant
- stromal (endometrial) C54.1
  - isthmus C54.0
- synovial — *see also* Neoplasm, connective tissue, malignant
  - biphasic — *see* Neoplasm, connective tissue, malignant
  - epithelioid cell — *see* Neoplasm, connective tissue, malignant
  - spindle cell — *see* Neoplasm, connective tissue, malignant

Sarcomatosis
- meningeal — *see* Neoplasm, meninges, malignant
- specified site NEC — *see* Neoplasm, connective tissue, malignant
- unspecified site C80.1

Sarcopenia (age-related) M62.84

Sarcosinemia E72.59

Sarcosporidiosis (intestinal) A07.8

SARS-CoV-2 — *see also* COVID-19
- sequelae (post acute) U09.9

Satiety, early R68.81

Saturnine — *see* condition

Saturnism
- overdose or wrong substance given or taken — *see* Table of Drugs and Chemicals, by drug, poisoning

Satyriasis F52.8

Sauriasis — *see* Ichthyosis

SBE (subacute bacterial endocarditis) I33.0

Scabies (any site) B86

Scabs R23.4

Scaglietti-Dagnini syndrome E22.0

Scald — *see* Burn

Scalenus anticus (anterior) **syndrome** G54.0

Scales R23.4

Scaling, skin R23.4

Scalp — *see* condition

Scapegoating affecting child Z62.3

Scaphocephaly Q75.0

Scapulalgia M89.8X1

Scapulohumeral myopathy G71.02

Scar, scarring — *see also* Cicatrix L90.5
- adherent L90.5
- atrophic L90.5
- cervix
  - in pregnancy or childbirth — *see* Pregnancy, complicated by, abnormal cervix
- cheloid L91.0
- chorioretinal H31.00- ☑
  - posterior pole macula H31.01- ☑
  - postsurgical H59.81- ☑
  - solar retinopathy H31.02- ☑
  - specified type NEC H31.09- ☑
- choroid — *see* Scar, chorioretinal
- conjunctiva H11.24- ☑
- cornea H17.9
  - xerophthalmic — *see also* Opacity, cornea
    - vitamin A deficiency E50.6
- defect (isthmocele) O34.22
- duodenum, obstructive K31.5
- hypertrophic L91.0
- keloid L91.0
- labia N90.89
- lung (base) J98.4
- macula — *see* Scar, chorioretinal, posterior pole
- muscle M62.89
- myocardium, myocardial I25.2
- painful L90.5
- posterior pole (eye) — *see* Scar, chorioretinal, posterior pole
- retina — *see* Scar, chorioretinal
- trachea J39.8
- transmural uterine, in pregnancy O34.29
- uterus N85.8
  - in pregnancy O34.29
- vagina N89.8
  - postoperative N99.2
- vulva N90.89

Scarabiasis B88.2

Scarlatina (anginosa) (maligna) A38.9
- myocarditis (acute) A38.1
  - old — *see* Myocarditis
- otitis media A38.0
- ulcerosa A38.8

Scarlet fever (albuminuria) (angina) A38.9

Schamberg's disease (progressive pigmentary dermatosis) L81.7

Schatzki's ring (acquired) (esophagus) (lower) K22.2
- congenital Q39.3

Schaufenster krankheit I20.8

Schaumann's
- benign lymphogranulomatosis D86.1
- disease or syndrome — *see* Sarcoidosis

Scheie's syndrome E76.03

Schenck's disease B42.1

Scheuermann's disease or osteochondrosis — *see* Osteochondrosis, juvenile, spine

Schilder (-Flatau) **disease** G37.0

Schilling-type monocytic leukemia C93.0- ☑

Schimmelbusch's disease, cystic mastitis, or hyperplasia — *see* Mastopathy, cystic

Schistosoma infestation — *see* Infestation, Schistosoma

Schistosomiasis B65.9
- with muscle disorder B65.9 *[M63.80]*
  - ankle B65.9 *[M63.87-]* ☑
  - foot B65.9 *[M63.87-]* ☑
  - forearm B65.9 *[M63.83-]* ☑
  - hand B65.9 *[M63.84-]* ☑
  - lower leg B65.9 *[M63.86-]* ☑
  - multiple sites B65.9 *[M63.89]*

☑ **Additional Character Required** — Refer to the Tabular List for Character Selection   ▽ **Subterms under main terms may continue to next column or page**

Schistosomiasis — *continued*
 with muscle disorder — *continued*
  pelvic region B65.9 *[M63.85-]* ☑
  shoulder region B65.9 *[M63.81-]* ☑
  specified site NEC B65.9 *[M63.88]*
  thigh B65.9 *[M63.85-]* ☑
  upper arm B65.9 *[M63.82-]* ☑
 Asiatic B65.2
 bladder B65.Ø
 chestermani B65.8
 colon B65.1
 cutaneous B65.3
 due to
  S. haematobium B65.Ø
  S. japonicum B65.2
  S. mansoni B65.1
  S. mattheii B65.8
 Eastern B65.2
 genitourinary tract B65.Ø
 intestinal B65.1
 lung NEC B65.9 *[J99]*
  pneumonia B65.9 *[J17]*
 Manson's (intestinal) B65.1
 oriental B65.2
 pulmonary NEC B65.9 *[J99]*
  pneumonia B65.9
 Schistosoma
  haematobium B65.Ø
  japonicum B65.2
  mansoni B65.1
 specified type NEC B65.8
 urinary B65.Ø
 vesical B65.Ø
Schizencephaly Q04.6
Schizoaffective psychosis F25.9
Schizodontia KØØ.2
Schizoid personality F6Ø.1
Schizophrenia, schizophrenic F2Ø.9
 acute (brief) (undifferentiated) F23
 atypical (form) F2Ø.3
 borderline F21
 catalepsy F2Ø.2
 catatonic (type) (excited) (withdrawn) F2Ø.2
 cenesthopathic, cenesthesiopathic F2Ø.89
 childhood type F84.5
 chronic undifferentiated F2Ø.9
 cyclic F25.Ø
 disorganized (type) F2Ø.1
 flexibilitas cerea F2Ø.2
 hebephrenic (type) F2Ø.1
 incipient F21
 latent F21
 negative type F2Ø.5
 paranoid (type) F2Ø.Ø
 paraphrenic F2Ø.Ø
 post-psychotic depression F32.89
 prepsychotic F21
 prodromal F21
 pseudoneurotic F21
 pseudopsychopathic F21
 reaction F23
 residual (state) (type) F2Ø.5
 restzustand F2Ø.5
 schizoaffective (type) — *see* Psychosis, schizoaffective
 simple (type) F2Ø.89
 simplex F2Ø.89
 specified type NEC F2Ø.89
 spectrum and other psychotic disorder F29
  specified NEC F28
 stupor F2Ø.2
 syndrome of childhood F84.5
 undifferentiated (type) F2Ø.3
  chronic F2Ø.5
Schizothymia (persistent) F6Ø.1
Schlatter-Osgood disease or osteochondrosis M92.52- ☑
Schlatter's tibia — *see* Osteochondrosis, juvenile, tibia
Schmidt's syndrome (polyglandular, autoimmune) E31.Ø
Schmincke's carcinoma or tumor — *see* Neoplasm, nasopharynx, malignant
Schmitz (-Stutzer) **dysentery** AØ3.Ø
Schmorl's disease or nodes
 lumbar region M51.46
 lumbosacral region M51.47
 sacrococcygeal region M53.3
 thoracic region M51.44
 thoracolumbar region M51.45

Schneiderian
 papilloma — *see* Neoplasm, nasopharynx, benign
  specified site — *see* Neoplasm, benign, by site
  unspecified site D14.Ø
 specified site — *see* Neoplasm, malignant, by site
  unspecified site C3Ø.Ø
Scholte's syndrome (malignant carcinoid) E34.Ø
Scholz (-Bielchowsky-Henneberg) **disease or syndrome** E75.25
Schönlein (-Henoch) disease or purpura (primary) (rheumatic) D69.Ø
Schottmuller's disease AØ1.4
Schroeder's syndrome (endocrine hypertensive) E27.Ø
Schüller-Christian disease or syndrome C96.5
Schultze's type acroparesthesia, simple I73.89
Schultz's disease or syndrome — *see* Agranulocytosis
Schwalbe-Ziehen-Oppenheim disease G24.1
Schwannoma — *see also* Neoplasm, nerve, benign
 malignant — *see also* Neoplasm, nerve, malignant
  with rhabdomyoblastic differentiation — *see* Neoplasm, nerve, malignant
 melanocytic — *see* Neoplasm, nerve, benign
 pigmented — *see* Neoplasm, nerve, benign
Schwannomatosis Q85.Ø3
Schwartz (-Jampel) **syndrome** G71.13
Schwartz-Bartter syndrome E22.2
Schweniger-Buzzi anetoderma L9Ø.1
Sciatic — *see* condition
Sciatica (infective) M54.3 ☑
 with lumbago M54.4- ☑
  due to intervertebral disc disorder — *see* Disorder, disc, with, radiculopathy
  due to displacement of intervertebral disc (with lumbago) — *see* Disorder, disc, with, radiculopathy
 wallet M54.3- ☑
Scimitar syndrome Q26.8
Sclera — *see* condition
Sclerectasia H15.84- ☑
Scleredema
 adultorum — *see* Sclerosis, systemic
 Buschke's — *see* Sclerosis, systemic
 newborn P83.Ø
Sclerema (adiposum) (edematosum) (neonatorum) (newborn) P83.Ø
 adultorum — *see* Sclerosis, systemic
Scleriasis — *see* Scleroderma
Scleritis H15.ØØ- ☑
 with corneal involvement H15.Ø4- ☑
 anterior H15.Ø1- ☑
 brawny H15.Ø2- ☑
 in (due to) zoster BØ2.34
 posterior H15.Ø3- ☑
 specified type NEC H15.Ø9- ☑
 syphilitic A52.71
 tuberculous (nodular) A18.51
Sclerochoroiditis H31.8
Scleroconjunctivitis — *see* Scleritis
Sclerocystic ovary syndrome E28.2
Sclerodactyly, sclerodactylia L94.3
Scleroderma, sclerodermia (acrosclerotic) (diffuse) (generalized) (progressive) (pulmonary) — *see also* Sclerosis, systemic M34.9
 circumscribed L94.Ø
 linear L94.1
 localized L94.Ø
 newborn P83.88
 systemic M34.9
Sclerokeratitis H16.8
 tuberculous A18.52
Scleroma nasi A48.8
Scleromalacia (perforans) H15.Ø5- ☑
Scleromyxedema L98.5
Sclérose en plaques G35
Sclerosis, sclerotic
 adrenal (gland) E27.8
 Alzheimer's — *see* Disease, Alzheimer's
 amyotrophic (lateral) G12.21
 aorta, aortic I7Ø.Ø
  valve — *see* Endocarditis, aortic
 artery, arterial, arteriolar, arteriovascular — *see* Arteriosclerosis
 ascending multiple G35
 brain (generalized) (lobular) G37.9
  artery, arterial I67.2
  diffuse G37.Ø
  disseminated G35
  insular G35

Sclerosis, sclerotic — *continued*
 brain — *continued*
  Krabbe's E75.23
  miliary G35
  multiple G35
  presenile (Alzheimer's) — *see* Disease, Alzheimer's, early onset
  senile (arteriosclerotic) I67.2
  stem, multiple G35
  tuberous Q85.1
 bulbar, multiple G35
 bundle of His I44.39
 cardiac — *see* Disease, heart, ischemic, atherosclerotic
 cardiorenal — *see* Hypertension, cardiorenal
 cardiovascular — *see also* Disease, cardiovascular
  renal — *see* Hypertension, cardiorenal
 cerebellar — *see* Sclerosis, brain
 cerebral — *see* Sclerosis, brain
 cerebrospinal (disseminated) (multiple) G35
 cerebrovascular I67.2
 choroid — *see* Degeneration, choroid
 combined (spinal cord) — *see also* Degeneration, combined
  multiple G35
 concentric (Balo) G37.5
 cornea — *see* Opacity, cornea
 coronary (artery) I25.1Ø
  with angina pectoris — *see* Arteriosclerosis, coronary (artery),
 corpus cavernosum
  female N9Ø.89
  male N48.6
 diffuse (brain) (spinal cord) G37.Ø
 disseminated G35
 dorsal G35
 dorsolateral (spinal cord) — *see* Degeneration, combined
 endometrium N85.5
 extrapyramidal G25.9
 eye, nuclear (senile) — *see* Cataract, senile, nuclear
 focal and segmental (glomerular) — *see also* NØØ-NØ7 with fourth character .1 NØ5.1
 Friedreich's (spinal cord) G11.11
 funicular (spermatic cord) N5Ø.89
 general (vascular) — *see* Arteriosclerosis
 gland (lymphatic) I89.8
 hepatic K74.1
  alcoholic K7Ø.2
 hereditary
  cerebellar G11.9
  spinal (Friedreich's ataxia) G11.11
 hippocampal G93.81
 insular G35
 kidney — *see* Sclerosis, renal
 larynx J38.7
 lateral (amyotrophic) (descending) (spinal) G12.21
  primary G12.23
 lens, senile nuclear — *see* Cataract, senile, nuclear
 liver K74.1
  with fibrosis K74.2
   alcoholic K7Ø.2
  alcoholic K7Ø.2
  cardiac K76.1
 lung — *see* Fibrosis, lung
 mastoid — *see* Mastoiditis, chronic
 mesial temporal G93.81
 mitral I05.8
 Mönckeberg's (medial) — *see* Arteriosclerosis, extremities
 multiple (brain stem) (cerebral) (generalized) (spinal cord) G35
 myocardium, myocardial — *see* Disease, heart, ischemic, atherosclerotic
 nuclear (senile), eye — *see* Cataract, senile, nuclear
 ovary N83.8
 pancreas K86.89
 penis N48.6
 peripheral arteries — *see* Arteriosclerosis, extremities
 plaques G35
 pluriglandular E31.8
 polyglandular E31.8
 posterolateral (spinal cord) — *see* Degeneration, combined
 presenile (Alzheimer's) — *see* Disease, Alzheimer's, early onset
 primary, lateral G12.23
 progressive, systemic M34.Ø
 pulmonary — *see* Fibrosis, lung

▼ **Subterms under main terms may continue to next column or page** ☑ **Additional Character Required** — Refer to the Tabular List for Character Selection

Sclerosis, sclerotic — *continued*
  pulmonary — *see* Fibrosis, lung — *continued*
    artery I27.0
    valve (heart) — *see* Endocarditis, pulmonary
  renal N26.9
    with
      cystine storage disease E72.09
      hypertensive heart disease (conditions in I11) — *see* Hypertension, cardiorenal
      arteriolar (hyaline) (hyperplastic) — *see* Hypertension, kidney
  retina (senile) (vascular) H35.00
  senile (vascular) — *see* Arteriosclerosis
  spinal (cord) (progressive) G95.89
    ascending G61.0
    combined — *see also* Degeneration, combined
      multiple G35
      syphilitic A52.11
    disseminated G35
    dorsolateral — *see* Degeneration, combined
    hereditary (Friedreich's) (mixed form) G11.11
    lateral (amyotrophic) G12.21
      progressive G12.23
    multiple G35
    posterior (syphilitic) A52.11
  stomach K31.89
  subendocardial, congenital I42.4
  systemic M34.9
    with
      lung involvement M34.81
      myopathy M34.82
      polyneuropathy M34.83
    drug-induced M34.2
    due to chemicals NEC M34.2
    progressive M34.0
    specified NEC M34.89
  temporal (mesial) G93.81
  tricuspid (heart) (valve) I07.8
  tuberous (brain) Q85.1
  tympanic membrane — *see* Disorder, tympanic membrane, specified NEC
  valve, valvular (heart) — *see* Endocarditis
  vascular — *see* Arteriosclerosis
  vein I87.8
Scoliosis (acquired) (postural) M41.9
  adolescent (idiopathic) — *see* Scoliosis, idiopathic, adolescent
  congenital Q67.5
    due to bony malformation Q76.3
    failure of segmentation (hemivertebra) Q76.3
    hemivertebra fusion Q76.3
    postural Q67.5
  degenerative M41.8- ☑
  idiopathic M41.20
    adolescent M41.129
      cervical region M41.122
      cervicothoracic region M41.123
      lumbar region M41.126
      lumbosacral region M41.127
      thoracic region M41.124
      thoracolumbar region M41.125
    cervical region M41.22
    cervicothoracic region M41.23
    infantile M41.00
      cervical region M41.02
      cervicothoracic region M41.03
      lumbar region M41.06
      lumbosacral region M41.07
      sacrococcygeal region M41.08
      thoracic region M41.04
      thoracolumbar region M41.05
    juvenile M41.119
      cervical region M41.112
      cervicothoracic region M41.113
      lumbar region M41.116
      lumbosacral region M41.117
      thoracic region M41.114
      thoracolumbar region M41.115
    lumbar region M41.26
    lumbosacral region M41.27
    thoracic region M41.24
    thoracolumbar region M41.25
  infantile — *see* Scoliosis, idiopathic, infantile
  neuromuscular M41.40
    cervical region M41.42
    cervicothoracic region M41.43
    lumbar region M41.46
    lumbosacral region M41.47

Scoliosis — *continued*
  neuromuscular — *continued*
    occipito-atlanto-axial region M41.41
    thoracic region M41.44
    thoracolumbar region M41.45
  paralytic — *see* Scoliosis, neuromuscular
  postradiation therapy M96.5
  rachitic (late effect or sequelae) E64.3 *[M49.80]*
    cervical region E64.3 *[M49.82]*
    cervicothoracic region E64.3 *[M49.83]*
    lumbar region E64.3 *[M49.86]*
    lumbosacral region E64.3 *[M49.87]*
    multiple sites E64.3 *[M49.89]*
    occipito-atlanto-axial region E64.3 *[M49.81]*
    sacrococcygeal region E64.3 *[M49.88]*
    thoracic region E64.3 *[M49.84]*
    thoracolumbar region E64.3 *[M49.85]*
  sciatic M54.4- ☑
  secondary (to) NEC M41.50
    cerebral palsy, Friedreich's ataxia, poliomyelitis, neuromuscular disorders — *see* Scoliosis, neuromuscular
    cervical region M41.52
    cervicothoracic region M41.53
    lumbar region M41.56
    lumbosacral region M41.57
    thoracic region M41.54
    thoracolumbar region M41.55
  specified form NEC M41.80
    cervical region M41.82
    cervicothoracic region M41.83
    lumbar region M41.86
    lumbosacral region M41.87
    thoracic region M41.84
    thoracolumbar region M41.85
  thoracogenic M41.30
    thoracic region M41.34
    thoracolumbar region M41.35
  tuberculous A18.01
Scoliotic pelvis
  with disproportion (fetopelvic) O33.0
    causing obstructed labor O65.0
Scorbutus, scorbutic — *see also* Scurvy
  anemia D53.2
Score, NIHSS (National Institutes of Health Stroke Scale) R29.7- ☑
Scotoma (arcuate) (Bjerrum) (central) (ring) — *see also* Defect, visual field, localized, scotoma
  scintillating H53.19
Scratch — *see* Abrasion
Scratchy throat R09.89
Screening (for) Z13.9
  alcoholism Z13.39
  anemia Z13.0
  anomaly, congenital Z13.89
  antenatal, of mother — *see also* Encounter, antenatal screening Z36.9
  arterial hypertension Z13.6
  arthropod-borne viral disease NEC Z11.59
  autism Z13.41
  bacteriuria, asymptomatic Z13.89
  behavioral disorder Z13.30
    specified NEC Z13.39
  brain injury, traumatic Z13.850
  bronchitis, chronic Z13.83
  brucellosis Z11.2
  cardiovascular disorder Z13.6
  cataract Z13.5
  chlamydial diseases Z11.8
  cholera Z11.0
  chromosomal abnormalities (nonprocreative) NEC Z13.79
  colonoscopy Z12.11
  congenital
    dislocation of hip Z13.89
    eye disorder Z13.5
    malformation or deformation Z13.89
  contamination NEC Z13.88
  coronavirus (disease) (novel) 2019 Z11.52
  COVID-19 Z11.52
  cystic fibrosis Z13.228
  dengue fever Z11.59
  dental disorder Z13.84
  depression (adult) (adolescent) (child) Z13.31
    maternal Z13.32
    perinatal Z13.32
  developmental
    delays Z13.40

Screening — *continued*
  developmental — *continued*
    delays — *continued*
      global (milestones) Z13.42
      specified NEC Z13.49
    handicap Z13.42
    in early childhood Z13.42
  diabetes mellitus Z13.1
  diphtheria Z11.2
  disability, intellectual Z13.39
  disease or disorder Z13.9
    bacterial NEC Z11.2
      intestinal infectious Z11.0
      respiratory tuberculosis Z11.1
    behavioral Z13.30
      specified NEC Z13.39
    blood or blood-forming organ Z13.0
    cardiovascular Z13.6
    Chagas' Z11.6
    chlamydial Z11.8
    coronavirus (novel) 2019 Z11.52
    COVID-19 Z11.52
    dental Z13.89
    developmental delays Z13.40
      global (milestones) Z13.42
      specified NEC Z13.49
    digestive tract NEC Z13.818
      lower GI Z13.811
      upper GI Z13.810
    ear Z13.5
    endocrine Z13.29
    eye Z13.5
    genitourinary Z13.89
    heart Z13.6
    human immunodeficiency virus (HIV) infection Z11.4
    immunity Z13.0
    infection
      intestinal Z11.0
        specified NEC Z11.6
    infectious Z11.9
    mental health and behavioral Z13.30
      specified NEC Z13.39
    metabolic Z13.228
    neurological Z13.89
    nutritional Z13.21
      metabolic Z13.228
        lipoid disorders Z13.220
    protozoal Z11.6
      intestinal Z11.0
    respiratory Z13.83
    rheumatic Z13.828
    rickettsial Z11.8
    sexually-transmitted NEC Z11.3
      human immunodeficiency virus (HIV) Z11.4
    sickle-cell (trait) Z13.0
    skin Z13.89
    specified NEC Z13.89
    spirochetal Z11.8
    thyroid Z13.29
    vascular Z13.6
    venereal Z11.3
    viral NEC Z11.59
      coronavirus (novel) 2019 Z11.52
      COVID-19 Z11.52
      human immunodeficiency virus (HIV) Z11.4
      intestinal Z11.0
      SARS-CoV-2 Z11.52
  elevated titer Z13.89
  emphysema Z13.83
  encephalitis, viral (mosquito- or tick-borne) Z11.59
  exposure to contaminants (toxic) Z13.88
  fever
    dengue Z11.59
    hemorrhagic Z11.59
    yellow Z11.59
  filariasis Z11.6
  galactosemia Z13.228
  gastrointestinal condition Z13.818
  genetic (nonprocreative) for procreative management — *see* Testing, genetic, for procreative management
    disease carrier status (nonprocreative) Z13.71
    specified NEC (nonprocreative) Z13.79
  genitourinary condition Z13.89
  glaucoma Z13.5
  gonorrhea Z11.3
  gout Z13.89
  helminthiasis (intestinal) Z11.6
  hematopoietic malignancy Z12.89

☑ **Additional Character Required** — Refer to the Tabular List for Character Selection   ▽ Subterms under main terms may continue to next column or page

Screening — *continued*
 hemoglobinopathies NEC Z13.0
 hemorrhagic fever Z11.59
 Hodgkin disease Z12.89
 human immunodeficiency virus (HIV) Z11.4
 human papillomavirus Z11.51
 hypertension Z13.6
 immunity disorders Z13.0
 infant or child (over 28 days old) Z00.129
  with abnormal findings Z00.121
 infection
  mycotic Z11.8
  parasitic Z11.8
 ingestion of radioactive substance Z13.88
 intellectual disability Z13.39
 intestinal
  helminthiasis Z11.6
  infectious disease Z11.0
 leishmaniasis Z11.6
 leprosy Z11.2
 leptospirosis Z11.8
 leukemia Z12.89
 lymphoma Z12.89
 malaria Z11.6
 malnutrition Z13.29
  metabolic Z13.228
  nutritional Z13.21
 measles Z11.59
 mental health disorder Z13.30
  specified NEC Z13.39
 metabolic errors, inborn Z13.228
 multiphasic Z13.89
 musculoskeletal disorder Z13.828
  osteoporosis Z13.820
 mycoses Z11.8
 myocardial infarction (acute) Z13.6
 neoplasm (malignant) (of) Z12.9
  bladder Z12.6
  blood Z12.89
  breast Z12.39
   routine mammogram Z12.31
  cervix Z12.4
  colon Z12.11
  genitourinary organs NEC Z12.79
   bladder Z12.6
   cervix Z12.4
   ovary Z12.73
   prostate Z12.5
   testis Z12.71
   vagina Z12.72
  hematopoietic system Z12.89
  intestinal tract Z12.10
   colon Z12.11
   rectum Z12.12
   small intestine Z12.13
  lung Z12.2
  lymph (glands) Z12.89
  nervous system Z12.82
  oral cavity Z12.81
  prostate Z12.5
  rectum Z12.12
  respiratory organs Z12.2
  skin Z12.83
  small intestine Z12.13
  specified site NEC Z12.89
  stomach Z12.0
 nephropathy Z13.89
 nervous system disorders NEC Z13.858
 neurological condition Z13.89
 osteoporosis Z13.820
 parasitic infestation Z11.9
  specified NEC Z11.8
 phenylketonuria Z13.228
 plague Z11.2
 poisoning (chemical) (heavy metal) Z13.88
 poliomyelitis Z11.59
 postnatal, chromosomal abnormalities Z13.89
 prenatal, of mother — *see also* Encounter, antenatal
   screening Z36.9
 protozoal disease Z11.6
  intestinal Z11.0
 pulmonary tuberculosis Z11.1
 radiation exposure Z13.88
 respiratory condition Z13.83
 respiratory tuberculosis Z11.1
 rheumatoid arthritis Z13.828
 rubella Z11.59
 SARS-CoV-2 Z11.52
 schistosomiasis Z11.6

Screening — *continued*
 sexually-transmitted disease NEC Z11.3
  human immunodeficiency virus (HIV) Z11.4
 sickle-cell disease or trait Z13.0
 skin condition Z13.89
 sleeping sickness Z11.6
 special Z13.9
  specified NEC Z13.89
 syphilis Z11.3
 tetanus Z11.2
 trachoma Z11.8
 traumatic brain injury Z13.850
 trypanosomiasis Z11.6
 tuberculosis, respiratory Z11.1
  active Z11.1
  latent Z11.7
 venereal disease Z11.3
 viral encephalitis (mosquito- or tick-borne) Z11.59
 whooping cough Z11.2
 worms, intestinal Z11.6
 yaws Z11.8
 yellow fever Z11.59
Scrofula, scrofulosis (tuberculosis of cervical lymph
   glands) A18.2
Scrofulide (primary) (tuberculous) A18.4
Scrofuloderma, scrofulodermia (any site) (primary)
   A18.4
Scrofulosus lichen (primary) (tuberculous) A18.4
Scrofulous — *see* condition
Scrotal tongue K14.5
Scrotum — *see* condition
Scurvy, scorbutic E54
 anemia D53.2
 gum E54
 infantile E54
 rickets E55.0 *[M90.80]*
Sealpox B08.62
Seasickness T75.3 ☑
Seatworm (infection) (infestation) B80
Sebaceous — *see also* condition
 cyst — *see* Cyst, sebaceous
Seborrhea, seborrheic L21.9
 capillitii R23.8
 capitis L21.0
 dermatitis L21.9
  infantile L21.1
 eczema L21.9
  infantile L21.1
 sicca L21.0
Seckel's syndrome Q87.19
Seclusion, pupil — *see* Membrane, pupillary
Second hand tobacco smoke exposure (acute)
   (chronic) Z77.22
 in the perinatal period P96.81
Secondary
 dentin (in pulp) K04.3
 neoplasm, secondaries — *see* Table of Neoplasms,
   secondary
Secretion
 antidiuretic hormone, inappropriate E22.2
 catecholamine, by pheochromocytoma E27.5
 hormone
  antidiuretic, inappropriate (syndrome) E22.2
  by
   carcinoid tumor E34.0
    pheochromocytoma E27.5
  ectopic NEC E34.2
 urinary
  excessive R35.89
  suppression R34
Section
 nerve, traumatic — *see* Injury, nerve
Sedative, hypnotic, or anxiolytic-induced
 anxiety disorder F13.980
 bipolar and related disorder F13.94
 delirium F13.921
 depressive disorder F13.94
 major neurocognitive disorder F13.97
 mild neurocognitive disorder F13.988
 psychotic disorder F13.959
 sexual dysfunction F13.981
 sleep disorder F13.982
Segmentation, incomplete (congenital) — *see also*
   Fusion
 bone NEC Q78.8
 lumbosacral (joint) (vertebra) Q76.49
Seitelberger's syndrome (infantile neuraxonal dystrophy) G31.89

Seizure(s) — *see also* Convulsions R56.9
 absence G40.A- ☑ (*following* G40.3)
 akinetic — *see* Epilepsy, generalized, specified NEC
 atonic — *see* Epilepsy, generalized, specified NEC
 autonomic (hysterical) F44.5
 convulsive — *see* Convulsions
 cortical (focal) (motor) — *see* Epilepsy, localization-related, symptomatic, with simple partial seizures
 disorder — *see also* Epilepsy G40.909
 due to stroke — *see* Sequelae (of), disease, cerebrovascular, by type, specified NEC
 epileptic — *see* Epilepsy
 febrile (simple) R56.00
  with status epilepticus G40.901
  complex (atypical) (complicated) R56.01
   with status epilepticus G40.901
 grand mal G40.409
  intractable G40.419
   with status epilepticus G40.411
   without status epilepticus G40.419
  not intractable G40.409
   with status epilepticus G40.401
   without status epilepticus G40.409
 heart — *see* Disease, heart
 hysterical F44.5
 intractable G40.919
  with status epilepticus G40.911
 Jacksonian (focal) (motor type) (sensory type) — *see*
   Epilepsy, localization-related, symptomatic, with
   simple partial seizures
 newborn P90
 nonspecific epileptic
  atonic — *see* Epilepsy, generalized, specified NEC
  clonic — *see* Epilepsy, generalized, specified NEC
  myoclonic — *see* Epilepsy, generalized, specified
    NEC
  tonic — *see* Epilepsy, generalized, specified NEC
  tonic-clonic — *see* Epilepsy, generalized, specified
    NEC
 partial, developing into secondarily generalized
   seizures
  complex — *see* Epilepsy, localization-related,
    symptomatic, with complex partial seizures
  simple — *see* Epilepsy, localization-related, symp-
    tomatic, with simple partial seizures
 petit mal G40.A- ☑ (*following* G40.3)
  intractable G40.A1- ☑ (*following* G40.3)
   with status epilepticus G40.A11 (*following* G40.3)
   without status epilepticus G40.A19 (*following*
     G40.3)
  not intractable G40.A0- ☑ (*following* G40.3)
   with status epilepticus G40.A01 (*following* G40.3)
   without status epilepticus G40.A09 (*following*
     G40.3)
 post traumatic R56.1
 recurrent G40.909
 specified NEC G40.89
 uncinate — *see* Epilepsy, localization-related, symptomatic, with complex partial seizures
Selenium deficiency, dietary E59
Self-damaging behavior (life-style) Z72.89
Self-harm (attempted)
 history (personal)
  in family Z81.8
  nonsuicidal Z91.52
  suicidal Z91.51
 nonsuicidal R45.88
Self-injury, nonsuicidal R45.88
 personal history Z91.52
Self-mutilation (attempted)
 history (personal)
  in family Z81.8
  nonsuicidal Z91.52
  suicidal Z91.51
 nonsuicidal R45.88
Self-poisoning
 history (personal) Z91.51
  in family Z81.8
 observation following (alleged) attempt Z03.6
Semicoma R40.1
Seminal vesiculitis N49.0
Seminoma C62.9- ☑
 specified site — *see* Neoplasm, malignant, by site
Senear-Usher disease or syndrome L10.4
Senectus R54
Senescence (without mention of psychosis) R54
Senile, senility — *see also* condition R41.81

Senile, senility — *continued*
  with
    acute confusional state F05
      mental changes NOS F03 ☑
      psychosis NEC — *see* Psychosis, senile
  asthenia R54
  cervix (atrophic) N88.8
  debility R54
  endometrium (atrophic) N85.8
  fallopian tube (atrophic) — *see* Atrophy, fallopian tube
  heart (failure) R54
  ovary (atrophic) — *see* Atrophy, ovary
  premature E34.8
  vagina, vaginitis (atrophic) N95.2
  wart L82.1

Sensation
  burning (skin) R20.8
    tongue K14.6
  loss of R20.8
  prickling (skin) R20.2
  tingling (skin) R20.2

Sense loss
  smell — *see* Disturbance, sensation, smell
  taste — *see* Disturbance, sensation, taste
  touch R20.8

Sensibility disturbance (cortical) (deep) (vibratory) R20.9

Sensitive, sensitivity — *see also* Allergy
  carotid sinus G90.01
  child (excessive) F93.8
  cold, autoimmune D59.12
  dentin K03.89
  gluten (non-celiac) K90.41
  latex Z91.040
  methemoglobin D74.8
  tuberculin, without clinical or radiological symptoms
    R76.11
  visual
    glare H53.71
    impaired contrast H53.72

Sensitiver Beziehungswahn F22

Sensitization, auto-erythrocytic D69.2

Separation
  anxiety, abnormal (of childhood) F93.0
  apophysis, traumatic — *code as* Fracture, by site
  choroid — *see* Detachment, choroid
  epiphysis, epiphyseal
    nontraumatic — *see also* Osteochondropathy,
      specified type NEC
      upper femoral — *see* Slipped, epiphysis, upper
        femoral
    traumatic — *code as* Fracture, by site
  fracture — *see* Fracture
  infundibulum cardiac from right ventricle by a partition
    Q24.3
  joint (traumatic) (current) — *code by* site under Dislo-
    cation
  muscle (nontraumatic) — *see* Diastasis, muscle
  pubic bone, obstetrical trauma O71.6
  retina, retinal — *see* Detachment, retina
  symphysis pubis, obstetrical trauma O71.6
  tracheal ring, incomplete, congenital Q32.1

Sepsis (generalized) (unspecified organism) A41.9
  with
    organ dysfunction (acute) (multiple) R65.20
      with septic shock R65.21
  actinomycotic A42.7
  adrenal hemorrhage syndrome (meningococcal) A39.1
  anaerobic A41.4
  Bacillus anthracis A22.7
  Brucella — *see also* Brucellosis A23.9
  candidal B37.7
  cryptogenic A41.9
  due to device, implant or graft T85.79 ☑
    arterial graft NEC T82.7 ☑
    breast (implant) T85.79 ☑
    catheter NEC T85.79 ☑
      dialysis (renal) T82.7 ☑
        intraperitoneal T85.71 ☑
      infusion NEC T82.7 ☑
        spinal (cranial) (epidural) (intrathecal) (spinal)
          (subarachnoid) (subdural) T85.735 ☑
      urethral indwelling T83.511 ☑
      urinary T83.518 ☑
    ectopic or molar pregnancy O08.82
    electronic (electrode) (pulse generator) (stimulator)
      bone T84.7 ☑
      cardiac T82.7 ☑

Sepsis — *continued*
  due to device, implant or graft — *continued*
    electronic — *continued*
      nervous system T85.738 ☑
        brain T85.731 ☑
        neurostimulator generator T85.734 ☑
        peripheral nerve T85.732 ☑
        spinal cord T85.733 ☑
      urinary T83.590 ☑
    fixation, internal (orthopedic) — *see* Complication,
      fixation device, infection
    gastrointestinal (bile duct) (esophagus) T85.79 ☑
      neurostimulator electrode (lead) T85.732 ☑
    genital T83.69 ☑
    heart NEC T82.7 ☑
      valve (prosthesis) T82.6 ☑
        graft T82.7 ☑
    joint prosthesis — *see* Complication, joint prosthe-
      sis, infection
    ocular (corneal graft) (orbital implant) T85.79 ☑
    orthopedic NEC T84.7 ☑
      fixation device, internal — *see* Complication,
        fixation device, infection
    specified NEC T85.79 ☑
    vascular T82.7 ☑
    ventricular intracranial (communicating) shunt
      T85.730 ☑
  during labor O75.3
  Enterococcus A41.81
  Erysipelothrix (rhusiopathiae) (erysipeloid) A26.7
  Escherichia coli (E. coli) A41.5 ☑
  extraintestinal yersiniosis A28.2
  following
    abortion (subsequent episode) O08.0
      current episode — *see* Abortion
    ectopic or molar pregnancy O08.82
    immunization T88.0 ☑
    infusion, therapeutic injection or transfusion NEC
      T80.29 ☑
    obstetrical procedure O86.04
  gangrenous A41.9
  gonococcal A54.86
  Gram-negative (organism) A41.5 ☑
    anaerobic A41.4
  Haemophilus influenzae A41.3
  herpesviral B00.7
  intra-abdominal K65.1
  intraocular — *see* Endophthalmitis, purulent
  Listeria monocytogenes A32.7
  localized — *code to* specific localized infection
    in operation wound T81.49 ☑
    skin — *see* Abscess
  malleus A24.0
  melioidosis A24.1
  meningeal — *see* Meningitis
  meningococcal A39.4
    acute A39.2
    chronic A39.3
  MSSA (Methicillin susceptible Staphylococcus aureus)
    A41.01
  newborn P36.9
    due to
      anaerobes NEC P36.5
      Escherichia coli P36.4
      Staphylococcus P36.30
        aureus P36.2
        specified NEC P36.39
      Streptococcus P36.10
        group B P36.0
        specified NEC P36.19
    specified NEC P36.8
  Pasteurella multocida A28.0
  pelvic, puerperal, postpartum, childbirth O85
  pneumococcal A40.3
  postprocedural T81.44 ☑
  puerperal, postpartum, childbirth (pelvic) O85
  Salmonella (arizonae) (cholerae-suis) (enteritidis) (ty-
    phimurium) A02.1
  severe R65.20
    with septic shock R65.21
  Shigella — *see also* Dysentery, bacillary A03.9
  skin, localized — *see* Abscess
  specified organism NEC A41.89
  Staphylococcus, staphylococcal A41.2
    aureus (methicillin susceptible) (MSSA) A41.01
      methicillin resistant (MRSA) A41.02
    coagulase-negative A41.1

Sepsis — *continued*
  Staphylococcus, staphylococcal — *continued*
    specified NEC A41.1
  Streptococcus, streptococcal A40.9
    agalactiae A40.1
    group
      A A40.0
      B A40.1
      D A41.81
    neonatal P36.10
      group B P36.0
      specified NEC P36.19
    pneumoniae A40.3
    pyogenes A40.0
    specified NEC A40.8
  tracheostomy stoma J95.02
  tularemic A21.7
  umbilical, umbilical cord (newborn) — *see* Sepsis,
    newborn
  Yersinia pestis A20.7

Septate — *see* Septum

Septic — *see* condition
  arm — *see* Cellulitis, upper limb
    with lymphangitis — *see* Lymphangitis, acute, upper
      limb
  embolus — *see* Embolism
  finger — *see* Cellulitis, digit
    with lymphangitis — *see* Lymphangitis, acute, digit
  foot — *see* Cellulitis, lower limb
    with lymphangitis — *see* Lymphangitis, acute,
      lower limb
  gallbladder (acute) K81.0
  hand — *see* Cellulitis, upper limb
    with lymphangitis — *see* Lymphangitis, acute, upper
      limb
  joint — *see* Arthritis, pyogenic or pyemic
  leg — *see* Cellulitis, lower limb
    with lymphangitis — *see* Lymphangitis, acute,
      lower limb
  nail — *see also* Cellulitis, digit
    with lymphangitis — *see* Lymphangitis, acute, digit
  sore — *see also* Abscess
    throat J02.0
      streptococcal J02.0
  spleen (acute) D73.89
  teeth, tooth (pulpal origin) K04.4
  throat — *see* Pharyngitis
  thrombus — *see* Thrombosis
  toe — *see* Cellulitis, digit
    with lymphangitis — *see* Lymphangitis, acute, digit
  tonsils, chronic J35.01
    with adenoiditis J35.03
  uterus — *see* Endometritis

Septicemia A41.9
  meaning sepsis — *see* Sepsis

Septum, septate (congenital) — *see also* Anomaly, by
  site
  anal Q42.3
    with fistula Q42.2
  aqueduct of Sylvius Q03.0
    with spina bifida — *see* Spina bifida, by site, with
      hydrocephalus
  uterus Q51.28
    complete Q51.21
    partial Q51.22
    specified NEC Q51.28
  vagina Q52.10
    in pregnancy — *see* Pregnancy, complicated by,
      abnormal vagina
    causing obstructed labor O65.5
    longitudinal Q52.129
      microperforate
        left side Q52.124
        right side Q52.123
      nonobstruction Q52.120
      obstructing Q52.129
        left side Q52.122
        right side Q52.121
    transverse Q52.11

Sequelae (of) — *see also* condition
  abscess, intracranial or intraspinal (conditions in G06)
    G09
  amputation — *code to* injury with seventh character
    S
  burn and corrosion — *code to* injury with seventh
    character S
  calcium deficiency E64.8

☑ **Additional Character Required — Refer to the Tabular List for Character Selection**   ⬇ **Subterms under main terms may continue to next column or page**

Sequelae — *continued*
  cerebrovascular disease — *see* Sequelae, disease, cerebrovascular
  childbirth O94
  contusion — *code to* injury with seventh character S
  corrosion — *see* Sequelae, burn and corrosion
  COVID-19 (post acute) U09.9
  crushing injury — *code to* injury with seventh character S
  disease
    cerebrovascular I69.90
      alteration of sensation I69.998
      aphasia I69.920
      apraxia I69.990
      ataxia I69.993
      cognitive deficits I69.91 ☑
      disturbance of vision I69.998
      dysarthria I69.922
      dysphagia I69.991
      dysphasia I69.921
      facial droop I69.992
      facial weakness I69.992
      fluency disorder I69.923
      hemiplegia I69.95- ☑
      hemorrhage
        intracerebral — *see* Sequelae, hemorrhage, intracerebral
        intracranial, nontraumatic NEC — *see* Sequelae, hemorrhage, intracranial, nontraumatic
        subarachnoid — *see* Sequelae, hemorrhage, subarachnoid
      language deficit I69.928
      monoplegia
        lower limb I69.94- ☑
        upper limb I69.93- ☑
      paralytic syndrome I69.96- ☑
      specified effect NEC I69.998
      specified type NEC I69.80
        alteration of sensation I69.898
        aphasia I69.820
        apraxia I69.890
        ataxia I69.893
        cognitive deficits I69.81 ☑
        disturbance of vision I69.898
        dysarthria I69.822
        dysphagia I69.891
        dysphasia I69.821
        facial droop I69.892
        facial weakness I69.892
        fluency disorder I69.823
        hemiplegia I69.85- ☑
        language deficit I69.828
        monoplegia
          lower limb I69.84- ☑
          upper limb I69.83- ☑
        paralytic syndrome I69.86- ☑
        specified effect NEC I69.898
      speech deficit I69.928
        speech deficit I69.828
    stroke NOS — *see* Sequelae, stroke NOS
  dislocation — *code to* injury with seventh character S
  encephalitis or encephalomyelitis (conditions in G04) G09
    in infectious disease NEC B94.8
    viral B94.1
  external cause — *code to* injury with seventh character S
  foreign body entering natural orifice — *code to* injury with seventh character S
  fracture — *code to* injury with seventh character S
  frostbite — *code to* injury with seventh character S
  Hansen's disease B92
  hemorrhage
    intracerebral I69.10
      alteration of sensation I69.198
      aphasia I69.120
      apraxia I69.190
      ataxia I69.193
      cognitive deficits I69.11 ☑
      disturbance of vision I69.198
      dysarthria I69.122
      dysphagia I69.191
      dysphasia I69.121
      facial droop I69.192
      facial weakness I69.192
      fluency disorder I69.123
      hemiplegia I69.15- ☑

Sequelae — *continued*
  hemorrhage — *continued*
    intracerebral — *continued*
      language deficit NEC I69.128
      monoplegia
        lower limb I69.14- ☑
        upper limb I69.13- ☑
      paralytic syndrome I69.16- ☑
      specified effect NEC I69.198
      speech deficit NEC I69.128
    intracranial, nontraumatic NEC I69.20
      alteration of sensation I69.298
      aphasia I69.220
      apraxia I69.290
      ataxia I69.293
      cognitive deficits I69.21 ☑
      disturbance of vision I69.298
      dysarthria I69.222
      dysphagia I69.291
      dysphasia I69.221
      facial droop I69.292
      facial weakness I69.292
      fluency disorder I69.223
      hemiplegia I69.25- ☑
      language deficit NEC I69.228
      monoplegia
        lower limb I69.24- ☑
        upper limb I69.23- ☑
      paralytic syndrome I69.26- ☑
      specified effect NEC I69.298
      speech deficit NEC I69.228
    subarachnoid I69.00
      alteration of sensation I69.098
      aphasia I69.020
      apraxia I69.090
      ataxia I69.093
      cognitive deficits — *see* subcategory I69.01- ☑
      disturbance of vision I69.098
      dysarthria I69.022
      dysphagia I69.091
      dysphasia I69.021
      facial droop I69.092
      facial weakness I69.092
      fluency disorder I69.023
      hemiplegia I69.05- ☑
      language deficit NEC I69.028
      monoplegia
        lower limb I69.04- ☑
        upper limb I69.03- ☑
      paralytic syndrome I69.06- ☑
      specified effect NEC I69.098
      speech deficit NEC I69.028
  hepatitis, viral B94.2
  hyperalimentation E68
  infarction
    cerebral I69.30
      alteration of sensation I69.398
      aphasia I69.320
      apraxia I69.390
      ataxia I69.393
      cognitive deficits I69.31 ☑
      disturbance of vision I69.398
      dysarthria I69.322
      dysphagia I69.391
      dysphasia I69.321
      facial droop I69.392
      facial weakness I69.392
      fluency disorder I69.323
      hemiplegia I69.35- ☑
      language deficit NEC I69.328
      monoplegia
        lower limb I69.34- ☑
        upper limb I69.33- ☑
      paralytic syndrome I69.36- ☑
      specified effect NEC I69.398
      speech deficit NEC I69.328
  infection, pyogenic, intracranial or intraspinal G09
  infectious disease B94.9
    specified NEC B94.8
  injury — *code to* injury with seventh character S
  leprosy B92
  meningitis
    bacterial (conditions in G00) G09
    other or unspecified cause (conditions in G03) G09
  muscle (and tendon) injury — *code to* injury with seventh character S
  myelitis — *see* Sequelae, encephalitis
  niacin deficiency E64.8

Sequelae — *continued*
  nutritional deficiency E64.9
    specified NEC E64.8
  obstetrical condition O94
  parasitic disease B94.9
  phlebitis or thrombophlebitis of intracranial or intraspinal venous sinuses and veins (conditions in G08) G09
  poisoning — *code to* poisoning with seventh character S
    nonmedicinal substance — *see* Sequelae, toxic effect, nonmedicinal substance
  poliomyelitis (acute) B91
  pregnancy O94
  protein-energy malnutrition E64.0
  puerperium O94
  rickets E64.3
  SARS-CoV-2 (post acute) U09.9
  selenium deficiency E64.8
  sprain and strain — *code to* injury with seventh character S
  stroke NOS I69.30
    alteration in sensation I69.398
    aphasia I69.320
    apraxia I69.390
    ataxia I69.393
    cognitive deficits I69.31 ☑
    disturbance of vision I69.398
    dysarthria I69.322
    dysphagia I69.391
    dysphasia I69.321
    facial droop I69.392
    facial weakness I69.392
    hemiplegia I69.35- ☑
    language deficit NEC I69.328
    monoplegia
      lower limb I69.34- ☑
      upper limb I69.33- ☑
    paralytic syndrome I69.36- ☑
    specified effect NEC I69.398
    speech deficit NEC I69.328
  tendon and muscle injury — *code to* injury with seventh character S
  thiamine deficiency E64.8
  trachoma B94.0
  tuberculosis B90.9
    bones and joints B90.2
    central nervous system B90.0
    genitourinary B90.1
    pulmonary (respiratory) B90.9
    specified organs NEC B90.8
  viral
    encephalitis B94.1
    hepatitis B94.2
  vitamin deficiency NEC E64.8
    A E64.1
    B E64.8
    C E64.2
  wound, open — *code to* injury with seventh character S

Sequestration — *see also* Sequestrum
  disc — *see* Displacement, intervertebral disc
  lung, congenital Q33.2

Sequestrum
  bone — *see* Osteomyelitis, chronic
  dental M27.2
  jaw bone M27.2
  orbit — *see* Osteomyelitis, orbit
  sinus (accessory) (nasal) — *see* Sinusitis

Sequoiosis lung or pneumonitis J67.8

Serology for syphilis
  doubtful
    with signs or symptoms — *code by* site and stage under Syphilis
    follow-up of latent syphilis — *see* Syphilis, latent
  negative, with signs or symptoms — *code by* site and stage under Syphilis
  positive A53.0
    with signs or symptoms — *code by* site and stage under Syphilis
  reactivated A53.0

Seroma — *see also* Hematoma
  postprocedural — *see* Complication, postprocedural, seroma
  traumatic, secondary and recurrent T79.2 ☑

Seropurulent — *see* condition

Serositis, multiple K65.8
  pericardial I31.1

Serositis, multiple — *continued*
  peritoneal K65.8
Serous — *see* condition
Sertoli cell
  adenoma
    specified site — *see* Neoplasm, benign, by site
    unspecified site
      female D27.9
      male D29.20
  carcinoma
    specified site — *see* Neoplasm, malignant, by site
    unspecified site (male) C62.9- ☑
      female C56.9
  tumor
    with lipid storage
      specified site — *see* Neoplasm, benign, by site
      unspecified site
        female D27.9
        male D29.20
    specified site — *see* Neoplasm, benign, by site
    unspecified site
      female D27.9
      male D29.20
Sertoli-Leydig cell tumor — *see* Neoplasm, benign, by site
  specified site — *see* Neoplasm, benign, by site
  unspecified site
    female D27.9
    male D29.20
Serum
  allergy, allergic reaction — *see also* Reaction, serum T80.69 ☑
    shock — *see also* Shock, anaphylactic T80.59 ☑
  arthritis — *see also* Reaction, serum T80.69 ☑
  complication or reaction NEC — *see also* Reaction, serum T80.69 ☑
  disease NEC — *see also* Reaction, serum T80.69 ☑
  hepatitis — *see also* Hepatitis, viral, type B
    carrier (suspected) of B18.1
  intoxication — *see also* Reaction, serum T80.69 ☑
  neuritis — *see also* Reaction, serum T80.69 ☑
  neuropathy G61.1
  poisoning NEC — *see also* Reaction, serum T80.69 ☑
  rash NEC — *see also* Reaction, serum T80.69 ☑
  reaction NEC — *see also* Reaction, serum T80.69 ☑
  sickness NEC — *see also* Reaction, serum T80.69 ☑
  urticaria — *see also* Reaction, serum T80.69 ☑
Sesamoiditis M25.8- ☑
Severe sepsis R65.20
  with septic shock R65.21
Sever's disease or osteochondrosis — *see* Osteochondrosis, juvenile, tarsus
Sex
  chromosome mosaics Q97.8
    lines with various numbers of X chromosomes Q97.2
  education Z70.8
  reassignment surgery status Z87.890
Sextuplet pregnancy — *see* Pregnancy, sextuplet
Sexual
  function, disorder of (psychogenic) F52.9
  immaturity (female) (male) E30.0
  impotence (psychogenic) organic origin NEC — *see* Dysfunction, sexual, male
  precocity (constitutional) (cryptogenic)(female) (idiopathic) (male) E30.1
Sexuality, pathologic — *see* Deviation, sexual
Sézary disease C84.1- ☑
Shadow, lung R91.8
Shaking palsy or paralysis — *see* Parkinsonism
Shallowness, acetabulum — *see* Derangement, joint, specified type NEC, hip
Shaver's disease J63.1
Sheath (tendon) — *see* condition
Sheathing, retinal vessels H35.01- ☑
Shedding
  nail L60.8
  premature, primary (deciduous) teeth K00.6
Sheehan's disease or syndrome E23.0
Shelf, rectal K62.89
Shell teeth K00.5
Shellshock (current) F43.0
  lasting state — *see* Disorder, post-traumatic stress
Shield kidney Q63.1
Shift
  auditory threshold (temporary) H93.24- ☑
  mediastinal R93.89
Shifting sleep-work schedule (affecting sleep) G47.26

Shiga (-Kruse) **dysentery** A03.0
Shiga's bacillus A03.0
Shigella (dysentery) — *see* Dysentery, bacillary
Shigellosis A03.9
  Group A A03.0
  Group B A03.1
  Group C A03.2
  Group D A03.3
Shin splints S86.89- ☑
Shingles — *see* Herpes, zoster
Shipyard disease or eye B30.0
Shirodkar suture, in pregnancy — *see* Pregnancy, complicated by, incompetent cervix
Shock R57.9
  with ectopic or molar pregnancy O08.3
  adrenal (cortical) (Addisonian) E27.2
  adverse food reaction (anaphylactic) — *see* Shock, anaphylactic, due to food
  allergic — *see* Shock, anaphylactic
  anaphylactic T78.2 ☑
    chemical — *see* Table of Drugs and Chemicals
    due to drug or medicinal substance
      correct substance properly administered T88.6 ☑
      overdose or wrong substance given or taken (by accident) — *see* Table of Drugs and Chemicals, by drug, poisoning
    due to food (nonpoisonous) T78.00 ☑
      additives T78.06 ☑
      dairy products T78.07 ☑
      eggs T78.08 ☑
      fish T78.03 ☑
        shellfish T78.02 ☑
      fruit T78.04 ☑
      milk T78.07 ☑
      nuts T78.05 ☑
        multiple types T78.05 ☑
        peanuts T78.01 ☑
      peanuts T78.01 ☑
      seeds T78.05 ☑
      specified type NEC T78.09 ☑
      vegetable T78.04 ☑
    following sting(s) — *see* Venom
    immunization T80.52 ☑
    serum T80.59 ☑
      blood and blood products T80.51 ☑
      immunization T80.52 ☑
      specified NEC T80.59 ☑
      vaccination T80.52 ☑
  anaphylactoid — *see* Shock, anaphylactic
  anesthetic
    correct substance properly administered T88.2 ☑
    overdose or wrong substance given or taken — *see* Table of Drugs and Chemicals, by drug, poisoning
    specified anesthetic — *see* Table of Drugs and Chemicals, by drug, poisoning
  cardiogenic R57.0
  chemical substance — *see* Table of Drugs and Chemicals
  complicating ectopic or molar pregnancy O08.3
  culture — *see* Disorder, adjustment
  drug
    due to correct substance properly administered T88.6
    overdose or wrong substance given or taken (by accident) — *see* Table of Drugs and Chemicals, by drug, poisoning
  during or after labor and delivery O75.1
  electric T75.4 ☑
    (taser) T75.4 ☑
  endotoxic R65.21
    postprocedural (resulting from a procedure, not elsewhere classified) T81.12 ☑
  following
    ectopic or molar pregnancy O08.3
    injury (immediate) (delayed) T79.4 ☑
    labor and delivery O75.1
  food (anaphylactic) — *see* Shock, anaphylactic, due to food
  from electroshock gun (taser) T75.4 ☑
  gram-negative R65.21
    postprocedural (resulting from a procedure, not elsewhere classified) T81.12 ☑
  hematologic R57.8
  hemorrhagic R57.8
    surgery (intraoperative) (postoperative) T81.19 ☑
    trauma T79.4 ☑

Shock — *continued*
  hypovolemic R57.1
    surgical T81.19 ☑
    traumatic T79.4 ☑
  insulin E15
    therapeutic misadventure — *see* subcategory T38.3 ☑
  kidney N17.0
    traumatic (following crushing) T79.5 ☑
  lightning T75.01 ☑
  liver K72.00
  lung J80
  obstetric O75.1
    with ectopic or molar pregnancy O08.3
    following ectopic or molar pregnancy O08.3
  pleural (surgical) T81.19 ☑
    due to trauma T79.4 ☑
  postprocedural (postoperative) T81.10 ☑
    with ectopic or molar pregnancy O08.3
    cardiogenic T81.11 ☑
    endotoxic T81.12 ☑
    following ectopic or molar pregnancy O08.3
    gram-negative T81.12 ☑
    hypovolemic T81.19 ☑
    septic T81.12 ☑
    specified type NEC T81.19 ☑
  psychic F43.0
  septic (due to severe sepsis) R65.21
  specified NEC R57.8
  surgical T81.10 ☑
  taser gun (taser) T75.4 ☑
  therapeutic misadventure NEC T81.10 ☑
  thyroxin
    overdose or wrong substance given or taken — *see* Table of Drugs and Chemicals, by drug, poisoning
  toxic, syndrome A48.3
  transfusion — *see* Complications, transfusion
  traumatic (immediate) (delayed) T79.4 ☑
Shoemaker's chest M95.4
Short, shortening, shortness
  arm (acquired) — *see also* Deformity, limb, unequal length
    congenital Q71.81- ☑
    forearm — *see* Deformity, limb, unequal length
  bowel syndrome K91.2
  breath R06.02
  cervical (complicating pregnancy) O26.87- ☑
    non-gravid uterus N88.3
  common bile duct, congenital Q44.5
  cord (umbilical), complicating delivery O69.3 ☑
  cystic duct, congenital Q44.5
  esophagus (congenital) Q39.8
  femur (acquired) — *see* Deformity, limb, unequal length, femur
    congenital — *see* Defect, reduction, lower limb, longitudinal, femur
  frenum, frenulum, linguae (congenital) Q38.1
  hip (acquired) — *see also* Deformity, limb, unequal length
    congenital Q65.89
  leg (acquired) — *see also* Deformity, limb, unequal length
    congenital Q72.81- ☑
    lower leg — *see also* Deformity, limb, unequal length
  limbed stature, with immunodeficiency D82.2
  lower limb (acquired) — *see also* Deformity, limb, unequal length
    congenital Q72.81- ☑
  organ or site, congenital NEC — *see* Distortion
  palate, congenital Q38.5
  radius (acquired) — *see also* Deformity, limb, unequal length
    congenital — *see* Defect, reduction, upper limb, longitudinal, radius
  rib syndrome Q77.2
  stature (child) (hereditary) (idiopathic) NEC R62.52
    constitutional E34.3
    due to endocrine disorder E34.3
    Laron-type E34.3
  tendon — *see also* Contraction, tendon
    with contracture of joint — *see* Contraction, joint
    Achilles (acquired) M67.0- ☑
      congenital Q66.89
    congenital Q79.8

Short, shortening, shortness — *continued*
thigh (acquired) — *see also* Deformity, limb, unequal
  length, femur
  congenital — *see* Defect, reduction, lower limb,
    longitudinal, femur
tibialis anterior (tendon) — *see* Contraction, tendon
umbilical cord
  complicating delivery O69.3 ☑
upper limb, congenital — *see* Defect, reduction, upper
  limb, specified type NEC
urethra N36.8
uvula, congenital Q38.5
vagina (congenital) Q52.4
Shortsightedness — *see* Myopia
Shoshin (acute fulminating beriberi) E51.11
Shoulder — *see* condition
Shovel-shaped incisors K00.2
Shower, thromboembolic — *see* Embolism
Shunt
arterial-venous (dialysis) Z99.2
arteriovenous, pulmonary (acquired) I28.0
  congenital Q25.72
cerebral ventricle (communicating) in situ Z98.2
surgical, prosthetic, with complications — *see* Compli-
  cations, cardiovascular, device or implant
Shutdown, renal N28.9
Shy-Drager syndrome G90.3
Sialadenitis, sialadenosis (any gland) (chronic) (period-
  ic) (suppurative) — *see* Sialoadenitis
Sialectasia K11.8
Sialidosis E77.1
Sialitis, silitis (any gland) (chronic) (suppurative) — *see*
  Sialoadenitis
Sialoadenitis (any gland) (periodic) (suppurative) K11.20
acute K11.21
  recurrent K11.22
chronic K11.23
Sialoadenopathy K11.9
Sialoangitis — *see* Sialoadenitis
Sialodochitis (fibrinosa) — *see* Sialoadenitis
Sialodocholithiasis K11.5
Sialolithiasis K11.5
Sialometaplasia, necrotizing K11.8
Sialorrhea — *see also* Ptyalism
periodic — *see* Sialoadenitis
Sialosis K11.7
Siamese twin Q89.4
Sibling rivalry Z62.891
Sicard's syndrome G52.7
Sicca syndrome — *see* Syndrome, Sjögren
Sick R69
or handicapped person in family Z63.79
  needing care at home Z63.6
sinus (syndrome) I49.5
Sick-euthyroid syndrome E07.81
Sickle-cell
anemia — *see* Disease, sickle-cell
beta plus — *see* Disease, sickle-cell, thalassemia, beta
  plus
beta zero — *see* Disease, sickle-cell, thalassemia, beta
  zero
trait D57.3
Sicklemia — *see also* Disease, sickle-cell
trait D57.3
Sickness
air (travel) T75.3 ☑
airplane T75.3 ☑
alpine T70.29 ☑
altitude T70.20 ☑
Andes T70.29 ☑
altitude T70.20 ☑
aviator's T70.29 ☑
balloon T70.29 ☑
car T75.3 ☑
compressed air T70.3 ☑
decompression T70.3 ☑
green D50.8
milk — *see* Poisoning, food, noxious
motion T75.3 ☑
mountain T70.29 ☑
  acute D75.1
protein — *see also* Reaction, serum T80.69 ☑
radiation T66 ☑
roundabout (motion) T75.3 ☑
sea T75.3 ☑
serum NEC — *see also* Reaction, serum T80.69 ☑
sleeping (African) B56.9
  by Trypanosoma B56.9

Sickness — *continued*
sleeping — *continued*
  by Trypanosoma — *continued*
    brucei
      gambiense B56.0
      rhodesiense B56.1
    East African B56.1
    Gambian B56.0
    Rhodesian B56.1
    West African B56.0
swing (motion) T75.3 ☑
train (railway) (travel) T75.3 ☑
travel (any vehicle) T75.3 ☑
Sideropenia — *see* Anemia, iron deficiency
Siderosilicosis J62.8
Siderosis (lung) J63.4
brain G93.89
eye (globe) — *see* Disorder, globe, degenerative,
  siderosis
Siemens' syndrome (ectodermal dysplasia) Q82.8
Sighing R06.89
psychogenic F45.8
Sigmoid — *see also* condition
flexure — *see* condition
kidney Q63.1
Sigmoiditis — *see also* Enteritis K52.9
infectious A09
noninfectious K52.9
Silfversköld's syndrome Q78.9
Silicosiderosis J62.8
Silicosis, silicotic (simple) (complicated) J62.8
with tuberculosis J65
Silicotuberculosis J65
Silo-fillers' disease J68.8
bronchitis J68.0
pneumonitis J68.0
pulmonary edema J68.1
Silver's syndrome Q87.19
Simian malaria B53.1
Simmonds' cachexia or disease E23.0
Simons' disease or syndrome (progressive lipodystro-
  phy) E88.1
Simple, simplex — *see* condition
Simulation, conscious (of illness) Z76.5
Simultanagnosia (asimultagnosia) R48.3
Sin Nombre virus disease (Hantavirus) (cardio)-pul-
  monary syndrome) B33.4
Sinding-Larsen disease or osteochondrosis — *see*
  Osteochondrosis, juvenile, patella
Singapore hemorrhagic fever A91
Singer's node or nodule J38.2
Single
atrium Q21.2
coronary artery Q24.5
umbilical artery Q27.0
ventricle Q20.4
Singultus R06.6
epidemicus B33.0
Sinus — *see also* Fistula
abdominal K63.89
arrest I45.5
arrhythmia I49.8
bradycardia R00.1
branchial cleft (internal) (external) Q18.0
coccygeal — *see* Sinus, pilonidal
dental K04.6
dermal (congenital) Q06.8
  with abscess Q06.8
  coccygeal, pilonidal — *see* Sinus, coccygeal
infected, skin NEC L08.89
marginal, ruptured or bleeding — *see* Hemorrhage,
  antepartum, specified cause NEC
medial, face and neck Q18.8
pause I45.5
pericranii Q01.9
pilonidal (infected) (rectum) L05.92
  with abscess L05.02
preauricular Q18.1
rectovaginal N82.3
Rokitansky-Aschoff (gallbladder) K82.8
sacrococcygeal (dermoid) (infected) — *see* Sinus, pilonidal
tachycardia R00.0
  paroxysmal I47.1
tarsi syndrome M25.57-
testis N50.89
tract (postinfective) — *see* Fistula
urachus Q64.4

Sinusitis (accessory) (chronic) (hyperplastic) (nasal)
  (nonpurulent) (purulent) J32.9
acute J01.90
  ethmoidal J01.20
    recurrent J01.21
  frontal J01.10
    recurrent J01.11
  involving more than one sinus, other than pansinusi-
    tis J01.80
    recurrent J01.81
  maxillary J01.00
    recurrent J01.01
  pansinusitis J01.40
    recurrent J01.41
  recurrent J01.91
  specified NEC J01.80
    recurrent J01.81
  sphenoidal J01.30
    recurrent J01.31
allergic — *see* Rhinitis, allergic
due to high altitude T70.1 ☑
ethmoidal J32.2
  acute J01.20
    recurrent J01.21
frontal J32.1
  acute J01.10
    recurrent J01.11
influenzal — *see* Influenza, with, respiratory manifestations NEC
involving more than one sinus but not pansinusitis
  J32.8
  acute J01.80
    recurrent J01.81
maxillary J32.0
  acute J01.00
    recurrent J01.01
sphenoidal J32.3
  acute J01.30
    recurrent J01.31
tuberculous, any sinus A15.8
Sinusitis-bronchiectasis-situs inversus (syndrome)
  (triad) Q89.3
Sipple's syndrome E31.22
Sirenomelia (syndrome) Q87.2
Siriasis T67.01 ☑
Sirkari's disease B55.0
Siti A65
Situation, psychiatric F99
Situational
disturbance (transient) — *see* Disorder, adjustment
  acute F43.0
maladjustment — *see* Disorder, adjustment
reaction — *see* Disorder, adjustment
  acute F43.0
Situs inversus or transversus (abdominalis) (thoracis)
  Q89.3
Sixth disease B08.20
due to human herpesvirus 6 B08.21
due to human herpesvirus 7 B08.22
Sjögren-Larsson syndrome Q87.19
Sjögren's syndrome or disease — *see* Syndrome, Sjögren
Skeletal — *see* condition
Skene's gland — *see* condition
Skenitis — *see* Urethritis
Skerljevo A65
Skevas-Zerfus disease — *see* Toxicity, venom, marine
  animal, sea anemone
Skin — *see also* condition
clammy R23.1
donor — *see* Donor, skin
dry L85.3
hidebound M35.9
Slate-dressers' or slate-miners' lung J62.8
Sleep
apnea — *see* Apnea, sleep
deprivation Z72.820
disorder or disturbance G47.9
  child F51.9
  nonorganic origin F51.9
  specified NEC G47.8
disturbance G47.9
  nonorganic origin F51.9
drunkenness F51.9
rhythm inversion G47.2- ☑
terrors F51.4
walking F51.3
  hysterical F44.89

Sleep hygiene
  abuse Z72.821
  inadequate Z72.821
  poor Z72.821
Sleeping sickness — *see* Sickness, sleeping
Sleeplessness — *see* Insomnia
  menopausal N95.1
Sleep-wake schedule disorder G47.20
Slim disease (in HIV infection) B20
Slipped, slipping
  epiphysis (traumatic) — *see also* Osteochondropathy,
    specified type NEC
    capital femoral (traumatic)
      acute (on chronic) S79.01- ☑
      current traumatic — *code as* Fracture, by site
      upper femoral (nontraumatic) M93.00- ☑
        acute M93.01- ☑
          on chronic M93.03- ☑
        chronic M93.02- ☑
  intervertebral disc — *see* Displacement, intervertebral
    disc
  ligature, umbilical P51.8
  patella — *see* Disorder, patella, derangement NEC
  rib M89.8X8
  sacroiliac joint — *see* subcategory M53.2 ☑
  tendon — *see* Disorder, tendon
  ulnar nerve, nontraumatic — *see* Lesion, nerve, ulnar
  vertebra NEC — *see* Spondylolisthesis
Slocumb's syndrome E27.0
Sloughing (multiple) (phagedena) (skin) — *see also*
    Gangrene
  abscess — *see* Abscess
  appendix K38.8
  fascia — *see* Disorder, soft tissue, specified type NEC
  scrotum N50.89
  tendon — *see* Disorder, tendon
  transplanted organ — *see* Rejection, transplant
  ulcer — *see* Ulcer, skin
Slow
  feeding, newborn P92.2
  flow syndrome, coronary I20.8
  heart (beat) R00.1
Slowing, urinary stream R39.198
Sluder's neuralgia (syndrome) G44.89
Slurred, slurring speech R47.81
Small (ness)
  for gestational age — *see* Small for dates
  introitus, vagina N89.6
  kidney (unknown cause) N27.9
    bilateral N27.1
    unilateral N27.0
  ovary (congenital) Q50.39
  pelvis
    with disproportion (fetopelvic) O33.1
      causing obstructed labor O65.1
  uterus N85.8
  white kidney N03.9
Small-and-light-for-dates — *see* Small for dates
Small-for-dates (infant) P05.10
  with weight of
    499 grams or less P05.11
    500-749 grams P05.12
    750-999 grams P05.13
    1000-1249 grams P05.14
    1250-1499 grams P05.15
    1500-1749 grams P05.16
    1750-1999 grams P05.17
    2000-2499 grams P05.18
    2500 grams and over P05.19
  specified NEC P05.19
Smallpox B03
Smearing, fecal R15.1
SMEI (severe myoclonic epilepsy in infancy) G40.83- ☑
Smith-Lemli-Opitz syndrome E78.72
Smith's fracture S52.54- ☑
Smoker — *see* Dependence, drug, nicotine
Smoker's
  bronchitis J41.0
  cough J41.0
  palate K13.24
  throat J31.2
  tongue K13.24
Smoking
  passive Z77.22
Smothering spells R06.81
Snaggle teeth, tooth M26.39

Snapping
  finger — *see* Trigger finger
  hip — *see* Derangement, joint, specified type NEC, hip
    involving the iliotibial band M76.3- ☑
  knee — *see* Derangement, knee
    involving the iliotibial band M76.3- ☑
Sneddon-Wilkinson disease or syndrome (sub-corneal
    pustular dermatosis) L13.1
Sneezing (intractable) R06.7
Sniffing
  cocaine
    abuse — *see* Abuse, drug, cocaine
    dependence — *see* Dependence, drug, cocaine
  gasoline
    abuse — *see* Abuse, drug, inhalant
    dependence — *see* Dependence, drug, inhalant
  glue (airplane)
    abuse — *see* Abuse, drug, inhalant
    drug dependence — *see* Dependence, drug, in-
      halant
Sniffles
  newborn P28.89
Snoring R06.83
Snow blindness — *see* Photokeratitis
Snuffles (non-syphilitic) R06.5
  newborn P28.89
  syphilitic (infant) A50.05 *[J99]*
Social
  exclusion Z60.4
    due to discrimination or persecution (perceived)
      Z60.5
  migrant Z59.00
    acculturation difficulty Z60.3
  rejection Z60.4
    due to discrimination or persecution Z60.5
  role conflict NEC Z73.5
  skills inadequacy NEC Z73.4
  transplantation Z60.3
Sodoku A25.0
Soemmerring's ring — *see* Cataract, secondary
Soft — *see also* condition
  nails L60.3
Softening
  bone — *see* Osteomalacia
  brain (necrotic) (progressive) G93.89
    congenital Q04.8
    embolic I63.4- ☑
    hemorrhagic — *see* Hemorrhage, intracranial, intrac-
      erebral
    occlusive I63.5- ☑
    thrombotic I63.3- ☑
  cartilage M94.2- ☑
    patella M22.4- ☑
  cerebellar — *see* Softening, brain
  cerebral — *see* Softening, brain
  cerebrospinal — *see* Softening, brain
  myocardial, heart — *see* Degeneration, myocardial
  spinal cord G95.89
  stomach K31.89
Soldier's
  heart F45.8
  patches I31.0
Solitary
  cyst, kidney N28.1
  kidney, congenital Q60.0
Solvent abuse — *see* Abuse, drug, inhalant
  dependence — *see* Dependence, drug, inhalant
Somatization reaction, somatic reaction — *see* Disor-
    der, somatoform
Somnambulism F51.3
  hysterical F44.89
Somnolence R40.0
  nonorganic origin F51.11
Sonne dysentery A03.3
Soor B37.0
Sore
  bed — *see* Ulcer, pressure, by site
  chiclero B55.1
  Delhi B55.1
  desert — *see* Ulcer, skin
  eye H57.1- ☑
  Lahore B55.1
  mouth K13.79
    canker K12.0
  muscle M79.10
  Naga — *see* Ulcer, skin
  of skin — *see* Ulcer, skin

Sore — *continued*
  oriental B55.1
  pressure — *see* Ulcer, pressure, by site
  skin L98.9
  soft A57
  throat (acute) — *see also* Pharyngitis
    with influenza, flu, or grippe — *see* Influenza, with,
      respiratory manifestations NEC
    chronic J31.2
    coxsackie (virus) B08.5
    diphtheritic A36.0
    herpesviral B00.2
    influenzal — *see* Influenza, with, respiratory mani-
      festations NEC
    septic J02.0
    streptococcal (ulcerative) J02.0
    viral NEC J02.8
      coxsackie B08.5
  tropical — *see* Ulcer, skin
  veldt — *see* Ulcer, skin
Soto's syndrome (cerebral gigantism) Q87.3
South African cardiomyopathy syndrome I42.8
Southeast Asian hemorrhagic fever A91
Spacing
  abnormal, tooth, teeth, fully erupted M26.30
  excessive, tooth, fully erupted M26.32
Spade-like hand (congenital) Q68.1
Spading nail L60.8
  congenital Q84.6
Spanish collar N47.1
Sparganosis B70.1
Spasm(s), **spastic, spasticity** — *see also* condition R25.2
  accommodation — *see* Spasm, of accommodation
  ampulla of Vater K83.4
  anus, ani (sphincter) (reflex) K59.4
    psychogenic F45.8
  artery I73.9
    cerebral G45.9
  Bell's G51.3- ☑
  bladder (sphincter, external or internal) N32.89
    psychogenic F45.8
  bronchus, bronchiole J98.01
  cardia K22.0
  cardiac I20.1
  carpopedal — *see* Tetany
  cerebral (arteries) (vascular) G45.9
  cervix, complicating delivery O62.4
  ciliary body (of accommodation) — *see* Spasm, of ac-
    commodation
  colon — *see also* Irritable, bowel K58.9
    with diarrhea K58.0
    psychogenic F45.8
  common duct K83.8
  compulsive — *see* Tic
  conjugate H51.8
  coronary (artery) I20.1
  diaphragm (reflex) R06.6
    epidemic B33.0
    psychogenic F45.8
  duodenum K59.89
  epidemic diaphragmatic (transient) B33.0
  esophagus (diffuse) K22.4
    psychogenic F45.8
  facial G51.3- ☑
  fallopian tube N83.8
  gastrointestinal (tract) K31.89
    psychogenic F45.8
  glottis J38.5
    hysterical F44.4
    psychogenic F45.8
      conversion reaction F44.4
    reflex through recurrent laryngeal nerve J38.5
  habit — *see* Tic
  heart I20.1
  hemifacial (clonic) G51.3- ☑
  hourglass — *see* Contraction, hourglass
  hysterical F44.4
  infantile — *see* Epilepsy, spasms
  inferior oblique, eye H51.8
  intestinal — *see also* Syndrome, irritable bowel K58.9
    psychogenic F45.8
  larynx, laryngeal J38.5
    hysterical F44.4
    psychogenic F45.8
      conversion reaction F44.4
  levator palpebrae superioris — *see* Disorder, eyelid
    function
  muscle NEC M62.838

Spasm(s), spastic, spasticity — *continued*
  muscle — *continued*
    back M62.830
  nerve, trigeminal G51.0
  nervous F45.8
  nodding F98.4
  occupational F48.8
  oculogyric H51.8
    psychogenic F45.8
  of accommodation H52.53- ☑
  ophthalmic artery — *see* Occlusion, artery, retina
  perineal, female N94.89
  peroneo-extensor — *see also* Deformity, limb, flat foot
  pharynx (reflex) J39.2
    hysterical F45.8
    psychogenic F45.8
  psychogenic F45.8
  pylorus NEC K31.3
    adult hypertrophic K31.89
    congenital or infantile Q40.0
    psychogenic F45.8
  rectum (sphincter) K59.4
    psychogenic F45.8
  retinal (artery) — *see* Occlusion, artery, retina
  sigmoid — *see also* Syndrome, irritable bowel K58.9
    psychogenic F45.8
  sphincter of Oddi K83.4
  stomach K31.89
    neurotic F45.8
  throat J39.2
    hysterical F45.8
    psychogenic F45.8
  tic F95.9
    chronic F95.1
    transient of childhood F95.0
  tongue K14.8
  torsion (progressive) G24.1
  trigeminal nerve — *see* Neuralgia, trigeminal
  ureter N13.5
  urethra (sphincter) N35.919
  uterus N85.8
    complicating labor O62.4
  vagina N94.2
    psychogenic F52.5
  vascular I73.9
  vasomotor I73.9
  vein NEC I87.8
  viscera — *see* Pain, abdominal
Spasmodic — *see* condition
Spasmophilia — *see* Tetany
Spasmus nutans F98.4
Spastic, spasticity — *see also* Spasm
  child (cerebral) (congenital) (paralysis) G80.1
Speaker's throat R49.8
Specific, specified — *see* condition
Speech
  defect, disorder, disturbance, impediment — *see* Disorder, speech R47.9
    psychogenic, in childhood and adolescence F98.8
    slurring R47.81
    specified NEC R47.89
Spencer's disease A08.19
Spens' syndrome (syncope with heart block) I45.9
Sperm counts (fertility testing) Z31.41
  postvasectomy Z30.8
    reversal Z31.42
Spermatic cord — *see* condition
Spermatocele N43.40
  congenital Q55.4
  multiple N43.42
  single N43.41
Spermatocystitis N49.0
Spermatocytoma C62.9- ☑
  specified site — *see* Neoplasm, malignant, by site
Spermatorrhea N50.89
Sphacelus — *see* Gangrene
Sphenoidal — *see* condition
Sphenoiditis (chronic) — *see* Sinusitis, sphenoidal
Sphenopalatine ganglion neuralgia G90.09
Sphericity, increased, lens (congenital) Q12.4
Spherocytosis (congenital) (familial) (hereditary) D58.0
  hemoglobin disease D58.0
  sickle-cell (disease) D57.8- ☑
Spherophakia Q12.4
Sphincter — *see* condition
Sphincteritis, sphincter of Oddi — *see* Cholangitis
Sphingolipidosis E75.3
  specified NEC E75.29

Sphingomyelinosis E75.3
Spicule tooth K00.2
Spider
  bite — *see* Toxicity, venom, spider
    nonvenomous — *see* Bite, by site, superficial, insect
  fingers — *see* Syndrome, Marfan's
  nevus I78.1
  toes — *see* Syndrome, Marfan's
  vascular I78.1
Spiegler-Fendt
  benign lymphocytoma L98.8
  sarcoid L08.89
Spielmeyer-Vogt disease E75.4
Spina bifida (aperta) Q05.9
  with hydrocephalus NEC Q05.4
  cervical Q05.5
    with hydrocephalus Q05.0
  dorsal Q05.6
    with hydrocephalus Q05.1
  lumbar Q05.7
    with hydrocephalus Q05.2
  lumbosacral Q05.7
    with hydrocephalus Q05.2
  occulta Q76.0
  sacral Q05.8
    with hydrocephalus Q05.3
  thoracic Q05.6
    with hydrocephalus Q05.1
  thoracolumbar Q05.6
    with hydrocephalus Q05.1
Spindle, Krukenberg's — *see* Pigmentation, cornea, posterior
Spine, spinal — *see* condition
Spiradenoma (eccrine) — *see* Neoplasm, skin, benign
Spirillosis A25.0
Spirillum
  minus A25.0
  obermeieri infection A68.0
Spirochetal — *see* condition
Spirochetosis A69.9
  arthritic, arthritica A69.9
  bronchopulmonary A69.8
  icterohemorrhagic A27.0
  lung A69.8
Spirometrosis B70.1
Spitting blood — *see* Hemoptysis
Splanchnoptosis K63.4
Spleen, splenic — *see* condition
Splenectasis — *see* Splenomegaly
Splenitis (interstitial) (malignant) (nonspecific) D73.89
  malarial — *see also* Malaria B54 *[D77]*
  tuberculous A18.85
Splenocele D73.89
Splenomegaly, splenomegalia (Bengal) (cryptogenic) (idiopathic) (tropical) R16.1
  with hepatomegaly R16.2
  cirrhotic D73.2
  congenital Q89.09
  congestive, chronic D73.2
  Egyptian B65.1
  Gaucher's E75.22
  malarial — *see also* Malaria B54 *[D77]*
  neutropenic D73.81
  Niemann-Pick — *see* Niemann-Pick disease or syndrome
  siderotic D73.2
  syphilitic A52.79
    congenital (early) A50.08 *[D77]*
Splenopathy D73.9
Splenoptosis D73.89
Splenosis D73.89
Splinter — *see* Foreign body, superficial, by site
Split, splitting
  foot Q72.7- ☑
  hand Q71.6 ☑
  heart sounds R01.2
  lip, congenital — *see* Cleft, lip
  nails L60.3
  urinary stream R39.13
Spondylarthrosis — *see* Spondylosis
Spondylitis (chronic) — *see also* Spondylopathy, inflammatory
  ankylopoietica — *see* Spondylitis, ankylosing
  ankylosing (chronic) M45.9
    with lung involvement M45.9 *[J99]*
    cervical region M45.2
    cervicothoracic region M45.3

Spondylitis — *continued*
  ankylosing — *continued*
    juvenile M08.1
    lumbar region M45.6
    lumbosacral region M45.7
    multiple sites M45.0
    occipito-atlanto-axial region M45.1
    sacrococcygeal region M45.8
    thoracic region M45.4
    thoracolumbar region M45.5
  atrophic (ligamentous) — *see* Spondylitis, ankylosing
  deformans (chronic) — *see* Spondylosis
  gonococcal A54.41
  gouty — *see also* Gout, by type, vertebrae M10.08
  in (due to)
    brucellosis A23.9 *[M49.80]*
      cervical region A23.9 *[M49.82]*
      cervicothoracic region A23.9 *[M49.83]*
      lumbar region A23.9 *[M49.86]*
      lumbosacral region A23.9 *[M49.87]*
      multiple sites A23.9 *[M49.89]*
      occipito-atlanto-axial region A23.9 *[M49.81]*
      sacrococcygeal region A23.9 *[M49.88]*
      thoracic region A23.9 *[M49.84]*
      thoracolumbar region A23.9 *[M49.85]*
    enterobacteria — *see also* subcategory M49.8 A04.9
    tuberculosis A18.01
  infectious NEC — *see* Spondylopathy, infective
  juvenile ankylosing (chronic) M08.1
  Kümmell's — *see* Spondylopathy, traumatic
  Marie-Strümpell — *see* Spondylitis, ankylosing
  muscularis — *see* Spondylopathy, specified NEC
  psoriatic L40.53
  rheumatoid — *see* Spondylitis, ankylosing
  rhizomelica — *see* Spondylitis, ankylosing
  sacroiliac NEC M46.1
  senescent, senile — *see* Spondylosis
  traumatic (chronic) or post-traumatic — *see* Spondylopathy, traumatic
  tuberculous A18.01
  typhosa A01.05
Spondyloarthritis
  axial — *see also* Spondlyitis, ankylosing
    non-radiographic M45.A0
      cervical M45.A2
      cervicothoracic M45.A3
      lumbar M45.A6
      lumbosacral M45.A7
      multiple sites M45.AB
      occipito-atlanto-axial region M45.A1
      sacral and sacrococcygeal M45.A8
      thoracic M45.A4
      thoracolumbar M45.A5
Spondylolisthesis (acquired) (degenerative) M43.10
  with disproportion (fetopelvic) O33.0
    causing obstructed labor O65.0
  cervical region M43.12
  cervicothoracic region M43.13
  congenital Q76.2
  lumbar region M43.16
  lumbosacral region M43.17
  multiple sites M43.19
  occipito-atlanto-axial region M43.11
  sacrococcygeal region M43.18
  thoracic region M43.14
  thoracolumbar region M43.15
  traumatic (old) M43.10
    acute
      fifth cervical (displaced) S12.430 ☑
        nondisplaced S12.431 ☑
        specified type NEC (displaced) S12.450 ☑
          nondisplaced S12.451 ☑
        type III S12.44 ☑
      fourth cervical (displaced) S12.330 ☑
        nondisplaced S12.331 ☑
        specified type NEC (displaced) S12.350 ☑
          nondisplaced S12.351 ☑
        type III S12.34 ☑
      second cervical (displaced) S12.130 ☑
        nondisplaced S12.131 ☑
        specified type NEC (displaced) S12.150 ☑
          nondisplaced S12.151 ☑
        type III S12.14 ☑
      seventh cervical (displaced) S12.630 ☑
        nondisplaced S12.631 ☑
        specified type NEC (displaced) S12.650 ☑
          nondisplaced S12.651 ☑

Subterms under main terms may continue to next column or page — ☑ Additional Character Required — Refer to the Tabular List for Character Selection — 293

Spasm — Spondylolisthesis

Spondylolisthesis — *continued*
  traumatic — *continued*
    acute — *continued*
      seventh cervical — *continued*
        type III S12.64 ☑
      sixth cervical (displaced) S12.530 ☑
        nondisplaced S12.531 ☑
        specified type NEC (displaced) S12.550 ☑
          nondisplaced S12.551 ☑
        type III S12.54 ☑
      third cervical (displaced) S12.230 ☑
        nondisplaced S12.231 ☑
        specified type NEC (displaced) S12.250 ☑
          nondisplaced S12.251 ☑
        type III S12.24 ☑
Spondylolysis (acquired) M43.00
  cervical region M43.02
  cervicothoracic region M43.03
  congenital Q76.2
  lumbar region M43.06
  lumbosacral region M43.07
    with disproportion (fetopelvic) O33.0
      causing obstructed labor O65.8
  multiple sites M43.09
  occipito-atlanto-axial region M43.01
  sacrococcygeal region M43.08
  thoracic region M43.04
  thoracolumbar region M43.05
Spondylopathy M48.9
  infective NEC M46.50
    cervical region M46.52
    cervicothoracic region M46.53
    lumbar region M46.56
    lumbosacral region M46.57
    multiple sites M46.59
    occipito-atlanto-axial region M46.51
    sacrococcygeal region M46.58
    thoracic region M46.54
    thoracolumbar region M46.55
  inflammatory M46.90
    cervical region M46.92
    cervicothoracic region M46.93
    lumbar region M46.96
    lumbosacral region M46.97
    multiple sites M46.99
    occipito-atlanto-axial region M46.91
    sacrococcygeal region M46.98
    specified type NEC M46.80
      cervical region M46.82
      cervicothoracic region M46.83
      lumbar region M46.86
      lumbosacral region M46.87
      multiple sites M46.89
      occipito-atlanto-axial region M46.81
      sacrococcygeal region M46.88
      thoracic region M46.84
      thoracolumbar region M46.85
    thoracic region M46.94
    thoracolumbar region M46.95
  neuropathic, in
    syringomyelia and syringobulbia G95.0
    tabes dorsalis A52.11
  specified NEC — *see* subcategory M48.8 ☑
  traumatic M48.30
    cervical region M48.32
    cervicothoracic region M48.33
    lumbar region M48.36
    lumbosacral region M48.37
    occipito-atlanto-axial region M48.31
    sacrococcygeal region M48.38
    thoracic region M48.34
    thoracolumbar region M48.35
Spondylosis M47.9
  with
    disproportion (fetopelvic) O33.0
      causing obstructed labor O65.0
    myelopathy NEC M47.10
      cervical region M47.12
      cervicothoracic region M47.13
      lumbar region M47.16
      occipito-atlanto-axial region M47.11
      thoracic region M47.14
      thoracolumbar region M47.15
    radiculopathy M47.20
      cervical region M47.22
      cervicothoracic region M47.23
      lumbar region M47.26
      lumbosacral region M47.27

Spondylosis — *continued*
  with — *continued*
    radiculopathy — *continued*
      occipito-atlanto-axial region M47.21
      sacrococcygeal region M47.28
      thoracic region M47.24
      thoracolumbar region M47.25
  specified NEC M47.899
    cervical region M47.892
    cervicothoracic region M47.893
    facet joint — *see also* Spondylosis M47.819
    lumbar region M47.896
    lumbosacral region M47.897
    occipito-atlanto-axial region M47.891
    sacrococcygeal region M47.898
    thoracic region M47.894
    thoracolumbar region M47.895
  traumatic — *see* Spondylopathy, traumatic
  without myelopathy or radiculopathy M47.819
    cervical region M47.812
    cervicothoracic region M47.813
    lumbar region M47.816
    lumbosacral region M47.817
    occipito-atlanto-axial region M47.811
    sacrococcygeal region M47.818
    thoracic region M47.814
    thoracolumbar region M47.815
Sponge
  inadvertently left in operation wound — *see* Foreign body, accidentally left during a procedure
  kidney (medullary) Q61.5
Sponge-diver's disease — *see* Toxicity, venom, marine animal, sea anemone
Spongioblastoma (any type) — *see* Neoplasm, malignant, by site
  specified site — *see* Neoplasm, malignant, by site
  unspecified site C71.9
Spongioneuroblastoma — *see* Neoplasm, malignant, by site
Spontaneous — *see also* condition
  fracture (cause unknown) — *see* Fracture, pathological
Spoon nail L60.3
  congenital Q84.6
Sporadic — *see* condition
Sporothrix schenckii infection — *see* Sporotrichosis
Sporotrichosis B42.9
  arthritis B42.82
  disseminated B42.7
  generalized B42.7
  lymphocutaneous (fixed) (progressive) B42.1
  pulmonary B42.0
  specified NEC B42.89
Spots, spotting (in) (of)
  Bitot's — *see also* Pigmentation, conjunctiva
    in the young child E50.1
    vitamin A deficiency E50.1
  café, au lait L81.3
  Cayenne pepper I78.1
  cotton wool, retina — *see* Occlusion, artery, retina
  de Morgan's (senile angiomas) I78.1
  Fuchs' black (myopic) — *see also* Myopia, degenerative H44.2- ☑
  intermenstrual (regular) N92.0
    irregular N92.1
  Koplik's B05.9
  liver L81.4
  pregnancy O26.85- ☑
  purpuric R23.3
  ruby I78.1
Spotted fever — *see* Fever, spotted A77.9
Sprain (joint) (ligament)
  acromioclavicular joint or ligament S43.5- ☑
  ankle S93.40- ☑
    calcaneofibular ligament S93.41- ☑
    deltoid ligament S93.42- ☑
    internal collateral ligament — *see* Sprain, ankle, specified ligament NEC
    specified ligament NEC S93.49- ☑
    talofibular ligament — *see* Sprain, ankle, specified ligament NEC
    tibiofibular ligament S93.43- ☑
  anterior longitudinal, cervical S13.4 ☑
  atlas, atlanto-axial, atlanto-occipital S13.4 ☑
  breast bone — *see* Sprain, sternum
  calcaneofibular — *see* Sprain, ankle
  carpal — *see* Sprain, wrist

Sprain — *continued*
  carpometacarpal — *see* Sprain, hand, specified site NEC
  cartilage
    costal S23.41 ☑
    semilunar (knee) — *see* Sprain, knee, specified site NEC
      with current tear — *see* Tear, meniscus
    thyroid region S13.5 ☑
    xiphoid — *see* Sprain, sternum
  cervical, cervicodorsal, cervicothoracic S13.4 ☑
  chondrosternal S23.421 ☑
  coracoclavicular S43.8- ☑
  coracohumeral S43.41- ☑
  coronary, knee — *see* Sprain, knee, specified site NEC
  costal cartilage S23.41 ☑
  cricoarytenoid articulation or ligament S13.5 ☑
  cricothyroid articulation S13.5 ☑
  cruciate, knee — *see* Sprain, knee, cruciate
  deltoid, ankle — *see* Sprain, ankle
  dorsal (spine) S23.3 ☑
  elbow S53.40- ☑
    radial collateral ligament S53.43- ☑
    radiohumeral S53.41- ☑
    rupture
      radial collateral ligament — *see* Rupture, traumatic, ligament, radial collateral
      ulnar collateral ligament — *see* Rupture, traumatic, ligament, ulnar collateral
    specified type NEC S53.49- ☑
    ulnar collateral ligament S53.44- ☑
    ulnohumeral S53.42- ☑
  femur, head — *see* Sprain, hip
  fibular collateral, knee — *see* Sprain, knee, collateral
  fibulocalcaneal — *see* Sprain, ankle
  finger(s) S63.61- ☑
    index S63.61- ☑
    interphalangeal (joint) S63.63- ☑
      index S63.63- ☑
      little S63.63- ☑
      middle S63.63- ☑
      ring S63.63- ☑
    little S63.61- ☑
    metacarpophalangeal (joint) S63.65- ☑
    middle S63.61- ☑
    ring S63.61- ☑
    specified site NEC S63.69- ☑
      index S63.69- ☑
      little S63.69- ☑
      middle S63.69- ☑
      ring S63.69- ☑
  foot S93.60- ☑
    specified ligament NEC S93.69- ☑
    tarsal ligament S93.61- ☑
    tarsometatarsal ligament S93.62- ☑
    toe — *see* Sprain, toe
  hand S63.9- ☑
    finger — *see* Sprain, finger
    specified site NEC — *see* subcategory S63.8 ☑
    thumb — *see* Sprain, thumb
  head S03.9 ☑
  hip S73.10- ☑
    iliofemoral ligament S73.11- ☑
    ischiocapsular (ligament) S73.12- ☑
    specified NEC S73.19- ☑
  iliofemoral — *see* Sprain, hip
  innominate
    acetabulum — *see* Sprain, hip
    sacral junction S33.6 ☑
  internal
    collateral, ankle — *see* Sprain, ankle
    semilunar cartilage — *see* Sprain, knee, specified site NEC
  interphalangeal
    finger — *see* Sprain, finger, interphalangeal (joint)
    toe — *see* Sprain, toe, interphalangeal joint
  ischiocapsular — *see* Sprain, hip
  ischiofemoral — *see* Sprain, hip
  jaw (articular disc) (cartilage) (meniscus) S03.4- ☑
    old M26.69
  knee S83.9- ☑
    collateral ligament S83.40- ☑
      lateral (fibular) S83.42- ☑
      medial (tibial) S83.41- ☑
    cruciate ligament S83.50- ☑
      anterior S83.51- ☑

☑ **Additional Character Required** — Refer to the Tabular List for Character Selection   ▽ **Subterms under main terms may continue to next column or page**

Sprain — *continued*
  knee — *continued*
    cruciate ligament — *continued*
      posterior S83.52- ☑
    lateral (fibular) collateral ligament S83.42- ☑
    medial (tibial) collateral ligament S83.41- ☑
    patellar ligament S76.11- ☑
    specified site NEC S83.8X- ☑
    superior tibiofibular joint (ligament) S83.6- ☑
  lateral collateral, knee — *see* Sprain, knee, collateral
  lumbar (spine) S33.5 ☑
  lumbosacral S33.9 ☑
  mandible (articular disc) S03.4- ☑
    old M26.69
  medial collateral, knee — *see* Sprain, knee, collateral
  meniscus
    jaw S03.4- ☑
      old M26.69
    knee — *see* Sprain, knee, specified site NEC
      with current tear — *see* Tear, meniscus
        old — *see* Derangement, knee, meniscus, due to old tear
    mandible S03.4- ☑
      old M26.69
  metacarpal (distal) (proximal) — *see* Sprain, hand, specified site NEC
  metacarpophalangeal — *see* Sprain, finger, metacarpophalangeal (joint)
  metatarsophalangeal — *see* Sprain, toe, metatarsophalangeal joint
  midcarpal — *see* Sprain, hand, specified site NEC
  midtarsal — *see* Sprain, foot, specified site NEC
  neck S13.9 ☑
    anterior longitudinal cervical ligament S13.4 ☑
    atlanto-axial joint S13.4 ☑
    atlanto-occipital joint S13.4 ☑
    cervical spine S13.4 ☑
    cricoarytenoid ligament S13.5 ☑
    cricothyroid ligament S13.5 ☑
    specified site NEC S13.8 ☑
    thyroid region (cartilage) S13.5 ☑
  nose S03.8 ☑
  orbicular, hip — *see* Sprain, hip
  patella — *see* Sprain, knee, specified site NEC
  patellar ligament S76.11- ☑
  pelvis NEC S33.8 ☑
  phalanx
    finger — *see* Sprain, finger
    toe — *see* Sprain, toe
  pubofemoral — *see* Sprain, hip
  radiocarpal — *see* Sprain, wrist
  radiohumeral — *see* Sprain, elbow
  radius, collateral — *see* Rupture, traumatic, ligament, radial collateral
  rib (cage) S23.41 ☑
  rotator cuff (capsule) S43.42- ☑
  sacroiliac (region)
    chronic or old — *see* subcategory M53.2 ☑
    joint S33.6 ☑
  scaphoid (hand) — *see* Sprain, hand, specified site NEC
  scapula (r) — *see* Sprain, shoulder girdle, specified site NEC
  semilunar cartilage (knee) — *see* Sprain, knee, specified site NEC
    with current tear — *see* Tear, meniscus
      old — *see* Derangement, knee, meniscus, due to old tear
  shoulder joint S43.40- ☑
    acromioclavicular joint (ligament) — *see* Sprain, acromioclavicular joint
    blade — *see* Sprain, shoulder, girdle, specified site NEC
    coracoclavicular joint (ligament) — *see* Sprain, coracoclavicular joint
    coracohumeral ligament — *see* Sprain, coracohumeral joint
    girdle S43.9- ☑
      specified site NEC S43.8- ☑
    rotator cuff — *see* Sprain, rotator cuff
    specified site NEC S43.49- ☑
    sternoclavicular joint (ligament) — *see* Sprain, sternoclavicular joint
  spine
    cervical S13.4 ☑
    lumbar S33.5 ☑
    thoracic S23.3 ☑

Sprain — *continued*
  sternoclavicular joint S43.6- ☑
  sternum S23.429 ☑
    chondrosternal joint S23.421 ☑
    specified site NEC S23.428 ☑
    sternoclavicular (joint) (ligament) S23.420 ☑
  symphysis
    jaw S03.4- ☑
      old M26.69
    mandibular S03.4- ☑
      old M26.69
  talofibular — *see* Sprain, ankle
  tarsal — *see* Sprain, foot, specified site NEC
  tarsometatarsal — *see* Sprain, foot, specified site NEC
  temporomandibular S03.4- ☑
    old M26.69
  thorax S23.9 ☑
    ribs S23.41 ☑
    specified site NEC S23.8 ☑
    spine S23.3 ☑
    sternum — *see* Sprain, sternum
  thumb S63.60- ☑
    interphalangeal (joint) S63.62- ☑
    metacarpophalangeal (joint) S63.64- ☑
    specified site NEC S63.68- ☑
  thyroid cartilage or region S13.5 ☑
  tibia (proximal end) — *see* Sprain, knee, specified site NEC
  tibial collateral, knee — *see* Sprain, knee, collateral
  tibiofibular
    distal — *see* Sprain, ankle
    superior — *see* Sprain, knee, specified site NEC
  toe(s) S93.50- ☑
    great S93.50- ☑
    interphalangeal joint S93.51- ☑
      great S93.51- ☑
      lesser S93.51- ☑
    lesser S93.50- ☑
    metatarsophalangeal joint S93.52- ☑
      great S93.52- ☑
      lesser S93.52- ☑
  ulna, collateral — *see* Rupture, traumatic, ligament, ulnar collateral
  ulnohumeral — *see* Sprain, elbow
  wrist S63.50- ☑
    carpal S63.51- ☑
    radiocarpal S63.52- ☑
    specified site NEC S63.59- ☑
  xiphoid cartilage — *see* Sprain, sternum
Sprengel's deformity (congenital) Q74.0
Sprue (tropical) K90.1
  celiac K90.0
  idiopathic K90.49
  meaning thrush B37.0
  nontropical K90.0
Spur, bone — *see also* Enthesopathy
  calcaneal M77.3- ☑
  iliac crest M76.2- ☑
  nose (septum) J34.89
Spurway's syndrome Q78.0
Sputum
  abnormal (amount) (color) (odor) (purulent) R09.3
  blood-stained R04.2
  excessive (cause unknown) R09.3
Squamous — *see also* condition
  epithelium in
    cervical canal (congenital) Q51.828
    uterine mucosa (congenital) Q51.818
Squashed nose M95.0
  congenital Q67.4
Squeeze, diver's T70.3 ☑
Squint — *see also* Strabismus
  accommodative — *see* Strabismus, convergent concomitant
SSADHD (succinic semialdehyde dehydrogenase deficiency) E72.81
St. Hubert's disease A82.9
Stab — *see also* Laceration
  internal organs — *see* Injury, by site
Stafne's cyst or cavity M27.0
Staggering gait R26.0
  hysterical F44.4
Staghorn calculus — *see* Calculus, kidney
Stähli's line (cornea) (pigment) — *see* Pigmentation, cornea, anterior

Stain, staining
  meconium (newborn) P96.83
  port wine Q82.5
  tooth, teeth (hard tissues) (extrinsic) K03.6
    due to
      accretions K03.6
      deposits (betel) (black) (green) (materia alba) (orange) (soft) (tobacco) K03.6
      metals (copper) (silver) K03.7
      nicotine K03.6
      pulpal bleeding K03.7
      tobacco K03.6
    intrinsic K00.8
Stammering — *see also* Disorder, fluency F80.81
Standstill
  auricular I45.5
  cardiac — *see* Arrest, cardiac
  sinoatrial I45.5
  ventricular — *see* Arrest, cardiac
Stannosis J63.5
Stanton's disease — *see* Melioidosis
Staphylitis (acute) (catarrhal) (chronic) (gangrenous) (membranous) (suppurative) (ulcerative) K12.2
Staphylococcal scalded skin syndrome L00
Staphylococcemia A41.2
Staphylococcus, staphylococcal — *see also* condition
  as cause of disease classified elsewhere B95.8
    aureus (methicillin susceptible) (MSSA) B95.61
      methicillin resistant (MRSA) B95.62
    specified NEC, as cause of disease classified elsewhere B95.7
Staphyloma (sclera)
  cornea H18.72- ☑
  equatorial H15.81- ☑
  localized (anterior) H15.82- ☑
  posticum H15.83- ☑
  ring H15.85- ☑
Stargardt's disease — *see* Dystrophy, retina
Starvation (inanition) (due to lack of food) T73.0 ☑
  edema — *see* Malnutrition, severe
Stasis
  bile (noncalculous) K83.1
  bronchus J98.09
    with infection — *see* Bronchitis
  cardiac — *see* Failure, heart, congestive
  cecum K59.89
  colon K59.89
  dermatitis I87.2
    with
      varicose ulcer — *see* Varix, leg, with ulcer, with inflammation
      varicose veins — *see* Varix, leg, with, inflammation
    due to postthrombotic syndrome — *see* Syndrome, postthrombotic
  duodenal K31.5
  eczema — *see* Varix, leg, with, inflammation
  edema — *see* Hypertension, venous (chronic), idiopathic
  foot T69.0- ☑
  ileocecal coil K59.89
  ileum K59.89
  intestinal K59.89
  jejunum K59.89
  kidney N19
  liver (cirrhotic) K76.1
  lymphatic I89.8
  pneumonia J18.2
  pulmonary — *see* Edema, lung
  rectal K59.89
  renal N19
    tubular N17.0
  ulcer — *see* Varix, leg, with, ulcer
    without varicose veins I87.2
  urine — *see* Retention, urine
  venous I87.8
State (of)
  affective and paranoid, mixed, organic psychotic F06.8
  agitated R45.1
    acute reaction to stress F43.0
  anxiety (neurotic) F41.1
  apprehension F41.1
  burn-out Z73.0
  climacteric, female Z78.0
    symptomatic N95.1
  compulsive F42.8
    mixed with obsessional thoughts F42.2
  confusional (psychogenic) F44.89

State — *continued*
  confusional — *continued*
    acute — *see also* Delirium
      with
        arteriosclerotic dementia F01.50
          with behavioral disturbance F01.51
        senility or dementia F05
      alcoholic F10.231
      epileptic F05
      reactive (from emotional stress, psychological trauma) F44.89
    subacute — *see* Delirium
  convulsive — *see* Convulsions
  crisis F43.0
  depressive F32.A
    neurotic F34.1
  dissociative F44.9
  emotional shock (stress) R45.7
  hypercoagulation — *see* Hypercoagulable
  locked-in G83.5
  menopausal Z78.0
    symptomatic N95.1
  neurotic F48.9
    with depersonalization F48.1
  obsessional F42.8
  oneiroid (schizophrenia-like) F23
  organic
    hallucinatory (nonalcoholic) F06.0
    paranoid (-hallucinatory) F06.2
  panic F41.0
  paranoid F22
    climacteric F22
    involutional F22
    menopausal F22
    organic F06.2
    senile F03 ☑
    simple F22
  persistent vegetative R40.3
  phobic F40.9
  postleukotomy F07.0
  pregnant
    gestational carrier Z33.3
    incidental Z33.1
  psychogenic, twilight F44.89
  psychopathic (constitutional) F60.2
  psychotic, organic — *see also* Psychosis, organic
    mixed paranoid and affective F06.8
    senile or presenile F03 ☑
    transient NEC F06.8
      with
        depression F06.31
        hallucinations F06.0
  residual schizophrenic F20.5
  restlessness R45.1
  stress (emotional) R45.7
  tension (mental) F48.9
    specified NEC F48.8
  transient organic psychotic NEC F06.8
    depressive type F06.31
    hallucinatory type F06.0
  twilight
    epileptic F05
    psychogenic F44.89
  vegetative, persistent R40.3
  vital exhaustion Z73.0
  withdrawal, — *see* Withdrawal, state
Status (post) — *see also* Presence (of)
  absence, epileptic — *see* Epilepsy, by type, with status epilepticus
  administration of tPA (rtPA) in a different facility within the last 24 hours prior to admission to current facility Z92.82
  adrenalectomy (unilateral) (bilateral) E89.6
  anastomosis Z98.0
  anginosus I20.9
  angioplasty (peripheral) Z98.62
    with implant Z95.820
    coronary artery Z98.61
      with implant Z95.5
  aortocoronary bypass Z95.1
  arthrodesis Z98.1
  artificial opening (of) Z93.9
    gastrointestinal tract Z93.4
    specified NEC Z93.8
    urinary tract Z93.6
    vagina Z93.8
  asthmaticus — *see* Asthma, by type, with status asthmaticus

Status — *continued*
  awaiting organ transplant Z76.82
  bariatric surgery Z98.84
  bed confinement Z74.01
  bleb, filtering (vitreous), after glaucoma surgery Z98.83
  breast implant Z98.82
    removal Z98.86
  cataract extraction Z98.4- ☑
  cholecystectomy Z90.49
  clitorectomy N90.811
    with excision of labia minora N90.812
  colectomy (complete) (partial) Z90.49
  colonization — *see* Carrier (suspected) of
  colostomy Z93.3
  convulsivus idiopathicus — *see* Epilepsy, by type, with status epilepticus
  coronary artery angioplasty — *see* Status, angioplasty, coronary artery
  coronary artery bypass graft Z95.1
  cystectomy (urinary bladder) Z90.6
  cystostomy Z93.50
    appendico-vesicostomy Z93.52
    cutaneous Z93.51
    specified NEC Z93.59
  delinquent immunization Z28.3
  dental Z98.818
    crown Z98.811
    fillings Z98.811
    restoration Z98.811
    sealant Z98.810
    specified NEC Z98.818
  deployment (current) (military) Z56.82
  dialysis (hemodialysis) (peritoneal) Z99.2
  do not resuscitate (DNR) Z66
  donor — *see* Donor
  embedded fragments — *see* Retained, foreign body fragments (type of)
  embedded splinter — *see* Retained, foreign body fragments (type of)
  enterostomy Z93.4
  epileptic, epilepticus — *see also* Epilepsy, by type, with status epilepticus G40.901
  estrogen receptor
    negative Z17.1
    positive Z17.0
  female genital cutting — *see* Female genital mutilation status
  female genital mutilation — *see* Female genital mutilation status
  filtering (vitreous) bleb after glaucoma surgery Z98.83
  gastrectomy (complete) (partial) Z90.3
  gastric banding Z98.84
  gastric bypass for obesity Z98.84
  gastrostomy Z93.1
  human immunodeficiency virus (HIV) infection, asymptomatic Z21
  hysterectomy (complete) (total) Z90.710
    partial (with remaining cervial stump) Z90.711
  ileostomy Z93.2
  implant
    breast Z98.82
  infibulation N90.813
  intestinal bypass Z98.0
  jejunostomy Z93.4
  lapsed immunization schedule Z28.3
  laryngectomy Z90.02
  lymphaticus E32.8
  malignancy
    castrate resistant prostate Z19.2
    hormone resistant Z19.2
    hormone sensitive Z19.1
  marmoratus G80.3
  mastectomy (unilateral) (bilateral) Z90.1- ☑
  military deployment status (current) Z56.82
    in theater or in support of military war, peacekeeping and humanitarian operations Z56.82
  nephrectomy (unilateral) (bilateral) Z90.5
  nephrostomy Z93.6
  obesity surgery Z98.84
  oophorectomy
    bilateral Z90.722
    unilateral Z90.721
  organ replacement
    by artificial or mechanical device or prosthesis of
      artery Z95.828
      bladder Z96.0
      blood vessel Z95.828
      breast Z97.8

Status — *continued*
  organ replacement — *continued*
    by artificial or mechanical device or prosthesis of — *continued*
      eye globe Z97.0
      heart Z95.812
        valve Z95.2
      intestine Z97.8
      joint Z96.60
        hip — *see* Presence, hip joint implant
        knee — *see* Presence, knee joint implant
        specified site NEC Z96.698
      kidney Z97.8
      larynx Z96.3
      lens Z96.1
      limbs — *see* Presence, artificial, limb
      liver Z97.8
      lung Z97.8
      pancreas Z97.8
    by organ transplant (heterologous)(homologous) — *see* Transplant
  pacemaker
    brain Z96.89
    cardiac Z95.0
    specified NEC Z96.89
  pancreatectomy Z90.410
    complete Z90.410
    partial Z90.411
    total Z90.410
  physical restraint Z78.1
  pneumonectomy (complete) (partial) Z90.2
  pneumothorax, therapeutic Z98.3
  postcommotio cerebri F07.81
  postoperative (postprocedural) NEC Z98.890
    breast implant Z98.82
    dental Z98.818
      crown Z98.811
      fillings Z98.811
      restoration Z98.811
      sealant Z98.810
      specified NEC Z98.818
    pneumothorax, therapeutic Z98.3
    uterine scar Z98.891
  postpartum (routine follow-up) Z39.2
    care immediately after delivery Z39.0
  postsurgical (postprocedural) NEC Z98.890
    pneumothorax, therapeutic Z98.3
  pregnancy, incidental Z33.1
  prosthesis coronary angioplasty Z95.5
  pseudophakia Z96.1
  renal dialysis (hemodialysis) (peritoneal) Z99.2
  retained foreign body — *see* Retained, foreign body fragments (type of)
  reversed jejunal transposition (for bypass) Z98.0
  salpingo-oophorectomy
    bilateral Z90.722
    unilateral Z90.721
  sex reassignment surgery status Z87.890
  shunt
    arteriovenous (for dialysis) Z99.2
    cerebrospinal fluid Z98.2
    ventricular (communicating) (for drainage) Z98.2
  splenectomy Z90.81
  thymicolymphaticus E32.8
  thymicus E32.8
  thymolymphaticus E32.8
  thyroidectomy (hypothyroidism) E89.0
  tooth (teeth) extraction — *see also* Absence, teeth, acquired K08.409
  tPA (rtPA) administration in a different facility within the last 24 hours prior to admission to current facility Z92.82
  tracheostomy Z93.0
  transplant — *see* Transplant
    organ removed Z98.85
  tubal ligation Z98.51
  underimmunization Z28.3
  ureterostomy Z93.6
  urethrostomy Z93.6
  vagina, artificial Z93.8
  vasectomy Z98.52
  wheelchair confinement Z99.3
Stealing
  child problem F91.8
    in company with others Z72.810
  pathological (compulsive) F63.2
Steam burn — *see* Burn
Steatocystoma multiplex L72.2

☑ **Additional Character Required** — Refer to the Tabular List for Character Selection   ▽ Subterms under main terms may continue to next column or page

Steatohepatitis (nonalcoholic) (NASH) K75.81
Steatoma L72.3
 eyelid (cystic) — *see* Dermatosis, eyelid
  infected — *see* Hordeolum
Steatorrhea (chronic) K90.9
 with lacteal obstruction K90.2
 idiopathic (adult) (infantile) K90.9
 pancreatic K90.3
 primary K90.0
 tropical K90.1
Steatosis E88.89
 heart — *see* Degeneration, myocardial
 kidney N28.89
 liver NEC K76.0
Steele-Richardson-Olszewski disease or syndrome
  G23.1
Steinbrocker's syndrome G90.8
Steinert's disease G71.11
Stein-Leventhal syndrome E28.2
Stein's syndrome E28.2
STEMI — *see also* Infarct, myocardium, ST elevation I21.3
Stenocardia I20.8
Stenocephaly Q75.8
Stenosis, stenotic (cicatricial) — *see also* Stricture
 ampulla of Vater K83.1
 anus, anal (canal) (sphincter) K62.4
  and rectum K62.4
  congenital Q42.3
   with fistula Q42.2
 aorta (ascending) (supraventricular) (congenital) Q25.1
  arteriosclerotic I70.0
  calcified I70.0
  supravalvular Q25.3
 aortic (valve) I35.0
  with insufficiency I35.2
  congenital Q23.0
  rheumatic I06.0
   with
    incompetency, insufficiency or regurgitation
     I06.2
     with mitral (valve) disease I08.0
      with tricuspid (valve) disease I08.3
    mitral (valve) disease I08.0
     with tricuspid (valve) disease I08.3
    tricuspid (valve) disease I08.2
     with mitral (valve) disease I08.3
  specified cause NEC I35.0
  syphilitic A52.03
 aqueduct of Sylvius (congenital) Q03.0
  with spina bifida — *see* Spina bifida, by site, with
   hydrocephalus
  acquired G91.1
 artery NEC — *see also* Arteriosclerosis I77.1
  celiac I77.4
  cerebral — *see* Occlusion, artery, cerebral
  extremities — *see* Arteriosclerosis, extremities
  precerebral — *see* Occlusion, artery, precerebral
  pulmonary (congenital) Q25.6
   acquired I28.8
  renal I70.1
  stent
   coronary T82.855 ☑
   peripheral T82.856 ☑
 bile duct (common) (hepatic) K83.1
  congenital Q44.3
 bladder-neck (acquired) N32.0
  congenital Q64.31
 brain G93.89
 bronchus J98.09
  congenital Q32.3
  syphilitic A52.72
 cardia (stomach) K22.2
  congenital Q39.3
 cardiovascular — *see* Disease, cardiovascular
 caudal M48.08
 cervix, cervical (canal) N88.2
  congenital Q51.828
  in pregnancy or childbirth — *see* Pregnancy, com-
    plicated by, abnormal cervix
 colon — *see also* Obstruction, intestine
  congenital Q42.9
   specified NEC Q42.8
 colostomy K94.03
 common (bile) duct K83.1
  congenital Q44.3
 coronary (artery) — *see* Disease, heart, ischemic,
   atherosclerotic
 cystic duct — *see* Obstruction, gallbladder

Stenosis, stenotic — *continued*
 due to presence of device, implant or graft — *see also*
   Complications, by site and type, specified NEC
   T85.858 ☑
  arterial graft NEC T82.858 ☑
  breast (implant) T85.858 ☑
  catheter T85.858 ☑
   dialysis (renal) T82.858 ☑
    intraperitoneal T85.858 ☑
   infusion NEC T82.858 ☑
    spinal (epidural) (subdural) T85.850 ☑
   urinary (indwelling) T83.85 ☑
  fixation, internal (orthopedic) NEC T84.85 ☑
  gastrointestinal (bile duct) (esophagus) T85.858 ☑
  genital NEC T83.85 ☑
  heart NEC T82.857 ☑
  joint prosthesis T84.85 ☑
  ocular (corneal graft) (orbital implant) NEC
   T85.858 ☑
  orthopedic NEC T84.85 ☑
  specified NEC T85.858 ☑
  urinary NEC T83.85 ☑
  vascular NEC T82.858 ☑
  ventricular intracranial shunt T85.850 ☑
 duodenum K31.5
  congenital Q41.0
 ejaculatory duct NEC N50.89
  stent
   vascular
    end stent
     adjacent to stent — *see* Arteriosclerosis
     within the stent
      coronary T82.855 ☑
      peripheral T82.856 ☑
    in stent
     coronary vessel T82.855 ☑
     peripheral vessel T82.856 ☑
 endocervical os — *see* Stenosis, cervix
 enterostomy K94.13
 esophagus K22.2
  congenital Q39.3
  syphilitic A52.79
   congenital A50.59 *[K23]*
 eustachian tube — *see* Obstruction, eustachian tube
 external ear canal (acquired) H61.30- ☑
  congenital Q16.1
  due to
   inflammation H61.32- ☑
   trauma H61.31- ☑
  postprocedural H95.81- ☑
  specified cause NEC H61.39- ☑
 gallbladder — *see* Obstruction, gallbladder
 glottis J38.6
 heart valve — *see also* Endocarditis I38
  aortic — *see* Stenosis, aortic
  congenital Q24.8
  mitral — *see* Stenosis, mitral
  pulmonary — *see* Stenosis, pulmonary valve
  tricuspid — *see* Stenosis, tricuspid Q22.4
 hepatic duct K83.1
 hymen N89.6
 hypertrophic subaortic (idiopathic) I42.1
 ileum — *see also* Obstruction, intestine, specified NEC
   K56.699
  congenital Q41.2
 infundibulum cardia Q24.3
 intervertebral foramina — *see also* Lesion, biomechanical, specified NEC
  connective tissue M99.79
   abdomen M99.79
   cervical region M99.71
   cervicothoracic M99.71
   head region M99.70
   lumbar region M99.73
   lumbosacral M99.73
   occipitocervical M99.70
   sacral region M99.74
   sacrococcygeal M99.74
   sacroiliac M99.74
   specified NEC M99.79
   thoracic region M99.72
   thoracolumbar M99.72
  disc M99.79
   abdomen M99.79
   cervical region M99.71
   cervicothoracic M99.71
   head region M99.70

Stenosis, stenotic — *continued*
 intervertebral foramina — *see also* Lesion, biomechanical, specified — *continued*
  disc — *continued*
   lower extremity M99.76
   lumbar region M99.73
   lumbosacral M99.73
   occipitocervical M99.70
   pelvic M99.75
   rib cage M99.78
   sacral region M99.74
   sacrococcygeal M99.74
   sacroiliac M99.74
   specified NEC M99.79
   thoracic region M99.72
   thoracolumbar M99.72
   upper extremity M99.77
  osseous M99.69
   abdomen M99.69
   cervical region M99.61
   cervicothoracic M99.61
   head region M99.60
   lower extremity M99.66
   lumbar region M99.63
   lumbosacral M99.63
   occipitocervical M99.60
   pelvic M99.65
   rib cage M99.68
   sacral region M99.64
   sacrococcygeal M99.64
   sacroiliac M99.64
   specified NEC M99.69
   thoracic region M99.62
   thoracolumbar M99.62
   upper extremity M99.67
  subluxation — *see* Stenosis, intervertebral foramina,
    osseous
 intestine — *see also* Obstruction, intestine
  congenital (small) Q41.9
   large Q42.9
    specified NEC Q42.8
   specified NEC Q41.8
 jejunum — *see also* Obstruction, intestine, specified
   NEC K56.699
  congenital Q41.1
 lacrimal (passage)
  canaliculi H04.54- ☑
   congenital Q10.5
  duct H04.55- ☑
  punctum H04.56- ☑
  sac H04.57- ☑
 lacrimonasal duct — *see* Stenosis, lacrimal, duct
  congenital Q10.5
 larynx J38.6
  congenital NEC Q31.8
   subglottic Q31.1
  syphilitic A52.73
   congenital A50.59 *[J99]*
 mitral (chronic) (inactive) (valve) I05.0
  with
   aortic valve disease I08.0
   incompetency, insufficiency or regurgitation
    I05.2
  active or acute I01.1
   with rheumatic or Sydenham's chorea I02.0
  congenital Q23.2
  specified cause, except rheumatic I34.2
  syphilitic A52.03
 myocardium, myocardial — *see also* Degeneration,
   myocardial
  hypertrophic subaortic (idiopathic) I42.1
 nares (anterior) (posterior) J34.89
  congenital Q30.0
 nasal duct — *see also* Stenosis, lacrimal, duct
  congenital Q10.5
 nasolacrimal duct — *see also* Stenosis, lacrimal, duct
  congenital Q10.5
 neural canal — *see also* Lesion, biomechanical, specified NEC
  connective tissue M99.49
   abdomen M99.49
   cervical region M99.41
   cervicothoracic M99.41
   head region M99.40
   lower extremity M99.46
   lumbar region M99.43
   lumbosacral M99.43
   occipitocervical M99.40

Stenosis, stenotic — *continued*
neural canal — *see also* Lesion, biomechanical, specified — *continued*
  connective tissue — *continued*
    pelvic M99.45
    rib cage M99.48
    sacral region M99.44
    sacrococcygeal M99.44
    sacroiliac M99.44
    specified NEC M99.49
    thoracic region M99.42
    thoracolumbar M99.42
    upper extremity M99.47
  intervertebral disc M99.59
    abdomen M99.59
    cervical region M99.51
    cervicothoracic M99.51
    head region M99.50
    lower extremity M99.56
    lumbar region M99.53
    lumbosacral M99.53
    occipitocervical M99.50
    pelvic M99.55
    rib cage M99.58
    sacral region M99.54
    sacrococcygeal M99.54
    sacroiliac M99.54
    specified NEC M99.59
    thoracic region M99.52
    thoracolumbar M99.52
    upper extremity M99.57
  osseous M99.39
    abdomen M99.39
    cervical region M99.31
    cervicothoracic M99.31
    head region M99.30
    lower extremity M99.36
    lumbar region M99.33
    lumbosacral M99.33
    occipitocervical M99.30
    pelvic M99.35
    rib cage M99.38
    sacral region M99.34
    sacrococcygeal M99.34
    sacroiliac M99.34
    specified NEC M99.39
    thoracic region M99.32
    thoracolumbar M99.32
    upper extremity M99.37
  subluxation M99.29
    cervical region M99.21
    cervicothoracic M99.21
    head region M99.20
    lower extremity M99.26
    lumbar region M99.23
    lumbosacral M99.23
    occipitocervical M99.20
    pelvic M99.25
    rib cage M99.28
    sacral region M99.24
    sacrococcygeal M99.24
    sacroiliac M99.24
    specified NEC M99.29
    thoracic region M99.22
    thoracolumbar M99.22
    upper extremity M99.27
organ or site, congenital NEC — *see* Atresia, by site
papilla of Vater K83.1
pulmonary (artery) (congenital) Q25.6
  with ventricular septal defect, transposition of aorta, and hypertrophy of right ventricle Q21.3
  acquired I28.8
  in tetralogy of Fallot Q21.3
  infundibular Q24.3
  subvalvular Q24.3
  supravalvular Q25.6
  valve I37.0
    with insufficiency I37.2
    congenital Q22.1
    rheumatic I09.89
      with aortic, mitral or tricuspid (valve) disease I08.8
  vein, acquired I28.8
  vessel NEC I28.8
pulmonic (congenital) Q22.1
  infundibular Q24.3
  subvalvular Q24.3
pylorus (hypertrophic) (acquired) K31.1
  adult K31.1

Stenosis, stenotic — *continued*
pylorus — *continued*
  congenital Q40.0
  infantile Q40.0
rectum (sphincter) — *see* Stricture, rectum
renal artery I70.1
  congenital Q27.1
salivary duct (any) K11.8
sphincter of Oddi K83.1
spinal M48.00
  cervical region M48.02
  cervicothoracic region M48.03
  lumbar region (NOS) (without neurogenic claudication) M48.061
    with neurogenic claudication M48.062
  lumbosacral region M48.07
  occipito-atlanto-axial region M48.01
  sacrococcygeal region M48.08
  thoracic region M48.04
  thoracolumbar region M48.05
stomach, hourglass K31.2
subaortic (congenital) Q24.4
  hypertrophic (idiopathic) I42.1
subglottic J38.6
  congenital Q31.1
  postprocedural J95.5
trachea J39.8
  congenital Q32.1
  syphilitic A52.73
  tuberculous NEC A15.5
tracheostomy J95.03
tricuspid (valve) I07.0
  with
    aortic (valve) disease I08.2
    incompetency, insufficiency or regurgitation I07.2
      with aortic (valve) disease I08.2
        with mitral (valve) disease I08.3
    mitral (valve) disease I08.1
      with aortic (valve) disease I08.3
  congenital Q22.4
  nonrheumatic I36.0
    with insufficiency I36.2
tubal N97.1
ureter — *see* Atresia, ureter
ureteropelvic junction, congenital Q62.11
ureterovesical orifice, congenital Q62.12
urethra (valve) *see also* Stricture, urethra
  congenital Q64.32
urinary meatus, congenital Q64.33
vagina N89.5
  congenital Q52.4
  in pregnancy — *see* Pregnancy, complicated by, abnormal vagina
    causing obstructed labor O65.5
valve (cardiac) (heart) — *see also* Endocarditis I38
  congenital Q24.8
    aortic Q23.0
    mitral Q23.2
    pulmonary Q22.1
    tricuspid Q22.4
vena cava (inferior) (superior) I87.1
  congenital Q26.0
vesicourethral orifice Q64.31
vulva N90.5
Stent jail T82.897 ☑
Stercolith (impaction) K56.41
  appendix K38.1
Stercoraceous, stercoral ulcer K63.3
anus or rectum K62.6
Stereotypies NEC F98.4
Sterility — *see* Infertility
Sterilization — *see* Encounter (for), sterilization
Sternalgia — *see* Angina
Sternopagus Q89.4
Sternum bifidum Q76.7
Steroid
effects (adverse) (adrenocortical) (iatrogenic)
  cushingoid E24.2
    correct substance properly administered — *see* Table of Drugs and Chemicals, by drug, adverse effect
    overdose or wrong substance given or taken — *see* Table of Drugs and Chemicals, by drug, poisoning
  diabetes — *see* subcategory E09 ☑

Steroid — *continued*
effects — *continued*
  diabetes — *see* subcategory — *continued*
    correct substance properly administered — *see* Table of Drugs and Chemicals, by drug, adverse effect
    overdose or wrong substance given or taken — *see* Table of Drugs and Chemicals, by drug, poisoning
  fever R50.2
  insufficiency E27.3
    correct substance properly administered — *see* Table of Drugs and Chemicals, by drug, adverse effect
    overdose or wrong substance given or taken — *see* Table of Drugs and Chemicals, by drug, poisoning
  responder H40.04- ☑
Stevens-Johnson disease or syndrome L51.1
  toxic epidermal necrolysis overlap L51.3
Stewart-Morel syndrome M85.2
Sticker's disease B08.3
Sticky eye — *see* Conjunctivitis, acute, mucopurulent
Stieda's disease — *see* Bursitis, tibial collateral
Stiff neck — *see* Torticollis
Stiff-man syndrome G25.82
Stiffness, joint NEC M25.60
  ankle M25.67- ☑
  ankylosis — *see* Ankylosis, joint
  contracture — *see* Contraction, joint
  elbow M25.62- ☑
  foot M25.67- ☑
  hand M25.64- ☑
  hip M25.65- ☑
  knee M25.66- ☑
  shoulder M25.61- ☑
  specified site NEC M25.69
  wrist M25.63- ☑
Stigmata congenital syphilis A50.59
Stillbirth P95
Still-Felty syndrome — *see* Felty's syndrome
Still's disease or syndrome (juvenile) M08.20
  adult-onset M06.1
  ankle M08.27- ☑
  elbow M08.22- ☑
  foot joint M08.27- ☑
  hand joint M08.24- ☑
  hip M08.25- ☑
  knee M08.26- ☑
  multiple site M08.29
  shoulder M08.21- ☑
  specified site NEC M08.2A
  vertebra M08.28
  wrist M08.23- ☑
Stimulation, ovary E28.1
Sting (venomous) (with allergic or anaphylactic shock) — *see* Table of Drugs and Chemicals, by animal or substance, poisoning
Stippled epiphyses Q78.8
Stitch
  abscess T81.41 ☑
  burst (in operation wound) — *see* Disruption, wound, operation
Stokes' disease E05.00
  with thyroid storm E05.01
Stokes-Adams disease or syndrome I45.9
Stokvis (-Talma) **disease** D74.8
Stoma malfunction
  colostomy K94.03
  enterostomy K94.13
  gastrostomy K94.23
  ileostomy K94.13
  tracheostomy J95.03
Stomach — *see* condition
Stomatitis (denture) (ulcerative) K12.1
  angular K13.0
    due to dietary or vitamin deficiency E53.0
  aphthous K12.0
  bovine B08.61
  candidal B37.0
  catarrhal K12.1
  diphtheritic A36.89
  due to
    dietary deficiency E53.0
    thrush B37.0
    vitamin deficiency
      B group NEC E53.9

Stomatitis — *continued*
　due to — *continued*
　　vitamin deficiency — *continued*
　　　B2 (riboflavin) E53.0
　epidemic B08.8
　epizootic B08.8
　follicular K12.1
　gangrenous A69.0
　Geotrichum B48.3
　herpesviral, herpetic B00.2
　herpetiformis K12.0
　malignant K12.1
　membranous acute K12.1
　monilial B37.0
　mycotic B37.0
　necrotizing ulcerative A69.0
　parasitic B37.0
　septic K12.1
　spirochetal A69.1
　suppurative (acute) K12.2
　ulceromembranous A69.1
　vesicular K12.1
　　with exanthem (enteroviral) B08.4
　　virus disease A93.8
　Vincent's A69.1
Stomatocytosis D58.8
Stomatomycosis B37.0
Stomatorrhagia K13.79
Stone(s) — *see also* Calculus
　bladder (diverticulum) N21.0
　cystine E72.09
　heart syndrome I50.1
　kidney N20.0
　prostate N42.0
　pulpal (dental) K04.2
　renal N20.0
　salivary gland or duct (any) K11.5
　urethra (impacted) N21.1
　urinary (duct) (impacted) (passage) N20.9
　　bladder (diverticulum) N21.0
　　lower tract N21.9
　　specified NEC N21.8
　xanthine E79.8 *[N22]*
Stonecutter's lung J62.8
Stonemason's asthma, disease, lung or pneumoco-niosis J62.8
Stoppage
　heart — *see* Arrest, cardiac
　urine — *see* Retention, urine
Storm, thyroid — *see* Thyrotoxicosis
Strabismus (congenital) (nonparalytic) H50.9
　concomitant H50.40
　　convergent — *see* Strabismus, convergent concomi-tant
　　divergent — *see* Strabismus, divergent concomitant
　convergent concomitant H50.00
　　accommodative component H50.43
　　alternating H50.05
　　　with
　　　　A pattern H50.06
　　　　specified nonconcomitances NEC H50.08
　　　　V pattern H50.07
　　monocular H50.01- ☑
　　　with
　　　　A pattern H50.02- ☑
　　　　specified nonconcomitances NEC H50.04- ☑
　　　　V pattern H50.03- ☑
　　　intermittent H50.31- ☑
　　　　alternating H50.32
　cyclotropia H50.41 ☑
　divergent concomitant H50.10
　　alternating H50.15
　　　with
　　　　A pattern H50.16
　　　　specified nonconcomitances NEC H50.18
　　　　V pattern H50.17
　　monocular H50.11- ☑
　　　with
　　　　A pattern H50.12- ☑
　　　　specified nonconcomitances NEC H50.14- ☑
　　　　V pattern H50.13- ☑
　　　intermittent H50.33
　　　　alternating H50.34
　Duane's syndrome H50.81- ☑
　due to adhesions, scars H50.69
　heterophoria H50.50
　　alternating H50.55
　　cyclophoria H50.54

Strabismus — *continued*
　heterophoria — *continued*
　　esophoria H50.51
　　exophoria H50.52
　　vertical H50.53
　heterotropia H50.40
　　intermittent H50.30
　hypertropia H50.2- ☑
　hypotropia — *see* Hypertropia
　latent H50.50
　mechanical H50.60
　　Brown's sheath syndrome H50.61- ☑
　　specified type NEC H50.69
　monofixation syndrome H50.42
　paralytic H49.9
　　abducens nerve H49.2- ☑
　　fourth nerve H49.1- ☑
　　Kearns-Sayre syndrome H49.81- ☑
　　ophthalmoplegia (external)
　　　progressive H49.4- ☑
　　　　with pigmentary retinopathy H49.81- ☑
　　　total H49.3- ☑
　　sixth nerve H49.2- ☑
　　specified type NEC H49.88- ☑
　　third nerve H49.0- ☑
　　trochlear nerve H49.1- ☑
　specified type NEC H50.89
　vertical H50.2- ☑
Strain
　back S39.012 ☑
　cervical S16.1 ☑
　eye NEC — *see* Disturbance, vision, subjective
　heart — *see* Disease, heart
　low back S39.012 ☑
　mental NOS Z73.3
　　work-related Z56.6
　muscle (tendon) — *see* Injury, muscle, by site, strain
　neck S16.1 ☑
　physical NOS Z73.3
　　work-related Z56.6
　postural — *see also* Disorder, soft tissue, due to use
　psychological NEC Z73.3
　tendon — *see* Injury, muscle, by site, strain
Straining, on urination R39.16
Strand, vitreous — *see* Opacity, vitreous, membranes and strands
Strangulation, strangulated — *see also* Asphyxia, traumatic
　appendix K38.8
　bladder-neck N32.0
　bowel or colon K56.2
　food or foreign body — *see* Foreign body, by site
　hemorrhoids — *see* Hemorrhoids, with complication
　hernia — *see also* Hernia, by site, with obstruction
　　with gangrene — *see* Hernia, by site, with gangrene
　intestine (large) (small) K56.2
　　with hernia — *see also* Hernia, by site, with obstruc-tion
　　　with gangrene — *see* Hernia, by site, with gan-grene
　mesentery K56.2
　mucus — *see* Asphyxia, mucus
　omentum K56.2
　organ or site, congenital NEC — *see* Atresia, by site
　ovary — *see* Torsion, ovary
　penis N48.89
　　foreign body T19.4 ☑
　rupture — *see* Hernia, by site, with obstruction
　stomach due to hernia — *see also* Hernia, by site, with obstruction
　　with gangrene — *see* Hernia, by site, with gangrene
　vesicourethral orifice N32.0
Strangury R30.0
Straw itch B88.0
Strawberry
　gallbladder K82.4
　mark Q82.5
　tongue (red) (white) K14.3
Streak(s)
　macula, angioid H35.33
　ovarian Q50.32
Strephosymbolia F81.0
　secondary to organic lesion R48.8
Streptobacillary fever A25.1
Streptobacillosis A25.1
Streptobacillus moniliformis A25.1
Streptococcus, streptococcal — *see also* condition

Streptococcus, streptococcal — *continued*
　as cause of disease classified elsewhere B95.5
　group
　　A, as cause of disease classified elsewhere B95.0
　　B, as cause of disease classified elsewhere B95.1
　　D, as cause of disease classified elsewhere B95.2
　　pneumoniae, as cause of disease classified elsewhere B95.3
　　specified NEC, as cause of disease classified elsewhere B95.4
Streptomycosis B47.1
Streptotrichosis A48.8
Stress F43.9
　family — *see* Disruption, family
　fetal P84
　　complicating pregnancy O77.9
　　due to drug administration O77.1
　mental NEC Z73.3
　　work-related Z56.6
　physical NEC Z73.3
　　work-related Z56.6
　polycythemia D75.1
　reaction — *see also* Reaction, stress F43.9
　work schedule Z56.3
Stretching, nerve — *see* Injury, nerve
Striae albicantes, atrophicae or distensae (cutis) L90.6
Stricture — *see also* Stenosis
　ampulla of Vater K83.1
　anus (sphincter) K62.4
　　congenital Q42.3
　　　with fistula Q42.2
　　infantile Q42.3
　　　with fistula Q42.2
　aorta (ascending) (congenital) Q25.1
　　arteriosclerotic I70.0
　　calcified I70.0
　　supravalvular, congenital Q25.3
　aortic (valve) — *see* Stenosis, aortic
　aqueduct of Sylvius (congenital) Q03.0
　　with spina bifida — *see* Spina bifida, by site, with hydrocephalus
　　acquired G91.1
　artery I77.1
　　basilar — *see* Occlusion, artery, basilar
　　carotid — *see* Occlusion, artery, carotid
　　celiac I77.4
　　congenital (peripheral) Q27.8
　　　cerebral Q28.3
　　　coronary Q24.5
　　　digestive system Q27.8
　　　lower limb Q27.8
　　　retinal Q14.1
　　　specified site NEC Q27.8
　　　umbilical Q27.0
　　　upper limb Q27.8
　　coronary — *see* Disease, heart, ischemic, atherosclerotic
　　　congenital Q24.5
　　precerebral — *see* Occlusion, artery, precerebral
　　pulmonary (congenital) Q25.6
　　　acquired I28.8
　　renal I70.1
　　vertebral — *see* Occlusion, artery, vertebral
　auditory canal (external) (congenital)
　　acquired — *see* Stenosis, external ear canal
　bile duct (common) (hepatic) K83.1
　　congenital Q44.3
　　postoperative K91.89
　bladder N32.89
　　neck N32.0
　bowel — *see* Obstruction, intestine
　brain G93.89
　bronchus J98.09
　　congenital Q32.3
　　syphilitic A52.72
　cardia (stomach) K22.2
　　congenital Q39.3
　cardiac — *see also* Disease, heart
　　orifice (stomach) K22.2
　cecum — *see* Obstruction, intestine
　cervix, cervical (canal) N88.2
　　congenital Q51.828
　　in pregnancy — *see* Pregnancy, complicated by, abnormal cervix
　　　causing obstructed labor O65.5
　colon — *see also* Obstruction, intestine
　　congenital Q42.9
　　　specified NEC Q42.8

Stricture — *continued*
colostomy K94.03
common (bile) duct K83.1
coronary (artery) — *see* Disease, heart, ischemic, atherosclerotic
cystic duct — *see* Obstruction, gallbladder
digestive organs NEC, congenital Q45.8
duodenum K31.5
congenital Q41.0
ear canal (external) (congenital) Q16.1
acquired — *see* Stricture, auditory canal, acquired
ejaculatory duct N50.89
enterostomy K94.13
esophagus K22.2
congenital Q39.3
syphilitic A52.79
congenital A50.59 *[K23]*
eustachian tube — *see also* Obstruction, eustachian tube
congenital Q17.8
fallopian tube N97.1
gonococcal A54.24
tuberculous A18.17
gallbladder — *see* Obstruction, gallbladder
glottis J38.6
heart — *see also* Disease, heart
valve — *see also* Endocarditis I38
aortic Q23.0
mitral Q23.2
pulmonary Q22.1
tricuspid Q22.4
hepatic duct K83.1
hourglass, of stomach K31.2
hymen N89.6
hypopharynx J39.2
ileum — *see also* Obstruction, intestine, specified NEC K56.699
congenital Q41.2
intestine — *see also* Obstruction, intestine
congenital (small) Q41.9
large Q42.9
specified NEC Q42.8
specified NEC Q41.8
ischemic K55.1
jejunum — *see also* Obstruction, intestine, specified NEC K56.699
congenital Q41.1
lacrimal passages — *see also* Stenosis, lacrimal
congenital Q10.5
larynx J38.6
congenital NEC Q31.8
subglottic Q31.1
syphilitic A52.73
congenital A50.59 *[J99]*
meatus
ear (congenital) Q16.1
acquired — *see* Stricture, auditory canal, acquired
osseous (ear) (congenital) Q16.1
acquired — *see* Stricture, auditory canal, acquired
urinarius — *see also* Stricture, urethra
congenital Q64.33
mitral (valve) — *see* Stenosis, mitral
myocardium, myocardial I51.5
hypertrophic subaortic (idiopathic) I42.1
nares (anterior) (posterior) J34.89
congenital Q30.0
nasal duct — *see also* Stenosis, lacrimal, duct
congenital Q10.5
nasolacrimal duct — *see also* Stenosis, lacrimal, duct
congenital Q10.5
nasopharynx J39.2
syphilitic A52.73
nose J34.89
congenital Q30.0
nostril (anterior) (posterior) J34.89
congenital Q30.0
syphilitic A52.73
congenital A50.59 *[J99]*
organ or site, congenital NEC — *see* Atresia, by site
os uteri — *see* Stricture, cervix
osseous meatus (ear) (congenital) Q16.1
acquired — *see* Stricture, auditory canal, acquired
oviduct — *see* Stricture, fallopian tube
pelviureteric junction (congenital) Q62.11
acquired, with hydronephrosis N13.0
penis, by foreign body T19.4 ☑

Stricture — *continued*
pharynx J39.2
prostate N42.89
pulmonary, pulmonic
artery (congenital) Q25.6
acquired I28.8
noncongenital I28.8
infundibulum (congenital) Q24.3
valve I37.0
congenital Q22.1
vein, acquired I28.8
vessel NEC I28.8
punctum lacrimale — *see also* Stenosis, lacrimal, punctum
congenital Q10.5
pylorus (hypertrophic) K31.1
adult K31.1
congenital Q40.0
infantile Q40.0
rectosigmoid — *see also* Obstruction, intestine, specified NEC K56.699
rectum (sphincter) K62.4
congenital Q42.1
with fistula Q42.0
due to
chlamydial lymphogranuloma A55
irradiation K91.89
lymphogranuloma venereum A55
gonococcal A54.6
inflammatory (chlamydial) A55
syphilitic A52.74
tuberculous A18.32
renal artery I70.1
congenital Q27.1
salivary duct or gland (any) K11.8
sigmoid (flexure) — *see* Obstruction, intestine
spermatic cord N50.89
stoma (following) (of)
colostomy K94.03
enterostomy K94.13
gastrostomy K94.23
ileostomy K94.13
tracheostomy J95.03
stomach K31.89
congenital Q40.2
hourglass K31.2
subaortic Q24.4
hypertrophic (acquired) (idiopathic) I42.1
subglottic J38.6
syphilitic NEC A52.79
trachea J39.8
congenital Q32.1
syphilitic A52.73
tuberculous NEC A15.5
tracheostomy J95.03
tricuspid (valve) — *see* Stenosis, tricuspid
tunica vaginalis N50.89
ureter (postoperative) N13.5
with
hydronephrosis N13.1
with infection N13.6
pyelonephritis (chronic) N11.1
congenital — *see* Atresia, ureter
tuberculous A18.11
ureteropelvic junction (congenital) Q62.11
acquired, with hydronephrosis N13.0
ureterovesical orifice N13.5
with infection N13.6
urethra (organic) (spasmodic) — *see also* Stricture, urethra, male N35.919
associated with schistosomiasis B65.0 *[N37]*
congenital Q64.39
valvular (posterior) Q64.2
due to
infection — *see* Stricture, urethra, postinfective
trauma — *see* Stricture, urethra, post-traumatic
female N35.92
gonococcal, gonorrheal A54.01
infective NEC — *see* Stricture, urethra, postinfective
late effect (sequelae) of injury — *see* Stricture, urethra, post-traumatic
male N35.919
anterior urethra N35.914
bulbous urethra N35.912
meatal N35.911
membranous urethra N35.913
overlapping sites N35.916

Stricture — *continued*
urethra — *see also* Stricture, urethra, male — *continued*
postcatheterization — *see* Stricture, urethra, postprocedural
postinfective NEC
female N35.12
male N35.119
anterior urethra N35.114
bulbous urethra N35.112
meatal N35.111
membranous urethra N35.113
overlapping sites N35.116
postobstetric N35.021
postoperative — *see* Stricture, urethra, postprocedural
postprocedural
female N99.12
male N99.114
anterior bulbous urethra N99.113
bulbous urethra N99.111
fossa navicularis N99.115
meatal N99.110
membranous urethra N99.112
overlapping sites N99.116
post-traumatic
female N35.028
due to childbirth N35.021
male N35.014
anterior urethra N35.013
bulbous urethra N35.011
meatal N35.010
membranous urethra N35.012
overlapping sites N35.016
sequela (late effect) of
childbirth N35.021
injury — *see* Stricture, urethra, post-traumatic
specified cause NEC
female N35.82
male N35.819
anterior urethra N35.814
bulbous urethra N35.812
meatal N35.811
membranous urethra N35.813
overlapping sites N35.816
syphilitic A52.76
traumatic — *see* Stricture, urethra, post-traumatic
valvular (posterior), congenital Q64.2
urinary meatus — *see* Stricture, urethra
uterus, uterine (synechiae) N85.6
os (external) (internal) — *see* Stricture, cervix
vagina (outlet) — *see* Stenosis, vagina
valve (cardiac) (heart) — *see also* Endocarditis
congenital
aortic Q23.0
mitral Q23.2
pulmonary Q22.1
tricuspid Q22.4
vas deferens N50.89
congenital Q55.4
vein I87.1
vena cava (inferior) (superior) NEC I87.1
congenital Q26.0
vesicourethral orifice N32.0
congenital Q64.31
vulva (acquired) N90.5
Stridor R06.1
congenital (larynx) P28.89
Stridulous — *see* condition
Stroke (apoplectic) (brain) (embolic) (ischemic) (paralytic) (thrombotic) I63.9
cerebral, perinatal P91.82- ☑
cryptogenic — *see also* infarction, cerebral I63.9
epileptic — *see* Epilepsy
heat T67.01 ☑
exertional T67.02 ☑
specified NEC T67.09 ☑
in evolution I63.9
intraoperative
during cardiac surgery I97.810
during other surgery I97.811
ischemic, perinatal arterial P91.82- ☑
lightning — *see* Lightning
meaning
cerebral hemorrhage — *code to* Hemorrhage, intracranial
cerebral infarction — *code to* Infarction, cerebral
neonatal P91.82- ☑

Stroke — *continued*
  postprocedural
    following cardiac surgery I97.820
    following other surgery I97.821
  sun T67.01 ☑
    specified NEC T67.09 ☑
  unspecified (NOS) I63.9
Stromatosis, endometrial D39.0
Strongyloidiasis, strongyloidosis B78.9
  cutaneous B78.1
  disseminated B78.7
  intestinal B78.0
Strophulus pruriginosus L28.2
Struck by lightning — *see* Lightning
Struma — *see also* Goiter
  Hashimoto E06.3
  lymphomatosa E06.3
  nodosa (simplex) E04.9
    endemic E01.2
      multinodular E01.1
    multinodular E04.2
      iodine-deficiency related E01.1
    toxic or with hyperthyroidism E05.20
      with thyroid storm E05.21
      multinodular E05.20
        with thyroid storm E05.21
      uninodular E05.10
        with thyroid storm E05.11
    toxicosa E05.20
      with thyroid storm E05.21
      multinodular E05.20
        with thyroid storm E05.21
      uninodular E05.10
        with thyroid storm E05.11
    uninodular E04.1
  ovarii D27.- ☑
  Riedel's E06.5
Strumipriva cachexia E03.4
Strümpell-Marie spine — *see* Spondylitis, ankylosing
Strümpell-Westphal pseudosclerosis E83.01
Stuart deficiency disease (factor X) D68.2
Stuart-Prower factor deficiency (factor X) D68.2
Student's elbow — *see* Bursitis, elbow, olecranon
Stump — *see* Amputation
Stunting, nutritional E45
Stupor (catatonic) R40.1
  depressive (single episode) F32.89
    recurrent episode F33.8
  dissociative F44.2
  manic F30.2
  manic-depressive F31.89
  psychogenic (anergic) F44.2
  reaction to exceptional stress (transient) F43.0
Sturge (-Weber) (-Dimitri) (-Kalischer) **disease or syndrome** Q85.8
Stuttering F80.81
  adult onset F98.5
  childhood onset F80.81
  following cerebrovascular disease — *see* Disorder, fluency. following cerebrovascular disease
  in conditions classified elsewhere R47.82
Sty, stye (external) (internal) (meibomian) (zeisian) — *see* Hordeolum
Subacidity, gastric K31.89
  psychogenic F45.8
Subacute — *see* condition
Subarachnoid — *see* condition
Subcortical — *see* condition
Subcostal syndrome, nerve compression — *see* Mononeuropathy, upper limb, specified site NEC
Subcutaneous, subcuticular — *see* condition
Subdural — *see* condition
Subendocardium — *see* condition
Subependymoma
  specified site — *see* Neoplasm, uncertain behavior, by site
  unspecified site D43.2
Suberosis J67.3
Subglossitis — *see* Glossitis
Subhemophilia D66
Subinvolution
  breast (postlactational) (postpuerperal) N64.89
  puerperal O90.89
  uterus (chronic) (nonpuerperal) N85.3
    puerperal O90.89
Sublingual — *see* condition
Sublinguitis — *see* Sialoadenitis

Subluxatable hip Q65.6
Subluxation — *see also* Dislocation
  acromioclavicular S43.11- ☑
  ankle S93.0- ☑
  atlantoaxial, recurrent M43.4
    with myelopathy M43.3
  carpometacarpal (joint) NEC S63.05- ☑
    thumb S63.04- ☑
  complex, vertebral — *see* Complex, subluxation
  congenital — *see also* Malposition, congenital
    hip — *see* Dislocation, hip, congenital, partial
    joint (excluding hip)
      lower limb Q68.8
      shoulder Q68.8
      upper limb Q68.8
  elbow (traumatic) S53.10- ☑
    anterior S53.11- ☑
    lateral S53.14- ☑
    medial S53.13- ☑
    posterior S53.12- ☑
    specified type NEC S53.19- ☑
  finger S63.20- ☑
    index S63.20- ☑
    interphalangeal S63.22- ☑
      distal S63.24- ☑
        index S63.24- ☑
        little S63.24- ☑
        middle S63.24- ☑
        ring S63.24- ☑
      index S63.22- ☑
      little S63.22- ☑
      middle S63.22- ☑
      proximal S63.23- ☑
        index S63.23- ☑
        little S63.23- ☑
        middle S63.23- ☑
        ring S63.23- ☑
      ring S63.22- ☑
    little S63.20- ☑
    metacarpophalangeal S63.21- ☑
      index S63.21- ☑
      little S63.21- ☑
      middle S63.21- ☑
      ring S63.21- ☑
    middle S63.20- ☑
    ring S63.20- ☑
  foot S93.30- ☑
    specified site NEC S93.33- ☑
    tarsal joint S93.31- ☑
    tarsometatarsal joint S93.32- ☑
    toe — *see* Subluxation, toe
  hip S73.00- ☑
    anterior S73.03- ☑
      obturator S73.02- ☑
    central S73.04- ☑
    posterior S73.01- ☑
  interphalangeal (joint)
    finger S63.22- ☑
      distal joint S63.24- ☑
        index S63.24- ☑
        little S63.24- ☑
        middle S63.24- ☑
        ring S63.24- ☑
      index S63.22- ☑
      little S63.22- ☑
      middle S63.22- ☑
      proximal joint S63.23- ☑
        index S63.23- ☑
        little S63.23- ☑
        middle S63.23- ☑
        ring S63.23- ☑
      ring S63.22- ☑
    thumb S63.12- ☑
    toe S93.13- ☑
      great S93.13- ☑
      lesser S93.13- ☑
  joint prosthesis — *see* Complications, joint prosthesis, mechanical, displacement, by site
  knee S83.10- ☑
    cap — *see* Subluxation, patella
    patella — *see* Subluxation, patella
    proximal tibia
      anteriorly S83.11- ☑
      laterally S83.14- ☑
      medially S83.13- ☑
      posteriorly S83.12- ☑

Subluxation — *continued*
  knee — *continued*
    specified type NEC S83.19- ☑
  lens — *see* Dislocation, lens, partial
  ligament, traumatic — *see* Sprain, by site
  metacarpal (bone)
    proximal end S63.06- ☑
  metacarpophalangeal (joint)
    finger S63.21- ☑
      index S63.21- ☑
      little S63.21- ☑
      middle S63.21- ☑
      ring S63.21- ☑
      thumb S63.11- ☑
  metatarsophalangeal joint S93.14- ☑
    great toe S93.14- ☑
    lesser toe S93.14- ☑
  midcarpal (joint) S63.03- ☑
  patella S83.00- ☑
    lateral S83.01- ☑
    recurrent (nontraumatic) — *see* Dislocation, patella, recurrent, incomplete
    specified type NEC S83.09- ☑
  pathological — *see* Dislocation, pathological
  radial head S53.00- ☑
    anterior S53.01- ☑
    nursemaid's elbow S53.03- ☑
    posterior S53.02- ☑
    specified type NEC S53.09- ☑
  radiocarpal (joint) S63.02- ☑
  radioulnar (joint)
    distal S63.01- ☑
    proximal — *see* Subluxation, elbow
  shoulder
    congenital Q68.8
    girdle S43.30- ☑
      scapula S43.31- ☑
      specified site NEC S43.39- ☑
    traumatic S43.00- ☑
      anterior S43.01- ☑
      inferior S43.03- ☑
      posterior S43.02- ☑
      specified type NEC S43.08- ☑
  sternoclavicular (joint) S43.20- ☑
    anterior S43.21- ☑
    posterior S43.22- ☑
  symphysis (pubis)
  thumb S63.103 ☑
    interphalangeal joint — *see* Subluxation, interphalangeal (joint), thumb
    metacarpophalangeal joint — *see* Subluxation, metacarpophalangeal (joint), thumb
  toe(s) S93.10- ☑
    great S93.10- ☑
      interphalangeal joint S93.13- ☑
      metatarsophalangeal joint S93.14- ☑
    interphalangeal joint S93.13- ☑
    lesser S93.10- ☑
      interphalangeal joint S93.13- ☑
      metatarsophalangeal joint S93.14- ☑
    metatarsophalangeal joint S93.149 ☑
  ulna
    distal end S63.07- ☑
    proximal end — *see* Subluxation, elbow
  ulnohumeral joint — *see* Subluxation, elbow
  vertebral
    recurrent NEC — *see* subcategory M43.5 ☑
    traumatic
      cervical S13.100 ☑
        atlantoaxial joint S13.120 ☑
        atlantooccipital joint S13.110 ☑
        atloidooccipital joint S13.110 ☑
        joint between
          C0 and C1 S13.110 ☑
          C1 and C2 S13.120 ☑
          C2 and C3 S13.130 ☑
          C3 and C4 S13.140 ☑
          C4 and C5 S13.150 ☑
          C5 and C6 S13.160 ☑
          C6 and C7 S13.170 ☑
          C7 and T1 S13.180 ☑
        occipitoatloid joint S13.110 ☑
      lumbar S33.100 ☑
        joint between
          L1 and L2 S33.110 ☑
          L2 and L3 S33.120 ☑

Subluxation — continued
  vertebral — continued
    traumatic — continued
      lumbar — continued
        joint between — continued
          L3 and L4 S33.130 ☑
          L4 and L5 S33.140 ☑
      thoracic S23.100 ☑
        joint between
          T1 and T2 S23.110 ☑
          T2 and T3 S23.120 ☑
          T3 and T4 S23.122 ☑
          T4 and T5 S23.130 ☑
          T5 and T6 S23.132 ☑
          T6 and T7 S23.140 ☑
          T7 and T8 S23.142 ☑
          T8 and T9 S23.150 ☑
          T9 and T10 S23.152 ☑
          T10 and T11 S23.160 ☑
          T11 and T12 S23.162 ☑
          T12 and L1 S23.170 ☑
  wrist (carpal bone) S63.00- ☑
    carpometacarpal joint — see Subluxation, carpometacarpal (joint)
    distal radioulnar joint — see Subluxation, radioulnar (joint), distal
    metacarpal bone, proximal — see Subluxation, metacarpal (bone), proximal end
    midcarpal — see Subluxation, midcarpal (joint)
    radiocarpal joint — see Subluxation, radiocarpal (joint)
    recurrent — see Dislocation, recurrent, wrist
    specified site NEC S63.09- ☑
    ulna — see Subluxation, ulna, distal end
Submaxillary — see condition
Submersion (fatal) (nonfatal) T75.1 ☑
Submucous — see condition
Subnormal, subnormality
  accommodation (old age) H52.4
  mental — see Disability, intellectual
  temperature (accidental) T68 ☑
Subphrenic — see condition
Subscapular nerve — see condition
Subseptus uterus Q51.28
Subsiding appendicitis K36
Substance (other psychoactive) **-induced**
  anxiety disorder F19.980
  bipolar and related disorder F19.94
  delirium F19.921
  depressive disorder F19.94
  major neurocognitive disorder F19.97
  mild neurocognitive disorder F19.988
  obsessive-compulsive and related disorder F19.988
  psychotic disorder F19.959
  sexual dysfunction F19.981
  sleep disorder F19.982
Substernal thyroid E04.9
  congenital Q89.2
Substitution disorder F44.9
Subtentorial — see condition
Subthyroidism (acquired) — see also Hypothyroidism
  congenital E03.1
Succenturiate placenta O43.19- ☑
Sucking thumb, child (excessive) F98.8
Sudamen, sudamina L74.1
Sudanese kala-azar B55.0
Sudden
  hearing loss — see Deafness, sudden
  heart failure — see Failure, heart
Sudeck's atrophy, disease, or syndrome — see Algoneurodystrophy
Suffocation — see Asphyxia, traumatic
Sugar
  blood
    high (transient) R73.9
    low (transient) E16.2
  in urine R81
Suicide, suicidal (attempted) T14.91 ☑
  by poisoning — see Table of Drugs and Chemicals
  history of (personal) Z91.51
    in family Z81.8
  ideation — see Ideation, suicidal
  risk
    meaning personal history of attempted suicide Z91.51
    meaning suicidal ideation — see Ideation, suicidal

Suicide, suicidal — continued
  tendencies
    meaning personal history of attempted suicide Z91.51
    meaning suicidal ideation — see Ideation, suicidal
  trauma — see nature of injury by site
Suipestifer infection — see Infection, salmonella
Sulfhemoglobinemia, sulphemoglobinemia (acquired) (with methemoglobinemia) D74.8
Sumatran mite fever A75.3
Summer — see condition
Sunburn L55.9
  due to
    tanning bed (acute) L56.8
      chronic L57.8
    ultraviolet radiation (acute) L56.8
      chronic L57.8
  first degree L55.0
  second degree L55.1
  third degree L55.2
SUNCT (short lasting unilateral neuralgiform headache with conjunctival injection and tearing) G44.059
  intractable G44.051
  not intractable G44.059
Sundowning F05
Sunken acetabulum — see Derangement, joint, specified type NEC, hip
Sunstroke T67.01 ☑
  specified NEC T67.09 ☑
Superfecundation — see Pregnancy, multiple
Superfetation — see Pregnancy, multiple
Superinvolution (uterus) N85.8
Supernumerary (congenital)
  aortic cusps Q23.8
  auditory ossicles Q16.3
  bone Q79.8
  breast Q83.1
  carpal bones Q74.0
  cusps, heart valve NEC Q24.8
    aortic Q23.8
    mitral Q23.2
    pulmonary Q22.3
  digit(s) Q69.9
  ear (lobule) Q17.0
  fallopian tube Q50.6
  finger Q69.0
  hymen Q52.4
  kidney Q63.0
  lacrimonasal duct Q10.6
  lobule (ear) Q17.0
  mitral cusps Q23.2
  muscle Q79.8
  nipple(s) Q83.3
  organ or site not listed — see Accessory
  ossicles, auditory Q16.3
  ovary Q50.31
  oviduct Q50.6
  pulmonary, pulmonic cusps Q22.3
  rib Q76.6
    cervical or first (syndrome) Q76.5
  roots (of teeth) K00.2
  spleen Q89.09
  tarsal bones Q74.2
  teeth K00.1
  testis Q55.29
  thumb Q69.1
  toe Q69.2
  uterus Q51.28
  vagina Q52.1 ☑
  vertebra Q76.49
Supervision (of)
  contraceptive — see Prescription, contraceptives
  dietary (for) Z71.3
    allergy (food) Z71.3
    colitis Z71.3
    diabetes mellitus Z71.3
    food allergy or intolerance Z71.3
    gastritis Z71.3
    hypercholesterolemia Z71.3
    hypoglycemia Z71.3
    intolerance (food) Z71.3
    obesity Z71.3
    specified NEC Z71.3
  healthy infant or child Z76.2
    foundling Z76.1
  high-risk pregnancy — see Pregnancy, complicated by, high, risk
  lactation Z39.1

Supervision — continued
  pregnancy — see Pregnancy, supervision of
Supplemental teeth K00.1
Suppression
  binocular vision H53.34
  lactation O92.5
  menstruation N94.89
  ovarian secretion E28.39
  renal N28.9
  urine, urinary secretion R34
Suppuration, suppurative — see also condition
  accessory sinus (chronic) — see Sinusitis
  adrenal gland
  antrum (chronic) — see Sinusitis, maxillary
  bladder — see Cystitis
  brain G06.0
    sequelae G09
  breast N61.1
    puerperal, postpartum or gestational — see Mastitis, obstetric, purulent
  dental periosteum M27.3
  ear (middle) — see also Otitis, media
    external NEC — see Otitis, externa, infective
    internal — see subcategory H83.0 ☑
  ethmoidal (chronic) (sinus) — see Sinusitis, ethmoidal
  fallopian tube — see Salpingo-oophoritis
  frontal (chronic) (sinus) — see Sinusitis, frontal
  gallbladder (acute) K81.0
  gum K05.20
    generalized — see Periodontitis, aggressive, generalized
    localized — see Periodontitis, aggressive, localized
  intracranial G06.0
  joint — see Arthritis, pyogenic or pyemic
  labyrinthine — see subcategory H83.0 ☑
  lung — see Abscess, lung
  mammary gland N61.1
    puerperal, postpartum O91.12
      associated with lactation O91.13
  maxilla, maxillary M27.2
    sinus (chronic) — see Sinusitis, maxillary
  muscle — see Myositis, infective
  nasal sinus (chronic) — see Sinusitis
  pancreas, acute — see also Pancreatitis, acute K85.80
  parotid gland — see Sialoadenitis
  pelvis, pelvic
    female — see Disease, pelvis, inflammatory
    male K65.0
  pericranial — see Osteomyelitis
  salivary duct or gland (any) — see Sialoadenitis
  sinus (accessory) (chronic) (nasal) — see Sinusitis
  sphenoidal sinus (chronic) — see Sinusitis, sphenoidal
  thymus (gland) E32.1
  thyroid (gland) E06.0
  tonsil — see Tonsillitis
  uterus — see Endometritis
Supraeruption of tooth (teeth) M26.34
Supraglottitis J04.30
  with obstruction J04.31
Suprarenal (gland) — see condition
Suprascapular nerve — see condition
Suprasellar — see condition
Surfer's knots or nodules S89.8- ☑
Surgical
  emphysema T81.82 ☑
  procedures, complication or misadventure — see Complications, surgical procedures
  shock T81.10 ☑
Surveillance (of) (for) — see also Observation
  alcohol abuse Z71.41
  contraceptive — see Prescription, contraceptives
  dietary Z71.3
  drug abuse Z71.51
Susceptibility to disease, genetic Z15.89
  malignant neoplasm Z15.09
    breast Z15.01
    endometrium Z15.04
    ovary Z15.02
    prostate Z15.03
    specified NEC Z15.09
  multiple endocrine neoplasia Z15.81
Suspected condition, ruled out — see also Observation, suspected
  amniotic cavity and membrane Z03.71
  cervical shortening Z03.75
  fetal anomaly Z03.73
  fetal growth Z03.74

☑ Additional Character Required — Refer to the Tabular List for Character Selection   ▽ Subterms under main terms may continue to next column or page

Suspected condition, ruled out — *continued*
  maternal and fetal conditions NEC Z03.79
  newborn — *see also* Observation, newborn, suspected
    condition ruled out Z05.9
  oligohydramnios Z03.71
  placental problem Z03.72
  polyhydramnios Z03.71
Suspended uterus
  in pregnancy or childbirth — *see* Pregnancy, compli-
    cated by, abnormal uterus
Sutton's nevus D22.9
Suture
  burst (in operation wound) T81.31 ☑
    external operation wound T81.31 ☑
    internal operation wound T81.32 ☑
  inadvertently left in operation wound — *see* Foreign
    body, accidentally left during a procedure
  removal Z48.02
Swab inadvertently left in operation wound — *see*
    Foreign body, accidentally left during a procedure
Swallowed, swallowing
  difficulty — *see* Dysphagia
  foreign body — *see* Foreign body, alimentary tract
Swan-neck deformity (finger) — *see* Deformity, finger,
    swan-neck
Swearing, compulsive F42.8
  in Gilles de la Tourette's syndrome F95.2
Sweat, sweats
  fetid L75.0
  night R61
Sweating, excessive R61
Sweeley-Klionsky disease E75.21
Sweet's disease or dermatosis L98.2
Swelling (of) R60.9
  abdomen, abdominal (not referable to any particular
    organ) — *see* Mass, abdominal
  ankle — *see* Effusion, joint, ankle
  arm M79.89
    forearm M79.89
  breast — *see also* Lump, breast N63.0
  Calabar B74.3
  cervical gland R59.0
  chest, localized R22.2
  ear H93.8- ☑
  extremity (lower) (upper) — *see* Disorder, soft tissue,
    specified type NEC
  finger M79.89
  foot M79.89
  glands R59.9
    generalized R59.1
    localized R59.0
  hand M79.89
  head (localized) R22.0
  inflammatory — *see* Inflammation
  intra-abdominal — *see* Mass, abdominal
  joint — *see* Effusion, joint
  leg M79.89
    lower M79.89
  limb — *see* Disorder, soft tissue, specified type NEC
  localized (skin) R22.9
    chest R22.2
    head R22.0
    limb
      lower — *see* Mass, localized, limb, lower
      upper — *see* Mass, localized, limb, upper
    neck R22.1
    trunk R22.2
  neck (localized) R22.1
  pelvic — *see* Mass, abdominal
  scrotum N50.89
  splenic — *see* Splenomegaly
  testis N50.89
  toe M79.89
  umbilical R19.09
  wandering, due to Gnathostoma (spinigerum) B83.1
  white — *see* Tuberculosis, arthritis
Swift (-Feer) **disease**
  overdose or wrong substance given or taken — *see*
    Table of Drugs and Chemicals, by drug, poisoning
Swimmer's
  cramp T75.1 ☑
  ear H60.33- ☑
  itch B65.3
Swimming in the head R42
Swollen — *see* Swelling
Swyer syndrome Q99.1
Sycosis L73.8

Sycosis — *continued*
  barbae (not parasitic) L73.8
  contagiosa (mycotic) B35.0
  lupoides L73.8
  mycotic B35.0
  parasitic B35.0
  vulgaris L73.8
Sydenham's chorea — *see* Chorea, Sydenham's
Sylvatic yellow fever A95.0
Sylvest's disease B33.0
Symblepharon H11.23- ☑
  congenital Q10.3
Symond's syndrome G93.2
Sympathetic — *see* condition
Sympatheticotonia G90.8
Sympathicoblastoma
  specified site — *see* Neoplasm, malignant, by site
  unspecified site C74.90
Sympathogonioma — *see* Sympathicoblastoma
Symphalangy (fingers) (toes) Q70.9
Symptoms NEC R68.89
  breast NEC N64.59
  cold J00
  development NEC R63.8
  factitious, self-induced — *see* Disorder, factitious
  genital organs, female R10.2
  involving
    abdomen NEC R19.8
    appearance NEC R46.89
    awareness R41.9
      altered mental status R41.82
      amnesia — *see* Amnesia
      borderline intellectual functioning R41.83
      coma — *see* Coma
      disorientation R41.0
      neurologic neglect syndrome R41.4
      senile cognitive decline R41.81
      specified symptom NEC R41.89
    behavior NEC R46.89
    cardiovascular system NEC R09.89
    chest NEC R09.89
    circulatory system NEC R09.89
    cognitive functions R41.9
      altered mental status R41.82
      amnesia — *see* Amnesia
      borderline intellectual functioning R41.83
      coma — *see* Coma
      disorientation R41.0
      neurologic neglect syndrome R41.4
      senile cognitive decline R41.81
      specified symptom NEC R41.89
    development NEC R62.50
    digestive system NEC R19.8
    emotional state NEC R45.89
      emotional lability R45.86
    food and fluid intake R63.8
    general perceptions and sensations R44.9
      specified NEC R44.8
    musculoskeletal system R29.91
      specified NEC R29.898
    nervous system R29.90
      specified NEC R29.818
    pelvis NEC R19.8
    respiratory system NEC R09.89
    skin and integument R23.9
    urinary system R39.9
  menopausal N95.1
  metabolism NEC R63.8
  neurotic F48.8
  of infancy R68.19
  pelvis NEC, female R10.2
  skin and integument NEC R23.9
  subcutaneous tissue NEC R23.9
  viral cold J00
Sympus Q74.2
Syncephalus Q89.4
Synchondrosis
  abnormal (congenital) Q78.8
  ischiopubic M91.0
Synchysis (scintillans) (senile) (vitreous body) H43.89
Syncope (near) (pre-) R55
  anginosa I20.8
  bradycardia R00.1
  cardiac R55
  carotid sinus G90.01
  due to spinal (lumbar) puncture G97.1
  heart R55
  heat T67.1 ☑

Syncope — *continued*
  laryngeal R05.4
  psychogenic F48.8
  tussive R05.8
  vasoconstriction R55
  vasodepressor R55
  vasomotor R55
  vasovagal R55
Syndactylism, syndactyly Q70.9
  complex (with synostosis)
    fingers Q70.0- ☑
    toes Q70.2- ☑
  simple (without synostosis)
    fingers Q70.1- ☑
    toes Q70.3- ☑
Syndrome — *see also* Disease
  5q minus NOS D46.C (*following* D46.2)
  48,XXXX Q97.1
  49,XXXXX Q97.1
  abdominal
    acute R10.0
    muscle deficiency Q79.4
  abnormal innervation H02.519
    left H02.516
      lower H02.515
      upper H02.514
    right H02.513
      lower H02.512
      upper H02.511
  abstinence, neonatal P96.1
  acid pulmonary aspiration, obstetric O74.0
  acquired immunodeficiency — *see* Human, immunod-
    eficiency virus (HIV) disease
  acute abdominal R10.0
  acute respiratory distress (adult) (child) J80
    idiopathic J84.114
  Adair-Dighton Q78.0
  Adams-Stokes (-Morgagni) I45.9
  adiposogenital E23.6
  adrenal
    hemorrhage (meningococcal) A39.1
    meningococcic A39.1
  adrenocortical — *see* Cushing's, syndrome
  adrenogenital E25.9
    congenital, associated with enzyme deficiency E25.0
  afferent loop NEC K91.89
  Alagille's Q44.7
  alcohol withdrawal (without convulsions) — *see* De-
    pendence, alcohol, with, withdrawal
  Alder's D72.0
  Aldrich (-Wiskott) D82.0
  alien hand R41.4
  Alport Q87.81
  alveolar hypoventilation E66.2
  alveolocapillary block J84.10
  amnesic, amnestic (confabulatory) (due to) — *see* Dis-
    order, amnesic
  amyostatic (Wilson's disease) E83.01
  androgen insensitivity E34.50
    complete E34.51
    partial E34.52
  androgen resistance — *see also* Syndrome, androgen
    insensitivity E34.50
  Angelman Q93.51
  anginal — *see* Angina
  ankyloglossia superior Q38.1
  anterior
    chest wall R07.89
    cord G83.82
    spinal artery G95.19
      compression M47.019
        cervical region M47.012
        cervicothoracic region M47.013
        lumbar region M47.016
        occipito-atlanto-axial region M47.011
        thoracic region M47.014
        thoracolumbar region M47.015
      tibial M76.81- ☑
  antibody deficiency D80.9
    agammaglobulinemic D80.1
      hereditary D80.0
    congenital D80.0
    hypogammaglobulinemic D80.1
      hereditary D80.0
  anticardiolipin (-antibody) D68.61
  antidepressant discontinuation T43.205 ☑
  antiphospholipid (-antibody) D68.61

▽ **Subterms under main terms may continue to next column or page**   ☑ **Additional Character Required** — **Refer to the Tabular List for Character Selection**   **303**

Suspected condition, ruled out — Syndrome

Syndrome — *continued*
- aortic
  - arch M31.4
  - bifurcation I74.09
- aortomesenteric duodenum occlusion K31.5
- apical ballooning (transient left ventricular) I51.81
- arcuate ligament I77.4
- argentaffin, argintaffinoma E34.0
- Arnold-Chiari — *see* Arnold-Chiari disease
- Arrillaga-Ayerza I27.0
- arterial tortuosity Q87.82
- arteriovenous steal T82.898- ☑
- Asherman's N85.6
- aspiration, of newborn — *see* Aspiration, by substance, with pneumonia
  - meconium P24.01
- ataxia-telangiectasia G11.3
- auriculotemporal G50.8
- autoerythrocyte sensitization (Gardner-Diamond) D69.2
- autoimmune lymphoproliferative [ALPS] D89.82
- autoimmune polyglandular E31.0
- autoinflammatory M04.9
  - specified type NEC M04.8
- autosomal — *see* Abnormal, autosomes
- Avellis' G46.8
- Ayerza (-Arrillaga) I27.0
- Babinski-Nageotte G83.89
- Bakwin-Krida Q78.5
- bare lymphocyte D81.6
- Barré-Guillain G61.0
- Barré-Liéou M53.0
- Barrett's — *see* Barrett's, esophagus
- Barsony-Polgar K22.4
- Bársony-Teschendorf K22.4
- Barth E78.71
- Bartter's E26.81
- basal cell nevus Q87.89
- Basedow's E05.00
  - with thyroid storm E05.01
- basilar artery G45.0
- Batten-Steinert G71.11
- battered
  - baby or child — *see* Maltreatment, child, physical abuse
  - spouse — *see* Maltreatment, adult, physical abuse
- Beals Q87.40
- Beau's I51.5
- Beck's I65.8
- Benedikt's G46.3
- Béquez César (-Steinbrinck-Chédiak-Higashi) E70.330
- Bernhardt-Roth — *see* Meralgia paresthetica
- Bernheim's — *see* Failure, heart, right
- big spleen D73.1
- bilateral polycystic ovarian E28.2
- Bing-Horton's — *see* Horton's headache
- Birt-Hogg-Dube syndrome Q87.89
- Björck (-Thorsen) E34.0
- black
  - lung J60
  - widow spider bite — *see* Toxicity, venom, spider, black widow
- Blackfan-Diamond D61.01
- Blau M04.8
- blind loop K90.2
  - congenital Q43.8
  - postsurgical K91.2
- blue sclera Q78.0
- blue toe I75.02- ☑
- Boder-Sedgewick G11.3
- Boerhaave's K22.3
- Borjeson Forssman Lehmann Q89.8
- Bouillaud's I01.9
- Bourneville (-Pringle) Q85.1
- Bouveret (-Hoffman) I47.9
- brachial plexus G54.0
- bradycardia-tachycardia I49.5
- brain (nonpsychotic) F09
  - with psychosis, psychotic reaction F09
  - acute or subacute — *see* Delirium
  - congenital — *see* Disability, intellectual
  - organic F09
    - post-traumatic (nonpsychotic) F07.81
      - psychotic F09
  - personality change F07.0
  - postcontusional F07.81
  - post-traumatic, nonpsychotic F07.81
  - psycho-organic F09
  - psychotic F06.8

Syndrome — *continued*
- brain stem stroke G46.3
- Brandt's (acrodermatitis enteropathica) E83.2
- broad ligament laceration N83.8
- Brock's J98.11
- bronze baby P83.88
- Brown-Sequard G83.81
- Brugada I49.8
- bubbly lung P27.0
- Buchem's M85.2
- Budd-Chiari I82.0
- bulbar (progressive) G12.22
- Bürger-Grütz E78.3
- Burke's K86.89
- Burnett's (milk-alkali) E83.52
- burning feet E53.9
- Bywaters' T79.5 ☑
- Call-Fleming I67.841
- carbohydrate-deficient glycoprotein (CDGS) E77.8
- carcinogenic thrombophlebitis I82.1
- carcinoid E34.0
- cardiac asthma I50.1
- cardiacos negros I27.0
- cardiofaciocutaneous Q87.89
- cardiopulmonary-obesity E66.2
- cardiorenal — *see* Hypertension, cardiorenal
- cardiorespiratory distress (idiopathic), newborn P22.0
- cardiovascular renal — *see* Hypertension, cardiorenal
- carotid
  - artery (hemispheric) (internal) G45.1
  - body G90.01
  - sinus G90.01
- carpal tunnel G56.0- ☑
- Cassidy (-Scholte) E34.0
- cat cry Q93.4
- cat eye Q92.8
- cauda equina G83.4
- causalgia — *see* Causalgia
- celiac K90.0
  - artery compression I77.4
  - axis I77.4
- central pain G89.0
- cerebellar
  - hereditary G11.9
  - stroke G46.4
- cerebellomedullary malformation — *see* Spina bifida
- cerebral
  - artery
    - anterior G46.1
    - middle G46.0
    - posterior G46.2
  - gigantism E22.0
- cervical (root) M53.1
  - disc — *see* Disorder, disc, cervical, with neuritis
  - fusion Q76.1
  - posterior, sympathicus M53.0
  - rib Q76.5
  - sympathetic paralysis G90.2
- cervicobrachial (diffuse) M53.1
- cervicocranial M53.0
- cervicodorsal outlet G54.2
- cervicothoracic outlet G54.0
- Céstan (-Raymond) I65.8
- Charcot's (angina cruris) (intermittent claudication) I73.9
- Charcot-Weiss-Baker G90.09
- CHARGE Q89.8
- Chédiak-Higashi (-Steinbrinck) E70.330
- chest wall R07.1
- Chiari's (hepatic vein thrombosis) I82.0
- Chilaiditi's Q43.3
- child maltreatment — *see* Maltreatment, child
- chondrocostal junction M94.0
- chondroectodermal dysplasia Q77.6
- chromosome 4 short arm deletion Q93.3
- chromosome 5 short arm deletion Q93.4
- chronic
  - infantile neurological, cutaneous and articular (CINCA) M04.2
  - pain G89.4
    - personality F68.8
- Churg-Strauss M30.1
- Clarke-Hadfield K86.89
- Clerambault's automatism G93.89
- Clouston's (hidrotic ectodermal dysplasia) Q82.4
- clumsiness, clumsy child F82
- cluster headache G44.009
  - intractable G44.001

Syndrome — *continued*
- cluster headache — *continued*
  - not intractable G44.009
- Coffin-Lowry Q89.8
- cold injury (newborn) P80.0
- combined immunity deficiency D81.9
- compartment (deep) (posterior) (traumatic) T79.A0 ☑ (*following* T79.7)
  - abdomen T79.A3 ☑ (*following* T79.7)
  - lower extremity (hip, buttock, thigh, leg, foot, toes) T79.A2 ☑ (*following* T79.7)
  - nontraumatic
    - abdomen M79.A3 (*following* M79.7)
    - lower extremity (hip, buttock, thigh, leg, foot, toes) M79.A2- ☑ (*following* M79.7)
    - specified site NEC M79.A9 (*following* M79.7)
    - upper extremity (shoulder, arm, forearm, wrist, hand, fingers) M79.A1- ☑ (*following* M79.7)
  - postprocedural — *see* Syndrome, compartment, nontraumatic
  - specified site NEC T79.A9 ☑ (*following* T79.7)
  - upper extremity (shoulder, arm, forearm, wrist, hand, fingers) T79.A1 ☑ (*following* T79.7)
- complex regional pain — *see* Syndrome, pain, complex regional
- compression T79.5 ☑
  - anterior spinal — *see* Syndrome, anterior, spinal artery, compression
  - cauda equina G83.4
  - celiac artery I77.4
  - vertebral artery M47.029
    - cervical region M47.022
    - occipito-atlanto-axial region M47.021
- concussion F07.81
- congenital
  - affecting multiple systems NEC Q87.89
  - central alveolar hypoventilation G47.35
  - facial diplegia Q87.0
  - muscular hypertrophy-cerebral Q87.89
  - oculo-auriculovertebral Q87.0
  - oculofacial diplegia (Moebius) Q87.0
  - rubella (manifest) P35.0
- congestion-fibrosis (pelvic), female N94.89
- congestive dysmenorrhea N94.6
- connective tissue M35.9
  - overlap NEC M35.1
- Conn's E26.01
- conus medullaris G95.81
- cord
  - anterior G83.82
  - posterior G83.83
- coronary
  - acute NEC I24.9
  - insufficiency or intermediate I20.0
  - slow flow I20.8
- Costen's (complex) M26.69
- costochondral junction M94.0
- costoclavicular G54.0
- costovertebral E22.0
- Cowden Q85.8
- craniovertebral M53.0
- Creutzfeldt-Jakob — *see* Creutzfeldt-Jakob disease or syndrome
- crib death R99
- cricopharyngeal — *see* Dysphagia
- cri-du-chat Q93.4
- croup J05.0
- CRPS I — *see* Syndrome, pain, complex regional I
- crush T79.5 ☑
- cryopyrin-associated perodic M04.2
- cryptophthalmos Q87.0
- cubital tunnel — *see* Lesion, nerve, ulnar
- Curschmann (-Batten) (-Steinert) G71.11
- Cushing's E24.9
  - alcohol-induced E24.4
  - due to
    - alcohol
      - drugs E24.2
    - ectopic ACTH E24.3
    - overproduction of pituitary ACTH E24.0
  - drug-induced E24.2
  - overdose or wrong substance given or taken — *see* Table of Drugs and Chemicals, by drug, poisoning
  - pituitary-dependent E24.0
  - specified type NEC E24.8
- cystic duct stump K91.5

Syndrome — continued

cytokine release D89.839
   grade 1 D89.831
   grade 2 D89.832
   grade 3 D89.833
   grade 4 D89.834
   grade 5 D89.835
Dana-Putnam D51.0
Danbolt (-Cross) (acrodermatitis enteropathica) E83.2
Dandy-Walker Q03.1
   with spina bifida Q07.01
Danlos' — see also Syndrome, Ehlers-Danlos Q79.60
De Quervain E34.51
de Toni-Fanconi (-Debré) E72.09
   with cystinosis E72.04
de Vivo syndrome E74.810
defibrination — see also Fibrinolysis
   with
      antepartum hemorrhage — see Hemorrhage,
         antepartum, with coagulation defect
      intrapartum hemorrhage — see Hemorrhage,
         complicating, delivery
   newborn P60
   postpartum O72.3
Degos' I77.89
Déjérine-Roussy G89.0
delayed sleep phase G47.21
demyelinating G37.9
dependence — see F10-F19 with fourth character .2
depersonalization (-derealization) F48.1
di George's D82.1
diabetes mellitus in newborn infant P70.2
diabetes mellitus-hypertension-nephrosis — see Diabetes, nephrosis
diabetes-nephrosis — see Diabetes, nephrosis
diabetic amyotrophy — see Diabetes, amyotrophy
dialysis associated steal T82.898- ☑
Diamond-Blackfan D61.01
Diamond-Gardener D69.2
DIC (diffuse or disseminated intravascular coagulopathy) D65
Dighton's Q78.0
disequilibrium E87.8
Döhle body-panmyelopathic D72.0
dorsolateral medullary G46.4
double athetosis G80.3
Down — see also Down syndrome Q90.9
Dravet (intractable) G40.834
   with status epilepticus G40.833
   without status epilepticus G40.834
Dresbach's (elliptocytosis) D58.1
DRESS (drug rash with eosinophilia and systemic symptoms) D72.12
Dressler's (postmyocardial infarction) I24.1
   postcardiotomy I97.0
drug rash with eosinophilia and systemic symptoms (DRESS) D72.12
drug withdrawal, infant of dependent mother P96.1
dry eye H04.12- ☑
due to abnormality
   chromosomal Q99.9
      sex
         female phenotype Q97.9
         male phenotype Q98.9
         specified NEC Q99.8
dumping (postgastrectomy) K91.1
   nonsurgical K31.89
Dupré's (meningism) R29.1
dysmetabolic X E88.81
dyspraxia, developmental F82
Eagle-Barrett Q79.4
Eaton-Lambert — see Syndrome, Lambert-Eaton
Ebstein's Q22.5
ectopic ACTH E24.3
eczema-thrombocytopenia D82.0
Eddowes' Q78.0
effort (psychogenic) F45.8
Ehlers-Danlos Q79.60
   classical (cEDS) (classical EDS) Q79.61
   hypermobile (hEDS) (hypermobile EDS) Q79.62
   specified NEC Q79.69
   vascular (vascular EDS) (vEDS) Q79.63
Eisenmenger's I27.83
Ekman's Q78.0
electric feet E53.8
Ellis-van Creveld Q77.6
empty nest Z60.0
endocrine-hypertensive E27.0

Syndrome — continued

entrapment — see Neuropathy, entrapment
eosinophilia-myalgia M35.89
epileptic — see also Epilepsy, by type
   absence G40.A09 (following G40.3)
      intractable G40.A19 (following G40.3)
         with status epilepticus G40.A11 (following G40.3)
         without status epilepticus G40.A19 (following G40.3)
      not intractable G40.A09 (following G40.3)
         with status epilepticus G40.A01 (following G40.3)
         without status epilepticus G40.A09 (following G40.3)
Erdheim-Chester (ECD) E88.89
Erdheim's E22.0
erythrocyte fragmentation D59.4
Evans D69.41
exhaustion F48.8
extrapyramidal G25.9
   specified NEC G25.89
eye retraction — see Strabismus
eyelid-malar-mandible Q87.0
Faber's D50.9
facet M47.89- ☑
facet joint — see also Spondylosis M47.819
facial pain, paroxysmal G50.0
Fallot's Q21.3
familial cold autoinflammatory M04.2
familial eczema-thrombocytopenia (Wiskott-Aldrich) D82.0
Fanconi (-de Toni) (-Debré) E72.09
   with cystinosis E72.04
Fanconi's (anemia) (congenital pancytopenia) D61.09
fatigue
   chronic R53.82
   psychogenic F48.8
faulty bowel habit K59.39
Feil-Klippel (brevicollis) Q76.1
Felty's — see Felty's syndrome
fertile eunuch E23.0
fetal
   alcohol (dysmorphic) Q86.0
   hydantoin Q86.1
Fiedler's I40.1
first arch Q87.0
fish odor E72.89
Fisher's G61.0
Fitzhugh-Curtis
   due to
      Chlamydia trachomatis A74.81
      Neisseria gonorrhorea (gonococcal peritonitis) A54.85
Fitz's — see also Pancreatitis, acute K85.80
Flajani (-Basedow) E05.00
   with thyroid storm E05.01
flatback — see Flatback syndrome
floppy
   baby P94.2
   iris (intraoeprative) (IFIS) H21.81
   mitral valve I34.1
flush E34.0
Foix-Alajouanine G95.19
Fong's Q87.2
food protein-induced enterocolitis (FPIES) K52.21
foramen magnum G93.5
Foster-Kennedy H47.14- ☑
Foville's (peduncular) G46.3
fragile X Q99.2
Franceschetti Q75.4
Frey's
   auriculotemporal G50.8
   hyperhidrosis L74.52
Friderichsen-Waterhouse A39.1
Froin's G95.89
frontal lobe F07.0
Fukuhara E88.49
functional
   bowel K59.9
   prepubertal castrate E29.1
Gaisböck's D75.1
ganglion (basal ganglia brain) G25.9
   geniculi G51.1
Gardner-Diamond D69.2
gastroesophageal
   junction K22.0
   laceration-hemorrhage K22.6

Syndrome — continued

gastrojejunal loop obstruction K91.89
Gee-Herter-Heubner K90.0
Gelineau's G47.419
   with cataplexy G47.411
genito-anorectal A55
Gerstmann-Sträussler-Scheinker (GSS) A81.82
Gianotti-Crosti L44.4
giant platelet (Bernard-Soulier) D69.1
Gilles de la Tourette's F95.2
Glass Q87.89
Gleich's D72.118
goiter-deafness E07.1
Goldberg Q89.8
Goldberg-Maxwell E34.51
Good's D83.8
Gopalan's (burning feet) E53.8
Gorlin's Q87.89
Gougerot-Blum L81.7
Gouley's I31.1
Gower's R55
gray or grey (newborn) P93.0
   platelet D69.1
Gubler-Millard G46.3
Guillain-Barré (-Strohl) G61.0
gustatory sweating G50.8
Hadfield-Clarke K86.89
hair tourniquet — see Constriction, external, by site
Hamman's J98.19
hand-foot L27.1
hand-shoulder G90.8
hantavirus (cardio)-pulmonary (HPS) (HCPS) B33.4
happy puppet Q93.51
Harada's H30.81- ☑
Hayem-Faber D50.9
headache NEC G44.89
   complicated NEC G44.59
Heberden's I20.8
Hedinger's E34.0
Hegglin's D72.0
HELLP (hemolysis, elevated liver enzymes and low platelet count) O14.2- ☑
   complicating
      childbirth O14.24
      puerperium O14.25
hemolytic-uremic D59.3
hemophagocytic, infection-associated D76.2
Henoch-Schönlein D69.0
hepatic flexure K59.89
hepatopulmonary K76.81
hepatorenal K76.7
   following delivery O90.4
   postoperative or postprocedural K91.83
   postpartum, puerperal O90.4
hepatourologic K76.7
Herter (-Gee) (nontropical sprue) K90.0
Heubner-Herter K90.0
Heyd's K76.7
Hilger's G90.09
histamine-like (fish poisoning) — see Poisoning, fish
histiocytic D76.3
histiocytosis NEC D76.3
HIV infection, acute B20
Hoffmann-Werdnig G12.0
Hollander-Simons E88.1
Hoppe-Goldflam G70.00
   with exacerbation (acute) G70.01
   in crisis G70.01
Horner's G90.2
hungry bone E83.81
hunterian glossitis D51.0
Hutchinson's triad A50.53
hyperabduction G54.0
hyperammonemia-hyperornithinemia-homocitrullinemia E72.4
hypereosinophilic (HES) D72.119
   idiopathic (IHES) D72.110
   lymphocytic variant (LHES) D72.111
   myeloid D72.118
   specified NEC D72.118
hyperimmunoglobulin D M04.1
hyperimmunoglobulin E (IgE) D82.4
hyperkalemic E87.5
hyperkinetic — see Hyperkinesia
hypermobility M35.7
hypernatremia E87.0
hyperosmolarity E87.0
hyperperfusion G97.82

Syndrome — *continued*
- hypersplenic D73.1
- hypertransfusion, newborn P61.1
- hyperventilation F45.8
- hyperviscosity (of serum)
  - polycythemic D75.1
  - sclerothymic D58.8
- hypoglycemic (familial) (neonatal) E16.2
- hypokalemic E87.6
- hyponatremic E87.1
- hypopituitarism E23.0
- hypoplastic left-heart Q23.4
- hypopotassemia E87.6
- hyposmolality E87.1
- hypotension, maternal O26.5- ☑
- hypothenar hammer I73.89
- hypoventilation, obesity (OHS) E66.2
- ICF (intravascular coagulation-fibrinolysis) D65
- idiopathic
  - cardiorespiratory distress, newborn P22.0
  - nephrotic (infantile) N04.9
- iliotibial band M76.3- ☑
- immobility, immobilization (paraplegic) M62.3
- immune effector cell-associated neurotoxicity (ICANS) G92.00
  - grade
    - 1 G92.01
    - 2 G92.02
    - 3 G92.03
    - 4 G92.04
    - 5 G92.05
    - unspecified G92.00
- immune reconstitution D89.3
- immune reconstitution inflammatory [IRIS] D89.3
- immunity deficiency, combined D81.9
- immunodeficiency
  - acquired — *see* Human, immunodeficiency virus (HIV) disease
  - combined D81.9
- impending coronary I20.0
- impingement, shoulder M75.4- ☑
- inappropriate secretion of antidiuretic hormone E22.2
- infant
  - gestational diabetes P70.0
  - of diabetic mother P70.1
- infantilism (pituitary) E23.0
- inferior vena cava I87.1
- inspissated bile (newborn) P59.1
- institutional (childhood) F94.2
- insufficient sleep F51.12
- intermediate coronary (artery) I20.0
- interspinous ligament — *see* Spondylopathy, specified NEC
- intestinal
  - carcinoid E34.0
  - knot K56.2
- intravascular coagulation-fibrinolysis (ICF) D65
- iodine-deficiency, congenital E00.9
  - type
    - mixed E00.2
    - myxedematous E00.1
    - neurological E00.0
- IRDS (idiopathic respiratory distress, newborn) P22.0
- irritable
  - bowel K58.9
    - with
      - constipation K58.1
      - diarrhea K58.0
    - mixed K58.2
    - psychogenic F45.8
    - specified NEC K58.8
  - heart (psychogenic) F45.8
  - weakness F48.8
- ischemic
  - bowel (transient) K55.9
    - chronic K55.1
    - due to mesenteric artery insufficiency K55.1
  - steal T82.898 ☑
- IVC (intravascular coagulopathy) D65
- Ivemark's Q89.01
- Jaccoud's — *see* Arthropathy, postrheumatic, chronic
- Jackson's G83.89
- Jakob-Creutzfeldt — *see* Creutzfeldt-Jakob disease or syndrome
- jaw-winking Q07.8
- Jervell-Lange-Nielsen I45.81
- jet lag G47.25
- Job's D71

Syndrome — *continued*
- Joseph-Diamond-Blackfan D61.01
- jugular foramen G52.7
- Kabuki Q89.8
- Kanner's (autism) F84.0
- Kartagener's Q89.3
- Kelly's D50.1
- Kimmelstiel-Wilson — *see* Diabetes, specified type, with Kimmelstiel-Wilson disease
- Klein (e)-Levine G47.13
- Klippel-Feil (brevicollis) Q76.1
- Köhler-Pellegrini-Steida — *see* Bursitis, tibial collateral
- König's K59.89
- Korsakoff (-Wernicke) (nonalcoholic) F04
  - alcoholic F10.26
- Kostmann's D70.0
- Krabbe's congenital muscle hypoplasia Q79.8
- labyrinthine — *see* subcategory H83.2
- lacunar NEC G46.7
- Lambert-Eaton G70.80
  - in
    - neoplastic disease G73.1
    - specified disease NEC G70.81
- Landau-Kleffner — *see* Epilepsy, specified NEC
- Larsen's Q74.8
- lateral
  - cutaneous nerve of thigh G57.1- ☑
  - medullary G46.4
- Launois' E22.0
- lazy
  - leukocyte D70.8
  - posture M62.3
- Lemiere I80.8
- Lennox-Gastaut G40.812
  - intractable G40.814
    - with status epilepticus G40.813
    - without status epilepticus G40.814
  - not intractable G40.812
    - with status epilepticus G40.811
    - without status epilepticus G40.812
- lenticular, progressive E83.01
- Leopold-Levi's E05.90
- Lev's I44.2
- Lichtheim's D51.0
- Li-Fraumeni Z15.01
- Lightwood's N25.89
- Lignac (de Toni) (-Fanconi) (-Debré) E72.09
  - with cystinosis E72.04
- Likoff's I20.8
- limbic epilepsy personality F07.0
- liver-kidney K76.7
- lobotomy F07.0
- Löffler's J82.89
- long arm 18 or 21 deletion Q93.89
- long QT I45.81
- Louis-Barré G11.3
- low
  - atmospheric pressure T70.29 ☑
  - back M54.50
  - output (cardiac) I50.9
- lower radicular, newborn (birth injury) P14.8
- Luetscher's (dehydration) E86.0
- Lupus anticoagulant D68.62
- Lutembacher's Q21.1
- macrophage activation D76.1
  - due to infection D76.2
- magnesium-deficiency R29.0
- Majeed M04.8
- Mal de Debarquement R42
- malabsorption K90.9
  - postsurgical K91.2
- malformation, congenital, due to
  - alcohol Q86.0
  - exogenous cause NEC Q86.8
  - hydantoin Q86.1
  - warfarin Q86.2
- malignant
  - carcinoid E34.0
  - neuroleptic G21.0
- Mallory-Weiss K22.6
- mandibulofacial dysostosis Q75.4
- manic-depressive — *see* Disorder, bipolar
- maple-syrup-urine E71.0
- Marable's I77.4
- Marfan's Q87.40
  - with
    - cardiovascular manifestations Q87.418
      - aortic dilation Q87.410

Syndrome — *continued*
- Marfan's — *continued*
  - with — *continued*
    - ocular manifestations Q87.42
    - skeletal manifestations Q87.43
- Marie's (acromegaly) E22.0
- mast cell activation — *see* Activation, mast cell
- maternal hypotension — *see* Syndrome, hypotension, maternal
- May (-Hegglin) D72.0
- McArdle (-Schmidt) (-Pearson) E74.04
- McQuarrie's E16.2
- meconium plug (newborn) P76.0
- median arcuate ligament I77.4
- Meekeren-Ehlers-Danlos Q79.6 ☑
- megavitamin-B6 E67.2
- Meige G24.4
- MELAS E88.41
- Mendelson's O74.0
- MERRF (myoclonic epilepsy associated with ragged-red fibers) E88.42
- mesenteric
  - artery (superior) K55.1
  - vascular insufficiency K55.1
- metabolic E88.81
- metastatic carcinoid E34.0
- micrognathia-glossoptosis Q87.0
- midbrain NEC G93.89
- middle lobe (lung) J98.19
- middle radicular G54.0
- migraine — *see also* Migraine G43.909
- Mikulicz' K11.8
- milk-alkali E83.52
- Millard-Gubler G46.3
- Miller-Dieker Q93.88
- Miller-Fisher G61.0
- Minkowski-Chauffard D58.0
- Mirizzi's K83.1
- MNGIE (Mitochondrial Neurogastrointestinal Encephalopathy) E88.49
- Möbius, ophthalmoplegic migraine — *see* Migraine, ophthalmoplegic
- monofixation H50.42
- Morel-Moore M85.2
- Morel-Morgagni M85.2
- Morgagni (-Morel) (-Stewart) M85.2
- Morgagni-Adams-Stokes I45.9
- Mounier-Kuhn Q32.4
  - with bronchiectasis J47.9
    - with
      - exacerbation (acute) J47.1
      - lower respiratory infection J47.0
    - acquired J98.09
      - with bronchiectasis J47.9
        - with
          - exacerbation (acute) J47.1
          - lower respiratory infection J47.0
- Muckle-Wells M04.2
- mucocutaneous lymph node (acute febrile) (MCLS) M30.3
- multiple endocrine neoplasia (MEN) — *see* Neoplasia, endocrine, multiple (MEN)
- multiple operations — *see* Disorder, factitious
- multisystem inflammatory (in adults) (in children) M35.81
- myasthenic G70.9
  - in
    - diabetes mellitus — *see* Diabetes, amyotrophy
    - endocrine disease NEC E34.9 *[G73.3]*
    - neoplastic disease — *see also* Neoplasm D49.9 *[G73.3]*
    - thyrotoxicosis (hyperthyroidism) E05.90 *[G73.3]*
      - with thyroid storm E05.91 *[G73.3]*
- myelodysplastic D46.9
  - with
    - 5q deletion D46.C *(following D46.2)*
    - isolated del (5q) chromosomal abnormality D46.C *(following D46.2)*
    - multilineage dysplasia D46.A *(following D46.2)*
      - with ringed sideroblasts D46.B *(following D46.2)*
  - lesions, low grade D46.20
  - specified NEC D46.Z *(following D46.4)*
- myeloid hypereosinophilic D72.118
- myelopathic pain G89.0
- myeloproliferative (chronic) D47.1
- myofascial pain M79.18
- Naffziger's G54.0

Syndrome — *continued*

nail patella Q87.2
NARP (Neuropathy, Ataxia and Retinitis pigmentosa) E88.49
neonatal abstinence P96.1
nephritic — *see also* Nephritis
   with edema — *see* Nephrosis
   acute N00.9
   chronic N03.9
   rapidly progressive N01.9
nephrotic (congenital) — *see also* Nephrosis N04.9
   with
      C3
         glomerulonephritis N04.A
         glomerulopathy N04.A
            with dense deposit disease N04.6
         dense deposit disease N04.6
         diffuse
            crescentic glomerulonephritis N04.7
            endocapillary proliferative glomerulonephritis N04.4
            membranous glomerulonephritis N04.2
            mesangial proliferative glomerulonephritis N04.3
            mesangiocapillary glomerulonephritis N04.5
         focal and segmental glomerular lesions N04.1
         minor glomerular abnormality N04.0
         specified morphological changes NEC N04.8
   diabetic — *see* Diabetes, nephrosis
neurologic neglect R41.4
Nezelof's D81.4
Nonne-Milroy-Meige Q82.0
Nothnagel's vasomotor acroparesthesia I73.89
obesity hypoventilation (OHS) E66.2
oculomotor H51.9
Ogilvie K59.81
ophthalmoplegia-cerebellar ataxia — *see* Strabismus, paralytic, third nerve
oral allergy T78.1
oral-facial-digital Q87.0
organic
   affective F06.30
   amnesic (not alcohol- or drug-induced) F04
   brain F09
   depressive F06.31
   hallucinosis F06.0
   personality F07.0
Ormond's N13.5
oro-facial-digital Q87.0
os trigonum Q68.8
Osler-Weber-Rendu I78.0
osteoporosis-osteomalacia M83.8
Osterreicher-Turner Q87.2
otolith — *see* subcategory H81.8 ☑
oto-palatal-digital Q87.0
outlet (thoracic) G54.0
ovary
   polycystic E28.2
   resistant E28.39
   sclerocystic E28.2
Owren's D68.2
Paget-Schroetter I82.890
pain — *see also* Pain
   complex regional I G90.50
      lower limb G90.52- ☑
      specified site NEC G90.59
      upper limb G90.51- ☑
   complex regional II — *see* Causalgia
painful
   bruising D69.2
   feet E53.8
   prostate N42.81
paralysis agitans — *see* Parkinsonism
paralytic G83.9
   specified NEC G83.89
Parinaud's H51.0
parkinsonian — *see* Parkinsonism
Parkinson's — *see* Parkinsonism
paroxysmal facial pain G50.0
Parry's E05.00
   with thyroid storm E05.01
Parsonage (-Aldren)-Turner G54.5
patella clunk M25.86- ☑
Paterson (-Brown) (-Kelly) D50.1
pectoral girdle I77.89
pectoralis minor I77.89

Syndrome — *continued*

pediatric autoimmune neuropsychiatric disorders associated with streptococcal infections (PANDAS) D89.89
pediatric inflammatory multisystem M35.81
Pelger-Huet D72.0
pellagra-cerebellar ataxia-renal aminoaciduria E72.02
pellagroid E52
Pellegrini-Stieda — *see* Bursitis, tibial collateral
pelvic congestion-fibrosis, female N94.89
penta X Q97.1
peptic ulcer — *see* Ulcer, peptic
perabduction I77.89
periodic fever M04.1
periodic fever, aphthous stomatitis, pharyngitis, and adenopathy [PFAPA] M04.8
periodic headache, in adults and children — *see* Headache, periodic syndromes in adults and children
periurethral fibrosis N13.5
phantom limb (without pain) G54.7
   with pain G54.6
pharyngeal pouch D82.1
Pick's — *see* Disease, Pick's
Pickwickian E66.2
PIE (pulmonary infiltration with eosinophilia) — *see also* Eosinophilia, pulmonary J82.89
pigmentary pallidal degeneration (progressive) G23.0
pineal E34.8
pituitary E22.0
placental transfusion — *see* Pregnancy, complicated by, placental transfusion syndromes
plantar fascia M72.2
plateau iris (post-iridectomy) (postprocedural) H21.82
Plummer-Vinson D50.1
pluricarential of infancy E40
plurideficiency E40
pluriglandular (compensatory) E31.8
   autoimmune E31.0
pneumatic hammer T75.21 ☑
polyangiitis overlap M30.8
polycarential of infancy E40
polyglandular E31.8
   autoimmune E31.0
polysplenia Q89.09
pontine NEC G93.89
popliteal
   artery entrapment I77.89
   web Q87.89
post chemoembolization — *code to* associated conditions
post endometrial ablation N99.85
postcardiac injury
   postcardiotomy I97.0
   postmyocardial infarction I24.1
postcardiotomy I97.0
postcholecystectomy K91.5
postcommissurotomy I97.0
postconcussional F07.81
postcontusional F07.81
post-COVID (-19) U09.9
postencephalitic F07.89
posterior
   cervical sympathetic M53.0
   cord G83.83
   fossa compression G93.5
   reversible encephalopathy (PRES) I67.83
postgastrectomy (dumping) K91.1
postgastric surgery K91.1
postinfarction I24.1
postlaminectomy NEC M96.1
postleukotomy F07.0
postmastectomy lymphedema I97.2
postmyocardial infarction I24.1
postoperative NEC T81.9 ☑
   blind loop K90.2
postpartum panhypopituitary (Sheehan) E23.0
postpolio (myelitic) G14
postthrombotic I87.009
   with
      inflammation I87.02- ☑
         with ulcer I87.03- ☑
      specified complication NEC I87.09- ☑
      ulcer I87.01- ☑
         with inflammation I87.03- ☑
   asymptomatic I87.00- ☑
postvagotomy K91.1
postvalvulotomy I97.0

Syndrome — *continued*

postviral NEC G93.3
   fatigue G93.3
Potain's K31.0
potassium intoxication E87.5
Prader-Willi Q87.11
Prader-Willi-like Q87.19
precerebral artery (multiple) (bilateral) G45.2
preinfarction I20.0
preleukemic D46.9
premature senility E34.8
premenstrual dysphoric F32.81
premenstrual tension N94.3
Prinzmetal-Massumi R07.1
prune belly Q79.4
pseudo -Turner's Q87.19
pseudocarpal tunnel (sublimis) — *see* Syndrome, carpal tunnel
pseudoparalytica G70.00
   with exacerbation (acute) G70.01
   in crisis G70.01
psycho-organic (nonpsychotic severity) F07.9
   acute or subacute F05
   depressive type F06.31
   hallucinatory type F06.0
   nonpsychotic severity F07.0
   specified NEC F07.89
pulmonary
   arteriosclerosis I27.0
   dysmaturity (Wilson-Mikity) P27.0
   hypoperfusion (idiopathic) P22.0
   renal (hemorrhagic) (Goodpasture's) M31.0
pure
   motor lacunar G46.5
   sensory lacunar G46.6
Putnam-Dana D51.0
pyogenic arthritis, pyoderma gangrenosum, and acne [PAPA] M04.8
pyramidopallidonigral G20
pyriformis — *see* Lesion, nerve, sciatic
QT interval prolongation I45.81
radicular NEC — *see* Radiculopathy
   upper limbs, newborn (birth injury) P14.3
rapid time-zone change G47.25
Rasmussen G04.81
Raymond (-Céstan) I65.8
Raynaud's I73.00
   with gangrene I73.01
RDS (respiratory distress syndrome, newborn) P22.0
reactive airways dysfunction J68.3
Refsum's G60.1
Reifenstein E34.52
renal glomerulohyalinosis-diabetic — *see* Diabetes, nephrosis
Rendu-Osler-Weber I78.0
residual ovary N99.83
resistant ovary E28.39
respiratory
   distress
      acute J80
         adult J80
         child J80
         idiopathic J84.114
      newborn (idiopathic) (type I) P22.0
         type II P22.1
restless legs G25.81
retinoblastoma (familial) C69.2 ☑
retroperitoneal fibrosis N13.5
retroviral seroconversion (acute) Z21
Reye's G93.7
Richter — *see* Leukemia, chronic lymphocytic, B-cell type
Ridley's I50.1
right
   heart, hypoplastic Q22.6
   ventricular obstruction — *see* Failure, heart, right
Romano-Ward (prolonged QT interval) I45.81
rotator cuff, shoulder — *see also* Tear, rotator cuff M75.10- ☑
Rotes Quérol — *see* Hyperostosis, ankylosing
Roth — *see* Meralgia paresthetica
rubella (congenital) P35.0
Ruvalcaba-Myhre-Smith E71.440
Rytand-Lipsitch I44.2
salt
   depletion E87.1
      due to heat NEC T67.8 ☑

Syndrome — *continued*
  salt — *continued*
    depletion — *continued*
      due to heat — *continued*
        causing heat exhaustion or prostration
          T67.4 ☑
      low E87.1
  salt-losing N28.89
  SATB2-associated Q87.89
  Scaglietti-Dagnini E22.0
  scalenus anticus (anterior) G54.0
  scapulocostal — *see* Mononeuropathy, upper limb,
    specified site NEC
  scapuloperoneal G71.09
  schizophrenic, of childhood NEC F84.5
  Schnitzler D47.2
  Scholte's E34.0
  Schroeder's E27.0
  Schüller-Christian C96.5
  Schwachman's — *see* Syndrome, Shwachman's
  Schwartz (-Jampel) G71.13
  Schwartz-Bartter E22.2
  scimitar Q26.8
  sclerocystic ovary E28.2
  Seitelberger's G31.89
  septicemic adrenal hemorrhage A39.1
  seroconversion, retroviral (acute) Z21
  serous meningitis G93.2
  severe acute respiratory (SARS) J12.81
    coronavirus 2 (*see also* COVID-19) U07.1
    pneumonia J12.82
  shaken infant T74.4 ☑
  shock (traumatic) T79.4 ☑
    kidney N17.0
    following crush injury T79.5 ☑
    toxic A48.3
  shock-lung J80
  Shone's — *code to* specific anomalies
  short
    bowel K91.2
    rib Q77.2
  shoulder-hand — *see* Algoneurodystrophy
  Shwachman's D70.4
  sicca — *see* Syndrome, Sjögren
  sick
    cell E87.1
    sinus I49.5
  sick-euthyroid E07.81
  sideropenic D50.1
  Siemens' ectodermal dysplasia Q82.4
  Silfversköld's Q78.9
  Simons' E88.1
  sinus tarsi M25.57- ☑
  sinusitis-bronchiectasis-situs inversus Q89.3
  Sipple's E31.22
  sirenomelia Q87.2
  Sjögren M35.00
    with
      central nervous system involvement M35.07
      dental involvement M35.0C
      gastrointestinal involvement M35.08
      glomerular disease M35.0A
      inflammatory arthritis M35.05
      keratoconjunctivitis M35.01
      lung involvement M35.02
      myopathy M35.03
      peripheral nervous system involvement M35.06
      renal tubular acidosis M35.04
      specified organ involvement, NEC M35.09
      tubulo-interstitial nephropathy M35.04
      vasculitis M35.0B
  Slocumb's E27.0
  slow flow, coronary I20.8
  Sluder's G44.89
  Smith-Magenis Q93.88
  Sneddon-Wilkinson L13.1
  Sotos' Q87.3
  South African cardiomyopathy I42.8
  spasmodic
    upward movement, eyes H51.8
    winking F95.8
  Spen's I45.9
  splenic
    agenesis Q89.01
    flexure K59.89
    neutropenia D73.81
  Spurway's Q78.0
  staphylococcal scalded skin L00

Syndrome — *continued*
  steal
    arteriovenous T82.898- ☑
    ischemic T82.898- ☑
    subclavian G45.8
  Stein-Leventhal E28.2
  Stein's E28.2
  Stevens-Johnson syndrome L51.1
    toxic epidermal necrolysis overlap L51.3
  Stewart-Morel M85.2
  Stickler Q89.8
  stiff baby Q89.8
  stiff man G25.82
  Still-Felty — *see* Felty's syndrome
  Stokes (-Adams) I45.9
  stone heart I50.1
  straight back, congenital Q76.49
  subclavian steal G45.8
  subcoracoid-pectoralis minor G54.0
  subcostal nerve compression I77.89
  subphrenic interposition Q43.3
  superior
    cerebellar artery I63.89
    mesenteric artery K55.1
    semi-circular canal dehiscence H83.8X- ☑
    vena cava I87.1
  supine hypotensive (maternal) — *see* Syndrome, hy-
    potension, maternal
  suprarenal cortical E27.0
  supraspinatus — *see also* Tear, rotator cuff M75.10- ☑
  Susac G93.49
  swallowed blood P78.2
  sweat retention L74.0
  Swyer Q99.1
  Symond's G93.2
  sympathetic
    cervical paralysis G90.2
    pelvic, female N94.89
  systemic inflammatory response (SIRS), of non-infec-
    tious origin (without organ dysfunction) R65.10
    with acute organ dysfunction R65.11
  tachycardia-bradycardia I49.5
  takotsubo I51.81
  TAR (thrombocytopenia with absent radius) Q87.2
  tarsal tunnel G57.5- ☑
  teething K00.7
  tegmental G93.89
  telangiectasic-pigmentation-cataract Q82.8
  temporal pyramidal apex — *see* Otitis, media, suppu-
    rative, acute
  temporomandibular joint-pain-dysfunction M26.62- ☑
  Terry's — *see also* Myopia, degenerative H44.2- ☑
  testicular feminization — *see also* Syndrome, androgen
    insensitivity E34.51
  thalamic pain (hyperesthetic) G89.0
  thoracic outlet (compression) G54.0
  Thorson-Björck E34.0
  thrombocytopenia with absent radius (TAR) Q87.2
  thyroid-adrenocortical insufficiency E31.0
  tibial
    anterior M76.81- ☑
    posterior M76.82- ☑
  Tietze's M94.0
  time-zone (rapid) G47.25
  Toni-Fanconi E72.09
    with cystinosis E72.04
  Touraine's Q79.8
  tourniquet — *see* Constriction, external, by site
  toxic shock A48.3
  transient left ventricular apical ballooning I51.81
  traumatic vasospastic T75.22 ☑
  Treacher Collins Q75.4
  triple X, female Q97.0
  trisomy Q92.9
    13 Q91.7
      meiotic nondisjunction Q91.4
      mitotic nondisjunction Q91.5
      mosaicism Q91.5
      translocation Q91.6
    18 Q91.3
      meiotic nondisjunction Q91.0
      mitotic nondisjunction Q91.1
      mosaicism Q91.1
      translocation Q91.2
    20 (q)(p) Q92.8
    21 Q90.9
      meiotic nondisjunction Q90.0
      mitotic nondisjunction Q90.1

Syndrome — *continued*
  trisomy — *continued*
    21 — *continued*
      mosaicism Q90.1
      translocation Q90.2
    22 Q92.8
  tropical wet feet T69.0- ☑
  Trousseau's I82.1
  tumor lysis (following antineoplastic chemotherapy)
    (spontaneous) NEC E88.3
  tumor necrosis factor receptor associated periodic
    (TRAPS) M04.1
  Twiddler's (due to)
    automatic implantable defibrillator T82.198 ☑
    cardiac pacemaker T82.198 ☑
  Unverricht (-Lundborg) — *see* Epilepsy, generalized,
    idiopathic
  upward gaze H51.8
  uremia, chronic — *see also* Disease, kidney, chronic
    N18.9
  urethral N34.3
  urethro-oculo-articular — *see* Reiter's disease
  urohepatic K76.7
  vago-hypoglossal G52.7
  van Buchem's M85.2
  van der Hoeve's Q78.0
  vascular NEC in cerebrovascular disease G46.8
  vasoconstriction, reversible cerebrovascular I67.841
  vasomotor I73.9
  vasospastic (traumatic) T75.22 ☑
  vasovagal R55
  VATER Q87.2
  velo-cardio-facial Q93.81
  vena cava (inferior) (superior) (obstruction) I87.1
  vertebral
    artery G45.0
      compression — *see* Syndrome, anterior, spinal
        artery, compression
    steal G45.0
  vertebro-basilar artery G45.0
  vertebrogenic (pain) — *see also* Pain, vertebrogenic
    M54.89
  vertiginous — *see* Disorder, vestibular function
  Vinson-Plummer D50.1
  virus B34.9
  visceral larva migrans B83.0
  visual disorientation H53.8
  vitamin B6 deficiency E53.1
  vitreal corneal H59.01- ☑
  vitreous (touch) H59.01- ☑
  Vogt-Koyanagi H20.82- ☑
  Volkmann's T79.6 ☑
  von Schroetter's I82.890
  von Willebrand (-Jürgen) D68.0
  Waldenström-Kjellberg D50.1
  Wallenberg's G46.3
  water retention E87.79
  Waterhouse (-Friderichsen) A39.1
  Weber-Gubler G46.3
  Weber-Leyden G46.3
  Weber's G46.3
  Wegener's M31.30
    with
      kidney involvement M31.31
      lung involvement M31.30
        with kidney involvement M31.31
  Weingarten's (tropical eosinophilia) J82.89
  Weiss-Baker G90.09
  Werdnig-Hoffman G12.0
  Wermer's E31.21
  Werner's E34.8
  Wernicke-Korsakoff (nonalcoholic) F04
    alcoholic F10.26
  Westphal-Strümpell E83.01
  West's — *see* Epilepsy, spasms
  wet
    feet (maceration) (tropical) T69.0- ☑
    lung, newborn P22.1
  whiplash S13.4 ☑
  whistling face Q87.0
  Wilkie's K55.1
  Wilkinson-Sneddon L13.1
  Willebrand (-Jürgens) D68.0
  Williams Q93.82
  Wilson's (hepatolenticular degeneration) E83.01
  Wiskott-Aldrich D82.0
  withdrawal — *see* Withdrawal, state

☑ **Additional Character Required** — Refer to the Tabular List for Character Selection   ⬇ Subterms under main terms may continue to next column or page

Syndrome — continued
　withdrawal — see Withdrawal, state — continued
　　drug
　　　infant of dependent mother P96.1
　　　therapeutic use, newborn P96.2
　Woakes' (ethmoiditis) J33.1
　Wright's (hyperabduction) G54.0
　X I20.9
　XXXX Q97.1
　XXXXX Q97.1
　XXXXY Q98.1
　XXY Q98.0
　Yao M04.8
　yellow nail L60.5
　Zahorsky's B08.5
　Zellweger syndrome E71.510
　Zellweger-like syndrome E71.541
Synechia (anterior) (iris) (posterior) (pupil) — see also
　　Adhesions, iris
　intra-uterine (traumatic) N85.6
Synesthesia R20.8
Syngamiasis, syngamosis B83.3
Synodontia K00.2
Synorchidism, synorchism Q55.1
Synostosis (congenital) Q78.8
　astragalo-scaphoid Q74.2
　radioulnar Q74.0
Synovial sarcoma — see Neoplasm, connective tissue,
　　malignant
Synovioma (malignant) — see also Neoplasm, connective
　　tissue, malignant
　benign — see Neoplasm, connective tissue, benign
Synoviosarcoma — see Neoplasm, connective tissue,
　　malignant
Synovitis — see also Tenosynovitis M65.9
　crepitant
　　hand M70.0- ☑
　　wrist M70.03- ☑
　gonococcal A54.49
　gouty — see Gout
　in (due to)
　　crystals M65.8- ☑
　　gonorrhea A54.49
　　syphilis (late) A52.78
　use, overuse, pressure — see Disorder, soft tissue,
　　　due to use
　infective NEC — see Tenosynovitis, infective NEC
　specified NEC — see Tenosynovitis, specified type NEC
　syphilitic A52.78
　　congenital (early) A50.02
　toxic — see Synovitis, transient
　transient M67.3- ☑
　　ankle M67.37- ☑
　　elbow M67.32- ☑
　　foot joint M67.37- ☑
　　hand joint M67.34- ☑
　　hip M67.35- ☑
　　knee M67.36- ☑
　　multiple site M67.39
　　pelvic region M67.35- ☑
　　shoulder M67.31- ☑
　　specified joint NEC M67.38
　　wrist M67.33- ☑
　traumatic, current — see Sprain
　tuberculous — see Tuberculosis, synovitis
　villonodular (pigmented) M12.2- ☑
　　ankle M12.27- ☑
　　elbow M12.22- ☑
　　foot joint M12.27- ☑
　　hand joint M12.24- ☑
　　hip M12.25- ☑
　　knee M12.26- ☑
　　multiple site M12.29
　　pelvic region M12.25- ☑
　　shoulder M12.21- ☑
　　specified joint NEC M12.28
　　vertebrae M12.28
　　wrist M12.23- ☑
Syphilid A51.39
　congenital A50.06
　newborn A50.06
　tubercular (late) A52.79
Syphilis, syphilitic (acquired) A53.9
　abdomen (late) A52.79
　acoustic nerve A52.15
　adenopathy (secondary) A51.49
　adrenal (gland) (with cortical hypofunction) A52.79

Syphilis, syphilitic — continued
　age under 2 years NOS — see also Syphilis, congenital,
　　early
　　acquired A51.9
　alopecia (secondary) A51.32
　anemia (late) A52.79 [D63.8]
　aneurysm (aorta) (ruptured) A52.01
　　central nervous system A52.05
　　congenital A50.54 [I79.0]
　anus (late) A52.74
　　primary A51.1
　　secondary A51.39
　aorta (arch) (abdominal) (thoracic) A52.02
　　aneurysm A52.01
　aortic (insufficiency) (regurgitation) (stenosis) A52.03
　　aneurysm A52.01
　arachnoid (adhesive) (cerebral) (spinal) A52.13
　asymptomatic — see Syphilis, latent
　ataxia (locomotor) A52.11
　atrophoderma maculatum A51.39
　auricular fibrillation A52.06
　bladder (late) A52.76
　bone A52.77
　　secondary A51.46
　brain A52.17
　breast (late) A52.79
　bronchus (late) A52.72
　bubo (primary) A51.0
　bulbar palsy A52.19
　bursa (late) A52.78
　cardiac decompensation A52.06
　cardiovascular A52.00
　central nervous system (late) (recurrent) (relapse) (ter-
　　tiary) A52.3
　　with
　　　ataxia A52.11
　　　general paralysis A52.17
　　　　juvenile A50.45
　　　paresis (general) A52.17
　　　　juvenile A50.45
　　　tabes (dorsalis) A52.11
　　　　juvenile A50.45
　　　taboparesis A52.17
　　　　juvenile A50.45
　　aneurysm A52.05
　　congenital A50.40
　　juvenile A50.40
　　remission in (sustained) A52.3
　　serology doubtful, negative, or positive A52.3
　　specified nature or site NEC A52.19
　　vascular A52.05
　cerebral A52.17
　　meningovascular A52.13
　　nerves (multiple palsies) A52.15
　　sclerosis A52.17
　　thrombosis A52.05
　cerebrospinal (tabetic type) A52.12
　cerebrovascular A52.05
　cervix (late) A52.76
　chancre (multiple) A51.0
　　extragenital A51.2
　　Rollet's A51.0
　Charcot's joint A52.16
　chorioretinitis A51.43
　　congenital A50.01
　　late A52.71
　　prenatal A50.01
　choroiditis — see Syphilitic chorioretinitis
　choroidoretinitis — see Syphilitic chorioretinitis
　ciliary body (secondary) A51.43
　　late A52.71
　colon (late) A52.74
　combined spinal sclerosis A52.11
　condyloma (latum) A51.31
　congenital A50.9
　　with
　　　paresis (general) A50.45
　　　tabes (dorsalis) A50.45
　　　taboparesis A50.45
　　chorioretinitis, choroiditis A50.01 [H32]
　　early, or less than 2 years after birth NEC A50.2
　　　with manifestations — see Syphilis, congenital,
　　　　early, symptomatic
　　　latent (without manifestations) A50.1
　　　　negative spinal fluid test A50.1
　　　　serology positive A50.1
　　　symptomatic A50.09
　　　　cutaneous A50.06

Syphilis, syphilitic — continued
　congenital — continued
　　early, or less than 2 years after birth — continued
　　　symptomatic — continued
　　　　mucocutaneous A50.07
　　　　oculopathy A50.01
　　　　osteochondropathy A50.02
　　　　pharyngitis A50.03
　　　　pneumonia A50.04
　　　　rhinitis A50.05
　　　　visceral A50.08
　　　interstitial keratitis A50.31
　　　juvenile neurosyphilis A50.45
　　　late, or 2 years or more after birth NEC A50.7
　　　　chorioretinitis, choroiditis A50.32
　　　　interstitial keratitis A50.31
　　　　juvenile neurosyphilis A50.45
　　　　latent (without manifestations) A50.6
　　　　　negative spinal fluid test A50.6
　　　　　serology positive A50.6
　　　　symptomatic or with manifestations NEC A50.59
　　　　　arthropathy A50.55
　　　　　cardiovascular A50.54
　　　　　Clutton's joints A50.51
　　　　　Hutchinson's teeth A50.52
　　　　　Hutchinson's triad A50.53
　　　　　osteochondropathy A50.56
　　　　　saddle nose A50.57
　conjugal A53.9
　　tabes A52.11
　conjunctiva (late) A52.71
　contact Z20.2
　cord bladder A52.19
　cornea, late A52.71
　coronary (artery) (sclerosis) A52.06
　coryza, congenital A50.05
　cranial nerve A52.15
　　multiple palsies A52.15
　cutaneous — see Syphilis, skin
　dacryocystitis (late) A52.71
　degeneration, spinal cord A52.12
　dementia paralytica A52.17
　　juvenilis A50.45
　destruction of bone A52.77
　dilatation, aorta A52.01
　due to blood transfusion A53.9
　dura mater A52.13
　ear A52.79
　　inner A52.79
　　　nerve (eighth) A52.15
　　　neurorecurrence A52.15
　early A51.9
　　cardiovascular A52.00
　　central nervous system A52.3
　　latent (without manifestations) (less than 2 years
　　　after infection) A51.5
　　　negative spinal fluid test A51.5
　　　serological relapse after treatment A51.5
　　　serology positive A51.5
　　relapse (treated, untreated) A51.9
　　skin A51.39
　　symptomatic A51.9
　　　extragenital chancre A51.2
　　　primary, except extragenital chancre A51.0
　　　secondary — see also Syphilis, secondary A51.39
　　　　relapse (treated, untreated) A51.49
　　ulcer A51.39
　eighth nerve (neuritis) A52.15
　endemic A65
　endocarditis A52.03
　　aortic A52.03
　　pulmonary A52.03
　epididymis (late) A52.76
　epiglottis (late) A52.73
　epiphysitis (congenital) (early) A50.02
　episcleritis (late) A52.71
　esophagus A52.79
　eustachian tube A52.73
　exposure to Z20.2
　eye A52.71
　eyelid (late) (with gumma) A52.71
　fallopian tube (late) A52.76
　fracture A52.77
　gallbladder (late) A52.74
　gastric (polyposis) (late) A52.74
　general A53.9
　　paralysis A52.17
　　　juvenile A50.45
　genital (primary) A51.0

Syphilis, syphilitic — *continued*
glaucoma A52.71
gumma NEC A52.79
  cardiovascular system A52.00
  central nervous system A52.3
  congenital A50.59
heart (block) (decompensation) (disease) (failure) A52.06 *[I52]*
  valve NEC A52.03
hemianesthesia A52.19
hemianopsia A52.71
hemiparesis A52.17
hemiplegia A52.17
hepatic artery A52.09
hepatis A52.74
hepatomegaly, congenital A50.08
hereditaria tarda — *see* Syphilis, congenital, late
hereditary — *see* Syphilis, congenital
Hutchinson's teeth A50.52
hyalitis A52.71
inactive — *see* Syphilis, latent
infantum — *see* Syphilis, congenital
inherited — *see* Syphilis, congenital
internal ear A52.79
intestine (late) A52.74
iris, iritis (secondary) A51.43
  late A52.71
joint (late) A52.77
keratitis (congenital) (interstitial) (late) A50.31
kidney (late) A52.75
lacrimal passages (late) A52.71
larynx (late) A52.73
late A52.9
  cardiovascular A52.00
  central nervous system A52.3
  kidney A52.75
  latent or 2 years or more after infection (without manifestations) A52.8
    negative spinal fluid test A52.8
    serology positive A52.8
  paresis A52.17
  specified site NEC A52.79
  symptomatic or with manifestations A52.79
  tabes A52.11
latent A53.0
  with signs or symptoms — *code by* site and stage under Syphilis
  central nervous system A52.2
  date of infection unspecified A53.0
  early, or less than 2 years after infection A51.5
  follow-up of latent syphilis A53.0
    date of infection unspecified A53.0
    late, or 2 years or more after infection A52.8
  late, or 2 years or more after infection A52.8
  positive serology (only finding) A53.0
    date of infection unspecified A53.0
    early, or less than 2 years after infection A51.5
    late, or 2 years or more after infection A52.8
lens (late) A52.71
leukoderma A51.39
  late A52.79
lienitis A52.79
lip A51.39
  chancre (primary) A51.2
  late A52.79
Lissauer's paralysis A52.17
liver A52.74
locomotor ataxia A52.11
lung A52.72
lymph gland (early) (secondary) A51.49
  late A52.79
lymphadenitis (secondary) A51.49
macular atrophy of skin A51.39
  striated A52.79
mediastinum (late) A52.73
meninges (adhesive) (brain) (spinal cord) A52.13
meningitis A52.13
  acute (secondary) A51.41
  congenital A50.41
meningoencephalitis A52.14
meningovascular A52.13
  congenital A50.41
mesarteritis A52.09
  brain A52.04
middle ear A52.77
mitral stenosis A52.03
monoplegia A52.17
mouth (secondary) A51.39

Syphilis, syphilitic — *continued*
mouth — *continued*
  late A52.79
mucocutaneous (secondary) A51.39
  late A52.79
mucous
  membrane (secondary) A51.39
    late A52.79
  patches A51.39
    congenital A50.07
mulberry molars A50.52
muscle A52.78
myocardium A52.06
nasal sinus (late) A52.73
neonatorum — *see* Syphilis, congenital
nephrotic syndrome (secondary) A51.44
nerve palsy (any cranial nerve) A52.15
  multiple A52.15
nervous system, central A52.3
neuritis A52.15
  acoustic A52.15
neurorecidive of retina A52.19
neuroretinitis A52.19
newborn — *see* Syphilis, congenital
nodular superficial (late) A52.79
nonvenereal A65
nose (late) A52.73
  saddle back deformity A50.57
occlusive arterial disease A52.09
oculopathy A52.71
ophthalmic (late) A52.71
optic nerve (atrophy) (neuritis) (papilla) A52.15
orbit (late) A52.71
organic A53.9
osseous (late) A52.77
osteochondritis (congenital) (early) A50.02 *[M90.80]*
osteoporosis A52.77
ovary (late) A52.76
oviduct (late) A52.76
palate (late) A52.79
pancreas (late) A52.74
paralysis A52.17
  general A52.17
    juvenile A50.45
paresis (general) A52.17
  juvenile A50.45
paresthesia A52.19
Parkinson's disease or syndrome A52.19
paroxysmal tachycardia A52.06
pemphigus (congenital) A50.06
penis (chancre) A51.0
  late A52.76
pericardium A52.06
perichondritis, larynx (late) A52.73
periosteum (late) A52.77
  congenital (early) A50.02 *[M90.80]*
  early (secondary) A51.46
peripheral nerve A52.79
petrous bone (late) A52.77
pharynx (late) A52.73
  secondary A51.39
pituitary (gland) A52.79
pleura (late) A52.73
pneumonia, white A50.04
pontine lesion A52.17
portal vein A52.09
primary A51.0
  anal A51.1
  and secondary — *see* Syphilis, secondary
  central nervous system A52.3
  extragenital chancre NEC A51.2
  fingers A51.2
  genital A51.0
  lip A51.2
  specified site NEC A51.2
  tonsils A51.2
prostate (late) A52.76
ptosis (eyelid) A52.71
pulmonary (late) A52.72
  artery A52.09
pyelonephritis (late) A52.75
recently acquired, symptomatic A51.9
rectum (late) A52.74
respiratory tract (late) A52.73
retina, late A52.71
retrobulbar neuritis A52.15
salpingitis A52.76
sclera (late) A52.71

Syphilis, syphilitic — *continued*
sclerosis
  cerebral A52.17
  coronary A52.06
  multiple A52.11
scotoma (central) A52.71
scrotum (late) A52.76
secondary (and primary) A51.49
  adenopathy A51.49
  anus A51.39
  bone A51.46
  chorioretinitis, choroiditis A51.43
  hepatitis A51.45
  liver A51.45
  lymphadenitis A51.49
  meningitis (acute) A51.41
  mouth A51.39
  mucous membranes A51.39
  periosteum, periostitis A51.46
  pharynx A51.39
  relapse (treated, untreated) A51.49
  skin A51.39
  specified form NEC A51.49
  tonsil A51.39
  ulcer A51.39
  viscera NEC A51.49
  vulva A51.39
seminal vesicle (late) A52.76
seronegative with signs or symptoms — *code by* site and stage under Syphilis
seropositive
  with signs or symptoms — *code by* site and stage under Syphilis
  follow-up of latent syphilis — *see* Syphilis, latent
  only finding — *see* Syphilis, latent
seventh nerve (paralysis) A52.15
sinus, sinusitis (late) A52.73
skeletal system A52.77
skin (with ulceration) (early) (secondary) A51.39
  late or tertiary A52.79
small intestine A52.74
spastic spinal paralysis A52.17
spermatic cord (late) A52.76
spinal (cord) A52.12
spleen A52.79
splenomegaly A52.79
spondylitis A52.77
staphyloma A52.71
stigmata (congenital) A50.59
stomach A52.74
synovium A52.78
tabes dorsalis (late) A52.11
  juvenile A50.45
tabetic type A52.11
  juvenile A50.45
taboparesis A52.17
  juvenile A50.45
tachycardia A52.06
tendon (late) A52.78
tertiary A52.9
  with symptoms NEC A52.79
  cardiovascular A52.00
  central nervous system A52.3
  multiple NEC A52.79
  specified site NEC A52.79
testis A52.76
thorax A52.73
throat A52.73
thymus (gland) (late) A52.79
thyroid (late) A52.79
tongue (late) A52.79
tonsil (lingual) (late) A52.73
  primary A51.2
  secondary A51.39
trachea (late) A52.73
tunica vaginalis (late) A52.76
ulcer (any site) (early) (secondary) A51.39
  late A52.79
  perforating A52.79
    foot A52.11
urethra (late) A52.76
urogenital (late) A52.76
uterus (late) A52.76
uveal tract (secondary) A51.43
  late A52.71
uveitis (secondary) A51.43
  late A52.71
uvula (late) (perforated) A52.79
vagina A51.0

☑ **Additional Character Required** — Refer to the Tabular List for Character Selection   ▽ Subterms under main terms may continue to next column or page

Syphilis, syphilitic — *continued*
  vagina — *continued*
    late A52.76
  valvulitis NEC A52.03
  vascular A52.00
    brain (cerebral) A52.05
  ventriculi A52.74
  vesicae urinariae (late) A52.76
  viscera (abdominal) (late) A52.74
    secondary A51.49
  vitreous (opacities) (late) A52.71
    hemorrhage A52.71
  vulva A51.0
    late A52.76

Syphilis, syphilitic — *continued*
  vulva — *continued*
    secondary A51.39
Syphiloma A52.79
  cardiovascular system A52.00
  central nervous system A52.3
  circulatory system A52.00
  congenital A50.59
Syphilophobia F45.29
Syringadenoma — *see also* Neoplasm, skin, benign
  papillary — *see* Neoplasm, skin, benign
Syringobulbia G95.0
Syringocystadenoma — *see* Neoplasm, skin, benign
  papillary — *see* Neoplasm, skin, benign

Syringoma — *see also* Neoplasm, skin, benign
  chondroid — *see* Neoplasm, skin, benign
Syringomyelia G95.0
Syringomyelitis — *see* Encephalitis
Syringomyelocele — *see* Spina bifida
Syringopontia G95.0
System, systemic — *see also* condition
  disease, combined — *see* Degeneration, combined
  inflammatory response syndrome (SIRS) of non-infec-
    tious origin (without organ dysfunction) R65.10
    with acute organ dysfunction R65.11
  lupus erythematosus M32.9
    inhibitor present D68.62

T

Tabacism, tabacosis, tabagism — *see also* Poisoning, tobacco
  meaning dependence (without remission) F17.200
    with
      disorder F17.299
        in remission F17.211
        specified disorder NEC F17.298
        withdrawal F17.203
Tabardillo A75.9
  flea-borne A75.2
  louse-borne A75.0
Tabes, tabetic A52.10
  with
    central nervous system syphilis A52.10
    Charcot's joint A52.16
    cord bladder A52.19
    crisis, viscera (any) A52.19
    paralysis, general A52.17
    paresis (general) A52.17
    perforating ulcer (foot) A52.19
  arthropathy (Charcot) A52.16
  bladder A52.19
  bone A52.11
  cerebrospinal A52.12
  congenital A50.45
  conjugal A52.10
  dorsalis A52.11
    juvenile A50.49
  juvenile A50.49
  latent A52.19
  mesenterica A18.39
  paralysis, insane, general A52.17
  spasmodic A52.17
  syphilis (cerebrospinal) A52.12
Taboparalysis A52.17
Taboparesis (remission) A52.17
  juvenile A50.45
TAC (trigeminal autonomic cephalgia) **NEC** G44.099
  intractable G44.091
  not intractable G44.099
Tache noir S60.22- ☑
Tachyalimentation K91.2
Tachyarrhythmia, tachyrhythmia — *see* Tachycardia
Tachycardia R00.0
  atrial (paroxysmal) I47.1
  auricular I47.1
  AV nodal re-entry (re-entrant) I47.1
  junctional (paroxysmal) I47.1
  newborn P29.11
  nodal (paroxysmal) I47.1
  non-paroxysmal AV nodal I45.89
  paroxysmal (sustained) (nonsustained) I47.9
    with sinus bradycardia I49.5
    atrial (PAT) I47.1
    atrioventricular (AV) (re-entrant) I47.1
      psychogenic F54
    junctional I47.1
      ectopic I47.1
    nodal I47.1
    psychogenic (atrial) (supraventricular) (ventricular) F54
    supraventricular (sustained) I47.1
      psychogenic F54
    ventricular I47.2
      psychogenic F54
  psychogenic F45.8
  sick sinus I49.5
  sinoauricular NOS R00.0
    paroxysmal I47.1
  sinus [sinusal] NOS R00.0
    paroxysmal I47.1
  supraventricular I47.1
  ventricular (paroxysmal) (sustained) I47.2
    psychogenic F54
Tachygastria K31.89
Tachypnea R06.82
  hysterical F45.8
  newborn (idiopathic) (transitory) P22.1
  psychogenic F45.8
  transitory, of newborn P22.1
TACO (transfusion associated circulatory overload) E87.71
Taenia (infection) (infestation) B68.9
  diminuta B71.0
  echinococcal infestation B67.90
  mediocanellata B68.1

Taenia — *continued*
  nana B71.0
  saginata B68.1
  solium (intestinal form) B68.0
    larval form — *see* Cysticercosis
Taeniasis (intestine) — *see* Taenia
Tag (hypertrophied skin) (infected) L91.8
  adenoid J35.8
  anus K64.4
  hemorrhoidal K64.4
  hymen N89.8
  perineal N90.89
  preauricular Q17.0
  sentinel K64.4
  skin L91.8
    accessory (congenital) Q82.8
    anus K64.4
    congenital Q82.8
    preauricular Q17.0
  tonsil J35.8
  urethra, urethral N36.8
  vulva N90.89
Tahyna fever B33.8
Takahara's disease E80.3
Takayasu's disease or syndrome M31.4
Talaromycosis B48.4
Talcosis (pulmonary) J62.0
Talipes (congenital) Q66.89
  acquired, planus — *see* Deformity, limb, flat foot
  asymmetric Q66.89
  calcaneovalgus Q66.4- ☑
  calcaneovarus Q66.1- ☑
  calcaneus Q66.89
  cavus Q66.7- ☑
  equinovalgus Q66.6
  equinovarus Q66.0- ☑
  equinus Q66.89
  percavus Q66.7- ☑
  planovalgus Q66.6
  planus (acquired) (any degree) — *see also* Deformity, limb, flat foot
    congenital Q66.5- ☑
    due to rickets (sequelae) E64.3
  valgus Q66.6
  varus Q66.3- ☑
Tall stature, constitutional E34.4
Talma's disease M62.89
Talon noir S90.3- ☑
  hand S60.22- ☑
  heel S90.3- ☑
  toe S90.1- ☑
Tamponade, heart I31.4
Tanapox (virus disease) B08.71
Tangier disease E78.6
Tantrum, child problem F91.8
Tapeworm (infection) (infestation) — *see* Infestation, tapeworm
Tapia's syndrome G52.7
TAR (thrombocytopenia with absent radius) **syndrome** Q87.2
Tarral-Besnier disease L44.0
Tarsal tunnel syndrome — *see* Syndrome, tarsal tunnel
Tarsalgia — *see* Pain, limb, lower
Tarsitis (eyelid) H01.8
  syphilitic A52.71
  tuberculous A18.4
Tartar (teeth) (dental calculus) K03.6
Tattoo (mark) L81.8
Tauri's disease E74.09
Taurodontism K00.2
Taussig-Bing syndrome Q20.1
Taybi's syndrome Q87.2
Tay-Sachs amaurotic familial idiocy or disease E75.02
TBI (traumatic brain injury) S06.9 ☑
Teacher's node or nodule J38.2
Tear, torn (traumatic) — *see also* Laceration
  with abortion — *see* Abortion
  annular fibrosis M51.35
  anus, anal (sphincter) S31.831 ☑
    complicating delivery
      with third degree perineal laceration — *see also* Delivery, complicated, by, laceration, perineum, third degree O70.20
        with mucosa O70.3
      without third degree perineal laceration O70.4
    nontraumatic (healed) (old) K62.81

Tear, torn — *continued*
  articular cartilage, old — *see* Derangement, joint, articular cartilage, by site
  bladder
    with ectopic or molar pregnancy O08.6
    following ectopic or molar pregnancy O08.6
    obstetrical O71.5
    traumatic — *see* Injury, bladder
  bowel
    with ectopic or molar pregnancy O08.6
    following ectopic or molar pregnancy O08.6
    obstetrical trauma O71.5
  broad ligament
    with ectopic or molar pregnancy O08.6
    following ectopic or molar pregnancy O08.6
    obstetrical trauma O71.6
  bucket handle (knee) (meniscus) — *see* Tear, meniscus
  capsule, joint — *see* Sprain
  cartilage — *see also* Sprain
    articular, old — *see* Derangement, joint, articular cartilage, by site
  cervix
    with ectopic or molar pregnancy O08.6
    following ectopic or molar pregnancy O08.6
    obstetrical trauma (current) O71.3
    old N88.1
    traumatic — *see* Injury, uterus
  dural G97.41
    nontraumatic G96.11
  internal organ — *see* Injury, by site
  knee cartilage
    articular (current) S83.3- ☑
    old — *see* Derangement, knee, meniscus, due to old tear
  ligament — *see* Sprain
  meniscus (knee) (current injury) S83.209 ☑
    bucket-handle S83.20- ☑
    lateral
      bucket-handle S83.25- ☑
      complex S83.27- ☑
      peripheral S83.26- ☑
      specified type NEC S83.28- ☑
    medial
      bucket-handle S83.21- ☑
      complex S83.23- ☑
      peripheral S83.22- ☑
      specified type NEC S83.24- ☑
    old — *see* Derangement, knee, meniscus, due to old tear
    site other than knee — *code as* Sprain
    specified type NEC S83.20- ☑
  muscle — *see* Strain
  pelvic
    floor, complicating delivery O70.1
    organ NEC, obstetrical trauma O71.5
      with ectopic or molar pregnancy O08.6
      following ectopic or molar pregnancy O08.6
  perineal, secondary O90.1
  periurethral tissue, obstetrical trauma O71.82
    with ectopic or molar pregnancy O08.6
    following ectopic or molar pregnancy O08.6
  rectovaginal septum — *see* Laceration, vagina
  retina, retinal (without detachment) (horseshoe) — *see also* Break, retina, horseshoe
    with detachment — *see* Detachment, retina, with retinal, break
  rotator cuff (nontraumatic) M75.10- ☑
    complete M75.12- ☑
    incomplete M75.11- ☑
    traumatic S46.01- ☑
      capsule S43.42- ☑
  semilunar cartilage, knee — *see* Tear, meniscus
  supraspinatus (complete) (incomplete) (nontraumatic) — *see also* Tear, rotator cuff M75.10- ☑
  tendon — *see* Strain
  tentorial, at birth P10.4
  umbilical cord
    complicating delivery O69.89 ☑
  urethra
    with ectopic or molar pregnancy O08.6
    following ectopic or molar pregnancy O08.6
    obstetrical trauma O71.5
  uterus — *see* Injury, uterus
  vagina — *see* Laceration, vagina
  vessel, from catheter — *see* Puncture, accidental complicating surgery
  vulva, complicating delivery O70.0

Tear-stone — *see* Dacryolith
Teeth — *see also* condition
  grinding
    psychogenic F45.8
    sleep related G47.63
Teething (syndrome) K00.7
Telangiectasia, telangiectasis (verrucous) I78.1
  ataxic (cerebellar) (Louis-Bar) G11.3
  familial I78.0
  hemorrhagic, hereditary (congenital) (senile) I78.0
  hereditary, hemorrhagic (congenital) (senile) I78.0
  juxtafoveal H35.07- ☑
  macular H35.07- ☑
  macularis eruptiva perstans D47.01
  parafoveal H35.07- ☑
  retinal (idiopathic) (juxtafoveal) (macular) (parafoveal)
    H35.07- ☑
  spider I78.1
Telephone scatologia F65.89
Telescoped bowel or intestine K56.1
  congenital Q43.8
Temperature
  body, high (of unknown origin) R50.9
  cold, trauma from T69.9 ☑
    newborn P80.0
    specified effect NEC T69.8 ☑
Temple — *see* condition
Temporal — *see* condition
**Temporomandibular joint pain-dysfunction syn-
  drome** M26.62- ☑
Temporosphenoidal — *see* condition
Tendency
  bleeding — *see* Defect, coagulation
  suicide
    meaning personal history of attempted suicide
      Z91.51
    meaning suicidal ideation — *see* Ideation, suicidal
  to fall R29.6
Tenderness, abdominal R10.819
  epigastric R10.816
  generalized R10.817
  left lower quadrant R10.814
  left upper quadrant R10.812
  periumbilic R10.815
  rebound R10.829
    epigastric R10.826
    generalized R10.827
    left lower quadrant R10.824
    left upper quadrant R10.822
    periumbilic R10.825
    right lower quadrant R10.823
    right upper quadrant R10.821
  right lower quadrant R10.813
  right upper quadrant R10.811
Tendinitis, tendonitis — *see also* Enthesopathy
  Achilles M76.6- ☑
  adhesive — *see* Tenosynovitis, specified type NEC
    shoulder — *see* Capsulitis, adhesive
  bicipital M75.2- ☑
  calcific M65.2- ☑
    ankle M65.27- ☑
    foot M65.27- ☑
    forearm M65.23- ☑
    hand M65.24- ☑
    lower leg M65.26- ☑
    multiple sites M65.29
    pelvic region M65.25- ☑
    shoulder M75.3- ☑
    specified site NEC M65.28
    thigh M65.25- ☑
    upper arm M65.22- ☑
  due to use, overuse, pressure — *see also* Disorder, soft
    tissue, due to use
    specified NEC — *see* Disorder, soft tissue, due to
      use, specified NEC
  gluteal M76.0- ☑
  patellar M76.5- ☑
  peroneal M76.7- ☑
  psoas M76.1- ☑
  tibial (posterior) M76.82- ☑
    anterior M76.81- ☑
  trochanteric — *see* Bursitis, hip, trochanteric
Tendon — *see* condition
Tendosynovitis — *see* Tenosynovitis
Tenesmus (rectal) R19.8
  vesical R30.1
Tennis elbow — *see* Epicondylitis, lateral

Tenonitis — *see also* Tenosynovitis
  eye (capsule) H05.04- ☑
Tenontosynovitis — *see* Tenosynovitis
Tenontothecitis — *see* Tenosynovitis
Tenophyte — *see* Disorder, synovium, specified type NEC
Tenosynovitis — *see also* Synovitis M65.9
  adhesive — *see* Tenosynovitis, specified type NEC
    shoulder — *see* Capsulitis, adhesive
  bicipital (calcifying) — *see* Tendinitis, bicipital
  gonococcal A54.49
  in (due to)
    crystals M65.8- ☑
    gonorrhea A54.49
    syphilis (late) A52.78
    use, overuse, pressure — *see also* Disorder, soft tis-
      sue, due to use
      specified NEC — *see* Disorder, soft tissue, due to
        use, specified NEC
  infective NEC M65.1- ☑
    ankle M65.17- ☑
    foot M65.17- ☑
    forearm M65.13- ☑
    hand M65.14- ☑
    lower leg M65.16- ☑
    multiple sites M65.19
    pelvic region M65.15- ☑
    shoulder region M65.11- ☑
    specified site NEC M65.18
    thigh M65.15- ☑
    upper arm M65.12- ☑
  radial styloid M65.4
  shoulder region M65.81- ☑
    adhesive — *see* Capsulitis, adhesive
  specified type NEC M65.88
    ankle M65.87- ☑
    foot M65.87- ☑
    forearm M65.83- ☑
    hand M65.84- ☑
    lower leg M65.86- ☑
    multiple sites M65.89
    pelvic region M65.85- ☑
    shoulder region M65.81- ☑
    specified site NEC M65.88
    thigh M65.85- ☑
    upper arm M65.82- ☑
  tuberculous — *see* Tuberculosis, tenosynovitis
Tenovaginitis — *see* Tenosynovitis
Tension
  arterial, high — *see also* Hypertension
    without diagnosis of hypertension R03.0
  headache G44.209
    intractable G44.201
    not intractable G44.209
  nervous R45.0
  pneumothorax J93.0
  premenstrual N94.3
  state (mental) F48.9
Tentorium — *see* condition
Teratencephalus Q89.8
Teratism Q89.7
Teratoblastoma (malignant) — *see* Neoplasm, malignant, by site
Teratocarcinoma — *see also* Neoplasm, malignant, by
  site
  liver C22.7
Teratoma (solid) — *see also* Neoplasm, uncertain behavior, by site
  with embryonal carcinoma, mixed — *see* Neoplasm,
    malignant, by site
  with malignant transformation — *see* Neoplasm, ma-
    lignant, by site
  adult (cystic) — *see* Neoplasm, benign, by site
  benign — *see* Neoplasm, benign, by site
  combined with choriocarcinoma — *see* Neoplasm,
    malignant, by site
  cystic (adult) — *see* Neoplasm, benign, by site
  differentiated — *see* Neoplasm, benign, by site
  embryonal — *see also* Neoplasm, malignant, by site
    liver C22.7
  immature — *see* Neoplasm, malignant, by site
  liver C22.7
    adult, benign, cystic, differentiated type or mature
      D13.4
  malignant — *see also* Neoplasm, malignant, by site
    anaplastic — *see* Neoplasm, malignant, by site
    intermediate — *see* Neoplasm, malignant, by site

Teratoma — *continued*
  malignant — *see also* Neoplasm, malignant, by site —
    continued
    intermediate — *see* Neoplasm, malignant, by site
      — *continued*
      specified site — *see* Neoplasm, malignant, by
        site
    unspecified site C62.90
    undifferentiated — *see* Neoplasm, malignant, by
      site
  mature — *see* Neoplasm, uncertain behavior, by site
    malignant — *see* Neoplasm, by site, malignant, by
      site
  ovary D27.- ☑
    embryonal, immature or malignant C56- ☑
  solid — *see* Neoplasm, uncertain behavior, by site
  testis C62.9- ☑
    adult, benign, cystic, differentiated type or mature
      D29.2- ☑
    scrotal C62.1- ☑
    undescended C62.0- ☑
Termination
  anomalous — *see also* Malposition, congenital
    right pulmonary vein Q26.3
  pregnancy, elective Z33.2
Ternidens diminutus infestation B81.8
Ternidensiasis B81.8
Terror(s) night (child) F51.4
Terrorism, victim of Z65.4
Terry's syndrome — *see also* Myopia, degenerative
  H44.2- ☑
Tertiary — *see* condition
Test, tests, testing (for)
  adequacy (for dialysis)
    hemodialysis Z49.31
    peritoneal Z49.32
  blood pressure Z01.30
    abnormal reading — *see* Blood, pressure
  blood typing Z01.83
    Rh typing Z01.83
  blood-alcohol Z02.83
    positive — *see* Findings, abnormal, in blood
  blood-drug Z02.83
    positive — *see* Findings, abnormal, in blood
  cardiac pulse generator (battery) Z45.010
  fertility Z31.41
  genetic
    disease carrier status for procreative management
      female Z31.430
      male Z31.440
    male partner of patient with recurrent pregnancy
      loss Z31.441
    procreative management NEC
      female Z31.438
      male Z31.448
  hearing Z01.10
    with abnormal findings NEC Z01.118
    infant or child (over 28 days old) Z00.129
      with abnormal findings Z00.121
  HIV (human immunodeficiency virus)
    nonconclusive (in infants) R75
    positive Z21
    seropositive Z21
  immunity status Z01.84
  intelligence NEC Z01.89
  laboratory (as part of a general medical examination)
    Z00.00
    with abnormal finding Z00.01
    for medicolegal reason NEC Z04.89
  male partner of patient with recurrent pregnancy loss
    Z31.441
  Mantoux (for tuberculosis) Z11.1
    abnormal result R76.11
  pregnancy, positive first pregnancy — *see* Pregnancy,
    normal, first
  procreative Z31.49
    fertility Z31.41
  skin, diagnostic
    allergy Z01.82
      special screening examination — *see* Screening,
        by name of disease
    Mantoux Z11.1
    tuberculin Z11.1
  specified NEC Z01.89
  tuberculin Z11.1
    abnormal result R76.11
  vision Z01.00
    with abnormal findings Z01.01

▽ Subterms under main terms may continue to next column or page   ☑ Additional Character Required — Refer to the Tabular List for Character Selection   313

Tear-stone — Test, tests, testing

Test, tests, testing — *continued*
 vision — *continued*
  following failed vision screening Z01.020
   with abnormal findings Z01.021
  infant or child (over 28 days old) Z00.129
   with abnormal findings Z00.121
  Wassermann Z11.3
  positive — *see* Serology for syphilis, positive
Testicle, testicular, testis — *see also* condition
 feminization syndrome — *see also* Syndrome, androgen insensitivity E34.51
 migrans Q55.29
Tetanus, tetanic (cephalic) (convulsions) A35
 with
  abortion A34
  ectopic or molar pregnancy O08.0
 following ectopic or molar pregnancy O08.0
 inoculation reaction (due to serum) — *see* Complications, vaccination
 neonatorum A33
 obstetrical A34
 puerperal, postpartum, childbirth A34
Tetany (due to) R29.0
 alkalosis E87.3
 associated with rickets E55.0
 convulsions R29.0
  hysterical F44.5
 functional (hysterical) F44.5
 hyperkinetic R29.0
  hysterical F44.5
 hyperpnea R06.4
  hysterical F44.5
  psychogenic F45.8
 hyperventilation — *see also* Hyperventilation R06.4
  hysterical F44.5
 neonatal (without calcium or magnesium deficiency) P71.3
 parathyroid (gland) E20.9
 parathyroprival E89.2
 post- (para)thyroidectomy E89.2
 postoperative E89.2
 pseudotetany R29.0
 psychogenic (conversion reaction) F44.5
Tetralogy of Fallot Q21.3
Tetraplegia (chronic) — *see also* Quadriplegia G82.50
Thailand hemorrhagic fever A91
Thalassanemia — *see* Thalassemia
Thalassemia (anemia) (disease) D56.9
 with other hemoglobinopathy D56.8
 alpha (major) (severe) (triple gene defect) D56.0
  minor D56.3
  silent carrier D56.3
  trait D56.3
 beta (severe) D56.1
  homozygous D56.1
  major D56.1
  minor D56.3
  trait D56.3
 delta-beta (homozygous) D56.2
  minor D56.3
  trait D56.3
 dominant D56.8
 hemoglobin
  C D56.8
  E-beta D56.5
 intermedia D56.1
 major D56.1
 minor D56.3
 mixed D56.8
 sickle-cell — *see* Disease, sickle-cell, thalassemia
 specified type NEC D56.8
 trait D56.3
 variants D56.8
Thanatophoric dwarfism or short stature Q77.1
Thaysen-Gee disease (nontropical sprue) K90.0
Thaysen's disease K90.0
Thecoma D27- ☑
 luteinized D27- ☑
 malignant C56- ☑
Thelarche, premature E30.8
Thelaziasis B83.8
Thelitis N61.0
 puerperal, postpartum or gestational — *see* Infection, nipple
Therapeutic — *see* condition

Therapy
 drug, long-term (current) (prophylactic)
  agents affecting estrogen receptors and estrogen levels NEC Z79.818
  anastrozole (Arimidex) Z79.811
  antibiotics Z79.2
   short-term use — *omit code*
  anticoagulants Z79.01
  anti-inflammatory Z79.1
  antiplatelet Z79.02
  antithrombotics Z79.02
  aromatase inhibitors Z79.811
  aspirin Z79.82
  birth control pill or patch Z79.3
  bisphosphonates Z79.83
  contraceptive, oral Z79.3
  drug, specified NEC Z79.899
  estrogen receptor downregulators Z79.818
  Evista Z79.810
  exemestane (Aromasin) Z79.811
  Fareston Z79.810
  fulvestrant (Faslodex) Z79.818
  gonadotropin-releasing hormone (GnRH) agonist Z79.818
  goserelin acetate (Zoladex) Z79.818
  hormone replacement Z79.890
  insulin Z79.4
  letrozole (Femara) Z79.811
  leuprolide acetate (leuprorelin) (Lupron) Z79.818
  megestrol acetate (Megace) Z79.818
  methadone
   for pain management Z79.891
   maintenance therapy F11.20
  Nolvadex Z79.810
  opiate analgesic Z79.891
  oral contraceptive Z79.3
  raloxifene (Evista) Z79.810
  selective estrogen receptor modulators (SERMs) Z79.810
  short term — *omit code*
  steroids
   inhaled Z79.51
   systemic Z79.52
  tamoxifen (Nolvadex) Z79.810
  toremifene (Fareston) Z79.810
Thermic — *see* condition
Thermography (abnormal) — *see also* Abnormal, diagnostic imaging R93.89
 breast R92.8
Thermoplegia T67.01 ☑
Thesaurismosis, glycogen — *see* Disease, glycogen storage
Thiamin deficiency E51.9
 specified NEC E51.8
Thiaminic deficiency with beriberi E51.11
Thibierge-Weissenbach syndrome — *see* Sclerosis, systemic
Thickening
 bone — *see* Hypertrophy, bone
 breast N64.59
 endometrium R93.89
 epidermal L85.9
  specified NEC L85.8
 hymen N89.6
 larynx J38.7
 nail L60.2
  congenital Q84.5
 periosteal — *see* Hypertrophy, bone
 pleura J92.9
  with asbestos J92.0
 skin R23.4
 subepiglottic J38.7
 tongue K14.8
 valve, heart — *see* Endocarditis
Thigh — *see* condition
Thinning vertebra — *see* Spondylopathy, specified NEC
Thirst, excessive R63.1
 due to deprivation of water T73.1 ☑
Thomsen disease G71.12
Thoracic — *see also* condition
 kidney Q63.2
 outlet syndrome G54.0
Thoracogastroschisis (congenital) Q79.8
Thoracopagus Q89.4
Thorax — *see* condition
Thorn's syndrome N28.89
Thorson-Björck syndrome E34.0
Threadworm (infection) (infestation) B80

Threatened
 abortion O20.0
  with subsequent abortion O03.9
 job loss, anxiety concerning Z56.2
 labor (without delivery) O47.9
  at or after 37 completed weeks of gestation O47.1
  before 37 completed weeks of gestation O47.0- ☑
 loss of job, anxiety concerning Z56.2
 miscarriage O20.0
 unemployment, anxiety concerning Z56.2
Three-day fever A93.1
Threshers' lung J67.0
Thrix annulata (congenital) Q84.1
Throat — *see* condition
Thrombasthenia (Glanzmann) (hemorrhagic) (hereditary) D69.1
Thromboangiitis I73.1
 obliterans (general) I73.1
  cerebral I67.89
  vessels
   brain I67.89
   spinal cord I67.89
Thromboarteritis — *see* Arteritis
Thromboasthenia (Glanzmann) (hemorrhagic) (hereditary) D69.1
Thrombocytasthenia (Glanzmann) D69.1
Thrombocythemia (hemorrhagic) *see also* Thrombocytosis D75.839
 essential D47.3
 idiopathic D47.3
 primary D47.3
Thrombocytopathy (dystrophic) (granulopenic) D69.1
Thrombocytopenia, thrombocytopenic D69.6
 with absent radius (TAR) Q87.2
 congenital D69.42
 dilutional D69.59
 due to
  (massive) blood transfusion D69.59
  drugs D69.59
  extracorporeal circulation of blood D69.59
  platelet alloimmunization D69.59
 essential D69.3
 heparin induced (HIT) D75.82
 hereditary D69.42
 idiopathic D69.3
 neonatal, transitory P61.0
  due to
   exchange transfusion P61.0
   idiopathic maternal thrombocytopenia P61.0
   isoimmunization P61.0
 primary NEC D69.49
  idiopathic D69.3
 puerperal, postpartum O72.3
 secondary D69.59
 transient neonatal P61.0
Thrombocytosis D75.839
 essential D47.3
 idiopathic D47.3
 primary D47.3
 reactive D75.838
 secondary D75.838
 specified NEC D75.838
Thromboembolism — *see* Embolism
Thrombopathy (Bernard-Soulier) D69.1
 constitutional D68.0
 Willebrand-Jurgens D68.0
Thrombopenia — *see* Thrombocytopenia
Thrombophilia D68.59
 primary NEC D68.59
 secondary NEC D68.69
 specified NEC D68.69
Thrombophlebitis I80.9
 antepartum O22.2- ☑
  deep O22.3- ☑
  superficial O22.2- ☑
 calf muscular vein (NOS) I80.25- ☑
 cavernous (venous) sinus G08
  complicating pregnancy O22.5- ☑
  nonpyogenic I67.6
 cerebral (sinus) (vein) G08
  nonpyogenic I67.6
  sequelae G09
 due to implanted device — *see* Complications, by site and type, specified NEC
 during or resulting from a procedure NEC T81.72 ☑
 femoral vein (superficial) I80.1- ☑
 femoropopliteal vein I80.0- ☑
 gastrocnemial vein I80.25- ☑

☑ **Additional Character Required** — Refer to the Tabular List for Character Selection ▽ Subterms under main terms may continue to next column or page

Thrombophlebitis — *continued*
- hepatic (vein) I80.8
- idiopathic, recurrent I82.1
- iliac vein (common) (external) (internal) I80.21- ☑
- iliofemoral I80.1- ☑
- intracranial venous sinus (any) G08
  - nonpyogenic I67.6
  - sequelae G09
- intraspinal venous sinuses and veins G08
  - nonpyogenic G95.19
- lateral (venous) sinus G08
  - nonpyogenic I67.6
- leg I80.3
  - superficial I80.0- ☑
- longitudinal (venous) sinus G08
  - nonpyogenic I67.6
- lower extremity I80.299
- migrans, migrating I82.1
- pelvic
  - with ectopic or molar pregnancy O08.0
  - following ectopic or molar pregnancy O08.0
  - puerperal O87.1
- peroneal vein I80.24- ☑
- popliteal vein — *see* Phlebitis, leg, deep, popliteal
- portal (vein) K75.1
- postoperative T81.72 ☑
- pregnancy — *see* Thrombophlebitis, antepartum
- puerperal, postpartum, childbirth O87.0
  - deep O87.1
  - pelvic O87.1
  - septic O86.81
  - superficial O87.0
- saphenous (greater) (lesser) I80.0- ☑
- sinus (intracranial) G08
  - nonpyogenic I67.6
- soleal vein I80.25- ☑
- specified site NEC I80.8
- tibial vein (anterior) (posterior) I80.23- ☑

Thrombosis, thrombotic (bland) (multiple) (progressive) (silent) (vessel) I82.90
- anal K64.5
- antepartum — *see* Thrombophlebitis, antepartum
- aorta, aortic I74.10
  - abdominal I74.09
    - saddle I74.01
  - bifurcation I74.09
  - saddle I74.01
  - specified site NEC I74.19
  - terminal I74.09
  - thoracic I74.11
  - valve — *see* Endocarditis, aortic
- apoplexy I63.3- ☑
- artery, arteries (postinfectional) I74.9
  - auditory, internal — *see* Occlusion, artery, precerebral, specified NEC
  - basilar — *see* Occlusion, artery, basilar
  - carotid (common) (internal) — *see* Occlusion, artery, carotid
  - cerebellar (anterior inferior) (posterior inferior) (superior) — *see* Occlusion, artery, cerebellar
  - cerebral — *see* Occlusion, artery, cerebral
  - choroidal (anterior) — *see* Occlusion, artery, precerebral, specified NEC
  - communicating, posterior — *see* Occlusion, artery, precerebral, specified NEC
  - coronary — *see also* Infarct, myocardium
    - not resulting in infarction I24.0
  - hepatic I74.8
  - hypophyseal — *see* Occlusion, artery, precerebral, specified NEC
  - iliac I74.5
  - limb I74.4
    - lower I74.3
    - upper I74.2
  - meningeal, anterior or posterior — *see* Occlusion, artery, cerebral, specified NEC
  - mesenteric (with gangrene) — *see also* Infarct, intestine K55.069
  - ophthalmic — *see* Occlusion, artery, retina
  - pontine — *see* Occlusion, artery, precerebral, specified NEC
  - precerebral — *see* Occlusion, artery, precerebral
  - pulmonary (iatrogenic) — *see* Embolism, pulmonary
  - renal N28.0
  - retinal — *see* Occlusion, artery, retina
  - spinal, anterior or posterior G95.11
  - traumatic NEC T14.8 ☑
  - vertebral — *see* Occlusion, artery, vertebral

Thrombosis, thrombotic — *continued*
- atrium, auricular — *see also* Infarct, myocardium
  - following acute myocardial infarction (current complication) I23.6
  - not resulting in infarction I51.3
  - old I51.3
- basilar (artery) — *see* Occlusion, artery, basilar
- brain (artery) (stem) — *see also* Occlusion, artery, cerebral
  - due to syphilis A52.05
  - puerperal O99.43
  - sinus — *see* Thrombosis, intracranial venous sinus
- capillary I78.8
- cardiac — *see also* Infarct, myocardium
  - not resulting in infarction I51.3
  - old I51.3
  - valve — *see* Endocarditis
- carotid (artery) (common) (internal) — *see* Occlusion, artery, carotid
- cavernous (venous) sinus — *see* Thrombosis, intracranial venous sinus
- cerebellar artery (anterior inferior) (posterior inferior) (superior) I66.3
- cerebral (artery) — *see* Occlusion, artery, cerebral
- cerebrovenous sinus — *see also* Thrombosis, intracranial venous sinus
  - puerperium O87.3
- chronic I82.91
- coronary (artery) (vein) — *see also* Infarct, myocardium
  - not resulting in infarction I24.0
- corpus cavernosum N48.89
- cortical I66.9
- deep — *see* Embolism, vein, lower extremity
- due to device, implant or graft — *see also* Complications, by site and type, specified NEC T85.868 ☑
  - arterial graft NEC T82.868 ☑
  - breast (implant) T85.868 ☑
  - catheter NEC T85.868 ☑
    - dialysis (renal) T82.868 ☑
      - intraperitoneal T85.868 ☑
    - infusion NEC T82.868 ☑
      - spinal (epidural) (subdural) T85.860 ☑
    - urinary (indwelling) T83.86 ☑
  - electronic (electrode) (pulse generator) (stimulator)
    - bone T84.86 ☑
    - cardiac T82.867 ☑
    - nervous system (brain) (peripheral nerve) (spinal) T85.860 ☑
    - urinary T83.86 ☑
  - fixation, internal (orthopedic) NEC T84.86 ☑
  - gastrointestinal (bile duct) (esophagus) T85.868 ☑
  - genital NEC T83.86 ☑
  - heart T82.867 ☑
  - joint prosthesis T84.86 ☑
  - ocular (corneal graft) (orbital implant) NEC T85.868 ☑
  - orthopedic NEC T84.86 ☑
  - specified NEC T85.868 ☑
  - urinary NEC T83.86 ☑
  - vascular NEC T82.868 ☑
  - ventricular intracranial shunt T85.860 ☑
- during the puerperium — *see* Thrombosis, puerperal
- endocardial — *see also* Infarct, myocardium
  - not resulting in infarction I51.3
- eye — *see* Occlusion, retina
- genital organ
  - female NEC N94.89
    - pregnancy — *see* Thrombophlebitis, antepartum
  - male N50.1
- gestational — *see* Phlebopathy, gestational
- heart (chamber) — *see also* Infarct, myocardium
  - not resulting in infarction I51.3
  - old I51.3
- hepatic (vein) I82.0
  - artery I74.8
- history (of) Z86.718
- intestine (with gangrene) — *see also* Infarct, intestine K55.069
- intracardiac NEC (apical) (atrial) (auricular) (ventricular) (old) I51.3
- intracranial (arterial) I66.9
  - venous sinus (any) G08
    - nonpyogenic origin I67.6
    - puerperium O87.3
- intramural — *see also* Infarct, myocardium
  - not resulting in infarction I51.3
  - old I51.3

Thrombosis, thrombotic — *continued*
- intraspinal venous sinuses and veins G08
  - nonpyogenic G95.19
- kidney (artery) N28.0
- lateral (venous) sinus — *see* Thrombosis, intracranial venous sinus
- leg — *see* Thrombosis, vein, lower extremity
  - arterial I74.3
- liver (venous) I82.0
  - artery I74.8
  - portal vein I81
- longitudinal (venous) sinus — *see* Thrombosis, intracranial venous sinus
- lower limb — *see* Thrombosis, vein, lower extremity
- lung (iatrogenic) (postoperative) — *see* Embolism, pulmonary
- meninges (brain) (arterial) I66.8
- mesenteric (artery) (with gangrene) — *see also* Infarct, intestine K55.069
  - vein (inferior) (superior) K55.0- ☑
- mitral I34.8
- mural — *see also* Infarct, myocardium
  - due to syphilis A52.06
  - not resulting in infarction I51.3
  - old I51.3
- omentum (with gangrene) — *see also* Infarct, intestine K55.069
- ophthalmic — *see* Occlusion, retina
- pampiniform plexus (male) N50.1
- parietal — *see also* Infarct, myocardium
  - not resulting in infarction I24.0
- penis, superficial vein N48.81
- perianal venous K64.5
- peripheral arteries I74.4
  - upper I74.2
- personal history (of) Z86.718
- portal I81
  - due to syphilis A52.09
- precerebral artery — *see* Occlusion, artery, precerebral
- puerperal, postpartum O87.0
  - brain (artery) O99.43
    - venous (sinus) O87.3
  - cardiac O99.43
  - cerebral (artery) O99.43
    - venous (sinus) O87.3
  - superficial O87.0
- pulmonary (artery) (iatrogenic) (postoperative) (vein) — *see* Embolism, pulmonary
- renal (artery) N28.0
  - vein I82.3
- resulting from presence of device, implant or graft — *see* Complications, by site and type, specified NEC
- retina, retinal — *see* Occlusion, retina
- scrotum N50.1
- seminal vesicle N50.1
- sigmoid (venous) sinus — *see* Thrombosis, intracranial venous sinus
- sinus, intracranial (any) — *see* Thrombosis, intracranial venous sinus
- specified site NEC I82.890
  - chronic I82.891
- spermatic cord N50.1
- spinal cord (arterial) G95.11
  - due to syphilis A52.09
  - pyogenic origin G06.1
- spleen, splenic D73.5
  - artery I74.8
- testis N50.1
- traumatic NEC T14.8 ☑
- tricuspid I07.8
- tumor — *see* Neoplasm, unspecified behavior, by site
- tunica vaginalis N50.1
- umbilical cord (vessels), complicating delivery O69.5 ☑
- vas deferens N50.1
- vein (acute) I82.90
  - antecubital I82.61- ☑
    - chronic I82.71- ☑
  - axillary I82.A1- ☑ *(following I82.7)*
    - chronic I82.A2- ☑ *(following I82.7)*
  - basilic I82.61- ☑
    - chronic I82.71- ☑
  - brachial I82.62- ☑
    - chronic I82.72- ☑
  - brachiocephalic (innominate) I82.290
    - chronic I82.291
  - cephalic I82.61- ☑
    - chronic I82.71- ☑

▽ Subterms under main terms may continue to next column or page   ☑ **Additional Character Required** — Refer to the Tabular List for Character Selection   **315**

Thrombophlebitis — Thrombosis, thrombotic

Thrombosis, thrombotic — *continued*
  vein — *continued*
    cerebral, nonpyogenic I67.6
    chronic I82.91
    deep (DVT) I82.40- ☑
      calf I82.4Z- ☑
        chronic I82.5Z- ☑
      lower leg I82.4Z- ☑
        chronic I82.5Z- ☑
      thigh I82.4Y- ☑
        chronic I82.5Y- ☑
      upper leg I82.4Y- ☑
        chronic I82.5Y- ☑
    femoral I82.41- ☑
      chronic I82.51- ☑
    iliac (iliofemoral) I82.42- ☑
      chronic I82.52- ☑
    innominate I82.290
      chronic I82.291
    internal jugular I82.C1- ☑ (*following* I82.7)
      chronic I82.C2- ☑ (*following* I82.7)
    lower extremity
      deep I82.40- ☑
        chronic I82.50- ☑
        specified NEC I82.49- ☑
          chronic NEC I82.59- ☑
      distal
        deep I82.4Z- ☑
      proximal
        deep I82.4Y- ☑
          chronic I82.5Y- ☑
      superficial I82.81- ☑
    perianal K64.5
    popliteal I82.43- ☑
      chronic I82.53- ☑
    radial I82.62- ☑
      chronic I82.72- ☑
    renal I82.3
    saphenous (greater) (lesser) I82.81- ☑
    specified NEC I82.890
      chronic NEC I82.891
    subclavian I82.B1- ☑ (*following* I82.7)
      chronic I82.B2- ☑ (*following* I82.7)
    thoracic NEC I82.290
      chronic I82.291
    tibial I82.44- ☑
      chronic I82.54- ☑
    ulnar I82.62- ☑
      chronic I82.72- ☑
    upper extremity I82.60- ☑
      chronic I82.70- ☑
      deep I82.62- ☑
        chronic I82.72- ☑
      superficial I82.61- ☑
        chronic I82.71- ☑
  vena cava
    inferior I82.220
      chronic I82.221
    superior I82.210
      chronic I82.211
  venous, perianal K64.5
  ventricle — *see also* Infarct, myocardium
    following acute myocardial infarction (current complication) I23.6
    not resulting in infarction I24.0
    old I51.3
Thrombus — *see* Thrombosis
Thrush — *see also* Candidiasis
  newborn P37.5
  oral B37.0
  vaginal B37.3
Thumb — *see also* condition
  sucking (child problem) F98.8
Thymitis E32.8
Thymoma — *see also* Neoplasm, thymus, by type
  malignant C37
  metaplastic C37
  microscopic D15.0
  sclerosing C37
  type A C37
  type AB C37
  type B1 C37
  type B2 C37
  type B3 C37
Thymus, thymic (gland) — *see* condition
Thyrocele — *see* Goiter
Thyroglossal — *see also* condition

Thyroglossal — *continued*
  cyst Q89.2
  duct, persistent Q89.2
Thyroid (gland) (body) — *see also* condition
  hormone resistance E07.89
  lingual Q89.2
  nodule (cystic) (nontoxic) (single) E04.1
Thyroiditis E06.9
  acute (nonsuppurative) (pyogenic) (suppurative) E06.0
  autoimmune E06.3
  chronic (nonspecific) (sclerosing) E06.5
    with thyrotoxicosis, transient E06.2
    fibrous E06.5
    lymphadenoid E06.3
    lymphocytic E06.3
    lymphoid E06.3
  de Quervain's E06.1
  drug-induced E06.4
  fibrous (chronic) E06.5
  giant-cell (follicular) E06.1
  granulomatous (de Quervain) (subacute) E06.1
  Hashimoto's (struma lymphomatosa) E06.3
  iatrogenic E06.4
  ligneous E06.5
  lymphocytic (chronic) E06.3
  lymphoid E06.3
  lymphomatous E06.3
  nonsuppurative E06.1
  postpartum, puerperal O90.5
  pseudotuberculous E06.1
  pyogenic E06.0
  radiation E06.4
  Riedel's E06.5
  subacute (granulomatous) E06.1
  suppurative E06.0
  tuberculous A18.81
  viral E06.1
  woody E06.5
Thyrolingual duct, persistent Q89.2
Thyromegaly E01.0
Thyrotoxic
  crisis — *see* Thyrotoxicosis
  heart disease or failure — *see also* Thyrotoxicosis E05.90 [I43]
    with thyroid storm E05.91 [I43]
  storm — *see* Thyrotoxicosis
Thyrotoxicosis (recurrent) E05.90
  with
    goiter (diffuse) E05.00
      with thyroid storm E05.01
      adenomatous uninodular E05.10
        with thyroid storm E05.11
      multinodular E05.20
        with thyroid storm E05.21
      nodular E05.20
        with thyroid storm E05.21
      uninodular E05.10
        with thyroid storm E05.11
    infiltrative
      dermopathy E05.00
        with thyroid storm E05.01
      ophthalmopathy E05.00
        with thyroid storm E05.01
    single thyroid nodule E05.10
      with thyroid storm E05.11
    thyroid storm E05.91
  due to
    ectopic thyroid nodule or tissue E05.30
      with thyroid storm E05.31
    ingestion of (excessive) thyroid material E05.40
      with thyroid storm E05.41
    overproduction of thyroid-stimulating hormone E05.80
      with thyroid storm E05.81
    specified cause NEC E05.80
      with thyroid storm E05.81
  factitia E05.40
    with thyroid storm E05.41
  heart — *see also* Failure, heart, high-output E05.90 [I43]
    with thyroid storm — *see also* Failure, heart, high-output E05.91 [I43]
    failure — *see also* Failure, heart, high-output E05.90 [I43]
  neonatal (transient) P72.1
  transient with chronic thyroiditis E06.2
Tibia vara M92.51- ☑
Tic (disorder) F95.9
  breathing F95.8

Tic — *continued*
  child problem F95.0
  compulsive F95.1
  de la Tourette F95.2
  degenerative (generalized) (localized) G25.69
    facial G25.69
  disorder
    chronic
      motor F95.1
      vocal F95.1
    combined vocal and multiple motor F95.2
    transient F95.0
  douloureux G50.0
    atypical G50.1
    postherpetic, postzoster B02.22
  drug-induced G25.61
  eyelid F95.8
  habit F95.9
    chronic F95.1
    transient of childhood F95.0
  lid, transient of childhood F95.0
  motor-verbal F95.2
  occupational F48.8
  orbicularis F95.8
    transient of childhood F95.0
  organic origin G25.69
  postchoreic G25.69
  provisional F95.0
  psychogenic, compulsive F95.1
  salaam R25.8
  spasm (motor or vocal) F95.9
    chronic F95.1
    transient of childhood F95.0
  specified NEC F95.8
Tick-borne — *see* condition
Tietze's disease or syndrome M94.0
Tight, tightness
  anus K62.89
  chest R07.89
  fascia (lata) M62.89
  foreskin (congenital) N47.1
  hymen, hymenal ring N89.6
  introitus (acquired) (congenital) N89.6
  rectal sphincter K62.89
  tendon — *see* Short, tendon
  urethral sphincter N35.919
Tilting vertebra — *see* Dorsopathy, deforming, specified NEC
Timidity, child F93.8
Tinea (intersecta) (tarsi) B35.9
  amiantacea L44.8
  asbestina B35.0
  barbae B35.0
  beard B35.0
  black dot B35.0
  blanca B36.2
  capitis B35.0
  corporis B35.4
  cruris B35.6
  flava B36.0
  foot B35.3
  furfuracea B36.0
  imbricata (Tokelau) B35.5
  kerion B35.0
  manuum B35.2
  microsporic — *see* Dermatophytosis
  nigra B36.1
  nodosa — *see* Piedra
  pedis B35.3
  scalp B35.0
  specified NEC B35.8
  sycosis B35.0
  tonsurans B35.0
  trichophytic — *see* Dermatophytosis
  unguium B35.1
  versicolor B36.0
Tingling sensation (skin) R20.2
Tin-miner's lung J63.5
Tinnitus NOS H93.1- ☑
  audible H93.1- ☑
  aurium H93.1- ☑
  pulsatile H93.A- ☑
  subjective H93.1- ☑
Tipped tooth (teeth) M26.33
Tipping
  pelvis M95.5
    with disproportion (fetopelvic) O33.0
      causing obstructed labor O65.0

☑ Additional Character Required — Refer to the Tabular List for Character Selection   ▽ Subterms under main terms may continue to next column or page

Tipping — *continued*
  tooth (teeth), fully erupted M26.33
Tiredness R53.83
Tissue — *see* condition
Tobacco (nicotine)
  abuse — *see* Tobacco, use
  dependence — *see* Dependence, drug, nicotine
  harmful use Z72.0
  heart — *see* Tobacco, toxic effect
  maternal use, affecting newborn P04.2
  toxic effect — *see* Table of Drugs and Chemicals, by
      substance, poisoning
    chewing tobacco — *see* Table of Drugs and Chemi-
        cals, by substance, poisoning
    cigarettes — *see* Table of Drugs and Chemicals, by
        substance, poisoning
  use Z72.0
    complicating
      childbirth O99.334 ☑
      pregnancy O99.33- ☑
      puerperium O99.335
    counseling and surveillance Z71.6
    history Z87.891
  withdrawal state — *see also* Dependence, drug, nico-
      tine F17.203
Tocopherol deficiency E56.0
Todd's
  cirrhosis K74.3
  paralysis (postepileptic) (transitory) G83.84
Toe — *see* condition
Toilet, artificial opening — *see* Attention to, artificial,
    opening
Tokelau (ringworm) B35.5
Tollwut — *see* Rabies
Tommaselli's disease R31.9
  correct substance properly administered — *see* Table
      of Drugs and Chemicals, by drug, adverse effect
  overdose or wrong substance given or taken — *see*
      Table of Drugs and Chemicals, by drug, poisoning
Tongue — *see also* condition
  tie Q38.1
Tonic pupil — *see* Anomaly, pupil, function, tonic pupil
Toni-Fanconi syndrome (cystinosis) E72.09
  with cystinosis E72.04
Tonsil — *see* condition
Tonsillitis (acute) (catarrhal) (croupous) (follicular) (gan-
    grenous) (infective) (lacunar) (lingual) (malignant)
    (membranous) (parenchymatous) (phlegmonous)
    (pseudomembranous) (purulent) (septic) (subacute)
    (suppurative) (toxic) (ulcerative) (vesicular) (viral)
    J03.90
  chronic J35.01
    with adenoiditis J35.03
  diphtheritic A36.0
  hypertrophic J35.01
    with adenoiditis J35.03
  recurrent J03.91
  specified organism NEC J03.80
    recurrent J03.81
  staphylococcal J03.80
    recurrent J03.81
  streptococcal J03.00
    recurrent J03.01
  tuberculous A15.8
  Vincent's A69.1
Tooth, teeth — *see* condition
Toothache K08.89
Topagnosis R20.8
Tophi — *see* Gout, chronic
TORCH infection — *see* Infection, congenital
  without active infection P00.2
Torn — *see* Tear
Tornwaldt's cyst or disease J39.2
Torsion
  accessory tube — *see* Torsion, fallopian tube
  adnexa (female) — *see* Torsion, fallopian tube
  aorta, acquired I77.1
  appendix epididymis N44.04
  appendix testis N44.03
  bile duct (common) (hepatic) K83.8
    congenital Q44.5
  bowel, colon or intestine K56.2
  cervix — *see* Malposition, uterus
  cystic duct K82.8
  dystonia — *see* Dystonia, torsion
  epididymis (appendix) N44.04
  fallopian tube N83.52- ☑

Torsion — *continued*
  fallopian tube — *continued*
    with ovary N83.53
  gallbladder K82.8
    congenital Q44.1
  hydatid of Morgagni
    female N83.52- ☑
    male N44.03
  kidney (pedicle) (leading to infarction) N28.0
  Meckel's diverticulum (congenital) Q43.0
    malignant — *see* Table of Neoplasms, small intes-
        tine, malignant
  mesentery K56.2
  omentum K56.2
  organ or site, congenital NEC — *see* Anomaly, by site
  ovary (pedicle) N83.51- ☑
    with fallopian tube N83.53
    congenital Q50.2
  oviduct — *see* Torsion, fallopian tube
  penis (acquired) N48.82
    congenital Q55.63
  spasm — *see* Dystonia, torsion
  spermatic cord N44.02
    extravaginal N44.01
    intravaginal N44.02
  spleen D73.5
  testis, testicle N44.00
    appendix N44.03
  tibia — *see* Deformity, limb, specified type NEC, lower
      leg
  uterus — *see* Malposition, uterus
Torticollis (intermittent) (spastic) M43.6
  congenital (sternomastoid) Q68.0
    due to birth injury P15.8
  hysterical F44.4
  ocular R29.891
  psychogenic F45.8
    conversion reaction F44.4
  rheumatic M43.6
  rheumatoid M06.88
  spasmodic G24.3
  traumatic, current S13.4 ☑
Tortipelvis G24.1
Tortuous
  aortic arch Q25.46
  artery I77.1
  organ or site, congenital NEC — *see* Distortion
  retinal vessel, congenital Q14.1
  ureter N13.8
  urethra N36.8
  vein — *see* Varix
Torture, victim of Z65.4
Torula, torular (histolytica) (infection) — *see* Cryptococ-
    cosis
Torulosis — *see* Cryptococcosis
Torus (mandibularis) (palatinus) M27.0
  fracture — *see* Fracture, by site, torus
Touraine's syndrome Q79.8
Tourette's syndrome F95.2
Tourniquet syndrome — *see* Constriction, external, by
    site
Tower skull Q75.0
  with exophthalmos Q87.0
Toxemia R68.89
  bacterial — *see* Sepsis
  burn — *see* Burn
  eclamptic (with pre-existing hypertension) — *see*
      Eclampsia
  erysipelatous — *see* Erysipelas
  fatigue R68.89
  food — *see* Poisoning, food
  gastrointestinal K52.1
  intestinal K52.1
  kidney — *see* Uremia
  malarial — *see* Malaria
  myocardial — *see* Myocarditis, toxic
  of pregnancy — *see* Pre-eclampsia
  pre-eclamptic — *see* Pre-eclampsia
  small intestine K52.1
  staphylococcal, due to food A05.0
  stasis R68.89
  uremic — *see* Uremia
  urinary — *see* Uremia
Toxemica cerebropathia psychica (nonalcoholic) F04
  alcoholic — *see* Alcohol, amnestic disorder
Toxic (poisoning) — *see also* condition T65.91 ☑

Toxic — *continued*
  effect — *see* Table of Drugs and Chemicals, by sub-
      stance, poisoning
  shock syndrome A48.3
  thyroid (gland) — *see* Thyrotoxicosis
Toxicemia — *see* Toxemia
Toxicity — *see* Table of Drugs and Chemicals, by sub-
      stance, poisoning
  fava bean D55.0
  food, noxious — *see* Poisoning, food
  from drug or nonmedicinal substance — *see* Table of
      Drugs and Chemicals, by drug
Toxicosis — *see also* Toxemia
  capillary, hemorrhagic D69.0
Toxinfection, gastrointestinal K52.1
Toxocariasis B83.0
Toxoplasma, toxoplasmosis (acquired) B58.9
  with
    hepatitis B58.1
    meningoencephalitis B58.2
    ocular involvement B58.00
    other organ involvement B58.89
    pneumonia, pneumonitis B58.3
  congenital (acute) (subacute) (chronic) P37.1
  maternal, manifest toxoplasmosis in infant (acute)
      (subacute) (chronic) P37.1
tPA (rtPA) **administation in a different facility within
    the last 24 hours prior to admission to current
    facility** Z92.82
Trabeculation, bladder N32.89
Trachea — *see* condition
Tracheitis (catarrhal) (infantile) (membranous) (plastic)
    (septal) (suppurative) (viral) J04.10
  with
    bronchitis (15 years of age and above) J40
      acute or subacute — *see* Bronchitis, acute
      chronic J42
      tuberculous NEC A15.5
      under 15 years of age J20.9
    laryngitis (acute) J04.2
      chronic J37.1
      tuberculous NEC A15.5
  acute J04.10
    with obstruction J04.11
  chronic J42
    with
      bronchitis (chronic) J42
      laryngitis (chronic) J37.1
  diphtheritic (membranous) A36.89
  due to external agent — *see* Inflammation, respiratory,
      upper, due to
  syphilitic A52.73
  tuberculous A15.5
Trachelitis (nonvenereal) — *see* Cervicitis
Tracheobronchial — *see* condition
Tracheobronchitis (15 years of age and above) — *see
    also* Bronchitis
  due to
    Bordetella bronchiseptica A37.80
      with pneumonia A37.81
    Francisella tularensis A21.8
Tracheobronchomegaly Q32.4
  with bronchiectasis J47.9
    with
      exacerbation (acute) J47.1
      lower respiratory infection J47.0
  acquired J98.09
    with bronchiectasis J47.9
      with
        exacerbation (acute) J47.1
        lower respiratory infection J47.0
Tracheobronchopneumonitis — *see* Pneumonia,
    broncho-
Tracheocele (external) (internal) J39.8
  congenital Q32.1
Tracheomalacia J39.8
  congenital Q32.0
Tracheopharyngitis (acute) J06.9
  chronic J42
  due to external agent — *see* Inflammation, respiratory,
      upper, due to
Tracheostenosis J39.8
Tracheostomy
  complication — *see* Complication, tracheostomy
  status Z93.0
    attention to Z43.0
    malfunctioning J95.03
Trachoma, trachomatous A71.9

Trachoma, trachomatous — *continued*
- active (stage) A71.1
  - contraction of conjunctiva A71.1
- dubium A71.0
- healed or sequelae B94.0
- initial (stage) A71.0
- pannus A71.1
- Türck's J37.0

Traction, vitreomacular H43.82- ☑
Train sickness T75.3 ☑
Trait(s)
- Hb-S D57.3
- hemoglobin
  - abnormal NEC D58.2
    - with thalassemia D56.3
  - C — *see* Disease, hemoglobin C
  - S (Hb-S) D57.3
- Lepore D56.3
- personality, accentuated Z73.1
- sickle-cell D57.3
  - with elliptocytosis or spherocytosis D57.3
- type A personality Z73.1

Tramp Z59.00
Trance R41.89
- hysterical F44.89

Transaminasemia R74.01
Transection
- abdomen (partial) S38.3 ☑
- aorta (incomplete) — *see also* Injury, aorta
  - complete — *see* Injury, aorta, laceration, major
- carotid artery (incomplete) — *see also* Injury, blood vessel, carotid, laceration
  - complete — *see* Injury, blood vessel, carotid, laceration, major
- celiac artery (incomplete) S35.211 ☑
  - branch (incomplete) S35.291 ☑
    - complete S35.292 ☑
  - complete S35.212 ☑
- innominate
  - artery (incomplete) — *see also* Injury, blood vessel, thoracic, innominate, artery, laceration
    - complete — *see* Injury, blood vessel, thoracic, innominate, artery, laceration, major
  - vein (incomplete) — *see also* Injury, blood vessel, thoracic, innominate, vein, laceration
    - complete — *see* Injury, blood vessel, thoracic, innominate, vein, laceration, major
- jugular vein (external) (incomplete) — *see also* Injury, blood vessel, jugular vein, laceration
  - complete — *see* Injury, blood vessel, jugular vein, laceration, major
  - internal (incomplete) — *see also* Injury, blood vessel, jugular vein, internal, laceration
    - complete — *see* Injury, blood vessel, jugular vein, internal, laceration, major
- mesenteric artery (incomplete) — *see also* Injury, mesenteric, artery, laceration
  - complete — *see* Injury, mesenteric artery, laceration, major
- pulmonary vessel (incomplete) — *see also* Injury, blood vessel, thoracic, pulmonary, laceration
  - complete — *see* Injury, blood vessel, thoracic, pulmonary, laceration, major
- subclavian — *see* Transection, innominate
- vena cava (incomplete) — *see also* Injury, vena cava
  - complete — *see* Injury, vena cava, laceration, major
- vertebral artery (incomplete) — *see also* Injury, blood vessel, vertebral, laceration
  - complete — *see* Injury, blood vessel, vertebral, laceration, major

Transfusion
- associated (red blood cell) hemochromatosis E83.111
- blood
  - ABO incompatible — *see* Complication(s), transfusion, incompatibility reaction, ABO
  - minor blood group (Duffy) (E) (K) (Kell) (Kidd) (Lewis) (M) (N) (P) (S) T80.89 ☑
  - reaction or complication — *see* Complications, transfusion
- fetomaternal (mother) — *see* Pregnancy, complicated by, placenta, transfusion syndrome
- maternofetal (mother) — *see* Pregnancy, complicated by, placenta, transfusion syndrome
- placental (syndrome) (mother) — *see* Pregnancy, complicated by, placenta, transfusion syndrome
- reaction (adverse) — *see* Complications, transfusion
- related acute lung injury (TRALI) J95.84

Transfusion — *continued*
- twin-to-twin — *see* Pregnancy, complicated by, placenta, transfusion syndrome, fetus to fetus

Transient (meaning homeless) — *see also* condition Z59.00
Translocation
- balanced autosomal Q95.9
  - in normal individual Q95.0
- chromosomes NEC Q99.8
  - balanced and insertion in normal individual Q95.0
- Down syndrome Q90.2
- trisomy
  - 13 Q91.6
  - 18 Q91.2
  - 21 Q90.2

Translucency, iris — *see* Degeneration, iris
Transmission of chemical substances through the placenta — *see* Absorption, chemical, through placenta
Transparency, lung, unilateral J43.0
Transplant (ed) (status) Z94.9
- awaiting organ Z76.82
- bone Z94.6
  - marrow Z94.81
- candidate Z76.82
- complication — *see* Complication, transplant
- cornea Z94.7
- heart Z94.1
  - and lung(s) Z94.3
  - valve Z95.2
    - prosthetic Z95.2
    - specified NEC Z95.4
    - xenogenic Z95.3
- intestine Z94.82
- kidney Z94.0
- liver Z94.4
- lung(s) Z94.2
  - and heart Z94.3
- organ (failure) (infection) (rejection) Z94.9
  - removal status Z98.85
- pancreas Z94.83
- skin Z94.5
- social Z60.3
- specified organ or tissue NEC Z94.89
- stem cells Z94.84
- tissue Z94.9

Transplants, ovarian, endometrial N80.1
Transposed — *see* Transposition
Transposition (congenital) — *see also* Malposition, congenital
- abdominal viscera Q89.3
- aorta (dextra) Q20.3
- appendix Q43.8
- colon Q43.8
- corrected Q20.5
- great vessels (complete) (partial) Q20.3
- heart Q24.0
  - with complete transposition of viscera Q89.3
- intestine (large) (small) Q43.8
- reversed jejunal (for bypass) (status) Z98.0
- scrotum Q55.23
- stomach Q40.2
  - with general transposition of viscera Q89.3
- tooth, teeth, fully erupted M26.30
- vessels, great (complete) (partial) Q20.3
- viscera (abdominal) (thoracic) Q89.3

Transsexualism F64.0
Transverse — *see also* condition
- arrest (deep), in labor O64.0 ☑
- lie (mother) O32.2 ☑
  - causing obstructed labor O64.8 ☑

Transvestism, transvestitism (dual-role) F64.1
- fetishistic F65.1

Trapped placenta (with hemorrhage) O72.0
- without hemorrhage O73.0

TRAPS (tumor necrosis factor receptor associated periodic syndrome) M04.1
Trauma, traumatism — *see also* Injury
- acoustic — *see* subcategory H83.3 ☑
- birth — *see* Birth, injury
- complicating ectopic or molar pregnancy O08.6
- during delivery O71.9
- following ectopic or molar pregnancy O08.6
- obstetric O71.9
  - specified NEC O71.89
- occlusal
  - primary K08.81
  - secondary K08.82

Traumatic — *see also* condition
- brain injury S06.9 ☑

Treacher Collins syndrome Q75.4
Treitz's hernia — *see* Hernia, abdomen, specified site NEC
Trematode infestation — *see* Infestation, fluke
Trematodiasis — *see* Infestation, fluke
Trembling paralysis — *see* Parkinsonism
Tremor(s) R25.1
- drug induced G25.1
- essential (benign) G25.0
- familial G25.0
- hereditary G25.0
- hysterical F44.4
- intention G25.2
- medication induced postural G25.1
- mercurial — *see* subcategory T56.1 ☑
- Parkinson's — *see* Parkinsonism
- psychogenic (conversion reaction) F44.4
- senilis R54
- specified type NEC G25.2

Trench
- fever A79.0
- foot — *see* Immersion, foot
- mouth A69.1

Treponema pallidum infection — *see* Syphilis
Treponematosis
- due to
  - T. pallidum — *see* Syphilis
  - T. pertenue — *see* Yaws

Triad
- Hutchinson's (congenital syphilis) A50.53
- Kartagener's Q89.3
- Saint's — *see* Hernia, diaphragm

Trichiasis (eyelid) H02.059
- with entropion — *see* Entropion
- left H02.056
  - lower H02.055
  - upper H02.054
- right H02.053
  - lower H02.052
  - upper H02.051

Trichinella spiralis (infection) (infestation) B75
Trichinellosis, trichiniasis, trichinelliasis, trichinosis B75
- with muscle disorder B75 *[M63.80]*
  - ankle B75 *[M63.87-]* ☑
  - foot B75 *[M63.87-]* ☑
  - forearm B75 *[M63.83-]* ☑
  - hand B75 *[M63.84-]* ☑
  - lower leg B75 *[M63.86-]* ☑
  - multiple sites B75 *[M63.89]*
  - pelvic region B75 *[M63.85-]* ☑
  - shoulder region B75 *[M63.81-]* ☑
  - specified site NEC B75 *[M63.88]*
  - thigh B75 *[M63.85-]* ☑
  - upper arm B75 *[M63.82-]* ☑

Trichobezoar T18.9 ☑
- intestine T18.3 ☑
- stomach T18.2 ☑

Trichocephaliasis, trichocephalosis B79
Trichocephalus infestation B79
Trichoclasis L67.8
Trichoepithelioma — *see also* Neoplasm, skin, benign
- malignant — *see* Neoplasm, skin, malignant

Trichofolliculoma — *see* Neoplasm, skin, benign
Tricholemmoma — *see* Neoplasm, skin, benign
Trichomoniasis A59.9
- bladder A59.03
- cervix A59.09
- intestinal A07.8
- prostate A59.02
- seminal vesicles A59.09
- specified site NEC A59.8
- urethra A59.03
- urogenitalis A59.00
- vagina A59.01
- vulva A59.01

Trichomycosis
- axillaris A48.8
- nodosa, nodularis B36.8

Trichonodosis L67.8
Trichophytid, trichophyton infection — *see* Dermatophytosis
Trichophytobezoar T18.9 ☑
- intestine T18.3 ☑
- stomach T18.2 ☑

  ☑ **Additional Character Required — Refer to the Tabular List for Character Selection**   ▽ **Subterms under main terms may continue to next column or page**

Trichophytosis — *see* Dermatophytosis
Trichoptilosis L67.8
Trichorrhexis (nodosa) (invaginata) L67.0
Trichosis axillaris A48.8
Trichosporosis nodosa B36.2
Trichostasis spinulosa (congenital) Q84.1
Trichostrongyliasis, trichostrongylosis (small intestine) B81.2
Trichostrongylus infection B81.2
Trichotillomania F63.3
Trichromat, trichromatopsia, anomalous (congenital) H53.55
Trichuriasis B79
Trichuris trichiura (infection) (infestation) (any site) B79
Tricuspid (valve) — *see* condition
Trifid — *see also* Accessory
  kidney (pelvis) Q63.8
  tongue Q38.3
Trigeminal neuralgia — *see* Neuralgia, trigeminal
Trigeminy R00.8
Trigger finger (acquired) M65.30
  congenital Q74.0
  index finger M65.32- ☑
  little finger M65.35- ☑
  middle finger M65.33- ☑
  ring finger M65.34- ☑
  thumb M65.31- ☑
Trigonitis (bladder) (chronic) (pseudomembranous) N30.30
  with hematuria N30.31
Trigonocephaly Q75.0
Trilocular heart — *see* Cor triloculare
Trimethylaminuria E72.52
Tripartite placenta O43.19- ☑
Triphalangeal thumb Q74.0
Triple — *see also* Accessory
  kidneys Q63.0
  uteri Q51.818
  X, female Q97.0
Triple I O41.12- ☑
Triplegia G83.89
  congenital G80.8
Triplet (newborn) — *see also* Newborn, triplet
  complicating pregnancy — *see* Pregnancy, triplet
Triplication — *see* Accessory
Triploidy Q92.7
Trismus R25.2
  neonatorum A33
  newborn A33
Trisomy (syndrome) Q92.9
  13 (partial) Q91.7
    meiotic nondisjunction Q91.4
    mitotic nondisjunction Q91.5
    mosaicism Q91.5
    translocation Q91.6
  18 (partial) Q91.3
    meiotic nondisjunction Q91.0
    mitotic nondisjunction Q91.1
    mosaicism Q91.1
    translocation Q91.2
  20 Q92.8
  21 (partial) Q90.9
    meiotic nondisjunction Q90.0
    mitotic nondisjunction Q90.1
    mosaicism Q90.1
    translocation Q90.2
  22 Q92.8
  autosomes Q92.9
  chromosome specified NEC Q92.8
    partial Q92.2
      due to unbalanced translocation Q92.5
    specified NEC Q92.8
    whole (nonsex chromosome)
      meiotic nondisjunction Q92.0
      mitotic nondisjunction Q92.1
      mosaicism Q92.1
  due to
    dicentrics — *see* Extra, marker chromosomes
    extra rings — *see* Extra, marker chromosomes
    isochromosomes — *see* Extra, marker chromosomes
  specified NEC Q92.8
  whole chromosome Q92.9
    meiotic nondisjunction Q92.0
    mitotic nondisjunction Q92.1
    mosaicism Q92.1
    partial Q92.9
    specified NEC Q92.8

Tritanomaly, tritanopia H53.55
Trombiculosis, trombiculiasis, trombidiosis B88.0
Trophedema (congenital) (hereditary) Q82.0
Trophoblastic disease — *see also* Mole, hydatidiform O01.9
Tropholymphedema Q82.0
Trophoneurosis NEC G96.89
  disseminated M34.9
Tropical — *see* condition
Trouble — *see also* Disease
  heart — *see* Disease, heart
  kidney — *see* Disease, renal
  nervous R45.0
  sinus — *see* Sinusitis
Trousseau's syndrome (thrombophlebitis migrans) I82.1
Truancy, childhood
  from school Z72.810
Truncus
  arteriosus (persistent) Q20.0
  communis Q20.0
Trunk — *see* condition
Trypanosomiasis
  African B56.9
    by Trypanosoma brucei
      gambiense B56.0
      rhodesiense B56.1
  American — *see* Chagas' disease
  Brazilian — *see* Chagas' disease
  by Trypanosoma
    brucei gambiense B56.0
    brucei rhodesiense B56.1
    cruzi — *see* Chagas' disease
  gambiensis, Gambian B56.0
  rhodesiensis, Rhodesian B56.1
  South American — *see* Chagas' disease
  where
    African trypanosomiasis is prevalent B56.9
    Chagas' disease is prevalent B57.2
Tryptasemia, hereditary alpha D89.44
T-shaped incisors K00.2
Tsutsugamushi (disease) (fever) A75.3
Tube, tubal, tubular — *see* condition
Tubercle — *see also* Tuberculosis
  brain, solitary A17.81
  Darwin's Q17.8
  Ghon, primary infection A15.7
Tuberculid, tuberculide (indurating, subcutaneous) (lichenoid) (miliary) (papulonecrotic) (primary) (skin) A18.4
Tuberculoma — *see also* Tuberculosis
  brain A17.81
  meninges (cerebral) (spinal) A17.1
  spinal cord A17.81
Tuberculosis, tubercular, tuberculous (calcification) (calcified) (caseous) (chromogenic acid-fast bacilli) (degeneration) (fibrocaseous) (fistula) (interstitial) (isolated circumscribed lesions) (necrosis) (parenchymatous) (ulcerative) A15.9
  with pneumoconiosis (any condition in J60-J64) J65
  abdomen (lymph gland) A18.39
  abscess (respiratory) A15.9
    bone A18.03
      hip A18.02
      knee A18.02
      sacrum A18.01
      specified site NEC A18.03
      spinal A18.01
      vertebra A18.01
    brain A17.81
    breast A18.89
    Cowper's gland A18.15
    dura (mater) (cerebral) (spinal) A17.81
    epidural (cerebral) (spinal) A17.81
    female pelvis A18.17
    frontal sinus A15.8
    genital organs NEC A18.10
    genitourinary A18.10
    gland (lymphatic) — *see* Tuberculosis, lymph gland
    hip A18.02
    intestine A18.32
    ischiorectal A18.32
    joint NEC A18.02
      hip A18.02
      knee A18.02
      specified NEC A18.02
      vertebral A18.01
    kidney A18.11
    knee A18.02

Tuberculosis, tubercular, tuberculous — *continued*
  abscess — *continued*
    latent Z22.7
    lumbar (spine) A18.01
    lung — *see* Tuberculosis, pulmonary
    meninges (cerebral) (spinal) A17.0
    muscle A18.09
    perianal (fistula) A18.32
    perinephritic A18.11
    perirectal A18.32
    rectum A18.32
    retropharyngeal A15.8
    sacrum A18.01
    scrofulous A18.2
    scrotum A18.15
    skin (primary) A18.4
    spinal cord A17.81
    spine or vertebra (column) A18.01
    subdiaphragmatic A18.31
    testis A18.15
    urinary A18.13
    uterus A18.17
  accessory sinus — *see* Tuberculosis, sinus
  Addison's disease A18.7
  adenitis — *see* Tuberculosis, lymph gland
  adenoids A15.8
  adenopathy — *see* Tuberculosis, lymph gland
  adherent pericardium A18.84
  adnexa (uteri) A18.17
  adrenal (capsule) (gland) A18.7
  alimentary canal A18.32
  anemia A18.89
  ankle (joint) (bone) A18.02
  anus A18.32
  apex, apical — *see* Tuberculosis, pulmonary
  appendicitis, appendix A18.32
  arachnoid A17.0
  artery, arteritis A18.89
    cerebral A18.89
  arthritis (chronic) (synovial) A18.02
    spine or vertebra (column) A18.01
  articular — *see* Tuberculosis, joint
  ascites A18.31
  asthma — *see* Tuberculosis, pulmonary
  axilla, axillary (gland) A18.2
  bladder A18.12
  bone A18.03
    hip A18.02
    knee A18.02
    limb NEC A18.03
    sacrum A18.01
    spine or vertebral column A18.01
  bowel (miliary) A18.32
  brain A17.81
  breast A18.89
  broad ligament A18.17
  bronchi, bronchial, bronchus A15.5
    ectasia, ectasis (bronchiectasis) — *see* Tuberculosis, pulmonary
    fistula A15.5
      primary (progressive) A15.7
    gland or node A15.4
      primary (progressive) A15.7
    lymph gland or node A15.4
      primary (progressive) A15.7
  bronchiectasis — *see* Tuberculosis, pulmonary
  bronchitis A15.5
  bronchopleural A15.6
  bronchopneumonia, bronchopneumonic — *see* Tuberculosis, pulmonary
  bronchorrhagia A15.5
  bronchotracheal A15.5
  bronze disease A18.7
  buccal cavity A18.83
  bulbourethral gland A18.15
  bursa A18.09
  cachexia A15.9
  cardiomyopathy A18.84
  caries — *see* Tuberculosis, bone
  cartilage A18.02
    intervertebral A18.01
  catarrhal — *see* Tuberculosis, respiratory
  cecum A18.32
  cellulitis (primary) A18.4
  cerebellum A17.81
  cerebral, cerebrum A17.81
  cerebrospinal A17.81
    meninges A17.0

Tuberculosis, tubercular, tuberculous — *continued*
- cervical (lymph gland or node) A18.2
- cervicitis, cervix (uteri) A18.16
- chest — *see* Tuberculosis, respiratory
- chorioretinitis A18.53
- choroid, choroiditis A18.53
- ciliary body A18.54
- colitis A18.32
- collier's J65
- colliquativa (primary) A18.4
- colon A18.32
- complex, primary A15.7
- congenital P37.0
- conjunctiva A18.59
- connective tissue (systemic) A18.89
- contact Z20.1
- cornea (ulcer) A18.52
- Cowper's gland A18.15
- coxae A18.02
- coxalgia A18.02
- cul-de-sac of Douglas A18.17
- curvature, spine A18.01
- cutis (colliquativa) (primary) A18.4
- cyst, ovary A18.18
- cystitis A18.12
- dactylitis A18.03
- diarrhea A18.32
- diffuse — *see* Tuberculosis, miliary
- digestive tract A18.32
- disseminated — *see* Tuberculosis, miliary
- duodenum A18.32
- dura (mater) (cerebral) (spinal) A17.0
  - abscess (cerebral) (spinal) A17.81
- dysentery A18.32
- ear (inner) (middle) A18.6
  - bone A18.03
  - external (primary) A18.4
  - skin (primary) A18.4
- elbow A18.02
- emphysema — *see* Tuberculosis, pulmonary
- empyema A15.6
- encephalitis A17.82
- endarteritis A18.89
- endocarditis A18.84
  - aortic A18.84
  - mitral A18.84
  - pulmonary A18.84
  - tricuspid A18.84
- endocrine glands NEC A18.82
- endometrium A18.17
- enteric, enterica, enteritis A18.32
- enterocolitis A18.32
- epididymis, epididymitis A18.15
- epidural abscess (cerebral) (spinal) A17.81
- epiglottis A15.5
- episcleritis A18.51
- erythema (induratum) (nodosum) (primary) A18.4
- esophagus A18.83
- eustachian tube A18.6
- exposure (to) Z20.1
- exudative — *see* Tuberculosis, pulmonary
- eye A18.50
- eyelid (primary) (lupus) A18.4
- fallopian tube (acute) (chronic) A18.17
- fascia A18.09
- fauces A15.8
- female pelvic inflammatory disease A18.17
- finger A18.03
- first infection A15.7
- gallbladder A18.83
- ganglion A18.09
- gastritis A18.83
- gastrocolic fistula A18.32
- gastroenteritis A18.32
- gastrointestinal tract A18.32
- general, generalized — *see* Tuberculosis, miliary
- genital organs A18.10
- genitourinary A18.10
- genu A18.02
- glandula suprarenalis A18.7
- glandular, general A18.2
- glottis A15.5
- grinder's J65
- gum A18.83
- hand A18.03
- heart A18.84
- hematogenous — *see* Tuberculosis, miliary
- hemoptysis — *see* Tuberculosis, pulmonary

Tuberculosis, tubercular, tuberculous — *continued*
- hemorrhage NEC — *see* Tuberculosis, pulmonary
- hemothorax A15.6
- hepatitis A18.83
- hilar lymph nodes A15.4
  - primary (progressive) A15.7
- hip (joint) (disease) (bone) A18.02
- hydropneumothorax A15.6
- hydrothorax A15.6
- hypoadrenalism A18.7
- hypopharynx A15.8
- ileocecal (hyperplastic) A18.32
- ileocolitis A18.32
- ileum A18.32
- iliac spine (superior) A18.03
- immunological findings only A15.7
- indurativa (primary) A18.4
- infantile A15.7
- infection A15.9
  - without clinical manifestations A15.7
- infraclavicular gland A18.2
- inguinal gland A18.2
- inguinalis A18.2
- intestine (any part) A18.32
- iridocyclitis A18.54
- iris, iritis A18.54
- ischiorectal A18.32
- jaw A18.03
- jejunum A18.32
- joint A18.02
  - vertebral A18.01
- keratitis (interstitial) A18.52
- keratoconjunctivitis A18.52
- kidney A18.11
- knee (joint) A18.02
- kyphosis, kyphoscoliosis A18.01
- laryngitis A15.5
- larynx A15.5
- latent Z22.7
- leptomeninges, leptomeningitis (cerebral) (spinal) A17.0
- lichenoides (primary) A18.4
- linguae A18.83
- lip A18.83
- liver A18.83
- lordosis A18.01
- lung — *see* Tuberculosis, pulmonary
- lupus vulgaris A18.4
- lymph gland or node (peripheral) A18.2
  - abdomen A18.39
  - bronchial A15.4
    - primary (progressive) A15.7
  - cervical A18.2
  - hilar A15.4
    - primary (progressive) A15.7
  - intrathoracic A15.4
    - primary (progressive) A15.7
  - mediastinal A15.4
    - primary (progressive) A15.7
  - mesenteric A18.39
  - retroperitoneal A18.39
  - tracheobronchial A15.4
    - primary (progressive) A15.7
- lymphadenitis — *see* Tuberculosis, lymph gland
- lymphangitis — *see* Tuberculosis, lymph gland
- lymphatic (gland) (vessel) — *see* Tuberculosis, lymph gland
- mammary gland A18.89
- marasmus A15.9
- mastoiditis A18.03
- mediastinal lymph gland or node A15.4
  - primary (progressive) A15.7
- mediastinitis A15.8
  - primary (progressive) A15.7
- mediastinum A15.8
  - primary (progressive) A15.7
- medulla A17.81
- melanosis, Addisonian A18.7
- meninges, meningitis (basilar) (cerebral) (cerebrospinal) (spinal) A17.0
- meningoencephalitis A17.82
- mesentery, mesenteric (gland or node) A18.39
- miliary A19.9
  - acute A19.2
    - multiple sites A19.1
    - single specified site A19.0
  - chronic A19.8
  - specified NEC A19.8
- millstone makers' J65

Tuberculosis, tubercular, tuberculous — *continued*
- miner's J65
- molder's J65
- mouth A18.83
- multiple A19.9
  - acute A19.1
  - chronic A19.8
- muscle A18.09
- myelitis A17.82
- myocardium, myocarditis A18.84
- nasal (passage) (sinus) A15.8
- nasopharynx A15.8
- neck gland A18.2
- nephritis A18.11
- nerve (mononeuropathy) A17.83
- nervous system A17.9
- nose (septum) A15.8
- ocular A18.50
- omentum A18.31
- oophoritis (acute) (chronic) A18.17
- optic (nerve trunk) (papilla) A18.59
- orbit A18.59
- orchitis A18.15
- organ, specified NEC A18.89
- osseous — *see* Tuberculosis, bone
- osteitis — *see* Tuberculosis, bone
- osteomyelitis — *see* Tuberculosis, bone
- otitis media A18.6
- ovary, ovaritis (acute) (chronic) A18.17
- oviduct (acute) (chronic) A18.17
- pachymeningitis A17.0
- palate (soft) A18.83
- pancreas A18.83
- papulonecrotic (a) (primary) A18.4
- parathyroid glands A18.82
- paronychia (primary) A18.4
- parotid gland or region A18.83
- pelvis (bony) A18.03
- penis A18.15
- peribronchitis A15.5
- pericardium, pericarditis A18.84
- perichondritis, larynx A15.5
- periostitis — *see* Tuberculosis, bone
- perirectal fistula A18.32
- peritoneum NEC A18.31
- peritonitis A18.31
- pharynx, pharyngitis A15.8
- phlyctenulosis (keratoconjunctivitis) A18.52
- phthisis NEC — *see* Tuberculosis, pulmonary
- pituitary gland A18.82
- pleura, pleural, pleurisy, pleuritis (fibrinous) (obliterative) (purulent) (simple plastic) (with effusion) A15.6
  - primary (progressive) A15.7
- pneumonia, pneumonic — *see* Tuberculosis, pulmonary
- pneumothorax (spontaneous) (tense valvular) — *see* Tuberculosis, pulmonary
- polyneuropathy A17.89
- polyserositis A19.9
  - acute A19.1
  - chronic A19.8
- potter's J65
- prepuce A18.15
- primary (complex) A15.7
- proctitis A18.32
- prostate, prostatitis A18.14
- pulmonalis — *see* Tuberculosis, pulmonary
- pulmonary (cavitated) (fibrotic) (infiltrative) (nodular) A15.0
  - childhood type or first infection A15.7
  - primary (complex) A15.7
- pyelitis A18.11
- pyelonephritis A18.11
- pyemia — *see* Tuberculosis, miliary
- pyonephrosis A18.11
- pyopneumothorax A15.6
- pyothorax A15.6
- rectum (fistula) (with abscess) A18.32
- reinfection stage — *see* Tuberculosis, pulmonary
- renal A18.11
- renis A18.11
- respiratory A15.9
  - primary A15.7
  - specified NEC A15.8
- retina, retinitis A18.53
- retroperitoneal (lymph gland or node) A18.39
- rheumatism NEC A18.09

☑ **Additional Character Required** — Refer to the Tabular List for Character Selection   ▽ **Subterms under main terms may continue to next column or page**

Tuberculosis, tubercular, tuberculous — continued
  rhinitis A15.8
  sacroiliac (joint) A18.01
  sacrum A18.01
  salivary gland A18.83
  salpingitis (acute) (chronic) A18.17
  sandblaster's J65
  sclera A18.51
  scoliosis A18.01
  scrofulous A18.2
  scrotum A18.15
  seminal tract or vesicle A18.15
  senile A15.9
  septic — see Tuberculosis, miliary
  shoulder (joint) A18.02
    blade A18.03
  sigmoid A18.32
  sinus (any nasal) A15.8
    bone A18.03
    epididymis A18.15
  skeletal NEC A18.03
  skin (any site) (primary) A18.4
  small intestine A18.32
  soft palate A18.83
  spermatic cord A18.15
  spine, spinal (column) A18.01
    cord A17.81
    medulla A17.81
    membrane A17.0
    meninges A17.0
  spleen, splenitis A18.85
  spondylitis A18.01
  sternoclavicular joint A18.02
  stomach A18.83
  stonemason's J65
  subcutaneous tissue (cellular) (primary) A18.4
  subcutis (primary) A18.4
  subdeltoid bursa A18.83
  submaxillary (region) A18.83
  supraclavicular gland A18.2
  suprarenal (capsule) (gland) A18.7
  swelling, joint (see also category M01) — see also Tuberculosis, joint A18.02
  symphysis pubis A18.02
  synovitis A18.09
    articular A18.02
    spine or vertebra A18.01
  systemic — see Tuberculosis, miliary
  tarsitis A18.4
  tendon (sheath) — see Tuberculosis, tenosynovitis
  tenosynovitis A18.09
    spine or vertebra A18.01
  testis A18.15
  throat A15.8
  thymus gland A18.82
  thyroid gland A18.81
  tongue A18.83
  tonsil, tonsillitis A15.8
  trachea, tracheal A15.5
    lymph gland or node A15.4
      primary (progressive) A15.7
  tracheobronchial A15.5
    lymph gland or node A15.4
      primary (progressive) A15.7
  tubal (acute) (chronic) A18.17
  tunica vaginalis A18.15
  ulcer (skin) (primary) A18.4
    bowel or intestine A18.32
    specified NEC — see Tuberculosis, by site
  unspecified site A15.9
  ureter A18.11
  urethra, urethral (gland) A18.13
  urinary organ or tract A18.13
  uterus A18.17
  uveal tract A18.54
  uvula A18.83
  vagina A18.18
  vas deferens A18.15
  verruca, verrucosa (cutis) (primary) A18.4
  vertebra (column) A18.01
  vesiculitis A18.15
  vulva A18.18
  wrist (joint) A18.02
Tuberculum
  Carabelli — see Excludes Note at K00.2
  occlusal — see Excludes Note at K00.2
  paramolare K00.2
Tuberosity, enitre maxillary M26.07

Tuberous sclerosis (brain) Q85.1
Tubo-ovarian — see condition
Tuboplasty, after previous sterilization Z31.0
  aftercare Z31.42
Tubotympanitis, catarrhal (chronic) — see Otitis, media, nonsuppurative, chronic, serous
Tularemia A21.9
  with
    conjunctivitis A21.1
    pneumonia A21.2
  abdominal A21.3
  bronchopneumonic A21.2
  conjunctivitis A21.1
  cryptogenic A21.3
  enteric A21.3
  gastrointestinal A21.3
  generalized A21.7
  ingestion A21.3
  intestinal A21.3
  oculoglandular A21.1
  ophthalmic A21.1
  pneumonia (any), pneumonic A21.2
  pulmonary A21.2
  sepsis A21.7
  specified NEC A21.8
  typhoidal A21.7
  ulceroglandular A21.0
Tularensis conjunctivitis A21.1
Tumefaction — see also Swelling
  liver — see Hypertrophy, liver
Tumor — see also Neoplasm, unspecified behavior, by site
  acinar cell — see Neoplasm, uncertain behavior, by site
  acinic cell — see Neoplasm, uncertain behavior, by site
  adenocarcinoid — see Neoplasm, malignant, by site
  adenomatoid — see also Neoplasm, benign, by site
    odontogenic — see Cyst, calcifying odontogenic
  adnexal (skin) — see Neoplasm, skin, benign, by site
  adrenal
    cortical (benign) D35.0- ☑
      malignant C74.0- ☑
    rest — see Neoplasm, benign, by site
  alpha-cell
    malignant
      pancreas C25.4
      specified site NEC — see Neoplasm, malignant, by site
      unspecified site C25.4
    pancreas D13.7
    specified site NEC — see Neoplasm, benign, by site
    unspecified site D13.7
  aneurysmal — see Aneurysm
  aortic body D44.7
    malignant C75.5
  Askin's — see Neoplasm, connective tissue, malignant
  basal cell — see also Neoplasm, skin, uncertain behavior D48.5
  Bednar — see Neoplasm, skin, malignant
  benign (unclassified) — see Neoplasm, benign, by site
  beta-cell
    malignant
      pancreas C25.4
      specified site NEC — see Neoplasm, malignant, by site
      unspecified site C25.4
    pancreas D13.7
    specified site NEC — see Neoplasm, benign, by site
    unspecified site D13.7
  Brenner D27.9
    borderline malignancy D39.1- ☑
    malignant C56- ☑
    proliferating D39.1- ☑
  bronchial alveolar, intravascular D38.1
  Brooke's — see Neoplasm, skin, benign
  brown fat — see Lipoma
  Burkitt — see Lymphoma, Burkitt
  calcifying epithelial odontogenic — see Cyst, calcifying odontogenic
  carcinoid D3A.00 (following D36)
    benign D3A.00 (following D36)
      appendix D3A.020 (following D36)
      ascending colon D3A.022 (following D36)
      bronchus (lung) D3A.090 (following D36)
      cecum D3A.021 (following D36)
      colon D3A.029 (following D36)
      descending colon D3A.024 (following D36)
      duodenum D3A.010 (following D36)
      foregut NOS D3A.094 (following D36)

Tumor — continued
  carcinoid — continued
    benign — continued
      hindgut NOS D3A.096 (following D36)
      ileum D3A.012 (following D36)
      jejunum D3A.011 (following D36)
      kidney D3A.093 (following D36)
      large intestine D3A.029 (following D36)
      lung (bronchus) D3A.090 (following D36)
      midgut NOS D3A.095 (following D36)
      rectum D3A.026 (following D36)
      sigmoid colon D3A.025 (following D36)
      small intestine D3A.019 (following D36)
      specified NEC D3A.098 (following D36)
      stomach D3A.092 (following D36)
      thymus D3A.091 (following D36)
      transverse colon D3A.023 (following D36)
    malignant C7A.00 (following C75)
      appendix C7A.020 (following C75)
      ascending colon C7A.022 (following C75)
      bronchus (lung) C7A.090 (following C75)
      cecum C7A.021 (following C75)
      colon C7A.029 (following C75)
      descending colon C7A.024 (following C75)
      duodenum C7A.010 (following C75)
      foregut NOS C7A.094 (following C75)
      hindgut NOS C7A.096 (following C75)
      ileum C7A.012 (following C75)
      jejunum C7A.011 (following C75)
      kidney C7A.093 (following C75)
      large intestine C7A.029 (following C75)
      lung (bronchus) C7A.090 (following C75)
      midgut NOS C7A.095 (following C75)
      rectum C7A.026 (following C75)
      sigmoid colon C7A.025 (following C75)
      small intestine C7A.019 (following C75)
      specified NEC C7A.098 (following C75)
      stomach C7A.092 (following C75)
      thymus C7A.091 (following C75)
      transverse colon C7A.023 (following C75)
    mesentery metastasis C7B.04 (following C75)
    secondary C7B.00 (following C75)
      bone C7B.03 (following C75)
      distant lymph nodes C7B.01 (following C75)
      liver C7B.02 (following C75)
      peritoneum C7B.04 (following C75)
      specified NEC C7B.09 (following C75)
  carotid body D44.6
    malignant C75.4
  cells — see also Neoplasm, unspecified behavior, by site
    benign — see Neoplasm, benign, by site
    malignant — see Neoplasm, malignant, by site
    uncertain whether benign or malignant — see Neoplasm, uncertain behavior, by site
  cervix, in pregnancy or childbirth — see Pregnancy, complicated by, tumor, cervix
  chondromatous giant cell — see Neoplasm, bone, benign
  chromaffin — see also Neoplasm, benign, by site
    malignant — see Neoplasm, malignant, by site
  Cock's peculiar L72.3
  Codman's — see Neoplasm, bone, benign
  dentigerous, mixed — see Cyst, calcifying odontogenic
  dermoid — see Neoplasm, benign, by site
    with malignant transformation C56- ☑
  desmoid (extra-abdominal) — see also Neoplasm, connective tissue, uncertain behavior
    abdominal — see Neoplasm, connective tissue, uncertain behavior
  embolus — see Neoplasm, secondary, by site
  embryonal (mixed) — see also Neoplasm, uncertain behavior, by site
    liver C22.7
  endodermal sinus
    specified site — see Neoplasm, malignant, by site
    unspecified site
      female C56.- ☑
      male C62.90
  epithelial
    benign — see Neoplasm, benign, by site
    malignant — see Neoplasm, malignant, by site
  Ewing's — see Neoplasm, bone, malignant, by site
  fatty — see Lipoma
  fibroid — see Leiomyoma
  G cell
    malignant
      pancreas C25.4

Tumor — *continued*
  G cell — *continued*
    malignant — *continued*
      specified site NEC — *see* Neoplasm, malignant, by site
      unspecified site C25.4
    specified site — *see* Neoplasm, uncertain behavior, by site
    unspecified site D37.8
  germ cell — *see also* Neoplasm, malignant, by site
    mixed — *see* Neoplasm, malignant, by site
  ghost cell, odontogenic — *see* Cyst, calcifying odontogenic
  giant cell — *see also* Neoplasm, uncertain behavior, by site
    bone D48.0
      malignant — *see* Neoplasm, bone, malignant
    chondromatous — *see* Neoplasm, bone, benign
    malignant — *see* Neoplasm, malignant, by site
    soft parts — *see* Neoplasm, connective tissue, uncertain behavior
      malignant — *see* Neoplasm, connective tissue, malignant
  glomus D18.00
    intra-abdominal D18.03
    intracranial D18.02
    jugulare D44.7
      malignant C75.5
    skin D18.01
    specified site NEC D18.09
  gonadal stromal — *see* Neoplasm, uncertain behavior, by site
  granular cell — *see also* Neoplasm, connective tissue, benign
    malignant — *see* Neoplasm, connective tissue, malignant
  granulosa cell D39.1- ☑
    juvenile D39.1- ☑
    malignant C56- ☑
  granulosa cell-theca cell D39.1- ☑
    malignant C56- ☑
  Grawitz's C64- ☑
  hemorrhoidal — *see* Hemorrhoids
  hilar cell D27- ☑
  hilus cell D27- ☑
  Hurthle cell (benign) D34
    malignant C73
  hydatid — *see* Echinococcus
  hypernephroid — *see also* Neoplasm, uncertain behavior, by site
  interstitial cell — *see also* Neoplasm, uncertain behavior, by site
    benign — *see* Neoplasm, benign, by site
    malignant — *see* Neoplasm, malignant, by site
  intravascular bronchial alveolar D38.1
  islet cell — *see* Neoplasm, benign, by site
    malignant — *see* Neoplasm, malignant, by site
      pancreas C25.4
      specified site NEC — *see* Neoplasm, malignant, by site
      unspecified site C25.4
    pancreas D13.7
    specified site NEC — *see* Neoplasm, benign, by site
    unspecified site D13.7
  juxtaglomerular D41.0- ☑
  Klatskin's C22.1
  Krukenberg's C79.6- ☑
  Leydig cell — *see* Neoplasm, uncertain behavior, by site
    benign — *see* Neoplasm, benign, by site
      specified site — *see* Neoplasm, benign, by site
      unspecified site
        female D27.9
        male D29.20
    malignant — *see* Neoplasm, malignant, by site
      specified site — *see* Neoplasm, malignant, by site
      unspecified site
        female C56.9
        male C62.90
    specified site — *see* Neoplasm, uncertain behavior, by site
    unspecified site
      female D39.10
      male D40.10
  lipid cell, ovary D27- ☑
  lipoid cell, ovary D27- ☑

Tumor — *continued*
  malignant — *see also* Neoplasm, malignant, by site C80.1
    fusiform cell (type) C80.1
    giant cell (type) C80.1
    localized, plasma cell — *see* Plasmacytoma, solitary
    mixed NEC C80.1
    small cell (type) C80.1
    spindle cell (type) C80.1
    unclassified C80.1
  mast cell D47.09
  melanotic, neuroectodermal — *see* Neoplasm, benign, by site
  Merkel cell — *see* Carcinoma, Merkel cell
  mesenchymal
    malignant — *see* Neoplasm, connective tissue, malignant
    mixed — *see* Neoplasm, connective tissue, uncertain behavior
  mesodermal, mixed — *see also* Neoplasm, malignant, by site
    liver C22.4
  mesonephric — *see also* Neoplasm, uncertain behavior, by site
    malignant — *see* Neoplasm, malignant, by site
  metastatic
    from specified site — *see* Neoplasm, malignant, by site
    of specified site — *see* Neoplasm, malignant, by site
    to specified site — *see* Neoplasm, secondary, by site
  mixed NEC — *see also* Neoplasm, benign, by site
    malignant — *see* Neoplasm, malignant, by site
  mucinous of low malignant potential
    specified site — *see* Neoplasm, malignant, by site
    unspecified site C56.9
  mucocarcinoid
    specified site — *see* Neoplasm, malignant, by site
    unspecified site C18.1
  mucoepidermoid — *see* Neoplasm, uncertain behavior, by site
  Müllerian, mixed
    specified site — *see* Neoplasm, malignant, by site
    unspecified site C54.9
  myoepithelial — *see* Neoplasm, benign, by site
  neuroectodermal (peripheral) — *see* Neoplasm, malignant, by site
    primitive
      specified site — *see* Neoplasm, malignant, by site
      unspecified site C71.9
  neuroendocrine D3A.8 (*following* D36)
    malignant poorly differentiated C7A.1 (*following* C75)
    secondary NEC C7B.8 (*following* C75)
    specified NEC C7A.8 (*following* C75)
  neurogenic olfactory C30.0
  nonencapsulated sclerosing C73
  odontogenic (adenomatoid) (benign) (calcifying epithelial) (keratocystic) (squamous) — *see* Cyst, calcifying odontogenic
    malignant C41.1
      upper jaw (bone) C41.0
  ovarian stromal D39.1- ☑
  ovary, in pregnancy — *see* Pregnancy, complicated by
  pacinian — *see* Neoplasm, skin, benign
  Pancoast's — *see* Pancoast's syndrome
  papillary — *see also* Papilloma
    cystic D37.9
    mucinous of low malignant potential C56- ☑
      specified site — *see* Neoplasm, malignant, by site
      unspecified site C56.9
    serous of low malignant potential
      specified site — *see* Neoplasm, malignant, by site
      unspecified site C56.9
  pelvic, in pregnancy or childbirth — *see* Pregnancy, complicated by
  phantom F45.8
  phyllodes D48.6- ☑
    benign D24- ☑
    malignant — *see* Neoplasm, breast, malignant
  Pindborg — *see* Cyst, calcifying odontogenic
  placental site trophoblastic D39.2
  plasma cell (malignant) (localized) — *see* Plasmacytoma, solitary
  polyvesicular vitelline
    specified site — *see* Neoplasm, malignant, by site

Tumor — *continued*
  polyvesicular vitelline — *continued*
    unspecified site
      female C56.9
      male C62.90
  Pott's puffy — *see* Osteomyelitis, specified NEC
  Rathke's pouch D44.3
  retinal anlage — *see* Neoplasm, benign, by site
  salivary gland type, mixed — *see* Neoplasm, salivary gland, benign
    malignant — *see* Neoplasm, salivary gland, malignant
  Sampson's N80.1
  Schmincke's — *see* Neoplasm, nasopharynx, malignant
  sclerosing stromal D27- ☑
  sebaceous — *see* Cyst, sebaceous
  secondary — *see* Neoplasm, secondary, by site
    carcinoid C7B.00 (*following* C75)
      bone C7B.03 (*following* C75)
      distant lymph nodes C7B.01 (*following* C75)
      liver C7B.02 (*following* C75)
      peritoneum C7B.04 (*following* C75)
      specified NEC C7B.09 (*following* C75)
    neuroendocrine NEC C7B.8 (*following* C75)
  serous of low malignant potential
    specified site — *see* Neoplasm, malignant, by site
    unspecified site C56.9
  Sertoli cell — *see* Neoplasm, benign, by site
    with lipid storage
      specified site — *see* Neoplasm, benign, by site
      unspecified site
        female D27.9
        male D29.20
    specified site — *see* Neoplasm, benign, by site
    unspecified site
      female D27.9
      male D29.20
  Sertoli-Leydig cell — *see* Neoplasm, benign, by site
    specified site — *see* Neoplasm, benign, by site
    unspecified site
      female D27.9
      male D29.20
  sex cord (-stromal) — *see* Neoplasm, uncertain behavior, by site
    with annular tubules D39.1- ☑
  skin appendage — *see* Neoplasm, skin, benign
  smooth muscle — *see* Neoplasm, connective tissue, uncertain behavior
  soft tissue
    benign — *see* Neoplasm, connective tissue, benign
    malignant — *see* Neoplasm, connective tissue, malignant
  sternomastoid (congenital) Q68.0
  stromal
    endometrial D39.0
    gastric D48.1
      benign D21.4
      malignant C16.9
      uncertain behavior D48.1
    gastrointestinal C49.A- ☑
      benign D21.4
      esophagus C49.A1
      malignant C49.A0
        colon C49.A4
        duodenum C49.A3
        esophagus C49.A1
        ileum C49.A3
        jejunum C49.A3
        large intestine C49.A4
        Meckel diverticulum C49.A3
        omentum C49.A9
        peritoneum C49.A9
        rectum C49.A5
        small intestine C49.A3
        specified site NEC C49.A9
        stomach C49.A2
      rectum C49.A5
      small intestine C49.A3
      specified site NEC C49.A9
      stomach C49.A2
      uncertain behavior D48.1
    intestine
      benign D21.4
      malignant
        large C49.A4
        small C49.A3
      uncertain behavior D48.1
    ovarian D39.1- ☑

☑ Additional Character Required — Refer to the Tabular List for Character Selection   ▽ Subterms under main terms may continue to next column or page

Tumor — *continued*
  stromal — *continued*
    stomach C49.A2
      benign D21.4
      malignant C49.A2
      uncertain behavior D48.1
    sweat gland — *see also* Neoplasm, skin, uncertain behavior
      benign — *see* Neoplasm, skin, benign
      malignant — *see* Neoplasm, skin, malignant
  syphilitic, brain A52.17
  testicular D40.10
  testicular stromal D40.1- ☑
  theca cell D27.- ☑
  theca cell-granulosa cell D39.1- ☑
  Triton, malignant — *see* Neoplasm, nerve, malignant
  trophoblastic, placental site D39.2
  turban D23.4
  uterus (body), in pregnancy or childbirth — *see* Pregnancy, complicated by, tumor, uterus
  vagina, in pregnancy or childbirth — *see* Pregnancy, complicated by
  varicose — *see* Varix
  von Recklinghausen's — *see* Neurofibromatosis
  vulva or perineum, in pregnancy or childbirth — *see* Pregnancy, complicated by
    causing obstructed labor O65.5
  Warthin's — *see* Neoplasm, salivary gland, benign
  Wilms' C64- ☑
  yolk sac — *see* Neoplasm, malignant, by site
    specified site — *see* Neoplasm, malignant, by site
    unspecified site
      female C56.9
      male C62.90
Tumor lysis syndrome (following antineoplastic chemotherapy) (spontaneous) NEC E88.3
Tumorlet — *see* Neoplasm, uncertain behavior, by site
Tungiasis B88.1
Tunica vasculosa lentis Q12.2
Turban tumor D23.4
Türck's trachoma J37.0
Turner-Kieser syndrome Q87.2
Turner-like syndrome Q87.19
Turner's
  hypoplasia (tooth) K00.4
  syndrome Q96.9
    specified NEC Q96.8
  tooth K00.4
Turner-Ullrich syndrome Q96.9
Tussis convulsiva — *see* Whooping cough
Twiddler's syndrome (due to)
  automatic implantable defibrillator T82.198
  cardiac pacemaker T82.198 ☑
Twilight state
  epileptic F05
  psychogenic F44.89
Twin (newborn) — *see also* Newborn, twin
  conjoined Q89.4
  pregnancy — *see* Pregnancy, twin
Twinning, teeth K00.2
Twist, twisted
  bowel, colon or intestine K56.2
  hair (congenital) Q84.1
  mesentery K56.2
  omentum K56.2
  organ or site, congenital NEC — *see* Anomaly, by site
  ovarian pedicle — *see* Torsion, ovary
Twitching R25.3
Tylosis (acquired) L84
  buccalis K13.29
  linguae K13.29
  palmaris et plantaris (congenital) (inherited) Q82.8
    acquired L85.1
Tympanism R14.0
Tympanites (abdominal) (intestinal) R14.0
Tympanitis — *see* Myringitis
Tympanosclerosis H74.0 ☑
Tympanum — *see* condition
Tympany
  abdomen R14.0
  chest R09.89
Type A behavior pattern Z73.1
Typhlitis — *see* Appendicitis
Typhoenteritis — *see* Typhoid
Typhoid (abortive) (ambulant) (any site) (clinical) (fever) (hemorrhagic) (infection) (intermittent) (malignant) (rheumatic) (Widal negative) A01.00

Typhoid — *continued*
  with pneumonia A01.03
  abdominal A01.09
  arthritis A01.04
  carrier (suspected) of Z22.0
  cholecystitis (current) A01.09
  endocarditis A01.02
  heart involvement A01.02
  inoculation reaction — *see* Complications, vaccination
  meningitis A01.01
  mesenteric lymph nodes A01.09
  myocarditis A01.02
  osteomyelitis A01.05
  perichondritis, larynx A01.09
  pneumonia A01.03
  specified NEC A01.09
  spine A01.05
  ulcer (perforating) A01.09
Typhomalaria (fever) — *see* Malaria
Typhomania A01.00
Typhoperitonitis A01.09
Typhus (fever) A75.9
  abdominal, abdominalis — *see* Typhoid
  African tick A77.1
  amarillic A95.9
  brain A75.9 *[G94]*
  cerebral A75.9 *[G94]*
  classical A75.0
  due to Rickettsia
    prowazekii A75.0
      recrudescent A75.1
    tsutsugamushi A75.3
    typhi A75.2
  endemic (flea-borne) A75.2
  epidemic (louse-borne) A75.0
  exanthematicus SAI A75.0
    brillii SAI A75.1
    mexicanus SAI A75.2
    typhus murinus A75.2
  exanthematic NEC A75.0
  flea-borne A75.2
  India tick A77.1
  Kenya (tick) A77.1
  louse-borne A75.0
  Mexican A75.2
  mite-borne A75.3
  murine A75.2
  North Asian tick-borne A77.2
  Orientia Tsutsugamushi (scrub typhus) A75.3
  petechial A75.9
  Queensland tick A77.3
  rat A75.2
  recrudescent A75.1
  recurrens — *see* Fever, relapsing
  Sao Paulo A77.0
  scrub (China) (India) (Malaysia) (New Guinea) A75.3
  shop (of Malaysia) A75.2
  Siberian tick A77.2
  tick-borne A77.9
  tropical (mite-borne) A75.3
Tyrosinemia E70.21
  newborn, transitory P74.5
Tyrosinosis E70.21
Tyrosinuria E70.29

U

Uhl's anomaly or disease Q24.8
Ulcer, ulcerated, ulcerating, ulceration, ulcerative
  alveolar process M27.3
  amebic (intestine) A06.1
    skin A06.7
  anastomotic — *see* Ulcer, gastrojejunal
  anorectal K62.6
  antral — *see* Ulcer, stomach
  anus (sphincter) (solitary) K62.6
  aorta — *see* Aneurysm
  aphthous (oral) (recurrent) K12.0
    genital organ(s)
      female N76.6
      male N50.89
  artery I77.2
  atrophic — *see* Ulcer, skin
    decubitus — *see* Ulcer, pressure, by site
  back L98.429
    with
      bone involvement without evidence of necrosis L98.426

Ulcer, ulcerated, ulcerating, ulceration, ulcerative — *continued*
  back — *continued*
    with — *continued*
      bone necrosis L98.424
      exposed fat layer L98.422
      muscle involvement without evidence of necrosis L98.425
      muscle necrosis L98.423
      skin breakdown only L98.421
      specified severity NEC L98.428
  Barrett's (esophagus) K22.10
    with bleeding K22.11
  bile duct (common) (hepatic) K83.8
  bladder (solitary) (sphincter) NEC N32.89
    bilharzial B65.9 *[N33]*
    in schistosomiasis (bilharzial) B65.9 *[N33]*
    submucosal — *see* Cystitis, interstitial
    tuberculous A18.12
  bleeding K27.4
  bone — *see* Osteomyelitis, specified type NEC
  bowel — *see* Ulcer, intestine
  breast N61.1
  bronchus J98.09
  buccal (cavity) (traumatic) K12.1
  Buruli A31.1
  buttock L98.419
    with
      bone involvement without evidence of necrosis L98.416
      bone necrosis L98.414
      exposed fat layer L98.412
      muscle involvement without evidence of necrosis L98.415
      muscle necrosis L98.413
      skin breakdown only L98.411
      specified severity NEC L98.418
  cancerous — *see* Neoplasm, malignant, by site
  cardia K22.10
    with bleeding K22.11
  cardioesophageal (peptic) K22.10
    with bleeding K22.11
  cecum — *see* Ulcer, intestine
  cervix (uteri) (decubitus) (trophic) N86
    with cervicitis N72
  chancroidal A57
  chiclero B55.1
  chronic (cause unknown) — *see* Ulcer, skin
  Cochin-China B55.1
  colon — *see* Ulcer, intestine
  conjunctiva H10.89
  cornea H16.00- ☑
    with hypopyon H16.03- ☑
    central H16.01- ☑
    dendritic (herpes simplex) B00.52
    marginal H16.04- ☑
    Mooren's H16.05- ☑
    mycotic H16.06- ☑
    perforated H16.07- ☑
    ring H16.02- ☑
    tuberculous (phlyctenular) A18.52
  corpus cavernosum (chronic) N48.5
  crural — *see* Ulcer, lower limb
  Curling's — *see* Ulcer, peptic, acute
  Cushing's — *see* Ulcer, peptic, acute
  cystic duct K82.8
  cystitis (interstitial) — *see* Cystitis, interstitial
  decubitus — *see* Ulcer, pressure, by site
  dendritic, cornea (herpes simplex) B00.52
  diabetes, diabetic — *see* Diabetes, ulcer
  Dieulafoy's K25.0
  due to
    infection NEC — *see* Ulcer, skin
    radiation NEC L59.8
    trophic disturbance (any region) — *see* Ulcer, skin
    X-ray L58.1
  duodenum, duodenal (eroded) (peptic) K26.9
    with
      hemorrhage K26.4
        and perforation K26.6
      perforation K26.5
      acute K26.3
        with
          hemorrhage K26.0
            and perforation K26.2
          perforation K26.1
      chronic K26.7

Ulcer, ulcerated, ulcerating, ulceration, ulcerative
— *continued*
- duodenum, duodenal — *continued*
  - chronic — *continued*
    - with
      - hemorrhage K26.4
        - and perforation K26.6
      - perforation K26.5
  - dysenteric A09
  - elusive — *see* Cystitis, interstitial
  - endocarditis (acute) (chronic) (subacute) I28.8
  - epiglottis J38.7
  - esophagus (peptic) K22.10
    - with bleeding K22.11
    - due to
      - aspirin K22.10
        - with bleeding K22.11
      - gastrointestinal reflux disease (without bleeding) K21.00
        - with bleeding K21.01
      - ingestion of chemical or medicament K22.10
        - with bleeding K22.11
    - fungal K22.10
      - with bleeding K22.11
    - infective K22.10
      - with bleeding K22.11
    - varicose — *see* Varix, esophagus
  - eyelid (region) H01.8
  - fauces J39.2
  - Fenwick (-Hunner) (solitary) — *see* Cystitis, interstitial
  - fistulous — *see* Ulcer, skin
  - foot (indolent) (trophic) — *see* Ulcer, lower limb
  - frambesial, initial A66.0
  - frenum (tongue) K14.0
  - gallbladder or duct K82.8
  - gangrenous — *see* Gangrene
  - gastric — *see* Ulcer, stomach
  - gastrocolic — *see* Ulcer, gastrojejunal
  - gastroduodenal — *see* Ulcer, peptic
  - gastroesophageal — *see* Ulcer, stomach
  - gastrointestinal — *see* Ulcer, gastrojejunal
  - gastrojejunal (peptic) K28.9
    - with
      - hemorrhage K28.4
        - and perforation K28.6
      - perforation K28.5
    - acute K28.3
      - with
        - hemorrhage K28.0
          - and perforation K28.2
        - perforation K28.1
    - chronic K28.7
      - with
        - hemorrhage K28.4
          - and perforation K28.6
        - perforation K28.5
  - gastrojejunocolic — *see* Ulcer, gastrojejunal
  - gingiva K06.8
  - gingivitis K05.10
    - nonplaque induced K05.11
    - plaque induced K05.10
  - glottis J38.7
  - granuloma of pudenda A58
  - gum K06.8
  - gumma, due to yaws A66.4
  - heel — *see* Ulcer, lower limb
  - hemorrhoid — *see also* Hemorrhoids, by degree K64.8
  - Hunner's — *see* Cystitis, interstitial
  - hypopharynx J39.2
  - hypopyon (chronic) (subacute) — *see* Ulcer, cornea, with hypopyon
  - hypostaticum — *see* Ulcer, varicose
  - ileum — *see* Ulcer, intestine
  - intestine, intestinal K63.3
    - with perforation K63.1
    - amebic A06.1
    - duodenal — *see* Ulcer, duodenum
    - granulocytopenic (with hemorrhage) — *see* Neutropenia
    - marginal — *see* Ulcer, gastrojejunal
    - perforating K63.1
      - newborn P78.0
    - primary, small intestine K63.3
  - rectum K62.6
  - stercoraceous, stercoral K63.3
  - tuberculous A18.32
  - typhoid (fever) — *see* Typhoid
  - varicose I86.8

Ulcer, ulcerated, ulcerating, ulceration, ulcerative
— *continued*
- jejunum, jejunal — *see* Ulcer, gastrojejunal
- keratitis — *see* Ulcer, cornea
- knee — *see* Ulcer, lower limb
- labium (majus) (minus) N76.6
- laryngitis — *see* Laryngitis
- larynx (aphthous) (contact) J38.7
  - diphtheritic A36.2
- leg — *see* Ulcer, lower limb
- lip K13.0
- Lipschütz's N76.6
- lower limb (atrophic) (chronic) (neurogenic) (perforating) (pyogenic) (trophic) (tropical) L97.909
  - with
    - bone involvement without evidence of necrosis L97.906
    - bone necrosis L97.904
    - exposed fat layer L97.902
    - muscle involvement without evidence of necrosis L97.905
    - muscle necrosis L97.903
    - skin breakdown only L97.901
    - specified severity NEC L97.908
  - ankle L97.309
    - with
      - bone involvement without evidence of necrosis L97.306
      - bone necrosis L97.304
      - exposed fat layer L97.302
      - muscle involvement without evidence of necrosis L97.305
      - muscle necrosis L97.303
      - skin breakdown only L97.301
      - specified severity NEC L97.308
    - left L97.329
      - with
        - bone involvement without evidence of necrosis L97.326
        - bone necrosis L97.324
        - exposed fat layer L97.322
        - muscle involvement without evidence of necrosis L97.325
        - muscle necrosis L97.323
        - skin breakdown only L97.321
        - specified severity NEC L97.328
    - right L97.319
      - with
        - bone involvement without evidence of necrosis L97.316
        - bone necrosis L97.314
        - exposed fat layer L97.312
        - muscle involvement without evidence of necrosis L97.315
        - muscle necrosis L97.313
        - skin breakdown only L97.311
        - specified severity NEC L97.318
  - calf L97.209
    - with
      - bone involvement without evidence of necrosis L97.206
      - bone necrosis L97.204
      - exposed fat layer L97.202
      - muscle involvement without evidence of necrosis L97.205
      - muscle necrosis L97.203
      - skin breakdown only L97.201
      - specified severity NEC L97.208
    - left L97.229
      - with
        - bone involvement without evidence of necrosis L97.226
        - bone necrosis L97.224
        - exposed fat layer L97.222
        - muscle involvement without evidence of necrosis L97.225
        - muscle necrosis L97.223
        - skin breakdown only L97.221
        - specified severity NEC L97.228
    - right L97.219
      - with
        - bone involvement without evidence of necrosis L97.216
        - bone necrosis L97.214
        - exposed fat layer L97.212
        - muscle involvement without evidence of necrosis L97.215
        - muscle necrosis L97.213
        - skin breakdown only L97.211

Ulcer, ulcerated, ulcerating, ulceration, ulcerative
— *continued*
- lower limb — *continued*
  - calf — *continued*
    - right — *continued*
      - with — *continued*
        - specified severity NEC L97.218
    - decubitus — *see* Ulcer, pressure, by site
    - foot specified NEC L97.509
      - with
        - bone involvement without evidence of necrosis L97.506
        - bone necrosis L97.504
        - exposed fat layer L97.502
        - muscle involvement without evidence of necrosis L97.505
        - muscle necrosis L97.503
        - skin breakdown only L97.501
        - specified severity NEC L97.508
      - left L97.529
        - with
          - bone involvement without evidence of necrosis L97.526
          - bone necrosis L97.524
          - exposed fat layer L97.522
          - muscle involvement without evidence of necrosis L97.525
          - muscle necrosis L97.523
          - skin breakdown only L97.521
          - specified severity NEC L97.528
      - right L97.519
        - with
          - bone involvement without evidence of necrosis L97.516
          - bone necrosis L97.514
          - exposed fat layer L97.512
          - muscle involvement without evidence of necrosis L97.515
          - muscle necrosis L97.513
          - skin breakdown only L97.511
          - specified severity NEC L97.518
    - heel L97.409
      - with
        - bone involvement without evidence of necrosis L97.406
        - bone necrosis L97.404
        - exposed fat layer L97.402
        - muscle involvement without evidence of necrosis L97.405
        - muscle necrosis L97.403
        - skin breakdown only L97.401
        - specified severity NEC L97.408
      - left L97.429
        - with
          - bone involvement without evidence of necrosis L97.426
          - bone necrosis L97.424
          - exposed fat layer L97.422
          - muscle involvement without evidence of necrosis L97.425
          - muscle necrosis L97.423
          - skin breakdown only L97.421
          - specified severity NEC L97.428
      - right L97.419
        - with
          - bone involvement without evidence of necrosis L97.416
          - bone necrosis L97.414
          - exposed fat layer L97.412
          - muscle involvement without evidence of necrosis L97.415
          - muscle necrosis L97.413
          - skin breakdown only L97.411
          - specified severity NEC L97.418
    - left L97.929
      - with
        - bone involvement without evidence of necrosis L97.926
        - bone necrosis L97.924
        - exposed fat layer L97.922
        - muscle involvement without evidence of necrosis L97.925
        - muscle necrosis L97.923
        - skin breakdown only L97.921
        - specified severity NEC L97.928
    - leprous A30.1
    - lower leg NOS L97.909

☑ **Additional Character Required** — Refer to the Tabular List for Character Selection   ▽ Subterms under main terms may continue to next column or page

Ulcer, ulcerated, ulcerating, ulceration, ulcerative	Ulcer, ulcerated, ulcerating, ulceration, ulcerative	Ulcer, ulcerated, ulcerating, ulceration, ulcerative

— continued
lower limb — continued
  lower leg — continued
    with
      bone involvement without evidence of
        necrosis L97.906
      bone necrosis L97.904
      exposed fat layer L97.902
      muscle involvement without evidence of
        necrosis L97.905
      muscle necrosis L97.903
      skin breakdown only L97.901
      specified severity NEC L97.908
    left L97.929
      with
        bone involvement without evidence of
          necrosis L97.926
        bone necrosis L97.924
        exposed fat layer L97.922
        muscle involvement without evidence of
          necrosis L97.925
        muscle necrosis L97.923
        skin breakdown only L97.921
        specified severity NEC L97.928
    right L97.919
      with
        bone involvement without evidence of
          necrosis L97.916
        bone necrosis L97.914
        exposed fat layer L97.912
        muscle involvement without evidence of
          necrosis L97.915
        muscle necrosis L97.913
        skin breakdown only L97.911
        specified severity NEC L97.918
  specified site NEC L97.809
    with
      bone involvement without evidence of
        necrosis L97.806
      bone necrosis L97.804
      exposed fat layer L97.802
      muscle involvement without evidence of
        necrosis L97.805
      muscle necrosis L97.803
      skin breakdown only L97.801
      specified severity NEC L97.808
    left L97.829
      with
        bone involvement without evidence
          of necrosis L97.826
        bone necrosis L97.824
        exposed fat layer L97.822
        muscle involvement without evidence
          of necrosis L97.825
        muscle necrosis L97.823
        skin breakdown only L97.821
        specified severity NEC L97.828
    right L97.819
      with
        bone involvement without evidence
          of necrosis L97.816
        bone necrosis L97.814
        exposed fat layer L97.812
        muscle involvement without evidence
          of necrosis L97.815
        muscle necrosis L97.813
        skin breakdown only L97.811
        specified severity NEC L97.818
  midfoot L97.409
    with
      bone involvement without evidence of
        necrosis L97.406
      bone necrosis L97.404
      exposed fat layer L97.402
      muscle involvement without evidence of
        necrosis L97.405
      muscle necrosis L97.403
      skin breakdown only L97.401
      specified severity NEC L97.408
    left L97.429
      with
        bone involvement without evidence of
          necrosis L97.426
        bone necrosis L97.424
        exposed fat layer L97.422
        muscle involvement without evidence of
          necrosis L97.425
        muscle necrosis L97.423

— continued
lower limb — continued
  midfoot — continued
    left — continued
      with — continued
        skin breakdown only L97.421
        specified severity NEC L97.428
    right L97.419
      with
        bone involvement without evidence of
          necrosis L97.416
        bone necrosis L97.414
        exposed fat layer L97.412
        muscle involvement without evidence of
          necrosis L97.415
        muscle necrosis L97.413
        skin breakdown only L97.411
        specified severity NEC L97.418
  right L97.919
    with
      bone involvement without evidence of
        necrosis L97.916
      bone necrosis L97.914
      exposed fat layer L97.912
      muscle involvement without evidence of
        necrosis L97.915
      muscle necrosis L97.913
      skin breakdown only L97.911
      specified severity NEC L97.918
syphilitic A52.19
thigh L97.109
  with
    bone involvement without evidence of
      necrosis L97.106
    bone necrosis L97.104
    exposed fat layer L97.102
    muscle involvement without evidence of
      necrosis L97.105
    muscle necrosis L97.103
    skin breakdown only L97.101
    specified severity NEC L97.108
  left L97.129
    with
      bone involvement without evidence of
        necrosis L97.126
      bone necrosis L97.124
      exposed fat layer L97.122
      muscle involvement without evidence of
        necrosis L97.125
      muscle necrosis L97.123
      skin breakdown only L97.121
      specified severity NEC L97.128
  right L97.119
    with
      bone involvement without evidence of
        necrosis L97.116
      bone necrosis L97.114
      exposed fat layer L97.112
      muscle involvement without evidence of
        necrosis L97.115
      muscle necrosis L97.113
      skin breakdown only L97.111
      specified severity NEC L97.118
toe L97.509
  with
    bone involvement without evidence of
      necrosis L97.506
    bone necrosis L97.504
    exposed fat layer L97.502
    muscle involvement without evidence of
      necrosis L97.505
    muscle necrosis L97.503
    skin breakdown only L97.501
    specified severity NEC L97.508
  left L97.529
    with
      bone involvement without evidence of
        necrosis L97.526
      bone necrosis L97.524
      exposed fat layer L97.522
      muscle involvement without evidence of
        necrosis L97.525
      muscle necrosis L97.523
      skin breakdown only L97.521
      specified severity NEC L97.528
  right L97.519

— continued
lower limb — continued
  toe — continued
    right — continued
      with
        bone involvement without evidence of
          necrosis L97.516
        bone necrosis L97.514
        exposed fat layer L97.512
        muscle involvement without evidence of
          necrosis L97.515
        muscle necrosis L97.513
        skin breakdown only L97.511
        specified severity NEC L97.518
  varicose — see Varix, leg, with, ulcer
luetic — see Ulcer, syphilitic
lung J98.4
  tuberculous — see Tuberculosis, pulmonary
malignant — see Neoplasm, malignant, by site
marginal NEC — see Ulcer, gastrojejunal
meatus (urinarius) N34.2
Meckel's diverticulum Q43.0
  malignant — see Table of Neoplasms, small intes-
    tine, malignant
Meleney's (chronic undermining) — see Ulcer, skin
Mooren's (cornea) — see Ulcer, cornea, Mooren's
mycobacterial (skin) A31.1
nasopharynx J39.2
neck, uterus N86
neurogenic NEC — see Ulcer, skin
nose, nasal (passage) (infective) (septum) J34.0
  skin — see Ulcer, skin
  spirochetal A69.8
  varicose (bleeding) I86.8
oral mucosa (traumatic) K12.1
palate (soft) K12.1
penis (chronic) N48.5
peptic (site unspecified) K27.9
  with
    hemorrhage K27.4
      and perforation K27.6
    perforation K27.5
  acute K27.3
    with
      hemorrhage K27.0
        and perforation K27.2
      perforation K27.1
  chronic K27.7
    with
      hemorrhage K27.4
        and perforation K27.6
      perforation K27.5
  esophagus K22.10
    with bleeding K22.11
  newborn P78.82
perforating K27.5
  skin — see Ulcer, skin
peritonsillar J35.8
phagedenic (tropical) — see Ulcer, skin
pharynx J39.2
phlebitis — see Phlebitis
plaster — see Ulcer, pressure, by site
popliteal space — see Ulcer, lower limb
postpyloric — see Ulcer, duodenum
prepuce N47.7
prepyloric — see Ulcer, stomach
pressure (pressure area) L89.9- ☑
  ankle L89.5- ☑
  back L89.1- ☑
  buttock L89.3- ☑
  coccyx L89.15- ☑
  contiguous site of back, buttock, hip L89.4- ☑
  elbow L89.0- ☑
  face L89.81- ☑
  head L89.81- ☑
  heel L89.6- ☑
  hip L89.2- ☑
  sacral region (tailbone) L89.15- ☑
  specified site NEC L89.89- ☑
  stage 1 (healing) (pre-ulcer skin changes limited to
    persistent focal edema)
    ankle L89.5- ☑
    back L89.1- ☑
    buttock L89.3- ☑
    coccyx L89.15- ☑
    contiguous site of back, buttock, hip L89.4- ☑

Ulcer, ulcerated, ulcerating, ulceration, ulcerative

— *continued*
- pressure — *continued*
  - stage 1 — *continued*
    - elbow L89.0- ☑
    - face L89.81- ☑
    - head L89.81- ☑
    - heel L89.6- ☑
    - hip L89.2- ☑
    - sacral region (tailbone) L89.15- ☑
    - specified site NEC L89.89- ☑
  - stage 2 (healing) (abrasion, blister, partial thickness skin loss involving epidermis and/or dermis)
    - ankle L89.5- ☑
    - back L89.1- ☑
    - buttock L89.3- ☑
    - coccyx L89.15- ☑
    - contiguous site of back, buttock, hip L89.4- ☑
    - elbow L89.0- ☑
    - face L89.81- ☑
    - head L89.81- ☑
    - heel L89.6- ☑
    - hip L89.2- ☑
    - sacral region (tailbone) L89.15- ☑
    - specified site NEC L89.89- ☑
  - stage 3 (healing) (full thickness skin loss involving damage or necrosis of subcutaneous tissue)
    - ankle L89.5- ☑
    - back L89.1- ☑
    - buttock L89.3- ☑
    - coccyx L89.15- ☑
    - contiguous site of back, buttock, hip L89.4- ☑
    - elbow L89.0- ☑
    - face L89.81- ☑
    - head L89.81- ☑
    - heel L89.6- ☑
    - hip L89.2- ☑
    - sacral region (tailbone) L89.15- ☑
    - specified site NEC L89.89- ☑
  - stage 4 (healing) (necrosis of soft tissues through to underlying muscle, tendon, or bone)
    - ankle L89.5- ☑
    - back L89.1- ☑
    - buttock L89.3- ☑
    - coccyx L89.15- ☑
    - contiguous site of back, buttock, hip L89.4- ☑
    - elbow L89.0- ☑
    - face L89.81- ☑
    - head L89.81- ☑
    - heel L89.6- ☑
    - hip L89.2- ☑
    - sacral region (tailbone) L89.15- ☑
    - specified site NEC L89.89- ☑
  - unspecified stage
    - ankle L89.5- ☑
    - back L89.1- ☑
    - buttock L89.3- ☑
    - coccyx L89.15- ☑
    - contiguous site of back, buttock, hip L89.4- ☑
    - elbow L89.0- ☑
    - face L89.81- ☑
    - head L89.81- ☑
    - heel L89.6- ☑
    - hip L89.2- ☑
    - sacral region (tailbone) L89.15- ☑
    - specified site NEC L89.89- ☑
  - unstageable
    - ankle L89.5- ☑
    - back L89.1- ☑
    - buttock L89.3- ☑
    - coccyx L89.15- ☑
    - contiguous site of back, buttock, hip L89.4- ☑
    - elbow L89.0- ☑
    - face L89.81- ☑
    - head L89.81- ☑
    - heel L89.6- ☑
    - hip L89.2- ☑
    - sacral region (tailbone) L89.15- ☑
    - specified site NEC L89.89- ☑
- primary of intestine K63.3
  - with perforation K63.1
- prostate N41.9
- pyloric — *see* Ulcer, stomach
- rectosigmoid K63.3
  - with perforation K63.1
- rectum (sphincter) (solitary) K62.6
  - stercoraceous, stercoral K62.6
- retina — *see* Inflammation, chorioretinal
- rodent — *see also* Neoplasm, skin, malignant
- sclera — *see* Scleritis
- scrofulous (tuberculous) A18.2
- scrotum N50.89
  - tuberculous A18.15
  - varicose I86.1
- seminal vesicle N50.89
- sigmoid — *see* Ulcer, intestine
- skin (atrophic) (chronic) (neurogenic) (non-healing) (perforating) (pyogenic) (trophic) (tropical) L98.499
  - with gangrene — *see* Gangrene
  - amebic A06.7
  - back — *see* Ulcer, back
  - buttock — *see* Ulcer, buttock
  - decubitus — *see* Ulcer, pressure
  - lower limb — *see* Ulcer, lower limb
  - mycobacterial A31.1
  - specified site NEC L98.499
    - with
      - bone involvement without evidence of necrosis L98.496
      - bone necrosis L98.494
      - exposed fat layer L98.492
      - muscle involvement without evidence of necrosis L98.495
      - muscle necrosis L98.493
      - skin breakdown only L98.491
      - specified severity NEC L98.498
  - tuberculous (primary) A18.4
  - varicose — *see* Ulcer, varicose
- sloughing — *see* Ulcer, skin
- solitary, anus or rectum (sphincter) K62.6
- sore throat J02.9
  - streptococcal J02.0
- spermatic cord N50.89
- spine (tuberculous) A18.01
- stasis (venous) — *see* Varix, leg, with, ulcer
  - without varicose veins I87.2
- stercoraceous, stercoral K63.3
  - with perforation K63.1
  - anus or rectum K62.6
- stoma, stomal — *see* Ulcer, gastrojejunal
- stomach (eroded) (peptic) (round) K25.9
  - with
    - hemorrhage K25.4
      - and perforation K25.6
    - perforation K25.5
  - acute K25.3
    - with
      - hemorrhage K25.0
        - and perforation K25.2
      - perforation K25.1
  - chronic K25.7
    - with
      - hemorrhage K25.4
        - and perforation K25.6
      - perforation K25.5
- stomal — *see* Ulcer, gastrojejunal
- stomatitis K12.1
- stress — *see* Ulcer, peptic
- strumous (tuberculous) A18.2
- submucosal, bladder — *see* Cystitis, interstitial
- syphilitic (any site) (early) (secondary) A51.39
  - late A52.79
  - perforating A52.79
    - foot A52.11
- testis N50.89
- thigh — *see* Ulcer, lower limb
- throat J39.2
  - diphtheritic A36.0
- toe — *see* Ulcer, lower limb
- tongue (traumatic) K14.0
- tonsil J35.8
  - diphtheritic A36.0
- trachea J39.8
- trophic — *see* Ulcer, skin
- tropical — *see* Ulcer, skin
- tuberculous — *see* Tuberculosis, ulcer
- tunica vaginalis N50.89
- turbinate J34.89
- typhoid (perforating) — *see* Typhoid
- unspecified site — *see* Ulcer, skin
- urethra (meatus) — *see* Urethritis
- uterus N85.8
  - cervix N86
    - with cervicitis N72
  - neck N86
    - with cervicitis N72
- vagina N76.5
  - in Behçet's disease M35.2 *[N77.0]*
  - pessary N89.8
- valve, heart I33.0
- varicose (lower limb, any part) — *see also* Varix, leg, with, ulcer
  - broad ligament I86.2
  - esophagus — *see* Varix, esophagus
  - inflamed or infected — *see* Varix, leg, with ulcer, with inflammation
  - nasal septum I86.8
  - perineum I86.3
  - scrotum I86.1
  - specified site NEC I86.8
  - sublingual I86.0
  - vulva I86.3
- vas deferens N50.89
- vulva (acute) (infectional) N76.6
  - in (due to)
    - Behçet's disease M35.2 *[N77.0]*
    - herpesviral (herpes simplex) infection A60.04
    - tuberculosis A18.18
- vulvobuccal, recurring N76.6
- X-ray L58.1
- yaws A66.4

Ulcerosa scarlatina A38.8

Ulcus — *see also* Ulcer
- cutis tuberculosum A18.4
- duodeni — *see* Ulcer, duodenum
- durum (syphilitic) A51.0
  - extragenital A51.2
- gastrojejunale — *see* Ulcer, gastrojejunal
- hypostaticum — *see* Ulcer, varicose
- molle (cutis) (skin) A57
- serpens corneae — *see* Ulcer, cornea, central
- ventriculi — *see* Ulcer, stomach

Ulegyria Q04.8

Ulerythema
- ophryogenes, congenital Q84.2
- sycosiforme L73.8

Ullrich (-Bonnevie)(-Turner) **syndrome** — *see also* Turner's syndrome Q87.19

Ullrich-Feichtiger syndrome Q87.0

Ulnar — *see* condition

Ulorrhagia, ulorrhea K06.8

Umbilicus, umbilical — *see* condition

Unacceptable
- contours of tooth K08.54
- morphology of tooth K08.54

Unavailability (of)
- bed at medical facility Z75.1
- health service-related agencies Z75.4
- medical facilities (at) Z75.3
  - due to
    - investigation by social service agency Z75.2
    - lack of services at home Z75.0
    - remoteness from facility Z75.3
    - waiting list Z75.1
  - home Z75.0
  - outpatient clinic Z75.3
- schooling Z55.1
- social service agencies Z75.4

Uncinaria americana infestation B76.1

Uncinariasis B76.9

Uncongenial work Z56.5

Unconscious (ness) — *see* Coma

Under observation — *see* Observation

Underachievement in school Z55.3

Underdevelopment — *see also* Undeveloped
- nose Q30.1
- sexual E30.0

Underdosing — *see also* Table of Drugs and Chemicals, categories T36-T50, with final character 6 Z91.14
- intentional NEC Z91.128
  - due to financial hardship of patient Z91.120
- unintentional NEC Z91.138
  - due to patient's age related debility Z91.130

Underfeeding, newborn P92.3

Underfill, endodontic M27.53

Underimmunization status Z28.3

☑ Additional Character Required — Refer to the Tabular List for Character Selection ⬭ Subterms under main terms may continue to next column or page

Undernourishment — see Malnutrition
Undernutrition — see Malnutrition
Underweight R63.6
  for gestational age — see Light for dates
Underwood's disease P83.0
Undescended — see also Malposition, congenital
  cecum Q43.3
  colon Q43.3
  testicle — see Cryptorchid
Undeveloped, undevelopment — see also Hypoplasia
  brain (congenital) Q02
  cerebral (congenital) Q02
  heart Q24.8
  lung Q33.6
  testis E29.1
  uterus E30.0
Undiagnosed (disease) R69
Undulant fever — see Brucellosis
Unemployment, anxiety concerning Z56.0
  threatened Z56.2
Unequal length (acquired) (limb) — see also Deformity,
    limb, unequal length
  leg — see also Deformity, limb, unequal length
    congenital Q72.9- ☑
Unextracted dental root K08.3
Unguis incarnatus L60.0
Unhappiness R45.2
Unicornate uterus Q51.4
  in pregnancy or childbirth O34.00
Unilateral — see also condition
  development, breast N64.89
  organ or site, congenital NEC — see Agenesis, by site
Unilocular heart Q20.8
Union, abnormal — see also Fusion
  larynx and trachea Q34.8
Universal mesentery Q43.3
**Unrepairable overhanging of dental restorative
    materials** K08.52
Unsatisfactory
  restoration of tooth K08.50
    specified NEC K08.59
  sample of cytologic smear
    anus R85.615
    cervix R87.615
    vagina R87.625
  surroundings Z59.1
  work Z56.5
Unsoundness of mind — see Psychosis
Unstable
  back NEC — see Instability, joint, spine
  hip (congenital) Q65.6
    acquired — see Derangement, joint, specified type
      NEC, hip
  joint — see Instability, joint
    secondary to removal of joint prosthesis M96.89
  lie (mother) O32.0 ☑
  lumbosacral joint (congenital) — see subcategory
    M53.2
  sacroiliac — see subcategory M53.2 ☑
  spine NEC — see Instability, joint, spine
Unsteadiness on feet R26.81
Untruthfulness, child problem F91.8
Unverricht (-Lundborg) **disease or epilepsy** — see
    Epilepsy, generalized, idiopathic
Unwanted
  multiple moves in the last 12 months Z59.81- ☑
  pregnancy Z64.0
Upbringing, institutional Z62.22
  away from parents NEC Z62.29
  in care of non-parental family member Z62.21
  in foster care Z62.21
  in orphanage or group home Z62.22
  in welfare custody Z62.21
Upper respiratory — see condition
Upset
  gastric K30
  gastrointestinal K30
    psychogenic F45.8
  intestinal (large) (small) K59.9
    psychogenic F45.8
  menstruation N93.9
  mental F48.9
  stomach K30
    psychogenic F45.8
Urachus — see also condition
  patent or persistent Q64.4

Urbach-Oppenheim disease (necrobiosis lipoidica dia-
    beticorum) — see E08-E13 with .620
Urbach's lipoid proteinosis E78.89
Urbach-Wiethe disease E78.89
Urban yellow fever A95.1
Urea
  blood, high — see Uremia
  cycle metabolism disorder — see Disorder, urea cycle
    metabolism
Uremia, uremic N19
  with
    ectopic or molar pregnancy O08.4
    polyneuropathy N18.9 [G63]
  chronic NOS — see also Disease, kidney, chronic N18.9
    due to hypertension — see Hypertensive, kidney
  complicating
    ectopic or molar pregnancy O08.4
  congenital P96.0
  extrarenal R39.2
  following ectopic or molar pregnancy O08.4
  newborn P96.0
  prerenal R39.2
Ureter, ureteral — see condition
Ureteralgia N23
Ureterectasis — see Hydroureter
Ureteritis N28.89
  cystica N28.86
  due to calculus N20.1
    with calculus, kidney N20.2
      with hydronephrosis N13.2
  gonococcal (acute) (chronic) A54.21
  nonspecific N28.89
Ureterocele N28.89
  congenital (orthotopic) Q62.31
    ectopic Q62.32
Ureterolith, ureterolithiasis — see Calculus, ureter
Ureterostomy
  attention to Z43.6
  status Z93.6
Urethra, urethral — see condition
Urethralgia R39.89
Urethritis (anterior) (posterior) N34.2
  calculous N21.1
  candidal B37.41
  chlamydial A56.01
  diplococcal (gonococcal) A54.01
    with abscess (accessory gland) (periurethral) A54.1
  gonococcal A54.01
    with abscess (accessory gland) (periurethral) A54.1
  nongonococcal N34.1
    Reiter's — see Reiter's disease
  nonspecific N34.1
  nonvenereal N34.1
  postmenopausal N34.2
  puerperal O86.22
  Reiter's — see Reiter's disease
  specified NEC N34.2
  trichomonal or due to Trichomonas (vaginalis) A59.03
Urethrocele N81.0
  with
    cystocele — see Cystocele
    prolapse of uterus — see Prolapse, uterus
Urethrolithiasis (with colic or infection) N21.1
Urethrorectal — see condition
Urethrorrhagia N36.8
Urethrorrhea R36.9
Urethrostomy
  attention to Z43.6
  status Z93.6
Urethrotrigonitis — see Trigonitis
Urethrovaginal — see condition
Urgency
  fecal R15.2
  hypertensive — see Hypertension
  urinary R39.15
Urhidrosis, uridrosis L74.8
Uric acid in blood (increased) E79.0
Uricacidemia (asymptomatic) E79.0
Uricemia (asymptomatic) E79.0
Uricosuria R82.998
Urinary — see condition
Urination
  frequent R35.0
  painful R30.9
Urine
  blood in — see Hematuria
  discharge, excessive R35.89

Urine — continued
  enuresis, nonorganic origin F98.0
  extravasation R39.0
  frequency R35.0
  incontinence R32
    nonorganic origin F98.0
  intermittent stream R39.198
  pus in N39.0
  retention or stasis R33.9
    organic R33.8
      drug-induced R33.0
    psychogenic F45.8
  secretion
    deficient R34
    excessive R35.89
    frequency R35.0
  stream
    intermittent R39.198
    slowing R39.198
    splitting R39.13
    weak R39.12
Urinemia — see Uremia
Urinoma, urethra N36.8
Uroarthritis, infectious (Reiter's) — see Reiter's disease
Urodialysis R34
Urolithiasis — see Calculus, urinary
Uronephrosis — see Hydronephrosis
Uropathy N39.9
  obstructive N13.9
    specified NEC N13.8
  reflux N13.9
    specified NEC N13.8
  vesicoureteral reflux-associated — see Reflux, vesi-
    coureteral
Urosepsis — code to condition
Urticaria L50.9
  with angioneurotic edema T78.3 ☑
    hereditary D84.1
  allergic L50.0
  cholinergic L50.5
  chronic L50.8
  cold, familial L50.2
  contact L50.6
  dermatographic L50.3
  due to
    cold or heat L50.2
    drugs L50.0
    food L50.0
    inhalants L50.0
    plants L50.6
    serum — see also Reaction, serum T80.69 ☑
  factitial L50.3
  familial cold M04.2
  giant T78.3 ☑
    hereditary D84.1
  gigantea T78.3 ☑
  idiopathic L50.1
  larynx T78.3 ☑
    hereditary D84.1
  neonatorum P83.88
  nonallergic L50.1
  papulosa (Hebra) L28.2
  pigmentosa D47.01
    congenital Q82.2
    of neonatal onset Q82.2
    of newborn onset Q82.2
  recurrent periodic L50.8
  serum — see also Reaction, serum T80.69 ☑
  solar L56.3
  specified type NEC L50.8
  thermal (cold) (heat) L50.2
  vibratory L50.4
  xanthelasmoidea — see Urticaria pigmentosa
Use (of)
  alcohol Z72.89
    with
      intoxication F10.929
      sleep disorder F10.982
      withdrawal F10.939
        with
          perceptual disturbance F10.932
          delirium F10.931
          uncomplicated F10.930
      harmful — see Abuse, alcohol
    amphetamines — see Use, stimulant NEC
    caffeine — see Use, stimulant NEC
    cannabis F12.90

☟ **Subterms under main terms may continue to next column or page**   ☑ **Additional Character Required** — Refer to the Tabular List for Character Selection

Use — *continued*
  cannabis — *continued*
    with
      anxiety disorder F12.980
      intoxication F12.929
        with
          delirium F12.921
          perceptual disturbance F12.922
          uncomplicated F12.920
      other specified disorder F12.988
      psychosis F12.959
        delusions F12.950
        hallucinations F12.951
      unspecified disorder F12.99
      withdrawal F12.93
  cocaine F14.90
    with
      anxiety disorder F14.980
      intoxication F14.929
        with
          delirium F14.921
          perceptual disturbance F14.922
          uncomplicated F14.920
      other specified disorder F14.988
      psychosis F14.959
        delusions F14.950
        hallucinations F14.951
      sexual dysfunction F14.981
      sleep disorder F14.982
      unspecified disorder F14.99
      withdrawal F14.93
    harmful — *see* Abuse, drug, cocaine
  drug(s) NEC F19.90
    with sleep disorder F19.982
    harmful — *see* Abuse, drug, by type
  hallucinogen NEC F16.90
    with
      anxiety disorder F16.980
      intoxication F16.929
        with
          delirium F16.921
        uncomplicated F16.920
      mood disorder F16.94
      other specified disorder F16.988
      perception disorder (flashbacks) F16.983
      psychosis F16.959
        delusions F16.950
        hallucinations F16.951
      unspecified disorder F16.99
    harmful — *see* Abuse, drug, hallucinogen NEC
  inhalants F18.90
    with
      anxiety disorder F18.980
      intoxication F18.929
        with delirium F18.921
        uncomplicated F18.920
      mood disorder F18.94
      other specified disorder F18.988
      persisting dementia F18.97
      psychosis F18.959
        delusions F18.950
        hallucinations F18.951
      unspecified disorder F18.99
    harmful — *see* Abuse, drug, inhalant
  methadone — *see* Use, opioid
  nonprescribed drugs F19.90
    harmful — *see* Abuse, non-psychoactive substance
  opioid F11.90
    with
      disorder F11.99
        mood F11.94
        sleep F11.982
        specified type NEC F11.988
      intoxication F11.929
        with
          delirium F11.921
          perceptual disturbance F11.922
          uncomplicated F11.920
      withdrawal F11.93
    harmful — *see* Abuse, drug, opioid
  patent medicines F19.90
    harmful — *see* Abuse, non-psychoactive substance
  psychoactive drug NEC F19.90
    with
      anxiety disorder F19.980
      intoxication F19.929
        with
          delirium F19.921

Use — *continued*
  psychoactive drug — *continued*
    with — *continued*
      intoxication — *continued*
        with — *continued*
          perceptual disturbance F19.922
        uncomplicated F19.920
      mood disorder F19.94
      other specified disorder F19.988
      persisting
        amnestic disorder F19.96
        dementia F19.97
      psychosis F19.959
        delusions F19.950
        hallucinations F19.951
      sexual dysfunction F19.981
      sleep disorder F19.982
      unspecified disorder F19.99
      withdrawal F19.939
        with
          delirium F19.931
          perceptual disturbance F19.932
        uncomplicated F19.930
    harmful — *see* Abuse, drug NEC, psychoactive NEC
  sedative, hypnotic, or anxiolytic F13.90
    with
      anxiety disorder F13.980
      intoxication F13.929
        with
          delirium F13.921
        uncomplicated F13.920
      other specified disorder F13.988
      persisting
        amnestic disorder F13.96
        dementia F13.97
      psychosis F13.959
        delusions F13.950
        hallucinations F13.951
      sexual dysfunction F13.981
      sleep disorder F13.982
      unspecified disorder F13.99
    harmful — *see* Abuse, drug, sedative, hypnotic, or anxiolytic
  stimulant NEC F15.90
    with
      anxiety disorder F15.980
      intoxication F15.929
        with
          delirium F15.921
          perceptual disturbance F15.922
        uncomplicated F15.920
      mood disorder F15.94
      other specified disorder F15.988
      psychosis F15.959
        delusions F15.950
        hallucinations F15.951
      sexual dysfunction F15.981
      sleep disorder F15.982
      unspecified disorder F15.99
      withdrawal F15.93
    harmful — *see* Abuse, drug, stimulant NEC
  tobacco Z72.0
    with dependence — *see* Dependence, drug, nicotine
  volatile solvents — *see also* Use, inhalant F18.90
    harmful — *see* Abuse, drug, inhalant
Usher-Senear disease or syndrome L10.4
Uta B55.1
Uteromegaly N85.2
Uterovaginal — *see* condition
Uterovesical — *see* condition
Uveal — *see* condition
Uveitis (anterior) — *see also* Iridocyclitis
  acute — *see* Iridocyclitis, acute
  chronic — *see* Iridocyclitis, chronic
  due to toxoplasmosis (acquired) B58.09
    congenital P37.1
  granulomatous — *see* Iridocyclitis, chronic
  heterochromic — *see* Cyclitis, Fuchs' heterochromic
  lens-induced — *see* Iridocyclitis, lens-induced
  posterior — *see* Chorioretinitis
  sympathetic H44.13- ☑
  syphilitic (secondary) A51.43
    congenital (early) A50.01
    late A52.71
  tuberculous A18.54
Uveoencephalitis — *see* Inflammation, chorioretinal
Uveokeratitis — *see* Iridocyclitis
Uveoparotitis D86.89

Uvula — *see* condition
Uvulitis (acute) (catarrhal) (chronic) (membranous) (suppurative) (ulcerative) K12.2

V

Vaccination (prophylactic)
  complication or reaction — *see* Complications, vaccination
  delayed Z28.9
  encounter for Z23
  not done — *see* Immunization, not done, because (of)
Vaccinia (generalized) (localized) T88.1 ☑
  congenital P35.8
  without vaccination B08.011
Vacuum, in sinus (accessory) (nasal) J34.89
Vagabond, vagabondage Z59.00
Vagabond's disease B85.1
Vagina, vaginal — *see* condition
Vaginalitis (tunica) (testis) N49.1
Vaginismus (reflex) N94.2
  functional F52.5
  nonorganic F52.5
  psychogenic F52.5
  secondary N94.2
Vaginitis (acute) (circumscribed) (diffuse) (emphysematous) (nonvenereal) (ulcerative) N76.0
  with ectopic or molar pregnancy O08.0
  amebic A06.82
  atrophic, postmenopausal N95.2
  bacterial N76.0
  blennorrhagic (gonococcal) A54.02
  candidal B37.3
  chlamydial A56.02
  chronic N76.1
  due to Trichomonas (vaginalis) A59.01
  following ectopic or molar pregnancy O08.0
  gonococcal A54.02
    with abscess (accessory gland) (periurethral) A54.1
  granuloma A58
  in (due to)
    candidiasis B37.3
    herpesviral (herpes simplex) infection A60.04
    pinworm infection B80 [N77.1]
  monilial B37.3
  mycotic (candidal) B37.3
  postmenopausal atrophic N95.2
  puerperal (postpartum) O86.13
  senile (atrophic) N95.2
  subacute or chronic N76.1
  syphilitic (early) A51.0
    late A52.76
  trichomonal A59.01
  tuberculous A18.18
Vaginosis — *see* Vaginitis
Vagotonia G52.2
Vagrancy Z59.00
VAIN — *see* Neoplasia, intraepithelial, vagina
Vallecula — *see* condition
Valley fever B38.0
Valsuani's disease — *see* Anemia, obstetric
Valve, valvular (formation) — *see also* condition
  cerebral ventricle (communicating) in situ Z98.2
  cervix, internal os Q51.828
  congenital NEC — *see* Atresia, by site
  ureter (pelvic junction) (vesical orifice) Q62.39
  urethra (congenital) (posterior) Q64.2
Valvulitis (chronic) — *see* Endocarditis
Valvulopathy — *see* Endocarditis
Van Bogaert's leukoencephalopathy (sclerosing) (subacute) A81.1
Van Bogaert-Scherer-Epstein disease or syndrome E75.5
Van Buchem's syndrome M85.2
Van Creveld-von Gierke disease E74.01
Van der Hoeve (-de Kleyn) **syndrome** Q78.0
Van der Woude's syndrome Q38.0
Van Neck's disease or osteochondrosis M91.0
Vanishing lung J44.9
Vapor asphyxia or suffocation T59.9 ☑
  specified agent — *see* Table of Drugs and Chemicals
Variance, lethal ball, prosthetic heart valve T82.09 ☑
Variants, thalassemic D56.8
Variations in hair color L67.1
Varicella B01.9
  with
    complications NEC B01.89

☑ **Additional Character Required** — Refer to the Tabular List for Character Selection   ▼ Subterms under main terms may continue to next column or page

Varicella — *continued*
  with — *continued*
    encephalitis B01.11
    encephalomyelitis B01.11
    meningitis B01.0
    myelitis B01.12
    pneumonia B01.2
  congenital P35.8
Varices — *see* Varix
Varicocele (scrotum) (thrombosed) I86.1
  ovary I86.2
  perineum I86.3
  spermatic cord (ulcerated) I86.1
Varicose
  aneurysm (ruptured) I77.0
  dermatitis — *see* Varix, leg, with, inflammation
  eczema — *see* Varix, leg, with, inflammation
  phlebitis — *see* Varix, with, inflammation
  tumor — *see* Varix
  ulcer (lower limb, any part) — *see also* Varix, leg, with, ulcer
    anus — *see also* Hemorrhoids K64.8
    esophagus — *see* Varix, esophagus
    inflamed or infected — *see* Varix, leg, with ulcer, with inflammation
    nasal septum I86.8
    perineum I86.3
    scrotum I86.1
    specified site NEC I86.8
  vein — *see* Varix
  vessel — *see* Varix, leg
Varicosis, varicosities, varicosity — *see* Varix
Variola (major) (minor) B03
Varioloid B03
Varix (lower limb) I83.90
  with
    bleeding I83.899
    edema I83.899
    inflammation I83.10
      with ulcer (venous) I83.209
    pain I83.819
    rupture I83.899
    specified complication NEC I83.899
    stasis dermatitis I83.10
      with ulcer (venous) I83.209
    swelling I83.899
    ulcer I83.009
      with inflammation I83.209
  aneurysmal I77.0
  asymptomatic I83.9- ☑
  bladder I86.2
  broad ligament I86.2
  complicating
    childbirth (lower extremity) O87.4
      anus or rectum O87.2
      genital (vagina, vulva or perineum) O87.8
    pregnancy (lower extremity) O22.0- ☑
      anus or rectum O22.4- ☑
      genital (vagina, vulva or perineum) O22.1- ☑
    puerperium (lower extremity) O87.4
      anus or rectum O87.2
      genital (vagina, vulva, perineum) O87.8
  congenital (any site) Q27.8
  esophagus (idiopathic) (primary) (ulcerated) I85.00
    bleeding I85.01
    congenital Q27.8
    in (due to)
      alcoholic liver disease I85.10
        bleeding I85.11
      cirrhosis of liver I85.10
        bleeding I85.11
      portal hypertension I85.10
        bleeding I85.11
      schistosomiasis I85.10
        bleeding I85.11
      toxic liver disease I85.10
        bleeding I85.11
    secondary I85.10
      bleeding I85.11
  gastric I86.4
  inflamed or infected I83.10
    ulcerated I83.209
  labia (majora) I86.3
  leg (asymptomatic) I83.9- ☑
    with
      edema I83.899
      inflammation I83.10

Varix — *continued*
  leg — *continued*
    with — *continued*
      inflammation — *continued*
        with ulcer — *see* Varix, leg, with, ulcer, with inflammation by site
      pain I83.819
      specified complication NEC I83.899
      swelling I83.899
      ulcer I83.0- ☑
        with inflammation I83.2- ☑
        ankle I83.003
          with inflammation I83.203
        calf I83.002
          with inflammation I83.202
        foot NEC I83.005
          with inflammation I83.205
        heel I83.004
          with inflammation I83.204
        lower leg NEC I83.008
          with inflammation I83.208
        midfoot I83.004
          with inflammation I83.204
        thigh I83.001
          with inflammation I83.201
    bilateral (asymptomatic) I83.93
      with
        edema I83.893
        pain I83.813
        specified complication NEC I83.893
        swelling I83.893
        ulcer I83.0- ☑
          with inflammation I83.209
    left (asymptomatic) I83.92
      with
        edema I83.892
        inflammation I83.12
          with ulcer — *see* Varix, leg, with, ulcer, with inflammation by site
        pain I83.812
        specified complication NEC I83.892
        swelling I83.892
        ulcer I83.029
          with inflammation I83.229
          ankle I83.023
            with inflammation I83.223
          calf I83.022
            with inflammation I83.222
          foot NEC I83.025
            with inflammation I83.225
          heel I83.024
            with inflammation I83.224
          lower leg NEC I83.028
            with inflammation I83.228
          midfoot I83.024
            with inflammation I83.224
          thigh I83.021
            with inflammation I83.221
    right (asymptomatic) I83.91
      with
        edema I83.891
        inflammation I83.11
          with ulcer — *see* Varix, leg, with, ulcer, with inflammation by site
        pain I83.811
        specified complication NEC I83.891
        swelling I83.891
        ulcer I83.019
          with inflammation I83.219
          ankle I83.013
            with inflammation I83.213
          calf I83.012
            with inflammation I83.212
          foot NEC I83.015
            with inflammation I83.215
          heel I83.014
            with inflammation I83.214
          lower leg NEC I83.018
            with inflammation I83.218
          midfoot I83.014
            with inflammation I83.214
          thigh I83.011
            with inflammation I83.211
  nasal septum I86.8
  orbit I86.8
    congenital Q27.8
  ovary I86.2
  papillary I78.1

Varix — *continued*
  pelvis I86.2
  perineum I86.3
  pharynx I86.8
  placenta O43.89- ☑
  renal papilla I86.8
  retina H35.09
  scrotum (ulcerated) I86.1
  sigmoid colon I86.8
  specified site NEC I86.8
  spinal (cord) (vessels) I86.8
  spleen, splenic (vein) (with phlebolith) I86.8
  stomach I86.4
  sublingual I86.0
  ulcerated I83.009
    inflamed or infected I83.209
  uterine ligament I86.2
  vagina I86.8
  vocal cord I86.8
  vulva I86.3
Vas deferens — *see* condition
Vas deferentitis N49.1
Vasa previa O69.4 ☑
  hemorrhage from, affecting newborn P50.0
Vascular — *see also* condition
  loop on optic papilla Q14.2
  spasm I73.9
  spider I78.1
Vascularization, cornea — *see* Neovascularization, cornea
Vasculitis I77.6
  allergic D69.0
  cryoglobulinemic D89.1
  disseminated I77.6
  hypocomplementemic M31.8
  kidney I77.89
  leukocytoclastic M31.0
  livedoid L95.0
  nodular L95.8
  retina H35.06- ☑
  rheumatic — *see* Fever, rheumatic
  rheumatoid — *see* Rheumatoid, vasculitis
  skin (limited to) L95.9
    specified NEC L95.8
  systemic M31.8
Vasculopathy, necrotizing M31.9
  cardiac allograft T86.290
  specified NEC M31.8
Vasitis (nodosa) N49.1
  tuberculous A18.15
Vasodilation I73.9
Vasomotor — *see* condition
Vasoplasty, after previous sterilization Z31.0
  aftercare Z31.42
Vasospasm (vasoconstriction) I73.9
  cerebral (cerebrovascular) (artery) I67.848
    reversible I67.841
  coronary I20.1
  nerve
    arm — *see* Mononeuropathy, upper limb
    brachial plexus G54.0
    cervical plexus G54.2
    leg — *see* Mononeuropathy, lower limb
  peripheral NOS I73.9
  retina (artery) — *see* Occlusion, artery, retina
Vasospastic — *see* condition
Vasovagal attack (paroxysmal) R55
  psychogenic F45.8
VATER syndrome Q87.2
Vater's ampulla — *see* condition
Vegetation, vegetative
  adenoid (nasal fossa) J35.8
  endocarditis (acute) (any valve) (subacute) I33.0
  heart (mycotic) (valve) I33.0
Veil
  Jackson's Q43.3
Vein, venous — *see* condition
Veldt sore — *see* Ulcer, skin
Velpeau's hernia — *see* Hernia, femoral
Venereal
  bubo A55
  disease A64
  granuloma inguinale A58
  lymphogranuloma (Durand-Nicolas-Favre) A55
Venofibrosis I87.8
Venom, venomous — *see* Table of Drugs and Chemicals, by animal or substance, poisoning
Venous — *see* condition

Ventilator lung, newborn P27.8
Ventral — *see* condition
Ventricle, ventricular — *see also* condition
　escape I49.3
　inversion Q20.5
Ventriculitis (cerebral) — *see also* Encephalitis G04.90
Ventriculostomy status Z98.2
Vernet's syndrome G52.7
Verneuil's disease (syphilitic bursitis) A52.78
Verruca (due to HPV) (filiformis) (simplex) (viral) (vulgaris)
　B07.9
　acuminata A63.0
　necrogenica (primary) (tuberculosa) A18.4
　plana B07.8
　plantaris B07.0
　seborrheica L82.1
　　inflamed L82.0
　senile (seborrheic) L82.1
　　inflamed L82.0
　tuberculosa (primary) A18.4
　venereal A63.0
Verrucosities — *see* Verruca
Verruga peruana, peruviana A44.1
Version
　cervix — *see* Malposition, uterus
　uterus (postinfectional) (postpartal, old) — *see* Malposition, uterus
Vertebra, vertebral — *see* condition
Vertical talus (congenital) Q66.80
　left foot Q66.82
　right foot Q66.81
Vertigo R42
　auditory — *see* Vertigo, aural
　aural H81.31- ☑
　benign paroxysmal (positional) H81.1- ☑
　central (origin) H81.4
　cerebral H81.4
　Dix and Hallpike (epidemic) — *see* Neuronitis, vestibular
　due to infrasound T75.23 ☑
　epidemic A88.1
　　Dix and Hallpike — *see* Neuronitis, vestibular
　　Pedersen's — *see* Neuronitis, vestibular
　　vestibular neuronitis — *see* Neuronitis, vestibular
　hysterical F44.89
　infrasound T75.23 ☑
　labyrinthine — *see* subcategory H81.0 ☑
　laryngeal R05.4
　malignant positional H81.4
　Ménière's — *see* subcategory H81.0 ☑
　menopausal N95.1
　otogenic — *see* Vertigo, aural
　paroxysmal positional, benign — *see* Vertigo, benign paroxysmal
　Pedersen's (epidemic) — *see* Neuronitis, vestibular
　peripheral NEC H81.39- ☑
　positional
　　benign paroxysmal — *see* Vertigo, benign paroxysmal
　　malignant H81.4
Very-low-density-lipoprotein-type (VLDL) **hyperlipoproteinemia** E78.1
Vesania — *see* Psychosis
Vesical — *see* condition
Vesicle
　cutaneous R23.8
　seminal — *see* condition
　skin R23.8
Vesicocolic — *see* condition
Vesicoperineal — *see* condition
Vesicorectal — *see* condition
Vesicourethrorectal — *see* condition
Vesicovaginal — *see* condition
Vesicular — *see* condition
Vesiculitis (seminal) N49.0
　amebic A06.82
　gonorrheal (acute) (chronic) A54.23
　trichomonal A59.09
　tuberculous A18.15
Vestibulitis (ear) — *see also* subcategory H83.0 ☑
　nose (external) J34.89
　vulvar N94.810
Vestibulopathy , acute peripheral (recurrent) — *see* Neuronitis, vestibular
Vestige, vestigial — *see also* Persistence
　branchial Q18.0
　structures in vitreous Q14.0

Vibration
　adverse effects T75.20 ☑
　　pneumatic hammer syndrome T75.21 ☑
　　specified effect NEC T75.29 ☑
　　vasospastic syndrome T75.22 ☑
　　vertigo from infrasound T75.23 ☑
　exposure (occupational) Z57.7
　vertigo T75.23 ☑
Vibriosis A28.9
Victim (of)
　crime Z65.4
　disaster Z65.5
　terrorism Z65.4
　torture Z65.4
　war Z65.5
Vidal's disease L28.0
Villaret's syndrome G52.7
Villous — *see* condition
VIN — *see* Neoplasia, intraepithelial, vulva
Vincent's infection (angina) (gingivitis) A69.1
　stomatitis NEC A69.1
Vinson-Plummer syndrome D50.1
Violence, physical R45.6
Viosterol deficiency — *see* Deficiency, calciferol
Vipoma — *see* Neoplasm, malignant, by site
Viremia B34.9
Virilism (adrenal) E25.9
　congenital E25.0
Virilization (female) (suprarenal) E25.9
　congenital E25.0
　isosexual E28.2
Virulent bubo A57
Virus, viral — *see also* condition
　as cause of disease classified elsewhere B97.89
　　respiratory syncytial virus (RSV) — *see* Virus, respiratory syncytial (RSV)
　cytomegalovirus B25.9
　human immunodeficiency (HIV) — *see* Human, immunodeficiency virus (HIV) disease
　infection — *see* Infection, virus
　respiratory syncytial (RSV)
　　as cause of disease classified elsewhere B97.4
　　bronchiolitis J21.0
　　bronchitis J20.5
　　bronchopneumonia J12.1
　　otitis media H65.- ☑ *[B97.4]*
　　pneumonia J12.1
　　upper respiratory infection J06.9 *[B97.4]*
　specified NEC B34.8
　swine influenza (viruses that normally cause infections in pigs) — *see also* Influenza, due to, identified novel influenza A virus J09.X2
　West Nile (fever) A92.30
　　with
　　　complications NEC A92.39
　　　cranial nerve disorders A92.32
　　　encephalitis A92.31
　　　encephalomyelitis A92.31
　　　neurologic manifestation NEC A92.32
　　　optic neuritis A92.32
　　　polyradiculitis A92.32
Viscera, visceral — *see* condition
Visceroptosis K63.4
Visible peristalsis R19.2
Vision, visual
　binocular, suppression H53.34
　blurred, blurring H53.8
　　hysterical F44.6
　defect, defective NEC H54.7
　disorientation (syndrome) H53.8
　disturbance H53.9
　　hysterical F44.6
　double H53.2
　examination Z01.00
　　with abnormal findings Z01.01
　　following failed vision screening Z01.020
　　　with abnormal findings Z01.021
　field, limitation (defect) — *see* Defect, visual field
　hallucinations R44.1
　halos H53.19
　loss — *see* Loss, vision
　　sudden — *see* Disturbance, vision, subjective, loss, sudden
　low (both eyes) — *see* Low, vision
　perception, simultaneous without fusion H53.33
Vitality, lack or want of R53.83
　newborn P96.89

Vitamin deficiency — *see* Deficiency, vitamin
Vitelline duct, persistent Q43.0
Vitiligo L80
　eyelid H02.739
　　left H02.736
　　　lower H02.735
　　　upper H02.734
　　right H02.733
　　　lower H02.732
　　　upper H02.731
　pinta A67.2
　vulva N90.89
Vitreal corneal syndrome H59.01- ☑
Vitreoretinopathy, proliferative — *see also* Retinopathy, proliferative
　with retinal detachment — *see* Detachment, retina, traction
Vitreous — *see also* condition
　touch syndrome — *see* Complication, postprocedural, following cataract surgery
Vocal cord — *see* condition
Vogt-Koyanagi syndrome H20.82- ☑
Vogt's disease or syndrome G80.3
Vogt-Spielmeyer amaurotic idiocy or disease E75.4
Voice
　change R49.9
　　specified NEC R49.8
　loss — *see* Aphonia
Volhynian fever A79.0
Volkmann's ischemic contracture or paralysis (complicating trauma) T79.6 ☑
Volvulus (bowel) (colon) (intestine) K56.2
　with perforation K56.2
　congenital Q43.8
　duodenum K31.5
　fallopian tube — *see* Torsion, fallopian tube
　oviduct — *see* Torsion, fallopian tube
　stomach (due to absence of gastrocolic ligament) K31.89
Vomiting R11.10
　with nausea R11.2
　asphyxia — *see* Foreign body, by site, causing asphyxia, gastric contents
　bilious (cause unknown) R11.14
　　following gastro-intestinal surgery K91.0
　　in newborn P92.01
　blood — *see* Hematemesis
　causing asphyxia, choking, or suffocation — *see* Foreign body, by site
　cyclical, in migraine G43.A0 (*following* G43.7)
　　with refractory migraine G43.A1 (*following* G43.7)
　　intractable G43.A1 (*following* G43.7)
　　not intractable G43.A0 (*following* G43.7)
　　psychogenic F50.89
　　without refractory migraine G43.A0 (*following* G43.7)
　cyclical syndrome NOS (unrelated to migraine) R11.15
　fecal mater R11.13
　following gastrointestinal surgery K91.0
　　psychogenic F50.89
　functional K31.89
　hysterical F50.89
　nervous F50.89
　neurotic F50.89
　newborn NEC P92.09
　　bilious P92.01
　periodic R11.10
　　psychogenic F50.89
　persistent R11.15
　projectile R11.12
　psychogenic F50.89
　uremic — *see* Uremia
　without nausea R11.11
Vomito negro — *see* Fever, yellow
Von Bezold's abscess — *see* Mastoiditis, acute
Von Economo-Cruchet disease A85.8
Von Eulenburg's disease G71.19
Von Gierke's disease E74.01
Von Hippel (-Lindau) **disease or syndrome** Q85.8
Von Jaksch's anemia or disease D64.89
Von Recklinghausen
　disease (neurofibromatosis) Q85.01
　bones E21.0
Von Schroetter's syndrome I82.890
Von Willebrand (-Jurgens)(-Minot) **disease or syndrome** D68.0
Von Zumbusch's disease L40.1
Voyeurism F65.3

☑ **Additional Character Required** — Refer to the Tabular List for Character Selection　　☵ Subterms under main terms may continue to next column or page

Vrolik's disease Q78.0
Vulva — *see* condition
Vulvismus N94.2
Vulvitis (acute) (allergic) (atrophic) (hypertrophic) (intertriginous) (senile) N76.2
  with ectopic or molar pregnancy O08.0
  adhesive, congenital Q52.79
  blennorrhagic (gonococcal) A54.02
  candidal B37.3
  chlamydial A56.02
  due to Haemophilus ducreyi A57
  following ectopic or molar pregnancy O08.0
  gonococcal A54.02
    with abscess (accessory gland) (periurethral) A54.1
  herpesviral A60.04
  leukoplakic N90.4
  monilial B37.3
  puerperal (postpartum) O86.19
  subacute or chronic N76.3
  syphilitic (early) A51.0
    late A52.76
  trichomonal A59.01
  tuberculous A18.18
Vulvodynia N94.819
  specified NEC N94.818
Vulvorectal — *see* condition
Vulvovaginitis (acute) — *see* Vaginitis

W

Waiting list, person on Z75.1
  for organ transplant Z76.82
  undergoing social agency investigation Z75.2
Waldenström
  hypergammaglobulinemia D89.0
  syndrome or macroglobulinemia C88.0
Waldenström-Kjellberg syndrome D50.1
Walking
  difficulty R26.2
    psychogenic F44.4
  sleep F51.3
    hysterical F44.89
Wall, abdominal — *see* condition
Wallenberg's disease or syndrome G46.3
Wallgren's disease I87.8
Wandering
  gallbladder, congenital Q44.1
  in diseases classified elsewhere Z91.83
  kidney, congenital Q63.8
  organ or site, congenital NEC — *see* Malposition, congenital, by site
  pacemaker (heart) I49.8
  spleen D73.89
War neurosis F48.8
Wart (due to HPV) (filiform) (infectious) (viral) B07.9
  anogenital region (venereal) A63.0
  common B07.8
  external genital organs (venereal) A63.0
  flat B07.8
  Hassal-Henle's (of cornea) H18.49
  Peruvian A44.1
  plantar B07.0
  prosector (tuberculous) A18.4
  seborrheic L82.1
    inflamed L82.0
  senile (seborrheic) L82.1
    inflamed L82.0
  tuberculous A18.4
  venereal A63.0
Warthin's tumor — *see* Neoplasm, salivary gland, benign
Wassilieff's disease A27.0
Wasting
  disease R64
    due to malnutrition E43
      with marasmus E41
  extreme (due to malnutrition) E43
    with marasmus E41
  muscle NEC — *see* Atrophy, muscle
Water
  clefts (senile cataract) — *see* Cataract, senile, incipient
  deprivation of T73.1 ☑
  intoxication E87.79
  itch B76.9
  lack of T73.1 ☑
    safe drinking Z58.6
  loading E87.70
  on
    brain — *see* Hydrocephalus

Water — *continued*
  on — *continued*
    chest J94.8
    poisoning E87.79
Waterbrash R12
Waterhouse (-Friderichsen) **syndrome or disease** (meningococcal) A39.1
Water-losing nephritis N25.89
Watermelon stomach K31.819
  with hemorrhage K31.811
  without hemorrhage K31.819
Watsoniasis B66.8
Wax in ear — *see* Impaction, cerumen
Weak, weakening, weakness (generalized) R53.1
  arches (acquired) — *see also* Deformity, limb, flat foot
  bladder (sphincter) R32
  facial R29.810
    following
      cerebrovascular disease I69.992
        cerebral infarction I69.392
        intracerebral hemorrhage I69.192
        nontraumatic intracranial hemorrhage NEC I69.292
        specified disease NEC I69.892
        stroke I69.392
        subarachnoid hemorrhage I69.092
  foot (double) — *see also* Weak, arches
  heart, cardiac — *see* Failure, heart
  mind F70
  muscle M62.81
  myocardium — *see* Failure, heart
  newborn P96.89
  pelvic fundus N81.89
  pubocervical tissue N81.82
  rectovaginal tissue N81.83
  senile R54
  urinary stream R39.12
  valvular — *see* Endocarditis
Wear, worn (with normal or routine use)
  articular bearing surface of internal joint prosthesis — *see* Complications, joint prosthesis, mechanical, wear of articular bearing surface, by site
  device, implant or graft — *see* Complications, by site, mechanical complication
  tooth, teeth (approximal) (hard tissues) (interproximal) (occlusal) K03.0
Weather, weathered
  effects of
    cold T69.9 ☑
      specified effect NEC T69.8 ☑
    hot — *see* Heat
    skin L57.8
Weaver's syndrome Q87.3
Web, webbed (congenital)
  duodenal Q43.8
  esophagus Q39.4
  fingers Q70.1- ☑
  larynx (glottic) (subglottic) Q31.0
  neck (pterygium colli) Q18.3
  Paterson-Kelly D50.1
  popliteal syndrome Q87.89
  toes Q70.3- ☑
Weber-Christian disease M35.6
Weber-Cockayne syndrome (epidermolysis bullosa) Q81.8
Weber-Gubler syndrome G46.3
Weber-Leyden syndrome G46.3
Weber-Osler syndrome I78.0
Weber's paralysis or syndrome G46.3
Wedge-shaped or wedging vertebra — *see* Collapse, vertebra NEC
Wegener's granulomatosis or syndrome M31.30
  with
    kidney involvement M31.31
    lung involvement M31.30
      with kidney involvement M31.31
Wegner's disease A50.02
Weight
  1000-2499 grams at birth (low) — *see* Low, birthweight
  999 grams or less at birth (extremely low) — *see* Low, birthweight, extreme
  and length below 10th percentile for gestational age P05.1- ☑
    below but length above 10th percentile for gestational age P05.0- ☑
  gain (abnormal) (excessive) R63.5

Weight — *continued*
  gain — *continued*
    in pregnancy — *see* Pregnancy, complicated by, excessive weight gain
      low — *see* Pregnancy, complicated by, insufficient, weight gain
  loss (abnormal) (cause unknown) R63.4
Weightlessness (effect of) T75.82 ☑
Weil (I)-**Marchesani syndrome** Q87.19
Weil's disease A27.0
Weingarten's syndrome J82.89
Weir Mitchell's disease I73.81
Weiss-Baker syndrome G90.09
Wells' disease L98.3
Wen — *see* Cyst, sebaceous
Wenckebach's block or phenomenon I44.1
Werdnig-Hoffmann syndrome (muscular atrophy) G12.0
Werlhof's disease D69.3
Wermer's disease or syndrome E31.21
Werner-His disease A79.0
Werner's disease or syndrome E34.8
Wernicke-Korsakoff's syndrome or psychosis (alcoholic) F10.96
  with dependence F10.26
  drug-induced
    due to drug abuse — *see* Abuse, drug, by type, with amnestic disorder
    due to drug dependence — *see* Dependence, drug, by type, with amnestic disorder
  nonalcoholic F04
Wernicke-Posadas disease B38.9
Wernicke's
  developmental aphasia F80.2
  disease or syndrome E51.2
  encephalopathy E51.2
  polioencephalitis, superior E51.2
West African fever B50.8
Westphal-Strümpell syndrome E83.01
West's syndrome — *see* Epilepsy, spasms
Wet
  feet, tropical (maceration) (syndrome) — *see* Immersion, foot
  lung (syndrome), newborn P22.1
Wharton's duct — *see* condition
Wheal — *see* Urticaria
Wheezing R06.2
Whiplash injury S13.4 ☑
Whipple's disease — *see also* subcategory M14.8- K90.81
Whipworm (disease) (infection) (infestation) B79
Whistling face Q87.0
White — *see also* condition
  kidney, small N03.9
  leg, puerperal, postpartum, childbirth O87.1
  mouth B37.0
  patches of mouth K13.29
  spot lesions, teeth
    chewing surface K02.51
    pit and fissure surface K02.51
    smooth surface K02.61
Whitehead L70.0
Whitlow — *see also* Cellulitis, digit
  with lymphangitis — *see* Lymphangitis, acute, digit
  herpesviral B00.89
Whitmore's disease or fever — *see* Melioidosis
Whooping cough A37.90
  with pneumonia A37.91
    due to Bordetella
      bronchiseptica A37.81
      parapertussis A37.11
      pertussis A37.01
    specified organism NEC A37.81
  due to
    Bordetella
      bronchiseptica A37.80
        with pneumonia A37.81
      parapertussis A37.10
        with pneumonia A37.11
      pertussis A37.00
        with pneumonia A37.01
    specified NEC A37.80
      with pneumonia A37.81
Wichman's asthma J38.5
Wide cranial sutures, newborn P96.3
Widening aorta — *see* Ectasia, aorta
  with aneurysm — *see* Aneurysm, aorta
Wilkie's disease or syndrome K55.1

Wilkinson-Sneddon disease or syndrome L13.1
Willebrand (-Jürgens) **thrombopathy** D68.0
Williams syndrome Q93.82
Willige-Hunt disease or syndrome G23.1
Wilms' tumor C64- ☑
Wilson-Mikity syndrome P27.0
Wilson's
  disease or syndrome E83.01
  hepatolenticular degeneration E83.01
  lichen ruber L43.9
Window — *see also* Imperfect, closure
  aorticopulmonary Q21.4
Winter — *see* condition
Wiskott-Aldrich syndrome D82.0
Withdrawal state — *see also* Dependence, drug by type, with withdrawal
  alcohol
    with perceptual disturbances F10.232
    without perceptual disturbances F10.239
  caffeine F15.93
  cannabis F12.23
  newborn
    correct therapeutic substance properly administered P96.2
    infant of dependent mother P96.1
  therapeutic substance, neonatal P96.2
Witts' anemia D50.8
Witzelsucht F07.0
Woakes' ethmoiditis or syndrome J33.1
Wolff-Hirschhorn syndrome Q93.3
Wolff-Parkinson-White syndrome I45.6
Wolhynian fever A79.0
Wolman's disease E75.5
Wood lung or pneumonitis J67.8
Woolly, wooly hair (congenital) (nevus) Q84.1
Woolsorter's disease A22.1
Word
  blindness (congenital) (developmental) F81.0
  deafness (congenital) (developmental) H93.25
Worm(s) (infection) (infestation) — *see also* Infestation, helminth
  guinea B72
  in intestine NEC B82.0
Worm-eaten soles A66.3
Worn out — *see* Exhaustion
  cardiac
    defibrillator (with synchronous cardiac pacemaker) Z45.02
    pacemaker
      battery Z45.010
      lead Z45.018
  device, implant or graft — *see* Complications, by site, mechanical
Worried well Z71.1
Worries R45.82
Wound check Z48.0- ☑
  due to injury — *code to* Injury, by site, using appropriate seventh character for subsequent encounter
Wound, open T14.8- ☑
  abdomen, abdominal
    wall S31.109 ☑
      with penetration into peritoneal cavity S31.609 ☑
      bite — *see* Bite, abdomen, wall
      epigastric region S31.102 ☑
        with penetration into peritoneal cavity S31.602 ☑
        bite — *see* Bite, abdomen, wall, epigastric region
        laceration — *see* Laceration, abdomen, wall, epigastric region
        puncture — *see* Puncture, abdomen, wall, epigastric region
      laceration — *see* Laceration, abdomen, wall
      left
        lower quadrant S31.104 ☑
          with penetration into peritoneal cavity S31.604 ☑
          bite — *see* Bite, abdomen, wall, left, lower quadrant
          laceration — *see* Laceration, abdomen, wall, left, lower quadrant
          puncture — *see* Puncture, abdomen, wall, left, lower quadrant
        upper quadrant S31.101 ☑
          with penetration into peritoneal cavity S31.601 ☑

Wound, open — *continued*
  abdomen, abdominal — *continued*
    wall — *continued*
      left — *continued*
        upper quadrant — *continued*
          bite — *see* Bite, abdomen, wall, left, upper quadrant
          laceration — *see* Laceration, abdomen, wall, left, upper quadrant
          puncture — *see* Puncture, abdomen, wall, left, upper quadrant
      periumbilic region S31.105 ☑
        with penetration into peritoneal cavity S31.605 ☑
        bite — *see* Bite, abdomen, wall, periumbilic region
        laceration — *see* Laceration, abdomen, wall, periumbilic region
        puncture — *see* Puncture, abdomen, wall, periumbilic region
      puncture — *see* Puncture, abdomen, wall
      right
        lower quadrant S31.103 ☑
          with penetration into peritoneal cavity S31.603 ☑
          bite — *see* Bite, abdomen, wall, right, lower quadrant
          laceration — *see* Laceration, abdomen, wall, right, lower quadrant
          puncture — *see* Puncture, abdomen, wall, right, lower quadrant
        upper quadrant S31.100 ☑
          with penetration into peritoneal cavity S31.600 ☑
          bite — *see* Bite, abdomen, wall, right, upper quadrant
          laceration — *see* Laceration, abdomen, wall, right, upper quadrant
          puncture — *see* Puncture, abdomen, wall, right, upper quadrant
  alveolar (process) — *see* Wound, open, oral cavity
  ankle S91.00- ☑
    bite — *see* Bite, ankle
    laceration — *see* Laceration, ankle
    puncture — *see* Puncture, ankle
  antecubital space — *see* Wound, open, elbow
  anterior chamber, eye — *see* Wound, open, ocular
  anus S31.839 ☑
    bite S31.835 ☑
    laceration — *see* Laceration, anus
    puncture — *see* Puncture, anus
  arm (upper) S41.10- ☑
    with amputation — *see* Amputation, traumatic, arm
    bite — *see* Bite, arm
    forearm — *see* Wound, open, forearm
    laceration — *see* Laceration, arm
    puncture — *see* Puncture, arm
  auditory canal (external) (meatus) — *see* Wound, open, ear
  auricle, ear — *see* Wound, open, ear
  axilla — *see* Wound, open, arm
  back — *see also* Wound, open, thorax, back
    lower S31.000 ☑
      with penetration into retroperitoneal space S31.001 ☑
      bite — *see* Bite, back, lower
      laceration — *see* Laceration, back, lower
      puncture — *see* Puncture, back, lower
  bite — *see* Bite
  blood vessel — *see* Injury, blood vessel
  breast S21.0- ☑
    with amputation — *see* Amputation, traumatic, breast
    bite — *see* Bite, breast
    laceration — *see* Laceration, breast
    puncture — *see* Puncture, breast
  buttock S31.809 ☑
    bite — *see* Bite, buttock
    laceration — *see* Laceration, buttock
    left S31.829 ☑
    puncture — *see* Puncture, buttock
    right S31.819 ☑
  calf — *see* Wound, open, leg
  canaliculus lacrimalis — *see* Wound, open, eyelid
  canthus, eye — *see* Wound, open, eyelid
  cervical esophagus S11.20 ☑
    bite S11.25 ☑

Wound, open — *continued*
  cervical esophagus — *continued*
    laceration — *see* Laceration, esophagus, traumatic, cervical
    puncture — *see* Puncture, cervical esophagus
  cheek (external) S01.40- ☑
    bite — *see* Bite, cheek
    internal — *see* Wound, open, oral cavity
    laceration — *see* Laceration, cheek
    puncture — *see* Puncture, cheek
  chest wall — *see* Wound, open, thorax
  chin — *see* Wound, open, head, specified site NEC
  choroid — *see* Wound, open, ocular
  ciliary body (eye) — *see* Wound, open, ocular
  clitoris S31.40 ☑
    with amputation — *see* Amputation, traumatic, clitoris
    bite S31.45 ☑
    laceration — *see* Laceration, vulva
    puncture — *see* Puncture, vulva
  conjunctiva — *see* Wound, open, ocular
  cornea — *see* Wound, open, ocular
  costal region — *see* Wound, open, thorax
  Descemet's membrane — *see* Wound, open, ocular
  digit(s)
    foot — *see* Wound, open, toe
    hand — *see* Wound, open, finger
  ear (canal) (external) S01.30- ☑
    with amputation — *see* Amputation, traumatic, ear
    bite — *see* Bite, ear
    drum S09.2- ☑
    laceration — *see* Laceration, ear
    puncture — *see* Puncture, ear
  elbow S51.00- ☑
    bite — *see* Bite, elbow
    laceration — *see* Laceration, elbow
    puncture — *see* Puncture, elbow
  epididymis — *see* Wound, open, testis
  epigastric region S31.102 ☑
    with penetration into peritoneal cavity S31.602 ☑
    bite — *see* Bite, abdomen, wall, epigastric region
    laceration — *see* Laceration, abdomen, wall, epigastric region
    puncture — *see* Puncture, abdomen, wall, epigastric region
  epiglottis — *see* Wound, open, neck, specified site NEC
  esophagus (thoracic) S27.819 ☑
    cervical — *see* Wound, open, cervical esophagus
    laceration S27.813 ☑
    specified type NEC S27.818 ☑
  eye — *see* Wound, open, ocular
  eyeball — *see* Wound, open, ocular
  eyebrow — *see* Wound, open, eyelid
  eyelid S01.10- ☑
    bite — *see* Bite, eyelid
    laceration — *see* Laceration, eyelid
    puncture — *see* Puncture, eyelid
  face NEC — *see* Wound, open, head, specified site NEC
  finger(s) S61.209 ☑
    with
      amputation — *see* Amputation, traumatic, finger
      damage to nail S61.309 ☑
    bite — *see* Bite, finger
    index S61.208 ☑
      with
        damage to nail S61.308 ☑
      left S61.201 ☑
        with
          damage to nail S61.301 ☑
      right S61.200 ☑
        with
          damage to nail S61.300 ☑
    laceration — *see* Laceration, finger
    little S61.208 ☑
      with
        damage to nail S61.308 ☑
      left S61.207 ☑
        with damage to nail S61.307 ☑
      right S61.206 ☑
        with damage to nail S61.306 ☑
    middle S61.208 ☑
      with
        damage to nail S61.308 ☑
      left S61.203 ☑
        with damage to nail S61.303 ☑
      right S61.202 ☑

☑ **Additional Character Required** — Refer to the Tabular List for Character Selection   ▽ **Subterms under main terms may continue to next column or page**

Wound, open — *continued*
  right — *continued*
    upper quadrant — *continued*
      laceration — *see* Laceration, abdomen, wall, right, upper quadrant
      puncture — *see* Puncture, abdomen, wall, right, upper quadrant
  sacral region — *see* Wound, open, back, lower
  sacroiliac region — *see* Wound, open, back, lower
  salivary gland — *see* Wound, open, oral cavity
  scalp S01.00 ☑
    bite S01.05 ☑
    laceration — *see* Laceration, scalp
    puncture — *see* Puncture, scalp
  scalpel, newborn (birth injury) P15.8
  scapular region — *see* Wound, open, shoulder
  sclera — *see* Wound, open, ocular
  scrotum S31.30 ☑
    with amputation — *see* Amputation, traumatic, scrotum
    bite S31.35 ☑
    laceration — *see* Laceration, scrotum
    puncture — *see* Puncture, scrotum
  shin — *see* Wound, open, leg
  shoulder S41.00- ☑
    with amputation — *see* Amputation, traumatic, arm
    bite — *see* Bite, shoulder
    laceration — *see* Laceration, shoulder
    puncture — *see* Puncture, shoulder
  skin NOS T14.8 ☑
  spermatic cord — *see* Wound, open, testis
  sternal region — *see* Wound, open, thorax, front wall
  submaxillary region — *see* Wound, open, head, specified site NEC
  submental region — *see* Wound, open, head, specified site NEC
  subungual
    finger(s) — *see* Wound, open, finger
    toe(s) — *see* Wound, open, toe
  supraclavicular region — *see* Wound, open, neck, specified site NEC
  temple, temporal region — *see* Wound, open, head, specified site NEC
  temporomandibular area — *see* Wound, open, cheek
  testis S31.30 ☑
    with amputation — *see* Amputation, traumatic, testes
    bite S31.35 ☑
    laceration — *see* Laceration, testis
    puncture — *see* Puncture, testis
  thigh S71.10- ☑
    with amputation — *see* Amputation, traumatic, hip
    bite — *see* Bite, thigh
    laceration — *see* Laceration, thigh
    puncture — *see* Puncture, thigh
  thorax, thoracic (wall) S21.90 ☑
    back S21.20- ☑
      with penetration S21.40 ☑
    bite — *see* Bite, thorax
    breast — *see* Wound, open, breast
    front S21.10- ☑
      with penetration S21.30 ☑
    laceration — *see* Laceration, thorax
    puncture — *see* Puncture, thorax
  throat — *see* Wound, open, neck
  thumb S61.009 ☑
    with
      amputation — *see* Amputation, traumatic, thumb
      damage to nail S61.109 ☑
    bite — *see* Bite, thumb
    laceration — *see* Laceration, thumb
    left S61.002 ☑
      with
        damage to nail S61.102 ☑
    puncture — *see* Puncture, thumb
    right S61.001 ☑
      with
        damage to nail S61.101 ☑
  thyroid (gland) — *see* Wound, open, neck, thyroid
  toe(s) S91.109 ☑
    with
      amputation — *see* Amputation, traumatic, toe
      damage to nail S91.209 ☑
    bite — *see* Bite, toe
    great S91.103 ☑

Wound, open — *continued*
  toe(s) — *continued*
    great — *continued*
      with
        damage to nail S91.203 ☑
      left S91.102 ☑
        with
          damage to nail S91.202 ☑
      right S91.101 ☑
        with
          damage to nail S91.201 ☑
      laceration — *see* Laceration, toe
    lesser S91.106 ☑
      with
        damage to nail S91.206 ☑
      left S91.105 ☑
        with
          damage to nail S91.205 ☑
      right S91.104 ☑
        with
          damage to nail S91.204 ☑
    puncture — *see* Puncture, toe
  tongue — *see* Wound, open, oral cavity
  trachea (cervical region) — *see* Wound, open, neck, trachea
  tunica vaginalis — *see* Wound, open, testis
  tympanum, tympanic membrane S09.2- ☑
    laceration — *see* Laceration, ear, drum
    puncture — *see* Puncture, tympanum
  umbilical region — *see* Wound, open, abdomen, wall, periumbilic region
  uvula — *see* Wound, open, oral cavity
  vagina S31.40 ☑
    bite S31.45 ☑
    laceration — *see* Laceration, vagina
    puncture — *see* Puncture, vagina
  vitreous (humor) — *see* Wound, open, ocular
  vocal cord S11.039 ☑
    bite — *see* Bite, vocal cord
    laceration S11.031 ☑
      with foreign body S11.032 ☑
    puncture S11.033 ☑
      with foreign body S11.034 ☑
  vulva S31.40 ☑
    with amputation — *see* Amputation, traumatic, vulva
    bite S31.45 ☑
    laceration — *see* Laceration, vulva
    puncture — *see* Puncture, vulva
  wrist S61.50- ☑
    bite — *see* Bite, wrist
    laceration — *see* Laceration, wrist
    puncture — *see* Puncture, wrist
Wound, superficial — *see* Injury — *see also* specified injury type
Wright's syndrome G54.0
Wrist — *see* condition
Wrong drug (by accident) (given in error) — *see* Table of Drugs and Chemicals, by drug, poisoning
Wry neck — *see* Torticollis
Wuchereria (bancrofti) **infestation** B74.0
Wuchereriasis B74.0
Wuchernde Struma Langhans C73

X

Xanthelasma (eyelid) (palpebrarum) H02.60
  left H02.66
    lower H02.65
    upper H02.64
  right H02.63
    lower H02.62
    upper H02.61
Xanthelasmatosis (essential) E78.2
Xanthinuria, hereditary E79.8
Xanthoastrocytoma
  specified site — *see* Neoplasm, malignant, by site
  unspecified site C71.9
Xanthofibroma — *see* Neoplasm, connective tissue, benign
Xanthogranuloma D76.3
Xanthoma(s), xanthomatosis (primary) (familial) (hereditary) E75.5
  with
    hyperlipoproteinemia
      Type I E78.3
      Type III E78.2

Xanthoma(s), xanthomatosis — *continued*
  with — *continued*
    hyperlipoproteinemia — *continued*
      Type IV E78.1
      Type V E78.3
  bone (generalisata) C96.5
  cerebrotendinous E75.5
  cutaneotendinous E75.5
  disseminatum (skin) E78.2
  eruptive E78.2
  hypercholesterinemic E78.00
  hypercholesterolemic E78.00
  hyperlipidemic E78.5
  joint E75.5
  multiple (skin) E78.2
  tendon (sheath) E75.5
  tuberosum E78.2
  tuberous E78.2
  tubo-eruptive E78.2
  verrucous, oral mucosa K13.4
Xanthosis R23.8
Xenophobia F40.10
Xeroderma — *see also* Ichthyosis
  acquired L85.0
    eyelid H01.149
      left H01.146
        lower H01.145
        upper H01.144
      right H01.143
        lower H01.142
        upper H01.141
  pigmentosum Q82.1
  vitamin A deficiency E50.8
Xerophthalmia (vitamin A deficiency) E50.7
  unrelated to vitamin A deficiency — *see* Keratoconjunctivitis
Xerosis
  conjunctiva H11.14- ☑
    with Bitot's spots — *see also* Pigmentation, conjunctiva
      vitamin A deficiency E50.1
    vitamin A deficiency E50.0
  cornea H18.89- ☑
    with ulceration — *see* Ulcer, cornea
      vitamin A deficiency E50.3
    vitamin A deficiency E50.2
  cutis (dry skin) L85.3
  skin L85.3
Xerostomia K11.7
Xiphopagus Q89.4
XO syndrome Q96.9
X-ray (of)
  abnormal findings — *see* Abnormal, diagnostic imaging
  breast (mammogram) (routine) Z12.31
  chest
    routine (as part of a general medical examination) Z00.00
      with abnormal findings Z00.01
  routine (as part of a general medical examination) Z00.00
    with abnormal findings Z00.01
XXXXY syndrome Q98.1
XXY syndrome Q98.0

Y

Yaba pox (virus disease) B08.72
Yatapoxvirus B08.70
  specified NEC B08.79
Yawning R06.89
  psychogenic F45.8
Yaws A66.9
  bone lesions A66.6
  butter A66.1
  chancre A66.0
  cutaneous, less than five years after infection A66.2
  early (cutaneous) (macular) (maculopapular) (micropapular) (papular) A66.2
    frambeside A66.2
    skin lesions NEC A66.2
  eyelid A66.2
  ganglion A66.6
  gangosis, gangosa A66.5
  gumma, gummata A66.4
    bone A66.6
  gummatous
    frambeside A66.4
    osteitis A66.6

☑ Additional Character Required — Refer to the Tabular List for Character Selection   ▽ Subterms under main terms may continue to next column or page

Yaws — *continued*
  gummatous — *continued*
    periostitis A66.6
  hydrarthrosis — *see also* subcategory M14.8- A66.6
  hyperkeratosis (early) (late) A66.3
  initial lesions A66.0
  joint lesions — *see also* subcategory M14.8- A66.6
  juxta-articular nodules A66.7
  late nodular (ulcerated) A66.4
  latent (without clinical manifestations) (with positive
    serology) A66.8
  mother A66.0
  mucosal A66.7
  multiple papillomata A66.1
  nodular, late (ulcerated) A66.4
  osteitis A66.6
  papilloma, plantar or palmar A66.1
  periostitis (hypertrophic) A66.6

Yaws — *continued*
  specified NEC A66.7
  ulcers A66.4
  wet crab A66.1
Yeast infection — *see also* Candidiasis B37.9
Yellow
  atrophy (liver) — *see* Failure, hepatic
  fever — *see* Fever, yellow
  jack — *see* Fever, yellow
  jaundice — *see* Jaundice
  nail syndrome L60.5
Yersiniosis — *see also* Infection, Yersinia
  extraintestinal A28.2
  intestinal A04.6

Z

Zahorsky's syndrome (herpangina) B08.5

Zellweger's syndrome E71.510
Zenker's diverticulum (esophagus) K22.5
Ziehen-Oppenheim disease G24.1
Zieve's syndrome K70.0
Zika NOS A92.5
  congenital P35.4
Zinc
  deficiency, dietary E60
  metabolism disorder E83.2
Zollinger-Ellison syndrome E16.4
Zona — *see* Herpes, zoster
Zoophobia F40.218
Zoster (herpes) — *see* Herpes, zoster
Zygomycosis B46.9
  specified NEC B46.8
Zymotic — *see* condition

⬡ **Subterms under main terms may continue to next column or page**   ☑ **Additional Character Required — Refer to the Tabular List for Character Selection**   335

Yaws — Zymotic

Neoplasm Table

Note: The list below gives the code number for neoplasms by anatomical site. For each site there are six possible code numbers according to whether the neoplasm in question is malignant, benign, in situ, of uncertain behavior, or of unspecified nature. The description of the neoplasm will often indicate which of the six columns is appropriate; e.g., malignant melanoma of skin, benign fibroadenoma of breast, carcinoma in situ of cervix uteri. Where such descriptors are not present, the remainder of the Index should be consulted where guidance is given to the appropriate column for each morphological (histological) variety listed; e.g., Mesonephroma – see Neoplasm, malignant; Embryoma — see also Neoplasm, uncertain behavior; Disease, Bowen's – see Neoplasm, skin, in situ. However, the guidance in the Index can be overridden if one of the descriptors mentioned above is present; e.g., malignant adenoma of colon is coded to C18.9 and not to D12.6 as the adjective "malignant" overrides the Index entry "Adenoma — see also Neoplasm, benign, by site." Codes listed with a dash -, following the code have a required additional character for laterality. The tabular list must be reviewed for the complete code.

	Malignant Primary	Malignant Secondary	Ca in situ	Benign	Uncertain Behavior	Unspecified Behavior
Neoplasm, neoplastic	C80.1	C79.9	D09.9	D36.9	D48.9	D49.9
abdomen,						
abdominal	C76.2	C79.8-☑	D09.8	D36.7	D48.7	D49.89
cavity	C76.2	C79.8-☑	D09.8	D36.7	D48.7	D49.89
organ	C76.2	C79.8-☑	D09.8	D36.7	D48.7	D49.89
viscera	C76.2	C79.8-☑	D09.8	D36.7	D48.7	D49.89
wall — see also Neoplasm, abdomen, wall, skin						
connective tissue	C49.4	C79.8-☑	—	D21.4	D48.1	D49.2
skin	C44.509	C79.2	D04.5	D23.5	D48.5	D49.2
basal cell carcinoma	C44.519	—	—	—	—	—
specified type NEC	C44.599	—	—	—	—	—
squamous cell carcinoma	C44.529	—	—	—	—	—
abdominopelvic	C76.8	C79.8-☑		D36.7	D48.7	D49.89
accessory sinus — see Neoplasm, sinus						
acoustic nerve	C72.4-☑	C79.49	—	D33.3	D43.3	D49.7
adenoid (pharynx) (tissue)	C11.1	C79.89	D00.08	D10.6	D37.05	D49.0
adipose tissue — see also Neoplasm, connective tissue	C49.4	C79.89	—	D21.9	D48.1	D49.2
adnexa (uterine)	C57.4	C79.89	D07.39	D28.7	D39.8	D49.59
adrenal	C74.9-☑	C79.7-☑	D09.3	D35.0-☑	D44.1-☑	D49.7
capsule	C74.9-☑	C79.7-☑	D09.3	D35.0-☑	D44.1-☑	D49.7
cortex	C74.0-☑	C79.7-☑	D09.3	D35.0-☑	D44.1-☑	D49.7
gland	C74.9-☑	C79.7-☑	D09.3	D35.0-☑	D44.1-☑	D49.7
medulla	C74.1-☑	C79.7-☑	D09.3	D35.0-☑	D44.1-☑	D49.7
ala nasi (external) — see also Neoplasm, skin, nose	C44.301	C79.2	D04.39	D23.39	D48.5	D49.2
alimentary canal or tract NEC	C26.9	C78.80	D01.9	D13.9	D37.9	D49.0
alveolar	C03.9	C79.89	D00.03	D10.39	D37.09	D49.0
mucosa	C03.9	C79.89	D00.03	D10.39	D37.09	D49.0
lower	C03.1	C79.89	D00.03	D10.39	D37.09	D49.0
upper	C03.0	C79.89	D00.03	D10.39	D37.09	D49.0
ridge or process	C41.1	C79.51	—	D16.5	D48.0	D49.2
carcinoma	C03.9	C79.8-☑	—	—	—	—
lower	C03.1	C79.8-☑	—	—	—	—
upper	C03.0	C79.8-☑	—	—	—	—
lower	C41.1	C79.51	—	D16.5	D48.0	D49.2
mucosa	C03.9	C79.89	D00.03	D10.39	D37.09	D49.0
lower	C03.1	C79.89	D00.03	D10.39	D37.09	D49.0
upper	C03.0	C79.89	D00.03	D10.39	D37.09	D49.0
upper	C41.0	C79.51	—	D16.4	D48.0	D49.2
sulcus	C06.1	C79.89	D00.02	D10.39	D37.09	D49.0
alveolus	C03.9	C79.89	D00.03	D10.39	D37.09	D49.0
lower	C03.1	C79.89	D00.03	D10.39	D37.09	D49.0
upper	C03.0	C79.89	D00.03	D10.39	D37.09	D49.0
ampulla of Vater	C24.1	C78.89	D01.5	D13.5	D37.6	D49.0
ankle NEC	C76.5-☑	C79.89	D04.7-☑	D36.7	D48.7	D49.89
anorectum, anorectal (junction)	C21.8	C78.5	D01.3	D12.9	D37.8	D49.0
antecubital fossa or space	C76.4-☑	C79.89	D04.6-☑	D36.7	D48.7	D49.89

	Malignant Primary	Malignant Secondary	Ca in situ	Benign	Uncertain Behavior	Unspecified Behavior
Neoplasm, neoplastic						
— continued						
antrum (Highmore) (maxillary)	C31.0	C78.39	D02.3	D14.0	D38.5	D49.1
pyloric	C16.3	C78.89	D00.2	D13.1	D37.1	D49.0
tympanicum	C30.1	C78.39	D02.3	D14.0	D38.5	D49.1
anus, anal	C21.0	C78.5	D01.3	D12.9	D37.8	D49.0
canal	C21.1	C78.5	D01.3	D12.9	D37.8	D49.0
cloacogenic zone	C21.2	C78.5	D01.3	D12.9	D37.8	D49.0
margin — see also Neoplasm, anus, skin	C44.500	C79.2	D04.5	D23.5	D48.5	D49.2
overlapping lesion with rectosigmoid junction or rectum	C21.8	—	—	—	—	—
skin	C44.500	C79.2	D04.5	D23.5	D48.5	D49.2
basal cell carcinoma	C44.510	—	—	—	—	—
specified type NEC	C44.590	—	—	—	—	—
squamous cell carcinoma	C44.520	—	—	—	—	—
sphincter	C21.1	C78.5	D01.3	D12.9	D37.8	D49.0
aorta (thoracic)	C49.3	C79.89	—	D21.3	D48.1	D49.2
abdominal	C49.4	C79.89	—	D21.4	D48.1	D49.2
aortic body	C75.5	C79.89	—	D35.6	D44.7	D49.7
aponeurosis	C49.9	C79.89	—	D21.9	D48.1	D49.2
palmar	C49.1-☑	C79.89	—	D21.1-☑	D48.1	D49.2
plantar	C49.2-☑	C79.89	—	D21.2-☑	D48.1	D49.2
appendix	C18.1	C78.5	D01.0	D12.1	D37.3	D49.0
arachnoid	C70.9	C79.49	—	D32.9	D42.9	D49.7
cerebral	C70.0	C79.32	—	D32.0	D42.0	D49.7
spinal	C70.1	C79.49	—	D32.1	D42.1	D49.7
areola	C50.0-☑	C79.81	D05-☑	D24-☑	D48.6-☑	D49.3
arm NEC	C76.4-☑	C79.89	D04.6-☑	D36.7	D48.7	D49.89
artery — see Neoplasm, connective tissue						
aryepiglottic fold	C13.1	C79.89	D00.08	D10.7	D37.05	D49.0
hypopharyngeal aspect	C13.1	C79.89	D00.08	D10.7	D37.05	D49.0
laryngeal aspect	C32.1	C78.39	D02.0	D14.1	D38.0	D49.1
marginal zone	C13.1	C79.89	D00.08	D10.7	D37.05	D49.0
arytenoid (cartilage)	C32.3	C78.39	D02.0	D14.1	D38.0	D49.1
fold — see Neoplasm, aryepiglottic						
associated with transplanted organ	C80.2	—		—	—	—
atlas	C41.2	C79.51	—	D16.6	D48.0	D49.2
atrium, cardiac	C38.0	C79.89	—	D15.1	D48.7	D49.89
auditory						
canal (external) (skin)	C44.20-☑	C79.2	D04.2-☑	D23.2-☑	D48.5	D49.2
internal	C30.1	C78.39	D02.3	D14.0	D38.5	D49.1
nerve	C72.4-☑	C79.49	—	D33.3	D43.3	D49.7
tube	C30.1	C78.39	D02.3	D14.0	D38.5	D49.1
opening	C11.2	C79.89	D00.08	D10.6	D37.05	D49.0
auricle, ear — see also Neoplasm, skin, ear	C44.20-☑	C79.2	D04.2-☑	D23.2-☑	D48.5	D49.2
auricular canal (external) — see also Neoplasm, skin, ear	C44.20-☑	C79.2	D04.2-☑	D23.2-☑	D48.5	D49.2
internal	C30.1	C78.39	D02.3	D14.0	D38.5	D49.2
autonomic nerve or nervous system NEC (see Neoplasm, nerve, peripheral)						
axilla, axillary	C76.1	C79.89	D09.8	D36.7	D48.7	D49.89
fold — see also Neoplasm, skin, trunk	C44.509	C79.2	D04.5	D23.5	D48.5	D49.2
back NEC	C76.8	C79.89	D04.5	D36.7	D48.7	D49.89
Bartholin's gland	C51.0	C79.82	D07.1	D28.0	D39.8	D49.59
basal ganglia	C71.0	C79.31	—	D33.0	D43.0	D49.6
basis pedunculi	C71.7	C79.31	—	D33.1	D43.1	D49.6
bile or biliary (tract)	C24.9	C78.89	D01.5	D13.5	D37.6	D49.0

☑ Additional Character Required — Refer to the Tabular List for Character Selection   ▽ Subterms under main terms may continue to next column or page

Neoplasm, abdomen, abdominal — Neoplasm, bile or biliary

Neoplasm, neoplastic — continued	Malignant Primary	Malignant Secondary	Ca in situ	Benign	Uncertain Behavior	Unspecified Behavior
bile or biliary — continued						
canaliculi (biliferi) (intrahepatic)	C22.1	C78.7	D01.5	D13.4	D37.6	D49.0
canals, interlobular	C22.1	C78.89	D01.5	D13.4	D37.6	D49.0
duct or passage (common) (cystic) (extrahepatic)	C24.0	C78.89	D01.5	D13.5	D37.6	D49.0
interlobular	C22.1	C78.89	D01.5	D13.4	D37.6	D49.0
intrahepatic	C22.1	C78.7	D01.5	D13.4	D37.6	D49.0
and extrahepatic	C24.8	C78.89	D01.5	D13.5	D37.6	D49.0
bladder (urinary)	C67.9	C79.11	D09.0	D30.3	D41.4	D49.4
dome	C67.1	C79.11	D09.0	D30.3	D41.4	D49.4
neck	C67.5	C79.11	D09.0	D30.3	D41.4	D49.4
orifice	C67.9	C79.11	D09.0	D30.3	D41.4	D49.4
ureteric	C67.6	C79.11	D09.0	D30.3	D41.4	D49.4
urethral	C67.5	C79.11	D09.0	D30.3	D41.4	D49.4
overlapping lesion	C67.8	—	—	—	—	—
sphincter	C67.8	C79.11	D09.0	D30.3	D41.4	D49.4
trigone	C67.0	C79.11	D09.0	D30.3	D41.4	D49.4
urachus	C67.7	C79.11	D09.0	D30.3	D41.4	D49.4
wall	C67.9	C79.11	D09.0	D30.3	D41.4	D49.4
anterior	C67.3	C79.11	D09.0	D30.3	D41.4	D49.4
lateral	C67.2	C79.11	D09.0	D30.3	D41.4	D49.4
posterior	C67.4	C79.11	D09.0	D30.3	D41.4	D49.4
blood vessel — see Neoplasm, connective tissue						
bone (periosteum)	C41.9	C79.51	—	D16.9-	D48.0	D49.2
acetabulum	C40.3-☑	C79.51	—	D16.3-☑	—	—
ankle	C40.3-☑	C79.51	—	D16.3-☑	—	—
arm NEC	C40.0-☑	C79.51	—	D16.0-☑	—	—
astragalus	C40.3-☑	C79.51	—	D16.3-☑	—	—
atlas	C41.2	C79.51	—	D16.6	D48.0	D49.2
axis	C41.2	C79.51	—	D16.6	D48.0	D49.2
back NEC	C41.2	C79.51	—	D16.6	D48.0	D49.2
calcaneus	C40.3-☑	C79.51	—	D16.3-☑	—	—
calvarium	C41.0	C79.51	—	D16.4	D48.0	D49.2
carpus (any)	C40.1-☑	C79.51	—	D16.1-☑	—	—
cartilage NEC	C41.9	C79.51	—	D16.9	D48.0	D49.2
clavicle	C41.3	C79.51	—	D16.7	D48.0	D49.2
clivus	C41.0	C79.51	—	D16.4	D48.0	D49.2
coccygeal vertebra	C41.4	C79.51	—	D16.8	D48.0	D49.2
coccyx	C41.4	C79.51	—	D16.8	D48.0	D49.2
costal cartilage	C41.3	C79.51	—	D16.7	D48.0	D49.2
costovertebral joint	C41.3	C79.51	—	D16.7	D48.0	D49.2
cranial	C41.0	C79.51	—	D16.4	D48.0	D49.2
cuboid	C40.3-☑	C79.51	—	D16.3-☑	—	—
cuneiform	C41.9	C79.51	—	D16.9	D48.0	D49.2
elbow	C40.0-☑	C79.51	—	D16.0-☑	—	—
ethmoid (labyrinth)	C41.0	C79.51	—	D16.4	D48.0	D49.2
face	C41.0	C79.51	—	D16.4	D48.0	D49.2
femur (any part)	C40.2-☑	C79.51	—	D16.2-☑	—	—
fibula (any part)	C40.2-☑	C79.51	—	D16.2-☑	—	—
finger (any)	C40.1-☑	C79.51	—	D16.1-☑	—	—
foot	C40.3-☑	C79.51	—	D16.3-☑	—	—
forearm	C40.0-☑	C79.51	—	D16.0-☑	—	—
frontal	C41.0	C79.51	—	D16.4	D48.0	D49.2
hand	C40.1-☑	C79.51	—	D16.1-☑	—	—
heel	C40.3-☑	C79.51	—	D16.3-☑	—	—
hip	C41.4	C79.51	—	D16.8	D48.0	D49.2
humerus (any part)	C40.0-☑	C79.51	—	D16.0-☑	—	—
hyoid	C41.0	C79.51	—	D16.4	D48.0	D49.2
ilium	C41.4	C79.51	—	D16.8	D48.0	D49.2
innominate	C41.4	C79.51	—	D16.8	D48.0	D49.2
intervertebral cartilage or disc	C41.2	C79.51	—	D16.6	D48.0	D49.2
ischium	C41.4	C79.51	—	D16.8	D48.0	D49.2
jaw (lower)	C41.1	C79.51	—	D16.5	D48.0	D49.2
knee	C40.2-☑	C79.51	—	D16.2-☑	—	—
leg NEC	C40.2-☑	C79.51	—	D16.2-☑	—	—
limb NEC	C40.9-☑	C79.51	—	D16.9	—	—

Neoplasm, neoplastic — continued	Malignant Primary	Malignant Secondary	Ca in situ	Benign	Uncertain Behavior	Unspecified Behavior
bone — continued						
limb — continued						
lower (long bones)	C40.2-☑	C79.51	—	D16.2-☑	—	—
short bones	C40.3-☑	C79.51	—	D16.3-☑	—	—
upper (long bones)	C40.0-☑	C79.51	—	D16.0-☑	—	—
short bones	C40.1-☑	C79.51	—	D16.1-☑	—	—
malar	C41.0	C79.51	—	D16.4	D48.0	D49.2
mandible	C41.1	C79.51	—	D16.5	D48.0	D49.2
marrow NEC (any bone)	C96.9	C79.52	—	—	D47.9	D49.89
mastoid	C41.0	C79.51	—	D16.4	D48.0	D49.2
maxilla, maxillary (superior)	C41.0	C79.51	—	D16.4	D48.0	D49.2
inferior	C41.1	C79.51	—	D16.5	D48.0	D49.2
metacarpus (any)	C40.1-☑	C79.51	—	D16.1-☑	—	—
metatarsus (any)	C40.3-☑	C79.51	—	D16.3-☑	—	—
navicular						
ankle	C40.3-☑	C79.51	—	—	—	—
hand	C40.1-☑	C79.51	—	—	—	—
nose, nasal	C41.0	C79.51	—	D16.4	D48.0	D49.2
occipital	C41.0	C79.51	—	D16.4	D48.0	D49.2
orbit	C41.0	C79.51	—	D16.4	D48.0	D49.2
overlapping sites	C40.8-☑	—	—	—	—	—
parietal	C41.0	C79.51	—	D16.4	D48.0	D49.2
patella	C40.2-☑	C79.51	—	—	—	—
pelvic	C41.4	C79.51	—	D16.8	D48.0	D49.2
phalanges						
foot	C40.3-☑	C79.51	—	—	—	—
hand	C40.1-☑	C79.51	—	—	—	—
pubic	C41.4	C79.51	—	D16.8	D48.0	D49.2
radius (any part)	C40.0-☑	C79.51	—	D16.0-☑	—	—
rib	C41.3	C79.51	—	D16.7	D48.0	D49.2
sacral vertebra	C41.4	C79.51	—	D16.8	D48.0	D49.2
sacrum	C41.4	C79.51	—	D16.8	D48.0	D49.2
scaphoid						
of ankle	C40.3-☑	C79.51	—	—	—	—
of hand	C40.1-☑	C79.51	—	—	—	—
scapula (any part)	C40.0-☑	C79.51	—	D16.0-☑	—	—
sella turcica	C41.0	C79.51	—	D16.4	D48.0	D49.2
shoulder	C40.0-☑	C79.51	—	D16.0-☑	—	—
skull	C41.0	C79.51	—	D16.4	D48.0	D49.2
sphenoid	C41.0	C79.51	—	D16.4	D48.0	D49.2
spine, spinal (column)	C41.2	C79.51	—	D16.6	D48.0	D49.2
coccyx	C41.4	C79.51	—	D16.8	D48.0	D49.2
sacrum	C41.4	C79.51	—	D16.8	D48.0	D49.2
sternum	C41.3	C79.51	—	D16.7	D48.0	D49.2
tarsus (any)	C40.3-☑	C79.51	—	—	—	—
temporal	C41.0	C79.51	—	D16.4	D48.0	D49.2
thumb	C40.1-☑	C79.51	—	—	—	—
tibia (any part)	C40.2-☑	C79.51	—	—	—	—
toe (any)	C40.3-☑	C79.51	—	—	—	—
trapezium	C40.1-☑	C79.51	—	—	—	—
trapezoid	C40.1-☑	C79.51	—	—	—	—
turbinate	C41.0	C79.51	—	D16.4	D48.0	D49.2
ulna (any part)	C40.0-☑	C79.51	—	D16.0-☑	—	—
unciform	C40.1-☑	C79.51	—	—	—	—
vertebra (column)	C41.2	C79.51	—	D16.6	D48.0	D49.2
coccyx	C41.4	C79.51	—	D16.8	D48.0	D49.2
sacrum	C41.4	C79.51	—	D16.8	D48.0	D49.2
vomer	C41.0	C79.51	—	D16.4	D48.0	D49.2
wrist	C40.1-☑	C79.51	—	—	—	—
xiphoid process	C41.3	C79.51	—	D16.7	D48.0	D49.2
zygomatic	C41.0	C79.51	—	D16.4	D48.0	D49.2
book-leaf (mouth) — ventral surface of tongue and floor of mouth	C06.89	C79.89	D00.00	D10.39	D37.09	D49.0
bowel — see Neoplasm, intestine						
brachial plexus	C47.1-☑	C79.89	—	D36.12	D48.2	D49.2
brain NEC	C71.9	C79.31	—	D33.2	D43.2	D49.6

Neoplasm, neoplastic	Malignant Primary	Malignant Secondary	Ca in situ	Benign	Uncertain Behavior	Unspecified Behavior
— continued						
brain — continued						
basal ganglia	C71.0	C79.31	—	D33.0	D43.0	D49.6
cerebellopontine angle	C71.6	C79.31	—	D33.1	D43.1	D49.6
cerebellum NOS	C71.6	C79.31	—	D33.1	D43.1	D49.6
cerebrum	C71.0	C79.31	—	D33.0	D43.0	D49.6
choroid plexus	C71.7	C79.31	—	D33.1	D43.1	D49.6
corpus callosum	C71.8	C79.31	—	D33.2	D43.2	D49.6
corpus striatum	C71.0	C79.31	—	D33.0	D43.0	D49.6
cortex (cerebral)	C71.0	C79.31	—	D33.0	D43.0	D49.6
frontal lobe	C71.1	C79.31	—	D33.0	D43.0	D49.6
globus pallidus	C71.0	C79.31	—	D33.0	D43.0	D49.6
hippocampus	C71.2	C79.31	—	D33.0	D43.0	D49.6
hypothalamus	C71.0	C79.31	—	D33.0	D43.0	D49.6
internal capsule	C71.0	C79.31	—	D33.0	D43.0	D49.6
medulla oblongata	C71.7	C79.31	—	D33.1	D43.1	D49.6
meninges	C70.0	C79.32	—	D32.0	D42.0	D49.7
midbrain	C71.7	C79.31	—	D33.1	D43.1	D49.6
occipital lobe	C71.4	C79.31	—	D33.0	D43.0	D49.6
overlapping lesion	C71.8	C79.31	—	—	—	—
parietal lobe	C71.3	C79.31	—	D33.0	D43.0	D49.6
peduncle	C71.7	C79.31	—	D33.1	D43.1	D49.6
pons	C71.7	C79.31	—	D33.1	D43.1	D49.6
stem	C71.7	C79.31	—	D33.1	D43.1	D49.6
tapetum	C71.8	C79.31	—	D33.2	D43.2	D49.6
temporal lobe	C71.2	C79.31	—	D33.0	D43.0	D49.6
thalamus	C71.0	C79.31	—	D33.0	D43.0	D49.6
uncus	C71.2	C79.31	—	D33.0	D43.0	D49.6
ventricle (floor)	C71.5	C79.31	—	D33.0	D43.0	D49.6
fourth	C71.7	C79.31	—	D33.1	D43.1	D49.6
branchial (cleft) (cyst) (vestiges)	C10.4	C79.89	D00.08	D10.5	D37.05	D49.0
breast (connective tissue) (glandular tissue) (soft parts)	C50.9-☑	C79.81	D05.-☑	D24.-☑	D48.6-☑	D49.3
areola	C50.0-☑	C79.81	D05.-☑	D24.-☑	D48.6-☑	D49.3
axillary tail	C50.6-☑	C79.81	D05.-☑	D24.-☑	D48.6-☑	D49.3
central portion	C50.1-☑	C79.81	D05.-☑	D24.-☑	D48.6-☑	D49.3
inner	C50.8-☑	C79.81	D05.-☑	D24.-☑	D48.6-☑	D49.3
lower	C50.8-☑	C79.81	D05.-☑	D24.-☑	D48.6-☑	D49.3
lower-inner quadrant	C50.3-☑	C79.81	D05.-☑	D24.-☑	D48.6-☑	D49.3
lower-outer quadrant	C50.5-☑	C79.81	D05.-☑	D24.-☑	D48.6-☑	D49.3
mastectomy site (skin) — see also Neoplasm, breast, skin	C44.501	C79.2	—	—	—	—
specified as breast tissue	C50.8-☑	C79.81	D05.-☑	D24.-☑	D48.6-☑	D49.3
midline	C50.8-☑	C79.81	D05.-☑	D24.-☑	D48.6-☑	D49.3
nipple	C50.0-☑	C79.81	D05.-☑	D24.-☑	D48.6-☑	D49.3
outer	C50.8-☑	C79.81	D05.-☑	D24.-☑	D48.6-☑	D49.3
overlapping lesion	C50.8-☑	—	—	—	—	—
skin	C44.501	C79.2	D04.5	D23.5	D48.5	D49.2
basal cell carcinoma	C44.511	—	—	—	—	—
specified type NEC	C44.591	—	—	—	—	—
squamous cell carcinoma	C44.521	—	—	—	—	—
tail (axillary)	C50.6-☑	C79.81	D05.-☑	D24.-☑	D48.6-☑	D49.3
upper	C50.8-☑	C79.81	D05.-☑	D24.-☑	D48.6-☑	D49.3
upper-inner quadrant	C50.2-☑	C79.81	D05.-☑	D24.-☑	D48.6-☑	D49.3
upper-outer quadrant	C50.4-☑	C79.81	D05.-☑	D24.-☑	D48.6-☑	D49.3
broad ligament	C57.1-☑	C79.82	D07.39	D28.2	D39.8	D49.59
bronchiogenic, bronchogenic (lung)	C34.9-☑	C78.0-☑	D02.2-☑	D14.3-☑	D38.1	D49.1
bronchiole	C34.9-☑	C78.0-☑	D02.2-☑	D14.3-☑	D38.1	D49.1
bronchus	C34.9-☑	C78.0-☑	D02.2-☑	D14.3-☑	D38.1	D49.1
carina	C34.0-☑	C78.0-☑	D02.2-☑	D14.3-☑	D38.1	D49.1
lower lobe of lung	C34.3-☑	C78.0-☑	D02.2-☑	D14.3-☑	D38.1	D49.1

Neoplasm, neoplastic	Malignant Primary	Malignant Secondary	Ca in situ	Benign	Uncertain Behavior	Unspecified Behavior
— continued						
bronchus — continued						
main	C34.0-☑	C78.0-☑	D02.2-☑	D14.3-☑	D38.1	D49.1
middle lobe of lung	C34.2	C78.0-☑	D02.21	D14.31	D38.1	D49.1
overlapping lesion	C34.8-☑	—	—	—	—	—
upper lobe of lung	C34.1-☑	C78.0-☑	D02.2-☑	D14.3-☑	D38.1	D49.1
brow	C44.309	C79.2	D04.39	D23.39	D48.5	D49.2
basal cell carcinoma	C44.319	—	—	—	—	—
specified type NEC	C44.399	—	—	—	—	—
squamous cell carcinoma	C44.329	—	—	—	—	—
buccal (cavity)	C06.9	C79.89	D00.00	D10.39	D37.09	D49.0
commissure	C06.0	C79.89	D00.02	D10.39	D37.09	D49.0
groove (lower) (upper)	C06.1	C79.89	D00.02	D10.39	D37.09	D49.0
mucosa	C06.0	C79.89	D00.02	D10.39	D37.09	D49.0
sulcus (lower) (upper)	C06.1	C79.89	D00.02	D10.39	D37.09	D49.0
bulbourethral gland	C68.0	C79.19	D09.19	D30.4	D41.3	D49.59
bursa — see Neoplasm, connective tissue						
buttock NEC	C76.3	C79.89	D04.5	D36.7	D48.7	D49.89
calf	C76.5-☑	C79.89	D04.7-☑	D36.7	D48.7	D49.89
calvarium	C41.0	C79.51	—	D16.4	D48.0	D49.2
calyx, renal	C65.-☑	C79.0-☑	D09.19	D30.1-☑	D41.1-☑	D49.51-☑
canal						
anal	C21.1	C78.5	D01.3	D12.9	D37.8	D49.0
auditory (external) — see also Neoplasm, skin, ear	C44.20-☑	C79.2	D04.2-☑	D23.2-☑	D48.5	D49.2
auricular (external) — see also Neoplasm, skin, ear	C44.20-☑	C79.2	D04.2-☑	D23.2-☑	D48.5	D49.2
canaliculi, biliary (biliferi) (intrahepatic)	C22.1	C78.7	D01.5	D13.4	D37.6	D49.0
canthus (eye) (inner) (outer)	C44.10-☑	C79.2	D04.1-☑	D23.1-☑	D48.5	D49.2
basal cell carcinoma	C44.11-☑	—	—	—	—	—
sebaceous cell	C44.13-☑	—	—	—	—	—
specified type NEC	C44.19-☑	—	—	—	—	—
squamous cell carcinoma	C44.12-☑	—	—	—	—	—
capillary — see Neoplasm, connective tissue						
caput coli	C18.0	C78.5	D01.0	D12.0	D37.4	D49.0
carcinoid — see Tumor, carcinoid						
cardia (gastric)	C16.0	C78.89	D00.2	D13.1	D37.1	D49.0
cardiac orifice (stomach)	C16.0	C78.89	D00.2	D13.1	D37.1	D49.0
cardio-esophageal junction	C16.0	C78.89	D00.2	D13.1	D37.1	D49.0
cardio-esophagus	C16.0	C78.89	D00.2	D13.1	D37.1	D49.0
carina (bronchus)	C34.0-☑	C78.0-☑	D02.2-☑	D14.3-☑	D38.1	D49.1
carotid (artery)	C49.0	C79.89	—	D21.0	D48.1	D49.2
body	C75.4	C79.89	—	D35.5	D44.6	D49.7
carpus (any bone)	C40.1-☑	C79.51	—	D16.1-☑	D48.0	D49.2
cartilage (articular) (joint) NEC — see also Neoplasm, bone						
bone	C41.9	C79.51	—	D16.9	D48.0	D49.2
arytenoid	C32.3	C78.39	D02.0	D14.1	D38.0	D49.1
auricular	C49.0	C79.89	—	D21.0	D48.1	D49.2
bronchi	C34.0-☑	C78.39	—	D14.3-☑	D38.1	D49.1
costal	C41.3	C79.51	—	D16.7	D48.0	D49.2
cricoid	C32.3	C78.39	D02.0	D14.1	D38.0	D49.1
cuneiform	C32.3	C78.39	D02.0	D14.1	D38.0	D49.1
ear (external)	C49.0	C79.89	—	D21.0	D48.1	D49.2
ensiform	C41.3	C79.51	—	D16.7	D48.0	D49.2
epiglottis	C32.1	C78.39	D02.0	D14.1	D38.0	D49.1

☑ Additional Character Required — Refer to the Tabular List for Character Selection   ▽ Subterms under main terms may continue to next column or page

Neoplasm, neoplastic	Malignant Primary	Malignant Secondary	Ca in situ	Benign	Uncertain Behavior	Unspecified Behavior
— continued						
cartilage — see also						
Neoplasm, bone —						
continued						
epiglottis —						
continued						
anterior						
surface	C10.1	C79.89	D00.08	D10.5	D37.05	D49.0
eyelid	C49.0	C79.89	—	D21.0	D48.1	D49.2
intervertebral	C41.2	C79.51	—	D16.6	D48.0	D49.2
larynx, laryngeal	C32.3	C78.39	D02.0	D14.1	D38.0	D49.1
nose, nasal	C30.0	C78.39	D02.3	D14.0	D38.5	D49.1
pinna	C49.0	C79.89	—	D21.0	D48.1	D49.2
rib	C41.3	C79.51	—	D16.7	D48.0	D49.2
semilunar						
(knee)	C40.2-☑	C79.51	—	D16.2-☑	D48.0	D49.2
thyroid	C32.3	C78.39	D02.0	D14.1	D38.0	D49.1
trachea	C33	C78.39	D02.1	D14.2	D38.1	D49.1
cauda equina	C72.1	C79.49	—	D33.4	D43.4	D49.7
cavity						
buccal	C06.9	C79.89	D00.00	D10.30	D37.09	D49.0
nasal	C30.0	C78.39	D02.3	D14.0	D38.5	D49.1
oral	C06.9	C79.89	D00.00	D10.30	D37.09	D49.0
peritoneal	C48.2	C78.6	—	D20.1	D48.4	D49.0
tympanic	C30.1	C78.39	D02.3	D14.0	D38.5	D49.1
cecum	C18.0	C78.5	D01.0	D12.0	D37.4	D49.0
central nervous						
system	C72.9	C79.40	—	—	—	—
cerebellopontine						
(angle)	C71.6	C79.31	—	D33.1	D43.1	D49.6
cerebellum,						
cerebellar	C71.6	C79.31	—	D33.1	D43.1	D49.6
cerebrum, cerebra						
(cortex)						
(hemisphere)						
(white matter)	C71.0	C79.31	—	D33.0	D43.0	D49.6
meninges	C70.0	C79.32	—	D32.0	D42.0	D49.7
peduncle	C71.7	C79.31	—	D33.1	D43.1	D49.6
ventricle	C71.5	C79.31	—	D33.0	D43.0	D49.6
fourth	C71.7	C79.31	—	D33.1	D43.1	D49.6
cervical region	C76.0	C79.89	D09.8	D36.7	D48.7	D49.89
cervix (cervical) (uteri)						
(uterus)	C53.9	C79.82	D06.9	D26.0	D39.0	D49.59
canal	C53.0	C79.82	D06.0	D26.0	D39.0	D49.59
endocervix (canal)						
(gland)	C53.0	C79.82	D06.0	D26.0	D39.0	D49.59
exocervix	C53.1	C79.82	D06.1	D26.0	D39.0	D49.59
external os	C53.1	C79.82	D06.1	D26.0	D39.0	D49.59
internal os	C53.0	C79.82	D06.0	D26.0	D39.0	D49.59
nabothian gland	C53.0	C79.82	D06.0	D26.0	D39.0	D49.59
overlapping						
lesion	C53.8	—	—	—	—	—
squamocolumnar						
junction	C53.8	C79.82	D06.7	D26.0	D39.0	D49.59
stump	C53.8	C79.82	D06.7	D26.0	D39.0	D49.59
cheek	C76.0	C79.89	D09.8	D36.7	D48.7	D49.89
external	C44.309	C79.2	D04.39	D23.39	D48.5	D49.2
basal cell						
carcinoma	C44.319	—	—	—	—	—
specified type						
NEC	C44.399	—	—	—	—	—
squamous cell						
carcinoma	C44.329	—	—	—	—	—
inner aspect	C06.0	C79.89	D00.02	D10.39	D37.09	D49.0
internal	C06.0	C79.89	D00.02	D10.39	D37.09	D49.0
mucosa	C06.0	C79.89	D00.02	D10.39	D37.09	D49.0
chest (wall) NEC	C76.1	C79.89	D09.8	D36.7	D48.7	D49.89
chiasma opticum	C72.3-☑	C79.49	—	D33.3	D43.3	D49.7
chin	C44.309	C79.2	D04.39	D23.39	D48.5	D49.2
basal cell						
carcinoma	C44.319	—	—	—	—	—
specified type						
NEC	C44.399	—	—	—	—	—
squamous cell						
carcinoma	C44.329	—	—	—	—	—
choana	C11.3	C79.89	D00.08	D10.6	D37.05	D49.0
cholangiole	C22.1	C78.89	D01.5	D13.4	D37.6	D49.0
choledochal duct	C24.0	C78.89	D01.5	D13.5	D37.6	D49.0
choroid	C69.3-☑	C79.49	D09.2-☑	D31.3-☑	D48.7	D49.81
plexus	C71.5	C79.31	—	D33.0	D43.0	D49.6
ciliary body	C69.4-☑	C79.49	D09.2-☑	D31.4-☑	D48.7	D49.89
clavicle	C41.3	C79.51	—	D16.7	D48.0	D49.2

Neoplasm, neoplastic	Malignant Primary	Malignant Secondary	Ca in situ	Benign	Uncertain Behavior	Unspecified Behavior
— continued						
clitoris	C51.2	C79.82	D07.1	D28.0	D39.8	D49.59
clivus	C41.0	C79.51	—	D16.4	D48.0	D49.2
cloacogenic zone	C21.2	C78.5	D01.3	D12.9	D37.8	D49.0
coccygeal						
body or glomus	C49.5	C79.89	—	D21.5	D48.1	D49.2
vertebra	C41.4	C79.51	—	D16.8	D48.0	D49.2
coccyx	C41.4	C79.51	—	D16.8	D48.0	D49.2
colon — see also						
Neoplasm,						
intestine,						
large	C18.9	C78.5	—	—	—	—
with rectum	C19	C78.5	D01.1	D12.7	D37.5	D49.0
columnella — see also						
Neoplasm, skin,						
face	C44.390	C79.2	D04.39	D23.39	D48.5	D49.2
column, spinal — see						
Neoplasm, spine						
commissure						
labial, lip	C00.6	C79.89	D00.01	D10.39	D37.01	D49.0
laryngeal	C32.0	C78.39	D02.0	D14.1	D38.0	D49.1
common (bile)						
duct	C24.0	C78.89	D01.5	D13.5	D37.6	D49.0
concha — see also						
Neoplasm, skin,						
ear	C44.20-☑	C79.2	D04.2-☑	D23.2-☑	D48.5	D49.2
nose	C30.0	C78.39	D02.3	D14.0	D38.5	D49.1
conjunctiva	C69.0-☑	C79.49	D09.2-☑	D31.0-☑	D48.7	D49.89
connective tissue						
NEC	C49.9	C79.89	—	D21.9	D48.1	D49.2

Note: For neoplasms of connective tissue (blood vessel, bursa, fascia, ligament, muscle, peripheral nerves, sympathetic and parasympathetic nerves and ganglia, synovia, tendon, etc.) or of morphological types that indicate connective tissue, code according to the list under "Neoplasm, connective tissue". For sites that do not appear in this list, code to neoplasm of that site; e.g., fibrosarcoma, pancreas (C25.9)

Note: Morphological types that indicate connective tissue appear in their proper place in the alphabetic index with the instruction "see Neoplasm, connective tissue ...."

	Malignant Primary	Malignant Secondary	Ca in situ	Benign	Uncertain Behavior	Unspecified Behavior
abdomen	C49.4	C79.89	—	D21.4	D48.1	D49.2
abdominal wall	C49.4	C79.89	—	D21.4	D48.1	D49.2
ankle	C49.2-☑	C79.89	—	D21.2-☑	D48.1	D49.2
antecubital fossa or						
space	C49.1-☑	C79.89	—	D21.1-☑	D48.1	D49.2
arm	C49.1-☑	C79.89	—	D21.1-☑	D48.1	D49.2
auricle (ear)	C49.0	C79.89	—	D21.0	D48.1	D49.2
axilla	C49.3	C79.89	—	D21.3	D48.1	D49.2
back	C49.6	C79.89	—	D21.6	D48.1	D49.2
breast — see						
Neoplasm,						
breast						
buttock	C49.5	C79.89	—	D21.5	D48.1	D49.2
calf	C49.2-☑	C79.89	—	D21.2-☑	D48.1	D49.2
cervical region	C49.0	C79.89	—	D21.0	D48.1	D49.2
cheek	C49.0	C79.89	—	D21.0	D48.1	D49.2
chest (wall)	C49.3	C79.89	—	D21.3	D48.1	D49.2
chin	C49.0	C79.89	—	D21.0	D48.1	D49.2
diaphragm	C49.3	C79.89	—	D21.3	D48.1	D49.2
ear (external)	C49.0	C79.89	—	D21.0	D48.1	D49.2
elbow	C49.1-☑	C79.89	—	D21.1-☑	D48.1	D49.2
extrarectal	C49.5	C79.89	—	D21.5	D48.1	D49.2
extremity	C49.9	C79.89	—	D21.9	D48.1	D49.2
lower	C49.2-☑	C79.89	—	D21.2-☑	D48.1	D49.2
upper	C49.1-☑	C79.89	—	D21.1-☑	D48.1	D49.2
eyelid	C49.0	C79.89	—	D21.0	D48.1	D49.2
face	C49.0	C79.89	—	D21.0	D48.1	D49.2
finger	C49.1-☑	C79.89	—	D21.1-☑	D48.1	D49.2
flank	C49.6	C79.89	—	D21.6	D48.1	D49.2
foot	C49.2-☑	C79.89	—	D21.2-☑	D48.1	D49.2
forearm	C49.1-☑	C79.89	—	D21.1-☑	D48.1	D49.2
forehead	C49.0	C79.89	—	D21.0	D48.1	D49.2
gastric	C49.4	C79.89	—	D21.4	D48.1	D49.2
gastrointestinal	C49.4	C79.89	—	D21.4	D48.1	D49.2
gluteal region	C49.5	C79.89	—	D21.5	D48.1	D49.2
great vessels						
NEC	C49.3	C79.89	—	D21.3	D48.1	D49.2
groin	C49.5	C79.89	—	D21.5	D48.1	D49.2
hand	C49.1-☑	C79.89	—	D21.1-☑	D48.1	D49.2
head	C49.0	C79.89	—	D21.0	D48.1	D49.2

Neoplasm, neoplastic — continued

	Malignant Primary	Malignant Secondary	Ca in situ	Benign	Uncertain Behavior	Unspecified Behavior
connective tissue — continued						
heel	C49.2-☑	C79.89	—	D21.2-☑	D48.1	D49.2
hip	C49.2-☑	C79.89	—	D21.2-☑	D48.1	D49.2
hypochondrium	C49.4	C79.89	—	D21.4	D48.1	D49.2
iliopsoas muscle	C49.5	C79.89	—	D21.5	D48.1	D49.2
infraclavicular region	C49.3	C79.89	—	D21.3	D48.1	D49.2
inguinal (canal) (region)	C49.5	C79.89	—	D21.5	D48.1	D49.2
intestinal	C49.4	C79.89	—	D21.4	D48.1	D49.2
intrathoracic	C49.3	C79.89	—	D21.3	D48.1	D49.2
ischiorectal fossa	C49.5	C79.89	—	D21.5	D48.1	D49.2
jaw	C03.9	C79.89	D00.03	D10.39	D48.1	D49.0
knee	C49.2-☑	C79.89	—	D21.2-☑	D48.1	D49.2
leg	C49.2-☑	C79.89	—	D21.2-☑	D48.1	D49.2
limb NEC	C49.9	C79.89	—	D21.9	D48.1	D49.2
lower	C49.2-☑	C79.89	—	D21.2-☑	D48.1	D49.2
upper	C49.1-☑	C79.89	—	D21.1-☑	D48.1	D49.2
nates	C49.5	C79.89	—	D21.5	D48.1	D49.2
neck	C49.0	C79.89	—	D21.0	D48.1	D49.2
orbit	C69.6-☑	C79.49	D09.2-☑	D31.6-☑	D48.1	D49.89
overlapping lesion	C49.8	—	—	—	—	—
pararectal	C49.5	C79.89	—	D21.5	D48.1	D49.2
para-urethral	C49.5	C79.89	—	D21.5	D48.1	D49.2
paravaginal	C49.5	C79.89	—	D21.5	D48.1	D49.2
pelvis (floor)	C49.5	C79.89	—	D21.5	D48.1	D49.2
pelvo-abdominal	C49.8	C79.89	—	D21.6	D48.1	D49.2
perineum	C49.5	C79.89	—	D21.5	D48.1	D49.2
perirectal (tissue)	C49.5	C79.89	—	D21.5	D48.1	D49.2
periurethral (tissue)	C49.5	C79.89	—	D21.5	D48.1	D49.2
popliteal fossa or space	C49.2-☑	C79.89	—	D21.2-☑	D48.1	D49.2
presacral	C49.5	C79.89	—	D21.5	D48.1	D49.2
psoas muscle	C49.4	C79.89	—	D21.4	D48.1	D49.2
pterygoid fossa	C49.0	C79.89	—	D21.0	D48.1	D49.2
rectovaginal septum or wall	C49.5	C79.89	—	D21.5	D48.1	D49.2
rectovesical	C49.5	C79.89	—	D21.5	D48.1	D49.2
retroperitoneum	C48.0	C78.6	—	D20.0	D48.3	D49.0
sacrococcygeal region	C49.5	C79.89	—	D21.5	D48.1	D49.2
scalp	C49.0	C79.89	—	D21.0	D48.1	D49.2
scapular region	C49.3	C79.89	—	D21.3	D48.1	D49.2
shoulder	C49.1-☑	C79.89	—	D21.1-☑	D48.1	D49.2
skin (dermis) NEC — see also Neoplasm, skin, by site	C44.90	C79.2	D04.9	D23.9	D48.5	D49.2
stomach	C49.4	C79.89	—	D21.4	D48.1	D49.2
submental	C49.0	C79.89	—	D21.0	D48.1	D49.2
supraclavicular region	C49.0	C79.89	—	D21.0	D48.1	D49.2
temple	C49.0	C79.89	—	D21.0	D48.1	D49.2
temporal region	C49.0	C79.89	—	D21.0	D48.1	D49.2
thigh	C49.2-☑	C79.89	—	D21.2-☑	D48.1	D49.2
thoracic (duct) (wall)	C49.3	C79.89	—	D21.3	D48.1	D49.2
thorax	C49.3	C79.89	—	D21.3	D48.1	D49.2
thumb	C49.1-☑	C79.89	—	D21.1-☑	D48.1	D49.2
toe	C49.2-☑	C79.89	—	D21.2-☑	D48.1	D49.2
trunk	C49.6	C79.89	—	D21.6	D48.1	D49.2
umbilicus	C49.4	C79.89	—	D21.4	D48.1	D49.2
vesicorectal	C49.5	C79.89	—	D21.5	D48.1	D49.2
wrist	C49.1-☑	C79.89	—	D21.1-☑	D48.1	D49.2
conus medullaris	C72.0	C79.49	—	D33.4	D43.4	D49.7
cord (true) (vocal)	C32.0	C78.39	D02.0	D14.1	D38.0	D49.1
false	C32.1	C78.39	D02.0	D14.1	D38.0	D49.1
spermatic	C63.1-☑	C79.82	D07.69	D29.8	D40.8	D49.59
spinal (cervical) (lumbar) (thoracic)	C72.0	C79.49	—	D33.4	D43.4	D49.7
cornea (limbus)	C69.1-☑	C79.49	D09.2-☑	D31.1-☑	D48.7	D49.89
corpus						
albicans	C56.-☑	C79.6-☑	D07.39	D27.-☑	D39.1-☑	D49.59
callosum, brain	C71.0	C79.31	—	D33.2	D43.2	D49.6

Neoplasm, neoplastic — continued

	Malignant Primary	Malignant Secondary	Ca in situ	Benign	Uncertain Behavior	Unspecified Behavior
corpus — continued						
cavernosum	C60.2	C79.82	D07.4	D29.0	D40.8	D49.59
gastric	C16.2	C78.89	D00.2	D13.1	D37.1	D49.0
overlapping sites	C54.8	—	—	—	—	—
penis	C60.2	C79.82	D07.4	D29.0	D40.8	D49.59
striatum, cerebrum	C71.0	C79.31	—	D33.0	D43.0	D49.6
uteri	C54.9	C79.82	D07.0	D26.1	D39.0	D49.59
isthmus	C54.0	C79.82	D07.0	D26.1	D39.0	D49.59
cortex						
adrenal	C74.0-☑	C79.7-☑	D09.3	D35.0-☑	D44.1-☑	D49.7
cerebral	C71.0	C79.31	—	D33.0	D43.0	D49.6
costal cartilage	C41.3	C79.51	—	D16.7	D48.0	D49.2
costovertebral joint	C41.3	C79.51	—	D16.7	D48.0	D49.2
Cowper's gland	C68.0	C79.19	D09.19	D30.4	D41.3	D49.59
cranial (fossa, any)	C71.9	C79.31	—	D33.2	D43.2	D49.6
meninges	C70.0	C79.32	—	D32.0	D42.0	D49.7
nerve	C72.50	C79.49	—	D33.3	D43.3	D49.7
specified NEC	C72.59	C79.49	—	D33.3	D43.3	D49.7
craniobuccal pouch	C75.2	C79.89	D09.3	D35.2	D44.3	D49.7
craniopharyngeal (duct) (pouch)	C75.2	C79.89	D09.3	D35.3	D44.4	D49.7
cricoid	C13.0	C79.89	D00.08	D10.7	D37.05	D49.0
cartilage	C32.3	C78.39	D02.0	D14.1	D38.0	D49.1
cricopharynx	C13.0	C79.89	D00.08	D10.7	D37.05	D49.0
crypt of Morgagni	C21.8	C78.5	D01.3	D12.9	D37.8	D49.0
crystalline lens	C69.4-☑	C79.49	D09.2-☑	D31.4-☑	D48.7	D49.89
cul-de-sac (Douglas')	C48.1	C78.6	—	D20.1	D48.4	D49.0
cuneiform cartilage	C32.3	C78.39	D02.0	D14.1	D38.0	D49.1
cutaneous — see Neoplasm, skin						
cutis — see Neoplasm, skin						
cystic (bile) duct (common)	C24.0	C78.89	D01.5	D13.5	D37.6	D49.0
dermis — see Neoplasm, skin						
diaphragm	C49.3	C79.89	—	D21.3	D48.1	D49.2
digestive organs, system, tube, or tract NEC	C26.9	C78.89	D01.9	D13.9	D37.9	D49.0
disc, intervertebral	C41.2	C79.51	—	D16.6	D48.0	D49.2
disease,						
generalized	C80.0	—	—	—	—	—
disseminated	C80.0	—	—	—	—	—
Douglas' cul-de-sac or pouch	C48.1	C78.6	—	D20.1	D48.4	D49.0
duodenojejunal junction	C17.8	C78.4	D01.49	D13.39	D37.2	D49.0
duodenum	C17.0	C78.4	D01.49	D13.2	D37.2	D49.0
dura (cranial) (mater)	C70.9	C79.49	—	D32.9	D42.9	D49.7
cerebral	C70.0	C79.32	—	D32.0	D42.0	D49.7
spinal	C70.1	C79.49	—	D32.1	D42.1	D49.7
ear (external) — see also Neoplasm, skin, ear	C44.20-☑	C79.2	D04.2-☑	D23.2-☑	D48.5	D49.2
auricle or auris — see also Neoplasm, skin, ear	C44.20-☑	C79.2	D04.2-☑	D23.2-☑	D48.5	D49.2
canal, external — see also Neoplasm, skin, ear	C44.20-☑	C79.2	D04.2-☑	D23.2-☑	D48.5	D49.2
cartilage	C49.0	C79.89	—	D21.0	D48.1	D49.2
external meatus — see also Neoplasm, skin, ear	C44.20-☑	C79.2	D04.2-☑	D23.2-☑	D48.5	D49.2
inner	C30.1	C78.39	D02.3	D14.0	D38.5	D49.1
lobule — see also Neoplasm, skin, ear	C44.20-☑	C79.2	D04.2-☑	D23.2-☑	D48.5	D49.2
middle	C30.1	C78.39	D02.3	D14.0	D38.5	D49.1
overlapping lesion with accessory sinuses	C31.8	—	—	—	—	—

	Malignant Primary	Malignant Secondary	Ca in situ	Benign	Uncertain Behavior	Unspecified Behavior
Neoplasm, neoplastic						
— *continued*						
ear — *see also*						
Neoplasm, skin, ear						
— *continued*						
skin	C44.20-☑	C79.2	D04.2-☑	D23.2-☑	D48.5	D49.2
basal cell						
carcinoma	C44.21-☑	—	—	—	—	—
specified type						
NEC	C44.29-☑	—	—	—	—	—
squamous cell						
carcinoma	C44.22-☑					
earlobe	C44.20-☑	C79.2	D04.2-☑	D23.2-☑	D48.5	D49.2
basal cell						
carcinoma	C44.21-☑	—	—	—	—	—
specified type						
NEC	C44.29-☑	—	—	—	—	—
squamous cell						
carcinoma	C44.22-☑	—	—	—	—	—
ejaculatory duct	C63.7	C79.82	D07.69	D29.8	D40.8	D49.59
elbow NEC	C76.4-☑	C79.89	D04.6-☑	D36.7	D48.7	D49.89
endocardium	C38.0	C79.89		D15.1	D48.7	D49.89
endocervix (canal)						
(gland)	C53.0	C79.82	D06.0	D26.0	D39.0	D49.59
endocrine gland						
NEC	C75.9	C79.89	D09.3	D35.9	D44.9	D49.7
pluriglandular	C75.8	C79.89	D09.3	D35.7	D44.9	D49.7
endometrium (gland)						
(stroma)	C54.1	C79.82	D07.0	D26.1	D39.0	D49.59
ensiform cartilage	C41.3	C79.51		D16.7	D48.0	D49.2
enteric — *see*						
Neoplasm,						
intestine						
ependyma (brain)	C71.5	C79.31	—	D33.0	D43.0	D49.6
fourth ventricle	C71.7	C79.31	—	D33.1	D43.1	D49.6
epicardium	C38.0	C79.89	—	D15.1	D48.7	D49.89
epididymis	C63.0-☑	C79.82	D07.69	D29.3-☑	D40.8	D49.59
epidural	C72.9	C79.49		D33.9	D43.9	D49.7
epiglottis	C32.1	C78.39	D02.0	D14.1	D38.0	D49.1
anterior aspect or						
surface	C10.1	C79.89	D00.08	D10.5	D37.05	D49.0
cartilage	C32.3	C78.39	D02.0	D14.1	D38.0	D49.1
free border						
(margin)	C10.1	C79.89	D00.08	D10.5	D37.05	D49.0
junctional						
region	C10.8	C79.89	D00.08	D10.5	D37.05	D49.0
posterior (laryngeal)						
surface	C32.1	C78.39	D02.0	D14.1	D38.0	D49.1
suprahyoid						
portion	C32.1	C78.39	D02.0	D14.1	D38.0	D49.1
esophagogastric						
junction	C16.0	C78.89	D00.2	D13.1	D37.1	D49.0
esophagus	C15.9	C78.89	D00.1	D13.0	D37.8	D49.0
abdominal	C15.5	C78.89	D00.1	D13.0	D37.8	D49.0
cervical	C15.3	C78.89	D00.1	D13.0	D37.8	D49.0
distal (third)	C15.5	C78.89	D00.1	D13.0	D37.8	D49.0
lower (third)	C15.5	C78.89	D00.1	D13.0	D37.8	D49.0
middle (third)	C15.4	C78.89	D00.1	D13.0	D37.8	D49.0
overlapping						
lesion	C15.8	—	—	—	—	—
proximal (third)	C15.3	C78.89	D00.1	D13.0	D37.8	D49.0
thoracic	C15.4	C78.89	D00.1	D13.0	D37.8	D49.0
upper (third)	C15.3	C78.89	D00.1	D13.0	D37.8	D49.0
ethmoid (sinus)	C31.1	C78.39	D02.3	D14.0	D38.5	D49.1
bone or						
labyrinth	C41.0	C79.51	—	D16.4	D48.0	D49.2
eustachian tube	C30.1	C78.39	D02.3	D14.0	D38.5	D49.1
exocervix	C53.1	C79.82	D06.1	D26.0	D39.0	D49.59
external						
meatus (ear) — *see*						
also Neoplasm,						
skin, ear	C44.20-☑	C79.2	D04.2-☑	D23.2-☑	D48.5	D49.2
os, cervix uteri	C53.1	C79.82	D06.1	D26.0	D39.0	D49.59
extradural	C72.9	C79.49		D33.9	D43.9	D49.7
extrahepatic (bile)						
duct	C24.0	C78.89	D01.5	D13.5	D37.6	D49.0
overlapping lesion						
with						
gallbladder	C24.8	—	—	—	—	—
extraocular						
muscle	C69.6-☑	C79.49	D09.2-☑	D31.6-☑	D48.7	D49.89
extrarectal	C76.3	C79.89	D09.8	D36.7	D48.7	D49.89
extremity	C76.8	C79.89	D04.8	D36.7	D48.7	D49.89

	Malignant Primary	Malignant Secondary	Ca in situ	Benign	Uncertain Behavior	Unspecified Behavior
Neoplasm, neoplastic						
— *continued*						
extremity — *continued*						
lower	C76.5-☑	C79.89	D04.7-☑	D36.7	D48.7	D49.89
upper	C76.4-☑	C79.89	D04.6-☑	D36.7	D48.7	D49.89
eyeball	C69.9-☑	C79.49	D09.2-☑	D31.9-☑	D48.7	D49.89
eyebrow	C44.309	C79.2	D04.39	D23.39	D48.5	D49.2
basal cell						
carcinoma	C44.319	—	—	—	—	—
specified type						
NEC	C44.399	—	—	—	—	—
squamous cell						
carcinoma	C44.329	—	—	—	—	—
eyelid (lower) (skin)						
(upper)	C44.10-☑	—	—	—	—	—
basal cell						
carcinoma	C44.11-☑	—	—	—	—	—
cartilage	C49.0	C79.89		D21.0	D48.1	D49.2
sebaceous cell	C44.13-☑	—	—	—	—	—
specified type						
NEC	C44.19-☑	—	—	—	—	—
squamous cell						
carcinoma	C44.12-☑	—	—	—	—	—
eye NEC	C69.9-☑	C79.49	D09.2-☑	D31.9-☑	D48.7	D49.89
overlapping						
sites	C69.8-☑					
face NEC	C76.0	C79.89	D04.39	D36.7	D48.7	D49.89
fallopian tube						
(accessory)	C57.0-☑	C79.82	D07.39	D28.2	D39.8	D49.59.
falx (cerebella)						
(cerebri)	C70.0	C79.32		D32.0	D42.0	D49.7
fascia — *see also*						
Neoplasm,						
connective tissue						
palmar	C49.1-☑	C79.89	—	D21.1-☑	D48.1	D49.2
plantar	C49.2-☑	C79.89	—	D21.2-☑	D48.1	D49.2
fatty tissue — *see*						
Neoplasm,						
connective tissue						
fauces, faucial NEC	C10.9	C79.89	D00.08	D10.5	D37.05	D49.0
pillars	C09.1	C79.89	D00.08	D10.5	D37.05	D49.0
tonsil	C09.9	C79.89	D00.08	D10.4	D37.05	D49.0
femur (any part)	C40.2-☑	—	—	D16.2-☑	—	—
fetal membrane	C58	C79.82	D07.0	D26.7	D39.2	D49.59
fibrous tissue — *see*						
Neoplasm,						
connective tissue						
fibula (any part)	C40.2-☑	C79.51	—	D16.2-☑	—	—
filum terminale	C72.0	C79.49	—	D33.4	D43.4	D49.7
finger NEC	C76.4-☑	C79.89	D04.6-☑	D36.7	D48.7	D49.89
flank NEC	C76.8	C79.89	D04.5	D36.7	D48.7	D49.89
follicle, nabothian	C53.0	C79.82	D06.0	D26.0	D39.0	D49.59
foot NEC	C76.5-☑	C79.89	D04.7-☑	D36.7	D48.7	D49.89
forearm NEC	C76.4-☑	C79.89	D04.6-☑	D36.7	D48.7	D49.89
forehead (skin)	C44.309	C79.2	D04.39	D23.39	D48.5	D49.2
basal cell						
carcinoma	C44.319	—	—	—	—	—
specified type						
NEC	C44.399	—	—	—	—	—
squamous cell						
carcinoma	C44.329	—	—	—	—	—
foreskin	C60.0	C79.82	D07.4	D29.0	D40.8	D49.59
fornix						
pharyngeal	C11.3	C79.89	D00.08	D10.6	D37.05	D49.0
vagina	C52	C79.82	D07.2	D28.1	D39.8	D49.59
fossa (of)						
anterior (cranial)	C71.9	C79.31	—	D33.2	D43.2	D49.6
cranial	C71.9	C79.31	—	D33.2	D43.2	D49.6
ischiorectal	C76.3	C79.89	D09.8	D36.7	D48.7	D49.89
middle (cranial)	C71.9	C79.31	—	D33.2	D43.2	D49.6
piriform	C12	C79.89	D00.08	D10.7	D37.05	D49.0
pituitary	C75.1	C79.89	D09.3	D35.2	D44.3	D49.7
posterior						
(cranial)	C71.9	C79.31	—	D33.2	D43.2	D49.6
pterygoid	C49.0	C79.89	—	D21.0	D48.1	D49.2
pyriform	C12	C79.89	D00.08	D10.7	D37.05	D49.0
Rosenmuller	C11.2	C79.89	D00.08	D10.6	D37.05	D49.0
tonsillar	C09.0	C79.89	D00.08	D10.5	D37.05	D49.0
fourchette	C51.9	C79.82	D07.1	D28.0	D39.8	D49.59
frenulum						
labii — *see*						
Neoplasm, lip,						
internal						

▽ Subterms under main terms may continue to next column or page　　　☑ Additional Character Required — Refer to the Tabular List for Character Selection

Neoplasm, neoplastic — continued

	Malignant Primary	Malignant Secondary	Ca in situ	Benign	Uncertain Behavior	Unspecified Behavior
frenulum — continued						
linguae	C02.2	C79.89	D00.07	D10.1	D37.02	D49.0
frontal						
bone	C41.0	C79.51	—	D16.4	D48.0	D49.2
lobe, brain	C71.1	C79.31	—	D33.0	D43.0	D49.6
pole	C71.1	C79.31	—	D33.0	D43.0	D49.6
sinus	C31.2	C78.39	D02.3	D14.0	D38.5	D49.1
fundus						
stomach	C16.1	C78.89	D00.2	D13.1	D37.1	D49.0
uterus	C54.3	C79.82	D07.0	D26.1	D39.0	D49.59
gallbladder	C23	C78.89	D01.5	D13.5	D37.6	D49.0
overlapping lesion with extrahepatic bile ducts	C24.8	—	—	—	—	—
gall duct (extrahepatic)	C24.0	C78.89	D01.5	D13.5	D37.6	D49.0
intrahepatic	C22.1	C78.7	D01.5	D13.4	D37.6	D49.0
ganglia — see also Neoplasm, nerve, peripheral	C47.9	C79.89	—	D36.10	D48.2	D49.2
basal	C71.0	C79.31	—	D33.0	D43.0	D49.6
cranial nerve	C72.50	C79.49	—	D33.3	D43.3	D49.7
Gartner's duct	C52	C79.82	D07.2	D28.1	D39.8	D49.59
gastric — see Neoplasm, stomach						
gastrocolic	C26.9	C78.89	D01.9	D13.9	D37.9	D49.0
gastroesophageal junction	C16.0	C78.89	D00.2	D13.1	D37.1	D49.0
gastrointestinal (tract) NEC	C26.9	C78.89	D01.9	D13.9	D37.9	D49.0
generalized	C80.0	—	—	—	—	—
genital organ or tract						
female NEC	C57.9	C79.82	D07.30	D28.9	D39.9	D49.59
overlapping lesion	C57.8	—	—	—	—	—
specified site NEC	C57.7	C79.82	D07.39	D28.7	D39.8	D49.59
male NEC	C63.9	C79.82	D07.60	D29.9	D40.9	D49.59
overlapping lesion	C63.8	—	—	—	—	—
specified site NEC	C63.7	C79.82	D07.69	D29.8	D40.8	D49.59
genitourinary tract						
female	C57.9	C79.82	D07.30	D28.9	D39.9	D49.59
male	C63.9	C79.82	D07.60	D29.9	D40.9	D49.59
gingiva (alveolar) (marginal)	C03.9	C79.89	D00.03	D10.39	D37.09	D49.0
lower	C03.1	C79.89	D00.03	D10.39	D37.09	D49.0
mandibular	C03.1	C79.89	D00.03	D10.39	D37.09	D49.0
maxillary	C03.0	C79.89	D00.03	D10.39	D37.09	D49.0
upper	C03.0	C79.89	D00.03	D10.39	D37.09	D49.0
gland, glandular (lymphatic) (system) — see also Neoplasm, lymph gland						
endocrine NEC	C75.9	C79.89	D09.3	D35.9	D44.9	D49.7
salivary — see Neoplasm, salivary gland						
glans penis	C60.1	C79.82	D07.4	D29.0	D40.8	D49.59
globus pallidus	C71.0	C79.31	—	D33.0	D43.0	D49.6
glomus						
coccygeal	C49.5	C79.89	—	D21.5	D48.1	D49.2
jugularis	C75.5	C79.89	—	D35.6	D44.7	D49.7
glosso-epiglottic fold(s)	C10.1	C79.89	D00.08	D10.5	D37.05	D49.0
glossopalatine fold	C09.1	C79.89	D00.08	D10.5	D37.05	D49.0
glossopharyngeal sulcus	C09.0	C79.89	D00.08	D10.5	D37.05	D49.0
glottis	C32.0	C78.39	D02.0	D14.1	D38.0	D49.1
gluteal region	C76.3	C79.89	D04.5	D36.7	D48.7	D49.89
great vessels NEC	C49.3	C79.89	—	D21.3	D48.1	D49.2
groin NEC	C76.3	C79.89	D04.5	D36.7	D48.7	D49.89
gum	C03.9	C79.89	D00.03	D10.39	D37.09	D49.0
lower	C03.1	C79.89	D00.03	D10.39	D37.09	D49.0
upper	C03.0	C79.89	D00.03	D10.39	D37.09	D49.0
hand NEC	C76.4-✓	C79.89	D04.6-✓	D36.7	D48.7	D49.89
head NEC	C76.0	C79.89	D04.4	D36.7	D48.7	D49.89
heart	C38.0	C79.89	—	D15.1	D48.7	D49.89

Neoplasm, neoplastic — continued

	Malignant Primary	Malignant Secondary	Ca in situ	Benign	Uncertain Behavior	Unspecified Behavior
heel NEC	C76.5-✓	C79.89	D04.7-✓	D36.7	D48.7	D49.89
helix — see also Neoplasm, skin, ear	C44.20-✓	C79.2	D04.2-✓	D23.2-✓	D48.5	D49.2
hematopoietic, hemopoietic tissue NEC	C96.9	—	—	—	—	—
specified NEC	C96.Z	—	—	—	—	—
hemisphere, cerebral	C71.0	C79.31	—	D33.0	D43.0	D49.6
hemorrhoidal zone	C21.1	C78.5	D01.3	D12.9	D37.8	D49.0
hepatic — see also Index to disease, by histology	C22.9	C78.7	D01.5	D13.4	D37.6	D49.0
duct (bile)	C24.0	C78.89	D01.5	D13.5	D37.6	D49.0
flexure (colon)	C18.3	C78.5	D01.0	D12.3	D37.4	D49.0
primary	C22.8	C78.7	D01.5	D13.4	D37.6	D49.0
hepatobiliary	C24.9	C78.89	D01.5	D13.5	D37.6	D49.0
hepatoblastoma	C22.2	C78.7	D01.5	D13.4	D37.6	D49.0
hepatoma	C22.0	C78.7	D01.5	D13.4	D37.6	D49.0
hilus of lung	C34.0-✓	C78.0-✓	D02.2-✓	D14.3-✓	D38.1	D49.1
hippocampus, brain	C71.2	C79.31	—	D33.0	D43.0	D49.6
hip NEC	C76.5-✓	C79.89	D04.7-✓	D36.7	D48.7	D49.89
humerus (any part)	C40.0-✓	C79.51	—	D16.0-✓	—	—
hymen	C52	C79.82	D07.2	D28.1	D39.8	D49.59
hypopharynx, hypopharyngeal NEC	C13.9	C79.89	D00.08	D10.7	D37.05	D49.0
overlapping lesion	C13.8	—	—	—	—	—
postcricoid region	C13.0	C79.89	D00.08	D10.7	D37.05	D49.0
posterior wall	C13.2	C79.89	D00.08	D10.7	D37.05	D49.0
pyriform fossa (sinus)	C12	C79.89	D00.08	D10.7	D37.05	D49.0
hypophysis	C75.1	C79.89	D09.3	D35.2	D44.3	D49.7
hypothalamus	C71.0	C79.31	—	D33.0	D43.0	D49.6
ileocecum, ileocecal (coil) (junction) (valve)	C18.0	C78.5	D01.0	D12.0	D37.4	D49.0
ileum	C17.2	C78.4	D01.49	D13.39	D37.2	D49.0
ilium	C41.4	C79.51	—	D16.8	D48.0	D49.2
immunoproliferative NEC	C88.9	—	—	—	—	—
infraclavicular (region)	C76.1	C79.89	D04.5	D36.7	D48.7	D49.89
inguinal (region)	C76.3	C79.89	D04.5	D36.7	D48.7	D49.89
insula	C71.0	C79.31	—	D33.0	D43.0	D49.6
insular tissue (pancreas)	C25.4	C78.89	D01.7	D13.7	D37.8	D49.0
brain	C71.0	C79.31	—	D33.0	D43.0	D49.6
interarytenoid fold	C13.1	C78.39	D00.08	D10.7	D37.05	D49.0
hypopharyngeal aspect	C13.1	C79.89	D00.08	D10.7	D37.05	D49.0
laryngeal aspect	C32.1	C78.39	D02.0	D14.1	D38.0	D49.1
marginal zone	C13.1	C79.89	D00.08	D10.7	D37.05	D49.0
interdental papillae	C03.9	C79.89	D00.03	D10.39	D37.09	D49.0
lower	C03.1	C79.89	D00.03	D10.39	D37.09	D49.0
upper	C03.0	C79.89	D00.03	D10.39	D37.09	D49.0
internal						
capsule	C71.0	C79.31	—	D33.0	D43.0	D49.6
os (cervix)	C53.0	C79.82	D06.0	D26.0	D39.0	D49.59
intervertebral cartilage or disc	C41.2	C79.51	—	D16.6	D48.0	D49.2
intestine, intestinal	C26.0	C78.80	D01.40	D13.9	D37.8	D49.0
large	C18.9	C78.5	D01.0	D12.6	D37.4	D49.0
appendix	C18.1	C78.5	D01.0	D12.1	D37.3	D49.0
caput coli	C18.0	C78.5	D01.0	D12.0	D37.4	D49.0
cecum	C18.0	C78.5	D01.0	D12.0	D37.4	D49.0
colon	C18.9	C78.5	D01.0	D12.6	D37.4	D49.0
and rectum	C19	C78.5	D01.1	D12.7	D37.5	D49.0
ascending	C18.2	C78.5	D01.0	D12.2	D37.4	D49.0
caput	C18.0	C78.5	D01.0	D12.0	D37.4	D49.0
descending	C18.6	C78.5	D01.0	D12.4	D37.4	D49.0
distal	C18.6	C78.5	D01.0	D12.4	D37.4	D49.0

✓ Additional Character Required — Refer to the Tabular List for Character Selection   ⬮ Subterms under main terms may continue to next column or page

	Malignant Primary	Malignant Secondary	Ca in situ	Benign	Uncertain Behavior	Unspecified Behavior
Neoplasm, neoplastic						
— *continued*						
intestine, intestinal — *continued*						
large — *continued*						
colon — *continued*						
left	C18.6	C78.5	D01.0	D12.4	D37.4	D49.0
overlapping lesion	C18.8	—		—	—	—
pelvic	C18.7	C78.5	D01.0	D12.5	D37.4	D49.0
right	C18.2	C78.5	D01.0	D12.2	D37.4	D49.0
sigmoid (flexure)	C18.7	C78.5	D01.0	D12.5	D37.4	D49.0
transverse	C18.4	C78.5	D01.0	D12.3	D37.4	D49.0
hepatic flexure	C18.3	C78.5	D01.0	D12.3	D37.4	D49.0
ileocecum, ileocecal (coil) (valve)	C18.0	C78.5	D01.0	D12.0	D37.4	D49.0
overlapping lesion	C18.8	—		—	—	—
sigmoid flexure (lower) (upper)	C18.7	C78.5	D01.0	D12.5	D37.4	D49.0
splenic flexure	C18.5	C78.5	D01.0	D12.3	D37.4	D49.0
small	C17.9	C78.4	D01.40	D13.30	D37.2	D49.0
duodenum	C17.0	C78.4	D01.49	D13.2	D37.2	D49.0
ileum	C17.2	C78.4	D01.49	D13.39	D37.2	D49.0
jejunum	C17.1	C78.4	D01.49	D13.39	D37.2	D49.0
overlapping lesion	C17.8			—	—	—
tract NEC	C26.0	C78.89	D01.40	D13.9	D37.8	D49.0
intra-abdominal	C76.2	C79.89	D09.8	D36.7	D48.7	D49.89
intracranial NEC	C71.9	C79.31	—	D33.2	D43.2	D49.6
intrahepatic (bile) duct	C22.1	C78.7	D01.5	D13.4	D37.6	D49.0
intraocular	C69.9-✓	C79.49	D09.2-✓	D31.9-✓	D48.7	D49.89
intraorbital	C69.6-✓	C79.49	D09.2-✓	D31.6-✓	D48.7	D49.89
intrasellar	C75.1	C79.89	D09.3	D35.2	D44.3	D49.7
intrathoracic (cavity) (organs)	C76.1	C79.89	D09.8	D15.9	D48.7	D49.89
specified NEC	C76.1	C79.89	D09.8	D15.7	—	—
iris	C69.4-✓	C79.49	D09.2-✓	D31.4-✓	D48.7	D49.89
ischiorectal (fossa)	C76.3	C79.89	D09.8	D36.7	D48.7	D49.89
ischium	C41.4	C79.51	—	D16.8	D48.0	D49.2
island of Reil	C71.0	C79.31	—	D33.0	D43.0	D49.6
islands or islets of Langerhans	C25.4	C78.89	D01.7	D13.7	D37.8	D49.0
isthmus uteri	C54.0	C79.82	D07.0	D26.1	D39.0	D49.59
jaw	C76.0	C79.89	D09.8	D36.7	D48.7	D49.89
bone	C41.1	C79.51	—	D16.5	D48.0	D49.2
lower	C41.1	C79.51	—	D16.5	—	—
upper	C41.0	C79.51	—	D16.4	—	—
carcinoma (any type) (lower)						
(upper)	C76.0	C79.89		—	—	—
skin — *see also* Neoplasm, skin, face	C44.309	C79.2	D04.39	D23.39	D48.5	D49.2
soft tissues	C03.9	C79.89	D00.03	D10.39	D37.09	D49.0
lower	C03.1	C79.89	D00.03	D10.39	D37.09	D49.0
upper	C03.0	C79.89	D00.03	D10.39	D37.09	D49.0
jejunum	C17.1	C78.4	D01.49	D13.39	D37.2	D49.0
joint NEC — *see also* Neoplasm, bone	C41.9	C79.51	—	D16.9	D48.0	D49.2
acromioclavicular	C40.0-✓	C79.51		D16.0-✓	—	—
bursa or synovial membrane — *see* Neoplasm, connective tissue						
costovertebral	C41.3	C79.51		D16.7	D48.0	D49.2
sternocostal	C41.3	C79.51		D16.7	D48.0	D49.2
temporomandibular	C41.1	C79.51		D16.5	D48.0	D49.2
junction						
anorectal	C21.8	C78.5	D01.3	D12.9	D37.8	D49.0
cardioesophageal	C16.0	C78.89	D00.2	D13.1	D37.1	D49.0
esophagogastric	C16.0	C78.89	D00.2	D13.1	D37.1	D49.0
gastroesophageal	C16.0	C78.89	D00.2	D13.1	D37.1	D49.0
hard and soft palate	C05.9	C79.89	D00.00	D10.39	D37.09	D49.0
ileocecal	C18.0	C78.5	D01.0	D12.0	D37.4	D49.0
Neoplasm, neoplastic						
— *continued*						
junction — *continued*						
pelvirectal	C19	C78.5	D01.1	D12.7	D37.5	D49.0
pelviureteric	C65.-✓	C79.0-✓	D09.19	D30.1-✓	D41.1-✓	D49.59
rectosigmoid	C19	C78.5	D01.1	D12.7	D37.5	D49.0
squamocolumnar, of cervix	C53.8	C79.82	D06.7	D26.0	D39.0	D49.59
Kaposi's sarcoma — *see* Kaposi's, sarcoma						
kidney (parenchymal)	C64.-✓	C79.0-✓	D09.19	D30.0-✓	D41.0-✓	D49.51-✓
calyx	C65.-✓	C79.0-✓	D09.19	D30.1-✓	D41.1-✓	D49.51-✓
hilus	C65.-✓	C79.0-✓	D09.19	D30.1-✓	D41.1-✓	D49.51-✓
pelvis	C65.-✓	C79.0-✓	D09.19	D30.1-✓	D41.1-✓	D49.51-✓
knee NEC	C76.5-✓	C79.89	D04.7-✓	D36.7	D48.7	D49.89
labia (skin)	C51.9	C79.82	D07.1	D28.0	D39.8	D49.59
majora	C51.0	C79.82	D07.1	D28.0	D39.8	D49.59
minora	C51.1	C79.82	D07.1	D28.0	D39.8	D49.59
labial — *see also* Neoplasm, lip	C00.9	C79.89	D00.01	D10.0	D37.01	D49.0
sulcus (lower) (upper)	C06.1	C79.89	D00.02	D10.39	D37.09	D49.0
labium (skin)	C51.9	C79.82	D07.1	D28.0	D39.8	D49.59
majus	C51.0	C79.82	D07.1	D28.0	D39.8	D49.59
minus	C51.1	C79.82	D07.1	D28.0	D39.8	D49.59
lacrimal						
canaliculi	C69.5-✓	C79.49	D09.2-✓	D31.5-✓	D48.7	D49.89
duct (nasal)	C69.5-✓	C79.49	D09.2-✓	D31.5-✓	D48.7	D49.89
gland	C69.5-✓	C79.49	D09.2-✓	D31.5-✓	D48.7	D49.89
punctum	C69.5-✓	C79.49	D09.2-✓	D31.5-✓	D48.7	D49.89
sac	C69.5-✓	C79.49	D09.2-✓	D31.5-✓	D48.7	D49.89
Langerhans, islands or islets	C25.4	C78.89	D01.7	D13.7	D37.8	D49.0
laryngopharynx	C13.9	C79.89	D00.08	D10.7	D37.05	D49.0
larynx, laryngeal NEC	C32.9	C78.39	D02.0	D14.1	D38.0	D49.1
aryepiglottic fold	C32.1	C78.39	D02.0	D14.1	D38.0	D49.1
cartilage (arytenoid) (cricoid) (cuneiform) (thyroid)	C32.3	C78.39	D02.0	D14.1	D38.0	D49.1
commissure (anterior) (posterior)	C32.0	C78.39	D02.0	D14.1	D38.0	D49.1
extrinsic NEC	C32.1	C78.39	D02.0	D14.1	D38.0	D49.1
meaning hypopharynx	C13.9	C79.89	D00.08	D10.7	D37.05	D49.0
interarytenoid fold	C32.1	C78.39	D02.0	D14.1	D38.0	D49.1
intrinsic	C32.0	C78.39	D02.0	D14.1	D38.0	D49.1
overlapping lesion	C32.8	—		—	—	—
ventricular band	C32.1	C78.39	D02.0	D14.1	D38.0	D49.1
leg NEC	C76.5-✓	C79.89	D04.7-✓	D36.7	D48.7	D49.89
lens, crystalline	C69.4-✓	C79.49	D09.2-✓	D31.4-✓	D48.7	D49.89
lid (lower) (upper)	C44.10-✓	C79.2	D04.1-✓	D23.1-✓	D48.5	D49.2
basal cell carcinoma	C44.11-✓	—	—	—	—	—
sebaceous cell	C44.13-✓	—	—	—	—	—
specified type NEC	C44.19-✓	—	—	—	—	—
squamous cell carcinoma	C44.12-✓	—	—	—	—	—
ligament — *see also* Neoplasm, connective tissue						
broad	C57.1-✓	C79.82	D07.39	D28.2	D39.8	D49.59
Mackenrodt's	C57.7	C79.82	D07.39	D28.7	D39.8	D49.59
non-uterine — *see* Neoplasm, connective tissue						
round	C57.2-✓	C79.82	—	D28.2	D39.8	D49.59
sacro-uterine	C57.3	C79.82	—	D28.2	D39.8	D49.59
uterine	C57.3	C79.82	—	D28.2	D39.8	D49.59
utero-ovarian	C57.7	C79.82	D07.39	D28.2	D39.8	D49.59
uterosacral	C57.3	C79.82	—	D28.2	D39.8	D49.59
limb	C76.8	C79.89	D04.8	D36.7	D48.7	D49.89
lower	C76.5-✓	C79.89	D04.7-✓	D36.7	D48.7	D49.89
upper	C76.4-✓	C79.89	D04.6-✓	D36.7	D48.7	D49.89
limbus of cornea	C69.1-✓	C79.49	D09.2-✓	D31.1-✓	D48.7	D49.89

Neoplasm, neoplastic	Malignant Primary	Malignant Secondary	Ca in situ	Benign	Uncertain Behavior	Unspecified Behavior
— continued						
lingual NEC — see also Neoplasm, tongue	C02.9	C79.89	D00.07	D10.1	D37.02	D49.0
lingula, lung	C34.1-☑	C78.0-☑	D02.2-☑	D14.3-☑	D38.1	D49.1
lip	C00.9	C79.89	D00.01	D10.0	D37.01	D49.0
buccal aspect — see Neoplasm, lip, internal						
commissure	C00.6	C79.89	D00.01	D10.0	D37.01	D49.0
external	C00.2	C79.89	D00.01	D10.0	D37.01	D49.0
lower	C00.1	C79.89	D00.01	D10.0	D37.01	D49.0
upper	C00.0	C79.89	D00.01	D10.0	D37.01	D49.0
frenulum — see Neoplasm, lip, internal						
inner aspect — see Neoplasm, lip, internal						
internal	C00.5	C79.89	D00.01	D10.0	D37.01	D49.0
lower	C00.4	C79.89	D00.01	D10.0	D37.01	D49.0
upper	C00.3	C79.89	D00.01	D10.0	D37.01	D49.0
lipstick area	C00.2	C79.89	D00.01	D10.0	D37.01	D49.0
lower	C00.1	C79.89	D00.01	D10.0	D37.01	D49.0
upper	C00.0	C79.89	D00.01	D10.0	D37.01	D49.0
lower	C00.1	C79.89	D00.01	D10.0	D37.01	D49.0
internal	C00.4	C79.89	D00.01	D10.0	D37.01	D49.0
mucosa — see Neoplasm, lip, internal						
oral aspect — see Neoplasm, lip, internal						
overlapping lesion	C00.8	—	—	—	—	—
with oral cavity or pharynx	C14.8					
skin (commissure) (lower) (upper)	C44.00	C79.2	D04.0	D23.0	D48.5	D49.2
basal cell carcinoma	C44.01	—	—	—	—	—
specified type NEC	C44.09	—	—	—	—	—
squamous cell carcinoma	C44.02	—	—	—	—	—
upper	C00.0	C79.89	D00.01	D10.0	D37.01	D49.0
internal	C00.3	C79.89	D00.01	D10.0	D37.01	D49.0
vermilion border	C00.2	C79.89	D00.01	D10.0	D37.01	D49.0
lower	C00.1	C79.89	D00.01	D10.0	D37.01	D49.0
upper	C00.0	C79.89	D00.01	D10.0	D37.01	D49.0
lipomatous — see Lipoma, by site						
liver — see also Index to disease, by histology	C22.9	C78.7	D01.5	D13.4	D37.6	D49.0
primary	C22.8	C78.7	D01.5	D13.4	D37.6	D49.0
lumbosacral plexus	C47.5	C79.89	—	D36.16	D48.2	D49.2
lung	C34.9-☑	C78.0-☑	D02.2-☑	D14.3-☑	D38.1	D49.1
azygos lobe	C34.1-☑	C78.0-☑	D02.2-☑	D14.3-☑	D38.1	D49.1
carina	C34.0-☑	C78.0-☑	D02.2-☑	D14.3-☑	D38.1	D49.1
hilus	C34.0-☑	C78.0-☑	D02.2-☑	D14.3-☑	D38.1	D49.1
lingula	C34.1-☑	C78.0-☑	D02.2-☑	D14.3-☑	D38.1	D49.1
lobe NEC	C34.9-☑	C78.0-☑	D02.2-☑	D14.3-☑	D38.1	D49.1
lower lobe	C34.3-☑	C78.0-☑	D02.2-☑	D14.3-☑	D38.1	D49.1
main bronchus	C34.0-☑	C78.0-☑	D02.2-☑	D14.3-☑	D38.1	D49.1
mesothelioma — see Mesothelioma						
middle lobe	C34.2	C78.0-☑	D02.21	D14.31·	D38.1	D49.1
overlapping lesion	C34.8-☑	—	—	—	—	—
upper lobe	C34.1-☑	C78.0-☑	D02.2-☑	D14.3-☑	D38.1	D49.1
lymph, lymphatic channel NEC	C49.9	C79.89	—	D21.9	D48.1	D49.2
gland						
(secondary)	—	C77.9	—	D36.0	D48.7	D49.89
abdominal	—	C77.2	—	D36.0	D48.7	D49.89
aortic	—	C77.2	—	D36.0	D48.7	D49.89
arm	—	C77.3	—	D36.0	D48.7	D49.89

Neoplasm, neoplastic	Malignant Primary	Malignant Secondary	Ca in situ	Benign	Uncertain Behavior	Unspecified Behavior
— continued						
lymph, lymphatic channel — continued						
gland — continued						
auricular (anterior) (posterior)	—	C77.0	—	D36.0	D48.7	D49.89
axilla, axillary	—	C77.3	—	D36.0	D48.7	D49.89
brachial	—	C77.3	—	D36.0	D48.7	D49.89
bronchial	—	C77.1	—	D36.0	D48.7	D49.89
bronchopulmonary	—	C77.1	—	D36.0	D48.7	D49.89
celiac	—	C77.2	—	D36.0	D48.7	D49.89
cervical	—	C77.0	—	D36.0	D48.7	D49.89
cervicofacial	—	C77.0	—	D36.0	D48.7	D49.89
Cloquet	—	C77.4	—	D36.0	D48.7	D49.89
colic	—	C77.2	—	D36.0	D48.7	D49.89
common duct	—	C77.2	—	D36.0	D48.7	D49.89
cubital	—	C77.3	—	D36.0	D48.7	D49.89
diaphragmatic	—	C77.1	—	D36.0	D48.7	D49.89
epigastric, inferior	—	C77.1	—	D36.0	D48.7	D49.89
epitrochlear	—	C77.3	—	D36.0	D48.7	D49.89
esophageal	—	C77.1	—	D36.0	D48.7	D49.89
face	—	C77.0	—	D36.0	D48.7	D49.89
femoral	—	C77.4	—	D36.0	D48.7	D49.89
gastric	—	C77.2	—	D36.0	D48.7	D49.89
groin	—	C77.4	—	D36.0	D48.7	D49.89
head	—	C77.0	—	D36.0	D48.7	D49.89
hepatic	—	C77.2	—	D36.0	D48.7	D49.89
hilar (pulmonary)	—	C77.1	—	D36.0	D48.7	D49.89
splenic	—	C77.2	—	D36.0	D48.7	D49.89
hypogastric	—	C77.5	—	D36.0	D48.7	D49.89
ileocolic	—	C77.2	—	D36.0	D48.7	D49.89
iliac	—	C77.5	—	D36.0	D48.7	D49.89
infraclavicular	—	C77.3	—	D36.0	D48.7	D49.89
inguina, inguinal	—	C77.4	—	D36.0	D48.7	D49.89
innominate	—	C77.1	—	D36.0	D48.7	D49.89
intercostal	—	C77.1	—	D36.0	D48.7	D49.89
intestinal	—	C77.2	—	D36.0	D48.7	D49.89
intrabdominal	—	C77.2	—	D36.0	D48.7	D49.89
intrapelvic	—	C77.5	—	D36.0	D48.7	D49.89
intrathoracic	—	C77.1	—	D36.0	D48.7	D49.89
jugular	—	C77.0	—	D36.0	D48.7	D49.89
leg	—	C77.4	—	D36.0	D48.7	D49.89
limb						
lower	—	C77.4	—	D36.0	D48.7	D49.89
upper	—	C77.3	—	D36.0	D48.7	D49.89
lower limb	—	C77.4	—	D36.0	D48.7	D49.89
lumbar	—	C77.2	—	D36.0	D48.7	D49.89
mandibular	—	C77.0	—	D36.0	D48.7	D49.89
mediastinal	—	C77.1	—	D36.0	D48.7	D49.89
mesenteric (inferior) (superior)	—	C77.2	—	D36.0	D48.7	D49.89
midcolic	—	C77.2	—	D36.0	D48.7	D49.89
multiple sites in categories C77.0 - C77.5	—	C77.8	—	D36.0	D48.7	D49.89
neck	—	C77.0	—	D36.0	D48.7	D49.89
obturator	—	C77.5	—	D36.0	D48.7	D49.89
occipital	—	C77.0	—	D36.0	D48.7	D49.89
pancreatic	—	C77.2	—	D36.0	D48.7	D49.89
para-aortic	—	C77.2	—	D36.0	D48.7	D49.89
paracervical	—	C77.5	—	D36.0	D48.7	D49.89
parametrial	—	C77.5	—	D36.0	D48.7	D49.89
parasternal	—	C77.1	—	D36.0	D48.7	D49.89
parotid	—	C77.0	—	D36.0	D48.7	D49.89
pectoral	—	C77.3	—	D36.0	D48.7	D49.89
pelvic	—	C77.5	—	D36.0	D48.7	D49.89
peri-aortic	—	C77.2	—	D36.0	D48.7	D49.89
peripancreatic	—	C77.2	—	D36.0	D48.7	D49.89
popliteal	—	C77.4	—	D36.0	D48.7	D49.89
porta hepatis	—	C77.2	—	D36.0	D48.7	D49.89
portal	—	C77.2	—	D36.0	D48.7	D49.89
preauricular	—	C77.0	—	D36.0	D48.7	D49.89
prelaryngeal	—	C77.0	—	D36.0	D48.7	D49.89
presymphysial	—	C77.5	—	D36.0	D48.7	D49.89
pretracheal	—	C77.0	—	D36.0	D48.7	D49.89
primary (any site) NEC	C96.9	—	—	—	—	—

☑ Additional Character Required — Refer to the Tabular List for Character Selection   ▽ Subterms under main terms may continue to next column or page

Neoplasm, neoplastic — continued

Neoplasm, neoplastic — continued	Malignant Primary	Malignant Secondary	Ca in situ	Benign	Uncertain Behavior	Unspecified Behavior
lymph, lymphatic channel — continued						
gland — continued						
pulmonary (hiler)	—	C77.1	—	D36.0	D48.7	D49.89
pyloric	—	C77.2	—	D36.0	D48.7	D49.89
retroperitoneal	—	C77.2	—	D36.0	D48.7	D49.89
retropharyngeal	—	C77.0	—	D36.0	D48.7	D49.89
Rosenmuller's	—	C77.4	—	D36.0	D48.7	D49.89
sacral	—	C77.5	—	D36.0	D48.7	D49.89
scalene	—	C77.0	—	D36.0	D48.7	D49.89
site NEC	—	C77.9	—	D36.0	D48.7	D49.89
splenic (hilar)	—	C77.2	—	D36.0	D48.7	D49.89
subclavicular	—	C77.3	—	D36.0	D48.7	D49.89
subinguinal	—	C77.4	—	D36.0	D48.7	D49.89
sublingual	—	C77.0	—	D36.0	D48.7	D49.89
submandibular	—	C77.0	—	D36.0	D48.7	D49.89
submaxillary	—	C77.0	—	D36.0	D48.7	D49.89
submental	—	C77.0	—	D36.0	D48.7	D49.89
subscapular	—	C77.3	—	D36.0	D48.7	D49.89
supraclavicular	—	C77.0	—	D36.0	D48.7	D49.89
thoracic	—	C77.1	—	D36.0	D48.7	D49.89
tibial	—	C77.4	—	D36.0	D48.7	D49.89
tracheal	—	C77.1	—	D36.0	D48.7	D49.89
tracheobronchial	—	C77.1	—	D36.0	D48.7	D49.89
upper limb	—	C77.3	—	D36.0	D48.7	D49.89
Virchow's	—	C77.0	—	D36.0	D48.7	D49.89
node — see also Neoplasm, lymph gland						
primary NEC	C96.9	—	—	—	—	—
vessel — see also Neoplasm, connective tissue	C49.9	C79.89	—	D21.9	D48.1	D49.2
Mackenrodt's ligament	C57.7	C79.82	D07.39	D28.7	D39.8	D49.59
malar	C41.0	C79.51	—	D16.4	D48.0	D49.2
region — see Neoplasm, cheek						
mammary gland — see Neoplasm, breast						
mandible	C41.1	C79.51	—	D16.5	D48.0	D49.2
alveolar						
mucosa (carcinoma)	C03.1	C79.89	D00.03	D10.39	D37.09	D49.0
ridge or process	C41.1	C79.51	—	D16.5	D48.0	D49.2
marrow (bone) NEC	C96.9	C79.52	—	—	D47.9	D49.89
mastectomy site (skin) — see also Neoplasm, breast, skin	C44.501	C79.2	—	—	—	—
specified as breast tissue	C50.8-☑	C79.81	—	—	—	—
mastoid (air cells) (antrum)	C30.1	C78.39	D02.3	D14.0	D38.5	D49.1
bone or process	C41.0	C79.51	—	D16.4	D48.0	D49.2
maxilla, maxillary (superior)	C41.0	C79.51	—	D16.4	D48.0	D49.2
alveolar						
mucosa	C03.0	C79.89	D00.03	D10.39	D37.09	D49.0
ridge or process (carcinoma)	C41.0	C79.51	—	D16.4	D48.0	D49.2
antrum	C31.0	C78.39	D02.3	D14.0	D38.5	D49.1
carcinoma	C03.0	C79.51	—	—	—	—
inferior — see Neoplasm, mandible						
sinus	C31.0	C78.39	D02.3	D14.0	D38.5	D49.1
meatus external (ear) — see also Neoplasm, skin, ear	C44.20-☑	C79.2	D04.2-☑	D23.2-☑	D48.5	D49.2
Meckel diverticulum, malignant	C17.3	C78.4	D01.49	D13.39	D37.2	D49.0
mediastinum, mediastinal	C38.3	C78.1	—	D15.2	D38.3	D49.89
anterior	C38.1	C78.1	—	D15.2	D38.3	D49.89

Neoplasm, neoplastic — continued

Neoplasm, neoplastic — continued	Malignant Primary	Malignant Secondary	Ca in situ	Benign	Uncertain Behavior	Unspecified Behavior
mediastinum, mediastinal — continued						
posterior	C38.2	C78.1	—	D15.2	D38.3	D49.89
medulla						
adrenal	C74.1-☑	C79.7-☑	D09.3	D35.0-☑	D44.1-☑	D49.7
oblongata	C71.7	C79.31	—	D33.1	D43.1	D49.6
meibomian gland	C44.10-☑	C79.2	D04.1-☑	D23.1-☑	D48.5	D49.2
basal cell carcinoma	C44.11-☑	—	—	—	—	—
sebaceous cell	C44.13-☑	—	—	—	—	—
specified type NEC	C44.19-☑	—	—	—	—	—
squamous cell carcinoma	C44.12-☑	—	—	—	—	—
melanoma — see Melanoma						
meninges	C70.9	C79.49	—	D32.9	D42.9	D49.7
brain	C70.0	C79.32	—	D32.0	D42.0	D49.7
cerebral	C70.0	C79.32	—	D32.0	D42.0	D49.7
crainial	C70.0	C79.32	—	D32.0	D42.0	D49.7
intracranial	C70.0	C79.32	—	D32.0	D42.0	D49.7
spinal (cord)	C70.1	C79.49	—	D32.1	D42.1	D49.7
meniscus, knee joint (lateral) (medial)	C40.2-☑	C79.51	—	D16.2-☑	D48.0	D49.2
Merkel cell — see Carcinoma, Merkel cell						
mesentery, mesenteric	C48.1	C78.6	—	D20.1	D48.4	D49.0
mesoappendix	C48.1	C78.6	—	D20.1	D48.4	D49.0
mesocolon	C48.1	C78.6	—	D20.1	D48.4	D49.0
mesopharynx — see Neoplasm, oropharynx						
mesosalpinx	C57.1-☑	C79.82	D07.39	D28.2	D39.8	D49.59
mesothelial tissue — see Mesothelioma						
mesothelioma — see Mesothelioma						
mesovarium	C57.1-☑	C79.82	D07.39	D28.2	D39.8	D49.59
metacarpus (any bone)	C40.1-☑	C79.51	—	D16.1-☑	—	—
metastatic NEC — see also Neoplasm, by site, secondary	—	C79.9	—	—	—	—
metatarsus (any bone)	C40.3-☑	C79.51	—	D16.3-☑	—	—
midbrain	C71.7	C79.31	—	D33.1	D43.1	D49.6
milk duct — see Neoplasm, breast						
mons						
pubis	C51.9	C79.82	D07.1	D28.0	D39.8	D49.59
veneris	C51.9	C79.82	D07.1	D28.0	D39.8	D49.59
motor tract	C72.9	C79.49	—	D33.9	D43.9	D49.7
brain	C71.9	C79.31	—	D33.2	D43.2	D49.6
cauda equina	C72.1	C79.49	—	D33.4	D43.4	D49.7
spinal	C72.0	C79.49	—	D33.4	D43.4	D49.7
mouth	C06.9	C79.89	D00.00	D10.30	D37.09	D49.0
book-leaf	C06.89	C79.89	—	—	—	—
floor	C04.9	C79.89	D00.06	D10.2	D37.09	D49.0
anterior portion	C04.0	C79.89	D00.06	D10.2	D37.09	D49.0
lateral portion	C04.1	C79.89	D00.06	D10.2	D37.09	D49.0
overlapping lesion	C04.8	—	—	—	—	—
overlapping NEC	C06.80	—	—	—	—	—
roof	C05.9	C79.89	D00.00	D10.39	D37.09	D49.0
specified part NEC	C06.89	C79.89	D00.00	D10.39	D37.09	D49.0
vestibule	C06.1	C79.89	D00.00	D10.39	D37.09	D49.0
mucosa						
alveolar (ridge or process)	C03.9	C79.89	D00.03	D10.39	D37.09	D49.0
lower	C03.1	C79.89	D00.03	D10.39	D37.09	D49.0
upper	C03.0	C79.89	D00.03	D10.39	D37.09	D49.0
buccal	C06.0	C79.89	D00.02	D10.39	D37.09	D49.0
cheek	C06.0	C79.89	D00.02	D10.39	D37.09	D49.0

Neoplasm, neoplastic — continued	Malignant Primary	Malignant Secondary	Ca in situ	Benign	Uncertain Behavior	Unspecified Behavior
mucosa — continued						
lip — see Neoplasm, lip, internal						
nasal	C30.0	C78.39	D02.3	D14.0	D38.5	D49.1
oral	C06.0	C79.89	D00.02	D10.39	D37.09	D49.0
Mullerian duct						
female	C57.7	C79.82	D07.39	D28.7	D39.8	D49.59
male	C63.7	C79.82	D07.69	D29.8	D40.8	D49.59
muscle — see also Neoplasm, connective tissue						
extraocular	C69.6-☑	C79.49	D09.2-☑	D31.6-☑	D48.7	D49.89
myocardium	C38.0	C79.89	—	D15.1	D48.7	D49.89
myometrium	C54.2	C79.82	D07.0	D26.1	D39.0	D49.59
myopericardium	C38.0	C79.89	—	D15.1	D48.7	D49.89
nabothian gland (follicle)	C53.0	C79.82	D06.0	D26.0	D39.0	D49.59
nail — see also Neoplasm, skin, limb	C44.90	C79.2	D04.9	D23.9	D48.5	D49.2
finger — see also Neoplasm, skin, limb, upper	C44.60-☑	C79.2	D04.6-☑	D23.6-☑	D48.5	D49.2
toe — see also Neoplasm, skin, limb, lower	C44.70-☑	C79.2	D04.7-☑	D23.7-☑	D48.5	D49.2
nares, naris (anterior) (posterior)	C30.0	C78.39	D02.3	D14.0	D38.5	D49.1
nasal — see Neoplasm, nose						
nasolabial groove — see also Neoplasm, skin, face	C44.309	C79.2	D04.39	D23.39	D48.5	D49.2
nasolacrimal duct	C69.5-☑	C79.49	D09.2-☑	D31.5-☑	D48.7	D49.89
nasopharynx, nasopharyngeal	C11.9	C79.89	D00.08	D10.6	D37.05	D49.0
floor	C11.3	C79.89	D00.08	D10.6	D37.05	D49.0
overlapping lesion	C11.8	—	—	—	—	—
roof	C11.0	C79.89	D00.08	D10.6	D37.05	D49.0
wall	C11.9	C79.89	D00.08	D10.6	D37.05	D49.0
anterior	C11.3	C79.89	D00.08	D10.6	D37.05	D49.0
lateral	C11.2	C79.89	D00.08	D10.6	D37.05	D49.0
posterior	C11.1	C79.89	D00.08	D10.6	D37.05	D49.0
superior	C11.0	C79.89	D00.08	D10.6	D37.05	D49.0
nates — see also Neoplasm, skin, trunk	C44.509	C79.2	D04.5	D23.5	D48.5	D49.2
neck NEC	C76.0	C79.89	D09.8	D36.7	D48.7	D49.89
skin	C44.40	—	—	—	—	—
basal cell carcinoma	C44.41	—	—	—	—	—
specified type NEC	C44.49	—	—	—	—	—
squamous cell carcinoma	C44.42	—	—	—	—	—
nerve (ganglion)	C47.9	C79.89	—	D36.10	D48.2	D49.2
abducens	C72.59	C79.49	—	D33.3	D43.3	D49.7
accessory (spinal)	C72.59	C79.49	—	D33.3	D43.3	D49.7
acoustic	C72.4-☑	C79.49	—	D33.3	D43.3	D49.7
auditory	C72.4-☑	C79.49	—	D33.3	D43.3	D49.7
autonomic NEC — see also Neoplasm, nerve, peripheral	C47.9	C79.89	—	D36.10	D48.2	D49.2
brachial	C47.1-☑	C79.89	—	D36.12	D48.2	D49.2
cranial	C72.50	C79.49	—	D33.3	D43.3	D49.7
specified NEC	C72.59	C79.49	—	D33.3	D43.3	D49.7
facial	C72.59	C79.49	—	D33.3	D43.3	D49.7
femoral	C47.2-☑	C79.89	—	D36.13	D48.2	D49.2
ganglion NEC — see also Neoplasm, nerve, peripheral	C47.9	C79.89	—	D36.10	D48.2	D49.2
glossopharyngeal	C72.59	C79.49	—	D33.3	D43.3	D49.7
hypoglossal	C72.59	C79.49	—	D33.3	D43.3	D49.7
intercostal	C47.3	C79.89	—	D36.14	D48.2	D49.2
lumbar	C47.6	C79.89	—	D36.17	D48.2	D49.2
median	C47.1-☑	C79.89	—	D36.12	D48.2	D49.2
obturator	C47.2-☑	C79.89	—	D36.13	D48.2	D49.2

Neoplasm, neoplastic — continued	Malignant Primary	Malignant Secondary	Ca in situ	Benign	Uncertain Behavior	Unspecified Behavior
nerve — continued						
oculomotor	C72.59	C79.49	—	D33.3	D43.3	D49.7
olfactory	C47.2-☑	C79.49	—	D33.3	D43.3	D49.7
optic	C72.3-☑	C79.49	—	D33.3	D43.3	D49.7
parasympathetic NEC	C47.9	C79.89	—	D36.10	D48.2	D49.2
peripheral NEC	C47.9	C79.89	—	D36.10	D48.2	D49.2
abdomen	C47.4	C79.89	—	D36.15	D48.2	D49.2
abdominal wall	C47.4	C79.89	—	D36.15	D48.2	D49.2
ankle	C47.2-☑	C79.89	—	D36.13	D48.2	D49.2
antecubital fossa or space	C47.1-☑	C79.89	—	D36.12	D48.2	D49.2
arm	C47.1-☑	C79.89	—	D36.12	D48.2	D49.2
auricle (ear)	C47.0	C79.89	—	D36.11	D48.2	D49.2
axilla	C47.3	C79.89	—	D36.12	D48.2	D49.2
back	C47.6	C79.89	—	D36.17	D48.2	D49.2
buttock	C47.5	C79.89	—	D36.16	D48.2	D49.2
calf	C47.2-☑	C79.89	—	D36.13	D48.2	D49.2
cervical region	C47.0	C79.89	—	D36.11	D48.2	D49.2
cheek	C47.0	C79.89	—	D36.11	D48.2	D49.2
chest (wall)	C47.3	C79.89	—	D36.14	D48.2	D49.2
chin	C47.0	C79.89	—	D36.11	D48.2	D49.2
ear (external)	C47.0	C79.89	—	D36.11	D48.2	D49.2
elbow	C47.1-☑	C79.89	—	D36.12	D48.2	D49.2
extrarectal	C47.5	C79.89	—	D36.16	D48.2	D49.2
extremity	C47.9	C79.89	—	D36.10	D48.2	D49.2
lower	C47.2-☑	C79.89	—	D36.13	D48.2	D49.2
upper	C47.1-☑	C79.89	—	D36.12	D48.2	D49.2
eyelid	C47.0	C79.89	—	D36.11	D48.2	D49.2
face	C47.0	C79.89	—	D36.11	D48.2	D49.2
finger	C47.1-☑	C79.89	—	D36.12	D48.2	D49.2
flank	C47.6	C79.89	—	D36.17	D48.2	D49.2
foot	C47.2-☑	C79.89	—	D36.13	D48.2	D49.2
forearm	C47.1-☑	C79.89	—	D36.12	D48.2	D49.2
forehead	C47.0	C79.89	—	D36.11	D48.2	D49.2
gluteal region	C47.5	C79.89	—	D36.16	D48.2	D49.2
groin	C47.5	C79.89	—	D36.16	D48.2	D49.2
hand	C47.1-☑	C79.89	—	D36.12	D48.2	D49.2
head	C47.0	C79.89	—	D36.11	D48.2	D49.2
heel	C47.2-☑	C79.89	—	D36.13	D48.2	D49.2
hip	C47.2-☑	C79.89	—	D36.13	D48.2	D49.2
infraclavicular region	C47.3	C79.89	—	D36.14	D48.2	D49.2
inguinal (canal) (region)	C47.5	C79.89	—	D36.16	D48.2	D49.2
intrathoracic	C47.3	C79.89	—	D36.14	D48.2	D49.2
ischiorectal fossa	C47.5	C79.89	—	D36.16	D48.2	D49.2
knee	C47.2-☑	C79.89	—	D36.13	D48.2	D49.2
leg	C47.2-☑	C79.89	—	D36.13	D48.2	D49.2
limb NEC	C47.9	C79.89	—	D36.10	D48.2	D49.2
lower	C47.2-☑	C79.89	—	D36.13	D48.2	D49.2
upper	C47.1-☑	C79.89	—	D36.12	D48.2	D49.2
nates	C47.5	C79.89	—	D36.16	D48.2	D49.2
neck	C47.0	C79.89	—	D36.11	D48.2	D49.2
orbit	C69.6-☑	C79.49	—	D31.6-☑	D48.7	D49.2
pararectal	C47.5	C79.89	—	D36.16	D48.2	D49.2
paraurethral	C47.5	C79.89	—	D36.16	D48.2	D49.2
paravaginal	C47.5	C79.89	—	D36.16	D48.2	D49.2
pelvis (floor)	C47.5	C79.89	—	D36.16	D48.2	D49.2
pelvoabdominal	C47.8	C79.89	—	D36.17	D48.2	D49.2
perineum	C47.5	C79.89	—	D36.16	D48.2	D49.2
perirectal (tissue)	C47.5	C79.89	—	D36.16	D48.2	D49.2
periurethral (tissue)	C47.5	C79.89	—	D36.16	D48.2	D49.2
popliteal fossa or space	C47.2-☑	C79.89	—	D36.13	D48.2	D49.2
presacral	C47.5	C79.89	—	D36.16	D48.2	D49.2
pterygoid fossa	C47.0	C79.89	—	D36.11	D48.2	D49.2
rectovaginal septum or wall	C47.5	C79.89	—	D36.16	D48.2	D49.2
rectovesical	C47.5	C79.89	—	D36.16	D48.2	D49.2
sacrococcygeal region	C47.5	C79.89	—	D36.16	D48.2	D49.2
scalp	C47.0	C79.89	—	D36.11	D48.2	D49.2

☑ Additional Character Required — Refer to the Tabular List for Character Selection ⬙ Subterms under main terms may continue to next column or page

Neoplasm, neoplastic — continued	Malignant Primary	Malignant Secondary	Ca in situ	Benign	Uncertain Behavior	Unspecified Behavior
nerve — *continued*						
peripheral — *continued*						
scapular region	C47.3	C79.89	—	D36.14	D48.2	D49.2
shoulder	C47.1-☑	C79.89		D36.12	D48.2	D49.2
submental	C47.0	C79.89		D36.11	D48.2	D49.2
supraclavicular region	C47.0	C79.89	—	D36.11	D48.2	D49.2
temple	C47.0	C79.89		D36.11	D48.2	D49.2
temporal region	C47.0	C79.89		D36.11	D48.2	D49.2
thigh	C47.2-☑	C79.89		D36.13	D48.2	D49.2
thoracic (duct) (wall)	C47.3	C79.89		D36.14	D48.2	D49.2
thorax	C47.3	C79.89		D36.14	D48.2	D49.2
thumb	C47.1-☑	C79.89		D36.12	D48.2	D49.2
toe	C47.2-☑	C79.89		D36.13	D48.2	D49.2
trunk	C47.6	C79.89		D36.17	D48.2	D49.2
umbilicus	C47.4	C79.89		D36.15	D48.2	D49.2
vesicorectal	C47.5	C79.89		D36.16	D48.2	D49.2
wrist	C47.1-☑	C79.89		D36.12	D48.2	D49.2
radial	C47.1-☑	C79.89		D36.12	D48.2	D49.2
sacral	C47.5	C79.89		D36.16	D48.2	D49.2
sciatic	C47.2-☑	C79.89		D36.13	D48.2	D49.2
spinal NEC	C47.9	C79.89		D36.10	D48.2	D49.2
accessory	C72.59	C79.49	—	D33.3	D43.3	D49.7
sympathetic NEC — *see also* Neoplasm, nerve, peripheral	C47.9	C79.89		D36.10	D48.2	D49.2
trigeminal	C72.59	C79.49		D33.3	D43.3	D49.7
trochlear	C72.59	C79.49		D33.3	D43.3	D49.7
ulnar	C47.1-☑	C79.89		D36.12	D48.2	D49.2
vagus	C72.59	C79.49		D33.3	D43.3	D49.7
nervous system (central)	C72.9	C79.40		D33.9	D43.9	D49.7
autonomic — *see* Neoplasm, nerve, peripheral						
parasympathetic — *see* Neoplasm, nerve, peripheral						
specified site NEC	—	C79.49	—	D33.7	D43.8	—
sympathetic — *see* Neoplasm, nerve, peripheral						
nevus — *see* Nevus						
nipple	C50.0-☑	C79.81	D05.-☑	D24.-☑	—	
nose, nasal	C76.0	C79.89	D09.8	D36.7	D48.7	D49.89
ala (external) (nasi) — *see also* Neoplasm, nose, skin	C44.301	C79.2	D04.39	D23.39	D48.5	D49.2
bone	C41.0	C79.51	—	D16.4	D48.0	D49.2
cartilage	C30.0	C78.39	D02.3	D14.0	D38.5	D49.1
cavity	C30.0	C78.39	D02.3	D14.0	D38.5	D49.1
choana	C11.3	C79.89	D00.08	D10.6	D37.05	D49.0
external (skin) — *see also* Neoplasm, nose, skin	C44.301	C79.2	D04.39	D23.39	D48.5	D49.2
fossa	C30.0	C78.39	D02.3	D14.0	D38.5	D49.1
internal	C30.0	C78.39	D02.3	D14.0	D38.5	D49.1
mucosa	C30.0	C78.39	D02.3	D14.0	D38.5	D49.1
septum	C30.0	C78.39	D02.3	D14.0	D38.5	D49.1
posterior margin	C11.3	C79.89	D00.08	D10.6	D37.05	D49.0
sinus — *see* Neoplasm, sinus						
skin	C44.301	C79.2	D04.39	D23.39	D48.5	D49.2
basal cell carcinoma	C44.311	—	—	—	—	—
specified type NEC	C44.391	—	—	—	—	—
squamous cell carcinoma	C44.321	—	—	—	—	—
turbinate (mucosa)	C30.0	C78.39	D02.3	D14.0	D38.5	D49.1
bone	C41.0	C79.51		D16.4	D48.0	D49.2
vestibule	C30.0	C78.39	D02.3	D14.0	D38.5	D49.1

Neoplasm, neoplastic — continued	Malignant Primary	Malignant Secondary	Ca in situ	Benign	Uncertain Behavior	Unspecified Behavior
nostril	C30.0	C78.39	D02.3	D14.0	D38.5	D49.1
nucleus pulposus	C41.2	C79.51	—	D16.6	D48.0	D49.2
occipital bone	C41.0	C79.51	—	D16.4	D48.0	D49.2
lobe or pole, brain	C71.4	C79.31		D33.0	D43.0	D49.6
odontogenic — *see* Neoplasm, jaw bone						
olfactory nerve or bulb	C72.2-☑	C79.49	—	D33.3	D43.3	D49.7
olive (brain)	C71.7	C79.31		D33.1	D43.1	D49.6
omentum	C48.1	C78.6		D20.1	D48.4	D49.0
operculum (brain)	C71.0	C79.31		D33.0	D43.0	D49.6
optic nerve, chiasm, or tract	C72.3-☑	C79.49	—	D33.3	D43.3	D49.7
oral (cavity)	C06.9	C79.89	D00.00	D10.30	D37.09	D49.0
ill-defined	C14.8	C79.89	D00.00	D10.30	D37.09	D49.0
mucosa	C06.0	C79.89	D00.02	D10.39	D37.09	D49.0
orbit	C69.6-☑	C79.49	D09.2-☑	D31.6-☑	D48.7	D49.89
autonomic nerve	C69.6-☑	C79.49	—	D31.6-☑	D48.7	D49.2
bone	C41.0	C79.51	—	D16.4	D48.0	D49.2
eye	C69.6-☑	C79.49	D09.2-☑	D31.6-☑	D48.7	D49.2
peripheral nerves	C69.6-☑	C79.49	—	D31.6-☑	D48.7	D49.2
soft parts	C69.6-☑	C79.49	D09.2-☑	D31.6-☑	D48.7	D49.89
organ of Zuckerkandl	C75.5	C79.89	—	D35.6	D44.7	D49.7
oropharynx	C10.9	C79.89	D00.08	D10.5	D37.05	D49.0
branchial cleft (vestige)	C10.4	C79.89	D00.08	D10.5	D37.05	D49.0
junctional region	C10.8	C79.89	D00.08	D10.5	D37.05	D49.0
lateral wall	C10.2	C79.89	D00.08	D10.5	D37.05	D49.0
overlapping lesion	C10.8	—	—	—	—	—
pillars or fauces	C09.1	C79.89	D00.08	D10.5	D37.05	D49.0
posterior wall	C10.3	C79.89	D00.08	D10.5	D37.05	D49.0
vallecula	C10.0	C79.89	D00.08	D10.5	D37.05	D49.0
os external	C53.1	C79.82	D06.1	D26.0	D39.0	D49.59
internal	C53.0	C79.82	D06.0	D26.0	D39.0	D49.59
ovary	C56.-☑	C79.6-☑	D07.39	D27.-☑	D39.1-☑	D49.59
oviduct	C57.0-☑	C79.82	D07.39	D28.2	D39.8	D49.59
palate	C05.9	C79.89	D00.00	D10.39	D37.09	D49.0
hard	C05.0	C79.89	D00.05	D10.39	D37.09	D49.0
junction of hard and soft palate	C05.9	C79.89	D00.00	D10.39	D37.09	D49.0
overlapping lesions	C05.8	—	—	—	—	—
soft	C05.1	C79.89	D00.04	D10.39	D37.09	D49.0
nasopharyngeal surface	C11.3	C79.89	D00.08	D10.6	D37.05	D49.0
posterior surface	C11.3	C79.89	D00.08	D10.6	D37.05	D49.0
superior surface	C11.3	C79.89	D00.08	D10.6	D37.05	D49.0
palatoglossal arch	C09.1	C79.89	D00.00	D10.5	D37.09	D49.0
palatopharyngeal arch	C09.1	C79.89	D00.00	D10.5	D37.09	D49.0
pallium	C71.0	C79.31		D33.0	D43.0	D49.6
palpebra	C44.10-☑	C79.2	D04.1-☑	D23.1-☑	D48.5	D49.2
basal cell carcinoma	C44.11-☑	—	—	—	—	—
sebaceous cell	C44.13-☑	—	—	—	—	—
specified type NEC	C44.19-☑	—	—	—	—	—
squamous cell carcinoma	C44.12-☑	—	—	—	—	—
pancreas	C25.9	C78.89	D01.7	D13.6	D37.8	D49.0
body	C25.1	C78.89	D01.7	D13.6	D37.8	D49.0
duct (of Santorini) (of Wirsung)	C25.3	C78.89	D01.7	D13.6	D37.8	D49.0
ectopic tissue	C25.7	C78.89	—	D13.6	D37.8	D49.0
head	C25.0	C78.89	D01.7	D13.6	D37.8	D49.0
islet cells	C25.4	C78.89	D01.7	D13.7	D37.8	D49.0
neck	C25.7	C78.89	D01.7	D13.6	D37.8	D49.0
overlapping lesion	C25.8	—	—	—	—	—
tail	C25.2	C78.89	D01.7	D13.6	D37.8	D49.0

Neoplasm, neoplastic	Malignant Primary	Malignant Secondary	Ca in situ	Benign	Uncertain Behavior	Unspecified Behavior
— continued						
para-aortic body	C75.5	C79.89	—	D35.6	D44.7	D49.7
paraganglion NEC	C75.5	C79.89	—	D35.6	D44.7	D49.7
parametrium	C57.3	C79.82	—	D28.2	D39.8	D49.59
paranephric	C48.0	C78.6	—	D20.0	D48.3	D49.0
pararectal	C76.3	C79.89	—	D36.7	D48.7	D49.89
parasagittal (region)	C76.0	C79.89	D09.8	D36.7	D48.7	D49.89
parasellar	C72.9	C79.49	—	D33.9	D43.8	D49.7
parathyroid (gland)	C75.0	C79.89	D09.3	D35.1	D44.2	D49.7
paraurethral	C76.3	C79.89	—	D36.7	D48.7	D49.89
gland	C68.1	C79.19	D09.19	D30.8	D41.8	D49.59
paravaginal	C76.3	C79.89	—	D36.7	D48.7	D49.89
parenchyma, kidney	C64.-✓	C79.0-✓	D09.19	D30.0-✓	D41.0-✓	D49.51-✓
parietal bone	C41.0	C79.51	—	D16.4	D48.0	D49.2
lobe, brain	C71.3	C79.31	—	D33.0	D43.0	D49.6
paroophoron	C57.1-✓	C79.82	D07.39	D28.2	D39.8	D49.59
parotid (duct) (gland)	C07	C79.89	D00.00	D11.0	D37.030	D49.0
parovarium	C57.1-✓	C79.82	D07.39	D28.2	D39.8	D49.59
patella	C40.20	C79.51	—	—	—	—
peduncle, cerebral	C71.7	C79.31	—	D33.1	D43.1	D49.6
pelvirectal junction	C19	C78.5	D01.1	D12.7	D37.5	D49.0
pelvis, pelvic	C76.3	C79.89	D09.8	D36.7	D48.7	D49.89
bone	C41.4	C79.51	—	D16.8	D48.0	D49.2
floor	C76.3	C79.89	D09.8	D36.7	D48.7	D49.89
renal	C65.-✓	C79.0-✓	D09.19	D30.1-✓	D41.1-✓	D49.51-✓
viscera	C76.3	C79.89	D09.8	D36.7	D48.7	D49.89
wall	C76.3	C79.89	D09.8	D36.7	D48.7	D49.89
pelvo-abdominal	C76.8	C79.89	D09.8	D36.7	D48.7	D49.89
penis	C60.9	C79.82	D07.4	D29.0	D40.8	D49.59
body	C60.2	C79.82	D07.4	D29.0	D40.8	D49.59
corpus (cavernosum)	C60.2	C79.82	D07.4	D29.0	D40.8	D49.59
glans	C60.1	C79.82	D07.4	D29.0	D40.8	D49.59
overlapping sites	C60.8	—	—	—	—	—
skin NEC	C60.9	C79.82	D07.4	D29.0	D40.8	D49.59
periadrenal (tissue)	C48.0	C78.6	—	D20.0	D48.3	D49.0
perianal (skin) — see also Neoplasm, anus, skin	C44.500	C79.2	D04.5	D23.5	D48.5	D49.2
pericardium	C38.0	C79.89	—	D15.1	D48.7	D49.89
perinephric	C48.0	C78.6	—	D20.0	D48.3	D49.0
perineum	C76.3	C79.89	D09.8	D36.7	D48.7	D49.89
periodontal tissue NEC	C03.9	C79.89	D00.03	D10.39	D37.09	D49.0
periosteum — see Neoplasm, bone						
peripancreatic	C48.0	C78.6	—	D20.0	D48.3	D49.0
peripheral nerve NEC	C47.9	C79.89	—	D36.10	D48.2	D49.2
perirectal (tissue)	C76.3	C79.89	—	D36.7	D48.7	D49.89
perirenal (tissue)	C48.0	C78.6	—	D20.0	D48.3	D49.0
peritoneum, peritoneal (cavity)	C48.2	C78.6	—	D20.1	D48.4	D49.0
benign mesothelial tissue — see Mesothelioma, benign						
overlapping lesion	C48.8	—	—	—	—	—
with digestive organs	C26.9	—	—	—	—	—
parietal	C48.1	C78.6	—	D20.1	D48.4	D49.0
pelvic	C48.1	C78.6	—	D20.1	D48.4	D49.0
specified part NEC	C48.1	C78.6	—	D20.1	D48.4	D49.0
peritonsillar (tissue)	C76.0	C79.89	D09.8	D36.7	D48.7	D49.89
periurethral tissue	C76.3	C79.89	—	D36.7	D48.7	D49.89
phalanges foot	C40.3-✓	C79.51	—	D16.3-✓	—	—
hand	C40.1-✓	C79.51	—	D16.1-✓	—	—
pharynx, pharyngeal	C14.0	C79.89	D00.08	D10.9	D37.05	D49.0
bursa	C11.1	C79.89	D00.08	D10.6	D37.05	D49.0
Neoplasm, neoplastic						
— continued						
pharynx, pharyngeal — continued						
fornix	C11.3	C79.89	D00.08	D10.6	D37.05	D49.0
recess	C11.2	C79.89	D00.08	D10.6	D37.05	D49.0
region	C14.0	C79.89	D00.08	D10.9	D37.05	D49.0
tonsil	C11.1	C79.89	D00.08	D10.6	D37.05	D49.0
wall (lateral) (posterior)	C14.0	C79.89	D00.08	D10.9	D37.05	D49.0
pia mater	C70.9	C79.40	—	D32.9	D42.9	D49.7
cerebral	C70.0	C79.32	—	D32.0	D42.0	D49.7
cranial	C70.0	C79.32	—	D32.0	D42.0	D49.7
spinal	C70.1	C79.49	—	D32.1	D42.1	D49.7
pillars of fauces	C09.1	C79.89	D00.08	D10.5	D37.05	D49.0
pineal (body) (gland)	C75.3	C79.89	D09.3	D35.4	D44.5	D49.7
pinna (ear) NEC — see also Neoplasm, skin, ear	C44.20-✓	C79.2	D04.2-✓	D23.2-✓	D48.5	D49.2
piriform fossa or sinus	C12	C79.89	D00.08	D10.7	D37.05	D49.0
pituitary (body) (fossa) (gland) (lobe)	C75.1	C79.89	D09.3	D35.2	D44.3	D49.7
placenta	C58	C79.82	D07.0	D26.7	D39.2	D49.59
pleura, pleural (cavity)	C38.4	C78.2	—	D19.0	D38.2	D49.1
overlapping lesion with heart or mediastinum	C38.8	—	—	—	—	—
parietal	C38.4	C78.2	—	D19.0	D38.2	D49.1
visceral	C38.4	C78.2	—	D19.0	D38.2	D49.1
plexus brachial	C47.1-✓	C79.89	—	D36.12	D48.2	D49.2
cervical	C47.0	C79.89	—	D36.11	D48.2	D49.2
choroid	C71.5	C79.31	—	D33.0	D43.0	D49.6
lumbosacral	C47.5	C79.89	—	D36.16	D48.2	D49.2
sacral	C47.5	C79.89	—	D36.16	D48.2	D49.2
pluriendocrine	C75.8	C79.89	D09.3	D35.7	D44.9	D49.7
pole frontal	C71.1	C79.31	—	D33.0	D43.0	D49.6
occipital	C71.4	C79.31	—	D33.0	D43.0	D49.6
pons (varolii)	C71.7	C79.31	—	D33.1	D43.1	D49.6
popliteal fossa or space	C76.5-✓	C79.89	D04.7-✓	D36.7	D48.7	D49.89
postcricoid (region)	C13.0	C79.89	D00.08	D10.7	D37.05	D49.0
posterior fossa (cranial)	C71.9	C79.31	—	D33.2	D43.2	D49.6
postnasal space	C11.9	C79.89	D00.08	D10.6	D37.05	D49.0
prepuce	C60.0	C79.82	D07.4	D29.0	D40.8	D49.59
prepylorus	C16.4	C78.89	D00.2	D13.1	D37.1	D49.0
presacral (region)	C76.3	C79.89	—	D36.7	D48.7	D49.89
prostate (gland)	C61	C79.82	D07.5	D29.1	D40.0	D49.59
utricle	C68.0	C79.19	D09.19	D30.4	D41.3	D49.59
pterygoid fossa	C49.0	C79.89	—	D21.0	D48.1	D49.2
pubic bone	C41.4	C79.51	—	D16.8	D48.0	D49.2
pudenda, pudendum (female)	C51.9	C79.82	D07.1	D28.0	D39.8	D49.59
pulmonary — see also Neoplasm, lung	C34.9-✓	C78.0-✓	D02.2-✓	D14.3-✓	D38.1	D49.1
putamen	C71.0	C79.31	—	D33.0	D43.0	D49.6
pyloric antrum	C16.3	C78.89	D00.2	D13.1	D37.1	D49.0
canal	C16.4	C78.89	D00.2	D13.1	D37.1	D49.0
pylorus	C16.4	C78.89	D00.2	D13.1	D37.1	D49.0
pyramid (brain)	C71.7	C79.31	—	D33.1	D43.1	D49.6
pyriform fossa or sinus	C12	C79.89	D00.08	D10.7	D37.05	D49.0
radius (any part)	C40.0-✓	C79.51	—	D16.0-✓	—	—
Rathke's pouch	C75.1	C79.89	D09.3	D35.2	D44.3	D49.7
rectosigmoid (junction)	C19	C78.5	D01.1	D12.7	D37.5	D49.0
overlapping lesion with anus or rectum	C21.8	—	—	—	—	—
rectouterine pouch	C48.1	C78.6	—	D20.1	D48.4	D49.0
rectovaginal septum or wall	C76.3	C79.89	D09.8	D36.7	D48.7	D49.89
rectovesical septum	C76.3	C79.89	D09.8	D36.7	D48.7	D49.89
rectum (ampulla)	C20	C78.5	D01.2	D12.8	D37.5	D49.0

348

☑ Additional Character Required — Refer to the Tabular List for Character Selection   ▽ Subterms under main terms may continue to next column or page

	Malignant Primary	Malignant Secondary	Ca in situ	Benign	Uncertain Behavior	Unspecified Behavior
Neoplasm, neoplastic — *continued*						
rectum — *continued*						
and colon	C19	C78.5	D01.1	D12.7	D37.5	D49.0
overlapping lesion with anus or rectosigmoid junction	C21.8	—	—	—	—	—
renal	C64.-☑	C79.0-☑	D09.19	D30.0-☑	D41.0-☑	D49.51-☑
calyx	C65.-☑	C79.0-☑	D09.19	D30.1-☑	D41.1-☑	D49.51-☑
hilus	C65.-☑	C79.0-☑	D09.19	D30.1-☑	D41.1-☑	D49.51-☑
parenchyma	C64.-☑	C79.0-☑	D09.19	D30.0-☑	D41.0-☑	D49.51-☑
pelvis	C65.-☑	C79.0-☑	D09.19	D30.1-☑	D41.1-☑	D49.51-☑
respiratory						
organs or system NEC	C39.9	C78.30	D02.4	D14.4	D38.6	D49.1
tract NEC	C39.9	C78.30	D02.4	D14.4	D38.5	D49.1
upper	C39.0	C78.30	D02.4	D14.4	D38.5	D49.1
retina	C69.2-☑	C79.49	D09.2-☑	D31.2-☑	D48.7	D49.81
retrobulbar	C69.6-☑	C79.49	—	D31.6-☑	D48.7	D49.89
retrocecal	C48.0	C78.6	—	D20.0	D48.3	D49.0
retromolar (area) (triangle) (trigone)	C06.2	C79.89	D00.00	D10.39	D37.09	D49.0
retro-orbital	C76.0	C79.89	D09.8	D36.7	D48.7	D49.89
retroperitoneal (space) (tissue)	C48.0	C78.6	—	D20.0	D48.3	D49.0
retroperitoneum	C48.0	C78.6	—	D20.0	D48.3	D49.0
retropharyngeal	C14.0	C79.89	D00.08	D10.9	D37.05	D49.0
retrovesical (septum)	C76.3	C79.89	D09.8	D36.7	D48.7	D49.89
rhinencephalon	C71.0	C79.31	—	D33.0	D43.0	D49.6
rib	C41.3	C79.51	—	D16.7	D48.0	D49.2
Rosenmuller's fossa	C11.2	C79.89	D00.08	D10.6	D37.05	D49.0
round ligament	C57.2-☑	C79.82	—	D28.2	D39.8	D49.59
sacrococcyx, sacrococcygeal	C41.4	C79.51	—	D16.8	D48.0	D49.2
region	C76.3	C79.89	D09.8	D36.7	D48.7	D49.89
sacrouterine ligament	C57.3	C79.82	—	D28.2	D39.8	D49.59
sacrum, sacral (vertebra)	C41.4	C79.51	—	D16.8	D48.0	D49.2
salivary gland or duct (major)	C08.9	C79.89	D00.00	D11.9	D37.039	D49.0
minor NEC	C06.9	C79.89	D00.00	D10.39	D37.04	D49.0
overlapping lesion	C08.9	—	—	—	—	—
parotid	C07	C79.89	D00.00	D11.0	D37.030	D49.0
pluriglandular	C08.9	C79.89	D00.00	D11.9	D37.039	D49.0
sublingual	C08.1	C79.89	D00.00	D11.7	D37.031	D49.0
submandibular	C08.0	C79.89	D00.00	D11.7	D37.032	D49.0
submaxillary	C08.0	C79.89	D00.00	D11.7	D37.032	D49.0
salpinx (uterine)	C57.0-☑	C79.82	D07.39	D28.2	D39.8	D49.59
Santorini's duct	C25.3	C78.89	D01.7	D13.6	D37.8	D49.0
scalp	C44.40	C79.2	D04.4	D23.4	D48.5	D49.2
basal cell carcinoma	C44.41	—	—	—	—	—
specified type NEC	C44.49	—	—	—	—	—
squamous cell carcinoma	C44.42	—	—	—	—	—
scapula (any part)	C40.0-☑	C79.51	—	D16.0-☑	—	—
scapular region	C76.1	C79.89	D09.8	D36.7	D48.7	D49.89
scar NEC — *see also* Neoplasm, skin, by site	C44.90	C79.2	D04.9	D23.9	D48.5	D49.2
sciatic nerve	C47.2-☑	C79.89	—	D36.13	D48.2	D49.2
sclera	C69.4-☑	C79.49	D09.2-☑	D31.4-☑	D48.7	D49.89
scrotum (skin)	C63.2	C79.82	D07.61	D29.4	D40.8	D49.59
sebaceous gland — *see* Neoplasm, skin						
sella turcica	C75.1	C79.89	D09.3	D35.2	D44.3	D49.7
bone	C41.0	C79.51	—	D16.4	D48.0	D49.2
semilunar cartilage (knee)	C40.2-☑	C79.51	—	D16.2-☑	D48.0	D49.2
seminal vesicle	C63.7	C79.82	D07.69	D29.8	D40.8	D49.59
septum						
nasal	C30.0	C78.39	D02.3	D14.0	D38.5	D49.1
posterior margin	C11.3	C79.89	D00.08	D10.6	D37.05	D49.0
rectovaginal	C76.3	C79.89	D09.8	D36.7	D48.7	D49.89
rectovesical	C76.3	C79.89	D09.8	D36.7	D48.7	D49.89

	Malignant Primary	Malignant Secondary	Ca in situ	Benign	Uncertain Behavior	Unspecified Behavior
Neoplasm, neoplastic — *continued*						
septum — *continued*						
urethrovaginal	C57.9	C79.82	D07.30	D28.9	D39.9	D49.59
vesicovaginal	C57.9	C79.82	D07.30	D28.9	D39.9	D49.59
shoulder NEC	C76.4-☑	C79.89	D04.6-☑	D36.7	D48.7	D49.89
sigmoid flexure (lower) (upper)	C18.7	C78.5	D01.0	D12.5	D37.4	D49.0
sinus (accessory)	C31.9	C78.39	D02.3	D14.0	D38.5	D49.1
bone (any)	C41.0	C79.51	—	D16.4	D48.0	D49.2
ethmoidal	C31.1	C78.39	D02.3	D14.0	D38.5	D49.1
frontal	C31.2	C78.39	D02.3	D14.0	D38.5	D49.1
maxillary	C31.0	C78.39	D02.3	D14.0	D38.5	D49.1
nasal, paranasal NEC	C31.9	C78.39	D02.3	D14.0	D38.5	D49.1
overlapping lesion	C31.8	—	—	—	—	—
pyriform	C12	C79.89	D00.08	D10.7	D37.05	D49.0
sphenoid	C31.3	C78.39	D02.3	D14.0	D38.5	D49.1
skeleton, skeletal NEC	C41.9	C79.51	—	D16.9	D48.0	D49.2
Skene's gland	C68.1	C79.19	D09.19	D30.8	D41.8	D49.59
skin NOS	C44.90	C79.2	D04.9	D23.9	D48.5	D49.2
abdominal wall	C44.509	C79.2	D04.5	D23.5	D48.5	D49.2
basal cell carcinoma	C44.519	—	—	—	—	—
specified type NEC	C44.599	—	—	—	—	—
squamous cell carcinoma	C44.529	—	—	—	—	—
ala nasi — *see also* Neoplasm, nose, skin	C44.301	C79.2	D04.39	D23.39	D48.5	D49.2
ankle — *see also* Neoplasm, skin, limb, lower	C44.70-☑	C79.2	D04.7-☑	D23.7-☑	D48.5	D49.2
antecubital space — *see also* Neoplasm, skin, limb, upper	C44.60-☑	C79.2	D04.6-☑	D23.6-☑	D48.5	D49.2
anus	C44.500	C79.2	D04.5	D23.5	D48.5	D49.2
basal cell carcinoma	C44.510	—	—	—	—	—
specified type NEC	C44.590	—	—	—	—	—
squamous cell carcinoma	C44.520	—	—	—	—	—
arm — *see also* Neoplasm, skin, limb, upper	C44.60-☑	C79.2	D04.6-☑	D23.6-☑	D48.5	D49.2
auditory canal (external) — *see also* Neoplasm, skin, ear	C44.20-☑	C79.2	D04.2-☑	D23.2-☑	D48.5	D49.2
auricle (ear) — *see also* Neoplasm, skin, ear	C44.20-☑	C79.2	D04.2-☑	D23.2-☑	D48.5	D49.2
auricular canal (external) — *see also* Neoplasm, skin, ear	C44.20-☑	C79.2	D04.2-☑	D23.2-☑	D48.5	D49.2
axilla, axillary fold — *see also* Neoplasm, skin, trunk	C44.509	C79.2	D04.5	D23.5	D48.5	D49.2
back — *see also* Neoplasm, skin, trunk	C44.509	C79.2	D04.5	D23.5	D48.5	D49.2
basal cell carcinoma	C44.91	—	—	—	—	—
breast	C44.501	C79.2	D04.5	D23.5	D48.5	D49.2
basal cell carcinoma	C44.511	—	—	—	—	—
specified type NEC	C44.591	—	—	—	—	—
squamous cell carcinoma	C44.521	—	—	—	—	—
brow — *see also* Neoplasm, skin, face	C44.309	C79.2	D04.39	D23.39	D48.5	D49.2
buttock — *see also* Neoplasm, skin, trunk	C44.509	C79.2	D04.5	D23.5	D48.5	D49.2

Neoplasm, neoplastic — continued
skin — continued

	Malignant Primary	Malignant Secondary	Ca in situ	Benign	Uncertain Behavior	Unspecified Behavior
calf — see also Neoplasm, skin, limb, lower	C44.70-☑	C79.2	D04.7-☑	D23.7-☑	D48.5	D49.2
canthus (eye) (inner) (outer)	C44.10-☑	C79.2	D04.1-☑	D23.1-☑	D48.5	D49.2
basal cell carcinoma	C44.11-☑	—	—	—	—	—
sebaceous cell	C44.13-☑	—	—	—	—	—
specified type NEC	C44.19-☑	—	—	—	—	—
squamous cell carcinoma	C44.12-☑	—	—	—	—	—
cervical region — see also Neoplasm, skin, neck	C44.40	C79.2	D04.4	D23.4	D48.5	D49.2
cheek (external) — see also Neoplasm, skin, face	C44.309	C79.2	D04.39	D23.39	D48.5	D49.2
chest (wall) — see also Neoplasm, skin, trunk	C44.509	C79.2	D04.5	D23.5	D48.5	D49.2
chin — see also Neoplasm, skin, face	C44.309	C79.2	D04.39	D23.39	D48.5	D49.2
clavicular area — see also Neoplasm, skin, trunk	C44.509	C79.2	D04.5	D23.5	D48.5	D49.2
clitoris	C51.2	C79.82	D07.1	D28.0	D39.8	D49.59
columnella — see also Neoplasm, skin, face	C44.309	C79.2	D04.39	D23.39	D48.5	D49.2
concha — see also Neoplasm, skin, ear	C44.20-☑	C79.2	D04.2-☑	D23.2-☑	D48.5	D49.2
ear (external)	C44.20-☑	C79.2	D04.2-☑	D23.2-☑	D48.5	D49.2
basal cell carcinoma	C44.21-☑	—	—	—	—	—
specified type NEC	C44.29-☑	—	—	—	—	—
squamous cell carcinoma	C44.22-☑	—	—	—	—	—
elbow — see also Neoplasm, skin, limb, upper	C44.60-☑	C79.2	D04.6-☑	D23.6-☑	D48.5	D49.2
eyebrow — see also Neoplasm, skin, face	C44.309	C79.2	D04.39	D23.39	D48.5	D49.2
eyelid	C44.10-☑	C79.2	D04.1-☑	D23.1-☑	D48.5	D49.2
basal cell carcinoma	C44.11-☑	—	—	—	—	—
sebaceous cell	C44.13-☑	—	—	—	—	—
specified type NEC	C44.19-☑	—	—	—	—	—
squamous cell carcinoma	C44.12-☑	—	—	—	—	—
face NOS	C44.300	C79.2	D04.30	D23.30	D48.5	D49.2
basal cell carcinoma	C44.310	—	—	—	—	—
specified type NEC	C44.390	—	—	—	—	—
squamous cell carcinoma	C44.320	—	—	—	—	—
female genital organs (external)	C51.9	C79.82	D07.1	D28.0	D39.8	D49.59
clitoris	C51.2	C79.82	D07.1	D28.0	D39.8	D49.59
labium NEC	C51.9	C79.82	D07.1	D28.0	D39.8	D49.59
majus	C51.0	C79.82	D07.1	D28.0	D39.8	D49.59
minus	C51.1	C79.82	D07.1	D28.0	D39.8	D49.59
pudendum	C51.9	C79.82	D07.1	D28.0	D39.8	D49.59
vulva	C51.9	C79.82	D07.1	D28.0	D39.8	D49.59
finger — see also Neoplasm, skin, limb, upper	C44.60-☑	C79.2	D04.6-☑	D23.6-☑	D48.5	D49.2
flank — see also Neoplasm, skin, trunk	C44.509	C79.2	D04.5	D23.5	D48.5	D49.2
foot — see also Neoplasm, skin, limb, lower	C44.70-☑	C79.2	D04.7-☑	D23.7-☑	D48.5	D49.2

Neoplasm, neoplastic — continued
skin — continued

	Malignant Primary	Malignant Secondary	Ca in situ	Benign	Uncertain Behavior	Unspecified Behavior
forearm — see also Neoplasm, skin, limb, upper	C44.60-☑	C79.2	D04.6-☑	D23.6-☑	D48.5	D49.2
forehead — see also Neoplasm, skin, face	C44.309	C79.2	D04.39	D23.39	D48.5	D49.2
glabella — see also Neoplasm, skin, face	C44.309	C79.2	D04.39	D23.39	D48.5	D49.2
gluteal region — see also Neoplasm, skin, trunk	C44.509	C79.2	D04.5	D23.5	D48.5	D49.2
groin — see also Neoplasm, skin, trunk	C44.509	C79.2	D04.5	D23.5	D48.5	D49.2
hand — see also Neoplasm, skin, limb, upper	C44.60-☑	C79.2	D04.6-☑	D23.6-☑	D48.5	D49.2
head NEC — see also Neoplasm, skin, scalp	C44.40	C79.2	D04.4	D23.4	D48.5	D49.2
heel — see also Neoplasm, skin, limb, lower	C44.70-☑	C79.2	D04.7-☑	D23.7-☑	D48.5	D49.2
helix — see also Neoplasm, skin, ear	C44.20-☑	C79.2	D04.2-☑	D23.2-☑	D48.5	D49.2
hip — see also Neoplasm, skin, limb, lower	C44.70-☑	C79.2	D04.7-☑	D23.7-☑	D48.5	D49.2
infraclavicular region — see also Neoplasm, skin, trunk	C44.509	C79.2	D04.5	D23.5	D48.5	D49.2
inguinal region — see also Neoplasm, skin, trunk	C44.509	C79.2	D04.5	D23.5	D48.5	D49.2
jaw — see also Neoplasm, skin, face	C44.309	C79.2	D04.39	D23.39	D48.5	D49.2
Kaposi's sarcoma — see Kaposi's, sarcoma, skin						
knee — see also Neoplasm, skin, limb, lower	C44.70-☑	C79.2	D04.7-☑	D23.7-☑	D48.5	D49.2
labia						
majora	C51.0	C79.82	D07.1	D28.0	D39.8	D49.59
minora	C51.1	C79.82	D07.1	D28.0	D39.8	D49.59
leg — see also Neoplasm, skin, limb, lower	C44.70-☑	C79.2	D04.7-☑	D23.7-☑	D48.5	D49.2
lid (lower) (upper)	C44.10-☑	C79.2	D04.1-☑	D23.1-☑	D48.5	D49.2
basal cell carcinoma	C44.11-☑	—	—	—	—	—
sebaceous cell	C44.13-☑	—	—	—	—	—
specified type NEC	C44.19-☑	—	—	—	—	—
squamous cell carcinoma	C44.12-☑	—	—	—	—	—
limb NEC	C44.90	C79.2	D04.9	D23.9	D48.5	D49.2
basal cell carcinoma	C44.91	—	—	—	—	—
lower	C44.70-☑	C79.2	D04.7-☑	D23.7-☑	D48.5	D49.2
basal cell carcinoma	C44.71-☑	—	—	—	—	—
specified type NEC	C44.79-☑	—	—	—	—	—
squamous cell carcinoma	C44.72-☑	—	—	—	—	—
upper	C44.60-☑	C79.2	D04.6-☑	D23.6-☑	D48.5	D49.2
basal cell carcinoma	C44.61-☑	—	—	—	—	—
specified type NEC	C44.69-☑	—	—	—	—	—
squamous cell carcinoma	C44.62-☑	—	—	—	—	—
lip (lower) (upper)	C44.00	C79.2	D04.0	D23.0	D48.5	D49.2

☑ **Additional Character Required — Refer to the Tabular List for Character Selection**   ▽ **Subterms under main terms may continue to next column or page**

	Malignant Primary	Malignant Secondary	Ca in situ	Benign	Uncertain Behavior	Unspecified Behavior
Neoplasm, neoplastic						
— *continued*						
skin — *continued*						
lip — *continued*						
basal cell carcinoma	C44.01	—	—	—	—	—
specified type NEC	C44.09					
squamous cell carcinoma	C44.02	—	—	—	—	—
male genital organs	C63.9	C79.82	D07.60	D29.9	D40.8	D49.59
penis	C60.9	C79.82	D07.4	D29.0	D40.8	D49.59
prepuce	C60.0	C79.82	D07.4	D29.0	D40.8	D49.59
scrotum	C63.2	C79.82	D07.61	D29.4	D40.8	D49.59
mastectomy site (skin) — *see also* Neoplasm, skin, breast	C44.501	C79.2				
specified as breast tissue	C50.8-☑	C79.81	—	—	—	—
meatus, acoustic (external) — *see also* Neoplasm, skin, ear	C44.20-☑	C79.2	D04.2-☑	D23.2-☑	D48.5	D49.2
melanotic — *see* Melanoma						
Merkel cell — *see* Carcinoma, Merkel cell						
nates — *see also* Neoplasm, skin, trunk	C44.509	C79.2	D04.5	D23.5	D48.5	D49.2
neck	C44.40	C79.2	D04.4	D23.4	D48.5	D49.2
basal cell carcinoma	C44.41	—	—	—	—	—
specified type NEC	C44.49	—	—	—	—	—
squamous cell carcinoma	C44.42	—	—	—	—	—
nevus — *see* Nevus, skin						
nose (external) — *see also* Neoplasm, nose, skin	C44.301	C79.2	D04.39	D23.39	D48.5	D49.2
overlapping lesion	C44.80	—	—	—	—	—
basal cell carcinoma	C44.81	—	—	—	—	—
specified type NEC	C44.89	—	—	—	—	—
squamous cell carcinoma	C44.82	—	—	—	—	—
palm — *see also* Neoplasm, skin, limb, upper	C44.60-☑	C79.2	D04.6-☑	D23.6-☑	D48.5	D49.2
palpebra	C44.10-☑	C79.2	D04.1-☑	D23.1-☑	D48.5	D49.2
basal cell carcinoma	C44.11-☑	—	—	—	—	—
sebaceous cell	C44.13-☑	—	—	—	—	—
specified type NEC	C44.19-☑	—	—	—	—	—
squamous cell carcinoma	C44.12-☑	—	—	—	—	—
penis NEC	C60.9	C79.82	D07.4	D29.0	D40.8	D49.59
perianal — *see also* Neoplasm, skin, anus	C44.500	C79.2	D04.5	D23.5	D48.5	D49.2
perineum — *see also* Neoplasm, skin, anus	C44.500	C79.2	D04.5	D23.5	D48.5	D49.2
pinna — *see also* Neoplasm, skin, ear	C44.20-☑	C79.2	D04.2-☑	D23.2-☑	D48.5	D49.2
plantar — *see also* Neoplasm, skin, limb, lower	C44.70-☑	C79.2	D04.7-☑	D23.7-☑	D48.5	D49.2
popliteal fossa or space — *see also* Neoplasm, skin, limb, lower	C44.70-☑	C79.2	D04.7-☑	D23.7-☑	D48.5	D49.2
prepuce	C60.0	C79.82	D07.4	D29.0	D40.8	D49.59

	Malignant Primary	Malignant Secondary	Ca in situ	Benign	Uncertain Behavior	Unspecified Behavior
Neoplasm, neoplastic						
— *continued*						
skin — *continued*						
pubes — *see also* Neoplasm, skin, trunk	C44.509	C79.2	D04.5	D23.5	D48.5	D49.2
sacrococcygeal region — *see also* Neoplasm, skin, trunk	C44.509	C79.2	D04.5	D23.5	D48.5	D49.2
scalp	C44.40	C79.2	D04.4	D23.4	D48.5	D49.2
basal cell carcinoma	C44.41	—	—	—	—	—
specified type NEC	C44.49	—	—	—	—	—
squamous cell carcinoma	C44.42	—	—	—	—	—
scapular region — *see also* Neoplasm, skin, trunk	C44.509	C79.2	D04.5	D23.5	D48.5	D49.2
scrotum	C63.2	C79.82	D07.61	D29.4	D40.8	D49.59
shoulder — *see also* Neoplasm, skin, limb, upper	C44.60-☑	C79.2	D04.6-☑	D23.6-☑	D48.5	D49.2
sole (foot) — *see also* Neoplasm, skin, limb, lower	C44.70-☑	C79.2	D04.7-☑	D23.7-☑	D48.5	D49.2
specified sites NEC	C44.80	C79.2	D04.8	D23.9	D48.5	D49.2
basal cell carcinoma	C44.81	—	—	—	—	—
specified type NEC	C44.89	—	—	—	—	—
squamous cell carcinoma	C44.82	—	—	—	—	—
specified type NEC	C44.99	—	—	—	—	—
squamous cell carcinoma	C44.92	—	—	—	—	—
submammary fold — *see also* Neoplasm, skin, trunk	C44.509	C79.2	D04.5	D23.5	D48.5	D49.2
supraclavicular region — *see also* Neoplasm, skin, neck	C44.40	C79.2	D04.4	D23.4	D48.5	D49.2
temple — *see also* Neoplasm, skin, face	C44.309	C79.2	D04.39	D23.39	D48.5	D49.2
thigh — *see also* Neoplasm, skin, limb, lower	C44.70-☑	C79.2	D04.7-☑	D23.7-☑	D48.5	D49.2
thoracic wall — *see also* Neoplasm, skin, trunk	C44.509	C79.2	D04.5	D23.5	D48.5	D49.2
thumb — *see also* Neoplasm, skin, limb, upper	C44.60-☑	C79.2	D04.6-☑	D23.6-☑	D48.5	D49.2
toe — *see also* Neoplasm, skin, limb, lower	C44.70-☑	C79.2	D04.7-☑	D23.7-☑	D48.5	D49.2
tragus — *see also* Neoplasm, skin, ear	C44.20-☑	C79.2	D04.2-☑	D23.2-☑	D48.5	D49.2
trunk	C44.509	C79.2	D04.5	D23.5	D48.5	D49.2
basal cell carcinoma	C44.519	—	—	—	—	—
specified type NEC	C44.599	—	—	—	—	—
squamous cell carcinoma	C44.529	—	—	—	—	—
umbilicus — *see also* Neoplasm, skin, trunk	C44.509	C79.2	D04.5	D23.5	D48.5	D49.2
vulva	C51.9	C79.82	D07.1	D28.0	D39.8	D49.59
overlapping lesion	C51.8					
wrist — *see also* Neoplasm, skin, limb, upper	C44.60-☑	C79.2	D04.6-☑	D23.6-☑	D48.5	D49.2
skull	C41.0	C79.51	—	D16.4	D48.0	D49.2

Neoplasm, neoplastic	Malignant Primary	Malignant Secondary	Ca in situ	Benign	Uncertain Behavior	Unspecified Behavior
— continued						
soft parts or tissues — see Neoplasm, connective tissue						
specified site NEC	C76.8	C79.89	D09.8	D36.7	D48.7	D49.89
spermatic cord	C63.1-☑	C79.82	D07.69	D29.8	D40.8	D49.59
sphenoid	C31.3	C78.39	D02.3	D14.0	D38.5	D49.1
bone	C41.0	C79.51	—	D16.4	D48.0	D49.2
sinus	C31.3	C78.39	D02.3	D14.0	D38.5	D49.1
sphincter						
anal	C21.1	C78.5	D01.3	D12.9	D37.8	D49.0
of Oddi	C24.0	C78.89	D01.5	D13.5	D37.6	D49.0
spine, spinal						
(column)	C41.2	C79.51	—	D16.6	D48.0	D49.2
bulb	C71.7	C79.31	—	D33.1	D43.1	D49.6
coccyx	C41.4	C79.51	—	D16.8	D48.0	D49.2
cord (cervical) (lumbar) (sacral) (thoracic)	C72.0	C79.49	—	D33.4	D43.4	D49.7
dura mater	C70.1	C79.49	—	D32.1	D42.1	D49.7
lumbosacral	C41.2	C79.51	—	D16.6	D48.0	D49.2
marrow NEC	C96.9	C79.52	—	—	D47.9	D49.89
membrane	C70.1	C79.49	—	D32.1	D42.1	D49.7
meninges	C70.1	C79.49	—	D32.1	D42.1	D49.7
nerve (root)	C47.9	C79.89	—	D36.10	D48.2	D49.2
pia mater	C70.1	C79.49	—	D32.1	D42.1	D49.7
root	C47.9	C79.89	—	D36.10	D48.2	D49.2
sacrum	C41.4	C79.51	—	D16.8	D48.0	D49.2
spleen, splenic NEC	C26.1	C78.89	D01.7	D13.9	D37.8	D49.0
flexure (colon)	C18.5	C78.5	D01.0	D12.3	D37.4	D49.0
stem, brain	C71.7	C79.31	—	D33.1	D43.1	D49.6
Stensen's duct	C07	C79.89	D00.00	D11.0	D37.030	
sternum	C41.3	C79.51	—	D16.7	D48.0	D49.2
stomach	C16.9	C78.89	D00.2	D13.1	D37.1	D49.0
antrum (pyloric)	C16.3	C78.89	D00.2	D13.1	D37.1	D49.0
body	C16.2	C78.89	D00.2	D13.1	D37.1	D49.0
cardia	C16.0	C78.89	D00.2	D13.1	D37.1	D49.0
cardiac orifice	C16.0	C78.89	D00.2	D13.1	D37.1	D49.0
corpus	C16.2	C78.89	D00.2	D13.1	D37.1	D49.0
fundus	C16.1	C78.89	D00.2	D13.1	D37.1	D49.0
greater curvature NEC	C16.6	C78.89	D00.2	D13.1	D37.1	D49.0
lesser curvature NEC	C16.5	C78.89	D00.2	D13.1	D37.1	D49.0
overlapping lesion	C16.8	—	—	—	—	—
prepylorus	C16.4	C78.89	D00.2	D13.1	D37.1	D49.0
pylorus	C16.4	C78.89	D00.2	D13.1	D37.1	D49.0
wall NEC	C16.9	C78.89	D00.2	D13.1	D37.1	D49.0
anterior NEC	C16.8	C78.89	D00.2	D13.1	D37.1	D49.0
posterior NEC	C16.8	C78.89	D00.2	D13.1	D37.1	D49.0
stroma, endometrial	C54.1	C79.82	D07.0	D26.1	D39.0	D49.59
stump, cervical	C53.8	C79.82	D06.7	D26.0	D39.0	D49.59
subcutaneous (nodule) (tissue) NEC — see Neoplasm, connective tissue						
subdural	C70.9	C79.32	—	D32.9	D42.9	D49.7
subglottis, subglottic	C32.2	C78.39	D02.0	D14.1	D38.0	D49.1
sublingual	C04.9	C79.89	D00.06	D10.2	D37.09	D49.0
gland or duct	C08.1	C79.89	D00.00	D11.7	D37.031	D49.0
submandibular gland	C08.0	C79.89	D00.00	D11.7	D37.032	D49.0
submaxillary gland or duct	C08.0	C79.89	D00.00	D11.7	D37.032	D49.0
submental	C76.0	C79.89	D09.8	D36.7	D48.7	D49.89
subpleural	C34.9-☑	C78.0-☑	D02.2-☑	D14.3-☑	D38.1	D49.1
substernal	C38.1	C78.1		D15.2	D38.3	D49.89
sudoriferous, sudoriparous gland, site unspecified	C44.90	C79.2	D04.9	D23.9	D48.5	D49.2
specified site — see Neoplasm, skin						
supraclavicular region	C76.0	C79.89	D09.8	D36.7	D48.7	D49.89
supraglottis	C32.1	C78.39	D02.0	D14.1	D38.0	D49.1
suprarenal	C74.9-☑	C79.7-☑	D09.3	D35.0-☑	D44.1-☑	D49.7
capsule	C74.9-☑	C79.7-☑	D09.3	D35.0-☑	D44.1-☑	D49.7

Neoplasm, neoplastic	Malignant Primary	Malignant Secondary	Ca in situ	Benign	Uncertain Behavior	Unspecified Behavior
— continued						
suprarenal — continued						
cortex	C74.0-☑	C79.7-☑	D09.3	D35.0-☑	D44.1-☑	D49.7
gland	C74.9-☑	C79.7-☑	D09.3	D35.0-☑	D44.1-☑	D49.7
medulla	C74.1-☑	C79.7-☑	D09.3	D35.0-☑	D44.1-☑	D49.7
suprasellar (region)	C71.9	C79.31	—	D33.2	D43.2	D49.6
supratentorial (brain) NEC	C71.0	C79.31	—	D33.0	D43.0	D49.6
sweat gland (apocrine) (eccrine), site unspecified	C44.90	C79.2	D04.9	D23.9	D48.5	D49.2
specified site — see Neoplasm, skin						
sympathetic nerve or nervous system NEC	C47.9	C79.89	—	D36.10	D48.2	D49.2
symphysis pubis	C41.4	C79.51	—	D16.8	D48.0	D49.2
synovial membrane — see Neoplasm, connective tissue						
tapetum, brain	C71.8	C79.31	—	D33.2	D43.2	D49.6
tarsus (any bone)	C40.3-☑	C79.51	—	D16.3-☑	—	
temple (skin) — see also Neoplasm, skin, face	C44.309	C79.2	D04.39	D23.39	D48.5	D49.2
temporal						
bone	C41.0	C79.51	—	D16.4	D48.0	D49.2
lobe or pole	C71.2	C79.31	—	D33.0	D43.0	D49.6
region	C76.0	C79.89	D09.8	D36.7	D48.7	D49.89
skin — see also Neoplasm, skin, face	C44.309	C79.2	D04.39	D23.39	D48.5	D49.2
tendon (sheath) — see Neoplasm, connective tissue						
tentorium (cerebelli)	C70.0	C79.32	—	D32.0	D42.0	D49.7
testis, testes	C62.9-☑	C79.82	D07.69	D29.2-☑	D40.1-☑	D49.59
descended	C62.1-☑	C79.82	D07.69	D29.2-☑	D40.1-☑	D49.59
ectopic	C62.0-☑	C79.82	D07.69	D29.2-☑	D40.1-☑	D49.59
retained	C62.0-☑	C79.82	D07.69	D29.2-☑	D40.1-☑	D49.59
scrotal	C62.1-☑	C79.82	D07.69	D29.2-☑	D40.1-☑	D49.59
undescended	C62.0-☑	C79.82	D07.69	D29.2-☑	D40.1-☑	D49.59
unspecified whether descended or undescended	C62.9-☑	C79.82	D07.69	D29.2-☑	D40.1-☑	D49.59
thalamus	C71.0	C79.31	—	D33.0	D43.0	D49.6
thigh NEC	C76.5-☑	C79.89	D04.7-☑	D36.7	D48.7	D49.89
thorax, thoracic (cavity) (organs NEC)	C76.1	C79.89	D09.8	D36.7	D48.7	D49.89
duct	C49.3	C79.89	—	D21.3	D48.1	D49.2
wall NEC	C76.1	C79.89	D09.8	D36.7	D48.7	D49.89
throat	C14.0	C79.89	D00.08	D10.9	D37.05	D49.0
thumb NEC	C76.4-☑	C79.89	D04.6-☑	D36.7	D48.7	D49.89
thymus (gland)	C37	C79.89	D09.3	D15.0	D38.4	D49.89
thyroglossal duct	C73	C79.89	D09.3	D34	D44.0	D49.7
thyroid (gland)	C73	C79.89	D09.3	D34	D44.0	D49.7
cartilage	C32.3	C78.39	D02.0	D14.1	D38.0	D49.1
tibia (any part)	C40.2-☑	C79.51	—	D16.2-☑	—	—
toe NEC	C76.5-☑	C79.89	D04.7-☑	D36.7	D48.7	D49.89
tongue	C02.9	C79.89	D00.07	D10.1	D37.02	D49.0
anterior (two-thirds) NEC	C02.3	C79.89	D00.07	D10.1	D37.02	D49.0
dorsal surface	C02.0	C79.89	D00.07	D10.1	D37.02	D49.0
ventral surface	C02.2	C79.89	D00.07	D10.1	D37.02	D49.0
base (dorsal surface)	C01	C79.89	D00.07	D10.1	D37.02	D49.0
border (lateral)	C02.1	C79.89	D00.07	D10.1	D37.02	D49.0
dorsal surface NEC	C02.0	C79.89	D00.07	D10.1	D37.02	D49.0
fixed part NEC	C01	C79.89	D00.07	D10.1	D37.02	D49.0
foreamen cecum	C02.0	C79.89	D00.07	D10.1	D37.02	D49.0
frenulum linguae	C02.2	C79.89	D00.07	D10.1	D37.02	D49.0
junctional zone	C02.8	C79.89	D00.07	D10.1	D37.02	D49.0
margin (lateral)	C02.1	C79.89	D00.07	D10.1	D37.02	D49.0
midline NEC	C02.1	C79.89	D00.07	D10.1	D37.02	D49.0
mobile part NEC	C02.3	C79.89	D00.07	D10.1	D37.02	D49.0

☑ Additional Character Required — Refer to the Tabular List for Character Selection   ▽ Subterms under main terms may continue to next column or page

	Malignant Primary	Malignant Secondary	Ca in situ	Benign	Uncertain Behavior	Unspecified Behavior
Neoplasm, neoplastic						
— *continued*						
tongue — *continued*						
overlapping						
lesion	C02.8	—	—	—	—	—
posterior (third)	C01	C79.89	D00.07	D10.1	D37.02	D49.0
root	C01	C79.89	D00.07	D10.1	D37.02	D49.0
surface (dorsal)	C02.0	C79.89	D00.07	D10.1	D37.02	D49.0
base	C01	C79.89	D00.07	D10.1	D37.02	D49.0
ventral	C02.2	C79.89	D00.07	D10.1	D37.02	D49.0
tip	C02.1	C79.89	D00.07	D10.1	D37.02	D49.0
tonsil	C02.4	C79.89	D00.07	D10.1	D37.02	D49.0
tonsil	C09.9	C79.89	D00.08	D10.4	D37.05	D49.0
fauces, faucial	C09.9	C79.89	D00.08	D10.4	D37.05	D49.0
lingual	C02.4	C79.89	D00.07	D10.1	D37.02	D49.0
overlapping						
sites	C09.8	—	—	—	—	—
palatine	C09.9	C79.89	D00.08	D10.4	D37.05	D49.0
pharyngeal	C11.1	C79.89	D00.08	D10.6	D37.05	D49.0
pillar (anterior)						
(posterior)	C09.1	C79.89	D00.08	D10.5	D37.05	D49.0
tonsillar fossa	C09.0	C79.89	D00.08	D10.5	D37.05	D49.0
tooth socket NEC	C03.9	C79.89	D00.03	D10.39	D37.09	D49.0
trachea (cartilage)						
(mucosa)	C33	C78.39	D02.1	D14.2	D38.1	D49.1
overlapping lesion						
with bronchus or						
lung	C34.8-☑	—	—	—	—	—
tracheobronchial	C34.8-☑	C78.39	D02.1	D14.2	D38.1	D49.1
overlapping lesion						
with lung	C34.8-☑	—	—	—	—	—
tragus — *see also*						
Neoplasm, skin,						
ear	C44.20-☑	C79.2	D04.2-☑	D23.2-☑	D48.5	D49.2
trunk NEC	C76.8	C79.89	D04.5	D36.7	D48.7	D49.89
tubo-ovarian	C57.8	C79.82	D07.39	D28.7	D39.8	D49.59
tunica vaginalis	C63.7	C79.82	D07.69	D29.8	D40.8	D49.59
turbinate (bone)	C41.0	C79.51		D16.4	D48.0	D49.2
nasal	C30.0	C78.39	D02.3	D14.0	D38.5	D49.1
tympanic cavity	C30.1	C78.39	D02.3	D14.0	D38.5	D49.1
ulna (any part)	C40.0-☑	C79.51	—	D16.0-☑	—	—
umbilicus, umbilical —						
see also Neoplasm,						
skin, trunk	C44.509	C79.2	D04.5	D23.5	D48.5	D49.2
uncus, brain	C71.2	C79.31	—	D33.0	D43.0	D49.6
unknown site or						
unspecified	C80.1	C79.9	D09.9	D36.9	D48.9	D49.9
urachus	C67.7	C79.11	D09.0	D30.3	D41.4	D49.4
ureter-bladder						
(junction)	C67.6	C79.11	D09.0	D30.3	D41.4	D49.4
ureter, ureteral	C66.-☑	C79.19	D09.19	D30.2-☑	D41.2-☑	D49.59
orifice (bladder)	C67.6	C79.11	D09.0	D30.3	D41.4	D49.4
urethra, urethral						
(gland)	C68.0	C79.19	D09.19	D30.4	D41.3	D49.59
orifice, internal	C67.5	C79.11	D09.0	D30.3	D41.4	D49.4
urethrovaginal						
(septum)	C57.9	C79.82	D07.30	D28.9	D39.8	D49.59
urinary organ or						
system	C68.9	C79.10	D09.10	D30.9	D41.9	D49.59
bladder — *see*						
Neoplasm,						
bladder						
overlapping						
lesion	C68.8	—	—	—	—	—
specified sites						
NEC	C68.8	C79.19	D09.19	D30.8	D41.8	D49.59
utero-ovarian	C57.8	C79.82	D07.39	D28.7	D39.8	D49.59
ligament	C57.1-☑	C79.82	D07.39	D28.2	D39.8	D49.59
uterosacral						
ligament	C57.3	C79.82	—	D28.2	D39.8	D49.59
uterus, uteri,						
uterine	C55	C79.82	D07.0	D26.9	D39.0	D49.59
adnexa NEC	C57.4	C79.82	D07.39	D28.7	D39.8	D49.59
body	C54.9	C79.82	D07.0	D26.1	D39.0	D49.59
cervix	C53.9	C79.82	D06.9	D26.0	D39.0	D49.59
cornu	C54.9	C79.82	D07.0	D26.1	D39.0	D49.59
corpus	C54.9	C79.82	D07.0	D26.1	D39.0	D49.59
endocervix (canal)						
(gland)	C53.0	C79.82	D06.0	D26.0	D39.0	D49.59
endometrium	C54.1	C79.82	D07.0	D26.1	D39.0	D49.59
exocervix	C53.1	C79.82	D06.1	D26.0	D39.0	D49.59
external os	C53.1	C79.82	D06.1	D26.0	D39.0	D49.59
fundus	C54.3	C79.82	D07.0	D26.1	D39.0	D49.59

	Malignant Primary	Malignant Secondary	Ca in situ	Benign	Uncertain Behavior	Unspecified Behavior
Neoplasm, neoplastic						
— *continued*						
uterus, uteri, uterine						
— *continued*						
internal os	C53.0	C79.82	D06.0	D26.0	D39.0	D49.59
isthmus	C54.0	C79.82	D07.0	D26.1	D39.0	D49.59
ligament	C57.3	C79.82	—	D28.2	D39.8	D49.59
broad	C57.1-☑	C79.82	D07.39	D28.2	D39.8	D49.59
round	C57.2-☑	C79.82	—	D28.2	D39.8	D49.59
lower segment	C54.0	C79.82	D07.0	D26.1	D39.0	D49.59
myometrium	C54.2	C79.82	D07.0	D26.1	D39.0	D49.59
overlapping						
sites	C54.8	—	—	—	—	—
squamocolumnar						
junction	C53.8	C79.82	D06.7	D26.0	D39.0	D49.59
tube	C57.0-☑	C79.82	D07.39	D28.2	D39.8	D49.59
utricle, prostatic	C68.0	C79.19	D09.19	D30.4	D41.3	D49.59
uveal tract	C69.4-☑	C79.49	D09.2-☑	D31.4-☑	D48.7	D49.89
uvula	C05.2	C79.89	D00.04	D10.39	D37.09	D49.0
vagina, vaginal (fornix)						
(vault) (wall)	C52	C79.82	D07.2	D28.1	D39.8	D49.59
vaginovesical	C57.9	C79.82	D07.30	D28.9	D39.9	D49.59
septum	C57.9	C79.82	D07.30	D28.9	D39.9	D49.59
vallecula						
(epiglottis)	C10.0	C79.89	D00.08	D10.5	D37.05	D49.0
vascular — *see*						
Neoplasm,						
connective tissue						
vas deferens	C63.1-☑	C79.82	D07.69	D29.8	D40.8	D49.59
Vater's ampulla	C24.1	C78.89	D01.5	D13.5	D37.6	D49.0
vein, venous — *see*						
Neoplasm,						
connective tissue						
vena cava (abdominal)						
(inferior)	C49.4	C79.89	—	D21.4	D48.1	D49.2
superior	C49.3	C79.89	—	D21.3	D48.1	D49.2
ventricle (cerebral)						
(floor) (lateral)						
(third)	C71.5	C79.31	—	D33.0	D43.0	D49.6
cardiac (left)						
(right)	C38.0	C79.89	—	D15.1	D48.7	D49.89
fourth	C71.7	C79.31	—	D33.1	D43.1	D49.6
ventricular band of						
larynx	C32.1	C78.39	D02.0	D14.1	D38.0	D49.1
ventriculus — *see*						
Neoplasm,						
stomach						
vermillion border —						
see Neoplasm, lip						
vermis,						
cerebellum	C71.6	C79.31	—	D33.1	D43.1	D49.6
vertebra (column)	C41.2	C79.51	—	D16.6	D48.0	D49.2
coccyx	C41.4	C79.51	—	D16.8	D48.0	D49.2
marrow NEC	C96.9	C79.52	—	—	D47.9	D49.89
sacrum	C41.4	C79.51	—	D16.8	D48.0	D49.2
vesical — *see*						
Neoplasm, bladder						
vesicle, seminal	C63.7	C79.82	D07.69	D29.8	D40.8	D49.59
vesicocervical						
tissue	C57.9	C79.82	D07.30	D28.9	D39.9	D49.59
vesicorectal	C76.3	C79.82	D09.8	D36.7	D48.7	D49.89
vesicovaginal	C57.9	C79.82	D07.30	D28.9	D39.9	D49.59
septum	C57.9	C79.82	D07.30	D28.9	D39.8	D49.59
vessel (blood) — *see*						
Neoplasm,						
connective tissue						
vestibular gland,						
greater	C51.0	C79.82	D07.1	D28.0	D39.8	D49.59
vestibule						
mouth	C06.1	C79.89	D00.00	D10.39	D37.09	D49.0
nose	C30.0	C78.39	D02.3	D14.0	D38.5	D49.1
Virchow's gland	C77.0	C77.0	—	D36.0	D48.7	D49.89
viscera NEC	C76.8	C79.89	D09.8	D36.7	D48.7	D49.89
vocal cords (true)	C32.0	C78.39	D02.0	D14.1	D38.0	D49.1
false	C32.1	C78.39	D02.0	D14.1	D38.0	D49.1
vomer	C41.0	C79.51	—	D16.4	D48.0	D49.2
vulva	C51.9	C79.82	D07.1	D28.0	D39.8	D49.59
vulvovaginal						
gland	C51.0	C79.82	D07.1	D28.0	D39.8	D49.59
Waldeyer's ring	C14.2	C79.89	D00.08	D10.9	D37.05	D49.0
Wharton's duct	C08.0	C79.89	D00.00	D11.7	D37.032	D49.0
white matter (central)						
(cerebral)	C71.0	C79.31	—	D33.0	D43.0	D49.6

	Malignant Primary	Malignant Secondary	Ca in situ	Benign	Uncertain Behavior	Unspecified Behavior
Neoplasm, neoplastic						
— *continued*						
windpipe	C33	C78.39	D02.1	D14.2	D38.1	D49.1
Wirsung's duct	C25.3	C78.89	D01.7	D13.6	D37.8	D49.0
wolffian (body) (duct)						
female	C57.7	C79.82	D07.39	D28.7	D39.8	D49.59
male	C63.7	C79.82	D07.69	D29.8	D40.8	D49.59
womb — *see*						
Neoplasm, uterus						
wrist NEC	C76.4-☑	C79.89	D04.6-☑	D36.7	D48.7	D49.89
xiphoid process	C41.3	C79.51	—	D16.7	D48.0	D49.2
Zuckerkandl						
organ	C75.5	C79.89	—	D35.6	D44.7	D49.7

☑ **Additional Character Required — Refer to the Tabular List for Character Selection**   ▽ **Subterms under main terms may continue to next column or page**

Table of Drugs and Chemicals

Substance	Poisoning, Accidental (unintentional)	Poisoning, Intentional Self-harm	Poisoning, Assault	Poisoning, Undetermined	Adverse Effect	Underdosing
14-hydroxydihydro-morphinone	T40.2X1	T40.2X2	T40.2X3	T40.2X4	—	—
1-Propanol	T51.3X1	T51.3X2	T51.3X3	T51.3X4	—	—
2,3,7,8-Tetrachlorodibenzo-p-dioxin	T53.7X1	T53.7X2	T53.7X3	T53.7X4	—	—
2,4,5-T (trichloro-phenoxyacetic acid)	T60.1X1	T60.1X2	T60.1X3	T60.1X4	—	—
2,4,5-Trichlorophen-oxyacetic acid	T60.3X1	T60.3X2	T60.3X3	T60.3X4	—	—
2,4-D (dichlorophen-oxyacetic acid)	T60.3X1	T60.3X2	T60.3X3	T60.3X4	—	—
2,4-Toluene diisocyanate	T65.0X1	T65.0X2	T65.0X3	T65.0X4	—	—
2-Deoxy-5-fluorouridine	T45.1X1	T45.1X2	T45.1X3	T45.1X4	T45.1X5	T45.1X6
2-Ethoxyethanol	T52.3X1	T52.3X2	T52.3X3	T52.3X4	—	—
2-Methoxyethanol	T52.3X1	T52.3X2	T52.3X3	T52.3X4	—	—
2-Propanol	T51.2X1	T51.2X2	T51.2X3	T51.2X4	—	—
3,4-methylenedioxymeth-amphetamine	T43.641	T43.642	T43.643	T43.644	—	—
4-Aminobutyric acid	T43.8X1	T43.8X2	T43.8X3	T43.8X4	T43.8X5	T43.8X6
4-Aminophenol	T39.1X1	T39.1X2	T39.1X3	T39.1X4	T39.1X5	T39.1X6
derivatives						
5-Deoxy-5-fluorouridine	T45.1X1	T45.1X2	T45.1X3	T45.1X4	T45.1X5	T45.1X6
5-Methoxypsoralen (5-MOP)	T50.991	T50.992	T50.993	T50.994	T50.995	T50.996
8-Aminoquinoline drugs	T37.2X1	T37.2X2	T37.2X3	T37.2X4	T37.2X5	T37.2X6
8-Methoxypsoralen (8-MOP)	T50.991	T50.992	T50.993	T50.994	T50.995	T50.996
ABOB	T37.5X1	T37.5X2	T37.5X3	T37.5X4	T37.5X5	T37.5X6
Abrine	T62.2X1	T62.2X2	T62.2X3	T62.2X4	—	—
Abrus (seed)	T62.2X1	T62.2X2	T62.2X3	T62.2X4	—	—
Absinthe	T51.0X1	T51.0X2	T51.0X3	T51.0X4	—	—
beverage	T51.0X1	T51.0X2	T51.0X3	T51.0X4	—	—
Acaricide	T60.8X1	T60.8X2	T60.8X3	T60.8X4	—	—
Acebutolol	T44.7X1	T44.7X2	T44.7X3	T44.7X4	T44.7X5	T44.7X6
Acecarbromal	T42.6X1	T42.6X2	T42.6X3	T42.6X4	T42.6X5	T42.6X6
Aceclidine	T44.1X1	T44.1X2	T44.1X3	T44.1X4	T44.1X5	T44.1X6
Acedapsone	T37.0X1	T37.0X2	T37.0X3	T37.0X4	T37.0X5	T37.0X6
Acefylline piperazine	T48.6X1	T48.6X2	T48.6X3	T48.6X4	T48.6X5	T48.6X6
Acemorphan	T40.2X1	T40.2X2	T40.2X3	T40.2X4	T40.2X5	T40.2X6
Acenocoumarin	T45.511	T45.512	T45.513	T45.514	T45.515	T45.516
Acenocoumarol	T45.511	T45.512	T45.513	T45.514	T45.515	T45.516
Acepifylline	T48.6X1	T48.6X2	T48.6X3	T48.6X4	T48.6X5	T48.6X6
Acepromazine	T43.3X1	T43.3X2	T43.3X3	T43.3X4	T43.3X5	T43.3X6
Acesulfamethoxypyridazine	T37.0X1	T37.0X2	T37.0X3	T37.0X4	T37.0X5	T37.0X6
Acetal	T52.8X1	T52.8X2	T52.8X3	T52.8X4	—	—
Acetaldehyde (vapor)	T52.8X1	T52.8X2	T52.8X3	T52.8X4	—	—
liquid	T65.891	T65.892	T65.893	T65.894	—	—
Acetaminophen	T39.1X1	T39.1X2	T39.1X3	T39.1X4	T39.1X5	T39.1X6
Acetaminosalol	T39.1X1	T39.1X2	T39.1X3	T39.1X4	T39.1X5	T39.1X6
Acetanilide	T39.1X1	T39.1X2	T39.1X3	T39.1X4	T39.1X5	T39.1X6
Acetarsol	T37.3X1	T37.3X2	T37.3X3	T37.3X4	T37.3X5	T37.3X6
Acetazolamide	T50.2X1	T50.2X2	T50.2X3	T50.2X4	T50.2X5	T50.2X6
Acetiamine	T45.2X1	T45.2X2	T45.2X3	T45.2X4	T45.2X5	T45.2X6
Acetic						
acid	T54.2X1	T54.2X2	T54.2X3	T54.2X4	—	—
with sodium acetate (ointment)	T49.3X1	T49.3X2	T49.3X3	T49.3X4	T49.3X5	T49.3X6
ester (solvent)(vapor)	T52.8X1	T52.8X2	T52.8X3	T52.8X4	—	—
irrigating solution	T50.3X1	T50.3X2	T50.3X3	T50.3X4	T50.3X5	T50.3X6
medicinal (lotion)	T49.2X1	T49.2X2	T49.2X3	T49.2X4	T49.2X5	T49.2X6
anhydride	T65.891	T65.892	T65.893	T65.894	—	—
ether (vapor)	T52.8X1	T52.8X2	T52.8X3	T52.8X4	—	—
Acetohexamide	T38.3X1	T38.3X2	T38.3X3	T38.3X4	T38.3X5	T38.3X6
Acetohydroxamic acid	T50.991	T50.992	T50.993	T50.994	T50.995	T50.996
Acetomenaphthone	T45.7X1	T45.7X2	T45.7X3	T45.7X4	T45.7X5	T45.7X6
Acetomorphine	T40.1X1	T40.1X2	T40.1X3	T40.1X4	—	—
Acetone (oils)	T52.4X1	T52.4X2	T52.4X3	T52.4X4	—	—
chlorinated	T52.4X1	T52.4X2	T52.4X3	T52.4X4	—	—
vapor	T52.4X1	T52.4X2	T52.4X3	T52.4X4	—	—
Acetonitrile	T52.8X1	T52.8X2	T52.8X3	T52.8X4	—	—
Acetophenazine	T43.3X1	T43.3X2	T43.3X3	T43.3X4	T43.3X5	T43.3X6
Acetophenetedin	T39.1X1	T39.1X2	T39.1X3	T39.1X4	T39.1X5	T39.1X6
Acetophenone	T52.4X1	T52.4X2	T52.4X3	T52.4X4	—	—
Acetorphine	T40.2X1	T40.2X2	T40.2X3	T40.2X4	—	—
Acetosulfone (sodium)	T37.1X1	T37.1X2	T37.1X3	T37.1X4	T37.1X5	T37.1X6
Acetrizoate (sodium)	T50.8X1	T50.8X2	T50.8X3	T50.8X4	T50.8X5	T50.8X6
Acetrizoic acid	T50.8X1	T50.8X2	T50.8X3	T50.8X4	T50.8X5	T50.8X6
Acetyl						
bromide	T53.6X1	T53.6X2	T53.6X3	T53.6X4	—	—
chloride	T53.6X1	T53.6X2	T53.6X3	T53.6X4	—	—
Acetylcarbromal	T42.6X1	T42.6X2	T42.6X3	T42.6X4	T42.6X5	T42.6X6
Acetylcholine						
chloride	T44.1X1	T44.1X2	T44.1X3	T44.1X4	T44.1X5	T44.1X6
derivative	T44.1X1	T44.1X2	T44.1X3	T44.1X4	T44.1X5	T44.1X6
Acetylcysteine	T48.4X1	T48.4X2	T48.4X3	T48.4X4	T48.4X5	T48.4X6
Acetyldigitoxin	T46.0X1	T46.0X2	T46.0X3	T46.0X4	T46.0X5	T46.0X6
Acetyldigoxin	T46.0X1	T46.0X2	T46.0X3	T46.0X4	T46.0X5	T46.0X6
Acetyldihydrocodeine	T40.2X1	T40.2X2	T40.2X3	T40.2X4	—	—
Acetyldihydrocodeinone	T40.2X1	T40.2X2	T40.2X3	T40.2X4	—	—
Acetylene (gas)	T59.891	T59.892	T59.893	T59.894	—	—
dichloride	T53.6X1	T53.6X2	T53.6X3	T53.6X4	—	—
incomplete combustion of	T58.11	T58.12	T58.13	T58.14	—	—
industrial	T59.891	T59.892	T59.893	T59.894	—	—
tetrachloride	T53.6X1	T53.6X2	T53.6X3	T53.6X4	—	—
vapor	T53.6X1	T53.6X2	T53.6X3	T53.6X4	—	—
Acetylpheneturide	T42.6X1	T42.6X2	T42.6X3	T42.6X4	T42.6X5	T42.6X6
Acetylphenylhydrazine	T39.8X1	T39.8X2	T39.8X3	T39.8X4	T39.8X5	T39.8X6
Acetylsalicylic acid (salts)	T39.011	T39.012	T39.013	T39.014	T39.015	T39.016
enteric coated	T39.011	T39.012	T39.013	T39.014	T39.015	T39.016
Acetylsulfamethoxypyridazine	T37.0X1	T37.0X2	T37.0X3	T37.0X4	T37.0X5	T37.0X6
Achromycin	T36.4X1	T36.4X2	T36.4X3	T36.4X4	T36.4X5	T36.4X6
ophthalmic preparation	T49.5X1	T49.5X2	T49.5X3	T49.5X4	T49.5X5	T49.5X6
topical NEC	T49.0X1	T49.0X2	T49.0X3	T49.0X4	T49.0X5	T49.0X6
Aciclovir	T37.5X1	T37.5X2	T37.5X3	T37.5X4	T37.5X5	T37.5X6
Acidifying agent NEC	T50.901	T50.902	T50.903	T50.904	T50.905	T50.906
Acid (corrosive) NEC	T54.2X1	T54.2X2	T54.2X3	T54.2X4	—	—
Acipimox	T46.6X1	T46.6X2	T46.6X3	T46.6X4	T46.6X5	T46.6X6
Acitretin	T50.991	T50.992	T50.993	T50.994	T50.995	T50.996
Aclarubicin	T45.1X1	T45.1X2	T45.1X3	T45.1X4	T45.1X5	T45.1X6
Aclatonium napadisilate	T48.1X1	T48.1X2	T48.1X3	T48.1X4	T48.1X5	T48.1X6
Aconite (wild)	T46.991	T46.992	T46.993	T46.994	T46.995	T46.996
Aconitine	T46.991	T46.992	T46.993	T46.994	T46.995	T46.996
Aconitum ferox	T46.991	T46.992	T46.993	T46.994	T46.995	T46.996
Acridine	T65.6X1	T65.6X2	T65.6X3	T65.6X4	—	—
vapor	T59.891	T59.892	T59.893	T59.894	—	—
Acriflavine	T37.91	T37.92	T37.93	T37.94	T37.95	T37.96
Acriflavinium chloride	T49.0X1	T49.0X2	T49.0X3	T49.0X4	T49.0X5	T49.0X6
Acrinol	T49.0X1	T49.0X2	T49.0X3	T49.0X4	T49.0X5	T49.0X6
Acrisorcin	T49.0X1	T49.0X2	T49.0X3	T49.0X4	T49.0X5	T49.0X6
Acrivastine	T45.0X1	T45.0X2	T45.0X3	T45.0X4	T45.0X5	T45.0X6
Acrolein (gas)	T59.891	T59.892	T59.893	T59.894	—	—
liquid	T54.1X1	T54.1X2	T54.1X3	T54.1X4	—	—
Acrylamide	T65.891	T65.892	T65.893	T65.894	—	—
Acrylic resin	T49.3X1	T49.3X2	T49.3X3	T49.3X4	T49.3X5	T49.3X6
Acrylonitrile	T65.891	T65.892	T65.893	T65.894	—	—
Actaea spicata	T62.2X1	T62.2X2	T62.2X3	T62.2X4	—	—
berry	T62.1X1	T62.1X2	T62.1X3	T62.1X4	—	—
Acterol	T37.3X1	T37.3X2	T37.3X3	T37.3X4	T37.3X5	T37.3X6
ACTH	T38.811	T38.812	T38.813	T38.814	T38.815	T38.816
Actinomycin C	T45.1X1	T45.1X2	T45.1X3	T45.1X4	T45.1X5	T45.1X6
Actinomycin D	T45.1X1	T45.1X2	T45.1X3	T45.1X4	T45.1X5	T45.1X6
Activated charcoal — see also Charcoal, medicinal	T47.6X1	T47.6X2	T47.6X3	T47.6X4	T47.6X5	T47.6X6
Acyclovir	T37.5X1	T37.5X2	T37.5X3	T37.5X4	T37.5X5	T37.5X6
Adenine	T45.2X1	T45.2X2	T45.2X3	T45.2X4	T45.2X5	T45.2X6
arabinoside	T37.5X1	T37.5X2	T37.5X3	T37.5X4	T37.5X5	T37.5X6
Adenosine (phosphate)	T46.2X1	T46.2X2	T46.2X3	T46.2X4	T46.2X5	T46.2X6
ADH	T38.891	T38.892	T38.893	T38.894	T38.895	T38.896
Adhesive NEC	T65.891	T65.892	T65.893	T65.894	—	—
Adicillin	T36.0X1	T36.0X2	T36.0X3	T36.0X4	T36.0X5	T36.0X6
Adiphenine	T44.3X1	T44.3X2	T44.3X3	T44.3X4	T44.3X5	T44.3X6
Adipiodone	T50.8X1	T50.8X2	T50.8X3	T50.8X4	T50.8X5	T50.8X6
Adjunct, pharmaceutical	T50.901	T50.902	T50.903	T50.904	T50.905	T50.906
Adrenal (extract, cortex or medulla) (glucocorticoids) (hormones) (mineralocorticoids)	T38.0X1	T38.0X2	T38.0X3	T38.0X4	T38.0X5	T38.0X6
ENT agent	T49.6X1	T49.6X2	T49.6X3	T49.6X4	T49.6X5	T49.6X6
ophthalmic preparation	T49.5X1	T49.5X2	T49.5X3	T49.5X4	T49.5X5	T49.5X6
topical NEC	T49.0X1	T49.0X2	T49.0X3	T49.0X4	T49.0X5	T49.0X6
Adrenalin — see Adrenaline						
Adrenaline	T44.5X1	T44.5X2	T44.5X3	T44.5X4	T44.5X5	T44.5X6
Adrenergic NEC	T44.901	T44.902	T44.903	T44.904	T44.905	T44.906
blocking agent NEC	T44.8X1	T44.8X2	T44.8X3	T44.8X4	T44.8X5	T44.8X6
beta, heart	T44.7X1	T44.7X2	T44.7X3	T44.7X4	T44.7X5	T44.7X6
specified NEC	T44.991	T44.992	T44.993	T44.994	T44.995	T44.996
Adrenochrome						
derivative	T46.991	T46.992	T46.993	T46.994	T46.995	T46.996
(mono) semicarbazone	T46.991	T46.992	T46.993	T46.994	T46.995	T46.996
Adrenocorticotrophic hormone	T38.811	T38.812	T38.813	T38.814	T38.815	T38.816
Adrenocorticotrophin	T38.811	T38.812	T38.813	T38.814	T38.815	T38.816
Adriamycin	T45.1X1	T45.1X2	T45.1X3	T45.1X4	T45.1X5	T45.1X6
Aerosol spray NEC	T65.91	T65.92	T65.93	T65.94	—	—
Aerosporin	T36.8X1	T36.8X2	T36.8X3	T36.8X4	T36.8X5	T36.8X6
ENT agent	T49.6X1	T49.6X2	T49.6X3	T49.6X4	T49.6X5	T49.6X6
ophthalmic preparation	T49.5X1	T49.5X2	T49.5X3	T49.5X4	T49.5X5	T49.5X6

Table of Drugs and Chemicals

14-hydroxydihydro-morphinone — Aerosporin

Substance	Poisoning, Accidental (unintentional)	Poisoning, Intentional Self-harm	Poisoning, Assault	Poisoning, Undetermined	Adverse Effect	Under-dosing
Aerosporin — *continued*						
topical NEC	T49.ØX1	T49.ØX2	T49.ØX3	T49.ØX4	T49.ØX5	T49.ØX6
Aethusa cynapium	T62.2X1	T62.2X2	T62.2X3	T62.2X4	—	—
Afghanistan black	T4Ø.711	T4Ø.712	T4Ø.713	T4Ø.714	T4Ø.715	T4Ø.716
Aflatoxin	T64.Ø1	T64.Ø2	T64.Ø3	T64.Ø4	—	—
Afloqualone	T42.8X1	T42.8X2	T42.8X3	T42.8X4	T42.8X5	T42.8X6
African boxwood	T62.2X1	T62.2X2	T62.2X3	T62.2X4	—	—
Agar	T47.4X1	T47.4X2	T47.4X3	T47.4X4	T47.4X5	T47.4X6
Agonist						
predominantly						
alpha-adrenoreceptor	T44.4X1	T44.4X2	T44.4X3	T44.4X4	T44.4X5	T44.4X6
beta-adrenoreceptor	T44.5X1	T44.5X2	T44.5X3	T44.5X4	T44.5X5	T44.5X6
Agricultural agent NEC	T65.91	T65.92	T65.93	T65.94	—	—
Agrypnal	T42.3X1	T42.3X2	T42.3X3	T42.3X4	T42.3X5	T42.3X6
AHLG	T5Ø.Z11	T5Ø.Z12	T5Ø.Z13	T5Ø.Z14	T5Ø.Z15	T5Ø.Z16
Air contaminant(s), **source/type NOS**	T65.91	T65.92	T65.93	T65.94	—	—
Ajmaline	T46.2X1	T46.2X2	T46.2X3	T46.2X4	T46.2X5	T46.2X6
Akee	T62.1X1	T62.1X2	T62.1X3	T62.1X4	—	—
Akrinol	T49.ØX1	T49.ØX2	T49.ØX3	T49.ØX4	T49.ØX5	T49.ØX6
Akritoin	T37.8X1	T37.8X2	T37.8X3	T37.8X4	T37.8X5	T37.8X6
Alacepril	T46.4X1	T46.4X2	T46.4X3	T46.4X4	T46.4X5	T46.4X6
Alantolactone	T37.4X1	T37.4X2	T37.4X3	T37.4X4	T37.4X5	T37.4X6
Albamycin	T36.8X1	T36.8X2	T36.8X3	T36.8X4	T36.8X5	T36.8X6
Albendazole	T37.4X1	T37.4X2	T37.4X3	T37.4X4	T37.4X5	T37.4X6
Albumin						
bovine	T45.8X1	T45.8X2	T45.8X3	T45.8X4	T45.8X5	T45.8X6
human serum	T45.8X1	T45.8X2	T45.8X3	T45.8X4	T45.8X5	T45.8X6
salt-poor	T45.8X1	T45.8X2	T45.8X3	T45.8X4	T45.8X5	T45.8X6
normal human serum	T45.8X1	T45.8X2	T45.8X3	T45.8X4	T45.8X5	T45.8X6
Albuterol	T48.6X1	T48.6X2	T48.6X3	T48.6X4	T48.6X5	T48.6X6
Albutoin	T42.ØX1	T42.ØX2	T42.ØX3	T42.ØX4	T42.ØX5	T42.ØX6
Alclometasone	T49.ØX1	T49.ØX2	T49.ØX3	T49.ØX4	T49.ØX5	T49.ØX6
Alcohol	T51.91	T51.92	T51.93	T51.94	—	—
absolute	T51.ØX1	T51.ØX2	T51.ØX3	T51.ØX4	—	—
beverage	T51.ØX1	T51.ØX2	T51.ØX3	T51.ØX4	—	—
allyl	T51.8X1	T51.8X2	T51.8X3	T51.8X4	—	—
amyl	T51.3X1	T51.3X2	T51.3X3	T51.3X4	—	—
antifreeze	T51.1X1	T51.1X2	T51.1X3	T51.1X4	—	—
beverage	T51.ØX1	T51.ØX2	T51.ØX3	T51.ØX4	—	—
butyl	T51.3X1	T51.3X2	T51.3X3	T51.3X4	—	—
dehydrated	T51.ØX1	T51.ØX2	T51.ØX3	T51.ØX4	—	—
beverage	T51.ØX1	T51.ØX2	T51.ØX3	T51.ØX4	—	—
denatured	T51.ØX1	T51.ØX2	T51.ØX3	T51.ØX4	—	—
deterrent NEC	T5Ø.6X1	T5Ø.6X2	T5Ø.6X3	T5Ø.6X4	T5Ø.6X5	T5Ø.6X6
diagnostic (gastric function)	T5Ø.8X1	T5Ø.8X2	T5Ø.8X3	T5Ø.8X4	T5Ø.8X5	T5Ø.8X6
ethyl	T51.ØX1	T51.ØX2	T51.ØX3	T51.ØX4	—	—
beverage	T51.ØX1	T51.ØX2	T51.ØX3	T51.ØX4	—	—
grain	T51.ØX1	T51.ØX2	T51.ØX3	T51.ØX4	—	—
beverage	T51.ØX1	T51.ØX2	T51.ØX3	T51.ØX4	—	—
industrial	T51.ØX1	T51.ØX2	T51.ØX3	T51.ØX4	—	—
isopropyl	T51.2X1	T51.2X2	T51.2X3	T51.2X4	—	—
methyl	T51.1X1	T51.1X2	T51.1X3	T51.1X4	—	—
preparation for consumption	T51.ØX1	T51.ØX2	T51.ØX3	T51.ØX4	—	—
propyl	T51.3X1	T51.3X2	T51.3X3	T51.3X4	—	—
secondary	T51.2X1	T51.2X2	T51.2X3	T51.2X4	—	—
radiator	T51.1X1	T51.1X2	T51.1X3	T51.1X4	—	—
rubbing	T51.2X1	T51.2X2	T51.2X3	T51.2X4	—	—
specified type NEC	T51.8X1	T51.8X2	T51.8X3	T51.8X4	—	—
surgical	T51.ØX1	T51.ØX2	T51.ØX3	T51.ØX4	—	—
vapor (from any type of Alcohol)	T59.891	T59.892	T59.893	T59.894	—	—
wood	T51.1X1	T51.1X2	T51.1X3	T51.1X4	—	—
Alcuronium (chloride)	T48.1X1	T48.1X2	T48.1X3	T48.1X4	T48.1X5	T48.1X6
Aldactone	T5Ø.ØX1	T5Ø.ØX2	T5Ø.ØX3	T5Ø.ØX4	T5Ø.ØX5	T5Ø.ØX6
Aldesulfone sodium	T37.1X1	T37.1X2	T37.1X3	T37.1X4	T37.1X5	T37.1X6
Aldicarb	T6Ø.ØX1	T6Ø.ØX2	T6Ø.ØX3	T6Ø.ØX4	—	—
Aldomet	T46.5X1	T46.5X2	T46.5X3	T46.5X4	T46.5X5	T46.5X6
Aldosterone	T5Ø.ØX1	T5Ø.ØX2	T5Ø.ØX3	T5Ø.ØX4	T5Ø.ØX5	T5Ø.ØX6
Aldrin (dust)	T6Ø.1X1	T6Ø.1X2	T6Ø.1X3	T6Ø.1X4	—	—
Aleve — *see* Naproxen						
Alexitol sodium	T47.1X1	T47.1X2	T47.1X3	T47.1X4	T47.1X5	T47.1X6
Alfacalcidol	T45.2X1	T45.2X2	T45.2X3	T45.2X4	T45.2X5	T45.2X6
Alfadolone	T41.1X1	T41.1X2	T41.1X3	T41.1X4	T41.1X5	T41.1X6
Alfaxalone	T41.1X1	T41.1X2	T41.1X3	T41.1X4	T41.1X5	T41.1X6
Alfentanil	T4Ø.411	T4Ø.412	T4Ø.413	T4Ø.414	T4Ø.415	T4Ø.416
Alfuzosin (hydrochloride)	T44.8X1	T44.8X2	T44.8X3	T44.8X4	T44.8X5	T44.8X6
Algae (harmful) (toxin)	T65.821	T65.822	T65.823	T65.824	—	—
Algeldrate	T47.1X1	T47.1X2	T47.1X3	T47.1X4	T47.1X5	T47.1X6
Algin	T47.8X1	T47.8X2	T47.8X3	T47.8X4	T47.8X5	T47.8X6
Alglucerase	T45.3X1	T45.3X2	T45.3X3	T45.3X4	T45.3X5	T45.3X6
Alidase	T45.3X1	T45.3X2	T45.3X3	T45.3X4	T45.3X5	T45.3X6
Alimemazine	T43.3X1	T43.3X2	T43.3X3	T43.3X4	T43.3X5	T43.3X6
Aliphatic thiocyanates	T65.ØX1	T65.ØX2	T65.ØX3	T65.ØX4	—	—
Alizapride	T45.ØX1	T45.ØX2	T45.ØX3	T45.ØX4	T45.ØX5	T45.ØX6
Alkali (caustic)	T54.3X1	T54.3X2	T54.3X3	T54.3X4	—	—
Alkaline antiseptic solution (aromatic)	T49.6X1	T49.6X2	T49.6X3	T49.6X4	T49.6X5	T49.6X6
Alkalinizing agents (medicinal)	T5Ø.9Ø1	T5Ø.9Ø2	T5Ø.9Ø3	T5Ø.9Ø4	T5Ø.9Ø5	T5Ø.9Ø6
Alkalizing agent NEC	T5Ø.9Ø1	T5Ø.9Ø2	T5Ø.9Ø3	T5Ø.9Ø4	T5Ø.9Ø5	T5Ø.9Ø6
Alka-seltzer	T39.Ø11	T39.Ø12	T39.Ø13	T39.Ø14	T39.Ø15	T39.Ø16
Alkavervir	T46.5X1	T46.5X2	T46.5X3	T46.5X4	T46.5X5	T46.5X6
Alkonium (bromide)	T49.ØX1	T49.ØX2	T49.ØX3	T49.ØX4	T49.ØX5	T49.ØX6
Alkylating drug NEC	T45.1X1	T45.1X2	T45.1X3	T45.1X4	T45.1X5	T45.1X6
antimyeloproliferative	T45.1X1	T45.1X2	T45.1X3	T45.1X4	T45.1X5	T45.1X6
lymphatic	T45.1X1	T45.1X2	T45.1X3	T45.1X4	T45.1X5	T45.1X6
Alkylisocyanate	T65.ØX1	T65.ØX2	T65.ØX3	T65.ØX4	—	—
Allantoin	T49.4X1	T49.4X2	T49.4X3	T49.4X4	T49.4X5	T49.4X6
Allegron	T43.Ø11	T43.Ø12	T43.Ø13	T43.Ø14	T43.Ø15	T43.Ø16
Allethrin	T49.ØX1	T49.ØX2	T49.ØX3	T49.ØX4	T49.ØX5	T49.ØX6
Allobarbital	T42.3X1	T42.3X2	T42.3X3	T42.3X4	T42.3X5	T42.3X6
Allopurinol	T5Ø.4X1	T5Ø.4X2	T5Ø.4X3	T5Ø.4X4	T5Ø.4X5	T5Ø.4X6
Allyl						
alcohol	T51.8X1	T51.8X2	T51.8X3	T51.8X4	—	—
disulfide	T46.6X1	T46.6X2	T46.6X3	T46.6X4	T46.6X5	T46.6X6
Allylestrenol	T38.5X1	T38.5X2	T38.5X3	T38.5X4	T38.5X5	T38.5X6
Allylisopropylacetylurea	T42.6X1	T42.6X2	T42.6X3	T42.6X4	T42.6X5	T42.6X6
Allylisopropylmalonylurea	T42.3X1	T42.3X2	T42.3X3	T42.3X4	T42.3X5	T42.3X6
Allylthiourea	T49.3X1	T49.3X2	T49.3X3	T49.3X4	T49.3X5	T49.3X6
Allyltribromide	T42.6X1	T42.6X2	T42.6X3	T42.6X4	T42.6X5	T42.6X6
Allypropymal	T42.3X1	T42.3X2	T42.3X3	T42.3X4	T42.3X5	T42.3X6
Almagate	T47.1X1	T47.1X2	T47.1X3	T47.1X4	T47.1X5	T47.1X6
Almasilate	T47.1X1	T47.1X2	T47.1X3	T47.1X4	T47.1X5	T47.1X6
Almitrine	T5Ø.7X1	T5Ø.7X2	T5Ø.7X3	T5Ø.7X4	T5Ø.7X5	T5Ø.7X6
Aloes	T47.2X1	T47.2X2	T47.2X3	T47.2X4	T47.2X5	T47.2X6
Aloglutamol	T47.1X1	T47.1X2	T47.1X3	T47.1X4	T47.1X5	T47.1X6
Aloin	T47.2X1	T47.2X2	T47.2X3	T47.2X4	T47.2X5	T47.2X6
Aloxidone	T42.2X1	T42.2X2	T42.2X3	T42.2X4	T42.2X5	T42.2X6
Alpha						
acetyldigoxin	T46.ØX1	T46.ØX2	T46.ØX3	T46.ØX4	T46.ØX5	T46.ØX6
adrenergic blocking drug	T44.6X1	T44.6X2	T44.6X3	T44.6X4	T44.6X5	T44.6X6
amylase	T45.3X1	T45.3X2	T45.3X3	T45.3X4	T45.3X5	T45.3X6
tocoferol (acetate)	T45.2X1	T45.2X2	T45.2X3	T45.2X4	T45.2X5	T45.2X6
tocopherol	T45.2X1	T45.2X2	T45.2X3	T45.2X4	T45.2X5	T45.2X6
Alphadolone	T41.1X1	T41.1X2	T41.1X3	T41.1X4	T41.1X5	T41.1X6
Alphaprodine	T4Ø.491	T4Ø.492	T4Ø.493	T4Ø.494	T4Ø.495	T4Ø.496
Alphaxalone	T41.1X1	T41.1X2	T41.1X3	T41.1X4	T41.1X5	T41.1X6
Alprazolam	T42.4X1	T42.4X2	T42.4X3	T42.4X4	T42.4X5	T42.4X6
Alprenolol	T44.7X1	T44.7X2	T44.7X3	T44.7X4	T44.7X5	T44.7X6
Alprostadil	T46.7X1	T46.7X2	T46.7X3	T46.7X4	T46.7X5	T46.7X6
Alsactide	T38.811	T38.812	T38.813	T38.814	T38.815	T38.816
Alseroxylon	T46.5X1	T46.5X2	T46.5X3	T46.5X4	T46.5X5	T46.5X6
Alteplase	T45.611	T45.612	T45.613	T45.614	T45.615	T45.616
Altizide	T5Ø.2X1	T5Ø.2X2	T5Ø.2X3	T5Ø.2X4	T5Ø.2X5	T5Ø.2X6
Altretamine	T45.1X1	T45.1X2	T45.1X3	T45.1X4	T45.1X5	T45.1X6
Alum (medicinal)	T49.4X1	T49.4X2	T49.4X3	T49.4X4	T49.4X5	T49.4X6
nonmedicinal (ammonium) (potassium)	T56.891	T56.892	T56.893	T56.894	—	—
Aluminium, aluminum						
acetate	T49.2X1	T49.2X2	T49.2X3	T49.2X4	T49.2X5	T49.2X6
solution	T49.ØX1	T49.ØX2	T49.ØX3	T49.ØX4	T49.ØX5	T49.ØX6
aspirin	T39.Ø11	T39.Ø12	T39.Ø13	T39.Ø14	T39.Ø15	T39.Ø16
bis (acetylsalicylate)	T39.Ø11	T39.Ø12	T39.Ø13	T39.Ø14	T39.Ø15	T39.Ø16
carbonate (gel, basic)	T47.1X1	T47.1X2	T47.1X3	T47.1X4	T47.1X5	T47.1X6
chlorhydroxide-complex	T47.1X1	T47.1X2	T47.1X3	T47.1X4	T47.1X5	T47.1X6
chloride	T49.2X1	T49.2X2	T49.2X3	T49.2X4	T49.2X5	T49.2X6
clofibrate	T46.6X1	T46.6X2	T46.6X3	T46.6X4	T46.6X5	T46.6X6
diacetate	T49.2X1	T49.2X2	T49.2X3	T49.2X4	T49.2X5	T49.2X6
glycinate	T47.1X1	T47.1X2	T47.1X3	T47.1X4	T47.1X5	T47.1X6
hydroxide (gel)	T47.1X1	T47.1X2	T47.1X3	T47.1X4	T47.1X5	T47.1X6
hydroxide-magnesium carb. gel	T47.1X1	T47.1X2	T47.1X3	T47.1X4	T47.1X5	T47.1X6
magnesium silicate	T47.1X1	T47.1X2	T47.1X3	T47.1X4	T47.1X5	T47.1X6
nicotinate	T46.7X1	T46.7X2	T46.7X3	T46.7X4	T46.7X5	T46.7X6
ointment (surgical) (topical)	T49.3X1	T49.3X2	T49.3X3	T49.3X4	T49.3X5	T49.3X6
phosphate	T47.1X1	T47.1X2	T47.1X3	T47.1X4	T47.1X5	T47.1X6
salicylate	T39.Ø91	T39.Ø92	T39.Ø93	T39.Ø94	T39.Ø95	T39.Ø96
silicate	T47.1X1	T47.1X2	T47.1X3	T47.1X4	T47.1X5	T47.1X6
sodium silicate	T47.1X1	T47.1X2	T47.1X3	T47.1X4	T47.1X5	T47.1X6
subacetate	T49.2X1	T49.2X2	T49.2X3	T49.2X4	T49.2X5	T49.2X6
sulfate	T49.ØX1	T49.ØX2	T49.ØX3	T49.ØX4	T49.ØX5	T49.ØX6
tannate	T47.6X1	T47.6X2	T47.6X3	T47.6X4	T47.6X5	T47.6X6

Aerosporin — Aluminium, aluminum

356 **Additional Character May Be Required — Refer to the Tabular List for Character Selection** **Subterms under main terms may continue to next column or page**

Substance	Poisoning, Accidental (unintentional)	Poisoning, Intentional Self-harm	Poisoning, Assault	Poisoning, Undetermined	Adverse Effect	Under-dosing
Aluminium, aluminum — *continued*						
topical NEC	T49.3X1	T49.3X2	T49.3X3	T49.3X4	T49.3X5	T49.3X6
Alurate	T42.3X1	T42.3X2	T42.3X3	T42.3X4	T42.3X5	T42.3X6
Alverine	T44.3X1	T44.3X2	T44.3X3	T44.3X4	T44.3X5	T44.3X6
Alvodine	T4Ø.2X1	T4Ø.2X2	T4Ø.2X3	T4Ø.2X4	T4Ø.2X5	T4Ø.2X6
Amanita phalloides	T62.ØX1	T62.ØX2	T62.ØX3	T62.ØX4	—	—
Amanitine	T62.ØX1	T62.ØX2	T62.ØX3	T62.ØX4	—	—
Amantadine	T42.8X1	T42.8X2	T42.8X3	T42.8X4	T42.8X5	T42.8X6
Ambazone	T49.6X1	T49.6X2	T49.6X3	T49.6X4	T49.6X5	T49.6X6
Ambenonium (chloride)	T44.ØX1	T44.ØX2	T44.ØX3	T44.ØX4	T44.ØX5	T44.ØX6
Ambroxol	T48.4X1	T48.4X2	T48.4X3	T48.4X4	T48.4X5	T48.4X6
Ambuphylline	T48.6X1	T48.6X2	T48.6X3	T48.6X4	T48.6X5	T48.6X6
Ambutonium bromide	T44.3X1	T44.3X2	T44.3X3	T44.3X4	T44.3X5	T44.3X6
Amcinonide	T49.ØX1	T49.ØX2	T49.ØX3	T49.ØX4	T49.ØX5	T49.ØX6
Amdinocilline	T36.ØX1	T36.ØX2	T36.ØX3	T36.ØX4	T36.ØX5	T36.ØX6
Ametazole	T5Ø.8X1	T5Ø.8X2	T5Ø.8X3	T5Ø.8X4	T5Ø.8X5	T5Ø.8X6
Amethocaine	T41.3X1	T41.3X2	T41.3X3	T41.3X4	T41.3X5	T41.3X6
regional	T41.3X1	T41.3X2	T41.3X3	T41.3X4	T41.3X5	T41.3X6
spinal	T41.3X1	T41.3X2	T41.3X3	T41.3X4	T41.3X5	T41.3X6
Amethopterin	T45.1X1	T45.1X2	T45.1X3	T45.1X4	T45.1X5	T45.1X6
Amezinium metilsulfate	T44.991	T44.992	T44.993	T44.994	T44.995	T44.996
Amfebutamone	T43.291	T43.292	T43.293	T43.294	T43.295	T43.296
Amfepramone	T5Ø.5X1	T5Ø.5X2	T5Ø.5X3	T5Ø.5X4	T5Ø.5X5	T5Ø.5X6
Amfetamine	T43.621	T43.622	T43.623	T43.624	T43.625	T43.626
Amfetaminil	T43.621	T43.622	T43.623	T43.624	T43.625	T43.626
Amfomycin	T36.8X1	T36.8X2	T36.8X3	T36.8X4	T36.8X5	T36.8X6
Amidefrine mesilate	T48.5X1	T48.5X2	T48.5X3	T48.5X4	T48.5X5	T48.5X6
Amidone	T4Ø.3X1	T4Ø.3X2	T4Ø.3X3	T4Ø.3X4	T4Ø.3X5	T4Ø.3X6
Amidopyrine	T39.2X1	T39.2X2	T39.2X3	T39.2X4	T39.2X5	T39.2X6
Amidotrizoate	T5Ø.8X1	T5Ø.8X2	T5Ø.8X3	T5Ø.8X4	T5Ø.8X5	T5Ø.8X6
Amiflamine	T43.1X1	T43.1X2	T43.1X3	T43.1X4	T43.1X5	T43.1X6
Amikacin	T36.5X1	T36.5X2	T36.5X3	T36.5X4	T36.5X5	T36.5X6
Amikhelline	T46.3X1	T46.3X2	T46.3X3	T46.3X4	T46.3X5	T46.3X6
Amiloride	T5Ø.2X1	T5Ø.2X2	T5Ø.2X3	T5Ø.2X4	T5Ø.2X5	T5Ø.2X6
Aminacrine	T49.ØX1	T49.ØX2	T49.ØX3	T49.ØX4	T49.ØX5	T49.ØX6
Amineptine	T43.Ø11	T43.Ø12	T43.Ø13	T43.Ø14	T43.Ø15	T43.Ø16
Aminitrozole	T37.3X1	T37.3X2	T37.3X3	T37.3X4	T37.3X5	T37.3X6
Aminoacetic acid (derivatives)	T5Ø.3X1	T5Ø.3X2	T5Ø.3X3	T5Ø.3X4	T5Ø.3X5	T5Ø.3X6
Amino acids	T5Ø.3X1	T5Ø.3X2	T5Ø.3X3	T5Ø.3X4	T5Ø.3X5	T5Ø.3X6
Aminoacridine	T49.ØX1	T49.ØX2	T49.ØX3	T49.ØX4	T49.ØX5	T49.ØX6
Aminobenzoic acid (-p)	T49.3X1	T49.3X2	T49.3X3	T49.3X4	T49.3X5	T49.3X6
Aminocaproic acid	T45.621	T45.622	T45.623	T45.624	T45.625	T45.626
Aminoethylisothiourium	T45.8X1	T45.8X2	T45.8X3	T45.8X4	T45.8X5	T45.8X6
Aminofenazone	T39.2X1	T39.2X2	T39.2X3	T39.2X4	T39.2X5	T39.2X6
Aminoglutethimide	T45.1X1	T45.1X2	T45.1X3	T45.1X4	T45.1X5	T45.1X6
Aminohippuric acid	T5Ø.8X1	T5Ø.8X2	T5Ø.8X3	T5Ø.8X4	T5Ø.8X5	T5Ø.8X6
Aminomethylbenzoic acid	T45.691	T45.692	T45.693	T45.694	T45.695	T45.696
Aminometradine	T5Ø.2X1	T5Ø.2X2	T5Ø.2X3	T5Ø.2X4	T5Ø.2X5	T5Ø.2X6
Aminopentamide	T44.3X1	T44.3X2	T44.3X3	T44.3X4	T44.3X5	T44.3X6
Aminophenazone	T39.2X1	T39.2X2	T39.2X3	T39.2X4	T39.2X5	T39.2X6
Aminophenol	T54.ØX1	T54.ØX2	T54.ØX3	T54.ØX4	—	—
Aminophenylpyridone	T43.591	T43.592	T43.593	T43.594	T43.595	T43.596
Aminophylline	T48.6X1	T48.6X2	T48.6X3	T48.6X4	T48.6X5	T48.6X6
Aminopterin sodium	T45.1X1	T45.1X2	T45.1X3	T45.1X4	T45.1X5	T45.1X6
Aminopyrine	T39.2X1	T39.2X2	T39.2X3	T39.2X4	T39.2X5	T39.2X6
Aminorex	T5Ø.5X1	T5Ø.5X2	T5Ø.5X3	T5Ø.5X4	T5Ø.5X5	T5Ø.5X6
Aminosalicylic acid	T37.1X1	T37.1X2	T37.1X3	T37.1X4	T37.1X5	T37.1X6
Aminosalylum	T37.1X1	T37.1X2	T37.1X3	T37.1X4	T37.1X5	T37.1X6
Amiodarone	T46.2X1	T46.2X2	T46.2X3	T46.2X4	T46.2X5	T46.2X6
Amiphenazole	T5Ø.7X1	T5Ø.7X2	T5Ø.7X3	T5Ø.7X4	T5Ø.7X5	T5Ø.7X6
Amiquinsin	T46.5X1	T46.5X2	T46.5X3	T46.5X4	T46.5X5	T46.5X6
Amisometradine	T5Ø.2X1	T5Ø.2X2	T5Ø.2X3	T5Ø.2X4	T5Ø.2X5	T5Ø.2X6
Amisulpride	T43.591	T43.592	T43.593	T43.594	T43.595	T43.596
Amitriptyline	T43.Ø11	T43.Ø12	T43.Ø13	T43.Ø14	T43.Ø15	T43.Ø16
Amitriptylinoxide	T43.Ø11	T43.Ø12	T43.Ø13	T43.Ø14	T43.Ø15	T43.Ø16
Amlexanox	T48.6X1	T48.6X2	T48.6X3	T48.6X4	T48.6X5	T48.6X6
Ammonia (fumes) (gas) (vapor)	T59.891	T59.892	T59.893	T59.894	—	—
aromatic spirit	T48.991	T48.992	T48.993	T48.994	T48.995	T48.996
liquid (household)	T54.3X1	T54.3X2	T54.3X3	T54.3X4	—	—
Ammoniated mercury	T49.ØX1	T49.ØX2	T49.ØX3	T49.ØX4	T49.ØX5	T49.ØX6
Ammonium						
acid tartrate	T49.5X1	T49.5X2	T49.5X3	T49.5X4	T49.5X5	T49.5X6
bromide	T42.6X1	T42.6X2	T42.6X3	T42.6X4	T42.6X5	T42.6X6
carbonate	T54.3X1	T54.3X2	T54.3X3	T54.3X4	—	—
chloride	T5Ø.991	T5Ø.992	T5Ø.993	T5Ø.994	T5Ø.995	T5Ø.996
expectorant	T48.4X1	T48.4X2	T48.4X3	T48.4X4	T48.4X5	T48.4X6
compounds (household) NEC	T54.3X1	T54.3X2	T54.3X3	T54.3X4	—	—
fumes (any usage)	T59.891	T59.892	T59.893	T59.894	—	—
industrial	T54.3X1	T54.3X2	T54.3X3	T54.3X4	—	—

Substance	Poisoning, Accidental (unintentional)	Poisoning, Intentional Self-harm	Poisoning, Assault	Poisoning, Undetermined	Adverse Effect	Under-dosing
Ammonium — *continued*						
ichthyosulronate	T49.4X1	T49.4X2	T49.4X3	T49.4X4	T49.4X5	T49.4X6
mandelate	T37.91	T37.92	T37.93	T37.94	T37.95	T37.96
sulfamate	T6Ø.3X1	T6Ø.3X2	T6Ø.3X3	T6Ø.3X4	—	—
sulfonate resin	T47.8X1	T47.8X2	T47.8X3	T47.8X4	T47.8X5	T47.8X6
Amobarbital (sodium)	T42.3X1	T42.3X2	T42.3X3	T42.3X4	T42.3X5	T42.3X6
Amodiaquine	T37.2X1	T37.2X2	T37.2X3	T37.2X4	T37.2X5	T37.2X6
Amopyroquin (e)	T37.2X1	T37.2X2	T37.2X3	T37.2X4	T37.2X5	T37.2X6
Amoxapine	T43.Ø11	T43.Ø12	T43.Ø13	T43.Ø14	T43.Ø15	T43.Ø16
Amoxicillin	T36.ØX1	T36.ØX2	T36.ØX3	T36.ØX4	T36.ØX5	T36.ØX6
Amperozide	T43.591	T43.592	T43.593	T43.594	T43.595	T43.596
Amphenidone	T43.591	T43.592	T43.593	T43.594	T43.595	T43.596
Amphetamine NEC	T43.621	T43.622	T43.623	T43.624	T43.625	T43.626
Amphomycin	T36.8X1	T36.8X2	T36.8X3	T36.8X4	T36.8X5	T36.8X6
Amphotalide	T37.4X1	T37.4X2	T37.4X3	T37.4X4	T37.4X5	T37.4X6
Amphotericin B	T36.7X1	T36.7X2	T36.7X3	T36.7X4	T36.7X5	T36.7X6
topical	T49.ØX1	T49.ØX2	T49.ØX3	T49.ØX4	T49.ØX5	T49.ØX6
Ampicillin	T36.ØX1	T36.ØX2	T36.ØX3	T36.ØX4	T36.ØX5	T36.ØX6
Amprotropine	T44.3X1	T44.3X2	T44.3X3	T44.3X4	T44.3X5	T44.3X6
Amsacrine	T45.1X1	T45.1X2	T45.1X3	T45.1X4	T45.1X5	T45.1X6
Amygdaline	T62.2X1	T62.2X2	T62.2X3	T62.2X4	—	—
Amyl						
acetate	T52.8X1	T52.8X2	T52.8X3	T52.8X4	—	—
vapor	T59.891	T59.892	T59.893	T59.894	—	—
alcohol	T51.3X1	T51.3X2	T51.3X3	T51.3X4	—	—
chloride	T53.6X1	T53.6X2	T53.6X3	T53.6X4	—	—
formate	T52.8X1	T52.8X2	T52.8X3	T52.8X4	—	—
nitrite	T46.3X1	T46.3X2	T46.3X3	T46.3X4	T46.3X5	T46.3X6
propionate	T65.891	T65.892	T65.893	T65.894	—	—
Amylase	T47.5X1	T47.5X2	T47.5X3	T47.5X4	T47.5X5	T47.5X6
Amyleine, regional	T41.3X1	T41.3X2	T41.3X3	T41.3X4	T41.3X5	T41.3X6
Amylene						
dichloride	T53.6X1	T53.6X2	T53.6X3	T53.6X4	—	—
hydrate	T51.3X1	T51.3X2	T51.3X3	T51.3X4	—	—
Amylmetacresol	T49.6X1	T49.6X2	T49.6X3	T49.6X4	T49.6X5	T49.6X6
Amylobarbitone	T42.3X1	T42.3X2	T42.3X3	T42.3X4	T42.3X5	T42.3X6
Amylocaine, regional	T41.3X1	T41.3X2	T41.3X3	T41.3X4	T41.3X5	T41.3X6
infiltration (subcutaneous)	T41.3X1	T41.3X2	T41.3X3	T41.3X4	T41.3X5	T41.3X6
nerve block (peripheral) (plexus)	T41.3X1	T41.3X2	T41.3X3	T41.3X4	T41.3X5	T41.3X6
spinal	T41.3X1	T41.3X2	T41.3X3	T41.3X4	T41.3X5	T41.3X6
topical (surface)	T41.3X1	T41.3X2	T41.3X3	T41.3X4	T41.3X5	T41.3X6
Amylopectin	T47.6X1	T47.6X2	T47.6X3	T47.6X4	T47.6X5	T47.6X6
Amytal (sodium)	T42.3X1	T42.3X2	T42.3X3	T42.3X4	T42.3X5	T42.3X6
Anabolic steroid	T38.7X1	T38.7X2	T38.7X3	T38.7X4	T38.7X5	T38.7X6
Analeptic NEC	T5Ø.7X1	T5Ø.7X2	T5Ø.7X3	T5Ø.7X4	T5Ø.7X5	T5Ø.7X6
Analgesic	T39.91	T39.92	T39.93	T39.94	T39.95	T39.96
anti-inflammatory NEC	T39.91	T39.92	T39.93	T39.94	T39.95	T39.96
propionic acid derivative	T39.311	T39.312	T39.313	T39.314	T39.315	T39.316
antirheumatic NEC	T39.4X1	T39.4X2	T39.4X3	T39.4X4	T39.4X5	T39.4X6
aromatic NEC	T39.1X1	T39.1X2	T39.1X3	T39.1X4	T39.1X5	T39.1X6
narcotic NEC	T4Ø.6Ø1	T4Ø.6Ø2	T4Ø.6Ø3	T4Ø.6Ø4	T4Ø.6Ø5	T4Ø.6Ø6
combination	T4Ø.6Ø1	T4Ø.6Ø2	T4Ø.6Ø3	T4Ø.6Ø4	T4Ø.6Ø5	T4Ø.6Ø6
obstetric	T4Ø.6Ø1	T4Ø.6Ø2	T4Ø.6Ø3	T4Ø.6Ø4	T4Ø.6Ø5	T4Ø.6Ø6
non-narcotic NEC	T39.91	T39.92	T39.93	T39.94	T39.95	T39.96
combination	T39.91	T39.92	T39.93	T39.94	T39.95	T39.96
pyrazole	T39.2X1	T39.2X2	T39.2X3	T39.2X4	T39.2X5	T39.2X6
specified NEC	T39.8X1	T39.8X2	T39.8X3	T39.8X4	T39.8X5	T39.8X6
Analgin	T39.2X1	T39.2X2	T39.2X3	T39.2X4	T39.2X5	T39.2X6
Anamirta cocculus	T62.1X1	T62.1X2	T62.1X3	T62.1X4	—	—
Ancillin	T36.ØX1	T36.ØX2	T36.ØX3	T36.ØX4	T36.ØX5	T36.ØX6
Ancrod	T45.691	T45.692	T45.693	T45.694	T45.695	T45.696
Androgen	T38.7X1	T38.7X2	T38.7X3	T38.7X4	T38.7X5	T38.7X6
Androgen-estrogen mixture	T38.7X1	T38.7X2	T38.7X3	T38.7X4	T38.7X5	T38.7X6
Androstalone	T38.7X1	T38.7X2	T38.7X3	T38.7X4	T38.7X5	T38.7X6
Androstanolone	T38.7X1	T38.7X2	T38.7X3	T38.7X4	T38.7X5	T38.7X6
Androsterone	T38.7X1	T38.7X2	T38.7X3	T38.7X4	T38.7X5	T38.7X6
Anemone pulsatilla	T62.2X1	T62.2X2	T62.2X3	T62.2X4	—	—
Anesthesia						
caudal	T41.3X1	T41.3X2	T41.3X3	T41.3X4	T41.3X5	T41.3X6
endotracheal	T41.ØX1	T41.ØX2	T41.ØX3	T41.ØX4	T41.ØX5	T41.ØX6
epidural	T41.3X1	T41.3X2	T41.3X3	T41.3X4	T41.3X5	T41.3X6
inhalation	T41.ØX1	T41.ØX2	T41.ØX3	T41.ØX4	T41.ØX5	T41.ØX6
local	T41.3X1	T41.3X2	T41.3X3	T41.3X4	T41.3X5	T41.3X6
mucosal	T41.3X1	T41.3X2	T41.3X3	T41.3X4	T41.3X5	T41.3X6
muscle relaxation	T48.1X1	T48.1X2	T48.1X3	T48.1X4	T48.1X5	T48.1X6
nerve blocking	T41.3X1	T41.3X2	T41.3X3	T41.3X4	T41.3X5	T41.3X6
plexus blocking	T41.3X1	T41.3X2	T41.3X3	T41.3X4	T41.3X5	T41.3X6
potentiated	T41.2Ø1	T41.2Ø2	T41.2Ø3	T41.2Ø4	T41.2Ø5	T41.2Ø6
rectal	T41.2Ø1	T41.2Ø2	T41.2Ø3	T41.2Ø4	T41.2Ø5	T41.2Ø6
general	T41.2Ø1	T41.2Ø2	T41.2Ø3	T41.2Ø4	T41.2Ø5	T41.2Ø6
local	T41.3X1	T41.3X2	T41.3X3	T41.3X4	T41.3X5	T41.3X6

Anesthesia ICD-10-CM 2022

Table of Drugs and Chemicals

Substance	Poisoning, Accidental (unintentional)	Poisoning, Intentional Self-harm	Poisoning, Assault	Poisoning, Undetermined	Adverse Effect	Under-dosing
Anesthesia — *continued*						
regional	T41.3X1	T41.3X2	T41.3X3	T41.3X4	T41.3X5	T41.3X6
surface	T41.3X1	T41.3X2	T41.3X3	T41.3X4	T41.3X5	T41.3X6
Anesthetic NEC — *see also* Anesthesia	T41.41	T41.42	T41.43	T41.44	T41.45	T41.46
with muscle relaxant	T41.201	T41.202	T41.203	T41.204	T41.205	T41.206
general	T41.201	T41.202	T41.203	T41.204	T41.205	T41.206
local	T41.3X1	T41.3X2	T41.3X3	T41.3X4	T41.3X5	T41.3X6
gaseous NEC	T41.0X1	T41.0X2	T41.0X3	T41.0X4	T41.0X5	T41.0X6
general NEC	T41.201	T41.202	T41.203	T41.204	T41.205	T41.206
halogenated hydrocarbon derivatives NEC	T41.0X1	T41.0X2	T41.0X3	T41.0X4	T41.0X5	T41.0X6
infiltration NEC	T41.3X1	T41.3X2	T41.3X3	T41.3X4	T41.3X5	T41.3X6
intravenous NEC	T41.1X1	T41.1X2	T41.1X3	T41.1X4	T41.1X5	T41.1X6
local NEC	T41.3X1	T41.3X2	T41.3X3	T41.3X4	T41.3X5	T41.3X6
rectal	T41.201	T41.202	T41.203	T41.204	T41.205	T41.206
general	T41.201	T41.202	T41.203	T41.204	T41.205	T41.206
local	T41.3X1	T41.3X2	T41.3X3	T41.3X4	T41.3X5	T41.3X6
regional NEC	T41.3X1	T41.3X2	T41.3X3	T41.3X4	T41.3X5	T41.3X6
spinal NEC	T41.3X1	T41.3X2	T41.3X3	T41.3X4	T41.3X5	T41.3X6
thiobarbiturate	T41.1X1	T41.1X2	T41.1X3	T41.1X4	T41.1X5	T41.1X6
topical	T41.3X1	T41.3X2	T41.3X3	T41.3X4	T41.3X5	T41.3X6
Aneurine	T45.2X1	T45.2X2	T45.2X3	T45.2X4	T45.2X5	T45.2X6
Angio-Conray	T50.8X1	T50.8X2	T50.8X3	T50.8X4	T50.8X5	T50.8X6
Angiotensin	T44.5X1	T44.5X2	T44.5X3	T44.5X4	T44.5X5	T44.5X6
Angiotensinamide	T44.991	T44.992	T44.993	T44.994	T44.995	T44.996
Anhydrohydroxy-progesterone	T38.5X1	T38.5X2	T38.5X3	T38.5X4	T38.5X5	T38.5X6
Anhydron	T50.2X1	T50.2X2	T50.2X3	T50.2X4	T50.2X5	T50.2X6
Anileridine	T40.491	T40.492	T40.493	T40.494	T40.495	T40.496
Aniline (dye) (liquid)	T65.3X1	T65.3X2	T65.3X3	T65.3X4	—	—
analgesic	T39.1X1	T39.1X2	T39.1X3	T39.1X4	T39.1X5	T39.1X6
derivatives, therapeutic NEC	T39.1X1	T39.1X2	T39.1X3	T39.1X4	T39.1X5	T39.1X6
vapor	T65.3X1	T65.3X2	T65.3X3	T65.3X4	—	—
Aniscoropine	T44.3X1	T44.3X2	T44.3X3	T44.3X4	T44.3X5	T44.3X6
Anise oil	T47.5X1	T47.5X2	T47.5X3	T47.5X4	T47.5X5	T47.5X6
Anisidine	T65.3X1	T65.3X2	T65.3X3	T65.3X4	—	—
Anisindione	T45.511	T45.512	T45.513	T45.514	T45.515	T45.516
Anisotropine methyl-bromide	T44.3X1	T44.3X2	T44.3X3	T44.3X4	T44.3X5	T44.3X6
Anistreplase	T45.611	T45.612	T45.613	T45.614	T45.615	T45.616
Anorexiant (central)	T50.5X1	T50.5X2	T50.5X3	T50.5X4	T50.5X5	T50.5X6
Anorexic agents	T50.5X1	T50.5X2	T50.5X3	T50.5X4	T50.5X5	T50.5X6
Ansamycin	T36.6X1	T36.6X2	T36.6X3	T36.6X4	T36.6X5	T36.6X6
Ant (bite) (sting)	T63.421	T63.422	T63.423	T63.424	—	—
Antabuse	T50.6X1	T50.6X2	T50.6X3	T50.6X4	T50.6X5	T50.6X6
Antacid NEC	T47.1X1	T47.1X2	T47.1X3	T47.1X4	T47.1X5	T47.1X6
Antagonist						
Aldosterone	T50.0X1	T50.0X2	T50.0X3	T50.0X4	T50.0X5	T50.0X6
alpha-adrenoreceptor	T44.6X1	T44.6X2	T44.6X3	T44.6X4	T44.6X5	T44.6X6
anticoagulant	T45.7X1	T45.7X2	T45.7X3	T45.7X4	T45.7X5	T45.7X6
beta-adrenoreceptor	T44.7X1	T44.7X2	T44.7X3	T44.7X4	T44.7X5	T44.7X6
extrapyramidal NEC	T44.3X1	T44.3X2	T44.3X3	T44.3X4	T44.3X5	T44.3X6
folic acid	T45.1X1	T45.1X2	T45.1X3	T45.1X4	T45.1X5	T45.1X6
H2 receptor	T47.0X1	T47.0X2	T47.0X3	T47.0X4	T47.0X5	T47.0X6
heavy metal	T45.8X1	T45.8X2	T45.8X3	T45.8X4	T45.8X5	T45.8X6
narcotic analgesic	T50.7X1	T50.7X2	T50.7X3	T50.7X4	T50.7X5	T50.7X6
opiate	T50.7X1	T50.7X2	T50.7X3	T50.7X4	T50.7X5	T50.7X6
pyrimidine	T45.1X1	T45.1X2	T45.1X3	T45.1X4	T45.1X5	T45.1X6
serotonin	T46.5X1	T46.5X2	T46.5X3	T46.5X4	T46.5X5	T46.5X6
Antazolin (e)	T45.0X1	T45.0X2	T45.0X3	T45.0X4	T45.0X5	T45.0X6
Anterior pituitary hormone NEC	T38.811	T38.812	T38.813	T38.814	T38.815	T38.816
Anthelmintic NEC	T37.4X1	T37.4X2	T37.4X3	T37.4X4	T37.4X5	T37.4X6
Anthiolimine	T37.4X1	T37.4X2	T37.4X3	T37.4X4	T37.4X5	T37.4X6
Anthralin	T49.4X1	T49.4X2	T49.4X3	T49.4X4	T49.4X5	T49.4X6
Anthramycin	T45.1X1	T45.1X2	T45.1X3	T45.1X4	T45.1X5	T45.1X6
Antiadrenergic NEC	T44.8X1	T44.8X2	T44.8X3	T44.8X4	T44.8X5	T44.8X6
Antiallergic NEC	T45.0X1	T45.0X2	T45.0X3	T45.0X4	T45.0X5	T45.0X6
Antiandrogen NEC	T38.6X1	T38.6X2	T38.6X3	T38.6X4	T38.6X5	T38.6X6
Anti-anemic (drug) (preparation)	T45.8X1	T45.8X2	T45.8X3	T45.8X4	T45.8X5	T45.8X6
Antianxiety drug NEC	T43.501	T43.502	T43.503	T43.504	T43.505	T43.506
Antiaris toxicaria	T65.891	T65.892	T65.893	T65.894	—	—
Antiarteriosclerotic drug	T46.6X1	T46.6X2	T46.6X3	T46.6X4	T46.6X5	T46.6X6
Antiasthmatic drug NEC	T48.6X1	T48.6X2	T48.6X3	T48.6X4	T48.6X5	T48.6X6
Antibiotic NEC	T36.91	T36.92	T36.93	T36.94	T36.95	T36.96
aminoglycoside	T36.5X1	T36.5X2	T36.5X3	T36.5X4	T36.5X5	T36.5X6
anticancer	T45.1X1	T45.1X2	T45.1X3	T45.1X4	T45.1X5	T45.1X6
antifungal	T36.7X1	T36.7X2	T36.7X3	T36.7X4	T36.7X5	T36.7X6
antimycobacterial	T36.5X1	T36.5X2	T36.5X3	T36.5X4	T36.5X5	T36.5X6
antineoplastic	T45.1X1	T45.1X2	T45.1X3	T45.1X4	T45.1X5	T45.1X6
b-lactam NEC	T36.1X1	T36.1X2	T36.1X3	T36.1X4	T36.1X5	T36.1X6

Substance	Poisoning, Accidental (unintentional)	Poisoning, Intentional Self-harm	Poisoning, Assault	Poisoning, Undetermined	Adverse Effect	Under-dosing
Antibiotic — *continued*						
cephalosporin (group)	T36.1X1	T36.1X2	T36.1X3	T36.1X4	T36.1X5	T36.1X6
chloramphenicol (group)	T36.2X1	T36.2X2	T36.2X3	T36.2X4	T36.2X5	T36.2X6
ENT	T49.6X1	T49.6X2	T49.6X3	T49.6X4	T49.6X5	T49.6X6
eye	T49.5X1	T49.5X2	T49.5X3	T49.5X4	T49.5X5	T49.5X6
fungicidal (local)	T49.0X1	T49.0X2	T49.0X3	T49.0X4	T49.0X5	T49.0X6
intestinal	T36.8X1	T36.8X2	T36.8X3	T36.8X4	T36.8X5	T36.8X6
local	T49.0X1	T49.0X2	T49.0X3	T49.0X4	T49.0X5	T49.0X6
macrolides	T36.3X1	T36.3X2	T36.3X3	T36.3X4	T36.3X5	T36.3X6
polypeptide	T36.8X1	T36.8X2	T36.8X3	T36.8X4	T36.8X5	T36.8X6
specified NEC	T36.8X1	T36.8X2	T36.8X3	T36.8X4	T36.8X5	T36.8X6
tetracycline (group)	T36.4X1	T36.4X2	T36.4X3	T36.4X4	T36.4X5	T36.4X6
throat	T49.6X1	T49.6X2	T49.6X3	T49.6X4	T49.6X5	T49.6X6
Anticancer agents NEC	T45.1X1	T45.1X2	T45.1X3	T45.1X4	T45.1X5	T45.1X6
Anticholesterolemic drug NEC	T46.6X1	T46.6X2	T46.6X3	T46.6X4	T46.6X5	T46.6X6
Anticholinergic NEC	T44.3X1	T44.3X2	T44.3X3	T44.3X4	T44.3X5	T44.3X6
Anticholinesterase	T44.0X1	T44.0X2	T44.0X3	T44.0X4	T44.0X5	T44.0X6
organophosphorus	T44.0X1	T44.0X2	T44.0X3	T44.0X4	T44.0X5	T44.0X6
insecticide	T60.0X1	T60.0X2	T60.0X3	T60.0X4	—	—
nerve gas	T59.891	T59.892	T59.893	T59.894	—	—
reversible	T44.0X1	T44.0X2	T44.0X3	T44.0X4	T44.0X5	T44.0X6
ophthalmological	T49.5X1	T49.5X2	T49.5X3	T49.5X4	T49.5X5	T49.5X6
Anticoagulant NEC	T45.511	T45.512	T45.513	T45.514	T45.515	T45.516
Antagonist	T45.7X1	T45.7X2	T45.7X3	T45.7X4	T45.7X5	T45.7X6
Anti-common-cold drug NEC	T48.5X1	T48.5X2	T48.5X3	T48.5X4	T48.5X5	T48.5X6
Anticonvulsant	T42.71	T42.72	T42.73	T42.74	T42.75	T42.76
barbiturate	T42.3X1	T42.3X2	T42.3X3	T42.3X4	T42.3X5	T42.3X6
combination (with barbiturate)	T42.3X1	T42.3X2	T42.3X3	T42.3X4	T42.3X5	T42.3X6
hydantoin	T42.0X1	T42.0X2	T42.0X3	T42.0X4	T42.0X5	T42.0X6
hypnotic NEC	T42.6X1	T42.6X2	T42.6X3	T42.6X4	T42.6X5	T42.6X6
oxazolidinedione	T42.2X1	T42.2X2	T42.2X3	T42.2X4	T42.2X5	T42.2X6
pyrimidinedione	T42.6X1	T42.6X2	T42.6X3	T42.6X4	T42.6X5	T42.6X6
specified NEC	T42.6X1	T42.6X2	T42.6X3	T42.6X4	T42.6X5	T42.6X6
succinimide	T42.2X1	T42.2X2	T42.2X3	T42.2X4	T42.2X5	T42.2X6
Antidepressant	T43.201	T43.202	T43.203	T43.204	T43.205	T43.206
monoamine oxidase inhibitor	T43.1X1	T43.1X2	T43.1X3	T43.1X4	T43.1X5	T43.1X6
selective serotonin norepinephrine reuptake inhibitor	T43.211	T43.212	T43.213	T43.214	T43.215	T43.216
selective serotonin reuptake inhibitor	T43.221	T43.222	T43.223	T43.224	T43.225	T43.226
specified NEC	T43.291	T43.292	T43.293	T43.294	T43.295	T43.296
tetracyclic	T43.021	T43.022	T43.023	T43.024	T43.025	T43.026
triazolopyridine	T43.211	T43.212	T43.213	T43.214	T43.215	T43.216
tricyclic	T43.011	T43.012	T43.013	T43.014	T43.015	T43.016
Antidiabetic NEC	T38.3X1	T38.3X2	T38.3X3	T38.3X4	T38.3X5	T38.3X6
biguanide	T38.3X1	T38.3X2	T38.3X3	T38.3X4	T38.3X5	T38.3X6
and sulfonyl combined	T38.3X1	T38.3X2	T38.3X3	T38.3X4	T38.3X5	T38.3X6
combined	T38.3X1	T38.3X2	T38.3X3	T38.3X4	T38.3X5	T38.3X6
sulfonylurea	T38.3X1	T38.3X2	T38.3X3	T38.3X4	T38.3X5	T38.3X6
Antidiarrheal drug NEC	T47.6X1	T47.6X2	T47.6X3	T47.6X4	T47.6X5	T47.6X6
absorbent	T47.6X1	T47.6X2	T47.6X3	T47.6X4	T47.6X5	T47.6X6
Anti-D immunoglobulin (human)	T50.Z11	T50.Z12	T50.Z13	T50.Z14	T50.Z15	T50.Z16
Antidiphtheria serum	T50.Z11	T50.Z12	T50.Z13	T50.Z14	T50.Z15	T50.Z16
Antidiuretic hormone	T38.891	T38.892	T38.893	T38.894	T38.895	T38.896
Antidote NEC	T50.6X1	T50.6X2	T50.6X3	T50.6X4	T50.6X5	T50.6X6
heavy metal	T45.8X1	T45.8X2	T45.8X3	T45.8X4	T45.8X5	T45.8X6
Antidysrhythmic NEC	T46.2X1	T46.2X2	T46.2X3	T46.2X4	T46.2X5	T46.2X6
Antiemetic drug	T45.0X1	T45.0X2	T45.0X3	T45.0X4	T45.0X5	T45.0X6
Antiepilepsy agent	T42.71	T42.72	T42.73	T42.74	T42.75	T42.76
combination	T42.5X1	T42.5X2	T42.5X3	T42.5X4	T42.5X5	T42.5X6
mixed	T42.5X1	T42.5X2	T42.5X3	T42.5X4	T42.5X5	T42.5X6
specified, NEC	T42.6X1	T42.6X2	T42.6X3	T42.6X4	T42.6X5	T42.6X6
Antiestrogen NEC	T38.6X1	T38.6X2	T38.6X3	T38.6X4	T38.6X5	T38.6X6
Antifertility pill	T38.4X1	T38.4X2	T38.4X3	T38.4X4	T38.4X5	T38.4X6
Antifibrinolytic drug	T45.621	T45.622	T45.623	T45.624	T45.625	T45.626
Antifilarial drug	T37.4X1	T37.4X2	T37.4X3	T37.4X4	T37.4X5	T37.4X6
Antiflatulent	T47.5X1	T47.5X2	T47.5X3	T47.5X4	T47.5X5	T47.5X6
Antifreeze	T65.91	T65.92	T65.93	T65.94	—	—
alcohol	T51.1X1	T51.1X2	T51.1X3	T51.1X4	—	—
ethylene glycol	T51.8X1	T51.8X2	T51.8X3	T51.8X4	—	—
Antifungal						
antibiotic (systemic)	T36.7X1	T36.7X2	T36.7X3	T36.7X4	T36.7X5	T36.7X6
anti-infective NEC	T37.91	T37.92	T37.93	T37.94	T37.95	T37.96
disinfectant, local	T49.0X1	T49.0X2	T49.0X3	T49.0X4	T49.0X5	T49.0X6
nonmedicinal (spray)	T60.3X1	T60.3X2	T60.3X3	T60.3X4	—	—
topical	T49.0X1	T49.0X2	T49.0X3	T49.0X4	T49.0X5	T49.0X6

Anesthesia — Antifungal

358 Additional Character May Be Required — Refer to the Tabular List for Character Selection Subterms under main terms may continue to next column or page

Substance	Poisoning, Accidental (unintentional)	Poisoning, Intentional Self-harm	Poisoning, Assault	Poisoning, Undetermined	Adverse Effect	Under-dosing
Anti-gastric-secretion drug NEC	T47.1X1	T47.1X2	T47.1X3	T47.1X4	T47.1X5	T47.1X6
Antigonadotrophin NEC	T38.6X1	T38.6X2	T38.6X3	T38.6X4	T38.6X5	T38.6X6
Antihallucinogen	T43.501	T43.502	T43.503	T43.504	T43.505	T43.506
Antihelmintics	T37.4X1	T37.4X2	T37.4X3	T37.4X4	T37.4X5	T37.4X6
Antihemophilic						
factor	T45.8X1	T45.8X2	T45.8X3	T45.8X4	T45.8X5	T45.8X6
fraction	T45.8X1	T45.8X2	T45.8X3	T45.8X4	T45.8X5	T45.8X6
globulin concentrate	T45.7X1	T45.7X2	T45.7X3	T45.7X4	T45.7X5	T45.7X6
human plasma	T45.8X1	T45.8X2	T45.8X3	T45.8X4	T45.8X5	T45.8X6
plasma, dried	T45.7X1	T45.7X2	T45.7X3	T45.7X4	T45.7X5	T45.7X6
Antihemorrhoidal preparation	T49.2X1	T49.2X2	T49.2X3	T49.2X4	T49.2X5	T49.2X6
Antiheparin drug	T45.7X1	T45.7X2	T45.7X3	T45.7X4	T45.7X5	T45.7X6
Antihistamine	T45.0X1	T45.0X2	T45.0X3	T45.0X4	T45.0X5	T45.0X6
Antihookworm drug	T37.4X1	T37.4X2	T37.4X3	T37.4X4	T37.4X5	T37.4X6
Anti-human lymphocytic globulin	T50.Z11	T50.Z12	T50.Z13	T50.Z14	T50.Z15	T50.Z16
Antihyperlipidemic drug	T46.6X1	T46.6X2	T46.6X3	T46.6X4	T46.6X5	T46.6X6
Antihypertensive drug NEC	T46.5X1	T46.5X2	T46.5X3	T46.5X4	T46.5X5	T46.5X6
Anti-infective NEC	T37.91	T37.92	T37.93	T37.94	T37.95	T37.96
anthelmintic	T37.4X1	T37.4X2	T37.4X3	T37.4X4	T37.4X5	T37.4X6
antibiotics	T36.91	T36.92	T36.93	T36.94	T36.95	T36.96
specified NEC	T36.8X1	T36.8X2	T36.8X3	T36.8X4	T36.8X5	T36.8X6
antimalarial	T37.2X1	T37.2X2	T37.2X3	T37.2X4	T37.2X5	T37.2X6
antimycobacterial NEC	T37.1X1	T37.1X2	T37.1X3	T37.1X4	T37.1X5	T37.1X6
antibiotics	T36.5X1	T36.5X2	T36.5X3	T36.5X4	T36.5X5	T36.5X6
antiprotozoal NEC	T37.3X1	T37.3X2	T37.3X3	T37.3X4	T37.3X5	T37.3X6
blood	T37.2X1	T37.2X2	T37.2X3	T37.2X4	T37.2X5	T37.2X6
antiviral	T37.5X1	T37.5X2	T37.5X3	T37.5X4	T37.5X5	T37.5X6
arsenical	T37.8X1	T37.8X2	T37.8X3	T37.8X4	T37.8X5	T37.8X6
bismuth, local	T49.0X1	T49.0X2	T49.0X3	T49.0X4	T49.0X5	T49.0X6
ENT	T49.6X1	T49.6X2	T49.6X3	T49.6X4	T49.6X5	T49.6X6
eye NEC	T49.5X1	T49.5X2	T49.5X3	T49.5X4	T49.5X5	T49.5X6
heavy metals NEC	T37.8X1	T37.8X2	T37.8X3	T37.8X4	T37.8X5	T37.8X6
local NEC	T49.0X1	T49.0X2	T49.0X3	T49.0X4	T49.0X5	T49.0X6
specified NEC	T49.0X1	T49.0X2	T49.0X3	T49.0X4	T49.0X5	T49.0X6
mixed	T37.91	T37.92	T37.93	T37.94	T37.95	T37.96
ophthalmic preparation	T49.5X1	T49.5X2	T49.5X3	T49.5X4	T49.5X5	T49.5X6
topical NEC	T49.0X1	T49.0X2	T49.0X3	T49.0X4	T49.0X5	T49.0X6
Anti-inflammatory drug NEC	T39.391	T39.392	T39.393	T39.394	T39.395	T39.396
local	T49.0X1	T49.0X2	T49.0X3	T49.0X4	T49.0X5	T49.0X6
nonsteroidal NEC	T39.391	T39.392	T39.393	T39.394	T39.395	T39.396
propionic acid derivative	T39.311	T39.312	T39.313	T39.314	T39.315	T39.316
specified NEC	T39.391	T39.392	T39.393	T39.394	T39.395	T39.396
Antikaluretic	T50.3X1	T50.3X2	T50.3X3	T50.3X4	T50.3X5	T50.3X6
Antiknock (tetraethyl lead)	T56.0X1	T56.0X2	T56.0X3	T56.0X4	—	—
Antilipemic drug NEC	T46.6X1	T46.6X2	T46.6X3	T46.6X4	T46.6X5	T46.6X6
Antimalarial	T37.2X1	T37.2X2	T37.2X3	T37.2X4	T37.2X5	T37.2X6
prophylactic NEC	T37.2X1	T37.2X2	T37.2X3	T37.2X4	T37.2X5	T37.2X6
pyrimidine derivative	T37.2X1	T37.2X2	T37.2X3	T37.2X4	T37.2X5	T37.2X6
Antimetabolite	T45.1X1	T45.1X2	T45.1X3	T45.1X4	T45.1X5	T45.1X6
Antimitotic agent	T45.1X1	T45.1X2	T45.1X3	T45.1X4	T45.1X5	T45.1X6
Antimony (compounds) (vapor) NEC	T56.891	T56.892	T56.893	T56.894	—	—
anti-infectives	T37.8X1	T37.8X2	T37.8X3	T37.8X4	T37.8X5	T37.8X6
dimercaptosuccinate	T37.3X1	T37.3X2	T37.3X3	T37.3X4	T37.3X5	T37.3X6
hydride	T56.891	T56.892	T56.893	T56.894	—	—
pesticide (vapor)	T60.8X1	T60.8X2	T60.8X3	T60.8X4	—	—
potassium (sodium) tartrate	T37.8X1	T37.8X2	T37.8X3	T37.8X4	T37.8X5	T37.8X6
sodium dimercaptosuccinate	T37.3X1	T37.3X2	T37.3X3	T37.3X4	T37.3X5	T37.3X6
tartrated	T37.8X1	T37.8X2	T37.8X3	T37.8X4	T37.8X5	T37.8X6
Antimuscarinic NEC	T44.3X1	T44.3X2	T44.3X3	T44.3X4	T44.3X5	T44.3X6
Antimycobacterial drug NEC	T37.1X1	T37.1X2	T37.1X3	T37.1X4	T37.1X5	T37.1X6
antibiotics	T36.5X1	T36.5X2	T36.5X3	T36.5X4	T36.5X5	T36.5X6
combination	T37.1X1	T37.1X2	T37.1X3	T37.1X4	T37.1X5	T37.1X6
Antinausea drug	T45.0X1	T45.0X2	T45.0X3	T45.0X4	T45.0X5	T45.0X6
Antinematode drug	T37.4X1	T37.4X2	T37.4X3	T37.4X4	T37.4X5	T37.4X6
Antineoplastic NEC	T45.1X1	T45.1X2	T45.1X3	T45.1X4	T45.1X5	T45.1X6
alkaloidal	T45.1X1	T45.1X2	T45.1X3	T45.1X4	T45.1X5	T45.1X6
antibiotics	T45.1X1	T45.1X2	T45.1X3	T45.1X4	T45.1X5	T45.1X6
combination	T45.1X1	T45.1X2	T45.1X3	T45.1X4	T45.1X5	T45.1X6
estrogen	T38.5X1	T38.5X2	T38.5X3	T38.5X4	T38.5X5	T38.5X6
steroid	T38.7X1	T38.7X2	T38.7X3	T38.7X4	T38.7X5	T38.7X6
Antiparasitic drug (systemic)	T37.91	T37.92	T37.93	T37.94	T37.95	T37.96
local	T49.0X1	T49.0X2	T49.0X3	T49.0X4	T49.0X5	T49.0X6
specified NEC	T37.8X1	T37.8X2	T37.8X3	T37.8X4	T37.8X5	T37.8X6
Antiparkinsonism drug NEC	T42.8X1	T42.8X2	T42.8X3	T42.8X4	T42.8X5	T42.8X6
Antiperspirant NEC	T49.2X1	T49.2X2	T49.2X3	T49.2X4	T49.2X5	T49.2X6
Antiphlogistic NEC	T39.4X1	T39.4X2	T39.4X3	T39.4X4	T39.4X5	T39.4X6
Antiplatyhelmintic drug	T37.4X1	T37.4X2	T37.4X3	T37.4X4	T37.4X5	T37.4X6
Antiprotozoal drug NEC	T37.3X1	T37.3X2	T37.3X3	T37.3X4	T37.3X5	T37.3X6
blood	T37.2X1	T37.2X2	T37.2X3	T37.2X4	T37.2X5	T37.2X6
local	T49.0X1	T49.0X2	T49.0X3	T49.0X4	T49.0X5	T49.0X6
Antipruritic drug NEC	T49.1X1	T49.1X2	T49.1X3	T49.1X4	T49.1X5	T49.1X6
Antipsychotic drug	T43.501	T43.502	T43.503	T43.504	T43.505	T43.506
specified NEC	T43.591	T43.592	T43.593	T43.594	T43.595	T43.596
Antipyretic	T39.91	T39.92	T39.93	T39.94	T39.95	T39.96
specified NEC	T39.8X1	T39.8X2	T39.8X3	T39.8X4	T39.8X5	T39.8X6
Antipyrine	T39.2X1	T39.2X2	T39.2X3	T39.2X4	T39.2X5	T39.2X6
Antirabies hyperimmune serum	T50.Z11	T50.Z12	T50.Z13	T50.Z14	T50.Z15	T50.Z16
Antirheumatic NEC	T39.4X1	T39.4X2	T39.4X3	T39.4X4	T39.4X5	T39.4X6
Antirigidity drug NEC	T42.8X1	T42.8X2	T42.8X3	T42.8X4	T42.8X5	T42.8X6
Antischistosomal drug	T37.4X1	T37.4X2	T37.4X3	T37.4X4	T37.4X5	T37.4X6
Antiscorpion sera	T50.Z11	T50.Z12	T50.Z13	T50.Z14	T50.Z15	T50.Z16
Antiseborrheics	T49.4X1	T49.4X2	T49.4X3	T49.4X4	T49.4X5	T49.4X6
Antiseptics (external) (medicinal)	T49.0X1	T49.0X2	T49.0X3	T49.0X4	T49.0X5	T49.0X6
Antistine	T45.0X1	T45.0X2	T45.0X3	T45.0X4	T45.0X5	T45.0X6
Antitapeworm drug	T37.4X1	T37.4X2	T37.4X3	T37.4X4	T37.4X5	T37.4X6
Antitetanus immunoglobulin	T50.Z11	T50.Z12	T50.Z13	T50.Z14	T50.Z15	T50.Z16
Antithrombotic	T45.521	T45.522	T45.523	T45.524	T45.525	T45.526
Antithyroid drug NEC	T38.2X1	T38.2X2	T38.2X3	T38.2X4	T38.2X5	T38.2X6
Antitoxin	T50.Z11	T50.Z12	T50.Z13	T50.Z14	T50.Z15	T50.Z16
diphtheria	T50.Z11	T50.Z12	T50.Z13	T50.Z14	T50.Z15	T50.Z16
gas gangrene	T50.Z11	T50.Z12	T50.Z13	T50.Z14	T50.Z15	T50.Z16
tetanus	T50.Z11	T50.Z12	T50.Z13	T50.Z14	T50.Z15	T50.Z16
Antitrichomonal drug	T37.3X1	T37.3X2	T37.3X3	T37.3X4	T37.3X5	T37.3X6
Antituberculars	T37.1X1	T37.1X2	T37.1X3	T37.1X4	T37.1X5	T37.1X6
antibiotics	T36.5X1	T36.5X2	T36.5X3	T36.5X4	T36.5X5	T36.5X6
Antitussive NEC	T48.3X1	T48.3X2	T48.3X3	T48.3X4	T48.3X5	T48.3X6
codeine mixture	T40.2X1	T40.2X2	T40.2X3	T40.2X4	T40.2X5	T40.2X6
opiate	T40.2X1	T40.2X2	T40.2X3	T40.2X4	T40.2X5	T40.2X6
Antivaricose drug	T46.8X1	T46.8X2	T46.8X3	T46.8X4	T46.8X5	T46.8X6
Antivenin, antivenom (sera)						
crotaline	T50.Z11	T50.Z12	T50.Z13	T50.Z14	T50.Z15	T50.Z16
spider bite	T50.Z11	T50.Z12	T50.Z13	T50.Z14	T50.Z15	T50.Z16
Antivertigo drug	T45.0X1	T45.0X2	T45.0X3	T45.0X4	T45.0X5	T45.0X6
Antiviral drug NEC	T37.5X1	T37.5X2	T37.5X3	T37.5X4	T37.5X5	T37.5X6
eye	T49.5X1	T49.5X2	T49.5X3	T49.5X4	T49.5X5	T49.5X6
Antiwhipworm drug	T37.4X1	T37.4X2	T37.4X3	T37.4X4	T37.4X5	T37.4X6
Ant poison — see Insecticide						
Antrol — see also by specific chemical substance	T60.91	T60.92	T60.93	T60.94	—	—
fungicide	T60.91	T60.92	T60.93	T60.94	—	—
ANTU (alpha naphthylthiourea)	T60.4X1	T60.4X2	T60.4X3	T60.4X4	—	—
Apalcillin	T36.0X1	T36.0X2	T36.0X3	T36.0X4	T36.0X5	T36.0X6
APC	T48.5X1	T48.5X2	T48.5X3	T48.5X4	T48.5X5	T48.5X6
Aplonidine	T44.4X1	T44.4X2	T44.4X3	T44.4X4	T44.4X5	T44.4X6
Apomorphine	T47.7X1	T47.7X2	T47.7X3	T47.7X4	T47.7X5	T47.7X6
Appetite depressants, central	T50.5X1	T50.5X2	T50.5X3	T50.5X4	T50.5X5	T50.5X6
Apraclonidine (hydrochloride)	T44.4X1	T44.4X2	T44.4X3	T44.4X4	T44.4X5	T44.4X6
Apresoline	T46.5X1	T46.5X2	T46.5X3	T46.5X4	T46.5X5	T46.5X6
Aprindine	T46.2X1	T46.2X2	T46.2X3	T46.2X4	T46.2X5	T46.2X6
Aprobarbital	T42.3X1	T42.3X2	T42.3X3	T42.3X4	T42.3X5	T42.3X6
Apronalide	T42.6X1	T42.6X2	T42.6X3	T42.6X4	T42.6X5	T42.6X6
Aprotinin	T45.621	T45.622	T45.623	T45.624	T45.625	T45.626
Aptocaine	T41.3X1	T41.3X2	T41.3X3	T41.3X4	T41.3X5	T41.3X6
Aqua fortis	T54.2X1	T54.2X2	T54.2X3	T54.2X4	—	—
Ara-A	T37.5X1	T37.5X2	T37.5X3	T37.5X4	T37.5X5	T37.5X6
Ara-C	T45.1X1	T45.1X2	T45.1X3	T45.1X4	T45.1X5	T45.1X6
Arachis oil	T49.3X1	T49.3X2	T49.3X3	T49.3X4	T49.3X5	T49.3X6
cathartic	T47.4X1	T47.4X2	T47.4X3	T47.4X4	T47.4X5	T47.4X6
Aralen	T37.2X1	T37.2X2	T37.2X3	T37.2X4	T37.2X5	T37.2X6
Arecoline	T44.1X1	T44.1X2	T44.1X3	T44.1X4	T44.1X5	T44.1X6
Arginine	T50.991	T50.992	T50.993	T50.994	T50.995	T50.996
glutamate	T50.991	T50.992	T50.993	T50.994	T50.995	T50.996
Argyrol	T49.0X1	T49.0X2	T49.0X3	T49.0X4	T49.0X5	T49.0X6
ENT agent	T49.6X1	T49.6X2	T49.6X3	T49.6X4	T49.6X5	T49.6X6
ophthalmic preparation	T49.5X1	T49.5X2	T49.5X3	T49.5X4	T49.5X5	T49.5X6
Aristocort	T38.0X1	T38.0X2	T38.0X3	T38.0X4	T38.0X5	T38.0X6
ENT agent	T49.6X1	T49.6X2	T49.6X3	T49.6X4	T49.6X5	T49.6X6
ophthalmic preparation	T49.5X1	T49.5X2	T49.5X3	T49.5X4	T49.5X5	T49.5X6

Aristocort ICD-10-CM 2022

Table of Drugs and Chemicals

Substance	Poisoning, Accidental (unintentional)	Poisoning, Intentional Self-harm	Poisoning, Assault	Poisoning, Undetermined	Adverse Effect	Under-dosing
Aristocort — *continued*						
topical NEC	T49.ØX1	T49.ØX2	T49.ØX3	T49.ØX4	T49.ØX5	T49.ØX6
Aromatics, corrosive	T54.1X1	T54.1X2	T54.1X3	T54.1X4	—	—
disinfectants	T54.1X1	T54.1X2	T54.1X3	T54.1X4	—	—
Arsenate of lead	T57.ØX1	T57.ØX2	T57.ØX3	T57.ØX4	—	—
herbicide	T57.ØX1	T57.ØX2	T57.ØX3	T57.ØX4	—	—
Arsenic, arsenicals (compounds) (dust) (vapor) **NEC**	T57.ØX1	T57.ØX2	T57.ØX3	T57.ØX4	—	—
anti-infectives	T37.8X1	T37.8X2	T37.8X3	T37.8X4	T37.8X5	T37.8X6
pesticide (dust) (fumes)	T57.ØX1	T57.ØX2	T57.ØX3	T57.ØX4	—	—
Arsine (gas)	T57.ØX1	T57.ØX2	T57.ØX3	T57.ØX4	—	—
Arsphenamine (silver)	T37.8X1	T37.8X2	T37.8X3	T37.8X4	T37.8X5	T37.8X6
Arsthinol	T37.3X1	T37.3X2	T37.3X3	T37.3X4	T37.3X5	T37.3X6
Artane	T44.3X1	T44.3X2	T44.3X3	T44.3X4	T44.3X5	T44.3X6
Arthropod (venomous) **NEC**	T63.481	T63.482	T63.483	T63.484	—	—
Articaine	T41.3X1	T41.3X2	T41.3X3	T41.3X4	T41.3X5	T41.3X6
Asbestos	T57.8X1	T57.8X2	T57.8X3	T57.8X4	—	—
Ascaridole	T37.4X1	T37.4X2	T37.4X3	T37.4X4	T37.4X5	T37.4X6
Ascorbic acid	T45.2X1	T45.2X2	T45.2X3	T45.2X4	T45.2X5	T45.2X6
Asiaticoside	T49.ØX1	T49.ØX2	T49.ØX3	T49.ØX4	T49.ØX5	T49.ØX6
Asparaginase	T45.1X1	T45.1X2	T45.1X3	T45.1X4	T45.1X5	T45.1X6
Aspidium (oleoresin)	T37.4X1	T37.4X2	T37.4X3	T37.4X4	T37.4X5	T37.4X6
Aspirin (aluminum) (soluble)	T39.Ø11	T39.Ø12	T39.Ø13	T39.Ø14	T39.Ø15	T39.Ø16
Aspoxicillin	T36.ØX1	T36.ØX2	T36.ØX3	T36.ØX4	T36.ØX5	T36.ØX6
Astemizole	T45.ØX1	T45.ØX2	T45.ØX3	T45.ØX4	T45.ØX5	T45.ØX6
Astringent (local)	T49.2X1	T49.2X2	T49.2X3	T49.2X4	T49.2X5	T49.2X6
specified NEC	T49.2X1	T49.2X2	T49.2X3	T49.2X4	T49.2X5	T49.2X6
Astromicin	T36.5X1	T36.5X2	T36.5X3	T36.5X4	T36.5X5	T36.5X6
Ataractic drug NEC	T43.5Ø1	T43.5Ø2	T43.5Ø3	T43.5Ø4	T43.5Ø5	T43.5Ø6
Atenolol	T44.7X1	T44.7X2	T44.7X3	T44.7X4	T44.7X5	T44.7X6
Atonia drug, intestinal	T47.4X1	T47.4X2	T47.4X3	T47.4X4	T47.4X5	T47.4X6
Atophan	T5Ø.4X1	T5Ø.4X2	T5Ø.4X3	T5Ø.4X4	T5Ø.4X5	T5Ø.4X6
Atracurium besilate	T48.1X1	T48.1X2	T48.1X3	T48.1X4	T48.1X5	T48.1X6
Atropine	T44.3X1	T44.3X2	T44.3X3	T44.3X4	T44.3X5	T44.3X6
derivative	T44.3X1	T44.3X2	T44.3X3	T44.3X4	T44.3X5	T44.3X6
methonitrate	T44.3X1	T44.3X2	T44.3X3	T44.3X4	T44.3X5	T44.3X6
Attapulgite	T47.6X1	T47.6X2	T47.6X3	T47.6X4	T47.6X5	T47.6X6
Auramine	T65.891	T65.892	T65.893	T65.894	—	—
dye	T65.6X1	T65.6X2	T65.6X3	T65.6X4	—	—
fungicide	T6Ø.3X1	T6Ø.3X2	T6Ø.3X3	T6Ø.3X4	—	—
Auranofin	T39.4X1	T39.4X2	T39.4X3	T39.4X4	T39.4X5	T39.4X6
Aurantiin	T46.991	T46.992	T46.993	T46.994	T46.995	T46.996
Aureomycin	T36.4X1	T36.4X2	T36.4X3	T36.4X4	T36.4X5	T36.4X6
ophthalmic preparation	T49.5X1	T49.5X2	T49.5X3	T49.5X4	T49.5X5	T49.5X6
topical NEC	T49.ØX1	T49.ØX2	T49.ØX3	T49.ØX4	T49.ØX5	T49.ØX6
Aurothioglucose	T39.4X1	T39.4X2	T39.4X3	T39.4X4	T39.4X5	T39.4X6
Aurothioglycanide	T39.4X1	T39.4X2	T39.4X3	T39.4X4	T39.4X5	T39.4X6
Aurothiomalate sodium	T39.4X1	T39.4X2	T39.4X3	T39.4X4	T39.4X5	T39.4X6
Aurotioprol	T39.4X1	T39.4X2	T39.4X3	T39.4X4	T39.4X5	T39.4X6
Automobile fuel	T52.ØX1	T52.ØX2	T52.ØX3	T52.ØX4	—	—
Autonomic nervous system agent NEC	T44.9Ø1	T44.9Ø2	T44.9Ø3	T44.9Ø4	T44.9Ø5	T44.9Ø6
Avlosulfon	T37.1X1	T37.1X2	T37.1X3	T37.1X4	T37.1X5	T37.1X6
Avomine	T42.6X1	T42.6X2	T42.6X3	T42.6X4	T42.6X5	T42.6X6
Axerophthol	T45.2X1	T45.2X2	T45.2X3	T45.2X4	T45.2X5	T45.2X6
Azacitidine	T45.1X1	T45.1X2	T45.1X3	T45.1X4	T45.1X5	T45.1X6
Azacyclonol	T43.591	T43.592	T43.593	T43.594	T43.595	T43.596
Azadirachta	T6Ø.2X1	T6Ø.2X2	T6Ø.2X3	T6Ø.2X4	—	—
Azanidazole	T37.3X1	T37.3X2	T37.3X3	T37.3X4	T37.3X5	T37.3X6
Azapetine	T46.7X1	T46.7X2	T46.7X3	T46.7X4	T46.7X5	T46.7X6
Azapropazone	T39.2X1	T39.2X2	T39.2X3	T39.2X4	T39.2X5	T39.2X6
Azaribine	T45.1X1	T45.1X2	T45.1X3	T45.1X4	T45.1X5	T45.1X6
Azaserine	T45.1X1	T45.1X2	T45.1X3	T45.1X4	T45.1X5	T45.1X6
Azatadine	T45.ØX1	T45.ØX2	T45.ØX3	T45.ØX4	T45.ØX5	T45.ØX6
Azatepa	T45.1X1	T45.1X2	T45.1X3	T45.1X4	T45.1X5	T45.1X6
Azathioprine	T45.1X1	T45.1X2	T45.1X3	T45.1X4	T45.1X5	T45.1X6
Azelaic acid	T49.ØX1	T49.ØX2	T49.ØX3	T49.ØX4	T49.ØX5	T49.ØX6
Azelastine	T45.ØX1	T45.ØX2	T45.ØX3	T45.ØX4	T45.ØX5	T45.ØX6
Azidocillin	T36.ØX1	T36.ØX2	T36.ØX3	T36.ØX4	T36.ØX5	T36.ØX6
Azidothymidine	T37.5X1	T37.5X2	T37.5X3	T37.5X4	T37.5X5	T37.5X6
Azinphos (ethyl) (methyl)	T6Ø.ØX1	T6Ø.ØX2	T6Ø.ØX3	T6Ø.ØX4	—	—
Aziridine (chelating)	T54.1X1	T54.1X2	T54.1X3	T54.1X4	—	—
Azithromycin	T36.3X1	T36.3X2	T36.3X3	T36.3X4	T36.3X5	T36.3X6
Azlocillin	T36.ØX1	T36.ØX2	T36.ØX3	T36.ØX4	T36.ØX5	T36.ØX6
Azobenzene smoke	T65.3X1	T65.3X2	T65.3X3	T65.3X4	—	—
acaricide	T6Ø.8X1	T6Ø.8X2	T6Ø.8X3	T6Ø.8X4	—	—
Azosulfamide	T37.ØX1	T37.ØX2	T37.ØX3	T37.ØX4	T37.ØX5	T37.ØX6
AZT	T37.5X1	T37.5X2	T37.5X3	T37.5X4	T37.5X5	T37.5X6
Aztreonam	T36.1X1	T36.1X2	T36.1X3	T36.1X4	T36.1X5	T36.1X6
Azulfidine	T37.ØX1	T37.ØX2	T37.ØX3	T37.ØX4	T37.ØX5	T37.ØX6
Azuresin	T5Ø.8X1	T5Ø.8X2	T5Ø.8X3	T5Ø.8X4	T5Ø.8X5	T5Ø.8X6
b-acetyldigoxin	T46.ØX1	T46.ØX2	T46.ØX3	T46.ØX4	T46.ØX5	T46.ØX6

Substance	Poisoning, Accidental (unintentional)	Poisoning, Intentional Self-harm	Poisoning, Assault	Poisoning, Undetermined	Adverse Effect	Under-dosing
P-Acetamidophenol	T39.1X1	T39.1X2	T39.1X3	T39.1X4	T39.1X5	T39.1X6
Bacampicillin	T36.ØX1	T36.ØX2	T36.ØX3	T36.ØX4	T36.ØX5	T36.ØX6
Bacillus						
lactobacillus	T47.8X1	T47.8X2	T47.8X3	T47.8X4	T47.8X5	T47.8X6
subtilis	T47.6X1	T47.6X2	T47.6X3	T47.6X4	T47.6X5	T47.6X6
Bacimycin	T49.ØX1	T49.ØX2	T49.ØX3	T49.ØX4	T49.ØX5	T49.ØX6
ophthalmic preparation	T49.5X1	T49.5X2	T49.5X3	T49.5X4	T49.5X5	T49.5X6
Bacitracin zinc	T49.ØX1	T49.ØX2	T49.ØX3	T49.ØX4	T49.ØX5	T49.ØX6
with neomycin	T49.ØX1	T49.ØX2	T49.ØX3	T49.ØX4	T49.ØX5	T49.ØX6
ENT agent	T49.6X1	T49.6X2	T49.6X3	T49.6X4	T49.6X5	T49.6X6
ophthalmic preparation	T49.5X1	T49.5X2	T49.5X3	T49.5X4	T49.5X5	T49.5X6
topical NEC	T49.ØX1	T49.ØX2	T49.ØX3	T49.ØX4	T49.ØX5	T49.ØX6
Baclofen	T42.8X1	T42.8X2	T42.8X3	T42.8X4	T42.8X5	T42.8X6
Baking soda	T5Ø.991	T5Ø.992	T5Ø.993	T5Ø.994	T5Ø.995	T5Ø.996
BAL	T45.8X1	T45.8X2	T45.8X3	T45.8X4	T45.8X5	T45.8X6
Bambuterol	T48.6X1	T48.6X2	T48.6X3	T48.6X4	T48.6X5	T48.6X6
Bamethan (sulfate)	T46.7X1	T46.7X2	T46.7X3	T46.7X4	T46.7X5	T46.7X6
Bamifylline	T48.6X1	T48.6X2	T48.6X3	T48.6X4	T48.6X5	T48.6X6
Bamipine	T45.ØX1	T45.ØX2	T45.ØX3	T45.ØX4	T45.ØX5	T45.ØX6
Baneberry — *see* Actaea spicata						
Banewort — *see* Belladonna						
Barbenyl	T42.3X1	T42.3X2	T42.3X3	T42.3X4	T42.3X5	T42.3X6
Barbexaclone	T42.6X1	T42.6X2	T42.6X3	T42.6X4	T42.6X5	T42.6X6
Barbital	T42.3X1	T42.3X2	T42.3X3	T42.3X4	T42.3X5	T42.3X6
sodium	T42.3X1	T42.3X2	T42.3X3	T42.3X4	T42.3X5	T42.3X6
Barbitone	T42.3X1	T42.3X2	T42.3X3	T42.3X4	T42.3X5	T42.3X6
Barbiturate NEC	T42.3X1	T42.3X2	T42.3X3	T42.3X4	T42.3X5	T42.3X6
with tranquilizer	T42.3X1	T42.3X2	T42.3X3	T42.3X4	T42.3X5	T42.3X6
anesthetic (intravenous)	T41.1X1	T41.1X2	T41.1X3	T41.1X4	T41.1X5	T41.1X6
Barium (carbonate) (chloride) (sulfite)	T57.8X1	T57.8X2	T57.8X3	T57.8X4	—	—
diagnostic agent	T5Ø.8X1	T5Ø.8X2	T5Ø.8X3	T5Ø.8X4	T5Ø.8X5	T5Ø.8X6
pesticide	T6Ø.4X1	T6Ø.4X2	T6Ø.4X3	T6Ø.4X4	—	—
rodenticide	T6Ø.4X1	T6Ø.4X2	T6Ø.4X3	T6Ø.4X4	—	—
sulfate (medicinal)	T5Ø.8X1	T5Ø.8X2	T5Ø.8X3	T5Ø.8X4	T5Ø.8X5	T5Ø.8X6
Barrier cream	T49.3X1	T49.3X2	T49.3X3	T49.3X4	T49.3X5	T49.3X6
Basic fuchsin	T49.ØX1	T49.ØX2	T49.ØX3	T49.ØX4	T49.ØX5	T49.ØX6
Battery acid or fluid	T54.2X1	T54.2X2	T54.2X3	T54.2X4	—	—
Bay rum	T51.8X1	T51.8X2	T51.8X3	T51.8X4	—	—
b-benzalbutyramide	T46.6X1	T46.6X2	T46.6X3	T46.6X4	T46.6X5	T46.6X6
BCG (vaccine)	T5Ø.A91	T5Ø.A92	T5Ø.A93	T5Ø.A94	T5Ø.A95	T5Ø.A96
BCNU	T45.1X1	T45.1X2	T45.1X3	T45.1X4	T45.1X5	T45.1X6
Bearsfoot	T62.2X1	T62.2X2	T62.2X3	T62.2X4	—	—
Beclamide	T42.6X1	T42.6X2	T42.6X3	T42.6X4	T42.6X5	T42.6X6
Beclomethasone	T44.5X1	T44.5X2	T44.5X3	T44.5X4	T44.5X5	T44.5X6
Bee (sting) (venom)	T63.441	T63.442	T63.443	T63.444	—	—
Befunolol	T49.5X1	T49.5X2	T49.5X3	T49.5X4	T49.5X5	T49.5X6
Bekanamycin	T36.5X1	T36.5X2	T36.5X3	T36.5X4	T36.5X5	T36.5X6
Belladonna — *see also* Nightshade						
alkaloids	T44.3X1	T44.3X2	T44.3X3	T44.3X4	T44.3X5	T44.3X6
extract	T44.3X1	T44.3X2	T44.3X3	T44.3X4	T44.3X5	T44.3X6
herb	T44.3X1	T44.3X2	T44.3X3	T44.3X4	T44.3X5	T44.3X6
Bemegride	T5Ø.7X1	T5Ø.7X2	T5Ø.7X3	T5Ø.7X4	T5Ø.7X5	T5Ø.7X6
Benactyzine	T44.3X1	T44.3X2	T44.3X3	T44.3X4	T44.3X5	T44.3X6
Benadryl	T45.ØX1	T45.ØX2	T45.ØX3	T45.ØX4	T45.ØX5	T45.ØX6
Benaprizine	T44.3X1	T44.3X2	T44.3X3	T44.3X4	T44.3X5	T44.3X6
Benazepril	T46.4X1	T46.4X2	T46.4X3	T46.4X4	T46.4X5	T46.4X6
Bencyclane	T46.7X1	T46.7X2	T46.7X3	T46.7X4	T46.7X5	T46.7X6
Bendazol	T46.3X1	T46.3X2	T46.3X3	T46.3X4	T46.3X5	T46.3X6
Bendrofluazide	T5Ø.2X1	T5Ø.2X2	T5Ø.2X3	T5Ø.2X4	T5Ø.2X5	T5Ø.2X6
Bendroflumethiazide	T5Ø.2X1	T5Ø.2X2	T5Ø.2X3	T5Ø.2X4	T5Ø.2X5	T5Ø.2X6
Benemid	T5Ø.4X1	T5Ø.4X2	T5Ø.4X3	T5Ø.4X4	T5Ø.4X5	T5Ø.4X6
Benethamine penicillin	T36.ØX1	T36.ØX2	T36.ØX3	T36.ØX4	T36.ØX5	T36.ØX6
Benexate	T47.1X1	T47.1X2	T47.1X3	T47.1X4	T47.1X5	T47.1X6
Benfluorex	T46.6X1	T46.6X2	T46.6X3	T46.6X4	T46.6X5	T46.6X6
Benfotiamine	T45.2X1	T45.2X2	T45.2X3	T45.2X4	T45.2X5	T45.2X6
Benisone	T49.ØX1	T49.ØX2	T49.ØX3	T49.ØX4	T49.ØX5	T49.ØX6
Benomyl	T6Ø.ØX1	T6Ø.ØX2	T6Ø.ØX3	T6Ø.ØX4	—	—
Benoquin	T49.8X1	T49.8X2	T49.8X3	T49.8X4	T49.8X5	T49.8X6
Benoxinate	T41.3X1	T41.3X2	T41.3X3	T41.3X4	T41.3X5	T41.3X6
Benperidol	T43.4X1	T43.4X2	T43.4X3	T43.4X4	T43.4X5	T43.4X6
Benproperine	T48.3X1	T48.3X2	T48.3X3	T48.3X4	T48.3X5	T48.3X6
Benserazide	T42.8X1	T42.8X2	T42.8X3	T42.8X4	T42.8X5	T42.8X6
Bentazepam	T42.4X1	T42.4X2	T42.4X3	T42.4X4	T42.4X5	T42.4X6
Bentiromide	T5Ø.8X1	T5Ø.8X2	T5Ø.8X3	T5Ø.8X4	T5Ø.8X5	T5Ø.8X6
Bentonite	T49.3X1	T49.3X2	T49.3X3	T49.3X4	T49.3X5	T49.3X6
Benzalbutyramide	T46.6X1	T46.6X2	T46.6X3	T46.6X4	T46.6X5	T46.6X6
Benzalkonium (chloride)	T49.ØX1	T49.ØX2	T49.ØX3	T49.ØX4	T49.ØX5	T49.ØX6
ophthalmic preparation	T49.5X1	T49.5X2	T49.5X3	T49.5X4	T49.5X5	T49.5X6
Benzamidosalicylate (calcium)	T37.1X1	T37.1X2	T37.1X3	T37.1X4	T37.1X5	T37.1X6
Benzamine	T41.3X1	T41.3X2	T41.3X3	T41.3X4	T41.3X5	T41.3X6

Substance	Poisoning, Accidental (unintentional)	Poisoning, Intentional Self-harm	Poisoning, Assault	Poisoning, Undetermined	Adverse Effect	Under-dosing
Benzamine — continued						
lactate	T49.1X1	T49.1X2	T49.1X3	T49.1X4	T49.1X5	T49.1X6
Benzamphetamine	T50.5X1	T50.5X2	T50.5X3	T50.5X4	T50.5X5	T50.5X6
Benzapril hydrochloride	T46.5X1	T46.5X2	T46.5X3	T46.5X4	T46.5X5	T46.5X6
Benzathine	T36.0X1	T36.0X2	T36.0X3	T36.0X4	T36.0X5	T36.0X6
benzylpenicillin						
Benzathine penicillin	T36.0X1	T36.0X2	T36.0X3	T36.0X4	T36.0X5	T36.0X6
Benzatropine	T42.8X1	T42.8X2	T42.8X3	T42.8X4	T42.8X5	T42.8X6
Benzbromarone	T50.4X1	T50.4X2	T50.4X3	T50.4X4	T50.4X5	T50.4X6
Benzcarbimine	T45.1X1	T45.1X2	T45.1X3	T45.1X4	T45.1X5	T45.1X6
Benzedrex	T44.991	T44.992	T44.993	T44.994	T44.995	T44.996
Benzedrine (amphetamine)	T43.621	T43.622	T43.623	T43.624	T43.625	T43.626
Benzenamine	T65.3X1	T65.3X2	T65.3X3	T65.3X4	—	—
Benzene	T52.1X1	T52.1X2	T52.1X3	T52.1X4	—	—
homologues (acetyl) (dimethyl) (methyl) (solvent)	T52.2X1	T52.2X2	T52.2X3	T52.2X4	—	—
Benzethonium (chloride)	T49.0X1	T49.0X2	T49.0X3	T49.0X4	T49.0X5	T49.0X6
Benzfetamine	T50.5X1	T50.5X2	T50.5X3	T50.5X4	T50.5X5	T50.5X6
Benzhexol	T44.3X1	T44.3X2	T44.3X3	T44.3X4	T44.3X5	T44.3X6
Benzhydramine (chloride)	T45.0X1	T45.0X2	T45.0X3	T45.0X4	T45.0X5	T45.0X6
Benzidine	T65.891	T65.892	T65.893	T65.894	—	—
Benzilonium bromide	T44.3X1	T44.3X2	T44.3X3	T44.3X4	T44.3X5	T44.3X6
Benzimidazole	T60.3X1	T60.3X2	T60.3X3	T60.3X4	—	—
Benzin (e) — see Ligroin						
Benziodarone	T46.3X1	T46.3X2	T46.3X3	T46.3X4	T46.3X5	T46.3X6
Benznidazole	T37.3X1	T37.3X2	T37.3X3	T37.3X4	T37.3X5	T37.3X6
Benzocaine	T41.3X1	T41.3X2	T41.3X3	T41.3X4	T41.3X5	T41.3X6
Benzodiapin	T42.4X1	T42.4X2	T42.4X3	T42.4X4	T42.4X5	T42.4X6
Benzodiazepine NEC	T42.4X1	T42.4X2	T42.4X3	T42.4X4	T42.4X5	T42.4X6
Benzoic acid	T49.0X1	T49.0X2	T49.0X3	T49.0X4	T49.0X5	T49.0X6
with salicylic acid	T49.0X1	T49.0X2	T49.0X3	T49.0X4	T49.0X5	T49.0X6
Benzoin (tincture)	T48.5X1	T48.5X2	T48.5X3	T48.5X4	T48.5X5	T48.5X6
Benzol (benzene)	T52.1X1	T52.1X2	T52.1X3	T52.1X4	—	—
vapor	T52.0X1	T52.0X2	T52.0X3	T52.0X4	—	—
Benzomorphan	T40.2X1	T40.2X2	T40.2X3	T40.2X4	T40.2X5	T40.2X6
Benzonatate	T48.3X1	T48.3X2	T48.3X3	T48.3X4	T48.3X5	T48.3X6
Benzophenones	T49.3X1	T49.3X2	T49.3X3	T49.3X4	T49.3X5	T49.3X6
Benzopyrone	T46.991	T46.992	T46.993	T46.994	T46.995	T46.996
Benzothiadiazides	T50.2X1	T50.2X2	T50.2X3	T50.2X4	T50.2X5	T50.2X6
Benzoxonium chloride	T49.0X1	T49.0X2	T49.0X3	T49.0X4	T49.0X5	T49.0X6
Benzoylpas calcium	T37.1X1	T37.1X2	T37.1X3	T37.1X4	T37.1X5	T37.1X6
Benzoyl peroxide	T49.0X1	T49.0X2	T49.0X3	T49.0X4	T49.0X5	T49.0X6
Benzperidin	T43.591	T43.592	T43.593	T43.594	T43.595	T43.596
Benzperidol	T43.591	T43.592	T43.593	T43.594	T43.595	T43.596
Benzphetamine	T50.5X1	T50.5X2	T50.5X3	T50.5X4	T50.5X5	T50.5X6
Benzpyrinium bromide	T44.1X1	T44.1X2	T44.1X3	T44.1X4	T44.1X5	T44.1X6
Benzquinamide	T45.0X1	T45.0X2	T45.0X3	T45.0X4	T45.0X5	T45.0X6
Benzthiazide	T50.2X1	T50.2X2	T50.2X3	T50.2X4	T50.2X5	T50.2X6
Benztropine						
anticholinergic	T44.3X1	T44.3X2	T44.3X3	T44.3X4	T44.3X5	T44.3X6
antiparkinson	T42.8X1	T42.8X2	T42.8X3	T42.8X4	T42.8X5	T42.8X6
Benzydamine	T49.0X1	T49.0X2	T49.0X3	T49.0X4	T49.0X5	T49.0X6
Benzyl						
acetate	T52.8X1	T52.8X2	T52.8X3	T52.8X4	—	—
alcohol	T49.0X1	T49.0X2	T49.0X3	T49.0X4	T49.0X5	T49.0X6
benzoate	T49.0X1	T49.0X2	T49.0X3	T49.0X4	T49.0X5	T49.0X6
Benzoic acid	T49.0X1	T49.0X2	T49.0X3	T49.0X4	T49.0X5	T49.0X6
morphine	T40.2X1	T40.2X2	T40.2X3	T40.2X4	—	—
nicotinate	T46.6X1	T46.6X2	T46.6X3	T46.6X4	T46.6X5	T46.6X6
penicillin	T36.0X1	T36.0X2	T36.0X3	T36.0X4	T36.0X5	T36.0X6
Benzylhydrochlorthiazide	T50.2X1	T50.2X2	T50.2X3	T50.2X4	T50.2X5	T50.2X6
Benzylpenicillin	T36.0X1	T36.0X2	T36.0X3	T36.0X4	T36.0X5	T36.0X6
Benzylthiouracil	T38.2X1	T38.2X2	T38.2X3	T38.2X4	T38.2X5	T38.2X6
Bephenium	T37.4X1	T37.4X2	T37.4X3	T37.4X4	T37.4X5	T37.4X6
hydroxynaphthoate						
Bepridil	T46.1X1	T46.1X2	T46.1X3	T46.1X4	T46.1X5	T46.1X6
Bergamot oil	T65.891	T65.892	T65.893	T65.894	—	—
Bergapten	T50.991	T50.992	T50.993	T50.994	T50.995	T50.996
Berries, poisonous	T62.1X1	T62.1X2	T62.1X3	T62.1X4	—	—
Beryllium (compounds)	T56.7X1	T56.7X2	T56.7X3	T56.7X4	—	—
beta adrenergic blocking agent, heart	T44.7X1	T44.7X2	T44.7X3	T44.7X4	T44.7X5	T44.7X6
Betacarotene	T45.2X1	T45.2X2	T45.2X3	T45.2X4	T45.2X5	T45.2X6
Beta-Chlor	T42.6X1	T42.6X2	T42.6X3	T42.6X4	T42.6X5	T42.6X6
Betahistine	T46.7X1	T46.7X2	T46.7X3	T46.7X4	T46.7X5	T46.7X6
Betaine	T47.5X1	T47.5X2	T47.5X3	T47.5X4	T47.5X5	T47.5X6
Betamethasone	T49.0X1	T49.0X2	T49.0X3	T49.0X4	T49.0X5	T49.0X6
topical	T49.0X1	T49.0X2	T49.0X3	T49.0X4	T49.0X5	T49.0X6
Betamicin	T36.8X1	T36.8X2	T36.8X3	T36.8X4	T36.8X5	T36.8X6
Betanidine	T46.5X1	T46.5X2	T46.5X3	T46.5X4	T46.5X5	T46.5X6
Betaxolol	T44.7X1	T44.7X2	T44.7X3	T44.7X4	T44.7X5	T44.7X6
Betazole	T50.8X1	T50.8X2	T50.8X3	T50.8X4	T50.8X5	T50.8X6
Bethanechol	T44.1X1	T44.1X2	T44.1X3	T44.1X4	T44.1X5	T44.1X6

Substance	Poisoning, Accidental (unintentional)	Poisoning, Intentional Self-harm	Poisoning, Assault	Poisoning, Undetermined	Adverse Effect	Under-dosing
Bethanechol — continued						
chloride	T44.1X1	T44.1X2	T44.1X3	T44.1X4	T44.1X5	T44.1X6
Bethanidine	T46.5X1	T46.5X2	T46.5X3	T46.5X4	T46.5X5	T46.5X6
Betoxycaine	T41.3X1	T41.3X2	T41.3X3	T41.3X4	T41.3X5	T41.3X6
Betula oil	T49.3X1	T49.3X2	T49.3X3	T49.3X4	T49.3X5	T49.3X6
Bevantolol	T44.7X1	T44.7X2	T44.7X3	T44.7X4	T44.7X5	T44.7X6
Bevonium metilsulfate	T44.3X1	T44.3X2	T44.3X3	T44.3X4	T44.3X5	T44.3X6
Bezafibrate	T46.6X1	T46.6X2	T46.6X3	T46.6X4	T46.6X5	T46.6X6
Bezitramide	T40.491	T40.492	T40.493	T40.494	T40.495	T40.496
BHA	T50.991	T50.992	T50.993	T50.994	T50.995	T50.996
Bhang	T40.711	T40.712	T40.713	T40.714	T40.715	T40.716
BHC (medicinal)	T49.0X1	T49.0X2	T49.0X3	T49.0X4	T49.0X5	T49.0X6
nonmedicinal (vapor)	T53.6X1	T53.6X2	T53.6X3	T53.6X4	—	—
Bialamicol	T37.3X1	T37.3X2	T37.3X3	T37.3X4	T37.3X5	T37.3X6
Bibenzonium bromide	T48.3X1	T48.3X2	T48.3X3	T48.3X4	T48.3X5	T48.3X6
Bibrocathol	T49.5X1	T49.5X2	T49.5X3	T49.5X4	T49.5X5	T49.5X6
Bichloride of mercury — see Mercury, chloride						
Bichromates (calcium) (potassium)(sodium) (crystals)	T57.8X1	T57.8X2	T57.8X3	T57.8X4	—	—
fumes	T56.2X1	T56.2X2	T56.2X3	T56.2X4	—	—
Biclotymol	T49.6X1	T49.6X2	T49.6X3	T49.6X4	T49.6X5	T49.6X6
Bicucculine	T50.7X1	T50.7X2	T50.7X3	T50.7X4	T50.7X5	T50.7X6
Bifemelane	T43.291	T43.292	T43.293	T43.294	T43.295	T43.296
Biguanide derivatives, oral	T38.3X1	T38.3X2	T38.3X3	T38.3X4	T38.3X5	T38.3X6
Bile salts	T47.5X1	T47.5X2	T47.5X3	T47.5X4	T47.5X5	T47.5X6
Biligrafin	T50.8X1	T50.8X2	T50.8X3	T50.8X4	T50.8X5	T50.8X6
Bilopaque	T50.8X1	T50.8X2	T50.8X3	T50.8X4	T50.8X5	T50.8X6
Binifibrate	T46.6X1	T46.6X2	T46.6X3	T46.6X4	T46.6X5	T46.6X6
Binitrobenzol	T65.3X1	T65.3X2	T65.3X3	T65.3X4	—	—
Bioflavonoid(s)	T46.991	T46.992	T46.993	T46.994	T46.995	T46.996
Biological substance NEC	T50.901	T50.902	T50.903	T50.904	T50.905	T50.906
Biotin	T45.2X1	T45.2X2	T45.2X3	T45.2X4	T45.2X5	T45.2X6
Biperiden	T44.3X1	T44.3X2	T44.3X3	T44.3X4	T44.3X5	T44.3X6
Bisacodyl	T47.2X1	T47.2X2	T47.2X3	T47.2X4	T47.2X5	T47.2X6
Bisbentiamine	T45.2X1	T45.2X2	T45.2X3	T45.2X4	T45.2X5	T45.2X6
Bisbutiamine	T45.2X1	T45.2X2	T45.2X3	T45.2X4	T45.2X5	T45.2X6
Bisdequalinium (salts) (diacetate)	T49.6X1	T49.6X2	T49.6X3	T49.6X4	T49.6X5	T49.6X6
Bishydroxycoumarin	T45.511	T45.512	T45.513	T45.514	T45.515	T45.516
Bismarsen	T37.8X1	T37.8X2	T37.8X3	T37.8X4	T37.8X5	T37.8X6
Bismuth salts	T47.6X1	T47.6X2	T47.6X3	T47.6X4	T47.6X5	T47.6X6
aluminate	T47.1X1	T47.1X2	T47.1X3	T47.1X4	T47.1X5	T47.1X6
anti-infectives	T37.8X1	T37.8X2	T37.8X3	T37.8X4	T37.8X5	T37.8X6
formic iodide	T49.0X1	T49.0X2	T49.0X3	T49.0X4	T49.0X5	T49.0X6
glycolylarsenate	T49.0X1	T49.0X2	T49.0X3	T49.0X4	T49.0X5	T49.0X6
nonmedicinal (compounds) NEC	T65.91	T65.92	T65.93	T65.94	—	—
subcarbonate	T47.6X1	T47.6X2	T47.6X3	T47.6X4	T47.6X5	T47.6X6
subsalicylate	T37.8X1	T37.8X2	T37.8X3	T37.8X4	T37.8X5	T37.8X6
sulfarsphenamine	T37.8X1	T37.8X2	T37.8X3	T37.8X4	T37.8X5	T37.8X6
Bisoprolol	T44.7X1	T44.7X2	T44.7X3	T44.7X4	T44.7X5	T44.7X6
Bisoxatin	T47.2X1	T47.2X2	T47.2X3	T47.2X4	T47.2X5	T47.2X6
Bisulepin (hydrochloride)	T45.0X1	T45.0X2	T45.0X3	T45.0X4	T45.0X5	T45.0X6
Bithionol	T37.8X1	T37.8X2	T37.8X3	T37.8X4	T37.8X5	T37.8X6
anthelminthic	T37.4X1	T37.4X2	T37.4X3	T37.4X4	T37.4X5	T37.4X6
Bitolterol	T48.6X1	T48.6X2	T48.6X3	T48.6X4	T48.6X5	T48.6X6
Bitoscanate	T37.4X1	T37.4X2	T37.4X3	T37.4X4	T37.4X5	T37.4X6
Bitter almond oil	T62.8X1	T62.8X2	T62.8X3	T62.8X4	—	—
Bittersweet	T62.2X1	T62.2X2	T62.2X3	T62.2X4	—	—
Black						
flag	T60.91	T60.92	T60.93	T60.94	—	—
henbane	T62.2X1	T62.2X2	T62.2X3	T62.2X4	—	—
leaf (40)	T60.91	T60.92	T60.93	T60.94	—	—
widow spider (bite)	T63.311	T63.312	T63.313	T63.314	—	—
antivenin	T50.Z11	T50.Z12	T50.Z13	T50.Z14	T50.Z15	T50.Z16
Blast furnace gas (carbon monoxide from)	T58.8X1	T58.8X2	T58.8X3	T58.8X4	—	—
Bleach	T54.91	T54.92	T54.93	T54.94	—	—
Bleaching agent (medicinal)	T49.4X1	T49.4X2	T49.4X3	T49.4X4	T49.4X5	T49.4X6
Bleomycin	T45.1X1	T45.1X2	T45.1X3	T45.1X4	T45.1X5	T45.1X6
Blockain	T41.3X1	T41.3X2	T41.3X3	T41.3X4	T41.3X5	T41.3X6
infiltration (subcutaneous)	T41.3X1	T41.3X2	T41.3X3	T41.3X4	T41.3X5	T41.3X6
nerve block (peripheral) (plexus)	T41.3X1	T41.3X2	T41.3X3	T41.3X4	T41.3X5	T41.3X6
topical (surface)	T41.3X1	T41.3X2	T41.3X3	T41.3X4	T41.3X5	T41.3X6
Blockers, calcium channel	T46.1X1	T46.1X2	T46.1X3	T46.1X4	T46.1X5	T46.1X6
Blood (derivatives) (natural) (plasma) (whole)	T45.8X1	T45.8X2	T45.8X3	T45.8X4	T45.8X5	T45.8X6
dried	T45.8X1	T45.8X2	T45.8X3	T45.8X4	T45.8X5	T45.8X6

Substance	Poisoning, Accidental (unintentional)	Poisoning, Intentional Self-harm	Poisoning, Assault	Poisoning, Undetermined	Adverse Effect	Under-dosing
Blood — *continued*						
drug affecting NEC	T45.91	T45.92	T45.93	T45.94	T45.95	T45.96
expander NEC	T45.8X1	T45.8X2	T45.8X3	T45.8X4	T45.8X5	T45.8X6
fraction NEC	T45.8X1	T45.8X2	T45.8X3	T45.8X4	T45.8X5	T45.8X6
substitute (macromolecular)	T45.8X1	T45.8X2	T45.8X3	T45.8X4	T45.8X5	T45.8X6
Blue velvet	T4Ø.2X1	T4Ø.2X2	T4Ø.2X3	T4Ø.2X4	—	—
Bone meal	T62.8X1	T62.8X2	T62.8X3	T62.8X4	—	—
Bonine	T45.ØX1	T45.ØX2	T45.ØX3	T45.ØX4	T45.ØX5	T45.ØX6
Bopindolol	T44.7X1	T44.7X2	T44.7X3	T44.7X4	T44.7X5	T44.7X6
Boracic acid	T49.ØX1	T49.ØX2	T49.ØX3	T49.ØX4	T49.ØX5	T49.ØX6
ENT agent	T49.6X1	T49.6X2	T49.6X3	T49.6X4	T49.6X5	T49.6X6
ophthalmic preparation	T49.5X1	T49.5X2	T49.5X3	T49.5X4	T49.5X5	T49.5X6
Borane complex	T57.8X1	T57.8X2	T57.8X3	T57.8X4	—	—
Borate(s)	T57.8X1	T57.8X2	T57.8X3	T57.8X4	—	—
buffer	T5Ø.991	T5Ø.992	T5Ø.993	T5Ø.994	T5Ø.995	T5Ø.996
cleanser	T54.91	T54.92	T54.93	T54.94	—	—
sodium	T57.8X1	T57.8X2	T57.8X3	T57.8X4	—	—
Borax (cleanser)	T54.91	T54.92	T54.93	T54.94	—	—
Bordeaux mixture	T6Ø.3X1	T6Ø.3X2	T6Ø.3X3	T6Ø.3X4	—	—
Boric acid	T49.ØX1	T49.ØX2	T49.ØX3	T49.ØX4	T49.ØX5	T49.ØX6
ENT agent	T49.6X1	T49.6X2	T49.6X3	T49.6X4	T49.6X5	T49.6X6
ophthalmic preparation	T49.5X1	T49.5X2	T49.5X3	T49.5X4	T49.5X5	T49.5X6
Bornaprine	T44.3X1	T44.3X2	T44.3X3	T44.3X4	T44.3X5	T44.3X6
Boron	T57.8X1	T57.8X2	T57.8X3	T57.8X4	—	—
hydride NEC	T57.8X1	T57.8X2	T57.8X3	T57.8X4	—	—
fumes or gas	T57.8X1	T57.8X2	T57.8X3	T57.8X4	—	—
trifluoride	T59.891	T59.892	T59.893	T59.894	—	—
Botox	T48.291	T48.292	T48.293	T48.294	T48.295	T48.296
Botulinus anti-toxin (type A, B)	T5Ø.Z11	T5Ø.Z12	T5Ø.Z13	T5Ø.Z14	T5Ø.Z15	T5Ø.Z16
Brake fluid vapor	T59.891	T59.892	T59.893	T59.894	—	—
Brallobarbital	T42.3X1	T42.3X2	T42.3X3	T42.3X4	T42.3X5	T42.3X6
Bran (wheat)	T47.4X1	T47.4X2	T47.4X3	T47.4X4	T47.4X5	T47.4X6
Brass (fumes)	T56.891	T56.892	T56.893	T56.894	—	—
Brasso	T52.ØX1	T52.ØX2	T52.ØX3	T52.ØX4	—	—
Bretylium tosilate	T46.2X1	T46.2X2	T46.2X3	T46.2X4	T46.2X5	T46.2X6
Brevital (sodium)	T41.1X1	T41.1X2	T41.1X3	T41.1X4	T41.1X5	T41.1X6
Brinase	T45.3X1	T45.3X2	T45.3X3	T45.3X4	T45.3X5	T45.3X6
British antilewisite	T45.8X1	T45.8X2	T45.8X3	T45.8X4	T45.8X5	T45.8X6
Brodifacoum	T6Ø.4X1	T6Ø.4X2	T6Ø.4X3	T6Ø.4X4	—	—
Bromal (hydrate)	T42.6X1	T42.6X2	T42.6X3	T42.6X4	T42.6X5	T42.6X6
Bromazepam	T42.4X1	T42.4X2	T42.4X3	T42.4X4	T42.4X5	T42.4X6
Bromazine	T45.ØX1	T45.ØX2	T45.ØX3	T45.ØX4	T45.ØX5	T45.ØX6
Brombenzylcyanide	T59.3X1	T59.3X2	T59.3X3	T59.3X4	—	—
Bromelains	T45.3X1	T45.3X2	T45.3X3	T45.3X4	T45.3X5	T45.3X6
Bromethalin	T6Ø.4X1	T6Ø.4X2	T6Ø.4X3	T6Ø.4X4	—	—
Bromhexine	T48.4X1	T48.4X2	T48.4X3	T48.4X4	T48.4X5	T48.4X6
Bromide salts	T42.6X1	T42.6X2	T42.6X3	T42.6X4	T42.6X5	T42.6X6
Bromindione	T45.511	T45.512	T45.513	T45.514	T45.515	T45.516
Bromine						
compounds (medicinal)	T42.6X1	T42.6X2	T42.6X3	T42.6X4	T42.6X5	T42.6X6
sedative	T42.6X1	T42.6X2	T42.6X3	T42.6X4	T42.6X5	T42.6X6
vapor	T59.891	T59.892	T59.893	T59.894	—	—
Bromisoval	T42.6X1	T42.6X2	T42.6X3	T42.6X4	T42.6X5	T42.6X6
Bromisovalum	T42.6X1	T42.6X2	T42.6X3	T42.6X4	T42.6X5	T42.6X6
Bromobenzylcyanide	T59.3X1	T59.3X2	T59.3X3	T59.3X4	—	—
Bromochlorosalicylani-lide	T49.ØX1	T49.ØX2	T49.ØX3	T49.ØX4	T49.ØX5	T49.ØX6
Bromocriptine	T42.8X1	T42.8X2	T42.8X3	T42.8X4	T42.8X5	T42.8X6
Bromodiphenhydramine	T45.ØX1	T45.ØX2	T45.ØX3	T45.ØX4	T45.ØX5	T45.ØX6
Bromoform	T42.6X1	T42.6X2	T42.6X3	T42.6X4	T42.6X5	T42.6X6
Bromophenol blue reagent	T5Ø.991	T5Ø.992	T5Ø.993	T5Ø.994	T5Ø.995	T5Ø.996
Bromopride	T47.8X1	T47.8X2	T47.8X3	T47.8X4	T47.8X5	T47.8X6
Bromosalicylchloranitide	T49.ØX1	T49.ØX2	T49.ØX3	T49.ØX4	T49.ØX5	T49.ØX6
Bromosalicylhydroxamic acid	T37.1X1	T37.1X2	T37.1X3	T37.1X4	T37.1X5	T37.1X6
Bromo-seltzer	T39.1X1	T39.1X2	T39.1X3	T39.1X4	T39.1X5	T39.1X6
Bromoxynil	T6Ø.3X1	T6Ø.3X2	T6Ø.3X3	T6Ø.3X4	—	—
Bromperidol	T43.4X1	T43.4X2	T43.4X3	T43.4X4	T43.4X5	T43.4X6
Brompheniramine	T45.ØX1	T45.ØX2	T45.ØX3	T45.ØX4	T45.ØX5	T45.ØX6
Bromsulfophthalein	T5Ø.8X1	T5Ø.8X2	T5Ø.8X3	T5Ø.8X4	T5Ø.8X5	T5Ø.8X6
Bromural	T42.6X1	T42.6X2	T42.6X3	T42.6X4	T42.6X5	T42.6X6
Bromvaletone	T42.6X1	T42.6X2	T42.6X3	T42.6X4	T42.6X5	T42.6X6
Bronchodilator NEC	T48.6X1	T48.6X2	T48.6X3	T48.6X4	T48.6X5	T48.6X6
Brotizolam	T42.4X1	T42.4X2	T42.4X3	T42.4X4	T42.4X5	T42.4X6
Brovincamine	T46.7X1	T46.7X2	T46.7X3	T46.7X4	T46.7X5	T46.7X6
Brown recluse spider (bite) (venom)	T63.331	T63.332	T63.333	T63.334	—	—
Brown spider (bite) (venom)	T63.391	T63.392	T63.393	T63.394	—	—
Broxaterol	T48.6X1	T48.6X2	T48.6X3	T48.6X4	T48.6X5	T48.6X6
Broxuridine	T45.1X1	T45.1X2	T45.1X3	T45.1X4	T45.1X5	T45.1X6

Substance	Poisoning, Accidental (unintentional)	Poisoning, Intentional Self-harm	Poisoning, Assault	Poisoning, Undetermined	Adverse Effect	Under-dosing
Broxyquinoline	T37.8X1	T37.8X2	T37.8X3	T37.8X4	T37.8X5	T37.8X6
Bruceine	T48.291	T48.292	T48.293	T48.294	T48.295	T48.296
Brucia	T62.2X1	T62.2X2	T62.2X3	T62.2X4	—	—
Brucine	T65.1X1	T65.1X2	T65.1X3	T65.1X4	—	—
Brunswick green — *see* Copper						
Bruten — *see* Ibuprofen						
Bryonia	T47.2X1	T47.2X2	T47.2X3	T47.2X4	T47.2X5	T47.2X6
Buclizine	T45.ØX1	T45.ØX2	T45.ØX3	T45.ØX4	T45.ØX5	T45.ØX6
Buclosamide	T49.ØX1	T49.ØX2	T49.ØX3	T49.ØX4	T49.ØX5	T49.ØX6
Budesonide	T44.5X1	T44.5X2	T44.5X3	T44.5X4	T44.5X5	T44.5X6
Budralazine	T46.5X1	T46.5X2	T46.5X3	T46.5X4	T46.5X5	T46.5X6
Bufferin	T39.Ø11	T39.Ø12	T39.Ø13	T39.Ø14	T39.Ø15	T39.Ø16
Buflomedil	T46.7X1	T46.7X2	T46.7X3	T46.7X4	T46.7X5	T46.7X6
Buformin	T38.3X1	T38.3X2	T38.3X3	T38.3X4	T38.3X5	T38.3X6
Bufotenine	T4Ø.991	T4Ø.992	T4Ø.993	T4Ø.994	—	—
Bufrolin	T48.6X1	T48.6X2	T48.6X3	T48.6X4	T48.6X5	T48.6X6
Bufylline	T48.6X1	T48.6X2	T48.6X3	T48.6X4	T48.6X5	T48.6X6
Bulk filler	T5Ø.5X1	T5Ø.5X2	T5Ø.5X3	T5Ø.5X4	T5Ø.5X5	T5Ø.5X6
cathartic	T47.4X1	T47.4X2	T47.4X3	T47.4X4	T47.4X5	T47.4X6
Bumetanide	T5Ø.1X1	T5Ø.1X2	T5Ø.1X3	T5Ø.1X4	T5Ø.1X5	T5Ø.1X6
Bunaftine	T46.2X1	T46.2X2	T46.2X3	T46.2X4	T46.2X5	T46.2X6
Bunamiodyl	T5Ø.8X1	T5Ø.8X2	T5Ø.8X3	T5Ø.8X4	T5Ø.8X5	T5Ø.8X6
Bunazosin	T44.6X1	T44.6X2	T44.6X3	T44.6X4	T44.6X5	T44.6X6
Bunitrolol	T44.7X1	T44.7X2	T44.7X3	T44.7X4	T44.7X5	T44.7X6
Buphenine	T46.7X1	T46.7X2	T46.7X3	T46.7X4	T46.7X5	T46.7X6
Bupivacaine	T41.3X1	T41.3X2	T41.3X3	T41.3X4	T41.3X5	T41.3X6
infiltration (subcutaneous)	T41.3X1	T41.3X2	T41.3X3	T41.3X4	T41.3X5	T41.3X6
nerve block (peripheral) (plexus)	T41.3X1	T41.3X2	T41.3X3	T41.3X4	T41.3X5	T41.3X6
spinal	T41.3X1	T41.3X2	T41.3X3	T41.3X4	T41.3X5	T41.3X6
Bupranolol	T44.7X1	T44.7X2	T44.7X3	T44.7X4	T44.7X5	T44.7X6
Buprenorphine	T4Ø.491	T4Ø.492	T4Ø.493	T4Ø.494	T4Ø.495	T4Ø.496
Bupropion	T43.291	T43.292	T43.293	T43.294	T43.295	T43.296
Burimamide	T47.1X1	T47.1X2	T47.1X3	T47.1X4	T47.1X5	T47.1X6
Buserelin	T38.891	T38.892	T38.893	T38.894	T38.895	T38.896
Buspirone	T43.591	T43.592	T43.593	T43.594	T43.595	T43.596
Busulfan, busulphan	T45.1X1	T45.1X2	T45.1X3	T45.1X4	T45.1X5	T45.1X6
Butabarbital (sodium)	T42.3X1	T42.3X2	T42.3X3	T42.3X4	T42.3X5	T42.3X6
Butabarbitone	T42.3X1	T42.3X2	T42.3X3	T42.3X4	T42.3X5	T42.3X6
Butabarpal	T42.3X1	T42.3X2	T42.3X3	T42.3X4	T42.3X5	T42.3X6
Butacaine	T41.3X1	T41.3X2	T41.3X3	T41.3X4	T41.3X5	T41.3X6
Butalamine	T46.7X1	T46.7X2	T46.7X3	T46.7X4	T46.7X5	T46.7X6
Butalbital	T42.3X1	T42.3X2	T42.3X3	T42.3X4	T42.3X5	T42.3X6
Butallylonal	T42.3X1	T42.3X2	T42.3X3	T42.3X4	T42.3X5	T42.3X6
Butamben	T41.3X1	T41.3X2	T41.3X3	T41.3X4	T41.3X5	T41.3X6
Butamirate	T48.3X1	T48.3X2	T48.3X3	T48.3X4	T48.3X5	T48.3X6
Butane (distributed in mobile container)	T59.891	T59.892	T59.893	T59.894	—	—
distributed through pipes	T59.891	T59.892	T59.893	T59.894	—	—
incomplete combustion	T58.11	T58.12	T58.13	T58.14	—	—
Butanilicaine	T41.3X1	T41.3X2	T41.3X3	T41.3X4	T41.3X5	T41.3X6
Butanol	T51.3X1	T51.3X2	T51.3X3	T51.3X4	—	—
Butanone, 2-butanone	T52.4X1	T52.4X2	T52.4X3	T52.4X4	—	—
Butantrone	T49.4X1	T49.4X2	T49.4X3	T49.4X4	T49.4X5	T49.4X6
Butaperazine	T43.3X1	T43.3X2	T43.3X3	T43.3X4	T43.3X5	T43.3X6
Butazolidin	T39.2X1	T39.2X2	T39.2X3	T39.2X4	T39.2X5	T39.2X6
Butetamate	T48.6X1	T48.6X2	T48.6X3	T48.6X4	T48.6X5	T48.6X6
Butethal	T42.3X1	T42.3X2	T42.3X3	T42.3X4	T42.3X5	T42.3X6
Butethamate	T44.3X1	T44.3X2	T44.3X3	T44.3X4	T44.3X5	T44.3X6
Buthalitone (sodium)	T41.1X1	T41.1X2	T41.1X3	T41.1X4	T41.1X5	T41.1X6
Butisol (sodium)	T42.3X1	T42.3X2	T42.3X3	T42.3X4	T42.3X5	T42.3X6
Butizide	T5Ø.2X1	T5Ø.2X2	T5Ø.2X3	T5Ø.2X4	T5Ø.2X5	T5Ø.2X6
Butobarbital	T42.3X1	T42.3X2	T42.3X3	T42.3X4	T42.3X5	T42.3X6
sodium	T42.3X1	T42.3X2	T42.3X3	T42.3X4	T42.3X5	T42.3X6
Butobarbitone	T42.3X1	T42.3X2	T42.3X3	T42.3X4	T42.3X5	T42.3X6
Butoconazole (nitrate)	T49.ØX1	T49.ØX2	T49.ØX3	T49.ØX4	T49.ØX5	T49.ØX6
Butorphanol	T4Ø.491	T4Ø.492	T4Ø.493	T4Ø.494	T4Ø.495	T4Ø.496
Butriptyline	T43.Ø11	T43.Ø12	T43.Ø13	T43.Ø14	T43.Ø15	T43.Ø16
Butropium bromide	T44.3X1	T44.3X2	T44.3X3	T44.3X4	T44.3X5	T44.3X6
Buttercups	T62.2X1	T62.2X2	T62.2X3	T62.2X4	—	—
Butter of antimony — *see* Antimony						
Butyl						
acetate (secondary)	T52.8X1	T52.8X2	T52.8X3	T52.8X4	—	—
alcohol	T51.3X1	T51.3X2	T51.3X3	T51.3X4	—	—
aminobenzoate	T41.3X1	T41.3X2	T41.3X3	T41.3X4	T41.3X5	T41.3X6
butyrate	T52.8X1	T52.8X2	T52.8X3	T52.8X4	—	—
carbinol	T51.3X1	T51.3X2	T51.3X3	T51.3X4	—	—
carbitol	T52.3X1	T52.3X2	T52.3X3	T52.3X4	—	—
cellosolve	T52.3X1	T52.3X2	T52.3X3	T52.3X4	—	—
chloral (hydrate)	T42.6X1	T42.6X2	T42.6X3	T42.6X4	T42.6X5	T42.6X6
formate	T52.8X1	T52.8X2	T52.8X3	T52.8X4	—	—
lactate	T52.8X1	T52.8X2	T52.8X3	T52.8X4	—	—

362 Additional Character May Be Required — Refer to the Tabular List for Character Selection

Subterms under main terms may continue to next column or page

Substance	Poisoning, Accidental (unintentional)	Poisoning, Intentional Self-harm	Poisoning, Assault	Poisoning, Undetermined	Adverse Effect	Under-dosing
Butyl — *continued*						
propionate	T52.8X1	T52.8X2	T52.8X3	T52.8X4	—	—
scopolamine bromide	T44.3X1	T44.3X2	T44.3X3	T44.3X4	T44.3X5	T44.3X6
thiobarbital sodium	T41.1X1	T41.1X2	T41.1X3	T41.1X4	T41.1X5	T41.1X6
Butylated hydroxyanisole	T50.991	T50.992	T50.993	T50.994	T50.995	T50.996
Butylchloral hydrate	T42.6X1	T42.6X2	T42.6X3	T42.6X4	T42.6X5	T42.6X6
Butyltoluene	T52.2X1	T52.2X2	T52.2X3	T52.2X4	—	—
Butyn	T41.3X1	T41.3X2	T41.3X3	T41.3X4	T41.3X5	T41.3X6
Butyrophenone (-based tranquilizers)	T43.4X1	T43.4X2	T43.4X3	T43.4X4	T43.4X5	T43.4X6
Cabergoline	T42.8X1	T42.8X2	T42.8X3	T42.8X4	T42.8X5	T42.8X6
Cacodyl, cacodylic acid	T57.0X1	T57.0X2	T57.0X3	T57.0X4	—	—
Cactinomycin	T45.1X1	T45.1X2	T45.1X3	T45.1X4	T45.1X5	T45.1X6
Cade oil	T49.4X1	T49.4X2	T49.4X3	T49.4X4	T49.4X5	T49.4X6
Cadexomer iodine	T49.0X1	T49.0X2	T49.0X3	T49.0X4	T49.0X5	T49.0X6
Cadmium (chloride) (fumes) (oxide)	T56.3X1	T56.3X2	T56.3X3	T56.3X4	—	—
sulfide (medicinal) NEC	T49.4X1	T49.4X2	T49.4X3	T49.4X4	T49.4X5	T49.4X6
Cadralazine	T46.5X1	T46.5X2	T46.5X3	T46.5X4	T46.5X5	T46.5X6
Caffeine	T43.611	T43.612	T43.613	T43.614	T43.615	T43.616
Calabar bean	T62.2X1	T62.2X2	T62.2X3	T62.2X4	—	—
Caladium seguinum	T62.2X1	T62.2X2	T62.2X3	T62.2X4	—	—
Calamine (lotion)	T49.3X1	T49.3X2	T49.3X3	T49.3X4	T49.3X5	T49.3X6
Calcifediol	T45.2X1	T45.2X2	T45.2X3	T45.2X4	T45.2X5	T45.2X6
Calciferol	T45.2X1	T45.2X2	T45.2X3	T45.2X4	T45.2X5	T45.2X6
Calcitonin	T50.991	T50.992	T50.993	T50.994	T50.995	T50.996
Calcitriol	T45.2X1	T45.2X2	T45.2X3	T45.2X4	T45.2X5	T45.2X6
Calcium	T50.3X1	T50.3X2	T50.3X3	T50.3X4	T50.3X5	T50.3X6
actylsalicylate	T39.011	T39.012	T39.013	T39.014	T39.015	T39.016
benzamidosalicylate	T37.1X1	T37.1X2	T37.1X3	T37.1X4	T37.1X5	T37.1X6
bromide	T42.6X1	T42.6X2	T42.6X3	T42.6X4	T42.6X5	T42.6X6
bromolactobionate	T42.6X1	T42.6X2	T42.6X3	T42.6X4	T42.6X5	T42.6X6
carbaspirin	T39.011	T39.012	T39.013	T39.014	T39.015	T39.016
carbimide	T50.6X1	T50.6X2	T50.6X3	T50.6X4	T50.6X5	T50.6X6
carbonate	T47.1X1	T47.1X2	T47.1X3	T47.1X4	T47.1X5	T47.1X6
chloride	T50.991	T50.992	T50.993	T50.994	T50.995	T50.996
anhydrous	T50.991	T50.992	T50.993	T50.994	T50.995	T50.996
cyanide	T57.8X1	T57.8X2	T57.8X3	T57.8X4	—	—
dioctyl sulfosuccinate	T47.4X1	T47.4X2	T47.4X3	T47.4X4	T47.4X5	T47.4X6
disodium edathamil	T45.8X1	T45.8X2	T45.8X3	T45.8X4	T45.8X5	T45.8X6
disodium edetate	T45.8X1	T45.8X2	T45.8X3	T45.8X4	T45.8X5	T45.8X6
dobesilate	T46.991	T46.992	T46.993	T46.994	T46.995	T46.996
EDTA	T45.8X1	T45.8X2	T45.8X3	T45.8X4	T45.8X5	T45.8X6
ferrous citrate	T45.4X1	T45.4X2	T45.4X3	T45.4X4	T45.4X5	T45.4X6
folinate	T45.8X1	T45.8X2	T45.8X3	T45.8X4	T45.8X5	T45.8X6
glubionate	T50.3X1	T50.3X2	T50.3X3	T50.3X4	T50.3X5	T50.3X6
gluconate	T50.3X1	T50.3X2	T50.3X3	T50.3X4	T50.3X5	T50.3X6
gluconogalactogluconate	T50.3X1	T50.3X2	T50.3X3	T50.3X4	T50.3X5	T50.3X6
hydrate, hydroxide	T54.3X1	T54.3X2	T54.3X3	T54.3X4	—	—
hypochlorite	T54.3X1	T54.3X2	T54.3X3	T54.3X4	—	—
iodide	T48.4X1	T48.4X2	T48.4X3	T48.4X4	T48.4X5	T48.4X6
ipodate	T50.8X1	T50.8X2	T50.8X3	T50.8X4	T50.8X5	T50.8X6
lactate	T50.3X1	T50.3X2	T50.3X3	T50.3X4	T50.3X5	T50.3X6
leucovorin	T45.8X1	T45.8X2	T45.8X3	T45.8X4	T45.8X5	T45.8X6
mandelate	T37.91	T37.92	T37.93	T37.94	T37.95	T37.96
oxide	T54.3X1	T54.3X2	T54.3X3	T54.3X4	—	—
pantothenate	T45.2X1	T45.2X2	T45.2X3	T45.2X4	T45.2X5	T45.2X6
phosphate	T50.3X1	T50.3X2	T50.3X3	T50.3X4	T50.3X5	T50.3X6
salicylate	T39.091	T39.092	T39.093	T39.094	T39.095	T39.096
salts	T50.3X1	T50.3X2	T50.3X3	T50.3X4	T50.3X5	T50.3X6
Calculus-dissolving drug	T50.991	T50.992	T50.993	T50.994	T50.995	T50.996
Calomel	T49.0X1	T49.0X2	T49.0X3	T49.0X4	T49.0X5	T49.0X6
Caloric agent	T50.3X1	T50.3X2	T50.3X3	T50.3X4	T50.3X5	T50.3X6
Calusterone	T38.7X1	T38.7X2	T38.7X3	T38.7X4	T38.7X5	T38.7X6
Camazepam	T42.4X1	T42.4X2	T42.4X3	T42.4X4	T42.4X5	T42.4X6
Camomile	T49.0X1	T49.0X2	T49.0X3	T49.0X4	T49.0X5	T49.0X6
Camoquin	T37.2X1	T37.2X2	T37.2X3	T37.2X4	T37.2X5	T37.2X6
Camphor						
insecticide	T60.2X1	T60.2X2	T60.2X3	T60.2X4	—	—
medicinal	T49.8X1	T49.8X2	T49.8X3	T49.8X4	T49.8X5	T49.8X6
Camylofin	T44.3X1	T44.3X2	T44.3X3	T44.3X4	T44.3X5	T44.3X6
Cancer chemotherapy drug regimen	T45.1X1	T45.1X2	T45.1X3	T45.1X4	T45.1X5	T45.1X6
Candeptin	T49.0X1	T49.0X2	T49.0X3	T49.0X4	T49.0X5	T49.0X6
Candicidin	T49.0X1	T49.0X2	T49.0X3	T49.0X4	T49.0X5	T49.0X6
Cannabinoids, synthetic	T40.721	T40.722	T40.723	T40.724	T40.725	T40.726
Cannabinol	T40.711	T40.712	T40.713	T40.714	T40.715	T40.716
Cannabis (derivatives)	T40.711	T40.712	T40.713	T40.714	T40.715	T40.716
Canned heat	T51.1X1	T51.1X2	T51.1X3	T51.1X4	—	—
Canrenoic acid	T50.0X1	T50.0X2	T50.0X3	T50.0X4	T50.0X5	T50.0X6
Canrenone	T50.0X1	T50.0X2	T50.0X3	T50.0X4	T50.0X5	T50.0X6
Cantharides, cantharidin, cantharis	T49.8X1	T49.8X2	T49.8X3	T49.8X4	T49.8X5	T49.8X6

Substance	Poisoning, Accidental (unintentional)	Poisoning, Intentional Self-harm	Poisoning, Assault	Poisoning, Undetermined	Adverse Effect	Under-dosing
Canthaxanthin	T50.991	T50.992	T50.993	T50.994	T50.995	T50.996
Capillary-active drug NEC	T46.901	T46.902	T46.903	T46.904	T46.905	T46.906
Capreomycin	T36.8X1	T36.8X2	T36.8X3	T36.8X4	T36.8X5	T36.8X6
Capsicum	T49.4X1	T49.4X2	T49.4X3	T49.4X4	T49.4X5	T49.4X6
Captafol	T60.3X1	T60.3X2	T60.3X3	T60.3X4	—	—
Captan	T60.3X1	T60.3X2	T60.3X3	T60.3X4	—	—
Captodiame, captodiamine	T43.591	T43.592	T43.593	T43.594	T43.595	T43.596
Captopril	T46.4X1	T46.4X2	T46.4X3	T46.4X4	T46.4X5	T46.4X6
Caramiphen	T44.3X1	T44.3X2	T44.3X3	T44.3X4	T44.3X5	T44.3X6
Carazolol	T44.7X1	T44.7X2	T44.7X3	T44.7X4	T44.7X5	T44.7X6
Carbachol	T44.1X1	T44.1X2	T44.1X3	T44.1X4	T44.1X5	T44.1X6
Carbacrylamine (resin)	T50.3X1	T50.3X2	T50.3X3	T50.3X4	T50.3X5	T50.3X6
Carbamate (insecticide)	T60.0X1	T60.0X2	T60.0X3	T60.0X4	—	—
Carbamate (sedative)	T42.6X1	T42.6X2	T42.6X3	T42.6X4	T42.6X5	T42.6X6
herbicide	T60.0X1	T60.0X2	T60.0X3	T60.0X4	—	—
insecticide	T60.0X1	T60.0X2	T60.0X3	T60.0X4	—	—
Carbamazepine	T42.1X1	T42.1X2	T42.1X3	T42.1X4	T42.1X5	T42.1X6
Carbamide	T47.3X1	T47.3X2	T47.3X3	T47.3X4	T47.3X5	T47.3X6
peroxide	T49.0X1	T49.0X2	T49.0X3	T49.0X4	T49.0X5	T49.0X6
topical	T49.8X1	T49.8X2	T49.8X3	T49.8X4	T49.8X5	T49.8X6
Carbamylcholine chloride	T44.1X1	T44.1X2	T44.1X3	T44.1X4	T44.1X5	T44.1X6
Carbaril	T60.0X1	T60.0X2	T60.0X3	T60.0X4	—	—
Carbarsone	T37.3X1	T37.3X2	T37.3X3	T37.3X4	T37.3X5	T37.3X6
Carbaryl	T60.0X1	T60.0X2	T60.0X3	T60.0X4	—	—
Carbaspirin	T39.011	T39.012	T39.013	T39.014	T39.015	T39.016
Carbazochrome (salicylate) (sodium sulfonate)	T49.4X1	T49.4X2	T49.4X3	T49.4X4	T49.4X5	T49.4X6
Carbenicillin	T36.0X1	T36.0X2	T36.0X3	T36.0X4	T36.0X5	T36.0X6
Carbenoxolone	T47.1X1	T47.1X2	T47.1X3	T47.1X4	T47.1X5	T47.1X6
Carbetapentane	T48.3X1	T48.3X2	T48.3X3	T48.3X4	T48.3X5	T48.3X6
Carbethyl salicylate	T39.091	T39.092	T39.093	T39.094	T39.095	T39.096
Carbidopa (with levodopa)	T42.8X1	T42.8X2	T42.8X3	T42.8X4	T42.8X5	T42.8X6
Carbimazole	T38.2X1	T38.2X2	T38.2X3	T38.2X4	T38.2X5	T38.2X6
Carbinol	T51.1X1	T51.1X2	T51.1X3	T51.1X4	—	—
Carbinoxamine	T45.0X1	T45.0X2	T45.0X3	T45.0X4	T45.0X5	T45.0X6
Carbiphene	T39.8X1	T39.8X2	T39.8X3	T39.8X4	T39.8X5	T39.8X6
Carbitol	T52.3X1	T52.3X2	T52.3X3	T52.3X4	—	—
Carbocaine	T41.3X1	T41.3X2	T41.3X3	T41.3X4	T41.3X5	T41.3X6
infiltration (subcutaneous)	T41.3X1	T41.3X2	T41.3X3	T41.3X4	T41.3X5	T41.3X6
nerve block (peripheral) (plexus)	T41.3X1	T41.3X2	T41.3X3	T41.3X4	T41.3X5	T41.3X6
topical (surface)	T41.3X1	T41.3X2	T41.3X3	T41.3X4	T41.3X5	T41.3X6
Carbocisteine	T48.4X1	T48.4X2	T48.4X3	T48.4X4	T48.4X5	T48.4X6
Carbocromen	T46.3X1	T46.3X2	T46.3X3	T46.3X4	T46.3X5	T46.3X6
Carbol fuchsin	T49.0X1	T49.0X2	T49.0X3	T49.0X4	T49.0X5	T49.0X6
Carbolic acid — *see also* Phenol	T54.0X1	T54.0X2	T54.0X3	T54.0X4	—	—
Carbolonium (bromide)	T48.1X1	T48.1X2	T48.1X3	T48.1X4	T48.1X5	T48.1X6
Carbo medicinalis	T47.6X1	T47.6X2	T47.6X3	T47.6X4	T47.6X5	T47.6X6
Carbomycin	T36.8X1	T36.8X2	T36.8X3	T36.8X4	T36.8X5	T36.8X6
Carbon						
bisulfide (liquid)	T65.4X1	T65.4X2	T65.4X3	T65.4X4	—	—
vapor	T65.4X1	T65.4X2	T65.4X3	T65.4X4	—	—
dioxide (gas)	T59.7X1	T59.7X2	T59.7X3	T59.7X4	—	—
medicinal	T41.5X1	T41.5X2	T41.5X3	T41.5X4	T41.5X5	T41.5X6
nonmedicinal	T59.7X1	T59.7X2	T59.7X3	T59.7X4	—	—
snow	T49.4X1	T49.4X2	T49.4X3	T49.4X4	T49.4X5	T49.4X6
disulfide (liquid)	T65.4X1	T65.4X2	T65.4X3	T65.4X4	—	—
vapor	T65.4X1	T65.4X2	T65.4X3	T65.4X4	—	—
monoxide (from incomplete combustion)	T58.91	T58.92	T58.93	T58.94	—	—
blast furnace gas	T58.8X1	T58.8X2	T58.8X3	T58.8X4	—	—
butane (distributed in mobile container)	T58.11	T58.12	T58.13	T58.14	—	—
distributed through pipes	T58.11	T58.12	T58.13	T58.14	—	—
charcoal fumes	T58.2X1	T58.2X2	T58.2X3	T58.2X4	—	—
coal	T58.2X1	T58.2X2	T58.2X3	T58.2X4	—	—
coke (in domestic stoves, fireplaces)	T58.2X1	T58.2X2	T58.2X3	T58.2X4	—	—
exhaust gas (motor) not in transit	T58.01	T58.02	T58.03	T58.04	—	—
combustion engine, any not in watercraft	T58.01	T58.02	T58.03	T58.04	—	—
farm tractor, not in transit	T58.01	T58.02	T58.03	T58.04	—	—
gas engine	T58.01	T58.02	T58.03	T58.04	—	—
motor pump	T58.01	T58.02	T58.03	T58.04	—	—
motor vehicle, not in transit	T58.01	T58.02	T58.03	T58.04	—	—
fuel (in domestic use)	T58.2X1	T58.2X2	T58.2X3	T58.2X4	—	—
gas (piped)	T58.11	T58.12	T58.13	T58.14	—	—

Subterms under main terms may continue to next column or page
Additional Character May Be Required — Refer to the Tabular List for Character Selection
363

Table of Drugs and Chemicals

Carbon — Central nervous system

Substance	Poisoning, Accidental (unintentional)	Poisoning, Intentional Self-harm	Poisoning, Assault	Poisoning, Undetermined	Adverse Effect	Under-dosing
Carbon — *continued*						
monoxide — *continued*						
fuel — *continued*						
gas — *continued*						
in mobile container	T58.11	T58.12	T58.13	T58.14	—	—
piped (natural)	T58.11	T58.12	T58.13	T58.14	—	—
utility	T58.11	T58.12	T58.13	T58.14	—	—
in mobile container	T58.11	T58.12	T58.13	T58.14	—	—
gas (piped)	T58.11	T58.12	T58.13	T58.14	—	—
illuminating gas	T58.11	T58.12	T58.13	T58.14	—	—
industrial fuels or gases, any	T58.8X1	T58.8X2	T58.8X3	T58.8X4	—	—
kerosene (in domestic stoves, fireplaces)	T58.2X1	T58.2X2	T58.2X3	T58.2X4	—	—
kiln gas or vapor	T58.8X1	T58.8X2	T58.8X3	T58.8X4	—	—
motor exhaust gas, not in transit	T58.01	T58.02	T58.03	T58.04	—	—
piped gas (manufactured) (natural)	T58.11	T58.12	T58.13	T58.14	—	—
producer gas	T58.8X1	T58.8X2	T58.8X3	T58.8X4	—	—
propane (distributed in mobile container)	T58.11	T58.12	T58.13	T58.14	—	—
distributed through pipes	T58.11	T58.12	T58.13	T58.14	—	—
solid (in domestic stoves, fireplaces)	T58.2X1	T58.2X2	T58.2X3	T58.2X4	—	—
specified source NEC	T58.8X1	T58.8X2	T58.8X3	T58.8X4	—	—
stove gas	T58.11	T58.12	T58.13	T58.14	—	—
piped	T58.11	T58.12	T58.13	T58.14	—	—
utility gas	T58.11	T58.12	T58.13	T58.14	—	—
piped	T58.11	T58.12	T58.13	T58.14	—	—
water gas	T58.11	T58.12	T58.13	T58.14	—	—
wood (in domestic stoves, fireplaces)	T58.2X1	T58.2X2	T58.2X3	T58.2X4	—	—
tetrachloride (vapor) NEC	T53.0X1	T53.0X2	T53.0X3	T53.0X4	—	—
liquid (cleansing agent) NEC	T53.0X1	T53.0X2	T53.0X3	T53.0X4	—	—
solvent	T53.0X1	T53.0X2	T53.0X3	T53.0X4	—	—
Carbonic acid gas	T59.7X1	T59.7X2	T59.7X3	T59.7X4	—	—
anhydrase inhibitor NEC	T50.2X1	T50.2X2	T50.2X3	T50.2X4	T50.2X5	T50.2X6
Carbophenothion	T60.0X1	T60.0X2	T60.0X3	T60.0X4	—	—
Carboplatin	T45.1X1	T45.1X2	T45.1X3	T45.1X4	T45.1X5	T45.1X6
Carboprost	T48.0X1	T48.0X2	T48.0X3	T48.0X4	T48.0X5	T48.0X6
Carboquone	T45.1X1	T45.1X2	T45.1X3	T45.1X4	T45.1X5	T45.1X6
Carbowax	T49.3X1	T49.3X2	T49.3X3	T49.3X4	T49.3X5	T49.3X6
Carboxymethylcellulose	T47.4X1	T47.4X2	T47.4X3	T47.4X4	T47.4X5	T47.4X6
Carbrital	T42.3X1	T42.3X2	T42.3X3	T42.3X4	T42.3X5	T42.3X6
Carbromal	T42.6X1	T42.6X2	T42.6X3	T42.6X4	T42.6X5	T42.6X6
Carbutamide	T38.3X1	T38.3X2	T38.3X3	T38.3X4	T38.3X5	T38.3X6
Carbuterol	T48.6X1	T48.6X2	T48.6X3	T48.6X4	T48.6X5	T48.6X6
Cardiac						
depressants	T46.2X1	T46.2X2	T46.2X3	T46.2X4	T46.2X5	T46.2X6
rhythm regulator	T46.2X1	T46.2X2	T46.2X3	T46.2X4	T46.2X5	T46.2X6
specified NEC	T46.2X1	T46.2X2	T46.2X3	T46.2X4	T46.2X5	T46.2X6
Cardiografin	T50.8X1	T50.8X2	T50.8X3	T50.8X4	T50.8X5	T50.8X6
Cardiogreen	T50.8X1	T50.8X2	T50.8X3	T50.8X4	T50.8X5	T50.8X6
Cardiotonic (glycoside) **NEC**	T46.0X1	T46.0X2	T46.0X3	T46.0X4	T46.0X5	T46.0X6
Cardiovascular drug NEC	T46.901	T46.902	T46.903	T46.904	T46.905	T46.906
Cardrase	T50.2X1	T50.2X2	T50.2X3	T50.2X4	T50.2X5	T50.2X6
Carfecillin	T36.0X1	T36.0X2	T36.0X3	T36.0X4	T36.0X5	T36.0X6
Carfenazine	T43.3X1	T43.3X2	T43.3X3	T43.3X4	T43.3X5	T43.3X6
Carfusin	T49.0X1	T49.0X2	T49.0X3	T49.0X4	T49.0X5	T49.0X6
Carindacillin	T36.0X1	T36.0X2	T36.0X3	T36.0X4	T36.0X5	T36.0X6
Carisoprodol	T42.8X1	T42.8X2	T42.8X3	T42.8X4	T42.8X5	T42.8X6
Carmellose	T47.4X1	T47.4X2	T47.4X3	T47.4X4	T47.4X5	T47.4X6
Carminative	T47.5X1	T47.5X2	T47.5X3	T47.5X4	T47.5X5	T47.5X6
Carmofur	T45.1X1	T45.1X2	T45.1X3	T45.1X4	T45.1X5	T45.1X6
Carmustine	T45.1X1	T45.1X2	T45.1X3	T45.1X4	T45.1X5	T45.1X6
Carotene	T45.2X1	T45.2X2	T45.2X3	T45.2X4	T45.2X5	T45.2X6
Carphenazine	T43.3X1	T43.3X2	T43.3X3	T43.3X4	T43.3X5	T43.3X6
Carpipramine	T42.4X1	T42.4X2	T42.4X3	T42.4X4	T42.4X5	T42.4X6
Carprofen	T39.311	T39.312	T39.313	T39.314	T39.315	T39.316
Carpronium chloride	T44.3X1	T44.3X2	T44.3X3	T44.3X4	T44.3X5	T44.3X6
Carrageenan	T47.8X1	T47.8X2	T47.8X3	T47.8X4	T47.8X5	T47.8X6
Carteolol	T44.7X1	T44.7X2	T44.7X3	T44.7X4	T44.7X5	T44.7X6
Carter's Little Pills	T47.2X1	T47.2X2	T47.2X3	T47.2X4	T47.2X5	T47.2X6
Cascara (sagrada)	T47.2X1	T47.2X2	T47.2X3	T47.2X4	T47.2X5	T47.2X6
Cassava	T62.2X1	T62.2X2	T62.2X3	T62.2X4	—	—
Castellani's paint	T49.0X1	T49.0X2	T49.0X3	T49.0X4	T49.0X5	T49.0X6
Castor						
bean	T62.2X1	T62.2X2	T62.2X3	T62.2X4	—	—
oil	T47.2X1	T47.2X2	T47.2X3	T47.2X4	T47.2X5	T47.2X6
Catalase	T45.3X1	T45.3X2	T45.3X3	T45.3X4	T45.3X5	T45.3X6

Substance	Poisoning, Accidental (unintentional)	Poisoning, Intentional Self-harm	Poisoning, Assault	Poisoning, Undetermined	Adverse Effect	Under-dosing
Caterpillar (sting)	T63.431	T63.432	T63.433	T63.434	—	—
Catha (edulis) (tea)	T43.691	T43.692	T43.693	T43.694	—	—
Cathartic NEC	T47.4X1	T47.4X2	T47.4X3	T47.4X4	T47.4X5	T47.4X6
anthacene derivative	T47.2X1	T47.2X2	T47.2X3	T47.2X4	T47.2X5	T47.2X6
bulk	T47.4X1	T47.4X2	T47.4X3	T47.4X4	T47.4X5	T47.4X6
contact	T47.2X1	T47.2X2	T47.2X3	T47.2X4	T47.2X5	T47.2X6
emollient NEC	T47.4X1	T47.4X2	T47.4X3	T47.4X4	T47.4X5	T47.4X6
irritant NEC	T47.2X1	T47.2X2	T47.2X3	T47.2X4	T47.2X5	T47.2X6
mucilage	T47.4X1	T47.4X2	T47.4X3	T47.4X4	T47.4X5	T47.4X6
saline	T47.3X1	T47.3X2	T47.3X3	T47.3X4	T47.3X5	T47.3X6
vegetable	T47.2X1	T47.2X2	T47.2X3	T47.2X4	T47.2X5	T47.2X6
Cathine	T50.5X1	T50.5X2	T50.5X3	T50.5X4	T50.5X5	T50.5X6
Cathomycin	T36.8X1	T36.8X2	T36.8X3	T36.8X4	T36.8X5	T36.8X6
Cation exchange resin	T50.3X1	T50.3X2	T50.3X3	T50.3X4	T50.3X5	T50.3X6
Caustic(s) NEC	T54.91	T54.92	T54.93	T54.94	—	—
alkali	T54.3X1	T54.3X2	T54.3X3	T54.3X4	—	—
hydroxide	T54.3X1	T54.3X2	T54.3X3	T54.3X4	—	—
potash	T54.3X1	T54.3X2	T54.3X3	T54.3X4	—	—
soda	T54.3X1	T54.3X2	T54.3X3	T54.3X4	—	—
specified NEC	T54.91	T54.92	T54.93	T54.94	—	—
Ceepryn	T49.0X1	T49.0X2	T49.0X3	T49.0X4	T49.0X5	T49.0X6
ENT agent	T49.6X1	T49.6X2	T49.6X3	T49.6X4	T49.6X5	T49.6X6
lozenges	T49.6X1	T49.6X2	T49.6X3	T49.6X4	T49.6X5	T49.6X6
Cefacetrile	T36.1X1	T36.1X2	T36.1X3	T36.1X4	T36.1X5	T36.1X6
Cefaclor	T36.1X1	T36.1X2	T36.1X3	T36.1X4	T36.1X5	T36.1X6
Cefadroxil	T36.1X1	T36.1X2	T36.1X3	T36.1X4	T36.1X5	T36.1X6
Cefalexin	T36.1X1	T36.1X2	T36.1X3	T36.1X4	T36.1X5	T36.1X6
Cefaloglycin	T36.1X1	T36.1X2	T36.1X3	T36.1X4	T36.1X5	T36.1X6
Cefaloridine	T36.1X1	T36.1X2	T36.1X3	T36.1X4	T36.1X5	T36.1X6
Cefalosporins	T36.1X1	T36.1X2	T36.1X3	T36.1X4	T36.1X5	T36.1X6
Cefalotin	T36.1X1	T36.1X2	T36.1X3	T36.1X4	T36.1X5	T36.1X6
Cefamandole	T36.1X1	T36.1X2	T36.1X3	T36.1X4	T36.1X5	T36.1X6
Cefamycin antibiotic	T36.1X1	T36.1X2	T36.1X3	T36.1X4	T36.1X5	T36.1X6
Cefapirin	T36.1X1	T36.1X2	T36.1X3	T36.1X4	T36.1X5	T36.1X6
Cefatrizine	T36.1X1	T36.1X2	T36.1X3	T36.1X4	T36.1X5	T36.1X6
Cefazedone	T36.1X1	T36.1X2	T36.1X3	T36.1X4	T36.1X5	T36.1X6
Cefazolin	T36.1X1	T36.1X2	T36.1X3	T36.1X4	T36.1X5	T36.1X6
Cefbuperazone	T36.1X1	T36.1X2	T36.1X3	T36.1X4	T36.1X5	T36.1X6
Cefetamet	T36.1X1	T36.1X2	T36.1X3	T36.1X4	T36.1X5	T36.1X6
Cefixime	T36.1X1	T36.1X2	T36.1X3	T36.1X4	T36.1X5	T36.1X6
Cefmenoxime	T36.1X1	T36.1X2	T36.1X3	T36.1X4	T36.1X5	T36.1X6
Cefmetazole	T36.1X1	T36.1X2	T36.1X3	T36.1X4	T36.1X5	T36.1X6
Cefminox	T36.1X1	T36.1X2	T36.1X3	T36.1X4	T36.1X5	T36.1X6
Cefonicid	T36.1X1	T36.1X2	T36.1X3	T36.1X4	T36.1X5	T36.1X6
Cefoperazone	T36.1X1	T36.1X2	T36.1X3	T36.1X4	T36.1X5	T36.1X6
Ceforanide	T36.1X1	T36.1X2	T36.1X3	T36.1X4	T36.1X5	T36.1X6
Cefotaxime	T36.1X1	T36.1X2	T36.1X3	T36.1X4	T36.1X5	T36.1X6
Cefotetan	T36.1X1	T36.1X2	T36.1X3	T36.1X4	T36.1X5	T36.1X6
Cefotiam	T36.1X1	T36.1X2	T36.1X3	T36.1X4	T36.1X5	T36.1X6
Cefoxitin	T36.1X1	T36.1X2	T36.1X3	T36.1X4	T36.1X5	T36.1X6
Cefpimizole	T36.1X1	T36.1X2	T36.1X3	T36.1X4	T36.1X5	T36.1X6
Cefpiramide	T36.1X1	T36.1X2	T36.1X3	T36.1X4	T36.1X5	T36.1X6
Cefradine	T36.1X1	T36.1X2	T36.1X3	T36.1X4	T36.1X5	T36.1X6
Cefroxadine	T36.1X1	T36.1X2	T36.1X3	T36.1X4	T36.1X5	T36.1X6
Cefsulodin	T36.1X1	T36.1X2	T36.1X3	T36.1X4	T36.1X5	T36.1X6
Ceftazidime	T36.1X1	T36.1X2	T36.1X3	T36.1X4	T36.1X5	T36.1X6
Cefteram	T36.1X1	T36.1X2	T36.1X3	T36.1X4	T36.1X5	T36.1X6
Ceftezole	T36.1X1	T36.1X2	T36.1X3	T36.1X4	T36.1X5	T36.1X6
Ceftizoxime	T36.1X1	T36.1X2	T36.1X3	T36.1X4	T36.1X5	T36.1X6
Ceftriaxone	T36.1X1	T36.1X2	T36.1X3	T36.1X4	T36.1X5	T36.1X6
Cefuroxime	T36.1X1	T36.1X2	T36.1X3	T36.1X4	T36.1X5	T36.1X6
Cefuzonam	T36.1X1	T36.1X2	T36.1X3	T36.1X4	T36.1X5	T36.1X6
Celestone	T38.0X1	T38.0X2	T38.0X3	T38.0X4	T38.0X5	T38.0X6
topical	T49.0X1	T49.0X2	T49.0X3	T49.0X4	T49.0X5	T49.0X6
Celiprolol	T44.7X1	T44.7X2	T44.7X3	T44.7X4	T44.7X5	T44.7X6
Cellosolve	T52.91	T52.92	T52.93	T52.94	—	—
Cell stimulants and proliferants	T49.8X1	T49.8X2	T49.8X3	T49.8X4	T49.8X5	T49.8X6
Cellulose						
cathartic	T47.4X1	T47.4X2	T47.4X3	T47.4X4	T47.4X5	T47.4X6
hydroxyethyl	T47.4X1	T47.4X2	T47.4X3	T47.4X4	T47.4X5	T47.4X6
nitrates (topical)	T49.3X1	T49.3X2	T49.3X3	T49.3X4	T49.3X5	T49.3X6
oxidized	T49.4X1	T49.4X2	T49.4X3	T49.4X4	T49.4X5	T49.4X6
Centipede (bite)	T63.411	T63.412	T63.413	T63.414	—	—
Central nervous system						
depressants	T42.71	T42.72	T42.73	T42.74	T42.75	T42.76
anesthetic (general) NEC	T41.201	T41.202	T41.203	T41.204	T41.205	T41.206
gases NEC	T41.0X1	T41.0X2	T41.0X3	T41.0X4	T41.0X5	T41.0X6
intravenous	T41.1X1	T41.1X2	T41.1X3	T41.1X4	T41.1X5	T41.1X6
barbiturates	T42.3X1	T42.3X2	T42.3X3	T42.3X4	T42.3X5	T42.3X6
benzodiazepines	T42.4X1	T42.4X2	T42.4X3	T42.4X4	T42.4X5	T42.4X6
bromides	T42.6X1	T42.6X2	T42.6X3	T42.6X4	T42.6X5	T42.6X6
cannabis sativa	T40.711	T40.712	T40.713	T40.714	T40.715	T40.716

Additional Character May Be Required — Refer to the Tabular List for Character Selection   ▽ **Subterms under main terms may continue to next column or page**

Substance	Poisoning, Accidental (unintentional)	Poisoning, Intentional Self-harm	Poisoning, Assault	Poisoning, Undetermined	Adverse Effect	Under-dosing
Central nervous system — *continued*						
depressants — *continued*						
chloral hydrate	T42.6X1	T42.6X2	T42.6X3	T42.6X4	T42.6X5	T42.6X6
ethanol	T51.ØX1	T51.ØX2	T51.ØX3	T51.ØX4	—	—
hallucinogenics	T4Ø.9Ø1	T4Ø.9Ø2	T4Ø.9Ø3	T4Ø.9Ø4	T4Ø.9Ø5	T4Ø.9Ø6
hypnotics	T42.71	T42.72	T42.73	T42.74	T42.75	T42.76
specified NEC	T42.6X1	T42.6X2	T42.6X3	T42.6X4	T42.6X5	T42.6X6
muscle relaxants	T42.8X1	T42.8X2	T42.8X3	T42.8X4	T42.8X5	T42.8X6
paraldehyde	T42.6X1	T42.6X2	T42.6X3	T42.6X4	T42.6X5	T42.6X6
sedatives; sedative-hypnotics	T42.71	T42.72	T42.73	T42.74	T42.75	T42.76
mixed NEC	T42.6X1	T42.6X2	T42.6X3	T42.6X4	T42.6X5	T42.6X6
specified NEC	T42.6X1	T42.6X2	T42.6X3	T42.6X4	T42.6X5	T42.6X6
muscle-tone depressants	T42.8X1	T42.8X2	T42.8X3	T42.8X4	T42.8X5	T42.8X6
stimulants	T43.6Ø1	T43.6Ø2	T43.6Ø3	T43.6Ø4	T43.6Ø5	T43.6Ø6
amphetamines	T43.621	T43.622	T43.623	T43.624	T43.625	T43.626
analeptics	T5Ø.7X1	T5Ø.7X2	T5Ø.7X3	T5Ø.7X4	T5Ø.7X5	T5Ø.7X6
antidepressants	T43.2Ø1	T43.2Ø2	T43.2Ø3	T43.2Ø4	T43.2Ø5	T43.2Ø6
opiate antagonists	T5Ø.7X1	T5Ø.7X2	T5Ø.7X3	T5Ø.7X4	T5Ø.7X5	T5Ø.7X6
specified NEC	T43.691	T43.692	T43.693	T43.694	T43.695	T43.696
Cephalexin	T36.1X1	T36.1X2	T36.1X3	T36.1X4	T36.1X5	T36.1X6
Cephaloglycin	T36.1X1	T36.1X2	T36.1X3	T36.1X4	T36.1X5	T36.1X6
Cephaloridine	T36.1X1	T36.1X2	T36.1X3	T36.1X4	T36.1X5	T36.1X6
Cephalosporins	T36.1X1	T36.1X2	T36.1X3	T36.1X4	T36.1X5	T36.1X6
N (adicillin)	T36.ØX1	T36.ØX2	T36.ØX3	T36.ØX4	T36.ØX5	T36.ØX6
Cephalothin	T36.1X1	T36.1X2	T36.1X3	T36.1X4	T36.1X5	T36.1X6
Cephalotin	T36.1X1	T36.1X2	T36.1X3	T36.1X4	T36.1X5	T36.1X6
Cephradine	T36.1X1	T36.1X2	T36.1X3	T36.1X4	T36.1X5	T36.1X6
Cerbera (odallam)	T62.2X1	T62.2X2	T62.2X3	T62.2X4	—	—
Cerberin	T46.ØX1	T46.ØX2	T46.ØX3	T46.ØX4	T46.ØX5	T46.ØX6
Cerebral stimulants	T43.6Ø1	T43.6Ø2	T43.6Ø3	T43.6Ø4	T43.6Ø5	T43.6Ø6
psychotherapeutic	T43.6Ø1	T43.6Ø2	T43.6Ø3	T43.6Ø4	T43.6Ø5	T43.6Ø6
specified NEC	T43.691	T43.692	T43.693	T43.694	T43.695	T43.696
Cerium oxalate	T45.ØX1	T45.ØX2	T45.ØX3	T45.ØX4	T45.ØX5	T45.ØX6
Cerous oxalate	T45.ØX1	T45.ØX2	T45.ØX3	T45.ØX4	T45.ØX5	T45.ØX6
Ceruletide	T5Ø.8X1	T5Ø.8X2	T5Ø.8X3	T5Ø.8X4	T5Ø.8X5	T5Ø.8X6
Cetalkonium (chloride)	T49.ØX1	T49.ØX2	T49.ØX3	T49.ØX4	T49.ØX5	T49.ØX6
Cethexonium chloride	T49.ØX1	T49.ØX2	T49.ØX3	T49.ØX4	T49.ØX5	T49.ØX6
Cetiedil	T46.7X1	T46.7X2	T46.7X3	T46.7X4	T46.7X5	T46.7X6
Cetirizine	T45.ØX1	T45.ØX2	T45.ØX3	T45.ØX4	T45.ØX5	T45.ØX6
Cetomacrogol	T5Ø.991	T5Ø.992	T5Ø.993	T5Ø.994	T5Ø.995	T5Ø.996
Cetotiamine	T45.2X1	T45.2X2	T45.2X3	T45.2X4	T45.2X5	T45.2X6
Cetoxime	T45.ØX1	T45.ØX2	T45.ØX3	T45.ØX4	T45.ØX5	T45.ØX6
Cetraxate	T47.1X1	T47.1X2	T47.1X3	T47.1X4	T47.1X5	T47.1X6
Cetrimide	T49.ØX1	T49.ØX2	T49.ØX3	T49.ØX4	T49.ØX5	T49.ØX6
Cetrimonium (bromide)	T49.ØX1	T49.ØX2	T49.ØX3	T49.ØX4	T49.ØX5	T49.ØX6
Cetylpyridinium chloride	T49.ØX1	T49.ØX2	T49.ØX3	T49.ØX4	T49.ØX5	T49.ØX6
ENT agent	T49.6X1	T49.6X2	T49.6X3	T49.6X4	T49.6X5	T49.6X6
lozenges	T49.6X1	T49.6X2	T49.6X3	T49.6X4	T49.6X5	T49.6X6
Cevadilla — *see* Sabadilla						
Cevitamic acid	T45.2X1	T45.2X2	T45.2X3	T45.2X4	T45.2X5	T45.2X6
Chalk, precipitated	T47.1X1	T47.1X2	T47.1X3	T47.1X4	T47.1X5	T47.1X6
Chamomile	T49.ØX1	T49.ØX2	T49.ØX3	T49.ØX4	T49.ØX5	T49.ØX6
Ch'an su	T46.ØX1	T46.ØX2	T46.ØX3	T46.ØX4	T46.ØX5	T46.ØX6
Charcoal	T47.6X1	T47.6X2	T47.6X3	T47.6X4	T47.6X5	T47.6X6
activated — *see also* Charcoal, medicinal	T47.6X1	T47.6X2	T47.6X3	T47.6X4	T47.6X5	T47.6X6
fumes (Carbon monoxide)	T58.2X1	T58.2X2	T58.2X3	T58.2X4	—	—
industrial	T58.8X1	T58.8X2	T58.8X3	T58.8X4	—	—
medicinal (activated)	T47.6X1	T47.6X2	T47.6X3	T47.6X4	T47.6X5	T47.6X6
antidiarrheal	T47.6X1	T47.6X2	T47.6X3	T47.6X4	T47.6X5	T47.6X6
poison control	T47.8X1	T47.8X2	T47.8X3	T47.8X4	T47.8X5	T47.8X6
specified use other than for diarrhea	T47.8X1	T47.8X2	T47.8X3	T47.8X4	T47.8X5	T47.8X6
topical	T49.8X1	T49.8X2	T49.8X3	T49.8X4	T49.8X5	T49.8X6
Chaulmosulfone	T37.1X1	T37.1X2	T37.1X3	T37.1X4	T37.1X5	T37.1X6
Chelating agent NEC	T5Ø.6X1	T5Ø.6X2	T5Ø.6X3	T5Ø.6X4	T5Ø.6X5	T5Ø.6X6
Chelidonium majus	T62.2X1	T62.2X2	T62.2X3	T62.2X4	—	—
Chemical substance NEC	T65.91	T65.92	T65.93	T65.94	—	—
Chenodeoxycholic acid	T47.5X1	T47.5X2	T47.5X3	T47.5X4	T47.5X5	T47.5X6
Chenodiol	T47.5X1	T47.5X2	T47.5X3	T47.5X4	T47.5X5	T47.5X6
Chenopodium	T37.4X1	T37.4X2	T37.4X3	T37.4X4	T37.4X5	T37.4X6
Cherry laurel	T62.2X1	T62.2X2	T62.2X3	T62.2X4	—	—
Chinidin (e)	T46.2X1	T46.2X2	T46.2X3	T46.2X4	T46.2X5	T46.2X6
Chiniofon	T37.8X1	T37.8X2	T37.8X3	T37.8X4	T37.8X5	T37.8X6
Chlophedianol	T48.3X1	T48.3X2	T48.3X3	T48.3X4	T48.3X5	T48.3X6
Chloral	T42.6X1	T42.6X2	T42.6X3	T42.6X4	T42.6X5	T42.6X6
derivative	T42.6X1	T42.6X2	T42.6X3	T42.6X4	T42.6X5	T42.6X6
hydrate	T42.6X1	T42.6X2	T42.6X3	T42.6X4	T42.6X5	T42.6X6
Chloralamide	T42.6X1	T42.6X2	T42.6X3	T42.6X4	T42.6X5	T42.6X6
Chloralodol	T42.6X1	T42.6X2	T42.6X3	T42.6X4	T42.6X5	T42.6X6
Chloralose	T6Ø.4X1	T6Ø.4X2	T6Ø.4X3	T6Ø.4X4	—	—

Substance	Poisoning, Accidental (unintentional)	Poisoning, Intentional Self-harm	Poisoning, Assault	Poisoning, Undetermined	Adverse Effect	Under-dosing
Chlorambucil	T45.1X1	T45.1X2	T45.1X3	T45.1X4	T45.1X5	T45.1X6
Chloramine	T57.8X1	T57.8X2	T57.8X3	T57.8X4	—	—
T	T49.ØX1	T49.ØX2	T49.ØX3	T49.ØX4	T49.ØX5	T49.ØX6
topical	T49.ØX1	T49.ØX2	T49.ØX3	T49.ØX4	T49.ØX5	T49.ØX6
Chloramphenicol	T36.2X1	T36.2X2	T36.2X3	T36.2X4	T36.2X5	T36.2X6
ENT agent	T49.6X1	T49.6X2	T49.6X3	T49.6X4	T49.6X5	T49.6X6
ophthalmic preparation	T49.5X1	T49.5X2	T49.5X3	T49.5X4	T49.5X5	T49.5X6
topical NEC	T49.ØX1	T49.ØX2	T49.ØX3	T49.ØX4	T49.ØX5	T49.ØX6
Chlorate (potassium) (sodium) **NEC**	T6Ø.3X1	T6Ø.3X2	T6Ø.3X3	T6Ø.3X4	—	—
herbicide	T6Ø.3X1	T6Ø.3X2	T6Ø.3X3	T6Ø.3X4	—	—
Chlorazanil	T5Ø.2X1	T5Ø.2X2	T5Ø.2X3	T5Ø.2X4	T5Ø.2X5	T5Ø.2X6
Chlorbenzene, chlorbenzol	T53.7X1	T53.7X2	T53.7X3	T53.7X4	—	—
Chlorbenzoxamine	T44.3X1	T44.3X2	T44.3X3	T44.3X4	T44.3X5	T44.3X6
Chlorbutol	T42.6X1	T42.6X2	T42.6X3	T42.6X4	T42.6X5	T42.6X6
Chlorcyclizine	T45.ØX1	T45.ØX2	T45.ØX3	T45.ØX4	T45.ØX5	T45.ØX6
Chlordan (e) (dust)	T6Ø.1X1	T6Ø.1X2	T6Ø.1X3	T6Ø.1X4	—	—
Chlordantoin	T49.ØX1	T49.ØX2	T49.ØX3	T49.ØX4	T49.ØX5	T49.ØX6
Chlordiazepoxide	T42.4X1	T42.4X2	T42.4X3	T42.4X4	T42.4X5	T42.4X6
Chlordiethyl benzamide	T49.3X1	T49.3X2	T49.3X3	T49.3X4	T49.3X5	T49.3X6
Chloresium	T49.8X1	T49.8X2	T49.8X3	T49.8X4	T49.8X5	T49.8X6
Chlorethiazol	T42.6X1	T42.6X2	T42.6X3	T42.6X4	T42.6X5	T42.6X6
Chlorethyl — *see* Ethyl chloride						
Chloretone	T42.6X1	T42.6X2	T42.6X3	T42.6X4	T42.6X5	T42.6X6
Chlorex	T53.6X1	T53.6X2	T53.6X3	T53.6X4	—	—
insecticide	T6Ø.1X1	T6Ø.1X2	T6Ø.1X3	T6Ø.1X4	—	—
Chlorfenvinphos	T6Ø.ØX1	T6Ø.ØX2	T6Ø.ØX3	T6Ø.ØX4	—	—
Chlorhexadol	T42.6X1	T42.6X2	T42.6X3	T42.6X4	T42.6X5	T42.6X6
Chlorhexamide	T45.1X1	T45.1X2	T45.1X3	T45.1X4	T45.1X5	T45.1X6
Chlorhexidine	T49.ØX1	T49.ØX2	T49.ØX3	T49.ØX4	T49.ØX5	T49.ØX6
Chlorhydroxyquinolin	T49.ØX1	T49.ØX2	T49.ØX3	T49.ØX4	T49.ØX5	T49.ØX6
Chloride of lime (bleach)	T54.3X1	T54.3X2	T54.3X3	T54.3X4	—	—
Chlorimipramine	T43.Ø11	T43.Ø12	T43.Ø13	T43.Ø14	T43.Ø15	T43.Ø16
Chlorinated						
camphene	T53.6X1	T53.6X2	T53.6X3	T53.6X4	—	—
diphenyl	T53.7X1	T53.7X2	T53.7X3	T53.7X4	—	—
hydrocarbons NEC	T53.91	T53.92	T53.93	T53.94	—	—
solvents	T53.91	T53.92	T53.93	T53.94	—	—
lime (bleach)	T54.3X1	T54.3X2	T54.3X3	T54.3X4	—	—
and boric acid solution	T49.ØX1	T49.ØX2	T49.ØX3	T49.ØX4	T49.ØX5	T49.ØX6
naphthalene (insecticide)	T6Ø.1X1	T6Ø.1X2	T6Ø.1X3	T6Ø.1X4	—	—
industrial (non-pesticide)	T53.7X1	T53.7X2	T53.7X3	T53.7X4	—	—
pesticide NEC	T6Ø.8X1	T6Ø.8X2	T6Ø.8X3	T6Ø.8X4	—	—
soda — *see also* sodium hypochlorite						
solution	T49.ØX1	T49.ØX2	T49.ØX3	T49.ØX4	T49.ØX5	T49.ØX6
Chlorine (fumes) (gas)	T59.4X1	T59.4X2	T59.4X3	T59.4X4	—	—
bleach	T54.3X1	T54.3X2	T54.3X3	T54.3X4	—	—
compound gas NEC	T59.4X1	T59.4X2	T59.4X3	T59.4X4	—	—
disinfectant	T59.4X1	T59.4X2	T59.4X3	T59.4X4	—	—
releasing agents NEC	T59.4X1	T59.4X2	T59.4X3	T59.4X4	—	—
Chlorisondamine chloride	T46.991	T46.992	T46.993	T46.994	T46.995	T46.996
Chlormadinone	T38.5X1	T38.5X2	T38.5X3	T38.5X4	T38.5X5	T38.5X6
Chlormephos	T6Ø.ØX1	T6Ø.ØX2	T6Ø.ØX3	T6Ø.ØX4	—	—
Chlormerodrin	T5Ø.2X1	T5Ø.2X2	T5Ø.2X3	T5Ø.2X4	T5Ø.2X5	T5Ø.2X6
Chlormethiazole	T42.6X1	T42.6X2	T42.6X3	T42.6X4	T42.6X5	T42.6X6
Chlormethine	T45.1X1	T45.1X2	T45.1X3	T45.1X4	T45.1X5	T45.1X6
Chlormethylenecycline	T36.4X1	T36.4X2	T36.4X3	T36.4X4	T36.4X5	T36.4X6
Chlormezanone	T42.6X1	T42.6X2	T42.6X3	T42.6X4	T42.6X5	T42.6X6
Chloroacetic acid	T6Ø.3X1	T6Ø.3X2	T6Ø.3X3	T6Ø.3X4	—	—
Chloroacetone	T59.3X1	T59.3X2	T59.3X3	T59.3X4	—	—
Chloroacetophenone	T59.3X1	T59.3X2	T59.3X3	T59.3X4	—	—
Chloroaniline	T53.7X1	T53.7X2	T53.7X3	T53.7X4	—	—
Chlorobenzene, chlorobenzol	T53.7X1	T53.7X2	T53.7X3	T53.7X4	—	—
Chlorobromomethane (fire extinguisher)	T53.6X1	T53.6X2	T53.6X3	T53.6X4	—	—
Chlorobutanol	T49.ØX1	T49.ØX2	T49.ØX3	T49.ØX4	T49.ØX5	T49.ØX6
Chlorocresol	T49.ØX1	T49.ØX2	T49.ØX3	T49.ØX4	T49.ØX5	T49.ØX6
Chlorodehydromethyltestosterone	T38.7X1	T38.7X2	T38.7X3	T38.7X4	T38.7X5	T38.7X6
Chlorodinitrobenzene	T53.7X1	T53.7X2	T53.7X3	T53.7X4	—	—
dust or vapor	T53.7X1	T53.7X2	T53.7X3	T53.7X4	—	—
Chlorodiphenyl	T53.7X1	T53.7X2	T53.7X3	T53.7X4	—	—
Chloroethane — *see* Ethyl chloride						
Chloroethylene	T53.6X1	T53.6X2	T53.6X3	T53.6X4	—	—
Chlorofluorocarbons	T53.5X1	T53.5X2	T53.5X3	T53.5X4	—	—
Chloroform (fumes) (vapor)	T53.1X1	T53.1X2	T53.1X3	T53.1X4	—	—
anesthetic	T41.ØX1	T41.ØX2	T41.ØX3	T41.ØX4	T41.ØX5	T41.ØX6
solvent	T53.1X1	T53.1X2	T53.1X3	T53.1X4	—	—
water, concentrated	T41.ØX1	T41.ØX2	T41.ØX3	T41.ØX4	T41.ØX5	T41.ØX6

Subterms under main terms may continue to next column or page   Additional Character May Be Required — Refer to the Tabular List for Character Selection   365

Substance	Poisoning, Accidental (unintentional)	Poisoning, Intentional Self-harm	Poisoning, Assault	Poisoning, Undetermined	Adverse Effect	Under-dosing
Chloroguanide	T37.2X1	T37.2X2	T37.2X3	T37.2X4	T37.2X5	T37.2X6
Chloromycetin	T36.2X1	T36.2X2	T36.2X3	T36.2X4	T36.2X5	T36.2X6
ENT agent	T49.6X1	T49.6X2	T49.6X3	T49.6X4	T49.6X5	T49.6X6
ophthalmic preparation	T49.5X1	T49.5X2	T49.5X3	T49.5X4	T49.5X5	T49.5X6
otic solution	T49.6X1	T49.6X2	T49.6X3	T49.6X4	T49.6X5	T49.6X6
topical NEC	T49.ØX1	T49.ØX2	T49.ØX3	T49.ØX4	T49.ØX5	T49.ØX6
Chloronitrobenzene	T53.7X1	T53.7X2	T53.7X3	T53.7X4	—	—
dust or vapor	T53.7X1	T53.7X2	T53.7X3	T53.7X4	—	—
Chlorophacinone	T6Ø.4X1	T6Ø.4X2	T6Ø.4X3	T6Ø.4X4	—	—
Chlorophenol	T53.7X1	T53.7X2	T53.7X3	T53.7X4	—	—
Chlorophenothane	T6Ø.1X1	T6Ø.1X2	T6Ø.1X3	T6Ø.1X4	—	—
Chlorophyll	T5Ø.991	T5Ø.992	T5Ø.993	T5Ø.994	T5Ø.995	T5Ø.996
Chloropicrin (fumes)	T53.6X1	T53.6X2	T53.6X3	T53.6X4	—	—
fumigant	T6Ø.8X1	T6Ø.8X2	T6Ø.8X3	T6Ø.8X4	—	—
fungicide	T6Ø.3X1	T6Ø.3X2	T6Ø.3X3	T6Ø.3X4	—	—
pesticide	T6Ø.8X1	T6Ø.8X2	T6Ø.8X3	T6Ø.8X4	—	—
Chloroprocaine	T41.3X1	T41.3X2	T41.3X3	T41.3X4	T41.3X5	T41.3X6
infiltration (subcutaneous)	T41.3X1	T41.3X2	T41.3X3	T41.3X4	T41.3X5	T41.3X6
nerve block (peripheral) (plexus)	T41.3X1	T41.3X2	T41.3X3	T41.3X4	T41.3X5	T41.3X6
spinal	T41.3X1	T41.3X2	T41.3X3	T41.3X4	T41.3X5	T41.3X6
Chloroptic	T49.5X1	T49.5X2	T49.5X3	T49.5X4	T49.5X5	T49.5X6
Chloropurine	T45.1X1	T45.1X2	T45.1X3	T45.1X4	T45.1X5	T45.1X6
Chloropyramine	T45.ØX1	T45.ØX2	T45.ØX3	T45.ØX4	T45.ØX5	T45.ØX6
Chloropyrifos	T6Ø.ØX1	T6Ø.ØX2	T6Ø.ØX3	T6Ø.ØX4	—	—
Chloropyrilene	T45.ØX1	T45.ØX2	T45.ØX3	T45.ØX4	T45.ØX5	T45.ØX6
Chloroquine	T37.2X1	T37.2X2	T37.2X3	T37.2X4	T37.2X5	T37.2X6
Chlorothalonil	T6Ø.3X1	T6Ø.3X2	T6Ø.3X3	T6Ø.3X4	—	—
Chlorothen	T45.ØX1	T45.ØX2	T45.ØX3	T45.ØX4	T45.ØX5	T45.ØX6
Chlorothiazide	T5Ø.2X1	T5Ø.2X2	T5Ø.2X3	T5Ø.2X4	T5Ø.2X5	T5Ø.2X6
Chlorothymol	T49.4X1	T49.4X2	T49.4X3	T49.4X4	T49.4X5	T49.4X6
Chlorotrianisene	T38.5X1	T38.5X2	T38.5X3	T38.5X4	T38.5X5	T38.5X6
Chlorovinyldichloroarsine, not in war	T57.ØX1	T57.ØX2	T57.ØX3	T57.ØX4	—	—
Chloroxine	T49.4X1	T49.4X2	T49.4X3	T49.4X4	T49.4X5	T49.4X6
Chloroxylenol	T49.ØX1	T49.ØX2	T49.ØX3	T49.ØX4	T49.ØX5	T49.ØX6
Chlorphenamine	T45.ØX1	T45.ØX2	T45.ØX3	T45.ØX4	T45.ØX5	T45.ØX6
Chlorphenesin	T42.8X1	T42.8X2	T42.8X3	T42.8X4	T42.8X5	T42.8X6
topical (antifungal)	T49.ØX1	T49.ØX2	T49.ØX3	T49.ØX4	T49.ØX5	T49.ØX6
Chlorpheniramine	T45.ØX1	T45.ØX2	T45.ØX3	T45.ØX4	T45.ØX5	T45.ØX6
Chlorphenoxamine	T45.ØX1	T45.ØX2	T45.ØX3	T45.ØX4	T45.ØX5	T45.ØX6
Chlorphentermine	T5Ø.5X1	T5Ø.5X2	T5Ø.5X3	T5Ø.5X4	T5Ø.5X5	T5Ø.5X6
Chlorprocaine — *see* Chloroprocaine						
Chlorproguanil	T37.2X1	T37.2X2	T37.2X3	T37.2X4	T37.2X5	T37.2X6
Chlorpromazine	T43.3X1	T43.3X2	T43.3X3	T43.3X4	T43.3X5	T43.3X6
Chlorpropamide	T38.3X1	T38.3X2	T38.3X3	T38.3X4	T38.3X5	T38.3X6
Chlorprothixene	T43.4X1	T43.4X2	T43.4X3	T43.4X4	T43.4X5	T43.4X6
Chlorquinaldol	T49.ØX1	T49.ØX2	T49.ØX3	T49.ØX4	T49.ØX5	T49.ØX6
Chlorquinol	T49.ØX1	T49.ØX2	T49.ØX3	T49.ØX4	T49.ØX5	T49.ØX6
Chlortalidone	T5Ø.2X1	T5Ø.2X2	T5Ø.2X3	T5Ø.2X4	T5Ø.2X5	T5Ø.2X6
Chlortetracycline	T36.4X1	T36.4X2	T36.4X3	T36.4X4	T36.4X5	T36.4X6
Chlorthalidone	T5Ø.2X1	T5Ø.2X2	T5Ø.2X3	T5Ø.2X4	T5Ø.2X5	T5Ø.2X6
Chlorthion	T6Ø.ØX1	T6Ø.ØX2	T6Ø.ØX3	T6Ø.ØX4	—	—
Chlorthiophos	T6Ø.ØX1	T6Ø.ØX2	T6Ø.ØX3	T6Ø.ØX4	—	—
Chlortrianisene	T38.5X1	T38.5X2	T38.5X3	T38.5X4	T38.5X5	T38.5X6
Chlor-Trimeton	T45.ØX1	T45.ØX2	T45.ØX3	T45.ØX4	T45.ØX5	T45.ØX6
Chlorzoxazone	T42.8X1	T42.8X2	T42.8X3	T42.8X4	T42.8X5	T42.8X6
Choke damp	T59.7X1	T59.7X2	T59.7X3	T59.7X4	—	—
Cholagogues	T47.5X1	T47.5X2	T47.5X3	T47.5X4	T47.5X5	T47.5X6
Cholebrine	T5Ø.8X1	T5Ø.8X2	T5Ø.8X3	T5Ø.8X4	T5Ø.8X5	T5Ø.8X6
Cholecalciferol	T45.2X1	T45.2X2	T45.2X3	T45.2X4	T45.2X5	T45.2X6
Cholecystokinin	T5Ø.8X1	T5Ø.8X2	T5Ø.8X3	T5Ø.8X4	T5Ø.8X5	T5Ø.8X6
Cholera vaccine	T5Ø.A91	T5Ø.A92	T5Ø.A93	T5Ø.A94	T5Ø.A95	T5Ø.A96
Choleretic	T47.5X1	T47.5X2	T47.5X3	T47.5X4	T47.5X5	T47.5X6
Cholesterol-lowering agents	T46.6X1	T46.6X2	T46.6X3	T46.6X4	T46.6X5	T46.6X6
Cholestyramine (resin)	T46.6X1	T46.6X2	T46.6X3	T46.6X4	T46.6X5	T46.6X6
Cholic acid	T47.5X1	T47.5X2	T47.5X3	T47.5X4	T47.5X5	T47.5X6
Choline	T48.6X1	T48.6X2	T48.6X3	T48.6X4	T48.6X5	T48.6X6
chloride	T5Ø.991	T5Ø.992	T5Ø.993	T5Ø.994	T5Ø.995	T5Ø.996
dihydrogen citrate	T5Ø.991	T5Ø.992	T5Ø.993	T5Ø.994	T5Ø.995	T5Ø.996
salicylate	T39.Ø91	T39.Ø92	T39.Ø93	T39.Ø94	T39.Ø95	T39.Ø96
theophyllinate	T48.6X1	T48.6X2	T48.6X3	T48.6X4	T48.6X5	T48.6X6
Cholinergic (drug) **NEC**	T44.1X1	T44.1X2	T44.1X3	T44.1X4	T44.1X5	T44.1X6
muscle tone enhancer	T44.1X1	T44.1X2	T44.1X3	T44.1X4	T44.1X5	T44.1X6
organophosphorus	T44.ØX1	T44.ØX2	T44.ØX3	T44.ØX4	T44.ØX5	T44.ØX6
insecticide	T6Ø.ØX1	T6Ø.ØX2	T6Ø.ØX3	T6Ø.ØX4	—	—
nerve gas	T59.891	T59.892	T59.893	T59.894	—	—
trimethyl ammonium propanediol	T44.1X1	T44.1X2	T44.1X3	T44.1X4	T44.1X5	T44.1X6
Cholinesterase reactivator	T5Ø.6X1	T5Ø.6X2	T5Ø.6X3	T5Ø.6X4	T5Ø.6X5	T5Ø.6X6
Cholografin	T5Ø.8X1	T5Ø.8X2	T5Ø.8X3	T5Ø.8X4	T5Ø.8X5	T5Ø.8X6

Substance	Poisoning, Accidental (unintentional)	Poisoning, Intentional Self-harm	Poisoning, Assault	Poisoning, Undetermined	Adverse Effect	Under-dosing
Chorionic gonadotropin	T38.891	T38.892	T38.893	T38.894	T38.895	T38.896
Chromate	T56.2X1	T56.2X2	T56.2X3	T56.2X4	—	—
dust or mist	T56.2X1	T56.2X2	T56.2X3	T56.2X4	—	—
lead — *see also* lead	T56.ØX1	T56.ØX2	T56.ØX3	T56.ØX4	—	—
paint	T56.ØX1	T56.ØX2	T56.ØX3	T56.ØX4	—	—
Chromic						
acid	T56.2X1	T56.2X2	T56.2X3	T56.2X4	—	—
dust or mist	T56.2X1	T56.2X2	T56.2X3	T56.2X4	—	—
phosphate 32P	T45.1X1	T45.1X2	T45.1X3	T45.1X4	T45.1X5	T45.1X6
Chromium	T56.2X1	T56.2X2	T56.2X3	T56.2X4	—	—
compounds — *see* Chromate						
sesquioxide	T5Ø.8X1	T5Ø.8X2	T5Ø.8X3	T5Ø.8X4	T5Ø.8X5	T5Ø.8X6
Chromomycin A3	T45.1X1	T45.1X2	T45.1X3	T45.1X4	T45.1X5	T45.1X6
Chromonar	T46.3X1	T46.3X2	T46.3X3	T46.3X4	T46.3X5	T46.3X6
Chromyl chloride	T56.2X1	T56.2X2	T56.2X3	T56.2X4	—	—
Chrysarobin	T49.4X1	T49.4X2	T49.4X3	T49.4X4	T49.4X5	T49.4X6
Chrysazin	T47.2X1	T47.2X2	T47.2X3	T47.2X4	T47.2X5	T47.2X6
Chymar	T45.3X1	T45.3X2	T45.3X3	T45.3X4	T45.3X5	T45.3X6
ophthalmic preparation	T49.5X1	T49.5X2	T49.5X3	T49.5X4	T49.5X5	T49.5X6
Chymopapain	T45.3X1	T45.3X2	T45.3X3	T45.3X4	T45.3X5	T45.3X6
Chymotrypsin	T45.3X1	T45.3X2	T45.3X3	T45.3X4	T45.3X5	T45.3X6
ophthalmic preparation	T49.5X1	T49.5X2	T49.5X3	T49.5X4	T49.5X5	T49.5X6
Cianidanol	T5Ø.991	T5Ø.992	T5Ø.993	T5Ø.994	T5Ø.995	T5Ø.996
Cianopramine	T43.Ø11	T43.Ø12	T43.Ø13	T43.Ø14	T43.Ø15	T43.Ø16
Cibenzoline	T46.2X1	T46.2X2	T46.2X3	T46.2X4	T46.2X5	T46.2X6
Ciclacillin	T36.ØX1	T36.ØX2	T36.ØX3	T36.ØX4	T36.ØX5	T36.ØX6
Ciclobarbital — *see* Hexobarbital						
Ciclonicate	T46.7X1	T46.7X2	T46.7X3	T46.7X4	T46.7X5	T46.7X6
Ciclopirox (olamine)	T49.ØX1	T49.ØX2	T49.ØX3	T49.ØX4	T49.ØX5	T49.ØX6
Ciclosporin	T45.1X1	T45.1X2	T45.1X3	T45.1X4	T45.1X5	T45.1X6
Cicuta maculata or virosa	T62.2X1	T62.2X2	T62.2X3	T62.2X4	—	—
Cicutoxin	T62.2X1	T62.2X2	T62.2X3	T62.2X4	—	—
Cigarette lighter fluid	T52.ØX1	T52.ØX2	T52.ØX3	T52.ØX4	—	—
Cigarettes (tobacco)	T65.221	T65.222	T65.223	T65.224	—	—
Ciguatoxin	T61.Ø1	T61.Ø2	T61.Ø3	T61.Ø4	—	—
Cilazapril	T46.4X1	T46.4X2	T46.4X3	T46.4X4	T46.4X5	T46.4X6
Cimetidine	T47.ØX1	T47.ØX2	T47.ØX3	T47.ØX4	T47.ØX5	T47.ØX6
Cimetropium bromide	T44.3X1	T44.3X2	T44.3X3	T44.3X4	T44.3X5	T44.3X6
Cinchocaine	T41.3X1	T41.3X2	T41.3X3	T41.3X4	T41.3X5	T41.3X6
topical (surface)	T41.3X1	T41.3X2	T41.3X3	T41.3X4	T41.3X5	T41.3X6
Cinchona	T37.2X1	T37.2X2	T37.2X3	T37.2X4	T37.2X5	T37.2X6
Cinchonine alkaloids	T37.2X1	T37.2X2	T37.2X3	T37.2X4	T37.2X5	T37.2X6
Cinchophen	T5Ø.4X1	T5Ø.4X2	T5Ø.4X3	T5Ø.4X4	T5Ø.4X5	T5Ø.4X6
Cinepazide	T46.7X1	T46.7X2	T46.7X3	T46.7X4	T46.7X5	T46.7X6
Cinnamedrine	T48.5X1	T48.5X2	T48.5X3	T48.5X4	T48.5X5	T48.5X6
Cinnarizine	T45.ØX1	T45.ØX2	T45.ØX3	T45.ØX4	T45.ØX5	T45.ØX6
Cinoxacin	T37.8X1	T37.8X2	T37.8X3	T37.8X4	T37.8X5	T37.8X6
Ciprofibrate	T46.6X1	T46.6X2	T46.6X3	T46.6X4	T46.6X5	T46.6X6
Ciprofloxacin	T36.8X1	T36.8X2	T36.8X3	T36.8X4	T36.8X5	T36.8X6
Cisapride	T47.8X1	T47.8X2	T47.8X3	T47.8X4	T47.8X5	T47.8X6
Cisplatin	T45.1X1	T45.1X2	T45.1X3	T45.1X4	T45.1X5	T45.1X6
Citalopram	T43.221	T43.222	T43.223	T43.224	T43.225	T43.226
Citanest	T41.3X1	T41.3X2	T41.3X3	T41.3X4	T41.3X5	T41.3X6
infiltration (subcutaneous)	T41.3X1	T41.3X2	T41.3X3	T41.3X4	T41.3X5	T41.3X6
nerve block (peripheral) (plexus)	T41.3X1	T41.3X2	T41.3X3	T41.3X4	T41.3X5	T41.3X6
Citric acid	T47.5X1	T47.5X2	T47.5X3	T47.5X4	T47.5X5	T47.5X6
Citrovorum (factor)	T45.8X1	T45.8X2	T45.8X3	T45.8X4	T45.8X5	T45.8X6
Claviceps purpurea	T62.2X1	T62.2X2	T62.2X3	T62.2X4	—	—
Clavulanic acid	T36.1X1	T36.1X2	T36.1X3	T36.1X4	T36.1X5	T36.1X6
Cleaner, cleansing agent, type not specified	T65.891	T65.892	T65.893	T65.894	—	—
of paint or varnish	T52.91	T52.92	T52.93	T52.94	—	—
specified type NEC	T65.891	T65.892	T65.893	T65.894	—	—
Clebopride	T47.8X1	T47.8X2	T47.8X3	T47.8X4	T47.8X5	T47.8X6
Clefamide	T37.3X1	T37.3X2	T37.3X3	T37.3X4	T37.3X5	T37.3X6
Clemastine	T45.ØX1	T45.ØX2	T45.ØX3	T45.ØX4	T45.ØX5	T45.ØX6
Clematis vitalba	T62.2X1	T62.2X2	T62.2X3	T62.2X4	—	—
Clemizole	T45.ØX1	T45.ØX2	T45.ØX3	T45.ØX4	T45.ØX5	T45.ØX6
penicillin	T36.ØX1	T36.ØX2	T36.ØX3	T36.ØX4	T36.ØX5	T36.ØX6
Clenbuterol	T48.6X1	T48.6X2	T48.6X3	T48.6X4	T48.6X5	T48.6X6
Clidinium bromide	T44.3X1	T44.3X2	T44.3X3	T44.3X4	T44.3X5	T44.3X6
Clindamycin	T36.8X1	T36.8X2	T36.8X3	T36.8X4	T36.8X5	T36.8X6
Clinofibrate	T46.6X1	T46.6X2	T46.6X3	T46.6X4	T46.6X5	T46.6X6
Clioquinol	T37.8X1	T37.8X2	T37.8X3	T37.8X4	T37.8X5	T37.8X6
Cliradon	T4Ø.2X1	T4Ø.2X2	T4Ø.2X3	T4Ø.2X4	—	—
Clobazam	T42.4X1	T42.4X2	T42.4X3	T42.4X4	T42.4X5	T42.4X6
Clobenzorex	T5Ø.5X1	T5Ø.5X2	T5Ø.5X3	T5Ø.5X4	T5Ø.5X5	T5Ø.5X6
Clobetasol	T49.ØX1	T49.ØX2	T49.ØX3	T49.ØX4	T49.ØX5	T49.ØX6
Clobetasone	T49.ØX1	T49.ØX2	T49.ØX3	T49.ØX4	T49.ØX5	T49.ØX6
Clobutinol	T48.3X1	T48.3X2	T48.3X3	T48.3X4	T48.3X5	T48.3X6
Clocortolone	T38.ØX1	T38.ØX2	T38.ØX3	T38.ØX4	T38.ØX5	T38.ØX6

Chloroguanide — Clocortolone

366 Additional Character May Be Required — Refer to the Tabular List for Character Selection Subterms under main terms may continue to next column or page

Substance	Poisoning, Accidental (unintentional)	Poisoning, Intentional Self-harm	Poisoning, Assault	Poisoning, Undetermined	Adverse Effect	Under-dosing
Clodantoin	T49.0X1	T49.0X2	T49.0X3	T49.0X4	T49.0X5	T49.0X6
Clodronic acid	T50.991	T50.992	T50.993	T50.994	T50.995	T50.996
Clofazimine	T37.1X1	T37.1X2	T37.1X3	T37.1X4	T37.1X5	T37.1X6
Clofedanol	T48.3X1	T48.3X2	T48.3X3	T48.3X4	T48.3X5	T48.3X6
Clofenamide	T50.2X1	T50.2X2	T50.2X3	T50.2X4	T50.2X5	T50.2X6
Clofenotane	T49.0X1	T49.0X2	T49.0X3	T49.0X4	T49.0X5	T49.0X6
Clofezone	T39.2X1	T39.2X2	T39.2X3	T39.2X4	T39.2X5	T39.2X6
Clofibrate	T46.6X1	T46.6X2	T46.6X3	T46.6X4	T46.6X5	T46.6X6
Clofibride	T46.6X1	T46.6X2	T46.6X3	T46.6X4	T46.6X5	T46.6X6
Cloforex	T50.5X1	T50.5X2	T50.5X3	T50.5X4	T50.5X5	T50.5X6
Clomethiazole	T42.6X1	T42.6X2	T42.6X3	T42.6X4	T42.6X5	T42.6X6
Clometocillin	T36.0X1	T36.0X2	T36.0X3	T36.0X4	T36.0X5	T36.0X6
Clomifene	T38.5X1	T38.5X2	T38.5X3	T38.5X4	T38.5X5	T38.5X6
Clomiphene	T38.5X1	T38.5X2	T38.5X3	T38.5X4	T38.5X5	T38.5X6
Clomipramine	T43.011	T43.012	T43.013	T43.014	T43.015	T43.016
Clomocycline	T36.4X1	T36.4X2	T36.4X3	T36.4X4	T36.4X5	T36.4X6
Clonazepam	T42.4X1	T42.4X2	T42.4X3	T42.4X4	T42.4X5	T42.4X6
Clonidine	T46.5X1	T46.5X2	T46.5X3	T46.5X4	T46.5X5	T46.5X6
Clonixin	T39.8X1	T39.8X2	T39.8X3	T39.8X4	T39.8X5	T39.8X6
Clopamide	T50.2X1	T50.2X2	T50.2X3	T50.2X4	T50.2X5	T50.2X6
Clopenthixol	T43.4X1	T43.4X2	T43.4X3	T43.4X4	T43.4X5	T43.4X6
Cloperastine	T48.3X1	T48.3X2	T48.3X3	T48.3X4	T48.3X5	T48.3X6
Clophedianol	T48.3X1	T48.3X2	T48.3X3	T48.3X4	T48.3X5	T48.3X6
Cloponone	T36.2X1	T36.2X2	T36.2X3	T36.2X4	T36.2X5	T36.2X6
Cloprednol	T38.0X1	T38.0X2	T38.0X3	T38.0X4	T38.0X5	T38.0X6
Cloral betaine	T42.6X1	T42.6X2	T42.6X3	T42.6X4	T42.6X5	T42.6X6
Cloramfenicol	T36.2X1	T36.2X2	T36.2X3	T36.2X4	T36.2X5	T36.2X6
Clorazepate (dipotassium)	T42.4X1	T42.4X2	T42.4X3	T42.4X4	T42.4X5	T42.4X6
Clorexolone	T50.2X1	T50.2X2	T50.2X3	T50.2X4	T50.2X5	T50.2X6
Clorfenamine	T45.0X1	T45.0X2	T45.0X3	T45.0X4	T45.0X5	T45.0X6
Clorgiline	T43.1X1	T43.1X2	T43.1X3	T43.1X4	T43.1X5	T43.1X6
Clorotepine	T44.3X1	T44.3X2	T44.3X3	T44.3X4	T44.3X5	T44.3X6
Clorox (bleach)	T54.91	T54.92	T54.93	T54.94	—	—
Clorprenaline	T48.6X1	T48.6X2	T48.6X3	T48.6X4	T48.6X5	T48.6X6
Clortermine	T50.5X1	T50.5X2	T50.5X3	T50.5X4	T50.5X5	T50.5X6
Clotiapine	T43.591	T43.592	T43.593	T43.594	T43.595	T43.596
Clotiazepam	T42.4X1	T42.4X2	T42.4X3	T42.4X4	T42.4X5	T42.4X6
Clotibric acid	T46.6X1	T46.6X2	T46.6X3	T46.6X4	T46.6X5	T46.6X6
Clotrimazole	T49.0X1	T49.0X2	T49.0X3	T49.0X4	T49.0X5	T49.0X6
Cloxacillin	T36.0X1	T36.0X2	T36.0X3	T36.0X4	T36.0X5	T36.0X6
Cloxazolam	T42.4X1	T42.4X2	T42.4X3	T42.4X4	T42.4X5	T42.4X6
Cloxiquine	T49.0X1	T49.0X2	T49.0X3	T49.0X4	T49.0X5	T49.0X6
Clozapine	T42.4X1	T42.4X2	T42.4X3	T42.4X4	T42.4X5	T42.4X6
Coagulant NEC	T45.7X1	T45.7X2	T45.7X3	T45.7X4	T45.7X5	T45.7X6
Coal (carbon monoxide from) — see also Carbon, monoxide, coal	T58.2X1	T58.2X2	T58.2X3	T58.2X4		
oil — see Kerosene						
tar	T49.1X1	T49.1X2	T49.1X3	T49.1X4	T49.1X5	T49.1X6
fumes	T59.891	T59.892	T59.893	T59.894		
medicinal (ointment)	T49.4X1	T49.4X2	T49.4X3	T49.4X4	T49.4X5	T49.4X6
analgesics NEC	T39.2X1	T39.2X2	T39.2X3	T39.2X4	T39.2X5	T39.2X6
naphtha (solvent)	T52.0X1	T52.0X2	T52.0X3	T52.0X4		
Cobalamine	T45.2X1	T45.2X2	T45.2X3	T45.2X4	T45.2X5	T45.2X6
Cobalt (nonmedicinal) (fumes) (industrial)	T56.891	T56.892	T56.893	T56.894	—	—
medicinal (trace) (chloride)	T45.8X1	T45.8X2	T45.8X3	T45.8X4	T45.8X5	T45.8X6
Cobra (venom)	T63.041	T63.042	T63.043	T63.044	—	—
Coca (leaf)	T40.5X1	T40.5X2	T40.5X3	T40.5X4	T40.5X5	T40.5X6
Cocaine	T40.5X1	T40.5X2	T40.5X3	T40.5X4	T40.5X5	T40.5X6
topical anesthetic	T41.3X1	T41.3X2	T41.3X3	T41.3X4	T41.3X5	T41.3X6
Cocarboxylase	T45.3X1	T45.3X2	T45.3X3	T45.3X4	T45.3X5	T45.3X6
Coccidioidin	T50.8X1	T50.8X2	T50.8X3	T50.8X4	T50.8X5	T50.8X6
Cocculus indicus	T62.1X1	T62.1X2	T62.1X3	T62.1X4	—	—
Cochineal	T65.6X1	T65.6X2	T65.6X3	T65.6X4	—	—
medicinal products	T50.991	T50.992	T50.993	T50.994	T50.995	T50.996
Codeine	T40.2X1	T40.2X2	T40.2X3	T40.2X4	T40.2X5	T40.2X6
Cod-liver oil	T45.2X1	T45.2X2	T45.2X3	T45.2X4	T45.2X5	T45.2X6
Coenzyme A	T50.991	T50.992	T50.993	T50.994	T50.995	T50.996
Coffee	T62.8X1	T62.8X2	T62.8X3	T62.8X4	—	—
Cogalactoisomerase	T50.991	T50.992	T50.993	T50.994	T50.995	T50.996
Cogentin	T44.3X1	T44.3X2	T44.3X3	T44.3X4	T44.3X5	T44.3X6
Coke fumes or gas (carbon monoxide)	T58.2X1	T58.2X2	T58.2X3	T58.2X4		
industrial use	T58.8X1	T58.8X2	T58.8X3	T58.8X4	—	—
Colace	T47.4X1	T47.4X2	T47.4X3	T47.4X4	T47.4X5	T47.4X6
Colaspase	T45.1X1	T45.1X2	T45.1X3	T45.1X4	T45.1X5	T45.1X6
Colchicine	T50.4X1	T50.4X2	T50.4X3	T50.4X4	T50.4X5	T50.4X6
Colchicum	T62.2X1	T62.2X2	T62.2X3	T62.2X4	—	—
Cold cream	T49.3X1	T49.3X2	T49.3X3	T49.3X4	T49.3X5	T49.3X6
Colecalciferol	T45.2X1	T45.2X2	T45.2X3	T45.2X4	T45.2X5	T45.2X6
Colestipol	T46.6X1	T46.6X2	T46.6X3	T46.6X4	T46.6X5	T46.6X6
Colestyramine	T46.6X1	T46.6X2	T46.6X3	T46.6X4	T46.6X5	T46.6X6

Substance	Poisoning, Accidental (unintentional)	Poisoning, Intentional Self-harm	Poisoning, Assault	Poisoning, Undetermined	Adverse Effect	Under-dosing
Colimycin	T36.8X1	T36.8X2	T36.8X3	T36.8X4	T36.8X5	T36.8X6
Colistimethate	T36.8X1	T36.8X2	T36.8X3	T36.8X4	T36.8X5	T36.8X6
Colistin	T36.8X1	T36.8X2	T36.8X3	T36.8X4	T36.8X5	T36.8X6
sulfate (eye preparation)	T49.5X1	T49.5X2	T49.5X3	T49.5X4	T49.5X5	T49.5X6
Collagen	T50.991	T50.992	T50.993	T50.994	T50.995	T50.996
Collagenase	T49.4X1	T49.4X2	T49.4X3	T49.4X4	T49.4X5	T49.4X6
Collodion	T49.3X1	T49.3X2	T49.3X3	T49.3X4	T49.3X5	T49.3X6
Colocynth	T47.2X1	T47.2X2	T47.2X3	T47.2X4	T47.2X5	T47.2X6
Colophony adhesive	T49.3X1	T49.3X2	T49.3X3	T49.3X4	T49.3X5	T49.3X6
Colorant — see also Dye	T50.991	T50.992	T50.993	T50.994	T50.995	T50.996
Coloring matter — see Dye(s)						
Combustion gas (after combustion) — see Carbon, monoxide						
prior to combustion	T59.891	T59.892	T59.893	T59.894	—	—
Compazine	T43.3X1	T43.3X2	T43.3X3	T43.3X4	T43.3X5	T43.3X6
Compound						
1080 (sodium fluoroacetate)	T60.4X1	T60.4X2	T60.4X3	T60.4X4		
269 (endrin)	T60.1X1	T60.1X2	T60.1X3	T60.1X4		
3422 (parathion)	T60.0X1	T60.0X2	T60.0X3	T60.0X4		
3911 (phorate)	T60.0X1	T60.0X2	T60.0X3	T60.0X4		
3956 (toxaphene)	T60.1X1	T60.1X2	T60.1X3	T60.1X4		
4049 (malathion)	T60.0X1	T60.0X2	T60.0X3	T60.0X4		
4069 (malathion)	T60.0X1	T60.0X2	T60.0X3	T60.0X4		
4124 (dicapthon)	T60.0X1	T60.0X2	T60.0X3	T60.0X4		
42 (warfarin)	T60.4X1	T60.4X2	T60.4X3	T60.4X4		
497 (dieldrin)	T60.1X1	T60.1X2	T60.1X3	T60.1X4		
E (cortisone)	T38.0X1	T38.0X2	T38.0X3	T38.0X4	T38.0X5	T38.0X6
F (hydrocortisone)	T38.0X1	T38.0X2	T38.0X3	T38.0X4	T38.0X5	T38.0X6
Congener, anabolic	T38.7X1	T38.7X2	T38.7X3	T38.7X4	T38.7X5	T38.7X6
Congo red	T50.8X1	T50.8X2	T50.8X3	T50.8X4	T50.8X5	T50.8X6
Coniine, conine	T62.2X1	T62.2X2	T62.2X3	T62.2X4		
Conium (maculatum)	T62.2X1	T62.2X2	T62.2X3	T62.2X4		
Conjugated estrogenic substances	T38.5X1	T38.5X2	T38.5X3	T38.5X4	T38.5X5	T38.5X6
Contac	T48.5X1	T48.5X2	T48.5X3	T48.5X4	T48.5X5	T48.5X6
Contact lens solution	T49.5X1	T49.5X2	T49.5X3	T49.5X4	T49.5X5	T49.5X6
Contraceptive (oral)	T38.4X1	T38.4X2	T38.4X3	T38.4X4	T38.4X5	T38.4X6
vaginal	T49.8X1	T49.8X2	T49.8X3	T49.8X4	T49.8X5	T49.8X6
Contrast medium, radiography	T50.8X1	T50.8X2	T50.8X3	T50.8X4	T50.8X5	T50.8X6
Convallaria glycosides	T46.0X1	T46.0X2	T46.0X3	T46.0X4	T46.0X5	T46.0X6
Convallaria majalis	T62.2X1	T62.2X2	T62.2X3	T62.2X4	—	—
berry	T62.1X1	T62.1X2	T62.1X3	T62.1X4	—	—
Copperhead snake (bite) (venom)	T63.061	T63.062	T63.063	T63.064	—	—
Copper (dust) (fumes) (nonmedicinal) NEC	T56.4X1	T56.4X2	T56.4X3	T56.4X4	—	—
arsenate, arsenite	T57.0X1	T57.0X2	T57.0X3	T57.0X4		
insecticide	T60.2X1	T60.2X2	T60.2X3	T60.2X4		
emetic	T47.7X1	T47.7X2	T47.7X3	T47.7X4	T47.7X5	T47.7X6
fungicide	T60.3X1	T60.3X2	T60.3X3	T60.3X4		
gluconate	T49.0X1	T49.0X2	T49.0X3	T49.0X4	T49.0X5	T49.0X6
insecticide	T60.2X1	T60.2X2	T60.2X3	T60.2X4		
medicinal (trace)	T45.8X1	T45.8X2	T45.8X3	T45.8X4	T45.8X5	T45.8X6
oleate	T49.0X1	T49.0X2	T49.0X3	T49.0X4	T49.0X5	T49.0X6
sulfate	T56.4X1	T56.4X2	T56.4X3	T56.4X4		
cupric	T56.4X1	T56.4X2	T56.4X3	T56.4X4		
fungicide	T60.3X1	T60.3X2	T60.3X3	T60.3X4		
medicinal						
ear	T49.6X1	T49.6X2	T49.6X3	T49.6X4	T49.6X5	T49.6X6
emetic	T47.7X1	T47.7X2	T47.7X3	T47.7X4	T47.7X5	T47.7X6
eye	T49.5X1	T49.5X2	T49.5X3	T49.5X4	T49.5X5	T49.5X6
cuprous	T56.4X1	T56.4X2	T56.4X3	T56.4X4		
fungicide	T60.3X1	T60.3X2	T60.3X3	T60.3X4		
medicinal						
ear	T49.6X1	T49.6X2	T49.6X3	T49.6X4	T49.6X5	T49.6X6
emetic	T47.7X1	T47.7X2	T47.7X3	T47.7X4	T47.7X5	T47.7X6
eye	T49.5X1	T49.5X2	T49.5X3	T49.5X4	T49.5X5	T49.5X6
Coral (sting)	T63.691	T63.692	T63.693	T63.694	—	—
snake (bite) (venom)	T63.021	T63.022	T63.023	T63.024	—	—
Corbadrine	T49.6X1	T49.6X2	T49.6X3	T49.6X4	T49.6X5	T49.6X6
Cordite	T65.891	T65.892	T65.893	T65.894	—	—
vapor	T59.891	T59.892	T59.893	T59.894		
Cordran	T49.0X1	T49.0X2	T49.0X3	T49.0X4	T49.0X5	T49.0X6
Corn cures	T49.4X1	T49.4X2	T49.4X3	T49.4X4	T49.4X5	T49.4X6
Cornhusker's lotion	T49.3X1	T49.3X2	T49.3X3	T49.3X4	T49.3X5	T49.3X6
Corn starch	T49.3X1	T49.3X2	T49.3X3	T49.3X4	T49.3X5	T49.3X6
Coronary vasodilator NEC	T46.3X1	T46.3X2	T46.3X3	T46.3X4	T46.3X5	T46.3X6
Corrosive NEC	T54.91	T54.92	T54.93	T54.94	—	—
acid NEC	T54.2X1	T54.2X2	T54.2X3	T54.2X4	—	—
aromatics	T54.1X1	T54.1X2	T54.1X3	T54.1X4	—	—

Corrosive NEC

ICD-10-CM 2022

Table of Drugs and Chemicals

Substance	Poisoning, Accidental (unintentional)	Poisoning, Intentional Self-harm	Poisoning, Assault	Poisoning, Undetermined	Adverse Effect	Under-dosing
Corrosive — *continued*						
aromatics — *continued*						
disinfectant	T54.1X1	T54.1X2	T54.1X3	T54.1X4	—	—
fumes NEC	T54.91	T54.92	T54.93	T54.94	—	—
specified NEC	T54.91	T54.92	T54.93	T54.94	—	—
sublimate	T56.1X1	T56.1X2	T56.1X3	T56.1X4	—	—
Cortate	T38.ØX1	T38.ØX2	T38.ØX3	T38.ØX4	T38.ØX5	T38.ØX6
Cort-Dome	T38.ØX1	T38.ØX2	T38.ØX3	T38.ØX4	T38.ØX5	T38.ØX6
ENT agent	T49.6X1	T49.6X2	T49.6X3	T49.6X4	T49.6X5	T49.6X6
ophthalmic preparation	T49.5X1	T49.5X2	T49.5X3	T49.5X4	T49.5X5	T49.5X6
topical NEC	T49.ØX1	T49.ØX2	T49.ØX3	T49.ØX4	T49.ØX5	T49.ØX6
Cortef	T38.ØX1	T38.ØX2	T38.ØX3	T38.ØX4	T38.ØX5	T38.ØX6
ENT agent	T49.6X1	T49.6X2	T49.6X3	T49.6X4	T49.6X5	T49.6X6
ophthalmic preparation	T49.5X1	T49.5X2	T49.5X3	T49.5X4	T49.5X5	T49.5X6
topical NEC	T49.ØX1	T49.ØX2	T49.ØX3	T49.ØX4	T49.ØX5	T49.ØX6
Corticosteroid	T38.ØX1	T38.ØX2	T38.ØX3	T38.ØX4	T38.ØX5	T38.ØX6
ENT agent	T49.6X1	T49.6X2	T49.6X3	T49.6X4	T49.6X5	T49.6X6
mineral	T5Ø.ØX1	T5Ø.ØX2	T5Ø.ØX3	T5Ø.ØX4	T5Ø.ØX5	T5Ø.ØX6
ophthalmic	T49.5X1	T49.5X2	T49.5X3	T49.5X4	T49.5X5	T49.5X6
topical NEC	T49.ØX1	T49.ØX2	T49.ØX3	T49.ØX4	T49.ØX5	T49.ØX6
Corticotropin	T38.811	T38.812	T38.813	T38.814	T38.815	T38.816
Cortisol	T49.ØX1	T49.ØX2	T49.ØX3	T49.ØX4	T49.ØX5	T49.ØX6
ENT agent	T49.6X1	T49.6X2	T49.6X3	T49.6X4	T49.6X5	T49.6X6
ophthalmic preparation	T49.5X1	T49.5X2	T49.5X3	T49.5X4	T49.5X5	T49.5X6
topical NEC	T49.ØX1	T49.ØX2	T49.ØX3	T49.ØX4	T49.ØX5	T49.ØX6
Cortisone (acetate)	T38.ØX1	T38.ØX2	T38.ØX3	T38.ØX4	T38.ØX5	T38.ØX6
ENT agent	T49.6X1	T49.6X2	T49.6X3	T49.6X4	T49.6X5	T49.6X6
ophthalmic preparation	T49.5X1	T49.5X2	T49.5X3	T49.5X4	T49.5X5	T49.5X6
topical NEC	T49.ØX1	T49.ØX2	T49.ØX3	T49.ØX4	T49.ØX5	T49.ØX6
Cortivazol	T38.ØX1	T38.ØX2	T38.ØX3	T38.ØX4	T38.ØX5	T38.ØX6
Cortogen	T38.ØX1	T38.ØX2	T38.ØX3	T38.ØX4	T38.ØX5	T38.ØX6
ENT agent	T49.6X1	T49.6X2	T49.6X3	T49.6X4	T49.6X5	T49.6X6
ophthalmic preparation	T49.5X1	T49.5X2	T49.5X3	T49.5X4	T49.5X5	T49.5X6
Cortone	T38.ØX1	T38.ØX2	T38.ØX3	T38.ØX4	T38.ØX5	T38.ØX6
ENT agent	T49.6X1	T49.6X2	T49.6X3	T49.6X4	T49.6X5	T49.6X6
ophthalmic preparation	T49.5X1	T49.5X2	T49.5X3	T49.5X4	T49.5X5	T49.5X6
Cortril	T38.ØX1	T38.ØX2	T38.ØX3	T38.ØX4	T38.ØX5	T38.ØX6
ENT agent	T49.6X1	T49.6X2	T49.6X3	T49.6X4	T49.6X5	T49.6X6
ophthalmic preparation	T49.5X1	T49.5X2	T49.5X3	T49.5X4	T49.5X5	T49.5X6
topical NEC	T49.ØX1	T49.ØX2	T49.ØX3	T49.ØX4	T49.ØX5	T49.ØX6
Corynebacterium parvum	T45.1X1	T45.1X2	T45.1X3	T45.1X4	T45.1X5	T45.1X6
Cosmetic preparation	T49.8X1	T49.8X2	T49.8X3	T49.8X4	T49.8X5	T49.8X6
Cosmetics	T49.8X1	T49.8X2	T49.8X3	T49.8X4	T49.8X5	T49.8X6
Cosyntropin	T38.811	T38.812	T38.813	T38.814	T38.815	T38.816
Cotarnine	T45.7X1	T45.7X2	T45.7X3	T45.7X4	T45.7X5	T45.7X6
Co-trimoxazole	T36.8X1	T36.8X2	T36.8X3	T36.8X4	T36.8X5	T36.8X6
Cottonseed oil	T49.3X1	T49.3X2	T49.3X3	T49.3X4	T49.3X5	T49.3X6
Cough mixture (syrup)	T48.4X1	T48.4X2	T48.4X3	T48.4X4	T48.4X5	T48.4X6
containing opiates	T4Ø.2X1	T4Ø.2X2	T4Ø.2X3	T4Ø.2X4	T4Ø.2X5	T4Ø.2X6
expectorants	T48.4X1	T48.4X2	T48.4X3	T48.4X4	T48.4X5	T48.4X6
Coumadin	T45.511	T45.512	T45.513	T45.514	T45.515	T45.516
rodenticide	T6Ø.4X1	T6Ø.4X2	T6Ø.4X3	T6Ø.4X4	—	—
Coumaphos	T6Ø.ØX1	T6Ø.ØX2	T6Ø.ØX3	T6Ø.ØX4	—	—
Coumarin	T45.511	T45.512	T45.513	T45.514	T45.515	T45.516
Coumetarol	T45.511	T45.512	T45.513	T45.514	T45.515	T45.516
Cowbane	T62.2X1	T62.2X2	T62.2X3	T62.2X4	—	—
Cozyme	T45.2X1	T45.2X2	T45.2X3	T45.2X4	T45.2X5	T45.2X6
Crack	T4Ø.5X1	T4Ø.5X2	T4Ø.5X3	T4Ø.5X4	—	—
Crataegus extract	T46.ØX1	T46.ØX2	T46.ØX3	T46.ØX4	T46.ØX5	T46.ØX6
Creolin	T54.1X1	T54.1X2	T54.1X3	T54.1X4	—	—
disinfectant	T54.1X1	T54.1X2	T54.1X3	T54.1X4	—	—
Creosol (compound)	T49.ØX1	T49.ØX2	T49.ØX3	T49.ØX4	T49.ØX5	T49.ØX6
Creosote (coal tar) (beechwood)	T49.ØX1	T49.ØX2	T49.ØX3	T49.ØX4	T49.ØX5	T49.ØX6
medicinal (expectorant)	T48.4X1	T48.4X2	T48.4X3	T48.4X4	T48.4X5	T48.4X6
syrup	T48.4X1	T48.4X2	T48.4X3	T48.4X4	T48.4X5	T48.4X6
Cresol(s)	T49.ØX1	T49.ØX2	T49.ØX3	T49.ØX4	T49.ØX5	T49.ØX6
and soap solution	T49.ØX1	T49.ØX2	T49.ØX3	T49.ØX4	T49.ØX5	T49.ØX6
Cresyl acetate	T49.ØX1	T49.ØX2	T49.ØX3	T49.ØX4	T49.ØX5	T49.ØX6
Cresylic acid	T49.ØX1	T49.ØX2	T49.ØX3	T49.ØX4	T49.ØX5	T49.ØX6
Crimidine	T6Ø.4X1	T6Ø.4X2	T6Ø.4X3	T6Ø.4X4	—	—
Croconazole	T37.8X1	T37.8X2	T37.8X3	T37.8X4	T37.8X5	T37.8X6
Cromoglicic acid	T48.6X1	T48.6X2	T48.6X3	T48.6X4	T48.6X5	T48.6X6
Cromolyn	T48.6X1	T48.6X2	T48.6X3	T48.6X4	T48.6X5	T48.6X6
Cromonar	T46.3X1	T46.3X2	T46.3X3	T46.3X4	T46.3X5	T46.3X6
Cropropamide	T39.8X1	T39.8X2	T39.8X3	T39.8X4	T39.8X5	T39.8X6
with crotethamide	T5Ø.7X1	T5Ø.7X2	T5Ø.7X3	T5Ø.7X4	T5Ø.7X5	T5Ø.7X6
Crotamiton	T49.ØX1	T49.ØX2	T49.ØX3	T49.ØX4	T49.ØX5	T49.ØX6
Crotethamide	T39.8X1	T39.8X2	T39.8X3	T39.8X4	T39.8X5	T39.8X6
with cropropamide	T5Ø.7X1	T5Ø.7X2	T5Ø.7X3	T5Ø.7X4	T5Ø.7X5	T5Ø.7X6
Croton (oil)	T47.2X1	T47.2X2	T47.2X3	T47.2X4	T47.2X5	T47.2X6
chloral	T42.6X1	T42.6X2	T42.6X3	T42.6X4	T42.6X5	T42.6X6
Crude oil	T52.ØX1	T52.ØX2	T52.ØX3	T52.ØX4	—	—
Cryogenine	T39.8X1	T39.8X2	T39.8X3	T39.8X4	T39.8X5	T39.8X6
Cryolite (vapor)	T6Ø.1X1	T6Ø.1X2	T6Ø.1X3	T6Ø.1X4	—	—
insecticide	T6Ø.1X1	T6Ø.1X2	T6Ø.1X3	T6Ø.1X4	—	—
Cryptenamine (tannates)	T46.5X1	T46.5X2	T46.5X3	T46.5X4	T46.5X5	T46.5X6
Crystal violet	T49.ØX1	T49.ØX2	T49.ØX3	T49.ØX4	T49.ØX5	T49.ØX6
Cuckoopint	T62.2X1	T62.2X2	T62.2X3	T62.2X4	—	—
Cumetharol	T45.511	T45.512	T45.513	T45.514	T45.515	T45.516
Cupric						
acetate	T6Ø.3X1	T6Ø.3X2	T6Ø.3X3	T6Ø.3X4	—	—
acetoarsenite	T57.ØX1	T57.ØX2	T57.ØX3	T57.ØX4	—	—
arsenate	T57.ØX1	T57.ØX2	T57.ØX3	T57.ØX4	—	—
gluconate	T49.ØX1	T49.ØX2	T49.ØX3	T49.ØX4	T49.ØX5	T49.ØX6
oleate	T49.ØX1	T49.ØX2	T49.ØX3	T49.ØX4	T49.ØX5	T49.ØX6
sulfate	T56.4X1	T56.4X2	T56.4X3	T56.4X4	—	—
Cuprous sulfate — *see also* Copper sulfate	T56.4X1	T56.4X2	T56.4X3	T56.4X4	—	—
Curare, curarine	T48.1X1	T48.1X2	T48.1X3	T48.1X4	T48.1X5	T48.1X6
Cyamemazine	T43.3X1	T43.3X2	T43.3X3	T43.3X4	T43.3X5	T43.3X6
Cyamopsis tetragonoloba	T46.6X1	T46.6X2	T46.6X3	T46.6X4	T46.6X5	T46.6X6
Cyanacetyl hydrazide	T37.1X1	T37.1X2	T37.1X3	T37.1X4	T37.1X5	T37.1X6
Cyanic acid (gas)	T59.891	T59.892	T59.893	T59.894	—	—
Cyanide(s) (compounds) (potassium) (sodium) **NEC**	T65.ØX1	T65.ØX2	T65.ØX3	T65.ØX4	—	—
dust or gas (inhalation) NEC	T57.3X1	T57.3X2	T57.3X3	T57.3X4	—	—
fumigant	T65.ØX1	T65.ØX2	T65.ØX3	T65.ØX4	—	—
hydrogen	T57.3X1	T57.3X2	T57.3X3	T57.3X4	—	—
mercuric — *see* Mercury						
pesticide (dust) (fumes)	T65.ØX1	T65.ØX2	T65.ØX3	T65.ØX4	—	—
Cyanoacrylate adhesive	T49.3X1	T49.3X2	T49.3X3	T49.3X4	T49.3X5	T49.3X6
Cyanocobalamin	T45.8X1	T45.8X2	T45.8X3	T45.8X4	T45.8X5	T45.8X6
Cyanogen (chloride) (gas) **NEC**	T59.891	T59.892	T59.893	T59.894	—	—
Cyclacillin	T36.ØX1	T36.ØX2	T36.ØX3	T36.ØX4	T36.ØX5	T36.ØX6
Cyclaine	T41.3X1	T41.3X2	T41.3X3	T41.3X4	T41.3X5	T41.3X6
Cyclamate	T5Ø.991	T5Ø.992	T5Ø.993	T5Ø.994	T5Ø.995	T5Ø.996
Cyclamen europaeum	T62.2X1	T62.2X2	T62.2X3	T62.2X4	—	—
Cyclandelate	T46.7X1	T46.7X2	T46.7X3	T46.7X4	T46.7X5	T46.7X6
Cyclazocine	T5Ø.7X1	T5Ø.7X2	T5Ø.7X3	T5Ø.7X4	T5Ø.7X5	T5Ø.7X6
Cyclizine	T45.ØX1	T45.ØX2	T45.ØX3	T45.ØX4	T45.ØX5	T45.ØX6
Cyclobarbital	T42.3X1	T42.3X2	T42.3X3	T42.3X4	T42.3X5	T42.3X6
Cyclobarbitone	T42.3X1	T42.3X2	T42.3X3	T42.3X4	T42.3X5	T42.3X6
Cyclobenzaprine	T48.1X1	T48.1X2	T48.1X3	T48.1X4	T48.1X5	T48.1X6
Cyclodrine	T44.3X1	T44.3X2	T44.3X3	T44.3X4	T44.3X5	T44.3X6
Cycloguanil embonate	T37.2X1	T37.2X2	T37.2X3	T37.2X4	T37.2X5	T37.2X6
Cyclohexane	T52.8X1	T52.8X2	T52.8X3	T52.8X4	—	—
Cyclohexanol	T51.8X1	T51.8X2	T51.8X3	T51.8X4	—	—
Cyclohexanone	T52.4X1	T52.4X2	T52.4X3	T52.4X4	—	—
Cycloheximide	T6Ø.3X1	T6Ø.3X2	T6Ø.3X3	T6Ø.3X4	—	—
Cyclohexyl acetate	T52.8X1	T52.8X2	T52.8X3	T52.8X4	—	—
Cycloleucin	T45.1X1	T45.1X2	T45.1X3	T45.1X4	T45.1X5	T45.1X6
Cyclomethycaine	T41.3X1	T41.3X2	T41.3X3	T41.3X4	T41.3X5	T41.3X6
Cyclopentamine	T44.4X1	T44.4X2	T44.4X3	T44.4X4	T44.4X5	T44.4X6
Cyclopenthiazide	T5Ø.2X1	T5Ø.2X2	T5Ø.2X3	T5Ø.2X4	T5Ø.2X5	T5Ø.2X6
Cyclopentolate	T44.3X1	T44.3X2	T44.3X3	T44.3X4	T44.3X5	T44.3X6
Cyclophosphamide	T45.1X1	T45.1X2	T45.1X3	T45.1X4	T45.1X5	T45.1X6
Cycloplegic drug	T49.5X1	T49.5X2	T49.5X3	T49.5X4	T49.5X5	T49.5X6
Cyclopropane	T41.291	T41.292	T41.293	T41.294	T41.295	T41.296
Cyclopyrabital	T39.8X1	T39.8X2	T39.8X3	T39.8X4	T39.8X5	T39.8X6
Cycloserine	T37.1X1	T37.1X2	T37.1X3	T37.1X4	T37.1X5	T37.1X6
Cyclosporin	T45.1X1	T45.1X2	T45.1X3	T45.1X4	T45.1X5	T45.1X6
Cyclothiazide	T5Ø.2X1	T5Ø.2X2	T5Ø.2X3	T5Ø.2X4	T5Ø.2X5	T5Ø.2X6
Cycrimine	T44.3X1	T44.3X2	T44.3X3	T44.3X4	T44.3X5	T44.3X6
Cyhalothrin	T6Ø.1X1	T6Ø.1X2	T6Ø.1X3	T6Ø.1X4	—	—
Cymarin	T46.ØX1	T46.ØX2	T46.ØX3	T46.ØX4	T46.ØX5	T46.ØX6
Cypermethrin	T6Ø.1X1	T6Ø.1X2	T6Ø.1X3	T6Ø.1X4	—	—
Cyphenothrin	T6Ø.2X1	T6Ø.2X2	T6Ø.2X3	T6Ø.2X4	—	—
Cyproheptadine	T45.ØX1	T45.ØX2	T45.ØX3	T45.ØX4	T45.ØX5	T45.ØX6
Cyproterone	T38.6X1	T38.6X2	T38.6X3	T38.6X4	T38.6X5	T38.6X6
Cysteamine	T5Ø.6X1	T5Ø.6X2	T5Ø.6X3	T5Ø.6X4	T5Ø.6X5	T5Ø.6X6
Cytarabine	T45.1X1	T45.1X2	T45.1X3	T45.1X4	T45.1X5	T45.1X6
Cytisus						
laburnum	T62.2X1	T62.2X2	T62.2X3	T62.2X4	—	—
scoparius	T62.2X1	T62.2X2	T62.2X3	T62.2X4	—	—
Cytochrome C	T47.5X1	T47.5X2	T47.5X3	T47.5X4	T47.5X5	T47.5X6
Cytomel	T38.1X1	T38.1X2	T38.1X3	T38.1X4	T38.1X5	T38.1X6
Cytosine arabinoside	T45.1X1	T45.1X2	T45.1X3	T45.1X4	T45.1X5	T45.1X6
Cytoxan	T45.1X1	T45.1X2	T45.1X3	T45.1X4	T45.1X5	T45.1X6
Cytozyme	T45.7X1	T45.7X2	T45.7X3	T45.7X4	T45.7X5	T45.7X6
S-Carboxymethylcysteine	T48.4X1	T48.4X2	T48.4X3	T48.4X4	T48.4X5	T48.4X6
Dacarbazine	T45.1X1	T45.1X2	T45.1X3	T45.1X4	T45.1X5	T45.1X6
Dactinomycin	T45.1X1	T45.1X2	T45.1X3	T45.1X4	T45.1X5	T45.1X6

Corrosive NEC — Dactinomycin

368

Additional Character May Be Required — Refer to the Tabular List for Character Selection

Subterms under main terms may continue to next column or page

Substance	Poisoning, Accidental (unintentional)	Poisoning, Intentional Self-harm	Poisoning, Assault	Poisoning, Undetermined	Adverse Effect	Under-dosing
DADPS	T37.1X1	T37.1X2	T37.1X3	T37.1X4	T37.1X5	T37.1X6
Dakin's solution	T49.0X1	T49.0X2	T49.0X3	T49.0X4	T49.0X5	T49.0X6
Dalapon (sodium)	T60.3X1	T60.3X2	T60.3X3	T60.3X4	—	—
Dalmane	T42.4X1	T42.4X2	T42.4X3	T42.4X4	T42.4X5	T42.4X6
Danazol	T38.6X1	T38.6X2	T38.6X3	T38.6X4	T38.6X5	T38.6X6
Danilone	T45.511	T45.512	T45.513	T45.514	T45.515	T45.516
Danthron	T47.2X1	T47.2X2	T47.2X3	T47.2X4	T47.2X5	T47.2X6
Dantrolene	T42.8X1	T42.8X2	T42.8X3	T42.8X4	T42.8X5	T42.8X6
Dantron	T47.2X1	T47.2X2	T47.2X3	T47.2X4	T47.2X5	T47.2X6
Daphne (gnidium) (mezereum)	T62.2X1	T62.2X2	T62.2X3	T62.2X4	—	—
berry	T62.1X1	T62.1X2	T62.1X3	T62.1X4	—	—
Dapsone	T37.1X1	T37.1X2	T37.1X3	T37.1X4	T37.1X5	T37.1X6
Daraprim	T37.2X1	T37.2X2	T37.2X3	T37.2X4	T37.2X5	T37.2X6
Darnel	T62.2X1	T62.2X2	T62.2X3	T62.2X4	—	—
Darvon	T39.8X1	T39.8X2	T39.8X3	T39.8X4	T39.8X5	T39.8X6
Daunomycin	T45.1X1	T45.1X2	T45.1X3	T45.1X4	T45.1X5	T45.1X6
Daunorubicin	T45.1X1	T45.1X2	T45.1X3	T45.1X4	T45.1X5	T45.1X6
DBI	T38.3X1	T38.3X2	T38.3X3	T38.3X4	T38.3X5	T38.3X6
D-Con	T60.91	T60.92	T60.93	T60.94	—	—
insecticide	T60.2X1	T60.2X2	T60.2X3	T60.2X4	—	—
rodenticide	T60.4X1	T60.4X2	T60.4X3	T60.4X4	—	—
DDAVP	T38.891	T38.892	T38.893	T38.894	T38.895	T38.896
DDE (bis(chlorophenyl)-dichloroethylene)	T60.2X1	T60.2X2	T60.2X3	T60.2X4	—	—
DDS	T37.1X1	T37.1X2	T37.1X3	T37.1X4	T37.1X5	T37.1X6
DDT (dust)	T60.1X1	T60.1X2	T60.1X3	T60.1X4	—	—
Deadly nightshade — see also Belladonna	T62.2X1	T62.2X2	T62.2X3	T62.2X4	—	—
berry	T62.1X1	T62.1X2	T62.1X3	T62.1X4	—	—
Deamino-D-arginine vasopressin	T38.891	T38.892	T38.893	T38.894	T38.895	T38.896
Deanol (aceglumate)	T50.991	T50.992	T50.993	T50.994	T50.995	T50.996
Debrisoquine	T46.5X1	T46.5X2	T46.5X3	T46.5X4	T46.5X5	T46.5X6
Decaborane	T57.8X1	T57.8X2	T57.8X3	T57.8X4	—	—
fumes	T59.891	T59.892	T59.893	T59.894	—	—
Decadron	T38.0X1	T38.0X2	T38.0X3	T38.0X4	T38.0X5	T38.0X6
ENT agent	T49.6X1	T49.6X2	T49.6X3	T49.6X4	T49.6X5	T49.6X6
ophthalmic preparation	T49.5X1	T49.5X2	T49.5X3	T49.5X4	T49.5X5	T49.5X6
topical NEC	T49.0X1	T49.0X2	T49.0X3	T49.0X4	T49.0X5	T49.0X6
Decahydronaphthalene	T52.8X1	T52.8X2	T52.8X3	T52.8X4	—	—
Decalin	T52.8X1	T52.8X2	T52.8X3	T52.8X4	—	—
Decamethonium (bromide)	T48.1X1	T48.1X2	T48.1X3	T48.1X4	T48.1X5	T48.1X6
Decholin	T47.5X1	T47.5X2	T47.5X3	T47.5X4	T47.5X5	T47.5X6
Declomycin	T36.4X1	T36.4X2	T36.4X3	T36.4X4	T36.4X5	T36.4X6
Decongestant, nasal (mucosa)	T48.5X1	T48.5X2	T48.5X3	T48.5X4	T48.5X5	T48.5X6
combination	T48.5X1	T48.5X2	T48.5X3	T48.5X4	T48.5X5	T48.5X6
Deet	T60.8X1	T60.8X2	T60.8X3	T60.8X4	—	—
Deferoxamine	T45.8X1	T45.8X2	T45.8X3	T45.8X4	T45.8X5	T45.8X6
Deflazacort	T38.0X1	T38.0X2	T38.0X3	T38.0X4	T38.0X5	T38.0X6
Deglycyrrhizinized extract of licorice	T48.4X1	T48.4X2	T48.4X3	T48.4X4	T48.4X5	T48.4X6
Dehydrocholic acid	T47.5X1	T47.5X2	T47.5X3	T47.5X4	T47.5X5	T47.5X6
Dehydroemetine	T37.3X1	T37.3X2	T37.3X3	T37.3X4	T37.3X5	T37.3X6
Dekalin	T52.8X1	T52.8X2	T52.8X3	T52.8X4	—	—
Delalutin	T38.5X1	T38.5X2	T38.5X3	T38.5X4	T38.5X5	T38.5X6
Delorazepam	T42.4X1	T42.4X2	T42.4X3	T42.4X4	T42.4X5	T42.4X6
Delphinium	T62.2X1	T62.2X2	T62.2X3	T62.2X4	—	—
Deltamethrin	T60.1X1	T60.1X2	T60.1X3	T60.1X4	—	—
Deltasone	T38.0X1	T38.0X2	T38.0X3	T38.0X4	T38.0X5	T38.0X6
Deltra	T38.0X1	T38.0X2	T38.0X3	T38.0X4	T38.0X5	T38.0X6
Delvinal	T42.3X1	T42.3X2	T42.3X3	T42.3X4	T42.3X5	T42.3X6
Demecarium (bromide)	T49.5X1	T49.5X2	T49.5X3	T49.5X4	T49.5X5	T49.5X6
Demeclocycline	T36.4X1	T36.4X2	T36.4X3	T36.4X4	T36.4X5	T36.4X6
Demecolcine	T45.1X1	T45.1X2	T45.1X3	T45.1X4	T45.1X5	T45.1X6
Demegestone	T38.5X1	T38.5X2	T38.5X3	T38.5X4	T38.5X5	T38.5X6
Demelanizing agents	T49.8X1	T49.8X2	T49.8X3	T49.8X4	T49.8X5	T49.8X6
Demephion -O and -S	T60.0X1	T60.0X2	T60.0X3	T60.0X4	—	—
Demerol	T40.2X1	T40.2X2	T40.2X3	T40.2X4	T40.2X5	T40.2X6
Demethylchlortetracycline	T36.4X1	T36.4X2	T36.4X3	T36.4X4	T36.4X5	T36.4X6
Demethyltetracycline	T36.4X1	T36.4X2	T36.4X3	T36.4X4	T36.4X5	T36.4X6
Demeton -O and -S	T60.0X1	T60.0X2	T60.0X3	T60.0X4	—	—
Demulcent (external)	T49.3X1	T49.3X2	T49.3X3	T49.3X4	T49.3X5	T49.3X6
specified NEC	T49.3X1	T49.3X2	T49.3X3	T49.3X4	T49.3X5	T49.3X6
Demulen	T38.4X1	T38.4X2	T38.4X3	T38.4X4	T38.4X5	T38.4X6
Denatured alcohol	T51.0X1	T51.0X2	T51.0X3	T51.0X4	—	—
Dendrid	T49.5X1	T49.5X2	T49.5X3	T49.5X4	T49.5X5	T49.5X6
Dental drug, topical application NEC	T49.7X1	T49.7X2	T49.7X3	T49.7X4	T49.7X5	T49.7X6
Dentifrice	T49.7X1	T49.7X2	T49.7X3	T49.7X4	T49.7X5	T49.7X6
Deodorant spray (feminine hygiene)	T49.8X1	T49.8X2	T49.8X3	T49.8X4	T49.8X5	T49.8X6

Substance	Poisoning, Accidental (unintentional)	Poisoning, Intentional Self-harm	Poisoning, Assault	Poisoning, Undetermined	Adverse Effect	Under-dosing
Deoxycortone	T50.0X1	T50.0X2	T50.0X3	T50.0X4	T50.0X5	T50.0X6
Deoxyribonuclease (pancreatic)	T45.3X1	T45.3X2	T45.3X3	T45.3X4	T45.3X5	T45.3X6
Depilatory	T49.4X1	T49.4X2	T49.4X3	T49.4X4	T49.4X5	T49.4X6
Deprenalin	T42.8X1	T42.8X2	T42.8X3	T42.8X4	T42.8X5	T42.8X6
Deprenyl	T42.8X1	T42.8X2	T42.8X3	T42.8X4	T42.8X5	T42.8X6
Depressant						
appetite (central)	T50.5X1	T50.5X2	T50.5X3	T50.5X4	T50.5X5	T50.5X6
cardiac	T46.2X1	T46.2X2	T46.2X3	T46.2X4	T46.2X5	T46.2X6
central nervous system (anesthetic) — see also Central nervous system, depressants	T42.71	T42.72	T42.73	T42.74	T42.75	T42.76
general anesthetic	T41.201	T41.202	T41.203	T41.204	T41.205	T41.206
muscle tone	T42.8X1	T42.8X2	T42.8X3	T42.8X4	T42.8X5	T42.8X6
muscle tone, central	T42.8X1	T42.8X2	T42.8X3	T42.8X4	T42.8X5	T42.8X6
psychotherapeutic	T43.501	T43.502	T43.503	T43.504	T43.505	T43.506
Depressant, appetite	T50.5X1	T50.5X2	T50.5X3	T50.5X4	T50.5X5	T50.5X6
Deptropine	T45.0X1	T45.0X2	T45.0X3	T45.0X4	T45.0X5	T45.0X6
Dequalinium (chloride)	T49.0X1	T49.0X2	T49.0X3	T49.0X4	T49.0X5	T49.0X6
Derris root	T60.2X1	T60.2X2	T60.2X3	T60.2X4	—	—
Deserpidine	T46.5X1	T46.5X2	T46.5X3	T46.5X4	T46.5X5	T46.5X6
Desferrioxamine	T45.8X1	T45.8X2	T45.8X3	T45.8X4	T45.8X5	T45.8X6
Desipramine	T43.011	T43.012	T43.013	T43.014	T43.015	T43.016
Deslanoside	T46.0X1	T46.0X2	T46.0X3	T46.0X4	T46.0X5	T46.0X6
Desloughing agent	T49.4X1	T49.4X2	T49.4X3	T49.4X4	T49.4X5	T49.4X6
Desmethylimipramine	T43.011	T43.012	T43.013	T43.014	T43.015	T43.016
Desmopressin	T38.891	T38.892	T38.893	T38.894	T38.895	T38.896
Desocodeine	T40.2X1	T40.2X2	T40.2X3	T40.2X4	T40.2X5	T40.2X6
Desogestrel	T38.5X1	T38.5X2	T38.5X3	T38.5X4	T38.5X5	T38.5X6
Desomorphine	T40.2X1	T40.2X2	T40.2X3	T40.2X4	—	—
Desonide	T49.0X1	T49.0X2	T49.0X3	T49.0X4	T49.0X5	T49.0X6
Desoximetasone	T49.0X1	T49.0X2	T49.0X3	T49.0X4	T49.0X5	T49.0X6
Desoxycorticosteroid	T50.0X1	T50.0X2	T50.0X3	T50.0X4	T50.0X5	T50.0X6
Desoxycortone	T50.0X1	T50.0X2	T50.0X3	T50.0X4	T50.0X5	T50.0X6
Desoxyephedrine	T43.621	T43.622	T43.623	T43.624	T43.625	T43.626
Detaxtran	T46.6X1	T46.6X2	T46.6X3	T46.6X4	T46.6X5	T46.6X6
Detergent	T49.2X1	T49.2X2	T49.2X3	T49.2X4	T49.2X5	T49.2X6
external medication	T49.2X1	T49.2X2	T49.2X3	T49.2X4	T49.2X5	T49.2X6
local	T49.2X1	T49.2X2	T49.2X3	T49.2X4	T49.2X5	T49.2X6
medicinal	T49.2X1	T49.2X2	T49.2X3	T49.2X4	T49.2X5	T49.2X6
nonmedicinal	T55.1X1	T55.1X2	T55.1X3	T55.1X4	—	—
specified NEC	T55.1X1	T55.1X2	T55.1X3	T55.1X4	—	—
Deterrent, alcohol	T50.6X1	T50.6X2	T50.6X3	T50.6X4	T50.6X5	T50.6X6
Detoxifying agent	T50.6X1	T50.6X2	T50.6X3	T50.6X4	T50.6X5	T50.6X6
Detrothyronine	T38.1X1	T38.1X2	T38.1X3	T38.1X4	T38.1X5	T38.1X6
Dettol (external medication)	T49.0X1	T49.0X2	T49.0X3	T49.0X4	T49.0X5	T49.0X6
Dexamethasone	T38.0X1	T38.0X2	T38.0X3	T38.0X4	T38.0X5	T38.0X6
ENT agent	T49.6X1	T49.6X2	T49.6X3	T49.6X4	T49.6X5	T49.6X6
ophthalmic preparation	T49.5X1	T49.5X2	T49.5X3	T49.5X4	T49.5X5	T49.5X6
topical NEC	T49.0X1	T49.0X2	T49.0X3	T49.0X4	T49.0X5	T49.0X6
Dexamfetamine	T43.621	T43.622	T43.623	T43.624	T43.625	T43.626
Dexamphetamine	T43.621	T43.622	T43.623	T43.624	T43.625	T43.626
Dexbrompheniramine	T45.0X1	T45.0X2	T45.0X3	T45.0X4	T45.0X5	T45.0X6
Dexchlorpheniramine	T45.0X1	T45.0X2	T45.0X3	T45.0X4	T45.0X5	T45.0X6
Dexedrine	T43.621	T43.622	T43.623	T43.624	T43.625	T43.626
Dexetimide	T44.3X1	T44.3X2	T44.3X3	T44.3X4	T44.3X5	T44.3X6
Dexfenfluramine	T50.5X1	T50.5X2	T50.5X3	T50.5X4	T50.5X5	T50.5X6
Dexpanthenol	T45.2X1	T45.2X2	T45.2X3	T45.2X4	T45.2X5	T45.2X6
Dextran (40) (70) (150)	T45.8X1	T45.8X2	T45.8X3	T45.8X4	T45.8X5	T45.8X6
Dextriferron	T45.4X1	T45.4X2	T45.4X3	T45.4X4	T45.4X5	T45.4X6
Dextroamphetamine	T43.621	T43.622	T43.623	T43.624	T43.625	T43.626
Dextro calcium pantothenate	T45.2X1	T45.2X2	T45.2X3	T45.2X4	T45.2X5	T45.2X6
Dextromethorphan	T48.3X1	T48.3X2	T48.3X3	T48.3X4	T48.3X5	T48.3X6
Dextromoramide	T40.491	T40.492	T40.493	T40.494	—	—
topical	T49.8X1	T49.8X2	T49.8X3	T49.8X4	T49.8X5	T49.8X6
Dextro pantothenyl alcohol	T45.2X1	T45.2X2	T45.2X3	T45.2X4	T45.2X5	T45.2X6
Dextropropoxyphene	T40.491	T40.492	T40.493	T40.494	T40.495	T40.496
Dextrorphan	T40.2X1	T40.2X2	T40.2X3	T40.2X4	T40.2X5	T40.2X6
Dextrose	T50.3X1	T50.3X2	T50.3X3	T50.3X4	T50.3X5	T50.3X6
concentrated solution, intravenous	T46.8X1	T46.8X2	T46.8X3	T46.8X4	T46.8X5	T46.8X6
Dextrothyroxin	T38.1X1	T38.1X2	T38.1X3	T38.1X4	T38.1X5	T38.1X6
Dextrothyroxine sodium	T38.1X1	T38.1X2	T38.1X3	T38.1X4	T38.1X5	T38.1X6
DFP	T44.0X1	T44.0X2	T44.0X3	T44.0X4	T44.0X5	T44.0X6
DHE	T37.3X1	T37.3X2	T37.3X3	T37.3X4	T37.3X5	T37.3X6
45	T46.5X1	T46.5X2	T46.5X3	T46.5X4	T46.5X5	T46.5X6
Diabinese	T38.3X1	T38.3X2	T38.3X3	T38.3X4	T38.3X5	T38.3X6
Diacetone alcohol	T52.4X1	T52.4X2	T52.4X3	T52.4X4	—	—
Diacetyl monoxime	T50.991	T50.992	T50.993	T50.994	—	—
Diacetylmorphine	T40.1X1	T40.1X2	T40.1X3	T40.1X4	—	—

Substance	Poisoning, Accidental (unintentional)	Poisoning, Intentional Self-harm	Poisoning, Assault	Poisoning, Undetermined	Adverse Effect	Under-dosing
Diachylon plaster	T49.4X1	T49.4X2	T49.4X3	T49.4X4	T49.4X5	T49.4X6
Diaethylstilboestrolum	T38.5X1	T38.5X2	T38.5X3	T38.5X4	T38.5X5	T38.5X6
Diagnostic agent NEC	T5Ø.8X1	T5Ø.8X2	T5Ø.8X3	T5Ø.8X4	T5Ø.8X5	T5Ø.8X6
Dial (soap)	T49.2X1	T49.2X2	T49.2X3	T49.2X4	T49.2X5	T49.2X6
sedative	T42.3X1	T42.3X2	T42.3X3	T42.3X4	T42.3X5	T42.3X6
Dialkyl carbonate	T52.91	T52.92	T52.93	T52.94	—	—
Diallylbarbituric acid	T42.3X1	T42.3X2	T42.3X3	T42.3X4	T42.3X5	T42.3X6
Diallymal	T42.3X1	T42.3X2	T42.3X3	T42.3X4	T42.3X5	T42.3X6
Dialysis solution (intraperitoneal)	T5Ø.3X1	T5Ø.3X2	T5Ø.3X3	T5Ø.3X4	T5Ø.3X5	T5Ø.3X6
Diaminodiphenylsulfone	T37.1X1	T37.1X2	T37.1X3	T37.1X4	T37.1X5	T37.1X6
Diamorphine	T4Ø.1X1	T4Ø.1X2	T4Ø.1X3	T4Ø.1X4	—	—
Diamox	T5Ø.2X1	T5Ø.2X2	T5Ø.2X3	T5Ø.2X4	T5Ø.2X5	T5Ø.2X6
Diamthazole	T49.ØX1	T49.ØX2	T49.ØX3	T49.ØX4	T49.ØX5	T49.ØX6
Dianthone	T47.2X1	T47.2X2	T47.2X3	T47.2X4	T47.2X5	T47.2X6
Diaphenylsulfone	T37.ØX1	T37.ØX2	T37.ØX3	T37.ØX4	T37.ØX5	T37.ØX6
Diasone (sodium)	T37.1X1	T37.1X2	T37.1X3	T37.1X4	T37.1X5	T37.1X6
Diastase	T47.5X1	T47.5X2	T47.5X3	T47.5X4	T47.5X5	T47.5X6
Diatrizoate	T5Ø.8X1	T5Ø.8X2	T5Ø.8X3	T5Ø.8X4	T5Ø.8X5	T5Ø.8X6
Diazepam	T42.4X1	T42.4X2	T42.4X3	T42.4X4	T42.4X5	T42.4X6
Diazinon	T6Ø.ØX1	T6Ø.ØX2	T6Ø.ØX3	T6Ø.ØX4	—	—
Diazomethane (gas)	T59.891	T59.892	T59.893	T59.894	—	—
Diazoxide	T46.5X1	T46.5X2	T46.5X3	T46.5X4	T46.5X5	T46.5X6
Dibekacin	T36.5X1	T36.5X2	T36.5X3	T36.5X4	T36.5X5	T36.5X6
Dibenamine	T44.6X1	T44.6X2	T44.6X3	T44.6X4	T44.6X5	T44.6X6
Dibenzepin	T43.Ø11	T43.Ø12	T43.Ø13	T43.Ø14	T43.Ø15	T43.Ø16
Dibenzheptropine	T45.ØX1	T45.ØX2	T45.ØX3	T45.ØX4	T45.ØX5	T45.ØX6
Dibenzyline	T44.6X1	T44.6X2	T44.6X3	T44.6X4	T44.6X5	T44.6X6
Diborane (gas)	T59.891	T59.892	T59.893	T59.894	—	—
Dibromochloropropane	T6Ø.8X1	T6Ø.8X2	T6Ø.8X3	T6Ø.8X4	—	—
Dibromodulcitol	T45.1X1	T45.1X2	T45.1X3	T45.1X4	T45.1X5	T45.1X6
Dibromoethane	T53.6X1	T53.6X2	T53.6X3	T53.6X4	—	—
Dibromomannitol	T45.1X1	T45.1X2	T45.1X3	T45.1X4	T45.1X5	T45.1X6
Dibromopropamidine isethionate	T49.ØX1	T49.ØX2	T49.ØX3	T49.ØX4	T49.ØX5	T49.ØX6
Dibrompropamidine	T49.ØX1	T49.ØX2	T49.ØX3	T49.ØX4	T49.ØX5	T49.ØX6
Dibucaine	T41.3X1	T41.3X2	T41.3X3	T41.3X4	T41.3X5	T41.3X6
topical (surface)	T41.3X1	T41.3X2	T41.3X3	T41.3X4	T41.3X5	T41.3X6
Dibunate sodium	T48.3X1	T48.3X2	T48.3X3	T48.3X4	T48.3X5	T48.3X6
Dibutoline sulfate	T44.3X1	T44.3X2	T44.3X3	T44.3X4	T44.3X5	T44.3X6
Dicamba	T6Ø.3X1	T6Ø.3X2	T6Ø.3X3	T6Ø.3X4	—	—
Dicapthon	T6Ø.ØX1	T6Ø.ØX2	T6Ø.ØX3	T6Ø.ØX4	—	—
Dichlobenil	T6Ø.3X1	T6Ø.3X2	T6Ø.3X3	T6Ø.3X4	—	—
Dichlone	T6Ø.3X1	T6Ø.3X2	T6Ø.3X3	T6Ø.3X4	—	—
Dichloralphenozone	T42.6X1	T42.6X2	T42.6X3	T42.6X4	T42.6X5	T42.6X6
Dichlorbenzidine	T65.3X1	T65.3X2	T65.3X3	T65.3X4	—	—
Dichlorhydrin	T52.8X1	T52.8X2	T52.8X3	T52.8X4	—	—
Dichlorhydroxyquinoline	T37.8X1	T37.8X2	T37.8X3	T37.8X4	T37.8X5	T37.8X6
Dichlorobenzene	T53.7X1	T53.7X2	T53.7X3	T53.7X4	—	—
Dichlorobenzyl alcohol	T49.6X1	T49.6X2	T49.6X3	T49.6X4	T49.6X5	T49.6X6
Dichlorodifluoromethane	T53.5X1	T53.5X2	T53.5X3	T53.5X4	—	—
Dichloroethane	T52.8X1	T52.8X2	T52.8X3	T52.8X4	—	—
Dichloroethylene	T53.6X1	T53.6X2	T53.6X3	T53.6X4	—	—
Dichloroethyl sulfide, not in war	T59.891	T59.892	T59.893	T59.894	—	—
Dichloroformoxine, not in war	T59.891	T59.892	T59.893	T59.894	—	—
Dichlorohydrin, alpha-dichlorohydrin	T52.8X1	T52.8X2	T52.8X3	T52.8X4	—	—
Dichloromethane (solvent)	T53.4X1	T53.4X2	T53.4X3	T53.4X4	—	—
vapor	T53.4X1	T53.4X2	T53.4X3	T53.4X4	—	—
Dichloronaphthoquinone	T6Ø.3X1	T6Ø.3X2	T6Ø.3X3	T6Ø.3X4	—	—
Dichlorophen	T37.4X1	T37.4X2	T37.4X3	T37.4X4	T37.4X5	T37.4X6
Dichloropropene	T6Ø.3X1	T6Ø.3X2	T6Ø.3X3	T6Ø.3X4	—	—
Dichloropropionic acid	T6Ø.3X1	T6Ø.3X2	T6Ø.3X3	T6Ø.3X4	—	—
Dichlorphenamide	T5Ø.2X1	T5Ø.2X2	T5Ø.2X3	T5Ø.2X4	T5Ø.2X5	T5Ø.2X6
Dichlorvos	T6Ø.ØX1	T6Ø.ØX2	T6Ø.ØX3	T6Ø.ØX4	—	—
Diclofenac	T39.391	T39.392	T39.393	T39.394	T39.395	T39.396
Diclofenamide	T5Ø.2X1	T5Ø.2X2	T5Ø.2X3	T5Ø.2X4	T5Ø.2X5	T5Ø.2X6
Diclofensine	T43.291	T43.292	T43.293	T43.294	T43.295	T43.296
Diclonixine	T39.8X1	T39.8X2	T39.8X3	T39.8X4	T39.8X5	T39.8X6
Dicloxacillin	T36.ØX1	T36.ØX2	T36.ØX3	T36.ØX4	T36.ØX5	T36.ØX6
Dicophane	T49.ØX1	T49.ØX2	T49.ØX3	T49.ØX4	T49.ØX5	T49.ØX6
Dicoumarol, dicoumarin, dicumarol	T45.511	T45.512	T45.513	T45.514	T45.515	T45.516
Dicrotophos	T6Ø.ØX1	T6Ø.ØX2	T6Ø.ØX3	T6Ø.ØX4	—	—
Dicyanogen (gas)	T65.ØX1	T65.ØX2	T65.ØX3	T65.ØX4	—	—
Dicyclomine	T44.3X1	T44.3X2	T44.3X3	T44.3X4	T44.3X5	T44.3X6
Dicycloverine	T44.3X1	T44.3X2	T44.3X3	T44.3X4	T44.3X5	T44.3X6
Dideoxycytidine	T37.5X1	T37.5X2	T37.5X3	T37.5X4	T37.5X5	T37.5X6
Dideoxyinosine	T37.5X1	T37.5X2	T37.5X3	T37.5X4	T37.5X5	T37.5X6
Dieldrin (vapor)	T6Ø.1X1	T6Ø.1X2	T6Ø.1X3	T6Ø.1X4	—	—
Diemal	T42.3X1	T42.3X2	T42.3X3	T42.3X4	T42.3X5	T42.3X6

Substance	Poisoning, Accidental (unintentional)	Poisoning, Intentional Self-harm	Poisoning, Assault	Poisoning, Undetermined	Adverse Effect	Under-dosing
Dienestrol	T38.5X1	T38.5X2	T38.5X3	T38.5X4	T38.5X5	T38.5X6
Dienoestrol	T38.5X1	T38.5X2	T38.5X3	T38.5X4	T38.5X5	T38.5X6
Dietetic drug NEC	T5Ø.9Ø1	T5Ø.9Ø2	T5Ø.9Ø3	T5Ø.9Ø4	T5Ø.9Ø5	T5Ø.9Ø6
Diethazine	T42.8X1	T42.8X2	T42.8X3	T42.8X4	T42.8X5	T42.8X6
Diethyl						
barbituric acid	T42.3X1	T42.3X2	T42.3X3	T42.3X4	T42.3X5	T42.3X6
carbamazine	T37.4X1	T37.4X2	T37.4X3	T37.4X4	T37.4X5	T37.4X6
carbinol	T51.3X1	T51.3X2	T51.3X3	T51.3X4	—	—
carbonate	T52.8X1	T52.8X2	T52.8X3	T52.8X4	—	—
ether (vapor) — *see also* ether	T41.ØX1	T41.ØX2	T41.ØX3	T41.ØX4	T41.ØX5	T41.ØX6
oxide	T52.8X1	T52.8X2	T52.8X3	T52.8X4	—	—
propion	T5Ø.5X1	T5Ø.5X2	T5Ø.5X3	T5Ø.5X4	T5Ø.5X5	T5Ø.5X6
stilbestrol	T38.5X1	T38.5X2	T38.5X3	T38.5X4	T38.5X5	T38.5X6
toluamide (nonmedicinal)	T6Ø.8X1	T6Ø.8X2	T6Ø.8X3	T6Ø.8X4	—	—
medicinal	T49.3X1	T49.3X2	T49.3X3	T49.3X4	T49.3X5	T49.3X6
Diethylcarbamazine	T37.4X1	T37.4X2	T37.4X3	T37.4X4	T37.4X5	T37.4X6
Diethylene						
dioxide	T52.8X1	T52.8X2	T52.8X3	T52.8X4	—	—
glycol (monoacetate) (monobutyl ether) (monoethyl ether)	T52.3X1	T52.3X2	T52.3X3	T52.3X4	—	—
Diethylhexylphthalate	T65.891	T65.892	T65.893	T65.894	—	—
Diethylpropion	T5Ø.5X1	T5Ø.5X2	T5Ø.5X3	T5Ø.5X4	T5Ø.5X5	T5Ø.5X6
Diethylstilbestrol	T38.5X1	T38.5X2	T38.5X3	T38.5X4	T38.5X5	T38.5X6
Diethylstilboestrol	T38.5X1	T38.5X2	T38.5X3	T38.5X4	T38.5X5	T38.5X6
Diethylsulfone-diethylmethane	T42.6X1	T42.6X2	T42.6X3	T42.6X4	T42.6X5	T42.6X6
Diethyltoluamide	T49.ØX1	T49.ØX2	T49.ØX3	T49.ØX4	T49.ØX5	T49.ØX6
Diethyltryptamine (DET)	T4Ø.991	T4Ø.992	T4Ø.993	T4Ø.994	—	—
Difebarbamate	T42.3X1	T42.3X2	T42.3X3	T42.3X4	T42.3X5	T42.3X6
Difencloxazine	T4Ø.2X1	T4Ø.2X2	T4Ø.2X3	T4Ø.2X4	T4Ø.2X5	T4Ø.2X6
Difenidol	T45.ØX1	T45.ØX2	T45.ØX3	T45.ØX4	T45.ØX5	T45.ØX6
Difenoxin	T47.6X1	T47.6X2	T47.6X3	T47.6X4	T47.6X5	T47.6X6
Difetarsone	T37.3X1	T37.3X2	T37.3X3	T37.3X4	T37.3X5	T37.3X6
Diffusin	T45.3X1	T45.3X2	T45.3X3	T45.3X4	T45.3X5	T45.3X6
Diflorasone	T49.ØX1	T49.ØX2	T49.ØX3	T49.ØX4	T49.ØX5	T49.ØX6
Diflos	T44.ØX1	T44.ØX2	T44.ØX3	T44.ØX4	T44.ØX5	T44.ØX6
Diflubenzuron	T6Ø.1X1	T6Ø.1X2	T6Ø.1X3	T6Ø.1X4	—	—
Diflucortolone	T49.ØX1	T49.ØX2	T49.ØX3	T49.ØX4	T49.ØX5	T49.ØX6
Diflunisal	T39.Ø91	T39.Ø92	T39.Ø93	T39.Ø94	T39.Ø95	T39.Ø96
Difluoromethyldopa	T42.8X1	T42.8X2	T42.8X3	T42.8X4	T42.8X5	T42.8X6
Difluorophate	T44.ØX1	T44.ØX2	T44.ØX3	T44.ØX4	T44.ØX5	T44.ØX6
Digestant NEC	T47.5X1	T47.5X2	T47.5X3	T47.5X4	T47.5X5	T47.5X6
Digitalin (e)	T46.ØX1	T46.ØX2	T46.ØX3	T46.ØX4	T46.ØX5	T46.ØX6
Digitalis (leaf)(glycoside)	T46.ØX1	T46.ØX2	T46.ØX3	T46.ØX4	T46.ØX5	T46.ØX6
lanata	T46.ØX1	T46.ØX2	T46.ØX3	T46.ØX4	T46.ØX5	T46.ØX6
purpurea	T46.ØX1	T46.ØX2	T46.ØX3	T46.ØX4	T46.ØX5	T46.ØX6
Digitoxin	T46.ØX1	T46.ØX2	T46.ØX3	T46.ØX4	T46.ØX5	T46.ØX6
Digitoxose	T46.ØX1	T46.ØX2	T46.ØX3	T46.ØX4	T46.ØX5	T46.ØX6
Digoxin	T46.ØX1	T46.ØX2	T46.ØX3	T46.ØX4	T46.ØX5	T46.ØX6
Digoxine	T46.ØX1	T46.ØX2	T46.ØX3	T46.ØX4	T46.ØX5	T46.ØX6
Dihydralazine	T46.5X1	T46.5X2	T46.5X3	T46.5X4	T46.5X5	T46.5X6
Dihydrazine	T46.5X1	T46.5X2	T46.5X3	T46.5X4	T46.5X5	T46.5X6
Dihydrocodeine	T4Ø.2X1	T4Ø.2X2	T4Ø.2X3	T4Ø.2X4	T4Ø.2X5	T4Ø.2X6
Dihydrocodeinone	T4Ø.2X1	T4Ø.2X2	T4Ø.2X3	T4Ø.2X4	T4Ø.2X5	T4Ø.2X6
Dihydroergocornine	T46.7X1	T46.7X2	T46.7X3	T46.7X4	T46.7X5	T46.7X6
Dihydroergocristine (mesilate)	T46.7X1	T46.7X2	T46.7X3	T46.7X4	T46.7X5	T46.7X6
Dihydroergokryptine	T46.7X1	T46.7X2	T46.7X3	T46.7X4	T46.7X5	T46.7X6
Dihydroergotamine	T46.5X1	T46.5X2	T46.5X3	T46.5X4	T46.5X5	T46.5X6
Dihydroergotoxine	T46.7X1	T46.7X2	T46.7X3	T46.7X4	T46.7X5	T46.7X6
mesilate	T46.7X1	T46.7X2	T46.7X3	T46.7X4	T46.7X5	T46.7X6
Dihydrohydroxycodeinone	T4Ø.2X1	T4Ø.2X2	T4Ø.2X3	T4Ø.2X4	T4Ø.2X5	T4Ø.2X6
Dihydrohydroxymorphinone	T4Ø.2X1	T4Ø.2X2	T4Ø.2X3	T4Ø.2X4	T4Ø.2X5	T4Ø.2X6
Dihydroisocodeine	T4Ø.2X1	T4Ø.2X2	T4Ø.2X3	T4Ø.2X4	T4Ø.2X5	T4Ø.2X6
Dihydromorphine	T4Ø.2X1	T4Ø.2X2	T4Ø.2X3	T4Ø.2X4	—	—
Dihydromorphinone	T4Ø.2X1	T4Ø.2X2	T4Ø.2X3	T4Ø.2X4	T4Ø.2X5	T4Ø.2X6
Dihydrostreptomycin	T36.5X1	T36.5X2	T36.5X3	T36.5X4	T36.5X5	T36.5X6
Dihydrotachysterol	T45.2X1	T45.2X2	T45.2X3	T45.2X4	T45.2X5	T45.2X6
Dihydroxyaluminum aminoacetate	T47.1X1	T47.1X2	T47.1X3	T47.1X4	T47.1X5	T47.1X6
Dihydroxyaluminum sodium carbonate	T47.1X1	T47.1X2	T47.1X3	T47.1X4	T47.1X5	T47.1X6
Dihydroxyanthraquinone	T47.2X1	T47.2X2	T47.2X3	T47.2X4	T47.2X5	T47.2X6
Dihydroxycodeinone	T4Ø.2X1	T4Ø.2X2	T4Ø.2X3	T4Ø.2X4	T4Ø.2X5	T4Ø.2X6
Dihydroxypropyl theophylline	T5Ø.2X1	T5Ø.2X2	T5Ø.2X3	T5Ø.2X4	T5Ø.2X5	T5Ø.2X6
Diiodohydroxyquin	T37.8X1	T37.8X2	T37.8X3	T37.8X4	T37.8X5	T37.8X6
topical	T49.ØX1	T49.ØX2	T49.ØX3	T49.ØX4	T49.ØX5	T49.ØX6
Diiodohydroxyquinoline	T37.8X1	T37.8X2	T37.8X3	T37.8X4	T37.8X5	T37.8X6
Diiodotyrosine	T38.2X1	T38.2X2	T38.2X3	T38.2X4	T38.2X5	T38.2X6
Diisopromine	T44.3X1	T44.3X2	T44.3X3	T44.3X4	T44.3X5	T44.3X6
Diisopropylamine	T46.3X1	T46.3X2	T46.3X3	T46.3X4	T46.3X5	T46.3X6

Diachylon plaster — Diisopropylamine

370

Additional Character May Be Required — Refer to the Tabular List for Character Selection

Subterms under main terms may continue to next column or page

Substance	Poisoning, Accidental (unintentional)	Poisoning, Intentional Self-harm	Poisoning, Assault	Poisoning, Undetermined	Adverse Effect	Under-dosing
Diisopropylfluorophosphonate	T44.0X1	T44.0X2	T44.0X3	T44.0X4	T44.0X5	T44.0X6
Dilantin	T42.0X1	T42.0X2	T42.0X3	T42.0X4	T42.0X5	T42.0X6
Dilaudid	T40.2X1	T40.2X2	T40.2X3	T40.2X4	T40.2X5	T40.2X6
Dilazep	T46.3X1	T46.3X2	T46.3X3	T46.3X4	T46.3X5	T46.3X6
Dill	T47.5X1	T47.5X2	T47.5X3	T47.5X4	T47.5X5	T47.5X6
Diloxanide	T37.3X1	T37.3X2	T37.3X3	T37.3X4	T37.3X5	T37.3X6
Diltiazem	T46.1X1	T46.1X2	T46.1X3	T46.1X4	T46.1X5	T46.1X6
Dimazole	T49.0X1	T49.0X2	T49.0X3	T49.0X4	T49.0X5	T49.0X6
Dimefline	T50.7X1	T50.7X2	T50.7X3	T50.7X4	T50.7X5	T50.7X6
Dimefox	T60.0X1	T60.0X2	T60.0X3	T60.0X4	—	—
Dimemorfan	T48.3X1	T48.3X2	T48.3X3	T48.3X4	T48.3X5	T48.3X6
Dimenhydrinate	T45.0X1	T45.0X2	T45.0X3	T45.0X4	T45.0X5	T45.0X6
Dimercaprol (British anti-lewisite)	T45.8X1	T45.8X2	T45.8X3	T45.8X4	T45.8X5	T45.8X6
Dimercaptopropanol	T45.8X1	T45.8X2	T45.8X3	T45.8X4	T45.8X5	T45.8X6
Dimestrol	T38.5X1	T38.5X2	T38.5X3	T38.5X4	T38.5X5	T38.5X6
Dimetane	T45.0X1	T45.0X2	T45.0X3	T45.0X4	T45.0X5	T45.0X6
Dimethicone	T47.1X1	T47.1X2	T47.1X3	T47.1X4	T47.1X5	T47.1X6
Dimethindene	T45.0X1	T45.0X2	T45.0X3	T45.0X4	T45.0X5	T45.0X6
Dimethisoquin	T49.1X1	T49.1X2	T49.1X3	T49.1X4	T49.1X5	T49.1X6
Dimethisterone	T38.5X1	T38.5X2	T38.5X3	T38.5X4	T38.5X5	T38.5X6
Dimethoate	T60.0X1	T60.0X2	T60.0X3	T60.0X4	—	—
Dimethocaine	T41.3X1	T41.3X2	T41.3X3	T41.3X4	T41.3X5	T41.3X6
Dimethoxanate	T48.3X1	T48.3X2	T48.3X3	T48.3X4	T48.3X5	T48.3X6
Dimethyl						
arsine, arsinic acid	T57.0X1	T57.0X2	T57.0X3	T57.0X4	—	—
carbinol	T51.2X1	T51.2X2	T51.2X3	T51.2X4	—	—
carbonate	T52.8X1	T52.8X2	T52.8X3	T52.8X4	—	—
diguanide	T38.3X1	T38.3X2	T38.3X3	T38.3X4	T38.3X5	T38.3X6
ketone	T52.4X1	T52.4X2	T52.4X3	T52.4X4	—	—
vapor	T52.4X1	T52.4X2	T52.4X3	T52.4X4	—	—
meperidine	T40.2X1	T40.2X2	T40.2X3	T40.2X4	T40.2X5	T40.2X6
parathion	T60.0X1	T60.0X2	T60.0X3	T60.0X4	—	—
phthlate	T49.3X1	T49.3X2	T49.3X3	T49.3X4	T49.3X5	T49.3X6
polysiloxane	T47.8X1	T47.8X2	T47.8X3	T47.8X4	T47.8X5	T47.8X6
sulfate (fumes)	T59.891	T59.892	T59.893	T59.894	—	—
liquid	T65.891	T65.892	T65.893	T65.894	—	—
sulfoxide (nonmedicinal)	T52.8X1	T52.8X2	T52.8X3	T52.8X4	—	—
medicinal	T49.4X1	T49.4X2	T49.4X3	T49.4X4	T49.4X5	T49.4X6
tryptamine	T40.991	T40.992	T40.993	T40.994	—	—
tubocurarine	T48.1X1	T48.1X2	T48.1X3	T48.1X4	T48.1X5	T48.1X6
Dimethylamine sulfate	T49.4X1	T49.4X2	T49.4X3	T49.4X4	—	—
Dimethylformamide	T52.8X1	T52.8X2	T52.8X3	T52.8X4	—	—
Dimethyltubocurarinium chloride	T48.1X1	T48.1X2	T48.1X3	T48.1X4	T48.1X5	T48.1X6
Dimeticone	T47.1X1	T47.1X2	T47.1X3	T47.1X4	T47.1X5	T47.1X6
Dimetilan	T60.0X1	T60.0X2	T60.0X3	T60.0X4	—	—
Dimetindene	T45.0X1	T45.0X2	T45.0X3	T45.0X4	T45.0X5	T45.0X6
Dimetotiazine	T43.3X1	T43.3X2	T43.3X3	T43.3X4	T43.3X5	T43.3X6
Dimorpholamine	T50.7X1	T50.7X2	T50.7X3	T50.7X4	T50.7X5	T50.7X6
Dimoxyline	T46.3X1	T46.3X2	T46.3X3	T46.3X4	T46.3X5	T46.3X6
Dinitrobenzene	T65.3X1	T65.3X2	T65.3X3	T65.3X4	—	—
vapor	T59.891	T59.892	T59.893	T59.894	—	—
Dinitrobenzol	T65.3X1	T65.3X2	T65.3X3	T65.3X4	—	—
vapor	T59.891	T59.892	T59.893	T59.894	—	—
Dinitrobutylphenol	T65.3X1	T65.3X2	T65.3X3	T65.3X4	—	—
Dinitro (-ortho-)cresol (pesticide) (spray)	T65.3X1	T65.3X2	T65.3X3	T65.3X4	—	—
Dinitrocyclohexylphenol	T65.3X1	T65.3X2	T65.3X3	T65.3X4	—	—
Dinitrophenol	T65.3X1	T65.3X2	T65.3X3	T65.3X4	—	—
Dinoprost	T48.0X1	T48.0X2	T48.0X3	T48.0X4	T48.0X5	T48.0X6
Dinoprostone	T48.0X1	T48.0X2	T48.0X3	T48.0X4	T48.0X5	T48.0X6
Dinoseb	T60.3X1	T60.3X2	T60.3X3	T60.3X4	—	—
Dioctyl sulfosuccinate (calcium) (sodium)	T47.4X1	T47.4X2	T47.4X3	T47.4X4	—	T47.4X6
Diodone	T50.8X1	T50.8X2	T50.8X3	T50.8X4	T50.8X5	T50.8X6
Diodoquin	T37.8X1	T37.8X2	T37.8X3	T37.8X4	T37.8X5	T37.8X6
Dionin	T40.2X1	T40.2X2	T40.2X3	T40.2X4	T40.2X5	T40.2X6
Diosmin	T46.991	T46.992	T46.993	T46.994	T46.995	T46.996
Dioxane	T52.8X1	T52.8X2	T52.8X3	T52.8X4	—	—
Dioxathion	T60.0X1	T60.0X2	T60.0X3	T60.0X4	—	—
Dioxin	T53.7X1	T53.7X2	T53.7X3	T53.7X4	—	—
Dioxopromethazine	T43.3X1	T43.3X2	T43.3X3	T43.3X4	T43.3X5	T43.3X6
Dioxyline	T46.3X1	T46.3X2	T46.3X3	T46.3X4	T46.3X5	T46.3X6
Dipentene	T52.8X1	T52.8X2	T52.8X3	T52.8X4	—	—
Diperodon	T41.3X1	T41.3X2	T41.3X3	T41.3X4	T41.3X5	T41.3X6
Diphacinone	T60.4X1	T60.4X2	T60.4X3	T60.4X4	—	—
Diphemanil	T44.3X1	T44.3X2	T44.3X3	T44.3X4	T44.3X5	T44.3X6
metilsulfate	T44.3X1	T44.3X2	T44.3X3	T44.3X4	T44.3X5	T44.3X6
Diphenadione	T45.511	T45.512	T45.513	T45.514	T45.515	T45.516
rodenticide	T60.4X1	T60.4X2	T60.4X3	T60.4X4	—	—
Diphenhydramine	T45.0X1	T45.0X2	T45.0X3	T45.0X4	T45.0X5	T45.0X6
Diphenidol	T45.0X1	T45.0X2	T45.0X3	T45.0X4	T45.0X5	T45.0X6
Diphenoxylate	T47.6X1	T47.6X2	T47.6X3	T47.6X4	T47.6X5	T47.6X6
Diphenylamine	T65.3X1	T65.3X2	T65.3X3	T65.3X4	—	—
Diphenylbutazone	T39.2X1	T39.2X2	T39.2X3	T39.2X4	T39.2X5	T39.2X6
Diphenylchloroarsine, not in war	T57.0X1	T57.0X2	T57.0X3	T57.0X4	—	—
Diphenylhydantoin	T42.0X1	T42.0X2	T42.0X3	T42.0X4	T42.0X5	T42.0X6
Diphenylmethane dye	T52.1X1	T52.1X2	T52.1X3	T52.1X4	—	—
Diphenylpyraline	T45.0X1	T45.0X2	T45.0X3	T45.0X4	T45.0X5	T45.0X6
Diphtheria						
antitoxin	T50.Z11	T50.Z12	T50.Z13	T50.Z14	T50.Z15	T50.Z16
toxoid	T50.A91	T50.A92	T50.A93	T50.A94	T50.A95	T50.A96
with tetanus toxoid	T50.A21	T50.A22	T50.A23	T50.A24	T50.A25	T50.A26
with pertussis component	T50.A11	T50.A12	T50.A13	T50.A14	T50.A15	T50.A16
vaccine	T50.A91	T50.A92	T50.A93	T50.A94	T50.A95	T50.A96
combination						
without pertussis	T50.A21	T50.A22	T50.A23	T50.A24	T50.A25	T50.A26
including pertussis	T50.A11	T50.A12	T50.A13	T50.A14	T50.A15	T50.A16
Diphylline	T50.2X1	T50.2X2	T50.2X3	T50.2X4	T50.2X5	T50.2X6
Dipipanone	T40.491	T40.492	T40.493	T40.494	—	—
Dipivefrine	T49.5X1	T49.5X2	T49.5X3	T49.5X4	T49.5X5	T49.5X6
Diplovax	T50.B91	T50.B92	T50.B93	T50.B94	T50.B95	T50.B96
Diprophylline	T50.2X1	T50.2X2	T50.2X3	T50.2X4	T50.2X5	T50.2X6
Dipropyline	T48.291	T48.292	T48.293	T48.294	T48.295	T48.296
Dipyridamole	T46.3X1	T46.3X2	T46.3X3	T46.3X4	T46.3X5	T46.3X6
Dipyrone	T39.2X1	T39.2X2	T39.2X3	T39.2X4	T39.2X5	T39.2X6
Diquat (dibromide)	T60.3X1	T60.3X2	T60.3X3	T60.3X4	—	—
Disinfectant	T65.891	T65.892	T65.893	T65.894	—	—
alkaline	T54.3X1	T54.3X2	T54.3X3	T54.3X4	—	—
aromatic	T54.1X1	T54.1X2	T54.1X3	T54.1X4	—	—
intestinal	T37.8X1	T37.8X2	T37.8X3	T37.8X4	T37.8X5	T37.8X6
Disipal	T42.8X1	T42.8X2	T42.8X3	T42.8X4	T42.8X5	T42.8X6
Disodium edetate	T50.6X1	T50.6X2	T50.6X3	T50.6X4	T50.6X5	T50.6X6
Disoprofol	T41.291	T41.292	T41.293	T41.294	T41.295	T41.296
Disopyramide	T46.2X1	T46.2X2	T46.2X3	T46.2X4	T46.2X5	T46.2X6
Distigmine (bromide)	T44.0X1	T44.0X2	T44.0X3	T44.0X4	T44.0X5	T44.0X6
Disulfamide	T50.2X1	T50.2X2	T50.2X3	T50.2X4	T50.2X5	T50.2X6
Disulfanilamide	T37.0X1	T37.0X2	T37.0X3	T37.0X4	T37.0X5	T37.0X6
Disulfiram	T50.6X1	T50.6X2	T50.6X3	T50.6X4	T50.6X5	T50.6X6
Disulfoton	T60.0X1	T60.0X2	T60.0X3	T60.0X4	—	—
Dithiazanine iodide	T37.4X1	T37.4X2	T37.4X3	T37.4X4	T37.4X5	T37.4X6
Dithiocarbamate	T60.0X1	T60.0X2	T60.0X3	T60.0X4	—	—
Dithranol	T49.4X1	T49.4X2	T49.4X3	T49.4X4	T49.4X5	T49.4X6
Diucardin	T50.2X1	T50.2X2	T50.2X3	T50.2X4	T50.2X5	T50.2X6
Diupres	T50.2X1	T50.2X2	T50.2X3	T50.2X4	T50.2X5	T50.2X6
Diuretic NEC	T50.2X1	T50.2X2	T50.2X3	T50.2X4	T50.2X5	T50.2X6
benzothiadiazine	T50.2X1	T50.2X2	T50.2X3	T50.2X4	T50.2X5	T50.2X6
carbonic acid anhydrase inhibitors	T50.2X1	T50.2X2	T50.2X3	T50.2X4	T50.2X5	T50.2X6
furfuryl NEC	T50.2X1	T50.2X2	T50.2X3	T50.2X4	T50.2X5	T50.2X6
loop (high-ceiling)	T50.1X1	T50.1X2	T50.1X3	T50.1X4	T50.1X5	T50.1X6
mercurial NEC	T50.2X1	T50.2X2	T50.2X3	T50.2X4	T50.2X5	T50.2X6
osmotic	T50.2X1	T50.2X2	T50.2X3	T50.2X4	T50.2X5	T50.2X6
purine NEC	T50.2X1	T50.2X2	T50.2X3	T50.2X4	T50.2X5	T50.2X6
saluretic NEC	T50.2X1	T50.2X2	T50.2X3	T50.2X4	T50.2X5	T50.2X6
sulfonamide	T50.2X1	T50.2X2	T50.2X3	T50.2X4	T50.2X5	T50.2X6
thiazide NEC	T50.2X1	T50.2X2	T50.2X3	T50.2X4	T50.2X5	T50.2X6
xanthine	T50.2X1	T50.2X2	T50.2X3	T50.2X4	T50.2X5	T50.2X6
Diurgin	T50.2X1	T50.2X2	T50.2X3	T50.2X4	T50.2X5	T50.2X6
Diuril	T50.2X1	T50.2X2	T50.2X3	T50.2X4	T50.2X5	T50.2X6
Diuron	T60.3X1	T60.3X2	T60.3X3	T60.3X4	—	—
Divalproex	T42.6X1	T42.6X2	T42.6X3	T42.6X4	T42.6X5	T42.6X6
Divinyl ether	T41.0X1	T41.0X2	T41.0X3	T41.0X4	T41.0X5	T41.0X6
Dixanthogen	T49.0X1	T49.0X2	T49.0X3	T49.0X4	T49.0X5	T49.0X6
Dixyrazine	T43.3X1	T43.3X2	T43.3X3	T43.3X4	T43.3X5	T43.3X6
D-lysergic acid diethylamide	T40.8X1	T40.8X2	T40.8X3	T40.8X4	—	—
DMCT	T36.4X1	T36.4X2	T36.4X3	T36.4X4	T36.4X5	T36.4X6
DMSO — see Dimethyl sulfoxide						
DNBP	T60.3X1	T60.3X2	T60.3X3	T60.3X4	—	—
DNOC	T65.3X1	T65.3X2	T65.3X3	T65.3X4	—	—
Dobutamine	T44.5X1	T44.5X2	T44.5X3	T44.5X4	T44.5X5	T44.5X6
DOCA	T38.0X1	T38.0X2	T38.0X3	T38.0X4	T38.0X5	T38.0X6
Docusate sodium	T47.4X1	T47.4X2	T47.4X3	T47.4X4	T47.4X5	T47.4X6
Dodicin	T49.0X1	T49.0X2	T49.0X3	T49.0X4	T49.0X5	T49.0X6
Dofamium chloride	T49.0X1	T49.0X2	T49.0X3	T49.0X4	T49.0X5	T49.0X6
Dolophine	T40.3X1	T40.3X2	T40.3X3	T40.3X4	T40.3X5	T40.3X6
Doloxene	T39.8X1	T39.8X2	T39.8X3	T39.8X4	T39.8X5	T39.8X6
Domestic gas (after combustion) — see Gas, utility						
prior to combustion	T59.891	T59.892	T59.893	T59.894	—	—
Domiodol	T48.4X1	T48.4X2	T48.4X3	T48.4X4	T48.4X5	T48.4X6
Domiphen (bromide)	T49.0X1	T49.0X2	T49.0X3	T49.0X4	T49.0X5	T49.0X6

Substance	Poisoning, Accidental (unintentional)	Poisoning, Intentional Self-harm	Poisoning, Assault	Poisoning, Undetermined	Adverse Effect	Under-dosing
Domperidone	T45.ØX1	T45.ØX2	T45.ØX3	T45.ØX4	T45.ØX5	T45.ØX6
Dopa	T42.8X1	T42.8X2	T42.8X3	T42.8X4	T42.8X5	T42.8X6
Dopamine	T44.991	T44.992	T44.993	T44.994	T44.995	T44.996
Doriden	T42.6X1	T42.6X2	T42.6X3	T42.6X4	T42.6X5	T42.6X6
Dormiral	T42.3X1	T42.3X2	T42.3X3	T42.3X4	T42.3X5	T42.3X6
Dormison	T42.6X1	T42.6X2	T42.6X3	T42.6X4	T42.6X5	T42.6X6
Dornase	T48.4X1	T48.4X2	T48.4X3	T48.4X4	T48.4X5	T48.4X6
Dorsacaine	T41.3X1	T41.3X2	T41.3X3	T41.3X4	T41.3X5	T41.3X6
Dosulepin	T43.Ø11	T43.Ø12	T43.Ø13	T43.Ø14	T43.Ø15	T43.Ø16
Dothiepin	T43.Ø11	T43.Ø12	T43.Ø13	T43.Ø14	T43.Ø15	T43.Ø16
Doxantrazole	T48.6X1	T48.6X2	T48.6X3	T48.6X4	T48.6X5	T48.6X6
Doxapram	T5Ø.7X1	T5Ø.7X2	T5Ø.7X3	T5Ø.7X4	T5Ø.7X5	T5Ø.7X6
Doxazosin	T44.6X1	T44.6X2	T44.6X3	T44.6X4	T44.6X5	T44.6X6
Doxepin	T43.Ø11	T43.Ø12	T43.Ø13	T43.Ø14	T43.Ø15	T43.Ø16
Doxifluridine	T45.1X1	T45.1X2	T45.1X3	T45.1X4	T45.1X5	T45.1X6
Doxorubicin	T45.1X1	T45.1X2	T45.1X3	T45.1X4	T45.1X5	T45.1X6
Doxycycline	T36.4X1	T36.4X2	T36.4X3	T36.4X4	T36.4X5	T36.4X6
Doxylamine	T45.ØX1	T45.ØX2	T45.ØX3	T45.ØX4	T45.ØX5	T45.ØX6
Dramamine	T45.ØX1	T45.ØX2	T45.ØX3	T45.ØX4	T45.ØX5	T45.ØX6
Drano (drain cleaner)	T54.3X1	T54.3X2	T54.3X3	T54.3X4	—	—
Dressing, live pulp	T49.7X1	T49.7X2	T49.7X3	T49.7X4	T49.7X5	T49.7X6
Drocode	T4Ø.2X1	T4Ø.2X2	T4Ø.2X3	T4Ø.2X4	T4Ø.2X5	T4Ø.2X6
Dromoran	T4Ø.2X1	T4Ø.2X2	T4Ø.2X3	T4Ø.2X4	T4Ø.2X5	T4Ø.2X6
Dromostanolone	T38.7X1	T38.7X2	T38.7X3	T38.7X4	T38.7X5	T38.7X6
Dronabinol	T4Ø.711	T4Ø.712	T4Ø.713	T4Ø.714	T4Ø.715	T4Ø.716
Droperidol	T43.591	T43.592	T43.593	T43.594	T43.595	T43.596
Dropropizine	T48.3X1	T48.3X2	T48.3X3	T48.3X4	T48.3X5	T48.3X6
Drostanolone	T38.7X1	T38.7X2	T38.7X3	T38.7X4	T38.7X5	T38.7X6
Drotaverine	T44.3X1	T44.3X2	T44.3X3	T44.3X4	T44.3X5	T44.3X6
Drotrecogin alfa	T45.511	T45.512	T45.513	T45.514	T45.515	T45.516
Drug NEC	T5Ø.9Ø1	T5Ø.9Ø2	T5Ø.9Ø3	T5Ø.9Ø4	T5Ø.9Ø5	T5Ø.9Ø6
specified NEC	T5Ø.991	T5Ø.992	T5Ø.993	T5Ø.994	T5Ø.995	T5Ø.996
DTIC	T45.1X1	T45.1X2	T45.1X3	T45.1X4	T45.1X5	T45.1X6
Duboisine	T44.3X1	T44.3X2	T44.3X3	T44.3X4	T44.3X5	T44.3X6
Dulcolax	T47.2X1	T47.2X2	T47.2X3	T47.2X4	T47.2X5	T47.2X6
Duponol (C) (EP)	T49.2X1	T49.2X2	T49.2X3	T49.2X4	T49.2X5	T49.2X6
Durabolin	T38.7X1	T38.7X2	T38.7X3	T38.7X4	T38.7X5	T38.7X6
Dyclone	T41.3X1	T41.3X2	T41.3X3	T41.3X4	T41.3X5	T41.3X6
Dyclonine	T41.3X1	T41.3X2	T41.3X3	T41.3X4	T41.3X5	T41.3X6
Dydrogesterone	T38.5X1	T38.5X2	T38.5X3	T38.5X4	T38.5X5	T38.5X6
Dye NEC	T65.6X1	T65.6X2	T65.6X3	T65.6X4	—	—
antiseptic	T49.ØX1	T49.ØX2	T49.ØX3	T49.ØX4	T49.ØX5	T49.ØX6
diagnostic agents	T5Ø.8X1	T5Ø.8X2	T5Ø.8X3	T5Ø.8X4	T5Ø.8X5	T5Ø.8X6
pharmaceutical NEC	T5Ø.9Ø1	T5Ø.9Ø2	T5Ø.9Ø3	T5Ø.9Ø4	T5Ø.9Ø5	T5Ø.9Ø6
Dyflos	T44.ØX1	T44.ØX2	T44.ØX3	T44.ØX4	T44.ØX5	T44.ØX6
Dymelor	T38.3X1	T38.3X2	T38.3X3	T38.3X4	T38.3X5	T38.3X6
Dynamite	T65.3X1	T65.3X2	T65.3X3	T65.3X4	—	—
fumes	T59.891	T59.892	T59.893	T59.894	—	—
Dyphylline	T44.3X1	T44.3X2	T44.3X3	T44.3X4	T44.3X5	T44.3X6
b-eucaine	T49.1X1	T49.1X2	T49.1X3	T49.1X4	T49.1X5	T49.1X6
Ear drug NEC	T49.6X1	T49.6X2	T49.6X3	T49.6X4	T49.6X5	T49.6X6
Ear preparations	T49.6X1	T49.6X2	T49.6X3	T49.6X4	T49.6X5	T49.6X6
Echothiophate, echothiopate, ecothiopate	T49.5X1	T49.5X2	T49.5X3	T49.5X4	T49.5X5	T49.5X6
Econazole	T49.ØX1	T49.ØX2	T49.ØX3	T49.ØX4	T49.ØX5	T49.ØX6
Ecothiopate iodide	T49.5X1	T49.5X2	T49.5X3	T49.5X4	T49.5X5	T49.5X6
Ecstasy	T43.641	T43.642	T43.643	T43.644	—	—
Ectylurea	T42.6X1	T42.6X2	T42.6X3	T42.6X4	T42.6X5	T42.6X6
Edathamil disodium	T45.8X1	T45.8X2	T45.8X3	T45.8X4	T45.8X5	T45.8X6
Edecrin	T5Ø.1X1	T5Ø.1X2	T5Ø.1X3	T5Ø.1X4	T5Ø.1X5	T5Ø.1X6
Edetate, disodium (calcium)	T45.8X1	T45.8X2	T45.8X3	T45.8X4	T45.8X5	T45.8X6
Edoxudine	T49.5X1	T49.5X2	T49.5X3	T49.5X4	T49.5X5	T49.5X6
Edrophonium	T44.ØX1	T44.ØX2	T44.ØX3	T44.ØX4	T44.ØX5	T44.ØX6
chloride	T44.ØX1	T44.ØX2	T44.ØX3	T44.ØX4	T44.ØX5	T44.ØX6
EDTA	T5Ø.6X1	T5Ø.6X2	T5Ø.6X3	T5Ø.6X4	T5Ø.6X5	T5Ø.6X6
Eflornithine	T37.2X1	T37.2X2	T37.2X3	T37.2X4	T37.2X5	T37.2X6
Efloxate	T46.3X1	T46.3X2	T46.3X3	T46.3X4	T46.3X5	T46.3X6
Elase	T49.8X1	T49.8X2	T49.8X3	T49.8X4	T49.8X5	T49.8X6
Elastase	T47.5X1	T47.5X2	T47.5X3	T47.5X4	T47.5X5	T47.5X6
Elaterium	T47.2X1	T47.2X2	T47.2X3	T47.2X4	T47.2X5	T47.2X6
Elcatonin	T5Ø.991	T5Ø.992	T5Ø.993	T5Ø.994	T5Ø.995	T5Ø.996
Elder	T62.2X1	T62.2X2	T62.2X3	T62.2X4	—	—
berry, (unripe)	T62.1X1	T62.1X2	T62.1X3	T62.1X4	—	—
Electrolyte balance drug	T5Ø.3X1	T5Ø.3X2	T5Ø.3X3	T5Ø.3X4	T5Ø.3X5	T5Ø.3X6
Electrolytes NEC	T5Ø.3X1	T5Ø.3X2	T5Ø.3X3	T5Ø.3X4	T5Ø.3X5	T5Ø.3X6
Electrolytic agent NEC	T5Ø.3X1	T5Ø.3X2	T5Ø.3X3	T5Ø.3X4	T5Ø.3X5	T5Ø.3X6
Elemental diet	T5Ø.9Ø1	T5Ø.9Ø2	T5Ø.9Ø3	T5Ø.9Ø4	T5Ø.9Ø5	T5Ø.9Ø6
Elliptinium acetate	T45.1X1	T45.1X2	T45.1X3	T45.1X4	T45.1X5	T45.1X6
Embramine	T45.ØX1	T45.ØX2	T45.ØX3	T45.ØX4	T45.ØX5	T45.ØX6
Emepronium (salts)	T44.3X1	T44.3X2	T44.3X3	T44.3X4	T44.3X5	T44.3X6
bromide	T44.3X1	T44.3X2	T44.3X3	T44.3X4	T44.3X5	T44.3X6
Emetic NEC	T47.7X1	T47.7X2	T47.7X3	T47.7X4	T47.7X5	T47.7X6

Substance	Poisoning, Accidental (unintentional)	Poisoning, Intentional Self-harm	Poisoning, Assault	Poisoning, Undetermined	Adverse Effect	Under-dosing
Emetine	T37.3X1	T37.3X2	T37.3X3	T37.3X4	T37.3X5	T37.3X6
Emollient NEC	T49.3X1	T49.3X2	T49.3X3	T49.3X4	T49.3X5	T49.3X6
Emorfazone	T39.8X1	T39.8X2	T39.8X3	T39.8X4	T39.8X5	T39.8X6
Emylcamate	T43.591	T43.592	T43.593	T43.594	T43.595	T43.596
Enalapril	T46.4X1	T46.4X2	T46.4X3	T46.4X4	T46.4X5	T46.4X6
Enalaprilat	T46.4X1	T46.4X2	T46.4X3	T46.4X4	T46.4X5	T46.4X6
Encainide	T46.2X1	T46.2X2	T46.2X3	T46.2X4	T46.2X5	T46.2X6
Endocaine	T41.3X1	T41.3X2	T41.3X3	T41.3X4	T41.3X5	T41.3X6
Endosulfan	T6Ø.2X1	T6Ø.2X2	T6Ø.2X3	T6Ø.2X4	—	—
Endothall	T6Ø.3X1	T6Ø.3X2	T6Ø.3X3	T6Ø.3X4	—	—
Endralazine	T46.5X1	T46.5X2	T46.5X3	T46.5X4	T46.5X5	T46.5X6
Endrin	T6Ø.1X1	T6Ø.1X2	T6Ø.1X3	T6Ø.1X4	—	—
Enflurane	T41.ØX1	T41.ØX2	T41.ØX3	T41.ØX4	T41.ØX5	T41.ØX6
Enhexymal	T42.3X1	T42.3X2	T42.3X3	T42.3X4	T42.3X5	T42.3X6
Enocitabine	T45.1X1	T45.1X2	T45.1X3	T45.1X4	T45.1X5	T45.1X6
Enovid	T38.4X1	T38.4X2	T38.4X3	T38.4X4	T38.4X5	T38.4X6
Enoxacin	T36.8X1	T36.8X2	T36.8X3	T36.8X4	T36.8X5	T36.8X6
Enoxaparin (sodium)	T45.511	T45.512	T45.513	T45.514	T45.515	T45.516
Enpiprazole	T43.591	T43.592	T43.593	T43.594	T43.595	T43.596
Enprofylline	T48.6X1	T48.6X2	T48.6X3	T48.6X4	T48.6X5	T48.6X6
Enprostil	T47.1X1	T47.1X2	T47.1X3	T47.1X4	T47.1X5	T47.1X6
Enterogastrone	T38.891	T38.892	T38.893	T38.894	T38.895	T38.896
ENT preparations (anti-infectives)	T49.6X1	T49.6X2	T49.6X3	T49.6X4	T49.6X5	T49.6X6
Enviomycin	T36.8X1	T36.8X2	T36.8X3	T36.8X4	T36.8X5	T36.8X6
Enzodase	T45.3X1	T45.3X2	T45.3X3	T45.3X4	T45.3X5	T45.3X6
Enzyme NEC	T45.3X1	T45.3X2	T45.3X3	T45.3X4	T45.3X5	T45.3X6
depolymerizing	T49.8X1	T49.8X2	T49.8X3	T49.8X4	T49.8X5	T49.8X6
fibrolytic	T45.3X1	T45.3X2	T45.3X3	T45.3X4	T45.3X5	T45.3X6
gastric	T47.5X1	T47.5X2	T47.5X3	T47.5X4	T47.5X5	T47.5X6
intestinal	T47.5X1	T47.5X2	T47.5X3	T47.5X4	T47.5X5	T47.5X6
local action	T49.4X1	T49.4X2	T49.4X3	T49.4X4	T49.4X5	T49.4X6
proteolytic	T49.4X1	T49.4X2	T49.4X3	T49.4X4	T49.4X5	T49.4X6
thrombolytic	T45.3X1	T45.3X2	T45.3X3	T45.3X4	T45.3X5	T45.3X6
EPAB	T41.3X1	T41.3X2	T41.3X3	T41.3X4	T41.3X5	T41.3X6
Epanutin	T42.ØX1	T42.ØX2	T42.ØX3	T42.ØX4	T42.ØX5	T42.ØX6
Ephedra	T44.991	T44.992	T44.993	T44.994	T44.995	T44.996
Ephedrine	T44.991	T44.992	T44.993	T44.994	T44.995	T44.996
Epichlorhydrin, epichlorohydrin	T52.8X1	T52.8X2	T52.8X3	T52.8X4	—	—
Epicillin	T36.ØX1	T36.ØX2	T36.ØX3	T36.ØX4	T36.ØX5	T36.ØX6
Epiestriol	T38.5X1	T38.5X2	T38.5X3	T38.5X4	T38.5X5	T38.5X6
Epilim — *see* Sodium valproate						
Epimestrol	T38.5X1	T38.5X2	T38.5X3	T38.5X4	T38.5X5	T38.5X6
Epinephrine	T44.5X1	T44.5X2	T44.5X3	T44.5X4	T44.5X5	T44.5X6
Epirubicin	T45.1X1	T45.1X2	T45.1X3	T45.1X4	T45.1X5	T45.1X6
Epitiostanol	T38.7X1	T38.7X2	T38.7X3	T38.7X4	T38.7X5	T38.7X6
Epitizide	T5Ø.2X1	T5Ø.2X2	T5Ø.2X3	T5Ø.2X4	T5Ø.2X5	T5Ø.2X6
EPN	T6Ø.ØX1	T6Ø.ØX2	T6Ø.ØX3	T6Ø.ØX4	—	—
EPO	T45.8X1	T45.8X2	T45.8X3	T45.8X4	T45.8X5	T45.8X6
Epoetin alpha	T45.8X1	T45.8X2	T45.8X3	T45.8X4	T45.8X5	T45.8X6
Epomediol	T5Ø.991	T5Ø.992	T5Ø.993	T5Ø.994	T5Ø.995	T5Ø.996
Epoprostenol	T45.521	T45.522	T45.523	T45.524	T45.525	T45.526
Epoxy resin	T65.891	T65.892	T65.893	T65.894	—	—
Eprazinone	T48.4X1	T48.4X2	T48.4X3	T48.4X4	T48.4X5	T48.4X6
Epsilon aminocaproic acid	T45.621	T45.622	T45.623	T45.624	T45.625	T45.626
Epsom salt	T47.3X1	T47.3X2	T47.3X3	T47.3X4	T47.3X5	T47.3X6
Eptazocine	T4Ø.491	T4Ø.492	T4Ø.493	T4Ø.494	T4Ø.495	T4Ø.496
Equanil	T43.591	T43.592	T43.593	T43.594	T43.595	T43.596
Equisetum	T62.2X1	T62.2X2	T62.2X3	T62.2X4	—	—
diuretic	T5Ø.2X1	T5Ø.2X2	T5Ø.2X3	T5Ø.2X4	T5Ø.2X5	T5Ø.2X6
Ergobasine	T48.ØX1	T48.ØX2	T48.ØX3	T48.ØX4	T48.ØX5	T48.ØX6
Ergocalciferol	T45.2X1	T45.2X2	T45.2X3	T45.2X4	T45.2X5	T45.2X6
Ergoloid mesylates	T46.7X1	T46.7X2	T46.7X3	T46.7X4	T46.7X5	T46.7X6
Ergometrine	T48.ØX1	T48.ØX2	T48.ØX3	T48.ØX4	T48.ØX5	T48.ØX6
Ergonovine	T48.ØX1	T48.ØX2	T48.ØX3	T48.ØX4	T48.ØX5	T48.ØX6
Ergotamine	T46.5X1	T46.5X2	T46.5X3	T46.5X4	T46.5X5	T46.5X6
Ergotocine	T48.ØX1	T48.ØX2	T48.ØX3	T48.ØX4	T48.ØX5	T48.ØX6
Ergotrate	T48.ØX1	T48.ØX2	T48.ØX3	T48.ØX4	T48.ØX5	T48.ØX6
Ergot NEC	T64.81	T64.82	T64.83	T64.84	—	—
derivative	T48.ØX1	T48.ØX2	T48.ØX3	T48.ØX4	T48.ØX5	T48.ØX6
medicinal (alkaloids)	T48.ØX1	T48.ØX2	T48.ØX3	T48.ØX4	T48.ØX5	T48.ØX6
prepared	T48.ØX1	T48.ØX2	T48.ØX3	T48.ØX4	T48.ØX5	T48.ØX6
Eritrityl tetranitrate	T46.3X1	T46.3X2	T46.3X3	T46.3X4	T46.3X5	T46.3X6
Erythrityl tetranitrate	T46.3X1	T46.3X2	T46.3X3	T46.3X4	T46.3X5	T46.3X6
Erythrol tetranitrate	T46.3X1	T46.3X2	T46.3X3	T46.3X4	T46.3X5	T46.3X6
Erythromycin (salts)	T36.3X1	T36.3X2	T36.3X3	T36.3X4	T36.3X5	T36.3X6
ophthalmic preparation	T49.5X1	T49.5X2	T49.5X3	T49.5X4	T49.5X5	T49.5X6
topical NEC	T49.ØX1	T49.ØX2	T49.ØX3	T49.ØX4	T49.ØX5	T49.ØX6
Erythropoietin	T45.8X1	T45.8X2	T45.8X3	T45.8X4	T45.8X5	T45.8X6
human	T45.8X1	T45.8X2	T45.8X3	T45.8X4	T45.8X5	T45.8X6
Escin	T46.991	T46.992	T46.993	T46.994	T46.995	T46.996
Esculin	T45.2X1	T45.2X2	T45.2X3	T45.2X4	T45.2X5	T45.2X6

Substance	Poisoning, Accidental (unintentional)	Poisoning, Intentional Self-harm	Poisoning, Assault	Poisoning, Undetermined	Adverse Effect	Under-dosing
Esculoside	T45.2X1	T45.2X2	T45.2X3	T45.2X4	T45.2X5	T45.2X6
ESDT (ether-soluble tar distillate)	T49.1X1	T49.1X2	T49.1X3	T49.1X4	T49.1X5	T49.1X6
Eserine	T49.5X1	T49.5X2	T49.5X3	T49.5X4	T49.5X5	T49.5X6
Esflurbiprofen	T39.311	T39.312	T39.313	T39.314	T39.315	T39.316
Eskabarb	T42.3X1	T42.3X2	T42.3X3	T42.3X4	T42.3X5	T42.3X6
Eskalith	T43.8X1	T43.8X2	T43.8X3	T43.8X4	T43.8X5	T43.8X6
Esmolol	T44.7X1	T44.7X2	T44.7X3	T44.7X4	T44.7X5	T44.7X6
Estanozolol	T38.7X1	T38.7X2	T38.7X3	T38.7X4	T38.7X5	T38.7X6
Estazolam	T42.4X1	T42.4X2	T42.4X3	T42.4X4	T42.4X5	T42.4X6
Estradiol	T38.5X1	T38.5X2	T38.5X3	T38.5X4	T38.5X5	T38.5X6
with testosterone	T38.7X1	T38.7X2	T38.7X3	T38.7X4	T38.7X5	T38.7X6
benzoate	T38.5X1	T38.5X2	T38.5X3	T38.5X4	T38.5X5	T38.5X6
Estramustine	T45.1X1	T45.1X2	T45.1X3	T45.1X4	T45.1X5	T45.1X6
Estriol	T38.5X1	T38.5X2	T38.5X3	T38.5X4	T38.5X5	T38.5X6
Estrogen	T38.5X1	T38.5X2	T38.5X3	T38.5X4	T38.5X5	T38.5X6
with progesterone	T38.5X1	T38.5X2	T38.5X3	T38.5X4	T38.5X5	T38.5X6
conjugated	T38.5X1	T38.5X2	T38.5X3	T38.5X4	T38.5X5	T38.5X6
Estrone	T38.5X1	T38.5X2	T38.5X3	T38.5X4	T38.5X5	T38.5X6
Estropipate	T38.5X1	T38.5X2	T38.5X3	T38.5X4	T38.5X5	T38.5X6
Etacrynate sodium	T5Ø.1X1	T5Ø.1X2	T5Ø.1X3	T5Ø.1X4	T5Ø.1X5	T5Ø.1X6
Etacrynic acid	T5Ø.1X1	T5Ø.1X2	T5Ø.1X3	T5Ø.1X4	T5Ø.1X5	T5Ø.1X6
Etafedrine	T48.6X1	T48.6X2	T48.6X3	T48.6X4	T48.6X5	T48.6X6
Etafenone	T46.3X1	T46.3X2	T46.3X3	T46.3X4	T46.3X5	T46.3X6
Etambutol	T37.1X1	T37.1X2	T37.1X3	T37.1X4	T37.1X5	T37.1X6
Etamiphyllin	T48.6X1	T48.6X2	T48.6X3	T48.6X4	T48.6X5	T48.6X6
Etamivan	T5Ø.7X1	T5Ø.7X2	T5Ø.7X3	T5Ø.7X4	T5Ø.7X5	T5Ø.7X6
Etamsylate	T45.7X1	T45.7X2	T45.7X3	T45.7X4	T45.7X5	T45.7X6
Etebenecid	T5Ø.4X1	T5Ø.4X2	T5Ø.4X3	T5Ø.4X4	T5Ø.4X5	T5Ø.4X6
Ethacridine	T49.ØX1	T49.ØX2	T49.ØX3	T49.ØX4	T49.ØX5	T49.ØX6
Ethacrynic acid	T5Ø.1X1	T5Ø.1X2	T5Ø.1X3	T5Ø.1X4	T5Ø.1X5	T5Ø.1X6
Ethadione	T42.2X1	T42.2X2	T42.2X3	T42.2X4	T42.2X5	T42.2X6
Ethambutol	T37.1X1	T37.1X2	T37.1X3	T37.1X4	T37.1X5	T37.1X6
Ethamide	T5Ø.2X1	T5Ø.2X2	T5Ø.2X3	T5Ø.2X4	T5Ø.2X5	T5Ø.2X6
Ethamivan	T5Ø.7X1	T5Ø.7X2	T5Ø.7X3	T5Ø.7X4	T5Ø.7X5	T5Ø.7X6
Ethamsylate	T45.7X1	T45.7X2	T45.7X3	T45.7X4	T45.7X5	T45.7X6
Ethanol	T51.ØX1	T51.ØX2	T51.ØX3	T51.ØX4	—	—
beverage	T51.ØX1	T51.ØX2	T51.ØX3	T51.ØX4	—	—
Ethanolamine oleate	T46.8X1	T46.8X2	T46.8X3	T46.8X4	T46.8X5	T46.8X6
Ethaverine	T44.3X1	T44.3X2	T44.3X3	T44.3X4	T44.3X5	T44.3X6
Ethchlorvynol	T42.6X1	T42.6X2	T42.6X3	T42.6X4	T42.6X5	T42.6X6
Ethebenecid	T5Ø.4X1	T5Ø.4X2	T5Ø.4X3	T5Ø.4X4	T5Ø.4X5	T5Ø.4X6
Ether (vapor)	T41.ØX1	T41.ØX2	T41.ØX3	T41.ØX4	T41.ØX5	T41.ØX6
anesthetic	T41.ØX1	T41.ØX2	T41.ØX3	T41.ØX4	T41.ØX5	T41.ØX6
divinyl	T41.ØX1	T41.ØX2	T41.ØX3	T41.ØX4	T41.ØX5	T41.ØX6
ethyl (medicinal)	T41.ØX1	T41.ØX2	T41.ØX3	T41.ØX4	T41.ØX5	T41.ØX6
nonmedicinal	T52.8X1	T52.8X2	T52.8X3	T52.8X4	—	—
petroleum — *see* Ligroin						
solvent	T52.8X1	T52.8X2	T52.8X3	T52.8X4	—	—
Ethiazide	T5Ø.2X1	T5Ø.2X2	T5Ø.2X3	T5Ø.2X4	T5Ø.2X5	T5Ø.2X6
Ethidium chloride (vapor)	T59.891	T59.892	T59.893	T59.894	—	—
Ethinamate	T42.6X1	T42.6X2	T42.6X3	T42.6X4	T42.6X5	T42.6X6
Ethinylestradiol, ethinyloestradiol	T38.5X1	T38.5X2	T38.5X3	T38.5X4	T38.5X5	T38.5X6
with						
levonorgestrel	T38.4X1	T38.4X2	T38.4X3	T38.4X4	T38.4X5	T38.4X6
norethisterone	T38.4X1	T38.4X2	T38.4X3	T38.4X4	T38.4X5	T38.4X6
Ethiodized oil (131 I)	T5Ø.8X1	T5Ø.8X2	T5Ø.8X3	T5Ø.8X4	T5Ø.8X5	T5Ø.8X6
Ethion	T6Ø.ØX1	T6Ø.ØX2	T6Ø.ØX3	T6Ø.ØX4	—	—
Ethionamide	T37.1X1	T37.1X2	T37.1X3	T37.1X4	T37.1X5	T37.1X6
Ethioniamide	T37.1X1	T37.1X2	T37.1X3	T37.1X4	T37.1X5	T37.1X6
Ethisterone	T38.5X1	T38.5X2	T38.5X3	T38.5X4	T38.5X5	T38.5X6
Ethobral	T42.3X1	T42.3X2	T42.3X3	T42.3X4	T42.3X5	T42.3X6
Ethocaine (infiltration) (topical)	T41.3X1	T41.3X2	T41.3X3	T41.3X4	T41.3X5	T41.3X6
nerve block (peripheral) (plexus)	T41.3X1	T41.3X2	T41.3X3	T41.3X4	T41.3X5	T41.3X6
spinal	T41.3X1	T41.3X2	T41.3X3	T41.3X4	T41.3X5	T41.3X6
Ethoheptazine	T4Ø.491	T4Ø.492	T4Ø.493	T4Ø.494	T4Ø.495	T4Ø.496
Ethopropazine	T44.3X1	T44.3X2	T44.3X3	T44.3X4	T44.3X5	T44.3X6
Ethosuximide	T42.2X1	T42.2X2	T42.2X3	T42.2X4	T42.2X5	T42.2X6
Ethotoin	T42.ØX1	T42.ØX2	T42.ØX3	T42.ØX4	T42.ØX5	T42.ØX6
Ethoxazene	T37.91	T37.92	T37.93	T37.94	T37.95	T37.96
Ethoxazorutoside	T46.991	T46.992	T46.993	T46.994	T46.995	T46.996
Ethoxzolamide	T5Ø.2X1	T5Ø.2X2	T5Ø.2X3	T5Ø.2X4	T5Ø.2X5	T5Ø.2X6
Ethyl						
acetate	T52.8X1	T52.8X2	T52.8X3	T52.8X4	—	—
alcohol	T51.ØX1	T51.ØX2	T51.ØX3	T51.ØX4	—	—
beverage	T51.ØX1	T51.ØX2	T51.ØX3	T51.ØX4	—	—
aldehyde (vapor)	T59.891	T59.892	T59.893	T59.894	—	—
liquid	T52.8X1	T52.8X2	T52.8X3	T52.8X4	—	—
aminobenzoate	T41.3X1	T41.3X2	T41.3X3	T41.3X4	T41.3X5	T41.3X6
aminophenothiazine	T43.3X1	T43.3X2	T43.3X3	T43.3X4	T43.3X5	T43.3X6

Substance	Poisoning, Accidental (unintentional)	Poisoning, Intentional Self-harm	Poisoning, Assault	Poisoning, Undetermined	Adverse Effect	Under-dosing
Ethyl — *continued*						
benzoate	T52.8X1	T52.8X2	T52.8X3	T52.8X4	—	—
biscoumacetate	T45.511	T45.512	T45.513	T45.514	T45.515	T45.516
bromide (anesthetic)	T41.ØX1	T41.ØX2	T41.ØX3	T41.ØX4	T41.ØX5	T41.ØX6
carbamate	T45.1X1	T45.1X2	T45.1X3	T45.1X4	T45.1X5	T45.1X6
carbinol	T51.3X1	T51.3X2	T51.3X3	T51.3X4	—	—
carbonate	T52.8X1	T52.8X2	T52.8X3	T52.8X4	—	—
chaulmoograte	T37.1X1	T37.1X2	T37.1X3	T37.1X4	T37.1X5	T37.1X6
chloride (anesthetic)	T41.ØX1	T41.ØX2	T41.ØX3	T41.ØX4	T41.ØX5	T41.ØX6
anesthetic (local)	T41.3X1	T41.3X2	T41.3X3	T41.3X4	T41.3X5	T41.3X6
inhaled	T41.ØX1	T41.ØX2	T41.ØX3	T41.ØX4	T41.ØX5	T41.ØX6
local	T49.4X1	T49.4X2	T49.4X3	T49.4X4	T49.4X5	T49.4X6
solvent	T53.6X1	T53.6X2	T53.6X3	T53.6X4	—	—
dibunate	T48.3X1	T48.3X2	T48.3X3	T48.3X4	T48.3X5	T48.3X6
dichloroarsine (vapor)	T57.ØX1	T57.ØX2	T57.ØX3	T57.ØX4	—	—
estranol	T38.7X1	T38.7X2	T38.7X3	T38.7X4	T38.7X5	T38.7X6
ether — *see also* ether	T52.8X1	T52.8X2	T52.8X3	T52.8X4	—	—
formate NEC (solvent)	T52.ØX1	T52.ØX2	T52.ØX3	T52.ØX4	—	—
fumarate	T49.4X1	T49.4X2	T49.4X3	T49.4X4	T49.4X5	T49.4X6
hydroxyisobutyrate NEC (solvent)	T52.8X1	T52.8X2	T52.8X3	T52.8X4	—	—
iodoacetate	T59.3X1	T59.3X2	T59.3X3	T59.3X4	—	—
lactate NEC (solvent)	T52.8X1	T52.8X2	T52.8X3	T52.8X4	—	—
loflazepate	T42.4X1	T42.4X2	T42.4X3	T42.4X4	T42.4X5	T42.4X6
mercuric chloride	T56.1X1	T56.1X2	T56.1X3	T56.1X4	—	—
methylcarbinol	T51.8X1	T51.8X2	T51.8X3	T51.8X4	—	—
morphine	T4Ø.2X1	T4Ø.2X2	T4Ø.2X3	T4Ø.2X4	T4Ø.2X5	T4Ø.2X6
noradrenaline	T48.6X1	T48.6X2	T48.6X3	T48.6X4	T48.6X5	T48.6X6
oxybutyrate NEC (solvent)	T52.8X1	T52.8X2	T52.8X3	T52.8X4	—	—
Ethylene (gas)	T59.891	T59.892	T59.893	T59.894	—	—
anesthetic (general)	T41.ØX1	T41.ØX2	T41.ØX3	T41.ØX4	T41.ØX5	T41.ØX6
chlorohydrin	T52.8X1	T52.8X2	T52.8X3	T52.8X4	—	—
vapor	T53.6X1	T53.6X2	T53.6X3	T53.6X4	—	—
dichloride	T52.8X1	T52.8X2	T52.8X3	T52.8X4	—	—
vapor	T53.6X1	T53.6X2	T53.6X3	T53.6X4	—	—
dinitrate	T52.3X1	T52.3X2	T52.3X3	T52.3X4	—	—
glycol(s)	T52.8X1	T52.8X2	T52.8X3	T52.8X4	—	—
dinitrate	T52.3X1	T52.3X2	T52.3X3	T52.3X4	—	—
monobutyl ether	T52.3X1	T52.3X2	T52.3X3	T52.3X4	—	—
imine	T54.1X1	T54.1X2	T54.1X3	T54.1X4	—	—
oxide (fumigant) (nonmedicinal)	T59.891	T59.892	T59.893	T59.894	—	—
medicinal	T49.ØX1	T49.ØX2	T49.ØX3	T49.ØX4	T49.ØX5	T49.ØX6
Ethylenediaminetetra-acetic acid	T5Ø.6X1	T5Ø.6X2	T5Ø.6X3	T5Ø.6X4	T5Ø.6X5	T5Ø.6X6
Ethylenediamine theophylline	T48.6X1	T48.6X2	T48.6X3	T48.6X4	T48.6X5	T48.6X6
Ethylenedinitrilotetra-acetate	T5Ø.6X1	T5Ø.6X2	T5Ø.6X3	T5Ø.6X4	T5Ø.6X5	T5Ø.6X6
Ethylestrenol	T38.7X1	T38.7X2	T38.7X3	T38.7X4	T38.7X5	T38.7X6
Ethylhydroxycellulose	T47.4X1	T47.4X2	T47.4X3	T47.4X4	T47.4X5	T47.4X6
Ethylidene						
chloride NEC	T53.6X1	T53.6X2	T53.6X3	T53.6X4	—	—
diacetate	T6Ø.3X1	T6Ø.3X2	T6Ø.3X3	T6Ø.3X4	—	—
dicoumarin	T45.511	T45.512	T45.513	T45.514	T45.515	T45.516
dicoumarol	T45.511	T45.512	T45.513	T45.514	T45.515	T45.516
diethyl ether	T52.ØX1	T52.ØX2	T52.ØX3	T52.ØX4	—	—
Ethylmorphine	T4Ø.2X1	T4Ø.2X2	T4Ø.2X3	T4Ø.2X4	T4Ø.2X5	T4Ø.2X6
Ethylnorepinephrine	T48.6X1	T48.6X2	T48.6X3	T48.6X4	T48.6X5	T48.6X6
Ethylparachlorophen-oxyisobutyrate	T46.6X1	T46.6X2	T46.6X3	T46.6X4	T46.6X5	T46.6X6
Ethynodiol	T38.4X1	T38.4X2	T38.4X3	T38.4X4	T38.4X5	T38.4X6
with mestranol diacetate	T38.4X1	T38.4X2	T38.4X3	T38.4X4	T38.4X5	T38.4X6
Etidocaine	T41.3X1	T41.3X2	T41.3X3	T41.3X4	T41.3X5	T41.3X6
infiltration (subcutaneous)	T41.3X1	T41.3X2	T41.3X3	T41.3X4	T41.3X5	T41.3X6
nerve (peripheral) (plexus)	T41.3X1	T41.3X2	T41.3X3	T41.3X4	T41.3X5	T41.3X6
Etidronate	T5Ø.991	T5Ø.992	T5Ø.993	T5Ø.994	T5Ø.995	T5Ø.996
Etidronic acid (disodium salt)	T5Ø.991	T5Ø.992	T5Ø.993	T5Ø.994	T5Ø.995	T5Ø.996
Etifoxine	T42.6X1	T42.6X2	T42.6X3	T42.6X4	T42.6X5	T42.6X6
Etilefrine	T44.4X1	T44.4X2	T44.4X3	T44.4X4	T44.4X5	T44.4X6
Etilfen	T42.3X1	T42.3X2	T42.3X3	T42.3X4	T42.3X5	T42.3X6
Etinodiol	T38.4X1	T38.4X2	T38.4X3	T38.4X4	T38.4X5	T38.4X6
Etiroxate	T46.6X1	T46.6X2	T46.6X3	T46.6X4	T46.6X5	T46.6X6
Etizolam	T42.4X1	T42.4X2	T42.4X3	T42.4X4	T42.4X5	T42.4X6
Etodolac	T39.391	T39.392	T39.393	T39.394	T39.395	T39.396
Etofamide	T37.3X1	T37.3X2	T37.3X3	T37.3X4	T37.3X5	T37.3X6
Etofibrate	T46.6X1	T46.6X2	T46.6X3	T46.6X4	T46.6X5	T46.6X6
Etofylline	T46.7X1	T46.7X2	T46.7X3	T46.7X4	T46.7X5	T46.7X6
clofibrate	T46.6X1	T46.6X2	T46.6X3	T46.6X4	T46.6X5	T46.6X6
Etoglucid	T45.1X1	T45.1X2	T45.1X3	T45.1X4	T45.1X5	T45.1X6
Etomidate	T41.1X1	T41.1X2	T41.1X3	T41.1X4	T41.1X5	T41.1X6
Etomide	T39.8X1	T39.8X2	T39.8X3	T39.8X4	T39.8X5	T39.8X6
Etomidoline	T44.3X1	T44.3X2	T44.3X3	T44.3X4	T44.3X5	T44.3X6

Subterms under main terms may continue to next column or page

Additional Character May Be Required — Refer to the Tabular List for Character Selection

373

Substance	Poisoning, Accidental (unintentional)	Poisoning, Intentional Self-harm	Poisoning, Assault	Poisoning, Undetermined	Adverse Effect	Under-dosing
Etoposide	T45.1X1	T45.1X2	T45.1X3	T45.1X4	T45.1X5	T45.1X6
Etorphine	T40.2X1	T40.2X2	T40.2X3	T40.2X4	T40.2X5	T40.2X6
Etoval	T42.3X1	T42.3X2	T42.3X3	T42.3X4	T42.3X5	T42.3X6
Etozolin	T50.1X1	T50.1X2	T50.1X3	T50.1X4	T50.1X5	T50.1X6
Etretinate	T50.991	T50.992	T50.993	T50.994	T50.995	T50.996
Etryptamine	T43.691	T43.692	T43.693	T43.694	T43.695	T43.696
Etybenzatropine	T44.3X1	T44.3X2	T44.3X3	T44.3X4	T44.3X5	T44.3X6
Etynodiol	T38.4X1	T38.4X2	T38.4X3	T38.4X4	T38.4X5	T38.4X6
Eucaine	T41.3X1	T41.3X2	T41.3X3	T41.3X4	T41.3X5	T41.3X6
Eucalyptus oil	T49.7X1	T49.7X2	T49.7X3	T49.7X4	T49.7X5	T49.7X6
Eucatropine	T49.5X1	T49.5X2	T49.5X3	T49.5X4	T49.5X5	T49.5X6
Eucodal	T40.2X1	T40.2X2	T40.2X3	T40.2X4	T40.2X5	T40.2X6
Euneryl	T42.3X1	T42.3X2	T42.3X3	T42.3X4	T42.3X5	T42.3X6
Euphthalmine	T44.3X1	T44.3X2	T44.3X3	T44.3X4	T44.3X5	T44.3X6
Eurax	T49.0X1	T49.0X2	T49.0X3	T49.0X4	T49.0X5	T49.0X6
Euresol	T49.4X1	T49.4X2	T49.4X3	T49.4X4	T49.4X5	T49.4X6
Euthroid	T38.1X1	T38.1X2	T38.1X3	T38.1X4	T38.1X5	T38.1X6
Evans blue	T50.8X1	T50.8X2	T50.8X3	T50.8X4	T50.8X5	T50.8X6
Evipal	T42.3X1	T42.3X2	T42.3X3	T42.3X4	T42.3X5	T42.3X6
sodium	T41.1X1	T41.1X2	T41.1X3	T41.1X4	T41.1X5	T41.1X6
Evipan	T42.3X1	T42.3X2	T42.3X3	T42.3X4	T42.3X5	T42.3X6
sodium	T41.1X1	T41.1X2	T41.1X3	T41.1X4	T41.1X5	T41.1X6
Exalamide	T49.0X1	T49.0X2	T49.0X3	T49.0X4	T49.0X5	T49.0X6
Exalgin	T39.1X1	T39.1X2	T39.1X3	T39.1X4	T39.1X5	T39.1X6
Excipients, pharmaceutical	T50.901	T50.902	T50.903	T50.904	T50.905	T50.906
Exhaust gas (engine) (motor vehicle)	T58.01	T58.02	T58.03	T58.04	—	—
Ex-Lax (phenolphthalein)	T47.2X1	T47.2X2	T47.2X3	T47.2X4	T47.2X5	T47.2X6
Expectorant NEC	T48.4X1	T48.4X2	T48.4X3	T48.4X4	T48.4X5	T48.4X6
Extended insulin zinc suspension	T38.3X1	T38.3X2	T38.3X3	T38.3X4	T38.3X5	T38.3X6
External medications (skin) (mucous membrane)	T49.91	T49.92	T49.93	T49.94	T49.95	T49.96
dental agent	T49.7X1	T49.7X2	T49.7X3	T49.7X4	T49.7X5	T49.7X6
ENT agent	T49.6X1	T49.6X2	T49.6X3	T49.6X4	T49.6X5	T49.6X6
ophthalmic preparation	T49.5X1	T49.5X2	T49.5X3	T49.5X4	T49.5X5	T49.5X6
specified NEC	T49.8X1	T49.8X2	T49.8X3	T49.8X4	T49.8X5	T49.8X6
Extrapyramidal antagonist NEC	T44.3X1	T44.3X2	T44.3X3	T44.3X4	T44.3X5	T44.3X6
Eye agents (anti-infective)	T49.5X1	T49.5X2	T49.5X3	T49.5X4	T49.5X5	T49.5X6
Eye drug NEC	T49.5X1	T49.5X2	T49.5X3	T49.5X4	T49.5X5	T49.5X6
FAC (fluorouracil + doxorubicin + cyclophosphamide)	T45.1X1	T45.1X2	T45.1X3	T45.1X4	T45.1X5	T45.1X6
Factor						
I (fibrinogen)	T45.8X1	T45.8X2	T45.8X3	T45.8X4	T45.8X5	T45.8X6
III (thromboplastin)	T45.8X1	T45.8X2	T45.8X3	T45.8X4	T45.8X5	T45.8X6
IX complex	T45.7X1	T45.7X2	T45.7X3	T45.7X4	T45.7X5	T45.7X6
human	T45.8X1	T45.8X2	T45.8X3	T45.8X4	T45.8X5	T45.8X6
VIII (antihemophilic Factor) (concentrate)	T45.8X1	T45.8X2	T45.8X3	T45.8X4	T45.8X5	T45.8X6
Famotidine	T47.0X1	T47.0X2	T47.0X3	T47.0X4	T47.0X5	T47.0X6
Fat suspension, intravenous	T50.991	T50.992	T50.993	T50.994	T50.995	T50.996
Fazadinium bromide	T48.1X1	T48.1X2	T48.1X3	T48.1X4	T48.1X5	T48.1X6
Febarbamate	T42.3X1	T42.3X2	T42.3X3	T42.3X4	T42.3X5	T42.3X6
Fecal softener	T47.4X1	T47.4X2	T47.4X3	T47.4X4	T47.4X5	T47.4X6
Fedrilate	T48.3X1	T48.3X2	T48.3X3	T48.3X4	T48.3X5	T48.3X6
Felodipine	T46.1X1	T46.1X2	T46.1X3	T46.1X4	T46.1X5	T46.1X6
Felypressin	T38.891	T38.892	T38.893	T38.894	T38.895	T38.896
Femoxetine	T43.221	T43.222	T43.223	T43.224	T43.225	T43.226
Fenalcomine	T46.3X1	T46.3X2	T46.3X3	T46.3X4	T46.3X5	T46.3X6
Fenamisal	T37.1X1	T37.1X2	T37.1X3	T37.1X4	T37.1X5	T37.1X6
Fenazone	T39.2X1	T39.2X2	T39.2X3	T39.2X4	T39.2X5	T39.2X6
Fenbendazole	T37.4X1	T37.4X2	T37.4X3	T37.4X4	T37.4X5	T37.4X6
Fenbutrazate	T50.5X1	T50.5X2	T50.5X3	T50.5X4	T50.5X5	T50.5X6
Fencamfamine	T43.691	T43.692	T43.693	T43.694	T43.695	T43.696
Fendiline	T46.1X1	T46.1X2	T46.1X3	T46.1X4	T46.1X5	T46.1X6
Fenetylline	T43.691	T43.692	T43.693	T43.694	T43.695	T43.696
Fenflumizole	T39.391	T39.392	T39.393	T39.394	T39.395	T39.396
Fenfluramine	T50.5X1	T50.5X2	T50.5X3	T50.5X4	T50.5X5	T50.5X6
Fenobarbital	T42.3X1	T42.3X2	T42.3X3	T42.3X4	T42.3X5	T42.3X6
Fenofibrate	T46.6X1	T46.6X2	T46.6X3	T46.6X4	T46.6X5	T46.6X6
Fenoprofen	T39.311	T39.312	T39.313	T39.314	T39.315	T39.316
Fenoterol	T48.6X1	T48.6X2	T48.6X3	T48.6X4	T48.6X5	T48.6X6
Fenoverine	T44.3X1	T44.3X2	T44.3X3	T44.3X4	T44.3X5	T44.3X6
Fenoxazoline	T48.5X1	T48.5X2	T48.5X3	T48.5X4	T48.5X5	T48.5X6
Fenproporex	T50.5X1	T50.5X2	T50.5X3	T50.5X4	T50.5X5	T50.5X6
Fenquizone	T50.2X1	T50.2X2	T50.2X3	T50.2X4	T50.2X5	T50.2X6
Fentanyl (analogs)	T40.411	T40.412	T40.413	T40.414	T40.415	T40.416
Fentazin	T43.3X1	T43.3X2	T43.3X3	T43.3X4	T43.3X5	T43.3X6
Fenthion	T60.0X1	T60.0X2	T60.0X3	T60.0X4	—	—
Fenticlor	T49.0X1	T49.0X2	T49.0X3	T49.0X4	T49.0X5	T49.0X6
Fenylbutazone	T39.2X1	T39.2X2	T39.2X3	T39.2X4	T39.2X5	T39.2X6
Feprazone	T39.2X1	T39.2X2	T39.2X3	T39.2X4	T39.2X5	T39.2X6
Fer de lance (bite) (venom)	T63.061	T63.062	T63.063	T63.064	—	—
Ferric — *see also* Iron						
chloride	T45.4X1	T45.4X2	T45.4X3	T45.4X4	T45.4X5	T45.4X6
citrate	T45.4X1	T45.4X2	T45.4X3	T45.4X4	T45.4X5	T45.4X6
hydroxide						
colloidal	T45.4X1	T45.4X2	T45.4X3	T45.4X4	T45.4X5	T45.4X6
polymaltose	T45.4X1	T45.4X2	T45.4X3	T45.4X4	T45.4X5	T45.4X6
pyrophosphate	T45.4X1	T45.4X2	T45.4X3	T45.4X4	T45.4X5	T45.4X6
Ferritin	T45.4X1	T45.4X2	T45.4X3	T45.4X4	T45.4X5	T45.4X6
Ferrocholinate	T45.4X1	T45.4X2	T45.4X3	T45.4X4	T45.4X5	T45.4X6
Ferrodextrane	T45.4X1	T45.4X2	T45.4X3	T45.4X4	T45.4X5	T45.4X6
Ferropolimaler	T45.4X1	T45.4X2	T45.4X3	T45.4X4	T45.4X5	T45.4X6
Ferrous — *see also* Iron						
phosphate	T45.4X1	T45.4X2	T45.4X3	T45.4X4	T45.4X5	T45.4X6
salt	T45.4X1	T45.4X2	T45.4X3	T45.4X4	T45.4X5	T45.4X6
with folic acid	T45.4X1	T45.4X2	T45.4X3	T45.4X4	T45.4X5	T45.4X6
Ferrous fumerate, gluconate, lactate, salt NEC, sulfate (medicinal)	T45.4X1	T45.4X2	T45.4X3	T45.4X4	T45.4X5	T45.4X6
Ferrovanadium (fumes)	T59.891	T59.892	T59.893	T59.894	—	—
Ferrum — *see* Iron						
Fertilizers NEC	T65.891	T65.892	T65.893	T65.894	—	—
with herbicide mixture	T60.3X1	T60.3X2	T60.3X3	T60.3X4	—	—
Fetoxilate	T47.6X1	T47.6X2	T47.6X3	T47.6X4	T47.6X5	T47.6X6
Fiber, dietary	T47.4X1	T47.4X2	T47.4X3	T47.4X4	T47.4X5	T47.4X6
Fiberglass	T65.831	T65.832	T65.833	T65.834	—	—
Fibrinogen (human)	T45.8X1	T45.8X2	T45.8X3	T45.8X4	T45.8X5	T45.8X6
Fibrinolysin (human)	T45.691	T45.692	T45.693	T45.694	T45.695	T45.696
Fibrinolysis						
affecting drug	T45.601	T45.602	T45.603	T45.604	T45.605	T45.606
inhibitor NEC	T45.621	T45.622	T45.623	T45.624	T45.625	T45.626
Fibrinolytic drug	T45.611	T45.612	T45.613	T45.614	T45.615	T45.616
Filix mas	T37.4X1	T37.4X2	T37.4X3	T37.4X4	T37.4X5	T37.4X6
Filtering cream	T49.3X1	T49.3X2	T49.3X3	T49.3X4	T49.3X5	T49.3X6
Fiorinal	T39.011	T39.012	T39.013	T39.014	T39.015	T39.016
Firedamp	T59.891	T59.892	T59.893	T59.894	—	—
Fish, noxious, nonbacterial	T61.91	T61.92	T61.93	T61.94	—	—
ciguatera	T61.01	T61.02	T61.03	T61.04	—	—
scombroid	T61.11	T61.12	T61.13	T61.14	—	—
shell	T61.781	T61.782	T61.783	T61.784	—	—
specified NEC	T61.771	T61.772	T61.773	T61.774	—	—
Flagyl	T37.3X1	T37.3X2	T37.3X3	T37.3X4	T37.3X5	T37.3X6
Flavine adenine dinucleotide	T45.2X1	T45.2X2	T45.2X3	T45.2X4	T45.2X5	T45.2X6
Flavodic acid	T46.991	T46.992	T46.993	T46.994	T46.995	T46.996
Flavoxate	T44.3X1	T44.3X2	T44.3X3	T44.3X4	T44.3X5	T44.3X6
Flaxedil	T48.1X1	T48.1X2	T48.1X3	T48.1X4	T48.1X5	T48.1X6
Flaxseed (medicinal)	T49.3X1	T49.3X2	T49.3X3	T49.3X4	T49.3X5	T49.3X6
Flecainide	T46.2X1	T46.2X2	T46.2X3	T46.2X4	T46.2X5	T46.2X6
Fleroxacin	T36.8X1	T36.8X2	T36.8X3	T36.8X4	T36.8X5	T36.8X6
Floctafenine	T39.8X1	T39.8X2	T39.8X3	T39.8X4	T39.8X5	T39.8X6
Flomax	T44.6X1	T44.6X2	T44.6X3	T44.6X4	T44.6X5	T44.6X6
Flomoxef	T36.1X1	T36.1X2	T36.1X3	T36.1X4	T36.1X5	T36.1X6
Flopropione	T44.3X1	T44.3X2	T44.3X3	T44.3X4	T44.3X5	T44.3X6
Florantyrone	T47.5X1	T47.5X2	T47.5X3	T47.5X4	T47.5X5	T47.5X6
Floraquin	T37.8X1	T37.8X2	T37.8X3	T37.8X4	T37.8X5	T37.8X6
Florinef	T38.0X1	T38.0X2	T38.0X3	T38.0X4	T38.0X5	T38.0X6
ENT agent	T49.6X1	T49.6X2	T49.6X3	T49.6X4	T49.6X5	T49.6X6
ophthalmic preparation	T49.5X1	T49.5X2	T49.5X3	T49.5X4	T49.5X5	T49.5X6
topical NEC	T49.0X1	T49.0X2	T49.0X3	T49.0X4	T49.0X5	T49.0X6
Flowers of sulfur	T49.4X1	T49.4X2	T49.4X3	T49.4X4	T49.4X5	T49.4X6
Floxuridine	T45.1X1	T45.1X2	T45.1X3	T45.1X4	T45.1X5	T45.1X6
Fluanisone	T43.4X1	T43.4X2	T43.4X3	T43.4X4	T43.4X5	T43.4X6
Flubendazole	T37.4X1	T37.4X2	T37.4X3	T37.4X4	T37.4X5	T37.4X6
Fluclorolone acetonide	T49.0X1	T49.0X2	T49.0X3	T49.0X4	T49.0X5	T49.0X6
Flucloxacillin	T36.0X1	T36.0X2	T36.0X3	T36.0X4	T36.0X5	T36.0X6
Fluconazole	T37.8X1	T37.8X2	T37.8X3	T37.8X4	T37.8X5	T37.8X6
Flucytosine	T37.8X1	T37.8X2	T37.8X3	T37.8X4	T37.8X5	T37.8X6
Fludeoxyglucose (18F)	T50.8X1	T50.8X2	T50.8X3	T50.8X4	T50.8X5	T50.8X6
Fludiazepam	T42.4X1	T42.4X2	T42.4X3	T42.4X4	T42.4X5	T42.4X6
Fludrocortisone	T50.0X1	T50.0X2	T50.0X3	T50.0X4	T50.0X5	T50.0X6
ENT agent	T49.6X1	T49.6X2	T49.6X3	T49.6X4	T49.6X5	T49.6X6
ophthalmic preparation	T49.5X1	T49.5X2	T49.5X3	T49.5X4	T49.5X5	T49.5X6
topical NEC	T49.0X1	T49.0X2	T49.0X3	T49.0X4	T49.0X5	T49.0X6
Fludroxycortide	T49.0X1	T49.0X2	T49.0X3	T49.0X4	T49.0X5	T49.0X6
Flufenamic acid	T39.391	T39.392	T39.393	T39.394	T39.395	T39.396
Fluindione	T45.511	T45.512	T45.513	T45.514	T45.515	T45.516
Flumequine	T37.8X1	T37.8X2	T37.8X3	T37.8X4	T37.8X5	T37.8X6
Flumethasone	T49.0X1	T49.0X2	T49.0X3	T49.0X4	T49.0X5	T49.0X6
Flumethiazide	T50.2X1	T50.2X2	T50.2X3	T50.2X4	T50.2X5	T50.2X6

Substance	Poisoning, Accidental (unintentional)	Poisoning, Intentional Self-harm	Poisoning, Assault	Poisoning, Undetermined	Adverse Effect	Under-dosing
Flumidin	T37.5X1	T37.5X2	T37.5X3	T37.5X4	T37.5X5	T37.5X6
Flunarizine	T46.7X1	T46.7X2	T46.7X3	T46.7X4	T46.7X5	T46.7X6
Flunidazole	T37.8X1	T37.8X2	T37.8X3	T37.8X4	T37.8X5	T37.8X6
Flunisolide	T48.6X1	T48.6X2	T48.6X3	T48.6X4	T48.6X5	T48.6X6
Flunitrazepam	T42.4X1	T42.4X2	T42.4X3	T42.4X4	T42.4X5	T42.4X6
Fluocinolone (acetonide)	T49.0X1	T49.0X2	T49.0X3	T49.0X4	T49.0X5	T49.0X6
Fluocinonide	T49.0X1	T49.0X2	T49.0X3	T49.0X4	T49.0X5	T49.0X6
Fluocortin (butyl)	T49.0X1	T49.0X2	T49.0X3	T49.0X4	T49.0X5	T49.0X6
Fluocortolone	T49.0X1	T49.0X2	T49.0X3	T49.0X4	T49.0X5	T49.0X6
Fluohydrocortisone	T38.0X1	T38.0X2	T38.0X3	T38.0X4	T38.0X5	T38.0X6
ENT agent	T49.6X1	T49.6X2	T49.6X3	T49.6X4	T49.6X5	T49.6X6
ophthalmic preparation	T49.5X1	T49.5X2	T49.5X3	T49.5X4	T49.5X5	T49.5X6
topical NEC	T49.0X1	T49.0X2	T49.0X3	T49.0X4	T49.0X5	T49.0X6
Fluonid	T49.0X1	T49.0X2	T49.0X3	T49.0X4	T49.0X5	T49.0X6
Fluopromazine	T43.3X1	T43.3X2	T43.3X3	T43.3X4	T43.3X5	T43.3X6
Fluoracetate	T60.8X1	T60.8X2	T60.8X3	T60.8X4	—	—
Fluorescein	T50.8X1	T50.8X2	T50.8X3	T50.8X4	T50.8X5	T50.8X6
Fluorhydrocortisone	T50.0X1	T50.0X2	T50.0X3	T50.0X4	T50.0X5	T50.0X6
Fluoride (nonmedicinal) (pesticide) (sodium) **NEC**	T60.8X1	T60.8X2	T60.8X3	T60.8X4	—	—
hydrogen — *see* Hydrofluoric acid						
medicinal NEC	T50.991	T50.992	T50.993	T50.994	T50.995	T50.996
dental use	T49.7X1	T49.7X2	T49.7X3	T49.7X4	T49.7X5	T49.7X6
not pesticide NEC	T54.91	T54.92	T54.93	T54.94		
stannous	T49.7X1	T49.7X2	T49.7X3	T49.7X4	T49.7X5	T49.7X6
Fluorinated corticosteroids	T38.0X1	T38.0X2	T38.0X3	T38.0X4	T38.0X5	T38.0X6
Fluorine (gas)	T59.5X1	T59.5X2	T59.5X3	T59.5X4	—	—
salt — *see* Fluoride(s)						
Fluoristan	T49.7X1	T49.7X2	T49.7X3	T49.7X4	T49.7X5	T49.7X6
Fluormetholone	T49.0X1	T49.0X2	T49.0X3	T49.0X4	T49.0X5	T49.0X6
Fluoroacetate	T60.8X1	T60.8X2	T60.8X3	T60.8X4	—	—
Fluorocarbon monomer	T53.6X1	T53.6X2	T53.6X3	T53.6X4	—	—
Fluorocytosine	T37.8X1	T37.8X2	T37.8X3	T37.8X4	T37.8X5	T37.8X6
Fluorodeoxyuridine	T45.1X1	T45.1X2	T45.1X3	T45.1X4	T45.1X5	T45.1X6
Fluorometholone	T49.0X1	T49.0X2	T49.0X3	T49.0X4	T49.0X5	T49.0X6
ophthalmic preparation	T49.5X1	T49.5X2	T49.5X3	T49.5X4	T49.5X5	T49.5X6
Fluorophosphate insecticide	T60.0X1	T60.0X2	T60.0X3	T60.0X4	—	—
Fluorosol	T46.3X1	T46.3X2	T46.3X3	T46.3X4	T46.3X5	T46.3X6
Fluorouracil	T45.1X1	T45.1X2	T45.1X3	T45.1X4	T45.1X5	T45.1X6
Fluorphenylalanine	T49.5X1	T49.5X2	T49.5X3	T49.5X4	T49.5X5	T49.5X6
Fluothane	T41.0X1	T41.0X2	T41.0X3	T41.0X4	T41.0X5	T41.0X6
Fluoxetine	T43.221	T43.222	T43.223	T43.224	T43.225	T43.226
Fluoxymesterone	T38.7X1	T38.7X2	T38.7X3	T38.7X4	T38.7X5	T38.7X6
Flupenthixol	T43.4X1	T43.4X2	T43.4X3	T43.4X4	T43.4X5	T43.4X6
Flupentixol	T43.4X1	T43.4X2	T43.4X3	T43.4X4	T43.4X5	T43.4X6
Fluphenazine	T43.3X1	T43.3X2	T43.3X3	T43.3X4	T43.3X5	T43.3X6
Fluprednidene	T49.0X1	T49.0X2	T49.0X3	T49.0X4	T49.0X5	T49.0X6
Fluprednisolone	T38.0X1	T38.0X2	T38.0X3	T38.0X4	T38.0X5	T38.0X6
Fluradoline	T39.8X1	T39.8X2	T39.8X3	T39.8X4	T39.8X5	T39.8X6
Flurandrenolide	T49.0X1	T49.0X2	T49.0X3	T49.0X4	T49.0X5	T49.0X6
Flurandrenolone	T49.0X1	T49.0X2	T49.0X3	T49.0X4	T49.0X5	T49.0X6
Flurazepam	T42.4X1	T42.4X2	T42.4X3	T42.4X4	T42.4X5	T42.4X6
Flurbiprofen	T39.311	T39.312	T39.313	T39.314	T39.315	T39.316
Flurobate	T49.0X1	T49.0X2	T49.0X3	T49.0X4	T49.0X5	T49.0X6
Fluroxene	T41.0X1	T41.0X2	T41.0X3	T41.0X4	T41.0X5	T41.0X6
Fluspirilene	T43.591	T43.592	T43.593	T43.594	T43.595	T43.596
Flutamide	T38.6X1	T38.6X2	T38.6X3	T38.6X4	T38.6X5	T38.6X6
Flutazolam	T42.4X1	T42.4X2	T42.4X3	T42.4X4	T42.4X5	T42.4X6
Fluticasone propionate	T38.0X1	T38.0X2	T38.0X3	T38.0X4	T38.0X5	T38.0X6
Flutoprazepam	T42.4X1	T42.4X2	T42.4X3	T42.4X4	T42.4X5	T42.4X6
Flutropium bromide	T48.6X1	T48.6X2	T48.6X3	T48.6X4	T48.6X5	T48.6X6
Fluvoxamine	T43.221	T43.222	T43.223	T43.224	T43.225	T43.226
Folacin	T45.8X1	T45.8X2	T45.8X3	T45.8X4	T45.8X5	T45.8X6
Folic acid	T45.8X1	T45.8X2	T45.8X3	T45.8X4	T45.8X5	T45.8X6
with ferrous salt	T45.2X1	T45.2X2	T45.2X3	T45.2X4	T45.2X5	T45.2X6
antagonist	T45.1X1	T45.1X2	T45.1X3	T45.1X4	T45.1X5	T45.1X6
Folinic acid	T45.8X1	T45.8X2	T45.8X3	T45.8X4	T45.8X5	T45.8X6
Folium stramoniae	T48.6X1	T48.6X2	T48.6X3	T48.6X4	T48.6X5	T48.6X6
Follicle-stimulating hormone, human	T38.811	T38.812	T38.813	T38.814	T38.815	T38.816
Folpet	T60.3X1	T60.3X2	T60.3X3	T60.3X4	—	—
Fominoben	T48.3X1	T48.3X2	T48.3X3	T48.3X4	T48.3X5	T48.3X6
Food, foodstuffs, noxious, nonbacterial, NEC	T62.91	T62.92	T62.93	T62.94	—	—
berries	T62.1X1	T62.1X2	T62.1X3	T62.1X4	—	—
fish — *see also* Fish	T61.91	T61.92	T61.93	T61.94	—	—
mushrooms	T62.0X1	T62.0X2	T62.0X3	T62.0X4	—	—
plants	T62.2X1	T62.2X2	T62.2X3	T62.2X4	—	—
seafood	T61.91	T61.92	T61.93	T61.94	—	—
specified NEC	T61.8X1	T61.8X2	T61.8X3	T61.8X4	—	—

Substance	Poisoning, Accidental (unintentional)	Poisoning, Intentional Self-harm	Poisoning, Assault	Poisoning, Undetermined	Adverse Effect	Under-dosing
Food, foodstuffs, noxious, nonbacterial, — *continued*						
seeds	T62.2X1	T62.2X2	T62.2X3	T62.2X4	—	—
shellfish	T61.781	T61.782	T61.783	T61.784	—	—
specified NEC	T62.8X1	T62.8X2	T62.8X3	T62.8X4	—	—
Fool's parsley	T62.2X1	T62.2X2	T62.2X3	T62.2X4	—	—
Formaldehyde (solution), gas or vapor	T59.2X1	T59.2X2	T59.2X3	T59.2X4	—	—
fungicide	T60.3X1	T60.3X2	T60.3X3	T60.3X4	—	—
Formalin	T59.2X1	T59.2X2	T59.2X3	T59.2X4	—	—
fungicide	T60.3X1	T60.3X2	T60.3X3	T60.3X4	—	—
vapor	T59.2X1	T59.2X2	T59.2X3	T59.2X4	—	—
Formic acid	T54.2X1	T54.2X2	T54.2X3	T54.2X4	—	—
vapor	T59.891	T59.892	T59.893	T59.894	—	—
Foscarnet sodium	T37.5X1	T37.5X2	T37.5X3	T37.5X4	T37.5X5	T37.5X6
Fosfestrol	T38.5X1	T38.5X2	T38.5X3	T38.5X4	T38.5X5	T38.5X6
Fosfomycin	T36.8X1	T36.8X2	T36.8X3	T36.8X4	T36.8X5	T36.8X6
Fosfonet sodium	T37.5X1	T37.5X2	T37.5X3	T37.5X4	T37.5X5	T37.5X6
Fosinopril	T46.4X1	T46.4X2	T46.4X3	T46.4X4	T46.4X5	T46.4X6
sodium	T46.4X1	T46.4X2	T46.4X3	T46.4X4	T46.4X5	T46.4X6
Fowler's solution	T57.0X1	T57.0X2	T57.0X3	T57.0X4	—	—
Foxglove	T62.2X1	T62.2X2	T62.2X3	T62.2X4	—	—
Framycetin	T36.5X1	T36.5X2	T36.5X3	T36.5X4	T36.5X5	T36.5X6
Frangula	T47.2X1	T47.2X2	T47.2X3	T47.2X4	T47.2X5	T47.2X6
extract	T47.2X1	T47.2X2	T47.2X3	T47.2X4	T47.2X5	T47.2X6
Frei antigen	T50.8X1	T50.8X2	T50.8X3	T50.8X4	T50.8X5	T50.8X6
Freon	T53.5X1	T53.5X2	T53.5X3	T53.5X4	—	—
Fructose	T50.3X1	T50.3X2	T50.3X3	T50.3X4	T50.3X5	T50.3X6
Frusemide	T50.1X1	T50.1X2	T50.1X3	T50.1X4	T50.1X5	T50.1X6
FSH	T38.811	T38.812	T38.813	T38.814	T38.815	T38.816
Ftorafur	T45.1X1	T45.1X2	T45.1X3	T45.1X4	T45.1X5	T45.1X6
Fuel						
automobile	T52.0X1	T52.0X2	T52.0X3	T52.0X4	—	—
exhaust gas, not in transit	T58.01	T58.02	T58.03	T58.04	—	—
vapor NEC	T52.0X1	T52.0X2	T52.0X3	T52.0X4	—	—
gas (domestic use) — *see also* Carbon, monoxide, fuel, utility	T59.891	T59.892	T59.893	T59.894	—	—
utility	T59.891	T59.892	T59.893	T59.894	—	—
incomplete combustion of — *see* Carbon, monoxide, fuel, utility						
in mobile container	T59.891	T59.892	T59.893	T59.894	—	—
piped (natural)	T59.891	T59.892	T59.893	T59.894	—	—
industrial, incomplete combustion	T58.8X1	T58.8X2	T58.8X3	T58.8X4	—	—
Fugillin	T36.8X1	T36.8X2	T36.8X3	T36.8X4	T36.8X5	T36.8X6
Fulminate of mercury	T56.1X1	T56.1X2	T56.1X3	T56.1X4	—	—
Fulvicin	T36.7X1	T36.7X2	T36.7X3	T36.7X4	T36.7X5	T36.7X6
Fumadil	T36.8X1	T36.8X2	T36.8X3	T36.8X4	T36.8X5	T36.8X6
Fumagillin	T36.8X1	T36.8X2	T36.8X3	T36.8X4	T36.8X5	T36.8X6
Fumaric acid	T49.4X1	T49.4X2	T49.4X3	T49.4X4	T49.4X5	T49.4X6
Fumes (from)	T59.91	T59.92	T59.93	T59.94	—	—
carbon monoxide — *see* Carbon, monoxide						
charcoal (domestic use) — *see* Charcoal, fumes						
chloroform — *see* Chloroform						
coke (in domestic stoves, fireplaces) — *see* Coke fumes						
corrosive NEC	T54.91	T54.92	T54.93	T54.94	—	—
ether — *see* ether						
freons	T53.5X1	T53.5X2	T53.5X3	T53.5X4	—	—
hydrocarbons	T59.891	T59.892	T59.893	T59.894	—	—
petroleum (liquefied)	T59.891	T59.892	T59.893	T59.894	—	—
distributed through pipes (pure or mixed with air)	T59.891	T59.892	T59.893	T59.894	—	—
lead — *see* lead						
metal — *see* Metals, or the specified metal						
nitrogen dioxide	T59.0X1	T59.0X2	T59.0X3	T59.0X4	—	—
pesticides — *see* Pesticides						
petroleum (liquefied)	T59.891	T59.892	T59.893	T59.894	—	—
distributed through pipes (pure or mixed with air)	T59.891	T59.892	T59.893	T59.894	—	—
polyester	T59.891	T59.892	T59.893	T59.894	—	—
specified source NEC — *see also* substance specified	T59.891	T59.892	T59.893	T59.894	—	—
sulfur dioxide	T59.1X1	T59.1X2	T59.1X3	T59.1X4	—	—

▼ Subterms under main terms may continue to next column or page   Additional Character May Be Required — Refer to the Tabular List for Character Selection   375

Flumidin — Fumes

Substance	Poisoning, Accidental (unintentional)	Poisoning, Intentional Self-harm	Poisoning, Assault	Poisoning, Undetermined	Adverse Effect	Under-dosing
Fumigant NEC	T60.91	T60.92	T60.93	T60.94	—	—
Fungicide NEC	T60.3X1	T60.3X2	T60.3X3	T60.3X4	—	—
(nonmedicinal)						
Fungi, noxious, used as food	T62.0X1	T62.0X2	T62.0X3	T62.0X4		
Fungizone	T36.7X1	T36.7X2	T36.7X3	T36.7X4	T36.7X5	T36.7X6
topical	T49.0X1	T49.0X2	T49.0X3	T49.0X4	T49.0X5	T49.0X6
Furacin	T49.0X1	T49.0X2	T49.0X3	T49.0X4	T49.0X5	T49.0X6
Furadantin	T37.91	T37.92	T37.93	T37.94	T37.95	T37.96
Furazolidone	T37.8X1	T37.8X2	T37.8X3	T37.8X4	T37.8X5	T37.8X6
Furazolium chloride	T49.0X1	T49.0X2	T49.0X3	T49.0X4	T49.0X5	T49.0X6
Furfural	T52.8X1	T52.8X2	T52.8X3	T52.8X4	—	—
Furnace (coal burning) (domestic), gas from	T58.2X1	T58.2X2	T58.2X3	T58.2X4	—	—
industrial	T58.8X1	T58.8X2	T58.8X3	T58.8X4	—	—
Furniture polish	T65.891	T65.892	T65.893	T65.894	—	—
Furosemide	T50.1X1	T50.1X2	T50.1X3	T50.1X4	T50.1X5	T50.1X6
Furoxone	T37.91	T37.92	T37.93	T37.94	T37.95	T37.96
Fursultiamine	T45.2X1	T45.2X2	T45.2X3	T45.2X4	T45.2X5	T45.2X6
Fusafungine	T36.8X1	T36.8X2	T36.8X3	T36.8X4	T36.8X5	T36.8X6
Fusel oil (any) (amyl) (butyl) (propyl), vapor	T51.3X1	T51.3X2	T51.3X3	T51.3X4	—	—
Fusidate (ethanolamine) (sodium)	T36.8X1	T36.8X2	T36.8X3	T36.8X4	T36.8X5	T36.8X6
Fusidic acid	T36.8X1	T36.8X2	T36.8X3	T36.8X4	T36.8X5	T36.8X6
Fytic acid, nonasodium	T50.6X1	T50.6X2	T50.6X3	T50.6X4	T50.6X5	T50.6X6
b-Galactosidase	T47.5X1	T47.5X2	T47.5X3	T47.5X4	T47.5X5	T47.5X6
GABA	T43.8X1	T43.8X2	T43.8X3	T43.8X4	T43.8X5	T43.8X6
Gadopentetic acid	T50.8X1	T50.8X2	T50.8X3	T50.8X4	T50.8X5	T50.8X6
Galactose	T50.3X1	T50.3X2	T50.3X3	T50.3X4	T50.3X5	T50.3X6
Galantamine	T44.0X1	T44.0X2	T44.0X3	T44.0X4	T44.0X5	T44.0X6
Gallamine (triethiodide)	T48.1X1	T48.1X2	T48.1X3	T48.1X4	T48.1X5	T48.1X6
Gallium citrate	T50.991	T50.992	T50.993	T50.994	T50.995	T50.996
Gallopamil	T46.1X1	T46.1X2	T46.1X3	T46.1X4	T46.1X5	T46.1X6
Gamboge	T47.2X1	T47.2X2	T47.2X3	T47.2X4	T47.2X5	T47.2X6
Gamimune	T50.Z11	T50.Z12	T50.Z13	T50.Z14	T50.Z15	T50.Z16
Gamma-aminobutyric acid	T43.8X1	T43.8X2	T43.8X3	T43.8X4	T43.8X5	T43.8X6
Gamma-benzene hexachloride (medicinal)	T49.0X1	T49.0X2	T49.0X3	T49.0X4	T49.0X5	T49.0X6
nonmedicinal, vapor	T53.6X1	T53.6X2	T53.6X3	T53.6X4	—	—
Gamma-BHC (medicinal) — see also Gamma-benzene hexachloride	T49.0X1	T49.0X2	T49.0X3	T49.0X4	T49.0X5	T49.0X6
Gamma globulin	T50.Z11	T50.Z12	T50.Z13	T50.Z14	T50.Z15	T50.Z16
Gamulin	T50.Z11	T50.Z12	T50.Z13	T50.Z14	T50.Z15	T50.Z16
Ganciclovir (sodium)	T37.5X1	T37.5X2	T37.5X3	T37.5X4	T37.5X5	T37.5X6
Ganglionic blocking drug NEC	T44.2X1	T44.2X2	T44.2X3	T44.2X4	T44.2X5	T44.2X6
specified NEC	T44.2X1	T44.2X2	T44.2X3	T44.2X4	T44.2X5	T44.2X6
Ganja	T40.711	T40.712	T40.713	T40.714	T40.715	T40.716
Garamycin	T36.5X1	T36.5X2	T36.5X3	T36.5X4	T36.5X5	T36.5X6
ophthalmic preparation	T49.5X1	T49.5X2	T49.5X3	T49.5X4	T49.5X5	T49.5X6
topical NEC	T49.0X1	T49.0X2	T49.0X3	T49.0X4	T49.0X5	T49.0X6
Gardenal	T42.3X1	T42.3X2	T42.3X3	T42.3X4	T42.3X5	T42.3X6
Gardepanyl	T42.3X1	T42.3X2	T42.3X3	T42.3X4	T42.3X5	T42.3X6
Gaseous substance — see Gas						
Gasoline	T52.0X1	T52.0X2	T52.0X3	T52.0X4	—	—
vapor	T52.0X1	T52.0X2	T52.0X3	T52.0X4	—	—
Gastric enzymes	T47.5X1	T47.5X2	T47.5X3	T47.5X4	T47.5X5	T47.5X6
Gastrografin	T50.8X1	T50.8X2	T50.8X3	T50.8X4	T50.8X5	T50.8X6
Gastrointestinal drug	T47.91	T47.92	T47.93	T47.94	T47.95	T47.96
biological	T47.8X1	T47.8X2	T47.8X3	T47.8X4	T47.8X5	T47.8X6
specified NEC	T47.8X1	T47.8X2	T47.8X3	T47.8X4	T47.8X5	T47.8X6
Gas NEC	T59.91	T59.92	T59.93	T59.94	—	—
acetylene	T59.891	T59.892	T59.893	T59.894	—	—
incomplete combustion of	T58.11	T58.12	T58.13	T58.14	—	—
air contaminants, source or type not specified	T59.91	T59.92	T59.93	T59.94	—	—
anesthetic	T41.0X1	T41.0X2	T41.0X3	T41.0X4	T41.0X5	T41.0X6
blast furnace	T58.8X1	T58.8X2	T58.8X3	T58.8X4	—	—
butane — see butane						
carbon monoxide — see Carbon, monoxide						
chlorine	T59.4X1	T59.4X2	T59.4X3	T59.4X4	—	—
coal	T58.2X1	T58.2X2	T58.2X3	T58.2X4	—	—
cyanide	T57.3X1	T57.3X2	T57.3X3	T57.3X4	—	—
dicyanogen	T65.0X1	T65.0X2	T65.0X3	T65.0X4	—	—
domestic — see Domestic gas						
exhaust	T58.01	T58.02	T58.03	T58.04		
from utility (for cooking, heating, or lighting) (after						

Substance	Poisoning, Accidental (unintentional)	Poisoning, Intentional Self-harm	Poisoning, Assault	Poisoning, Undetermined	Adverse Effect	Under-dosing
Gas — continued						
from utility — see Carbon, monoxide, fuel, utility — continued						
combustion) — see Carbon, monoxide, fuel, utility						
prior to combustion	T59.891	T59.892	T59.893	T59.894	—	—
from wood- or coal-burning stove or fireplace	T58.2X1	T58.2X2	T58.2X3	T58.2X4		
fuel (domestic use) (after combustion) — see also Carbon, monoxide, fuel						
industrial use	T58.8X1	T58.8X2	T58.8X3	T58.8X4		
prior to combustion	T59.891	T59.892	T59.893	T59.894		
utility	T59.891	T59.892	T59.893	T59.894		
incomplete combustion of — see Carbon, monoxide, fuel, utility						
in mobile container	T59.891	T59.892	T59.893	T59.894		
piped (natural)	T59.891	T59.892	T59.893	T59.894		
garage	T58.01	T58.02	T58.03	T58.04	—	—
hydrocarbon NEC	T59.891	T59.892	T59.893	T59.894		
incomplete combustion of — see Carbon, monoxide, fuel, utility						
liquefied — see butane						
piped	T59.891	T59.892	T59.893	T59.894		
hydrocyanic acid	T65.0X1	T65.0X2	T65.0X3	T65.0X4	—	—
illuminating (after combustion)	T58.11	T58.12	T58.13	T58.14		
prior to combustion	T59.891	T59.892	T59.893	T59.894		
incomplete combustion, any — see Carbon, monoxide						
kiln	T58.8X1	T58.8X2	T58.8X3	T58.8X4	—	—
lacrimogenic	T59.3X1	T59.3X2	T59.3X3	T59.3X4	—	—
liquefied petroleum — see butane						
marsh	T59.891	T59.892	T59.893	T59.894	—	—
motor exhaust, not in transit	T58.01	T58.02	T58.03	T58.04	—	—
mustard, not in war	T59.891	T59.892	T59.893	T59.894	—	—
natural	T59.891	T59.892	T59.893	T59.894	—	—
nerve, not in war	T59.91	T59.92	T59.93	T59.94	—	—
oil	T52.0X1	T52.0X2	T52.0X3	T52.0X4	—	—
petroleum (liquefied) (distributed in mobile containers)	T59.891	T59.892	T59.893	T59.894	—	—
piped (pure or mixed with air)	T59.891	T59.892	T59.893	T59.894	—	—
piped (manufactured) (natural) NEC	T59.891	T59.892	T59.893	T59.894	—	—
producer	T58.8X1	T58.8X2	T58.8X3	T58.8X4	—	—
propane — see propane						
refrigerant (chlorofluoro-carbon)	T53.5X1	T53.5X2	T53.5X3	T53.5X4	—	—
not chlorofluoro-carbon	T59.891	T59.892	T59.893	T59.894	—	—
sewer	T59.91	T59.92	T59.93	T59.94	—	—
specified source NEC	T59.91	T59.92	T59.93	T59.94	—	—
stove (after combustion)	T58.11	T58.12	T58.13	T58.14	—	—
prior to combustion	T59.891	T59.892	T59.893	T59.894	—	—
tear	T59.3X1	T59.3X2	T59.3X3	T59.3X4	—	—
therapeutic	T41.5X1	T41.5X2	T41.5X3	T41.5X4	T41.5X5	T41.5X6
utility (for cooking, heating, or lighting) (piped) NEC	T59.891	T59.892	T59.893	T59.894	—	—
incomplete combustion of — see Carbon, monoxide, fuel, utilty						
in mobile container	T59.891	T59.892	T59.893	T59.894	—	—
piped (natural)	T59.891	T59.892	T59.893	T59.894	—	—
water	T58.11	T58.12	T58.13	T58.14	—	—
incomplete combustion of — see Carbon, monoxide, fuel, utility						
Gaultheria procumbens	T62.2X1	T62.2X2	T62.2X3	T62.2X4	—	—
Gefarnate	T44.3X1	T44.3X2	T44.3X3	T44.3X4	T44.3X5	T44.3X6
Gelatin (intravenous)	T45.8X1	T45.8X2	T45.8X3	T45.8X4	T45.8X5	T45.8X6
absorbable (sponge)	T45.7X1	T45.7X2	T45.7X3	T45.7X4	T45.7X5	T45.7X6
Gelfilm	T49.8X1	T49.8X2	T49.8X3	T49.8X4	T49.8X5	T49.8X6
Gelfoam	T45.7X1	T45.7X2	T45.7X3	T45.7X4	T45.7X5	T45.7X6
Gelsemine	T50.991	T50.992	T50.993	T50.994	T50.995	T50.996
Gelsemium (sempervirens)	T62.2X1	T62.2X2	T62.2X3	T62.2X4	—	—
Gemeprost	T48.0X1	T48.0X2	T48.0X3	T48.0X4	T48.0X5	T48.0X6
Gemfibrozil	T46.6X1	T46.6X2	T46.6X3	T46.6X4	T46.6X5	T46.6X6

Additional Character May Be Required — Refer to the Tabular List for Character Selection   ▼ Subterms under main terms may continue to next column or page

Substance	Poisoning, Accidental (unintentional)	Poisoning, Intentional Self-harm	Poisoning, Assault	Poisoning, Undetermined	Adverse Effect	Under-dosing
Gemonil	T42.3X1	T42.3X2	T42.3X3	T42.3X4	T42.3X5	T42.3X6
Gentamicin	T36.5X1	T36.5X2	T36.5X3	T36.5X4	T36.5X5	T36.5X6
ophthalmic preparation	T49.5X1	T49.5X2	T49.5X3	T49.5X4	T49.5X5	T49.5X6
topical NEC	T49.0X1	T49.0X2	T49.0X3	T49.0X4	T49.0X5	T49.0X6
Gentian	T47.5X1	T47.5X2	T47.5X3	T47.5X4	T47.5X5	T47.5X6
violet	T49.0X1	T49.0X2	T49.0X3	T49.0X4	T49.0X5	T49.0X6
Gepefrine	T44.4X1	T44.4X2	T44.4X3	T44.4X4	T44.4X5	T44.4X6
Gestonorone caproate	T38.5X1	T38.5X2	T38.5X3	T38.5X4	T38.5X5	T38.5X6
Gexane	T49.0X1	T49.0X2	T49.0X3	T49.0X4	T49.0X5	T49.0X6
Gila monster (venom)	T63.111	T63.112	T63.113	T63.114	—	—
Ginger	T47.5X1	T47.5X2	T47.5X3	T47.5X4	T47.5X5	T47.5X6
Jamaica — see Jamaica, ginger						
Gitalin	T46.0X1	T46.0X2	T46.0X3	T46.0X4	T46.0X5	T46.0X6
amorphous	T46.0X1	T46.0X2	T46.0X3	T46.0X4	T46.0X5	T46.0X6
Gitaloxin	T46.0X1	T46.0X2	T46.0X3	T46.0X4	T46.0X5	T46.0X6
Gitoxin	T46.0X1	T46.0X2	T46.0X3	T46.0X4	T46.0X5	T46.0X6
Glafenine	T39.8X1	T39.8X2	T39.8X3	T39.8X4	T39.8X5	T39.8X6
Glandular extract (medicinal) NEC	T50.Z91	T50.Z92	T50.Z93	T50.Z94	T50.Z95	T50.Z96
Glaucarubin	T37.3X1	T37.3X2	T37.3X3	T37.3X4	T37.3X5	T37.3X6
Glibenclamide	T38.3X1	T38.3X2	T38.3X3	T38.3X4	T38.3X5	T38.3X6
Glibornuride	T38.3X1	T38.3X2	T38.3X3	T38.3X4	T38.3X5	T38.3X6
Gliclazide	T38.3X1	T38.3X2	T38.3X3	T38.3X4	T38.3X5	T38.3X6
Glimidine	T38.3X1	T38.3X2	T38.3X3	T38.3X4	T38.3X5	T38.3X6
Glipizide	T38.3X1	T38.3X2	T38.3X3	T38.3X4	T38.3X5	T38.3X6
Gliquidone	T38.3X1	T38.3X2	T38.3X3	T38.3X4	T38.3X5	T38.3X6
Glisolamide	T38.3X1	T38.3X2	T38.3X3	T38.3X4	T38.3X5	T38.3X6
Glisoxepide	T38.3X1	T38.3X2	T38.3X3	T38.3X4	T38.3X5	T38.3X6
Globin zinc insulin	T38.3X1	T38.3X2	T38.3X3	T38.3X4	T38.3X5	T38.3X6
Globulin						
antilymphocytic	T50.Z11	T50.Z12	T50.Z13	T50.Z14	T50.Z15	T50.Z16
antirhesus	T50.Z11	T50.Z12	T50.Z13	T50.Z14	T50.Z15	T50.Z16
antivenin	T50.Z11	T50.Z12	T50.Z13	T50.Z14	T50.Z15	T50.Z16
antiviral	T50.Z11	T50.Z12	T50.Z13	T50.Z14	T50.Z15	T50.Z16
Glucagon	T38.3X1	T38.3X2	T38.3X3	T38.3X4	T38.3X5	T38.3X6
Glucocorticoids	T38.0X1	T38.0X2	T38.0X3	T38.0X4	T38.0X5	T38.0X6
Glucocorticosteroid	T38.0X1	T38.0X2	T38.0X3	T38.0X4	T38.0X5	T38.0X6
Gluconic acid	T50.991	T50.992	T50.993	T50.994	T50.995	T50.996
Glucosamine sulfate	T39.4X1	T39.4X2	T39.4X3	T39.4X4	T39.4X5	T39.4X6
Glucose	T50.3X1	T50.3X2	T50.3X3	T50.3X4	T50.3X5	T50.3X6
with sodium chloride	T50.3X1	T50.3X2	T50.3X3	T50.3X4	T50.3X5	T50.3X6
Glucosulfone sodium	T37.1X1	T37.1X2	T37.1X3	T37.1X4	T37.1X5	T37.1X6
Glucurolactone	T47.8X1	T47.8X2	T47.8X3	T47.8X4	T47.8X5	T47.8X6
Glue NEC	T52.8X1	T52.8X2	T52.8X3	T52.8X4	—	—
Glutamic acid	T47.5X1	T47.5X2	T47.5X3	T47.5X4	T47.5X5	T47.5X6
Glutaral (medicinal)	T49.0X1	T49.0X2	T49.0X3	T49.0X4	T49.0X5	T49.0X6
nonmedicinal	T65.891	T65.892	T65.893	T65.894	—	—
Glutaraldehyde	T65.891	T65.892	T65.893	T65.894	—	—
(nonmedicinal)						
medicinal	T49.0X1	T49.0X2	T49.0X3	T49.0X4	T49.0X5	T49.0X6
Glutathione	T50.6X1	T50.6X2	T50.6X3	T50.6X4	T50.6X5	T50.6X6
Glutethimide	T42.6X1	T42.6X2	T42.6X3	T42.6X4	T42.6X5	T42.6X6
Glyburide	T38.3X1	T38.3X2	T38.3X3	T38.3X4	T38.3X5	T38.3X6
Glycerin	T47.4X1	T47.4X2	T47.4X3	T47.4X4	T47.4X5	T47.4X6
Glycerol	T47.4X1	T47.4X2	T47.4X3	T47.4X4	T47.4X5	T47.4X6
borax	T49.6X1	T49.6X2	T49.6X3	T49.6X4	T49.6X5	T49.6X6
intravenous	T50.3X1	T50.3X2	T50.3X3	T50.3X4	T50.3X5	T50.3X6
iodinated	T48.4X1	T48.4X2	T48.4X3	T48.4X4	T48.4X5	T48.4X6
Glycerophosphate	T50.991	T50.992	T50.993	T50.994	T50.995	T50.996
Glyceryl						
gualacolate	T48.4X1	T48.4X2	T48.4X3	T48.4X4	T48.4X5	T48.4X6
nitrate	T46.3X1	T46.3X2	T46.3X3	T46.3X4	T46.3X5	T46.3X6
triacetate (topical)	T49.0X1	T49.0X2	T49.0X3	T49.0X4	T49.0X5	T49.0X6
trinitrate	T46.3X1	T46.3X2	T46.3X3	T46.3X4	T46.3X5	T46.3X6
Glycine	T50.3X1	T50.3X2	T50.3X3	T50.3X4	T50.3X5	T50.3X6
Glyclopyramide	T38.3X1	T38.3X2	T38.3X3	T38.3X4	T38.3X5	T38.3X6
Glycobiarsol	T37.3X1	T37.3X2	T37.3X3	T37.3X4	T37.3X5	T37.3X6
Glycols (ether)	T52.3X1	T52.3X2	T52.3X3	T52.3X4	—	—
Glyconiazide	T37.1X1	T37.1X2	T37.1X3	T37.1X4	T37.1X5	T37.1X6
Glycopyrrolate	T44.3X1	T44.3X2	T44.3X3	T44.3X4	T44.3X5	T44.3X6
Glycopyrronium	T44.3X1	T44.3X2	T44.3X3	T44.3X4	T44.3X5	T44.3X6
bromide	T44.3X1	T44.3X2	T44.3X3	T44.3X4	T44.3X5	T44.3X6
Glycoside, cardiac	T46.0X1	T46.0X2	T46.0X3	T46.0X4	T46.0X5	T46.0X6
(stimulant)						
Glycyclamide	T38.3X1	T38.3X2	T38.3X3	T38.3X4	T38.3X5	T38.3X6
Glycyrrhiza extract	T48.4X1	T48.4X2	T48.4X3	T48.4X4	T48.4X5	T48.4X6
Glycyrrhizic acid	T48.4X1	T48.4X2	T48.4X3	T48.4X4	T48.4X5	T48.4X6
Glycyrrhizinate potassium	T48.4X1	T48.4X2	T48.4X3	T48.4X4	T48.4X5	T48.4X6
Glymidine sodium	T38.3X1	T38.3X2	T38.3X3	T38.3X4	T38.3X5	T38.3X6
Glyphosate	T60.3X1	T60.3X2	T60.3X3	T60.3X4	—	—
Glyphylline	T48.6X1	T48.6X2	T48.6X3	T48.6X4	T48.6X5	T48.6X6
Gold						
colloidal (I98Au)	T45.1X1	T45.1X2	T45.1X3	T45.1X4	T45.1X5	T45.1X6

Substance	Poisoning, Accidental (unintentional)	Poisoning, Intentional Self-harm	Poisoning, Assault	Poisoning, Undetermined	Adverse Effect	Under-dosing
Gold — continued						
salts	T39.4X1	T39.4X2	T39.4X3	T39.4X4	T39.4X5	T39.4X6
Golden sulfide of antimony	T56.891	T56.892	T56.893	T56.894	—	—
Goldylocks	T62.2X1	T62.2X2	T62.2X3	T62.2X4	—	—
Gonadal tissue extract	T38.901	T38.902	T38.903	T38.904	T38.905	T38.906
female	T38.5X1	T38.5X2	T38.5X3	T38.5X4	T38.5X5	T38.5X6
male	T38.7X1	T38.7X2	T38.7X3	T38.7X4	T38.7X5	T38.7X6
Gonadorelin	T38.891	T38.892	T38.893	T38.894	T38.895	T38.896
Gonadotropin	T38.891	T38.892	T38.893	T38.894	T38.895	T38.896
chorionic	T38.891	T38.892	T38.893	T38.894	T38.895	T38.896
pituitary	T38.811	T38.812	T38.813	T38.814	T38.815	T38.816
Goserelin	T45.1X1	T45.1X2	T45.1X3	T45.1X4	T45.1X5	T45.1X6
Grain alcohol	T51.0X1	T51.0X2	T51.0X3	T51.0X4	—	—
Gramicidin	T49.0X1	T49.0X2	T49.0X3	T49.0X4	T49.0X5	T49.0X6
Granisetron	T45.0X1	T45.0X2	T45.0X3	T45.0X4	T45.0X5	T45.0X6
Gratiola officinalis	T62.2X1	T62.2X2	T62.2X3	T62.2X4	—	—
Grease	T65.891	T65.892	T65.893	T65.894	—	—
Green hellebore	T62.2X1	T62.2X2	T62.2X3	T62.2X4	—	—
Green soap	T49.2X1	T49.2X2	T49.2X3	T49.2X4	T49.2X5	T49.2X6
Grifulvin	T36.7X1	T36.7X2	T36.7X3	T36.7X4	T36.7X5	T36.7X6
Griseofulvin	T36.7X1	T36.7X2	T36.7X3	T36.7X4	T36.7X5	T36.7X6
Growth hormone	T38.811	T38.812	T38.813	T38.814	T38.815	T38.816
Guaiacol derivatives	T48.4X1	T48.4X2	T48.4X3	T48.4X4	T48.4X5	T48.4X6
Guaiac reagent	T50.991	T50.992	T50.993	T50.994	T50.995	T50.996
Guaifenesin	T48.4X1	T48.4X2	T48.4X3	T48.4X4	T48.4X5	T48.4X6
Guaimesal	T48.4X1	T48.4X2	T48.4X3	T48.4X4	T48.4X5	T48.4X6
Guaiphenesin	T48.4X1	T48.4X2	T48.4X3	T48.4X4	T48.4X5	T48.4X6
Guamecycline	T36.4X1	T36.4X2	T36.4X3	T36.4X4	T36.4X5	T36.4X6
Guanabenz	T46.5X1	T46.5X2	T46.5X3	T46.5X4	T46.5X5	T46.5X6
Guanacline	T46.5X1	T46.5X2	T46.5X3	T46.5X4	T46.5X5	T46.5X6
Guanadrel	T46.5X1	T46.5X2	T46.5X3	T46.5X4	T46.5X5	T46.5X6
Guanatol	T37.2X1	T37.2X2	T37.2X3	T37.2X4	T37.2X5	T37.2X6
Guanethidine	T46.5X1	T46.5X2	T46.5X3	T46.5X4	T46.5X5	T46.5X6
Guanfacine	T46.5X1	T46.5X2	T46.5X3	T46.5X4	T46.5X5	T46.5X6
Guano	T65.891	T65.892	T65.893	T65.894	—	—
Guanochlor	T46.5X1	T46.5X2	T46.5X3	T46.5X4	T46.5X5	T46.5X6
Guanoclor	T46.5X1	T46.5X2	T46.5X3	T46.5X4	T46.5X5	T46.5X6
Guanoctine	T46.5X1	T46.5X2	T46.5X3	T46.5X4	T46.5X5	T46.5X6
Guanoxabenz	T46.5X1	T46.5X2	T46.5X3	T46.5X4	T46.5X5	T46.5X6
Guanoxan	T46.5X1	T46.5X2	T46.5X3	T46.5X4	T46.5X5	T46.5X6
Guar gum (medicinal)	T46.6X1	T46.6X2	T46.6X3	T46.6X4	T46.6X5	T46.6X6
Hachimycin	T36.7X1	T36.7X2	T36.7X3	T36.7X4	T36.7X5	T36.7X6
Hair						
dye	T49.4X1	T49.4X2	T49.4X3	T49.4X4	T49.4X5	T49.4X6
preparation NEC	T49.4X1	T49.4X2	T49.4X3	T49.4X4	T49.4X5	T49.4X6
Halazepam	T42.4X1	T42.4X2	T42.4X3	T42.4X4	T42.4X5	T42.4X6
Halcinolone	T49.0X1	T49.0X2	T49.0X3	T49.0X4	T49.0X5	T49.0X6
Halcinonide	T49.0X1	T49.0X2	T49.0X3	T49.0X4	T49.0X5	T49.0X6
Halethazole	T49.0X1	T49.0X2	T49.0X3	T49.0X4	T49.0X5	T49.0X6
Hallucinogen NOS	T40.901	T40.902	T40.903	T40.904	T40.905	T40.906
specified NEC	T40.991	T40.992	T40.993	T40.994	T40.995	T40.996
Halofantrine	T37.2X1	T37.2X2	T37.2X3	T37.2X4	T37.2X5	T37.2X6
Halofenate	T46.6X1	T46.6X2	T46.6X3	T46.6X4	T46.6X5	T46.6X6
Halometasone	T49.0X1	T49.0X2	T49.0X3	T49.0X4	T49.0X5	T49.0X6
Haloperidol	T43.4X1	T43.4X2	T43.4X3	T43.4X4	T43.4X5	T43.4X6
Haloprogin	T49.0X1	T49.0X2	T49.0X3	T49.0X4	T49.0X5	T49.0X6
Halotex	T49.0X1	T49.0X2	T49.0X3	T49.0X4	T49.0X5	T49.0X6
Halothane	T41.0X1	T41.0X2	T41.0X3	T41.0X4	T41.0X5	T41.0X6
Haloxazolam	T42.4X1	T42.4X2	T42.4X3	T42.4X4	T42.4X5	T42.4X6
Halquinols	T49.0X1	T49.0X2	T49.0X3	T49.0X4	T49.0X5	T49.0X6
Hamamelis	T49.2X1	T49.2X2	T49.2X3	T49.2X4	T49.2X5	T49.2X6
Haptendextran	T45.8X1	T45.8X2	T45.8X3	T45.8X4	T45.8X5	T45.8X6
Harmonyl	T46.5X1	T46.5X2	T46.5X3	T46.5X4	T46.5X5	T46.5X6
Hartmann's solution	T50.3X1	T50.3X2	T50.3X3	T50.3X4	T50.3X5	T50.3X6
Hashish	T40.711	T40.712	T40.713	T40.714	T40.715	T40.716
Hawaiian Woodrose seeds	T40.991	T40.992	T40.993	T40.994	—	—
HCB	T60.3X1	T60.3X2	T60.3X3	T60.3X4	—	—
HCH	T53.6X1	T53.6X2	T53.6X3	T53.6X4	—	—
medicinal	T49.0X1	T49.0X2	T49.0X3	T49.0X4	T49.0X5	T49.0X6
HCN	T57.3X1	T57.3X2	T57.3X3	T57.3X4	—	—
Headache cures, drugs, powders NEC	T50.901	T50.902	T50.903	T50.904	T50.905	T50.906
Heavenly Blue (morning glory)	T40.991	T40.992	T40.993	T40.994	—	—
Heavy metal antidote	T45.8X1	T45.8X2	T45.8X3	T45.8X4	T45.8X5	T45.8X6
Hedaquinium	T49.0X1	T49.0X2	T49.0X3	T49.0X4	T49.0X5	T49.0X6
Hedge hyssop	T62.2X1	T62.2X2	T62.2X3	T62.2X4	—	—
Heet	T49.8X1	T49.8X2	T49.8X3	T49.8X4	T49.8X5	T49.8X6
Helenin	T37.4X1	T37.4X2	T37.4X3	T37.4X4	T37.4X5	T37.4X6
Helium (nonmedicinal) NEC	T59.891	T59.892	T59.893	T59.894	—	—
medicinal	T48.991	T48.992	T48.993	T48.994	T48.995	T48.996

▽ Subterms under main terms may continue to next column or page   Additional Character May Be Required — Refer to the Tabular List for Character Selection   377

Gemonil — Helium

Table of Drugs and Chemicals

Hellebore — Hydrocyanic acid

Substance	Poisoning, Accidental (unintentional)	Poisoning, Intentional Self-harm	Poisoning, Assault	Poisoning, Undetermined	Adverse Effect	Under-dosing
Hellebore (black) (green) (white)	T62.2X1	T62.2X2	T62.2X3	T62.2X4	—	—
Hematin	T45.8X1	T45.8X2	T45.8X3	T45.8X4	T45.8X5	T45.8X6
Hematinic preparation	T45.8X1	T45.8X2	T45.8X3	T45.8X4	T45.8X5	T45.8X6
Hematological agent	T45.91	T45.92	T45.93	T45.94	T45.95	T45.96
specified NEC	T45.8X1	T45.8X2	T45.8X3	T45.8X4	T45.8X5	T45.8X6
Hemlock	T62.2X1	T62.2X2	T62.2X3	T62.2X4	—	—
Hemostatic	T45.621	T45.622	T45.623	T45.624	T45.625	T45.626
drug, systemic	T45.621	T45.622	T45.623	T45.624	T45.625	T45.626
Hemostyptic	T49.4X1	T49.4X2	T49.4X3	T49.4X4	T49.4X5	T49.4X6
Henbane	T62.2X1	T62.2X2	T62.2X3	T62.2X4	—	—
Heparin (sodium)	T45.511	T45.512	T45.513	T45.514	T45.515	T45.516
action reverser	T45.7X1	T45.7X2	T45.7X3	T45.7X4	T45.7X5	T45.7X6
Heparin-fraction	T45.511	T45.512	T45.513	T45.514	T45.515	T45.516
Heparinoid (systemic)	T45.511	T45.512	T45.513	T45.514	T45.515	T45.516
Hepatic secretion stimulant	T47.8X1	T47.8X2	T47.8X3	T47.8X4	T47.8X5	T47.8X6
Hepatitis B						
immune globulin	T50.Z11	T50.Z12	T50.Z13	T50.Z14	T50.Z15	T50.Z16
vaccine	T50.B91	T50.B92	T50.B93	T50.B94	T50.B95	T50.B96
Hepronicate	T46.7X1	T46.7X2	T46.7X3	T46.7X4	T46.7X5	T46.7X6
Heptabarb	T42.3X1	T42.3X2	T42.3X3	T42.3X4	T42.3X5	T42.3X6
Heptabarbital	T42.3X1	T42.3X2	T42.3X3	T42.3X4	T42.3X5	T42.3X6
Heptabarbitone	T42.3X1	T42.3X2	T42.3X3	T42.3X4	T42.3X5	T42.3X6
Heptachlor	T60.1X1	T60.1X2	T60.1X3	T60.1X4	—	—
Heptalgin	T40.2X1	T40.2X2	T40.2X3	T40.2X4	T40.2X5	T40.2X6
Heptaminol	T46.3X1	T46.3X2	T46.3X3	T46.3X4	T46.3X5	T46.3X6
Herbicide NEC	T60.3X1	T60.3X2	T60.3X3	T60.3X4	—	—
Heroin	T40.1X1	T40.1X2	T40.1X3	T40.1X4	—	—
Herplex	T49.5X1	T49.5X2	T49.5X3	T49.5X4	T49.5X5	T49.5X6
HES	T45.8X1	T45.8X2	T45.8X3	T45.8X4	T45.8X5	T45.8X6
Hesperidin	T46.991	T46.992	T46.993	T46.994	T46.995	T46.996
Hetacillin	T36.0X1	T36.0X2	T36.0X3	T36.0X4	T36.0X5	T36.0X6
Hetastarch	T45.8X1	T45.8X2	T45.8X3	T45.8X4	T45.8X5	T45.8X6
HETP	T60.0X1	T60.0X2	T60.0X3	T60.0X4	—	—
Hexachlorobenzene (vapor)	T60.3X1	T60.3X2	T60.3X3	T60.3X4	—	—
Hexachlorocyclohexane	T53.6X1	T53.6X2	T53.6X3	T53.6X4	—	—
Hexachlorophene	T49.0X1	T49.0X2	T49.0X3	T49.0X4	T49.0X5	T49.0X6
Hexadiline	T46.3X1	T46.3X2	T46.3X3	T46.3X4	T46.3X5	T46.3X6
Hexadimethrine (bromide)	T45.7X1	T45.7X2	T45.7X3	T45.7X4	T45.7X5	T45.7X6
Hexadylamine	T46.3X1	T46.3X2	T46.3X3	T46.3X4	T46.3X5	T46.3X6
Hexaethyl tetraphosphate	T60.0X1	T60.0X2	T60.0X3	T60.0X4	—	—
Hexafluorenium bromide	T48.1X1	T48.1X2	T48.1X3	T48.1X4	T48.1X5	T48.1X6
Hexafluronium (bromide)	T48.1X1	T48.1X2	T48.1X3	T48.1X4	T48.1X5	T48.1X6
Hexa-germ	T49.2X1	T49.2X2	T49.2X3	T49.2X4	T49.2X5	T49.2X6
Hexahydrobenzol	T52.8X1	T52.8X2	T52.8X3	T52.8X4	—	—
Hexahydrocresol(s)	T51.8X1	T51.8X2	T51.8X3	T51.8X4	—	—
arsenide	T57.0X1	T57.0X2	T57.0X3	T57.0X4	—	—
arseniurated	T57.0X1	T57.0X2	T57.0X3	T57.0X4	—	—
cyanide	T57.3X1	T57.3X2	T57.3X3	T57.3X4	—	—
gas	T59.891	T59.892	T59.893	T59.894	—	—
Fluoride (liquid)	T57.8X1	T57.8X2	T57.8X3	T57.8X4	—	—
vapor	T59.891	T59.892	T59.893	T59.894	—	—
phophorated	T60.0X1	T60.0X2	T60.0X3	T60.0X4	—	—
sulfate	T57.8X1	T57.8X2	T57.8X3	T57.8X4	—	—
sulfide (gas)	T59.6X1	T59.6X2	T59.6X3	T59.6X4	—	—
arseniurated	T57.0X1	T57.0X2	T57.0X3	T57.0X4	—	—
sulfurated	T57.8X1	T57.8X2	T57.8X3	T57.8X4	—	—
Hexahydrophenol	T51.8X1	T51.8X2	T51.8X3	T51.8X4	—	—
Hexalen	T51.8X1	T51.8X2	T51.8X3	T51.8X4	—	—
Hexamethonium bromide	T44.2X1	T44.2X2	T44.2X3	T44.2X4	T44.2X5	T44.2X6
Hexamethylene	T52.8X1	T52.8X2	T52.8X3	T52.8X4	—	—
Hexamethylmelamine	T45.1X1	T45.1X2	T45.1X3	T45.1X4	T45.1X5	T45.1X6
Hexamidine	T49.0X1	T49.0X2	T49.0X3	T49.0X4	T49.0X5	T49.0X6
Hexamine (mandelate)	T37.8X1	T37.8X2	T37.8X3	T37.8X4	T37.8X5	T37.8X6
Hexanone, 2-hexanone	T52.4X1	T52.4X2	T52.4X3	T52.4X4	—	—
Hexanuorenium	T48.1X1	T48.1X2	T48.1X3	T48.1X4	T48.1X5	T48.1X6
Hexapropymate	T42.6X1	T42.6X2	T42.6X3	T42.6X4	T42.6X5	T42.6X6
Hexasonium iodide	T44.3X1	T44.3X2	T44.3X3	T44.3X4	T44.3X5	T44.3X6
Hexcarbacholine bromide	T48.1X1	T48.1X2	T48.1X3	T48.1X4	T48.1X5	T48.1X6
Hexemal	T42.3X1	T42.3X2	T42.3X3	T42.3X4	T42.3X5	T42.3X6
Hexestrol	T38.5X1	T38.5X2	T38.5X3	T38.5X4	T38.5X5	T38.5X6
Hexethal (sodium)	T42.3X1	T42.3X2	T42.3X3	T42.3X4	T42.3X5	T42.3X6
Hexetidine	T37.8X1	T37.8X2	T37.8X3	T37.8X4	T37.8X5	T37.8X6
Hexobarbital	T42.3X1	T42.3X2	T42.3X3	T42.3X4	T42.3X5	T42.3X6
rectal	T41.291	T41.292	T41.293	T41.294	T41.295	T41.296
sodium	T41.1X1	T41.1X2	T41.1X3	T41.1X4	T41.1X5	T41.1X6
Hexobendine	T46.3X1	T46.3X2	T46.3X3	T46.3X4	T46.3X5	T46.3X6
Hexocyclium	T44.3X1	T44.3X2	T44.3X3	T44.3X4	T44.3X5	T44.3X6
metilsulfate	T44.3X1	T44.3X2	T44.3X3	T44.3X4	T44.3X5	T44.3X6
Hexoestrol	T38.5X1	T38.5X2	T38.5X3	T38.5X4	T38.5X5	T38.5X6
Hexone	T52.4X1	T52.4X2	T52.4X3	T52.4X4	—	—
Hexoprenaline	T48.6X1	T48.6X2	T48.6X3	T48.6X4	T48.6X5	T48.6X6
Hexylcaine	T41.3X1	T41.3X2	T41.3X3	T41.3X4	T41.3X5	T41.3X6
Hexylresorcinol	T52.2X1	T52.2X2	T52.2X3	T52.2X4	—	—
HGH (human growth hormone)	T38.811	T38.812	T38.813	T38.814	T38.815	T38.816
Hinkle's pills	T47.2X1	T47.2X2	T47.2X3	T47.2X4	T47.2X5	T47.2X6
Histalog	T50.8X1	T50.8X2	T50.8X3	T50.8X4	T50.8X5	T50.8X6
Histamine (phosphate)	T50.8X1	T50.8X2	T50.8X3	T50.8X4	T50.8X5	T50.8X6
Histoplasmin	T50.8X1	T50.8X2	T50.8X3	T50.8X4	T50.8X5	T50.8X6
Holly berries	T62.2X1	T62.2X2	T62.2X3	T62.2X4	—	—
Homatropine	T44.3X1	T44.3X2	T44.3X3	T44.3X4	T44.3X5	T44.3X6
methylbromide	T44.3X1	T44.3X2	T44.3X3	T44.3X4	T44.3X5	T44.3X6
Homochlorcyclizine	T45.0X1	T45.0X2	T45.0X3	T45.0X4	T45.0X5	T45.0X6
Homosalate	T49.3X1	T49.3X2	T49.3X3	T49.3X4	T49.3X5	T49.3X6
Homo-tet	T50.Z11	T50.Z12	T50.Z13	T50.Z14	T50.Z15	T50.Z16
Hormone	T38.801	T38.802	T38.803	T38.804	T38.805	T38.806
adrenal cortical steroids	T38.0X1	T38.0X2	T38.0X3	T38.0X4	T38.0X5	T38.0X6
androgenic	T38.7X1	T38.7X2	T38.7X3	T38.7X4	T38.7X5	T38.7X6
anterior pituitary NEC	T38.811	T38.812	T38.813	T38.814	T38.815	T38.816
antidiabetic agents	T38.3X1	T38.3X2	T38.3X3	T38.3X4	T38.3X5	T38.3X6
antidiuretic	T38.891	T38.892	T38.893	T38.894	T38.895	T38.896
cancer therapy	T45.1X1	T45.1X2	T45.1X3	T45.1X4	T45.1X5	T45.1X6
follicle stimulating	T38.811	T38.812	T38.813	T38.814	T38.815	T38.816
gonadotropic	T38.891	T38.892	T38.893	T38.894	T38.895	T38.896
pituitary	T38.811	T38.812	T38.813	T38.814	T38.815	T38.816
growth	T38.811	T38.812	T38.813	T38.814	T38.815	T38.816
luteinizing	T38.811	T38.812	T38.813	T38.814	T38.815	T38.816
ovarian	T38.5X1	T38.5X2	T38.5X3	T38.5X4	T38.5X5	T38.5X6
oxytocic	T48.0X1	T48.0X2	T48.0X3	T48.0X4	T48.0X5	T48.0X6
parathyroid (derivatives)	T50.991	T50.992	T50.993	T50.994	T50.995	T50.996
pituitary (posterior) NEC	T38.891	T38.892	T38.893	T38.894	T38.895	T38.896
anterior	T38.811	T38.812	T38.813	T38.814	T38.815	T38.816
specified, NEC	T38.891	T38.892	T38.893	T38.894	T38.895	T38.896
thyroid	T38.1X1	T38.1X2	T38.1X3	T38.1X4	T38.1X5	T38.1X6
Hornet (sting)	T63.451	T63.452	T63.453	T63.454	—	—
Horse anti-human lymphocytic serum	T50.Z11	T50.Z12	T50.Z13	T50.Z14	T50.Z15	T50.Z16
Horticulture agent NEC	T65.91	T65.92	T65.93	T65.94	—	—
with pesticide	T60.91	T60.92	T60.93	T60.94	—	—
Human						
albumin	T45.8X1	T45.8X2	T45.8X3	T45.8X4	T45.8X5	T45.8X6
growth hormone (HGH)	T38.811	T38.812	T38.813	T38.814	T38.815	T38.816
immune serum	T50.Z11	T50.Z12	T50.Z13	T50.Z14	T50.Z15	T50.Z16
Hyaluronidase	T45.3X1	T45.3X2	T45.3X3	T45.3X4	T45.3X5	T45.3X6
Hyazyme	T45.3X1	T45.3X2	T45.3X3	T45.3X4	T45.3X5	T45.3X6
Hycodan	T40.2X1	T40.2X2	T40.2X3	T40.2X4	T40.2X5	T40.2X6
Hydantoin derivative NEC	T42.0X1	T42.0X2	T42.0X3	T42.0X4	T42.0X5	T42.0X6
Hydeltra	T38.0X1	T38.0X2	T38.0X3	T38.0X4	T38.0X5	T38.0X6
Hydergine	T44.6X1	T44.6X2	T44.6X3	T44.6X4	T44.6X5	T44.6X6
Hydrabamine penicillin	T36.0X1	T36.0X2	T36.0X3	T36.0X4	T36.0X5	T36.0X6
Hydralazine	T46.5X1	T46.5X2	T46.5X3	T46.5X4	T46.5X5	T46.5X6
Hydrargaphen	T49.0X1	T49.0X2	T49.0X3	T49.0X4	T49.0X5	T49.0X6
Hydrargyri aminochloridum	T49.0X1	T49.0X2	T49.0X3	T49.0X4	T49.0X5	T49.0X6
Hydrastine	T48.291	T48.292	T48.293	T48.294	T48.295	T48.296
Hydrazine	T54.1X1	T54.1X2	T54.1X3	T54.1X4	—	—
monoamine oxidase inhibitors	T43.1X1	T43.1X2	T43.1X3	T43.1X4	T43.1X5	T43.1X6
Hydrazoic acid, azides	T54.2X1	T54.2X2	T54.2X3	T54.2X4	—	—
Hydriodic acid	T48.4X1	T48.4X2	T48.4X3	T48.4X4	T48.4X5	T48.4X6
Hydrocarbon gas	T59.891	T59.892	T59.893	T59.894	—	—
incomplete combustion of — see Carbon, monoxide, fuel, utility						
liquefied (mobile container)	T59.891	T59.892	T59.893	T59.894	—	—
piped (natural)	T59.891	T59.892	T59.893	T59.894	—	—
Hydrochloric acid (liquid)	T54.2X1	T54.2X2	T54.2X3	T54.2X4	—	—
medicinal (digestant)	T47.5X1	T47.5X2	T47.5X3	T47.5X4	T47.5X5	T47.5X6
vapor	T59.891	T59.892	T59.893	T59.894	—	—
Hydrochlorothiazide	T50.2X1	T50.2X2	T50.2X3	T50.2X4	T50.2X5	T50.2X6
Hydrocodone	T40.2X1	T40.2X2	T40.2X3	T40.2X4	T40.2X5	T40.2X6
Hydrocortisone (derivatives)	T38.0X1	T38.0X2	T38.0X3	T38.0X4	T38.0X5	T38.0X6
aceponate	T49.0X1	T49.0X2	T49.0X3	T49.0X4	T49.0X5	T49.0X6
ENT agent	T49.6X1	T49.6X2	T49.6X3	T49.6X4	T49.6X5	T49.6X6
ophthalmic preparation	T49.5X1	T49.5X2	T49.5X3	T49.5X4	T49.5X5	T49.5X6
topical NEC	T49.0X1	T49.0X2	T49.0X3	T49.0X4	T49.0X5	T49.0X6
Hydrocortone	T38.0X1	T38.0X2	T38.0X3	T38.0X4	T38.0X5	T38.0X6
ENT agent	T49.6X1	T49.6X2	T49.6X3	T49.6X4	T49.6X5	T49.6X6
ophthalmic preparation	T49.5X1	T49.5X2	T49.5X3	T49.5X4	T49.5X5	T49.5X6
topical NEC	T49.0X1	T49.0X2	T49.0X3	T49.0X4	T49.0X5	T49.0X6
Hydrocyanic acid (liquid)	T57.3X1	T57.3X2	T57.3X3	T57.3X4	—	—

Substance	Poisoning, Accidental (unintentional)	Poisoning, Intentional Self-harm	Poisoning, Assault	Poisoning, Undetermined	Adverse Effect	Under-dosing
Hydrocyanic acid — *continued*						
gas	T65.ØX1	T65.ØX2	T65.ØX3	T65.ØX4	—	—
Hydroflumethiazide	T50.2X1	T5Ø.2X2	T5Ø.2X3	T5Ø.2X4	T5Ø.2X5	T5Ø.2X6
Hydrofluoric acid (liquid)	T54.2X1	T54.2X2	T54.2X3	T54.2X4	—	—
vapor	T59.891	T59.892	T59.893	T59.894	—	—
Hydrogen	T59.891	T59.892	T59.893	T59.894	—	—
arsenide	T57.ØX1	T57.ØX2	T57.ØX3	T57.ØX4	—	—
arseniureted	T57.ØX1	T57.ØX2	T57.ØX3	T57.ØX4	—	—
chloride	T57.8X1	T57.8X2	T57.8X3	T57.8X4	—	—
cyanide (salts)	T57.3X1	T57.3X2	T57.3X3	T57.3X4	—	—
gas	T57.3X1	T57.3X2	T57.3X3	T57.3X4	—	—
Fluoride	T59.5X1	T59.5X2	T59.5X3	T59.5X4	—	—
vapor	T59.5X1	T59.5X2	T59.5X3	T59.5X4	—	—
peroxide	T49.ØX1	T49.ØX2	T49.ØX3	T49.ØX4	T49.ØX5	T49.ØX6
phosphureted	T57.1X1	T57.1X2	T57.1X3	T57.1X4	—	—
sulfide	T59.6X1	T59.6X2	T59.6X3	T59.6X4	—	—
arseniureted	T57.ØX1	T57.ØX2	T57.ØX3	T57.ØX4	—	—
sulfureted	T59.6X1	T59.6X2	T59.6X3	T59.6X4	—	—
Hydromethylpyridine	T46.7X1	T46.7X2	T46.7X3	T46.7X4	T46.7X5	T46.7X6
Hydromorphinol	T4Ø.2X1	T4Ø.2X2	T4Ø.2X3	T4Ø.2X4	—	—
Hydromorphinone	T4Ø.2X1	T4Ø.2X2	T4Ø.2X3	T4Ø.2X4	T4Ø.2X5	T4Ø.2X6
Hydromorphone	T4Ø.2X1	T4Ø.2X2	T4Ø.2X3	T4Ø.2X4	T4Ø.2X5	T4Ø.2X6
Hydromox	T5Ø.2X1	T5Ø.2X2	T5Ø.2X3	T5Ø.2X4	T5Ø.2X5	T5Ø.2X6
Hydrophilic lotion	T49.3X1	T49.3X2	T49.3X3	T49.3X4	T49.3X5	T49.3X6
Hydroquinidine	T46.2X1	T46.2X2	T46.2X3	T46.2X4	T46.2X5	T46.2X6
Hydroquinone	T52.2X1	T52.2X2	T52.2X3	T52.2X4	—	—
vapor	T59.891	T59.892	T59.893	T59.894	—	—
Hydrosulfuric acid (gas)	T59.6X1	T59.6X2	T59.6X3	T59.6X4	—	—
Hydrotalcite	T47.1X1	T47.1X2	T47.1X3	T47.1X4	T47.1X5	T47.1X6
Hydrous wool fat	T49.3X1	T49.3X2	T49.3X3	T49.3X4	T49.3X5	T49.3X6
Hydroxide, caustic	T54.3X1	T54.3X2	T54.3X3	T54.3X4	—	—
Hydroxocobalamin	T45.8X1	T45.8X2	T45.8X3	T45.8X4	T45.8X5	T45.8X6
Hydroxyamphetamine	T49.5X1	T49.5X2	T49.5X3	T49.5X4	T49.5X5	T49.5X6
Hydroxycarbamide	T45.1X1	T45.1X2	T45.1X3	T45.1X4	T45.1X5	T45.1X6
Hydroxychloroquine	T37.8X1	T37.8X2	T37.8X3	T37.8X4	T37.8X5	T37.8X6
Hydroxydihydrocodeinone	T4Ø.2X1	T4Ø.2X2	T4Ø.2X3	T4Ø.2X4	T4Ø.2X5	T4Ø.2X6
Hydroxyestrone	T38.5X1	T38.5X2	T38.5X3	T38.5X4	T38.5X5	T38.5X6
Hydroxyethyl starch	T45.8X1	T45.8X2	T45.8X3	T45.8X4	T45.8X5	T45.8X6
Hydroxymethylpentanone	T52.4X1	T52.4X2	T52.4X3	T52.4X4	—	—
Hydroxyphenamate	T43.591	T43.592	T43.593	T43.594	T43.595	T43.596
Hydroxyphenylbutazone	T39.2X1	T39.2X2	T39.2X3	T39.2X4	T39.2X5	T39.2X6
Hydroxyprogesterone	T38.5X1	T38.5X2	T38.5X3	T38.5X4	T38.5X5	T38.5X6
caproate	T38.5X1	T38.5X2	T38.5X3	T38.5X4	T38.5X5	T38.5X6
Hydroxyquinoline (derivatives) **NEC**	T37.8X1	T37.8X2	T37.8X3	T37.8X4	T37.8X5	T37.8X6
Hydroxystilbamidine	T37.3X1	T37.3X2	T37.3X3	T37.3X4	T37.3X5	T37.3X6
Hydroxytoluene (nonmedicinal)	T54.ØX1	T54.ØX2	T54.ØX3	T54.ØX4	—	—
medicinal	T49.ØX1	T49.ØX2	T49.ØX3	T49.ØX4	T49.ØX5	T49.ØX6
Hydroxyurea	T45.1X1	T45.1X2	T45.1X3	T45.1X4	T45.1X5	T45.1X6
Hydroxyzine	T43.591	T43.592	T43.593	T43.594	T43.595	T43.596
Hyoscine	T44.3X1	T44.3X2	T44.3X3	T44.3X4	T44.3X5	T44.3X6
Hyoscyamine	T44.3X1	T44.3X2	T44.3X3	T44.3X4	T44.3X5	T44.3X6
Hyoscyamus	T44.3X1	T44.3X2	T44.3X3	T44.3X4	T44.3X5	T44.3X6
dry extract	T44.3X1	T44.3X2	T44.3X3	T44.3X4	T44.3X5	T44.3X6
Hypaque	T5Ø.8X1	T5Ø.8X2	T5Ø.8X3	T5Ø.8X4	T5Ø.8X5	T5Ø.8X6
Hypertussis	T5Ø.Z11	T5Ø.Z12	T5Ø.Z13	T5Ø.Z14	T5Ø.Z15	T5Ø.Z16
Hypnotic	T42.71	T42.72	T42.73	T42.74	T42.75	T42.76
anticonvulsant	T42.71	T42.72	T42.73	T42.74	T42.75	T42.76
specified NEC	T42.6X1	T42.6X2	T42.6X3	T42.6X4	T42.6X5	T42.6X6
Hypochlorite	T49.ØX1	T49.ØX2	T49.ØX3	T49.ØX4	T49.ØX5	T49.ØX6
Hypophysis, posterior	T38.891	T38.892	T38.893	T38.894	T38.895	T38.896
Hypotensive NEC	T46.5X1	T46.5X2	T46.5X3	T46.5X4	T46.5X5	T46.5X6
Hypromellose	T49.5X1	T49.5X2	T49.5X3	T49.5X4	T49.5X5	T49.5X6
Ibacitabine	T37.5X1	T37.5X2	T37.5X3	T37.5X4	T37.5X5	T37.5X6
Ibopamine	T44.991	T44.992	T44.993	T44.994	T44.995	T44.996
Ibufenac	T39.311	T39.312	T39.313	T39.314	T39.315	T39.316
Ibuprofen	T39.311	T39.312	T39.313	T39.314	T39.315	T39.316
Ibuproxam	T39.311	T39.312	T39.313	T39.314	T39.315	T39.316
Ibuterol	T48.6X1	T48.6X2	T48.6X3	T48.6X4	T48.6X5	T48.6X6
Ichthammol	T49.ØX1	T49.ØX2	T49.ØX3	T49.ØX4	T49.ØX5	T49.ØX6
Ichthyol	T49.4X1	T49.4X2	T49.4X3	T49.4X4	T49.4X5	T49.4X6
Idarubicin	T45.1X1	T45.1X2	T45.1X3	T45.1X4	T45.1X5	T45.1X6
Idrocilamide	T42.8X1	T42.8X2	T42.8X3	T42.8X4	T42.8X5	T42.8X6
Ifenprodil	T46.7X1	T46.7X2	T46.7X3	T46.7X4	T46.7X5	T46.7X6
Ifosfamide	T45.1X1	T45.1X2	T45.1X3	T45.1X4	T45.1X5	T45.1X6
Iletin	T38.3X1	T38.3X2	T38.3X3	T38.3X4	T38.3X5	T38.3X6
Ilex	T62.2X1	T62.2X2	T62.2X3	T62.2X4	—	—
Illuminating gas (after combustion)	T58.11	T58.12	T58.13	T58.14	—	—
prior to combustion	T59.891	T59.892	T59.893	T59.894	—	—
Ilopan	T45.2X1	T45.2X2	T45.2X3	T45.2X4	T45.2X5	T45.2X6
Iloprost	T46.7X1	T46.7X2	T46.7X3	T46.7X4	T46.7X5	T46.7X6

Substance	Poisoning, Accidental (unintentional)	Poisoning, Intentional Self-harm	Poisoning, Assault	Poisoning, Undetermined	Adverse Effect	Under-dosing
Ilotycin	T36.3X1	T36.3X2	T36.3X3	T36.3X4	T36.3X5	T36.3X6
ophthalmic preparation	T49.5X1	T49.5X2	T49.5X3	T49.5X4	T49.5X5	T49.5X6
topical NEC	T49.ØX1	T49.ØX2	T49.ØX3	T49.ØX4	T49.ØX5	T49.ØX6
Imidazole-4-carboxamide	T45.1X1	T45.1X2	T45.1X3	T45.1X4	T45.1X5	T45.1X6
Iminostilbene	T42.1X1	T42.1X2	T42.1X3	T42.1X4	T42.1X5	T42.1X6
Imipenem	T36.ØX1	T36.ØX2	T36.ØX3	T36.ØX4	T36.ØX5	T36.ØX6
Imipramine	T43.Ø11	T43.Ø12	T43.Ø13	T43.Ø14	T43.Ø15	T43.Ø16
Immu-G	T5Ø.Z11	T5Ø.Z12	T5Ø.Z13	T5Ø.Z14	T5Ø.Z15	T5Ø.Z16
Immuglobin	T5Ø.Z11	T5Ø.Z12	T5Ø.Z13	T5Ø.Z14	T5Ø.Z15	T5Ø.Z16
Immune						
globulin	T5Ø.Z11	T5Ø.Z12	T5Ø.Z13	T5Ø.Z14	T5Ø.Z15	T5Ø.Z16
serum globulin	T5Ø.Z11	T5Ø.Z12	T5Ø.Z13	T5Ø.Z14	T5Ø.Z15	T5Ø.Z16
Immunoglobin human (intravenous) (normal)	T5Ø.Z11	T5Ø.Z12	T5Ø.Z13	T5Ø.Z14	T5Ø.Z15	T5Ø.Z16
unmodified	T5Ø.Z11	T5Ø.Z12	T5Ø.Z13	T5Ø.Z14	T5Ø.Z15	T5Ø.Z16
Immunosuppressive drug	T45.1X1	T45.1X2	T45.1X3	T45.1X4	T45.1X5	T45.1X6
Immu-tetanus	T5Ø.Z11	T5Ø.Z12	T5Ø.Z13	T5Ø.Z14	T5Ø.Z15	T5Ø.Z16
Indalpine	T43.221	T43.222	T43.223	T43.224	T43.225	T43.226
Indanazoline	T48.5X1	T48.5X2	T48.5X3	T48.5X4	T48.5X5	T48.5X6
Indandione (derivatives)	T45.511	T45.512	T45.513	T45.514	T45.515	T45.516
Indapamide	T46.5X1	T46.5X2	T46.5X3	T46.5X4	T46.5X5	T46.5X6
Indendione (derivatives)	T45.511	T45.512	T45.513	T45.514	T45.515	T45.516
Indenolol	T44.7X1	T44.7X2	T44.7X3	T44.7X4	T44.7X5	T44.7X6
Inderal	T44.7X1	T44.7X2	T44.7X3	T44.7X4	T44.7X5	T44.7X6
Indian						
hemp	T4Ø.711	T4Ø.712	T4Ø.713	T4Ø.714	T4Ø.715	T4Ø.716
tobacco	T62.2X1	T62.2X2	T62.2X3	T62.2X4	—	—
Indigo carmine	T5Ø.8X1	T5Ø.8X2	T5Ø.8X3	T5Ø.8X4	T5Ø.8X5	T5Ø.8X6
Indobufen	T45.521	T45.522	T45.523	T45.524	T45.525	T45.526
Indocin	T39.2X1	T39.2X2	T39.2X3	T39.2X4	T39.2X5	T39.2X6
Indocyanine green	T5Ø.8X1	T5Ø.8X2	T5Ø.8X3	T5Ø.8X4	T5Ø.8X5	T5Ø.8X6
Indometacin	T39.391	T39.392	T39.393	T39.394	T39.395	T39.396
Indomethacin	T39.391	T39.392	T39.393	T39.394	T39.395	T39.396
farnesil	T39.4X1	T39.4X2	T39.4X3	T39.4X4	T39.4X5	T39.4X6
Indoramin	T44.6X1	T44.6X2	T44.6X3	T44.6X4	T44.6X5	T44.6X6
Industrial						
alcohol	T51.ØX1	T51.ØX2	T51.ØX3	T51.ØX4	—	—
fumes	T59.891	T59.892	T59.893	T59.894	—	—
solvents (fumes) (vapors)	T52.91	T52.92	T52.93	T52.94	—	—
Influenza vaccine	T5Ø.B91	T5Ø.B92	T5Ø.B93	T5Ø.B94	T5Ø.B95	T5Ø.B96
Ingested substance NEC	T65.91	T65.92	T65.93	T65.94	—	—
INH	T37.1X1	T37.1X2	T37.1X3	T37.1X4	T37.1X5	T37.1X6
Inhalation, gas (noxious) — *see* Gas						
Inhibitor						
angiotensin-converting enzyme	T46.4X1	T46.4X2	T46.4X3	T46.4X4	T46.4X5	T46.4X6
carbonic anhydrase	T5Ø.2X1	T5Ø.2X2	T5Ø.2X3	T5Ø.2X4	T5Ø.2X5	T5Ø.2X6
fibrinolysis	T45.621	T45.622	T45.623	T45.624	T45.625	T45.626
monoamine oxidase NEC	T43.1X1	T43.1X2	T43.1X3	T43.1X4	T43.1X5	T43.1X6
hydrazine	T43.1X1	T43.1X2	T43.1X3	T43.1X4	T43.1X5	T43.1X6
postsynaptic	T43.8X1	T43.8X2	T43.8X3	T43.8X4	T43.8X5	T43.8X6
prothrombin synthesis	T45.511	T45.512	T45.513	T45.514	T45.515	T45.516
Ink	T65.891	T65.892	T65.893	T65.894	—	—
Inorganic substance NEC	T57.91	T57.92	T57.93	T57.94	—	—
Inosine pranobex	T37.5X1	T37.5X2	T37.5X3	T37.5X4	T37.5X5	T37.5X6
Inositol	T5Ø.991	T5Ø.992	T5Ø.993	T5Ø.994	T5Ø.995	T5Ø.996
nicotinate	T46.7X1	T46.7X2	T46.7X3	T46.7X4	T46.7X5	T46.7X6
Inproquone	T45.1X1	T45.1X2	T45.1X3	T45.1X4	T45.1X5	T45.1X6
Insecticide NEC	T6Ø.91	T6Ø.92	T6Ø.93	T6Ø.94	—	—
carbamate	T6Ø.ØX1	T6Ø.ØX2	T6Ø.ØX3	T6Ø.ØX4	—	—
chlorinated	T6Ø.1X1	T6Ø.1X2	T6Ø.1X3	T6Ø.1X4	—	—
mixed	T6Ø.91	T6Ø.92	T6Ø.93	T6Ø.94	—	—
organochlorine	T6Ø.1X1	T6Ø.1X2	T6Ø.1X3	T6Ø.1X4	—	—
organophosphorus	T6Ø.ØX1	T6Ø.ØX2	T6Ø.ØX3	T6Ø.ØX4	—	—
Insect (sting), venomous	T63.481	T63.482	T63.483	T63.484	—	—
ant	T63.421	T63.422	T63.423	T63.424	—	—
bee	T63.441	T63.442	T63.443	T63.444	—	—
caterpillar	T63.431	T63.432	T63.433	T63.434	—	—
hornet	T63.451	T63.452	T63.453	T63.454	—	—
wasp	T63.461	T63.462	T63.463	T63.464	—	—
Insular tissue extract	T38.3X1	T38.3X2	T38.3X3	T38.3X4	T38.3X5	T38.3X6
Insulin (amorphous) (globin) (isophane) (Lente) (NPH) (Semilente) (Ultralente)	T38.3X1	T38.3X2	T38.3X3	T38.3X4	T38.3X5	T38.3X6
defalan	T38.3X1	T38.3X2	T38.3X3	T38.3X4	T38.3X5	T38.3X6
human	T38.3X1	T38.3X2	T38.3X3	T38.3X4	T38.3X5	T38.3X6
injection, soluble	T38.3X1	T38.3X2	T38.3X3	T38.3X4	T38.3X5	T38.3X6
biphasic	T38.3X1	T38.3X2	T38.3X3	T38.3X4	T38.3X5	T38.3X6
intermediate acting	T38.3X1	T38.3X2	T38.3X3	T38.3X4	T38.3X5	T38.3X6
protamine zinc	T38.3X1	T38.3X2	T38.3X3	T38.3X4	T38.3X5	T38.3X6
slow acting	T38.3X1	T38.3X2	T38.3X3	T38.3X4	T38.3X5	T38.3X6
zinc						

Subterms under main terms may continue to next column or page

Additional Character May Be Required — Refer to the Tabular List for Character Selection

379

Substance	Poisoning, Accidental (unintentional)	Poisoning, Intentional Self-harm	Poisoning, Assault	Poisoning, Undetermined	Adverse Effect	Under-dosing
Insulin — *continued*						
zinc — *continued*						
protamine injection	T38.3X1	T38.3X2	T38.3X3	T38.3X4	T38.3X5	T38.3X6
suspension (amorphous) (crystalline)	T38.3X1	T38.3X2	T38.3X3	T38.3X4	T38.3X5	T38.3X6
Interferon (alpha) (beta) (gamma)	T37.5X1	T37.5X2	T37.5X3	T37.5X4	T37.5X5	T37.5X6
Intestinal motility control drug	T47.6X1	T47.6X2	T47.6X3	T47.6X4	T47.6X5	T47.6X6
biological	T47.8X1	T47.8X2	T47.8X3	T47.8X4	T47.8X5	T47.8X6
Intranarcon	T41.1X1	T41.1X2	T41.1X3	T41.1X4	T41.1X5	T41.1X6
Intravenous						
amino acids	T5Ø.991	T5Ø.992	T5Ø.993	T5Ø.994	T5Ø.995	T5Ø.996
fat suspension	T5Ø.991	T5Ø.992	T5Ø.993	T5Ø.994	T5Ø.995	T5Ø.996
Inulin	T5Ø.8X1	T5Ø.8X2	T5Ø.8X3	T5Ø.8X4	T5Ø.8X5	T5Ø.8X6
Invert sugar	T5Ø.3X1	T5Ø.3X2	T5Ø.3X3	T5Ø.3X4	T5Ø.3X5	T5Ø.3X6
Inza — *see* Naproxen						
Iobenzamic acid	T5Ø.8X1	T5Ø.8X2	T5Ø.8X3	T5Ø.8X4	T5Ø.8X5	T5Ø.8X6
Iocarmic acid	T5Ø.8X1	T5Ø.8X2	T5Ø.8X3	T5Ø.8X4	T5Ø.8X5	T5Ø.8X6
Iocetamic acid	T5Ø.8X1	T5Ø.8X2	T5Ø.8X3	T5Ø.8X4	T5Ø.8X5	T5Ø.8X6
Iodamide	T5Ø.8X1	T5Ø.8X2	T5Ø.8X3	T5Ø.8X4	T5Ø.8X5	T5Ø.8X6
Iodide NEC — *see also* Iodine	T49.ØX1	T49.ØX2	T49.ØX3	T49.ØX4	T49.ØX5	T49.ØX6
mercury (ointment)	T49.ØX1	T49.ØX2	T49.ØX3	T49.ØX4	T49.ØX5	T49.ØX6
methylate	T49.ØX1	T49.ØX2	T49.ØX3	T49.ØX4	T49.ØX5	T49.ØX6
potassium (expectorant) NEC	T48.4X1	T48.4X2	T48.4X3	T48.4X4	T48.4X5	T48.4X6
Iodinated						
contrast medium	T5Ø.8X1	T5Ø.8X2	T5Ø.8X3	T5Ø.8X4	T5Ø.8X5	T5Ø.8X6
glycerol	T48.4X1	T48.4X2	T48.4X3	T48.4X4	T48.4X5	T48.4X6
human serum albumin (131I)	T5Ø.8X1	T5Ø.8X2	T5Ø.8X3	T5Ø.8X4	T5Ø.8X5	T5Ø.8X6
Iodine (antiseptic, external) (tincture) **NEC**	T49.ØX1	T49.ØX2	T49.ØX3	T49.ØX4	T49.ØX5	T49.ØX6
125 — *see also* Radiation sickness, and Exposure to radioactivce isotopes	T5Ø.8X1	T5Ø.8X2	T5Ø.8X3	T5Ø.8X4	T5Ø.8X5	T5Ø.8X6
therapeutic	T5Ø.991	T5Ø.992	T5Ø.993	T5Ø.994	T5Ø.995	T5Ø.996
131 — *see also* Radiation sickness, and Exposure to radioactivce isotopes	T5Ø.8X1	T5Ø.8X2	T5Ø.8X3	T5Ø.8X4	T5Ø.8X5	T5Ø.8X6
therapeutic	T38.2X1	T38.2X2	T38.2X3	T38.2X4	T38.2X5	T38.2X6
diagnostic	T5Ø.8X1	T5Ø.8X2	T5Ø.8X3	T5Ø.8X4	T5Ø.8X5	T5Ø.8X6
for thyroid conditions (antithyroid)	T38.2X1	T38.2X2	T38.2X3	T38.2X4	T38.2X5	T38.2X6
solution	T49.ØX1	T49.ØX2	T49.ØX3	T49.ØX4	T49.ØX5	T49.ØX6
vapor	T59.891	T59.892	T59.893	T59.894	—	—
Iodipamide	T5Ø.8X1	T5Ø.8X2	T5Ø.8X3	T5Ø.8X4	T5Ø.8X5	T5Ø.8X6
Iodized (poppy seed) oil	T5Ø.8X1	T5Ø.8X2	T5Ø.8X3	T5Ø.8X4	T5Ø.8X5	T5Ø.8X6
Iodobismitol	T37.8X1	T37.8X2	T37.8X3	T37.8X4	T37.8X5	T37.8X6
Iodochlorhydroxyquin	T37.8X1	T37.8X2	T37.8X3	T37.8X4	T37.8X5	T37.8X6
topical	T49.ØX1	T49.ØX2	T49.ØX3	T49.ØX4	T49.ØX5	T49.ØX6
Iodochlorhydroxyquinoline	T37.8X1	T37.8X2	T37.8X3	T37.8X4	T37.8X5	T37.8X6
Iodocholesterol (131I)	T5Ø.8X1	T5Ø.8X2	T5Ø.8X3	T5Ø.8X4	T5Ø.8X5	T5Ø.8X6
Iodoform	T49.ØX1	T49.ØX2	T49.ØX3	T49.ØX4	T49.ØX5	T49.ØX6
Iodohippuric acid	T5Ø.8X1	T5Ø.8X2	T5Ø.8X3	T5Ø.8X4	T5Ø.8X5	T5Ø.8X6
Iodopanoic acid	T5Ø.8X1	T5Ø.8X2	T5Ø.8X3	T5Ø.8X4	T5Ø.8X5	T5Ø.8X6
Iodophthalein (sodium)	T5Ø.8X1	T5Ø.8X2	T5Ø.8X3	T5Ø.8X4	T5Ø.8X5	T5Ø.8X6
Iodopyracet	T5Ø.8X1	T5Ø.8X2	T5Ø.8X3	T5Ø.8X4	T5Ø.8X5	T5Ø.8X6
Iodoquinol	T37.8X1	T37.8X2	T37.8X3	T37.8X4	T37.8X5	T37.8X6
Iodoxamic acid	T5Ø.8X1	T5Ø.8X2	T5Ø.8X3	T5Ø.8X4	T5Ø.8X5	T5Ø.8X6
Iofendylate	T5Ø.8X1	T5Ø.8X2	T5Ø.8X3	T5Ø.8X4	T5Ø.8X5	T5Ø.8X6
Ioglycamic acid	T5Ø.8X1	T5Ø.8X2	T5Ø.8X3	T5Ø.8X4	T5Ø.8X5	T5Ø.8X6
Iohexol	T5Ø.8X1	T5Ø.8X2	T5Ø.8X3	T5Ø.8X4	T5Ø.8X5	T5Ø.8X6
Ion exchange resin						
anion	T47.8X1	T47.8X2	T47.8X3	T47.8X4	T47.8X5	T47.8X6
cation	T5Ø.3X1	T5Ø.3X2	T5Ø.3X3	T5Ø.3X4	T5Ø.3X5	T5Ø.3X6
cholestyramine	T46.6X1	T46.6X2	T46.6X3	T46.6X4	T46.6X5	T46.6X6
intestinal	T47.8X1	T47.8X2	T47.8X3	T47.8X4	T47.8X5	T47.8X6
Iopamidol	T5Ø.8X1	T5Ø.8X2	T5Ø.8X3	T5Ø.8X4	T5Ø.8X5	T5Ø.8X6
Iopanoic acid	T5Ø.8X1	T5Ø.8X2	T5Ø.8X3	T5Ø.8X4	T5Ø.8X5	T5Ø.8X6
Iophenoic acid	T5Ø.8X1	T5Ø.8X2	T5Ø.8X3	T5Ø.8X4	T5Ø.8X5	T5Ø.8X6
Iopodate, sodium	T5Ø.8X1	T5Ø.8X2	T5Ø.8X3	T5Ø.8X4	T5Ø.8X5	T5Ø.8X6
Iopodic acid	T5Ø.8X1	T5Ø.8X2	T5Ø.8X3	T5Ø.8X4	T5Ø.8X5	T5Ø.8X6
Iopromide	T5Ø.8X1	T5Ø.8X2	T5Ø.8X3	T5Ø.8X4	T5Ø.8X5	T5Ø.8X6
Iopydol	T5Ø.8X1	T5Ø.8X2	T5Ø.8X3	T5Ø.8X4	T5Ø.8X5	T5Ø.8X6
Iotalamic acid	T5Ø.8X1	T5Ø.8X2	T5Ø.8X3	T5Ø.8X4	T5Ø.8X5	T5Ø.8X6
Iothalamate	T5Ø.8X1	T5Ø.8X2	T5Ø.8X3	T5Ø.8X4	T5Ø.8X5	T5Ø.8X6
Iothiouracil	T38.2X1	T38.2X2	T38.2X3	T38.2X4	T38.2X5	T38.2X6
Iotrol	T5Ø.8X1	T5Ø.8X2	T5Ø.8X3	T5Ø.8X4	T5Ø.8X5	T5Ø.8X6
Iotrolan	T5Ø.8X1	T5Ø.8X2	T5Ø.8X3	T5Ø.8X4	T5Ø.8X5	T5Ø.8X6
Iotroxate	T5Ø.8X1	T5Ø.8X2	T5Ø.8X3	T5Ø.8X4	T5Ø.8X5	T5Ø.8X6
Iotroxic acid	T5Ø.8X1	T5Ø.8X2	T5Ø.8X3	T5Ø.8X4	T5Ø.8X5	T5Ø.8X6
Ioversol	T5Ø.8X1	T5Ø.8X2	T5Ø.8X3	T5Ø.8X4	T5Ø.8X5	T5Ø.8X6
Ioxaglate	T5Ø.8X1	T5Ø.8X2	T5Ø.8X3	T5Ø.8X4	T5Ø.8X5	T5Ø.8X6
Ioxaglic acid	T5Ø.8X1	T5Ø.8X2	T5Ø.8X3	T5Ø.8X4	T5Ø.8X5	T5Ø.8X6
Ioxitalamic acid	T5Ø.8X1	T5Ø.8X2	T5Ø.8X3	T5Ø.8X4	T5Ø.8X5	T5Ø.8X6
Ipecac	T47.7X1	T47.7X2	T47.7X3	T47.7X4	T47.7X5	T47.7X6
Ipecacuanha	T48.4X1	T48.4X2	T48.4X3	T48.4X4	T48.4X5	T48.4X6
Ipodate, calcium	T5Ø.8X1	T5Ø.8X2	T5Ø.8X3	T5Ø.8X4	T5Ø.8X5	T5Ø.8X6
Ipral	T42.3X1	T42.3X2	T42.3X3	T42.3X4	T42.3X5	T42.3X6
Ipratropium (bromide)	T48.6X1	T48.6X2	T48.6X3	T48.6X4	T48.6X5	T48.6X6
Ipriflavone	T46.3X1	T46.3X2	T46.3X3	T46.3X4	T46.3X5	T46.3X6
Iprindole	T43.Ø11	T43.Ø12	T43.Ø13	T43.Ø14	T43.Ø15	T43.Ø16
Iproclozide	T43.1X1	T43.1X2	T43.1X3	T43.1X4	T43.1X5	T43.1X6
Iprofenin	T5Ø.8X1	T5Ø.8X2	T5Ø.8X3	T5Ø.8X4	T5Ø.8X5	T5Ø.8X6
Iproheptine	T49.2X1	T49.2X2	T49.2X3	T49.2X4	T49.2X5	T49.2X6
Iproniazid	T43.1X1	T43.1X2	T43.1X3	T43.1X4	T43.1X5	T43.1X6
Iproplatin	T45.1X1	T45.1X2	T45.1X3	T45.1X4	T45.1X5	T45.1X6
Iproveratril	T46.1X1	T46.1X2	T46.1X3	T46.1X4	T46.1X5	T46.1X6
Iron (compounds) (medicinal) **NEC**	T45.4X1	T45.4X2	T45.4X3	T45.4X4	T45.4X5	T45.4X6
ammonium	T45.4X1	T45.4X2	T45.4X3	T45.4X4	T45.4X5	T45.4X6
dextran injection	T45.4X1	T45.4X2	T45.4X3	T45.4X4	T45.4X5	T45.4X6
nonmedicinal	T56.891	T56.892	T56.893	T56.894	—	—
salts	T45.4X1	T45.4X2	T45.4X3	T45.4X4	T45.4X5	T45.4X6
sorbitex	T45.4X1	T45.4X2	T45.4X3	T45.4X4	T45.4X5	T45.4X6
sorbitol citric acid complex	T45.4X1	T45.4X2	T45.4X3	T45.4X4	T45.4X5	T45.4X6
Irrigating fluid (vaginal)	T49.8X1	T49.8X2	T49.8X3	T49.8X4	T49.8X5	T49.8X6
eye	T49.5X1	T49.5X2	T49.5X3	T49.5X4	T49.5X5	T49.5X6
Isepamicin	T36.5X1	T36.5X2	T36.5X3	T36.5X4	T36.5X5	T36.5X6
Isoaminile (citrate)	T48.3X1	T48.3X2	T48.3X3	T48.3X4	T48.3X5	T48.3X6
Isoamyl nitrite	T46.3X1	T46.3X2	T46.3X3	T46.3X4	T46.3X5	T46.3X6
Isobenzan	T6Ø.1X1	T6Ø.1X2	T6Ø.1X3	T6Ø.1X4	—	—
Isobutyl acetate	T52.8X1	T52.8X2	T52.8X3	T52.8X4	—	—
Isocarboxazid	T43.1X1	T43.1X2	T43.1X3	T43.1X4	T43.1X5	T43.1X6
Isoconazole	T49.ØX1	T49.ØX2	T49.ØX3	T49.ØX4	T49.ØX5	T49.ØX6
Isocyanate	T65.ØX1	T65.ØX2	T65.ØX3	T65.ØX4	—	—
Isoephedrine	T44.991	T44.992	T44.993	T44.994	T44.995	T44.996
Isoetarine	T48.6X1	T48.6X2	T48.6X3	T48.6X4	T48.6X5	T48.6X6
Isoethadione	T42.2X1	T42.2X2	T42.2X3	T42.2X4	T42.2X5	T42.2X6
Isoetharine	T44.5X1	T44.5X2	T44.5X3	T44.5X4	T44.5X5	T44.5X6
Isoflurane	T41.ØX1	T41.ØX2	T41.ØX3	T41.ØX4	T41.ØX5	T41.ØX6
Isoflurophate	T44.ØX1	T44.ØX2	T44.ØX3	T44.ØX4	T44.ØX5	T44.ØX6
Isomaltose, ferric complex	T45.4X1	T45.4X2	T45.4X3	T45.4X4	T45.4X5	T45.4X6
Isometheptene	T44.3X1	T44.3X2	T44.3X3	T44.3X4	T44.3X5	T44.3X6
Isoniazid	T37.1X1	T37.1X2	T37.1X3	T37.1X4	T37.1X5	T37.1X6
with						
rifampicin	T36.6X1	T36.6X2	T36.6X3	T36.6X4	T36.6X5	T36.6X6
thioacetazone	T37.1X1	T37.1X2	T37.1X3	T37.1X4	T37.1X5	T37.1X6
Isonicotinic acid hydrazide	T37.1X1	T37.1X2	T37.1X3	T37.1X4	T37.1X5	T37.1X6
Isonipecaine	T4Ø.491	T4Ø.492	T4Ø.493	T4Ø.494	T4Ø.495	T4Ø.496
Isopentaquine	T37.2X1	T37.2X2	T37.2X3	T37.2X4	T37.2X5	T37.2X6
Isophane insulin	T38.3X1	T38.3X2	T38.3X3	T38.3X4	T38.3X5	T38.3X6
Isophorone	T65.891	T65.892	T65.893	T65.894	—	—
Isophosphamide	T45.1X1	T45.1X2	T45.1X3	T45.1X4	T45.1X5	T45.1X6
Isopregnenone	T38.5X1	T38.5X2	T38.5X3	T38.5X4	T38.5X5	T38.5X6
Isoprenaline	T48.6X1	T48.6X2	T48.6X3	T48.6X4	T48.6X5	T48.6X6
Isopromethazine	T43.3X1	T43.3X2	T43.3X3	T43.3X4	T43.3X5	T43.3X6
Isopropamide	T44.3X1	T44.3X2	T44.3X3	T44.3X4	T44.3X5	T44.3X6
iodide	T44.3X1	T44.3X2	T44.3X3	T44.3X4	T44.3X5	T44.3X6
Isopropanol	T51.2X1	T51.2X2	T51.2X3	T51.2X4	—	—
Isopropyl						
acetate	T52.8X1	T52.8X2	T52.8X3	T52.8X4	—	—
alcohol	T51.2X1	T51.2X2	T51.2X3	T51.2X4	—	—
medicinal	T49.4X1	T49.4X2	T49.4X3	T49.4X4	T49.4X5	T49.4X6
ether	T52.8X1	T52.8X2	T52.8X3	T52.8X4	—	—
Isopropylaminophenazone	T39.2X1	T39.2X2	T39.2X3	T39.2X4	T39.2X5	T39.2X6
Isoproterenol	T48.6X1	T48.6X2	T48.6X3	T48.6X4	T48.6X5	T48.6X6
Isosorbide dinitrate	T46.3X1	T46.3X2	T46.3X3	T46.3X4	T46.3X5	T46.3X6
Isothipendyl	T45.ØX1	T45.ØX2	T45.ØX3	T45.ØX4	T45.ØX5	T45.ØX6
Isotretinoin	T5Ø.991	T5Ø.992	T5Ø.993	T5Ø.994	T5Ø.995	T5Ø.996
Isoxazolyl penicillin	T36.ØX1	T36.ØX2	T36.ØX3	T36.ØX4	T36.ØX5	T36.ØX6
Isoxicam	T39.391	T39.392	T39.393	T39.394	T39.395	T39.396
Isoxsuprine	T46.7X1	T46.7X2	T46.7X3	T46.7X4	T46.7X5	T46.7X6
Ispagula	T47.4X1	T47.4X2	T47.4X3	T47.4X4	T47.4X5	T47.4X6
husk	T47.4X1	T47.4X2	T47.4X3	T47.4X4	T47.4X5	T47.4X6
Isradipine	T46.1X1	T46.1X2	T46.1X3	T46.1X4	T46.1X5	T46.1X6
I-thyroxine sodium	T38.1X1	T38.1X2	T38.1X3	T38.1X4	T38.1X5	T38.1X6
Itraconazole	T37.8X1	T37.8X2	T37.8X3	T37.8X4	T37.8X5	T37.8X6
Itramin tosilate	T46.3X1	T46.3X2	T46.3X3	T46.3X4	T46.3X5	T46.3X6
Ivermectin	T37.4X1	T37.4X2	T37.4X3	T37.4X4	T37.4X5	T37.4X6
Izoniazid	T37.1X1	T37.1X2	T37.1X3	T37.1X4	T37.1X5	T37.1X6
with thioacetazone	T37.1X1	T37.1X2	T37.1X3	T37.1X4	T37.1X5	T37.1X6
Jalap	T47.2X1	T47.2X2	T47.2X3	T47.2X4	T47.2X5	T47.2X6

Insulin — Jamaica

380

Additional Character May Be Required — Refer to the Tabular List for Character Selection

Subterms under main terms may continue to next column or page

Substance	Poisoning, Accidental (unintentional)	Poisoning, Intentional Self-harm	Poisoning, Assault	Poisoning, Undetermined	Adverse Effect	Under-dosing
Jamaica						
dogwood (bark)	T39.8X1	T39.8X2	T39.8X3	T39.8X4	T39.8X5	T39.8X6
ginger	T65.891	T65.892	T65.893	T65.894	—	—
root	T62.2X1	T62.2X2	T62.2X3	T62.2X4	—	—
Jatropha	T62.2X1	T62.2X2	T62.2X3	T62.2X4	—	—
curcas	T62.2X1	T62.2X2	T62.2X3	T62.2X4	—	—
Jectofer	T45.4X1	T45.4X2	T45.4X3	T45.4X4	T45.4X5	T45.4X6
Jellyfish (sting)	T63.621	T63.622	T63.623	T63.624	—	—
Jequirity (bean)	T62.2X1	T62.2X2	T62.2X3	T62.2X4	—	—
Jimson weed (stramonium)	T62.2X1	T62.2X2	T62.2X3	T62.2X4	—	—
seeds	T62.2X1	T62.2X2	T62.2X3	T62.2X4	—	—
Josamycin	T36.3X1	T36.3X2	T36.3X3	T36.3X4	T36.3X5	T36.3X6
Juniper tar	T49.1X1	T49.1X2	T49.1X3	T49.1X4	T49.1X5	T49.1X6
Kallidinogenase	T46.7X1	T46.7X2	T46.7X3	T46.7X4	T46.7X5	T46.7X6
Kallikrein	T46.7X1	T46.7X2	T46.7X3	T46.7X4	T46.7X5	T46.7X6
Kanamycin	T36.5X1	T36.5X2	T36.5X3	T36.5X4	T36.5X5	T36.5X6
Kantrex	T36.5X1	T36.5X2	T36.5X3	T36.5X4	T36.5X5	T36.5X6
Kaolin	T47.6X1	T47.6X2	T47.6X3	T47.6X4	T47.6X5	T47.6X6
light	T47.6X1	T47.6X2	T47.6X3	T47.6X4	T47.6X5	T47.6X6
Karaya (gum)	T47.4X1	T47.4X2	T47.4X3	T47.4X4	T47.4X5	T47.4X6
Kebuzone	T39.2X1	T39.2X2	T39.2X3	T39.2X4	T39.2X5	T39.2X6
Kelevan	T60.1X1	T60.1X2	T60.1X3	T60.1X4	—	—
Kemithal	T41.1X1	T41.1X2	T41.1X3	T41.1X4	T41.1X5	T41.1X6
Kenacort	T38.0X1	T38.0X2	T38.0X3	T38.0X4	T38.0X5	T38.0X6
Keratolytic drug NEC	T49.4X1	T49.4X2	T49.4X3	T49.4X4	T49.4X5	T49.4X6
anthracene	T49.4X1	T49.4X2	T49.4X3	T49.4X4	T49.4X5	T49.4X6
Keratoplastic NEC	T49.4X1	T49.4X2	T49.4X3	T49.4X4	T49.4X5	T49.4X6
Kerosene, kerosine (fuel) (solvent) **NEC**	T52.0X1	T52.0X2	T52.0X3	T52.0X4	—	—
insecticide	T52.0X1	T52.0X2	T52.0X3	T52.0X4	—	—
vapor	T52.0X1	T52.0X2	T52.0X3	T52.0X4	—	—
Ketamine	T41.291	T41.292	T41.293	T41.294	T41.295	T41.296
Ketazolam	T42.4X1	T42.4X2	T42.4X3	T42.4X4	T42.4X5	T42.4X6
Ketazon	T39.2X1	T39.2X2	T39.2X3	T39.2X4	T39.2X5	T39.2X6
Ketobemidone	T40.491	T40.492	T40.493	T40.494	—	—
Ketoconazole	T49.0X1	T49.0X2	T49.0X3	T49.0X4	T49.0X5	T49.0X6
Ketols	T52.4X1	T52.4X2	T52.4X3	T52.4X4	—	—
Ketone oils	T52.4X1	T52.4X2	T52.4X3	T52.4X4	—	—
Ketoprofen	T39.311	T39.312	T39.313	T39.314	T39.315	T39.316
Ketorolac	T39.8X1	T39.8X2	T39.8X3	T39.8X4	T39.8X5	T39.8X6
Ketotifen	T45.0X1	T45.0X2	T45.0X3	T45.0X4	T45.0X5	T45.0X6
Khat	T43.691	T43.692	T43.693	T43.694	—	—
Khellin	T46.3X1	T46.3X2	T46.3X3	T46.3X4	T46.3X5	T46.3X6
Khelloside	T46.3X1	T46.3X2	T46.3X3	T46.3X4	T46.3X5	T46.3X6
Kiln gas or vapor (carbon monoxide)	T58.8X1	T58.8X2	T58.8X3	T58.8X4	—	—
Kitasamycin	T36.3X1	T36.3X2	T36.3X3	T36.3X4	T36.3X5	T36.3X6
Konsyl	T47.4X1	T47.4X2	T47.4X3	T47.4X4	T47.4X5	T47.4X6
Kosam seed	T62.2X1	T62.2X2	T62.2X3	T62.2X4	—	—
Krait (venom)	T63.091	T63.092	T63.093	T63.094	—	—
Kwell (insecticide)	T60.1X1	T60.1X2	T60.1X3	T60.1X4	—	—
anti-infective (topical)	T49.0X1	T49.0X2	T49.0X3	T49.0X4	T49.0X5	T49.0X6
Labetalol	T44.8X1	T44.8X2	T44.8X3	T44.8X4	T44.8X5	T44.8X6
Laburnum (seeds)	T62.2X1	T62.2X2	T62.2X3	T62.2X4	—	—
leaves	T62.2X1	T62.2X2	T62.2X3	T62.2X4	—	—
Lachesine	T49.5X1	T49.5X2	T49.5X3	T49.5X4	T49.5X5	T49.5X6
Lacidipine	T46.5X1	T46.5X2	T46.5X3	T46.5X4	T46.5X5	T46.5X6
Lacquer	T65.6X1	T65.6X2	T65.6X3	T65.6X4	—	—
Lacrimogenic gas	T59.3X1	T59.3X2	T59.3X3	T59.3X4	—	—
Lactated potassic saline	T50.3X1	T50.3X2	T50.3X3	T50.3X4	T50.3X5	T50.3X6
Lactic acid	T49.8X1	T49.8X2	T49.8X3	T49.8X4	T49.8X5	T49.8X6
Lactobacillus						
acidophilus	T47.6X1	T47.6X2	T47.6X3	T47.6X4	T47.6X5	T47.6X6
compound	T47.6X1	T47.6X2	T47.6X3	T47.6X4	T47.6X5	T47.6X6
bifidus, lyophilized	T47.6X1	T47.6X2	T47.6X3	T47.6X4	T47.6X5	T47.6X6
bulgaricus	T47.6X1	T47.6X2	T47.6X3	T47.6X4	T47.6X5	T47.6X6
sporogenes	T47.6X1	T47.6X2	T47.6X3	T47.6X4	T47.6X5	T47.6X6
Lactoflavin	T45.2X1	T45.2X2	T45.2X3	T45.2X4	T45.2X5	T45.2X6
Lactose (as excipient)	T50.901	T50.902	T50.903	T50.904	T50.905	T50.906
Lactuca (virosa) (extract)	T42.6X1	T42.6X2	T42.6X3	T42.6X4	T42.6X5	T42.6X6
Lactucarium	T42.6X1	T42.6X2	T42.6X3	T42.6X4	T42.6X5	T42.6X6
Lactulose	T47.3X1	T47.3X2	T47.3X3	T47.3X4	T47.3X5	T47.3X6
Laevo — see Levo-						
Lanatosides	T46.0X1	T46.0X2	T46.0X3	T46.0X4	T46.0X5	T46.0X6
Lanolin	T49.3X1	T49.3X2	T49.3X3	T49.3X4	T49.3X5	T49.3X6
Largactil	T43.3X1	T43.3X2	T43.3X3	T43.3X4	T43.3X5	T43.3X6
Larkspur	T62.2X1	T62.2X2	T62.2X3	T62.2X4	—	—
Laroxyl	T43.011	T43.012	T43.013	T43.014	T43.015	T43.016
Lasix	T50.1X1	T50.1X2	T50.1X3	T50.1X4	T50.1X5	T50.1X6
Lassar's paste	T49.4X1	T49.4X2	T49.4X3	T49.4X4	T49.4X5	T49.4X6
Latamoxef	T36.1X1	T36.1X2	T36.1X3	T36.1X4	T36.1X5	T36.1X6
Latex	T65.811	T65.812	T65.813	T65.814	—	—
Lathyrus (seed)	T62.2X1	T62.2X2	T62.2X3	T62.2X4	—	—

Substance	Poisoning, Accidental (unintentional)	Poisoning, Intentional Self-harm	Poisoning, Assault	Poisoning, Undetermined	Adverse Effect	Under-dosing
Laudanum	T40.0X1	T40.0X2	T40.0X3	T40.0X4	T40.0X5	T40.0X6
Laudexium	T48.1X1	T48.1X2	T48.1X3	T48.1X4	T48.1X5	T48.1X6
Laughing gas	T41.0X1	T41.0X2	T41.0X3	T41.0X4	T41.0X5	T41.0X6
Laurel, black or cherry	T62.2X1	T62.2X2	T62.2X3	T62.2X4	—	—
Laurolinium	T49.0X1	T49.0X2	T49.0X3	T49.0X4	T49.0X5	T49.0X6
Lauryl sulfoacetate	T49.2X1	T49.2X2	T49.2X3	T49.2X4	T49.2X5	T49.2X6
Laxative NEC	T47.4X1	T47.4X2	T47.4X3	T47.4X4	T47.4X5	T47.4X6
osmotic	T47.3X1	T47.3X2	T47.3X3	T47.3X4	T47.3X5	T47.3X6
saline	T47.3X1	T47.3X2	T47.3X3	T47.3X4	T47.3X5	T47.3X6
stimulant	T47.2X1	T47.2X2	T47.2X3	T47.2X4	T47.2X5	T47.2X6
L-dopa	T42.8X1	T42.8X2	T42.8X3	T42.8X4	T42.8X5	T42.8X6
Lead (dust) (fumes) (vapor) **NEC**	T56.0X1	T56.0X2	T56.0X3	T56.0X4	—	—
acetate	T49.2X1	T49.2X2	T49.2X3	T49.2X4	T49.2X5	T49.2X6
alkyl (fuel additive)	T56.0X1	T56.0X2	T56.0X3	T56.0X4	—	—
anti-infectives	T37.8X1	T37.8X2	T37.8X3	T37.8X4	T37.8X5	T37.8X6
antiknock compound (tetraethyl)	T56.0X1	T56.0X2	T56.0X3	T56.0X4	—	—
arsenate, arsenite (dust)(herbicide) (insecticide) (vapor)	T57.0X1	T57.0X2	T57.0X3	T57.0X4	—	—
carbonate	T56.0X1	T56.0X2	T56.0X3	T56.0X4	—	—
paint	T56.0X1	T56.0X2	T56.0X3	T56.0X4	—	—
chromate	T56.0X1	T56.0X2	T56.0X3	T56.0X4	—	—
paint	T56.0X1	T56.0X2	T56.0X3	T56.0X4	—	—
dioxide	T56.0X1	T56.0X2	T56.0X3	T56.0X4	—	—
inorganic	T56.0X1	T56.0X2	T56.0X3	T56.0X4	—	—
iodide	T56.0X1	T56.0X2	T56.0X3	T56.0X4	—	—
pigment (paint)	T56.0X1	T56.0X2	T56.0X3	T56.0X4	—	—
monoxide (dust)	T56.0X1	T56.0X2	T56.0X3	T56.0X4	—	—
paint	T56.0X1	T56.0X2	T56.0X3	T56.0X4	—	—
organic	T56.0X1	T56.0X2	T56.0X3	T56.0X4	—	—
oxide	T56.0X1	T56.0X2	T56.0X3	T56.0X4	—	—
paint	T56.0X1	T56.0X2	T56.0X3	T56.0X4	—	—
paint	T56.0X1	T56.0X2	T56.0X3	T56.0X4	—	—
salts	T56.0X1	T56.0X2	T56.0X3	T56.0X4	—	—
specified compound NEC	T56.0X1	T56.0X2	T56.0X3	T56.0X4	—	—
tetra-ethyl	T56.0X1	T56.0X2	T56.0X3	T56.0X4	—	—
Lebanese red	T40.711	T40.712	T40.713	T40.714	T40.715	T40.716
Lefetamine	T39.8X1	T39.8X2	T39.8X3	T39.8X4	T39.8X5	T39.8X6
Lenperone	T43.4X1	T43.4X2	T43.4X3	T43.4X4	T43.4X5	T43.4X6
Lente lietin (insulin)	T38.3X1	T38.3X2	T38.3X3	T38.3X4	T38.3X5	T38.3X6
Leptazol	T50.7X1	T50.7X2	T50.7X3	T50.7X4	T50.7X5	T50.7X6
Leptophos	T60.0X1	T60.0X2	T60.0X3	T60.0X4	—	—
Leritine	T40.2X1	T40.2X2	T40.2X3	T40.2X4	T40.2X5	T40.2X6
Letosteine	T48.4X1	T48.4X2	T48.4X3	T48.4X4	T48.4X5	T48.4X6
Letter	T38.1X1	T38.1X2	T38.1X3	T38.1X4	T38.1X5	T38.1X6
Lettuce opium	T42.6X1	T42.6X2	T42.6X3	T42.6X4	T42.6X5	T42.6X6
Leucinocaine	T41.3X1	T41.3X2	T41.3X3	T41.3X4	T41.3X5	T41.3X6
Leucocianidol	T46.991	T46.992	T46.993	T46.994	T46.995	T46.996
Leucovorin (factor)	T45.8X1	T45.8X2	T45.8X3	T45.8X4	T45.8X5	T45.8X6
Leukeran	T45.1X1	T45.1X2	T45.1X3	T45.1X4	T45.1X5	T45.1X6
Leuprolide	T38.891	T38.892	T38.893	T38.894	T38.895	T38.896
Levalbuterol	T48.6X1	T48.6X2	T48.6X3	T48.6X4	T48.6X5	T48.6X6
Levallorphan	T50.7X1	T50.7X2	T50.7X3	T50.7X4	T50.7X5	T50.7X6
Levamisole	T37.4X1	T37.4X2	T37.4X3	T37.4X4	T37.4X5	T37.4X6
Levanil	T42.6X1	T42.6X2	T42.6X3	T42.6X4	T42.6X5	T42.6X6
Levarterenol	T44.4X1	T44.4X2	T44.4X3	T44.4X4	T44.4X5	T44.4X6
Levdropropizine	T48.3X1	T48.3X2	T48.3X3	T48.3X4	T48.3X5	T48.3X6
Levobunolol	T49.5X1	T49.5X2	T49.5X3	T49.5X4	T49.5X5	T49.5X6
Levocabastine (hydrochloride)	T45.0X1	T45.0X2	T45.0X3	T45.0X4	T45.0X5	T45.0X6
Levocarnitine	T50.991	T50.992	T50.993	T50.994	T50.995	T50.996
Levodopa	T42.8X1	T42.8X2	T42.8X3	T42.8X4	T42.8X5	T42.8X6
with carbidopa	T42.8X1	T42.8X2	T42.8X3	T42.8X4	T42.8X5	T42.8X6
Levo-dromoran	T40.2X1	T40.2X2	T40.2X3	T40.2X4	T40.2X5	T40.2X6
Levoglutamide	T50.991	T50.992	T50.993	T50.994	T50.995	T50.996
Levoid	T38.1X1	T38.1X2	T38.1X3	T38.1X4	T38.1X5	T38.1X6
Levo-isomethadone	T40.3X1	T40.3X2	T40.3X3	T40.3X4	T40.3X5	T40.3X6
Levomepromazine	T43.3X1	T43.3X2	T43.3X3	T43.3X4	T43.3X5	T43.3X6
Levonordefrin	T49.6X1	T49.6X2	T49.6X3	T49.6X4	T49.6X5	T49.6X6
Levonorgestrel	T38.4X1	T38.4X2	T38.4X3	T38.4X4	T38.4X5	T38.4X6
with ethinylestradiol	T38.5X1	T38.5X2	T38.5X3	T38.5X4	T38.5X5	T38.5X6
Levopromazine	T43.3X1	T43.3X2	T43.3X3	T43.3X4	T43.3X5	T43.3X6
Levoprome	T42.6X1	T42.6X2	T42.6X3	T42.6X4	T42.6X5	T42.6X6
Levopropoxyphene	T40.491	T40.492	T40.493	T40.494	T40.495	T40.496
Levopropylhexedrine	T50.5X1	T50.5X2	T50.5X3	T50.5X4	T50.5X5	T50.5X6
Levoproxyphylline	T48.6X1	T48.6X2	T48.6X3	T48.6X4	T48.6X5	T48.6X6
Levorphanol	T40.491	T40.492	T40.493	T40.494	T40.495	T40.496
Levothyroxine	T38.1X1	T38.1X2	T38.1X3	T38.1X4	T38.1X5	T38.1X6
sodium	T38.1X1	T38.1X2	T38.1X3	T38.1X4	T38.1X5	T38.1X6
Levsin	T44.3X1	T44.3X2	T44.3X3	T44.3X4	T44.3X5	T44.3X6
Levulose	T50.3X1	T50.3X2	T50.3X3	T50.3X4	T50.3X5	T50.3X6

Subterms under main terms may continue to next column or page
Additional Character May Be Required — Refer to the Tabular List for Character Selection
381
Jamaica — Levulose

Substance	Poisoning, Accidental (unintentional)	Poisoning, Intentional Self-harm	Poisoning, Assault	Poisoning, Undetermined	Adverse Effect	Under-dosing
Lewisite (gas), not in war	T57.ØX1	T57.ØX2	T57.ØX3	T57.ØX4	—	—
Librium	T42.4X1	T42.4X2	T42.4X3	T42.4X4	T42.4X5	T42.4X6
Lidex	T49.ØX1	T49.ØX2	T49.ØX3	T49.ØX4	T49.ØX5	T49.ØX6
Lidocaine	T41.3X1	T41.3X2	T41.3X3	T41.3X4	T41.3X5	T41.3X6
regional	T41.3X1	T41.3X2	T41.3X3	T41.3X4	T41.3X5	T41.3X6
spinal	T41.3X1	T41.3X2	T41.3X3	T41.3X4	T41.3X5	T41.3X6
Lidofenin	T5Ø.8X1	T5Ø.8X2	T5Ø.8X3	T5Ø.8X4	T5Ø.8X5	T5Ø.8X6
Lidoflazine	T46.1X1	T46.1X2	T46.1X3	T46.1X4	T46.1X5	T46.1X6
Lighter fluid	T52.ØX1	T52.ØX2	T52.ØX3	T52.ØX4	—	—
Lignin hemicellulose	T47.6X1	T47.6X2	T47.6X3	T47.6X4	T47.6X5	T47.6X6
Lignocaine	T41.3X1	T41.3X2	T41.3X3	T41.3X4	T41.3X5	T41.3X6
regional	T41.3X1	T41.3X2	T41.3X3	T41.3X4	T41.3X5	T41.3X6
spinal	T41.3X1	T41.3X2	T41.3X3	T41.3X4	T41.3X5	T41.3X6
Ligroin (e) (solvent)	T52.ØX1	T52.ØX2	T52.ØX3	T52.ØX4	—	—
vapor	T59.891	T59.892	T59.893	T59.894	—	—
Ligustrum vulgare	T62.2X1	T62.2X2	T62.2X3	T62.2X4	—	—
Lily of the valley	T62.2X1	T62.2X2	T62.2X3	T62.2X4	—	—
Lime (chloride)	T54.3X1	T54.3X2	T54.3X3	T54.3X4	—	—
Limonene	T52.8X1	T52.8X2	T52.8X3	T52.8X4	—	—
Lincomycin	T36.8X1	T36.8X2	T36.8X3	T36.8X4	T36.8X5	T36.8X6
Lindane (insecticide) (nonmedicinal) (vapor)	T53.6X1	T53.6X2	T53.6X3	T53.6X4	—	—
medicinal	T49.ØX1	T49.ØX2	T49.ØX3	T49.ØX4	T49.ØX5	T49.ØX6
Liniments NEC	T49.91	T49.92	T49.93	T49.94	T49.95	T49.96
Linoleic acid	T46.6X1	T46.6X2	T46.6X3	T46.6X4	T46.6X5	T46.6X6
Linolenic acid	T46.6X1	T46.6X2	T46.6X3	T46.6X4	T46.6X5	T46.6X6
Linseed	T47.4X1	T47.4X2	T47.4X3	T47.4X4	T47.4X5	T47.4X6
Liothyronine	T38.1X1	T38.1X2	T38.1X3	T38.1X4	T38.1X5	T38.1X6
Liotrix	T38.1X1	T38.1X2	T38.1X3	T38.1X4	T38.1X5	T38.1X6
Lipancreatin	T47.5X1	T47.5X2	T47.5X3	T47.5X4	T47.5X5	T47.5X6
Lipo-alprostadil	T46.7X1	T46.7X2	T46.7X3	T46.7X4	T46.7X5	T46.7X6
Lipo-Lutin	T38.5X1	T38.5X2	T38.5X3	T38.5X4	T38.5X5	T38.5X6
Lipotropic drug NEC	T5Ø.9Ø1	T5Ø.9Ø2	T5Ø.9Ø3	T5Ø.9Ø4	T5Ø.9Ø5	T5Ø.9Ø6
Liquefied petroleum gases	T59.891	T59.892	T59.893	T59.894	—	—
piped (pure or mixed with air)	T59.891	T59.892	T59.893	T59.894	—	—
Liquid						
paraffin	T47.4X1	T47.4X2	T47.4X3	T47.4X4	T47.4X5	T47.4X6
petrolatum	T47.4X1	T47.4X2	T47.4X3	T47.4X4	T47.4X5	T47.4X6
topical	T49.3X1	T49.3X2	T49.3X3	T49.3X4	T49.3X5	T49.3X6
specified NEC	T65.891	T65.892	T65.893	T65.894	—	—
substance	T65.91	T65.92	T65.93	T65.94	—	—
Liquor creosolis compositus	T65.891	T65.892	T65.893	T65.894	—	—
Liquorice	T48.4X1	T48.4X2	T48.4X3	T48.4X4	T48.4X5	T48.4X6
extract	T47.8X1	T47.8X2	T47.8X3	T47.8X4	T47.8X5	T47.8X6
Lisinopril	T46.4X1	T46.4X2	T46.4X3	T46.4X4	T46.4X5	T46.4X6
Lisuride	T42.8X1	T42.8X2	T42.8X3	T42.8X4	T42.8X5	T42.8X6
Lithane	T43.8X1	T43.8X2	T43.8X3	T43.8X4	T43.8X5	T43.8X6
Lithium	T56.891	T56.892	T56.893	T56.894	—	—
gluconate	T43.591	T43.592	T43.593	T43.594	T43.595	T43.596
salts (carbonate)	T43.591	T43.592	T43.593	T43.594	T43.595	T43.596
Lithonate	T43.8X1	T43.8X2	T43.8X3	T43.8X4	T43.8X5	T43.8X6
Liver						
extract	T45.8X1	T45.8X2	T45.8X3	T45.8X4	T45.8X5	T45.8X6
for parenteral use	T45.8X1	T45.8X2	T45.8X3	T45.8X4	T45.8X5	T45.8X6
fraction 1	T45.8X1	T45.8X2	T45.8X3	T45.8X4	T45.8X5	T45.8X6
hydrolysate	T45.8X1	T45.8X2	T45.8X3	T45.8X4	T45.8X5	T45.8X6
Lizard (bite) (venom)	T63.121	T63.122	T63.123	T63.124	—	—
LMD	T45.8X1	T45.8X2	T45.8X3	T45.8X4	T45.8X5	T45.8X6
Lobelia	T62.2X1	T62.2X2	T62.2X3	T62.2X4	—	—
Lobeline	T5Ø.7X1	T5Ø.7X2	T5Ø.7X3	T5Ø.7X4	T5Ø.7X5	T5Ø.7X6
Local action drug NEC	T49.8X1	T49.8X2	T49.8X3	T49.8X4	T49.8X5	T49.8X6
Locorten	T49.ØX1	T49.ØX2	T49.ØX3	T49.ØX4	T49.ØX5	T49.ØX6
Lofepramine	T43.Ø11	T43.Ø12	T43.Ø13	T43.Ø14	T43.Ø15	T43.Ø16
Lolium temulentum	T62.2X1	T62.2X2	T62.2X3	T62.2X4	—	—
Lomotil	T47.6X1	T47.6X2	T47.6X3	T47.6X4	T47.6X5	T47.6X6
Lomustine	T45.1X1	T45.1X2	T45.1X3	T45.1X4	T45.1X5	T45.1X6
Lonidamine	T45.1X1	T45.1X2	T45.1X3	T45.1X4	T45.1X5	T45.1X6
Loperamide	T47.6X1	T47.6X2	T47.6X3	T47.6X4	T47.6X5	T47.6X6
Loprazolam	T42.4X1	T42.4X2	T42.4X3	T42.4X4	T42.4X5	T42.4X6
Lorajmine	T46.2X1	T46.2X2	T46.2X3	T46.2X4	T46.2X5	T46.2X6
Loratidine	T45.ØX1	T45.ØX2	T45.ØX3	T45.ØX4	T45.ØX5	T45.ØX6
Lorazepam	T42.4X1	T42.4X2	T42.4X3	T42.4X4	T42.4X5	T42.4X6
Lorcainide	T46.2X1	T46.2X2	T46.2X3	T46.2X4	T46.2X5	T46.2X6
Lormetazepam	T42.4X1	T42.4X2	T42.4X3	T42.4X4	T42.4X5	T42.4X6
Lotions NEC	T49.91	T49.92	T49.93	T49.94	T49.95	T49.96
Lotusate	T42.3X1	T42.3X2	T42.3X3	T42.3X4	T42.3X5	T42.3X6
Lovastatin	T46.6X1	T46.6X2	T46.6X3	T46.6X4	T46.6X5	T46.6X6
Lowila	T49.2X1	T49.2X2	T49.2X3	T49.2X4	T49.2X5	T49.2X6
Loxapine	T43.591	T43.592	T43.593	T43.594	T43.595	T43.596
Lozenges (throat)	T49.6X1	T49.6X2	T49.6X3	T49.6X4	T49.6X5	T49.6X6
LSD	T4Ø.8X1	T4Ø.8X2	T4Ø.8X3	T4Ø.8X4	—	—

Substance	Poisoning, Accidental (unintentional)	Poisoning, Intentional Self-harm	Poisoning, Assault	Poisoning, Undetermined	Adverse Effect	Under-dosing
L-Tryptophan — *see* amino acid						
Lubricant, eye	T49.5X1	T49.5X2	T49.5X3	T49.5X4	T49.5X5	T49.5X6
Lubricating oil NEC	T52.ØX1	T52.ØX2	T52.ØX3	T52.ØX4	—	—
Lucanthone	T37.4X1	T37.4X2	T37.4X3	T37.4X4	T37.4X5	T37.4X6
Luminal	T42.3X1	T42.3X2	T42.3X3	T42.3X4	T42.3X5	T42.3X6
Lung irritant (gas) **NEC**	T59.91	T59.92	T59.93	T59.94	—	—
Luteinizing hormone	T38.811	T38.812	T38.813	T38.814	T38.815	T38.816
Lutocylol	T38.5X1	T38.5X2	T38.5X3	T38.5X4	T38.5X5	T38.5X6
Lutromone	T38.5X1	T38.5X2	T38.5X3	T38.5X4	T38.5X5	T38.5X6
Lututrin	T48.291	T48.292	T48.293	T48.294	T48.295	T48.296
Lye (concentrated)	T54.3X1	T54.3X2	T54.3X3	T54.3X4	—	—
Lygranum (skin test)	T5Ø.8X1	T5Ø.8X2	T5Ø.8X3	T5Ø.8X4	T5Ø.8X5	T5Ø.8X6
Lymecycline	T36.4X1	T36.4X2	T36.4X3	T36.4X4	T36.4X5	T36.4X6
Lymphogranuloma venereum antigen	T5Ø.8X1	T5Ø.8X2	T5Ø.8X3	T5Ø.8X4	T5Ø.8X5	T5Ø.8X6
Lynestrenol	T38.4X1	T38.4X2	T38.4X3	T38.4X4	T38.4X5	T38.4X6
Lyovac Sodium Edecrin	T5Ø.1X1	T5Ø.1X2	T5Ø.1X3	T5Ø.1X4	T5Ø.1X5	T5Ø.1X6
Lypressin	T38.891	T38.892	T38.893	T38.894	T38.895	T38.896
Lysergic acid diethylamide	T4Ø.8X1	T4Ø.8X2	T4Ø.8X3	T4Ø.8X4	—	—
Lysergide	T4Ø.8X1	T4Ø.8X2	T4Ø.8X3	T4Ø.8X4	—	—
Lysine vasopressin	T38.891	T38.892	T38.893	T38.894	T38.895	T38.896
Lysol	T54.1X1	T54.1X2	T54.1X3	T54.1X4	—	—
Lysozyme	T49.ØX1	T49.ØX2	T49.ØX3	T49.ØX4	T49.ØX5	T49.ØX6
Lytta (vitatta)	T49.8X1	T49.8X2	T49.8X3	T49.8X4	T49.8X5	T49.8X6
Mace	T59.3X1	T59.3X2	T59.3X3	T59.3X4	—	—
Macrogol	T5Ø.991	T5Ø.992	T5Ø.993	T5Ø.994	T5Ø.995	T5Ø.996
Macrolide						
anabolic drug	T38.7X1	T38.7X2	T38.7X3	T38.7X4	T38.7X5	T38.7X6
antibiotic	T36.3X1	T36.3X2	T36.3X3	T36.3X4	T36.3X5	T36.3X6
Mafenide	T49.ØX1	T49.ØX2	T49.ØX3	T49.ØX4	T49.ØX5	T49.ØX6
Magaldrate	T47.1X1	T47.1X2	T47.1X3	T47.1X4	T47.1X5	T47.1X6
Magic mushroom	T4Ø.991	T4Ø.992	T4Ø.993	T4Ø.994	—	—
Magnamycin	T36.8X1	T36.8X2	T36.8X3	T36.8X4	T36.8X5	T36.8X6
Magnesia magma	T47.1X1	T47.1X2	T47.1X3	T47.1X4	T47.1X5	T47.1X6
Magnesium NEC	T56.891	T56.892	T56.893	T56.894	—	—
carbonate	T47.1X1	T47.1X2	T47.1X3	T47.1X4	T47.1X5	T47.1X6
citrate	T47.4X1	T47.4X2	T47.4X3	T47.4X4	T47.4X5	T47.4X6
hydroxide	T47.1X1	T47.1X2	T47.1X3	T47.1X4	T47.1X5	T47.1X6
oxide	T47.1X1	T47.1X2	T47.1X3	T47.1X4	T47.1X5	T47.1X6
peroxide	T49.ØX1	T49.ØX2	T49.ØX3	T49.ØX4	T49.ØX5	T49.ØX6
salicylate	T39.Ø91	T39.Ø92	T39.Ø93	T39.Ø94	T39.Ø95	T39.Ø96
silicofluoride	T5Ø.3X1	T5Ø.3X2	T5Ø.3X3	T5Ø.3X4	T5Ø.3X5	T5Ø.3X6
sulfate	T47.4X1	T47.4X2	T47.4X3	T47.4X4	T47.4X5	T47.4X6
thiosulfate	T45.ØX1	T45.ØX2	T45.ØX3	T45.ØX4	T45.ØX5	T45.ØX6
trisilicate	T47.1X1	T47.1X2	T47.1X3	T47.1X4	T47.1X5	T47.1X6
Malathion (medicinal)	T49.ØX1	T49.ØX2	T49.ØX3	T49.ØX4	T49.ØX5	T49.ØX6
insecticide	T6Ø.ØX1	T6Ø.ØX2	T6Ø.ØX3	T6Ø.ØX4	—	—
Male fern extract	T37.4X1	T37.4X2	T37.4X3	T37.4X4	T37.4X5	T37.4X6
M-AMSA	T45.1X1	T45.1X2	T45.1X3	T45.1X4	T45.1X5	T45.1X6
Mandelic acid	T37.8X1	T37.8X2	T37.8X3	T37.8X4	T37.8X5	T37.8X6
Manganese (dioxide) (salts)	T57.2X1	T57.2X2	T57.2X3	T57.2X4	—	—
medicinal	T5Ø.991	T5Ø.992	T5Ø.993	T5Ø.994	T5Ø.995	T5Ø.996
Mannitol	T47.3X1	T47.3X2	T47.3X3	T47.3X4	T47.3X5	T47.3X6
hexanitrate	T46.3X1	T46.3X2	T46.3X3	T46.3X4	T46.3X5	T46.3X6
Mannomustine	T45.1X1	T45.1X2	T45.1X3	T45.1X4	T45.1X5	T45.1X6
MAO inhibitors	T43.1X1	T43.1X2	T43.1X3	T43.1X4	T43.1X5	T43.1X6
Mapharsen	T37.8X1	T37.8X2	T37.8X3	T37.8X4	T37.8X5	T37.8X6
Maphenide	T49.ØX1	T49.ØX2	T49.ØX3	T49.ØX4	T49.ØX5	T49.ØX6
Maprotiline	T43.Ø21	T43.Ø22	T43.Ø23	T43.Ø24	T43.Ø25	T43.Ø26
Marcaine	T41.3X1	T41.3X2	T41.3X3	T41.3X4	T41.3X5	T41.3X6
infiltration (subcutaneous)	T41.3X1	T41.3X2	T41.3X3	T41.3X4	T41.3X5	T41.3X6
nerve block (peripheral) (plexus)	T41.3X1	T41.3X2	T41.3X3	T41.3X4	T41.3X5	T41.3X6
Marezine	T45.ØX1	T45.ØX2	T45.ØX3	T45.ØX4	T45.ØX5	T45.ØX6
Marihuana	T4Ø.711	T4Ø.712	T4Ø.713	T4Ø.714	T4Ø.715	T4Ø.716
Marijuana	T4Ø.711	T4Ø.712	T4Ø.713	T4Ø.714	T4Ø.715	T4Ø.716
Marine (sting)	T63.691	T63.692	T63.693	T63.694	—	—
animals (sting)	T63.691	T63.692	T63.693	T63.694	—	—
plants (sting)	T63.711	T63.712	T63.713	T63.714	—	—
Marplan	T43.1X1	T43.1X2	T43.1X3	T43.1X4	T43.1X5	T43.1X6
Marsh gas	T59.891	T59.892	T59.893	T59.894	—	—
Marsilid	T43.1X1	T43.1X2	T43.1X3	T43.1X4	T43.1X5	T43.1X6
Matulane	T45.1X1	T45.1X2	T45.1X3	T45.1X4	T45.1X5	T45.1X6
Mazindol	T5Ø.5X1	T5Ø.5X2	T5Ø.5X3	T5Ø.5X4	T5Ø.5X5	T5Ø.5X6
MCPA	T6Ø.3X1	T6Ø.3X2	T6Ø.3X3	T6Ø.3X4	—	—
MDMA	T43.641	T43.642	T43.643	T43.644	—	—
Meadow saffron	T62.2X1	T62.2X2	T62.2X3	T62.2X4	—	—
Measles virus vaccine (attenuated)	T5Ø.B91	T5Ø.B92	T5Ø.B93	T5Ø.B94	T5Ø.B95	T5Ø.B96
Meat, noxious	T62.8X1	T62.8X2	T62.8X3	T62.8X4	—	—
Meballymal	T42.3X1	T42.3X2	T42.3X3	T42.3X4	T42.3X5	T42.3X6
Mebanazine	T43.1X1	T43.1X2	T43.1X3	T43.1X4	T43.1X5	T43.1X6
Mebaral	T42.3X1	T42.3X2	T42.3X3	T42.3X4	T42.3X5	T42.3X6

382

Additional Character May Be Required — Refer to the Tabular List for Character Selection

Subterms under main terms may continue to next column or page

Substance	Poisoning, Accidental (unintentional)	Poisoning, Intentional Self-harm	Poisoning, Assault	Poisoning, Undetermined	Adverse Effect	Under-dosing
Mebendazole	T37.4X1	T37.4X2	T37.4X3	T37.4X4	T37.4X5	T37.4X6
Mebeverine	T44.3X1	T44.3X2	T44.3X3	T44.3X4	T44.3X5	T44.3X6
Mebhydrolin	T45.0X1	T45.0X2	T45.0X3	T45.0X4	T45.0X5	T45.0X6
Mebumal	T42.3X1	T42.3X2	T42.3X3	T42.3X4	T42.3X5	T42.3X6
Mebutamate	T43.591	T43.592	T43.593	T43.594	T43.595	T43.596
Mecamylamine	T44.2X1	T44.2X2	T44.2X3	T44.2X4	T44.2X5	T44.2X6
Mechlorethamine	T45.1X1	T45.1X2	T45.1X3	T45.1X4	T45.1X5	T45.1X6
Mecillinam	T36.0X1	T36.0X2	T36.0X3	T36.0X4	T36.0X5	T36.0X6
Meclizine (hydrochloride)	T45.0X1	T45.0X2	T45.0X3	T45.0X4	T45.0X5	T45.0X6
Meclocycline	T36.4X1	T36.4X2	T36.4X3	T36.4X4	T36.4X5	T36.4X6
Meclofenamate	T39.391	T39.392	T39.393	T39.394	T39.395	T39.396
Meclofenamic acid	T39.391	T39.392	T39.393	T39.394	T39.395	T39.396
Meclofenoxate	T43.691	T43.692	T43.693	T43.694	T43.695	T43.696
Meclozine	T45.0X1	T45.0X2	T45.0X3	T45.0X4	T45.0X5	T45.0X6
Mecobalamin	T45.8X1	T45.8X2	T45.8X3	T45.8X4	T45.8X5	T45.8X6
Mecoprop	T60.3X1	T60.3X2	T60.3X3	T60.3X4	—	—
Mecrilate	T49.3X1	T49.3X2	T49.3X3	T49.3X4	T49.3X5	T49.3X6
Mecysteine	T48.4X1	T48.4X2	T48.4X3	T48.4X4	T48.4X5	T48.4X6
Medazepam	T42.4X1	T42.4X2	T42.4X3	T42.4X4	T42.4X5	T42.4X6
Medicament NEC	T50.901	T50.902	T50.903	T50.904	T50.905	T50.906
Medinal	T42.3X1	T42.3X2	T42.3X3	T42.3X4	T42.3X5	T42.3X6
Medomin	T42.3X1	T42.3X2	T42.3X3	T42.3X4	T42.3X5	T42.3X6
Medrogestone	T38.5X1	T38.5X2	T38.5X3	T38.5X4	T38.5X5	T38.5X6
Medroxalol	T44.8X1	T44.8X2	T44.8X3	T44.8X4	T44.8X5	T44.8X6
Medroxyprogesterone acetate (depot)	T38.5X1	T38.5X2	T38.5X3	T38.5X4	T38.5X5	T38.5X6
Medrysone	T49.0X1	T49.0X2	T49.0X3	T49.0X4	T49.0X5	T49.0X6
Mefenamic acid	T39.391	T39.392	T39.393	T39.394	T39.395	T39.396
Mefenorex	T50.5X1	T50.5X2	T50.5X3	T50.5X4	T50.5X5	T50.5X6
Mefloquine	T37.2X1	T37.2X2	T37.2X3	T37.2X4	T37.2X5	T37.2X6
Mefruside	T50.2X1	T50.2X2	T50.2X3	T50.2X4	T50.2X5	T50.2X6
Megahallucinogen	T40.901	T40.902	T40.903	T40.904	T40.905	T40.906
Megestrol	T38.5X1	T38.5X2	T38.5X3	T38.5X4	T38.5X5	T38.5X6
Meglumine						
antimoniate	T37.8X1	T37.8X2	T37.8X3	T37.8X4	T37.8X5	T37.8X6
diatrizoate	T50.8X1	T50.8X2	T50.8X3	T50.8X4	T50.8X5	T50.8X6
iodipamide	T50.8X1	T50.8X2	T50.8X3	T50.8X4	T50.8X5	T50.8X6
iotroxate	T50.8X1	T50.8X2	T50.8X3	T50.8X4	T50.8X5	T50.8X6
MEK (methyl ethyl ketone)	T52.4X1	T52.4X2	T52.4X3	T52.4X4	—	—
Meladinin	T49.3X1	T49.3X2	T49.3X3	T49.3X4	T49.3X5	T49.3X6
Meladrazine	T44.3X1	T44.3X2	T44.3X3	T44.3X4	T44.3X5	T44.3X6
Melaleuca alternifolia oil	T49.0X1	T49.0X2	T49.0X3	T49.0X4	T49.0X5	T49.0X6
Melanizing agents	T49.3X1	T49.3X2	T49.3X3	T49.3X4	T49.3X5	T49.3X6
Melanocyte-stimulating hormone	T38.891	T38.892	T38.893	T38.894	T38.895	T38.896
Melarsonyl potassium	T37.3X1	T37.3X2	T37.3X3	T37.3X4	T37.3X5	T37.3X6
Melarsoprol	T37.3X1	T37.3X2	T37.3X3	T37.3X4	T37.3X5	T37.3X6
Melia azedarach	T62.2X1	T62.2X2	T62.2X3	T62.2X4		
Melitracen	T43.011	T43.012	T43.013	T43.014	T43.015	T43.016
Mellaril	T43.3X1	T43.3X2	T43.3X3	T43.3X4	T43.3X5	T43.3X6
Meloxine	T49.3X1	T49.3X2	T49.3X3	T49.3X4	T49.3X5	T49.3X6
Melperone	T43.4X1	T43.4X2	T43.4X3	T43.4X4	T43.4X5	T43.4X6
Melphalan	T45.1X1	T45.1X2	T45.1X3	T45.1X4	T45.1X5	T45.1X6
Memantine	T43.8X1	T43.8X2	T43.8X3	T43.8X4	T43.8X5	T43.8X6
Menadiol	T45.7X1	T45.7X2	T45.7X3	T45.7X4	T45.7X5	T45.7X6
sodium sulfate	T45.7X1	T45.7X2	T45.7X3	T45.7X4	T45.7X5	T45.7X6
Menadione	T45.7X1	T45.7X2	T45.7X3	T45.7X4	T45.7X5	T45.7X6
sodium bisulfite	T45.7X1	T45.7X2	T45.7X3	T45.7X4	T45.7X5	T45.7X6
Menaphthone	T45.7X1	T45.7X2	T45.7X3	T45.7X4	T45.7X5	T45.7X6
Menaquinone	T45.7X1	T45.7X2	T45.7X3	T45.7X4	T45.7X5	T45.7X6
Menatetrenone	T45.7X1	T45.7X2	T45.7X3	T45.7X4	T45.7X5	T45.7X6
Meningococcal vaccine	T50.A91	T50.A92	T50.A93	T50.A94	T50.A95	T50.A96
Menningovax (-AC) (-C)	T50.A91	T50.A92	T50.A93	T50.A94	T50.A95	T50.A96
Menotropins	T38.811	T38.812	T38.813	T38.814	T38.815	T38.816
Menthol	T48.5X1	T48.5X2	T48.5X3	T48.5X4	T48.5X5	T48.5X6
Mepacrine	T37.2X1	T37.2X2	T37.2X3	T37.2X4	T37.2X5	T37.2X6
Meparfynol	T42.6X1	T42.6X2	T42.6X3	T42.6X4	T42.6X5	T42.6X6
Mepartricin	T36.7X1	T36.7X2	T36.7X3	T36.7X4	T36.7X5	T36.7X6
Mepazine	T43.3X1	T43.3X2	T43.3X3	T43.3X4	T43.3X5	T43.3X6
Mepenzolate	T44.3X1	T44.3X2	T44.3X3	T44.3X4	T44.3X5	T44.3X6
bromide	T44.3X1	T44.3X2	T44.3X3	T44.3X4	T44.3X5	T44.3X6
Meperidine	T40.491	T40.492	T40.493	T40.494	T40.495	T40.496
Mephebarbital	T42.3X1	T42.3X2	T42.3X3	T42.3X4	T42.3X5	T42.3X6
Mephenamin (e)	T42.8X1	T42.8X2	T42.8X3	T42.8X4	T42.8X5	T42.8X6
Mephenesin	T42.8X1	T42.8X2	T42.8X3	T42.8X4	T42.8X5	T42.8X6
Mephenhydramine	T45.0X1	T45.0X2	T45.0X3	T45.0X4	T45.0X5	T45.0X6
Mephenoxalone	T42.8X1	T42.8X2	T42.8X3	T42.8X4	T42.8X5	T42.8X6
Mephentermine	T44.991	T44.992	T44.993	T44.994	T44.995	T44.996
Mephenytoin	T42.0X1	T42.0X2	T42.0X3	T42.0X4	T42.0X5	T42.0X6
with phenobarbital	T42.3X1	T42.3X2	T42.3X3	T42.3X4	T42.3X5	T42.3X6
Mephobarbital	T42.3X1	T42.3X2	T42.3X3	T42.3X4	T42.3X5	T42.3X6
Mephosfolan	T60.0X1	T60.0X2	T60.0X3	T60.0X4	—	—
Mepindolol	T44.7X1	T44.7X2	T44.7X3	T44.7X4	T44.7X5	T44.7X6

Substance	Poisoning, Accidental (unintentional)	Poisoning, Intentional Self-harm	Poisoning, Assault	Poisoning, Undetermined	Adverse Effect	Under-dosing
Mepiperphenidol	T44.3X1	T44.3X2	T44.3X3	T44.3X4	T44.3X5	T44.3X6
Mepitiostane	T38.7X1	T38.7X2	T38.7X3	T38.7X4	T38.7X5	T38.7X6
Mepivacaine	T41.3X1	T41.3X2	T41.3X3	T41.3X4	T41.3X5	T41.3X6
epidural	T41.3X1	T41.3X2	T41.3X3	T41.3X4	T41.3X5	T41.3X6
Meprednisone	T38.0X1	T38.0X2	T38.0X3	T38.0X4	T38.0X5	T38.0X6
Meprobam	T43.591	T43.592	T43.593	T43.594	T43.595	T43.596
Meprobamate	T43.591	T43.592	T43.593	T43.594	T43.595	T43.596
Meproscillarin	T46.0X1	T46.0X2	T46.0X3	T46.0X4	T46.0X5	T46.0X6
Meprylcaine	T41.3X1	T41.3X2	T41.3X3	T41.3X4	T41.3X5	T41.3X6
Meptazinol	T39.8X1	T39.8X2	T39.8X3	T39.8X4	T39.8X5	T39.8X6
Mepyramine	T45.0X1	T45.0X2	T45.0X3	T45.0X4	T45.0X5	T45.0X6
Mequitazine	T43.3X1	T43.3X2	T43.3X3	T43.3X4	T43.3X5	T43.3X6
Meralluride	T50.2X1	T50.2X2	T50.2X3	T50.2X4	T50.2X5	T50.2X6
Merbaphen	T50.2X1	T50.2X2	T50.2X3	T50.2X4	T50.2X5	T50.2X6
Merbromin	T49.0X1	T49.0X2	T49.0X3	T49.0X4	T49.0X5	T49.0X6
Mercaptobenzothiazole salts	T49.0X1	T49.0X2	T49.0X3	T49.0X4	T49.0X5	T49.0X6
Mercaptomerin	T50.2X1	T50.2X2	T50.2X3	T50.2X4	T50.2X5	T50.2X6
Mercaptopurine	T45.1X1	T45.1X2	T45.1X3	T45.1X4	T45.1X5	T45.1X6
Mercumatilin	T50.2X1	T50.2X2	T50.2X3	T50.2X4	T50.2X5	T50.2X6
Mercuramide	T50.2X1	T50.2X2	T50.2X3	T50.2X4	T50.2X5	T50.2X6
Mercurochrome	T49.0X1	T49.0X2	T49.0X3	T49.0X4	T49.0X5	T49.0X6
Mercurophylline	T50.2X1	T50.2X2	T50.2X3	T50.2X4	T50.2X5	T50.2X6
Mercury, mercurial, mercuric, mercurous (compounds) (cyanide) (fumes) (nonmedicinal) (vapor) NEC	T56.1X1	T56.1X2	T56.1X3	T56.1X4	—	—
ammoniated	T49.0X1	T49.0X2	T49.0X3	T49.0X4	T49.0X5	T49.0X6
anti-infective						
local	T49.0X1	T49.0X2	T49.0X3	T49.0X4	T49.0X5	T49.0X6
systemic	T37.8X1	T37.8X2	T37.8X3	T37.8X4	T37.8X5	T37.8X6
topical	T49.0X1	T49.0X2	T49.0X3	T49.0X4	T49.0X5	T49.0X6
chloride (ammoniated)	T49.0X1	T49.0X2	T49.0X3	T49.0X4	T49.0X5	T49.0X6
fungicide	T56.1X1	T56.1X2	T56.1X3	T56.1X4	—	—
diuretic NEC	T50.2X1	T50.2X2	T50.2X3	T50.2X4	T50.2X5	T50.2X6
fungicide	T56.1X1	T56.1X2	T56.1X3	T56.1X4	—	—
organic (fungicide)	T56.1X1	T56.1X2	T56.1X3	T56.1X4	—	—
oxide, yellow	T49.0X1	T49.0X2	T49.0X3	T49.0X4	T49.0X5	T49.0X6
Mersalyl	T50.2X1	T50.2X2	T50.2X3	T50.2X4	T50.2X5	T50.2X6
Merthiolate	T49.0X1	T49.0X2	T49.0X3	T49.0X4	T49.0X5	T49.0X6
ophthalmic preparation	T49.5X1	T49.5X2	T49.5X3	T49.5X4	T49.5X5	T49.5X6
Meruvax	T50.B91	T50.B92	T50.B93	T50.B94	T50.B95	T50.B96
Mesalazine	T47.8X1	T47.8X2	T47.8X3	T47.8X4	T47.8X5	T47.8X6
Mescal buttons	T40.991	T40.992	T40.993	T40.994	—	—
Mescaline	T40.991	T40.992	T40.993	T40.994	—	—
Mesna	T48.4X1	T48.4X2	T48.4X3	T48.4X4	T48.4X5	T48.4X6
Mesoglycan	T46.6X1	T46.6X2	T46.6X3	T46.6X4	T46.6X5	T46.6X6
Mesoridazine	T43.3X1	T43.3X2	T43.3X3	T43.3X4	T43.3X5	T43.3X6
Mestanolone	T38.7X1	T38.7X2	T38.7X3	T38.7X4	T38.7X5	T38.7X6
Mesterolone	T38.7X1	T38.7X2	T38.7X3	T38.7X4	T38.7X5	T38.7X6
Mestranol	T38.5X1	T38.5X2	T38.5X3	T38.5X4	T38.5X5	T38.5X6
Mesulergine	T42.8X1	T42.8X2	T42.8X3	T42.8X4	T42.8X5	T42.8X6
Mesulfen	T49.0X1	T49.0X2	T49.0X3	T49.0X4	T49.0X5	T49.0X6
Mesuximide	T42.2X1	T42.2X2	T42.2X3	T42.2X4	T42.2X5	T42.2X6
Metabutethamine	T41.3X1	T41.3X2	T41.3X3	T41.3X4	T41.3X5	T41.3X6
Metactesylacetate	T49.0X1	T49.0X2	T49.0X3	T49.0X4	T49.0X5	T49.0X6
Metacycline	T36.4X1	T36.4X2	T36.4X3	T36.4X4	T36.4X5	T36.4X6
Metaldehyde (snail killer) NEC	T60.8X1	T60.8X2	T60.8X3	T60.8X4	—	—
Metals (heavy) (nonmedicinal)	T56.91	T56.92	T56.93	T56.94	—	—
dust, fumes, or vapor NEC	T56.91	T56.92	T56.93	T56.94	—	—
light NEC	T56.91	T56.92	T56.93	T56.94	—	—
dust, fumes, or vapor NEC	T56.91	T56.92	T56.93	T56.94	—	—
specified NEC	T56.891	T56.892	T56.893	T56.894	—	—
thallium	T56.811	T56.812	T56.813	T56.814	—	—
Metamfetamine	T43.621	T43.622	T43.623	T43.624	T43.625	T43.626
Metamizole sodium	T39.2X1	T39.2X2	T39.2X3	T39.2X4	T39.2X5	T39.2X6
Metampicillin	T36.0X1	T36.0X2	T36.0X3	T36.0X4	T36.0X5	T36.0X6
Metamucil	T47.4X1	T47.4X2	T47.4X3	T47.4X4	T47.4X5	T47.4X6
Metandienone	T38.7X1	T38.7X2	T38.7X3	T38.7X4	T38.7X5	T38.7X6
Metandrostenolone	T38.7X1	T38.7X2	T38.7X3	T38.7X4	T38.7X5	T38.7X6
Metaphen	T49.0X1	T49.0X2	T49.0X3	T49.0X4	T49.0X5	T49.0X6
Metaphos	T60.0X1	T60.0X2	T60.0X3	T60.0X4	—	—
Metapramine	T43.011	T43.012	T43.013	T43.014	T43.015	T43.016
Metaproterenol	T48.291	T48.292	T48.293	T48.294	T48.295	T48.296
Metaraminol	T44.4X1	T44.4X2	T44.4X3	T44.4X4	T44.4X5	T44.4X6
Metaxalone	T42.8X1	T42.8X2	T42.8X3	T42.8X4	T42.8X5	T42.8X6
Metenolone	T38.7X1	T38.7X2	T38.7X3	T38.7X4	T38.7X5	T38.7X6
Metergoline	T42.8X1	T42.8X2	T42.8X3	T42.8X4	T42.8X5	T42.8X6
Metescufylline	T46.991	T46.992	T46.993	T46.994	T46.995	T46.996

Substance	Poisoning, Accidental (unintentional)	Poisoning, Intentional Self-harm	Poisoning, Assault	Poisoning, Undetermined	Adverse Effect	Under-dosing
Metetoin	T42.ØX1	T42.ØX2	T42.ØX3	T42.ØX4	T42.ØX5	T42.ØX6
Metformin	T38.3X1	T38.3X2	T38.3X3	T38.3X4	T38.3X5	T38.3X6
Methacholine	T44.1X1	T44.1X2	T44.1X3	T44.1X4	T44.1X5	T44.1X6
Methacycline	T36.4X1	T36.4X2	T36.4X3	T36.4X4	T36.4X5	T36.4X6
Methadone	T4Ø.3X1	T4Ø.3X2	T4Ø.3X3	T4Ø.3X4	T4Ø.3X5	T4Ø.3X6
Methallenestril	T38.5X1	T38.5X2	T38.5X3	T38.5X4	T38.5X5	T38.5X6
Methallenoestril	T38.5X1	T38.5X2	T38.5X3	T38.5X4	T38.5X5	T38.5X6
Methamphetamine	T43.621	T43.622	T43.623	T43.624	T43.625	T43.626
Methampyrone	T39.2X1	T39.2X2	T39.2X3	T39.2X4	T39.2X5	T39.2X6
Methandienone	T38.7X1	T38.7X2	T38.7X3	T38.7X4	T38.7X5	T38.7X6
Methandriol	T38.7X1	T38.7X2	T38.7X3	T38.7X4	T38.7X5	T38.7X6
Methandrostenolone	T38.7X1	T38.7X2	T38.7X3	T38.7X4	T38.7X5	T38.7X6
Methane	T59.891	T59.892	T59.893	T59.894	—	—
Methanethiol	T59.891	T59.892	T59.893	T59.894	—	—
Methaniazide	T37.1X1	T37.1X2	T37.1X3	T37.1X4	T37.1X5	T37.1X6
Methanol (vapor)	T51.1X1	T51.1X2	T51.1X3	T51.1X4	—	—
Methantheline	T44.3X1	T44.3X2	T44.3X3	T44.3X4	T44.3X5	T44.3X6
Methanthelinium bromide	T44.3X1	T44.3X2	T44.3X3	T44.3X4	T44.3X5	T44.3X6
Methaphenilene	T45.ØX1	T45.ØX2	T45.ØX3	T45.ØX4	T45.ØX5	T45.ØX6
Methapyrilene	T45.ØX1	T45.ØX2	T45.ØX3	T45.ØX4	T45.ØX5	T45.ØX6
Methaqualone (compound)	T42.6X1	T42.6X2	T42.6X3	T42.6X4	T42.6X5	T42.6X6
Metharbital	T42.3X1	T42.3X2	T42.3X3	T42.3X4	T42.3X5	T42.3X6
Methazolamide	T5Ø.2X1	T5Ø.2X2	T5Ø.2X3	T5Ø.2X4	T5Ø.2X5	T5Ø.2X6
Methdilazine	T43.3X1	T43.3X2	T43.3X3	T43.3X4	T43.3X5	T43.3X6
Methedrine	T43.621	T43.622	T43.623	T43.624	T43.625	T43.626
Methenamine (mandelate)	T37.8X1	T37.8X2	T37.8X3	T37.8X4	T37.8X5	T37.8X6
Methenolone	T38.7X1	T38.7X2	T38.7X3	T38.7X4	T38.7X5	T38.7X6
Methergine	T48.ØX1	T48.ØX2	T48.ØX3	T48.ØX4	T48.ØX5	T48.ØX6
Methetoin	T42.ØX1	T42.ØX2	T42.ØX3	T42.ØX4	T42.ØX5	T42.ØX6
Methiacil	T38.2X1	T38.2X2	T38.2X3	T38.2X4	T38.2X5	T38.2X6
Methicillin	T36.ØX1	T36.ØX2	T36.ØX3	T36.ØX4	T36.ØX5	T36.ØX6
Methimazole	T38.2X1	T38.2X2	T38.2X3	T38.2X4	T38.2X5	T38.2X6
Methiodal sodium	T5Ø.8X1	T5Ø.8X2	T5Ø.8X3	T5Ø.8X4	T5Ø.8X5	T5Ø.8X6
Methionine	T5Ø.991	T5Ø.992	T5Ø.993	T5Ø.994	T5Ø.995	T5Ø.996
Methisazone	T37.5X1	T37.5X2	T37.5X3	T37.5X4	T37.5X5	T37.5X6
Methisoprinol	T37.5X1	T37.5X2	T37.5X3	T37.5X4	T37.5X5	T37,5X6
Methitural	T42.3X1	T42.3X2	T42.3X3	T42.3X4	T42.3X5	T42.3X6
Methixene	T44.3X1	T44.3X2	T44.3X3	T44.3X4	T44.3X5	T44.3X6
Methobarbital, methobarbitone	T42.3X1	T42.3X2	T42.3X3	T42.3X4	T42.3X5	T42.3X6
Methocarbamol	T42.8X1	T42.8X2	T42.8X3	T42.8X4	T42.8X5	T42.8X6
skeletal muscle relaxant	T48.1X1	T48.1X2	T48.1X3	T48.1X4	T48.1X5	T48.1X6
Methohexital	T41.1X1	T41.1X2	T41.1X3	T41.1X4	T41.1X5	T41.1X6
Methohexitone	T41.1X1	T41.1X2	T41.1X3	T41.1X4	T41.1X5	T41.1X6
Methoin	T42.ØX1	T42.ØX2	T42.ØX3	T42.ØX4	T42.ØX5	T42.ØX6
Methopholine	T39.8X1	T39.8X2	T39.8X3	T39.8X4	T39.8X5	T39.8X6
Methopromazine	T43.3X1	T43.3X2	T43.3X3	T43.3X4	T43.3X5	T43.3X6
Methorate	T48.3X1	T48.3X2	T48.3X3	T48.3X4	T48.3X5	T48.3X6
Methoserpidine	T46.5X1	T46.5X2	T46.5X3	T46.5X4	T46.5X5	T46.5X6
Methotrexate	T45.1X1	T45.1X2	T45.1X3	T45.1X4	T45.1X5	T45.1X6
Methotrimeprazine	T43.3X1	T43.3X2	T43.3X3	T43.3X4	T43.3X5	T43.3X6
Methoxa-Dome	T49.3X1	T49.3X2	T49.3X3	T49.3X4	T49.3X5	T49.3X6
Methoxamine	T44.4X1	T44.4X2	T44.4X3	T44.4X4	T44.4X5	T44.4X6
Methoxsalen	T5Ø.991	T5Ø.992	T5Ø.993	T5Ø.994	T5Ø.995	T5Ø.996
Methoxyaniline	T65.3X1	T65.3X2	T65.3X3	T65.3X4	—	—
Methoxybenzyl penicillin	T36.ØX1	T36.ØX2	T36.ØX3	T36.ØX4	T36.ØX5	T36.ØX6
Methoxychlor	T53.7X1	T53.7X2	T53.7X3	T53.7X4	—	—
Methoxy-DDT	T53.7X1	T53.7X2	T53.7X3	T53.7X4	—	—
Methoxyflurane	T41.ØX1	T41.ØX2	T41.ØX3	T41.ØX4	T41.ØX5	T41.ØX6
Methoxyphenamine	T48.6X1	T48.6X2	T48.6X3	T48.6X4	T48.6X5	T48.6X6
Methoxypromazine	T43.3X1	T43.3X2	T43.3X3	T43.3X4	T43.3X5	T43.3X6
Methscopolamine bromide	T44.3X1	T44.3X2	T44.3X3	T44.3X4	T44.3X5	T44.3X6
Methsuximide	T42.2X1	T42.2X2	T42.2X3	T42.2X4	T42.2X5	T42.2X6
Methyclothiazide	T5Ø.2X1	T5Ø.2X2	T5Ø.2X3	T5Ø.2X4	T5Ø.2X5	T5Ø.2X6
Methyl						
acetate	T52.4X1	T52.4X2	T52.4X3	T52.4X4	—	—
acetone	T52.4X1	T52.4X2	T52.4X3	T52.4X4	—	—
acrylate	T65.891	T65.892	T65.893	T65.894	—	—
alcohol	T51.1X1	T51.1X2	T51.1X3	T51.1X4	—	—
aminophenol	T65.3X1	T65.3X2	T65.3X3	T65.3X4	—	—
amphetamine	T43.621	T43.622	T43.623	T43.624	T43.625	T43.626
androstanolone	T38.7X1	T38.7X2	T38.7X3	T38.7X4	T38.7X5	T38.7X6
atropine	T44.3X1	T44.3X2	T44.3X3	T44.3X4	T44.3X5	T44.3X6
benzene	T52.2X1	T52.2X2	T52.2X3	T52.2X4	—	—
benzoate	T52.8X1	T52.8X2	T52.8X3	T52.8X4	—	—
benzol	T52.2X1	T52.2X2	T52.2X3	T52.2X4	—	—
bromide (gas)	T59.891	T59.892	T59.893	T59.894	—	—
fumigant	T6Ø.8X1	T6Ø.8X2	T6Ø.8X3	T6Ø.8X4	—	—
butanol	T51.3X1	T51.3X2	T51.3X3	T51.3X4	—	—
carbinol	T51.1X1	T51.1X2	T51.1X3	T51.1X4	—	—
carbonate	T52.8X1	T52.8X2	T52.8X3	T52.8X4	—	—
CCNU	T45.1X1	T45.1X2	T45.1X3	T45.1X4	T45.1X5	T45.1X6

Substance	Poisoning, Accidental (unintentional)	Poisoning, Intentional Self-harm	Poisoning, Assault	Poisoning, Undetermined	Adverse Effect	Under-dosing
Methyl — *continued*						
cellosolve	T52.91	T52.92	T52.93	T52.94	—	—
cellulose	T47.4X1	T47.4X2	T47.4X3	T47.4X4	T47.4X5	T47.4X6
chloride (gas)	T59.891	T59.892	T59.893	T59.894	—	—
chloroformate	T59.3X1	T59.3X2	T59.3X3	T59.3X4	—	—
cyclohexane	T52.8X1	T52.8X2	T52.8X3	T52.8X4	—	—
cyclohexanol	T51.8X1	T51.8X2	T51.8X3	T51.8X4	—	—
cyclohexanone	T52.8X1	T52.8X2	T52.8X3	T52.8X4	—	—
cyclohexyl acetate	T52.8X1	T52.8X2	T52.8X3	T52.8X4	—	—
demeton	T6Ø.ØX1	T6Ø.ØX2	T6Ø.ØX3	T6Ø.ØX4	—	—
dihydromorphinone	T4Ø.2X1	T4Ø.2X2	T4Ø.2X3	T4Ø.2X4	T4Ø.2X5	T4Ø.2X6
ergometrine	T48.ØX1	T48.ØX2	T48.ØX3	T48.ØX4	T48.ØX5	T48.ØX6
ergonovine	T48.ØX1	T48.ØX2	T48.ØX3	T48.ØX4	T48.ØX5	T48.ØX6
ethyl ketone	T52.4X1	T52.4X2	T52.4X3	T52.4X4	—	—
glucamine antimonate	T37.8X1	T37.8X2	T37.8X3	T37.8X4	T37.8X5	T37.8X6
hydrazine	T65.891	T65.892	T65.893	T65.894	—	—
iodide	T65.891	T65.892	T65.893	T65.894	—	—
isobutyl ketone	T52.4X1	T52.4X2	T52.4X3	T52.4X4	—	—
isothiocyanate	T6Ø.3X1	T6Ø.3X2	T6Ø.3X3	T6Ø.3X4	—	—
mercaptan	T59.891	T59.892	T59.893	T59.894	—	—
morphine NEC	T4Ø.2X1	T4Ø.2X2	T4Ø.2X3	T4Ø.2X4	T4Ø.2X5	T4Ø.2X6
nicotinate	T49.4X1	T49.4X2	T49.4X3	T49.4X4	T49.4X5	T49.4X6
paraben	T49.ØX1	T49.ØX2	T49.ØX3	T49.ØX4	T49.ØX5	T49.ØX6
parafynol	T42.6X1	T42.6X2	T42.6X3	T42.6X4	T42.6X5	T42.6X6
parathion	T6Ø.ØX1	T6Ø.ØX2	T6Ø.ØX3	T6Ø.ØX4	—	—
peridol	T43.4X1	T43.4X2	T43.4X3	T43.4X4	T43.4X5	T43.4X6
phenidate	T43.631	T43.632	T43.633	T43.634	T43.635	T43.636
prednisolone	T38.ØX1	T38.ØX2	T38.ØX3	T38.ØX4	T38.ØX5	T38.ØX6
ENT agent	T49.6X1	T49.6X2	T49.6X3	T49.6X4	T49.6X5	T49.6X6
ophthalmic preparation	T49.5X1	T49.5X2	T49.5X3	T49.5X4	T49.5X5	T49.5X6
topical NEC	T49.ØX1	T49.ØX2	T49.ØX3	T49.ØX4	T49.ØX5	T49.ØX6
propylcarbinol	T51.3X1	T51.3X2	T51.3X3	T51.3X4	—	—
rosaniline NEC	T49.ØX1	T49.ØX2	T49.ØX3	T49.ØX4	T49.ØX5	T49.ØX6
salicylate	T49.2X1	T49.2X2	T49.2X3	T49.2X4	T49.2X5	T49.2X6
sulfate (fumes)	T59.891	T59.892	T59.893	T59.894	—	—
liquid	T52.8X1	T52.8X2	T52.8X3	T52.8X4	—	—
sulfonal	T42.6X1	T42.6X2	T42.6X3	T42.6X4	T42.6X5	T42.6X6
testosterone	T38.7X1	T38.7X2	T38.7X3	T38.7X4	T38.7X5	T38.7X6
thiouracil	T38.2X1	T38.2X2	T38.2X3	T38.2X4	T38.2X5	T38.2X6
Methylamphetamine	T43.621	T43.622	T43.623	T43.624	T43.625	T43.626
Methylated spirit	T51.1X1	T51.1X2	T51.1X3	T51.1X4	—	—
Methylatropine nitrate	T44.3X1	T44.3X2	T44.3X3	T44.3X4	T44.3X5	T44.3X6
Methylbenactyzium bromide	T44.3X1	T44.3X2	T44.3X3	T44.3X4	T44.3X5	T44.3X6
Methylbenzethonium chloride	T49.ØX1	T49.ØX2	T49.ØX3	T49.ØX4	T49.ØX5	T49.ØX6
Methylcellulose	T47.4X1	T47.4X2	T47.4X3	T47.4X4	T47.4X5	T47.4X6
laxative	T47.4X1	T47.4X2	T47.4X3	T47.4X4	T47.4X5	T47.4X6
Methylchlorophenoxyacetic acid	T6Ø.3X1	T6Ø.3X2	T6Ø.3X3	T6Ø.3X4	—	—
Methyldopa	T46.5X1	T46.5X2	T46.5X3	T46.5X4	T46.5X5	T46.5X6
Methyldopate	T46.5X1	T46.5X2	T46.5X3	T46.5X4	T46.5X5	T46.5X6
Methylene						
blue	T5Ø.6X1	T5Ø.6X2	T5Ø.6X3	T5Ø.6X4	T5Ø.6X5	T5Ø.6X6
chloride or dichloride (solvent) NEC	T53.4X1	T53.4X2	T53.4X3	T53.4X4	—	—
Methylenedioxyamphetamine	T43.621	T43.622	T43.623	T43.624	T43.625	T43.626
Methylenedioxymeth-amphetamine	T43.641	T43.642	T43.643	T43.644	—	—
Methylergometrine	T48.ØX1	T48.ØX2	T48.ØX3	T48.ØX4	T48.ØX5	T48.ØX6
Methylergonovine	T48.ØX1	T48.ØX2	T48.ØX3	T48.ØX4	T48.ØX5	T48.ØX6
Methylestrenolone	T38.5X1	T38.5X2	T38.5X3	T38.5X4	T38.5X5	T38.5X6
Methylethyl cellulose	T5Ø.991	T5Ø.992	T5Ø.993	T5Ø.994	T5Ø.995	T5Ø.996
Methylhexabital	T42.3X1	T42.3X2	T42.3X3	T42.3X4	T42.3X5	T42.3X6
Methylmorphine	T4Ø.2X1	T4Ø.2X2	T4Ø.2X3	T4Ø.2X4	T4Ø.2X5	T4Ø.2X6
Methylparaben (ophthalmic)	T49.5X1	T49.5X2	T49.5X3	T49.5X4	T49.5X5	T49.5X6
Methylparafynol	T42.6X1	T42.6X2	T42.6X3	T42.6X4	T42.6X5	T42.6X6
Methylpentynol, methylpenthynol	T42.6X1	T42.6X2	T42.6X3	T42.6X4	T42.6X5	T42.6X6
Methylphenidate	T43.631	T43.632	T43.633	T43.634	T43.635	T43.636
Methylphenobarbital	T42.3X1	T42.3X2	T42.3X3	T42.3X4	T42.3X5	T42.3X6
Methylpolysiloxane	T47.1X1	T47.1X2	T47.1X3	T47.1X4	T47.1X5	T47.1X6
Methylprednisolone — *see* Methyl, prednisolone						
Methylrosaniline	T49.ØX1	T49.ØX2	T49.ØX3	T49.ØX4	T49.ØX5	T49.ØX6
Methylrosanilinium chloride	T49.ØX1	T49.ØX2	T49.ØX3	T49.ØX4	T49.ØX5	T49.ØX6
Methyltestosterone	T38.7X1	T38.7X2	T38.7X3	T38.7X4	T38.7X5	T38.7X6
Methylthionine chloride	T5Ø.6X1	T5Ø.6X2	T5Ø.6X3	T5Ø.6X4	T5Ø.6X5	T5Ø.6X6
Methylthioninium chloride	T5Ø.6X1	T5Ø.6X2	T5Ø.6X3	T5Ø.6X4	T5Ø.6X5	T5Ø.6X6
Methylthiouracil	T38.2X1	T38.2X2	T38.2X3	T38.2X4	T38.2X5	T38.2X6

384
Additional Character May Be Required — Refer to the Tabular List for Character Selection
Subterms under main terms may continue to next column or page

Substance	Poisoning, Accidental (unintentional)	Poisoning, Intentional Self-harm	Poisoning, Assault	Poisoning, Undetermined	Adverse Effect	Under-dosing
Methyprylon	T42.6X1	T42.6X2	T42.6X3	T42.6X4	T42.6X5	T42.6X6
Methysergide	T46.5X1	T46.5X2	T46.5X3	T46.5X4	T46.5X5	T46.5X6
Metiamide	T47.1X1	T47.1X2	T47.1X3	T47.1X4	T47.1X5	T47.1X6
Meticillin	T36.0X1	T36.0X2	T36.0X3	T36.0X4	T36.0X5	T36.0X6
Meticrane	T50.2X1	T50.2X2	T50.2X3	T50.2X4	T50.2X5	T50.2X6
Metildigoxin	T46.0X1	T46.0X2	T46.0X3	T46.0X4	T46.0X5	T46.0X6
Metipranolol	T49.5X1	T49.5X2	T49.5X3	T49.5X4	T49.5X5	T49.5X6
Metirosine	T46.5X1	T46.5X2	T46.5X3	T46.5X4	T46.5X5	T46.5X6
Metisazone	T37.5X1	T37.5X2	T37.5X3	T37.5X4	T37.5X5	T37.5X6
Metixene	T44.3X1	T44.3X2	T44.3X3	T44.3X4	T44.3X5	T44.3X6
Metizoline	T48.5X1	T48.5X2	T48.5X3	T48.5X4	T48.5X5	T48.5X6
Metoclopramide	T45.0X1	T45.0X2	T45.0X3	T45.0X4	T45.0X5	T45.0X6
Metofenazate	T43.3X1	T43.3X2	T43.3X3	T43.3X4	T43.3X5	T43.3X6
Metofoline	T39.8X1	T39.8X2	T39.8X3	T39.8X4	T39.8X5	T39.8X6
Metolazone	T50.2X1	T50.2X2	T50.2X3	T50.2X4	T50.2X5	T50.2X6
Metopon	T40.2X1	T40.2X2	T40.2X3	T40.2X4	T40.2X5	T40.2X6
Metoprine	T45.1X1	T45.1X2	T45.1X3	T45.1X4	T45.1X5	T45.1X6
Metoprolol	T44.7X1	T44.7X2	T44.7X3	T44.7X4	T44.7X5	T44.7X6
Metrifonate	T60.0X1	T60.0X2	T60.0X3	T60.0X4	—	—
Metrizamide	T50.8X1	T50.8X2	T50.8X3	T50.8X4	T50.8X5	T50.8X6
Metrizoic acid	T50.8X1	T50.8X2	T50.8X3	T50.8X4	T50.8X5	T50.8X6
Metronidazole	T37.8X1	T37.8X2	T37.8X3	T37.8X4	T37.8X5	T37.8X6
Metycaine	T41.3X1	T41.3X2	T41.3X3	T41.3X4	T41.3X5	T41.3X6
infiltration (subcutaneous)	T41.3X1	T41.3X2	T41.3X3	T41.3X4	T41.3X5	T41.3X6
nerve block (peripheral) (plexus)	T41.3X1	T41.3X2	T41.3X3	T41.3X4	T41.3X5	T41.3X6
topical (surface)	T41.3X1	T41.3X2	T41.3X3	T41.3X4	T41.3X5	T41.3X6
Metyrapone	T50.8X1	T50.8X2	T50.8X3	T50.8X4	T50.8X5	T50.8X6
Mevinphos	T60.0X1	T60.0X2	T60.0X3	T60.0X4	—	—
Mexazolam	T42.4X1	T42.4X2	T42.4X3	T42.4X4	T42.4X5	T42.4X6
Mexenone	T49.3X1	T49.3X2	T49.3X3	T49.3X4	T49.3X5	T49.3X6
Mexiletine	T46.2X1	T46.2X2	T46.2X3	T46.2X4	T46.2X5	T46.2X6
Mezereon	T62.2X1	T62.2X2	T62.2X3	T62.2X4	—	—
berries	T62.1X1	T62.1X2	T62.1X3	T62.1X4	—	—
Mezlocillin	T36.0X1	T36.0X2	T36.0X3	T36.0X4	T36.0X5	T36.0X6
Mianserin	T43.021	T43.022	T43.023	T43.024	T43.025	T43.026
Micatin	T49.0X1	T49.0X2	T49.0X3	T49.0X4	T49.0X5	T49.0X6
Miconazole	T49.0X1	T49.0X2	T49.0X3	T49.0X4	T49.0X5	T49.0X6
Micronomicin	T36.5X1	T36.5X2	T36.5X3	T36.5X4	T36.5X5	T36.5X6
Midazolam	T42.4X1	T42.4X2	T42.4X3	T42.4X4	T42.4X5	T42.4X6
Midecamycin	T36.3X1	T36.3X2	T36.3X3	T36.3X4	T36.3X5	T36.3X6
Mifepristone	T38.6X1	T38.6X2	T38.6X3	T38.6X4	T38.6X5	T38.6X6
Milk of magnesia	T47.1X1	T47.1X2	T47.1X3	T47.1X4	T47.1X5	T47.1X6
Millipede (tropical)	T63.411	T63.412	T63.413	T63.414	—	—
(venomous)						
Miltown	T43.591	T43.592	T43.593	T43.594	T43.595	T43.596
Milverine	T44.3X1	T44.3X2	T44.3X3	T44.3X4	T44.3X5	T44.3X6
Minaprine	T43.291	T43.292	T43.293	T43.294	T43.295	T43.296
Minaxolone	T41.291	T41.292	T41.293	T41.294	T41.295	T41.296
Mineral						
acids	T54.2X1	T54.2X2	T54.2X3	T54.2X4	—	—
oil (laxative)(medicinal)	T47.4X1	T47.4X2	T47.4X3	T47.4X4	T47.4X5	T47.4X6
emulsion	T47.2X1	T47.2X2	T47.2X3	T47.2X4	T47.2X5	T47.2X6
nonmedicinal	T52.0X1	T52.0X2	T52.0X3	T52.0X4	—	—
topical	T49.3X1	T49.3X2	T49.3X3	T49.3X4	T49.3X5	T49.3X6
salt NEC	T50.3X1	T50.3X2	T50.3X3	T50.3X4	T50.3X5	T50.3X6
spirits	T52.0X1	T52.0X2	T52.0X3	T52.0X4	—	—
Mineralocorticosteroid	T50.0X1	T50.0X2	T50.0X3	T50.0X4	T50.0X5	T50.0X6
Minocycline	T36.4X1	T36.4X2	T36.4X3	T36.4X4	T36.4X5	T36.4X6
Minoxidil	T46.7X1	T46.7X2	T46.7X3	T46.7X4	T46.7X5	T46.7X6
Miokamycin	T36.3X1	T36.3X2	T36.3X3	T36.3X4	T36.3X5	T36.3X6
Miotic drug	T49.5X1	T49.5X2	T49.5X3	T49.5X4	T49.5X5	T49.5X6
Mipafox	T60.0X1	T60.0X2	T60.0X3	T60.0X4	—	—
Mirex	T60.1X1	T60.1X2	T60.1X3	T60.1X4	—	—
Mirtazapine	T43.021	T43.022	T43.023	T43.024	T43.025	T43.026
Misonidazole	T37.3X1	T37.3X2	T37.3X3	T37.3X4	T37.3X5	T37.3X6
Misoprostol	T47.1X1	T47.1X2	T47.1X3	T47.1X4	T47.1X5	T47.1X6
Mithramycin	T45.1X1	T45.1X2	T45.1X3	T45.1X4	T45.1X5	T45.1X6
Mitobronitol	T45.1X1	T45.1X2	T45.1X3	T45.1X4	T45.1X5	T45.1X6
Mitoguazone	T45.1X1	T45.1X2	T45.1X3	T45.1X4	T45.1X5	T45.1X6
Mitolactol	T45.1X1	T45.1X2	T45.1X3	T45.1X4	T45.1X5	T45.1X6
Mitomycin	T45.1X1	T45.1X2	T45.1X3	T45.1X4	T45.1X5	T45.1X6
Mitopodozide	T45.1X1	T45.1X2	T45.1X3	T45.1X4	T45.1X5	T45.1X6
Mitotane	T45.1X1	T45.1X2	T45.1X3	T45.1X4	T45.1X5	T45.1X6
Mitoxantrone	T45.1X1	T45.1X2	T45.1X3	T45.1X4	T45.1X5	T45.1X6
Mivacurium chloride	T48.1X1	T48.1X2	T48.1X3	T48.1X4	T48.1X5	T48.1X6
Miyari bacteria	T47.6X1	T47.6X2	T47.6X3	T47.6X4	T47.6X5	T47.6X6
Moclobemide	T43.1X1	T43.1X2	T43.1X3	T43.1X4	T43.1X5	T43.1X6
Moderil	T46.5X1	T46.5X2	T46.5X3	T46.5X4	T46.5X5	T46.5X6
Mofebutazone	T39.2X1	T39.2X2	T39.2X3	T39.2X4	T39.2X5	T39.2X6
Mogadon — see Nitrazepam						
Molindone	T43.591	T43.592	T43.593	T43.594	T43.595	T43.596
Molsidomine	T46.3X1	T46.3X2	T46.3X3	T46.3X4	T46.3X5	T46.3X6

Substance	Poisoning, Accidental (unintentional)	Poisoning, Intentional Self-harm	Poisoning, Assault	Poisoning, Undetermined	Adverse Effect	Under-dosing
Mometasone	T49.0X1	T49.0X2	T49.0X3	T49.0X4	T49.0X5	T49.0X6
Monistat	T49.0X1	T49.0X2	T49.0X3	T49.0X4	T49.0X5	T49.0X6
Monkshood	T62.2X1	T62.2X2	T62.2X3	T62.2X4	—	—
Monoamine oxidase inhibitor NEC	T43.1X1	T43.1X2	T43.1X3	T43.1X4	T43.1X5	T43.1X6
hydrazine	T43.1X1	T43.1X2	T43.1X3	T43.1X4	T43.1X5	T43.1X6
Monobenzone	T49.4X1	T49.4X2	T49.4X3	T49.4X4	T49.4X5	T49.4X6
Monochloroacetic acid	T60.3X1	T60.3X2	T60.3X3	T60.3X4	—	—
Monochlorobenzene	T53.7X1	T53.7X2	T53.7X3	T53.7X4	—	—
Monoethanolamine	T46.8X1	T46.8X2	T46.8X3	T46.8X4	T46.8X5	T46.8X6
oleate	T46.8X1	T46.8X2	T46.8X3	T46.8X4	T46.8X5	T46.8X6
Monooctanoin	T50.991	T50.992	T50.993	T50.994	T50.995	T50.996
Monophenylbutazone	T39.2X1	T39.2X2	T39.2X3	T39.2X4	T39.2X5	T39.2X6
Monosodium glutamate	T65.891	T65.892	T65.893	T65.894	—	—
Monosulfiram	T49.0X1	T49.0X2	T49.0X3	T49.0X4	T49.0X5	T49.0X6
Monoxide, carbon — see Carbon, monoxide						
Monoxidine hydrochloride	T46.1X1	T46.1X2	T46.1X3	T46.1X4	T46.1X5	T46.1X6
Monuron	T60.3X1	T60.3X2	T60.3X3	T60.3X4	—	—
Moperone	T43.4X1	T43.4X2	T43.4X3	T43.4X4	T43.4X5	T43.4X6
Mopidamol	T45.1X1	T45.1X2	T45.1X3	T45.1X4	T45.1X5	T45.1X6
MOPP (mechloreth-amine + vincristine + prednisone + procarba-zine)	T45.1X1	T45.1X2	T45.1X3	T45.1X4	T45.1X5	T45.1X6
Morfin	T40.2X1	T40.2X2	T40.2X3	T40.2X4	T40.2X5	T40.2X6
Morinamide	T37.1X1	T37.1X2	T37.1X3	T37.1X4	T37.1X5	T37.1X6
Morning glory seeds	T40.991	T40.992	T40.993	T40.994	—	—
Moroxydine	T37.5X1	T37.5X2	T37.5X3	T37.5X4	T37.5X5	T37.5X6
Morphazinamide	T37.1X1	T37.1X2	T37.1X3	T37.1X4	T37.1X5	T37.1X6
Morphine	T40.2X1	T40.2X2	T40.2X3	T40.2X4	T40.2X5	T40.2X6
antagonist	T50.7X1	T50.7X2	T50.7X3	T50.7X4	T50.7X5	T50.7X6
Morpholinylethylmorphine	T40.2X1	T40.2X2	T40.2X3	T40.2X4	—	—
Morsuximide	T42.2X1	T42.2X2	T42.2X3	T42.2X4	T42.2X5	T42.2X6
Mosapramine	T43.591	T43.592	T43.593	T43.594	T43.595	T43.596
Moth balls — see also Pesticides	T60.2X1	T60.2X2	T60.2X3	T60.2X4	—	—
naphthalene	T60.2X1	T60.2X2	T60.2X3	T60.2X4	—	—
paradichlorobenzene	T60.1X1	T60.1X2	T60.1X3	T60.1X4	—	—
Motor exhaust gas	T58.01	T58.02	T58.03	T58.04	—	—
Mouthwash (antiseptic) (zinc chloride)	T49.6X1	T49.6X2	T49.6X3	T49.6X4	T49.6X5	T49.6X6
Moxastine	T45.0X1	T45.0X2	T45.0X3	T45.0X4	T45.0X5	T45.0X6
Moxaverine	T44.3X1	T44.3X2	T44.3X3	T44.3X4	T44.3X5	T44.3X6
Moxisylyte	T46.7X1	T46.7X2	T46.7X3	T46.7X4	T46.7X5	T46.7X6
Mucilage, plant	T47.4X1	T47.4X2	T47.4X3	T47.4X4	T47.4X5	T47.4X6
Mucolytic drug	T48.4X1	T48.4X2	T48.4X3	T48.4X4	T48.4X5	T48.4X6
Mucomyst	T48.4X1	T48.4X2	T48.4X3	T48.4X4	T48.4X5	T48.4X6
Mucous membrane agents (external)	T49.91	T49.92	T49.93	T49.94	T49.95	T49.96
specified NEC	T49.8X1	T49.8X2	T49.8X3	T49.8X4	T49.8X5	T49.8X6
Multiple unspecified drugs, medicaments and biological substances	T50.911	T50.912	T50.913	T50.914	T50.915	T50.916
Mumps						
immune globulin (human)	T50.Z11	T50.Z12	T50.Z13	T50.Z14	T50.Z15	T50.Z16
skin test antigen	T50.8X1	T50.8X2	T50.8X3	T50.8X4	T50.8X5	T50.8X6
vaccine	T50.B91	T50.B92	T50.B93	T50.B94	T50.B95	T50.B96
Mumpsvax	T50.B91	T50.B92	T50.B93	T50.B94	T50.B95	T50.B96
Mupirocin	T49.0X1	T49.0X2	T49.0X3	T49.0X4	T49.0X5	T49.0X6
Muriatic acid — see Hydrochloric acid						
Muromonab-CD3	T45.1X1	T45.1X2	T45.1X3	T45.1X4	T45.1X5	T45.1X6
Muscle-action drug NEC	T48.201	T48.202	T48.203	T48.204	T48.205	T48.206
Muscle affecting agents NEC	T48.201	T48.202	T48.203	T48.204	T48.205	T48.206
oxytocic	T48.0X1	T48.0X2	T48.0X3	T48.0X4	T48.0X5	T48.0X6
relaxants	T48.201	T48.202	T48.203	T48.204	T48.205	T48.206
central nervous system	T42.8X1	T42.8X2	T42.8X3	T42.8X4	T42.8X5	T42.8X6
skeletal	T48.1X1	T48.1X2	T48.1X3	T48.1X4	T48.1X5	T48.1X6
smooth	T44.3X1	T44.3X2	T44.3X3	T44.3X4	T44.3X5	T44.3X6
Muscle relaxant — see Relaxant, muscle						
Muscle-tone depressant, central NEC	T42.8X1	T42.8X2	T42.8X3	T42.8X4	T42.8X5	T42.8X6
specified NEC	T42.8X1	T42.8X2	T42.8X3	T42.8X4	T42.8X5	T42.8X6
Mushroom, noxious	T62.0X1	T62.0X2	T62.0X3	T62.0X4	—	—
Mussel, noxious	T61.781	T61.782	T61.783	T61.784	—	—
Mustard (emetic)	T47.7X1	T47.7X2	T47.7X3	T47.7X4	T47.7X5	T47.7X6
black	T47.7X1	T47.7X2	T47.7X3	T47.7X4	T47.7X5	T47.7X6
gas, not in war	T59.91	T59.92	T59.93	T59.94	—	—
nitrogen	T45.1X1	T45.1X2	T45.1X3	T45.1X4	T45.1X5	T45.1X6
Mustine	T45.1X1	T45.1X2	T45.1X3	T45.1X4	T45.1X5	T45.1X6
M-vac	T45.1X1	T45.1X2	T45.1X3	T45.1X4	T45.1X5	T45.1X6

Substance	Poisoning, Accidental (unintentional)	Poisoning, Intentional Self-harm	Poisoning, Assault	Poisoning, Undetermined	Adverse Effect	Under-dosing
Mycifradin	T36.5X1	T36.5X2	T36.5X3	T36.5X4	T36.5X5	T36.5X6
topical	T49.ØX1	T49.ØX2	T49.ØX3	T49.ØX4	T49.ØX5	T49.ØX6
Mycitracin	T36.8X1	T36.8X2	T36.8X3	T36.8X4	T36.8X5	T36.8X6
ophthalmic preparation	T49.5X1	T49.5X2	T49.5X3	T49.5X4	T49.5X5	T49.5X6
Mycostatin	T36.7X1	T36.7X2	T36.7X3	T36.7X4	T36.7X5	T36.7X6
topical	T49.ØX1	T49.ØX2	T49.ØX3	T49.ØX4	T49.ØX5	T49.ØX6
Mycotoxins	T64.81	T64.82	T64.83	T64.84	—	—
aflatoxin	T64.Ø1	T64.Ø2	T64.Ø3	T64.Ø4	—	—
specified NEC	T64.81	T64.82	T64.83	T64.84	—	—
Mydriacyl	T44.3X1	T44.3X2	T44.3X3	T44.3X4	T44.3X5	T44.3X6
Mydriatic drug	T49.5X1	T49.5X2	T49.5X3	T49.5X4	T49.5X5	T49.5X6
Myelobromal	T45.1X1	T45.1X2	T45.1X3	T45.1X4	T45.1X5	T45.1X6
Myleran	T45.1X1	T45.1X2	T45.1X3	T45.1X4	T45.1X5	T45.1X6
Myochrysin (e)	T39.2X1	T39.2X2	T39.2X3	T39.2X4	T39.2X5	T39.2X6
Myoneural blocking agents	T48.1X1	T48.1X2	T48.1X3	T48.1X4	T48.1X5	T48.1X6
Myralact	T49.ØX1	T49.ØX2	T49.ØX3	T49.ØX4	T49.ØX5	T49.ØX6
Myristica fragrans	T62.2X1	T62.2X2	T62.2X3	T62.2X4	—	—
Myristicin	T65.891	T65.892	T65.893	T65.894	—	—
Mysoline	T42.3X1	T42.3X2	T42.3X3	T42.3X4	T42.3X5	T42.3X6
Nabilone	T4Ø.711	T4Ø.712	T4Ø.713	T4Ø.714	T4Ø.715	T4Ø.716
Nabumetone	T39.391	T39.392	T39.393	T39.394	T39.395	T39.396
Nadolol	T44.7X1	T44.7X2	T44.7X3	T44.7X4	T44.7X5	T44.7X6
Nafcillin	T36.ØX1	T36.ØX2	T36.ØX3	T36.ØX4	T36.ØX5	T36.ØX6
Nafoxidine	T38.6X1	T38.6X2	T38.6X3	T38.6X4	T38.6X5	T38.6X6
Naftazone	T46.991	T46.992	T46.993	T46.994	T46.995	T46.996
Naftidrofuryl (oxalate)	T46.7X1	T46.7X2	T46.7X3	T46.7X4	T46.7X5	T46.7X6
Naftifine	T49.ØX1	T49.ØX2	T49.ØX3	T49.ØX4	T49.ØX5	T49.ØX6
Nail polish remover	T52.91	T52.92	T52.93	T52.94	—	—
Nalbuphine	T4Ø.491	T4Ø.492	T4Ø.493	T4Ø.494	T4Ø.495	T4Ø.496
Naled	T6Ø.ØX1	T6Ø.ØX2	T6Ø.ØX3	T6Ø.ØX4	—	—
Nalidixic acid	T37.8X1	T37.8X2	T37.8X3	T37.8X4	T37.8X5	T37.8X6
Nalorphine	T5Ø.7X1	T5Ø.7X2	T5Ø.7X3	T5Ø.7X4	T5Ø.7X5	T5Ø.7X6
Naloxone	T5Ø.7X1	T5Ø.7X2	T5Ø.7X3	T5Ø.7X4	T5Ø.7X5	T5Ø.7X6
Naltrexone	T5Ø.7X1	T5Ø.7X2	T5Ø.7X3	T5Ø.7X4	T5Ø.7X5	T5Ø.7X6
Namenda	T43.8X1	T43.8X2	T43.8X3	T43.8X4	T43.8X5	T43.8X6
Nandrolone	T38.7X1	T38.7X2	T38.7X3	T38.7X4	T38.7X5	T38.7X6
Naphazoline	T48.5X1	T48.5X2	T48.5X3	T48.5X4	T48.5X5	T48.5X6
Naphtha (painters') (petroleum)	T52.ØX1	T52.ØX2	T52.ØX3	T52.ØX4	—	—
solvent	T52.ØX1	T52.ØX2	T52.ØX3	T52.ØX4	—	—
vapor	T52.ØX1	T52.ØX2	T52.ØX3	T52.ØX4	—	—
Naphthalene (non-chlorinated)	T6Ø.2X1	T6Ø.2X2	T6Ø.2X3	T6Ø.2X4	—	—
chlorinated	T6Ø.1X1	T6Ø.1X2	T6Ø.1X3	T6Ø.1X4	—	—
vapor	T6Ø.1X1	T6Ø.1X2	T6Ø.1X3	T6Ø.1X4	—	—
insecticide or moth repellent	T6Ø.2X1	T6Ø.2X2	T6Ø.2X3	T6Ø.2X4	—	—
chlorinated	T6Ø.1X1	T6Ø.1X2	T6Ø.1X3	T6Ø.1X4	—	—
vapor	T6Ø.2X1	T6Ø.2X2	T6Ø.2X3	T6Ø.2X4	—	—
chlorinated	T6Ø.1X1	T6Ø.1X2	T6Ø.1X3	T6Ø.1X4	—	—
Naphthol	T65.891	T65.892	T65.893	T65.894	—	—
Naphthylamine	T65.891	T65.892	T65.893	T65.894	—	—
Naphthylthiourea (ANTU)	T6Ø.4X1	T6Ø.4X2	T6Ø.4X3	T6Ø.4X4	—	—
Naprosyn — *see* Naproxen						
Naproxen	T39.311	T39.312	T39.313	T39.314	T39.315	T39.316
Narcotic (drug)	T4Ø.6Ø1	T4Ø.6Ø2	T4Ø.6Ø3	T4Ø.6Ø4	T4Ø.6Ø5	T4Ø.6Ø6
analgesic NEC	T4Ø.6Ø1	T4Ø.6Ø2	T4Ø.6Ø3	T4Ø.6Ø4	T4Ø.6Ø5	T4Ø.6Ø6
antagonist	T5Ø.7X1	T5Ø.7X2	T5Ø.7X3	T5Ø.7X4	T5Ø.7X5	T5Ø.7X6
specified NEC	T4Ø.691	T4Ø.692	T4Ø.693	T4Ø.694	T4Ø.695	T4Ø.696
synthetic	T4Ø.491	T4Ø.492	T4Ø.493	T4Ø.494	T4Ø.495	T4Ø.496
Narcotine	T48.3X1	T48.3X2	T48.3X3	T48.3X4	T48.3X5	T48.3X6
Nardil	T43.1X1	T43.1X2	T43.1X3	T43.1X4	T43.1X5	T43.1X6
Nasal drug NEC	T49.6X1	T49.6X2	T49.6X3	T49.6X4	T49.6X5	T49.6X6
Natamycin	T49.ØX1	T49.ØX2	T49.ØX3	T49.ØX4	T49.ØX5	T49.ØX6
Natrium cyanide — *see* Cyanide(s)						
Natural						
blood (product)	T45.8X1	T45.8X2	T45.8X3	T45.8X4	T45.8X5	T45.8X6
gas (piped)	T59.891	T59.892	T59.893	T59.894	—	—
incomplete combustion	T58.11	T58.12	T58.13	T58.14	—	—
Nealbarbital	T42.3X1	T42.3X2	T42.3X3	T42.3X4	T42.3X5	T42.3X6
Nectadon	T48.3X1	T48.3X2	T48.3X3	T48.3X4	T48.3X5	T48.3X6
Nedocromil	T48.6X1	T48.6X2	T48.6X3	T48.6X4	T48.6X5	T48.6X6
Nefopam	T39.8X1	T39.8X2	T39.8X3	T39.8X4	T39.8X5	T39.8X6
Nematocyst (sting)	T63.691	T63.692	T63.693	T63.694	—	—
Nembutal	T42.3X1	T42.3X2	T42.3X3	T42.3X4	T42.3X5	T42.3X6
Nemonapride	T43.591	T43.592	T43.593	T43.594	T43.595	T43.596
Neoarsphenamine	T37.8X1	T37.8X2	T37.8X3	T37.8X4	T37.8X5	T37.8X6
Neocinchophen	T5Ø.4X1	T5Ø.4X2	T5Ø.4X3	T5Ø.4X4	T5Ø.4X5	T5Ø.4X6
Neomycin (derivatives)	T36.5X1	T36.5X2	T36.5X3	T36.5X4	T36.5X5	T36.5X6
with						
bacitracin	T49.ØX1	T49.ØX2	T49.ØX3	T49.ØX4	T49.ØX5	T49.ØX6
Neomycin — *continued*						
with — *continued*						
neostigmine	T44.ØX1	T44.ØX2	T44.ØX3	T44.ØX4	T44.ØX5	T44.ØX6
ENT agent	T49.6X1	T49.6X2	T49.6X3	T49.6X4	T49.6X5	T49.6X6
ophthalmic preparation	T49.5X1	T49.5X2	T49.5X3	T49.5X4	T49.5X5	T49.5X6
topical NEC	T49.ØX1	T49.ØX2	T49.ØX3	T49.ØX4	T49.ØX5	T49.ØX6
Neonal	T42.3X1	T42.3X2	T42.3X3	T42.3X4	T42.3X5	T42.3X6
Neoprontosil	T37.ØX1	T37.ØX2	T37.ØX3	T37.ØX4	T37.ØX5	T37.ØX6
Neosalvarsan	T37.8X1	T37.8X2	T37.8X3	T37.8X4	T37.8X5	T37.8X6
Neosilversalvarsan	T37.8X1	T37.8X2	T37.8X3	T37.8X4	T37.8X5	T37.8X6
Neosporin	T36.8X1	T36.8X2	T36.8X3	T36.8X4	T36.8X5	T36.8X6
ENT agent	T49.6X1	T49.6X2	T49.6X3	T49.6X4	T49.6X5	T49.6X6
opthalmic preparation	T49.5X1	T49.5X2	T49.5X3	T49.5X4	T49.5X5	T49.5X6
topical NEC	T49.ØX1	T49.ØX2	T49.ØX3	T49.ØX4	T49.ØX5	T49.ØX6
Neostigmine bromide	T44.ØX1	T44.ØX2	T44.ØX3	T44.ØX4	T44.ØX5	T44.ØX6
Neraval	T42.3X1	T42.3X2	T42.3X3	T42.3X4	T42.3X5	T42.3X6
Neravan	T42.3X1	T42.3X2	T42.3X3	T42.3X4	T42.3X5	T42.3X6
Nerium oleander	T62.2X1	T62.2X2	T62.2X3	T62.2X4	—	—
Nerve gas, not in war	T59.91	T59.92	T59.93	T59.94	—	—
Nesacaine	T41.3X1	T41.3X2	T41.3X3	T41.3X4	T41.3X5	T41.3X6
infiltration (subcutaneous)	T41.3X1	T41.3X2	T41.3X3	T41.3X4	T41.3X5	T41.3X6
nerve block (peripheral) (plexus)	T41.3X1	T41.3X2	T41.3X3	T41.3X4	T41.3X5	T41.3X6
Netilmicin	T36.5X1	T36.5X2	T36.5X3	T36.5X4	T36.5X5	T36.5X6
Neurobarb	T42.3X1	T42.3X2	T42.3X3	T42.3X4	T42.3X5	T42.3X6
Neuroleptic drug NEC	T43.5Ø1	T43.5Ø2	T43.5Ø3	T43.5Ø4	T43.5Ø5	T43.5Ø6
Neuromuscular blocking drug	T48.1X1	T48.1X2	T48.1X3	T48.1X4	T48.1X5	T48.1X6
Neutral insulin injection	T38.3X1	T38.3X2	T38.3X3	T38.3X4	T38.3X5	T38.3X6
Neutral spirits	T51.ØX1	T51.ØX2	T51.ØX3	T51.ØX4	—	—
beverage	T51.ØX1	T51.ØX2	T51.ØX3	T51.ØX4	—	—
Niacin	T46.7X1	T46.7X2	T46.7X3	T46.7X4	T46.7X5	T46.7X6
Niacinamide	T45.2X1	T45.2X2	T45.2X3	T45.2X4	T45.2X5	T45.2X6
Nialamide	T43.1X1	T43.1X2	T43.1X3	T43.1X4	T43.1X5	T43.1X6
Niaprazine	T42.6X1	T42.6X2	T42.6X3	T42.6X4	T42.6X5	T42.6X6
Nicametate	T46.7X1	T46.7X2	T46.7X3	T46.7X4	T46.7X5	T46.7X6
Nicardipine	T46.1X1	T46.1X2	T46.1X3	T46.1X4	T46.1X5	T46.1X6
Nicergoline	T46.7X1	T46.7X2	T46.7X3	T46.7X4	T46.7X5	T46.7X6
Nickel (carbonyl) (tetra-carbonyl) (fumes) (vapor)	T56.891	T56.892	T56.893	T56.894	—	—
Nickelocene	T56.891	T56.892	T56.893	T56.894	—	—
Niclosamide	T37.4X1	T37.4X2	T37.4X3	T37.4X4	T37.4X5	T37.4X6
Nicofuranose	T46.7X1	T46.7X2	T46.7X3	T46.7X4	T46.7X5	T46.7X6
Nicomorphine	T4Ø.2X1	T4Ø.2X2	T4Ø.2X3	T4Ø.2X4	—	—
Nicorandil	T46.3X1	T46.3X2	T46.3X3	T46.3X4	T46.3X5	T46.3X6
Nicotiana (plant)	T62.2X1	T62.2X2	T62.2X3	T62.2X4	—	—
Nicotinamide	T45.2X1	T45.2X2	T45.2X3	T45.2X4	T45.2X5	T45.2X6
Nicotine (insecticide) (spray) (sulfate) **NEC**	T6Ø.2X1	T6Ø.2X2	T6Ø.2X3	T6Ø.2X4	—	—
from tobacco	T65.291	T65.292	T65.293	T65.294	—	—
cigarettes	T65.221	T65.222	T65.223	T65.224	—	—
not insecticide	T65.291	T65.292	T65.293	T65.294	—	—
Nicotinic acid	T46.7X1	T46.7X2	T46.7X3	T46.7X4	T46.7X5	T46.7X6
Nicotinyl alcohol	T46.7X1	T46.7X2	T46.7X3	T46.7X4	T46.7X5	T46.7X6
Nicoumalone	T45.511	T45.512	T45.513	T45.514	T45.515	T45.516
Nifedipine	T46.1X1	T46.1X2	T46.1X3	T46.1X4	T46.1X5	T46.1X6
Nifenazone	T39.2X1	T39.2X2	T39.2X3	T39.2X4	T39.2X5	T39.2X6
Nifuraldezone	T37.91	T37.92	T37.93	T37.94	T37.95	T37.96
Nifuratel	T37.8X1	T37.8X2	T37.8X3	T37.8X4	T37.8X5	T37.8X6
Nifurtimox	T37.3X1	T37.3X2	T37.3X3	T37.3X4	T37.3X5	T37.3X6
Nifurtoinol	T37.8X1	T37.8X2	T37.8X3	T37.8X4	T37.8X5	T37.8X6
Nightshade, deadly (solanum) — *see also* Belladonna	T62.2X1	T62.2X2	T62.2X3	T62.2X4	—	—
berry	T62.1X1	T62.1X2	T62.1X3	T62.1X4	—	—
Nikethamide	T5Ø.7X1	T5Ø.7X2	T5Ø.7X3	T5Ø.7X4	T5Ø.7X5	T5Ø.7X6
Nilstat	T36.7X1	T36.7X2	T36.7X3	T36.7X4	T36.7X5	T36.7X6
topical	T49.ØX1	T49.ØX2	T49.ØX3	T49.ØX4	T49.ØX5	T49.ØX6
Nilutamide	T38.6X1	T38.6X2	T38.6X3	T38.6X4	T38.6X5	T38.6X6
Nimesulide	T39.391	T39.392	T39.393	T39.394	T39.395	T39.396
Nimetazepam	T42.4X1	T42.4X2	T42.4X3	T42.4X4	T42.4X5	T42.4X6
Nimodipine	T46.1X1	T46.1X2	T46.1X3	T46.1X4	T46.1X5	T46.1X6
Nimorazole	T37.3X1	T37.3X2	T37.3X3	T37.3X4	T37.3X5	T37.3X6
Nimustine	T45.1X1	T45.1X2	T45.1X3	T45.1X4	T45.1X5	T45.1X6
Niridazole	T37.4X1	T37.4X2	T37.4X3	T37.4X4	T37.4X5	T37.4X6
Nisentil	T4Ø.2X1	T4Ø.2X2	T4Ø.2X3	T4Ø.2X4	T4Ø.2X5	T4Ø.2X6
Nisoldipine	T46.1X1	T46.1X2	T46.1X3	T46.1X4	T46.1X5	T46.1X6
Nitramine	T65.3X1	T65.3X2	T65.3X3	T65.3X4	—	—
Nitrate, organic	T46.3X1	T46.3X2	T46.3X3	T46.3X4	T46.3X5	T46.3X6
Nitrazepam	T42.4X1	T42.4X2	T42.4X3	T42.4X4	T42.4X5	T42.4X6
Nitrefazole	T5Ø.6X1	T5Ø.6X2	T5Ø.6X3	T5Ø.6X4	T5Ø.6X5	T5Ø.6X6
Nitrendipine	T46.1X1	T46.1X2	T46.1X3	T46.1X4	T46.1X5	T46.1X6
Nitric						
acid (liquid)	T54.2X1	T54.2X2	T54.2X3	T54.2X4	—	—

Mycifradin — Nitric

386

Additional Character May Be Required — Refer to the Tabular List for Character Selection

Subterms under main terms may continue to next column or page

Substance	Poisoning, Accidental (unintentional)	Poisoning, Intentional Self-harm	Poisoning, Assault	Poisoning, Undetermined	Adverse Effect	Under-dosing
Nitric — *continued*						
acid — *continued*						
vapor	T59.891	T59.892	T59.893	T59.894	—	—
oxide (gas)	T59.ØX1	T59.ØX2	T59.ØX3	T59.ØX4	—	—
Nitrimidazine	T37.3X1	T37.3X2	T37.3X3	T37.3X4	T37.3X5	T37.3X6
Nitrite, amyl (medicinal) (vapor)	T46.3X1	T46.3X2	T46.3X3	T46.3X4	T46.3X5	T46.3X6
Nitroaniline	T65.3X1	T65.3X2	T65.3X3	T65.3X4	—	—
vapor	T59.891	T59.892	T59.893	T59.894	—	—
Nitrobenzene, nitrobenzol	T65.3X1	T65.3X2	T65.3X3	T65.3X4	—	—
vapor	T65.3X1	T65.3X2	T65.3X3	T65.3X4	—	—
Nitrocellulose	T65.891	T65.892	T65.893	T65.894	—	—
lacquer	T65.891	T65.892	T65.893	T65.894	—	—
Nitrodiphenyl	T65.3X1	T65.3X2	T65.3X3	T65.3X4	—	—
Nitrofural	T49.ØX1	T49.ØX2	T49.ØX3	T49.ØX4	T49.ØX5	T49.ØX6
Nitrofurantoin	T37.8X1	T37.8X2	T37.8X3	T37.8X4	T37.8X5	T37.8X6
Nitrofurazone	T49.ØX1	T49.ØX2	T49.ØX3	T49.ØX4	T49.ØX5	T49.ØX6
Nitrogen	T59.ØX1	T59.ØX2	T59.ØX3	T59.ØX4	—	—
mustard	T45.1X1	T45.1X2	T45.1X3	T45.1X4	T45.1X5	T45.1X6
Nitroglycerin, nitroglycerol (medicinal)	T46.3X1	T46.3X2	T46.3X3	T46.3X4	T46.3X5	T46.3X6
nonmedicinal	T65.5X1	T65.5X2	T65.5X3	T65.5X4	—	—
fumes	T65.5X1	T65.5X2	T65.5X3	T65.5X4	—	—
Nitroglycol	T52.3X1	T52.3X2	T52.3X3	T52.3X4	—	—
Nitrohydrochloric acid	T54.2X1	T54.2X2	T54.2X3	T54.2X4	—	—
Nitromersol	T49.ØX1	T49.ØX2	T49.ØX3	T49.ØX4	T49.ØX5	T49.ØX6
Nitronaphthalene	T65.891	T65.892	T65.893	T65.894	—	—
Nitrophenol	T54.ØX1	T54.ØX2	T54.ØX3	T54.ØX4	—	—
Nitropropane	T52.8X1	T52.8X2	T52.8X3	T52.8X4	—	—
Nitroprusside	T46.5X1	T46.5X2	T46.5X3	T46.5X4	T46.5X5	T46.5X6
Nitrosodimethylamine	T65.3X1	T65.3X2	T65.3X3	T65.3X4	—	—
Nitrothiazol	T37.4X1	T37.4X2	T37.4X3	T37.4X4	T37.4X5	T37.4X6
Nitrotoluene, nitrotoluol	T65.3X1	T65.3X2	T65.3X3	T65.3X4	—	—
vapor	T65.3X1	T65.3X2	T65.3X3	T65.3X4	—	—
Nitrous						
acid (liquid)	T54.2X1	T54.2X2	T54.2X3	T54.2X4	—	—
fumes	T59.891	T59.892	T59.893	T59.894	—	—
ether spirit	T46.3X1	T46.3X2	T46.3X3	T46.3X4	T46.3X5	T46.3X6
oxide	T41.ØX1	T41.ØX2	T41.ØX3	T41.ØX4	T41.ØX5	T41.ØX6
Nitroxoline	T37.8X1	T37.8X2	T37.8X3	T37.8X4	T37.8X5	T37.8X6
Nitrozone	T49.ØX1	T49.ØX2	T49.ØX3	T49.ØX4	T49.ØX5	T49.ØX6
Nizatidine	T47.ØX1	T47.ØX2	T47.ØX3	T47.ØX4	T47.ØX5	T47.ØX6
Nizofenone	T43.8X1	T43.8X2	T43.8X3	T43.8X4	T43.8X5	T43.8X6
Noctec	T42.6X1	T42.6X2	T42.6X3	T42.6X4	T42.6X5	T42.6X6
Noludar	T42.6X1	T42.6X2	T42.6X3	T42.6X4	T42.6X5	T42.6X6
Nomegestrol	T38.5X1	T38.5X2	T38.5X3	T38.5X4	T38.5X5	T38.5X6
Nomifensine	T43.291	T43.292	T43.293	T43.294	T43.295	T43.296
Nonoxinol	T49.8X1	T49.8X2	T49.8X3	T49.8X4	T49.8X5	T49.8X6
Nonylphenoxy (polyethoxyethanol)	T49.8X1	T49.8X2	T49.8X3	T49.8X4	T49.8X5	T49.8X6
Noptil	T42.3X1	T42.3X2	T42.3X3	T42.3X4	T42.3X5	T42.3X6
Noradrenaline	T44.4X1	T44.4X2	T44.4X3	T44.4X4	T44.4X5	T44.4X6
Noramidopyrine	T39.2X1	T39.2X2	T39.2X3	T39.2X4	T39.2X5	T39.2X6
methanesulfonate sodium	T39.2X1	T39.2X2	T39.2X3	T39.2X4	T39.2X5	T39.2X6
Norbormide	T60.4X1	T60.4X2	T60.4X3	T60.4X4	—	—
Nordazepam	T42.4X1	T42.4X2	T42.4X3	T42.4X4	T42.4X5	T42.4X6
Norepinephrine	T44.4X1	T44.4X2	T44.4X3	T44.4X4	T44.4X5	T44.4X6
Norethandrolone	T38.7X1	T38.7X2	T38.7X3	T38.7X4	T38.7X5	T38.7X6
Norethindrone	T38.4X1	T38.4X2	T38.4X3	T38.4X4	T38.4X5	T38.4X6
Norethisterone (acetate) (enantate)	T38.4X1	T38.4X2	T38.4X3	T38.4X4	T38.4X5	T38.4X6
with ethinylestradiol	T38.5X1	T38.5X2	T38.5X3	T38.5X4	T38.5X5	T38.5X6
Noretynodrel	T38.5X1	T38.5X2	T38.5X3	T38.5X4	T38.5X5	T38.5X6
Norfenefrine	T44.4X1	T44.4X2	T44.4X3	T44.4X4	T44.4X5	T44.4X6
Norfloxacin	T36.8X1	T36.8X2	T36.8X3	T36.8X4	T36.8X5	T36.8X6
Norgestrel	T38.4X1	T38.4X2	T38.4X3	T38.4X4	T38.4X5	T38.4X6
Norgestrienone	T38.4X1	T38.4X2	T38.4X3	T38.4X4	T38.4X5	T38.4X6
Norlestrin	T38.4X1	T38.4X2	T38.4X3	T38.4X4	T38.4X5	T38.4X6
Norlutin	T38.4X1	T38.4X2	T38.4X3	T38.4X4	T38.4X5	T38.4X6
Normal serum albumin (human), salt-poor	T45.8X1	T45.8X2	T45.8X3	T45.8X4	T45.8X5	T45.8X6
Normethandrone	T38.5X1	T38.5X2	T38.5X3	T38.5X4	T38.5X5	T38.5X6
Normison — *see* Benzodiazepines						
Normorphine	T40.2X1	T40.2X2	T40.2X3	T40.2X4	—	—
Norpseudoephedrine	T50.5X1	T50.5X2	T50.5X3	T50.5X4	T50.5X5	T50.5X6
Nortestosterone (furanpropionate)	T38.7X1	T38.7X2	T38.7X3	T38.7X4	T38.7X5	T38.7X6
Nortriptyline	T43.Ø11	T43.Ø12	T43.Ø13	T43.Ø14	T43.Ø15	T43.Ø16
Noscapine	T48.3X1	T48.3X2	T48.3X3	T48.3X4	T48.3X5	T48.3X6
Nose preparations	T49.6X1	T49.6X2	T49.6X3	T49.6X4	T49.6X5	T49.6X6
Novobiocin	T36.5X1	T36.5X2	T36.5X3	T36.5X4	T36.5X5	T36.5X6

Substance	Poisoning, Accidental (unintentional)	Poisoning, Intentional Self-harm	Poisoning, Assault	Poisoning, Undetermined	Adverse Effect	Under-dosing
Novocain (infiltration) (topical)	T41.3X1	T41.3X2	T41.3X3	T41.3X4	T41.3X5	T41.3X6
nerve block (peripheral) (plexus)	T41.3X1	T41.3X2	T41.3X3	T41.3X4	T41.3X5	T41.3X6
spinal	T41.3X1	T41.3X2	T41.3X3	T41.3X4	T41.3X5	T41.3X6
Noxious foodstuff	T62.91	T62.92	T62.93	T62.94	—	—
specified NEC	T62.8X1	T62.8X2	T62.8X3	T62.8X4	—	—
Noxiptiline	T43.Ø11	T43.Ø12	T43.Ø13	T43.Ø14	T43.Ø15	T43.Ø16
Noxytiolin	T49.ØX1	T49.ØX2	T49.ØX3	T49.ØX4	T49.ØX5	T49.ØX6
NPH Iletin (insulin)	T38.3X1	T38.3X2	T38.3X3	T38.3X4	T38.3X5	T38.3X6
Numorphan	T40.2X1	T40.2X2	T40.2X3	T40.2X4	T40.2X5	T40.2X6
Nunol	T42.3X1	T42.3X2	T42.3X3	T42.3X4	T42.3X5	T42.3X6
Nupercaine (spinal anesthetic)	T41.3X1	T41.3X2	T41.3X3	T41.3X4	T41.3X5	T41.3X6
topical (surface)	T41.3X1	T41.3X2	T41.3X3	T41.3X4	T41.3X5	T41.3X6
Nutmeg oil (liniment)	T49.3X1	T49.3X2	T49.3X3	T49.3X4	T49.3X5	T49.3X6
Nutritional supplement	T50.901	T50.902	T50.903	T50.904	T50.905	T50.906
Nux vomica	T65.1X1	T65.1X2	T65.1X3	T65.1X4	—	—
Nydrazid	T37.1X1	T37.1X2	T37.1X3	T37.1X4	T37.1X5	T37.1X6
Nylidrin	T46.7X1	T46.7X2	T46.7X3	T46.7X4	T46.7X5	T46.7X6
Nystatin	T36.7X1	T36.7X2	T36.7X3	T36.7X4	T36.7X5	T36.7X6
topical	T49.ØX1	T49.ØX2	T49.ØX3	T49.ØX4	T49.ØX5	T49.ØX6
Nytol	T45.ØX1	T45.ØX2	T45.ØX3	T45.ØX4	T45.ØX5	T45.ØX6
Obidoxime chloride	T50.6X1	T50.6X2	T50.6X3	T50.6X4	T50.6X5	T50.6X6
Octafonium (chloride)	T49.3X1	T49.3X2	T49.3X3	T49.3X4	T49.3X5	T49.3X6
Octamethyl pyrophosphoramide	T60.ØX1	T60.ØX2	T60.ØX3	T60.ØX4	—	—
Octanoin	T50.991	T50.992	T50.993	T50.994	T50.995	T50.996
Octatropine methylbromide	T44.3X1	T44.3X2	T44.3X3	T44.3X4	T44.3X5	T44.3X6
Octotiamine	T45.2X1	T45.2X2	T45.2X3	T45.2X4	T45.2X5	T45.2X6
Octoxinol (9)	T49.8X1	T49.8X2	T49.8X3	T49.8X4	T49.8X5	T49.8X6
Octreotide	T38.991	T38.992	T38.993	T38.994	T38.995	T38.996
Octyl nitrite	T46.3X1	T46.3X2	T46.3X3	T46.3X4	T46.3X5	T46.3X6
Oestradiol	T38.5X1	T38.5X2	T38.5X3	T38.5X4	T38.5X5	T38.5X6
Oestriol	T38.5X1	T38.5X2	T38.5X3	T38.5X4	T38.5X5	T38.5X6
Oestrogen	T38.5X1	T38.5X2	T38.5X3	T38.5X4	T38.5X5	T38.5X6
Oestrone	T38.5X1	T38.5X2	T38.5X3	T38.5X4	T38.5X5	T38.5X6
Ofloxacin	T36.8X1	T36.8X2	T36.8X3	T36.8X4	T36.8X5	T36.8X6
Oil (of)	T65.891	T65.892	T65.893	T65.894	—	—
bitter almond	T62.8X1	T62.8X2	T62.8X3	T62.8X4	—	—
cloves	T49.7X1	T49.7X2	T49.7X3	T49.7X4	T49.7X5	T49.7X6
colors	T65.6X1	T65.6X2	T65.6X3	T65.6X4	—	—
fumes	T59.891	T59.892	T59.893	T59.894	—	—
lubricating	T52.ØX1	T52.ØX2	T52.ØX3	T52.ØX4	—	—
Niobe	T52.8X1	T52.8X2	T52.8X3	T52.8X4	—	—
vitriol (liquid)	T54.2X1	T54.2X2	T54.2X3	T54.2X4	—	—
fumes	T54.2X1	T54.2X2	T54.2X3	T54.2X4	—	—
wintergreen (bitter) NEC	T49.3X1	T49.3X2	T49.3X3	T49.3X4	T49.3X5	T49.3X6
Oily preparation (for skin)	T49.3X1	T49.3X2	T49.3X3	T49.3X4	T49.3X5	T49.3X6
Ointment NEC	T49.3X1	T49.3X2	T49.3X3	T49.3X4	T49.3X5	T49.3X6
Olanzapine	T43.591	T43.592	T43.593	T43.594	T43.595	T43.596
Oleander	T62.2X1	T62.2X2	T62.2X3	T62.2X4	—	—
Oleandomycin	T36.3X1	T36.3X2	T36.3X3	T36.3X4	T36.3X5	T36.3X6
Oleandrin	T46.ØX1	T46.ØX2	T46.ØX3	T46.ØX4	T46.ØX5	T46.ØX6
Oleic acid	T46.6X1	T46.6X2	T46.6X3	T46.6X4	T46.6X5	T46.6X6
Oleovitamin A	T45.2X1	T45.2X2	T45.2X3	T45.2X4	T45.2X5	T45.2X6
Oleum ricini	T47.2X1	T47.2X2	T47.2X3	T47.2X4	T47.2X5	T47.2X6
Olive oil (medicinal) **NEC**	T47.4X1	T47.4X2	T47.4X3	T47.4X4	T47.4X5	T47.4X6
Olivomycin	T45.1X1	T45.1X2	T45.1X3	T45.1X4	T45.1X5	T45.1X6
Olsalazine	T47.8X1	T47.8X2	T47.8X3	T47.8X4	T47.8X5	T47.8X6
Omeprazole	T47.1X1	T47.1X2	T47.1X3	T47.1X4	T47.1X5	T47.1X6
OMPA	T60.ØX1	T60.ØX2	T60.ØX3	T60.ØX4	—	—
Oncovin	T45.1X1	T45.1X2	T45.1X3	T45.1X4	T45.1X5	T45.1X6
Ondansetron	T45.ØX1	T45.ØX2	T45.ØX3	T45.ØX4	T45.ØX5	T45.ØX6
Ophthaine	T41.3X1	T41.3X2	T41.3X3	T41.3X4	T41.3X5	T41.3X6
Ophthetic	T41.3X1	T41.3X2	T41.3X3	T41.3X4	T41.3X5	T41.3X6
Opiate NEC	T40.601	T40.602	T40.603	T40.604	T40.605	T40.606
antagonists	T50.7X1	T50.7X2	T50.7X3	T50.7X4	T50.7X5	T50.7X6
Opioid NEC	T40.2X1	T40.2X2	T40.2X3	T40.2X4	T40.2X5	T40.2X6
Opipramol	T43.Ø11	T43.Ø12	T43.Ø13	T43.Ø14	T43.Ø15	T43.Ø16
Opium alkaloids (total)	T40.ØX1	T40.ØX2	T40.ØX3	T40.ØX4	T40.ØX5	T40.ØX6
standardized powdered	T40.ØX1	T40.ØX2	T40.ØX3	T40.ØX4	T40.ØX5	T40.ØX6
tincture (camphorated)	T40.ØX1	T40.ØX2	T40.ØX3	T40.ØX4	T40.ØX5	T40.ØX6
Oracon	T38.4X1	T38.4X2	T38.4X3	T38.4X4	T38.4X5	T38.4X6
Oragrafin	T50.8X1	T50.8X2	T50.8X3	T50.8X4	T50.8X5	T50.8X6
Oral contraceptives	T38.4X1	T38.4X2	T38.4X3	T38.4X4	T38.4X5	T38.4X6
Oral rehydration salts	T50.3X1	T50.3X2	T50.3X3	T50.3X4	T50.3X5	T50.3X6
Orazamide	T50.991	T50.992	T50.993	T50.994	T50.995	T50.996
Orciprenaline	T48.291	T48.292	T48.293	T48.294	T48.295	T48.296
Organidin	T48.4X1	T48.4X2	T48.4X3	T48.4X4	T48.4X5	T48.4X6
Organonitrate NEC	T46.3X1	T46.3X2	T46.3X3	T46.3X4	T46.3X5	T46.3X6
Organophosphates	T60.ØX1	T60.ØX2	T60.ØX3	T60.ØX4	—	—

Substance	Poisoning, Accidental (unintentional)	Poisoning, Intentional Self-harm	Poisoning, Assault	Poisoning, Undetermined	Adverse Effect	Underdosing
Orimune	T50.B91	T50.B92	T50.B93	T50.B94	T50.B95	T50.B96
Orinase	T38.3X1	T38.3X2	T38.3X3	T38.3X4	T38.3X5	T38.3X6
Ormeloxifene	T38.6X1	T38.6X2	T38.6X3	T38.6X4	T38.6X5	T38.6X6
Ornidazole	T37.3X1	T37.3X2	T37.3X3	T37.3X4	T37.3X5	T37.3X6
Ornithine aspartate	T50.991	T50.992	T50.993	T50.994	T50.995	T50.996
Ornoprostil	T47.1X1	T47.1X2	T47.1X3	T47.1X4	T47.1X5	T47.1X6
Orphenadrine (hydrochloride)	T42.8X1	T42.8X2	T42.8X3	T42.8X4	T42.8X5	T42.8X6
Ortal (sodium)	T42.3X1	T42.3X2	T42.3X3	T42.3X4	T42.3X5	T42.3X6
Orthoboric acid	T49.0X1	T49.0X2	T49.0X3	T49.0X4	T49.0X5	T49.0X6
ENT agent	T49.6X1	T49.6X2	T49.6X3	T49.6X4	T49.6X5	T49.6X6
ophthalmic preparation	T49.5X1	T49.5X2	T49.5X3	T49.5X4	T49.5X5	T49.5X6
Orthocaine	T41.3X1	T41.3X2	T41.3X3	T41.3X4	T41.3X5	T41.3X6
Orthodichlorobenzene	T53.7X1	T53.7X2	T53.7X3	T53.7X4	—	—
Ortho-Novum	T38.4X1	T38.4X2	T38.4X3	T38.4X4	T38.4X5	T38.4X6
Orthotolidine (reagent)	T54.2X1	T54.2X2	T54.2X3	T54.2X4	—	—
Osmic acid (liquid)	T54.2X1	T54.2X2	T54.2X3	T54.2X4	—	—
fumes	T54.2X1	T54.2X2	T54.2X3	T54.2X4	—	—
Osmotic diuretics	T50.2X1	T50.2X2	T50.2X3	T50.2X4	T50.2X5	T50.2X6
Otilonium bromide	T44.3X1	T44.3X2	T44.3X3	T44.3X4	T44.3X5	T44.3X6
Otorhinolaryngological drug NEC	T49.6X1	T49.6X2	T49.6X3	T49.6X4	T49.6X5	T49.6X6
Ouabain (e)	T46.0X1	T46.0X2	T46.0X3	T46.0X4	T46.0X5	T46.0X6
Ovarian						
hormone	T38.5X1	T38.5X2	T38.5X3	T38.5X4	T38.5X5	T38.5X6
stimulant	T38.5X1	T38.5X2	T38.5X3	T38.5X4	T38.5X5	T38.5X6
Ovral	T38.4X1	T38.4X2	T38.4X3	T38.4X4	T38.4X5	T38.4X6
Ovulen	T38.4X1	T38.4X2	T38.4X3	T38.4X4	T38.4X5	T38.4X6
Oxacillin	T36.0X1	T36.0X2	T36.0X3	T36.0X4	T36.0X5	T36.0X6
Oxalic acid	T54.2X1	T54.2X2	T54.2X3	T54.2X4	—	—
ammonium salt	T50.991	T50.992	T50.993	T50.994	T50.995	T50.996
Oxamniquine	T37.4X1	T37.4X2	T37.4X3	T37.4X4	T37.4X5	T37.4X6
Oxanamide	T43.591	T43.592	T43.593	T43.594	T43.595	T43.596
Oxandrolone	T38.7X1	T38.7X2	T38.7X3	T38.7X4	T38.7X5	T38.7X6
Oxantel	T37.4X1	T37.4X2	T37.4X3	T37.4X4	T37.4X5	T37.4X6
Oxapium iodide	T44.3X1	T44.3X2	T44.3X3	T44.3X4	T44.3X5	T44.3X6
Oxaprotiline	T43.021	T43.022	T43.023	T43.024	T43.025	T43.026
Oxaprozin	T39.311	T39.312	T39.313	T39.314	T39.315	T39.316
Oxatomide	T45.0X1	T45.0X2	T45.0X3	T45.0X4	T45.0X5	T45.0X6
Oxazepam	T42.4X1	T42.4X2	T42.4X3	T42.4X4	T42.4X5	T42.4X6
Oxazimedrine	T50.5X1	T50.5X2	T50.5X3	T50.5X4	T50.5X5	T50.5X6
Oxazolam	T42.4X1	T42.4X2	T42.4X3	T42.4X4	T42.4X5	T42.4X6
Oxazolidine derivatives	T42.2X1	T42.2X2	T42.2X3	T42.2X4	T42.2X5	T42.2X6
Oxazolidinedione (derivative)	T42.2X1	T42.2X2	T42.2X3	T42.2X4	T42.2X5	T42.2X6
Ox bile extract	T47.5X1	T47.5X2	T47.5X3	T47.5X4	T47.5X5	T47.5X6
Oxcarbazepine	T42.1X1	T42.1X2	T42.1X3	T42.1X4	T42.1X5	T42.1X6
Oxedrine	T44.4X1	T44.4X2	T44.4X3	T44.4X4	T44.4X5	T44.4X6
Oxeladin (citrate)	T48.3X1	T48.3X2	T48.3X3	T48.3X4	T48.3X5	T48.3X6
Oxendolone	T38.5X1	T38.5X2	T38.5X3	T38.5X4	T38.5X5	T38.5X6
Oxetacaine	T41.3X1	T41.3X2	T41.3X3	T41.3X4	T41.3X5	T41.3X6
Oxethazine	T41.3X1	T41.3X2	T41.3X3	T41.3X4	T41.3X5	T41.3X6
Oxetorone	T39.8X1	T39.8X2	T39.8X3	T39.8X4	T39.8X5	T39.8X6
Oxiconazole	T49.0X1	T49.0X2	T49.0X3	T49.0X4	T49.0X5	T49.0X6
Oxidizing agent NEC	T54.91	T54.92	T54.93	T54.94	—	—
Oxipurinol	T50.4X1	T50.4X2	T50.4X3	T50.4X4	T50.4X5	T50.4X6
Oxitriptan	T43.291	T43.292	T43.293	T43.294	T43.295	T43.296
Oxitropium bromide	T48.6X1	T48.6X2	T48.6X3	T48.6X4	T48.6X5	T48.6X6
Oxodipine	T46.1X1	T46.1X2	T46.1X3	T46.1X4	T46.1X5	T46.1X6
Oxolamine	T48.3X1	T48.3X2	T48.3X3	T48.3X4	T48.3X5	T48.3X6
Oxolinic acid	T37.8X1	T37.8X2	T37.8X3	T37.8X4	T37.8X5	T37.8X6
Oxomemazine	T43.3X1	T43.3X2	T43.3X3	T43.3X4	T43.3X5	T43.3X6
Oxophenarsine	T37.3X1	T37.3X2	T37.3X3	T37.3X4	T37.3X5	T37.3X6
Oxprenolol	T44.7X1	T44.7X2	T44.7X3	T44.7X4	T44.7X5	T44.7X6
Oxsoralen	T49.3X1	T49.3X2	T49.3X3	T49.3X4	T49.3X5	T49.3X6
Oxtriphylline	T48.6X1	T48.6X2	T48.6X3	T48.6X4	T48.6X5	T48.6X6
Oxybate sodium	T41.291	T41.292	T41.293	T41.294	T41.295	T41.296
Oxybuprocaine	T41.3X1	T41.3X2	T41.3X3	T41.3X4	T41.3X5	T41.3X6
Oxybutynin	T44.3X1	T44.3X2	T44.3X3	T44.3X4	T44.3X5	T44.3X6
Oxychlorosene	T49.0X1	T49.0X2	T49.0X3	T49.0X4	T49.0X5	T49.0X6
Oxycodone	T40.2X1	T40.2X2	T40.2X3	T40.2X4	T40.2X5	T40.2X6
Oxyfedrine	T46.3X1	T46.3X2	T46.3X3	T46.3X4	T46.3X5	T46.3X6
Oxygen	T41.5X1	T41.5X2	T41.5X3	T41.5X4	T41.5X5	T41.5X6
Oxylone	T49.0X1	T49.0X2	T49.0X3	T49.0X4	T49.0X5	T49.0X6
ophthalmic preparation	T49.5X1	T49.5X2	T49.5X3	T49.5X4	T49.5X5	T49.5X6
Oxymesterone	T38.7X1	T38.7X2	T38.7X3	T38.7X4	T38.7X5	T38.7X6
Oxymetazoline	T48.5X1	T48.5X2	T48.5X3	T48.5X4	T48.5X5	T48.5X6
Oxymetholone	T38.7X1	T38.7X2	T38.7X3	T38.7X4	T38.7X5	T38.7X6
Oxymorphone	T40.2X1	T40.2X2	T40.2X3	T40.2X4	T40.2X5	T40.2X6
Oxypertine	T43.591	T43.592	T43.593	T43.594	T43.595	T43.596
Oxyphenbutazone	T39.2X1	T39.2X2	T39.2X3	T39.2X4	T39.2X5	T39.2X6
Oxyphencyclimine	T44.3X1	T44.3X2	T44.3X3	T44.3X4	T44.3X5	T44.3X6
Oxyphenisatine	T47.2X1	T47.2X2	T47.2X3	T47.2X4	T47.2X5	T47.2X6

Substance	Poisoning, Accidental (unintentional)	Poisoning, Intentional Self-harm	Poisoning, Assault	Poisoning, Undetermined	Adverse Effect	Underdosing
Oxyphenonium bromide	T44.3X1	T44.3X2	T44.3X3	T44.3X4	T44.3X5	T44.3X6
Oxypolygelatin	T45.8X1	T45.8X2	T45.8X3	T45.8X4	T45.8X5	T45.8X6
Oxyquinoline (derivatives)	T37.8X1	T37.8X2	T37.8X3	T37.8X4	T37.8X5	T37.8X6
Oxytetracycline	T36.4X1	T36.4X2	T36.4X3	T36.4X4	T36.4X5	T36.4X6
Oxytocic drug NEC	T48.0X1	T48.0X2	T48.0X3	T48.0X4	T48.0X5	T48.0X6
Oxytocin (synthetic)	T48.0X1	T48.0X2	T48.0X3	T48.0X4	T48.0X5	T48.0X6
Ozone	T59.891	T59.892	T59.893	T59.894	—	—
PABA	T49.3X1	T49.3X2	T49.3X3	T49.3X4	T49.3X5	T49.3X6
Packed red cells	T45.8X1	T45.8X2	T45.8X3	T45.8X4	T45.8X5	T45.8X6
Padimate	T49.3X1	T49.3X2	T49.3X3	T49.3X4	T49.3X5	T49.3X6
Paint NEC	T65.6X1	T65.6X2	T65.6X3	T65.6X4	—	—
cleaner	T52.91	T52.92	T52.93	T52.94	—	—
fumes NEC	T59.891	T59.892	T59.893	T59.894	—	—
lead (fumes)	T56.0X1	T56.0X2	T56.0X3	T56.0X4	—	—
solvent NEC	T52.8X1	T52.8X2	T52.8X3	T52.8X4	—	—
stripper	T52.8X1	T52.8X2	T52.8X3	T52.8X4	—	—
Palfium	T40.2X1	T40.2X2	T40.2X3	T40.2X4	—	—
Palm kernel oil	T50.991	T50.992	T50.993	T50.994	T50.995	T50.996
Paludrine	T37.2X1	T37.2X2	T37.2X3	T37.2X4	T37.2X5	T37.2X6
PAM (pralidoxime)	T50.6X1	T50.6X2	T50.6X3	T50.6X4	T50.6X5	T50.6X6
Pamaquine (naphthoute)	T37.2X1	T37.2X2	T37.2X3	T37.2X4	T37.2X5	T37.2X6
Panadol	T39.1X1	T39.1X2	T39.1X3	T39.1X4	T39.1X5	T39.1X6
Pancreatic digestive secretion stimulant	T47.8X1	T47.8X2	T47.8X3	T47.8X4	T47.8X5	T47.8X6
dornase	T45.3X1	T45.3X2	T45.3X3	T45.3X4	T45.3X5	T45.3X6
Pancreatin	T47.5X1	T47.5X2	T47.5X3	T47.5X4	T47.5X5	T47.5X6
Pancrelipase	T47.5X1	T47.5X2	T47.5X3	T47.5X4	T47.5X5	T47.5X6
Pancuronium (bromide)	T48.1X1	T48.1X2	T48.1X3	T48.1X4	T48.1X5	T48.1X6
Pangamic acid	T45.2X1	T45.2X2	T45.2X3	T45.2X4	T45.2X5	T45.2X6
Panthenol	T45.2X1	T45.2X2	T45.2X3	T45.2X4	T45.2X5	T45.2X6
topical	T49.8X1	T49.8X2	T49.8X3	T49.8X4	T49.8X5	T49.8X6
Pantopon	T40.0X1	T40.0X2	T40.0X3	T40.0X4	T40.0X5	T40.0X6
Pantothenic acid	T45.2X1	T45.2X2	T45.2X3	T45.2X4	T45.2X5	T45.2X6
Panwarfin	T45.511	T45.512	T45.513	T45.514	T45.515	T45.516
Papain	T47.5X1	T47.5X2	T47.5X3	T47.5X4	T47.5X5	T47.5X6
digestant	T47.5X1	T47.5X2	T47.5X3	T47.5X4	T47.5X5	T47.5X6
Papaveretum	T40.0X1	T40.0X2	T40.0X3	T40.0X4	T40.0X5	T40.0X6
Papaverine	T44.3X1	T44.3X2	T44.3X3	T44.3X4	T44.3X5	T44.3X6
Para-acetamidophenol	T39.1X1	T39.1X2	T39.1X3	T39.1X4	T39.1X5	T39.1X6
Para-aminobenzoic acid	T49.3X1	T49.3X2	T49.3X3	T49.3X4	T49.3X5	T49.3X6
Para-aminophenol derivatives	T39.1X1	T39.1X2	T39.1X3	T39.1X4	T39.1X5	T39.1X6
Para-aminosalicylic acid	T37.1X1	T37.1X2	T37.1X3	T37.1X4	T37.1X5	T37.1X6
Paracetaldehyde	T42.6X1	T42.6X2	T42.6X3	T42.6X4	T42.6X5	T42.6X6
Paracetamol	T39.1X1	T39.1X2	T39.1X3	T39.1X4	T39.1X5	T39.1X6
Parachlorophenol (camphorated)	T49.0X1	T49.0X2	T49.0X3	T49.0X4	T49.0X5	T49.0X6
Paracodin	T40.2X1	T40.2X2	T40.2X3	T40.2X4	T40.2X5	T40.2X6
Paradione	T42.2X1	T42.2X2	T42.2X3	T42.2X4	T42.2X5	T42.2X6
Paraffin(s) (wax)	T52.0X1	T52.0X2	T52.0X3	T52.0X4	—	—
liquid (medicinal)	T47.4X1	T47.4X2	T47.4X3	T47.4X4	T47.4X5	T47.4X6
nonmedicinal	T52.0X1	T52.0X2	T52.0X3	T52.0X4	—	—
Paraformaldehyde	T60.3X1	T60.3X2	T60.3X3	T60.3X4	—	—
Paraldehyde	T42.6X1	T42.6X2	T42.6X3	T42.6X4	T42.6X5	T42.6X6
Paramethadione	T42.2X1	T42.2X2	T42.2X3	T42.2X4	T42.2X5	T42.2X6
Paramethasone	T38.0X1	T38.0X2	T38.0X3	T38.0X4	T38.0X5	T38.0X6
acetate	T49.0X1	T49.0X2	T49.0X3	T49.0X4	T49.0X5	T49.0X6
Paraoxon	T60.0X1	T60.0X2	T60.0X3	T60.0X4	—	—
Paraquat	T60.3X1	T60.3X2	T60.3X3	T60.3X4	—	—
Parasympatholytic NEC	T44.3X1	T44.3X2	T44.3X3	T44.3X4	T44.3X5	T44.3X6
Parasympathomimetic drug NEC	T44.1X1	T44.1X2	T44.1X3	T44.1X4	T44.1X5	T44.1X6
Parathion	T60.0X1	T60.0X2	T60.0X3	T60.0X4	—	—
Parathormone	T50.991	T50.992	T50.993	T50.994	T50.995	T50.996
Parathyroid extract	T50.991	T50.992	T50.993	T50.994	T50.995	T50.996
Paratyphoid vaccine	T50.A91	T50.A92	T50.A93	T50.A94	T50.A95	T50.A96
Paredrine	T44.4X1	T44.4X2	T44.4X3	T44.4X4	T44.4X5	T44.4X6
Paregoric	T40.0X1	T40.0X2	T40.0X3	T40.0X4	T40.0X5	T40.0X6
Pargyline	T46.5X1	T46.5X2	T46.5X3	T46.5X4	T46.5X5	T46.5X6
Paris green	T57.0X1	T57.0X2	T57.0X3	T57.0X4	—	—
insecticide	T57.0X1	T57.0X2	T57.0X3	T57.0X4	—	—
Parnate	T43.1X1	T43.1X2	T43.1X3	T43.1X4	T43.1X5	T43.1X6
Paromomycin	T36.5X1	T36.5X2	T36.5X3	T36.5X4	T36.5X5	T36.5X6
Paroxypropione	T45.1X1	T45.1X2	T45.1X3	T45.1X4	T45.1X5	T45.1X6
Parzone	T40.2X1	T40.2X2	T40.2X3	T40.2X4	T40.2X5	T40.2X6
PAS	T37.1X1	T37.1X2	T37.1X3	T37.1X4	T37.1X5	T37.1X6
Pasiniazid	T37.1X1	T37.1X2	T37.1X3	T37.1X4	T37.1X5	T37.1X6
PBB (polybrominated biphenyls)	T65.891	T65.892	T65.893	T65.894	—	—
PCB	T65.891	T65.892	T65.893	T65.894	—	—

Additional Character May Be Required — Refer to the Tabular List for Character Selection   ▽ Subterms under main terms may continue to next column or page

Substance	Poisoning, Accidental (unintentional)	Poisoning, Intentional Self-harm	Poisoning, Assault	Poisoning, Undetermined	Adverse Effect	Under-dosing
PCP						
meaning pentachlorophenol	T6Ø.1X1	T6Ø.1X2	T6Ø.1X3	T6Ø.1X4	—	—
fungicide	T6Ø.3X1	T6Ø.3X2	T6Ø.3X3	T6Ø.3X4	—	—
herbicide	T6Ø.3X1	T6Ø.3X2	T6Ø.3X3	T6Ø.3X4	—	—
insecticide	T6Ø.1X1	T6Ø.1X2	T6Ø.1X3	T6Ø.1X4	—	—
meaning phencyclidine	T4Ø.991	T4Ø.992	T4Ø.993	T4Ø.994	—	—
Peach kernel oil (emulsion)	T47.4X1	T47.4X2	T47.4X3	T47.4X4	T47.4X5	T47.4X6
Peanut oil (emulsion) **NEC**	T47.4X1	T47.4X2	T47.4X3	T47.4X4	T47.4X5	T47.4X6
topical	T49.3X1	T49.3X2	T49.3X3	T49.3X4	T49.3X5	T49.3X6
Pearly Gates (morning glory seeds)	T4Ø.991	T4Ø.992	T4Ø.993	T4Ø.994	—	—
Pecazine	T43.3X1	T43.3X2	T43.3X3	T43.3X4	T43.3X5	T43.3X6
Pectin	T47.6X1	T47.6X2	T47.6X3	T47.6X4	T47.6X5	T47.6X6
Pefloxacin	T37.8X1	T37.8X2	T37.8X3	T37.8X4	T37.8X5	T37.8X6
Pegademase, bovine	T5Ø.Z91	T5Ø.Z92	T5Ø.Z93	T5Ø.Z94	T5Ø.Z95	T5Ø.Z96
Pelletierine tannate	T37.4X1	T37.4X2	T37.4X3	T37.4X4	T37.4X5	T37.4X6
Pemirolast (potassium)	T48.6X1	T48.6X2	T48.6X3	T48.6X4	T48.6X5	T48.6X6
Pemoline	T5Ø.7X1	T5Ø.7X2	T5Ø.7X3	T5Ø.7X4	T5Ø.7X5	T5Ø.7X6
Pempidine	T44.2X1	T44.2X2	T44.2X3	T44.2X4	T44.2X5	T44.2X6
Penamecillin	T36.ØX1	T36.ØX2	T36.ØX3	T36.ØX4	T36.ØX5	T36.ØX6
Penbutolol	T44.7X1	T44.7X2	T44.7X3	T44.7X4	T44.7X5	T44.7X6
Penethamate	T36.ØX1	T36.ØX2	T36.ØX3	T36.ØX4	T36.ØX5	T36.ØX6
Penfluridol	T43.591	T43.592	T43.593	T43.594	T43.595	T43.596
Penflutizide	T5Ø.2X1	T5Ø.2X2	T5Ø.2X3	T5Ø.2X4	T5Ø.2X5	T5Ø.2X6
Pengitoxin	T46.ØX1	T46.ØX2	T46.ØX3	T46.ØX4	T46.ØX5	T46.ØX6
Penicillamine	T5Ø.6X1	T5Ø.6X2	T5Ø.6X3	T5Ø.6X4	T5Ø.6X5	T5Ø.6X6
Penicillin (any)	T36.ØX1	T36.ØX2	T36.ØX3	T36.ØX4	T36.ØX5	T36.ØX6
Penicillinase	T45.3X1	T45.3X2	T45.3X3	T45.3X4	T45.3X5	T45.3X6
Penicilloyl polylysine	T5Ø.8X1	T5Ø.8X2	T5Ø.8X3	T5Ø.8X4	T5Ø.8X5	T5Ø.8X6
Penimepicycline	T36.4X1	T36.4X2	T36.4X3	T36.4X4	T36.4X5	T36.4X6
Pentachloroethane	T53.6X1	T53.6X2	T53.6X3	T53.6X4	—	—
Pentachloronaphthalene	T53.7X1	T53.7X2	T53.7X3	T53.7X4	—	—
Pentachlorophenol (pesticide)	T6Ø.1X1	T6Ø.1X2	T6Ø.1X3	T6Ø.1X4	—	—
fungicide	T6Ø.3X1	T6Ø.3X2	T6Ø.3X3	T6Ø.3X4	—	—
herbicide	T6Ø.3X1	T6Ø.3X2	T6Ø.3X3	T6Ø.3X4	—	—
insecticide	T6Ø.1X1	T6Ø.1X2	T6Ø.1X3	T6Ø.1X4	—	—
Pentaerythritol	T46.3X1	T46.3X2	T46.3X3	T46.3X4	T46.3X5	T46.3X6
chloral	T42.6X1	T42.6X2	T42.6X3	T42.6X4	T42.6X5	T42.6X6
tetranitrate NEC	T46.3X1	T46.3X2	T46.3X3	T46.3X4	T46.3X5	T46.3X6
Pentaerythrityl tetranitrate	T46.3X1	T46.3X2	T46.3X3	T46.3X4	T46.3X5	T46.3X6
Pentagastrin	T5Ø.8X1	T5Ø.8X2	T5Ø.8X3	T5Ø.8X4	T5Ø.8X5	T5Ø.8X6
Pentalin	T53.6X1	T53.6X2	T53.6X3	T53.6X4	—	—
Pentamethonium bromide	T44.2X1	T44.2X2	T44.2X3	T44.2X4	T44.2X5	T44.2X6
Pentamidine	T37.3X1	T37.3X2	T37.3X3	T37.3X4	T37.3X5	T37.3X6
Pentanol	T51.3X1	T51.3X2	T51.3X3	T51.3X4	—	—
Pentapyrrolinium (bitartrate)	T44.2X1	T44.2X2	T44.2X3	T44.2X4	T44.2X5	T44.2X6
Pentaquine	T37.2X1	T37.2X2	T37.2X3	T37.2X4	T37.2X5	T37.2X6
Pentazocine	T4Ø.491	T4Ø.492	T4Ø.493	T4Ø.494	T4Ø.495	T4Ø.496
Pentetrazole	T5Ø.7X1	T5Ø.7X2	T5Ø.7X3	T5Ø.7X4	T5Ø.7X5	T5Ø.7X6
Penthienate bromide	T44.3X1	T44.3X2	T44.3X3	T44.3X4	T44.3X5	T44.3X6
Pentifylline	T46.7X1	T46.7X2	T46.7X3	T46.7X4	T46.7X5	T46.7X6
Pentobarbital	T42.3X1	T42.3X2	T42.3X3	T42.3X4	T42.3X5	T42.3X6
sodium	T42.3X1	T42.3X2	T42.3X3	T42.3X4	T42.3X5	T42.3X6
Pentobarbitone	T42.3X1	T42.3X2	T42.3X3	T42.3X4	T42.3X5	T42.3X6
Pentolonium tartrate	T44.2X1	T44.2X2	T44.2X3	T44.2X4	T44.2X5	T44.2X6
Pentosan polysulfate (sodium)	T39.8X1	T39.8X2	T39.8X3	T39.8X4	T39.8X5	T39.8X6
Pentostatin	T45.1X1	T45.1X2	T45.1X3	T45.1X4	T45.1X5	T45.1X6
Pentothal	T41.1X1	T41.1X2	T41.1X3	T41.1X4	T41.1X5	T41.1X6
Pentoxifylline	T46.7X1	T46.7X2	T46.7X3	T46.7X4	T46.7X5	T46.7X6
Pentoxyverine	T48.3X1	T48.3X2	T48.3X3	T48.3X4	T48.3X5	T48.3X6
Pentrinat	T46.3X1	T46.3X2	T46.3X3	T46.3X4	T46.3X5	T46.3X6
Pentylenetetrazole	T5Ø.7X1	T5Ø.7X2	T5Ø.7X3	T5Ø.7X4	T5Ø.7X5	T5Ø.7X6
Pentylsalicylamide	T37.1X1	T37.1X2	T37.1X3	T37.1X4	T37.1X5	T37.1X6
Pentymal	T42.3X1	T42.3X2	T42.3X3	T42.3X4	T42.3X5	T42.3X6
Peplomycin	T45.1X1	T45.1X2	T45.1X3	T45.1X4	T45.1X5	T45.1X6
Peppermint (oil)	T47.5X1	T47.5X2	T47.5X3	T47.5X4	T47.5X5	T47.5X6
Pepsin	T47.5X1	T47.5X2	T47.5X3	T47.5X4	T47.5X5	T47.5X6
digestant	T47.5X1	T47.5X2	T47.5X3	T47.5X4	T47.5X5	T47.5X6
Pepstatin	T47.1X1	T47.1X2	T47.1X3	T47.1X4	T47.1X5	T47.1X6
Peptavlon	T5Ø.8X1	T5Ø.8X2	T5Ø.8X3	T5Ø.8X4	T5Ø.8X5	T5Ø.8X6
Perazine	T43.3X1	T43.3X2	T43.3X3	T43.3X4	T43.3X5	T43.3X6
Percaine (spinal)	T41.3X1	T41.3X2	T41.3X3	T41.3X4	T41.3X5	T41.3X6
topical (surface)	T41.3X1	T41.3X2	T41.3X3	T41.3X4	T41.3X5	T41.3X6
Perchloroethylene	T53.3X1	T53.3X2	T53.3X3	T53.3X4	—	—
medicinal	T37.4X1	T37.4X2	T37.4X3	T37.4X4	T37.4X5	T37.4X6
vapor	T53.3X1	T53.3X2	T53.3X3	T53.3X4	—	—
Percodan	T4Ø.2X1	T4Ø.2X2	T4Ø.2X3	T4Ø.2X4	T4Ø.2X5	T4Ø.2X6

Substance	Poisoning, Accidental (unintentional)	Poisoning, Intentional Self-harm	Poisoning, Assault	Poisoning, Undetermined	Adverse Effect	Under-dosing
Percogesic — *see also* acetaminophen	T45.ØX1	T45.ØX2	T45.ØX3	T45.ØX4	T45.ØX5	T45.ØX6
Percorten	T38.ØX1	T38.ØX2	T38.ØX3	T38.ØX4	T38.ØX5	T38.ØX6
Pergolide	T42.8X1	T42.8X2	T42.8X3	T42.8X4	T42.8X5	T42.8X6
Pergonal	T38.811	T38.812	T38.813	T38.814	T38.815	T38.816
Perhexilene	T46.3X1	T46.3X2	T46.3X3	T46.3X4	T46.3X5	T46.3X6
Perhexiline (maleate)	T46.3X1	T46.3X2	T46.3X3	T46.3X4	T46.3X5	T46.3X6
Periactin	T45.ØX1	T45.ØX2	T45.ØX3	T45.ØX4	T45.ØX5	T45.ØX6
Periciazine	T43.3X1	T43.3X2	T43.3X3	T43.3X4	T43.3X5	T43.3X6
Periclor	T42.6X1	T42.6X2	T42.6X3	T42.6X4	T42.6X5	T42.6X6
Perindopril	T46.4X1	T46.4X2	T46.4X3	T46.4X4	T46.4X5	T46.4X6
Perisoxal	T39.8X1	T39.8X2	T39.8X3	T39.8X4	T39.8X5	T39.8X6
Peritoneal dialysis solution	T5Ø.3X1	T5Ø.3X2	T5Ø.3X3	T5Ø.3X4	T5Ø.3X5	T5Ø.3X6
Peritrate	T46.3X1	T46.3X2	T46.3X3	T46.3X4	T46.3X5	T46.3X6
Perlapine	T42.4X1	T42.4X2	T42.4X3	T42.4X4	T42.4X5	T42.4X6
Permanganate	T65.891	T65.892	T65.893	T65.894	—	—
Permethrin	T6Ø.1X1	T6Ø.1X2	T6Ø.1X3	T6Ø.1X4	—	—
Pernocton	T42.3X1	T42.3X2	T42.3X3	T42.3X4	T42.3X5	T42.3X6
Pernoston	T42.3X1	T42.3X2	T42.3X3	T42.3X4	T42.3X5	T42.3X6
Peronine	T4Ø.2X1	T4Ø.2X2	T4Ø.2X3	T4Ø.2X4	—	—
Perphenazine	T43.3X1	T43.3X2	T43.3X3	T43.3X4	T43.3X5	T43.3X6
Pertofrane	T43.Ø11	T43.Ø12	T43.Ø13	T43.Ø14	T43.Ø15	T43.Ø16
Pertussis						
immune serum (human)	T5Ø.Z11	T5Ø.Z12	T5Ø.Z13	T5Ø.Z14	T5Ø.Z15	T5Ø.Z16
vaccine (with diphtheria toxoid) (with tetanus toxoid)	T5Ø.A11	T5Ø.A12	T5Ø.A13	T5Ø.A14	T5Ø.A15	T5Ø.A16
Peruvian balsam	T49.ØX1	T49.ØX2	T49.ØX3	T49.ØX4	T49.ØX5	T49.ØX6
Peruvoside	T46.ØX1	T46.ØX2	T46.ØX3	T46.ØX4	T46.ØX5	T46.ØX6
Pesticide (dust) (fumes) (vapor) **NEC**	T6Ø.91	T6Ø.92	T6Ø.93	T6Ø.94	—	—
arsenic	T57.ØX1	T57.ØX2	T57.ØX3	T57.ØX4	—	—
chlorinated	T6Ø.1X1	T6Ø.1X2	T6Ø.1X3	T6Ø.1X4	—	—
cyanide	T65.ØX1	T65.ØX2	T65.ØX3	T65.ØX4	—	—
kerosene	T52.ØX1	T52.ØX2	T52.ØX3	T52.ØX4	—	—
mixture (of compounds)	T6Ø.91	T6Ø.92	T6Ø.93	T6Ø.94	—	—
naphthalene	T6Ø.2X1	T6Ø.2X2	T6Ø.2X3	T6Ø.2X4	—	—
organochlorine (compounds)	T6Ø.1X1	T6Ø.1X2	T6Ø.1X3	T6Ø.1X4	—	—
petroleum (distillate) (products) NEC	T6Ø.8X1	T6Ø.8X2	T6Ø.8X3	T6Ø.8X4	—	—
specified ingredient NEC	T6Ø.8X1	T6Ø.8X2	T6Ø.8X3	T6Ø.8X4	—	—
strychnine	T65.1X1	T65.1X2	T65.1X3	T65.1X4	—	—
thallium	T6Ø.4X1	T6Ø.4X2	T6Ø.4X3	T6Ø.4X4	—	—
Pethidine	T4Ø.491	T4Ø.492	T4Ø.493	T4Ø.494	T4Ø.495	T4Ø.496
Petrichloral	T42.6X1	T42.6X2	T42.6X3	T42.6X4	T42.6X5	T42.6X6
Petrol	T52.ØX1	T52.ØX2	T52.ØX3	T52.ØX4	—	—
vapor	T52.ØX1	T52.ØX2	T52.ØX3	T52.ØX4	—	—
Petrolatum	T49.3X1	T49.3X2	T49.3X3	T49.3X4	T49.3X5	T49.3X6
hydrophilic	T49.3X1	T49.3X2	T49.3X3	T49.3X4	T49.3X5	T49.3X6
liquid	T47.4X1	T47.4X2	T47.4X3	T47.4X4	T47.4X5	T47.4X6
topical	T49.3X1	T49.3X2	T49.3X3	T49.3X4	T49.3X5	T49.3X6
nonmedicinal	T52.ØX1	T52.ØX2	T52.ØX3	T52.ØX4	—	—
red veterinary	T49.3X1	T49.3X2	T49.3X3	T49.3X4	T49.3X5	T49.3X6
white	T49.3X1	T49.3X2	T49.3X3	T49.3X4	T49.3X5	T49.3X6
Petroleum (products) **NEC**	T52.ØX1	T52.ØX2	T52.ØX3	T52.ØX4	—	—
benzine(s) — *see* Ligroin						
ether — *see* Ligroin						
jelly — *see* Petrolatum						
naphtha — *see* Ligroin						
pesticide	T6Ø.8X1	T6Ø.8X2	T6Ø.8X3	T6Ø.8X4	—	—
solids	T52.ØX1	T52.ØX2	T52.ØX3	T52.ØX4	—	—
solvents	T52.ØX1	T52.ØX2	T52.ØX3	T52.ØX4	—	—
vapor	T52.ØX1	T52.ØX2	T52.ØX3	T52.ØX4	—	—
Peyote	T4Ø.991	T4Ø.992	T4Ø.993	T4Ø.994	—	—
Phanodorm, phanodorn	T42.3X1	T42.3X2	T42.3X3	T42.3X4	T42.3X5	T42.3X6
Phanquinone	T37.3X1	T37.3X2	T37.3X3	T37.3X4	T37.3X5	T37.3X6
Phanquone	T37.3X1	T37.3X2	T37.3X3	T37.3X4	T37.3X5	T37.3X6
Pharmaceutical						
adjunct NEC	T5Ø.9Ø1	T5Ø.9Ø2	T5Ø.9Ø3	T5Ø.9Ø4	T5Ø.9Ø5	T5Ø.9Ø6
excipient NEC	T5Ø.9Ø1	T5Ø.9Ø2	T5Ø.9Ø3	T5Ø.9Ø4	T5Ø.9Ø5	T5Ø.9Ø6
sweetener	T5Ø.9Ø1	T5Ø.9Ø2	T5Ø.9Ø3	T5Ø.9Ø4	T5Ø.9Ø5	T5Ø.9Ø6
viscous agent	T5Ø.9Ø1	T5Ø.9Ø2	T5Ø.9Ø3	T5Ø.9Ø4	T5Ø.9Ø5	T5Ø.9Ø6
Phemitone	T42.3X1	T42.3X2	T42.3X3	T42.3X4	T42.3X5	T42.3X6
Phenacaine	T41.3X1	T41.3X2	T41.3X3	T41.3X4	T41.3X5	T41.3X6
Phenacemide	T42.6X1	T42.6X2	T42.6X3	T42.6X4	T42.6X5	T42.6X6
Phenacetin	T39.1X1	T39.1X2	T39.1X3	T39.1X4	T39.1X5	T39.1X6
Phenadoxone	T4Ø.2X1	T4Ø.2X2	T4Ø.2X3	T4Ø.2X4	—	—
Phenaglycodol	T43.591	T43.592	T43.593	T43.594	T43.595	T43.596
Phenantoin	T42.ØX1	T42.ØX2	T42.ØX3	T42.ØX4	T42.ØX5	T42.ØX6
Phenaphthazine reagent	T5Ø.991	T5Ø.992	T5Ø.993	T5Ø.994	T5Ø.995	T5Ø.996
Phenazocine	T4Ø.491	T4Ø.492	T4Ø.493	T4Ø.494	T4Ø.495	T4Ø.496
Phenazone	T39.2X1	T39.2X2	T39.2X3	T39.2X4	T39.2X5	T39.2X6

Subterms under main terms may continue to next column or page Additional Character May Be Required — Refer to the Tabular List for Character Selection 389

Substance	Poisoning, Accidental (unintentional)	Poisoning, Intentional Self-harm	Poisoning, Assault	Poisoning, Undetermined	Adverse Effect	Under-dosing
Phenazopyridine	T39.8X1	T39.8X2	T39.8X3	T39.8X4	T39.8X5	T39.8X6
Phenbenicillin	T36.ØX1	T36.ØX2	T36.ØX3	T36.ØX4	T36.ØX5	T36.ØX6
Phenbutrazate	T5Ø.5X1	T5Ø.5X2	T5Ø.5X3	T5Ø.5X4	T5Ø.5X5	T5Ø.5X6
Phencyclidine	T4Ø.991	T4Ø.992	T4Ø.993	T4Ø.994	T4Ø.995	T4Ø.996
Phendimetrazine	T5Ø.5X1	T5Ø.5X2	T5Ø.5X3	T5Ø.5X4	T5Ø.5X5	T5Ø.5X6
Phenelzine	T43.1X1	T43.1X2	T43.1X3	T43.1X4	T43.1X5	T43.1X6
Phenemal	T42.3X1	T42.3X2	T42.3X3	T42.3X4	T42.3X5	T42.3X6
Phenergan	T42.6X1	T42.6X2	T42.6X3	T42.6X4	T42.6X5	T42.6X6
Pheneticillin	T36.ØX1	T36.ØX2	T36.ØX3	T36.ØX4	T36.ØX5	T36.ØX6
Pheneturide	T42.6X1	T42.6X2	T42.6X3	T42.6X4	T42.6X5	T42.6X6
Phenformin	T38.3X1	T38.3X2	T38.3X3	T38.3X4	T38.3X5	T38.3X6
Phenglutarimide	T44.3X1	T44.3X2	T44.3X3	T44.3X4	T44.3X5	T44.3X6
Phenicarbazide	T39.8X1	T39.8X2	T39.8X3	T39.8X4	T39.8X5	T39.8X6
Phenindamine	T45.ØX1	T45.ØX2	T45.ØX3	T45.ØX4	T45.ØX5	T45.ØX6
Phenindione	T45.511	T45.512	T45.513	T45.514	T45.515	T45.516
Pheniprazine	T43.1X1	T43.1X2	T43.1X3	T43.1X4	T43.1X5	T43.1X6
Pheniramine	T45.ØX1	T45.ØX2	T45.ØX3	T45.ØX4	T45.ØX5	T45.ØX6
Phenisatin	T47.2X1	T47.2X2	T47.2X3	T47.2X4	T47.2X5	T47.2X6
Phenmetrazine	T5Ø.5X1	T5Ø.5X2	T5Ø.5X3	T5Ø.5X4	T5Ø.5X5	T5Ø.5X6
Phenobal	T42.3X1	T42.3X2	T42.3X3	T42.3X4	T42.3X5	T42.3X6
Phenobarbital	T42.3X1	T42.3X2	T42.3X3	T42.3X4	T42.3X5	T42.3X6
with						
mephenytoin	T42.3X1	T42.3X2	T42.3X3	T42.3X4	T42.3X5	T42.3X6
phenytoin	T42.3X1	T42.3X2	T42.3X3	T42.3X4	T42.3X5	T42.3X6
sodium	T42.3X1	T42.3X2	T42.3X3	T42.3X4	T42.3X5	T42.3X6
Phenobarbitone	T42.3X1	T42.3X2	T42.3X3	T42.3X4	T42.3X5	T42.3X6
Phenobutiodil	T5Ø.8X1	T5Ø.8X2	T5Ø.8X3	T5Ø.8X4	T5Ø.8X5	T5Ø.8X6
Phenoctide	T49.ØX1	T49.ØX2	T49.ØX3	T49.ØX4	T49.ØX5	T49.ØX6
Phenol	T49.ØX1	T49.ØX2	T49.ØX3	T49.ØX4	T49.ØX5	T49.ØX6
disinfectant	T54.ØX1	T54.ØX2	T54.ØX3	T54.ØX4	—	—
in oil injection	T46.8X1	T46.8X2	T46.8X3	T46.8X4	T46.8X5	T46.8X6
medicinal	T49.1X1	T49.1X2	T49.1X3	T49.1X4	T49.1X5	T49.1X6
nonmedicinal NEC	T54.ØX1	T54.ØX2	T54.ØX3	T54.ØX4	—	—
pesticide	T6Ø.8X1	T6Ø.8X2	T6Ø.8X3	T6Ø.8X4	—	—
red	T5Ø.8X1	T5Ø.8X2	T5Ø.8X3	T5Ø.8X4	T5Ø.8X5	T5Ø.8X6
Phenolic preparation	T49.1X1	T49.1X2	T49.1X3	T49.1X4	T49.1X5	T49.1X6
Phenolphthalein	T47.2X1	T47.2X2	T47.2X3	T47.2X4	T47.2X5	T47.2X6
Phenolsulfonphthalein	T5Ø.8X1	T5Ø.8X2	T5Ø.8X3	T5Ø.8X4	T5Ø.8X5	T5Ø.8X6
Phenomorphan	T4Ø.2X1	T4Ø.2X2	T4Ø.2X3	T4Ø.2X4	—	—
Phenonyl	T42.3X1	T42.3X2	T42.3X3	T42.3X4	T42.3X5	T42.3X6
Phenoperidine	T4Ø.491	T4Ø.492	T4Ø.493	T4Ø.494	—	—
Phenopyrazone	T46.991	T46.992	T46.993	T46.994	T46.995	T46.996
Phenoquin	T5Ø.4X1	T5Ø.4X2	T5Ø.4X3	T5Ø.4X4	T5Ø.4X5	T5Ø.4X6
Phenothiazine (psychotropic) **NEC**	T43.3X1	T43.3X2	T43.3X3	T43.3X4	T43.3X5	T43.3X6
insecticide	T6Ø.2X1	T6Ø.2X2	T6Ø.2X3	T6Ø.2X4	—	—
Phenothrin	T49.ØX1	T49.ØX2	T49.ØX3	T49.ØX4	T49.ØX5	T49.ØX6
Phenoxybenzamine	T46.7X1	T46.7X2	T46.7X3	T46.7X4	T46.7X5	T46.7X6
Phenoxyethanol	T49.ØX1	T49.ØX2	T49.ØX3	T49.ØX4	T49.ØX5	T49.ØX6
Phenoxymethyl penicillin	T36.ØX1	T36.ØX2	T36.ØX3	T36.ØX4	T36.ØX5	T36.ØX6
Phenprobamate	T42.8X1	T42.8X2	T42.8X3	T42.8X4	T42.8X5	T42.8X6
Phenprocoumon	T45.511	T45.512	T45.513	T45.514	T45.515	T45.516
Phensuximide	T42.2X1	T42.2X2	T42.2X3	T42.2X4	T42.2X5	T42.2X6
Phentermine	T5Ø.5X1	T5Ø.5X2	T5Ø.5X3	T5Ø.5X4	T5Ø.5X5	T5Ø.5X6
Phenthicillin	T36.ØX1	T36.ØX2	T36.ØX3	T36.ØX4	T36.ØX5	T36.ØX6
Phentolamine	T46.7X1	T46.7X2	T46.7X3	T46.7X4	T46.7X5	T46.7X6
Phenyl						
butazone	T39.2X1	T39.2X2	T39.2X3	T39.2X4	T39.2X5	T39.2X6
enediamine	T65.3X1	T65.3X2	T65.3X3	T65.3X4	—	—
hydrazine	T65.3X1	T65.3X2	T65.3X3	T65.3X4	—	—
antineoplastic	T45.1X1	T45.1X2	T45.1X3	T45.1X4	T45.1X5	T45.1X6
mercuric compounds — *see* Mercury						
salicylate	T49.3X1	T49.3X2	T49.3X3	T49.3X4	T49.3X5	T49.3X6
Phenylalanine mustard	T45.1X1	T45.1X2	T45.1X3	T45.1X4	T45.1X5	T45.1X6
Phenylbutazone	T39.2X1	T39.2X2	T39.2X3	T39.2X4	T39.2X5	T39.2X6
Phenylenediamine	T65.3X1	T65.3X2	T65.3X3	T65.3X4	—	—
Phenylephrine	T44.4X1	T44.4X2	T44.4X3	T44.4X4	T44.4X5	T44.4X6
Phenylethylbiguanide	T38.3X1	T38.3X2	T38.3X3	T38.3X4	T38.3X5	T38.3X6
Phenylmercuric						
acetate	T49.ØX1	T49.ØX2	T49.ØX3	T49.ØX4	T49.ØX5	T49.ØX6
borate	T49.ØX1	T49.ØX2	T49.ØX3	T49.ØX4	T49.ØX5	T49.ØX6
nitrate	T49.ØX1	T49.ØX2	T49.ØX3	T49.ØX4	T49.ØX5	T49.ØX6
Phenylmethylbarbitone	T42.3X1	T42.3X2	T42.3X3	T42.3X4	T42.3X5	T42.3X6
Phenylpropanol	T47.5X1	T47.5X2	T47.5X3	T47.5X4	T47.5X5	T47.5X6
Phenylpropanolamine	T44.991	T44.992	T44.993	T44.994	T44.995	T44.996
Phenylsulfthion	T6Ø.ØX1	T6Ø.ØX2	T6Ø.ØX3	T6Ø.ØX4	—	—
Phenyltoloxamine	T45.ØX1	T45.ØX2	T45.ØX3	T45.ØX4	T45.ØX5	T45.ØX6
Phenyramidol, phenyramidon	T39.8X1	T39.8X2	T39.8X3	T39.8X4	T39.8X5	T39.8X6
Phenytoin	T42.ØX1	T42.ØX2	T42.ØX3	T42.ØX4	T42.ØX5	T42.ØX6
with Phenobarbital	T42.3X1	T42.3X2	T42.3X3	T42.3X4	T42.3X5	T42.3X6
pHisoHex	T49.2X1	T49.2X2	T49.2X3	T49.2X4	T49.2X5	T49.2X6

Substance	Poisoning, Accidental (unintentional)	Poisoning, Intentional Self-harm	Poisoning, Assault	Poisoning, Undetermined	Adverse Effect	Under-dosing
Pholcodine	T48.3X1	T48.3X2	T48.3X3	T48.3X4	T48.3X5	T48.3X6
Pholedrine	T46.991	T46.992	T46.993	T46.994	T46.995	T46.996
Phorate	T6Ø.ØX1	T6Ø.ØX2	T6Ø.ØX3	T6Ø.ØX4	—	—
Phosdrin	T6Ø.ØX1	T6Ø.ØX2	T6Ø.ØX3	T6Ø.ØX4	—	—
Phosfolan	T6Ø.ØX1	T6Ø.ØX2	T6Ø.ØX3	T6Ø.ØX4	—	—
Phosgene (gas)	T59.891	T59.892	T59.893	T59.894	—	—
Phosphamidon	T6Ø.ØX1	T6Ø.ØX2	T6Ø.ØX3	T6Ø.ØX4	—	—
Phosphate	T65.891	T65.892	T65.893	T65.894	—	—
laxative	T47.4X1	T47.4X2	T47.4X3	T47.4X4	T47.4X5	T47.4X6
organic	T6Ø.ØX1	T6Ø.ØX2	T6Ø.ØX3	T6Ø.ØX4	—	—
solvent	T52.91	T52.92	T52.93	T52.94	—	—
tricresyl	T65.891	T65.892	T65.893	T65.894	—	—
Phosphine	T57.1X1	T57.1X2	T57.1X3	T57.1X4	—	—
fumigant	T57.1X1	T57.1X2	T57.1X3	T57.1X4	—	—
Phospholine	T49.5X1	T49.5X2	T49.5X3	T49.5X4	T49.5X5	T49.5X6
Phosphoric acid	T54.2X1	T54.2X2	T54.2X3	T54.2X4	—	—
Phosphorus (compound) **NEC**	T57.1X1	T57.1X2	T57.1X3	T57.1X4	—	—
pesticide	T6Ø.ØX1	T6Ø.ØX2	T6Ø.ØX3	T6Ø.ØX4	—	—
Phthalates	T65.891	T65.892	T65.893	T65.894	—	—
Phthalic anhydride	T65.891	T65.892	T65.893	T65.894	—	—
Phthalimidoglutarimide	T42.6X1	T42.6X2	T42.6X3	T42.6X4	T42.6X5	T42.6X6
Phthalylsulfathiazole	T37.ØX1	T37.ØX2	T37.ØX3	T37.ØX4	T37.ØX5	T37.ØX6
Phylloquinone	T45.7X1	T45.7X2	T45.7X3	T45.7X4	T45.7X5	T45.7X6
Physeptone	T4Ø.3X1	T4Ø.3X2	T4Ø.3X3	T4Ø.3X4	T4Ø.3X5	T4Ø.3X6
Physostigma venenosum	T62.2X1	T62.2X2	T62.2X3	T62.2X4	—	—
Physostigmine	T49.5X1	T49.5X2	T49.5X3	T49.5X4	T49.5X5	T49.5X6
Phytolacca decandra	T62.2X1	T62.2X2	T62.2X3	T62.2X4	—	—
berries	T62.1X1	T62.1X2	T62.1X3	T62.1X4	—	—
Phytomenadione	T45.7X1	T45.7X2	T45.7X3	T45.7X4	T45.7X5	T45.7X6
Phytonadione	T45.7X1	T45.7X2	T45.7X3	T45.7X4	T45.7X5	T45.7X6
Picoperine	T48.3X1	T48.3X2	T48.3X3	T48.3X4	T48.3X5	T48.3X6
Picosulfate (sodium)	T47.2X1	T47.2X2	T47.2X3	T47.2X4	T47.2X5	T47.2X6
Picric (acid)	T54.2X1	T54.2X2	T54.2X3	T54.2X4	—	—
Picrotoxin	T5Ø.7X1	T5Ø.7X2	T5Ø.7X3	T5Ø.7X4	T5Ø.7X5	T5Ø.7X6
Piketoprofen	T49.ØX1	T49.ØX2	T49.ØX3	T49.ØX4	T49.ØX5	T49.ØX6
Pilocarpine	T44.1X1	T44.1X2	T44.1X3	T44.1X4	T44.1X5	T44.1X6
Pilocarpus (jaborandi) extract	T44.1X1	T44.1X2	T44.1X3	T44.1X4	T44.1X5	T44.1X6
Pilsicainide (hydrochloride)	T46.2X1	T46.2X2	T46.2X3	T46.2X4	T46.2X5	T46.2X6
Pimaricin	T36.7X1	T36.7X2	T36.7X3	T36.7X4	T36.7X5	T36.7X6
Pimeclone	T5Ø.7X1	T5Ø.7X2	T5Ø.7X3	T5Ø.7X4	T5Ø.7X5	T5Ø.7X6
Pimelic ketone	T52.8X1	T52.8X2	T52.8X3	T52.8X4	—	—
Pimethixene	T45.ØX1	T45.ØX2	T45.ØX3	T45.ØX4	T45.ØX5	T45.ØX6
Piminodine	T4Ø.2X1	T4Ø.2X2	T4Ø.2X3	T4Ø.2X4	T4Ø.2X5	T4Ø.2X6
Pimozide	T43.591	T43.592	T43.593	T43.594	T43.595	T43.596
Pinacidil	T46.5X1	T46.5X2	T46.5X3	T46.5X4	T46.5X5	T46.5X6
Pinaverium bromide	T44.3X1	T44.3X2	T44.3X3	T44.3X4	T44.3X5	T44.3X6
Pinazepam	T42.4X1	T42.4X2	T42.4X3	T42.4X4	T42.4X5	T42.4X6
Pindolol	T44.7X1	T44.7X2	T44.7X3	T44.7X4	T44.7X5	T44.7X6
Pindone	T6Ø.4X1	T6Ø.4X2	T6Ø.4X3	T6Ø.4X4	—	—
Pine oil (disinfectant)	T65.891	T65.892	T65.893	T65.894	—	—
Pinkroot	T37.4X1	T37.4X2	T37.4X3	T37.4X4	T37.4X5	T37.4X6
Pipadone	T4Ø.2X1	T4Ø.2X2	T4Ø.2X3	T4Ø.2X4	—	—
Pipamazine	T45.ØX1	T45.ØX2	T45.ØX3	T45.ØX4	T45.ØX5	T45.ØX6
Pipamperone	T43.4X1	T43.4X2	T43.4X3	T43.4X4	T43.4X5	T43.4X6
Pipazetate	T48.3X1	T48.3X2	T48.3X3	T48.3X4	T48.3X5	T48.3X6
Pipemidic acid	T37.8X1	T37.8X2	T37.8X3	T37.8X4	T37.8X5	T37.8X6
Pipenzolate bromide	T44.3X1	T44.3X2	T44.3X3	T44.3X4	T44.3X5	T44.3X6
Piperacetazine	T43.3X1	T43.3X2	T43.3X3	T43.3X4	T43.3X5	T43.3X6
Piperacillin	T36.ØX1	T36.ØX2	T36.ØX3	T36.ØX4	T36.ØX5	T36.ØX6
Piperazine	T37.4X1	T37.4X2	T37.4X3	T37.4X4	T37.4X5	T37.4X6
estrone sulfate	T38.5X1	T38.5X2	T38.5X3	T38.5X4	T38.5X5	T38.5X6
Piper cubeba	T62.2X1	T62.2X2	T62.2X3	T62.2X4	—	—
Piperidione	T48.3X1	T48.3X2	T48.3X3	T48.3X4	T48.3X5	T48.3X6
Piperidolate	T44.3X1	T44.3X2	T44.3X3	T44.3X4	T44.3X5	T44.3X6
Piperocaine	T41.3X1	T41.3X2	T41.3X3	T41.3X4	T41.3X5	T41.3X6
infiltration (subcutaneous)	T41.3X1	T41.3X2	T41.3X3	T41.3X4	T41.3X5	T41.3X6
nerve block (peripheral) (plexus)	T41.3X1	T41.3X2	T41.3X3	T41.3X4	T41.3X5	T41.3X6
topical (surface)	T41.3X1	T41.3X2	T41.3X3	T41.3X4	T41.3X5	T41.3X6
Piperonyl butoxide	T6Ø.8X1	T6Ø.8X2	T6Ø.8X3	T6Ø.8X4	—	—
Pipethanate	T44.3X1	T44.3X2	T44.3X3	T44.3X4	T44.3X5	T44.3X6
Pipobroman	T45.1X1	T45.1X2	T45.1X3	T45.1X4	T45.1X5	T45.1X6
Pipotiazine	T43.3X1	T43.3X2	T43.3X3	T43.3X4	T43.3X5	T43.3X6
Pipoxizine	T45.ØX1	T45.ØX2	T45.ØX3	T45.ØX4	T45.ØX5	T45.ØX6
Pipradrol	T43.691	T43.692	T43.693	T43.694	T43.695	T43.696
Piprinhydrinate	T45.ØX1	T45.ØX2	T45.ØX3	T45.ØX4	T45.ØX5	T45.ØX6
Pirarubicin	T45.1X1	T45.1X2	T45.1X3	T45.1X4	T45.1X5	T45.1X6
Pirazinamide	T37.1X1	T37.1X2	T37.1X3	T37.1X4	T37.1X5	T37.1X6
Pirbuterol	T48.6X1	T48.6X2	T48.6X3	T48.6X4	T48.6X5	T48.6X6
Pirenzepine	T47.1X1	T47.1X2	T47.1X3	T47.1X4	T47.1X5	T47.1X6
Piretanide	T5Ø.1X1	T5Ø.1X2	T5Ø.1X3	T5Ø.1X4	T5Ø.1X5	T5Ø.1X6

390 Additional Character May Be Required — Refer to the Tabular List for Character Selection ▽ Subterms under main terms may continue to next column or page

Substance	Poisoning, Accidental (unintentional)	Poisoning, Intentional Self-harm	Poisoning, Assault	Poisoning, Undetermined	Adverse Effect	Under-dosing
Piribedil	T42.8X1	T42.8X2	T42.8X3	T42.8X4	T42.8X5	T42.8X6
Piridoxilate	T46.3X1	T46.3X2	T46.3X3	T46.3X4	T46.3X5	T46.3X6
Piritramide	T4Ø.491	T4Ø.492	T4Ø.493	T4Ø.494	—	—
Piromidic acid	T37.8X1	T37.8X2	T37.8X3	T37.8X4	T37.8X5	T37.8X6
Piroxicam	T39.391	T39.392	T39.393	T39.394	T39.395	T39.396
beta-cyclodextrin complex	T39.8X1	T39.8X2	T39.8X3	T39.8X4	T39.8X5	T39.8X6
Pirozadil	T46.6X1	T46.6X2	T46.6X3	T46.6X4	T46.6X5	T46.6X6
Piscidia (bark) (erythrina)	T39.8X1	T39.8X2	T39.8X3	T39.8X4	T39.8X5	T39.8X6
Pitch	T65.891	T65.892	T65.893	T65.894	—	—
Pitkin's solution	T41.3X1	T41.3X2	T41.3X3	T41.3X4	T41.3X5	T41.3X6
Pitocin	T48.ØX1	T48.ØX2	T48.ØX3	T48.ØX4	T48.ØX5	T48.ØX6
Pitressin (tannate)	T38.891	T38.892	T38.893	T38.894	T38.895	T38.896
Pituitary extracts (posterior)	T38.891	T38.892	T38.893	T38.894	T38.895	T38.896
anterior	T38.811	T38.812	T38.813	T38.814	T38.815	T38.816
Pituitrin	T38.891	T38.892	T38.893	T38.894	T38.895	T38.896
Pivampicillin	T36.ØX1	T36.ØX2	T36.ØX3	T36.ØX4	T36.ØX5	T36.ØX6
Pivmecillinam	T36.ØX1	T36.ØX2	T36.ØX3	T36.ØX4	T36.ØX5	T36.ØX6
Placental hormone	T38.891	T38.892	T38.893	T38.894	T38.895	T38.896
Placidyl	T42.6X1	T42.6X2	T42.6X3	T42.6X4	T42.6X5	T42.6X6
Plague vaccine	T5Ø.A91	T5Ø.A92	T5Ø.A93	T5Ø.A94	T5Ø.A95	T5Ø.A96
Plant						
food or fertilizer NEC	T65.891	T65.892	T65.893	T65.894	—	—
containing herbicide	T6Ø.3X1	T6Ø.3X2	T6Ø.3X3	T6Ø.3X4	—	—
noxious, used as food	T62.2X1	T62.2X2	T62.2X3	T62.2X4	—	—
berries	T62.1X1	T62.1X2	T62.1X3	T62.1X4	—	—
seeds	T62.2X1	T62.2X2	T62.2X3	T62.2X4	—	—
specified type NEC	T62.2X1	T62.2X2	T62.2X3	T62.2X4	—	—
Plasma	T45.8X1	T45.8X2	T45.8X3	T45.8X4	T45.8X5	T45.8X6
expander NEC	T45.8X1	T45.8X2	T45.8X3	T45.8X4	T45.8X5	T45.8X6
protein fraction (human)	T45.8X1	T45.8X2	T45.8X3	T45.8X4	T45.8X5	T45.8X6
Plasmanate	T45.8X1	T45.8X2	T45.8X3	T45.8X4	T45.8X5	T45.8X6
Plasminogen (tissue) activator	T45.611	T45.612	T45.613	T45.614	T45.615	T45.616
Plaster dressing	T49.3X1	T49.3X2	T49.3X3	T49.3X4	T49.3X5	T49.3X6
Plastic dressing	T49.3X1	T49.3X2	T49.3X3	T49.3X4	T49.3X5	T49.3X6
Plegicil	T43.3X1	T43.3X2	T43.3X3	T43.3X4	T43.3X5	T43.3X6
Plicamycin	T45.1X1	T45.1X2	T45.1X3	T45.1X4	T45.1X5	T45.1X6
Podophyllotoxin	T49.8X1	T49.8X2	T49.8X3	T49.8X4	T49.8X5	T49.8X6
Podophyllum (resin)	T49.4X1	T49.4X2	T49.4X3	T49.4X4	T49.4X5	T49.4X6
Poisonous berries	T62.1X1	T62.1X2	T62.1X3	T62.1X4	—	—
Poison NEC	T65.91	T65.92	T65.93	T65.94	—	—
Pokeweed (any part)	T62.2X1	T62.2X2	T62.2X3	T62.2X4	—	—
Poldine metilsulfate	T44.3X1	T44.3X2	T44.3X3	T44.3X4	T44.3X5	T44.3X6
Polidexide (sulfate)	T46.6X1	T46.6X2	T46.6X3	T46.6X4	T46.6X5	T46.6X6
Polidocanol	T46.8X1	T46.8X2	T46.8X3	T46.8X4	T46.8X5	T46.8X6
Poliomyelitis vaccine	T5Ø.B91	T5Ø.B92	T5Ø.B93	T5Ø.B94	T5Ø.B95	T5Ø.B96
Polish (car) (floor) (furniture) (metal) (porcelain) (silver)	T65.891	T65.892	T65.893	T65.894	—	—
abrasive	T65.891	T65.892	T65.893	T65.894	—	—
porcelain	T65.891	T65.892	T65.893	T65.894	—	—
Poloxalkol	T47.4X1	T47.4X2	T47.4X3	T47.4X4	T47.4X5	T47.4X6
Poloxamer	T47.4X1	T47.4X2	T47.4X3	T47.4X4	T47.4X5	T47.4X6
Polyaminostyrene resins	T5Ø.3X1	T5Ø.3X2	T5Ø.3X3	T5Ø.3X4	T5Ø.3X5	T5Ø.3X6
Polycarbophil	T47.4X1	T47.4X2	T47.4X3	T47.4X4	T47.4X5	T47.4X6
Polychlorinated biphenyl	T65.891	T65.892	T65.893	T65.894	—	—
Polycycline	T36.4X1	T36.4X2	T36.4X3	T36.4X4	T36.4X5	T36.4X6
Polyester fumes	T59.891	T59.892	T59.893	T59.894	—	—
Polyester resin hardener	T52.91	T52.92	T52.93	T52.94	—	—
fumes	T59.891	T59.892	T59.893	T59.894	—	—
Polyestradiol phosphate	T38.5X1	T38.5X2	T38.5X3	T38.5X4	T38.5X5	T38.5X6
Polyethanolamine alkyl sulfate	T49.2X1	T49.2X2	T49.2X3	T49.2X4	T49.2X5	T49.2X6
Polyethylene adhesive	T49.3X1	T49.3X2	T49.3X3	T49.3X4	T49.3X5	T49.3X6
Polyferose	T45.4X1	T45.4X2	T45.4X3	T45.4X4	T45.4X5	T45.4X6
Polygeline	T45.8X1	T45.8X2	T45.8X3	T45.8X4	T45.8X5	T45.8X6
Polymyxin	T36.8X1	T36.8X2	T36.8X3	T36.8X4	T36.8X5	T36.8X6
B	T36.8X1	T36.8X2	T36.8X3	T36.8X4	T36.8X5	T36.8X6
ENT agent	T49.6X1	T49.6X2	T49.6X3	T49.6X4	T49.6X5	T49.6X6
ophthalmic preparation	T49.5X1	T49.5X2	T49.5X3	T49.5X4	T49.5X5	T49.5X6
topical NEC	T49.ØX1	T49.ØX2	T49.ØX3	T49.ØX4	T49.ØX5	T49.ØX6
E sulfate (eye preparation)	T49.5X1	T49.5X2	T49.5X3	T49.5X4	T49.5X5	T49.5X6
Polynoxylin	T49.ØX1	T49.ØX2	T49.ØX3	T49.ØX4	T49.ØX5	T49.ØX6
Polyoestradiol phosphate	T38.5X1	T38.5X2	T38.5X3	T38.5X4	T38.5X5	T38.5X6
Polyoxymethyleneurea	T49.ØX1	T49.ØX2	T49.ØX3	T49.ØX4	T49.ØX5	T49.ØX6
Polysilane	T47.8X1	T47.8X2	T47.8X3	T47.8X4	T47.8X5	T47.8X6
Polytetrafluoroethylene (inhaled)	T59.891	T59.892	T59.893	T59.894	—	—
Polythiazide	T5Ø.2X1	T5Ø.2X2	T5Ø.2X3	T5Ø.2X4	T5Ø.2X5	T5Ø.2X6
Polyvidone	T45.8X1	T45.8X2	T45.8X3	T45.8X4	T45.8X5	T45.8X6
Polyvinylpyrrolidone	T45.8X1	T45.8X2	T45.8X3	T45.8X4	T45.8X5	T45.8X6
Pontocaine (hydrochloride) (infiltration) (topical)	T41.3X1	T41.3X2	T41.3X3	T41.3X4	T41.3X5	T41.3X6
nerve block (peripheral) (plexus)	T41.3X1	T41.3X2	T41.3X3	T41.3X4	T41.3X5	T41.3X6
spinal	T41.3X1	T41.3X2	T41.3X3	T41.3X4	T41.3X5	T41.3X6
Porfiromycin	T45.1X1	T45.1X2	T45.1X3	T45.1X4	T45.1X5	T45.1X6
Posterior pituitary hormone NEC	T38.891	T38.892	T38.893	T38.894	T38.895	T38.896
Pot	T4Ø.711	T4Ø.712	T4Ø.713	T4Ø.714	T4Ø.715	T4Ø.716
Potash (caustic)	T54.3X1	T54.3X2	T54.3X3	T54.3X4	—	—
Potassic saline injection (lactated)	T5Ø.3X1	T5Ø.3X2	T5Ø.3X3	T5Ø.3X4	T5Ø.3X5	T5Ø.3X6
Potassium (salts) **NEC**	T5Ø.3X1	T5Ø.3X2	T5Ø.3X3	T5Ø.3X4	T5Ø.3X5	T5Ø.3X6
aminobenzoate	T45.8X1	T45.8X2	T45.8X3	T45.8X4	T45.8X5	T45.8X6
aminosalicylate	T37.1X1	T37.1X2	T37.1X3	T37.1X4	T37.1X5	T37.1X6
antimony 'tartrate'	T37.8X1	T37.8X2	T37.8X3	T37.8X4	T37.8X5	T37.8X6
arsenite (solution)	T57.ØX1	T57.ØX2	T57.ØX3	T57.ØX4	—	—
bichromate	T56.2X1	T56.2X2	T56.2X3	T56.2X4	—	—
bisulfate	T47.3X1	T47.3X2	T47.3X3	T47.3X4	T47.3X5	T47.3X6
bromide	T42.6X1	T42.6X2	T42.6X3	T42.6X4	T42.6X5	T42.6X6
canrenoate	T5Ø.ØX1	T5Ø.ØX2	T5Ø.ØX3	T5Ø.ØX4	T5Ø.ØX5	T5Ø.ØX6
carbonate	T54.3X1	T54.3X2	T54.3X3	T54.3X4	—	—
chlorate NEC	T65.891	T65.892	T65.893	T65.894	—	—
chloride	T5Ø.3X1	T5Ø.3X2	T5Ø.3X3	T5Ø.3X4	T5Ø.3X5	T5Ø.3X6
citrate	T5Ø.991	T5Ø.992	T5Ø.993	T5Ø.994	T5Ø.995	T5Ø.996
cyanide	T65.ØX1	T65.ØX2	T65.ØX3	T65.ØX4	—	—
ferric hexacyanoferrate (medicinal)	T5Ø.6X1	T5Ø.6X2	T5Ø.6X3	T5Ø.6X4	T5Ø.6X5	T5Ø.6X6
nonmedicinal	T65.891	T65.892	T65.893	T65.894	—	—
Fluoride	T57.8X1	T57.8X2	T57.8X3	T57.8X4	—	—
glucaldrate	T47.1X1	T47.1X2	T47.1X3	T47.1X4	T47.1X5	T47.1X6
hydroxide	T54.3X1	T54.3X2	T54.3X3	T54.3X4	—	—
iodate	T49.ØX1	T49.ØX2	T49.ØX3	T49.ØX4	T49.ØX5	T49.ØX6
iodide	T48.4X1	T48.4X2	T48.4X3	T48.4X4	T48.4X5	T48.4X6
nitrate	T57.8X1	T57.8X2	T57.8X3	T57.8X4	—	—
oxalate	T65.891	T65.892	T65.893	T65.894	—	—
perchlorate (nonmedicinal) NEC	T65.891	T65.892	T65.893	T65.894	—	—
antithyroid	T38.2X1	T38.2X2	T38.2X3	T38.2X4	T38.2X5	T38.2X6
medicinal	T38.2X1	T38.2X2	T38.2X3	T38.2X4	T38.2X5	T38.2X6
Permanganate (nonmedicinal)	T65.891	T65.892	T65.893	T65.894	—	—
medicinal	T49.ØX1	T49.ØX2	T49.ØX3	T49.ØX4	T49.ØX5	T49.ØX6
sulfate	T47.2X1	T47.2X2	T47.2X3	T47.2X4	T47.2X5	T47.2X6
Potassium-removing resin	T5Ø.3X1	T5Ø.3X2	T5Ø.3X3	T5Ø.3X4	T5Ø.3X5	T5Ø.3X6
Potassium-retaining drug	T5Ø.3X1	T5Ø.3X2	T5Ø.3X3	T5Ø.3X4	T5Ø.3X5	T5Ø.3X6
Povidone	T45.8X1	T45.8X2	T45.8X3	T45.8X4	T45.8X5	T45.8X6
iodine	T49.ØX1	T49.ØX2	T49.ØX3	T49.ØX4	T49.ØX5	T49.ØX6
Practolol	T44.7X1	T44.7X2	T44.7X3	T44.7X4	T44.7X5	T44.7X6
Prajmalium bitartrate	T46.2X1	T46.2X2	T46.2X3	T46.2X4	T46.2X5	T46.2X6
Pralidoxime (iodide)	T5Ø.6X1	T5Ø.6X2	T5Ø.6X3	T5Ø.6X4	T5Ø.6X5	T5Ø.6X6
chloride	T5Ø.6X1	T5Ø.6X2	T5Ø.6X3	T5Ø.6X4	T5Ø.6X5	T5Ø.6X6
Pramiverine	T44.3X1	T44.3X2	T44.3X3	T44.3X4	T44.3X5	T44.3X6
Pramocaine	T49.1X1	T49.1X2	T49.1X3	T49.1X4	T49.1X5	T49.1X6
Pramoxine	T49.1X1	T49.1X2	T49.1X3	T49.1X4	T49.1X5	T49.1X6
Prasterone	T38.7X1	T38.7X2	T38.7X3	T38.7X4	T38.7X5	T38.7X6
Pravastatin	T46.6X1	T46.6X2	T46.6X3	T46.6X4	T46.6X5	T46.6X6
Prazepam	T42.4X1	T42.4X2	T42.4X3	T42.4X4	T42.4X5	T42.4X6
Praziquantel	T37.4X1	T37.4X2	T37.4X3	T37.4X4	T37.4X5	T37.4X6
Prazitone	T43.291	T43.292	T43.293	T43.294	T43.295	T43.296
Prazosin	T44.6X1	T44.6X2	T44.6X3	T44.6X4	T44.6X5	T44.6X6
Prednicarbate	T49.ØX1	T49.ØX2	T49.ØX3	T49.ØX4	T49.ØX5	T49.ØX6
Prednimustine	T45.1X1	T45.1X2	T45.1X3	T45.1X4	T45.1X5	T45.1X6
Prednisolone	T38.ØX1	T38.ØX2	T38.ØX3	T38.ØX4	T38.ØX5	T38.ØX6
ENT agent	T49.6X1	T49.6X2	T49.6X3	T49.6X4	T49.6X5	T49.6X6
ophthalmic preparation	T49.5X1	T49.5X2	T49.5X3	T49.5X4	T49.5X5	T49.5X6
steaglate	T49.ØX1	T49.ØX2	T49.ØX3	T49.ØX4	T49.ØX5	T49.ØX6
topical NEC	T49.ØX1	T49.ØX2	T49.ØX3	T49.ØX4	T49.ØX5	T49.ØX6
Prednisone	T38.ØX1	T38.ØX2	T38.ØX3	T38.ØX4	T38.ØX5	T38.ØX6
Prednylidene	T38.ØX1	T38.ØX2	T38.ØX3	T38.ØX4	T38.ØX5	T38.ØX6
Pregnandiol	T38.5X1	T38.5X2	T38.5X3	T38.5X4	T38.5X5	T38.5X6
Pregneninolone	T38.5X1	T38.5X2	T38.5X3	T38.5X4	T38.5X5	T38.5X6
Preludin	T43.691	T43.692	T43.693	T43.694	T43.695	T43.696
Premarin	T38.5X1	T38.5X2	T38.5X3	T38.5X4	T38.5X5	T38.5X6
Premedication anesthetic	T41.2Ø1	T41.2Ø2	T41.2Ø3	T41.2Ø4	T41.2Ø5	T41.2Ø6
Prenalterol	T44.5X1	T44.5X2	T44.5X3	T44.5X4	T44.5X5	T44.5X6
Prenoxdiazine	T48.3X1	T48.3X2	T48.3X3	T48.3X4	T48.3X5	T48.3X6
Prenylamine	T46.3X1	T46.3X2	T46.3X3	T46.3X4	T46.3X5	T46.3X6
Preparation H	T49.8X1	T49.8X2	T49.8X3	T49.8X4	T49.8X5	T49.8X6
Preparation, local	T49.4X1	T49.4X2	T49.4X3	T49.4X4	T49.4X5	T49.4X6
Preservative (nonmedicinal)	T65.891	T65.892	T65.893	T65.894	—	—
medicinal	T5Ø.9Ø1	T5Ø.9Ø2	T5Ø.9Ø3	T5Ø.9Ø4	T5Ø.9Ø5	T5Ø.9Ø6

Subterms under main terms may continue to next column or page

Additional Character May Be Required — Refer to the Tabular List for Character Selection

391

Substance	Poisoning, Accidental (unintentional)	Poisoning, Intentional Self-harm	Poisoning, Assault	Poisoning, Undetermined	Adverse Effect	Under-dosing
Preservative — *continued*						
wood	T6Ø.91	T6Ø.92	T6Ø.93	T6Ø.94	—	—
Prethcamide	T5Ø.7X1	T5Ø.7X2	T5Ø.7X3	T5Ø.7X4	T5Ø.7X5	T5Ø.7X6
Pride of China	T62.2X1	T62.2X2	T62.2X3	T62.2X4	—	—
Pridinol	T44.3X1	T44.3X2	T44.3X3	T44.3X4	T44.3X5	T44.3X6
Prifinium bromide	T44.3X1	T44.3X2	T44.3X3	T44.3X4	T44.3X5	T44.3X6
Prilocaine	T41.3X1	T41.3X2	T41.3X3	T41.3X4	T41.3X5	T41.3X6
infiltration (subcutaneous)	T41.3X1	T41.3X2	T41.3X3	T41.3X4	T41.3X5	T41.3X6
nerve block (peripheral) (plexus)	T41.3X1	T41.3X2	T41.3X3	T41.3X4	T41.3X5	T41.3X6
regional	T41.3X1	T41.3X2	T41.3X3	T41.3X4	T41.3X5	T41.3X6
Primaquine	T37.2X1	T37.2X2	T37.2X3	T37.2X4	T37.2X5	T37.2X6
Primidone	T42.6X1	T42.6X2	T42.6X3	T42.6X4	T42.6X5	T42.6X6
Primula (veris)	T62.2X1	T62.2X2	T62.2X3	T62.2X4	—	—
Prinadol	T4Ø.2X1	T4Ø.2X2	T4Ø.2X3	T4Ø.2X4	T4Ø.2X5	T4Ø.2X6
Priscol, Priscoline	T44.6X1	T44.6X2	T44.6X3	T44.6X4	T44.6X5	T44.6X6
Pristinamycin	T36.3X1	T36.3X2	T36.3X3	T36.3X4	T36.3X5	T36.3X6
Privet	T62.2X1	T62.2X2	T62.2X3	T62.2X4	—	—
berries	T62.1X1	T62.1X2	T62.1X3	T62.1X4	—	—
Privine	T44.4X1	T44.4X2	T44.4X3	T44.4X4	T44.4X5	T44.4X6
Pro-Banthine	T44.3X1	T44.3X2	T44.3X3	T44.3X4	T44.3X5	T44.3X6
Probarbital	T42.3X1	T42.3X2	T42.3X3	T42.3X4	T42.3X5	T42.3X6
Probenecid	T5Ø.4X1	T5Ø.4X2	T5Ø.4X3	T5Ø.4X4	T5Ø.4X5	T5Ø.4X6
Probucol	T46.6X1	T46.6X2	T46.6X3	T46.6X4	T46.6X5	T46.6X6
Procainamide	T46.2X1	T46.2X2	T46.2X3	T46.2X4	T46.2X5	T46.2X6
Procaine	T41.3X1	T41.3X2	T41.3X3	T41.3X4	T41.3X5	T41.3X6
benzylpenicillin	T36.ØX1	T36.ØX2	T36.ØX3	T36.ØX4	T36.ØX5	T36.ØX6
nerve block (periphreal) (plexus)	T41.3X1	T41.3X2	T41.3X3	T41.3X4	T41.3X5	T41.3X6
penicillin G	T36.ØX1	T36.ØX2	T36.ØX3	T36.ØX4	T36.ØX5	T36.ØX6
regional	T41.3X1	T41.3X2	T41.3X3	T41.3X4	T41.3X5	T41.3X6
spinal	T41.3X1	T41.3X2	T41.3X3	T41.3X4	T41.3X5	T41.3X6
Procalmidol	T43.591	T43.592	T43.593	T43.594	T43.595	T43.596
Procarbazine	T45.1X1	T45.1X2	T45.1X3	T45.1X4	T45.1X5	T45.1X6
Procaterol	T44.5X1	T44.5X2	T44.5X3	T44.5X4	T44.5X5	T44.5X6
Prochlorperazine	T43.3X1	T43.3X2	T43.3X3	T43.3X4	T43.3X5	T43.3X6
Procyclidine	T44.3X1	T44.3X2	T44.3X3	T44.3X4	T44.3X5	T44.3X6
Producer gas	T58.8X1	T58.8X2	T58.8X3	T58.8X4	—	—
Profadol	T4Ø.491	T4Ø.492	T4Ø.493	T4Ø.494	T4Ø.495	T4Ø.496
Profenamine	T44.3X1	T44.3X2	T44.3X3	T44.3X4	T44.3X5	T44.3X6
Profenil	T44.3X1	T44.3X2	T44.3X3	T44.3X4	T44.3X5	T44.3X6
Proflavine	T49.ØX1	T49.ØX2	T49.ØX3	T49.ØX4	T49.ØX5	T49.ØX6
Progabide	T42.6X1	T42.6X2	T42.6X3	T42.6X4	T42.6X5	T42.6X6
Progesterone	T38.5X1	T38.5X2	T38.5X3	T38.5X4	T38.5X5	T38.5X6
Progestin	T38.5X1	T38.5X2	T38.5X3	T38.5X4	T38.5X5	T38.5X6
oral contraceptive	T38.4X1	T38.4X2	T38.4X3	T38.4X4	T38.4X5	T38.4X6
Progestogen NEC	T38.5X1	T38.5X2	T38.5X3	T38.5X4	T38.5X5	T38.5X6
Progestone	T38.5X1	T38.5X2	T38.5X3	T38.5X4	T38.5X5	T38.5X6
Proglumide	T47.1X1	T47.1X2	T47.1X3	T47.1X4	T47.1X5	T47.1X6
Proguanil	T37.2X1	T37.2X2	T37.2X3	T37.2X4	T37.2X5	T37.2X6
Prolactin	T38.811	T38.812	T38.813	T38.814	T38.815	T38.816
Prolintane	T43.691	T43.692	T43.693	T43.694	T43.695	T43.696
Proloid	T38.1X1	T38.1X2	T38.1X3	T38.1X4	T38.1X5	T38.1X6
Proluton	T38.5X1	T38.5X2	T38.5X3	T38.5X4	T38.5X5	T38.5X6
Promacetin	T37.1X1	T37.1X2	T37.1X3	T37.1X4	T37.1X5	T37.1X6
Promazine	T43.3X1	T43.3X2	T43.3X3	T43.3X4	T43.3X5	T43.3X6
Promedol	T4Ø.2X1	T4Ø.2X2	T4Ø.2X3	T4Ø.2X4	—	—
Promegestone	T38.5X1	T38.5X2	T38.5X3	T38.5X4	T38.5X5	T38.5X6
Promethazine (teoclate)	T43.3X1	T43.3X2	T43.3X3	T43.3X4	T43.3X5	T43.3X6
Promin	T37.1X1	T37.1X2	T37.1X3	T37.1X4	T37.1X5	T37.1X6
Pronase	T45.3X1	T45.3X2	T45.3X3	T45.3X4	T45.3X5	T45.3X6
Pronestyl (hydrochloride)	T46.2X1	T46.2X2	T46.2X3	T46.2X4	T46.2X5	T46.2X6
Pronetalol	T44.7X1	T44.7X2	T44.7X3	T44.7X4	T44.7X5	T44.7X6
Prontosil	T37.ØX1	T37.ØX2	T37.ØX3	T37.ØX4	T37.ØX5	T37.ØX6
Propachlor	T6Ø.3X1	T6Ø.3X2	T6Ø.3X3	T6Ø.3X4	—	—
Propafenone	T46.2X1	T46.2X2	T46.2X3	T46.2X4	T46.2X5	T46.2X6
Propallylonal	T42.3X1	T42.3X2	T42.3X3	T42.3X4	T42.3X5	T42.3X6
Propamidine	T49.ØX1	T49.ØX2	T49.ØX3	T49.ØX4	T49.ØX5	T49.ØX6
Propane (distributed in mobile container)	T59.891	T59.892	T59.893	T59.894	—	—
distributed through pipes	T59.891	T59.892	T59.893	T59.894	—	—
incomplete combustion	T58.11	T58.12	T58.13	T58.14	—	—
Propanidid	T41.291	T41.292	T41.293	T41.294	T41.295	T41.296
Propanil	T6Ø.3X1	T6Ø.3X2	T6Ø.3X3	T6Ø.3X4	—	—
Propantheline	T44.3X1	T44.3X2	T44.3X3	T44.3X4	T44.3X5	T44.3X6
bromide	T44.3X1	T44.3X2	T44.3X3	T44.3X4	T44.3X5	T44.3X6
Proparacaine	T41.3X1	T41.3X2	T41.3X3	T41.3X4	T41.3X5	T41.3X6
Propatylnitrate	T46.3X1	T46.3X2	T46.3X3	T46.3X4	T46.3X5	T46.3X6
Propicillin	T36.ØX1	T36.ØX2	T36.ØX3	T36.ØX4	T36.ØX5	T36.ØX6
Propiolactone	T49.ØX1	T49.ØX2	T49.ØX3	T49.ØX4	T49.ØX5	T49.ØX6
Propiomazine	T45.ØX1	T45.ØX2	T45.ØX3	T45.ØX4	T45.ØX5	T45.ØX6
Propionaldehyde (medicinal)	T42.6X1	T42.6X2	T42.6X3	T42.6X4	T42.6X5	T42.6X6

Substance	Poisoning, Accidental (unintentional)	Poisoning, Intentional Self-harm	Poisoning, Assault	Poisoning, Undetermined	Adverse Effect	Under-dosing
Propionate (calcium) (sodium)	T49.ØX1	T49.ØX2	T49.ØX3	T49.ØX4	T49.ØX5	T49.ØX6
Propion gel	T49.ØX1	T49.ØX2	T49.ØX3	T49.ØX4	T49.ØX5	T49.ØX6
Propitocaine	T41.3X1	T41.3X2	T41.3X3	T41.3X4	T41.3X5	T41.3X6
infiltration (subcutaneous)	T41.3X1	T41.3X2	T41.3X3	T41.3X4	T41.3X5	T41.3X6
nerve block (peripheral) (plexus)	T41.3X1	T41.3X2	T41.3X3	T41.3X4	T41.3X5	T41.3X6
Propofol	T41.291	T41.292	T41.293	T41.294	T41.295	T41.296
Propoxur	T6Ø.ØX1	T6Ø.ØX2	T6Ø.ØX3	T6Ø.ØX4	—	—
Propoxycaine	T41.3X1	T41.3X2	T41.3X3	T41.3X4	T41.3X5	T41.3X6
infiltration (subcutaneous)	T41.3X1	T41.3X2	T41.3X3	T41.3X4	T41.3X5	T41.3X6
nerve block (peripheral) (plexus)	T41.3X1	T41.3X2	T41.3X3	T41.3X4	T41.3X5	T41.3X6
topical (surface)	T41.3X1	T41.3X2	T41.3X3	T41.3X4	T41.3X5	T41.3X6
Propoxyphene	T4Ø.491	T4Ø.492	T4Ø.493	T4Ø.494	T4Ø.495	T4Ø.496
Propranolol	T44.7X1	T44.7X2	T44.7X3	T44.7X4	T44.7X5	T44.7X6
Propyl						
alcohol	T51.3X1	T51.3X2	T51.3X3	T51.3X4	—	—
carbinol	T51.3X1	T51.3X2	T51.3X3	T51.3X4	—	—
hexadrine	T44.4X1	T44.4X2	T44.4X3	T44.4X4	T44.4X5	T44.4X6
iodone	T5Ø.8X1	T5Ø.8X2	T5Ø.8X3	T5Ø.8X4	T5Ø.8X5	T5Ø.8X6
thiouracil	T38.2X1	T38.2X2	T38.2X3	T38.2X4	T38.2X5	T38.2X6
Propylaminophenothiazine	T43.3X1	T43.3X2	T43.3X3	T43.3X4	T43.3X5	T43.3X6
Propylene	T59.891	T59.892	T59.893	T59.894	—	—
Propylhexedrine	T48.5X1	T48.5X2	T48.5X3	T48.5X4	T48.5X5	T48.5X6
Propyliodone	T5Ø.8X1	T5Ø.8X2	T5Ø.8X3	T5Ø.8X4	T5Ø.8X5	T5Ø.8X6
Propylparaben (ophthalmic)	T49.5X1	T49.5X2	T49.5X3	T49.5X4	T49.5X5	T49.5X6
Propylthiouracil	T38.2X1	T38.2X2	T38.2X3	T38.2X4	T38.2X5	T38.2X6
Propyphenazone	T39.2X1	T39.2X2	T39.2X3	T39.2X4	T39.2X5	T39.2X6
Proquazone	T39.391	T39.392	T39.393	T39.394	T39.395	T39.396
Proscillaridin	T46.ØX1	T46.ØX2	T46.ØX3	T46.ØX4	T46.ØX5	T46.ØX6
Prostacyclin	T45.521	T45.522	T45.523	T45.524	T45.525	T45.526
Prostaglandin (I2)	T45.521	T45.522	T45.523	T45.524	T45.525	T45.526
E1	T46.7X1	T46.7X2	T46.7X3	T46.7X4	T46.7X5	T46.7X6
E2	T48.ØX1	T48.ØX2	T48.ØX3	T48.ØX4	T48.ØX5	T48.ØX6
F2 alpha	T48.ØX1	T48.ØX2	T48.ØX3	T48.ØX4	T48.ØX5	T48.ØX6
Prostigmin	T44.ØX1	T44.ØX2	T44.ØX3	T44.ØX4	T44.ØX5	T44.ØX6
Prosultiamine	T45.2X1	T45.2X2	T45.2X3	T45.2X4	T45.2X5	T45.2X6
Protamine sulfate	T45.7X1	T45.7X2	T45.7X3	T45.7X4	T45.7X5	T45.7X6
zinc insulin	T38.3X1	T38.3X2	T38.3X3	T38.3X4	T38.3X5	T38.3X6
Protease	T47.5X1	T47.5X2	T47.5X3	T47.5X4	T47.5X5	T47.5X6
Protectant, skin NEC	T49.3X1	T49.3X2	T49.3X3	T49.3X4	T49.3X5	T49.3X6
Protein hydrolysate	T5Ø.991	T5Ø.992	T5Ø.993	T5Ø.994	T5Ø.995	T5Ø.996
Prothiaden — *see* Dothiepin hydrochloride						
Prothionamide	T37.1X1	T37.1X2	T37.1X3	T37.1X4	T37.1X5	T37.1X6
Prothipendyl	T43.591	T43.592	T43.593	T43.594	T43.595	T43.596
Prothoate	T6Ø.ØX1	T6Ø.ØX2	T6Ø.ØX3	T6Ø.ØX4	—	—
Prothrombin						
activator	T45.7X1	T45.7X2	T45.7X3	T45.7X4	T45.7X5	T45.7X6
synthesis inhibitor	T45.511	T45.512	T45.513	T45.514	T45.515	T45.516
Protionamide	T37.1X1	T37.1X2	T37.1X3	T37.1X4	T37.1X5	T37.1X6
Protirelin	T38.891	T38.892	T38.893	T38.894	T38.895	T38.896
Protokylol	T48.6X1	T48.6X2	T48.6X3	T48.6X4	T48.6X5	T48.6X6
Protopam	T5Ø.6X1	T5Ø.6X2	T5Ø.6X3	T5Ø.6X4	T5Ø.6X5	T5Ø.6X6
Protoveratrine(s) (A) (B)	T46.5X1	T46.5X2	T46.5X3	T46.5X4	T46.5X5	T46.5X6
Protriptyline	T43.Ø11	T43.Ø12	T43.Ø13	T43.Ø14	T43.Ø15	T43.Ø16
Provera	T38.5X1	T38.5X2	T38.5X3	T38.5X4	T38.5X5	T38.5X6
Provitamin A	T45.2X1	T45.2X2	T45.2X3	T45.2X4	T45.2X5	T45.2X6
Proxibarbal	T42.3X1	T42.3X2	T42.3X3	T42.3X4	T42.3X5	T42.3X6
Proxymetacaine	T41.3X1	T41.3X2	T41.3X3	T41.3X4	T41.3X5	T41.3X6
Proxyphylline	T48.6X1	T48.6X2	T48.6X3	T48.6X4	T48.6X5	T48.6X6
Prozac — *see* Fluoxetine hydrochloride						
Prunus						
laurocerasus	T62.2X1	T62.2X2	T62.2X3	T62.2X4	—	—
virginiana	T62.2X1	T62.2X2	T62.2X3	T62.2X4	—	—
Prussian blue						
commercial	T65.891	T65.892	T65.893	T65.894	—	—
therapeutic	T5Ø.6X1	T5Ø.6X2	T5Ø.6X3	T5Ø.6X4	T5Ø.6X5	T5Ø.6X6
Prussic acid	T65.ØX1	T65.ØX2	T65.ØX3	T65.ØX4	—	—
vapor	T57.3X1	T57.3X2	T57.3X3	T57.3X4	—	—
Pseudoephedrine	T44.991	T44.992	T44.993	T44.994	T44.995	T44.996
Psilocin	T4Ø.991	T4Ø.992	T4Ø.993	T4Ø.994	—	—
Psilocybin	T4Ø.991	T4Ø.992	T4Ø.993	T4Ø.994	—	—
Psilocybine	T4Ø.991	T4Ø.992	T4Ø.993	T4Ø.994	—	—
Psoralene (nonmedicinal)	T65.891	T65.892	T65.893	T65.894	—	—
Psoralens (medicinal)	T5Ø.991	T5Ø.992	T5Ø.993	T5Ø.994	T5Ø.995	T5Ø.996
PSP (phenolsulfonphthalein)	T5Ø.8X1	T5Ø.8X2	T5Ø.8X3	T5Ø.8X4	T5Ø.8X5	T5Ø.8X6
Psychodysleptic drug NOS	T4Ø.9Ø1	T4Ø.9Ø2	T4Ø.9Ø3	T4Ø.9Ø4	T4Ø.9Ø5	T4Ø.9Ø6
specified NEC	T4Ø.991	T4Ø.992	T4Ø.993	T4Ø.994	T4Ø.995	T4Ø.996

Preservative — Psychodysleptic drug NOS
392 Additional Character May Be Required — Refer to the Tabular List for Character Selection
Subterms under main terms may continue to next column or page

Substance	Poisoning, Accidental (unintentional)	Poisoning, Intentional Self-harm	Poisoning, Assault	Poisoning, Undetermined	Adverse Effect	Under-dosing
Psychostimulant	T43.6Ø1	T43.6Ø2	T43.6Ø3	T43.6Ø4	T43.6Ø5	T43.6Ø6
amphetamine	T43.621	T43.622	T43.623	T43.624	T43.625	T43.626
caffeine	T43.611	T43.612	T43.613	T43.614	T43.615	T43.616
methylphenidate	T43.631	T43.632	T43.633	T43.634	T43.635	T43.636
specified NEC	T43.691	T43.692	T43.693	T43.694	T43.695	T43.696
Psychotherapeutic drug NEC	T43.91	T43.92	T43.93	T43.94	T43.95	T43.96
antidepressants — *see also* Antidepressant	T43.2Ø1	T43.2Ø2	T43.2Ø3	T43.2Ø4	T43.2Ø5	T43.2Ø6
specified NEC	T43.8X1	T43.8X2	T43.8X3	T43.8X4	T43.8X5	T43.8X6
tranquilizers NEC	T43.5Ø1	T43.5Ø2	T43.5Ø3	T43.5Ø4	T43.5Ø5	T43.5Ø6
Psychotomimetic agents	T4Ø.9Ø1	T4Ø.9Ø2	T4Ø.9Ø3	T4Ø.9Ø4	T4Ø.9Ø5	T4Ø.9Ø6
Psychotropic drug NEC	T43.91	T43.92	T43.93	T43.94	T43.95	T43.96
specified NEC	T43.8X1	T43.8X2	T43.8X3	T43.8X4	T43.8X5	T43.8X6
Psyllium hydrophilic mucilloid	T47.4X1	T47.4X2	T47.4X3	T47.4X4	T47.4X5	T47.4X6
Pteroylglutamic acid	T45.8X1	T45.8X2	T45.8X3	T45.8X4	T45.8X5	T45.8X6
Pteroyltriglutamate	T45.1X1	T45.1X2	T45.1X3	T45.1X4	T45.1X5	T45.1X6
PTFE — *see* Polytetrafluoroethylene						
Pulp						
devitalizing paste	T49.7X1	T49.7X2	T49.7X3	T49.7X4	T49.7X5	T49.7X6
dressing	T49.7X1	T49.7X2	T49.7X3	T49.7X4	T49.7X5	T49.7X6
Pulsatilla	T62.2X1	T62.2X2	T62.2X3	T62.2X4	—	—
Pumpkin seed extract	T37.4X1	T37.4X2	T37.4X3	T37.4X4	T37.4X5	T37.4X6
Purex (bleach)	T54.91	T54.92	T54.93	T54.94	—	—
Purgative NEC — *see also* Cathartic	T47.4X1	T47.4X2	T47.4X3	T47.4X4	T47.4X5	T47.4X6
Purine analogue (antineoplastic)	T45.1X1	T45.1X2	T45.1X3	T45.1X4	T45.1X5	T45.1X6
Purine diuretics	T5Ø.2X1	T5Ø.2X2	T5Ø.2X3	T5Ø.2X4	T5Ø.2X5	T5Ø.2X6
Purinethol	T45.1X1	T45.1X2	T45.1X3	T45.1X4	T45.1X5	T45.1X6
PVP	T45.8X1	T45.8X2	T45.8X3	T45.8X4	T45.8X5	T45.8X6
Pyrabital	T39.8X1	T39.8X2	T39.8X3	T39.8X4	T39.8X5	T39.8X6
Pyramidon	T39.2X1	T39.2X2	T39.2X3	T39.2X4	T39.2X5	T39.2X6
Pyrantel	T37.4X1	T37.4X2	T37.4X3	T37.4X4	T37.4X5	T37.4X6
Pyrathiazine	T45.ØX1	T45.ØX2	T45.ØX3	T45.ØX4	T45.ØX5	T45.ØX6
Pyrazinamide	T37.1X1	T37.1X2	T37.1X3	T37.1X4	T37.1X5	T37.1X6
Pyrazinoic acid (amide)	T37.1X1	T37.1X2	T37.1X3	T37.1X4	T37.1X5	T37.1X6
Pyrazole (derivatives)	T39.2X1	T39.2X2	T39.2X3	T39.2X4	T39.2X5	T39.2X6
Pyrazolone analgesic NEC	T39.2X1	T39.2X2	T39.2X3	T39.2X4	T39.2X5	T39.2X6
Pyrethrin, pyrethrum (nonmedicinal)	T6Ø.2X1	T6Ø.2X2	T6Ø.2X3	T6Ø.2X4	—	—
Pyrethrum extract	T49.ØX1	T49.ØX2	T49.ØX3	T49.ØX4	T49.ØX5	T49.ØX6
Pyribenzamine	T45.ØX1	T45.ØX2	T45.ØX3	T45.ØX4	T45.ØX5	T45.ØX6
Pyridine	T52.8X1	T52.8X2	T52.8X3	T52.8X4	—	—
aldoxime methiodide	T5Ø.6X1	T5Ø.6X2	T5Ø.6X3	T5Ø.6X4	T5Ø.6X5	T5Ø.6X6
aldoxime methyl chloride	T5Ø.6X1	T5Ø.6X2	T5Ø.6X3	T5Ø.6X4	T5Ø.6X5	T5Ø.6X6
vapor	T59.891	T59.892	T59.893	T59.894	—	—
Pyridium	T39.8X1	T39.8X2	T39.8X3	T39.8X4	T39.8X5	T39.8X6
Pyridostigmine bromide	T44.ØX1	T44.ØX2	T44.ØX3	T44.ØX4	T44.ØX5	T44.ØX6
Pyridoxal phosphate	T45.2X1	T45.2X2	T45.2X3	T45.2X4	T45.2X5	T45.2X6
Pyridoxine	T45.2X1	T45.2X2	T45.2X3	T45.2X4	T45.2X5	T45.2X6
Pyrilamine	T45.ØX1	T45.ØX2	T45.ØX3	T45.ØX4	T45.ØX5	T45.ØX6
Pyrimethamine	T37.2X1	T37.2X2	T37.2X3	T37.2X4	T37.2X5	T37.2X6
with sulfadoxine	T37.2X1	T37.2X2	T37.2X3	T37.2X4	T37.2X5	T37.2X6
Pyrimidine antagonist	T45.1X1	T45.1X2	T45.1X3	T45.1X4	T45.1X5	T45.1X6
Pyriminil	T6Ø.4X1	T6Ø.4X2	T6Ø.4X3	T6Ø.4X4	—	—
Pyrithione zinc	T49.4X1	T49.4X2	T49.4X3	T49.4X4	T49.4X5	T49.4X6
Pyrithyldione	T42.6X1	T42.6X2	T42.6X3	T42.6X4	T42.6X5	T42.6X6
Pyrogallic acid	T49.ØX1	T49.ØX2	T49.ØX3	T49.ØX4	T49.ØX5	T49.ØX6
Pyrogallol	T49.ØX1	T49.ØX2	T49.ØX3	T49.ØX4	T49.ØX5	T49.ØX6
Pyroxylin	T49.3X1	T49.3X2	T49.3X3	T49.3X4	T49.3X5	T49.3X6
Pyrrobutamine	T45.ØX1	T45.ØX2	T45.ØX3	T45.ØX4	T45.ØX5	T45.ØX6
Pyrrolizidine alkaloids	T62.8X1	T62.8X2	T62.8X3	T62.8X4	—	—
Pyrvinium chloride	T37.4X1	T37.4X2	T37.4X3	T37.4X4	T37.4X5	T37.4X6
PZI	T38.3X1	T38.3X2	T38.3X3	T38.3X4	T38.3X5	T38.3X6
Quaalude	T42.6X1	T42.6X2	T42.6X3	T42.6X4	T42.6X5	T42.6X6
Quarternary ammonium						
anti-infective	T49.ØX1	T49.ØX2	T49.ØX3	T49.ØX4	T49.ØX5	T49.ØX6
ganglion blocking	T44.2X1	T44.2X2	T44.2X3	T44.2X4	T44.2X5	T44.2X6
parasympatholytic	T44.3X1	T44.3X2	T44.3X3	T44.3X4	T44.3X5	T44.3X6
Quazepam	T42.4X1	T42.4X2	T42.4X3	T42.4X4	T42.4X5	T42.4X6
Quicklime	T54.3X1	T54.3X2	T54.3X3	T54.3X4	—	—
Quillaja extract	T48.4X1	T48.4X2	T48.4X3	T48.4X4	T48.4X5	T48.4X6
Quinacrine	T37.2X1	T37.2X2	T37.2X3	T37.2X4	T37.2X5	T37.2X6
Quinaglute	T46.2X1	T46.2X2	T46.2X3	T46.2X4	T46.2X5	T46.2X6
Quinalbarbital	T42.3X1	T42.3X2	T42.3X3	T42.3X4	T42.3X5	T42.3X6
Quinalbarbitone sodium	T42.3X1	T42.3X2	T42.3X3	T42.3X4	T42.3X5	T42.3X6
Quinalphos	T6Ø.ØX1	T6Ø.ØX2	T6Ø.ØX3	T6Ø.ØX4	—	—
Quinapril	T46.4X1	T46.4X2	T46.4X3	T46.4X4	T46.4X5	T46.4X6
Quinestradiol	T38.5X1	T38.5X2	T38.5X3	T38.5X4	T38.5X5	T38.5X6
Quinestradol	T38.5X1	T38.5X2	T38.5X3	T38.5X4	T38.5X5	T38.5X6
Quinestrol	T38.5X1	T38.5X2	T38.5X3	T38.5X4	T38.5X5	T38.5X6
Quinethazone	T5Ø.2X1	T5Ø.2X2	T5Ø.2X3	T5Ø.2X4	T5Ø.2X5	T5Ø.2X6
Quingestanol	T38.4X1	T38.4X2	T38.4X3	T38.4X4	T38.4X5	T38.4X6
Quinidine	T46.2X1	T46.2X2	T46.2X3	T46.2X4	T46.2X5	T46.2X6
Quinine	T37.2X1	T37.2X2	T37.2X3	T37.2X4	T37.2X5	T37.2X6
Quiniobine	T37.8X1	T37.8X2	T37.8X3	T37.8X4	T37.8X5	T37.8X6
Quinisocaine	T49.1X1	T49.1X2	T49.1X3	T49.1X4	T49.1X5	T49.1X6
Quinocide	T37.2X1	T37.2X2	T37.2X3	T37.2X4	T37.2X5	T37.2X6
Quinoline (derivatives) **NEC**	T37.8X1	T37.8X2	T37.8X3	T37.8X4	T37.8X5	T37.8X6
Quinupramine	T43.Ø11	T43.Ø12	T43.Ø13	T43.Ø14	T43.Ø15	T43.Ø16
Quotane	T41.3X1	T41.3X2	T41.3X3	T41.3X4	T41.3X5	T41.3X6
Rabies						
immune globulin (human)	T5Ø.Z11	T5Ø.Z12	T5Ø.Z13	T5Ø.Z14	T5Ø.Z15	T5Ø.Z16
vaccine	T5Ø.B91	T5Ø.B92	T5Ø.B93	T5Ø.B94	T5Ø.B95	T5Ø.B96
Racemoramide	T4Ø.2X1	T4Ø.2X2	T4Ø.2X3	T4Ø.2X4	—	—
Racemorphan	T4Ø.2X1	T4Ø.2X2	T4Ø.2X3	T4Ø.2X4	T4Ø.2X5	T4Ø.2X6
Racepinefrin	T44.5X1	T44.5X2	T44.5X3	T44.5X4	T44.5X5	T44.5X6
Raclopride	T43.591	T43.592	T43.593	T43.594	T43.595	T43.596
Radiator alcohol	T51.1X1	T51.1X2	T51.1X3	T51.1X4	—	—
Radioactive drug NEC	T5Ø.8X1	T5Ø.8X2	T5Ø.8X3	T5Ø.8X4	T5Ø.8X5	T5Ø.8X6
Radio-opaque (drugs) (materials)	T5Ø.8X1	T5Ø.8X2	T5Ø.8X3	T5Ø.8X4	T5Ø.8X5	T5Ø.8X6
Ramifenazone	T39.2X1	T39.2X2	T39.2X3	T39.2X4	T39.2X5	T39.2X6
Ramipril	T46.4X1	T46.4X2	T46.4X3	T46.4X4	T46.4X5	T46.4X6
Ranitidine	T47.ØX1	T47.ØX2	T47.ØX3	T47.ØX4	T47.ØX5	T47.ØX6
Ranunculus	T62.2X1	T62.2X2	T62.2X3	T62.2X4	—	—
Rat poison NEC	T6Ø.4X1	T6Ø.4X2	T6Ø.4X3	T6Ø.4X4	—	—
Rattlesnake (venom)	T63.Ø11	T63.Ø12	T63.Ø13	T63.Ø14	—	—
Raubasine	T46.7X1	T46.7X2	T46.7X3	T46.7X4	T46.7X5	T46.7X6
Raudixin	T46.5X1	T46.5X2	T46.5X3	T46.5X4	T46.5X5	T46.5X6
Rautensin	T46.5X1	T46.5X2	T46.5X3	T46.5X4	T46.5X5	T46.5X6
Rautina	T46.5X1	T46.5X2	T46.5X3	T46.5X4	T46.5X5	T46.5X6
Rautotal	T46.5X1	T46.5X2	T46.5X3	T46.5X4	T46.5X5	T46.5X6
Rauwiloid	T46.5X1	T46.5X2	T46.5X3	T46.5X4	T46.5X5	T46.5X6
Rauwoldin	T46.5X1	T46.5X2	T46.5X3	T46.5X4	T46.5X5	T46.5X6
Rauwolfia (alkaloids)	T46.5X1	T46.5X2	T46.5X3	T46.5X4	T46.5X5	T46.5X6
Razoxane	T45.1X1	T45.1X2	T45.1X3	T45.1X4	T45.1X5	T45.1X6
Realgar	T57.ØX1	T57.ØX2	T57.ØX3	T57.ØX4	—	—
Recombinant (R) — *see* specific protein						
Red blood cells, packed	T45.8X1	T45.8X2	T45.8X3	T45.8X4	T45.8X5	T45.8X6
Red squill (scilliroside)	T6Ø.4X1	T6Ø.4X2	T6Ø.4X3	T6Ø.4X4	—	—
Reducing agent, industrial NEC	T65.891	T65.892	T65.893	T65.894	—	—
Refrigerant gas (chlorofluorocarbon)	T53.5X1	T53.5X2	T53.5X3	T53.5X4	—	—
not chlorofluorocarbon	T59.891	T59.892	T59.893	T59.894	—	—
Regroton	T5Ø.2X1	T5Ø.2X2	T5Ø.2X3	T5Ø.2X4	T5Ø.2X5	T5Ø.2X6
Rehydration salts (oral)	T5Ø.3X1	T5Ø.3X2	T5Ø.3X3	T5Ø.3X4	T5Ø.3X5	T5Ø.3X6
Rela	T42.8X1	T42.8X2	T42.8X3	T42.8X4	T42.8X5	T42.8X6
Relaxant, muscle						
anesthetic	T48.1X1	T48.1X2	T48.1X3	T48.1X4	T48.1X5	T48.1X6
central nervous system	T42.8X1	T42.8X2	T42.8X3	T42.8X4	T42.8X5	T42.8X6
skeletal NEC	T48.1X1	T48.1X2	T48.1X3	T48.1X4	T48.1X5	T48.1X6
smooth NEC	T44.3X1	T44.3X2	T44.3X3	T44.3X4	T44.3X5	T44.3X6
Remoxipride	T43.591	T43.592	T43.593	T43.594	T43.595	T43.596
Renese	T5Ø.2X1	T5Ø.2X2	T5Ø.2X3	T5Ø.2X4	T5Ø.2X5	T5Ø.2X6
Renografin	T5Ø.8X1	T5Ø.8X2	T5Ø.8X3	T5Ø.8X4	T5Ø.8X5	T5Ø.8X6
Replacement solution	T5Ø.3X1	T5Ø.3X2	T5Ø.3X3	T5Ø.3X4	T5Ø.3X5	T5Ø.3X6
Reproterol	T48.6X1	T48.6X2	T48.6X3	T48.6X4	T48.6X5	T48.6X6
Rescinnamine	T46.5X1	T46.5X2	T46.5X3	T46.5X4	T46.5X5	T46.5X6
Reserpin (e)	T46.5X1	T46.5X2	T46.5X3	T46.5X4	T46.5X5	T46.5X6
Resorcin, resorcinol (nonmedicinal)	T65.891	T65.892	T65.893	T65.894	—	—
medicinal	T49.4X1	T49.4X2	T49.4X3	T49.4X4	T49.4X5	T49.4X6
Respaire	T48.4X1	T48.4X2	T48.4X3	T48.4X4	T48.4X5	T48.4X6
Respiratory drug NEC	T48.9Ø1	T48.9Ø2	T48.9Ø3	T48.9Ø4	T48.9Ø5	T48.9Ø6
antiasthmatic NEC	T48.6X1	T48.6X2	T48.6X3	T48.6X4	T48.6X5	T48.6X6
anti-common-cold NEC	T48.5X1	T48.5X2	T48.5X3	T48.5X4	T48.5X5	T48.5X6
expectorant NEC	T48.4X1	T48.4X2	T48.4X3	T48.4X4	T48.4X5	T48.4X6
stimulant	T48.9Ø1	T48.9Ø2	T48.9Ø3	T48.9Ø4	T48.9Ø5	T48.9Ø6
Retinoic acid	T49.ØX1	T49.ØX2	T49.ØX3	T49.ØX4	T49.ØX5	T49.ØX6
Retinol	T45.2X1	T45.2X2	T45.2X3	T45.2X4	T45.2X5	T45.2X6
Rh (D) **immune globulin** (human)	T5Ø.Z11	T5Ø.Z12	T5Ø.Z13	T5Ø.Z14	T5Ø.Z15	T5Ø.Z16
Rhodine	T39.Ø11	T39.Ø12	T39.Ø13	T39.Ø14	T39.Ø15	T39.Ø16
RhoGAM	T5Ø.Z11	T5Ø.Z12	T5Ø.Z13	T5Ø.Z14	T5Ø.Z15	T5Ø.Z16
Rhubarb						
dry extract	T47.2X1	T47.2X2	T47.2X3	T47.2X4	T47.2X5	T47.2X6
tincture, compound	T47.2X1	T47.2X2	T47.2X3	T47.2X4	T47.2X5	T47.2X6
Ribavirin	T37.5X1	T37.5X2	T37.5X3	T37.5X4	T37.5X5	T37.5X6
Riboflavin	T45.2X1	T45.2X2	T45.2X3	T45.2X4	T45.2X5	T45.2X6
Ribostamycin	T36.5X1	T36.5X2	T36.5X3	T36.5X4	T36.5X5	T36.5X6

Substance	Poisoning, Accidental (unintentional)	Poisoning, Intentional Self-harm	Poisoning, Assault	Poisoning, Undetermined	Adverse Effect	Under-dosing
Ricin	T62.2X1	T62.2X2	T62.2X3	T62.2X4	—	—
Ricinus communis	T62.2X1	T62.2X2	T62.2X3	T62.2X4	—	—
Rickettsial vaccine NEC	T5Ø.A91	T5Ø.A92	T5Ø.A93	T5Ø.A94	T5Ø.A95	T5Ø.A96
Rifabutin	T36.6X1	T36.6X2	T36.6X3	T36.6X4	T36.6X5	T36.6X6
Rifamide	T36.6X1	T36.6X2	T36.6X3	T36.6X4	T36.6X5	T36.6X6
Rifampicin	T36.6X1	T36.6X2	T36.6X3	T36.6X4	T36.6X5	T36.6X6
with isoniazid	T37.1X1	T37.1X2	T37.1X3	T37.1X4	T37.1X5	T37.1X6
Rifampin	T36.6X1	T36.6X2	T36.6X3	T36.6X4	T36.6X5	T36.6X6
Rifamycin	T36.6X1	T36.6X2	T36.6X3	T36.6X4	T36.6X5	T36.6X6
Rifaximin	T36.6X1	T36.6X2	T36.6X3	T36.6X4	T36.6X5	T36.6X6
Rimantadine	T37.5X1	T37.5X2	T37.5X3	T37.5X4	T37.5X5	T37.5X6
Rimazolium metilsulfate	T39.8X1	T39.8X2	T39.8X3	T39.8X4	T39.8X5	T39.8X6
Rimifon	T37.1X1	T37.1X2	T37.1X3	T37.1X4	T37.1X5	T37.1X6
Rimiterol	T48.6X1	T48.6X2	T48.6X3	T48.6X4	T48.6X5	T48.6X6
Ringer (lactate) **solution**	T5Ø.3X1	T5Ø.3X2	T5Ø.3X3	T5Ø.3X4	T5Ø.3X5	T5Ø.3X6
Ristocetin	T36.8X1	T36.8X2	T36.8X3	T36.8X4	T36.8X5	T36.8X6
Ritalin	T43.631	T43.632	T43.633	T43.634	T43.635	T43.636
Ritodrine	T44.5X1	T44.5X2	T44.5X3	T44.5X4	T44.5X5	T44.5X6
Roach killer — *see* Insecticide						
Rociverine	T44.3X1	T44.3X2	T44.3X3	T44.3X4	T44.3X5	T44.3X6
Rocky Mountain spotted fever vaccine	T5Ø.A91	T5Ø.A92	T5Ø.A93	T5Ø.A94	T5Ø.A95	T5Ø.A96
Rodenticide NEC	T6Ø.4X1	T6Ø.4X2	T6Ø.4X3	T6Ø.4X4	—	—
Rohypnol	T42.4X1	T42.4X2	T42.4X3	T42.4X4	T42.4X5	T42.4X6
Rokitamycin	T36.3X1	T36.3X2	T36.3X3	T36.3X4	T36.3X5	T36.3X6
Rolaids	T47.1X1	T47.1X2	T47.1X3	T47.1X4	T47.1X5	T47.1X6
Rolitetracycline	T36.4X1	T36.4X2	T36.4X3	T36.4X4	T36.4X5	T36.4X6
Romilar	T48.3X1	T48.3X2	T48.3X3	T48.3X4	T48.3X5	T48.3X6
Ronifibrate	T46.6X1	T46.6X2	T46.6X3	T46.6X4	T46.6X5	T46.6X6
Rosaprostol	T47.1X1	T47.1X2	T47.1X3	T47.1X4	T47.1X5	T47.1X6
Rose bengal sodium (131I)	T5Ø.8X1	T5Ø.8X2	T5Ø.8X3	T5Ø.8X4	T5Ø.8X5	T5Ø.8X6
Rose water ointment	T49.3X1	T49.3X2	T49.3X3	T49.3X4	T49.3X5	T49.3X6
Rosoxacin	T37.8X1	T37.8X2	T37.8X3	T37.8X4	T37.8X5	T37.8X6
Rotenone	T6Ø.2X1	T6Ø.2X2	T6Ø.2X3	T6Ø.2X4	—	—
Rotoxamine	T45.ØX1	T45.ØX2	T45.ØX3	T45.ØX4	T45.ØX5	T45.ØX6
Rough-on-rats	T6Ø.4X1	T6Ø.4X2	T6Ø.4X3	T6Ø.4X4	—	—
Roxatidine	T47.ØX1	T47.ØX2	T47.ØX3	T47.ØX4	T47.ØX5	T47.ØX6
Roxithromycin	T36.3X1	T36.3X2	T36.3X3	T36.3X4	T36.3X5	T36.3X6
Rt-PA	T45.611	T45.612	T45.613	T45.614	T45.615	T45.616
Rubbing alcohol	T51.2X1	T51.2X2	T51.2X3	T51.2X4	—	—
Rubefacient	T49.4X1	T49.4X2	T49.4X3	T49.4X4	T49.4X5	T49.4X6
Rubella vaccine	T5Ø.B91	T5Ø.B92	T5Ø.B93	T5Ø.B94	T5Ø.B95	T5Ø.B96
Rubeola vaccine	T5Ø.B91	T5Ø.B92	T5Ø.B93	T5Ø.B94	T5Ø.B95	T5Ø.B96
Rubidium chloride Rb82	T5Ø.8X1	T5Ø.8X2	T5Ø.8X3	T5Ø.8X4	T5Ø.8X5	T5Ø.8X6
Rubidomycin	T45.1X1	T45.1X2	T45.1X3	T45.1X4	T45.1X5	T45.1X6
Rue	T62.2X1	T62.2X2	T62.2X3	T62.2X4	—	—
Rufocromomycin	T45.1X1	T45.1X2	T45.1X3	T45.1X4	T45.1X5	T45.1X6
Russel's viper venin	T45.7X1	T45.7X2	T45.7X3	T45.7X4	T45.7X5	T45.7X6
Ruta (graveolens)	T62.2X1	T62.2X2	T62.2X3	T62.2X4	—	—
Rutinum	T46,991	T46.992	T46.993	T46.994	T46.995	T46.996
Rutoside	T46.991	T46.992	T46.993	T46.994	T46.995	T46.996
b-sitosterol(s)	T46.6X1	T46.6X2	T46.6X3	T46.6X4	T46.6X5	T46.6X6
Sabadilla (plant)	T62.2X1	T62.2X2	T62.2X3	T62.2X4	—	—
pesticide	T6Ø.2X1	T6Ø.2X2	T6Ø.2X3	T6Ø.2X4	—	—
Saccharated iron oxide	T45.8X1	T45.8X2	T45.8X3	T45.8X4	T45.8X5	T45.8X6
Saccharin	T5Ø.9Ø1	T5Ø.9Ø2	T5Ø.9Ø3	T5Ø.9Ø4	T5Ø.9Ø5	T5Ø.9Ø6
Saccharomyces boulardii	T47.6X1	T47.6X2	T47.6X3	T47.6X4	T47.6X5	T47.6X6
Safflower oil	T46.6X1	T46.6X2	T46.6X3	T46.6X4	T46.6X5	T46.6X6
Safrazine	T43.1X1	T43.1X2	T43.1X3	T43.1X4	T43.1X5	T43.1X6
Salazosulfapyridine	T37.ØX1	T37.ØX2	T37.ØX3	T37.ØX4	T37.ØX5	T37.ØX6
Salbutamol	T48.6X1	T48.6X2	T48.6X3	T48.6X4	T48.6X5	T48.6X6
Salicylamide	T39.Ø91	T39.Ø92	T39.Ø93	T39.Ø94	T39.Ø95	T39.Ø96
Salicylate NEC	T39.Ø91	T39.Ø92	T39.Ø93	T39.Ø94	T39.Ø95	T39.Ø96
methyl	T49.3X1	T49.3X2	T49.3X3	T49.3X4	T49.3X5	T49.3X6
theobromine calcium	T5Ø.2X1	T5Ø.2X2	T5Ø.2X3	T5Ø.2X4	T5Ø.2X5	T5Ø.2X6
Salicylazosulfapyridine	T37.ØX1	T37.ØX2	T37.ØX3	T37.ØX4	T37.ØX5	T37.ØX6
Salicylhydroxamic acid	T49.ØX1	T49.ØX2	T49.ØX3	T49.ØX4	T49.ØX5	T49.ØX6
Salicylic acid	T49.4X1	T49.4X2	T49.4X3	T49.4X4	T49.4X5	T49.4X6
with benzoic acid	T49.4X1	T49.4X2	T49.4X3	T49.4X4	T49.4X5	T49.4X6
congeners	T39.Ø91	T39.Ø92	T39.Ø93	T39.Ø94	T39.Ø95	T39.Ø96
derivative	T39.Ø91	T39.Ø92	T39.Ø93	T39.Ø94	T39.Ø95	T39.Ø96
salts	T39.Ø91	T39.Ø92	T39.Ø93	T39.Ø94	T39.Ø95	T39.Ø96
Salinazid	T37.1X1	T37.1X2	T37.1X3	T37.1X4	T37.1X5	T37.1X6
Salmeterol	T48.6X1	T48.6X2	T48.6X3	T48.6X4	T48.6X5	T48.6X6
Salol	T49.3X1	T49.3X2	T49.3X3	T49.3X4	T49.3X5	T49.3X6
Salsalate	T39.Ø91	T39.Ø92	T39.Ø93	T39.Ø94	T39.Ø95	T39.Ø96
Salt-replacing drug	T5Ø.9Ø1	T5Ø.9Ø2	T5Ø.9Ø3	T5Ø.9Ø4	T5Ø.9Ø5	T5Ø.9Ø6
Salt-retaining mineralocorticoid	T5Ø.ØX1	T5Ø.ØX2	T5Ø.ØX3	T5Ø.ØX4	T5Ø.ØX5	T5Ø.ØX6
Salt substitute	T5Ø.9Ø1	T5Ø.9Ø2	T5Ø.9Ø3	T5Ø.9Ø4	T5Ø.9Ø5	T5Ø.9Ø6
Saluretic NEC	T5Ø.2X1	T5Ø.2X2	T5Ø.2X3	T5Ø.2X4	T5Ø.2X5	T5Ø.2X6
Saluron	T5Ø.2X1	T5Ø.2X2	T5Ø.2X3	T5Ø.2X4	T5Ø.2X5	T5Ø.2X6
Salvarsan 606 (neosilver) (silver)	T37.8X1	T37.8X2	T37.8X3	T37.8X4	T37.8X5	T37.8X6
Sambucus canadensis	T62.2X1	T62.2X2	T62.2X3	T62.2X4	—	—
berry	T62.1X1	T62.1X2	T62.1X3	T62.1X4	—	—
Sandril	T46.5X1	T46.5X2	T46.5X3	T46.5X4	T46.5X5	T46.5X6
Sanguinaria canadensis	T62.2X1	T62.2X2	T62.2X3	T62.2X4	—	—
Saniflush (cleaner)	T54.2X1	T54.2X2	T54.2X3	T54.2X4	—	—
Santonin	T37.4X1	T37.4X2	T37.4X3	T37.4X4	T37.4X5	T37.4X6
Santyl	T49.8X1	T49.8X2	T49.8X3	T49.8X4	T49.8X5	T49.8X6
Saralasin	T46.5X1	T46.5X2	T46.5X3	T46.5X4	T46.5X5	T46.5X6
Sarcolysin	T45.1X1	T45.1X2	T45.1X3	T45.1X4	T45.1X5	T45.1X6
Sarkomycin	T45.1X1	T45.1X2	T45.1X3	T45.1X4	T45.1X5	T45.1X6
Saroten	T43.Ø11	T43.Ø12	T43.Ø13	T43.Ø14	T43.Ø15	T43.Ø16
Saturnine — *see* Lead						
Savin (oil)	T49.4X1	T49.4X2	T49.4X3	T49.4X4	T49.4X5	T49.4X6
Scammony	T47.2X1	T47.2X2	T47.2X3	T47.2X4	T47.2X5	T47.2X6
Scarlet red	T49.8X1	T49.8X2	T49.8X3	T49.8X4	T49.8X5	T49.8X6
Scheele's green	T57.ØX1	T57.ØX2	T57.ØX3	T57.ØX4	—	—
insecticide	T57.ØX1	T57.ØX2	T57.ØX3	T57.ØX4	—	—
Schizontozide (blood) (tissue)	T37.2X1	T37.2X2	T37.2X3	T37.2X4	T37.2X5	T37.2X6
Schradan	T6Ø.ØX1	T6Ø.ØX2	T6Ø.ØX3	T6Ø.ØX4	—	—
Schweinfurth green	T57.ØX1	T57.ØX2	T57.ØX3	T57.ØX4	—	—
insecticide	T57.ØX1	T57.ØX2	T57.ØX3	T57.ØX4	—	—
Scilla, rat poison	T6Ø.4X1	T6Ø.4X2	T6Ø.4X3	T6Ø.4X4	—	—
Scillaren	T6Ø.4X1	T6Ø.4X2	T6Ø.4X3	T6Ø.4X4	—	—
Sclerosing agent	T46.8X1	T46.8X2	T46.8X3	T46.8X4	T46.8X5	T46.8X6
Scombrotoxin	T61.11	T61.12	T61.13	T61.14	—	—
Scopolamine	T44.3X1	T44.3X2	T44.3X3	T44.3X4	T44.3X5	T44.3X6
Scopolia extract	T44.3X1	T44.3X2	T44.3X3	T44.3X4	T44.3X5	T44.3X6
Scouring powder	T65.891	T65.892	T65.893	T65.894	—	—
Sea						
anemone (sting)	T63.631	T63.632	T63.633	T63.634	—	—
cucumber (sting)	T63.691	T63.692	T63.693	T63.694	—	—
snake (bite) (venom)	T63.Ø91	T63.Ø92	T63.Ø93	T63.Ø94	—	—
urchin spine (puncture)	T63.691	T63.692	T63.693	T63.694	—	—
Seafood	T61.91	T61.92	T61.93	T61.94	—	—
specified NEC	T61.8X1	T61.8X2	T61.8X3	T61.8X4	—	—
Secbutabarbital	T42.3X1	T42.3X2	T42.3X3	T42.3X4	T42.3X5	T42.3X6
Secbutabarbitone	T42.3X1	T42.3X2	T42.3X3	T42.3X4	T42.3X5	T42.3X6
Secnidazole	T37.3X1	T37.3X2	T37.3X3	T37.3X4	T37.3X5	T37.3X6
Secobarbital	T42.3X1	T42.3X2	T42.3X3	T42.3X4	T42.3X5	T42.3X6
Seconal	T42.3X1	T42.3X2	T42.3X3	T42.3X4	T42.3X5	T42.3X6
Secretin	T5Ø.8X1	T5Ø.8X2	T5Ø.8X3	T5Ø.8X4	T5Ø.8X5	T5Ø.8X6
Sedative NEC	T42.71	T42.72	T42.73	T42.74	T42.75	T42.76
mixed NEC	T42.6X1	T42.6X2	T42.6X3	T42.6X4	T42.6X5	T42.6X6
Sedormid	T42.6X1	T42.6X2	T42.6X3	T42.6X4	T42.6X5	T42.6X6
Seed disinfectant or dressing	T6Ø.8X1	T6Ø.8X2	T6Ø.8X3	T6Ø.8X4	—	—
Seeds (poisonous)	T62.2X1	T62.2X2	T62.2X3	T62.2X4	—	—
Selegiline	T42.8X1	T42.8X2	T42.8X3	T42.8X4	T42.8X5	T42.8X6
Selenium NEC	T56.891	T56.892	T56.893	T56.894	—	—
disulfide or sulfide	T49.4X1	T49.4X2	T49.4X3	T49.4X4	T49.4X5	T49.4X6
fumes	T59.891	T59.892	T59.893	T59.894	—	—
sulfide	T49.4X1	T49.4X2	T49.4X3	T49.4X4	T49.4X5	T49.4X6
Selenomethionine (75Se)	T5Ø.8X1	T5Ø.8X2	T5Ø.8X3	T5Ø.8X4	T5Ø.8X5	T5Ø.8X6
Selsun	T49.4X1	T49.4X2	T49.4X3	T49.4X4	T49.4X5	T49.4X6
Semustine	T45.1X1	T45.1X2	T45.1X3	T45.1X4	T45.1X5	T45.1X6
Senega syrup	T48.4X1	T48.4X2	T48.4X3	T48.4X4	T48.4X5	T48.4X6
Senna	T47.2X1	T47.2X2	T47.2X3	T47.2X4	T47.2X5	T47.2X6
Sennoside A+B	T47.2X1	T47.2X2	T47.2X3	T47.2X4	T47.2X5	T47.2X6
Septisol	T49.2X1	T49.2X2	T49.2X3	T49.2X4	T49.2X5	T49.2X6
Seractide	T38.811	T38.812	T38.813	T38.814	T38.815	T38.816
Serax	T42.4X1	T42.4X2	T42.4X3	T42.4X4	T42.4X5	T42.4X6
Serenesil	T42.6X1	T42.6X2	T42.6X3	T42.6X4	T42.6X5	T42.6X6
Serenium (hydrochloride)	T37.91	T37.92	T37.93	T37.94	T37.95	T37.96
Serepax — *see* Oxazepam						
Sermorelin	T38.891	T38.892	T38.893	T38.894	T38.895	T38.896
Sernyl	T41.1X1	T41.1X2	T41.1X3	T41.1X4	T41.1X5	T41.1X6
Serotonin	T5Ø.991	T5Ø.992	T5Ø.993	T5Ø.994	T5Ø.995	T5Ø.996
Serpasil	T46.5X1	T46.5X2	T46.5X3	T46.5X4	T46.5X5	T46.5X6
Serrapeptase	T45.3X1	T45.3X2	T45.3X3	T45.3X4	T45.3X5	T45.3X6
Serum						
antibotulinus	T5Ø.Z11	T5Ø.Z12	T5Ø.Z13	T5Ø.Z14	T5Ø.Z15	T5Ø.Z16
anticytotoxic	T5Ø.Z11	T5Ø.Z12	T5Ø.Z13	T5Ø.Z14	T5Ø.Z15	T5Ø.Z16
antidiphtheria	T5Ø.Z11	T5Ø.Z12	T5Ø.Z13	T5Ø.Z14	T5Ø.Z15	T5Ø.Z16
antimeningococcus	T5Ø.Z11	T5Ø.Z12	T5Ø.Z13	T5Ø.Z14	T5Ø.Z15	T5Ø.Z16
anti-Rh	T5Ø.Z11	T5Ø.Z12	T5Ø.Z13	T5Ø.Z14	T5Ø.Z15	T5Ø.Z16
anti-snake-bite	T5Ø.Z11	T5Ø.Z12	T5Ø.Z13	T5Ø.Z14	T5Ø.Z15	T5Ø.Z16
antitetanic	T5Ø.Z11	T5Ø.Z12	T5Ø.Z13	T5Ø.Z14	T5Ø.Z15	T5Ø.Z16
antitoxic	T5Ø.Z11	T5Ø.Z12	T5Ø.Z13	T5Ø.Z14	T5Ø.Z15	T5Ø.Z16
complement (inhibitor)	T45.8X1	T45.8X2	T45.8X3	T45.8X4	T45.8X5	T45.8X6
convalescent	T5Ø.Z11	T5Ø.Z12	T5Ø.Z13	T5Ø.Z14	T5Ø.Z15	T5Ø.Z16

Substance	Poisoning, Accidental (unintentional)	Poisoning, Intentional Self-harm	Poisoning, Assault	Poisoning, Undetermined	Adverse Effect	Under-dosing
Serum — *continued*						
hemolytic complement	T45.8X1	T45.8X2	T45.8X3	T45.8X4	T45.8X5	T45.8X6
immune (human)	T5Ø.Z11	T5Ø.Z12	T5Ø.Z13	T5Ø.Z14	T5Ø.Z15	T5Ø.Z16
protective NEC	T5Ø.Z11	T5Ø.Z12	T5Ø.Z13	T5Ø.Z14	T5Ø.Z15	T5Ø.Z16
Setastine	T45.ØX1	T45.ØX2	T45.ØX3	T45.ØX4	T45.ØX5	T45.ØX6
Setoperone	T43.591	T43.592	T43.593	T43.594	T43.595	T43.596
Sewer gas	T59.91	T59.92	T59.93	T59.94	—	—
Shampoo	T55.ØX1	T55.ØX2	T55.ØX3	T55.ØX4	—	—
Shellfish, noxious, nonbacterial	T61.781	T61.782	T61.783	T61.784	—	—
Sildenafil	T46.7X1	T46.7X2	T46.7X3	T46.7X4	T46.7X5	T46.7X6
Silibinin	T5Ø.991	T5Ø.992	T5Ø.993	T5Ø.994	T5Ø.995	T5Ø.996
Silicone NEC	T65.891	T65.892	T65.893	T65.894	—	—
medicinal	T49.3X1	T49.3X2	T49.3X3	T49.3X4	T49.3X5	T49.3X6
Silvadene	T49.ØX1	T49.ØX2	T49.ØX3	T49.ØX4	T49.ØX5	T49.ØX6
Silver	T49.ØX1	T49.ØX2	T49.ØX3	T49.ØX4	T49.ØX5	T49.ØX6
anti-infectives	T49.ØX1	T49.ØX2	T49.ØX3	T49.ØX4	T49.ØX5	T49.ØX6
arsphenamine	T37.8X1	T37.8X2	T37.8X3	T37.8X4	T37.8X5	T37.8X6
colloidal	T49.ØX1	T49.ØX2	T49.ØX3	T49.ØX4	T49.ØX5	T49.ØX6
nitrate	T49.ØX1	T49.ØX2	T49.ØX3	T49.ØX4	T49.ØX5	T49.ØX6
ophthalmic preparation	T49.5X1	T49.5X2	T49.5X3	T49.5X4	T49.5X5	T49.5X6
toughened (keratolytic)	T49.4X1	T49.4X2	T49.4X3	T49.4X4	T49.4X5	T49.4X6
nonmedicinal (dust)	T56.891	T56.892	T56.893	T56.894	—	—
protein	T49.5X1	T49.5X2	T49.5X3	T49.5X4	T49.5X5	T49.5X6
salvarsan	T37.8X1	T37.8X2	T37.8X3	T37.8X4	T37.8X5	T37.8X6
sulfadiazine	T49.4X1	T49.4X2	T49.4X3	T49.4X4	T49.4X5	T49.4X6
Silymarin	T5Ø.991	T5Ø.992	T5Ø.993	T5Ø.994	T5Ø.995	T5Ø.996
Simaldrate	T47.1X1	T47.1X2	T47.1X3	T47.1X4	T47.1X5	T47.1X6
Simazine	T6Ø.3X1	T6Ø.3X2	T6Ø.3X3	T6Ø.3X4	—	—
Simethicone	T47.1X1	T47.1X2	T47.1X3	T47.1X4	T47.1X5	T47.1X6
Simfibrate	T46.6X1	T46.6X2	T46.6X3	T46.6X4	T46.6X5	T46.6X6
Simvastatin	T46.6X1	T46.6X2	T46.6X3	T46.6X4	T46.6X5	T46.6X6
Sincalide	T5Ø.8X1	T5Ø.8X2	T5Ø.8X3	T5Ø.8X4	T5Ø.8X5	T5Ø.8X6
Sinequan	T43.Ø11	T43.Ø12	T43.Ø13	T43.Ø14	T43.Ø15	T43.Ø16
Singoserp	T46.5X1	T46.5X2	T46.5X3	T46.5X4	T46.5X5	T46.5X6
Sintrom	T45.511	T45.512	T45.513	T45.514	T45.515	T45.516
Sisomicin	T36.5X1	T36.5X2	T36.5X3	T36.5X4	T36.5X5	T36.5X6
Sitosterols	T46.6X1	T46.6X2	T46.6X3	T46.6X4	T46.6X5	T46.6X6
Skeletal muscle relaxants	T48.1X1	T48.1X2	T48.1X3	T48.1X4	T48.1X5	T48.1X6
Skin						
agents (external)	T49.91	T49.92	T49.93	T49.94	T49.95	T49.96
specified NEC	T49.8X1	T49.8X2	T49.8X3	T49.8X4	T49.8X5	T49.8X6
test antigen	T5Ø.8X1	T5Ø.8X2	T5Ø.8X3	T5Ø.8X4	T5Ø.8X5	T5Ø.8X6
Sleep-eze	T45.ØX1	T45.ØX2	T45.ØX3	T45.ØX4	T45.ØX5	T45.ØX6
Sleeping draught, pill	T42.71	T42.72	T42.73	T42.74	T42.75	T42.76
Smallpox vaccine	T5Ø.B11	T5Ø.B12	T5Ø.B13	T5Ø.B14	T5Ø.B15	T5Ø.B16
Smelter fumes NEC	T56.91	T56.92	T56.93	T56.94	—	—
Smog	T59.1X1	T59.1X2	T59.1X3	T59.1X4	—	—
Smoke NEC	T59.811	T59.812	T59.813	T59.814	—	—
Smooth muscle relaxant	T44.3X1	T44.3X2	T44.3X3	T44.3X4	T44.3X5	T44.3X6
Snail killer NEC	T6Ø.8X1	T6Ø.8X2	T6Ø.8X3	T6Ø.8X4	—	—
Snake venom or bite	T63.ØØ1	T63.ØØ2	T63.ØØ3	T63.ØØ4	—	—
hemocoagulase	T45.7X1	T45.7X2	T45.7X3	T45.7X4	T45.7X5	T45.7X6
Snuff	T65.211	T65.212	T65.213	T65.214	—	—
Soap (powder) (product)	T55.ØX1	T55.ØX2	T55.ØX3	T55.ØX4	—	—
enema	T47.4X1	T47.4X2	T47.4X3	T47.4X4	T47.4X5	T47.4X6
medicinal, soft	T49.2X1	T49.2X2	T49.2X3	T49.2X4	T49.2X5	T49.2X6
superfatted	T49.2X1	T49.2X2	T49.2X3	T49.2X4	T49.2X5	T49.2X6
Sobrerol	T48.4X1	T48.4X2	T48.4X3	T48.4X4	T48.4X5	T48.4X6
Soda (caustic)	T54.3X1	T54.3X2	T54.3X3	T54.3X4	—	—
bicarb	T47.1X1	T47.1X2	T47.1X3	T47.1X4	T47.1X5	T47.1X6
chlorinated — *see* Sodium, hypochlorite						
Sodium						
acetosulfone	T37.1X1	T37.1X2	T37.1X3	T37.1X4	T37.1X5	T37.1X6
acetrizoate	T5Ø.8X1	T5Ø.8X2	T5Ø.8X3	T5Ø.8X4	T5Ø.8X5	T5Ø.8X6
acid phosphate	T5Ø.3X1	T5Ø.3X2	T5Ø.3X3	T5Ø.3X4	T5Ø.3X5	T5Ø.3X6
alginate	T47.8X1	T47.8X2	T47.8X3	T47.8X4	T47.8X5	T47.8X6
amidotrizoate	T5Ø.8X1	T5Ø.8X2	T5Ø.8X3	T5Ø.8X4	T5Ø.8X5	T5Ø.8X6
aminopterin	T45.1X1	T45.1X2	T45.1X3	T45.1X4	T45.1X5	T45.1X6
amylosulfate	T47.8X1	T47.8X2	T47.8X3	T47.8X4	T47.8X5	T47.8X6
amytal	T42.3X1	T42.3X2	T42.3X3	T42.3X4	T42.3X5	T42.3X6
antimony gluconate	T37.3X1	T37.3X2	T37.3X3	T37.3X4	T37.3X5	T37.3X6
arsenate	T57.ØX1	T57.ØX2	T57.ØX3	T57.ØX4	—	—
aurothiomalate	T39.4X1	T39.4X2	T39.4X3	T39.4X4	T39.4X5	T39.4X6
aurothiosulfate	T39.4X1	T39.4X2	T39.4X3	T39.4X4	T39.4X5	T39.4X6
barbiturate	T42.3X1	T42.3X2	T42.3X3	T42.3X4	T42.3X5	T42.3X6
basic phosphate	T47.4X1	T47.4X2	T47.4X3	T47.4X4	T47.4X5	T47.4X6
bicarbonate	T47.1X1	T47.1X2	T47.1X3	T47.1X4	T47.1X5	T47.1X6
bichromate	T57.8X1	T57.8X2	T57.8X3	T57.8X4	—	—
biphosphate	T5Ø.3X1	T5Ø.3X2	T5Ø.3X3	T5Ø.3X4	T5Ø.3X5	T5Ø.3X6
bisulfate	T65.891	T65.892	T65.893	T65.894	—	—
borate						

Substance	Poisoning, Accidental (unintentional)	Poisoning, Intentional Self-harm	Poisoning, Assault	Poisoning, Undetermined	Adverse Effect	Under-dosing
Sodium — *continued*						
borate — *continued*						
cleanser	T57.8X1	T57.8X2	T57.8X3	T57.8X4	—	—
eye	T49.5X1	T49.5X2	T49.5X3	T49.5X4	T49.5X5	T49.5X6
therapeutic	T49.8X1	T49.8X2	T49.8X3	T49.8X4	T49.8X5	T49.8X6
bromide	T42.6X1	T42.6X2	T42.6X3	T42.6X4	T42.6X5	T42.6X6
cacodylate (nonmedicinal) NEC	T5Ø.8X1	T5Ø.8X2	T5Ø.8X3	T5Ø.8X4	T5Ø.8X5	T5Ø.8X6
anti-infective	T37.8X1	T37.8X2	T37.8X3	T37.8X4	T37.8X5	T37.8X6
herbicide	T6Ø.3X1	T6Ø.3X2	T6Ø.3X3	T6Ø.3X4	—	—
calcium edetate	T45.8X1	T45.8X2	T45.8X3	T45.8X4	T45.8X5	T45.8X6
carbonate NEC	T54.3X1	T54.3X2	T54.3X3	T54.3X4	—	—
chlorate NEC	T65.891	T65.892	T65.893	T65.894	—	—
herbicide	T54.91	T54.92	T54.93	T54.94	—	—
chloride	T5Ø.3X1	T5Ø.3X2	T5Ø.3X3	T5Ø.3X4	T5Ø.3X5	T5Ø.3X6
with glucose	T5Ø.3X1	T5Ø.3X2	T5Ø.3X3	T5Ø.3X4	T5Ø.3X5	T5Ø.3X6
chromate	T65.891	T65.892	T65.893	T65.894	—	—
citrate	T5Ø.991	T5Ø.992	T5Ø.993	T5Ø.994	T5Ø.995	T5Ø.996
cromoglicate	T48.6X1	T48.6X2	T48.6X3	T48.6X4	T48.6X5	T48.6X6
cyanide	T65.ØX1	T65.ØX2	T65.ØX3	T65.ØX4	—	—
cyclamate	T5Ø.3X1	T5Ø.3X2	T5Ø.3X3	T5Ø.3X4	T5Ø.3X5	T5Ø.3X6
dehydrocholate	T45.8X1	T45.8X2	T45.8X3	T45.8X4	T45.8X5	T45.8X6
diatrizoate	T5Ø.8X1	T5Ø.8X2	T5Ø.8X3	T5Ø.8X4	T5Ø.8X5	T5Ø.8X6
dibunate	T48.4X1	T48.4X2	T48.4X3	T48.4X4	T48.4X5	T48.4X6
dioctyl sulfosuccinate	T47.4X1	T47.4X2	T47.4X3	T47.4X4	T47.4X5	T47.4X6
dipantoyl ferrate	T45.8X1	T45.8X2	T45.8X3	T45.8X4	T45.8X5	T45.8X6
edetate	T45.8X1	T45.8X2	T45.8X3	T45.8X4	T45.8X5	T45.8X6
ethacrynate	T5Ø.1X1	T5Ø.1X2	T5Ø.1X3	T5Ø.1X4	T5Ø.1X5	T5Ø.1X6
feredetate	T45.8X1	T45.8X2	T45.8X3	T45.8X4	T45.8X5	T45.8X6
Fluoride — *see* Fluoride						
fluoroacetate (dust) (pesticide)	T6Ø.4X1	T6Ø.4X2	T6Ø.4X3	T6Ø.4X4	—	—
free salt	T5Ø.3X1	T5Ø.3X2	T5Ø.3X3	T5Ø.3X4	T5Ø.3X5	T5Ø.3X6
fusidate	T36.8X1	T36.8X2	T36.8X3	T36.8X4	T36.8X5	T36.8X6
glucaldrate	T47.1X1	T47.1X2	T47.1X3	T47.1X4	T47.1X5	T47.1X6
glucosulfone	T37.1X1	T37.1X2	T37.1X3	T37.1X4	T37.1X5	T37.1X6
glutamate	T45.8X1	T45.8X2	T45.8X3	T45.8X4	T45.8X5	T45.8X6
hydrogen carbonate	T5Ø.3X1	T5Ø.3X2	T5Ø.3X3	T5Ø.3X4	T5Ø.3X5	T5Ø.3X6
hydroxide	T54.3X1	T54.3X2	T54.3X3	T54.3X4	—	—
hypochlorite (bleach) NEC	T54.3X1	T54.3X2	T54.3X3	T54.3X4	—	—
disinfectant	T54.3X1	T54.3X2	T54.3X3	T54.3X4	—	—
medicinal (anti-infective) (external)	T49.ØX1	T49.ØX2	T49.ØX3	T49.ØX4	T49.ØX5	T49.ØX6
vapor	T54.3X1	T54.3X2	T54.3X3	T54.3X4	—	—
hyposulfite	T49.ØX1	T49.ØX2	T49.ØX3	T49.ØX4	T49.ØX5	T49.ØX6
indigotin disulfonate	T5Ø.8X1	T5Ø.8X2	T5Ø.8X3	T5Ø.8X4	T5Ø.8X5	T5Ø.8X6
iodide	T5Ø.991	T5Ø.992	T5Ø.993	T5Ø.994	T5Ø.995	T5Ø.996
I-131	T5Ø.8X1	T5Ø.8X2	T5Ø.8X3	T5Ø.8X4	T5Ø.8X5	T5Ø.8X6
therapeutic	T38.2X1	T38.2X2	T38.2X3	T38.2X4	T38.2X5	T38.2X6
iodohippurate (131I)	T5Ø.8X1	T5Ø.8X2	T5Ø.8X3	T5Ø.8X4	T5Ø.8X5	T5Ø.8X6
iopodate	T5Ø.8X1	T5Ø.8X2	T5Ø.8X3	T5Ø.8X4	T5Ø.8X5	T5Ø.8X6
iothalamate	T5Ø.8X1	T5Ø.8X2	T5Ø.8X3	T5Ø.8X4	T5Ø.8X5	T5Ø.8X6
iron edetate	T45.4X1	T45.4X2	T45.4X3	T45.4X4	T45.4X5	T45.4X6
lactate (compound solution)	T45.8X1	T45.8X2	T45.8X3	T45.8X4	T45.8X5	T45.8X6
lauryl (sulfate)	T49.2X1	T49.2X2	T49.2X3	T49.2X4	T49.2X5	T49.2X6
L-triiodothyronine	T38.1X1	T38.1X2	T38.1X3	T38.1X4	T38.1X5	T38.1X6
magnesium citrate	T5Ø.991	T5Ø.992	T5Ø.993	T5Ø.994	T5Ø.995	T5Ø.996
mersalate	T5Ø.2X1	T5Ø.2X2	T5Ø.2X3	T5Ø.2X4	T5Ø.2X5	T5Ø.2X6
metasilicate	T65.891	T65.892	T65.893	T65.894	—	—
metrizoate	T5Ø.8X1	T5Ø.8X2	T5Ø.8X3	T5Ø.8X4	T5Ø.8X5	T5Ø.8X6
monofluoroacetate (pesticide)	T6Ø.1X1	T6Ø.1X2	T6Ø.1X3	T6Ø.1X4	—	—
morrhuate	T46.8X1	T46.8X2	T46.8X3	T46.8X4	T46.8X5	T46.8X6
nafcillin	T36.ØX1	T36.ØX2	T36.ØX3	T36.ØX4	T36.ØX5	T36.ØX6
nitrate (oxidizing agent)	T65.891	T65.892	T65.893	T65.894	—	—
nitrite	T5Ø.6X1	T5Ø.6X2	T5Ø.6X3	T5Ø.6X4	T5Ø.6X5	T5Ø.6X6
nitroferricyanide	T46.5X1	T46.5X2	T46.5X3	T46.5X4	T46.5X5	T46.5X6
nitroprusside	T46.5X1	T46.5X2	T46.5X3	T46.5X4	T46.5X5	T46.5X6
oxalate	T65.891	T65.892	T65.893	T65.894	—	—
oxide/peroxide	T65.891	T65.892	T65.893	T65.894	—	—
oxybate	T41.291	T41.292	T41.293	T41.294	T41.295	T41.296
para-aminohippurate	T5Ø.8X1	T5Ø.8X2	T5Ø.8X3	T5Ø.8X4	T5Ø.8X5	T5Ø.8X6
perborate (nonmedicinal) NEC	T65.891	T65.892	T65.893	T65.894	—	—
medicinal	T49.ØX1	T49.ØX2	T49.ØX3	T49.ØX4	T49.ØX5	T49.ØX6
soap	T55.ØX1	T55.ØX2	T55.ØX3	T55.ØX4	—	—
percarbonate — *see* Sodium, perborate						
pertechnetate Tc99m	T5Ø.8X1	T5Ø.8X2	T5Ø.8X3	T5Ø.8X4	T5Ø.8X5	T5Ø.8X6
phosphate						
cellulose	T45.8X1	T45.8X2	T45.8X3	T45.8X4	T45.8X5	T45.8X6
dibasic	T47.2X1	T47.2X2	T47.2X3	T47.2X4	T47.2X5	T47.2X6

Subterms under main terms may continue to next column or page | Additional Character May Be Required — Refer to the Tabular List for Character Selection | 395

Substance	Poisoning, Accidental (unintentional)	Poisoning, Intentional Self-harm	Poisoning, Assault	Poisoning, Undetermined	Adverse Effect	Under-dosing
Sodium — *continued*						
phosphate — *continued*						
monobasic	T47.2X1	T47.2X2	T47.2X3	T47.2X4	T47.2X5	T47.2X6
phytate	T50.6X1	T50.6X2	T50.6X3	T50.6X4	T50.6X5	T50.6X6
picosulfate	T47.2X1	T47.2X2	T47.2X3	T47.2X4	T47.2X5	T47.2X6
polyhydroxyaluminium monocarbonate	T47.1X1	T47.1X2	T47.1X3	T47.1X4	T47.1X5	T47.1X6
polystyrene sulfonate	T50.3X1	T50.3X2	T50.3X3	T50.3X4	T50.3X5	T50.3X6
propionate	T49.0X1	T49.0X2	T49.0X3	T49.0X4	T49.0X5	T49.0X6
propyl hydroxybenzoate	T50.991	T50.992	T50.993	T50.994	T50.995	T50.996
psylliate	T46.8X1	T46.8X2	T46.8X3	T46.8X4	T46.8X5	T46.8X6
removing resins	T50.3X1	T50.3X2	T50.3X3	T50.3X4	T50.3X5	T50.3X6
salicylate	T39.091	T39.092	T39.093	T39.094	T39.095	T39.096
salt NEC	T50.3X1	T50.3X2	T50.3X3	T50.3X4	T50.3X5	T50.3X6
selenate	T60.2X1	T60.2X2	T60.2X3	T60.2X4	—	—
stibogluconate	T37.3X1	T37.3X2	T37.3X3	T37.3X4	T37.3X5	T37.3X6
sulfate	T47.4X1	T47.4X2	T47.4X3	T47.4X4	T47.4X5	T47.4X6
sulfoxone	T37.1X1	T37.1X2	T37.1X3	T37.1X4	T37.1X5	T37.1X6
tetradecyl sulfate	T46.8X1	T46.8X2	T46.8X3	T46.8X4	T46.8X5	T46.8X6
thiopental	T41.1X1	T41.1X2	T41.1X3	T41.1X4	T41.1X5	T41.1X6
thiosalicylate	T39.091	T39.092	T39.093	T39.094	T39.095	T39.096
thiosulfate	T50.6X1	T50.6X2	T50.6X3	T50.6X4	T50.6X5	T50.6X6
tolbutamide	T38.3X1	T38.3X2	T38.3X3	T38.3X4	T38.3X5	T38.3X6
(L)-triiodothyronine	T38.1X1	T38.1X2	T38.1X3	T38.1X4	T38.1X5	T38.1X6
tyropanoate	T50.8X1	T50.8X2	T50.8X3	T50.8X4	T50.8X5	T50.8X6
valproate	T42.6X1	T42.6X2	T42.6X3	T42.6X4	T42.6X5	T42.6X6
versenate	T50.6X1	T50.6X2	T50.6X3	T50.6X4	T50.6X5	T50.6X6
Sodium-free salt	T50.901	T50.902	T50.903	T50.904	T50.905	T50.906
Sodium-removing resin	T50.3X1	T50.3X2	T50.3X3	T50.3X4	T50.3X5	T50.3X6
Soft soap	T55.0X1	T55.0X2	T55.0X3	T55.0X4	—	—
Solanine	T62.2X1	T62.2X2	T62.2X3	T62.2X4	—	—
berries	T62.1X1	T62.1X2	T62.1X3	T62.1X4	—	—
Solanum dulcamara	T62.2X1	T62.2X2	T62.2X3	T62.2X4	—	—
berries	T62.1X1	T62.1X2	T62.1X3	T62.1X4	—	—
Solapsone	T37.1X1	T37.1X2	T37.1X3	T37.1X4	T37.1X5	T37.1X6
Solar lotion	T49.3X1	T49.3X2	T49.3X3	T49.3X4	T49.3X5	T49.3X6
Solasulfone	T37.1X1	T37.1X2	T37.1X3	T37.1X4	T37.1X5	T37.1X6
Soldering fluid	T65.891	T65.892	T65.893	T65.894	—	—
Solid substance	T65.91	T65.92	T65.93	T65.94	—	—
specified NEC	T65.891	T65.892	T65.893	T65.894	—	—
Solvent, industrial NEC	T52.91	T52.92	T52.93	T52.94	—	—
naphtha	T52.0X1	T52.0X2	T52.0X3	T52.0X4	—	—
petroleum	T52.0X1	T52.0X2	T52.0X3	T52.0X4	—	—
specified NEC	T52.8X1	T52.8X2	T52.8X3	T52.8X4	—	—
Soma	T42.8X1	T42.8X2	T42.8X3	T42.8X4	T42.8X5	T42.8X6
Somatorelin	T38.891	T38.892	T38.893	T38.894	T38.895	T38.896
Somatostatin	T38.991	T38.992	T38.993	T38.994	T38.995	T38.996
Somatotropin	T38.811	T38.812	T38.813	T38.814	T38.815	T38.816
Somatrem	T38.811	T38.812	T38.813	T38.814	T38.815	T38.816
Somatropin	T38.811	T38.812	T38.813	T38.814	T38.815	T38.816
Sominex	T45.0X1	T45.0X2	T45.0X3	T45.0X4	T45.0X5	T45.0X6
Somnos	T42.6X1	T42.6X2	T42.6X3	T42.6X4	T42.6X5	T42.6X6
Somonal	T42.3X1	T42.3X2	T42.3X3	T42.3X4	T42.3X5	T42.3X6
Soneryl	T42.3X1	T42.3X2	T42.3X3	T42.3X4	T42.3X5	T42.3X6
Soothing syrup	T50.901	T50.902	T50.903	T50.904	T50.905	T50.906
Sopor	T42.6X1	T42.6X2	T42.6X3	T42.6X4	T42.6X5	T42.6X6
Soporific	T42.71	T42.72	T42.73	T42.74	T42.75	T42.76
Soporific drug	T42.71	T42.72	T42.73	T42.74	T42.75	T42.76
specified type NEC	T42.6X1	T42.6X2	T42.6X3	T42.6X4	T42.6X5	T42.6X6
Sorbide nitrate	T46.3X1	T46.3X2	T46.3X3	T46.3X4	T46.3X5	T46.3X6
Sorbitol	T47.4X1	T47.4X2	T47.4X3	T47.4X4	T47.4X5	T47.4X6
Sotalol	T44.7X1	T44.7X2	T44.7X3	T44.7X4	T44.7X5	T44.7X6
Sotradecol	T46.8X1	T46.8X2	T46.8X3	T46.8X4	T46.8X5	T46.8X6
Soysterol	T46.6X1	T46.6X2	T46.6X3	T46.6X4	T46.6X5	T46.6X6
Spacoline	T44.3X1	T44.3X2	T44.3X3	T44.3X4	T44.3X5	T44.3X6
Spanish fly	T49.8X1	T49.8X2	T49.8X3	T49.8X4	T49.8X5	T49.8X6
Sparine	T43.3X1	T43.3X2	T43.3X3	T43.3X4	T43.3X5	T43.3X6
Sparteine	T48.0X1	T48.0X2	T48.0X3	T48.0X4	T48.0X5	T48.0X6
Spasmolytic						
anticholinergics	T44.3X1	T44.3X2	T44.3X3	T44.3X4	T44.3X5	T44.3X6
autonomic	T44.3X1	T44.3X2	T44.3X3	T44.3X4	T44.3X5	T44.3X6
bronchial NEC	T48.6X1	T48.6X2	T48.6X3	T48.6X4	T48.6X5	T48.6X6
quaternary ammonium	T44.3X1	T44.3X2	T44.3X3	T44.3X4	T44.3X5	T44.3X6
skeletal muscle NEC	T48.1X1	T48.1X2	T48.1X3	T48.1X4	T48.1X5	T48.1X6
Spectinomycin	T36.5X1	T36.5X2	T36.5X3	T36.5X4	T36.5X5	T36.5X6
Speed	T43.621	T43.622	T43.623	T43.624	T43.625	T43.626
Spermicide	T49.8X1	T49.8X2	T49.8X3	T49.8X4	T49.8X5	T49.8X6
Spider (bite) (venom)	T63.391	T63.392	T63.393	T63.394	—	—
antivenin	T50.Z11	T50.Z12	T50.Z13	T50.Z14	T50.Z15	T50.Z16
Spigelia (root)	T37.4X1	T37.4X2	T37.4X3	T37.4X4	T37.4X5	T37.4X6
Spindle inactivator	T50.4X1	T50.4X2	T50.4X3	T50.4X4	T50.4X5	T50.4X6
Spiperone	T43.4X1	T43.4X2	T43.4X3	T43.4X4	T43.4X5	T43.4X6
Spiramycin	T36.3X1	T36.3X2	T36.3X3	T36.3X4	T36.3X5	T36.3X6
Spirapril	T46.4X1	T46.4X2	T46.4X3	T46.4X4	T46.4X5	T46.4X6
Spirilene	T43.591	T43.592	T43.593	T43.594	T43.595	T43.596
Spirit(s) (neutral) **NEC**	T51.0X1	T51.0X2	T51.0X3	T51.0X4	—	—
beverage	T51.0X1	T51.0X2	T51.0X3	T51.0X4	—	—
industrial	T51.0X1	T51.0X2	T51.0X3	T51.0X4	—	—
mineral	T52.0X1	T52.0X2	T52.0X3	T52.0X4	—	—
of salt — *see* Hydrochloric acid						
surgical	T51.0X1	T51.0X2	T51.0X3	T51.0X4	—	—
Spironolactone	T50.0X1	T50.0X2	T50.0X3	T50.0X4	T50.0X5	T50.0X6
Spiroperidol	T43.4X1	T43.4X2	T43.4X3	T43.4X4	T43.4X5	T43.4X6
Sponge, absorbable (gelatin)	T45.7X1	T45.7X2	T45.7X3	T45.7X4	T45.7X5	T45.7X6
Sporostacin	T49.0X1	T49.0X2	T49.0X3	T49.0X4	T49.0X5	T49.0X6
Spray (aerosol)	T65.91	T65.92	T65.93	T65.94	—	—
cosmetic	T65.891	T65.892	T65.893	T65.894	—	—
medicinal NEC	T50.901	T50.902	T50.903	T50.904	T50.905	T50.906
pesticides — *see* Pesticides						
specified content — *see* specific substance						
Spurge flax	T62.2X1	T62.2X2	T62.2X3	T62.2X4	—	—
Spurges	T62.2X1	T62.2X2	T62.2X3	T62.2X4	—	—
Sputum viscosity-lowering drug	T48.4X1	T48.4X2	T48.4X3	T48.4X4	T48.4X5	T48.4X6
Squill	T46.0X1	T46.0X2	T46.0X3	T46.0X4	T46.0X5	T46.0X6
rat poison	T60.4X1	T60.4X2	T60.4X3	T60.4X4	—	—
Squirting cucumber (cathartic)	T47.2X1	T47.2X2	T47.2X3	T47.2X4	T47.2X5	T47.2X6
Stains	T65.6X1	T65.6X2	T65.6X3	T65.6X4	—	—
Stannous fluoride	T49.7X1	T49.7X2	T49.7X3	T49.7X4	T49.7X5	T49.7X6
Stanolone	T38.7X1	T38.7X2	T38.7X3	T38.7X4	T38.7X5	T38.7X6
Stanozolol	T38.7X1	T38.7X2	T38.7X3	T38.7X4	T38.7X5	T38.7X6
Staphisagria or stavesacre (pediculicide)	T49.0X1	T49.0X2	T49.0X3	T49.0X4	T49.0X5	T49.0X6
Starch	T50.901	T50.902	T50.903	T50.904	T50.905	T50.906
Stelazine	T43.3X1	T43.3X2	T43.3X3	T43.3X4	T43.3X5	T43.3X6
Stemetil	T43.3X1	T43.3X2	T43.3X3	T43.3X4	T43.3X5	T43.3X6
Stepronin	T48.4X1	T48.4X2	T48.4X3	T48.4X4	T48.4X5	T48.4X6
Sterculia	T47.4X1	T47.4X2	T47.4X3	T47.4X4	T47.4X5	T47.4X6
Sternutator gas	T59.891	T59.892	T59.893	T59.894	—	—
Steroid	T38.0X1	T38.0X2	T38.0X3	T38.0X4	T38.0X5	T38.0X6
anabolic	T38.7X1	T38.7X2	T38.7X3	T38.7X4	T38.7X5	T38.7X6
androgenic	T38.7X1	T38.7X2	T38.7X3	T38.7X4	T38.7X5	T38.7X6
antineoplastic, hormone	T38.7X1	T38.7X2	T38.7X3	T38.7X4	T38.7X5	T38.7X6
estrogen	T38.5X1	T38.5X2	T38.5X3	T38.5X4	T38.5X5	T38.5X6
ENT agent	T49.6X1	T49.6X2	T49.6X3	T49.6X4	T49.6X5	T49.6X6
ophthalmic preparation	T49.5X1	T49.5X2	T49.5X3	T49.5X4	T49.5X5	T49.5X6
topical NEC	T49.0X1	T49.0X2	T49.0X3	T49.0X4	T49.0X5	T49.0X6
Stibine	T56.891	T56.892	T56.893	T56.894	—	—
Stibogluconate	T37.3X1	T37.3X2	T37.3X3	T37.3X4	T37.3X5	T37.3X6
Stibophen	T37.4X1	T37.4X2	T37.4X3	T37.4X4	T37.4X5	T37.4X6
Stilbamidine (isetionate)	T37.3X1	T37.3X2	T37.3X3	T37.3X4	T37.3X5	T37.3X6
Stilbestrol	T38.5X1	T38.5X2	T38.5X3	T38.5X4	T38.5X5	T38.5X6
Stilboestrol	T38.5X1	T38.5X2	T38.5X3	T38.5X4	T38.5X5	T38.5X6
Stimulant						
central nervous system — *see also* Psychostimulant	T43.601	T43.602	T43.603	T43.604	T43.605	T43.606
analeptics	T50.7X1	T50.7X2	T50.7X3	T50.7X4	T50.7X5	T50.7X6
opiate antagonist	T50.7X1	T50.7X2	T50.7X3	T50.7X4	T50.7X5	T50.7X6
psychotherapeutic NEC — *see also* Psychotherapeutic drug	T43.601	T43.602	T43.603	T43.604	T43.605	T43.606
specified NEC	T43.691	T43.692	T43.693	T43.694	T43.695	T43.696
respiratory	T48.901	T48.902	T48.903	T48.904	T48.905	T48.906
Stone-dissolving drug	T50.901	T50.902	T50.903	T50.904	T50.905	T50.906
Storage battery (cells) (acid)	T54.2X1	T54.2X2	T54.2X3	T54.2X4	—	—
Stovaine	T41.3X1	T41.3X2	T41.3X3	T41.3X4	T41.3X5	T41.3X6
infiltration (subcutaneous)	T41.3X1	T41.3X2	T41.3X3	T41.3X4	T41.3X5	T41.3X6
nerve block (peripheral) (plexus)	T41.3X1	T41.3X2	T41.3X3	T41.3X4	T41.3X5	T41.3X6
spinal	T41.3X1	T41.3X2	T41.3X3	T41.3X4	T41.3X5	T41.3X6
topical (surface)	T41.3X1	T41.3X2	T41.3X3	T41.3X4	T41.3X5	T41.3X6
Stovarsal	T37.8X1	T37.8X2	T37.8X3	T37.8X4	T37.8X5	T37.8X6
Stove gas — *see* Gas, stove						
Stoxil	T49.5X1	T49.5X2	T49.5X3	T49.5X4	T49.5X5	T49.5X6
Stramonium	T48.6X1	T48.6X2	T48.6X3	T48.6X4	T48.6X5	T48.6X6
natural state	T62.2X1	T62.2X2	T62.2X3	T62.2X4	—	—
Streptodornase	T45.3X1	T45.3X2	T45.3X3	T45.3X4	T45.3X5	T45.3X6
Streptoducin	T36.5X1	T36.5X2	T36.5X3	T36.5X4	T36.5X5	T36.5X6
Streptokinase	T45.611	T45.612	T45.613	T45.614	T45.615	T45.616
Streptomycin (derivative)	T36.5X1	T36.5X2	T36.5X3	T36.5X4	T36.5X5	T36.5X6
Streptonivicin	T36.5X1	T36.5X2	T36.5X3	T36.5X4	T36.5X5	T36.5X6
Streptovarycin	T36.5X1	T36.5X2	T36.5X3	T36.5X4	T36.5X5	T36.5X6

396 Additional Character May Be Required — Refer to the Tabular List for Character Selection

Subterms under main terms may continue to next column or page

Substance	Poisoning, Accidental (unintentional)	Poisoning, Intentional Self-harm	Poisoning, Assault	Poisoning, Undetermined	Adverse Effect	Under-dosing
Streptozocin	T45.1X1	T45.1X2	T45.1X3	T45.1X4	T45.1X5	T45.1X6
Streptozotocin	T45.1X1	T45.1X2	T45.1X3	T45.1X4	T45.1X5	T45.1X6
Stripper (paint) (solvent)	T52.8X1	T52.8X2	T52.8X3	T52.8X4	—	—
Strobane	T60.1X1	T60.1X2	T60.1X3	T60.1X4	—	—
Strofantina	T46.0X1	T46.0X2	T46.0X3	T46.0X4	T46.0X5	T46.0X6
Strophanthin (g) (k)	T46.0X1	T46.0X2	T46.0X3	T46.0X4	T46.0X5	T46.0X6
Strophanthus	T46.0X1	T46.0X2	T46.0X3	T46.0X4	T46.0X5	T46.0X6
Strophantin	T46.0X1	T46.0X2	T46.0X3	T46.0X4	T46.0X5	T46.0X6
Strophantin-g	T46.0X1	T46.0X2	T46.0X3	T46.0X4	T46.0X5	T46.0X6
Strychnine (nonmedicinal) (pesticide) (salts)	T65.1X1	T65.1X2	T65.1X3	T65.1X4	—	—
medicinal	T48.291	T48.292	T48.293	T48.294	T48.295	T48.296
Strychnos (ignatii) — see Strychnine						
Styramate	T42.8X1	T42.8X2	T42.8X3	T42.8X4	T42.8X5	T42.8X6
Styrene	T65.891	T65.892	T65.893	T65.894	—	—
Succinimide, antiepileptic or anticonvulsant	T42.2X1	T42.2X2	T42.2X3	T42.2X4	T42.2X5	T42.2X6
mercuric — see Mercury						
Succinylcholine	T48.1X1	T48.1X2	T48.1X3	T48.1X4	T48.1X5	T48.1X6
Succinylsulfathiazole	T37.0X1	T37.0X2	T37.0X3	T37.0X4	T37.0X5	T37.0X6
Sucralfate	T47.1X1	T47.1X2	T47.1X3	T47.1X4	T47.1X5	T47.1X6
Sucrose	T50.3X1	T50.3X2	T50.3X3	T50.3X4	T50.3X5	T50.3X6
Sufentanil	T40.411	T40.412	T40.413	T40.414	T40.415	T40.416
Sulbactam	T36.0X1	T36.0X2	T36.0X3	T36.0X4	T36.0X5	T36.0X6
Sulbenicillin	T36.0X1	T36.0X2	T36.0X3	T36.0X4	T36.0X5	T36.0X6
Sulbentine	T49.0X1	T49.0X2	T49.0X3	T49.0X4	T49.0X5	T49.0X6
Sulfacetamide	T49.0X1	T49.0X2	T49.0X3	T49.0X4	T49.0X5	T49.0X6
ophthalmic preparation	T49.5X1	T49.5X2	T49.5X3	T49.5X4	T49.5X5	T49.5X6
Sulfachlorpyridazine	T37.0X1	T37.0X2	T37.0X3	T37.0X4	T37.0X5	T37.0X6
Sulfacitine	T37.0X1	T37.0X2	T37.0X3	T37.0X4	T37.0X5	T37.0X6
Sulfadiasulfone sodium	T37.0X1	T37.0X2	T37.0X3	T37.0X4	T37.0X5	T37.0X6
Sulfadiazine	T37.0X1	T37.0X2	T37.0X3	T37.0X4	T37.0X5	T37.0X6
silver (topical)	T49.0X1	T49.0X2	T49.0X3	T49.0X4	T49.0X5	T49.0X6
Sulfadimethoxine	T37.0X1	T37.0X2	T37.0X3	T37.0X4	T37.0X5	T37.0X6
Sulfadimidine	T37.0X1	T37.0X2	T37.0X3	T37.0X4	T37.0X5	T37.0X6
Sulfadoxine	T37.0X1	T37.0X2	T37.0X3	T37.0X4	T37.0X5	T37.0X6
with pyrimethamine	T37.2X1	T37.2X2	T37.2X3	T37.2X4	T37.2X5	T37.2X6
Sulfaethidole	T37.0X1	T37.0X2	T37.0X3	T37.0X4	T37.0X5	T37.0X6
Sulfafurazole	T37.0X1	T37.0X2	T37.0X3	T37.0X4	T37.0X5	T37.0X6
Sulfaguanidine	T37.0X1	T37.0X2	T37.0X3	T37.0X4	T37.0X5	T37.0X6
Sulfalene	T37.0X1	T37.0X2	T37.0X3	T37.0X4	T37.0X5	T37.0X6
Sulfaloxate	T37.0X1	T37.0X2	T37.0X3	T37.0X4	T37.0X5	T37.0X6
Sulfaloxic acid	T37.0X1	T37.0X2	T37.0X3	T37.0X4	T37.0X5	T37.0X6
Sulfamazone	T39.2X1	T39.2X2	T39.2X3	T39.2X4	T39.2X5	T39.2X6
Sulfamerazine	T37.0X1	T37.0X2	T37.0X3	T37.0X4	T37.0X5	T37.0X6
Sulfameter	T37.0X1	T37.0X2	T37.0X3	T37.0X4	T37.0X5	T37.0X6
Sulfamethazine	T37.0X1	T37.0X2	T37.0X3	T37.0X4	T37.0X5	T37.0X6
Sulfamethizole	T37.0X1	T37.0X2	T37.0X3	T37.0X4	T37.0X5	T37.0X6
Sulfamethoxazole	T37.0X1	T37.0X2	T37.0X3	T37.0X4	T37.0X5	T37.0X6
with trimethoprim	T36.8X1	T36.8X2	T36.8X3	T36.8X4	T36.8X5	T36.8X6
Sulfamethoxydiazine	T37.0X1	T37.0X2	T37.0X3	T37.0X4	T37.0X5	T37.0X6
Sulfamethoxypyridazine	T37.0X1	T37.0X2	T37.0X3	T37.0X4	T37.0X5	T37.0X6
Sulfamethylthiazole	T37.0X1	T37.0X2	T37.0X3	T37.0X4	T37.0X5	T37.0X6
Sulfametoxydiazine	T37.0X1	T37.0X2	T37.0X3	T37.0X4	T37.0X5	T37.0X6
Sulfamidopyrine	T39.2X1	T39.2X2	T39.2X3	T39.2X4	T39.2X5	T39.2X6
Sulfamonomethoxine	T37.0X1	T37.0X2	T37.0X3	T37.0X4	T37.0X5	T37.0X6
Sulfamoxole	T37.0X1	T37.0X2	T37.0X3	T37.0X4	T37.0X5	T37.0X6
Sulfamylon	T49.0X1	T49.0X2	T49.0X3	T49.0X4	T49.0X5	T49.0X6
Sulfan blue (diagnostic dye)	T50.8X1	T50.8X2	T50.8X3	T50.8X4	T50.8X5	T50.8X6
Sulfanilamide	T37.0X1	T37.0X2	T37.0X3	T37.0X4	T37.0X5	T37.0X6
Sulfanilylguanidine	T37.0X1	T37.0X2	T37.0X3	T37.0X4	T37.0X5	T37.0X6
Sulfaperin	T37.0X1	T37.0X2	T37.0X3	T37.0X4	T37.0X5	T37.0X6
Sulfaphenazole	T37.0X1	T37.0X2	T37.0X3	T37.0X4	T37.0X5	T37.0X6
Sulfaphenylthiazole	T37.0X1	T37.0X2	T37.0X3	T37.0X4	T37.0X5	T37.0X6
Sulfaproxyline	T37.0X1	T37.0X2	T37.0X3	T37.0X4	T37.0X5	T37.0X6
Sulfapyridine	T37.0X1	T37.0X2	T37.0X3	T37.0X4	T37.0X5	T37.0X6
Sulfapyrimidine	T37.0X1	T37.0X2	T37.0X3	T37.0X4	T37.0X5	T37.0X6
Sulfarsphenamine	T37.8X1	T37.8X2	T37.8X3	T37.8X4	T37.8X5	T37.8X6
Sulfasalazine	T37.0X1	T37.0X2	T37.0X3	T37.0X4	T37.0X5	T37.0X6
Sulfasuxidine	T37.0X1	T37.0X2	T37.0X3	T37.0X4	T37.0X5	T37.0X6
Sulfasymazine	T37.0X1	T37.0X2	T37.0X3	T37.0X4	T37.0X5	T37.0X6
Sulfated amylopectin	T47.8X1	T47.8X2	T47.8X3	T47.8X4	T47.8X5	T47.8X6
Sulfathiazole	T37.0X1	T37.0X2	T37.0X3	T37.0X4	T37.0X5	T37.0X6
Sulfatostearate	T49.2X1	T49.2X2	T49.2X3	T49.2X4	T49.2X5	T49.2X6
Sulfinpyrazone	T50.4X1	T50.4X2	T50.4X3	T50.4X4	T50.4X5	T50.4X6
Sulfiram	T49.0X1	T49.0X2	T49.0X3	T49.0X4	T49.0X5	T49.0X6
Sulfisomidine	T37.0X1	T37.0X2	T37.0X3	T37.0X4	T37.0X5	T37.0X6
Sulfisoxazole	T37.0X1	T37.0X2	T37.0X3	T37.0X4	T37.0X5	T37.0X6
ophthalmic preparation	T49.5X1	T49.5X2	T49.5X3	T49.5X4	T49.5X5	T49.5X6
Sulfobromophthalein (sodium)	T50.8X1	T50.8X2	T50.8X3	T50.8X4	T50.8X5	T50.8X6
Sulfobromphthalein	T50.8X1	T50.8X2	T50.8X3	T50.8X4	T50.8X5	T50.8X6

Substance	Poisoning, Accidental (unintentional)	Poisoning, Intentional Self-harm	Poisoning, Assault	Poisoning, Undetermined	Adverse Effect	Under-dosing
Sulfogaiacol	T48.4X1	T48.4X2	T48.4X3	T48.4X4	T48.4X5	T48.4X6
Sulfomyxin	T36.8X1	T36.8X2	T36.8X3	T36.8X4	T36.8X5	T36.8X6
Sulfonal	T42.6X1	T42.6X2	T42.6X3	T42.6X4	T42.6X5	T42.6X6
Sulfonamide NEC	T37.0X1	T37.0X2	T37.0X3	T37.0X4	T37.0X5	T37.0X6
eye	T49.5X1	T49.5X2	T49.5X3	T49.5X4	T49.5X5	T49.5X6
Sulfonazide	T37.1X1	T37.1X2	T37.1X3	T37.1X4	T37.1X5	T37.1X6
Sulfones	T37.1X1	T37.1X2	T37.1X3	T37.1X4	T37.1X5	T37.1X6
Sulfonethylmethane	T42.6X1	T42.6X2	T42.6X3	T42.6X4	T42.6X5	T42.6X6
Sulfonmethane	T42.6X1	T42.6X2	T42.6X3	T42.6X4	T42.6X5	T42.6X6
Sulfonphthal, sulfonphthol	T50.8X1	T50.8X2	T50.8X3	T50.8X4	T50.8X5	T50.8X6
Sulfonylurea derivatives, oral	T38.3X1	T38.3X2	T38.3X3	T38.3X4	T38.3X5	T38.3X6
Sulforidazine	T43.3X1	T43.3X2	T43.3X3	T43.3X4	T43.3X5	T43.3X6
Sulfoxone	T37.1X1	T37.1X2	T37.1X3	T37.1X4	T37.1X5	T37.1X6
Sulfuric acid	T54.2X1	T54.2X2	T54.2X3	T54.2X4	—	—
Sulfur, sulfurated, sulfuric, sulfurous, sulfuryl (compounds NEC) (medicinal)	T49.4X1	T49.4X2	T49.4X3	T49.4X4	T49.4X5	T49.4X6
acid	T54.2X1	T54.2X2	T54.2X3	T54.2X4	—	—
dioxide (gas)	T59.1X1	T59.1X2	T59.1X3	T59.1X4	—	—
ether — see Ether(s)						
hydrogen	T59.6X1	T59.6X2	T59.6X3	T59.6X4	—	—
medicinal (keratolytic) (ointment) NEC	T49.4X1	T49.4X2	T49.4X3	T49.4X4	T49.4X5	T49.4X6
ointment	T49.0X1	T49.0X2	T49.0X3	T49.0X4	T49.0X5	T49.0X6
pesticide (vapor)	T60.91	T60.92	T60.93	T60.94		
vapor NEC	T59.891	T59.892	T59.893	T59.894	—	—
Sulglicotide	T47.1X1	T47.1X2	T47.1X3	T47.1X4	T47.1X5	T47.1X6
Sulindac	T39.391	T39.392	T39.393	T39.394	T39.395	T39.396
Sulisatin	T47.2X1	T47.2X2	T47.2X3	T47.2X4	T47.2X5	T47.2X6
Sulisobenzone	T49.3X1	T49.3X2	T49.3X3	T49.3X4	T49.3X5	T49.3X6
Sulkowitch's reagent	T50.8X1	T50.8X2	T50.8X3	T50.8X4	T50.8X5	T50.8X6
Sulmetozine	T44.3X1	T44.3X2	T44.3X3	T44.3X4	T44.3X5	T44.3X6
Suloctidil	T46.7X1	T46.7X2	T46.7X3	T46.7X4	T46.7X5	T46.7X6
Sulph- — see also Sulf-						
Sulphadiazine	T37.0X1	T37.0X2	T37.0X3	T37.0X4	T37.0X5	T37.0X6
Sulphadimethoxine	T37.0X1	T37.0X2	T37.0X3	T37.0X4	T37.0X5	T37.0X6
Sulphadimidine	T37.0X1	T37.0X2	T37.0X3	T37.0X4	T37.0X5	T37.0X6
Sulphadione	T37.1X1	T37.1X2	T37.1X3	T37.1X4	T37.1X5	T37.1X6
Sulphafurazole	T37.0X1	T37.0X2	T37.0X3	T37.0X4	T37.0X5	T37.0X6
Sulphamethizole	T37.0X1	T37.0X2	T37.0X3	T37.0X4	T37.0X5	T37.0X6
Sulphamethoxazole	T37.0X1	T37.0X2	T37.0X3	T37.0X4	T37.0X5	T37.0X6
Sulphan blue	T50.8X1	T50.8X2	T50.8X3	T50.8X4	T50.8X5	T50.8X6
Sulphaphenazole	T37.0X1	T37.0X2	T37.0X3	T37.0X4	T37.0X5	T37.0X6
Sulphapyridine	T37.0X1	T37.0X2	T37.0X3	T37.0X4	T37.0X5	T37.0X6
Sulphasalazine	T37.0X1	T37.0X2	T37.0X3	T37.0X4	T37.0X5	T37.0X6
Sulphinpyrazone	T50.4X1	T50.4X2	T50.4X3	T50.4X4	T50.4X5	T50.4X6
Sulpiride	T43.591	T43.592	T43.593	T43.594	T43.595	T43.596
Sulprostone	T48.0X1	T48.0X2	T48.0X3	T48.0X4	T48.0X5	T48.0X6
Sulpyrine	T39.2X1	T39.2X2	T39.2X3	T39.2X4	T39.2X5	T39.2X6
Sultamicillin	T36.0X1	T36.0X2	T36.0X3	T36.0X4	T36.0X5	T36.0X6
Sulthiame	T42.6X1	T42.6X2	T42.6X3	T42.6X4	T42.6X5	T42.6X6
Sultiame	T42.6X1	T42.6X2	T42.6X3	T42.6X4	T42.6X5	T42.6X6
Sultopride	T43.591	T43.592	T43.593	T43.594	T43.595	T43.596
Sumatriptan	T39.8X1	T39.8X2	T39.8X3	T39.8X4	T39.8X5	T39.8X6
Sunflower seed oil	T46.6X1	T46.6X2	T46.6X3	T46.6X4	T46.6X5	T46.6X6
Superinone	T48.4X1	T48.4X2	T48.4X3	T48.4X4	T48.4X5	T48.4X6
Suprofen	T39.311	T39.312	T39.313	T39.314	T39.315	T39.316
Suramin (sodium)	T37.4X1	T37.4X2	T37.4X3	T37.4X4	T37.4X5	T37.4X6
Surfacaine	T41.3X1	T41.3X2	T41.3X3	T41.3X4	T41.3X5	T41.3X6
Surital	T41.1X1	T41.1X2	T41.1X3	T41.1X4	T41.1X5	T41.1X6
Sutilains	T45.3X1	T45.3X2	T45.3X3	T45.3X4	T45.3X5	T45.3X6
Suxamethonium (chloride)	T48.1X1	T48.1X2	T48.1X3	T48.1X4	T48.1X5	T48.1X6
Suxethonium (chloride)	T48.1X1	T48.1X2	T48.1X3	T48.1X4	T48.1X5	T48.1X6
Suxibuzone	T39.2X1	T39.2X2	T39.2X3	T39.2X4	T39.2X5	T39.2X6
Sweetener	T50.901	T50.902	T50.903	T50.904	T50.905	T50.906
Sweet niter spirit	T46.3X1	T46.3X2	T46.3X3	T46.3X4	T46.3X5	T46.3X6
Sweet oil (birch)	T49.3X1	T49.3X2	T49.3X3	T49.3X4	T49.3X5	T49.3X6
Sym-dichloroethyl ether	T53.6X1	T53.6X2	T53.6X3	T53.6X4	—	—
Sympatholytic NEC	T44.8X1	T44.8X2	T44.8X3	T44.8X4	T44.8X5	T44.8X6
haloalkylamine	T44.8X1	T44.8X2	T44.8X3	T44.8X4	T44.8X5	T44.8X6
Sympathomimetic NEC	T44.901	T44.902	T44.903	T44.904	T44.905	T44.906
anti-common-cold	T48.5X1	T48.5X2	T48.5X3	T48.5X4	T48.5X5	T48.5X6
bronchodilator	T48.6X1	T48.6X2	T48.6X3	T48.6X4	T48.6X5	T48.6X6
specified NEC	T44.991	T44.992	T44.993	T44.994	T44.995	T44.996
Synagis	T50.B91	T50.B92	T50.B93	T50.B94	T50.B95	T50.B96
Synalar	T49.0X1	T49.0X2	T49.0X3	T49.0X4	T49.0X5	T49.0X6
Synthetic cannabinoids	T40.721	T40.722	T40.723	T40.724	T40.725	T40.726
Synthroid	T38.1X1	T38.1X2	T38.1X3	T38.1X4	T38.1X5	T38.1X6
Syntocinon	T48.0X1	T48.0X2	T48.0X3	T48.0X4	T48.0X5	T48.0X6
Syrosingopine	T46.5X1	T46.5X2	T46.5X3	T46.5X4	T46.5X5	T46.5X6

Substance	Poisoning, Accidental (unintentional)	Poisoning, Intentional Self-harm	Poisoning, Assault	Poisoning, Undetermined	Adverse Effect	Under-dosing
Systemic drug	T45.91	T45.92	T45.93	T45.94	T45.95	T45.96
specified NEC	T45.8X1	T45.8X2	T45.8X3	T45.8X4	T45.8X5	T45.8X6
Tablets — see also specified substance	T50.901	T50.902	T50.903	T50.904	T50.905	T50.906
Tace	T38.5X1	T38.5X2	T38.5X3	T38.5X4	T38.5X5	T38.5X6
Tacrine	T44.0X1	T44.0X2	T44.0X3	T44.0X4	T44.0X5	T44.0X6
Tadalafil	T46.7X1	T46.7X2	T46.7X3	T46.7X4	T46.7X5	T46.7X6
Talampicillin	T36.0X1	T36.0X2	T36.0X3	T36.0X4	T36.0X5	T36.0X6
Talbutal	T42.3X1	T42.3X2	T42.3X3	T42.3X4	T42.3X5	T42.3X6
Talc powder	T49.3X1	T49.3X2	T49.3X3	T49.3X4	T49.3X5	T49.3X6
Talcum	T49.3X1	T49.3X2	T49.3X3	T49.3X4	T49.3X5	T49.3X6
Taleranol	T38.6X1	T38.6X2	T38.6X3	T38.6X4	T38.6X5	T38.6X6
Tamoxifen	T38.6X1	T38.6X2	T38.6X3	T38.6X4	T38.6X5	T38.6X6
Tamsulosin	T44.6X1	T44.6X2	T44.6X3	T44.6X4	T44.6X5	T44.6X6
Tandearil, tanderil	T39.2X1	T39.2X2	T39.2X3	T39.2X4	T39.2X5	T39.2X6
Tannic acid	T49.2X1	T49.2X2	T49.2X3	T49.2X4	T49.2X5	T49.2X6
medicinal (astringent)	T49.2X1	T49.2X2	T49.2X3	T49.2X4	T49.2X5	T49.2X6
Tannin — see Tannic acid						
Tansy	T62.2X1	T62.2X2	T62.2X3	T62.2X4	—	—
TAO	T36.3X1	T36.3X2	T36.3X3	T36.3X4	T36.3X5	T36.3X6
Tapazole	T38.2X1	T38.2X2	T38.2X3	T38.2X4	T38.2X5	T38.2X6
Taractan	T43.591	T43.592	T43.593	T43.594	T43.595	T43.596
Tarantula (venomous)	T63.321	T63.322	T63.323	T63.324		
Tartar emetic	T37.8X1	T37.8X2	T37.8X3	T37.8X4	T37.8X5	T37.8X6
Tartaric acid	T65.891	T65.892	T65.893	T65.894	—	—
Tartrated antimony (anti-infective)	T37.8X1	T37.8X2	T37.8X3	T37.8X4	T37.8X5	T37.8X6
Tartrate, laxative	T47.4X1	T47.4X2	T47.4X3	T47.4X4	T47.4X5	T47.4X6
Tar NEC	T52.0X1	T52.0X2	T52.0X3	T52.0X4	—	—
camphor	T60.1X1	T60.1X2	T60.1X3	T60.1X4	—	—
distillate	T49.1X1	T49.1X2	T49.1X3	T49.1X4	T49.1X5	T49.1X6
fumes	T59.891	T59.892	T59.893	T59.894	—	—
medicinal	T49.1X1	T49.1X2	T49.1X3	T49.1X4	T49.1X5	T49.1X6
ointment	T49.1X1	T49.1X2	T49.1X3	T49.1X4	T49.1X5	T49.1X6
Tauromustine	T45.1X1	T45.1X2	T45.1X3	T45.1X4	T45.1X5	T45.1X6
TCA — see Trichloroacetic acid						
TCDD	T53.7X1	T53.7X2	T53.7X3	T53.7X4	—	—
TDI (vapor)	T65.0X1	T65.0X2	T65.0X3	T65.0X4	—	—
Tear						
gas	T59.3X1	T59.3X2	T59.3X3	T59.3X4	—	—
solution	T49.5X1	T49.5X2	T49.5X3	T49.5X4	T49.5X5	T49.5X6
Teclothiazide	T50.2X1	T50.2X2	T50.2X3	T50.2X4	T50.2X5	T50.2X6
Teclozan	T37.3X1	T37.3X2	T37.3X3	T37.3X4	T37.3X5	T37.3X6
Tegafur	T45.1X1	T45.1X2	T45.1X3	T45.1X4	T45.1X5	T45.1X6
Tegretol	T42.1X1	T42.1X2	T42.1X3	T42.1X4	T42.1X5	T42.1X6
Teicoplanin	T36.8X1	T36.8X2	T36.8X3	T36.8X4	T36.8X5	T36.8X6
Telepaque	T50.8X1	T50.8X2	T50.8X3	T50.8X4	T50.8X5	T50.8X6
Tellurium	T56.891	T56.892	T56.893	T56.894	—	—
fumes	T56.891	T56.892	T56.893	T56.894	—	—
TEM	T45.1X1	T45.1X2	T45.1X3	T45.1X4	T45.1X5	T45.1X6
Temazepam	T42.4X1	T42.4X2	T42.4X3	T42.4X4	T42.4X5	T42.4X6
Temocillin	T36.0X1	T36.0X2	T36.0X3	T36.0X4	T36.0X5	T36.0X6
Tenamfetamine	T43.621	T43.622	T43.623	T43.624	T43.625	T43.626
Teniposide	T45.1X1	T45.1X2	T45.1X3	T45.1X4	T45.1X5	T45.1X6
Tenitramine	T46.3X1	T46.3X2	T46.3X3	T46.3X4	T46.3X5	T46.3X6
Tenoglicin	T48.4X1	T48.4X2	T48.4X3	T48.4X4	T48.4X5	T48.4X6
Tenonitrozole	T37.3X1	T37.3X2	T37.3X3	T37.3X4	T37.3X5	T37.3X6
Tenoxicam	T39.391	T39.392	T39.393	T39.394	T39.395	T39.396
TEPA	T45.1X1	T45.1X2	T45.1X3	T45.1X4	T45.1X5	T45.1X6
TEPP	T60.0X1	T60.0X2	T60.0X3	T60.0X4	—	—
Teprotide	T46.5X1	T46.5X2	T46.5X3	T46.5X4	T46.5X5	T46.5X6
Terazosin	T44.6X1	T44.6X2	T44.6X3	T44.6X4	T44.6X5	T44.6X6
Terbufos	T60.0X1	T60.0X2	T60.0X3	T60.0X4	—	—
Terbutaline	T48.6X1	T48.6X2	T48.6X3	T48.6X4	T48.6X5	T48.6X6
Terconazole	T49.0X1	T49.0X2	T49.0X3	T49.0X4	T49.0X5	T49.0X6
Terfenadine	T45.0X1	T45.0X2	T45.0X3	T45.0X4	T45.0X5	T45.0X6
Teriparatide (acetate)	T50.991	T50.992	T50.993	T50.994	T50.995	T50.996
Terizidone	T37.1X1	T37.1X2	T37.1X3	T37.1X4	T37.1X5	T37.1X6
Terlipressin	T38.891	T38.892	T38.893	T38.894	T38.895	T38.896
Terodiline	T46.3X1	T46.3X2	T46.3X3	T46.3X4	T46.3X5	T46.3X6
Teroxalene	T37.4X1	T37.4X2	T37.4X3	T37.4X4	T37.4X5	T37.4X6
Terpin (cis) hydrate	T48.4X1	T48.4X2	T48.4X3	T48.4X4	T48.4X5	T48.4X6
Terramycin	T36.4X1	T36.4X2	T36.4X3	T36.4X4	T36.4X5	T36.4X6
Tertatolol	T44.7X1	T44.7X2	T44.7X3	T44.7X4	T44.7X5	T44.7X6
Tessalon	T48.3X1	T48.3X2	T48.3X3	T48.3X4	T48.3X5	T48.3X6
Testolactone	T38.7X1	T38.7X2	T38.7X3	T38.7X4	T38.7X5	T38.7X6
Testosterone	T38.7X1	T38.7X2	T38.7X3	T38.7X4	T38.7X5	T38.7X6
Tetanus toxoid or vaccine	T50.A91	T50.A92	T50.A93	T50.A94	T50.A95	T50.A96
antitoxin	T50.Z11	T50.Z12	T50.Z13	T50.Z14	T50.Z15	T50.Z16
immune globulin (human)	T50.Z11	T50.Z12	T50.Z13	T50.Z14	T50.Z15	T50.Z16
toxoid	T50.A91	T50.A92	T50.A93	T50.A94	T50.A95	T50.A96
with diphtheria toxoid	T50.A21	T50.A22	T50.A23	T50.A24	T50.A25	T50.A26
with pertussis	T50.A11	T50.A12	T50.A13	T50.A14	T50.A15	T50.A16

Substance	Poisoning, Accidental (unintentional)	Poisoning, Intentional Self-harm	Poisoning, Assault	Poisoning, Undetermined	Adverse Effect	Under-dosing
Tetrabenazine	T43.591	T43.592	T43.593	T43.594	T43.595	T43.596
Tetracaine	T41.3X1	T41.3X2	T41.3X3	T41.3X4	T41.3X5	T41.3X6
nerve block (peripheral) (plexus)	T41.3X1	T41.3X2	T41.3X3	T41.3X4	T41.3X5	T41.3X6
regional	T41.3X1	T41.3X2	T41.3X3	T41.3X4	T41.3X5	T41.3X6
spinal	T41.3X1	T41.3X2	T41.3X3	T41.3X4	T41.3X5	T41.3X6
Tetrachlorethylene — see Tetrachloroethylene						
Tetrachlormethiazide	T50.2X1	T50.2X2	T50.2X3	T50.2X4	T50.2X5	T50.2X6
Tetrachloroethane	T53.6X1	T53.6X2	T53.6X3	T53.6X4	—	—
vapor	T53.6X1	T53.6X2	T53.6X3	T53.6X4	—	—
paint or varnish	T53.6X1	T53.6X2	T53.6X3	T53.6X4	—	—
Tetrachloroethylene (liquid)	T53.3X1	T53.3X2	T53.3X3	T53.3X4	—	—
medicinal	T37.4X1	T37.4X2	T37.4X3	T37.4X4	T37.4X5	T37.4X6
vapor	T53.3X1	T53.3X2	T53.3X3	T53.3X4	—	—
Tetrachloromethane — see Carbon tetrachloride						
Tetracosactide	T38.811	T38.812	T38.813	T38.814	T38.815	T38.816
Tetracosactrin	T38.811	T38.812	T38.813	T38.814	T38.815	T38.816
Tetracycline	T36.4X1	T36.4X2	T36.4X3	T36.4X4	T36.4X5	T36.4X6
ophthalmic preparation	T49.5X1	T49.5X2	T49.5X3	T49.5X4	T49.5X5	T49.5X6
topical NEC	T49.0X1	T49.0X2	T49.0X3	T49.0X4	T49.0X5	T49.0X6
Tetradifon	T60.8X1	T60.8X2	T60.8X3	T60.8X4	—	—
Tetradotoxin	T61.771	T61.772	T61.773	T61.774	—	—
Tetraethyl						
lead	T56.0X1	T56.0X2	T56.0X3	T56.0X4	—	—
pyrophosphate	T60.0X1	T60.0X2	T60.0X3	T60.0X4	—	—
Tetraethylammonium chloride	T44.2X1	T44.2X2	T44.2X3	T44.2X4	T44.2X5	T44.2X6
Tetraethylthiuram disulfide	T50.6X1	T50.6X2	T50.6X3	T50.6X4	T50.6X5	T50.6X6
Tetrahydroaminoacridine	T44.0X1	T44.0X2	T44.0X3	T44.0X4	T44.0X5	T44.0X6
Tetrahydrocannabinol	T40.711	T40.712	T40.713	T40.714	T40.715	T40.716
Tetrahydrofuran	T52.8X1	T52.8X2	T52.8X3	T52.8X4	—	—
Tetrahydronaphthalene	T52.8X1	T52.8X2	T52.8X3	T52.8X4	—	—
Tetrahydrozoline	T49.5X1	T49.5X2	T49.5X3	T49.5X4	T49.5X5	T49.5X6
Tetralin	T52.8X1	T52.8X2	T52.8X3	T52.8X4	—	—
Tetramethrin	T60.2X1	T60.2X2	T60.2X3	T60.2X4	—	—
Tetramethylthiuram (disulfide) NEC	T60.3X1	T60.3X2	T60.3X3	T60.3X4	—	—
medicinal	T49.0X1	T49.0X2	T49.0X3	T49.0X4	T49.0X5	T49.0X6
Tetramisole	T37.4X1	T37.4X2	T37.4X3	T37.4X4	T37.4X5	T37.4X6
Tetranicotinoyl fructose	T46.7X1	T46.7X2	T46.7X3	T46.7X4	T46.7X5	T46.7X6
Tetrazepam	T42.4X1	T42.4X2	T42.4X3	T42.4X4	T42.4X5	T42.4X6
Tetronal	T42.6X1	T42.6X2	T42.6X3	T42.6X4	T42.6X5	T42.6X6
Tetryl	T65.3X1	T65.3X2	T65.3X3	T65.3X4	—	—
Tetrylammonium chloride	T44.2X1	T44.2X2	T44.2X3	T44.2X4	T44.2X5	T44.2X6
Tetryzoline	T49.5X1	T49.5X2	T49.5X3	T49.5X4	T49.5X5	T49.5X6
Thalidomide	T45.1X1	T45.1X2	T45.1X3	T45.1X4	T45.1X5	T45.1X6
Thallium (compounds) (dust) NEC	T56.811	T56.812	T56.813	T56.814	—	—
pesticide	T60.4X1	T60.4X2	T60.4X3	T60.4X4	—	—
THC	T40.711	T40.712	T40.713	T40.714	T40.715	T40.716
Thebacon	T48.3X1	T48.3X2	T48.3X3	T48.3X4	T48.3X5	T48.3X6
Thebaine	T40.2X1	T40.2X2	T40.2X3	T40.2X4	T40.2X5	T40.2X6
Thenoic acid	T49.6X1	T49.6X2	T49.6X3	T49.6X4	T49.6X5	T49.6X6
Thenyldiamine	T45.0X1	T45.0X2	T45.0X3	T45.0X4	T45.0X5	T45.0X6
Theobromine (calcium salicylate)	T48.6X1	T48.6X2	T48.6X3	T48.6X4	T48.6X5	T48.6X6
sodium salicylate	T48.6X1	T48.6X2	T48.6X3	T48.6X4	T48.6X5	T48.6X6
Theophyllamine	T48.6X1	T48.6X2	T48.6X3	T48.6X4	T48.6X5	T48.6X6
Theophylline	T48.6X1	T48.6X2	T48.6X3	T48.6X4	T48.6X5	T48.6X6
aminobenzoic acid	T48.6X1	T48.6X2	T48.6X3	T48.6X4	T48.6X5	T48.6X6
ethylenediamine	T48.6X1	T48.6X2	T48.6X3	T48.6X4	T48.6X5	T48.6X6
piperazine p-amino-benzoate	T48.6X1	T48.6X2	T48.6X3	T48.6X4	T48.6X5	T48.6X6
Thiabendazole	T37.4X1	T37.4X2	T37.4X3	T37.4X4	T37.4X5	T37.4X6
Thialbarbital	T41.1X1	T41.1X2	T41.1X3	T41.1X4	T41.1X5	T41.1X6
Thiamazole	T38.2X1	T38.2X2	T38.2X3	T38.2X4	T38.2X5	T38.2X6
Thiambutosine	T37.1X1	T37.1X2	T37.1X3	T37.1X4	T37.1X5	T37.1X6
Thiamine	T45.2X1	T45.2X2	T45.2X3	T45.2X4	T45.2X5	T45.2X6
Thiamphenicol	T36.2X1	T36.2X2	T36.2X3	T36.2X4	T36.2X5	T36.2X6
Thiamylal	T41.1X1	T41.1X2	T41.1X3	T41.1X4	T41.1X5	T41.1X6
sodium	T41.1X1	T41.1X2	T41.1X3	T41.1X4	T41.1X5	T41.1X6
Thiazesim	T43.291	T43.292	T43.293	T43.294	T43.295	T43.296
Thiazides (diuretics)	T50.2X1	T50.2X2	T50.2X3	T50.2X4	T50.2X5	T50.2X6
Thiazinamium metilsulfate	T43.3X1	T43.3X2	T43.3X3	T43.3X4	T43.3X5	T43.3X6
Thiethylperazine	T43.3X1	T43.3X2	T43.3X3	T43.3X4	T43.3X5	T43.3X6
Thimerosal	T49.0X1	T49.0X2	T49.0X3	T49.0X4	T49.0X5	T49.0X6
ophthalmic preparation	T49.5X1	T49.5X2	T49.5X3	T49.5X4	T49.5X5	T49.5X6
Thioacetazone	T37.1X1	T37.1X2	T37.1X3	T37.1X4	T37.1X5	T37.1X6

Additional Character May Be Required — Refer to the Tabular List for Character Selection   Subterms under main terms may continue to next column or page

Substance	Poisoning, Accidental (unintentional)	Poisoning, Intentional Self-harm	Poisoning, Assault	Poisoning, Undetermined	Adverse Effect	Under-dosing
Thioacetazone — continued						
with isoniazid	T37.1X1	T37.1X2	T37.1X3	T37.1X4	T37.1X5	T37.1X6
Thiobarbital sodium	T41.1X1	T41.1X2	T41.1X3	T41.1X4	T41.1X5	T41.1X6
Thiobarbiturate anesthetic	T41.1X1	T41.1X2	T41.1X3	T41.1X4	T41.1X5	T41.1X6
Thiobismol	T37.8X1	T37.8X2	T37.8X3	T37.8X4	T37.8X5	T37.8X6
Thiobutabarbital sodium	T41.1X1	T41.1X2	T41.1X3	T41.1X4	T41.1X5	T41.1X6
Thiocarbamate (insecticide)	T60.0X1	T60.0X2	T60.0X3	T60.0X4	—	—
Thiocarbamide	T38.2X1	T38.2X2	T38.2X3	T38.2X4	T38.2X5	T38.2X6
Thiocarbarsone	T37.8X1	T37.8X2	T37.8X3	T37.8X4	T37.8X5	T37.8X6
Thiocarlide	T37.1X1	T37.1X2	T37.1X3	T37.1X4	T37.1X5	T37.1X6
Thioctamide	T50.991	T50.992	T50.993	T50.994	T50.995	T50.996
Thioctic acid	T50.991	T50.992	T50.993	T50.994	T50.995	T50.996
Thiofos	T60.0X1	T60.0X2	T60.0X3	T60.0X4	—	—
Thioglycolate	T49.4X1	T49.4X2	T49.4X3	T49.4X4	T49.4X5	T49.4X6
Thioglycolic acid	T65.891	T65.892	T65.893	T65.894	—	—
Thioguanine	T45.1X1	T45.1X2	T45.1X3	T45.1X4	T45.1X5	T45.1X6
Thiomercaptomerin	T50.2X1	T50.2X2	T50.2X3	T50.2X4	T50.2X5	T50.2X6
Thiomerin	T50.2X1	T50.2X2	T50.2X3	T50.2X4	T50.2X5	T50.2X6
Thiomersal	T49.0X1	T49.0X2	T49.0X3	T49.0X4	T49.0X5	T49.0X6
Thionazin	T60.0X1	T60.0X2	T60.0X3	T60.0X4	—	—
Thiopental (sodium)	T41.1X1	T41.1X2	T41.1X3	T41.1X4	T41.1X5	T41.1X6
Thiopentone (sodium)	T41.1X1	T41.1X2	T41.1X3	T41.1X4	T41.1X5	T41.1X6
Thiopropazate	T43.3X1	T43.3X2	T43.3X3	T43.3X4	T43.3X5	T43.3X6
Thioproperazine	T43.3X1	T43.3X2	T43.3X3	T43.3X4	T43.3X5	T43.3X6
Thioridazine	T43.3X1	T43.3X2	T43.3X3	T43.3X4	T43.3X5	T43.3X6
Thiosinamine	T49.3X1	T49.3X2	T49.3X3	T49.3X4	T49.3X5	T49.3X6
Thiotepa	T45.1X1	T45.1X2	T45.1X3	T45.1X4	T45.1X5	T45.1X6
Thiothixene	T43.4X1	T43.4X2	T43.4X3	T43.4X4	T43.4X5	T43.4X6
Thiouracil (benzyl) (methyl) (propyl)	T38.2X1	T38.2X2	T38.2X3	T38.2X4	T38.2X5	T38.2X6
Thiourea	T38.2X1	T38.2X2	T38.2X3	T38.2X4	T38.2X5	T38.2X6
Thiphenamil	T44.3X1	T44.3X2	T44.3X3	T44.3X4	T44.3X5	T44.3X6
Thiram	T60.3X1	T60.3X2	T60.3X3	T60.3X4	—	—
medicinal	T49.2X1	T49.2X2	T49.2X3	T49.2X4	T49.2X5	T49.2X6
Thonzylamine (systemic)	T45.0X1	T45.0X2	T45.0X3	T45.0X4	T45.0X5	T45.0X6
mucosal decongestant	T48.5X1	T48.5X2	T48.5X3	T48.5X4	T48.5X5	T48.5X6
Thorazine	T43.3X1	T43.3X2	T43.3X3	T43.3X4	T43.3X5	T43.3X6
Thorium dioxide suspension	T50.8X1	T50.8X2	T50.8X3	T50.8X4	T50.8X5	T50.8X6
Thornapple	T62.2X1	T62.2X2	T62.2X3	T62.2X4	—	—
Throat drug NEC	T49.6X1	T49.6X2	T49.6X3	T49.6X4	T49.6X5	T49.6X6
Thrombin	T45.7X1	T45.7X2	T45.7X3	T45.7X4	T45.7X5	T45.7X6
Thrombolysin	T45.611	T45.612	T45.613	T45.614	T45.615	T45.616
Thromboplastin	T45.7X1	T45.7X2	T45.7X3	T45.7X4	T45.7X5	T45.7X6
Thurfyl nicotinate	T46.7X1	T46.7X2	T46.7X3	T46.7X4	T46.7X5	T46.7X6
Thymol	T49.0X1	T49.0X2	T49.0X3	T49.0X4	T49.0X5	T49.0X6
Thymopentin	T37.5X1	T37.5X2	T37.5X3	T37.5X4	T37.5X5	T37.5X6
Thymoxamine	T46.7X1	T46.7X2	T46.7X3	T46.7X4	T46.7X5	T46.7X6
Thymus extract	T38.891	T38.892	T38.893	T38.894	T38.895	T38.896
Thyreotrophic hormone	T38.811	T38.812	T38.813	T38.814	T38.815	T38.816
Thyroglobulin	T38.1X1	T38.1X2	T38.1X3	T38.1X4	T38.1X5	T38.1X6
Thyroid (hormone)	T38.1X1	T38.1X2	T38.1X3	T38.1X4	T38.1X5	T38.1X6
Thyrolar	T38.1X1	T38.1X2	T38.1X3	T38.1X4	T38.1X5	T38.1X6
Thyrotrophin	T38.811	T38.812	T38.813	T38.814	T38.815	T38.816
Thyrotropic hormone	T38.811	T38.812	T38.813	T38.814	T38.815	T38.816
Thyroxine	T38.1X1	T38.1X2	T38.1X3	T38.1X4	T38.1X5	T38.1X6
Tiabendazole	T37.4X1	T37.4X2	T37.4X3	T37.4X4	T37.4X5	T37.4X6
Tiamizide	T50.2X1	T50.2X2	T50.2X3	T50.2X4	T50.2X5	T50.2X6
Tianeptine	T43.291	T43.292	T43.293	T43.294	T43.295	T43.296
Tiapamil	T46.1X1	T46.1X2	T46.1X3	T46.1X4	T46.1X5	T46.1X6
Tiapride	T43.591	T43.592	T43.593	T43.594	T43.595	T43.596
Tiaprofenic acid	T39.311	T39.312	T39.313	T39.314	T39.315	T39.316
Tiaramide	T39.8X1	T39.8X2	T39.8X3	T39.8X4	T39.8X5	T39.8X6
Ticarcillin	T36.0X1	T36.0X2	T36.0X3	T36.0X4	T36.0X5	T36.0X6
Ticlatone	T49.0X1	T49.0X2	T49.0X3	T49.0X4	T49.0X5	T49.0X6
Ticlopidine	T45.521	T45.522	T45.523	T45.524	T45.525	T45.526
Ticrynafen	T50.1X1	T50.1X2	T50.1X3	T50.1X4	T50.1X5	T50.1X6
Tidiacic	T50.991	T50.992	T50.993	T50.994	T50.995	T50.996
Tiemonium	T44.3X1	T44.3X2	T44.3X3	T44.3X4	T44.3X5	T44.3X6
iodide	T44.3X1	T44.3X2	T44.3X3	T44.3X4	T44.3X5	T44.3X6
Tienilic acid	T50.1X1	T50.1X2	T50.1X3	T50.1X4	T50.1X5	T50.1X6
Tifenamil	T44.3X1	T44.3X2	T44.3X3	T44.3X4	T44.3X5	T44.3X6
Tigan	T45.0X1	T45.0X2	T45.0X3	T45.0X4	T45.0X5	T45.0X6
Tigloidine	T44.3X1	T44.3X2	T44.3X3	T44.3X4	T44.3X5	T44.3X6
Tilactase	T47.5X1	T47.5X2	T47.5X3	T47.5X4	T47.5X5	T47.5X6
Tiletamine	T41.291	T41.292	T41.293	T41.294	T41.295	T41.296
Tilidine	T40.491	T40.492	T40.493	T40.494	—	—
Timepidium bromide	T44.3X1	T44.3X2	T44.3X3	T44.3X4	T44.3X5	T44.3X6
Timiperone	T43.4X1	T43.4X2	T43.4X3	T43.4X4	T43.4X5	T43.4X6
Timolol	T44.7X1	T44.7X2	T44.7X3	T44.7X4	T44.7X5	T44.7X6
Tincture, iodine — see Iodine						
Tindal	T43.3X1	T43.3X2	T43.3X3	T43.3X4	T43.3X5	T43.3X6
Tinidazole	T37.3X1	T37.3X2	T37.3X3	T37.3X4	T37.3X5	T37.3X6
Tin (chloride) (dust) (oxide)	T56.6X1	T56.6X2	T56.6X3	T56.6X4	—	—
NEC anti-infectives	T37.8X1	T37.8X2	T37.8X3	T37.8X4	T37.8X5	T37.8X6
Tinoridine	T39.8X1	T39.8X2	T39.8X3	T39.8X4	T39.8X5	T39.8X6
Tiocarlide	T37.1X1	T37.1X2	T37.1X3	T37.1X4	T37.1X5	T37.1X6
Tioclomarol	T45.511	T45.512	T45.513	T45.514	T45.515	T45.516
Tioconazole	T49.0X1	T49.0X2	T49.0X3	T49.0X4	T49.0X5	T49.0X6
Tioguanine	T45.1X1	T45.1X2	T45.1X3	T45.1X4	T45.1X5	T45.1X6
Tiopronin	T50.991	T50.992	T50.993	T50.994	T50.995	T50.996
Tiotixene	T43.4X1	T43.4X2	T43.4X3	T43.4X4	T43.4X5	T43.4X6
Tioxolone	T49.4X1	T49.4X2	T49.4X3	T49.4X4	T49.4X5	T49.4X6
Tipepidine	T48.3X1	T48.3X2	T48.3X3	T48.3X4	T48.3X5	T48.3X6
Tiquizium bromide	T44.3X1	T44.3X2	T44.3X3	T44.3X4	T44.3X5	T44.3X6
Tiratricol	T38.1X1	T38.1X2	T38.1X3	T38.1X4	T38.1X5	T38.1X6
Tisopurine	T50.4X1	T50.4X2	T50.4X3	T50.4X4	T50.4X5	T50.4X6
Titanium (compounds) (vapor)	T56.891	T56.892	T56.893	T56.894	—	—
dioxide	T49.3X1	T49.3X2	T49.3X3	T49.3X4	T49.3X5	T49.3X6
ointment	T49.3X1	T49.3X2	T49.3X3	T49.3X4	T49.3X5	T49.3X6
oxide	T49.3X1	T49.3X2	T49.3X3	T49.3X4	T49.3X5	T49.3X6
tetrachloride	T56.891	T56.892	T56.893	T56.894	—	—
Titanocene	T56.891	T56.892	T56.893	T56.894	—	—
Titroid	T38.1X1	T38.1X2	T38.1X3	T38.1X4	T38.1X5	T38.1X6
Tizanidine	T42.8X1	T42.8X2	T42.8X3	T42.8X4	T42.8X5	T42.8X6
TMTD	T60.3X1	T60.3X2	T60.3X3	T60.3X4	—	—
TNT (fumes)	T65.3X1	T65.3X2	T65.3X3	T65.3X4	—	—
Toadstool	T62.0X1	T62.0X2	T62.0X3	T62.0X4	—	—
Tobacco NEC	T65.291	T65.292	T65.293	T65.294	—	—
cigarettes	T65.221	T65.222	T65.223	T65.224	—	—
Indian	T62.2X1	T62.2X2	T62.2X3	T62.2X4	—	—
smoke, second-hand	T65.221	T65.222	T65.223	T65.224	—	—
Tobramycin	T36.5X1	T36.5X2	T36.5X3	T36.5X4	T36.5X5	T36.5X6
Tocainide	T46.2X1	T46.2X2	T46.2X3	T46.2X4	T46.2X5	T46.2X6
Tocoferol	T45.2X1	T45.2X2	T45.2X3	T45.2X4	T45.2X5	T45.2X6
Tocopherol	T45.2X1	T45.2X2	T45.2X3	T45.2X4	T45.2X5	T45.2X6
acetate	T45.2X1	T45.2X2	T45.2X3	T45.2X4	T45.2X5	T45.2X6
Tocosamine	T48.0X1	T48.0X2	T48.0X3	T48.0X4	T48.0X5	T48.0X6
Todralazine	T46.5X1	T46.5X2	T46.5X3	T46.5X4	T46.5X5	T46.5X6
Tofisopam	T42.4X1	T42.4X2	T42.4X3	T42.4X4	T42.4X5	T42.4X6
Tofranil	T43.011	T43.012	T43.013	T43.014	T43.015	T43.016
Toilet deodorizer	T65.891	T65.892	T65.893	T65.894	—	—
Tolamolol	T44.7X1	T44.7X2	T44.7X3	T44.7X4	T44.7X5	T44.7X6
Tolazamide	T38.3X1	T38.3X2	T38.3X3	T38.3X4	T38.3X5	T38.3X6
Tolazoline	T46.7X1	T46.7X2	T46.7X3	T46.7X4	T46.7X5	T46.7X6
Tolbutamide (sodium)	T38.3X1	T38.3X2	T38.3X3	T38.3X4	T38.3X5	T38.3X6
Tolciclate	T49.0X1	T49.0X2	T49.0X3	T49.0X4	T49.0X5	T49.0X6
Tolmetin	T39.391	T39.392	T39.393	T39.394	T39.395	T39.396
Tolnaftate	T49.0X1	T49.0X2	T49.0X3	T49.0X4	T49.0X5	T49.0X6
Tolonidine	T46.5X1	T46.5X2	T46.5X3	T46.5X4	T46.5X5	T46.5X6
Toloxatone	T42.6X1	T42.6X2	T42.6X3	T42.6X4	T42.6X5	T42.6X6
Tolperisone	T44.3X1	T44.3X2	T44.3X3	T44.3X4	T44.3X5	T44.3X6
Tolserol	T42.8X1	T42.8X2	T42.8X3	T42.8X4	T42.8X5	T42.8X6
Toluene (liquid)	T52.2X1	T52.2X2	T52.2X3	T52.2X4	—	—
diisocyanate	T65.0X1	T65.0X2	T65.0X3	T65.0X4	—	—
Toluidine	T65.891	T65.892	T65.893	T65.894	—	—
vapor	T59.891	T59.892	T59.893	T59.894	—	—
Toluol (liquid)	T52.2X1	T52.2X2	T52.2X3	T52.2X4	—	—
Toluylenediamine	T65.3X1	T65.3X2	T65.3X3	T65.3X4	—	—
Tolylene-2,4-diisocyanate	T65.0X1	T65.0X2	T65.0X3	T65.0X4	—	—
Tonic NEC	T50.901	T50.902	T50.903	T50.904	T50.905	T50.906
Topical action drug NEC	T49.91	T49.92	T49.93	T49.94	T49.95	T49.96
ear, nose or throat	T49.6X1	T49.6X2	T49.6X3	T49.6X4	T49.6X5	T49.6X6
eye	T49.5X1	T49.5X2	T49.5X3	T49.5X4	T49.5X5	T49.5X6
skin	T49.91	T49.92	T49.93	T49.94	T49.95	T49.96
specified NEC	T49.8X1	T49.8X2	T49.8X3	T49.8X4	T49.8X5	T49.8X6
Toquizine	T44.3X1	T44.3X2	T44.3X3	T44.3X4	T44.3X5	T44.3X6
Toremifene	T38.6X1	T38.6X2	T38.6X3	T38.6X4	T38.6X5	T38.6X6
Tosylchloramide sodium	T49.8X1	T49.8X2	T49.8X3	T49.8X4	T49.8X5	T49.8X6
Toxaphene (dust) (spray)	T60.1X1	T60.1X2	T60.1X3	T60.1X4	—	—
Toxin, diphtheria (Schick Test)	T50.8X1	T50.8X2	T50.8X3	T50.8X4	T50.8X5	T50.8X6
Toxoid combined	T50.A21	T50.A22	T50.A23	T50.A24	T50.A25	T50.A26
diphtheria	T50.A91	T50.A92	T50.A93	T50.A94	T50.A95	T50.A96
tetanus	T50.A91	T50.A92	T50.A93	T50.A94	T50.A95	T50.A96
Trace element NEC	T45.8X1	T45.8X2	T45.8X3	T45.8X4	T45.8X5	T45.8X6
Tractor fuel NEC	T52.0X1	T52.0X2	T52.0X3	T52.0X4	—	—
Tragacanth	T50.991	T50.992	T50.993	T50.994	T50.995	T50.996
Tramadol	T40.421	T40.422	T40.423	T40.424	T40.425	T40.426
Tramazoline	T48.5X1	T48.5X2	T48.5X3	T48.5X4	T48.5X5	T48.5X6

Substance	Poisoning, Accidental (unintentional)	Poisoning, Intentional Self-harm	Poisoning, Assault	Poisoning, Undetermined	Adverse Effect	Under-dosing
Tranexamic acid	T45.621	T45.622	T45.623	T45.624	T45.625	T45.626
Tranilast	T45.ØX1	T45.ØX2	T45.ØX3	T45.ØX4	T45.ØX5	T45.ØX6
Tranquilizer NEC	T43.5Ø1	T43.5Ø2	T43.5Ø3	T43.5Ø4	T43.5Ø5	T43.5Ø6
with hypnotic or sedative	T42.6X1	T42.6X2	T42.6X3	T42.6X4	T42.6X5	T42.6X6
benzodiazepine NEC	T42.4X1	T42.4X2	T42.4X3	T42.4X4	T42.4X5	T42.4X6
butyrophenone NEC	T43.4X1	T43.4X2	T43.4X3	T43.4X4	T43.4X5	T43.4X6
carbamate	T43.591	T43.592	T43.593	T43.594	T43.595	T43.596
dimethylamine	T43.3X1	T43.3X2	T43.3X3	T43.3X4	T43.3X5	T43.3X6
ethylamine	T43.3X1	T43.3X2	T43.3X3	T43.3X4	T43.3X5	T43.3X6
hydroxyzine	T43.591	T43.592	T43.593	T43.594	T43.595	T43.596
major NEC	T43.5Ø1	T43.5Ø2	T43.5Ø3	T43.5Ø4	T43.5Ø5	T43.5Ø6
penothiazine NEC	T43.3X1	T43.3X2	T43.3X3	T43.3X4	T43.3X5	T43.3X6
phenothiazine-based	T43.3X1	T43.3X2	T43.3X3	T43.3X4	T43.3X5	T43.3X6
piperazine NEC	T43.3X1	T43.3X2	T43.3X3	T43.3X4	T43.3X5	T43.3X6
piperidine	T43.3X1	T43.3X2	T43.3X3	T43.3X4	T43.3X5	T43.3X6
propylamine	T43.3X1	T43.3X2	T43.3X3	T43.3X4	T43.3X5	T43.3X6
specified NEC	T43.591	T43.592	T43.593	T43.594	T43.595	T43.596
thioxanthene NEC	T43.591	T43.592	T43.593	T43.594	T43.595	T43.596
Tranxene	T42.4X1	T42.4X2	T42.4X3	T42.4X4	T42.4X5	T42.4X6
Tranylcypromine	T43.1X1	T43.1X2	T43.1X3	T43.1X4	T43.1X5	T43.1X6
Trapidil	T46.3X1	T46.3X2	T46.3X3	T46.3X4	T46.3X5	T46.3X6
Trasentine	T44.3X1	T44.3X2	T44.3X3	T44.3X4	T44.3X5	T44.3X6
Travert	T5Ø.3X1	T5Ø.3X2	T5Ø.3X3	T5Ø.3X4	T5Ø.3X5	T5Ø.3X6
Trazodone	T43.211	T43.212	T43.213	T43.214	T43.215	T43.216
Trecator	T37.1X1	T37.1X2	T37.1X3	T37.1X4	T37.1X5	T37.1X6
Treosulfan	T45.1X1	T45.1X2	T45.1X3	T45.1X4	T45.1X5	T45.1X6
Tretamine	T45.1X1	T45.1X2	T45.1X3	T45.1X4	T45.1X5	T45.1X6
Tretinoin	T49.ØX1	T49.ØX2	T49.ØX3	T49.ØX4	T49.ØX5	T49.ØX6
Tretoquinol	T48.6X1	T48.6X2	T48.6X3	T48.6X4	T48.6X5	T48.6X6
Triacetin	T49.ØX1	T49.ØX2	T49.ØX3	T49.ØX4	T49.ØX5	T49.ØX6
Triacetoxyanthracene	T49.4X1	T49.4X2	T49.4X3	T49.4X4	T49.4X5	T49.4X6
Triacetyloleandomycin	T36.3X1	T36.3X2	T36.3X3	T36.3X4	T36.3X5	T36.3X6
Triamcinolone	T38.ØX1	T38.ØX2	T38.ØX3	T38.ØX4	T38.ØX5	T38.ØX6
ENT agent	T49.6X1	T49.6X2	T49.6X3	T49.6X4	T49.6X5	T49.6X6
hexacetonide	T49.ØX1	T49.ØX2	T49.ØX3	T49.ØX4	T49.ØX5	T49.ØX6
ophthalmic preparation	T49.5X1	T49.5X2	T49.5X3	T49.5X4	T49.5X5	T49.5X6
topical NEC	T49.ØX1	T49.ØX2	T49.ØX3	T49.ØX4	T49.ØX5	T49.ØX6
Triampyzine	T44.3X1	T44.3X2	T44.3X3	T44.3X4	T44.3X5	T44.3X6
Triamterene	T5Ø.2X1	T5Ø.2X2	T5Ø.2X3	T5Ø.2X4	T5Ø.2X5	T5Ø.2X6
Triazine (herbicide)	T6Ø.3X1	T6Ø.3X2	T6Ø.3X3	T6Ø.3X4	—	—
Triaziquone	T45.1X1	T45.1X2	T45.1X3	T45.1X4	T45.1X5	T45.1X6
Triazolam	T42.4X1	T42.4X2	T42.4X3	T42.4X4	T42.4X5	T42.4X6
Triazole (herbicide)	T6Ø.3X1	T6Ø.3X2	T6Ø.3X3	T6Ø.3X4	—	—
Tribenoside	T46.991	T46.992	T46.993	T46.994	T46.995	T46.996
Tribromacetaldehyde	T42.6X1	T42.6X2	T42.6X3	T42.6X4	T42.6X5	T42.6X6
Tribromoethanol, rectal	T41.291	T41.292	T41.293	T41.294	T41.295	T41.296
Tribromomethane	T42.6X1	T42.6X2	T42.6X3	T42.6X4	T42.6X5	T42.6X6
Trichlorethane	T53.2X1	T53.2X2	T53.2X3	T53.2X4	—	—
Trichlorethylene	T53.2X1	T53.2X2	T53.2X3	T53.2X4	—	—
Trichlorfon	T6Ø.ØX1	T6Ø.ØX2	T6Ø.ØX3	T6Ø.ØX4	—	—
Trichlormethiazide	T5Ø.2X1	T5Ø.2X2	T5Ø.2X3	T5Ø.2X4	T5Ø.2X5	T5Ø.2X6
Trichlormethine	T45.1X1	T45.1X2	T45.1X3	T45.1X4	T45.1X5	T45.1X6
Trichloroacetic acid, Trichloracetic acid	T54.2X1	T54.2X2	T54.2X3	T54.2X4	—	—
medicinal	T49.4X1	T49.4X2	T49.4X3	T49.4X4	T49.4X5	T49.4X6
Trichloroethane	T53.2X1	T53.2X2	T53.2X3	T53.2X4	—	—
Trichloroethanol	T42.6X1	T42.6X2	T42.6X3	T42.6X4	T42.6X5	T42.6X6
Trichloroethylene (liquid) (vapor)	T53.2X1	T53.2X2	T53.2X3	T53.2X4	—	—
anesthetic (gas)	T41.ØX1	T41.ØX2	T41.ØX3	T41.ØX4	T41.ØX5	T41.ØX6
vapor NEC	T53.2X1	T53.2X2	T53.2X3	T53.2X4	—	—
Trichloroethyl phosphate	T42.6X1	T42.6X2	T42.6X3	T42.6X4	T42.6X5	T42.6X6
Trichlorofluoromethane NEC	T53.5X1	T53.5X2	T53.5X3	T53.5X4	—	—
Trichloronate	T6Ø.ØX1	T6Ø.ØX2	T6Ø.ØX3	T6Ø.ØX4	—	—
Trichloropropane	T53.6X1	T53.6X2	T53.6X3	T53.6X4	—	—
Trichlorotriethylamine	T45.1X1	T45.1X2	T45.1X3	T45.1X4	T45.1X5	T45.1X6
Trichomonacides NEC	T37.3X1	T37.3X2	T37.3X3	T37.3X4	T37.3X5	T37.3X6
Trichomycin	T36.7X1	T36.7X2	T36.7X3	T36.7X4	T36.7X5	T36.7X6
Triclobisonium chloride	T49.ØX1	T49.ØX2	T49.ØX3	T49.ØX4	T49.ØX5	T49.ØX6
Triclocarban	T49.ØX1	T49.ØX2	T49.ØX3	T49.ØX4	T49.ØX5	T49.ØX6
Triclofos	T42.6X1	T42.6X2	T42.6X3	T42.6X4	T42.6X5	T42.6X6
Triclosan	T49.ØX1	T49.ØX2	T49.ØX3	T49.ØX4	T49.ØX5	T49.ØX6
Tricresyl phosphate	T65.891	T65.892	T65.893	T65.894	—	—
solvent	T52.91	T52.92	T52.93	T52.94	—	—
Tricyclamol chloride	T44.3X1	T44.3X2	T44.3X3	T44.3X4	T44.3X5	T44.3X6
Tridesilon	T49.ØX1	T49.ØX2	T49.ØX3	T49.ØX4	T49.ØX5	T49.ØX6
Tridihexethyl iodide	T44.3X1	T44.3X2	T44.3X3	T44.3X4	T44.3X5	T44.3X6
Tridione	T42.2X1	T42.2X2	T42.2X3	T42.2X4	T42.2X5	T42.2X6
Trientine	T45.8X1	T45.8X2	T45.8X3	T45.8X4	T45.8X5	T45.8X6
Triethanolamine NEC	T54.3X1	T54.3X2	T54.3X3	T54.3X4	—	—
detergent	T54.3X1	T54.3X2	T54.3X3	T54.3X4	—	—
trinitrate (biphosphate)	T46.3X1	T46.3X2	T46.3X3	T46.3X4	T46.3X5	T46.3X6

Substance	Poisoning, Accidental (unintentional)	Poisoning, Intentional Self-harm	Poisoning, Assault	Poisoning, Undetermined	Adverse Effect	Under-dosing
Triethanomelamine	T45.1X1	T45.1X2	T45.1X3	T45.1X4	T45.1X5	T45.1X6
Triethylenemelamine	T45.1X1	T45.1X2	T45.1X3	T45.1X4	T45.1X5	T45.1X6
Triethylenephosphoramide	T45.1X1	T45.1X2	T45.1X3	T45.1X4	T45.1X5	T45.1X6
Triethylenethiophosphoramide	T45.1X1	T45.1X2	T45.1X3	T45.1X4	T45.1X5	T45.1X6
Trifluoperazine	T43.3X1	T43.3X2	T43.3X3	T43.3X4	T43.3X5	T43.3X6
Trifluoroethyl vinyl ether	T41.ØX1	T41.ØX2	T41.ØX3	T41.ØX4	T41.ØX5	T41.ØX6
Trifluperidol	T43.4X1	T43.4X2	T43.4X3	T43.4X4	T43.4X5	T43.4X6
Triflupromazine	T43.3X1	T43.3X2	T43.3X3	T43.3X4	T43.3X5	T43.3X6
Trifluridine	T37.5X1	T37.5X2	T37.5X3	T37.5X4	T37.5X5	T37.5X6
Triflusal	T45.521	T45.522	T45.523	T45.524	T45.525	T45.526
Trihexyphenidyl	T44.3X1	T44.3X2	T44.3X3	T44.3X4	T44.3X5	T44.3X6
Triiodothyronine	T38.1X1	T38.1X2	T38.1X3	T38.1X4	T38.1X5	T38.1X6
Trilene	T41.ØX1	T41.ØX2	T41.ØX3	T41.ØX4	T41.ØX5	T41.ØX6
Trilostane	T38.991	T38.992	T38.993	T38.994	T38.995	T38.996
Trimebutine	T44.3X1	T44.3X2	T44.3X3	T44.3X4	T44.3X5	T44.3X6
Trimecaine	T41.3X1	T41.3X2	T41.3X3	T41.3X4	T41.3X5	T41.3X6
Trimeprazine (tartrate)	T44.3X1	T44.3X2	T44.3X3	T44.3X4	T44.3X5	T44.3X6
Trimetaphan camsilate	T44.2X1	T44.2X2	T44.2X3	T44.2X4	T44.2X5	T44.2X6
Trimetazidine	T46.7X1	T46.7X2	T46.7X3	T46.7X4	T46.7X5	T46.7X6
Trimethadione	T42.2X1	T42.2X2	T42.2X3	T42.2X4	T42.2X5	T42.2X6
Trimethaphan	T44.2X1	T44.2X2	T44.2X3	T44.2X4	T44.2X5	T44.2X6
Trimethidinium	T44.2X1	T44.2X2	T44.2X3	T44.2X4	T44.2X5	T44.2X6
Trimethobenzamide	T45.ØX1	T45.ØX2	T45.ØX3	T45.ØX4	T45.ØX5	T45.ØX6
Trimethoprim	T37.8X1	T37.8X2	T37.8X3	T37.8X4	T37.8X5	T37.8X6
with sulfamethoxazole	T36.8X1	T36.8X2	T36.8X3	T36.8X4	T36.8X5	T36.8X6
Trimethylcarbinol	T51.3X1	T51.3X2	T51.3X3	T51.3X4	—	—
Trimethylpsoralen	T49.3X1	T49.3X2	T49.3X3	T49.3X4	T49.3X5	T49.3X6
Trimeton	T45.ØX1	T45.ØX2	T45.ØX3	T45.ØX4	T45.ØX5	T45.ØX6
Trimetrexate	T45.1X1	T45.1X2	T45.1X3	T45.1X4	T45.1X5	T45.1X6
Trimipramine	T43.Ø11	T43.Ø12	T43.Ø13	T43.Ø14	T43.Ø15	T43.Ø16
Trimustine	T45.1X1	T45.1X2	T45.1X3	T45.1X4	T45.1X5	T45.1X6
Trinitrine	T46.3X1	T46.3X2	T46.3X3	T46.3X4	T46.3X5	T46.3X6
Trinitrobenzol	T65.3X1	T65.3X2	T65.3X3	T65.3X4	—	—
Trinitrophenol	T65.3X1	T65.3X2	T65.3X3	T65.3X4	—	—
Trinitrotoluene (fumes)	T65.3X1	T65.3X2	T65.3X3	T65.3X4	—	—
Trional	T42.6X1	T42.6X2	T42.6X3	T42.6X4	T42.6X5	T42.6X6
Triorthocresyl phosphate	T65.891	T65.892	T65.893	T65.894	—	—
Trioxide of arsenic	T57.ØX1	T57.ØX2	T57.ØX3	T57.ØX4	—	—
Trioxysalen	T49.4X1	T49.4X2	T49.4X3	T49.4X4	T49.4X5	T49.4X6
Tripamide	T5Ø.2X1	T5Ø.2X2	T5Ø.2X3	T5Ø.2X4	T5Ø.2X5	T5Ø.2X6
Triparanol	T46.6X1	T46.6X2	T46.6X3	T46.6X4	T46.6X5	T46.6X6
Tripelennamine	T45.ØX1	T45.ØX2	T45.ØX3	T45.ØX4	T45.ØX5	T45.ØX6
Triperiden	T44.3X1	T44.3X2	T44.3X3	T44.3X4	T44.3X5	T44.3X6
Triperidol	T43.4X1	T43.4X2	T43.4X3	T43.4X4	T43.4X5	T43.4X6
Triphenylphosphate	T65.891	T65.892	T65.893	T65.894	—	—
Triple						
bromides	T42.6X1	T42.6X2	T42.6X3	T42.6X4	T42.6X5	T42.6X6
carbonate	T47.1X1	T47.1X2	T47.1X3	T47.1X4	T47.1X5	T47.1X6
vaccine						
DPT	T5Ø.A11	T5Ø.A12	T5Ø.A13	T5Ø.A14	T5Ø.A15	T5Ø.A16
including pertussis	T5Ø.A11	T5Ø.A12	T5Ø.A13	T5Ø.A14	T5Ø.A15	T5Ø.A16
MMR	T5Ø.B91	T5Ø.B92	T5Ø.B93	T5Ø.B94	T5Ø.B95	T5Ø.B96
Triprolidine	T45.ØX1	T45.ØX2	T45.ØX3	T45.ØX4	T45.ØX5	T45.ØX6
Trisodium hydrogen edetate	T5Ø.6X1	T5Ø.6X2	T5Ø.6X3	T5Ø.6X4	T5Ø.6X5	T5Ø.6X6
Trisoralen	T49.3X1	T49.3X2	T49.3X3	T49.3X4	T49.3X5	T49.3X6
Trisulfapyrimidines	T37.ØX1	T37.ØX2	T37.ØX3	T37.ØX4	T37.ØX5	T37.ØX6
Trithiozine	T44.3X1	T44.3X2	T44.3X3	T44.3X4	T44.3X5	T44.3X6
Tritiozine	T44.3X1	T44.3X2	T44.3X3	T44.3X4	T44.3X5	T44.3X6
Tritoqualine	T45.ØX1	T45.ØX2	T45.ØX3	T45.ØX4	T45.ØX5	T45.ØX6
Trofosfamide	T45.1X1	T45.1X2	T45.1X3	T45.1X4	T45.1X5	T45.1X6
Troleandomycin	T36.3X1	T36.3X2	T36.3X3	T36.3X4	T36.3X5	T36.3X6
Trolnitrate (phosphate)	T46.3X1	T46.3X2	T46.3X3	T46.3X4	T46.3X5	T46.3X6
Tromantadine	T37.5X1	T37.5X2	T37.5X3	T37.5X4	T37.5X5	T37.5X6
Trometamol	T5Ø.2X1	T5Ø.2X2	T5Ø.2X3	T5Ø.2X4	T5Ø.2X5	T5Ø.2X6
Tromethamine	T5Ø.2X1	T5Ø.2X2	T5Ø.2X3	T5Ø.2X4	T5Ø.2X5	T5Ø.2X6
Tronothane	T41.3X1	T41.3X2	T41.3X3	T41.3X4	T41.3X5	T41.3X6
Tropacine	T44.3X1	T44.3X2	T44.3X3	T44.3X4	T44.3X5	T44.3X6
Tropatepine	T44.3X1	T44.3X2	T44.3X3	T44.3X4	T44.3X5	T44.3X6
Tropicamide	T44.3X1	T44.3X2	T44.3X3	T44.3X4	T44.3X5	T44.3X6
Trospium chloride	T44.3X1	T44.3X2	T44.3X3	T44.3X4	T44.3X5	T44.3X6
Troxerutin	T46.991	T46.992	T46.993	T46.994	T46.995	T46.996
Troxidone	T42.2X1	T42.2X2	T42.2X3	T42.2X4	T42.2X5	T42.2X6
Tryparsamide	T37.3X1	T37.3X2	T37.3X3	T37.3X4	T37.3X5	T37.3X6
Trypsin	T45.3X1	T45.3X2	T45.3X3	T45.3X4	T45.3X5	T45.3X6
Tryptizol	T43.Ø11	T43.Ø12	T43.Ø13	T43.Ø14	T43.Ø15	T43.Ø16
TSH	T38.811	T38.812	T38.813	T38.814	T38.815	T38.816
Tuaminoheptane	T48.5X1	T48.5X2	T48.5X3	T48.5X4	T48.5X5	T48.5X6
Tuberculin, purified protein derivative (PPD)	T5Ø.8X1	T5Ø.8X2	T5Ø.8X3	T5Ø.8X4	T5Ø.8X5	T5Ø.8X6
Tubocurare	T48.1X1	T48.1X2	T48.1X3	T48.1X4	T48.1X5	T48.1X6
Tubocurarine (chloride)	T48.1X1	T48.1X2	T48.1X3	T48.1X4	T48.1X5	T48.1X6
Tulobuterol	T48.6X1	T48.6X2	T48.6X3	T48.6X4	T48.6X5	T48.6X6

400 Additional Character May Be Required — Refer to the Tabular List for Character Selection

Subterms under main terms may continue to next column or page

Substance	Poisoning, Accidental (unintentional)	Poisoning, Intentional Self-harm	Poisoning, Assault	Poisoning, Undetermined	Adverse Effect	Under-dosing
Turpentine (spirits of)	T52.8X1	T52.8X2	T52.8X3	T52.8X4	—	—
vapor	T52.8X1	T52.8X2	T52.8X3	T52.8X4	—	—
Tybamate	T43.591	T43.592	T43.593	T43.594	T43.595	T43.596
Tyloxapol	T48.4X1	T48.4X2	T48.4X3	T48.4X4	T48.4X5	T48.4X6
Tymazoline	T48.5X1	T48.5X2	T48.5X3	T48.5X4	T48.5X5	T48.5X6
Typhoid-paratyphoid vaccine	T50.A91	T50.A92	T50.A93	T50.A94	T50.A95	T50.A96
Typhus vaccine	T50.A91	T50.A92	T50.A93	T50.A94	T50.A95	T50.A96
Tyropanoate	T50.8X1	T50.8X2	T50.8X3	T50.8X4	T50.8X5	T50.8X6
Tyrothricin	T49.6X1	T49.6X2	T49.6X3	T49.6X4	T49.6X5	T49.6X6
ENT agent	T49.6X1	T49.6X2	T49.6X3	T49.6X4	T49.6X5	T49.6X6
ophthalmic preparation	T49.5X1	T49.5X2	T49.5X3	T49.5X4	T49.5X5	T49.5X6
Ufenamate	T39.391	T39.392	T39.393	T39.394	T39.395	T39.396
Ultraviolet light protectant	T49.3X1	T49.3X2	T49.3X3	T49.3X4	T49.3X5	T49.3X6
Undecenoic acid	T49.0X1	T49.0X2	T49.0X3	T49.0X4	T49.0X5	T49.0X6
Undecoylium	T49.0X1	T49.0X2	T49.0X3	T49.0X4	T49.0X5	T49.0X6
Undecylenic acid (derivatives)	T49.0X1	T49.0X2	T49.0X3	T49.0X4	T49.0X5	T49.0X6
Unna's boot	T49.3X1	T49.3X2	T49.3X3	T49.3X4	T49.3X5	T49.3X6
Unsaturated fatty acid	T46.6X1	T46.6X2	T46.6X3	T46.6X4	T46.6X5	T46.6X6
Uracil mustard	T45.1X1	T45.1X2	T45.1X3	T45.1X4	T45.1X5	T45.1X6
Uramustine	T45.1X1	T45.1X2	T45.1X3	T45.1X4	T45.1X5	T45.1X6
Urapidil	T46.5X1	T46.5X2	T46.5X3	T46.5X4	T46.5X5	T46.5X6
Urari	T48.1X1	T48.1X2	T48.1X3	T48.1X4	T48.1X5	T48.1X6
Urate oxidase	T50.4X1	T50.4X2	T50.4X3	T50.4X4	T50.4X5	T50.4X6
Urea	T47.3X1	T47.3X2	T47.3X3	T47.3X4	T47.3X5	T47.3X6
peroxide	T49.0X1	T49.0X2	T49.0X3	T49.0X4	T49.0X5	T49.0X6
stibamine	T37.4X1	T37.4X2	T37.4X3	T37.4X4	T37.4X5	T37.4X6
topical	T49.8X1	T49.8X2	T49.8X3	T49.8X4	T49.8X5	T49.8X6
Urethane	T45.1X1	T45.1X2	T45.1X3	T45.1X4	T45.1X5	T45.1X6
Urginea (maritima) (scilla) — *see* Squill						
Uric acid metabolism drug NEC	T50.4X1	T50.4X2	T50.4X3	T50.4X4	T50.4X5	T50.4X6
Uricosuric agent	T50.4X1	T50.4X2	T50.4X3	T50.4X4	T50.4X5	T50.4X6
Urinary anti-infective	T37.8X1	T37.8X2	T37.8X3	T37.8X4	T37.8X5	T37.8X6
Urofollitropin	T38.811	T38.812	T38.813	T38.814	T38.815	T38.816
Urokinase	T45.611	T45.612	T45.613	T45.614	T45.615	T45.616
Urokon	T50.8X1	T50.8X2	T50.8X3	T50.8X4	T50.8X5	T50.8X6
Ursodeoxycholic acid	T50.991	T50.992	T50.993	T50.994	T50.995	T50.996
Ursodiol	T50.991	T50.992	T50.993	T50.994	T50.995	T50.996
Urtica	T62.2X1	T62.2X2	T62.2X3	T62.2X4	—	—
Utility gas — *see* Gas, utility						
Vaccine NEC	T50.Z91	T50.Z92	T50.Z93	T50.Z94	T50.Z95	T50.Z96
antineoplastic	T50.Z91	T50.Z92	T50.Z93	T50.Z94	T50.Z95	T50.Z96
bacterial NEC	T50.A91	T50.A92	T50.A93	T50.A94	T50.A95	T50.A96
with						
other bacterial component	T50.A21	T50.A22	T50.A23	T50.A24	T50.A25	T50.A26
pertussis component	T50.A11	T50.A12	T50.A13	T50.A14	T50.A15	T50.A16
viral-rickettsial component	T50.A21	T50.A22	T50.A23	T50.A24	T50.A25	T50.A26
mixed NEC	T50.A21	T50.A22	T50.A23	T50.A24	T50.A25	T50.A26
BCG	T50.A91	T50.A92	T50.A93	T50.A94	T50.A95	T50.A96
cholera	T50.A91	T50.A92	T50.A93	T50.A94	T50.A95	T50.A96
diphtheria	T50.A91	T50.A92	T50.A93	T50.A94	T50.A95	T50.A96
with tetanus	T50.A21	T50.A22	T50.A23	T50.A24	T50.A25	T50.A26
and pertussis	T50.A11	T50.A12	T50.A13	T50.A14	T50.A15	T50.A16
influenza	T50.B91	T50.B92	T50.B93	T50.B94	T50.B95	T50.B96
measles	T50.B91	T50.B92	T50.B93	T50.B94	T50.B95	T50.B96
with mumps and rubella	T50.B91	T50.B92	T50.B93	T50.B94	T50.B95	T50.B96
meningococcal	T50.A91	T50.A92	T50.A93	T50.A94	T50.A95	T50.A96
mumps	T50.B91	T50.B92	T50.B93	T50.B94	T50.B95	T50.B96
paratyphoid	T50.A91	T50.A92	T50.A93	T50.A94	T50.A95	T50.A96
pertussis	T50.A11	T50.A12	T50.A13	T50.A14	T50.A15	T50.A16
with diphtheria	T50.A11	T50.A12	T50.A13	T50.A14	T50.A15	T50.A16
and tetanus	T50.A11	T50.A12	T50.A13	T50.A14	T50.A15	T50.A16
with other component	T50.A11	T50.A12	T50.A13	T50.A14	T50.A15	T50.A16
plague	T50.A91	T50.A92	T50.A93	T50.A94	T50.A95	T50.A96
poliomyelitis	T50.B91	T50.B92	T50.B93	T50.B94	T50.B95	T50.B96
poliovirus	T50.B91	T50.B92	T50.B93	T50.B94	T50.B95	T50.B96
rabies	T50.B91	T50.B92	T50.B93	T50.B94	T50.B95	T50.B96
respiratory syncytial virus	T50.B91	T50.B92	T50.B93	T50.B94	T50.B95	T50.B96
rickettsial NEC	T50.A91	T50.A92	T50.A93	T50.A94	T50.A95	T50.A96
with						
bacterial component	T50.A21	T50.A22	T50.A23	T50.A24	T50.A25	T50.A26
Rocky Mountain spotted fever	T50.A91	T50.A92	T50.A93	T50.A94	T50.A95	T50.A96
rubella	T50.B91	T50.B92	T50.B93	T50.B94	T50.B95	T50.B96
sabin oral	T50.B91	T50.B92	T50.B93	T50.B94	T50.B95	T50.B96
smallpox	T50.B11	T50.B12	T50.B13	T50.B14	T50.B15	T50.B16
TAB	T50.A91	T50.A92	T50.A93	T50.A94	T50.A95	T50.A96

Substance	Poisoning, Accidental (unintentional)	Poisoning, Intentional Self-harm	Poisoning, Assault	Poisoning, Undetermined	Adverse Effect	Under-dosing
Vaccine — *continued*						
tetanus	T50.A91	T50.A92	T50.A93	T50.A94	T50.A95	T50.A96
typhoid	T50.A91	T50.A92	T50.A93	T50.A94	T50.A95	T50.A96
typhus	T50.A91	T50.A92	T50.A93	T50.A94	T50.A95	T50.A96
viral NEC	T50.B91	T50.B92	T50.B93	T50.B94	T50.B95	T50.B96
yellow fever	T50.B91	T50.B92	T50.B93	T50.B94	T50.B95	T50.B96
Vaccinia immune globulin	T50.Z11	T50.Z12	T50.Z13	T50.Z14	T50.Z15	T50.Z16
Vaginal contraceptives	T49.8X1	T49.8X2	T49.8X3	T49.8X4	T49.8X5	T49.8X6
Valerian						
root	T42.6X1	T42.6X2	T42.6X3	T42.6X4	T42.6X5	T42.6X6
tincture	T42.6X1	T42.6X2	T42.6X3	T42.6X4	T42.6X5	T42.6X6
Valethamate bromide	T44.3X1	T44.3X2	T44.3X3	T44.3X4	T44.3X5	T44.3X6
Valisone	T49.0X1	T49.0X2	T49.0X3	T49.0X4	T49.0X5	T49.0X6
Valium	T42.4X1	T42.4X2	T42.4X3	T42.4X4	T42.4X5	T42.4X6
Valmid	T42.6X1	T42.6X2	T42.6X3	T42.6X4	T42.6X5	T42.6X6
Valnoctamide	T42.6X1	T42.6X2	T42.6X3	T42.6X4	T42.6X5	T42.6X6
Valproate (sodium)	T42.6X1	T42.6X2	T42.6X3	T42.6X4	T42.6X5	T42.6X6
Valproic acid	T42.6X1	T42.6X2	T42.6X3	T42.6X4	T42.6X5	T42.6X6
Valpromide	T42.6X1	T42.6X2	T42.6X3	T42.6X4	T42.6X5	T42.6X6
Vanadium	T56.891	T56.892	T56.893	T56.894	—	—
Vancomycin	T36.8X1	T36.8X2	T36.8X3	T36.8X4	T36.8X5	T36.8X6
Vapor — *see also* Gas	T59.91	T59.92	T59.93	T59.94	—	—
kiln (carbon monoxide)	T58.8X1	T58.8X2	T58.8X3	T58.8X4	—	—
lead — *see* lead						
specified source NEC	T59.891	T59.892	T59.893	T59.894	—	—
Vardenafil	T46.7X1	T46.7X2	T46.7X3	T46.7X4	T46.7X5	T46.7X6
Varicose reduction drug	T46.8X1	T46.8X2	T46.8X3	T46.8X4	T46.8X5	T46.8X6
Varnish	T65.4X1	T65.4X2	T65.4X3	T65.4X4	—	—
cleaner	T52.91	T52.92	T52.93	T52.94	—	—
Vaseline	T49.3X1	T49.3X2	T49.3X3	T49.3X4	T49.3X5	T49.3X6
Vasodilan	T46.7X1	T46.7X2	T46.7X3	T46.7X4	T46.7X5	T46.7X6
Vasodilator						
coronary NEC	T46.3X1	T46.3X2	T46.3X3	T46.3X4	T46.3X5	T46.3X6
peripheral NEC	T46.7X1	T46.7X2	T46.7X3	T46.7X4	T46.7X5	T46.7X6
Vasopressin	T38.891	T38.892	T38.893	T38.894	T38.895	T38.896
Vasopressor drugs	T38.891	T38.892	T38.893	T38.894	T38.895	T38.896
Vecuronium bromide	T48.1X1	T48.1X2	T48.1X3	T48.1X4	T48.1X5	T48.1X6
Vegetable extract, astringent	T49.2X1	T49.2X2	T49.2X3	T49.2X4	T49.2X5	T49.2X6
Venlafaxine	T43.211	T43.212	T43.213	T43.214	T43.215	T43.216
Venom, venomous (bite) (sting)	T63.91	T63.92	T63.93	T63.94	—	—
amphibian NEC	T63.831	T63.832	T63.833	T63.834	—	—
animal NEC	T63.891	T63.892	T63.893	T63.894	—	—
ant	T63.421	T63.422	T63.423	T63.424	—	—
arthropod NEC	T63.481	T63.482	T63.483	T63.484	—	—
bee	T63.441	T63.442	T63.443	T63.444	—	—
centipede	T63.411	T63.412	T63.413	T63.414	—	—
fish	T63.591	T63.592	T63.593	T63.594	—	—
frog	T63.811	T63.812	T63.813	T63.814	—	—
hornet	T63.451	T63.452	T63.453	T63.454	—	—
insect NEC	T63.481	T63.482	T63.483	T63.484	—	—
lizard	T63.121	T63.122	T63.123	T63.124	—	—
marine						
animals	T63.691	T63.692	T63.693	T63.694	—	—
bluebottle	T63.611	T63.612	T63.613	T63.614	—	—
jellyfish NEC	T63.621	T63.622	T63.623	T63.624	—	—
Portuguese Man-o-war	T63.611	T63.612	T63.613	T63.614	—	—
sea anemone	T63.631	T63.632	T63.633	T63.634	—	—
specified NEC	T63.691	T63.692	T63.693	T63.694	—	—
fish	T63.591	T63.592	T63.593	T63.594	—	—
plants	T63.711	T63.712	T63.713	T63.714	—	—
sting ray	T63.511	T63.512	T63.513	T63.514	—	—
millipede (tropical)	T63.411	T63.412	T63.413	T63.414	—	—
plant NEC	T63.791	T63.792	T63.793	T63.794	—	—
marine	T63.711	T63.712	T63.713	T63.714	—	—
reptile	T63.191	T63.192	T63.193	T63.194	—	—
gila monster	T63.111	T63.112	T63.113	T63.114	—	—
lizard NEC	T63.121	T63.122	T63.123	T63.124	—	—
scorpion	T63.2X1	T63.2X2	T63.2X3	T63.2X4	—	—
snake	T63.001	T63.002	T63.003	T63.004	—	—
African NEC	T63.081	T63.082	T63.083	T63.084	—	—
American (North) (South) NEC	T63.061	T63.062	T63.063	T63.064	—	—
Asian	T63.081	T63.082	T63.083	T63.084	—	—
Australian	T63.071	T63.072	T63.073	T63.074	—	—
cobra	T63.041	T63.042	T63.043	T63.044	—	—
coral snake	T63.021	T63.022	T63.023	T63.024	—	—
rattlesnake	T63.011	T63.012	T63.013	T63.014	—	—
specified NEC	T63.091	T63.092	T63.093	T63.094	—	—
taipan	T63.031	T63.032	T63.033	T63.034	—	—
specified NEC	T63.891	T63.892	T63.893	T63.894	—	—
spider	T63.301	T63.302	T63.303	T63.304	—	—

⚕ Subterms under main terms may continue to next column or page   Additional Character May Be Required — Refer to the Tabular List for Character Selection   401

Turpentine — Venom, venomous

Substance	Poisoning, Accidental (unintentional)	Poisoning, Intentional Self-harm	Poisoning, Assault	Poisoning, Undetermined	Adverse Effect	Under-dosing
Venom, venomous — continued						
spider — continued						
black widow	T63.311	T63.312	T63.313	T63.314	—	—
brown recluse	T63.331	T63.332	T63.333	T63.334	—	—
specified NEC	T63.391	T63.392	T63.393	T63.394	—	—
tarantula	T63.321	T63.322	T63.323	T63.324	—	—
sting ray	T63.511	T63.512	T63.513	T63.514	—	—
toad	T63.821	T63.822	T63.823	T63.824	—	—
wasp	T63.461	T63.462	T63.463	T63.464	—	—
Venous sclerosing drug NEC	T46.8X1	T46.8X2	T46.8X3	T46.8X4	T46.8X5	T46.8X6
Ventolin — see Albuterol						
Veramon	T42.3X1	T42.3X2	T42.3X3	T42.3X4	T42.3X5	T42.3X6
Verapamil	T46.1X1	T46.1X2	T46.1X3	T46.1X4	T46.1X5	T46.1X6
Veratrine	T46.5X1	T46.5X2	T46.5X3	T46.5X4	T46.5X5	T46.5X6
Veratrum						
album	T62.2X1	T62.2X2	T62.2X3	T62.2X4	—	—
alkaloids	T46.5X1	T46.5X2	T46.5X3	T46.5X4	T46.5X5	T46.5X6
viride	T62.2X1	T62.2X2	T62.2X3	T62.2X4	—	—
Verdigris	T60.3X1	T60.3X2	T60.3X3	T60.3X4	—	—
Veronal	T42.3X1	T42.3X2	T42.3X3	T42.3X4	T42.3X5	T42.3X6
Veroxil	T37.4X1	T37.4X2	T37.4X3	T37.4X4	T37.4X5	T37.4X6
Versenate	T50.6X1	T50.6X2	T50.6X3	T50.6X4	T50.6X5	T50.6X6
Versidyne	T39.8X1	T39.8X2	T39.8X3	T39.8X4	T39.8X5	T39.8X6
Vetrabutine	T48.0X1	T48.0X2	T48.0X3	T48.0X4	T48.0X5	T48.0X6
Vidarabine	T37.5X1	T37.5X2	T37.5X3	T37.5X4	T37.5X5	T37.5X6
Vienna						
green	T57.0X1	T57.0X2	T57.0X3	T57.0X4	—	—
insecticide	T60.2X1	T60.2X2	T60.2X3	T60.2X4	—	—
red	T57.0X1	T57.0X2	T57.0X3	T57.0X4	—	—
pharmaceutical dye	T50.991	T50.992	T50.993	T50.994	T50.995	T50.996
Vigabatrin	T42.6X1	T42.6X2	T42.6X3	T42.6X4	T42.6X5	T42.6X6
Viloxazine	T43.291	T43.292	T43.293	T43.294	T43.295	T43.296
Viminol	T39.8X1	T39.8X2	T39.8X3	T39.8X4	T39.8X5	T39.8X6
Vinbarbital, vinbarbitone	T42.3X1	T42.3X2	T42.3X3	T42.3X4	T42.3X5	T42.3X6
Vinblastine	T45.1X1	T45.1X2	T45.1X3	T45.1X4	T45.1X5	T45.1X6
Vinburnine	T46.7X1	T46.7X2	T46.7X3	T46.7X4	T46.7X5	T46.7X6
Vincamine	T45.1X1	T45.1X2	T45.1X3	T45.1X4	T45.1X5	T45.1X6
Vincristine	T45.1X1	T45.1X2	T45.1X3	T45.1X4	T45.1X5	T45.1X6
Vindesine	T45.1X1	T45.1X2	T45.1X3	T45.1X4	T45.1X5	T45.1X6
Vinesthene, vinethene	T41.0X1	T41.0X2	T41.0X3	T41.0X4	T41.0X5	T41.0X6
Vinorelbine tartrate	T45.1X1	T45.1X2	T45.1X3	T45.1X4	T45.1X5	T45.1X6
Vinpocetine	T46.7X1	T46.7X2	T46.7X3	T46.7X4	T46.7X5	T46.7X6
Vinyl						
acetate	T65.891	T65.892	T65.893	T65.894	—	—
bital	T42.3X1	T42.3X2	T42.3X3	T42.3X4	T42.3X5	T42.3X6
bromide	T65.891	T65.892	T65.893	T65.894	—	—
chloride	T59.891	T59.892	T59.893	T59.894	—	—
ether	T41.0X1	T41.0X2	T41.0X3	T41.0X4	T41.0X5	T41.0X6
Vinylbital	T42.3X1	T42.3X2	T42.3X3	T42.3X4	T42.3X5	T42.3X6
Vinylidene chloride	T65.891	T65.892	T65.893	T65.894	—	—
Vioform	T37.8X1	T37.8X2	T37.8X3	T37.8X4	T37.8X5	T37.8X6
topical	T49.0X1	T49.0X2	T49.0X3	T49.0X4	T49.0X5	T49.0X6
Viomycin	T36.8X1	T36.8X2	T36.8X3	T36.8X4	T36.8X5	T36.8X6
Viosterol	T45.2X1	T45.2X2	T45.2X3	T45.2X4	T45.2X5	T45.2X6
Viper (venom)	T63.091	T63.092	T63.093	T63.094	—	—
Viprynium	T37.4X1	T37.4X2	T37.4X3	T37.4X4	T37.4X5	T37.4X6
Viquidil	T46.7X1	T46.7X2	T46.7X3	T46.7X4	T46.7X5	T46.7X6
Viral vaccine NEC	T50.B91	T50.B92	T50.B93	T50.B94	T50.B95	T50.B96
Virginiamycin	T36.8X1	T36.8X2	T36.8X3	T36.8X4	T36.8X5	T36.8X6
Virugon	T37.5X1	T37.5X2	T37.5X3	T37.5X4	T37.5X5	T37.5X6
Viscous agent	T50.901	T50.902	T50.903	T50.904	T50.905	T50.906
Visine	T49.5X1	T49.5X2	T49.5X3	T49.5X4	T49.5X5	T49.5X6
Visnadine	T46.3X1	T46.3X2	T46.3X3	T46.3X4	T46.3X5	T46.3X6
Vitamin NEC	T45.2X1	T45.2X2	T45.2X3	T45.2X4	T45.2X5	T45.2X6
A	T45.2X1	T45.2X2	T45.2X3	T45.2X4	T45.2X5	T45.2X6
B1	T45.2X1	T45.2X2	T45.2X3	T45.2X4	T45.2X5	T45.2X6
B2	T45.2X1	T45.2X2	T45.2X3	T45.2X4	T45.2X5	T45.2X6
B6	T45.2X1	T45.2X2	T45.2X3	T45.2X4	T45.2X5	T45.2X6
B12	T45.2X1	T45.2X2	T45.2X3	T45.2X4	T45.2X5	T45.2X6
B15	T45.2X1	T45.2X2	T45.2X3	T45.2X4	T45.2X5	T45.2X6
B NEC	T45.2X1	T45.2X2	T45.2X3	T45.2X4	T45.2X5	T45.2X6
nicotinic acid	T46.7X1	T46.7X2	T46.7X3	T46.7X4	T46.7X5	T46.7X6
C	T45.2X1	T45.2X2	T45.2X3	T45.2X4	T45.2X5	T45.2X6
D	T45.2X1	T45.2X2	T45.2X3	T45.2X4	T45.2X5	T45.2X6
D2	T45.2X1	T45.2X2	T45.2X3	T45.2X4	T45.2X5	T45.2X6
D3	T45.2X1	T45.2X2	T45.2X3	T45.2X4	T45.2X5	T45.2X6
E	T45.2X1	T45.2X2	T45.2X3	T45.2X4	T45.2X5	T45.2X6
E acetate	T45.2X1	T45.2X2	T45.2X3	T45.2X4	T45.2X5	T45.2X6
hematopoietic	T45.8X1	T45.8X2	T45.8X3	T45.8X4	T45.8X5	T45.8X6
K1	T45.7X1	T45.7X2	T45.7X3	T45.7X4	T45.7X5	T45.7X6
K2	T45.7X1	T45.7X2	T45.7X3	T45.7X4	T45.7X5	T45.7X6
K NEC	T45.7X1	T45.7X2	T45.7X3	T45.7X4	T45.7X5	T45.7X6
Vitamin — continued						
PP	T45.2X1	T45.2X2	T45.2X3	T45.2X4	T45.2X5	T45.2X6
ulceroprotectant	T47.1X1	T47.1X2	T47.1X3	T47.1X4	T47.1X5	T47.1X6
Vleminckx's solution	T49.4X1	T49.4X2	T49.4X3	T49.4X4	T49.4X5	T49.4X6
Voltaren — see Diclofenac						
sodium						
Warfarin	T45.511	T45.512	T45.513	T45.514	T45.515	T45.516
rodenticide	T60.4X1-	T60.4X2-	T60.4X3-	T60.4X4-	—	—
sodium	T45.511	T45.512	T45.513	T45.514	T45.515	T45.516
Wasp (sting)	T63.461	T63.462	T63.463	T63.464	—	—
Water						
balance drug	T50.3X1	T50.3X2	T50.3X3	T50.3X4	T50.3X5	T50.3X6
distilled	T50.3X1	T50.3X2	T50.3X3	T50.3X4	T50.3X5	T50.3X6
gas — see Gas, water						
incomplete combustion of — see Carbon, monoxide, fuel, utility						
hemlock	T62.2X1	T62.2X2	T62.2X3	T62.2X4	—	—
moccasin (venom)	T63.061	T63.062	T63.063	T63.064	—	—
purified	T50.3X1	T50.3X2	T50.3X3	T50.3X4	T50.3X5	T50.3X6
Wax (paraffin) (petroleum)	T52.0X1	T52.0X2	T52.0X3	T52.0X4	—	—
automobile	T65.891	T65.892	T65.893	T65.894	—	—
floor	T52.0X1	T52.0X2	T52.0X3	T52.0X4	—	—
Weed killers NEC	T60.3X1	T60.3X2	T60.3X3	T60.3X4	—	—
Welldorm	T42.6X1	T42.6X2	T42.6X3	T42.6X4	T42.6X5	T42.6X6
White						
arsenic	T57.0X1	T57.0X2	T57.0X3	T57.0X4	—	—
hellebore	T62.2X1	T62.2X2	T62.2X3	T62.2X4	—	—
lotion (keratolytic)	T49.4X1	T49.4X2	T49.4X3	T49.4X4	T49.4X5	T49.4X6
spirit	T52.0X1	T52.0X2	T52.0X3	T52.0X4	—	—
Whitewash	T65.891	T65.892	T65.893	T65.894	—	—
Whole blood (human)	T45.8X1	T45.8X2	T45.8X3	T45.8X4	T45.8X5	T45.8X6
Wild						
black cherry	T62.2X1	T62.2X2	T62.2X3	T62.2X4	—	—
poisonous plants NEC	T62.2X1	T62.2X2	T62.2X3	T62.2X4	—	—
Window cleaning fluid	T65.891	T65.892	T65.893	T65.894	—	—
Wintergreen (oil)	T49.3X1	T49.3X2	T49.3X3	T49.3X4	T49.3X5	T49.3X6
Wisterine	T62.2X1	T62.2X2	T62.2X3	T62.2X4	—	—
Witch hazel	T49.2X1	T49.2X2	T49.2X3	T49.2X4	T49.2X5	T49.2X6
Wood alcohol or spirit	T51.1X1	T51.1X2	T51.1X3	T51.1X4	—	—
Wool fat (hydrous)	T49.3X1	T49.3X2	T49.3X3	T49.3X4	T49.3X5	T49.3X6
Woorali	T48.1X1	T48.1X2	T48.1X3	T48.1X4	T48.1X5	T48.1X6
Wormseed, American	T37.4X1	T37.4X2	T37.4X3	T37.4X4	T37.4X5	T37.4X6
Xamoterol	T44.5X1	T44.5X2	T44.5X3	T44.5X4	T44.5X5	T44.5X6
Xanthine diuretics	T50.2X1	T50.2X2	T50.2X3	T50.2X4	T50.2X5	T50.2X6
Xanthinol nicotinate	T46.7X1	T46.7X2	T46.7X3	T46.7X4	T46.7X5	T46.7X6
Xanthotoxin	T49.3X1	T49.3X2	T49.3X3	T49.3X4	T49.3X5	T49.3X6
Xantinol nicotinate	T46.7X1	T46.7X2	T46.7X3	T46.7X4	T46.7X5	T46.7X6
Xantocillin	T36.0X1	T36.0X2	T36.0X3	T36.0X4	T36.0X5	T36.0X6
Xenon (127Xe) (133Xe)	T50.8X1	T50.8X2	T50.8X3	T50.8X4	T50.8X5	T50.8X6
Xenysalate	T49.4X1	T49.4X2	T49.4X3	T49.4X4	T49.4X5	T49.4X6
Xibornol	T37.8X1	T37.8X2	T37.8X3	T37.8X4	T37.8X5	T37.8X6
Xigris	T45.511	T45.512	T45.513	T45.514	T45.515	T45.516
Xipamide	T50.2X1	T50.2X2	T50.2X3	T50.2X4	T50.2X5	T50.2X6
Xylene (vapor)	T52.2X1	T52.2X2	T52.2X3	T52.2X4	—	—
Xylocaine (infiltration) (topical)	T41.3X1	T41.3X2	T41.3X3	T41.3X4	T41.3X5	T41.3X6
nerve block (peripheral) (plexus)	T41.3X1	T41.3X2	T41.3X3	T41.3X4	T41.3X5	T41.3X6
spinal	T41.3X1	T41.3X2	T41.3X3	T41.3X4	T41.3X5	T41.3X6
Xylol (vapor)	T52.2X1	T52.2X2	T52.2X3	T52.2X4	—	—
Xylometazoline	T48.5X1	T48.5X2	T48.5X3	T48.5X4	T48.5X5	T48.5X6
Yeast	T45.2X1	T45.2X2	T45.2X3	T45.2X4	T45.2X5	T45.2X6
dried	T45.2X1	T45.2X2	T45.2X3	T45.2X4	T45.2X5	T45.2X6
Yellow						
fever vaccine	T50.B91	T50.B92	T50.B93	T50.B94	T50.B95	T50.B96
jasmine	T62.2X1	T62.2X2	T62.2X3	T62.2X4	—	—
phenolphthalein	T47.2X1	T47.2X2	T47.2X3	T47.2X4	T47.2X5	T47.2X6
Yew	T62.2X1	T62.2X2	T62.2X3	T62.2X4	—	—
Yohimbic acid	T40.991	T40.992	T40.993	T40.994	T40.995	T40.996
Zactane	T39.8X1	T39.8X2	T39.8X3	T39.8X4	T39.8X5	T39.8X6
Zalcitabine	T37.5X1	T37.5X2	T37.5X3	T37.5X4	T37.5X5	T37.5X6
Zaroxolyn	T50.2X1	T50.2X2	T50.2X3	T50.2X4	T50.2X5	T50.2X6
Zephiran (topical)	T49.0X1	T49.0X2	T49.0X3	T49.0X4	T49.0X5	T49.0X6
ophthalmic preparation	T49.5X1	T49.5X2	T49.5X3	T49.5X4	T49.5X5	T49.5X6
Zeranol	T38.7X1	T38.7X2	T38.7X3	T38.7X4	T38.7X5	T38.7X6
Zerone	T51.1X1	T51.1X2	T51.1X3	T51.1X4	—	—
Zidovudine	T37.5X1	T37.5X2	T37.5X3	T37.5X4	T37.5X5	T37.5X6
Zimeldine	T43.221	T43.222	T43.223	T43.224	T43.225	T43.226
Zinc (compounds) (fumes) (vapor) NEC	T56.5X1	T56.5X2	T56.5X3	T56.5X4	—	—
anti-infectives	T49.0X1	T49.0X2	T49.0X3	T49.0X4	T49.0X5	T49.0X6
antivaricose	T46.8X1	T46.8X2	T46.8X3	T46.8X4	T46.8X5	T46.8X6

Substance	Poisoning, Accidental (unintentional)	Poisoning, Intentional Self-harm	Poisoning, Assault	Poisoning, Undetermined	Adverse Effect	Under-dosing
Zinc (compounds) (fumes) (vapor) **NEC** — *continued*						
bacitracin	T49.0X1	T49.0X2	T49.0X3	T49.0X4	T49.0X5	T49.0X6
chloride (mouthwash)	T49.6X1	T49.6X2	T49.6X3	T49.6X4	T49.6X5	T49.6X6
chromate	T56.5X1	T56.5X2	T56.5X3	T56.5X4	—	—
gelatin	T49.3X1	T49.3X2	T49.3X3	T49.3X4	T49.3X5	T49.3X6
oxide	T49.3X1	T49.3X2	T49.3X3	T49.3X4	T49.3X5	T49.3X6
plaster	T49.3X1	T49.3X2	T49.3X3	T49.3X4	T49.3X5	T49.3X6
peroxide	T49.0X1	T49.0X2	T49.0X3	T49.0X4	T49.0X5	T49.0X6
pesticides	T56.5X1	T56.5X2	T56.5X3	T56.5X4	—	—
phosphide	T60.4X1	T60.4X2	T60.4X3	T60.4X4	—	—
pyrithionate	T49.4X1	T49.4X2	T49.4X3	T49.4X4	T49.4X5	T49.4X6
stearate	T49.3X1	T49.3X2	T49.3X3	T49.3X4	T49.3X5	T49.3X6
sulfate	T49.5X1	T49.5X2	T49.5X3	T49.5X4	T49.5X5	T49.5X6
ENT agent	T49.6X1	T49.6X2	T49.6X3	T49.6X4	T49.6X5	T49.6X6
ophthalmic solution	T49.5X1	T49.5X2	T49.5X3	T49.5X4	T49.5X5	T49.5X6
topical NEC	T49.0X1	T49.0X2	T49.0X3	T49.0X4	T49.0X5	T49.0X6
undecylenate	T49.0X1	T49.0X2	T49.0X3	T49.0X4	T49.0X5	T49.0X6
Zineb	T60.0X1	T60.0X2	T60.0X3	T60.0X4	—	—
Zinostatin	T45.1X1	T45.1X2	T45.1X3	T45.1X4	T45.1X5	T45.1X6
Zipeprol	T48.3X1	T48.3X2	T48.3X3	T48.3X4	T48.3X5	T48.3X6
Zofenopril	T46.4X1	T46.4X2	T46.4X3	T46.4X4	T46.4X5	T46.4X6
Zolpidem	T42.6X1	T42.6X2	T42.6X3	T42.6X4	T42.6X5	T42.6X6
Zomepirac	T39.391	T39.392	T39.393	T39.394	T39.395	T39.396
Zopiclone	T42.6X1	T42.6X2	T42.6X3	T42.6X4	T42.6X5	T42.6X6
Zorubicin	T45.1X1	T45.1X2	T45.1X3	T45.1X4	T45.1X5	T45.1X6
Zotepine	T43.591	T43.592	T43.593	T43.594	T43.595	T43.596
Zovant	T45.511	T45.512	T45.513	T45.514	T45.515	T45.516
Zoxazolamine	T42.8X1	T42.8X2	T42.8X3	T42.8X4	T42.8X5	T42.8X6
Zuclopenthixol	T43.4X1	T43.4X2	T43.4X3	T43.4X4	T43.4X5	T43.4X6
Zygadenus (venenosus)	T62.2X1	T62.2X2	T62.2X3	T62.2X4	—	—
Zyprexa	T43.591	T43.592	T43.593	T43.594	T43.595	T43.596

▽ Subterms under main terms may continue to next column or page   Additional Character May Be Required — Refer to the Tabular List for Character Selection   403

Zinc — Zyprexa

A

Abandonment (causing exposure to weather conditions)
(with intent to injure or kill) NEC X58 ☑
Abuse (adult) (child) (mental) (physical) (sexual) X58 ☑
Accident (to) X58 ☑
  aircraft (in transit) (powered) — *see also* Accident,
    transport, aircraft
    due to, caused by cataclysm — *see* Forces of nature,
      by type
  animal-drawn vehicle — *see* Accident, transport, ani-
    mal-drawn vehicle occupant
  animal-rider — *see* Accident, transport, animal-rider
  automobile — *see* Accident, transport, car occupant
  bare foot water skier V94.4 ☑
  boat, boating — *see also* Accident, watercraft
    striking swimmer
      powered V94.11 ☑
      unpowered V94.12 ☑
  bus — *see* Accident, transport, bus occupant
  cable car, not on rails V98.0 ☑
    on rails — *see* Accident, transport, streetcar occu-
      pant
  car — *see* Accident, transport, car occupant
  caused by, due to
    animal NEC W64 ☑
    chain hoist W24.0 ☑
    cold (excessive) — *see* Exposure, cold
    corrosive liquid, substance — *see* Table of Drugs
      and Chemicals
    cutting or piercing instrument — *see* Contact, with,
      by type of instrument
    drive belt W24.0 ☑
    electric
      current — *see* Exposure, electric current
      motor — *see also* Contact, with, by type of ma-
        chine W31.3 ☑
      current (of) W86.8 ☑
    environmental factor NEC X58 ☑
    explosive material — *see* Explosion
    fire, flames — *see* Exposure, fire
    firearm missile — *see* Discharge, firearm by type
    heat (excessive) — *see* Heat
    hot — *see* Contact, with, hot
    ignition — *see* Ignition
    lifting device W24.0 ☑
    lightning — *see* subcategory T75.0 ☑
      causing fire — *see* Exposure, fire
    machine, machinery — *see* Contact, with, by type
      of machine
    natural factor NEC X58 ☑
    pulley (block) W24.0 ☑
    radiation — *see* Radiation
    steam X13.1 ☑
      inhalation X13.0 ☑
      pipe X16 ☑
    thunderbolt — *see* subcategory T75.0 ☑
      causing fire — *see* Exposure, fire
    transmission device W24.1 ☑
  coach — *see* Accident, transport, bus occupant
  coal car — *see* Accident, transport, industrial vehicle
    occupant
  diving — *see also* Fall, into, water
    with
      drowning or submersion — *see* Drowning
  forklift — *see* Accident, transport, industrial vehicle
    occupant
  heavy transport vehicle NOS — *see* Accident, transport,
    truck occupant
  ice yacht V98.2 ☑
  in
    medical, surgical procedure
      as, or due to misadventure — *see* Misadventure
      causing an abnormal reaction or later complica-
        tion without mention of misadventure —
        see also Complication of or following, by
        type of procedure Y84.9
  land yacht V98.1 ☑
  late effect of — *see* W00-X58 with 7th character S
  logging car — *see* Accident, transport, industrial vehicle
    occupant
  machine, machinery — *see also* Contact, with, by type
    of machine
    on board watercraft V93.69 ☑
      explosion — *see* Explosion, in, watercraft

Accident — *continued*
  machine, machinery — *see also* Contact, with, by type
    of machine — *continued*
    on board watercraft — *continued*
      fire — *see* Burn, on board watercraft
      powered craft V93.63 ☑
        ferry boat V93.61 ☑
        fishing boat V93.62 ☑
        jetskis V93.63 ☑
        liner V93.61 ☑
        merchant ship V93.60 ☑
        passenger ship V93.61 ☑
        sailboat V93.64 ☑
    mine tram — *see* Accident, transport, industrial vehicle
      occupant
  mobility scooter (motorized) — *see* Accident, transport,
    pedestrian, conveyance, specified type NEC
  motor scooter — *see* Accident, transport, motorcyclist
  motor vehicle NOS (traffic) — *see also* Accident, trans-
    port V89.2 ☑
    nontraffic V89.0 ☑
    three-wheeled NOS — *see* Accident, transport,
      three-wheeled motor vehicle occupant
  motorcycle NOS — *see* Accident, transport, motorcyclist
  nonmotor vehicle NOS (nontraffic) — *see also* Accident,
    transport V89.1 ☑
    traffic NOS V89.3 ☑
  nontraffic (victim's mode of transport NOS) V88.9 ☑
    collision (between) V88.7 ☑
      bus and truck V88.5 ☑
      car and:
        bus V88.3 ☑
        pickup V88.2 ☑
        three-wheeled motor vehicle V88.0 ☑
        train V88.6 ☑
        truck V88.4 ☑
        two-wheeled motor vehicle V88.0 ☑
        van V88.2 ☑
      specified vehicle NEC and:
        three-wheeled motor vehicle V88.1 ☑
        two-wheeled motor vehicle V88.1 ☑
    known mode of transport — *see* Accident, transport,
      by type of vehicle
    noncollision V88.8 ☑
  on board watercraft V93.89 ☑
    powered craft V93.83 ☑
      ferry boat V93.81 ☑
      fishing boat V93.82 ☑
      jetskis V93.83 ☑
      liner V93.81 ☑
      merchant ship V93.80 ☑
      passenger ship V93.81 ☑
    unpowered craft V93.88 ☑
      canoe V93.85 ☑
      inflatable V93.86 ☑
        in tow
          recreational V94.31 ☑
          specified NEC V94.32 ☑
      kayak V93.85 ☑
      sailboat V93.84 ☑
      surf-board V93.88 ☑
      water skis V93.87 ☑
      windsurfer V93.88 ☑
  parachutist V97.29 ☑
    entangled in object V97.21 ☑
    injured on landing V97.22 ☑
  pedal cycle — *see* Accident, transport, pedal cyclist
  pedestrian (on foot)
    with
      another pedestrian W51 ☑
        on pedestrian conveyance NEC V00.09 ☑
        with fall W03 ☑
          due to ice or snow W00.0 ☑
      rider of
        hoverboard V00.038 ☑
        Segway V00.038 ☑
        standing
          electric scooter V00.031 ☑
          micro-mobility pedestrian conveyance
            NEC V00.038 ☑
      roller skater (in-line) V00.01 ☑
      skate boarder V00.02 ☑
    transport vehicle — *see* Accident, transport
    on pedestrian conveyance — *see* Accident, trans-
      port, pedestrian, conveyance

Accident — *continued*
  pick-up truck or van — *see* Accident, transport, pickup
    truck occupant
  quarry truck — *see* Accident, transport, industrial vehi-
    cle occupant
  railway vehicle (any) (in motion) — *see* Accident,
    transport, railway vehicle occupant
    due to cataclysm — *see* Forces of nature, by type
  scooter (non-motorized) — *see* Accident, transport,
    pedestrian, conveyance, scooter
  sequelae of — *see* categories W00-X58 with 7th charac-
    ter S
  skateboard — *see* Accident, transport, pedestrian,
    conveyance, skateboard
  ski(ing) — *see* Accident, transport, pedestrian, con-
    veyance
    lift V98.3 ☑
  specified cause NEC X58 ☑
  streetcar — *see* Accident, transport, streetcar occupant
  traffic (victim's mode of transport NOS) V87.9 ☑
    collision (between) V87.7 ☑
      bus and truck V87.5 ☑
      car and:
        bus V87.3 ☑
        pickup V87.2 ☑
        three-wheeled motor vehicle V87.0 ☑
        train V87.6 ☑
        truck V87.4 ☑
        two-wheeled motor vehicle V87.0 ☑
        van V87.2 ☑
      specified vehicle NEC V86.39 ☑
        and
          three-wheeled motor vehicle V87.1 ☑
          two-wheeled motor vehicle V87.1 ☑
        driver V86.09 ☑
        passenger V86.19 ☑
        person on outside V86.29 ☑
        while boarding or alighting V86.49 ☑
    known mode of transport — *see* Accident, transport,
      by type of vehicle
    noncollision V87.8 ☑
  transport (involving injury to) V99 ☑
    18 wheeler — *see* Accident, transport, truck occu-
      pant
    agricultural vehicle occupant (nontraffic) V84.9 ☑
      driver V84.5 ☑
      hanger-on V84.7 ☑
      passenger V84.6 ☑
      traffic V84.3 ☑
        driver V84.0 ☑
        hanger-on V84.2 ☑
        passenger V84.1 ☑
      while boarding or alighting V84.4 ☑
    aircraft NEC V97.89 ☑
      military NEC V97.818 ☑
        civilian injured by V97.811 ☑
        with civilian aircraft V97.810 ☑
      occupant injured (in)
        nonpowered craft accident V96.9 ☑
          balloon V96.00 ☑
            collision V96.03 ☑
            crash V96.01 ☑
            explosion V96.05 ☑
            fire V96.04 ☑
            forced landing V96.02 ☑
            specified type NEC V96.09 ☑
          glider V96.20 ☑
            collision V96.23 ☑
            crash V96.21 ☑
            explosion V96.25 ☑
            fire V96.24 ☑
            forced landing V96.22 ☑
            specified type NEC V96.29 ☑
          hang glider V96.10 ☑
            collision V96.13 ☑
            crash V96.11 ☑
            explosion V96.15 ☑
            fire V96.14 ☑
            forced landing V96.12 ☑
            specified type NEC V96.19 ☑
          specified craft NEC V96.8 ☑
        powered craft accident V95.9 ☑
          fixed wing NEC
            commercial V95.30 ☑
              collision V95.33 ☑
              crash V95.31 ☑

☑ **Additional Character Required** — Refer to the Tabular List for Character Selection   ▽ **Subterms under main terms may continue to next column or page**

Accident — *continued*
  transport — *continued*
    aircraft — *continued*
      occupant injured — *continued*
        powered craft accident — *continued*
          fixed wing — *continued*
            commercial — *continued*
              explosion V95.35 ☑
              fire V95.34 ☑
              forced landing V95.32 ☑
              specified type NEC V95.39 ☑
            private V95.20 ☑
              collision V95.23 ☑
              crash V95.21 ☑
              explosion V95.25 ☑
              fire V95.24 ☑
              forced landing V95.22 ☑
              specified type NEC V95.29 ☑
          glider V95.10 ☑
            collision V95.13 ☑
            crash V95.11 ☑
            explosion V95.15 ☑
            fire V95.14 ☑
            forced landing V95.12 ☑
            specified type NEC V95.19 ☑
          helicopter V95.00 ☑
            collision V95.03 ☑
            crash V95.01 ☑
            explosion V95.05 ☑
            fire V95.04 ☑
            forced landing V95.02 ☑
            specified type NEC V95.09 ☑
          spacecraft V95.40 ☑
            collision V95.43 ☑
            crash V95.41 ☑
            explosion V95.45 ☑
            fire V95.44 ☑
            forced landing V95.42 ☑
            specified type NEC V95.49 ☑
          specified craft NEC V95.8 ☑
          ultralight V95.10 ☑
            collision V95.13 ☑
            crash V95.11 ☑
            explosion V95.15 ☑
            fire V95.14 ☑
            forced landing V95.12 ☑
            specified type NEC V95.19 ☑
        specified accident NEC V97.0 ☑
        while boarding or alighting V97.1 ☑
      person (injured by)
        falling from, in or on aircraft V97.0 ☑
        machinery on aircraft V97.89 ☑
        on ground with aircraft involvement
          V97.39 ☑
        rotating propeller V97.32 ☑
        struck by object falling from aircraft V97.31 ☑
        sucked into aircraft jet V97.33 ☑
        while boarding or alighting aircraft V97.1 ☑
    airport (battery-powered) passenger vehicle — *see* Accident, transport, industrial vehicle occupant
    all-terrain vehicle occupant (nontraffic) V86.95 ☑
      driver V86.55 ☑
      dune buggy — *see* Accident, transport, dune buggy occupant
      hanger-on V86.75 ☑
      passenger V86.65 ☑
      snowmobile — *see* Accident, transport, snowmobile occupant
      specified type NEC V86.99 ☑
        driver V86.59 ☑
        passenger V86.69 ☑
        person on outside V86.79 ☑
      traffic V86.35 ☑
        driver V86.05 ☑
        hanger-on V86.25 ☑
        passenger V86.15 ☑
      while boarding or alighting V86.45 ☑
    ambulance occupant (traffic) V86.31 ☑
      driver V86.01 ☑
      hanger-on V86.21 ☑
      nontraffic V86.91 ☑
        driver V86.51 ☑
        hanger-on V86.71 ☑
        passenger V86.61 ☑
      passenger V86.11 ☑

Accident — *continued*
  transport — *continued*
    ambulance occupant — *continued*
      while boarding or alighting V86.41 ☑
    animal-drawn vehicle occupant (in) V80.929 ☑
      collision (with)
        animal V80.12 ☑
          being ridden V80.711 ☑
        animal-drawn vehicle V80.721 ☑
        bus V80.42 ☑
        car V80.42 ☑
        fixed or stationary object V80.82 ☑
        military vehicle V80.920 ☑
        nonmotor vehicle V80.791 ☑
        pedal cycle V80.22 ☑
        pedestrian V80.12 ☑
        pickup V80.42 ☑
        railway train or vehicle V80.62 ☑
        specified motor vehicle NEC V80.52 ☑
        streetcar V80.731 ☑
        truck V80.42 ☑
        two- or three-wheeled motor vehicle V80.32 ☑
        van V80.42 ☑
      noncollision V80.02 ☑
      specified circumstance NEC V80.928 ☑
    animal-rider V80.919 ☑
      collision (with)
        animal V80.11 ☑
          being ridden V80.710 ☑
        animal-drawn vehicle V80.720 ☑
        bus V80.41 ☑
        car V80.41 ☑
        fixed or stationary object V80.81 ☑
        military vehicle V80.910 ☑
        nonmotor vehicle V80.790 ☑
        pedal cycle V80.21 ☑
        pedestrian V80.11 ☑
        pickup V80.41 ☑
        railway train or vehicle V80.61 ☑
        specified motor vehicle NEC V80.51 ☑
        streetcar V80.730 ☑
        truck V80.41 ☑
        two- or three-wheeled motor vehicle V80.31 ☑
        van V80.41 ☑
      noncollision V80.018 ☑
        specified as horse rider V80.010 ☑
      specified circumstance NEC V80.918 ☑
    armored car — *see* Accident, transport, truck occupant
    battery-powered truck (baggage) (mail) — *see* Accident, transport, industrial vehicle occupant
    bus occupant V79.9 ☑
      collision (with)
        animal (traffic) V70.9 ☑
          being ridden (traffic) V76.9 ☑
            nontraffic V76.3 ☑
            while boarding or alighting V76.4 ☑
          nontraffic V70.3 ☑
          while boarding or alighting V70.4 ☑
        animal-drawn vehicle (traffic) V76.9 ☑
          nontraffic V76.3 ☑
          while boarding or alighting V76.4 ☑
        bus (traffic) V74.9 ☑
          nontraffic V74.3 ☑
          while boarding or alighting V74.4 ☑
        car (traffic) V73.9 ☑
          nontraffic V73.3 ☑
          while boarding or alighting V73.4 ☑
        motor vehicle NOS (traffic) V79.60 ☑
          nontraffic V79.20 ☑
          specified type NEC (traffic) V79.69 ☑
            nontraffic V79.29 ☑
        pedal cycle (traffic) V71.9 ☑
          nontraffic V71.3 ☑
          while boarding or alighting V71.4 ☑
        pickup truck (traffic) V73.9 ☑
          nontraffic V73.3 ☑
          while boarding or alighting V73.4 ☑
        railway vehicle (traffic) V75.9 ☑
          nontraffic V75.3 ☑
          while boarding or alighting V75.4 ☑
        specified vehicle NEC (traffic) V76.9 ☑
          nontraffic V76.3 ☑
          while boarding or alighting V76.4 ☑

Accident — *continued*
  transport — *continued*
    bus occupant — *continued*
      collision — *continued*
        stationary object (traffic) V77.9 ☑
          nontraffic V77.3 ☑
          while boarding or alighting V77.4 ☑
        streetcar (traffic) V76.9 ☑
          nontraffic V76.3 ☑
          while boarding or alighting V76.4 ☑
        three wheeled motor vehicle (traffic) V72.9 ☑
          nontraffic V72.3 ☑
          while boarding or alighting V72.4 ☑
        truck (traffic) V74.9 ☑
          nontraffic V74.3 ☑
          while boarding or alighting V74.4 ☑
        two wheeled motor vehicle (traffic) V72.9 ☑
          nontraffic V72.3 ☑
          while boarding or alighting V72.4 ☑
        van (traffic) V73.9 ☑
          nontraffic V73.3 ☑
          while boarding or alighting V73.4 ☑
      driver
        collision (with)
          animal (traffic) V70.5 ☑
            being ridden (traffic) V76.5 ☑
              nontraffic V76.0 ☑
            nontraffic V70.0 ☑
          animal-drawn vehicle (traffic) V76.5 ☑
            nontraffic V76.0 ☑
          bus (traffic) V74.5 ☑
            nontraffic V74.0 ☑
          car (traffic) V73.5 ☑
            nontraffic V73.0 ☑
          motor vehicle NOS (traffic) V79.40 ☑
            nontraffic V79.00 ☑
            specified type NEC (traffic) V79.49 ☑
              nontraffic V79.09 ☑
          pedal cycle (traffic) V71.5 ☑
            nontraffic V71.0 ☑
          pickup truck (traffic) V73.5 ☑
            nontraffic V73.0 ☑
          railway vehicle (traffic) V75.5 ☑
            nontraffic V75.0 ☑
          specified vehicle NEC (traffic) V76.5 ☑
            nontraffic V76.0 ☑
          stationary object (traffic) V77.5 ☑
            nontraffic V77.0 ☑
          streetcar (traffic) V76.5 ☑
            nontraffic V76.0 ☑
          three wheeled motor vehicle (traffic) V72.5 ☑
            nontraffic V72.0 ☑
          truck (traffic) V74.5 ☑
            nontraffic V74.0 ☑
          two wheeled motor vehicle (traffic) V72.5 ☑
            nontraffic V72.0 ☑
          van (traffic) V73.5 ☑
            nontraffic V73.0 ☑
        noncollision accident (traffic) V78.5 ☑
          nontraffic V78.0 ☑
      hanger-on
        collision (with)
          animal (traffic) V70.7 ☑
            being ridden (traffic) V76.7 ☑
              nontraffic V76.2 ☑
            nontraffic V70.2 ☑
          animal-drawn vehicle (traffic) V76.7 ☑
            nontraffic V76.2 ☑
          bus (traffic) V74.7 ☑
            nontraffic V74.2 ☑
          car (traffic) V73.7 ☑
            nontraffic V73.2 ☑
          pedal cycle (traffic) V71.7 ☑
            nontraffic V71.2 ☑
          pickup truck (traffic) V73.7 ☑
            nontraffic V73.2 ☑
          railway vehicle (traffic) V75.7 ☑
            nontraffic V75.2 ☑
          specified vehicle NEC (traffic) V76.7 ☑
            nontraffic V76.2 ☑
          stationary object (traffic) V77.7 ☑
            nontraffic V77.2 ☑
          streetcar (traffic) V76.7 ☑
            nontraffic V76.2 ☑

Accident — *continued*
  transport — *continued*
    bus occupant — *continued*
      hanger-on — *continued*
        collision — *continued*
          three wheeled motor vehicle (traffic)
            V72.7 ☑
            nontraffic V74.2 ☑
          truck (traffic) V74.7 ☑
            nontraffic V74.2 ☑
          two wheeled motor vehicle (traffic)
            V72.7 ☑
            nontraffic V72.2 ☑
          van (traffic) V73.7 ☑
            nontraffic V73.2 ☑
        noncollision accident (traffic) V78.7 ☑
          nontraffic V78.2 ☑
      noncollision accident (traffic) V78.9 ☑
        nontraffic V78.3 ☑
        while boarding or alighting V78.4 ☑
      nontraffic V79.3 ☑
    passenger
      collision (with)
        animal (traffic) V70.6 ☑
          being ridden (traffic) V76.6 ☑
            nontraffic V76.1 ☑
          nontraffic V70.1 ☑
        animal-drawn vehicle (traffic) V76.6 ☑
          nontraffic V76.1 ☑
        bus (traffic) V74.6 ☑
          nontraffic V74.1 ☑
        car (traffic) V73.6 ☑
          nontraffic V73.1 ☑
        motor vehicle NOS (traffic) V79.50 ☑
          nontraffic V79.10 ☑
          specified type NEC (traffic) V79.59 ☑
            nontraffic V79.19 ☑
        pedal cycle (traffic) V71.6 ☑
          nontraffic V71.1 ☑
        pickup truck (traffic) V73.6 ☑
          nontraffic V73.1 ☑
        railway vehicle (traffic) V75.6 ☑
          nontraffic V75.1 ☑
        specified vehicle NEC (traffic) V76.6 ☑
          nontraffic V76.1 ☑
        stationary object (traffic) V77.6 ☑
          nontraffic V77.1 ☑
        streetcar (traffic) V76.6 ☑
          nontraffic V76.1 ☑
        three wheeled motor vehicle (traffic)
            V72.6 ☑
          nontraffic V72.1 ☑
        truck (traffic) V74.6 ☑
          nontraffic V74.1 ☑
        two wheeled motor vehicle (traffic)
            V72.6 ☑
          nontraffic V72.1 ☑
        van (traffic) V73.6 ☑
          nontraffic V73.1 ☑
      noncollision accident (traffic) V78.6 ☑
        nontraffic V78.1 ☑
      specified type NEC V79.88 ☑
      military vehicle V79.81 ☑
  cable car, not on rails V98.0 ☑
    on rails — *see* Accident, transport, streetcar occupant
  car occupant V49.9 ☑
    ambulance occupant — *see* Accident, transport, ambulance occupant
    collision (with)
      animal (traffic) V40.9 ☑
        being ridden (traffic) V46.9 ☑
          nontraffic V46.3 ☑
          while boarding or alighting V46.4 ☑
        nontraffic V40.3 ☑
        while boarding or alighting V40.4 ☑
      animal-drawn vehicle (traffic) V46.9 ☑
        nontraffic V46.3 ☑
        while boarding or alighting V46.4 ☑
      bus (traffic) V44.9 ☑
        nontraffic V44.3 ☑
        while boarding or alighting V44.4 ☑
      car (traffic) V43.92 ☑
        nontraffic V43.32 ☑
        while boarding or alighting V43.42 ☑
      motor vehicle NOS (traffic) V49.60 ☑

Accident — *continued*
  transport — *continued*
    car occupant — *continued*
      collision — *continued*
        motor vehicle — *continued*
          nontraffic V49.20 ☑
          specified type NEC (traffic) V49.69 ☑
            nontraffic V49.29 ☑
        pedal cycle (traffic) V41.9 ☑
          nontraffic V41.3 ☑
          while boarding or alighting V41.4 ☑
        pickup truck (traffic) V43.93 ☑
          nontraffic V43.33 ☑
          while boarding or alighting V43.43 ☑
        railway vehicle (traffic) V45.9 ☑
          nontraffic V45.3 ☑
          while boarding or alighting V45.4 ☑
        specified vehicle NEC (traffic) V46.9 ☑
          nontraffic V46.3 ☑
          while boarding or alighting V46.4 ☑
        sport utility vehicle (traffic) V43.91 ☑
          nontraffic V43.31 ☑
          while boarding or alighting V43.41 ☑
        stationary object (traffic) V47.9 ☑
          nontraffic V47.3 ☑
          while boarding or alighting V47.4 ☑
        streetcar (traffic) V46.9 ☑
          nontraffic V46.3 ☑
          while boarding or alighting V46.4 ☑
        three wheeled motor vehicle (traffic) V42.9 ☑
          nontraffic V42.3 ☑
          while boarding or alighting V42.4 ☑
        truck (traffic) V44.9 ☑
          nontraffic V44.3 ☑
          while boarding or alighting V44.4 ☑
        two wheeled motor vehicle (traffic) V42.9 ☑
          nontraffic V42.3 ☑
          while boarding or alighting V42.4 ☑
        van (traffic) V43.94 ☑
          nontraffic V43.34 ☑
          while boarding or alighting V43.44 ☑
      driver
        collision (with)
          animal (traffic) V40.5 ☑
            being ridden (traffic) V46.5 ☑
              nontraffic V46.0 ☑
            nontraffic V40.0 ☑
          animal-drawn vehicle (traffic) V46.5 ☑
            nontraffic V46.0 ☑
          bus (traffic) V44.5 ☑
            nontraffic V44.0 ☑
          car (traffic) V43.52 ☑
            nontraffic V43.02 ☑
          motor vehicle NOS (traffic) V49.40 ☑
            nontraffic V49.00 ☑
            specified type NEC (traffic) V49.49 ☑
              nontraffic V49.09 ☑
          pedal cycle (traffic) V41.5 ☑
            nontraffic V41.0 ☑
          pickup truck (traffic) V43.53 ☑
            nontraffic V43.03 ☑
          railway vehicle (traffic) V45.5 ☑
            nontraffic V45.0 ☑
          specified vehicle NEC (traffic) V46.5 ☑
            nontraffic V46.0 ☑
          sport utility vehicle (traffic) V43.51 ☑
            nontraffic V43.01 ☑
          stationary object (traffic) V47.5 ☑
            nontraffic V47.0 ☑
          streetcar (traffic) V46.5 ☑
            nontraffic V46.0 ☑
          three wheeled motor vehicle (traffic)
              V42.5 ☑
            nontraffic V42.0 ☑
          truck (traffic) V44.5 ☑
            nontraffic V44.0 ☑
          two wheeled motor vehicle (traffic)
              V42.5 ☑
            nontraffic V42.0 ☑
          van (traffic) V43.54 ☑
            nontraffic V43.04 ☑
        noncollision accident (traffic) V48.5 ☑
          nontraffic V48.0 ☑
      hanger-on
        collision (with)
          animal (traffic) V40.7 ☑

Accident — *continued*
  transport — *continued*
    car occupant — *continued*
      hanger-on — *continued*
        collision — *continued*
          animal — *continued*
            being ridden (traffic) V46.7 ☑
              nontraffic V46.2 ☑
            nontraffic V40.2 ☑
          animal-drawn vehicle (traffic) V46.7 ☑
            nontraffic V46.2 ☑
          bus (traffic) V44.7 ☑
            nontraffic V44.2 ☑
          car (traffic) V43.72 ☑
            nontraffic V43.22 ☑
          pedal cycle (traffic) V41.7 ☑
            nontraffic V41.2 ☑
          pickup truck (traffic) V43.73 ☑
            nontraffic V43.23 ☑
          railway vehicle (traffic) V45.7 ☑
            nontraffic V45.2 ☑
          specified vehicle NEC (traffic) V46.7 ☑
            nontraffic V46.2 ☑
          sport utility vehicle (traffic) V43.71 ☑
            nontraffic V43.21 ☑
          stationary object (traffic) V47.7 ☑
            nontraffic V47.2 ☑
          streetcar (traffic) V46.7 ☑
            nontraffic V46.2 ☑
          three wheeled motor vehicle (traffic)
              V42.7 ☑
            nontraffic V42.2 ☑
          truck (traffic) V44.7 ☑
            nontraffic V44.2 ☑
          two wheeled motor vehicle (traffic)
              V42.7 ☑
            nontraffic V42.2 ☑
          van (traffic) V43.74 ☑
            nontraffic V43.24 ☑
        noncollision accident (traffic) V48.7 ☑
          nontraffic V48.2 ☑
      noncollision accident (traffic) V48.9 ☑
        nontraffic V48.3 ☑
        while boarding or alighting V48.4 ☑
      nontraffic V49.3 ☑
      passenger
        collision (with)
          animal (traffic) V40.6 ☑
            being ridden (traffic) V46.6 ☑
              nontraffic V46.1 ☑
            nontraffic V40.1 ☑
          animal-drawn vehicle (traffic) V46.6 ☑
            nontraffic V46.1 ☑
          bus (traffic) V44.6 ☑
            nontraffic V44.1 ☑
          car (traffic) V43.62 ☑
            nontraffic V43.12 ☑
          motor vehicle NOS (traffic) V49.50 ☑
            nontraffic V49.10 ☑
            specified type NEC (traffic) V49.59 ☑
              nontraffic V49.19 ☑
          pedal cycle (traffic) V41.6 ☑
            nontraffic V41.1 ☑
          pickup truck (traffic) V43.63 ☑
            nontraffic V43.13 ☑
          railway vehicle (traffic) V45.6 ☑
            nontraffic V45.1 ☑
          specified vehicle NEC (traffic) V46.6 ☑
            nontraffic V46.1 ☑
          sport utility vehicle (traffic) V43.61 ☑
            nontraffic V43.11 ☑
          stationary object (traffic) V47.6 ☑
            nontraffic V47.1 ☑
          streetcar (traffic) V46.6 ☑
            nontraffic V46.1 ☑
          three wheeled motor vehicle (traffic)
              V42.6 ☑
            nontraffic V42.1 ☑
          truck (traffic) V44.6 ☑
            nontraffic V44.1 ☑
          two wheeled motor vehicle (traffic)
              V42.6 ☑
            nontraffic V42.1 ☑
          van (traffic) V43.64 ☑
            nontraffic V43.14 ☑
        noncollision accident (traffic) V48.6 ☑

☑ **Additional Character Required** — **Refer to the Tabular List for Character Selection**   ▽ **Subterms under main terms may continue to next column or page**

Accident — *continued*
　transport — *continued*
　　car occupant — *continued*
　　　passenger — *continued*
　　　　noncollision accident — *continued*
　　　　　nontraffic V48.1 ☑
　　　　specified type NEC V49.88 ☑
　　　　military vehicle V49.81 ☑
　　coal car — *see* Accident, transport, industrial vehicle
　　　　occupant
　　construction vehicle occupant (nontraffic) V85.9 ☑
　　　driver V85.5 ☑
　　　hanger-on V85.7 ☑
　　　passenger V85.6 ☑
　　　traffic V85.3 ☑
　　　　driver V85.0 ☑
　　　　hanger-on V85.2 ☑
　　　　passenger V85.1 ☑
　　　while boarding or alighting V85.4 ☑
　　dirt bike rider (nontraffic) V86.96 ☑
　　　driver V86.56 ☑
　　　hanger-on V86.76 ☑
　　　passenger V86.66 ☑
　　　traffic V86.36 ☑
　　　　driver V86.06 ☑
　　　　hanger-on V86.26 ☑
　　　　passenger V86.16 ☑
　　　while boarding or alighting V86.46 ☑
　　due to cataclysm — *see* Forces of nature, by type
　　dune buggy occupant (nontraffic) V86.93 ☑
　　　driver V86.53 ☑
　　　hanger-on V86.73 ☑
　　　passenger V86.63 ☑
　　　traffic V86.33 ☑
　　　　driver V86.03 ☑
　　　　hanger-on V86.23 ☑
　　　　passenger V86.13 ☑
　　　while boarding or alighting V86.43 ☑
　　forklift — *see* Accident, transport, industrial vehicle
　　　　occupant
　　go cart — *see* Accident, transport, all-terrain vehicle
　　　　occupant
　　golf cart — *see* Accident, transport, all-terrain vehicle occupant
　　heavy transport vehicle occupant — *see* Accident,
　　　　transport, truck occupant
　　hoverboard V00.848 ☑
　　ice yacht V98.2 ☑
　　industrial vehicle occupant (nontraffic) V83.9 ☑
　　　driver V83.5 ☑
　　　hanger-on V83.7 ☑
　　　passenger V83.6 ☑
　　　traffic V83.3 ☑
　　　　driver V83.0 ☑
　　　　hanger-on V83.2 ☑
　　　　passenger V83.1 ☑
　　　while boarding or alighting V83.4 ☑
　　interurban electric car — *see* Accident, transport,
　　　　streetcar
　　land yacht V98.1 ☑
　　logging car — *see* Accident, transport, industrial
　　　　vehicle occupant
　　military vehicle occupant (traffic) V86.34 ☑
　　　driver V86.04 ☑
　　　hanger-on V86.24 ☑
　　　nontraffic V86.94 ☑
　　　　driver V86.54 ☑
　　　　hanger-on V86.74 ☑
　　　　passenger V86.64 ☑
　　　passenger V86.14 ☑
　　　while boarding or alighting V86.44 ☑
　　mine tram — *see* Accident, transport, industrial ve-
　　　　hicle occupant
　　motor vehicle NEC occupant (traffic) V89.2 ☑
　　motorcoach — *see* Accident, transport, bus occu-
　　　　pant
　　motor/cross bike rider — *see also* Accident, trans-
　　　　port, dirt bike rider V86.96 ☑
　　motorcyclist V29.9 ☑
　　　collision (with)
　　　　animal (traffic) V20.9 ☑
　　　　　being ridden (traffic) V26.9 ☑
　　　　　　nontraffic V26.2 ☑
　　　　　　while boarding or alighting V26.3 ☑
　　　　　nontraffic V20.2 ☑
　　　　　while boarding or alighting V20.3 ☑

Accident — *continued*
　transport — *continued*
　　motorcyclist — *continued*
　　　collision — *continued*
　　　　animal-drawn vehicle (traffic) V26.9 ☑
　　　　　nontraffic V26.2 ☑
　　　　　while boarding or alighting V26.3 ☑
　　　　bus (traffic) V24.9 ☑
　　　　　nontraffic V24.2 ☑
　　　　　while boarding or alighting V24.3 ☑
　　　　car (traffic) V23.9 ☑
　　　　　nontraffic V23.2 ☑
　　　　　while boarding or alighting V23.3 ☑
　　　　motor vehicle NOS (traffic) V29.60 ☑
　　　　　nontraffic V29.20 ☑
　　　　　specified type NEC (traffic) V29.69 ☑
　　　　　　nontraffic V29.29 ☑
　　　　pedal cycle (traffic) V21.9 ☑
　　　　　nontraffic V21.2 ☑
　　　　　while boarding or alighting V21.3 ☑
　　　　pickup truck (traffic) V23.9 ☑
　　　　　nontraffic V23.2 ☑
　　　　　while boarding or alighting V23.3 ☑
　　　　railway vehicle (traffic) V25.9 ☑
　　　　　nontraffic V25.2 ☑
　　　　　while boarding or alighting V25.3 ☑
　　　　specified vehicle NEC (traffic) V26.9 ☑
　　　　　nontraffic V26.2 ☑
　　　　　while boarding or alighting V26.3 ☑
　　　　stationary object (traffic) V27.9 ☑
　　　　　nontraffic V27.2 ☑
　　　　　while boarding or alighting V27.3 ☑
　　　　streetcar (traffic) V26.9 ☑
　　　　　nontraffic V26.2 ☑
　　　　　while boarding or alighting V26.3 ☑
　　　　three wheeled motor vehicle (traffic) V22.9 ☑
　　　　　nontraffic V22.2 ☑
　　　　　while boarding or alighting V22.3 ☑
　　　　truck (traffic) V24.9 ☑
　　　　　nontraffic V24.2 ☑
　　　　　while boarding or alighting V24.3 ☑
　　　　two wheeled motor vehicle (traffic) V22.9 ☑
　　　　　nontraffic V22.2 ☑
　　　　　while boarding or alighting V22.3 ☑
　　　　van (traffic) V23.9 ☑
　　　　　nontraffic V23.2 ☑
　　　　　while boarding or alighting V23.3 ☑
　　　driver
　　　　collision (with)
　　　　　animal (traffic) V20.4 ☑
　　　　　　being ridden (traffic) V26.4 ☑
　　　　　　　nontraffic V26.0 ☑
　　　　　　nontraffic V20.0 ☑
　　　　　animal-drawn vehicle (traffic) V26.4 ☑
　　　　　　nontraffic V26.0 ☑
　　　　　bus (traffic) V24.4 ☑
　　　　　　nontraffic V24.0 ☑
　　　　　car (traffic) V23.4 ☑
　　　　　　nontraffic V23.0 ☑
　　　　　motor vehicle NOS (traffic) V29.40 ☑
　　　　　　nontraffic V29.00 ☑
　　　　　　specified type NEC (traffic) V29.49 ☑
　　　　　　　nontraffic V29.09 ☑
　　　　　pedal cycle (traffic) V21.4 ☑
　　　　　　nontraffic V21.0 ☑
　　　　　pickup truck (traffic) V23.4 ☑
　　　　　　nontraffic V23.0 ☑
　　　　　railway vehicle (traffic) V25.4 ☑
　　　　　　nontraffic V25.0 ☑
　　　　　specified vehicle NEC (traffic) V26.4 ☑
　　　　　　nontraffic V26.0 ☑
　　　　　stationary object (traffic) V27.4 ☑
　　　　　　nontraffic V27.0 ☑
　　　　　streetcar (traffic) V26.4 ☑
　　　　　　nontraffic V26.0 ☑
　　　　　three wheeled motor vehicle (traffic)
　　　　　　V22.4 ☑
　　　　　　nontraffic V22.0 ☑
　　　　　truck (traffic) V24.4 ☑
　　　　　　nontraffic V24.0 ☑
　　　　　two wheeled motor vehicle (traffic)
　　　　　　V22.4 ☑
　　　　　　nontraffic V22.0 ☑
　　　　　van (traffic) V23.4 ☑
　　　　　　nontraffic V23.0 ☑
　　　　noncollision accident (traffic) V28.4 ☑

Accident — *continued*
　transport — *continued*
　　motorcyclist — *continued*
　　　driver — *continued*
　　　　noncollision accident — *continued*
　　　　　nontraffic V28.0 ☑
　　　　noncollision accident (traffic) V28.9 ☑
　　　　　nontraffic V28.2 ☑
　　　　　while boarding or alighting V28.3 ☑
　　　nontraffic V29.3 ☑
　　　passenger
　　　　collision (with)
　　　　　animal (traffic) V20.5 ☑
　　　　　　being ridden (traffic) V26.5 ☑
　　　　　　　nontraffic V26.1 ☑
　　　　　　nontraffic V20.1 ☑
　　　　　animal-drawn vehicle (traffic) V26.5 ☑
　　　　　　nontraffic V26.1 ☑
　　　　　bus (traffic) V24.5 ☑
　　　　　　nontraffic V24.1 ☑
　　　　　car (traffic) V23.5 ☑
　　　　　　nontraffic V23.1 ☑
　　　　　motor vehicle NOS (traffic) V29.50 ☑
　　　　　　nontraffic V29.10 ☑
　　　　　　specified type NEC (traffic) V29.59 ☑
　　　　　　　nontraffic V29.19 ☑
　　　　　pedal cycle (traffic) V21.5 ☑
　　　　　　nontraffic V21.1 ☑
　　　　　pickup truck (traffic) V23.5 ☑
　　　　　　nontraffic V23.1 ☑
　　　　　railway vehicle (traffic) V25.5 ☑
　　　　　　nontraffic V25.1 ☑
　　　　　specified vehicle NEC (traffic) V26.5 ☑
　　　　　　nontraffic V26.1 ☑
　　　　　stationary object (traffic) V27.5 ☑
　　　　　　nontraffic V27.1 ☑
　　　　　streetcar (traffic) V26.5 ☑
　　　　　　nontraffic V26.1 ☑
　　　　　three wheeled motor vehicle (traffic)
　　　　　　V22.5 ☑
　　　　　　nontraffic V22.1 ☑
　　　　　truck (traffic) V24.5 ☑
　　　　　　nontraffic V24.1 ☑
　　　　　two wheeled motor vehicle (traffic)
　　　　　　V22.5 ☑
　　　　　　nontraffic V22.1 ☑
　　　　　van (traffic) V23.5 ☑
　　　　　　nontraffic V23.1 ☑
　　　　noncollision accident (traffic) V28.5 ☑
　　　　　nontraffic V28.1 ☑
　　　specified type NEC V29.88 ☑
　　　military vehicle V29.81 ☑
　　occupant (of)
　　　aircraft (powered) V95.9 ☑
　　　　fixed wing
　　　　　commercial — *see* Accident, transport,
　　　　　　aircraft, occupant, powered, fixed
　　　　　　wing, commercial
　　　　　private — *see* Accident, transport, air-
　　　　　　craft, occupant, powered, fixed
　　　　　　wing, private
　　　　nonpowered V96.9 ☑
　　　　specified NEC V95.8 ☑
　　　airport battery-powered vehicle — *see* Accident,
　　　　　transport, industrial vehicle occupant
　　　all-terrain vehicle (ATV) — *see* Accident, trans-
　　　　　port, all-terrain vehicle occupant
　　　animal-drawn vehicle — *see* Accident, transport,
　　　　　animal-drawn vehicle occupant
　　　automobile — *see* Accident, transport, car occu-
　　　　　pant
　　　balloon V96.00 ☑
　　　battery-powered vehicle — *see* Accident, trans-
　　　　　port, industrial vehicle occupant
　　　bicycle — *see* Accident, transport, pedal cyclist
　　　　motorized — *see* Accident, transport, motor-
　　　　　cycle rider
　　　boat NEC — *see* Accident, watercraft
　　　bulldozer — *see* Accident, transport, construction
　　　　　vehicle occupant
　　　bus — *see* Accident, transport, bus occupant
　　　cable car (on rails) — *see also* Accident, transport,
　　　　　streetcar occupant
　　　　not on rails V98.0 ☑
　　　car — *see also* Accident, transport, car occupant

Accident — *continued*
 transport — *continued*
  occupant — *continued*
   car — *see also* Accident, transport, car occupant — *continued*
    cable (on rails) — *see also* Accident, transport, streetcar occupant
     not on rails V98.0 ☑
    coach — *see* Accident, transport, bus occupant
    coal-car — *see* Accident, transport, industrial vehicle occupant
    digger — *see* Accident, transport, construction vehicle occupant
    dump truck — *see* Accident, transport, construction vehicle occupant
    earth-leveler — *see* Accident, transport, construction vehicle occupant
    farm machinery (self-propelled) — *see* Accident, transport, agricultural vehicle occupant
    forklift — *see* Accident, transport, industrial vehicle occupant
    glider (unpowered) V96.20 ☑
     hang V96.10 ☑
     powered (microlight) (ultralight) — *see* Accident, transport, aircraft, occupant, powered, glider
    glider (unpowered) NEC V96.20 ☑
    hang-glider V96.10 ☑
    harvester — *see* Accident, transport, agricultural vehicle occupant
    heavy (transport) vehicle — *see* Accident, transport, truck occupant
    helicopter — *see* Accident, transport, aircraft, occupant, helicopter
    ice-yacht V98.2 ☑
    kite (carrying person) V96.8 ☑
    land-yacht V98.1 ☑
    logging car — *see* Accident, transport, industrial vehicle occupant
    mechanical shovel — *see* Accident, transport, construction vehicle occupant
    microlight — *see* Accident, transport, aircraft, occupant, powered, glider
    minibus — *see* Accident, transport, pickup truck occupant
    minivan — *see* Accident, transport, pickup truck occupant
    moped — *see* Accident, transport, motorcycle
    motor scooter — *see* Accident, transport, motorcycle
    motorcycle (with sidecar) — *see* Accident, transport, motorcycle
    off-road motor-vehicle — *see also* Accident, transport, all-terrain vehicle occupant V86.99 ☑
    pedal cycle — *see also* Accident, transport, pedal cyclist
    pick-up (truck) — *see* Accident, transport, pickup truck occupant
    railway (train) (vehicle) (subterranean) (elevated) — *see* Accident, transport, railway vehicle occupant
    rickshaw — *see* Accident, transport, pedal cycle
     motorized — *see* Accident, transport, three-wheeled motor vehicle
     pedal driven — *see* Accident, transport, pedal cyclist
    road-roller — *see* Accident, transport, construction vehicle occupant
    ship NOS V94.9 ☑
    ski-lift (chair) (gondola) V98.3 ☑
    snowmobile — *see* Accident, transport, snowmobile occupant
    spacecraft, spaceship — *see* Accident, transport, aircraft, occupant, spacecraft
    sport utility vehicle — *see* Accident, transport, pickup truck occupant
    streetcar (interurban) (operating on public street or highway) — *see* Accident, transport, streetcar occupant
    SUV — *see* Accident, transport, pickup truck occupant
    téléférique V98.0 ☑
    three-wheeled vehicle (motorized) — *see also* Accident, transport, three-wheeled motor vehicle occupant

Accident — *continued*
 transport — *continued*
  occupant — *continued*
   three-wheeled vehicle — *see also* Accident, transport, three-wheeled motor vehicle occupant — *continued*
    nonmotorized — *see* Accident, transport, pedal cycle
   tractor (farm) (and trailer) — *see* Accident, transport, agricultural vehicle occupant
   train — *see* Accident, transport, railway vehicle occupant
   tram — *see* Accident, transport, streetcar occupant
    in mine or quarry — *see* Accident, transport, industrial vehicle occupant
   tricycle — *see* Accident, transport, pedal cycle
    motorized — *see* Accident, transport, three-wheeled motor vehicle
   trolley — *see* Accident, transport, streetcar occupant
    in mine or quarry — *see* Accident, transport, industrial vehicle occupant
   tub, in mine or quarry — *see* Accident, transport, industrial vehicle occupant
   ultralight — *see* Accident, transport, aircraft, occupant, powered, glider
   van — *see* Accident, transport, van occupant
   vehicle NEC V89.9 ☑
    heavy transport — *see* Accident, transport, truck occupant
    motor (traffic) NEC V89.2 ☑
     nontraffic NEC V89.0 ☑
   watercraft NOS V94.9 ☑
    causing drowning — *see* Drowning, resulting from accident to boat
  off-road motor-vehicle — *see also* Accident, transport, all-terrain vehicle occupant V86.99 ☑
  parachutist V97.29 ☑
   after accident to aircraft — *see* Accident, transport, aircraft
   entangled in object V97.21 ☑
   injured on landing V97.22 ☑
  pedal cyclist V19.9 ☑
   collision (with)
    animal (traffic) V10.9 ☑
     being ridden (traffic) V16.9 ☑
      nontraffic V16.2 ☑
      while boarding or alighting V16.3 ☑
     nontraffic V10.2 ☑
     while boarding or alighting V10.3 ☑
    animal-drawn vehicle (traffic) V16.9 ☑
     nontraffic V16.2 ☑
     while boarding or alighting V16.3 ☑
    bus (traffic) V14.9 ☑
     nontraffic V14.2 ☑
     while boarding or alighting V14.3 ☑
    car (traffic) V13.9 ☑
     nontraffic V13.2 ☑
     while boarding or alighting V13.3 ☑
    motor vehicle NOS (traffic) V19.60 ☑
     nontraffic V19.20 ☑
     specified type NEC (traffic) V19.69 ☑
      nontraffic V19.29 ☑
    pedal cycle (traffic) V11.9 ☑
     nontraffic V11.2 ☑
     while boarding or alighting V11.3 ☑
    pickup truck (traffic) V13.9 ☑
     nontraffic V13.2 ☑
     while boarding or alighting V13.3 ☑
    railway vehicle (traffic) V15.9 ☑
     nontraffic V15.2 ☑
     while boarding or alighting V15.3 ☑
    specified vehicle NEC (traffic) V16.9 ☑
     nontraffic V16.2 ☑
     while boarding or alighting V16.3 ☑
    stationary object (traffic) V17.9 ☑
     nontraffic V17.2 ☑
     while boarding or alighting V17.3 ☑
    streetcar (traffic) V16.9 ☑
     nontraffic V16.2 ☑
     while boarding or alighting V16.3 ☑
    three wheeled motor vehicle (traffic) V12.9 ☑
     nontraffic V12.2 ☑
     while boarding or alighting V12.3 ☑
    truck (traffic) V14.9 ☑

Accident — *continued*
 transport — *continued*
  pedal cyclist — *continued*
   collision — *continued*
    truck — *continued*
     nontraffic V14.2 ☑
     while boarding or alighting V14.3 ☑
    two wheeled motor vehicle (traffic) V12.9 ☑
     nontraffic V12.2 ☑
     while boarding or alighting V12.3 ☑
    van (traffic) V13.9 ☑
     nontraffic V13.2 ☑
     while boarding or alighting V13.3 ☑
   driver
    collision (with)
     animal (traffic) V10.4 ☑
      being ridden (traffic) V16.4 ☑
       nontraffic V16.0 ☑
      nontraffic V10.0 ☑
     animal-drawn vehicle (traffic) V16.4 ☑
      nontraffic V16.0 ☑
     bus (traffic) V14.4 ☑
      nontraffic V14.0 ☑
     car (traffic) V13.4 ☑
      nontraffic V13.0 ☑
     motor vehicle NOS (traffic) V19.40 ☑
      nontraffic V19.00 ☑
      specified type NEC (traffic) V19.49 ☑
       nontraffic V19.09 ☑
     pedal cycle (traffic) V11.4 ☑
      nontraffic V11.0 ☑
     pickup truck (traffic) V13.4 ☑
      nontraffic V13.0 ☑
     railway vehicle (traffic) V15.4 ☑
      nontraffic V15.0 ☑
     specified vehicle NEC (traffic) V16.4 ☑
      nontraffic V16.0 ☑
     stationary object (traffic) V17.4 ☑
      nontraffic V17.0 ☑
     streetcar (traffic) V16.4 ☑
      nontraffic V16.0 ☑
     three wheeled motor vehicle (traffic) V12.4 ☑
      nontraffic V12.0 ☑
     truck (traffic) V14.4 ☑
      nontraffic V14.0 ☑
     two wheeled motor vehicle (traffic) V12.4 ☑
      nontraffic V12.0 ☑
     van (traffic) V13.4 ☑
      nontraffic V13.0 ☑
    noncollision accident (traffic) V18.4 ☑
     nontraffic V18.0 ☑
   noncollision accident (traffic) V18.9 ☑
    nontraffic V18.2 ☑
    while boarding or alighting V18.3 ☑
   nontraffic V19.3 ☑
   passenger
    collision (with)
     animal (traffic) V10.5 ☑
      being ridden (traffic) V16.5 ☑
       nontraffic V16.1 ☑
      nontraffic V10.1 ☑
     animal-drawn vehicle (traffic) V16.5 ☑
      nontraffic V16.1 ☑
     bus (traffic) V14.5 ☑
      nontraffic V14.1 ☑
     car (traffic) V13.5 ☑
      nontraffic V13.1 ☑
     motor vehicle NOS (traffic) V19.50 ☑
      nontraffic V19.10 ☑
      specified type NEC (traffic) V19.59 ☑
       nontraffic V19.19 ☑
     pedal cycle (traffic) V11.5 ☑
      nontraffic V11.1 ☑
     pickup truck (traffic) V13.5 ☑
      nontraffic V13.1 ☑
     railway vehicle (traffic) V15.5 ☑
      nontraffic V15.1 ☑
     specified vehicle NEC (traffic) V16.5 ☑
      nontraffic V16.1 ☑
     stationary object (traffic) V17.5 ☑
      nontraffic V17.1 ☑
     streetcar (traffic) V16.5 ☑
      nontraffic V16.1 ☑

☑ Additional Character Required — Refer to the Tabular List for Character Selection   ▽ Subterms under main terms may continue to next column or page

Accident — *continued*
  transport — *continued*
    pedal cyclist — *continued*
      passenger — *continued*
        collision — *continued*
          three wheeled motor vehicle (traffic)
            V12.5 ☑
            nontraffic V12.1 ☑
          truck (traffic) V14.5 ☑
            nontraffic V14.1 ☑
          two wheeled motor vehicle (traffic)
            V12.5 ☑
            nontraffic V12.1 ☑
          van (traffic) V13.5 ☑
            nontraffic V13.1 ☑
        noncollision accident (traffic) V18.5 ☑
          nontraffic V18.1 ☑
      specified type NEC V19.88 ☑
        military vehicle V19.81 ☑
    pedestrian
      conveyance (occupant) V09.9 ☑
        baby stroller V00.828 ☑
          collision (with) V09.9 ☑
            animal being ridden or animal drawn
              vehicle V06.99 ☑
              nontraffic V06.09 ☑
              traffic V06.19 ☑
            bus or heavy transport V04.99 ☑
              nontraffic V04.09 ☑
              traffic V04.19 ☑
            car V03.99 ☑
              nontraffic V03.09 ☑
              traffic V03.19 ☑
            pedal cycle V01.99 ☑
              nontraffic V01.09 ☑
              traffic V01.19 ☑
            pick-up truck or van V03.99 ☑
              nontraffic V03.09 ☑
              traffic V03.19 ☑
            railway (train) (vehicle) V05.99 ☑
              nontraffic V05.09 ☑
              traffic V05.19 ☑
            stationary object V00.822 ☑
            streetcar V06.99 ☑
              nontraffic V06.09 ☑
              traffic V06.19 ☑
            two- or three-wheeled motor vehicle
              V02.99 ☑
              nontraffic V02.09 ☑
              traffic V02.19 ☑
            vehicle V09.9 ☑
              animal-drawn V06.99 ☑
                nontraffic V06.09 ☑
                traffic V06.19 ☑
              motor
                nontraffic V09.00 ☑
                traffic V09.20 ☑
         fall V00.821 ☑
        nontraffic V09.1 ☑
          involving motor vehicle NEC V09.00 ☑
        traffic V09.3 ☑
          involving motor vehicle NEC V09.20 ☑
        flat-bottomed NEC V00.388 ☑
          collision (with) V09.9 ☑
            animal being ridden or animal drawn
              vehicle V06.99 ☑
              nontraffic V06.09 ☑
              traffic V06.19 ☑
            bus or heavy transport V04.99 ☑
              nontraffic V04.09 ☑
              traffic V04.19 ☑
            car V03.99 ☑
              nontraffic V03.09 ☑
              traffic V03.19 ☑
            pedal cycle V01.99 ☑
              nontraffic V01.09 ☑
              traffic V01.19 ☑
            pick-up truck or van V03.99 ☑
              nontraffic V03.09 ☑
              traffic V03.19 ☑
            railway (train) (vehicle) V05.99 ☑
              nontraffic V05.09 ☑
              traffic V05.19 ☑
            stationary object V00.382 ☑
            streetcar V06.99 ☑
              nontraffic V06.09 ☑

Accident — *continued*
  transport — *continued*
    pedestrian — *continued*
      conveyance — *continued*
        flat-bottomed — *continued*
          collision — *continued*
           streetcar — *continued*
              traffic V06.19 ☑
           two- or three-wheeled motor vehicle
              V02.99 ☑
              nontraffic V02.09 ☑
              traffic V02.19 ☑
            vehicle V09.9 ☑
              animal-drawn V06.99 ☑
                nontraffic V06.09 ☑
                traffic V06.19 ☑
              motor
                nontraffic V09.00 ☑
                traffic V09.20 ☑
        fall V00.381 ☑
        nontraffic V09.1 ☑
          involving motor vehicle NEC V09.00 ☑
        snow
          board — *see* Accident, transport,
            pedestrian, conveyance, snow
            board
          ski — *see* Accident, transport, pedes-
            trian, conveyance, skis (snow)
        traffic V09.3 ☑
          involving motor vehicle NEC V09.20 ☑
      gliding type NEC V00.288 ☑
        collision (with) V09.9 ☑
          animal being ridden or animal drawn
            vehicle V06.99 ☑
              nontraffic V06.09 ☑
              traffic V06.19 ☑
           bus or heavy transport V04.99 ☑
              nontraffic V04.09 ☑
              traffic V04.19 ☑
           car V03.99 ☑
              nontraffic V03.09 ☑
              traffic V03.19 ☑
           pedal cycle V01.99 ☑
              nontraffic V01.09 ☑
              traffic V01.19 ☑
           pick-up truck or van V03.99 ☑
              nontraffic V03.09 ☑
              traffic V03.19 ☑
           railway (train) (vehicle) V05.99 ☑
              nontraffic V05.09 ☑
              traffic V05.19 ☑
           stationary object V00.282 ☑
           streetcar V06.99 ☑
              nontraffic V06.09 ☑
              traffic V02.19 ☑
           two- or three-wheeled motor vehicle
              V02.99 ☑
              nontraffic V02.09 ☑
            vehicle V09.9 ☑
              animal-drawn V06.99 ☑
                nontraffic V06.09 ☑
                traffic V06.19 ☑
              motor
                nontraffic V09.00 ☑
                traffic V09.20 ☑
        fall V00.281 ☑
        heelies — *see* Accident, transport,
          pedestrian, conveyance, heelies
        ice skate — *see* Accident, transport,
          pedestrian, conveyance, ice skate
        nontraffic V09.1 ☑
          involving motor vehicle NEC V09.00 ☑
        sled — *see* Accident, transport, pedestri-
          an, conveyance, sled
        traffic V09.3 ☑
          involving motor vehicle NEC V09.20 ☑
        wheelies — *see* Accident, transport,
          pedestrian, conveyance, heelies
      heelies V00.158 ☑
        colliding with stationary object
          V00.152 ☑
        fall V00.151 ☑

Accident — *continued*
  transport — *continued*
    pedestrian — *continued*
      conveyance — *continued*
        hoverboard
          collision with
           animal being ridden or animal drawn
            vehicle V06.938 ☑
              nontraffic V06.038 ☑
              traffic V06.138 ☑
           bus or heavy transport V04.938 ☑
              nontraffic V04.038 ☑
              traffic V04.138 ☑
           car V03.938 ☑
              nontraffic V03.038 ☑
              traffic V03.138 ☑
           pedal cycle V01.938 ☑
              nontraffic V01.038 ☑
              traffic V01.138 ☑
           pick-up or van V03.938 ☑
              nontraffic V03.038 ☑
              traffic V03.138 ☑
           railway (train) (vehicle) V05.938 ☑
              nontraffic V05.038 ☑
              traffic V05.138 ☑
           streetcar V06.938 ☑
              nontraffic V06.038 ☑
              traffic V06.138 ☑
           three-wheeled motor vehicle
              V02.938 ☑
              nontraffic V02.038 ☑
              traffic V02.138 ☑
           two-wheeled motor vehicle
              V02.938 ☑
              nontraffic V02.038 ☑
              traffic V02.138 ☑
           vehicle, nonmotor, specified NEC
              V06.938 ☑
              nontraffic V06.038 ☑
              traffic V06.138 ☑
          fall V00.848 ☑
        ice skates V00.218 ☑
          collision (with) V09.9 ☑
           animal being ridden or animal drawn
            vehicle V06.99 ☑
              nontraffic V06.09 ☑
              traffic V06.19 ☑
           bus or heavy transport V04.99 ☑
              nontraffic V04.09 ☑
              traffic V04.19 ☑
           car V03.99 ☑
              nontraffic V03.09 ☑
              traffic V03.19 ☑
           pedal cycle V01.99 ☑
              nontraffic V01.09 ☑
              traffic V01.19 ☑
           pick-up truck or van V03.99 ☑
              nontraffic V03.09 ☑
              traffic V03.19 ☑
           railway (train) (vehicle) V05.99 ☑
              nontraffic V05.09 ☑
              traffic V05.19 ☑
           stationary object V00.212 ☑
           streetcar V06.99 ☑
              nontraffic V06.09 ☑
              traffic V06.19 ☑
           two- or three-wheeled motor vehicle
              V02.99 ☑
              nontraffic V02.09 ☑
              traffic V02.19 ☑
           vehicle V09.9 ☑
            animal-drawn V06.99 ☑
              nontraffic V06.09 ☑
              traffic V06.19 ☑
            motor
              nontraffic V09.00 ☑
              traffic V09.20 ☑
         fall V00.211 ☑
        nontraffic V09.1 ☑
          involving motor vehicle NEC V09.00 ☑
        traffic V09.3 ☑
          involving motor vehicle NEC V09.20 ☑
      motorized mobility scooter V00.838 ☑
        collision with stationary object
          V00.832 ☑
        fall from V00.831 ☑

Accident — *continued*
  transport — *continued*
    pedestrian — *continued*
      conveyance — *continued*
        nontraffic V09.1 ☑
          involving motor vehicle V09.00 ☑
            military V09.01 ☑
            specified type NEC V09.09 ☑
        roller skates (non in-line) V00.128 ☑
          collision (with) V09.9 ☑
            animal being ridden or animal drawn
              vehicle V06.91 ☑
              nontraffic V06.01 ☑
              traffic V06.11 ☑
            bus or heavy transport V04.91 ☑
              nontraffic V04.01 ☑
              traffic V04.11 ☑
            car V03.91 ☑
              nontraffic V03.01 ☑
              traffic V03.11 ☑
            pedal cycle V01.91 ☑
              nontraffic V01.01 ☑
              traffic V01.11 ☑
            pick-up truck or van V03.91 ☑
              nontraffic V03.01 ☑
              traffic V03.11 ☑
            railway (train) (vehicle) V05.91 ☑
              nontraffic V05.01 ☑
              traffic V05.11 ☑
            stationary object V00.122 ☑
            streetcar V06.91 ☑
              nontraffic V06.01 ☑
              traffic V06.11 ☑
            two- or three-wheeled motor vehicle
              V02.91 ☑
              nontraffic V02.01 ☑
              traffic V02.11 ☑
            vehicle V09.9 ☑
              animal-drawn V06.91 ☑
                nontraffic V06.01 ☑
                traffic V06.11 ☑
              motor
                nontraffic V09.00 ☑
                traffic V09.20 ☑
        fall V00.121 ☑
        in-line V00.118 ☑
          collision — *see also* Accident, transport, pedestrian, conveyance occupant, roller skates, collision with stationary object V00.112 ☑
            fall V00.111 ☑
          nontraffic V09.1 ☑
            involving motor vehicle NEC V09.00 ☑
          traffic V09.3 ☑
            involving motor vehicle NEC V09.20 ☑
        rolling shoes V00.158 ☑
          colliding with stationary object V00.152 ☑
          fall V00.151 ☑
        rolling type NEC V00.188 ☑
          collision (with) V09.9 ☑
            animal being ridden or animal drawn
              vehicle V06.99 ☑
              nontraffic V06.09 ☑
              traffic V06.19 ☑
            bus or heavy transport V04.99 ☑
              nontraffic V04.09 ☑
              traffic V04.19 ☑
            car V03.99 ☑
              nontraffic V03.09 ☑
              traffic V03.19 ☑
            pedal cycle V01.99 ☑
              nontraffic V01.09 ☑
              traffic V01.19 ☑
            pick-up truck or van V03.99 ☑
              nontraffic V03.09 ☑
              traffic V03.19 ☑
            railway (train) (vehicle) V05.99 ☑
              nontraffic V05.09 ☑
              traffic V05.19 ☑
            stationary object V00.182 ☑
            streetcar V06.99 ☑
              nontraffic V06.09 ☑
              traffic V06.19 ☑
            two- or three-wheeled motor vehicle
              V02.99 ☑

Accident — *continued*
  transport — *continued*
    pedestrian — *continued*
      conveyance — *continued*
        rolling type — *continued*
          collision — *continued*
            two- or three-wheeled motor vehicle — *continued*
              nontraffic V02.09 ☑
              traffic V02.19 ☑
            vehicle V09.9 ☑
              animal-drawn V06.99 ☑
                nontraffic V06.09 ☑
                traffic V06.19 ☑
              motor
                nontraffic V09.00 ☑
                traffic V09.20 ☑
        fall V00.181 ☑
        in-line roller skate — *see* Accident, transport, pedestrian, conveyance, roller skate, in-line
        nontraffic V09.1 ☑
          involving motor vehicle NEC V09.00 ☑
        roller skate — *see* Accident, transport, pedestrian, conveyance, roller skate
        scooter (non-motorized) — *see* Accident, transport, pedestrian, conveyance, scooter
        skateboard — *see* Accident, transport, pedestrian, conveyance, skateboard
        traffic V09.3 ☑
          involving motor vehicle NEC V09.20 ☑
      scooter (non-motorized) V00.148 ☑
        collision (with) V09.9 ☑
          animal being ridden or animal drawn
            vehicle V06.99 ☑
            nontraffic V06.09 ☑
            traffic V06.19 ☑
          bus or heavy transport V04.99 ☑
            nontraffic V04.09 ☑
            traffic V04.19 ☑
          car V03.99 ☑
            nontraffic V03.09 ☑
            traffic V03.19 ☑
          pedal cycle V01.99 ☑
            nontraffic V01.09 ☑
            traffic V01.19 ☑
          pick-up truck or van V03.99 ☑
            nontraffic V03.09 ☑
            traffic V03.19 ☑
          railway (train) (vehicle) V05.99 ☑
            nontraffic V05.09 ☑
            traffic V05.19 ☑
          stationary object V00.142 ☑
          streetcar V06.99 ☑
            nontraffic V06.09 ☑
            traffic V06.19 ☑
          two- or three-wheeled motor vehicle
            V02.99 ☑
            nontraffic V02.09 ☑
            traffic V02.19 ☑
          vehicle V09.9 ☑
            animal-drawn V06.99 ☑
              nontraffic V06.09 ☑
              traffic V06.19 ☑
            motor
              nontraffic V09.00 ☑
              traffic V09.20 ☑
        fall V00.141 ☑
        nontraffic V09.1 ☑
          involving motor vehicle NEC V09.00 ☑
        traffic V09.3 ☑
          involving motor vehicle NEC V09.20 ☑
      Segway
        collision with
          animal being ridden or animal drawn
            vehicle V06.938 ☑
            nontraffic V06.038 ☑
            traffic V06.138 ☑
          bus or heavy transport V04.938 ☑
            nontraffic V04.038 ☑
            traffic V04.138 ☑
          car V03.938 ☑
            nontraffic V03.038 ☑

Accident — *continued*
  transport — *continued*
    pedestrian — *continued*
      conveyance — *continued*
        Segway — *continued*
          collision with — *continued*
            car — *continued*
              traffic V03.138 ☑
            pedal cycle V01.938 ☑
              nontraffic V01.038 ☑
              traffic V01.138 ☑
            pick-up or van V03.938 ☑
              nontraffic V03.038 ☑
              traffic V03.138 ☑
            railway (train) (vehicle) V05.938 ☑
              nontraffic V05.038 ☑
              traffic V05.138 ☑
            streetcar V06.938 ☑
              nontraffic V06.038 ☑
              traffic V06.138 ☑
            three-wheeled vehicle V02.938 ☑
              nontraffic V02.038 ☑
              traffic V02.138 ☑
            two-wheeled vehicle V02.938 ☑
              nontraffic V02.038 ☑
              traffic V02.138 ☑
            vehicle, nonmotor, specified NEC
              V06.938 ☑
              nontraffic V06.038 ☑
              traffic V06.138 ☑
          fall V00.848 ☑
        skate board V00.138 ☑
          collision (with) V09.9 ☑
            animal being ridden or animal drawn
              vehicle V06.92 ☑
              nontraffic V06.02 ☑
              traffic V06.12 ☑
            bus or heavy transport V04.92 ☑
              nontraffic V04.02 ☑
              traffic V04.12 ☑
            car V03.92 ☑
              nontraffic V03.02 ☑
              traffic V03.12 ☑
            pedal cycle V01.92 ☑
              nontraffic V01.02 ☑
              traffic V01.12 ☑
            pick-up truck or van V03.92 ☑
              nontraffic V03.02 ☑
              traffic V03.12 ☑
            railway (train) (vehicle) V05.92 ☑
              nontraffic V05.02 ☑
              traffic V05.12 ☑
            stationary object V00.132 ☑
            streetcar V06.92 ☑
              nontraffic V06.02 ☑
              traffic V06.12 ☑
            two- or three-wheeled motor vehicle
              V02.92 ☑
              nontraffic V02.02 ☑
              traffic V02.12 ☑
            vehicle V09.9 ☑
              animal-drawn V06.92 ☑
                nontraffic V06.02 ☑
                traffic V06.12 ☑
              motor
                nontraffic V09.00 ☑
                traffic V09.20 ☑
         fall V00.131 ☑
        nontraffic V09.1 ☑
          involving motor vehicle NEC V09.00 ☑
        traffic V09.3 ☑
          involving motor vehicle NEC V09.20 ☑
        skis (snow) V00.328 ☑
          collision (with) V09.9 ☑
            animal being ridden or animal drawn
              vehicle V06.99 ☑
              nontraffic V06.09 ☑
              traffic V06.19 ☑
            bus or heavy transport V04.99 ☑
              nontraffic V04.09 ☑
              traffic V04.19 ☑
            car V03.99 ☑
              nontraffic V03.09 ☑
              traffic V03.19 ☑
            pedal cycle V01.99 ☑
              nontraffic V01.09 ☑

     ☑ **Additional Character Required** — **Refer to the Tabular List for Character Selection**   ▽ **Subterms under main terms may continue to next column or page**

Accident — *continued*
  transport — *continued*
    pedestrian — *continued*
      conveyance — *continued*
        skis — *continued*
          collision — *continued*
            pedal cycle — *continued*
              traffic V01.19 ☑
            pick-up truck or van V03.99 ☑
              nontraffic V03.09 ☑
              traffic V03.19 ☑
            railway (train) (vehicle) V05.99 ☑
              nontraffic V05.09 ☑
              traffic V05.19 ☑
            stationary object V00.322 ☑
            streetcar V06.99 ☑
              nontraffic V06.09 ☑
              traffic V06.19 ☑
            two- or three-wheeled motor vehicle V02.99 ☑
              nontraffic V02.09 ☑
              traffic V02.19 ☑
            vehicle V09.9
              animal-drawn V06.99 ☑
                nontraffic V06.09 ☑
                traffic V06.19 ☑
              motor
                nontraffic V09.00 ☑
                traffic V09.20 ☑
           fall V00.321 ☑
          nontraffic V09.1 ☑
            involving motor vehicle NEC V09.00 ☑
          traffic V09.3 ☑
            involving motor vehicle NEC V09.20 ☑
        sled V00.228 ☑
          collision (with) V09.9
            animal being ridden or animal drawn vehicle V06.99 ☑
              nontraffic V06.09 ☑
              traffic V06.19 ☑
            bus or heavy transport V04.99 ☑
              nontraffic V04.09 ☑
              traffic V04.19 ☑
            car V03.99 ☑
              nontraffic V03.09 ☑
              traffic V03.19 ☑
            pedal cycle V01.99 ☑
              nontraffic V01.09 ☑
              traffic V01.19 ☑
            pick-up truck or van V03.99 ☑
              nontraffic V03.09 ☑
              traffic V03.19 ☑
            railway (train) (vehicle) V05.99 ☑
              nontraffic V05.09 ☑
              traffic V05.19 ☑
            stationary object V00.222 ☑
            streetcar V06.99 ☑
              nontraffic V06.09 ☑
              traffic V06.19 ☑
            two- or three-wheeled motor vehicle V02.99 ☑
              nontraffic V02.09 ☑
              traffic V02.19 ☑
            vehicle V09.9 ☑
              animal-drawn V06.99 ☑
                nontraffic V06.09 ☑
                traffic V06.19 ☑
              motor
                nontraffic V09.00 ☑
                traffic V09.20 ☑
           fall V00.221 ☑
          nontraffic V09.1 ☑
            involving motor vehicle NEC V09.00 ☑
          traffic V09.3 ☑
            involving motor vehicle NEC V09.20 ☑
        snow board V00.318 ☑
          collision (with) V09.9 ☑
            animal being ridden or animal drawn vehicle V06.99 ☑
              nontraffic V06.09 ☑
              traffic V06.19 ☑
            bus or heavy transport V04.99 ☑
              nontraffic V04.09 ☑
              traffic V04.19 ☑
            car V03.99 ☑
              nontraffic V03.09 ☑

Accident — *continued*
  transport — *continued*
    pedestrian — *continued*
      conveyance — *continued*
        snow board — *continued*
          collision — *continued*
            car — *continued*
              traffic V03.19 ☑
            pedal cycle V01.99 ☑
              nontraffic V01.09 ☑
              traffic V01.19 ☑
            pick-up truck or van V03.99 ☑
              nontraffic V03.09 ☑
              traffic V03.19 ☑
            railway (train) (vehicle) V05.99 ☑
              nontraffic V05.09 ☑
              traffic V05.19 ☑
            stationary object V00.312 ☑
            streetcar V06.99 ☑
              nontraffic V06.09 ☑
              traffic V06.19 ☑
            two- or three-wheeled motor vehicle V02.99 ☑
              nontraffic V02.09 ☑
              traffic V02.19 ☑
            vehicle V09.9
              animal-drawn V06.99 ☑
                nontraffic V06.09 ☑
                traffic V06.19 ☑
              motor
                nontraffic V09.00 ☑
                traffic V09.20 ☑
           fall V00.311 ☑
          nontraffic V09.1 ☑
            involving motor vehicle NEC V09.00 ☑
          traffic V09.3 ☑
            involving motor vehicle NEC V09.20 ☑
        specified type NEC V00.898 ☑
          collision (with) V09.9 ☑
            animal being ridden or animal drawn vehicle V06.99 ☑
              nontraffic V06.09 ☑
              traffic V06.19 ☑
            bus or heavy transport V04.99 ☑
              nontraffic V04.09 ☑
              traffic V04.19 ☑
            car V03.99 ☑
              nontraffic V03.09 ☑
              traffic V03.19 ☑
            pedal cycle V01.99 ☑
              nontraffic V01.09 ☑
              traffic V01.19 ☑
            pick-up truck or van V03.99 ☑
              nontraffic V03.09 ☑
              traffic V03.19 ☑
            railway (train) (vehicle) V05.99 ☑
              nontraffic V05.09 ☑
              traffic V05.19 ☑
            stationary object V00.892 ☑
            streetcar V06.99 ☑
              nontraffic V06.09 ☑
              traffic V06.19 ☑
            two- or three-wheeled motor vehicle V02.99 ☑
              nontraffic V02.09 ☑
              traffic V02.19 ☑
            vehicle V09.9 ☑
              animal-drawn V06.99 ☑
                nontraffic V06.09 ☑
                traffic V06.19 ☑
              motor
                nontraffic V09.00 ☑
                traffic V09.20 ☑
           fall V00.891 ☑
          nontraffic V09.1 ☑
            involving motor vehicle NEC V09.00 ☑
          traffic V09.3 ☑
            involving motor vehicle NEC V09.20 ☑
      standing
        electric scooter
          collsion with
            animal being ridden or animal drawn vehicle V06.931 ☑
              nontraffic V06.031 ☑
              traffic V06.131 ☑
            bus or heavy transport V04.931 ☑

Accident — *continued*
  transport — *continued*
    pedestrian — *continued*
      conveyance — *continued*
        standing — *continued*
          electric scooter — *continued*
            collsion with — *continued*
              bus or heavy transport — *continued*
                nontraffic V04.031 ☑
                traffic V04.131 ☑
              car V03.931 ☑
                nontraffic V04.031 ☑
                traffic V04.131 ☑
              pedal cycle V01.931 ☑
                nontraffic V01.031 ☑
                traffic V01.131 ☑
              pick-up or van V03.931 ☑
                nontraffic V03.031 ☑
                traffic V03.131 ☑
              railway (train) (vehicle) V05.931 ☑
                nontraffic V05.031 ☑
                traffic V05.131 ☑
              streetcar V06.931 ☑
                nontraffic V06.031 ☑
                traffic V06.131 ☑
              three-wheeled motor vehicle V02.931 ☑
                nontraffic V02.031 ☑
                traffic V02.131 ☑
              two-wheeled motor vehicle V02.931 ☑
                nontraffic V02.031 ☑
                traffic V02.131 ☑
              vehicle, nonmotor, specified NEC V06.931 ☑
                nontraffic V06.031 ☑
                traffic V06.131 ☑
           fall V00.841 ☑
          micro-mobility pedestrian conveyance collision with
            animal being ridden or animal drawn vehicle V06.938 ☑
              nontraffic V06.038 ☑
              traffic V06.138 ☑
            bus or heavy transport V04.938 ☑
              nontraffic V04.038 ☑
              traffic V04.138 ☑
            car V03.938 ☑
              nontraffic V03.038 ☑
              traffic V03.138 ☑
            pedal cycle V01.938 ☑
              nontraffic V01.038 ☑
              traffic V01.138 ☑
            pick-up or van V03.938 ☑
              nontraffic V03.038 ☑
              traffic V03.138 ☑
            railway (train) (vehicle) V05.938 ☑
              nontraffic V05.038 ☑
              traffic V05.138 ☑
            stationary object V00.842 ☑
            streetcar V06.938 ☑
              nontraffic V06.038 ☑
              traffic V06.138 ☑
            three-wheeled motor vehicle V02.938 ☑
              nontraffic V02.038 ☑
              traffic V02.138 ☑
            two-wheeled motor vehicle V02.938 ☑
              nontraffic V02.038 ☑
              traffic V02.138 ☑
            vehicle, nonmotor, specified NEC V06.938 ☑
              nontraffic V06.038 ☑
              traffic V06.138 ☑
          fall V00.848 ☑
        traffic V09.3 ☑
          involving motor vehicle V09.20 ☑
            military V09.21 ☑
            specified type NEC V09.29 ☑
        wheelchair (powered) V00.818 ☑
          collision (with) V09.9
            animal being ridden or animal drawn vehicle V06.99 ☑
              nontraffic V06.09 ☑

Accident — *continued*
  transport — *continued*
    pedestrian — *continued*
      conveyance — *continued*
        wheelchair — *continued*
          collision — *continued*
            animal being ridden or animal drawn
              vehicle — *continued*
              traffic V06.19 ☑
            bus or heavy transport V04.99 ☑
              nontraffic V04.09 ☑
              traffic V04.19 ☑
            car V03.99 ☑
              nontraffic V03.09 ☑
              traffic V03.19 ☑
            pedal cycle V01.99 ☑
              nontraffic V01.09 ☑
              traffic V01.19 ☑
            pick-up truck or van V03.99 ☑
              nontraffic V03.09 ☑
              traffic V03.19 ☑
            railway (train) (vehicle) V05.99 ☑
              nontraffic V05.09 ☑
              traffic V05.19 ☑
            stationary object V00.812 ☑
            streetcar V06.99 ☑
              nontraffic V06.09 ☑
              traffic V06.19 ☑
            two- or three-wheeled motor vehicle
              V02.99 ☑
              nontraffic V02.09 ☑
              traffic V02.19 ☑
            vehicle V09.9 ☑
              animal-drawn V06.99 ☑
                nontraffic V06.09 ☑
                traffic V06.19 ☑
              motor
                nontraffic V09.00 ☑
                traffic V09.20 ☑
           fall V00.811 ☑
          nontraffic V09.1 ☑
            involving motor vehicle NEC V09.00 ☑
          traffic V09.3 ☑
            involving motor vehicle NEC V09.20 ☑
         wheeled shoe V00.158 ☑
          colliding with stationary object
            V00.152 ☑
          fall V00.151 ☑
      on foot — *see also* Accident, pedestrian
        collision (with)
          animal being ridden or animal drawn ve-
            hicle V06.90 ☑
            nontraffic V06.00 ☑
            traffic V06.10 ☑
          bus or heavy transport V04.90 ☑
            nontraffic V04.00 ☑
            traffic V04.10 ☑
          car V03.90 ☑
            nontraffic V03.00 ☑
            traffic V03.10 ☑
          pedal cycle V01.90 ☑
            nontraffic V01.00 ☑
            traffic V01.10 ☑
          pick-up truck or van V03.90 ☑
            nontraffic V03.00 ☑
            traffic V03.10 ☑
          railway (train) (vehicle) V05.90 ☑
            nontraffic V05.00 ☑
            traffic V05.10 ☑
          streetcar V06.90 ☑
            nontraffic V06.00 ☑
            traffic V06.10 ☑
          two- or three-wheeled motor vehicle
            V02.90 ☑
            nontraffic V02.00 ☑
            traffic V02.10 ☑
          vehicle V09.9 ☑
            animal-drawn V06.90 ☑
              nontraffic V06.00 ☑
              traffic V06.10 ☑
            motor
        nontraffic V09.1 ☑
          involving motor vehicle V09.00 ☑
            military V09.01 ☑
            specified type NEC V09.09 ☑
        traffic V09.3 ☑

Accident — *continued*
  transport — *continued*
    pedestrian — *continued*
      on foot — *see also* Accident, pedestrian — con-
        tinued
        traffic — *continued*
          involving motor vehicle V09.20 ☑
            military V09.21 ☑
            specified type NEC V09.29 ☑
      person NEC (unknown way or transportation) V99 ☑
      collision (between)
        bus (with)
          heavy transport vehicle (traffic) V87.5 ☑
            nontraffic V88.5 ☑
        car (with)
          bus (traffic) V87.3 ☑
            nontraffic V88.3 ☑
          heavy transport vehicle (traffic) V87.4 ☑
            nontraffic V88.4 ☑
          nontraffic V88.5 ☑
          pick-up truck or van (traffic) V87.2 ☑
            nontraffic V88.2 ☑
          train or railway vehicle (traffic) V87.6 ☑
            nontraffic V88.6 ☑
          two-or three-wheeled motor vehicle
            (traffic) V87.0 ☑
            nontraffic V88.0 ☑
        motor vehicle (traffic) NEC V87.7 ☑
          nontraffic V88.7 ☑
        two-or three-wheeled vehicle (with) (traffic)
          motor vehicle NEC V87.1 ☑
            nontraffic V88.1 ☑
        nonmotor vehicle (collision) (noncollision) (traf-
         fic) V87.9 ☑
          nontraffic V88.9 ☑
    pickup truck occupant V59.9 ☑
      collision (with)
        animal (traffic) V50.9 ☑
          being ridden (traffic) V56.9 ☑
            nontraffic V56.3 ☑
            while boarding or alighting V56.4 ☑
          nontraffic V50.3 ☑
          while boarding or alighting V50.4 ☑
        animal-drawn vehicle (traffic) V56.9 ☑
          nontraffic V56.3 ☑
          while boarding or alighting V56.4 ☑
        bus (traffic) V54.9 ☑
          nontraffic V54.3 ☑
          while boarding or alighting V54.4 ☑
        car (traffic) V53.9 ☑
          nontraffic V53.3 ☑
          while boarding or alighting V53.4 ☑
        motor vehicle NOS (traffic) V59.60 ☑
          nontraffic V59.20 ☑
          specified type NEC (traffic) V59.69 ☑
            nontraffic V59.29 ☑
        pedal cycle (traffic) V51.9 ☑
          nontraffic V51.3 ☑
          while boarding or alighting V51.4 ☑
        pickup truck (traffic) V53.9 ☑
          nontraffic V53.3 ☑
          while boarding or alighting V53.4 ☑
        railway vehicle (traffic) V55.9 ☑
          nontraffic V55.3 ☑
          while boarding or alighting V55.4 ☑
        specified vehicle NEC (traffic) V56.9 ☑
          nontraffic V56.3 ☑
          while boarding or alighting V56.4 ☑
        stationary object (traffic) V57.9 ☑
          nontraffic V57.3 ☑
          while boarding or alighting V57.4 ☑
        streetcar (traffic) V56.9 ☑
          nontraffic V56.3 ☑
          while boarding or alighting V56.4 ☑
        three wheeled motor vehicle (traffic) V52.9 ☑
          nontraffic V52.3 ☑
          while boarding or alighting V52.4 ☑
        truck (traffic) V54.9 ☑
          nontraffic V54.3 ☑
          while boarding or alighting V54.4 ☑
        two wheeled motor vehicle (traffic) V52.9 ☑
          nontraffic V52.3 ☑
          while boarding or alighting V52.4 ☑
        van (traffic) V53.9 ☑
          nontraffic V53.3 ☑
          while boarding or alighting V53.4 ☑

Accident — *continued*
  transport — *continued*
    pickup truck occupant — *continued*
      driver
        collision (with)
          animal (traffic) V50.5 ☑
            being ridden (traffic) V56.5 ☑
              nontraffic V56.0 ☑
            nontraffic V50.0 ☑
          animal-drawn vehicle (traffic) V56.5 ☑
            nontraffic V56.0 ☑
          bus (traffic) V54.5 ☑
            nontraffic V54.0 ☑
          car (traffic) V53.5 ☑
            nontraffic V53.0 ☑
          motor vehicle NOS (traffic) V59.40 ☑
            nontraffic V59.00 ☑
            specified type NEC (traffic) V59.49 ☑
              nontraffic V59.09 ☑
          pedal cycle (traffic) V51.5 ☑
            nontraffic V51.0 ☑
          pickup truck (traffic) V53.5 ☑
            nontraffic V53.0 ☑
          railway vehicle (traffic) V55.5 ☑
            nontraffic V55.0 ☑
          specified vehicle NEC (traffic) V56.5 ☑
            nontraffic V56.0 ☑
          stationary object (traffic) V57.5 ☑
            nontraffic V57.0 ☑
          streetcar (traffic) V56.5 ☑
            nontraffic V56.0 ☑
          three wheeled motor vehicle (traffic)
            V52.5 ☑
            nontraffic V52.0 ☑
          truck (traffic) V54.5 ☑
            nontraffic V54.0 ☑
          two wheeled motor vehicle (traffic)
            V52.5 ☑
            nontraffic V52.0 ☑
          van (traffic) V53.5 ☑
            nontraffic V53.0 ☑
        noncollision accident (traffic) V58.5 ☑
          nontraffic V58.0 ☑
      hanger-on
        collision (with)
          animal (traffic) V50.7 ☑
            being ridden (traffic) V56.7 ☑
              nontraffic V56.2 ☑
            nontraffic V50.2 ☑
          animal-drawn vehicle (traffic) V56.7 ☑
            nontraffic V56.2 ☑
          bus (traffic) V54.7 ☑
            nontraffic V54.2 ☑
          car (traffic) V53.7 ☑
            nontraffic V53.2 ☑
          pedal cycle (traffic) V51.7 ☑
            nontraffic V51.2 ☑
          pickup truck (traffic) V53.7 ☑
            nontraffic V53.2 ☑
          railway vehicle (traffic) V55.7 ☑
            nontraffic V55.2 ☑
          specified vehicle NEC (traffic) V56.7 ☑
            nontraffic V56.2 ☑
          stationary object (traffic) V57.7 ☑
            nontraffic V57.2 ☑
          streetcar (traffic) V56.7 ☑
            nontraffic V56.2 ☑
          three wheeled motor vehicle (traffic)
            V52.7 ☑
            nontraffic V52.2 ☑
          truck (traffic) V54.7 ☑
            nontraffic V54.2 ☑
          two wheeled motor vehicle (traffic)
            V52.7 ☑
            nontraffic V52.2 ☑
          van (traffic) V53.7 ☑
            nontraffic V53.2 ☑
        noncollision accident (traffic) V58.7 ☑
          nontraffic V58.2 ☑
      noncollision accident (traffic) V58.9 ☑
        nontraffic V58.3 ☑
        while boarding or alighting V58.4 ☑
      nontraffic V59.3 ☑
      passenger
        collision (with)
          animal (traffic) V50.6 ☑

☑ **Additional Character Required** — Refer to the Tabular List for Character Selection
🔻 **Subterms under main terms may continue to next column or page**

Accident — *continued*
  transport — *continued*
    pickup truck occupant — *continued*
      passenger — *continued*
        collision — *continued*
          animal — *continued*
            being ridden (traffic) V56.6 ☑
              nontraffic V56.1 ☑
              nontraffic V50.1 ☑
            animal-drawn vehicle (traffic) V56.6 ☑
              nontraffic V56.1 ☑
            bus (traffic) V54.6 ☑
              nontraffic V54.1 ☑
            car (traffic) V53.6 ☑
              nontraffic V53.1 ☑
            motor vehicle NOS (traffic) V59.50 ☑
              nontraffic V59.10 ☑
              specified type NEC (traffic) V59.59 ☑
                nontraffic V59.19 ☑
            pedal cycle (traffic) V51.6 ☑
              nontraffic V51.1 ☑
            pickup truck (traffic) V53.6 ☑
              nontraffic V53.1 ☑
            railway vehicle (traffic) V55.6 ☑
              nontraffic V55.1 ☑
            specified vehicle NEC (traffic) V56.6 ☑
              nontraffic V56.1 ☑
            stationary object (traffic) V57.6 ☑
              nontraffic V57.1 ☑
            streetcar (traffic) V56.6 ☑
              nontraffic V56.1 ☑
            three wheeled motor vehicle (traffic) V52.6 ☑
              nontraffic V52.1 ☑
            truck (traffic) V54.6 ☑
              nontraffic V54.1 ☑
            two wheeled motor vehicle (traffic) V52.6 ☑
              nontraffic V52.1 ☑
            van (traffic) V53.6 ☑
              nontraffic V53.1 ☑
        noncollision accident (traffic) V58.6 ☑
          nontraffic V58.1 ☑
      specified type NEC V59.88 ☑
      military vehicle V59.81 ☑
    quarry truck — *see* Accident, transport, industrial vehicle occupant
    race car — *see* Accident, transport, motor vehicle NEC occupant
    railway vehicle occupant V81.9 ☑
      collision (with) V81.3 ☑
        motor vehicle (non-military) (traffic) V81.1 ☑
          military V81.83 ☑
          nontraffic V81.0 ☑
        rolling stock V81.2 ☑
        specified object NEC V81.3 ☑
      during derailment V81.7 ☑
        with antecedent collision — *see* Accident, transport, railway vehicle occupant, collision
      explosion V81.81 ☑
      fall (in railway vehicle) V81.5 ☑
        during derailment V81.7 ☑
          with antecedent collision — *see* Accident, transport, railway vehicle occupant, collision
        from railway vehicle V81.6 ☑
          during derailment V81.7 ☑
            with antecedent collision — *see* Accident, transport, railway vehicle occupant, collision
        while boarding or alighting V81.4 ☑
      fire V81.81 ☑
      object falling onto train V81.82 ☑
      specified type NEC V81.89 ☑
      while boarding or alighting V81.4 ☑
    Segway V00.848 ☑
    ski lift V98.3 ☑
    snowmobile occupant (nontraffic) V86.92 ☑
      driver V86.52 ☑
      hanger-on V86.72 ☑
      passenger V86.62 ☑
      traffic V86.32 ☑
        driver V86.02 ☑
        hanger-on V86.22 ☑
        passenger V86.12 ☑

Accident — *continued*
  transport — *continued*
    snowmobile occupant — *continued*
      while boarding or alighting V86.42 ☑
    specified NEC V98.8 ☑
    sport utility vehicle occupant — *see also* Accident, transport, pickup truck occupant
    streetcar occupant V82.9 ☑
      collision (with) V82.3 ☑
        motor vehicle (traffic) V82.1 ☑
          nontraffic V82.0 ☑
        rolling stock V82.2 ☑
      during derailment V82.7 ☑
        with antecedent collision — *see* Accident, transport, streetcar occupant, collision
      fall (in streetcar) V82.5 ☑
        during derailment V82.7 ☑
          with antecedent collision — *see* Accident, transport, streetcar occupant, collision
        from streetcar V82.6 ☑
          during derailment V82.7 ☑
            with antecedent collision — *see* Accident, transport, streetcar occupant, collision
          while boarding or alighting V82.4 ☑
        while boarding or alighting V82.4 ☑
      specified type NEC V82.8 ☑
      while boarding or alighting V82.4 ☑
    three-wheeled motor vehicle occupant V39.9 ☑
      collision (with)
        animal (traffic) V30.9 ☑
          being ridden (traffic) V36.9 ☑
            nontraffic V36.3 ☑
            while boarding or alighting V36.4 ☑
          nontraffic V30.3 ☑
          while boarding or alighting V30.4 ☑
        animal-drawn vehicle (traffic) V36.9 ☑
          nontraffic V36.3 ☑
          while boarding or alighting V36.4 ☑
        bus (traffic) V34.9 ☑
          nontraffic V34.3 ☑
          while boarding or alighting V34.4 ☑
        car (traffic) V33.9 ☑
          nontraffic V33.3 ☑
          while boarding or alighting V33.4 ☑
        motor vehicle NOS (traffic) V39.60 ☑
          nontraffic V39.20 ☑
          specified type NEC (traffic) V39.69 ☑
            nontraffic V39.29 ☑
        pedal cycle (traffic) V31.9 ☑
          nontraffic V31.3 ☑
          while boarding or alighting V31.4 ☑
        pickup truck (traffic) V33.9 ☑
          nontraffic V33.3 ☑
          while boarding or alighting V33.4 ☑
        railway vehicle (traffic) V35.9 ☑
          nontraffic V35.3 ☑
          while boarding or alighting V35.4 ☑
        specified vehicle NEC (traffic) V36.9 ☑
          nontraffic V36.3 ☑
          while boarding or alighting V36.4 ☑
        stationary object (traffic) V37.9 ☑
          nontraffic V37.3 ☑
          while boarding or alighting V37.4 ☑
        streetcar (traffic) V36.9 ☑
          nontraffic V36.3 ☑
          while boarding or alighting V36.4 ☑
        three wheeled motor vehicle (traffic) V32.9 ☑
          nontraffic V32.3 ☑
          while boarding or alighting V32.4 ☑
        truck (traffic) V34.9 ☑
          nontraffic V34.3 ☑
          while boarding or alighting V34.4 ☑
        two wheeled motor vehicle (traffic) V32.9 ☑
          nontraffic V32.3 ☑
          while boarding or alighting V32.4 ☑
        van (traffic) V33.9 ☑
          nontraffic V33.3 ☑
          while boarding or alighting V33.4 ☑
      driver
        collision (with)
          animal (traffic) V30.5 ☑
            being ridden (traffic) V36.5 ☑
              nontraffic V36.0 ☑
            nontraffic V30.0 ☑

Accident — *continued*
  transport — *continued*
    three-wheeled motor vehicle occupant — *continued*
      driver — *continued*
        collision — *continued*
          animal-drawn vehicle (traffic) V36.5 ☑
            nontraffic V36.0 ☑
          bus (traffic) V34.5 ☑
            nontraffic V34.0 ☑
          car (traffic) V33.5 ☑
            nontraffic V33.0 ☑
          motor vehicle NOS (traffic) V39.40 ☑
            nontraffic V39.00 ☑
            specified type NEC (traffic) V39.49 ☑
              nontraffic V39.09 ☑
          pedal cycle (traffic) V31.5 ☑
            nontraffic V31.0 ☑
          pickup truck (traffic) V33.5 ☑
            nontraffic V33.0 ☑
          railway vehicle (traffic) V35.5 ☑
            nontraffic V35.0 ☑
          specified vehicle NEC (traffic) V36.5 ☑
            nontraffic V36.0 ☑
          stationary object (traffic) V37.5 ☑
            nontraffic V37.0 ☑
          streetcar (traffic) V36.5 ☑
            nontraffic V36.0 ☑
          three wheeled motor vehicle (traffic) V32.5 ☑
            nontraffic V32.0 ☑
          truck (traffic) V34.5 ☑
            nontraffic V34.0 ☑
          two wheeled motor vehicle (traffic) V32.5 ☑
            nontraffic V32.0 ☑
          van (traffic) V33.5 ☑
            nontraffic V33.0 ☑
        noncollision accident (traffic) V38.5 ☑
          nontraffic V38.0 ☑
      hanger-on
        collision (with)
          animal (traffic) V30.7 ☑
            being ridden (traffic) V36.7 ☑
              nontraffic V36.2 ☑
            nontraffic V30.2 ☑
          animal-drawn vehicle (traffic) V36.7 ☑
            nontraffic V36.2 ☑
          bus (traffic) V34.7 ☑
            nontraffic V34.2 ☑
          car (traffic) V33.7 ☑
            nontraffic V33.2 ☑
          pedal cycle (traffic) V31.7 ☑
            nontraffic V31.2 ☑
          pickup truck (traffic) V33.7 ☑
            nontraffic V33.2 ☑
          railway vehicle (traffic) V35.7 ☑
            nontraffic V35.2 ☑
          specified vehicle NEC (traffic) V36.7 ☑
            nontraffic V36.2 ☑
          stationary object (traffic) V37.7 ☑
            nontraffic V37.2 ☑
          streetcar (traffic) V36.7 ☑
            nontraffic V36.2 ☑
          three wheeled motor vehicle (traffic) V32.7 ☑
            nontraffic V32.2 ☑
          truck (traffic) V34.7 ☑
            nontraffic V34.2 ☑
          two wheeled motor vehicle (traffic) V32.7 ☑
            nontraffic V32.2 ☑
          van (traffic) V33.7 ☑
            nontraffic V33.2 ☑
        noncollision accident (traffic) V38.7 ☑
          nontraffic V38.2 ☑
      noncollision accident (traffic) V38.9 ☑
        nontraffic V38.3 ☑
        while boarding or alighting V38.4 ☑
      nontraffic V39.3 ☑
      passenger
        collision (with)
          animal (traffic) V30.6 ☑
            being ridden (traffic) V36.6 ☑
              nontraffic V36.1 ☑
            nontraffic V30.1 ☑

Accident — *continued*
transport — *continued*
three-wheeled motor vehicle occupant — *continued*
passenger — *continued*
collision — *continued*
animal-drawn vehicle (traffic) V36.6 ☑
nontraffic V36.1 ☑
bus (traffic) V34.6 ☑
nontraffic V34.1 ☑
car (traffic) V33.6 ☑
nontraffic V33.1 ☑
motor vehicle NOS (traffic) V39.50 ☑
nontraffic V39.10 ☑
specified type NEC (traffic) V39.59 ☑
nontraffic V39.19 ☑
pedal cycle (traffic) V31.6 ☑
nontraffic V31.1 ☑
pickup truck (traffic) V33.6 ☑
nontraffic V33.1 ☑
railway vehicle (traffic) V35.6 ☑
nontraffic V35.1 ☑
specified vehicle NEC (traffic) V36.6 ☑
nontraffic V36.1 ☑
stationary object (traffic) V37.6 ☑
nontraffic V37.1 ☑
streetcar (traffic) V36.6 ☑
nontraffic V36.1 ☑
three wheeled motor vehicle (traffic) V32.6 ☑
nontraffic V32.1 ☑
truck (traffic) V34.6 ☑
nontraffic V34.1 ☑
two wheeled motor vehicle (traffic) V32.6 ☑
nontraffic V32.1 ☑
van (traffic) V33.6 ☑
nontraffic V33.1 ☑
noncollision accident (traffic) V38.6 ☑
nontraffic V38.1 ☑
specified type NEC V39.89 ☑
military vehicle V39.81 ☑
tractor (farm) (and trailer) — *see* Accident, transport, agricultural vehicle occupant
tram — *see* Accident, transport, streetcar
in mine or quarry — *see* Accident, transport, industrial vehicle occupant
trolley — *see* Accident, transport, streetcar
in mine or quarry — *see* Accident, transport, industrial vehicle occupant
truck (heavy) occupant V69.9 ☑
collision (with)
animal (traffic) V60.9 ☑
being ridden (traffic) V66.9 ☑
nontraffic V66.3 ☑
while boarding or alighting V66.4 ☑
nontraffic V60.3 ☑
while boarding or alighting V60.4 ☑
animal-drawn vehicle (traffic) V66.9 ☑
nontraffic V66.3 ☑
while boarding or alighting V66.4 ☑
bus (traffic) V64.9 ☑
nontraffic V64.3 ☑
while boarding or alighting V64.4 ☑
car (traffic) V63.9 ☑
nontraffic V63.3 ☑
while boarding or alighting V63.4 ☑
motor vehicle NOS (traffic) V69.60 ☑
nontraffic V69.20 ☑
specified type NEC (traffic) V69.69 ☑
nontraffic V69.29 ☑
pedal cycle (traffic) V61.9 ☑
nontraffic V61.3 ☑
while boarding or alighting V61.4 ☑
pickup truck (traffic) V63.9 ☑
nontraffic V63:3 ☑
while boarding or alighting V63.4 ☑
railway vehicle (traffic) V65.9 ☑
nontraffic V65.3 ☑
while boarding or alighting V65.4 ☑
specified vehicle NEC (traffic) V66.9 ☑
nontraffic V66.3 ☑
while boarding or alighting V66.4 ☑
stationary object (traffic) V67.9 ☑
nontraffic V67.3 ☑
while boarding or alighting V67.4 ☑

Accident — *continued*
transport — *continued*
truck occupant — *continued*
collision — *continued*
streetcar (traffic) V66.9 ☑
nontraffic V66.3 ☑
while boarding or alighting V66.4 ☑
three wheeled motor vehicle (traffic) V62.9 ☑
nontraffic V62.3 ☑
while boarding or alighting V62.4 ☑
truck (traffic) V64.9 ☑
nontraffic V64.3 ☑
while boarding or alighting V64.4 ☑
two wheeled motor vehicle (traffic) V62.9 ☑
nontraffic V62.3 ☑
while boarding or alighting V62.4 ☑
van (traffic) V63.9 ☑
nontraffic V63.3 ☑
while boarding or alighting V63.4 ☑
driver
collision (with)
animal (traffic) V60.5 ☑
being ridden (traffic) V66.5 ☑
nontraffic V66.0 ☑
nontraffic V60.0 ☑
animal-drawn vehicle (traffic) V66.5 ☑
nontraffic V66.0 ☑
bus (traffic) V64.5 ☑
nontraffic V64.0 ☑
car (traffic) V63.5 ☑
nontraffic V63.0 ☑
motor vehicle NOS (traffic) V69.40 ☑
nontraffic V69.00 ☑
specified type NEC (traffic) V69.49 ☑
nontraffic V69.09 ☑
pedal cycle (traffic) V61.5 ☑
nontraffic V61.0 ☑
pickup truck (traffic) V63.5 ☑
nontraffic V63.0 ☑
railway vehicle (traffic) V65.5 ☑
nontraffic V65.0 ☑
specified vehicle NEC (traffic) V66.5 ☑
nontraffic V66.0 ☑
stationary object (traffic) V67.5 ☑
nontraffic V67.0 ☑
streetcar (traffic) V66.5 ☑
nontraffic V66.0 ☑
three wheeled motor vehicle (traffic) V62.5 ☑
nontraffic V62.0 ☑
truck (traffic) V64.5 ☑
nontraffic V64.0 ☑
two wheeled motor vehicle (traffic) V62.5 ☑
nontraffic V62.0 ☑
van (traffic) V63.5 ☑
nontraffic V63.0 ☑
noncollision accident (traffic) V68.5 ☑
nontraffic V68.0 ☑
dump — *see* Accident, transport, construction vehicle occupant
hanger-on
collision (with)
animal (traffic) V60.7 ☑
being ridden (traffic) V66.7 ☑
nontraffic V66.2 ☑
nontraffic V60.2 ☑
animal-drawn vehicle (traffic) V66.7 ☑
nontraffic V66.2 ☑
bus (traffic) V64.7 ☑
nontraffic V64.2 ☑
car (traffic) V63.7 ☑
nontraffic V63.2 ☑
pedal cycle (traffic) V61.7 ☑
nontraffic V61.2 ☑
pickup truck (traffic) V63.7 ☑
nontraffic V63.2 ☑
railway vehicle (traffic) V65.7 ☑
nontraffic V65.2 ☑
specified vehicle NEC (traffic) V66.7 ☑
nontraffic V66.2 ☑
stationary object (traffic) V67.7 ☑
nontraffic V67.2 ☑
streetcar (traffic) V66.7 ☑
nontraffic V66.2 ☑

Accident — *continued*
transport — *continued*
truck occupant — *continued*
hanger-on — *continued*
collision — *continued*
three wheeled motor vehicle (traffic) V62.7 ☑
nontraffic V62.2 ☑
truck (traffic) V64.7 ☑
nontraffic V64.2 ☑
two wheeled motor vehicle (traffic) V62.7 ☑
nontraffic V62.2 ☑
van (traffic) V63.7 ☑
nontraffic V63.2 ☑
noncollision accident (traffic) V68.7 ☑
nontraffic V68.2 ☑
noncollision accident (traffic) V68.9 ☑
nontraffic V68.3 ☑
while boarding or alighting V68.4 ☑
nontraffic V69.3 ☑
passenger
collision (with)
animal (traffic) V60.6 ☑
being ridden (traffic) V66.6 ☑
nontraffic V66.1- ☑
nontraffic V60.1 ☑
animal-drawn vehicle (traffic) V66.6 ☑
nontraffic V66.1 ☑
bus (traffic) V64.6 ☑
nontraffic V64.1 ☑
car (traffic) V63.6 ☑
nontraffic V63.1 ☑
motor vehicle NOS (traffic) V69.50 ☑
nontraffic V69.10 ☑
specified type NEC (traffic) V69.59 ☑
nontraffic V69.19 ☑
pedal cycle (traffic) V61.6 ☑
nontraffic V61.1 ☑
pickup truck (traffic) V63.6 ☑
nontraffic V63.1 ☑
railway vehicle (traffic) V65.6 ☑
nontraffic V65.1 ☑
specified vehicle NEC (traffic) V66.6 ☑
nontraffic V66.1 ☑
stationary object (traffic) V67.6 ☑
nontraffic V67.1 ☑
streetcar (traffic) V66.6 ☑
nontraffic V66.1 ☑
three wheeled motor vehicle (traffic) V62.6 ☑
nontraffic V62.1 ☑
truck (traffic) V64.6 ☑
nontraffic V64.1 ☑
two wheeled motor vehicle (traffic) V62.6 ☑
nontraffic V62.1 ☑
van (traffic) V63.6 ☑
nontraffic V63.1 ☑
noncollision accident (traffic) V68.6 ☑
nontraffic V68.1 ☑
pickup — *see* Accident, transport, pickup truck occupant
specified type NEC V69.88 ☑
military vehicle V69.81 ☑
van occupant V59.9 ☑
collision (with)
animal (traffic) V50.9 ☑
being ridden (traffic) V56.9 ☑
nontraffic V56.3 ☑
while boarding or alighting V56.4 ☑
nontraffic V50.3 ☑
while boarding or alighting V50.4 ☑
animal-drawn vehicle (traffic) V56.9 ☑
nontraffic V56.3 ☑
while boarding or alighting V56.4 ☑
bus (traffic) V54.9 ☑
nontraffic V54.3 ☑
while boarding or alighting V54.4 ☑
car (traffic) V53.9 ☑
nontraffic V53.3 ☑
while boarding or alighting V53.4 ☑
motor vehicle NOS (traffic) V59.60 ☑
nontraffic V59.20 ☑
specified type NEC (traffic) V59.69 ☑
nontraffic V59.29 ☑

☑ **Additional Character Required — Refer to the Tabular List for Character Selection**   ▽ **Subterms under main terms may continue to next column or page**

Accident — *continued*
  transport — *continued*
    van occupant — *continued*
      collision — *continued*
        pedal cycle (traffic) V51.9 ☑
          nontraffic V51.3 ☑
          while boarding or alighting V51.4 ☑
        pickup truck (traffic) V53.9 ☑
          nontraffic V53.3 ☑
          while boarding or alighting V53.4 ☑
        railway vehicle (traffic) V55.9 ☑
          nontraffic V55.3 ☑
          while boarding or alighting V55.4 ☑
        specified vehicle NEC (traffic) V56.9 ☑
          nontraffic V56.3 ☑
          while boarding or alighting V56.4 ☑
        stationary object (traffic) V57.9 ☑
          nontraffic V57.3 ☑
          while boarding or alighting V57.4 ☑
        streetcar (traffic) V56.9 ☑
          nontraffic V56.3 ☑
          while boarding or alighting V56.4 ☑
        three wheeled motor vehicle (traffic) V52.9 ☑
          nontraffic V52.3 ☑
          while boarding or alighting V52.4 ☑
        truck (traffic) V54.9 ☑
          nontraffic V54.3 ☑
          while boarding or alighting V54.4 ☑
        two wheeled motor vehicle (traffic) V52.9 ☑
          nontraffic V52.3 ☑
          while boarding or alighting V52.4 ☑
        van (traffic) V53.9 ☑
          nontraffic V53.3 ☑
          while boarding or alighting V53.4 ☑
    driver
      collision (with)
        animal (traffic) V50.5 ☑
          being ridden (traffic) V56.5 ☑
            nontraffic V56.0 ☑
          nontraffic V50.0 ☑
        animal-drawn vehicle (traffic) V56.5 ☑
          nontraffic V56.0 ☑
        bus (traffic) V54.5 ☑
          nontraffic V54.0 ☑
        car (traffic) V53.5 ☑
          nontraffic V53.0 ☑
        motor vehicle NOS (traffic) V59.40 ☑
          nontraffic V59.00 ☑
          specified type NEC (traffic) V59.49 ☑
            nontraffic V59.09 ☑
        pedal cycle (traffic) V51.5 ☑
          nontraffic V51.0 ☑
        pickup truck (traffic) V53.5 ☑
          nontraffic V53.0 ☑
        railway vehicle (traffic) V55.5 ☑
          nontraffic V55.0 ☑
        specified vehicle NEC (traffic) V56.5 ☑
          nontraffic V56.0 ☑
        stationary object (traffic) V57.5 ☑
          nontraffic V57.0 ☑
        streetcar (traffic) V56.5 ☑
          nontraffic V56.0 ☑
        three wheeled motor vehicle (traffic) V52.5 ☑
          nontraffic V52.0 ☑
        truck (traffic) V54.5 ☑
          nontraffic V54.0 ☑
        two wheeled motor vehicle (traffic) V52.5 ☑
          nontraffic V52.0 ☑
        van (traffic) V53.5 ☑
          nontraffic V53.0 ☑
      noncollision accident (traffic) V58.5 ☑
        nontraffic V58.0 ☑
    hanger-on
      collision (with)
        animal (traffic) V50.7 ☑
          being ridden (traffic) V56.7 ☑
            nontraffic V56.2 ☑
          nontraffic V50.2 ☑
        animal-drawn vehicle (traffic) V56.7 ☑
          nontraffic V56.2 ☑
        bus (traffic) V54.7 ☑
          nontraffic V54.2 ☑
        car (traffic) V53.7 ☑
          nontraffic V53.2 ☑

Accident — *continued*
  transport — *continued*
    van occupant — *continued*
      hanger-on — *continued*
        collision — *continued*
          pedal cycle (traffic) V51.7 ☑
            nontraffic V51.2 ☑
          pickup truck (traffic) V53.7 ☑
            nontraffic V53.2 ☑
          railway vehicle (traffic) V55.7 ☑
            nontraffic V55.2 ☑
          specified vehicle NEC (traffic) V56.7 ☑
            nontraffic V56.2 ☑
          stationary object (traffic) V57.7 ☑
            nontraffic V57.2 ☑
          streetcar (traffic) V56.7 ☑
            nontraffic V56.2 ☑
          three wheeled motor vehicle (traffic) V52.7 ☑
            nontraffic V52.2 ☑
          truck (traffic) V54.7 ☑
            nontraffic V54.2 ☑
          two wheeled motor vehicle (traffic) V52.7 ☑
            nontraffic V52.2 ☑
          van (traffic) V53.7 ☑
            nontraffic V53.2 ☑
        noncollision accident (traffic) V58.7 ☑
          nontraffic V58.2 ☑
      noncollision accident (traffic) V58.9 ☑
        nontraffic V58.3 ☑
        while boarding or alighting V58.4 ☑
      nontraffic V59.3 ☑
      passenger
        collision (with)
          animal (traffic) V50.6 ☑
            being ridden (traffic) V56.6 ☑
            nontraffic V56.1 ☑
            nontraffic V50.1 ☑
          animal-drawn vehicle (traffic) V56.6 ☑
            nontraffic V56.1 ☑
          bus (traffic) V54.6 ☑
            nontraffic V54.1 ☑
          car (traffic) V53.6 ☑
            nontraffic V53.1 ☑
          motor vehicle NOS (traffic) V59.50 ☑
            nontraffic V59.10 ☑
            specified type NEC (traffic) V59.59 ☑
              nontraffic V59.19 ☑
          pedal cycle (traffic) V51.6 ☑
            nontraffic V51.1 ☑
          pickup truck (traffic) V53.6 ☑
            nontraffic V53.1 ☑
          railway vehicle (traffic) V55.6 ☑
            nontraffic V55.1 ☑
          specified vehicle NEC (traffic) V56.6 ☑
            nontraffic V56.1 ☑
          stationary object (traffic) V57.6 ☑
            nontraffic V57.1 ☑
          streetcar (traffic) V56.6 ☑
            nontraffic V56.1 ☑
          three wheeled motor vehicle (traffic) V52.6 ☑
            nontraffic V52.1 ☑
          truck (traffic) V54.6 ☑
            nontraffic V54.1 ☑
          two wheeled motor vehicle (traffic) V52.6 ☑
            nontraffic V52.1 ☑
          van (traffic) V53.6 ☑
            nontraffic V53.1 ☑
        noncollision accident (traffic) V58.6 ☑
          nontraffic V58.1 ☑
      specified type NEC V59.88 ☑
      military vehicle V59.81 ☑
    watercraft occupant — *see* Accident, watercraft
    vehicle NEC V89.9 ☑
      animal-drawn NEC — *see* Accident, transport, animal-drawn vehicle occupant
      special
        agricultural — *see* Accident, transport, agricultural vehicle occupant
        construction — *see* Accident, transport, construction vehicle occupant
        industrial — *see* Accident, transport, industrial vehicle occupant

Accident — *continued*
  vehicle — *continued*
    three-wheeled NEC (motorized) — *see* Accident, transport, three-wheeled motor vehicle occupant
  watercraft V94.9 ☑
    causing
      drowning — *see* Drowning, due to, accident to, watercraft
      injury NEC V91.89 ☑
        crushed between craft and object V91.19 ☑
          powered craft V91.13 ☑
            ferry boat V91.11 ☑
            fishing boat V91.12 ☑
            jetskis V91.13 ☑
            liner V91.11 ☑
            merchant ship V91.10 ☑
            passenger ship V91.11 ☑
          unpowered craft V91.18 ☑
            canoe V91.15 ☑
            inflatable V91.16 ☑
            kayak V91.15 ☑
            sailboat V91.14 ☑
            surf-board V91.18 ☑
            windsurfer V91.18 ☑
        fall on board V91.29 ☑
          powered craft V91.23 ☑
            ferry boat V91.21 ☑
            fishing boat V91.22 ☑
            jetskis V91.23 ☑
            liner V91.21 ☑
            merchant ship V91.20 ☑
            passenger ship V91.21 ☑
          unpowered craft
            canoe V91.25 ☑
            inflatable V91.26 ☑
            kayak V91.25 ☑
            sailboat V91.24 ☑
        fire on board causing burn V91.09 ☑
          powered craft V91.03 ☑
            ferry boat V91.01 ☑
            fishing boat V91.02 ☑
            jetskis V91.03 ☑
            liner V91.01 ☑
            merchant ship V91.00 ☑
            passenger ship V91.01 ☑
          unpowered craft V91.08 ☑
            canoe V91.05 ☑
            inflatable V91.06 ☑
            kayak V91.05 ☑
            sailboat V91.04 ☑
            surf-board V91.08 ☑
            water skis V91.07 ☑
            windsurfer V91.08 ☑
        hit by falling object V91.39 ☑
          powered craft V91.33 ☑
            ferry boat V91.31 ☑
            fishing boat V91.32 ☑
            jetskis V91.33 ☑
            liner V91.31 ☑
            merchant ship V91.30 ☑
            passenger ship V91.31 ☑
          unpowered craft V91.38 ☑
            canoe V91.35 ☑
            inflatable V91.36 ☑
            kayak V91.35 ☑
            sailboat V91.34 ☑
            surf-board V91.38 ☑
            water skis V91.37 ☑
            windsurfer V91.38 ☑
        specified type NEC V91.89 ☑
          powered craft V91.83 ☑
            ferry boat V91.81 ☑
            fishing boat V91.82 ☑
            jetskis V91.83 ☑
            liner V91.81 ☑
            merchant ship V91.80 ☑
            passenger ship V91.81 ☑
          unpowered craft V91.88 ☑
            canoe V91.85 ☑
            inflatable V91.86 ☑
            kayak V91.85 ☑
            sailboat V91.84 ☑
            surf-board V91.88 ☑
            water skis V91.87 ☑
            windsurfer V91.88 ☑

Accident — *continued*
  watercraft — *continued*
    due to, caused by cataclysm — *see* Forces of nature, by type
    military NEC V94.818 ☑
      civilian in water injured by V94.811 ☑
      with civilian watercraft V94.810 ☑
    nonpowered, struck by
      nonpowered vessel V94.22 ☑
      powered vessel V94.21 ☑
    specified type NEC V94.89 ☑
    striking swimmer
      powered V94.11 ☑
      unpowered V94.12 ☑

Acid throwing (assault) Y08.89 ☑

Activity (involving) (of victim at time of event) Y93.9
  aerobic and step exercise (class) Y93.A3 (*following* Y93.7)
  alpine skiing Y93.23
  animal care NEC Y93.K9 (*following* Y93.7)
  arts and handcrafts NEC Y93.D9 (*following* Y93.7)
  athletics played as a team or group NEC Y93.69
  athletics played individually NEC Y93.59
  athletics NEC Y93.79
  baking Y93.G3 (*following* Y93.7)
  ballet Y93.41
  barbells Y93.B3 (*following* Y93.7)
  BASE (Building, Antenna, Span, Earth) jumping Y93.33
  baseball Y93.64
  basketball Y93.67
  bathing (personal) Y93.E1 (*following* Y93.7)
  beach volleyball Y93.68
  bike riding Y93.55
  blackout game Y93.85
  boogie boarding Y93.18
  bowling Y93.54
  boxing Y93.71
  brass instrument playing Y93.J4 (*following* Y93.7)
  building construction Y93.H3 (*following* Y93.7)
  bungee jumping Y93.34
  calisthenics Y93.A2 (*following* Y93.7)
  canoeing (in calm and turbulent water) Y93.16
  capture the flag Y93.6A
  cardiorespiratory exercise NEC Y93.A9 (*following* Y93.7)
  caregiving (providing) NEC Y93.F9 (*following* Y93.7)
    bathing Y93.F1 (*following* Y93.7)
    lifting Y93.F2 (*following* Y93.7)
  cellular
    communication device Y93.C2 (*following* Y93.7)
    telephone Y93.C2 (*following* Y93.7)
  challenge course Y93.A5 (*following* Y93.7)
  cheerleading Y93.45
  choking game Y93.85
  circuit training Y93.A4 (*following* Y93.7)
  cleaning
    floor Y93.E5 (*following* Y93.7)
  climbing NEC Y93.39
    mountain Y93.31
    rock Y93.31
    wall Y93.31
  clothing care and maintenance NEC Y93.E9 (*following* Y93.7)
  combatives Y93.75
  computer
    keyboarding Y93.C1 (*following* Y93.7)
    technology NEC Y93.C9 (*following* Y93.7)
  confidence course Y93.A5 (*following* Y93.7)
  construction (building) Y93.H3 (*following* Y93.7)
  cooking and baking Y93.G3 (*following* Y93.7)
  cool down exercises Y93.A2 (*following* Y93.7)
  cricket Y93.69
  crocheting Y93.D1 (*following* Y93.7)
  cross country skiing Y93.24
  dancing (all types) Y93.41
  digging
    dirt Y93.H1 (*following* Y93.7)
  dirt digging Y93.H1 (*following* Y93.7)
  dishwashing Y93.G1 (*following* Y93.7)
  diving (platform) (springboard) Y93.12
    underwater Y93.15
  dodge ball Y93.6A
  downhill skiing Y93.23
  drum playing Y93.J2 (*following* Y93.7)
  dumbbells Y93.B3 (*following* Y93.7)
  electronic
    devices NEC Y93.C9 (*following* Y93.7)
      hand held interactive Y93.C2 (*following* Y93.7)

Activity — *continued*
  electronic — *continued*
    game playing (using) (with)
      interactive device Y93.C2 (*following* Y93.7)
      keyboard or other stationary device Y93.C1 (*following* Y93.7)
  elliptical machine Y93.A1 (*following* Y93.7)
  exercise(s)
    machines ((primarily) for)
      cardiorespiratory conditioning Y93.A1 (*following* Y93.7)
      muscle strengthening Y93.B1 (*following* Y93.7)
    muscle strengthening (non-machine) NEC Y93.B9 (*following* Y93.7)
  external motion NEC Y93.I9 (*following* Y93.7)
    rollercoaster Y93.I1 (*following* Y93.7)
  fainting game Y93.85
  field hockey Y93.65
  figure skating (pairs) (singles) Y93.21
  flag football Y93.62
  floor mopping and cleaning Y93.E5 (*following* Y93.7)
  food preparation and clean up Y93.G1 (*following* Y93.7)
  football (American) NOS Y93.61
    flag Y93.62
    tackle Y93.61
    touch Y93.62
  four square Y93.6A
  free weights Y93.B3 (*following* Y93.7)
  frisbee (ultimate) Y93.74
  furniture
    building Y93.D3 (*following* Y93.7)
    finishing Y93.D3 (*following* Y93.7)
    repair Y93.D3 (*following* Y93.7)
  game playing (electronic)
    using interactive device Y93.C2 (*following* Y93.7)
    using keyboard or other stationary device Y93.C1 (*following* Y93.7)
  gardening Y93.H2 (*following* Y93.7)
  golf Y93.53
  grass drills Y93.A6 (*following* Y93.7)
  grilling and smoking food Y93.G2 (*following* Y93.7)
  grooming and shearing an animal Y93.K3 (*following* Y93.7)
  guerilla drills Y93.A6 (*following* Y93.7)
  gymnastics (rhythmic) Y93.43
  hand held interactive electronic device Y93.C2 (*following* Y93.7)
  handball Y93.73
  handcrafts NEC Y93.D9 (*following* Y93.7)
  hang gliding Y93.35
  hiking (on level or elevated terrain) Y93.Ø1
  hockey (ice) Y93.22
    field Y93.65
  horseback riding Y93.52
  household (interior) maintenance NEC Y93.E9 (*following* Y93.7)
  ice NEC Y93.29
    dancing Y93.21
    hockey Y93.22
    skating Y93.21
  inline roller skating Y93.51
  ironing Y93.E4 (*following* Y93.7)
  judo Y93.75
  jumping jacks Y93.A2 (*following* Y93.7)
  jumping rope Y93.56
  jumping (off) NEC Y93.39
    BASE (Building, Antenna, Span, Earth) Y93.33
    bungee Y93.34
    jacks Y93.A2 (*following* Y93.7)
    rope Y93.56
  karate Y93.75
  kayaking (in calm and turbulent water) Y93.16
  keyboarding (computer) Y93.C1 (*following* Y93.7)
  kickball Y93.6A
  knitting Y93.D1 (*following* Y93.7)
  lacrosse Y93.65
  land maintenance NEC Y93.H9 (*following* Y93.7)
  landscaping Y93.H2 (*following* Y93.7)
  laundry Y93.E2 (*following* Y93.7)
  machines (exercise)
    primarily for cardiorespiratory conditioning Y93.A1 (*following* Y93.7)
    primarily for muscle strengthening Y93.B1 (*following* Y93.7)
  maintenance
    exterior building NEC Y93.H9 (*following* Y93.7)
    household (interior) NEC Y93.E9 (*following* Y93.7)
    land Y93.H9 (*following* Y93.7)
    property Y93.H9 (*following* Y93.7)

Activity — *continued*
  marching (on level or elevated terrain) Y93.Ø1
  martial arts Y93.75
  microwave oven Y93.G3 (*following* Y93.7)
  milking an animal Y93.K2 (*following* Y93.7)
  mopping (floor) Y93.E5 (*following* Y93.7)
  mountain climbing Y93.31
  muscle strengthening
    exercises (non-machine) NEC Y93.B9 (*following* Y93.7)
    machines Y93.B1 (*following* Y93.7)
  musical keyboard (electronic) playing Y93.J1 (*following* Y93.7)
  nordic skiing Y93.24
  obstacle course Y93.A5 (*following* Y93.7)
  oven (microwave) Y93.G3 (*following* Y93.7)
  packing up and unpacking in moving to a new residence Y93.E6 (*following* Y93.7)
  parasailing Y93.19
  pass out game Y93.85
  percussion instrument playing NEC Y93.J2 (*following* Y93.7)
  personal
    bathing and showering Y93.E1 (*following* Y93.7)
    hygiene NEC Y93.E8 (*following* Y93.7)
    showering Y93.E1 (*following* Y93.7)
  physical games generally associated with school recess, summer camp and children Y93.6A
  physical training NEC Y93.A9 (*following* Y93.7)
  piano playing Y93.J1 (*following* Y93.7)
  pilates Y93.B4 (*following* Y93.7)
  platform diving Y93.12
  playing musical instrument
    brass instrument Y93.J4 (*following* Y93.7)
    drum Y93.J2 (*following* Y93.7)
    musical keyboard (electronic) Y93.J1 (*following* Y93.7)
    percussion instrument NEC Y93.J2 (*following* Y93.7)
    piano Y93.J1 (*following* Y93.7)
    string instrument Y93.J3 (*following* Y93.7)
    winds instrument Y93.J4 (*following* Y93.7)
  property maintenance
    exterior NEC Y93.H9 (*following* Y93.7)
    interior NEC Y93.E9 (*following* Y93.7)
  pruning (garden and lawn) Y93.H2 (*following* Y93.7)
  pull-ups Y93.B2 (*following* Y93.7)
  push-ups Y93.B2 (*following* Y93.7)
  racquetball Y93.73
  rafting (in calm and turbulent water) Y93.16
  raking (leaves) Y93.H1 (*following* Y93.7)
  rappelling Y93.32
  refereeing a sports activity Y93.81
  residential relocation Y93.E6 (*following* Y93.7)
  rhythmic gymnastics Y93.43
  rhythmic movement NEC Y93.49
  riding
    horseback Y93.52
    rollercoaster Y93.I1 (*following* Y93.7)
  rock climbing Y93.31
  roller skating (inline) Y93.51
  rollercoaster riding Y93.I1 (*following* Y93.7)
  rough housing and horseplay Y93.83
  rowing (in calm and turbulent water) Y93.16
  rugby Y93.63
  running Y93.Ø2
  SCUBA diving Y93.15
  sewing Y93.D2 (*following* Y93.7)
  shoveling Y93.H1 (*following* Y93.7)
    dirt Y93.H1 (*following* Y93.7)
    snow Y93.H1 (*following* Y93.7)
  showering (personal) Y93.E1 (*following* Y93.7)
  sit-ups Y93.B2 (*following* Y93.7)
  skateboarding Y93.51
  skating (ice) Y93.21
    roller Y93.51
  skiing (alpine) (downhill) Y93.23
    cross country Y93.24
    nordic Y93.24
    water Y93.17
  sledding (snow) Y93.23
  sleeping (sleep) Y93.84
  smoking and grilling food Y93.G2 (*following* Y93.7)
  snorkeling Y93.15
  snow NEC Y93.29
    boarding Y93.23
    shoveling Y93.H1 (*following* Y93.7)
    sledding Y93.23
    tubing Y93.23
  soccer Y93.66

☑ Additional Character Required — Refer to the Tabular List for Character Selection   ▽ Subterms under main terms may continue to next column or page

Activity — *continued*
softball Y93.64
specified NEC Y93.89
spectator at an event Y93.82
sports NEC Y93.79
   sports played as a team or group NEC Y93.69
   sports played individually NEC Y93.59
springboard diving Y93.12
squash Y93.73
stationary bike Y93.A1 (*following* Y93.7)
step (stepping) exercise (class) Y93.A3 (*following* Y93.7)
stepper machine Y93.A1 (*following* Y93.7)
stove Y93.G3 (*following* Y93.7)
string instrument playing Y93.J3 (*following* Y93.7)
surfing Y93.18
   wind Y93.18
swimming Y93.11
tackle football Y93.61
tap dancing Y93.41
tennis Y93.73
tobogganing Y93.23
touch football Y93.62
track and field events (non-running) Y93.57
   running Y93.02
trampoline Y93.44
treadmill Y93.A1 (*following* Y93.7)
trimming shrubs Y93.H2 (*following* Y93.7)
tubing (in calm and turbulent water) Y93.16
   snow Y93.23
ultimate frisbee Y93.74
underwater diving Y93.15
unpacking in moving to a new residence Y93.E6 (*following* Y93.7)
use of stove, oven and microwave oven Y93.G3 (*following* Y93.7)
vacuuming Y93.E3 (*following* Y93.7)
volleyball (beach) (court) Y93.68
wake boarding Y93.17
walking (on level or elevated terrain) Y93.01
   an animal Y93.K1 (*following* Y93.7)
walking an animal Y93.K1 (*following* Y93.7)
wall climbing Y93.31
warm up and cool down exercises Y93.A2 (*following* Y93.7)
water NEC Y93.19
   aerobics Y93.14
   craft NEC Y93.19
   exercise Y93.14
   polo Y93.13
   skiing Y93.17
   sliding Y93.18
   survival training and testing Y93.19
weeding (garden and lawn) Y93.H2 (*following* Y93.7)
wind instrument playing Y93.J4 (*following* Y93.7)
windsurfing Y93.18
wrestling Y93.72
yoga Y93.42
Adverse effect of drugs — *see* Table of Drugs and Chemicals
Aerosinusitis — *see* Air, pressure
After-effect, late — *see* Sequelae
Air
blast in war operations — *see* War operations, air blast
pressure
   change, rapid
      during
         ascent W94.29 ☑
            while (in) (surfacing from)
               aircraft W94.23 ☑
               deep water diving W94.21 ☑
               underground W94.22 ☑
         descent W94.39 ☑
            in
               aircraft W94.31 ☑
               water W94.32 ☑
   high, prolonged W94.0 ☑
   low, prolonged W94.12 ☑
      due to residence or long visit at high altitude W94.11 ☑
Alpine sickness W94.11 ☑
Altitude sickness W94.11 ☑
Anaphylactic shock, anaphylaxis — *see* Table of Drugs and Chemicals
Andes disease W94.11 ☑
Arachnidism, arachnoidism X58 ☑
Arson (with intent to injure or kill) X97 ☑

Asphyxia, asphyxiation
by
   food (bone) (seed) — *see* categories T17 and T18 ☑
   gas — *see also* Table of Drugs and Chemicals
      legal
         execution — *see* Legal, intervention, gas
         intervention — *see* Legal, intervention, gas
from
   fire — *see also* Exposure, fire
      in war operations — *see* War operations, fire
   ignition — *see* Ignition
   vomitus T17.81 ☑
in war operations — *see* War operations, restriction of airway
Aspiration
food (any type) (into respiratory tract) (with asphyxia, obstruction respiratory tract, suffocation) — *see* categories T17 and T18 ☑
foreign body — *see* Foreign body, aspiration
vomitus (with asphyxia, obstruction respiratory tract, suffocation) T17.81 ☑
Assassination (attempt) — *see* Assault
Assault (homicidal) (by) (in) Y09
arson X97 ☑
bite (of human being) Y04.1 ☑
bodily force Y04.8 ☑
   bite Y04.1 ☑
   bumping into Y04.2 ☑
   sexual — *see* subcategories T74.0, T76.0 ☑
   unarmed fight Y04.0 ☑
bomb X96.9 ☑
   antipersonnel X96.0 ☑
   fertilizer X96.3 ☑
   gasoline X96.1 ☑
   letter X96.2 ☑
   petrol X96.1 ☑
   pipe X96.3 ☑
   specified NEC X96.8 ☑
brawl (hand) (fists) (foot) (unarmed) Y04.0 ☑
burning, burns (by fire) NEC X97 ☑
   acid Y08.89 ☑
   caustic, corrosive substance Y08.89 ☑
   chemical from swallowing caustic, corrosive substance — *see* Table of Drugs and Chemicals
   cigarette(s) X97 ☑
   hot object X98.9 ☑
      fluid NEC X98.2 ☑
      household appliance X98.3 ☑
      specified NEC X98.8 ☑
      steam X98.0 ☑
      tap water X98.1 ☑
      vapors X98.0 ☑
   scalding — *see* Assault, burning
   steam X98.0 ☑
   vitriol Y08.89 ☑
caustic, corrosive substance (gas) Y08.89 ☑
crashing of
   aircraft Y08.81 ☑
   motor vehicle Y03.8 ☑
      pushed in front of Y02.0 ☑
      run over Y03.0 ☑
      specified NEC Y03.8 ☑
cutting or piercing instrument X99.9 ☑
   dagger X99.2 ☑
   glass X99.0 ☑
   knife X99.1 ☑
   specified NEC X99.8 ☑
   sword X99.2 ☑
dagger X99.2 ☑
drowning (in) X92.9 ☑
   bathtub X92.0 ☑
   natural water X92.3 ☑
   specified NEC X92.8 ☑
   swimming pool X92.1 ☑
      following fall X92.2 ☑
dynamite X96.8 ☑
explosive(s) (material) X96.9 ☑
fight (hand) (fists) (foot) (unarmed) Y04.0 ☑
   with weapon — *see* Assault, by type of weapon
fire X97 ☑
firearm X95.9 ☑
   airgun X95.01 ☑
   handgun X93 ☑
   hunting rifle X94.1 ☑
   larger X94.9 ☑
      specified NEC X94.8 ☑

Assault — *continued*
firearm — *continued*
   machine gun X94.2 ☑
   shotgun X94.0 ☑
   specified NEC X95.8 ☑
from high place Y01 ☑
gunshot (wound) NEC — *see* Assault, firearm, by type
incendiary device X97 ☑
injury Y09
   to child due to criminal abortion attempt NEC Y08.89 ☑
knife X99.1 ☑
late effect of — *see* categories X92-Y08 with 7th character S
placing before moving object NEC Y02.8 ☑
   motor vehicle Y02.0 ☑
poisoning — *see* categories T36-T65 with 7th character S
puncture, any part of body — *see* Assault, cutting or piercing instrument
pushing
   before moving object NEC Y02.8 ☑
      motor vehicle Y02.0 ☑
      subway train Y02.1 ☑
      train Y02.1 ☑
   from high place Y01 ☑
rape T74.2- ☑
scalding — *see* Assault, burning
sequelae of — *see* categories X92-Y08 with 7th character S
sexual (by bodily force) T74.2- ☑
shooting — *see* Assault, firearm
specified means NEC Y08.89 ☑
stab, any part of body — *see* Assault, cutting or piercing instrument
steam X98.0 ☑
striking against
   other person Y04.2 ☑
   sports equipment Y08.09 ☑
      baseball bat Y08.02 ☑
      hockey stick Y08.01 ☑
struck by
   sports equipment Y08.09 ☑
      baseball bat Y08.02 ☑
      hockey stick Y08.01 ☑
submersion — *see* Assault, drowning
violence Y09
weapon Y09
   blunt Y00 ☑
   cutting or piercing — *see* Assault, cutting or piercing instrument
   firearm — *see* Assault, firearm
wound Y09
   cutting — *see* Assault, cutting or piercing instrument
   gunshot — *see* Assault, firearm
   knife X99.1 ☑
   piercing — *see* Assault, cutting or piercing instrument
   puncture — *see* Assault, cutting or piercing instrument
   stab — *see* Assault, cutting or piercing instrument
Attack by mammals NEC W55.89 ☑
Avalanche — *see* Landslide
Aviator's disease — *see* Air, pressure

B

Barotitis, barodontalgia, barosinusitis, barotrauma (otitic) (sinus) — *see* Air, pressure
Battered (baby) (child) (person) (syndrome) X58 ☑
Bayonet wound W26.1 ☑
in
   legal intervention — *see* Legal, intervention, sharp object, bayonet
   war operations — *see* War operations, combat
stated as undetermined whether accidental or intentional Y28.8 ☑
suicide (attempt) X78.2 ☑
Bean in nose — *see* categories T17 and T18 ☑
Bed set on fire NEC — *see* Exposure, fire, uncontrolled, building, bed
Beheading (by guillotine)
homicide X99.9 ☑
legal execution — *see* Legal, intervention
Bending, injury in (prolonged) (static) X50.1 ☑

Bends — *see* Air, pressure, change
Bite, bitten by
  alligator W58.01 ☑
  arthropod (nonvenomous) NEC W57 ☑
  bull W55.21 ☑
  cat W55.01 ☑
  cow W55.21 ☑
  crocodile W58.11 ☑
  dog W54.0 ☑
  goat W55.31 ☑
  hoof stock NEC W55.31 ☑
  horse W55.11 ☑
  human being (accidentally) W50.3 ☑
    with intent to injure or kill Y04.1 ☑
    as, or caused by, a crowd or human stampede (with fall) W52 ☑
    assault Y04.1 ☑
    homicide (attempt) Y04.1 ☑
    in
      fight Y04.1 ☑
  insect (nonvenomous) W57 ☑
  lizard (nonvenomous) W59.01 ☑
  mammal NEC W55.81 ☑
    marine W56.31 ☑
  marine animal (nonvenomous) W56.81 ☑
  millipede W57 ☑
  moray eel W56.51 ☑
  mouse W53.01 ☑
  person(s) (accidentally) W50.3 ☑
    with intent to injure or kill Y04.1 ☑
    as, or caused by, a crowd or human stampede (with fall) W52 ☑
    assault Y04.1 ☑
    homicide (attempt) Y04.1 ☑
    in
      fight Y04.1 ☑
  pig W55.41 ☑
  raccoon W55.51 ☑
  rat W53.11 ☑
  reptile W59.81 ☑
    lizard W59.01 ☑
    snake W59.11 ☑
    turtle W59.21 ☑
      terrestrial W59.81 ☑
  rodent W53.81 ☑
    mouse W53.01 ☑
    rat W53.11 ☑
    specified NEC W53.81 ☑
    squirrel W53.21 ☑
  shark W56.41 ☑
  sheep W55.31 ☑
  snake (nonvenomous) W59.11 ☑
  spider (nonvenomous) W57 ☑
  squirrel W53.21 ☑
Blast (air) in war operations — *see* War operations, blast
Blizzard X37.2 ☑
Blood alcohol level Y90.9
  less than 20mg/100ml Y90.0
  presence in blood, level not specified Y90.9
  20-39mg/100ml Y90.1
  40-59mg/100ml Y90.2
  60-79mg/100ml Y90.3
  80-99mg/100ml Y90.4
  100-119mg/100ml Y90.5
  120-199mg/100ml Y90.6
  200-239mg/100ml Y90.7
Blow X58 ☑
  by law-enforcing agent, police (on duty) — *see* Legal, intervention, manhandling
    blunt object — *see* Legal, intervention, blunt object
Blowing up — *see* Explosion
Brawl (hand) (fists) (foot) Y04.0 ☑
Breakage (accidental) (part of)
  ladder (causing fall) W11 ☑
  scaffolding (causing fall) W12 ☑
Broken
  glass, contact with — *see* Contact, with, glass
  power line (causing electric shock) W85 ☑
Bumping against, into (accidentally)
  object NEC W22.8 ☑
    caused by crowd or human stampede (with fall) W52 ☑
    sports equipment W21.9 ☑
    with fall — *see* Fall, due to, bumping against, object
  person(s) W51 ☑
    with fall W03 ☑

Bumping against, into — *continued*
  person(s) — *continued*
    with fall — *continued*
      due to ice or snow W00.0 ☑
    assault Y04.2 ☑
    caused by, a crowd or human stampede (with fall) W52 ☑
    homicide (attempt) Y04.2 ☑
  sports equipment W21.9 ☑
Burn, burned, burning (accidental) (by) (from) (on)
  acid NEC — *see* Table of Drugs and Chemicals
  bed linen — *see* Exposure, fire, uncontrolled, in building, bed
  blowtorch X08.8 ☑
    with ignition of clothing NEC X06.2 ☑
      nightwear X05 ☑
  bonfire, campfire (controlled) — *see also* Exposure, fire, controlled, not in building
    uncontrolled — *see* Exposure, fire, uncontrolled, not in building
  candle X08.8 ☑
    with ignition of clothing NEC X06.2 ☑
      nightwear X05 ☑
  caustic liquid, substance (external) (internal) NEC — *see* Table of Drugs and Chemicals
  chemical (external) (internal) — *see also* Table of Drugs and Chemicals
    in war operations — *see* War operations. fire
  cigar(s) or cigarette(s) X08.8 ☑
    with ignition of clothing NEC X06.2 ☑
      nightwear X05 ☑
  clothes, clothing NEC (from controlled fire) X06.2 ☑
    with conflagration — *see* Exposure, fire, uncontrolled, building
      not in building or structure — *see* Exposure, fire, uncontrolled, not in building
  cooker (hot) X15.8 ☑
    stated as undetermined whether accidental or intentional Y27.3 ☑
    suicide (attempt) X77.3 ☑
  electric blanket X16 ☑
  engine (hot) X17 ☑
  fire, flames — *see* Exposure, fire
  flare, Very pistol — *see* Discharge, firearm NEC
  heat
    from appliance (electrical) (household) X15.8 ☑
      cooker X15.8 ☑
      hotplate X15.2 ☑
      kettle X15.8 ☑
      light bulb X15.8 ☑
      saucepan X15.3 ☑
      skillet X15.3 ☑
      stated as undetermined whether accidental or intentional Y27.3 ☑
      stove X15.0 ☑
      suicide (attempt) X77.3 ☑
      toaster X15.1 ☑
    in local application or packing during medical or surgical procedure Y63.5
  heating
    appliance, radiator or pipe X16 ☑
  homicide (attempt) — *see* Assault, burning
  hot
    air X14.1 ☑
    cooker X15.8 ☑
    drink X10.0 ☑
    engine X17 ☑
    fat X10.2 ☑
    fluid NEC X12 ☑
    food X10.1 ☑
    gases X14.1 ☑
    heating appliance X16 ☑
    household appliance NEC X15.8 ☑
    kettle X15.8 ☑
    liquid NEC X12 ☑
    machinery X17 ☑
    metal (molten) (liquid) NEC X18 ☑
    object (not producing fire or flames) NEC X19 ☑
    oil (cooking) X10.2 ☑
    pipe(s) X16 ☑
    radiator X16 ☑
    saucepan (glass) (metal) X15.3 ☑
    stove (kitchen) X15.0 ☑
    substance NEC X19 ☑
      caustic or corrosive NEC — *see* Table of Drugs and Chemicals

Burn, burned, burning — *continued*
  hot — *continued*
    toaster X15.1 ☑
    tool X17 ☑
    vapor X13.1 ☑
    water (tap) — *see* Contact, with, hot, tap water
  hotplate X15.2 ☑
    suicide (attempt) X77.3 ☑
  ignition — *see* Ignition
  in war operations — *see* War operations, fire
  inflicted by other person X97 ☑
    by hot objects, hot vapor, and steam — *see* Assault, burning, hot object
  internal, from swallowed caustic, corrosive liquid, substance — *see* Table of Drugs and Chemicals
  iron (hot) X15.8 ☑
    stated as undetermined whether accidental or intentional Y27.3 ☑
    suicide (attempt) X77.3 ☑
  kettle (hot) X15.8 ☑
    stated as undetermined whether accidental or intentional Y27.3 ☑
    suicide (attempt) X77.3 ☑
  lamp (flame) X08.8 ☑
    with ignition of clothing NEC X06.2 ☑
      nightwear X05 ☑
  lighter (cigar) (cigarette) X08.8 ☑
    with ignition of clothing NEC X06.2 ☑
      nightwear X05 ☑
  lightning — *see* subcategory T75.0 ☑
    causing fire — *see* Exposure, fire
  liquid (boiling) (hot) NEC X12 ☑
    stated as undetermined whether accidental or intentional Y27.2 ☑
    suicide (attempt) X77.2 ☑
  local application of externally applied substance in medical or surgical care Y63.5
  machinery (hot) X17 ☑
  matches X08.8 ☑
    with ignition of clothing NEC X06.2 ☑
      nightwear X05 ☑
  mattress — *see* Exposure, fire, uncontrolled, building, bed
  medicament, externally applied Y63.5
  metal (hot) (liquid) (molten) NEC X18 ☑
  nightwear (nightclothes, nightdress, gown, pajamas, robe) X05 ☑
  object (hot) NEC X19 ☑
  on board watercraft
    due to
      accident to watercraft V91.09 ☑
        powered craft V91.03 ☑
          ferry boat V91.01 ☑
          fishing boat V91.02 ☑
          jetskis V91.03 ☑
          liner V91.01 ☑
          merchant ship V91.00 ☑
          passenger ship V91.01 ☑
        unpowered craft V91.08 ☑
          canoe V91.05 ☑
          inflatable V91.06 ☑
          kayak V91.05 ☑
          sailboat V91.04 ☑
          surf-board V91.08 ☑
          water skis V91.07 ☑
          windsurfer V91.08 ☑
      fire on board V93.09 ☑
        ferry boat V93.01 ☑
        fishing boat V93.02 ☑
        jetskis V93.03 ☑
        liner V93.01 ☑
        merchant ship V93.00 ☑
        passenger ship V93.01 ☑
        powered craft NEC V93.03 ☑
        sailboat V93.04 ☑
      specified heat source NEC on board V93.19 ☑
        ferry boat V93.11 ☑
        fishing boat V93.12 ☑
        jetskis V93.13 ☑
        liner V93.11 ☑
        merchant ship V93.10 ☑
        passenger ship V93.11 ☑
        powered craft NEC V93.13 ☑
        sailboat V93.14 ☑
  pipe (hot) X16 ☑
    smoking X08.8 ☑

☑ **Additional Character Required — Refer to the Tabular List for Character Selection** ▽ **Subterms under main terms may continue to next column or page**

Burn, burned, burning — *continued*
  pipe — *continued*
    smoking — *continued*
      with ignition of clothing NEC X06.2 ☑
        nightwear X05 ☑
  powder — *see* Powder burn
  radiator (hot) X16 ☑
  saucepan (hot) (glass) (metal) X15.3 ☑
    stated as undetermined whether accidental or intentional Y27.3 ☑
    suicide (attempt) X77.3 ☑
  self-inflicted X76 ☑
    stated as undetermined whether accidental or intentional Y26 ☑
  stated as undetermined whether accidental or intentional Y27.0 ☑
  steam X13.1 ☑
    pipe X16 ☑
      stated as undetermined whether accidental or intentional Y27.8 ☑
    stated as undetermined whether accidental or intentional Y27.0 ☑
    suicide (attempt) X77.0 ☑
  stove (hot) (kitchen) X15.0 ☑
    stated as undetermined whether accidental or intentional Y27.3 ☑
    suicide (attempt) X77.3 ☑
  substance (hot) NEC X19 ☑
    boiling X12 ☑
      stated as undetermined whether accidental or intentional Y27.2 ☑
      suicide (attempt) X77.2 ☑
    molten (metal) X18 ☑
  suicide (attempt) NEC X76 ☑
    hot
      household appliance X77.3 ☑
      object X77.9 ☑
  therapeutic misadventure
    heat in local application or packing during medical or surgical procedure Y63.5
    overdose of radiation Y63.2
  toaster (hot) X15.1 ☑
    stated as undetermined whether accidental or intentional Y27.3 ☑
    suicide (attempt) X77.3 ☑
  tool (hot) X17 ☑
  torch, welding X08.8 ☑
    with ignition of clothing NEC X06.2 ☑
      nightwear X05 ☑
  trash fire (controlled) — *see* Exposure, fire, controlled, not in building
    uncontrolled — *see* Exposure, fire, uncontrolled, not in building
  vapor (hot) X13.1 ☑
    stated as undetermined whether accidental or intentional Y27.0 ☑
    suicide (attempt) X77.0 ☑
  Very pistol — *see* Discharge, firearm NEC
Butted by animal W55.82 ☑
  bull W55.22 ☑
  cow W55.22 ☑
  goat W55.32 ☑
  horse W55.12 ☑
  pig W55.42 ☑
  sheep W55.32 ☑

C

Caisson disease — *see* Air, pressure, change
Campfire (exposure to) (controlled) — *see also* Exposure, fire, controlled, not in building
  uncontrolled — *see* Exposure, fire, uncontrolled, not in building
Capital punishment (any means) — *see* Legal, intervention
Car sickness T75.3 ☑
Casualty (not due to war) NEC X58 ☑
  war — *see* War operations
Cat
  bite W55.01 ☑
  scratch W55.03 ☑
Cataclysm, cataclysmic (any injury) NEC — *see* Forces of nature
Catching fire — *see* Exposure, fire

Caught
  between
    folding object W23.0 ☑
    objects (moving) (stationary and moving) W23.0 ☑
      and machinery — *see* Contact, with, by type of machine
      stationary W23.1 ☑
    sliding door and door frame W23.0 ☑
  by, in
    machinery (moving parts of) — *see* Contact, with, by type of machine
    washing-machine wringer W23.0 ☑
    under packing crate (due to losing grip) W23.1 ☑
Cave-in caused by cataclysmic earth surface movement or eruption — *see* Landslide
Change(s) in air pressure — *see* Air, pressure, change
Choked, choking (on) (any object except food or vomitus)
  food (bone) (seed) — *see* categories T17 and T18 ☑
  vomitus T17.81- ☑
Civil insurrection — *see* War operations
Cloudburst (any injury) X37.8 ☑
Cold, exposure to (accidental) (excessive) (extreme) (natural) (place) NEC — *see* Exposure, cold
Collapse
  building W20.1 ☑
    burning (uncontrolled fire) X00.2 ☑
  dam or man-made structure (causing earth movement) X36.0 ☑
  machinery — *see* Contact, with, by type of machine
  structure W20.1 ☑
    burning (uncontrolled fire) X00.2 ☑
Collision (accidental) NEC — *see also* Accident, transport V89.9 ☑
  pedestrian W51 ☑
    with fall W03 ☑
      due to ice or snow W00.0 ☑
      involving pedestrian conveyance — *see* Accident, transport, pedestrian, conveyance
    and
      crowd or human stampede (with fall) W52 ☑
      object W22.8 ☑
        with fall — *see* Fall, due to, bumping against, object
  person(s) — *see* Collision, pedestrian
  transport vehicle NEC V89.9 ☑
    and
      avalanche, fallen or not moving — *see* Accident, transport
        falling or moving — *see* Landslide
      landslide, fallen or not moving — *see* Accident, transport
        falling or moving — *see* Landslide
    due to cataclysm — *see* Forces of nature, by type
    intentional, purposeful suicide (attempt) — *see* Suicide, collision
Combustion, spontaneous — *see* Ignition
Complication (delayed) of or following (medical or surgical procedure) Y84.9
  with misadventure — *see* Misadventure
  amputation of limb(s) Y83.5
  anastomosis (arteriovenous) (blood vessel) (gastrojejunal) (tendon) (natural or artificial material) Y83.2
  aspiration (of fluid) Y84.4
    tissue Y84.8
  biopsy Y84.8
  blood
    sampling Y84.7
    transfusion
      procedure Y84.8
  bypass Y83.2
  catheterization (urinary) Y84.6
    cardiac Y84.0
  colostomy Y83.3
  cystostomy Y83.3
  dialysis (kidney) Y84.1
  drug — *see* Table of Drugs and Chemicals
  due to misadventure — *see* Misadventure
  duodenostomy Y83.3
  electroshock therapy Y84.3
  external stoma, creation of Y83.3
  formation of external stoma Y83.3
  gastrostomy Y83.3
  graft Y83.2
  hypothermia (medically-induced) Y84.8

Complication (delayed) of or following — *continued*
  implant, implantation (of)
    artificial
      internal device (cardiac pacemaker) (electrodes in brain) (heart valve prosthesis) (orthopedic) Y83.1
      material or tissue (for anastomosis or bypass) Y83.2
        with creation of external stoma Y83.3
    natural tissues (for anastomosis or bypass) Y83.2
      with creation of external stoma Y83.3
  infusion
    procedure Y84.8
  injection — *see* Table of Drugs and Chemicals
    procedure Y84.8
  insertion of gastric or duodenal sound Y84.5
  insulin-shock therapy Y84.3
  paracentesis (abdominal) (thoracic) (aspirative) Y84.4
  procedures other than surgical operation — *see* Complication of or following, by type of procedure
  radiological procedure or therapy Y84.2
  removal of organ (partial) (total) NEC Y83.6
  sampling
    blood Y84.7
    fluid NEC Y84.4
    tissue Y84.8
  shock therapy Y84.3
  surgical operation NEC — *see also* Complication of or following, by type of operation Y83.9
    reconstructive NEC Y83.4
      with
        anastomosis, bypass or graft Y83.2
        formation of external stoma Y83.3
    specified NEC Y83.8
  transfusion — *see also* Table of Drugs and Chemicals
    procedure Y84.8
  transplant, transplantation (heart) (kidney) (liver) (whole organ, any) Y83.0
    partial organ Y83.4
  ureterostomy Y83.3
  vaccination — *see also* Table of Drugs and Chemicals
    procedure Y84.8
Compression
  divers' squeeze — *see* Air, pressure, change
  trachea by
    food (lodged in esophagus) — *see* categories T17 and T18 ☑
    vomitus (lodged in esophagus) T17.81- ☑
Conflagration — *see* Exposure, fire, uncontrolled
Constriction (external)
  hair W49.01 ☑
  jewelry W49.04 ☑
  ring W49.04 ☑
  rubber band W49.03 ☑
  specified item NEC W49.09 ☑
  string W49.02 ☑
  thread W49.02 ☑
Contact (accidental)
  with
    abrasive wheel (metalworking) W31.1 ☑
    alligator W58.09 ☑
      bite W58.01 ☑
      crushing W58.03 ☑
      strike W58.02 ☑
    amphibian W62.9 ☑
      frog W62.0 ☑
      toad W62.1 ☑
    animal (nonvenomous) NEC W64 ☑
      marine W56.89 ☑
        bite W56.81 ☑
        dolphin — *see* Contact, with, dolphin
        fish NEC — *see* Contact, with, fish
        mammal — *see* Contact, with, mammal, marine
        orca — *see* Contact, with, orca
        sea lion — *see* Contact, with, sea lion
        shark — *see* Contact, with, shark
        strike W56.82 ☑
    animate mechanical force NEC W64 ☑
    arrow W21.89 ☑
      not thrown, projected or falling W45.8 ☑
    arthropods (nonvenomous) W57 ☑
    axe W27.0 ☑
    band-saw (industrial) W31.2 ☑
    bayonet — *see* Bayonet wound
    bee(s) X58 ☑

Contact — *continued*
with — *continued*
  bench-saw (industrial) W31.2 ☑
  bird W61.99 ☑
    bite W61.91 ☑
    chicken — *see* Contact, with, chicken
    duck — *see* Contact, with, duck
    goose — *see* Contact, with, goose
    macaw — *see* Contact, with, macaw
    parrot — *see* Contact, with, parrot
    psittacine — *see* Contact, with, psittacine
    strike W61.92 ☑
    turkey — *see* Contact, with, turkey
  blender W29.0 ☑
  boiling water X12 ☑
    stated as undetermined whether accidental or
      intentional Y27.2 ☑
    suicide (attempt) X77.2 ☑
  bore, earth-drilling or mining (land) (seabed)
    W31.0 ☑
  buffalo — *see* Contact, with, hoof stock NEC
  bull W55.29 ☑
    bite W55.21 ☑
    gored W55.22 ☑
    strike W55.22 ☑
  bumper cars W31.81 ☑
  camel — *see* Contact, with, hoof stock NEC
  can
    lid W26.8 ☑
    opener W27.4 ☑
      powered W29.0 ☑
  cat W55.09 ☑
    bite W55.01 ☑
    scratch W55.03 ☑
  caterpillar (venomous) X58 ☑
  centipede (venomous) X58 ☑
  chain
    hoist W24.0 ☑
      agricultural operations W30.89 ☑
    saw W29.3 ☑
  chicken W61.39 ☑
    peck W61.33 ☑
    strike W61.32 ☑
  chisel W27.0 ☑
  circular saw W31.2 ☑
  cobra X58 ☑
  combine (harvester) W30.0 ☑
  conveyer belt W24.1 ☑
  cooker (hot) X15.8 ☑
    stated as undetermined whether accidental or
      intentional Y27.3 ☑
    suicide (attempt) X77.3 ☑
  coral X58 ☑
  cotton gin W31.82 ☑
  cow W55.29 ☑
    bite W55.21 ☑
    strike W55.22 ☑
  crane W24.0 ☑
    agricultural operations W30.89 ☑
  crocodile W58.19 ☑
    bite W58.11 ☑
    crushing W58.13 ☑
    strike W58.12 ☑
  dagger W26.1 ☑
    stated as undetermined whether accidental or
      intentional Y28.2 ☑
    suicide (attempt) X78.2 ☑
  dairy equipment W31.82 ☑
  dart W21.89 ☑
    not thrown, projected or falling W45.8 ☑
  deer — *see* Contact, with, hoof stock NEC
  derrick W24.0 ☑
    agricultural operations W30.89 ☑
      hay W30.2 ☑
  dog W54.8 ☑
    bite W54.0 ☑
    strike W54.1 ☑
  dolphin W56.09 ☑
    bite W56.01 ☑
    strike W56.02 ☑
  donkey — *see* Contact, with, hoof stock NEC
  drill (powered) W29.8 ☑
    earth (land) (seabed) W31.0 ☑
    nonpowered W27.8 ☑
  drive belt W24.0 ☑
    agricultural operations W30.89 ☑

Contact — *continued*
with — *continued*
  dry ice — *see* Exposure, cold, man-made
  dryer (clothes) (powered) (spin) W29.2 ☑
  duck W61.69 ☑
    bite W61.61 ☑
    strike W61.62 ☑
  earth (-)
    drilling machine (industrial) W31.0 ☑
    scraping machine in stationary use W31.83 ☑
  edge of stiff paper W26.2 ☑
  electric
    beater W29.0 ☑
    blanket X16 ☑
    fan W29.2 ☑
      commercial W31.82 ☑
    knife W29.1 ☑
    mixer W29.0 ☑
  elevator (building) W24.0 ☑
    agricultural operations W30.89 ☑
    grain W30.3 ☑
  engine(s), hot NEC X17 ☑
  excavating machine W31.0 ☑
  farm machine W30.9 ☑
  feces — *see* Contact, with, by type of animal
  fer de lance X58 ☑
  fish W56.59 ☑
    bite W56.51 ☑
    shark — *see* Contact, with, shark
    strike W56.52 ☑
  flying horses W31.81 ☑
  forging (metalworking) machine W31.1 ☑
  fork W27.4 ☑
  forklift (truck) W24.0 ☑
    agricultural operations W30.89 ☑
  frog W62.0 ☑
  garden
    cultivator (powered) W29.3 ☑
      riding W30.89 ☑
    fork W27.1 ☑
  gas turbine W31.3 ☑
  Gila monster X58 ☑
  giraffe — *see* Contact, with, hoof stock NEC
  glass (sharp) (broken) W25 ☑
    assault X99.0 ☑
    due to fall — *see* Fall, by type
    stated as undetermined whether accidental or
      intentional Y28.0 ☑
    suicide (attempt) X78.0 ☑
    with subsequent fall W18.02 ☑
  goat W55.39 ☑
    bite W55.31 ☑
    strike W55.32 ☑
  goose W61.59 ☑
    bite W61.51 ☑
    strike W61.52 ☑
  hand
    saw W27.0 ☑
    tool (not powered) NEC W27.8 ☑
      powered W29.8 ☑
  harvester W30.0 ☑
  hay-derrick W30.2 ☑
  heating
    appliance (hot) X16 ☑
    pad (electric) X16 ☑
  heat NEC X19 ☑
    from appliance (electrical) (household) — *see*
      Contact, with, hot, household appliance
    heating appliance X16 ☑
  hedge-trimmer (powered) W29.3 ☑
  hoe W27.1 ☑
  hoist (chain) (shaft) NEC W24.0 ☑
    agricultural W30.89 ☑
  hoof stock NEC W55.39 ☑
    bite W55.31 ☑
    strike W55.32 ☑
  hornet(s) X58 ☑
  horse W55.19 ☑
    bite W55.11 ☑
    strike W55.12 ☑
  hot
    air X14.1 ☑
      inhalation X14.0 ☑
    cooker X15.8 ☑
    drinks X10.0 ☑
    engine X17 ☑

Contact — *continued*
with — *continued*
  hot — *continued*
    fats X10.2 ☑
    fluids NEC X12 ☑
      assault X98.2 ☑
      suicide (attempt) X77.2 ☑
      undetermined whether accidental or inten-
        tional Y27.2 ☑
    food X10.1 ☑
    gases X14.1 ☑
      inhalation X14.0 ☑
    heating appliance X16 ☑
    household appliance X15.8 ☑
      assault X98.3 ☑
      cooker X15.8 ☑
      hotplate X15.2 ☑
      kettle X15.8 ☑
      light bulb X15.8 ☑
      object NEC X19 ☑
        assault X98.8 ☑
        stated as undetermined whether acciden-
          tal or intentional Y27.9 ☑
        suicide (attempt) X77.8 ☑
      saucepan X15.3 ☑
      skillet X15.3 ☑
      stated as undetermined whether accidental
        or intentional Y27.3 ☑
      stove X15.0 ☑
      suicide (attempt) X77.3 ☑
      toaster X15.1 ☑
    kettle X15.8 ☑
    light bulb X15.8 ☑
    liquid NEC — *see also* Burn X12 ☑
      drinks X10.0 ☑
      stated as undetermined whether accidental
        or intentional Y27.2 ☑
      suicide (attempt) X77.2 ☑
      tap water X11.8 ☑
      stated as undetermined whether acciden-
        tal or intentional Y27.1 ☑
      suicide (attempt) X77.1 ☑
    machinery X17 ☑
    metal (molten) (liquid) NEC X18 ☑
    object (not producing fire or flames) NEC X19 ☑
    oil (cooking) X10.2 ☑
    pipe X16 ☑
    plate X15.2 ☑
    radiator X16 ☑
    saucepan (glass) (metal) X15.3 ☑
    skillet X15.3 ☑
    stove (kitchen) X15.0 ☑
    substance NEC X19 ☑
    tap-water X11.8 ☑
      assault X98.1 ☑
      heated on stove X12 ☑
      stated as undetermined whether acciden-
        tal or intentional Y27.2 ☑
      suicide (attempt) X77.2 ☑
      in bathtub X11.0 ☑
      running X11.1 ☑
      stated as undetermined whether accidental
        or intentional Y27.1 ☑
      suicide (attempt) X77.1 ☑
    toaster X15.1 ☑
    tool X17 ☑
    vapors X13.1 ☑
      inhalation X13.0 ☑
    water (tap) X11.8 ☑
      boiling X12 ☑
      stated as undetermined whether acciden-
        tal or intentional Y27.2 ☑
      suicide (attempt) X77.2 ☑
      heated on stove X12 ☑
      stated as undetermined whether acciden-
        tal or intentional Y27.2 ☑
      suicide (attempt) X77.2 ☑
      in bathtub X11.0 ☑
      running X11.1 ☑
      stated as undetermined whether accidental
        or intentional Y27.1 ☑
      suicide (attempt) X77.1 ☑
  hotplate X15.2 ☑
  ice-pick W27.4 ☑
  insect (nonvenomous) NEC W57 ☑
  kettle (hot) X15.8 ☑

Contact — *continued*
  with — *continued*
    knife W26.0 ☑
      assault X99.1 ☑
      electric W29.1 ☑
      stated as undetermined whether accidental or
        intentional Y28.1 ☑
      suicide (attempt) X78.1 ☑
    lathe (metalworking) W31.1 ☑
      turnings W45.8 ☑
      woodworking W31.2 ☑
    lawnmower (powered) (ridden) W28 ☑
      causing electrocution W86.8 ☑
        suicide (attempt) X83.1 ☑
      unpowered W27.1 ☑
    lift, lifting (devices) W24.0 ☑
      agricultural operations W30.89 ☑
      shaft W24.0 ☑
    liquefied gas — *see* Exposure, cold, man-made
    liquid air, hydrogen, nitrogen — *see* Exposure, cold,
      man-made
    lizard (nonvenomous) W59.09 ☑
      bite W59.01 ☑
      strike W59.02 ☑
    llama — *see* Contact, with, hoof stock NEC
    macaw W61.19 ☑
      bite W61.11 ☑
      strike W61.12 ☑
    machine, machinery W31.9 ☑
      abrasive wheel W31.1 ☑
      agricultural including animal-powered W30.9 ☑
        combine harvester W30.0 ☑
        grain storage elevator W30.3 ☑
        hay derrick W30.2 ☑
        power take-off device W30.1 ☑
        reaper W30.0 ☑
        specified NEC W30.89 ☑
        thresher W30.0 ☑
        transport vehicle, stationary W30.81 ☑
      band saw W31.2 ☑
      bench saw W31.2 ☑
      circular saw W31.2 ☑
      commercial NEC W31.82 ☑
      drilling, metal (industrial) W31.1 ☑
      earth-drilling W31.0 ☑
      earthmoving or scraping W31.89 ☑
      excavating W31.89 ☑
      forging machine W31.1 ☑
      gas turbine W31.3 ☑
      hot X17 ☑
      internal combustion engine W31.3 ☑
      land drill W31.0 ☑
      lathe W31.1 ☑
      lifting (devices) W24.0 ☑
      metal drill W31.1 ☑
      metalworking (industrial) W31.1 ☑
      milling, metal W31.1 ☑
      mining W31.0 ☑
      molding W31.2 ☑
      overhead plane W31.2 ☑
      power press, metal W31.1 ☑
      prime mover W31.3 ☑
      printing W31.89 ☑
      radial saw W31.2 ☑
      recreational W31.81 ☑
      roller-coaster W31.81 ☑
      rolling mill, metal W31.1 ☑
      sander W31.2 ☑
      seabed drill W31.0 ☑
      shaft
        hoist W31.0 ☑
        lift W31.0 ☑
      specified NEC W31.89 ☑
      spinning W31.89 ☑
      steam engine W31.3 ☑
      transmission W24.1 ☑
      undercutter W31.0 ☑
      water driven turbine W31.3 ☑
      weaving W31.89 ☑
      woodworking or forming (industrial) W31.2 ☑
    mammal (feces) (urine) W55.89 ☑
      bull — *see* Contact, with, bull
      cat — *see* Contact, with, cat
      cow — *see* Contact, with, cow
      goat — *see* Contact, with, goat
      hoof stock — *see* Contact, with, hoof stock

Contact — *continued*
  with — *continued*
    mammal — *continued*
      horse — *see* Contact, with, horse
      marine W56.39 ☑
        dolphin — *see* Contact, with, dolphin
        orca — *see* Contact, with, orca
        sea lion — *see* Contact, with, sea lion
        specified NEC W56.39 ☑
          bite W56.31 ☑
          strike W56.32 ☑
      pig — *see* Contact, with, pig
      raccoon — *see* Contact, with, raccoon
      rodent — *see* Contact, with, rodent
      sheep — *see* Contact, with, sheep
      specified NEC W55.89 ☑
        bite W55.81 ☑
        strike W55.82 ☑
    marine
      animal W56.89 ☑
        bite W56.81 ☑
        dolphin — *see* Contact, with, dolphin
        fish NEC — *see* Contact, with, fish
        mammal — *see* Contact, with, mammal, marine
        orca — *see* Contact, with, orca
        sea lion — *see* Contact, with, sea lion
        shark — *see* Contact, with, shark
        strike W56.82 ☑
    meat
      grinder (domestic) W29.0 ☑
        industrial W31.82 ☑
        nonpowered W27.4 ☑
      slicer (domestic) W29.0 ☑
        industrial W31.82 ☑
    merry go round W31.81 ☑
    metal, hot (liquid) (molten) NEC X18 ☑
    millipede W57 ☑
    nail W45.0 ☑
      gun W29.4 ☑
    needle (sewing) W27.3 ☑
      hypodermic W46.0 ☑
        contaminated W46.1 ☑
    object (blunt) NEC
      hot NEC X19 ☑
      legal intervention — *see* Legal, intervention,
        blunt object
      sharp NEC W45.8 ☑
        inflicted by other person NEC W45.8 ☑
          stated as
            intentional homicide (attempt) — *see*
              Assault, cutting or piercing instrument
        legal intervention — *see* Legal, intervention,
          sharp object
        self-inflicted X78.9 ☑
    orca W56.29 ☑
      bite W56.21 ☑
      strike W56.22 ☑
    overhead plane W31.2 ☑
    paper (as sharp object) W26.2 ☑
    paper-cutter W27.5 ☑
    parrot W61.09 ☑
      bite W61.01 ☑
      strike W61.02 ☑
    pig W55.49 ☑
      bite W55.41 ☑
      strike W55.42 ☑
    pipe, hot X16 ☑
    pitchfork W27.1 ☑
    plane (metal) (wood) W27.0 ☑
      overhead W31.2 ☑
    plant thorns, spines, sharp leaves or other mechanisms W60 ☑
    powered
      garden cultivator W29.3 ☑
      household appliance, implement, or machine
        W29.8 ☑
      saw (industrial) W31.2 ☑
        hand W29.8 ☑
    printing machine W31.89 ☑
    psittacine bird W61.29 ☑
      bite W61.21 ☑
      macaw — *see* Contact, with, macaw
      parrot — *see* Contact, with, parrot
      strike W61.22 ☑

Contact — *continued*
  with — *continued*
    pulley (block) (transmission) W24.0 ☑
      agricultural operations W30.89 ☑
    raccoon W55.59 ☑
      bite W55.51 ☑
      strike W55.52 ☑
    radial-saw (industrial) W31.2 ☑
    radiator (hot) X16 ☑
    rake W27.1 ☑
    rattlesnake X58 ☑
    reaper W30.0 ☑
    reptile W59.89 ☑
      lizard — *see* Contact, with, lizard
      snake — *see* Contact, with, snake
      specified NEC W59.89 ☑
        bite W59.81 ☑
        crushing W59.83 ☑
        strike W59.82 ☑
      turtle — *see* Contact, with, turtle
    rivet gun (powered) W29.4 ☑
    road scraper — *see* Accident, transport, construction
      vehicle
    rodent (feces) (urine) W53.89 ☑
      bite W53.81 ☑
      mouse W53.09 ☑
        bite W53.01 ☑
      rat W53.19 ☑
        bite W53.11 ☑
      specified NEC W53.89 ☑
        bite W53.81 ☑
      squirrel W53.29 ☑
        bite W53.21 ☑
    roller coaster W31.81 ☑
    rope NEC W24.0 ☑
      agricultural operations W30.89 ☑
    saliva — *see* Contact, with, by type of animal
    sander W29.8 ☑
      industrial W31.2 ☑
    saucepan (hot) (glass) (metal) X15.3 ☑
    saw W27.0 ☑
      band (industrial) W31.2 ☑
      bench (industrial) W31.2 ☑
      chain W29.3 ☑
      hand W27.0 ☑
    sawing machine, metal W31.1 ☑
    scissors W27.2 ☑
    scorpion X58 ☑
    screwdriver W27.0 ☑
      powered W29.8 ☑
    sea
      anemone, cucumber or urchin (spine) X58 ☑
      lion W56.19 ☑
        bite W56.11 ☑
        strike W56.12 ☑
    serpent — *see* Contact, with, snake, by type
    sewing-machine (electric) (powered) W29.2 ☑
      not powered W27.8 ☑
    shaft (hoist) (lift) (transmission) NEC W24.0 ☑
      agricultural W30.89 ☑
    shark W56.49 ☑
      bite W56.41 ☑
      strike W56.42 ☑
    sharp object(s) W26.9 ☑
      specified NEC W26.8 ☑
    shears (hand) W27.2 ☑
      powered (industrial) W31.1 ☑
        domestic W29.2 ☑
    sheep W55.39 ☑
      bite W55.31 ☑
      strike W55.32 ☑
    shovel W27.8 ☑
      steam — *see* Accident, transport, construction
        vehicle
    snake (nonvenomous) W59.19 ☑
      bite W59.11 ☑
      crushing W59.13 ☑
      strike W59.12 ☑
    spade W27.1 ☑
    spider (venomous) X58 ☑
    spin-drier W29.2 ☑
    spinning machine W31.89 ☑
    splinter W45.8 ☑
    sports equipment W21.9 ☑
    staple gun (powered) W29.8 ☑
    steam X13.1 ☑

Contact — *continued*
  with — *continued*
    steam — *continued*
      engine W31.3 ☑
      inhalation X13.0 ☑
      pipe X16 ☑
      shovel W31.89 ☑
    stove (hot) (kitchen) X15.0 ☑
    substance, hot NEC X19 ☑
      molten (metal) X18 ☑
    sword W26.1 ☑
      assault X99.2 ☑
      stated as undetermined whether accidental or
        intentional Y28.2 ☑
      suicide (attempt) X78.2 ☑
    tarantula X58 ☑
    thresher W30.0 ☑
    tin can lid W26.8 ☑
    toad W62.1 ☑
    toaster (hot) X15.1 ☑
    tool W27.8 ☑
      hand (not powered) W27.8 ☑
        auger W27.0 ☑
        axe W27.0 ☑
        can opener W27.4 ☑
        chisel W27.0 ☑
        fork W27.4 ☑
        garden W27.1 ☑
        handsaw W27.0 ☑
        hoe W27.1 ☑
        ice-pick W27.4 ☑
        kitchen utensil W27.4 ☑
        manual
          lawn mower W27.1 ☑
          sewing machine W27.8 ☑
        meat grinder W27.4 ☑
        needle (sewing) W27.3 ☑
          hypodermic W46.0 ☑
            contaminated W46.1 ☑
        paper cutter W27.5 ☑
        pitchfork W27.1 ☑
        rake W27.1 ☑
        scissors W27.2 ☑
        screwdriver W27.0 ☑
        specified NEC W27.8 ☑
        workbench W27.0 ☑
      hot X17 ☑
      powered W29.8 ☑
        blender W29.0 ☑
          commercial W31.82 ☑
        can opener W29.0 ☑
          commercial W31.82 ☑
        chainsaw W29.3 ☑
        clothes dryer W29.2 ☑
          commercial W31.82 ☑
        dishwasher W29.2 ☑
          commercial W31.82 ☑
        edger W29.3 ☑
        electric fan W29.2 ☑
          commercial W31.82 ☑
        electric knife W29.1 ☑
        food processor W29.0 ☑
          commercial W31.82 ☑
        garbage disposal W29.0 ☑
          commercial W31.82 ☑
        garden tool W29.3 ☑
        hedge trimmer W29.3 ☑
        ice maker W29.0 ☑
          commercial W31.82 ☑
        kitchen appliance W29.0 ☑
          commercial W31.82 ☑
        lawn mower W28 ☑
        meat grinder W29.0 ☑
          commercial W31.82 ☑
        mixer W29.0 ☑
          commercial W31.82 ☑
        rototiller W29.3 ☑
        sewing machine W29.2 ☑
          commercial W31.82 ☑
        washing machine W29.2 ☑
          commercial W31.82 ☑
    transmission device (belt, cable, chain, gear, pinion,
      shaft) W24.1 ☑
      agricultural operations W30.89 ☑
    turbine (gas) (water-driven) W31.3 ☑
    turkey W61.49 ☑

Contact — *continued*
  with — *continued*
    turkey — *continued*
      peck W61.43 ☑
      strike W61.42 ☑
    turtle (nonvenomous) W59.29 ☑
      bite W59.21 ☑
      strike W59.22 ☑
      terrestrial W59.89 ☑
        bite W59.81 ☑
        crushing W59.83 ☑
        strike W59.82 ☑
    under-cutter W31.0 ☑
    urine — *see* Contact, with, by type of animal
    vehicle
      agricultural use (transport) — *see* Accident,
        transport, agricultural vehicle
        not on public highway W30.81 ☑
      industrial use (transport) — *see* Accident, trans-
        port, industrial vehicle
        not on public highway W31.83 ☑
      off-road use (transport) — *see* Accident, trans-
        port, all-terrain or off-road vehicle
        not on public highway W31.83 ☑
      special construction use (transport) — *see* Acci-
        dent, transport, construction vehicle
        not on public highway W31.83 ☑
    venomous
      animal X58 ☑
      arthropods X58 ☑
      lizard X58 ☑
      marine animal NEC X58 ☑
      marine plant NEC X58 ☑
      millipedes (tropical) X58 ☑
      plant(s) X58 ☑
      snake X58 ☑
      spider X58 ☑
      viper X58 ☑
    washing-machine (powered) W29.2 ☑
    wasp X58 ☑
    weaving-machine W31.89 ☑
    winch W24.0 ☑
      agricultural operations W30.89 ☑
    wire NEC W24.0 ☑
      agricultural operations W30.89 ☑
    wood slivers W45.8 ☑
    yellow jacket X58 ☑
    zebra — *see* Contact, with, hoof stock NEC
  pressure X50.9 ☑
  stress X50.9 ☑
Coup de soleil X32 ☑
Crash
  aircraft (in transit) (powered) V95.9 ☑
    balloon V96.01 ☑
    fixed wing NEC (private) V95.21 ☑
      commercial V95.31 ☑
    glider V96.21 ☑
      hang V96.11 ☑
      powered V95.11 ☑
    helicopter V95.01 ☑
    in war operations — *see* War operations, destruction
      of aircraft
    microlight V95.11 ☑
    nonpowered V96.9 ☑
      specified NEC V96.8 ☑
    powered NEC V95.8 ☑
    stated as
      homicide (attempt) Y08.81 ☑
      suicide (attempt) X83.0 ☑
    ultralight V95.11 ☑
  spacecraft V95.41 ☑
  transport vehicle NEC — *see also* Accident, transport
    V89.9 ☑
    homicide (attempt) Y03.8 ☑
    motor NEC (traffic) V89.2 ☑
      homicide (attempt) Y03.8 ☑
      suicide (attempt) — *see* Suicide, collision
Cruelty (mental) (physical) (sexual) X58 ☑
Crushed (accidentally) X58 ☑
  between objects (moving) (stationary and moving)
    W23.0 ☑
  stationary W23.1 ☑
  by
    alligator W58.03 ☑
    avalanche NEC — *see* Landslide
    cave-in W20.0 ☑

Crushed — *continued*
  by — *continued*
    cave-in — *continued*
      caused by cataclysmic earth surface movement
        — *see* Landslide
    crocodile W58.13 ☑
    crowd or human stampede W52 ☑
    falling
      aircraft V97.39 ☑
        in war operations — *see* War operations, de-
          struction of aircraft
      earth, material W20.0 ☑
        caused by cataclysmic earth surface move-
          ment — *see* Landslide
      object NEC W20.8 ☑
    landslide NEC — *see* Landslide
    lizard (nonvenomous) W59.09 ☑
    machinery — *see* Contact, with, by type of machine
    reptile NEC W59.89 ☑
    snake (nonvenomous) W59.13 ☑
  in
    machinery — *see* Contact, with, by type of machine
Cut, cutting (any part of body) (accidental) — *see also*
  Contact, with, by object or machine
  during medical or surgical treatment as misadventure
    — *see* Index to Diseases and Injuries, Complica-
    tions
  homicide (attempt) — *see* Assault, cutting or piercing
    instrument
  inflicted by other person — *see* Assault, cutting or
    piercing instrument
  legal
    execution — *see* Legal, intervention
    intervention — *see* Legal, intervention, sharp object
  machine NEC — *see also* Contact, with, by type of ma-
    chine W31.9 ☑
  self-inflicted — *see* Suicide, cutting or piercing instru-
    ment
  suicide (attempt) — *see* Suicide, cutting or piercing
    instrument
Cyclone (any injury) X37.1 ☑

D

Decapitation (accidental circumstances) NEC X58 ☑
  homicide X99.9 ☑
  legal execution — *see* Legal, intervention
Dehydration from lack of water X58 ☑
Deprivation X58 ☑
Derailment (accidental)
  railway (rolling stock) (train) (vehicle) (without an-
    tecedent collision) V81.7 ☑
    with antecedent collision — *see* Accident, transport,
      railway vehicle occupant
  streetcar (without antecedent collision) V82.7 ☑
    with antecedent collision — *see* Accident, transport,
      streetcar occupant
Descent
  parachute (voluntary) (without accident to aircraft)
    V97.29 ☑
    due to accident to aircraft — *see* Accident, transport,
      aircraft
Desertion X58 ☑
Destitution X58 ☑
Disability, late effect or sequela of injury — *see* Se-
  quelae
Discharge (accidental)
  airgun W34.010 ☑
    assault X95.01 ☑
    homicide (attempt) X95.01 ☑
    stated as undetermined whether accidental or inten-
      tional Y24.0 ☑
    suicide (attempt) X74.01 ☑
  BB gun — *see* Discharge, airgun
  firearm (accidental) W34.00 ☑
    assault X95.9 ☑
    handgun (pistol) (revolver) W32.0 ☑
      assault X93 ☑
      homicide (attempt) X93 ☑
      legal intervention — *see* Legal, intervention,
        firearm, handgun
      stated as undetermined whether accidental or
        intentional Y22 ☑
      suicide (attempt) X72 ☑
    homicide (attempt) X95.9 ☑
    hunting rifle W33.02 ☑

☑ **Additional Character Required — Refer to the Tabular List for Character Selection**   ▽ **Subterms under main terms may continue to next column or page**

Discharge — *continued*
　firearm — *continued*
　　hunting rifle — *continued*
　　　assault X94.1
　　　homicide (attempt) X94.1 ☑
　　　legal intervention
　　　　injuring
　　　　　bystander Y35.032 ☑
　　　　　law enforcement personnel Y35.031 ☑
　　　　　suspect Y35.033 ☑
　　　　　unspecified person Y35.039 ☑
　　　　stated as undetermined whether accidental or intentional Y23.1 ☑
　　　suicide (attempt) X73.1 ☑
　　larger W33.00 ☑
　　　assault X94.9 ☑
　　　homicide (attempt) X94.9 ☑
　　　hunting rifle — *see* Discharge, firearm, hunting rifle
　　　legal intervention — *see* Legal, intervention, firearm by type of firearm
　　　machine gun — *see* Discharge, firearm, machine gun
　　　shotgun — *see* Discharge, firearm, shotgun
　　　specified NEC W33.09 ☑
　　　　assault X94.8 ☑
　　　　homicide (attempt) X94.8 ☑
　　　　legal intervention
　　　　　injuring
　　　　　　bystander Y35.092 ☑
　　　　　　law enforcement personnel Y35.091 ☑
　　　　　　suspect Y35.093 ☑
　　　　　　unspecified person Y35.099 ☑
　　　　　stated as undetermined whether accidental or intentional Y23.8 ☑
　　　　suicide (attempt) X73.8 ☑
　　　stated as undetermined whether accidental or intentional Y23.9 ☑
　　　suicide (attempt) X73.9 ☑
　　legal intervention
　　　injuring
　　　　bystander Y35.002 ☑
　　　　law enforcement personnel Y35.001 ☑
　　　　suspect Y35.03 ☑
　　　　unspecified person Y35.009 ☑
　　　using rubber bullet
　　　　injuring
　　　　　bystander Y35.042 ☑
　　　　　law enforcement personnel Y35.041 ☑
　　　　　suspect Y35.043 ☑
　　　　　unspecified person Y35.049 ☑
　　machine gun W33.03 ☑
　　　assault X94.2 ☑
　　　homicide (attempt) X94.2 ☑
　　　legal intervention — *see* Legal, intervention, firearm, machine gun
　　　stated as undetermined whether accidental or intentional Y23.3 ☑
　　　suicide (attempt) X73.2 ☑
　　pellet gun — *see* Discharge, airgun
　　shotgun W33.01 ☑
　　　assault X94.0 ☑
　　　homicide (attempt) X94.0 ☑
　　　legal intervention — *see* Legal, intervention, firearm, specified NEC
　　　stated as undetermined whether accidental or intentional Y23.0 ☑
　　　suicide (attempt) X73.0 ☑
　　specified NEC W34.09 ☑
　　　assault X95.8 ☑
　　　homicide (attempt) X95.8 ☑
　　　legal intervention — *see* Legal, intervention, firearm, specified NEC
　　　stated as undetermined whether accidental or intentional Y24.8 ☑
　　　suicide (attempt) X74.8 ☑
　　stated as undetermined whether accidental or intentional Y24.9 ☑
　　suicide (attempt) X74.9 ☑
　　Very pistol W34.09 ☑
　　　assault X95.8 ☑
　　　homicide (attempt) X95.8 ☑
　　　stated as undetermined whether accidental or intentional Y24.8 ☑
　　　suicide (attempt) X74.8 ☑

Discharge — *continued*
　firework(s) W39 ☑
　　stated as undetermined whether accidental or intentional Y25 ☑
　gas-operated gun NEC W34.018 ☑
　　airgun — *see* Discharge, airgun
　　assault X95.09 ☑
　　homicide (attempt) X95.09 ☑
　　paintball gun — *see* Discharge, paintball gun
　　stated as undetermined whether accidental or intentional Y24.8 ☑
　　suicide (attempt) X74.09 ☑
　gun NEC — *see also* Discharge, firearm NEC
　　air — *see* Discharge, airgun
　　BB — *see* Discharge, airgun
　　for single hand use — *see* Discharge, firearm, handgun
　　hand — *see* Discharge, firearm, handgun
　　machine — *see* Discharge, firearm, machine gun
　　other specified — *see* Discharge, firearm NEC
　　paintball — *see* Discharge, paintball gun
　　pellet — *see* Discharge, airgun
　handgun — *see* Discharge, firearm, handgun
　machine gun — *see* Discharge, firearm, machine gun
　paintball gun W34.011 ☑
　　assault X95.02 ☑
　　homicide (attempt) X95.02 ☑
　　stated as undetermined whether accidental or intentional Y24.8 ☑
　　suicide (attempt) X74.02 ☑
　pistol — *see* Discharge, firearm, handgun
　　flare — *see* Discharge, firearm, Very pistol
　　pellet — *see* Discharge, airgun
　　Very — *see* Discharge, firearm, Very pistol
　revolver — *see* Discharge, firearm, handgun
　rifle (hunting) — *see* Discharge, firearm, hunting rifle
　shotgun — *see* Discharge, firearm, shotgun
　spring-operated gun NEC W34.018 ☑
　　assault X95.09 ☑
　　homicide (attempt) X95.09 ☑
　　stated as undetermined whether accidental or intentional Y24.8 ☑
　　suicide (attempt) X74.09 ☑

Disease
　Andes W94.11 ☑
　aviator's — *see* Air, pressure
　range W94.11 ☑
Diver's disease, palsy, paralysis, squeeze — *see* Air, pressure
Diving (into water) — *see* Accident, diving
Dog bite W54.0 ☑
Dragged by transport vehicle NEC — *see also* Accident, transport V09.9 ☑
Drinking poison (accidental) — *see* Table of Drugs and Chemicals
Dropped (accidentally) **while being carried or supported by other person** W04 ☑
Drowning (accidental) W74 ☑
　assault X92.9 ☑
　due to
　　accident (to)
　　　machinery — *see* Contact, with, by type of machine
　　　watercraft V90.89 ☑
　　　　burning V90.29 ☑
　　　　　powered V90.23 ☑
　　　　　　fishing boat V90.22 ☑
　　　　　　jetskis V90.23 ☑
　　　　　　merchant ship V90.20 ☑
　　　　　　passenger ship V90.21 ☑
　　　　　unpowered V90.28 ☑
　　　　　　canoe V90.25 ☑
　　　　　　inflatable V90.26 ☑
　　　　　　kayak V90.25 ☑
　　　　　　sailboat V90.24 ☑
　　　　　　water skis V90.27 ☑
　　　　crushed V90.39 ☑
　　　　　powered V90.33 ☑
　　　　　　fishing boat V90.32 ☑
　　　　　　jetskis V90.33 ☑
　　　　　　merchant ship V90.30 ☑
　　　　　　passenger ship V90.31 ☑
　　　　　unpowered V90.38 ☑
　　　　　　canoe V90.35 ☑
　　　　　　inflatable V90.36 ☑
　　　　　　kayak V90.35 ☑

Drowning — *continued*
　due to — *continued*
　　accident — *continued*
　　　watercraft — *continued*
　　　　crushed — *continued*
　　　　　unpowered — *continued*
　　　　　　sailboat V90.34 ☑
　　　　　　water skis V90.37 ☑
　　　　overturning V90.09 ☑
　　　　　powered V90.03 ☑
　　　　　　fishing boat V90.02 ☑
　　　　　　jetskis V90.03 ☑
　　　　　　merchant ship V90.00 ☑
　　　　　　passenger ship V90.01 ☑
　　　　　unpowered V90.08 ☑
　　　　　　canoe V90.05 ☑
　　　　　　inflatable V90.06 ☑
　　　　　　kayak V90.05 ☑
　　　　　　sailboat V90.04 ☑
　　　　sinking V90.19 ☑
　　　　　powered V90.13 ☑
　　　　　　fishing boat V90.12 ☑
　　　　　　jetskis V90.13 ☑
　　　　　　merchant ship V90.10 ☑
　　　　　　passenger ship V90.11 ☑
　　　　　unpowered V90.18 ☑
　　　　　　canoe V90.15 ☑
　　　　　　inflatable V90.16 ☑
　　　　　　kayak V90.15 ☑
　　　　　　sailboat V90.14 ☑
　　　　specified type NEC V90.89 ☑
　　　　　powered V90.83 ☑
　　　　　　fishing boat V90.82 ☑
　　　　　　jetskis V90.83 ☑
　　　　　　merchant ship V90.80 ☑
　　　　　　passenger ship V90.81 ☑
　　　　　unpowered V90.88 ☑
　　　　　　canoe V90.85 ☑
　　　　　　inflatable V90.86 ☑
　　　　　　kayak V90.85 ☑
　　　　　　sailboat V90.84 ☑
　　　　　　water skis V90.87 ☑
　　avalanche — *see* Landslide
　　cataclysmic
　　　earth surface movement NEC — *see* Forces of nature, earth movement
　　　storm — *see* Forces of nature, cataclysmic storm
　　cloudburst X37.8 ☑
　　cyclone X37.1 ☑
　　fall overboard (from) V92.09 ☑
　　　powered craft V92.03 ☑
　　　　ferry boat V92.01 ☑
　　　　fishing boat V92.02 ☑
　　　　jetskis V92.03 ☑
　　　　liner V92.01 ☑
　　　　merchant ship V92.00 ☑
　　　　passenger ship V92.01 ☑
　　resulting from
　　　accident to watercraft — *see* Drowning, due to, accident to, watercraft
　　　being washed overboard (from) V92.29 ☑
　　　　powered craft V92.23 ☑
　　　　　ferry boat V92.21 ☑
　　　　　fishing boat V92.22 ☑
　　　　　jetskis V92.23 ☑
　　　　　liner V92.21 ☑
　　　　　merchant ship V92.20 ☑
　　　　　passenger ship V92.21 ☑
　　　　unpowered craft V92.28 ☑
　　　　　canoe V92.25 ☑
　　　　　inflatable V92.26 ☑
　　　　　kayak V92.25 ☑
　　　　　sailboat V92.24 ☑
　　　　　surf-board V92.28 ☑
　　　　　water skis V92.27 ☑
　　　　　windsurfer V92.28 ☑
　　　motion of watercraft V92.19 ☑
　　　　powered craft V92.13 ☑
　　　　　ferry boat V92.11 ☑
　　　　　fishing boat V92.12 ☑
　　　　　jetskis V92.13 ☑
　　　　　liner V92.11 ☑
　　　　　merchant ship V92.10 ☑
　　　　　passenger ship V92.11 ☑
　　　　unpowered craft
　　　　　canoe V92.15 ☑

Drowning — continued
  due to — continued
    fall overboard — continued
      resulting from — continued
        motion of watercraft — continued
          unpowered craft — continued
            inflatable V92.16 ☑
            kayak V92.15 ☑
            sailboat V92.14 ☑
          unpowered craft V92.08 ☑
            canoe V92.05 ☑
            inflatable V92.06 ☑
            kayak V92.05 ☑
            sailboat V92.04 ☑
            surf-board V92.08 ☑
            water skis V92.07 ☑
            windsurfer V92.08 ☑
      hurricane X37.0 ☑
      jumping into water from watercraft (involved in accident) — see also Drowning, due to, accident to, watercraft
        without accident to or on watercraft W16.711 ☑
      tidal wave NEC — see Forces of nature, tidal wave
      torrential rain X37.8 ☑
  following
    fall
      into
        bathtub W16.211 ☑
        bucket W16.221 ☑
        fountain — see Drowning, following, fall, into, water, specified NEC
        quarry — see Drowning, following, fall, into, water, specified NEC
        reservoir — see Drowning, following, fall, into, water, specified NEC
        swimming-pool W16.011 ☑
          stated as undetermined whether accidental or intentional Y21.3 ☑
          striking
            bottom W16.021 ☑
            wall W16.031 ☑
          suicide (attempt) X71.2 ☑
        water NOS W16.41 ☑
          natural (lake) (open sea) (river) (stream) (pond) W16.111 ☑
            striking
              bottom W16.121 ☑
              side W16.131 ☑
          specified NEC W16.311 ☑
            striking
              bottom W16.321 ☑
              wall W16.331 ☑
      overboard NEC — see Drowning, due to, fall overboard
    jump or dive
      from boat W16.711 ☑
        striking bottom W16.721 ☑
      into
        fountain — see Drowning, following, jump or dive, into, water, specified NEC
        quarry — see Drowning, following, jump or dive, into, water, specified NEC
        reservoir — see Drowning, following, jump or dive, into, water, specified NEC
        swimming-pool W16.511 ☑
          striking
            bottom W16.521 ☑
            wall W16.531 ☑
          suicide (attempt) X71.2 ☑
        water NOS W16.91 ☑
          natural (lake) (open sea) (river) (stream) (pond) W16.611 ☑
          specified NEC W16.811 ☑
            bottom W16.821 ☑
            striking
              bottom W16.821 ☑
              wall W16.831 ☑
            striking
              bottom W16.821 ☑
              wall W16.831 ☑
          striking bottom W16.621 ☑
  homicide (attempt) X92.9 ☑
  in
    bathtub (accidental) W65 ☑
      assault X92.0 ☑
      following fall W16.211 ☑

Drowning — continued
  in — continued
    bathtub — continued
      following fall — continued
        stated as undetermined whether accidental or intentional Y21.1 ☑
      stated as undetermined whether accidental or intentional Y21.0 ☑
      suicide (attempt) X71.0 ☑
    lake — see Drowning, in, natural water
    natural water (lake) (open sea) (river) (stream) (pond) W69 ☑
      assault X92.3
      following
        dive or jump W16.611 ☑
          striking bottom W16.621 ☑
        fall W16.111 ☑
          striking
            bottom W16.121 ☑
            side W16.131 ☑
      stated as undetermined whether accidental or intentional Y21.4 ☑
      suicide (attempt) X71.3 ☑
    quarry — see Drowning, in, specified place NEC
    quenching tank — see Drowning, in, specified place NEC
    reservoir — see Drowning, in, specified place NEC
    river — see Drowning, in, natural water
    sea — see Drowning, in, natural water
    specified place NEC W73 ☑
      assault X92.8 ☑
      following
        dive or jump W16.811 ☑
          striking
            bottom W16.821 ☑
            wall W16.831 ☑
        fall W16.311 ☑
          striking
            bottom W16.321 ☑
            wall W16.331 ☑
      stated as undetermined whether accidental or intentional Y21.8 ☑
      suicide (attempt) X71.8 ☑
    stream — see Drowning, in, natural water
    swimming-pool W67 ☑
      assault X92.1 ☑
        following fall X92.2 ☑
      following
        dive or jump W16.511 ☑
          striking
            bottom W16.521 ☑
            wall W16.531 ☑
        fall W16.011 ☑
          striking
            bottom W16.021 ☑
            wall W16.031 ☑
      stated as undetermined whether accidental or intentional Y21.2 ☑
        following fall Y21.3 ☑
      suicide (attempt) X71.1 ☑
        following fall X71.2 ☑
    war operations — see War operations, restriction of airway
  resulting from accident to watercraft — see Drowning, due to, accident, watercraft
  self-inflicted X71.9 ☑
  stated as undetermined whether accidental or intentional Y21.9 ☑
  suicide (attempt) X71.9 ☑

E

Earth falling (on) W20.0 ☑
  caused by cataclysmic earth surface movement or eruption — see Landslide
Earth (surface) movement NEC — see Forces of nature, earth movement
Earthquake (any injury) X34 ☑
Effect(s) (adverse) of
  air pressure (any) — see Air, pressure
  cold, excessive (exposure to) — see Exposure, cold
  heat (excessive) — see Heat
  hot place (weather) — see Heat
  insolation X30 ☑
  late — see Sequelae
  motion — see Motion

Effect(s) (adverse) of — continued
  nuclear explosion or weapon in war operations — see War operations, nuclear weapon
  radiation — see Radiation
  travel — see Travel
Electric shock (accidental) (by) (in) — see Exposure, electric current
Electrocution (accidental) — see Exposure, electric current
Endotracheal tube wrongly placed during anesthetic procedure
Entanglement
  in
    bed linen, causing suffocation T71 ☑
    wheel of pedal cycle V19.88 ☑
Entry of foreign body or material — see Foreign body
Environmental pollution related condition — see category Z57 ☑
Execution, legal (any method) — see Legal, intervention
Exhaustion
  cold — see Exposure, cold
  due to excessive exertion — see also Overexertion X50.9 ☑
  heat — see Heat
Explosion (accidental) (of) (with secondary fire) W40.9 ☑
  acetylene W40.1 ☑
  aerosol can W36.1 ☑
  air tank (compressed) (in machinery) W36.2 ☑
  aircraft (in transit) (powered) NEC V95.9 ☑
    balloon V96.05 ☑
    fixed wing NEC (private) V95.25 ☑
      commercial V95.35 ☑
    glider V96.25 ☑
      hang V96.15 ☑
      powered V95.15 ☑
    helicopter V95.05 ☑
    in war operations — see War operations, destruction of aircraft
    microlight V95.15 ☑
    nonpowered V96.9 ☑
      specified NEC V96.8 ☑
    powered NEC V95.8 ☑
    stated as
      homicide (attempt) Y03.8 ☑
      suicide (attempt) X83.0 ☑
    ultralight V95.15 ☑
  anesthetic gas in operating room W40.1 ☑
  antipersonnel bomb W40.8 ☑
    assault X96.0 ☑
    homicide (attempt) X96.0 ☑
    suicide (attempt) X75 ☑
  assault X96.9 ☑
  bicycle tire W37.0 ☑
  blasting (cap) (materials) W40.0 ☑
  boiler (machinery), not on transport vehicle W35 ☑
    on watercraft — see Explosion, in, watercraft
  butane W40.1 ☑
  caused by other person X96.9 ☑
  coal gas W40.1 ☑
  detonator W40.0 ☑
  dump (munitions) W40.8 ☑
  dynamite W40.0 ☑
    in
      assault X96.8 ☑
      homicide (attempt) X96.8 ☑
      legal intervention
        injuring
          bystander Y35.112 ☑
          law enforcement personnel Y35.111 ☑
          suspect Y35.113 ☑
          unspecified person Y35.119 ☑
      suicide (attempt) X75 ☑
  explosive (material) W40.9 ☑
    gas W40.1 ☑
    in blasting operation W40.0 ☑
    specified NEC W40.8 ☑
      in
        assault X96.8 ☑
        homicide (attempt) X96.8 ☑
        legal intervention
          injuring
            bystander Y35.192 ☑
            law enforcement personnel Y35.191 ☑
            suspect Y35.193 ☑
            unspecified person Y35.199

☑ Additional Character Required — Refer to the Tabular List for Character Selection
▽ Subterms under main terms may continue to next column or page

Explosion — *continued*
  explosive — *continued*
    specified — *continued*
      in — *continued*
        suicide (attempt) X75 ☑
  factory (munitions) W40.8 ☑
  fertilizer bomb W40.8 ☑
    assault X96.3 ☑
    homicide (attempt) X96.3 ☑
    suicide (attempt) X75 ☑
  firearm (parts) NEC W34.19 ☑
    airgun W34.110 ☑
    BB gun W34.110 ☑
    gas, air or spring-operated gun NEC W34.118 ☑
    hangun W32.1 ☑
    hunting rifle W33.12 ☑
    larger firearm W33.10 ☑
      specified NEC W33.19 ☑
    machine gun W33.13 ☑
    paintball gun W34.111 ☑
    pellet gun W34.110 ☑
    shotgun W33.11 ☑
    Very pistol [flare] W34.19 ☑
  fire-damp W40.1 ☑
  fireworks W39 ☑
  gas (coal) (explosive) W40.1 ☑
    cylinder W36.9 ☑
      aerosol can W36.1 ☑
      air tank W36.2 ☑
      pressurized W36.3 ☑
      specified NEC W36.8 ☑
  gasoline (fumes) (tank) not in moving motor vehicle
    W40.1 ☑
    bomb W40.8 ☑
      assault X96.1 ☑
      homicide (attempt) X96.1 ☑
      suicide (attempt) X75 ☑
    in motor vehicle — *see* Accident, transport, by type
      of vehicle
  grain store W40.8 ☑
  grenade W40.8 ☑
    in
      assault X96.8 ☑
      homicide (attempt) X96.8 ☑
      legal intervention
        injuring
          bystander Y35.192 ☑
          law enforcement personnel Y35.191 ☑
          suspect Y35.193 ☑
          unspecified person Y35.199 ☑
      suicide (attempt) X75 ☑
  handgun (parts) — *see* Explosion, firearm, hangun
    (parts)
  homicide (attempt) X96.9 ☑
    antipersonnel bomb — *see* Explosion, antipersonnel
      bomb
    fertilizer bomb — *see* Explosion, fertilizer bomb
    gasoline bomb — *see* Explosion, gasoline bomb
    letter bomb — *see* Explosion, letter bomb
    pipe bomb — *see* Explosion, pipe bomb
    specified NEC X96.8 ☑
  hose, pressurized W37.8 ☑
  hot water heater, tank (in machinery) W35 ☑
    on watercraft — *see* Explosion, in, watercraft
  in, on
    dump W40.8 ☑
    factory W40.8 ☑
    mine (of explosive gases) NEC W40.1 ☑
    watercraft V93.59 ☑
      powered craft V93.53 ☑
        ferry boat V93.51 ☑
        fishing boat V93.52 ☑
        jetskis V93.53 ☑
        liner V93.51 ☑
        merchant ship V93.50 ☑
        passenger ship V93.51 ☑
        sailboat V93.54 ☑
  letter bomb W40.8 ☑
    assault X96.2 ☑
    homicide (attempt) X96.2 ☑
    suicide (attempt) X75 ☑
  machinery — *see also* Contact, with, by type of ma-
    chine
    on board watercraft — *see* Explosion, in, watercraft
    pressure vessel — *see* Explosion, by type of vessel
  methane W40.1 ☑

Explosion — *continued*
  mine W40.1 ☑
  missile NEC W40.8 ☑
  mortar bomb W40.8 ☑
    in
      assault X96.8 ☑
      homicide (attempt) X96.8 ☑
      legal intervention
        injuring
          bystander Y35.192 ☑
          law enforcement personnel Y35.191 ☑
          suspect Y35.193 ☑
          unspecified person Y35.199 ☑
      suicide (attempt) X75 ☑
  munitions (dump) (factory) W40.8 ☑
  pipe, pressurized W37.8 ☑
    bomb W40.8 ☑
      assault X96.4 ☑
      homicide (attempt) X96.4 ☑
      suicide (attempt) X75 ☑
  pressure, pressurized
    cooker W38 ☑
    gas tank (in machinery) W36.3 ☑
    hose W37.8 ☑
    pipe W37.8 ☑
    specified device NEC W38 ☑
    tire W37.8 ☑
      bicycle W37.0 ☑
    vessel (in machinery) W38 ☑
  propane W40.1 ☑
  self-inflicted X75 ☑
  shell (artillery) NEC W40.8 ☑
    during war operations — *see* War operations, explo-
      sion
    in
      legal intervention
        injuring
          bystander Y35.122 ☑
          law enforcement personnel Y35.121 ☑
          suspect Y35.123 ☑
          unspecified person Y35.129 ☑
    war — *see* War operations, explosion
  spacecraft V95.45 ☑
  stated as undetermined whether accidental or inten-
    tional Y25 ☑
  steam or water lines (in machinery) W37.8 ☑
  stove W40.9 ☑
  suicide (attempt) X75 ☑
  tire, pressurized W37.8 ☑
    bicycle W37.0 ☑
  undetermined whether accidental or intentional Y25 ☑
  vehicle tire NEC W37.8 ☑
    bicycle W37.0 ☑
  war operations — *see* War operations, explosion

Exposure (to) X58 ☑
  air pressure change — *see* Air, pressure
  cold (accidental) (excessive) (extreme) (natural) (place)
    X31 ☑
    assault Y08.89 ☑
    due to
      man-made conditions W93.8 ☑
        dry ice (contact) W93.01 ☑
          inhalation W93.02 ☑
        liquid air (contact) (hydrogen) (nitrogen)
          W93.11 ☑
          inhalation W93.12 ☑
        refrigeration unit (deep freeze) W93.2 ☑
        suicide (attempt) X83.2 ☑
      weather (conditions) X31 ☑
    homicide (attempt) Y08.89 ☑
    self-inflicted X83.2 ☑
  due to abandonment or neglect X58 ☑
  electric current W86.8 ☑
    appliance (faulty) W86.8 ☑
      domestic W86.0 ☑
    caused by other person Y08.89 ☑
    conductor (faulty) W86.1 ☑
    control apparatus (faulty) W86.1 ☑
    electric power generating plant, distribution station
      W86.1 ☑
    electroshock gun — *see* Exposure, electric current,
      taser
    high-voltage cable W85 ☑
    homicide (attempt) Y08.89 ☑
    legal execution — *see* Legal, intervention, specified
      means NEC

Exposure — *continued*
  electric current — *continued*
    lightning — *see* subcategory T75.0 ☑
    live rail W86.8 ☑
    misadventure in medical or surgical procedure in
      electroshock therapy Y63.4
    motor (electric) (faulty) W86.8 ☑
      domestic W86.0 ☑
    self-inflicted X83.1 ☑
    specified NEC W86.8 ☑
      domestic W86.0 ☑
    stun gun — *see* Exposure, electric current, taser
    suicide (attempt) X83.1 ☑
    taser W86.8 ☑
      assault Y08.89 ☑
      legal intervention — *see* category Y35 ☑
      self-harm (intentional) X83.8 ☑
      undetermined intent Y33 ☑
    third rail W86.8 ☑
    transformer (faulty) W86.1 ☑
    transmission lines W85 ☑
  environmental tobacco smoke X58 ☑
  excessive
    cold — *see* Exposure, cold
    heat (natural) NEC X30 ☑
      man-made W92 ☑
  factor(s) NOS X58 ☑
    environmental NEC X58 ☑
    man-made NEC W99 ☑
    natural NEC — *see* Forces of nature
    specified NEC X58 ☑
  fire, flames (accidental) X08.8 ☑
    assault X97 ☑
    campfire — *see* Exposure, fire, controlled, not in
      building
    controlled (in)
      with ignition (of) clothing — *see also* Ignition,
        clothes X06.2 ☑
        nightwear X05 ☑
      bonfire — *see* Exposure, fire, controlled, not in
        building
      brazier (in building or structure) — *see also* Ex-
        posure, fire, controlled, building
        not in building or structure — *see* Exposure,
          fire, controlled, not in building
      building or structure X02.0 ☑
        with
          fall from building X02.3 ☑
          from building X02.5 ☑
          injury due to building collapse X02.2 ☑
          smoke inhalation X02.1 ☑
        hit by object from building X02.4 ☑
        specified mode of injury NEC X02.8 ☑
      fireplace, furnace or stove — *see* Exposure, fire,
        controlled, building
      not in building or structure X03.0 ☑
        with
          fall X03.3 ☑
          smoke inhalation X03.1 ☑
        hit by object X03.4 ☑
        specified mode of injury NEC X03.8 ☑
      trash — *see* Exposure, fire, controlled, not in
        building
    fireplace — *see* Exposure, fire, controlled, building
    fittings or furniture (in building or structure) (uncon-
      trolled) — *see* Exposure, fire, uncontrolled,
      building
    forest (uncontrolled) — *see* Exposure, fire, uncon-
      trolled, not in building
    grass (uncontrolled) — *see* Exposure, fire, uncon-
      trolled, not in building
    hay (uncontrolled) — *see* Exposure, fire, uncon-
      trolled, not in building
    homicide (attempt) X97 ☑
    ignition of highly flammable material X04 ☑
    in, of, on, starting in
      machinery — *see* Contact, with, by type of ma-
        chine
      motor vehicle (in motion) — *see also* Accident,
        transport, occupant by type of vehicle
        V87.8 ☑
        with collision — *see* Collision
      railway rolling stock, train, vehicle V81.81 ☑
        with collision — *see* Accident, transport, rail-
          way vehicle occupant
      street car (in motion) V82.8 ☑

Exposure — continued
  fire, flames — continued
    in, of, on, starting in — continued
      street car — continued
        with collision — see Accident, transport,
          streetcar occupant
      transport vehicle NEC — see also Accident,
        transport
        with collision — see Collision
      war operations — see also War operations, fire
        from nuclear explosion — see War operations,
          nuclear weapons
      watercraft (in transit) (not in transit) V91.09 ☑
        localized — see Burn, on board watercraft,
          due to, fire on board
        powered craft V91.03 ☑
          ferry boat V91.01 ☑
          fishing boat V91.02 ☑
          jet skis V91.03 ☑
          liner V91.01 ☑
          merchant ship V91.00 ☑
          passenger ship V91.01 ☑
        unpowered craft V91.08 ☑
          canoe V91.05 ☑
          inflatable V91.06 ☑
          kayak V91.05 ☑
          sailboat V91.04 ☑
          surf-board V91.08 ☑
          waterskis V91.07 ☑
          windsurfer V91.08 ☑
    lumber (uncontrolled) — see Exposure, fire, uncon-
      trolled, not in building
    mine (uncontrolled) — see Exposure, fire, uncon-
      trolled, not in building
    prairie (uncontrolled) — see Exposure, fire, uncon-
      trolled, not in building
    resulting from
      explosion — see Explosion
      lightning X08.8 ☑
    self-inflicted X76 ☑
    specified NEC X08.8 ☑
    started by other person X97 ☑
    stated as undetermined whether accidental or inten-
      tional Y26 ☑
    stove — see Exposure, fire, controlled, building
    suicide (attempt) X76 ☑
    tunnel (uncontrolled) — see Exposure, fire, uncon-
      trolled, not in building
    uncontrolled
      in building or structure X00.0 ☑
        with
          fall from building X00.3 ☑
          injury due to building collapse X00.2 ☑
          jump from building X00.5 ☑
          smoke inhalation X00.1 ☑
        bed X08.00 ☑
          due to
            cigarette X08.01 ☑
            specified material NEC X08.09 ☑
        furniture NEC X08.20 ☑
          due to
            cigarette X08.21 ☑
            specified material NEC X08.29 ☑
        hit by object from building X00.4 ☑
        sofa X08.10 ☑
          due to
            cigarette X08.11 ☑
            specified material NEC X08.19 ☑
        specified mode of injury NEC X00.8 ☑
      not in building or structure (any) X01.0 ☑
        with
          fall X01.3 ☑
          smoke inhalation X01.1 ☑
        hit by object X01.4 ☑
        specified mode of injury NEC X01.8 ☑
      undetermined whether accidental or intentional
        Y26 ☑
  forces of nature NEC — see Forces of nature
  G-forces (abnormal) W49.9 ☑
  gravitational forces (abnormal) W49.9 ☑
  heat (natural) NEC — see Heat
  high-pressure jet (hydraulic) (pneumatic) W49.9 ☑
  hydraulic jet W49.9 ☑
  inanimate mechanical force W49.9 ☑
  jet, high-pressure (hydraulic) (pneumatic) W49.9 ☑
  lightning — see subcategory T75.0 ☑

Exposure — continued
  lightning — see subcategory — continued
    causing fire — see Exposure, fire
  mechanical forces NEC W49.9 ☑
    animate NEC W64 ☑
    inanimate NEC W49.9 ☑
  noise W42.9 ☑
    supersonic W42.0 ☑
  noxious substance — see Table of Drugs and Chemicals
  pneumatic jet W49.9 ☑
  prolonged in deep-freeze unit or refrigerator W93.2 ☑
  radiation — see Radiation
  smoke — see also Exposure, fire
    tobacco, second hand Z77.22
  specified factors NEC X58 ☑
  sunlight X32 ☑
    man-made (sun lamp) W89.8 ☑
      tanning bed W89.1 ☑
  supersonic waves W42.0 ☑
  transmission line(s), electric W85 ☑
  vibration W49.9 ☑
  waves
    infrasound W49.9 ☑
    sound W42.9 ☑
    supersonic W42.0 ☑
  weather NEC — see Forces of nature

External cause status Y99.9 ☑
  child assisting in compensated work for family Y99.8
  civilian activity done for financial or other compensa-
    tion Y99.0
  civilian activity done for income or pay Y99.0
  family member assisting in compensated work for
    other family member Y99.8
  hobby not done for income Y99.8
  leisure activity Y99.8
  military activity Y99.1
  off-duty activity of military personnel Y99.8
  recreation or sport not for income or while a student
    Y99.8
  specified NEC Y99.8
  student activity Y99.8
  volunteer activity Y99.2

F

Factors, supplemental
  alcohol
    blood level
      less than 20mg/100ml Y90.0
      presence in blood, level not specified Y90.9
      20-39mg/100ml Y90.1
      40-59mg/100ml Y90.2
      60-79mg/100ml Y90.3
      80-99mg/100ml Y90.4
      100-119mg/100ml Y90.5
      120-199mg/100ml Y90.6
      200-239mg/100ml Y90.7
      240mg/100ml or more Y90.8
    presence in blood, but level not specified Y90.9
  environmental-pollution-related condition- see Z57 ☑
  nosocomial condition Y95
  work-related condition Y99.0

Failure
  in suture or ligature during surgical procedure Y65.2
  mechanical, of instrument or apparatus (any) (during
    any medical or surgical procedure) Y65.8
  sterile precautions (during medical and surgical care)
    — see Misadventure, failure, sterile precautions,
    by type of procedure
  to
    introduce tube or instrument Y65.4
      endotracheal tube during anesthesia Y65.3
    make curve (transport vehicle) NEC — see Accident,
      transport
    remove tube or instrument Y65.4

Fall, falling (accidental) W19 ☑
  building W20.1 ☑
    burning (uncontrolled fire) X00.3 ☑
  down
    embankment W17.81 ☑
    escalator W10.0 ☑
    hill W17.81 ☑
    ladder W11 ☑
    ramp W10.2 ☑
    stairs, steps W10.9 ☑

Fall, falling — continued
  due to
    bumping against
      object W18.00 ☑
        sharp glass W18.02 ☑
        specified NEC W18.09 ☑
        sports equipment W18.01 ☑
      person W03 ☑
        due to ice or snow W00.0 ☑
        on pedestrian conveyance — see Accident,
          transport, pedestrian, conveyance
    collision with another person W03 ☑
      due to ice or snow W00.0 ☑
      involving pedestrian conveyance — see Acci-
        dent, transport, pedestrian, conveyance
    grocery cart tipping over W17.82 ☑
    ice or snow W00.9 ☑
      from one level to another W00.2 ☑
      on stairs or steps W00.1 ☑
      involving pedestrian conveyance — see Acci-
        dent, transport, pedestrian, conveyance
      on same level W00.0 ☑
    slipping (on moving sidewalk) W01.0 ☑
      with subsequent striking against object
        W01.10 ☑
        furniture W01.190 ☑
        sharp object W01.119 ☑
          glass W01.110 ☑
          power tool or machine W01.111 ☑
          specified NEC W01.118 ☑
        specified NEC W01.198 ☑
    striking against
      object W18.00 ☑
        sharp glass W18.02 ☑
        specified NEC W18.09 ☑
        sports equipment W18.01 ☑
      person W03 ☑
        due to ice or snow W00.0 ☑
        on pedestrian conveyance — see Accident,
          transport, pedestrian, conveyance
  earth (with asphyxia or suffocation (by pressure)) —
    see Earth, falling
  from, off, out of
    aircraft NEC (with accident to aircraft NEC) V97.0 ☑
      while boarding or alighting V97.1 ☑
    balcony W13.0 ☑
    bed W06 ☑
    boat, ship, watercraft NEC (with drowning or sub-
      mersion) — see Drowning, due to, fall over-
      board
      with hitting bottom or object V94.0 ☑
    bridge W13.1 ☑
    building W13.9 ☑
      burning (uncontrolled fire) X00.3 ☑
    cavity W17.2 ☑
    chair W07 ☑
    cherry picker W17.89 ☑
    cliff W15 ☑
    dock W17.4 ☑
    embankment W17.81 ☑
    escalator W10.0 ☑
    flagpole W13.8 ☑
    furniture NEC W08 ☑
    grocery cart W17.82 ☑
    haystack W17.89 ☑
    high place NEC W17.89 ☑
      stated as undetermined whether accidental or
        intentional Y30 ☑
    hole W17.2 ☑
    incline W10.2 ☑
    ladder W11 ☑
    lifting device W17.89 ☑
    machine, machinery — see also Contact, with, by
      type of machine
      not in operation W17.89 ☑
    manhole W17.1 ☑
    mobile elevated work platform [MEWP] W17.89 ☑
    motorized mobility scooter W05.2 ☑
    one level to another NEC W17.89 ☑
      intentional, purposeful, suicide (attempt) X80 ☑
      stated as undetermined whether accidental or
        intentional Y30 ☑
    pit W17.2 ☑
    playground equipment W09.8 ☑
      jungle gym W09.2 ☑
      slide W09.0 ☑

Fall, falling — *continued*
  from, off, out of — *continued*
    playground equipment — *continued*
      swing W09.1 ☑
    quarry W17.89 ☑
    railing W13.9 ☑
    ramp W10.2 ☑
    roof W13.2 ☑
    scaffolding W12 ☑
    scooter (nonmotorized) W05.1 ☑
      motorized mobility W05.2 ☑
    sky lift W17.89 ☑
    stairs, steps W10.9 ☑
      curb W10.1 ☑
      due to ice or snow W00.1 ☑
      escalator W10.0 ☑
      incline W10.2 ☑
      ramp W10.2 ☑
      sidewalk curb W10.1 ☑
      specified NEC W10.8 ☑
      standing
        electric scooter V00.841 ☑
        micro-mobility pedestrian conveyance V00.848 ☑
    stepladder W11 ☑
    storm drain W17.1 ☑
    streetcar NEC V82.6 ☑
      while boarding or alighting V82.4 ☑
      with antecedent collision — *see* Accident, transport, streetcar occupant
    structure NEC W13.8 ☑
      burning (uncontrolled fire) X00.3 ☑
    table W08 ☑
    toilet W18.11 ☑
      with subsequent striking against object W18.12 ☑
    train NEC V81.6 ☑
      during derailment (without antecedent collision) V81.7 ☑
      with antecedent collision — *see* Accident, transport, railway vehicle occupant
      while boarding or alighting V81.4 ☑
    transport vehicle after collision — *see* Accident, transport, by type of vehicle, collision
    tree W14 ☑
    vehicle (in motion) NEC — *see also* Accident, transport V89.9 ☑
      motor NEC — *see also* Accident, transport, occupant, by type of vehicle V87.8 ☑
      stationary W17.89 ☑
      while boarding or alighting — *see* Accident, transport, by type of vehicle, while boarding or alighting
    viaduct W13.8 ☑
    wall W13.8 ☑
    watercraft — *see also* Drowning, due to, fall overboard
      with hitting bottom or object V94.0 ☑
    well W17.0 ☑
    wheelchair, non-moving W05.0 ☑
      powered — *see* Accident, transport, pedestrian, conveyance occupant, specified type NEC
    window W13.4 ☑
  in, on
    aircraft NEC V97.0 ☑
      while boarding or alighting V97.1 ☑
      with accident to aircraft V97.0 ☑
    bathtub (empty) W18.2 ☑
      filled W16.212 ☑
        causing drowning W16.211 ☑
    escalator W10.0 ☑
    incline W10.2 ☑
    ladder W11 ☑
    machine, machinery — *see* Contact, with, by type of machine
    object, edged, pointed or sharp (with cut) — *see* Fall, by type
    playground equipment W09.8 ☑
      jungle gym W09.2 ☑
      slide W09.0 ☑
      swing W09.1 ☑
    ramp W10.2 ☑
    scaffolding W12 ☑
    shower W18.2 ☑
      causing drowning W16.211 ☑
    staircase, stairs, steps W10.9 ☑

Fall, falling — *continued*
  in, on — *continued*
    staircase, stairs, steps — *continued*
      curb W10.1 ☑
      due to ice or snow W00.1 ☑
      escalator W10.0 ☑
      incline W10.2 ☑
      specified NEC W10.8 ☑
    streetcar (without antecedent collision) V82.5 ☑
      with antecedent collision — *see* Accident, transport, streetcar occupant
      while boarding or alighting V82.4 ☑
    train (without antecedent collision) V81.5 ☑
      with antecedent collision — *see* Accident, transport, railway vehicle occupant
      during derailment (without antecedent collision) V81.7 ☑
        with antecedent collision — *see* Accident, transport, railway vehicle occupant
      while boarding or alighting V81.4 ☑
    transport vehicle after collision — *see* Accident, transport, by type of vehicle, collision
    watercraft V93.39 ☑
      due to
        accident to craft V91.29 ☑
          powered craft V91.23 ☑
            ferry boat V91.21 ☑
            fishing boat V91.22 ☑
            jetskis V91.23 ☑
            liner V91.21 ☑
            merchant ship V91.20 ☑
            passenger ship V91.21 ☑
          unpowered craft
            canoe V91.25 ☑
            inflatable V91.26 ☑
            kayak V91.25 ☑
            sailboat V91.24 ☑
        powered craft V93.33 ☑
          ferry boat V93.31 ☑
          fishing boat V93.32 ☑
          jetskis V93.33 ☑
          liner V93.31 ☑
          merchant ship V93.30 ☑
          passenger ship V93.31 ☑
        unpowered craft V93.38 ☑
          canoe V93.35 ☑
          inflatable V93.36 ☑
          kayak V93.35 ☑
          sailboat V93.34 ☑
          surf-board V93.38 ☑
          windsurfer V93.38 ☑
  into
    cavity W17.2 ☑
    dock W17.4 ☑
    fire — *see* Exposure, fire, by type
    haystack W17.89 ☑
    hole W17.2 ☑
    lake — *see* Fall, into, water
    manhole W17.1 ☑
    moving part of machinery — *see* Contact, with, by type of machine
    ocean — *see* Fall, into, water
    opening in surface NEC W17.89 ☑
    pit W17.2 ☑
    pond — *see* Fall, into, water
    quarry W17.89 ☑
    river — *see* Fall, into, water
    shaft W17.89 ☑
    storm drain W17.1 ☑
    stream — *see* Fall, into, water
    swimming pool — *see also* Fall, into, water, in, swimming pool
      empty W17.3 ☑
    tank W17.89 ☑
    water W16.42 ☑
      causing drowning W16.41 ☑
      from watercraft — *see* Drowning, due to, fall overboard
      hitting diving board W21.4 ☑
      in
        bathtub W16.212 ☑
          causing drowning W16.211 ☑
        bucket W16.222 ☑
          causing drowning W16.221 ☑
        natural body of water W16.112 ☑
          causing drowning W16.111 ☑

Fall, falling — *continued*
  into — *continued*
    water — *continued*
      in — *continued*
        natural body of water — *continued*
          striking
            bottom W16.122 ☑
              causing drowning W16.121 ☑
            side W16.132 ☑
              causing drowning W16.131 ☑
        specified water NEC W16.312 ☑
          causing drowning W16.311 ☑
          striking
            bottom W16.322 ☑
              causing drowning W16.321 ☑
            wall W16.332 ☑
              causing drowning W16.331 ☑
        swimming pool W16.012 ☑
          causing drowning W16.011 ☑
          striking
            bottom W16.022 ☑
              causing drowning W16.031 ☑
            wall W16.032 ☑
              causing drowning W16.021 ☑
        utility bucket W16.222 ☑
          causing drowning W16.221 ☑
    well W17.0 ☑
  involving
    bed W06 ☑
    chair W07 ☑
    furniture NEC W08 ☑
    glass — *see* Fall, by type
    playground equipment W09.8 ☑
      jungle gym W09.2 ☑
      slide W09.0 ☑
      swing W09.1 ☑
    roller blades — *see* Accident, transport, pedestrian, conveyance
    skateboard(s) — *see* Accident, transport, pedestrian, conveyance
    skates (ice) (in line) (roller) — *see* Accident, transport, pedestrian, conveyance
    skis — *see* Accident, transport, pedestrian, conveyance
    table W08 ☑
    wheelchair, non-moving W05.0 ☑
      powered — *see* Accident, transport, pedestrian, conveyance, specified type NEC
  object — *see* Struck by, object, falling
  off
    toilet W18.11 ☑
      with subsequent striking against object W18.12 ☑
  on same level W18.30 ☑
    due to
      specified NEC W18.39 ☑
      stepping on an object W18.31 ☑
  out of
    bed W06 ☑
    building NEC W13.8 ☑
    chair W07 ☑
    furniture NEC W08 ☑
    wheelchair, non-moving W05.0 ☑
      powered — *see* Accident, transport, pedestrian, conveyance, specified type NEC
    window W13.4 ☑
  over
    animal W01.0 ☑
    cliff W15 ☑
    embankment W17.81 ☑
    small object W01.0 ☑
  rock W20.8 ☑
  same level W18.30 ☑
    from
      being crushed, pushed, or stepped on by a crowd or human stampede W52 ☑
      collision, pushing, shoving, by or with other person W03 ☑
      slipping, stumbling, tripping W01.0 ☑
    involving ice or snow W00.0 ☑
      involving skates (ice) (roller), skateboard, skis — *see* Accident, transport, pedestrian, conveyance
  snowslide (avalanche) — *see* Landslide
  stone W20.8 ☑
  structure W20.1 ☑

Fall, falling — *continued*
structure — *continued*
burning (uncontrolled fire) X00.3 ☑
through
bridge W13.1 ☑
floor W13.3 ☑
roof W13.2 ☑
wall W13.8 ☑
window W13.4 ☑
timber W20.8 ☑
tree (caused by lightning) W20.8 ☑
while being carried or supported by other person(s) W04 ☑
Fallen on by
animal (not being ridden) NEC W55.89 ☑
Felo-de-se — *see* Suicide
Fight (hand) (fists) (foot) — *see* Assault, fight
Fire (accidental) — *see* Exposure, fire
Firearm discharge — *see* Discharge, firearm
Fireball effects from nuclear explosion in war operations — *see* War operations, nuclear weapons
Fireworks (explosion) W39
Flash burns from explosion — *see* Explosion
Flood (any injury) (caused by) X38 ☑
collapse of man-made structure causing earth movement X36.0 ☑
tidal wave — *see* Forces of nature, tidal wave
Food (any type) **in**
air passages (with asphyxia, obstruction, or suffocation) — *see* categories T17 and T18 ☑
alimentary tract causing asphyxia (due to compression of trachea) — *see* categories T17 and T18 ☑
Forces of nature X39.8 ☑
avalanche X36.1 ☑
causing transport accident — *see* Accident, transport, by type of vehicle
blizzard X37.2 ☑
cataclysmic storm X37.9 ☑
with flood X38 ☑
blizzard X37.2 ☑
cloudburst X37.8 ☑
cyclone X37.1 ☑
dust storm X37.3 ☑
hurricane X37.0 ☑
specified storm NEC X37.8 ☑
storm surge X37.0 ☑
tornado X37.1 ☑
twister X37.1 ☑
typhoon X37.0 ☑
cloudburst X37.8 ☑
cold (natural) X31 ☑
cyclone X37.1 ☑
dam collapse causing earth movement X36.0 ☑
dust storm X37.3 ☑
earth movement X36.1 ☑
caused by dam or structure collapse X36.0 ☑
earthquake X34 ☑
earthquake X34 ☑
flood (caused by) X38 ☑
dam collapse X36.0 ☑
tidal wave — *see* Forces of nature, tidal wave
heat (natural) X30 ☑
hurricane X37.0 ☑
landslide X36.1 ☑
causing transport accident — *see* Accident, transport, by type of vehicle
lightning — *see* subcategory T75.0 ☑
causing fire — *see* Exposure, fire
mudslide X36.1 ☑
causing transport accident — *see* Accident, transport, by type of vehicle
radiation (natural) X39.08 ☑
radon X39.01 ☑
radon X39.01 ☑
specified force NEC X39.8 ☑
storm surge X37.0 ☑
structure collapse causing earth movement X36.0 ☑
sunlight X32 ☑
tidal wave X37.41 ☑
due to
earthquake X37.41 ☑
landslide X37.43 ☑
storm X37.42 ☑
volcanic eruption X37.41 ☑
tornado X37.1 ☑
tsunami X37.41 ☑

Forces of nature — *continued*
twister X37.1 ☑
typhoon X37.0 ☑
volcanic eruption X35 ☑
Foreign body
aspiration — *see* Index to Diseases and Injuries, Foreign body, respiratory tract
embedded in skin W45 ☑
entering through skin W45.8 ☑
can lid W26.8 ☑
nail W45.0 ☑
paper W26.2 ☑
specified NEC W45.8 ☑
splinter W45.8 ☑
Forest fire (exposure to) — *see* Exposure, fire, uncontrolled, not in building
Found injured X58 ☑
from exposure (to) — *see* Exposure
on
highway, road(way), street V89.9 ☑
railway right of way V81.9 ☑
Fracture (circumstances unknown or unspecified) X58 ☑
due to specified cause NEC X58 ☑
Freezing — *see* Exposure, cold
Frostbite X31 ☑
due to man-made conditions — *see* Exposure, cold, man-made
Frozen — *see* Exposure, cold

G

Gored by bull W55.22 ☑
Gunshot wound W34.00 ☑

H

Hailstones, injured by X39.8 ☑
Hanged herself or himself — *see* Hanging, self-inflicted
Hanging (accidental) — *see also* category T71 ☑
legal execution — *see* Legal, intervention, specified means NEC
Heat (effects of) (excessive) X30 ☑
due to
man-made conditions W92 ☑
on board watercraft V93.29 ☑
fishing boat V93.22 ☑
merchant ship V93.20 ☑
passenger ship V93.21 ☑
sailboat V93.24 ☑
specified powered craft NEC V93.23 ☑
weather (conditions) X30 ☑
from
electric heating apparatus causing burning X16 ☑
nuclear explosion in war operations — *see* War operations, nuclear weapons
inappropriate in local application or packing in medical or surgical procedure Y63.5
Hemorrhage
delayed following medical or surgical treatment without mention of misadventure — *see* Index to Diseases and Injuries, Complication(s)
during medical or surgical treatment as misadventure — *see* Index to Diseases and Injuries, Complication(s)
High
altitude (effects) — *see* Air, pressure, low
level of radioactivity, effects — *see* Radiation
pressure (effects) — *see* Air, pressure, high
temperature, effects — *see* Heat
Hit, hitting (accidental) by — *see* Struck by
Hitting against — *see* Striking against
Homicide (attempt) (justifiable) — *see* Assault
Hot
place, effects — *see also* Heat
weather, effects X30 ☑
House fire (uncontrolled) — *see* Exposure, fire, uncontrolled, building
Humidity, causing problem X39.8 ☑
Hunger X58 ☑
Hurricane (any injury) X37.0 ☑
Hypobarism, hypobaropathy — *see* Air, pressure, low

I

Ictus
caloris — *see also* Heat

Ictus — *continued*
solaris X30 ☑
Ignition (accidental) — *see also* Exposure, fire X08.8 ☑
anesthetic gas in operating room W40.1 ☑
apparel X06.2 ☑
from highly flammable material X04 ☑
nightwear X05 ☑
bed linen (sheets) (spreads) (pillows) (mattress) — *see* Exposure, fire, uncontrolled, building, bed
benzine X04 ☑
clothes, clothing NEC (from controlled fire) X06.2 ☑
from
highly flammable material X04 ☑
ether X04 ☑
in operating room W40.1 ☑
explosive material — *see* Explosion
gasoline X04 ☑
jewelry (plastic) (any) X06.0 ☑
kerosene X04 ☑
material
explosive — *see* Explosion
highly flammable with secondary explosion X04 ☑
nightwear X05 ☑
paraffin X04 ☑
petrol X04 ☑
Immersion (accidental) — *see also* Drowning
hand or foot due to cold (excessive) X31 ☑
Implantation of quills of porcupine W55.89 ☑
Inanition (from) (hunger) X58 ☑
thirst X58 ☑
Inappropriate operation performed
correct operation on wrong side or body part (wrong side) (wrong site) Y65.53
operation intended for another patient done on wrong patient Y65.52
wrong operation performed on correct patient Y65.51
Inattention after, at birth (homicidal intent) (infanticidal intent) X58 ☑
Incident, adverse
device
anesthesiology Y70.8
accessory Y70.2
diagnostic Y70.0
miscellaneous Y70.8
monitoring Y70.0
prosthetic Y70.2
rehabilitative Y70.1
surgical Y70.3
therapeutic Y70.1
cardiovascular Y71.8
accessory Y71.2
diagnostic Y71.0
miscellaneous Y71.8
monitoring Y71.0
prosthetic Y71.2
rehabilitative Y71.1
surgical Y71.3
therapeutic Y71.1
gastroenterology Y73.8
accessory Y73.2
diagnostic Y73.0
miscellaneous Y73.8
monitoring Y73.0
prosthetic Y73.2
rehabilitative Y73.1
surgical Y73.3
therapeutic Y73.1
general
hospital Y74.8
accessory Y74.2
diagnostic Y74.0
miscellaneous Y74.8
monitoring Y74.0
prosthetic Y74.2
rehabilitative Y74.1
surgical Y74.3
therapeutic Y74.1
surgical Y81.8
accessory Y81.2
diagnostic Y81.0
miscellaneous Y81.8
monitoring Y81.0
prosthetic Y81.2
rehabilitative Y81.1
surgical Y81.3
therapeutic Y81.1
gynecological Y76.8
accessory Y76.2

Incident, adverse — *continued*
  device — *continued*
    gynecological — *continued*
      diagnostic Y76.0
      miscellaneous Y76.8
      monitoring Y76.0
      prosthetic Y76.2
      rehabilitative Y76.1
      surgical Y76.3
      therapeutic Y76.1
    medical Y82.9
      specified type NEC Y82.8
    neurological Y75.8
      accessory Y75.2
      diagnostic Y75.0
      miscellaneous Y75.8
      monitoring Y75.0
      prosthetic Y75.2
      rehabilitative Y75.1
      surgical Y75.3
      therapeutic Y75.1
    obstetrical Y76.8
      accessory Y76.2
      diagnostic Y76.0
      miscellaneous Y76.8
      monitoring Y76.0
      prosthetic Y76.2
      rehabilitative Y76.1
      surgical Y76.3
      therapeutic Y76.1
    ophthalmic Y77.8
      accessory Y77.2
      contact lens (rigid gas permeable) (soft (hy-drophilic)) Y77.11
      diagnostic Y77.0
      miscellaneous Y77.8
      monitoring Y77.0
      prosthetic Y77.2
      rehabilitative Y77.19
      surgical Y77.3
      therapeutic Y77.19
    orthopedic Y79.8
      accessory Y79.2
      diagnostic Y79.0
      miscellaneous Y79.8
      monitoring Y79.0
      prosthetic Y79.2
      rehabilitative Y79.1
      surgical Y79.3
      therapeutic Y79.1
    otorhinolaryngological Y72.8
      accessory Y72.2
      diagnostic Y72.0
      miscellaneous Y72.8
      monitoring Y72.0
      prosthetic Y72.2
      rehabilitative Y72.1
      surgical Y72.3
      therapeutic Y72.1
    personal use Y74.8
      accessory Y74.2
      diagnostic Y74.0
      miscellaneous Y74.8
      monitoring Y74.0
      prosthetic Y74.2
      rehabilitative Y74.1
      surgical Y74.3
      therapeutic Y74.1
    physical medicine Y80.8
      accessory Y80.2
      diagnostic Y80.0
      miscellaneous Y80.8
      monitoring Y80.0
      prosthetic Y80.2
      rehabilitative Y80.1
      surgical Y80.3
      therapeutic Y80.1
    plastic surgical Y81.8
      accessory Y81.2
      diagnostic Y81.0
      miscellaneous Y81.8
      monitoring Y81.0
      prosthetic Y81.2
      rehabilitative Y81.1
      surgical Y81.3
      therapeutic Y81.1
    radiological Y78.8
      accessory Y78.2
      diagnostic Y78.0

Incident, adverse — *continued*
  device — *continued*
    radiological — *continued*
      miscellaneous Y78.8
      monitoring Y78.0
      prosthetic Y78.2
      rehabilitative Y78.1
      surgical Y78.3
      therapeutic Y78.1
    urology Y73.8
      accessory Y73.2
      diagnostic Y73.0
      miscellaneous Y73.8
      monitoring Y73.0
      prosthetic Y73.2
      rehabilitative Y73.1
      surgical Y73.3
      therapeutic Y73.1
Incineration (accidental) — *see* Exposure, fire
Infanticide — *see* Assault
Infrasound waves (causing injury) W49.9 ☑
Ingestion
  foreign body (causing injury) (with obstruction) — *see* Foreign body, alimentary canal
  poisonous
    plant(s) X58 ☑
    substance NEC — *see* Table of Drugs and Chemicals
Inhalation
  excessively cold substance, man-made — *see* Exposure, cold, man-made
  food (any type) (into respiratory tract) (with asphyxia, obstruction respiratory tract, suffocation) — *see* categories T17 and T18 ☑
  foreign body — *see* Foreign body, aspiration
  gastric contents (with asphyxia, obstruction respiratory passage, suffocation) T17.81- ☑
  hot air or gases X14.0 ☑
  liquid air, hydrogen, nitrogen W93.12 ☑
    suicide (attempt) X83.2 ☑
  steam X13.0 ☑
    assault X98.0 ☑
    stated as undetermined whether accidental or intentional Y27.0 ☑
    suicide (attempt) X77.0 ☑
  toxic gas — *see* Table of Drugs and Chemicals
  vomitus (with asphyxia, obstruction respiratory passage, suffocation) T17.81- ☑
Injury, injured (accidental(ly)) NOS X58 ☑
  by, caused by, from
    assault — *see* Assault
    law-enforcing agent, police, in course of legal intervention — *see* Legal intervention
    suicide (attempt) X83.8 ☑
  due to, in
    civil insurrection — *see* War operations
    fight — *see also* Assault, fight Y04.0 ☑
    war operations — *see* War operations
  homicide — *see also* Assault Y09
  inflicted (by)
    in course of arrest (attempted), suppression of disturbance, maintenance of order, by law-enforcing agents — *see* Legal intervention
    other person
      stated as
        accidental X58 ☑
        intentional, homicide (attempt) — *see* Assault
        undetermined whether accidental or intentional Y33 ☑
  purposely (inflicted) by other person(s) — *see* Assault
  self-inflicted X83.8 ☑
    stated as accidental X58 ☑
  specified cause NEC X58 ☑
  undetermined whether accidental or intentional Y33 ☑
Insolation, effects X30 ☑
Insufficient nourishment X58 ☑
Interruption of respiration (by)
  food (lodged in esophagus) — *see* categories T17 and T18 ☑
  vomitus (lodged in esophagus) T17.81- ☑
Intervention, legal — *see* Legal intervention
Intoxication
  drug — *see* Table of Drugs and Chemicals
  poison — *see* Table of Drugs and Chemicals

J

Jammed (accidentally)
  between objects (moving) (stationary and moving) W23.0 ☑
    stationary W23.1 ☑
Jumped, jumping
  before moving object NEC X81.8 ☑
    motor vehicle X81.0 ☑
    subway train X81.1 ☑
    train X81.1 ☑
    undetermined whether accidental or intentional Y31 ☑
  from
    boat (into water) voluntarily, without accident (to or on boat) W16.712 ☑
      striking bottom W16.722 ☑
        causing drowning W16.721 ☑
      with
        accident to or on boat — *see* Accident, water-craft
        drowning or submersion W16.711 ☑
          suicide (attempt) X71.3 ☑
    building — *see also* Jumped, from, high place W13.9 ☑
      burning (uncontrolled fire) X00.5 ☑
    high place NEC W17.89 ☑
      suicide (attempt) X80 ☑
      undetermined whether accidental or intentional Y30 ☑
    structure — *see also* Jumped, from, high place W13.9 ☑
      burning (uncontrolled fire) X00.5 ☑
  into water W16.92 ☑
    causing drowning W16.91 ☑
    from, off watercraft — *see* Jumped, from, boat
    in
      natural body W16.612 ☑
        causing drowning W16.611 ☑
        striking bottom W16.622 ☑
          causing drowning W16.621 ☑
      specified place NEC W16.812 ☑
        causing drowning W16.811 ☑
        striking
          bottom W16.822 ☑
            causing drowning W16.821 ☑
          wall W16.832 ☑
            causing drowning W16.831 ☑
      swimming pool W16.512 ☑
        causing drowning W16.511 ☑
        striking
          bottom W16.522 ☑
            causing drowning W16.521 ☑
          wall W16.532 ☑
            causing drowning W16.531 ☑
  suicide (attempt) X71.3 ☑

K

Kicked by
  animal NEC W55.82 ☑
  person(s) (accidentally) W50.1 ☑
    with intent to injure or kill Y04.0 ☑
    as, or caused by, a crowd or human stampede (with fall) W52 ☑
    assault Y04.0 ☑
    homicide (attempt) Y04.0 ☑
    in
      fight Y04.0 ☑
      legal intervention
        injuring
          bystander Y35.812 ☑
          law enforcement personnel Y35.811 ☑
          suspect Y35.813 ☑
          unspecified person Y35.819 ☑
Kicking
  against
    object W22.8 ☑
      sports equipment W21.9 ☑
      stationary W22.09 ☑
        sports equipment W21.89 ☑
    person — *see* Striking against, person
    sports equipment W21.9 ☑
  carpet stretcher with knee X50.3 ☑
Killed, killing (accidentally) NOS — *see also* Injury X58 ☑

Killed, killing — *continued*
  in
    action — *see* War operations
    brawl, fight (hand) (fists) (foot) Y04.0 ☑
      by weapon — *see also* Assault
        cutting, piercing — *see* Assault, cutting or piercing instrument
        firearm — *see* Discharge, firearm, by type, homicide
    self
      stated as
        accident NOS X58 ☑
        suicide — *see* Suicide
        undetermined whether accidental or intentional Y33 ☑
Kneeling (prolonged) (static) X50.1 ☑
Knocked down (accidentally) (by) NOS X58 ☑
  animal (not being ridden) NEC — *see also* Struck by, by type of animal
  crowd or human stampede W52 ☑
  person W51 ☑
    in brawl, fight Y04.0 ☑
  transport vehicle NEC — *see also* Accident, transport V09.9 ☑

L

Laceration NEC — *see* Injury
Lack of
  care (helpless person) (infant) (newborn) X58 ☑
  food except as result of abandonment or neglect X58 ☑
    due to abandonment or neglect X58 ☑
  water except as result of transport accident X58 ☑
    due to transport accident — *see* Accident, transport, by type
  helpless person, infant, newborn X58 ☑
Landslide (falling on transport vehicle) X36.1 ☑
  caused by collapse of man-made structure X36.0 ☑
Late effect — *see* Sequelae
Legal
  execution (any method) — *see* Legal, intervention
  intervention (by)
    baton — *see* Legal, intervention, blunt object, baton
    bayonet — *see* Legal, intervention, sharp object, bayonet
    blow — *see* Legal, intervention, manhandling
    blunt object
      baton
        injuring
          bystander Y35.312 ☑
          law enforcement personnel Y35.311 ☑
          suspect Y35.313 ☑
          unspecified person Y35.319 ☑
      injuring
        bystander Y35.302 ☑
        law enforcement personnel Y35.301 ☑
        suspect Y35.303 ☑
        unspecified person Y35.309 ☑
      specified NEC
        injuring
          bystander Y35.392 ☑
          law enforcement personnel Y35.391 ☑
          suspect Y35.393 ☑
          unspecified person Y35.399 ☑
      stave
        injuring
          bystander Y35.392 ☑
          law enforcement personnel Y35.391 ☑
          suspect Y35.393 ☑
          unspecified person Y35.399 ☑
    bomb — *see* Legal, intervention, explosive
    conducted energy device
      injuring
        bystander Y35.832 ☑
        law enforcement personnel Y35.831 ☑
        suspect Y35.833 ☑
        unspecified person Y35.839 ☑
    cutting or piercing instrument — *see* Legal, intervention, sharp object
    dynamite — *see* Legal, intervention, explosive, dynamite
    electroshock device (taser)
      injuring
        bystander Y35.832 ☑
        law enforcement personnel Y35.831 ☑

Legal — *continued*
  intervention — *continued*
    electroshock device — *continued*
      injuring — *continued*
        suspect Y35.833 ☑
        unspecified person Y35.839 ☑
    explosive(s)
      dynamite
        injuring
          bystander Y35.112 ☑
          law enforcement personnel Y35.111 ☑
          suspect Y35.113 ☑
          unspecified person Y35.119 ☑
      grenade
        injuring
          bystander Y35.192 ☑
          law enforcement personnel Y35.191 ☑
          suspect Y35.193 ☑
          unspecified person Y35.199 ☑
      injuring
        bystander Y35.102 ☑
        law enforcement personnel Y35.101 ☑
        suspect Y35.103 ☑
        unspecified person Y35.109 ☑
      mortar bomb
        injuring
          bystander Y35.192 ☑
          law enforcement personnel Y35.191 ☑
          suspect Y35.193 ☑
          unspecified person Y35.199 ☑
      shell
        injuring
          bystander Y35.122 ☑
          law enforcement personnel Y35.121 ☑
          suspect Y35.123 ☑
          unspecified person Y35.129 ☑
      specified NEC
        injuring
          bystander Y35.192 ☑
          law enforcement personnel Y35.191 ☑
          suspect Y35.193 ☑
          unspecified person Y35.199 ☑
    firearm(s) (discharge)
      handgun
        injuring
          bystander Y35.022 ☑
          law enforcement personnel Y35.021 ☑
          suspect Y35.023 ☑
          unspecified person Y35.029 ☑
      injuring
        bystander Y35.002 ☑
        law enforcement personnel Y35.001 ☑
        suspect Y35.003 ☑
        unspecified person Y35.009 ☑
      machine gun
        injuring
          bystander Y35.012 ☑
          law enforcement personnel Y35.011 ☑
          suspect Y35.013 ☑
          unspecified person Y35.019 ☑
      rifle pellet
        injuring
          bystander Y35.032 ☑
          law enforcement personnel Y35.031 ☑
          suspect Y35.033 ☑
          unspecified person Y35.039 ☑
      rubber bullet
        injuring
          bystander Y35.042 ☑
          law enforcement personnel Y35.041 ☑
          suspect Y35.043 ☑
          unspecified person Y35.049 ☑
      shotgun — *see* Legal, intervention, firearm, specified NEC
      specified NEC
        injuring
          bystander Y35.092 ☑
          law enforcement personnel Y35.091 ☑
          suspect Y35.093 ☑
          unspecified person Y35.099 ☑
    gas (asphyxiation) (poisoning)
      injuring
        bystander Y35.202 ☑
        law enforcement personnel Y35.201 ☑
        suspect Y35.203 ☑
        unspecified person Y35.209 ☑

Legal — *continued*
  intervention — *continued*
    gas — *continued*
      specified NEC
        injuring
          bystander Y35.292 ☑
          law enforcement personnel Y35.291 ☑
          suspect Y35.293 ☑
          unspecified person Y35.299 ☑
      tear gas
        injuring
          bystander Y35.212 ☑
          law enforcement personnel Y35.211 ☑
          suspect Y35.213 ☑
          unspecified person Y35.219 ☑
    grenade — *see* Legal, intervention, explosive, grenade
    injuring
      bystander Y35.92 ☑
      law enforcement personnel Y35.91 ☑
      suspect Y35.93 ☑
      unspecified person Y35.99 ☑
    late effect (of) — *see* with 7th character S Y35 ☑
    manhandling
      injuring
        bystander Y35.812 ☑
        law enforcement personnel Y35.811 ☑
        suspect Y35.813 ☑
        unspecified person Y35.819 ☑
    sequelae (of) — *see* with 7th character S Y35 ☑
    sharp objects
      bayonet
        injuring
          bystander Y35.412 ☑
          law enforcement personnel Y35.411 ☑
          suspect Y35.413 ☑
          unspecified person Y35.419 ☑
      injuring
        bystander Y35.402 ☑
        law enforcement personnel Y35.401 ☑
        suspect Y35.403 ☑
        unspecified person Y35.409 ☑
      specified NEC
        injuring
          bystander Y35.492 ☑
          law enforcement personnel Y35.491 ☑
          suspect Y35.493 ☑
          unspecified person Y35.499 ☑
    specified means NEC
      injuring
        bystander Y35.892 ☑
        law enforcement personnel Y35.891 ☑
        suspect Y35.893 ☑
        unspecified person Y35.899 ☑
    stabbing — *see* Legal, intervention, sharp object
    stave — *see* Legal, intervention, blunt object, stave
    stun gun
      injuring
        bystander Y35.832 ☑
        law enforcement personnel Y35.831 ☑
        suspect Y35.833 ☑
        unspecified person Y35.839 ☑
    taser
      injuring
        bystander Y35.832 ☑
        law enforcement personnel Y35.831 ☑
        suspect Y35.833 ☑
        unspecified person Y35.839 ☑
    tear gas — *see* Legal, intervention, gas, tear gas
    truncheon — *see* Legal, intervention, blunt object, stave
Lifting — *see also* Overexertion
  heavy objects X50.0 ☑
  weights X50.0 ☑
Lightning (shock) (stroke) (struck by) — *see* subcategory T75.0 ☑
  causing fire — *see* Exposure, fire
Loss of control (transport vehicle) NEC — *see* Accident, transport
Lost at sea NOS — *see* Drowning, due to, fall overboard
Low
  pressure (effects) — *see* Air, pressure, low
  temperature (effects) — *see* Exposure, cold
Lying before train, vehicle or other moving object X81.8 ☑
  subway train X81.1 ☑

Lying before train, vehicle or other moving object — *continued*
- train X81.1 ☑
- undetermined whether accidental or intentional Y31 ☑

Lynching — *see* Assault

M

Malfunction (mechanism or component) (of)
- firearm W34.10 ☑
  - airgun W34.110 ☑
  - BB gun W34.110 ☑
  - gas, air or spring-operated gun NEC W34.118 ☑
  - handgun W32.1 ☑
  - hunting rifle W33.12 ☑
  - larger firearm W33.10 ☑
    - specified NEC W33.19 ☑
  - machine gun W33.13 ☑
  - paintball gun W34.111 ☑
  - pellet gun W34.110 ☑
  - shotgun W33.11 ☑
  - specified NEC W34.19 ☑
  - Very pistol [flare] W34.19 ☑
- handgun — *see* Malfunction, firearm, handgun

Maltreatment — *see* Perpetrator
Mangled (accidentally) NOS X58 ☑
Manhandling (in brawl, fight) Y04.0 ☑
- legal intervention — *see* Legal, intervention, manhandling

Manslaughter (nonaccidental) — *see* Assault
Mauled by animal NEC W55.89 ☑
Medical procedure, complication of (delayed or as an abnormal reaction without mention of misadventure) — *see* Complication of or following, by specified type of procedure
- due to or as a result of misadventure — *see* Misadventure

Melting (due to fire) — *see also* Exposure, fire
- apparel NEC X06.3 ☑
- clothes, clothing NEC X06.3 ☑
  - nightwear X05 ☑
- fittings or furniture (burning building) (uncontrolled fire) X00.8 ☑
- nightwear X05 ☑
- plastic jewelry X06.1 ☑

Mental cruelty X58 ☑
Military operations (injuries to military and civilians occuring during peacetime on military property and during routine military exercises and operations) (by) (from) (involving) Y37.90- ☑
- air blast Y37.20- ☑
- aircraft
  - destruction — *see* Military operations, destruction of aircraft
  - airway restriction — *see* Military operations, restriction of airways
  - asphyxiation — *see* Military operations, restriction of airways
- biological weapons Y37.6X- ☑
- blast Y37.20- ☑
- blast fragments Y37.20- ☑
- blast wave Y37.20- ☑
- blast wind Y37.20- ☑
- bomb Y37.20- ☑
  - dirty Y37.50- ☑
  - gasoline Y37.31- ☑
  - incendiary Y37.31- ☑
  - petrol Y37.31- ☑
- bullet Y37.43- ☑
  - incendiary Y37.32- ☑
  - rubber Y37.41- ☑
- chemical weapons Y37.7X- ☑
- combat
  - hand to hand (unarmed) combat Y37.44- ☑
  - using blunt or piercing object Y37.45- ☑
- conflagration — *see* Military operations, fire
- conventional warfare NEC Y37.49- ☑
- depth-charge Y37.01- ☑
- destruction of aircraft Y37.10- ☑
  - due to
    - air to air missile Y37.11- ☑
    - collision with other aircraft Y37.12- ☑
    - detonation (accidental) of onboard munitions and explosives Y37.14- ☑
    - enemy fire or explosives Y37.11- ☑
    - explosive placed on aircraft Y37.11- ☑

Military operations — *continued*
- destruction of aircraft — *continued*
  - due to — *continued*
    - onboard fire Y37.13- ☑
    - rocket propelled grenade [RPG] Y37.11- ☑
    - small arms fire Y37.11- ☑
    - surface to air missile Y37.11- ☑
    - specified NEC Y37.19- ☑
- detonation (accidental) of
  - onboard marine weapons Y37.05- ☑
  - own munitions or munitions launch device Y37.24- ☑
- dirty bomb Y37.50- ☑
- explosion (of) Y37.20- ☑
  - aerial bomb Y37.21- ☑
  - bomb NOS — *see also* Military operations, bomb(s) Y37.20- ☑
  - fragments Y37.20- ☑
  - grenade Y37.29- ☑
  - guided missile Y37.22- ☑
  - improvised explosive device [IED] (person-borne) (roadside) (vehicle-borne) Y37.23- ☑
  - land mine Y37.29- ☑
  - marine mine (at sea) (in harbor) Y37.02- ☑
  - marine weapon Y37.00- ☑
    - specified NEC Y37.09- ☑
  - own munitions or munitions launch device (accidental) Y37.24- ☑
  - sea-based artillery shell Y37.03- ☑
  - specified NEC Y37.29- ☑
  - torpedo Y37.04- ☑
- fire Y37.30- ☑
  - specified NEC Y37.39- ☑
- firearms
  - discharge Y37.43- ☑
  - pellets Y37.42- ☑
- flamethrower Y37.33- ☑
- fragments (from) (of)
  - improvised explosive device [IED] (person-borne) (roadside) (vehicle-borne) Y37.26- ☑
  - munitions Y37.25- ☑
  - specified NEC Y37.29- ☑
  - weapons Y37.27- ☑
- friendly fire Y37.92- ☑
- hand to hand (unarmed) combat Y37.44- ☑
- hot substances — *see* Military operations, fire
- incendiary bullet Y37.32- ☑
- nuclear weapon (effects of) Y37.50- ☑
  - acute radiation exposure Y37.54- ☑
  - blast pressure Y37.51- ☑
  - direct blast Y37.51- ☑
  - direct heat Y37.53- ☑
  - fallout exposure Y37.54- ☑
  - fireball Y37.53- ☑
  - indirect blast (struck or crushed by blast debris) (being thrown by blast) Y37.52- ☑
  - ionizing radiation (immediate exposure) Y37.54- ☑
  - nuclear radiation Y37.54- ☑
  - radiation
    - ionizing (immediate exposure) Y37.54- ☑
    - nuclear Y37.54- ☑
    - thermal Y37.53- ☑
  - secondary effects Y37.54- ☑
  - specified NEC Y37.59- ☑
  - thermal radiation Y37.53- ☑
- restriction of air (airway)
  - intentional Y37.46- ☑
  - unintentional Y37.47- ☑
- rubber bullets Y37.41- ☑
- shrapnel NOS Y37.29- ☑
- suffocation — *see* Military operations, restriction of airways
- unconventional warfare NEC Y37.7X- ☑
- underwater blast NOS Y37.00- ☑
- warfare
  - conventional NEC Y37.49- ☑
  - unconventional NEC Y37.7X- ☑
- weapon of mass destruction [WMD] Y37.91- ☑
- weapons
  - biological weapons Y37.6X- ☑
  - chemical Y37.7X- ☑
  - nuclear (effects of) Y37.50- ☑
    - acute radiation exposure Y37.54- ☑
    - blast pressure Y37.51- ☑
    - direct blast Y37.51- ☑
    - direct heat Y37.53- ☑

Military operations — *continued*
- weapons — *continued*
  - nuclear — *continued*
    - fallout exposure Y37.54- ☑
    - fireball Y37.53- ☑
    - radiation
      - ionizing (immediate exposure) Y37.54- ☑
      - nuclear Y37.54- ☑
      - thermal Y37.53- ☑
    - secondary effects Y37.54- ☑
    - specified NEC Y37.59- ☑
  - of mass destruction [WMD] Y37.91- ☑

Misadventure(s) to patient(s) during surgical or medical care Y69
- contaminated medical or biological substance (blood, drug, fluid) Y64.9
  - administered (by) NEC Y64.9
    - immunization Y64.1
    - infusion Y64.0
    - injection Y64.1
    - specified means NEC Y64.8
    - transfusion Y64.0
    - vaccination Y64.1
- excessive amount of blood or other fluid during transfusion or infusion Y63.0
- failure
  - in dosage Y63.9
    - electroshock therapy Y63.4
    - inappropriate temperature (too hot or too cold) in local application and packing Y63.5
    - infusion
      - excessive amount of fluid Y63.0
      - incorrect dilution of fluid Y63.1
    - insulin-shock therapy Y63.4
    - nonadministration of necessary drug or biological substance Y63.6
    - overdose — *see* Table of Drugs and Chemicals
    - radiation, in therapy Y63.2
    - radiation
      - overdose Y63.2
    - specified procedure NEC Y63.8
    - transfusion
      - excessive amount of blood Y63.0
  - mechanical, of instrument or apparatus (any) (during any procedure) Y65.8
  - sterile precautions (during procedure) Y62.9
    - aspiration of fluid or tissue (by puncture or catheterization, except heart) Y62.6
    - biopsy (except needle aspiration) Y62.8
      - needle (aspirating) Y62.6
    - blood sampling Y62.6
    - catheterization Y62.6
      - heart Y62.5
    - dialysis (kidney) Y62.2
    - endoscopic examination Y62.4
    - enema Y62.8
    - immunization Y62.3
    - infusion Y62.1
    - injection Y62.3
    - needle biopsy Y62.6
    - paracentesis (abdominal) (thoracic) Y62.6
    - perfusion Y62.2
    - puncture (lumbar) Y62.6
    - removal of catheter or packing Y62.8
    - specified procedure NEC Y62.8
    - surgical operation Y62.0
    - transfusion Y62.1
    - vaccination Y62.3
  - suture or ligature during surgical procedure Y65.2
  - to introduce or to remove tube or instrument — *see* Failure, to
- hemorrhage — *see* Index to Diseases and Injuries, Complication(s)
- inadvertent exposure of patient to radiation Y63.3
- inappropriate
  - operation performed — *see* Inappropriate operation performed
  - temperature (too hot or too cold) in local application or packing Y63.5
- infusion — *see also* Misadventure, by type, infusion Y69
  - excessive amount of fluid Y63.0
  - incorrect dilution of fluid Y63.1
  - wrong fluid Y65.1
- mismatched blood in transfusion Y65.0
- nonadministration of necessary drug or biological substance Y63.6
- overdose — *see* Table of Drugs and Chemicals

Misadventure(s) **to patient**(s) **during surgical or medical care** — continued
  overdose — see Table of Drugs and Chemicals — continued
    radiation (in therapy) Y63.2
  perforation — see Index to Diseases and Injuries, Complication(s)
  performance of inappropriate operation — see Inappropriate operation performed
  puncture — see Index to Diseases and Injuries, Complication(s)
  specified type NEC Y65.8
    failure
      suture or ligature during surgical operation Y65.2
      to introduce or to remove tube or instrument — see Failure, to
    infusion of wrong fluid Y65.1
    performance of inappropriate operation — see Inappropriate operation performed
    transfusion of mismatched blood Y65.0
    wrong
      fluid in infusion Y65.1
      placement of endotracheal tube during anesthetic procedure Y65.3
  transfusion — see Misadventure, by type, transfusion
    excessive amount of blood Y63.0
    mismatched blood Y65.0
  wrong
    drug given in error — see Table of Drugs and Chemicals
    fluid in infusion Y65.1
    placement of endotracheal tube during anesthetic procedure Y65.3
Mismatched blood in transfusion Y65.0
Motion sickness T75.3 ☑
Mountain sickness W94.11 ☑
Mudslide (of cataclysmic nature) — see Landslide
Murder (attempt) — see Assault

N

Nail
  contact with W45.0 ☑
    gun W29.4 ☑
  embedded in skin W45.0 ☑
Neglect (criminal) (homicidal intent) X58 ☑
Noise (causing injury) (pollution) W42.9 ☑
  supersonic W42.0 ☑
Nonadministration (of)
  drug or biological substance (necessary) Y63.6
  surgical and medical care Y66
Nosocomial condition Y95

O

Object
  falling
    from, in, on, hitting
      machinery — see Contact, with, by type of machine
  set in motion by
    accidental explosion or rupture of pressure vessel W38 ☑
    firearm — see Discharge, firearm, by type
    machine(ry) — see Contact, with, by type of machine
Overdose (drug) — see Table of Drugs and Chemicals
  radiation Y63.2
Overexertion X50.9 ☑
  from
    prolonged static or awkward postures X50.1 ☑
    repetitive movements X50.3 ☑
    specified strenuous movements or postures NEC X50.9 ☑
    strenuous movement or load X50.0 ☑
Overexposure (accidental) (to)
  cold — see also Exposure, cold X31 ☑
    due to man-made conditions — see Exposure, cold, man-made
  heat — see also Heat X30 ☑
  radiation — see Radiation
  radioactivity W88.0 ☑
  sun (sunburn) X32 ☑
  weather NEC — see Forces of nature
  wind NEC — see Forces of nature
Overheated — see Heat

Overturning (accidental)
  machinery — see Contact, with, by type of machine
  transport vehicle NEC — see also Accident, transport V89.9 ☑
  watercraft (causing drowning, submersion) — see also Drowning, due to, accident to, watercraft, overturning
    causing injury except drowning or submersion — see Accident, watercraft, causing, injury NEC

P

Parachute descent (voluntary) (without accident to aircraft) V97.29 ☑
  due to accident to aircraft — see Accident, transport, aircraft
Pecked by bird W61.99 ☑
Perforation during medical or surgical treatment as misadventure — see Index to Diseases and Injuries, Complication(s)
Perpetrator, perpetration, of assault, maltreatment and neglect (by) Y07.9
  boyfriend Y07.03
  brother Y07.410
    stepbrother Y07.435
  coach Y07.53
  cousin
    female Y07.491
    male Y07.490
  daycare provider Y07.519
    at-home
      adult care Y07.512
      childcare Y07.510
    care center
      adult care Y07.513
      childcare Y07.511
  family member NEC Y07.499
  father Y07.11
    adoptive Y07.13
    foster Y07.420
    stepfather Y07.430
  foster father Y07.420
  foster mother Y07.421
  girl friend Y07.04
  healthcare provider Y07.529
    mental health Y07.521
    specified NEC Y07.528
  husband Y07.01
  instructor Y07.53
  mother Y07.12
    adoptive Y07.14
    foster Y07.421
    stepmother Y07.433
  multiple perpetrators Y07.6
  nonfamily member Y07.50
    specified NEC Y07.59
  nurse Y07.528
  occupational therapist Y07.528
  partner of parent
    female Y07.434
    male Y07.432
  physical therapist Y07.528
  sister Y07.411
  speech therapist Y07.528
  stepbrother Y07.435
  stepfather Y07.430
  stepmother Y07.433
  stepsister Y07.436
  teacher Y07.53
  wife Y07.02
Piercing — see Contact, with, by type of object or machine
Pinched
  between objects (moving) (stationary and moving) W23.0 ☑
  stationary W23.1 ☑
Pinned under machine(ry) — see Contact, with, by type of machine
Place of occurrence Y92.9
  abandoned house Y92.89
  airplane Y92.813
  airport Y92.520
  ambulatory health services establishment NEC Y92.538
  ambulatory surgery center Y92.530
  amusement park Y92.831
  apartment (co-op) — see Place of occurrence, residence, apartment
  assembly hall Y92.29

Place of occurrence — continued
  bank Y92.510
  barn Y92.71
  baseball field Y92.320
  basketball court Y92.310
  beach Y92.832
  boarding house — see Place of occurrence, residence, boarding house
  boat Y92.814
  bowling alley Y92.39
  bridge Y92.89
  building under construction Y92.61
  bus Y92.811
    station Y92.521
  cafe Y92.511
  campsite Y92.833
  campus — see Place of occurrence, school
  canal Y92.89
  car Y92.810
  casino Y92.59
  children's home — see Place of occurrence, residence, institutional, orphanage
  church Y92.22
  cinema Y92.26
  clubhouse Y92.29
  coal pit Y92.64
  college (community) Y92.214
  condominium — see Place of occurrence, residence, apartment
  construction area — see Place of occurrence, industrial and construction area
  convalescent home — see Place of occurrence, residence, institutional, nursing home
  court-house Y92.240
  cricket ground Y92.328
  cultural building Y92.258
    art gallery Y92.250
    museum Y92.251
    music hall Y92.252
    opera house Y92.253
    specified NEC Y92.258
    theater Y92.254
  dancehall Y92.252
  day nursery Y92.210
  dentist office Y92.531
  derelict house Y92.89
  desert Y92.820
  dockyard Y92.62
  dock NOS Y92.89
  doctor's office Y92.531
  dormitory — see Place of occurrence, residence, institutional, school dormitory
  dry dock Y92.62
  factory (building) (premises) Y92.63
  farm (land under cultivation) (outbuildings) Y92.79
    barn Y92.71
    chicken coop Y92.72
    field Y92.73
    hen house Y92.72
    house — see Place of occurrence, residence, house
    orchard Y92.74
    specified NEC Y92.79
  football field Y92.321
  forest Y92.821
  freeway Y92.411
  gallery Y92.250
  garage (commercial) Y92.59
    boarding house Y92.044
    military base Y92.135
    mobile home Y92.025
    nursing home Y92.124
    orphanage Y92.114
    private house Y92.015
    reform school Y92.155
  gas station Y92.524
  gasworks Y92.69
  golf course Y92.39
  gravel pit Y92.64
  grocery Y92.512
  gymnasium Y92.39
  handball court Y92.318
  harbor Y92.89
  harness racing course Y92.39
  healthcare provider office Y92.531
  highway (interstate) Y92.411
  hill Y92.828
  hockey rink Y92.330
  home — see Place of occurrence, residence

Place of occurrence — continued

hospice — *see* Place of occurrence, residence, institutional, nursing home
hospital Y92.239
  cafeteria Y92.233
  corridor Y92.232
  operating room Y92.234
  patient
    bathroom Y92.231
    room Y92.230
  specified NEC Y92.238
hotel Y92.59
house — *see also* Place of occurrence, residence
  abandoned Y92.89
  under construction Y92.61
industrial and construction area (yard) Y92.69
  building under construction Y92.61
  dock Y92.62
  dry dock Y92.62
  factory Y92.63
  gasworks Y92.69
  mine Y92.64
  oil rig Y92.65
  pit Y92.64
  power station Y92.69
  shipyard Y92.62
  specified NEC Y92.69
  tunnel under construction Y92.69
  workshop Y92.69
kindergarten Y92.211
lacrosse field Y92.328
lake Y92.828
library Y92.241
mall Y92.59
market Y92.512
marsh Y92.828
military
  base — *see* Place of occurrence, residence, institutional, military base
  training ground Y92.84
mine Y92.64
mosque Y92.22
motel Y92.59
motorway (interstate) Y92.411
mountain Y92.828
movie-house Y92.26
museum Y92.251
music-hall Y92.252
not applicable Y92.9
nuclear power station Y92.69
nursing home — *see* Place of occurrence, residence, institutional, nursing home
office building Y92.59
offshore installation Y92.65
oil rig Y92.65
old people's home — *see* Place of occurrence, residence, institutional, specified NEC
opera-house Y92.253
orphanage — *see* Place of occurrence, residence, institutional, orphanage
outpatient surgery center Y92.530
park (public) Y92.830
  amusement Y92.831
parking garage Y92.89
  lot Y92.481
pavement Y92.480
physician office Y92.531
polo field Y92.328
pond Y92.828
post office Y92.242
power station Y92.69
prairie Y92.828
prison — *see* Place of occurrence, residence, institutional, prison
public
  administration building Y92.248
    city hall Y92.243
    courthouse Y92.240
    library Y92.241
    post office Y92.242
    specified NEC Y92.248
  building NEC Y92.29
  hall Y92.29
  place NOS Y92.89
race course Y92.39
radio station Y92.59
railway line (bridge) Y92.85
ranch (outbuildings) — *see* Place of occurrence, farm

Place of occurrence — continued

recreation area Y92.838
  amusement park Y92.831
  beach Y92.832
  campsite Y92.833
  park (public) Y92.830
  seashore Y92.832
  specified NEC Y92.838
reform school - — *see* Place of occurrence, residence, institutional, reform school
religious institution Y92.22
residence (non-institutional) (private) Y92.009
  apartment Y92.039
    bathroom Y92.031
    bedroom Y92.032
    kitchen Y92.030
    specified NEC Y92.038
  bathroom Y92.002
  bedroom Y92.003
  boarding house Y92.049
    bathroom Y92.041
    bedroom Y92.042
    driveway Y92.043
    garage Y92.044
    garden Y92.046
    kitchen Y92.040
    specified NEC Y92.048
    swimming pool Y92.045
    yard Y92.046
  dining room Y92.001
  garden Y92.007
  home Y92.009
  house, single family Y92.019
    bathroom Y92.012
    bedroom Y92.013
    dining room Y92.011
    driveway Y92.014
    garage Y92.015
    garden Y92.017
    kitchen Y92.010
    specified NEC Y92.018
    swimming pool Y92.016
    yard Y92.017
  institutional Y92.10
    children's home — *see* Place of occurrence, residence, institutional, orphanage
    hospice — *see* Place of occurrence, residence, institutional, nursing home
    military base Y92.139
      barracks Y92.133
      garage Y92.135
      garden Y92.137
      kitchen Y92.130
      mess hall Y92.131
      specified NEC Y92.138
      swimming pool Y92.136
      yard Y92.137
    nursing home Y92.129
      bathroom Y92.121
      bedroom Y92.122
      driveway Y92.123
      garage Y92.124
      garden Y92.126
      kitchen Y92.120
      specified NEC Y92.128
      swimming pool Y92.125
      yard Y92.126
    orphanage Y92.119
      bathroom Y92.111
      bedroom Y92.112
      driveway Y92.113
      garage Y92.114
      garden Y92.116
      kitchen Y92.110
      specified NEC Y92.118
      swimming pool Y92.115
      yard Y92.116
    prison Y92.149
      bathroom Y92.142
      cell Y92.143
      courtyard Y92.147
      dining room Y92.141
      kitchen Y92.140
      specified NEC Y92.148
      swimming pool Y92.146
    reform school Y92.159
      bathroom Y92.152
      bedroom Y92.153
      dining room Y92.151

Place of occurrence — continued

residence — *continued*
  institutional — *continued*
    reform school — *continued*
      driveway Y92.154
      garage Y92.155
      garden Y92.157
      kitchen Y92.150
      specified NEC Y92.158
      swimming pool Y92.156
      yard Y92.157
    school dormitory Y92.169
      bathroom Y92.162
      bedroom Y92.163
      dining room Y92.161
      kitchen Y92.160
      specified NEC Y92.168
    specified NEC Y92.199
      bathroom Y92.192
      bedroom Y92.193
      dining room Y92.191
      driveway Y92.194
      garage Y92.195
      garden Y92.197
      kitchen Y92.190
      specified NEC Y92.198
      swimming pool Y92.196
      yard Y92.197
  kitchen Y92.000
  mobile home Y92.029
    bathroom Y92.022
    bedroom Y92.023
    dining room Y92.021
    driveway Y92.024
    garage Y92.025
    garden Y92.027
    kitchen Y92.020
    specified NEC Y92.028
    swimming pool Y92.026
    yard Y92.027
  specified place in residence NEC Y92.008
  specified residence type NEC Y92.099
    bathroom Y92.091
    bedroom Y92.092
    driveway Y92.093
    garage Y92.094
    garden Y92.096
    kitchen Y92.090
    specified NEC Y92.098
    swimming pool Y92.095
    yard Y92.096
restaurant Y92.511
riding school Y92.39
river Y92.828
road Y92.410
rodeo ring Y92.39
rugby field Y92.328
same day surgery center Y92.530
sand pit Y92.64
school (private) (public) (state) Y92.219
  college Y92.214
  daycare center Y92.210
  elementary school Y92.211
  high school Y92.213
  kindergarten Y92.211
  middle school Y92.212
  specified NEC Y92.218
  trace school Y92.215
  university Y92.214
  vocational school Y92.215
sea (shore) Y92.832
senior citizen center Y92.29
service area
  airport Y92.520
  bus station Y92.521
  gas station Y92.524
  highway rest stop Y92.523
  railway station Y92.522
shipyard Y92.62
shop (commercial) Y92.513
sidewalk Y92.480
silo Y92.79
skating rink (roller) Y92.331
  ice Y92.330
slaughter house Y92.86
soccer field Y92.322
specified place NEC Y92.89
sports area Y92.39

Place of occurrence — *continued*
  sports area — *continued*
    athletic
      court Y92.318
        basketball Y92.310
        specified NEC Y92.318
        squash Y92.311
        tennis Y92.312
      field Y92.328
        baseball Y92.320
        cricket ground Y92.328
        football Y92.321
        hockey Y92.328
        soccer Y92.322
        specified NEC Y92.328
    golf course Y92.39
    gymnasium Y92.39
    riding school Y92.39
    skating rink (roller) Y92.331
      ice Y92.330
    stadium Y92.39
    swimming pool Y92.34
  squash court Y92.311
  stadium Y92.39
  steeplechasing course Y92.39
  store Y92.512
  stream Y92.828
  street and highway Y92.410
    bike path Y92.482
    freeway Y92.411
    highway ramp Y92.415
    interstate highway Y92.411
    local residential or business street Y92.414
    motorway Y92.411
    parking lot Y92.481
    parkway Y92.412
    sidewalk Y92.480
    specified NEC Y92.488
    state road Y92.413
  subway car Y92.816
  supermarket Y92.512
  swamp Y92.828
  swimming pool (public) Y92.34
    private (at) Y92.095
      boarding house Y92.045
      military base Y92.136
      mobile home Y92.026
      nursing home Y92.125
      orphanage Y92.115
      prison Y92.146
      reform school Y92.156
      single family residence Y92.016
  synagogue Y92.22
  television station Y92.59
  tennis court Y92.312
  theater Y92.254
  trade area Y92.59
    bank Y92.510
    cafe Y92.511
    casino Y92.59
    garage Y92.59
    hotel Y92.59
    market Y92.512
    office building Y92.59
    radio station Y92.59
    restaurant Y92.511
    shop Y92.513
    shopping mall Y92.59
    store Y92.512
    supermarket Y92.512
    television station Y92.59
    warehouse Y92.59
  trailer park, residential — *see* Place of occurrence, residence, mobile home
  trailer site NOS Y92.89
  train Y92.815
    station Y92.522
  truck Y92.812
  tunnel under construction Y92.69
  university Y92.214
  urgent (health) care center Y92.532
  vehicle (transport) Y92.818
    airplane Y92.813
    boat Y92.814
    bus Y92.811
    car Y92.810
    specified NEC Y92.818
    subway car Y92.816
    train Y92.815

Place of occurrence — *continued*
  vehicle — *continued*
    truck Y92.812
  warehouse Y92.59
  water reservoir Y92.89
  wilderness area Y92.828
    desert Y92.820
    forest Y92.821
    marsh Y92.828
    mountain Y92.828
    prairie Y92.828
    specified NEC Y92.828
    swamp Y92.828
  workshop Y92.69
  yard, private Y92.096
    boarding house Y92.046
    mobile home Y92.027
    single family house Y92.017
  youth center Y92.29
  zoo (zoological garden) Y92.834
Plumbism — *see* Table of Drugs and Chemicals, lead
Poisoning (accidental) (by) — *see also* Table of Drugs and Chemicals
  by plant, thorns, spines, sharp leaves or other mechanisms NEC X58 ☑
  carbon monoxide
    generated by
      motor.vehicle — *see* Accident, transport
      watercraft (in transit) (not in transit) V93.89 ☑
        ferry boat V93.81 ☑
        fishing boat V93.82 ☑
        jet skis V93.83 ☑
        liner V93.81 ☑
        merchant ship V93.80 ☑
        passenger ship V93.81 ☑
        powered craft NEC V93.83 ☑
  caused by injection of poisons into skin by plant thorns, spines, sharp leaves X58 ☑
  marine or sea plants (venomous) X58 ☑
  execution — *see* Legal, intervention, gas
  intervention
    by gas — *see* Legal, intervention, gas
    other specified means — *see* Legal, intervention, specified means NEC
  exhaust gas
    generated by
      motor vehicle — *see* Accident, transport
      watercraft (in transit) (not in transit) V93.89 ☑
        ferry boat V93.81 ☑
        fishing boat V93.82 ☑
        jet skis V93.83 ☑
        liner V93.81 ☑
        merchant ship V93.80 ☑
        passenger ship V93.81 ☑
        powered craft NEC V93.83 ☑
  fumes or smoke due to
    explosion — *see also* Explosion W40.9 ☑
    fire — *see* Exposure, fire
    ignition — *see* Ignition
  gas
    in legal intervention — *see* Legal, intervention, gas
    legal execution — *see* Legal, intervention, gas
  in war operations — *see* War operations
  legal
Powder burn (by) (from)
  airgun W34.110 ☑
  BB gun W34.110 ☑
  firearm NEC W34.19 ☑
  gas, air or spring-operated gun NEC W34.118 ☑
  handgun W32.1 ☑
  hunting rifle W33.12 ☑
  larger firearm W33.10 ☑
    specified NEC W33.19 ☑
  machine gun W33.13 ☑
  paintball gun W34.111 ☑
  pellet gun W34.110 ☑
  shotgun W33.11 ☑
  Very pistol [flare] W34.19 ☑
Premature cessation (of) **surgical and medical care** Y66
Privation (food) (water) X58 ☑
Procedure (operation)
  correct, on wrong side or body part (wrong side) (wrong site) Y65.53
  intended for another patient done on wrong patient Y65.52
  performed on patient not scheduled for surgery Y65.52

Procedure — *continued*
  performed on wrong patient Y65.52
  wrong, performed on correct patient Y65.51
Prolonged
  sitting in transport vehicle — *see* Travel, by type of vehicle
  stay in
    high altitude as cause of anoxia, barodontalgia, barotitis or hypoxia W94.11 ☑
    weightless environment X52 ☑
Pulling, excessive — *see also* Overexertion X50.9- ☑
Puncture, puncturing — *see also* Contact, with, by type of object or machine
  by
    plant thorns, spines, sharp leaves or other mechanisms NEC W60 ☑
    during medical or surgical treatment as misadventure — *see* Index to Diseases and Injuries, Complication(s)
Pushed, pushing (accidental) (injury in)
  by other person(s) (accidental) W51 ☑
    as, or caused by, a crowd or human stampede (with fall) W52 ☑
    before moving object NEC Y02.8 ☑
      motor vehicle Y02.0 ☑
      subway train Y02.1 ☑
      train Y02.1 ☑
    from
      high place NEC
        in accidental circumstances W17.89 ☑
        stated as
          intentional, homicide (attempt) Y01 ☑
          undetermined whether accidental or intentional Y30 ☑
      transport vehicle NEC — *see also* Accident, transport V89.9 ☑
        stated as
          intentional, homicide (attempt) Y08.89 ☑
    with fall W03 ☑
      due to ice or snow W00.0 ☑
  overexertion X50.9 ☑

R

Radiation (exposure to)
  arc lamps W89.0 ☑
  atomic power plant (malfunction) NEC W88.1 ☑
  complication of or abnormal reaction to medical radiotherapy Y84.2
  electromagnetic, ionizing W88.0 ☑
  gamma rays W88.1 ☑
  in
    war operations (from or following nuclear explosion) — *see* War operations
  inadvertent exposure of patient (receiving test or therapy) Y63.3
  infrared (heaters and lamps) W90.1 ☑
    excessive heat from W92 ☑
  ionized, ionizing (particles, artificially accelerated)
    radioisotopes W88.1 ☑
    specified NEC W88.8 ☑
    x-rays W88.0 ☑
  isotopes, radioactive — *see* Radiation, radioactive isotopes
  laser(s) W90.2 ☑
    in war operations — *see* War operations
    misadventure in medical care Y63.2
  light sources (man-made visible and ultraviolet) W89.9 ☑
    natural X32 ☑
    specified NEC W89.8 ☑
    tanning bed W89.1 ☑
    welding light W89.0 ☑
  man-made visible light W89.9 ☑
    specified NEC W89.8 ☑
    tanning bed W89.1 ☑
    welding light W89.0 ☑
  microwave W90.8 ☑
  misadventure in medical or surgical procedure Y63.2
  natural NEC X39.08 ☑
    radon X39.01 ☑
  overdose (in medical or surgical procedure) Y63.2
  radar W90.0 ☑
  radioactive isotopes (any) W88.1 ☑
    atomic power plant malfunction W88.1 ☑
    misadventure in medical or surgical treatment Y63.2

Radiation — *continued*
  radiofrequency W90.0 ☑
  radium NEC W88.1 ☑
  sun X32 ☑
  ultraviolet (light) (man-made) W89.9 ☑
    natural X32 ☑
    specified NEC W89.8 ☑
    tanning bed W89.1 ☑
    welding light W89.0 ☑
  welding arc, torch, or light W89.0 ☑
    excessive heat from W92 ☑
  x-rays (hard) (soft) W88.0 ☑
Range disease W94.11 ☑
Rape (attempted) T74.2- ☑
Rat bite W53.11 ☑
Reaching (prolonged) (static) X50.1 ☑
Reaction, abnormal to medical procedure — *see also*
    Complication of or following, by type of procedure
    Y84.9
  biologicals — *see* Table of Drugs and Chemicals
  drugs — *see* Table of Drugs and Chemicals
  vaccine — *see* Table of Drugs and Chemicals
  with misadventure — *see* Misadventure
Recoil
  airgun W34.110 ☑
  BB gun W34.110 ☑
  firearm NEC W34.19 ☑
  gas, air or spring-operated gun NEC W34.118 ☑
  handgun W32.1 ☑
  hunting rifle W33.12 ☑
  larger firearm W33.10 ☑
    specified NEC W33.19 ☑
  machine gun W33.13 ☑
  paintball gun W34.111 ☑
  pellet W34.110 ☑
  shotgun W33.11 ☑
  Very pistol [flare] W34.19 ☑
Reduction in
  atmospheric pressure — *see* Air, pressure, change
Rock falling on or hitting (accidentally) (person)
    W20.8 ☑
  in cave-in W20.0 ☑
Run over (accidentally) (by)
  animal (not being ridden) NEC W55.89 ☑
  machinery — *see* Contact, with, by specified type of
    machine
  transport vehicle NEC — *see also* Accident, transport
    V09.9 ☑
    intentional homicide (attempt) Y03.0 ☑
    motor NEC V09.20 ☑
      intentional homicide (attempt) Y03.0 ☑
Running
  before moving object X81.8 ☑
    motor vehicle X81.0 ☑
Running off, away
  animal (being ridden) — *see also* Accident, transport
    V80.918 ☑
    not being ridden W55.89 ☑
  animal-drawn vehicle NEC — *see also* Accident, trans-
    port V80.928 ☑
  highway, road(way), street
    transport vehicle NEC — *see also* Accident, transport
    V89.9 ☑
Rupture pressurized devices — *see* Explosion, by type
    of device

S

Saturnism — *see* Table of Drugs and Chemicals, lead
Scald, scalding (accidental) (by) (from) (in) X19 ☑
  air (hot) X14.1 ☑
  gases (hot) X14.1 ☑
  homicide (attempt) — *see* Assault, burning, hot object
  inflicted by other person
    stated as intentional, homicide (attempt) — *see*
      Assault, burning, hot object
  liquid (boiling) (hot) NEC X12 ☑
    stated as undetermined whether accidental or inten-
      tional Y27.2 ☑
    suicide (attempt) X77.2 ☑
  local application of externally applied substance in
    medical or surgical care Y63.5
  metal (molten) (liquid) (hot) NEC X18 ☑
  self-inflicted X77.9 ☑
    stated as undetermined whether accidental or inten-
      tional Y27.8 ☑

Scald, scalding — *continued*
  steam X13.1 ☑
    assault X98.0 ☑
    stated as undetermined whether accidental or inten-
      tional Y27.0 ☑
    suicide (attempt) X77.0 ☑
  suicide (attempt) X77.9 ☑
  vapor (hot) X13.1 ☑
    assault X98.0 ☑
    stated as undetermined whether accidental or inten-
      tional Y27.0 ☑
    suicide (attempt) X77.0 ☑
Scratched by
  cat W55.03 ☑
  person(s) (accidentally) W50.4 ☑
    with intent to injure or kill Y04.0 ☑
    as, or caused by, a crowd or human stampede (with
      fall) W52
    assault Y04.0 ☑
    homicide (attempt) Y04.0 ☑
    in
      fight Y04.0 ☑
      legal intervention
        injuring
          bystander Y35.892 ☑
          law enforcement personnel Y35.891 ☑
          suspect Y35.893 ☑
          unspecified person Y35.899 ☑
Seasickness T75.3 ☑
Self-harm NEC — *see also* External cause by type, unde-
    termined whether accidental or intentional
  intentional — *see* Suicide
  poisoning NEC — *see* Table of Drugs and Chemicals,
    poisoning, accidental
Self-inflicted (injury) **NEC** — *see also* External cause by
    type, undetermined whether accidental or intention-
    al
  intentional — *see* Suicide
  poisoning NEC — *see* Table of Drugs and Chemicals,
    poisoning, accidental
Sequelae (of)
  accident NEC — *see* W00-X58 with 7th character S
  assault (homicidal) (any means) — *see* X92-Y08 with
    7th character S
  homicide, attempt (any means) — *see* X92-Y08 with
    7th character S
  injury undetermined whether accidentally or purposely
    inflicted — *see* Y21-Y33 with 7th character S
  intentional self-harm (classifiable to X71-X83) — *see*
    X71-X83 with 7th character S
  legal intervention — *see* with 7th character S Y35
  motor vehicle accident — *see* V00-V99 with 7th char-
    acter S
  suicide, attempt (any means) — *see* X71-X83 with 7th
    character S
  transport accident — *see* V00-V99 with 7th character
    S
  war operations — *see* War operations
Shock
  electric — *see* Exposure, electric current
  from electric appliance (any) (faulty) W86.8 ☑
    domestic W86.0 ☑
    suicide (attempt) X83.1 ☑
Shooting, shot (accidental(ly)) — *see also* Discharge,
    firearm, by type
  herself or himself — *see* Discharge, firearm by type,
    self-inflicted
  homicide (attempt) — *see* Discharge, firearm by type,
    homicide
  in war operations — *see* War operations
  inflicted by other person — *see* Discharge, firearm by
    type, homicide
    accidental — *see* Discharge, firearm, by type of
      firearm
  legal
    execution — *see* Legal, intervention, firearm
    intervention — *see* Legal, intervention, firearm
  self-inflicted — *see* Discharge, firearm by type, suicide
    accidental — *see* Discharge, firearm, by type of
      firearm
  suicide (attempt) — *see* Discharge, firearm by type,
    suicide
Shoving (accidentally) **by other person** — *see* Pushed,
    by other person
Sickness
  alpine W94.11 ☑
  motion — *see* Motion

Sickness — *continued*
  mountain W94.11 ☑
Sinking (accidental)
  watercraft (causing drowning, submersion) — *see also*
    Drowning, due to, accident to, watercraft, sinking
  causing injury except drowning or submersion —
    see Accident, watercraft, causing, injury NEC
Siriasis X32 ☑
Sitting (prolonged) (static) X50.1 ☑
Slashed wrists — *see* Cut, self-inflicted
Slipping (accidental) (on same level) (with fall) W01.0 ☑
  on
    ice W00.0 ☑
      with skates — *see* Accident, transport, pedestri-
        an, conveyance
    mud W01.0 ☑
    oil W01.0 ☑
    snow W00.0 ☑
      with skis — *see* Accident, transport, pedestrian,
        conveyance
    surface (slippery) (wet) NEC W01.0 ☑
  without fall W18.40 ☑
    due to
      specified NEC W18.49 ☑
      stepping from one level to another W18.43 ☑
      stepping into hole or opening W18.42 ☑
      stepping on object W18.41 ☑
Sliver, wood, contact with W45.8 ☑
Smoldering (due to fire) — *see* Exposure, fire
Sodomy (attempted) **by force** T74.2 ☑
Sound waves (causing injury) W42.9 ☑
  supersonic W42.0 ☑
Splinter, contact with W45.8 ☑
Stab, stabbing — *see* Cut
Standing (prolonged) (static) X50.1 ☑
Starvation X58 ☑
Status of external cause Y99.9
  child assisting in compensated work for family Y99.8
  civilian activity done for financial or other compensa-
    tion Y99.0
  civilian activity done for income or pay Y99.0
  family member assisting in compensated work for
    other family member Y99.8
  hobby not done for income Y99.8
  leisure activity Y99.8
  military activity Y99.1
  off-duty activity of military personnel Y99.8
  recreation or sport not for income or while a student
    Y99.8
  specified NEC Y99.8
  student activity Y99.8
  volunteer activity Y99.2
Stepped on
  by
    animal (not being ridden) NEC W55.89 ☑
    crowd or human stampede W52 ☑
    person W50.0 ☑
Stepping on
  object W22.8 ☑
    sports equipment W21.9 ☑
    stationary W22.09 ☑
      sports equipment W21.89 ☑
    with fall W18.31 ☑
  person W51 ☑
    by crowd or human stampede W52 ☑
  sports equipment W21.9 ☑
Sting
  arthropod, nonvenomous W57 ☑
  insect, nonvenomous W57 ☑
Storm (cataclysmic) — *see* Forces of nature, cataclysmic
    storm
Straining, excessive — *see also* Overexertion X50.9 ☑
Strangling — *see* Strangulation
Strangulation (accidental) T71 ☑
Strenuous movements — *see also* Overexertion
    X50.9 ☑
Striking against
  airbag (automobile) W22.10 ☑
    driver side W22.11 ☑
    front passenger side W22.12 ☑
    specified NEC W22.19 ☑
  bottom when
    diving or jumping into water (in) W16.822 ☑
      causing drowning W16.821 ☑
    from boat W16.722 ☑
      causing drowning W16.721 ☑

Striking against — *continued*
  bottom when — *continued*
    diving or jumping into water — *continued*
      natural body W16.622 ✔
        causing drowning W16.821 ✔
      swimming pool W16.522 ✔
        causing drowning W16.521 ✔
    falling into water (in) W16.322 ✔
      causing drowning W16.321 ✔
      fountain — *see* Striking against, bottom when,
        falling into water, specified NEC
      natural body W16.122 ✔
        causing drowning W16.121 ✔
      reservoir — *see* Striking against, bottom when,
        falling into water, specified NEC
      specified NEC W16.322 ✔
        causing drowning W16.321 ✔
      swimming pool W16.022 ✔
        causing drowning W16.021 ✔
  diving board (swimming-pool) W21.4 ✔
  object W22.8 ✔
    caused by crowd or human stampede (with fall)
      W52 ✔
    furniture W22.03 ✔
    lamppost W22.02 ✔
    sports equipment W21.9 ✔
    stationary W22.09 ✔
      sports equipment W21.89 ✔
    wall W22.01 ✔
    with
      drowning or submersion — *see* Drowning
      fall — *see* Fall, due to, bumping against, object
  person(s) W51 ✔
    as, or caused by, a crowd or human stampede (with
      fall) W52 ✔
    assault Y04.2 ✔
    homicide (attempt) Y04.2 ✔
    with fall W03 ✔
      due to ice or snow W00.0 ✔
  sports equipment W21.9 ✔
  wall (when) W22.01 ✔
    diving or jumping into water (in) W16.832 ✔
      causing drowning W16.831 ✔
      swimming pool W16.532 ✔
        causing drowning W16.531 ✔
    falling into water (in) W16.332 ✔
      causing drowning W16.331 ✔
      fountain — *see* Striking against, wall when,
        falling into water, specified NEC
      natural body W16.132 ✔
        causing drowning W16.131 ✔
      reservoir — *see* Striking against, wall when,
        falling into water, specified NEC
      specified NEC W16.332 ✔
        causing drowning W16.331 ✔
      swimming pool W16.032 ✔
        causing drowning W16.031 ✔
    swimming pool (when) W22.042 ✔
      causing drowning W22.041 ✔
      diving or jumping into water W16.532 ✔
        causing drowning W16.531 ✔
      falling into water W16.032 ✔
        causing drowning W16.031 ✔

Struck (accidentally) **by**
  airbag (automobile) W22.10 ✔
    driver side W22.11 ✔
    front passenger side W22.12 ✔
    specified NEC W22.19 ✔
  alligator W58.02 ✔
  animal (not being ridden) NEC W55.89 ✔
  avalanche — *see* Landslide
  ball (hit) (thrown) W21.00 ✔
    assault Y08.09 ✔
    baseball W21.03 ✔
    basketball W21.05 ✔
    football W21.01 ✔
    golf ball W21.04 ✔
    soccer W21.02 ✔
    softball W21.07 ✔
    specified NEC W21.09 ✔
    volleyball W21.06 ✔
  bat or racquet
    baseball bat W21.11 ✔
      assault Y08.02 ✔
    golf club W21.13 ✔
      assault Y08.09 ✔

Struck (accidentally) **by** — *continued*
  bat or racquet — *continued*
    specified NEC W21.19 ✔
      assault Y08.09 ✔
    tennis racquet W21.12 ✔
      assault Y08.09 ✔
  bullet — *see also* Discharge, firearm by type
    in war operations — *see* War operations
  crocodile W58.12 ✔
  dog W54.1 ✔
  flare, Very pistol — *see* Discharge, firearm NEC
  hailstones X39.8 ✔
  hockey (ice)
    field
      puck W21.221 ✔
      stick W21.211 ✔
    puck W21.220 ✔
    stick W21.210 ✔
      assault Y08.01 ✔
  landslide — *see* Landslide
  law-enforcement agent (on duty) — *see* Legal, inter-
    vention, manhandling
    with blunt object — *see* Legal, intervention, blunt
      object
  lightning T75.0 ✔
    causing fire — *see* Exposure, fire
  machine — *see* Contact, with, by type of machine
  mammal NEC W55.89 ✔
    marine W56.32 ✔
  marine animal W56.82 ✔
  missile
    firearm — *see* Discharge, firearm by type
    in war operations — *see* War operations, missile
  object W22.8 ✔
    blunt W22.8 ✔
      assault Y00 ✔
      suicide (attempt) X79 ✔
      undetermined whether accidental or intentional
        Y29 ✔
    falling W20.8 ✔
      from, in, on
        building W20.1 ✔
          burning (uncontrolled fire) X00.4 ✔
        cataclysmic
          earth surface movement NEC — *see*
            Landslide
          storm — *see* Forces of nature, cataclysmic
            storm
        cave-in W20.0 ✔
        earthquake X34 ✔
        machine (in operation) — *see* Contact, with,
          by type of machine
        structure W20.1 ✔
          burning X00.4 ✔
        transport vehicle (in motion) — *see* Accident,
          transport, by type of vehicle
        watercraft V93.49 ✔
          due to
            accident to craft V91.39 ✔
              powered craft V91.33 ✔
                ferry boat V91.31 ✔
                fishing boat V91.32 ✔
                jetskis V91.33 ✔
                liner V91.31 ✔
                merchant ship V91.30 ✔
                passenger ship V91.31 ✔
              unpowered craft V91.38 ✔
                canoe V91.35 ✔
                inflatable V91.36 ✔
                kayak V91.35 ✔
                sailboat V91.34 ✔
                surf-board V91.38 ✔
                windsurfer V91.38 ✔
            powered craft V93.43 ✔
              ferry boat V93.41 ✔
              fishing boat V93.42 ✔
              jetskis V93.43 ✔
              liner V93.41 ✔
              merchant ship V93.40 ✔
              passenger ship V93.41 ✔
            unpowered craft V93.48 ✔
              sailboat V93.44 ✔
              surf-board V93.48 ✔
              windsurfer V93.48 ✔
    moving NEC W20.8 ✔
    projected W20.8 ✔

Struck (accidentally) **by** — *continued*
  object — *continued*
    projected — *continued*
      assault Y00 ✔
      in sports W21.9 ✔
        assault Y08.09 ✔
        ball W21.00 ✔
          baseball W21.03 ✔
          basketball W21.05 ✔
          football W21.01 ✔
          golf ball W21.04 ✔
          soccer W21.02 ✔
          softball W21.07 ✔
          specified NEC W21.09 ✔
          volleyball W21.06 ✔
        bat or racquet
          baseball bat W21.11 ✔
            assault Y08.02 ✔
          golf club W21.13 ✔
            assault Y08.09 ✔
          specified NEC W21.19 ✔
            assault Y08.09 ✔
          tennis racquet W21.12 ✔
            assault Y08.09 ✔
        hockey (ice)
          field
            puck W21.221 ✔
            stick W21.211 ✔
          puck W21.220 ✔
          stick W21.210 ✔
            assault Y08.01 ✔
        specified NEC W21.89 ✔
    set in motion by explosion — *see* Explosion
    thrown W20.8 ✔
      assault Y00 ✔
      in sports W21.9 ✔
        assault Y08.09 ✔
        ball W21.00 ✔
          baseball W21.03 ✔
          basketball W21.05 ✔
          football W21.01 ✔
          golf ball W21.04 ✔
          soccer W21.02 ✔
          soft ball W21.07 ✔
          specified NEC W21.09 ✔
          volleyball W21.06 ✔
        bat or racquet
          baseball bat W21.11 ✔
            assault Y08.02 ✔
          golf club W21.13 ✔
            assault Y08.09 ✔
          specified NEC W21.19 ✔
            assault Y08.09 ✔
          tennis racquet W21.12 ✔
            assault Y08.09 ✔
        hockey (ice)
          field
            puck W21.221 ✔
            stick W21.211 ✔
          puck W21.220 ✔
          stick W21.210 ✔
            assault Y08.01 ✔
        specified NEC W21.89 ✔
  other person(s) W50.0 ✔
    with
      blunt object W22.8 ✔
        intentional, homicide (attempt) Y00 ✔
      sports equipment W21.9 ✔
      undetermined whether accidental or inten-
        tional Y29 ✔
    fall W03 ✔
      due to ice or snow W00.0 ✔
    as, or caused by, a crowd or human stampede (with
      fall) W52 ✔
    assault Y04.2 ✔
    homicide (attempt) Y04.2 ✔
    in legal intervention
      injuring
        bystander Y35.812 ✔
        law enforcement personnel Y35.811 ✔
        suspect Y35.813 ✔
        unspecified person Y35.819 ✔
    sports equipment W21.9 ✔
  police (on duty) — *see* Legal, intervention, manhan-
    dling

Struck (accidentally) **by** — *continued*
  police — *see* Legal, intervention, manhandling — *continued*
    with blunt object — *see* Legal, intervention, blunt object
  sports equipment W21.9 ☑
    assault Y08.09 ☑
    ball W21.00 ☑
      baseball W21.03 ☑
      basketball W21.05 ☑
      football W21.01 ☑
      golf ball W21.04 ☑
      soccer W21.02 ☑
      soft ball W21.07 ☑
      specified NEC W21.09 ☑
      volleyball W21.06 ☑
    bat or racquet
      baseball bat W21.11 ☑
        assault Y08.02 ☑
      golf club W21.13 ☑
        assault Y08.09 ☑
      specified NEC W21.19 ☑
      tennis racquet W21.12 ☑
        assault Y08.09 ☑
    cleats (shoe) W21.31 ☑
    foot wear NEC W21.39 ☑
    football helmet W21.81 ☑
    hockey (ice)
      field
        puck W21.221 ☑
        stick W21.211 ☑
      puck W21.220 ☑
      stick W21.210 ☑
        assault Y08.01 ☑
    skate blades W21.32 ☑
    specified NEC W21.89 ☑
      assault Y08.09 ☑
  thunderbolt — *see* subcategory T75.0
    causing fire — *see* Exposure, fire
  transport vehicle NEC — *see also* Accident, transport V09.9 ☑
    intentional, homicide (attempt) Y03.0 ☑
    motor NEC — *see also* Accident, transport V09.20 ☑
      homicide Y03.0 ☑
  vehicle (transport) NEC — *see* Accident, transport, by type of vehicle
    stationary (falling from jack, hydraulic lift, ramp) W20.8 ☑

Stumbling
  over
    animal NEC W01.0 ☑
      with fall W18.09 ☑
    carpet, rug or (small) object W22.8 ☑
      with fall W18.09 ☑
    person W51 ☑
      with fall W03 ☑
        due to ice or snow W00.0 ☑
  without fall W18.40 ☑
    due to
      specified NEC W18.49 ☑
      stepping from one level to another W18.43 ☑
      stepping into hole or opening W18.42 ☑
      stepping on object W18.41 ☑
Submersion (accidental) — *see* Drowning
Suffocation (accidental) (by external means) (by pressure) (mechanical) — *see also* category T71 ☑
  due to, by
    avalanche — *see* Landslide
    explosion — *see* Explosion
    fire — *see* Exposure, fire
    food, any type (aspiration) (ingestion) (inhalation) — *see* categories T17 and T18 ☑
    ignition — *see* Ignition
    landslide — *see* Landslide
    machine(ry) — *see* Contact, with, by type of machine
    vomitus (aspiration) (inhalation) T17.81- ☑
  in
    burning building X00.8 ☑
Suicide, suicidal (attempted) (by) X83.8 ☑
  blunt object X79 ☑
  burning, burns X76 ☑
    hot object X77.9 ☑
      fluid NEC X77.2 ☑
      household appliance X77.3 ☑
      specified NEC X77.8 ☑

Suicide, suicidal — *continued*
  burning, burns — *continued*
    hot object — *continued*
      steam X77.0 ☑
      tap water X77.1 ☑
      vapors X77.0 ☑
  caustic substance — *see* Table of Drugs and Chemicals
  cold, extreme X83.2 ☑
  collision of motor vehicle with
    motor vehicle X82.0 ☑
    specified NEC X82.8 ☑
    train X82.1 ☑
    tree X82.2 ☑
  crashing of aircraft X83.0 ☑
  cut (any part of body) X78.9 ☑
  cutting or piercing instrument X78.9 ☑
    dagger X78.2 ☑
    glass X78.0 ☑
    knife X78.1 ☑
    specified NEC X78.8 ☑
    sword X78.2 ☑
  drowning (in) X71.9 ☑
    bathtub X71.0 ☑
    natural water X71.3 ☑
    specified NEC X71.8 ☑
    swimming pool X71.1 ☑
      following fall X71.2 ☑
  electrocution X83.1 ☑
  explosive(s) (material) X75 ☑
  fire, flames X76 ☑
  firearm X74.9 ☑
    airgun X74.01 ☑
    handgun X72 ☑
    hunting rifle X73.1 ☑
    larger X73.9 ☑
      specified NEC X73.8 ☑
    machine gun X73.2 ☑
    shotgun X73.0 ☑
    specified NEC X74.8 ☑
  hanging X83.8 ☑
  hot object — *see* Suicide, burning, hot object
  jumping
    before moving object X81.8 ☑
      motor vehicle X81.0 ☑
      subway train X81.1 ☑
      train X81.1 ☑
    from high place X80 ☑
  late effect of attempt — *see* X71-X83 with 7th character S
  lying before moving object, train, vehicle X81.8 ☑
  poisoning — *see* Table of Drugs and Chemicals
  puncture (any part of body) — *see* Suicide, cutting or piercing instrument
  scald — *see* Suicide, burning, hot object
  sequelae of attempt — *see* X71-X83 with 7th character S
  sharp object (any) — *see* Suicide, cutting or piercing instrument
  shooting — *see* Suicide, firearm
  specified means NEC X83.8 ☑
  stab (any part of body) — *see* Suicide, cutting or piercing instrument
  steam, hot vapors X77.0 ☑
  strangulation X83.8 ☑
  submersion — *see* Suicide, drowning
  suffocation X83.8 ☑
  wound NEC X83.8 ☑
Sunstroke X32 ☑
Supersonic waves (causing injury) W42.0 ☑
Surgical procedure, complication of (delayed or as an abnormal reaction without mention of misadventure) — *see also* Complication of or following, by type of procedure
  due to or as a result of misadventure — *see* Misadventure
Swallowed, swallowing
  foreign body — *see* Foreign body, alimentary canal
  poison — *see* Table of Drugs and Chemicals
  substance
    caustic or corrosive — *see* Table of Drugs and Chemicals
    poisonous — *see* Table of Drugs and Chemicals

T

Tackle in sport W03 ☑

Terrorism (involving) Y38.80 ☑
  biological weapons Y38.6X- ☑
  chemical weapons Y38.7X- ☑
  conflagration Y38.3X- ☑
  drowning and submersion Y38.89- ☑
  explosion Y38.2X- ☑
    destruction of aircraft Y38.1X- ☑
    marine weapons Y38.0X- ☑
  fire Y38.3X- ☑
  firearms Y38.4X- ☑
  hot substances Y38.3X- ☑
  lasers Y38.89- ☑
  nuclear weapons Y38.5X- ☑
  piercing or stabbing instruments Y38.89- ☑
  secondary effects Y38.9X- ☑
  specified method NEC Y38.89- ☑
  suicide bomber Y38.81- ☑
Thirst X58 ☑
Threat to breathing
  aspiration — *see* Aspiration
  due to cave-in, falling earth or substance NEC T71 ☑
Thrown (accidentally)
  against part (any) of or object in transport vehicle (in motion) NEC — *see also* Accident, transport
  from
    high place, homicide (attempt) Y01 ☑
    machinery — *see* Contact, with, by type of machine
    transport vehicle NEC — *see also* Accident, transport V89.9 ☑
  off — *see* Thrown, from
Thunderbolt — *see* subcategory T75.0 ☑
  causing fire — *see* Exposure, fire
Tidal wave (any injury) **NEC** — *see* Forces of nature, tidal wave
Took
  overdose (drug) — *see* Table of Drugs and Chemicals
  poison — *see* Table of Drugs and Chemicals
Tornado (any injury) X37.1 ☑
Torrential rain (any injury) X37.8 ☑
Torture X58 ☑
Trampled by animal NEC W55.89 ☑
Trapped (accidentally)
  between objects (moving) (stationary and moving) — *see* Caught
  by part (any) of
    motorcycle V29.88 ☑
    pedal cycle V19.88 ☑
    transport vehicle NEC — *see also* Accident, transport V89.9 ☑
Travel (effects) (sickness) T75.3 ☑
Tree falling on or hitting (accidentally) (person) W20.8 ☑
Tripping
  over
    animal W01.0 ☑
      with fall W01.0 ☑
    carpet, rug or (small) object W22.8 ☑
      with fall W18.09 ☑
    person W51 ☑
      with fall W03 ☑
        due to ice or snow W00.0 ☑
  without fall W18.40 ☑
    due to
      specified NEC W18.49 ☑
      stepping from one level to another W18.43 ☑
      stepping into hole or opening W18.42 ☑
      stepping on object W18.41 ☑
Twisted by person(s) (accidentally) W50.2 ☑
  with intent to injure or kill Y04.0 ☑
  as, or caused by, a crowd or human stampede (with fall) W52 ☑
  assault Y04.0 ☑
  homicide (attempt) Y04.0 ☑
  in
    fight Y04.0 ☑
    legal intervention — *see* Legal, intervention, manhandling
Twisting (prolonged) (static) X50.1- ☑

U

Underdosing of necessary drugs, medicaments or biological substances Y63.6
Undetermined intent (contact) (exposure)
  automobile collision Y32 ☑
  blunt object Y29 ☑

◷ **Subterms under main terms may continue to next column or page**   ☑ **Additional Character Required — Refer to the Tabular List for Character Selection**   **437**

Struck — Undetermined intent

Undetermined intent — *continued*
 drowning (submersion) (in) Y21.9 ☑
  bathtub Y21.0 ☑
   after fall Y21.1 ☑
  natural water (lake) (ocean) (pond) (river) (stream) Y21.4 ☑
  specified place NEC Y21.8 ☑
  swimming pool Y21.2 ☑
   after fall Y21.3 ☑
 explosive material Y25 ☑
 fall, jump or push from high place Y30 ☑
 falling, lying or running before moving object Y31 ☑
 fire Y26 ☑
 firearm discharge Y24.9 ☑
  airgun (BB) (pellet) Y24.0 ☑
  handgun (pistol) (revolver) Y22 ☑
  hunting rifle Y23.1 ☑
  larger Y23.9 ☑
   hunting rifle Y23.1 ☑
   machine gun Y23.3 ☑
   military Y23.2 ☑
   shotgun Y23.0 ☑
   specified type NEC Y23.8 ☑
  machine gun Y23.3 ☑
  military Y23.2 ☑
  shotgun Y23.0 ☑
  specified type NEC Y24.8 ☑
  Very pistol Y24.8 ☑
 hot object Y27.9 ☑
  fluid NEC Y27.2 ☑
  household appliance Y27.3 ☑
  specified object NEC Y27.8 ☑
  steam Y27.0 ☑
  tap water Y27.1 ☑
  vapor Y27.0 ☑
 jump, fall or push from high place Y30 ☑
 lying, falling or running before moving object Y31 ☑
 motor vehicle crash Y32 ☑
 push, fall or jump from high place Y30 ☑
 running, falling or lying before moving object Y31 ☑
 sharp object Y28.9 ☑
  dagger Y28.2 ☑
  glass Y28.0 ☑
  knife Y28.1 ☑
  specified object NEC Y28.8 ☑
  sword Y28.2 ☑
 smoke Y26 ☑
 specified event NEC Y33 ☑
Use of hand as hammer X50.3 ☑

V

Vibration (causing injury) W49.9 ☑
Victim (of)
 avalanche — *see* Landslide
 earth movements NEC — *see* Forces of nature, earth movement
 earthquake X34 ☑
 flood — *see* Flood
 landslide — *see* Landslide
 lightning — *see* subcategory T75.0 ☑
  causing fire — *see* Exposure, fire
 storm (cataclysmic) NEC — *see* Forces of nature, cataclysmic storm
 volcanic eruption X35 ☑
Volcanic eruption (any injury) X35 ☑
Vomitus, gastric contents in air passages (with asphyxia, obstruction or suffocation) T17.81- ☑

W

Walked into stationary object (any) W22.09 ☑
 furniture W22.03 ☑
 lamppost W22.02 ☑
 wall W22.01 ☑
War operations (injuries to military personnel and civilians during war, civil insurrection and peacekeeping missions) (by) (from) (involving) Y36.90 ☑

War operations — *continued*
 after cessation of hostilities Y36.89- ☑
  explosion (of)
   bomb placed during war operations Y36.82- ☑
   mine placed during war operations Y36.81- ☑
  specified NEC Y36.88- ☑
 air blast Y36.20- ☑
 aircraft
  destruction — *see* War operations, destruction of aircraft
  airway restriction — *see* War operations, restriction of airways
  asphyxiation — *see* War operations, restriction of airways
 biological weapons Y36.6X- ☑
 blast Y36.20- ☑
 blast fragments Y36.20- ☑
 blast wave Y36.20- ☑
 blast wind Y36.20- ☑
 bomb Y36.20- ☑
  dirty Y36.50- ☑
  gasoline Y36.31- ☑
  incendiary Y36.31- ☑
  petrol Y36.31- ☑
 bullet Y36.43- ☑
  incendiary Y36.32- ☑
  rubber Y36.41- ☑
 chemical weapons Y36.7X- ☑
 combat
  hand to hand (unarmed) combat Y36.44- ☑
  using blunt or piercing object Y36.45- ☑
 conflagration — *see* War operations, fire
 conventional warfare NEC Y36.49- ☑
 depth-charge Y36.01- ☑
 destruction of aircraft Y36.10- ☑
  due to
   air to air missile Y36.11- ☑
   collision with other aircraft Y36.12- ☑
   detonation (accidental) of onboard munitions and explosives Y36.14- ☑
   enemy fire or explosives Y36.11- ☑
   explosive placed on aircraft Y36.11- ☑
   onboard fire Y36.13- ☑
   rocket propelled grenade [RPG] Y36.11- ☑
   small arms fire Y36.11- ☑
   surface to air missile Y36.11- ☑
  specified NEC Y36.19- ☑
 detonation (accidental) of
  onboard marine weapons Y36.05- ☑
  own munitions or munitions launch device Y36.24- ☑
 dirty bomb Y36.50- ☑
 explosion (of) Y36.20- ☑
  aerial bomb Y36.21- ☑
  after cessation of
   bomb placed during war operations Y36.82- ☑
   mine placed during war operations Y36.81- ☑
  bomb NOS — *see also* War operations, bomb(s) Y36.20- ☑
  fragments Y36.20- ☑
  grenade Y36.29- ☑
  guided missile Y36.22- ☑
  improvised explosive device [IED] (person-borne) (roadside) (vehicle-borne) Y36.23- ☑
  land mine Y36.29- ☑
  marine mine (at sea) (in harbor) Y36.02- ☑
  marine weapon Y36.00- ☑
   specified NEC Y36.09- ☑
  own munitions or munitions launch device (accidental) Y36.24- ☑
  sea-based artillery shell Y36.03- ☑
  specified NEC Y36.29- ☑
  torpedo Y36.04- ☑
 fire Y36.30- ☑
  specified NEC Y36.39- ☑
 firearms
  discharge Y36.43- ☑
  pellets Y36.42- ☑

War operations — *continued*
 flamethrower Y36.33- ☑
 fragments (from) (of)
  improvised explosive device [IED] (person-borne) (roadside) (vehicle-borne) Y36.26- ☑
  munitions Y36.25- ☑
  specified NEC Y36.29- ☑
  weapons Y36.27- ☑
 friendly fire Y36.92 ☑
 hand to hand (unarmed) combat Y36.44- ☑
 hot substances — *see* War operations, fire
 incendiary bullet Y36.32- ☑
 nuclear weapon (effects of) Y36.50- ☑
  acute radiation exposure Y36.54- ☑
  blast pressure Y36.51- ☑
  direct blast Y36.51- ☑
  direct heat Y36.53- ☑
  fallout exposure Y36.54- ☑
  fireball Y36.53- ☑
  indirect blast (struck or crushed by blast debris) (being thrown by blast) Y36.52- ☑
  ionizing radiation (immediate exposure) Y36.54- ☑
  nuclear radiation Y36.54- ☑
  radiation
   ionizing (immediate exposure) Y36.54- ☑
   nuclear Y36.54- ☑
   thermal Y36.53- ☑
  secondary effects Y36.54- ☑
  specified NEC Y36.59- ☑
  thermal radiation Y36.53- ☑
 restriction of air (airway)
  intentional Y36.46- ☑
  unintentional Y36.47- ☑
 rubber bullets Y36.41- ☑
 shrapnel NOS Y36.29- ☑
 suffocation — *see* War operations, restriction of airways
 unconventional warfare NEC Y36.7X- ☑
 underwater blast NOS Y36.00- ☑
 warfare
  conventional NEC Y36.49- ☑
  unconventional NEC Y36.7X- ☑
 weapon of mass destruction [WMD] Y36.91 ☑
 weapons
  biological weapons Y36.6X- ☑
  chemical Y36.7X- ☑
  nuclear (effects of) Y36.50- ☑
   acute radiation exposure Y36.54- ☑
   blast pressure Y36.51- ☑
   direct blast Y36.51- ☑
   direct heat Y36.53- ☑
   fallout exposure Y36.54- ☑
   fireball Y36.53- ☑
   radiation
    ionizing (immediate exposure) Y36.54- ☑
    nuclear Y36.54- ☑
    thermal Y36.53- ☑
   secondary effects Y36.54- ☑
   specified NEC Y36.59- ☑
 of mass destruction [WMD] Y36.91 ☑
Washed
 away by flood — *see* Flood
 off road by storm (transport vehicle) — *see* Forces of nature, cataclysmic storm
Weather exposure NEC — *see* Forces of nature
Weightlessness (causing injury) (effects of) (in spacecraft, real or simulated) X52 ☑
Work related condition Y99.0
Wound (accidental) NEC — *see also* Injury X58 ☑
 battle — *see also* War operations Y36.90 ☑
 gunshot — *see* Discharge, firearm by type
Wreck transport vehicle NEC — *see also* Accident, transport V89.9 ☑
Wrong
 device implanted into correct surgical site Y65.51
 fluid in infusion Y65.1
 patient, procedure performed on Y65.52
 procedure (operation) on correct patient Y65.51

Chapter 1. Certain Infectious and Parasitic Diseases (A00–B99)

Chapter-specific Guidelines with Coding Examples

The chapter-specific guidelines from the ICD-10-CM Official Guidelines for Coding and Reporting have been provided below. Along with these guidelines are coding examples, contained in the shaded boxes, that have been developed to help illustrate the coding and/or sequencing guidance found in these guidelines.

a. Human immunodeficiency virus (HIV) infections

1) Code only confirmed cases

Code only confirmed cases of HIV infection/illness. This is an exception to the hospital inpatient guideline Section II, H.

In this context, "confirmation" does not require documentation of positive serology or culture for HIV; the provider's diagnostic statement that the patient is HIV positive or has an HIV-related illness is sufficient.

> Patient admitted with anemia with possible HIV infection
>
> **D64.9   Anemia, unspecified**
>
> *Explanation:* Only the anemia is coded in this scenario because it has not been confirmed that an HIV infection is present. This is an exception to the guideline Section II, H for hospital inpatient coding.

2) Selection and sequencing of HIV codes

(a) Patient admitted for HIV-related condition

If a patient is admitted for an HIV-related condition, the principal diagnosis should be B20, Human immunodeficiency virus [HIV] disease followed by additional diagnosis codes for all reported HIV-related conditions.

(b) Patient with HIV disease admitted for unrelated condition

If a patient with HIV disease is admitted for an unrelated condition (such as a traumatic injury), the code for the unrelated condition (e.g., the nature of injury code) should be the principal diagnosis. Other diagnoses would be B20 followed by additional diagnosis codes for all reported HIV-related conditions.

> Unstable angina, native coronary artery atherosclerosis, HIV
>
> **I25.110   Atherosclerotic heart disease of native coronary artery with unstable angina pectoris**
>
> **B20   Human immunodeficiency virus [HIV] disease**
>
> *Explanation:* The arteriosclerotic coronary artery disease and the unstable angina are not related to HIV, so those conditions are reported first using a combination code, and HIV is reported secondarily.

(c) Whether the patient is newly diagnosed

Whether the patient is newly diagnosed or has had previous admissions/encounters for HIV conditions is irrelevant to the sequencing decision.

(d) Asymptomatic human immunodeficiency virus

Z21, Asymptomatic human immunodeficiency virus [HIV] infection status, is to be applied when the patient without any documentation of symptoms is listed as being "HIV positive," "known HIV," "HIV test positive," or similar terminology. Do not use this code if the term "AIDS" or "HIV disease" is used or if the patient is treated for any HIV-related illness or is described as having any condition(s) resulting from his/her HIV positive status; use B20 in these cases.

(e) Patients with inconclusive HIV serology

Patients with inconclusive HIV serology, but no definitive diagnosis or manifestations of the illness, may be assigned code R75, Inconclusive laboratory evidence of human immunodeficiency virus [HIV].

(f) Previously diagnosed HIV-related illness

Patients with any known prior diagnosis of an HIV-related illness should be coded to B20. Once a patient has developed an HIV-related illness, the patient should always be assigned code B20 on every subsequent admission/encounter. Patients previously diagnosed with any HIV illness (B20) should never be assigned to R75 or Z21, Asymptomatic human immunodeficiency virus [HIV] infection status.

(g) HIV infection in pregnancy, childbirth and the puerperium

During pregnancy, childbirth or the puerperium, a patient admitted (or presenting for a health care encounter) because of an HIV-related illness should receive a principal diagnosis code of O98.7-, Human immunodeficiency [HIV] disease complicating pregnancy, childbirth and the puerperium, followed by B20 and the code(s) for the HIV-related illness(es). Codes from Chapter 15 always take sequencing priority.

Patients with asymptomatic HIV infection status admitted (or presenting for a health care encounter) during pregnancy, childbirth, or the puerperium should receive codes of O98.7- and Z21.

(h) Encounters for testing for HIV

If a patient is being seen to determine his/her HIV status, use code Z11.4, Encounter for screening for human immunodeficiency virus [HIV]. Use additional codes for any associated high-risk behavior, **if applicable**.

If a patient with signs or symptoms is being seen for HIV testing, code the signs and symptoms. An additional counseling code Z71.7, Human immunodeficiency virus [HIV] counseling, may be used if counseling is provided during the encounter for the test.

When a patient returns to be informed of his/her HIV test results and the test result is negative, use code Z71.7, Human immunodeficiency virus [HIV] counseling.

If the results are positive, see previous guidelines and assign codes as appropriate.

(i) History of HIV managed by medication

If a patient with documented history of HIV disease is currently managed on antiretroviral medications, assign code B20, Human immunodeficiency virus [HIV] disease. Code Z79.899, Other long term (current) drug therapy, may be assigned as an additional code to identify the long-term (current) use of antiretroviral medications.

b. Infectious agents as the cause of diseases classified to other chapters

Certain infections are classified in chapters other than Chapter 1 and no organism is identified as part of the infection code. In these instances, it is necessary to use an additional code from Chapter 1 to identify the organism. A code from category B95, Streptococcus, Staphylococcus, and Enterococcus as the cause of diseases classified to other chapters, B96, Other bacterial agents as the cause of diseases classified to other chapters, or B97, Viral agents as the cause of diseases classified to other chapters, is to be used as an additional code to identify the organism. An instructional note will be found at the infection code advising that an additional organism code is required.

c. Infections resistant to antibiotics

Many bacterial infections are resistant to current antibiotics. It is necessary to identify all infections documented as antibiotic resistant. Assign a code from category Z16, Resistance to antimicrobial drugs, following the infection code only if the infection code does not identify drug resistance.

d. Sepsis, severe sepsis, and septic shock

1) Coding of sepsis and severe sepsis

(a) Sepsis

For a diagnosis of sepsis, assign the appropriate code for the underlying systemic infection. If the type of infection or causal organism is not further specified, assign code A41.9, Sepsis, unspecified organism.

A code from subcategory R65.2, Severe sepsis, should not be assigned unless severe sepsis or an associated acute organ dysfunction is documented.

(i) Negative or inconclusive blood cultures and sepsis

Negative or inconclusive blood cultures do not preclude a diagnosis of sepsis in patients with clinical evidence of the condition; however, the provider should be queried.

(ii) Urosepsis

The term urosepsis is a nonspecific term. It is not to be considered synonymous with sepsis. It has no default code in the Alphabetic Index. Should a provider use this term, he/she must be queried for clarification.

(iii) Sepsis with organ dysfunction

If a patient has sepsis and associated acute organ dysfunction or multiple organ dysfunction (MOD), follow the instructions for coding severe sepsis.

(iv) Acute organ dysfunction that is not clearly associated with the sepsis

If a patient has sepsis and an acute organ dysfunction, but the medical record documentation indicates that the acute organ dysfunction is related to a medical condition other than the sepsis, do not assign a code from subcategory R65.2, Severe sepsis. An acute organ dysfunction must be associated with the sepsis in order to assign the severe sepsis code. If the documentation is not clear as to whether an acute organ dysfunction is related to the sepsis or another medical condition, query the provider.

Sepsis and acute respiratory failure due to COPD exacerbation	
A41.9	Sepsis, unspecified organism
J44.1	Chronic obstructive pulmonary disease with (acute) exacerbation
J96.00	Acute respiratory failure, unspecified whether with hypoxia or hypercapnia

Explanation: Although acute organ dysfunction is present in the form of acute respiratory failure, severe sepsis (R65.2) is not coded in this example, as the acute respiratory failure is attributed to the COPD exacerbation rather than the sepsis. Sequencing of these codes would be determined by the circumstances of the admission.

(b) Severe sepsis

The coding of severe sepsis requires a minimum of 2 codes: first a code for the underlying systemic infection, followed by a code from subcategory R65.2, Severe sepsis. If the causal organism is not documented, assign code A41.9, Sepsis, unspecified organism, for the infection. Additional code(s) for the associated acute organ dysfunction are also required.

Due to the complex nature of severe sepsis, some cases may require querying the provider prior to assignment of the codes.

2) Septic shock

Septic shock generally refers to circulatory failure associated with severe sepsis, and therefore, it represents a type of acute organ dysfunction.

For cases of septic shock, the code for the systemic infection should be sequenced first, followed by code R65.21, Severe sepsis with septic shock or code T81.12, Postprocedural septic shock. Any additional codes for the other acute organ dysfunctions should also be assigned. As noted in the sequencing instructions in the Tabular List, the code for septic shock cannot be assigned as a principal diagnosis.

Sepsis with septic shock	
A41.9	Sepsis, unspecified organism
R65.21	Severe sepsis with septic shock

Explanation: Documentation of septic shock automatically implies severe sepsis as it is a form of acute organ dysfunction. Septic shock is not coded as the principal diagnosis; it is always preceded by the code for the systemic infection.

3) Sequencing of severe sepsis

If severe sepsis is present on admission, and meets the definition of principal diagnosis, the underlying systemic infection should be assigned as principal diagnosis followed by the appropriate code from subcategory R65.2 as required by the sequencing rules in the Tabular List. A code from subcategory R65.2 can never be assigned as a principal diagnosis.

When severe sepsis develops during an encounter (it was not present on admission), the underlying systemic infection and the appropriate code from subcategory R65.2 should be assigned as secondary diagnoses.

Severe sepsis may be present on admission, but the diagnosis may not be confirmed until sometime after admission. If the documentation is not clear whether severe sepsis was present on admission, the provider should be queried.

4) Sepsis or severe sepsis with a localized infection

If the reason for admission is sepsis or severe sepsis and a localized infection, such as pneumonia or cellulitis, a code(s) for the underlying systemic infection should be assigned first and the code for the localized infection should be assigned as a secondary diagnosis. If the patient has severe sepsis, a code from subcategory R65.2 should also be assigned as a secondary diagnosis. If the patient is admitted with a localized infection, such as pneumonia, and sepsis/severe sepsis doesn't develop until after admission, the localized infection should be assigned first, followed by the appropriate sepsis/severe sepsis codes.

Patient presents with acute renal failure due to severe sepsis from *Pseudomonas* pneumonia	
A41.52	Sepsis due to Pseudomonas
J15.1	Pneumonia due to Pseudomonas
R65.20	Severe sepsis without septic shock
N17.9	Acute kidney failure, unspecified

Explanation: If all conditions are present on admission, the systemic infection (sepsis) is sequenced first followed by the codes for the localized infection (pneumonia), severe sepsis and any organ dysfunction. If only the pneumonia was present on admission with the sepsis and resulting renal failure developing later in the admission, then the pneumonia would be sequenced first.

5) Sepsis due to a postprocedural infection

(a) Documentation of causal relationship

As with all postprocedural complications, code assignment is based on the provider's documentation of the relationship between the infection and the procedure.

(b) Sepsis due to a postprocedural infection

For infections following a procedure, a code from T81.40, to T81.43 Infection following a procedure, or a code from O86.00 to O86.03, Infection of obstetric surgical wound, that identifies the site of the infection should be coded first, if known. Assign an additional code for sepsis following a procedure (T81.44) or sepsis following an obstetrical procedure (O86.04). Use an additional code to identify the infectious agent. If the patient has severe sepsis, the appropriate code from subcategory R65.2 should also be assigned with the additional code(s) for any acute organ dysfunction.

For infections following infusion, transfusion, therapeutic injection, or immunization, a code from subcategory T80.2, Infections following infusion, transfusion, and therapeutic injection, or code T88.0-, Infection following immunization, should be coded first, followed by the code for the specific infection. If the patient has severe sepsis, the appropriate code from subcategory R65.2 should also be assigned, with the additional codes(s) for any acute organ dysfunction.

(c) Postprocedural infection and postprocedural septic shock

If a postprocedural infection has resulted in postprocedural septic shock, assign the codes indicated above for sepsis due to a postprocedural infection, followed by code T81.12-, Postprocedural septic shock. Do not assign code R65.21, Severe sepsis with septic shock. Additional code(s) should be assigned for any acute organ dysfunction.

Septic shock following abdominal procedure with intramuscular abscess	
T81.42XA	Infection following a procedure, deep incisional surgical site, initial encounter
T81.44XA	Sepsis following a procedure, initial encounter
A41.9	Sepsis, unspecified organism
T81.12XA	Postprocedural septic shock, initial encounter

Explanation: The first code reported identifies the site of the postprocedural infection with intramuscular abscess coded to "deep incisional surgical site." If sepsis occurred as a result of the postprocedural infection, code T81.44- should be coded as a secondary diagnosis, followed by a code for the specific type of sepsis. Postprocedural septic shock is captured by code T81.12- and not with code R65.21. If any other acute organ dysfunction was documented as associated with the postprocedural sepsis, additional codes could be assigned to represent those conditions.

6) Sepsis and severe sepsis associated with a noninfectious process (condition)

In some cases, a noninfectious process (condition) such as trauma, may lead to an infection which can result in sepsis or severe sepsis. If sepsis or severe sepsis is documented as associated with a noninfectious condition, such as a burn or serious injury, and this condition meets the definition for principal diagnosis, the code for the noninfectious condition should be sequenced first, followed by the code for the resulting infection. If severe sepsis is present, a code from subcategory R65.2 should also be assigned with any associated organ dysfunction(s) codes. It is not necessary to assign a code from subcategory R65.1, Systemic inflammatory response syndrome (SIRS) of non-infectious origin, for these cases.

If the infection meets the definition of principal diagnosis, it should be sequenced before the non-infectious condition. When both the associated non-infectious condition and the infection meet the definition of principal diagnosis, either may be assigned as principal diagnosis.

Only one code from category R65, Symptoms and signs specifically associated with systemic inflammation and infection, should be assigned. Therefore, when a non-infectious condition leads to an infection resulting in severe sepsis, assign the appropriate code from subcategory R65.2, Severe sepsis. Do not additionally assign a code from subcategory R65.1, Systemic inflammatory response syndrome (SIRS) of non-infectious origin.

See Section I.C.18. SIRS due to non-infectious process

Patient admitted with multiple third-degree burns of right upper arm develops severe MSSA sepsis with septic shock, three days into admission

T22.391A	Burn of third degree of multiple sites of right shoulder and upper arm limb, except wrist and hand, initial encounter
A41.01	Sepsis due to Methicillin susceptible Staphylococcus aureus
R65.21	Severe sepsis with septic shock

Explanation: Severe sepsis is coded rather than SIRS from R65 because it is documented as a severe systemic infectious response with septic shock to a noninfectious condition. The code for the systemic infection is not used as the principal diagnosis because it was not present on admission. The patient was admitted for the burn injury.

---

7) Sepsis and septic shock complicating abortion, pregnancy, childbirth, and the puerperium

See Section I.C.15. Sepsis and septic shock complicating abortion, pregnancy, childbirth and the puerperium

8) Newborn sepsis

See Section I.C.16. f. Bacterial sepsis of Newborn

e. Methicillin resistant Staphylococcus aureus (MRSA) conditions

1) Selection and sequencing of MRSA codes

(a) Combination codes for MRSA infection

When a patient is diagnosed with an infection that is due to methicillin resistant *Staphylococcus aureus* (MRSA), and that infection has a combination code that includes the causal organism (e.g., sepsis, pneumonia) assign the appropriate combination code for the condition (e.g., code A41.02, Sepsis due to Methicillin resistant Staphylococcus aureus or code J15.212, Pneumonia due to Methicillin resistant Staphylococcus aureus). Do not assign code B95.62, Methicillin resistant Staphylococcus aureus infection as the cause of diseases classified elsewhere, as an additional code, because the combination code includes the type of infection and the MRSA organism. Do not assign a code from subcategory Z16.11, Resistance to penicillins, as an additional diagnosis.

See Section C.1. for instructions on coding and sequencing of sepsis and severe sepsis.

(b) Other codes for MRSA infection

When there is documentation of a current infection (e.g., wound infection, stitch abscess, urinary tract infection) due to MRSA, and that infection does not have a combination code that includes the causal organism, assign the appropriate code to identify the condition along with code B95.62, Methicillin resistant Staphylococcus aureus infection as the cause of diseases classified elsewhere for the MRSA infection. Do not assign a code from subcategory Z16.11, Resistance to penicillins.

(c) Methicillin susceptible Staphylococcus aureus (MSSA) and MRSA colonization

The condition or state of being colonized or carrying MSSA or MRSA is called colonization or carriage, while an individual person is described as being colonized or being a carrier.

Colonization means that MSSA or MSRA is present on or in the body without necessarily causing illness. A positive MRSA colonization test might be documented by the provider as "MRSA screen positive" or "MRSA nasal swab positive".

Assign code Z22.322, Carrier or suspected carrier of Methicillin resistant Staphylococcus aureus, for patients documented as having MRSA colonization. Assign code Z22.321, Carrier or suspected carrier of Methicillin susceptible Staphylococcus aureus, for patients documented as having MSSA colonization. Colonization is not necessarily indicative of a disease process or as the cause of a specific condition the patient may have unless documented as such by the provider.

(d) MRSA colonization and infection

If a patient is documented as having both MRSA colonization and infection during a hospital admission, code Z22.322, Carrier or suspected carrier of Methicillin resistant Staphylococcus aureus, and a code for the MRSA infection may both be assigned.

f. Zika virus infections

1) Code only confirmed cases

Code only a confirmed diagnosis of Zika virus (A92.5, Zika virus disease) as documented by the provider. This is an exception to the hospital inpatient guideline Section II, H. In this context, "confirmation" does not require documentation of the type of test performed; the provider's diagnostic statement that the condition is confirmed is sufficient. This code should be assigned regardless of the stated mode of transmission.

If the provider documents "suspected", "possible" or "probable" Zika, do not assign code A92.5. Assign a code(s) explaining the reason for encounter (such as fever, rash, or joint pain) or Z20.821, Contact with and (suspected) exposure to Zika virus.

g. Coronavirus infections

1) COVID-19 infection (infection due to SARS-CoV-2)

(a) Code only confirmed cases

Code only a confirmed diagnosis of the 2019 novel coronavirus disease (COVID-19) as documented by the provider, or documentation of a positive COVID-19 test result. For a confirmed diagnosis, assign code U07.1, COVID-19. This is an exception to the hospital inpatient guideline Section II, H. In this context, "confirmation" does not require documentation of a positive test result for COVID-19; the provider's documentation that the individual has COVID-19 is sufficient.

If the provider documents "suspected," "possible," "probable," or "inconclusive" COVID-19, do not assign code U07.1. Instead, code the signs and symptoms reported. See guideline I.C.1.g.1.g.

An elderly patient who is a former smoker is admitted with a productive cough, fatigue, and chest discomfort. CXR and PFTs indicate acute bronchitis. Treatment includes cough suppressants and anti-inflammatory medication, along with isolation precautions. The provider documents acute bronchitis likely due to COVID-19. Laboratory tests were inconclusive.

J20.9	Acute bronchitis, unspecified
Z87.891	History of tobacco dependence

Explanation: Because the COVID-19 diagnosis was documented as likely by the provider, code U07.1 cannot be assigned. Instead a code explaining the reason for the encounter is used, in this case the acute bronchitis. Code J20.9 Acute bronchitis, unspecified, is used because the causative organism, specifically that which causes COVID-19, is not confirmed. Without further documentation of COVID-19 or another causative organism being present, code J20.8 Acute bronchitis due to other specified organisms, does not apply.

A 75-year-old male from a nursing home presents with shortness of breath and fever of 102.7. Patient was diagnosed with pneumonia, confirmed on CXR. Laboratory tests come back positive for COVID-19.

U07.1	COVID-19
J12.82	Pneumonia due to coronavirus disease 2019

Explanation: The provider does not need to explicitly link the test result to the respiratory condition, nor does the provider need to explicitly document a diagnosis of COVID-19; the positive test result alone can be used to assign code U07.1. This advice is limited to laboratory tests for COVID-19 only. The significance of all other laboratory test results must be documented by the provider. According to guideline I.C.1.b, code U07.1 should be sequenced before the pneumonia code.

(b) Sequencing of codes

When COVID-19 meets the definition of principal diagnosis, code U07.1, COVID-19, should be sequenced first, followed by the appropriate codes for associated manifestations, except when another guideline requires that certain codes be sequenced first, such as obstetrics, sepsis, or transplant complications.

The patient presents with acute hypoxic respiratory failure due to sepsis from COVID-19 related pneumonia.

A41.89	Other specified sepsis
U07.1	COVID-19
J12.82	Pneumonia due to coronavirus disease 2019
J96.01	Acute respiratory failure with hypoxia
R65.20	Severe sepsis without septic shock

Explanation: If all conditions are present on admission, the systemic infection (sepsis) is sequenced first, followed by the code(s) for the localized infection (COVID-19 and pneumonia). The acute respiratory failure (acute organ dysfunction) is clearly documented as being associated with the sepsis, and therefore a severe sepsis code from subcategory R65.2- can also be assigned. If the sepsis had developed later in the admission, with or without any associated respiratory failure, the COVID-19 code would be sequenced first.

For a COVID-19 infection that progresses to sepsis, see Section I.C.1.d. Sepsis, Severe Sepsis, and Septic Shock

See Section I.C.15.s. for COVID-19 infection in pregnancy, childbirth, and the puerperium

See Section I.C.16.h. for COVID-19 infection in newborn

For a COVID-19 infection in a lung transplant patient, see Section I.C.19.g.3.a. Transplant complications other than kidney.

(c) Acute respiratory manifestations of COVID-19

When the reason for the encounter/admission is a respiratory manifestation of COVID-19, assign code U07.1, COVID-19, as the principal/first-listed diagnosis and assign code(s) for the respiratory manifestation(s) as additional diagnoses.

The following conditions are examples of common respiratory manifestations of COVID-19.

(i) Pneumonia

For a patient with pneumonia confirmed as due to COVID-19, assign codes U07.1, COVID-19, and J12.82, Pneumonia due to coronavirus disease 2019.

(ii) Acute bronchitis

For a patient with acute bronchitis confirmed as due to COVID-19, assign codes U07.1, and J20.8, Acute bronchitis due to other specified organisms.

Bronchitis not otherwise specified (NOS) due to COVID-19 should be coded using code U07.1 and J40, Bronchitis, not specified as acute or chronic.

(iii) Lower respiratory infection

If the COVID-19 is documented as being associated with a lower respiratory infection, not otherwise specified (NOS), or an acute respiratory infection, NOS, codes U07.1 and J22, Unspecified acute lower respiratory infection, should be assigned.

If the COVID-19 is documented as being associated with a respiratory infection, NOS, codes U07.1 and J98.8, Other specified respiratory disorders, should be assigned.

(iv) Acute respiratory distress syndrome

For acute respiratory distress syndrome (ARDS) due to COVID-19, assign codes U07.1, and J80, Acute respiratory distress syndrome.

(v) Acute respiratory failure

For acute respiratory failure due to COVID-19, assign code U07.1, and code J96.0-, Acute respiratory failure.

(d) Non-respiratory manifestations of COVID-19

When the reason for the encounter/admission is a non-respiratory manifestation (e.g., viral enteritis) of COVID-19, assign code U07.1, COVID-19, as the principal/first-listed diagnosis and assign code(s) for the manifestation(s) as additional diagnoses.

(e) Exposure to COVID-19

For asymptomatic individuals with actual or suspected exposure to COVID-19, assign code Z20.822, Contact with and (suspected) exposure to COVID-19.

For symptomatic individuals with actual or suspected exposure to COVID-19 and the infection has been ruled out, or test results are inconclusive or unknown, assign code Z20.822, Contact with and (suspected) exposure to COVID-19. See guideline I.C.21.c.1, Contact/Exposure, for additional guidance regarding the use of category Z20 codes.

If COVID-19 is confirmed, see guideline I.C.1.g.1.a.

(f) Screening for COVID-19

During the COVID-19 pandemic, a screening code is generally not appropriate. Do not assign code Z11.52, Encounter for screening for COVID-19. For encounters for COVID-19 testing, including

preoperative testing, code as exposure to COVID-19 (guideline I.C.1.g.1.e).

Coding guidance will be updated as new information concerning any changes in the pandemic status becomes available.

(g) Signs and symptoms without definitive diagnosis of COVID-19

For patients presenting with any signs/symptoms associated with COVID-19 (such as fever, etc.) but a definitive diagnosis has not been established, assign the appropriate code(s) for each of the presenting signs and symptoms such as:

- **R05.1, Acute** cough, **or R05.9, Cough, unspecified**
- R06.02 Shortness of breath
- R50.9 Fever, unspecified

If a patient with signs/symptoms associated with COVID-19 also has an actual or suspected contact with or exposure to COVID-19, assign Z20.822, Contact with and (suspected) exposure to COVID19, as an additional code.

(h) Asymptomatic individuals who test positive for COVID-19

For asymptomatic individuals who test positive for COVID-19, see guideline I.C.1.g.1.a. Although the individual is asymptomatic, the individual has tested positive and is considered to have the COVID-19 infection.

(i) Personal history of COVID-19

For patients with a history of COVID-19, assign code Z86.16, Personal history of COVID-19.

(j) Follow-up visits after COVID-19 infection has resolved

For individuals who previously had COVID-19, **without residual symptom(s) or condition(s),** and are being seen for follow-up evaluation, and COVID-19 test results are negative, assign codes Z09, Encounter for follow-up examination after completed treatment for conditions other than malignant neoplasm, and Z86.16, Personal history of COVID-19.

For follow-up visits for individuals with symptom(s) or condition(s) related to a previous COVID-19 infection, see guideline I.C.1.g.1.m.

See Section I.C.21.c.8, Factors influencing health states and contact with health services, Follow-up

(k) Encounter for antibody testing

For an encounter for antibody testing that is not being performed to confirm a current COVID-19 infection, nor is a follow-up test after resolution of COVID-19, assign Z01.84, Encounter for antibody response examination.

Follow the applicable guidelines above if the individual is being tested to confirm a current COVID-19 infection.

For follow-up testing after a COVID-19 infection, see guideline I.C.1.g.1.j.

(l) Multisystem inflammatory syndrome

For individuals with multisystem inflammatory syndrome (MIS) and COVID-19, assign code U07.1, COVID-19, as the principal/first-listed diagnosis and assign code M35.81, Multisystem inflammatory syndrome, as an additional diagnosis.

If an individual with a history of COVID-19 develops MIS, assign codes M35.81, Multisystem inflammatory syndrome, and **U09.9, Post COVID-19 condition, unspecified**.

If an individual with a known or suspected exposure to COVID-19, and no current COVID-19 infection or history of COVID-19, develops MIS, assign codes M35.81, Multisystem inflammatory syndrome, and Z20.822, Contact with and (suspected) exposure to COVID-19.

Additional codes should be assigned for any associated complications of MIS.

(m) Post COVID-19 condition

For sequela of COVID-19, or associated symptoms or conditions that develop following a previous COVID-19 infection, assign a code(s) for the specific symptom(s) or condition(s) related to the previous COVID-19 infection, if known, and code U09.9, Post COVID-19 condition, unspecified.

Code U09.9 should not be assigned for manifestations of an active (current) COVID-19 infection.

If a patient has a condition(s) associated with a previous COVID-19 infection and develops a new active (current) COVID-19 infection, code U09.9 may be assigned in conjunction with code U07.1, COVID-19, to identify that the patient also has a condition(s) associated with a previous COVID-19 infection. Code(s) for the specific condition(s) associated with the previous COVID-19 infection and code(s) for manifestation(s) of the new active (current) COVID-19 infection should also be assigned.

Chapter 1. Certain Infectious and Parasitic Diseases (A00-B99)

INCLUDES diseases generally recognized as communicable or transmissible
Use additional code to identify resistance to antimicrobial drugs (Z16.-)
EXCLUDES 1 certain localized infections - see body system-related chapters
EXCLUDES 2 carrier or suspected carrier of infectious disease (Z22.-)
infectious and parasitic diseases complicating pregnancy, childbirth and the puerperium (O98.-)
infectious and parasitic diseases specific to the perinatal period (P35-P39)
influenza and other acute respiratory infections (J00-J22)

This chapter contains the following blocks:

A00-A09	Intestinal infectious diseases
A15-A19	Tuberculosis
A20-A28	Certain zoonotic bacterial diseases
A30-A49	Other bacterial diseases
A50-A64	Infections with a predominantly sexual mode of transmission
A65-A69	Other spirochetal diseases
A70-A74	Other diseases caused by chlamydiae
A75-A79	Rickettsioses
A80-A89	Viral and prion infections of the central nervous system
A90-A99	Arthropod-borne viral fevers and viral hemorrhagic fevers
B00-B09	Viral infections characterized by skin and mucous membrane lesions
B10	Other human herpesviruses
B15-B19	Viral hepatitis
B20	Human immunodeficiency virus [HIV] disease
B25-B34	Other viral diseases
B35-B49	Mycoses
B50-B64	Protozoal diseases
B65-B83	Helminthiases
B85-B89	Pediculosis, acariasis and other infestations
B90-B94	Sequelae of infectious and parasitic diseases
B95-B97	Bacterial and viral infectious agents
B99	Other infectious diseases

Intestinal infectious diseases (A00-A09)

A00 Cholera
  DEF: Acute infection of the bowel due to *Vibrio cholerae* that presents with profuse diarrhea, cramps, and vomiting, resulting in severe dehydration, electrolyte imbalance, and death. It is spread through ingestion of food or water contaminated with feces of infected persons.

  A00.0 Cholera due to Vibrio cholerae 01, biovar cholerae CC
    Classical cholera

  A00.1 Cholera due to Vibrio cholerae 01, biovar eltor CC
    Cholera eltor

  A00.9 Cholera, unspecified CC

A01 Typhoid and paratyphoid fevers
  DEF: Typhoid fever: Acute generalized illness caused by *Salmonella typhi.* Clinical features include fever, headache, abdominal pain, cough, toxemia, leukopenia, abnormal pulse, rose spots on the skin, bacteremia, hyperplasia of intestinal lymph nodes, mesenteric lymphadenopathy, and Peyer's patches in the intestines.
  DEF: Paratyphoid fever: Prolonged febrile illness, caused by *Salmonella* serotypes other than *S. typhi,* especially *S. enterica* serotypes paratyphi A, B, and C.

  A01.0 Typhoid fever
    Infection due to Salmonella typhi

    A01.00 Typhoid fever, unspecified CC
    A01.01 Typhoid meningitis CC
    A01.02 Typhoid fever with heart involvement CC
      Typhoid endocarditis
      Typhoid myocarditis
    A01.03 Typhoid pneumonia CC HCC
    A01.04 Typhoid arthritis CC HCC
    A01.05 Typhoid osteomyelitis CC HCC
    A01.09 Typhoid fever with other complications CC
  A01.1 Paratyphoid fever A CC
  A01.2 Paratyphoid fever B CC
  A01.3 Paratyphoid fever C CC
  A01.4 Paratyphoid fever, unspecified CC
    Infection due to Salmonella paratyphi NOS

A02 Other salmonella infections
  INCLUDES infection or foodborne intoxication due to any Salmonella species other than S. typhi and S. paratyphi

  A02.0 Salmonella enteritis CC
    Salmonellosis
    TIP: Dehydration (E86.0) is a complication of salmonella enteritis and may be reported separately.
  A02.1 Salmonella sepsis HIV MCC HCC
  A02.2 Localized salmonella infections

    A02.20 Localized salmonella infection, unspecified HIV
    A02.21 Salmonella meningitis HIV MCC
    A02.22 Salmonella pneumonia HIV MCC HCC
    A02.23 Salmonella arthritis HIV CC HCC
    A02.24 Salmonella osteomyelitis HIV CC HCC
    A02.25 Salmonella pyelonephritis HIV CC
      Salmonella tubulo-interstitial nephropathy
    A02.29 Salmonella with other localized infection HIV CC
  A02.8 Other specified salmonella infections HIV CC
  A02.9 Salmonella infection, unspecified HIV CC

A03 Shigellosis
  DEF: Infection caused by the genus *Shigella*, of the family *Enterobacteriaceae* that is known to cause an acute dysenteric infection of the bowel with fever, drowsiness, anorexia, nausea, vomiting, bloody diarrhea, abdominal cramps, and distention.

  A03.0 Shigellosis due to Shigella dysenteriae CC
    Group A shigellosis [Shiga-Kruse dysentery]
  A03.1 Shigellosis due to Shigella flexneri
    Group B shigellosis
  A03.2 Shigellosis due to Shigella boydii
    Group C shigellosis
  A03.3 Shigellosis due to Shigella sonnei
    Group D shigellosis
  A03.8 Other shigellosis
  A03.9 Shigellosis, unspecified
    Bacillary dysentery NOS

A04 Other bacterial intestinal infections
  EXCLUDES 1 bacterial foodborne intoxications, NEC (A05.-)
    tuberculous enteritis (A18.32)
  DEF: *Escherichia coli*: Gram-negative, anaerobic bacteria of the family *Enterobacteriaceae* found in the large intestine of warm-blooded animals, generally as a nonpathologic entity aiding in digestion. They become pathogenic when an opportunity to grow somewhere outside this relationship presents itself, such as ingestion of fecal-contaminated food or water.

  A04.0 Enteropathogenic Escherichia coli infection CC
  A04.1 Enterotoxigenic Escherichia coli infection CC
  A04.2 Enteroinvasive Escherichia coli infection CC
  A04.3 Enterohemorrhagic Escherichia coli infection CC
    DEF: *E. coli* infection penetrating the intestinal mucosa, producing microscopic ulceration and bleeding.
  A04.4 Other intestinal Escherichia coli infections CC
    Escherichia coli enteritis NOS
  A04.5 Campylobacter enteritis CC
    TIP: For Guillain-Barre syndrome occurring as a sequela of *Campylobacter enteritis*, assign code G61.0 as the first-listed diagnosis followed by B94.8 for the sequelae.
  A04.6 Enteritis due to Yersinia enterocolitica CC
    EXCLUDES 1 extraintestinal yersiniosis (A28.2)
  A04.7 Enterocolitis due to Clostridium difficile
    Foodborne intoxication by Clostridium difficile
    Pseudomembraneous colitis
    AHA: 2017,4Q,4
    A04.71 Enterocolitis due to Clostridium difficile, recurrent CC
      AHA: 2020,1Q,18
    A04.72 Enterocolitis due to Clostridium difficile, not specified as recurrent CC
  A04.8 Other specified bacterial intestinal infections CC
  A04.9 Bacterial intestinal infection, unspecified CC
    Bacterial enteritis NOS

✓ Additional Character Required   ✓x7th Placeholder   Questionable PDx   Manifestation   Unspecified Dx   UPD Unacceptable PDx   H1-H14 HAC   HCC CMS-HCC Dx   HIV HIV Dx

ICD-10-CM 2022   443

Chapter 1. Certain Infectious and Parasitic Diseases

A05–A09

✓4ᵗʰ A05   Other bacterial foodborne intoxications, not elsewhere classified

EXCLUDES 1   Clostridium difficile foodborne intoxication and infection (A04.7-)

Escherichia coli infection (A04.0-A04.4)

listeriosis (A32.-)

salmonella foodborne intoxication and infection (A02.-)

toxic effect of noxious foodstuffs (T61-T62)

A05.0   **Foodborne staphylococcal intoxication**   `CC`

TIP: Assign code A04.8 to report a staphylococcal infection when it is caused by the ingestion of contaminated food but not caused by *S. aureus* toxins.

A05.1   **Botulism food poisoning**   `CC`

Botulism NOS

Classical foodborne intoxication due to Clostridium botulinum

EXCLUDES 1   infant botulism (A48.51)

wound botulism (A48.52)

DEF: Muscle-paralyzing neurotoxic disease caused by ingesting pre-formed toxin from the bacterium *Clostridium botulinum*. It causes vomiting and diarrhea, vision problems, slurred speech, difficulty swallowing, paralysis, and death.

A05.2   **Foodborne Clostridium perfringens [Clostridium welchii] intoxication**   `CC`

Enteritis necroticans

Pig-bel

A05.3   **Foodborne Vibrio parahaemolyticus intoxication**   `CC`

A05.4   **Foodborne Bacillus cereus intoxication**   `CC`

A05.5   **Foodborne Vibrio vulnificus intoxication**   `CC`

A05.8   **Other specified bacterial foodborne intoxications**   `CC`

A05.9   **Bacterial foodborne intoxication, unspecified**

✓4ᵗʰ A06   Amebiasis

INCLUDES   infection due to Entamoeba histolytica

EXCLUDES 1   other protozoal intestinal diseases (A07.-)

EXCLUDES 2   acanthamebiasis (B60.1-)

Naegleriasis (B60.2)

DEF: Infection with a single cell protozoan known as the amoeba. Transmission occurs through ingestion of feces, contaminated food or water, use of human feces as fertilizer, or person-to-person contact.

A06.0   **Acute amebic dysentery**   `CC`

Acute amebiasis

Intestinal amebiasis NOS

A06.1   **Chronic intestinal amebiasis**   `CC`

A06.2   **Amebic nondysenteric colitis**   `CC`

A06.3   **Ameboma of intestine**   `CC`

Ameboma NOS

A06.4   **Amebic liver abscess**   `MCC`

Hepatic amebiasis

A06.5   **Amebic lung abscess**   `MCC` `HCC`

Amebic abscess of lung (and liver)

A06.6   **Amebic brain abscess**   `MCC`

Amebic abscess of brain (and liver) (and lung)

A06.7   **Cutaneous amebiasis**

✓5ᵗʰ A06.8   **Amebic infection of other sites**

A06.81   **Amebic cystitis**   `CC`

A06.82   **Other amebic genitourinary infections**   `CC`

Amebic balanitis

Amebic vesiculitis

Amebic vulvovaginitis

A06.89   **Other amebic infections**   `CC`

Amebic appendicitis

Amebic splenic abscess

A06.9   **Amebiasis, unspecified**

✓4ᵗʰ A07   Other protozoal intestinal diseases

DEF: Protozoa: Group comprised of the simplest, single celled organisms, ranging in size from micro to macroscopic. They can live alone or in colonies, and do not show any differentiation in tissues. Most are motile and can live free in nature, but some are parasitic, causing disease in the variety of hosts they inhabit.

A07.0   **Balantidiasis**

Balantidial dysentery

A07.1   **Giardiasis [lambliasis]**   `CC`

DEF: Infection caused by the flagellate protozoan *Giardia lamblia* causing gastrointestinal problems such as vomiting, chronic diarrhea, and weight loss. The most common parasite in the U.S., this is usually transmitted by ingesting contaminated water while in the cyst state, after which it latches onto the wall of the small intestine.

A07.2   **Cryptosporidiosis**   `CC` `HCC`

DEF: Microscopic parasite found in water and one of the most common causes of waterborne gastrointestinal infectious disease in the United States. It is usually transmitted by ingesting contaminated drinking water or recreational water and causes profuse watery diarrhea, flatulence, abdominal pain, and cramping.

A07.3   **Isosporiasis**   `HIV` `CC`

Infection due to Isospora belli and Isospora hominis

Intestinal coccidiosis

Isosporosis

A07.4   **Cyclosporiasis**   `CC`

A07.8   **Other specified protozoal intestinal diseases**   `CC`

Intestinal microsporidiosis

Intestinal trichomoniasis

Sarcocystosis

Sarcosporidiosis

A07.9   **Protozoal intestinal disease, unspecified**   `CC`

Flagellate diarrhea

Protozoal colitis

Protozoal diarrhea

Protozoal dysentery

✓4ᵗʰ A08   Viral and other specified intestinal infections

EXCLUDES 1   influenza with involvement of gastrointestinal tract (J09.X3, J10.2, J11.2)

A08.0   **Rotaviral enteritis**   `CC`

✓5ᵗʰ A08.1   **Acute gastroenteropathy due to Norwalk agent and other small round viruses**

A08.11   **Acute gastroenteropathy due to Norwalk agent**   `CC`

Acute gastroenteropathy due to Norovirus

Acute gastroenteropathy due to Norwalk-like agent

A08.19   **Acute gastroenteropathy due to other small round viruses**   `CC`

Acute gastroenteropathy due to small round virus [SRV] NOS

A08.2   **Adenoviral enteritis**   `CC`

✓5ᵗʰ A08.3   **Other viral enteritis**

A08.31   **Calicivirus enteritis**   `CC`

A08.32   **Astrovirus enteritis**   `CC`

A08.39   **Other viral enteritis**   `CC`

Coxsackie virus enteritis

Echovirus enteritis

Enterovirus enteritis NEC

Torovirus enteritis

A08.4   **Viral intestinal infection, unspecified**

Viral enteritis NOS

Viral gastroenteritis NOS

Viral gastroenteropathy NOS

AHA: 2016,3Q,12

A08.8   **Other specified intestinal infections**

A09   **Infectious gastroenteritis and colitis, unspecified**   `CC`

Infectious colitis NOS

Infectious enteritis NOS

Infectious gastroenteritis NOS

EXCLUDES 1   colitis NOS (K52.9)

diarrhea NOS (R19.7)

enteritis NOS (K52.9)

gastroenteritis NOS (K52.9)

noninfective gastroenteritis and colitis, unspecified (K52.9)

DEF: Colitis: Inflammation of mucous membranes of the colon.

DEF: Enteritis: Inflammation of mucous membranes of the small intestine.

DEF: Gastroenteritis: Inflammation of mucous membranes of the stomach and intestines.

`N` Newborn: 0   `P` Pediatric: 0-17   `M` Maternity: 9-64   `A` Adult: 15-124   `MCC` Major Complication/Comorbidity   `CC` Complication/Comorbidity   `SW` Severe Wound Dx

444   ICD-10-CM 2022

Tuberculosis (A15-A19)

INCLUDES	infections due to Mycobacterium tuberculosis and Mycobacterium bovis

EXCLUDES 1
congenital tuberculosis (P37.0)
nonspecific reaction to test for tuberculosis without active tuberculosis (R76.1-)
pneumoconiosis associated with tuberculosis, any type in A15 (J65)
positive PPD (R76.11)
positive tuberculin skin test without active tuberculosis (R76.11)
sequelae of tuberculosis (B90.-)
silicotuberculosis (J65)

DEF: Bacterial infection that typically spreads by inhalation of an airborne agent that usually attacks the lungs, but may also affect other organs.

✓4ᵗʰ **A15   Respiratory tuberculosis**

A15.0   Tuberculosis of lung   `HIV` `CC`
Tuberculous bronchiectasis
Tuberculous fibrosis of lung
Tuberculous pneumonia
Tuberculous pneumothorax

Tuberculosis of Lung

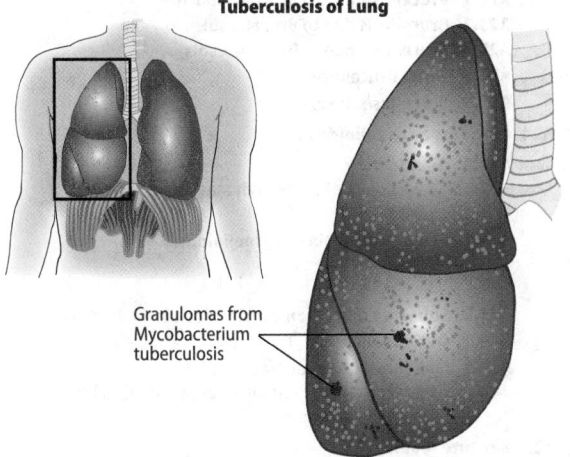

Granulomas from Mycobacterium tuberculosis

A15.4   Tuberculosis of intrathoracic lymph nodes   `HIV` `CC`
Tuberculosis of hilar lymph nodes
Tuberculosis of mediastinal lymph nodes
Tuberculosis of tracheobronchial lymph nodes
EXCLUDES 1   tuberculosis specified as primary (A15.7)

A15.5   Tuberculosis of larynx, trachea and bronchus   `HIV` `CC`
Tuberculosis of bronchus
Tuberculosis of glottis
Tuberculosis of larynx
Tuberculosis of trachea

A15.6   Tuberculous pleurisy   `HIV` `CC`
Tuberculosis of pleura Tuberculous empyema
EXCLUDES 1   primary respiratory tuberculosis (A15.7)

A15.7   Primary respiratory tuberculosis   `HIV` `CC`

A15.8   Other respiratory tuberculosis   `HIV` `CC`
Mediastinal tuberculosis
Nasopharyngeal tuberculosis
Tuberculosis of nose
Tuberculosis of sinus [any nasal]

A15.9   Respiratory tuberculosis unspecified   `HIV` `CC`

✓4ᵗʰ **A17   Tuberculosis of nervous system**

A17.0   Tuberculous meningitis   `HIV` `MCC`
Tuberculosis of meninges (cerebral)(spinal)
Tuberculous leptomeningitis
EXCLUDES 1   tuberculous meningoencephalitis (A17.82)

A17.1   Meningeal tuberculoma   `HIV` `MCC`
Tuberculoma of meninges (cerebral) (spinal)
EXCLUDES 2   tuberculoma of brain and spinal cord (A17.81)

✓5ᵗʰ **A17.8   Other tuberculosis of nervous system**

A17.81   Tuberculoma of brain and spinal cord   `HIV` `MCC`
Tuberculous abscess of brain and spinal cord

A17.82   Tuberculous meningoencephalitis   `HIV` `MCC`
Tuberculous myelitis

A17.83   Tuberculous neuritis   `HIV` `MCC`
Tuberculous mononeuropathy

A17.89   Other tuberculosis of nervous system   `HIV` `MCC`
Tuberculous polyneuropathy

A17.9   Tuberculosis of nervous system, unspecified   `HIV` `CC`

✓4ᵗʰ **A18   Tuberculosis of other organs**

✓5ᵗʰ **A18.0   Tuberculosis of bones and joints**

A18.01   Tuberculosis of spine   `HIV` `CC`
Pott's disease or curvature of spine
Tuberculous arthritis
Tuberculous osteomyelitis of spine
Tuberculous spondylitis

A18.02   Tuberculous arthritis of other joints   `HIV` `CC`
Tuberculosis of hip (joint)
Tuberculosis of knee (joint)

A18.03   Tuberculosis of other bones   `HIV` `CC`
Tuberculous mastoiditis
Tuberculous osteomyelitis

A18.09   Other musculoskeletal tuberculosis   `HIV` `CC`
Tuberculous myositis
Tuberculous synovitis
Tuberculous tenosynovitis

✓5ᵗʰ **A18.1   Tuberculosis of genitourinary system**

A18.10   Tuberculosis of genitourinary system, unspecified   `HIV` `CC`

A18.11   Tuberculosis of kidney and ureter   `HIV` `CC`

A18.12   Tuberculosis of bladder   `HIV` `CC`

A18.13   Tuberculosis of other urinary organs   `HIV` `CC`
Tuberculosis urethritis

A18.14   Tuberculosis of prostate   `HIV` `CC` `A` ♂

A18.15   Tuberculosis of other male genital organs   `HIV` `CC` ♂

A18.16   Tuberculosis of cervix   `HIV` `CC` ♀

A18.17   Tuberculous female pelvic inflammatory disease   `HIV` `CC` ♀
Tuberculous endometritis
Tuberculous oophoritis and salpingitis

A18.18   Tuberculosis of other female genital organs   `HIV` `CC` ♀
Tuberculous ulceration of vulva

A18.2   Tuberculous peripheral lymphadenopathy   `HIV` `CC`
Tuberculous adenitis
EXCLUDES 2   tuberculosis of bronchial and mediastinal lymph nodes (A15.4)
tuberculosis of mesenteric and retroperitoneal lymph nodes (A18.39)
tuberculous tracheobronchial adenopathy (A15.4)

✓5ᵗʰ **A18.3   Tuberculosis of intestines, peritoneum and mesenteric glands**

A18.31   Tuberculous peritonitis   `HIV` `MCC`
Tuberculous ascites
DEF: Tuberculous inflammation of the membrane lining the abdomen.

A18.32   Tuberculous enteritis   `HIV` `CC`
Tuberculosis of anus and rectum
Tuberculosis of intestine (large) (small)

A18.39   Retroperitoneal tuberculosis   `HIV` `CC`
Tuberculosis of mesenteric glands
Tuberculosis of retroperitoneal (lymph glands)

A18.4   Tuberculosis of skin and subcutaneous tissue   `HIV` `CC`
Erythema induratum, tuberculous
Lupus excedens
Lupus vulgaris NOS
Lupus vulgaris of eyelid
Scrofuloderma
Tuberculosis of external ear
EXCLUDES 2   lupus erythematosus (L93.-)
systemic lupus erythematosus (M32.-)

✓5ᵗʰ **A18.5   Tuberculosis of eye**
EXCLUDES 2   lupus vulgaris of eyelid (A18.4)

A18.50   Tuberculosis of eye, unspecified   `HIV` `CC`

A18.51   Tuberculous episcleritis   `HIV` `CC`

A18.52 **Tuberculous keratitis** `HIV` `CC`
Tuberculous interstitial keratitis
Tuberculous keratoconjunctivitis (interstitial) (phlyctenular)

A18.53 **Tuberculous chorioretinitis** `HIV` `CC`

A18.54 **Tuberculous iridocyclitis** `HIV` `CC`

A18.59 **Other tuberculosis of eye** `HIV` `CC`
Tuberculous conjunctivitis

A18.6 **Tuberculosis of (inner) (middle) ear** `HIV` `CC`
Tuberculous otitis media
EXCLUDES 2   tuberculosis of external ear (A18.4)
tuberculous mastoiditis (A18.03)

A18.7 **Tuberculosis of adrenal glands** `HIV` `CC`
Tuberculous Addison's disease

✓5th **A18.8** **Tuberculosis of other specified organs**

A18.81 **Tuberculosis of thyroid gland** `HIV` `CC`

A18.82 **Tuberculosis of other endocrine glands** `HIV` `CC`
Tuberculosis of pituitary gland
Tuberculosis of thymus gland

A18.83 **Tuberculosis of digestive tract organs, not elsewhere classified** `HIV` `CC`
EXCLUDES 1   tuberculosis of intestine (A18.32)

A18.84 **Tuberculosis of heart** `HIV` `CC`
Tuberculous cardiomyopathy
Tuberculous endocarditis
Tuberculous myocarditis
Tuberculous pericarditis

A18.85 **Tuberculosis of spleen** `HIV` `CC`

A18.89 **Tuberculosis of other sites** `HIV` `CC`
Tuberculosis of muscle
Tuberculous cerebral arteritis

✓4th **A19** **Miliary tuberculosis**
INCLUDES   disseminated tuberculosis
generalized tuberculosis
tuberculous polyserositis

A19.0 **Acute miliary tuberculosis of a single specified site** `HIV` `MCC`

A19.1 **Acute miliary tuberculosis of multiple sites** `HIV` `MCC`

A19.2 **Acute miliary tuberculosis, unspecified** `HIV` `MCC`

A19.8 **Other miliary tuberculosis** `HIV` `MCC`

A19.9 **Miliary tuberculosis, unspecified** `HIV` `MCC`

Certain zoonotic bacterial diseases (A20-A28)

✓4th **A20** **Plague**
INCLUDES   infection due to Yersinia pestis

A20.0 **Bubonic plague** `MCC`

A20.1 **Cellulocutaneous plague** `MCC`

A20.2 **Pneumonic plague** `MCC` `HCC`

A20.3 **Plague meningitis** `MCC`

A20.7 **Septicemic plague** `MCC` `HCC`

A20.8 **Other forms of plague** `MCC`
Abortive plague
Asymptomatic plague
Pestis minor

A20.9 **Plague, unspecified** `MCC`

✓4th **A21** **Tularemia**
INCLUDES   deer-fly fever
infection due to Francisella tularensis
rabbit fever
DEF: Febrile disease transmitted to humans by the bites of deer flies, fleas, and ticks, by inhaling aerosolized *F. tularensis*, or by ingesting contaminated food or water. Patients quickly develop fever, chills, weakness, headache, backache, and malaise.

A21.0 **Ulceroglandular tularemia** `CC`

A21.1 **Oculoglandular tularemia** `CC`
Ophthalmic tularemia

A21.2 **Pulmonary tularemia** `CC` `HCC`

A21.3 **Gastrointestinal tularemia** `CC`
Abdominal tularemia

A21.7 **Generalized tularemia** `CC`

A21.8 **Other forms of tularemia** `CC`

A21.9 **Tularemia, unspecified** `CC`

✓4th **A22** **Anthrax**
INCLUDES   infection due to Bacillus anthracis

A22.0 **Cutaneous anthrax** `CC`
Malignant carbuncle
Malignant pustule

A22.1 **Pulmonary anthrax** `MCC` `HCC`
Inhalation anthrax
Ragpicker's disease
Woolsorter's disease

A22.2 **Gastrointestinal anthrax** `CC`

A22.7 **Anthrax sepsis** `MCC` `HCC`

A22.8 **Other forms of anthrax** `CC`
Anthrax meningitis

A22.9 **Anthrax, unspecified** `CC`

✓4th **A23** **Brucellosis**
INCLUDES   Malta fever
Mediterranean fever
undulant fever

A23.0 **Brucellosis due to Brucella melitensis**

A23.1 **Brucellosis due to Brucella abortus**

A23.2 **Brucellosis due to Brucella suis**

A23.3 **Brucellosis due to Brucella canis**

A23.8 **Other brucellosis** `CC`

A23.9 **Brucellosis, unspecified** `CC`

✓4th **A24** **Glanders and melioidosis**

A24.0 **Glanders** `CC`
Infection due to Pseudomonas mallei
Malleus

A24.1 **Acute and fulminating melioidosis** `CC`
Melioidosis pneumonia
Melioidosis sepsis

A24.2 **Subacute and chronic melioidosis** `CC`

A24.3 **Other melioidosis** `CC`

A24.9 **Melioidosis, unspecified** `CC`
Infection due to Pseudomonas pseudomallei NOS
Whitmore's disease

✓4th **A25** **Rat-bite fevers**

A25.0 **Spirillosis** `CC`
Sodoku

A25.1 **Streptobacillosis** `CC`
Epidemic arthritic erythema
Haverhill fever
Streptobacillary rat-bite fever

A25.9 **Rat-bite fever, unspecified** `CC`

✓4th **A26** **Erysipeloid**
DEF: Acute cutaneous infection typically caused by trauma to the skin. Presenting as cellulitis, it may become systemic, affecting other organs. It is a gram-positive bacillus and mainly acquired by those who routinely handle meat.

A26.0 **Cutaneous erysipeloid**
Erythema migrans

A26.7 **Erysipelothrix sepsis** `MCC` `HCC`

A26.8 **Other forms of erysipeloid**

A26.9 **Erysipeloid, unspecified**

✓4th **A27** **Leptospirosis**

A27.0 **Leptospirosis icterohemorrhagica** `CC`
Leptospiral or spirochetal jaundice (hemorrhagic)
Weil's disease

✓5th **A27.8** **Other forms of leptospirosis**

A27.81 **Aseptic meningitis in leptospirosis** `MCC`

A27.89 **Other forms of leptospirosis** `CC`

A27.9 **Leptospirosis, unspecified** `CC`

✓4th **A28** **Other zoonotic bacterial diseases, not elsewhere classified**

A28.0 **Pasteurellosis** `CC`

A28.1 **Cat-scratch disease** `CC`
Cat-scratch fever

A28.2 **Extraintestinal yersiniosis** `CC`
EXCLUDES 1   enteritis due to Yersinia enterocolitica (A04.6)
plague (A20.-)

A28.8 **Other specified zoonotic bacterial diseases, not elsewhere classified** `CC`

A28.9 **Zoonotic bacterial disease, unspecified** `CC`

Other bacterial diseases (A30-A49)

AHA: 2016,3Q,8-14

☑4ᵗʰ **A30 Leprosy [Hansen's disease]**
  INCLUDES   infection due to Mycobacterium leprae
  EXCLUDES 1   sequelae of leprosy (B92)

  A30.0 Indeterminate **leprosy**   CC
          I leprosy

  A30.1 Tuberculoid **leprosy**   CC
          TT leprosy

  A30.2 Borderline tuberculoid **leprosy**   CC
          BT leprosy

  A30.3 Borderline **leprosy**   CC
          BB leprosy

  A30.4 Borderline lepromatous **leprosy**   CC
          BL leprosy

  A30.5 Lepromatous **leprosy**   CC
          LL leprosy

  A30.8 Other forms of leprosy   CC

  A30.9 Leprosy, unspecified   CC

☑4ᵗʰ **A31 Infection due to other mycobacteria**
  EXCLUDES 2   leprosy (A30.-)
             tuberculosis (A15-A19)

  A31.0 Pulmonary **mycobacterial infection**   CC HCC
          Infection due to Mycobacterium avium
          Infection due to Mycobacterium intracellulare [Battey bacillus]
          Infection due to Mycobacterium kansasii

  A31.1 Cutaneous **mycobacterial infection**   CC
          Buruli ulcer
          Infection due to Mycobacterium marinum
          Infection due to Mycobacterium ulcerans

  A31.2 Disseminated **mycobacterium avium-intracellulare complex (DMAC)**   HIV CC HCC
          MAC sepsis

  A31.8 Other mycobacterial infections   HIV CC

  A31.9 Mycobacterial infection, unspecified   HIV CC
          Atypical mycobacterial infection NOS
          Mycobacteriosis NOS

☑4ᵗʰ **A32 Listeriosis**
  INCLUDES   listerial foodborne infection
  EXCLUDES 1   neonatal (disseminated) listeriosis (P37.2)

  A32.0 Cutaneous **listeriosis**   CC

☑5ᵗʰ **A32.1** Listerial **meningitis and meningoencephalitis**
      A32.11 Listerial **meningitis**   CC
      A32.12 Listerial **meningoencephalitis**   CC

  A32.7 Listerial **sepsis**   MCC HCC

☑5ᵗʰ **A32.8** Other forms of listeriosis
      A32.81 Oculoglandular **listeriosis**   CC
      A32.82 Listerial **endocarditis**   CC
      A32.89 Other forms of listeriosis   CC
              Listerial cerebral arteritis

  A32.9 Listeriosis, unspecified   CC

A33 Tetanus neonatorum   MCC N

A34 Obstetrical tetanus   CC M ♀

A35 Other tetanus   MCC
      Tetanus NOS
      EXCLUDES 1   obstetrical tetanus (A34)
                 tetanus neonatorum (A33)
      DEF: Tetanus: Acute, often fatal, infectious disease caused by the anaerobic, spore-forming bacillus Clostridium tetani. The bacillus enters the body through a contaminated wound, burns, surgical wounds, or cutaneous ulcers. Symptoms include lockjaw, spasms, seizures, and paralysis.

☑4ᵗʰ **A36 Diphtheria**
  A36.0 Pharyngeal **diphtheria**   CC
          Diphtheritic membranous angina
          Tonsillar diphtheria

  A36.1 Nasopharyngeal **diphtheria**   CC

  A36.2 Laryngeal **diphtheria**   CC
          Diphtheritic laryngotracheitis

  A36.3 Cutaneous **diphtheria**   CC
          EXCLUDES 2   erythrasma (L08.1)

☑5ᵗʰ **A36.8** Other diphtheria
      A36.81 Diphtheritic **cardiomyopathy**   CC HCC
              Diphtheritic myocarditis

      A36.82 Diphtheritic **radiculomyelitis**   CC
      A36.83 Diphtheritic **polyneuritis**   CC
      A36.84 Diphtheritic **tubulo-interstitial nephropathy**   CC
      A36.85 Diphtheritic **cystitis**   CC
      A36.86 Diphtheritic **conjunctivitis**   CC
      A36.89 Other **diphtheritic complications**   CC
              Diphtheritic peritonitis

  A36.9 Diphtheria, unspecified   CC

☑4ᵗʰ **A37 Whooping cough**
      DEF: Acute, highly contagious respiratory tract infection caused by Bordetella pertussis and B. bronchiseptica. Whooping cough is known by its characteristic paroxysmal cough.

☑5ᵗʰ **A37.0** Whooping cough due to Bordetella pertussis
      A37.00 Whooping cough due to Bordetella pertussis without pneumonia   CC
              ▶Paroxysmal cough due to Bordetella pertussis without pneumonia◀

      A37.01 Whooping cough due to Bordetella pertussis with pneumonia   MCC
              ▶Paroxysmal cough due to Bordetella pertussis with pneumonia◀

☑5ᵗʰ **A37.1** Whooping cough due to Bordetella parapertussis
      A37.10 Whooping cough due to Bordetella parapertussis without pneumonia   CC
      A37.11 Whooping cough due to Bordetella parapertussis with pneumonia   MCC

☑5ᵗʰ **A37.8** Whooping cough due to other Bordetella species
      A37.80 Whooping cough due to other Bordetella species without pneumonia   CC
      A37.81 Whooping cough due to other Bordetella species with pneumonia   MCC

☑5ᵗʰ **A37.9** Whooping cough, unspecified species
      A37.90 Whooping cough, unspecified species without pneumonia   CC
      A37.91 Whooping cough, unspecified species with pneumonia   MCC

☑4ᵗʰ **A38 Scarlet fever**
  INCLUDES   scarlatina
  EXCLUDES 2   streptococcal sore throat (J02.0)
      DEF: Acute contagious disease caused by Group A bacteria, the same bacterium that causes strep throat. Individuals with strep throat can develop scarlet fever particularly if the infection is not treated with antibiotics. It is characterized by a red blush to the skin of the chest and abdomen and swelling of the nose, throat, and mouth.

  A38.0 Scarlet fever with **otitis media**   CC
  A38.1 Scarlet fever with **myocarditis**   CC
  A38.8 Scarlet fever with other **complications**   CC
  A38.9 Scarlet fever, **uncomplicated**   CC
          Scarlet fever, NOS

☑4ᵗʰ **A39 Meningococcal infection**
      DEF: Condition caused by Neisseria meningitidis, a bacteria that may invade the spinal cord, brain, heart, joints, optic nerve, or bloodstream.

  A39.0 Meningococcal **meningitis**   MCC

  A39.1 Waterhouse-Friderichsen **syndrome**   MCC HCC
          Meningococcal hemorrhagic adrenalitis
          Meningococcic adrenal syndrome

  A39.2 Acute **meningococcemia**   MCC HCC
  A39.3 Chronic **meningococcemia**   MCC HCC
  A39.4 Meningococcemia, unspecified   MCC HCC

☑5ᵗʰ **A39.5** Meningococcal **heart disease**
      A39.50 Meningococcal **carditis, unspecified**   MCC
      A39.51 Meningococcal **endocarditis**   MCC
      A39.52 Meningococcal **myocarditis**   MCC
      A39.53 Meningococcal **pericarditis**   MCC

☑5ᵗʰ **A39.8** Other meningococcal infections
      A39.81 Meningococcal **encephalitis**   MCC
      A39.82 Meningococcal **retrobulbar neuritis** CC
      A39.83 Meningococcal **arthritis**   CC HCC
      A39.84 Postmeningococcal **arthritis**   CC HCC

A39.89 Other meningococcal infections `CC`
　Meningococcal conjunctivitis

A39.9 Meningococcal infection, unspecified `CC`
　Meningococcal disease NOS

✓4ᵗʰ **A40 Streptococcal sepsis**
　Code first:
　　postprocedural streptococcal sepsis (T81.4-)
　　streptococcal sepsis during labor (O75.3)
　　streptococcal sepsis following abortion or ectopic or molar pregnancy (O03-O07, O08.0)
　　streptococcal sepsis following immunization (T88.0)
　　streptococcal sepsis following infusion, transfusion or therapeutic injection (T80.2-)

　　EXCLUDES 1   neonatal (P36.0-P36.1)
　　　　　　　　 puerperal sepsis (O85)
　　　　　　　　 sepsis due to Streptococcus, group D (A41.81)

　　AHA: 2020,2Q,8,28; 2019,4Q,65; 2018,4Q,89; 2018,1Q,16; 2016,1Q,32

A40.0 Sepsis due to streptococcus, group A `MCC` `HCC`

A40.1 Sepsis due to streptococcus, group B `MCC` `HCC`
　AHA: 2019,1Q,14

A40.3 Sepsis due to Streptococcus pneumoniae `MCC` `HCC`
　Pneumococcal sepsis

A40.8 Other streptococcal sepsis `MCC` `HCC`

A40.9 Streptococcal sepsis, unspecified `HIV` `MCC` `HCC`

✓4ᵗʰ **A41 Other sepsis**
　Code first:
　　postprocedural sepsis (T81.4-)
　　sepsis during labor (O75.3)
　　sepsis following abortion, ectopic or molar pregnancy (O03-O07, O08.0)
　　sepsis following immunization (T88.0)
　　sepsis following infusion, transfusion or therapeutic injection (T80.2-)

　　EXCLUDES 1   bacteremia NOS (R78.81)
　　　　　　　　 neonatal (P36.-)
　　　　　　　　 puerperal sepsis (O85)
　　　　　　　　 streptococcal sepsis (A40.-)

　　EXCLUDES 2   sepsis (due to) (in) actinomycotic (A42.7)
　　　　　　　　 sepsis (due to) (in) anthrax (A22.7)
　　　　　　　　 sepsis (due to) (in) candidal (B37.7)
　　　　　　　　 sepsis (due to) (in) Erysipelothrix (A26.7)
　　　　　　　　 sepsis (due to) (in) extraintestinal yersiniosis (A28.2)
　　　　　　　　 sepsis (due to) (in) gonococcal (A54.86)
　　　　　　　　 sepsis (due to) (in) herpesviral (B00.7)
　　　　　　　　 sepsis (due to) (in) listerial (A32.7)
　　　　　　　　 sepsis (due to) (in) melioidosis (A24.1)
　　　　　　　　 sepsis (due to) (in) meningococcal (A39.2-A39.4)
　　　　　　　　 sepsis (due to) (in) plague (A20.7)
　　　　　　　　 sepsis (due to) (in) tularemia (A21.7)
　　　　　　　　 toxic shock syndrome (A48.3)

　　AHA: 2020,2Q,8,28; 2019,4Q,65; 2019,3Q,17; 2018,4Q,18; 2018,1Q,16; 2016,1Q,32; 2014,2Q,13

✓5ᵗʰ **A41.0 Sepsis due to Staphylococcus aureus**

A41.01 Sepsis due to Methicillin susceptible Staphylococcus aureus `HIV` `MCC` `HCC`
　MSSA sepsis
　Staphylococcus aureus sepsis NOS
　AHA: 2020,2Q,17

A41.02 Sepsis due to Methicillin resistant Staphylococcus aureus `HIV` `MCC` `HCC`

A41.1 Sepsis due to other specified staphylococcus `HIV` `MCC` `HCC`
　Coagulase negative staphylococcus sepsis

A41.2 Sepsis due to unspecified staphylococcus `HIV` `MCC` `HCC`

A41.3 Sepsis due to Hemophilus influenzae `HIV` `MCC` `HCC`

A41.4 Sepsis due to anaerobes `HIV` `MCC` `HCC`
　EXCLUDES 1   gas gangrene (A48.0)

✓5ᵗʰ **A41.5 Sepsis due to other Gram-negative organisms**

A41.50 Gram-negative sepsis, unspecified `HIV` `MCC` `HCC`
　Gram-negative sepsis NOS
　AHA: 2020,2Q,28

A41.51 Sepsis due to Escherichia coli [E. coli] `HIV` `MCC` `HCC`
　AHA: 2020,2Q,17

A41.52 Sepsis due to Pseudomonas `HIV` `MCC` `HCC`
　Pseudomonas aeroginosa

A41.53 Sepsis due to Serratia `HIV` `MCC` `HCC`

A41.59 Other Gram-negative sepsis `HIV` `MCC` `HCC`

✓5ᵗʰ **A41.8 Other specified sepsis**

A41.81 Sepsis due to Enterococcus `HIV` `MCC` `HCC`
　TIP: E. faecium, is a species of Enterococcus that is highly resistant to multiple antibiotics. Assign a code from category Z16 when resistance to antimicrobial drugs is documented.

A41.89 Other specified sepsis `HIV` `MCC` `HCC`
　AHA: 2020,2Q,8; 2017,1Q,51; 2016,3Q,8-14
　TIP: Viral sepsis is coded here; assign an additional code to identify the specific viral agent or illness.

A41.9 Sepsis, unspecified organism `HIV` `MCC` `HCC`
　Septicemia NOS
　AHA: 2020,2Q,28

✓4ᵗʰ **A42 Actinomycosis**
　EXCLUDES 1   actinomycetoma (B47.1)

A42.0 Pulmonary actinomycosis `HIV` `CC` `HCC`

A42.1 Abdominal actinomycosis `HIV` `CC`

A42.2 Cervicofacial actinomycosis `HIV` `CC`

A42.7 Actinomycotic sepsis `HIV` `MCC` `HCC`

✓5ᵗʰ **A42.8 Other forms of actinomycosis**

A42.81 Actinomycotic meningitis `HIV` `CC`

A42.82 Actinomycotic encephalitis `HIV` `CC`

A42.89 Other forms of actinomycosis `HIV` `CC`

A42.9 Actinomycosis, unspecified `HIV` `CC`

✓4ᵗʰ **A43 Nocardiosis**
　DEF: Rare bacterial infection occurring most often in those with weakened immune systems. Can be acquired in soil, decaying plants, or standing water. It typically begins in the lungs and has a tendency to spread to other body systems.

A43.0 Pulmonary nocardiosis `HIV` `CC` `HCC`

A43.1 Cutaneous nocardiosis `HIV` `CC`

A43.8 Other forms of nocardiosis `HIV` `CC`

A43.9 Nocardiosis, unspecified `HIV` `CC`

✓4ᵗʰ **A44 Bartonellosis**

A44.0 Systemic bartonellosis `CC`
　Oroya fever

A44.1 Cutaneous and mucocutaneous bartonellosis `CC`
　Verruga peruana

A44.8 Other forms of bartonellosis `CC`

A44.9 Bartonellosis, unspecified `CC`

A46 Erysipelas
　EXCLUDES 1   postpartum or puerperal erysipelas (O86.89)
　DEF: Skin infection affecting the upper dermis and superficial dermal lymphatics. Lesion edges are well-demarcated with distinct raised borders. It is often caused by group A Streptococci.

✓4ᵗʰ **A48 Other bacterial diseases, not elsewhere classified**
　EXCLUDES 1   actinomycetoma (B47.1)

A48.0 Gas gangrene `MCC` `HCC`
　Clostridial cellulitis
　Clostridial myonecrosis
　AHA: 2017,4Q,102

A48.1 Legionnaires' disease `HIV` `MCC` `HCC`
　DEF: Severe and often fatal infection by Legionella pneumophila. Symptoms include high fever, gastrointestinal pain, headache, myalgia, dry cough, and pneumonia and it is usually transmitted through airborne water droplets via air conditioning systems or hot tubs.

A48.2 Nonpneumonic Legionnaires' disease [Pontiac fever]

A48.3 Toxic shock syndrome `MCC` `HCC`
　Use additional code to identify the organism (B95, B96)
　EXCLUDES 1   endotoxic shock NOS (R57.8)
　　　　　　　　 sepsis NOS (A41.9)
　DEF: Bacteria producing an endotoxin, such as Staphylococci, flood the body with the toxins producing a high fever, vomiting and diarrhea, decreasing blood pressure, a skin rash, and shock. Synonym(s): TSS.

A48.4 Brazilian purpuric fever
　Systemic Hemophilus aegyptius infection

✓5ᵗʰ **A48.5 Other specified botulism**
　Non-foodborne intoxication due to toxins of Clostridium botulinum [C. botulinum]
　EXCLUDES 1   food poisoning due to toxins of Clostridium botulinum (A05.1)

A48.51 Infant botulism `CC` `P`

N Newborn: 0   P Pediatric: 0-17   M Maternity: 9-64   A Adult: 15-124   MCC Major Complication/Comorbidity   CC Complication/Comorbidity   SW Severe Wound Dx

448   ICD-10-CM 2022

A48.52 Wound botulism `CC`
Non-foodborne botulism NOS
Use additional code for associated wound

A48.8 Other specified bacterial diseases

☑4ᵗʰ **A49 Bacterial infection of unspecified site**
> EXCLUDES 1   *bacterial agents as the cause of diseases classified elsewhere (B95-B96)*
> *chlamydial infection NOS (A74.9)*
> *meningococcal infection NOS (A39.9)*
> *rickettsial infection NOS (A79.9)*
> *spirochetal infection NOS (A69.9)*

☑5ᵗʰ **A49.0 Staphylococcal infection, unspecified site**

A49.01 Methicillin susceptible Staphylococcus aureus infection, unspecified site
Methicillin susceptible Staphylococcus aureus (MSSA) infection
Staphylococcus aureus infection NOS

A49.02 Methicillin resistant Staphylococcus aureus infection, unspecified site
Methicillin resistant Staphylococcus aureus (MRSA) infection

A49.1 Streptococcal infection, unspecified site
A49.2 Hemophilus influenzae infection, unspecified site
A49.3 Mycoplasma infection, unspecified site
A49.8 Other bacterial infections of unspecified site
A49.9 Bacterial infection, unspecified
> EXCLUDES 1   *bacteremia NOS (R78.81)*

Infections with a predominantly sexual mode of transmission (A50-A64)

> EXCLUDES 1   *human immunodeficiency virus [HIV] disease (B20)*
> *nonspecific and nongonococcal urethritis (N34.1)*
> *Reiter's disease (M02.3-)*

AHA: 2021,2Q,6

☑4ᵗʰ **A50 Congenital syphilis**

☑5ᵗʰ **A50.0 Early congenital syphilis, symptomatic**
Any congenital syphilitic condition specified as early or manifest less than two years after birth.

A50.01 Early congenital syphilitic oculopathy `CC`
A50.02 Early congenital syphilitic osteochondropathy `CC`
A50.03 Early congenital syphilitic pharyngitis `CC`
Early congenital syphilitic laryngitis
A50.04 Early congenital syphilitic pneumonia `CC`
A50.05 Early congenital syphilitic rhinitis `CC`
A50.06 Early cutaneous congenital syphilis `CC`
A50.07 Early mucocutaneous congenital syphilis `CC`
A50.08 Early visceral congenital syphilis `CC`
A50.09 Other early congenital syphilis, symptomatic `CC`

A50.1 Early congenital syphilis, latent
Congenital syphilis without clinical manifestations, with positive serological reaction and negative spinal fluid test, less than two years after birth.

A50.2 Early congenital syphilis, unspecified `CC`
Congenital syphilis NOS less than two years after birth.

☑5ᵗʰ **A50.3 Late congenital syphilitic oculopathy**
> EXCLUDES 1   *Hutchinson's triad (A50.53)*

A50.30 Late congenital syphilitic oculopathy, unspecified `CC`
A50.31 Late congenital syphilitic interstitial keratitis `CC`
A50.32 Late congenital syphilitic chorioretinitis `CC`
A50.39 Other late congenital syphilitic oculopathy `CC`

☑5ᵗʰ **A50.4 Late congenital neurosyphilis [juvenile neurosyphilis]**
Use additional code to identify any associated mental disorder
> EXCLUDES 1   *Hutchinson's triad (A50.53)*

A50.40 Late congenital neurosyphilis, unspecified `CC`
Juvenile neurosyphilis NOS
A50.41 Late congenital syphilitic meningitis `MCC`
A50.42 Late congenital syphilitic encephalitis `MCC`
A50.43 Late congenital syphilitic polyneuropathy `CC`
A50.44 Late congenital syphilitic optic nerve atrophy `CC`

A50.45 Juvenile general paresis `CC`
Dementia paralytica juvenilis
Juvenile tabetoparetic neurosyphilis
A50.49 Other late congenital neurosyphilis `CC`
Juvenile tabes dorsalis

☑5ᵗʰ **A50.5 Other late congenital syphilis, symptomatic**
Any congenital syphilitic condition specified as late or manifest two years or more after birth.

A50.51 Clutton's joints `CC`
A50.52 Hutchinson's teeth `CC`
A50.53 Hutchinson's triad `CC`
A50.54 Late congenital cardiovascular syphilis `CC`
A50.55 Late congenital syphilitic arthropathy `CC` `HCC`
A50.56 Late congenital syphilitic osteochondropathy `CC`
A50.57 Syphilitic saddle nose `CC`
A50.59 Other late congenital syphilis, symptomatic `CC`

A50.6 Late congenital syphilis, latent
Congenital syphilis without clinical manifestations, with positive serological reaction and negative spinal fluid test, two years or more after birth.

A50.7 Late congenital syphilis, unspecified
Congenital syphilis NOS two years or more after birth.

A50.9 Congenital syphilis, unspecified

☑4ᵗʰ **A51 Early syphilis**
DEF: Syphilis: Sexually transmitted disease caused by the *Treponema pallidum* spirochete. Syphilis usually exhibits cutaneous manifestations and may exist for years without symptoms.

A51.0 Primary genital syphilis
Syphilitic chancre NOS
A51.1 Primary anal syphilis
A51.2 Primary syphilis of other sites

☑5ᵗʰ **A51.3 Secondary syphilis of skin and mucous membranes**
DEF: Transitory or chronic cutaneous eruptions that present within two to 10 weeks following an initial syphilis infection that may include nontender lymphadenopathy along with alopecia and condylomata lata.

A51.31 Condyloma latum `CC`
A51.32 Syphilitic alopecia `CC`
A51.39 Other secondary syphilis of skin `CC`
Syphilitic leukoderma
Syphilitic mucous patch
> EXCLUDES 1   *late syphilitic leukoderma (A52.79)*

☑5ᵗʰ **A51.4 Other secondary syphilis**
A51.41 Secondary syphilitic meningitis `MCC`
A51.42 Secondary syphilitic female pelvic disease `CC` ♀
A51.43 Secondary syphilitic oculopathy `CC`
Secondary syphilitic chorioretinitis
Secondary syphilitic iridocyclitis, iritis
Secondary syphilitic uveitis
A51.44 Secondary syphilitic nephritis `CC`
A51.45 Secondary syphilitic hepatitis `CC`
A51.46 Secondary syphilitic osteopathy `CC`
A51.49 Other secondary syphilitic conditions `CC`
Secondary syphilitic lymphadenopathy
Secondary syphilitic myositis

A51.5 Early syphilis, latent
Syphilis (acquired) without clinical manifestations, with positive serological reaction and negative spinal fluid test, less than two years after infection.

A51.9 Early syphilis, unspecified

☑4ᵗʰ **A52 Late syphilis**
☑5ᵗʰ **A52.0 Cardiovascular and cerebrovascular syphilis**
A52.00 Cardiovascular syphilis, unspecified `CC`
A52.01 Syphilitic aneurysm of aorta `CC`
A52.02 Syphilitic aortitis `CC`
A52.03 Syphilitic endocarditis `CC`
Syphilitic aortic valve incompetence or stenosis
Syphilitic mitral valve stenosis
Syphilitic pulmonary valve regurgitation
A52.04 Syphilitic cerebral arteritis `CC`

A52.05 **Other cerebrovascular syphilis** `CC`
Syphilitic cerebral aneurysm (ruptured) (non-ruptured)
Syphilitic cerebral thrombosis

A52.06 **Other syphilitic heart involvement** `CC`
Syphilitic coronary artery disease
Syphilitic myocarditis
Syphilitic pericarditis

A52.09 **Other cardiovascular syphilis** `CC`

✓5ᵗʰ **A52.1** **Symptomatic neurosyphilis**

A52.10 **Symptomatic neurosyphilis, unspecified** `CC`

A52.11 **Tabes dorsalis** `CC`
Locomotor ataxia (progressive)
Tabetic neurosyphilis

A52.12 **Other cerebrospinal syphilis** `CC`

A52.13 **Late syphilitic meningitis** `MCC`

A52.14 **Late syphilitic encephalitis** `MCC`

A52.15 **Late syphilitic neuropathy** `CC`
Late syphilitic acoustic neuritis
Late syphilitic optic (nerve) atrophy
Late syphilitic polyneuropathy
Late syphilitic retrobulbar neuritis

A52.16 **Charcôt's arthropathy (tabetic)** `CC`
DEF: Progressive neurologic arthropathy in which chronic degeneration of joints in the weight-bearing areas with peripheral hypertrophy occurs as a complication of a neuropathy disorder. Supporting structures relax from a loss of sensation resulting in chronic joint instability.

A52.17 **General paresis** `CC`
Dementia paralytica

A52.19 **Other symptomatic neurosyphilis** `CC`
Syphilitic parkinsonism

A52.2 **Asymptomatic neurosyphilis** `CC`

A52.3 **Neurosyphilis, unspecified** `CC`
Gumma (syphilitic)
Syphilis (late)
Syphiloma
AHA: 2021,2Q,6

✓5ᵗʰ **A52.7** **Other symptomatic late syphilis**

A52.71 **Late syphilitic oculopathy** `CC`
Late syphilitic chorioretinitis
Late syphilitic episcleritis

A52.72 **Syphilis of lung and bronchus** `CC`

A52.73 **Symptomatic late syphilis of other respiratory organs** `CC`

A52.74 **Syphilis of liver and other viscera** `CC`
Late syphilitic peritonitis

A52.75 **Syphilis of kidney and ureter** `CC`
Syphilitic glomerular disease

A52.76 **Other genitourinary symptomatic late syphilis** `CC`
Late syphilitic female pelvic inflammatory disease

A52.77 **Syphilis of bone and joint** `CC`

A52.78 **Syphilis of other musculoskeletal tissue** `CC`
Late syphilitic bursitis
Syphilis [stage unspecified] of bursa
Syphilis [stage unspecified] of muscle
Syphilis [stage unspecified] of synovium
Syphilis [stage unspecified] of tendon

A52.79 **Other symptomatic late syphilis** `CC`
Late syphilitic leukoderma
Syphilis of adrenal gland
Syphilis of pituitary gland
Syphilis of thyroid gland
Syphilitic splenomegaly
EXCLUDES 1 syphilitic leukoderma (secondary) (A51.39)

A52.8 **Late syphilis, latent**
Syphilis (acquired) without clinical manifestations, with positive serological reaction and negative spinal fluid test, two years or more after infection

A52.9 **Late syphilis, unspecified**

✓4ᵗʰ **A53** **Other and unspecified syphilis**

A53.0 **Latent syphilis, unspecified as early or late**
Latent syphilis NOS
Positive serological reaction for syphilis

A53.9 **Syphilis, unspecified**
Infection due to Treponema pallidum NOS
Syphilis (acquired) NOS
EXCLUDES 1 syphilis NOS under two years of age (A50.2)

✓4ᵗʰ **A54** **Gonococcal infection**
DEF: Sexually transmitted bacterial infection caused by *Neisseria gonorrhoeae*. Women are often asymptomatic, while men tend to develop urinary symptoms quickly.

✓5ᵗʰ **A54.0** **Gonococcal infection of lower genitourinary tract without periurethral or accessory gland abscess**
EXCLUDES 1 gonococcal infection with genitourinary gland abscess (A54.1)
gonococcal infection with periurethral abscess (A54.1)

A54.00 **Gonococcal infection of lower genitourinary tract, unspecified** `CC`

A54.01 **Gonococcal cystitis and urethritis, unspecified** `CC`

A54.02 **Gonococcal vulvovaginitis, unspecified** `CC` ♀

A54.03 **Gonococcal cervicitis, unspecified** `CC` ♀

A54.09 **Other gonococcal infection of lower genitourinary tract** `CC`

A54.1 **Gonococcal infection of lower genitourinary tract with periurethral and accessory gland abscess** `CC`
Gonococcal Bartholin's gland abscess

✓5ᵗʰ **A54.2** **Gonococcal pelviperitonitis and other gonococcal genitourinary infection**

A54.21 **Gonococcal infection of kidney and ureter** `CC`

A54.22 **Gonococcal prostatitis** `CC` ♂

A54.23 **Gonococcal infection of other male genital organs** `CC` ♂
Gonococcal epididymitis
Gonococcal orchitis

A54.24 **Gonococcal female pelvic inflammatory disease** `CC` ♀
Gonococcal pelviperitonitis
EXCLUDES 1 gonococcal peritonitis (A54.85)

A54.29 **Other gonococcal genitourinary infections** `CC`

✓5ᵗʰ **A54.3** **Gonococcal infection of eye**

A54.30 **Gonococcal infection of eye, unspecified** `CC`

A54.31 **Gonococcal conjunctivitis** `CC`
Ophthalmia neonatorum due to gonococcus

A54.32 **Gonococcal iridocyclitis** `CC`

A54.33 **Gonococcal keratitis** `CC`

A54.39 **Other gonococcal eye infection** `CC`
Gonococcal endophthalmia

✓5ᵗʰ **A54.4** **Gonococcal infection of musculoskeletal system**

A54.40 **Gonococcal infection of musculoskeletal system, unspecified** `CC` `HCC`

A54.41 **Gonococcal spondylopathy** `CC` `HCC`

A54.42 **Gonococcal arthritis** `CC` `HCC`
EXCLUDES 2 gonococcal infection of spine (A54.41)

A54.43 **Gonococcal osteomyelitis** `CC` `HCC`
EXCLUDES 2 gonococcal infection of spine (A54.41)

A54.49 **Gonococcal infection of other musculoskeletal tissue** `CC` `HCC`
Gonococcal bursitis
Gonococcal myositis
Gonococcal synovitis
Gonococcal tenosynovitis

A54.5 **Gonococcal pharyngitis**

A54.6 **Gonococcal infection of anus and rectum**

✓5ᵗʰ **A54.8** **Other gonococcal infections**

A54.81 **Gonococcal meningitis** `MCC`

A54.82 **Gonococcal brain abscess** `CC`

A54.83 **Gonococcal heart infection** `CC`
Gonococcal endocarditis
Gonococcal myocarditis
Gonococcal pericarditis

A54.84 **Gonococcal pneumonia** `CC` `HCC`

A54.85 **Gonococcal** peritonitis   `CC` `HCC`
         EXCLUDES 1   *gonococcal pelviperitonitis (A54.24)*

A54.86 **Gonococcal** sepsis   `MCC` `HCC`

A54.89 **Other gonococcal infections**   `CC`
         Gonococcal keratoderma
         Gonococcal lymphadenitis

A54.9 **Gonococcal infection, unspecified**   `CC`

A55 Chlamydial lymphogranuloma (venereum)
     Climatic or tropical bubo
     Durand-Nicolas-Favre disease
     Esthiomene
     Lymphogranuloma inguinale

✓4ᵗʰ A56 Other sexually transmitted chlamydial diseases
     INCLUDES   sexually transmitted diseases due to Chlamydia
                 trachomatis
     EXCLUDES 1   *neonatal chlamydial conjunctivitis (P39.1)*
                 neonatal chlamydial pneumonia (P23.1)
     EXCLUDES 2   *chlamydial lymphogranuloma (A55)*
                 conditions classified to A74.-
     DEF: *Chlamydia trachomatis*: Bacterium that causes a common venereal disease. Symptoms of chlamydia are usually mild or absent, however, serious complications may cause irreversible damage, including cystitis, pelvic inflammatory disease, and infertility in women and discharge from the penis, prostatitis, and infertility in men. Genital chlamydial infection can cause arthritis, skin lesions, and inflammation of the eye and urethra.
     Synonym(s): *Reiter's syndrome.*

   ✓5ᵗʰ **A56.0 Chlamydial infection of** lower genitourinary tract
       A56.00 **Chlamydial infection of lower genitourinary tract, unspecified**
       A56.01 **Chlamydial** cystitis and urethritis
       A56.02 **Chlamydial** vulvovaginitis   ♀
       A56.09 **Other chlamydial infection of lower genitourinary tract**
          Chlamydial cervicitis

   ✓5ᵗʰ **A56.1 Chlamydial infection of** pelviperitoneum **and other** genitourinary organs
       A56.11 **Chlamydial** female pelvic inflammatory disease   ♀
       A56.19 **Other chlamydial genitourinary infection**
          Chlamydial epididymitis
          Chlamydial orchitis

   A56.2 **Chlamydial infection of genitourinary tract, unspecified**
   A56.3 **Chlamydial infection of** anus and rectum
   A56.4 **Chlamydial infection of** pharynx
   A56.8 **Sexually transmitted chlamydial infection of other sites**

A57 Chancroid
     Ulcus molle
     DEF: Localized infection by *Haemophilus ducreyi*, causing genital ulcers and infecting the inguinal lymph nodes.

A58 Granuloma inguinale
     Donovanosis

✓4ᵗʰ A59 Trichomoniasis
     EXCLUDES 2   *intestinal trichomoniasis (A07.8)*
     DEF: Infection with the parasitic, flagellated protozoa of the genus *Trichomonas*. This protozoon is found in the intestinal and genitourinary tracts of humans and in the mouth around tartar, cavities, and areas of periodontal disease.

   ✓5ᵗʰ **A59.0 Urogenital trichomoniasis**
       A59.00 **Urogenital trichomoniasis, unspecified**
          Fluor (vaginalis) due to Trichomonas
          Leukorrhea (vaginalis) due to Trichomonas
       A59.01 **Trichomonal** vulvovaginitis   ♀
       A59.02 **Trichomonal** prostatitis   ♂
       A59.03 **Trichomonal** cystitis and urethritis
       A59.09 **Other urogenital trichomoniasis**
          Trichomonas cervicitis

   A59.8 **Trichomoniasis of other sites**
   A59.9 **Trichomoniasis, unspecified**

✓4ᵗʰ A60 Anogenital herpesviral [herpes simplex] infections
   ✓5ᵗʰ **A60.0 Herpesviral infection of** genitalia and urogenital tract
       A60.00 **Herpesviral infection of urogenital system, unspecified**   `HIV`
       A60.01 **Herpesviral infection of** penis   `HIV` ♂
       A60.02 **Herpesviral infection of other** male genital organs   ♂

       A60.03 **Herpesviral** cervicitis   ♀
       A60.04 **Herpesviral** vulvovaginitis   `HIV` ♀
          Herpesviral [herpes simplex] ulceration
          Herpesviral [herpes simplex] vaginitis
          Herpesviral [herpes simplex] vulvitis
       A60.09 **Herpesviral infection of other urogenital tract**   `HIV`
          AHA: 2020,1Q,20

   A60.1 **Herpesviral infection of** perianal skin and rectum   `HIV`
   A60.9 **Anogenital herpesviral infection, unspecified**   `HIV`

✓4ᵗʰ A63 Other predominantly sexually transmitted diseases, not elsewhere classified
     EXCLUDES 2   *molluscum contagiosum (B08.1)*
                 papilloma of cervix (D26.0)

   A63.0 **Anogenital (venereal) warts**
       Anogenital warts due to (human) papillomavirus [HPV]
       Condyloma acuminatum

   A63.8 **Other specified predominantly sexually transmitted diseases**

A64 Unspecified sexually transmitted disease

Other spirochetal diseases (A65-A69)

     EXCLUDES 2   *leptospirosis (A27.-)*
                 syphilis (A50-A53)

A65 Nonvenereal syphilis
     Bejel
     Endemic syphilis
     Njovera

✓4ᵗʰ A66 Yaws
     INCLUDES   bouba
                 frambesia (tropica)
                 pian

   A66.0 **Initial lesions of yaws**
       Chancre of yaws
       Frambesia, initial or primary
       Initial frambesial ulcer
       Mother yaw

   A66.1 **Multiple papillomata and wet crab yaws**
       Frambesioma
       Pianoma
       Plantar or palmar papilloma of yaws

   A66.2 **Other early skin lesions of yaws**
       Cutaneous yaws, less than five years after infection
       Early yaws (cutaneous) (macular) (maculopapular) (micropapular) (papular)
       Frambeside of early yaws

   A66.3 **Hyperkeratosis of yaws**
       Ghoul hand
       Hyperkeratosis, palmar or plantar (early) (late) due to yaws
       Worm-eaten soles

   A66.4 **Gummata and ulcers of yaws**
       Gummatous frambeside
       Nodular late yaws (ulcerated)

   A66.5 **Gangosa**
       Rhinopharyngitis mutilans

   A66.6 **Bone and joint lesions of yaws**   `HCC`
       Yaws ganglion
       Yaws goundou
       Yaws gumma, bone
       Yaws gummatous osteitis or periostitis
       Yaws hydrarthrosis
       Yaws osteitis
       Yaws periostitis (hypertrophic)

   A66.7 **Other manifestations of yaws**
       Juxta-articular nodules of yaws
       Mucosal yaws

   A66.8 **Latent yaws**
       Yaws without clinical manifestations, with positive serology

   A66.9 **Yaws, unspecified**

✓4ᵗʰ A67 Pinta [carate]
   A67.0 **Primary lesions of pinta**
       Chancre (primary) of pinta
       Papule (primary) of pinta

A67.1 **Intermediate lesions of pinta**
Erythematous plaques of pinta
Hyperchromic lesions of pinta
Hyperkeratosis of pinta
Pintids

A67.2 **Late lesions of pinta**
Achromic skin lesions of pinta
Cicatricial skin lesions of pinta
Dyschromic skin lesions of pinta

A67.3 **Mixed lesions of pinta**
Achromic with hyperchromic skin lesions of pinta [carate]

A67.9 **Pinta, unspecified**

✓4ᵗʰ **A68** **Relapsing fevers**

INCLUDES recurrent fever
EXCLUDES 2 *Lyme disease (A69.2-)*

A68.0 **Louse-borne relapsing fever**   CC
Relapsing fever due to Borrelia recurrentis

A68.1 **Tick-borne relapsing fever**   CC
Relapsing fever due to any Borrelia species other than Borrelia recurrentis

A68.9 **Relapsing fever, unspecified**   CC

✓4ᵗʰ **A69** **Other spirochetal infections**

A69.0 **Necrotizing ulcerative stomatitis**
Cancrum oris
Fusospirochetal gangrene
Noma
Stomatitis gangrenosa

A69.1 **Other Vincent's infections**   CC
Fusospirochetal pharyngitis
Necrotizing ulcerative (acute) gingivitis
Necrotizing ulcerative (acute) gingivostomatitis
Spirochetal stomatitis
Trench mouth
Vincent's angina
Vincent's gingivitis

✓5ᵗʰ **A69.2** **Lyme disease**
Erythema chronicum migrans due to Borrelia burgdorferi
DEF: Recurrent multisystem disorder through tick bites that begins with lesions of erythema chronicum migrans and is followed by arthritis of the large joints, myalgia, malaise, and neurological and cardiac manifestations.

A69.20 **Lyme disease, unspecified**   CC
A69.21 **Meningitis due to Lyme disease**   CC
A69.22 **Other neurologic disorders in Lyme disease**   CC
Cranial neuritis
Meningoencephalitis
Polyneuropathy
A69.23 **Arthritis due to Lyme disease**   CC HCC
A69.29 **Other conditions associated with Lyme disease**   CC
Myopericarditis due to Lyme disease
AHA: 2016,3Q,12

A69.8 **Other specified spirochetal infections**
A69.9 **Spirochetal infection, unspecified**

Other diseases caused by chlamydiae (A70-A74)

EXCLUDES 1 *sexually transmitted chlamydial diseases (A55-A56)*

A70 **Chlamydia psittaci infections**   CC
Ornithosis
Parrot fever
Psittacosis

✓4ᵗʰ **A71** **Trachoma**

EXCLUDES 1 *sequelae of trachoma (B94.0)*

A71.0 **Initial stage of trachoma**
Trachoma dubium

A71.1 **Active stage of trachoma**
Granular conjunctivitis (trachomatous)
Trachomatous follicular conjunctivitis
Trachomatous pannus

A71.9 **Trachoma, unspecified**

✓4ᵗʰ **A74** **Other diseases caused by chlamydiae**

EXCLUDES 1 *neonatal chlamydial conjunctivitis (P39.1)*
neonatal chlamydial pneumonia (P23.1)
Reiter's disease (M02.3-)
sexually transmitted chlamydial diseases (A55-A56)
EXCLUDES 2 *chlamydial pneumonia (J16.0)*

A74.0 **Chlamydial conjunctivitis**
Paratrachoma

✓5ᵗʰ **A74.8** **Other chlamydial diseases**

A74.81 **Chlamydial peritonitis**
A74.89 **Other chlamydial diseases**
A74.9 **Chlamydial infection, unspecified**
Chlamydiosis NOS

Rickettsioses (A75-A79)

DEF: Rickettsia: Condition caused by bacteria that live in lice/ticks transmitted to humans through bites.

✓4ᵗʰ **A75** **Typhus fever**

EXCLUDES 1 *rickettsiosis due to Ehrlichia sennetsu (A79.81)*

A75.0 **Epidemic louse-borne typhus fever due to Rickettsia prowazekii**   CC
Classical typhus (fever)
Epidemic (louse-borne) typhus

A75.1 **Recrudescent typhus [Brill's disease]**   CC
Brill-Zinsser disease

A75.2 **Typhus fever due to Rickettsia typhi**   CC
Murine (flea-borne) typhus

A75.3 **Typhus fever due to Rickettsia tsutsugamushi**   CC
Scrub (mite-borne) typhus
Tsutsugamushi fever
Typhus fever due to Orientia Tsutsugamushi (scrub typhus)

A75.9 **Typhus fever, unspecified**   CC
Typhus (fever) NOS

✓4ᵗʰ **A77** **Spotted fever [tick-borne rickettsioses]**

A77.0 **Spotted fever due to Rickettsia rickettsii**   CC
Rocky Mountain spotted fever
Sao Paulo fever

A77.1 **Spotted fever due to Rickettsia conorii**   CC
African tick typhus
Boutonneuse fever
India tick typhus
Kenya tick typhus
Marseilles fever
Mediterranean tick fever

A77.2 **Spotted fever due to Rickettsia siberica**   CC
North Asian tick fever
Siberian tick typhus

A77.3 **Spotted fever due to Rickettsia australis**   CC
Queensland tick typhus

✓5ᵗʰ **A77.4** **Ehrlichiosis**

EXCLUDES 1 ▶*anaplasmosis [A. phagocytophilum] (A79.82)*◀
▶*rickettsiosis due to Ehrlichia sennetsu*◀ *(A79.81)*

A77.40 **Ehrlichiosis, unspecified**   CC
A77.41 **Ehrlichiosis chafeensis [E. chafeensis]**   CC
A77.49 **Other ehrlichiosis**
Ehrlichiosis due to E. ewingii
Ehrlichiosis due to E. muris euclairensis

A77.8 **Other spotted fevers**   CC
Rickettsia 364D/R. philipii (Pacific Coast tick fever)
Spotted fever due to Rickettsia africae (African tick bite fever)
Spotted fever due to Rickettsia parkeri

A77.9 **Spotted fever, unspecified**   CC
Tick-borne typhus NOS

A78 **Q fever**   CC
Infection due to Coxiella burnetii
Nine Mile fever
Quadrilateral fever

✓4ᵗʰ **A79** **Other rickettsioses**

A79.0 **Trench fever**   CC
Quintan fever
Wolhynian fever

A79.1   **Rickettsialpox due to** Rickettsia akari   `CC`
Kew Garden fever
Vesicular rickettsiosis

✓5ᵗʰ **A79.8**   **Other specified rickettsioses**

    A79.81   **Rickettsiosis due to** Ehrlichia sennetsu   `CC`
        Rickettsiosis due to Neorickettsia sennetsu

●   **A79.82**   **Anaplasmosis [A. phagocytophilum]**   `CC`
        Transfusion transmitted A. phagocytophilum

    A79.89   **Other specified rickettsioses**   `CC`

    A79.9   **Rickettsiosis, unspecified**   `CC`
        Rickettsial infection NOS

Viral and prion infections of the central nervous system (A80-A89)

`EXCLUDES 1`   postpolio syndrome (G14)
           sequelae of poliomyelitis (B91)
           sequelae of viral encephalitis (B94.1)

✓4ᵗʰ **A80**   **Acute poliomyelitis**

    `EXCLUDES 1` ▶acute flaccid myelitis (G04.82)◀

    A80.0   **Acute paralytic poliomyelitis, vaccine-associated**   `MCC`
    A80.1   **Acute paralytic poliomyelitis, wild virus, imported**   `MCC`
    A80.2   **Acute paralytic poliomyelitis, wild virus, indigenous**   `MCC`
✓5ᵗʰ **A80.3**   **Acute paralytic poliomyelitis, other and unspecified**

       A80.30   **Acute paralytic poliomyelitis, unspecified**   `MCC`
       A80.39   **Other acute paralytic poliomyelitis**   `MCC`

    A80.4   **Acute nonparalytic poliomyelitis**
    A80.9   **Acute poliomyelitis, unspecified**

✓4ᵗʰ **A81**   **Atypical virus infections of central nervous system**

    `INCLUDES`   diseases of the central nervous system caused by prions
    Use additional code to identify:
       dementia with behavioral disturbance (F02.81)
       dementia without behavioral disturbance (F02.80)

✓5ᵗʰ **A81.0**   **Creutzfeldt-Jakob disease**

       DEF: Communicable, rare spongiform encephalopathy occurring later in life with progressive destruction of the pyramidal and extrapyramidal systems eventually leading to death. Progressive dementia, wasting of muscles, tremor, and other symptoms are present.

       A81.00   **Creutzfeldt-Jakob disease, unspecified**   `CC` `HCC`
          Jakob-Creutzfeldt disease, unspecified

       A81.01   **Variant Creutzfeldt-Jakob disease**   `CC` `HCC`
          vCJD

       A81.09   **Other Creutzfeldt-Jakob disease**   `CC` `HCC`
          CJD
          Familial Creutzfeldt-Jakob disease
          Iatrogenic Creutzfeldt-Jakob disease
          Sporadic Creutzfeldt-Jakob disease
          Subacute spongiform encephalopathy (with dementia)

    A81.1   **Subacute sclerosing panencephalitis**   `CC` `HCC`
       Dawson's inclusion body encephalitis
       Van Bogaert's sclerosing leukoencephalopathy

    A81.2   **Progressive multifocal leukoencephalopathy**   `HIV` `CC` `HCC`
       Multifocal leukoencephalopathy NOS

✓5ᵗʰ **A81.8**   **Other atypical virus infections of central nervous system**

       A81.81   **Kuru**   `CC` `HCC`
       A81.82   **Gerstmann-Sträussler-Scheinker syndrome**   `HIV` `CC` `HCC`
          GSS syndrome
       A81.83   **Fatal familial insomnia**   `HIV` `CC` `HCC`
          FFI
       A81.89   **Other atypical virus infections of central nervous system**   `HIV` `CC` `HCC`

    A81.9   **Atypical virus infection of central nervous system, unspecified**   `HIV` `CC` `HCC`
       Prion diseases of the central nervous system NOS

✓4ᵗʰ **A82**   **Rabies**

    A82.0   **Sylvatic rabies**   `CC`
    A82.1   **Urban rabies**   `CC`
    A82.9   **Rabies, unspecified**   `CC`

✓4ᵗʰ **A83**   **Mosquito-borne viral encephalitis**

    `INCLUDES`   mosquito-borne viral meningoencephalitis
    `EXCLUDES 2`   Venezuelan equine encephalitis (A92.2)
            West Nile fever (A92.3-)
            West Nile virus (A92.3-)

    A83.0   **Japanese encephalitis**   `MCC`
    A83.1   **Western equine encephalitis**   `MCC`
    A83.2   **Eastern equine encephalitis**   `MCC`
    A83.3   **St Louis encephalitis**   `MCC`
    A83.4   **Australian encephalitis**   `MCC`
       Kunjin virus disease
    A83.5   **California encephalitis**   `MCC`
       California meningoencephalitis
       La Crosse encephalitis
    A83.6   **Rocio virus disease**   `MCC`
    A83.8   **Other mosquito-borne viral encephalitis**   `MCC`
    A83.9   **Mosquito-borne viral encephalitis, unspecified**   `MCC`

✓4ᵗʰ **A84**   **Tick-borne viral encephalitis**

    `INCLUDES`   tick-borne viral meningoencephalitis

    A84.0   **Far Eastern tick-borne encephalitis [Russian spring-summer encephalitis]**   `MCC`
    A84.1   **Central European tick-borne encephalitis**   `MCC`
✓5ᵗʰ **A84.8**   **Other tick-borne viral encephalitis**

       AHA: 2020,4Q,4-5

       A84.81   **Powassan virus disease**   `MCC`
       A84.89   **Other tick-borne viral encephalitis**   `MCC`
          Louping ill
          Code first, if applicable, transfusion related infection (T80.22-)

    A84.9   **Tick-borne viral encephalitis, unspecified**   `MCC`

✓4ᵗʰ **A85**   **Other viral encephalitis, not elsewhere classified**

    `INCLUDES`   specified viral encephalomyelitis NEC
            specified viral meningoencephalitis NEC
    `EXCLUDES 1`   benign myalgic encephalomyelitis (G93.3)
            encephalitis due to cytomegalovirus (B25.8)
            encephalitis due to herpesvirus NEC (B10.0-)
            encephalitis due to herpesvirus [herpes simplex] (B00.4)
            encephalitis due to measles virus (B05.0)
            encephalitis due to mumps virus (B26.2)
            encephalitis due to poliomyelitis virus (A80.-)
            encephalitis due to zoster (B02.0)
            lymphocytic choriomeningitis (A87.2)

    A85.0   **Enteroviral encephalitis**   `HIV` `CC`
       Enteroviral encephalomyelitis
    A85.1   **Adenoviral encephalitis**   `HIV` `CC`
       Adenoviral meningoencephalitis
    A85.2   **Arthropod-borne viral encephalitis, unspecified**   `MCC`
       `EXCLUDES 1`   West nile virus with encephalitis (A92.31)
    A85.8   **Other specified viral encephalitis**   `HIV` `CC`
       Encephalitis lethargica
       Von Economo-Cruchet disease

    A86   **Unspecified viral encephalitis**   `HIV` `CC`
       Viral encephalomyelitis NOS
       Viral meningoencephalitis NOS

✓4ᵗʰ **A87**   **Viral meningitis**

    `EXCLUDES 1`   meningitis due to herpesvirus [herpes simplex] (B00.3)
            meningitis due to measles virus (B05.1)
            meningitis due to mumps virus (B26.1)
            meningitis due to poliomyelitis virus (A80.-)
            meningitis due to zoster (B02.1)

    DEF: Meningitis: Inflammation of the meningeal layers of the brain and spine.

    A87.0   **Enteroviral meningitis**   `CC`
       Coxsackievirus meningitis
       Echovirus meningitis
    A87.1   **Adenoviral meningitis**   `CC`
    A87.2   **Lymphocytic choriomeningitis**   `CC`
       Lymphocytic meningoencephalitis
    A87.8   **Other viral meningitis**   `CC`
    A87.9   **Viral meningitis, unspecified**   `CC`

✓ Additional Character Required   ✓x7ᵗʰ Placeholder   Questionable PDx   Manifestation   Unspecified Dx   `UPD` Unacceptable PDx   `H1`-`H14` HAC   `HCC` CMS-HCC Dx   `HIV` HIV Dx

ICD-10-CM 2022   **453**

A79.1–A87.9

✓4ᵗʰ A88 Other viral infections of central nervous system, not elsewhere classified
> EXCLUDES 1   viral encephalitis NOS (A86)
> viral meningitis NOS (A87.9)

A88.0 Enteroviral exanthematous fever [Boston exanthem] `CC`

A88.1 Epidemic vertigo

A88.8 Other specified viral infections of central nervous system `HIV` `CC`

A89 Unspecified viral infection of central nervous system `HIV` `CC`

Arthropod-borne viral fevers and viral hemorrhagic fevers (A90-A99)

A90 Dengue fever [classical dengue] `CC`
> EXCLUDES 1   dengue hemorrhagic fever (A91)

AHA: 2016,3Q,13

A91 Dengue hemorrhagic fever `CC`

✓4ᵗʰ A92 Other mosquito-borne viral fevers
> EXCLUDES 1   Ross River disease (B33.1)

A92.0 Chikungunya virus disease `CC`
Chikungunya (hemorrhagic) fever

A92.1 O'nyong-nyong fever `CC`

A92.2 Venezuelan equine fever `CC`
Venezuelan equine encephalitis
Venezuelan equine encephalomyelitis virus disease

✓5ᵗʰ A92.3 West Nile virus infection
West Nile fever
AHA: 2016,3Q,12

A92.30 West Nile virus infection, unspecified `MCC`
West Nile fever NOS
West Nile fever without complications
West Nile virus NOS

A92.31 West Nile virus infection with encephalitis `MCC`
West Nile encephalitis
West Nile encephalomyelitis

A92.32 West Nile virus infection with other neurologic manifestation `MCC`
Use additional code to specify the neurologic manifestation

A92.39 West Nile virus infection with other complications `MCC`
Use additional code to specify the other conditions

A92.4 Rift Valley fever `CC`

A92.5 Zika virus disease `CC`
Zika virus fever
Zika virus infection
Zika NOS
> EXCLUDES 1   congenital Zika virus disease (P35.4)

AHA: 2016,4Q,4-7
DEF: Virus transmitted via a bite from an infected Aedes species mosquito. Common symptoms of the virus include fever, rash, joint pain, and conjunctivitis; they are usually mild in nature and may last from several days to a week. Most people who have the Zika virus do not require medical attention; however, in pregnant women, the Zika virus can cause a serious birth defect called microcephaly, as well as other severe fetal brain defects.
TIP: Code only confirmed diagnoses of Zika virus; documentation by the physician that the disease is confirmed is sufficient.

A92.8 Other specified mosquito-borne viral fevers `CC`

A92.9 Mosquito-borne viral fever, unspecified `CC`

✓4ᵗʰ A93 Other arthropod-borne viral fevers, not elsewhere classified

A93.0 Oropouche virus disease `CC`
Oropouche fever

A93.1 Sandfly fever `CC`
Pappataci fever
Phlebotomus fever

A93.2 Colorado tick fever `CC`

A93.8 Other specified arthropod-borne viral fevers `CC`
Piry virus disease
Vesicular stomatitis virus disease [Indiana fever]

A94 Unspecified arthropod-borne viral fever `CC`
Arboviral fever NOS
Arbovirus infection NOS

✓4ᵗʰ A95 Yellow fever

A95.0 Sylvatic yellow fever `CC`
Jungle yellow fever

A95.1 Urban yellow fever `CC`

A95.9 Yellow fever, unspecified `CC`

✓4ᵗʰ A96 Arenaviral hemorrhagic fever

A96.0 Junin hemorrhagic fever `CC`
Argentinian hemorrhagic fever

A96.1 Machupo hemorrhagic fever `CC`
Bolivian hemorrhagic fever

A96.2 Lassa fever

A96.8 Other arenaviral hemorrhagic fevers `CC`

A96.9 Arenaviral hemorrhagic fever, unspecified `CC`

✓4ᵗʰ A98 Other viral hemorrhagic fevers, not elsewhere classified
> EXCLUDES 1   chikungunya hemorrhagic fever (A92.0)
> dengue hemorrhagic fever (A91)

A98.0 Crimean-Congo hemorrhagic fever `CC`
Central Asian hemorrhagic fever

A98.1 Omsk hemorrhagic fever `CC`

A98.2 Kyasanur Forest disease `CC`

A98.3 Marburg virus disease

A98.4 Ebola virus disease

A98.5 Hemorrhagic fever with renal syndrome `CC`
Epidemic hemorrhagic fever
Korean hemorrhagic fever
Russian hemorrhagic fever
Hantaan virus disease
Hantavirus disease with renal manifestations
Nephropathia epidemica
Songo fever
> EXCLUDES 1   hantavirus (cardio)-pulmonary syndrome (B33.4)

A98.8 Other specified viral hemorrhagic fevers `CC`

A99 Unspecified viral hemorrhagic fever `CC`

Viral infections characterized by skin and mucous membrane lesions (B00-B09)

✓4ᵗʰ B00 Herpesviral [herpes simplex] infections
> EXCLUDES 1   congenital herpesviral infections (P35.2)
> EXCLUDES 2   anogenital herpesviral infection (A60.-)
> gammaherpesviral mononucleosis (B27.0-)
> herpangina (B08.5)

B00.0 Eczema herpeticum `HIV`
Kaposi's varicelliform eruption

B00.1 Herpesviral vesicular dermatitis `HIV`
Herpes simplex facialis
Herpes simplex labialis
Herpes simplex otitis externa
Vesicular dermatitis of ear
Vesicular dermatitis of lip

B00.2 Herpesviral gingivostomatitis and pharyngotonsillitis `HIV` `CC`
Herpesviral pharyngitis

B00.3 Herpesviral meningitis `HIV` `MCC`

B00.4 Herpesviral encephalitis `HIV` `MCC`
Herpesviral meningoencephalitis
Simian B disease
> EXCLUDES 1   herpesviral encephalitis due to herpesvirus 6 and 7 (B10.01, B10.09)
> non-simplex herpesviral encephalitis (B10.0-)

✓5ᵗʰ B00.5 Herpesviral ocular disease

B00.50 Herpesviral ocular disease, unspecified `HIV` `CC`

B00.51 Herpesviral iridocyclitis `HIV` `CC`
Herpesviral iritis
Herpesviral uveitis, anterior

B00.52 Herpesviral keratitis `HIV` `CC`
Herpesviral keratoconjunctivitis

B00.53 Herpesviral conjunctivitis `HIV` `CC`

B00.59 Other herpesviral disease of eye `HIV` `CC`
Herpesviral dermatitis of eyelid

B00.7 Disseminated herpesviral disease `HIV` `MCC` `HCC`
Herpesviral sepsis

✓5ᵗʰ B00.8 Other forms of herpesviral infections

B00.81 Herpesviral hepatitis `HIV` `CC`

       B00.82   **Herpes simplex** myelitis   `MCC` `HCC`

       B00.89   **Other herpesviral infection**   `HIV` `CC`

           Herpesviral whitlow

     B00.9   **Herpesviral infection, unspecified**   `HIV`

       Herpes simplex infection NOS

`✓4ᵗʰ` **B01**   **Varicella [chickenpox]**

     B01.0   **Varicella** meningitis   `CC`

   `✓5ᵗʰ` **B01.1**   **Varicella** encephalitis, myelitis and encephalomyelitis

       Postchickenpox encephalitis, myelitis and encephalomyelitis

       B01.11   **Varicella** encephalitis and encephalomyelitis   `MCC`

          Postchickenpox encephalitis and encephalomyelitis

       B01.12   **Varicella** myelitis   `MCC` `HCC`

          Postchickenpox myelitis

     B01.2   **Varicella** pneumonia   `MCC`

   `✓5ᵗʰ` **B01.8**   **Varicella with other complications**

       B01.81   **Varicella** keratitis   `CC`

       B01.89   **Other varicella complications**   `CC`

     B01.9   **Varicella without complication**   `CC`

       Varicella NOS

`✓4ᵗʰ` **B02**   **Zoster [herpes zoster]**

     `INCLUDES`   shingles

           zona

     B02.0   **Zoster** encephalitis   `HIV` `CC`

       Zoster meningoencephalitis

     B02.1   **Zoster** meningitis   `HIV` `MCC`

       AHA: 2019,1Q,18

   `✓5ᵗʰ` **B02.2**   **Zoster with other nervous system involvement**

       B02.21   **Postherpetic** geniculate ganglionitis   `HIV` `CC`

       B02.22   **Postherpetic** trigeminal neuralgia   `HIV` `CC`

       B02.23   **Postherpetic** polyneuropathy   `HIV` `CC`

       B02.24   **Postherpetic** myelitis   `MCC` `HCC`

          Herpes zoster myelitis

       B02.29   **Other postherpetic nervous system involvement**   `HIV` `CC`

          Postherpetic radiculopathy

   `✓5ᵗʰ` **B02.3**   **Zoster** ocular **disease**

       B02.30   **Zoster ocular disease, unspecified**   `HIV` `CC`

       B02.31   **Zoster** conjunctivitis   `HIV` `CC`

       B02.32   **Zoster** iridocyclitis   `HIV` `CC`

       B02.33   **Zoster** keratitis   `HIV` `CC`

          Herpes zoster keratoconjunctivitis

       B02.34   **Zoster** scleritis   `HIV` `CC`

       B02.39   **Other herpes zoster eye disease**   `HIV` `CC`

          Zoster blepharitis

     B02.7   **Disseminated** zoster   `HIV` `CC`

     B02.8   **Zoster with other complications**   `HIV` `CC`

       Herpes zoster otitis externa

     B02.9   **Zoster without complications**   `HIV`

       Zoster NOS

   B03   **Smallpox**   `CC`

     `NOTE`   In 1980 the 33rd World Health Assembly declared that smallpox had been eradicated.

          The classification is maintained for surveillance purposes.

   B04   **Monkeypox**   `CC`

`✓4ᵗʰ` **B05**   **Measles**

     `INCLUDES`   morbilli

     `EXCLUDES 1`   *subacute sclerosing panencephalitis (A81.1)*

     B05.0   **Measles complicated by** encephalitis   `MCC`

       Postmeasles encephalitis

     B05.1   **Measles complicated by** meningitis   `CC`

       Postmeasles meningitis

     B05.2   **Measles complicated by** pneumonia   `MCC`

       Postmeasles pneumonia

     B05.3   **Measles complicated by** otitis media

       Postmeasles otitis media

     B05.4   **Measles with** intestinal **complications**   `CC`

   `✓5ᵗʰ` **B05.8**   **Measles with other complications**

       B05.81   **Measles** keratitis **and keratoconjunctivitis**   `CC`

       B05.89   **Other measles complications**   `CC`

     B05.9   **Measles without complication**

       Measles NOS

`✓4ᵗʰ` **B06**   **Rubella [German measles]**

     `EXCLUDES 1`   *congenital rubella (P35.0)*

     DEF: Highly contagious virus in which the symptoms are mild and short-lived in most people. Rubella during pregnancy, however, can result in abortion, stillbirth, or congenital defects.

   `✓5ᵗʰ` **B06.0**   **Rubella with** neurological **complications**

       B06.00   **Rubella with neurological complication, unspecified**   `CC`

       B06.01   **Rubella** encephalitis   `MCC`

          Rubella meningoencephalitis

       B06.02   **Rubella** meningitis   `CC`

       B06.09   **Other neurological complications of rubella**   `CC`

   `✓5ᵗʰ` **B06.8**   **Rubella with other complications**

       B06.81   **Rubella** pneumonia   `CC`

       B06.82   **Rubella** arthritis   `CC` `HCC`

       B06.89   **Other rubella complications**   `CC`

     B06.9   **Rubella without complication**

       Rubella NOS

`✓4ᵗʰ` **B07**   **Viral warts**

     `INCLUDES`   verruca simplex

           verruca vulgaris

           viral warts due to human papillomavirus

     `EXCLUDES 2`   *anogenital (venereal) warts (A63.0)*

           papilloma of bladder (D41.4)

           papilloma of cervix (D26.0)

           papilloma larynx (D14.1)

     B07.0   **Plantar** wart

       Verruca plantaris

     B07.8   **Other viral warts**

       Common wart

       Flat wart

       Verruca plana

     B07.9   **Viral wart, unspecified**

`✓4ᵗʰ` **B08**   **Other viral infections characterized by skin and mucous membrane lesions, not elsewhere classified**

     `EXCLUDES 1`   *vesicular stomatitis virus disease (A93.8)*

   `✓5ᵗʰ` **B08.0**   **Other orthopoxvirus infections**

     `EXCLUDES 2`   *monkeypox (B04)*

     `✓6ᵗʰ` **B08.01**   **Cowpox and vaccinia not from vaccine**

       B08.010   **Cowpox**

          DEF: Disease contracted by milking infected cows. The vesicles usually appear on the fingers, hands, and adjacent areas and usually disappear without scarring. Other symptoms include local edema, lymphangitis, and regional lymphadenitis with or without fever.

       B08.011   **Vaccinia not from vaccine**

          `EXCLUDES 1`   *vaccinia (from vaccination) (generalized) (T88.1)*

     B08.02   **Orf virus disease**

       Contagious pustular dermatitis

       Ecthyma contagiosum

     B08.03   **Pseudocowpox [milker's node]**

     B08.04   **Paravaccinia, unspecified**

     B08.09   **Other orthopoxvirus infections**

       Orthopoxvirus infection NOS

     B08.1   **Molluscum contagiosum**

       DEF: Benign poxvirus infection causing small bumps on the skin or conjunctiva, transmitted by close contact.

   `✓5ᵗʰ` **B08.2**   **Exanthema subitum [sixth disease]**

       Roseola infantum

       B08.20   **Exanthema subitum [sixth disease], unspecified**   `P`

          Roseola infantum, unspecified

       B08.21   **Exanthema subitum [sixth disease] due to human herpesvirus 6**   `P`

          Roseola infantum due to human herpesvirus 6

       B08.22   **Exanthema subitum [sixth disease] due to human herpesvirus 7**   `P`

          Roseola infantum due to human herpesvirus 7

☑ Additional Character Required   `✓x7ᵗʰ` Placeholder   Questionable PDx   Manifestation   Unspecified Dx   `UPD` Unacceptable PDx   `H1`-`H14` HAC   `HCC` CMS-HCC Dx   `HIV` HIV Dx

ICD-10-CM 2022   **455**

B08.3 **Erythema infectiosum [fifth disease]** `CC`
DEF: Infection with human parvovirus B19, mainly occurring in children. Symptoms include a low-grade fever, malaise, or a "cold" a few days before the appearance of a mild rash illness that presents as a "slapped-cheek" rash on the face and a lacy red rash on the trunk and limbs.

B08.4 **Enteroviral vesicular stomatitis with exanthem**
Hand, foot and mouth disease

B08.5 **Enteroviral vesicular pharyngitis**
Herpangina
DEF: Acute infectious Coxsackie virus infection causing throat lesions, fever, and vomiting that generally affects children in the summer.

√5ᵗʰ **B08.6** **Parapoxvirus infections**
    B08.60 **Parapoxvirus infection, unspecified**
    B08.61 **Bovine stomatitis**
    B08.62 **Sealpox**
    B08.69 **Other parapoxvirus infections**

√5ᵗʰ **B08.7** **Yatapoxvirus infections**
    B08.70 **Yatapoxvirus infection, unspecified**
    B08.71 **Tanapox virus disease** `CC`
    B08.72 **Yaba pox virus disease**
        Yaba monkey tumor disease
    B08.79 **Other yatapoxvirus infections**

B08.8 **Other specified viral infections characterized by skin and mucous membrane lesions**
Enteroviral lymphonodular pharyngitis
Foot-and-mouth disease
Poxvirus NEC

B09 **Unspecified viral infection characterized by skin and mucous membrane lesions**
Viral enanthema NOS
Viral exanthema NOS

Other human herpesviruses (B10)

√4ᵗʰ **B10** **Other human herpesviruses**
   EXCLUDES 2   cytomegalovirus (B25.9)
        Epstein-Barr virus (B27.0-)
        herpes NOS (B00.9)
        herpes simplex (B00.-)
        herpes zoster (B02.-)
        human herpesvirus NOS (B00.-)
        human herpesvirus 1 and 2 (B00.-)
        human herpesvirus 3 (B01.-, B02.-)
        human herpesvirus 4 (B27.0-)
        human herpesvirus 5 (B25.-)
        varicella (B01.-)
        zoster (B02.-)

√5ᵗʰ **B10.0** **Other human herpesvirus encephalitis**
   EXCLUDES 2   herpes encephalitis NOS (B00.4)
        herpes simplex encephalitis (B00.4)
        human herpesvirus encephalitis (B00.4)
        simian B herpes virus encephalitis (B00.4)
    B10.01 **Human herpesvirus 6 encephalitis** `HIV` `MCC`
    B10.09 **Other human herpesvirus encephalitis** `HIV` `MCC`
        Human herpesvirus 7 encephalitis

√5ᵗʰ **B10.8** **Other human herpesvirus infection**
    B10.81 **Human herpesvirus 6 infection**
    B10.82 **Human herpesvirus 7 infection**
    B10.89 **Other human herpesvirus infection**
        Human herpesvirus 8 infection
        Kaposi's sarcoma-associated herpesvirus infection

Viral hepatitis (B15-B19)

EXCLUDES 1   sequelae of viral hepatitis (B94.2)
EXCLUDES 2   cytomegaloviral hepatitis (B25.1)
        herpesviral [herpes simplex] hepatitis (B00.81)
DEF: Hepatitis A: HAV infection that is self-limiting with flulike symptoms. Transmission is fecal-oral.
DEF: Hepatitis B: HBV infection that can be chronic and systemic. Transmission is bodily fluids.
DEF: Hepatitis C: HCV infection that can be chronic and systemic. Transmission is blood transfusion and unidentified agents.
DEF: Hepatitis D (delta): HDV that occurs only in the presence of hepatitis B virus. Transmission is contaminated blood in contact with mucous membranes.
DEF: Hepatitis E: HEV is an epidemic form. Transmission is fecal-oral, most often from contaminated water.

√4ᵗʰ **B15** **Acute hepatitis A**
    B15.0 **Hepatitis A with hepatic coma** `MCC`
    B15.9 **Hepatitis A without hepatic coma** `CC`
        Hepatitis A (acute)(viral) NOS

√4ᵗʰ **B16** **Acute hepatitis B**
    AHA: 2016,3Q,13
    B16.0 **Acute hepatitis B with delta-agent with hepatic coma** `MCC`
    B16.1 **Acute hepatitis B with delta-agent without hepatic coma** `CC`
    B16.2 **Acute hepatitis B without delta-agent with hepatic coma** `MCC`
    B16.9 **Acute hepatitis B without delta-agent and without hepatic coma** `CC`
        Hepatitis B (acute) (viral) NOS

√4ᵗʰ **B17** **Other acute viral hepatitis**
    B17.0 **Acute delta-(super) infection of hepatitis B carrier** `CC`
   √5ᵗʰ **B17.1** **Acute hepatitis C**
       B17.10 **Acute hepatitis C without hepatic coma** `CC`
         Acute hepatitis C NOS
       B17.11 **Acute hepatitis C with hepatic coma** `MCC`
    B17.2 **Acute hepatitis E** `CC`
    B17.8 **Other specified acute viral hepatitis** `CC`
        Hepatitis non-A non-B (acute) (viral) NEC
    B17.9 **Acute viral hepatitis, unspecified** `CC`
        Acute hepatitis NOS
        Acute infectious hepatitis NOS

√4ᵗʰ **B18** **Chronic viral hepatitis**
   INCLUDES   carrier of viral hepatitis
    AHA: 2017,1Q,41
    B18.0 **Chronic viral hepatitis B with delta-agent** `CC` `HCC`
    B18.1 **Chronic viral hepatitis B without delta-agent** `CC` `HCC`
        Carrier of viral hepatitis B
        Chronic (viral) hepatitis B
    B18.2 **Chronic viral hepatitis C** `HCC`
        Carrier of viral hepatitis C
        AHA: 2018,1Q,4
    B18.8 **Other chronic viral hepatitis** `CC` `HCC`
        Carrier of other viral hepatitis
    B18.9 **Chronic viral hepatitis, unspecified** `CC` `HCC`
        Carrier of unspecified viral hepatitis

√4ᵗʰ **B19** **Unspecified viral hepatitis**
    B19.0 **Unspecified viral hepatitis with hepatic coma** `MCC`
   √5ᵗʰ **B19.1** **Unspecified viral hepatitis B**
       B19.10 **Unspecified viral hepatitis B without hepatic coma** `CC`
         Unspecified viral hepatitis B NOS
       B19.11 **Unspecified viral hepatitis B with hepatic coma** `MCC`
   √5ᵗʰ **B19.2** **Unspecified viral hepatitis C**
       B19.20 **Unspecified viral hepatitis C without hepatic coma** `CC`
         Viral hepatitis C NOS
       B19.21 **Unspecified viral hepatitis C with hepatic coma** `MCC`
    B19.9 **Unspecified viral hepatitis without hepatic coma** `CC`
        Viral hepatitis NOS

Human immunodeficiency virus [HIV] disease (B20)

B20   **Human immunodeficiency virus [HIV] disease**   `CC` `HCC`

> **INCLUDES**   acquired immune deficiency syndrome [AIDS]
> AIDS-related complex [ARC]
> HIV infection, symptomatic

Code first Human immunodeficiency virus [HIV] disease complicating pregnancy, childbirth and the puerperium, if applicable (O98.7-)
Use additional code(s) to identify all manifestations of HIV infection

> **EXCLUDES 1**   *asymptomatic human immunodeficiency virus [HIV] infection status (Z21)*
> *exposure to HIV virus (Z20.6)*
> *inconclusive serologic evidence of HIV (R75)*

AHA: 2021,2Q,6; 2021,1Q,52; 2020,4Q,97; 2020,2Q,12; 2019,1Q,8-11

Other viral diseases (B25-B34)

✓4ᵗʰ B25   **Cytomegaloviral disease**

> **EXCLUDES 1**   *congenital cytomegalovirus infection (P35.1)*
> *cytomegaloviral mononucleosis (B27.1-)*

B25.0   **Cytomegaloviral** pneumonitis   `MCC` `HCC`
B25.1   **Cytomegaloviral** hepatitis   `CC` `HCC`
B25.2   **Cytomegaloviral** pancreatitis   `MCC` `HCC`
B25.8   **Other cytomegaloviral diseases**   `HIV` `CC` `HCC`
     Cytomegaloviral encephalitis
B25.9   **Cytomegaloviral disease, unspecified**   `HIV` `CC` `HCC`

✓4ᵗʰ B26   **Mumps**

> **INCLUDES**   epidemic parotitis
> infectious parotitis

B26.0   **Mumps** orchitis   `CC` ♂
B26.1   **Mumps** meningitis   `MCC`
B26.2   **Mumps** encephalitis   `MCC`
B26.3   **Mumps** pancreatitis   `CC`
✓5ᵗʰ B26.8   **Mumps with other complications**
     B26.81   **Mumps** hepatitis   `CC`
     B26.82   **Mumps** myocarditis   `CC`
     B26.83   **Mumps** nephritis   `CC`
     B26.84   **Mumps** polyneuropathy   `CC`
     B26.85   **Mumps** arthritis   `CC` `HCC`
     B26.89   **Other mumps complications**   `CC`
B26.9   **Mumps without complication**
     Mumps NOS
     Mumps parotitis NOS

✓4ᵗʰ B27   **Infectious mononucleosis**

> **INCLUDES**   glandular fever
> monocytic angina
> Pfeiffer's disease

✓5ᵗʰ B27.0   **Gammaherpesviral mononucleosis**
     Mononucleosis due to Epstein-Barr virus
     B27.00   **Gammaherpesviral mononucleosis** without complication
     B27.01   **Gammaherpesviral mononucleosis** with polyneuropathy
     B27.02   **Gammaherpesviral mononucleosis** with meningitis
     B27.09   **Gammaherpesviral mononucleosis** with other complications
         Hepatomegaly in gammaherpesviral mononucleosis
✓5ᵗʰ B27.1   **Cytomegaloviral mononucleosis**
     B27.10   **Cytomegaloviral mononucleosis** without complications
     B27.11   **Cytomegaloviral mononucleosis** with polyneuropathy
     B27.12   **Cytomegaloviral mononucleosis** with meningitis
     B27.19   **Cytomegaloviral mononucleosis** with other complication
         Hepatomegaly in cytomegaloviral mononucleosis
✓5ᵗʰ B27.8   **Other infectious mononucleosis**
     B27.80   **Other infectious mononucleosis** without complication
     B27.81   **Other infectious mononucleosis** with polyneuropathy
     B27.82   **Other infectious mononucleosis** with meningitis

     B27.89   **Other infectious mononucleosis with other complication**
         Hepatomegaly in other infectious mononucleosis
✓5ᵗʰ B27.9   **Infectious mononucleosis, unspecified**
     B27.90   **Infectious mononucleosis, unspecified** without complication
     B27.91   **Infectious mononucleosis, unspecified** with polyneuropathy
     B27.92   **Infectious mononucleosis, unspecified** with meningitis
     B27.99   **Infectious mononucleosis, unspecified** with other complication
         Hepatomegaly in unspecified infectious mononucleosis

✓4ᵗʰ B30   **Viral conjunctivitis**

> **EXCLUDES 1**   *herpesviral [herpes simplex] ocular disease (B00.5)*
> *ocular zoster (B02.3)*

Viral Conjunctivitis

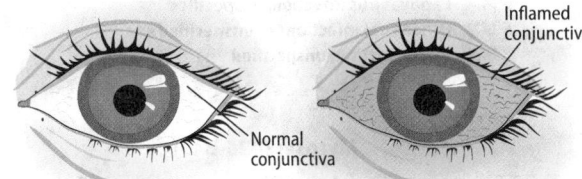

Normal conjunctiva   Inflamed conjunctiva

B30.0   **Keratoconjunctivitis due to adenovirus**
     Epidemic keratoconjunctivitis
     Shipyard eye
B30.1   **Conjunctivitis due to adenovirus**
     Acute adenoviral follicular conjunctivitis
     Swimming-pool conjunctivitis
B30.2   **Viral pharyngoconjunctivitis**
B30.3   **Acute epidemic hemorrhagic conjunctivitis (enteroviral)**
     Conjunctivitis due to coxsackievirus 24
     Conjunctivitis due to enterovirus 70
     Hemorrhagic conjunctivitis (acute)(epidemic)
B30.8   **Other viral conjunctivitis**
     Newcastle conjunctivitis
B30.9   **Viral conjunctivitis, unspecified**

✓4ᵗʰ B33   **Other viral diseases, not elsewhere classified**

B33.0   **Epidemic myalgia**
     Bornholm disease
B33.1   **Ross River disease**   `CC`
     Epidemic polyarthritis and exanthema
     Ross River fever
✓5ᵗʰ B33.2   **Viral carditis**
     Coxsackie (virus) carditis
     B33.20   **Viral carditis, unspecified**   `CC`
     B33.21   **Viral** endocarditis   `CC`
     B33.22   **Viral** myocarditis   `CC`
     B33.23   **Viral** pericarditis   `CC`
     B33.24   **Viral** cardiomyopathy   `HCC`
B33.3   **Retrovirus infections, not elsewhere classified**
     Retrovirus infection NOS
B33.4   **Hantavirus (cardio)-pulmonary syndrome [HPS] [HCPS]**   `CC`
     Hantavirus disease with pulmonary manifestations
     Sin nombre virus disease
     Use additional code to identify any associated acute kidney failure (N17.9)

> **EXCLUDES 1**   *hantavirus disease with renal manifestations (A98.5)*
> *hemorrhagic fever with renal manifestations (A98.5)*

B33.8   **Other specified viral diseases**

> **EXCLUDES 1**   *anogenital human papillomavirus infection (A63.0)*
> *viral warts due to human papillomavirus infection (B07)*

✓4ᵗʰ **B34 Viral infection of unspecified site**

> EXCLUDES 1   anogenital human papillomavirus infection (A63.0)
> cytomegaloviral disease NOS (B25.9)
> herpesvirus [herpes simplex] infection NOS (B00.9)
> retrovirus infection NOS (B33.3)
> viral agents as the cause of diseases classified elsewhere (B97.-)
> viral warts due to human papillomavirus infection (B07)

B34.0 Adenovirus infection, unspecified

B34.1 Enterovirus infection, unspecified
Coxsackievirus infection NOS
Echovirus infection NOS

B34.2 Coronavirus infection, unspecified
> EXCLUDES 1   COVID-19 (U07.1)
> pneumonia due to SARS-associated coronavirus (J12.81)

AHA: 2020,1Q,34-36

B34.3 Parvovirus infection, unspecified   CC

B34.4 Papovavirus infection, unspecified

B34.8 Other viral infections of unspecified site

B34.9 Viral infection, unspecified
Viremia NOS
AHA: 2016,3Q,10

Mycoses (B35-B49)

> EXCLUDES 2   hypersensitivity pneumonitis due to organic dust (J67.-)
> mycosis fungoides (C84.0-)

✓4ᵗʰ **B35 Dermatophytosis**

> INCLUDES   favus
> infections due to species of Epidermophyton, Micro-sporum and Trichophyton
> tinea, any type except those in B36.-

DEF: Contagious superficial fungal infection of the skin that invades and grows in dead keratin.

B35.0 Tinea barbae and tinea capitis
Beard ringworm
Kerion
Scalp ringworm
Sycosis, mycotic

B35.1 Tinea unguium
Dermatophytic onychia
Dermatophytosis of nail
Onychomycosis
Ringworm of nails

B35.2 Tinea manuum
Dermatophytosis of hand
Hand ringworm

B35.3 Tinea pedis
Athlete's foot
Dermatophytosis of foot
Foot ringworm

B35.4 Tinea corporis
Ringworm of the body

B35.5 Tinea imbricata
Tokelau

B35.6 Tinea cruris
Dhobi itch
Groin ringworm
Jock itch

B35.8 Other dermatophytoses
Disseminated dermatophytosis
Granulomatous dermatophytosis

B35.9 Dermatophytosis, unspecified
Ringworm NOS

✓4ᵗʰ **B36 Other superficial mycoses**

B36.0 Pityriasis versicolor
Tinea flava
Tinea versicolor

B36.1 Tinea nigra
Keratomycosis nigricans palmaris
Microsporosis nigra
Pityriasis nigra

B36.2 White piedra
Tinea blanca

B36.3 Black piedra

B36.8 Other specified superficial mycoses

B36.9 Superficial mycosis, unspecified

✓4ᵗʰ **B37 Candidiasis**

> INCLUDES   candidosis
> moniliasis
> EXCLUDES 1   neonatal candidiasis (P37.5)

DEF: Candida: Genus of yeast-like fungi that are commonly found in the mouth, skin, intestinal tract, and vagina. It may cause a white, cheesy discharge.

B37.0 Candidal stomatitis   HIV CC
Oral thrush

B37.1 Pulmonary candidiasis   HIV MCC HCC
Candidal bronchitis
Candidal pneumonia

B37.2 Candidiasis of skin and nail   HIV
Candidal onychia
Candidal paronychia
> EXCLUDES 2   diaper dermatitis (L22)

B37.3 Candidiasis of vulva and vagina   ♀
Candidal vulvovaginitis
Monilial vulvovaginitis
Vaginal thrush

✓5ᵗʰ **B37.4 Candidiasis of other urogenital sites**

B37.41 Candidal cystitis and urethritis   CC H6

B37.42 Candidal balanitis   ♂

B37.49 Other urogenital candidiasis   CC H6
Candidal pyelonephritis

B37.5 Candidal meningitis   HIV MCC

B37.6 Candidal endocarditis   HIV MCC

B37.7 Candidal sepsis   MCC HCC
Disseminated candidiasis
Systemic candidiasis
AHA: 2014,4Q,46
TIP: This code is assigned when sepsis is documented as due to any Candida type. If the nonspecific term "non-Candida albicans" is documented, code B48.8 Other specified mycoses, is assigned.

✓5ᵗʰ **B37.8 Candidiasis of other sites**

B37.81 Candidal esophagitis   HIV CC HCC

B37.82 Candidal enteritis   HIV CC
Candidal proctitis

B37.83 Candidal cheilitis   HIV CC

B37.84 Candidal otitis externa   HIV CC

B37.89 Other sites of candidiasis   HIV CC
Candidal osteomyelitis

B37.9 Candidiasis, unspecified   HIV
Thrush NOS

✓4ᵗʰ **B38 Coccidioidomycosis**

B38.0 Acute pulmonary coccidioidomycosis   HIV CC HCC

B38.1 Chronic pulmonary coccidioidomycosis   HIV CC HCC

B38.2 Pulmonary coccidioidomycosis, unspecified   HIV CC HCC

B38.3 Cutaneous coccidioidomycosis   HIV CC

B38.4 Coccidioidomycosis meningitis   HIV MCC
DEF: Coccidioides immitis infection of the lining of the brain and/or spinal cord.

B38.7 Disseminated coccidioidomycosis   HIV CC
Generalized coccidioidomycosis

✓5ᵗʰ **B38.8 Other forms of coccidioidomycosis**

B38.81 Prostatic coccidioidomycosis   HIV CC ♂

B38.89 Other forms of coccidioidomycosis   HIV CC

B38.9 Coccidioidomycosis, unspecified   HIV CC

✓4ᵗʰ **B39 Histoplasmosis**

Code first associated AIDS (B2Ø)

Use additional code for any associated manifestations, such as:

    endocarditis (I39)

    meningitis (GØ2)

    pericarditis (I32)

    retinitis (H32)

DEF: Type of lung infection caused by breathing in fungal spores often found in the droppings of bats and birds or soil contaminated by their droppings.

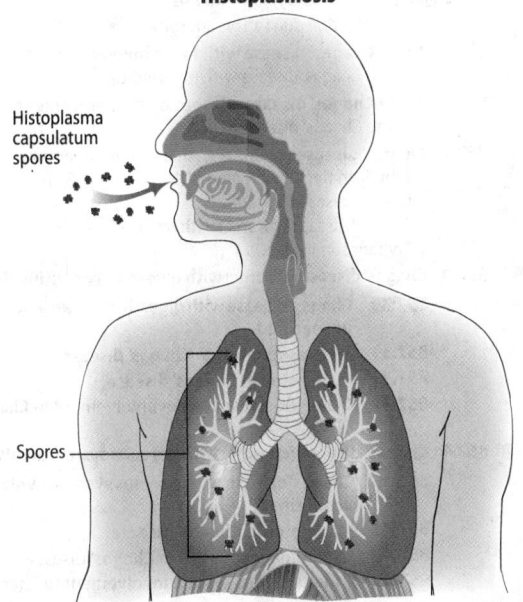

Histoplasmosis

Histoplasma capsulatum spores

Spores

B39.Ø Acute pulmonary **histoplasmosis capsulati**	HIV MCC HCC
B39.1 Chronic pulmonary **histoplasmosis capsulati**	HIV MCC HCC
B39.2 **Pulmonary histoplasmosis capsulati, unspecified**	HIV MCC HCC
B39.3 Disseminated **histoplasmosis capsulati**	HIV CC
Generalized histoplasmosis capsulati	
B39.4 **Histoplasmosis capsulati, unspecified**	HIV
American histoplasmosis	
B39.5 **Histoplasmosis** duboisii	HIV
African histoplasmosis	
B39.9 **Histoplasmosis, unspecified**	HIV

✓4ᵗʰ **B4Ø Blastomycosis**

    EXCLUDES 1   *Brazilian blastomycosis (B41.-)*

               keloidal blastomycosis (B48.Ø)

B4Ø.Ø Acute pulmonary **blastomycosis**	CC HCC
B4Ø.1 Chronic pulmonary **blastomycosis**	CC HCC
B4Ø.2 **Pulmonary blastomycosis, unspecified**	CC HCC
B4Ø.3 **Cutaneous** blastomycosis	CC
B4Ø.7 Disseminated **blastomycosis**	CC
Generalized blastomycosis	

✓6ᵗʰ **B4Ø.8** Other forms of blastomycosis

B4Ø.81 **Blastomycotic** meningoencephalitis	CC
Meningomyelitis due to blastomycosis	
B4Ø.89 Other forms of blastomycosis	CC
B4Ø.9 **Blastomycosis, unspecified**	CC

✓4ᵗʰ **B41 Paracoccidioidomycosis**

    INCLUDES   Brazilian blastomycosis

               Lutz' disease

B41.Ø **Pulmonary paracoccidioidomycosis**	CC HCC
B41.7 **Disseminated paracoccidioidomycosis**	CC
Generalized paracoccidioidomycosis	
B41.8 Other forms of paracoccidioidomycosis	CC
B41.9 **Paracoccidioidomycosis, unspecified**	CC

✓4ᵗʰ **B42 Sporotrichosis**

B42.Ø **Pulmonary** sporotrichosis	
B42.1 **Lymphocutaneous** sporotrichosis	

B42.7 Disseminated **sporotrichosis**	
Generalized sporotrichosis	

✓5ᵗʰ **B42.8** Other forms of sporotrichosis

B42.81 **Cerebral** sporotrichosis	
Meningitis due to sporotrichosis	
B42.82 **Sporotrichosis** arthritis	HCC
B42.89 **Other forms of sporotrichosis**	
B42.9 **Sporotrichosis, unspecified**	

✓4ᵗʰ **B43 Chromomycosis and pheomycotic abscess**

B43.Ø **Cutaneous** chromomycosis	
Dermatitis verrucosa	
B43.1 **Pheomycotic** brain abscess	
Cerebral chromomycosis	
B43.2 **Subcutaneous pheomycotic** abscess and cyst	
B43.8 Other forms of chromomycosis	
B43.9 **Chromomycosis, unspecified**	

✓4ᵗʰ **B44 Aspergillosis**

    INCLUDES   aspergilloma

B44.Ø **Invasive pulmonary aspergillosis**	MCC HCC
B44.1 **Other pulmonary aspergillosis**	CC HCC
B44.2 **Tonsillar** aspergillosis	CC HCC
B44.7 Disseminated **aspergillosis**	CC HCC
Generalized aspergillosis	

✓5ᵗʰ **B44.8** Other forms of aspergillosis

B44.81 **Allergic bronchopulmonary** aspergillosis	CC HCC
B44.89 **Other forms of aspergillosis**	CC HCC
B44.9 **Aspergillosis, unspecified**	CC HCC

✓4ᵗʰ **B45 Cryptococcosis**

B45.Ø **Pulmonary cryptococcosis**	HIV CC HCC
B45.1 **Cerebral** cryptococcosis	MCC HCC
Cryptococcal meningitis	
Cryptococcosis meningocerebralis	
B45.2 **Cutaneous** cryptococcosis	HIV CC HCC
B45.3 **Osseous** cryptococcosis	HIV CC HCC
B45.7 Disseminated **cryptococcosis**	HIV CC HCC
Generalized cryptococcosis	
B45.8 Other forms of cryptococcosis	HIV CC HCC
B45.9 **Cryptococcosis, unspecified**	HIV CC HCC

✓4ᵗʰ **B46 Zygomycosis**

B46.Ø **Pulmonary mucormycosis**	MCC HCC
B46.1 **Rhinocerebral mucormycosis**	MCC HCC
B46.2 **Gastrointestinal mucormycosis**	MCC HCC
B46.3 **Cutaneous mucormycosis**	MCC HCC
Subcutaneous mucormycosis	
B46.4 Disseminated **mucormycosis**	MCC HCC
Generalized mucormycosis	
B46.5 **Mucormycosis, unspecified**	MCC HCC
B46.8 Other zygomycoses	
Entomophthoromycosis	
B46.9 **Zygomycosis, unspecified**	MCC HCC
Phycomycosis NOS	

✓4ᵗʰ **B47 Mycetoma**

B47.Ø **Eumycetoma**	CC
Madura foot, mycotic	
Maduromycosis	
B47.1 **Actinomycetoma**	HIV CC
B47.9 **Mycetoma, unspecified**	HIV CC
Madura foot NOS	

✓4ᵗʰ **B48 Other mycoses, not elsewhere classified**

B48.Ø **Lobomycosis**	
Keloidal blastomycosis	
Lobo's disease	
B48.1 **Rhinosporidiosis**	
B48.2 **Allescheriasis**	CC
Infection due to Pseudallescheria boydii	
EXCLUDES 1 *eumycetoma (B47.Ø)*	
B48.3 **Geotrichosis**	CC
Geotrichum stomatitis	
B48.4 **Penicillosis**	CC HCC
Talaromycosis	

✓ Additional Character Required   ✓x7ᵗʰ Placeholder   Questionable PDx   Manifestation   Unspecified Dx   UPD Unacceptable PDx   H1 - H14 HAC   HCC CMS-HCC Dx   HIV HIV Dx

ICD-10-CM 2022   **459**

Chapter 1. Certain Infectious and Parasitic Diseases

B48.8   **Other specified mycoses**   HIV CC HCC
Adiaspiromycosis
Infection of tissue and organs by Alternaria
Infection of tissue and organs by Drechslera
Infection of tissue and organs by Fusarium
Infection of tissue and organs by saprophytic fungi NEC
AHA: 2014,4Q,46; 2014,2Q,13
TIP: This code is assigned when the nonspecific term "non-*Candida albicans*" sepsis is documented. If sepsis is documented as due to any *Candida* type, code B37.7 Candidal sepsis, is assigned.

B49   **Unspecified mycosis**   CC
Fungemia NOS

Protozoal diseases (B5Ø-B64)

EXCLUDES 1   amebiasis (AØ6.-)
other protozoal intestinal diseases (AØ7.-)

✓4ᵗʰ **B5Ø**   **Plasmodium falciparum malaria**
INCLUDES   mixed infections of Plasmodium falciparum with any other Plasmodium species

B5Ø.Ø   **Plasmodium falciparum malaria with cerebral complications**   CC
Cerebral malaria NOS

B5Ø.8   **Other severe and complicated Plasmodium falciparum malaria**   CC
Severe or complicated Plasmodium falciparum malaria NOS

B5Ø.9   **Plasmodium falciparum malaria, unspecified**   MCC

✓4ᵗʰ **B51**   **Plasmodium vivax malaria**
INCLUDES   mixed infections of Plasmodium vivax with other Plasmodium species, except Plasmodium falciparum
EXCLUDES 1   Plasmodium vivax with Plasmodium falciparum (B5Ø.-)

B51.Ø   **Plasmodium vivax malaria with rupture of spleen**   CC

B51.8   **Plasmodium vivax malaria with other complications**   CC

B51.9   **Plasmodium vivax malaria without complication**   CC
Plasmodium vivax malaria NOS

✓4ᵗʰ **B52**   **Plasmodium malariae malaria**
INCLUDES   mixed infections of Plasmodium malariae with other Plasmodium species, except Plasmodium falciparum and Plasmodium vivax
EXCLUDES 1   Plasmodium falciparum (B5Ø.-)
Plasmodium vivax (B51.-)

B52.Ø   **Plasmodium malariae malaria with nephropathy**

B52.8   **Plasmodium malariae malaria with other complications**   CC

B52.9   **Plasmodium malariae malaria without complication**   CC
Plasmodium malariae malaria NOS

✓4ᵗʰ **B53**   **Other specified malaria**

B53.Ø   **Plasmodium ovale malaria**   CC
EXCLUDES 1   Plasmodium ovale with Plasmodium falciparum (B5Ø.-)
Plasmodium ovale with Plasmodium malariae (B52.-)
Plasmodium ovale with Plasmodium vivax (B51.-)

B53.1   **Malaria due to simian plasmodia**   CC
EXCLUDES 1   malaria due to simian plasmodia with Plasmodium falciparum (B5Ø.-)
malaria due to simian plasmodia with Plasmodium malariae (B52.-)
malaria due to simian plasmodia with Plasmodium ovale (B53.Ø)
malaria due to simian plasmodia with Plasmodium vivax (B51.-)

B53.8   **Other malaria, not elsewhere classified**   CC

B54   **Unspecified malaria**   CC

✓4ᵗʰ **B55**   **Leishmaniasis**

B55.Ø   **Visceral leishmaniasis**   CC
Kala-azar
Post-kala-azar dermal leishmaniasis

B55.1   **Cutaneous leishmaniasis**   CC

B55.2   **Mucocutaneous leishmaniasis**   CC

B55.9   **Leishmaniasis, unspecified**   CC

✓4ᵗʰ **B56**   **African trypanosomiasis**

B56.Ø   **Gambiense trypanosomiasis**   CC
Infection due to Trypanosoma brucei gambiense
West African sleeping sickness

B56.1   **Rhodesiense trypanosomiasis**   CC
East African sleeping sickness
Infection due to Trypanosoma brucei rhodesiense

B56.9   **African trypanosomiasis, unspecified**   CC
Sleeping sickness NOS

✓4ᵗʰ **B57**   **Chagas' disease**
INCLUDES   American trypanosomiasis
infection due to Trypanosoma cruzi

B57.Ø   **Acute Chagas' disease with heart involvement**   CC
Acute Chagas' disease with myocarditis

B57.1   **Acute Chagas' disease without heart involvement**   CC
Acute Chagas' disease NOS

B57.2   **Chagas' disease (chronic) with heart involvement**   CC
American trypanosomiasis NOS
Chagas' disease (chronic) NOS
Chagas' disease (chronic) with myocarditis
Trypanosomiasis NOS

✓5ᵗʰ **B57.3**   **Chagas' disease (chronic) with digestive system involvement**

B57.3Ø   **Chagas' disease with digestive system involvement, unspecified**   CC

B57.31   **Megaesophagus in Chagas' disease**   CC

B57.32   **Megacolon in Chagas' disease**   CC

B57.39   **Other digestive system involvement in Chagas' disease**   CC

✓5ᵗʰ **B57.4**   **Chagas' disease (chronic) with nervous system involvement**

B57.4Ø   **Chagas' disease with nervous system involvement, unspecified**   CC

B57.41   **Meningitis in Chagas' disease**   CC

B57.42   **Meningoencephalitis in Chagas' disease**   CC

B57.49   **Other nervous system involvement in Chagas' disease**   CC

B57.5   **Chagas' disease (chronic) with other organ involvement**   CC

✓4ᵗʰ **B58**   **Toxoplasmosis**
INCLUDES   infection due to Toxoplasma gondii
EXCLUDES 1   congenital toxoplasmosis (P37.1)

✓5ᵗʰ **B58.Ø**   **Toxoplasma oculopathy**

B58.ØØ   **Toxoplasma oculopathy, unspecified**   HIV CC

B58.Ø1   **Toxoplasma chorioretinitis**   HIV CC

B58.Ø9   **Other toxoplasma oculopathy**   HIV CC
Toxoplasma uveitis

B58.1   **Toxoplasma hepatitis**   HIV CC

B58.2   **Toxoplasma meningoencephalitis**   HIV MCC HCC

B58.3   **Pulmonary toxoplasmosis**   HIV MCC HCC

✓5ᵗʰ **B58.8**   **Toxoplasmosis with other organ involvement**

B58.81   **Toxoplasma myocarditis**   HIV MCC

B58.82   **Toxoplasma myositis**   HIV CC

B58.83   **Toxoplasma tubulo-interstitial nephropathy**   HIV CC
Toxoplasma pyelonephritis

B58.89   **Toxoplasmosis with other organ involvement**   HIV CC

B58.9   **Toxoplasmosis, unspecified**   HIV CC

B59   **Pneumocystosis**   HIV MCC HCC
Pneumonia due to Pneumocystis carinii
Pneumonia due to Pneumocystis jiroveci

✓4ᵗʰ **B6Ø**   **Other protozoal diseases, not elsewhere classified**
EXCLUDES 1   cryptosporidiosis (AØ7.2)
intestinal microsporidiosis (AØ7.8)
isosporiasis (AØ7.3)

✓5ᵗʰ **B6Ø.Ø**   **Babesiosis**
AHA: 2020,4Q,5-6

B6Ø.ØØ   **Babesiosis, unspecified**   CC
Babesiosis due to unspecified Babesia species
Piroplasmosis, unspecified

B6Ø.Ø1   **Babesiosis due to Babesia microti**   CC
Infection due to B. microti

B60.02 **Babesiosis due to** Babesia duncani   `CC`
Infection due to B. duncani and B. duncani-type species

B60.03 **Babesiosis due to** Babesia divergens   `CC`
Babesiosis due to Babesia MO-1
Infection due to B. divergens and B. divergens-like strains

B60.09 **Other babesiosis**   `CC`
Babesiosis due to Babesia KO-1
Babesiosis due to Babesia venatorum
Infection due to other Babesia species
Infection due to other protozoa of the order Piroplasmida
Other piroplasmosis

✓5ᵗʰ B60.1 **Acanthamebiasis**

B60.10 **Acanthamebiasis, unspecified**   `CC`

B60.11 Meningoencephalitis **due to Acanthamoeba (culbertsoni)**

B60.12 Conjunctivitis **due to Acanthamoeba**

B60.13 Keratoconjunctivitis **due to Acanthamoeba**

B60.19 **Other acanthamebic disease**   `CC`

B60.2 **Naegleriasis**   `CC`
Primary amebic meningoencephalitis

B60.8 **Other specified protozoal diseases**   `HIV`
Microsporidiosis

B64 **Unspecified protozoal disease**

Helminthiases (B65-B83)

✓4ᵗʰ B65 **Schistosomiasis [bilharziasis]**

`INCLUDES`   snail fever

B65.0 **Schistosomiasis due to** Schistosoma haematobium **[urinary schistosomiasis]**   `CC`

B65.1 **Schistosomiasis due to** Schistosoma mansoni **[intestinal schistosomiasis]**   `CC`

B65.2 **Schistosomiasis due to** Schistosoma japonicum   `CC`
Asiatic schistosomiasis

B65.3 Cercarial dermatitis   `CC`
Swimmer's itch

B65.8 **Other schistosomiasis**   `CC`
Infection due to Schistosoma intercalatum
Infection due to Schistosoma mattheei
Infection due to Schistosoma mekongi

B65.9 **Schistosomiasis, unspecified**   `CC`

✓4ᵗʰ B66 **Other fluke infections**

B66.0 **Opisthorchiasis**   `CC`
Infection due to cat liver fluke
Infection due to Opisthorchis (felineus)(viverrini)

B66.1 **Clonorchiasis**   `CC`
Chinese liver fluke disease
Infection due to Clonorchis sinensis
Oriental liver fluke disease

B66.2 **Dicroceliasis**   `CC`
Infection due to Dicrocoelium dendriticum
Lancet fluke infection

B66.3 **Fascioliasis**   `CC`
Infection due to Fasciola gigantica
Infection due to Fasciola hepatica
Infection due to Fasciola indica
Sheep liver fluke disease

B66.4 **Paragonimiasis**   `CC` `HCC`
Infection due to Paragonimus species
Lung fluke disease
Pulmonary distomiasis

B66.5 **Fasciolopsiasis**   `CC`
Infection due to Fasciolopsis buski
Intestinal distomiasis

B66.8 **Other specified fluke infections**   `CC`
Echinostomiasis
Heterophyiasis
Metagonimiasis
Nanophyetiasis
Watsoniasis

B66.9 **Fluke infection, unspecified**

✓4ᵗʰ B67 **Echinococcosis**

`INCLUDES`   hydatidosis

B67.0 **Echinococcus granulosus infection of** liver   `CC`

B67.1 **Echinococcus granulosus infection of** lung   `CC` `HCC`

B67.2 **Echinococcus granulosus infection of** bone   `CC`

✓5ᵗʰ B67.3 **Echinococcus granulosus infection, other and multiple sites**

B67.31 **Echinococcus granulosus infection,** thyroid gland   `CC`

B67.32 **Echinococcus granulosus infection,** multiple sites   `CC`

B67.39 **Echinococcus granulosus infection,** other sites   `CC`

B67.4 **Echinococcus granulosus infection, unspecified**   `CC`
Dog tapeworm (infection)

B67.5 **Echinococcus** multilocularis **infection of** liver   `CC`

✓5ᵗʰ B67.6 **Echinococcus** multilocularis **infection, other and multiple sites**

B67.61 **Echinococcus multilocularis infection,** multiple sites   `CC`

B67.69 **Echinococcus multilocularis infection, other sites**   `CC`

B67.7 **Echinococcus** multilocularis **infection, unspecified**   `CC`

B67.8 **Echinococcosis, unspecified, of** liver   `CC`

✓5ᵗʰ B67.9 **Echinococcosis, other and unspecified**

B67.90 **Echinococcosis, unspecified**   `CC`
Echinococcosis NOS

B67.99 **Other echinococcosis**   `CC`

✓4ᵗʰ B68 **Taeniasis**

`EXCLUDES 1`   *cysticercosis (B69.-)*

B68.0 **Taenia** solium **taeniasis**   `CC`
Pork tapeworm (infection)

B68.1 **Taenia** saginata **taeniasis**   `CC`
Beef tapeworm (infection)
Infection due to adult tapeworm Taenia saginata

B68.9 **Taeniasis, unspecified**   `CC`

✓4ᵗʰ B69 **Cysticercosis**

`INCLUDES`   cysticerciasis infection due to larval form of Taenia solium
DEF: Condition that is developed when larvae or eggs of the tapeworm *Taenia solium* are ingested, most commonly in fecally contaminated water or undercooked pork.

B69.0 **Cysticercosis of** central nervous system   `CC`

B69.1 **Cysticercosis of** eye   `CC`

✓5ᵗʰ B69.8 **Cysticercosis of other sites**

B69.81 Myositis **in cysticercosis**   `CC`

B69.89 **Cysticercosis of other sites**   `CC`

B69.9 **Cysticercosis, unspecified**   `CC`

✓4ᵗʰ B70 **Diphyllobothriasis and sparganosis**

B70.0 **Diphyllobothriasis**   `HCC`
Diphyllobothrium (adult) (latum) (pacificum) infection
Fish tapeworm (infection)
`EXCLUDES 2`   *larval diphyllobothriasis (B70.1)*

B70.1 **Sparganosis**   `CC`
Infection due to Sparganum (mansoni) (proliferum)
Infection due to Spirometra larva
Larval diphyllobothriasis
Spirometrosis

✓4ᵗʰ B71 **Other cestode infections**

B71.0 **Hymenolepiasis**   `CC`
Dwarf tapeworm infection
Rat tapeworm (infection)

B71.1 **Dipylidiasis**   `CC`

B71.8 **Other specified cestode infections**   `CC`
Coenurosis

B71.9 **Cestode infection, unspecified**
Tapeworm (infection) NOS

B72 **Dracunculiasis**   `CC`
`INCLUDES`   guinea worm infection
infection due to Dracunculus medinensis

✓4ᵗʰ **B73 Onchocerciasis**

INCLUDES   onchocerca volvulus infection
onchocercosis
river blindness

  ✓5ᵗʰ **B73.0 Onchocerciasis** with eye disease

    B73.00 Onchocerciasis with eye involvement, unspecified   CC

    B73.01 Onchocerciasis with endophthalmitis   CC

    B73.02 Onchocerciasis with glaucoma   CC

    B73.09 Onchocerciasis with other eye involvement   CC
      Infestation of eyelid due to onchocerciasis

  B73.1 Onchocerciasis without eye disease   CC

✓4ᵗʰ **B74 Filariasis**

EXCLUDES 2   onchocerciasis (B73)
    tropical (pulmonary) eosinophilia NOS ▶(J82.89)◀

  B74.0 Filariasis due to Wuchereria bancrofti   CC
    Bancroftian elephantiasis
    Bancroftian filariasis

  B74.1 Filariasis due to Brugia malayi   CC

  B74.2 Filariasis due to Brugia timori   CC

  B74.3 Loiasis   CC
    Calabar swelling
    Eyeworm disease of Africa
    Loa loa infection

  B74.4 Mansonelliasis   CC
    Infection due to Mansonella ozzardi
    Infection due to Mansonella perstans
    Infection due to Mansonella streptocerca

  B74.8 Other filariases   CC
    Dirofilariasis

  B74.9 Filariasis, unspecified   CC

B75 Trichinellosis   CC

INCLUDES   infection due to Trichinella species
trichiniasis

DEF: Infection by *Trichinella spiralis*, the smallest of the parasitic nematodes, that is transmitted by eating undercooked pork or bear meat. *Synonym(s): Trichinosis.*

✓4ᵗʰ **B76 Hookworm diseases**

INCLUDES   uncinariasis

  B76.0 Ancylostomiasis   CC
    Infection due to Ancylostoma species

  B76.1 Necatoriasis   CC
    Infection due to Necator americanus

  B76.8 Other hookworm diseases   CC

  B76.9 Hookworm disease, unspecified   CC
    Cutaneous larva migrans NOS

✓4ᵗʰ **B77 Ascariasis**

INCLUDES   ascaridiasis
roundworm infection

  B77.0 Ascariasis with intestinal complications   CC

  ✓5ᵗʰ **B77.8 Ascariasis with other complications**

    B77.81 Ascariasis pneumonia   MCC

    B77.89 Ascariasis with other complications   CC

  B77.9 Ascariasis, unspecified   CC

✓4ᵗʰ **B78 Strongyloidiasis**

EXCLUDES 1   trichostrongyliasis (B81.2)

  B78.0 Intestinal strongyloidiasis   HIV CC

  B78.1 Cutaneous strongyloidiasis

  B78.7 Disseminated strongyloidiasis   HIV CC

  B78.9 Strongyloidiasis, unspecified   HIV CC

B79 Trichuriasis   CC

INCLUDES   trichocephaliasis
whipworm (disease)(infection)

B80 Enterobiasis   CC

INCLUDES   oxyuriasis
pinworm infection
threadworm infection

✓4ᵗʰ **B81 Other intestinal helminthiases, not elsewhere classified**

EXCLUDES 1   angiostrongyliasis due to:
    angiostrongylus cantonensis (B83.2)
    parastrongylus cantonensis (B83.2)

  B81.0 Anisakiasis   CC
    Infection due to Anisakis larva

  B81.1 Intestinal capillariasis   CC
    Capillariasis NOS
    Infection due to Capillaria philippinensis
    EXCLUDES 2   hepatic capillariasis (B83.8)

  B81.2 Trichostrongyliasis   CC

  B81.3 Intestinal angiostrongyliasis
    Angiostrongyliasis due to:
    Angiostrongylus costaricensis
    Parastrongylus costaricensis

  B81.4 Mixed intestinal helminthiases   CC
    Infection due to intestinal helminths classified to more than one of the categories B65.0-B81.3 and B81.8
    Mixed helminthiasis NOS

  B81.8 Other specified intestinal helminthiases   CC
    Infection due to Oesophagostomum species [esophagostomiasis]
    Infection due to Ternidens diminutus [ternidensiasis]

✓4ᵗʰ **B82 Unspecified intestinal parasitism**

  B82.0 Intestinal helminthiasis, unspecified   CC

  B82.9 Intestinal parasitism, unspecified

✓4ᵗʰ **B83 Other helminthiases**

EXCLUDES 1   capillariasis NOS (B81.1)
EXCLUDES 2   intestinal capillariasis (B81.1)

  B83.0 Visceral larva migrans
    Toxocariasis

  B83.1 Gnathostomiasis
    Wandering swelling

  B83.2 Angiostrongyliasis due to Parastrongylus cantonensis
    Eosinophilic meningoencephalitis due to Parastrongylus cantonensis
    EXCLUDES 2   intestinal angiostrongyliasis (B81.3)

  B83.3 Syngamiasis
    Syngamosis

  B83.4 Internal hirudiniasis
    EXCLUDES 2   external hirudiniasis (B88.3)

  B83.8 Other specified helminthiases
    Acanthocephaliasis
    Gongylonemiasis
    Hepatic capillariasis
    Metastrongyliasis
    Thelaziasis

  B83.9 Helminthiasis, unspecified
    Worms NOS
    EXCLUDES 1   intestinal helminthiasis NOS (B82.0)

Pediculosis, acariasis and other infestations (B85-B89)

✓4ᵗʰ **B85 Pediculosis and phthiriasis**

  B85.0 Pediculosis due to Pediculus humanus capitis
    Head-louse infestation

  B85.1 Pediculosis due to Pediculus humanus corporis
    Body-louse infestation

  B85.2 Pediculosis, unspecified

  B85.3 Phthiriasis
    Infestation by crab-louse
    Infestation by Phthirus pubis

  B85.4 Mixed pediculosis and phthiriasis
    Infestation classifiable to more than one of the categories B85.0-B85.3

B86 Scabies
  Sarcoptic itch
  DEF: Mite infestation that is caused by *Sarcoptes scabiei*. Scabies causes intense itching and sometimes secondary infection.

✓4ᵗʰ **B87 Myiasis**

INCLUDES   infestation by larva of flies

  B87.0 Cutaneous myiasis
    Creeping myiasis

N Newborn: 0   P Pediatric: 0-17   M Maternity: 9-64   A Adult: 15-124   MCC Major Complication/Comorbidity   CC Complication/Comorbidity   SW Severe Wound Dx

462   ICD-10-CM 2022

B87.1 **Wound** myiasis
　Traumatic myiasis

B87.2 **Ocular** myiasis

B87.3 **Nasopharyngeal** myiasis
　Laryngeal myiasis

B87.4 **Aural** myiasis

✓5ᵗʰ **B87.8** **Myiasis of other sites**

　B87.81 **Genitourinary** myiasis

　B87.82 **Intestinal** myiasis

　B87.89 **Myiasis of other sites**

B87.9 **Myiasis, unspecified**

✓4ᵗʰ **B88** **Other infestations**

B88.0 **Other acariasis**
　Acarine dermatitis
　Dermatitis due to Demodex species
　Dermatitis due to Dermanyssus gallinae
　Dermatitis due to Liponyssoides sanguineus
　Trombiculosis
　EXCLUDES 2　scabies (B86)

B88.1 **Tungiasis [sandflea infestation]**

B88.2 **Other arthropod infestations**
　Scarabiasis

B88.3 **External hirudiniasis**
　Leech infestation NOS
　EXCLUDES 2　internal hirudiniasis (B83.4)

B88.8 **Other specified infestations**
　Ichthyoparasitism due to Vandellia cirrhosa
　Linguatulosis
　Porocephaliasis

B88.9 **Infestation, unspecified**
　Infestation (skin) NOS
　Infestation by mites NOS
　Skin parasites NOS

B89 **Unspecified parasitic disease**

Sequelae of infectious and parasitic diseases (B90-B94)

NOTE　Categories B90-B94 are to be used to indicate conditions in categories A00-B89 as the cause of sequelae, which are themselves classified elsewhere. The "sequelae" include conditions specified as such; they also include residuals of diseases classifiable to the above categories if there is evidence that the disease itself is no longer present. Codes from these categories are not to be used for chronic infections. Code chronic current infections to active infectious disease as appropriate.

Code first condition resulting from (sequela) the infectious or parasitic disease

✓4ᵗʰ **B90** **Sequelae of** tuberculosis

B90.0 **Sequelae of** central nervous system **tuberculosis**

B90.1 **Sequelae of** genitourinary **tuberculosis**

B90.2 **Sequelae of tuberculosis of** bones and joints

B90.8 **Sequelae of tuberculosis of other organs**
　EXCLUDES 2　sequelae of respiratory tuberculosis (B90.9)

B90.9 **Sequelae of** respiratory **and unspecified tuberculosis**
　Sequelae of tuberculosis NOS

B91 **Sequelae of** poliomyelitis
　EXCLUDES 1　postpolio syndrome (G14)

B92 **Sequelae of** leprosy

✓4ᵗʰ **B94** **Sequelae of other and unspecified infectious and parasitic diseases**

B94.0 **Sequelae of** trachoma

B94.1 **Sequelae of** viral encephalitis

B94.2 **Sequelae of** viral hepatitis

B94.8 **Sequelae of other specified infectious and parasitic diseases**
　AHA: 2021,1Q,25-30,31-49; 2020,3Q,10-14; 2017,4Q,109

B94.9 **Sequelae of unspecified infectious and parasitic disease**
　EXCLUDES 2　▶post COVID-19 condition (U09.9)◀

Bacterial and viral infectious agents (B95-B97)

NOTE　These categories are provided for use as supplementary or additional codes to identify the infectious agent(s) in diseases classified elsewhere.

AHA: 2020,2Q,18; 2018,4Q,34; 2018,1Q,16

✓4ᵗʰ **B95** **Streptococcus, Staphylococcus, and Enterococcus as the cause of diseases classified elsewhere**

B95.0 **Streptococcus, group A, as the cause of diseases classified elsewhere** UPD

B95.1 **Streptococcus, group B, as the cause of diseases classified elsewhere** UPD
　AHA: 2020,1Q,10; 2019,2Q,8-10

B95.2 **Enterococcus as the cause of diseases classified elsewhere** UPD

B95.3 **Streptococcus pneumoniae as the cause of diseases classified elsewhere** UPD

B95.4 **Other streptococcus as the cause of diseases classified elsewhere** UPD

B95.5 **Unspecified streptococcus as the cause of diseases classified elsewhere** UPD

✓5ᵗʰ **B95.6** **Staphylococcus aureus as the cause of diseases classified elsewhere**

　B95.61 **Methicillin susceptible Staphylococcus aureus infection as the cause of diseases classified elsewhere** UPD
　　Methicillin susceptible Staphylococcus aureus (MSSA) infection as the cause of diseases classified elsewhere
　　Staphylococcus aureus infection NOS as the cause of diseases classified elsewhere

　B95.62 **Methicillin resistant Staphylococcus aureus infection as the cause of diseases classified elsewhere** UPD
　　Methicillin resistant staphylococcus aureus (MRSA) infection as the cause of diseases classified elsewhere
　　AHA: 2016,1Q,12

B95.7 **Other staphylococcus as the cause of diseases classified elsewhere** UPD

B95.8 **Unspecified staphylococcus as the cause of diseases classified elsewhere** UPD

✓4ᵗʰ **B96** **Other bacterial agents as the cause of diseases classified elsewhere**

B96.0 **Mycoplasma pneumoniae [M. pneumoniae] as the cause of diseases classified elsewhere** UPD
　Pleuro-pneumonia-like-organism [PPLO]

B96.1 **Klebsiella pneumoniae [K. pneumoniae] as the cause of diseases classified elsewhere** UPD

✓5ᵗʰ **B96.2** **Escherichia coli [E. coli] as the cause of diseases classified elsewhere**

　B96.20 **Unspecified Escherichia coli [E. coli] as the cause of diseases classified elsewhere** UPD
　　Escherichia coli [E. coli] NOS

　B96.21 **Shiga toxin-producing Escherichia coli [E. coli] [STEC] O157 as the cause of diseases classified elsewhere** UPD
　　E. coli O157:H- (nonmotile) with confirmation of Shiga toxin
　　E. coli O157 with confirmation of Shiga toxin when H antigen is unknown, or is not H7
　　O157:H7 Escherichia coli [E.coli] with or without confirmation of Shiga toxin-production
　　Shiga toxin-producing Escherichia coli [E.coli] O157:H7 with or without confirmation of Shiga toxin-production
　　STEC O157:H7 with or without confirmation of Shiga toxin-production

　B96.22 **Other specified Shiga toxin-producing Escherichia coli [E. coli] [STEC] as the cause of diseases classified elsewhere** UPD
　　Non-O157 Shiga toxin-producing Escherichia coli [E.coli]
　　Non-O157 Shiga toxin-producing Escherichia coli [E.coli] with known O group

　B96.23 **Unspecified Shiga toxin-producing Escherichia coli [E. coli] [STEC] as the cause of diseases classified elsewhere** UPD
　　Shiga toxin-producing Escherichia coli [E. coli] with unspecified O group
　　STEC NOS

　B96.29 **Other Escherichia coli [E. coli] as the cause of diseases classified elsewhere** UPD
　　Non-Shiga toxin-producing E. coli

B96.3 **Hemophilus influenzae [H. influenzae] as the cause of diseases classified elsewhere** UPD

B96.4 **Proteus (mirabilis) (morganii) as the cause of diseases classified elsewhere** UPD

✔ Additional Character Required　✓x7ᵗʰ Placeholder　Questionable PDx　Manifestation　Unspecified Dx　UPD Unacceptable PDx　H1-H14 HAC　HCC CMS-HCC Dx　HIV HIV Dx

ICD-10-CM 2022　　463

B96.5   **Pseudomonas (aeruginosa) (mallei) (pseudomallei) as the cause of diseases classified elsewhere** `UPD`
     AHA: 2015,1Q,18

B96.6   **Bacteroides fragilis [B. fragilis] as the cause of diseases classified elsewhere** `UPD`

B96.7   **Clostridium perfringens [C. perfringens] as the cause of diseases classified elsewhere** `UPD`

✓5ᵗʰ **B96.8**   **Other specified bacterial agents as the cause of diseases classified elsewhere**

     B96.81   Helicobacter pylori [H. pylori] as the cause of diseases classified elsewhere `UPD`

     B96.82   Vibrio vulnificus as the cause of diseases classified elsewhere `UPD`

     B96.89   Other specified bacterial agents as the cause of diseases classified elsewhere `UPD`

✓4ᵗʰ **B97**   **Viral agents as the cause of diseases classified elsewhere**
     AHA: 2016,3Q,8-10,14

B97.0   **Adenovirus as the cause of diseases classified elsewhere** `UPD`

✓5ᵗʰ **B97.1**   **Enterovirus as the cause of diseases classified elsewhere**

     B97.10   Unspecified enterovirus as the cause of diseases classified elsewhere `UPD`

     B97.11   Coxsackievirus as the cause of diseases classified elsewhere `UPD`

     B97.12   Echovirus as the cause of diseases classified elsewhere `UPD`

     B97.19   Other enterovirus as the cause of diseases classified elsewhere `UPD`

✓5ᵗʰ **B97.2**   **Coronavirus as the cause of diseases classified elsewhere**
     TIP: Do not report a code from this subcategory for COVID-19; refer to U07.1.

     B97.21   SARS-associated coronavirus as the cause of diseases classified elsewhere `CC` `UPD`
        EXCLUDES 1   pneumonia due to SARS-associated coronavirus (J12.81)

     B97.29   Other coronavirus as the cause of diseases classified elsewhere `UPD`
        AHA: 2020,2Q,5; 2020,1Q,34-36

✓5ᵗʰ **B97.3**   **Retrovirus as the cause of diseases classified elsewhere**
     EXCLUDES 1   human immunodeficiency virus [HIV] disease (B20)

     B97.30   Unspecified retrovirus as the cause of diseases classified elsewhere `UPD`

     B97.31   Lentivirus as the cause of diseases classified elsewhere `UPD`

     B97.32   Oncovirus as the cause of diseases classified elsewhere `UPD`

     B97.33   Human T-cell lymphotrophic virus, type I [HTLV-I] as the cause of diseases classified elsewhere `CC` `UPD`

     B97.34   Human T-cell lymphotrophic virus, type II [HTLV-II] as the cause of diseases classified elsewhere `CC` `UPD`

     B97.35   Human immunodeficiency virus, type 2 [HIV 2] as the cause of diseases classified elsewhere `CC` `UPD` `HCC`

     B97.39   Other retrovirus as the cause of diseases classified elsewhere `UPD`

B97.4   **Respiratory syncytial virus as the cause of diseases classified elsewhere** `UPD`
     RSV as the cause of diseases classified elsewhere
     Code first related disorders, such as:
        otitis media (H65.-)
        upper respiratory infection (J06.9)
     EXCLUDES 1   ►acute bronchiolitis due to respiratory syncytial virus (RSV) (J21.0)◄
        ►acute bronchitis due to respiratory syncytial virus (RSV) (J20.5)◄
        ►respiratory syncytial virus (RSV) pneumonia (J12.1)◄
     EXCLUDES 2   ~~acute bronchiolitis due to respiratory syncytial virus (RSV) (J21.0)~~
        ~~acute bronchitis due to respiratory syncytial virus (RSV) (J20.5)~~
        ~~respiratory syncytial virus (RSV) pneumonia (J12.1)~~

B97.5   **Reovirus as the cause of diseases classified elsewhere** `UPD`

B97.6   **Parvovirus as the cause of diseases classified elsewhere** `UPD`

B97.7   **Papillomavirus as the cause of diseases classified elsewhere** `UPD`

✓5ᵗʰ **B97.8**   **Other viral agents as the cause of diseases classified elsewhere**

     B97.81   Human metapneumovirus as the cause of diseases classified elsewhere `UPD`

     B97.89   Other viral agents as the cause of diseases classified elsewhere `UPD`

Other infectious diseases (B99)

✓4ᵗʰ **B99**   **Other and unspecified infectious diseases**

     B99.8   **Other infectious disease** `HIV`

     B99.9   **Unspecified infectious disease**

Chapter 2. Neoplasms (C00–D49)

Chapter-specific Guidelines with Coding Examples

The chapter-specific guidelines from the ICD-10-CM Official Guidelines for Coding and Reporting have been provided below. Along with these guidelines are coding examples, contained in the shaded boxes, that have been developed to help illustrate the coding and/or sequencing guidance found in these guidelines.

General guidelines

Chapter 2 of the ICD-10-CM contains the codes for most benign and all malignant neoplasms. Certain benign neoplasms, such as prostatic adenomas, may be found in the specific body system chapters. To properly code a neoplasm, it is necessary to determine from the record if the neoplasm is benign, in-situ, malignant, or of uncertain histologic behavior. If malignant, any secondary (metastatic) sites should also be determined.

Primary malignant neoplasms overlapping site boundaries

A primary malignant neoplasm that overlaps two or more contiguous (next to each other) sites should be classified to the subcategory/code .8 ('overlapping lesion'), unless the combination is specifically indexed elsewhere. For multiple neoplasms of the same site that are not contiguous such as tumors in different quadrants of the same breast, codes for each site should be assigned.

> A 73-year-old white female with a large rapidly growing malignant tumor in the left breast extending from the upper outer quadrant into the axillary tail
>
> **C50.812**   **Malignant neoplasm of overlapping sites of left female breast**
>
> *Explanation*: Because this is a single large tumor that overlaps two contiguous sites, a single code for overlapping sites is assigned.

> A 52-year old white female with two distinct lesions of the right breast, one (0.5 cm) in the upper outer quadrant and a second (1.5 cm) in the lower outer quadrant; path report indicates both lesions are malignant
>
> **C50.411**   **Malignant neoplasm of upper-outer quadrant of right female breast**
>
> **C50.511**   **Malignant neoplasm of lower-outer quadrant of right female breast**
>
> *Explanation*: This patient has two distinct malignant lesions of right breast in adjacent quadrants. Because the lesions are not contiguous, two codes are reported.

Malignant neoplasm of ectopic tissue

Malignant neoplasms of ectopic tissue are to be coded to the site of origin mentioned, e.g., ectopic pancreatic malignant neoplasms involving the stomach are coded to malignant neoplasm of pancreas, unspecified (C25.9).

The neoplasm table in the Alphabetic Index should be referenced first. However, if the histological term is documented, that term should be referenced first, rather than going immediately to the Neoplasm Table, in order to determine which column in the Neoplasm Table is appropriate. For example, if the documentation indicates "adenoma," refer to the term in the Alphabetic Index to review the entries under this term and the instructional note to "see also neoplasm, by site, benign." The table provides the proper code based on the type of neoplasm and the site. It is important to select the proper column in the table that corresponds to the type of neoplasm. The Tabular List should then be referenced to verify that the correct code has been selected from the table and that a more specific site code does not exist.

See Section I.C.21. Factors influencing health status and contact with health services, Status, for information regarding Z15.0, codes for genetic susceptibility to cancer.

a. Treatment directed at the malignancy

If the treatment is directed at the malignancy, designate the malignancy as the principal diagnosis.

The only exception to this guideline is if a patient admission/encounter is solely for the administration of chemotherapy, immunotherapy or external beam radiation therapy, assign the appropriate Z51.-- code as the first-listed or principal diagnosis, and the diagnosis or problem for which the service is being performed as a secondary diagnosis.

b. Treatment of secondary site

When a patient is admitted because of a primary neoplasm with metastasis and treatment is directed toward the secondary site only, the secondary neoplasm is designated as the principal diagnosis even though the primary malignancy is still present.

> Patient with primary prostate cancer with metastasis to lungs admitted for wedge resection of mass in right lung
>
> **C78.01**   **Secondary malignant neoplasm of right lung**
>
> **C61**   **Malignant neoplasm of prostate**
>
> *Explanation*: Since the admission is for treatment of the lung metastasis, the secondary lung metastasis is sequenced before the primary prostate cancer.

c. Coding and sequencing of complications

Coding and sequencing of complications associated with the malignancies or with the therapy thereof are subject to the following guidelines:

1) Anemia associated with malignancy

When admission/encounter is for management of an anemia associated with the malignancy, and the treatment is only for anemia, the appropriate code for the malignancy is sequenced as the principal or first-listed diagnosis followed by the appropriate code for the anemia (such as code D63.0, Anemia in neoplastic disease).

> Patient is admitted for treatment of anemia in advanced colon cancer
>
> **C18.9**   **Malignant neoplasm of colon, unspecified**
>
> **D63.0**   **Anemia in neoplastic disease**
>
> *Explanation*: Even though the admission was solely to treat the anemia, this guideline indicates that the code for the malignancy is sequenced first.

2) Anemia associated with chemotherapy, immunotherapy and radiation therapy

When the admission/encounter is for management of an anemia associated with an adverse effect of the administration of chemotherapy or immunotherapy and the only treatment is for the anemia, the anemia code is sequenced first followed by the appropriate codes for the neoplasm and the adverse effect (T45.1X5, Adverse effect of antineoplastic and immunosuppressive drugs).

> A 56-year-old Hispanic male with grade II follicular lymphoma involving multiple lymph node sites referred for blood transfusion to treat anemia due to chemotherapy
>
> **D64.81**   **Anemia due to antineoplastic chemotherapy**
>
> **C82.18**   **Follicular lymphoma grade II, lymph nodes of multiple sites**
>
> **T45.1X5A**   **Adverse effect of antineoplastic and immunosuppressive drugs, initial encounter**
>
> *Explanation*: The code for the anemia is sequenced first followed by the code for the malignant neoplasm and lastly the code for the adverse effect.

When the admission/encounter is for management of an anemia associated with an adverse effect of radiotherapy, the anemia code should be sequenced first, followed by the appropriate neoplasm code and code Y84.2, Radiological procedure and radiotherapy as the cause of abnormal reaction of the patient, or of later complication, without mention of misadventure at the time of the procedure.

A 55-year-old male with a large malignant rectal tumor has been receiving external radiation therapy to shrink the tumor prior to planned surgery. He is admitted today for a blood transfusion to treat anemia related to radiation therapy.

D64.89   **Other specified anemias**

C20   **Malignant neoplasm of rectum**

Y84.2   **Radiological procedure and radiotherapy as the cause of abnormal reaction of the patient, or of later complication, without mention of misadventure at the time of the procedure**

Explanation: The code for the anemia is sequenced first, followed by the code for the malignancy, and lastly the code for the abnormal reaction due to radiotherapy.

3) Management of dehydration due to the malignancy

When the admission/encounter is for management of dehydration due to the malignancy and only the dehydration is being treated (intravenous rehydration), the dehydration is sequenced first, followed by the code(s) for the malignancy.

4) Treatment of a complication resulting from a surgical procedure

When the admission/encounter is for treatment of a complication resulting from a surgical procedure, designate the complication as the principal or first-listed diagnosis if treatment is directed at resolving the complication.

d. Primary malignancy previously excised

When a primary malignancy has been previously excised or eradicated from its site and there is no further treatment directed to that site and there is no evidence of any existing primary malignancy at that site, a code from category Z85, Personal history of malignant neoplasm, should be used to indicate the former site of the malignancy. Any mention of extension, invasion, or metastasis to another site is coded as a secondary malignant neoplasm to that site. The secondary site may be the principal or first-listed diagnosis with the Z85 code used as a secondary code.

History of breast cancer, left radical mastectomy 18 months ago with no current treatment; bronchoscopy with lung biopsy shows metastatic disease in the right lung

C78.01   **Secondary malignant neoplasm of right lung**

Z85.3   **Personal history of malignant neoplasm of breast**

Explanation: The patient has undergone a diagnostic procedure that revealed metastatic breast cancer in the right lung. The code for the secondary (metastatic) site is sequenced first followed by a personal history code to identify the former site of the primary malignancy.

e. Admissions/encounters involving chemotherapy, immunotherapy and radiation therapy

1) Episode of care involves surgical removal of neoplasm

When an episode of care involves the surgical removal of a neoplasm, primary or secondary site, followed by adjunct chemotherapy or radiation treatment during the same episode of care, the code for the neoplasm should be assigned as principal or first-listed diagnosis.

2) Patient admission/encounter solely for administration of chemotherapy, immunotherapy and radiation therapy

If a patient admission/encounter is solely for the administration of chemotherapy, immunotherapy or external beam radiation therapy assign code Z51.0, Encounter for antineoplastic radiation therapy, or Z51.11, Encounter for antineoplastic chemotherapy, or Z51.12, Encounter for antineoplastic immunotherapy as the first-listed or principal diagnosis. If a patient receives more than one of these therapies during the same admission more than one of these codes may be assigned, in any sequence.

The malignancy for which the therapy is being administered should be assigned as a secondary diagnosis.

If a patient admission/encounter is for the insertion or implantation of radioactive elements (e.g., brachytherapy) the appropriate code for the malignancy is sequenced as the principal or first-listed diagnosis. Code Z51.0 should not be assigned.

3) Patient admitted for radiation therapy, chemotherapy or immunotherapy and develops complications

When a patient is admitted for the purpose of external beam radiotherapy, immunotherapy or chemotherapy and develops complications such as uncontrolled nausea and vomiting or dehydration, the principal or first-listed diagnosis is Z51.0, Encounter for antineoplastic radiation therapy, or Z51.11, Encounter for antineoplastic chemotherapy, or Z51.12, Encounter for antineoplastic immunotherapy followed by any codes for the complications.

When a patient is admitted for the purpose of insertion or implantation of radioactive elements (e.g., brachytherapy) and develops complications such as uncontrolled nausea and vomiting or dehydration, the principal or first-listed diagnosis is the appropriate code for the malignancy followed by any codes for the complications.

A patient with prostate cancer was admitted for brachytherapy seed implantation and consequently developed urinary retention.

C61   **Malignant neoplasm of prostate**

R33.9   **Retention of urine, unspecified**

Explanation: A code for the malignancy should be listed as the principal diagnosis when insertion of a radioactive element is the reason for admission, even when a complication related to that radioactive element occurs. Codes describing the complications should be listed as secondary codes.

f. Admission/encounter to determine extent of malignancy

When the reason for admission/encounter is to determine the extent of the malignancy, or for a procedure such as paracentesis or thoracentesis, the primary malignancy or appropriate metastatic site is designated as the principal or first-listed diagnosis, even though chemotherapy or radiotherapy is administered.

Patient with left lung cancer with malignant pleural effusion admitted for paracentesis and initiation/administration of chemotherapy

C34.92   **Malignant neoplasm of unspecified part of left bronchus or lung**

J91.0   **Malignant pleural effusion**

Z51.11   **Encounter for antineoplastic chemotherapy**

Explanation: The lung cancer is sequenced before the chemotherapy in this instance because the paracentesis for the malignant effusion is also being performed. An instructional note under the malignant effusion instructs that the lung cancer be sequenced first.

g. Symptoms, signs, and abnormal findings listed in Chapter 18 associated with neoplasms

Symptoms, signs, and ill-defined conditions listed in Chapter 18 characteristic of, or associated with, an existing primary or secondary site malignancy cannot be used to replace the malignancy as principal or first-listed diagnosis, regardless of the number of admissions or encounters for treatment and care of the neoplasm.

See Section I.C.21. Factors influencing health status and contact with health services, Encounter for prophylactic organ removal.

h. Admission/encounter for pain control/management

See Section I.C.6. for information on coding admission/encounter for pain control/management.

i. Malignancy in two or more noncontiguous sites

A patient may have more than one malignant tumor in the same organ. These tumors may represent different primaries or metastatic disease, depending on the site. Should the documentation be unclear, the provider should be queried as to the status of each tumor so that the correct codes can be assigned.

j. Disseminated malignant neoplasm, unspecified

Code C80.0, Disseminated malignant neoplasm, unspecified, is for use only in those cases where the patient has advanced metastatic disease and no known primary or secondary sites are specified. It should not be used in place of assigning codes for the primary site and all known secondary sites.

Patient who has had no medical care for many years is seen today and diagnosed with carcinomatosis

C80.0   **Disseminated malignant neoplasm, unspecified**

Explanation: Carcinomatosis NOS is an "includes" note under this code. Should seldom be used but is available for use in cases such as this.

k. Malignant neoplasm without specification of site

Code C80.1, Malignant (primary) neoplasm, unspecified, equates to Cancer, unspecified. This code should only be used when no determination can be made as to the primary site of a malignancy. This code should rarely be used in the inpatient setting.

l. Sequencing of neoplasm codes

1) Encounter for treatment of primary malignancy

If the reason for the encounter is for treatment of a primary malignancy, assign the malignancy as the principal/first-listed diagnosis. The primary site is to be sequenced first, followed by any metastatic sites.

2) Encounter for treatment of secondary malignancy

When an encounter is for a primary malignancy with metastasis and treatment is directed toward the metastatic (secondary) site(s) only, the metastatic site(s) is designated as the principal/first-listed diagnosis. The primary malignancy is coded as an additional code.

Patient has primary colon cancer with metastasis to rib and is evaluated for possible excision of portion of rib bone

C79.51   **Secondary malignant neoplasm of bone**

C18.9   **Malignant neoplasm of colon, unspecified**

Explanation: The treatment for this encounter is focused on the metastasis to the rib bone rather than the primary colon cancer, thus indicating that the bone metastasis is sequenced as the first-listed code.

3) Malignant neoplasm in a pregnant patient

When a pregnant **patient** has a malignant neoplasm, a code from subcategory O9A.1-, Malignant neoplasm complicating pregnancy, childbirth, and the puerperium, should be sequenced first, followed by the appropriate code from Chapter 2 to indicate the type of neoplasm.

A 30-year-old pregnant female in second trimester evaluated for thyroid malignancy

O9A.112   **Malignant neoplasm complicating pregnancy, second trimester**

C73   **Malignant neoplasm of thyroid gland**

Explanation: Codes from chapter 15 describing complications of pregnancy are sequenced as first-listed codes, further specified by codes from other chapters such as neoplastic, unless the pregnancy is documented as incidental to the condition. See also guideline 1.C.15.a.1.

4) Encounter for complication associated with a neoplasm

When an encounter is for management of a complication associated with a neoplasm, such as dehydration, and the treatment is only for the complication, the complication is coded first, followed by the appropriate code(s) for the neoplasm.

The exception to this guideline is anemia. When the admission/encounter is for management of an anemia associated with the malignancy, and the treatment is only for anemia, the appropriate code for the malignancy is sequenced as the principal or first-listed diagnosis followed by code D63.0, Anemia in neoplastic disease.

Patient with pancreatic cancer is seen for initiation of TPN for cancer-related moderate protein-calorie malnutrition

E44.0   **Moderate protein-calorie malnutrition**

C25.9   **Malignant neoplasm of pancreas, unspecified**

Explanation: The encounter is to initiate treatment for malnutrition, a common complication of many types of neoplasms, and is sequenced first.

5) Complication from surgical procedure for treatment of a neoplasm

When an encounter is for treatment of a complication resulting from a surgical procedure performed for the treatment of the neoplasm, designate the complication as the principal/first-listed diagnosis. See the guideline regarding the coding of a current malignancy versus personal history to determine if the code for the neoplasm should also be assigned.

6) Pathologic fracture due to a neoplasm

When an encounter is for a pathological fracture due to a neoplasm, and the focus of treatment is the fracture, a code from subcategory M84.5, Pathological fracture in neoplastic disease, should be sequenced first, followed by the code for the neoplasm.

If the focus of treatment is the neoplasm with an associated pathological fracture, the neoplasm code should be sequenced first, followed by a code from M84.5 for the pathological fracture.

m. Current malignancy versus personal history of malignancy

When a primary malignancy has been excised but further treatment, such as an additional surgery for the malignancy, radiation therapy or chemotherapy is directed to that site, the primary malignancy code should be used until treatment is completed.

Female patient with ongoing chemotherapy after right mastectomy for breast cancer

C50.911   **Malignant neoplasm of unspecified site of right female breast**

Z90.11   **Acquired absence of right breast and nipple**

Explanation: Even though the breast has been removed, the breast cancer is still being treated with chemotherapy and therefore is still coded as a current condition rather than personal history.

When a primary malignancy has been previously excised or eradicated from its site, there is no further treatment (of the malignancy) directed to that site, and there is no evidence of any existing primary malignancy at that site, a code from category Z85, Personal history of malignant neoplasm, should be used to indicate the former site of the malignancy.

Codes from subcategories Z85.0 – Z85.85 should only be assigned for the former site of a primary malignancy, not the site of a secondary malignancy. Code Z85.89 may be assigned for the former site(s) of either a primary or secondary malignancy.

See Section I.C.21. Factors influencing health status and contact with health services, History (of)

n. Leukemia, multiple myeloma, and malignant plasma cell neoplasms in remission versus personal history

The categories for leukemia, and category C90, Multiple myeloma and malignant plasma cell neoplasms, have codes indicating whether or not the leukemia has achieved remission. There are also codes Z85.6, Personal history of leukemia, and Z85.79, Personal history of other malignant neoplasms of lymphoid, hematopoietic and related tissues. If the documentation is unclear as to whether the leukemia has achieved remission, the provider should be queried.

See Section I.C.21. Factors influencing health status and contact with health services, History (of)

o. Aftercare following surgery for neoplasm

See Section I.C.21. Factors influencing health status and contact with health services, Aftercare

p. Follow-up care for completed treatment of a malignancy

See Section I.C.21. Factors influencing health status and contact with health services, Follow-up

q. Prophylactic organ removal for prevention of malignancy

See Section I.C. 21, Factors influencing health status and contact with health services, Prophylactic organ removal

r. Malignant neoplasm associated with transplanted organ

A malignant neoplasm of a transplanted organ should be coded as a transplant complication. Assign first the appropriate code from category T86.-, Complications of transplanted organs and tissue, followed by code C80.2, Malignant neoplasm associated with transplanted organ. Use an additional code for the specific malignancy.

s. Breast implant associated anaplastic large cell lymphoma

Breast implant associated anaplastic large cell lymphoma (BIA-ALCL) is a type of lymphoma that can develop around breast implants. Assign code C84.7A, Anaplastic large cell lymphoma, ALK-negative, breast, for BIA-ALCL. Do not assign a complication code from chapter 19.

Chapter 2. Neoplasms (C00-D49)

NOTE

Functional activity

All neoplasms are classified in this chapter, whether they are functionally active or not. An additional code from Chapter 4 may be used, to identify functional activity associated with any neoplasm.

Morphology [Histology]

Chapter 2 classifies neoplasms primarily by site (topography), with broad groupings for behavior, malignant, in situ, benign, etc. The Table of Neoplasms should be used to identify the correct topography code. In a few cases, such as for malignant melanoma and certain neuroendocrine tumors, the morphology (histologic type) is included in the category and codes.

Primary malignant neoplasms overlapping site boundaries

A primary malignant neoplasm that overlaps two or more contiguous (next to each other) sites should be classified to the subcategory/code .8 ("overlapping lesion"), unless the combination is specifically indexed elsewhere. For multiple neoplasms of the same site that are not contiguous, such as tumors in different quadrants of the same breast, codes for each site should be assigned.

Malignant neoplasm of ectopic tissue

Malignant neoplasms of ectopic tissue are to be coded to the site mentioned, e.g., ectopic pancreatic malignant neoplasms are coded to pancreas, unspecified (C25.9).

AHA: 2017,4Q,103; 2017,1Q,4,5-6,8

This chapter contains the following blocks:

C00-C14	Malignant neoplasms of lip, oral cavity and pharynx
C15-C26	Malignant neoplasms of digestive organs
C30-C39	Malignant neoplasms of respiratory and intrathoracic organs
C40-C41	Malignant neoplasms of bone and articular cartilage
C43-C44	Melanoma and other malignant neoplasms of skin
C45-C49	Malignant neoplasms of mesothelial and soft tissue
C50	Malignant neoplasms of breast
C51-C58	Malignant neoplasms of female genital organs
C60-C63	Malignant neoplasms of male genital organs
C64-C68	Malignant neoplasms of urinary tract
C69-C72	Malignant neoplasms of eye, brain and other parts of central nervous system
C73-C75	Malignant neoplasms of thyroid and other endocrine glands
C7A	Malignant neuroendocrine tumors
C7B	Secondary neuroendocrine tumors
C76-C80	Malignant neoplasms of ill-defined, other secondary and unspecified sites
C81-C96	Malignant neoplasms of lymphoid, hematopoietic and related tissue
D00-D09	In situ neoplasms
D10-D36	Benign neoplasms, except benign neuroendocrine tumors
D3A	Benign neuroendocrine tumors
D37-D48	Neoplasms of uncertain behavior, polycythemia vera and myelodysplastic syndromes
D49	Neoplasms of unspecified behavior

MALIGNANT NEOPLASMS(C00-C96)

Malignant neoplasms, stated or presumed to be primary (of specified sites), and certain specified histologies, except neuroendocrine, and of lymphoid, hematopoietic and related tissue (C00-C75).

Malignant neoplasms of lip, oral cavity and pharynx (C00-C14)

☑4ᵗʰ C00 Malignant neoplasm of lip

Use additional code to identify:
- alcohol abuse and dependence (F10.-)
- history of tobacco dependence (Z87.891)
- tobacco dependence (F17.-)
- tobacco use (Z72.0)

   EXCLUDES 1   *malignant melanoma of lip (C43.0)*

                      Merkel cell carcinoma of lip (C4A.0)

                      other and unspecified malignant neoplasm of skin of lip (C44.0-)

C00.0 Malignant neoplasm of external upper lip
Malignant neoplasm of lipstick area of upper lip
Malignant neoplasm of upper lip NOS
Malignant neoplasm of vermilion border of upper lip

C00.1 Malignant neoplasm of external lower lip
Malignant neoplasm of lower lip NOS
Malignant neoplasm of lipstick area of lower lip
Malignant neoplasm of vermilion border of lower lip

C00.2 Malignant neoplasm of external lip, unspecified
Malignant neoplasm of vermilion border of lip NOS

C00.3 Malignant neoplasm of upper lip, inner aspect
Malignant neoplasm of buccal aspect of upper lip
Malignant neoplasm of frenulum of upper lip
Malignant neoplasm of mucosa of upper lip
Malignant neoplasm of oral aspect of upper lip

C00.4 Malignant neoplasm of lower lip, inner aspect
Malignant neoplasm of buccal aspect of lower lip
Malignant neoplasm of frenulum of lower lip
Malignant neoplasm of mucosa of lower lip
Malignant neoplasm of oral aspect of lower lip

C00.5 Malignant neoplasm of lip, unspecified, inner aspect
Malignant neoplasm of buccal aspect of lip, unspecified
Malignant neoplasm of frenulum of lip, unspecified
Malignant neoplasm of mucosa of lip, unspecified
Malignant neoplasm of oral aspect of lip, unspecified

C00.6 Malignant neoplasm of commissure of lip, unspecified

C00.8 Malignant neoplasm of overlapping sites of lip

C00.9 Malignant neoplasm of lip, unspecified

C01 Malignant neoplasm of base of tongue   **HCC**
Malignant neoplasm of dorsal surface of base of tongue
Malignant neoplasm of fixed part of tongue NOS
Malignant neoplasm of posterior third of tongue
Use additional code to identify:
- alcohol abuse and dependence (F10.-)
- history of tobacco dependence (Z87.891)
- tobacco dependence (F17.-)
- tobacco use (Z72.0)

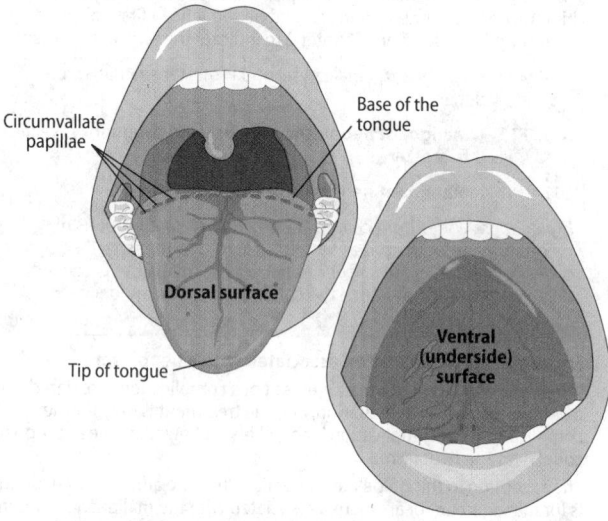

Malignant Neoplasm of Tongue

Circumvallate papillae
Base of the tongue
Dorsal surface
Tip of tongue
Ventral (underside) surface

☑4ᵗʰ C02 Malignant neoplasm of other and unspecified parts of tongue

Use additional code to identify:
- alcohol abuse and dependence (F10.-)
- history of tobacco dependence (Z87.891)
- tobacco dependence (F17.-)
- tobacco use (Z72.0)

C02.0 Malignant neoplasm of dorsal surface of tongue   **HCC**
Malignant neoplasm of anterior two-thirds of tongue, dorsal surface
   EXCLUDES 2   *malignant neoplasm of dorsal surface of base of tongue (C01)*

C02.1 Malignant neoplasm of border of tongue   **HCC**
Malignant neoplasm of tip of tongue

C02.2 Malignant neoplasm of ventral surface of tongue   **HCC**
Malignant neoplasm of anterior two-thirds of tongue, ventral surface
Malignant neoplasm of frenulum linguae

C02.3 Malignant neoplasm of anterior two-thirds of tongue, part unspecified   **HCC**
Malignant neoplasm of middle third of tongue NOS
Malignant neoplasm of mobile part of tongue NOS

C02.4 Malignant neoplasm of lingual tonsil   **HCC**
   EXCLUDES 2   *malignant neoplasm of tonsil NOS (C09.9)*

N Newborn: 0   **P** Pediatric: 0-17   **M** Maternity: 9-64   **A** Adult: 15-124   **MCC** Major Complication/Comorbidity   **CC** Complication/Comorbidity   **SW** Severe Wound Dx

468   ICD-10-CM 2022

C02.8   **Malignant neoplasm of** overlapping sites **of tongue**   `HCC`
     Malignant neoplasm of two or more contiguous sites of tongue

C02.9   **Malignant neoplasm of tongue, unspecified**   `HCC`

☑4ᵗʰ **C03**   **Malignant neoplasm of** gum

    `INCLUDES`   malignant neoplasm of alveolar (ridge) mucosa
               malignant neoplasm of gingiva

Use additional code to identify:
   alcohol abuse and dependence (F10.-)
   history of tobacco dependence (Z87.891)
   tobacco dependence (F17.-)
   tobacco use (Z72.0)

    `EXCLUDES 2`   *malignant odontogenic neoplasms (C41.0-C41.1)*

C03.0   **Malignant neoplasm of** upper gum   `HCC`

C03.1   **Malignant neoplasm of** lower gum   `HCC`

C03.9   **Malignant neoplasm of gum, unspecified**   `HCC`

☑4ᵗʰ **C04**   **Malignant neoplasm of** floor of mouth

Use additional code to identify:
   alcohol abuse and dependence (F10.-)
   history of tobacco dependence (Z87.891)
   tobacco dependence (F17.-)
   tobacco use (Z72.0)

C04.0   **Malignant neoplasm of** anterior **floor of mouth**   `HCC`
     Malignant neoplasm of anterior to the premolar-canine junction

C04.1   **Malignant neoplasm of** lateral **floor of mouth**   `HCC`

C04.8   **Malignant neoplasm of** overlapping sites **of floor of mouth**   `HCC`

C04.9   **Malignant neoplasm of floor of mouth, unspecified**   `HCC`

☑4ᵗʰ **C05**   **Malignant neoplasm of** palate

Use additional code to identify:
   alcohol abuse and dependence (F10.-)
   history of tobacco dependence (Z87.891)
   tobacco dependence (F17.-)
   tobacco use (Z72.0)

    `EXCLUDES 1`   *Kaposi's sarcoma of palate (C46.2)*

C05.0   **Malignant neoplasm of** hard palate   `HCC`

C05.1   **Malignant neoplasm of** soft palate   `HCC`
    `EXCLUDES 2`   *malignant neoplasm of nasopharyngeal surface of soft palate (C11.3)*

C05.2   **Malignant neoplasm of** uvula   `HCC`

C05.8   **Malignant neoplasm of** overlapping sites **of palate**   `HCC`

C05.9   **Malignant neoplasm of palate, unspecified**   `HCC`
     Malignant neoplasm of roof of mouth

☑4ᵗʰ **C06**   **Malignant neoplasm of** other and unspecified parts of mouth

Use additional code to identify:
   alcohol abuse and dependence (F10.-)
   history of tobacco dependence (Z87.891)
   tobacco dependence (F17.-)
   tobacco use (Z72.0)

C06.0   **Malignant neoplasm of** cheek mucosa   `HCC`
     Malignant neoplasm of buccal mucosa NOS
     Malignant neoplasm of internal cheek

C06.1   **Malignant neoplasm of** vestibule **of mouth**   `HCC`
     Malignant neoplasm of buccal sulcus (upper) (lower)
     Malignant neoplasm of labial sulcus (upper) (lower)

C06.2   **Malignant neoplasm of** retromolar area   `HCC`

☑5ᵗʰ **C06.8**   **Malignant neoplasm of** overlapping sites **of other and unspecified parts of mouth**

   C06.80   **Malignant neoplasm of overlapping sites of unspecified parts of mouth**   `HCC`

   C06.89   **Malignant neoplasm of overlapping sites of other parts of mouth**   `HCC`
       "book leaf" neoplasm [ventral surface of tongue and floor of mouth]

C06.9   **Malignant neoplasm of mouth, unspecified**   `HCC`
     Malignant neoplasm of minor salivary gland, unspecified site
     Malignant neoplasm of oral cavity NOS

C07   **Malignant neoplasm of** parotid gland   `HCC`

Use additional code to identify:
   alcohol abuse and dependence (F10.-)
   exposure to environmental tobacco smoke (Z77.22)
   exposure to tobacco smoke in the perinatal period (P96.81)
   history of tobacco dependence (Z87.891)
   occupational exposure to environmental tobacco smoke (Z57.31)
   tobacco dependence (F17.-)
   tobacco use (Z72.0)

☑4ᵗʰ **C08**   **Malignant neoplasm of** other and unspecified major salivary glands

    `INCLUDES`   malignant neoplasm of salivary ducts

Use additional code to identify:
   alcohol abuse and dependence (F10.-)
   exposure to environmental tobacco smoke (Z77.22)
   exposure to tobacco smoke in the perinatal period (P96.81)
   history of tobacco dependence (Z87.891)
   occupational exposure to environmental tobacco smoke (Z57.31)
   tobacco dependence (F17.-)
   tobacco use (Z72.0)

    `EXCLUDES 1`   *malignant neoplasms of specified minor salivary glands which are classified according to their anatomical location*

    `EXCLUDES 2`   *malignant neoplasms of minor salivary glands NOS (C06.9)*
                 malignant neoplasm of parotid gland (C07)

C08.0   **Malignant neoplasm of** submandibular **gland**   `HCC`
     Malignant neoplasm of submaxillary gland

C08.1   **Malignant neoplasm of** sublingual **gland**   `HCC`

C08.9   **Malignant neoplasm of** major salivary gland, **unspecified**   `HCC`
     Malignant neoplasm of salivary gland (major) NOS

☑4ᵗʰ **C09**   **Malignant neoplasm of** tonsil

Use additional code to identify:
   alcohol abuse and dependence (F10.-)
   exposure to environmental tobacco smoke (Z77.22)
   exposure to tobacco smoke in the perinatal period (P96.81)
   history of tobacco dependence (Z87.891)
   occupational exposure to environmental tobacco smoke (Z57.31)
   tobacco dependence (F17.-)
   tobacco use (Z72.0)

    `EXCLUDES 2`   *malignant neoplasm of lingual tonsil (C02.4)*
                 malignant neoplasm of pharyngeal tonsil (C11.1)

C09.0   **Malignant neoplasm of** tonsillar fossa   `HCC`

C09.1   **Malignant neoplasm of** tonsillar pillar (anterior) (posterior)   `HCC`

C09.8   **Malignant neoplasm of** overlapping sites **of tonsil**   `HCC`

C09.9   **Malignant neoplasm of tonsil, unspecified**   `HCC`
     Malignant neoplasm of tonsil NOS
     Malignant neoplasm of faucial tonsils
     Malignant neoplasm of palatine tonsils

☑4ᵗʰ **C10**   **Malignant neoplasm of** oropharynx

Use additional code to identify:
   alcohol abuse and dependence (F10.-)
   exposure to environmental tobacco smoke (Z77.22)
   exposure to tobacco smoke in the perinatal period (P96.81)
   history of tobacco dependence (Z87.891)
   occupational exposure to environmental tobacco smoke (Z57.31)
   tobacco dependence (F17.-)
   tobacco use (Z72.0)

    `EXCLUDES 2`   *malignant neoplasm of tonsil (C09.-)*

DEF: Oropharynx: Middle portion of pharynx (throat); communicates with the oral cavity, nasopharynx and laryngopharynx.

C10.0   **Malignant neoplasm of** vallecula   `HCC`

C10.1   **Malignant neoplasm of** anterior surface of epiglottis   `HCC`
     Malignant neoplasm of epiglottis, free border [margin]
     Malignant neoplasm of glossoepiglottic fold(s)
    `EXCLUDES 2`   *malignant neoplasm of epiglottis (suprahyoid portion) NOS (C32.1)*

C10.2   **Malignant neoplasm of** lateral wall **of oropharynx**   `HCC`

C10.3   **Malignant neoplasm of** posterior wall **of oropharynx**   `HCC`

C10.4   **Malignant neoplasm of** branchial cleft   `HCC`
     Malignant neoplasm of branchial cyst [site of neoplasm]

C10.8   **Malignant neoplasm of** overlapping sites **of oropharynx**   `HCC`
     Malignant neoplasm of junctional region of oropharynx

C10.9   **Malignant neoplasm of oropharynx, unspecified**   `HCC`

✓4ᵗʰ C11 Malignant neoplasm of nasopharynx
Use additional code to identify:
exposure to environmental tobacco smoke (Z77.22)
exposure to tobacco smoke in the perinatal period (P96.81)
history of tobacco dependence (Z87.891)
occupational exposure to environmental tobacco smoke (Z57.31)
tobacco dependence (F17.-)
tobacco use (Z72.0)
DEF: Nasopharynx: Upper portion of pharynx (throat); communicates with the nasal cavities, oropharynx and tympanic cavities.

C11.0 Malignant neoplasm of superior wall of nasopharynx HCC
Malignant neoplasm of roof of nasopharynx

C11.1 Malignant neoplasm of posterior wall of nasopharynx HCC
Malignant neoplasm of adenoid
Malignant neoplasm of pharyngeal tonsil

C11.2 Malignant neoplasm of lateral wall of nasopharynx HCC
Malignant neoplasm of fossa of Rosenmüller
Malignant neoplasm of opening of auditory tube
Malignant neoplasm of pharyngeal recess

C11.3 Malignant neoplasm of anterior wall of nasopharynx HCC
Malignant neoplasm of floor of nasopharynx
Malignant neoplasm of nasopharyngeal (anterior) (posterior) surface of soft palate
Malignant neoplasm of posterior margin of nasal choana
Malignant neoplasm of posterior margin of nasal septum

C11.8 Malignant neoplasm of overlapping sites of nasopharynx HCC

C11.9 Malignant neoplasm of nasopharynx, unspecified HCC
Malignant neoplasm of nasopharyngeal wall NOS

C12 Malignant neoplasm of pyriform sinus HCC
Malignant neoplasm of pyriform fossa
Use additional code to identify:
exposure to environmental tobacco smoke (Z77.22)
exposure to tobacco smoke in the perinatal period (P96.81)
history of tobacco dependence (Z87.891)
occupational exposure to environmental tobacco smoke (Z57.31)
tobacco dependence (F17.-)
tobacco use (Z72.0)

✓4ᵗʰ C13 Malignant neoplasm of hypopharynx
Use additional code to identify:
exposure to environmental tobacco smoke (Z77.22)
exposure to tobacco smoke in the perinatal period (P96.81)
history of tobacco dependence (Z87.891)
occupational exposure to environmental tobacco smoke (Z57.31)
tobacco dependence (F17.-)
tobacco use (Z72.0)
EXCLUDES 2 malignant neoplasm of pyriform sinus (C12)
DEF: Hypopharynx: Lower portion of pharynx (throat); communicates with the oropharynx and the esophagus. **Synonym(s):** laryngopharynx.

C13.0 Malignant neoplasm of postcricoid region HCC

C13.1 Malignant neoplasm of aryepiglottic fold, hypopharyngeal aspect HCC
Malignant neoplasm of aryepiglottic fold, marginal zone
Malignant neoplasm of aryepiglottic fold NOS
Malignant neoplasm of interarytenoid fold, marginal zone
Malignant neoplasm of interarytenoid fold NOS
EXCLUDES 2 malignant neoplasm of aryepiglottic fold or interarytenoid fold, laryngeal aspect (C32.1)

C13.2 Malignant neoplasm of posterior wall of hypopharynx HCC

C13.8 Malignant neoplasm of overlapping sites of hypopharynx HCC

C13.9 Malignant neoplasm of hypopharynx, unspecified HCC
Malignant neoplasm of hypopharyngeal wall NOS

✓4ᵗʰ C14 Malignant neoplasm of other and ill-defined sites in the lip, oral cavity and pharynx
Use additional code to identify:
alcohol abuse and dependence (F10.-)
exposure to environmental tobacco smoke (Z77.22)
exposure to tobacco smoke in the perinatal period (P96.81)
history of tobacco dependence (Z87.891)
occupational exposure to environmental tobacco smoke (Z57.31)
tobacco dependence (F17.-)
tobacco use (Z72.0)
EXCLUDES 1 malignant neoplasm of oral cavity NOS (C06.9)

C14.0 Malignant neoplasm of pharynx, unspecified HCC

C14.2 Malignant neoplasm of Waldeyer's ring HCC
DEF: Waldeyer's ring: Ring of lymphoid tissue that is made up of the two palatine tonsils, the pharyngeal tonsil (adenoid), and the lingual tonsil. It functions as the defense against infection and assists with the development of the immune system.

C14.8 Malignant neoplasm of overlapping sites of lip, oral cavity and pharynx HCC
Primary malignant neoplasm of two or more contiguous sites of lip, oral cavity and pharynx
EXCLUDES 1 "book leaf" neoplasm [ventral surface of tongue and floor of mouth] (C06.89)

Malignant neoplasms of digestive organs (C15-C26)

EXCLUDES 1 Kaposi's sarcoma of gastrointestinal sites (C46.4)
EXCLUDES 2 gastrointestinal stromal tumors (C49.A-)

✓4ᵗʰ C15 Malignant neoplasm of esophagus
Use additional code to identify:
alcohol abuse and dependence (F10.-)

C15.3 Malignant neoplasm of upper third of esophagus CC HCC

C15.4 Malignant neoplasm of middle third of esophagus CC HCC

C15.5 Malignant neoplasm of lower third of esophagus CC HCC
EXCLUDES 1 malignant neoplasm of cardio-esophageal junction (C16.0)

C15.8 Malignant neoplasm of overlapping sites of esophagus CC HCC

C15.9 Malignant neoplasm of esophagus, unspecified CC HCC

✓4ᵗʰ C16 Malignant neoplasm of stomach
Use additional code to identify:
alcohol abuse and dependence (F10.-)
EXCLUDES 2 malignant carcinoid tumor of the stomach (C7A.092)

C16.0 Malignant neoplasm of cardia CC HCC
Malignant neoplasm of cardiac orifice
Malignant neoplasm of cardio-esophageal junction
Malignant neoplasm of esophagus and stomach
Malignant neoplasm of gastro-esophageal junction

C16.1 Malignant neoplasm of fundus of stomach CC HCC

C16.2 Malignant neoplasm of body of stomach CC HCC

C16.3 Malignant neoplasm of pyloric antrum CC HCC
Malignant neoplasm of gastric antrum

C16.4 Malignant neoplasm of pylorus CC HCC
Malignant neoplasm of prepylorus
Malignant neoplasm of pyloric canal

C16.5 Malignant neoplasm of lesser curvature of stomach, unspecified CC HCC
Malignant neoplasm of lesser curvature of stomach, not classifiable to C16.1-C16.4

C16.6 Malignant neoplasm of greater curvature of stomach, unspecified CC HCC
Malignant neoplasm of greater curvature of stomach, not classifiable to C16.0-C16.4

C16.8 Malignant neoplasm of overlapping sites of stomach CC HCC

C16.9 Malignant neoplasm of stomach, unspecified CC HCC
Gastric cancer NOS

✓4ᵗʰ C17 Malignant neoplasm of small intestine
EXCLUDES 1 malignant carcinoid tumors of the small intestine (C7A.01)
AHA: 2016,1Q,19

C17.0 Malignant neoplasm of duodenum CC HCC

C17.1 Malignant neoplasm of jejunum CC HCC

C17.2 Malignant neoplasm of ileum CC HCC
EXCLUDES 1 malignant neoplasm of ileocecal valve (C18.0)

C17.3 Meckel's diverticulum, malignant CC HCC
EXCLUDES 1 Meckel's diverticulum, congenital (Q43.0)
DEF: Congenital, abnormal remnant of embryonic digestive system development that leaves a sacculation or outpouching from the wall of the small intestine near the terminal part of the ileum made of acid-secreting tissue as in the stomach.

C17.8 Malignant neoplasm of overlapping sites of small intestine CC HCC

C17.9 Malignant neoplasm of small intestine, unspecified CC HCC

✓4ᵗʰ C18 Malignant neoplasm of colon

> **EXCLUDES 1** *malignant carcinoid tumors of the colon (C7A.Ø2-)*

Colon

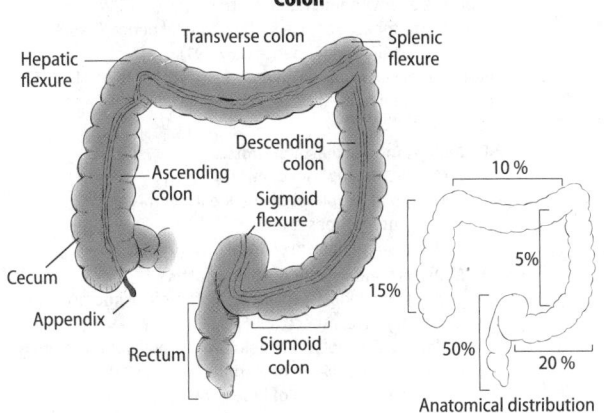

Transverse colon
Splenic flexure
Hepatic flexure
Descending colon
Ascending colon
Sigmoid flexure
Cecum
Appendix
Rectum
Sigmoid colon

10 %
5%
15%
50%
20 %

Anatomical distribution of large bowel cancers

C18.Ø Malignant neoplasm of cecum `CC` `HCC`
Malignant neoplasm of ileocecal valve

C18.1 Malignant neoplasm of appendix `CC` `HCC`

C18.2 Malignant neoplasm of ascending colon `CC` `HCC`

C18.3 Malignant neoplasm of hepatic flexure `CC` `HCC`

C18.4 Malignant neoplasm of transverse colon `CC` `HCC`

C18.5 Malignant neoplasm of splenic flexure `CC` `HCC`

C18.6 Malignant neoplasm of descending colon `CC` `HCC`

C18.7 Malignant neoplasm of sigmoid colon `CC` `HCC`
Malignant neoplasm of sigmoid (flexure)
> **EXCLUDES 1** *malignant neoplasm of rectosigmoid junction (C19)*

C18.8 Malignant neoplasm of overlapping sites of colon `CC` `HCC`

C18.9 Malignant neoplasm of colon, unspecified `CC` `HCC`
Malignant neoplasm of large intestine NOS

C19 Malignant neoplasm of rectosigmoid junction `CC` `HCC`
Malignant neoplasm of colon with rectum
Malignant neoplasm of rectosigmoid (colon)
> **EXCLUDES 1** *malignant carcinoid tumors of the colon (C7A.Ø2-)*

C20 Malignant neoplasm of rectum `CC` `HCC`
Malignant neoplasm of rectal ampulla
> **EXCLUDES 1** *malignant carcinoid tumor of the rectum (C7A.Ø26)*

✓4ᵗʰ C21 Malignant neoplasm of anus and anal canal

> **EXCLUDES 2** *malignant carcinoid tumors of the anus (C7A.Ø2-)*
> *malignant melanoma of anal margin (C43.51)*
> *malignant melanoma of anal skin (C43.51)*
> *malignant melanoma of perianal skin (C43.51)*
> *other and unspecified malignant neoplasm of anal margin (C44.5ØØ, C44.51Ø, C44.52Ø, C44.59Ø)*
> *other and unspecified malignant neoplasm of anal skin (C44.5ØØ, C44.51Ø, C44.52Ø, C44.59Ø)*
> *other and unspecified malignant neoplasm of perianal skin (C44.5ØØ, C44.51Ø, C44.52Ø, C44.59Ø)*

C21.Ø Malignant neoplasm of anus, unspecified `CC` `HCC`

C21.1 Malignant neoplasm of anal canal `CC` `HCC`
Malignant neoplasm of anal sphincter

C21.2 Malignant neoplasm of cloacogenic zone `CC` `HCC`

C21.8 Malignant neoplasm of overlapping sites of rectum, anus and anal canal `CC` `HCC`
Malignant neoplasm of anorectal junction
Malignant neoplasm of anorectum
Primary malignant neoplasm of two or more contiguous sites of rectum, anus and anal canal

✓4ᵗʰ C22 Malignant neoplasm of liver and intrahepatic bile ducts

> **EXCLUDES 1** *malignant neoplasm of biliary tract NOS (C24.9)*
> *secondary malignant neoplasm of liver and intrahepatic bile duct (C78.7)*

Use additional code to identify:
alcohol abuse and dependence (F1Ø.-)
hepatitis B (B16.-, B18.Ø-B18.1)
hepatitis C (B17.1-, B18.2)

C22.Ø Liver cell carcinoma `CC` `HCC`
Hepatocellular carcinoma
Hepatoma
AHA: 2016,1Q,18

C22.1 Intrahepatic bile duct carcinoma `CC` `HCC`
Cholangiocarcinoma
> **EXCLUDES 1** *malignant neoplasm of hepatic duct (C24.Ø)*

C22.2 Hepatoblastoma `CC` `HCC`

C22.3 Angiosarcoma of liver `CC` `HCC`
Kupffer cell sarcoma

C22.4 Other sarcomas of liver `CC` `HCC`

C22.7 Other specified carcinomas of liver `CC` `HCC`

C22.8 Malignant neoplasm of liver, primary, unspecified as to type `CC` `HCC`

C22.9 Malignant neoplasm of liver, not specified as primary or secondary `CC` `HCC`

C23 Malignant neoplasm of gallbladder `CC` `HCC`

✓4ᵗʰ C24 Malignant neoplasm of other and unspecified parts of biliary tract

> **EXCLUDES 1** *malignant neoplasm of intrahepatic bile duct (C22.1)*

C24.Ø Malignant neoplasm of extrahepatic bile duct `CC` `HCC`
Malignant neoplasm of biliary duct or passage NOS
Malignant neoplasm of common bile duct
Malignant neoplasm of cystic duct
Malignant neoplasm of hepatic duct

C24.1 Malignant neoplasm of ampulla of Vater `CC` `HCC`
DEF: Malignant neoplasm in the area of dilation at the juncture of the common bile and pancreatic ducts near the opening into the lumen of the duodenum.

C24.8 Malignant neoplasm of overlapping sites of biliary tract `CC` `HCC`
Malignant neoplasm involving both intrahepatic and extrahepatic bile ducts
Primary malignant neoplasm of two or more contiguous sites of biliary tract

C24.9 Malignant neoplasm of biliary tract, unspecified `CC` `HCC`

✓4ᵗʰ C25 Malignant neoplasm of pancreas

▶Code also if applicable exocrine pancreatic insufficiency◀ (K86.81)
Use additional code to identify:
alcohol abuse and dependence (F1Ø.-)

Pancreas

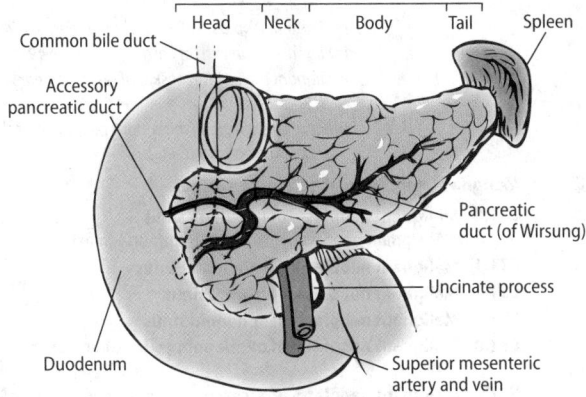

Common bile duct
Accessory pancreatic duct
Head
Neck
Body
Tail
Spleen
Pancreatic duct (of Wirsung)
Uncinate process
Duodenum
Superior mesenteric artery and vein

C25.Ø Malignant neoplasm of head of pancreas `CC` `HCC`

C25.1 Malignant neoplasm of body of pancreas `CC` `HCC`

C25.2 Malignant neoplasm of tail of pancreas `CC` `HCC`

C25.3 Malignant neoplasm of pancreatic duct `CC` `HCC`

C25.4 Malignant neoplasm of endocrine pancreas `CC` `HCC`
Malignant neoplasm of islets of Langerhans
Use additional code to identify any functional activity

✔ Additional Character Required ✓x7ᵗʰ Placeholder Questionable PDx Manifestation Unspecified Dx UPD Unacceptable PDx H1-H14 HAC HCC CMS-HCC Dx HIV HIV Dx

ICD-10-CM 2022 **471**

C25.7   **Malignant neoplasm of other parts of pancreas**   `CC` `HCC`
Malignant neoplasm of neck of pancreas

C25.8   **Malignant neoplasm of overlapping sites of pancreas**   `CC` `HCC`

C25.9   **Malignant neoplasm of pancreas, unspecified**   `CC` `HCC`

✓4ᵗʰ **C26**   **Malignant neoplasm of other and ill-defined digestive organs**

> `EXCLUDES 1`   *malignant neoplasm of peritoneum and retroperitoneum (C48.-)*

C26.0   **Malignant neoplasm of intestinal tract, part unspecified**   `HCC`
Malignant neoplasm of intestine NOS

C26.1   **Malignant neoplasm of spleen**   `HCC`
> `EXCLUDES 1`   *Hodgkin lymphoma (C81.-)*
> *non-Hodgkin lymphoma (C82-C85)*

C26.9   **Malignant neoplasm of ill-defined sites within the digestive system**   `HCC`
Malignant neoplasm of alimentary canal or tract NOS
Malignant neoplasm of gastrointestinal tract NOS
> `EXCLUDES 1`   *malignant neoplasm of abdominal NOS (C76.2)*
> *malignant neoplasm of intra-abdominal NOS (C76.2)*

Malignant neoplasms of respiratory and intrathoracic organs (C30-C39)

> `INCLUDES`   malignant neoplasm of middle ear
> `EXCLUDES 1`   mesothelioma (C45.-)

✓4ᵗʰ **C30**   **Malignant neoplasm of nasal cavity and middle ear**

C30.0   **Malignant neoplasm of nasal cavity**   `HCC`
Malignant neoplasm of cartilage of nose
Malignant neoplasm of nasal concha
Malignant neoplasm of internal nose
Malignant neoplasm of septum of nose
Malignant neoplasm of vestibule of nose
> `EXCLUDES 1`   *malignant neoplasm of nasal bone (C41.0)*
> *malignant neoplasm of nose NOS (C76.0)*
> *malignant neoplasm of olfactory bulb (C72.2-)*
> *malignant neoplasm of posterior margin of nasal septum and choana (C11.3)*
> *malignant melanoma of skin of nose (C43.31)*
> *malignant neoplasm of turbinates (C41.0)*
> *other and unspecified malignant neoplasm of skin of nose (C44.301, C44.311, C44.321, C44.391)*

C30.1   **Malignant neoplasm of middle ear**   `HCC`
Malignant neoplasm of antrum tympanicum
Malignant neoplasm of auditory tube
Malignant neoplasm of eustachian tube
Malignant neoplasm of inner ear
Malignant neoplasm of mastoid air cells
Malignant neoplasm of tympanic cavity
> `EXCLUDES 1`   *malignant neoplasm of auricular canal (external) (C43.2-,C44.2-)*
> *malignant neoplasm of bone of ear (meatus) (C41.0)*
> *malignant neoplasm of cartilage of ear (C49.0)*
> *malignant melanoma of skin of (external) ear (C43.2-)*
> *other and unspecified malignant neoplasm of skin of (external) ear (C44.2-)*

✓4ᵗʰ **C31**   **Malignant neoplasm of accessory sinuses**

C31.0   **Malignant neoplasm of maxillary sinus**   `HCC`
Malignant neoplasm of antrum (Highmore) (maxillary)

C31.1   **Malignant neoplasm of ethmoidal sinus**   `HCC`

C31.2   **Malignant neoplasm of frontal sinus**   `HCC`

C31.3   **Malignant neoplasm of sphenoid sinus**   `HCC`

C31.8   **Malignant neoplasm of overlapping sites of accessory sinuses**   `HCC`

C31.9   **Malignant neoplasm of accessory sinus, unspecified**   `HCC`

✓4ᵗʰ **C32**   **Malignant neoplasm of larynx**
Use additional code to identify:
alcohol abuse and dependence (F10.-)
exposure to environmental tobacco smoke (Z77.22)
exposure to tobacco smoke in the perinatal period (P96.81)
history of tobacco dependence (Z87.891)
occupational exposure to environmental tobacco smoke (Z57.31)
tobacco dependence (F17.-)
tobacco use (Z72.0)

C32.0   **Malignant neoplasm of glottis**   `HCC`
Malignant neoplasm of intrinsic larynx
Malignant neoplasm of laryngeal commissure (anterior)(posterior)
Malignant neoplasm of vocal cord (true) NOS

C32.1   **Malignant neoplasm of supraglottis**   `HCC`
Malignant neoplasm of aryepiglottic fold or interarytenoid fold, laryngeal aspect
Malignant neoplasm of epiglottis (suprahyoid portion) NOS
Malignant neoplasm of extrinsic larynx
Malignant neoplasm of false vocal cord
Malignant neoplasm of posterior (laryngeal) surface of epiglottis
Malignant neoplasm of ventricular bands
> `EXCLUDES 2`   *malignant neoplasm of anterior surface of epiglottis (C10.1)*
> *malignant neoplasm of aryepiglottic fold or interarytenoid fold, hypopharyngeal aspect (C13.1)*
> *malignant neoplasm of aryepiglottic fold or interarytenoid fold, marginal zone (C13.1)*
> *malignant neoplasm of aryepiglottic fold or interarytenoid fold NOS (C13.1)*

C32.2   **Malignant neoplasm of subglottis**   `HCC`

C32.3   **Malignant neoplasm of laryngeal cartilage**   `HCC`

C32.8   **Malignant neoplasm of overlapping sites of larynx**   `HCC`

C32.9   **Malignant neoplasm of larynx, unspecified**   `HCC`

C33   **Malignant neoplasm of trachea**   `CC` `HCC`
Use additional code to identify:
exposure to environmental tobacco smoke (Z77.22)
exposure to tobacco smoke in the perinatal period (P96.81)
history of tobacco dependence (Z87.891)
occupational exposure to environmental tobacco smoke (Z57.31)
tobacco dependence (F17.-)
tobacco use (Z72.0)

✓4ᵗʰ **C34**   **Malignant neoplasm of bronchus and lung**
Use additional code to identify:
exposure to environmental tobacco smoke (Z77.22)
exposure to tobacco smoke in the perinatal period (P96.81)
history of tobacco dependence (Z87.891)
occupational exposure to environmental tobacco smoke (Z57.31)
tobacco dependence (F17.-)
tobacco use (Z72.0)
> `EXCLUDES 1`   *Kaposi's sarcoma of lung (C46.5-)*
> *malignant carcinoid tumor of the bronchus and lung (C7A.090)*

AHA: 2019,1Q,16
TIP: When documented, assign code I31.3 for associated malignant pericardial effusion. If the sole reason for admission is to treat the effusion with no treatment of the lung malignancy rendered, code I31.3 may be sequenced first.

✓5ᵗʰ **C34.0**   **Malignant neoplasm of main bronchus**
Malignant neoplasm of carina
Malignant neoplasm of hilus (of lung)

C34.00   **Malignant neoplasm of unspecified main bronchus**   `CC` `HCC`

C34.01   **Malignant neoplasm of right main bronchus**   `CC` `HCC`

C34.02   **Malignant neoplasm of left main bronchus**   `CC` `HCC`

✓5ᵗʰ **C34.1**   **Malignant neoplasm of upper lobe, bronchus or lung**

C34.10   **Malignant neoplasm of upper lobe, unspecified bronchus or lung**   `CC` `HCC`

C34.11   **Malignant neoplasm of upper lobe, right bronchus or lung**   `CC` `HCC`

C34.12   **Malignant neoplasm of upper lobe, left bronchus or lung**   `CC` `HCC`

C34.2   **Malignant neoplasm of middle lobe, bronchus or lung**   `CC` `HCC`

√5ᵗʰ **C34.3** Malignant neoplasm of lower lobe, bronchus or lung

C34.30 Malignant neoplasm of lower lobe, unspecified bronchus or lung　CC HCC

C34.31 Malignant neoplasm of lower lobe, right bronchus or lung　CC HCC

C34.32 Malignant neoplasm of lower lobe, left bronchus or lung　CC HCC

√5ᵗʰ **C34.8** Malignant neoplasm of overlapping sites of bronchus and lung

C34.80 Malignant neoplasm of overlapping sites of unspecified bronchus and lung　CC HCC

C34.81 Malignant neoplasm of overlapping sites of right bronchus and lung　CC HCC

C34.82 Malignant neoplasm of overlapping sites of left bronchus and lung　CC HCC

√5ᵗʰ **C34.9** Malignant neoplasm of unspecified part of bronchus or lung

C34.90 Malignant neoplasm of unspecified part of unspecified bronchus or lung　CC HCC
Lung cancer NOS

C34.91 Malignant neoplasm of unspecified part of right bronchus or lung　CC HCC

C34.92 Malignant neoplasm of unspecified part of left bronchus or lung　CC HCC

C37 Malignant neoplasm of thymus　CC HCC
　EXCLUDES 1　malignant carcinoid tumor of the thymus (C7A.091)

√4ᵗʰ **C38** Malignant neoplasm of heart, mediastinum and pleura
　EXCLUDES 1　mesothelioma (C45.-)

C38.0 Malignant neoplasm of heart
Malignant neoplasm of pericardium
　EXCLUDES 1　malignant neoplasm of great vessels (C49.3)

C38.1 Malignant neoplasm of anterior mediastinum　CC HCC

C38.2 Malignant neoplasm of posterior mediastinum　CC HCC

C38.3 Malignant neoplasm of mediastinum, part unspecified　CC HCC

C38.4 Malignant neoplasm of pleura　CC HCC

C38.8 Malignant neoplasm of overlapping sites of heart, mediastinum and pleura　CC HCC

√4ᵗʰ **C39** Malignant neoplasm of other and ill-defined sites in the respiratory system and intrathoracic organs
Use additional code to identify:
exposure to environmental tobacco smoke (Z77.22)
exposure to tobacco smoke in the perinatal period (P96.81)
history of tobacco dependence (Z87.891)
occupational exposure to environmental tobacco smoke (Z57.31)
tobacco dependence (F17.-)
tobacco use (Z72.0)
　EXCLUDES 1　intrathoracic malignant neoplasm NOS (C76.1)
　　thoracic malignant neoplasm NOS (C76.1)

C39.0 Malignant neoplasm of upper respiratory tract, part unspecified　HCC

C39.9 Malignant neoplasm of lower respiratory tract, part unspecified　HCC
Malignant neoplasm of respiratory tract NOS

Malignant neoplasms of bone and articular cartilage (C40-C41)

INCLUDES　malignant neoplasm of cartilage (articular) (joint)
　　malignant neoplasm of periosteum
EXCLUDES 1　malignant neoplasm of bone marrow NOS (C96.9)
　　malignant neoplasm of synovia (C49.-)

√4ᵗʰ **C40** Malignant neoplasm of bone and articular cartilage of limbs
Use additional code to identify major osseous defect, if applicable (M89.7-)

√5ᵗʰ **C40.0** Malignant neoplasm of scapula and long bones of upper limb

C40.00 Malignant neoplasm of scapula and long bones of unspecified upper limb　CC HCC

C40.01 Malignant neoplasm of scapula and long bones of right upper limb　CC HCC

C40.02 Malignant neoplasm of scapula and long bones of left upper limb　CC HCC

√5ᵗʰ **C40.1** Malignant neoplasm of short bones of upper limb

C40.10 Malignant neoplasm of short bones of unspecified upper limb　CC HCC

C40.11 Malignant neoplasm of short bones of right upper limb　CC HCC

C40.12 Malignant neoplasm of short bones of left upper limb　CC HCC

√5ᵗʰ **C40.2** Malignant neoplasm of long bones of lower limb

C40.20 Malignant neoplasm of long bones of unspecified lower limb　CC HCC

C40.21 Malignant neoplasm of long bones of right lower limb　CC HCC

C40.22 Malignant neoplasm of long bones of left lower limb　CC HCC

√5ᵗʰ **C40.3** Malignant neoplasm of short bones of lower limb

C40.30 Malignant neoplasm of short bones of unspecified lower limb　CC HCC

C40.31 Malignant neoplasm of short bones of right lower limb　CC HCC

C40.32 Malignant neoplasm of short bones of left lower limb　CC HCC

√5ᵗʰ **C40.8** Malignant neoplasm of overlapping sites of bone and articular cartilage of limb

C40.80 Malignant neoplasm of overlapping sites of bone and articular cartilage of unspecified limb　CC HCC

C40.81 Malignant neoplasm of overlapping sites of bone and articular cartilage of right limb　CC HCC

C40.82 Malignant neoplasm of overlapping sites of bone and articular cartilage of left limb　CC HCC

√5ᵗʰ **C40.9** Malignant neoplasm of unspecified bones and articular cartilage of limb

C40.90 Malignant neoplasm of unspecified bones and articular cartilage of unspecified limb　CC HCC

C40.91 Malignant neoplasm of unspecified bones and articular cartilage of right limb　CC HCC

C40.92 Malignant neoplasm of unspecified bones and articular cartilage of left limb　CC HCC

√4ᵗʰ **C41** Malignant neoplasm of bone and articular cartilage of other and unspecified sites
　EXCLUDES 1　malignant neoplasm of bones of limbs (C40.-)
　　malignant neoplasm of cartilage of ear (C49.0)
　　malignant neoplasm of cartilage of eyelid (C49.0)
　　malignant neoplasm of cartilage of larynx (C32.3)
　　malignant neoplasm of cartilage of limbs (C40.-)
　　malignant neoplasm of cartilage of nose (C30.0)

C41.0 Malignant neoplasm of bones of skull and face　CC HCC
Malignant neoplasm of maxilla (superior)
Malignant neoplasm of orbital bone
　EXCLUDES 2　carcinoma, any type except intraosseous or odontogenic of:
　　maxillary sinus (C31.0)
　　upper jaw (C03.0)
　　malignant neoplasm of jaw bone (lower) (C41.1)

C41.1 Malignant neoplasm of mandible　CC HCC
Malignant neoplasm of inferior maxilla
Malignant neoplasm of lower jaw bone
　EXCLUDES 2　carcinoma, any type except intraosseous or odontogenic of:
　　jaw NOS (C03.9)
　　lower (C03.1)
　　malignant neoplasm of upper jaw bone (C41.0)

C41.2 Malignant neoplasm of vertebral column　CC HCC
　EXCLUDES 1　malignant neoplasm of sacrum and coccyx (C41.4)

C41.3 Malignant neoplasm of ribs, sternum and clavicle　CC HCC

C41.4 Malignant neoplasm of pelvic bones, sacrum and coccyx　CC HCC

C41.9 Malignant neoplasm of bone and articular cartilage, unspecified　CC HCC

Melanoma and other malignant neoplasms of skin (C43-C44)

√4ᵗʰ **C43** Malignant melanoma of skin
　EXCLUDES 1　melanoma in situ (D03.-)
　EXCLUDES 2　malignant melanoma of skin of genital organs (C51-C52, C60.-, C63.-)
　　Merkel cell carcinoma (C4A.-)
　　sites other than skin - code to malignant neoplasm of the site

C43.0 Malignant melanoma of lip　HCC
　EXCLUDES 1　malignant neoplasm of vermilion border of lip (C00.0-C00.2)

✔ Additional Character Required　√x7ᵗʰ Placeholder　Questionable PDx　Manifestation　Unspecified Dx　UPD Unacceptable PDx　H1-H14 HAC　HCC CMS-HCC Dx　HIV HIV Dx

ICD-10-CM 2022　　　　　　　　　　　　　　473

☑5ᵗʰ **C43.1 Malignant melanoma of** eyelid, including canthus
    AHA: 2018,4Q,4

  C43.10 Malignant melanoma of unspecified eyelid, including canthus HCC

☑6ᵗʰ **C43.11 Malignant melanoma of** right **eyelid, including canthus**

    C43.111 Malignant melanoma of right upper **eyelid, including canthus**

    C43.112 Malignant melanoma of right lower **eyelid, including canthus** HCC

☑6ᵗʰ **C43.12 Malignant melanoma of** left **eyelid, including canthus**

    C43.121 Malignant melanoma of left upper **eyelid, including canthus**

    C43.122 Malignant melanoma of left lower **eyelid, including canthus** HCC

☑5ᵗʰ **C43.2 Malignant melanoma of** ear and external auricular canal

  C43.20 Malignant melanoma of unspecified ear and external auricular canal HCC

  C43.21 Malignant melanoma of right **ear and external auricular canal**

  C43.22 Malignant melanoma of left **ear and external auricular canal** HCC

☑5ᵗʰ **C43.3 Malignant melanoma of other and unspecified** parts of face

  C43.30 Malignant melanoma of unspecified part of face HCC

  C43.31 Malignant melanoma of nose HCC

  C43.39 Malignant melanoma of other parts of face HCC

C43.4 Malignant melanoma of scalp and neck HCC

☑5ᵗʰ **C43.5 Malignant melanoma of** trunk

    EXCLUDES 2   *malignant neoplasm of anus NOS (C21.0)*
         malignant neoplasm of scrotum (C63.2)

  C43.51 Malignant melanoma of anal skin HCC
    Malignant melanoma of anal margin
    Malignant melanoma of perianal skin

  C43.52 Malignant melanoma of skin of breast HCC

  C43.59 Malignant melanoma of other part of trunk HCC

☑5ᵗʰ **C43.6 Malignant melanoma of** upper limb, including shoulder

  C43.60 Malignant melanoma of unspecified upper limb, including shoulder HCC

  C43.61 Malignant melanoma of right **upper limb, including shoulder** HCC

  C43.62 Malignant melanoma of left **upper limb, including shoulder** HCC

☑5ᵗʰ **C43.7 Malignant melanoma of** lower limb, including hip

  C43.70 Malignant melanoma of unspecified lower limb, including hip HCC

  C43.71 Malignant melanoma of right **lower limb, including hip** HCC

  C43.72 Malignant melanoma of left **lower limb, including hip** HCC

C43.8 Malignant melanoma of overlapping sites of skin HCC

C43.9 Malignant melanoma of skin, unspecified HCC
  Malignant melanoma of unspecified site of skin
  Melanoma (malignant) NOS

☑4ᵗʰ **C4A Merkel cell carcinoma**

  DEF: Malignant cutaneous cancer predominantly found in elderly patients with sun exposure that usually presents as a flesh-colored or bluish-red lump typically seen on the neck, head, and face.

C4A.0 Merkel cell carcinoma of lip HCC

    EXCLUDES 1   *malignant neoplasm of vermilion border of lip (C00.0-C00.2)*

☑5ᵗʰ **C4A.1 Merkel cell carcinoma of** eyelid, including canthus

    AHA: 2018,4Q,4

  C4A.10 Merkel cell carcinoma of unspecified eyelid, including canthus HCC

☑6ᵗʰ **C4A.11 Merkel cell carcinoma of** right **eyelid, including canthus**

    C4A.111 Merkel cell carcinoma of right upper **eyelid, including canthus**

    C4A.112 Merkel cell carcinoma of right lower **eyelid, including canthus** HCC

☑6ᵗʰ **C4A.12 Merkel cell carcinoma of** left **eyelid, including canthus**

    C4A.121 Merkel cell carcinoma of left upper **eyelid, including canthus** HCC

    C4A.122 Merkel cell carcinoma of left lower **eyelid, including canthus** HCC

☑5ᵗʰ **C4A.2 Merkel cell carcinoma of** ear and external auricular canal

  C4A.20 Merkel cell carcinoma of unspecified ear and external auricular canal HCC

  C4A.21 Merkel cell carcinoma of right **ear and external auricular canal** HCC

  C4A.22 Merkel cell carcinoma of left **ear and external auricular canal**

☑5ᵗʰ **C4A.3 Merkel cell carcinoma of other and unspecified** parts of face

  C4A.30 Merkel cell carcinoma of unspecified part of face HCC

  C4A.31 Merkel cell carcinoma of nose HCC

  C4A.39 Merkel cell carcinoma of other parts of face HCC

C4A.4 Merkel cell carcinoma of scalp and neck HCC

☑5ᵗʰ **C4A.5 Merkel cell carcinoma of** trunk

    EXCLUDES 2   *malignant neoplasm of anus NOS (C21.0)*
         malignant neoplasm of scrotum (C63.2)

  C4A.51 Merkel cell carcinoma of anal skin HCC
    Merkel cell carcinoma of anal margin
    Merkel cell carcinoma of perianal skin

  C4A.52 Merkel cell carcinoma of skin of breast HCC

  C4A.59 Merkel cell carcinoma of other part of trunk HCC

☑5ᵗʰ **C4A.6 Merkel cell carcinoma of** upper limb, including shoulder

  C4A.60 Merkel cell carcinoma of unspecified upper limb, including shoulder HCC

  C4A.61 Merkel cell carcinoma of right **upper limb, including shoulder** HCC

  C4A.62 Merkel cell carcinoma of left **upper limb, including shoulder** HCC

☑5ᵗʰ **C4A.7 Merkel cell carcinoma of** lower limb, including hip

  C4A.70 Merkel cell carcinoma of unspecified lower limb, including hip HCC

  C4A.71 Merkel cell carcinoma of right **lower limb, including hip** HCC

  C4A.72 Merkel cell carcinoma of left **lower limb, including hip** HCC

C4A.8 Merkel cell carcinoma of overlapping sites HCC

C4A.9 Merkel cell carcinoma, unspecified HCC
  Merkel cell carcinoma of unspecified site
  Merkel cell carcinoma NOS

☑4ᵗʰ **C44 Other and unspecified malignant neoplasm** of skin

    INCLUDES   malignant neoplasm of sebaceous glands
         malignant neoplasm of sweat glands

    EXCLUDES 1   *Kaposi's sarcoma of skin (C46.0)*
         malignant melanoma of skin (C43.-)
         malignant neoplasm of skin of genital organs (C51-C52, C60.-, C63.2)
         Merkel cell carcinoma (C4A.-)

  DEF: Basal cell carcinoma: Abnormal growth of skin cells that arises from the deepest layer of the epidermis and may present as an open sore, red patches, pink growth, or scar. Typically caused by sun exposure, it is one of the most common forms of skin cancer.

  DEF: Squamous cell carcinoma: Uncontrolled growth of abnormal skin cells that arises from the outer layers of the skin (epidermis) and may present as an open sore. It is characterized by a firm, red nodule, elevated growth with a central depression, or a flat sore with a scaly crust.

☑5ᵗʰ **C44.0 Other and unspecified malignant neoplasm of skin of** lip

    EXCLUDES 1   *malignant neoplasm of lip (C00.-)*

  C44.00 Unspecified malignant neoplasm of skin of lip

  C44.01 Basal cell carcinoma of skin of lip

  C44.02 Squamous cell carcinoma of skin of lip

  C44.09 Other specified malignant neoplasm of skin of lip

☑5ᵗʰ **C44.1 Other and unspecified malignant neoplasm of skin of** eyelid, including canthus

    EXCLUDES 1   *connective tissue of eyelid (C49.0)*

    AHA: 2018,4Q,4

☑6ᵗʰ **C44.10 Unspecified malignant neoplasm of skin of eyelid, including canthus**

  C44.101 Unspecified malignant neoplasm of skin of unspecified eyelid, including canthus

☑7ᵗʰ **C44.102 Unspecified malignant neoplasm of skin of** right **eyelid, including canthus**

  C44.1021 Unspecified malignant neoplasm of skin of right upper **eyelid, including canthus**

N Newborn: 0   P Pediatric: 0-17   M Maternity: 9-64   A Adult: 15-124   MCC Major Complication/Comorbidity   CC Complication/Comorbidity   SW Severe Wound Dx

474

ICD-10-CM 2022

C44.1022   Unspecified malignant neoplasm of skin of right lower eyelid, including canthus

✓7ᵗʰ C44.109   Unspecified malignant neoplasm of skin of left eyelid, including canthus

    C44.1091   Unspecified malignant neoplasm of skin of left upper eyelid, including canthus

    C44.1092   Unspecified malignant neoplasm of skin of left lower eyelid, including canthus

✓6ᵗʰ C44.11   Basal cell carcinoma of skin of eyelid, including canthus

    C44.111   Basal cell carcinoma of skin of unspecified eyelid, including canthus

   ✓7ᵗʰ C44.112   Basal cell carcinoma of skin of right eyelid, including canthus

     C44.1121   Basal cell carcinoma of skin of right upper eyelid, including canthus

     C44.1122   Basal cell carcinoma of skin of right lower eyelid, including canthus

   ✓7ᵗʰ C44.119   Basal cell carcinoma of skin of left eyelid, including canthus

     C44.1191   Basal cell carcinoma of skin of left upper eyelid, including canthus

     C44.1192   Basal cell carcinoma of skin of left lower eyelid, including canthus

✓6ᵗʰ C44.12   Squamous cell carcinoma of skin of eyelid, including canthus

    C44.121   Squamous cell carcinoma of skin of unspecified eyelid, including canthus

   ✓7ᵗʰ C44.122   Squamous cell carcinoma of skin of right eyelid, including canthus

     C44.1221   Squamous cell carcinoma of skin of right upper eyelid, including canthus

     C44.1222   Squamous cell carcinoma of skin of right lower eyelid, including canthus

   ✓7ᵗʰ C44.129   Squamous cell carcinoma of skin of left eyelid, including canthus

     C44.1291   Squamous cell carcinoma of skin of left upper eyelid, including canthus

     C44.1292   Squamous cell carcinoma of skin of left lower eyelid, including canthus

✓6ᵗʰ C44.13   Sebaceous cell carcinoma of skin of eyelid, including canthus

    C44.131   Sebaceous cell carcinoma of skin of unspecified eyelid, including canthus

   ✓7ᵗʰ C44.132   Sebaceous cell carcinoma of skin of right eyelid, including canthus

     C44.1321   Sebaceous cell carcinoma of skin of right upper eyelid, including canthus

     C44.1322   Sebaceous cell carcinoma of skin of right lower eyelid, including canthus

   ✓7ᵗʰ C44.139   Sebaceous cell carcinoma of skin of left eyelid, including canthus

     C44.1391   Sebaceous cell carcinoma of skin of left upper eyelid, including canthus

     C44.1392   Sebaceous cell carcinoma of skin of left lower eyelid, including canthus

✓6ᵗʰ C44.19   Other specified malignant neoplasm of skin of eyelid, including canthus

    C44.191   Other specified malignant neoplasm of skin of unspecified eyelid, including canthus

   ✓7ᵗʰ C44.192   Other specified malignant neoplasm of skin of right eyelid, including canthus

     C44.1921   Other specified malignant neoplasm of skin of right upper eyelid, including canthus

     C44.1922   Other specified malignant neoplasm of skin of right lower eyelid, including canthus

   ✓7ᵗʰ C44.199   Other specified malignant neoplasm of skin of left eyelid, including canthus

     C44.1991   Other specified malignant neoplasm of skin of left upper eyelid, including canthus

     C44.1992   Other specified malignant neoplasm of skin of left lower eyelid, including canthus

✓5ᵗʰ C44.2   Other and unspecified malignant neoplasm of skin of ear and external auricular canal

    EXCLUDES 1   connective tissue of ear (C49.0)

   ✓6ᵗʰ C44.20   Unspecified malignant neoplasm of skin of ear and external auricular canal

    C44.201   Unspecified malignant neoplasm of skin of unspecified ear and external auricular canal

    C44.202   Unspecified malignant neoplasm of skin of right ear and external auricular canal

    C44.209   Unspecified malignant neoplasm of skin of left ear and external auricular canal

   ✓6ᵗʰ C44.21   Basal cell carcinoma of skin of ear and external auricular canal

    C44.211   Basal cell carcinoma of skin of unspecified ear and external auricular canal

    C44.212   Basal cell carcinoma of skin of right ear and external auricular canal

    C44.219   Basal cell carcinoma of skin of left ear and external auricular canal

   ✓6ᵗʰ C44.22   Squamous cell carcinoma of skin of ear and external auricular canal

    C44.221   Squamous cell carcinoma of skin of unspecified ear and external auricular canal

    C44.222   Squamous cell carcinoma of skin of right ear and external auricular canal

    C44.229   Squamous cell carcinoma of skin of left ear and external auricular canal

   ✓6ᵗʰ C44.29   Other specified malignant neoplasm of skin of ear and external auricular canal

    C44.291   Other specified malignant neoplasm of skin of unspecified ear and external auricular canal

    C44.292   Other specified malignant neoplasm of skin of right ear and external auricular canal

    C44.299   Other specified malignant neoplasm of skin of left ear and external auricular canal

✓5ᵗʰ C44.3   Other and unspecified malignant neoplasm of skin of other and unspecified parts of face

   ✓6ᵗʰ C44.30   Unspecified malignant neoplasm of skin of other and unspecified parts of face

    C44.300   Unspecified malignant neoplasm of skin of unspecified part of face

    C44.301   Unspecified malignant neoplasm of skin of nose

    C44.309   Unspecified malignant neoplasm of skin of other parts of face

   ✓6ᵗʰ C44.31   Basal cell carcinoma of skin of other and unspecified parts of face

    C44.310   Basal cell carcinoma of skin of unspecified parts of face

    C44.311   Basal cell carcinoma of skin of nose

    C44.319   Basal cell carcinoma of skin of other parts of face

   ✓6ᵗʰ C44.32   Squamous cell carcinoma of skin of other and unspecified parts of face

    C44.320   Squamous cell carcinoma of skin of unspecified parts of face

    C44.321   Squamous cell carcinoma of skin of nose

    C44.329   Squamous cell carcinoma of skin of other parts of face

   ✓6ᵗʰ C44.39   Other specified malignant neoplasm of skin of other and unspecified parts of face

    C44.390   Other specified malignant neoplasm of skin of unspecified parts of face

    C44.391   Other specified malignant neoplasm of skin of nose

    C44.399   Other specified malignant neoplasm of skin of other parts of face

✔ Additional Character Required   ✓x7ᵗʰ Placeholder   Questionable PDx   Manifestation   Unspecified Dx   **UPD** Unacceptable PDx   **H1**-**H14** HAC   **HCC** CMS-HCC Dx   **HIV** HIV Dx

ICD-10-CM 2022   475

Chapter 2. Neoplasms

C44.4–C45.7

✓5ᵗʰ **C44.4** **Other and unspecified malignant neoplasm of skin of** scalp and neck

    C44.40 Unspecified malignant neoplasm of skin of scalp and neck

    C44.41 Basal cell carcinoma of skin of scalp and neck

    C44.42 Squamous cell carcinoma of skin of scalp and neck

    C44.49 Other specified malignant neoplasm of skin of scalp and neck

✓5ᵗʰ **C44.5** **Other and unspecified malignant neoplasm of** skin of trunk

    EXCLUDES 1   anus NOS (C21.0)

                   scrotum (C63.2)

  ✓6ᵗʰ **C44.50** Unspecified malignant neoplasm of skin of trunk

    C44.500 Unspecified malignant neoplasm of anal skin

            Unspecified malignant neoplasm of anal margin

            Unspecified malignant neoplasm of perianal skin

    C44.501 Unspecified malignant neoplasm of skin of breast

    C44.509 Unspecified malignant neoplasm of skin of other part of trunk

  ✓6ᵗʰ **C44.51** Basal cell carcinoma of skin of trunk

    C44.510 Basal cell carcinoma of anal skin

            Basal cell carcinoma of anal margin

            Basal cell carcinoma of perianal skin

    C44.511 Basal cell carcinoma of skin of breast

    C44.519 Basal cell carcinoma of skin of other part of trunk

  ✓6ᵗʰ **C44.52** Squamous cell carcinoma of skin of trunk

    C44.520 Squamous cell carcinoma of anal skin

            Squamous cell carcinoma of anal margin

            Squamous cell carcinoma of perianal skin

    C44.521 Squamous cell carcinoma of skin of breast

    C44.529 Squamous cell carcinoma of skin of other part of trunk

  ✓6ᵗʰ **C44.59** Other specified malignant neoplasm of skin of trunk

    C44.590 Other specified malignant neoplasm of anal skin

            Other specified malignant neoplasm of anal margin

            Other specified malignant neoplasm of perianal skin

    C44.591 Other specified malignant neoplasm of skin of breast

    C44.599 Other specified malignant neoplasm of skin of other part of trunk

✓5ᵗʰ **C44.6** **Other and unspecified malignant neoplasm of skin of** upper limb, including shoulder

  ✓6ᵗʰ **C44.60** Unspecified malignant neoplasm of skin of upper limb, including shoulder

    C44.601 Unspecified malignant neoplasm of skin of unspecified upper limb, including shoulder

    C44.602 Unspecified malignant neoplasm of skin of right upper limb, including shoulder

    C44.609 Unspecified malignant neoplasm of skin of left upper limb, including shoulder

  ✓6ᵗʰ **C44.61** Basal cell carcinoma of skin of upper limb, including shoulder

    C44.611 Basal cell carcinoma of skin of unspecified upper limb, including shoulder

    C44.612 Basal cell carcinoma of skin of right upper limb, including shoulder

    C44.619 Basal cell carcinoma of skin of left upper limb, including shoulder

  ✓6ᵗʰ **C44.62** Squamous cell carcinoma of skin of upper limb, including shoulder

    C44.621 Squamous cell carcinoma of skin of unspecified upper limb, including shoulder

    C44.622 Squamous cell carcinoma of skin of right upper limb, including shoulder

    C44.629 Squamous cell carcinoma of skin of left upper limb, including shoulder

  ✓6ᵗʰ **C44.69** Other specified malignant neoplasm of skin of upper limb, including shoulder

    C44.691 Other specified malignant neoplasm of skin of unspecified upper limb, including shoulder

    C44.692 Other specified malignant neoplasm of skin of right upper limb, including shoulder

    C44.699 Other specified malignant neoplasm of skin of left upper limb, including shoulder

✓5ᵗʰ **C44.7** **Other and unspecified malignant neoplasm of skin of** lower limb, including hip

  ✓6ᵗʰ **C44.70** Unspecified malignant neoplasm of skin of lower limb, including hip

    C44.701 Unspecified malignant neoplasm of skin of unspecified lower limb, including hip

    C44.702 Unspecified malignant neoplasm of skin of right lower limb, including hip

    C44.709 Unspecified malignant neoplasm of skin of left lower limb, including hip

  ✓6ᵗʰ **C44.71** Basal cell carcinoma of skin of lower limb, including hip

    C44.711 Basal cell carcinoma of skin of unspecified lower limb, including hip

    C44.712 Basal cell carcinoma of skin of right lower limb, including hip

    C44.719 Basal cell carcinoma of skin of left lower limb, including hip

  ✓6ᵗʰ **C44.72** Squamous cell carcinoma of skin of lower limb, including hip

    C44.721 Squamous cell carcinoma of skin of unspecified lower limb, including hip

    C44.722 Squamous cell carcinoma of skin of right lower limb, including hip

    C44.729 Squamous cell carcinoma of skin of left lower limb, including hip

  ✓6ᵗʰ **C44.79** Other specified malignant neoplasm of skin of lower limb, including hip

    C44.791 Other specified malignant neoplasm of skin of unspecified lower limb, including hip

    C44.792 Other specified malignant neoplasm of skin of right lower limb, including hip

    C44.799 Other specified malignant neoplasm of skin of left lower limb, including hip

✓5ᵗʰ **C44.8** **Other and unspecified malignant neoplasm of** overlapping sites of skin

    C44.80 Unspecified malignant neoplasm of overlapping sites of skin

    C44.81 Basal cell carcinoma of overlapping sites of skin

    C44.82 Squamous cell carcinoma of overlapping sites of skin

    C44.89 Other specified malignant neoplasm of overlapping sites of skin

✓5ᵗʰ **C44.9** **Other and unspecified malignant neoplasm of skin, unspecified**

    C44.90 Unspecified malignant neoplasm of skin, unspecified

            Malignant neoplasm of unspecified site of skin

    C44.91 Basal cell carcinoma of skin, unspecified

    C44.92 Squamous cell carcinoma of skin, unspecified

    C44.99 Other specified malignant neoplasm of skin, unspecified

Malignant neoplasms of mesothelial and soft tissue (C45-C49)

✓4ᵗʰ **C45** **Mesothelioma**

    DEF: Rare type of cancer that forms in the thin layer of protective tissue that covers the majority of internal organs (mesothelium).

  C45.0 **Mesothelioma of** pleura   CC HCC

    EXCLUDES 1   other malignant neoplasm of pleura (C38.4)

    AHA: 2017,2Q,11

    TIP: For pleural mesothelioma that has metastasized to the chest wall, assign this code for the primary site along with C79.89 for metastatic cancer in the chest wall.

  C45.1 **Mesothelioma of** peritoneum   CC HCC

    Mesothelioma of cul-de-sac

    Mesothelioma of mesentery

    Mesothelioma of mesocolon

    Mesothelioma of omentum

    Mesothelioma of peritoneum (parietal) (pelvic)

    EXCLUDES 1   other malignant neoplasm of soft tissue of peritoneum (C48.-)

  C45.2 **Mesothelioma of** pericardium   CC HCC

    EXCLUDES 1   other malignant neoplasm of pericardium (C38.0)

  C45.7 **Mesothelioma of other sites**   HCC

N Newborn: 0   P Pediatric: 0-17   M Maternity: 9-64   A Adult: 15-124   MCC Major Complication/Comorbidity   CC Complication/Comorbidity   SW Severe Wound Dx

476   ICD-10-CM 2022

C45.9 **Mesothelioma, unspecified**   HCC

✓4ᵗʰ **C46 Kaposi's sarcoma**

Code first any human immunodeficiency virus [HIV] disease (B20)

DEF: Malignant neoplasm that causes patches of abnormal tissue to grow under the skin, in the lining of the mouth, nose, and throat, in lymph nodes, or in other visceral organs. Kaposi's sarcoma is caused by human herpesvirus8 (HHV8).

C46.0 **Kaposi's sarcoma of** skin   HIV CC HCC

C46.1 **Kaposi's sarcoma of** soft tissue   HIV CC HCC

Kaposi's sarcoma of blood vessel

Kaposi's sarcoma of connective tissue

Kaposi's sarcoma of fascia

Kaposi's sarcoma of ligament

Kaposi's sarcoma of lymphatic(s) NEC

Kaposi's sarcoma of muscle

EXCLUDES 2 *Kaposi's sarcoma of lymph glands and nodes (C46.3)*

C46.2 **Kaposi's sarcoma of** palate   HIV CC HCC

C46.3 **Kaposi's sarcoma of** lymph nodes   HIV CC HCC

C46.4 **Kaposi's sarcoma of** gastrointestinal sites   HIV CC HCC

✓5ᵗʰ **C46.5** **Kaposi's sarcoma of** lung

AHA: 2019,1Q,16

TIP: When associated malignant pericardial effusion is documented, assign code I31.3. If the sole reason for admission is to treat the effusion with no treatment of the lung malignancy rendered, code I31.3 may be sequenced first.

C46.50 **Kaposi's sarcoma of unspecified lung**   HIV CC HCC

C46.51 **Kaposi's sarcoma of** right **lung**   HIV CC HCC

C46.52 **Kaposi's sarcoma of** left **lung**   HIV CC HCC

C46.7 **Kaposi's sarcoma of other sites**   HIV CC HCC

C46.9 **Kaposi's sarcoma, unspecified**   HIV CC HCC

Kaposi's sarcoma of unspecified site

✓4ᵗʰ **C47 Malignant neoplasm of peripheral nerves and autonomic nervous system**

INCLUDES malignant neoplasm of sympathetic and parasympathetic nerves and ganglia

EXCLUDES 1 *Kaposi's sarcoma of soft tissue (C46.1)*

C47.0 **Malignant neoplasm of peripheral nerves of** head, face and neck   CC HCC

EXCLUDES 1 *malignant neoplasm of peripheral nerves of orbit (C69.6-)*

✓5ᵗʰ **C47.1** **Malignant neoplasm of peripheral nerves of** upper limb, including shoulder

C47.10 **Malignant neoplasm of peripheral nerves of unspecified upper limb, including shoulder**   CC HCC

C47.11 **Malignant neoplasm of peripheral nerves of** right **upper limb, including shoulder**   CC HCC

C47.12 **Malignant neoplasm of peripheral nerves of** left **upper limb, including shoulder**   CC HCC

✓5ᵗʰ **C47.2** **Malignant neoplasm of peripheral nerves of** lower limb, including hip

C47.20 **Malignant neoplasm of peripheral nerves of unspecified lower limb, including hip**   CC HCC

C47.21 **Malignant neoplasm of peripheral nerves of** right **lower limb, including hip**   CC HCC

C47.22 **Malignant neoplasm of peripheral nerves of** left **lower limb, including hip**   CC HCC

C47.3 **Malignant neoplasm of peripheral nerves of** thorax   CC HCC

C47.4 **Malignant neoplasm of peripheral nerves of** abdomen   CC HCC

C47.5 **Malignant neoplasm of peripheral nerves of** pelvis   CC HCC

C47.6 **Malignant neoplasm of peripheral nerves of** trunk, unspecified   CC HCC

Malignant neoplasm of peripheral nerves of unspecified part of trunk

C47.8 **Malignant neoplasm of** overlapping sites **of peripheral nerves and autonomic nervous system**   CC HCC

C47.9 **Malignant neoplasm of peripheral nerves and autonomic nervous system, unspecified**   CC HCC

Malignant neoplasm of unspecified site of peripheral nerves and autonomic nervous system

✓4ᵗʰ **C48 Malignant neoplasm of** retroperitoneum and peritoneum

EXCLUDES 1 *Kaposi's sarcoma of connective tissue (C46.1)*
mesothelioma (C45.-)

C48.0 **Malignant neoplasm of** retroperitoneum   CC HCC

C48.1 **Malignant neoplasm of** specified parts of peritoneum   CC HCC

Malignant neoplasm of cul-de-sac

Malignant neoplasm of mesentery

Malignant neoplasm of mesocolon

Malignant neoplasm of omentum

Malignant neoplasm of parietal peritoneum

Malignant neoplasm of pelvic peritoneum

C48.2 **Malignant neoplasm of** peritoneum, unspecified   CC HCC

C48.8 **Malignant neoplasm of** overlapping sites **of retroperitoneum and peritoneum**   CC HCC

✓4ᵗʰ **C49 Malignant neoplasm of** other connective and soft tissue

INCLUDES malignant neoplasm of blood vessel

malignant neoplasm of bursa

malignant neoplasm of cartilage

malignant neoplasm of fascia

malignant neoplasm of fat

malignant neoplasm of ligament, except uterine

malignant neoplasm of lymphatic vessel

malignant neoplasm of muscle

malignant neoplasm of synovia

malignant neoplasm of tendon (sheath)

EXCLUDES 1 *malignant neoplasm of cartilage (of):*
articular (C40-C41)
larynx (C32.3)
nose (C30.0)
malignant neoplasm of connective tissue of breast (C50.-)

EXCLUDES 2 *Kaposi's sarcoma of soft tissue (C46.1)*
malignant neoplasm of heart (C38.0)
malignant neoplasm of peripheral nerves and autonomic nervous system (C47.-)
malignant neoplasm of peritoneum (C48.2)
malignant neoplasm of retroperitoneum (C48.0)
malignant neoplasm of uterine ligament (C57.3)
mesothelioma (C45.-)

C49.0 **Malignant neoplasm of connective and soft tissue of** head, face and neck   CC HCC

Malignant neoplasm of connective tissue of ear

Malignant neoplasm of connective tissue of eyelid

EXCLUDES 1 *connective tissue of orbit (C69.6-)*

✓5ᵗʰ **C49.1** **Malignant neoplasm of connective and soft tissue of** upper limb, including shoulder

C49.10 **Malignant neoplasm of connective and soft tissue of unspecified upper limb, including shoulder**   CC HCC

C49.11 **Malignant neoplasm of connective and soft tissue of** right **upper limb, including shoulder**   CC HCC

C49.12 **Malignant neoplasm of connective and soft tissue of** left **upper limb, including shoulder**   CC HCC

✓5ᵗʰ **C49.2** **Malignant neoplasm of connective and soft tissue of** lower limb, including hip

C49.20 **Malignant neoplasm of connective and soft tissue of unspecified lower limb, including hip**   CC HCC

C49.21 **Malignant neoplasm of connective and soft tissue of** right **lower limb, including hip**   CC HCC

C49.22 **Malignant neoplasm of connective and soft tissue of** left **lower limb, including hip**   CC HCC

C49.3 **Malignant neoplasm of connective and soft tissue of** thorax   CC HCC

Malignant neoplasm of axilla

Malignant neoplasm of diaphragm

Malignant neoplasm of great vessels

EXCLUDES 1 *malignant neoplasm of breast (C50.-)*
malignant neoplasm of heart (C38.0)
malignant neoplasm of mediastinum (C38.1-C38.3)
malignant neoplasm of thymus (C37)

AHA: 2015,3Q,19

C49.4 **Malignant neoplasm of connective and soft tissue of** abdomen   CC HCC

Malignant neoplasm of abdominal wall

Malignant neoplasm of hypochondrium

C49.5 **Malignant neoplasm of connective and soft tissue of** pelvis   CC HCC

Malignant neoplasm of buttock

Malignant neoplasm of groin

Malignant neoplasm of perineum

C49.6 Malignant neoplasm of connective and soft tissue of trunk, unspecified　CC HCC
Malignant neoplasm of back NOS

C49.8 Malignant neoplasm of overlapping sites of connective and soft tissue　CC HCC
Primary malignant neoplasm of two or more contiguous sites of connective and soft tissue

C49.9 Malignant neoplasm of connective and soft tissue, unspecified　CC HCC

√5ᵗʰ **C49.A** Gastrointestinal stromal tumor
AHA: 2016,4Q,8
DEF: Uncommon malignant tumor found in the GI tract that originates from interstitial cells of the autonomic nervous system. Most occur in the stomach or small intestine but can originate anywhere in the GI tract.

C49.A0 Gastrointestinal stromal tumor, unspecified site　CC HCC

C49.A1 Gastrointestinal stromal tumor of esophagus

C49.A2 Gastrointestinal stromal tumor of stomach　CC HCC

C49.A3 Gastrointestinal stromal tumor of small intestine　CC HCC

C49.A4 Gastrointestinal stromal tumor of large intestine　CC HCC

C49.A5 Gastrointestinal stromal tumor of rectum　CC HCC

C49.A9 Gastrointestinal stromal tumor of other sites　CC HCC

Malignant neoplasms of breast (C50)

√4ᵗʰ **C50** Malignant neoplasm of breast
INCLUDES　connective tissue of breast
Paget's disease of breast
Paget's disease of nipple
Use additional code to identify estrogen receptor status (Z17.0, Z17.1)
EXCLUDES 1　skin of breast (C44.501, C44.511, C44.521, C44.591)
AHA: 2017,4Q,19

Female Breast

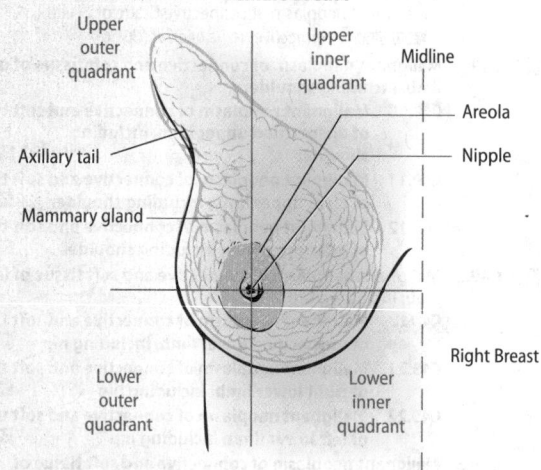

√5ᵗʰ **C50.0** Malignant neoplasm of nipple and areola
√6ᵗʰ **C50.01** Malignant neoplasm of nipple and areola, female
C50.011 Malignant neoplasm of nipple and areola, right female breast　HCC ♀
C50.012 Malignant neoplasm of nipple and areola, left female breast　HCC ♀
C50.019 Malignant neoplasm of nipple and areola, unspecified female breast　HCC ♀
√6ᵗʰ **C50.02** Malignant neoplasm of nipple and areola, male
C50.021 Malignant neoplasm of nipple and areola, right male breast　HCC ♂
C50.022 Malignant neoplasm of nipple and areola, left male breast　HCC ♂
C50.029 Malignant neoplasm of nipple and areola, unspecified male breast　HCC ♂

√5ᵗʰ **C50.1** Malignant neoplasm of central portion of breast
√6ᵗʰ **C50.11** Malignant neoplasm of central portion of breast, female
C50.111 Malignant neoplasm of central portion of right female breast　HCC ♀
C50.112 Malignant neoplasm of central portion of left female breast　HCC ♀
C50.119 Malignant neoplasm of central portion of unspecified female breast　HCC ♀
√6ᵗʰ **C50.12** Malignant neoplasm of central portion of breast, male
C50.121 Malignant neoplasm of central portion of right male breast　HCC ♂
C50.122 Malignant neoplasm of central portion of left male breast　HCC ♂
C50.129 Malignant neoplasm of central portion of unspecified male breast　HCC ♂

√5ᵗʰ **C50.2** Malignant neoplasm of upper-inner quadrant of breast
√6ᵗʰ **C50.21** Malignant neoplasm of upper-inner quadrant of breast, female
C50.211 Malignant neoplasm of upper-inner quadrant of right female breast　HCC ♀
C50.212 Malignant neoplasm of upper-inner quadrant of left female breast　HCC ♀
C50.219 Malignant neoplasm of upper-inner quadrant of unspecified female breast　HCC ♀
√6ᵗʰ **C50.22** Malignant neoplasm of upper-inner quadrant of breast, male
C50.221 Malignant neoplasm of upper-inner quadrant of right male breast　HCC ♂
C50.222 Malignant neoplasm of upper-inner quadrant of left male breast　HCC ♂
C50.229 Malignant neoplasm of upper-inner quadrant of unspecified male breast　HCC ♂

√5ᵗʰ **C50.3** Malignant neoplasm of lower-inner quadrant of breast
√6ᵗʰ **C50.31** Malignant neoplasm of lower-inner quadrant of breast, female
C50.311 Malignant neoplasm of lower-inner quadrant of right female breast　HCC ♀
C50.312 Malignant neoplasm of lower-inner quadrant of left female breast　HCC ♀
C50.319 Malignant neoplasm of lower-inner quadrant of unspecified female breast　HCC ♀
√6ᵗʰ **C50.32** Malignant neoplasm of lower-inner quadrant of breast, male
C50.321 Malignant neoplasm of lower-inner quadrant of right male breast　HCC ♂
C50.322 Malignant neoplasm of lower-inner quadrant of left male breast　HCC ♂
C50.329 Malignant neoplasm of lower-inner quadrant of unspecified male breast　HCC ♂

√5ᵗʰ **C50.4** Malignant neoplasm of upper-outer quadrant of breast
√6ᵗʰ **C50.41** Malignant neoplasm of upper-outer quadrant of breast, female
C50.411 Malignant neoplasm of upper-outer quadrant of right female breast　HCC ♀
C50.412 Malignant neoplasm of upper-outer quadrant of left female breast　HCC ♀
C50.419 Malignant neoplasm of upper-outer quadrant of unspecified female breast　HCC ♀
√6ᵗʰ **C50.42** Malignant neoplasm of upper-outer quadrant of breast, male
C50.421 Malignant neoplasm of upper-outer quadrant of right male breast　HCC ♂
C50.422 Malignant neoplasm of upper-outer quadrant of left male breast　HCC ♂
C50.429 Malignant neoplasm of upper-outer quadrant of unspecified male breast　HCC ♂

√5ᵗʰ **C50.5** Malignant neoplasm of lower-outer quadrant of breast
√6ᵗʰ **C50.51** Malignant neoplasm of lower-outer quadrant of breast, female
C50.511 Malignant neoplasm of lower-outer quadrant of right female breast　HCC ♀
C50.512 Malignant neoplasm of lower-outer quadrant of left female breast　HCC ♀

         C50.519 Malignant neoplasm of lower-outer quadrant of unspecified female breast   HCC ♀

     √6th **C50.52** Malignant neoplasm of lower-outer quadrant of breast, male

         C50.521 Malignant neoplasm of lower-outer quadrant of right male breast   HCC ♂

         C50.522 Malignant neoplasm of lower-outer quadrant of left male breast   HCC ♂

         C50.529 Malignant neoplasm of lower-outer quadrant of unspecified male breast   HCC ♂

   √5th **C50.6** Malignant neoplasm of axillary tail of breast

     √6th **C50.61** Malignant neoplasm of axillary tail of breast, female

         C50.611 Malignant neoplasm of axillary tail of right female breast   HCC ♀

         C50.612 Malignant neoplasm of axillary tail of left female breast   HCC ♀

         C50.619 Malignant neoplasm of axillary tail of unspecified female breast   HCC ♀

     √6th **C50.62** Malignant neoplasm of axillary tail of breast, male

         C50.621 Malignant neoplasm of axillary tail of right male breast   HCC ♂

         C50.622 Malignant neoplasm of axillary tail of left male breast   HCC ♂

         C50.629 Malignant neoplasm of axillary tail of unspecified male breast   HCC ♂

   √5th **C50.8** Malignant neoplasm of overlapping sites of breast

     √6th **C50.81** Malignant neoplasm of overlapping sites of breast, female

         C50.811 Malignant neoplasm of overlapping sites of right female breast   HCC ♀

         C50.812 Malignant neoplasm of overlapping sites of left female breast   HCC ♀

         C50.819 Malignant neoplasm of overlapping sites of unspecified female breast   HCC ♀

     √6th **C50.82** Malignant neoplasm of overlapping sites of breast, male

         C50.821 Malignant neoplasm of overlapping sites of right male breast   HCC ♂

         C50.822 Malignant neoplasm of overlapping sites of left male breast   HCC ♂

         C50.829 Malignant neoplasm of overlapping sites of unspecified male breast   HCC ♂

   √5th **C50.9** Malignant neoplasm of breast of unspecified site

     √6th **C50.91** Malignant neoplasm of breast of unspecified site, female

         C50.911 Malignant neoplasm of unspecified site of right female breast   HCC ♀

         C50.912 Malignant neoplasm of unspecified site of left female breast   HCC ♀

         C50.919 Malignant neoplasm of unspecified site of unspecified female breast   HCC ♀

     √6th **C50.92** Malignant neoplasm of breast of unspecified site, male

         C50.921 Malignant neoplasm of unspecified site of right male breast   HCC ♂

         C50.922 Malignant neoplasm of unspecified site of left male breast   HCC ♂

         C50.929 Malignant neoplasm of unspecified site of unspecified male breast   HCC ♂

Malignant neoplasms of female genital organs (C51-C58)

   INCLUDES   malignant neoplasm of skin of female genital organs

√4th **C51 Malignant neoplasm of vulva**

     EXCLUDES 1   carcinoma in situ of vulva (D07.1)

   C51.0 Malignant neoplasm of labium majus   HCC ♀
     Malignant neoplasm of Bartholin's [greater vestibular] gland

   C51.1 Malignant neoplasm of labium minus   HCC ♀

   C51.2 Malignant neoplasm of clitoris   HCC ♀

   C51.8 Malignant neoplasm of overlapping sites of vulva   HCC ♀

   C51.9 Malignant neoplasm of vulva, unspecified   HCC ♀
     Malignant neoplasm of external female genitalia NOS
     Malignant neoplasm of pudendum

C52 Malignant neoplasm of vagina   HCC ♀
     EXCLUDES 1   carcinoma in situ of vagina (D07.2)

√4th **C53 Malignant neoplasm of cervix uteri**

   EXCLUDES 1   carcinoma in situ of cervix uteri (D06.-)

   AHA: 2017,4Q,103

   C53.0 Malignant neoplasm of endocervix   HCC ♀

   C53.1 Malignant neoplasm of exocervix   HCC ♀

   C53.8 Malignant neoplasm of overlapping sites of cervix uteri   ♀

   C53.9 Malignant neoplasm of cervix uteri, unspecified   HCC ♀

√4th **C54 Malignant neoplasm of corpus uteri**

   C54.0 Malignant neoplasm of isthmus uteri   HCC ♀
     Malignant neoplasm of lower uterine segment

   C54.1 Malignant neoplasm of endometrium   HCC ♀

   C54.2 Malignant neoplasm of myometrium   HCC ♀

   C54.3 Malignant neoplasm of fundus uteri   HCC ♀

   C54.8 Malignant neoplasm of overlapping sites of corpus uteri   HCC ♀

   C54.9 Malignant neoplasm of corpus uteri, unspecified   HCC ♀

C55 Malignant neoplasm of uterus, part unspecified   HCC ♀

√4th **C56 Malignant neoplasm of ovary**

   Use additional code to identify any functional activity

   C56.1 Malignant neoplasm of right ovary   CC HCC ♀

   C56.2 Malignant neoplasm of left ovary   CC HCC ♀

●   **C56.3** Malignant neoplasm of bilateral ovaries   CC

   C56.9 Malignant neoplasm of unspecified ovary   CC HCC ♀

√4th **C57 Malignant neoplasm of other and unspecified female genital organs**

   √5th **C57.0** Malignant neoplasm of fallopian tube
     Malignant neoplasm of oviduct
     Malignant neoplasm of uterine tube

     C57.00 Malignant neoplasm of unspecified fallopian tube   HCC ♀

     C57.01 Malignant neoplasm of right fallopian tube   HCC ♀

     C57.02 Malignant neoplasm of left fallopian tube   HCC ♀

   √5th **C57.1** Malignant neoplasm of broad ligament

     C57.10 Malignant neoplasm of unspecified broad ligament   HCC ♀

     C57.11 Malignant neoplasm of right broad ligament   ♀

     C57.12 Malignant neoplasm of left broad ligament   HCC ♀

   √5th **C57.2** Malignant neoplasm of round ligament

     C57.20 Malignant neoplasm of unspecified round ligament   HCC ♀

     C57.21 Malignant neoplasm of right round ligament   HCC ♀

     C57.22 Malignant neoplasm of left round ligament   HCC ♀

   C57.3 Malignant neoplasm of parametrium   HCC ♀
     Malignant neoplasm of uterine ligament NOS

   C57.4 Malignant neoplasm of uterine adnexa, unspecified   HCC ♀

   C57.7 Malignant neoplasm of other specified female genital organs   HCC ♀
     Malignant neoplasm of wolffian body or duct

   C57.8 Malignant neoplasm of overlapping sites of female genital organs   HCC ♀
     Primary malignant neoplasm of two or more contiguous sites of the female genital organs whose point of origin cannot be determined
     Primary tubo-ovarian malignant neoplasm whose point of origin cannot be determined
     Primary utero-ovarian malignant neoplasm whose point of origin cannot be determined

   C57.9 Malignant neoplasm of female genital organ, unspecified   HCC ♀
     Malignant neoplasm of female genitourinary tract NOS

✔ Additional Character Required   √x7th Placeholder   Questionable PDx   Manifestation   Unspecified Dx   UPD Unacceptable PDx   H1-H4 HAC   HCC CMS-HCC Dx   HIV HIV Dx

ICD-10-CM 2022   479

Chapter 2. Neoplasms

C58 Malignant neoplasm of placenta HCC M ♀
INCLUDES choriocarcinoma NOS
chorionepithelioma NOS
EXCLUDES 1 chorioadenoma (destruens) (D39.2)
hydatidiform mole NOS (O01.9)
invasive hydatidiform mole (D39.2)
male choriocarcinoma NOS (C62.9-)
malignant hydatidiform mole (D39.2)

Malignant neoplasms of male genital organs (C60-C63)

INCLUDES malignant neoplasm of skin of male genital organs

√4th **C60 Malignant neoplasm of penis**

    C60.0 Malignant neoplasm of prepuce HCC ♂
Malignant neoplasm of foreskin

    C60.1 Malignant neoplasm of glans penis HCC ♂

    C60.2 Malignant neoplasm of body of penis HCC ♂
Malignant neoplasm of corpus cavernosum

    C60.8 Malignant neoplasm of overlapping sites of penis HCC ♂

    C60.9 Malignant neoplasm of penis, unspecified HCC ♂
Malignant neoplasm of skin of penis NOS

C61 Malignant neoplasm of prostate HCC ♂
Use additional code to identify:
hormone sensitivity status (Z19.1-Z19.2)
rising PSA following treatment for malignant neoplasm of prostate (R97.21)
EXCLUDES 1 malignant neoplasm of seminal vesicle (C63.7)
AHA: 2017,1Q,17

√4th **C62 Malignant neoplasm of testis**
Use additional code to identify any functional activity

   √5th **C62.0 Malignant neoplasm of undescended testis**
Malignant neoplasm of ectopic testis
Malignant neoplasm of retained testis

    C62.00 Malignant neoplasm of unspecified undescended testis HCC ♂

    C62.01 Malignant neoplasm of undescended right testis HCC ♂

    C62.02 Malignant neoplasm of undescended left testis HCC ♂

   √5th **C62.1 Malignant neoplasm of descended testis**
Malignant neoplasm of scrotal testis

    C62.10 Malignant neoplasm of unspecified descended testis HCC ♂

    C62.11 Malignant neoplasm of descended right testis HCC ♂

    C62.12 Malignant neoplasm of descended left testis HCC ♂

   √5th **C62.9 Malignant neoplasm of testis, unspecified whether descended or undescended**

    C62.90 Malignant neoplasm of unspecified testis, unspecified whether descended or undescended HCC ♂
Malignant neoplasm of testis NOS

    C62.91 Malignant neoplasm of right testis, unspecified whether descended or undescended HCC ♂

    C62.92 Malignant neoplasm of left testis, unspecified whether descended or undescended HCC ♂

√4th **C63 Malignant neoplasm of other and unspecified male genital organs**

   √5th **C63.0 Malignant neoplasm of epididymis**

    C63.00 Malignant neoplasm of unspecified epididymis HCC ♂

    C63.01 Malignant neoplasm of right epididymis HCC ♂

    C63.02 Malignant neoplasm of left epididymis HCC ♂

   √5th **C63.1 Malignant neoplasm of spermatic cord**

    C63.10 Malignant neoplasm of unspecified spermatic cord HCC ♂

    C63.11 Malignant neoplasm of right spermatic cord HCC ♂

    C63.12 Malignant neoplasm of left spermatic cord HCC ♂

    C63.2 Malignant neoplasm of scrotum HCC ♂
Malignant neoplasm of skin of scrotum

    C63.7 Malignant neoplasm of other specified male genital organs HCC ♂
Malignant neoplasm of seminal vesicle
Malignant neoplasm of tunica vaginalis

    C63.8 Malignant neoplasm of overlapping sites of male genital organs HCC ♂
Primary malignant neoplasm of two or more contiguous sites of male genital organs whose point of origin cannot be determined

    C63.9 Malignant neoplasm of male genital organ, unspecified HCC ♂
Malignant neoplasm of male genitourinary tract NOS

Malignant neoplasms of urinary tract (C64-C68)

√4th **C64 Malignant neoplasm of kidney, except renal pelvis**
EXCLUDES 1 malignant carcinoid tumor of the kidney (C7A.093)
malignant neoplasm of renal calyces (C65.-)
malignant neoplasm of renal pelvis (C65.-)

    C64.1 Malignant neoplasm of right kidney, except renal pelvis CC HCC

    C64.2 Malignant neoplasm of left kidney, except renal pelvis CC HCC

    C64.9 Malignant neoplasm of unspecified kidney, except renal pelvis CC HCC

√4th **C65 Malignant neoplasm of renal pelvis**
INCLUDES malignant neoplasm of pelviureteric junction
malignant neoplasm of renal calyces

    C65.1 Malignant neoplasm of right renal pelvis CC HCC

    C65.2 Malignant neoplasm of left renal pelvis CC HCC

    C65.9 Malignant neoplasm of unspecified renal pelvis CC HCC

√4th **C66 Malignant neoplasm of ureter**
EXCLUDES 1 malignant neoplasm of ureteric orifice of bladder (C67.6)

    C66.1 Malignant neoplasm of right ureter CC HCC

    C66.2 Malignant neoplasm of left ureter CC HCC

    C66.9 Malignant neoplasm of unspecified ureter CC HCC

√4th **C67 Malignant neoplasm of bladder**

    C67.0 Malignant neoplasm of trigone of bladder HCC

    C67.1 Malignant neoplasm of dome of bladder HCC

    C67.2 Malignant neoplasm of lateral wall of bladder HCC

    C67.3 Malignant neoplasm of anterior wall of bladder HCC

    C67.4 Malignant neoplasm of posterior wall of bladder HCC

    C67.5 Malignant neoplasm of bladder neck HCC
Malignant neoplasm of internal urethral orifice

    C67.6 Malignant neoplasm of ureteric orifice HCC

    C67.7 Malignant neoplasm of urachus HCC

    C67.8 Malignant neoplasm of overlapping sites of bladder HCC

    C67.9 Malignant neoplasm of bladder, unspecified HCC
AHA: 2016,1Q,19

√4th **C68 Malignant neoplasm of other and unspecified urinary organs**
EXCLUDES 1 malignant neoplasm of female genitourinary tract NOS (C57.9)
malignant neoplasm of male genitourinary tract NOS (C63.9)

    C68.0 Malignant neoplasm of urethra CC HCC
EXCLUDES 1 malignant neoplasm of urethral orifice of bladder (C67.5)

    C68.1 Malignant neoplasm of paraurethral glands CC HCC

    C68.8 Malignant neoplasm of overlapping sites of urinary organs CC HCC
Primary malignant neoplasm of two or more contiguous sites of urinary organs whose point of origin cannot be determined

    C68.9 Malignant neoplasm of urinary organ, unspecified CC HCC
Malignant neoplasm of urinary system NOS

Malignant neoplasms of eye, brain and other parts of central nervous system (C69-C72)

✓4ᵗʰ **C69 Malignant neoplasm of** eye and adnexa

> EXCLUDES 1   *malignant neoplasm of connective tissue of eyelid (C49.0)*
> *malignant neoplasm of eyelid (skin) (C43.1-, C44.1-)*
> *malignant neoplasm of optic nerve (C72.3-)*

✓5ᵗʰ **C69.0 Malignant neoplasm of** conjunctiva

   C69.00 Malignant neoplasm of unspecified conjunctiva HCC
   C69.01 Malignant neoplasm of right **conjunctiva** HCC
   C69.02 Malignant neoplasm of left **conjunctiva** HCC

✓5ᵗʰ **C69.1 Malignant neoplasm of** cornea

   C69.10 Malignant neoplasm of unspecified cornea HCC
   C69.11 Malignant neoplasm of right **cornea** HCC
   C69.12 Malignant neoplasm of left **cornea** HCC

✓5ᵗʰ **C69.2 Malignant neoplasm of** retina

> EXCLUDES 1   *dark area on retina (D49.81)*
> *neoplasm of unspecified behavior of retina and choroid (D49.81)*
> *retinal freckle (D49.81)*

   C69.20 Malignant neoplasm of unspecified retina HCC
   C69.21 Malignant neoplasm of right **retina** HCC
   C69.22 Malignant neoplasm of left **retina** HCC

✓5ᵗʰ **C69.3 Malignant neoplasm of** choroid

   C69.30 Malignant neoplasm of unspecified choroid HCC
   C69.31 Malignant neoplasm of right **choroid** HCC
   C69.32 Malignant neoplasm of left **choroid** HCC

✓5ᵗʰ **C69.4 Malignant neoplasm of** ciliary body

   C69.40 Malignant neoplasm of unspecified ciliary body HCC
   C69.41 Malignant neoplasm of right **ciliary body** HCC
   C69.42 Malignant neoplasm of left **ciliary body** HCC

✓5ᵗʰ **C69.5 Malignant neoplasm of** lacrimal gland and duct

   Malignant neoplasm of lacrimal sac
   Malignant neoplasm of nasolacrimal duct

   C69.50 Malignant neoplasm of unspecified lacrimal gland and duct HCC
   C69.51 Malignant neoplasm of right **lacrimal gland and duct** HCC
   C69.52 Malignant neoplasm of left **lacrimal gland and duct** HCC

✓5ᵗʰ **C69.6 Malignant neoplasm of** orbit

   Malignant neoplasm of connective tissue of orbit
   Malignant neoplasm of extraocular muscle
   Malignant neoplasm of peripheral nerves of orbit
   Malignant neoplasm of retrobulbar tissue
   Malignant neoplasm of retro-ocular tissue

> EXCLUDES 1   *malignant neoplasm of orbital bone (C41.0)*

   C69.60 Malignant neoplasm of unspecified orbit HCC
   C69.61 Malignant neoplasm of right **orbit** HCC
   C69.62 Malignant neoplasm of left **orbit** HCC

✓5ᵗʰ **C69.8 Malignant neoplasm of** overlapping **sites of eye and adnexa**

   C69.80 Malignant neoplasm of overlapping sites of unspecified eye and adnexa HCC
   C69.81 Malignant neoplasm of overlapping sites of right **eye and adnexa** HCC
   C69.82 Malignant neoplasm of overlapping sites of left **eye and adnexa** HCC

✓5ᵗʰ **C69.9 Malignant neoplasm of unspecified site of eye**

   Malignant neoplasm of eyeball

   C69.90 Malignant neoplasm of unspecified site of unspecified eye HCC
   C69.91 Malignant neoplasm of unspecified site of right **eye** HCC
   C69.92 Malignant neoplasm of unspecified site of left **eye** HCC

✓4ᵗʰ **C70 Malignant neoplasm of** meninges

   C70.0 Malignant neoplasm of cerebral **meninges** CC HCC
   C70.1 Malignant neoplasm of spinal **meninges** CC HCC
   C70.9 Malignant neoplasm of meninges, unspecified CC HCC

✓4ᵗʰ **C71 Malignant neoplasm of** brain

> EXCLUDES 1   *malignant neoplasm of cranial nerves (C72.2-C72.5)*
> *retrobulbar malignant neoplasm (C69.6-)*

Lobes of the Brain

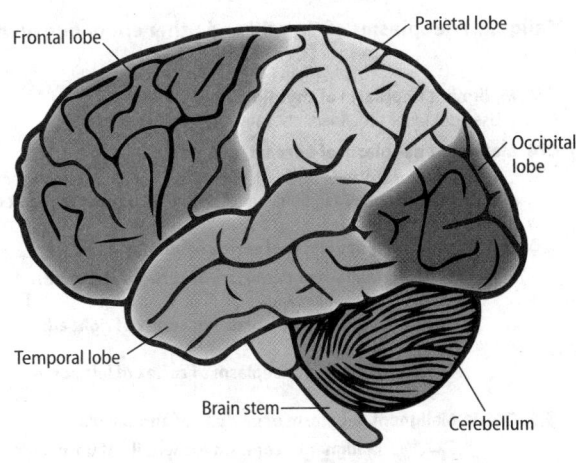

C71.0 **Malignant neoplasm of** cerebrum, except lobes and ventricles CC HCC
   Malignant neoplasm of supratentorial NOS

C71.1 **Malignant neoplasm of** frontal **lobe** CC HCC
C71.2 **Malignant neoplasm of** temporal **lobe** CC HCC
C71.3 **Malignant neoplasm of** parietal **lobe** CC HCC
C71.4 **Malignant neoplasm of** occipital **lobe** CC HCC
C71.5 **Malignant neoplasm of** cerebral **ventricle** CC HCC

> EXCLUDES 1   *malignant neoplasm of fourth cerebral ventricle (C71.7)*

C71.6 **Malignant neoplasm of** cerebellum CC HCC
C71.7 **Malignant neoplasm of** brain stem CC HCC
   Malignant neoplasm of fourth cerebral ventricle
   Infratentorial malignant neoplasm NOS

C71.8 **Malignant neoplasm of** overlapping sites **of brain** CC HCC
C71.9 **Malignant neoplasm of brain, unspecified** CC HCC
   AHA: 2014,3Q,3

✓4ᵗʰ **C72 Malignant neoplasm of** spinal cord, cranial nerves **and other parts of** central nervous system

> EXCLUDES 1   *malignant neoplasm of meninges (C70.-)*
> *malignant neoplasm of peripheral nerves and autonomic nervous system (C47.-)*

C72.0 **Malignant neoplasm of** spinal cord CC HCC
C72.1 **Malignant neoplasm of** cauda equina CC HCC

✓5ᵗʰ C72.2 **Malignant neoplasm of** olfactory nerve

   Malignant neoplasm of olfactory bulb

   C72.20 Malignant neoplasm of unspecified olfactory nerve CC HCC
   C72.21 Malignant neoplasm of right **olfactory nerve** CC HCC
   C72.22 Malignant neoplasm of left **olfactory nerve** CC HCC

✓5ᵗʰ C72.3 **Malignant neoplasm of** optic nerve

   C72.30 Malignant neoplasm of unspecified optic nerve CC HCC
   C72.31 Malignant neoplasm of right **optic nerve** CC HCC
   C72.32 Malignant neoplasm of left **optic nerve** CC HCC

✓5ᵗʰ C72.4 **Malignant neoplasm of** acoustic nerve

   C72.40 Malignant neoplasm of unspecified acoustic nerve CC HCC
   C72.41 Malignant neoplasm of right **acoustic nerve** CC HCC
   C72.42 Malignant neoplasm of left **acoustic nerve** CC HCC

✓5ᵗʰ C72.5 **Malignant neoplasm of other and unspecified** cranial nerves

   C72.50 Malignant neoplasm of unspecified cranial nerve CC HCC
     Malignant neoplasm of cranial nerve NOS
   C72.59 Malignant neoplasm of other cranial nerves CC HCC

☑ Additional Character Required   ✓x7ᵗʰ Placeholder   Questionable PDx   Manifestation   Unspecified Dx   UPD Unacceptable PDx   H1-H14 HAC   HCC CMS-HCC Dx   HIV HIV Dx

ICD-10-CM 2022   481

Chapter 2. Neoplasms

   C72.9   **Malignant neoplasm of central nervous system, unspecified**   `CC` `HCC`

        Malignant neoplasm of unspecified site of central nervous system

        Malignant neoplasm of nervous system NOS

Malignant neoplasms of thyroid and other endocrine glands (C73-C75)

C73   **Malignant neoplasm of thyroid gland**   `HCC`

      Use additional code to identify any functional activity

✓4ᵗʰ   **C74**   **Malignant neoplasm of adrenal gland**

      TIP: If an adrenal gland tumor is described as functioning (producing too much of a hormone), additional codes should be assigned to report the functional activity.

  ✓5ᵗʰ   **C74.Ø**   **Malignant neoplasm of cortex of adrenal gland**

     C74.ØØ   **Malignant neoplasm of cortex of unspecified adrenal gland**   `CC` `HCC`

     C74.Ø1   **Malignant neoplasm of cortex of right adrenal gland**   `CC` `HCC`

     C74.Ø2   **Malignant neoplasm of cortex of left adrenal gland**   `CC` `HCC`

  ✓5ᵗʰ   **C74.1**   **Malignant neoplasm of medulla of adrenal gland**

     C74.1Ø   **Malignant neoplasm of medulla of unspecified adrenal gland**   `CC` `HCC`

     C74.11   **Malignant neoplasm of medulla of right adrenal gland**   `CC` `HCC`

     C74.12   **Malignant neoplasm of medulla of left adrenal gland**   `CC` `HCC`

  ✓5ᵗʰ   **C74.9**   **Malignant neoplasm of unspecified part of adrenal gland**

     C74.9Ø   **Malignant neoplasm of unspecified part of unspecified adrenal gland**   `CC` `HCC`

     C74.91   **Malignant neoplasm of unspecified part of right adrenal gland**   `CC` `HCC`

     C74.92   **Malignant neoplasm of unspecified part of left adrenal gland**   `CC` `HCC`

✓4ᵗʰ   **C75**   **Malignant neoplasm of other endocrine glands and related structures**

      EXCLUDES 1   malignant carcinoid tumors (C7A.Ø-)

            malignant neoplasm of adrenal gland (C74.-)

            malignant neoplasm of endocrine pancreas (C25.4)

            malignant neoplasm of islets of Langerhans (C25.4)

            malignant neoplasm of ovary (C56.-)

            malignant neoplasm of testis (C62.-)

            malignant neoplasm of thymus (C37)

            malignant neoplasm of thyroid gland (C73)

            malignant neuroendocrine tumors (C7A.-)

   C75.Ø   **Malignant neoplasm of parathyroid gland**   `CC` `HCC`

   C75.1   **Malignant neoplasm of pituitary gland**   `CC` `HCC`

   C75.2   **Malignant neoplasm of craniopharyngeal duct**   `CC` `HCC`

   C75.3   **Malignant neoplasm of pineal gland**   `CC` `HCC`

   C75.4   **Malignant neoplasm of carotid body**   `CC` `HCC`

   C75.5   **Malignant neoplasm of aortic body and other paraganglia**   `CC` `HCC`

   C75.8   **Malignant neoplasm with pluriglandular involvement, unspecified**   `CC` `HCC`

   C75.9   **Malignant neoplasm of endocrine gland, unspecified**   `CC` `HCC`

Malignant neuroendocrine tumors (C7A)

✓4ᵗʰ   **C7A**   **Malignant neuroendocrine tumors**

      Code also any associated multiple endocrine neoplasia [MEN] syndromes (E31.2-)

      Use additional code to identify any associated endocrine syndrome, such as:

      carcinoid syndrome (E34.Ø)

      EXCLUDES 2   malignant pancreatic islet cell tumors (C25.4)

             Merkel cell carcinoma (C4A.-)

      AHA: 2019,3Q,7

      DEF: Tumors comprised of cells that are capable of producing hormonal syndromes in which the normal hormonal balance required to support body system function is adversely affected.

  ✓5ᵗʰ   **C7A.Ø**   **Malignant carcinoid tumors**

      AHA: 2019,3Q,7

      DEF: Specific type of slow-growing neuroendocrine tumors. Carcinoid tumors occur most commonly in the hormone producing cells of the gastrointestinal tracts and can also occur in the pancreas, testes, ovaries, or lungs.

     C7A.ØØ   **Malignant carcinoid tumor of unspecified site**   `CC` `HCC`

  ✓6ᵗʰ   **C7A.Ø1**   **Malignant carcinoid tumors of the small intestine**

     C7A.Ø1Ø   **Malignant carcinoid tumor of the duodenum**   `CC` `HCC`

     C7A.Ø11   **Malignant carcinoid tumor of the jejunum**   `CC` `HCC`

     C7A.Ø12   **Malignant carcinoid tumor of the ileum**   `CC` `HCC`

     C7A.Ø19   **Malignant carcinoid tumor of the small intestine, unspecified portion**   `CC` `HCC`

  ✓6ᵗʰ   **C7A.Ø2**   **Malignant carcinoid tumors of the appendix, large intestine, and rectum**

     C7A.Ø2Ø   **Malignant carcinoid tumor of the appendix**   `CC` `HCC`

     C7A.Ø21   **Malignant carcinoid tumor of the cecum**   `CC` `HCC`

     C7A.Ø22   **Malignant carcinoid tumor of the ascending colon**   `CC` `HCC`

     C7A.Ø23   **Malignant carcinoid tumor of the transverse colon**   `CC` `HCC`

     C7A.Ø24   **Malignant carcinoid tumor of the descending colon**   `CC` `HCC`

     C7A.Ø25   **Malignant carcinoid tumor of the sigmoid colon**   `CC` `HCC`

     C7A.Ø26   **Malignant carcinoid tumor of the rectum**   `CC` `HCC`

     C7A.Ø29   **Malignant carcinoid tumor of the large intestine, unspecified portion**   `CC` `HCC`

        Malignant carcinoid tumor of the colon NOS

  ✓6ᵗʰ   **C7A.Ø9**   **Malignant carcinoid tumors of other sites**

     C7A.Ø9Ø   **Malignant carcinoid tumor of the bronchus and lung**   `CC` `HCC`

        AHA: 2019,1Q,16

        TIP: When associated malignant pericardial effusion is documented, assign code I31.3. If the sole reason for admission is to treat the effusion with no treatment of the lung malignancy rendered, code I31.3 may be sequenced first.

     C7A.Ø91   **Malignant carcinoid tumor of the thymus**   `CC` `HCC`

     C7A.Ø92   **Malignant carcinoid tumor of the stomach**   `CC` `HCC`

     C7A.Ø93   **Malignant carcinoid tumor of the kidney**   `CC` `HCC`

     C7A.Ø94   **Malignant carcinoid tumor of the foregut, unspecified**   `CC` `HCC`

     C7A.Ø95   **Malignant carcinoid tumor of the midgut, unspecified**   `CC` `HCC`

     C7A.Ø96   **Malignant carcinoid tumor of the hindgut, unspecified**   `CC` `HCC`

     C7A.Ø98   **Malignant carcinoid tumors of other sites**   `CC` `HCC`

N Newborn: 0   P Pediatric: 0-17   M Maternity: 9-64   A Adult: 15-124   MCC Major Complication/Comorbidity   CC Complication/Comorbidity   SW Severe Wound Dx

482   ICD-10-CM 2022

C7A.1 **Malignant** poorly differentiated **neuroendocrine tumors** `CC` `HCC`

Malignant poorly differentiated neuroendocrine tumor NOS

Malignant poorly differentiated neuroendocrine carcinoma, any site

High grade neuroendocrine carcinoma, any site

C7A.8 **Other malignant neuroendocrine tumors** `CC` `HCC`
AHA: 2019,3Q,7

Secondary neuroendocrine tumors (C7B)

✓4ᵗʰ **C7B** Secondary **neuroendocrine tumors**

Use additional code to identify any functional activity

✓5ᵗʰ **C7B.Ø** **Secondary** carcinoid tumors

AHA: 2019,3Q,7
DEF: Specific type of slow-growing neuroendocrine tumors. Carcinoid tumors occur most commonly in the hormone producing cells of the gastrointestinal tracts and can also occur in the pancreas, testes, ovaries, or lungs.

C7B.ØØ **Secondary carcinoid tumors, unspecified site** `HCC`

C7B.Ø1 **Secondary carcinoid tumors of** distant lymph nodes `CC` `HCC`

C7B.Ø2 **Secondary carcinoid tumors of** liver `CC` `HCC`

C7B.Ø3 **Secondary carcinoid tumors of** bone `CC` `HCC`

C7B.Ø4 **Secondary carcinoid tumors of** peritoneum `CC` `HCC`

Mesentary metastasis of carcinoid tumor

C7B.Ø9 **Secondary carcinoid tumors of other sites** `CC` `HCC`

C7B.1 **Secondary** Merkel cell carcinoma `HCC`

Merkel cell carcinoma nodal presentation

Merkel cell carcinoma visceral metastatic presentation

C7B.8 **Other secondary neuroendocrine tumors** `CC` `HCC`
AHA: 2019,3Q,7

Malignant neoplasms of ill-defined, other secondary and unspecified sites (C76-C8Ø)

✓4ᵗʰ **C76** **Malignant neoplasm of other and ill-defined sites**

EXCLUDES 1   *malignant neoplasm of female genitourinary tract NOS (C57.9)*

malignant neoplasm of male genitourinary tract NOS (C63.9)

malignant neoplasm of lymphoid, hematopoietic and related tissue (C81-C96)

malignant neoplasm of skin (C44.-)

malignant neoplasm of unspecified site NOS (C80.1)

C76.Ø **Malignant neoplasm of** head, face and neck `HCC`

Malignant neoplasm of cheek NOS

Malignant neoplasm of nose NOS

C76.1 **Malignant neoplasm of** thorax `HCC`

Intrathoracic malignant neoplasm NOS

Malignant neoplasm of axilla NOS

Thoracic malignant neoplasm NOS

C76.2 **Malignant neoplasm of** abdomen `HCC`

C76.3 **Malignant neoplasm of** pelvis `HCC`

Malignant neoplasm of groin NOS

Malignant neoplasm of sites overlapping systems within the pelvis

Rectovaginal (septum) malignant neoplasm

Rectovesical (septum) malignant neoplasm

✓5ᵗʰ C76.4 **Malignant neoplasm of** upper limb

C76.4Ø **Malignant neoplasm of unspecified upper limb** `HCC`

C76.41 **Malignant neoplasm of** right upper limb `HCC`

C76.42 **Malignant neoplasm of** left upper limb `HCC`

✓5ᵗʰ C76.5 **Malignant neoplasm of** lower limb

C76.5Ø **Malignant neoplasm of unspecified lower limb** `HCC`

C76.51 **Malignant neoplasm of** right lower limb `HCC`

C76.52 **Malignant neoplasm of** left lower limb `HCC`

C76.8 **Malignant neoplasm of other** specified ill-defined sites `HCC`

Malignant neoplasm of overlapping ill-defined sites

✓4ᵗʰ **C77** Secondary **and unspecified malignant neoplasm of** lymph nodes

EXCLUDES 1   *malignant neoplasm of lymph nodes, specified as primary (C81-C86, C88, C96.-)*

mesentary metastasis of carcinoid tumor (C7B.Ø4)

secondary carcinoid tumors of distant lymph nodes (C7B.Ø1)

C77.Ø **Secondary and unspecified malignant neoplasm of lymph nodes of** head, face and neck `CC` `HCC`

Secondary and unspecified malignant neoplasm of supraclavicular lymph nodes

C77.1 **Secondary and unspecified malignant neoplasm of** intrathoracic **lymph nodes** `CC` `HCC`

C77.2 **Secondary and unspecified malignant neoplasm of** intra-abdominal **lymph nodes** `CC` `HCC`

C77.3 **Secondary and unspecified malignant neoplasm of** axilla and upper limb **lymph nodes** `CC` `HCC`

Secondary and unspecified malignant neoplasm of pectoral lymph nodes

C77.4 **Secondary and unspecified malignant neoplasm of** inguinal and lower limb **lymph nodes** `CC` `HCC`

C77.5 **Secondary and unspecified malignant neoplasm of** intrapelvic **lymph nodes** `CC` `HCC`

C77.8 **Secondary and unspecified malignant neoplasm of lymph nodes of** multiple regions `CC` `HCC`

C77.9 **Secondary and unspecified malignant neoplasm of lymph node, unspecified** `CC` `HCC`

✓4ᵗʰ **C78** Secondary **malignant neoplasm of** respiratory and digestive **organs**

EXCLUDES 1   *secondary carcinoid tumors of liver (C7B.Ø2)*

secondary carcinoid tumors of peritoneum (C7B.Ø4)

EXCLUDES 2   *lymph node metastases (C77.Ø)*

✓5ᵗʰ C78.Ø **Secondary malignant neoplasm of** lung

AHA: 2019,1Q,16

C78.ØØ **Secondary malignant neoplasm of unspecified lung** `CC` `HCC`

C78.Ø1 **Secondary malignant neoplasm of** right lung `CC` `HCC`

C78.Ø2 **Secondary malignant neoplasm of** left lung `CC` `HCC`

C78.1 **Secondary malignant neoplasm of** mediastinum `CC` `HCC`

C78.2 **Secondary malignant neoplasm of** pleura `CC` `HCC`

✓5ᵗʰ C78.3 **Secondary malignant neoplasm of other and unspecified respiratory organs**

C78.3Ø **Secondary malignant neoplasm of unspecified respiratory organ** `CC` `HCC`

C78.39 **Secondary malignant neoplasm of other respiratory organs** `CC` `HCC`

C78.4 **Secondary malignant neoplasm of** small intestine `CC` `HCC`

C78.5 **Secondary malignant neoplasm of** large intestine and rectum `CC` `HCC`

C78.6 **Secondary malignant neoplasm of** retroperitoneum and peritoneum `CC` `HCC`

AHA: 2017,2Q,12

C78.7 **Secondary malignant neoplasm of** liver and intrahepatic bile duct `CC` `HCC`

✓5ᵗʰ C78.8 **Secondary malignant neoplasm of other and unspecified digestive organs**

C78.8Ø **Secondary malignant neoplasm of unspecified digestive organ** `CC` `HCC`

C78.89 **Secondary malignant neoplasm of other digestive organs** `CC` `HCC`

Code also exocrine pancreatic insufficiency (K86.81)

✓4ᵗʰ **C79** Secondary **malignant neoplasm of other and unspecified sites**

EXCLUDES 1   *secondary carcinoid tumors (C7B.-)*

secondary neuroendocrine tumors (C7B.-)

✓5ᵗʰ C79.Ø **Secondary malignant neoplasm of** kidney and renal pelvis

C79.ØØ **Secondary malignant neoplasm of unspecified kidney and renal pelvis** `CC` `HCC`

C79.Ø1 **Secondary malignant neoplasm of** right kidney and renal pelvis `CC` `HCC`

C79.Ø2 **Secondary malignant neoplasm of** left kidney and renal pelvis `CC` `HCC`

✓5ᵗʰ C79.1 **Secondary malignant neoplasm of** bladder **and other and unspecified** urinary organs

C79.1Ø **Secondary malignant neoplasm of unspecified urinary organs** `CC` `HCC`

✓ Additional Character Required   ✓x7ᵗʰ Placeholder   Questionable PDx   Manifestation   Unspecified Dx   `UPD` Unacceptable PDx   `H1`-`H14` HAC   `HCC` CMS-HCC Dx   `HIV` HIV Dx

ICD-10-CM 2022   483

C79.11 **Secondary malignant neoplasm of bladder** `CC` `HCC`
    EXCLUDES 2 *lymph node metastases (C77.0)*

C79.19 **Secondary malignant neoplasm of other urinary organs** `CC` `HCC`

C79.2 **Secondary malignant neoplasm of skin** `CC` `HCC`
    EXCLUDES 1 *secondary Merkel cell carcinoma (C7B.1)*

√5ᵗʰ **C79.3** **Secondary malignant neoplasm of brain and cerebral meninges**

  C79.31 **Secondary malignant neoplasm of brain** `CC` `HCC`

  C79.32 **Secondary malignant neoplasm of cerebral meninges** `CC` `HCC`
    AHA: 2020,1Q,13

√5ᵗʰ **C79.4** **Secondary malignant neoplasm of other and unspecified parts of nervous system**

  C79.40 **Secondary malignant neoplasm of unspecified part of nervous system** `CC` `HCC`

  C79.49 **Secondary malignant neoplasm of other parts of nervous system** `CC` `HCC`

√5ᵗʰ **C79.5** **Secondary malignant neoplasm of bone and bone marrow**
    EXCLUDES 1 *secondary carcinoid tumors of bone (C7B.03)*

  C79.51 **Secondary malignant neoplasm of bone** `CC` `HCC`
    TIP: Do not assign in addition to a code from subcategory C90.0 when multiple myeloma is described as metastatic to the bone; bone involvement is integral to multiple myeloma.

  C79.52 **Secondary malignant neoplasm of bone marrow** `CC` `HCC`

√5ᵗʰ **C79.6** **Secondary malignant neoplasm of ovary**

  C79.60 **Secondary malignant neoplasm of unspecified ovary** `CC` `HCC` ♀

  C79.61 **Secondary malignant neoplasm of right ovary** `CC` `HCC` ♀

  C79.62 **Secondary malignant neoplasm of left ovary** `CC` `HCC` ♀

  C79.63 **Secondary malignant neoplasm of bilateral ovaries** `CC`

√5ᵗʰ **C79.7** **Secondary malignant neoplasm of adrenal gland**

  C79.70 **Secondary malignant neoplasm of unspecified adrenal gland** `CC` `HCC`

  C79.71 **Secondary malignant neoplasm of right adrenal gland** `CC` `HCC`

  C79.72 **Secondary malignant neoplasm of left adrenal gland** `CC` `HCC`

√5ᵗʰ **C79.8** **Secondary malignant neoplasm of other specified sites**

  C79.81 **Secondary malignant neoplasm of breast** `CC` `HCC`

  C79.82 **Secondary malignant neoplasm of genital organs** `CC` `HCC`

  C79.89 **Secondary malignant neoplasm of other specified sites** `CC` `HCC`
    AHA: 2017,2Q,11

C79.9 **Secondary malignant neoplasm of unspecified site** `CC` `HCC`
  Metastatic cancer NOS
  Metastatic disease NOS
    EXCLUDES 1 *carcinomatosis NOS (C80.0)*
        generalized cancer NOS (C80.0)
        malignant (primary) neoplasm of unspecified site (C80.1)

√4ᵗʰ **C80** **Malignant neoplasm without specification of site**
    EXCLUDES 1 *malignant carcinoid tumor of unspecified site (C7A.00)*
        malignant neoplasm of specified multiple sites - code to each site

C80.0 **Disseminated malignant neoplasm, unspecified** `CC` `HCC`
  Carcinomatosis NOS
  Generalized cancer, unspecified site (primary) (secondary)
  Generalized malignancy, unspecified site (primary) (secondary)

C80.1 **Malignant (primary) neoplasm, unspecified** `HCC`
  Cancer NOS
  Cancer unspecified site (primary)
  Carcinoma unspecified site (primary)
  Malignancy unspecified site (primary)
    EXCLUDES 1 *secondary malignant neoplasm of unspecified site (C79.9)*

C80.2 **Malignant neoplasm associated with transplanted organ** `CC` `UPD` `HCC`
  Code first complication of transplanted organ (T86.-)
  Use additional code to identify the specific malignancy

Malignant neoplasms of lymphoid, hematopoietic and related tissue (C81-C96)

    EXCLUDES 2 *Kaposi's sarcoma of lymph nodes (C46.3)*
        secondary and unspecified neoplasm of lymph nodes (C77.-)
        secondary neoplasm of bone marrow (C79.52)
        secondary neoplasm of spleen (C78.89)

√4ᵗʰ **C81** **Hodgkin lymphoma**
    EXCLUDES 1 *personal history of Hodgkin lymphoma (Z85.71)*
  DEF: Malignant disorder of lymphoid cells characterized by the presence of progressively swollen lymph nodes and spleen that may also involve the liver. A diagnosis of Hodgkin's lymphoma can be confirmed by the presence of Reed-Sternberg cells. **Synonym(s):** *Hodgkin disease.*

√5ᵗʰ **C81.0** **Nodular lymphocyte predominant Hodgkin lymphoma**

  C81.00 **Nodular lymphocyte predominant Hodgkin lymphoma, unspecified site** `CC` `HCC`

  C81.01 **Nodular lymphocyte predominant Hodgkin lymphoma, lymph nodes of head, face, and neck** `CC` `HCC`

  C81.02 **Nodular lymphocyte predominant Hodgkin lymphoma, intrathoracic lymph nodes** `CC` `HCC`

  C81.03 **Nodular lymphocyte predominant Hodgkin lymphoma, intra-abdominal lymph nodes** `CC` `HCC`

  C81.04 **Nodular lymphocyte predominant Hodgkin lymphoma, lymph nodes of axilla and upper limb** `CC` `HCC`

  C81.05 **Nodular lymphocyte predominant Hodgkin lymphoma, lymph nodes of inguinal region and lower limb** `CC` `HCC`

  C81.06 **Nodular lymphocyte predominant Hodgkin lymphoma, intrapelvic lymph nodes** `CC` `HCC`

  C81.07 **Nodular lymphocyte predominant Hodgkin lymphoma, spleen** `CC` `HCC`

  C81.08 **Nodular lymphocyte predominant Hodgkin lymphoma, lymph nodes of multiple sites** `CC` `HCC`

  C81.09 **Nodular lymphocyte predominant Hodgkin lymphoma, extranodal and solid organ sites** `CC` `HCC`

√5ᵗʰ **C81.1** **Nodular sclerosis Hodgkin lymphoma**
  Nodular sclerosis classical Hodgkin lymphoma

  C81.10 **Nodular sclerosis Hodgkin lymphoma, unspecified site** `CC` `HCC`

  C81.11 **Nodular sclerosis Hodgkin lymphoma, lymph nodes of head, face, and neck** `CC` `HCC`

  C81.12 **Nodular sclerosis Hodgkin lymphoma, intrathoracic lymph nodes** `CC` `HCC`

  C81.13 **Nodular sclerosis Hodgkin lymphoma, intra-abdominal lymph nodes** `CC` `HCC`

  C81.14 **Nodular sclerosis Hodgkin lymphoma, lymph nodes of axilla and upper limb** `CC` `HCC`

  C81.15 **Nodular sclerosis Hodgkin lymphoma, lymph nodes of inguinal region and lower limb** `CC` `HCC`

  C81.16 **Nodular sclerosis Hodgkin lymphoma, intrapelvic lymph nodes** `CC` `HCC`

  C81.17 **Nodular sclerosis Hodgkin lymphoma, spleen** `CC` `HCC`

  C81.18 **Nodular sclerosis Hodgkin lymphoma, lymph nodes of multiple sites** `CC` `HCC`

  C81.19 **Nodular sclerosis Hodgkin lymphoma, extranodal and solid organ sites** `CC` `HCC`

√5ᵗʰ **C81.2** **Mixed cellularity Hodgkin lymphoma**
  Mixed cellularity classical Hodgkin lymphoma

  C81.20 **Mixed cellularity Hodgkin lymphoma, unspecified site** `CC` `HCC`

  C81.21 **Mixed cellularity Hodgkin lymphoma, lymph nodes of head, face, and neck** `CC` `HCC`

  C81.22 **Mixed cellularity Hodgkin lymphoma, intrathoracic lymph nodes** `CC` `HCC`

  C81.23 **Mixed cellularity Hodgkin lymphoma, intra-abdominal lymph nodes** `CC` `HCC`

  C81.24 **Mixed cellularity Hodgkin lymphoma, lymph nodes of axilla and upper limb** `CC` `HCC`

  C81.25 **Mixed cellularity Hodgkin lymphoma, lymph nodes of inguinal region and lower limb** `CC` `HCC`

C81.26   **Mixed cellularity Hodgkin lymphoma, intrapelvic lymph nodes** `CC` `HCC`

C81.27   **Mixed cellularity Hodgkin lymphoma, spleen** `CC` `HCC`

C81.28   **Mixed cellularity Hodgkin lymphoma, lymph nodes of multiple sites** `CC` `HCC`

C81.29   **Mixed cellularity Hodgkin lymphoma, extranodal and solid organ sites** `CC` `HCC`

✓5ᵗʰ **C81.3**   **Lymphocyte depleted Hodgkin lymphoma**

Lymphocyte depleted classical Hodgkin lymphoma

C81.30   **Lymphocyte depleted Hodgkin lymphoma, unspecified site** `CC` `HCC`

C81.31   **Lymphocyte depleted Hodgkin lymphoma, lymph nodes of head, face, and neck** `CC` `HCC`

C81.32   **Lymphocyte depleted Hodgkin lymphoma, intrathoracic lymph nodes** `CC` `HCC`

C81.33   **Lymphocyte depleted Hodgkin lymphoma, intra-abdominal lymph nodes** `CC` `HCC`

C81.34   **Lymphocyte depleted Hodgkin lymphoma, lymph nodes of axilla and upper limb** `CC` `HCC`

C81.35   **Lymphocyte depleted Hodgkin lymphoma, lymph nodes of inguinal region and lower limb** `CC` `HCC`

C81.36   **Lymphocyte depleted Hodgkin lymphoma, intrapelvic lymph nodes** `CC` `HCC`

C81.37   **Lymphocyte depleted Hodgkin lymphoma, spleen** `CC` `HCC`

C81.38   **Lymphocyte depleted Hodgkin lymphoma, lymph nodes of multiple sites** `CC` `HCC`

C81.39   **Lymphocyte depleted Hodgkin lymphoma, extranodal and solid organ sites** `CC` `HCC`

✓5ᵗʰ **C81.4**   **Lymphocyte-rich Hodgkin lymphoma**

Lymphocyte-rich classical Hodgkin lymphoma

EXCLUDES 1   nodular lymphocyte predominant Hodgkin lymphoma (C81.0-)

C81.40   **Lymphocyte-rich Hodgkin lymphoma, unspecified site** `CC` `HCC`

C81.41   **Lymphocyte-rich Hodgkin lymphoma, lymph nodes of head, face, and neck** `CC` `HCC`

C81.42   **Lymphocyte-rich Hodgkin lymphoma, intrathoracic lymph nodes** `CC` `HCC`

C81.43   **Lymphocyte-rich Hodgkin lymphoma, intra-abdominal lymph nodes** `CC` `HCC`

C81.44   **Lymphocyte-rich Hodgkin lymphoma, lymph nodes of axilla and upper limb** `CC` `HCC`

C81.45   **Lymphocyte-rich Hodgkin lymphoma, lymph nodes of inguinal region and lower limb** `CC` `HCC`

C81.46   **Lymphocyte-rich Hodgkin lymphoma, intrapelvic lymph nodes** `CC` `HCC`

C81.47   **Lymphocyte-rich Hodgkin lymphoma, spleen** `CC` `HCC`

C81.48   **Lymphocyte-rich Hodgkin lymphoma, lymph nodes of multiple sites** `CC` `HCC`

C81.49   **Lymphocyte-rich Hodgkin lymphoma, extranodal and solid organ sites** `CC` `HCC`

✓5ᵗʰ **C81.7**   **Other Hodgkin lymphoma**

Classical Hodgkin lymphoma NOS
Other classical Hodgkin lymphoma

C81.70   **Other Hodgkin lymphoma, unspecified site** `CC` `HCC`

C81.71   **Other Hodgkin lymphoma, lymph nodes of head, face, and neck** `CC` `HCC`

C81.72   **Other Hodgkin lymphoma, intrathoracic lymph nodes** `CC` `HCC`

C81.73   **Other Hodgkin lymphoma, intra-abdominal lymph nodes** `CC` `HCC`

C81.74   **Other Hodgkin lymphoma, lymph nodes of axilla and upper limb** `CC` `HCC`

C81.75   **Other Hodgkin lymphoma, lymph nodes of inguinal region and lower limb** `CC` `HCC`

C81.76   **Other Hodgkin lymphoma, intrapelvic lymph nodes** `CC` `HCC`

C81.77   **Other Hodgkin lymphoma, spleen** `CC` `HCC`

C81.78   **Other Hodgkin lymphoma, lymph nodes of multiple sites** `CC` `HCC`

C81.79   **Other Hodgkin lymphoma, extranodal and solid organ sites** `CC` `HCC`

✓6ᵗʰ **C81.9**   **Hodgkin lymphoma, unspecified**

C81.90   **Hodgkin lymphoma, unspecified, unspecified site** `CC` `HCC`

C81.91   **Hodgkin lymphoma, unspecified, lymph nodes of head, face, and neck** `CC` `HCC`

C81.92   **Hodgkin lymphoma, unspecified, intrathoracic lymph nodes** `CC` `HCC`

C81.93   **Hodgkin lymphoma, unspecified, intra-abdominal lymph nodes** `CC` `HCC`

C81.94   **Hodgkin lymphoma, unspecified, lymph nodes of axilla and upper limb** `CC` `HCC`

C81.95   **Hodgkin lymphoma, unspecified, lymph nodes of inguinal region and lower limb** `CC` `HCC`

C81.96   **Hodgkin lymphoma, unspecified, intrapelvic lymph nodes** `CC` `HCC`

C81.97   **Hodgkin lymphoma, unspecified, spleen** `CC` `HCC`

C81.98   **Hodgkin lymphoma, unspecified, lymph nodes of multiple sites** `CC` `HCC`

C81.99   **Hodgkin lymphoma, unspecified, extranodal and solid organ sites** `CC` `HCC`

✓4ᵗʰ **C82**   **Follicular lymphoma**

INCLUDES   follicular lymphoma with or without diffuse areas

EXCLUDES 1   mature T/NK-cell lymphomas (C84.-)
personal history of non-Hodgkin lymphoma (Z85.72)

DEF: Most common subgroup of non-Hodgkin lymphomas (NHL), accounting for 20 to 30 percent of all NHLs. NHL is a B-cell lymphoma that is slow growing and characterized by the circular pattern of malignant cell growth with the cells clustered into identifiable nodules or follicles.

✓5ᵗʰ **C82.0**   **Follicular lymphoma grade I**

C82.00   **Follicular lymphoma grade I, unspecified site** `CC` `HCC`

C82.01   **Follicular lymphoma grade I, lymph nodes of head, face, and neck** `CC` `HCC`

C82.02   **Follicular lymphoma grade I, intrathoracic lymph nodes** `CC` `HCC`

C82.03   **Follicular lymphoma grade I, intra-abdominal lymph nodes** `CC` `HCC`

C82.04   **Follicular lymphoma grade I, lymph nodes of axilla and upper limb** `CC` `HCC`

C82.05   **Follicular lymphoma grade I, lymph nodes of inguinal region and lower limb** `CC` `HCC`

C82.06   **Follicular lymphoma grade I, intrapelvic lymph nodes** `CC` `HCC`

C82.07   **Follicular lymphoma grade I, spleen** `CC` `HCC`

C82.08   **Follicular lymphoma grade I, lymph nodes of multiple sites** `CC` `HCC`

C82.09   **Follicular lymphoma grade I, extranodal and solid organ sites** `CC` `HCC`

✓5ᵗʰ **C82.1**   **Follicular lymphoma grade II**

C82.10   **Follicular lymphoma grade II, unspecified site** `CC` `HCC`

C82.11   **Follicular lymphoma grade II, lymph nodes of head, face, and neck** `CC` `HCC`

C82.12   **Follicular lymphoma grade II, intrathoracic lymph nodes** `CC` `HCC`

C82.13   **Follicular lymphoma grade II, intra-abdominal lymph nodes** `CC` `HCC`

C82.14   **Follicular lymphoma grade II, lymph nodes of axilla and upper limb** `CC` `HCC`

C82.15   **Follicular lymphoma grade II, lymph nodes of inguinal region and lower limb** `CC` `HCC`

C82.16   **Follicular lymphoma grade II, intrapelvic lymph nodes** `CC` `HCC`

C82.17   **Follicular lymphoma grade II, spleen** `CC` `HCC`

C82.18   **Follicular lymphoma grade II, lymph nodes of multiple sites** `CC` `HCC`

C82.19   **Follicular lymphoma grade II, extranodal and solid organ sites** `CC` `HCC`

✓5ᵗʰ **C82.2**   **Follicular lymphoma grade III, unspecified**

C82.20   **Follicular lymphoma grade III, unspecified, unspecified site** `CC` `HCC`

C82.21   **Follicular lymphoma grade III, unspecified, lymph nodes of head, face, and neck** `CC` `HCC`

C82.22   **Follicular lymphoma grade III, unspecified, intrathoracic lymph nodes** `CC` `HCC`

C82.23   **Follicular lymphoma grade III, unspecified, intra-abdominal lymph nodes** `CC` `HCC`

C82.24   **Follicular lymphoma grade III, unspecified, lymph nodes of axilla and upper limb** `CC` `HCC`

C82.25   **Follicular lymphoma grade III, unspecified, lymph nodes of inguinal region and lower limb** `CC` `HCC`

✔ Additional Character Required   ✓x7ᵗʰ Placeholder   Questionable PDx   Manifestation   Unspecified Dx   `UPD` Unacceptable PDx   `H1`-`H14` HAC   `HCC` CMS-HCC Dx   `HIV` HIV Dx

ICD-10-CM 2022   **485**

Chapter 2. Neoplasms

C82.26 Follicular lymphoma grade III, unspecified, intrapelvic lymph nodes   CC HCC

C82.27 Follicular lymphoma grade III, unspecified, spleen   CC HCC

C82.28 Follicular lymphoma grade III, unspecified, lymph nodes of multiple sites   CC HCC

C82.29 Follicular lymphoma grade III, unspecified, extranodal and solid organ sites   CC HCC

✓5ᵗʰ **C82.3** Follicular lymphoma grade IIIa

C82.30 Follicular lymphoma grade IIIa, unspecified site   CC HCC

C82.31 Follicular lymphoma grade IIIa, lymph nodes of head, face, and neck   CC HCC

C82.32 Follicular lymphoma grade IIIa, intrathoracic lymph nodes   CC HCC

C82.33 Follicular lymphoma grade IIIa, intra-abdominal lymph nodes   CC HCC

C82.34 Follicular lymphoma grade IIIa, lymph nodes of axilla and upper limb   CC HCC

C82.35 Follicular lymphoma grade IIIa, lymph nodes of inguinal region and lower limb   CC HCC

C82.36 Follicular lymphoma grade IIIa, intrapelvic lymph nodes   CC HCC

C82.37 Follicular lymphoma grade IIIa, spleen   CC HCC

C82.38 Follicular lymphoma grade IIIa, lymph nodes of multiple sites   CC HCC

C82.39 Follicular lymphoma grade IIIa, extranodal and solid organ sites   CC HCC

✓5ᵗʰ **C82.4** Follicular lymphoma grade IIIb

C82.40 Follicular lymphoma grade IIIb, unspecified site   CC HCC

C82.41 Follicular lymphoma grade IIIb, lymph nodes of head, face, and neck   CC HCC

C82.42 Follicular lymphoma grade IIIb, intrathoracic lymph nodes   CC HCC

C82.43 Follicular lymphoma grade IIIb, intra-abdominal lymph nodes   CC HCC

C82.44 Follicular lymphoma grade IIIb, lymph nodes of axilla and upper limb   CC HCC

C82.45 Follicular lymphoma grade IIIb, lymph nodes of inguinal region and lower limb   CC HCC

C82.46 Follicular lymphoma grade IIIb, intrapelvic lymph nodes   CC HCC

C82.47 Follicular lymphoma grade IIIb, spleen   CC HCC

C82.48 Follicular lymphoma grade IIIb, lymph nodes of multiple sites   CC HCC

C82.49 Follicular lymphoma grade IIIb, extranodal and solid organ sites   CC HCC

✓5ᵗʰ **C82.5** Diffuse follicle center lymphoma

C82.50 Diffuse follicle center lymphoma, unspecified site   HIV CC HCC

C82.51 Diffuse follicle center lymphoma, lymph nodes of head, face, and neck   HIV CC HCC

C82.52 Diffuse follicle center lymphoma, intrathoracic lymph nodes   HIV CC HCC

C82.53 Diffuse follicle center lymphoma, intra-abdominal lymph nodes   HIV CC HCC

C82.54 Diffuse follicle center lymphoma, lymph nodes of axilla and upper limb   HIV CC HCC

C82.55 Diffuse follicle center lymphoma, lymph nodes of inguinal region and lower limb   HIV CC HCC

C82.56 Diffuse follicle center lymphoma, intrapelvic lymph nodes   HIV CC HCC

C82.57 Diffuse follicle center lymphoma, spleen   HIV CC HCC

C82.58 Diffuse follicle center lymphoma, lymph nodes of multiple sites   HIV CC HCC

C82.59 Diffuse follicle center lymphoma, extranodal and solid organ sites   HIV CC HCC

✓5ᵗʰ **C82.6** Cutaneous follicle center lymphoma

C82.60 Cutaneous follicle center lymphoma, unspecified site   CC HCC

C82.61 Cutaneous follicle center lymphoma, lymph nodes of head, face, and neck   CC HCC

C82.62 Cutaneous follicle center lymphoma, intrathoracic lymph nodes   CC HCC

C82.63 Cutaneous follicle center lymphoma, intra-abdominal lymph nodes   CC HCC

C82.64 Cutaneous follicle center lymphoma, lymph nodes of axilla and upper limb   CC HCC

C82.65 Cutaneous follicle center lymphoma, lymph nodes of inguinal region and lower limb   CC HCC

C82.66 Cutaneous follicle center lymphoma, intrapelvic lymph nodes   CC HCC

C82.67 Cutaneous follicle center lymphoma, spleen   CC HCC

C82.68 Cutaneous follicle center lymphoma, lymph nodes of multiple sites   CC HCC

C82.69 Cutaneous follicle center lymphoma, extranodal and solid organ sites   CC HCC

✓5ᵗʰ **C82.8** Other types of follicular lymphoma

C82.80 Other types of follicular lymphoma, unspecified site   CC HCC

C82.81 Other types of follicular lymphoma, lymph nodes of head, face, and neck   CC HCC

C82.82 Other types of follicular lymphoma, intrathoracic lymph nodes   CC HCC

C82.83 Other types of follicular lymphoma, intra-abdominal lymph nodes   CC HCC

C82.84 Other types of follicular lymphoma, lymph nodes of axilla and upper limb   CC HCC

C82.85 Other types of follicular lymphoma, lymph nodes of inguinal region and lower limb   CC HCC

C82.86 Other types of follicular lymphoma, intrapelvic lymph nodes   CC HCC

C82.87 Other types of follicular lymphoma, spleen   CC HCC

C82.88 Other types of follicular lymphoma, lymph nodes of multiple sites   CC HCC

C82.89 Other types of follicular lymphoma, extranodal and solid organ sites   CC HCC

✓5ᵗʰ **C82.9** Follicular lymphoma, unspecified

C82.90 Follicular lymphoma, unspecified, unspecified site   CC HCC

C82.91 Follicular lymphoma, unspecified, lymph nodes of head, face, and neck   CC HCC

C82.92 Follicular lymphoma, unspecified, intrathoracic lymph nodes   CC HCC

C82.93 Follicular lymphoma, unspecified, intra-abdominal lymph nodes   CC HCC

C82.94 Follicular lymphoma, unspecified, lymph nodes of axilla and upper limb   CC HCC

C82.95 Follicular lymphoma, unspecified, lymph nodes of inguinal region and lower limb   CC HCC

C82.96 Follicular lymphoma, unspecified, intrapelvic lymph nodes   CC HCC

C82.97 Follicular lymphoma, unspecified, spleen   CC HCC

C82.98 Follicular lymphoma, unspecified, lymph nodes of multiple sites   CC HCC

C82.99 Follicular lymphoma, unspecified, extranodal and solid organ sites   CC HCC

✓4ᵗʰ **C83** Non-follicular lymphoma

EXCLUDES 1   personal history of non-Hodgkin lymphoma (Z85.72)

✓5ᵗʰ **C83.0** Small cell B-cell lymphoma

Lymphoplasmacytic lymphoma
Nodal marginal zone lymphoma
Non-leukemic variant of B-CLL
Splenic marginal zone lymphoma

EXCLUDES 1   chronic lymphocytic leukemia (C91.1)
     mature T/NK-cell lymphomas (C84.-)
     Waldenström macroglobulinemia (C88.0)

DEF: Nonfollicular lymphoma that is rare, slow growing, and usually found in the older population.

C83.00 Small cell B-cell lymphoma, unspecified site   HIV CC HCC

C83.01 Small cell B-cell lymphoma, lymph nodes of head, face, and neck   HIV CC HCC

C83.02 Small cell B-cell lymphoma, intrathoracic lymph nodes   HIV CC HCC

C83.03 Small cell B-cell lymphoma, intra-abdominal lymph nodes   HIV CC HCC

C83.04 Small cell B-cell lymphoma, lymph nodes of axilla and upper limb   HIV CC HCC

C83.05 Small cell B-cell lymphoma, lymph nodes of inguinal region and lower limb   HIV CC HCC

N Newborn: 0   P Pediatric: 0-17   M Maternity: 9-64   A Adult: 15-124   MCC Major Complication/Comorbidity   CC Complication/Comorbidity   SW Severe Wound Dx

486   ICD-10-CM 2022

C83.06   Small cell B-cell lymphoma, intrapelvic lymph nodes   HIV CC HCC

C83.07   Small cell B-cell lymphoma, spleen   HIV CC HCC

C83.08   Small cell B-cell lymphoma, lymph nodes of multiple sites   HIV CC HCC

C83.09   Small cell B-cell lymphoma, extranodal and solid organ sites   HIV CC HCC

✓5ᵗʰ **C83.1**   Mantle cell lymphoma

Centrocytic lymphoma

Malignant lymphomatous polyposis

DEF: Rare form of B-cell non-Hodgkin lymphoma named for the location of the tumor cell production, the mantle zone of the lymph nodes.

C83.10   Mantle cell lymphoma, unspecified site   HIV CC HCC

C83.11   Mantle cell lymphoma, lymph nodes of head, face, and neck   HIV CC HCC

C83.12   Mantle cell lymphoma, intrathoracic lymph nodes   HIV CC HCC

C83.13   Mantle cell lymphoma, intra-abdominal lymph nodes   HIV CC HCC

C83.14   Mantle cell lymphoma, lymph nodes of axilla and upper limb   HIV CC HCC

C83.15   Mantle cell lymphoma, lymph nodes of inguinal region and lower limb   HIV CC HCC

C83.16   Mantle cell lymphoma, intrapelvic lymph nodes   HIV CC HCC

C83.17   Mantle cell lymphoma, spleen   HIV CC HCC

C83.18   Mantle cell lymphoma, lymph nodes of multiple sites   HIV CC HCC

C83.19   Mantle cell lymphoma, extranodal and solid organ sites   HIV CC HCC

✓5ᵗʰ **C83.3**   Diffuse large B-cell lymphoma

Anaplastic diffuse large B-cell lymphoma

CD30-positive diffuse large B-cell lymphoma

Centroblastic diffuse large B-cell lymphoma

Diffuse large B-cell lymphoma, subtype not specified

Immunoblastic diffuse large B-cell lymphoma

Plasmablastic diffuse large B-cell lymphoma

T-cell rich diffuse large B-cell lymphoma

EXCLUDES 1   mediastinal (thymic) large B-cell lymphoma (C85.2-)

mature T/NK-cell lymphomas (C84.-)

DEF: Nonfollicular lymphoma that is one of the more common types of lymphoma. This cancer is fast growing and affects any age but is found mostly in the older population.

C83.30   Diffuse large B-cell lymphoma, unspecified site   HIV CC HCC

C83.31   Diffuse large B-cell lymphoma, lymph nodes of head, face, and neck   HIV CC HCC

C83.32   Diffuse large B-cell lymphoma, intrathoracic lymph nodes   HIV CC HCC

C83.33   Diffuse large B-cell lymphoma, intra-abdominal lymph nodes   HIV CC HCC

C83.34   Diffuse large B-cell lymphoma, lymph nodes of axilla and upper limb   HIV CC HCC

C83.35   Diffuse large B-cell lymphoma, lymph nodes of inguinal region and lower limb   HIV CC HCC

C83.36   Diffuse large B-cell lymphoma, intrapelvic lymph nodes   HIV CC HCC

C83.37   Diffuse large B-cell lymphoma, spleen   HIV CC HCC

C83.38   Diffuse large B-cell lymphoma, lymph nodes of multiple sites   HIV CC HCC

C83.39   Diffuse large B-cell lymphoma, extranodal and solid organ sites   HIV CC HCC

✓5ᵗʰ **C83.5**   Lymphoblastic (diffuse) lymphoma

B-precursor lymphoma

Lymphoblastic B-cell lymphoma

Lymphoblastic lymphoma NOS

Lymphoblastic T-cell lymphoma

T-precursor lymphoma

DEF: Type of non-Hodgkin lymphoma considered lymphoma or leukemia—the determination is made based on the amount of bone marrow involvement. The cells are small to medium immature T-cells that often originate in the thymus where many of the T-cells are made.

C83.50   Lymphoblastic (diffuse) lymphoma, unspecified site   CC HCC

C83.51   Lymphoblastic (diffuse) lymphoma, lymph nodes of head, face, and neck   CC HCC

C83.52   Lymphoblastic (diffuse) lymphoma, intrathoracic lymph nodes   CC HCC

C83.53   Lymphoblastic (diffuse) lymphoma, intra-abdominal lymph nodes   CC HCC

C83.54   Lymphoblastic (diffuse) lymphoma, lymph nodes of axilla and upper limb   CC HCC

C83.55   Lymphoblastic (diffuse) lymphoma, lymph nodes of inguinal region and lower limb   CC HCC

C83.56   Lymphoblastic (diffuse) lymphoma, intrapelvic lymph nodes   CC HCC

C83.57   Lymphoblastic (diffuse) lymphoma, spleen   CC HCC

C83.58   Lymphoblastic (diffuse) lymphoma, lymph nodes of multiple sites   CC HCC

C83.59   Lymphoblastic (diffuse) lymphoma, extranodal and solid organ sites   CC HCC

✓5ᵗʰ **C83.7**   Burkitt lymphoma

Atypical Burkitt lymphoma

Burkitt-like lymphoma

EXCLUDES 1   mature B-cell leukemia Burkitt type (C91.A-)

DEF: Malignancy of the lymphatic system, most often seen as a large bone-deteriorating lesion within the jaw or as an abdominal mass. It is a form of non-Hodgkin's lymphoma and is recognized as the fastest growing human tumor.

C83.70   Burkitt lymphoma, unspecified site   HIV CC HCC

C83.71   Burkitt lymphoma, lymph nodes of head, face, and neck   HIV CC HCC

C83.72   Burkitt lymphoma, intrathoracic lymph nodes   HIV CC HCC

C83.73   Burkitt lymphoma, intra-abdominal lymph nodes   HIV CC HCC

C83.74   Burkitt lymphoma, lymph nodes of axilla and upper limb   HIV CC HCC

C83.75   Burkitt lymphoma, lymph nodes of inguinal region and lower limb   HIV CC HCC

C83.76   Burkitt lymphoma, intrapelvic lymph nodes   HIV CC HCC

C83.77   Burkitt lymphoma, spleen   HIV CC HCC

C83.78   Burkitt lymphoma, lymph nodes of multiple sites   HIV CC HCC

C83.79   Burkitt lymphoma, extranodal and solid organ sites   HIV CC HCC

✓5ᵗʰ **C83.8**   Other non-follicular lymphoma

Intravascular large B-cell lymphoma

Lymphoid granulomatosis

Primary effusion B-cell lymphoma

EXCLUDES 1   mediastinal (thymic) large B-cell lymphoma (C85.2-)

T-cell rich B-cell lymphoma (C83.3-)

C83.80   Other non-follicular lymphoma, unspecified site   HIV CC HCC

C83.81   Other non-follicular lymphoma, lymph nodes of head, face, and neck   HIV CC HCC

C83.82   Other non-follicular lymphoma, intrathoracic lymph nodes   HIV CC HCC

C83.83   Other non-follicular lymphoma, intra-abdominal lymph nodes   HIV CC HCC

C83.84   Other non-follicular lymphoma, lymph nodes of axilla and upper limb   HIV CC HCC

C83.85   Other non-follicular lymphoma, lymph nodes of inguinal region and lower limb   HIV CC HCC

C83.86   Other non-follicular lymphoma, intrapelvic lymph nodes   HIV CC HCC

C83.87   Other non-follicular lymphoma, spleen   HIV CC HCC

C83.88   Other non-follicular lymphoma, lymph nodes of multiple sites   HIV CC HCC

C83.89   Other non-follicular lymphoma, extranodal and solid organ sites   HIV CC HCC

✓5ᵗʰ **C83.9**   Non-follicular (diffuse) lymphoma, unspecified

C83.90   Non-follicular (diffuse) lymphoma, unspecified, unspecified site   HIV CC HCC

C83.91   Non-follicular (diffuse) lymphoma, unspecified, lymph nodes of head, face, and neck   HIV CC HCC

C83.92   Non-follicular (diffuse) lymphoma, unspecified, intrathoracic lymph nodes   HIV CC HCC

C83.93   Non-follicular (diffuse) lymphoma, unspecified, intra-abdominal lymph nodes   HIV CC HCC

C83.94   Non-follicular (diffuse) lymphoma, unspecified, lymph nodes of axilla and upper limb   HIV CC HCC

☑ Additional Character Required   ✓7ᵗʰ Placeholder   Questionable PDx   Manifestation   Unspecified Dx   UPD Unacceptable PDx   H1-H14 HAC   HCC CMS-HCC Dx   HIV HIV Dx

ICD-10-CM 2022   487

C83.95 Non-follicular (diffuse) lymphoma, unspecified, lymph nodes of inguinal region and lower limb `HIV` `CC` `HCC`

C83.96 Non-follicular (diffuse) lymphoma, unspecified, intrapelvic lymph nodes `HIV` `CC` `HCC`

C83.97 Non-follicular (diffuse) lymphoma, unspecified, spleen `HIV` `CC` `HCC`

C83.98 Non-follicular (diffuse) lymphoma, unspecified, lymph nodes of multiple sites `HIV` `CC` `HCC`

C83.99 Non-follicular (diffuse) lymphoma, unspecified, extranodal and solid organ sites `HIV` `CC` `HCC`

√4ᵗʰ **C84 Mature T/NK-cell lymphomas**

EXCLUDES 1   *personal history of non-Hodgkin lymphoma (Z85.72)*

√5ᵗʰ **C84.0 Mycosis fungoides**

EXCLUDES 1   *peripheral T-cell lymphoma, not classified (C84.4-)*

DEF: Most common form of cutaneous T-cell lymphoma. A type of non-Hodgkin lymphoma in which white blood cells become cancerous and affect the skin and sometimes internal organs.

Synonym(s): *Alibert-Bazin syndrome.*

C84.00 Mycosis fungoides, unspecified site `CC` `HCC`

C84.01 Mycosis fungoides, lymph nodes of head, face, and neck `CC` `HCC`

C84.02 Mycosis fungoides, intrathoracic lymph nodes `CC` `HCC`

C84.03 Mycosis fungoides, intra-abdominal lymph nodes `CC` `HCC`

C84.04 Mycosis fungoides, lymph nodes of axilla and upper limb `CC` `HCC`

C84.05 Mycosis fungoides, lymph nodes of inguinal region and lower limb `CC` `HCC`

C84.06 Mycosis fungoides, intrapelvic lymph nodes `CC` `HCC`

C84.07 Mycosis fungoides, spleen `CC` `HCC`

C84.08 Mycosis fungoides, lymph nodes of multiple sites `CC` `HCC`

C84.09 Mycosis fungoides, extranodal and solid organ sites `CC` `HCC`

√5ᵗʰ **C84.1 Sézary disease**

DEF: Extension of mycosis fungoides that affects the blood and all of the skin, appearing as sunburn, rather than patches. It spreads to the lymph nodes and is often linked to a weakened immune system.

C84.10 Sézary disease, unspecified site `CC` `HCC`

C84.11 Sézary disease, lymph nodes of head, face, and neck `CC` `HCC`

C84.12 Sézary disease, intrathoracic lymph nodes `CC` `HCC`

C84.13 Sézary disease, intra-abdominal lymph nodes `CC` `HCC`

C84.14 Sézary disease, lymph nodes of axilla and upper limb `CC` `HCC`

C84.15 Sézary disease, lymph nodes of inguinal region and lower limb `CC` `HCC`

C84.16 Sézary disease, intrapelvic lymph nodes `CC` `HCC`

C84.17 Sézary disease, spleen `CC` `HCC`

C84.18 Sézary disease, lymph nodes of multiple sites `CC` `HCC`

C84.19 Sézary disease, extranodal and solid organ sites `CC` `HCC`

√5ᵗʰ **C84.4 Peripheral T-cell lymphoma, not classified**

Lennert's lymphoma

Lymphoepithelioid lymphoma

Mature T-cell lymphoma, not elsewhere classified

C84.40 Peripheral T-cell lymphoma, not classified, unspecified site `HIV` `CC` `HCC`

C84.41 Peripheral T-cell lymphoma, not classified, lymph nodes of head, face, and neck `HIV` `CC` `HCC`

C84.42 Peripheral T-cell lymphoma, not classified, intrathoracic lymph nodes `HIV` `CC` `HCC`

C84.43 Peripheral T-cell lymphoma, not classified, intra-abdominal lymph nodes `HIV` `CC` `HCC`

C84.44 Peripheral T-cell lymphoma, not classified, lymph nodes of axilla and upper limb `HIV` `CC` `HCC`

C84.45 Peripheral T-cell lymphoma, not classified, lymph nodes of inguinal region and lower limb `HIV` `CC` `HCC`

C84.46 Peripheral T-cell lymphoma, not classified, intrapelvic lymph nodes `HIV` `CC` `HCC`

C84.47 Peripheral T-cell lymphoma, not classified, spleen `HIV` `CC` `HCC`

C84.48 Peripheral T-cell lymphoma, not classified, lymph nodes of multiple sites `HIV` `CC` `HCC`

C84.49 Peripheral T-cell lymphoma, not classified, extranodal and solid organ sites `HIV` `CC` `HCC`

√5ᵗʰ **C84.6 Anaplastic large cell lymphoma, ALK-positive**

Anaplastic large cell lymphoma, CD30-positive

C84.60 Anaplastic large cell lymphoma, ALK-positive, unspecified site `HIV` `CC` `HCC`

C84.61 Anaplastic large cell lymphoma, ALK-positive, lymph nodes of head, face, and neck `HIV` `CC` `HCC`

C84.62 Anaplastic large cell lymphoma, ALK-positive, intrathoracic lymph nodes `HIV` `CC` `HCC`

C84.63 Anaplastic large cell lymphoma, ALK-positive, intra-abdominal lymph nodes `HIV` `CC` `HCC`

C84.64 Anaplastic large cell lymphoma, ALK-positive, lymph nodes of axilla and upper limb `HIV` `CC` `HCC`

C84.65 Anaplastic large cell lymphoma, ALK-positive, lymph nodes of inguinal region and lower limb `HIV` `CC` `HCC`

C84.66 Anaplastic large cell lymphoma, ALK-positive, intrapelvic lymph nodes `HIV` `CC` `HCC`

C84.67 Anaplastic large cell lymphoma, ALK-positive, spleen `HIV` `CC` `HCC`

C84.68 Anaplastic large cell lymphoma, ALK-positive, lymph nodes of multiple sites `HIV` `CC` `HCC`

C84.69 Anaplastic large cell lymphoma, ALK-positive, extranodal and solid organ sites `HIV` `CC` `HCC`

√5ᵗʰ **C84.7 Anaplastic large cell lymphoma, ALK-negative**

EXCLUDES 1   *primary cutaneous CD30-positive T-cell proliferations (C86.6-)*

C84.70 Anaplastic large cell lymphoma, ALK-negative, unspecified site `HIV` `CC` `HCC`

C84.71 Anaplastic large cell lymphoma, ALK-negative, lymph nodes of head, face, and neck `HIV` `CC` `HCC`

C84.72 Anaplastic large cell lymphoma, ALK-negative, intrathoracic lymph nodes `HIV` `CC` `HCC`

C84.73 Anaplastic large cell lymphoma, ALK-negative, intra-abdominal lymph nodes `HIV` `CC` `HCC`

C84.74 Anaplastic large cell lymphoma, ALK-negative, lymph nodes of axilla and upper limb `HIV` `CC` `HCC`

C84.75 Anaplastic large cell lymphoma, ALK-negative, lymph nodes of inguinal region and lower limb `HIV` `CC` `HCC`

C84.76 Anaplastic large cell lymphoma, ALK-negative, intrapelvic lymph nodes `HIV` `CC` `HCC`

C84.77 Anaplastic large cell lymphoma, ALK-negative, spleen `HIV` `CC` `HCC`

C84.78 Anaplastic large cell lymphoma, ALK-negative, lymph nodes of multiple sites `HIV` `CC` `HCC`

C84.79 Anaplastic large cell lymphoma, ALK-negative, extranodal and solid organ sites `HIV` `CC` `HCC`

C84.7A Anaplastic large cell lymphoma, ALK-negative, breast `CC`

Breast implant associated anaplastic large cell lymphoma (BIA-ALCL)

Use additional code to identify:

breast implant status (Z98.82)

personal history of breast implant removal (Z98.86)

√5ᵗʰ **C84.A Cutaneous T-cell lymphoma, unspecified**

AHA: 2021,2Q,6

C84.A0 Cutaneous T-cell lymphoma, unspecified, unspecified site `HIV` `CC` `HCC`

C84.A1 Cutaneous T-cell lymphoma, unspecified lymph nodes of head, face, and neck `HIV` `CC` `HCC`

C84.A2 Cutaneous T-cell lymphoma, unspecified, intrathoracic lymph nodes `HIV` `CC` `HCC`

C84.A3 Cutaneous T-cell lymphoma, unspecified, intra-abdominal lymph nodes `HIV` `CC` `HCC`

C84.A4 Cutaneous T-cell lymphoma, unspecified, lymph nodes of axilla and upper limb `HIV` `CC` `HCC`

C84.A5 Cutaneous T-cell lymphoma, unspecified, lymph nodes of inguinal region and lower limb `HIV` `CC` `HCC`

C84.A6 Cutaneous T-cell lymphoma, unspecified, intrapelvic lymph nodes `HIV` `CC` `HCC`

C84.A7 Cutaneous T-cell lymphoma, unspecified, spleen `HIV` `CC` `HCC`

`N` Newborn: 0   `P` Pediatric: 0-17   `M` Maternity: 9-64   `A` Adult: 15-124   `MCC` Major Complication/Comorbidity   `CC` Complication/Comorbidity   `SW` Severe Wound Dx

488   ICD-10-CM 2022

C84.A8   **Cutaneous T-cell lymphoma, unspecified, lymph nodes of multiple sites** `HIV` `CC` `HCC`

C84.A9   **Cutaneous T-cell lymphoma, unspecified, extranodal and solid organ sites** `HIV` `CC` `HCC`

√5ᵗʰ **C84.Z**   **Other mature T/NK-cell lymphomas**

> `NOTE` If T-cell lineage or involvement is mentioned in conjunction with a specific lymphoma, code to the more specific description.

> `EXCLUDES 1` angioimmunoblastic T-cell lymphoma (C86.5)
> blastic NK-cell lymphoma (C86.4)
> enteropathy-type T-cell lymphoma (C86.2)
> extranodal NK-cell lymphoma, nasal type (C86.0)
> hepatosplenic T-cell lymphoma (C86.1)
> primary cutaneous CD30-positive T-cell proliferations (C86.6)
> subcutaneous panniculitis-like T-cell lymphoma (C86.3)
> T-cell leukemia (C91.1-)

C84.Z0   **Other mature T/NK-cell lymphomas, unspecified site** `HIV` `CC` `HCC`

C84.Z1   **Other mature T/NK-cell lymphomas, lymph nodes of head, face, and neck** `HIV` `CC` `HCC`

C84.Z2   **Other mature T/NK-cell lymphomas, intrathoracic lymph nodes** `HIV` `CC` `HCC`

C84.Z3   **Other mature T/NK-cell lymphomas, intra-abdominal lymph nodes** `HIV` `CC` `HCC`

C84.Z4   **Other mature T/NK-cell lymphomas, lymph nodes of axilla and upper limb** `HIV` `CC` `HCC`

C84.Z5   **Other mature T/NK-cell lymphomas, lymph nodes of inguinal region and lower limb** `HIV` `CC` `HCC`

C84.Z6   **Other mature T/NK-cell lymphomas, intrapelvic lymph nodes** `HIV` `CC` `HCC`

C84.Z7   **Other mature T/NK-cell lymphomas, spleen** `HIV` `CC` `HCC`

C84.Z8   **Other mature T/NK-cell lymphomas, lymph nodes of multiple sites** `HIV` `CC` `HCC`

C84.Z9   **Other mature T/NK-cell lymphomas, extranodal and solid organ sites** `HIV` `CC` `HCC`

√5ᵗʰ **C84.9**   **Mature T/NK-cell lymphomas, unspecified**

> NK/T cell lymphoma NOS

> `EXCLUDES 1` mature T-cell lymphoma, not elsewhere classified (C84.4-)

C84.90   **Mature T/NK-cell lymphomas, unspecified, unspecified site** `HIV` `CC` `HCC`

C84.91   **Mature T/NK-cell lymphomas, unspecified, lymph nodes of head, face, and neck** `HIV` `CC` `HCC`

C84.92   **Mature T/NK-cell lymphomas, unspecified, intrathoracic lymph nodes** `HIV` `CC` `HCC`

C84.93   **Mature T/NK-cell lymphomas, unspecified, intra-abdominal lymph nodes** `HIV` `CC` `HCC`

C84.94   **Mature T/NK-cell lymphomas, unspecified, lymph nodes of axilla and upper limb** `HIV` `CC` `HCC`

C84.95   **Mature T/NK-cell lymphomas, unspecified, lymph nodes of inguinal region and lower limb** `HIV` `CC` `HCC`

C84.96   **Mature T/NK-cell lymphomas, unspecified, intrapelvic lymph nodes** `HIV` `CC` `HCC`

C84.97   **Mature T/NK-cell lymphomas, unspecified, spleen** `HIV` `CC` `HCC`

C84.98   **Mature T/NK-cell lymphomas, unspecified, lymph nodes of multiple sites** `HIV` `CC` `HCC`

C84.99   **Mature T/NK-cell lymphomas, unspecified, extranodal and solid organ sites** `HIV` `CC` `HCC`

√4ᵗʰ **C85**   **Other specified and unspecified types of non-Hodgkin lymphoma**

> `EXCLUDES 1` other specified types of T/NK-cell lymphoma (C86.-)
> personal history of non-Hodgkin lymphoma (Z85.72)

√5ᵗʰ **C85.1**   **Unspecified B-cell lymphoma**

> `NOTE` If B-cell lineage or involvement is mentioned in conjunction with a specific lymphoma, code to the more specific description.

C85.10   **Unspecified B-cell lymphoma, unspecified site** `HIV` `CC` `HCC`

C85.11   **Unspecified B-cell lymphoma, lymph nodes of head, face, and neck** `HIV` `CC` `HCC`

C85.12   **Unspecified B-cell lymphoma, intrathoracic lymph nodes** `HIV` `CC` `HCC`

C85.13   **Unspecified B-cell lymphoma, intra-abdominal lymph nodes** `HIV` `CC` `HCC`

C85.14   **Unspecified B-cell lymphoma, lymph nodes of axilla and upper limb** `HIV` `CC` `HCC`

C85.15   **Unspecified B-cell lymphoma, lymph nodes of inguinal region and lower limb** `HIV` `CC` `HCC`

C85.16   **Unspecified B-cell lymphoma, intrapelvic lymph nodes** `HIV` `CC` `HCC`

C85.17   **Unspecified B-cell lymphoma, spleen** `HIV` `CC` `HCC`

C85.18   **Unspecified B-cell lymphoma, lymph nodes of multiple sites** `HIV` `CC` `HCC`

C85.19   **Unspecified B-cell lymphoma, extranodal and solid organ sites** `HIV` `CC` `HCC`

√5ᵗʰ **C85.2**   **Mediastinal (thymic) large B-cell lymphoma**

C85.20   **Mediastinal (thymic) large B-cell lymphoma, unspecified site** `HIV` `CC` `HCC`

C85.21   **Mediastinal (thymic) large B-cell lymphoma, lymph nodes of head, face, and neck** `HIV` `CC` `HCC`

C85.22   **Mediastinal (thymic) large B-cell lymphoma, intrathoracic lymph nodes** `HIV` `CC` `HCC`

C85.23   **Mediastinal (thymic) large B-cell lymphoma, intra-abdominal lymph nodes** `HIV` `CC` `HCC`

C85.24   **Mediastinal (thymic) large B-cell lymphoma, lymph nodes of axilla and upper limb** `HIV` `CC` `HCC`

C85.25   **Mediastinal (thymic) large B-cell lymphoma, lymph nodes of inguinal region and lower limb** `HIV` `CC` `HCC`

C85.26   **Mediastinal (thymic) large B-cell lymphoma, intrapelvic lymph nodes** `HIV` `CC` `HCC`

C85.27   **Mediastinal (thymic) large B-cell lymphoma, spleen** `HIV` `CC` `HCC`

C85.28   **Mediastinal (thymic) large B-cell lymphoma, lymph nodes of multiple sites** `HIV` `CC` `HCC`

C85.29   **Mediastinal (thymic) large B-cell lymphoma, extranodal and solid organ sites** `HIV` `CC` `HCC`

√5ᵗʰ **C85.8**   **Other specified types of non-Hodgkin lymphoma**

C85.80   **Other specified types of non-Hodgkin lymphoma, unspecified site** `HIV` `CC` `HCC`

C85.81   **Other specified types of non-Hodgkin lymphoma, lymph nodes of head, face, and neck** `HIV` `CC` `HCC`

C85.82   **Other specified types of non-Hodgkin lymphoma, intrathoracic lymph nodes** `HIV` `CC` `HCC`

C85.83   **Other specified types of non-Hodgkin lymphoma, intra-abdominal lymph nodes** `HIV` `CC` `HCC`

C85.84   **Other specified types of non-Hodgkin lymphoma, lymph nodes of axilla and upper limb** `HIV` `CC` `HCC`

C85.85   **Other specified types of non-Hodgkin lymphoma, lymph nodes of inguinal region and lower limb** `HIV` `CC` `HCC`

C85.86   **Other specified types of non-Hodgkin lymphoma, intrapelvic lymph nodes** `HIV` `CC` `HCC`

C85.87   **Other specified types of non-Hodgkin lymphoma, spleen** `HIV` `CC` `HCC`

C85.88   **Other specified types of non-Hodgkin lymphoma, lymph nodes of multiple sites** `HIV` `CC` `HCC`

C85.89   **Other specified types of non-Hodgkin lymphoma, extranodal and solid organ sites** `HIV` `CC` `HCC`

√5ᵗʰ **C85.9**   **Non-Hodgkin lymphoma, unspecified**

> Lymphoma NOS
> Malignant lymphoma NOS
> Non-Hodgkin lymphoma NOS

C85.90   **Non-Hodgkin lymphoma, unspecified, unspecified site** `HIV` `CC` `HCC`

C85.91   **Non-Hodgkin lymphoma, unspecified, lymph nodes of head, face, and neck** `HIV` `CC` `HCC`

C85.92   **Non-Hodgkin lymphoma, unspecified, intrathoracic lymph nodes** `HIV` `CC` `HCC`

C85.93   **Non-Hodgkin lymphoma, unspecified, intra-abdominal lymph nodes** `HIV` `CC` `HCC`

C85.94   **Non-Hodgkin lymphoma, unspecified, lymph nodes of axilla and upper limb** `HIV` `CC` `HCC`

C85.95   **Non-Hodgkin lymphoma, unspecified, lymph nodes of inguinal region and lower limb** `HIV` `CC` `HCC`

C85.96   **Non-Hodgkin lymphoma, unspecified, intrapelvic lymph nodes** `HIV` `CC` `HCC`

C85.97   **Non-Hodgkin lymphoma, unspecified, spleen** `HIV` `CC` `HCC`

C85.98   **Non-Hodgkin lymphoma, unspecified, lymph nodes of multiple sites** `HIV` `CC` `HCC`

☑ Additional Character Required   √x7ᵗʰ Placeholder   Questionable PDx   Manifestation   Unspecified Dx   `UPD` Unacceptable PDx   `H1`-`H14` HAC   `HCC` CMS-HCC Dx   `HIV` HIV Dx

ICD-10-CM 2022   489

C85.99   **Non-Hodgkin lymphoma, unspecified,** extranodal and solid organ sites   `HIV` `CC` `HCC`

✓4ᵗʰ **C86**   **Other specified types of T/NK-cell lymphoma**

    EXCLUDES 1   anaplastic large cell lymphoma, ALK negative (C84.7-)
       anaplastic large cell lymphoma, ALK positive (C84.6-)
       mature T/NK-cell lymphomas (C84.-)
       other specified types of non-Hodgkin lymphoma (C85.8-)

C86.0   **Extranodal NK/T-cell lymphoma, nasal type**   `HIV` `CC` `HCC`

C86.1   **Hepatosplenic T-cell lymphoma**   `HIV` `CC` `HCC`
    Alpha-beta and gamma delta types

C86.2   **Enteropathy-type (intestinal) T-cell lymphoma**   `HIV` `CC` `HCC`
    Enteropathy associated T-cell lymphoma

C86.3   **Subcutaneous panniculitis-like T-cell lymphoma**   `HIV` `CC` `HCC`

C86.4   **Blastic NK-cell lymphoma**   `HIV` `CC` `HCC`
    Blastic plasmacytoid dendritic cell neoplasm (BPDCN)

C86.5   **Angioimmunoblastic T-cell lymphoma**   `HIV` `CC` `HCC`
    Angioimmunoblastic lymphadenopathy with dysproteinemia (AILD)

C86.6   **Primary cutaneous CD30-positive T-cell proliferations**   `HIV` `CC` `HCC`
    Lymphomatoid papulosis
    Primary cutaneous anaplastic large cell lymphoma
    Primary cutaneous CD30-positive large T-cell lymphoma

✓4ᵗʰ **C88**   **Malignant immunoproliferative diseases and certain other B-cell lymphomas**

    EXCLUDES 1   B-cell lymphoma, unspecified (C85.1-)
       personal history of other malignant neoplasms of lymphoid, hematopoietic and related tissues (Z85.79)

C88.0   **Waldenström macroglobulinemia**   `HCC`
    Lymphoplasmacytic lymphoma with IgM-production
    Macroglobulinemia (idiopathic) (primary)
    EXCLUDES 1   small cell B-cell lymphoma (C83.0)

C88.2   **Heavy chain disease**   `CC` `HCC`
    Franklin disease
    Gamma heavy chain disease
    Mu heavy chain disease

C88.3   **Immunoproliferative small intestinal disease**   `CC` `HCC`
    Alpha heavy chain disease
    Mediterranean lymphoma

C88.4   **Extranodal marginal zone B-cell lymphoma of mucosa-associated lymphoid tissue [MALT-lymphoma]**   `HIV` `CC` `HCC`
    Lymphoma of skin-associated lymphoid tissue [SALT-lymphoma]
    Lymphoma of bronchial-associated lymphoid tissue [BALT-lymphoma]
    EXCLUDES 1   high malignant (diffuse large B-cell) lymphoma (C83.3-)

C88.8   **Other malignant immunoproliferative diseases**   `CC` `HCC`

C88.9   **Malignant immunoproliferative disease, unspecified**   `CC` `HCC`
    Immunoproliferative disease NOS

✓4ᵗʰ **C90**   **Multiple myeloma and malignant plasma cell neoplasms**

    EXCLUDES 1   personal history of other malignant neoplasms of lymphoid, hematopoietic and related tissues (Z85.79)

    AHA: 2019,2Q,30

✓5ᵗʰ **C90.0**   **Multiple myeloma**
    Kahler's disease
    Medullary plasmacytoma
    Myelomatosis
    Plasma cell myeloma
    EXCLUDES 1   solitary myeloma (C90.3-)
       solitary plasmactyoma (C90.3-)
    TIP: Do not assign an additional code for bone metastasis (C79.51) when multiple myeloma is described as metastatic to the bone; bone involvement is integral to this disease process.

C90.00   **Multiple myeloma** not having achieved remission   `CC` `HCC`
    Multiple myeloma with failed remission
    Multiple myeloma NOS

C90.01   **Multiple myeloma** in remission   `CC` `HCC`

C90.02   **Multiple myeloma** in relapse   `CC` `HCC`

✓5ᵗʰ **C90.1**   **Plasma cell leukemia**
    Plasmacytic leukemia
    AHA: 2019,2Q,30

C90.10   **Plasma cell leukemia** not having achieved remission   `CC` `HCC`
    Plasma cell leukemia with failed remission
    Plasma cell leukemia NOS

C90.11   **Plasma cell leukemia** in remission   `CC` `HCC`

C90.12   **Plasma cell leukemia** in relapse   `CC` `HCC`

✓5ᵗʰ **C90.2**   **Extramedullary plasmacytoma**

C90.20   **Extramedullary plasmacytoma** not having achieved remission   `CC` `HCC`
    Extramedullary plasmacytoma with failed remission
    Extramedullary plasmacytoma NOS

C90.21   **Extramedullary plasmacytoma** in remission   `CC` `HCC`

C90.22   **Extramedullary plasmacytoma** in relapse   `CC` `HCC`

✓5ᵗʰ **C90.3**   **Solitary plasmacytoma**
    Localized malignant plasma cell tumor NOS
    Plasmacytoma NOS
    Solitary myeloma

C90.30   **Solitary plasmacytoma** not having achieved remission   `CC` `HCC`
    Solitary plasmacytoma with failed remission
    Solitary plasmacytoma NOS

C90.31   **Solitary plasmacytoma** in remission   `CC` `HCC`

C90.32   **Solitary plasmacytoma** in relapse   `CC` `HCC`

✓4ᵗʰ **C91**   **Lymphoid leukemia**

    EXCLUDES 1   personal history of leukemia (Z85.6)
    AHA: 2020,1Q,13
    DEF: Malignant proliferation of immature lymphocytes (white blood cells that make up lymphoid tissue), called lymphoblasts, that originate in the bone marrow. Can be acute (ALL) or chronic (CLL).

✓5ᵗʰ **C91.0**   **Acute lymphoblastic leukemia [ALL]**

    `NOTE`   Codes in subcategory C91.0- should only be used for T-cell and B-cell precursor leukemia

C91.00   **Acute lymphoblastic leukemia** not having achieved remission   `CC` `HCC`
    Acute lymphoblastic leukemia with failed remission
    Acute lymphoblastic leukemia NOS

C91.01   **Acute lymphoblastic leukemia,** in remission   `CC` `HCC`

C91.02   **Acute lymphoblastic leukemia,** in relapse   `CC` `HCC`

✓5ᵗʰ **C91.1**   **Chronic lymphocytic leukemia of B-cell type**
    Lymphoplasmacytic leukemia
    Richter syndrome
    EXCLUDES 1   lymphoplasmacytic lymphoma (C83.0-)

C91.10   **Chronic lymphocytic leukemia of B-cell type** not having achieved remission   `CC` `HCC`
    Chronic lymphocytic leukemia of B-cell type with failed remission
    Chronic lymphocytic leukemia of B-cell type NOS

C91.11   **Chronic lymphocytic leukemia of B-cell type** in remission   `CC` `HCC`

C91.12   **Chronic lymphocytic leukemia of B-cell type** in relapse   `CC` `HCC`

✓5ᵗʰ **C91.3**   **Prolymphocytic leukemia of B-cell type**

C91.30   **Prolymphocytic leukemia of B-cell type** not having achieved remission   `CC` `HCC`
    Prolymphocytic leukemia of B-cell type with failed remission
    Prolymphocytic leukemia of B-cell type NOS

C91.31   **Prolymphocytic leukemia of B-cell type,** in remission   `CC` `HCC`

C91.32   **Prolymphocytic leukemia of B-cell type,** in relapse   `CC` `HCC`

✓5ᵗʰ **C91.4** Hairy cell **leukemia**

Leukemic reticuloendotheliosis

DEF: Rare type of leukemia that is slow growing and often also considered a type of lymphoma. The small B-cell lymphocytes appear with "hairy" projections under a microscope and are found mostly in the bone marrow, spleen, and blood.

C91.40 **Hairy cell leukemia** not having achieved remission   CC HCC

Hairy cell leukemia with failed remission

Hairy cell leukemia NOS

C91.41 **Hairy cell leukemia, in remission**   CC HCC

C91.42 **Hairy cell leukemia, in relapse**   CC HCC

✓5ᵗʰ **C91.5** Adult T-cell **lymphoma/leukemia (HTLV-1-associated)**

Acute variant of adult T-cell lymphoma/leukemia (HTLV-1-associated)

Chronic variant of adult T-cell lymphoma/leukemia (HTLV-1-associated)

Lymphomatoid variant of adult T-cell lymphoma/leukemia (HTLV-1-associated)

Smouldering variant of adult T-cell lymphoma/leukemia (HTLV-1-associated)

C91.50 **Adult T-cell lymphoma/leukemia (HTLV-1-associated)** not having achieved remission   CC HCC A

Adult T-cell lymphoma/leukemia (HTLV-1-associated) with failed remission

Adult T-cell lymphoma/leukemia (HTLV-1-associated) NOS

C91.51 **Adult T-cell lymphoma/leukemia (HTLV-1-associated), in remission**   CC HCC A

C91.52 **Adult T-cell lymphoma/leukemia (HTLV-1-associated), in relapse**   CC HCC A

✓5ᵗʰ **C91.6** Prolymphocytic **leukemia of T-cell type**

C91.60 **Prolymphocytic leukemia of T-cell type** not having achieved remission   CC HCC

Prolymphocytic leukemia of T-cell type with failed remission

Prolymphocytic leukemia of T-cell type NOS

C91.61 **Prolymphocytic leukemia of T-cell type, in remission**   CC HCC

C91.62 **Prolymphocytic leukemia of T-cell type, in relapse**   CC HCC

✓5ᵗʰ **C91.A** Mature B-cell **leukemia** Burkitt-type

EXCLUDES 1   *Burkitt lymphoma (C83.7-)*

C91.A0 **Mature B-cell leukemia Burkitt-type** not having achieved remission   CC HCC

Mature B-cell leukemia Burkitt-type with failed remission

Mature B-cell leukemia Burkitt-type NOS

C91.A1 **Mature B-cell leukemia Burkitt-type, in remission**   CC HCC

C91.A2 **Mature B-cell leukemia Burkitt-type, in relapse**   CC HCC

✓5ᵗʰ **C91.Z** Other **lymphoid leukemia**

T-cell large granular lymphocytic leukemia (associated with rheumatoid arthritis)

C91.Z0 **Other lymphoid leukemia** not having achieved remission   CC HCC

Other lymphoid leukemia with failed remission

Other lymphoid leukemia NOS

C91.Z1 **Other lymphoid leukemia, in remission**   CC HCC

C91.Z2 **Other lymphoid leukemia, in relapse**   CC HCC

✓5ᵗʰ **C91.9** Lymphoid **leukemia, unspecified**

C91.90 **Lymphoid leukemia, unspecified** not having achieved remission   CC HCC

Lymphoid leukemia with failed remission

Lymphoid leukemia NOS

C91.91 **Lymphoid leukemia, unspecified, in remission**   CC HCC

C91.92 **Lymphoid leukemia, unspecified, in relapse**   CC HCC

✓4ᵗʰ **C92** Myeloid **leukemia**

INCLUDES   granulocytic leukemia

        myelogenous leukemia

EXCLUDES 1   *personal history of leukemia (Z85.6)*

AHA: 2020,1Q,13; 2019,1Q,16

DEF: Cancer that develops in immature myelocytes called myeloblasts. These are the cells that become white blood cells (except lymphocytes), red blood cells, or platelet-making cells. Can be acute (AML) or chronic (CML).

TIP: Pancytopenia, although common in some types of myeloid leukemias, is not always inherent. When it is documented, code D61.818 can be assigned in addition to a code from this category.

✓5ᵗʰ **C92.0** Acute myeloblastic **leukemia**

Acute myeloblastic leukemia, minimal differentiation

Acute myeloblastic leukemia (with maturation)

Acute myeloblastic leukemia 1/ETO

Acute myeloblastic leukemia M0

Acute myeloblastic leukemia M1

Acute myeloblastic leukemia M2

Acute myeloblastic leukemia with t(8;21)

Acute myeloblastic leukemia (without a FAB classification) NOS

Refractory anemia with excess blasts in transformation [RAEBT]

EXCLUDES 1   *acute exacerbation of chronic myeloid leukemia (C92.10)*

        refractory anemia with excess of blasts not in transformation (D46.2-)

AHA: 2018,4Q,87

C92.00 **Acute myeloblastic leukemia,** not having achieved remission   CC HCC

Acute myeloblastic leukemia with failed remission

Acute myeloblastic leukemia NOS

C92.01 **Acute myeloblastic leukemia, in remission**   CC HCC

C92.02 **Acute myeloblastic leukemia, in relapse**   CC HCC

✓5ᵗʰ **C92.1** Chronic **myeloid leukemia,** BCR/ABL-positive

Chronic myelogenous leukemia, Philadelphia chromosome (Ph1) positive

Chronic myelogenous leukemia, t(9;22) (q34;q11)

Chronic myelogenous leukemia with crisis of blast cells

EXCLUDES 1   *atypical chronic myeloid leukemia BCR/ABL-negative (C92.2-)*

        chronic myelomonocytic leukemia (C93.1-)

        chronic myeloproliferative disease (D47.1)

C92.10 **Chronic myeloid leukemia, BCR/ABL-positive,** not having achieved remission   CC HCC

Chronic myeloid leukemia, BCR/ABL-positive with failed remission

Chronic myeloid leukemia, BCR/ABL-positive NOS

C92.11 **Chronic myeloid leukemia, BCR/ABL-positive, in remission**   CC HCC

C92.12 **Chronic myeloid leukemia, BCR/ABL-positive, in relapse**   CC HCC

✓5ᵗʰ **C92.2** Atypical chronic **myeloid leukemia, BCR/ABL-negative**

C92.20 **Atypical chronic myeloid leukemia, BCR/ABL-negative,** not having achieved remission   CC HCC

Atypical chronic myeloid leukemia, BCR/ABL-negative with failed remission

Atypical chronic myeloid leukemia, BCR/ABL-negative NOS

C92.21 **Atypical chronic myeloid leukemia, BCR/ABL-negative, in remission**   CC HCC

C92.22 **Atypical chronic myeloid leukemia, BCR/ABL-negative, in relapse**   CC HCC

✓5ᵗʰ **C92.3** Myeloid **sarcoma**

A malignant tumor of immature myeloid cells

Chloroma

Granulocytic sarcoma

C92.30 **Myeloid sarcoma,** not having achieved remission   CC HCC

Myeloid sarcoma with failed remission

Myeloid sarcoma NOS

C92.31 **Myeloid sarcoma, in remission**   CC HCC

C92.32 **Myeloid sarcoma, in relapse**   CC HCC

✓ Additional Character Required   ✓x7ᵗʰ Placeholder   Questionable PDx   Manifestation   Unspecified Dx   UPD Unacceptable PDx   H1-H4 HAC   HCC CMS-HCC Dx   HIV HIV Dx

ICD-10-CM 2022   491

√5ᵗʰ C92.4 Acute promyelocytic leukemia

AML M3
AML Me with t(15;17) and variants

C92.40 Acute promyelocytic leukemia, not having achieved remission `CC` `HCC`

Acute promyelocytic leukemia with failed remission
Acute promyelocytic leukemia NOS

C92.41 Acute promyelocytic leukemia, in remission `CC` `HCC`

C92.42 Acute promyelocytic leukemia, in relapse `CC` `HCC`

√5ᵗʰ C92.5 Acute myelomonocytic leukemia

AML M4
AML M4 Eo with inv(16) or t(16;16)

C92.50 Acute myelomonocytic leukemia, not having achieved remission `CC` `HCC`

Acute myelomonocytic leukemia with failed remission
Acute myelomonocytic leukemia NOS

C92.51 Acute myelomonocytic leukemia, in remission `CC` `HCC`

C92.52 Acute myelomonocytic leukemia, in relapse `CC` `HCC`

√5ᵗʰ C92.6 Acute myeloid leukemia with 11q23-abnormality

Acute myeloid leukemia with variation of MLL-gene

C92.60 Acute myeloid leukemia with 11q23-abnormality not having achieved remission `CC` `HCC`

Acute myeloid leukemia with 11q23-abnormality with failed remission
Acute myeloid leukemia with 11q23-abnormality NOS

C92.61 Acute myeloid leukemia with 11q23-abnormality in remission `CC` `HCC`

C92.62 Acute myeloid leukemia with 11q23-abnormality in relapse `CC` `HCC`

√5ᵗʰ C92.A Acute myeloid leukemia with multilineage dysplasia

Acute myeloid leukemia with dysplasia of remaining hematopoesis and/or myelodysplastic disease in its history

C92.A0 Acute myeloid leukemia with multilineage dysplasia, not having achieved remission `CC` `HCC`

Acute myeloid leukemia with multilineage dysplasia with failed remission
Acute myeloid leukemia with multilineage dysplasia NOS

C92.A1 Acute myeloid leukemia with multilineage dysplasia, in remission `CC` `HCC`

C92.A2 Acute myeloid leukemia with multilineage dysplasia, in relapse `CC` `HCC`

√5ᵗʰ C92.Z Other myeloid leukemia

C92.Z0 Other myeloid leukemia not having achieved remission `CC` `HCC`

Myeloid leukemia NEC with failed remission
Myeloid leukemia NEC

C92.Z1 Other myeloid leukemia, in remission `CC` `HCC`

C92.Z2 Other myeloid leukemia, in relapse `CC` `HCC`

√5ᵗʰ C92.9 Myeloid leukemia, unspecified

C92.90 Myeloid leukemia, unspecified, not having achieved remission `CC` `HCC`

Myeloid leukemia, unspecified with failed remission
Myeloid leukemia, unspecified NOS

C92.91 Myeloid leukemia, unspecified in remission `CC` `HCC`

C92.92 Myeloid leukemia, unspecified in relapse `CC` `HCC`

√4ᵗʰ C93 Monocytic leukemia

`INCLUDES` monocytoid leukemia
`EXCLUDES 1` personal history of leukemia (Z85.6)
AHA: 2020,1Q,13

√5ᵗʰ C93.0 Acute monoblastic/monocytic leukemia

AML M5
AML M5a
AML M5b

C93.00 Acute monoblastic/monocytic leukemia, not having achieved remission `CC` `HCC`

Acute monoblastic/monocytic leukemia with failed remission
Acute monoblastic/monocytic leukemia NOS

C93.01 Acute monoblastic/monocytic leukemia, in remission `CC` `HCC`

C93.02 Acute monoblastic/monocytic leukemia, in relapse `CC` `HCC`

√5ᵗʰ C93.1 Chronic myelomonocytic leukemia

Chronic monocytic leukemia
CMML-1
CMML-2
CMML with eosinophilia
Code also, if applicable, eosinophilia (D72.18)

C93.10 Chronic myelomonocytic leukemia not having achieved remission `CC` `HCC`

Chronic myelomonocytic leukemia with failed remission
Chronic myelomonocytic leukemia NOS

C93.11 Chronic myelomonocytic leukemia, in remission `CC` `HCC`

C93.12 Chronic myelomonocytic leukemia, in relapse `CC` `HCC`

√5ᵗʰ C93.3 Juvenile myelomonocytic leukemia

C93.30 Juvenile myelomonocytic leukemia, not having achieved remission `CC` `HCC` `P`

Juvenile myelomonocytic leukemia with failed remission
Juvenile myelomonocytic leukemia NOS

C93.31 Juvenile myelomonocytic leukemia, in remission `CC` `HCC` `P`

C93.32 Juvenile myelomonocytic leukemia, in relapse `CC` `HCC` `P`

√5ᵗʰ C93.Z Other monocytic leukemia

C93.Z0 Other monocytic leukemia, not having achieved remission `CC` `HCC`

Other monocytic leukemia NOS

C93.Z1 Other monocytic leukemia, in remission `CC` `HCC`

C93.Z2 Other monocytic leukemia, in relapse `CC` `HCC`

√5ᵗʰ C93.9 Monocytic leukemia, unspecified

C93.90 Monocytic leukemia, unspecified, not having achieved remission `CC` `HCC`

Monocytic leukemia, unspecified with failed remission
Monocytic leukemia, unspecified NOS

C93.91 Monocytic leukemia, unspecified in remission `CC` `HCC`

C93.92 Monocytic leukemia, unspecified in relapse `CC` `HCC`

√4ᵗʰ C94 Other leukemias of specified cell type

`EXCLUDES 1` leukemic reticuloendotheliosis (C91.4-)
myelodysplastic syndromes (D46.-)
personal history of leukemia (Z85.6)
plasma cell leukemia (C90.1-)
AHA: 2020,1Q,13

√5ᵗʰ C94.0 Acute erythroid leukemia

Acute myeloid leukemia M6(a)(b)
Erythroleukemia
DEF: Erythroleukemia: Malignant blood dyscrasia (a myeloproliferative disorder).

C94.00 Acute erythroid leukemia, not having achieved remission `CC` `HCC`

Acute erythroid leukemia with failed remission
Acute erythroid leukemia NOS

C94.01 Acute erythroid leukemia, in remission `CC` `HCC`

C94.02 Acute erythroid leukemia, in relapse `CC` `HCC`

√5ᵗʰ C94.2 Acute megakaryoblastic leukemia

Acute myeloid leukemia M7
Acute megakaryocytic leukemia

C94.20 Acute megakaryoblastic leukemia not having achieved remission `CC` `HCC`

Acute megakaryoblastic leukemia with failed remission
Acute megakaryoblastic leukemia NOS

C94.21 Acute megakaryoblastic leukemia, in remission `CC` `HCC`

C94.22 Acute megakaryoblastic leukemia, in relapse `CC` `HCC`

`N` Newborn: 0   `P` Pediatric: 0-17   `M` Maternity: 9-64   `A` Adult: 15-124   `MCC` Major Complication/Comorbidity   `CC` Complication/Comorbidity   `SW` Severe Wound Dx

492   ICD-10-CM 2022

✓5th C94.3 Mast cell leukemia
    AHA: 2017,4Q,5

    C94.30 Mast cell leukemia not having achieved remission CC HCC
        Mast cell leukemia with failed remission
        Mast cell leukemia NOS

    C94.31 Mast cell leukemia, in remission CC HCC

    C94.32 Mast cell leukemia, in relapse CC HCC

✓5th C94.4 Acute panmyelosis with myelofibrosis
    Acute myelofibrosis
    EXCLUDES 1   *myelofibrosis NOS (D75.81)*
           secondary myelofibrosis NOS (D75.81)

    C94.40 Acute panmyelosis with myelofibrosis not having achieved remission CC HCC
        Acute myelofibrosis NOS
        Acute panmyelosis with myelofibrosis with failed remission
        Acute panmyelosis NOS

    C94.41 Acute panmyelosis with myelofibrosis, in remission CC HCC

    C94.42 Acute panmyelosis with myelofibrosis, in relapse CC HCC

C94.6 Myelodysplastic disease, not classified CC HCC
    Myeloproliferative disease, not classified

✓5th C94.8 Other specified leukemias
    Aggressive NK-cell leukemia
    Acute basophilic leukemia

    C94.80 Other specified leukemias not having achieved remission CC HCC
        Other specified leukemia with failed remission
        Other specified leukemias NOS

    C94.81 Other specified leukemias, in remission CC HCC

    C94.82 Other specified leukemias, in relapse CC HCC

✓4th C95 Leukemia of unspecified cell type
    EXCLUDES 1   *personal history of leukemia (Z85.6)*
    AHA: 2020,1Q,13

✓5th C95.0 Acute leukemia of unspecified cell type
    Acute bilineal leukemia
    Acute mixed lineage leukemia
    Biphenotypic acute leukemia
    Stem cell leukemia of unclear lineage
    EXCLUDES 1   *acute exacerbation of unspecified chronic leukemia (C95.10)*

    C95.00 Acute leukemia of unspecified cell type not having achieved remission CC HCC
        Acute leukemia of unspecified cell type with failed remission
        Acute leukemia NOS

    C95.01 Acute leukemia of unspecified cell type, in remission CC HCC

    C95.02 Acute leukemia of unspecified cell type, in relapse CC HCC

✓5th C95.1 Chronic leukemia of unspecified cell type

    C95.10 Chronic leukemia of unspecified cell type not having achieved remission CC HCC
        Chronic leukemia of unspecified cell type with failed remission
        Chronic leukemia NOS

    C95.11 Chronic leukemia of unspecified cell type, in remission CC HCC

    C95.12 Chronic leukemia of unspecified cell type, in relapse CC HCC

✓5th C95.9 Leukemia, unspecified

    C95.90 Leukemia, unspecified not having achieved remission CC HCC
        Leukemia, unspecified with failed remission
        Leukemia NOS

    C95.91 Leukemia, unspecified, in remission CC HCC

    C95.92 Leukemia, unspecified, in relapse CC HCC

✓4th C96 Other and unspecified malignant neoplasms of lymphoid, hematopoietic and related tissue
    EXCLUDES 1   *personal history of other malignant neoplasms of lymphoid, hematopoietic and related tissues (Z85.79)*

C96.0 Multifocal and multisystemic (disseminated) Langerhans-cell histiocytosis CC HCC
    Histiocytosis X, multisystemic
    Letterer-Siwe disease
    EXCLUDES 1   *adult pulmonary Langerhans cell histiocytosis (J84.82)*
           multifocal and unisystemic Langerhans-cell histiocytosis (C96.5)
           unifocal Langerhans-cell histiocytosis (C96.6)

✓5th C96.2 Malignant mast cell neoplasm
    EXCLUDES 1   *indolent mastocytosis (D47.02)*
           mast cell leukemia (C94.30)
           mastocytosis (congenital) (cutaneous) (Q82.2)
    AHA: 2017,4Q,5
    DEF: Mast cell: Type of white blood cell found in the loose connective tissue of blood vessels and bronchioles responsible for acute hypersensitivity reactions, including anaphylactic shock. The IgE receptors on these cells bind with allergens causing cell degranulation and diffuse, widespread histamine release that results in airway constriction and vasodilation with decreased systemic blood pressure.

    C96.20 Malignant mast cell neoplasm, unspecified CC HCC

    C96.21 Aggressive systemic mastocytosis CC HCC

    C96.22 Mast cell sarcoma CC HCC

    C96.29 Other malignant mast cell neoplasm CC HCC

C96.4 Sarcoma of dendritic cells (accessory cells) CC HCC
    Follicular dendritic cell sarcoma
    Interdigitating dendritic cell sarcoma
    Langerhans cell sarcoma

C96.5 Multifocal and unisystemic Langerhans-cell histiocytosis CC HCC
    Hand-Schüller-Christian disease
    Histiocytosis X, multifocal
    EXCLUDES 1   *multifocal and multisystemic (disseminated) Langerhans-cell histiocytosis (C96.0)*
           unifocal Langerhans-cell histiocytosis (C96.6)

C96.6 Unifocal Langerhans-cell histiocytosis CC HCC
    Eosinophilic granuloma
    Histiocytosis X, unifocal
    Histiocytosis X NOS
    Langerhans-cell histiocytosis NOS
    EXCLUDES 1   *multifocal and multisysemic (disseminated) Langerhans-cell histiocytosis (C96.0)*
           multifocal and unisystemic Langerhans-cell histiocytosis (C96.5)

C96.A Histiocytic sarcoma CC HCC
    Malignant histiocytosis

C96.Z Other specified malignant neoplasms of lymphoid, hematopoietic and related tissue CC HCC

C96.9 Malignant neoplasm of lymphoid, hematopoietic and related tissue, unspecified CC HCC

✔ Additional Character Required   ✓x7th Placeholder   Questionable PDx   Manifestation   Unspecified Dx   UPD Unacceptable PDx   H1-H4 HAC   HCC CMS-HCC Dx   HIV HIV Dx

Chapter 2. Neoplasms

D00–D03.70

In situ neoplasms (D00-D09)

INCLUDES   Bowen's disease
erythroplasia
grade III intraepithelial neoplasia
Queyrat's erythroplasia

☑4ᵗʰ **D00**   **Carcinoma in situ of** oral cavity, esophagus and stomach
     EXCLUDES 1   *melanoma in situ (D03.-)*

☑5ᵗʰ   **D00.0**   **Carcinoma in situ of** lip, oral cavity and pharynx
Use additional code to identify:
exposure to environmental tobacco smoke (Z77.22)
exposure to tobacco smoke in the perinatal period (P96.81)
history of tobacco dependence (Z87.891)
occupational exposure to environmental tobacco smoke (Z57.31)
tobacco dependence (F17.-)
tobacco use (Z72.0)
     EXCLUDES 1   *carcinoma in situ of aryepiglottic fold or interarytenoid fold, laryngeal aspect (D02.0)*
carcinoma in situ of epiglottis NOS (D02.0)
carcinoma in situ of epiglottis suprahyoid portion (D02.0)
carcinoma in situ of skin of lip (D03.0, D04.0)

     D00.00   **Carcinoma in situ of oral cavity, unspecified site**
     D00.01   **Carcinoma in situ of** labial mucosa and vermilion border
     D00.02   **Carcinoma in situ of** buccal mucosa
     D00.03   **Carcinoma in situ of** gingiva and edentulous alveolar ridge
     D00.04   **Carcinoma in situ of** soft palate
     D00.05   **Carcinoma in situ of** hard palate
     D00.06   **Carcinoma in situ of** floor of mouth
     D00.07   **Carcinoma in situ of** tongue
     D00.08   **Carcinoma in situ of** pharynx
Carcinoma in situ of aryepiglottic fold NOS
Carcinoma in situ of hypopharyngeal aspect of aryepiglottic fold
Carcinoma in situ of marginal zone of aryepiglottic fold

  D00.1   **Carcinoma in situ of** esophagus
  D00.2   **Carcinoma in situ of** stomach

☑4ᵗʰ **D01**   **Carcinoma in situ of other and unspecified** digestive organs
     EXCLUDES 1   *melanoma in situ (D03.-)*

  D01.0   **Carcinoma in situ of** colon
     EXCLUDES 1   *carcinoma in situ of rectosigmoid junction (D01.1)*
  D01.1   **Carcinoma in situ of** rectosigmoid junction
  D01.2   **Carcinoma in situ of** rectum
  D01.3   **Carcinoma in situ of** anus and anal canal
Anal intraepithelial neoplasia III [AIN III]
Severe dysplasia of anus
     EXCLUDES 1   *anal intraepithelial neoplasia I and II [AIN I and AIN II] (K62.82)*
carcinoma in situ of anal margin (D04.5)
carcinoma in situ of anal skin (D04.5)
carcinoma in situ of perianal skin (D04.5)

☑5ᵗʰ   **D01.4**   **Carcinoma in situ of other and unspecified parts of** intestine
     EXCLUDES 1   *carcinoma in situ of ampulla of Vater (D01.5)*
     D01.40   **Carcinoma in situ of unspecified part of intestine**
     D01.49   **Carcinoma in situ of other parts of intestine**
  D01.5   **Carcinoma in situ of** liver, gallbladder and bile ducts
Carcinoma in situ of ampulla of Vater
  D01.7   **Carcinoma in situ of other specified** digestive organs
Carcinoma in situ of pancreas
  D01.9   **Carcinoma in situ of digestive organ, unspecified**

☑4ᵗʰ **D02**   **Carcinoma in situ of** middle ear and respiratory system
Use additional code to identify:
exposure to environmental tobacco smoke (Z77.22)
exposure to tobacco smoke in the perinatal period (P96.81)
history of tobacco dependence (Z87.891)
occupational exposure to environmental tobacco smoke (Z57.31)
tobacco dependence (F17.-)
tobacco use (Z72.0)
     EXCLUDES 1   *melanoma in situ (D03.-)*

  D02.0   **Carcinoma in situ of** larynx
Carcinoma in situ of aryepiglottic fold or interarytenoid fold, laryngeal aspect
Carcinoma in situ of epiglottis (suprahyoid portion)
     EXCLUDES 1   *carcinoma in situ of aryepiglottic fold or interarytenoid fold NOS (D00.08)*
carcinoma in situ of hypopharyngeal aspect (D00.08)
carcinoma in situ of marginal zone (D00.08)
  D02.1   **Carcinoma in situ of** trachea
☑5ᵗʰ   **D02.2**   **Carcinoma in situ of** bronchus and lung
     D02.20   **Carcinoma in situ of unspecified bronchus and lung**
     D02.21   **Carcinoma in situ of** right **bronchus and lung**
     D02.22   **Carcinoma in situ of** left **bronchus and lung**
  D02.3   **Carcinoma in situ of other parts of respiratory system**
Carcinoma in situ of accessory sinuses
Carcinoma in situ of middle ear
Carcinoma in situ of nasal cavities
     EXCLUDES 1   *carcinoma in situ of ear (external) (skin) (D04.2-)*
carcinoma in situ of nose NOS (D09.8)
carcinoma in situ of skin of nose (D04.3)
  D02.4   **Carcinoma in situ of respiratory system, unspecified**

☑4ᵗʰ **D03**   **Melanoma in situ**
  D03.0   **Melanoma in situ of** lip   HCC
☑5ᵗʰ   **D03.1**   **Melanoma in situ of** eyelid, including canthus
AHA: 2018,4Q,4
     D03.10   **Melanoma in situ of unspecified eyelid, including canthus**   HCC
   ☑6ᵗʰ   **D03.11**   **Melanoma in situ of** right **eyelid, including canthus**
     D03.111   **Melanoma in situ of right** upper **eyelid, including canthus**   HCC
     D03.112   **Melanoma in situ of right** lower **eyelid, including canthus**   HCC
   ☑6ᵗʰ   **D03.12**   **Melanoma in situ of** left **eyelid, including canthus**
     D03.121   **Melanoma in situ of left** upper **eyelid, including canthus**   HCC
     D03.122   **Melanoma in situ of left** lower **eyelid, including canthus**   HCC
☑5ᵗʰ   **D03.2**   **Melanoma in situ of** ear and external auricular canal
     D03.20   **Melanoma in situ of unspecified ear and external auricular canal**   HCC
     D03.21   **Melanoma in situ of** right **ear and external auricular canal**   HCC
     D03.22   **Melanoma in situ of** left **ear and external auricular canal**   HCC
☑5ᵗʰ   **D03.3**   **Melanoma in situ of other and unspecified parts of** face
     D03.30   **Melanoma in situ of unspecified part of face**   HCC
     D03.39   **Melanoma in situ of other parts of face**   HCC
  D03.4   **Melanoma in situ of** scalp and neck   HCC
☑5ᵗʰ   **D03.5**   **Melanoma in situ of** trunk
     D03.51   **Melanoma in situ of** anal skin   HCC
Melanoma in situ of anal margin
Melanoma in situ of perianal skin
     D03.52   **Melanoma in situ of** breast (skin) (soft tissue)   HCC
     D03.59   **Melanoma in situ of other part of trunk**   HCC
☑5ᵗʰ   **D03.6**   **Melanoma in situ of** upper limb, including shoulder
     D03.60   **Melanoma in situ of unspecified upper limb, including shoulder**   HCC
     D03.61   **Melanoma in situ of** right **upper limb, including shoulder**   HCC
     D03.62   **Melanoma in situ of** left **upper limb, including shoulder**   HCC
☑5ᵗʰ   **D03.7**   **Melanoma in situ of** lower limb, including hip
     D03.70   **Melanoma in situ of unspecified lower limb, including hip**   HCC

D03.71 Melanoma in situ of right lower limb, including hip   HCC

D03.72 Melanoma in situ of left lower limb, including hip   HCC

D03.8 Melanoma in situ of other sites   HCC
Melanoma in situ of scrotum
> EXCLUDES 1   carcinoma in situ of scrotum (D07.61)

D03.9 Melanoma in situ, unspecified   HCC

☑4ᵗʰ **D04** **Carcinoma in situ of skin**
> EXCLUDES 1   erythroplasia of Queyrat (penis) NOS (D07.4)
> melanoma in situ (D03.-)

D04.0 Carcinoma in situ of skin of lip
> EXCLUDES 2   carcinoma in situ of vermilion border of lip (D00.01)

☑5ᵗʰ **D04.1** Carcinoma in situ of skin of eyelid, including canthus
AHA: 2018,4Q,4

   D04.10 Carcinoma in situ of skin of unspecified eyelid, including canthus

   ☑6ᵗʰ **D04.11** Carcinoma in situ of skin of right eyelid, including canthus
     D04.111 Carcinoma in situ of skin of right upper eyelid, including canthus
     D04.112 Carcinoma in situ of skin of right lower eyelid, including canthus

   ☑6ᵗʰ **D04.12** Carcinoma in situ of skin of left eyelid, including canthus
     D04.121 Carcinoma in situ of skin of left upper eyelid, including canthus
     D04.122 Carcinoma in situ of skin of left lower eyelid, including canthus

☑5ᵗʰ **D04.2** Carcinoma in situ of skin of ear and external auricular canal

   D04.20 Carcinoma in situ of skin of unspecified ear and external auricular canal
   D04.21 Carcinoma in situ of skin of right ear and external auricular canal
   D04.22 Carcinoma in situ of skin of left ear and external auricular canal

☑5ᵗʰ **D04.3** Carcinoma in situ of skin of other and unspecified parts of face
   D04.30 Carcinoma in situ of skin of unspecified part of face
   D04.39 Carcinoma in situ of skin of other parts of face

D04.4 Carcinoma in situ of skin of scalp and neck

D04.5 Carcinoma in situ of skin of trunk
Carcinoma in situ of anal margin
Carcinoma in situ of anal skin
Carcinoma in situ of perianal skin
Carcinoma in situ of skin of breast
> EXCLUDES 1   carcinoma in situ of anus NOS (D01.3)
> carcinoma in situ of scrotum (D07.61)
> carcinoma in situ of skin of genital organs (D07.-)

☑5ᵗʰ **D04.6** Carcinoma in situ of skin of upper limb, including shoulder
   D04.60 Carcinoma in situ of skin of unspecified upper limb, including shoulder
   D04.61 Carcinoma in situ of skin of right upper limb, including shoulder
   D04.62 Carcinoma in situ of skin of left upper limb, including shoulder

☑5ᵗʰ **D04.7** Carcinoma in situ of skin of lower limb, including hip
   D04.70 Carcinoma in situ of skin of unspecified lower limb, including hip
   D04.71 Carcinoma in situ of skin of right lower limb, including hip
   D04.72 Carcinoma in situ of skin of left lower limb, including hip

D04.8 Carcinoma in situ of skin of other sites
D04.9 Carcinoma in situ of skin, unspecified

☑4ᵗʰ **D05** **Carcinoma in situ of breast**
> EXCLUDES 1   carcinoma in situ of skin of breast (D04.5)
> melanoma in situ of breast (skin) (D03.5)
> Paget's disease of breast or nipple (C50.-)

☑5ᵗʰ **D05.0** Lobular carcinoma in situ of breast
   D05.00 Lobular carcinoma in situ of unspecified breast
   D05.01 Lobular carcinoma in situ of right breast
   D05.02 Lobular carcinoma in situ of left breast

☑5ᵗʰ **D05.1** Intraductal carcinoma in situ of breast
   D05.10 Intraductal carcinoma in situ of unspecified breast
   D05.11 Intraductal carcinoma in situ of right breast

   D05.12 Intraductal carcinoma in situ of left breast

☑5ᵗʰ **D05.8** Other specified type of carcinoma in situ of breast
   D05.80 Other specified type of carcinoma in situ of unspecified breast
   D05.81 Other specified type of carcinoma in situ of right breast
   D05.82 Other specified type of carcinoma in situ of left breast

☑5ᵗʰ **D05.9** Unspecified type of carcinoma in situ of breast
   D05.90 Unspecified type of carcinoma in situ of unspecified breast
   D05.91 Unspecified type of carcinoma in situ of right breast
   D05.92 Unspecified type of carcinoma in situ of left breast

☑4ᵗʰ **D06** **Carcinoma in situ of cervix uteri**
> INCLUDES   cervical adenocarcinoma in situ
> cervical intraepithelial glandular neoplasia
> cervical intraepithelial neoplasia III [CIN III]
> severe dysplasia of cervix uteri
> EXCLUDES 1   cervical intraepithelial neoplasia II [CIN II] (N87.1)
> cytologic evidence of malignancy of cervix without histologic confirmation (R87.614)
> high grade squamous intraepithelial lesion (HGSIL) of cervix (R87.613)
> melanoma in situ of cervix (D03.5)
> moderate cervical dysplasia (N87.1)

D06.0 Carcinoma in situ of endocervix   ♀
D06.1 Carcinoma in situ of exocervix   ♀
D06.7 Carcinoma in situ of other parts of cervix   ♀
D06.9 Carcinoma in situ of cervix, unspecified   ♀

☑4ᵗʰ **D07** **Carcinoma in situ of other and unspecified genital organs**
> EXCLUDES 1   melanoma in situ of trunk (D03.5)

D07.0 Carcinoma in situ of endometrium   ♀
D07.1 Carcinoma in situ of vulva   ♀
Severe dysplasia of vulva
Vulvar intraepithelial neoplasia III [VIN III]
> EXCLUDES 1   moderate dysplasia of vulva (N90.1)
> vulvar intraepithelial neoplasia II [VIN II] (N90.1)

D07.2 Carcinoma in situ of vagina   ♀
Severe dysplasia of vagina
Vaginal intraepithelial neoplasia III [VAIN III]
> EXCLUDES 1   moderate dysplasia of vagina (N89.1)
> vaginal intraepithelial neoplasia II [VIN II] (N89.1)

☑5ᵗʰ **D07.3** Carcinoma in situ of other and unspecified female genital organs
   D07.30 Carcinoma in situ of unspecified female genital organs   ♀
   D07.39 Carcinoma in situ of other female genital organs   ♀

D07.4 Carcinoma in situ of penis   ♂
Erythroplasia of Queyrat NOS

D07.5 Carcinoma in situ of prostate   ♂
Prostatic intraepithelial neoplasia III (PIN III)
Severe dysplasia of prostate
> EXCLUDES 1   dysplasia (mild) (moderate) of prostate (N42.3-)
> prostatic intraepithelial neoplasia II [PIN II] (N42.3-)

☑5ᵗʰ **D07.6** Carcinoma in situ of other and unspecified male genital organs
   D07.60 Carcinoma in situ of unspecified male genital organs   ♂
   D07.61 Carcinoma in situ of scrotum   ♂
   D07.69 Carcinoma in situ of other male genital organs   ♂

☑4ᵗʰ **D09** **Carcinoma in situ of other and unspecified sites**
> EXCLUDES 1   melanoma in situ (D03.-)

D09.0 Carcinoma in situ of bladder

☑5ᵗʰ **D09.1** Carcinoma in situ of other and unspecified urinary organs
   D09.10 Carcinoma in situ of unspecified urinary organ
   D09.19 Carcinoma in situ of other urinary organs

☑5ᵗʰ **D09.2** Carcinoma in situ of eye
> EXCLUDES 1   carcinoma in situ of skin of eyelid (D04.1-)
   D09.20 Carcinoma in situ of unspecified eye
   D09.21 Carcinoma in situ of right eye
   D09.22 Carcinoma in situ of left eye

☑ Additional Character Required   ☑x7ᵗʰ Placeholder   Questionable PDx   Manifestation   Unspecified Dx   UPD Unacceptable PDx   H1-H14 HAC   HCC CMS-HCC Dx   HIV HIV Dx

ICD-10-CM 2022   495

D09.3   Carcinoma in situ of **thyroid** and other **endocrine glands**
> EXCLUDES 1   *carcinoma in situ of endocrine pancreas (D01.7)*
> *carcinoma in situ of ovary (D07.39)*
> *carcinoma in situ of testis (D07.69)*

D09.8   Carcinoma in situ of other specified sites

D09.9   Carcinoma in situ, unspecified

Benign neoplasms, except benign neuroendocrine tumors (D10-D36)

☑4ᵗʰ **D10**   Benign neoplasm of **mouth and pharynx**

D10.0   Benign neoplasm of **lip**
> Benign neoplasm of lip (frenulum) (inner aspect) (mucosa) (vermilion border)
> EXCLUDES 1   *benign neoplasm of skin of lip (D22.0, D23.0)*

D10.1   Benign neoplasm of **tongue**
> Benign neoplasm of lingual tonsil

D10.2   Benign neoplasm of **floor** of mouth

☑5ᵗʰ **D10.3**   Benign neoplasm **of other and unspecified parts of mouth**

     D10.30   Benign neoplasm of unspecified part of mouth
     D10.39   Benign neoplasm of other parts of mouth
> Benign neoplasm of minor salivary gland NOS
> EXCLUDES 1   *benign odontogenic neoplasms (D16.4-D16.5)*
> *benign neoplasm of mucosa of lip (D10.0)*
> *benign neoplasm of nasopharyngeal surface of soft palate (D10.6)*

D10.4   Benign neoplasm of **tonsil**
> Benign neoplasm of tonsil (faucial) (palatine)
> EXCLUDES 1   *benign neoplasm of lingual tonsil (D10.1)*
> *benign neoplasm of pharyngeal tonsil (D10.6)*
> *benign neoplasm of tonsillar fossa (D10.5)*
> *benign neoplasm of tonsillar pillars (D10.5)*

D10.5   Benign neoplasm of other parts of **oropharynx**
> Benign neoplasm of epiglottis, anterior aspect
> Benign neoplasm of tonsillar fossa
> Benign neoplasm of tonsillar pillars
> Benign neoplasm of vallecula
> EXCLUDES 1   *benign neoplasm of epiglottis NOS (D14.1)*
> *benign neoplasm of epiglottis, suprahyoid portion (D14.1)*
> **DEF:** Oropharynx: Middle portion of pharynx (throat); communicates with the oral cavity, nasopharynx and laryngopharynx.

D10.6   Benign neoplasm of **nasopharynx**
> Benign neoplasm of pharyngeal tonsil
> Benign neoplasm of posterior margin of septum and choanae
> **DEF:** Nasopharynx: Upper portion of pharynx (throat); communicates with the nasal cavities, oropharynx and tympanic cavities.

D10.7   Benign neoplasm of **hypopharynx**
> **DEF:** Hypopharynx: Lower portion of pharynx (throat); communicates with the oropharynx and the esophagus.
> ***Synonym(s):*** *laryngopharynx.*

D10.9   Benign neoplasm of pharynx, unspecified

☑4ᵗʰ **D11**   Benign neoplasm of **major salivary glands**
> EXCLUDES 1   *benign neoplasms of specified minor salivary glands which are classified according to their anatomical location*
> *benign neoplasms of minor salivary glands NOS (D10.39)*

D11.0   Benign neoplasm of **parotid gland**

D11.7   Benign neoplasm of other major salivary glands
> Benign neoplasm of sublingual salivary gland
> Benign neoplasm of submandibular salivary gland

D11.9   Benign neoplasm of major salivary gland, unspecified

☑4ᵗʰ **D12**   Benign neoplasm of **colon, rectum, anus and anal canal**
> EXCLUDES 1   *benign carcinoid tumors of the large intestine, and rectum (D3A.02-)*
> *polyp of colon NOS (K63.5)*
> **AHA:** 2018,2Q,14; 2017,1Q,15; 2015,2Q,14
> **TIP:** Code K63.5 Polyp of colon, is assigned when documentation states hyperplastic colon polyps, regardless of the site in the colon. Slow-growing, hyperplastic polyps are not precancerous and are classified differently from benign or adenomatous polyps.

D12.0   Benign neoplasm of **cecum**
> Benign neoplasm of ileocecal valve

D12.1   Benign neoplasm of **appendix**
> EXCLUDES 1   *benign carcinoid tumor of the appendix (D3A.020)*

D12.2   Benign neoplasm of **ascending colon**

D12.3   Benign neoplasm of **transverse colon**
> Benign neoplasm of hepatic flexure
> Benign neoplasm of splenic flexure
> **AHA:** 2017,1Q,16

D12.4   Benign neoplasm of **descending colon**

D12.5   Benign neoplasm of **sigmoid colon**

D12.6   Benign neoplasm of colon, unspecified
> Adenomatosis of colon
> Benign neoplasm of large intestine NOS
> Polyposis (hereditary) of colon
> EXCLUDES 1   *inflammatory polyp of colon (K51.4-)*

D12.7   Benign neoplasm of **rectosigmoid junction**

D12.8   Benign neoplasm of **rectum**
> EXCLUDES 1   *benign carcinoid tumor of the rectum (D3A.026)*
> **AHA:** 2018,1Q,6

D12.9   Benign neoplasm of **anus and anal canal**
> Benign neoplasm of anus NOS
> EXCLUDES 1   *benign neoplasm of anal margin (D22.5, D23.5)*
> *benign neoplasm of anal skin (D22.5, D23.5)*
> *benign neoplasm of perianal skin (D22.5, D23.5)*

☑4ᵗʰ **D13**   Benign neoplasm of other and ill-defined parts of **digestive system**
> EXCLUDES 1   *benign stromal tumors of digestive system (D21.4)*

D13.0   Benign neoplasm of **esophagus**

D13.1   Benign neoplasm of **stomach**
> EXCLUDES 1   *benign carcinoid tumor of the stomach (D3A.092)*

D13.2   Benign neoplasm of **duodenum**
> EXCLUDES 1   *benign carcinoid tumor of the duodenum (D3A.010)*

☑5ᵗʰ **D13.3**   Benign neoplasm of other and unspecified parts of **small intestine**
> EXCLUDES 1   *benign carcinoid tumors of the small intestine (D3A.01-)*
> *benign neoplasm of ileocecal valve (D12.0)*

     D13.30   Benign neoplasm of unspecified part of small intestine
     D13.39   Benign neoplasm of other parts of small intestine

D13.4   Benign neoplasm of **liver**
> Benign neoplasm of intrahepatic bile ducts

D13.5   Benign neoplasm of **extrahepatic bile ducts**

D13.6   Benign neoplasm of **pancreas**
> EXCLUDES 1   *benign neoplasm of endocrine pancreas (D13.7)*

D13.7   Benign neoplasm of **endocrine pancreas**
> Benign neoplasm of islets of Langerhans
> Islet cell tumor
> Use additional code to identify any functional activity

D13.9   Benign neoplasm of **ill-defined sites** within the digestive system
> Benign neoplasm of digestive system NOS
> Benign neoplasm of intestine NOS
> Benign neoplasm of spleen

☑4ᵗʰ **D14**   Benign neoplasm of **middle ear and respiratory system**

D14.0   Benign neoplasm of **middle ear, nasal cavity and accessory sinuses**
> Benign neoplasm of cartilage of nose
> EXCLUDES 1   *benign neoplasm of auricular canal (external) (D22.2-, D23.2-)*
> *benign neoplasm of bone of ear (D16.4)*
> *benign neoplasm of bone of nose (D16.4)*
> *benign neoplasm of cartilage of ear (D21.0)*
> *benign neoplasm of ear (external)(skin) (D22.2-, D23.2-)*
> *benign neoplasm of nose NOS (D36.7)*
> *benign neoplasm of skin of nose (D22.39, D23.39)*
> *benign neoplasm of olfactory bulb (D33.3)*
> *benign neoplasm of posterior margin of septum and choanae (D10.6)*
> *polyp of accessory sinus (J33.8)*
> *polyp of ear (middle) (H74.4)*
> *polyp of nasal (cavity) (J33.-)*

N Newborn: 0   P Pediatric: 0-17   M Maternity: 9-64   A Adult: 15-124   MCC Major Complication/Comorbidity   CC Complication/Comorbidity   SW Severe Wound Dx

496   ICD-10-CM 2022

D14.1   **Benign neoplasm of** larynx
Adenomatous polyp of larynx
Benign neoplasm of epiglottis (suprahyoid portion)
> EXCLUDES 1   *benign neoplasm of epiglottis, anterior aspect (D10.5)*
> *polyp (nonadenomatous) of vocal cord or larynx (J38.1)*

D14.2   **Benign neoplasm of** trachea

☑5ᵗʰ **D14.3**   **Benign neoplasm of** bronchus and lung
> EXCLUDES 1   *benign carcinoid tumor of the bronchus and lung (D3A.090)*

    D14.30   **Benign neoplasm of unspecified bronchus and lung**
    D14.31   **Benign neoplasm of** right **bronchus and lung**
    D14.32   **Benign neoplasm of** left **bronchus and lung**

D14.4   **Benign neoplasm of respiratory system, unspecified**

☑4ᵗʰ **D15**   **Benign neoplasm of other and unspecified** intrathoracic organs
> EXCLUDES 1   *benign neoplasm of mesothelial tissue (D19.-)*

D15.0   **Benign neoplasm of** thymus
> EXCLUDES 1   *benign carcinoid tumor of the thymus (D3A.091)*

D15.1   **Benign neoplasm of** heart
> EXCLUDES 1   *benign neoplasm of great vessels (D21.3)*

D15.2   **Benign neoplasm of** mediastinum
D15.7   **Benign neoplasm of other specified intrathoracic organs**
D15.9   **Benign neoplasm of intrathoracic organ, unspecified**

☑4ᵗʰ **D16**   **Benign neoplasm of** bone and articular cartilage
> EXCLUDES 1   *benign neoplasm of connective tissue of ear (D21.0)*
> *benign neoplasm of connective tissue of eyelid (D21.0)*
> *benign neoplasm of connective tissue of larynx (D14.1)*
> *benign neoplasm of connective tissue of nose (D14.0)*
> *benign neoplasm of synovia (D21.-)*

☑5ᵗʰ **D16.0**   **Benign neoplasm of** scapula and long bones of upper limb

    D16.00   **Benign neoplasm of scapula and long bones of unspecified upper limb**
    D16.01   **Benign neoplasm of scapula and long bones of** right **upper limb**
    D16.02   **Benign neoplasm of scapula and long bones of** left **upper limb**

☑5ᵗʰ **D16.1**   **Benign neoplasm of** short bones of upper limb

    D16.10   **Benign neoplasm of short bones of unspecified upper limb**
    D16.11   **Benign neoplasm of short bones of** right **upper limb**
    D16.12   **Benign neoplasm of short bones of** left **upper limb**

☑5ᵗʰ **D16.2**   **Benign neoplasm of** long bones of lower limb

    D16.20   **Benign neoplasm of long bones of unspecified lower limb**
    D16.21   **Benign neoplasm of long bones of** right **lower limb**
    D16.22   **Benign neoplasm of long bones of** left **lower limb**

☑5ᵗʰ **D16.3**   **Benign neoplasm of** short bones of lower limb

    D16.30   **Benign neoplasm of short bones of unspecified lower limb**
    D16.31   **Benign neoplasm of short bones of** right **lower limb**
    D16.32   **Benign neoplasm of short bones of** left **lower limb**

D16.4   **Benign neoplasm of bones of** skull and face
Benign neoplasm of maxilla (superior)
Benign neoplasm of orbital bone
Keratocyst of maxilla
Keratocystic odontogenic tumor of maxilla
> EXCLUDES 2   *benign neoplasm of lower jaw bone (D16.5)*

D16.5   **Benign neoplasm of** lower jaw bone
Keratocyst of mandible
Keratocystic odontogenic tumor of mandible

D16.6   **Benign neoplasm of** vertebral column
> EXCLUDES 1   *benign neoplasm of sacrum and coccyx (D16.8)*

D16.7   **Benign neoplasm of** ribs, sternum and clavicle
D16.8   **Benign neoplasm of** pelvic bones, sacrum and coccyx
D16.9   **Benign neoplasm of bone and articular cartilage, unspecified**

☑4ᵗʰ **D17**   **Benign** lipomatous **neoplasm**

D17.0   **Benign lipomatous neoplasm of** skin and subcutaneous tissue **of head, face and neck**

D17.1   **Benign lipomatous neoplasm of** skin and subcutaneous tissue **of trunk**

☑5ᵗʰ **D17.2**   **Benign lipomatous neoplasm of** skin and subcutaneous tissue **of limb**

    D17.20   **Benign lipomatous neoplasm of skin and subcutaneous tissue of unspecified limb**

    D17.21   **Benign lipomatous neoplasm of skin and subcutaneous tissue of** right **arm**
    D17.22   **Benign lipomatous neoplasm of skin and subcutaneous tissue of** left **arm**
    D17.23   **Benign lipomatous neoplasm of skin and subcutaneous tissue of** right **leg**
    D17.24   **Benign lipomatous neoplasm of skin and subcutaneous tissue of** left **leg**

☑5ᵗʰ **D17.3**   **Benign lipomatous neoplasm of** skin and subcutaneous tissue **of other and unspecified sites**

    D17.30   **Benign lipomatous neoplasm of skin and subcutaneous tissue of unspecified sites**
    D17.39   **Benign lipomatous neoplasm of skin and subcutaneous tissue of other sites**

D17.4   **Benign lipomatous neoplasm of** intrathoracic organs
D17.5   **Benign lipomatous neoplasm of** intra-abdominal organs
> EXCLUDES 1   *benign lipomatous neoplasm of peritoneum and retroperitoneum (D17.79)*

D17.6   **Benign lipomatous neoplasm of** spermatic cord   ♂

☑5ᵗʰ **D17.7**   **Benign lipomatous neoplasm of** other sites

    D17.71   **Benign lipomatous neoplasm of** kidney
    D17.72   **Benign lipomatous neoplasm of other** genitourinary organ
    D17.79   **Benign lipomatous neoplasm of other sites**
Benign lipomatous neoplasm of peritoneum
Benign lipomatous neoplasm of retroperitoneum

D17.9   **Benign lipomatous neoplasm, unspecified**
Lipoma NOS

☑4ᵗʰ **D18**   **Hemangioma and lymphangioma, any site**
> EXCLUDES 1   *benign neoplasm of glomus jugulare (D35.6)*
> *blue or pigmented nevus (D22.-)*
> *nevus NOS (D22.-)*
> *vascular nevus (Q82.5)*

☑5ᵗʰ **D18.0**   **Hemangioma**
Angioma NOS
Cavernous nevus
DEF: Common benign tumor usually occurring in infancy that is composed of newly formed blood vessels due to malformation of the angioblastic tissue.

    D18.00   **Hemangioma unspecified site**
    D18.01   **Hemangioma of** skin and subcutaneous tissue
    D18.02   **Hemangioma of** intracranial structures   HCC
    D18.03   **Hemangioma of** intra-abdominal structures
    D18.09   **Hemangioma of other sites**

D18.1   **Lymphangioma, any site**
AHA: 2018,3Q,31; 2018,2Q,13

☑4ᵗʰ **D19**   **Benign neoplasm of** mesothelial tissue

D19.0   **Benign neoplasm of mesothelial tissue of** pleura
D19.1   **Benign neoplasm of mesothelial tissue of** peritoneum
D19.7   **Benign neoplasm of mesothelial tissue of other sites**
D19.9   **Benign neoplasm of mesothelial tissue, unspecified**
Benign mesothelioma NOS

☑4ᵗʰ **D20**   **Benign neoplasm of soft tissue of** retroperitoneum and peritoneum
> EXCLUDES 1   *benign lipomatous neoplasm of peritoneum and retroperitoneum (D17.79)*
> *benign neoplasm of mesothelial tissue (D19.-)*

D20.0   **Benign neoplasm of soft tissue of** retroperitoneum
D20.1   **Benign neoplasm of soft tissue of** peritoneum

Chapter 2. Neoplasms

✓4ᵗʰ D21 Other benign neoplasms of connective and other soft tissue

INCLUDES benign neoplasm of blood vessel
benign neoplasm of bursa
benign neoplasm of cartilage
benign neoplasm of fascia
benign neoplasm of fat
benign neoplasm of ligament, except uterine
benign neoplasm of lymphatic channel
benign neoplasm of muscle
benign neoplasm of synovia
benign neoplasm of tendon (sheath)
benign stromal tumors

EXCLUDES 1 *benign neoplasm of articular cartilage (D16.-)*
benign neoplasm of cartilage of larynx (D14.1)
benign neoplasm of cartilage of nose (D14.0)
benign neoplasm of connective tissue of breast (D24.-)
benign neoplasm of peripheral nerves and autonomic nervous system (D36.1-)
benign neoplasm of peritoneum (D20.1)
benign neoplasm of retroperitoneum (D20.0)
benign neoplasm of uterine ligament, any (D28.2)
benign neoplasm of vascular tissue (D18.-)
hemangioma (D18.0-)
lipomatous neoplasm (D17.-)
lymphangioma (D18.1)
uterine leiomyoma (D25.-)

D21.0 Benign neoplasm of connective and other soft tissue of head, face and neck
Benign neoplasm of connective tissue of ear
Benign neoplasm of connective tissue of eyelid
EXCLUDES 1 *benign neoplasm of connective tissue of orbit (D31.6-)*

✓5ᵗʰ D21.1 Benign neoplasm of connective and other soft tissue of upper limb, including shoulder
D21.10 Benign neoplasm of connective and other soft tissue of unspecified upper limb, including shoulder
D21.11 Benign neoplasm of connective and other soft tissue of right upper limb, including shoulder
D21.12 Benign neoplasm of connective and other soft tissue of left upper limb, including shoulder

✓5ᵗʰ D21.2 Benign neoplasm of connective and other soft tissue of lower limb, including hip
D21.20 Benign neoplasm of connective and other soft tissue of unspecified lower limb, including hip
D21.21 Benign neoplasm of connective and other soft tissue of right lower limb, including hip
D21.22 Benign neoplasm of connective and other soft tissue of left lower limb, including hip

D21.3 Benign neoplasm of connective and other soft tissue of thorax
Benign neoplasm of axilla
Benign neoplasm of diaphragm
Benign neoplasm of great vessels
EXCLUDES 1 *benign neoplasm of heart (D15.1)*
benign neoplasm of mediastinum (D15.2)
benign neoplasm of thymus (D15.0)

D21.4 Benign neoplasm of connective and other soft tissue of abdomen
Benign stromal tumors of abdomen

D21.5 Benign neoplasm of connective and other soft tissue of pelvis
EXCLUDES 1 *benign neoplasm of any uterine ligament (D28.2)*
uterine leiomyoma (D25.-)

D21.6 Benign neoplasm of connective and other soft tissue of trunk, unspecified
Benign neoplasm of connective and other soft tissue of back NOS

D21.9 Benign neoplasm of connective and other soft tissue, unspecified

✓4ᵗʰ D22 Melanocytic nevi
INCLUDES atypical nevus
blue hairy pigmented nevus
nevus NOS

D22.0 Melanocytic nevi of lip

✓5ᵗʰ D22.1 Melanocytic nevi of eyelid, including canthus
AHA: 2018,4Q,4
D22.10 Melanocytic nevi of unspecified eyelid, including canthus

✓6ᵗʰ D22.11 Melanocytic nevi of right eyelid, including canthus
D22.111 Melanocytic nevi of right upper eyelid, including canthus
D22.112 Melanocytic nevi of right lower eyelid, including canthus
✓6ᵗʰ D22.12 Melanocytic nevi of left eyelid, including canthus
D22.121 Melanocytic nevi of left upper eyelid, including canthus
D22.122 Melanocytic nevi of left lower eyelid, including canthus

✓5ᵗʰ D22.2 Melanocytic nevi of ear and external auricular canal
D22.20 Melanocytic nevi of unspecified ear and external auricular canal
D22.21 Melanocytic nevi of right ear and external auricular canal
D22.22 Melanocytic nevi of left ear and external auricular canal

✓5ᵗʰ D22.3 Melanocytic nevi of other and unspecified parts of face
D22.30 Melanocytic nevi of unspecified part of face
D22.39 Melanocytic nevi of other parts of face

D22.4 Melanocytic nevi of scalp and neck

D22.5 Melanocytic nevi of trunk
Melanocytic nevi of anal margin
Melanocytic nevi of anal skin
Melanocytic nevi of perianal skin
Melanocytic nevi of skin of breast

✓5ᵗʰ D22.6 Melanocytic nevi of upper limb, including shoulder
D22.60 Melanocytic nevi of unspecified upper limb, including shoulder
D22.61 Melanocytic nevi of right upper limb, including shoulder
D22.62 Melanocytic nevi of left upper limb, including shoulder

✓5ᵗʰ D22.7 Melanocytic nevi of lower limb, including hip
D22.70 Melanocytic nevi of unspecified lower limb, including hip
D22.71 Melanocytic nevi of right lower limb, including hip
D22.72 Melanocytic nevi of left lower limb, including hip

D22.9 Melanocytic nevi, unspecified

✓4ᵗʰ D23 Other benign neoplasms of skin
INCLUDES benign neoplasm of hair follicles
benign neoplasm of sebaceous glands
benign neoplasm of sweat glands
EXCLUDES 1 *benign lipomatous neoplasms of skin (D17.0-D17.3)*
EXCLUDES 2 *melanocytic nevi (D22.-)*

D23.0 Other benign neoplasm of skin of lip
EXCLUDES 1 *benign neoplasm of vermilion border of lip (D10.0)*

✓5ᵗʰ D23.1 Other benign neoplasm of skin of eyelid, including canthus
AHA: 2018,4Q,4
D23.10 Other benign neoplasm of skin of unspecified eyelid, including canthus
✓6ᵗʰ D23.11 Other benign neoplasm of skin of right eyelid, including canthus
D23.111 Other benign neoplasm of skin of right upper eyelid, including canthus
D23.112 Other benign neoplasm of skin of right lower eyelid, including canthus
✓6ᵗʰ D23.12 Other benign neoplasm of skin of left eyelid, including canthus
D23.121 Other benign neoplasm of skin of left upper eyelid, including canthus
D23.122 Other benign neoplasm of skin of left lower eyelid, including canthus

✓5ᵗʰ D23.2 Other benign neoplasm of skin of ear and external auricular canal
D23.20 Other benign neoplasm of skin of unspecified ear and external auricular canal
D23.21 Other benign neoplasm of skin of right ear and external auricular canal
D23.22 Other benign neoplasm of skin of left ear and external auricular canal

✓5ᵗʰ D23.3 Other benign neoplasm of skin of other and unspecified parts of face
D23.30 Other benign neoplasm of skin of unspecified part of face
D23.39 Other benign neoplasm of skin of other parts of face

D23.4 Other benign neoplasm of skin of scalp and neck

D23.5   **Other benign neoplasm of skin of** trunk
     Other benign neoplasm of anal margin
     Other benign neoplasm of anal skin
     Other benign neoplasm of perianal skin
     Other benign neoplasm of skin of breast
     EXCLUDES 1   *benign neoplasm of anus NOS (D12.9)*

✓5th **D23.6**   **Other benign neoplasm of skin of** upper limb, including shoulder
   D23.60   **Other benign neoplasm of skin of unspecified upper limb, including shoulder**
   D23.61   **Other benign neoplasm of skin of** right **upper limb, including shoulder**
   D23.62   **Other benign neoplasm of skin of** left **upper limb, including shoulder**

✓5th **D23.7**   **Other benign neoplasm of skin of** lower limb, including hip
   D23.70   **Other benign neoplasm of skin of unspecified lower limb, including hip**
   D23.71   **Other benign neoplasm of skin of** right **lower limb, including hip**
   D23.72   **Other benign neoplasm of skin of** left **lower limb, including hip**

D23.9   **Other benign neoplasm of skin, unspecified**

✓4th **D24**   **Benign neoplasm of** breast
   INCLUDES   benign neoplasm of connective tissue of breast
     benign neoplasm of soft parts of breast
     fibroadenoma of breast
   EXCLUDES 2   *adenofibrosis of breast (N60.2)*
     benign cyst of breast (N60.-)
     benign mammary dysplasia (N60.-)
     benign neoplasm of skin of breast (D22.5, D23.5)
     fibrocystic disease of breast (N60.-)

   D24.1   **Benign neoplasm of** right **breast**
   D24.2   **Benign neoplasm of** left **breast**
   D24.9   **Benign neoplasm of unspecified breast**

✓4th **D25**   **Leiomyoma of uterus**
   INCLUDES   uterine fibroid
     uterine fibromyoma
     uterine myoma

Uterine Leiomyomas (Fibroids)

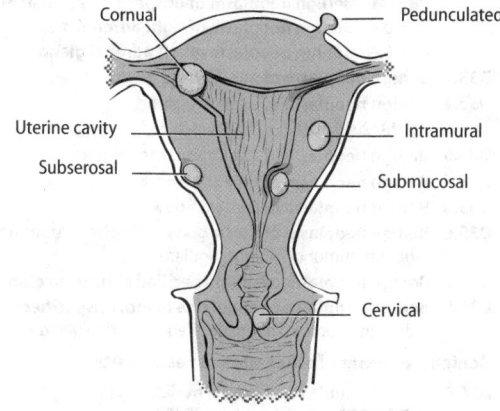

Cornual   Pedunculated
Uterine cavity   Intramural
Subserosal   Submucosal
Cervical

   D25.0   Submucous **leiomyoma of uterus**   ♀
   D25.1   Intramural **leiomyoma of uterus**   ♀
     Interstitial leiomyoma of uterus
   D25.2   Subserosal **leiomyoma of uterus**   ♀
     Subperitoneal leiomyoma of uterus
   D25.9   **Leiomyoma of uterus, unspecified**   ♀

✓4th **D26**   **Other benign neoplasms of** uterus
   D26.0   **Other benign neoplasm of** cervix uteri   ♀
   D26.1   **Other benign neoplasm of** corpus uteri   ♀
   D26.7   **Other benign neoplasm of other** parts **of uterus**   ♀
   D26.9   **Other benign neoplasm of uterus, unspecified**   ♀

✓4th **D27**   **Benign neoplasm of** ovary
   Use additional code to identify any functional activity
   EXCLUDES 2   *corpus albicans cyst (N83.2-)*
     corpus luteum cyst (N83.1-)
     endometrial cyst (N80.1)
     follicular (atretic) cyst (N83.0-)
     graafian follicle cyst (N83.0-)
     ovarian cyst NEC (N83.2-)
     ovarian retention cyst (N83.2-)

   D27.0   **Benign neoplasm of** right **ovary**   ♀
   D27.1   **Benign neoplasm of** left **ovary**   ♀
   D27.9   **Benign neoplasm of unspecified ovary**   ♀

✓4th **D28**   **Benign neoplasm of other and unspecified** female genital organs
   INCLUDES   adenomatous polyp
     benign neoplasm of skin of female genital organs
     benign teratoma
   EXCLUDES 1   *epoophoron cyst (Q50.5)*
     fimbrial cyst (Q50.4)
     Gartner's duct cyst (Q52.4)
     parovarian cyst (Q50.5)

   D28.0   **Benign neoplasm of** vulva   ♀
   D28.1   **Benign neoplasm of** vagina   ♀
   D28.2   **Benign neoplasm of** uterine tubes and ligaments   ♀
     Benign neoplasm of fallopian tube
     Benign neoplasm of uterine ligament (broad) (round)
   D28.7   **Benign neoplasm of other specified female genital organs**   ♀
   D28.9   **Benign neoplasm of female genital organ, unspecified**   ♀

✓4th **D29**   **Benign neoplasm of** male genital organs
   INCLUDES   benign neoplasm of skin of male genital organs
   D29.0   **Benign neoplasm of** penis   ♂
   D29.1   **Benign neoplasm of** prostate   ♂
     EXCLUDES 1   *enlarged prostate (N40.-)*

✓5th **D29.2**   **Benign neoplasm of** testis
     Use additional code to identify any functional activity
   D29.20   **Benign neoplasm of unspecified testis**   ♂
   D29.21   **Benign neoplasm of** right **testis**   ♂
   D29.22   **Benign neoplasm of** left **testis**   ♂

✓5th **D29.3**   **Benign neoplasm of** epididymis
   D29.30   **Benign neoplasm of unspecified epididymis**   ♂
   D29.31   **Benign neoplasm of** right **epididymis**   ♂
   D29.32   **Benign neoplasm of** left **epididymis**   ♂

   D29.4   **Benign neoplasm of** scrotum   ♂
     Benign neoplasm of skin of scrotum
   D29.8   **Benign neoplasm of other specified male genital organs**   ♂
     Benign neoplasm of seminal vesicle
     Benign neoplasm of spermatic cord
     Benign neoplasm of tunica vaginalis
   D29.9   **Benign neoplasm of male genital organ, unspecified**   ♂

✓4th **D30**   **Benign neoplasm of** urinary organs
✓5th **D30.0**   **Benign neoplasm of** kidney
     EXCLUDES 1   *benign carcinoid tumor of the kidney (D3A.093)*
     benign neoplasm of renal calyces (D30.1-)
     benign neoplasm of renal pelvis (D30.1-)
   D30.00   **Benign neoplasm of unspecified kidney**
   D30.01   **Benign neoplasm of** right **kidney**
   D30.02   **Benign neoplasm of** left **kidney**

✓5th **D30.1**   **Benign neoplasm of** renal pelvis
   D30.10   **Benign neoplasm of unspecified renal pelvis**
   D30.11   **Benign neoplasm of** right **renal pelvis**
   D30.12   **Benign neoplasm of** left **renal pelvis**

✓5th **D30.2**   **Benign neoplasm of** ureter
     EXCLUDES 1   *benign neoplasm of ureteric orifice of bladder (D30.3)*
   D30.20   **Benign neoplasm of unspecified ureter**
   D30.21   **Benign neoplasm of** right **ureter**
   D30.22   **Benign neoplasm of** left **ureter**

   D30.3   **Benign neoplasm of** bladder
     Benign neoplasm of ureteric orifice of bladder
     Benign neoplasm of urethral orifice of bladder

Chapter 2. Neoplasms

D23.5–D30.3

D30.4 **Benign neoplasm of** urethra
> **EXCLUDES 1** *benign neoplasm of urethral orifice of bladder (D30.3)*

D30.8 **Benign neoplasm of other specified urinary organs**
Benign neoplasm of paraurethral glands

D30.9 **Benign neoplasm of urinary organ, unspecified**
Benign neoplasm of urinary system NOS

✓4ᵗʰ **D31** **Benign neoplasm of** eye and adnexa
> **EXCLUDES 1** *benign neoplasm of connective tissue of eyelid (D21.0)*
> *benign neoplasm of optic nerve (D33.3)*
> *benign neoplasm of skin of eyelid (D22.1-, D23.1-)*

✓5ᵗʰ **D31.0** **Benign neoplasm of** conjunctiva
> **D31.00** **Benign neoplasm of unspecified conjunctiva**
> **D31.01** **Benign neoplasm of** right **conjunctiva**
> **D31.02** **Benign neoplasm of** left **conjunctiva**

✓5ᵗʰ **D31.1** **Benign neoplasm of** cornea
> **D31.10** **Benign neoplasm of unspecified cornea**
> **D31.11** **Benign neoplasm of** right **cornea**
> **D31.12** **Benign neoplasm of** left **cornea**

✓5ᵗʰ **D31.2** **Benign neoplasm of** retina
> **EXCLUDES 1** *dark area on retina (D49.81)*
> *hemangioma of retina (D49.81)*
> *neoplasm of unspecified behavior of retina and choroid (D49.81)*
> *retinal freckle (D49.81)*
> **D31.20** **Benign neoplasm of unspecified retina**
> **D31.21** **Benign neoplasm of** right **retina**
> **D31.22** **Benign neoplasm of** left **retina**

✓5ᵗʰ **D31.3** **Benign neoplasm of** choroid
> **D31.30** **Benign neoplasm of unspecified choroid**
> **D31.31** **Benign neoplasm of** right **choroid**
> **D31.32** **Benign neoplasm of** left **choroid**

✓5ᵗʰ **D31.4** **Benign neoplasm of** ciliary body
> **D31.40** **Benign neoplasm of unspecified ciliary body**
> **D31.41** **Benign neoplasm of** right **ciliary body**
> **D31.42** **Benign neoplasm of** left **ciliary body**

✓5ᵗʰ **D31.5** **Benign neoplasm of** lacrimal gland and duct
Benign neoplasm of lacrimal sac
Benign neoplasm of nasolacrimal duct
> **D31.50** **Benign neoplasm of unspecified lacrimal gland and duct**
> **D31.51** **Benign neoplasm of** right **lacrimal gland and duct**
> **D31.52** **Benign neoplasm of** left **lacrimal gland and duct**

✓5ᵗʰ **D31.6** **Benign neoplasm of unspecified site of** orbit
Benign neoplasm of connective tissue of orbit
Benign neoplasm of extraocular muscle
Benign neoplasm of peripheral nerves of orbit
Benign neoplasm of retrobulbar tissue
Benign neoplasm of retro-ocular tissue
> **EXCLUDES 1** *benign neoplasm of orbital bone (D16.4)*
> **D31.60** **Benign neoplasm of unspecified site of unspecified orbit**
> **D31.61** **Benign neoplasm of unspecified site of** right **orbit**
> **D31.62** **Benign neoplasm of unspecified site of** left **orbit**

✓5ᵗʰ **D31.9** **Benign neoplasm of unspecified** part of eye
Benign neoplasm of eyeball
> **D31.90** **Benign neoplasm of unspecified part of unspecified eye**
> **D31.91** **Benign neoplasm of unspecified part of** right **eye**
> **D31.92** **Benign neoplasm of unspecified part of** left **eye**

✓4ᵗʰ **D32** **Benign neoplasm of** meninges
D32.0 **Benign neoplasm of** cerebral **meninges** `HCC`
D32.1 **Benign neoplasm of** spinal **meninges** `HCC`
D32.9 **Benign neoplasm of meninges, unspecified** `HCC`
Meningioma NOS

✓4ᵗʰ **D33** **Benign neoplasm of** brain and other parts of central nervous system
> **EXCLUDES 1** *angioma (D18.0-)*
> *benign neoplasm of meninges (D32.-)*
> *benign neoplasm of peripheral nerves and autonomic nervous system (D36.1-)*
> *hemangioma (D18.0-)*
> *neurofibromatosis (Q85.0-)*
> *retro-ocular benign neoplasm (D31.6-)*

D33.0 **Benign neoplasm of** brain, supratentorial `HCC`
Benign neoplasm of cerebral ventricle
Benign neoplasm of cerebrum
Benign neoplasm of frontal lobe
Benign neoplasm of occipital lobe
Benign neoplasm of parietal lobe
Benign neoplasm of temporal lobe
> **EXCLUDES 1** *benign neoplasm of fourth ventricle (D33.1)*

D33.1 **Benign neoplasm of** brain, infratentorial `HCC`
Benign neoplasm of brain stem
Benign neoplasm of cerebellum
Benign neoplasm of fourth ventricle

D33.2 **Benign neoplasm of brain, unspecified** `HCC`

D33.3 **Benign neoplasm of** cranial nerves `HCC`
Benign neoplasm of olfactory bulb

D33.4 **Benign neoplasm of** spinal cord `HCC`

D33.7 **Benign neoplasm of other specified parts of central nervous system** `HCC`

D33.9 **Benign neoplasm of central nervous system, unspecified** `HCC`
Benign neoplasm of nervous system (central) NOS

D34 **Benign neoplasm of** thyroid gland
Use additional code to identify any functional activity

✓4ᵗʰ **D35** **Benign neoplasm of other and unspecified** endocrine glands
Use additional code to identify any functional activity
> **EXCLUDES 1** *benign neoplasm of endocrine pancreas (D13.7)*
> *benign neoplasm of ovary (D27.-)*
> *benign neoplasm of testis (D29.2.-)*
> *benign neoplasm of thymus (D15.0)*

✓5ᵗʰ **D35.0** **Benign neoplasm of** adrenal gland
> **D35.00** **Benign neoplasm of unspecified adrenal gland**
> **D35.01** **Benign neoplasm of** right **adrenal gland**
> **D35.02** **Benign neoplasm of** left **adrenal gland**

D35.1 **Benign neoplasm of** parathyroid gland
D35.2 **Benign neoplasm of** pituitary gland `HCC`
AHA: 2014,3Q,22
D35.3 **Benign neoplasm of** craniopharyngeal duct `HCC`
D35.4 **Benign neoplasm of** pineal gland `HCC`
D35.5 **Benign neoplasm of** carotid body
D35.6 **Benign neoplasm of** aortic body and other paraganglia
Benign tumor of glomus jugulare
D35.7 **Benign neoplasm of other specified endocrine glands**
D35.9 **Benign neoplasm of endocrine gland, unspecified**
Benign neoplasm of unspecified endocrine gland

✓4ᵗʰ **D36** **Benign neoplasm of other and unspecified sites**
D36.0 **Benign neoplasm of** lymph nodes
> **EXCLUDES 1** *lymphangioma (D18.1)*

✓5ᵗʰ **D36.1** **Benign neoplasm of** peripheral nerves and autonomic nervous system
> **EXCLUDES 1** *benign neoplasm of peripheral nerves of orbit (D31.6-)*
> *neurofibromatosis (Q85.0-)*
> **D36.10** **Benign neoplasm of peripheral nerves and autonomic nervous system, unspecified**
> **D36.11** **Benign neoplasm of peripheral nerves and autonomic nervous system of** face, head, and neck
> **D36.12** **Benign neoplasm of peripheral nerves and autonomic nervous system, upper limb, including shoulder**
> **D36.13** **Benign neoplasm of peripheral nerves and autonomic nervous system of** lower limb, including hip
> **D36.14** **Benign neoplasm of peripheral nerves and autonomic nervous system of** thorax
> **D36.15** **Benign neoplasm of peripheral nerves and autonomic nervous system of** abdomen

N Newborn: 0 **P** Pediatric: 0-17 **M** Maternity: 9-64 **A** Adult: 15-124 **MCC** Major Complication/Comorbidity **CC** Complication/Comorbidity **SW** Severe Wound Dx

500 ICD-10-CM 2022

D36.16   Benign neoplasm of peripheral nerves and autonomic nervous system of pelvis

D36.17   Benign neoplasm of peripheral nerves and autonomic nervous system of trunk, unspecified

D36.7   Benign neoplasm of other specified sites
Benign neoplasm of back NOS
Benign neoplasm of nose NOS

D36.9   Benign neoplasm, unspecified site

Benign neuroendocrine tumors (D3A)

✓4ᵗʰ **D3A**   **Benign neuroendocrine tumors**
Code also any associated multiple endocrine neoplasia [MEN] syndromes (E31.2-)
Use additional code to identify any associated endocrine syndrome, such as:
carcinoid syndrome (E34.0)
EXCLUDES 2   benign pancreatic islet cell tumors (D13.7)

✓5ᵗʰ **D3A.0**   **Benign carcinoid tumors**
DEF: Specific type of slow-growing neuroendocrine tumors. Carcinoid tumors occur most commonly in the hormone producing cells of the gastrointestinal tracts and can also occur in the pancreas, testes, ovaries, or lungs.

D3A.00   **Benign carcinoid tumor of unspecified site**
Carcinoid tumor NOS

✓6ᵗʰ **D3A.01**   **Benign carcinoid tumors of the** small intestine
D3A.010   Benign carcinoid tumor of the duodenum
D3A.011   Benign carcinoid tumor of the jejunum
D3A.012   Benign carcinoid tumor of the ileum
D3A.019   Benign carcinoid tumor of the small intestine, unspecified portion

✓6ᵗʰ **D3A.02**   **Benign carcinoid tumors of the** appendix, large intestine, and rectum
D3A.020   Benign carcinoid tumor of the appendix
D3A.021   Benign carcinoid tumor of the cecum
D3A.022   Benign carcinoid tumor of the ascending colon
D3A.023   Benign carcinoid tumor of the transverse colon
D3A.024   Benign carcinoid tumor of the descending colon
D3A.025   Benign carcinoid tumor of the sigmoid colon
D3A.026   Benign carcinoid tumor of the rectum
D3A.029   Benign carcinoid tumor of the large intestine, unspecified portion
Benign carcinoid tumor of the colon NOS

✓6ᵗʰ **D3A.09**   **Benign carcinoid tumors of other sites**
D3A.090   Benign carcinoid tumor of the bronchus and lung
D3A.091   Benign carcinoid tumor of the thymus
D3A.092   Benign carcinoid tumor of the stomach
D3A.093   Benign carcinoid tumor of the kidney
D3A.094   Benign carcinoid tumor of the foregut, unspecified
D3A.095   Benign carcinoid tumor of the midgut, unspecified
D3A.096   Benign carcinoid tumor of the hindgut, unspecified
D3A.098   Benign carcinoid tumors of other sites

D3A.8   **Other benign neuroendocrine tumors**
Neuroendocrine tumor NOS

Neoplasms of uncertain behavior, polycythemia vera and myelodysplastic syndromes (D37-D48)

NOTE   Categories D37-D44, and D48 classify by site neoplasms of uncertain behavior, i.e., histologic confirmation whether the neoplasm is malignant or benign cannot be made.
EXCLUDES 1   neoplasms of unspecified behavior (D49.-)

✓4ᵗʰ **D37**   **Neoplasm of uncertain behavior of** oral cavity and digestive organs
EXCLUDES 1   stromal tumors of uncertain behavior of digestive system (D48.1)

✓5ᵗʰ **D37.0**   **Neoplasm of uncertain behavior of** lip, oral cavity and pharynx
EXCLUDES 1   neoplasm of uncertain behavior of aryepiglottic fold or interarytenoid fold, laryngeal aspect (D38.0)
neoplasm of uncertain behavior of epiglottis NOS (D38.0)
neoplasm of uncertain behavior of skin of lip (D48.5)
neoplasm of uncertain behavior of suprahyoid portion of epiglottis (D38.0)

D37.01   **Neoplasm of uncertain behavior of** lip
Neoplasm of uncertain behavior of vermilion border of lip

D37.02   **Neoplasm of uncertain behavior of** tongue

✓6ᵗʰ **D37.03**   **Neoplasm of uncertain behavior of the** major salivary glands
D37.030   Neoplasm of uncertain behavior of the parotid salivary glands
D37.031   Neoplasm of uncertain behavior of the sublingual salivary glands
D37.032   Neoplasm of uncertain behavior of the submandibular salivary glands
D37.039   Neoplasm of uncertain behavior of the major salivary glands, unspecified

D37.04   **Neoplasm of uncertain behavior of the** minor salivary glands
Neoplasm of uncertain behavior of submucosal salivary glands of lip
Neoplasm of uncertain behavior of submucosal salivary glands of cheek
Neoplasm of uncertain behavior of submucosal salivary glands of hard palate
Neoplasm of uncertain behavior of submucosal salivary glands of soft palate

D37.05   **Neoplasm of uncertain behavior of** pharynx
Neoplasm of uncertain behavior of aryepiglottic fold of pharynx NOS
Neoplasm of uncertain behavior of hypopharyngeal aspect of aryepiglottic fold of pharynx
Neoplasm of uncertain behavior of marginal zone of aryepiglottic fold of pharynx

D37.09   **Neoplasm of uncertain behavior of other specified sites of the oral cavity**

D37.1   **Neoplasm of uncertain behavior of** stomach

D37.2   **Neoplasm of uncertain behavior of** small intestine

D37.3   **Neoplasm of uncertain behavior of** appendix

D37.4   **Neoplasm of uncertain behavior of** colon

D37.5   **Neoplasm of uncertain behavior of** rectum
Neoplasm of uncertain behavior of rectosigmoid junction

D37.6   **Neoplasm of uncertain behavior of** liver, gallbladder and bile ducts
Neoplasm of uncertain behavior of ampulla of Vater

D37.8   **Neoplasm of uncertain behavior of other specified digestive organs**
Neoplasm of uncertain behavior of anal canal
Neoplasm of uncertain behavior of anal sphincter
Neoplasm of uncertain behavior of anus NOS
Neoplasm of uncertain behavior of esophagus
Neoplasm of uncertain behavior of intestine NOS
Neoplasm of uncertain behavior of pancreas
EXCLUDES 1   neoplasm of uncertain behavior of anal margin (D48.5)
neoplasm of uncertain behavior of anal skin (D48.5)
neoplasm of uncertain behavior of perianal skin (D48.5)

D37.9   **Neoplasm of uncertain behavior of digestive organ, unspecified**

Chapter 2. Neoplasms

D38–D44.9

☑4ᵗʰ **D38 Neoplasm of uncertain behavior of middle ear and respiratory and intrathoracic organs**
    EXCLUDES 1   neoplasm of uncertain behavior of heart (D48.7)

   D38.Ø Neoplasm of uncertain behavior of larynx
     Neoplasm of uncertain behavior of aryepiglottic fold or interarytenoid fold, laryngeal aspect
     Neoplasm of uncertain behavior of epiglottis (suprahyoid portion)
     EXCLUDES 1   neoplasm of uncertain behavior of aryepiglottic fold or interarytenoid fold NOS (D37.Ø5)
        neoplasm of uncertain behavior of hypopharyngeal aspect of aryepiglottic fold (D37.Ø5)
        neoplasm of uncertain behavior of marginal zone of aryepiglottic fold (D37.Ø5)

   D38.1 Neoplasm of uncertain behavior of trachea, bronchus and lung

   D38.2 Neoplasm of uncertain behavior of pleura

   D38.3 Neoplasm of uncertain behavior of mediastinum

   D38.4 Neoplasm of uncertain behavior of thymus

   D38.5 Neoplasm of uncertain behavior of other respiratory organs
     Neoplasm of uncertain behavior of accessory sinuses
     Neoplasm of uncertain behavior of cartilage of nose
     Neoplasm of uncertain behavior of middle ear
     Neoplasm of uncertain behavior of nasal cavities
     EXCLUDES 1   neoplasm of uncertain behavior of ear (external) (skin) (D48.5)
        neoplasm of uncertain behavior of nose NOS (D48.7)
        neoplasm of uncertain behavior of skin of nose (D48.5)

   D38.6 Neoplasm of uncertain behavior of respiratory organ, unspecified

☑4ᵗʰ **D39 Neoplasm of uncertain behavior of female genital organs**

   D39.Ø Neoplasm of uncertain behavior of uterus ♀

   ☑5ᵗʰ **D39.1 Neoplasm of uncertain behavior of ovary** ♀
     Use additional code to identify any functional activity

     D39.1Ø Neoplasm of uncertain behavior of unspecified ovary ♀

     D39.11 Neoplasm of uncertain behavior of right ovary ♀

     D39.12 Neoplasm of uncertain behavior of left ovary ♀

   D39.2 Neoplasm of uncertain behavior of placenta M ♀
     Chorioadenoma destruens
     Invasive hydatidiform mole
     Malignant hydatidiform mole
     EXCLUDES 1   hydatidiform mole NOS (OØ1.9)

   D39.8 Neoplasm of uncertain behavior of other specified female genital organs ♀
     Neoplasm of uncertain behavior of skin of female genital organs

   D39.9 Neoplasm of uncertain behavior of female genital organ, unspecified ♀

☑4ᵗʰ **D4Ø Neoplasm of uncertain behavior of male genital organs**

   D4Ø.Ø Neoplasm of uncertain behavior of prostate ♂

   ☑5ᵗʰ **D4Ø.1 Neoplasm of uncertain behavior of testis**

     D4Ø.1Ø Neoplasm of uncertain behavior of unspecified testis ♂

     D4Ø.11 Neoplasm of uncertain behavior of right testis ♂

     D4Ø.12 Neoplasm of uncertain behavior of left testis ♂

   D4Ø.8 Neoplasm of uncertain behavior of other specified male genital organs ♂
     Neoplasm of uncertain behavior of skin of male genital organs

   D4Ø.9 Neoplasm of uncertain behavior of male genital organ, unspecified ♂

☑4ᵗʰ **D41 Neoplasm of uncertain behavior of urinary organs**

   ☑5ᵗʰ **D41.Ø Neoplasm of uncertain behavior of kidney**
     EXCLUDES 1   neoplasm of uncertain behavior of renal pelvis (D41.1-)

     D41.ØØ Neoplasm of uncertain behavior of unspecified kidney

     D41.Ø1 Neoplasm of uncertain behavior of right kidney

     D41.Ø2 Neoplasm of uncertain behavior of left kidney

   ☑5ᵗʰ **D41.1 Neoplasm of uncertain behavior of renal pelvis**

     D41.1Ø Neoplasm of uncertain behavior of unspecified renal pelvis

     D41.11 Neoplasm of uncertain behavior of right renal pelvis

     D41.12 Neoplasm of uncertain behavior of left renal pelvis

   ☑5ᵗʰ **D41.2 Neoplasm of uncertain behavior of ureter**

     D41.2Ø Neoplasm of uncertain behavior of unspecified ureter

     D41.21 Neoplasm of uncertain behavior of right ureter

     D41.22 Neoplasm of uncertain behavior of left ureter

   D41.3 Neoplasm of uncertain behavior of urethra

   D41.4 Neoplasm of uncertain behavior of bladder

   D41.8 Neoplasm of uncertain behavior of other specified urinary organs

   D41.9 Neoplasm of uncertain behavior of unspecified urinary organ

☑4ᵗʰ **D42 Neoplasm of uncertain behavior of meninges**

   D42.Ø Neoplasm of uncertain behavior of cerebral meninges HCC

   D42.1 Neoplasm of uncertain behavior of spinal meninges HCC

   D42.9 Neoplasm of uncertain behavior of meninges, unspecified HCC

☑4ᵗʰ **D43 Neoplasm of uncertain behavior of brain and central nervous system**
   EXCLUDES 1   neoplasm of uncertain behavior of peripheral nerves and autonomic nervous system (D48.2)

   D43.Ø Neoplasm of uncertain behavior of brain, supratentorial HCC
     Neoplasm of uncertain behavior of cerebral ventricle
     Neoplasm of uncertain behavior of cerebrum
     Neoplasm of uncertain behavior of frontal lobe
     Neoplasm of uncertain behavior of occipital lobe
     Neoplasm of uncertain behavior of parietal lobe
     Neoplasm of uncertain behavior of temporal lobe
     EXCLUDES 1   neoplasm of uncertain behavior of fourth ventricle (D43.1)

   D43.1 Neoplasm of uncertain behavior of brain, infratentorial HCC
     Neoplasm of uncertain behavior of brain stem
     Neoplasm of uncertain behavior of cerebellum
     Neoplasm of uncertain behavior of fourth ventricle

   D43.2 Neoplasm of uncertain behavior of brain, unspecified HCC

   D43.3 Neoplasm of uncertain behavior of cranial nerves HCC

   D43.4 Neoplasm of uncertain behavior of spinal cord HCC

   D43.8 Neoplasm of uncertain behavior of other specified parts of central nervous system HCC

   D43.9 Neoplasm of uncertain behavior of central nervous system, unspecified HCC
     Neoplasm of uncertain behavior of nervous system (central) NOS

☑4ᵗʰ **D44 Neoplasm of uncertain behavior of endocrine glands**
   EXCLUDES 1   multiple endocrine adenomatosis (E31.2-)
     multiple endocrine neoplasia (E31.2-)
     neoplasm of uncertain behavior of endocrine pancreas (D37.8)
     neoplasm of uncertain behavior of ovary (D39.1-)
     neoplasm of uncertain behavior of testis (D4Ø.1-)
     neoplasm of uncertain behavior of thymus (D38.4)

   D44.Ø Neoplasm of uncertain behavior of thyroid gland

   ☑5ᵗʰ **D44.1 Neoplasm of uncertain behavior of adrenal gland**
     Use additional code to identify any functional activity

     D44.1Ø Neoplasm of uncertain behavior of unspecified adrenal gland

     D44.11 Neoplasm of uncertain behavior of right adrenal gland

     D44.12 Neoplasm of uncertain behavior of left adrenal gland

   D44.2 Neoplasm of uncertain behavior of parathyroid gland

   D44.3 Neoplasm of uncertain behavior of pituitary gland HCC
     Use additional code to identify any functional activity

   D44.4 Neoplasm of uncertain behavior of craniopharyngeal duct HCC

   D44.5 Neoplasm of uncertain behavior of pineal gland HCC

   D44.6 Neoplasm of uncertain behavior of carotid body HCC

   D44.7 Neoplasm of uncertain behavior of aortic body and other paraganglia HCC
     AHA: 2021,2Q,7; 2016,4Q,26

   D44.9 Neoplasm of uncertain behavior of unspecified endocrine gland

D45 Polycythemia vera `HCC`
> EXCLUDES 1   *familial polycythemia (D75.0)*
>   *secondary polycythemia (D75.1)*

DEF: Abnormal proliferation of all bone marrow elements, increased red cell mass, and total blood volume. The etiology is unknown, but it is frequently associated with splenomegaly, leukocytosis, and thrombocythemia.

☑4ᵗʰ **D46 Myelodysplastic syndromes**
> Use additional code for adverse effect, if applicable, to identify drug (T36-T50 with fifth or sixth character 5)
> EXCLUDES 2   *drug-induced aplastic anemia (D61.1)*

D46.0 Refractory anemia without ring sideroblasts, so stated `HCC`
> Refractory anemia without sideroblasts, without excess of blasts

D46.1 Refractory anemia with ring sideroblasts `HCC`
> RARS

☑5ᵗʰ **D46.2 Refractory anemia with excess of blasts [RAEB]**

     D46.20 Refractory anemia with excess of blasts, unspecified `HCC`
>   RAEB NOS

     D46.21 Refractory anemia with excess of blasts 1 `HCC`
>   RAEB 1

     D46.22 Refractory anemia with excess of blasts 2 `CC` `HCC`
>   RAEB 2

D46.A Refractory cytopenia with multilineage dysplasia `HCC`

D46.B Refractory cytopenia with multilineage dysplasia and ring sideroblasts `HCC`
> RCMD RS

D46.C Myelodysplastic syndrome with isolated del(5q) chromosomal abnormality `CC` `HCC`
> Myelodysplastic syndrome with 5q deletion
> 5q minus syndrome NOS

D46.4 Refractory anemia, unspecified `HCC`

D46.Z Other myelodysplastic syndromes `HCC`
> EXCLUDES 1   *chronic myelomonocytic leukemia (C93.1-)*

D46.9 Myelodysplastic syndrome, unspecified `HCC`
> Myelodysplasia NOS

☑4ᵗʰ **D47 Other neoplasms of uncertain behavior of lymphoid, hematopoietic and related tissue**

☑5ᵗʰ **D47.0 Mast cell neoplasms of uncertain behavior**
> EXCLUDES 1   *congenital cutaneous mastocytosis (Q82.2)*
>   *histiocytic neoplasms of uncertain behavior (D47.Z9)*
>   *malignant mast cell neoplasm (C96.2-)*

AHA: 2017,4Q,5

     D47.01 Cutaneous mastocytosis `CC`
>   Diffuse cutaneous mastocytosis
>   Maculopapular cutaneous mastocytosis
>   Solitary mastocytoma
>   Telangiectasia macularis eruptiva perstans
>   Urticaria pigmentosa
>   EXCLUDES 1   *congenital (diffuse) (maculopapular) cutaneous mastocytosis (Q82.2)*
>   *congenital urticaria pigmentosa (Q82.2)*
>   *extracutaneous mastocytoma (D47.09)*

     D47.02 Systemic mastocytosis `CC`
>   Indolent systemic mastocytosis
>   Isolated bone marrow mastocytosis
>   Smoldering systemic mastocytosis
>   Systemic mastocytosis, with an associated hematological non-mast cell lineage disease (SM-AHNMD)
>   Code also, if applicable, any associated hematological non-mast cell lineage disease, such as:
>   acute myeloid leukemia (C92.6-, C92.A-)
>   chronic myelomonocytic leukemia (C93.1-)
>   essential thrombocytosis (D47.3)
>   hypereosinophilic syndrome (D72.1)
>   myelodysplastic syndrome (D46.9)
>   myeloproliferative syndrome (D47.1)
>   non-Hodgkin lymphoma (C82-C85)
>   plasma cell myeloma (C90.0-)
>   polycythemia vera (D45)
>   EXCLUDES 1   *aggressive systemic mastocytosis (C96.21)*
>   *mast cell leukemia (C94.3-)*

     D47.09 Other mast cell neoplasms of uncertain behavior `CC`
>   Extracutaneous mastocytoma
>   Mast cell tumor NOS
>   Mastocytoma NOS
>   Mastocytosis NOS

D47.1 Chronic myeloproliferative disease `CC` `HCC`
> Chronic neutrophilic leukemia
> Myeloproliferative disease, unspecified
> EXCLUDES 1   *atypical chronic myeloid leukemia BCR/ABL-negative (C92.2-)*
>   *chronic myeloid leukemia BCR/ABL-positive (C92.1-)*
>   *myelofibrosis NOS (D75.81)*
>   *myelophthisic anemia (D61.82)*
>   *myelophthisis (D61.82)*
>   *secondary myelofibrosis NOS (D75.81)*

D47.2 Monoclonal gammopathy
> Monoclonal gammopathy of undetermined significance [MGUS]

D47.3 Essential (hemorrhagic) thrombocythemia `HCC`
> Essential thrombocytosis
> Idiopathic hemorrhagic thrombocythemia
> ▶Primary thrombocytosis◀
> EXCLUDES 2   ▶*reactive thrombocytosis (D75.838)*◀
>   ▶*secondary thrombocytosis (D75.838)*◀
>   ▶*thrombocythemia NOS (D75.839)*◀
>   ▶*thrombocytosis NOS (D75.839)*◀

DEF: Chronic myeloproliferative neoplasm involving production of excess blood platelets that may result in abnormal clotting or hemorrhaging.

D47.4 Osteomyelofibrosis `HCC`
> Chronic idiopathic myelofibrosis
> Myelofibrosis (idiopathic) (with myeloid metaplasia)
> Myelosclerosis (megakaryocytic) with myeloid metaplasia
> Secondary myelofibrosis in myeloproliferative disease
> EXCLUDES 1   *acute myelofibrosis (C94.4-)*

☑5ᵗʰ **D47.Z Other specified neoplasms of uncertain behavior of lymphoid, hematopoietic and related tissue**
> AHA: 2016,4Q,8

     D47.Z1 Post-transplant lymphoproliferative disorder (PTLD) `CC` `UPD` `HCC`
>   Code first complications of transplanted organs and tissue (T86.-)
>   **DEF:** Excessive proliferation of B-cell lymphocytes following Epstein-Barr virus infection in organ transplant patients. It may progress to non-Hodgkin lymphoma.

     D47.Z2 Castleman disease `CC` `HCC`
>   ▶Code also, if applicable, human herpesvirus 8 infection◀ (B10.89)
>   EXCLUDES 2   *Kaposi's sarcoma (C46.-)*
>   **DEF:** Rare disease of the lymph nodes and lymphoid tissues that closely mimics lymphoma.

     D47.Z9 Other specified neoplasms of uncertain behavior of lymphoid, hematopoietic and related tissue `CC` `HCC`
>   Histiocytic tumors of uncertain behavior

D47.9 Neoplasm of uncertain behavior of lymphoid, hematopoietic and related tissue, unspecified `CC` `HCC`
> Lymphoproliferative disease NOS

☑4ᵗʰ **D48 Neoplasm of uncertain behavior of other and unspecified sites**
> EXCLUDES 1   *neurofibromatosis (nonmalignant) (Q85.0-)*

D48.0 Neoplasm of uncertain behavior of bone and articular cartilage
> EXCLUDES 1   *neoplasm of uncertain behavior of cartilage of ear (D48.1)*
>   *neoplasm of uncertain behavior of cartilage of larynx (D38.0)*
>   *neoplasm of uncertain behavior of cartilage of nose (D38.5)*
>   *neoplasm of uncertain behavior of connective tissue of eyelid (D48.1)*
>   *neoplasm of uncertain behavior of synovia (D48.1)*

☑ Additional Character Required   ☑x7ᵗʰ Placeholder   Questionable PDx   Manifestation   Unspecified Dx   `UPD` Unacceptable PDx   H1-H14 HAC   `HCC` CMS-HCC Dx   `HIV` HIV Dx

ICD-10-CM 2022   503

D48.1 Neoplasm of uncertain behavior of connective and other soft tissue

Neoplasm of uncertain behavior of connective tissue of ear
Neoplasm of uncertain behavior of connective tissue of eyelid
Stromal tumors of uncertain behavior of digestive system

> EXCLUDES 1 *neoplasm of uncertain behavior of articular cartilage (D48.0)*
> *neoplasm of uncertain behavior of cartilage of larynx (D38.0)*
> *neoplasm of uncertain behavior of cartilage of nose (D38.5)*
> *neoplasm of uncertain behavior of connective tissue of breast (D48.6-)*

D48.2 Neoplasm of uncertain behavior of peripheral nerves and autonomic nervous system

> EXCLUDES 1 *neoplasm of uncertain behavior of peripheral nerves of orbit (D48.7)*

D48.3 Neoplasm of uncertain behavior of retroperitoneum

D48.4 Neoplasm of uncertain behavior of peritoneum

D48.5 Neoplasm of uncertain behavior of skin

Neoplasm of uncertain behavior of anal margin
Neoplasm of uncertain behavior of anal skin
Neoplasm of uncertain behavior of perianal skin
Neoplasm of uncertain behavior of skin of breast

> EXCLUDES 1 *neoplasm of uncertain behavior of anus NOS (D37.8)*
> *neoplasm of uncertain behavior of skin of genital organs (D39.8, D40.8)*
> *neoplasm of uncertain behavior of vermilion border of lip (D37.0)*

√5th **D48.6 Neoplasm of uncertain behavior of** breast

Neoplasm of uncertain behavior of connective tissue of breast
Cystosarcoma phyllodes

> EXCLUDES 1 *neoplasm of uncertain behavior of skin of breast (D48.5)*

D48.60 Neoplasm of uncertain behavior of unspecified breast

D48.61 Neoplasm of uncertain behavior of right **breast**

D48.62 Neoplasm of uncertain behavior of left **breast**

D48.7 Neoplasm of uncertain behavior of other specified sites

Neoplasm of uncertain behavior of eye
Neoplasm of uncertain behavior of heart
Neoplasm of uncertain behavior of peripheral nerves of orbit

> EXCLUDES 1 *neoplasm of uncertain behavior of connective tissue (D48.1)*
> *neoplasm of uncertain behavior of skin of eyelid (D48.5)*

D48.9 Neoplasm of uncertain behavior, unspecified

Neoplasms of unspecified behavior (D49)

√4th **D49 Neoplasms of unspecified behavior**

> NOTE Category D49 classifies by site neoplasms of unspecified morphology and behavior. The term "mass", unless otherwise stated, is not to be regarded as a neoplastic growth.

> INCLUDES "growth" NOS
> neoplasm NOS
> new growth NOS
> tumor NOS

> EXCLUDES 1 *neoplasms of uncertain behavior (D37-D44, D48)*

D49.0 Neoplasm of unspecified behavior of digestive system

> EXCLUDES 1 *neoplasm of unspecified behavior of margin of anus (D49.2)*
> *neoplasm of unspecified behavior of perianal skin (D49.2)*
> *neoplasm of unspecified behavior of skin of anus (D49.2)*

D49.1 Neoplasm of unspecified behavior of respiratory system

D49.2 Neoplasm of unspecified behavior of bone, soft tissue, and skin

> EXCLUDES 1 *neoplasm of unspecified behavior of anal canal (D49.0)*
> *neoplasm of unspecified behavior of anus NOS (D49.0)*
> *neoplasm of unspecified behavior of bone marrow (D49.89)*
> *neoplasm of unspecified behavior of cartilage of larynx (D49.1)*
> *neoplasm of unspecified behavior of cartilage of nose (D49.1)*
> *neoplasm of unspecified behavior of connective tissue of breast (D49.3)*
> *neoplasm of unspecified behavior of skin of genital organs (D49.59)*
> *neoplasm of unspecified behavior of vermilion border of lip (D49.0)*

D49.3 Neoplasm of unspecified behavior of breast

> EXCLUDES 1 *neoplasm of unspecified behavior of skin of breast (D49.2)*

D49.4 Neoplasm of unspecified behavior of bladder

√5th **D49.5 Neoplasm of unspecified behavior of** other genitourinary organs

AHA: 2016,4Q,9

√6th **D49.51 Neoplasm of unspecified behavior of** kidney

D49.511 Neoplasm of unspecified behavior of right **kidney**

D49.512 Neoplasm of unspecified behavior of left **kidney**

D49.519 Neoplasm of unspecified behavior of unspecified kidney

D49.59 Neoplasm of unspecified behavior of other genitourinary organ

D49.6 Neoplasm of unspecified behavior of brain [HCC]

> EXCLUDES 1 *neoplasm of unspecified behavior of cerebral meninges (D49.7)*
> *neoplasm of unspecified behavior of cranial nerves (D49.7)*

D49.7 Neoplasm of unspecified behavior of endocrine glands and other parts of nervous system

> EXCLUDES 1 *neoplasm of unspecified behavior of peripheral, sympathetic, and parasympathetic nerves and ganglia (D49.2)*

√5th **D49.8 Neoplasm of unspecified behavior of other specified sites**

> EXCLUDES 1 *neoplasm of unspecified behavior of eyelid (skin) (D49.2)*
> *neoplasm of unspecified behavior of eyelid cartilage (D49.2)*
> *neoplasm of unspecified behavior of great vessels (D49.2)*
> *neoplasm of unspecified behavior of optic nerve (D49.7)*

D49.81 Neoplasm of unspecified behavior of retina and choroid

Dark area on retina
Retinal freckle

D49.89 Neoplasm of unspecified behavior of other specified sites

D49.9 Neoplasm of unspecified behavior of unspecified site

N Newborn: 0 P Pediatric: 0-17 M Maternity: 9-64 A Adult: 15-124 MCC Major Complication/Comorbidity CC Complication/Comorbidity SW Severe Wound Dx

504

ICD-10-CM 2022

Chapter 3. Diseases of the Blood and Blood-forming Organs and Certain Disorders Involving the Immune Mechanism (D5Ø–D89)

Chapter-specific Guidelines with Coding Examples
Reserved for future guideline expansion

Chapter 3. Diseases of the Blood and Blood-forming Organs *(vertical sidebar)*

Chapter 3. Diseases of the Blood and Blood-forming Organs and Certain Disorders Involving the Immune Mechanism (D5Ø-D89)

EXCLUDES 2
    autoimmune disease (systemic) NOS (M35.9)
    certain conditions originating in the perinatal period (PØØ-P96)
    complications of pregnancy, childbirth and the puerperium (OØØ-O9A)
    congenital malformations, deformations and chromosomal
      abnormalities (QØØ-Q99)
    endocrine, nutritional and metabolic diseases (EØØ-E88)
    human immunodeficiency virus [HIV] disease (B2Ø)
    injury, poisoning and certain other consequences of external causes
      (SØØ-T88)
    neoplasms (CØØ-D49)
    symptoms, signs and abnormal clinical and laboratory findings, not
      elsewhere classified (RØØ-R94)

This chapter contains the following blocks:

D50-D53   Nutritional anemias
D55-D59   Hemolytic anemias
D60-D64   Aplastic and other anemias and other bone marrow failure syndromes
D65-D69   Coagulation defects, purpura and other hemorrhagic conditions
D70-D77   Other disorders of blood and blood-forming organs
D78   Intraoperative and postprocedural complications of the spleen
D80-D89   Certain disorders involving the immune mechanism

Nutritional anemias (D5Ø-D53)

DEF: Nutritional anemia: The result of inadequate intake or absorption of a vitamin or mineral that impacts the production of red blood cells or causes them to develop abnormally affecting the size and shape.

TIP: Documentation must identify a link between anemia and the nutritional deficiency; low levels of a particular nutrient may occur concurrently with anemia but not cause the anemia.

✓4th D5Ø   Iron deficiency anemia

    INCLUDES   asiderotic anemia
                 hypochromic anemia

    D5Ø.Ø   Iron deficiency anemia secondary to blood loss (chronic)
        Posthemorrhagic anemia (chronic)
        EXCLUDES 1   *acute posthemorrhagic anemia (D62)*
                           congenital anemia from fetal blood loss (P61.3)
        AHA: 2019,3Q,17

    D5Ø.1   Sideropenic dysphagia
        Kelly-Paterson syndrome
        Plummer-Vinson syndrome

    D5Ø.8   Other iron deficiency anemias
        Iron deficiency anemia due to inadequate dietary iron intake

    D5Ø.9   Iron deficiency anemia, unspecified

✓4th D51   Vitamin B12 deficiency anemia

    EXCLUDES 1   *vitamin B12 deficiency (E53.8)*

    D51.Ø   Vitamin B12 deficiency anemia due to intrinsic factor deficiency
        Addison anemia
        Biermer anemia
        Pernicious (congenital) anemia
        Congenital intrinsic factor deficiency
        DEF: Chronic progressive anemia due to vitamin B12 malabsorption, caused by lack of secretion of intrinsic factor, which is produced by the gastric mucosa of the stomach.

    D51.1   Vitamin B12 deficiency anemia due to selective vitamin B12 malabsorption with proteinuria
        Imerslund (Gräsbeck) syndrome
        Megaloblastic hereditary anemia

    D51.2   Transcobalamin II deficiency

    D51.3   Other dietary vitamin B12 deficiency anemia
        Vegan anemia

    D51.8   Other vitamin B12 deficiency anemias

    D51.9   Vitamin B12 deficiency anemia, unspecified

✓4th D52   Folate deficiency anemia

    EXCLUDES 1   *folate deficiency without anemia (E53.8)*

    DEF: Deficiency in a B complex vitamin needed for the production of healthy red blood cells. Lack of folate, or folic acid, and other absorption conditions can cause anemia resulting in large, misshapen red blood cells called megaloblasts.

    D52.Ø   Dietary folate deficiency anemia
        Nutritional megaloblastic anemia
        DEF: Result of a poor diet with inadequate intake of folate, which is needed to produce healthy red blood cells.

    D52.1   Drug-induced folate deficiency anemia
        Use additional code for adverse effect, if applicable, to identify drug (T36-T5Ø with fifth or sixth character 5)

    D52.8   Other folate deficiency anemias

    D52.9   Folate deficiency anemia, unspecified
        Folic acid deficiency anemia NOS

✓4th D53   Other nutritional anemias

    INCLUDES   megaloblastic anemia unresponsive to vitamin B12 or folate therapy

    D53.Ø   Protein deficiency anemia
        Amino-acid deficiency anemia
        Orotaciduric anemia
        EXCLUDES 1   *Lesch-Nyhan syndrome (E79.1)*

    D53.1   Other megaloblastic anemias, not elsewhere classified
        Megaloblastic anemia NOS
        EXCLUDES 1   *Di Guglielmo's disease (C94.Ø)*

    D53.2   Scorbutic anemia
        EXCLUDES 1   *scurvy (E54)*

    D53.8   Other specified nutritional anemias
        Anemia associated with deficiency of copper
        Anemia associated with deficiency of molybdenum
        Anemia associated with deficiency of zinc
        EXCLUDES 1   *nutritional deficiencies without anemia, such as:*
                           copper deficiency NOS (E61.Ø)
                           molybdenum deficiency NOS (E61.5)
                           zinc deficiency NOS (E6Ø)

    D53.9   Nutritional anemia, unspecified
        Simple chronic anemia
        EXCLUDES 1   *anemia NOS (D64.9)*
        AHA: 2018,4Q,88

Hemolytic anemias (D55-D59)

✓4th D55   Anemia due to enzyme disorders

    EXCLUDES 1   *drug-induced enzyme deficiency anemia (D59.2)*

    D55.Ø   Anemia due to glucose-6-phosphate dehydrogenase [G6PD] deficiency   HCC
        Favism
        G6PD deficiency anemia
        EXCLUDES 1   *glucose-6-phosphate dehydrogenase (G6PD) deficiency without anemia (D75.A)*

    D55.1   Anemia due to other disorders of glutathione metabolism   HCC
        Anemia (due to) enzyme deficiencies, except G6PD, related to the hexose monophosphate [HMP] shunt pathway
        Anemia (due to) hemolytic nonspherocytic (hereditary), type I

▲   **✓6th D55.2   Anemia due to disorders of glycolytic enzymes**
        ~~Hemolytic nonspherocytic (hereditary) anemia, type II~~
        ~~Hexokinase deficiency anemia~~
        ~~Pyruvate kinase [PK] deficiency anemia~~
        ~~Triose-phosphate isomerase deficiency anemia~~
        EXCLUDES 1   *disorders of glycolysis not associated with anemia (E74.81-)*

●   **D55.21   Anemia due to pyruvate kinase deficiency**
            PK deficiency anemia
            Pyruvate kinase deficiency anemia

●   **D55.29   Anemia due to other disorders of glycolytic enzymes**
            Hexokinase deficiency anemia
            Triose-phosphate isomerase deficiency anemia

    D55.3   Anemia due to disorders of nucleotide metabolism   HCC

    D55.8   Other anemias due to enzyme disorders   HCC

    D55.9   Anemia due to enzyme disorder, unspecified   HCC

N Newborn: 0   P Pediatric: 0-17   M Maternity: 9-64   A Adult: 15-124   MCC Major Complication/Comorbidity   CC Complication/Comorbidity   SW Severe Wound Dx

506   ICD-10-CM 2022

☑️4ᵗʰ **D56 Thalassemia**

> EXCLUDES 1   *sickle-cell thalassemia (D57.4-)*
>
> **DEF:** Group of inherited disorders of hemoglobin metabolism causing mild to severe anemia. It is usually found in people of Mediterranean, African, Chinese, or Asian descent.

Thalassemia

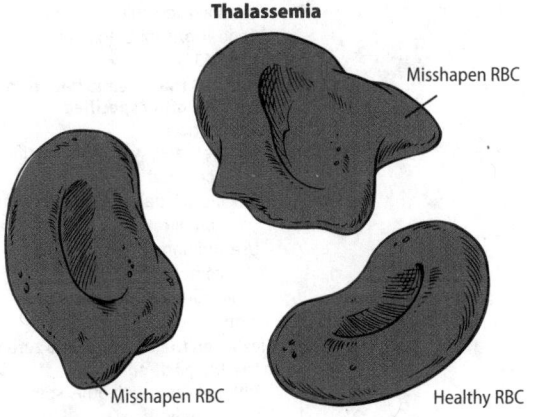

Misshapen RBC

Misshapen RBC   Healthy RBC

D56.0 Alpha thalassemia   HCC
> Alpha thalassemia major
> Hemoglobin H Constant Spring
> Hemoglobin H disease
> Hydrops fetalis due to alpha thalassemia
> Severe alpha thalassemia
> Triple gene defect alpha thalassemia
> Use additional code, if applicable, for hydrops fetalis due to alpha thalassemia (P56.99)
>> EXCLUDES 1   *alpha thalassemia trait or minor (D56.3)*
>> *asymptomatic alpha thalassemia (D56.3)*
>> *hydrops fetalis due to isoimmunization (P56.0)*
>> *hydrops fetalis not due to immune hemolysis (P83.2)*
>
> **DEF:** HBA1 and HBA2 genetic variant of chromosome 16 prevalent among those of African and Southeast Asian descent. Alpha thalassemia is associated with a wide spectrum of anemic presentation and includes hemoglobin H disease subtypes.

D56.1 Beta thalassemia   HCC
> Beta thalassemia major
> Cooley's anemia
> Homozygous beta thalassemia
> Severe beta thalassemia
> Thalassemia intermedia
> Thalassemia major
>> EXCLUDES 1   *beta thalassemia minor (D56.3)*
>> *beta thalassemia trait (D56.3)*
>> *delta-beta thalassemia (D56.2)*
>> *hemoglobin E-beta thalassemia (D56.5)*
>> *sickle-cell beta thalassemia (D57.4-)*

D56.2 Delta-beta thalassemia   HCC
> Homozygous delta-beta thalassemia
>> EXCLUDES 1   *delta-beta thalassemia minor (D56.3)*
>> *delta-beta thalassemia trait (D56.3)*

D56.3 Thalassemia minor
> Alpha thalassemia minor
> Alpha thalassemia silent carrier
> Alpha thalassemia trait
> Beta thalassemia minor
> Beta thalassemia trait
> Delta-beta thalassemia minor
> Delta-beta thalassemia trait
> Thalassemia trait NOS
>> EXCLUDES 1   *alpha thalassemia (D56.0)*
>> *beta thalassemia (D56.1)*
>> *delta-beta thalassemia (D56.2)*
>> *hemoglobin E-beta thalassemia (D56.5)*
>> *sickle-cell trait (D57.3)*
>
> **DEF:** Solitary abnormal gene that identifies a carrier of the disease, yet with an absence of symptoms or a clinically mild anemic presentation.

D56.4 Hereditary persistence of fetal hemoglobin [HPFH]   HCC

D56.5 Hemoglobin E-beta thalassemia   HCC
>> EXCLUDES 1   *beta thalassemia (D56.1)*
>> *beta thalassemia minor (D56.3)*
>> *beta thalassemia trait (D56.3)*
>> *delta-beta thalassemia (D56.2)*
>> *delta-beta thalassemia trait (D56.3)*
>> *hemoglobin E disease (D58.2)*
>> *other hemoglobinopathies (D58.2)*
>> *sickle-cell beta thalassemia (D57.4-)*

D56.8 Other thalassemias   HCC
> Dominant thalassemia
> Hemoglobin C thalassemia
> Mixed thalassemia
> Thalassemia with other hemoglobinopathy
>> EXCLUDES 1   *hemoglobin C disease (D58.2)*
>> *hemoglobin E disease (D58.2)*
>> *other hemoglobinopathies (D58.2)*
>> *sickle-cell anemia (D57.-)*
>> *sickle-cell thalassemia (D57.4)*

D56.9 Thalassemia, unspecified
> Mediterranean anemia (with other hemoglobinopathy)

☑️4ᵗʰ **D57 Sickle-cell disorders**

> Use additional code for any associated fever (R50.81)
>> EXCLUDES 1   *other hemoglobinopathies (D58.-)*
>
> **DEF:** Severe, chronic inherited diseases caused by a genetic variation in hemoglobin protein of the red blood cell. The gene mutation causes the red blood cell to become hard, sticky, and crescent or sickle shaped, making it harder for red blood cells to travel through the bloodstream, disrupting blood flow and decreasing oxygen transport to tissues.

Sickle cell

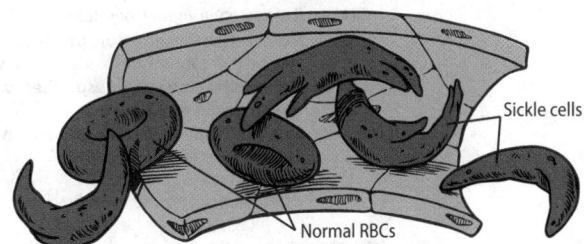

Sickle cells

Normal RBCs

☑️5ᵗʰ **D57.0 Hb-SS disease with crisis**
> Sickle-cell disease with crisis
> Hb-SS disease with vasoocclusive pain
> **AHA:** 2020,4Q,6-7

> **D57.00 Hb-SS disease with crisis, unspecified**   MCC HCC
>> Hb-SS disease with (painful) crisis NOS
>> Hb-SS disease with vasoocclusive pain NOS

> **D57.01 Hb-SS disease with acute chest syndrome**   MCC HCC

> **D57.02 Hb-SS disease with splenic sequestration**   MCC HCC

> **D57.03 Hb-SS disease with cerebral vascular involvement**   MCC HCC
>> Code also, if applicable, cerebral infarction (I63.-)

> **D57.09 Hb-SS disease with crisis with other specified complication**   MCC HCC
>> Use additional code to identify complications, such as:
>> cholelithiasis (K80.-)
>> priapism (N48.32)

D57.1 Sickle-cell disease without crisis   HCC
> Hb-SS disease without crisis
> Sickle-cell anemia NOS
> Sickle-cell disease NOS
> Sickle-cell disorder NOS

☑️5ᵗʰ **D57.2 Sickle-cell/Hb-C disease**
> Hb-SC disease
> Hb-S/Hb-C disease
> **AHA:** 2020,4Q,6-7

> **D57.20 Sickle-cell/Hb-C disease without crisis**   HCC

> ☑️6ᵗʰ **D57.21 Sickle-cell/Hb-C disease with crisis**

>> **D57.211 Sickle-cell/Hb-C disease with acute chest syndrome**   MCC HCC

✅ Additional Character Required   ☑️x7ᵗʰ Placeholder   Questionable PDx   Manifestation   Unspecified Dx   UPD Unacceptable PDx   H1-H14 HAC   HCC CMS-HCC Dx   HIV HIV Dx

ICD-10-CM 2022   **507**

D57.212 **Sickle-cell/Hb-C disease** with splenic sequestration `MCC` `HCC`

D57.213 **Sickle-cell/Hb-C disease** with cerebral vascular involvement `MCC` `HCC`

Code also, if applicable, cerebral infarction (I63.-)

D57.218 **Sickle-cell/Hb-C disease with crisis with other specified complication** `MCC` `HCC`

Use additional code to identify complications, such as:
cholelithiasis (K80.-)
priapism (N48.32)

D57.219 **Sickle-cell/Hb-C disease with crisis, unspecified** `MCC` `HCC`

Sickle-cell/Hb-C disease with crisis NOS
Sickle-cell/Hb-C disease with vasoocclusive pain NOS

D57.3 **Sickle-cell** trait `HCC`
Hb-S trait
Heterozygous hemoglobin S
DEF: Heterozygous genetic makeup characterized by one gene for normal hemoglobin and one for sickle-cell hemoglobin. The clinical disease is rarely present.

✓5ᵗʰ **D57.4** **Sickle-cell** thalassemia
Sickle-cell beta thalassemia
Thalassemia Hb-S disease
AHA: 2020,4Q,6-7

D57.40 **Sickle-cell thalassemia** without crisis `HCC`
Microdrepanocytosis
Sickle-cell thalassemia NOS

✓6ᵗʰ **D57.41** **Sickle-cell thalassemia, unspecified, with crisis**
Sickle-cell thalassemia with (painful) crisis NOS
Sickle-cell thalassemia with vasoocclusive pain NOS

D57.411 **Sickle-cell thalassemia, unspecified, with acute chest syndrome** `MCC` `HCC`

D57.412 **Sickle-cell thalassemia, unspecified, with splenic sequestration** `MCC` `HCC`

D57.413 **Sickle-cell thalassemia, unspecified, with cerebral vascular involvement** `MCC` `HCC`

Code also, if applicable cerebral infarction (I63.-)

D57.418 **Sickle-cell thalassemia, unspecified, with crisis with other specified complication** `MCC` `HCC`

Use additional code to identify complications, such as:
cholelithiasis (K80.-)
priapism (N48.32)

D57.419 **Sickle-cell thalassemia, unspecified, with crisis** `MCC` `HCC`

Sickle-cell thalassemia with (painful) crisis NOS
▶Sickle-cell thalassemia with vasoocclusive pain NOS◀

D57.42 **Sickle-cell thalassemia** beta zero without crisis `HCC`
HbS-beta zero without crisis
Sickle-cell beta zero without crisis

✓6ᵗʰ **D57.43** **Sickle-cell thalassemia** beta zero with crisis
HbS-beta zero with crisis
Sickle-cell beta zero with crisis

D57.431 **Sickle-cell thalassemia beta zero** with acute chest syndrome `MCC` `HCC`
HbS-beta zero with acute chest syndrome
Sickle-cell beta zero with acute chest syndrome

D57.432 **Sickle-cell thalassemia beta zero** with splenic sequestration `MCC` `HCC`
HbS-beta zero with splenic sequestration
Sickle-cell beta zero with splenic sequestration

D57.433 **Sickle-cell thalassemia beta zero** with cerebral vascular involvement `MCC` `HCC`
HbS-beta zero with cerebral vascular involvement
Sickle-cell beta zero with cerebral vascular involvement
Code also, if applicable cerebral infarction (I63.-)

D57.438 **Sickle-cell thalassemia beta zero with crisis with other specified complication** `MCC` `HCC`
HbS-beta zero with other specified complication
Sickle-cell beta zero with other specified complication
Use additional code to identify complications, such as:
cholelithiasis (K80.-)
priapism (N48.32)

D57.439 **Sickle-cell thalassemia beta zero with crisis, unspecified** `MCC` `HCC`
HbS-beta zero with other specified complication
Sickle-cell beta zero with crisis unspecified
Sickle-cell thalassemia beta zero with (painful) crisis NOS
▶Sickle-cell thalassemia beta zero with vasoocclusive pain NOS◀

D57.44 **Sickle-cell thalassemia** beta plus without crisis `HCC`
HbS-beta plus without crisis
Sickle-cell beta plus without crisis

✓6ᵗʰ **D57.45** **Sickle-cell thalassemia** beta plus with crisis
HbS-beta plus with crisis
Sickle-cell beta plus with crisis

D57.451 **Sickle-cell thalassemia beta plus** with acute chest syndrome `MCC` `HCC`
HbS-beta plus with acute chest syndrome
Sickle-cell beta plus with acute chest syndrome

D57.452 **Sickle-cell thalassemia beta plus** with splenic sequestration `MCC` `HCC`
HbS-beta plus with splenic sequestration
Sickle-cell beta plus with splenic sequestration

D57.453 **Sickle-cell thalassemia beta plus** with cerebral vascular involvement `MCC` `HCC`
HbS-beta plus with cerebral vascular involvement
Sickle-cell beta plus with cerebral vascular involvement
Code also, if applicable cerebral infarction (I63.-)

D57.458 **Sickle-cell thalassemia beta plus with crisis with other specified complication** `MCC` `HCC`
HbS-beta plus with crisis with other specified complication
Sickle-cell beta plus with crisis with other specified complication
Use additional code to identify complications, such as:
cholelithiasis (K80.-)
priapism (N48.32)

D57.459 **Sickle-cell thalassemia beta plus with crisis, unspecified** `MCC` `HCC`
HbS-beta plus with crisis with unspecified complication
Sickle-cell beta plus with crisis with unspecified complication
Sickle-cell thalassemia beta plus with (painful) crisis NOS
▶Sickle-cell thalassemia beta plus with vasoocclusive pain NOS◀

Ⓝ Newborn: 0   Ⓟ Pediatric: 0-17   Ⓜ Maternity: 9-64   Ⓐ Adult: 15-124   `MCC` Major Complication/Comorbidity   `CC` Complication/Comorbidity   `SW` Severe Wound Dx

508

ICD-10-CM 2022

✓5ᵗʰ **D57.8 Other sickle-cell disorders**
     Hb-SD disease
     Hb-SE disease
     AHA: 2020,4Q,6-7

     D57.80 Other sickle-cell disorders without crisis   HCC

✓6ᵗʰ   **D57.81 Other sickle-cell disorders** with crisis

        D57.811 Other sickle-cell disorders with acute chest syndrome   MCC HCC

        D57.812 Other sickle-cell disorders with splenic sequestration   MCC HCC

        D57.813 Other sickle-cell disorders with cerebral vascular involvement   MCC HCC
          Code also, if applicable: cerebral infarction (I63.-)

        D57.818 Other sickle-cell disorders with crisis with other specified complication   MCC HCC
          Use additional code to identify complications, such as:
            cholelithiasis (K80.-)
            priapism (N48.32)

        D57.819 Other sickle-cell disorders with crisis, unspecified   MCC HCC
          Other sickle-cell disorders with crisis NOS
          Other sickle-cell disorders with vasoocclusive pain NOS

✓4ᵗʰ **D58 Other** hereditary **hemolytic anemias**
     EXCLUDES 1   hemolytic anemia of the newborn (P55.-)

     D58.0 Hereditary spherocytosis   HCC
       Acholuric (familial) jaundice
       Congenital (spherocytic) hemolytic icterus
       Minkowski-Chauffard syndrome
       DEF: Inherited condition caused by mutations to genes responsible for the production of proteins that form the membranes of red blood cells. The shape and flexibility of the red blood cell membrane is altered, diminishing the cell's ability to traverse the spleen, therefore becoming trapped and destroyed before the red blood cell has reached maturity.

     D58.1 Hereditary elliptocytosis   HCC
       Elliptocytosis (congenital)
       Ovalocytosis (congenital) (hereditary)

     D58.2 Other hemoglobinopathies   HCC
       Abnormal hemoglobin NOS
       Congenital Heinz body anemia
       Hb-C disease
       Hb-D disease
       Hb-E disease
       Hemoglobinopathy NOS
       Unstable hemoglobin hemolytic disease
       EXCLUDES 1   familial polycythemia (D75.0)
           Hb-M disease (D74.0)
           hemoglobin E-beta thalassemia (D56.5)
           hereditary persistence of fetal hemoglobin [HPFH] (D56.4)
           high-altitude polycythemia (D75.1)
           methemoglobinemia (D74.-)
           other hemoglobinopathies with thalassemia (D56.8)

     D58.8 Other specified hereditary hemolytic anemias   CC HCC
       Stomatocytosis

     D58.9 Hereditary hemolytic anemia, unspecified   CC HCC

✓4ᵗʰ **D59 Acquired hemolytic anemia**
     DEF: Non-hereditary anemia characterized by premature destruction of red blood cells caused by infectious organisms, poisons, and physical agents.

     D59.0 Drug-induced autoimmune hemolytic anemia   CC HCC
       Use additional code for adverse effect, if applicable, to identify drug (T36-T50 with fifth or sixth character 5)

✓5ᵗʰ   **D59.1 Other** autoimmune **hemolytic anemias**
       EXCLUDES 2   Evans syndrome (D69.41)
           hemolytic disease of newborn (P55.-)
           paroxysmal cold hemoglobinuria (D59.6)
       AHA: 2020,4Q,7-8

       D59.10 Autoimmune hemolytic anemia, unspecified   CC HCC

       D59.11 Warm autoimmune hemolytic anemia   CC HCC
          Warm type (primary) (secondary) (symptomatic) autoimmune hemolytic anemia
          Warm type autoimmune hemolytic disease

       D59.12 Cold autoimmune hemolytic anemia   CC HCC
          Chronic cold hemagglutinin disease
          Cold agglutinin disease
          Cold agglutinin hemoglobinuria
          Cold type (primary) (secondary) (symptomatic) autoimmune hemolytic anemia
          Cold type autoimmune hemolytic disease

       D59.13 Mixed type autoimmune hemolytic anemia   CC HCC
          Mixed type autoimmune hemolytic disease
          Mixed type, cold and warm, (primary) (secondary) (symptomatic) autoimmune hemolytic anemia

       D59.19 Other autoimmune hemolytic anemia   CC HCC

     D59.2 Drug-induced nonautoimmune hemolytic anemia   CC HCC
       Drug-induced enzyme deficiency anemia
       Use additional code for adverse effect, if applicable, to identify drug (T36-T50 with fifth or sixth character 5)

     D59.3 Hemolytic-uremic syndrome   MCC HCC
       Use additional code to identify associated:
         E. coli infection (B96.2-)
         Pneumococcal pneumonia (J13)
         Shigella dysenteriae (A03.9)
       DEF: Condition typically precipitated by infection causing low platelets and destruction of red blood cells resulting in hemolytic anemia. This cell damage and blockage of renal capillaries lead to kidney failure. Mainly affects children.

     D59.4 Other nonautoimmune hemolytic anemias   CC HCC
       Mechanical hemolytic anemia
       Microangiopathic hemolytic anemia
       Toxic hemolytic anemia

     D59.5 Paroxysmal nocturnal hemoglobinuria [Marchiafava-Micheli]   HCC
       EXCLUDES 1   hemoglobinuria NOS (R82.3)

     D59.6 Hemoglobinuria due to hemolysis from other external causes   HCC
       Hemoglobinuria from exertion
       March hemoglobinuria
       Paroxysmal cold hemoglobinuria
       Use additional code (Chapter 20) to identify external cause
       EXCLUDES 1   hemoglobinuria NOS (R82.3)

     D59.8 Other acquired hemolytic anemias   HCC

     D59.9 Acquired hemolytic anemia, unspecified   CC HCC
       Idiopathic hemolytic anemia, chronic

Aplastic and other anemias and other bone marrow failure syndromes (D60-D64)

✓4ᵗʰ **D60 Acquired pure red cell aplasia [erythroblastopenia]**
     INCLUDES   red cell aplasia (acquired) (adult) (with thymoma)
     EXCLUDES 1   congenital red cell aplasia (D61.01)
     DEF: Bone marrow failure characterized by underproduction of red blood cells while white blood cell and platelet production remains normal.

     D60.0 Chronic acquired pure red cell aplasia   MCC HCC

     D60.1 Transient acquired pure red cell aplasia   MCC HCC

     D60.8 Other acquired pure red cell aplasias   MCC HCC

     D60.9 Acquired pure red cell aplasia, unspecified   MCC HCC

✓4ᵗʰ **D61 Other aplastic anemias and other bone marrow failure syndromes**
     EXCLUDES 2   neutropenia (D70.-)
     AHA: 2020,3Q,22; 2014,4Q,22
     DEF: Aplastic anemia: Bone marrow failure characterized by underproduction of red bloods cells, white blood cells and platelets.

✓5ᵗʰ   **D61.0 Constitutional aplastic anemia**

       D61.01 Constitutional (pure) red blood cell aplasia   CC HCC
          Blackfan-Diamond syndrome
          Congenital (pure) red cell aplasia
          Familial hypoplastic anemia
          Primary (pure) red cell aplasia
          Red cell (pure) aplasia of infants
          EXCLUDES 1   acquired red cell aplasia (D60.9)

D61.09   **Other constitutional aplastic anemia**   `CC` `HCC`
Fanconi's anemia
Pancytopenia with malformations

D61.1   **Drug-induced aplastic anemia**   `MCC` `HCC`
Use additional code for adverse effect, if applicable, to identify drug (T36-T50 with fifth or sixth character 5)

D61.2   **Aplastic anemia due to other external agents**   `MCC` `HCC`
Code first, if applicable, toxic effects of substances chiefly nonmedicinal as to source (T51-T65)

D61.3   **Idiopathic aplastic anemia**   `MCC` `HCC`

✓5th **D61.8**   **Other specified aplastic anemias and other bone marrow failure syndromes**

✓6th **D61.81**   **Pancytopenia**
> EXCLUDES 1   *pancytopenia (due to) (with) aplastic anemia (D61.9)*
> *pancytopenia (due to) (with) bone marrow infiltration (D61.82)*
> *pancytopenia (due to) (with) congenital (pure) red cell aplasia (D61.01)*
> *pancytopenia (due to) (with) hairy cell leukemia (C91.4-)*
> *pancytopenia (due to) (with) human immunodeficiency virus disease (B20)*
> *pancytopenia (due to) (with) leukoerythroblastic anemia (D61.82)*
> *pancytopenia (due to) (with) myeloproliferative disease (D47.1)*
> EXCLUDES 2   *pancytopenia (due to) (with) myelodysplastic syndromes (D46.-)*
>
> **DEF:** Shortage of all three blood cells: white, red, and platelets.

D61.810   **Antineoplastic chemotherapy induced pancytopenia**   `MCC` `HCC`
> EXCLUDES 2   *aplastic anemia due to antineoplastic chemotherapy (D61.1)*
>
> **AHA:** 2020,3Q,22

D61.811   **Other drug-induced pancytopenia**   `MCC` `HCC`
> EXCLUDES 2   *aplastic anemia due to drugs (D61.1)*

D61.818   **Other pancytopenia**   `CC` `HCC`
> **AHA:** 2020,3Q,24; 2019,1Q,16
> **TIP:** Assign this code in addition to myeloid leukemia codes (C92.-) when pancytopenia is documented. Although common in some types of myeloid leukemia, pancytopenia is not always inherent.

D61.82   **Myelophthisis**   `CC` `HCC`
Leukoerythroblastic anemia
Myelophthisic anemia
Panmyelophthisis
Code also the underlying disorder, such as:
malignant neoplasm of breast (C50.-)
tuberculosis (A15.-)
> EXCLUDES 1   *idiopathic myelofibrosis (D47.1)*
> *myelofibrosis NOS (D75.81)*
> *myelofibrosis with myeloid metaplasia (D47.4)*
> *primary myelofibrosis (D47.1)*
> *secondary myelofibrosis (D75.81)*
>
> **DEF:** Condition that occurs when normal hematopoietic tissue in the bone marrow is replaced with abnormal tissue, such as fibrous tissue or tumors. Most commonly seen during the advanced stages of cancer.

D61.89   **Other specified aplastic anemias and other bone marrow failure syndromes**   `MCC` `HCC`

D61.9   **Aplastic anemia, unspecified**   `CC` `HCC`
Hypoplastic anemia NOS
Medullary hypoplasia

D62   **Acute posthemorrhagic anemia**   `CC`
> EXCLUDES 1   *anemia due to chronic blood loss (D50.0)*
> *blood loss anemia NOS (D50.0)*
> *congenital anemia from fetal blood loss (P61.3)*
>
> **AHA:** 2019,3Q,11,17

✓4th **D63**   **Anemia in chronic diseases classified elsewhere**

D63.0   **Anemia in neoplastic disease**
Code first neoplasm (C00-D49)
> EXCLUDES 1   *aplastic anemia due to antineoplastic chemotherapy (D61.1)*
> EXCLUDES 2   *anemia due to antineoplastic chemotherapy (D64.81)*

D63.1   **Anemia in chronic kidney disease**
Erythropoietin resistant anemia (EPO resistant anemia)
Code first underlying chronic kidney disease (CKD) (N18.-)

D63.8   **Anemia in other chronic diseases classified elsewhere**
Code first underlying disease, such as:
diphyllobothriasis (B70.0)
hookworm disease (B76.0-B76.9)
hypothyroidism (E00.0-E03.9)
malaria (B50.0-B54)
symptomatic late syphilis (A52.79)
tuberculosis (A18.89)

✓4th **D64**   **Other anemias**
> EXCLUDES 1   *refractory anemia (D46.-)*
> *refractory anemia with excess blasts in transformation [RAEB T] (C92.0-)*
>
> **DEF:** Sideroblastic anemia: Hereditary or secondary disorder in which the red blood cells cannot effectively use iron, a nutrient needed to make hemoglobin. Although the iron can enter the red blood cell it is not assimilated into the hemoglobin molecule and builds up ringed sideroblasts around the cell nucleus.

D64.0   **Hereditary sideroblastic anemia**   `HCC`
Sex-linked hypochromic sideroblastic anemia

D64.1   **Secondary sideroblastic anemia due to disease**   `HCC`
Code first underlying disease

D64.2   **Secondary sideroblastic anemia due to drugs and toxins**   `HCC`
Code first poisoning due to drug or toxin, if applicable (T36-T65 with fifth or sixth character 1-4 or 6)
Use additional code for adverse effect, if applicable, to identify drug (T36-T50 with fifth or sixth character 5)

D64.3   **Other sideroblastic anemias**   `HCC`
Sideroblastic anemia NOS
Pyridoxine-responsive sideroblastic anemia NEC

D64.4   **Congenital dyserythropoietic anemia**
Dyshematopoietic anemia (congenital)
> EXCLUDES 1   *Blackfan-Diamond syndrome (D61.01)*
> *Di Guglielmo's disease (C94.0)*

✓5th **D64.8**   **Other specified anemias**

D64.81   **Anemia due to antineoplastic chemotherapy**
Antineoplastic chemotherapy induced anemia
> EXCLUDES 1   ~~aplastic anemia due to antineoplastic chemotherapy (D61.1)~~
> EXCLUDES 2   *anemia in neoplastic disease (D63.0)*
> ▶*aplastic anemia due to antineoplastic chemotherapy (D61.1)*◄
>
> **AHA:** 2014,4Q,22
> **DEF:** Reversible adverse effect of chemotherapy, causing inhibition of bone marrow production. A decrease in red blood cell production prevents adequate oxygenation of the tissues and organs causing fatigue, shortness of breath (SOB), and exacerbation of other medical conditions.

D64.89   **Other specified anemias**
Infantile pseudoleukemia

D64.9   **Anemia, unspecified**
> **AHA:** 2020,3Q,24; 2018,4Q,88; 2017,1Q,7

`N` Newborn: 0   `P` Pediatric: 0-17   `M` Maternity: 9-64   `A` Adult: 15-124   `MCC` Major Complication/Comorbidity   `CC` Complication/Comorbidity   `SW` Severe Wound Dx

510   ICD-10-CM 2022

Coagulation defects, purpura and other hemorrhagic conditions (D65-D69)

D65 Disseminated intravascular coagulation [defibrination syndrome] `MCC` `HCC`

Afibrinogenemia, acquired
Consumption coagulopathy
Diffuse or disseminated intravascular coagulation [DIC]
Fibrinolytic hemorrhage, acquired
Fibrinolytic purpura
Purpura fulminans

EXCLUDES 1   *disseminated intravascular coagulation (complicating):*
abortion or ectopic or molar pregnancy (O00-O07, O08.1)
in newborn (P60)
pregnancy, childbirth and the puerperium (O45.0, O46.0, O67.0, O72.3)

AHA: 2021,1Q,39

Coagulation

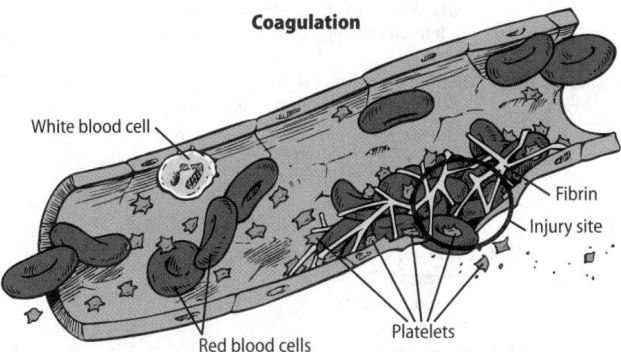

White blood cell
Fibrin
Injury site
Red blood cells
Platelets

D66 Hereditary factor VIII deficiency `MCC` `HCC`

Classical hemophilia
Deficiency factor VIII (with functional defect)
Hemophilia A
Hemophilia NOS

EXCLUDES 1   *factor VIII deficiency with vascular defect (D68.0)*

DEF: Hereditary, sex-linked lack of antihemophilic globulin (AHG) (factor VIII) that causes abnormal coagulation characterized by increased bleeding; large bruises of skin; bleeding in the mouth, nose, and gastrointestinal tract; and hemorrhages into joints, resulting in swelling and impaired function.

D67 Hereditary factor IX deficiency `MCC` `HCC`

Christmas disease
Factor IX deficiency (with functional defect)
Hemophilia B
Plasma thromboplastin component [PTC] deficiency

D68 Other coagulation defects √4ᵗʰ

EXCLUDES 1   *abnormal coagulation profile (R79.1)*
coagulation defects complicating abortion or ectopic or molar pregnancy (O00-O07, O08.1)
coagulation defects complicating pregnancy, childbirth and the puerperium (O45.0, O46.0, O67.0, O72.3)

AHA: 2016,1Q,14

D68.0 Von Willebrand's disease `CC` `HCC`

Angiohemophilia
Factor VIII deficiency with vascular defect
Vascular hemophilia

EXCLUDES 1   *capillary fragility (hereditary) (D69.8)*
factor VIII deficiency NOS (D66)
factor VIII deficiency with functional defect (D66)

DEF: Congenital, abnormal blood coagulation caused by deficient blood factor VII. Symptoms include excess or prolonged bleeding.

D68.1 Hereditary factor XI deficiency `CC` `HCC`

Hemophilia C
Plasma thromboplastin antecedent [PTA] deficiency
Rosenthal's disease

D68.2 Hereditary deficiency of other clotting factors `CC` `HCC`

AC globulin deficiency
Congenital afibrinogenemia
Deficiency of factor I [fibrinogen]
Deficiency of factor II [prothrombin]
Deficiency of factor V [labile]
Deficiency of factor VII [stable]
Deficiency of factor X [Stuart-Prower]
Deficiency of factor XII [Hageman]
Deficiency of factor XIII [fibrin stabilizing]
Dysfibrinogenemia (congenital)
Hypoproconvertinemia
Owren's disease
Proaccelerin deficiency

D68.3 Hemorrhagic disorder due to circulating anticoagulants √5ᵗʰ

D68.31 Hemorrhagic disorder due to intrinsic circulating anticoagulants, antibodies, or inhibitors √6ᵗʰ

D68.311 Acquired hemophilia `CC` `HCC`

Autoimmune hemophilia
Autoimmune inhibitors to clotting factors
Secondary hemophilia

D68.312 Antiphospholipid antibody with hemorrhagic disorder `CC` `HCC`

Lupus anticoagulant (LAC) with hemorrhagic disorder
Systemic lupus erythematosus [SLE] inhibitor with hemorrhagic disorder

EXCLUDES 1   *antiphospholipid antibody, finding without diagnosis (R76.0)*
antiphospholipid antibody syndrome (D68.61)
antiphospholipid antibody with hypercoagulable state (D68.61)
lupus anticoagulant (LAC) finding without diagnosis (R76.0)
lupus anticoagulant (LAC) with hypercoagulable state (D68.62)
systemic lupus erythematosus [SLE] inhibitor finding without diagnosis (R76.0)
systemic lupus erythematosus [SLE] inhibitor with hypercoagulable state (D68.62)

D68.318 Other hemorrhagic disorder due to intrinsic circulating anticoagulants, antibodies, or inhibitors `CC` `HCC`

Antithromboplastinemia
Antithromboplastinogenemia
Hemorrhagic disorder due to intrinsic increase in antithrombin
Hemorrhagic disorder due to intrinsic increase in anti-VIIIa
Hemorrhagic disorder due to intrinsic increase in anti-IXa
Hemorrhagic disorder due to intrinsic increase in anti-XIa

D68.32 Hemorrhagic disorder due to extrinsic circulating anticoagulants `CC` `HCC`

Drug-induced hemorrhagic disorder
Hemorrhagic disorder due to increase in anti-IIa
Hemorrhagic disorder due to increase in anti-Xa
Hyperheparinemia
Use additional code for adverse effect, if applicable, to identify drug (T45.515, T45.525)

AHA: 2021,1Q,4; 2016,1Q,14-15

TIP: Do not assign to identify routine therapeutic anticoagulation effects; assign only for documented adverse effects.

D68.4 Acquired coagulation factor deficiency `CC` `HCC`

Deficiency of coagulation factor due to liver disease
Deficiency of coagulation factor due to vitamin K deficiency

EXCLUDES 1   *vitamin K deficiency of newborn (P53)*

Chapter 3. Diseases of the Blood and Blood-forming Organs

D68.5–D69.9

✓5ᵗʰ **D68.5** **Primary thrombophilia**
Primary hypercoagulable states
EXCLUDES 1   *antiphospholipid syndrome (D68.61)*
lupus anticoagulant (D68.62)
secondary activated protein C resistance (D68.69)
secondary antiphospholipid antibody syndrome (D68.69)
secondary lupus anticoagulant with hypercoagulable state (D68.69)
secondary systemic lupus erythematosus [SLE] inhibitor with hypercoagulable state (D68.69)
systemic lupus erythematosus [SLE] inhibitor finding without diagnosis (R76.0)
systemic lupus erythematosus [SLE] inhibitor with hemorrhagic disorder (D68.312)
thrombotic thrombocytopenic purpura ▶(M31.19)◄
DEF: Thrombophilia: Increased tendency of the blood to clot, which can lead to thrombus or embolus formation.

D68.51 **Activated protein C resistance**   CC HCC
Factor V Leiden mutation

D68.52 **Prothrombin gene mutation**   CC HCC

D68.59 **Other primary thrombophilia**   CC HCC
Antithrombin III deficiency
Hypercoagulable state NOS
Primary hypercoagulable state NEC
Primary thrombophilia NEC
Protein C deficiency
Protein S deficiency
Thrombophilia NOS
AHA: 2021,2Q,8

✓5ᵗʰ **D68.6** **Other thrombophilia**
Other hypercoagulable states
EXCLUDES 1   *diffuse or disseminated intravascular coagulation [DIC] (D65)*
heparin induced thrombocytopenia (HIT) (D75.82)
hyperhomocysteinemia (E72.11)

D68.61 **Antiphospholipid syndrome**   CC HCC
Anticardiolipin syndrome
Antiphospholipid antibody syndrome
EXCLUDES 1   *anti-phospholipid antibody, finding without diagnosis (R76.0)*
anti-phospholipid antibody with hemorrhagic disorder (D68.312)
lupus anticoagulant syndrome (D68.62)

D68.62 **Lupus anticoagulant syndrome**   CC HCC
Lupus anticoagulant
Presence of systemic lupus erythematosus [SLE] inhibitor
EXCLUDES 1   *anticardiolipin syndrome (D68.61)*
antiphospholipid syndrome (D68.61)
lupus anticoagulant (LAC) finding without diagnosis (R76.0)
lupus anticoagulant (LAC) with hemorrhagic disorder (D68.312)

D68.69 **Other thrombophilia**   CC HCC
Hypercoagulable states NEC
Secondary hypercoagulable state NOS
AHA: 2021,2Q,8

D68.8 **Other specified coagulation defects**   CC HCC
EXCLUDES 1   *hemorrhagic disease of newborn (P53)*
AHA: 2021,1Q,39

D68.9 **Coagulation defect, unspecified**   CC HCC

✓4ᵗʰ **D69** **Purpura and other hemorrhagic conditions**
EXCLUDES 1   *benign hypergammaglobulinemic purpura (D89.0)*
cryoglobulinemic purpura (D89.1)
essential (hemorrhagic) thrombocythemia (D47.3)
hemorrhagic thrombocythemia (D47.3)
purpura fulminans (D65)
thrombotic thrombocytopenic purpura ▶(M31.19)◄
Waldenström hypergammaglobulinemic purpura (D89.0)

D69.0 **Allergic purpura**   CC HCC
Allergic vasculitis
Nonthrombocytopenic hemorrhagic purpura
Nonthrombocytopenic idiopathic purpura
Purpura anaphylactoid
Purpura Henoch(-Schönlein)
Purpura rheumatica
Vascular purpura
EXCLUDES 1   *thrombocytopenic hemorrhagic purpura (D69.3)*
AHA: 2020,3Q,26
DEF: Any hemorrhagic condition, thrombocytic or nonthrombocytopenic in origin, caused by a presumed allergic reaction.

D69.1 **Qualitative platelet defects**   HCC
Bernard-Soulier [giant platelet] syndrome
Glanzmann's disease
Grey platelet syndrome
Thromboasthenia (hemorrhagic) (hereditary)
Thrombocytopathy
EXCLUDES 1   *von Willebrand's disease (D68.0)*

D69.2 **Other nonthrombocytopenic purpura**   HCC
Purpura NOS
Purpura simplex
Senile purpura

D69.3 **Immune thrombocytopenic purpura**   CC HCC
Hemorrhagic (thrombocytopenic) purpura
Idiopathic thrombocytopenic purpura
Tidal platelet dysgenesis
DEF: Tidal platelet dysgenesis: Fluctuation of platelet counts from normal to very low within periods of 20 to 40 days and may involve autoimmune platelet destruction.

✓5ᵗʰ **D69.4** **Other primary thrombocytopenia**
EXCLUDES 1   *transient neonatal thrombocytopenia (P61.0)*
Wiskott-Aldrich syndrome (D82.0)

D69.41 **Evans syndrome**   CC HCC

D69.42 **Congenital and hereditary thrombocytopenia purpura**   CC HCC
Congenital thrombocytopenia
Hereditary thrombocytopenia
Code first congenital or hereditary disorder, such as: thrombocytopenia with absent radius (TAR syndrome) (Q87.2)

D69.49 **Other primary thrombocytopenia**   HCC
Megakaryocytic hypoplasia
Primary thrombocytopenia NOS

✓5ᵗʰ **D69.5** **Secondary thrombocytopenia**
EXCLUDES 1   *heparin induced thrombocytopenia (HIT) (D75.82)*
transient thrombocytopenia of newborn (P61.0)

D69.51 **Posttransfusion purpura**
Posttransfusion purpura from whole blood (fresh) or blood products
PTP

D69.59 **Other secondary thrombocytopenia**
AHA: 2014,4Q,22

D69.6 **Thrombocytopenia, unspecified**   HCC
AHA: 2020,3Q,24

D69.8 **Other specified hemorrhagic conditions**   HCC
Capillary fragility (hereditary)
Vascular pseudohemophilia

D69.9 **Hemorrhagic condition, unspecified**   HCC

Other disorders of blood and blood-forming organs (D70-D77)

✓4ᵗʰ **D70 Neutropenia**

INCLUDES   agranulocytosis
decreased absolute neurophile count (ANC)
Use additional code for any associated:
fever (R50.81)
mucositis (J34.81, K12.3-, K92.81, N76.81)

EXCLUDES 1   *neutropenic splenomegaly (D73.81)*
transient neonatal neutropenia (P61.5)

DEF: Abnormally low number of neutrophils. Neutrophils are phagocytic, meaning they surround and consume harmful pathogens, primarily bacteria. When neutrophil counts decrease the risk of infection increases.

D70.0 Congenital agranulocytosis   HCC
Congenital neutropenia
Infantile genetic agranulocytosis
Kostmann's disease

D70.1 Agranulocytosis secondary to cancer chemotherapy   HCC
Code also underlying neoplasm
Use additional code for adverse effect, if applicable, to identify drug (T45.1X5)
AHA: 2020,3Q,22; 2014,4Q,22

D70.2 Other drug-induced agranulocytosis   HCC
Use additional code for adverse effect, if applicable, to identify drug (T36-T50 with fifth or sixth character 5)

D70.3 Neutropenia due to infection   HCC

D70.4 Cyclic neutropenia   HCC
Cyclic hematopoiesis
Periodic neutropenia

D70.8 Other neutropenia   HCC

D70.9 Neutropenia, unspecified   HCC
AHA: 2020,3Q,24

D71 Functional disorders of polymorphonuclear neutrophils   HCC
Cell membrane receptor complex [CR3] defect
Chronic (childhood) granulomatous disease
Congenital dysphagocytosis
Progressive septic granulomatosis

✓4ᵗʰ **D72 Other disorders of white blood cells**

EXCLUDES 1   *basophilia (D72.824)*
immunity disorders (D80-D89)
neutropenia (D70)
preleukemia (syndrome) (D46.9)

D72.0 Genetic anomalies of leukocytes   HCC
Alder (granulation) (granulocyte) anomaly
Alder syndrome
Hereditary leukocytic hypersegmentation
Hereditary leukocytic hyposegmentation
Hereditary leukomelanopathy
May-Hegglin (granulation) (granulocyte) anomaly
May-Hegglin syndrome
Pelger-Huët (granulation) (granulocyte) anomaly
Pelger-Huët syndrome
EXCLUDES 1   *Chédiak (-Steinbrinck)-Higashi syndrome (E70.330)*

✓6ᵗʰ **D72.1 Eosinophilia**

EXCLUDES 2   *Löffler's syndrome ▶(J82.89)◄*
pulmonary eosinophilia ▶(J82.-)◄

AHA: 2020,4Q,8-10
DEF: Abnormally large accumulation or formation of eosinophils (nucleated, granular leukocytes) in the blood, characteristic of allergic states and infection.

D72.10 Eosinophilia, unspecified

✓6ᵗʰ **D72.11 Hypereosinophilic syndrome [HES]**

D72.110 Idiopathic hypereosinophilic syndrome [IHES]

D72.111 Lymphocytic Variant Hypereosinophilic Syndrome [LHES]
Lymphocyte variant hypereosinophilia
Code also, if applicable, any associated lymphocytic neoplastic disorder

D72.118 Other hypereosinophilic syndrome
Episodic angioedema with eosinophilia
Gleich's syndrome

D72.119 Hypereosinophilic syndrome [HES], unspecified

D72.12 Drug rash with eosinophilia and systemic symptoms syndrome
DRESS syndrome
Use additional code for adverse effect, if applicable, to identify drug (T36-T50 with fifth or sixth character 5)

D72.18 *Eosinophilia in diseases classified elsewhere*
Code first underlying disease, such as:
chronic myelomonocytic leukemia (C93.1-)

D72.19 Other eosinophilia
Familial eosinophilia
Hereditary eosinophilia

✓5ᵗʰ **D72.8 Other specified disorders of white blood cells**

EXCLUDES 1   *leukemia (C91-C95)*

✓6ᵗʰ **D72.81 Decreased white blood cell count**
EXCLUDES 1   *neutropenia (D70.-)*

D72.810 Lymphocytopenia
Decreased lymphocytes

D72.818 Other decreased white blood cell count
Basophilic leukopenia
Eosinophilic leukopenia
Monocytopenia
Other decreased leukocytes
Plasmacytopenia

D72.819 Decreased white blood cell count, unspecified
Decreased leukocytes, unspecified
Leukocytopenia, unspecified
Leukopenia
EXCLUDES 1   *malignant leukopenia (D70.9)*

✓6ᵗʰ **D72.82 Elevated white blood cell count**
EXCLUDES 1   *eosinophilia (D72.1)*

D72.820 Lymphocytosis (symptomatic)
Elevated lymphocytes

D72.821 Monocytosis (symptomatic)
EXCLUDES 1   *infectious mononucleosis (B27.-)*

D72.822 Plasmacytosis

D72.823 Leukemoid reaction
Basophilic leukemoid reaction
Leukemoid reaction NOS
Lymphocytic leukemoid reaction
Monocytic leukemoid reaction
Myelocytic leukemoid reaction
Neutrophilic leukemoid reaction

D72.824 Basophilia
DEF: Increase in the basophils of the blood, a type of white blood cell, often seen in conjunction with neoplastic disorders.

D72.825 Bandemia
Bandemia without diagnosis of specific infection
EXCLUDES 1   *confirmed infection - code to infection*
leukemia (C91.-, C92.-, C93.-, C94.-, C95.-)
DEF: Increase in early neutrophil cells, called band cells, that may indicate infection.

D72.828 Other elevated white blood cell count

D72.829 Elevated white blood cell count, unspecified
Elevated leukocytes, unspecified
Leukocytosis, unspecified

D72.89 Other specified disorders of white blood cells
Abnormality of white blood cells NEC

D72.9 Disorder of white blood cells, unspecified
Abnormal leukocyte differential NOS

✓4ᵗʰ **D73 Diseases of spleen**

D73.0 Hyposplenism
Atrophy of spleen
EXCLUDES 1   *asplenia (congenital) (Q89.01)*
postsurgical absence of spleen (Z90.81)

✔ Additional Character Required   ✔x7ᵗʰ Placeholder   Questionable PDx   Manifestation   Unspecified Dx   UPD Unacceptable PDx   H1-H14 HAC   HCC CMS-HCC Dx   HIV HIV Dx

ICD-10-CM 2022   513

Chapter 3. Diseases of the Blood and Blood-forming Organs

D73.1 Hypersplenism
EXCLUDES 1   *neutropenic splenomegaly (D73.81)*
primary splenic neutropenia (D73.81)
splenitis, splenomegaly in late syphilis (A52.79)
splenitis, splenomegaly in tuberculosis (A18.85)
splenomegaly NOS (R16.1)
splenomegaly congenital (Q89.0)

D73.2 Chronic congestive splenomegaly

D73.3 Abscess of spleen

D73.4 Cyst of spleen

D73.5 Infarction of spleen
Splenic rupture, nontraumatic
Torsion of spleen
EXCLUDES 1   *rupture of spleen due to Plasmodium vivax malaria (B51.0)*
traumatic rupture of spleen (S36.03-)

✓5ᵗʰ **D73.8 Other diseases of spleen**

D73.81 Neutropenic splenomegaly
Werner-Schultz disease

D73.89 Other diseases of spleen
Fibrosis of spleen NOS
Perisplenitis
Splenitis NOS

D73.9 Disease of spleen, unspecified

✓4ᵗʰ **D74 Methemoglobinemia**

D74.0 Congenital methemoglobinemia   CC
Congenital NADH-methemoglobin reductase deficiency
Hemoglobin-M [Hb-M] disease
Methemoglobinemia, hereditary

D74.8 Other methemoglobinemias   CC
Acquired methemoglobinemia (with sulfhemoglobinemia)
Toxic methemoglobinemia

D74.9 Methemoglobinemia, unspecified   CC

✓4ᵗʰ **D75 Other and unspecified diseases of blood and blood-forming organs**
EXCLUDES 2   *acute lymphadenitis (L04.-)*
chronic lymphadenitis (I88.1)
enlarged lymph nodes (R59.-)
hypergammaglobulinemia NOS (D89.2)
lymphadenitis NOS (I88.9)
mesenteric lymphadenitis (acute) (chronic) (I88.0)

D75.0 Familial erythrocytosis
Benign polycythemia
Familial polycythemia
EXCLUDES 1   *hereditary ovalocytosis (D58.1)*

D75.1 Secondary polycythemia
Acquired polycythemia
Emotional polycythemia
Erythrocytosis NOS
Hypoxemic polycythemia
Nephrogenous polycythemia
Polycythemia due to erythropoietin
Polycythemia due to fall in plasma volume
Polycythemia due to high altitude
Polycythemia due to stress
Polycythemia NOS
Relative polycythemia
EXCLUDES 1   *polycythemia neonatorum (P61.1)*
polycythemia vera (D45)
DEF: Elevated number of red blood cells in circulating blood as a result of reduced oxygen supply to the tissues.

✓5ᵗʰ **D75.8 Other specified diseases of blood and blood-forming organs**

D75.81 Myelofibrosis   CC   HCC
Myelofibrosis NOS
Secondary myelofibrosis NOS
Code first the underlying disorder, such as:
malignant neoplasm of breast (C50.-)
Use additional code, if applicable, for associated therapy-related myelodysplastic syndrome (D46.-)
Use additional code for adverse effect, if applicable, to identify drug (T45.1X5)
EXCLUDES 1   *acute myelofibrosis (C94.4-)*
idiopathic myelofibrosis (D47.1)
leukoerythroblastic anemia (D61.82)
myelofibrosis with myeloid metaplasia (D47.4)
myelophthisic anemia (D61.82)
myelophthisis (D61.82)
primary myelofibrosis (D47.1)

D75.82 Heparin induced thrombocytopenia (HIT)   HCC
DEF: Immune-mediated reaction to heparin therapy causing an abrupt fall in platelet count and serious complications such as pulmonary embolism, stroke, AMI, or DVT.

✓6ᵗʰ **D75.83 Thrombocytosis**
EXCLUDES 2   *essential thrombocythemia (D47.3)*

D75.838 Other thrombocytosis
Reactive thrombocytosis
Secondary thrombocytosis
Code also underlying condition, if known and applicable

D75.839 Thrombocytosis, unspecified
Thrombocythemia NOS
Thrombocytosis NOS

D75.89 Other specified diseases of blood and blood-forming organs

D75.9 Disease of blood and blood-forming organs, unspecified

D75.A Glucose-6-phosphate dehydrogenase (G6PD) deficiency without anemia
EXCLUDES 1   *glucose-6-phosphate dehydrogenase (G6PD) deficiency with anemia (D55.0)*
AHA: 2019,4Q,4-5

✓4ᵗʰ **D76 Other specified diseases with participation of lymphoreticular and reticulohistiocytic tissue**
EXCLUDES 1   *(Abt-) Letterer-Siwe disease (C96.0)*
eosinophilic granuloma (C96.6)
Hand-Schüller-Christian disease (C96.5)
histiocytic medullary reticulosis (C96.9)
histiocytic sarcoma (C96.A)
histiocytosis X, multifocal (C96.5)
histiocytosis X, unifocal (C96.6)
Langerhans-cell histiocytosis, multifocal (C96.5)
Langerhans-cell histiocytosis NOS (C96.6)
Langerhans-cell histiocytosis, unifocal (C96.6)
leukemic reticuloendotheliosis (C91.4-)
lipomelanotic reticulosis (I89.8)
malignant histiocytosis (C96.A)
malignant reticulosis (C86.0)
nonlipid reticuloendotheliosis (C96.0)

D76.1 Hemophagocytic lymphohistiocytosis   CC   HCC
Familial hemophagocytic reticulosis
Histiocytoses of mononuclear phagocytes

D76.2 Hemophagocytic syndrome, infection-associated   CC   HCC
Use additional code to identify infectious agent or disease

D76.3 Other histiocytosis syndromes   CC   HCC
Reticulohistiocytoma (giant-cell)
Sinus histiocytosis with massive lymphadenopathy
Xanthogranuloma

D77   *Other disorders of blood and blood-forming organs in diseases classified elsewhere*

     Code first underlying disease, such as:
       amyloidosis (E85.-)
       congenital early syphilis (A50.0)
       echinococcosis (B67.0-B67.9)
       malaria (B50.0-B54)
       schistosomiasis [bilharziasis] (B65.0-B65.9)
       vitamin C deficiency (E54)

       EXCLUDES 1   *rupture of spleen due to Plasmodium vivax malaria (B51.0)*
                    splenitis, splenomegaly in late syphilis (A52.79)
                    splenitis, splenomegaly in tuberculosis (A18.85)

Intraoperative and postprocedural complications of the spleen (D78)

D78   **Intraoperative and postprocedural complications of the spleen**

     AHA: 2016,4Q,9-10

     D78.0   Intraoperative hemorrhage and hematoma of the spleen complicating a procedure

       EXCLUDES 1   *intraoperative hemorrhage and hematoma of the spleen due to accidental puncture or laceration during a procedure (D78.1-)*

       D78.01   **Intraoperative hemorrhage and hematoma of the spleen complicating a procedure on the spleen**   cc

       D78.02   **Intraoperative hemorrhage and hematoma of the spleen complicating other procedure**   cc

     D78.1   Accidental puncture and laceration of the spleen during a procedure

       D78.11   **Accidental puncture and laceration of the spleen during a procedure on the spleen**   cc

       D78.12   **Accidental puncture and laceration of the spleen during other procedure**   cc

     D78.2   Postprocedural hemorrhage of the spleen following a procedure

       D78.21   **Postprocedural hemorrhage of the spleen following a procedure on the spleen**   cc

       D78.22   **Postprocedural hemorrhage of the spleen following other procedure**   cc

     D78.3   Postprocedural hematoma and seroma of the spleen following a procedure

       D78.31   **Postprocedural hematoma of the spleen following a procedure on the spleen**   cc

       D78.32   **Postprocedural hematoma of the spleen following other procedure**   cc

       D78.33   **Postprocedural seroma of the spleen following a procedure on the spleen**   cc

       D78.34   **Postprocedural seroma of the spleen following other procedure**   cc

     D78.8   Other intraoperative and postprocedural complications of the spleen

       Use additional code, if applicable, to further specify disorder

       D78.81   **Other intraoperative complications of the spleen**   cc

       D78.89   **Other postprocedural complications of the spleen**   cc

Certain disorders involving the immune mechanism (D80-D89)

     INCLUDES   defects in the complement system
               immunodeficiency disorders, except human immunodeficiency virus [HIV] disease
               sarcoidosis

     EXCLUDES 1   *autoimmune disease (systemic) NOS (M35.9)*
               functional disorders of polymorphonuclear neutrophils (D71)
               human immunodeficiency virus [HIV] disease (B20)

D80   **Immunodeficiency with predominantly antibody defects**

     D80.0   Hereditary hypogammaglobulinemia   cc HCC
       Autosomal recessive agammaglobulinemia (Swiss type)
       X-linked agammaglobulinemia [Bruton] (with growth hormone deficiency)

     D80.1   Nonfamilial hypogammaglobulinemia   cc HCC
       Agammaglobulinemia with immunoglobulin-bearing B-lymphocytes
       Common variable agammaglobulinemia [CVAgamma]
       Hypogammaglobulinemia NOS

     D80.2   Selective deficiency of immunoglobulin A [IgA]   cc HCC

     D80.3   Selective deficiency of immunoglobulin G [IgG] subclasses   cc HCC

     D80.4   Selective deficiency of immunoglobulin M [IgM]   cc HCC

     D80.5   Immunodeficiency with increased immunoglobulin M [IgM]   cc HCC

     D80.6   Antibody deficiency with near-normal immunoglobulins or with hyperimmunoglobulinemia   cc HCC

     D80.7   Transient hypogammaglobulinemia of infancy   cc HCC

     D80.8   Other immunodeficiencies with predominantly antibody defects   cc HCC
       Kappa light chain deficiency

     D80.9   Immunodeficiency with predominantly antibody defects, unspecified   cc HCC

D81   **Combined immunodeficiencies**

     EXCLUDES 1   *autosomal recessive agammaglobulinemia (Swiss type) (D80.0)*

     D81.0   Severe combined immunodeficiency [SCID] with reticular dysgenesis   cc HCC

     D81.1   Severe combined immunodeficiency [SCID] with low T- and B-cell numbers   cc HCC

     D81.2   Severe combined immunodeficiency [SCID] with low or normal B-cell numbers   cc HCC

     D81.3   Adenosine deaminase [ADA] deficiency

       AHA: 2019,4Q,5-6

       D81.30   **Adenosine deaminase deficiency, unspecified**   cc HCC
            ADA deficiency NOS

       D81.31   **Severe combined immunodeficiency due to adenosine deaminase deficiency**   cc HCC
            ADA deficiency with SCID
            Adenosine deaminase [ADA] deficiency with severe combined immunodeficiency

       D81.32   **Adenosine deaminase 2 deficiency**   cc HCC
            ADA2 deficiency
            Adenosine deaminase deficiency type 2
            Code also, if applicable, any associated manifestations, such as:
                polyarteritis nodosa (M30.0)
                stroke (I63.-)

       D81.39   **Other adenosine deaminase deficiency**   cc HCC
            Adenosine deaminase [ADA] deficiency type 1, NOS
            Adenosine deaminase [ADA] deficiency type 1, without SCID
            Adenosine deaminase [ADA] deficiency type 1, without severe combined immunodeficiency
            Partial ADA deficiency (type 1)
            Partial adenosine deaminase deficiency (type 1)

     D81.4   Nezelof's syndrome   cc HCC

     D81.5   Purine nucleoside phosphorylase [PNP] deficiency   cc HCC

     D81.6   Major histocompatibility complex class I deficiency   cc HCC
       Bare lymphocyte syndrome

     D81.7   Major histocompatibility complex class II deficiency   cc HCC

     D81.8   Other combined immunodeficiencies

       D81.81   **Biotin-dependent carboxylase deficiency**
            Multiple carboxylase deficiency

            EXCLUDES 1   *biotin-dependent carboxylase deficiency due to dietary deficiency of biotin (E53.8)*

            D81.810   **Biotinidase deficiency**
            D81.818   **Other biotin-dependent carboxylase deficiency**
                Holocarboxylase synthetase deficiency
                Other multiple carboxylase deficiency
            D81.819   **Biotin-dependent carboxylase deficiency, unspecified**
                Multiple carboxylase deficiency, unspecified

       D81.89   **Other combined immunodeficiencies**   cc HCC

     D81.9   Combined immunodeficiency, unspecified   cc HCC
       Severe combined immunodeficiency disorder [SCID] NOS

D82   **Immunodeficiency associated with other major defects**

     EXCLUDES 1   *ataxia telangiectasia [Louis-Bar] (G11.3)*

     D82.0   Wiskott-Aldrich syndrome   cc HCC
       Immunodeficiency with thrombocytopenia and eczema

✔ Additional Character Required   ✔x7th Placeholder   Questionable PDx   Manifestation   Unspecified Dx   UPD Unacceptable PDx   H1-H4 HAC   HCC CMS-HCC Dx   HIV HIV Dx

ICD-10-CM 2022   515

D82.1 Di George's syndrome `CC` `HCC`
Pharyngeal pouch syndrome
Thymic alymphoplasia
Thymic aplasia or hypoplasia with immunodeficiency
AHA: 2019,3Q,14

D82.2 Immunodeficiency with short-limbed stature `HCC`

D82.3 Immunodeficiency following hereditary defective response to Epstein-Barr virus `HCC`
X-linked lymphoproliferative disease

D82.4 Hyperimmunoglobulin E [IgE] syndrome `HCC`

D82.8 Immunodeficiency associated with other specified major defects `HCC`

D82.9 Immunodeficiency associated with major defect, unspecified `HCC`

✓4ᵗʰ **D83 Common variable immunodeficiency**

D83.0 Common variable immunodeficiency with predominant abnormalities of B-cell numbers and function `CC` `HCC`

D83.1 Common variable immunodeficiency with predominant immunoregulatory T-cell disorders `CC` `HCC`

D83.2 Common variable immunodeficiency with autoantibodies to B- or T-cells `CC` `HCC`

D83.8 Other common variable immunodeficiencies `CC` `HCC`

D83.9 Common variable immunodeficiency, unspecified `CC` `HCC`

✓4ᵗʰ **D84 Other immunodeficiencies**

D84.0 Lymphocyte function antigen-1 [LFA-1] defect `HCC`

D84.1 Defects in the complement system `HCC`
C1 esterase inhibitor [C1-INH] deficiency

✓5ᵗʰ **D84.8 Other specified immunodeficiencies**
AHA: 2020,4Q,10-12

 D84.81 Immunodeficiency due to conditions classified elsewhere `CC` `HCC`
  Code first underlying condition, such as:
  chromosomal abnormalities (Q90-Q99)
  diabetes mellitus (E08-E13)
  malignant neoplasms (C00-C96)
  `EXCLUDES 1` certain disorders involving the immune mechanism (D80-D83, D84.0, D84.1, D84.9)
   human immunodeficiency virus [HIV] disease (B20)
  AHA: 2021,1Q,52

✓6ᵗʰ **D84.82 Immunodeficiency due to drugs and external causes**

 D84.821 Immunodeficiency due to drugs `CC` `HCC`
  Immunodeficiency due to (current or past) medication
  Use additional code for adverse effect if applicable, to identify adverse effect of drug (T36-T50 with fifth or six character 5)
  Use additional code, if applicable, for associated long term (current) drug therapy drug or medication such as:
  long term (current) drug therapy systemic steroids (Z79.52)
  other long term (current) drug therapy (Z79.899)

 D84.822 Immunodeficiency due to external causes `CC` `HCC`
  Code also, if applicable, radiological procedure and radiotherapy (Y84.2)
  Use additional code for external cause such as:
  exposure to ionizing radiation (W88)

 D84.89 Other immunodeficiencies `CC` `HCC`

D84.9 Immunodeficiency, unspecified `CC` `HCC`
Immunocompromised NOS
Immunodeficient NOS
Immunosuppressed NOS
AHA: 2020,4Q,10

✓4ᵗʰ **D86 Sarcoidosis**
DEF: Clustering of immune cells resulting in granuloma formation. Often affects the lungs and lymphatic system but can occur in other body sites.

D86.0 Sarcoidosis of lung `HCC`

D86.1 Sarcoidosis of lymph nodes

D86.2 Sarcoidosis of lung with sarcoidosis of lymph nodes `HCC`

D86.3 Sarcoidosis of skin

✓5ᵗʰ **D86.8 Sarcoidosis of other sites**

 D86.81 Sarcoid meningitis

 D86.82 Multiple cranial nerve palsies in sarcoidosis `HCC`

 D86.83 Sarcoid iridocyclitis

 D86.84 Sarcoid pyelonephritis
  Tubulo-interstitial nephropathy in sarcoidosis

 D86.85 Sarcoid myocarditis

 D86.86 Sarcoid arthropathy
  Polyarthritis in sarcoidosis

 D86.87 Sarcoid myositis

 D86.89 Sarcoidosis of other sites
  Hepatic granuloma
  Uveoparotid fever [Heerfordt]

D86.9 Sarcoidosis, unspecified

✓4ᵗʰ **D89 Other disorders involving the immune mechanism, not elsewhere classified**
 `EXCLUDES 1` hyperglobulinemia NOS (R77.1)
  monoclonal gammopathy (of undetermined significance) (D47.2)
 `EXCLUDES 2` transplant failure and rejection (T86.-)

D89.0 Polyclonal hypergammaglobulinemia
Benign hypergammaglobulinemic purpura
Polyclonal gammopathy NOS

D89.1 Cryoglobulinemia `HCC`
Cryoglobulinemic purpura
Cryoglobulinemic vasculitis
Essential cryoglobulinemia
Idiopathic cryoglobulinemia
Mixed cryoglobulinemia
Primary cryoglobulinemia
Secondary cryoglobulinemia

D89.2 Hypergammaglobulinemia, unspecified

D89.3 Immune reconstitution syndrome `HCC`
Immune reconstitution inflammatory syndrome [IRIS]
Use additional code for adverse effect, if applicable, to identify drug (T36-T50 with fifth or sixth character 5)

✓5ᵗʰ **D89.4 Mast cell activation syndrome and related disorders**
 `EXCLUDES 1` aggressive systemic mastocytosis (C96.21)
  congenital cutaneous mastocytosis (Q82.2)
  (non-congenital) cutaneous mastocytosis (D47.01)
  (indolent) systemic mastocytosis (D47.02)
  malignant mast cell neoplasm (C96.2-)
  malignant mastocytoma (C96.29)
  mast cell leukemia (C94.3-)
  mast cell sarcoma (C96.22)
  mastocytoma NOS (D47.09)
  other mast cell neoplasms of uncertain behavior (D47.09)
  systemic mastocytosis associated with a clonal hematologic non-mast cell lineage disease (SM-AHNMD) (D47.02)
 AHA: 2016,4Q,11

 D89.40 Mast cell activation, unspecified `HCC`
  Mast cell activation disorder, unspecified
  Mast cell activation syndrome, NOS

 D89.41 Monoclonal mast cell activation syndrome `HCC`

 D89.42 Idiopathic mast cell activation syndrome `HCC`

 D89.43 Secondary mast cell activation `HCC`
  Secondary mast cell activation syndrome
  Code also underlying etiology, if known

 D89.44 Hereditary alpha tryptasemia
  Use additional code, if applicable, for:
  allergy status, other than to drugs and biological substances (Z91.0-)
  personal history of anaphylaxis (Z87.892)

 D89.49 Other mast cell activation disorder `HCC`
  Other mast cell activation syndrome

✓5ᵗʰ **D89.8** **Other specified disorders involving the immune mechanism, not elsewhere classified**

✓6ᵗʰ   **D89.81** **Graft-versus-host disease**

Code first underlying cause, such as:
    complications of transplanted organs and tissue (T86.-)
    complications of blood transfusion (T80.89)
Use additional code to identify associated manifestations, such as:
desquamative dermatitis (L30.8)
diarrhea (R19.7)
elevated bilirubin (R17)
hair loss (L65.9)

     D89.810 **Acute graft-versus-host disease** `CC` `UPD` `HCC`

     D89.811 **Chronic graft-versus-host disease** `CC` `UPD` `HCC`

     D89.812 **Acute on chronic graft-versus-host disease** `CC` `UPD` `HCC`

     D89.813 **Graft-versus-host disease, unspecified** `CC` `UPD` `HCC`

   D89.82 **Autoimmune lymphoproliferative syndrome [ALPS]** `HCC`

DEF: Rare genetic alteration of the Fas protein that impairs normal cellular apoptosis (normal cell death), causing abnormal accumulation of lymphocytes in the lymph glands, liver, and spleen. Symptoms include neutropenia, anemia, and thrombocytopenia.

✓6ᵗʰ   **D89.83** **Cytokine release syndrome**

Code first underlying cause, such as:
    complications following infusion, transfusion and therapeutic injection (T80.89-)
    complications of transplanted organs and tissue (T86.-)
Use additional code to identify associated manifestations

AHA: 2020,4Q,12-15

DEF: Form of systemic inflammatory response syndrome (SIRS) in which immune substances (cytokines) are released rapidly and in large amounts from the affected immune cells into the blood. The severity of associated symptoms or manifestations varies based on the underlying cause. This syndrome occurs as a complication of a disease, infection, or drug (often an adverse effect of immunotherapy in the form of treatment receiving monoclonal antibodies or Chimeric Antigen Receptor T [CAR-T] cells).

     D89.831 **Cytokine release syndrome, grade 1** `UPD`

     D89.832 **Cytokine release syndrome, grade 2** `UPD`

     D89.833 **Cytokine release syndrome, grade 3** `CC` `UPD`

     D89.834 **Cytokine release syndrome, grade 4** `CC` `UPD`

     D89.835 **Cytokine release syndrome, grade 5** `CC` `UPD`

     D89.839 **Cytokine release syndrome, grade unspecified** `UPD`

   D89.89 **Other specified disorders involving the immune mechanism, not elsewhere classified** `HCC`

     `EXCLUDES 1`   human immunodeficiency virus disease (B20)

     AHA: 2017,4Q,109

D89.9 **Disorder involving the immune mechanism, unspecified** `HCC`

Immune disease NOS
AHA: 2015,3Q,22

☑ Additional Character Required   ✓x7ᵗʰ Placeholder   Questionable PDx   **Manifestation**   Unspecified Dx   `UPD` Unacceptable PDx   `H1`-`H14` HAC   `HCC` CMS-HCC Dx   `HIV` HIV Dx

ICD-10-CM 2022   517

Chapter 4. Endocrine, Nutritional and Metabolic Diseases (E00–E89)

Chapter-specific Guidelines with Coding Examples

The chapter-specific guidelines from the ICD-10-CM Official Guidelines for Coding and Reporting have been provided below. Along with these guidelines are coding examples, contained in the shaded boxes, that have been developed to help illustrate the coding and/or sequencing guidance found in these guidelines.

a. Diabetes mellitus

The diabetes mellitus codes are combination codes that include the type of diabetes mellitus, the body system affected, and the complications affecting that body system. As many codes within a particular category as are necessary to describe all of the complications of the disease may be used. They should be sequenced based on the reason for a particular encounter. Assign as many codes from categories E08–E13 as needed to identify all of the associated conditions that the patient has.

> Patient is seen for poorly controlled diabetes, type 2, with diabetic polyneuropathy and diabetic retinopathy with macular edema
>
> **E11.65**   **Type 2 diabetes mellitus with hyperglycemia**
>
> **E11.311**   **Type 2 diabetes mellitus with unspecified diabetic retinopathy with macular edema**
>
> **E11.42**   **Type 2 diabetes mellitus with diabetic polyneuropathy**
>
> *Explanation*: Use as many codes to describe the diabetic complications as needed. Many are combination codes that describe more than one condition. Code first the reason for the encounter. "Poorly controlled" is described as "with hyperglycemia." Diabetes documented as "uncontrolled" is not assumed to be hyperglycemic but can be classified to either hyperglycemia or hypoglycemia. If documentation is not clear, the provider must be queried so that the appropriate code can be reported.

1) Type of diabetes

The age of a patient is not the sole determining factor, though most type 1 diabetics develop the condition before reaching puberty. For this reason, type 1 diabetes mellitus is also referred to as juvenile diabetes.

> A 45-year-old patient is diagnosed with type 1 diabetes
>
> **E10.9**   **Type 1 diabetes mellitus without complications**
>
> *Explanation*: Although most type 1 diabetics are diagnosed in childhood or adolescence, it can also begin in adults.

2) Type of diabetes mellitus not documented

If the type of diabetes mellitus is not documented in the medical record the default is E11.-, Type 2 diabetes mellitus.

> H & P lists diabetes and hypertension on patient problem list
>
> **E11.9**   **Type 2 diabetes mellitus without complications**
>
> **I10**   **Essential (primary) hypertension**
>
> *Explanation*: Since the type of diabetes was not documented and no complications were noted, the default code is E11.9.

3) Diabetes mellitus and the use of insulin, oral hypoglycemics, and injectable non-insulin drugs

If the documentation in a medical record does not indicate the type of diabetes but does indicate that the patient uses insulin, code E11-, Type 2 diabetes mellitus, should be assigned. **Additional** code(s) should be assigned from category Z79 to identify the long-term (current) use of insulin, oral hypoglycemic drugs, **or injectable non-insulin antidiabetic, as follows:**

If the patient is treated with both oral medications and insulin, **both code Z79.4, Long term (current) use of insulin, and code Z79.84, Long term (current) use of oral hypoglycemic drugs,** should be assigned.

If the patient is treated with both insulin and an injectable non-insulin antidiabetic drug, assign codes Z79.4, Long term (current) use of insulin, and Z79.899, Other long term (current) drug therapy.

If the patient is treated with both oral hypoglycemic drugs and an injectable non-insulin antidiabetic drug, assign codes Z79.84, Long term (current) use of oral hypoglycemic drugs, and Z79.899, Other long term (current) drug therapy.

Code Z79.4 should not be assigned if insulin is given temporarily to bring a type 2 patient's blood sugar under control during an encounter.

> Type 2 diabetic patient on daily metformin and Victoza is admitted in ketoacidosis, insulin given to stabilize blood sugars and discontinued at discharge
>
> **E11.10**   **Type 2 diabetes mellitus with ketoacidosis without coma**
>
> **Z79.84**   **Long term (current) use of oral hypoglycemic drugs**
>
> **Z79.899**   **Other long term (current) drug therapy**
>
> *Explanation*: Documentation indicates the patient is on an oral antidiabetic medication (metformin) and an injectable noninsulin antidiabetic medication (Victoza). Although insulin was given to the patient during the encounter, it was discontinued at discharge, indicating that the patient does not regularly use insulin. A Z code representing long-term use of the oral drug and long-term use of the injectable medication can be applied. Applying code Z79.4 to represent long-term use of insulin would be inappropriate.

4) Diabetes mellitus in pregnancy and gestational diabetes

See Section I.C.15. Diabetes mellitus in pregnancy.

See Section I.C.15. Gestational (pregnancy induced) diabetes

5) Complications due to insulin pump malfunction
(a) Underdose of insulin due to insulin pump failure

An underdose of insulin due to an insulin pump failure should be assigned to a code from subcategory T85.6, Mechanical complication of other specified internal and external prosthetic devices, implants and grafts, that specifies the type of pump malfunction, as the principal or first-listed code, followed by code T38.3X6-, Underdosing of insulin and oral hypoglycemic [antidiabetic] drugs. Additional codes for the type of diabetes mellitus and any associated complications due to the underdosing should also be assigned.

> A 24-year-old type 1 diabetic male treated in ED for hyperglycemia; insulin pump found to be malfunctioning and underdosing
>
> **T85.614A**   **Breakdown (mechanical) of insulin pump, initial encounter**
>
> **T38.3X6A**   **Underdosing of insulin and oral hypoglycemic [antidiabetic] drugs, initial encounter**
>
> **E10.65**   **Type 1 diabetes mellitus with hyperglycemia**
>
> *Explanation*: The complication code for the mechanical breakdown of the pump is sequenced first, followed by the underdosing code and type of diabetes with complication. Code all other diabetic complication codes necessary to describe the patient's condition.

(b) Overdose of insulin due to insulin pump failure

The principal or first-listed code for an encounter due to an insulin pump malfunction resulting in an overdose of insulin, should also be T85.6-, Mechanical complication of other specified internal and external prosthetic devices, implants and grafts, followed by code T38.3X1-, Poisoning by insulin and oral hypoglycemic [antidiabetic] drugs, accidental (unintentional).

> A 24-year-old type 1 diabetic male found down with diabetic coma, brought into ED and treated for hypoglycemia; insulin pump found to be malfunctioning and overdosing
>
> **T85.614A**   **Breakdown (mechanical) of insulin pump, initial encounter**
>
> **T38.3X1A**   **Poisoning by insulin and oral hypoglycemic [antidiabetic] drugs, accidental (unintentional), initial encounter**
>
> **E10.641**   **Type 1 diabetes mellitus with hypoglycemia with coma**
>
> *Explanation*: The complication code for the mechanical breakdown of the pump is sequenced first, followed by the poisoning code and type of diabetes with complication. All the characters in the combination code must be used to form a valid code and to fully describe the type of diabetes, the hypoglycemia, and the coma.

6) Secondary diabetes mellitus

Codes under categories E08, Diabetes mellitus due to underlying condition, E09, Drug or chemical induced diabetes mellitus, and E13, Other specified diabetes mellitus, identify complications/manifestations associated with secondary diabetes mellitus. Secondary diabetes is always caused by another condition or event (e.g., cystic fibrosis, malignant neoplasm of pancreas, pancreatectomy, adverse effect of drug, or poisoning).

(a) Secondary diabetes mellitus and the use of insulin or oral hypoglycemic drugs

For patients with secondary diabetes mellitus who routinely use insulin, oral hypoglycemic drugs, **or injectable non-insulin drugs,** additional code**(s)** from category Z79 should be assigned to identify the long-term (current) use of insulin, oral hypoglycemic drugs, **or non-injectable non-insulin drugs as follows:**

If the patient is treated with both oral medications and insulin, **both code Z79.4, Long term (current) use of insulin, and code Z79.84, Long term (current) use of oral hypoglycemic drugs,** should be assigned.

If the patient is treated with both insulin and an injectable non-insulin antidiabetic drug, assign codes Z79.4, Long- term (current) use of insulin, and Z79.899, Other long term (current) drug therapy.

If the patient is treated with both oral hypoglycemic drugs and an injectable non-insulin antidiabetic drug, assign codes Z79.84, Long-term (current) use of oral hypoglycemic drugs, and Z79.899, Other long-term (current) drug therapy.

Code Z79.4 should not be assigned if insulin is given temporarily to bring a secondary diabetic patient's blood sugar under control during an encounter

The patient, maintained on metformin and insulin, was admitted for treatment of diabetic gangrene. The patient developed diabetes secondary to Nelson's syndrome.

E24.1	**Nelson's syndrome**
E08.52	**Diabetes mellitus due to underlying condition with diabetic peripheral angiopathy with gangrene**
Z79.4	**Long term (current) use of insulin**
Z79.84	**Long term (current) use of oral hypoglycemic drugs**

Explanation: When diabetes is caused by an underlying condition, the underlying condition should always be sequenced before any codes representing the diabetes. Patients with secondary diabetes may be maintained on both insulin and an oral hypoglycemic. When maintained on both, report a code for the long term use of insulin and a code for the long term use of oral hypoglycemic.

(b) Assigning and sequencing secondary diabetes codes and its causes

The sequencing of the secondary diabetes codes in relationship to codes for the cause of the diabetes is based on the Tabular List instructions for categories E08, E09 and E13.

(i) Secondary diabetes mellitus due to pancreatectomy

For postpancreatectomy diabetes mellitus (lack of insulin due to the surgical removal of all or part of the pancreas), assign code E89.1, Postprocedural hypoinsulinemia. Assign a code from category E13 and a code from subcategory Z90.41, Acquired absence of pancreas, as additional codes.

Patient with newly diagnosed diabetes after surgical removal of part of pancreas is discharged with referral for consult to initiate insulin.

E89.1	**Postprocedural hypoinsulinemia**
E13.9	**Other specified diabetes mellitus without complications**
Z90.411	**Acquired partial absence of pancreas**

Explanation: Sequence the postprocedural complication of the hypoinsulinemia due to the partial removal of the pancreas as the first-listed code, followed by codes for other specified diabetes (NEC) without complications and partial acquired absence of the pancreas. Code Z79.4 Long term (current) use of insulin, is not added because the insulin has not yet been started.

(ii) Secondary diabetes due to drugs

Secondary diabetes may be caused by an adverse effect of correctly administered medications, poisoning or sequela of poisoning.

See section I.C.19.e for coding of adverse effects and poisoning, and section I.C.20 for external cause code reporting.

Initial encounter for corticosteroid-induced diabetes mellitus

E09.9	**Drug or chemical induced diabetes mellitus without complications**
T38.0X5A	**Adverse effect of glucocorticoids and synthetic analogues, initial encounter**

Explanation: If the diabetes is caused by an adverse effect of a drug, the diabetic condition is coded first. If it occurs from a poisoning or overdose, the poisoning code causing the diabetes is sequenced first.

Chapter 4. Endocrine, Nutritional and Metabolic Diseases (E00-E89)

NOTE All neoplasms, whether functionally active or not, are classified in Chapter 2. Appropriate codes in this chapter (i.e. E05.8, E07.0, E16-E31, E34.-) may be used as additional codes to indicate either functional activity by neoplasms and ectopic endocrine tissue or hyperfunction and hypofunction of endocrine glands associated with neoplasms and other conditions classified elsewhere.

EXCLUDES 1   *transitory endocrine and metabolic disorders specific to newborn (P70-P74)*

AHA: 2018,2Q,6

This chapter contains the following blocks:

E00-E07   Disorders of thyroid gland
E08-E13   Diabetes mellitus
E15-E16   Other disorders of glucose regulation and pancreatic internal secretion
E20-E35   Disorders of other endocrine glands
E36   Intraoperative complications of endocrine system
E40-E46   Malnutrition
E50-E64   Other nutritional deficiencies
E65-E68   Overweight, obesity and other hyperalimentation
E70-E88   Metabolic disorders
E89   Postprocedural endocrine and metabolic complications and disorders, not elsewhere classified

Disorders of thyroid gland (E00-E07)

√4ᵗʰ E00   Congenital iodine-deficiency syndrome

Use additional code (F70-F79) to identify associated intellectual disabilities

EXCLUDES 1   *subclinical iodine-deficiency hypothyroidism (E02)*

E00.0   Congenital iodine-deficiency syndrome, neurological type
Endemic cretinism, neurological type

E00.1   Congenital iodine-deficiency syndrome, myxedematous type
Endemic hypothyroid cretinism
Endemic cretinism, myxedematous type

E00.2   Congenital iodine-deficiency syndrome, mixed type
Endemic cretinism, mixed type

E00.9   Congenital iodine-deficiency syndrome, unspecified
Congenital iodine-deficiency hypothyroidism NOS
Endemic cretinism NOS

√4ᵗʰ E01   Iodine-deficiency related thyroid disorders and allied conditions

EXCLUDES 1   *congenital iodine-deficiency syndrome (E00.-)*
subclinical iodine-deficiency hypothyroidism (E02)

E01.0   Iodine-deficiency related diffuse (endemic) goiter

E01.1   Iodine-deficiency related multinodular (endemic) goiter
Iodine-deficiency related nodular goiter

E01.2   Iodine-deficiency related (endemic) goiter, unspecified
Endemic goiter NOS

E01.8   Other iodine-deficiency related thyroid disorders and allied conditions
Acquired iodine-deficiency hypothyroidism NOS

E02   Subclinical iodine-deficiency hypothyroidism
AHA: 2021,1Q,8

√4ᵗʰ E03   Other hypothyroidism

EXCLUDES 1   *iodine-deficiency related hypothyroidism (E00-E02)*
postprocedural hypothyroidism (E89.0)

DEF: Hypothyroidism: Underproduction of thyroid hormone.

E03.0   Congenital hypothyroidism with diffuse goiter
Congenital parenchymatous goiter (nontoxic)
Congenital goiter (nontoxic) NOS
EXCLUDES 1   *transitory congenital goiter with normal function (P72.0)*

E03.1   Congenital hypothyroidism without goiter
Aplasia of thyroid (with myxedema)
Congenital atrophy of thyroid
Congenital hypothyroidism NOS

E03.2   Hypothyroidism due to medicaments and other exogenous substances
Code first poisoning due to drug or toxin, if applicable (T36-T65 with fifth or sixth character 1-4 or 6)
Use additional code for adverse effect, if applicable, to identify drug (T36-T50 with fifth or sixth character 5)

E03.3   Postinfectious hypothyroidism

E03.4   Atrophy of thyroid (acquired)
EXCLUDES 1   *congenital atrophy of thyroid (E03.1)*

E03.5   Myxedema coma   **MCC** **HCC**

E03.8   Other specified hypothyroidism
AHA: 2021,1Q,8

E03.9   Hypothyroidism, unspecified
Myxedema NOS

√4ᵗʰ E04   Other nontoxic goiter

EXCLUDES 1   *congenital goiter (NOS) (diffuse) (parenchymatous) (E03.0)*
iodine-deficiency related goiter (E00-E02)

E04.0   Nontoxic diffuse goiter
Diffuse (colloid) nontoxic goiter
Simple nontoxic goiter

E04.1   Nontoxic single thyroid nodule
Colloid nodule (cystic) (thyroid)
Nontoxic uninodular goiter
Thyroid (cystic) nodule NOS
DEF: Enlarged thyroid, commonly due to decreased thyroid production, with a single nodule. No clinical hypothyroidism.

E04.2   Nontoxic multinodular goiter
Cystic goiter NOS
Multinodular (cystic) goiter NOS
DEF: Enlarged thyroid, commonly due to decreased thyroid production with multiple nodules. No clinical hypothyroidism.

E04.8   Other specified nontoxic goiter

E04.9   Nontoxic goiter, unspecified
Goiter NOS
Nodular goiter (nontoxic) NOS

√4ᵗʰ E05   Thyrotoxicosis [hyperthyroidism]

EXCLUDES 1   *chronic thyroiditis with transient thyrotoxicosis (E06.2)*
neonatal thyrotoxicosis (P72.1)

DEF: Excessive quantities of hormones from the thyroid gland caused by overproduction or loss of storage ability.

√5ᵗʰ E05.0   Thyrotoxicosis with diffuse goiter
Exophthalmic or toxic goiter NOS
Graves' disease
Toxic diffuse goiter
DEF: Diffuse thyroid enlargement accompanied by hyperthyroidism, bulging eyes, and dermopathy.

E05.00   Thyrotoxicosis with diffuse goiter without thyrotoxic crisis or storm

E05.01   Thyrotoxicosis with diffuse goiter with thyrotoxic crisis or storm   **MCC**

Goiter

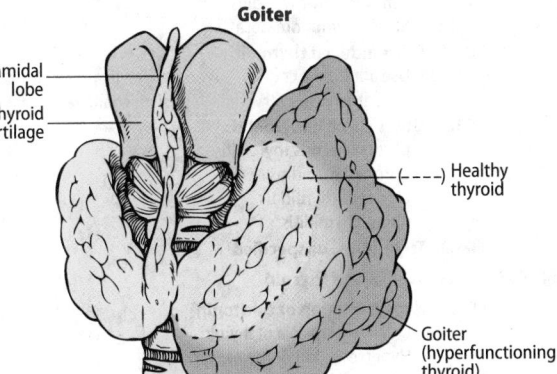

Pyramidal lobe
Thyroid cartilage
Healthy thyroid
Goiter (hyperfunctioning thyroid)

√5ᵗʰ E05.1   Thyrotoxicosis with toxic single thyroid nodule
Thyrotoxicosis with toxic uninodular goiter
DEF: Symptomatic hyperthyroidism with a single nodule on the enlarged thyroid gland. Onset of symptoms can be abrupt and include extreme nervousness, insomnia, weight loss, tremors, and psychosis or coma.

E05.10   Thyrotoxicosis with toxic single thyroid nodule without thyrotoxic crisis or storm

E05.11   Thyrotoxicosis with toxic single thyroid nodule with thyrotoxic crisis or storm   **MCC**

√5ᵗʰ E05.2   Thyrotoxicosis with toxic multinodular goiter
Toxic nodular goiter NOS

E05.20   Thyrotoxicosis with toxic multinodular goiter without thyrotoxic crisis or storm

E05.21   Thyrotoxicosis with toxic multinodular goiter with thyrotoxic crisis or storm   **MCC**

√5ᵗʰ E05.3   Thyrotoxicosis from ectopic thyroid tissue

E05.30   Thyrotoxicosis from ectopic thyroid tissue without thyrotoxic crisis or storm

✓ Additional Character Required   √x7ᵗʰ Placeholder   Questionable PDx   Manifestation   Unspecified Dx   UPD Unacceptable PDx   H1–H14 HAC   HCC CMS-HCC Dx   HIV HIV Dx

ICD-10-CM 2022   **521**

Chapter 4. Endocrine, Nutritional and Metabolic Diseases

    E05.31   **Thyrotoxicosis from ectopic thyroid tissue** with thyrotoxic crisis or storm   `MCC`

✓5ᵗʰ **E05.4**   **Thyrotoxicosis factitia**

    E05.40   **Thyrotoxicosis factitia** without thyrotoxic crisis or storm

    E05.41   **Thyrotoxicosis factitia** with thyrotoxic crisis or storm   `MCC`

✓5ᵗʰ **E05.8**   **Other thyrotoxicosis**

    Overproduction of thyroid-stimulating hormone

    E05.80   **Other thyrotoxicosis** without thyrotoxic crisis or storm

    E05.81   **Other thyrotoxicosis** with thyrotoxic crisis or storm   `MCC`

✓5ᵗʰ **E05.9**   **Thyrotoxicosis, unspecified**

    Hyperthyroidism NOS

    E05.90   **Thyrotoxicosis, unspecified** without thyrotoxic crisis or storm

    E05.91   **Thyrotoxicosis, unspecified** with thyrotoxic crisis or storm   `MCC`

✓4ᵗʰ **E06**   **Thyroiditis**

    EXCLUDES 1   postpartum thyroiditis (O90.5)

    DEF: Inflammation of the thyroid gland.

  E06.0   **Acute thyroiditis**   `CC`

    Abscess of thyroid

    Pyogenic thyroiditis

    Suppurative thyroiditis

    Use additional code (B95-B97) to identify infectious agent

  E06.1   **Subacute thyroiditis**

    de Quervain thyroiditis

    Giant-cell thyroiditis

    Granulomatous thyroiditis

    Nonsuppurative thyroiditis

    Viral thyroiditis

    EXCLUDES 1   autoimmune thyroiditis (E06.3)

  E06.2   **Chronic thyroiditis with transient thyrotoxicosis**

    EXCLUDES 1   autoimmune thyroiditis (E06.3)

  E06.3   **Autoimmune thyroiditis**

    Hashimoto's thyroiditis

    Hashitoxicosis (transient)

    Lymphadenoid goiter

    Lymphocytic thyroiditis

    Struma lymphomatosa

  E06.4   **Drug-induced thyroiditis**

    Use additional code for adverse effect, if applicable, to identify drug (T36-T50 with fifth or sixth character 5)

  E06.5   **Other chronic thyroiditis**

    Chronic fibrous thyroiditis

    Chronic thyroiditis NOS

    Ligneous thyroiditis

    Riedel thyroiditis

  E06.9   **Thyroiditis, unspecified**

✓4ᵗʰ **E07**   **Other disorders of thyroid**

  E07.0   **Hypersecretion of calcitonin**

    C-cell hyperplasia of thyroid

    Hypersecretion of thyrocalcitonin

  E07.1   **Dyshormonogenetic goiter**

    Familial dyshormonogenetic goiter

    Pendred's syndrome

    EXCLUDES 1   transitory congenital goiter with normal function (P72.0)

✓5ᵗʰ **E07.8**   **Other specified disorders of thyroid**

    E07.81   **Sick-euthyroid syndrome**

      Euthyroid sick-syndrome

      DEF: Thyroid dysfunction caused by abnormal levels of thyroid hormones T3 and/or T4. This syndrome is often associated with starvation or critical illness.

    E07.89   **Other specified disorders of thyroid**

      Abnormality of thyroid-binding globulin

      Hemorrhage of thyroid

      Infarction of thyroid

  E07.9   **Disorder of thyroid, unspecified**

Diabetes mellitus (E08-E13)

AHA: 2020,1Q,12; 2018,2Q,6; 2017,4Q,100-101; 2016,2Q,36; 2016,1Q,11-13; 2013,4Q,114; 2013,3Q,20

✓4ᵗʰ **E08**   **Diabetes mellitus** due to underlying condition

    Code first the underlying condition, such as:

      congenital rubella (P35.0)

      Cushing's syndrome (E24.-)

      cystic fibrosis (E84.-)

      malignant neoplasm (C00-C96)

      malnutrition (E40-E46)

      pancreatitis and other diseases of the pancreas (K85-K86.-)

    Use additional code to identify control using:

      insulin (Z79.4)

      oral antidiabetic drugs (Z79.84)

      oral hypoglycemic drugs (Z79.84)

    EXCLUDES 1   drug or chemical induced diabetes mellitus (E09.-)

      gestational diabetes (O24.4-)

      neonatal diabetes mellitus (P70.2)

      postpancreatectomy diabetes mellitus (E13.-)

      postprocedural diabetes mellitus (E13.-)

      secondary diabetes mellitus NEC (E13.-)

      type 1 diabetes mellitus (E10.-)

      type 2 diabetes mellitus (E11.-)

✓5ᵗʰ **E08.0**   **Diabetes mellitus due to underlying condition with hyperosmolarity**

    DEF: Diabetic hyperosmolarity: Extremely high levels of glucose in the blood without ketones.

    E08.00   ***Diabetes mellitus due to underlying condition with hyperosmolarity** without nonketotic hyperglycemic-hyperosmolar coma (NKHHC)*   `MCC` `H9` `HCC`

    E08.01   ***Diabetes mellitus due to underlying condition with hyperosmolarity** with coma*   `MCC` `H9` `HCC`

✓5ᵗʰ **E08.1**   **Diabetes mellitus due to underlying condition with ketoacidosis**

    DEF: Diabetic ketoacidosis: Potentially life-threatening complication due to a shortage of insulin in which the body switches to burning fatty acids and producing acidic ketone bodies.

    E08.10   ***Diabetes mellitus due to underlying condition with ketoacidosis** without coma*   `MCC` `H9` `HCC`

    E08.11   ***Diabetes mellitus due to underlying condition with ketoacidosis** with coma*   `MCC` `H9` `HCC`

✓5ᵗʰ **E08.2**   **Diabetes mellitus due to underlying condition with kidney complications**

    AHA: 2019,3Q,3; 2018,4Q,88

    E08.21   ***Diabetes mellitus due to underlying condition with diabetic** nephropathy*   `HCC`

      Diabetes mellitus due to underlying condition with intercapillary glomerulosclerosis

      Diabetes mellitus due to underlying condition with intracapillary glomerulonephrosis

      Diabetes mellitus due to underlying condition with Kimmelstiel-Wilson disease

    E08.22   ***Diabetes mellitus due to underlying condition with diabetic** chronic kidney disease*   `HCC`

      Use additional code to identify stage of chronic kidney disease (N18.1-N18.6)

    E08.29   ***Diabetes mellitus due to underlying condition with other diabetic kidney complication***   `HCC`

      Renal tubular degeneration in diabetes mellitus due to underlying condition

N Newborn: 0   P Pediatric: 0-17   M Maternity: 9-64   A Adult: 15-124   `MCC` Major Complication/Comorbidity   `CC` Complication/Comorbidity   `SW` Severe Wound Dx

522

ICD-10-CM 2022

✓5ᵗʰ **E08.3** **Diabetes mellitus due to underlying condition with ophthalmic complications**
    AHA: 2016,4Q,11-13

One of the following 7th characters is to be assigned to codes in subcategories E08.32, E08.33, E08.34, E08.35, and E08.37 to designate laterality of the disease:
1   right eye
2   left eye
3   bilateral
9   unspecified eye

✓6ᵗʰ **E08.31** **Diabetes mellitus due to underlying condition with unspecified diabetic retinopathy**
    DEF: Diabetic retinopathy: Diabetic complication from damage to the retinal vessels resulting in vision problems that can progress to blindness.

    E08.311 *Diabetes mellitus due to underlying condition with unspecified diabetic retinopathy with macular edema* HCC

    E08.319 *Diabetes mellitus due to underlying condition with unspecified diabetic retinopathy without macular edema* HCC

✓6ᵗʰ **E08.32** **Diabetes mellitus due to underlying condition with mild nonproliferative diabetic retinopathy**
    Diabetes mellitus due to underlying condition with nonproliferative diabetic retinopathy NOS

    ✓7ᵗʰ *E08.321* *Diabetes mellitus due to underlying condition with mild nonproliferative diabetic retinopathy with macular edema* HCC

    ✓7ᵗʰ *E08.329* *Diabetes mellitus due to underlying condition with mild nonproliferative diabetic retinopathy without macular edema* HCC

✓6ᵗʰ **E08.33** **Diabetes mellitus due to underlying condition with moderate nonproliferative diabetic retinopathy**

    ✓7ᵗʰ *E08.331* *Diabetes mellitus due to underlying condition with moderate nonproliferative diabetic retinopathy with macular edema* HCC

    ✓7ᵗʰ *E08.339* *Diabetes mellitus due to underlying condition with moderate nonproliferative diabetic retinopathy without macular edema* HCC

✓6ᵗʰ **E08.34** **Diabetes mellitus due to underlying condition with severe nonproliferative diabetic retinopathy**

    ✓7ᵗʰ *E08.341* *Diabetes mellitus due to underlying condition with severe nonproliferative diabetic retinopathy with macular edema* HCC

    ✓7ᵗʰ *E08.349* *Diabetes mellitus due to underlying condition with severe nonproliferative diabetic retinopathy without macular edema* HCC

✓6ᵗʰ **E08.35** **Diabetes mellitus due to underlying condition with proliferative diabetic retinopathy**

    ✓7ᵗʰ *E08.351* *Diabetes mellitus due to underlying condition with proliferative diabetic retinopathy with macular edema* HCC

    ✓7ᵗʰ *E08.352* *Diabetes mellitus due to underlying condition with proliferative diabetic retinopathy with traction retinal detachment involving the macula* HCC

    ✓7ᵗʰ *E08.353* *Diabetes mellitus due to underlying condition with proliferative diabetic retinopathy with traction retinal detachment not involving the macula* HCC

    ✓7ᵗʰ *E08.354* *Diabetes mellitus due to underlying condition with proliferative diabetic retinopathy with combined traction retinal detachment and rhegmatogenous retinal detachment* HCC

    ✓7ᵗʰ *E08.355* *Diabetes mellitus due to underlying condition with stable proliferative diabetic retinopathy* HCC

    ✓7ᵗʰ *E08.359* *Diabetes mellitus due to underlying condition with proliferative diabetic retinopathy without macular edema* HCC

E08.36 *Diabetes mellitus due to underlying condition with diabetic cataract* HCC
    AHA: 2019,2Q,30-31; 2016,4Q,142

✓x7ᵗʰ **E08.37** *Diabetes mellitus due to underlying condition with diabetic macular edema, resolved following treatment* HCC

E08.39 *Diabetes mellitus due to underlying condition with other diabetic ophthalmic complication* HCC
    Use additional code to identify manifestation, such as:
    diabetic glaucoma (H40-H42)

✓5ᵗʰ **E08.4** **Diabetes mellitus due to underlying condition with neurological complications**

E08.40 *Diabetes mellitus due to underlying condition with diabetic neuropathy, unspecified* HCC

E08.41 *Diabetes mellitus due to underlying condition with diabetic mononeuropathy* HCC

E08.42 *Diabetes mellitus due to underlying condition with diabetic polyneuropathy* HCC
    Diabetes mellitus due to underlying condition with diabetic neuralgia

E08.43 *Diabetes mellitus due to underlying condition with diabetic autonomic (poly)neuropathy* HCC
    Diabetes mellitus due to underlying condition with diabetic gastroparesis
    AHA: 2013,4Q,114

E08.44 *Diabetes mellitus due to underlying condition with diabetic amyotrophy* HCC

E08.49 *Diabetes mellitus due to underlying condition with other diabetic neurological complication* HCC

✓5ᵗʰ **E08.5** **Diabetes mellitus due to underlying condition with circulatory complications**

E08.51 *Diabetes mellitus due to underlying condition with diabetic peripheral angiopathy without gangrene* HCC
    AHA: 2018,3Q,3-4; 2018,2Q,7

E08.52 *Diabetes mellitus due to underlying condition with diabetic peripheral angiopathy with gangrene* CC HCC
    Diabetes mellitus due to underlying condition with diabetic gangrene
    AHA: 2020,2Q,18; 2018,3Q,3; 2018,2Q,7; 2017,4Q,102

E08.59 *Diabetes mellitus due to underlying condition with other circulatory complications* HCC

✓5ᵗʰ **E08.6** **Diabetes mellitus due to underlying condition with other specified complications**

✓6ᵗʰ **E08.61** **Diabetes mellitus due to underlying condition with diabetic arthropathy**

    E08.610 *Diabetes mellitus due to underlying condition with diabetic neuropathic arthropathy* HCC
    Diabetes mellitus due to underlying condition with Charcôt's joints
    DEF: Charcot's joint: Progressive neurologic arthropathy in which chronic degeneration of joints in the weight-bearing areas with peripheral hypertrophy occurs as a complication of a neuropathy disorder. Supporting structures relax from a loss of sensation resulting in chronic joint instability.

    E08.618 *Diabetes mellitus due to underlying condition with other diabetic arthropathy* HCC
    AHA: 2018,2Q,6

✓6ᵗʰ **E08.62** **Diabetes mellitus due to underlying condition with skin complications**

    E08.620 *Diabetes mellitus due to underlying condition with diabetic dermatitis* HCC
    Diabetes mellitus due to underlying condition with diabetic necrobiosis lipoidica

    E08.621 *Diabetes mellitus due to underlying condition with foot ulcer* HCC
    Use additional code to identify site of ulcer (L97.4-, L97.5-)
    AHA: 2020,2Q,19

☑ Additional Character Required ✓7ᵗʰ Placeholder Questionable PDx Manifestation Unspecified Dx UPD Unacceptable PDx H1-H14 HAC HCC CMS-HCC Dx HIV HIV Dx

ICD-10-CM 2022   523

E08.622 **Diabetes mellitus due to underlying condition with other skin ulcer** HCC
Use additional code to identify site of ulcer (L97.1-L97.9, L98.41-L98.49)
AHA: 2021,1Q,7; 2017,4Q,17

E08.628 **Diabetes mellitus due to underlying condition with other skin complications** HCC

✓6th **E08.63** **Diabetes mellitus due to underlying condition with oral complications**

E08.630 **Diabetes mellitus due to underlying condition with** periodontal disease HCC

E08.638 **Diabetes mellitus due to underlying condition with other oral complications** HCC

✓6th **E08.64** **Diabetes mellitus due to underlying condition with** hypoglycemia
AHA: 2017,1Q,42

E08.641 **Diabetes mellitus due to underlying condition with hypoglycemia** with coma MCC HCC

E08.649 **Diabetes mellitus due to underlying condition with hypoglycemia** without coma HCC
AHA: 2016,3Q,42; 2015,3Q,21

E08.65 **Diabetes mellitus due to underlying condition with** hyperglycemia HCC
AHA: 2017,1Q,42; 2013,3Q,20

E08.69 **Diabetes mellitus due to underlying condition with other specified complication** HCC
Use additional code to identify complication
AHA: 2016,4Q,141; 2016,1Q,13

E08.8 **Diabetes mellitus due to underlying condition with unspecified complications** HCC

E08.9 **Diabetes mellitus due to underlying condition** without complications HCC
AHA: 2020,2Q,18

✓4th **E09** **Drug or chemical induced diabetes mellitus**
Code first poisoning due to drug or toxin, if applicable (T36-T65 with fifth or sixth character 1-4 or 6)
Use additional code for adverse effect, if applicable, to identify drug (T36-T50 with fifth or sixth character 5)
Use additional code to identify control using:
  insulin (Z79.4)
  oral antidiabetic drugs (Z79.84)
  oral hypoglycemic drugs (Z79.84)
EXCLUDES 1   diabetes mellitus due to underlying condition (E08.-)
    gestational diabetes (O24.4-)
    neonatal diabetes mellitus (P70.2)
    postpancreatectomy diabetes mellitus (E13.-)
    postprocedural diabetes mellitus (E13.-)
    secondary diabetes mellitus NEC (E13.-)
    type 1 diabetes mellitus (E10.-)
    type 2 diabetes mellitus (E11.-)

✓5th **E09.0** **Drug or chemical induced diabetes mellitus with** hyperosmolarity
DEF: Diabetic hyperosmolarity: Extremely high levels of glucose in the blood without ketones.

E09.00 **Drug or chemical induced diabetes mellitus with hyperosmolarity** without nonketotic hyperglycemic-hyperosmolar coma (NKHHC) MCC H9 HCC

E09.01 **Drug or chemical induced diabetes mellitus with hyperosmolarity** with coma MCC H9 HCC

✓5th **E09.1** **Drug or chemical induced diabetes mellitus with** ketoacidosis
DEF: Diabetic ketoacidosis: Potentially life-threatening complication due to a shortage of insulin in which the body switches to burning fatty acids and producing acidic ketone bodies.

E09.10 **Drug or chemical induced diabetes mellitus with ketoacidosis** without coma MCC H9 HCC

E09.11 **Drug or chemical induced diabetes mellitus with ketoacidosis** with coma MCC H9 HCC

✓5th **E09.2** **Drug or chemical induced diabetes mellitus with** kidney complications
AHA: 2019,3Q,3; 2018,4Q,88

E09.21 **Drug or chemical induced diabetes mellitus with diabetic** nephropathy HCC
Drug or chemical induced diabetes mellitus with intercapillary glomerulosclerosis
Drug or chemical induced diabetes mellitus with intracapillary glomerulonephrosis
Drug or chemical induced diabetes mellitus with Kimmelstiel-Wilson disease

E09.22 **Drug or chemical induced diabetes mellitus with diabetic** chronic kidney disease HCC
Use additional code to identify stage of chronic kidney disease (N18.1-N18.6)

E09.29 **Drug or chemical induced diabetes mellitus with other diabetic kidney complication** HCC
Drug or chemical induced diabetes mellitus with renal tubular degeneration

✓5th **E09.3** **Drug or chemical induced diabetes mellitus with** ophthalmic complications
AHA: 2016,4Q,11-13

One of the following 7th characters is to be assigned to codes in subcategories E09.32, E09.33, E09.34, E09.35, and E09.37 to designate laterality of the disease:
1   right eye
2   left eye
3   bilateral
9   unspecified eye

✓6th **E09.31** **Drug or chemical induced diabetes mellitus with unspecified diabetic** retinopathy
DEF: Diabetic retinopathy: Diabetic complication from damage to the retinal vessels resulting in vision problems that can progress to blindness.

E09.311 **Drug or chemical induced diabetes mellitus with unspecified diabetic retinopathy** with macular edema HCC

E09.319 **Drug or chemical induced diabetes mellitus with unspecified diabetic retinopathy** without macular edema HCC

E09.32 **Drug or chemical induced diabetes mellitus with** mild nonproliferative **diabetic** retinopathy
Drug or chemical induced diabetes mellitus with nonproliferative diabetic retinopathy NOS

✓7th **E09.321** **Drug or chemical induced diabetes mellitus with mild nonproliferative diabetic retinopathy** with macular edema HCC

✓7th **E09.329** **Drug or chemical induced diabetes mellitus with mild nonproliferative diabetic retinopathy** without macular edema HCC

✓6th **E09.33** **Drug or chemical induced diabetes mellitus with** moderate nonproliferative **diabetic** retinopathy

✓7th **E09.331** **Drug or chemical induced diabetes mellitus with moderate nonproliferative diabetic retinopathy** with macular edema HCC

✓7th **E09.339** **Drug or chemical induced diabetes mellitus with moderate nonproliferative diabetic retinopathy** without macular edema HCC

✓6th **E09.34** **Drug or chemical induced diabetes mellitus with** severe nonproliferative **diabetic** retinopathy

✓7th **E09.341** **Drug or chemical induced diabetes mellitus with severe nonproliferative diabetic retinopathy** with macular edema HCC

✓7th **E09.349** **Drug or chemical induced diabetes mellitus with severe nonproliferative diabetic retinopathy** without macular edema HCC

✓6th **E09.35** **Drug or chemical induced diabetes mellitus with** proliferative **diabetic** retinopathy

✓7th **E09.351** **Drug or chemical induced diabetes mellitus with proliferative diabetic retinopathy** with macular edema HCC

✓7th **E09.352** **Drug or chemical induced diabetes mellitus with proliferative diabetic retinopathy** with traction retinal detachment involving the macula HCC

✓7ᵗʰ **E09.353 Drug or chemical induced diabetes mellitus with proliferative diabetic retinopathy** with traction retinal detachment not involving the macula   HCC

✓7ᵗʰ **E09.354 Drug or chemical induced diabetes mellitus with proliferative diabetic retinopathy** with combined traction retinal detachment and rhegmatogenous retinal detachment   HCC

✓7ᵗʰ **E09.355 Drug or chemical induced diabetes mellitus** with stable **proliferative diabetic retinopathy**   HCC

✓7ᵗʰ **E09.359 Drug or chemical induced diabetes mellitus with proliferative diabetic retinopathy** without macular edema   HCC

E09.36 Drug or chemical induced diabetes mellitus with diabetic cataract   HCC
AHA: 2019,2Q,30-31; 2016,4Q,142

✓x7ᵗʰ **E09.37 Drug or chemical induced diabetes mellitus with diabetic** macular edema, resolved following treatment   HCC

E09.39 Drug or chemical induced diabetes mellitus with other diabetic ophthalmic complication   HCC
Use additional code to identify manifestation, such as:
diabetic glaucoma (H40-H42)

✓5ᵗʰ **E09.4 Drug or chemical induced diabetes mellitus with** neurological complications

E09.40 Drug or chemical induced diabetes mellitus with neurological complications with diabetic neuropathy, unspecified   HCC

E09.41 Drug or chemical induced diabetes mellitus with neurological complications with diabetic mononeuropathy   HCC

E09.42 Drug or chemical induced diabetes mellitus with neurological complications with diabetic polyneuropathy   HCC
Drug or chemical induced diabetes mellitus with diabetic neuralgia

E09.43 Drug or chemical induced diabetes mellitus with neurological complications with diabetic autonomic (poly)neuropathy   HCC
Drug or chemical induced diabetes mellitus with diabetic gastroparesis
AHA: 2013,4Q,114

E09.44 Drug or chemical induced diabetes mellitus with neurological complications with diabetic amyotrophy   HCC

E09.49 Drug or chemical induced diabetes mellitus with neurological complications with other diabetic neurological complication   HCC

✓5ᵗʰ **E09.5 Drug or chemical induced diabetes mellitus with** circulatory complications

E09.51 Drug or chemical induced diabetes mellitus with diabetic peripheral angiopathy without gangrene   HCC
AHA: 2018,3Q,3-4; 2018,2Q,7

E09.52 Drug or chemical induced diabetes mellitus with diabetic peripheral angiopathy with gangrene   CC HCC
Drug or chemical induced diabetes mellitus with diabetic gangrene
AHA: 2020,2Q,18; 2018,3Q,3; 2018,2Q,7; 2017,4Q,102

E09.59 Drug or chemical induced diabetes mellitus with other circulatory complications   HCC

✓5ᵗʰ **E09.6 Drug or chemical induced diabetes mellitus with other specified complications**

✓6ᵗʰ **E09.61 Drug or chemical induced diabetes mellitus with** diabetic arthropathy

E09.610 Drug or chemical induced diabetes mellitus with diabetic neuropathic arthropathy   HCC
Drug or chemical induced diabetes mellitus with Charcôt's joints
DEF: Charcot's joint: Progressive neurologic arthropathy in which chronic degeneration of joints in the weight-bearing areas with peripheral hypertrophy occurs as a complication of a neuropathy disorder. Supporting structures relax from a loss of sensation resulting in chronic joint instability.

E09.618 Drug or chemical induced diabetes mellitus with other diabetic arthropathy   HCC
AHA: 2018,2Q,6

✓6ᵗʰ **E09.62 Drug or chemical induced diabetes mellitus with** skin complications

E09.620 Drug or chemical induced diabetes mellitus with diabetic dermatitis   HCC
Drug or chemical induced diabetes mellitus with diabetic necrobiosis lipoidica

E09.621 Drug or chemical induced diabetes mellitus with foot ulcer   HCC
Use additional code to identify site of ulcer (L97.4-, L97.5-)
AHA: 2020,2Q,19

E09.622 Drug or chemical induced diabetes mellitus with other skin ulcer   HCC
Use additional code to identify site of ulcer (L97.1-L97.9, L98.41-L98.49)
AHA: 2021,1Q,7; 2017,4Q,17

E09.628 Drug or chemical induced diabetes mellitus with other skin complications   HCC

✓6ᵗʰ **E09.63 Drug or chemical induced diabetes mellitus with** oral complications

E09.630 Drug or chemical induced diabetes mellitus with periodontal disease   HCC

E09.638 Drug or chemical induced diabetes mellitus with other oral complications   HCC

✓6ᵗʰ **E09.64 Drug or chemical induced diabetes mellitus with** hypoglycemia
AHA: 2017,1Q,42

E09.641 Drug or chemical induced diabetes mellitus with hypoglycemia with coma   MCC HCC

E09.649 Drug or chemical induced diabetes mellitus with hypoglycemia without coma   HCC
AHA: 2016,3Q,42; 2015,3Q,21

E09.65 Drug or chemical induced diabetes mellitus with hyperglycemia   HCC
AHA: 2017,1Q,42; 2013,3Q,20

E09.69 Drug or chemical induced diabetes mellitus with other specified complication   HCC
Use additional code to identify complication
AHA: 2016,4Q,141; 2016,1Q,13

E09.8 Drug or chemical induced diabetes mellitus with unspecified complications   HCC

E09.9 Drug or chemical induced diabetes mellitus without complications   HCC
AHA: 2020,2Q,18

Chapter 4. Endocrine, Nutritional and Metabolic Diseases

E09.353–E09.9

Chapter 4. Endocrine, Nutritional and Metabolic Diseases

E10–E10.59

✓4ᵗʰ **E10 Type 1 diabetes mellitus**

INCLUDES
- brittle diabetes (mellitus)
- diabetes (mellitus) due to autoimmune process
- diabetes (mellitus) due to immune mediated pancreatic islet beta-cell destruction
- idiopathic diabetes (mellitus)
- juvenile onset diabetes (mellitus)
- ketosis-prone diabetes (mellitus)

EXCLUDES 1
- *diabetes mellitus due to underlying condition (E08.-)*
- *drug or chemical induced diabetes mellitus (E09.-)*
- *gestational diabetes (O24.4-)*
- *hyperglycemia NOS (R73.9)*
- *neonatal diabetes mellitus (P70.2)*
- *postpancreatectomy diabetes mellitus (E13.-)*
- *postprocedural diabetes mellitus (E13.-)*
- *secondary diabetes mellitus NEC (E13.-)*
- *type 2 diabetes mellitus (E11.-)*

AHA: 2020,3Q,30

✓5ᵗʰ **E10.1 Type 1 diabetes mellitus with ketoacidosis**

AHA: 2013,3Q,20

DEF: Diabetic ketoacidosis: Potentially life-threatening complication due to a shortage of insulin in which the body switches to burning fatty acids and producing acidic ketone bodies.

E10.10 Type 1 diabetes mellitus with ketoacidosis without coma MCC H9 HCC

E10.11 Type 1 diabetes mellitus with ketoacidosis with coma MCC H9 HCC

✓5ᵗʰ **E10.2 Type 1 diabetes mellitus with kidney complications**

AHA: 2019,3Q,3; 2018,4Q,88

E10.21 Type 1 diabetes mellitus with diabetic nephropathy HCC

- Type 1 diabetes mellitus with intercapillary glomerulosclerosis
- Type 1 diabetes mellitus with intracapillary glomerulonephrosis
- Type 1 diabetes mellitus with Kimmelstiel-Wilson disease

E10.22 Type 1 diabetes mellitus with diabetic chronic kidney disease HCC

Use additional code to identify stage of chronic kidney disease (N18.1-N18.6)

E10.29 Type 1 diabetes mellitus with other diabetic kidney complication HCC

- Type 1 diabetes mellitus with renal tubular degeneration

AHA: 2016,1Q,13

✓5ᵗʰ **E10.3 Type 1 diabetes mellitus with ophthalmic complications**

AHA: 2016,4Q,11-13

One of the following 7th characters is to be assigned to codes in subcategories E10.32, E10.33, E10.34, E10.35, and E10.37 to designate laterality of the disease:
1. right eye
2. left eye
3. bilateral
9. unspecified eye

✓6ᵗʰ **E10.31 Type 1 diabetes mellitus with unspecified diabetic retinopathy**

DEF: Diabetic retinopathy: Diabetic complication from damage to the retinal vessels resulting in vision problems that can progress to blindness.

E10.311 Type 1 diabetes mellitus with unspecified diabetic retinopathy with macular edema HCC

E10.319 Type 1 diabetes mellitus with unspecified diabetic retinopathy without macular edema HCC

✓6ᵗʰ **E10.32 Type 1 diabetes mellitus with mild nonproliferative diabetic retinopathy**

- Type 1 diabetes mellitus with nonproliferative diabetic retinopathy NOS

✓7ᵗʰ **E10.321 Type 1 diabetes mellitus with mild nonproliferative diabetic retinopathy with macular edema** HCC

✓7ᵗʰ **E10.329 Type 1 diabetes mellitus with mild nonproliferative diabetic retinopathy without macular edema** HCC

✓6ᵗʰ **E10.33 Type 1 diabetes mellitus with moderate nonproliferative diabetic retinopathy**

✓7ᵗʰ **E10.331 Type 1 diabetes mellitus with moderate nonproliferative diabetic retinopathy with macular edema** HCC

✓7ᵗʰ **E10.339 Type 1 diabetes mellitus with moderate nonproliferative diabetic retinopathy without macular edema** HCC

✓6ᵗʰ **E10.34 Type 1 diabetes mellitus with severe nonproliferative diabetic retinopathy**

✓7ᵗʰ **E10.341 Type 1 diabetes mellitus with severe nonproliferative diabetic retinopathy with macular edema** HCC

✓7ᵗʰ **E10.349 Type 1 diabetes mellitus with severe nonproliferative diabetic retinopathy without macular edema** HCC

✓6ᵗʰ **E10.35 Type 1 diabetes mellitus with proliferative diabetic retinopathy**

✓7ᵗʰ **E10.351 Type 1 diabetes mellitus with proliferative diabetic retinopathy with macular edema** HCC

✓7ᵗʰ **E10.352 Type 1 diabetes mellitus with proliferative diabetic retinopathy with traction retinal detachment involving the macula** HCC

✓7ᵗʰ **E10.353 Type 1 diabetes mellitus with proliferative diabetic retinopathy with traction retinal detachment not involving the macula** HCC

✓7ᵗʰ **E10.354 Type 1 diabetes mellitus with proliferative diabetic retinopathy with combined traction retinal detachment and rhegmatogenous retinal detachment** HCC

✓7ᵗʰ **E10.355 Type 1 diabetes mellitus with stable proliferative diabetic retinopathy** HCC

✓7ᵗʰ **E10.359 Type 1 diabetes mellitus with proliferative diabetic retinopathy without macular edema** HCC

E10.36 Type 1 diabetes mellitus with diabetic cataract HCC

AHA: 2019,2Q,30-31; 2016,4Q,142

✓x7ᵗʰ **E10.37 Type 1 diabetes mellitus with diabetic macular edema, resolved following treatment** HCC

E10.39 Type 1 diabetes mellitus with other diabetic ophthalmic complication HCC

Use additional code to identify manifestation, such as:
- diabetic glaucoma (H40-H42)

✓5ᵗʰ **E10.4 Type 1 diabetes mellitus with neurological complications**

E10.40 Type 1 diabetes mellitus with diabetic neuropathy, unspecified HCC

E10.41 Type 1 diabetes mellitus with diabetic mononeuropathy HCC

E10.42 Type 1 diabetes mellitus with diabetic polyneuropathy HCC

- Type 1 diabetes mellitus with diabetic neuralgia

E10.43 Type 1 diabetes mellitus with diabetic autonomic (poly)neuropathy HCC

- Type 1 diabetes mellitus with diabetic gastroparesis

AHA: 2013,4Q,114

E10.44 Type 1 diabetes mellitus with diabetic amyotrophy HCC

E10.49 Type 1 diabetes mellitus with other diabetic neurological complication HCC

✓5ᵗʰ **E10.5 Type 1 diabetes mellitus with circulatory complications**

E10.51 Type 1 diabetes mellitus with diabetic peripheral angiopathy without gangrene HCC

AHA: 2018,3Q,3-4; 2018,2Q,7

E10.52 Type 1 diabetes mellitus with diabetic peripheral angiopathy with gangrene CC HCC

- Type 1 diabetes mellitus with diabetic gangrene

AHA: 2020,2Q,18; 2018,3Q,3; 2018,2Q,7; 2017,4Q,102

E10.59 Type 1 diabetes mellitus with other circulatory complications HCC

N Newborn: 0   P Pediatric: 0-17   M Maternity: 9-64   A Adult: 15-124   MCC Major Complication/Comorbidity   CC Complication/Comorbidity   SW Severe Wound Dx

526

ICD-10-CM 2022

✓5ᵗʰ **E10.6   Type 1 diabetes mellitus with other specified complications**

✓6ᵗʰ **E10.61   Type 1 diabetes mellitus with diabetic arthropathy**

E10.610   Type 1 diabetes mellitus with diabetic neuropathic arthropathy   HCC

Type 1 diabetes mellitus with Charcôt's joints

DEF: Charcot's joint: Progressive neurologic arthropathy in which chronic degeneration of joints in the weight-bearing areas with peripheral hypertrophy occurs as a complication of a neuropathy disorder. Supporting structures relax from a loss of sensation resulting in chronic joint instability.

E10.618   Type 1 diabetes mellitus with other diabetic arthropathy   HCC

AHA: 2018,2Q,6

✓6ᵗʰ **E10.62   Type 1 diabetes mellitus with skin complications**

E10.620   Type 1 diabetes mellitus with diabetic dermatitis   HCC

Type 1 diabetes mellitus with diabetic necrobiosis lipoidica

E10.621   Type 1 diabetes mellitus with foot ulcer   HCC

Use additional code to identify site of ulcer (L97.4-, L97.5-)

AHA: 2020,2Q,19

E10.622   Type 1 diabetes mellitus with other skin ulcer   HCC

Use additional code to identify site of ulcer (L97.1-L97.9, L98.41-L98.49)

AHA: 2021,1Q,7; 2017,4Q,17

E10.628   Type 1 diabetes mellitus with other skin complications   HCC

✓6ᵗʰ **E10.63   Type 1 diabetes mellitus with oral complications**

E10.630   Type 1 diabetes mellitus with periodontal disease   HCC

E10.638   Type 1 diabetes mellitus with other oral complications   HCC

✓6ᵗʰ **E10.64   Type 1 diabetes mellitus with hypoglycemia**

AHA: 2017,1Q,42

E10.641   Type 1 diabetes mellitus with hypoglycemia with coma   MCC HCC

E10.649   Type 1 diabetes mellitus with hypoglycemia without coma   HCC

AHA: 2016,3Q,42; 2016,1Q,13; 2015,3Q,21

E10.65   Type 1 diabetes mellitus with hyperglycemia   HCC

AHA: 2017,1Q,42; 2013,3Q,20

E10.69   Type 1 diabetes mellitus with other specified complication   HCC

Use additional code to identify complication

AHA: 2016,4Q,141; 2016,1Q,13

E10.8   Type 1 diabetes mellitus with unspecified complications   HCC

E10.9   Type 1 diabetes mellitus without complications   HCC

AHA: 2020,2Q,18

✓4ᵗʰ **E11   Type 2 diabetes mellitus**

INCLUDES   diabetes (mellitus) due to insulin secretory defect

diabetes NOS

insulin resistant diabetes (mellitus)

Use additional code to identify control using:

insulin (Z79.4)

oral antidiabetic drugs (Z79.84)

oral hypoglycemic drugs (Z79.84)

EXCLUDES 1   *diabetes mellitus due to underlying condition (E08.-)*

drug or chemical induced diabetes mellitus (E09.-)

gestational diabetes (O24.4-)

neonatal diabetes mellitus (P70.2)

postpancreatectomy diabetes mellitus (E13.-)

postprocedural diabetes mellitus (E13.-)

secondary diabetes mellitus NEC (E13.-)

type 1 diabetes mellitus (E10.-)

AHA: 2020,3Q,30; 2020,1Q,12; 2016,2Q,10; 2013,1Q,26

✓5ᵗʰ **E11.0   Type 2 diabetes mellitus with hyperosmolarity**

DEF: Diabetic hyperosmolarity: Extremely high levels of glucose in the blood without ketones.

E11.00   Type 2 diabetes mellitus with hyperosmolarity without nonketotic hyperglycemic-hyperosmolar coma (NKHHC)   MCC H9 HCC

E11.01   Type 2 diabetes mellitus with hyperosmolarity with coma   MCC H9 HCC

✓5ᵗʰ **E11.1   Type 2 diabetes mellitus with ketoacidosis**

AHA: 2017,4Q,6

DEF: Diabetic ketoacidosis: Potentially life-threatening complication due to a shortage of insulin in which the body switches to burning fatty acids and producing acidic ketone bodies.

E11.10   Type 2 diabetes mellitus with ketoacidosis without coma   MCC H9 HCC

E11.11   Type 2 diabetes mellitus with ketoacidosis with coma   MCC H9 HCC

✓5ᵗʰ **E11.2   Type 2 diabetes mellitus with kidney complications**

AHA: 2019,3Q,3; 2018,4Q,88

E11.21   Type 2 diabetes mellitus with diabetic nephropathy   HCC

Type 2 diabetes mellitus with intercapillary glomerulosclerosis

Type 2 diabetes mellitus with intracapillary glomerulonephrosis

Type 2 diabetes mellitus with Kimmelstiel-Wilson disease

E11.22   Type 2 diabetes mellitus with diabetic chronic kidney disease   HCC

Use additional code to identify stage of chronic kidney disease (N18.1-N18.6)

E11.29   Type 2 diabetes mellitus with other diabetic kidney complication   HCC

Type 2 diabetes mellitus with renal tubular degeneration

✓5ᵗʰ **E11.3   Type 2 diabetes mellitus with ophthalmic complications**

AHA: 2016,4Q,11-13

One of the following 7th characters is to be assigned to codes in subcategories E11.32, E11.33, E11.34, E11.35, and E11.37 to designate laterality of the disease:

1   right eye
2   left eye
3   bilateral
9   unspecified eye

✓6ᵗʰ **E11.31   Type 2 diabetes mellitus with unspecified diabetic retinopathy**

DEF: Diabetic retinopathy: Diabetic complication from damage to the retinal vessels resulting in vision problems that can progress to blindness.

E11.311   Type 2 diabetes mellitus with unspecified diabetic retinopathy with macular edema   HCC

E11.319   Type 2 diabetes mellitus with unspecified diabetic retinopathy without macular edema   HCC

☑ Additional Character Required   ✓x7ᵗʰ Placeholder   Questionable PDx   Manifestation   Unspecified Dx   UPD Unacceptable PDx   H1-H14 HAC   HCC CMS-HCC Dx   HIV HIV Dx

ICD-10-CM 2022   **527**

Chapter 4. Endocrine, Nutritional and Metabolic Diseases

E11.32–E11.9

✓6ᵗʰ **E11.32** **Type 2 diabetes mellitus with** mild nonproliferative diabetic retinopathy
Type 2 diabetes mellitus with nonproliferative diabetic retinopathy NOS

     ✓7ᵗʰ **E11.321** **Type 2 diabetes mellitus with mild nonproliferative diabetic retinopathy with macular edema** `HCC`

     ✓7ᵗʰ **E11.329** **Type 2 diabetes mellitus with mild nonproliferative diabetic retinopathy without macular edema** `HCC`

✓6ᵗʰ **E11.33** **Type 2 diabetes mellitus with** moderate nonproliferative diabetic retinopathy

     ✓7ᵗʰ **E11.331** **Type 2 diabetes mellitus with moderate nonproliferative diabetic retinopathy with macular edema** `HCC`

     ✓7ᵗʰ **E11.339** **Type 2 diabetes mellitus with moderate nonproliferative diabetic retinopathy without macular edema** `HCC`

✓6ᵗʰ **E11.34** **Type 2 diabetes mellitus with** severe nonproliferative diabetic retinopathy

     ✓7ᵗʰ **E11.341** **Type 2 diabetes mellitus with severe nonproliferative diabetic retinopathy with macular edema** `HCC`

     ✓7ᵗʰ **E11.349** **Type 2 diabetes mellitus with severe nonproliferative diabetic retinopathy without macular edema** `HCC`

✓6ᵗʰ **E11.35** **Type 2 diabetes mellitus with** proliferative **diabetic retinopathy**

     ✓7ᵗʰ **E11.351** **Type 2 diabetes mellitus with proliferative diabetic retinopathy with macular edema** `HCC`

     ✓7ᵗʰ **E11.352** **Type 2 diabetes mellitus with proliferative diabetic retinopathy with traction retinal detachment involving the macula** `HCC`

     ✓7ᵗʰ **E11.353** **Type 2 diabetes mellitus with proliferative diabetic retinopathy with traction retinal detachment not involving the macula** `HCC`

     ✓7ᵗʰ **E11.354** **Type 2 diabetes mellitus with proliferative diabetic retinopathy with combined traction retinal detachment and rhegmatogenous retinal detachment** `HCC`

     ✓7ᵗʰ **E11.355** **Type 2 diabetes mellitus with stable proliferative diabetic retinopathy** `HCC`

     ✓7ᵗʰ **E11.359** **Type 2 diabetes mellitus with proliferative diabetic retinopathy without macular edema** `HCC`

E11.36 **Type 2 diabetes mellitus with diabetic cataract** `HCC`
AHA: 2019,2Q,30-31; 2016,4Q,142

✓x7ᵗʰ **E11.37** **Type 2 diabetes mellitus with diabetic** macular edema, resolved following treatment `HCC`

E11.39 **Type 2 diabetes mellitus with other diabetic ophthalmic complication** `HCC`
Use additional code to identify manifestation, such as:
diabetic glaucoma (H40-H42)

✓5ᵗʰ **E11.4** **Type 2 diabetes mellitus with** neurological complications

     E11.40 **Type 2 diabetes mellitus with diabetic** neuropathy, unspecified `HCC`
AHA: 2013,4Q,129

     E11.41 **Type 2 diabetes mellitus with diabetic mononeuropathy** `HCC`

     E11.42 **Type 2 diabetes mellitus with diabetic polyneuropathy** `HCC`
Type 2 diabetes mellitus with diabetic neuralgia
AHA: 2020,1Q,12

     E11.43 **Type 2 diabetes mellitus with diabetic** autonomic (poly)neuropathy `HCC`
Type 2 diabetes mellitus with diabetic gastroparesis
AHA: 2013,4Q,114

     E11.44 **Type 2 diabetes mellitus with diabetic amyotrophy** `HCC`

     E11.49 **Type 2 diabetes mellitus with other diabetic neurological complication** `HCC`

✓5ᵗʰ **E11.5** **Type 2 diabetes mellitus with** circulatory complications

     E11.51 **Type 2 diabetes mellitus with diabetic** peripheral angiopathy without gangrene `HCC`
AHA: 2018,3Q,3-4; 2018,2Q,7

     E11.52 **Type 2 diabetes mellitus with diabetic** peripheral angiopathy with gangrene `CC` `HCC`
Type 2 diabetes mellitus with diabetic gangrene
AHA: 2020,2Q,18; 2018,3Q,3; 2018,2Q,7; 2017,4Q,102

     E11.59 **Type 2 diabetes mellitus with other circulatory complications** `HCC`

✓5ᵗʰ **E11.6** **Type 2 diabetes mellitus with other specified complications**

     ✓6ᵗʰ **E11.61** **Type 2 diabetes mellitus with diabetic** arthropathy

         E11.610 **Type 2 diabetes mellitus with diabetic** neuropathic **arthropathy** `HCC`
Type 2 diabetes mellitus with Charcôt's joints
DEF: Charcot's joint: Progressive neurologic arthropathy in which chronic degeneration of joints in the weight-bearing areas with peripheral hypertrophy occurs as a complication of a neuropathy disorder. Supporting structures relax from a loss of sensation resulting in chronic joint instability.

         E11.618 **Type 2 diabetes mellitus with other diabetic arthropathy** `HCC`
AHA: 2018,2Q,6

     ✓6ᵗʰ **E11.62** **Type 2 diabetes mellitus with** skin complications

         E11.620 **Type 2 diabetes mellitus with** diabetic dermatitis `HCC`
Type 2 diabetes mellitus with diabetic necrobiosis lipoidica

         E11.621 **Type 2 diabetes mellitus with** foot ulcer `HCC`
Use additional code to identify site of ulcer (L97.4-, L97.5-)
AHA: 2020,2Q,19; 2020,1Q,12

         E11.622 **Type 2 diabetes mellitus with other skin ulcer** `HCC`
Use additional code to identify site of ulcer (L97.1-L97.9, L98.41-L98.49)
AHA: 2021,1Q,7; 2017,4Q,17

         E11.628 **Type 2 diabetes mellitus with other skin complications** `HCC`

     ✓6ᵗʰ **E11.63** **Type 2 diabetes mellitus with** oral complications

         E11.630 **Type 2 diabetes mellitus with** periodontal disease `HCC`

         E11.638 **Type 2 diabetes mellitus with other oral complications** `HCC`

     ✓6ᵗʰ **E11.64** **Type 2 diabetes mellitus with** hypoglycemia
AHA: 2017,1Q,42

         E11.641 **Type 2 diabetes mellitus with hypoglycemia** with coma `MCC` `HCC`

         E11.649 **Type 2 diabetes mellitus with hypoglycemia** without coma `HCC`
AHA: 2016,3Q,42; 2015,3Q,21

     E11.65 **Type 2 diabetes mellitus with** hyperglycemia `HCC`
AHA: 2017,1Q,42; 2013,3Q,20

     E11.69 **Type 2 diabetes mellitus with other specified complication** `HCC`
Use additional code to identify complication
AHA: 2020,1Q,12; 2016,4Q,141; 2016,1Q,13

E11.8 **Type 2 diabetes mellitus with unspecified complications** `HCC`

E11.9 **Type 2 diabetes mellitus** without complications `HCC`
AHA: 2020,2Q,18

✓4ᵗʰ E13   Other specified diabetes mellitus

     INCLUDES   diabetes mellitus due to genetic defects of beta-cell function
                   diabetes mellitus due to genetic defects in insulin action
                   postpancreatectomy diabetes mellitus
                   postprocedural diabetes mellitus
                   secondary diabetes mellitus NEC

     Use additional code to identify control using:
         insulin (Z79.4)
         oral antidiabetic drugs (Z79.84)
         oral hypoglycemic drugs (Z79.84)

     EXCLUDES 1   *diabetes (mellitus) due to autoimmune process (E10.-)*
                   diabetes (mellitus) due to immune mediated pancreatic islet beta-cell destruction (E10.-)
                   diabetes mellitus due to underlying condition (E08.-)
                   drug or chemical induced diabetes mellitus (E09.-)
                   gestational diabetes (O24.4-)
                   neonatal diabetes mellitus (P70.2)
                   type 1 diabetes mellitus (E10.-)

     AHA: 2018,3Q,4; 2016,1Q,11-13

     TIP: Use this category when the diabetes is documented as diabetes type 1.5. Synonymous terms used in the documentation may also include combined diabetes type 1 and type 2, latent autoimmune diabetes of adults (LADA), slow-progressing type 1 diabetes, or double diabetes.

     TIP: When postprocedural or postpancreatectomy hypoinsulinemia (E89.1) is documented with postprocedural or postpancreatectomy diabetes mellitus (E13.-), code E89.1 should be sequenced first.

✓5ᵗʰ E13.0   Other specified diabetes mellitus with hyperosmolarity
     DEF: Diabetic hyperosmolarity: Extremely high levels of glucose in the blood without ketones.

     E13.00   Other specified diabetes mellitus with hyperosmolarity without nonketotic hyperglycemic-hyperosmolar coma (NKHHC)   MCC   H9   HCC
         EXCLUDES 2   *type 2 diabetes mellitus (E11.-)*

     E13.01   Other specified diabetes mellitus with hyperosmolarity with coma   MCC   H9   HCC

✓5ᵗʰ E13.1   Other specified diabetes mellitus with ketoacidosis
     AHA: 2016,2Q,10; 2013,1Q,26
     DEF: Diabetic ketoacidosis: Potentially life-threatening complication due to a shortage of insulin in which the body switches to burning fatty acids and producing acidic ketone bodies.

     E13.10   Other specified diabetes mellitus with ketoacidosis without coma   MCC   H9   HCC

     E13.11   Other specified diabetes mellitus with ketoacidosis with coma   MCC   H9   HCC

✓5ᵗʰ E13.2   Other specified diabetes mellitus with kidney complications
     AHA: 2019,3Q,3; 2018,4Q,88

     E13.21   Other specified diabetes mellitus with diabetic nephropathy   HCC
         Other specified diabetes mellitus with intercapillary glomerulosclerosis
         Other specified diabetes mellitus with intracapillary glomerulonephrosis
         Other specified diabetes mellitus with Kimmelstiel-Wilson disease

     E13.22   Other specified diabetes mellitus with diabetic chronic kidney disease   HCC
         Use additional code to identify stage of chronic kidney disease (N18.1-N18.6)

     E13.29   Other specified diabetes mellitus with other diabetic kidney complication   HCC
         Other specified diabetes mellitus with renal tubular degeneration

✓5ᵗʰ E13.3   Other specified diabetes mellitus with ophthalmic complications
     AHA: 2016,4Q,11-13

     One of the following 7th characters is to be assigned to codes in subcategories E13.32, E13.33, E13.34, E13.35, and E13.37 to designate laterality of the disease:
     1   right eye
     2   left eye
     3   bilateral
     9   unspecified eye

     ✓6ᵗʰ E13.31   Other specified diabetes mellitus with unspecified diabetic retinopathy
         DEF: Diabetic retinopathy: Diabetic complication from damage to the retinal vessels resulting in vision problems that can progress to blindness.

         E13.311   Other specified diabetes mellitus with unspecified diabetic retinopathy with macular edema   HCC

         E13.319   Other specified diabetes mellitus with unspecified diabetic retinopathy without macular edema   HCC

     ✓6ᵗʰ E13.32   Other specified diabetes mellitus with mild nonproliferative diabetic retinopathy
         Other specified diabetes mellitus with nonproliferative diabetic retinopathy NOS

         ✓7ᵗʰ E13.321   Other specified diabetes mellitus with mild nonproliferative diabetic retinopathy with macular edema   HCC

         ✓7ᵗʰ E13.329   Other specified diabetes mellitus with mild nonproliferative diabetic retinopathy without macular edema   HCC

     ✓6ᵗʰ E13.33   Other specified diabetes mellitus with moderate nonproliferative diabetic retinopathy

         ✓7ᵗʰ E13.331   Other specified diabetes mellitus with moderate nonproliferative diabetic retinopathy with macular edema   HCC

         ✓7ᵗʰ E13.339   Other specified diabetes mellitus with moderate nonproliferative diabetic retinopathy without macular edema   HCC

     ✓6ᵗʰ E13.34   Other specified diabetes mellitus with severe nonproliferative diabetic retinopathy

         ✓7ᵗʰ E13.341   Other specified diabetes mellitus with severe nonproliferative diabetic retinopathy with macular edema   HCC

         ✓7ᵗʰ E13.349   Other specified diabetes mellitus with severe nonproliferative diabetic retinopathy without macular edema   HCC

     ✓6ᵗʰ E13.35   Other specified diabetes mellitus with proliferative diabetic retinopathy

         ✓7ᵗʰ E13.351   Other specified diabetes mellitus with proliferative diabetic retinopathy with macular edema   HCC

         ✓7ᵗʰ E13.352   Other specified diabetes mellitus with proliferative diabetic retinopathy with traction retinal detachment involving the macula   HCC

         ✓7ᵗʰ E13.353   Other specified diabetes mellitus with proliferative diabetic retinopathy with traction retinal detachment not involving the macula   HCC

         ✓7ᵗʰ E13.354   Other specified diabetes mellitus with proliferative diabetic retinopathy with combined traction retinal detachment and rhegmatogenous retinal detachment   HCC

         ✓7ᵗʰ E13.355   Other specified diabetes mellitus with stable proliferative diabetic retinopathy   HCC

         ✓7ᵗʰ E13.359   Other specified diabetes mellitus with proliferative diabetic retinopathy without macular edema   HCC

     E13.36   Other specified diabetes mellitus with diabetic cataract   HCC
         AHA: 2019,2Q,30-31; 2016,4Q,142

     ✓x7ᵗʰ E13.37   Other specified diabetes mellitus with diabetic macular edema, resolved following treatment   HCC

Chapter 4. Endocrine, Nutritional and Metabolic Diseases

E13.39   Other specified diabetes mellitus with other diabetic ophthalmic complication   HCC
     Use additional code to identify manifestation, such as:
         diabetic glaucoma (H40-H42)

✓5ᵗʰ **E13.4   Other specified diabetes mellitus with neurological complications**

    E13.40   Other specified diabetes mellitus with diabetic neuropathy, unspecified   HCC

    E13.41   Other specified diabetes mellitus with diabetic mononeuropathy   HCC

    E13.42   Other specified diabetes mellitus with diabetic polyneuropathy   HCC
       Other specified diabetes mellitus with diabetic neuralgia

    E13.43   Other specified diabetes mellitus with diabetic autonomic (poly)neuropathy   HCC
       Other specified diabetes mellitus with diabetic gastroparesis
       AHA: 2013,4Q,114

    E13.44   Other specified diabetes mellitus with diabetic amyotrophy   HCC

    E13.49   Other specified diabetes mellitus with other diabetic neurological complication   HCC

✓5ᵗʰ **E13.5   Other specified diabetes mellitus with circulatory complications**

    E13.51   Other specified diabetes mellitus with diabetic peripheral angiopathy without gangrene   HCC
       AHA: 2018,3Q,3-4; 2018,2Q,7

    E13.52   Other specified diabetes mellitus with diabetic peripheral angiopathy with gangrene   CC HCC
       Other specified diabetes mellitus with diabetic gangrene
       AHA: 2020,2Q,18; 2018,3Q,3; 2018,2Q,7; 2017,4Q,102

    E13.59   Other specified diabetes mellitus with other circulatory complications   HCC

✓5ᵗʰ **E13.6   Other specified diabetes mellitus with other specified complications**

    ✓6ᵗʰ **E13.61   Other specified diabetes mellitus with diabetic arthropathy**

       E13.610   Other specified diabetes mellitus with diabetic neuropathic arthropathy   HCC
          Other specified diabetes mellitus with Charcôt's joints
          DEF: Charcôt's joint: Progressive neurologic arthropathy in which chronic degeneration of joints in the weight-bearing areas with peripheral hypertrophy occurs as a complication of a neuropathy disorder. Supporting structures relax from a loss of sensation resulting in chronic joint instability.

       E13.618   Other specified diabetes mellitus with other diabetic arthropathy   HCC
          AHA: 2018,2Q,6

    ✓6ᵗʰ **E13.62   Other specified diabetes mellitus with skin complications**

       E13.620   Other specified diabetes mellitus with diabetic dermatitis   HCC
          Other specified diabetes mellitus with diabetic necrobiosis lipoidica

       E13.621   Other specified diabetes mellitus with foot ulcer   HCC
          Use additional code to identify site of ulcer (L97.4-, L97.5-)
          AHA: 2020,2Q,19

       E13.622   Other specified diabetes mellitus with other skin ulcer   HCC
          Use additional code to identify site of ulcer (L97.1-L97.9, L98.41-L98.49)
          AHA: 2021,1Q,7; 2017,4Q,17

       E13.628   Other specified diabetes mellitus with other skin complications   HCC

    ✓6ᵗʰ **E13.63   Other specified diabetes mellitus with oral complications**

       E13.630   Other specified diabetes mellitus with periodontal disease   HCC

       E13.638   Other specified diabetes mellitus with other oral complications   HCC

    ✓6ᵗʰ **E13.64   Other specified diabetes mellitus with hypoglycemia**
       AHA: 2017,1Q,42

       E13.641   Other specified diabetes mellitus with hypoglycemia with coma   MCC HCC

       E13.649   Other specified diabetes mellitus with hypoglycemia without coma   HCC
          AHA: 2016,3Q,42; 2015,3Q,21

    E13.65   Other specified diabetes mellitus with hyperglycemia   HCC
       AHA: 2017,1Q,42; 2013,3Q,20

    E13.69   Other specified diabetes mellitus with other specified complication   HCC
       Use additional code to identify complication
       AHA: 2016,4Q,141; 2016,1Q,13

E13.8   Other specified diabetes mellitus with unspecified complications   HCC

E13.9   Other specified diabetes mellitus without complications   HCC
    AHA: 2020,2Q,18

Other disorders of glucose regulation and pancreatic internal secretion (E15-E16)

E15   Nondiabetic hypoglycemic coma   CC H9 HCC
    INCLUDES   drug-induced insulin coma in nondiabetic
                hyperinsulinism with hypoglycemic coma
                hypoglycemic coma NOS

✓4ᵗʰ **E16   Other disorders of pancreatic internal secretion**

    E16.0   Drug-induced hypoglycemia without coma
       EXCLUDES 1   diabetes with hypoglycemia without coma (E09.649)
       Use additional code for adverse effect, if applicable, to identify drug (T36-T50 with fifth or sixth character 5)

    E16.1   Other hypoglycemia
       Functional hyperinsulinism
       Functional nonhyperinsulinemic hypoglycemia
       Hyperinsulinism NOS
       Hyperplasia of pancreatic islet beta cells NOS
       EXCLUDES 1   diabetes with hypoglycemia (E08.649, E10.649, E11.649, E13.649)
               hypoglycemia in infant of diabetic mother (P70.1)
               neonatal hypoglycemia (P70.4)

    E16.2   Hypoglycemia, unspecified
       EXCLUDES 1   diabetes with hypoglycemia (E08.649, E10.649, E11.649, E13.649)
       AHA: 2016,3Q,42
       TIP: Assign for nondiabetic hypoglycemic encephalopathy not further clarified in the documentation.

    E16.3   Increased secretion of glucagon
       Hyperplasia of pancreatic endocrine cells with glucagon excess

    E16.4   Increased secretion of gastrin
       Hypergastrinemia
       Hyperplasia of pancreatic endocrine cells with gastrin excess
       Zollinger-Ellison syndrome

    E16.8   Other specified disorders of pancreatic internal secretion
       Increased secretion from endocrine pancreas of growth hormone-releasing hormone
       Increased secretion from endocrine pancreas of pancreatic polypeptide
       Increased secretion from endocrine pancreas of somatostatin
       Increased secretion from endocrine pancreas of vasoactive-intestinal polypeptide

    E16.9   Disorder of pancreatic internal secretion, unspecified
       Islet-cell hyperplasia NOS
       Pancreatic endocrine cell hyperplasia NOS

N Newborn: 0   P Pediatric: 0-17   M Maternity: 9-64   A Adult: 15-124   MCC Major Complication/Comorbidity   CC Complication/Comorbidity   SW Severe Wound Dx

530   ICD-10-CM 2022

Disorders of other endocrine glands (E20-E35)

EXCLUDES 1   galactorrhea (N64.3)
     gynecomastia (N62)

✓4th E20 Hypoparathyroidism

EXCLUDES 1   Di George's syndrome (D82.1)
     postprocedural hypoparathyroidism (E89.2)
     tetany NOS (R29.0)
     transitory neonatal hypoparathyroidism (P71.4)

E20.0 Idiopathic hypoparathyroidism   HCC
   DEF: Abnormally low secretion of parathyroid hormones, with unknown cause, which triggers decreased calcium and increased phosphorus in the blood that can result in cataracts, muscle cramps, tetany, tingling, or burning in the lips, fingers, and toes.

E20.1 Pseudohypoparathyroidism

E20.8 Other hypoparathyroidism   HCC

E20.9 Hypoparathyroidism, unspecified   HCC
   Parathyroid tetany

✓4th E21 Hyperparathyroidism and other disorders of parathyroid gland

EXCLUDES 1   adult osteomalacia (M83.-)
     ectopic hyperparathyroidism (E34.2)
     ~~familial hypocalciuric hypercalcemia (E83.52)~~
     hungry bone syndrome (E83.81)
     infantile and juvenile osteomalacia (E55.0)

EXCLUDES 2   ▶familial hypocalciuric hypercalcemia (E83.52)◀

E21.0 Primary hyperparathyroidism
   Hyperplasia of parathyroid
   Osteitis fibrosa cystica generalisata [von Recklinghausen's disease of bone]
   DEF: Parathyroid dysfunction commonly caused by hyperplasia of two or more glands. Symptoms include hypercalcemia and increased parathyroid hormone levels.

E21.1 Secondary hyperparathyroidism, not elsewhere classified   HCC
   EXCLUDES 1   secondary hyperparathyroidism of renal origin (N25.81)

E21.2 Other hyperparathyroidism   HCC
   Tertiary hyperparathyroidism
   EXCLUDES 1   familial hypocalciuric hypercalcemia (E83.52)

E21.3 Hyperparathyroidism, unspecified   HCC

E21.4 Other specified disorders of parathyroid gland   HCC

E21.5 Disorder of parathyroid gland, unspecified   HCC

✓4th E22 Hyperfunction of pituitary gland

EXCLUDES 1   Cushing's syndrome (E24.-)
     Nelson's syndrome (E24.1)
     overproduction of ACTH not associated with Cushing's disease (E27.0)
     overproduction of pituitary ACTH (E24.0)
     overproduction of thyroid-stimulating hormone (E05.8-)

E22.0 Acromegaly and pituitary gigantism   HCC
   Overproduction of growth hormone
   EXCLUDES 1   constitutional gigantism (E34.4)
      constitutional tall stature (E34.4)
      increased secretion from endocrine pancreas of growth hormone-releasing hormone (E16.8)
   DEF: Acromegaly: Chronic condition caused by overproduction of the pituitary growth hormone resulting in enlarged skeletal parts and facial features.

E22.1 Hyperprolactinemia   CC HCC
   Use additional code for adverse effect, if applicable, to identify drug (T36-T50 with fifth or sixth character 5)

E22.2 Syndrome of inappropriate secretion of antidiuretic hormone   CC HCC

E22.8 Other hyperfunction of pituitary gland   CC HCC
   Central precocious puberty

E22.9 Hyperfunction of pituitary gland, unspecified   CC HCC

✓4th E23 Hypofunction and other disorders of the pituitary gland

INCLUDES   the listed conditions whether the disorder is in the pituitary or the hypothalamus

EXCLUDES 1   postprocedural hypopituitarism (E89.3)

E23.0 Hypopituitarism   CC HCC
   Fertile eunuch syndrome
   Hypogonadotropic hypogonadism
   Idiopathic growth hormone deficiency
   Isolated deficiency of gonadotropin
   Isolated deficiency of growth hormone
   Isolated deficiency of pituitary hormone
   Kallmann's syndrome
   Lorain-Levi short stature
   Necrosis of pituitary gland (postpartum)
   Panhypopituitarism
   Pituitary cachexia
   Pituitary insufficiency NOS
   Pituitary short stature
   Sheehan's syndrome
   Simmonds' disease

E23.1 Drug-induced hypopituitarism   HCC
   Use additional code for adverse effect, if applicable, to identify drug (T36-T50 with fifth or sixth character 5)

E23.2 Diabetes insipidus   CC HCC
   EXCLUDES 1   nephrogenic diabetes insipidus (N25.1)

E23.3 Hypothalamic dysfunction, not elsewhere classified   HCC
   EXCLUDES 1   Prader-Willi syndrome (Q87.11)
      Russell-Silver syndrome (Q87.19)

E23.6 Other disorders of pituitary gland   HCC
   Abscess of pituitary
   Adiposogenital dystrophy

E23.7 Disorder of pituitary gland, unspecified   HCC

✓4th E24 Cushing's syndrome

EXCLUDES 1   congenital adrenal hyperplasia (E25.0)
   DEF: Abdominal striae, acne, hypertension, decreased carbohydrate tolerance, moon face, obesity, protein catabolism, and psychiatric disturbances resulting from increased adrenocortical secretion of cortisol caused by ACTH-dependent adrenocortical hyperplasia or tumor, or by steroid effects.

E24.0 Pituitary-dependent Cushing's disease   CC HCC
   Overproduction of pituitary ACTH
   Pituitary-dependent hypercorticalism

E24.1 Nelson's syndrome   HCC

E24.2 Drug-induced Cushing's syndrome   CC HCC
   Use additional code for adverse effect, if applicable, to identify drug (T36-T50 with fifth or sixth character 5)

E24.3 Ectopic ACTH syndrome   CC HCC

E24.4 Alcohol-induced pseudo-Cushing's syndrome   CC HCC

E24.8 Other Cushing's syndrome   CC HCC

E24.9 Cushing's syndrome, unspecified   CC HCC

✓4th E25 Adrenogenital disorders

INCLUDES   adrenogenital syndromes, virilizing or feminizing, whether acquired or due to adrenal hyperplasia
     consequent on inborn enzyme defects in hormone synthesis
     female adrenal pseudohermaphroditism
     female heterosexual precocious pseudopuberty
     male isosexual precocious pseudopuberty
     male macrogenitosomia praecox
     male sexual precocity with adrenal hyperplasia
     male virilization (female)

EXCLUDES 1   indeterminate sex and pseudohermaphroditism (Q56)
     chromosomal abnormalities (Q90-Q99)

E25.0 Congenital adrenogenital disorders associated with enzyme deficiency   HCC
   Congenital adrenal hyperplasia
   21-Hydroxylase deficiency
   Salt-losing congenital adrenal hyperplasia

E25.8 Other adrenogenital disorders   HCC
   Idiopathic adrenogenital disorder
   Use additional code for adverse effect, if applicable, to identify drug (T36-T50 with fifth or sixth character 5)

E25.9 Adrenogenital disorder, unspecified   HCC
   Adrenogenital syndrome NOS

☑ Additional Character Required   ✓x7th Placeholder   Questionable PDx   Manifestation   Unspecified Dx   UPD Unacceptable PDx   H1-H14 HAC   HCC CMS-HCC Dx   HIV HIV Dx

ICD-10-CM 2022   531

✓4ᵗʰ **E26 Hyperaldosteronism**

  ✓5ᵗʰ **E26.0 Primary hyperaldosteronism**

    E26.01 Conn's syndrome   HCC
       Code also adrenal adenoma (D35.0-)

    E26.02 Glucocorticoid-remediable aldosteronism   HCC
       Familial aldosteronism type I
       DEF: Rare autosomal dominant familial form of primary aldosteronism in which the secretion of aldosterone is under the influence of adrenocorticotrophic hormone (ACTH) rather than the renin-angiotensin mechanism. Moderate hypersecretion of aldosterone and suppressed plasma renin activity that are rapidly reversed by administration of glucosteroids. Symptoms include hypertension and mild hypokalemia.

    E26.09 Other primary hyperaldosteronism   HCC
       Primary aldosteronism due to adrenal hyperplasia (bilateral)

  E26.1 Secondary hyperaldosteronism   HCC

  ✓5ᵗʰ **E26.8 Other hyperaldosteronism**

    E26.81 Bartter's syndrome   HCC
    E26.89 Other hyperaldosteronism   HCC

  E26.9 Hyperaldosteronism, unspecified   HCC
    Aldosteronism NOS
    Hyperaldosteronism NOS

✓4ᵗʰ **E27 Other disorders of adrenal gland**

  E27.0 Other adrenocortical overactivity   CC HCC
    Overproduction of ACTH, not associated with Cushing's disease
    Premature adrenarche
    EXCLUDES 1   Cushing's syndrome (E24.-)

  E27.1 Primary adrenocortical insufficiency   CC HCC
    Addison's disease
    Autoimmune adrenalitis
    EXCLUDES 1   Addison only phenotype adrenoleukodystrophy (E71.528)
           amyloidosis (E85.-)
           tuberculous Addison's disease (A18.7)
           Waterhouse-Friderichsen syndrome (A39.1)

  E27.2 Addisonian crisis   CC HCC
    Adrenal crisis
    Adrenocortical crisis
    DEF: Life-threatening condition that occurs when there is not enough cortisol excreted from the adrenal glands. This condition may be due to injury to the adrenal glands or to the pituitary gland, which controls adrenal hormone secretion, or when a patient stops hydrocortisone treatment too quickly or too early.

  E27.3 Drug-induced adrenocortical insufficiency   CC HCC
    Use additional code for adverse effect, if applicable, to identify drug (T36-T50 with fifth or sixth character 5)

  ✓5ᵗʰ **E27.4 Other and unspecified adrenocortical insufficiency**
    EXCLUDES 1   adrenoleukodystrophy [Addison-Schilder] (E71.528)
           Waterhouse-Friderichsen syndrome (A39.1)

    E27.40 Unspecified adrenocortical insufficiency   CC HCC
       Adrenocortical insufficiency NOS
       Hypoaldosteronism

    E27.49 Other adrenocortical insufficiency   CC HCC
       Adrenal hemorrhage
       Adrenal infarction

  E27.5 Adrenomedullary hyperfunction   CC HCC
    Adrenomedullary hyperplasia
    Catecholamine hypersecretion

  E27.8 Other specified disorders of adrenal gland   HCC
    Abnormality of cortisol-binding globulin

  E27.9 Disorder of adrenal gland, unspecified   HCC

✓4ᵗʰ **E28 Ovarian dysfunction**

  EXCLUDES 1   isolated gonadotropin deficiency (E23.0)
           postprocedural ovarian failure (E89.4-)

  E28.0 Estrogen excess   ♀
    Use additional code for adverse effect, if applicable, to identify drug (T36-T50 with fifth or sixth character 5)

  E28.1 Androgen excess   ♀
    Hypersecretion of ovarian androgens
    Use additional code for adverse effect, if applicable, to identify drug (T36-T50 with fifth or sixth character 5)

  E28.2 Polycystic ovarian syndrome   ♀
    Sclerocystic ovary syndrome
    Stein-Leventhal syndrome
    DEF: Common hormonal disorder among women of reproductive age that involves enlarged ovaries with numerous small cysts located along the outer ovarian edge.

  ✓5ᵗʰ **E28.3 Primary ovarian failure**
    EXCLUDES 1   pure gonadal dysgenesis (Q99.1)
           Turner's syndrome (Q96.-)

    ✓6ᵗʰ **E28.31 Premature menopause**

      E28.310 Symptomatic premature menopause   A ♀
        Symptoms such as flushing, sleeplessness, headache, lack of concentration, associated with premature menopause

      E28.319 Asymptomatic premature menopause   A ♀
        Premature menopause NOS

    E28.39 Other primary ovarian failure   ♀
       Decreased estrogen
       Resistant ovary syndrome

  E28.8 Other ovarian dysfunction   ♀
    Ovarian hyperfunction NOS
    EXCLUDES 1   postprocedural ovarian failure (E89.4-)

  E28.9 Ovarian dysfunction, unspecified   ♀

✓4ᵗʰ **E29 Testicular dysfunction**

  EXCLUDES 1   androgen insensitivity syndrome (E34.5-)
           azoospermia or oligospermia NOS (N46.0-N46.1)
           isolated gonadotropin deficiency (E23.0)
           Klinefelter's syndrome (Q98.0-Q98.1, Q98.4)

  E29.0 Testicular hyperfunction   ♂
    Hypersecretion of testicular hormones

  E29.1 Testicular hypofunction   ♂
    Defective biosynthesis of testicular androgen NOS
    5-delta-Reductase deficiency (with male pseudohermaphroditism)
    Testicular hypogonadism NOS
    Use additional code for adverse effect, if applicable, to identify drug (T36-T50 with fifth or sixth character 5)
    EXCLUDES 1   postprocedural testicular hypofunction (E89.5)

  E29.8 Other testicular dysfunction   ♂

  E29.9 Testicular dysfunction, unspecified   ♂

✓4ᵗʰ **E30 Disorders of puberty, not elsewhere classified**

  E30.0 Delayed puberty
    Constitutional delay of puberty
    Delayed sexual development

  E30.1 Precocious puberty   P
    Precocious menstruation
    EXCLUDES 1   Albright (-McCune) (-Sternberg) syndrome (Q78.1)
           central precocious puberty (E22.8)
           congenital adrenal hyperplasia (E25.0)
           female heterosexual precocious pseudopuberty (E25.-)
           male isosexual precocious pseudopuberty (E25.-)

  E30.8 Other disorders of puberty   P
    Premature thelarche

  E30.9 Disorder of puberty, unspecified

✓4ᵗʰ **E31 Polyglandular dysfunction**

  EXCLUDES 1   ataxia telangiectasia [Louis-Bar] (G11.3)
           dystrophia myotonica [Steinert] (G71.11)
           pseudohypoparathyroidism (E20.1)

  E31.0 Autoimmune polyglandular failure   HCC
    Schmidt's syndrome

  E31.1 Polyglandular hyperfunction   HCC
    EXCLUDES 1   multiple endocrine adenomatosis (E31.2-)
           multiple endocrine neoplasia (E31.2-)

N Newborn: 0   P Pediatric: 0-17   M Maternity: 9-64   A Adult: 15-124   MCC Major Complication/Comorbidity   CC Complication/Comorbidity   SW Severe Wound Dx

532

ICD-10-CM 2022

✓5th **E31.2 Multiple endocrine neoplasia [MEN] syndromes**

Multiple endocrine adenomatosis

Code also any associated malignancies and other conditions associated with the syndromes

DEF: Group of conditions in which several endocrine glands grow excessively (such as in adenomatous hyperplasia) and/or develop benign or malignant tumors. Tumors and hyperplasia associated with MEN often produce excess hormones, which impede normal physiology. There is no comprehensive cure known for MEN syndrome. Treatment is directed at the hyperplasia or tumors in each individual gland. Tumors are usually surgically removed and oral medications or hormonal injections are used to correct hormone imbalances.

E31.20 Multiple endocrine neoplasia [MEN] syndrome, unspecified `HCC`

Multiple endocrine adenomatosis NOS

Multiple endocrine neoplasia [MEN] syndrome NOS

E31.21 Multiple endocrine neoplasia [MEN] type I `HCC`

Wermer's syndrome

E31.22 Multiple endocrine neoplasia [MEN] type IIA `HCC`

Sipple's syndrome

E31.23 Multiple endocrine neoplasia [MEN] type IIB `HCC`

E31.8 Other polyglandular dysfunction `HCC`

E31.9 Polyglandular dysfunction, unspecified `HCC`

✓4th **E32 Diseases of thymus**

EXCLUDES 1 aplasia or hypoplasia of thymus with immunodeficiency (D82.1)

myasthenia gravis (G70.0)

E32.0 Persistent hyperplasia of thymus `HCC`

Hypertrophy of thymus

E32.1 Abscess of thymus `CC` `HCC`

E32.8 Other diseases of thymus

EXCLUDES 1 aplasia or hypoplasia with immunodeficiency (D82.1)

thymoma (D15.0)

E32.9 Disease of thymus, unspecified `HCC`

✓4th **E34 Other endocrine disorders**

EXCLUDES 1 pseudohypoparathyroidism (E20.1)

E34.0 Carcinoid syndrome `CC` `HCC`

NOTE May be used as an additional code to identify functional activity associated with a carcinoid tumor.

E34.1 Other hypersecretion of intestinal hormones

E34.2 Ectopic hormone secretion, not elsewhere classified

EXCLUDES 1 ectopic ACTH syndrome (E24.3)

E34.3 Short stature due to endocrine disorder

Constitutional short stature

Laron-type short stature

EXCLUDES 1 achondroplastic short stature (Q77.4)

hypochondroplastic short stature (Q77.4)

nutritional short stature (E45)

pituitary short stature (E23.0)

progeria (E34.8)

renal short stature (N25.0)

Russell-Silver syndrome (Q87.19)

short-limbed stature with immunodeficiency (D82.2)

short stature in specific dysmorphic syndromes - code to syndrome - see Alphabetical Index

short stature NOS (R62.52)

E34.4 Constitutional tall stature `HCC`

Constitutional gigantism

✓5th **E34.5 Androgen insensitivity syndrome**

DEF: X-linked recessive condition in which individuals that are chromosomally male fail to develop normal male external genitalia due to an abnormality on the X chromosome that prohibits the body, completely or in part, from recognizing the androgens produced. **Synonym(s):** AIS

E34.50 Androgen insensitivity syndrome, unspecified

Androgen insensitivity NOS

E34.51 Complete androgen insensitivity syndrome

Complete androgen insensitivity

de Quervain syndrome

Goldberg-Maxwell syndrome

E34.52 Partial androgen insensitivity syndrome

Partial androgen insensitivity

Reifenstein syndrome

E34.8 Other specified endocrine disorders

Pineal gland dysfunction

Progeria

EXCLUDES 2 pseudohypoparathyroidism (E20.1)

E34.9 Endocrine disorder, unspecified

Endocrine disturbance NOS

Hormone disturbance NOS

E35 Disorders of endocrine glands in diseases classified elsewhere

Code first underlying disease, such as:

late congenital syphilis of thymus gland [Dubois disease] (A50.5)

Use additional code, if applicable, to identify:

sequelae of tuberculosis of other organs (B90.8)

EXCLUDES 1 Echinococcus granulosus infection of thyroid gland (B67.3)

meningococcal hemorrhagic adrenalitis (A39.1)

syphilis of endocrine gland (A52.79)

tuberculosis of adrenal gland, except calcification (A18.7)

tuberculosis of endocrine gland NEC (A18.82)

tuberculosis of thyroid gland (A18.81)

Waterhouse-Friderichsen syndrome (A39.1)

Intraoperative complications of endocrine system (E36)

✓4th **E36 Intraoperative complications of endocrine system**

EXCLUDES 2 postprocedural endocrine and metabolic complications and disorders, not elsewhere classified (E89.-)

✓5th **E36.0 Intraoperative hemorrhage and hematoma of an endocrine system organ or structure complicating a procedure**

EXCLUDES 1 intraoperative hemorrhage and hematoma of an endocrine system organ or structure due to accidental puncture or laceration during a procedure (E36.1-)

E36.01 Intraoperative hemorrhage and hematoma of an endocrine system organ or structure complicating an endocrine system procedure `CC`

AHA: 2020,1Q,19

E36.02 Intraoperative hemorrhage and hematoma of an endocrine system organ or structure complicating other procedure `CC`

✓5th **E36.1 Accidental puncture and laceration of an endocrine system organ or structure during a procedure**

E36.11 Accidental puncture and laceration of an endocrine system organ or structure during an endocrine system procedure `CC`

E36.12 Accidental puncture and laceration of an endocrine system organ or structure during other procedure `CC`

E36.8 Other intraoperative complications of endocrine system

Use additional code, if applicable, to further specify disorder

Malnutrition (E40-E46)

EXCLUDES 1 intestinal malabsorption (K90.-)

sequelae of protein-calorie malnutrition (E64.0)

EXCLUDES 2 nutritional anemias (D50-D53)

starvation (T73.0)

AHA: 2020,1Q,4-7; 2017,4Q,108; 2017,3Q,25

TIP: Assign additional code for BMI from category Z68, when documented. BMI can be based on documentation from clinicians who are not the patient's provider.

TIP: Malnutrition is not considered integral to cancer; assign the appropriate code in addition to the code for the specific type of cancer.

E40 Kwashiorkor `MCC` `HCC`

Severe malnutrition with nutritional edema with dyspigmentation of skin and hair

EXCLUDES 1 marasmic kwashiorkor (E42)

E41 Nutritional marasmus `MCC` `HCC`

Severe malnutrition with marasmus

EXCLUDES 1 marasmic kwashiorkor (E42)

AHA: 2017,3Q,24

DEF: Protein-calorie malabsorption or malnutrition in children characterized by tissue wasting, dehydration, and subcutaneous fat depletion. It may occur with infectious disease.

E42 Marasmic kwashiorkor `MCC` `HCC`

Intermediate form severe protein-calorie malnutrition

Severe protein-calorie malnutrition with signs of both kwashiorkor and marasmus

Chapter 4. Endocrine, Nutritional and Metabolic Diseases

E43   **Unspecified severe protein-calorie malnutrition** `MCC` `HCC`
Starvation edema
AHA: 2020,1Q,5,6; 2017,4Q,108
TIP: Assign code R64 when emaciation is documented without documentation of malnutrition.

√4th **E44**   **Protein-calorie malnutrition of moderate and mild degree**
AHA: 2020,1Q,5

     E44.0   **Moderate protein-calorie malnutrition** `CC` `HCC`
     E44.1   **Mild protein-calorie malnutrition** `CC` `HCC`

E45   **Retarded development following protein-calorie malnutrition** `CC` `HCC`
Nutritional short stature
Nutritional stunting
Physical retardation due to malnutrition

E46   **Unspecified protein-calorie malnutrition** `CC` `HCC`
Malnutrition NOS
Protein-calorie imbalance NOS
     EXCLUDES 1   nutritional deficiency NOS (E63.9)
AHA: 2018,4Q,82

Other nutritional deficiencies (E50-E64)

EXCLUDES 2   nutritional anemias (D50-D53)

√4th **E50**   **Vitamin A deficiency**
     EXCLUDES 1   sequelae of vitamin A deficiency (E64.1)

     E50.0   **Vitamin A deficiency with conjunctival xerosis**
     E50.1   **Vitamin A deficiency with Bitot's spot and conjunctival xerosis**
         Bitot's spot in the young child
         DEF: Vitamin A deficiency with conjunctival dryness and superficial spots of keratinized epithelium.
     E50.2   **Vitamin A deficiency with corneal xerosis**
     E50.3   **Vitamin A deficiency with corneal ulceration and xerosis**
     E50.4   **Vitamin A deficiency with keratomalacia**
         DEF: Vitamin A deficiency creating corneal dryness that progresses to corneal insensitivity, softness, and necrosis. It is usually bilateral.
     E50.5   **Vitamin A deficiency with night blindness**
     E50.6   **Vitamin A deficiency with xerophthalmic scars of cornea**
     E50.7   **Other ocular manifestations of vitamin A deficiency**
         Xerophthalmia NOS
     E50.8   **Other manifestations of vitamin A deficiency**
         Follicular keratosis
         Xeroderma
     E50.9   **Vitamin A deficiency, unspecified**
         Hypovitaminosis A NOS

√4th **E51**   **Thiamine deficiency**
     EXCLUDES 1   sequelae of thiamine deficiency (E64.8)

     √5th **E51.1**   **Beriberi**

         E51.11   **Dry beriberi** `CC`
             Beriberi NOS
             Beriberi with polyneuropathy
         E51.12   **Wet beriberi** `CC`
             Beriberi with cardiovascular manifestations
             Cardiovascular beriberi
             Shoshin disease

     E51.2   **Wernicke's encephalopathy** `CC`
         DEF: Deficiency of vitamin B1 resulting in a triad of acute mental confusion, ataxia, and ophthalmoplegia. The vast majority of affected patients are alcoholics.
     E51.8   **Other manifestations of thiamine deficiency** `CC`
     E51.9   **Thiamine deficiency, unspecified** `CC`

E52   **Niacin deficiency [pellagra]**
Niacin (-tryptophan) deficiency
Nicotinamide deficiency
Pellagra (alcoholic)
     EXCLUDES 1   sequelae of niacin deficiency (E64.8)

√4th **E53**   **Deficiency of other B group vitamins**
     EXCLUDES 1   sequelae of vitamin B deficiency (E64.8)

     E53.0   **Riboflavin deficiency** `CC`
         Ariboflavinosis
         Vitamin B2 deficiency
     E53.1   **Pyridoxine deficiency**
         Vitamin B6 deficiency
         EXCLUDES 1   pyridoxine-responsive sideroblastic anemia (D64.3)

     E53.8   **Deficiency of other specified B group vitamins**
         Biotin deficiency
         Cyanocobalamin deficiency
         Folate deficiency
         Folic acid deficiency
         Pantothenic acid deficiency
         Vitamin B12 deficiency
         EXCLUDES 1   folate deficiency anemia (D52.-)
                 vitamin B12 deficiency anemia (D51.-)

     E53.9   **Vitamin B deficiency, unspecified**

E54   **Ascorbic acid deficiency**
Deficiency of vitamin C
Scurvy
     EXCLUDES 1   scorbutic anemia (D53.2)
                 sequelae of vitamin C deficiency (E64.2)
DEF: Vitamin C deficiency causing swollen gums, myalgia, weight loss, and weakness.

√4th **E55**   **Vitamin D deficiency**
     EXCLUDES 1   adult osteomalacia (M83.-)
                 osteoporosis (M80.-)
                 sequelae of rickets (E64.3)

     E55.0   **Rickets, active** `CC`
         Infantile osteomalacia
         Juvenile osteomalacia
         EXCLUDES 1   celiac rickets (K90.0)
                 Crohn's rickets (K50.-)
                 hereditary vitamin D-dependent rickets (E83.32)
                 inactive rickets (E64.3)
                 renal rickets (N25.0)
                 sequelae of rickets (E64.3)
                 vitamin D-resistant rickets (E83.31)
         DEF: Rickets: Softening or weakening of the bones due to a lack of vitamin D, calcium, and phosphate.
     E55.9   **Vitamin D deficiency, unspecified**
         Avitaminosis D

√4th **E56**   **Other vitamin deficiencies**
     EXCLUDES 1   sequelae of other vitamin deficiencies (E64.8)

     E56.0   **Deficiency of vitamin E**
     E56.1   **Deficiency of vitamin K**
         EXCLUDES 1   deficiency of coagulation factor due to vitamin K deficiency (D68.4)
                 vitamin K deficiency of newborn (P53)
     E56.8   **Deficiency of other vitamins**
     E56.9   **Vitamin deficiency, unspecified**

E58   **Dietary calcium deficiency**
     EXCLUDES 1   disorders of calcium metabolism (E83.5-)
                 sequelae of calcium deficiency (E64.8)

E59   **Dietary selenium deficiency**
Keshan disease
     EXCLUDES 1   sequelae of selenium deficiency (E64.8)

E60   **Dietary zinc deficiency**

√4th **E61**   **Deficiency of other nutrient elements**
     Use additional code for adverse effect, if applicable, to identify drug (T36-T50 with fifth or sixth character 5)
     EXCLUDES 1   disorders of mineral metabolism (E83.-)
                 iodine deficiency related thyroid disorders (E00-E02)
                 sequelae of malnutrition and other nutritional deficiencies (E64.-)

     E61.0   **Copper deficiency**
     E61.1   **Iron deficiency**
         EXCLUDES 1   iron deficiency anemia (D50.-)
     E61.2   **Magnesium deficiency**
     E61.3   **Manganese deficiency**
     E61.4   **Chromium deficiency**
     E61.5   **Molybdenum deficiency**
     E61.6   **Vanadium deficiency**
     E61.7   **Deficiency of multiple nutrient elements**
     E61.8   **Deficiency of other specified nutrient elements**
     E61.9   **Deficiency of nutrient element, unspecified**

✓4ᵗʰ **E63 Other nutritional deficiencies**

> EXCLUDES 1   *dehydration (E86.0)*
> *failure to thrive, adult (R62.7)*
> *failure to thrive, child (R62.51)*
> *feeding problems in newborn (P92.-)*
> *sequelae of malnutrition and other nutritional deficiencies (E64.-)*

> EXCLUDES 2   ▶*dehydration (E86.0)*◀
> ▶*failure to thrive, adult (R62.7)*◀
> ▶*failure to thrive, child (R62.51)*◀
> ▶*feeding problems in newborn (P92.-)*◀
> ▶*sequelae of malnutrition and other nutritional deficiencies (E64.-)*◀

E63.0 Essential fatty acid [EFA] deficiency

E63.1 Imbalance of constituents of food intake

E63.8 Other specified nutritional deficiencies

E63.9 Nutritional deficiency, unspecified

✓4ᵗʰ **E64 Sequelae of malnutrition and other nutritional deficiencies**

> **NOTE**   This category is to be used to indicate conditions in categories E43, E44, E46, E50-E63 as the cause of sequelae, which are themselves classified elsewhere. The 'sequelae' include conditions specified as such; they also include the late effects of diseases classifiable to the above categories if the disease itself is no longer present

> Code first condition resulting from (sequela) of malnutrition and other nutritional deficiencies

E64.0 Sequelae of protein-calorie malnutrition   CC HCC

> EXCLUDES 2   *retarded development following protein-calorie malnutrition (E45)*

E64.1 Sequelae of vitamin A deficiency

E64.2 Sequelae of vitamin C deficiency

E64.3 Sequelae of rickets

E64.8 Sequelae of other nutritional deficiencies

E64.9 Sequelae of unspecified nutritional deficiency

Overweight, obesity and other hyperalimentation (E65-E68)

E65 Localized adiposity
> Fat pad

✓4ᵗʰ **E66 Overweight and obesity**

> Code first obesity complicating pregnancy, childbirth and the puerperium, if applicable (O99.21-)
> Use additional code to identify body mass index (BMI), if known (Z68.-)

> EXCLUDES 1   *adiposogenital dystrophy (E23.6)*
> *lipomatosis NOS (E88.2)*
> *lipomatosis dolorosa [Dercum] (E88.2)*
> *Prader-Willi syndrome (Q87.11)*

> **AHA:** 2018,4Q,77,79-80
> **TIP:** Do not assign a BMI code (Z68.-) when a pregnant patient is documented as being overweight or obese. Only a code from subcategory O99.21- and a code from this category should be assigned.

✓5ᵗʰ **E66.0 Obesity due to excess calories**

> **E66.01 Morbid (severe) obesity due to excess calories**   H11 HCC

> > EXCLUDES 1   *morbid (severe) obesity with alveolar hypoventilation (E66.2)*

> **E66.09 Other obesity due to excess calories**

E66.1 Drug-induced obesity

> Use additional code for adverse effect, if applicable, to identify drug (T36-T50 with fifth or sixth character 5)

E66.2 Morbid (severe) obesity with alveolar hypoventilation   CC HCC

> Obesity hypoventilation syndrome (OHS)
> Pickwickian syndrome

E66.3 Overweight

> **AHA:** 2018,4Q,78

E66.8 Other obesity

E66.9 Obesity, unspecified

> Obesity NOS
> **AHA:** 2021,2Q,10

✓4ᵗʰ **E67 Other hyperalimentation**

> EXCLUDES 1   *hyperalimentation NOS (R63.2)*
> *sequelae of hyperalimentation (E68)*

E67.0 Hypervitaminosis A

E67.1 Hypercarotenemia

> **DEF:** Elevated blood carotene level as a result of excessive carotenoid ingestion or an inability to convert carotenoids to vitamin A. Characteristics often include yellow discoloration of the skin, which may follow overeating of carotenoid-rich foods such as carrots, sweet potatoes, or squash.

E67.2 Megavitamin-B6 syndrome

E67.3 Hypervitaminosis D

E67.8 Other specified hyperalimentation

E68 Sequelae of hyperalimentation

> Code first condition resulting from (sequela) of hyperalimentation

Metabolic disorders (E70-E88)

> EXCLUDES 1   *androgen insensitivity syndrome (E34.5-)*
> *congenital adrenal hyperplasia (E25.0)*
> *Ehlers-Danlos syndromes (Q79.6-)*
> *hemolytic anemias attributable to enzyme disorders (D55.-)*
> *Marfan's syndrome (Q87.4)*
> *5-alpha-reductase deficiency (E29.1)*

> EXCLUDES 2   ▶*Ehlers-Danlos syndromes (Q79.6-)*◀
> **AHA:** 2018,2Q,6

✓4ᵗʰ **E70 Disorders of aromatic amino-acid metabolism**

E70.0 Classical phenylketonuria   CC HCC

E70.1 Other hyperphenylalaninemias   CC HCC

✓5ᵗʰ **E70.2 Disorders of tyrosine metabolism**

> EXCLUDES 1   *transitory tyrosinemia of newborn (P74.5)*

> **E70.20 Disorder of tyrosine metabolism, unspecified**   CC HCC

> **E70.21 Tyrosinemia**   CC HCC
> > Hypertyrosinemia

> **E70.29 Other disorders of tyrosine metabolism**   CC HCC
> > Alkaptonuria
> > Ochronosis

✓5ᵗʰ **E70.3 Albinism**

> **DEF:** Absence of pigment in skin, hair, and eyes. This genetic condition is often accompanied by astigmatism, photophobia, and nystagmus.

> **E70.30 Albinism, unspecified**   CC HCC

> ✓6ᵗʰ **E70.31 Ocular albinism**

> > **E70.310 X-linked ocular albinism**   CC HCC

> > **E70.311 Autosomal recessive ocular albinism**   CC HCC

> > **E70.318 Other ocular albinism**   CC HCC

> > **E70.319 Ocular albinism, unspecified**   CC HCC

> ✓6ᵗʰ **E70.32 Oculocutaneous albinism**

> > EXCLUDES 1   *Chediak-Higashi syndrome (E70.330)*
> > *Hermansky-Pudlak syndrome (E70.331)*

> > **E70.320 Tyrosinase negative oculocutaneous albinism**   CC HCC
> > > Albinism I
> > > Oculocutaneous albinism ty-neg

> > **E70.321 Tyrosinase positive oculocutaneous albinism**   CC HCC
> > > Albinism II
> > > Oculocutaneous albinism ty-pos

> > **E70.328 Other oculocutaneous albinism**   CC HCC
> > > Cross syndrome

> > **E70.329 Oculocutaneous albinism, unspecified**   CC HCC

> ✓6ᵗʰ **E70.33 Albinism with hematologic abnormality**

> > **E70.330 Chediak-Higashi syndrome**   CC HCC

> > **E70.331 Hermansky-Pudlak syndrome**   CC HCC

> > **E70.338 Other albinism with hematologic abnormality**   CC HCC

> > **E70.339 Albinism with hematologic abnormality, unspecified**   CC HCC

> **E70.39 Other specified albinism**   CC HCC
> > Piebaldism

✓5ᵗʰ **E70.4 Disorders of histidine metabolism**

> **E70.40 Disorders of histidine metabolism, unspecified**   CC HCC

> **E70.41 Histidinemia**   CC HCC

> **E70.49 Other disorders of histidine metabolism**   CC HCC

E70.5 Disorders of tryptophan metabolism   CC HCC

☑ Additional Character Required   ✓x7ᵗʰ Placeholder   Questionable PDx   Manifestation   Unspecified Dx   UPD Unacceptable PDx   H1-H14 HAC   HCC CMS-HCC Dx   HIV HIV Dx

ICD-10-CM 2022   535

✓5th **E70.8   Other disorders of aromatic amino-acid metabolism**
AHA: 2020,4Q,15-16

E70.81   **Aromatic L-amino acid decarboxylase deficiency**   CC HCC
AADC deficiency

E70.89   **Other disorders of aromatic amino-acid metabolism**   CC HCC

E70.9   Disorder of aromatic amino-acid metabolism, unspecified   CC HCC

✓4th **E71   Disorders of branched-chain amino-acid metabolism and fatty-acid metabolism**

E71.0   **Maple-syrup-urine disease**   CC HCC

✓5th **E71.1   Other disorders of branched-chain amino-acid metabolism**

✓6th   E71.11   **Branched-chain organic acidurias**

E71.110   **Isovaleric acidemia**   CC HCC

E71.111   **3-methylglutaconic aciduria**   CC HCC

E71.118   **Other branched-chain organic acidurias**   CC HCC

✓6th   E71.12   **Disorders of propionate metabolism**

E71.120   **Methylmalonic acidemia**   CC HCC

E71.121   **Propionic acidemia**   CC HCC

E71.128   **Other disorders of propionate metabolism**   CC HCC

E71.19   **Other disorders of branched-chain amino-acid metabolism**   CC HCC
Hyperleucine-isoleucinemia
Hypervalinemia

E71.2   Disorder of branched-chain amino-acid metabolism, unspecified   CC HCC

✓5th **E71.3   Disorders of fatty-acid metabolism**

EXCLUDES 1   *peroxisomal disorders (E71.5)*
Refsum's disease (G60.1)
Schilder's disease (G37.0)

EXCLUDES 2   *carnitine deficiency due to inborn error of metabolism (E71.42)*

E71.30   Disorder of fatty-acid metabolism, unspecified

✓6th   E71.31   **Disorders of fatty-acid oxidation**

E71.310   **Long chain/very long chain acyl CoA dehydrogenase deficiency**   CC HCC
LCAD
VLCAD

E71.311   **Medium chain acyl CoA dehydrogenase deficiency**   CC HCC
MCAD

E71.312   **Short chain acyl CoA dehydrogenase deficiency**   CC HCC
SCAD

E71.313   **Glutaric aciduria type II**   CC HCC
Glutaric aciduria type II A
Glutaric aciduria type II B
Glutaric aciduria type II C
EXCLUDES 1   *glutaric aciduria (type 1) NOS (E72.3)*

E71.314   **Muscle carnitine palmitoyltransferase deficiency**   CC HCC

E71.318   **Other disorders of fatty-acid oxidation**   CC HCC

E71.32   **Disorders of ketone metabolism**   CC HCC

E71.39   **Other disorders of fatty-acid metabolism**   CC HCC

✓5th **E71.4   Disorders of carnitine metabolism**

EXCLUDES 1   *muscle carnitine palmitoyltransferase deficiency (E71.314)*

E71.40   Disorder of carnitine metabolism, unspecified   HCC

E71.41   **Primary carnitine deficiency**   HCC

E71.42   **Carnitine deficiency due to inborn errors of metabolism**   HCC
Code also associated inborn error or metabolism

E71.43   **Iatrogenic carnitine deficiency**   HCC
Carnitine deficiency due to hemodialysis
Carnitine deficiency due to Valproic acid therapy

✓6th   E71.44   **Other secondary carnitine deficiency**

E71.440   **Ruvalcaba-Myhre-Smith syndrome**   HCC

E71.448   **Other secondary carnitine deficiency**   HCC

✓5th **E71.5   Peroxisomal disorders**

EXCLUDES 1   *Schilder's disease (G37.0)*

E71.50   Peroxisomal disorder, unspecified   CC HCC

✓6th   E71.51   **Disorders of peroxisome biogenesis**
Group 1 peroxisomal disorders
EXCLUDES 1   *Refsum's disease (G60.1)*

E71.510   **Zellweger syndrome**   CC HCC

E71.511   **Neonatal adrenoleukodystrophy**   CC HCC
EXCLUDES 1   *X-linked adrenoleukodystrophy (E71.42-)*

E71.518   **Other disorders of peroxisome biogenesis**   CC HCC

✓6th   E71.52   **X-linked adrenoleukodystrophy**

E71.520   **Childhood cerebral X-linked adrenoleukodystrophy**   CC HCC

E71.521   **Adolescent X-linked adrenoleukodystrophy**   CC HCC

E71.522   **Adrenomyeloneuropathy**   CC HCC

E71.528   **Other X-linked adrenoleukodystrophy**   CC HCC
Addison only phenotype adrenoleukodystrophy
Addison-Schilder adrenoleukodystrophy

E71.529   **X-linked adrenoleukodystrophy, unspecified type**   CC HCC

E71.53   **Other group 2 peroxisomal disorders**   CC HCC

✓6th   E71.54   **Other peroxisomal disorders**

E71.540   **Rhizomelic chondrodysplasia punctata**   CC HCC
EXCLUDES 1   *chondrodysplasia punctata NOS (Q77.3)*

E71.541   **Zellweger-like syndrome**   CC HCC

E71.542   **Other group 3 peroxisomal disorders**   CC HCC

E71.548   **Other peroxisomal disorders**   CC HCC

✓4th **E72   Other disorders of amino-acid metabolism**

EXCLUDES 1   *disorders of:*
aromatic amino-acid metabolism (E70.-)
branched-chain amino-acid metabolism (E71.0-E71.2)
fatty-acid metabolism (E71.3)
purine and pyrimidine metabolism (E79.-)
gout (M1A.-, M10.-)

✓5th **E72.0   Disorders of amino-acid transport**

EXCLUDES 1   *disorders of tryptophan metabolism (E70.5)*

E72.00   Disorders of amino-acid transport, unspecified   CC HCC

E72.01   **Cystinuria**   CC HCC

E72.02   **Hartnup's disease**   CC HCC

E72.03   **Lowe's syndrome**   CC HCC
Use additional code for associated glaucoma (H42)

E72.04   **Cystinosis**   CC HCC
Fanconi (-de Toni) (-Debré) syndrome with cystinosis
EXCLUDES 1   *Fanconi (-de Toni) (-Debré) syndrome without cystinosis (E72.09)*

E72.09   **Other disorders of amino-acid transport**   CC HCC
Fanconi (-de Toni) (-Debré) syndrome, unspecified

✓5th **E72.1   Disorders of sulfur-bearing amino-acid metabolism**

EXCLUDES 1   *cystinosis (E72.04)*
cystinuria (E72.01)
transcobalamin II deficiency (D51.2)

E72.10   Disorders of sulfur-bearing amino-acid metabolism, unspecified   CC HCC

E72.11   **Homocystinuria**   CC HCC
Cystathionine synthase deficiency

E72.12   **Methylenetetrahydrofolate reductase deficiency**   CC HCC

E72.19   **Other disorders of sulfur-bearing amino-acid metabolism**   CC HCC
Cystathioninuria
Methioninemia
Sulfite oxidase deficiency

✓5ᵗʰ **E72.2 Disorders of urea cycle metabolism**
> EXCLUDES 1 *disorders of ornithine metabolism (E72.4)*

E72.20 Disorder of urea cycle metabolism, unspecified cc HCC
Hyperammonemia
> EXCLUDES 1 *hyperammonemia- hyperornithinemia-homocitrullinemia syndrome E72.4*
> *transient hyperammonemia of newborn (P74.6)*

E72.21 Argininemia cc HCC
E72.22 Arginosuccinic aciduria cc HCC
E72.23 Citrullinemia cc HCC
E72.29 Other disorders of urea cycle metabolism cc HCC

E72.3 Disorders of lysine and hydroxylysine metabolism cc HCC
Glutaric aciduria NOS
Glutaric aciduria (type I)
Hydroxylysinemia
Hyperlysinemia
> EXCLUDES 1 *glutaric aciduria type II (E71.313)*
> *Refsum's disease (G60.1)*
> *Zellweger syndrome (E71.510)*

E72.4 Disorders of ornithine metabolism cc HCC
Hyperammonemia-Hyperornithinemia-Homocitrullinemia syndrome
Ornithinemia (types I, II)
Ornithine transcarbamylase deficiency
> EXCLUDES 1 *hereditary choroidal dystrophy (H31.2-)*

✓5ᵗʰ **E72.5 Disorders of glycine metabolism**

E72.50 Disorder of glycine metabolism, unspecified cc HCC
E72.51 Non-ketotic hyperglycinemia cc HCC
E72.52 Trimethylaminuria cc HCC
E72.53 Primary hyperoxaluria cc HCC
Oxalosis
Oxaluria
AHA: 2018,4Q,29
E72.59 Other disorders of glycine metabolism cc HCC
D-glycericacidemia
Hyperhydroxyprolinemia
Hyperprolinemia (types I, II)
Sarcosinemia

✓5ᵗʰ **E72.8 Other specified disorders of amino-acid metabolism**
AHA: 2018,4Q,5
E72.81 Disorders of gamma aminobutyric acid metabolism cc HCC
4-hydroxybutyric aciduria
Disorders of GABA metabolism
GABA metabolic defect
GABA transaminase deficiency
GABA-T deficiency
Gamma-hydroxybutyric aciduria
SSADHD
Succinic semialdehyde dehydrogenase deficiency
E72.89 Other specified disorders of amino-acid metabolism cc HCC
Disorders of beta-amino-acid metabolism
Disorders of gamma-glutamyl cycle

E72.9 Disorder of amino-acid metabolism, unspecified cc HCC

✓4ᵗʰ **E73 Lactose intolerance**
DEF: Inability to break down sugar in dairy products due to a deficiency in the enzyme lactase.
E73.0 Congenital lactase deficiency
E73.1 Secondary lactase deficiency
E73.8 Other lactose intolerance
E73.9 Lactose intolerance, unspecified

✓4ᵗʰ **E74 Other disorders of carbohydrate metabolism**
> EXCLUDES 1 *diabetes mellitus (E08-E13)*
> *hypoglycemia NOS (E16.2)*
> *increased secretion of glucagon (E16.3)*
> *mucopolysaccharidosis (E76.0-E76.3)*

✓5ᵗʰ **E74.0 Glycogen storage disease**

E74.00 Glycogen storage disease, unspecified cc HCC
E74.01 von Gierke disease cc HCC
Type I glycogen storage disease

E74.02 Pompe disease cc HCC
Cardiac glycogenosis
Type II glycogen storage disease
E74.03 Cori disease cc HCC
Forbes disease
Type III glycogen storage disease
E74.04 McArdle disease cc HCC
Type V glycogen storage disease
E74.09 Other glycogen storage disease cc HCC
Andersen disease
Hers disease
Tauri disease
Glycogen storage disease, types 0, IV, VI-XI
Liver phosphorylase deficiency
Muscle phosphofructokinase deficiency

✓5ᵗʰ **E74.1 Disorders of fructose metabolism**
> EXCLUDES 1 *muscle phosphofructokinase deficiency (E74.09)*

E74.10 Disorder of fructose metabolism, unspecified
E74.11 Essential fructosuria
Fructokinase deficiency
E74.12 Hereditary fructose intolerance
Fructosemia
E74.19 Other disorders of fructose metabolism
Fructose-1, 6-diphosphatase deficiency

✓5ᵗʰ **E74.2 Disorders of galactose metabolism**

E74.20 Disorders of galactose metabolism, unspecified cc HCC
E74.21 Galactosemia cc HCC
DEF: Any of three genetic disorders caused by a defective galactose metabolism. Symptoms include failure to thrive in infancy, jaundice, liver and spleen damage, cataracts, and mental retardation.
E74.29 Other disorders of galactose metabolism cc HCC
Galactokinase deficiency

✓5ᵗʰ **E74.3 Other disorders of intestinal carbohydrate absorption**
> EXCLUDES 2 *lactose intolerance (E73.-)*

E74.31 Sucrase-isomaltase deficiency
E74.39 Other disorders of intestinal carbohydrate absorption
Disorder of intestinal carbohydrate absorption NOS
Glucose-galactose malabsorption
Sucrase deficiency

E74.4 Disorders of pyruvate metabolism and gluconeogenesis cc HCC
Deficiency of phosphoenolpyruvate carboxykinase
Deficiency of pyruvate carboxylase
Deficiency of pyruvate dehydrogenase
> EXCLUDES 1 *disorders of pyruvate metabolism and gluconeogenesis with anemia (D55.-)*
> *Leigh's syndrome (G31.82)*

✓5ᵗʰ **E74.8 Other specified disorders of carbohydrate metabolism**
AHA: 2020,4Q,16
✓6ᵗʰ **E74.81 Disorders of glucose transport, not elsewhere classified**
E74.810 Glucose transporter protein type 1 deficiency cc HCC
De Vivo syndrome
Glucose transport defect, blood-brain barrier
Glut1 deficiency
GLUT1 deficiency syndrome 1, infantile onset
GLUT1 deficiency syndrome 2, childhood onset
E74.818 Other disorders of glucose transport cc HCC
(Familial) renal glycosuria
E74.819 Disorders of glucose transport, unspecified cc HCC
E74.89 Other specified disorders of carbohydrate metabolism cc HCC
Essential pentosuria
E74.9 Disorder of carbohydrate metabolism, unspecified HCC

✓4th E75　Disorders of sphingolipid metabolism and other lipid storage disorders

EXCLUDES 1　*mucolipidosis, types I–III (E77.0-E77.1)*
Refsum's disease (G60.1)

✓5th E75.0　GM2 gangliosidosis

E75.00　**GM2 gangliosidosis, unspecified**　CC HCC

E75.01　**Sandhoff disease**　CC HCC

E75.02　**Tay-Sachs disease**　CC HCC

DEF: Genetic mutation of the HEXA gene that inhibits the breakdown of a toxic substance called ganglioside. The accumulation of ganglioside results in destruction of the neurons in the brain and spinal cord.

Tay-Sachs Disease

Healthy neuron

Lysosome

Neuron affected by Tay-Sachs

Bulging lysosome

E75.09　**Other GM2 gangliosidosis**　CC HCC
Adult GM2 gangliosidosis
Juvenile GM2 gangliosidosis

✓5th E75.1　Other and unspecified gangliosidosis

E75.10　**Unspecified gangliosidosis**　CC HCC
Gangliosidosis NOS

E75.11　**Mucolipidosis IV**　CC HCC

E75.19　**Other gangliosidosis**　CC HCC
GM1 gangliosidosis
GM3 gangliosidosis

✓5th E75.2　Other sphingolipidosis

EXCLUDES 1　*adrenoleukodystrophy [Addison-Schilder] (E71.528)*

E75.21　**Fabry (-Anderson) disease**　HCC

E75.22　**Gaucher disease**　HCC

E75.23　**Krabbe disease**　CC HCC

✓6th E75.24　Niemann-Pick disease

▶Acid sphingomyelinase deficiency (ASMD)◀

E75.240　**Niemann-Pick disease type A**　HCC
▶Acid sphingomyelinase deficiency type A (ASMD type A)◀
▶Infantile neurovisceral acid sphingomyelinase deficiency◀

E75.241　**Niemann-Pick disease type B**　HCC
▶Acid sphingomyelinase deficiency type B (ASMD type B)◀
▶Chronic visceral acid sphingomyelinase deficiency◀

E75.242　**Niemann-Pick disease type C**　HCC

E75.243　**Niemann-Pick disease type D**　HCC

E75.244　**Niemann-Pick disease type A/B**
Acid sphingomyelinase deficiency type A/B (ASMD type A/B)
Chronic neurovisceral acid sphingomyelinase deficiency

E75.248　**Other Niemann-Pick disease**　HCC

E75.249　**Niemann-Pick disease, unspecified**　HCC
▶Acid sphingomyelinase deficiency (ASMD) NOS◀

E75.25　**Metachromatic leukodystrophy**　CC HCC

E75.26　**Sulfatase deficiency**　CC HCC
Multiple sulfatase deficiency (MSD)
AHA: 2018,4Q,5-6

E75.29　**Other sphingolipidosis**　CC HCC
Farber's syndrome
Sulfatide lipidosis

E75.3　**Sphingolipidosis, unspecified**　HCC

E75.4　**Neuronal ceroid lipofuscinosis**　CC HCC
Batten disease
Bielschowsky-Jansky disease
Kufs disease
Spielmeyer-Vogt disease

E75.5　**Other lipid storage disorders**
Cerebrotendinous cholesterosis [van Bogaert-Scherer-Epstein]
Wolman's disease

E75.6　**Lipid storage disorder, unspecified**

✓4th E76　Disorders of glycosaminoglycan metabolism

✓5th E76.0　Mucopolysaccharidosis, type I

E76.01　**Hurler's syndrome**　CC HCC

E76.02　**Hurler-Scheie syndrome**　CC HCC

E76.03　**Scheie's syndrome**　CC HCC

E76.1　**Mucopolysaccharidosis, type II**　CC HCC
Hunter's syndrome

✓5th E76.2　Other mucopolysaccharidoses

✓6th E76.21　Morquio mucopolysaccharidoses

E76.210　**Morquio A mucopolysaccharidoses**　CC HCC
Classic Morquio syndrome
Morquio syndrome A
Mucopolysaccharidosis, type IVA

E76.211　**Morquio B mucopolysaccharidoses**　CC HCC
Morquio-like mucopolysaccharidoses
Morquio-like syndrome
Morquio syndrome B
Mucopolysaccharidosis, type IVB

E76.219　**Morquio mucopolysaccharidoses, unspecified**　CC HCC
Morquio syndrome
Mucopolysaccharidosis, type IV

E76.22　**Sanfilippo mucopolysaccharidoses**　CC HCC
Mucopolysaccharidosis, type III (A) (B) (C) (D)
Sanfilippo A syndrome
Sanfilippo B syndrome
Sanfilippo C syndrome
Sanfilippo D syndrome

E76.29　**Other mucopolysaccharidoses**　CC HCC
beta-Glucuronidase deficiency
Maroteaux-Lamy (mild) (severe) syndrome
Mucopolysaccharidosis, types VI, VII

E76.3　**Mucopolysaccharidosis, unspecified**　CC HCC

E76.8　**Other disorders of glucosaminoglycan metabolism**　CC HCC

E76.9　**Glucosaminoglycan metabolism disorder, unspecified**　CC HCC

✓4th E77　Disorders of glycoprotein metabolism

E77.0　**Defects in post-translational modification of lysosomal enzymes**　HCC
Mucolipidosis II [I-cell disease]
Mucolipidosis III [pseudo-Hurler polydystrophy]

E77.1　**Defects in glycoprotein degradation**　HCC
Aspartylglucosaminuria
Fucosidosis
Mannosidosis
Sialidosis [mucolipidosis I]

E77.8　**Other disorders of glycoprotein metabolism**　HCC

E77.9　**Disorder of glycoprotein metabolism, unspecified**　HCC

✓4th **E78 Disorders of lipoprotein metabolism and other lipidemias**

> EXCLUDES 1   *sphingolipidosis (E75.0-E75.3)*

   ✓5th **E78.0 Pure hypercholesterolemia**

     AHA: 2016,4Q,13-14

     E78.00 Pure hypercholesterolemia, unspecified
       Fredrickson's hyperlipoproteinemia, type IIa
       Hyperbetalipoproteinemia
       Low-density-lipoprotein-type [LDL]
         hyperlipoproteinemia
       (Pure) hypercholesterolemia NOS

     E78.01 Familial hypercholesterolemia

   E78.1 Pure hyperglyceridemia
     Elevated fasting triglycerides
     Endogenous hyperglyceridemia
     Fredrickson's hyperlipoproteinemia, type IV
     Hyperlipidemia, group B
     Hyperprebetalipoproteinemia
     Very-low-density-lipoprotein-type [VLDL] hyperlipoproteinemia

   E78.2 Mixed hyperlipidemia
     Broad- or floating-betalipoproteinemia
     Combined hyperlipidemia NOS
     Elevated cholesterol with elevated triglycerides NEC
     Fredrickson's hyperlipoproteinemia, type IIb or III
     Hyperbetalipoproteinemia with prebetalipoproteinemia
     Hypercholesteremia with endogenous hyperglyceridemia
     Hyperlipidemia, group C
     Tubo-eruptive xanthoma
     Xanthoma tuberosum

> EXCLUDES 1   *cerebrotendinous cholesterosis [van Bogaert-Scherer-Epstein] (E75.5)*
>   *familial combined hyperlipidemia (E78.49)*

   E78.3 Hyperchylomicronemia
     Chylomicron retention disease
     Fredrickson's hyperlipoproteinemia, type I or V
     Hyperlipidemia, group D
     Mixed hyperglyceridemia

   ✓5th **E78.4 Other hyperlipidemia**

     AHA: 2018,4Q,6

     E78.41 Elevated Lipoprotein(a)
       Elevated Lp(a)

     E78.49 Other hyperlipidemia
       Familial combined hyperlipidemia

   E78.5 Hyperlipidemia, unspecified

   E78.6 Lipoprotein deficiency
     Abetalipoproteinemia
     Depressed HDL cholesterol
     High-density lipoprotein deficiency
     Hypoalphalipoproteinemia
     Hypobetalipoproteinemia (familial)
     Lecithin cholesterol acyltransferase deficiency
     Tangier disease

   ✓5th **E78.7 Disorders of bile acid and cholesterol metabolism**

> EXCLUDES 1   *Niemann-Pick disease type C (E75.242)*

     E78.70 Disorder of bile acid and cholesterol metabolism, unspecified

     E78.71 Barth syndrome   CC

     E78.72 Smith-Lemli-Opitz syndrome   CC

     E78.79 Other disorders of bile acid and cholesterol metabolism

   ✓5th **E78.8 Other disorders of lipoprotein metabolism**

     E78.81 Lipoid dermatoarthritis

     E78.89 Other lipoprotein metabolism disorders

   E78.9 Disorder of lipoprotein metabolism, unspecified

✓4th **E79 Disorders of purine and pyrimidine metabolism**

> EXCLUDES 1   *Ataxia-telangiectasia (Q87.19)*
>   *Bloom's syndrome (Q82.8)*
>   *Cockayne's syndrome (Q87.19)*
>   *calculus of kidney (N20.0)*
>   *combined immunodeficiency disorders (D81.-)*
>   *Fanconi's anemia (D61.09)*
>   *gout (M1A.-, M10.-)*
>   *orotaciduric anemia (D53.0)*
>   *progeria (E34.8)*
>   *Werner's syndrome (E34.8)*
>   *xeroderma pigmentosum (Q82.1)*

   E79.0 Hyperuricemia without signs of inflammatory arthritis and tophaceous disease
     Asymptomatic hyperuricemia

   E79.1 Lesch-Nyhan syndrome   CC   HCC
     HGPRT deficiency

   E79.2 Myoadenylate deaminase deficiency   CC   HCC

   E79.8 Other disorders of purine and pyrimidine metabolism   CC   HCC
     Hereditary xanthinuria

   E79.9 Disorder of purine and pyrimidine metabolism, unspecified   CC   HCC

✓4th **E80 Disorders of porphyrin and bilirubin metabolism**

> INCLUDES   defects of catalase and peroxidase

   E80.0 Hereditary erythropoietic porphyria   CC   HCC
     Congenital erythropoietic porphyria
     Erythropoietic protoporphyria

   E80.1 Porphyria cutanea tarda   CC   HCC

   ✓5th **E80.2 Other and unspecified porphyria**

     E80.20 Unspecified porphyria   CC   HCC
       Porphyria NOS

     E80.21 Acute intermittent (hepatic) porphyria   CC   HCC

     E80.29 Other porphyria
       Hereditary coproporphyria

   E80.3 Defects of catalase and peroxidase   CC   HCC
     Acatalasia [Takahara]

   E80.4 Gilbert syndrome

   E80.5 Crigler-Najjar syndrome

   E80.6 Other disorders of bilirubin metabolism
     Dubin-Johnson syndrome
     Rotor's syndrome

   E80.7 Disorder of bilirubin metabolism, unspecified

✓4th **E83 Disorders of mineral metabolism**

> EXCLUDES 1   *dietary mineral deficiency (E58-E61)*
>   *parathyroid disorders (E20-E21)*
>   *vitamin D deficiency (E55.-)*

   ✓5th **E83.0 Disorders of copper metabolism**

     E83.00 Disorder of copper metabolism, unspecified

     E83.01 Wilson's disease
       Code also associated Kayser Fleischer ring (H18.04-)

     E83.09 Other disorders of copper metabolism
       Menkes' (kinky hair) (steely hair) disease

   ✓5th **E83.1 Disorders of iron metabolism**

> EXCLUDES 1   *iron deficiency anemia (D50.-)*
>   *sideroblastic anemia (D64.0-D64.3)*

     E83.10 Disorder of iron metabolism, unspecified

     ✓6th **E83.11 Hemochromatosis**

> EXCLUDES 1   *GALD (P78.84)*
>   *gestational alloimmune liver disease (P78.84)*
>   *neonatal hemochromatosis (P78.84)*

       E83.110 Hereditary hemochromatosis   HCC
         Bronzed diabetes
         Pigmentary cirrhosis (of liver)
         Primary (hereditary) hemochromatosis

       E83.111 Hemochromatosis due to repeated red blood cell transfusions
         Iron overload due to repeated red blood cell transfusions
         Transfusion (red blood cell) associated hemochromatosis

       E83.118 Other hemochromatosis

       E83.119 Hemochromatosis, unspecified

✓ Additional Character Required   ✓x7th Placeholder   Questionable PDx   Manifestation   Unspecified Dx   UPD Unacceptable PDx   H1-H14 HAC   HCC CMS-HCC Dx   HIV HIV Dx

ICD-10-CM 2022   539

E83.19   **Other disorders of iron metabolism**
Use additional code, if applicable, for idiopathic pulmonary hemosiderosis (J84.03)

E83.2   **Disorders of zinc metabolism**
Acrodermatitis enteropathica

✓5ᵗʰ E83.3   **Disorders of phosphorus metabolism and phosphatases**
EXCLUDES 1   *adult osteomalacia (M83.-)*
osteoporosis (M80.-)

E83.30   **Disorder of phosphorus metabolism, unspecified**

E83.31   **Familial hypophosphatemia**
Vitamin D-resistant osteomalacia
Vitamin D-resistant rickets
EXCLUDES 1   *vitamin D-deficiency rickets (E55.0)*

E83.32   **Hereditary vitamin D-dependent rickets (type 1) (type 2)**
25-hydroxyvitamin D 1-alpha-hydroxylase deficiency
Pseudovitamin D deficiency
Vitamin D receptor defect

E83.39   **Other disorders of phosphorus metabolism**
Acid phosphatase deficiency
Hypophosphatasia

✓5ᵗʰ E83.4   **Disorders of magnesium metabolism**

E83.40   **Disorders of magnesium metabolism, unspecified**

E83.41   **Hypermagnesemia**
AHA: 2016,4Q,54

E83.42   **Hypomagnesemia**

E83.49   **Other disorders of magnesium metabolism**

✓5ᵗʰ E83.5   **Disorders of calcium metabolism**
EXCLUDES 1   *chondrocalcinosis (M11.1-M11.2)*
hungry bone syndrome (E83.81)
hyperparathyroidism (E21.0-E21.3)

E83.50   **Unspecified disorder of calcium metabolism**

E83.51   **Hypocalcemia**

E83.52   **Hypercalcemia**
Familial hypocalciuric hypercalcemia

E83.59   **Other disorders of calcium metabolism**

✓5ᵗʰ E83.8   **Other disorders of mineral metabolism**

E83.81   **Hungry bone syndrome**

E83.89   **Other disorders of mineral metabolism**

E83.9   **Disorder of mineral metabolism, unspecified**

✓4ᵗʰ **E84   Cystic fibrosis**
INCLUDES   mucoviscidosis
Code also exocrine pancreatic insufficiency (K86.81)
DEF: Genetic disorder affecting the respiratory, digestive, and reproductive systems in infants to young adults by disturbing exocrine gland function and causing chronic pulmonary disease with excess mucus production and pancreatic deficiency.

E84.0   **Cystic fibrosis with pulmonary manifestations**   `MCC` `HCC`
Use additional code to identify any infectious organism present, such as:
Pseudomonas (B96.5)
AHA: 2021,1Q,23

✓5ᵗʰ E84.1   **Cystic fibrosis with intestinal manifestations**

E84.11   **Meconium ileus in cystic fibrosis**   `MCC` `HCC` `N`
EXCLUDES 1   *meconium ileus not due to cystic fibrosis (P76.0)*

E84.19   **Cystic fibrosis with other intestinal manifestations**   `CC` `HCC`
Distal intestinal obstruction syndrome

E84.8   **Cystic fibrosis with other manifestations**   `CC` `HCC`

E84.9   **Cystic fibrosis, unspecified**   `CC` `HCC`

✓4ᵗʰ **E85   Amyloidosis**
EXCLUDES 2   *Alzheimer's disease (G30.0-)*
DEF: Conditions of diverse etiologies characterized by the accumulation of insoluble fibrillar proteins (amyloid) in various organs and tissues of the body, compromising vital functions.

E85.0   **Non-neuropathic heredofamilial amyloidosis**   `CC` `HCC`
Hereditary amyloid nephropathy
Code also associated disorders, such as:
autoinflammatory syndromes (M04.-)
EXCLUDES 2   *transthyretin-related (ATTR) familial amyloid cardiomyopathy (E85.4)*

E85.1   **Neuropathic heredofamilial amyloidosis**   `CC` `HCC`
Amyloid polyneuropathy (Portuguese)
Transthyretin-related (ATTR) familial amyloid polyneuropathy
AHA: 2012,4Q,99

E85.2   **Heredofamilial amyloidosis, unspecified**   `CC` `HCC`

E85.3   **Secondary systemic amyloidosis**   `CC` `HCC`
Hemodialysis-associated amyloidosis

E85.4   **Organ-limited amyloidosis**   `CC` `HCC`
Localized amyloidosis
Transthyretin-related (ATTR) familial amyloid cardiomyopathy

✓5ᵗʰ E85.8   **Other amyloidosis**
AHA: 2017,4Q,7

E85.81   **Light chain (AL) amyloidosis**   `CC` `HCC`

E85.82   **Wild-type transthyretin-related (ATTR) amyloidosis**   `CC` `HCC`
Senile systemic amyloidosis (SSA)

E85.89   **Other amyloidosis**   `CC` `HCC`

E85.9   **Amyloidosis, unspecified**   `CC` `HCC`

✓4ᵗʰ **E86   Volume depletion**
Use additional code(s) for any associated disorders of electrolyte and acid-base balance (E87.-)
EXCLUDES 1   *dehydration of newborn (P74.1)*
postprocedural hypovolemic shock (T81.19)
traumatic hypovolemic shock (T79.4)
EXCLUDES 2   *hypovolemic shock NOS (R57.1)*
AHA: 2019,2Q,7; 2018,2Q,6

E86.0   **Dehydration**
AHA: 2019,2Q,7; 2019,1Q,12; 2014,1Q,7
TIP: Can be assigned in addition to hypernatremia (E87.0) or hyponatremia (E87.1), when documented.

E86.1   **Hypovolemia**
Depletion of volume of plasma

E86.9   **Volume depletion, unspecified**
DEF: Depletion of total body water (dehydration) and/or contraction of total intravascular plasma (hypovolemia).

✓4ᵗʰ **E87   Other disorders of fluid, electrolyte and acid-base balance**
EXCLUDES 1   *diabetes insipidus (E23.2)*
electrolyte imbalance associated with hyperemesis gravidarum (O21.1)
electrolyte imbalance following ectopic or molar pregnancy (O08.5)
familial periodic paralysis (G72.3)
AHA: 2018,2Q,6

E87.0   **Hyperosmolality and hypernatremia**   `CC`
Sodium [Na] excess
Sodium [Na] overload
AHA: 2014,1Q,7
TIP: Assign an additional code for dehydration (E86.0), when documented.

E87.1   **Hypo-osmolality and hyponatremia**   `CC`
Sodium [Na] deficiency
EXCLUDES 1   *syndrome of inappropriate secretion of antidiuretic hormone (E22.2)*
AHA: 2014,1Q,7
TIP: Assign an additional code for dehydration (E86.0), when documented.

E87.2   **Acidosis**   `CC`
Acidosis NOS
Lactic acidosis
Metabolic acidosis
Respiratory acidosis
EXCLUDES 1   ▶*diabetic acidosis - see categories E08-E10, E11, E13 with ketoacidosis*◀
AHA: 2020,3Q,30
DEF: Reduction of alkaline in the blood and tissues caused by an increase in acid and decrease in bicarbonate.

E87.3   **Alkalosis**   `CC`
Alkalosis NOS
Metabolic alkalosis
Respiratory alkalosis

E87.4   **Mixed disorder of acid-base balance**   `CC`

E87.5   **Hyperkalemia**
Potassium [K] excess
Potassium [K] overload

E87.6   **Hypokalemia**
Potassium [K] deficiency

√5th   **E87.7**   **Fluid overload**

     EXCLUDES 1   *edema NOS (R60.9)*
            fluid retention (R60.9)

     E87.70   **Fluid overload, unspecified**

     E87.71   **Transfusion associated circulatory overload**
          Fluid overload due to transfusion (blood) (blood
             components)
          TACO

     E87.79   **Other fluid overload**

E87.8   **Other disorders of electrolyte and fluid balance, not elsewhere classified**
Electrolyte imbalance NOS
Hyperchloremia
Hypochloremia

√4th   **E88**   **Other and unspecified metabolic disorders**
Use additional codes for associated conditions
     EXCLUDES 1   *histiocytosis X (chronic) (C96.6)*

√5th   **E88.0**   **Disorders of plasma-protein metabolism, not elsewhere classified**

     EXCLUDES 1   *monoclonal gammopathy (of undetermined*
            significance) (D47.2)
            polyclonal hypergammaglobulinemia (D89.0)
            Waldenström macroglobulinemia (C88.0)

     EXCLUDES 2   *disorder of lipoprotein metabolism (E78.-)*

     E88.01   **Alpha-1-antitrypsin deficiency**   HCC
          AAT deficiency

     E88.02   **Plasminogen deficiency**   CC
          Dysplasminogenemia
          Hypoplasminogenemia
          Type 1 plasminogen deficiency
          Type 2 plasminogen deficiency
          Code also, if applicable, ligneous conjunctivitis
             (H10.51)
          Use additional code for associated findings, such as:
            hydrocephalus (G91.4)
            otitis media (H67.-)
            respiratory disorder related to plasminogen
             deficiency (J99)
          AHA: 2018,4Q,6-7

     E88.09   **Other disorders of plasma-protein metabolism, not elsewhere classified**
          Bisalbuminemia

E88.1   **Lipodystrophy, not elsewhere classified**
Lipodystrophy NOS
     EXCLUDES 1   *Whipple's disease (K90.81)*

E88.2   **Lipomatosis, not elsewhere classified**
Lipomatosis NOS
Lipomatosis (Check) dolorosa [Dercum]

E88.3   **Tumor lysis syndrome**   MCC
Tumor lysis syndrome (spontaneous)
Tumor lysis syndrome following antineoplastic drug
    chemotherapy
Use additional code for adverse effect, if applicable, to identify
    drug (T45.1X5)
AHA: 2020,1Q,37; 2019,2Q,24
DEF: Potentially fatal metabolic complication of tumor necrosis
caused by spontaneous or treatment-related accumulation of
byproducts from dying cancer cells. Symptoms include
hyperkalemia, hyperphosphatemia, hypocalcemia, hyperuricemia,
and hyperuricosuria.

√5th   **E88.4**   **Mitochondrial metabolism disorders**

     EXCLUDES 1   *disorders of pyruvate metabolism (E74.4)*
            Kearns-Sayre syndrome (H49.81)
            Leber's disease (H47.22)
            Leigh's encephalopathy (G31.82)
            mitochondrial myopathy, NEC (G71.3)
            Reye's syndrome (G93.7)

     E88.40   **Mitochondrial metabolism disorder,
            unspecified**   CC HCC

     E88.41   **MELAS syndrome**   CC HCC
          Mitochondrial myopathy, encephalopathy, lactic
             acidosis and stroke-like episodes

     E88.42   **MERRF syndrome**   CC HCC
          Myoclonic epilepsy associated with ragged-red fibers
          Code also progressive myoclonic epilepsy (G40.3-)

     E88.49   **Other mitochondrial metabolism
            disorders**   CC HCC

√5th   **E88.8**   **Other specified metabolic disorders**

     E88.81   **Metabolic syndrome**
          Dysmetabolic syndrome X
          Use additional codes for associated manifestations,
            such as:
            obesity (E66.-)
          DEF: Group of health risks that increase the likelihood
          of developing heart disease, stroke, and diabetes. These
          risks include certain parameters for blood pressure,
          cholesterol, and glucose levels.

     E88.89   **Other specified metabolic disorders**   HCC
          Launois-Bensaude adenolipomatosis
          EXCLUDES 1   *adult pulmonary Langerhans cell*
                histiocytosis (J84.82)

E88.9   **Metabolic disorder, unspecified**

Postprocedural endocrine and metabolic complications and disorders, not elsewhere classified (E89)

√4th   **E89**   **Postprocedural endocrine and metabolic complications and disorders, not elsewhere classified**
     EXCLUDES 2   *intraoperative complications of endocrine system organ or*
            structure (E36.0-, E36.1-, E36.8)

E89.0   **Postprocedural hypothyroidism**
Postirradiation hypothyroidism
Postsurgical hypothyroidism

E89.1   **Postprocedural hypoinsulinemia**   CC
Postpancreatectomy hyperglycemia
Postsurgical hypoinsulinemia
Use additional code, if applicable, to identify:
   acquired absence of pancreas (Z90.41-)
   diabetes mellitus (postpancreatectomy) (postprocedural)
     (E13.-)
   insulin use (Z79.4)
     EXCLUDES 1   *transient postprocedural hyperglycemia (R73.9)*
            transient postprocedural hypoglycemia (E16.2)

E89.2   **Postprocedural hypoparathyroidism**   HCC
Parathyroprival tetany

E89.3   **Postprocedural hypopituitarism**   HCC
Postirradiation hypopituitarism

√5th   **E89.4**   **Postprocedural ovarian failure**

     E89.40   **Asymptomatic postprocedural ovarian failure**   ♀
          Postprocedural ovarian failure NOS

     E89.41   **Symptomatic postprocedural ovarian failure**   ♀
          Symptoms such as flushing, sleeplessness, headache,
            lack of concentration, associated with
            postprocedural menopause

E89.5   **Postprocedural testicular hypofunction**   ♂

E89.6   **Postprocedural adrenocortical (-medullary) hypofunction**   CC HCC

√5th   **E89.8**   **Other postprocedural endocrine and metabolic complications and disorders**
AHA: 2016,4Q,9-10

     √6th   **E89.81**   **Postprocedural hemorrhage of an endocrine system organ or structure following a procedure**

          E89.810   **Postprocedural hemorrhage of an
                endocrine system organ or structure
                following an endocrine system
                procedure**   CC

          E89.811   **Postprocedural hemorrhage of an
                endocrine system organ or structure
                following other procedure**   CC

     √6th   **E89.82**   **Postprocedural hematoma and seroma of an endocrine system organ or structure**

          E89.820   **Postprocedural hematoma of an
                endocrine system organ or structure
                following an endocrine system
                procedure**   CC

          E89.821   **Postprocedural hematoma of an
                endocrine system organ or structure
                following other procedure**   CC

          E89.822   **Postprocedural seroma of an endocrine
                system organ or structure following an
                endocrine system procedure**   CC

E89.823 Postprocedural seroma of an endocrine system organ or structure following other procedure CC

E89.89 Other postprocedural endocrine and metabolic complications and disorders CC
Use additional code, if applicable, to further specify disorder

Chapter 5. Mental, Behavioral and Neurodevelopmental Disorders (F01–F99)

Chapter-specific Guidelines with Coding Examples

The chapter-specific guidelines from the ICD-10-CM Official Guidelines for Coding and Reporting have been provided below. Along with these guidelines are coding examples, contained in the shaded boxes, that have been developed to help illustrate the coding and/or sequencing guidance found in these guidelines.

a. Pain disorders related to psychological factors

Assign code F45.41, for pain that is exclusively related to psychological disorders. As indicated by the Excludes 1 note under category G89, a code from category G89 should not be assigned with code F45.41.

> Perceived abdominal pain determined to be persistent somatoform pain disorder
>
> **F45.41   Pain disorder exclusively related to psychological factors**
>
> *Explanation*: This pain was diagnosed as being exclusively psychological; therefore, no code from category G89 is added.

Code F45.42, Pain disorders with related psychological factors, should be used with a code from category G89, Pain, not elsewhere classified, if there is documentation of a psychological component for a patient with acute or chronic pain.

See Section I.C.6. Pain

b. Mental and behavioral disorders due to psychoactive substance use

1) In remission

Selection of codes for "in remission" for categories F10-F19, Mental and behavioral disorders due to psychoactive substance use (categories F10-F19 with -11, -.21) requires the provider's clinical judgment. The appropriate codes for "in remission" are assigned only on the basis of provider documentation (as defined in the Official Guidelines for Coding and Reporting), unless otherwise instructed by the classification.

Mild substance use disorders in early or sustained remission are classified to the appropriate codes for substance abuse in remission, and moderate or severe substance use disorders in early or sustained remission are classified to the appropriate codes for substance dependence in remission.

> Insomnia in patient with history of methamphetamine abuse; lab results indicate no current drug use
>
> **G47.00   Insomnia, unspecified**
>
> **F15.10   Other stimulant abuse, uncomplicated**
>
> *Explanation*: Insomnia is a common side-effect of stimulant use, such as methamphetamines. Although lab tests do not indicate that the patient is currently using methamphetamines, there is no specific documentation stating that the stimulant abuse is in remission. "History of" abuse does not equate to "in remission" in this instance.

2) Psychoactive substance use, abuse and dependence

When the provider documentation refers to use, abuse and dependence of the same substance (e.g. alcohol, opioid, cannabis, etc.), only one code should be assigned to identify the pattern of use based on the following hierarchy:

- If both use and abuse are documented, assign only the code for abuse
- If both abuse and dependence are documented, assign only the code for dependence
- If use, abuse and dependence are all documented, assign only the code for dependence
- If both use and dependence are documented, assign only the code for dependence.

> History and physical notes cannabis dependence; progress note says cannabis abuse
>
> **F12.20   Cannabis dependence, uncomplicated**
>
> *Explanation*: In the hierarchy, the dependence code is used if both abuse and dependence are documented.

> Discharge summary says cocaine abuse; progress notes list cocaine use
>
> **F14.10   Cocaine abuse, uncomplicated**
>
> *Explanation*: In the hierarchy, the abuse code is used if both abuse and use are documented.

3) Psychoactive substance use, unspecified

As with all other unspecified diagnoses, the codes for unspecified psychoactive substance use (F10.9-, F11.9-, F12.9-, F13.9-, F14.9-, F15.9-, F16.9-, F18.9-, F19.9-) should only be assigned based on provider documentation and when they meet the definition of a reportable diagnosis (see Section III, Reporting Additional Diagnoses). These codes are to be used only when the psychoactive substance use is associated with a **substance related** disorder (chapter 5 **disorders** such as sexual dysfunction, sleep disorder, or a mental or behavioral disorder) **or medical condition**, and such a relationship is documented by the provider.

4) Medical conditions due to psychoactive substance use, abuse and dependence

Medical conditions due to substance use, abuse, and dependence are not classified as substance-induced disorders. Assign the diagnosis code for the medical condition as directed by the Alphabetical Index along with the appropriate psychoactive substance use, abuse or dependence code. For example, for alcoholic pancreatitis due to alcohol dependence, assign the appropriate code from subcategory K85.2, Alcohol induced acute pancreatitis, and the appropriate code from subcategory F10.2, such as code F10.20, Alcohol dependence, uncomplicated. It would not be appropriate to assign code F10.288, Alcohol dependence with other alcohol-induced disorder.

5) Blood alcohol level

A code from category Y90, Evidence of alcohol involvement determined by blood alcohol level, may be assigned when this information is documented and the patient's provider has documented a condition classifiable to category F10, Alcohol related disorders. The blood alcohol level does not need to be documented by the patient's provider in order for it to be coded.

c. Factitious disorder

Factitious disorder imposed on self or Munchausen's syndrome is a disorder in which a person falsely reports or causes his or her own physical or psychological signs or symptoms. For patients with documented factitious disorder on self or Munchausen's syndrome, assign the appropriate code from subcategory F68.1-, Factitious disorder imposed on self.

Munchausen's syndrome by proxy (MSBP) is a disorder in which a caregiver (perpetrator) falsely reports or causes an illness or injury in another person (victim) under his or her care, such as a child, an elderly adult, or a person who has a disability. The condition is also referred to as "factitious disorder imposed on another" or "factitious disorder by proxy." The perpetrator, not the victim, receives this diagnosis. Assign code F68.A, Factitious disorder imposed on another, to the perpetrator's record. For the victim of a patient suffering from MSBP, assign the appropriate code from categories T74, Adult and child abuse, neglect and other maltreatment, confirmed, or T76, Adult and child abuse, neglect and other maltreatment, suspected.

See Section I.C.19.f. Adult and child abuse, neglect and other maltreatment

Chapter 5. Mental, Behavioral and Neurodevelopmental Disorders (F01-F99)

INCLUDES   disorders of psychological development
EXCLUDES 2   *symptoms, signs and abnormal clinical laboratory findings, not elsewhere classified (R00-R99)*

This chapter contains the following blocks:

F01-F09	Mental disorders due to known physiological conditions
F10-F19	Mental and behavioral disorders due to psychoactive substance use
F20-F29	Schizophrenia, schizotypal, delusional, and other non-mood psychotic disorders
F30-F39	Mood [affective] disorders
F40-F48	Anxiety, dissociative, stress-related, somatoform and other nonpsychotic mental disorders
F50-F59	Behavioral syndromes associated with physiological disturbances and physical factors
F60-F69	Disorders of adult personality and behavior
F70-F79	Intellectual disabilities
F80-F89	Pervasive and specific developmental disorders
F90-F98	Behavioral and emotional disorders with onset usually occurring in childhood and adolescence
F99	Unspecified mental disorder

Mental disorders due to known physiological conditions (F01-F09)

NOTE   This block comprises a range of mental disorders grouped together on the basis of their having in common a demonstrable etiology in cerebral disease, brain injury, or other insult leading to cerebral dysfunction. The dysfunction may be primary, as in diseases, injuries, and insults that affect the brain directly and selectively; or secondary, as in systemic diseases and disorders that attack the brain only as one of the multiple organs or systems of the body that are involved.

✓4ᵗʰ F01 Vascular dementia

Vascular dementia as a result of infarction of the brain due to vascular disease, including hypertensive cerebrovascular disease.

INCLUDES   arteriosclerotic dementia

Code first the underlying physiological condition or sequelae of cerebrovascular disease.

✓5ᵗʰ F01.5 Vascular dementia

F01.50 Vascular dementia without behavioral disturbance   HCC A

Major neurocognitive disorder without behavioral disturbance

AHA: 2021,2Q,4

F01.51 Vascular dementia with behavioral disturbance   CC HCC A

Major neurocognitive disorder due to vascular disease, with behavioral disturbance

Major neurocognitive disorder with aggressive behavior

Major neurocognitive disorder with combative behavior

Major neurocognitive disorder with violent behavior

Vascular dementia with aggressive behavior

Vascular dementia with combative behavior

Vascular dementia with violent behavior

Use additional code, if applicable, to identify wandering in vascular dementia (Z91.83)

✓4ᵗʰ F02 Dementia in other diseases classified elsewhere

INCLUDES   major neurocognitive disorder in other diseases classified elsewhere

Code first the underlying physiological condition, such as:
Alzheimer's (G30.-)
cerebral lipidosis (E75.4)
Creutzfeldt-Jakob disease (A81.0-)
dementia with Lewy bodies (G31.83)
dementia with Parkinsonism (G31.83)
epilepsy and recurrent seizures (G40.-)
frontotemporal dementia (G31.09)
hepatolenticular degeneration (E83.0)
human immunodeficiency virus [HIV] disease (B20)
Huntington's disease (G10)
hypercalcemia (E83.52)
hypothyroidism, acquired (E00-E03.-)
intoxications (T36-T65)
Jakob-Creutzfeldt disease (A81.0-)
multiple sclerosis (G35)
neurosyphilis (A52.17)
niacin deficiency [pellagra] (E52)
Parkinson's disease (G20)
Pick's disease (G31.01)
polyarteritis nodosa (M30.0)
prion disease (A81.9)
systemic lupus erythematosus (M32.-)
traumatic brain injury (S06.-)
trypanosomiasis (B56.-, B57.-)
vitamin B deficiency (E53.8)

EXCLUDES 2   *dementia in alcohol and psychoactive substance disorders (F10-F19, with .17, .27, .97)*
vascular dementia (F01.5-)

✓5ᵗʰ F02.8 Dementia in other diseases classified elsewhere

AHA: 2017,2Q,7; 2016,4Q,141; 2016,2Q,6
TIP: A code from this subcategory should always be assigned with a code from category G30 when Alzheimer's disease is documented, even in the absence of documented dementia.

F02.80 *Dementia in other diseases classified elsewhere without behavioral disturbance*   HCC

Dementia in other diseases classified elsewhere NOS

Major neurocognitive disorder in other diseases classified elsewhere

F02.81 *Dementia in other diseases classified elsewhere with behavioral disturbance*   CC HCC

Dementia in other diseases classified elsewhere with aggressive behavior

Dementia in other diseases classified elsewhere with combative behavior

Dementia in other diseases classified elsewhere with violent behavior

Major neurocognitive disorder in other diseases classified elsewhere with aggressive behavior

Major neurocognitive disorder in other diseases classified elsewhere with combative behavior

Major neurocognitive disorder in other diseases classified elsewhere with violent behavior

Use additional code, if applicable, to identify wandering in dementia in conditions classified elsewhere (Z91.83)

✓4ᵗʰ F03 Unspecified dementia

Presenile dementia NOS
Presenile psychosis NOS
Primary degenerative dementia NOS
Senile dementia NOS
Senile dementia depressed or paranoid type
Senile psychosis NOS

EXCLUDES 1   *senility NOS (R41.81)*

EXCLUDES 2   *mild memory disturbance due to known physiological condition (F06.8)*
senile dementia with delirium or acute confusional state (F05)

✓5ᵗʰ F03.9 Unspecified dementia

F03.90 Unspecified dementia without behavioral disturbance   HIV HCC A

Dementia NOS

AHA: 2021,2Q,4; 2012,4Q,92

N Newborn: 0   P Pediatric: 0-17   M Maternity: 9-64   A Adult: 15-124   MCC Major Complication/Comorbidity   CC Complication/Comorbidity   SW Severe Wound Dx

544   ICD-10-CM 2022

F03.91 **Unspecified dementia** with behavioral disturbance   `CC` `HCC` `A`
> Unspecified dementia with aggressive behavior
> Unspecified dementia with combative behavior
> Unspecified dementia with violent behavior
> Use additional code, if applicable, to identify wandering in unspecified dementia (Z91.83)

F04 **Amnestic disorder due to known physiological condition**   `HCC`
> Korsakov's psychosis or syndrome, nonalcoholic
> Code first the underlying physiological condition
> `EXCLUDES 1` *amnesia NOS (R41.3)*
> *anterograde amnesia (R41.1)*
> *dissociative amnesia (F44.0)*
> *retrograde amnesia (R41.2)*
> `EXCLUDES 2` *alcohol-induced or unspecified Korsakov's syndrome (F10.26, F10.96)*
> *Korsakov's syndrome induced by other psychoactive substances (F13.26, F13.96, F19.16, F19.26, F19.96)*

F05 **Delirium due to known physiological condition**   `CC`
> Acute or subacute brain syndrome
> Acute or subacute confusional state (nonalcoholic)
> Acute or subacute infective psychosis
> Acute or subacute organic reaction
> Acute or subacute psycho-organic syndrome
> Delirium of mixed etiology
> Delirium superimposed on dementia
> Sundowning
> Code first the underlying physiological condition
> `EXCLUDES 1` *delirium NOS (R41.0)*
> `EXCLUDES 2` *delirium tremens alcohol-induced or unspecified (F10.231, F10.921)*
>
> **AHA:** 2019,2Q,34

`✓4ᵗʰ` **F06** **Other mental disorders due to known physiological condition**
> `INCLUDES` mental disorders due to endocrine disorder
> mental disorders due to exogenous hormone
> mental disorders due to exogenous toxic substance
> mental disorders due to primary cerebral disease
> mental disorders due to somatic illness
> mental disorders due to systemic disease affecting the brain
> Code first the underlying physiological condition
> `EXCLUDES 1` *unspecified dementia (F03)*
> `EXCLUDES 2` *delirium due to known physiological condition (F05)*
> *dementia as classified in F01-F02*
> *other mental disorders associated with alcohol and other psychoactive substances (F10-F19)*

F06.0 **Psychotic disorder** with hallucinations **due to known physiological condition**   `CC`
> Organic hallucinatory state (nonalcoholic)
> `EXCLUDES 2` *hallucinations and perceptual disturbance induced by alcohol and other psychoactive substances (F10-F19 with .151, .251, .951)*
> *schizophrenia (F20.-)*

F06.1 **Catatonic disorder due to known physiological condition**
> Catatonia associated with another mental disorder
> Catatonia NOS
> `EXCLUDES 1` *catatonic stupor (R40.1)*
> *stupor NOS (R40.1)*
> `EXCLUDES 2` *catatonic schizophrenia (F20.2)*
> *dissociative stupor (F44.2)*
>
> **DEF:** Catatonic: Abnormal neuropsychiatric state characterized by stupor, immobility or purposeless movements, or unresponsiveness in a person who otherwise appears awake.

F06.2 **Psychotic disorder** with delusions **due to known physiological condition**   `CC`
> Paranoid and paranoid-hallucinatory organic states
> Schizophrenia-like psychosis in epilepsy
> `EXCLUDES 2` *alcohol and drug-induced psychotic disorder (F10-F19 with .150, .250, .950)*
> *brief psychotic disorder (F23)*
> *delusional disorder (F22)*
> *schizophrenia (F20.-)*

`✓5ᵗʰ` **F06.3** **Mood** disorder due to known physiological condition
> `EXCLUDES 2` *mood disorders due to alcohol and other psychoactive substances (F10-F19 with .14, .24, .94)*
> *mood disorders, not due to known physiological condition or unspecified (F30-F39)*

F06.30 **Mood disorder due to known physiological condition, unspecified**

F06.31 **Mood disorder due to known physiological condition with** depressive features
> Depressive disorder due to known physiological condition, with depressive features

F06.32 **Mood disorder due to known physiological condition with** major depressive-like episode
> Depressive disorder due to known physiological condition, with major depressive-like episode

F06.33 **Mood disorder due to known physiological condition with** manic features
> Bipolar and related disorder due to a known physiological condition, with manic features
> Bipolar and related disorder due to known physiological condition, with manic- or hypomanic-like episodes

F06.34 **Mood disorder due to known physiological condition with** mixed features
> Bipolar and related disorder due to known physiological condition, with mixed features
> Depressive disorder due to known physiological condition, with mixed features

F06.4 **Anxiety** disorder due to known physiological condition
> `EXCLUDES 2` *anxiety disorders due to alcohol and other psychoactive substances (F10-F19 with .180, .280, .980)*
> *anxiety disorders, not due to known physiological condition or unspecified (F40.-, F41.-)*

F06.8 **Other specified mental disorders due to known physiological condition**   `HIV`
> Epileptic psychosis NOS
> Obsessive-compulsive and related disorder due to a known physiological condition
> Organic dissociative disorder
> Organic emotionally labile [asthenic] disorder

`✓4ᵗʰ` **F07** **Personality and behavioral disorders due to known physiological condition**
> Code first the underlying physiological condition

F07.0 **Personality** change due to known physiological condition
> Frontal lobe syndrome
> Limbic epilepsy personality syndrome
> Lobotomy syndrome
> Organic personality disorder
> Organic pseudopsychopathic personality
> Organic pseudoretarded personality
> Postleucotomy syndrome
> Code first underlying physiological condition
> `EXCLUDES 1` *mild cognitive impairment (G31.84)*
> *postconcussional syndrome (F07.81)*
> *postencephalitic syndrome (F07.89)*
> *signs and symptoms involving emotional state (R45.-)*
> `EXCLUDES 2` *specific personality disorder (F60.-)*

`✓5ᵗʰ` **F07.8** **Other personality and behavioral disorders due to known physiological condition**

F07.81 **Postconcussional syndrome**
> Postcontusional syndrome (encephalopathy)
> Post-traumatic brain syndrome, nonpsychotic
> Use additional code to identify associated post-traumatic headache, if applicable (G44.3-)
> `EXCLUDES 1` *current concussion (brain) (S06.0-)*
> *postencephalitic syndrome (F07.89)*
>
> **DEF:** Concussion symptoms that persist for weeks or months after a head injury. These symptoms may include headache, giddiness, fatigue, insomnia, mood fluctuation, and a subjective feeling of impaired intellectual function with extreme reaction to normal stressors.

`✔` Additional Character Required   `✓x7ᵗʰ` Placeholder   Questionable PDx   Manifestation   Unspecified Dx   `UPD` Unacceptable PDx   `H1`-`H14` HAC   `HCC` CMS-HCC Dx   `HIV` HIV Dx

ICD-10-CM 2022   **545**

F07.89 Other personality and behavioral disorders due to known physiological condition **UPD**
  Postencephalitic syndrome
  Right hemispheric organic affective disorder

F07.9 Unspecified personality and behavioral disorder due to known physiological condition **HIV**
  Organic psychosyndrome

F09 Unspecified mental disorder due to known physiological condition **HIV**
  Mental disorder NOS due to known physiological condition
  Organic brain syndrome NOS
  Organic mental disorder NOS
  Organic psychosis NOS
  Symptomatic psychosis NOS
  Code first the underlying physiological condition
  EXCLUDES 1 psychosis NOS (F29)

Mental and behavioral disorders due to psychoactive substance use (F10-F19)

AHA: 2020,1Q,9; 2018,4Q,69-70; 2017,4Q,8; 2017,2Q,27
TIP: Psychoactive substance withdrawal can occur in individuals who do not have a diagnosis of dependence but who use the substance regularly (i.e., use or abuse) and then reduce or cease the use.

F10 Alcohol related disorders
  Use additional code for blood alcohol level, if applicable (Y90.-)
  AHA: 2019,3Q,8

F10.1 Alcohol abuse
    EXCLUDES 1 alcohol dependence (F10.2-)
      alcohol use, unspecified (F10.9-)
    AHA: 2018,1Q,16; 2015,2Q,15

  F10.10 Alcohol abuse, uncomplicated
    Alcohol use disorder, mild

  F10.11 Alcohol abuse, in remission
    Alcohol use disorder, mild, in early remission
    Alcohol use disorder, mild, in sustained remission

  F10.12 Alcohol abuse with intoxication
    F10.120 Alcohol abuse with intoxication, uncomplicated **HCC**
    F10.121 Alcohol abuse with intoxication delirium **CC HCC**
    F10.129 Alcohol abuse with intoxication, unspecified **HCC**

  F10.13 Alcohol abuse, with withdrawal
    AHA: 2020,4Q,16-17
    F10.130 Alcohol abuse with withdrawal, uncomplicated **CC HCC**
    F10.131 Alcohol abuse with withdrawal delirium **CC HCC**
    F10.132 Alcohol abuse with withdrawal with perceptual disturbance **CC HCC**
    F10.139 Alcohol abuse with withdrawal, unspecified **CC HCC**

  F10.14 Alcohol abuse with alcohol-induced mood disorder **CC HCC**
    Alcohol use disorder, mild, with alcohol-induced bipolar or related disorder
    Alcohol use disorder, mild, with alcohol-induced depressive disorder

  F10.15 Alcohol abuse with alcohol-induced psychotic disorder
    F10.150 Alcohol abuse with alcohol-induced psychotic disorder with delusions **HCC**
    F10.151 Alcohol abuse with alcohol-induced psychotic disorder with hallucinations **CC HCC**
      DEF: Psychosis lasting less than six months with slight or no clouding of consciousness in which auditory hallucinations predominate.
    F10.159 Alcohol abuse with alcohol-induced psychotic disorder, unspecified **CC HCC**

  F10.18 Alcohol abuse with other alcohol-induced disorders
    F10.180 Alcohol abuse with alcohol-induced anxiety disorder **CC HCC**
    F10.181 Alcohol abuse with alcohol-induced sexual dysfunction **CC HCC**
    F10.182 Alcohol abuse with alcohol-induced sleep disorder **HCC**

    F10.188 Alcohol abuse with other alcohol-induced disorder **CC HCC**
  F10.19 Alcohol abuse with unspecified alcohol-induced disorder **CC HCC**

F10.2 Alcohol dependence
    EXCLUDES 1 alcohol abuse (F10.1-)
      alcohol use, unspecified (F10.9-)
    EXCLUDES 2 toxic effect of alcohol (T51.0-)

  F10.20 Alcohol dependence, uncomplicated **HCC**
    Alcohol use disorder, moderate
    Alcohol use disorder, severe
    AHA: 2020,1Q,9

  F10.21 Alcohol dependence, in remission **HCC**
    Alcohol use disorder, moderate, in early remission
    Alcohol use disorder, moderate, in sustained remission
    Alcohol use disorder, severe, in early remission
    Alcohol use disorder, severe, in sustained remission

  F10.22 Alcohol dependence with intoxication
    Acute drunkenness (in alcoholism)
    EXCLUDES 2 alcohol dependence with withdrawal (F10.23-)
    F10.220 Alcohol dependence with intoxication, uncomplicated **HCC**
    F10.221 Alcohol dependence with intoxication delirium **CC HCC**
    F10.229 Alcohol dependence with intoxication, unspecified **HCC**

  F10.23 Alcohol dependence with withdrawal
    EXCLUDES 2 alcohol dependence with intoxication (F10.22-)
    AHA: 2018,1Q,16; 2015,2Q,15
    F10.230 Alcohol dependence with withdrawal, uncomplicated **CC HCC**
    F10.231 Alcohol dependence with withdrawal delirium **CC HCC**
    F10.232 Alcohol dependence with withdrawal with perceptual disturbance **CC HCC**
    F10.239 Alcohol dependence with withdrawal, unspecified **CC HCC**

  F10.24 Alcohol dependence with alcohol-induced mood disorder **CC HCC**
    Alcohol use disorder, moderate, with alcohol-induced bipolar or related disorder
    Alcohol use disorder, moderate, with alcohol-induced depressive disorder
    Alcohol use disorder, severe, with alcohol-induced bipolar or related disorder
    Alcohol use disorder, severe, with alcohol-induced depressive disorder

  F10.25 Alcohol dependence with alcohol-induced psychotic disorder
    F10.250 Alcohol dependence with alcohol-induced psychotic disorder with delusions **HCC**
    F10.251 Alcohol dependence with alcohol-induced psychotic disorder with hallucinations **CC HCC**
    F10.259 Alcohol dependence with alcohol-induced psychotic disorder, unspecified **CC HCC**

  F10.26 Alcohol dependence with alcohol-induced persisting amnestic disorder **HCC**
    Alcohol use disorder, moderate, with alcohol-induced major neurocognitive disorder, amnestic-confabulatory type
    Alcohol use disorder, severe, with alcohol-induced major neurocognitive disorder, amnestic-confabulatory type
    DEF: Prominent and lasting reduced memory span and disordered time appreciation and confabulation that occurs in alcoholics as sequel to acute alcoholic psychosis.

F10.27 Alcohol dependence with alcohol-induced persisting dementia `CC` `HCC`
     Alcohol use disorder, moderate, with alcohol-induced major neurocognitive disorder, nonamnestic-confabulatory type
     Alcohol use disorder, severe, with alcohol-induced major neurocognitive disorder, nonamnestic-confabulatory type

√6ᵗʰ **F10.28 Alcohol dependence with other alcohol-induced disorders**

     F10.280 Alcohol dependence with alcohol-induced anxiety disorder `CC` `HCC`

     F10.281 Alcohol dependence with alcohol-induced sexual dysfunction `CC` `HCC`

     F10.282 Alcohol dependence with alcohol-induced sleep disorder `HCC`

     F10.288 Alcohol dependence with other alcohol-induced disorder `CC` `HCC`
         Alcohol use disorder, moderate, with alcohol-induced mild neurocognitive disorder
         Alcohol use disorder, severe, with alcohol-induced mild neurocognitive disorder
         AHA: 2020,1Q,9

F10.29 Alcohol dependence with unspecified alcohol-induced disorder `CC` `HCC`

√5ᵗʰ **F10.9 Alcohol use, unspecified**
     `EXCLUDES 1`   *alcohol abuse (F10.1-)*
            alcohol dependence (F10.2-)
     AHA: 2018,2Q,10-11
     TIP: Assign a substance use code only when the provider documents a relationship between the use and an associated physical, mental, or behavioral disorder. As with all diagnoses, substance use codes must meet the definition of a reportable diagnosis.

√6ᵗʰ **F10.92 Alcohol use, unspecified with intoxication**

     F10.920 Alcohol use, unspecified with intoxication, uncomplicated `HCC`
         AHA: 2018,2Q,10-11

     F10.921 Alcohol use, unspecified with intoxication delirium `CC` `HCC`

     F10.929 Alcohol use, unspecified with intoxication, unspecified `HCC`

√6ᵗʰ **F10.93 Alcohol use, unspecified with withdrawal**
     AHA: 2020,4Q,16-17

     F10.930 Alcohol use, unspecified with withdrawal, uncomplicated `CC` `HCC`

     F10.931 Alcohol use, unspecified with withdrawal delirium `CC` `HCC`

     F10.932 Alcohol use, unspecified with withdrawal with perceptual disturbance `CC` `HCC`

     F10.939 Alcohol use, unspecified with withdrawal, unspecified `CC` `HCC`

F10.94 Alcohol use, unspecified with alcohol-induced mood disorder `CC` `HCC`
     Alcohol induced bipolar or related disorder, without use disorder
     Alcohol induced depressive disorder, without use disorder

√6ᵗʰ **F10.95 Alcohol use, unspecified with alcohol-induced psychotic disorder**

     F10.950 Alcohol use, unspecified with alcohol-induced psychotic disorder with delusions `HCC`

     F10.951 Alcohol use, unspecified with alcohol-induced psychotic disorder with hallucinations `CC` `HCC`

     F10.959 Alcohol use, unspecified with alcohol-induced psychotic disorder, unspecified `CC` `HCC`
         Alcohol-induced psychotic disorder without use disorder

F10.96 Alcohol use, unspecified with alcohol-induced persisting amnestic disorder `HCC`
     Alcohol-induced major neurocognitive disorder, amnestic-confabulatory type, without use disorder

F10.97 Alcohol use, unspecified with alcohol-induced persisting dementia `HCC`
     Alcohol-induced major neurocognitive disorder, nonamnestic-confabulatory type, without use disorder

√6ᵗʰ **F10.98 Alcohol use, unspecified with other alcohol-induced disorders**

     F10.980 Alcohol use, unspecified with alcohol-induced anxiety disorder `CC` `HCC`
         Alcohol induced anxiety disorder, without use disorder

     F10.981 Alcohol use, unspecified with alcohol-induced sexual dysfunction `CC` `HCC`
         Alcohol induced sexual dysfunction, without use disorder

     F10.982 Alcohol use, unspecified with alcohol-induced sleep disorder `HCC`
         Alcohol induced sleep disorder, without use disorder

     F10.988 Alcohol use, unspecified with other alcohol-induced disorder `CC` `HCC`
         Alcohol induced mild neurocognitive disorder, without use disorder

F10.99 Alcohol use, unspecified with unspecified alcohol-induced disorder `CC` `HCC`

√4ᵗʰ **F11 Opioid related disorders**

√5ᵗʰ **F11.1 Opioid abuse**
     `EXCLUDES 1`   *opioid dependence (F11.2-)*
            opioid use, unspecified (F11.9-)

     F11.10 Opioid abuse, uncomplicated `HCC`
         Opioid use disorder, mild

     F11.11 Opioid abuse, in remission `HCC`
         Opioid use disorder, mild, in early remission
         Opioid use disorder, mild, in sustained remission

√6ᵗʰ **F11.12 Opioid abuse with intoxication**

     F11.120 Opioid abuse with intoxication, uncomplicated `HCC`

     F11.121 Opioid abuse with intoxication delirium `CC` `HCC`

     F11.122 Opioid abuse with intoxication with perceptual disturbance `HCC`

     F11.129 Opioid abuse with intoxication, unspecified `HCC`

     F11.13 Opioid abuse with withdrawal `CC` `HCC`
         AHA: 2020,4Q,16-17

     F11.14 Opioid abuse with opioid-induced mood disorder `HCC`
         Opioid use disorder, mild, with opioid-induced depressive disorder

√6ᵗʰ **F11.15 Opioid abuse with opioid-induced psychotic disorder**

     F11.150 Opioid abuse with opioid-induced psychotic disorder with delusions `CC` `HCC`

     F11.151 Opioid abuse with opioid-induced psychotic disorder with hallucinations `CC` `HCC`

     F11.159 Opioid abuse with opioid-induced psychotic disorder, unspecified `HCC`

√6ᵗʰ **F11.18 Opioid abuse with other opioid-induced disorder**

     F11.181 Opioid abuse with opioid-induced sexual dysfunction `HCC`

     F11.182 Opioid abuse with opioid-induced sleep disorder `HCC`

     F11.188 Opioid abuse with other opioid-induced disorder `HCC`

F11.19 Opioid abuse with unspecified opioid-induced disorder `HCC`

Chapter 5. Mental, Behavioral and Neurodevelopmental Disorders

✓5th **F11.2 Opioid** dependence

     EXCLUDES 1   *opioid abuse (F11.1-)*
                    opioid use, unspecified (F11.9-)
     EXCLUDES 2   *opioid poisoning (T40.0-T40.2-)*

     F11.20 Opioid dependence, uncomplicated   CC HCC
         Opioid use disorder, moderate
         Opioid use disorder, severe

     F11.21 Opioid dependence, in remission   HCC
         Opioid use disorder, moderate, in early remission
         Opioid use disorder, moderate, in sustained remission
         Opioid use disorder, severe, in early remission
         Opioid use disorder, severe, in sustained remission

✓6th **F11.22 Opioid dependence with intoxication**

         EXCLUDES 1   *opioid dependence with withdrawal (F11.23)*

         F11.220 Opioid dependence with intoxication, uncomplicated   HCC

         F11.221 Opioid dependence with intoxication delirium   CC HCC

         F11.222 Opioid dependence with intoxication with perceptual disturbance   CC HCC

         F11.229 Opioid dependence with intoxication, unspecified   HCC

     F11.23 Opioid dependence with withdrawal   CC HCC

         EXCLUDES 1   *opioid dependence with intoxication (F11.22-)*

     F11.24 Opioid dependence with opioid-induced mood disorder   HCC
         Opioid use disorder, moderate, with opioid induced depressive disorder

✓6th **F11.25 Opioid dependence with opioid-induced psychotic disorder**

         F11.250 Opioid dependence with opioid-induced psychotic disorder with delusions   CC HCC

         F11.251 Opioid dependence with opioid-induced psychotic disorder with hallucinations   CC HCC

         F11.259 Opioid dependence with opioid-induced psychotic disorder, unspecified   CC HCC

✓6th **F11.28 Opioid dependence with other opioid-induced disorder**

         F11.281 Opioid dependence with opioid-induced sexual dysfunction   CC HCC

         F11.282 Opioid dependence with opioid-induced sleep disorder   CC HCC

         F11.288 Opioid dependence with other opioid-induced disorder   CC HCC

     F11.29 Opioid dependence with unspecified opioid-induced disorder   HCC

✓5th **F11.9 Opioid use, unspecified**

     EXCLUDES 1   *opioid abuse (F11.1-)*
                   opioid dependence (F11.2-)

     TIP: Assign a substance use code only when the provider documents a relationship between the use and an associated physical, mental, or behavioral disorder. As with all diagnoses, substance use codes must meet the definition of a reportable diagnosis.

     F11.90 Opioid use, unspecified, uncomplicated
         AHA: 2018,2Q,10-11

✓6th **F11.92 Opioid use, unspecified with intoxication**

         EXCLUDES 1   *opioid use, unspecified with withdrawal (F11.93)*

         F11.920 Opioid use, unspecified with intoxication, uncomplicated   HCC

         F11.921 Opioid use, unspecified with intoxication delirium   CC HCC
             Opioid-induced delirium

         F11.922 Opioid use, unspecified with intoxication with perceptual disturbance   HCC

         F11.929 Opioid use, unspecified with intoxication, unspecified   HCC

     F11.93 Opioid use, unspecified with withdrawal   CC HCC

         EXCLUDES 1   *opioid use, unspecified with intoxication (F11.92-)*

     F11.94 Opioid use, unspecified with opioid-induced mood disorder   HCC
         Opioid induced depressive disorder, without use disorder

✓6th **F11.95 Opioid use, unspecified with opioid-induced psychotic disorder**

         F11.950 Opioid use, unspecified with opioid-induced psychotic disorder with delusions   CC HCC

         F11.951 Opioid use, unspecified with opioid-induced psychotic disorder with hallucinations   CC HCC

         F11.959 Opioid use, unspecified with opioid-induced psychotic disorder, unspecified   HCC

✓6th **F11.98 Opioid use, unspecified with other specified opioid-induced disorder**

         F11.981 Opioid use, unspecified with opioid-induced sexual dysfunction   HCC
             Opioid induced sexual dysfunction, without use disorder

         F11.982 Opioid use, unspecified with opioid-induced sleep disorder   HCC
             Opioid induced sleep disorder, without use disorder

         F11.988 Opioid use, unspecified with other opioid-induced disorder   HCC
             Opioid induced anxiety disorder, without use disorder

     F11.99 Opioid use, unspecified with unspecified opioid-induced disorder   HCC

✓4th **F12 Cannabis related disorders**

     INCLUDES   marijuana
     AHA: 2020,1Q,8

✓5th **F12.1 Cannabis abuse**

     EXCLUDES 1   *cannabis dependence (F12.2-)*
                  cannabis use, unspecified (F12.9-)

     F12.10 Cannabis abuse, uncomplicated
         Cannabis use disorder, mild

     F12.11 Cannabis abuse, in remission
         Cannabis use disorder, mild, in early remission
         Cannabis use disorder, mild, in sustained remission

✓6th **F12.12 Cannabis abuse with intoxication**

         F12.120 Cannabis abuse with intoxication, uncomplicated   HCC

         F12.121 Cannabis abuse with intoxication delirium   CC HCC

         F12.122 Cannabis abuse with intoxication with perceptual disturbance   HCC

         F12.129 Cannabis abuse with intoxication, unspecified   HCC

     F12.13 Cannabis abuse with withdrawal   HCC
         AHA: 2020,4Q,16-17

✓6th **F12.15 Cannabis abuse with psychotic disorder**

         F12.150 Cannabis abuse with psychotic disorder with delusions   CC HCC

         F12.151 Cannabis abuse with psychotic disorder with hallucinations   CC HCC

         F12.159 Cannabis abuse with psychotic disorder, unspecified   HCC

✓6th **F12.18 Cannabis abuse with other cannabis-induced disorder**

         F12.180 Cannabis abuse with cannabis-induced anxiety disorder   HCC

         F12.188 Cannabis abuse with other cannabis-induced disorder   HCC
             Cannabis use disorder, mild, with cannabis-induced sleep disorder

     F12.19 Cannabis abuse with unspecified cannabis-induced disorder   HCC

N Newborn: 0   P Pediatric: 0-17   M Maternity: 9-64   A Adult: 15-124   MCC Major Complication/Comorbidity   CC Complication/Comorbidity   SW Severe Wound Dx

548   ICD-10-CM 2022

✓5ᵗʰ **F12.2 Cannabis** dependence

> EXCLUDES 1   *cannabis abuse (F12.1-)*
>   *cannabis use, unspecified (F12.9-)*
> EXCLUDES 2   *cannabis poisoning (T40.7-)*

F12.20 Cannabis dependence, uncomplicated   HCC
Cannabis use disorder, moderate
Cannabis use disorder, severe

F12.21 Cannabis dependence, in remission   HCC
Cannabis use disorder, moderate, in early remission
Cannabis use disorder, moderate, in sustained remission
Cannabis use disorder, severe, in early remission
Cannabis use disorder, severe, in sustained remission

✓6ᵗʰ **F12.22 Cannabis dependence with** intoxication

F12.220 Cannabis dependence with intoxication, uncomplicated   HCC

F12.221 Cannabis dependence with intoxication delirium   CC HCC

F12.222 Cannabis dependence with intoxication with perceptual disturbance   HCC

F12.229 Cannabis dependence with intoxication, unspecified   HCC

F12.23 Cannabis dependence with withdrawal   HCC
AHA: 2018,4Q,7

✓6ᵗʰ **F12.25 Cannabis dependence with** psychotic disorder

F12.250 Cannabis dependence with psychotic disorder with delusions   CC HCC

F12.251 Cannabis dependence with psychotic disorder with hallucinations   CC HCC

F12.259 Cannabis dependence with psychotic disorder, unspecified   HCC

✓6ᵗʰ **F12.28 Cannabis dependence with other cannabis-induced disorder**

F12.280 Cannabis dependence with cannabis-induced anxiety **disorder**   HCC

F12.288 Cannabis dependence with other cannabis-induced disorder   HCC
Cannabis use disorder, moderate, with cannabis-induced sleep disorder
Cannabis use disorder, severe, with cannabis-induced sleep disorder

F12.29 Cannabis dependence with unspecified cannabis-induced disorder   HCC

✓5ᵗʰ **F12.9 Cannabis use, unspecified**

> EXCLUDES 1   *cannabis abuse (F12.1-)*
>   *cannabis dependence (F12.2-)*

TIP: Assign a substance use code only when the provider documents a relationship between the use and an associated physical, mental, or behavioral disorder. As with all diagnoses, substance use codes must meet the definition of a reportable diagnosis.

F12.90 Cannabis use, unspecified, uncomplicated
AHA: 2018,2Q,10-11

✓6ᵗʰ **F12.92 Cannabis use, unspecified with** intoxication

F12.920 Cannabis use, unspecified with intoxication, uncomplicated   HCC

F12.921 Cannabis use, unspecified with intoxication delirium   CC HCC

F12.922 Cannabis use, unspecified with intoxication with perceptual disturbance   HCC

F12.929 Cannabis use, unspecified with intoxication, unspecified   HCC

F12.93 Cannabis use, unspecified with withdrawal   HCC
AHA: 2018,4Q,7

✓6ᵗʰ **F12.95 Cannabis use, unspecified with** psychotic disorder

F12.950 Cannabis use, unspecified with psychotic disorder with delusions   CC HCC

F12.951 Cannabis use, unspecified with psychotic disorder with hallucinations   CC HCC

F12.959 Cannabis use, unspecified with psychotic disorder, unspecified   HCC
Cannabis induced psychotic disorder, without use disorder

✓6ᵗʰ **F12.98 Cannabis use, unspecified with other cannabis-induced disorder**

F12.980 Cannabis use, unspecified with anxiety **disorder**   HCC
Cannabis induced anxiety disorder, without use disorder

F12.988 Cannabis use, unspecified with other cannabis-induced disorder   HCC
Cannabis induced sleep disorder, without use disorder

F12.99 Cannabis use, unspecified with unspecified cannabis-induced disorder   HCC

✓4ᵗʰ **F13 Sedative, hypnotic, or anxiolytic** related disorders

✓5ᵗʰ **F13.1 Sedative, hypnotic or anxiolytic-related** abuse

> EXCLUDES 1   *sedative, hypnotic or anxiolytic-related dependence (F13.2-)*
>   *sedative, hypnotic, or anxiolytic use, unspecified (F13.9-)*

F13.10 Sedative, hypnotic or anxiolytic abuse, uncomplicated   HCC
Sedative, hypnotic, or anxiolytic use disorder, mild

F13.11 Sedative, hypnotic or anxiolytic abuse, in remission   HCC
Sedative, hypnotic or anxiolytic use disorder, mild, in early remission
Sedative, hypnotic or anxiolytic use disorder, mild, in sustained remission

✓6ᵗʰ **F13.12 Sedative, hypnotic or anxiolytic abuse with intoxication**

F13.120 Sedative, hypnotic or anxiolytic abuse with intoxication, uncomplicated   HCC

F13.121 Sedative, hypnotic or anxiolytic abuse with intoxication delirium   CC HCC

F13.129 Sedative, hypnotic or anxiolytic abuse with intoxication, unspecified   HCC

✓6ᵗʰ **F13.13 Sedative, hypnotic or anxiolytic abuse with** withdrawal
AHA: 2020,4Q,16-17

F13.130 Sedative, hypnotic or anxiolytic abuse with withdrawal, uncomplicated   CC HCC

F13.131 Sedative, hypnotic or anxiolytic abuse with withdrawal delirium   CC HCC

F13.132 Sedative, hypnotic or anxiolytic abuse with withdrawal with perceptual disturbance   CC HCC

F13.139 Sedative, hypnotic or anxiolytic abuse with withdrawal, unspecified   CC HCC

F13.14 Sedative, hypnotic or anxiolytic abuse with sedative, hypnotic or anxiolytic-induced mood **disorder**   HCC
Sedative, hypnotic, or anxiolytic use disorder, mild, with sedative, hypnotic, or anxiolytic-induced bipolar or related disorder
Sedative, hypnotic, or anxiolytic use disorder, mild, with sedative, hypnotic, or anxiolytic-induced depressive disorder

✓6ᵗʰ **F13.15 Sedative, hypnotic or anxiolytic abuse with sedative, hypnotic or anxiolytic-induced** psychotic disorder

F13.150 Sedative, hypnotic or anxiolytic abuse with sedative, hypnotic or anxiolytic-induced psychotic disorder with delusions   CC HCC

F13.151 Sedative, hypnotic or anxiolytic abuse with sedative, hypnotic or anxiolytic-induced psychotic disorder with hallucinations   CC HCC

F13.159 Sedative, hypnotic or anxiolytic abuse with sedative, hypnotic or anxiolytic-induced psychotic disorder, unspecified   HCC

✓6ᵗʰ **F13.18 Sedative, hypnotic or anxiolytic abuse with other sedative, hypnotic or anxiolytic-induced disorders**

F13.180 Sedative, hypnotic or anxiolytic abuse with sedative, hypnotic or anxiolytic-induced anxiety **disorder**   HCC

Chapter 5. Mental, Behavioral and Neurodevelopmental Disorders

F13.181 Sedative, hypnotic or anxiolytic abuse with sedative, hypnotic or anxiolytic-induced sexual dysfunction `HCC`

F13.182 Sedative, hypnotic or anxiolytic abuse with sedative, hypnotic or anxiolytic-induced sleep disorder `HCC`

F13.188 Sedative, hypnotic or anxiolytic abuse with other sedative, hypnotic or anxiolytic-induced disorder `HCC`

F13.19 Sedative, hypnotic or anxiolytic abuse with unspecified sedative, hypnotic or anxiolytic-induced disorder `HCC`

✓5ᵗʰ **F13.2** Sedative, hypnotic or anxiolytic-related dependence

> *EXCLUDES 1* sedative, hypnotic or anxiolytic-related abuse (F13.1-)
> sedative, hypnotic, or anxiolytic use, unspecified (F13.9-)
>
> *EXCLUDES 2* sedative, hypnotic, or anxiolytic poisoning (T42.-)

F13.20 Sedative, hypnotic or anxiolytic dependence, uncomplicated `CC` `HCC`

F13.21 Sedative, hypnotic or anxiolytic dependence, in remission `HCC`

> Sedative, hypnotic or anxiolytic use disorder, moderate, in early remission
> Sedative, hypnotic or anxiolytic use disorder, moderate, in sustained remission
> Sedative, hypnotic or anxiolytic use disorder, severe, in early remission
> Sedative, hypnotic or anxiolytic use disorder, severe, in sustained remission

✓6ᵗʰ **F13.22** Sedative, hypnotic or anxiolytic dependence with intoxication

> *EXCLUDES 1* sedative, hypnotic or anxiolytic dependence with withdrawal (F13.23-)

F13.220 Sedative, hypnotic or anxiolytic dependence with intoxication, uncomplicated `HCC`

F13.221 Sedative, hypnotic or anxiolytic dependence with intoxication delirium `CC` `HCC`

F13.229 Sedative, hypnotic or anxiolytic dependence with intoxication, unspecified `HCC`

✓6ᵗʰ **F13.23** Sedative, hypnotic or anxiolytic dependence with withdrawal

> Sedative, hypnotic, or anxiolytic use disorder, moderate
> Sedative, hypnotic, or anxiolytic use disorder, severe
>
> *EXCLUDES 1* sedative, hypnotic or anxiolytic dependence with intoxication (F13.22-)

F13.230 Sedative, hypnotic or anxiolytic dependence with withdrawal, uncomplicated `CC` `HCC`

F13.231 Sedative, hypnotic or anxiolytic dependence with withdrawal delirium `CC` `HCC`

F13.232 Sedative, hypnotic or anxiolytic dependence with withdrawal with perceptual disturbance `CC` `HCC`

> Sedative, hypnotic, or anxiolytic withdrawal with perceptual disturbances

F13.239 Sedative, hypnotic or anxiolytic dependence with withdrawal, unspecified `CC` `HCC`

> Sedative, hypnotic, or anxiolytic withdrawal without perceptual disturbances

F13.24 Sedative, hypnotic or anxiolytic dependence with sedative, hypnotic or anxiolytic-induced mood disorder `HCC`

> Sedative, hypnotic, or anxiolytic use disorder, moderate, with sedative, hypnotic, or anxiolytic-induced bipolar or related disorder
> Sedative, hypnotic, or anxiolytic use disorder, moderate, with sedative, hypnotic, or anxiolytic-induced depressive disorder
> Sedative, hypnotic, or anxiolytic use disorder, severe, with sedative, hypnotic, or anxiolytic-induced bipolar or related disorder
> Sedative, hypnotic, or anxiolytic use disorder, severe, with sedative, hypnotic, or anxiolytic-induced depressive disorder

✓6ᵗʰ **F13.25** Sedative, hypnotic or anxiolytic dependence with sedative, hypnotic or anxiolytic-induced psychotic disorder

F13.250 Sedative, hypnotic or anxiolytic dependence with sedative, hypnotic or anxiolytic-induced psychotic disorder with delusions `CC` `HCC`

F13.251 Sedative, hypnotic or anxiolytic dependence with sedative, hypnotic or anxiolytic-induced psychotic disorder with hallucinations `CC` `HCC`

F13.259 Sedative, hypnotic or anxiolytic dependence with sedative, hypnotic or anxiolytic-induced psychotic disorder, unspecified `CC` `HCC`

F13.26 Sedative, hypnotic or anxiolytic dependence with sedative, hypnotic or anxiolytic-induced persisting amnestic disorder `CC` `HCC`

F13.27 Sedative, hypnotic or anxiolytic dependence with sedative, hypnotic or anxiolytic-induced persisting dementia `CC` `HCC`

> Sedative, hypnotic, or anxiolytic use disorder, moderate, with sedative, hypnotic, or anxiolytic induced major neurocognitive disorder
> Sedative, hypnotic, or anxiolytic use disorder, severe, with sedative, hypnotic, or anxiolytic-induced major neurocognitive disorder

✓6ᵗʰ **F13.28** Sedative, hypnotic or anxiolytic dependence with other sedative, hypnotic or anxiolytic-induced disorders

F13.280 Sedative, hypnotic or anxiolytic dependence with sedative, hypnotic or anxiolytic-induced anxiety disorder `CC` `HCC`

F13.281 Sedative, hypnotic or anxiolytic dependence with sedative, hypnotic or anxiolytic-induced sexual dysfunction `CC` `HCC`

F13.282 Sedative, hypnotic or anxiolytic dependence with sedative, hypnotic or anxiolytic-induced sleep disorder `CC` `HCC`

F13.288 Sedative, hypnotic or anxiolytic dependence with other sedative, hypnotic or anxiolytic-induced disorder `CC` `HCC`

> Sedative, hypnotic, or anxiolytic use disorder, moderate, with sedative, hypnotic, or anxiolytic-induced mild neurocognitive disorder
> Sedative, hypnotic, or anxiolytic use disorder, severe, with sedative, hypnotic, or anxiolytic-induced mild neurocognitive disorder

F13.29 Sedative, hypnotic or anxiolytic dependence with unspecified sedative, hypnotic or anxiolytic-induced disorder `HCC`

☑5ᵗʰ **F13.9 Sedative, hypnotic or anxiolytic-related use, unspecified**

> EXCLUDES 1   *sedative, hypnotic or anxiolytic-related abuse (F13.1-)*
> *sedative, hypnotic or anxiolytic-related dependence (F13.2-)*

TIP: Assign a substance use code only when the provider documents a relationship between the use and an associated physical, mental, or behavioral disorder. As with all diagnoses, substance use codes must meet the definition of a reportable diagnosis.

F13.90 Sedative, hypnotic, or anxiolytic use, unspecified, uncomplicated
> AHA: 2018,2Q,10-11

☑6ᵗʰ **F13.92 Sedative, hypnotic or anxiolytic use, unspecified with intoxication**

> EXCLUDES 1   *sedative, hypnotic or anxiolytic use, unspecified with withdrawal (F13.93-)*

F13.920 Sedative, hypnotic or anxiolytic use, unspecified with intoxication, uncomplicated HCC

F13.921 Sedative, hypnotic or anxiolytic use, unspecified with intoxication delirium CC HCC
> Sedative, hypnotic, or anxiolytic-induced delirium

F13.929 Sedative, hypnotic or anxiolytic use, unspecified with intoxication, unspecified HCC

☑6ᵗʰ **F13.93 Sedative, hypnotic or anxiolytic use, unspecified with withdrawal**

> EXCLUDES 1   *sedative, hypnotic or anxiolytic use, unspecified with intoxication (F13.92-)*

F13.930 Sedative, hypnotic or anxiolytic use, unspecified with withdrawal, uncomplicated CC HCC

F13.931 Sedative, hypnotic or anxiolytic use, unspecified with withdrawal delirium CC HCC

F13.932 Sedative, hypnotic or anxiolytic use, unspecified with withdrawal with perceptual disturbances CC HCC

F13.939 Sedative, hypnotic or anxiolytic use, unspecified with withdrawal, unspecified CC HCC

F13.94 Sedative, hypnotic or anxiolytic use, unspecified with sedative, hypnotic or anxiolytic-induced mood disorder HCC
> Sedative, hypnotic, or anxiolytic-induced bipolar or related disorder, without use disorder
> Sedative, hypnotic, or anxiolytic-induced depressive disorder, without use disorder

☑6ᵗʰ **F13.95 Sedative, hypnotic or anxiolytic use, unspecified with sedative, hypnotic or anxiolytic-induced psychotic disorder**

F13.950 Sedative, hypnotic or anxiolytic use, unspecified with sedative, hypnotic or anxiolytic-induced psychotic disorder with delusions CC HCC

F13.951 Sedative, hypnotic or anxiolytic use, unspecified with sedative, hypnotic or anxiolytic-induced psychotic disorder with hallucinations CC HCC

F13.959 Sedative, hypnotic or anxiolytic use, unspecified with sedative, hypnotic or anxiolytic-induced psychotic disorder, unspecified HCC
> Sedative, hypnotic, or anxiolytic-induced psychotic disorder, without use disorder

F13.96 Sedative, hypnotic or anxiolytic use, unspecified with sedative, hypnotic or anxiolytic-induced persisting amnestic disorder HCC

F13.97 Sedative, hypnotic or anxiolytic use, unspecified with sedative, hypnotic or anxiolytic-induced persisting dementia CC HCC
> Sedative, hypnotic, or anxiolytic-induced major neurocognitive disorder, without use disorder

☑6ᵗʰ **F13.98 Sedative, hypnotic or anxiolytic use, unspecified with other sedative, hypnotic or anxiolytic-induced disorders**

F13.980 Sedative, hypnotic or anxiolytic use, unspecified with sedative, hypnotic or anxiolytic-induced anxiety disorder HCC
> Sedative, hypnotic, or anxiolytic-induced anxiety disorder, without use disorder

F13.981 Sedative, hypnotic or anxiolytic use, unspecified with sedative, hypnotic or anxiolytic-induced sexual dysfunction HCC
> Sedative, hypnotic, or anxiolytic-induced sexual dysfunction disorder, without use disorder

F13.982 Sedative, hypnotic or anxiolytic use, unspecified with sedative, hypnotic or anxiolytic-induced sleep disorder HCC
> Sedative, hypnotic, or anxiolytic-induced sleep disorder, without use disorder

F13.988 Sedative, hypnotic or anxiolytic use, unspecified with other sedative, hypnotic or anxiolytic-induced disorder HCC
> Sedative, hypnotic, or anxiolytic-induced mild neurocognitive disorder

F13.99 Sedative, hypnotic or anxiolytic use, unspecified with unspecified sedative, hypnotic or anxiolytic-induced disorder HCC

☑4ᵗʰ **F14 Cocaine related disorders**

> EXCLUDES 2   *other stimulant-related disorders (F15.-)*

☑5ᵗʰ **F14.1 Cocaine abuse**

> EXCLUDES 1   *cocaine dependence (F14.2-)*
> *cocaine use, unspecified (F14.9-)*

F14.10 Cocaine abuse, uncomplicated HCC
> Cocaine use disorder, mild

F14.11 Cocaine abuse, in remission HCC
> Cocaine use disorder, mild, in early remission
> Cocaine use disorder, mild, in sustained remission

☑6ᵗʰ **F14.12 Cocaine abuse with intoxication**

F14.120 Cocaine abuse with intoxication, uncomplicated HCC

F14.121 Cocaine abuse with intoxication with delirium CC HCC

F14.122 Cocaine abuse with intoxication with perceptual disturbance HCC

F14.129 Cocaine abuse with intoxication, unspecified HCC

F14.13 Cocaine abuse, unspecified with withdrawal CC HCC
> AHA: 2020,4Q,16-17

F14.14 Cocaine abuse with cocaine-induced mood disorder HCC
> Cocaine use disorder, mild, with cocaine-induced bipolar or related disorder
> Cocaine use disorder, mild, with cocaine-induced depressive disorder

☑6ᵗʰ **F14.15 Cocaine abuse with cocaine-induced psychotic disorder**

F14.150 Cocaine abuse with cocaine-induced psychotic disorder with delusions CC HCC

F14.151 Cocaine abuse with cocaine-induced psychotic disorder with hallucinations CC HCC

F14.159 Cocaine abuse with cocaine-induced psychotic disorder, unspecified HCC

☑6ᵗʰ **F14.18 Cocaine abuse with other cocaine-induced disorder**

F14.180 Cocaine abuse with cocaine-induced anxiety disorder HCC

F14.181 Cocaine abuse with cocaine-induced sexual dysfunction HCC

F14.182 Cocaine abuse with cocaine-induced sleep disorder HCC

☑ Additional Character Required   ☑x7ᵗʰ Placeholder   Questionable PDx   Manifestation   Unspecified Dx   UPD Unacceptable PDx   H1-H14 HAC   HCC CMS-HCC Dx   HIV HIV Dx

ICD-10-CM 2022   551

F14.188 Cocaine abuse with other cocaine-induced disorder
Cocaine use disorder, mild, with cocaine-induced obsessive compulsive or related disorder

F14.19 Cocaine abuse with unspecified cocaine-induced disorder HCC

✓5ᵗʰ **F14.2 Cocaine dependence**
   EXCLUDES 1   *cocaine abuse (F14.1-)*
             cocaine use, unspecified (F14.9-)
   EXCLUDES 2   *cocaine poisoning (T40.5-)*

F14.20 Cocaine dependence, uncomplicated CC HCC
Cocaine use disorder, moderate
Cocaine use disorder, severe

F14.21 Cocaine dependence, in remission HCC
Cocaine use disorder, moderate, in early remission
Cocaine use disorder, moderate, in sustained remission
Cocaine use disorder, severe, in early remission
Cocaine use disorder, severe, in sustained remission

✓6ᵗʰ **F14.22 Cocaine dependence with intoxication**
   EXCLUDES 1   *cocaine dependence with withdrawal (F14.23)*

F14.220 Cocaine dependence with intoxication, uncomplicated HCC

F14.221 Cocaine dependence with intoxication delirium CC HCC

F14.222 Cocaine dependence with intoxication with perceptual disturbance CC HCC

F14.229 Cocaine dependence with intoxication, unspecified CC HCC

F14.23 Cocaine dependence with withdrawal CC HCC
   EXCLUDES 1   *cocaine dependence with intoxication (F14.22-)*

F14.24 Cocaine dependence with cocaine-induced mood disorder HCC
Cocaine use disorder, moderate, with cocaine-induced bipolar or related disorder
Cocaine use disorder, moderate, with cocaine-induced depressive disorder
Cocaine use disorder, severe, with cocaine-induced bipolar or related disorder
Cocaine use disorder, severe, with cocaine-induced depressive disorder

✓6ᵗʰ **F14.25 Cocaine dependence with cocaine-induced psychotic disorder**

F14.250 Cocaine dependence with cocaine-induced psychotic disorder with delusions CC HCC

F14.251 Cocaine dependence with cocaine-induced psychotic disorder with hallucinations CC HCC

F14.259 Cocaine dependence with cocaine-induced psychotic disorder, unspecified CC HCC

✓6ᵗʰ **F14.28 Cocaine dependence with other cocaine-induced disorder**

F14.280 Cocaine dependence with cocaine-induced anxiety disorder CC HCC

F14.281 Cocaine dependence with cocaine-induced sexual dysfunction CC HCC

F14.282 Cocaine dependence with cocaine-induced sleep disorder CC HCC

F14.288 Cocaine dependence with other cocaine-induced disorder CC HCC
Cocaine use disorder, moderate, with cocaine-induced obsessive compulsive or related disorder
Cocaine use disorder, severe, with cocaine-induced obsessive compulsive or related disorder

F14.29 Cocaine dependence with unspecified cocaine-induced disorder HCC

✓5ᵗʰ **F14.9 Cocaine use, unspecified**
   EXCLUDES 1   *cocaine abuse (F14.1-)*
             cocaine dependence (F14.2-)
TIP: Assign a substance use code only when the provider documents a relationship between the use and an associated physical, mental, or behavioral disorder. As with all diagnoses, substance use codes must meet the definition of a reportable diagnosis.

F14.90 Cocaine use, unspecified, uncomplicated
   AHA: 2018,2Q,10-11

✓6ᵗʰ **F14.92 Cocaine use, unspecified with intoxication**

F14.920 Cocaine use, unspecified with intoxication, uncomplicated HCC

F14.921 Cocaine use, unspecified with intoxication delirium CC HCC

F14.922 Cocaine use, unspecified with intoxication with perceptual disturbance HCC

F14.929 Cocaine use, unspecified with intoxication, unspecified HCC

F14.93 Cocaine use, unspecified with withdrawal CC HCC
   AHA: 2020,4Q,16-17

F14.94 Cocaine use, unspecified with cocaine-induced mood disorder HCC
Cocaine induced bipolar or related disorder, without use disorder
Cocaine induced depressive disorder, without use disorder

✓6ᵗʰ **F14.95 Cocaine use, unspecified with cocaine-induced psychotic disorder**

F14.950 Cocaine use, unspecified with cocaine-induced psychotic disorder with delusions CC HCC

F14.951 Cocaine use, unspecified with cocaine-induced psychotic disorder with hallucinations CC HCC

F14.959 Cocaine use, unspecified with cocaine-induced psychotic disorder, unspecified HCC
Cocaine induced psychotic disorder, without use disorder

✓6ᵗʰ **F14.98 Cocaine use, unspecified with other specified cocaine-induced disorder**

F14.980 Cocaine use, unspecified with cocaine-induced anxiety disorder HCC
Cocaine induced anxiety disorder, without use disorder

F14.981 Cocaine use, unspecified with cocaine-induced sexual dysfunction HCC
Cocaine induced sexual dysfunction, without use disorder

F14.982 Cocaine use, unspecified with cocaine-induced sleep disorder HCC
Cocaine induced sleep disorder, without use disorder

F14.988 Cocaine use, unspecified with other cocaine-induced disorder HCC
Cocaine induced obsessive compulsive or related disorder

F14.99 Cocaine use, unspecified with unspecified cocaine-induced disorder HCC

✓4ᵗʰ **F15 Other stimulant related disorders**
   INCLUDES   amphetamine-related disorders
             caffeine
   EXCLUDES 2   *cocaine-related disorders (F14.-)*

✓5ᵗʰ **F15.1 Other stimulant abuse**
   EXCLUDES 1   *other stimulant dependence (F15.2-)*
             other stimulant use, unspecified (F15.9-)

F15.10 Other stimulant abuse, uncomplicated HCC
Amphetamine type substance use disorder, mild
Other or unspecified stimulant use disorder, mild

F15.11 **Other stimulant abuse, in remission** `HCC`
Amphetamine type substance use disorder, mild, in early remission
Amphetamine type substance use disorder, mild, in sustained remission
Other or unspecified stimulant use disorder, mild, in early remission
Other or unspecified stimulant use disorder, mild, in sustained remission

✓6ᵗʰ F15.12 **Other stimulant abuse with intoxication**

F15.120 **Other stimulant abuse with intoxication, uncomplicated** `HCC`

F15.121 **Other stimulant abuse with intoxication delirium** `CC` `HCC`

F15.122 **Other stimulant abuse with intoxication with perceptual disturbance** `HCC`
Amphetamine or other stimulant use disorder, mild, with amphetamine or other stimulant intoxication, with perceptual disturbances

F15.129 **Other stimulant abuse with intoxication, unspecified** `HCC`
Amphetamine or other stimulant use disorder, mild, with amphetamine or other stimulant intoxication, without perceptual disturbances

F15.13 **Other stimulant abuse with withdrawal** `CC` `HCC`
AHA: 2020,4Q,16-17

F15.14 **Other stimulant abuse with stimulant-induced mood disorder** `HCC`
Amphetamine or other stimulant use disorder, mild, with amphetamine or other stimulant induced bipolar or related disorder
Amphetamine or other stimulant use disorder, mild, with amphetamine or other stimulant induced depressive disorder

✓6ᵗʰ F15.15 **Other stimulant abuse with stimulant-induced psychotic disorder**

F15.150 **Other stimulant abuse with stimulant-induced psychotic disorder with delusions** `CC` `HCC`

F15.151 **Other stimulant abuse with stimulant-induced psychotic disorder with hallucinations** `CC` `HCC`

F15.159 **Other stimulant abuse with stimulant-induced psychotic disorder, unspecified** `HCC`

✓6ᵗʰ F15.18 **Other stimulant abuse with other stimulant-induced disorder**

F15.180 **Other stimulant abuse with stimulant-induced anxiety disorder** `HCC`

F15.181 **Other stimulant abuse with stimulant-induced sexual dysfunction** `HCC`

F15.182 **Other stimulant abuse with stimulant-induced sleep disorder** `HCC`

F15.188 **Other stimulant abuse with other stimulant-induced disorder** `HCC`
Amphetamine or other stimulant use disorder, mild, with amphetamine or other stimulant induced obsessive-compulsive or related disorder

F15.19 **Other stimulant abuse with unspecified stimulant-induced disorder** `HCC`

✓5ᵗʰ F15.2 **Other stimulant dependence**
EXCLUDES 1 *other stimulant abuse (F15.1-)*
other stimulant use, unspecified (F15.9-)

F15.20 **Other stimulant dependence, uncomplicated** `CC` `HCC`
Amphetamine type substance use disorder, moderate
Amphetamine type substance use disorder, severe
Other or unspecified stimulant use disorder, moderate
Other or unspecified stimulant use disorder, severe

F15.21 **Other stimulant dependence, in remission** `HCC`
Amphetamine type substance use disorder, moderate, in early remission
Amphetamine type substance use disorder, moderate, in sustained remission
Amphetamine type substance use disorder, severe, in early remission
Amphetamine type substance use disorder, severe, in sustained remission
Other or unspecified stimulant use disorder, moderate, in early remission
Other or unspecified stimulant use disorder, moderate, in sustained remission
Other or unspecified stimulant use disorder, severe, in early remission
Other or unspecified stimulant use disorder, severe, in sustained remission

✓6ᵗʰ F15.22 **Other stimulant dependence with intoxication**
EXCLUDES 1 *other stimulant dependence with withdrawal (F15.23)*

F15.220 **Other stimulant dependence with intoxication, uncomplicated** `HCC`

F15.221 **Other stimulant dependence with intoxication delirium** `CC` `HCC`

F15.222 **Other stimulant dependence with intoxication with perceptual disturbance** `CC` `HCC`
Amphetamine or other stimulant use disorder, moderate, with amphetamine or other stimulant intoxication, with perceptual disturbances
Amphetamine or other stimulant use disorder, severe, with amphetamine or other stimulant intoxication, with perceptual disturbances

F15.229 **Other stimulant dependence with intoxication, unspecified** `HCC`
Amphetamine or other stimulant use disorder, moderate, with amphetamine or other stimulant intoxication, without perceptual disturbances
Amphetamine or other stimulant use disorder, severe, with amphetamine or other stimulant intoxication, without perceptual disturbances

F15.23 **Other stimulant dependence with withdrawal** `CC` `HCC`
Amphetamine or other stimulant withdrawal
EXCLUDES 1 *other stimulant dependence with intoxication (F15.22-)*

F15.24 **Other stimulant dependence with stimulant-induced mood disorder** `HCC`
Amphetamine or other stimulant use disorder, moderate, with amphetamine or other stimulant-induced bipolar or related disorder
Amphetamine or other stimulant use disorder, moderate, with amphetamine or other stimulant induced depressive disorder
Amphetamine or other stimulant use disorder, severe, with amphetamine or other stimulant-induced bipolar or related disorder
Amphetamine or other stimulant use disorder, severe, with amphetamine or other stimulant-induced depressive disorder

✓6ᵗʰ F15.25 **Other stimulant dependence with stimulant-induced psychotic disorder**

F15.250 **Other stimulant dependence with stimulant-induced psychotic disorder with delusions** `CC` `HCC`

F15.251 **Other stimulant dependence with stimulant-induced psychotic disorder with hallucinations** `CC` `HCC`

F15.259 **Other stimulant dependence with stimulant-induced psychotic disorder, unspecified** `CC` `HCC`

Chapter 5. Mental, Behavioral and Neurodevelopmental Disorders

F15.28–F16.159

√6ᵗʰ **F15.28** **Other stimulant dependence with other stimulant-induced disorder**

    F15.280 **Other stimulant dependence with stimulant-induced anxiety disorder** `CC` `HCC`

    F15.281 **Other stimulant dependence with stimulant-induced sexual dysfunction** `CC` `HCC`

    F15.282 **Other stimulant dependence with stimulant-induced sleep disorder** `CC` `HCC`

    F15.288 **Other stimulant dependence with other stimulant-induced disorder** `CC` `HCC`

        Amphetamine or other stimulant use disorder, moderate, with amphetamine orother stimulant induced obsessive compulsive or related disorder

        Amphetamine or other stimulant use disorder, severe, with amphetamine or otherstimulant induced obsessive compulsive or related disorder

    F15.29 **Other stimulant dependence with unspecified stimulant-induced disorder** `HCC`

√5ᵗʰ **F15.9** **Other stimulant use, unspecified**

    EXCLUDES 1   *other stimulant abuse (F15.1-)*

             other stimulant dependence (F15.2-)

    TIP: Assign a substance use code only when the provider documents a relationship between the use and an associated physical, mental, or behavioral disorder. As with all diagnoses, substance use codes must meet the definition of a reportable diagnosis.

    F15.90 **Other stimulant use, unspecified, uncomplicated**

        AHA: 2018,2Q,10-11

√6ᵗʰ   **F15.92** **Other stimulant use, unspecified with intoxication**

        EXCLUDES 1   *other stimulant use, unspecified with withdrawal (F15.93)*

    F15.920 **Other stimulant use, unspecified with intoxication, uncomplicated** `HCC`

    F15.921 **Other stimulant use, unspecified with intoxication delirium** `CC` `HCC`

        Amphetamine or other stimulant-induced delirium

    F15.922 **Other stimulant use, unspecified with intoxication with perceptual disturbance** `HCC`

    F15.929 **Other stimulant use, unspecified with intoxication, unspecified** `HCC`

        Caffeine intoxication

    F15.93 **Other stimulant use, unspecified with withdrawal** `CC` `HCC`

        Caffeine withdrawal

        EXCLUDES 1   *other stimulant use, unspecified with intoxication (F15.92-)*

√6ᵗʰ   **F15.94** **Other stimulant use, unspecified with stimulant-induced mood disorder** `HCC`

        Amphetamine or other stimulant-induced bipolar or related disorder, without use disorder

        Amphetamine or other stimulant-induced depressive disorder, without use disorder

√6ᵗʰ   **F15.95** **Other stimulant use, unspecified with stimulant-induced psychotic disorder**

    F15.950 **Other stimulant use, unspecified with stimulant-induced psychotic disorder with delusions** `CC` `HCC`

    F15.951 **Other stimulant use, unspecified with stimulant-induced psychotic disorder with hallucinations** `CC` `HCC`

    F15.959 **Other stimulant use, unspecified with stimulant-induced psychotic disorder, unspecified** `HCC`

        Amphetamine or other stimulant-induced psychotic disorder, without use disorder

√6ᵗʰ **F15.98** **Other stimulant use, unspecified with other stimulant-induced disorder**

    F15.980 **Other stimulant use, unspecified with stimulant-induced anxiety disorder** `HCC`

        Amphetamine or other stimulant-induced anxiety disorder, without use disorder

        Caffeine induced anxiety disorder, without use disorder

    F15.981 **Other stimulant use, unspecified with stimulant-induced sexual dysfunction** `HCC`

        Amphetamine or other stimulant-induced sexual dysfunction, without use disorder

    F15.982 **Other stimulant use, unspecified with stimulant-induced sleep disorder** `HCC`

        Amphetamine or other stimulant-induced sleep disorder, without use disorder

        Caffeine induced sleep disorder, without use disorder

    F15.988 **Other stimulant use, unspecified with other stimulant-induced disorder** `HCC`

        Amphetamine or other stimulant-induced obsessive compulsive or related disorder, without use disorder

    F15.99 **Other stimulant use, unspecified with unspecified stimulant-induced disorder** `HCC`

√4ᵗʰ **F16** **Hallucinogen related disorders**

    INCLUDES   ecstasy

            PCP

            phencyclidine

    AHA: 2018,4Q,31

√5ᵗʰ   **F16.1** **Hallucinogen abuse**

        EXCLUDES 1   *hallucinogen dependence (F16.2-)*

                      hallucinogen use, unspecified (F16.9-)

    F16.10 **Hallucinogen abuse, uncomplicated** `HCC`

        Other hallucinogen use disorder, mild

        Phencyclidine use disorder, mild

    F16.11 **Hallucinogen abuse, in remission** `HCC`

        Other hallucinogen use disorder, mild, in early remission

        Other hallucinogen use disorder, mild, in sustained remission

        Phencyclidine use disorder, mild, in early remission

        Phencyclidine use disorder, mild, in sustained remission

√6ᵗʰ   **F16.12** **Hallucinogen abuse with intoxication**

    F16.120 **Hallucinogen abuse with intoxication, uncomplicated** `HCC`

    F16.121 **Hallucinogen abuse with intoxication with delirium** `CC` `HCC`

    F16.122 **Hallucinogen abuse with intoxication with perceptual disturbance** `HCC`

    F16.129 **Hallucinogen abuse with intoxication, unspecified** `HCC`

    F16.14 **Hallucinogen abuse with hallucinogen-induced mood disorder** `HCC`

        Other hallucinogen use disorder, mild, with other hallucinogen induced bipolar or related disorder

        Other hallucinogen use disorder, mild, with other hallucinogen induced depressive disorder

        Phencyclidine use disorder, mild, with phencyclidine induced bipolar or related disorder

        Phencyclidine use disorder, mild, with phencyclidine induced depressive disorder

√6ᵗʰ   **F16.15** **Hallucinogen abuse with hallucinogen-induced psychotic disorder**

    F16.150 **Hallucinogen abuse with hallucinogen-induced psychotic disorder with delusions** `CC` `HCC`

    F16.151 **Hallucinogen abuse with hallucinogen-induced psychotic disorder with hallucinations** `CC` `HCC`

    F16.159 **Hallucinogen abuse with hallucinogen-induced psychotic disorder, unspecified** `HCC`

Ⓝ Newborn: 0   Ⓟ Pediatric: 0-17   Ⓜ Maternity: 9-64   Ⓐ Adult: 15-124   `MCC` Major Complication/Comorbidity   `CC` Complication/Comorbidity   `SW` Severe Wound Dx

554

ICD-10-CM 2022

√6ᵗʰ F16.18 Hallucinogen abuse with other hallucinogen-induced disorder

   F16.180 Hallucinogen abuse with hallucinogen-induced anxiety disorder `HCC`

   F16.183 Hallucinogen abuse with hallucinogen persisting perception disorder (flashbacks) `HCC`

   F16.188 Hallucinogen abuse with other hallucinogen-induced disorder `HCC`

F16.19 Hallucinogen abuse with unspecified hallucinogen-induced disorder `HCC`

√5ᵗʰ F16.2 Hallucinogen dependence

   EXCLUDES 1   *hallucinogen abuse (F16.1-)*
                  hallucinogen use, unspecified (F16.9-)

   F16.20 Hallucinogen dependence, uncomplicated `CC` `HCC`
      Other hallucinogen use disorder, moderate
      Other hallucinogen use disorder, severe
      Phencyclidine use disorder, moderate
      Phencyclidine use disorder, severe

   F16.21 Hallucinogen dependence, in remission `HCC`
      Other hallucinogen use disorder, moderate, in early remission
      Other hallucinogen use disorder, moderate, in sustained remission
      Other hallucinogen use disorder, severe, in early remission
      Other hallucinogen use disorder, severe, in sustained remission
      Phencyclidine use disorder, moderate, in early remission
      Phencyclidine use disorder, moderate, in sustained remission
      Phencyclidine use disorder, severe, in early remission
      Phencyclidine use disorder, severe, in sustained remission

   √6ᵗʰ F16.22 Hallucinogen dependence with intoxication

      F16.220 Hallucinogen dependence with intoxication, uncomplicated `HCC`

      F16.221 Hallucinogen dependence with intoxication with delirium `CC` `HCC`

      F16.229 Hallucinogen dependence with intoxication, unspecified `HCC`

   F16.24 Hallucinogen dependence with hallucinogen-induced mood disorder `HCC`
      Other hallucinogen use disorder, moderate, with other hallucinogen induced bipolar or related disorder
      Other hallucinogen use disorder, moderate, with other hallucinogen induced depressive disorder
      Other hallucinogen use disorder, severe, with other hallucinogen-induced bipolar or related disorder
      Other hallucinogen use disorder, severe, with other hallucinogen-induced depressive disorder
      Phencyclidine use disorder, moderate, with phencyclidine induced bipolar or related disorder
      Phencyclidine use disorder, moderate, with phencyclidine induced depressive disorder
      Phencyclidine use disorder, severe, with phencyclidine induced bipolar or related disorder
      Phencyclidine use disorder, severe, with phencyclidine-induced depressive disorder

   √6ᵗʰ F16.25 Hallucinogen dependence with hallucinogen-induced psychotic disorder

      F16.250 Hallucinogen dependence with hallucinogen-induced psychotic disorder with delusions `CC` `HCC`

      F16.251 Hallucinogen dependence with hallucinogen-induced psychotic disorder with hallucinations `CC` `HCC`

      F16.259 Hallucinogen dependence with hallucinogen-induced psychotic disorder, unspecified `CC` `HCC`

   √6ᵗʰ F16.28 Hallucinogen dependence with other hallucinogen-induced disorder

      F16.280 Hallucinogen dependence with hallucinogen-induced anxiety disorder `CC` `HCC`

      F16.283 Hallucinogen dependence with hallucinogen persisting perception disorder (flashbacks) `CC` `HCC`

      F16.288 Hallucinogen dependence with other hallucinogen-induced disorder `CC` `HCC`

F16.29 Hallucinogen dependence with unspecified hallucinogen-induced disorder `HCC`

√5ᵗʰ F16.9 Hallucinogen use, unspecified

   EXCLUDES 1   *hallucinogen abuse (F16.1-)*
                  hallucinogen dependence (F16.2-)

   TIP: Assign a substance use code only when the provider documents a relationship between the use and an associated physical, mental, or behavioral disorder. As with all diagnoses, substance use codes must meet the definition of a reportable diagnosis.

   F16.90 Hallucinogen use, unspecified, uncomplicated
      AHA: 2018,2Q,10-11

   √6ᵗʰ F16.92 Hallucinogen use, unspecified with intoxication

      F16.920 Hallucinogen use, unspecified with intoxication, uncomplicated `HCC`

      F16.921 Hallucinogen use, unspecified with intoxication with delirium `CC` `HCC`
         Other hallucinogen intoxication delirium

      F16.929 Hallucinogen use, unspecified with intoxication, unspecified `HCC`

   F16.94 Hallucinogen use, unspecified with hallucinogen-induced mood disorder `HCC`
      Other hallucinogen induced bipolar or related disorder, without use disorder
      Other hallucinogen induced depressive disorder, without use disorder
      Phencyclidine induced bipolar or related disorder, without use disorder
      Phencyclidine induced depressive disorder, without use disorder

   √6ᵗʰ F16.95 Hallucinogen use, unspecified with hallucinogen-induced psychotic disorder

      F16.950 Hallucinogen use, unspecified with hallucinogen-induced psychotic disorder with delusions `CC` `HCC`

      F16.951 Hallucinogen use, unspecified with hallucinogen-induced psychotic disorder with hallucinations `CC` `HCC`

      F16.959 Hallucinogen use, unspecified with hallucinogen-induced psychotic disorder, unspecified `HCC`
         Other hallucinogen induced psychotic disorder, without use disorder
         Phencyclidine induced psychotic disorder, without use disorder

   √6ᵗʰ F16.98 Hallucinogen use, unspecified with other specified hallucinogen-induced disorder

      F16.980 Hallucinogen use, unspecified with hallucinogen-induced anxiety disorder `HCC`
         Other hallucinogen-induced anxiety disorder, without use disorder
         Phencyclidine induced anxiety disorder, without use disorder

      F16.983 Hallucinogen use, unspecified with hallucinogen persisting perception disorder (flashbacks) `HCC`

      F16.988 Hallucinogen use, unspecified with other hallucinogen-induced disorder `HCC`

   F16.99 Hallucinogen use, unspecified with unspecified hallucinogen-induced disorder `HCC`

✔ Additional Character Required   √x7ᵗʰ Placeholder   Questionable PDx   Manifestation   Unspecified Dx   `UPD` Unacceptable PDx   `H1`-`H14` HAC   `HCC` CMS-HCC Dx   `HIV` HIV Dx

ICD-10-CM 2022   555

Chapter 5. Mental, Behavioral and Neurodevelopmental Disorders

✓4ᵗʰ **F17** Nicotine dependence

    EXCLUDES 1   history of tobacco dependence (Z87.891)
               tobacco use NOS (Z72.0)

    EXCLUDES 2   tobacco use (smoking) during pregnancy, childbirth and the puerperium (O99.33-)
               toxic effect of nicotine (T65.2-)

    AHA: 2013,4Q,108-109

✓5ᵗʰ **F17.2** Nicotine dependence

  ✓6ᵗʰ **F17.20** Nicotine dependence, unspecified

    F17.200 Nicotine dependence, unspecified, uncomplicated   UPD
         Tobacco use disorder, mild
         Tobacco use disorder, moderate
         Tobacco use disorder, severe
         AHA: 2016,1Q,36
         TIP: Assign when provider documentation indicates "smoker" without further specification.

    F17.201 Nicotine dependence, unspecified, in remission   UPD
         Tobacco use disorder, mild, in early remission
         Tobacco use disorder, mild, in sustained remission
         Tobacco use disorder, moderate, in early remission
         Tobacco use disorder, moderate, in sustained remission
         Tobacco use disorder, severe, in early remission
         Tobacco use disorder, severe, in sustained remission

    F17.203 Nicotine dependence unspecified, with withdrawal   CC
         Tobacco withdrawal

    F17.208 Nicotine dependence, unspecified, with other nicotine-induced disorders

    F17.209 Nicotine dependence, unspecified, with unspecified nicotine-induced disorders

  ✓6ᵗʰ **F17.21** Nicotine dependence, cigarettes

    F17.210 Nicotine dependence, cigarettes, uncomplicated   UPD
         AHA: 2017,2Q,28-29

    F17.211 Nicotine dependence, cigarettes, in remission   UPD
         Tobacco use disorder, cigarettes, mild, in early remission
         Tobacco use disorder, cigarettes, mild, in sustained remission
         Tobacco use disorder, cigarettes, moderate, in early remission
         Tobacco use disorder, cigarettes, moderate, in sustained remission
         Tobacco use disorder, cigarettes, severe, in early remission
         Tobacco use disorder, cigarettes, severe, in sustained remission

    F17.213 Nicotine dependence, cigarettes, with withdrawal   CC

    F17.218 Nicotine dependence, cigarettes, with other nicotine-induced disorders

    F17.219 Nicotine dependence, cigarettes, with unspecified nicotine-induced disorders

  ✓6ᵗʰ **F17.22** Nicotine dependence, chewing tobacco

    F17.220 Nicotine dependence, chewing tobacco, uncomplicated   UPD

    F17.221 Nicotine dependence, chewing tobacco, in remission   UPD
         Tobacco use disorder, chewing tobacco, mild, in early remission
         Tobacco use disorder, chewing tobacco, mild, in sustained remission
         Tobacco use disorder, chewing tobacco, moderate, in early remission
         Tobacco use disorder, chewing tobacco, moderate, in sustained remission
         Tobacco use disorder, chewing tobacco, severe, in early remission
         Tobacco use disorder, chewing tobacco, severe, in sustained remission

    F17.223 Nicotine dependence, chewing tobacco, with withdrawal   CC

    F17.228 Nicotine dependence, chewing tobacco, with other nicotine-induced disorders

    F17.229 Nicotine dependence, chewing tobacco, with unspecified nicotine-induced disorders

  ✓6ᵗʰ **F17.29** Nicotine dependence, other tobacco product

    F17.290 Nicotine dependence, other tobacco product, uncomplicated   UPD
         AHA: 2017,2Q,28-29

    F17.291 Nicotine dependence, other tobacco product, in remission   UPD
         Tobacco use disorder, other tobacco product, mild, in early remission
         Tobacco use disorder, other tobacco product, mild, in sustained remission
         Tobacco use disorder, other tobacco product, moderate, in early remission
         Tobacco use disorder, other tobacco product, moderate, in sustained remission
         Tobacco use disorder, other tobacco product, severe, in early remission
         Tobacco use disorder, other tobacco product, severe, in sustained remission

    F17.293 Nicotine dependence, other tobacco product, with withdrawal   CC

    F17.298 Nicotine dependence, other tobacco product, with other nicotine-induced disorders

    F17.299 Nicotine dependence, other tobacco product, with unspecified nicotine-induced disorders

✓4ᵗʰ **F18** Inhalant related disorders

    INCLUDES   volatile solvents

✓5ᵗʰ **F18.1** Inhalant abuse

    EXCLUDES 1   inhalant dependence (F18.2-)
               inhalant use, unspecified (F18.9-)

  F18.10 Inhalant abuse, uncomplicated   HCC
     Inhalant use disorder, mild

  F18.11 Inhalant abuse, in remission   HCC
     Inhalant use disorder, mild, in early remission
     Inhalant use disorder, mild, in sustained remission

  ✓6ᵗʰ **F18.12** Inhalant abuse with intoxication

    F18.120 Inhalant abuse with intoxication, uncomplicated   HCC

    F18.121 Inhalant abuse with intoxication delirium   CC HCC

    F18.129 Inhalant abuse with intoxication, unspecified   HCC

  F18.14 Inhalant abuse with inhalant-induced mood disorder   HCC
     Inhalant use disorder, mild, with inhalant induced depressive disorder

  ✓6ᵗʰ **F18.15** Inhalant abuse with inhalant-induced psychotic disorder

    F18.150 Inhalant abuse with inhalant-induced psychotic disorder with delusions   CC HCC

    F18.151 Inhalant abuse with inhalant-induced psychotic disorder with hallucinations   CC HCC

N Newborn: 0   P Pediatric: 0-17   M Maternity: 9-64   A Adult: 15-124   MCC Major Complication/Comorbidity   CC Complication/Comorbidity   SW Severe Wound Dx

556   ICD-10-CM 2022

F18.159 Inhalant abuse with inhalant-induced psychotic disorder, unspecified `HCC`

F18.17 Inhalant abuse with inhalant-induced dementia `CC` `HCC`
Inhalant use disorder, mild, with inhalant induced major neurocognitive disorder

✓6ᵗʰ **F18.18** Inhalant abuse with other inhalant-induced disorders
F18.180 Inhalant abuse with inhalant-induced anxiety disorder `HCC`
F18.188 Inhalant abuse with other inhalant-induced disorder
Inhalant use disorder, mild, with inhalant induced mild neurocognitive disorder

F18.19 Inhalant abuse with unspecified inhalant-induced disorder `HCC`

✓5ᵗʰ **F18.2** Inhalant dependence
`EXCLUDES 1` inhalant abuse (F18.1-)
inhalant use, unspecified (F18.9-)

F18.20 Inhalant dependence, uncomplicated `CC` `HCC`
Inhalant use disorder, moderate
Inhalant use disorder, severe

F18.21 Inhalant dependence, in remission `HCC`
Inhalant use disorder, moderate, in early remission
Inhalant use disorder, moderate, in sustained remission
Inhalant use disorder, severe, in early remission
Inhalant use disorder, severe, in sustained remission

✓6ᵗʰ **F18.22** Inhalant dependence with intoxication
F18.220 Inhalant dependence with intoxication, uncomplicated `HCC`
F18.221 Inhalant dependence with intoxication delirium `CC` `HCC`
F18.229 Inhalant dependence with intoxication, unspecified `HCC`

F18.24 Inhalant dependence with inhalant-induced mood disorder `HCC`
Inhalant use disorder, moderate, with inhalant induced depressive disorder
Inhalant use disorder, severe, with inhalant induced depressive disorder

✓6ᵗʰ **F18.25** Inhalant dependence with inhalant-induced psychotic disorder
F18.250 Inhalant dependence with inhalant-induced psychotic disorder with delusions `CC` `HCC`
F18.251 Inhalant dependence with inhalant-induced psychotic disorder with hallucinations `CC` `HCC`
F18.259 Inhalant dependence with inhalant-induced psychotic disorder, unspecified `CC` `HCC`

F18.27 Inhalant dependence with inhalant-induced dementia `CC` `HCC`
Inhalant use disorder, moderate, with inhalant induced major neurocognitive disorder
Inhalant use disorder, severe, with inhalant induced major neurocognitive disorder

✓6ᵗʰ **F18.28** Inhalant dependence with other inhalant-induced disorders
F18.280 Inhalant dependence with inhalant-induced anxiety disorder `CC` `HCC`
F18.288 Inhalant dependence with other inhalant-induced disorder `CC` `HCC`
Inhalant use disorder, moderate, with inhalant-induced mild neurocognitive disorder
Inhalant use disorder, severe, with inhalant-induced mild neurocognitive disorder

F18.29 Inhalant dependence with unspecified inhalant-induced disorder `HCC`

✓5ᵗʰ **F18.9** Inhalant use, unspecified
`EXCLUDES 1` inhalant abuse (F18.1-)
inhalant dependence (F18.2-)
TIP: Assign a substance use code only when the provider documents a relationship between the use and an associated physical, mental, or behavioral disorder. As with all diagnoses, substance use codes must meet the definition of a reportable diagnosis.

F18.90 Inhalant use, unspecified, uncomplicated
AHA: 2018,2Q,10-11

✓6ᵗʰ **F18.92** Inhalant use, unspecified with intoxication
F18.920 Inhalant use, unspecified with intoxication, uncomplicated `HCC`
F18.921 Inhalant use, unspecified with intoxication with delirium `CC` `HCC`
F18.929 Inhalant use, unspecified with intoxication, unspecified `HCC`

F18.94 Inhalant use, unspecified with inhalant-induced mood disorder `HCC`
Inhalant induced depressive disorder

✓6ᵗʰ **F18.95** Inhalant use, unspecified with inhalant-induced psychotic disorder
F18.950 Inhalant use, unspecified with inhalant-induced psychotic disorder with delusions `CC` `HCC`
F18.951 Inhalant use, unspecified with inhalant-induced psychotic disorder with hallucinations `CC` `HCC`
F18.959 Inhalant use, unspecified with inhalant-induced psychotic disorder, unspecified `HCC`

F18.97 Inhalant use, unspecified with inhalant-induced persisting dementia `CC` `HCC`
Inhalant-induced major neurocognitive disorder

✓6ᵗʰ **F18.98** Inhalant use, unspecified with other inhalant-induced disorders
F18.980 Inhalant use, unspecified with inhalant-induced anxiety disorder `HCC`
F18.988 Inhalant use, unspecified with other inhalant-induced disorder `HCC`
Inhalant-induced mild neurocognitive disorder

F18.99 Inhalant use, unspecified with unspecified inhalant-induced disorder `HCC`

✓4ᵗʰ **F19** Other psychoactive substance related disorders
`INCLUDES` polysubstance drug use (indiscriminate drug use)

✓5ᵗʰ **F19.1** Other psychoactive substance abuse
`EXCLUDES 1` other psychoactive substance dependence (F19.2-)
other psychoactive substance use, unspecified (F19.9-)

F19.10 Other psychoactive substance abuse, uncomplicated `HCC`
Other (or unknown) substance use disorder, mild

F19.11 Other psychoactive substance abuse, in remission `HCC`
Other (or unknown) substance use disorder, mild, in early remission
Other (or unknown) substance use disorder, mild, in sustained remission

✓6ᵗʰ **F19.12** Other psychoactive substance abuse with intoxication
F19.120 Other psychoactive substance abuse with intoxication, uncomplicated `HCC`
F19.121 Other psychoactive substance abuse with intoxication delirium `CC` `HCC`
F19.122 Other psychoactive substance abuse with intoxication with perceptual disturbances `HCC`
F19.129 Other psychoactive substance abuse with intoxication, unspecified `HCC`

✓6ᵗʰ **F19.13** Other psychoactive substance abuse with withdrawal
AHA: 2020,4Q,16-17
F19.130 Other psychoactive substance abuse with withdrawal, uncomplicated `CC` `HCC`
F19.131 Other psychoactive substance abuse with withdrawal delirium `CC` `HCC`

F19.132 Other psychoactive substance abuse with withdrawal with perceptual disturbance `CC` `HCC`

F19.139 Other psychoactive substance abuse with withdrawal, unspecified `CC` `HCC`

F19.14 Other psychoactive substance abuse with psychoactive substance-induced mood disorder `HCC`
  Other (or unknown) substance use disorder, mild, with other (or unknown) substance-induced bipolar or related disorder
  Other (or unknown) substance use disorder, mild, with other (or unknown) substance-induced depressive disorder

√6ᵗʰ **F19.15** Other psychoactive substance abuse with psychoactive substance-induced psychotic disorder

F19.150 Other psychoactive substance abuse with psychoactive substance-induced psychotic disorder with delusions `CC` `HCC`

F19.151 Other psychoactive substance abuse with psychoactive substance-induced psychotic disorder with hallucinations `CC` `HCC`

F19.159 Other psychoactive substance abuse with psychoactive substance-induced psychotic disorder, unspecified `HCC`

F19.16 Other psychoactive substance abuse with psychoactive substance-induced persisting amnestic disorder `HCC`

F19.17 Other psychoactive substance abuse with psychoactive substance-induced persisting dementia `CC` `HCC`
  Other (or unknown) substance use disorder, mild, with other (or unknown) substance-induced major neurocognitive disorder

√6ᵗʰ **F19.18** Other psychoactive substance abuse with other psychoactive substance-induced disorders

F19.180 Other psychoactive substance abuse with psychoactive substance-induced anxiety disorder `HCC`

F19.181 Other psychoactive substance abuse with psychoactive substance-induced sexual dysfunction `HCC`

F19.182 Other psychoactive substance abuse with psychoactive substance-induced sleep disorder `HCC`

F19.188 Other psychoactive substance abuse with other psychoactive substance-induced disorder `HCC`
  Other (or unknown) substance use disorder, mild, with other (or unknown) substance induced mild neurocognitive disorder
  Other (or unknown) substance use disorder, mild, with other (or unknown) substance induced obsessive-compulsive or related disorder

F19.19 Other psychoactive substance abuse with unspecified psychoactive substance-induced disorder `HCC`

√5ᵗʰ **F19.2** Other psychoactive substance dependence
  `EXCLUDES 1`   other psychoactive substance abuse (F19.1-)
    other psychoactive substance use, unspecified (F19.9-)

F19.20 Other psychoactive substance dependence, uncomplicated `CC` `HCC`
  Other (or unknown) substance use disorder, moderate
  Other (or unknown) substance use disorder, severe

F19.21 Other psychoactive substance dependence, in remission `HCC`
  Other (or unknown) substance use disorder, moderate, in early remission
  Other (or unknown) substance use disorder, moderate, in sustained remission
  Other (or unknown) substance use disorder, severe, in early remission
  Other (or unknown) substance use disorder, severe, in sustained remission

√6ᵗʰ **F19.22** Other psychoactive substance dependence with intoxication
  `EXCLUDES 1`   other psychoactive substance dependence with withdrawal (F19.23-)

F19.220 Other psychoactive substance dependence with intoxication, uncomplicated `HCC`

F19.221 Other psychoactive substance dependence with intoxication delirium `CC` `HCC`

F19.222 Other psychoactive substance dependence with intoxication with perceptual disturbance `CC` `HCC`

F19.229 Other psychoactive substance dependence with intoxication, unspecified `HCC`

√6ᵗʰ **F19.23** Other psychoactive substance dependence with withdrawal
  `EXCLUDES 1`   other psychoactive substance dependence with intoxication (F19.22-)

F19.230 Other psychoactive substance dependence with withdrawal, uncomplicated `CC` `HCC`

F19.231 Other psychoactive substance dependence with withdrawal delirium `CC` `HCC`

F19.232 Other psychoactive substance dependence with withdrawal with perceptual disturbance `CC` `HCC`

F19.239 Other psychoactive substance dependence with withdrawal, unspecified `CC` `HCC`

F19.24 Other psychoactive substance dependence with psychoactive substance-induced mood disorder `HCC`
  Other (or unknown) substance use disorder, moderate, with other (or unknown) substance induced bipolar or related disorder
  Other (or unknown) substance use disorder, moderate, with other (or unknown) substance induced depressive disorder
  Other (or unknown) substance use disorder, severe, with other (or unknown) substance induced bipolar or related disorder
  Other (or unknown) substance use disorder, severe, with other (or unknown) substance induced depressive disorder

√6ᵗʰ **F19.25** Other psychoactive substance dependence with psychoactive substance-induced psychotic disorder

F19.250 Other psychoactive substance dependence with psychoactive substance-induced psychotic disorder with delusions `CC` `HCC`

F19.251 Other psychoactive substance dependence with psychoactive substance-induced psychotic disorder with hallucinations `CC` `HCC`

F19.259 Other psychoactive substance dependence with psychoactive substance-induced psychotic disorder, unspecified `CC` `HCC`

F19.26 Other psychoactive substance dependence with psychoactive substance-induced persisting amnestic disorder `CC` `HCC`

F19.27 Other psychoactive substance dependence with psychoactive substance-induced persisting dementia `CC` `HCC`
  Other (or unknown) substance use disorder, moderate, with other (or unknown) substance induced major neurocognitive disorder
  Other (or unknown) substance use disorder, severe, with other (or unknown) substance induced major neurocognitive disorder

√6ᵗʰ **F19.28** Other psychoactive substance dependence with other psychoactive substance-induced disorders

F19.280 Other psychoactive substance dependence with psychoactive substance-induced anxiety disorder `CC` `HCC`

F19.281 Other psychoactive substance dependence with psychoactive substance-induced sexual dysfunction CC HCC

F19.282 Other psychoactive substance dependence with psychoactive substance-induced sleep disorder CC HCC

F19.288 Other psychoactive substance dependence with other psychoactive substance-induced disorder CC HCC

Other (or unknown) substance use disorder, moderate, with other (or unknown) substance induced mild neurocognitive disorder

Other (or unknown) substance use disorder, severe, with other (or unknown) substance induced mild neurocognitive disorder

Other (or unknown) substance use disorder, moderate, with other (or unknown) substance induced obsessive compulsive or related disorder

Other (or unknown) substance use disorder, severe, with other (or unknown) substance induced obsessive-compulsive or related disorder

F19.29 Other psychoactive substance dependence with unspecified psychoactive substance-induced disorder HCC

√5ᵗʰ F19.9 Other psychoactive substance use, unspecified

EXCLUDES 1   other psychoactive substance abuse (F19.1-)
other psychoactive substance dependence (F19.2-)

TIP: Assign a substance use code only when the provider documents a relationship between the use and an associated physical, mental, or behavioral disorder. As with all diagnoses, substance use codes must meet the definition of a reportable diagnosis.

F19.90 Other psychoactive substance use, unspecified, uncomplicated
AHA: 2018,2Q,10-11

√6ᵗʰ F19.92 Other psychoactive substance use, unspecified with intoxication

EXCLUDES 1   other psychoactive substance use, unspecified with withdrawal (F19.93)

F19.920 Other psychoactive substance use, unspecified with intoxication, uncomplicated HCC

F19.921 Other psychoactive substance use, unspecified with intoxication with delirium CC HCC
Other (or unknown) substance-induced delirium

F19.922 Other psychoactive substance use, unspecified with intoxication with perceptual disturbance HCC

F19.929 Other psychoactive substance use, unspecified with intoxication, unspecified HCC

√6ᵗʰ F19.93 Other psychoactive substance use, unspecified with withdrawal

EXCLUDES 1   other psychoactive substance use, unspecified with intoxication (F19.92-)

F19.930 Other psychoactive substance use, unspecified with withdrawal, uncomplicated CC HCC

F19.931 Other psychoactive substance use, unspecified with withdrawal delirium CC HCC

F19.932 Other psychoactive substance use, unspecified with withdrawal with perceptual disturbance CC HCC

F19.939 Other psychoactive substance use, unspecified with withdrawal, unspecified CC HCC

F19.94 Other psychoactive substance use, unspecified with psychoactive substance-induced mood disorder HCC
Other (or unknown) substance-induced bipolar or related disorder, without use disorder
Other (or unknown) substance-induced depressive disorder, without use disorder

√6ᵗʰ F19.95 Other psychoactive substance use, unspecified with psychoactive substance-induced psychotic disorder

F19.950 Other psychoactive substance use, unspecified with psychoactive substance-induced psychotic disorder with delusions CC HCC

F19.951 Other psychoactive substance use, unspecified with psychoactive substance-induced psychotic disorder with hallucinations CC HCC

F19.959 Other psychoactive substance use, unspecified with psychoactive substance-induced psychotic disorder, unspecified HCC
Other or unknown substance-induced psychotic disorder, without use disorder

F19.96 Other psychoactive substance use, unspecified with psychoactive substance-induced persisting amnestic disorder HCC

F19.97 Other psychoactive substance use, unspecified with psychoactive substance-induced persisting dementia CC HCC
Other (or unknown) substance-induced major neurocognitive disorder, without use disorder

√6ᵗʰ F19.98 Other psychoactive substance use, unspecified with other psychoactive substance-induced disorders

F19.980 Other psychoactive substance use, unspecified with psychoactive substance-induced anxiety disorder HCC
Other (or unknown) substance-induced anxiety disorder, without use disorder

F19.981 Other psychoactive substance use, unspecified with psychoactive substance-induced sexual dysfunction HCC
Other (or unknown) substance-induced sexual dysfunction, without use disorder

F19.982 Other psychoactive substance use, unspecified with psychoactive substance-induced sleep disorder HCC
Other (or unknown) substance-induced sleep disorder, without use disorder

F19.988 Other psychoactive substance use, unspecified with other psychoactive substance-induced disorder HCC
Other (or unknown) substance-induced mild neurocognitive disorder, without use disorder
Other (or unknown) substance-induced obsessive-compulsive or related disorder, without use disorder

F19.99 Other psychoactive substance use, unspecified with unspecified psychoactive substance-induced disorder HCC

Schizophrenia, schizotypal, delusional, and other non-mood psychotic disorders (F20-F29)

✓4ᵗʰ F20 Schizophrenia

> **EXCLUDES 1**   brief psychotic disorder (F23)
> cyclic schizophrenia (F25.0)
> mood [affective] disorders with psychotic symptoms (F30.2, F31.2, F31.5, F31.64, F32.3, F33.3)
> schizoaffective disorder (F25.-)
> schizophrenic reaction NOS (F23)
>
> **EXCLUDES 2**   schizophrenic reaction in:
>   alcoholism (F10.15-, F10.25-, F10.95-)
>   brain disease (F06.2)
>   epilepsy (F06.2)
>   psychoactive drug use (F11-F19 with .15. .25, .95)
>   schizotypal disorder (F21)

DEF: Group of disorders with disturbances in thought (delusions, hallucinations), mood (blunted, flattened, inappropriate affect), and sense of self. Schizophrenia also includes bizarre, purposeless behavior, repetitious activity, or inactivity.

F20.0 Paranoid schizophrenia `CC` `HCC`
Paraphrenic schizophrenia
> **EXCLUDES 1**   involutional paranoid state (F22)
>   paranoia (F22)

DEF: Preoccupied with delusional suspicions and auditory hallucinations related to a single theme. This type of schizophrenia is usually hostile, grandiose, threatening, persecutory, and occasionally hypochondriacal.

F20.1 Disorganized schizophrenia `CC` `HCC`
Hebephrenic schizophrenia
Hebephrenia

F20.2 Catatonic schizophrenia `CC` `HCC`
Schizophrenic catalepsy
Schizophrenic catatonia
Schizophrenic flexibilitas cerea
> **EXCLUDES 1**   catatonic stupor (R40.1)

DEF: Extreme changes in motor activity. One extreme is a decreased response or reaction to the environment and the other is spontaneous activity.

F20.3 Undifferentiated schizophrenia `HCC`
Atypical schizophrenia
> **EXCLUDES 1**   acute schizophrenia-like psychotic disorder (F23)
> **EXCLUDES 2**   post-schizophrenic depression (F32.89)

F20.5 Residual schizophrenia `CC` `HCC`
Restzustand (schizophrenic)
Schizophrenic residual state

✓5ᵗʰ F20.8 Other schizophrenia

> **F20.81 Schizophreniform disorder** `CC` `HCC`
> Schizophreniform psychosis NOS
>
> **F20.89 Other schizophrenia** `CC` `HCC`
> Cenesthopathic schizophrenia
> Simple schizophrenia

F20.9 Schizophrenia, unspecified `HCC`
AHA: 2019,2Q,32

F21 Schizotypal disorder `HCC`
Borderline schizophrenia
Latent schizophrenia
Latent schizophrenic reaction
Prepsychotic schizophrenia
Prodromal schizophrenia
Pseudoneurotic schizophrenia
Pseudopsychopathic schizophrenia
Schizotypal personality disorder
> **EXCLUDES 2**   Asperger's syndrome (F84.5)
>   schizoid personality disorder (F60.1)

DEF: Disorder characterized by various oddities of thinking, perception, communication, and behavior that may be manifested as magical thinking, ideas of reference, paranoid ideation, recurrent illusions and derealization (depersonalization), or social isolation.

F22 Delusional disorders `HCC`
Delusional dysmorphophobia
Involutional paranoid state
Paranoia
Paranoia querulans
Paranoid psychosis
Paranoid state
Paraphrenia (late)
Sensitiver Beziehungswahn
> **EXCLUDES 1**   mood [affective] disorders with psychotic symptoms (F30.2, F31.2, F31.5, F31.64, F32.3, F33.3)
>   paranoid schizophrenia (F20.0)
> **EXCLUDES 2**   paranoid personality disorder (F60.0)
>   paranoid psychosis, psychogenic (F23)
>   paranoid reaction (F23)

F23 Brief psychotic disorder `CC` `HCC`
Paranoid reaction
Psychogenic paranoid psychosis
> **EXCLUDES 2**   mood [affective] disorders with psychotic symptoms (F30.2, F31.2, F31.5, F31.64, F32.3, F33.3)

AHA: 2019,2Q,32

F24 Shared psychotic disorder `HCC`
Folie à deux
Induced paranoid disorder
Induced psychotic disorder

✓4ᵗʰ F25 Schizoaffective disorders

> **EXCLUDES 1**   mood [affective] disorders with psychotic symptoms (F30.2, F31.2, F31.5, F31.64, F32.3, F33.3)
>   schizophrenia (F20.-)

> **F25.0 Schizoaffective disorder, bipolar type** `HCC`
> Cyclic schizophrenia
> Schizoaffective disorder, manic type
> Schizoaffective disorder, mixed type
> Schizoaffective psychosis, bipolar type
>
> **F25.1 Schizoaffective disorder, depressive type** `HCC`
> Schizoaffective psychosis, depressive type
>
> **F25.8 Other schizoaffective disorders** `HCC`
>
> **F25.9 Schizoaffective disorder, unspecified** `HCC`
> Schizoaffective psychosis NOS

F28 Other psychotic disorder not due to a substance or known physiological condition `HIV` `HCC`
Chronic hallucinatory psychosis
Other specified schizophrenia spectrum and other psychotic disorder

F29 Unspecified psychosis not due to a substance or known physiological condition `HIV` `HCC`
Psychosis NOS
Unspecified schizophrenia spectrum and other psychotic disorder
> **EXCLUDES 1**   mental disorder NOS (F99)
>   unspecified mental disorder due to known physiological condition (F09)

Mood [affective] disorders (F30-F39)

✓4ᵗʰ F30 Manic episode

> **INCLUDES**   bipolar disorder, single manic episode
> mixed affective episode
> **EXCLUDES 1**   bipolar disorder (F31.-)
>   major depressive disorder, recurrent (F33.-)
>   major depressive disorder, single episode (F32.-)

DEF: Mania: Characterized by abnormal states of elation or excitement out of keeping with the individual's circumstances and varying from enhanced liveliness (hypomania) to violent, almost uncontrollable, excitement. Aggression and anger, flight of ideas, distractibility, impaired judgment, and grandiose ideas are common.

✓5ᵗʰ F30.1 Manic episode without psychotic symptoms

> **F30.10 Manic episode without psychotic symptoms, unspecified** `CC` `HCC`
>
> **F30.11 Manic episode without psychotic symptoms, mild** `CC` `HCC`
>
> **F30.12 Manic episode without psychotic symptoms, moderate** `CC` `HCC`
>
> **F30.13 Manic episode, severe, without psychotic symptoms** `CC` `HCC`

Ⓝ Newborn: 0   Ⓟ Pediatric: 0-17   Ⓜ Maternity: 9-64   Ⓐ Adult: 15-124   `MCC` Major Complication/Comorbidity   `CC` Complication/Comorbidity   `SW` Severe Wound Dx

560   ICD-10-CM 2022

F30.2 **Manic episode, severe with psychotic symptoms** `CC` `HCC`
Manic stupor
Mania with mood-congruent psychotic symptoms
Mania with mood-incongruent psychotic symptoms

F30.3 **Manic episode in partial remission** `HCC`

F30.4 **Manic episode in full remission** `HCC`

F30.8 **Other manic episodes** `HCC`
Hypomania

F30.9 **Manic episode, unspecified** `CC` `HCC`
Mania NOS

`✓4ᵗʰ` **F31** **Bipolar disorder**

  `INCLUDES` bipolar I disorder
          bipolar type I disorder
          manic-depressive illness
          manic-depressive psychosis
          manic-depressive reaction
  `EXCLUDES 1` *bipolar disorder, single manic episode (F30.-)*
          major depressive disorder, recurrent (F33.-)
          major depressive disorder, single episode (F32.-)
  `EXCLUDES 2` *cyclothymia (F34.0)*
  AHA: 2020,1Q,23

F31.0 **Bipolar disorder, current episode hypomanic** `CC` `HCC`

`✓5ᵗʰ` **F31.1** **Bipolar disorder, current episode manic without psychotic features**

  F31.10 **Bipolar disorder, current episode manic without psychotic features, unspecified** `CC` `HCC`

  F31.11 **Bipolar disorder, current episode manic without psychotic features, mild** `CC` `HCC`

  F31.12 **Bipolar disorder, current episode manic without psychotic features, moderate** `CC` `HCC`

  F31.13 **Bipolar disorder, current episode manic without psychotic features, severe** `CC` `HCC`

F31.2 **Bipolar disorder, current episode manic severe with psychotic features** `CC` `HCC`
Bipolar disorder, current episode manic with mood-congruent psychotic symptoms
Bipolar disorder, current episode manic with mood-incongruent psychotic symptoms
Bipolar I disorder, current or most recent episode manic with psychotic features

`✓5ᵗʰ` **F31.3** **Bipolar disorder, current episode depressed, mild or moderate severity**

  F31.30 **Bipolar disorder, current episode depressed, mild or moderate severity, unspecified** `CC` `HCC`

  F31.31 **Bipolar disorder, current episode depressed, mild** `CC` `HCC`

  F31.32 **Bipolar disorder, current episode depressed, moderate** `CC` `HCC`

F31.4 **Bipolar disorder, current episode depressed, severe, without psychotic features** `CC` `HCC`

F31.5 **Bipolar disorder, current episode depressed, severe, with psychotic features** `CC` `HCC`
Bipolar disorder, current episode depressed with mood-congruent psychotic symptoms
Bipolar disorder, current episode depressed with mood-incongruent psychotic symptoms
Bipolar I disorder, current or most recent episode depressed, with psychotic features

`✓5ᵗʰ` **F31.6** **Bipolar disorder, current episode mixed**

  F31.60 **Bipolar disorder, current episode mixed, unspecified** `CC` `HCC`

  F31.61 **Bipolar disorder, current episode mixed, mild** `CC` `HCC`

  F31.62 **Bipolar disorder, current episode mixed, moderate** `CC` `HCC`

  F31.63 **Bipolar disorder, current episode mixed, severe, without psychotic features** `CC` `HCC`

  F31.64 **Bipolar disorder, current episode mixed, severe, with psychotic features** `CC` `HCC`
Bipolar disorder, current episode mixed with mood-congruent psychotic symptoms
Bipolar disorder, current episode mixed with mood-incongruent psychotic symptoms

`✓5ᵗʰ` **F31.7** **Bipolar disorder, currently in remission**

  F31.70 **Bipolar disorder, currently in remission, most recent episode unspecified** `HCC`

F31.71 **Bipolar disorder, in partial remission, most recent episode hypomanic** `HCC`

F31.72 **Bipolar disorder, in full remission, most recent episode hypomanic** `HCC`

F31.73 **Bipolar disorder, in partial remission, most recent episode manic** `HCC`

F31.74 **Bipolar disorder, in full remission, most recent episode manic** `HCC`

F31.75 **Bipolar disorder, in partial remission, most recent episode depressed** `HCC`

F31.76 **Bipolar disorder, in full remission, most recent episode depressed** `HCC`

F31.77 **Bipolar disorder, in partial remission, most recent episode mixed** `HCC`

F31.78 **Bipolar disorder, in full remission, most recent episode mixed** `HCC`

`✓5ᵗʰ` **F31.8** **Other bipolar disorders**

  F31.81 **Bipolar II disorder** `CC` `HCC`
Bipolar disorder, type 2

  F31.89 **Other bipolar disorder** `CC` `HCC`
Recurrent manic episodes NOS

F31.9 **Bipolar disorder, unspecified** `HCC`
Manic depression
AHA: 2020,1Q,23

▲ `✓4ᵗʰ` **F32** **Depressive episode**

  `INCLUDES` single episode of agitated depression
          single episode of depressive reaction
          single episode of major depression
          single episode of psychogenic depression
          single episode of reactive depression
          single episode of vital depression
  `EXCLUDES 1` *bipolar disorder (F31.-)*
          manic episode (F30.-)
          recurrent depressive disorder (F33.-)
  `EXCLUDES 2` *adjustment disorder (F43.2)*
  AHA: 2020,1Q,23
  DEF: Mood disorder that produces depression that may exhibit as sadness, low self-esteem, or guilt feelings. Other manifestations may be withdrawal from friends and family and interrupted sleep.

F32.0 **Major depressive disorder, single episode, mild** `CC` `HCC`

F32.1 **Major depressive disorder, single episode, moderate** `CC` `HCC`

F32.2 **Major depressive disorder, single episode, severe without psychotic features** `CC` `HCC`

F32.3 **Major depressive disorder, single episode, severe with psychotic features** `CC` `HCC`
Single episode of major depression with mood-congruent psychotic symptoms
Single episode of major depression with mood-incongruent psychotic symptoms
Single episode of major depression with psychotic symptoms
Single episode of psychogenic depressive psychosis
Single episode of psychotic depression
Single episode of reactive depressive psychosis

F32.4 **Major depressive disorder, single episode, in partial remission** `HCC`

F32.5 **Major depressive disorder, single episode, in full remission** `HCC`

`✓5ᵗʰ` **F32.8** **Other depressive episodes**
  AHA: 2016,4Q,14

  F32.81 **Premenstrual dysphoric disorder** ♀
    `EXCLUDES 1` *premenstrual tension syndrome (N94.3)*
    DEF: Severe manifestation of premenstrual syndrome (PMS) that can be disabling and destructive to day-to-day activities. It can exacerbate pre-existing emotional disorders, like depression and anxiety, and cause feelings of loss of control, fatigue, and irritability.

  F32.89 **Other specified depressive episodes**
Atypical depression
Post-schizophrenic depression
Single episode of 'masked' depression NOS

F32.9 **Major depressive disorder, single episode, unspecified**
~~Depression NOS~~
~~Depressive disorder NOS~~
Major depression NOS
AHA: 2021,1Q,10; 2013,4Q,107

● **F32.A Depression, unspecified**
Depression NOS
Depressive disorder NOS

✓4ᵗʰ **F33 Major depressive disorder, recurrent**
INCLUDES recurrent episodes of depressive reaction
recurrent episodes of endogenous depression
recurrent episodes of major depression
recurrent episodes of psychogenic depression
recurrent episodes of reactive depression
recurrent episodes of seasonal depressive disorder
recurrent episodes of vital depression
EXCLUDES 1 bipolar disorder (F31.-)
manic episode (F30.-)
AHA: 2020,1Q,23
DEF: Mood disorder that produces depression that may exhibit as sadness, low self-esteem, or guilt feelings. Other manifestations may be withdrawal from friends and family and interrupted sleep.

F33.0 Major depressive disorder, recurrent, mild CC HCC

F33.1 Major depressive disorder, recurrent, moderate CC HCC

F33.2 Major depressive disorder, recurrent, severe without psychotic features CC HCC

F33.3 Major depressive disorder, recurrent, severe with psychotic symptoms CC HCC
Endogenous depression with psychotic symptoms
Major depressive disorder, recurrent, with psychotic features
Recurrent severe episodes of major depression with mood-congruent psychotic symptoms
Recurrent severe episodes of major depression with mood-incongruent psychotic symptoms
Recurrent severe episodes of major depression with psychotic symptoms
Recurrent severe episodes of psychogenic depressive psychosis
Recurrent severe episodes of psychotic depression
Recurrent severe episodes of reactive depressive psychosis

✓5ᵗʰ **F33.4 Major depressive disorder, recurrent, in remission**

F33.40 Major depressive disorder, recurrent, in remission, unspecified CC HCC

F33.41 Major depressive disorder, recurrent, in partial remission HCC

F33.42 Major depressive disorder, recurrent, in full remission HCC

F33.8 Other recurrent depressive disorders CC HCC
Recurrent brief depressive episodes

F33.9 Major depressive disorder, recurrent, unspecified CC HCC
Monopolar depression NOS

✓4ᵗʰ **F34 Persistent mood [affective] disorders**

F34.0 Cyclothymic disorder
Affective personality disorder
Cycloid personality
Cyclothymia
Cyclothymic personality
DEF: Mood disorder characterized by fast and repeated alterations between hypomanic and depressed moods.

F34.1 Dysthymic disorder
Depressive neurosis
Depressive personality disorder
Dysthymia
Neurotic depression
Persistent anxiety depression
Persistent depressive disorder
EXCLUDES 2 anxiety depression (mild or not persistent) (F41.8)
DEF: Depression without psychosis. It is a less severe but persistent depression and is considered a mild to moderate chronic form of depression.

✓6ᵗʰ **F34.8 Other persistent mood [affective] disorders**
AHA: 2016,4Q,14

F34.81 Disruptive mood dysregulation disorder CC HCC

F34.89 Other specified persistent mood disorders CC HCC

F34.9 Persistent mood [affective] disorder, unspecified CC HCC

F39 Unspecified mood [affective] disorder HCC
Affective psychosis NOS

Anxiety, dissociative, stress-related, somatoform and other nonpsychotic mental disorders (F40-F48)

✓4ᵗʰ **F40 Phobic anxiety disorders**
DEF: Phobia: Broad-range anxiety with abnormally intense dread of certain objects or specific situations that would not normally have that effect.

✓5ᵗʰ **F40.0 Agoraphobia**
DEF: Profound anxiety or fear of leaving familiar settings like home, or being in unfamiliar locations or with strangers or crowds. Agoraphobia may or may not be preceded by recurrent panic attacks.

F40.00 Agoraphobia, unspecified

F40.01 Agoraphobia with panic disorder
Panic disorder with agoraphobia
EXCLUDES 1 panic disorder without agoraphobia (F41.0)

F40.02 Agoraphobia without panic disorder

✓5ᵗʰ **F40.1 Social phobias**
Anthropophobia
Social anxiety disorder
Social anxiety disorder of childhood
Social neurosis

F40.10 Social phobia, unspecified

F40.11 Social phobia, generalized

✓5ᵗʰ **F40.2 Specific (isolated) phobias**
EXCLUDES 2 dysmorphophobia (nondelusional) (F45.22)
nosophobia (F45.22)

✓6ᵗʰ **F40.21 Animal type phobia**

F40.210 Arachnophobia
Fear of spiders

F40.218 Other animal type phobia

✓6ᵗʰ **F40.22 Natural environment type phobia**

F40.220 Fear of thunderstorms

F40.228 Other natural environment type phobia

✓6ᵗʰ **F40.23 Blood, injection, injury type phobia**

F40.230 Fear of blood

F40.231 Fear of injections and transfusions

F40.232 Fear of other medical care

F40.233 Fear of injury

✓6ᵗʰ **F40.24 Situational type phobia**

F40.240 Claustrophobia

F40.241 Acrophobia

F40.242 Fear of bridges

F40.243 Fear of flying

F40.248 Other situational type phobia

✓6ᵗʰ **F40.29 Other specified phobia**

F40.290 Androphobia
Fear of men

F40.291 Gynephobia
Fear of women

F40.298 Other specified phobia

F40.8 Other phobic anxiety disorders
Phobic anxiety disorder of childhood

F40.9 Phobic anxiety disorder, unspecified
Phobia NOS
Phobic state NOS

✓4ᵗʰ **F41 Other anxiety disorders**
EXCLUDES 2 anxiety in:
acute stress reaction (F43.0)
neurasthenia (F48.8)
psychophysiologic disorders (F45.-)
transient adjustment reaction (F43.2)
separation anxiety (F93.0)

F41.0 Panic disorder [episodic paroxysmal anxiety]
Panic attack
Panic state
EXCLUDES 1 panic disorder with agoraphobia (F40.01)
DEF: Neurotic disorder characterized by recurrent panic or anxiety, apprehension, fear, or terror. Symptoms include shortness of breath, palpitations, dizziness, and shakiness; fear of dying may persist.

F41.1   **Generalized anxiety disorder**
- Anxiety neurosis
- Anxiety reaction
- Anxiety state
- Overanxious disorder
  - *EXCLUDES 2*   *neurasthenia (F48.8)*

F41.3   **Other mixed anxiety disorders**

F41.8   **Other specified anxiety disorders**
- Anxiety depression (mild or not persistent)
- Anxiety hysteria
- Mixed anxiety and depressive disorder
- **AHA:** 2021,1Q,10

F41.9   **Anxiety disorder, unspecified**
- Anxiety NOS
- **AHA:** 2021,1Q,10

☑4ᵗʰ F42   Obsessive-compulsive disorder
- *EXCLUDES 2*   *obsessive-compulsive personality (disorder) (F60.5)*
  - *obsessive-compulsive symptoms occurring in depression (F32-F33)*
  - *obsessive-compulsive symptoms occurring in schizophrenia (F20.-)*

AHA: 2016,4Q,14-15

F42.2   **Mixed obsessional thoughts and acts**

F42.3   **Hoarding disorder**

F42.4   **Excoriation (skin-picking) disorder**
- *EXCLUDES 1*   *factitial dermatitis (L98.1)*
  - *other specified behavioral and emotional disorders with onset usually occurring in early childhood and adolescence (F98.8)*

F42.8   **Other obsessive-compulsive disorder**
- Anancastic neurosis
- Obsessive-compulsive neurosis

F42.9   **Obsessive-compulsive disorder, unspecified**

☑4ᵗʰ F43   Reaction to severe stress, and adjustment disorders

F43.0   **Acute stress reaction**
- Acute crisis reaction
- Acute reaction to stress
- Combat and operational stress reaction
- Combat fatigue
- Crisis state
- Psychic shock

☑5ᵗʰ F43.1   Post-traumatic stress disorder (PTSD)
- Traumatic neurosis
- **DEF:** Preoccupation with traumatic events beyond normal experience (i.e., rape, personal assault, etc.) that may also include recurring flashbacks of the trauma. Symptoms include difficulty remembering, sleeping, or concentrating, and guilt feelings for surviving.
  - **F43.10**   **Post-traumatic stress disorder, unspecified**
  - **F43.11**   **Post-traumatic stress disorder, acute**
  - **F43.12**   **Post-traumatic stress disorder, chronic**

☑5ᵗʰ F43.2   Adjustment disorders
- Culture shock
- Grief reaction
- Hospitalism in children
  - *EXCLUDES 2*   *separation anxiety disorder of childhood (F93.0)*
- **F43.20**   **Adjustment disorder, unspecified**
- **F43.21**   **Adjustment disorder with depressed mood**
  - **AHA:** 2014,1Q,25
- **F43.22**   **Adjustment disorder with anxiety**
- **F43.23**   **Adjustment disorder with mixed anxiety and depressed mood**
- **F43.24**   **Adjustment disorder with disturbance of conduct**
- **F43.25**   **Adjustment disorder with mixed disturbance of emotions and conduct**
- **F43.29**   **Adjustment disorder with other symptoms**

F43.8   **Other reactions to severe stress**
- Other specified trauma and stressor-related disorder

F43.9   **Reaction to severe stress, unspecified**
- Trauma and stressor-related disorder, NOS

☑4ᵗʰ F44   Dissociative and conversion disorders
- *INCLUDES*   conversion hysteria
  - conversion reaction
  - hysteria
  - hysterical psychosis
  - *EXCLUDES 2*   *malingering [conscious simulation] (Z76.5)*

F44.0   **Dissociative amnesia**   HCC
- *EXCLUDES 1*   *amnesia NOS (R41.3)*
  - *anterograde amnesia (R41.1)*
  - *dissociative amnesia with dissociative fugue (F44.1)*
  - *retrograde amnesia (R41.2)*
- *EXCLUDES 2*   *alcohol-or other psychoactive substance-induced amnestic disorder (F10, F13, F19 with .26, .96)*
  - *amnestic disorder due to known physiological condition (F04)*
  - *postictal amnesia in epilepsy (G40.-)*

F44.1   **Dissociative fugue**   HCC
- Dissociative amnesia with dissociative fugue
- *EXCLUDES 2*   *postictal fugue in epilepsy (G40.-)*
- **DEF:** Dissociative hysteria identified by memory loss and flight from familiar surroundings to a completely separate environment. Episodes may last hours or days. Conscious activity is not associated with perception of surroundings and there is no later memory of the episode.

F44.2   **Dissociative stupor**
- *EXCLUDES 1*   *catatonic stupor (R40.1)*
  - *stupor NOS (R40.1)*
- *EXCLUDES 2*   *catatonic disorder due to known physiological condition (F06.1)*
  - *depressive stupor (F32, F33)*
  - *manic stupor (F30, F31)*

F44.4   **Conversion disorder with motor symptom or deficit**
- Conversion disorder with abnormal movement
- Conversion disorder with speech symptoms
- Conversion disorder with swallowing symptoms
- Conversion disorder with weakness/paralysis
- Dissociative motor disorders
- Psychogenic aphonia
- Psychogenic dysphonia

F44.5   **Conversion disorder with seizures or convulsions**
- Conversion disorder with attacks or seizures
- Dissociative convulsions
- **AHA:** 2021,1Q,3; 2019,1Q,19

F44.6   **Conversion disorder with sensory symptom or deficit**
- Conversion disorder with anesthesia or sensory loss
- Conversion disorder with special sensory symptoms
- Dissociative anesthesia and sensory loss
- Psychogenic deafness

F44.7   **Conversion disorder with mixed symptom presentation**

☑5ᵗʰ F44.8   Other dissociative and conversion disorders
- **F44.81**   **Dissociative identity disorder**   HCC
  - Multiple personality disorder
- **F44.89**   **Other dissociative and conversion disorders**
  - Ganser's syndrome
  - Psychogenic confusion
  - Psychogenic twilight state
  - Trance and possession disorders

F44.9   **Dissociative and conversion disorder, unspecified**
- Dissociative disorder NOS

☑ Additional Character Required   ☑x7ᵗʰ Placeholder   Questionable PDx   Manifestation   Unspecified Dx   UPD Unacceptable PDx   H1 -H14 HAC   HCC CMS-HCC Dx   HIV HIV Dx

ICD-10-CM 2022   563

Chapter 5. Mental, Behavioral and Neurodevelopmental Disorders

F45–F51.09

✓4ᵗʰ **F45 Somatoform disorders**

    EXCLUDES 2   dissociative and conversion disorders (F44.-)
        factitious disorders (F68.1-, F68.A)
        hair-plucking (F63.3)
        lalling (F80.0)
        lisping (F80.0)
        malingering [conscious simulation] (Z76.5)
        nail-biting (F98.8)
        psychological or behavioral factors associated with disorders or diseases classified elsewhere (F54)
        sexual dysfunction, not due to a substance or known physiological condition (F52.-)
        thumb-sucking (F98.8)
        tic disorders (in childhood and adolescence) (F95.-)
        Tourette's syndrome (F95.2)
        trichotillomania (F63.3)

    DEF: Types of disorders causing inconsistent physical symptoms that cannot be explained.

    F45.0 Somatization disorder
        Briquet's disorder
        Multiple psychosomatic disorder

    F45.1 Undifferentiated somatoform disorder
        Somatic symptom disorder
        Undifferentiated psychosomatic disorder

✓5ᵗʰ **F45.2 Hypochondriacal disorders**
       EXCLUDES 2   delusional dysmorphophobia (F22)
                    fixed delusions about bodily functions or shape (F22)

       F45.20 Hypochondriacal disorder, unspecified

       F45.21 Hypochondriasis
            Hypochondriacal neurosis
            Illness anxiety disorder

       F45.22 Body dysmorphic disorder
            Dysmorphophobia (nondelusional)
            Nosophobia

       F45.29 Other hypochondriacal disorders

✓5ᵗʰ **F45.4 Pain disorders related to psychological factors**
       EXCLUDES 1   pain NOS (R52)

       F45.41 Pain disorder exclusively related to psychological factors
            Somatoform pain disorder (persistent)

       F45.42 Pain disorder with related psychological factors
            Code also associated acute or chronic pain (G89.-)

    F45.8 Other somatoform disorders
        Psychogenic dysmenorrhea
        Psychogenic dysphagia, including 'globus hystericus'
        Psychogenic pruritus
        Psychogenic torticollis
        Somatoform autonomic dysfunction
        Teeth grinding
       EXCLUDES 1   sleep related teeth grinding (G47.63)

    F45.9 Somatoform disorder, unspecified
        Psychosomatic disorder NOS

✓4ᵗʰ **F48 Other nonpsychotic mental disorders**

    F48.1 Depersonalization-derealization syndrome   `HCC`

    F48.2 Pseudobulbar affect
        Involuntary emotional expression disorder
        Code first underlying cause, if known, such as:
           amyotrophic lateral sclerosis (G12.21)
           multiple sclerosis (G35)
           sequelae of cerebrovascular disease (I69.-)
           sequelae of traumatic intracranial injury (S06.-)

    F48.8 Other specified nonpsychotic mental disorders
        Dhat syndrome
        Neurasthenia
        Occupational neurosis, including writer's cramp
        Psychasthenia
        Psychasthenic neurosis
        Psychogenic syncope

    F48.9 Nonpsychotic mental disorder, unspecified
        Neurosis NOS

Behavioral syndromes associated with physiological disturbances and physical factors (F50-F59)

✓4ᵗʰ **F50 Eating disorders**

    EXCLUDES 1   anorexia NOS (R63.0)
              ~~feeding difficulties (R63.3)~~
              feeding problems of newborn (P92.-)
              polyphagia (R63.2)
    EXCLUDES 2   ▶feeding difficulties (R63.3)◀
              feeding disorder in infancy or childhood (F98.2-)

    AHA: 2018,4Q,82

    TIP: Assign additional code for BMI from category Z68, when documented. BMI can be based on documentation from clinicians who are not the patient's provider.

✓5ᵗʰ **F50.0 Anorexia nervosa**
       EXCLUDES 1   loss of appetite (R63.0)
                  psychogenic loss of appetite (F50.89)

       DEF: Psychological eating disorder characterized by an intense fear of gaining weight and an unrealistic perception of body image that perpetuates the feeling of being fat or having too much fat. Avoidance of food and restrictive or unhealthy eating are common.

       F50.00 Anorexia nervosa, unspecified   `CC`

       F50.01 Anorexia nervosa, restricting type   `CC`

       F50.02 Anorexia nervosa, binge eating/purging type   `CC`
           EXCLUDES 1   bulimia nervosa (F50.2)

    F50.2 Bulimia nervosa   `CC`
        Bulimia NOS
        Hyperorexia nervosa
       EXCLUDES 1   anorexia nervosa, binge eating/purging type (F50.02)
       DEF: Episodic pattern of overeating (binge eating) followed by purging or extreme exercise accompanied by an awareness of the abnormal eating pattern with a fear of not being able to stop eating.

✓5ᵗʰ **F50.8 Other eating disorders**
       EXCLUDES 2   pica of infancy and childhood (F98.3)
       AHA: 2017,4Q,9; 2016,4Q,15-16

       F50.81 Binge eating disorder

       F50.82 Avoidant/restrictive food intake disorder

       F50.89 Other specified eating disorder
            Pica in adults
            Psychogenic loss of appetite

    F50.9 Eating disorder, unspecified
        Atypical anorexia nervosa
        Atypical bulimia nervosa
        Feeding or eating disorder, unspecified
        Other specified feeding disorder

✓4ᵗʰ **F51 Sleep disorders not due to a substance or known physiological condition**

    EXCLUDES 2   organic sleep disorders (G47.-)

✓5ᵗʰ **F51.0 Insomnia not due to a substance or known physiological condition**
       EXCLUDES 2   alcohol related insomnia (F10.182, F10.282, F10.982)
               drug-related insomnia (F11.182, F11.282, F11.982, F13.182, F13.282, F13.982, F14.182, F14.282, F14.982, F15.182, F15.282, F15.982, F19.182, F19.282, F19.982)
              insomnia NOS (G47.0-)
              insomnia due to known physiological condition (G47.0-)
              organic insomnia (G47.0-)
              sleep deprivation (Z72.820)

       F51.01 Primary insomnia
            Idiopathic insomnia

       F51.02 Adjustment insomnia

       F51.03 Paradoxical insomnia

       F51.04 Psychophysiologic insomnia

       F51.05 Insomnia due to other mental disorder
            Code also associated mental disorder

       F51.09 Other insomnia not due to a substance or known physiological condition

☒ Newborn: 0   ☒ Pediatric: 0-17   ☒ Maternity: 9-64   ☒ Adult: 15-124   `MCC` Major Complication/Comorbidity   `CC` Complication/Comorbidity   `SW` Severe Wound Dx

564
ICD-10-CM 2022

✓5ᵗʰ **F51.1 Hypersomnia not due to a substance or known physiological condition**
> EXCLUDES 2   *alcohol related hypersomnia (F10.182, F10.282, F10.982)*
> *drug-related hypersomnia (F11.182, F11.282, F11.982, F13.182, F13.282, F13.982, F14.182, F14.282, F14.982, F15.182, F15.282, F15.982, F19.182, F19.282, F19.982)*
> *hypersomnia NOS (G47.10)*
> *hypersomnia due to known physiological condition (G47.10)*
> *idiopathic hypersomnia (G47.11, G47.12)*
> *narcolepsy (G47.4-)*

F51.11 Primary hypersomnia

F51.12 Insufficient sleep syndrome
> EXCLUDES 1   *sleep deprivation (Z72.820)*

F51.13 Hypersomnia due to other mental disorder
Code also associated mental disorder

F51.19 Other hypersomnia not due to a substance or known physiological condition

F51.3 Sleepwalking [somnambulism]
Non-rapid eye movement sleep arousal disorders, sleepwalking type

F51.4 Sleep terrors [night terrors]
Non-rapid eye movement sleep arousal disorders, sleep terror type

F51.5 Nightmare disorder
Dream anxiety disorder

F51.8 Other sleep disorders not due to a substance or known physiological condition

F51.9 Sleep disorder not due to a substance or known physiological condition, unspecified
Emotional sleep disorder NOS

✓4ᵗʰ **F52 Sexual dysfunction not due to a substance or known physiological condition**
> EXCLUDES 2   *Dhat syndrome (F48.8)*

F52.0 Hypoactive sexual desire disorder
Lack or loss of sexual desire
Male hypoactive sexual desire disorder
Sexual anhedonia
> EXCLUDES 1   *decreased libido (R68.82)*

F52.1 Sexual aversion disorder
Sexual aversion and lack of sexual enjoyment

✓5ᵗʰ **F52.2 Sexual arousal disorders**
Failure of genital response

F52.21 Male erectile disorder   ♂
Erectile disorder
Psychogenic impotence
> EXCLUDES 1   *impotence of organic origin (N52.-)*
> *impotence NOS (N52.-)*

F52.22 Female sexual arousal disorder   ♀
Female sexual interest/arousal disorder

✓5ᵗʰ **F52.3 Orgasmic disorder**
Inhibited orgasm
Psychogenic anorgasmy

F52.31 Female orgasmic disorder   ♀

F52.32 Male orgasmic disorder   ♂
Delayed ejaculation

F52.4 Premature ejaculation   ♂

F52.5 Vaginismus not due to a substance or known physiological condition   ♀
Psychogenic vaginismus
> EXCLUDES 2   *vaginismus (due to a known physiological condition) (N94.2)*

DEF: Psychogenic response resulting in painful contractions of the vaginal canal muscles. This condition can be severe enough to prevent sexual intercourse.

F52.6 Dyspareunia not due to a substance or known physiological condition   ♀
Genito-pelvic pain penetration disorder
Psychogenic dyspareunia
> EXCLUDES 2   *dyspareunia (due to a known physiological condition) (N94.1-)*

F52.8 Other sexual dysfunction not due to a substance or known physiological condition
Excessive sexual drive
Nymphomania
Satyriasis

F52.9 Unspecified sexual dysfunction not due to a substance or known physiological condition   UPD
Sexual dysfunction NOS

✓4ᵗʰ **F53 Mental and behavioral disorders associated with the puerperium, not elsewhere classified**
> EXCLUDES 1   *mood disorders with psychotic features (F30.2, F31.2, F31.5, F31.64, F32.3, F33.3)*
> *postpartum dysphoria (O90.6)*
> *psychosis in schizophrenia, schizotypal, delusional, and other psychotic disorders (F20-F29)*

AHA: 2018,4Q,8

F53.0 Postpartum depression   M ♀
Postnatal depression, NOS
Postpartum depression, NOS

F53.1 Puerperal psychosis   HCC M ♀
Postpartum psychosis
Puerperal psychosis, NOS

F54 *Psychological and behavioral factors associated with disorders or diseases classified elsewhere*
Psychological factors affecting physical conditions
Code first the associated physical disorder, such as:
asthma (J45.-)
dermatitis (L23-L25)
gastric ulcer (K25.-)
mucous colitis (K58.-)
ulcerative colitis (K51.-)
urticaria (L50.-)
> EXCLUDES 2   *tension-type headache (G44.2)*

✓4ᵗʰ **F55 Abuse of non-psychoactive substances**
> EXCLUDES 2   *abuse of psychoactive substances (F10-F19)*

F55.0 Abuse of antacids
F55.1 Abuse of herbal or folk remedies
F55.2 Abuse of laxatives
F55.3 Abuse of steroids or hormones
F55.4 Abuse of vitamins
F55.8 Abuse of other non-psychoactive substances

F59 Unspecified behavioral syndromes associated with physiological disturbances and physical factors
Psychogenic physiological dysfunction NOS

Disorders of adult personality and behavior (F60-F69)

✓4ᵗʰ **F60 Specific personality disorders**

F60.0 Paranoid personality disorder   HCC
Expansive paranoid personality (disorder)
Fanatic personality (disorder)
Paranoid personality (disorder)
Querulant personality (disorder)
Sensitive paranoid personality (disorder)
> EXCLUDES 2   *paranoia (F22)*
> *paranoia querulans (F22)*
> *paranoid psychosis (F22)*
> *paranoid schizophrenia (F20.0)*
> *paranoid state (F22)*

F60.1 Schizoid personality disorder   HCC
> EXCLUDES 2   *Asperger's syndrome (F84.5)*
> *delusional disorder (F22)*
> *schizoid disorder of childhood (F84.5)*
> *schizophrenia (F20.-)*
> *schizotypal disorder (F21)*

F60.2 Antisocial personality disorder   HCC
Amoral personality (disorder)
Asocial personality (disorder)
Dissocial personality disorder
Psychopathic personality (disorder)
Sociopathic personality (disorder)
> EXCLUDES 1   *conduct disorders (F91.-)*
> EXCLUDES 2   *borderline personality disorder (F60.3)*

✓ Additional Character Required   ✓x7ᵗʰ Placeholder   Questionable PDx   Manifestation   Unspecified Dx   UPD Unacceptable PDx   H1 -H14 HAC   HCC CMS-HCC Dx   HIV HIV Dx

ICD-10-CM 2022   565

Chapter 5. Mental, Behavioral and Neurodevelopmental Disorders

F60.3–F69

F60.3 Borderline personal disorder `HCC`
Aggressive personality (disorder)
Emotionally unstable personality disorder
Explosive personality (disorder)
> `EXCLUDES 2`   antisocial personality disorder (F60.2)

F60.4 Histrionic personality disorder `HCC`
Hysterical personality (disorder)
Psychoinfantile personality (disorder)

F60.5 Obsessive-compulsive personality disorder `HCC`
Anankastic personality (disorder)
Compulsive personality (disorder)
Obsessional personality (disorder)
> `EXCLUDES 2`   obsessive-compulsive disorder (F42.-)

F60.6 Avoidant personality disorder `HCC`
Anxious personality disorder

F60.7 Dependent personality disorder `HCC`
Asthenic personality (disorder)
Inadequate personality (disorder)
Passive personality (disorder)
> **DEF:** Lack of self-confidence, fear of abandonment, and an obsessive need to be taken care of.

`✓5ᵗʰ` **F60.8 Other specific personality disorders**

     F60.81 Narcissistic personality disorder `HCC`
     F60.89 Other specific personality disorders `HCC`
         Eccentric personality disorder
         "Haltlose" type personality disorder
         Immature personality disorder
         Passive-aggressive personality disorder
         Psychoneurotic personality disorder
         Self-defeating personality disorder

F60.9 Personality disorder, unspecified `HCC`
Character disorder NOS
Character neurosis NOS
Pathological personality NOS

`✓4ᵗʰ` **F63 Impulse disorders**
> `EXCLUDES 2`   habitual excessive use of alcohol or psychoactive substances (F10-F19)
>   impulse disorders involving sexual behavior (F65.-)

F63.0 Pathological gambling
Compulsive gambling
Gambling disorder
> `EXCLUDES 1`   gambling and betting NOS (Z72.6)
> `EXCLUDES 2`   excessive gambling by manic patients (F30, F31)
>   gambling in antisocial personality disorder (F60.2)

F63.1 Pyromania
Pathological fire-setting
> `EXCLUDES 2`   fire-setting (by) (in):
>   adult with antisocial personality disorder (F60.2)
>   alcohol or psychoactive substance intoxication (F10-F19)
>   conduct disorders (F91.-)
>   mental disorders due to known physiological condition (F01-F09)
>   schizophrenia (F20.-)

F63.2 Kleptomania
Pathological stealing
> `EXCLUDES 1`   shoplifting as the reason for observation for suspected mental disorder (Z03.8)
> `EXCLUDES 2`   depressive disorder with stealing (F31-F33)
>   stealing due to underlying mental condition - code to mental condition
>   stealing in mental disorders due to known physiological condition (F01-F09)

F63.3 Trichotillomania
Hair plucking
> `EXCLUDES 2`   other stereotyped movement disorder (F98.4)

`✓5ᵗʰ` **F63.8 Other impulse disorders**
     F63.81 Intermittent explosive disorder
     F63.89 Other impulse disorders
F63.9 Impulse disorder, unspecified
Impulse control disorder NOS

`✓4ᵗʰ` **F64 Gender identity disorders**
> **AHA:** 2016,4Q,16

F64.0 Transsexualism
Gender identity disorder in adolescence and adulthood
Gender dysphoria in adolescents and adults

F64.1 Dual role transvestism
Use additional code to identify sex reassignment status (Z87.890)
> `EXCLUDES 1`   gender identity disorder in childhood (F64.2)
> `EXCLUDES 2`   fetishistic transvestism (F65.1)

F64.2 Gender identity disorder of childhood `P`
Gender dysphoria in children
> `EXCLUDES 1`   gender identity disorder in adolescence and adulthood (F64.0)
> `EXCLUDES 2`   sexual maturation disorder (F66)

F64.8 Other gender identity disorders
Other specified gender dysphoria

F64.9 Gender identity disorder, unspecified
Gender dysphoria, unspecified
Gender-role disorder NOS

`✓4ᵗʰ` **F65 Paraphilias**

F65.0 Fetishism
Fetishistic disorder

F65.1 Transvestic fetishism
Fetishistic transvestism
Transvestic disorder

F65.2 Exhibitionism
Exhibitionistic disorder

F65.3 Voyeurism
Voyeuristic disorder

F65.4 Pedophilia
Pedophilic disorder

`✓5ᵗʰ` **F65.5 Sadomasochism**
     F65.50 Sadomasochism, unspecified
     F65.51 Sexual masochism
         Sexual masochism disorder
     F65.52 Sexual sadism
         Sexual sadism disorder

`✓5ᵗʰ` **F65.8 Other paraphilias**
     F65.81 Frotteurism
         Frotteuristic disorder
     F65.89 Other paraphilias
         Necrophilia
         Other specified paraphilic disorder

F65.9 Paraphilia, unspecified
Paraphilic disorder, unspecified
Sexual deviation NOS

F66 Other sexual disorders
Sexual maturation disorder
Sexual relationship disorder

`✓4ᵗʰ` **F68 Other disorders of adult personality and behavior**
> **AHA:** 2018,4Q,9,65

`✓5ᵗʰ` **F68.1 Factitious disorder imposed on self**
Compensation neurosis
Elaboration of physical symptoms for psychological reasons
Hospital hopper syndrome
Münchausen's syndrome
Peregrinating patient
> `EXCLUDES 2`   factitial dermatitis (L98.1)
>   person feigning illness (with obvious motivation) (Z76.5)

     F68.10 Factitious disorder imposed on self, unspecified `CC`
     F68.11 Factitious disorder imposed on self, with predominantly psychological signs and symptoms
     F68.12 Factitious disorder imposed on self, with predominantly physical signs and symptoms `CC`
     F68.13 Factitious disorder imposed on self, with combined psychological and physical signs and symptoms

F68.A Factitious disorder imposed on another `CC`
Factitious disorder by proxy
Münchausen's by proxy

F68.8 Other specified disorders of adult personality and behavior

F69 Unspecified disorder of adult personality and behavior `A`

`N` Newborn: 0   `P` Pediatric: 0-17   `M` Maternity: 9-64   `A` Adult: 15-124   `MCC` Major Complication/Comorbidity   `CC` Complication/Comorbidity   `SW` Severe Wound Dx

566   ICD-10-CM 2022

Intellectual disabilities (F70-F79)

Code first any associated physical or developmental disorders

EXCLUDES 1   *borderline intellectual functioning, IQ above 70 to 84 (R41.83)*

F70   Mild intellectual disabilities
    IQ level 50-55 to approximately 70
    Mild mental subnormality

F71   Moderate intellectual disabilities
    IQ level 35-40 to 50-55
    Moderate mental subnormality

F72   Severe intellectual disabilities   `CC`
    IQ 20-25 to 35-40
    Severe mental subnormality

F73   Profound intellectual disabilities   `CC`
    IQ level below 20-25
    Profound mental subnormality

▲ ✓4ᵗʰ **F78   Other intellectual disabilities**

●   ✓5ᵗʰ **F78.A   Other genetic related intellectual disabilities**

●   **F78.A1   SYNGAP1-related intellectual disability**
       Code also, if applicable, any associated:
         autism spectrum disorder (F84.0)
         autistic disorder (F84.0)
         encephalopathy (G93.4-)
         epilepsy and recurrent seizures (G40.-)
         other pervasive developmental disorders (F84.8)
         pervasive developmental disorder, NOS (F84.9)

●   **F78.A9   Other genetic related intellectual disability**
       Code also, if applicable, any associated disorders

F79   Unspecified intellectual disabilities
    Mental deficiency NOS
    Mental subnormality NOS

Pervasive and specific developmental disorders (F80-F89)

✓4ᵗʰ **F80   Specific developmental disorders of speech and language**

F80.0   Phonological disorder
    Dyslalia
    Functional speech articulation disorder
    Lalling
    Lisping
    Phonological developmental disorder
    Speech articulation developmental disorder
    Speech-sound disorder
    EXCLUDES 1   *speech articulation impairment due to aphasia NOS (R47.01)*
             speech articulation impairment due to apraxia (R48.2)
    EXCLUDES 2   *speech articulation impairment due to hearing loss (F80.4)*
             speech articulation impairment due to intellectual disabilities (F70-F79)
             speech articulation impairment with expressive language developmental disorder (F80.1)
             speech articulation impairment with mixed receptive expressive language developmental disorder (F80.2)

F80.1   Expressive language disorder
    Developmental dysphasia or aphasia, expressive type
    EXCLUDES 1   *mixed receptive-expressive language disorder (F80.2)*
             dysphasia and aphasia NOS (R47.-)
    EXCLUDES 2   *acquired aphasia with epilepsy [Landau-Kleffner] (G40.80-)*
             selective mutism (F94.0)
             intellectual disabilities (F70-F79)
             pervasive developmental disorders (F84.-)

F80.2   Mixed receptive-expressive language disorder
    Developmental dysphasia or aphasia, receptive type
    Developmental Wernicke's aphasia
    EXCLUDES 1   *central auditory processing disorder (H93.25)*
             dysphasia or aphasia NOS (R47.-)
             expressive language disorder (F80.1)
             expressive type dysphasia or aphasia (F80.1)
             word deafness (H93.25)
    EXCLUDES 2   *acquired aphasia with epilepsy [Landau-Kleffner] (G40.80-)*
             pervasive developmental disorders (F84.-)
             selective mutism (F94.0)
             intellectual disabilities (F70-F79)

F80.4   Speech and language development delay due to hearing loss
    Code also type of hearing loss (H90.-, H91.-)

✓5ᵗʰ **F80.8   Other developmental disorders of speech and language**
    AHA: 2017,1Q,27

    F80.81   Childhood onset fluency disorder
       Cluttering NOS
       Stuttering NOS
       EXCLUDES 1   *adult onset fluency disorder (F98.5)*
              fluency disorder in conditions classified elsewhere (R47.82)
              fluency disorder (stuttering) following cerebrovascular disease (I69. with final characters -23)

    F80.82   Social pragmatic communication disorder
       EXCLUDES 1   *Asperger's syndrome (F84.5)*
              autistic disorder (F84.0)
       AHA: 2016,4Q,16

    F80.89   Other developmental disorders of speech and language

F80.9   Developmental disorder of speech and language, unspecified
    Communication disorder NOS
    Language disorder NOS

✓4ᵗʰ **F81   Specific developmental disorders of scholastic skills**

F81.0   Specific reading disorder
    "Backward reading"
    Developmental dyslexia
    Specific learning disorder, with impairment in reading
    Specific reading retardation
    EXCLUDES 1   *alexia NOS (R48.0)*
             dyslexia NOS (R48.0)
    DEF: Serious impairment of reading skills unexplained in relation to general intelligence and teaching processes.

F81.2   Mathematics disorder
    Developmental acalculia
    Developmental arithmetical disorder
    Developmental Gerstmann's syndrome
    Specific learning disorder, with impairment in mathematics
    EXCLUDES 1   *acalculia NOS (R48.8)*
    EXCLUDES 2   *arithmetical difficulties associated with a reading disorder (F81.0)*
             arithmetical difficulties associated with a spelling disorder (F81.81)
             arithmetical difficulties due to inadequate teaching (Z55.8)

✓5ᵗʰ **F81.8   Other developmental disorders of scholastic skills**

    F81.81   Disorder of written expression
       Specific learning disorder, with impairment in written expression
       Specific spelling disorder

    F81.89   Other developmental disorders of scholastic skills

F81.9   Developmental disorder of scholastic skills, unspecified   `UPD`
    Knowledge acquisition disability NOS
    Learning disability NOS
    Learning disorder NOS

✔ Additional Character Required   ✓ₓ7ᵗʰ Placeholder   Questionable PDx   Manifestation   Unspecified Dx   `UPD` Unacceptable PDx   H1-H14 HAC   HCC CMS-HCC Dx   HIV HIV Dx

ICD-10-CM 2022   567

F82　Specific developmental disorder of motor function
　　Clumsy child syndrome
　　Developmental coordination disorder
　　Developmental dyspraxia
　　EXCLUDES 1　*abnormalities of gait and mobility (R26.-)*
　　　　　　　　lack of coordination (R27.-)
　　EXCLUDES 2　*lack of coordination secondary to intellectual disabilities*
　　　　　　　　(F70-F79)

✓4ᵗʰ **F84　Pervasive developmental disorders**
　　▶Code also any associated medical condition and intellectual disabilities◀
　　~~Use additional code to identify any associated medical condition and~~
　　~~intellectual disabilities.~~

　　F84.0　Autistic disorder　　CC
　　　　Autism spectrum disorder
　　　　Infantile autism
　　　　Infantile psychosis
　　　　Kanner's syndrome
　　　　EXCLUDES 1　*Asperger's syndrome (F84.5)*
　　　　AHA: 2017,1Q,27

　　F84.2　Rett's syndrome　　CC
　　　　EXCLUDES 1　*Asperger's syndrome (F84.5)*
　　　　　　　　　autistic disorder (F84.0)
　　　　　　　　　other childhood disintegrative disorder (F84.3)

　　F84.3　Other childhood disintegrative disorder　　CC P
　　　　Dementia infantilis
　　　　Disintegrative psychosis
　　　　Heller's syndrome
　　　　Symbiotic psychosis
　　　　Use additional code to identify any associated neurological
　　　　　　condition
　　　　EXCLUDES 1　*Asperger's syndrome (F84.5)*
　　　　　　　　　autistic disorder (F84.0)
　　　　　　　　　Rett's syndrome (F84.2)

　　F84.5　Asperger's syndrome　　CC
　　　　Asperger's disorder
　　　　Autistic psychopathy
　　　　Schizoid disorder of childhood
　　　　DEF: High-functioning form of autism. Children with this
　　　　syndrome usually develop speech on schedule, are generally very
　　　　intelligent, and communicate well, but have considerable social
　　　　shortcomings. ***Synonym(s):*** AS.

　　F84.8　Other pervasive developmental disorders　　CC
　　　　Overactive disorder associated with intellectual disabilities and
　　　　　　stereotyped movements

　　F84.9　Pervasive developmental disorder, unspecified　　CC
　　　　Atypical autism

F88　Other disorders of psychological development
　　Developmental agnosia
　　Global developmental delay
　　Other specified neurodevelopmental disorder

F89　Unspecified disorder of psychological development
　　Developmental disorder NOS
　　Neurodevelopmental disorder NOS

Behavioral and emotional disorders with onset usually occurring in childhood and adolescence (F90-F98)

　　NOTE　　Codes within categories F90-F98 may be used regardless of the age
　　　　　　of a patient. These disorders generally have onset within the
　　　　　　childhood or adolescent years, but may continue throughout life
　　　　　　or not be diagnosed until adulthood

✓4ᵗʰ **F90　Attention-deficit hyperactivity disorders**
　　INCLUDES　　attention deficit disorder with hyperactivity
　　　　　　　　attention deficit syndrome with hyperactivity
　　EXCLUDES 2　*anxiety disorders (F40.-, F41.-)*
　　　　　　　　mood [affective] disorders (F30-F39)
　　　　　　　　pervasive developmental disorders (F84.-)
　　　　　　　　schizophrenia (F20.-)

　　**F90.0　Attention-deficit hyperactivity disorder, predominantly
　　　　　　inattentive type**
　　　　Attention-deficit/hyperactivity disorder, predominantly
　　　　　　inattentive presentation

　　**F90.1　Attention-deficit hyperactivity disorder, predominantly
　　　　　　hyperactive type**
　　　　Attention-deficit/hyperactivity disorder, predominantly
　　　　　　hyperactive impulsive presentation

　　F90.2　Attention-deficit hyperactivity disorder, combined type
　　　　Attention-deficit/hyperactivity disorder, combined presentation

　　F90.8　Attention-deficit hyperactivity disorder, other type

　　F90.9　Attention-deficit hyperactivity disorder, unspecified type
　　　　Attention-deficit hyperactivity disorder of childhood or
　　　　　　adolescence NOS
　　　　Attention-deficit hyperactivity disorder NOS

✓4ᵗʰ **F91　Conduct disorders**
　　EXCLUDES 1　*antisocial behavior (Z72.81-)*
　　　　　　　　antisocial personality disorder (F60.2)
　　EXCLUDES 2　*conduct problems associated with attention-deficit
　　　　　　　　　hyperactivity disorder (F90.-)*
　　　　　　　　mood [affective] disorders (F30-F39)
　　　　　　　　pervasive developmental disorders (F84.-)
　　　　　　　　schizophrenia (F20.-)

　　F91.0　Conduct disorder confined to family context

　　F91.1　Conduct disorder, childhood-onset type
　　　　Unsocialized conduct disorder
　　　　Conduct disorder, solitary aggressive type
　　　　Unsocialized aggressive disorder

　　F91.2　Conduct disorder, adolescent-onset type
　　　　Socialized conduct disorder
　　　　Conduct disorder, group type

　　F91.3　Oppositional defiant disorder

　　F91.8　Other conduct disorders
　　　　Other specified conduct disorder
　　　　Other specified disruptive disorder

　　F91.9　Conduct disorder, unspecified
　　　　Behavioral disorder NOS
　　　　Conduct disorder NOS
　　　　Disruptive behavior disorder NOS
　　　　Disruptive disorder NOS

✓4ᵗʰ **F93　Emotional disorders with onset specific to childhood**

　　F93.0　Separation anxiety disorder of childhood
　　　　EXCLUDES 2　*mood [affective] disorders (F30-F39)*
　　　　　　　　　nonpsychotic mental disorders (F40-F48)
　　　　　　　　　phobic anxiety disorder of childhood (F40.8)
　　　　　　　　　social phobia (F40.1)

　　F93.8　Other childhood emotional disorders
　　　　Identity disorder
　　　　EXCLUDES 2　*gender identity disorder of childhood (F64.2)*

　　F93.9　Childhood emotional disorder, unspecified

✓4ᵗʰ **F94　Disorders of social functioning with onset specific to childhood
　　　　and adolescence**

　　F94.0　Selective mutism
　　　　Elective mutism
　　　　EXCLUDES 2　*pervasive developmental disorders (F84.-)*
　　　　　　　　　schizophrenia (F20.-)
　　　　　　　　　*specific developmental disorders of speech and
　　　　　　　　　　language (F80.-)*
　　　　　　　　　*transient mutism as part of separation anxiety in
　　　　　　　　　　young children (F93.0)*

　　F94.1　Reactive attachment disorder of childhood
　　　　Use additional code to identify any associated failure to thrive
　　　　　　or growth retardation
　　　　EXCLUDES 1　*disinhibited attachment disorder of childhood (F94.2)*
　　　　　　　　　normal variation in pattern of selective attachment
　　　　EXCLUDES 2　*Asperger's syndrome (F84.5)*
　　　　　　　　　maltreatment syndromes (T74.-)
　　　　　　　　　*sexual or physical abuse in childhood, resulting in
　　　　　　　　　　psychosocial problems (Z62.81-)*

　　F94.2　Disinhibited attachment disorder of childhood
　　　　Affectionless psychopathy
　　　　Institutional syndrome
　　　　EXCLUDES 1　*reactive attachment disorder of childhood (F94.1)*
　　　　EXCLUDES 2　*Asperger's syndrome (F84.5)*
　　　　　　　　　attention-deficit hyperactivity disorders (F90.-)
　　　　　　　　　hospitalism in children (F43.2-)

　　F94.8　Other childhood disorders of social functioning

　　F94.9　Childhood disorder of social functioning, unspecified

✓4ᵗʰ **F95　Tic disorder**

　　F95.0　Transient tic disorder
　　　　Provisional tic disorder

　　F95.1　Chronic motor or vocal tic disorder

F95.2 Tourette's disorder
 Combined vocal and multiple motor tic disorder [de la Tourette]
 Tourette's syndrome

F95.8 **Other tic disorders**

F95.9 **Tic disorder, unspecified**
 Tic NOS

✓4ᵗʰ **F98** **Other behavioral and emotional disorders with onset usually occurring in childhood and adolescence**
 EXCLUDES 2 *breath-holding spells (R06.89)*
  gender identity disorder of childhood (F64.2)
  Kleine-Levin syndrome (G47.13)
  obsessive-compulsive disorder (F42.-)
  sleep disorders not due to a substance or known physiological condition (F51.-)

F98.0 **Enuresis not due to a substance or known physiological condition**
 Enuresis (primary) (secondary) of nonorganic origin
 Functional enuresis
 Psychogenic enuresis
 Urinary incontinence of nonorganic origin
 EXCLUDES 1 *enuresis NOS (R32)*

F98.1 **Encopresis not due to a substance or known physiological condition**
 Functional encopresis
 Incontinence of feces of nonorganic origin
 Psychogenic encopresis
 Use additional code to identify the cause of any coexisting constipation
 EXCLUDES 1 *encopresis NOS (R15.-)*

✓5ᵗʰ **F98.2** **Other feeding disorders of infancy and childhood**
 EXCLUDES 1 *feeding difficulties (R63.3)*
 EXCLUDES 2 *anorexia nervosa and other eating disorders (F50.-)*
  ▶*feeding difficulties (R63.3)*◀
  feeding problems of newborn (P92.-)
  pica of infancy or childhood (F98.3)

 F98.21 **Rumination disorder of infancy**

 F98.29 **Other feeding disorders of infancy and early childhood**

F98.3 **Pica of infancy and childhood**

F98.4 **Stereotyped movement disorders**
 Stereotype/habit disorder
 EXCLUDES 1 *abnormal involuntary movements (R25.-)*
 EXCLUDES 2 *compulsions in obsessive-compulsive disorder (F42.-)*
  hair plucking (F63.3)
  movement disorders of organic origin (G20-G25)
  nail-biting (F98.8)
  nose-picking (F98.8)
  stereotypies that are part of a broader psychiatric condition (F01-F95)
  thumb-sucking (F98.8)
  tic disorders (F95.-)
  trichotillomania (F63.3)

F98.5 **Adult onset fluency disorder**
 EXCLUDES 1 *childhood onset fluency disorder (F80.81)*
  dysphasia (R47.02)
  fluency disorder in conditions classified elsewhere (R47.82)
  fluency disorder (stuttering) following cerebrovascular disease (I69. with final characters -23)
  tic disorders (F95.-)

F98.8 **Other specified behavioral and emotional disorders with onset usually occurring in childhood and adolescence**
 Excessive masturbation
 Nail-biting
 Nose-picking
 Thumb-sucking

F98.9 **Unspecified behavioral and emotional disorders with onset usually occurring in childhood and adolescence**

Unspecified mental disorder (F99)

F99 **Mental disorder, not otherwise specified**
 Mental illness NOS
 EXCLUDES 1 *unspecified mental disorder due to known physiological condition (F09)*

Chapter 6. Diseases of the Nervous System (G00-G99)

Chapter-specific Guidelines with Coding Examples

The chapter-specific guidelines from the ICD-10-CM Official Guidelines for Coding and Reporting have been provided below. Along with these guidelines are coding examples, contained in the shaded boxes, that have been developed to help illustrate the coding and/or sequencing guidance found in these guidelines.

a. Dominant/nondominant side

Codes from category G81, Hemiplegia and hemiparesis, and subcategories G83.1, Monoplegia of lower limb, G83.2, Monoplegia of upper limb, and G83.3, Monoplegia, unspecified, identify whether the dominant or nondominant side is affected. Should the affected side be documented, but not specified as dominant or nondominant, and the classification system does not indicate a default, code selection is as follows:

- For ambidextrous patients, the default should be dominant.
- If the left side is affected, the default is non-dominant.
- If the right side is affected, the default is dominant.

> Hemiplegia affecting left side of ambidextrous patient
>
> **G81.92**   **Hemiplegia, unspecified affecting left dominant side**
>
> *Explanation*: Documentation states that the left side is affected and dominant is used for ambidextrous persons.

> Right spastic hemiplegia, unknown whether patient is right- or left-handed
>
> **G81.11**   **Spastic hemiplegia affecting right dominant side**
>
> *Explanation*: Since it is unknown whether the patient is right- or left-handed, if the right side is affected, the default is dominant.

b. Pain—category G89

1) General coding information

Codes in category G89, Pain, not elsewhere classified, may be used in conjunction with codes from other categories and chapters to provide more detail about acute or chronic pain and neoplasm-related pain, unless otherwise indicated below.

If the pain is not specified as acute or chronic, post-thoracotomy, postprocedural, or neoplasm-related, do not assign codes from category G89.

A code from category G89 should not be assigned if the underlying (definitive) diagnosis is known, unless the reason for the encounter is pain control/ management and not management of the underlying condition.

When an admission or encounter is for a procedure aimed at treating the underlying condition (e.g., spinal fusion, kyphoplasty), a code for the underlying condition (e.g., vertebral fracture, spinal stenosis) should be assigned as the principal diagnosis. No code from category G89 should be assigned.

> Elderly patient with back pain is admitted for kyphoplasty for age-related osteopathic compression fracture at vertebra T3
>
> **M80.08XA**   **Age-related osteoporosis with current pathological fracture, vertebra(e), initial encounter for fracture**
>
> *Explanation*: No code is assigned for the pain as it is inherent in the underlying condition being treated.

(a) Category G89 codes as principal or first-listed diagnosis

Category G89 codes are acceptable as principal diagnosis or the first-listed code:

- When pain control or pain management is the reason for the admission/encounter (e.g., a patient with displaced intervertebral disc, nerve impingement and severe back pain presents for injection of steroid into the spinal canal). The underlying cause of the pain should be reported as an additional diagnosis, if known.

- When a patient is admitted for the insertion of a neurostimulator for pain control, assign the appropriate pain code as the principal or first-listed diagnosis. When an admission or encounter is for a procedure aimed at treating the underlying condition and a neurostimulator is inserted for pain control during the same admission/encounter, a code for the underlying condition should be assigned as the principal diagnosis and the appropriate pain code should be assigned as a secondary diagnosis.

> Patient with chronic pain from lumbar spondylosis with radiculopathy not relieved by surgery is admitted for insertion of neurostimulator.
>
> **G89.29**   **Other chronic pain**
>
> **M47.26**   **Other spondylosis with radiculopathy, lumbar region**
>
> *Explanation*: Since the patient is admitted specifically for a neurostimulator implantation for pain management and not to treat the underlying spondylosis, the chronic pain code is sequenced first, followed by the underlying condition. Neither code M54.16 nor M54.5 is necessary because M47.26 describes the radiculopathy and the site.

(b) Use of category G89 codes in conjunction with site specific pain codes

(i) Assigning category G89 and site-specific pain codes

Codes from category G89 may be used in conjunction with codes that identify the site of pain (including codes from chapter 18) if the category G89 code provides additional information. For example, if the code describes the site of the pain, but does not fully describe whether the pain is acute or chronic, then both codes should be assigned.

> During hospital stay, patient is seen by orthopaedics to evaluate chronic left shoulder pain.
>
> **M25.512**   **Pain in left shoulder**
>
> **G89.29**   **Other chronic pain**
>
> *Explanation*: No underlying condition has been determined yet so the pain would be the reason for the visit. The M25 pain code in this instance does not fully describe the condition as it does not represent that the pain is chronic. The G89 chronic pain code is assigned to provide specificity.

(ii) Sequencing of category G89 codes with site-specific pain codes

The sequencing of category G89 codes with site-specific pain codes (including chapter 18 codes), is dependent on the circumstances of the encounter/admission as follows:

- If the encounter is for pain control or pain management, assign the code from category G89 followed by the code identifying the specific site of pain (e.g., encounter for pain management for acute neck pain from trauma is assigned code G89.11, Acute pain due to trauma, followed by code M54.2, Cervicalgia, to identify the site of pain).

> Management of acute, traumatic right knee pain
>
> **G89.11**   **Acute pain due to trauma**
>
> **M25.561**   **Pain in right knee**
>
> *Explanation*: The reason for the encounter is to manage or control the pain, not to treat or evaluate an underlying condition. The G89 pain code is assigned as the principal diagnosis but in this instance does not fully describe the condition as it does not include the site and laterality. The M25 pain code is added to provide this information.

Chapter 6. Diseases of the Nervous System

- If the encounter is for any other reason except pain control or pain management, and a related definitive diagnosis has not been established (confirmed) by the provider, assign the code for the specific site of pain first, followed by the appropriate code from category G89.

> Tests are performed to investigate the source of the patient's chronic epigastric abdominal pain
>
> **R1Ø.13   Epigastric pain**
>
> **G89.29   Other chronic pain**
>
> *Explanation*: In this instance the patient's epigastric pain is not being treated; rather the source of the pain is being investigated. A code from chapter 18 for epigastric pain is sequenced before the additional specificity of the G89 code for the chronic pain.

2) Pain due to devices, implants and grafts

See Section I.C.19. Pain due to medical devices

3) Postoperative pain

The provider's documentation should be used to guide the coding of postoperative pain, as well as *Section III. Reporting Additional Diagnoses* and *Section IV. Diagnostic Coding and Reporting in the Outpatient Setting*.

The default for post-thoracotomy and other postoperative pain not specified as acute or chronic is the code for the acute form.

Routine or expected postoperative pain immediately after surgery should not be coded.

> Pain pump dose is increased for the patient's unexpected, extreme pain post-thoracotomy
>
> **G89.12   Acute post-thoracotomy pain**
>
> *Explanation*: When acute or chronic is not documented, default to acute. The use of "unexpected, extreme" and the increase of medication dosage indicate that the pain was more than routine or expected.

(a) Postoperative pain not associated with specific postoperative complication

Postoperative pain not associated with a specific postoperative complication is assigned to the appropriate postoperative pain code in category G89.

(b) Postoperative pain associated with specific postoperative complication

Postoperative pain associated with a specific postoperative complication (such as painful wire sutures) is assigned to the appropriate code(s) found in Chapter 19, Injury, poisoning, and certain other consequences of external causes. If appropriate, use additional code(s) from category G89 to identify acute or chronic pain (G89.18 or G89.28).

4) Chronic pain

Chronic pain is classified to subcategory G89.2. There is no time frame defining when pain becomes chronic pain. The provider's documentation should be used to guide use of these codes.

5) Neoplasm related pain

Code G89.3 is assigned to pain documented as being related, associated or due to cancer, primary or secondary malignancy, or tumor. This code is assigned regardless of whether the pain is acute or chronic.

This code may be assigned as the principal or first-listed code when the stated reason for the admission/encounter is documented as pain control/pain management. The underlying neoplasm should be reported as an additional diagnosis.

> Pain medication adjustment for chronic pain from bone metastasis
>
> **G89.3   Neoplasm related pain (acute)(chronic)**
>
> **C79.51   Secondary malignant neoplasm of bone**
>
> *Explanation*: Since the encounter was for pain medication management, the pain, rather than the neoplasm, was the reason for the encounter and is sequenced first. This "neoplasm-related pain" code includes both acute and chronic pain.

When the reason for the admission/encounter is management of the neoplasm and the pain associated with the neoplasm is also documented, code G89.3 may be assigned as an additional diagnosis. It is not necessary to assign an additional code for the site of the pain.

See Section I.C.2 for instructions on the sequencing of neoplasms for all other stated reasons for the admission/encounter (except for pain control/pain management).

> Patient with lung cancer presents with acute hip pain and is evaluated and found to have iliac bone metastasis
>
> **C79.51   Secondary malignant neoplasm of bone**
>
> **C34.9Ø   Malignant neoplasm of unspecified part of unspecified bronchus or lung**
>
> **G89.3   Neoplasm related pain (acute)(chronic)**
>
> *Explanation*: The reason for the encounter was the evaluation and diagnosis of the bone metastasis, whose code would be assigned as first-listed, followed by codes for the primary neoplasm and the pain due to the iliac bone metastasis.

6) Chronic pain syndrome

Central pain syndrome (G89.Ø) and chronic pain syndrome (G89.4) are different than the term "chronic pain," and therefore codes should only be used when the provider has specifically documented this condition.

See Section I.C.5. Pain disorders related to psychological factors

Chapter 6. Diseases of the Nervous System (G00-G99)

EXCLUDES 2   certain conditions originating in the perinatal period (P04-P96)
certain infectious and parasitic diseases (A00-B99)
complications of pregnancy, childbirth and the puerperium (O00-O9A)
congenital malformations, deformations, and chromosomal abnormalities (Q00-Q99)
endocrine, nutritional and metabolic diseases (E00-E88)
injury, poisoning and certain other consequences of external causes (S00-T88)
neoplasms (C00-D49)
symptoms, signs and abnormal clinical and laboratory findings, not elsewhere classified (R00-R94)

This chapter contains the following blocks:

G00-G09   Inflammatory diseases of the central nervous system
G10-G14   Systemic atrophies primarily affecting the central nervous system
G20-G26   Extrapyramidal and movement disorders
G30-G32   Other degenerative diseases of the nervous system
G35-G37   Demyelinating diseases of the central nervous system
G40-G47   Episodic and paroxysmal disorders
G50-G59   Nerve, nerve root and plexus disorders
G60-G65   Polyneuropathies and other disorders of the peripheral nervous system
G70-G73   Diseases of myoneural junction and muscle
G80-G83   Cerebral palsy and other paralytic syndromes
G89-G99   Other disorders of the nervous system

Inflammatory diseases of the central nervous system (G00-G09)

✓4th G00   Bacterial meningitis, not elsewhere classified

INCLUDES   bacterial arachnoiditis
bacterial leptomeningitis
bacterial meningitis
bacterial pachymeningitis

EXCLUDES 1   bacterial meningoencephalitis (G04.2)
bacterial meningomyelitis (G04.2)

DEF: Inflammation of meningeal layers of the brain and spinal cord due to a bacterial infection.

G00.0   Hemophilus meningitis   `MCC`
Meningitis due to Hemophilus influenzae

G00.1   Pneumococcal meningitis   `MCC`
Meningtitis due to Streptococcal pneumoniae

G00.2   Streptococcal meningitis   `MCC`
Use additional code to further identify organism (B95.0-B95.5)

G00.3   Staphylococcal meningitis   `MCC`
Use additional code to further identify organism (B95.61-B95.8)

G00.8   Other bacterial meningitis   `MCC`
Meningitis due to Escherichia coli
Meningitis due to Friedländer's bacillus
Meningitis due to Klebsiella
Use additional code to further identify organism (B96.-)

G00.9   Bacterial meningitis, unspecified   `MCC`
Meningitis due to gram-negative bacteria, unspecified
Purulent meningitis NOS
Pyogenic meningitis NOS
Suppurative meningitis NOS

G01   *Meningitis in bacterial diseases classified elsewhere*   `MCC`

Code first underlying disease

EXCLUDES 1   meningitis (in):
gonococcal (A54.81)
leptospirosis (A27.81)
listeriosis (A32.11)
Lyme disease (A69.21)
meningococcal (A39.0)
neurosyphilis (A52.13)
tuberculosis (A17.0)
meningoencephalitis and meningomyelitis in bacterial diseases classified elsewhere (G05)

G02   *Meningitis in other infectious and parasitic diseases classified elsewhere*   `MCC`

Code first underlying disease, such as:
African trypanosomiasis (B56.-)
poliovirus infection (A80.-)

EXCLUDES 1   candidal meningitis (B37.5)
coccidioidomycosis meningitis (B38.4)
cryptococcal meningitis (B45.1)
herpesviral [herpes simplex] meningitis (B00.3)
infectious mononucleosis complicated by meningitis ▶(B27.- with fifth character 2)◀
measles complicated by meningitis (B05.1)
meningoencephalitis and meningomyelitis in other infectious and parasitic diseases classified elsewhere (G05)
mumps meningitis (B26.1)
rubella meningitis (B06.02)
varicella [chickenpox] meningitis (B01.0)
zoster meningitis (B02.1)

✓4th G03   Meningitis due to other and unspecified causes

INCLUDES   arachnoiditis NOS
leptomeningitis NOS
meningitis NOS
pachymeningitis NOS

EXCLUDES 1   meningoencephalitis (G04.-)
meningomyelitis (G04.-)

G03.0   Nonpyogenic meningitis   `MCC`
Aseptic meningitis
Nonbacterial meningitis
DEF: Type of meningitis where no bacterial, viral, or other infectious source exists that explains the meningitis symptomology.

G03.1   Chronic meningitis   `CC`

G03.2   Benign recurrent meningitis [Mollaret]   `CC`
DEF: Aseptic or noninfectious inflammation of the meninges with the presence of Mollaret cells in the spinal fluid. The patient experiences recurrent bouts of inflammation, lasting anywhere from two to five days.

G03.8   Meningitis due to other specified causes   `MCC`

G03.9   Meningitis, unspecified   `MCC`
Arachnoiditis (spinal) NOS

✓4th G04   Encephalitis, myelitis and encephalomyelitis

INCLUDES   acute ascending myelitis
meningoencephalitis
meningomyelitis

EXCLUDES 1   encephalopathy NOS (G93.40)

EXCLUDES 2   acute transverse myelitis (G37.3-)
alcoholic encephalopathy (G31.2)
benign myalgic encephalomyelitis (G93.3)
multiple sclerosis (G35)
subacute necrotizing myelitis (G37.4)
toxic encephalitis ▶(G92.8)◀
toxic encephalopathy ▶(G92.8)◀

DEF: Encephalitis: Inflammation of the brain, often caused by viral or bacterial infection.
DEF: Encephalomyelitis: Inflammatory disease, often viral in nature, that affects the brain and spinal cord.
DEF: Myelitis: Inflammation of the spinal cord.

✓5th G04.0   Acute disseminated encephalitis and encephalomyelitis (ADEM)

EXCLUDES 1   acute necrotizing hemorrhagic encephalopathy (G04.3-)
other noninfectious acute disseminated encephalomyelitis (noninfectious ADEM) (G04.81)

G04.00   Acute disseminated encephalitis and encephalomyelitis, unspecified   `MCC`

G04.01   Postinfectious acute disseminated encephalitis and encephalomyelitis (postinfectious ADEM)   `MCC`

EXCLUDES 1   post chickenpox encephalitis (B01.1)
post measles encephalitis (B05.0)
post measles myelitis (B05.1)

G04.02 **Postimmunization** acute disseminated encephalitis, myelitis and encephalomyelitis   `MCC`
  Encephalitis, post immunization
  Encephalomyelitis, post immunization
  Use additional code to identify the vaccine (T50.A-, T50.B-, T50.Z-)

G04.1 **Tropical spastic paraplegia**   `CC` `HCC`

G04.2 **Bacterial meningoencephalitis and meningomyelitis, not elsewhere classified**   `MCC`

✓5ᵗʰ **G04.3** **Acute necrotizing hemorrhagic encephalopathy**
  `EXCLUDES 1`   acute disseminated encephalitis and encephalomyelitis (G04.0-)

    G04.30 **Acute necrotizing hemorrhagic encephalopathy, unspecified**   `MCC`

    G04.31 **Postinfectious** acute necrotizing hemorrhagic encephalopathy   `MCC`

    G04.32 **Postimmunization** acute necrotizing hemorrhagic encephalopathy   `MCC`
    Use additional code to identify the vaccine (T50.A-, T50.B-, T50.Z-)

    G04.39 **Other acute necrotizing hemorrhagic encephalopathy**   `MCC`
    Code also underlying etiology, if applicable

✓5ᵗʰ **G04.8** **Other encephalitis, myelitis and encephalomyelitis**
  Code also any associated seizure (G40.-, R56.9)

    G04.81 **Other encephalitis and encephalomyelitis**   `HIV` `MCC`
    Noninfectious acute disseminated encephalomyelitis (noninfectious ADEM)

    G04.82 **Acute flaccid myelitis**   `MCC`
    `EXCLUDES 1`   transverse myelitis (G37.3)

    G04.89 **Other myelitis**   `HIV` `MCC` `HCC`
    AHA: 2020,1Q,14

✓5ᵗʰ **G04.9** **Encephalitis, myelitis and encephalomyelitis, unspecified**

    G04.90 **Encephalitis and encephalomyelitis, unspecified**   `HIV` `MCC`
    Ventriculitis (cerebral) NOS

    G04.91 **Myelitis, unspecified**   `HIV` `MCC` `HCC`

✓4ᵗʰ **G05** **Encephalitis, myelitis and encephalomyelitis in diseases classified elsewhere**
  Code first underlying disease, such as:
  ▶congenital toxoplasmosis encephalitis, myelitis and encephalomyelitis (P37.1)◀
  ▶cytomegaloviral encephalitis, myelitis and encephalomyelitis (B25.8)◀
  ▶encephalitis, myelitis and encephalomyelitis (in) systemic lupus erythematosus (M32.19)◀
  ▶eosinophilic meningoencephalitis (B83.2)◀
  human immunodeficiency virus [HIV] disease (B20)
  poliovirus (A80.-)
  suppurative otitis media (H66.01-H66.4)
  trichinellosis (B75)
  `EXCLUDES 1`   adenoviral encephalitis, myelitis and encephalomyelitis (A85.1)
    ~~congenital toxoplasmosis encephalitis, myelitis and encephalomyelitis (P37.1)~~
    ~~cytomegaloviral encephalitis, myelitis and encephalomyelitis (B25.8)~~
    encephalitis, myelitis and encephalomyelitis (in) measles (B05.0)
    ~~encephalitis, myelitis and encephalomyelitis (in) systemic lupus erythematosus (M32.19)~~
    enteroviral encephalitis, myelitis and encephalomyelitis (A85.0)
    ~~eosinophilic meningoencephalitis (B83.2)~~
    herpesviral [herpes simplex] encephalitis, myelitis and encephalomyelitis (B00.4)
    listerial encephalitis, myelitis and encephalomyelitis (A32.12)
    meningococcal encephalitis, myelitis and encephalomyelitis (A39.81)
    mumps encephalitis, myelitis and encephalomyelitis (B26.2)
    postchickenpox encephalitis, myelitis and encephalomyelitis (B01.1-)
    rubella encephalitis, myelitis and encephalomyelitis (B06.01)
    toxoplasmosis encephalitis, myelitis and encephalomyelitis (B58.2)
    zoster encephalitis, myelitis and encephalomyelitis (B02.0)

    G05.3 *Encephalitis and encephalomyelitis in diseases classified elsewhere*   `MCC`
    Meningoencephalitis in diseases classified elsewhere

    G05.4 *Myelitis in diseases classified elsewhere*   `MCC` `HCC`
    Meningomyelitis in diseases classified elsewhere

✓4ᵗʰ **G06** **Intracranial and intraspinal abscess and granuloma**
  Use additional code (B95-B97) to identify infectious agent
  DEF: Abscess: Circumscribed collection of pus resulting from bacteria, frequently associated with swelling and other signs of inflammation.
  DEF: Granuloma: Abnormal, dense collections of cells forming a mass or nodule of chronically inflamed tissue with granulations that is usually associated with an infective process.

    G06.0 **Intracranial abscess and granuloma**   `MCC`
    Brain [any part] abscess (embolic)
    Cerebellar abscess (embolic)
    Cerebral abscess (embolic)
    Intracranial epidural abscess or granuloma
    Intracranial extradural abscess or granuloma
    Intracranial subdural abscess or granuloma
    Otogenic abscess (embolic)
    `EXCLUDES 1`   tuberculous intracranial abscess and granuloma (A17.81)

    G06.1 **Intraspinal abscess and granuloma**   `MCC`
    Abscess (embolic) of spinal cord [any part]
    Intraspinal epidural abscess or granuloma
    Intraspinal extradural abscess or granuloma
    Intraspinal subdural abscess or granuloma
    `EXCLUDES 1`   tuberculous intraspinal abscess and granuloma (A17.81)

    G06.2 **Extradural and subdural abscess, unspecified**   `MCC`

`N` Newborn: 0   `P` Pediatric: 0-17   `M` Maternity: 9-64   `A` Adult: 15-124   `MCC` Major Complication/Comorbidity   `CC` Complication/Comorbidity   `SW` Severe Wound Dx

574   ICD-10-CM 2022

G07 *Intracranial and intraspinal abscess and granuloma in diseases classified elsewhere* `MCC`

Code first underlying disease, such as:

schistosomiasis granuloma of brain (B65.-)

> `EXCLUDES 1`　abscess of brain:
>> amebic (A06.6)
>> chromomycotic (B43.1)
>> gonococcal (A54.82)
>> tuberculous (A17.81)
>> tuberculoma of meninges (A17.1)

G08 **Intracranial and intraspinal phlebitis and thrombophlebitis** `MCC`

Septic embolism of intracranial or intraspinal venous sinuses and veins

Septic endophlebitis of intracranial or intraspinal venous sinuses and veins

Septic phlebitis of intracranial or intraspinal venous sinuses and veins

Septic thrombophlebitis of intracranial or intraspinal venous sinuses and veins

Septic thrombosis of intracranial or intraspinal venous sinuses and veins

> `EXCLUDES 1`　intracranial phlebitis and thrombophlebitis complicating:
>> abortion, ectopic or molar pregnancy (O00-O07, O08.7)
>> pregnancy, childbirth and the puerperium (O22.5, O87.3)
>> nonpyogenic intracranial phlebitis and thrombophlebitis (I67.6)
>
> `EXCLUDES 2`　intracranial phlebitis and thrombophlebitis complicating nonpyogenic intraspinal phlebitis and thrombophlebitis (G95.1)

DEF: Inflammation and formation of a blood clot in a vein within the brain or spine, or their linings.

G09 **Sequelae of inflammatory diseases of central nervous system**

> `NOTE`　Category G09 is to be used to indicate conditions whose primary classification is to G00-G08 as the cause of sequelae, themselves classifiable elsewhere. The "sequelae" include conditions specified as residuals.

Code first condition resulting from (sequela) of inflammatory diseases of central nervous system

Systemic atrophies primarily affecting the central nervous system (G10-G14)

G10 **Huntington's disease** `CC` `HCC`

Huntington's chorea

Huntington's dementia

Code also dementia in other diseases classified elsewhere without behavioral disturbance (F02.80)

DEF: Genetic disease caused by degeneration of nerve cells in the brain, characterized by chronic progressive mental deterioration. Dementia and death occur within 15 to 20 years of onset.

`✓4ᵗʰ` **G11** **Hereditary ataxia**

> `EXCLUDES 2`　cerebral palsy (G80.-)
>> hereditary and idiopathic neuropathy (G60.-)
>> metabolic disorders (E70-E88)

DEF: Ataxia: Defect in muscular control or coordination due to a central nervous system disorder, particularly when voluntary muscular movements are attempted.

G11.0 Congenital nonprogressive **ataxia** `CC` `HCC`

`✓5ᵗʰ` **G11.1** **Early-onset cerebellar ataxia**

　　AHA: 2020,4Q,17-18

G11.10 **Early-onset cerebellar ataxia, unspecified** `CC` `HCC`

G11.11 **Friedreich ataxia** `CC` `HCC`

Autosomal recessive Friedreich ataxia

Friedreich ataxia with retained reflexes

G11.19 **Other early-onset cerebellar ataxia** `CC` `HCC`

Early-onset cerebellar ataxia with essential tremor

Early-onset cerebellar ataxia with myoclonus [Hunt's ataxia]

Early-onset cerebellar ataxia with retained tendon reflexes

X-linked recessive spinocerebellar ataxia

G11.2 Late-onset cerebellar **ataxia** `CC` `HCC` `A`

G11.3 Cerebellar **ataxia** with defective DNA repair `CC` `HCC`

Ataxia telangiectasia [Louis-Bar]

> `EXCLUDES 2`　Cockayne's syndrome (Q87.19)
>> other disorders of purine and pyrimidine metabolism (E79.-)
>> xeroderma pigmentosum (Q82.1)

G11.4 Hereditary spastic paraplegia `CC` `HCC`

G11.8 Other hereditary ataxias `CC` `HCC`

G11.9 **Hereditary ataxia, unspecified** `CC` `HCC`

Hereditary cerebellar ataxia NOS

Hereditary cerebellar degeneration

Hereditary cerebellar disease

Hereditary cerebellar syndrome

`✓4ᵗʰ` **G12** **Spinal muscular atrophy and related syndromes**

G12.0 Infantile **spinal muscular atrophy, type I [Werdnig-Hoffman]** `CC` `HCC`

G12.1 **Other inherited spinal muscular atrophy** `CC` `HCC`

Adult form spinal muscular atrophy

Childhood form, type II spinal muscular atrophy

Distal spinal muscular atrophy

Juvenile form, type III spinal muscular atrophy [Kugelberg-Welander]

Progressive bulbar palsy of childhood [Fazio-Londe]

Scapuloperoneal form spinal muscular atrophy

`✓5ᵗʰ` **G12.2** Motor neuron disease

　　AHA: 2017,4Q,9-10

G12.20 **Motor neuron disease, unspecified** `CC` `HCC`

G12.21 **Amyotrophic lateral sclerosis** `CC` `HCC` `A`

G12.22 **Progressive bulbar palsy** `CC` `HCC`

G12.23 **Primary lateral sclerosis** `CC` `HCC`

G12.24 **Familial motor neuron disease** `CC` `HCC`

G12.25 **Progressive spinal muscle atrophy** `CC` `HCC`

G12.29 **Other motor neuron disease** `CC` `HCC`

G12.8 **Other spinal muscular atrophies and related syndromes** `CC` `HCC`

G12.9 Spinal muscular atrophy, unspecified `CC` `HCC`

`✓4ᵗʰ` **G13** **Systemic atrophies primarily affecting central nervous system in diseases classified elsewhere**

G13.0 *Paraneoplastic neuromyopathy and neuropathy* `HCC`

Carcinomatous neuromyopathy

Sensorial paraneoplastic neuropathy [Denny Brown]

Code first underlying neoplasm (C00-D49)

G13.1 *Other systemic atrophy primarily affecting central nervous system in neoplastic disease* `HCC`

Paraneoplastic limbic encephalopathy

Code first underlying neoplasm (C00-D49)

G13.2 *Systemic atrophy primarily affecting the central nervous system in myxedema* `HCC`

Code first underlying disease, such as:

hypothyroidism (E03.-)

myxedematous congenital iodine deficiency (E00.1)

G13.8 *Systemic atrophy primarily affecting central nervous system in other diseases classified elsewhere* `HCC`

Code first underlying disease

G14 **Postpolio syndrome**

> `INCLUDES`　postpolio myelitic syndrome
> `EXCLUDES 1`　sequelae of poliomyelitis (B91)

Extrapyramidal and movement disorders (G20-G26)

G20 **Parkinson's disease** `HCC`

Hemiparkinsonism

Idiopathic Parkinsonism or Parkinson's disease

Paralysis agitans

Parkinsonism or Parkinson's disease NOS

Primary Parkinsonism or Parkinson's disease

Use additional code to identify:

dementia with behavioral disturbance (F02.81)

dementia without behavioral disturbance (F02.80)

> `EXCLUDES 1`　dementia with Parkinsonism (G31.83)

AHA: 2017,2Q,7; 2016,2Q,6

TIP: Repeated falls (R29.6) are not integral to Parkinson's disease and can be separately coded.

`✓4ᵗʰ` **G21** **Secondary parkinsonism**

> `EXCLUDES 1`　dementia with Parkinsonism (G31.83)
>> Huntington's disease (G10)
>> Shy-Drager syndrome (G90.3)
>> syphilitic Parkinsonism (A52.19)

G21.0 Malignant neuroleptic **syndrome** `MCC`

Use additional code for adverse effect, if applicable, to identify drug (T43.3X5, T43.4X5, T43.505, T43.595)

> `EXCLUDES 1`　neuroleptic induced parkinsonism (G21.11)

✔ Additional Character Required　`✓x7ᵗʰ` Placeholder　Questionable PDx　Manifestation　Unspecified Dx　`UPD` Unacceptable PDx　`H1`-`H14` HAC　`HCC` CMS-HCC Dx　`HIV` HIV Dx

Chapter 6. Diseases of the Nervous System

G21.1–G26

✓5ᵗʰ **G21.1** **Other drug-induced secondary parkinsonism**

     G21.11 **Neuroleptic induced parkinsonism** `CC` `HCC`
         Use additional code for adverse effect, if applicable, to identify drug (T43.3X5, T43.4X5, T43.5Ø5, T43.595)
         EXCLUDES 1   *malignant neuroleptic syndrome (G21.Ø)*

     G21.19 **Other drug induced secondary parkinsonism** `CC` `HCC`
         Other medication-induced parkinsonism
         Use additional code for adverse effect, if applicable, to identify drug (T36-T5Ø with fifth or sixth character 5)

G21.2 **Secondary parkinsonism due to other external agents** `CC` `HCC`
     Code first (T51-T65) to identify external agent

G21.3 **Postencephalitic parkinsonism** `CC` `HCC`

G21.4 **Vascular parkinsonism** `HCC`

G21.8 **Other secondary parkinsonism** `CC` `HCC`

G21.9 **Secondary parkinsonism, unspecified** `CC` `HCC`

✓4ᵗʰ **G23** **Other degenerative diseases of basal ganglia**
     EXCLUDES 2   *multi-system degeneration of the autonomic nervous system (G90.3)*

G23.Ø **Hallervorden-Spatz disease** `CC` `HCC`
     Pigmentary pallidal degeneration

G23.1 **Progressive supranuclear ophthalmoplegia [Steele-Richardson-Olszewski]** `CC` `HCC`
     Progressive supranuclear palsy

G23.2 **Striatonigral degeneration** `CC` `HCC`

G23.8 **Other specified degenerative diseases of basal ganglia** `CC` `HCC`
     Calcification of basal ganglia

G23.9 **Degenerative disease of basal ganglia, unspecified** `CC` `HCC`

✓4ᵗʰ **G24** **Dystonia**
     INCLUDES   dyskinesia
     EXCLUDES 2   *athetoid cerebral palsy (G80.3)*
     DEF: Disorder of abnormal muscle tone, excessive or inadequate. Involuntary movements and prolonged muscle contractions result in tremors, abnormalities in posture, and twisting body motions that affect an isolated area or the whole body.

✓5ᵗʰ **G24.Ø** **Drug induced dystonia**
     Use additional code for adverse effect, if applicable, to identify drug (T36-T5Ø with fifth or sixth character 5)

     G24.Ø1 **Drug induced subacute dyskinesia**
         Drug induced blepharospasm
         Drug induced orofacial dyskinesia
         Neuroleptic induced tardive dyskinesia
         Tardive dyskinesia

     G24.Ø2 **Drug induced acute dystonia** `CC`
         Acute dystonic reaction to drugs
         Neuroleptic induced acute dystonia

     G24.Ø9 **Other drug induced dystonia** `CC`

G24.1 **Genetic torsion dystonia**
     Dystonia deformans progressiva
     Dystonia musculorum deformans
     Familial torsion dystonia
     Idiopathic familial dystonia
     Idiopathic (torsion) dystonia NOS
     (Schwalbe-) Ziehen-Oppenheim disease

G24.2 **Idiopathic nonfamilial dystonia** `CC`

G24.3 **Spasmodic torticollis**
     EXCLUDES 1   *congenital torticollis (Q68.Ø)*
                    hysterical torticollis (F44.4)
                    ocular torticollis (R29.891)
                    psychogenic torticollis (F45.8)
                    torticollis NOS (M43.6)
                    traumatic recurrent torticollis (S13.4)
     DEF: Twisted, unnatural position of the neck due to contracted cervical muscles that pull the head to one side or cause involuntary shaking of the head.

G24.4 **Idiopathic orofacial dystonia**
     Orofacial dyskinesia
     EXCLUDES 1   *drug induced orofacial dyskinesia (G24.Ø1)*

G24.5 **Blepharospasm**
     EXCLUDES 1   *drug induced blepharospasm (G24.Ø1)*
     DEF: Involuntary contraction of the orbicularis oculi muscle, resulting in the eyelids being completely closed.

G24.8 **Other dystonia** `CC`
     Acquired torsion dystonia NOS

G24.9 **Dystonia, unspecified**
     Dyskinesia NOS

✓4ᵗʰ **G25** **Other extrapyramidal and movement disorders**
     EXCLUDES 2   *sleep related movement disorders (G47.6-)*

G25.Ø **Essential tremor**
     Familial tremor
     EXCLUDES 1   *tremor NOS (R25.1)*

G25.1 **Drug-induced tremor**
     Use additional code for adverse effect, if applicable, to identify drug (T36-T5Ø with fifth or sixth character 5)

G25.2 **Other specified forms of tremor**
     Intention tremor

G25.3 **Myoclonus**
     Drug-induced myoclonus
     Palatal myoclonus
     Use additional code for adverse effect, if applicable, to identify drug (T36-T5Ø with fifth or sixth character 5)
     EXCLUDES 1   *facial myokymia (G51.4)*
                    myoclonic epilepsy (G40.-)
     DEF: Spasmodic, brief, involuntary muscle contractions that can be due to an undetermined etiology, drug-induced, or caused by a disease process.

G25.4 **Drug-induced chorea**
     Use additional code for adverse effect, if applicable, to identify drug (T36-T5Ø with fifth or sixth character 5)

G25.5 **Other chorea**
     Chorea NOS
     EXCLUDES 1   *chorea NOS with heart involvement (I02.0)*
                    Huntington's chorea (G10)
                    rheumatic chorea (I02.-)
                    Sydenham's chorea (I02.-)

✓5ᵗʰ **G25.6** **Drug induced tics and other tics of organic origin**

     G25.61 **Drug induced tics**
         Use additional code for adverse effect, if applicable, to identify drug (T36-T5Ø with fifth or sixth character 5)

     G25.69 **Other tics of organic origin**
         EXCLUDES 1   *habit spasm (F95.9)*
                      tic NOS (F95.9)
                      Tourette's syndrome (F95.2)

✓5ᵗʰ **G25.7** **Other and unspecified drug induced movement disorders**
     Use additional code for adverse effect, if applicable, to identify drug (T36-T5Ø with fifth or sixth character 5)

     G25.70 **Drug induced movement disorder, unspecified**

     G25.71 **Drug induced akathisia**
         Drug induced acathisia
         Neuroleptic induced acute akathisia
         Tardive akathisia

     G25.79 **Other drug induced movement disorders**

✓5ᵗʰ **G25.8** **Other specified extrapyramidal and movement disorders**

     G25.81 **Restless legs syndrome**
         DEF: Neurological disorder of unknown etiology creating an irresistible urge to move the legs, which may temporarily relieve the symptoms. This syndrome is accompanied by motor restlessness and sensations of pain, burning, prickling, or tingling.

     G25.82 **Stiff-man syndrome** `CC`

     G25.83 **Benign shuddering attacks**

     G25.89 **Other specified extrapyramidal and movement disorders**

G25.9 **Extrapyramidal and movement disorder, unspecified** `CC`

G26 ***Extrapyramidal and movement disorders in diseases classified elsewhere***
     Code first underlying disease

N Newborn: 0   P Pediatric: 0-17   M Maternity: 9-64   A Adult: 15-124   MCC Major Complication/Comorbidity   CC Complication/Comorbidity   SW Severe Wound Dx

576   ICD-10-CM 2022

Other degenerative diseases of the nervous system (G30-G32)

✓4ᵗʰ G30 Alzheimer's disease

INCLUDES   Alzheimer's dementia senile and presenile forms

Use additional code to identify:
- delirium, if applicable (F05)
- dementia with behavioral disturbance (F02.81)
- dementia without behavioral disturbance (F02.80)

EXCLUDES 1   senile degeneration of brain NEC (G31.1)
       senile dementia NOS (F03)
       senility NOS (R41.81)

AHA: 2017,1Q,43
TIP: A code from subcategory F02.8 should always be assigned with a code from this category, even in the absence of documented dementia.
TIP: Functional quadriplegia (R53.2) is not integral to Alzheimer's disease and can be coded in addition to codes from category G30.

G30.0 Alzheimer's disease with early onset   HCC
G30.1 Alzheimer's disease with late onset   HCC A
G30.8 Other Alzheimer's disease   HCC
G30.9 Alzheimer's disease, unspecified   HCC
     AHA: 2016,2Q,6; 2012,4Q,95

✓4ᵗʰ G31 Other degenerative diseases of nervous system, not elsewhere classified

For codes G31.0 - G31.83, G31.85 - G31.9, use additional code to identify:
- dementia with behavioral disturbance (F02.81)
- dementia without behavioral disturbance (F02.80)

EXCLUDES 2   Reye's syndrome (G93.7)

✓5ᵗʰ G31.0 Frontotemporal dementia

G31.01 Pick's disease   HCC
Primary progressive aphasia
Progressive isolated aphasia
DEF: Progressive frontotemporal dementia with asymmetrical atrophy of the frontal and temporal regions of the cerebral cortex and abnormal rounded brain cells called Pick cells with the presence of abnormal staining of protein (called tau). Symptoms include prominent apathy, behavioral changes such as disinhibition and restlessness, echolalia, impairment of language, memory, and intellect, increased carelessness, poor personal hygiene, and decreased attention span.

G31.09 Other frontotemporal dementia   HCC
Frontal dementia

G31.1 Senile degeneration of brain, not elsewhere classified   HCC
EXCLUDES 1   Alzheimer's disease (G30.-)
       senility NOS (R41.81)

G31.2 Degeneration of nervous system due to alcohol   HCC
Alcoholic cerebellar ataxia
Alcoholic cerebellar degeneration
Alcoholic cerebral degeneration
Alcoholic encephalopathy
Dysfunction of the autonomic nervous system due to alcohol
Code also associated alcoholism (F10.-)

✓5ᵗʰ G31.8 Other specified degenerative diseases of nervous system

G31.81 Alpers disease   CC HCC
Grey-matter degeneration

G31.82 Leigh's disease   CC HCC
Subacute necrotizing encephalopathy

G31.83 Dementia with Lewy bodies   HCC
Dementia with Parkinsonism
Lewy body dementia
Lewy body disease
AHA: 2017,2Q,7; 2016,4Q,141
DEF: Cerebral dementia with neurophysiologic changes, increased hippocampal volume, hypoperfusion in the occipital lobes, beta amyloid deposits with neurofibrillary tangles, and atrophy of the cortex and brainstem. Hallmark neuropsychological characteristics include fluctuating cognition with pronounced variation in attention and alertness, recurrent hallucinations, and Parkinsonism.

G31.84 Mild cognitive impairment, so stated
Mild neurocognitive disorder
EXCLUDES 1   age related cognitive decline (R41.81)
       altered mental status (R41.82)
       cerebral degeneration (G31.9)
       change in mental status (R41.82)
       cognitive deficits following (sequelae of) cerebral hemorrhage or infarction (I69.01-, I69.11-, I69.21-, I69.31-, I69.81-, I69.91-)
       cognitive impairment due to intracranial or head injury (S06.-)
       dementia (F01.-, F02.-, F03)
       mild memory disturbance (F06.8)
       neurologic neglect syndrome (R41.4)
       personality change, nonpsychotic (F68.8)

G31.85 Corticobasal degeneration   HCC

G31.89 Other specified degenerative diseases of nervous system   HCC

G31.9 Degenerative disease of nervous system, unspecified   HCC

✓4ᵗʰ G32 Other degenerative disorders of nervous system in diseases classified elsewhere

G32.0 *Subacute combined degeneration of spinal cord in diseases classified elsewhere*   CC HCC
Dana-Putnam syndrome
Sclerosis of spinal cord (combined) (dorsolateral) (posterolateral)
Code first underlying disease, such as:
- anemia (D51.9)
- dietary (D51.3)
- pernicious (D51.0)
- vitamin B12 deficiency (E53.8)

EXCLUDES 1   syphilitic combined degeneration of spinal cord (A52.11)

✓5ᵗʰ G32.8 Other specified degenerative disorders of nervous system in diseases classified elsewhere
Code first underlying disease, such as:
- amyloidosis cerebral degeneration (E85.-)
- cerebral degeneration (due to) hypothyroidism (E00.0-E03.9)
- cerebral degeneration (due to) neoplasm (C00-D49)
- cerebral degeneration (due to) vitamin B deficiency, except thiamine (E52-E53.-)

EXCLUDES 1   superior hemorrhagic polioencephalitis [Wernicke's encephalopathy] (E51.2)

G32.81 *Cerebellar ataxia in diseases classified elsewhere*   CC HCC
Code first underlying disease, such as:
- celiac disease (with gluten ataxia) (K90.0)
- cerebellar ataxia (in) neoplastic disease (paraneoplastic cerebellar degeneration) (C00-D49)
- non-celiac gluten ataxia (M35.9)

EXCLUDES 1   systemic atrophy primarily affecting the central nervous system in alcoholic cerebellar ataxia (G31.2)
       systemic atrophy primarily affecting the central nervous system in myxedema (G13.2)

G32.89 *Other specified degenerative disorders of nervous system in diseases classified elsewhere*
Degenerative encephalopathy in diseases classified elsewhere

Demyelinating diseases of the central nervous system (G35-G37)

G35 Multiple sclerosis   HCC
Disseminated multiple sclerosis
Generalized multiple sclerosis
Multiple sclerosis NOS
Multiple sclerosis of brain stem
Multiple sclerosis of cord
AHA: 2021,1Q,7

Chapter 6. Diseases of the Nervous System

G36–G40.201

✓4ᵗʰ G36 Other acute disseminated demyelination

> EXCLUDES 1   postinfectious encephalitis and encephalomyelitis NOS (G04.01)

> **DEF:** Demyelination: Abnormal loss of myelin, the protective white matter that insulates nerve endings and facilitates neuroreception and neurotransmission. When this substance is damaged, the nerve is short-circuited, resulting in impaired or loss of function.

G36.0 Neuromyelitis optica [Devic]   CC HCC
> Demyelination in optic neuritis
> EXCLUDES 1   optic neuritis NOS (H46)

G36.1 Acute and subacute hemorrhagic leukoencephalitis [Hurst]   CC HCC

G36.8 Other specified acute disseminated demyelination   CC HCC

G36.9 Acute disseminated demyelination, unspecified   HIV CC HCC

✓4ᵗʰ G37 Other demyelinating diseases of central nervous system

G37.0 Diffuse sclerosis of central nervous system   CC HCC
> Periaxial encephalitis
> Schilder's disease
> EXCLUDES 1   X linked adrenoleukodystrophy (E71.52-)

G37.1 Central demyelination of corpus callosum   CC HCC

G37.2 Central pontine myelinolysis   CC HCC

G37.3 Acute transverse myelitis in demyelinating disease of central nervous system   CC HCC
> Acute transverse myelitis NOS
> Acute transverse myelopathy
> EXCLUDES 1   ▶acute flaccid myelitis (G04.82)◀
>   multiple sclerosis (G35)
>   neuromyelitis optica [Devic] (G36.0)

G37.4 Subacute necrotizing myelitis of central nervous system   HIV MCC HCC

G37.5 Concentric sclerosis [Balo] of central nervous system   CC HCC

G37.8 Other specified demyelinating diseases of central nervous system   CC HCC

G37.9 Demyelinating disease of central nervous system, unspecified   HIV CC HCC

Episodic and paroxysmal disorders (G40-G47)

✓4ᵗʰ G40 Epilepsy and recurrent seizures

> NOTE   The following terms are to be considered equivalent to intractable: pharmacoresistant (pharmacologically resistant), treatment resistant, refractory (medically) and poorly controlled

> EXCLUDES 1   conversion disorder with seizures (F44.5)
>   convulsions NOS (R56.9)
>   post traumatic seizures (R56.1)
>   seizure (convulsive) NOS (R56.9)
>   seizure of newborn (P90)

> EXCLUDES 2   hippocampal sclerosis (G93.81)
>   mesial temporal sclerosis (G93.81)
>   temporal sclerosis (G93.81)
>   Todd's paralysis (G83.84)

✓5ᵗʰ G40.0 Localization-related (focal) (partial) idiopathic epilepsy and epileptic syndromes with seizures of localized onset
> Benign childhood epilepsy with centrotemporal EEG spikes
> Childhood epilepsy with occipital EEG paroxysms
> EXCLUDES 1   adult onset localization-related epilepsy (G40.1-, G40.2-)

✓6ᵗʰ G40.00 Localization-related (focal) (partial) idiopathic epilepsy and epileptic syndromes with seizures of localized onset, not intractable
> Localization-related (focal) (partial) idiopathic epilepsy and epileptic syndromes with seizures of localized onset without intractability

G40.001 Localization-related (focal) (partial) idiopathic epilepsy and epileptic syndromes with seizures of localized onset, not intractable, with status epilepticus   CC HCC

G40.009 Localization-related (focal) (partial) idiopathic epilepsy and epileptic syndromes with seizures of localized onset, not intractable, without status epilepticus   CC HCC
> Localization-related (focal) (partial) idiopathic epilepsy and epileptic syndromes with seizures of localized onset NOS

✓6ᵗʰ G40.01 Localization-related (focal) (partial) idiopathic epilepsy and epileptic syndromes with seizures of localized onset, intractable

G40.011 Localization-related (focal) (partial) idiopathic epilepsy and epileptic syndromes with seizures of localized onset, intractable, with status epilepticus   CC HCC

G40.019 Localization-related (focal) (partial) idiopathic epilepsy and epileptic syndromes with seizures of localized onset, intractable, without status epilepticus   CC HCC

✓5ᵗʰ G40.1 Localization-related (focal) (partial) symptomatic epilepsy and epileptic syndromes with simple partial seizures
> Attacks without alteration of consciousness
> Epilepsia partialis continua [Kozhevnikof]
> Simple partial seizures developing into secondarily generalized seizures

✓6ᵗʰ G40.10 Localization-related (focal) (partial) symptomatic epilepsy and epileptic syndromes with simple partial seizures, not intractable
> Localization-related (focal) (partial) symptomatic epilepsy and epileptic syndromes with simple partial seizures without intractability

G40.101 Localization-related (focal) (partial) symptomatic epilepsy and epileptic syndromes with simple partial seizures, not intractable, with status epilepticus   CC HCC

G40.109 Localization-related (focal) (partial) symptomatic epilepsy and epileptic syndromes with simple partial seizures, not intractable, without status epilepticus   CC HCC
> Localization-related (focal) (partial) symptomatic epilepsy and epileptic syndromes with simple partial seizures NOS

✓6ᵗʰ G40.11 Localization-related (focal) (partial) symptomatic epilepsy and epileptic syndromes with simple partial seizures, intractable

G40.111 Localization-related (focal) (partial) symptomatic epilepsy and epileptic syndromes with simple partial seizures, intractable, with status epilepticus   CC HCC

G40.119 Localization-related (focal) (partial) symptomatic epilepsy and epileptic syndromes with simple partial seizures, intractable, without status epilepticus   CC HCC

✓5ᵗʰ G40.2 Localization-related (focal) (partial) symptomatic epilepsy and epileptic syndromes with complex partial seizures
> Attacks with alteration of consciousness, often with automatisms
> Complex partial seizures developing into secondarily generalized seizures

✓6ᵗʰ G40.20 Localization-related (focal) (partial) symptomatic epilepsy and epileptic syndromes with complex partial seizures, not intractable
> Localization-related (focal) (partial) symptomatic epilepsy and epileptic syndromes with complex partial seizures without intractability

G40.201 Localization-related (focal) (partial) symptomatic epilepsy and epileptic syndromes with complex partial seizures, not intractable, with status epilepticus   CC HCC

N Newborn: 0   P Pediatric: 0-17   M Maternity: 9-64   A Adult: 15-124   MCC Major Complication/Comorbidity   CC Complication/Comorbidity   SW Severe Wound Dx

578   ICD-10-CM 2022

G36–G40.201

G40.209 Localization-related (focal) (partial) symptomatic epilepsy and epileptic syndromes with complex partial seizures, not intractable, without status epilepticus `CC` `HCC`

Localization-related (focal) symptomatic epilepsy and epileptic syndromes with complex partial seizures NOS

✓6ᵗʰ **G40.21** Localization-related (focal) (partial) symptomatic epilepsy and epileptic syndromes with complex partial seizures, intractable

G40.211 Localization-related (focal) (partial) symptomatic epilepsy and epileptic syndromes with complex partial seizures, intractable, with status epilepticus `CC` `HCC`

G40.219 Localization-related (focal) (partial) symptomatic epilepsy and epileptic syndromes with complex partial seizures, intractable, without status epilepticus `CC` `HCC`

✓5ᵗʰ **G40.3** Generalized idiopathic epilepsy and epileptic syndromes

Code also MERRF syndrome, if applicable (E88.42)

✓6ᵗʰ **G40.30** Generalized idiopathic epilepsy and epileptic syndromes, not intractable

Generalized idiopathic epilepsy and epileptic syndromes without intractability

G40.301 Generalized idiopathic epilepsy and epileptic syndromes, not intractable, with status epilepticus `MCC` `HCC`

G40.309 Generalized idiopathic epilepsy and epileptic syndromes, not intractable, without status epilepticus `HCC`

Generalized idiopathic epilepsy and epileptic syndromes NOS

✓6ᵗʰ **G40.31** Generalized idiopathic epilepsy and epileptic syndromes, intractable

G40.311 Generalized idiopathic epilepsy and epileptic syndromes, intractable, with status epilepticus `MCC` `HCC`

G40.319 Generalized idiopathic epilepsy and epileptic syndromes, intractable, without status epilepticus `MCC` `HCC`

✓5ᵗʰ **G40.A** Absence epileptic syndrome

Childhood absence epilepsy [pyknolepsy]
Juvenile absence epilepsy
Absence epileptic syndrome, NOS

✓6ᵗʰ **G40.A0** Absence epileptic syndrome, not intractable

G40.A01 Absence epileptic syndrome, not intractable, with status epilepticus `HCC`

G40.A09 Absence epileptic syndrome, not intractable, without status epilepticus `HCC`

✓6ᵗʰ **G40.A1** Absence epileptic syndrome, intractable

G40.A11 Absence epileptic syndrome, intractable, with status epilepticus `CC` `HCC`

G40.A19 Absence epileptic syndrome, intractable, without status epilepticus `CC` `HCC`

✓5ᵗʰ **G40.B** Juvenile myoclonic epilepsy [impulsive petit mal]

✓6ᵗʰ **G40.B0** Juvenile myoclonic epilepsy, not intractable

G40.B01 Juvenile myoclonic epilepsy, not intractable, with status epilepticus `CC` `HCC`

G40.B09 Juvenile myoclonic epilepsy, not intractable, without status epilepticus `CC` `HCC`

✓6ᵗʰ **G40.B1** Juvenile myoclonic epilepsy, intractable

G40.B11 Juvenile myoclonic epilepsy, intractable, with status epilepticus `CC` `HCC`

G40.B19 Juvenile myoclonic epilepsy, intractable, without status epilepticus `CC` `HCC`

✓5ᵗʰ **G40.4** Other generalized epilepsy and epileptic syndromes

Epilepsy with grand mal seizures on awakening
Epilepsy with myoclonic absences
Epilepsy with myoclonic-astatic seizures
Grand mal seizure NOS
Nonspecific atonic epileptic seizures
Nonspecific clonic epileptic seizures
Nonspecific myoclonic epileptic seizures
Nonspecific tonic epileptic seizures
Nonspecific tonic-clonic epileptic seizures
Symptomatic early myoclonic encephalopathy

✓6ᵗʰ **G40.40** Other generalized epilepsy and epileptic syndromes, not intractable

Other generalized epilepsy and epileptic syndromes without intractability
Other generalized epilepsy and epileptic syndromes NOS

G40.401 Other generalized epilepsy and epileptic syndromes, not intractable, with status epilepticus `HCC`

G40.409 Other generalized epilepsy and epileptic syndromes, not intractable, without status epilepticus `HCC`

✓6ᵗʰ **G40.41** Other generalized epilepsy and epileptic syndromes, intractable

G40.411 Other generalized epilepsy and epileptic syndromes, intractable, with status epilepticus `CC` `HCC`

G40.419 Other generalized epilepsy and epileptic syndromes, intractable, without status epilepticus `CC` `HCC`

G40.42 Cyclin-Dependent Kinase-Like 5 Deficiency Disorder `HCC`

CDKL5

Use additional code, if known, to identify associated manifestations, such as:
cortical blindness (H47.61-)
global development delay (F88)

AHA: 2020,4Q,18-19

✓5ᵗʰ **G40.5** Epileptic seizures related to external causes

Epileptic seizures related to alcohol
Epileptic seizures related to drugs
Epileptic seizures related to hormonal changes
Epileptic seizures related to sleep deprivation
Epileptic seizures related to stress

Code also, if applicable, associated epilepsy and recurrent seizures (G40.-)

Use additional code for adverse effect, if applicable, to identify drug (T36-T50 with fifth or sixth character 5)

✓6ᵗʰ **G40.50** Epileptic seizures related to external causes, not intractable

G40.501 Epileptic seizures related to external causes, not intractable, with status epilepticus `CC` `HCC`

G40.509 Epileptic seizures related to external causes, not intractable, without status epilepticus `CC` `HCC`

Epileptic seizures related to external causes, NOS

✓5ᵗʰ **G40.8** Other epilepsy and recurrent seizures

Epilepsies and epileptic syndromes undetermined as to whether they are focal or generalized
Landau-Kleffner syndrome

✓6ᵗʰ **G40.80** Other epilepsy

G40.801 Other epilepsy, not intractable, with status epilepticus `CC` `HCC`

Other epilepsy without intractability with status epilepticus

G40.802 Other epilepsy, not intractable, without status epilepticus `CC` `HCC`

Other epilepsy NOS
Other epilepsy without intractability without status epilepticus

G40.803 Other epilepsy, intractable, with status epilepticus `CC` `HCC`

G40.804 Other epilepsy, intractable, without status epilepticus `CC` `HCC`

✓ Additional Character Required   ✓x7ᵗʰ Placeholder   Questionable PDx   **Manifestation**   Unspecified Dx   `UPD` Unacceptable PDx   `H1`-`H14` HAC   `HCC` CMS-HCC Dx   `HIV` HIV Dx

ICD-10-CM 2022   579

✓6ᵗʰ G40.81 Lennox-Gastaut syndrome

> **DEF:** Severe form of epilepsy with usual onset in early childhood. Seizures are frequent and difficult to treat, causing falls and intellectual impairment.

> **G40.811 Lennox-Gastaut syndrome, not intractable, with status epilepticus** `CC` `HCC`

> **G40.812 Lennox-Gastaut syndrome, not intractable, without status epilepticus** `CC` `HCC`

> **G40.813 Lennox-Gastaut syndrome, intractable, with status epilepticus** `CC` `HCC`

> **G40.814 Lennox-Gastaut syndrome, intractable, without status epilepticus** `CC` `HCC`

✓6ᵗʰ G40.82 Epileptic spasms

> Infantile spasms
> Salaam attacks
> West's syndrome

> **G40.821 Epileptic spasms, not intractable, with status epilepticus** `CC` `HCC`

> **G40.822 Epileptic spasms, not intractable, without status epilepticus** `CC` `HCC`

> **G40.823 Epileptic spasms, intractable, with status epilepticus** `CC` `HCC`

> **G40.824 Epileptic spasms, intractable, without status epilepticus** `CC` `HCC`

✓6ᵗʰ G40.83 Dravet syndrome

> Polymorphic epilepsy in infancy (PMEI)
> Severe myoclonic epilepsy in infancy (SMEI)
> **AHA:** 2020,4Q,19

> **G40.833 Dravet syndrome, intractable, with status epilepticus** `CC` `HCC`

> **G40.834 Dravet syndrome, intractable, without status epilepticus** `CC` `HCC`
> > Dravet syndrome NOS

G40.89 Other seizures `CC` `HCC`

> **EXCLUDES 1**   post traumatic seizures (R56.1)
> > recurrent seizures NOS (G40.909)
> > seizure NOS (R56.9)

✓5ᵗʰ G40.9 Epilepsy, unspecified

> **AHA:** 2019,1Q,19

✓6ᵗʰ G40.90 Epilepsy, unspecified, not intractable

> Epilepsy, unspecified, without intractability

> **G40.901 Epilepsy, unspecified, not intractable, with status epilepticus** `HCC`

> **G40.909 Epilepsy, unspecified, not intractable, without status epilepticus** `HCC`
> > Epilepsy NOS
> > Epileptic convulsions NOS
> > Epileptic fits NOS
> > Epileptic seizures NOS
> > Recurrent seizures NOS
> > Seizure disorder NOS
> > **AHA:** 2021,2Q,3; 2021,1Q,3

✓6ᵗʰ G40.91 Epilepsy, unspecified, intractable

> Intractable seizure disorder NOS

> **G40.911 Epilepsy, unspecified, intractable, with status epilepticus** `CC` `HCC`

> **G40.919 Epilepsy, unspecified, intractable, without status epilepticus** `CC` `HCC`

✓4ᵗʰ G43 Migraine

> **NOTE**   The following terms are to be considered equivalent to intractable: pharmacoresistant (pharmacologically resistant), treatment resistant, refractory (medically) and poorly controlled

> Use additional code for adverse effect, if applicable, to identify drug (T36-T50 with fifth or sixth character 5)

> **EXCLUDES 1**   headache NOS (R51.9)
> > lower half migraine (G44.00)

> **EXCLUDES 2**   headache syndromes (G44.-)

> **DEF:** Headaches that occur periodically on one or both sides of the head that may be associated with nausea and vomiting, sensitivity to light and sound, dizziness, distorted vision, and cognitive disturbances.

✓5ᵗʰ G43.0 Migraine without aura

> Common migraine
> **EXCLUDES 1**   chronic migraine without aura (G43.7-)

✓6ᵗʰ G43.00 Migraine without aura, not intractable

> Migraine without aura without mention of refractory migraine

> **G43.001 Migraine without aura, not intractable, with status migrainosus**

> **G43.009 Migraine without aura, not intractable, without status migrainosus**
> > Migraine without aura NOS

✓6ᵗʰ G43.01 Migraine without aura, intractable

> Migraine without aura with refractory migraine

> **G43.011 Migraine without aura, intractable, with status migrainosus**

> **G43.019 Migraine without aura, intractable, without status migrainosus**

✓5ᵗʰ G43.1 Migraine with aura

> Basilar migraine
> Classical migraine
> Migraine equivalents
> Migraine preceded or accompanied by transient focal neurological phenomena
> Migraine triggered seizures
> Migraine with acute-onset aura
> Migraine with aura without headache (migraine equivalents)
> Migraine with prolonged aura
> Migraine with typical aura
> Retinal migraine
> Code also any associated seizure (G40.-, R56.9)
> **EXCLUDES 1**   persistent migraine aura (G43.5-, G43.6-)

✓6ᵗʰ G43.10 Migraine with aura, not intractable

> Migraine with aura without mention of refractory migraine

> **G43.101 Migraine with aura, not intractable, with status migrainosus**

> **G43.109 Migraine with aura, not intractable, without status migrainosus**
> > Migraine with aura NOS

✓6ᵗʰ G43.11 Migraine with aura, intractable

> Migraine with aura with refractory migraine

> **G43.111 Migraine with aura, intractable, with status migrainosus**

> **G43.119 Migraine with aura, intractable, without status migrainosus**

✓5ᵗʰ G43.4 Hemiplegic migraine

> Familial migraine
> Sporadic migraine

✓6ᵗʰ G43.40 Hemiplegic migraine, not intractable

> Hemiplegic migraine without refractory migraine

> **G43.401 Hemiplegic migraine, not intractable, with status migrainosus**

> **G43.409 Hemiplegic migraine, not intractable, without status migrainosus**
> > Hemiplegic migraine NOS

✓6ᵗʰ G43.41 Hemiplegic migraine, intractable

> Hemiplegic migraine with refractory migraine

> **G43.411 Hemiplegic migraine, intractable, with status migrainosus**

> **G43.419 Hemiplegic migraine, intractable, without status migrainosus**

Ⓝ Newborn: 0   Ⓟ Pediatric: 0-17   Ⓜ Maternity: 9-64   Ⓐ Adult: 15-124   `MCC` Major Complication/Comorbidity   `CC` Complication/Comorbidity   `SW` Severe Wound Dx

580   ICD-10-CM 2022

✓5ᵗʰ G43.5 Persistent migraine aura without cerebral infarction

    ✓6ᵗʰ G43.50 Persistent migraine aura without cerebral infarction, not intractable
        Persistent migraine aura without cerebral infarction, without refractory migraine

        G43.501 Persistent migraine aura without cerebral infarction, not intractable, with status migrainosus

        G43.509 Persistent migraine aura without cerebral infarction, not intractable, without status migrainosus
            Persistent migraine aura NOS

    ✓6ᵗʰ G43.51 Persistent migraine aura without cerebral infarction, intractable
        Persistent migraine aura without cerebral infarction, with refractory migraine

        G43.511 Persistent migraine aura without cerebral infarction, intractable, with status migrainosus

        G43.519 Persistent migraine aura without cerebral infarction, intractable, without status migrainosus

✓5ᵗʰ G43.6 Persistent migraine aura with cerebral infarction
    Code also the type of cerebral infarction (I63.-)

    ✓6ᵗʰ G43.60 Persistent migraine aura with cerebral infarction, not intractable
        Persistent migraine aura with cerebral infarction, without refractory migraine

        G43.601 Persistent migraine aura with cerebral infarction, not intractable, with status migrainosus `CC`

        G43.609 Persistent migraine aura with cerebral infarction, not intractable, without status migrainosus `CC`

    ✓6ᵗʰ G43.61 Persistent migraine aura with cerebral infarction, intractable
        Persistent migraine aura with cerebral infarction, with refractory migraine

        G43.611 Persistent migraine aura with cerebral infarction, intractable, with status migrainosus `CC`

        G43.619 Persistent migraine aura with cerebral infarction, intractable, without status migrainosus `CC`

✓5ᵗʰ G43.7 Chronic migraine without aura
    Transformed migraine
    EXCLUDES 1 *migraine without aura (G43.0-)*

    ✓6ᵗʰ G43.70 Chronic migraine without aura, not intractable
        Chronic migraine without aura, without refractory migraine

        G43.701 Chronic migraine without aura, not intractable, with status migrainosus

        G43.709 Chronic migraine without aura, not intractable, without status migrainosus
            Chronic migraine without aura NOS

    ✓6ᵗʰ G43.71 Chronic migraine without aura, intractable
        Chronic migraine without aura, with refractory migraine

        G43.711 Chronic migraine without aura, intractable, with status migrainosus

        G43.719 Chronic migraine without aura, intractable, without status migrainosus

✓5ᵗʰ G43.A Cyclical vomiting
    EXCLUDES 1 *cyclical vomiting syndrome unrelated to migraine (R11.15)*

    AHA: 2019,4Q,15

    G43.A0 Cyclical vomiting, in migraine, not intractable
        Cyclical vomiting, without refractory migraine

    G43.A1 Cyclical vomiting, in migraine, intractable
        Cyclical vomiting, with refractory migraine

✓5ᵗʰ G43.B Ophthalmoplegic migraine

    G43.B0 Ophthalmoplegic migraine, not intractable
        Ophthalmoplegic migraine, without refractory migraine

    G43.B1 Ophthalmoplegic migraine, intractable
        Ophthalmoplegic migraine, with refractory migraine

✓5ᵗʰ G43.C Periodic headache syndromes in child or adult

    G43.C0 Periodic headache syndromes in child or adult, not intractable
        Periodic headache syndromes in child or adult, without refractory migraine

    G43.C1 Periodic headache syndromes in child or adult, intractable
        Periodic headache syndromes in child or adult, with refractory migraine

✓5ᵗʰ G43.D Abdominal migraine

    G43.D0 Abdominal migraine, not intractable
        Abdominal migraine, without refractory migraine

    G43.D1 Abdominal migraine, intractable
        Abdominal migraine, with refractory migraine

✓5ᵗʰ G43.8 Other migraine

    ✓6ᵗʰ G43.80 Other migraine, not intractable
        Other migraine, without refractory migraine

        G43.801 Other migraine, not intractable, with status migrainosus

        G43.809 Other migraine, not intractable, without status migrainosus

    ✓6ᵗʰ G43.81 Other migraine, intractable
        Other migraine, with refractory migraine

        G43.811 Other migraine, intractable, with status migrainosus

        G43.819 Other migraine, intractable, without status migrainosus

    ✓6ᵗʰ G43.82 Menstrual migraine, not intractable
        Menstrual headache, not intractable
        Menstrual migraine, without refractory migraine
        Menstrually related migraine, not intractable
        Pre-menstrual headache, not intractable
        Pre-menstrual migraine, not intractable
        Pure menstrual migraine, not intractable
        Code also associated premenstrual tension syndrome (N94.3)

        G43.821 Menstrual migraine, not intractable, with status migrainosus ♀

        G43.829 Menstrual migraine, not intractable, without status migrainosus ♀
            Menstrual migraine NOS

    ✓6ᵗʰ G43.83 Menstrual migraine, intractable
        Menstrual headache, intractable
        Menstrual migraine, with refractory migraine
        Menstrually related migraine, intractable
        Pre-menstrual headache, intractable
        Pre-menstrual migraine, intractable
        Pure menstrual migraine, intractable
        Code also associated premenstrual tension syndrome (N94.3)

        G43.831 Menstrual migraine, intractable, with status migrainosus ♀

        G43.839 Menstrual migraine, intractable, without status migrainosus ♀

✓5ᵗʰ G43.9 Migraine, unspecified

    ✓6ᵗʰ G43.90 Migraine, unspecified, not intractable
        Migraine, unspecified, without refractory migraine

        G43.901 Migraine, unspecified, not intractable, with status migrainosus
            Status migrainosus NOS

        G43.909 Migraine, unspecified, not intractable, without status migrainosus
            Migraine NOS

    ✓6ᵗʰ G43.91 Migraine, unspecified, intractable
        Migraine, unspecified, with refractory migraine

        G43.911 Migraine, unspecified, intractable, with status migrainosus

        G43.919 Migraine, unspecified, intractable, without status migrainosus

✓ Additional Character Required   ✓x7ᵗʰ Placeholder   Questionable PDx   **Manifestation**   Unspecified Dx   **UPD** Unacceptable PDx   **H1-H14** HAC   **HCC** CMS-HCC Dx   **HIV** HIV Dx

ICD-10-CM 2022   581

Chapter 6. Diseases of the Nervous System

✓4th **G44 Other headache syndromes**
> EXCLUDES 1   headache NOS (R51.9)
> EXCLUDES 2   atypical facial pain (G50.1)
> headache due to lumbar puncture (G97.1)
> migraines (G43.-)
> trigeminal neuralgia (G50.0)

✓5th **G44.0 Cluster headaches and other trigeminal autonomic cephalgias (TAC)**
> **DEF:** Cluster headache: Characteristic grouping or clustering of headaches that can last for a number of weeks or months and then completely disappear for months or years. They are typically not associated with gastrointestinal upset or light sensitivity as experienced in migraines.

✓6th **G44.00 Cluster headache syndrome, unspecified**
> Ciliary neuralgia
> Cluster headache NOS
> Histamine cephalgia
> Lower half migraine
> Migrainous neuralgia

   G44.001 Cluster headache syndrome, unspecified, intractable

   G44.009 Cluster headache syndrome, unspecified, not intractable
> Cluster headache syndrome NOS

✓6th **G44.01 Episodic cluster headache**

   G44.011 Episodic cluster headache, intractable

   G44.019 Episodic cluster headache, not intractable
> Episodic cluster headache NOS

✓6th **G44.02 Chronic cluster headache**

   G44.021 Chronic cluster headache, intractable

   G44.029 Chronic cluster headache, not intractable
> Chronic cluster headache NOS

✓6th **G44.03 Episodic paroxysmal hemicrania**
> Paroxysmal hemicrania NOS

   G44.031 Episodic paroxysmal hemicrania, intractable

   G44.039 Episodic paroxysmal hemicrania, not intractable
> Episodic paroxysmal hemicrania NOS

✓6th **G44.04 Chronic paroxysmal hemicrania**

   G44.041 Chronic paroxysmal hemicrania, intractable

   G44.049 Chronic paroxysmal hemicrania, not intractable
> Chronic paroxysmal hemicrania NOS

✓6th **G44.05 Short lasting unilateral neuralgiform headache with conjunctival injection and tearing (SUNCT)**

   G44.051 Short lasting unilateral neuralgiform headache with conjunctival injection and tearing (SUNCT), intractable

   G44.059 Short lasting unilateral neuralgiform headache with conjunctival injection and tearing (SUNCT), not intractable
> Short lasting unilateral neuralgiform headache with conjunctival injection and tearing (SUNCT) NOS

✓6th **G44.09 Other trigeminal autonomic cephalgias (TAC)**

   G44.091 Other trigeminal autonomic cephalgias (TAC), intractable

   G44.099 Other trigeminal autonomic cephalgias (TAC), not intractable

G44.1 Vascular headache, not elsewhere classified
> EXCLUDES 2   cluster headache (G44.0)
> complicated headache syndromes (G44.5-)
> drug-induced headache (G44.4-)
> migraine (G43.-)
> other specified headache syndromes (G44.8-)
> post-traumatic headache (G44.3-)
> tension-type headache (G44.2-)

✓6th **G44.2 Tension-type headache**

✓6th **G44.20 Tension-type headache, unspecified**

   G44.201 Tension-type headache, unspecified, intractable

   G44.209 Tension-type headache, unspecified, not intractable
> Tension headache NOS

✓6th **G44.21 Episodic tension-type headache**

   G44.211 Episodic tension-type headache, intractable

   G44.219 Episodic tension-type headache, not intractable
> Episodic tension-type headache NOS

✓6th **G44.22 Chronic tension-type headache**

   G44.221 Chronic tension-type headache, intractable

   G44.229 Chronic tension-type headache, not intractable
> Chronic tension-type headache NOS

✓5th **G44.3 Post-traumatic headache**

✓6th **G44.30 Post-traumatic headache, unspecified**

   G44.301 Post-traumatic headache, unspecified, intractable

   G44.309 Post-traumatic headache, unspecified, not intractable
> Post-traumatic headache NOS

✓6th **G44.31 Acute post-traumatic headache**

   G44.311 Acute post-traumatic headache, intractable

   G44.319 Acute post-traumatic headache, not intractable
> Acute post-traumatic headache NOS

✓6th **G44.32 Chronic post-traumatic headache**

   G44.321 Chronic post-traumatic headache, intractable

   G44.329 Chronic post-traumatic headache, not intractable
> Chronic post-traumatic headache NOS

✓5th **G44.4 Drug-induced headache, not elsewhere classified**
> Medication overuse headache
> Use additional code for adverse effect, if applicable, to identify drug (T36-T50 with fifth or sixth character 5)

   G44.40 Drug-induced headache, not elsewhere classified, not intractable

   G44.41 Drug-induced headache, not elsewhere classified, intractable

✓5th **G44.5 Complicated headache syndromes**

   G44.51 Hemicrania continua
> **DEF:** Persistent primary headache of unknown causation occurring on one side of the face and head. May last for more than three months, with daily and continuous pain of moderate intensity with severe exacerbations.

   G44.52 New daily persistent headache (NDPH)

   G44.53 Primary thunderclap headache

   G44.59 Other complicated headache syndrome

✓5th **G44.8 Other specified headache syndromes**
> EXCLUDES 2   headache with orthostatic or positional component, not elsewhere classifed (R51.0)

   G44.81 Hypnic headache

   G44.82 Headache associated with sexual activity
> Orgasmic headache
> Preorgasmic headache

   G44.83 Primary cough headache

   G44.84 Primary exertional headache

   G44.85 Primary stabbing headache

   G44.86 Cervicogenic headache
> Code also associated cervical spinal condition, if known

   G44.89 Other headache syndrome

✓4th **G45 Transient cerebral ischemic attacks and related syndromes**
> EXCLUDES 1   neonatal cerebral ischemia (P91.0)
> transient retinal artery occlusion (H34.0-)

AHA: 2018,2Q,9

DEF: Transient cerebral ischemic attack: Intermittent or brief cerebral dysfunction from lack of oxygenation with no persistent neurological deficits associated with occlusive vascular disease. TIA may denote an impending cerebrovascular accident.

G45.0 Vertebro-basilar artery syndrome   CC

G45.1 Carotid artery syndrome (hemispheric)   CC

G45.2 Multiple and bilateral precerebral artery syndromes   CC

G45.3 Amaurosis fugax   CC

N Newborn: 0   P Pediatric: 0-17   M Maternity: 9-64   A Adult: 15-124   MCC Major Complication/Comorbidity   CC Complication/Comorbidity   SW Severe Wound Dx

582

ICD-10-CM 2022

G45.4 **Transient global amnesia**
     EXCLUDES 1   *amnesia NOS (R41.3)*

G45.8 **Other transient cerebral ischemic attacks and related syndromes**   `CC`

G45.9 **Transient cerebral ischemic attack, unspecified**   `CC`
     Spasm of cerebral artery
     TIA
     Transient cerebral ischemia NOS

√4th **G46** **Vascular syndromes of brain in cerebrovascular diseases**
     Code first underlying cerebrovascular disease (I60-I69)

G46.0 **Middle cerebral artery syndrome**   `CC`

G46.1 **Anterior cerebral artery syndrome**   `CC`

G46.2 **Posterior cerebral artery syndrome**   `CC`

G46.3 **Brain stem stroke syndrome**
     Benedikt syndrome
     Claude syndrome
     Foville syndrome
     Millard-Gubler syndrome
     Wallenberg syndrome
     Weber syndrome

G46.4 **Cerebellar stroke syndrome**

G46.5 **Pure motor lacunar syndrome**

G46.6 **Pure sensory lacunar syndrome**

G46.7 **Other lacunar syndromes**

G46.8 **Other vascular syndromes of brain in cerebrovascular diseases**

√4th **G47** **Sleep disorders**
     EXCLUDES 2   *nightmares (F51.5)*
                nonorganic sleep disorders (F51.-)
                sleep terrors (F51.4)
                sleepwalking (F51.3)

√5th **G47.0** **Insomnia**
     EXCLUDES 2   *alcohol related insomnia (F10.182, F10.282, F10.982)*
                drug-related insomnia (F11.182, F11.282, F11.982, F13.182, F13.282, F13.982, F14.182, F14.282, F14.982, F15.182, F15.282, F15.982, F19.182, F19.282, F19.982)
                idiopathic insomnia (F51.01)
                insomnia due to a mental disorder (F51.05)
                insomnia not due to a substance or known physiological condition (F51.0-)
                nonorganic insomnia (F51.0-)
                primary insomnia (F51.01)
                sleep apnea (G47.3-)

     G47.00 **Insomnia, unspecified**
         Insomnia NOS

     G47.01 **Insomnia due to medical condition**
         Code also associated medical condition

     G47.09 **Other insomnia**

√5th **G47.1** **Hypersomnia**
     EXCLUDES 2   *alcohol-related hypersomnia (F10.182, F10.282, F10.982)*
                drug-related hypersomnia (F11.182, F11.282, F11.982, F13.182, F13.282, F13.982, F14.182, F14.282, F14.982, F15.182, F15.282, F15.982, F19.182, F19.282, F19.982)
                hypersomnia due to a mental disorder (F51.13)
                hypersomnia not due to a substance or known physiological condition (F51.1-)
                primary hypersomnia (F51.11)
                sleep apnea (G47.3-)

     G47.10 **Hypersomnia, unspecified**
         Hypersomnia NOS

     G47.11 **Idiopathic hypersomnia with long sleep time**
         Idiopathic hypersomnia NOS

     G47.12 **Idiopathic hypersomnia without long sleep time**

     G47.13 **Recurrent hypersomnia**
         Kleine-Levin syndrome
         Menstrual related hypersomnia

     G47.14 **Hypersomnia due to medical condition**
         Code also associated medical condition

     G47.19 **Other hypersomnia**

√6th **G47.2** **Circadian rhythm sleep disorders**
     Disorders of the sleep wake schedule
     Inversion of nyctohemeral rhythm
     Inversion of sleep rhythm
     DEF: Circadian rhythm: Daily cycle (24-hour period) of physical, mental, and behavioral changes. It is largely influenced by environmental cues, such as changes in light or temperature. ***Synonym(s):*** *sleep/wake cycle.*

     G47.20 **Circadian rhythm sleep disorder, unspecified type**
         Sleep wake schedule disorder NOS

     G47.21 **Circadian rhythm sleep disorder, delayed sleep phase type**
         Delayed sleep phase syndrome

     G47.22 **Circadian rhythm sleep disorder, advanced sleep phase type**

     G47.23 **Circadian rhythm sleep disorder, irregular sleep wake type**
         Irregular sleep-wake pattern

     G47.24 **Circadian rhythm sleep disorder, free running type**
         Circadian rhythm sleep disorder, non-24-hour sleep-wake type

     G47.25 **Circadian rhythm sleep disorder, jet lag type**

     G47.26 **Circadian rhythm sleep disorder, shift work type**

     G47.27 *Circadian rhythm sleep disorder in conditions classified elsewhere*
         Code first underlying condition

     G47.29 **Other circadian rhythm sleep disorder**

√5th **G47.3** **Sleep apnea**
     Code also any associated underlying condition
     EXCLUDES 1   *apnea NOS (R06.81)*
                Cheyne-Stokes breathing (R06.3)
                pickwickian syndrome (E66.2)
                sleep apnea of newborn (P28.3)

     G47.30 **Sleep apnea, unspecified**
         Sleep apnea NOS

     G47.31 **Primary central sleep apnea**
         Idiopathic central sleep apnea

     G47.32 **High altitude periodic breathing**

     G47.33 **Obstructive sleep apnea (adult) (pediatric)**
         Obstructive sleep apnea hypopnea
         EXCLUDES 1   *obstructive sleep apnea of newborn (P28.3)*

     G47.34 **Idiopathic sleep related nonobstructive alveolar hypoventilation**
         Sleep related hypoxia

     G47.35 **Congenital central alveolar hypoventilation syndrome**

     G47.36 *Sleep related hypoventilation in conditions classified elsewhere*
         Sleep related hypoxemia in conditions classified elsewhere
         Code first underlying condition

     G47.37 *Central sleep apnea in conditions classified elsewhere*
         Code first underlying condition

     G47.39 **Other sleep apnea**

√5th **G47.4** **Narcolepsy and cataplexy**

     √6th **G47.41** **Narcolepsy**

         G47.411 **Narcolepsy with cataplexy**
         G47.419 **Narcolepsy without cataplexy**
             Narcolepsy NOS

     √6th **G47.42** **Narcolepsy in conditions classified elsewhere**
         Code first underlying condition

         G47.421 *Narcolepsy in conditions classified elsewhere with cataplexy*
         G47.429 *Narcolepsy in conditions classified elsewhere without cataplexy*

√5th **G47.5** **Parasomnia**
     EXCLUDES 1   *alcohol induced parasomnia (F10.182, F10.282, F10.982)*
                drug induced parasomnia (F11.182, F11.282, F11.982, F13.182, F13.282, F13.982, F14.182, F14.282, F14.982, F15.182, F15.282, F15.982, F19.182, F19.282, F19.982)
                parasomnia not due to a substance or known physiological condition (F51.8)

     G47.50 **Parasomnia, unspecified**
         Parasomnia NOS

     G47.51 **Confusional arousals**

☑ Additional Character Required   √x7th Placeholder   Questionable PDx   Manifestation   Unspecified Dx   UPD Unacceptable PDx   H1-H14 HAC   HCC CMS-HCC Dx   HIV HIV Dx

ICD-10-CM 2022   583

G47.52   **REM sleep behavior disorder**

G47.53   **Recurrent isolated sleep paralysis**

G47.54   *Parasomnia in conditions classified elsewhere*
     Code first underlying condition

G47.59   **Other parasomnia**

✓5ᵗʰ **G47.6   Sleep related movement disorders**
     EXCLUDES 2   *restless legs syndrome (G25.81)*

G47.61   **Periodic limb movement disorder**

G47.62   **Sleep related leg cramps**

G47.63   **Sleep related bruxism**
     EXCLUDES 1   *psychogenic bruxism (F45.8)*

G47.69   **Other sleep related movement disorders**

G47.8   Other sleep disorders
     Other specified sleep-wake disorder

G47.9   Sleep disorder, unspecified
     Sleep disorder NOS
     Unspecified sleep-wake disorder

Nerve, nerve root and plexus disorders (G50-G59)

EXCLUDES 1   *current traumatic nerve, nerve root and plexus disorders - see Injury, nerve by body region*
neuralgia NOS (M79.2)
neuritis NOS (M79.2)
peripheral neuritis in pregnancy (O26.82-)
radiculitis NOS (M54.1-)

✓4ᵗʰ **G50   Disorders of trigeminal nerve**
     INCLUDES   disorders of 5th cranial nerve

Trigeminal and Facial Nerve Branches

Supratrochlear nerve
Supraorbital nerve
V2 branch
Infraorbital nerve
V1 branch
Trigeminal nerve (CN V) branches in infratemporal fossa
V3 branch
Mental nerve
Mental foramen

G50.0   Trigeminal neuralgia
     Syndrome of paroxysmal facial pain
     Tic douloureux

G50.1   Atypical facial pain

G50.8   Other disorders of trigeminal nerve

G50.9   Disorder of trigeminal nerve, unspecified

✓4ᵗʰ **G51   Facial nerve disorders**
     INCLUDES   disorders of 7th cranial nerve

G51.0   Bell's palsy
     Facial palsy

G51.1   Geniculate ganglionitis
     EXCLUDES 1   *postherpetic geniculate ganglionitis (B02.21)*

G51.2   Melkersson's syndrome
     Melkersson-Rosenthal syndrome

✓5ᵗʰ **G51.3   Clonic hemifacial spasm**
     AHA: 2018,4Q,10

G51.31   **Clonic hemifacial spasm, right**

G51.32   **Clonic hemifacial spasm, left**

G51.33   **Clonic hemifacial spasm, bilateral**

G51.39   **Clonic hemifacial spasm, unspecified**

G51.4   Facial myokymia

G51.8   Other disorders of facial nerve

G51.9   Disorder of facial nerve, unspecified

✓4ᵗʰ **G52   Disorders of other cranial nerves**
     EXCLUDES 2   *disorders of acoustic [8th] nerve (H93.3)*
       disorders of optic [2nd] nerve (H46, H47.0)
       paralytic strabismus due to nerve palsy (H49.0-H49.2)

G52.0   Disorders of olfactory nerve
     Disorders of 1st cranial nerve

G52.1   Disorders of glossopharyngeal nerve
     Disorder of 9th cranial nerve
     Glossopharyngeal neuralgia

G52.2   Disorders of vagus nerve
     Disorders of pneumogastric [10th] nerve

G52.3   Disorders of hypoglossal nerve
     Disorders of 12th cranial nerve

G52.7   Disorders of multiple cranial nerves
     Polyneuritis cranialis

G52.8   Disorders of other specified cranial nerves

G52.9   Cranial nerve disorder, unspecified

G53   *Cranial nerve disorders in diseases classified elsewhere*
     Code first underlying disease, such as:
     neoplasm (C00-D49)
     EXCLUDES 1   *multiple cranial nerve palsy in sarcoidosis (D86.82)*
       multiple cranial nerve palsy in syphilis (A52.15)
       postherpetic geniculate ganglionitis (B02.21)
       postherpetic trigeminal neuralgia (B02.22)

✓4ᵗʰ **G54   Nerve root and plexus disorders**
     EXCLUDES 1   *current traumatic nerve root and plexus disorders - see nerve injury by body region*
       intervertebral disc disorders (M50-M51)
       neuralgia or neuritis NOS (M79.2)
       neuritis or radiculitis brachial NOS (M54.13)
       neuritis or radiculitis lumbar NOS (M54.16)
       neuritis or radiculitis lumbosacral NOS (M54.17)
       neuritis or radiculitis thoracic NOS (M54.14)
       radiculitis NOS (M54.10)
       radiculopathy NOS (M54.10)
       spondylosis (M47.-)

G54.0   Brachial plexus disorders
     Thoracic outlet syndrome
     DEF: Acquired disorder affecting the spinal nerves that send signals to the shoulder, arm, and hand, causing corresponding motor and sensory dysfunction. This disorder is characterized by regional paresthesia, pain, muscle weakness, and in severe cases paralysis.

G54.1   Lumbosacral plexus disorders

G54.2   Cervical root disorders, not elsewhere classified

G54.3   Thoracic root disorders, not elsewhere classified

G54.4   Lumbosacral root disorders, not elsewhere classified

G54.5   Neuralgic amyotrophy
     Parsonage-Aldren-Turner syndrome
     Shoulder-girdle neuritis
     EXCLUDES 1   *neuralgic amyotrophy in diabetes mellitus (E08-E13 with .44)*

G54.6   Phantom limb syndrome with pain   HCC

G54.7   Phantom limb syndrome without pain   HCC
     Phantom limb syndrome NOS

G54.8   Other nerve root and plexus disorders

G54.9   Nerve root and plexus disorder, unspecified

G55   *Nerve root and plexus compressions in diseases classified elsewhere*
     Code first underlying disease, such as:
     neoplasm (C00-D49)
     EXCLUDES 1   *nerve root compression (due to) (in) ankylosing spondylitis (M45.-)*
       nerve root compression (due to) (in) dorsopathies (M53.-, M54.-)
       nerve root compression (due to) (in) intervertebral disc disorders (M50.1-, M51.1-)
       nerve root compression (due to) (in) spondylopathies (M46.-, M48.-)
       nerve root compression (due to) (in) spondylosis ▶(M47.0-, M47.2-)◀

N Newborn: 0   P Pediatric: 0-17   M Maternity: 9-64   A Adult: 15-124   MCC Major Complication/Comorbidity   CC Complication/Comorbidity   SW Severe Wound Dx

584

ICD-10-CM 2022

✓4ᵗʰ **G56 Mononeuropathies of** upper limb

> EXCLUDES 1   *current traumatic nerve disorder - see nerve injury by body region*

AHA: 2016,4Q,17-18

Nerves of Upper Limb

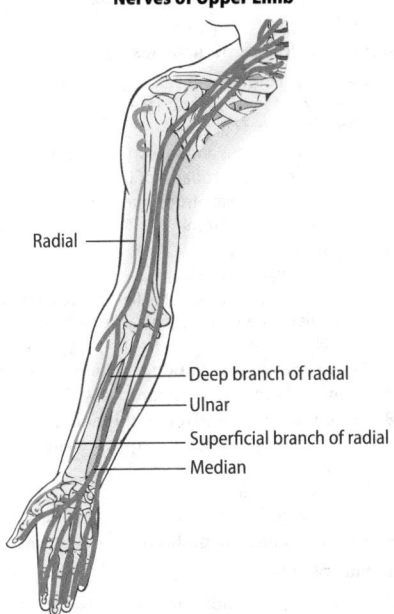

- Radial
- Deep branch of radial
- Ulnar
- Superficial branch of radial
- Median

✓5ᵗʰ **G56.0 Carpal tunnel syndrome**

> **DEF:** Swelling and inflammation in the tendons or bursa surrounding the median nerve caused by repetitive activity. The resulting compression on the nerve causes pain, numbness, and tingling especially to the palm, index, middle finger, and thumb.

G56.00	Carpal tunnel syndrome, **unspecified upper limb**
G56.01	Carpal tunnel syndrome, **right upper limb**
G56.02	Carpal tunnel syndrome, **left upper limb**
G56.03	Carpal tunnel syndrome, **bilateral upper limbs**

✓5ᵗʰ **G56.1 Other lesions of** median nerve

G56.10	Other lesions of median nerve, **unspecified upper limb**
G56.11	Other lesions of median nerve, **right upper limb**
G56.12	Other lesions of median nerve, **left upper limb**
G56.13	Other lesions of median nerve, **bilateral upper limbs**

✓5ᵗʰ **G56.2 Lesion of** ulnar nerve

> Tardy ulnar nerve palsy

G56.20	Lesion of ulnar nerve, **unspecified upper limb**
G56.21	Lesion of ulnar nerve, **right upper limb**
G56.22	Lesion of ulnar nerve, **left upper limb**
G56.23	Lesion of ulnar nerve, **bilateral upper limbs**

✓5ᵗʰ **G56.3 Lesion of** radial nerve

G56.30	Lesion of radial nerve, **unspecified upper limb**
G56.31	Lesion of radial nerve, **right upper limb**
G56.32	Lesion of radial nerve, **left upper limb**
G56.33	Lesion of radial nerve, **bilateral upper limbs**

✓5ᵗʰ **G56.4 Causalgia of upper limb**

> Complex regional pain syndrome II of upper limb

> EXCLUDES 1   *complex regional pain syndrome I of lower limb (G90.52-)*
> *complex regional pain syndrome I of upper limb (G90.51-)*
> *complex regional pain syndrome II of lower limb (G57.7-)*
> *reflex sympathetic dystrophy of lower limb (G90.52-)*
> *reflex sympathetic dystrophy of upper limb (G90.51-)*

G56.40	Causalgia of **unspecified upper limb**
G56.41	Causalgia of **right upper limb**
G56.42	Causalgia of **left upper limb**
G56.43	Causalgia of **bilateral upper limbs**

✓5ᵗʰ **G56.8 Other specified mononeuropathies of upper limb**

> Interdigital neuroma of upper limb

G56.80	Other specified mononeuropathies of **unspecified upper limb**

G56.81	Other specified mononeuropathies of **right upper limb**
G56.82	Other specified mononeuropathies of **left upper limb**
G56.83	Other specified mononeuropathies of **bilateral upper limbs**

✓5ᵗʰ **G56.9 Unspecified mononeuropathy of upper limb**

G56.90	Unspecified mononeuropathy of **unspecified upper limb**
G56.91	Unspecified mononeuropathy of **right upper limb**
G56.92	Unspecified mononeuropathy of **left upper limb**
G56.93	Unspecified mononeuropathy of **bilateral upper limbs**

✓4ᵗʰ **G57 Mononeuropathies of** lower limb

> EXCLUDES 1   *current traumatic nerve disorder - see nerve injury by body region*

AHA: 2016,4Q,17-18

Nerves of Lower Limb

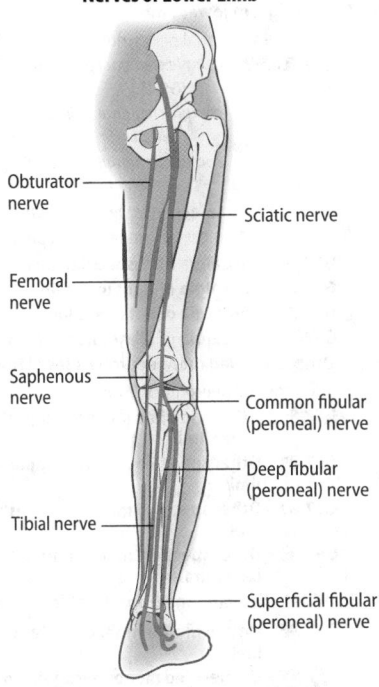

- Obturator nerve
- Sciatic nerve
- Femoral nerve
- Saphenous nerve
- Common fibular (peroneal) nerve
- Deep fibular (peroneal) nerve
- Tibial nerve
- Superficial fibular (peroneal) nerve

✓5ᵗʰ **G57.0 Lesion of** sciatic nerve

> EXCLUDES 1   *sciatica NOS (M54.3-)*
> EXCLUDES 2   *sciatica attributed to intervertebral disc disorder (M51.1.-)*

G57.00	Lesion of sciatic nerve, **unspecified lower limb**
G57.01	Lesion of sciatic nerve, **right lower limb**
G57.02	Lesion of sciatic nerve, **left lower limb**
G57.03	Lesion of sciatic nerve, **bilateral lower limbs**

✓5ᵗʰ **G57.1 Meralgia paresthetica**

> Lateral cutaneous nerve of thigh syndrome

G57.10	Meralgia paresthetica, **unspecified lower limb**
G57.11	Meralgia paresthetica, **right lower limb**
G57.12	Meralgia paresthetica, **left lower limb**
G57.13	Meralgia paresthetica, **bilateral lower limbs**

✓5ᵗʰ **G57.2 Lesion of** femoral nerve

G57.20	Lesion of femoral nerve, **unspecified lower limb**
G57.21	Lesion of femoral nerve, **right lower limb**
G57.22	Lesion of femoral nerve, **left lower limb**
G57.23	Lesion of femoral nerve, **bilateral lower limbs**

✓5ᵗʰ **G57.3 Lesion of** lateral popliteal nerve

> Peroneal nerve palsy
> AHA: 2020,3Q,12

G57.30	Lesion of lateral popliteal nerve, **unspecified lower limb**
G57.31	Lesion of lateral popliteal nerve, **right lower limb**
G57.32	Lesion of lateral popliteal nerve, **left lower limb**
G57.33	Lesion of lateral popliteal nerve, **bilateral lower limbs**

✔ Additional Character Required   ✓x7ᵗʰ Placeholder   Questionable PDx   Manifestation   Unspecified Dx   UPD Unacceptable PDx   H1-H14 HAC   HCC CMS-HCC Dx   HIV HIV Dx

ICD-10-CM 2022   585

Chapter 6. Diseases of the Nervous System

G57.4–G62.9

☑5ᵗʰ **G57.4 Lesion of** medial popliteal nerve

    G57.40 Lesion of medial popliteal nerve, unspecified lower limb

    G57.41 Lesion of medial popliteal nerve, right lower limb

    G57.42 Lesion of medial popliteal nerve, left lower limb

    G57.43 Lesion of medial popliteal nerve, bilateral lower limbs

☑5ᵗʰ **G57.5 Tarsal tunnel syndrome**

    G57.50 Tarsal tunnel syndrome, unspecified lower limb

    G57.51 Tarsal tunnel syndrome, right lower limb

    G57.52 Tarsal tunnel syndrome, left lower limb

    G57.53 Tarsal tunnel syndrome, bilateral lower limbs

☑5ᵗʰ **G57.6 Lesion of** plantar nerve

    Morton's metatarsalgia

    G57.60 Lesion of plantar nerve, unspecified lower limb

    G57.61 Lesion of plantar nerve, right lower limb

    G57.62 Lesion of plantar nerve, left lower limb

    G57.63 Lesion of plantar nerve, bilateral lower limbs

☑5ᵗʰ **G57.7 Causalgia of** lower limb

    Complex regional pain syndrome II of lower limb

    EXCLUDES 1   complex regional pain syndrome I of lower limb (G90.52-)

               complex regional pain syndrome I of upper limb (G90.51-)

               complex regional pain syndrome II of upper limb (G56.4-)

               reflex sympathetic dystrophy of lower limb (G90.52-)

               reflex sympathetic dystrophy of upper limb (G90.51-)

    G57.70 Causalgia of unspecified lower limb

    G57.71 Causalgia of right lower limb

    G57.72 Causalgia of left lower limb

    G57.73 Causalgia of bilateral lower limbs

☑5ᵗʰ **G57.8 Other specified mononeuropathies of lower limb**

    Interdigital neuroma of lower limb

    G57.80 Other specified mononeuropathies of unspecified lower limb

    G57.81 Other specified mononeuropathies of right lower limb

    G57.82 Other specified mononeuropathies of left lower limb

    G57.83 Other specified mononeuropathies of bilateral lower limbs

☑5ᵗʰ **G57.9 Unspecified mononeuropathy of lower limb**

    G57.90 Unspecified mononeuropathy of unspecified lower limb

    G57.91 Unspecified mononeuropathy of right lower limb

    G57.92 Unspecified mononeuropathy of left lower limb

    G57.93 Unspecified mononeuropathy of bilateral lower limbs

☑4ᵗʰ **G58 Other mononeuropathies**

    G58.0 Intercostal neuropathy

    G58.7 Mononeuritis multiplex

    G58.8 Other specified mononeuropathies

    G58.9 Mononeuropathy, unspecified

G59 Mononeuropathy in diseases classified elsewhere

    Code first underlying disease

    EXCLUDES 1   diabetic mononeuropathy (E08-E13 with .41)

               syphilitic nerve paralysis (A52.19)

               syphilitic neuritis (A52.15)

               tuberculous mononeuropathy (A17.83)

Polyneuropathies and other disorders of the peripheral nervous system (G60-G65)

EXCLUDES 1   neuralgia NOS (M79.2)

              neuritis NOS (M79.2)

              peripheral neuritis in pregnancy (O26.82-)

              radiculitis NOS (M54.10)

☑4ᵗʰ **G60 Hereditary and idiopathic** neuropathy

    G60.0 Hereditary motor and sensory **neuropathy**

        Charcôt-Marie-Tooth disease

        Déjérine-Sottas disease

        Hereditary motor and sensory neuropathy, types I-IV

        Hypertrophic neuropathy of infancy

        Peroneal muscular atrophy (axonal type) (hypertrophic type)

        Roussy-Levy syndrome

    G60.1 Refsum's disease   `CC`

        Infantile Refsum disease

        DEF: Genetic disorder of the lipid metabolism characterized by retinitis pigmentosa, degenerative nerve disease, ataxia, and dry, rough, scaly skin.

    G60.2 Neuropathy in association with hereditary ataxia

    G60.3 Idiopathic progressive **neuropathy**

    G60.8 Other hereditary and idiopathic neuropathies

        Dominantly inherited sensory neuropathy

        Morvan's disease

        Nelaton's syndrome

        Recessively inherited sensory neuropathy

    G60.9 Hereditary and idiopathic neuropathy, unspecified

☑4ᵗʰ **G61 Inflammatory** polyneuropathy

    G61.0 Guillain-Barre syndrome   `CC` `HCC`

        Acute (post-)infective polyneuritis

        Miller Fisher syndrome

        AHA: 2020,3Q,12; 2014,2Q,4

        DEF: Autoimmune disorder due to an immune response to foreign antigens with paraplegia of limbs, flaccid paralysis, ophthalmoplegia, ataxia, and areflexia. In most cases, this disorder is triggered by a mild viral infection, surgery, or following an immunization.

        TIP: Guillain-Barre syndrome can occur as a sequela of *Campylobacter* enteritis. Assign code B94.8 for the sequelae as an additional diagnosis.

    G61.1 Serum neuropathy   `HCC`

        Use additional code for adverse effect, if applicable, to identify serum (T50.-)

☑5ᵗʰ **G61.8 Other inflammatory polyneuropathies**

    G61.81 Chronic inflammatory demyelinating polyneuritis   `CC` `HCC`

    G61.82 Multifocal motor neuropathy   `HCC`

        MMN

        AHA: 2016,4Q,18

    G61.89 Other inflammatory polyneuropathies   `HCC`

    G61.9 Inflammatory polyneuropathy, unspecified   `HCC`

☑4ᵗʰ **G62 Other and unspecified polyneuropathies**

    G62.0 Drug-induced polyneuropathy   `HCC`

        Use additional code for adverse effect, if applicable, to identify drug (T36-T50 with fifth or sixth character 5)

    G62.1 Alcoholic polyneuropathy   `HCC`

        AHA: 2019,3Q,8

    G62.2 Polyneuropathy due to other toxic agents   `HCC`

        Code first (T51-T65) to identify toxic agent

☑5ᵗʰ **G62.8 Other specified polyneuropathies**

    G62.81 Critical illness polyneuropathy   `CC` `HCC`

        Acute motor neuropathy

    G62.82 Radiation-induced polyneuropathy   `HCC`

        Use additional external cause code (W88-W90, X39.0-) to identify cause

    G62.89 Other specified polyneuropathies

        AHA: 2016,2Q,11

    G62.9 Polyneuropathy, unspecified

        Neuropathy NOS

Ⓝ Newborn: 0   Ⓟ Pediatric: 0-17   Ⓜ Maternity: 9-64   Ⓐ Adult: 15-124   `MCC` Major Complication/Comorbidity   `CC` Complication/Comorbidity   `SW` Severe Wound Dx

586

ICD-10-CM 2022

G63 Polyneuropathy in diseases classified elsewhere `HCC`

Code first underlying disease, such as:
amyloidosis (E85.-)
endocrine disease, except diabetes (E00-E07, E15-E16, E20-E34)
metabolic diseases (E70-E88)
neoplasm (C00-D49)
nutritional deficiency (E40-E64)

`EXCLUDES 1`   polyneuropathy (in):
diabetes mellitus (E08-E13 with .42)
diphtheria (A36.83)
▶infectious mononucleosis complicated by polyneuropathy (B27.0-B27.9 with fifth character 1)◀
Lyme disease (A69.22)
mumps (B26.84)
postherpetic (B02.23)
rheumatoid arthritis (M05.5-)
scleroderma (M34.83)
systemic lupus erythematosus (M32.19)

AHA: 2021,1Q,7; 2012,4Q,99

G64 Other disorders of peripheral nervous system
Disorder of peripheral nervous system NOS

`✓4ᵗʰ` **G65 Sequelae of inflammatory and toxic polyneuropathies**
Code first condition resulting from (sequela) of inflammatory and toxic polyneuropathies

G65.0 Sequelae of Guillain-Barré syndrome `HCC`
G65.1 Sequelae of other inflammatory polyneuropathy `HCC`
G65.2 Sequelae of toxic polyneuropathy `HCC`

Diseases of myoneural junction and muscle (G70-G73)

`✓4ᵗʰ` **G70 Myasthenia gravis and other myoneural disorders**
`EXCLUDES 1`   botulism (A05.1, A48.51-A48.52)
transient neonatal myasthenia gravis (P94.0)

`✓5ᵗʰ` **G70.0 Myasthenia gravis**
DEF: Autoimmune neuromuscular disorder caused by antibodies to the acetylcholine receptors at the neuromuscular junction, interfering with proper binding of the neurotransmitter from the neuron to the target muscle, causing muscle weakness, fatigue, and exhaustion, without pain or atrophy.

G70.00 Myasthenia gravis without (acute) exacerbation `HCC`
Myasthenia gravis NOS

G70.01 Myasthenia gravis with (acute) exacerbation `MCC` `HCC`
Myasthenia gravis in crisis

G70.1 Toxic myoneural disorders `HCC`
Code first (T51-T65) to identify toxic agent

G70.2 Congenital and developmental myasthenia `HCC`

`✓5ᵗʰ` **G70.8 Other specified myoneural disorders**

G70.80 Lambert-Eaton syndrome, unspecified `CC` `HCC`
Lambert-Eaton syndrome NOS

G70.81 Lambert-Eaton syndrome in disease classified elsewhere `CC` `HCC`
Code first underlying disease
`EXCLUDES 1`   Lambert-Eaton syndrome in neoplastic disease (G73.1)

G70.89 Other specified myoneural disorders `HCC`
G70.9 Myoneural disorder, unspecified `HCC`

`✓4ᵗʰ` **G71 Primary disorders of muscles**
`EXCLUDES 2`   arthrogryposis multiplex congenita (Q74.3)
metabolic disorders (E70-E88)
myositis (M60.-)

`✓5ᵗʰ` **G71.0 Muscular dystrophy**
AHA: 2018,4Q,11-12

G71.00 Muscular dystrophy, unspecified `HCC`
G71.01 Duchenne or Becker muscular dystrophy `HCC`
Autosomal recessive, childhood type, muscular dystrophy resembling Duchenne or Becker muscular dystrophy
Benign [Becker] muscular dystrophy
Severe [Duchenne] muscular dystrophy

G71.02 Facioscapulohumeral muscular dystrophy `HCC`
Scapulohumeral muscular dystrophy

G71.09 Other specified muscular dystrophies `HCC`
Benign scapuloperoneal muscular dystrophy with early contractures [Emery-Dreifuss]
Congenital muscular dystrophy NOS
Congenital muscular dystrophy with specific morphological abnormalities of the muscle fiber
Distal muscular dystrophy
Limb-girdle muscular dystrophy
Ocular muscular dystrophy
Oculopharyngeal muscular dystrophy
Scapuloperoneal muscular dystrophy

`✓6ᵗʰ` **G71.1 Myotonic disorders**

G71.11 Myotonic muscular dystrophy `HCC`
Dystrophia myotonica [Steinert]
Myotonia atrophica
Myotonic dystrophy
Proximal myotonic myopathy (PROMM)
Steinert disease

G71.12 Myotonia congenita
Acetazolamide responsive myotonia congenita
Dominant myotonia congenita [Thomsen disease]
Myotonia levior
Recessive myotonia congenita [Becker disease]

G71.13 Myotonic chondrodystrophy
Chondrodystrophic myotonia
Congenital myotonic chondrodystrophy
Schwartz-Jampel disease

G71.14 Drug induced myotonia
Use additional code for adverse effect, if applicable, to identify drug (T36-T50 with fifth or sixth character 5)

G71.19 Other specified myotonic disorders
Myotonia fluctuans
Myotonia permanens
Neuromyotonia [Isaacs]
Paramyotonia congenita (of von Eulenburg)
Pseudomyotonia
Symptomatic myotonia

`✓5ᵗʰ` **G71.2 Congenital myopathies**
`EXCLUDES 2`   arthrogryposis multiplex congenita (Q74.3)
AHA: 2020,4Q,19-21

G71.20 Congenital myopathy, unspecified `CC` `HCC`
G71.21 Nemaline myopathy `CC` `HCC`
`✓6ᵗʰ` **G71.22 Centronuclear myopathy**

G71.220 X-linked myotubular myopathy `CC` `HCC`
Myotubular (centronuclear) myopathy

G71.228 Other centronuclear myopathy `CC` `HCC`
Autosomal centronuclear myopathy
Autosomal dominant centronuclear myopathy
Autosomal recessive centronuclear myopathy
Centronuclear myopathy, NOS

G71.29 Other congenital myopathy `CC` `HCC`
Central core disease
Minicore disease
Multicore disease
Multiminicore disease

G71.3 Mitochondrial myopathy, not elsewhere classified
`EXCLUDES 1`   Kearns-Sayre syndrome (H49.81)
Leber's disease (H47.21)
Leigh's encephalopathy (G31.82)
mitochondrial metabolism disorders (E88.4.-)
Reye's syndrome (G93.7)

G71.8 Other primary disorders of muscles
G71.9 Primary disorder of muscle, unspecified
Hereditary myopathy NOS

▲

`✓` Additional Character Required   `✓x7ᵗʰ` Placeholder   Questionable PDx   Manifestation   Unspecified Dx   `UPD` Unacceptable PDx   `H1`-`H4` HAC   `HCC` CMS-HCC Dx   `HIV` HIV Dx

ICD-10-CM 2022   587

Chapter 6. Diseases of the Nervous System

G72–G82.52

✓4ᵗʰ G72 Other and unspecified myopathies

EXCLUDES 1   arthrogryposis multiplex congenita (Q74.3)
dermatopolymyositis (M33.-)
ischemic infarction of muscle (M62.2-)
myositis (M60.-)
polymyositis (M33.2.-)

G72.0 Drug-induced myopathy   CC
Use additional code for adverse effect, if applicable, to identify drug (T36-T50 with fifth or sixth character 5)

G72.1 Alcoholic myopathy   CC
Use additional code to identify alcoholism (F10.-)

G72.2 Myopathy due to other toxic agents   CC
Code first (T51-T65) to identify toxic agent

G72.3 Periodic paralysis
Familial periodic paralysis
Hyperkalemic periodic paralysis (familial)
Hypokalemic periodic paralysis (familial)
Myotonic periodic paralysis (familial)
Normokalemic paralysis (familial)
Potassium sensitive periodic paralysis
EXCLUDES 1   paramyotonia congenita (of von Eulenburg) (G71.19)

✓5ᵗʰ G72.4 Inflammatory and immune myopathies, not elsewhere classified

G72.41 Inclusion body myositis [IBM]

G72.49 Other inflammatory and immune myopathies, not elsewhere classified
Inflammatory myopathy NOS

✓6ᵗʰ G72.8 Other specified myopathies

G72.81 Critical illness myopathy   CC
Acute necrotizing myopathy
Acute quadriplegic myopathy
Intensive care (ICU) myopathy
Myopathy of critical illness
AHA: 2020,3Q,12

G72.89 Other specified myopathies

G72.9 Myopathy, unspecified

✓4ᵗʰ G73 Disorders of myoneural junction and muscle in diseases classified elsewhere

G73.1 Lambert-Eaton syndrome in neoplastic disease   CC UPD HCC
Code first underlying neoplasm (C00-D49)
EXCLUDES 1   Lambert-Eaton syndrome not associated with neoplasm (G70.80-G70.81)

G73.3 Myasthenic syndromes in other diseases classified elsewhere   CC HCC
Code first underlying disease, such as:
neoplasm (C00-D49)
thyrotoxicosis (E05.-)

G73.7 Myopathy in diseases classified elsewhere
Code first underlying disease, such as:
hyperparathyroidism (E21.0, E21.3)
hypoparathyroidism (E20.-)
glycogen storage disease (E74.0)
lipid storage disorders (E75.-)
EXCLUDES 1   myopathy in:
rheumatoid arthritis (M05.32)
sarcoidosis (D86.87)
scleroderma (M34.82)
▶Sjögren syndrome◀ (M35.03)
systemic lupus erythematosus (M32.19)

Cerebral palsy and other paralytic syndromes (G80-G83)

✓4ᵗʰ G80 Cerebral palsy

EXCLUDES 1   hereditary spastic paraplegia (G11.4)

G80.0 Spastic quadriplegic cerebral palsy   MCC HCC
Congenital spastic paralysis (cerebral)

G80.1 Spastic diplegic cerebral palsy   CC HCC
Spastic cerebral palsy NOS

G80.2 Spastic hemiplegic cerebral palsy   CC HCC

G80.3 Athetoid cerebral palsy   CC HCC
Double athetosis (syndrome)
Dyskinetic cerebral palsy
Dystonic cerebral palsy
Vogt disease

G80.4 Ataxic cerebral palsy   HCC

G80.8 Other cerebral palsy   HCC
Mixed cerebral palsy syndromes

G80.9 Cerebral palsy, unspecified   HCC
Cerebral palsy NOS

✓4ᵗʰ G81 Hemiplegia and hemiparesis

NOTE   This category is to be used only when hemiplegia (complete)(incomplete) is reported without further specification, or is stated to be old or longstanding but of unspecified cause. The category is also for use in multiple coding to identify these types of hemiplegia resulting from any cause.

EXCLUDES 1   congenital cerebral palsy (G80.-)
hemiplegia and hemiparesis due to sequela of cerebrovascular disease (I69.05-, I69.15-, I69.25-, I69.35-, I69.85-, I69.95-)

AHA: 2015,1Q,25

TIP: If the documentation specifies the affected side but not whether it is the dominant or nondominant side, the default is as follows: for ambidextrous patients, the default is dominant; when the left side is affected, the default is nondominant; and when the right side is affected, the default is dominant.

✓5ᵗʰ G81.0 Flaccid hemiplegia

G81.00 Flaccid hemiplegia affecting unspecified side   CC HCC

G81.01 Flaccid hemiplegia affecting right dominant side   CC HCC

G81.02 Flaccid hemiplegia affecting left dominant side   CC HCC

G81.03 Flaccid hemiplegia affecting right nondominant side   CC HCC

G81.04 Flaccid hemiplegia affecting left nondominant side   CC HCC

✓5ᵗʰ G81.1 Spastic hemiplegia

G81.10 Spastic hemiplegia affecting unspecified side   CC HCC

G81.11 Spastic hemiplegia affecting right dominant side   CC HCC

G81.12 Spastic hemiplegia affecting left dominant side   CC HCC

G81.13 Spastic hemiplegia affecting right nondominant side   CC HCC

G81.14 Spastic hemiplegia affecting left nondominant side   CC HCC

✓5ᵗʰ G81.9 Hemiplegia, unspecified

AHA: 2014,1Q,23

G81.90 Hemiplegia, unspecified affecting unspecified side   CC HCC

G81.91 Hemiplegia, unspecified affecting right dominant side   CC HCC

G81.92 Hemiplegia, unspecified affecting left dominant side   CC HCC

G81.93 Hemiplegia, unspecified affecting right nondominant side   CC HCC

G81.94 Hemiplegia, unspecified affecting left nondominant side   CC HCC

✓4ᵗʰ G82 Paraplegia (paraparesis) and quadriplegia (quadriparesis)

NOTE   This category is to be used only when the listed conditions are reported without further specification, or are stated to be old or longstanding but of unspecified cause. The category is also for use in multiple coding to identify these conditions resulting from any cause

EXCLUDES 1   congenital cerebral palsy (G80.-)
functional quadriplegia (R53.2)
hysterical paralysis (F44.4)

✓5ᵗʰ G82.2 Paraplegia
Paralysis of both lower limbs NOS
Paraparesis (lower) NOS
Paraplegia (lower) NOS
AHA: 2017,3Q,3

G82.20 Paraplegia, unspecified   CC HCC

G82.21 Paraplegia, complete   CC HCC

G82.22 Paraplegia, incomplete   CC HCC

✓5ᵗʰ G82.5 Quadriplegia

G82.50 Quadriplegia, unspecified   MCC HCC

G82.51 Quadriplegia, C1-C4 complete   MCC HCC

G82.52 Quadriplegia, C1-C4 incomplete   MCC HCC

	G82.53	**Quadriplegia, C5-C7 complete**	`MCC` `HCC`
	G82.54	**Quadriplegia, C5-C7 incomplete**	`MCC` `HCC`

✓4ᵗʰ G83 Other paralytic syndromes

NOTE This category is to be used only when the listed conditions are reported without further specification, or are stated to be old or longstanding but of unspecified cause. The category is also for use in multiple coding to identify these conditions resulting from any cause.

INCLUDES paralysis (complete) (incomplete), except as in G80-G82

G83.0 Diplegia of upper limbs   `CC` `HCC`
Diplegia (upper)
Paralysis of both upper limbs

✓5ᵗʰ G83.1 Monoplegia of lower limb
Paralysis of lower limb
EXCLUDES 1 *monoplegia of lower limbs due to sequela of cerebrovascular disease (I69.04-, I69.14-, I69.24-, I69.34-, I69.84-, I69.94-)*

TIP: If the documentation specifies the affected side but not whether it is the dominant or nondominant side, the default is as follows: for ambidextrous patients, the default is dominant; when the left side is affected, the default is nondominant; and when the right side is affected, the default is dominant.

	G83.10	**Monoplegia of lower limb affecting unspecified side**	`HCC`
	G83.11	**Monoplegia of lower limb affecting** right dominant **side**	`HCC`
	G83.12	**Monoplegia of lower limb affecting** left dominant **side**	`HCC`
	G83.13	**Monoplegia of lower limb affecting** right nondominant **side**	`HCC`
	G83.14	**Monoplegia of lower limb affecting** left nondominant **side**	`HCC`

✓5ᵗʰ G83.2 Monoplegia of upper limb
Paralysis of upper limb
EXCLUDES 1 *monoplegia of upper limbs due to sequela of cerebrovascular disease (I69.03-, I69.13-, I69.23-, I69.33-, I69.83-, I69.93-)*

TIP: If the documentation specifies the affected side but not whether it is the dominant or nondominant side, the default is as follows: for ambidextrous patients, the default is dominant; when the left side is affected, the default is nondominant; and when the right side is affected, the default is dominant.

	G83.20	**Monoplegia of upper limb affecting unspecified side**	`HCC`
	G83.21	**Monoplegia of upper limb affecting** right dominant **side**	`HCC`
	G83.22	**Monoplegia of upper limb affecting** left dominant **side**	`HCC`
	G83.23	**Monoplegia of upper limb affecting** right nondominant **side**	`HCC`
	G83.24	**Monoplegia of upper limb affecting** left nondominant **side**	`HCC`

✓5ᵗʰ G83.3 Monoplegia, unspecified
TIP: If the documentation specifies the affected side but not whether it is the dominant or nondominant side, the default is as follows: for ambidextrous patients, the default is dominant; when the left side is affected, the default is nondominant; and when the right side is affected, the default is dominant.

	G83.30	**Monoplegia, unspecified affecting unspecified side**	`HCC`
	G83.31	**Monoplegia, unspecified affecting** right dominant **side**	`HCC`
	G83.32	**Monoplegia, unspecified affecting** left dominant **side**	`HCC`
	G83.33	**Monoplegia, unspecified affecting** right nondominant **side**	`HCC`
	G83.34	**Monoplegia, unspecified affecting** left nondominant **side**	`HCC`

G83.4 Cauda equina syndrome   `CC` `HCC`
Neurogenic bladder due to cauda equina syndrome
EXCLUDES 1 *cord bladder NOS (G95.89)*
neurogenic bladder NOS (N31.9)

AHA: 2020,3Q,24
DEF: Compression of the spinal nerve roots presenting with pain and tingling radiating down the buttocks, back of the thigh and calf, and into the foot in a sciatic manner with aching in the bladder, perineum, and sacrum. Loss of bowel and bladder control may also occur.

G83.5 Locked-in state   `MCC` `HCC`

✓5ᵗʰ G83.8 Other specified paralytic syndromes
EXCLUDES 1 *paralytic syndromes due to current spinal cord injury - code to spinal cord injury (S14, S24, S34)*

	G83.81	**Brown-Séquard syndrome**	`HCC`
	G83.82	**Anterior cord syndrome**	`HCC`
	G83.83	**Posterior cord syndrome**	`HCC`
	G83.84	**Todd's paralysis (postepileptic)**	`HCC`
	G83.89	**Other specified paralytic syndromes**	`HCC`

G83.9 Paralytic syndrome, unspecified   `HCC`

Other disorders of the nervous system (G89-G99)

✓4ᵗʰ G89 Pain, not elsewhere classified
Code also related psychological factors associated with pain (F45.42)
EXCLUDES 1 *generalized pain NOS (R52)*
pain disorders exclusively related to psychological factors (F45.41)
pain NOS (R52)
EXCLUDES 2 *atypical face pain (G50.1)*
headache syndromes (G44.-)
localized pain, unspecified type - code to pain by site, such as:
abdomen pain (R10.-)
back pain (M54.9)
breast pain (N64.4)
chest pain (R07.1-R07.9)
ear pain (H92.0-)
eye pain (H57.1)
headache (R51.9)
joint pain (M25.5-)
limb pain (M79.6-)
lumbar region pain ▶(M54.5-)◀
painful urination (R30.9)
pelvic and perineal pain (R10.2)
renal colic (N23)
shoulder pain (M25.51-)
spine pain (M54.-)
throat pain (R07.0)
tongue pain (K14.6)
tooth pain (K08.8)
migraines (G43.-)
myalgia (M79.1-)
pain from prosthetic devices, implants, and grafts (T82.84, T83.84, T84.84, T85.84-)
phantom limb syndrome with pain (G54.6)
vulvar vestibulitis (N94.810)
vulvodynia (N94.81-)

G89.0 Central pain syndrome
Déjérine-Roussy syndrome
Myelopathic pain syndrome
Thalamic pain syndrome (hyperesthetic)

✓5ᵗʰ G89.1 Acute pain, not elsewhere classified

	G89.11	**Acute pain** due to trauma
	G89.12	**Acute** post-thoracotomy **pain**
		Post-thoracotomy pain NOS
	G89.18	**Other acute** postprocedural **pain**
		Postoperative pain NOS
		Postprocedural pain NOS

✓ Additional Character Required   ✓x7ᵗʰ Placeholder   Questionable PDx   Manifestation   Unspecified Dx   `UPD` Unacceptable PDx   `H1`-`H4` HAC   `HCC` CMS-HCC Dx   `HIV` HIV Dx

ICD-10-CM 2022   589

✓5ᵗʰ **G89.2** **Chronic pain,** not elsewhere classified

   EXCLUDES 1   *causalgia, lower limb (G57.7-)*

               causalgia, upper limb (G56.4-)

               central pain syndrome (G89.0)

               chronic pain syndrome (G89.4)

               complex regional pain syndrome II, lower limb (G57.7-)

               complex regional pain syndrome II, upper limb (G56.4-)

               neoplasm related chronic pain (G89.3)

               reflex sympathetic dystrophy (G90.5-)

     G89.21 **Chronic pain due to** trauma

     G89.22 **Chronic** post-thoracotomy **pain**

     G89.28 **Other chronic** postprocedural **pain**

           Other chronic postoperative pain

     G89.29 **Other chronic pain**

G89.3 **Neoplasm related pain (acute) (chronic)**

      Cancer associated pain

      Pain due to malignancy (primary) (secondary)

      Tumor associated pain

G89.4 **Chronic pain syndrome**

      Chronic pain associated with significant psychosocial dysfunction

✓4ᵗʰ **G90** **Disorders of autonomic nervous system**

   EXCLUDES 1   *dysfunction of the autonomic nervous system due to alcohol (G31.2)*

✓5ᵗʰ **G90.0** **Idiopathic peripheral autonomic neuropathy**

     G90.01 **Carotid sinus syncope**

           Carotid sinus syndrome

           DEF: Vagal activation caused by pressure on the carotid sinus baroreceptors. Sympathetic nerve impulses may cause sinus arrest or AV block.

     G90.09 **Other idiopathic peripheral autonomic neuropathy**

           Idiopathic peripheral autonomic neuropathy NOS

G90.1 **Familial dysautonomia [Riley-Day]**   HCC

G90.2 **Horner's syndrome**

      Bernard(-Horner) syndrome

      Cervical sympathetic dystrophy or paralysis

G90.3 **Multi-system degeneration of the autonomic nervous system**   CC   HCC

      Neurogenic orthostatic hypotension [Shy-Drager]

     EXCLUDES 1   *orthostatic hypotension NOS (I95.1)*

G90.4 **Autonomic dysreflexia**

      Use additional code to identify the cause, such as:

         fecal impaction (K56.41)

         pressure ulcer (pressure area) (L89.-)

         urinary tract infection (N39.0)

✓5ᵗʰ **G90.5** **Complex regional pain syndrome I (CRPS I)**

      Reflex sympathetic dystrophy

     EXCLUDES 1   *causalgia of lower limb (G57.7-)*

                causalgia of upper limb (G56.4-)

                complex regional pain syndrome II of lower limb (G57.7-)

                complex regional pain syndrome II of upper limb (G56.4-)

     G90.50 **Complex regional pain syndrome I, unspecified**   CC

   ✓6ᵗʰ **G90.51** **Complex regional pain syndrome I of** upper limb

        G90.511 **Complex regional pain syndrome I of** right upper limb   CC

        G90.512 **Complex regional pain syndrome I of** left upper limb   CC

        G90.513 **Complex regional pain syndrome I of** upper limb, bilateral   CC

        G90.519 **Complex regional pain syndrome I of** unspecified upper limb   CC

   ✓6ᵗʰ **G90.52** **Complex regional pain syndrome I of** lower limb

        G90.521 **Complex regional pain syndrome I of** right lower limb   CC

        G90.522 **Complex regional pain syndrome I of** left lower limb   CC

        G90.523 **Complex regional pain syndrome I of** lower limb, bilateral   CC

        G90.529 **Complex regional pain syndrome I of** unspecified lower limb   CC

     G90.59 **Complex regional pain syndrome I of other specified site**   CC

G90.8 **Other disorders of autonomic nervous system**

G90.9 **Disorder of the autonomic nervous system, unspecified**

✓4ᵗʰ **G91** **Hydrocephalus**

   INCLUDES   acquired hydrocephalus

   EXCLUDES 1   *Arnold-Chiari syndrome with hydrocephalus (Q07.-)*

                congenital hydrocephalus (Q03.-)

                spina bifida with hydrocephalus (Q05.-)

   DEF: Abnormal buildup of cerebrospinal fluid in the brain causing dilation of the ventricles.

Hydrocephalus (Acquired)

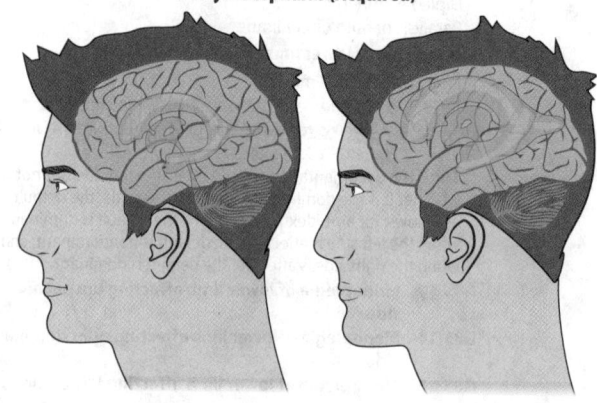

Normal ventricles   Hydrocephalic ventricles

G91.0 **Communicating hydrocephalus**   CC   HCC

      Secondary normal pressure hydrocephalus

G91.1 **Obstructive hydrocephalus**   CC   HCC

      DEF: Obstruction of the cerebrospinal fluid passage from the brain into the spinal canal characterized by headaches, drowsiness, poor coordination, urinary incontinence, nausea, vomiting, and papilledema.

G91.2 **(Idiopathic) normal pressure hydrocephalus**   CC   HCC

      Normal pressure hydrocephalus NOS

G91.3 **Post-traumatic hydrocephalus, unspecified**   CC   HCC

G91.4 *Hydrocephalus in diseases classified elsewhere*   HCC

      Code first underlying condition, such as:

         congenital syphilis (A50.4-)

         neoplasm (C00-D49)

         plasminogen deficiency (E88.02)

        EXCLUDES 1   *hydrocephalus due to congenital toxoplasmosis (P37.1)*

      AHA: 2014,3Q,3

G91.8 **Other hydrocephalus**   CC   HCC

G91.9 **Hydrocephalus, unspecified**   CC   HCC

▲ ✓4ᵗʰ **G92** **Toxic encephalopathy**

      ~~Toxic encephalitis~~

      ~~Toxic metabolic encephalopathy~~

      ~~Code first, if applicable, drug induced (T36-T50) or use (T51-T65) to identify toxic agent~~

      AHA: 2021,1Q,13; 2017,1Q,39-40

      DEF: Brain tissue degeneration due to a toxic substance.

 ● ✓5ᵗʰ **G92.0** **Immune effector cell-associated neurotoxicity syndrome**

       Code first underlying cause such as:

         complications of immune effector cellular therapy (T80.82)

       Code also associated signs and symptoms, such as seizures and cerebral edema

       Code also, if applicable:

         cerebral edema (G93.6)

         unspecified convulsions (R56.9)

 ●   **G92.00** **Immune effector cell-associated neurotoxicity syndrome, grade unspecified**

           ICANS, grade unspecified

 ●   **G92.01** **Immune effector cell-associated neurotoxicity syndrome,** grade 1

           ICANS, grade 1

 ●   **G92.02** **Immune effector cell-associated neurotoxicity syndrome,** grade 2

           ICANS, grade 2

N Newborn: 0   P Pediatric: 0-17   M Maternity: 9-64   A Adult: 15-124   MCC Major Complication/Comorbidity   CC Complication/Comorbidity   SW Severe Wound Dx

590

ICD-10-CM 2022

●   **G92.03**   **Immune effector cell-associated neurotoxicity syndrome, grade 3**   `CC`
          ICANS, grade 3

●   **G92.04**   **Immune effector cell-associated neurotoxicity syndrome, grade 4**   `CC`
          ICANS, grade 4

●   **G92.05**   **Immune effector cell-associated neurotoxicity syndrome, grade 5**   `CC`
          ICANS, grade 5

●   **G92.8**   **Other toxic encephalopathy**   `MCC`
        Toxic encephalitis
        Toxic metabolic encephalopathy
        Code first poisoning due to drug or toxin, if applicable, (T36-T65 with fifth or sixth character 1-4 or 6)
        Use additional code for adverse effect, if applicable, to identify drug (T36-T50 with fifth or sixth character 5)

●   **G92.9**   **Unspecified toxic encephalopathy**   `MCC`
        Code first poisoning due to drug or toxin, if applicable, (T36-T65 with fifth or sixth character 1-4 or 6)
        Use additional code for adverse effect, if applicable, to identify drug (T36-T50 with fifth or sixth character 5)

✓4ᵗʰ   **G93**   **Other disorders of brain**

     G93.0   **Cerebral cysts**
        Arachnoid cyst
        Porencephalic cyst, acquired
        `EXCLUDES 1`   *acquired periventricular cysts of newborn (P91.1)*
                   congenital cerebral cysts (Q04.6)

     G93.1   **Anoxic brain damage, not elsewhere classified**   `CC` `HCC`
        `EXCLUDES 1`   *cerebral anoxia due to anesthesia during labor and delivery (O74.3)*
                   cerebral anoxia due to anesthesia during the puerperium (O89.2)
                   neonatal anoxia (P84)
        DEF: Brain injury not resulting from birth trauma that is due to lack of oxygen. Brain cells, when deprived of oxygen, begin to expire after four minutes.

     G93.2   **Benign intracranial hypertension**
        Pseudotumor
        `EXCLUDES 1`   *hypertensive encephalopathy (I67.4)*
                   obstructive hydrocephalus (G91.1)

     G93.3   **Postviral fatigue syndrome**
        Benign myalgic encephalomyelitis
        `EXCLUDES 1`   *chronic fatigue syndrome NOS (R53.82)*

✓5ᵗʰ   **G93.4**   **Other and unspecified encephalopathy**
        `EXCLUDES 1`   *alcoholic encephalopathy (G31.2)*
                   encephalopathy in diseases classified elsewhere (G94)
                   hypertensive encephalopathy (I67.4)
        `EXCLUDES 2`   *toxic (metabolic) encephalopathy ▶(G92.8)◀*

        G93.40   **Encephalopathy, unspecified**   `HIV` `CC`
                AHA: 2017,2Q,8

        G93.41   **Metabolic encephalopathy**   `HIV` `MCC`
                Septic encephalopathy
                AHA: 2017,2Q,8; 2016,3Q,42; 2015,3Q,21
                TIP: Assign separately when documented with diabetic hypoglycemia (E08.649, E09.649, E10.649, E11.649, E13.649).

        G93.49   **Other encephalopathy**   `HIV` `CC`
                Encephalopathy NEC
                AHA: 2021,2Q,3; 2018,4Q,16; 2018,2Q,22,24; 2017,2Q,9

     G93.5   **Compression of brain**   `MCC` `HCC`
        Arnold-Chiari type 1 compression of brain
        Compression of brain (stem)
        Herniation of brain (stem)
        `EXCLUDES 1`   *diffuse traumatic compression of brain (S06.2-)*
                   focal traumatic compression of brain (S06.3-)
                   ▶*traumatic compression of brain (S06.A-)*◀
        AHA: 2020,2Q,31

     G93.6   **Cerebral edema**   `MCC` `HCC`
        `EXCLUDES 1`   *cerebral edema due to birth injury (P11.0)*
                   traumatic cerebral edema (S06.1-)

     G93.7   **Reye's syndrome**   `MCC` `HCC` `P`
        Code first poisoning due to salicylates, if applicable (T39.0-, with sixth character 1-4)
        Use additional code for adverse effect due to salicylates, if applicable (T39.0-, with sixth character 5)
        DEF: Rare childhood illness often developed after a viral upper respiratory infection. Symptoms include vomiting, elevated serum transaminase, brain swelling, disturbances of consciousness, seizures, and changes in liver and other viscera; it can be fatal.

✓5ᵗʰ   **G93.8**   **Other specified disorders of brain**

        G93.81   **Temporal sclerosis**
                Hippocampal sclerosis
                Mesial temporal sclerosis

        G93.82   **Brain death**   `MCC`

        G93.89   **Other specified disorders of brain**
                Postradiation encephalopathy
                AHA: 2020,2Q,24; 2019,3Q,8

     G93.9   **Disorder of brain, unspecified**   `HIV`

✓   **G94**   *Other disorders of brain in diseases classified elsewhere*
        Code first underlying disease
        `EXCLUDES 1`   *encephalopathy in congenital syphilis (A50.49)*
                   encephalopathy in influenza (J09.X9, J10.81, J11.81)
                   encephalopathy in syphilis (A52.19)
                   hydrocephalus in diseases classified elsewhere (G91.4)
        AHA: 2018,2Q,22; 2017,2Q,8-9

✓4ᵗʰ   **G95**   **Other and unspecified diseases of spinal cord**
        `EXCLUDES 2`   *myelitis (G04.-)*

     G95.0   **Syringomyelia and syringobulbia**   `CC` `HCC`

✓5ᵗʰ   **G95.1**   **Vascular myelopathies**
        `EXCLUDES 2`   *intraspinal phlebitis and thrombophlebitis, except non-pyogenic (G08)*

        G95.11   **Acute infarction of spinal cord (embolic) (nonembolic)**   `MCC` `HCC`
                Anoxia of spinal cord
                Arterial thrombosis of spinal cord

        G95.19   **Other vascular myelopathies**   `MCC` `HCC`
                Edema of spinal cord
                Hematomyelia
                Nonpyogenic intraspinal phlebitis and thrombophlebitis
                Subacute necrotic myelopathy

✓5ᵗʰ   **G95.2**   **Other and unspecified cord compression**

        G95.20   **Unspecified cord compression**   `HIV` `CC` `HCC`
        G95.29   **Other cord compression**   `HIV` `CC` `HCC`

✓5ᵗʰ   **G95.8**   **Other specified diseases of spinal cord**
        `EXCLUDES 1`   *neurogenic bladder NOS (N31.9)*
                   neurogenic bladder due to cauda equina syndrome (G83.4)
                   neuromuscular dysfunction of bladder without spinal cord lesion (N31.-)

        G95.81   **Conus medullaris syndrome**   `CC` `HCC`

        G95.89   **Other specified diseases of spinal cord**   `CC` `HCC`
                Cord bladder NOS
                Drug-induced myelopathy
                Radiation-induced myelopathy
                `EXCLUDES 1`   *myelopathy NOS (G95.9)*

     G95.9   **Disease of spinal cord, unspecified**   `HIV` `CC` `HCC`
        Myelopathy NOS

Chapter 6. Diseases of the Nervous System

✓4ᵗʰ **G96** **Other disorders of central nervous system**

✓5ᵗʰ **G96.0** **Cerebrospinal fluid leak**

Code also if applicable:
    intracranial hypotension (G96.81-)

EXCLUDES 1   *cerebrospinal fluid leak from spinal puncture (G97.0)*

AHA: 2020,4Q,21-22; 2018,2Q,13

DEF: Cerebrospinal fluid (CSF) leak occurs when the clear fluid surrounding and cushioning the brain or spinal cord escapes because of a hole or tear in the membranes surrounding these organs. Cranial CSF leaks present as otorrhea, rhinorrhea, or leakage from the skull base while spinal CSF leaks develop because of tears in the soft tissues surrounding the spinal cord. Although both may occur spontaneously, underlying causes can also include traumatic or postoperative events.

G96.00 **Cerebrospinal fluid leak, unspecified**   CC
Code also if applicable:
    head injury (S00.- to S09.-)

G96.01 **Cranial cerebrospinal fluid leak, spontaneous**   CC
Otorrhea due to spontaneous cerebrospinal fluid CSF leak
Rhinorrhea due to spontaneous cerebrospinal fluid CSF leak
Spontaneous cerebrospinal fluid leak from skull base

G96.02 **Spinal cerebrospinal fluid leak, spontaneous**   CC
Spontaneous cerebrospinal fluid leak from spine

G96.08 **Other cranial cerebrospinal fluid leak**   CC
Postoperative cranial cerebrospinal fluid leak
Traumatic cranial cerebrospinal fluid leak
Code also if applicable:
    head injury (S00.- to S09.-)

G96.09 **Other spinal cerebrospinal fluid leak**   CC
Other spinal CSF leak
Postoperative spinal cerebrospinal fluid leak
Traumatic spinal cerebrospinal fluid leak
Code also if applicable:
    head injury (S00.- to S09.-)

✓5ᵗʰ **G96.1** **Disorders of meninges, not elsewhere classified**

G96.11 **Dural tear**   CC
Code also intracranial hypotension, if applicable (G96.81-)

EXCLUDES 1   *accidental puncture or laceration of dura during a procedure (G97.41)*

AHA: 2014,4Q,24

G96.12 **Meningeal adhesions (cerebral) (spinal)**

✓6ᵗʰ **G96.19** **Other disorders of meninges, not elsewhere classified**

AHA: 2020,4Q,22

G96.191 **Perineural cyst**
Cervical nerve root cyst
Lumbar nerve root cyst
Sacral nerve root cyst
Tarlov cyst
Thoracic nerve root cyst

G96.198 **Other disorders of meninges, not elsewhere classified**

✓5ᵗʰ **G96.8** **Other specified disorders of central nervous system**

AHA: 2020,4Q,21,23-24

✓6ᵗʰ **G96.81** **Intracranial hypotension**

Code also any associated diagnoses, such as:
brachial amyotrophy (G54.5)
cerebrospinal fluid leak from spine (G96.02)
cranial nerve disorders in diseases classified elsewhere (G53)
nerve root and compressions in diseases classified elsewhere (G55)
nonpyogenic thrombosis of intracranial venous system (I67.6)
nontraumatic intracerebral hemorrhage (I61.-)
nontraumatic subdural hemorrhage (I62.0-)
other and unspecified cord compression (G95.2-)
other secondary parkinsonism (G21.8)
reversible cerebrovascular vasoconstriction syndrome (I67.841)
spinal cord herniation (G95.89)
stroke (I63.-)
syringomyelia (G95.0)

DEF: Central nervous system disorder resulting from a loss of cerebrospinal fluid (CSF) volume. More often associated with CSF leak at the level of the spine rather than the skull base, causes can be spontaneous, iatrogenic or traumatic spinal dura defects or holes, or overdrainage of CSF shunt devices. The most common symptom is headache.

G96.810 **Intracranial hypotension, unspecified**

G96.811 **Intracranial hypotension, spontaneous**

G96.819 **Other intracranial hypotension**

G96.89 **Other specified disorders of central nervous system**

G96.9 **Disorder of central nervous system, unspecified**   HIV

✓4ᵗʰ **G97** **Intraoperative and postprocedural complications and disorders of nervous system, not elsewhere classified**

EXCLUDES 2   *intraoperative and postprocedural cerebrovascular infarction (I97.81-, I97.82-)*

AHA: 2016,4Q,9-10

G97.0 **Cerebrospinal fluid leak from spinal puncture**   CC
Code also any associated diagnoses or complications, such as:
intracranial hypotension following a procedure (G97.83-G97.84)

Spinal Puncture

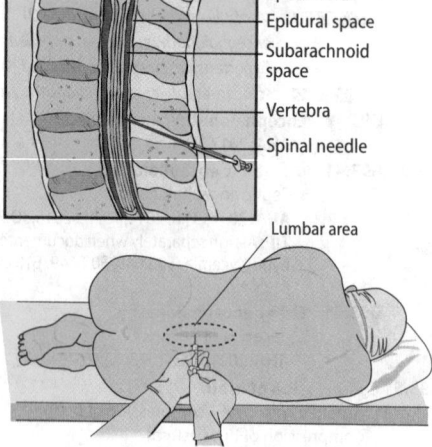

Spinal cord
Epidural space
Subarachnoid space
Vertebra
Spinal needle

Lumbar area

G97.1 **Other reaction to spinal and lumbar puncture**
Headache due to lumbar puncture
Other reaction to spinal dural puncture
Code also, if applicable, any associated headache with orthostatic component (R51.0)

G97.2 **Intracranial hypotension following ventricular shunting**   CC
Code also any associated diagnoses or complications

N Newborn: 0   P Pediatric: 0-17   M Maternity: 9-64   A Adult: 15-124   MCC Major Complication/Comorbidity   CC Complication/Comorbidity   SW Severe Wound Dx

G96–G97.2

592

ICD-10-CM 2022

✓5ᵗʰ **G97.3** Intraoperative hemorrhage and hematoma of a nervous system organ or structure complicating a procedure

     EXCLUDES 1   *intraoperative hemorrhage and hematoma of a nervous system organ or structure due to accidental puncture and laceration during a procedure (G97.4-)*

     G97.31 Intraoperative hemorrhage and hematoma of a nervous system organ or structure complicating a nervous system procedure   CC

     G97.32 Intraoperative hemorrhage and hematoma of a nervous system organ or structure complicating other procedure   CC

✓5ᵗʰ **G97.4** Accidental puncture and laceration of a nervous system organ or structure during a procedure

     G97.41 Accidental puncture or laceration of dura during a procedure   CC

       Incidental (inadvertent) durotomy

       Code also any associated diagnoses or complications

       AHA: 2014,4Q,24

     G97.48 Accidental puncture and laceration of other nervous system organ or structure during a nervous system procedure   CC

     G97.49 Accidental puncture and laceration of other nervous system organ or structure during other procedure   CC

✓5ᵗʰ **G97.5** Postprocedural hemorrhage of a nervous system organ or structure following a procedure

     G97.51 Postprocedural hemorrhage of a nervous system organ or structure following a nervous system procedure   CC

     G97.52 Postprocedural hemorrhage of a nervous system organ or structure following other procedure   CC

✓5ᵗʰ **G97.6** Postprocedural hematoma and seroma of a nervous system organ or structure following a procedure

     G97.61 Postprocedural hematoma of a nervous system organ or structure following a nervous system procedure   CC

       AHA: 2020,3Q,24

     G97.62 Postprocedural hematoma of a nervous system organ or structure following other procedure   CC

     G97.63 Postprocedural seroma of a nervous system organ or structure following a nervous system procedure   CC

     G97.64 Postprocedural seroma of a nervous system organ or structure following other procedure   CC

✓5ᵗʰ **G97.8** Other intraoperative and postprocedural complications and disorders of nervous system

     Use additional code to further specify disorder

     AHA: 2020,4Q,23

     G97.81 Other intraoperative complications of nervous system   CC

     G97.82 Other postprocedural complications and disorders of nervous system   CC

     G97.83 Intracranial hypotension following lumbar cerebrospinal fluid shunting   CC

       Code also any associated diagnoses or complications

     G97.84 Intracranial hypotension following other procedure   CC

       Code also, if applicable:

         accidental puncture or laceration of dura during a procedure (G97.41)

         cerebrospinal fluid leak from spinal puncture (G97.0)

✓4ᵗʰ **G98** Other disorders of nervous system not elsewhere classified

     INCLUDES   nervous system disorder NOS

G98.0 Neurogenic arthritis, not elsewhere classified

     Nonsyphilitic neurogenic arthropathy NEC

     Nonsyphilitic neurogenic spondylopathy NEC

     EXCLUDES 1   *spondylopathy (in):*

       syringomyelia and syringobulbia (G95.0)

       tabes dorsalis (A52.11)

G98.8 Other disorders of nervous system   HIV

     Nervous system disorder NOS

✓4ᵗʰ **G99** Other disorders of nervous system in diseases classified elsewhere

G99.0 *Autonomic neuropathy in diseases classified elsewhere*   CC

     Code first underlying disease, such as:

       amyloidosis (E85.-)

       gout (M1A.-, M10.-)

       hyperthyroidism (E05.-)

     EXCLUDES 1   *diabetic autonomic neuropathy (E08-E13 with .43)*

G99.2 *Myelopathy in diseases classified elsewhere*   CC   HCC

     Code first underlying disease, such as:

       neoplasm (C00-D49)

     EXCLUDES 1   *myelopathy in:*

       intervertebral disease (M50.0-, M51.0-)

       spondylosis (M47.0-, M47.1-)

     AHA: 2018,3Q,18-19

     TIP: Use this code in addition to a spondylolisthesis code (M43.1-) or a spinal stenosis code (M48.0-) when either of these disorders is documented as the cause of the myelopathy.

G99.8 *Other specified disorders of nervous system in diseases classified elsewhere*

     Code first underlying disorder, such as:

       amyloidosis (E85.-)

       avitaminosis (E56.9)

     EXCLUDES 1   *nervous system involvement in:*

       cysticercosis (B69.0)

       rubella (B06.0-)

       syphilis (A52.1-)

☑ Additional Character Required   ✓x7ᵗʰ Placeholder   Questionable PDx   Manifestation   Unspecified Dx   UPD Unacceptable PDx   H1-H14 HAC   HCC CMS-HCC Dx   HIV HIV Dx

ICD-10-CM 2022   593

Chapter 7. Diseases of the Eye and Adnexa (H00–H59)

Chapter-specific Guidelines with Coding Examples

The chapter-specific guidelines from the ICD-10-CM Official Guidelines for Coding and Reporting have been provided below. Along with these guidelines are coding examples, contained in the shaded boxes, that have been developed to help illustrate the coding and/or sequencing guidance found in these guidelines.

a. Glaucoma

1) Assigning glaucoma codes

Assign as many codes from category H40, Glaucoma, as needed to identify the type of glaucoma, the affected eye, and the glaucoma stage.

2) Bilateral glaucoma with same type and stage

When a patient has bilateral glaucoma and both eyes are documented as being the same type and stage, and there is a code for bilateral glaucoma, report only the code for the type of glaucoma, bilateral, with the seventh character for the stage.

> Bilateral severe stage pigmentary glaucoma
>
> **H40.1333   Pigmentary glaucoma, bilateral, severe stage**
>
> *Explanation*: In this scenario, the patient has the same type and stage of glaucoma in both eyes. As this type of glaucoma has a code for bilateral, assign only the code for the bilateral glaucoma with the seventh character for the stage.

When a patient has bilateral glaucoma and both eyes are documented as being the same type and stage, and the classification does not provide a code for bilateral glaucoma (i.e. subcategories H40.10 and H40.20) report only one code for the type of glaucoma with the appropriate seventh character for the stage.

> Bilateral open-angle glaucoma; not specified as to type and stage indeterminate in both eyes
>
> **H40.10X4   Unspecified open-angle glaucoma, indeterminate stage**
>
> *Explanation*: In this scenario, the patient has glaucoma of the same type and stage of both eyes, but there is no code specifically for bilateral glaucoma. Only one code is assigned with the appropriate seventh character for the stage.

3) Bilateral glaucoma stage with different types or stages

When a patient has bilateral glaucoma and each eye is documented as having a different type or stage, and the classification distinguishes laterality, assign the appropriate code for each eye rather than the code for bilateral glaucoma.

When a patient has bilateral glaucoma and each eye is documented as having a different type, and the classification does not distinguish laterality (i.e. subcategories H40.10 and H40.20), assign one code for each type of glaucoma with the appropriate seventh character for the stage.

> Documentation relates mild, unspecified primary angle-closure glaucoma of the left eye with mild unspecified open-angle glaucoma of the right eye
>
> **H40.20X1   Unspecified primary angle-closure glaucoma, mild stage**
>
> **H40.10X1   Unspecified open-angle glaucoma, mild stage**
>
> *Explanation*: In this scenario the patient has a different type of glaucoma in each eye and the classification does not distinguish laterality. A code for each type of glaucoma is assigned, each with the appropriate seventh character for the stage.

When a patient has bilateral glaucoma and each eye is documented as having the same type, but different stage, and the classification does not distinguish laterality (i.e. subcategories H40.10 and H40.20), assign a code for the type of glaucoma for each eye with the seventh character for the specific glaucoma stage documented for each eye.

> Bilateral open-angle glaucoma, not specified as to type; the right eye is documented to be in mild stage and the left eye as being in moderate stage
>
> **H40.10X1   Unspecified open-angle glaucoma, mild stage**
>
> **H40.10X2   Unspecified open-angle glaucoma, moderate stage**
>
> *Explanation*: In this scenario the patient has the same type of glaucoma in each eye but each eye is at a different stage, and the classification does not distinguish laterality at this subcategory level. Two codes are assigned; both codes represent the same type of glaucoma but each has a different seventh character identifying the appropriate stage for each eye.

4) Patient admitted with glaucoma and stage evolves during the admission

If a patient is admitted with glaucoma and the stage progresses during the admission, assign the code for highest stage documented.

> Patient admitted with mild low-tension glaucoma of the right eye, which progresses to moderate stage during the patient's stay
>
> **H40.1212   Low-tension glaucoma, right eye, moderate stage**
>
> *Explanation*: When the glaucoma stage progresses during an admission, assign only the code for the highest stage documented.

5) Indeterminate stage glaucoma

Assignment of the seventh character "4" for "indeterminate stage" should be based on the clinical documentation. The seventh character "4" is used for glaucomas whose stage cannot be clinically determined. This seventh character should not be confused with the seventh character "0", unspecified, which should be assigned when there is no documentation regarding the stage of the glaucoma.

b. Blindness

If "blindness" or "low vision" of both eyes is documented but the visual impairment category is not documented, assign code H54.3, Unqualified visual loss, both eyes. If "blindness" or "low vision" in one eye is documented but the visual impairment category is not documented, assign a code from H54.6-, Unqualified visual loss, one eye. If "blindness" or "visual loss" is documented without any information about whether one or both eyes are affected, assign code H54.7, Unspecified visual loss.

> Blindness in 89-year-old male
>
> **H54.7   Unspecified visual loss**
>
> *Explanation*: Blindness is stated, but there is no mention of whether one or both eyes are affected or the severity of this visual impairment.

Chapter 7. Diseases of the Eye and Adnexa (H00-H59)

NOTE   Use an external cause code following the code for the eye condition, if applicable, to identify the cause of the eye condition

EXCLUDES 2   *certain conditions originating in the perinatal period (P04-P96)*
certain infectious and parasitic diseases (A00-B99)
complications of pregnancy, childbirth and the puerperium (O00-O9A)
congenital malformations, deformations, and chromosomal abnormalities (Q00-Q99)
diabetes mellitus related eye conditions (E09.3-, E10.3-, E11.3-, E13.3-)
endocrine, nutritional and metabolic diseases (E00-E88)
injury (trauma) of eye and orbit (S05.-)
injury, poisoning and certain other consequences of external causes (S00-T88)
neoplasms (C00-D49)
symptoms, signs and abnormal clinical and laboratory findings, not elsewhere classified (R00-R94)
syphilis related eye disorders (A50.01, A50.3-, A51.43, A52.71)

This chapter contains the following blocks:

H00-H05	Disorders of eyelid, lacrimal system and orbit
H10-H11	Disorders of conjunctiva
H15-H22	Disorders of sclera, cornea, iris and ciliary body
H25-H28	Disorders of lens
H30-H36	Disorders of choroid and retina
H40-H42	Glaucoma
H43-H44	Disorders of vitreous body and globe
H46-H47	Disorders of optic nerve and visual pathways
H49-H52	Disorders of ocular muscles, binocular movement, accommodation and refraction
H53-H54	Visual disturbances and blindness
H55-H57	Other disorders of eye and adnexa
H59	Intraoperative and postprocedural complications and disorders of eye and adnexa, not elsewhere classified

Disorders of eyelid, lacrimal system and orbit (H00-H05)

EXCLUDES 2   *open wound of eyelid (S01.1-)*
superficial injury of eyelid (S00.1-, S00.2-)

✓4ᵗʰ **H00 Hordeolum and chalazion**

✓5ᵗʰ **H00.0 Hordeolum (externum) (internum) of eyelid**

    DEF: Acute localized infection of the gland of Zeis (external hordeolum) or Molt or of the meibomian glands (internal hordeolum) of the orbit.

✓6ᵗʰ **H00.01 Hordeolum externum**

    Hordeolum NOS
    Stye

    H00.011 Hordeolum externum right upper eyelid
    H00.012 Hordeolum externum right lower eyelid
    H00.013 Hordeolum externum right eye, unspecified eyelid
    H00.014 Hordeolum externum left upper eyelid
    H00.015 Hordeolum externum left lower eyelid
    H00.016 Hordeolum externum left eye, unspecified eyelid
    H00.019 Hordeolum externum unspecified eye, unspecified eyelid

✓6ᵗʰ **H00.02 Hordeolum internum**

    Infection of meibomian gland

    H00.021 Hordeolum internum right upper eyelid
    H00.022 Hordeolum internum right lower eyelid
    H00.023 Hordeolum internum right eye, unspecified eyelid
    H00.024 Hordeolum internum left upper eyelid
    H00.025 Hordeolum internum left lower eyelid
    H00.026 Hordeolum internum left eye, unspecified eyelid
    H00.029 Hordeolum internum unspecified eye, unspecified eyelid

✓6ᵗʰ **H00.03 Abscess of eyelid**

    Furuncle of eyelid

    H00.031 Abscess of right upper eyelid
    H00.032 Abscess of right lower eyelid
    H00.033 Abscess of eyelid right eye, unspecified eyelid
    H00.034 Abscess of left upper eyelid
    H00.035 Abscess of left lower eyelid
    H00.036 Abscess of eyelid left eye, unspecified eyelid
    H00.039 Abscess of eyelid unspecified eye, unspecified eyelid

✓5ᵗʰ **H00.1 Chalazion**

    Meibomian (gland) cyst

    EXCLUDES 2   *infected meibomian gland (H00.02-)*

    DEF: Noninfectious, obstructive mass in the oil gland of the eyelid that results in a small chronic lump or inflammation.

    H00.11 Chalazion right upper eyelid
    H00.12 Chalazion right lower eyelid
    H00.13 Chalazion right eye, unspecified eyelid
    H00.14 Chalazion left upper eyelid
    H00.15 Chalazion left lower eyelid
    H00.16 Chalazion left eye, unspecified eyelid
    H00.19 Chalazion unspecified eye, unspecified eyelid

✓4ᵗʰ **H01 Other inflammation of eyelid**

✓5ᵗʰ **H01.0 Blepharitis**

    EXCLUDES 1   *blepharoconjunctivitis (H10.5-)*

✓6ᵗʰ **H01.00 Unspecified blepharitis**

    AHA: 2018,4Q,13

    H01.001 Unspecified blepharitis right upper eyelid
    H01.002 Unspecified blepharitis right lower eyelid
    H01.003 Unspecified blepharitis right eye, unspecified eyelid
    H01.004 Unspecified blepharitis left upper eyelid
    H01.005 Unspecified blepharitis left lower eyelid
    H01.006 Unspecified blepharitis left eye, unspecified eyelid
    H01.009 Unspecified blepharitis unspecified eye, unspecified eyelid
    H01.00A Unspecified blepharitis right eye, upper and lower eyelids
    H01.00B Unspecified blepharitis left eye, upper and lower eyelids

✓6ᵗʰ **H01.01 Ulcerative blepharitis**

    AHA: 2018,4Q,13

    H01.011 Ulcerative blepharitis right upper eyelid
    H01.012 Ulcerative blepharitis right lower eyelid
    H01.013 Ulcerative blepharitis right eye, unspecified eyelid
    H01.014 Ulcerative blepharitis left upper eyelid
    H01.015 Ulcerative blepharitis left lower eyelid
    H01.016 Ulcerative blepharitis left eye, unspecified eyelid
    H01.019 Ulcerative blepharitis unspecified eye, unspecified eyelid
    H01.01A Ulcerative blepharitis right eye, upper and lower eyelids
    H01.01B Ulcerative blepharitis left eye, upper and lower eyelids

✓6ᵗʰ **H01.02 Squamous blepharitis**

    AHA: 2018,4Q,13

    H01.021 Squamous blepharitis right upper eyelid
    H01.022 Squamous blepharitis right lower eyelid
    H01.023 Squamous blepharitis right eye, unspecified eyelid
    H01.024 Squamous blepharitis left upper eyelid
    H01.025 Squamous blepharitis left lower eyelid
    H01.026 Squamous blepharitis left eye, unspecified eyelid
    H01.029 Squamous blepharitis unspecified eye, unspecified eyelid
    H01.02A Squamous blepharitis right eye, upper and lower eyelids
    H01.02B Squamous blepharitis left eye, upper and lower eyelids

✓5ᵗʰ **H01.1 Noninfectious dermatoses of eyelid**

✓6ᵗʰ **H01.11 Allergic dermatitis of eyelid**

    Contact dermatitis of eyelid

    H01.111 Allergic dermatitis of right upper eyelid
    H01.112 Allergic dermatitis of right lower eyelid
    H01.113 Allergic dermatitis of right eye, unspecified eyelid
    H01.114 Allergic dermatitis of left upper eyelid
    H01.115 Allergic dermatitis of left lower eyelid
    H01.116 Allergic dermatitis of left eye, unspecified eyelid
    H01.119 Allergic dermatitis of unspecified eye, unspecified eyelid

✓6ᵗʰ **H01.12** **Discoid lupus erythematosus of eyelid**

    H01.121 **Discoid lupus erythematosus of** right upper **eyelid**

    H01.122 **Discoid lupus erythematosus of** right lower **eyelid**

    H01.123 **Discoid lupus erythematosus of** right eye, unspecified **eyelid**

    H01.124 **Discoid lupus erythematosus of** left upper **eyelid**

    H01.125 **Discoid lupus erythematosus of** left lower **eyelid**

    H01.126 **Discoid lupus erythematosus of** left eye, unspecified **eyelid**

    H01.129 **Discoid lupus erythematosus of unspecified eye, unspecified eyelid**

✓6ᵗʰ **H01.13** **Eczematous dermatitis of eyelid**

    H01.131 **Eczematous dermatitis of** right upper **eyelid**

    H01.132 **Eczematous dermatitis of** right lower **eyelid**

    H01.133 **Eczematous dermatitis of** right eye, unspecified **eyelid**

    H01.134 **Eczematous dermatitis of** left upper **eyelid**

    H01.135 **Eczematous dermatitis of** left lower **eyelid**

    H01.136 **Eczematous dermatitis of** left eye, unspecified **eyelid**

    H01.139 **Eczematous dermatitis of unspecified eye, unspecified eyelid**

✓6ᵗʰ **H01.14** **Xeroderma of eyelid**

    H01.141 **Xeroderma of** right upper **eyelid**

    H01.142 **Xeroderma of** right lower **eyelid**

    H01.143 **Xeroderma of** right eye, unspecified **eyelid**

    H01.144 **Xeroderma of** left upper **eyelid**

    H01.145 **Xeroderma of** left lower **eyelid**

    H01.146 **Xeroderma of** left eye, unspecified **eyelid**

    H01.149 **Xeroderma of unspecified eye, unspecified eyelid**

H01.8 **Other specified inflammations of eyelid**

H01.9 **Unspecified inflammation of eyelid**
    Inflammation of eyelid NOS

✓4ᵗʰ **H02** **Other disorders of eyelid**

    EXCLUDES 1   *congenital malformations of eyelid (Q10.0-Q10.3)*

Entropion and Ectropion

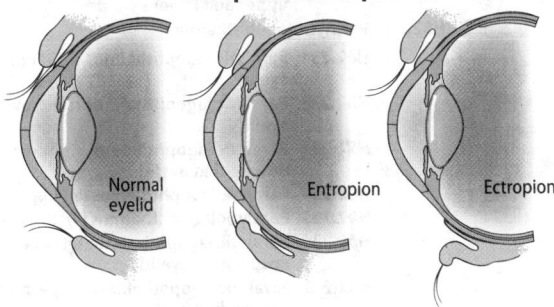

Normal eyelid   Entropion   Ectropion

✓5ᵗʰ **H02.0** **Entropion and trichiasis of eyelid**

    DEF: Entropion: Inversion of the eyelid, turning the edge in toward the eyeball and causing irritation from contact of the lashes with the surface of the eye.

    DEF: Trichiasis: Condition wherein the eyelid is in a normal position but lashes are ingrown or misdirected in their growth so that they irritate the tissues of the eye.

✓6ᵗʰ **H02.00** **Unspecified entropion of eyelid**

    H02.001 **Unspecified entropion of** right upper **eyelid**

    H02.002 **Unspecified entropion of** right lower **eyelid**

    H02.003 **Unspecified entropion of** right eye, unspecified **eyelid**

    H02.004 **Unspecified entropion of** left upper **eyelid**

    H02.005 **Unspecified entropion of** left lower **eyelid**

    H02.006 **Unspecified entropion of** left eye, unspecified **eyelid**

    H02.009 **Unspecified entropion of unspecified eye, unspecified eyelid**

✓6ᵗʰ **H02.01** **Cicatricial entropion of eyelid**

    H02.011 **Cicatricial entropion of** right upper **eyelid**

    H02.012 **Cicatricial entropion of** right lower **eyelid**

    H02.013 **Cicatricial entropion of** right eye, unspecified **eyelid**

    H02.014 **Cicatricial entropion of** left upper **eyelid**

    H02.015 **Cicatricial entropion of** left lower **eyelid**

    H02.016 **Cicatricial entropion of** left eye, unspecified **eyelid**

    H02.019 **Cicatricial entropion of unspecified eye, unspecified eyelid**

✓6ᵗʰ **H02.02** **Mechanical entropion of eyelid**

    H02.021 **Mechanical entropion of** right upper **eyelid**

    H02.022 **Mechanical entropion of** right lower **eyelid**

    H02.023 **Mechanical entropion of** right eye, unspecified **eyelid**

    H02.024 **Mechanical entropion of** left upper **eyelid**

    H02.025 **Mechanical entropion of** left lower **eyelid**

    H02.026 **Mechanical entropion of** left eye, unspecified **eyelid**

    H02.029 **Mechanical entropion of unspecified eye, unspecified eyelid**

✓6ᵗʰ **H02.03** **Senile entropion of eyelid**

    H02.031 **Senile entropion of** right upper **eyelid**   Ⓐ

    H02.032 **Senile entropion of** right lower **eyelid**   Ⓐ

    H02.033 **Senile entropion of** right eye, unspecified **eyelid**   Ⓐ

    H02.034 **Senile entropion of** left upper **eyelid**   Ⓐ

    H02.035 **Senile entropion of** left lower **eyelid**   Ⓐ

    H02.036 **Senile entropion of** left eye, unspecified **eyelid**   Ⓐ

    H02.039 **Senile entropion of unspecified eye, unspecified eyelid**   Ⓐ

✓6ᵗʰ **H02.04** **Spastic entropion of eyelid**

    H02.041 **Spastic entropion of** right upper **eyelid**

    H02.042 **Spastic entropion of** right lower **eyelid**

    H02.043 **Spastic entropion of** right eye, unspecified **eyelid**

    H02.044 **Spastic entropion of** left upper **eyelid**

    H02.045 **Spastic entropion of** left lower **eyelid**

    H02.046 **Spastic entropion of** left eye, unspecified **eyelid**

    H02.049 **Spastic entropion of unspecified eye, unspecified eyelid**

✓6ᵗʰ **H02.05** **Trichiasis without entropion**

    H02.051 **Trichiasis without entropion** right upper **eyelid**

    H02.052 **Trichiasis without entropion** right lower **eyelid**

    H02.053 **Trichiasis without entropion** right eye, unspecified **eyelid**

    H02.054 **Trichiasis without entropion** left upper **eyelid**

    H02.055 **Trichiasis without entropion** left lower **eyelid**

    H02.056 **Trichiasis without entropion** left eye, unspecified **eyelid**

    H02.059 **Trichiasis without entropion unspecified eye, unspecified eyelid**

✓5ᵗʰ **H02.1** **Ectropion of eyelid**

    DEF: Drooping of the lower eyelid away from the eye or outward turning or eversion of the edge of the eyelid, exposing the palpebral conjunctiva and causing irritation.

✓6ᵗʰ **H02.10** **Unspecified ectropion of eyelid**

    H02.101 **Unspecified ectropion of** right upper **eyelid**

    H02.102 **Unspecified ectropion of** right lower **eyelid**

    H02.103 **Unspecified ectropion of** right eye, unspecified **eyelid**

    H02.104 **Unspecified ectropion of** left upper **eyelid**

    H02.105 **Unspecified ectropion of** left lower **eyelid**

    H02.106 **Unspecified ectropion of** left eye, unspecified **eyelid**

✓ Additional Character Required   ✓x7ᵗʰ Placeholder   Questionable PDx   Manifestation   Unspecified Dx   UPD Unacceptable PDx   H1-H14 HAC   HCC CMS-HCC Dx   HIV HIV Dx

ICD-10-CM 2022   597

Chapter 7. Diseases of the Eye and Adnexa

H02.109 Unspecified ectropion of unspecified eye, unspecified eyelid

✓6ᵗʰ **H02.11** Cicatricial ectropion of eyelid

    H02.111 Cicatricial ectropion of right upper eyelid
    H02.112 Cicatricial ectropion of right lower eyelid
    H02.113 Cicatricial ectropion of right eye, unspecified eyelid
    H02.114 Cicatricial ectropion of left upper eyelid
    H02.115 Cicatricial ectropion of left lower eyelid
    H02.116 Cicatricial ectropion of left eye, unspecified eyelid
    H02.119 Cicatricial ectropion of unspecified eye, unspecified eyelid

✓6ᵗʰ **H02.12** Mechanical ectropion of eyelid

    H02.121 Mechanical ectropion of right upper eyelid
    H02.122 Mechanical ectropion of right lower eyelid
    H02.123 Mechanical ectropion of right eye, unspecified eyelid
    H02.124 Mechanical ectropion of left upper eyelid
    H02.125 Mechanical ectropion of left lower eyelid
    H02.126 Mechanical ectropion of left eye, unspecified eyelid
    H02.129 Mechanical ectropion of unspecified eye, unspecified eyelid

✓6ᵗʰ **H02.13** Senile ectropion of eyelid

    H02.131 Senile ectropion of right upper eyelid   Ⓐ
    H02.132 Senile ectropion of right lower eyelid   Ⓐ
    H02.133 Senile ectropion of right eye, unspecified eyelid   Ⓐ
    H02.134 Senile ectropion of left upper eyelid   Ⓐ
    H02.135 Senile ectropion of left lower eyelid   Ⓐ
    H02.136 Senile ectropion of left eye, unspecified eyelid   Ⓐ
    H02.139 Senile ectropion of unspecified eye, unspecified eyelid   Ⓐ

✓6ᵗʰ **H02.14** Spastic ectropion of eyelid

    H02.141 Spastic ectropion of right upper eyelid
    H02.142 Spastic ectropion of right lower eyelid
    H02.143 Spastic ectropion of right eye, unspecified eyelid
    H02.144 Spastic ectropion of left upper eyelid
    H02.145 Spastic ectropion of left lower eyelid
    H02.146 Spastic ectropion of left eye, unspecified eyelid
    H02.149 Spastic ectropion of unspecified eye, unspecified eyelid

✓6ᵗʰ **H02.15** Paralytic ectropion of eyelid

    AHA: 2018,4Q,13

    H02.151 Paralytic ectropion of right upper eyelid
    H02.152 Paralytic ectropion of right lower eyelid
    H02.153 Paralytic ectropion of right eye, unspecified eyelid
    H02.154 Paralytic ectropion of left upper eyelid
    H02.155 Paralytic ectropion of left lower eyelid
    H02.156 Paralytic ectropion of left eye, unspecified eyelid
    H02.159 Paralytic ectropion of unspecified eye, unspecified eyelid

✓5ᵗʰ **H02.2** Lagophthalmos

    AHA: 2018,4Q,14
    DEF: Condition of the eye that prevents it from closing completely.

✓6ᵗʰ **H02.20** Unspecified lagophthalmos

    H02.201 Unspecified lagophthalmos right upper eyelid
    H02.202 Unspecified lagophthalmos right lower eyelid
    H02.203 Unspecified lagophthalmos right eye, unspecified eyelid
    H02.204 Unspecified lagophthalmos left upper eyelid
    H02.205 Unspecified lagophthalmos left lower eyelid
    H02.206 Unspecified lagophthalmos left eye, unspecified eyelid
    H02.209 Unspecified lagophthalmos unspecified eye, unspecified eyelid

    H02.20A Unspecified lagophthalmos right eye, upper and lower eyelids
    H02.20B Unspecified lagophthalmos left eye, upper and lower eyelids
    H02.20C Unspecified lagophthalmos, bilateral, upper and lower eyelids

✓6ᵗʰ **H02.21** Cicatricial lagophthalmos

    H02.211 Cicatricial lagophthalmos right upper eyelid
    H02.212 Cicatricial lagophthalmos right lower eyelid
    H02.213 Cicatricial lagophthalmos right eye, unspecified eyelid
    H02.214 Cicatricial lagophthalmos left upper eyelid
    H02.215 Cicatricial lagophthalmos left lower eyelid
    H02.216 Cicatricial lagophthalmos left eye, unspecified eyelid
    H02.219 Cicatricial lagophthalmos unspecified eye, unspecified eyelid
    H02.21A Cicatricial lagophthalmos right eye, upper and lower eyelids
    H02.21B Cicatricial lagophthalmos left eye, upper and lower eyelids
    H02.21C Cicatricial lagophthalmos, bilateral, upper and lower eyelids

✓6ᵗʰ **H02.22** Mechanical lagophthalmos

    H02.221 Mechanical lagophthalmos right upper eyelid
    H02.222 Mechanical lagophthalmos right lower eyelid
    H02.223 Mechanical lagophthalmos right eye, unspecified eyelid
    H02.224 Mechanical lagophthalmos left upper eyelid
    H02.225 Mechanical lagophthalmos left lower eyelid
    H02.226 Mechanical lagophthalmos left eye, unspecified eyelid
    H02.229 Mechanical lagophthalmos unspecified eye, unspecified eyelid
    H02.22A Mechanical lagophthalmos right eye, upper and lower eyelids
    H02.22B Mechanical lagophthalmos left eye, upper and lower eyelids
    H02.22C Mechanical lagophthalmos, bilateral, upper and lower eyelids

✓6ᵗʰ **H02.23** Paralytic lagophthalmos

    H02.231 Paralytic lagophthalmos right upper eyelid
    H02.232 Paralytic lagophthalmos right lower eyelid
    H02.233 Paralytic lagophthalmos right eye, unspecified eyelid
    H02.234 Paralytic lagophthalmos left upper eyelid
    H02.235 Paralytic lagophthalmos left lower eyelid
    H02.236 Paralytic lagophthalmos left eye, unspecified eyelid
    H02.239 Paralytic lagophthalmos unspecified eye, unspecified eyelid
    H02.23A Paralytic lagophthalmos right eye, upper and lower eyelids
    H02.23B Paralytic lagophthalmos left eye, upper and lower eyelids
    H02.23C Paralytic lagophthalmos, bilateral, upper and lower eyelids

✓5ᵗʰ **H02.3** Blepharochalasis

    Pseudoptosis
    DEF: Loss of elasticity and relaxation of skin of the eyelid, thickened or indurated skin on the eyelid associated with recurrent episodes of edema, and intracellular atrophy.

    H02.30 Blepharochalasis unspecified eye, unspecified eyelid
    H02.31 Blepharochalasis right upper eyelid
    H02.32 Blepharochalasis right lower eyelid
    H02.33 Blepharochalasis right eye, unspecified eyelid
    H02.34 Blepharochalasis left upper eyelid
    H02.35 Blepharochalasis left lower eyelid
    H02.36 Blepharochalasis left eye, unspecified eyelid

Ⓝ Newborn: 0   Ⓟ Pediatric: 0-17   Ⓜ Maternity: 9-64   Ⓐ Adult: 15-124   ᴹᶜᶜ Major Complication/Comorbidity   ᶜᶜ Complication/Comorbidity   ˢʷ Severe Wound Dx

598

ICD-10-CM 2022

✓6th **H02.4 Ptosis of eyelid**

  ✓6th **H02.40 Unspecified ptosis of eyelid**

    H02.401 Unspecified ptosis of right eyelid

    H02.402 Unspecified ptosis of left eyelid

    H02.403 Unspecified ptosis of bilateral eyelids

    H02.409 Unspecified ptosis of unspecified eyelid

  ✓6th **H02.41 Mechanical ptosis of eyelid**

    H02.411 Mechanical ptosis of right eyelid

    H02.412 Mechanical ptosis of left eyelid

    H02.413 Mechanical ptosis of bilateral eyelids

    H02.419 Mechanical ptosis of unspecified eyelid

  ✓6th **H02.42 Myogenic ptosis of eyelid**

    H02.421 Myogenic ptosis of right eyelid

    H02.422 Myogenic ptosis of left eyelid

    H02.423 Myogenic ptosis of bilateral eyelids

    H02.429 Myogenic ptosis of unspecified eyelid

  ✓6th **H02.43 Paralytic ptosis of eyelid**

    Neurogenic ptosis of eyelid

    H02.431 Paralytic ptosis of right eyelid

    H02.432 Paralytic ptosis of left eyelid

    H02.433 Paralytic ptosis of bilateral eyelids

    H02.439 Paralytic ptosis unspecified eyelid

✓5th **H02.5 Other disorders affecting eyelid function**

  EXCLUDES 2   blepharospasm (G24.5)

    organic tic (G25.69)

    psychogenic tic (F95.-)

  ✓6th **H02.51 Abnormal innervation syndrome**

    H02.511 Abnormal innervation syndrome right upper eyelid

    H02.512 Abnormal innervation syndrome right lower eyelid

    H02.513 Abnormal innervation syndrome right eye, unspecified eyelid

    H02.514 Abnormal innervation syndrome left upper eyelid

    H02.515 Abnormal innervation syndrome left lower eyelid

    H02.516 Abnormal innervation syndrome left eye, unspecified eyelid

    H02.519 Abnormal innervation syndrome unspecified eye, unspecified eyelid

  ✓6th **H02.52 Blepharophimosis**

    Ankyloblepharon

    H02.521 Blepharophimosis right upper eyelid

    H02.522 Blepharophimosis right lower eyelid

    H02.523 Blepharophimosis right eye, unspecified eyelid

    H02.524 Blepharophimosis left upper eyelid

    H02.525 Blepharophimosis left lower eyelid

    H02.526 Blepharophimosis left eye, unspecified eyelid

    H02.529 Blepharophimosis unspecified eye, unspecified lid

  ✓6th **H02.53 Eyelid retraction**

    Eyelid lag

    H02.531 Eyelid retraction right upper eyelid

    H02.532 Eyelid retraction right lower eyelid

    H02.533 Eyelid retraction right eye, unspecified eyelid

    H02.534 Eyelid retraction left upper eyelid

    H02.535 Eyelid retraction left lower eyelid

    H02.536 Eyelid retraction left eye, unspecified eyelid

    H02.539 Eyelid retraction unspecified eye, unspecified lid

  H02.59 Other disorders affecting eyelid function

    Deficient blink reflex

    Sensory disorders

✓5th **H02.6 Xanthelasma of eyelid**

  DEF: Condition in which there are small yellow tumors that occur on the eyelid, usually appearing near the nose.

  H02.60 Xanthelasma of unspecified eye, unspecified eyelid

  H02.61 Xanthelasma of right upper eyelid

  H02.62 Xanthelasma of right lower eyelid

  H02.63 Xanthelasma of right eye, unspecified eyelid

  H02.64 Xanthelasma of left upper eyelid

  H02.65 Xanthelasma of left lower eyelid

  H02.66 Xanthelasma of left eye, unspecified eyelid

✓5th **H02.7 Other and unspecified degenerative disorders of eyelid and periocular area**

  H02.70 Unspecified degenerative disorders of eyelid and periocular area

  ✓6th **H02.71 Chloasma of eyelid and periocular area**

    Dyspigmentation of eyelid

    Hyperpigmentation of eyelid

    H02.711 Chloasma of right upper eyelid and periocular area

    H02.712 Chloasma of right lower eyelid and periocular area

    H02.713 Chloasma of right eye, unspecified eyelid and periocular area

    H02.714 Chloasma of left upper eyelid and periocular area

    H02.715 Chloasma of left lower eyelid and periocular area

    H02.716 Chloasma of left eye, unspecified eyelid and periocular area

    H02.719 Chloasma of unspecified eye, unspecified eyelid and periocular area

  ✓6th **H02.72 Madarosis of eyelid and periocular area**

    Hypotrichosis of eyelid

    H02.721 Madarosis of right upper eyelid and periocular area

    H02.722 Madarosis of right lower eyelid and periocular area

    H02.723 Madarosis of right eye, unspecified eyelid and periocular area

    H02.724 Madarosis of left upper eyelid and periocular area

    H02.725 Madarosis of left lower eyelid and periocular area

    H02.726 Madarosis of left eye, unspecified eyelid and periocular area

    H02.729 Madarosis of unspecified eye, unspecified eyelid and periocular area

  ✓6th **H02.73 Vitiligo of eyelid and periocular area**

    Hypopigmentation of eyelid

    H02.731 Vitiligo of right upper eyelid and periocular area

    H02.732 Vitiligo of right lower eyelid and periocular area

    H02.733 Vitiligo of right eye, unspecified eyelid and periocular area

    H02.734 Vitiligo of left upper eyelid and periocular area

    H02.735 Vitiligo of left lower eyelid and periocular area

    H02.736 Vitiligo of left eye, unspecified eyelid and periocular area

    H02.739 Vitiligo of unspecified eye, unspecified eyelid and periocular area

  H02.79 Other degenerative disorders of eyelid and periocular area

✓5th **H02.8 Other specified disorders of eyelid**

  ✓6th **H02.81 Retained foreign body in eyelid**

    Use additional code to identify the type of retained foreign body (Z18.-)

    EXCLUDES 1   laceration of eyelid with foreign body (S01.12-)

      retained intraocular foreign body (H44.6-, H44.7-)

      superficial foreign body of eyelid and periocular area (S00.25-)

    H02.811 Retained foreign body in right upper eyelid

    H02.812 Retained foreign body in right lower eyelid

    H02.813 Retained foreign body in right eye, unspecified eyelid

    H02.814 Retained foreign body in left upper eyelid

    H02.815 Retained foreign body in left lower eyelid

    H02.816 Retained foreign body in left eye, unspecified eyelid

    H02.819 Retained foreign body in unspecified eye, unspecified eyelid

  ✓6th **H02.82 Cysts of eyelid**

    Sebaceous cyst of eyelid

    H02.821 Cysts of right upper eyelid

    H02.822 Cysts of right lower eyelid

✓ Additional Character Required   ✓x7th Placeholder   Questionable PDx   Manifestation   Unspecified Dx   UPD Unacceptable PDx   H1 - H14 HAC   HCC CMS-HCC Dx   HIV HIV Dx

ICD-10-CM 2022   599

Chapter 7. Diseases of the Eye and Adnexa

H02.823–H04.151

H02.823   **Cysts of** right eye, unspecified **eyelid**
H02.824   **Cysts of** left upper **eyelid**
H02.825   **Cysts of** left lower **eyelid**
H02.826   **Cysts of** left eye, unspecified **eyelid**
H02.829   **Cysts of** unspecified eye, unspecified **eyelid**

✓6ᵗʰ   **H02.83   Dermatochalasis of eyelid**

    DEF: Acquired form of connective tissue disorder associated with decreased elastic tissue and abnormal elastin formation, resulting in loss of elasticity of the skin of the eyelid. It is generally associated with aging.

H02.831   **Dermatochalasis of** right upper **eyelid**
H02.832   **Dermatochalasis of** right lower **eyelid**
H02.833   **Dermatochalasis of** right eye, unspecified **eyelid**
H02.834   **Dermatochalasis of** left upper **eyelid**
H02.835   **Dermatochalasis of** left lower **eyelid**
H02.836   **Dermatochalasis of** left eye, unspecified **eyelid**
H02.839   **Dermatochalasis of** unspecified eye, unspecified **eyelid**

✓6ᵗʰ   **H02.84   Edema of eyelid**

    Hyperemia of eyelid

H02.841   **Edema of** right upper **eyelid**
H02.842   **Edema of** right lower **eyelid**
H02.843   **Edema of** right eye, unspecified **eyelid**
H02.844   **Edema of** left upper **eyelid**
H02.845   **Edema of** left lower **eyelid**
H02.846   **Edema of** left eye, unspecified **eyelid**
H02.849   **Edema of** unspecified eye, unspecified **eyelid**

✓6ᵗʰ   **H02.85   Elephantiasis of eyelid**

H02.851   **Elephantiasis of** right upper **eyelid**
H02.852   **Elephantiasis of** right lower **eyelid**
H02.853   **Elephantiasis of** right eye, unspecified **eyelid**
H02.854   **Elephantiasis of** left upper **eyelid**
H02.855   **Elephantiasis of** left lower **eyelid**
H02.856   **Elephantiasis of** left eye, unspecified **eyelid**
H02.859   **Elephantiasis of** unspecified eye, unspecified **eyelid**

✓6ᵗʰ   **H02.86   Hypertrichosis of eyelid**

H02.861   **Hypertrichosis of** right upper **eyelid**
H02.862   **Hypertrichosis of** right lower **eyelid**
H02.863   **Hypertrichosis of** right eye, unspecified **eyelid**
H02.864   **Hypertrichosis of** left upper **eyelid**
H02.865   **Hypertrichosis of** left lower **eyelid**
H02.866   **Hypertrichosis of** left eye, unspecified **eyelid**
H02.869   **Hypertrichosis of** unspecified eye, unspecified **eyelid**

✓6ᵗʰ   **H02.87   Vascular anomalies of eyelid**

H02.871   **Vascular anomalies of** right upper **eyelid**
H02.872   **Vascular anomalies of** right lower **eyelid**
H02.873   **Vascular anomalies of** right eye, unspecified **eyelid**
H02.874   **Vascular anomalies of** left upper **eyelid**
H02.875   **Vascular anomalies of** left lower **eyelid**
H02.876   **Vascular anomalies of** left eye, unspecified **eyelid**
H02.879   **Vascular anomalies of** unspecified eye, unspecified **eyelid**

✓6ᵗʰ   **H02.88   Meibomian gland dysfunction of eyelid**

    AHA: 2018,4Q,14-15

H02.881   **Meibomian gland dysfunction** right upper **eyelid**
H02.882   **Meibomian gland dysfunction** right lower **eyelid**
H02.883   **Meibomian gland dysfunction of** right eye, unspecified **eyelid**
H02.884   **Meibomian gland dysfunction** left upper **eyelid**
H02.885   **Meibomian gland dysfunction** left lower **eyelid**
H02.886   **Meibomian gland dysfunction of** left eye, unspecified **eyelid**
H02.889   **Meibomian gland dysfunction of** unspecified eye, unspecified **eyelid**

H02.88A   **Meibomian gland dysfunction** right eye, upper and lower **eyelids**
H02.88B   **Meibomian gland dysfunction** left eye, upper and lower **eyelids**

H02.89   **Other specified disorders of eyelid**

    Hemorrhage of eyelid

H02.9   Unspecified disorder of eyelid

    Disorder of eyelid NOS

✓4ᵗʰ   **H04   Disorders of lacrimal system**

    EXCLUDES 1   congenital malformations of lacrimal system (Q10.4-Q10.6)

✓5ᵗʰ   **H04.0   Dacryoadenitis**

    DEF: Inflammation of the lacrimal gland.

✓6ᵗʰ   **H04.00   Unspecified dacryoadenitis**

H04.001   **Unspecified dacryoadenitis,** right **lacrimal gland**
H04.002   **Unspecified dacryoadenitis,** left **lacrimal gland**
H04.003   **Unspecified dacryoadenitis,** bilateral **lacrimal glands**
H04.009   **Unspecified dacryoadenitis, unspecified lacrimal gland**

✓6ᵗʰ   **H04.01   Acute dacryoadenitis**

H04.011   **Acute dacryoadenitis,** right **lacrimal gland**
H04.012   **Acute dacryoadenitis,** left **lacrimal gland**
H04.013   **Acute dacryoadenitis,** bilateral **lacrimal glands**
H04.019   **Acute dacryoadenitis, unspecified lacrimal gland**

✓6ᵗʰ   **H04.02   Chronic dacryoadenitis**

H04.021   **Chronic dacryoadenitis,** right **lacrimal gland**
H04.022   **Chronic dacryoadenitis,** left **lacrimal gland**
H04.023   **Chronic dacryoadenitis,** bilateral **lacrimal gland**
H04.029   **Chronic dacryoadenitis, unspecified lacrimal gland**

✓6ᵗʰ   **H04.03   Chronic enlargement of lacrimal gland**

H04.031   **Chronic enlargement of** right **lacrimal gland**
H04.032   **Chronic enlargement of** left **lacrimal gland**
H04.033   **Chronic enlargement of** bilateral **lacrimal glands**
H04.039   **Chronic enlargement of unspecified lacrimal gland**

✓5ᵗʰ   **H04.1   Other disorders of lacrimal gland**

✓6ᵗʰ   **H04.11   Dacryops**

H04.111   **Dacryops of** right **lacrimal gland**
H04.112   **Dacryops of** left **lacrimal gland**
H04.113   **Dacryops of** bilateral **lacrimal glands**
H04.119   **Dacryops of unspecified lacrimal gland**

✓6ᵗʰ   **H04.12   Dry eye syndrome**

    Tear film insufficiency, NOS

H04.121   **Dry eye syndrome of** right **lacrimal gland**
H04.122   **Dry eye syndrome of** left **lacrimal gland**
H04.123   **Dry eye syndrome of** bilateral **lacrimal glands**
H04.129   **Dry eye syndrome of unspecified lacrimal gland**

✓6ᵗʰ   **H04.13   Lacrimal cyst**

    Lacrimal cystic degeneration

H04.131   **Lacrimal cyst,** right **lacrimal gland**
H04.132   **Lacrimal cyst,** left **lacrimal gland**
H04.133   **Lacrimal cyst,** bilateral **lacrimal glands**
H04.139   **Lacrimal cyst, unspecified lacrimal gland**

✓6ᵗʰ   **H04.14   Primary lacrimal gland atrophy**

H04.141   **Primary lacrimal gland atrophy,** right **lacrimal gland**
H04.142   **Primary lacrimal gland atrophy,** left **lacrimal gland**
H04.143   **Primary lacrimal gland atrophy,** bilateral **lacrimal glands**
H04.149   **Primary lacrimal gland atrophy, unspecified lacrimal gland**

✓6ᵗʰ   **H04.15   Secondary lacrimal gland atrophy**

H04.151   **Secondary lacrimal gland atrophy,** right **lacrimal gland**

Ⓝ Newborn: 0   Ⓟ Pediatric: 0-17   Ⓜ Maternity: 9-64   Ⓐ Adult: 15-124   **MCC** Major Complication/Comorbidity   **CC** Complication/Comorbidity   **SW** Severe Wound Dx

600

ICD-10-CM 2022

H04.152 **Secondary lacrimal gland atrophy**, left lacrimal gland

H04.153 **Secondary lacrimal gland atrophy**, bilateral **lacrimal glands**

H04.159 **Secondary lacrimal gland atrophy**, unspecified lacrimal gland

√6th H04.16 **Lacrimal gland dislocation**

H04.161 **Lacrimal gland dislocation**, right **lacrimal gland**

H04.162 **Lacrimal gland dislocation**, left **lacrimal gland**

H04.163 **Lacrimal gland dislocation**, bilateral **lacrimal glands**

H04.169 **Lacrimal gland dislocation**, unspecified **lacrimal gland**

H04.19 **Other specified disorders of lacrimal gland**

√5th H04.2 **Epiphora**

DEF: Excessive tearing or overflow of tears down the cheeks often due to a stricture in the lacrimal passages but can be caused by other conditions.

√6th H04.20 **Unspecified epiphora**

H04.201 **Unspecified epiphora**, right side

H04.202 **Unspecified epiphora**, left side

H04.203 **Unspecified epiphora**, bilateral

H04.209 **Unspecified epiphora**, unspecified side

√6th H04.21 **Epiphora** due to excess lacrimation

H04.211 **Epiphora due to excess lacrimation**, right lacrimal gland

H04.212 **Epiphora due to excess lacrimation**, left lacrimal gland

H04.213 **Epiphora due to excess lacrimation**, bilateral **lacrimal glands**

H04.219 **Epiphora due to excess lacrimation**, unspecified lacrimal gland

√6th H04.22 **Epiphora** due to insufficient drainage

H04.221 **Epiphora due to insufficient drainage**, right side

H04.222 **Epiphora due to insufficient drainage**, left side

H04.223 **Epiphora due to insufficient drainage**, bilateral

H04.229 **Epiphora due to insufficient drainage**, unspecified side

√5th H04.3 **Acute and unspecified inflammation of lacrimal passages**

EXCLUDES 1   *neonatal dacryocystitis (P39.1)*

√6th H04.30 **Unspecified dacryocystitis**

H04.301 **Unspecified dacryocystitis of** right lacrimal passage

H04.302 **Unspecified dacryocystitis of** left lacrimal passage

H04.303 **Unspecified dacryocystitis of** bilateral lacrimal passages

H04.309 **Unspecified dacryocystitis of** unspecified lacrimal passage

√6th H04.31 **Phlegmonous dacryocystitis**

H04.311 **Phlegmonous dacryocystitis of** right lacrimal passage

H04.312 **Phlegmonous dacryocystitis of** left lacrimal passage

H04.313 **Phlegmonous dacryocystitis of** bilateral lacrimal passages

H04.319 **Phlegmonous dacryocystitis of** unspecified lacrimal passage

√6th H04.32 **Acute dacryocystitis**

Acute dacryopericystitis

H04.321 **Acute dacryocystitis of** right lacrimal passage

H04.322 **Acute dacryocystitis of** left lacrimal passage

H04.323 **Acute dacryocystitis of** bilateral lacrimal passages

H04.329 **Acute dacryocystitis of** unspecified lacrimal passage

√6th H04.33 **Acute lacrimal canaliculitis**

H04.331 **Acute lacrimal canaliculitis of** right lacrimal passage

H04.332 **Acute lacrimal canaliculitis of** left lacrimal passage

H04.333 **Acute lacrimal canaliculitis of** bilateral lacrimal passages

H04.339 **Acute lacrimal canaliculitis of** unspecified lacrimal passage

√5th H04.4 **Chronic inflammation of lacrimal passages**

√6th H04.41 **Chronic dacryocystitis**

H04.411 **Chronic dacryocystitis of** right lacrimal passage

H04.412 **Chronic dacryocystitis of** left lacrimal passage

H04.413 **Chronic dacryocystitis of** bilateral lacrimal passages

H04.419 **Chronic dacryocystitis of** unspecified lacrimal passage

√6th H04.42 **Chronic lacrimal canaliculitis**

H04.421 **Chronic lacrimal canaliculitis of** right lacrimal passage

H04.422 **Chronic lacrimal canaliculitis of** left lacrimal passage

H04.423 **Chronic lacrimal canaliculitis of** bilateral lacrimal passages

H04.429 **Chronic lacrimal canaliculitis of** unspecified lacrimal passage

√6th H04.43 **Chronic lacrimal mucocele**

H04.431 **Chronic lacrimal mucocele of** right lacrimal passage

H04.432 **Chronic lacrimal mucocele of** left lacrimal passage

H04.433 **Chronic lacrimal mucocele of** bilateral lacrimal passages

H04.439 **Chronic lacrimal mucocele of** unspecified lacrimal passage

√5th H04.5 **Stenosis and insufficiency of lacrimal passages**

√6th H04.51 **Dacryolith**

H04.511 **Dacryolith of** right lacrimal passage

H04.512 **Dacryolith of** left lacrimal passage

H04.513 **Dacryolith of** bilateral lacrimal passages

H04.519 **Dacryolith of** unspecified lacrimal passage

√6th H04.52 **Eversion** of lacrimal punctum

H04.521 **Eversion of** right lacrimal punctum

H04.522 **Eversion of** left lacrimal punctum

H04.523 **Eversion of** bilateral lacrimal punctum

H04.529 **Eversion of** unspecified lacrimal punctum

√6th H04.53 **Neonatal obstruction** of nasolacrimal duct

EXCLUDES 1   *congenital stenosis and stricture of lacrimal duct (Q10.5)*

H04.531 **Neonatal obstruction of** right nasolacrimal duct   N

H04.532 **Neonatal obstruction of** left nasolacrimal duct   N

H04.533 **Neonatal obstruction of** bilateral nasolacrimal duct   N

H04.539 **Neonatal obstruction of** unspecified nasolacrimal duct   N

√6th H04.54 **Stenosis of lacrimal** canaliculi

H04.541 **Stenosis of** right lacrimal canaliculi

H04.542 **Stenosis of** left lacrimal canaliculi

H04.543 **Stenosis of** bilateral lacrimal canaliculi

H04.549 **Stenosis of** unspecified lacrimal canaliculi

√6th H04.55 **Acquired stenosis of nasolacrimal** duct

H04.551 **Acquired stenosis of** right nasolacrimal duct

H04.552 **Acquired stenosis of** left nasolacrimal duct

H04.553 **Acquired stenosis of** bilateral nasolacrimal duct

H04.559 **Acquired stenosis of** unspecified nasolacrimal duct

√6th H04.56 **Stenosis of lacrimal** punctum

H04.561 **Stenosis of** right lacrimal punctum

H04.562 **Stenosis of** left lacrimal punctum

H04.563 **Stenosis of** bilateral lacrimal punctum

H04.569 **Stenosis of** unspecified lacrimal punctum

√6th H04.57 **Stenosis of lacrimal** sac

H04.571 **Stenosis of** right lacrimal sac

H04.572 **Stenosis of** left lacrimal sac

H04.573 **Stenosis of** bilateral lacrimal sac

H04.579 **Stenosis of** unspecified lacrimal sac

✔ Additional Character Required   √x7th Placeholder   Questionable PDx   Manifestation   Unspecified Dx   UPD Unacceptable PDx   H1-H14 HAC   HCC CMS-HCC Dx   HIV HIV Dx

ICD-10-CM 2022   601

Chapter 7. Diseases of the Eye and Adnexa

H04.6–H05.422

√5ᵗʰ **H04.6** **Other changes of lacrimal passages**
    √6ᵗʰ **H04.61** **Lacrimal fistula**
        H04.611 Lacrimal fistula right lacrimal passage   SW
        H04.612 Lacrimal fistula left lacrimal passage   SW
        H04.613 Lacrimal fistula bilateral lacrimal passages   SW
        H04.619 Lacrimal fistula unspecified lacrimal passage   SW
    H04.69 Other changes of lacrimal passages
  √6ᵗʰ **H04.8** **Other disorders of lacrimal system**
    √6ᵗʰ **H04.81** **Granuloma of lacrimal passages**
        H04.811 Granuloma of right lacrimal passage
        H04.812 Granuloma of left lacrimal passage
        H04.813 Granuloma of bilateral lacrimal passages
        H04.819 Granuloma of unspecified lacrimal passage
    H04.89 Other disorders of lacrimal system
  H04.9 **Disorder of lacrimal system, unspecified**

√4ᵗʰ **H05** **Disorders of orbit**
    EXCLUDES 1   congenital malformation of orbit (Q10.7)
  √5ᵗʰ **H05.0** **Acute inflammation of orbit**
    H05.00 **Unspecified acute inflammation of orbit**
    √6ᵗʰ **H05.01** **Cellulitis of orbit**
        Abscess of orbit
        H05.011 **Cellulitis of right orbit**   CC
        H05.012 **Cellulitis of left orbit**   CC
        H05.013 **Cellulitis of bilateral orbits**   CC
        H05.019 **Cellulitis of unspecified orbit**   CC
    √6ᵗʰ **H05.02** **Osteomyelitis of orbit**
        H05.021 **Osteomyelitis of right orbit**   CC
        H05.022 **Osteomyelitis of left orbit**   CC
        H05.023 **Osteomyelitis of bilateral orbits**   CC
        H05.029 **Osteomyelitis of unspecified orbit**   CC
    √6ᵗʰ **H05.03** **Periostitis of orbit**
        H05.031 **Periostitis of right orbit**   CC
        H05.032 **Periostitis of left orbit**   CC
        H05.033 **Periostitis of bilateral orbits**   CC
        H05.039 **Periostitis of unspecified orbit**   CC
    √6ᵗʰ **H05.04** **Tenonitis of orbit**
        H05.041 **Tenonitis of right orbit**
        H05.042 **Tenonitis of left orbit**
        H05.043 **Tenonitis of bilateral orbits**
        H05.049 **Tenonitis of unspecified orbit**
  √5ᵗʰ **H05.1** **Chronic inflammatory disorders of orbit**
    H05.10 **Unspecified chronic inflammatory disorders of orbit**
    √6ᵗʰ **H05.11** **Granuloma of orbit**
        Pseudotumor (inflammatory) of orbit
        H05.111 **Granuloma of right orbit**
        H05.112 **Granuloma of left orbit**
        H05.113 **Granuloma of bilateral orbits**
        H05.119 **Granuloma of unspecified orbit**
    √6ᵗʰ **H05.12** **Orbital myositis**
        H05.121 **Orbital myositis, right orbit**
        H05.122 **Orbital myositis, left orbit**
        H05.123 **Orbital myositis, bilateral**
        H05.129 **Orbital myositis, unspecified orbit**
  √5ᵗʰ **H05.2** **Exophthalmic conditions**
    H05.20 **Unspecified exophthalmos**
    √6ᵗʰ **H05.21** **Displacement (lateral) of globe**
        H05.211 **Displacement (lateral) of globe, right eye**
        H05.212 **Displacement (lateral) of globe, left eye**
        H05.213 **Displacement (lateral) of globe, bilateral**
        H05.219 **Displacement (lateral) of globe, unspecified eye**
    √6ᵗʰ **H05.22** **Edema of orbit**
        Orbital congestion
        H05.221 **Edema of right orbit**
        H05.222 **Edema of left orbit**
        H05.223 **Edema of bilateral orbit**
        H05.229 **Edema of unspecified orbit**
    √6ᵗʰ **H05.23** **Hemorrhage of orbit**
        H05.231 **Hemorrhage of right orbit**

H05.232 **Hemorrhage of left orbit**
H05.233 **Hemorrhage of bilateral orbit**
H05.239 **Hemorrhage of unspecified orbit**
  √6ᵗʰ **H05.24** **Constant exophthalmos**
    H05.241 **Constant exophthalmos, right eye**
    H05.242 **Constant exophthalmos, left eye**
    H05.243 **Constant exophthalmos, bilateral**
    H05.249 **Constant exophthalmos, unspecified eye**
  √6ᵗʰ **H05.25** **Intermittent exophthalmos**
    H05.251 **Intermittent exophthalmos, right eye**
    H05.252 **Intermittent exophthalmos, left eye**
    H05.253 **Intermittent exophthalmos, bilateral**
    H05.259 **Intermittent exophthalmos, unspecified eye**
  √6ᵗʰ **H05.26** **Pulsating exophthalmos**
    H05.261 **Pulsating exophthalmos, right eye**
    H05.262 **Pulsating exophthalmos, left eye**
    H05.263 **Pulsating exophthalmos, bilateral**
    H05.269 **Pulsating exophthalmos, unspecified eye**
  √5ᵗʰ **H05.3** **Deformity of orbit**
    EXCLUDES 1   congenital deformity of orbit (Q10.7)
        hypertelorism (Q75.2)
    H05.30 **Unspecified deformity of orbit**
    √6ᵗʰ **H05.31** **Atrophy of orbit**
        H05.311 **Atrophy of right orbit**
        H05.312 **Atrophy of left orbit**
        H05.313 **Atrophy of bilateral orbit**
        H05.319 **Atrophy of unspecified orbit**
    √6ᵗʰ **H05.32** **Deformity of orbit due to bone disease**
        Code also associated bone disease
        H05.321 **Deformity of right orbit due to bone disease**
        H05.322 **Deformity of left orbit due to bone disease**
        H05.323 **Deformity of bilateral orbits due to bone disease**
        H05.329 **Deformity of unspecified orbit due to bone disease**
    √6ᵗʰ **H05.33** **Deformity of orbit due to trauma or surgery**
        H05.331 **Deformity of right orbit due to trauma or surgery**
        H05.332 **Deformity of left orbit due to trauma or surgery**
        H05.333 **Deformity of bilateral orbits due to trauma or surgery**
        H05.339 **Deformity of unspecified orbit due to trauma or surgery**
    √6ᵗʰ **H05.34** **Enlargement of orbit**
        H05.341 **Enlargement of right orbit**
        H05.342 **Enlargement of left orbit**
        H05.343 **Enlargement of bilateral orbits**
        H05.349 **Enlargement of unspecified orbit**
    √6ᵗʰ **H05.35** **Exostosis of orbit**
        H05.351 **Exostosis of right orbit**
        H05.352 **Exostosis of left orbit**
        H05.353 **Exostosis of bilateral orbits**
        H05.359 **Exostosis of unspecified orbit**
  √5ᵗʰ **H05.4** **Enophthalmos**
    √6ᵗʰ **H05.40** **Unspecified enophthalmos**
        H05.401 **Unspecified enophthalmos, right eye**
        H05.402 **Unspecified enophthalmos, left eye**
        H05.403 **Unspecified enophthalmos, bilateral**
        H05.409 **Unspecified enophthalmos, unspecified eye**
    √6ᵗʰ **H05.41** **Enophthalmos due to atrophy of orbital tissue**
        H05.411 **Enophthalmos due to atrophy of orbital tissue, right eye**
        H05.412 **Enophthalmos due to atrophy of orbital tissue, left eye**
        H05.413 **Enophthalmos due to atrophy of orbital tissue, bilateral**
        H05.419 **Enophthalmos due to atrophy of orbital tissue, unspecified eye**
    √6ᵗʰ **H05.42** **Enophthalmos due to trauma or surgery**
        H05.421 **Enophthalmos due to trauma or surgery, right eye**
        H05.422 **Enophthalmos due to trauma or surgery, left eye**

H05.423   **Enophthalmos due to trauma or surgery, bilateral**

H05.429   **Enophthalmos due to trauma or surgery, unspecified eye**

√5ᵗʰ H05.5   **Retained (old) foreign body following penetrating wound of orbit**

Retrobulbar foreign body

Use additional code to identify the type of retained foreign body (Z18.-)

EXCLUDES 1   *current penetrating wound of orbit (S05.4-)*

EXCLUDES 2   *retained foreign body of eyelid (H02.81-)*

retained intraocular foreign body (H44.6-, H44.7-)

H05.50   **Retained (old) foreign body following penetrating wound of unspecified orbit**

H05.51   **Retained (old) foreign body following penetrating wound of right orbit**

H05.52   **Retained (old) foreign body following penetrating wound of left orbit**

H05.53   **Retained (old) foreign body following penetrating wound of bilateral orbits**

√5ᵗʰ H05.8   **Other disorders of orbit**

√6ᵗʰ H05.81   **Cyst of orbit**

Encephalocele of orbit

H05.811   **Cyst of right orbit**

H05.812   **Cyst of left orbit**

H05.813   **Cyst of bilateral orbits**

H05.819   **Cyst of unspecified orbit**

√6ᵗʰ H05.82   **Myopathy of extraocular muscles**

H05.821   **Myopathy of extraocular muscles, right orbit**

H05.822   **Myopathy of extraocular muscles, left orbit**

H05.823   **Myopathy of extraocular muscles, bilateral**

H05.829   **Myopathy of extraocular muscles, unspecified orbit**

H05.89   **Other disorders of orbit**

H05.9   **Unspecified disorder of orbit**

Disorders of conjunctiva (H10-H11)

√4ᵗʰ **H10   Conjunctivitis**

EXCLUDES 1   *keratoconjunctivitis (H16.2-)*

√5ᵗʰ H10.0   **Mucopurulent conjunctivitis**

√6ᵗʰ H10.01   **Acute follicular conjunctivitis**

H10.011   **Acute follicular conjunctivitis, right eye**

H10.012   **Acute follicular conjunctivitis, left eye**

H10.013   **Acute follicular conjunctivitis, bilateral**

H10.019   **Acute follicular conjunctivitis, unspecified eye**

√6ᵗʰ H10.02   **Other mucopurulent conjunctivitis**

H10.021   **Other mucopurulent conjunctivitis, right eye**

H10.022   **Other mucopurulent conjunctivitis, left eye**

H10.023   **Other mucopurulent conjunctivitis, bilateral**

H10.029   **Other mucopurulent conjunctivitis, unspecified eye**

√5ᵗʰ H10.1   **Acute atopic conjunctivitis**

Acute papillary conjunctivitis

H10.10   **Acute atopic conjunctivitis, unspecified eye**

H10.11   **Acute atopic conjunctivitis, right eye**

H10.12   **Acute atopic conjunctivitis, left eye**

H10.13   **Acute atopic conjunctivitis, bilateral**

√5ᵗʰ H10.2   **Other acute conjunctivitis**

√6ᵗʰ H10.21   **Acute toxic conjunctivitis**

Acute chemical conjunctivitis

Code first (T51-T65) to identify chemical and intent

EXCLUDES 1   *burn and corrosion of eye and adnexa (T26.-)*

H10.211   **Acute toxic conjunctivitis, right eye**

H10.212   **Acute toxic conjunctivitis, left eye**

H10.213   **Acute toxic conjunctivitis, bilateral**

H10.219   **Acute toxic conjunctivitis, unspecified eye**

√6ᵗʰ H10.22   **Pseudomembranous conjunctivitis**

H10.221   **Pseudomembranous conjunctivitis, right eye**

H10.222   **Pseudomembranous conjunctivitis, left eye**

H10.223   **Pseudomembranous conjunctivitis, bilateral**

H10.229   **Pseudomembranous conjunctivitis, unspecified eye**

√6ᵗʰ H10.23   **Serous conjunctivitis, except viral**

EXCLUDES 1   *viral conjunctivitis (B30.-)*

H10.231   **Serous conjunctivitis, except viral, right eye**

H10.232   **Serous conjunctivitis, except viral, left eye**

H10.233   **Serous conjunctivitis, except viral, bilateral**

H10.239   **Serous conjunctivitis, except viral, unspecified eye**

√5ᵗʰ H10.3   **Unspecified acute conjunctivitis**

EXCLUDES 1   *ophthalmia neonatorum NOS (P39.1)*

H10.30   **Unspecified acute conjunctivitis, unspecified eye**

H10.31   **Unspecified acute conjunctivitis, right eye**

H10.32   **Unspecified acute conjunctivitis, left eye**

H10.33   **Unspecified acute conjunctivitis, bilateral**

√5ᵗʰ H10.4   **Chronic conjunctivitis**

√6ᵗʰ H10.40   **Unspecified chronic conjunctivitis**

H10.401   **Unspecified chronic conjunctivitis, right eye**

H10.402   **Unspecified chronic conjunctivitis, left eye**

H10.403   **Unspecified chronic conjunctivitis, bilateral**

H10.409   **Unspecified chronic conjunctivitis, unspecified eye**

√6ᵗʰ H10.41   **Chronic giant papillary conjunctivitis**

H10.411   **Chronic giant papillary conjunctivitis, right eye**

H10.412   **Chronic giant papillary conjunctivitis, left eye**

H10.413   **Chronic giant papillary conjunctivitis, bilateral**

H10.419   **Chronic giant papillary conjunctivitis, unspecified eye**

√6ᵗʰ H10.42   **Simple chronic conjunctivitis**

H10.421   **Simple chronic conjunctivitis, right eye**

H10.422   **Simple chronic conjunctivitis, left eye**

H10.423   **Simple chronic conjunctivitis, bilateral**

H10.429   **Simple chronic conjunctivitis, unspecified eye**

√6ᵗʰ H10.43   **Chronic follicular conjunctivitis**

H10.431   **Chronic follicular conjunctivitis, right eye**

H10.432   **Chronic follicular conjunctivitis, left eye**

H10.433   **Chronic follicular conjunctivitis, bilateral**

H10.439   **Chronic follicular conjunctivitis, unspecified eye**

H10.44   **Vernal conjunctivitis**

EXCLUDES 1   *vernal keratoconjunctivitis with limbar and corneal involvement (H16.26-)*

H10.45   **Other chronic allergic conjunctivitis**

√5ᵗʰ H10.5   **Blepharoconjunctivitis**

√6ᵗʰ H10.50   **Unspecified blepharoconjunctivitis**

H10.501   **Unspecified blepharoconjunctivitis, right eye**

H10.502   **Unspecified blepharoconjunctivitis, left eye**

H10.503   **Unspecified blepharoconjunctivitis, bilateral**

H10.509   **Unspecified blepharoconjunctivitis, unspecified eye**

√6ᵗʰ H10.51   **Ligneous conjunctivitis**

Code also underlying condition if known, such as: plasminogen deficiency (E88.02)

H10.511   **Ligneous conjunctivitis, right eye**

H10.512   **Ligneous conjunctivitis, left eye**

H10.513   **Ligneous conjunctivitis, bilateral**

H10.519   **Ligneous conjunctivitis, unspecified eye**

✔ Additional Character Required   √x7ᵗʰ Placeholder   Questionable PDx   Manifestation   Unspecified Dx   UPD Unacceptable PDx   H1-H14 HAC   HCC CMS-HCC Dx   HIV HIV Dx

ICD-10-CM 2022   603

✓6ᵗʰ **H10.52** Angular **blepharoconjunctivitis**
- H10.521 Angular blepharoconjunctivitis, **right eye**
- H10.522 Angular blepharoconjunctivitis, **left eye**
- H10.523 Angular blepharoconjunctivitis, **bilateral**
- H10.529 Angular blepharoconjunctivitis, **unspecified eye**

✓6ᵗʰ **H10.53** Contact **blepharoconjunctivitis**
- H10.531 Contact blepharoconjunctivitis, **right eye**
- H10.532 Contact blepharoconjunctivitis, **left eye**
- H10.533 Contact blepharoconjunctivitis, **bilateral**
- H10.539 Contact blepharoconjunctivitis, **unspecified eye**

✓5ᵗʰ **H10.8 Other conjunctivitis**

✓6ᵗʰ **H10.81 Pingueculitis**

    EXCLUDES 1   *pinguecula (H11.15-)*
- H10.811 Pingueculitis, **right eye**
- H10.812 Pingueculitis, **left eye**
- H10.813 Pingueculitis, **bilateral**
- H10.819 Pingueculitis, **unspecified eye**

✓6ᵗʰ **H10.82 Rosacea conjunctivitis**

    Code first underlying rosacea dermatitis (L71.-)

    AHA: 2018,4Q,15
- H10.821 Rosacea conjunctivitis, **right eye**
- H10.822 Rosacea conjunctivitis, **left eye**
- H10.823 Rosacea conjunctivitis, **bilateral**
- H10.829 Rosacea conjunctivitis, **unspecified eye**

   H10.89 **Other conjunctivitis**

   H10.9 Unspecified conjunctivitis

✓4ᵗʰ **H11 Other disorders of conjunctiva**

    EXCLUDES 1   *keratoconjunctivitis (H16.2-)*

✓5ᵗʰ **H11.0 Pterygium of eye**

    EXCLUDES 1   *pseudopterygium (H11.81-)*

    DEF: Benign, wedge-shaped, conjunctival thickening that advances from the inner corner of the eye toward the cornea.

Pterygium

Pterygium

✓6ᵗʰ **H11.00 Unspecified pterygium of eye**
- H11.001 Unspecified pterygium of **right eye**
- H11.002 Unspecified pterygium of **left eye**
- H11.003 Unspecified pterygium of eye, **bilateral**
- H11.009 Unspecified pterygium of unspecified eye

✓6ᵗʰ **H11.01 Amyloid pterygium**
- H11.011 Amyloid pterygium of **right eye**
- H11.012 Amyloid pterygium of **left eye**
- H11.013 Amyloid pterygium of eye, **bilateral**
- H11.019 Amyloid pterygium of unspecified eye

✓6ᵗʰ **H11.02 Central pterygium of eye**
- H11.021 Central pterygium of **right eye**
- H11.022 Central pterygium of **left eye**
- H11.023 Central pterygium of eye, **bilateral**
- H11.029 Central pterygium of unspecified eye

✓6ᵗʰ **H11.03 Double pterygium of eye**
- H11.031 Double pterygium of **right eye**
- H11.032 Double pterygium of **left eye**
- H11.033 Double pterygium of eye, **bilateral**
- H11.039 Double pterygium of unspecified eye

✓6ᵗʰ **H11.04 Peripheral pterygium of eye, stationary**
- H11.041 Peripheral pterygium, stationary, **right eye**
- H11.042 Peripheral pterygium, stationary, **left eye**
- H11.043 Peripheral pterygium, stationary, **bilateral**
- H11.049 Peripheral pterygium, stationary, **unspecified eye**

✓6ᵗʰ **H11.05 Peripheral pterygium of eye, progressive**
- H11.051 Peripheral pterygium, progressive, **right eye**
- H11.052 Peripheral pterygium, progressive, **left eye**
- H11.053 Peripheral pterygium, progressive, **bilateral**
- H11.059 Peripheral pterygium, progressive, **unspecified eye**

✓6ᵗʰ **H11.06 Recurrent pterygium of eye**
- H11.061 Recurrent pterygium of **right eye**
- H11.062 Recurrent pterygium of **left eye**
- H11.063 Recurrent pterygium of eye, **bilateral**
- H11.069 Recurrent pterygium of unspecified eye

✓5ᵗʰ **H11.1 Conjunctival degenerations and deposits**

    EXCLUDES 2   *pseudopterygium (H11.81)*

   H11.10 Unspecified conjunctival degenerations

✓6ᵗʰ **H11.11 Conjunctival deposits**
- H11.111 Conjunctival deposits, **right eye**
- H11.112 Conjunctival deposits, **left eye**
- H11.113 Conjunctival deposits, **bilateral**
- H11.119 Conjunctival deposits, **unspecified eye**

✓6ᵗʰ **H11.12 Conjunctival concretions**
- H11.121 Conjunctival concretions, **right eye**
- H11.122 Conjunctival concretions, **left eye**
- H11.123 Conjunctival concretions, **bilateral**
- H11.129 Conjunctival concretions, **unspecified eye**

✓6ᵗʰ **H11.13 Conjunctival pigmentations**

    Conjunctival argyrosis [argyria]
- H11.131 Conjunctival pigmentations, **right eye**
- H11.132 Conjunctival pigmentations, **left eye**
- H11.133 Conjunctival pigmentations, **bilateral**
- H11.139 Conjunctival pigmentations, **unspecified eye**

✓6ᵗʰ **H11.14 Conjunctival xerosis, unspecified**

    EXCLUDES 1   *xerosis of conjunctiva due to vitamin A deficiency (E50.0, E50.1)*

    DEF: Abnormal dryness of the conjunctiva due to lack of sufficient tears or conjunctival secretions.
- H11.141 Conjunctival xerosis, unspecified, **right eye**
- H11.142 Conjunctival xerosis, unspecified, **left eye**
- H11.143 Conjunctival xerosis, unspecified, **bilateral**
- H11.149 Conjunctival xerosis, unspecified, **unspecified eye**

✓6ᵗʰ **H11.15 Pinguecula**

    EXCLUDES 1   *pingueculitis (H10.81-)*

    DEF: Proliferation on the conjunctiva near the sclerocorneal junction, usually of the side of the nose and usually in older patients.

Pinguecula

Pinguecula
- H11.151 Pinguecula, **right eye**
- H11.152 Pinguecula, **left eye**
- H11.153 Pinguecula, **bilateral**
- H11.159 Pinguecula, **unspecified eye**

✓5ᵗʰ **H11.2 Conjunctival scars**

✓6ᵗʰ **H11.21 Conjunctival adhesions and strands (localized)**
- H11.211 Conjunctival adhesions and strands (localized), **right eye**
- H11.212 Conjunctival adhesions and strands (localized), **left eye**
- H11.213 Conjunctival adhesions and strands (localized), **bilateral**
- H11.219 Conjunctival adhesions and strands (localized), **unspecified eye**

N Newborn: 0   P Pediatric: 0-17   M Maternity: 9-64   A Adult: 15-124   MCC Major Complication/Comorbidity   CC Complication/Comorbidity   SW Severe Wound Dx

604   ICD-10-CM 2022

√6ᵗʰ **H11.22 Conjunctival** granuloma

     H11.221 Conjunctival granuloma, right eye

     H11.222 Conjunctival granuloma, left eye

     H11.223 Conjunctival granuloma, bilateral

     H11.229 Conjunctival granuloma, unspecified

√6ᵗʰ **H11.23 Symblepharon**

     H11.231 Symblepharon, right eye

     H11.232 Symblepharon, left eye

     H11.233 Symblepharon, bilateral

     H11.239 Symblepharon, unspecified eye

√6ᵗʰ **H11.24 Scarring of conjunctiva**

     H11.241 Scarring of conjunctiva, right eye

     H11.242 Scarring of conjunctiva, left eye

     H11.243 Scarring of conjunctiva, bilateral

     H11.249 Scarring of conjunctiva, unspecified eye

√5ᵗʰ **H11.3 Conjunctival hemorrhage**

     Subconjunctival hemorrhage

     H11.30 Conjunctival hemorrhage, unspecified eye

     H11.31 Conjunctival hemorrhage, right eye

     H11.32 Conjunctival hemorrhage, left eye

     H11.33 Conjunctival hemorrhage, bilateral

√5ᵗʰ **H11.4 Other conjunctival vascular disorders and cysts**

√6ᵗʰ **H11.41 Vascular abnormalities of conjunctiva**

     Conjunctival aneurysm

     H11.411 Vascular abnormalities of conjunctiva, right eye

     H11.412 Vascular abnormalities of conjunctiva, left eye

     H11.413 Vascular abnormalities of conjunctiva, bilateral

     H11.419 Vascular abnormalities of conjunctiva, unspecified eye

√6ᵗʰ **H11.42 Conjunctival edema**

     H11.421 Conjunctival edema, right eye

     H11.422 Conjunctival edema, left eye

     H11.423 Conjunctival edema, bilateral

     H11.429 Conjunctival edema, unspecified eye

√6ᵗʰ **H11.43 Conjunctival hyperemia**

     H11.431 Conjunctival hyperemia, right eye

     H11.432 Conjunctival hyperemia, left eye

     H11.433 Conjunctival hyperemia, bilateral

     H11.439 Conjunctival hyperemia, unspecified eye

√6ᵗʰ **H11.44 Conjunctival cysts**

     H11.441 Conjunctival cysts, right eye

     H11.442 Conjunctival cysts, left eye

     H11.443 Conjunctival cysts, bilateral

     H11.449 Conjunctival cysts, unspecified eye

√5ᵗʰ **H11.8 Other specified disorders of conjunctiva**

√6ᵗʰ **H11.81 Pseudopterygium of conjunctiva**

     H11.811 Pseudopterygium of conjunctiva, right eye

     H11.812 Pseudopterygium of conjunctiva, left eye

     H11.813 Pseudopterygium of conjunctiva, bilateral

     H11.819 Pseudopterygium of conjunctiva, unspecified eye

√6ᵗʰ **H11.82 Conjunctivochalasis**

     H11.821 Conjunctivochalasis, right eye

     H11.822 Conjunctivochalasis, left eye

     H11.823 Conjunctivochalasis, bilateral

     H11.829 Conjunctivochalasis, unspecified eye

     H11.89 Other specified disorders of conjunctiva

H11.9 Unspecified disorder of conjunctiva

Disorders of sclera, cornea, iris and ciliary body (H15-H22)

√4ᵗʰ **H15 Disorders of sclera**

√5ᵗʰ **H15.0 Scleritis**

√6ᵗʰ **H15.00 Unspecified scleritis**

     H15.001 Unspecified scleritis, right eye

     H15.002 Unspecified scleritis, left eye

     H15.003 Unspecified scleritis, bilateral

     H15.009 Unspecified scleritis, unspecified eye

√6ᵗʰ **H15.01 Anterior scleritis**

     H15.011 Anterior scleritis, right eye

     H15.012 Anterior scleritis, left eye

     H15.013 Anterior scleritis, bilateral

     H15.019 Anterior scleritis, unspecified eye

√6ᵗʰ **H15.02 Brawny scleritis**

     H15.021 Brawny scleritis, right eye

     H15.022 Brawny scleritis, left eye

     H15.023 Brawny scleritis, bilateral

     H15.029 Brawny scleritis, unspecified eye

√6ᵗʰ **H15.03 Posterior scleritis**

     Sclerotenonitis

     H15.031 Posterior scleritis, right eye

     H15.032 Posterior scleritis, left eye

     H15.033 Posterior scleritis, bilateral

     H15.039 Posterior scleritis, unspecified eye

√6ᵗʰ **H15.04 Scleritis with corneal involvement**

     H15.041 Scleritis with corneal involvement, right eye

     H15.042 Scleritis with corneal involvement, left eye

     H15.043 Scleritis with corneal involvement, bilateral

     H15.049 Scleritis with corneal involvement, unspecified eye

√6ᵗʰ **H15.05 Scleromalacia perforans**

     H15.051 Scleromalacia perforans, right eye

     H15.052 Scleromalacia perforans, left eye

     H15.053 Scleromalacia perforans, bilateral

     H15.059 Scleromalacia perforans, unspecified eye

√6ᵗʰ **H15.09 Other scleritis**

     Scleral abscess

     H15.091 Other scleritis, right eye

     H15.092 Other scleritis, left eye

     H15.093 Other scleritis, bilateral

     H15.099 Other scleritis, unspecified eye

√5ᵗʰ **H15.1 Episcleritis**

√6ᵗʰ **H15.10 Unspecified episcleritis**

     H15.101 Unspecified episcleritis, right eye

     H15.102 Unspecified episcleritis, left eye

     H15.103 Unspecified episcleritis, bilateral

     H15.109 Unspecified episcleritis, unspecified eye

√6ᵗʰ **H15.11 Episcleritis periodica fugax**

     H15.111 Episcleritis periodica fugax, right eye

     H15.112 Episcleritis periodica fugax, left eye

     H15.113 Episcleritis periodica fugax, bilateral

     H15.119 Episcleritis periodica fugax, unspecified eye

√6ᵗʰ **H15.12 Nodular episcleritis**

     H15.121 Nodular episcleritis, right eye

     H15.122 Nodular episcleritis, left eye

     H15.123 Nodular episcleritis, bilateral

     H15.129 Nodular episcleritis, unspecified eye

√5ᵗʰ **H15.8 Other disorders of sclera**

     EXCLUDES 2   blue sclera (Q13.5)

              degenerative myopia (H44.2-)

√6ᵗʰ **H15.81 Equatorial staphyloma**

     H15.811 Equatorial staphyloma, right eye

     H15.812 Equatorial staphyloma, left eye

     H15.813 Equatorial staphyloma, bilateral

     H15.819 Equatorial staphyloma, unspecified eye

√6ᵗʰ **H15.82 Localized anterior staphyloma**

     H15.821 Localized anterior staphyloma, right eye

     H15.822 Localized anterior staphyloma, left eye

     H15.823 Localized anterior staphyloma, bilateral

     H15.829 Localized anterior staphyloma, unspecified eye

√6ᵗʰ **H15.83 Staphyloma posticum**

     H15.831 Staphyloma posticum, right eye

     H15.832 Staphyloma posticum, left eye

     H15.833 Staphyloma posticum, bilateral

     H15.839 Staphyloma posticum, unspecified eye

√6ᵗʰ **H15.84 Scleral ectasia**

     H15.841 Scleral ectasia, right eye

     H15.842 Scleral ectasia, left eye

     H15.843 Scleral ectasia, bilateral

     H15.849 Scleral ectasia, unspecified eye

√6ᵗʰ **H15.85 Ring staphyloma**

     H15.851 Ring staphyloma, right eye

✓ Additional Character Required   √x7ᵗʰ Placeholder   Questionable PDx   Manifestation   Unspecified Dx   UPD Unacceptable PDx   H1-H14 HAC   HCC CMS-HCC Dx   HIV HIV Dx

Chapter 7. Diseases of the Eye and Adnexa

H15.852–H16.302

H15.852 **Ring staphyloma**, left eye
H15.853 **Ring staphyloma**, bilateral
H15.859 **Ring staphyloma, unspecified eye**
H15.89 **Other disorders of sclera**
H15.9 **Unspecified disorder of sclera**

☑4ᵗʰ **H16 Keratitis**
DEF: Condition in which the cornea becomes inflamed and irritated.

☑5ᵗʰ **H16.0 Corneal ulcer**

☑6ᵗʰ **H16.00 Unspecified corneal ulcer**
H16.001 **Unspecified corneal ulcer,** right **eye**
H16.002 **Unspecified corneal ulcer,** left **eye**
H16.003 **Unspecified corneal ulcer,** bilateral
H16.009 **Unspecified corneal ulcer, unspecified eye**

☑6ᵗʰ **H16.01 Central corneal ulcer**
H16.011 **Central corneal ulcer,** right **eye**
H16.012 **Central corneal ulcer,** left **eye**
H16.013 **Central corneal ulcer,** bilateral
H16.019 **Central corneal ulcer, unspecified eye**

☑6ᵗʰ **H16.02 Ring corneal ulcer**
H16.021 **Ring corneal ulcer,** right **eye**
H16.022 **Ring corneal ulcer,** left **eye**
H16.023 **Ring corneal ulcer,** bilateral
H16.029 **Ring corneal ulcer, unspecified eye**

☑6ᵗʰ **H16.03 Corneal ulcer** with hypopyon
H16.031 **Corneal ulcer with hypopyon,** right **eye**
H16.032 **Corneal ulcer with hypopyon,** left **eye**
H16.033 **Corneal ulcer with hypopyon,** bilateral
H16.039 **Corneal ulcer with hypopyon, unspecified eye**

☑6ᵗʰ **H16.04 Marginal corneal ulcer**
H16.041 **Marginal corneal ulcer,** right **eye**
H16.042 **Marginal corneal ulcer,** left **eye**
H16.043 **Marginal corneal ulcer,** bilateral
H16.049 **Marginal corneal ulcer, unspecified eye**

☑6ᵗʰ **H16.05 Mooren's corneal ulcer**
H16.051 **Mooren's corneal ulcer,** right **eye**
H16.052 **Mooren's corneal ulcer,** left **eye**
H16.053 **Mooren's corneal ulcer,** bilateral
H16.059 **Mooren's corneal ulcer, unspecified eye**

☑6ᵗʰ **H16.06 Mycotic corneal ulcer**
H16.061 **Mycotic corneal ulcer,** right **eye**
H16.062 **Mycotic corneal ulcer,** left **eye**
H16.063 **Mycotic corneal ulcer,** bilateral
H16.069 **Mycotic corneal ulcer, unspecified eye**

☑6ᵗʰ **H16.07 Perforated corneal ulcer**
H16.071 **Perforated corneal ulcer,** right **eye**
H16.072 **Perforated corneal ulcer,** left **eye**
H16.073 **Perforated corneal ulcer,** bilateral
H16.079 **Perforated corneal ulcer, unspecified eye**

☑5ᵗʰ **H16.1 Other and unspecified superficial keratitis without conjunctivitis**

☑6ᵗʰ **H16.10 Unspecified superficial keratitis**
H16.101 **Unspecified superficial keratitis,** right **eye**
H16.102 **Unspecified superficial keratitis,** left **eye**
H16.103 **Unspecified superficial keratitis,** bilateral
H16.109 **Unspecified superficial keratitis, unspecified eye**

☑6ᵗʰ **H16.11 Macular keratitis**
Areolar keratitis
Nummular keratitis
Stellate keratitis
Striate keratitis
H16.111 **Macular keratitis,** right **eye**
H16.112 **Macular keratitis,** left **eye**
H16.113 **Macular keratitis,** bilateral
H16.119 **Macular keratitis, unspecified eye**

☑6ᵗʰ **H16.12 Filamentary keratitis**
H16.121 **Filamentary keratitis,** right **eye**
H16.122 **Filamentary keratitis,** left **eye**
H16.123 **Filamentary keratitis,** bilateral
H16.129 **Filamentary keratitis, unspecified eye**

☑6ᵗʰ **H16.13 Photokeratitis**
Snow blindness
Welders keratitis
H16.131 **Photokeratitis,** right **eye**

H16.132 **Photokeratitis,** left **eye**
H16.133 **Photokeratitis,** bilateral
H16.139 **Photokeratitis, unspecified eye**

☑6ᵗʰ **H16.14 Punctate keratitis**
H16.141 **Punctate keratitis,** right **eye**
H16.142 **Punctate keratitis,** left **eye**
H16.143 **Punctate keratitis,** bilateral
H16.149 **Punctate keratitis, unspecified eye**

☑5ᵗʰ **H16.2 Keratoconjunctivitis**

☑6ᵗʰ **H16.20 Unspecified keratoconjunctivitis**
Superficial keratitis with conjunctivitis NOS
H16.201 **Unspecified keratoconjunctivitis,** right **eye**
H16.202 **Unspecified keratoconjunctivitis,** left **eye**
H16.203 **Unspecified keratoconjunctivitis,** bilateral
H16.209 **Unspecified keratoconjunctivitis, unspecified eye**

☑6ᵗʰ **H16.21 Exposure keratoconjunctivitis**
H16.211 **Exposure keratoconjunctivitis,** right **eye**
H16.212 **Exposure keratoconjunctivitis,** left **eye**
H16.213 **Exposure keratoconjunctivitis,** bilateral
H16.219 **Exposure keratoconjunctivitis, unspecified eye**

☑6ᵗʰ **H16.22 Keratoconjunctivitis** sicca, not specified as Sjögren's
EXCLUDES 1   *Sjögren's syndrome (M35.01)*
H16.221 **Keratoconjunctivitis sicca, not specified as Sjögren's,** right **eye**
H16.222 **Keratoconjunctivitis sicca, not specified as Sjögren's,** left **eye**
H16.223 **Keratoconjunctivitis sicca, not specified as Sjögren's,** bilateral
H16.229 **Keratoconjunctivitis sicca, not specified as Sjögren's, unspecified eye**

☑6ᵗʰ **H16.23 Neurotrophic keratoconjunctivitis**
H16.231 **Neurotrophic keratoconjunctivitis,** right **eye**
H16.232 **Neurotrophic keratoconjunctivitis,** left **eye**
H16.233 **Neurotrophic keratoconjunctivitis,** bilateral
H16.239 **Neurotrophic keratoconjunctivitis, unspecified eye**

☑6ᵗʰ **H16.24 Ophthalmia nodosa**
H16.241 **Ophthalmia nodosa,** right **eye**
H16.242 **Ophthalmia nodosa,** left **eye**
H16.243 **Ophthalmia nodosa,** bilateral
H16.249 **Ophthalmia nodosa, unspecified eye**

☑6ᵗʰ **H16.25 Phlyctenular keratoconjunctivitis**
H16.251 **Phlyctenular keratoconjunctivitis,** right **eye**
H16.252 **Phlyctenular keratoconjunctivitis,** left **eye**
H16.253 **Phlyctenular keratoconjunctivitis,** bilateral
H16.259 **Phlyctenular keratoconjunctivitis, unspecified eye**

☑6ᵗʰ **H16.26 Vernal keratoconjunctivitis, with limbar and corneal involvement**
EXCLUDES 1   *vernal conjunctivitis without limbar and corneal involvement (H10.44)*
H16.261 **Vernal keratoconjunctivitis, with limbar and corneal involvement,** right **eye**
H16.262 **Vernal keratoconjunctivitis, with limbar and corneal involvement,** left **eye**
H16.263 **Vernal keratoconjunctivitis, with limbar and corneal involvement,** bilateral
H16.269 **Vernal keratoconjunctivitis, with limbar and corneal involvement, unspecified eye**

☑6ᵗʰ **H16.29 Other keratoconjunctivitis**
H16.291 **Other keratoconjunctivitis,** right **eye**
H16.292 **Other keratoconjunctivitis,** left **eye**
H16.293 **Other keratoconjunctivitis,** bilateral
H16.299 **Other keratoconjunctivitis, unspecified eye**

☑5ᵗʰ **H16.3 Interstitial and deep keratitis**

☑6ᵗʰ **H16.30 Unspecified interstitial keratitis**
H16.301 **Unspecified interstitial keratitis,** right **eye**
H16.302 **Unspecified interstitial keratitis,** left **eye**

        H16.303 **Unspecified interstitial keratitis,** bilateral
        H16.309 **Unspecified interstitial keratitis, unspecified eye**

☑6ᵗʰ **H16.31** Corneal **abscess**
        H16.311 **Corneal abscess,** right **eye**
        H16.312 **Corneal abscess,** left **eye**
        H16.313 **Corneal abscess,** bilateral
        H16.319 **Corneal abscess, unspecified eye**

☑6ᵗʰ **H16.32** Diffuse **interstitial keratitis**
        Cogan's syndrome
        H16.321 **Diffuse interstitial keratitis,** right **eye**
        H16.322 **Diffuse interstitial keratitis,** left **eye**
        H16.323 **Diffuse interstitial keratitis,** bilateral
        H16.329 **Diffuse interstitial keratitis, unspecified eye**

☑6ᵗʰ **H16.33** Sclerosing **keratitis**
        H16.331 **Sclerosing keratitis,** right **eye**
        H16.332 **Sclerosing keratitis,** left **eye**
        H16.333 **Sclerosing keratitis,** bilateral
        H16.339 **Sclerosing keratitis, unspecified eye**

☑6ᵗʰ **H16.39** Other **interstitial and deep keratitis**
        H16.391 **Other interstitial and deep keratitis,** right **eye**
        H16.392 **Other interstitial and deep keratitis,** left **eye**
        H16.393 **Other interstitial and deep keratitis,** bilateral
        H16.399 **Other interstitial and deep keratitis, unspecified eye**

☑5ᵗʰ **H16.4** Corneal **neovascularization**

☑6ᵗʰ **H16.40** Unspecified **corneal neovascularization**
        H16.401 **Unspecified corneal neovascularization,** right **eye**
        H16.402 **Unspecified corneal neovascularization,** left **eye**
        H16.403 **Unspecified corneal neovascularization,** bilateral
        H16.409 **Unspecified corneal neovascularization, unspecified eye**

☑6ᵗʰ **H16.41** Ghost **vessels (corneal)**
        H16.411 **Ghost vessels (corneal),** right **eye**
        H16.412 **Ghost vessels (corneal),** left **eye**
        H16.413 **Ghost vessels (corneal),** bilateral
        H16.419 **Ghost vessels (corneal), unspecified eye**

☑6ᵗʰ **H16.42** Pannus **(corneal)**
        H16.421 **Pannus (corneal),** right **eye**
        H16.422 **Pannus (corneal),** left **eye**
        H16.423 **Pannus (corneal),** bilateral
        H16.429 **Pannus (corneal), unspecified eye**

☑6ᵗʰ **H16.43** Localized **vascularization of cornea**
        H16.431 **Localized vascularization of cornea,** right **eye**
        H16.432 **Localized vascularization of cornea,** left **eye**
        H16.433 **Localized vascularization of cornea,** bilateral
        H16.439 **Localized vascularization of cornea, unspecified eye**

☑6ᵗʰ **H16.44** Deep **vascularization of cornea**
        H16.441 **Deep vascularization of cornea,** right **eye**
        H16.442 **Deep vascularization of cornea,** left **eye**
        H16.443 **Deep vascularization of cornea,** bilateral
        H16.449 **Deep vascularization of cornea, unspecified eye**

H16.8 **Other keratitis**   UPD
H16.9 **Unspecified keratitis**

☑4ᵗʰ **H17** **Corneal scars and opacities**

☑5ᵗʰ **H17.0** **Adherent leukoma**
        H17.00 **Adherent leukoma, unspecified eye**
        H17.01 **Adherent leukoma,** right **eye**
        H17.02 **Adherent leukoma,** left **eye**
        H17.03 **Adherent leukoma,** bilateral

☑5ᵗʰ **H17.1** **Central corneal opacity**
        H17.10 **Central corneal opacity, unspecified eye**
        H17.11 **Central corneal opacity,** right **eye**
        H17.12 **Central corneal opacity,** left **eye**
        H17.13 **Central corneal opacity,** bilateral

☑5ᵗʰ **H17.8** **Other corneal scars and opacities**

☑6ᵗʰ **H17.81** Minor **opacity of cornea**
        Corneal nebula
        H17.811 **Minor opacity of cornea,** right **eye**
        H17.812 **Minor opacity of cornea,** left **eye**
        H17.813 **Minor opacity of cornea,** bilateral
        H17.819 **Minor opacity of cornea, unspecified eye**

☑6ᵗʰ **H17.82** Peripheral **opacity of cornea**
        H17.821 **Peripheral opacity of cornea,** right **eye**
        H17.822 **Peripheral opacity of cornea,** left **eye**
        H17.823 **Peripheral opacity of cornea,** bilateral
        H17.829 **Peripheral opacity of cornea, unspecified eye**

        H17.89 **Other corneal scars and opacities**

H17.9 **Unspecified corneal scar and opacity**

☑4ᵗʰ **H18** **Other disorders of cornea**

☑5ᵗʰ **H18.0** **Corneal pigmentations and deposits**

☑6ᵗʰ **H18.00** **Unspecified corneal deposit**
        H18.001 **Unspecified corneal deposit,** right **eye**
        H18.002 **Unspecified corneal deposit,** left **eye**
        H18.003 **Unspecified corneal deposit,** bilateral
        H18.009 **Unspecified corneal deposit, unspecified eye**

☑6ᵗʰ **H18.01** Anterior **corneal pigmentations**
        Staehli's line
        H18.011 **Anterior corneal pigmentations,** right **eye**
        H18.012 **Anterior corneal pigmentations,** left **eye**
        H18.013 **Anterior corneal pigmentations,** bilateral
        H18.019 **Anterior corneal pigmentations, unspecified eye**

☑6ᵗʰ **H18.02** Argentous **corneal deposits**
        H18.021 **Argentous corneal deposits,** right **eye**
        H18.022 **Argentous corneal deposits,** left **eye**
        H18.023 **Argentous corneal deposits,** bilateral
        H18.029 **Argentous corneal deposits, unspecified eye**

☑6ᵗʰ **H18.03** **Corneal deposits in** metabolic disorders
        Code also associated metabolic disorder
        H18.031 **Corneal deposits in metabolic disorders,** right **eye**
        H18.032 **Corneal deposits in metabolic disorders,** left **eye**
        H18.033 **Corneal deposits in metabolic disorders,** bilateral
        H18.039 **Corneal deposits in metabolic disorders, unspecified eye**

☑6ᵗʰ **H18.04** Kayser-Fleischer **ring**
        Code also associated Wilson's disease (E83.01)
        H18.041 **Kayser-Fleischer ring,** right **eye**
        H18.042 **Kayser-Fleischer ring,** left **eye**
        H18.043 **Kayser-Fleischer ring,** bilateral
        H18.049 **Kayser-Fleischer ring, unspecified eye**

☑6ᵗʰ **H18.05** Posterior **corneal pigmentations**
        Krukenberg's spindle
        H18.051 **Posterior corneal pigmentations,** right **eye**
        H18.052 **Posterior corneal pigmentations,** left **eye**
        H18.053 **Posterior corneal pigmentations,** bilateral
        H18.059 **Posterior corneal pigmentations, unspecified eye**

☑6ᵗʰ **H18.06** Stromal **corneal pigmentations**
        Hematocornea
        H18.061 **Stromal corneal pigmentations,** right **eye**
        H18.062 **Stromal corneal pigmentations,** left **eye**
        H18.063 **Stromal corneal pigmentations,** bilateral
        H18.069 **Stromal corneal pigmentations, unspecified eye**

☑5ᵗʰ **H18.1** **Bullous keratopathy**
        DEF: Corneal swelling due to a damaged corneal endothelium. Bullous keratopathy is characterized by recurring, rupturing epithelial blisters causing glaucoma, iridocyclitis, and Fuchs' dystrophy.
        H18.10 **Bullous keratopathy, unspecified eye**
        H18.11 **Bullous keratopathy,** right **eye**
        H18.12 **Bullous keratopathy,** left **eye**
        H18.13 **Bullous keratopathy,** bilateral

☑ Additional Character Required   √×7ᵗʰ Placeholder   Questionable PDx   Manifestation   Unspecified Dx   UPD Unacceptable PDx   H1-H14 HAC   HCC CMS-HCC Dx   HIV HIV Dx

ICD-10-CM 2022   607

✓5ᵗʰ **H18.2 Other and unspecified corneal edema**

H18.20 Unspecified corneal edema

✓6ᵗʰ **H18.21 Corneal edema** secondary to contact lens

> EXCLUDES 2 *other corneal disorders due to contact lens (H18.82-)*

H18.211 Corneal edema secondary to contact lens, right eye

H18.212 Corneal edema secondary to contact lens, left eye

H18.213 Corneal edema secondary to contact lens, bilateral

H18.219 Corneal edema secondary to contact lens, unspecified eye

✓6ᵗʰ **H18.22 Idiopathic corneal edema**

H18.221 Idiopathic corneal edema, right eye

H18.222 Idiopathic corneal edema, left eye

H18.223 Idiopathic corneal edema, bilateral

H18.229 Idiopathic corneal edema, unspecified eye

✓6ᵗʰ **H18.23 Secondary corneal edema**

H18.231 Secondary corneal edema, right eye

H18.232 Secondary corneal edema, left eye

H18.233 Secondary corneal edema, bilateral

H18.239 Secondary corneal edema, unspecified eye

✓5ᵗʰ **H18.3 Changes of corneal membranes**

H18.30 Unspecified corneal membrane change

✓6ᵗʰ **H18.31 Folds and rupture in** Bowman's membrane

H18.311 Folds and rupture in Bowman's membrane, right eye

H18.312 Folds and rupture in Bowman's membrane, left eye

H18.313 Folds and rupture in Bowman's membrane, bilateral

H18.319 Folds and rupture in Bowman's membrane, unspecified eye

✓6ᵗʰ **H18.32 Folds** in Descemet's membrane

H18.321 Folds in Descemet's membrane, right eye

H18.322 Folds in Descemet's membrane, left eye

H18.323 Folds in Descemet's membrane, bilateral

H18.329 Folds in Descemet's membrane, unspecified eye

✓6ᵗʰ **H18.33 Rupture** in Descemet's membrane

H18.331 Rupture in Descemet's membrane, right eye

H18.332 Rupture in Descemet's membrane, left eye

H18.333 Rupture in Descemet's membrane, bilateral

H18.339 Rupture in Descemet's membrane, unspecified eye

✓5ᵗʰ **H18.4 Corneal degeneration**

> EXCLUDES 1 *Mooren's ulcer (H16.0-)*
> *recurrent erosion of cornea (H18.83-)*

H18.40 Unspecified corneal degeneration

✓6ᵗʰ **H18.41 Arcus senilis**

Senile corneal changes

H18.411 Arcus senilis, right eye
H18.412 Arcus senilis, left eye
H18.413 Arcus senilis, bilateral
H18.419 Arcus senilis, unspecified eye

✓6ᵗʰ **H18.42 Band keratopathy**

H18.421 Band keratopathy, right eye
H18.422 Band keratopathy, left eye
H18.423 Band keratopathy, bilateral
H18.429 Band keratopathy, unspecified eye

H18.43 Other calcerous corneal degeneration

✓6ᵗʰ **H18.44 Keratomalacia**

> EXCLUDES 1 *keratomalacia due to vitamin A deficiency (E50.4)*

H18.441 Keratomalacia, right eye
H18.442 Keratomalacia, left eye
H18.443 Keratomalacia, bilateral
H18.449 Keratomalacia, unspecified eye

✓6ᵗʰ **H18.45 Nodular corneal degeneration**

H18.451 Nodular corneal degeneration, right eye
H18.452 Nodular corneal degeneration, left eye

H18.453 Nodular corneal degeneration, bilateral

H18.459 Nodular corneal degeneration, unspecified eye

✓6ᵗʰ **H18.46 Peripheral corneal degeneration**

H18.461 Peripheral corneal degeneration, right eye

H18.462 Peripheral corneal degeneration, left eye

H18.463 Peripheral corneal degeneration, bilateral

H18.469 Peripheral corneal degeneration, unspecified eye

H18.49 Other corneal degeneration

✓5ᵗʰ **H18.5 Hereditary corneal dystrophies**

AHA: 2020,4Q,24

✓6ᵗʰ **H18.50 Unspecified hereditary corneal dystrophies**

H18.501 Unspecified hereditary corneal dystrophies, right eye

H18.502 Unspecified hereditary corneal dystrophies, left eye

H18.503 Unspecified hereditary corneal dystrophies, bilateral

H18.509 Unspecified hereditary corneal dystrophies, unspecified eye

✓6ᵗʰ **H18.51 Endothelial corneal dystrophy**

Fuchs' dystrophy

H18.511 Endothelial corneal dystrophy, right eye

H18.512 Endothelial corneal dystrophy, left eye

H18.513 Endothelial corneal dystrophy, bilateral

H18.519 Endothelial corneal dystrophy, unspecified eye

✓6ᵗʰ **H18.52 Epithelial (juvenile) corneal dystrophy**

H18.521 Epithelial (juvenile) corneal dystrophy, right eye

H18.522 Epithelial (juvenile) corneal dystrophy, left eye

H18.523 Epithelial (juvenile) corneal dystrophy, bilateral

H18.529 Epithelial (juvenile) corneal dystrophy, unspecified eye

✓6ᵗʰ **H18.53 Granular corneal dystrophy**

H18.531 Granular corneal dystrophy, right eye
H18.532 Granular corneal dystrophy, left eye
H18.533 Granular corneal dystrophy, bilateral
H18.539 Granular corneal dystrophy, unspecified eye

✓6ᵗʰ **H18.54 Lattice corneal dystrophy**

H18.541 Lattice corneal dystrophy, right eye
H18.542 Lattice corneal dystrophy, left eye
H18.543 Lattice corneal dystrophy, bilateral
H18.549 Lattice corneal dystrophy, unspecified eye

✓6ᵗʰ **H18.55 Macular corneal dystrophy**

H18.551 Macular corneal dystrophy, right eye
H18.552 Macular corneal dystrophy, left eye
H18.553 Macular corneal dystrophy, bilateral
H18.559 Macular corneal dystrophy, unspecified eye

✓6ᵗʰ **H18.59 Other hereditary corneal dystrophies**

H18.591 Other hereditary corneal dystrophies, right eye

H18.592 Other hereditary corneal dystrophies, left eye

H18.593 Other hereditary corneal dystrophies, bilateral

H18.599 Other hereditary corneal dystrophies, unspecified eye

✓5ᵗʰ **H18.6 Keratoconus**

✓6ᵗʰ **H18.60 Keratoconus, unspecified**

H18.601 Keratoconus, unspecified, right eye
H18.602 Keratoconus, unspecified, left eye
H18.603 Keratoconus, unspecified, bilateral
H18.609 Keratoconus, unspecified, unspecified eye

✓6ᵗʰ **H18.61 Keratoconus, stable**

H18.611 Keratoconus, stable, right eye
H18.612 Keratoconus, stable, left eye
H18.613 Keratoconus, stable, bilateral
H18.619 Keratoconus, stable, unspecified eye

Ⓝ Newborn: 0   Ⓟ Pediatric: 0-17   Ⓜ Maternity: 9-64   Ⓐ Adult: 15-124   MCC Major Complication/Comorbidity   CC Complication/Comorbidity   SW Severe Wound Dx

608

ICD-10-CM 2022

✓6ᵗʰ **H18.62**   **Keratoconus,** unstable

     Acute hydrops

     H18.621   **Keratoconus, unstable,** right **eye**

     H18.622   **Keratoconus, unstable,** left **eye**

     H18.623   **Keratoconus, unstable,** bilateral

     H18.629   **Keratoconus, unstable, unspecified eye**

✓5ᵗʰ **H18.7**   **Other and unspecified corneal deformities**

     EXCLUDES 1   *congenital malformations of cornea (Q13.3-Q13.4)*

     H18.70   **Unspecified corneal deformity**

     ✓6ᵗʰ **H18.71**   **Corneal** ectasia

       H18.711   **Corneal ectasia,** right **eye**

       H18.712   **Corneal ectasia,** left **eye**

       H18.713   **Corneal ectasia,** bilateral

       H18.719   **Corneal ectasia, unspecified eye**

     ✓6ᵗʰ **H18.72**   **Corneal** staphyloma

       H18.721   **Corneal staphyloma,** right **eye**

       H18.722   **Corneal staphyloma,** left **eye**

       H18.723   **Corneal staphyloma,** bilateral

       H18.729   **Corneal staphyloma, unspecified eye**

     ✓6ᵗʰ **H18.73**   Descemetocele

       H18.731   **Descemetocele,** right **eye**

       H18.732   **Descemetocele,** left **eye**

       H18.733   **Descemetocele,** bilateral

       H18.739   **Descemetocele, unspecified eye**

     ✓6ᵗʰ **H18.79**   **Other corneal deformities**

       H18.791   **Other corneal deformities,** right **eye**

       H18.792   **Other corneal deformities,** left **eye**

       H18.793   **Other corneal deformities,** bilateral

       H18.799   **Other corneal deformities, unspecified eye**

✓5ᵗʰ **H18.8**   **Other specified disorders of cornea**

     ✓6ᵗʰ **H18.81**   **Anesthesia and hypoesthesia of cornea**

       H18.811   **Anesthesia and hypoesthesia of cornea,** right **eye**

       H18.812   **Anesthesia and hypoesthesia of cornea,** left **eye**

       H18.813   **Anesthesia and hypoesthesia of cornea,** bilateral

       H18.819   **Anesthesia and hypoesthesia of cornea, unspecified eye**

     ✓6ᵗʰ **H18.82**   **Corneal disorder due to contact lens**

       EXCLUDES 2   *corneal edema due to contact lens (H18.21-)*

       H18.821   **Corneal disorder due to contact lens,** right **eye**

       H18.822   **Corneal disorder due to contact lens,** left **eye**

       H18.823   **Corneal disorder due to contact lens,** bilateral

       H18.829   **Corneal disorder due to contact lens, unspecified eye**

     ✓6ᵗʰ **H18.83**   **Recurrent erosion of cornea**

       H18.831   **Recurrent erosion of cornea,** right **eye**

       H18.832   **Recurrent erosion of cornea,** left **eye**

       H18.833   **Recurrent erosion of cornea,** bilateral

       H18.839   **Recurrent erosion of cornea, unspecified eye**

     ✓6ᵗʰ **H18.89**   **Other specified disorders of cornea**

       H18.891   **Other specified disorders of cornea,** right **eye**

       H18.892   **Other specified disorders of cornea,** left **eye**

       H18.893   **Other specified disorders of cornea,** bilateral

       H18.899   **Other specified disorders of cornea, unspecified eye**

H18.9   **Unspecified disorder of cornea**

✓4ᵗʰ **H20**   **Iridocyclitis**

     ✓5ᵗʰ **H20.0**   **Acute and** subacute **iridocyclitis**

     Acute anterior uveitis

     Acute cyclitis

     Acute iritis

     Subacute anterior uveitis

     Subacute cyclitis

     Subacute iritis

     EXCLUDES 1   *iridocyclitis, iritis, uveitis (due to) (in) diabetes mellitus (E08-E13 with .39)*

       iridocyclitis, iritis, uveitis (due to) (in) diphtheria (A36.89)

       iridocyclitis, iritis, uveitis (due to) (in) gonococcal (A54.32)

       iridocyclitis, iritis, uveitis (due to) (in) herpes (simplex) (B00.51)

       iridocyclitis, iritis, uveitis (due to) (in) herpes zoster (B02.32)

       iridocyclitis, iritis, uveitis (due to) (in) late congenital syphilis (A50.39)

       iridocyclitis, iritis, uveitis (due to) (in) late syphilis (A52.71)

       iridocyclitis, iritis, uveitis (due to) (in) sarcoidosis (D86.83)

       iridocyclitis, iritis, uveitis (due to) (in) syphilis (A51.43)

       iridocyclitis, iritis, uveitis (due to) (in) toxoplasmosis (B58.09)

       iridocyclitis, iritis, uveitis (due to) (in) tuberculosis (A18.54)

       H20.00   **Unspecified acute and subacute iridocyclitis**   CC

     ✓6ᵗʰ **H20.01**   **Primary iridocyclitis**

       H20.011   **Primary iridocyclitis,** right **eye**   CC

       H20.012   **Primary iridocyclitis,** left **eye**   CC

       H20.013   **Primary iridocyclitis,** bilateral

       H20.019   **Primary iridocyclitis, unspecified eye**   CC

     ✓6ᵗʰ **H20.02**   **Recurrent acute iridocyclitis**

       H20.021   **Recurrent acute iridocyclitis,** right **eye**   CC

       H20.022   **Recurrent acute iridocyclitis,** left **eye**   CC

       H20.023   **Recurrent acute iridocyclitis,** bilateral   CC

       H20.029   **Recurrent acute iridocyclitis, unspecified eye**   CC

     ✓6ᵗʰ **H20.03**   **Secondary infectious iridocyclitis**

       H20.031   **Secondary infectious iridocyclitis,** right **eye**   CC

       H20.032   **Secondary infectious iridocyclitis,** left **eye**   CC

       H20.033   **Secondary infectious iridocyclitis,** bilateral   CC

       H20.039   **Secondary infectious iridocyclitis, unspecified eye**   CC

     ✓6ᵗʰ **H20.04**   **Secondary noninfectious iridocyclitis**

       H20.041   **Secondary noninfectious iridocyclitis,** right **eye**

       H20.042   **Secondary noninfectious iridocyclitis,** left **eye**

       H20.043   **Secondary noninfectious iridocyclitis,** bilateral

       H20.049   **Secondary noninfectious iridocyclitis, unspecified eye**

     ✓6ᵗʰ **H20.05**   Hypopyon

       H20.051   **Hypopyon,** right **eye**

       H20.052   **Hypopyon,** left **eye**

       H20.053   **Hypopyon,** bilateral

       H20.059   **Hypopyon, unspecified eye**

     ✓5ᵗʰ **H20.1**   **Chronic iridocyclitis**

       Use additional code for any associated cataract (H26.21-)

       EXCLUDES 2   *posterior cyclitis (H30.2-)*

       H20.10   **Chronic iridocyclitis, unspecified eye**

       H20.11   **Chronic iridocyclitis,** right **eye**

       H20.12   **Chronic iridocyclitis,** left **eye**

       H20.13   **Chronic iridocyclitis,** bilateral

     ✓6ᵗʰ **H20.2**   **Lens-induced iridocyclitis**

       H20.20   **Lens-induced iridocyclitis, unspecified eye**

☑ Additional Character Required   ✓x7ᵗʰ Placeholder   Questionable PDx   Manifestation   Unspecified Dx   UPD Unacceptable PDx   H1-H14 HAC   HCC CMS-HCC Dx   HIV HIV Dx

ICD-10-CM 2022   609

    H20.21   Lens-induced iridocyclitis, right eye
    H20.22   Lens-induced iridocyclitis, left eye
    H20.23   Lens-induced iridocyclitis, bilateral

✓5th **H20.8   Other iridocyclitis**

    EXCLUDES 2   glaucomatocyclitis crises (H40.4-)
         posterior cyclitis (H30.2-)
         sympathetic uveitis (H44.13-)

✓6th **H20.81   Fuchs' heterochromic cyclitis**

    H20.811   Fuchs' heterochromic cyclitis, right eye
    H20.812   Fuchs' heterochromic cyclitis, left eye
    H20.813   Fuchs' heterochromic cyclitis, bilateral
    H20.819   Fuchs' heterochromic cyclitis, unspecified eye

✓6th **H20.82   Vogt-Koyanagi syndrome**

    H20.821   Vogt-Koyanagi syndrome, right eye
    H20.822   Vogt-Koyanagi syndrome, left eye
    H20.823   Vogt-Koyanagi syndrome, bilateral
    H20.829   Vogt-Koyanagi syndrome, unspecified eye

H20.9   Unspecified iridocyclitis   CC
    Uveitis NOS

✓4th **H21   Other disorders of iris and ciliary body**

    EXCLUDES 2   sympathetic uveitis (H44.1-)

✓5th **H21.0   Hyphema**

    EXCLUDES 1   traumatic hyphema (S05.1-)

Hyphema

- Iris
- Cornea
- Hyphema

    H21.00   Hyphema, unspecified eye
    H21.01   Hyphema, right eye
    H21.02   Hyphema, left eye
    H21.03   Hyphema, bilateral

✓5th **H21.1   Other vascular disorders of iris and ciliary body**

    Neovascularization of iris or ciliary body
    Rubeosis iridis
    Rubeosis of iris

✓6th **H21.1X   Other vascular disorders of iris and ciliary body**

    H21.1X1   Other vascular disorders of iris and ciliary body, right eye
    H21.1X2   Other vascular disorders of iris and ciliary body, left eye
    H21.1X3   Other vascular disorders of iris and ciliary body, bilateral
    H21.1X9   Other vascular disorders of iris and ciliary body, unspecified eye

✓5th **H21.2   Degeneration of iris and ciliary body**

✓6th **H21.21   Degeneration of chamber angle**

    H21.211   Degeneration of chamber angle, right eye
    H21.212   Degeneration of chamber angle, left eye
    H21.213   Degeneration of chamber angle, bilateral
    H21.219   Degeneration of chamber angle, unspecified eye

✓6th **H21.22   Degeneration of ciliary body**

    H21.221   Degeneration of ciliary body, right eye
    H21.222   Degeneration of ciliary body, left eye
    H21.223   Degeneration of ciliary body, bilateral
    H21.229   Degeneration of ciliary body, unspecified eye

✓6th **H21.23   Degeneration of iris (pigmentary)**

    Translucency of iris
    H21.231   Degeneration of iris (pigmentary), right eye

    H21.232   Degeneration of iris (pigmentary), left eye
    H21.233   Degeneration of iris (pigmentary), bilateral
    H21.239   Degeneration of iris (pigmentary), unspecified eye

✓6th **H21.24   Degeneration of pupillary margin**

    H21.241   Degeneration of pupillary margin, right eye
    H21.242   Degeneration of pupillary margin, left eye
    H21.243   Degeneration of pupillary margin, bilateral
    H21.249   Degeneration of pupillary margin, unspecified eye

✓6th **H21.25   Iridoschisis**

    H21.251   Iridoschisis, right eye
    H21.252   Iridoschisis, left eye
    H21.253   Iridoschisis, bilateral
    H21.259   Iridoschisis, unspecified eye

✓6th **H21.26   Iris atrophy (essential) (progressive)**

    H21.261   Iris atrophy (essential) (progressive), right eye
    H21.262   Iris atrophy (essential) (progressive), left eye
    H21.263   Iris atrophy (essential) (progressive), bilateral
    H21.269   Iris atrophy (essential) (progressive), unspecified eye

✓6th **H21.27   Miotic pupillary cyst**

    H21.271   Miotic pupillary cyst, right eye
    H21.272   Miotic pupillary cyst, left eye
    H21.273   Miotic pupillary cyst, bilateral
    H21.279   Miotic pupillary cyst, unspecified eye

    H21.29   Other iris atrophy

✓5th **H21.3   Cyst of iris, ciliary body and anterior chamber**

    EXCLUDES 2   miotic pupillary cyst (H21.27-)

✓6th **H21.30   Idiopathic cysts of iris, ciliary body or anterior chamber**

    Cyst of iris, ciliary body or anterior chamber NOS
    H21.301   Idiopathic cysts of iris, ciliary body or anterior chamber, right eye
    H21.302   Idiopathic cysts of iris, ciliary body or anterior chamber, left eye
    H21.303   Idiopathic cysts of iris, ciliary body or anterior chamber, bilateral
    H21.309   Idiopathic cysts of iris, ciliary body or anterior chamber, unspecified eye

✓6th **H21.31   Exudative cysts of iris or anterior chamber**

    H21.311   Exudative cysts of iris or anterior chamber, right eye
    H21.312   Exudative cysts of iris or anterior chamber, left eye
    H21.313   Exudative cysts of iris or anterior chamber, bilateral
    H21.319   Exudative cysts of iris or anterior chamber, unspecified eye

✓6th **H21.32   Implantation cysts of iris, ciliary body or anterior chamber**

    H21.321   Implantation cysts of iris, ciliary body or anterior chamber, right eye
    H21.322   Implantation cysts of iris, ciliary body or anterior chamber, left eye
    H21.323   Implantation cysts of iris, ciliary body or anterior chamber, bilateral
    H21.329   Implantation cysts of iris, ciliary body or anterior chamber, unspecified eye

✓6th **H21.33   Parasitic cyst of iris, ciliary body or anterior chamber**

    H21.331   Parasitic cyst of iris, ciliary body or anterior chamber, right eye   CC
    H21.332   Parasitic cyst of iris, ciliary body or anterior chamber, left eye   CC
    H21.333   Parasitic cyst of iris, ciliary body or anterior chamber, bilateral   CC
    H21.339   Parasitic cyst of iris, ciliary body or anterior chamber, unspecified eye   CC

✓6th **H21.34   Primary cyst of pars plana**

    H21.341   Primary cyst of pars plana, right eye
    H21.342   Primary cyst of pars plana, left eye

N Newborn: 0   P Pediatric: 0-17   M Maternity: 9-64   A Adult: 15-124   MCC Major Complication/Comorbidity   CC Complication/Comorbidity   SW Severe Wound Dx

610   ICD-10-CM 2022

H21.343   **Primary cyst of pars plana**, bilateral
H21.349   **Primary cyst of pars plana, unspecified eye**

✓6ᵗʰ **H21.35**   Exudative **cyst of** pars plana

> **DEF:** Protein, fatty-filled bullous elevation of the nonpigmented outermost ciliary epithelium of pars plana, due to fluid leak from blood vessels.

H21.351   **Exudative cyst of pars plana**, right **eye**
H21.352   **Exudative cyst of pars plana**, left **eye**
H21.353   **Exudative cyst of pars plana**, bilateral
H21.359   **Exudative cyst of pars plana, unspecified eye**

✓5ᵗʰ **H21.4**   **Pupillary membranes**

Iris bombé
Pupillary occlusion
Pupillary seclusion
> EXCLUDES 1   *congenital pupillary membranes (Q13.8)*

H21.40   **Pupillary membranes, unspecified eye**
H21.41   **Pupillary membranes**, right **eye**
H21.42   **Pupillary membranes**, left **eye**
H21.43   **Pupillary membranes**, bilateral

✓5ᵗʰ **H21.5**   **Other and unspecified adhesions and disruptions of iris and ciliary body**
> EXCLUDES 1   *corectopia (Q13.2)*

✓6ᵗʰ **H21.50**   **Unspecified adhesions of iris**

Synechia (iris) NOS

H21.501   **Unspecified adhesions of iris**, right **eye**
H21.502   **Unspecified adhesions of iris**, left **eye**
H21.503   **Unspecified adhesions of iris**, bilateral
H21.509   **Unspecified adhesions of iris and ciliary body, unspecified eye**

✓6ᵗʰ **H21.51**   **Anterior synechiae (iris)**

H21.511   **Anterior synechiae (iris)**, right **eye**
H21.512   **Anterior synechiae (iris)**, left **eye**
H21.513   **Anterior synechiae (iris)**, bilateral
H21.519   **Anterior synechiae (iris), unspecified eye**

✓6ᵗʰ **H21.52**   **Goniosynechiae**

H21.521   **Goniosynechiae**, right **eye**
H21.522   **Goniosynechiae**, left **eye**
H21.523   **Goniosynechiae**, bilateral
H21.529   **Goniosynechiae, unspecified eye**

✓6ᵗʰ **H21.53**   **Iridodialysis**

H21.531   **Iridodialysis**, right **eye**
H21.532   **Iridodialysis**, left **eye**
H21.533   **Iridodialysis**, bilateral
H21.539   **Iridodialysis, unspecified eye**

✓6ᵗʰ **H21.54**   **Posterior synechiae (iris)**

H21.541   **Posterior synechiae (iris)**, right **eye**
H21.542   **Posterior synechiae (iris)**, left **eye**
H21.543   **Posterior synechiae (iris)**, bilateral
H21.549   **Posterior synechiae (iris), unspecified eye**

✓6ᵗʰ **H21.55**   **Recession of chamber angle**

H21.551   **Recession of chamber angle**, right **eye**
H21.552   **Recession of chamber angle**, left **eye**
H21.553   **Recession of chamber angle**, bilateral
H21.559   **Recession of chamber angle, unspecified eye**

✓6ᵗʰ **H21.56**   **Pupillary abnormalities**

Deformed pupil
Ectopic pupil
Rupture of sphincter, pupil
> EXCLUDES 1   *congenital deformity of pupil (Q13.2-)*

H21.561   **Pupillary abnormality**, right **eye**
H21.562   **Pupillary abnormality**, left **eye**
H21.563   **Pupillary abnormality**, bilateral
H21.569   **Pupillary abnormality, unspecified eye**

✓5ᵗʰ **H21.8**   **Other specified disorders of iris and ciliary body**

H21.81   **Floppy iris syndrome**

Intraoperative floppy iris syndrome (IFIS)
Use additional code for adverse effect, if applicable, to identify drug (T36-T50 with fifth or sixth character 5)

H21.82   **Plateau iris syndrome (post-iridectomy) (postprocedural)**
H21.89   **Other specified disorders of iris and ciliary body**

H21.9   **Unspecified disorder of iris and ciliary body**

H22   *Disorders of iris and ciliary body in diseases classified elsewhere*

Code first underlying disease, such as:
gout (M1A.-, M10.-)
leprosy (A30.-)
parasitic disease (B89)

Disorders of lens (H25-H28)

✓4ᵗʰ **H25**   **Age-related cataract**

Senile cataract
> EXCLUDES 2   *capsular glaucoma with pseudoexfoliation of lens (H40.1-)*

Cataracts

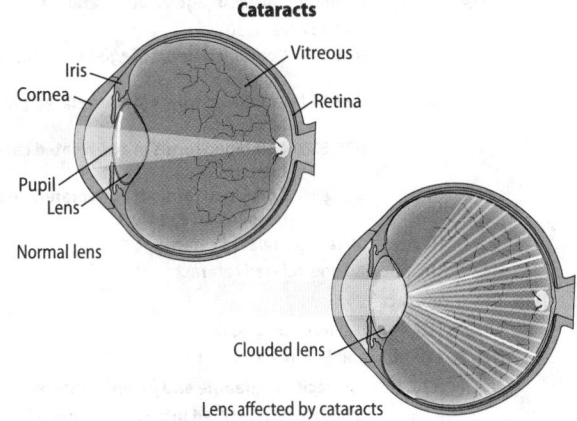

Iris — Vitreous
Cornea — Retina
Pupil
Lens
Normal lens
Clouded lens

Lens affected by cataracts

✓5ᵗʰ **H25.0**   **Age-related** incipient **cataract**

✓6ᵗʰ **H25.01**   Cortical **age-related cataract**

H25.011   **Cortical age-related cataract**, right **eye**   Ⓐ
H25.012   **Cortical age-related cataract**, left **eye**   Ⓐ
H25.013   **Cortical age-related cataract, bilateral**   Ⓐ
H25.019   **Cortical age-related cataract, unspecified eye**   Ⓐ

✓6ᵗʰ **H25.03**   Anterior subcapsular polar **age-related cataract**

H25.031   **Anterior subcapsular polar age-related cataract**, right **eye**   Ⓐ
H25.032   **Anterior subcapsular polar age-related cataract**, left **eye**   Ⓐ
H25.033   **Anterior subcapsular polar age-related cataract, bilateral**   Ⓐ
H25.039   **Anterior subcapsular polar age-related cataract, unspecified eye**   Ⓐ

✓6ᵗʰ **H25.04**   Posterior subcapsular polar **age-related cataract**

H25.041   **Posterior subcapsular polar age-related cataract**, right **eye**   Ⓐ
H25.042   **Posterior subcapsular polar age-related cataract**, left **eye**   Ⓐ
H25.043   **Posterior subcapsular polar age-related cataract, bilateral**   Ⓐ
H25.049   **Posterior subcapsular polar age-related cataract, unspecified eye**   Ⓐ

✓6ᵗʰ **H25.09**   **Other age-related incipient cataract**

Coronary age-related cataract
Punctate age-related cataract
Water clefts

H25.091   **Other age-related incipient cataract**, right **eye**   Ⓐ
H25.092   **Other age-related incipient cataract**, left **eye**   Ⓐ
H25.093   **Other age-related incipient cataract, bilateral**   Ⓐ
H25.099   **Other age-related incipient cataract, unspecified eye**   Ⓐ

✓5ᵗʰ **H25.1**   **Age-related** nuclear **cataract**

Cataracta brunescens
Nuclear sclerosis cataract
AHA: 2019,2Q,31; 2016,1Q,32

H25.10   **Age-related nuclear cataract, unspecified eye**   Ⓐ
H25.11   **Age-related nuclear cataract**, right **eye**   Ⓐ
H25.12   **Age-related nuclear cataract**, left **eye**   Ⓐ
H25.13   **Age-related nuclear cataract**, bilateral   Ⓐ

☑ Additional Character Required   ✓x7ᵗʰ Placeholder   Questionable PDx   Manifestation   Unspecified Dx   UPD Unacceptable PDx   H1-H14 HAC   HCC CMS-HCC Dx   HIV HIV Dx

ICD-10-CM 2022   611

Chapter 7. Diseases of the Eye and Adnexa

✓5th **H25.2** **Age-related cataract, morgagnian type**
     Age-related hypermature cataract
     H25.20 **Age-related cataract, morgagian type, unspecified eye** A
     H25.21 **Age-related cataract, morgagian type, right eye** A
     H25.22 **Age-related cataract, morgagian type, left eye** A
     H25.23 **Age-related cataract, morgagian type, bilateral** A

✓5th **H25.8** **Other age-related cataract**
   ✓6th **H25.81** **Combined forms of age-related cataract**
     AHA: 2019,2Q,30
     H25.811 **Combined forms of age-related cataract, right eye** A
     H25.812 **Combined forms of age-related cataract, left eye** A
     H25.813 **Combined forms of age-related cataract, bilateral** A
     H25.819 **Combined forms of age-related cataract, unspecified eye** A
   H25.89 **Other age-related cataract** A
   H25.9 **Unspecified age-related cataract** A

✓4th **H26** **Other cataract**
   EXCLUDES 1   congenital cataract (Q12.0)

✓5th **H26.0** **Infantile and juvenile cataract**
   ✓6th **H26.00** **Unspecified infantile and juvenile cataract**
     H26.001 **Unspecified infantile and juvenile cataract, right eye** P
     H26.002 **Unspecified infantile and juvenile cataract, left eye** P
     H26.003 **Unspecified infantile and juvenile cataract, bilateral** P
     H26.009 **Unspecified infantile and juvenile cataract, unspecified eye** P

   ✓6th **H26.01** **Infantile and juvenile cortical, lamellar, or zonular cataract**
     H26.011 **Infantile and juvenile cortical, lamellar, or zonular cataract, right eye** P
     H26.012 **Infantile and juvenile cortical, lamellar, or zonular cataract, left eye** P
     H26.013 **Infantile and juvenile cortical, lamellar, or zonular cataract, bilateral** P
     H26.019 **Infantile and juvenile cortical, lamellar, or zonular cataract, unspecified eye** P

   ✓6th **H26.03** **Infantile and juvenile nuclear cataract**
     H26.031 **Infantile and juvenile nuclear cataract, right eye** P
     H26.032 **Infantile and juvenile nuclear cataract, left eye** P
     H26.033 **Infantile and juvenile nuclear cataract, bilateral** P
     H26.039 **Infantile and juvenile nuclear cataract, unspecified eye** P

   ✓6th **H26.04** **Anterior subcapsular polar infantile and juvenile cataract**
     H26.041 **Anterior subcapsular polar infantile and juvenile cataract, right eye** P
     H26.042 **Anterior subcapsular polar infantile and juvenile cataract, left eye** P
     H26.043 **Anterior subcapsular polar infantile and juvenile cataract, bilateral** P
     H26.049 **Anterior subcapsular polar infantile and juvenile cataract, unspecified eye** P

   ✓6th **H26.05** **Posterior subcapsular polar infantile and juvenile cataract**
     H26.051 **Posterior subcapsular polar infantile and juvenile cataract, right eye** P
     H26.052 **Posterior subcapsular polar infantile and juvenile cataract, left eye** P
     H26.053 **Posterior subcapsular polar infantile and juvenile cataract, bilateral** P
     H26.059 **Posterior subcapsular polar infantile and juvenile cataract, unspecified eye** P

   ✓6th **H26.06** **Combined forms of infantile and juvenile cataract**
     H26.061 **Combined forms of infantile and juvenile cataract, right eye** P

     H26.062 **Combined forms of infantile and juvenile cataract, left eye** P
     H26.063 **Combined forms of infantile and juvenile cataract, bilateral** P
     H26.069 **Combined forms of infantile and juvenile cataract, unspecified eye** P
   H26.09 **Other infantile and juvenile cataract** P

✓5th **H26.1** **Traumatic cataract**
     Use additional code (Chapter 20) to identify external cause
   ✓6th **H26.10** **Unspecified traumatic cataract**
     H26.101 **Unspecified traumatic cataract, right eye**
     H26.102 **Unspecified traumatic cataract, left eye**
     H26.103 **Unspecified traumatic cataract, bilateral**
     H26.109 **Unspecified traumatic cataract, unspecified eye**

   ✓6th **H26.11** **Localized traumatic opacities**
     H26.111 **Localized traumatic opacities, right eye**
     H26.112 **Localized traumatic opacities, left eye**
     H26.113 **Localized traumatic opacities, bilateral**
     H26.119 **Localized traumatic opacities, unspecified eye**

   ✓6th **H26.12** **Partially resolved traumatic cataract**
     H26.121 **Partially resolved traumatic cataract, right eye**
     H26.122 **Partially resolved traumatic cataract, left eye**
     H26.123 **Partially resolved traumatic cataract, bilateral**
     H26.129 **Partially resolved traumatic cataract, unspecified eye**

   ✓6th **H26.13** **Total traumatic cataract**
     H26.131 **Total traumatic cataract, right eye**
     H26.132 **Total traumatic cataract, left eye**
     H26.133 **Total traumatic cataract, bilateral**
     H26.139 **Total traumatic cataract, unspecified eye**

✓5th **H26.2** **Complicated cataract**
     H26.20 **Unspecified complicated cataract**
     Cataracta complicata NOS
   ✓6th **H26.21** **Cataract with neovascularization**
     Code also associated condition, such as: chronic iridocyclitis (H20.1-)
     H26.211 **Cataract with neovascularization, right eye**
     H26.212 **Cataract with neovascularization, left eye**
     H26.213 **Cataract with neovascularization, bilateral**
     H26.219 **Cataract with neovascularization, unspecified eye**

   ✓6th **H26.22** **Cataract secondary to ocular disorders (degenerative) (inflammatory)**
     Code also associated ocular disorder
     H26.221 **Cataract secondary to ocular disorders (degenerative) (inflammatory), right eye**
     H26.222 **Cataract secondary to ocular disorders (degenerative) (inflammatory), left eye**
     H26.223 **Cataract secondary to ocular disorders (degenerative) (inflammatory), bilateral**
     H26.229 **Cataract secondary to ocular disorders (degenerative) (inflammatory), unspecified eye**

   ✓6th **H26.23** **Glaucomatous flecks (subcapsular)**
     Code first underlying glaucoma (H40-H42)
     H26.231 **Glaucomatous flecks (subcapsular), right eye**
     H26.232 **Glaucomatous flecks (subcapsular), left eye**
     H26.233 **Glaucomatous flecks (subcapsular), bilateral**
     H26.239 **Glaucomatous flecks (subcapsular), unspecified eye**

✓5th **H26.3** **Drug-induced cataract**
     Toxic cataract
     Use additional code for adverse effect, if applicable, to identify drug (T36-T50 with fifth or sixth character 5)
     H26.30 **Drug-induced cataract, unspecified eye**
     H26.31 **Drug-induced cataract, right eye**
     H26.32 **Drug-induced cataract, left eye**
     H26.33 **Drug-induced cataract, bilateral**

✓5ᵗʰ **H26.4** Secondary cataract

     H26.40 **Unspecified secondary cataract**

     ✓6ᵗʰ **H26.41** Soemmering's ring

         H26.411 **Soemmering's ring, right eye**

         H26.412 **Soemmering's ring, left eye**

         H26.413 **Soemmering's ring, bilateral**

         H26.419 **Soemmering's ring, unspecified eye**

     ✓6ᵗʰ **H26.49** **Other secondary cataract**

         AHA: 2018,2Q,14

         H26.491 **Other secondary cataract, right eye**

         H26.492 **Other secondary cataract, left eye**

         H26.493 **Other secondary cataract, bilateral**

         H26.499 **Other secondary cataract, unspecified eye**

   H26.8 **Other specified cataract**

   H26.9 **Unspecified cataract**

✓4ᵗʰ **H27** **Other disorders of lens**

     EXCLUDES 1   congenital lens malformations (Q12.-)

         mechanical complications of intraocular lens implant (T85.2)

         pseudophakia (Z96.1)

   ✓5ᵗʰ **H27.0** **Aphakia**

     Acquired absence of lens

     Acquired aphakia

     Aphakia due to trauma

       EXCLUDES 1   cataract extraction status (Z98.4-)

           congenital absence of lens (Q12.3)

           congenital aphakia (Q12.3)

     H27.00 **Aphakia, unspecified eye**

     H27.01 **Aphakia, right eye**

     H27.02 **Aphakia, left eye**

     H27.03 **Aphakia, bilateral**

   ✓5ᵗʰ **H27.1** **Dislocation of lens**

     H27.10 **Unspecified dislocation of lens**

     ✓6ᵗʰ **H27.11** **Subluxation of lens**

         H27.111 **Subluxation of lens, right eye**

         H27.112 **Subluxation of lens, left eye**

         H27.113 **Subluxation of lens, bilateral**

         H27.119 **Subluxation of lens, unspecified eye**

     ✓6ᵗʰ **H27.12** **Anterior dislocation of lens**

         H27.121 **Anterior dislocation of lens, right eye**

         H27.122 **Anterior dislocation of lens, left eye**

         H27.123 **Anterior dislocation of lens, bilateral**

         H27.129 **Anterior dislocation of lens, unspecified eye**

     ✓6ᵗʰ **H27.13** **Posterior dislocation of lens**

         H27.131 **Posterior dislocation of lens, right eye**

         H27.132 **Posterior dislocation of lens, left eye**

         H27.133 **Posterior dislocation of lens, bilateral**

         H27.139 **Posterior dislocation of lens, unspecified eye**

   H27.8 **Other specified disorders of lens**

   H27.9 **Unspecified disorder of lens**

H28 **Cataract in diseases classified elsewhere**

   Code first underlying disease, such as:

     hypoparathyroidism (E20.-)

     myotonia (G71.1-)

     myxedema (E03.-)

     protein-calorie malnutrition (E40-E46)

       EXCLUDES 1   cataract in diabetes mellitus (E08.36, E09.36, E10.36, E11.36, E13.36)

Disorders of choroid and retina (H30-H36)

✓4ᵗʰ **H30** **Chorioretinal inflammation**

   ✓5ᵗʰ **H30.0** Focal chorioretinal inflammation

     Focal chorioretinitis

     Focal choroiditis

     Focal retinitis

     Focal retinochoroiditis

     ✓6ᵗʰ **H30.00** **Unspecified focal chorioretinal inflammation**

         Focal chorioretinitis NOS

         Focal choroiditis NOS

         Focal retinitis NOS

         Focal retinochoroiditis NOS

         H30.001 **Unspecified focal chorioretinal inflammation, right eye**

         H30.002 **Unspecified focal chorioretinal inflammation, left eye**

         H30.003 **Unspecified focal chorioretinal inflammation, bilateral**

         H30.009 **Unspecified focal chorioretinal inflammation, unspecified eye**

     ✓6ᵗʰ **H30.01** **Focal chorioretinal inflammation, juxtapapillary**

         H30.011 **Focal chorioretinal inflammation, juxtapapillary, right eye**

         H30.012 **Focal chorioretinal inflammation, juxtapapillary, left eye**

         H30.013 **Focal chorioretinal inflammation, juxtapapillary, bilateral**

         H30.019 **Focal chorioretinal inflammation, juxtapapillary, unspecified eye**

     ✓6ᵗʰ **H30.02** **Focal chorioretinal inflammation of posterior pole**

         H30.021 **Focal chorioretinal inflammation of posterior pole, right eye**

         H30.022 **Focal chorioretinal inflammation of posterior pole, left eye**

         H30.023 **Focal chorioretinal inflammation of posterior pole, bilateral**

         H30.029 **Focal chorioretinal inflammation of posterior pole, unspecified eye**

     ✓6ᵗʰ **H30.03** **Focal chorioretinal inflammation, peripheral**

         H30.031 **Focal chorioretinal inflammation, peripheral, right eye**

         H30.032 **Focal chorioretinal inflammation, peripheral, left eye**

         H30.033 **Focal chorioretinal inflammation, peripheral, bilateral**

         H30.039 **Focal chorioretinal inflammation, peripheral, unspecified eye**

     ✓6ᵗʰ **H30.04** **Focal chorioretinal inflammation, macular or paramacular**

         H30.041 **Focal chorioretinal inflammation, macular or paramacular, right eye**

         H30.042 **Focal chorioretinal inflammation, macular or paramacular, left eye**

         H30.043 **Focal chorioretinal inflammation, macular or paramacular, bilateral**

         H30.049 **Focal chorioretinal inflammation, macular or paramacular, unspecified eye**

   ✓5ᵗʰ **H30.1** Disseminated chorioretinal inflammation

     Disseminated chorioretinitis

     Disseminated choroiditis

     Disseminated retinitis

     Disseminated retinochoroiditis

       EXCLUDES 2   exudative retinopathy (H35.02-)

     ✓6ᵗʰ **H30.10** **Unspecified disseminated chorioretinal inflammation**

         Disseminated chorioretinitis NOS

         Disseminated choroiditis NOS

         Disseminated retinitis NOS

         Disseminated retinochoroiditis NOS

         H30.101 **Unspecified disseminated chorioretinal inflammation, right eye** CC

         H30.102 **Unspecified disseminated chorioretinal inflammation, left eye** CC

         H30.103 **Unspecified disseminated chorioretinal inflammation, bilateral** CC

         H30.109 **Unspecified disseminated chorioretinal inflammation, unspecified eye** CC

     ✓6ᵗʰ **H30.11** **Disseminated chorioretinal inflammation of posterior pole**

         H30.111 **Disseminated chorioretinal inflammation of posterior pole, right eye** CC

         H30.112 **Disseminated chorioretinal inflammation of posterior pole, left eye** CC

         H30.113 **Disseminated chorioretinal inflammation of posterior pole, bilateral** CC

         H30.119 **Disseminated chorioretinal inflammation of posterior pole, unspecified eye** CC

     ✓6ᵗʰ **H30.12** **Disseminated chorioretinal inflammation, peripheral**

         H30.121 **Disseminated chorioretinal inflammation, peripheral right eye** CC

         H30.122 **Disseminated chorioretinal inflammation, peripheral, left eye** CC

         H30.123 **Disseminated chorioretinal inflammation, peripheral, bilateral** CC

✓ Additional Character Required   ✓x7ᵗʰ Placeholder   Questionable PDx   Manifestation   Unspecified Dx   UPD Unacceptable PDx   H1-H14 HAC   HCC CMS-HCC Dx   HIV HIV Dx

ICD-10-CM 2022   613

Chapter 7. Diseases of the Eye and Adnexa

H30.129–H31.329

H30.129 Disseminated chorioretinal inflammation, peripheral, unspecified eye   CC

✓6th **H30.13** Disseminated chorioretinal inflammation, generalized

   H30.131 Disseminated chorioretinal inflammation, generalized, right eye   CC

   H30.132 Disseminated chorioretinal inflammation, generalized, left eye   CC

   H30.133 Disseminated chorioretinal inflammation, generalized, bilateral   CC

   H30.139 Disseminated chorioretinal inflammation, generalized, unspecified eye   CC

✓6th **H30.14** Acute posterior multifocal placoid pigment epitheliopathy

   H30.141 Acute posterior multifocal placoid pigment epitheliopathy, right eye   CC

   H30.142 Acute posterior multifocal placoid pigment epitheliopathy, left eye   CC

   H30.143 Acute posterior multifocal placoid pigment epitheliopathy, bilateral   CC

   H30.149 Acute posterior multifocal placoid pigment epitheliopathy, unspecified eye   CC

✓5th **H30.2** Posterior cyclitis

   Pars planitis

   H30.20 Posterior cyclitis, unspecified eye

   H30.21 Posterior cyclitis, right eye

   H30.22 Posterior cyclitis, left eye

   H30.23 Posterior cyclitis, bilateral

✓5th **H30.8** Other chorioretinal inflammations

✓6th **H30.81** Harada's disease

   H30.811 Harada's disease, right eye

   H30.812 Harada's disease, left eye

   H30.813 Harada's disease, bilateral

   H30.819 Harada's disease, unspecified eye

✓6th **H30.89** Other chorioretinal inflammations

   H30.891 Other chorioretinal inflammations, right eye   CC

   H30.892 Other chorioretinal inflammations, left eye   CC

   H30.893 Other chorioretinal inflammations, bilateral   CC

   H30.899 Other chorioretinal inflammations, unspecified eye   CC

✓5th **H30.9** Unspecified chorioretinal inflammation

   Chorioretinitis NOS
   Choroiditis NOS
   Neuroretinitis NOS
   Retinitis NOS
   Retinochoroiditis NOS

   H30.90 Unspecified chorioretinal inflammation, unspecified eye   CC

   H30.91 Unspecified chorioretinal inflammation, right eye   CC

   H30.92 Unspecified chorioretinal inflammation, left eye   CC

   H30.93 Unspecified chorioretinal inflammation, bilateral   CC

✓4th **H31** Other disorders of choroid

✓5th **H31.0** Chorioretinal scars

   EXCLUDES 2   postsurgical chorioretinal scars (H59.81-)

✓6th **H31.00** Unspecified chorioretinal scars

   H31.001 Unspecified chorioretinal scars, right eye

   H31.002 Unspecified chorioretinal scars, left eye

   H31.003 Unspecified chorioretinal scars, bilateral

   H31.009 Unspecified chorioretinal scars, unspecified eye

✓6th **H31.01** Macula scars of posterior pole (postinflammatory) (post-traumatic)

   EXCLUDES 1   postprocedural chorioretinal scar (H59.81-)

   H31.011 Macula scars of posterior pole (postinflammatory) (post-traumatic), right eye

   H31.012 Macula scars of posterior pole (postinflammatory) (post-traumatic), left eye

   H31.013 Macula scars of posterior pole (postinflammatory) (post-traumatic), bilateral

   H31.019 Macula scars of posterior pole (postinflammatory) (post-traumatic), unspecified eye

✓6th **H31.02** Solar retinopathy

   H31.021 Solar retinopathy, right eye

   H31.022 Solar retinopathy, left eye

   H31.023 Solar retinopathy, bilateral

   H31.029 Solar retinopathy, unspecified eye

✓6th **H31.09** Other chorioretinal scars

   H31.091 Other chorioretinal scars, right eye

   H31.092 Other chorioretinal scars, left eye

   H31.093 Other chorioretinal scars, bilateral

   H31.099 Other chorioretinal scars, unspecified eye

✓5th **H31.1** Choroidal degeneration

   EXCLUDES 2   angioid streaks of macula (H35.33)

✓6th **H31.10** Unspecified choroidal degeneration

   Choroidal sclerosis NOS

   H31.101 Choroidal degeneration, unspecified, right eye

   H31.102 Choroidal degeneration, unspecified, left eye

   H31.103 Choroidal degeneration, unspecified, bilateral

   H31.109 Choroidal degeneration, unspecified, unspecified eye

✓6th **H31.11** Age-related choroidal atrophy

   H31.111 Age-related choroidal atrophy, right eye   A

   H31.112 Age-related choroidal atrophy, left eye   A

   H31.113 Age-related choroidal atrophy, bilateral   A

   H31.119 Age-related choroidal atrophy, unspecified eye   A

✓6th **H31.12** Diffuse secondary atrophy of choroid

   H31.121 Diffuse secondary atrophy of choroid, right eye

   H31.122 Diffuse secondary atrophy of choroid, left eye

   H31.123 Diffuse secondary atrophy of choroid, bilateral

   H31.129 Diffuse secondary atrophy of choroid, unspecified eye

✓5th **H31.2** Hereditary choroidal dystrophy

   EXCLUDES 2   hyperornithinemia (E72.4)
        ornithinemia (E72.4)

   H31.20 Hereditary choroidal dystrophy, unspecified

   H31.21 Choroideremia

   H31.22 Choroidal dystrophy (central areolar) (generalized) (peripapillary)

   H31.23 Gyrate atrophy, choroid

   H31.29 Other hereditary choroidal dystrophy

✓5th **H31.3** Choroidal hemorrhage and rupture

✓6th **H31.30** Unspecified choroidal hemorrhage

   H31.301 Unspecified choroidal hemorrhage, right eye

   H31.302 Unspecified choroidal hemorrhage, left eye

   H31.303 Unspecified choroidal hemorrhage, bilateral

   H31.309 Unspecified choroidal hemorrhage, unspecified eye

✓6th **H31.31** Expulsive choroidal hemorrhage

   H31.311 Expulsive choroidal hemorrhage, right eye

   H31.312 Expulsive choroidal hemorrhage, left eye

   H31.313 Expulsive choroidal hemorrhage, bilateral

   H31.319 Expulsive choroidal hemorrhage, unspecified eye

✓6th **H31.32** Choroidal rupture

   H31.321 Choroidal rupture, right eye   CC

   H31.322 Choroidal rupture, left eye   CC

   H31.323 Choroidal rupture, bilateral   CC

   H31.329 Choroidal rupture, unspecified eye   CC

N Newborn: 0   P Pediatric: 0-17   M Maternity: 9-64   A Adult: 15-124   MCC Major Complication/Comorbidity   CC Complication/Comorbidity   SW Severe Wound Dx

614   ICD-10-CM 2022

✓5ᵗʰ **H31.4　Choroidal** detachment

　✓6ᵗʰ **H31.40　Unspecified choroidal detachment**

　　　H31.401　Unspecified choroidal detachment, right eye　cc

　　　H31.402　Unspecified choroidal detachment, left eye　cc

　　　H31.403　Unspecified choroidal detachment, bilateral　cc

　　　H31.409　Unspecified choroidal detachment, unspecified eye　cc

　✓6ᵗʰ **H31.41　Hemorrhagic choroidal detachment**

　　　H31.411　Hemorrhagic choroidal detachment, right eye　cc

　　　H31.412　Hemorrhagic choroidal detachment, left eye　cc

　　　H31.413　Hemorrhagic choroidal detachment, bilateral　cc

　　　H31.419　Hemorrhagic choroidal detachment, unspecified eye　cc

　✓6ᵗʰ **H31.42　Serous choroidal detachment**

　　　H31.421　Serous choroidal detachment, right eye　cc

　　　H31.422　Serous choroidal detachment, left eye　cc

　　　H31.423　Serous choroidal detachment, bilateral　cc

　　　H31.429　Serous choroidal detachment, unspecified eye　cc

　H31.8　Other specified disorders of choroid

　H31.9　Unspecified disorder of choroid

H32　Chorioretinal disorders in diseases classified elsewhere

　Code first underlying disease, such as:
　　congenital toxoplasmosis (P37.1)
　　histoplasmosis (B39.-)
　　leprosy (A30.-)

　　EXCLUDES 1　chorioretinitis (in):
　　　　　　toxoplasmosis (acquired) (B58.01)
　　　　　　tuberculosis (A18.53)

✓4ᵗʰ **H33　Retinal detachments and breaks**

　EXCLUDES 1　detachment of retinal pigment epithelium (H35.72-, H35.73-)

Retinal Detachment

✓5ᵗʰ **H33.0　Retinal detachment** with retinal break

　Rhegmatogenous retinal detachment

　EXCLUDES 1　serous retinal detachment (without retinal break) (H33.2-)

　✓6ᵗʰ **H33.00　Unspecified retinal detachment with retinal break**

　　　H33.001　Unspecified retinal detachment with retinal break, right eye

　　　H33.002　Unspecified retinal detachment with retinal break, left eye

　　　H33.003　Unspecified retinal detachment with retinal break, bilateral

　　　H33.009　Unspecified retinal detachment with retinal break, unspecified eye

　✓6ᵗʰ **H33.01　Retinal detachment with** single break

　　　H33.011　Retinal detachment with single break, right eye

　　　H33.012　Retinal detachment with single break, left eye

　　　H33.013　Retinal detachment with single break, bilateral

　　　H33.019　Retinal detachment with single break, unspecified eye

　✓6ᵗʰ **H33.02　Retinal detachment with** multiple breaks

　　　H33.021　Retinal detachment with multiple breaks, right eye

　　　H33.022　Retinal detachment with multiple breaks, left eye

　　　H33.023　Retinal detachment with multiple breaks, bilateral

　　　H33.029　Retinal detachment with multiple breaks, unspecified eye

　✓6ᵗʰ **H33.03　Retinal detachment with** giant retinal tear

　　　H33.031　Retinal detachment with giant retinal tear, right eye

　　　H33.032　Retinal detachment with giant retinal tear, left eye

　　　H33.033　Retinal detachment with giant retinal tear, bilateral

　　　H33.039　Retinal detachment with giant retinal tear, unspecified eye

　✓6ᵗʰ **H33.04　Retinal detachment with** retinal dialysis

　　　H33.041　Retinal detachment with retinal dialysis, right eye

　　　H33.042　Retinal detachment with retinal dialysis, left eye

　　　H33.043　Retinal detachment with retinal dialysis, bilateral

　　　H33.049　Retinal detachment with retinal dialysis, unspecified eye

　✓6ᵗʰ **H33.05　Total retinal detachment**

　　　H33.051　Total retinal detachment, right eye

　　　H33.052　Total retinal detachment, left eye

　　　H33.053　Total retinal detachment, bilateral

　　　H33.059　Total retinal detachment, unspecified eye

✓5ᵗʰ **H33.1　Retinoschisis and retinal cysts**

　EXCLUDES 1　congenital retinoschisis (Q14.1)
　　　　　　microcystoid degeneration of retina (H35.42-)

　✓6ᵗʰ **H33.10　Unspecified retinoschisis**

　　　H33.101　Unspecified retinoschisis, right eye

　　　H33.102　Unspecified retinoschisis, left eye

　　　H33.103　Unspecified retinoschisis, bilateral

　　　H33.109　Unspecified retinoschisis, unspecified eye

　✓6ᵗʰ **H33.11　Cyst of ora serrata**

　　　H33.111　Cyst of ora serrata, right eye

　　　H33.112　Cyst of ora serrata, left eye

　　　H33.113　Cyst of ora serrata, bilateral

　　　H33.119　Cyst of ora serrata, unspecified eye

　✓6ᵗʰ **H33.12　Parasitic cyst of retina**

　　　H33.121　Parasitic cyst of retina, right eye　cc

　　　H33.122　Parasitic cyst of retina, left eye　cc

　　　H33.123　Parasitic cyst of retina, bilateral　cc

　　　H33.129　Parasitic cyst of retina, unspecified eye　cc

　✓6ᵗʰ **H33.19　Other retinoschisis and retinal cysts**

　　　Pseudocyst of retina

　　　H33.191　Other retinoschisis and retinal cysts, right eye

　　　H33.192　Other retinoschisis and retinal cysts, left eye

　　　H33.193　Other retinoschisis and retinal cysts, bilateral

　　　H33.199　Other retinoschisis and retinal cysts, unspecified eye

✓5ᵗʰ **H33.2　Serous retinal detachment**

　Retinal detachment NOS

　Retinal detachment without retinal break

　EXCLUDES 1　central serous chorioretinopathy (H35.71-)

　　H33.20　Serous retinal detachment, unspecified eye　cc

　　H33.21　Serous retinal detachment, right eye　cc

　　H33.22　Serous retinal detachment, left eye　cc

　　H33.23　Serous retinal detachment, bilateral　cc

✓5th **H33.3 Retinal breaks** without detachment

> EXCLUDES 1 chorioretinal scars after surgery for detachment (H59.81-)
> peripheral retinal degeneration without break (H35.4-)

✓6th **H33.30 Unspecified retinal break**

H33.301 Unspecified retinal break, right eye
H33.302 Unspecified retinal break, left eye
H33.303 Unspecified retinal break, bilateral
H33.309 Unspecified retinal break, unspecified eye

✓6th **H33.31 Horseshoe tear of retina without detachment**

Operculum of retina without detachment

H33.311 Horseshoe tear of retina without detachment, right eye
H33.312 Horseshoe tear of retina without detachment, left eye
H33.313 Horseshoe tear of retina without detachment, bilateral
H33.319 Horseshoe tear of retina without detachment, unspecified eye

✓6th **H33.32 Round hole of retina without detachment**

H33.321 Round hole, right eye
H33.322 Round hole, left eye
H33.323 Round hole, bilateral
H33.329 Round hole, unspecified eye

✓6th **H33.33 Multiple defects of retina without detachment**

H33.331 Multiple defects of retina without detachment, right eye
H33.332 Multiple defects of retina without detachment, left eye
H33.333 Multiple defects of retina without detachment, bilateral
H33.339 Multiple defects of retina without detachment, unspecified eye

✓5th **H33.4 Traction detachment of retina**

Proliferative vitreo-retinopathy with retinal detachment

H33.40 Traction detachment of retina, unspecified eye CC
H33.41 Traction detachment of retina, right eye CC
H33.42 Traction detachment of retina, left eye CC
H33.43 Traction detachment of retina, bilateral CC

H33.8 Other retinal detachments CC

✓4th **H34 Retinal vascular occlusions**

> EXCLUDES 1 amaurosis fugax (G45.3)

✓5th **H34.0 Transient retinal artery occlusion**

H34.00 Transient retinal artery occlusion, unspecified eye CC
H34.01 Transient retinal artery occlusion, right eye CC
H34.02 Transient retinal artery occlusion, left eye CC
H34.03 Transient retinal artery occlusion, bilateral CC

✓5th **H34.1 Central retinal artery occlusion**

H34.10 Central retinal artery occlusion, unspecified eye CC
H34.11 Central retinal artery occlusion, right eye CC
H34.12 Central retinal artery occlusion, left eye CC
H34.13 Central retinal artery occlusion, bilateral CC

✓5th **H34.2 Other retinal artery occlusions**

✓6th **H34.21 Partial retinal artery occlusion**

Hollenhorst's plaque
Retinal microembolism

H34.211 Partial retinal artery occlusion, right eye CC
H34.212 Partial retinal artery occlusion, left eye CC
H34.213 Partial retinal artery occlusion, bilateral CC
H34.219 Partial retinal artery occlusion, unspecified eye CC

✓6th **H34.23 Retinal artery branch occlusion**

H34.231 Retinal artery branch occlusion, right eye CC
H34.232 Retinal artery branch occlusion, left eye CC
H34.233 Retinal artery branch occlusion, bilateral CC

H34.239 Retinal artery branch occlusion, unspecified eye CC

✓5th **H34.8 Other retinal vascular occlusions**

AHA: 2016,4Q,19

✓6th **H34.81 Central retinal vein occlusion**

> One of the following 7th characters is to be assigned to codes in subcategory H34.81 to designate the severity of the occlusion:
> 0 with macular edema
> 1 with retinal neovascularization
> 2 stable
> old central retinal vein occlusion

✓7th **H34.811 Central retinal vein occlusion, right eye** CC
✓7th **H34.812 Central retinal vein occlusion, left eye** CC
✓7th **H34.813 Central retinal vein occlusion, bilateral** CC
✓7th **H34.819 Central retinal vein occlusion, unspecified eye** CC

✓6th **H34.82 Venous engorgement**

Incipient retinal vein occlusion
Partial retinal vein occlusion

H34.821 Venous engorgement, right eye
H34.822 Venous engorgement, left eye
H34.823 Venous engorgement, bilateral
H34.829 Venous engorgement, unspecified eye

✓6th **H34.83 Tributary (branch) retinal vein occlusion**

> One of the following 7th characters is to be assigned to codes in subcategory H34.83 to designate the severity of the occlusion:
> 0 with macular edema
> 1 with retinal neovascularization
> 2 stable
> old tributary (branch) retinal vein occlusion

✓7th **H34.831 Tributary (branch) retinal vein occlusion, right eye**
✓7th **H34.832 Tributary (branch) retinal vein occlusion, left eye**
✓7th **H34.833 Tributary (branch) retinal vein occlusion, bilateral**
✓7th **H34.839 Tributary (branch) retinal vein occlusion, unspecified eye**

H34.9 Unspecified retinal vascular occlusion CC

✓4th **H35 Other retinal disorders**

> EXCLUDES 2 diabetic retinal disorders (E08.311-E08.359, E09.311-E09.359, E10.311-E10.359, E11.311-E11.359, E13.311-E13.359)

✓5th **H35.0 Background retinopathy and retinal vascular changes**

Code also any associated hypertension ▶(I10)◄

H35.00 Unspecified background retinopathy

✓6th **H35.01 Changes in retinal vascular appearance**

Retinal vascular sheathing

H35.011 Changes in retinal vascular appearance, right eye
H35.012 Changes in retinal vascular appearance, left eye
H35.013 Changes in retinal vascular appearance, bilateral
H35.019 Changes in retinal vascular appearance, unspecified eye

✓6th **H35.02 Exudative retinopathy**

Coats retinopathy

H35.021 Exudative retinopathy, right eye
H35.022 Exudative retinopathy, left eye
H35.023 Exudative retinopathy, bilateral
H35.029 Exudative retinopathy, unspecified eye

✓6th **H35.03 Hypertensive retinopathy**

H35.031 Hypertensive retinopathy, right eye
H35.032 Hypertensive retinopathy, left eye
H35.033 Hypertensive retinopathy, bilateral
H35.039 Hypertensive retinopathy, unspecified eye

✓6th **H35.04 Retinal micro-aneurysms, unspecified**

H35.041 Retinal micro-aneurysms, unspecified, right eye
H35.042 Retinal micro-aneurysms, unspecified, left eye

N Newborn: 0   P Pediatric: 0-17   M Maternity: 9-64   A Adult: 15-124   MCC Major Complication/Comorbidity   CC Complication/Comorbidity   SW Severe Wound Dx

616   ICD-10-CM 2022

H35.043 Retinal micro-aneurysms, unspecified, bilateral

H35.049 Retinal micro-aneurysms, unspecified, unspecified eye

✓6th **H35.05** Retinal neovascularization, unspecified

H35.051 Retinal neovascularization, unspecified, right eye

H35.052 Retinal neovascularization, unspecified, left eye

H35.053 Retinal neovascularization, unspecified, bilateral

H35.059 Retinal neovascularization, unspecified, unspecified eye

✓6th **H35.06** Retinal vasculitis

Eales disease

Retinal perivasculitis

DEF: Sight-threatening intraocular inflammation of the retinal blood vessels that causes minimal, partial, or even complete blindness.

H35.061 Retinal vasculitis, right eye

H35.062 Retinal vasculitis, left eye

H35.063 Retinal vasculitis, bilateral

H35.069 Retinal vasculitis, unspecified eye

✓6th **H35.07** Retinal telangiectasis

H35.071 Retinal telangiectasis, right eye

H35.072 Retinal telangiectasis, left eye

H35.073 Retinal telangiectasis, bilateral

H35.079 Retinal telangiectasis, unspecified eye

H35.09 Other intraretinal microvascular abnormalities

Retinal varices

✓5th **H35.1** Retinopathy of prematurity

✓6th **H35.10** Retinopathy of prematurity, unspecified

Retinopathy of prematurity NOS

H35.101 Retinopathy of prematurity, unspecified, right eye

H35.102 Retinopathy of prematurity, unspecified, left eye

H35.103 Retinopathy of prematurity, unspecified, bilateral

H35.109 Retinopathy of prematurity, unspecified, unspecified eye

✓6th **H35.11** Retinopathy of prematurity, stage 0

H35.111 Retinopathy of prematurity, stage 0, right eye

H35.112 Retinopathy of prematurity, stage 0, left eye

H35.113 Retinopathy of prematurity, stage 0, bilateral

H35.119 Retinopathy of prematurity, stage 0, unspecified eye

✓6th **H35.12** Retinopathy of prematurity, stage 1

H35.121 Retinopathy of prematurity, stage 1, right eye

H35.122 Retinopathy of prematurity, stage 1, left eye

H35.123 Retinopathy of prematurity, stage 1, bilateral

H35.129 Retinopathy of prematurity, stage 1, unspecified eye

✓6th **H35.13** Retinopathy of prematurity, stage 2

H35.131 Retinopathy of prematurity, stage 2, right eye

H35.132 Retinopathy of prematurity, stage 2, left eye

H35.133 Retinopathy of prematurity, stage 2, bilateral

H35.139 Retinopathy of prematurity, stage 2, unspecified eye

✓6th **H35.14** Retinopathy of prematurity, stage 3

H35.141 Retinopathy of prematurity, stage 3, right eye

H35.142 Retinopathy of prematurity, stage 3, left eye

H35.143 Retinopathy of prematurity, stage 3, bilateral

H35.149 Retinopathy of prematurity, stage 3, unspecified eye

✓6th **H35.15** Retinopathy of prematurity, stage 4

H35.151 Retinopathy of prematurity, stage 4, right eye

H35.152 Retinopathy of prematurity, stage 4, left eye

H35.153 Retinopathy of prematurity, stage 4, bilateral

H35.159 Retinopathy of prematurity, stage 4, unspecified eye

✓6th **H35.16** Retinopathy of prematurity, stage 5

H35.161 Retinopathy of prematurity, stage 5, right eye

H35.162 Retinopathy of prematurity, stage 5, left eye

H35.163 Retinopathy of prematurity, stage 5, bilateral

H35.169 Retinopathy of prematurity, stage 5, unspecified eye

✓6th **H35.17** Retrolental fibroplasia

H35.171 Retrolental fibroplasia, right eye

H35.172 Retrolental fibroplasia, left eye

H35.173 Retrolental fibroplasia, bilateral

H35.179 Retrolental fibroplasia, unspecified eye

✓5th **H35.2** Other non-diabetic proliferative retinopathy

Proliferative vitreo-retinopathy

EXCLUDES 1   proliferative vitreo-retinopathy with retinal detachment (H33.4-)

H35.20 Other non-diabetic proliferative retinopathy, unspecified eye

H35.21 Other non-diabetic proliferative retinopathy, right eye

H35.22 Other non-diabetic proliferative retinopathy, left eye

H35.23 Other non-diabetic proliferative retinopathy, bilateral

✓5th **H35.3** Degeneration of macula and posterior pole

H35.30 Unspecified macular degeneration   A

Age-related macular degeneration

✓6th **H35.31** Nonexudative age-related macular degeneration

Atrophic age-related macular degeneration

Dry age-related macular degeneration

AHA: 2016,4Q,20-21

> One of the following 7th characters is to be assigned to each code in subcategory H35.31 to designate the stage of the disease:
> 0   stage unspecified
> 1   early dry stage
> 2   intermediate dry stage
> 3   advanced atrophic without subfoveal involvement
>   advanced dry stage
> 4   advanced atrophic with subfoveal involvement

✓7th **H35.311** Nonexudative age-related macular degeneration, right eye   A

✓7th **H35.312** Nonexudative age-related macular degeneration, left eye   A

✓7th **H35.313** Nonexudative age-related macular degeneration, bilateral   A

✓7th **H35.319** Nonexudative age-related macular degeneration, unspecified eye   A

✓6th **H35.32** Exudative age-related macular degeneration

Wet age-related macular degeneration

AHA: 2016,4Q,20-21

> One of the following 7th characters is to be assigned to each code in subcategory H35.32 to designate the stage of the disease:
> 0   stage unspecified
> 1   with active choroidal neovascularization
> 2   with inactive choroidal neovascularization
>   with involuted or regressed neovascularization
> 3   with inactive scar

✓7th **H35.321** Exudative age-related macular degeneration, right eye   HCC A

✓7th **H35.322** Exudative age-related macular degeneration, left eye   HCC A

✓7th **H35.323** Exudative age-related macular degeneration, bilateral   HCC A

✓7th **H35.329** Exudative age-related macular degeneration, unspecified eye   HCC A

☑ Additional Character Required   ✓x7th Placeholder   Questionable PDx   Manifestation   Unspecified Dx   UPD Unacceptable PDx   H1–H14 HAC   HCC CMS-HCC Dx   HIV HIV Dx

ICD-10-CM 2022   617

Chapter 7. Diseases of the Eye and Adnexa

H35.33 **Angioid streaks** of macula
> **DEF:** Degeneration of the choroid, characterized by broad, irregular, dark brown streaks radiating from the optic disc; occurs with pseudoxanthoma elasticum or Paget's disease.

√6ᵗʰ **H35.34** **Macular cyst, hole, or pseudohole**
- **H35.341** Macular cyst, hole, or pseudohole, **right eye**
- **H35.342** Macular cyst, hole, or pseudohole, **left eye**
- **H35.343** Macular cyst, hole, or pseudohole, **bilateral**
- **H35.349** Macular cyst, hole, or pseudohole, **unspecified eye**

√6ᵗʰ **H35.35** **Cystoid macular degeneration**
> **EXCLUDES 1** *cystoid macular edema following cataract surgery (H59.03-)*
- **H35.351** Cystoid macular degeneration, **right eye**
- **H35.352** Cystoid macular degeneration, **left eye**
- **H35.353** Cystoid macular degeneration, **bilateral**
- **H35.359** Cystoid macular degeneration, **unspecified eye**

√6ᵗʰ **H35.36** **Drusen (degenerative)** of macula
> **AHA:** 2017,1Q,51; 2016,4Q,21
- **H35.361** Drusen (degenerative) of macula, **right eye**
- **H35.362** Drusen (degenerative) of macula, **left eye**
- **H35.363** Drusen (degenerative) of macula, **bilateral**
- **H35.369** Drusen (degenerative) of macula, **unspecified eye**

√6ᵗʰ **H35.37** **Puckering of macula**
- **H35.371** Puckering of macula, **right eye**
- **H35.372** Puckering of macula, **left eye**
- **H35.373** Puckering of macula, **bilateral**
- **H35.379** Puckering of macula, **unspecified eye**

√6ᵗʰ **H35.38** **Toxic maculopathy**
> Code first poisoning due to drug or toxin, if applicable (T36-T65 with fifth or sixth character 1-4 or 6)
> Use additional code for adverse effect, if applicable, to identify drug (T36-T50 with fifth or sixth character 5)
- **H35.381** Toxic maculopathy, **right eye**
- **H35.382** Toxic maculopathy, **left eye**
- **H35.383** Toxic maculopathy, **bilateral**
- **H35.389** Toxic maculopathy, **unspecified eye**

√5ᵗʰ **H35.4** **Peripheral retinal degeneration**
> **EXCLUDES 1** *hereditary retinal degeneration (dystrophy) (H35.5-)*
> *peripheral retinal degeneration with retinal break (H33.3-)*

H35.40 **Unspecified peripheral retinal degeneration**

√6ᵗʰ **H35.41** **Lattice** degeneration of retina
> Palisade degeneration of retina
> **DEF:** Degeneration of the retina, often bilateral, that is usually benign. It is characterized by lines intersecting at irregular intervals in the peripheral retina. Retinal thinning and retinal holes may occur.
- **H35.411** Lattice degeneration of retina, **right eye**
- **H35.412** Lattice degeneration of retina, **left eye**
- **H35.413** Lattice degeneration of retina, **bilateral**
- **H35.419** Lattice degeneration of retina, **unspecified eye**

√6ᵗʰ **H35.42** **Microcystoid** degeneration of retina
- **H35.421** Microcystoid degeneration of retina, **right eye**
- **H35.422** Microcystoid degeneration of retina, **left eye**
- **H35.423** Microcystoid degeneration of retina, **bilateral**
- **H35.429** Microcystoid degeneration of retina, **unspecified eye**

√6ᵗʰ **H35.43** **Paving stone** degeneration of retina
- **H35.431** Paving stone degeneration of retina, **right eye**
- **H35.432** Paving stone degeneration of retina, **left eye**
- **H35.433** Paving stone degeneration of retina, **bilateral**

- **H35.439** Paving stone degeneration of retina, **unspecified eye**

√6ᵗʰ **H35.44** **Age-related reticular** degeneration of retina
- **H35.441** Age-related reticular degeneration of retina, **right eye** A
- **H35.442** Age-related reticular degeneration of retina, **left eye** A
- **H35.443** Age-related reticular degeneration of retina, **bilateral** A
- **H35.449** Age-related reticular degeneration of retina, **unspecified eye** A

√6ᵗʰ **H35.45** **Secondary pigmentary** degeneration
- **H35.451** Secondary pigmentary degeneration, **right eye**
- **H35.452** Secondary pigmentary degeneration, **left eye**
- **H35.453** Secondary pigmentary degeneration, **bilateral**
- **H35.459** Secondary pigmentary degeneration, **unspecified eye**

√6ᵗʰ **H35.46** **Secondary vitreoretinal** degeneration
- **H35.461** Secondary vitreoretinal degeneration, **right eye**
- **H35.462** Secondary vitreoretinal degeneration, **left eye**
- **H35.463** Secondary vitreoretinal degeneration, **bilateral**
- **H35.469** Secondary vitreoretinal degeneration, **unspecified eye**

√5ᵗʰ **H35.5** **Hereditary retinal dystrophy**
> **EXCLUDES 1** *dystrophies primarily involving Bruch's membrane (H31.1-)*

H35.50 **Unspecified hereditary retinal dystrophy**

H35.51 **Vitreoretinal** dystrophy

H35.52 **Pigmentary retinal dystrophy**
> Albipunctate retinal dystrophy
> Retinitis pigmentosa
> Tapetoretinal dystrophy

H35.53 **Other dystrophies primarily involving the sensory retina**
> Stargardt's disease

H35.54 **Dystrophies primarily involving the** retinal pigment epithelium
> Vitelliform retinal dystrophy

√5ᵗʰ **H35.6** **Retinal hemorrhage**
- **H35.60** **Retinal hemorrhage, unspecified eye**
- **H35.61** **Retinal hemorrhage, right eye**
- **H35.62** **Retinal hemorrhage, left eye**
- **H35.63** **Retinal hemorrhage, bilateral**

√5ᵗʰ **H35.7** **Separation of retinal layers**
> **EXCLUDES 1** *retinal detachment (serous) (H33.2-)*
> *rhegmatogenous retinal detachment (H33.0-)*

H35.70 **Unspecified separation of retinal layers** CC

√6ᵗʰ **H35.71** **Central serous** chorioretinopathy
- **H35.711** Central serous chorioretinopathy, **right eye**
- **H35.712** Central serous chorioretinopathy, **left eye**
- **H35.713** Central serous chorioretinopathy, **bilateral**
- **H35.719** Central serous chorioretinopathy, **unspecified eye**

√6ᵗʰ **H35.72** **Serous detachment** of retinal pigment epithelium
- **H35.721** Serous detachment of retinal pigment epithelium, **right eye** CC
- **H35.722** Serous detachment of retinal pigment epithelium, **left eye** CC
- **H35.723** Serous detachment of retinal pigment epithelium, **bilateral** CC
- **H35.729** Serous detachment of retinal pigment epithelium, **unspecified eye** CC

√6ᵗʰ **H35.73** **Hemorrhagic detachment** of retinal pigment epithelium
- **H35.731** Hemorrhagic detachment of retinal pigment epithelium, **right eye** CC
- **H35.732** Hemorrhagic detachment of retinal pigment epithelium, **left eye** CC
- **H35.733** Hemorrhagic detachment of retinal pigment epithelium, **bilateral** CC

N Newborn: 0　　P Pediatric: 0-17　　M Maternity: 9-64　　A Adult: 15-124　　MCC Major Complication/Comorbidity　　CC Complication/Comorbidity　　SW Severe Wound Dx

618　　ICD-10-CM 2022

H35.739 Hemorrhagic detachment of retinal pigment epithelium, unspecified eye `CC`

√5ᵗʰ **H35.8** Other specified retinal disorders

> EXCLUDES 2   *retinal hemorrhage (H35.6-)*

  H35.81 Retinal edema
    Retinal cotton wool spots

  H35.82 Retinal ischemia   `CC`

  H35.89 Other specified retinal disorders

H35.9 Unspecified retinal disorder

H36 *Retinal disorders in diseases classified elsewhere*

> Code first underlying disease, such as:
> lipid storage disorders (E75.-)
> sickle-cell disorders (D57.-)
>
> EXCLUDES 1   *arteriosclerotic retinopathy (H35.0-)*
> *diabetic retinopathy (E08.3-, E09.3-, E10.3-, E11.3-, E13.3-)*

Glaucoma (H40-H42)

√4ᵗʰ **H40** Glaucoma

> EXCLUDES 1   *absolute glaucoma (H44.51-)*
> *congenital glaucoma (Q15.0)*
> *traumatic glaucoma due to birth injury (P15.3)*

Open Angle/Angle Closure Glaucoma

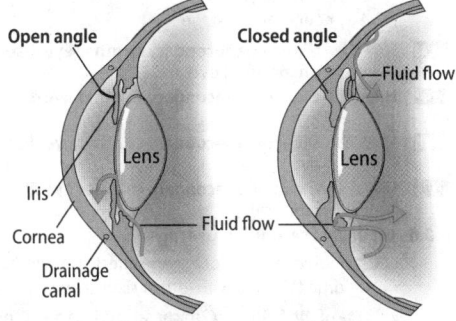

√5ᵗʰ **H40.0** Glaucoma suspect

√6ᵗʰ   **H40.00** Preglaucoma, unspecified

    H40.001 Preglaucoma, unspecified, right eye
    H40.002 Preglaucoma, unspecified, left eye
    H40.003 Preglaucoma, unspecified, bilateral
    H40.009 Preglaucoma, unspecified, unspecified eye

√6ᵗʰ   **H40.01** Open angle with borderline findings, low risk

    Open angle, low risk

    H40.011 Open angle with borderline findings, low risk, right eye
    H40.012 Open angle with borderline findings, low risk, left eye
    H40.013 Open angle with borderline findings, low risk, bilateral
    H40.019 Open angle with borderline findings, low risk, unspecified eye

√6ᵗʰ   **H40.02** Open angle with borderline findings, high risk

    Open angle, high risk

    H40.021 Open angle with borderline findings, high risk, right eye
    H40.022 Open angle with borderline findings, high risk, left eye
    H40.023 Open angle with borderline findings, high risk, bilateral
    H40.029 Open angle with borderline findings, high risk, unspecified eye

√6ᵗʰ   **H40.03** Anatomical narrow angle

    Primary angle closure suspect

    H40.031 Anatomical narrow angle, right eye
    H40.032 Anatomical narrow angle, left eye
    H40.033 Anatomical narrow angle, bilateral
    H40.039 Anatomical narrow angle, unspecified eye

√6ᵗʰ   **H40.04** Steroid responder

    H40.041 Steroid responder, right eye
    H40.042 Steroid responder, left eye
    H40.043 Steroid responder, bilateral

    H40.049 Steroid responder, unspecified eye

√6ᵗʰ **H40.05** Ocular hypertension

  H40.051 Ocular hypertension, right eye
  H40.052 Ocular hypertension, left eye
  H40.053 Ocular hypertension, bilateral
  H40.059 Ocular hypertension, unspecified eye

√6ᵗʰ **H40.06** Primary angle closure without glaucoma damage

  H40.061 Primary angle closure without glaucoma damage, right eye
  H40.062 Primary angle closure without glaucoma damage, left eye
  H40.063 Primary angle closure without glaucoma damage, bilateral
  H40.069 Primary angle closure without glaucoma damage, unspecified eye

√5ᵗʰ **H40.1** Open-angle glaucoma

> One of the following 7th characters is to be assigned to each code in subcategories H40.10, H40.11, H40.12, H40.13, and H40.14 to designate the stage of glaucoma.
> 0   stage unspecified
> 1   mild stage
> 2   moderate stage
> 3   severe stage
> 4   indeterminate stage

√x7ᵗʰ **H40.10** Unspecified open-angle glaucoma

> **TIP:** Only one code from this subcategory should be assigned when both left and right eyes are the same stage.

√6ᵗʰ **H40.11** Primary open-angle glaucoma

  Chronic simple glaucoma
  AHA: 2016,4Q,22

  √7ᵗʰ **H40.111** Primary open-angle glaucoma, right eye
  √7ᵗʰ **H40.112** Primary open-angle glaucoma, left eye
  √7ᵗʰ **H40.113** Primary open-angle glaucoma, bilateral
  √7ᵗʰ **H40.119** Primary open-angle glaucoma, unspecified eye

√6ᵗʰ **H40.12** Low-tension glaucoma

  √7ᵗʰ **H40.121** Low-tension glaucoma, right eye   `UPD`
  √7ᵗʰ **H40.122** Low-tension glaucoma, left eye   `UPD`
  √7ᵗʰ **H40.123** Low-tension glaucoma, bilateral   `UPD`
  √7ᵗʰ **H40.129** Low-tension glaucoma, unspecified eye   `UPD`

√6ᵗʰ **H40.13** Pigmentary glaucoma

  √7ᵗʰ **H40.131** Pigmentary glaucoma, right eye   `UPD`
  √7ᵗʰ **H40.132** Pigmentary glaucoma, left eye   `UPD`
  √7ᵗʰ **H40.133** Pigmentary glaucoma, bilateral   `UPD`
  √7ᵗʰ **H40.139** Pigmentary glaucoma, unspecified eye   `UPD`

√6ᵗʰ **H40.14** Capsular glaucoma with pseudoexfoliation of lens

  √7ᵗʰ **H40.141** Capsular glaucoma with pseudoexfoliation of lens, right eye
  √7ᵗʰ **H40.142** Capsular glaucoma with pseudoexfoliation of lens, left eye
  √7ᵗʰ **H40.143** Capsular glaucoma with pseudoexfoliation of lens, bilateral
  √7ᵗʰ **H40.149** Capsular glaucoma with pseudoexfoliation of lens, unspecified eye

√6ᵗʰ **H40.15** Residual stage of open-angle glaucoma

  H40.151 Residual stage of open-angle glaucoma, right eye   `UPD`
  H40.152 Residual stage of open-angle glaucoma, left eye   `UPD`
  H40.153 Residual stage of open-angle glaucoma, bilateral   `UPD`
  H40.159 Residual stage of open-angle glaucoma, unspecified eye   `UPD`

☑ Additional Character Required   √x7ᵗʰ Placeholder   Questionable PDx   **Manifestation**   Unspecified Dx   `UPD` Unacceptable PDx   `H1`-`H14` HAC   `HCC` CMS-HCC Dx   `HIV` HIV Dx

✓5th H40.2 Primary angle-closure glaucoma

> EXCLUDES 1   *aqueous misdirection (H40.83-)*
> *malignant glaucoma (H40.83-)*

> One of the following 7th characters is to be assigned to code H40.20 and H40.22 to designate the stage of glaucoma.
> 0   stage unspecified
> 1   mild stage
> 2   moderate stage
> 3   severe stage
> 4   indeterminate stage

✓x7th H40.20 Unspecified primary angle-closure glaucoma

> **TIP:** Only one code from this subcategory should be assigned when both left and right eyes are the same stage.

✓6th H40.21 Acute angle-closure glaucoma

> Acute angle-closure glaucoma attack
> Acute angle-closure glaucoma crisis

     H40.211 **Acute angle-closure glaucoma, right eye** `CC`

     H40.212 **Acute angle-closure glaucoma, left eye** `CC`

     H40.213 **Acute angle-closure glaucoma, bilateral** `CC`

     H40.219 **Acute angle-closure glaucoma, unspecified eye** `CC`

✓6th H40.22 Chronic angle-closure glaucoma

> Chronic primary angle closure glaucoma

     ✓7th H40.221 **Chronic angle-closure glaucoma, right eye**

     ✓7th H40.222 **Chronic angle-closure glaucoma, left eye**

     ✓7th H40.223 **Chronic angle-closure glaucoma, bilateral**

     ✓7th H40.229 **Chronic angle-closure glaucoma, unspecified eye**

✓6th H40.23 Intermittent angle-closure glaucoma

     H40.231 **Intermittent angle-closure glaucoma, right eye**

     H40.232 **Intermittent angle-closure glaucoma, left eye**

     H40.233 **Intermittent angle-closure glaucoma, bilateral**

     H40.239 **Intermittent angle-closure glaucoma, unspecified eye**

✓6th H40.24 Residual stage of angle-closure glaucoma

     H40.241 **Residual stage of angle-closure glaucoma, right eye**

     H40.242 **Residual stage of angle-closure glaucoma, left eye**

     H40.243 **Residual stage of angle-closure glaucoma, bilateral**

     H40.249 **Residual stage of angle-closure glaucoma, unspecified eye**

✓5th H40.3 Glaucoma secondary to eye trauma

> Code also underlying condition

> One of the following 7th characters is to be assigned to each code in subcategory H40.3 to designate the stage of glaucoma.
> 0   stage unspecified
> 1   mild stage
> 2   moderate stage
> 3   severe stage
> 4   indeterminate stage

✓x7th H40.30 Glaucoma secondary to eye trauma, unspecified eye

✓x7th H40.31 Glaucoma secondary to eye trauma, right eye

✓x7th H40.32 Glaucoma secondary to eye trauma, left eye

✓x7th H40.33 Glaucoma secondary to eye trauma, bilateral

✓5th H40.4 Glaucoma secondary to eye inflammation

> Code also underlying condition

> One of the following 7th characters is to be assigned to each code in subcategory H40.4 to designate the stage of glaucoma.
> 0   stage unspecified
> 1   mild stage
> 2   moderate stage
> 3   severe stage
> 4   indeterminate stage

✓x7th H40.40 Glaucoma secondary to eye inflammation, unspecified eye

✓x7th H40.41 Glaucoma secondary to eye inflammation, right eye

✓x7th H40.42 Glaucoma secondary to eye inflammation, left eye

✓x7th H40.43 Glaucoma secondary to eye inflammation, bilateral

✓5th H40.5 Glaucoma secondary to other eye disorders

> Code also underlying eye disorder

> One of the following 7th characters is to be assigned to each code in subcategory H40.5 to designate the stage of glaucoma.
> 0   stage unspecified
> 1   mild stage
> 2   moderate stage
> 3   severe stage
> 4   indeterminate stage

✓x7th H40.50 Glaucoma secondary to other eye disorders, unspecified eye

✓x7th H40.51 Glaucoma secondary to other eye disorders, right eye

✓x7th H40.52 Glaucoma secondary to other eye disorders, left eye

✓x7th H40.53 Glaucoma secondary to other eye disorders, bilateral

✓5th H40.6 Glaucoma secondary to drugs

> Use additional code for adverse effect, if applicable, to identify drug (T36-T50 with fifth or sixth character 5)

> One of the following 7th characters is to be assigned to each code in subcategory H40.6 to designate the stage of glaucoma
> 0   stage unspecified
> 1   mild stage
> 2   moderate stage
> 3   severe stage
> 4   indeterminate stage

✓x7th H40.60 Glaucoma secondary to drugs, unspecified eye

✓x7th H40.61 Glaucoma secondary to drugs, right eye

✓x7th H40.62 Glaucoma secondary to drugs, left eye

✓x7th H40.63 Glaucoma secondary to drugs, bilateral

✓5th H40.8 Other glaucoma

✓6th H40.81 Glaucoma with increased episcleral venous pressure

     H40.811 **Glaucoma with increased episcleral venous pressure, right eye**

     H40.812 **Glaucoma with increased episcleral venous pressure, left eye**

     H40.813 **Glaucoma with increased episcleral venous pressure, bilateral**

     H40.819 **Glaucoma with increased episcleral venous pressure, unspecified eye**

✓6th H40.82 Hypersecretion glaucoma

     H40.821 **Hypersecretion glaucoma, right eye**

     H40.822 **Hypersecretion glaucoma, left eye**

     H40.823 **Hypersecretion glaucoma, bilateral**

     H40.829 **Hypersecretion glaucoma, unspecified eye**

✓6th H40.83 Aqueous misdirection

> Malignant glaucoma

     H40.831 **Aqueous misdirection, right eye**

     H40.832 **Aqueous misdirection, left eye**

     H40.833 **Aqueous misdirection, bilateral**

     H40.839 **Aqueous misdirection, unspecified eye**

   H40.89 **Other specified glaucoma**

H40.9 Unspecified glaucoma

H42   *Glaucoma in diseases classified elsewhere*

> Code first underlying condition, such as:
> - amyloidosis (E85.-)
> - aniridia (Q13.1)
> - glaucoma (in) diabetes mellitus (E08.39, E09.39, E10.39, E11.39, E13.39)
> - Lowe's syndrome (E72.03)
> - Reiger's anomaly (Q13.81)
> - specified metabolic disorder (E70-E88)
>
> **EXCLUDES 1**   *glaucoma (in) onchocerciasis (B73.02)*
> *glaucoma (in) syphilis (A52.71)*
> *glaucoma (in) tuberculous (A18.59)*

Disorders of vitreous body and globe (H43-H44)

✓4ᵗʰ **H43**   **Disorders of vitreous body**

   ✓5ᵗʰ **H43.0**   **Vitreous** prolapse

     EXCLUDES 1   *traumatic vitreous prolapse (S05.2-)*
       vitreous syndrome following cataract surgery (H59.0-)

     H43.00   Vitreous prolapse, unspecified eye
     H43.01   Vitreous prolapse, right eye
     H43.02   Vitreous prolapse, left eye
     H43.03   Vitreous prolapse, bilateral

   ✓5ᵗʰ **H43.1**   **Vitreous** hemorrhage

     H43.10   Vitreous hemorrhage, unspecified eye   `HCC`
     H43.11   Vitreous hemorrhage, right eye   `HCC`
     H43.12   Vitreous hemorrhage, left eye   `HCC`
     H43.13   Vitreous hemorrhage, bilateral   `HCC`

   ✓5ᵗʰ **H43.2**   **Crystalline deposits** in vitreous body

     H43.20   Crystalline deposits in vitreous body, unspecified eye
     H43.21   Crystalline deposits in vitreous body, right eye
     H43.22   Crystalline deposits in vitreous body, left eye
     H43.23   Crystalline deposits in vitreous body, bilateral

   ✓5ᵗʰ **H43.3**   **Other vitreous opacities**

     ✓6ᵗʰ **H43.31**   **Vitreous** membranes and strands

       H43.311   Vitreous membranes and strands, right eye
       H43.312   Vitreous membranes and strands, left eye
       H43.313   Vitreous membranes and strands, bilateral
       H43.319   Vitreous membranes and strands, unspecified eye

     ✓6ᵗʰ **H43.39**   **Other vitreous opacities**
       Vitreous floaters
       H43.391   Other vitreous opacities, right eye
       H43.392   Other vitreous opacities, left eye
       H43.393   Other vitreous opacities, bilateral
       H43.399   Other vitreous opacities, unspecified eye

   ✓5ᵗʰ **H43.8**   **Other disorders of vitreous body**

     EXCLUDES 1   *proliferative vitreo-retinopathy with retinal detachment (H33.4-)*
     EXCLUDES 2   *vitreous abscess (H44.02-)*

     ✓6ᵗʰ **H43.81**   **Vitreous** degeneration
       Vitreous detachment
       H43.811   Vitreous degeneration, right eye
       H43.812   Vitreous degeneration, left eye
       H43.813   Vitreous degeneration, bilateral
       H43.819   Vitreous degeneration, unspecified eye

     ✓6ᵗʰ **H43.82**   **Vitreomacular** adhesion
       Vitreomacular traction
       H43.821   Vitreomacular adhesion, right eye   `A`
       H43.822   Vitreomacular adhesion, left eye   `A`
       H43.823   Vitreomacular adhesion, bilateral   `A`
       H43.829   Vitreomacular adhesion, unspecified eye   `A`

     H43.89   **Other disorders of vitreous body**

   H43.9   **Unspecified disorder of vitreous body**

✓4ᵗʰ **H44**   **Disorders of globe**

   INCLUDES   disorders affecting multiple structures of eye

   ✓5ᵗʰ **H44.0**   **Purulent endophthalmitis**

     Use additional code to identify organism
     EXCLUDES 1   *bleb associated endophthalmitis (H59.4-)*

     ✓6ᵗʰ **H44.00**   **Unspecified purulent endophthalmitis**
       H44.001   Unspecified purulent endophthalmitis, right eye   `CC`
       H44.002   Unspecified purulent endophthalmitis, left eye   `CC`
       H44.003   Unspecified purulent endophthalmitis, bilateral   `CC`
       H44.009   Unspecified purulent endophthalmitis, unspecified eye   `CC`

     ✓6ᵗʰ **H44.01**   **Panophthalmitis (acute)**
       H44.011   Panophthalmitis (acute), right eye   `CC`
       H44.012   Panophthalmitis (acute), left eye   `CC`
       H44.013   Panophthalmitis (acute), bilateral   `CC`
       H44.019   Panophthalmitis (acute), unspecified eye   `CC`

     ✓6ᵗʰ **H44.02**   **Vitreous abscess (chronic)**
       H44.021   Vitreous abscess (chronic), right eye   `CC`
       H44.022   Vitreous abscess (chronic), left eye   `CC`
       H44.023   Vitreous abscess (chronic), bilateral   `CC`
       H44.029   Vitreous abscess (chronic), unspecified eye   `CC`

   ✓5ᵗʰ **H44.1**   **Other endophthalmitis**

     EXCLUDES 1   *bleb associated endophthalmitis (H59.4-)*
     EXCLUDES 2   *ophthalmia nodosa (H16.2-)*

     ✓6ᵗʰ **H44.11**   **Panuveitis**
       DEF: Inflammation of all layers of the uvea of the eye, including the choroid, iris, and ciliary body. It also typically involves the lens, retina, optic nerve, and vitreous and causes reduced vision or blindness.
       H44.111   Panuveitis, right eye   `CC`
       H44.112   Panuveitis, left eye   `CC`
       H44.113   Panuveitis, bilateral   `CC`
       H44.119   Panuveitis, unspecified eye   `CC`

     ✓6ᵗʰ **H44.12**   **Parasitic endophthalmitis, unspecified**
       H44.121   Parasitic endophthalmitis, unspecified, right eye   `CC`
       H44.122   Parasitic endophthalmitis, unspecified, left eye   `CC`
       H44.123   Parasitic endophthalmitis, unspecified, bilateral   `CC`
       H44.129   Parasitic endophthalmitis, unspecified, unspecified eye   `CC`

     ✓6ᵗʰ **H44.13**   **Sympathetic uveitis**
       H44.131   Sympathetic uveitis, right eye   `CC`
       H44.132   Sympathetic uveitis, left eye   `CC`
       H44.133   Sympathetic uveitis, bilateral   `CC`
       H44.139   Sympathetic uveitis, unspecified   `CC`

     H44.19   **Other endophthalmitis**   `CC`

   ✓5ᵗʰ **H44.2**   **Degenerative myopia**

     Malignant myopia
     AHA: 2017,4Q,10-11

     H44.20   Degenerative myopia, unspecified eye
     H44.21   Degenerative myopia, right eye
     H44.22   Degenerative myopia, left eye
     H44.23   Degenerative myopia, bilateral

     ✓6ᵗʰ **H44.2A**   **Degenerative myopia with** choroidal neovascularization
       Use additional code for any associated choroid disorders (H31.-)
       H44.2A1   Degenerative myopia with choroidal neovascularization, right eye
       H44.2A2   Degenerative myopia with choroidal neovascularization, left eye
       H44.2A3   Degenerative myopia with choroidal neovascularization, bilateral eye
       H44.2A9   Degenerative myopia with choroidal neovascularization, unspecified eye

☑6ᵗʰ **H44.2B** **Degenerative myopia** with macular hole

H44.2B1 **Degenerative myopia with macular hole, right eye**

H44.2B2 **Degenerative myopia with macular hole, left eye**

H44.2B3 **Degenerative myopia with macular hole, bilateral eye**

H44.2B9 **Degenerative myopia with macular hole, unspecified eye**

☑6ᵗʰ **H44.2C** **Degenerative myopia** with retinal detachment

Use additional code to identify the retinal detachment (H33.-)

H44.2C1 **Degenerative myopia with retinal detachment, right eye**

H44.2C2 **Degenerative myopia with retinal detachment, left eye**

H44.2C3 **Degenerative myopia with retinal detachment, bilateral eye**

H44.2C9 **Degenerative myopia with retinal detachment, unspecified eye**

☑6ᵗʰ **H44.2D** **Degenerative myopia** with foveoschisis

H44.2D1 **Degenerative myopia with foveoschisis, right eye**

H44.2D2 **Degenerative myopia with foveoschisis, left eye**

H44.2D3 **Degenerative myopia with foveoschisis, bilateral eye**

H44.2D9 **Degenerative myopia with foveoschisis, unspecified eye**

☑6ᵗʰ **H44.2E** **Degenerative myopia with other maculopathy**

H44.2E1 **Degenerative myopia with other maculopathy, right eye**

H44.2E2 **Degenerative myopia with other maculopathy, left eye**

H44.2E3 **Degenerative myopia with other maculopathy, bilateral eye**

H44.2E9 **Degenerative myopia with other maculopathy, unspecified**

☑5ᵗʰ **H44.3** **Other and unspecified degenerative disorders of globe**

H44.30 **Unspecified degenerative disorder of globe**

☑6ᵗʰ **H44.31** **Chalcosis**

H44.311 **Chalcosis, right eye**

H44.312 **Chalcosis, left eye**

H44.313 **Chalcosis, bilateral**

H44.319 **Chalcosis, unspecified eye**

☑6ᵗʰ **H44.32** **Siderosis of eye**

DEF: Iron pigment deposits within tissue of the eyeball caused by high iron content of the blood. Symptoms include cataracts, rust-colored anterior subcapsular deposits, iris heterochromia, pupillary mydriasis, and depressed electroretinogram amplitudes.

H44.321 **Siderosis of eye, right eye**

H44.322 **Siderosis of eye, left eye**

H44.323 **Siderosis of eye, bilateral**

H44.329 **Siderosis of eye, unspecified eye**

☑6ᵗʰ **H44.39** **Other degenerative disorders of globe**

H44.391 **Other degenerative disorders of globe, right eye**

H44.392 **Other degenerative disorders of globe, left eye**

H44.393 **Other degenerative disorders of globe, bilateral**

H44.399 **Other degenerative disorders of globe, unspecified**

☑5ᵗʰ **H44.4** **Hypotony of eye**

H44.40 **Unspecified hypotony of eye**

☑6ᵗʰ **H44.41** **Flat anterior chamber** hypotony of eye

H44.411 **Flat anterior chamber hypotony of right eye**

H44.412 **Flat anterior chamber hypotony of left eye**

H44.413 **Flat anterior chamber hypotony of eye, bilateral**

H44.419 **Flat anterior chamber hypotony of unspecified eye**

☑6ᵗʰ **H44.42** **Hypotony of eye due to** ocular fistula

H44.421 **Hypotony of right eye due to ocular fistula**

H44.422 **Hypotony of left eye due to ocular fistula**

☑6ᵗʰ **H44.43** **Hypotony of eye due to other ocular disorders**

H44.423 **Hypotony of eye due to ocular fistula, bilateral**

H44.429 **Hypotony of unspecified eye due to ocular fistula**

☑6ᵗʰ **H44.43** **Hypotony of eye due to other ocular disorders**

H44.431 **Hypotony of eye due to other ocular disorders, right eye**

H44.432 **Hypotony of eye due to other ocular disorders, left eye**

H44.433 **Hypotony of eye due to other ocular disorders, bilateral**

H44.439 **Hypotony of eye due to other ocular disorders, unspecified eye**

☑6ᵗʰ **H44.44** **Primary hypotony of eye**

H44.441 **Primary hypotony of right eye**

H44.442 **Primary hypotony of left eye**

H44.443 **Primary hypotony of eye, bilateral**

H44.449 **Primary hypotony of unspecified eye**

☑5ᵗʰ **H44.5** **Degenerated conditions of globe**

H44.50 **Unspecified degenerated conditions of globe**

☑6ᵗʰ **H44.51** **Absolute glaucoma**

H44.511 **Absolute glaucoma, right eye**

H44.512 **Absolute glaucoma, left eye**

H44.513 **Absolute glaucoma, bilateral**

H44.519 **Absolute glaucoma, unspecified eye**

☑6ᵗʰ **H44.52** **Atrophy of globe**

Phthisis bulbi

H44.521 **Atrophy of globe, right eye**

H44.522 **Atrophy of globe, left eye**

H44.523 **Atrophy of globe, bilateral**

H44.529 **Atrophy of globe, unspecified eye**

☑6ᵗʰ **H44.53** **Leucocoria**

H44.531 **Leucocoria, right eye**

H44.532 **Leucocoria, left eye**

H44.533 **Leucocoria, bilateral**

H44.539 **Leucocoria, unspecified eye**

☑5ᵗʰ **H44.6** **Retained (old) intraocular foreign body,** magnetic

Use additional code to identify magnetic foreign body (Z18.11)

EXCLUDES 1 current intraocular foreign body (S05.-)

EXCLUDES 2 retained foreign body in eyelid (H02.81-)

retained (old) foreign body following penetrating wound of orbit (H05.5-)

retained (old) intraocular foreign body, nonmagnetic (H44.7-)

☑6ᵗʰ **H44.60** **Unspecified retained (old) intraocular foreign body, magnetic**

H44.601 **Unspecified retained (old) intraocular foreign body, magnetic, right eye**

H44.602 **Unspecified retained (old) intraocular foreign body, magnetic, left eye**

H44.603 **Unspecified retained (old) intraocular foreign body, magnetic, bilateral**

H44.609 **Unspecified retained (old) intraocular foreign body, magnetic, unspecified eye**

☑6ᵗʰ **H44.61** **Retained (old) magnetic foreign body in** anterior chamber

H44.611 **Retained (old) magnetic foreign body in anterior chamber, right eye**

H44.612 **Retained (old) magnetic foreign body in anterior chamber, left eye**

H44.613 **Retained (old) magnetic foreign body in anterior chamber, bilateral**

H44.619 **Retained (old) magnetic foreign body in anterior chamber, unspecified eye**

☑6ᵗʰ **H44.62** **Retained (old) magnetic foreign body in** iris or ciliary body

H44.621 **Retained (old) magnetic foreign body in iris or ciliary body, right eye**

H44.622 **Retained (old) magnetic foreign body in iris or ciliary body, left eye**

H44.623 **Retained (old) magnetic foreign body in iris or ciliary body, bilateral**

H44.629 **Retained (old) magnetic foreign body in iris or ciliary body, unspecified eye**

☑6ᵗʰ **H44.63** **Retained (old) magnetic foreign body in** lens

H44.631 **Retained (old) magnetic foreign body in lens, right eye**

H44.632 **Retained (old) magnetic foreign body in lens, left eye**

Ⓝ Newborn: 0   Ⓟ Pediatric: 0-17   Ⓜ Maternity: 9-64   Ⓐ Adult: 15-124   **MCC** Major Complication/Comorbidity   **CC** Complication/Comorbidity   **SW** Severe Wound Dx

622   ICD-10-CM 2022

H44.633 Retained (old) magnetic foreign body in lens, **bilateral**

H44.639 Retained (old) magnetic foreign body in lens, unspecified eye

√6ᵗʰ **H44.64** Retained (old) magnetic foreign body in **posterior wall of globe**

H44.641 Retained (old) magnetic foreign body in posterior wall of globe, **right eye**

H44.642 Retained (old) magnetic foreign body in posterior wall of globe, **left eye**

H44.643 Retained (old) magnetic foreign body in posterior wall of globe, **bilateral**

H44.649 Retained (old) magnetic foreign body in posterior wall of globe, unspecified eye

√6ᵗʰ **H44.65** Retained (old) magnetic foreign body in **vitreous body**

H44.651 Retained (old) magnetic foreign body in vitreous body, **right eye**

H44.652 Retained (old) magnetic foreign body in vitreous body, **left eye**

H44.653 Retained (old) magnetic foreign body in vitreous body, **bilateral**

H44.659 Retained (old) magnetic foreign body in vitreous body, unspecified eye

√6ᵗʰ **H44.69** Retained (old) intraocular foreign body, magnetic, in other or multiple sites

H44.691 Retained (old) intraocular foreign body, magnetic, in other or multiple sites, **right eye**

H44.692 Retained (old) intraocular foreign body, magnetic, in other or multiple sites, **left eye**

H44.693 Retained (old) intraocular foreign body, magnetic, in other or multiple sites, **bilateral**

H44.699 Retained (old) intraocular foreign body, magnetic, in other or multiple sites, unspecified eye

√5ᵗʰ **H44.7** Retained (old) intraocular foreign body, **nonmagnetic**

Use additional code to identify nonmagnetic foreign body (Z18.01-Z18.10, Z18.12, Z18.2-Z18.9)

> **EXCLUDES 1**   *current intraocular foreign body (S05.-)*

> **EXCLUDES 2**   *retained foreign body in eyelid (H02.81-)*
> *retained (old) foreign body following penetrating wound of orbit (H05.5-)*
> *retained (old) intraocular foreign body, magnetic (H44.6-)*

√6ᵗʰ **H44.70** Unspecified retained (old) intraocular foreign body, nonmagnetic

H44.701 Unspecified retained (old) intraocular foreign body, nonmagnetic, **right eye**

H44.702 Unspecified retained (old) intraocular foreign body, nonmagnetic, **left eye**

H44.703 Unspecified retained (old) intraocular foreign body, nonmagnetic, **bilateral**

H44.709 Unspecified retained (old) intraocular foreign body, nonmagnetic, unspecified eye

> Retained (old) intraocular foreign body NOS

√6ᵗʰ **H44.71** Retained (nonmagnetic) (old) foreign body in **anterior chamber**

H44.711 Retained (nonmagnetic) (old) foreign body in anterior chamber, **right eye**

H44.712 Retained (nonmagnetic) (old) foreign body in anterior chamber, **left eye**

H44.713 Retained (nonmagnetic) (old) foreign body in anterior chamber, **bilateral**

H44.719 Retained (nonmagnetic) (old) foreign body in anterior chamber, unspecified eye

√6ᵗʰ **H44.72** Retained (nonmagnetic) (old) foreign body in **iris or ciliary body**

H44.721 Retained (nonmagnetic) (old) foreign body in iris or ciliary body, **right eye**

H44.722 Retained (nonmagnetic) (old) foreign body in iris or ciliary body, **left eye**

H44.723 Retained (nonmagnetic) (old) foreign body in iris or ciliary body, **bilateral**

H44.729 Retained (nonmagnetic) (old) foreign body in iris or ciliary body, unspecified eye

√6ᵗʰ **H44.73** Retained (nonmagnetic) (old) foreign body in **lens**

H44.731 Retained (nonmagnetic) (old) foreign body in lens, **right eye**

H44.732 Retained (nonmagnetic) (old) foreign body in lens, **left eye**

H44.733 Retained (nonmagnetic) (old) foreign body in lens, **bilateral**

H44.739 Retained (nonmagnetic) (old) foreign body in lens, unspecified eye

√6ᵗʰ **H44.74** Retained (nonmagnetic) (old) foreign body in **posterior wall of globe**

H44.741 Retained (nonmagnetic) (old) foreign body in posterior wall of globe, **right eye**

H44.742 Retained (nonmagnetic) (old) foreign body in posterior wall of globe, **left eye**

H44.743 Retained (nonmagnetic) (old) foreign body in posterior wall of globe, **bilateral**

H44.749 Retained (nonmagnetic) (old) foreign body in posterior wall of globe, unspecified eye

√6ᵗʰ **H44.75** Retained (nonmagnetic) (old) foreign body in **vitreous body**

H44.751 Retained (nonmagnetic) (old) foreign body in vitreous body, **right eye**

H44.752 Retained (nonmagnetic) (old) foreign body in vitreous body, **left eye**

H44.753 Retained (nonmagnetic) (old) foreign body in vitreous body, **bilateral**

H44.759 Retained (nonmagnetic) (old) foreign body in vitreous body, unspecified eye

√6ᵗʰ **H44.79** Retained (old) intraocular foreign body, nonmagnetic, in other or multiple sites

H44.791 Retained (old) intraocular foreign body, nonmagnetic, in other or multiple sites, **right eye**

H44.792 Retained (old) intraocular foreign body, nonmagnetic, in other or multiple sites, **left eye**

H44.793 Retained (old) intraocular foreign body, nonmagnetic, in other or multiple sites, **bilateral**

H44.799 Retained (old) intraocular foreign body, nonmagnetic, in other or multiple sites, unspecified eye

√5ᵗʰ **H44.8** Other disorders of globe

√6ᵗʰ **H44.81** Hemophthalmos

> **DEF:** Pool of blood within the eyeball, not from a current injury.

H44.811 Hemophthalmos, **right eye**

H44.812 Hemophthalmos, **left eye**

H44.813 Hemophthalmos, **bilateral**

H44.819 Hemophthalmos, unspecified eye

√6ᵗʰ **H44.82** Luxation of globe

H44.821 Luxation of globe, **right eye**

H44.822 Luxation of globe, **left eye**

H44.823 Luxation of globe, **bilateral**

H44.829 Luxation of globe, unspecified eye

H44.89 Other disorders of globe

H44.9 Unspecified disorder of globe

Disorders of optic nerve and visual pathways (H46-H47)

√4ᵗʰ **H46** Optic neuritis

> **EXCLUDES 2**   *ischemic optic neuropathy (H47.01-)*
> *neuromyelitis optica [Devic] (G36.0)*

√5ᵗʰ **H46.0** Optic **papillitis**

H46.00 Optic papillitis, unspecified eye   CC

H46.01 Optic papillitis, **right eye**   CC

H46.02 Optic papillitis, **left eye**   CC

H46.03 Optic papillitis, **bilateral**   CC

√5ᵗʰ **H46.1** Retrobulbar neuritis

> Retrobulbar neuritis NOS
> **EXCLUDES 1**   *syphilitic retrobulbar neuritis (A52.15)*

H46.10 Retrobulbar neuritis, unspecified eye   CC

H46.11 Retrobulbar neuritis, **right eye**   CC

H46.12 Retrobulbar neuritis, **left eye**   CC

H46.13 Retrobulbar neuritis, **bilateral**   CC

H46.2 **Nutritional** optic neuropathy

✔ Additional Character Required   √x7ᵗʰ Placeholder   Questionable PDx   Manifestation   Unspecified Dx   UPD Unacceptable PDx   H1-H4 HAC   HCC CMS-HCC Dx   HIV HIV Dx

ICD-10-CM 2022   623

Chapter 7. Diseases of the Eye and Adnexa

H46.3 **Toxic optic neuropathy**
Code first (T51-T65) to identify cause

H46.8 **Other optic neuritis** CC

H46.9 **Unspecified optic neuritis** CC

✓4ᵗʰ H47 **Other disorders of optic [2nd] nerve and visual pathways**

  ✓5ᵗʰ H47.0 **Disorders of optic nerve, not elsewhere classified**

    ✓6ᵗʰ H47.01 **Ischemic optic neuropathy**

      H47.011 **Ischemic optic neuropathy, right eye**

      H47.012 **Ischemic optic neuropathy, left eye**

      H47.013 **Ischemic optic neuropathy, bilateral**

      H47.019 **Ischemic optic neuropathy, unspecified eye**

    ✓6ᵗʰ H47.02 **Hemorrhage in optic nerve sheath**

      H47.021 **Hemorrhage in optic nerve sheath, right eye**

      H47.022 **Hemorrhage in optic nerve sheath, left eye**

      H47.023 **Hemorrhage in optic nerve sheath, bilateral**

      H47.029 **Hemorrhage in optic nerve sheath, unspecified eye**

    ✓6ᵗʰ H47.03 **Optic nerve hypoplasia**

      H47.031 **Optic nerve hypoplasia, right eye**

      H47.032 **Optic nerve hypoplasia, left eye**

      H47.033 **Optic nerve hypoplasia, bilateral**

      H47.039 **Optic nerve hypoplasia, unspecified eye**

    ✓6ᵗʰ H47.09 **Other disorders of optic nerve, not elsewhere classified**
      Compression of optic nerve

      H47.091 **Other disorders of optic nerve, not elsewhere classified, right eye**

      H47.092 **Other disorders of optic nerve, not elsewhere classified, left eye**

      H47.093 **Other disorders of optic nerve, not elsewhere classified, bilateral**

      H47.099 **Other disorders of optic nerve, not elsewhere classified, unspecified eye**

  ✓5ᵗʰ H47.1 **Papilledema**
    DEF: Swelling of the optic papilla, the raised area connected to the optic disk made up of nerves that enter the eyeball. It may be caused by increased intracranial pressure, decreased ocular pressure, or a retinal disorder.

    H47.10 **Unspecified papilledema** CC

    H47.11 **Papilledema associated with increased intracranial pressure** CC

    H47.12 **Papilledema associated with decreased ocular pressure**

    H47.13 **Papilledema associated with retinal disorder**

    ✓6ᵗʰ H47.14 **Foster-Kennedy syndrome**

      H47.141 **Foster-Kennedy syndrome, right eye**

      H47.142 **Foster-Kennedy syndrome, left eye**

      H47.143 **Foster-Kennedy syndrome, bilateral**

      H47.149 **Foster-Kennedy syndrome, unspecified eye**

  ✓5ᵗʰ H47.2 **Optic atrophy**

    H47.20 **Unspecified optic atrophy**

    ✓6ᵗʰ H47.21 **Primary optic atrophy**

      H47.211 **Primary optic atrophy, right eye**

      H47.212 **Primary optic atrophy, left eye**

      H47.213 **Primary optic atrophy, bilateral**

      H47.219 **Primary optic atrophy, unspecified eye**

    H47.22 **Hereditary optic atrophy**
      Leber's optic atrophy

    ✓6ᵗʰ H47.23 **Glaucomatous optic atrophy**

      H47.231 **Glaucomatous optic atrophy, right eye**

      H47.232 **Glaucomatous optic atrophy, left eye**

      H47.233 **Glaucomatous optic atrophy, bilateral**

      H47.239 **Glaucomatous optic atrophy, unspecified eye**

    ✓6ᵗʰ H47.29 **Other optic atrophy**
      Temporal pallor of optic disc

      H47.291 **Other optic atrophy, right eye**

      H47.292 **Other optic atrophy, left eye**

      H47.293 **Other optic atrophy, bilateral**

      H47.299 **Other optic atrophy, unspecified eye**

✓5ᵗʰ H47.3 **Other disorders of optic disc**

  ✓6ᵗʰ H47.31 **Coloboma of optic disc**

    H47.311 **Coloboma of optic disc, right eye**

    H47.312 **Coloboma of optic disc, left eye**

    H47.313 **Coloboma of optic disc, bilateral**

    H47.319 **Coloboma of optic disc, unspecified eye**

  ✓6ᵗʰ H47.32 **Drusen of optic disc**

    H47.321 **Drusen of optic disc, right eye**

    H47.322 **Drusen of optic disc, left eye**

    H47.323 **Drusen of optic disc, bilateral**

    H47.329 **Drusen of optic disc, unspecified eye**

  ✓6ᵗʰ H47.33 **Pseudopapilledema of optic disc**

    H47.331 **Pseudopapilledema of optic disc, right eye**

    H47.332 **Pseudopapilledema of optic disc, left eye**

    H47.333 **Pseudopapilledema of optic disc, bilateral**

    H47.339 **Pseudopapilledema of optic disc, unspecified eye**

  ✓6ᵗʰ H47.39 **Other disorders of optic disc**

    H47.391 **Other disorders of optic disc, right eye**

    H47.392 **Other disorders of optic disc, left eye**

    H47.393 **Other disorders of optic disc, bilateral**

    H47.399 **Other disorders of optic disc, unspecified eye**

✓5ᵗʰ H47.4 **Disorders of optic chiasm**
  Code also underlying condition

  H47.41 **Disorders of optic chiasm in (due to) inflammatory disorders** CC

  H47.42 **Disorders of optic chiasm in (due to) neoplasm** CC

  H47.43 **Disorders of optic chiasm in (due to) vascular disorders** CC

  H47.49 **Disorders of optic chiasm in (due to) other disorders** CC

✓5ᵗʰ H47.5 **Disorders of other visual pathways**
  Disorders of optic tracts, geniculate nuclei and optic radiations
  Code also underlying condition

  ✓6ᵗʰ H47.51 **Disorders of visual pathways in (due to) inflammatory disorders**

    H47.511 **Disorders of visual pathways in (due to) inflammatory disorders, right side** CC

    H47.512 **Disorders of visual pathways in (due to) inflammatory disorders, left side** CC

    H47.519 **Disorders of visual pathways in (due to) inflammatory disorders, unspecified side**

  ✓6ᵗʰ H47.52 **Disorders of visual pathways in (due to) neoplasm**

    H47.521 **Disorders of visual pathways in (due to) neoplasm, right side** CC

    H47.522 **Disorders of visual pathways in (due to) neoplasm, left side** CC

    H47.529 **Disorders of visual pathways in (due to) neoplasm, unspecified side** CC

  ✓6ᵗʰ H47.53 **Disorders of visual pathways in (due to) vascular disorders**

    H47.531 **Disorders of visual pathways in (due to) vascular disorders, right side** CC

    H47.532 **Disorders of visual pathways in (due to) vascular disorders, left side** CC

    H47.539 **Disorders of visual pathways in (due to) vascular disorders, unspecified side** CC

✓5ᵗʰ H47.6 **Disorders of visual cortex**
  Code also underlying condition
  EXCLUDES 1 injury to visual cortex S04.04-

  ✓6ᵗʰ H47.61 **Cortical blindness**

    H47.611 **Cortical blindness, right side of brain**

    H47.612 **Cortical blindness, left side of brain**

    H47.619 **Cortical blindness, unspecified side of brain**

  ✓6ᵗʰ H47.62 **Disorders of visual cortex in (due to) inflammatory disorders**

    H47.621 **Disorders of visual cortex in (due to) inflammatory disorders, right side of brain** CC

    H47.622 **Disorders of visual cortex in (due to) inflammatory disorders, left side of brain** CC

N Newborn: 0   P Pediatric: 0-17   M Maternity: 9-64   A Adult: 15-124   MCC Major Complication/Comorbidity   CC Complication/Comorbidity   SW Severe Wound Dx

624

ICD-10-CM 2022

H47.629   Disorders of visual cortex in (due to) inflammatory disorders, unspecified side of brain   `CC`

✓6ᵗʰ H47.63   Disorders of visual cortex in (due to) neoplasm

    H47.631   Disorders of visual cortex in (due to) neoplasm, right side of brain   `CC`

    H47.632   Disorders of visual cortex in (due to) neoplasm, left side of brain   `CC`

    H47.639   Disorders of visual cortex in (due to) neoplasm, unspecified side of brain   `CC`

✓6ᵗʰ H47.64   Disorders of visual cortex in (due to) vascular disorders

    H47.641   Disorders of visual cortex in (due to) vascular disorders, right side of brain   `CC`

    H47.642   Disorders of visual cortex in (due to) vascular disorders, left side of brain   `CC`

    H47.649   Disorders of visual cortex in (due to) vascular disorders, unspecified side of brain   `CC`

H47.9   Unspecified disorder of visual pathways

Disorders of ocular muscles, binocular movement, accommodation and refraction (H49-H52)

EXCLUDES 2   nystagmus and other irregular eye movements (H55)

✓4ᵗʰ H49   Paralytic strabismus

    EXCLUDES 2   internal ophthalmoplegia (H52.51-)
          internuclear ophthalmoplegia (H51.2-)
          progressive supranuclear ophthalmoplegia (G23.1)

    DEF: Strabismus: Misalignment of the eyes with the inability to move and focus in the same direction due to conditions affecting the muscles controlling them.

✓5ᵗʰ H49.0   Third [oculomotor] nerve palsy

    H49.00   Third [oculomotor] nerve palsy, unspecified eye
    H49.01   Third [oculomotor] nerve palsy, right eye
    H49.02   Third [oculomotor] nerve palsy, left eye
    H49.03   Third [oculomotor] nerve palsy, bilateral

✓5ᵗʰ H49.1   Fourth [trochlear] nerve palsy

    H49.10   Fourth [trochlear] nerve palsy, unspecified eye
    H49.11   Fourth [trochlear] nerve palsy, right eye
    H49.12   Fourth [trochlear] nerve palsy, left eye
    H49.13   Fourth [trochlear] nerve palsy, bilateral

✓5ᵗʰ H49.2   Sixth [abducent] nerve palsy

    H49.20   Sixth [abducent] nerve palsy, unspecified eye
    H49.21   Sixth [abducent] nerve palsy, right eye
    H49.22   Sixth [abducent] nerve palsy, left eye
    H49.23   Sixth [abducent] nerve palsy, bilateral

✓5ᵗʰ H49.3   Total (external) ophthalmoplegia

    H49.30   Total (external) ophthalmoplegia, unspecified eye
    H49.31   Total (external) ophthalmoplegia, right eye
    H49.32   Total (external) ophthalmoplegia, left eye
    H49.33   Total (external) ophthalmoplegia, bilateral

✓5ᵗʰ H49.4   Progressive external ophthalmoplegia

    EXCLUDES 1   Kearns-Sayre syndrome (H49.81-)

    H49.40   Progressive external ophthalmoplegia, unspecified eye
    H49.41   Progressive external ophthalmoplegia, right eye
    H49.42   Progressive external ophthalmoplegia, left eye
    H49.43   Progressive external ophthalmoplegia, bilateral

✓5ᵗʰ H49.8   Other paralytic strabismus

✓6ᵗʰ H49.81   Kearns-Sayre syndrome

    Progressive external ophthalmoplegia with pigmentary retinopathy
    Use additional code for other manifestation, such as: heart block (I45.9)

    H49.811   Kearns-Sayre syndrome, right eye   `CC` `HCC`
    H49.812   Kearns-Sayre syndrome, left eye   `CC` `HCC`
    H49.813   Kearns-Sayre syndrome, bilateral   `CC` `HCC`
    H49.819   Kearns-Sayre syndrome, unspecified eye   `CC` `HCC`

✓6ᵗʰ H49.88   Other paralytic strabismus

    External ophthalmoplegia NOS

    H49.881   Other paralytic strabismus, right eye
    H49.882   Other paralytic strabismus, left eye
    H49.883   Other paralytic strabismus, bilateral
    H49.889   Other paralytic strabismus, unspecified eye

H49.9   Unspecified paralytic strabismus

✓4ᵗʰ H50   Other strabismus

    DEF: Strabismus: Misalignment of the eyes with the inability to move and focus in the same direction due to conditions affecting the muscles controlling them.

✓5ᵗʰ H50.0   Esotropia

    Convergent concomitant strabismus
    EXCLUDES 1   intermittent esotropia (H50.31-, H50.32)

    H50.00   Unspecified esotropia

✓6ᵗʰ H50.01   Monocular esotropia

    H50.011   Monocular esotropia, right eye
    H50.012   Monocular esotropia, left eye

✓6ᵗʰ H50.02   Monocular esotropia with A pattern

    H50.021   Monocular esotropia with A pattern, right eye
    H50.022   Monocular esotropia with A pattern, left eye

✓6ᵗʰ H50.03   Monocular esotropia with V pattern

    H50.031   Monocular esotropia with V pattern, right eye
    H50.032   Monocular esotropia with V pattern, left eye

✓6ᵗʰ H50.04   Monocular esotropia with other noncomitancies

    H50.041   Monocular esotropia with other noncomitancies, right eye
    H50.042   Monocular esotropia with other noncomitancies, left eye

    H50.05   Alternating esotropia
    H50.06   Alternating esotropia with A pattern
    H50.07   Alternating esotropia with V pattern
    H50.08   Alternating esotropia with other noncomitancies

Eye Muscle Diseases

R.   L.
Monocular (one eye only) esotropia (inward)

Monocular exotropia (outward)

Monocular hypertropia (upward)

✓5ᵗʰ H50.1   Exotropia

    Divergent concomitant strabismus
    EXCLUDES 1   intermittent exotropia (H50.33-, H50.34)

    H50.10   Unspecified exotropia

✓6ᵗʰ H50.11   Monocular exotropia

    H50.111   Monocular exotropia, right eye
    H50.112   Monocular exotropia, left eye

✓6ᵗʰ H50.12   Monocular exotropia with A pattern

    H50.121   Monocular exotropia with A pattern, right eye
    H50.122   Monocular exotropia with A pattern, left eye

✓6ᵗʰ H50.13   Monocular exotropia with V pattern

    H50.131   Monocular exotropia with V pattern, right eye
    H50.132   Monocular exotropia with V pattern, left eye

✔ Additional Character Required   ✓x7ᵗʰ Placeholder   Questionable PDx   Manifestation   Unspecified Dx   UPD Unacceptable PDx   H1-H14 HAC   HCC CMS-HCC Dx   HIV HIV Dx

ICD-10-CM 2022   625

Chapter 7. Diseases of the Eye and Adnexa

H50.14–H53.033

√6ᵗʰ **H50.14** **Monocular exotropia with other noncomitancies**
    H50.141 **Monocular exotropia with other noncomitancies, right eye**
    H50.142 **Monocular exotropia with other noncomitancies, left eye**
  H50.15 **Alternating exotropia**
  H50.16 **Alternating exotropia with A pattern**
  H50.17 **Alternating exotropia with V pattern**
  H50.18 **Alternating exotropia with other noncomitancies**

√5ᵗʰ **H50.2** **Vertical strabismus**
  Hypertropia
  H50.21 **Vertical strabismus, right eye**
  H50.22 **Vertical strabismus, left eye**

√5ᵗʰ **H50.3** **Intermittent heterotropia**
  H50.30 **Unspecified intermittent heterotropia**
  √6ᵗʰ **H50.31** **Intermittent monocular esotropia**
    H50.311 **Intermittent monocular esotropia, right eye**
    H50.312 **Intermittent monocular esotropia, left eye**
  H50.32 **Intermittent alternating esotropia**
  √6ᵗʰ **H50.33** **Intermittent monocular exotropia**
    H50.331 **Intermittent monocular exotropia, right eye**
    H50.332 **Intermittent monocular exotropia, left eye**
  H50.34 **Intermittent alternating exotropia**

√5ᵗʰ **H50.4** **Other and unspecified heterotropia**
  H50.40 **Unspecified heterotropia**
  √6ᵗʰ **H50.41** **Cyclotropia**
    H50.411 **Cyclotropia, right eye**
    H50.412 **Cyclotropia, left eye**
  H50.42 **Monofixation syndrome**
  H50.43 **Accommodative component in esotropia**

√5ᵗʰ **H50.5** **Heterophoria**
  H50.50 **Unspecified heterophoria**
  H50.51 **Esophoria**
  H50.52 **Exophoria**
  H50.53 **Vertical heterophoria**
  H50.54 **Cyclophoria**
  H50.55 **Alternating heterophoria**

√5ᵗʰ **H50.6** **Mechanical strabismus**
  H50.60 **Mechanical strabismus, unspecified**
  √6ᵗʰ **H50.61** **Brown's sheath syndrome**
    H50.611 **Brown's sheath syndrome, right eye**
    H50.612 **Brown's sheath syndrome, left eye**
  H50.69 **Other mechanical strabismus**
    Strabismus due to adhesions
    Traumatic limitation of duction of eye muscle

√5ᵗʰ **H50.8** **Other specified strabismus**
  √6ᵗʰ **H50.81** **Duane's syndrome**
    H50.811 **Duane's syndrome, right eye**
    H50.812 **Duane's syndrome, left eye**
  H50.89 **Other specified strabismus**
  H50.9 **Unspecified strabismus**

√4ᵗʰ **H51** **Other disorders of binocular movement**
  H51.0 **Palsy (spasm) of conjugate gaze**
  √5ᵗʰ **H51.1** **Convergence insufficiency and excess**
    H51.11 **Convergence insufficiency**
    H51.12 **Convergence excess**
  √5ᵗʰ **H51.2** **Internuclear ophthalmoplegia**
    H51.20 **Internuclear ophthalmoplegia, unspecified eye**
    H51.21 **Internuclear ophthalmoplegia, right eye**
    H51.22 **Internuclear ophthalmoplegia, left eye**
    H51.23 **Internuclear ophthalmoplegia, bilateral**
  H51.8 **Other specified disorders of binocular movement**
  H51.9 **Unspecified disorder of binocular movement**

√4ᵗʰ **H52** **Disorders of refraction and accommodation**
  √5ᵗʰ **H52.0** **Hypermetropia**
    H52.00 **Hypermetropia, unspecified eye**
    H52.01 **Hypermetropia, right eye**
    H52.02 **Hypermetropia, left eye**
    H52.03 **Hypermetropia, bilateral**

√5ᵗʰ **H52.1** **Myopia**
  EXCLUDES 1   degenerative myopia (H44.2-)
  H52.10 **Myopia, unspecified eye**
  H52.11 **Myopia, right eye**
  H52.12 **Myopia, left eye**
  H52.13 **Myopia, bilateral**

√5ᵗʰ **H52.2** **Astigmatism**
  √6ᵗʰ **H52.20** **Unspecified astigmatism**
    H52.201 **Unspecified astigmatism, right eye**
    H52.202 **Unspecified astigmatism, left eye**
    H52.203 **Unspecified astigmatism, bilateral**
    H52.209 **Unspecified astigmatism, unspecified eye**
  √6ᵗʰ **H52.21** **Irregular astigmatism**
    H52.211 **Irregular astigmatism, right eye**
    H52.212 **Irregular astigmatism, left eye**
    H52.213 **Irregular astigmatism, bilateral**
    H52.219 **Irregular astigmatism, unspecified eye**
  √6ᵗʰ **H52.22** **Regular astigmatism**
    H52.221 **Regular astigmatism, right eye**
    H52.222 **Regular astigmatism, left eye**
    H52.223 **Regular astigmatism, bilateral**
    H52.229 **Regular astigmatism, unspecified eye**

√5ᵗʰ **H52.3** **Anisometropia and aniseikonia**
  H52.31 **Anisometropia**
  H52.32 **Aniseikonia**
  H52.4 **Presbyopia**

√5ᵗʰ **H52.5** **Disorders of accommodation**
  √6ᵗʰ **H52.51** **Internal ophthalmoplegia (complete) (total)**
    H52.511 **Internal ophthalmoplegia (complete) (total), right eye**
    H52.512 **Internal ophthalmoplegia (complete) (total), left eye**
    H52.513 **Internal ophthalmoplegia (complete) (total), bilateral**
    H52.519 **Internal ophthalmoplegia (complete) (total), unspecified eye**
  √6ᵗʰ **H52.52** **Paresis of accommodation**
    H52.521 **Paresis of accommodation, right eye**
    H52.522 **Paresis of accommodation, left eye**
    H52.523 **Paresis of accommodation, bilateral**
    H52.529 **Paresis of accommodation, unspecified eye**
  √6ᵗʰ **H52.53** **Spasm of accommodation**
    H52.531 **Spasm of accommodation, right eye**
    H52.532 **Spasm of accommodation, left eye**
    H52.533 **Spasm of accommodation, bilateral**
    H52.539 **Spasm of accommodation, unspecified eye**
  H52.6 **Other disorders of refraction**
  H52.7 **Unspecified disorder of refraction**

Visual disturbances and blindness (H53-H54)

√4ᵗʰ **H53** **Visual disturbances**
  √5ᵗʰ **H53.0** **Amblyopia ex anopsia**
  EXCLUDES 1   amblyopia due to vitamin A deficiency (E50.5)
  √6ᵗʰ **H53.00** **Unspecified amblyopia**
    H53.001 **Unspecified amblyopia, right eye**
    H53.002 **Unspecified amblyopia, left eye**
    H53.003 **Unspecified amblyopia, bilateral**
    H53.009 **Unspecified amblyopia, unspecified eye**
  √6ᵗʰ **H53.01** **Deprivation amblyopia**
    H53.011 **Deprivation amblyopia, right eye**
    H53.012 **Deprivation amblyopia, left eye**
    H53.013 **Deprivation amblyopia, bilateral**
    H53.019 **Deprivation amblyopia, unspecified eye**
  √6ᵗʰ **H53.02** **Refractive amblyopia**
    H53.021 **Refractive amblyopia, right eye**
    H53.022 **Refractive amblyopia, left eye**
    H53.023 **Refractive amblyopia, bilateral**
    H53.029 **Refractive amblyopia, unspecified eye**
  √6ᵗʰ **H53.03** **Strabismic amblyopia**
  EXCLUDES 1   strabismus (H50.-)
    H53.031 **Strabismic amblyopia, right eye**
    H53.032 **Strabismic amblyopia, left eye**
    H53.033 **Strabismic amblyopia, bilateral**

H53.Ø39 **Strabismic amblyopia,** unspecified eye

√6ᵗʰ H53.Ø4 **Amblyopia** suspect

AHA: 2016,4Q,22-23

H53.Ø41 **Amblyopia suspect,** right eye

H53.Ø42 **Amblyopia suspect,** left eye

H53.Ø43 **Amblyopia suspect,** bilateral

H53.Ø49 **Amblyopia suspect,** unspecified eye

√5ᵗʰ H53.1 **Subjective visual disturbances**

EXCLUDES 1   subjective visual disturbances due to vitamin A deficiency (E5Ø.5)

visual hallucinations (R44.1)

H53.1Ø **Unspecified subjective visual disturbances**

H53.11 **Day blindness**

Hemeralopia

√6ᵗʰ H53.12 **Transient** visual loss

Scintillating scotoma

EXCLUDES 1   amaurosis fugax (G45.3-)

transient retinal artery occlusion (H34.Ø-)

H53.121 **Transient visual loss,** right eye   CC

H53.122 **Transient visual loss,** left eye   CC

H53.123 **Transient visual loss,** bilateral   CC

H53.129 **Transient visual loss,** unspecified eye   CC

√6ᵗʰ H53.13 **Sudden** visual loss

H53.131 **Sudden visual loss,** right eye   CC

H53.132 **Sudden visual loss,** left eye   CC

H53.133 **Sudden visual loss,** bilateral   CC

H53.139 **Sudden visual loss,** unspecified eye   CC

√6ᵗʰ H53.14 **Visual** discomfort

Asthenopia

Photophobia

H53.141 **Visual discomfort,** right eye

H53.142 **Visual discomfort,** left eye

H53.143 **Visual discomfort,** bilateral

H53.149 **Visual discomfort,** unspecified

H53.15 **Visual** distortions of shape and size

Metamorphopsia

H53.16 **Psychophysical** visual disturbances

H53.19 **Other subjective visual disturbances**

Visual halos

H53.2 **Diplopia**

Double vision

√5ᵗʰ H53.3 **Other and unspecified disorders of binocular vision**

H53.3Ø **Unspecified disorder of binocular vision**

H53.31 **Abnormal retinal correspondence**

H53.32 **Fusion with defective stereopsis**

H53.33 **Simultaneous visual perception without fusion**

H53.34 **Suppression of binocular vision**

√5ᵗʰ H53.4 **Visual field defects**

H53.4Ø **Unspecified visual field defects**

√6ᵗʰ H53.41 **Scotoma involving** central area

Central scotoma

H53.411 **Scotoma involving central area,** right eye

H53.412 **Scotoma involving central area,** left eye

H53.413 **Scotoma involving central area,** bilateral

H53.419 **Scotoma involving central area,** unspecified eye

√6ᵗʰ H53.42 **Scotoma of** blind spot area

Enlarged blind spot

H53.421 **Scotoma of blind spot area,** right eye

H53.422 **Scotoma of blind spot area,** left eye

H53.423 **Scotoma of blind spot area,** bilateral

H53.429 **Scotoma of blind spot area, unspecified eye**

√6ᵗʰ H53.43 **Sector or arcuate** defects

Arcuate scotoma

Bjerrum scotoma

H53.431 **Sector or arcuate defects,** right eye

H53.432 **Sector or arcuate defects,** left eye

H53.433 **Sector or arcuate defects,** bilateral

H53.439 **Sector or arcuate defects, unspecified eye**

√6ᵗʰ H53.45 **Other localized visual field defect**

Peripheral visual field defect

Ring scotoma NOS

Scotoma NOS

H53.451 **Other localized visual field defect,** right eye

H53.452 **Other localized visual field defect,** left eye

H53.453 **Other localized visual field defect,** bilateral

H53.459 **Other localized visual field defect,** unspecified eye

√6ᵗʰ H53.46 **Homonymous** bilateral field defects

Homonymous hemianopia

Homonymous hemianopsia

Quadrant anopia

Quadrant anopsia

H53.461 **Homonymous bilateral field defects,** right side

H53.462 **Homonymous bilateral field defects,** left side

H53.469 **Homonymous bilateral field defects,** unspecified side

Homonymous bilateral field defects NOS

H53.47 **Heteronymous** bilateral field defects

Heteronymous hemianop(s)ia

√6ᵗʰ H53.48 **Generalized contraction** of visual field

H53.481 **Generalized contraction of visual field,** right eye

H53.482 **Generalized contraction of visual field,** left eye

H53.483 **Generalized contraction of visual field,** bilateral

H53.489 **Generalized contraction of visual field,** unspecified eye

√5ᵗʰ H53.5 **Color vision deficiencies**

Color blindness

EXCLUDES 2   day blindness (H53.11)

H53.5Ø **Unspecified color vision deficiencies**

Color blindness NOS

H53.51 **Achromatopsia**

DEF: Nonprogressive genetic visual disorder characterized by complete color blindness, decreased vision, and light sensitivity.

H53.52 **Acquired color vision deficiency**

H53.53 **Deuteranomaly**

Deuteranopia

DEF: Male-only genetic disorder causing difficulty in distinguishing green and red; no shortened spectrum.

H53.54 **Protanomaly**

Protanopia

H53.55 **Tritanomaly**

Tritanopia

H53.59 **Other color vision deficiencies**

√5ᵗʰ H53.6 **Night blindness**

EXCLUDES 1   night blindness due to vitamin A deficiency (E5Ø.5)

H53.6Ø **Unspecified night blindness**

H53.61 **Abnormal dark adaptation curve**

H53.62 **Acquired** night blindness

H53.63 **Congenital** night blindness

H53.69 **Other night blindness**

√5ᵗʰ H53.7 **Vision** sensitivity deficiencies

H53.71 **Glare** sensitivity

H53.72 **Impaired contrast** sensitivity

H53.8 **Other visual disturbances**

H53.9 **Unspecified visual disturbance**

√4ᵗʰ H54 **Blindness and low vision**

NOTE   For definition of visual impairment categories see table below

Code first any associated underlying cause of the blindness

EXCLUDES 1   amaurosis fugax (G45.3)

AHA: 2017,4Q,11-12

√5ᵗʰ H54.Ø **Blindness,** both eyes

Visual impairment categories 3, 4, 5 in both eyes.

√6ᵗʰ H54.ØX **Blindness, both eyes, different category levels**

√7ᵗʰ H54.ØX3 **Blindness right eye, category 3**

✔ Additional Character Required   √x7ᵗʰ Placeholder   Questionable PDx   Manifestation   Unspecified Dx   UPD Unacceptable PDx   H1-H14 HAC   HCC CMS-HCC Dx   HIV HIV Dx

ICD-10-CM 2022   627

H54.0X33 Blindness right eye category 3, blindness left eye category 3

H54.0X34 Blindness right eye category 3, blindness left eye category 4

H54.0X35 Blindness right eye category 3, blindness left eye category 5

✓7th H54.0X4 Blindness right eye, category 4

H54.0X43 Blindness right eye category 4, blindness left eye category 3

H54.0X44 Blindness right eye category 4, blindness left eye category 4

H54.0X45 Blindness right eye category 4, blindness left eye category 5

✓7th H54.0X5 Blindness right eye, category 5

H54.0X53 Blindness right eye category 5, blindness left eye category 3

H54.0X54 Blindness right eye category 5, blindness left eye category 4

H54.0X55 Blindness right eye category 5, blindness left eye category 5

✓5th H54.1 Blindness, one eye, low vision other eye

Visual impairment categories 3, 4, 5 in one eye, with categories 1 or 2 in the other eye.

H54.10 Blindness, one eye, low vision other eye, unspecified eyes

✓6th H54.11 Blindness, right eye, low vision left eye

✓7th H54.113 Blindness right eye category 3, low vision left eye

H54.1131 Blindness right eye category 3, low vision left eye category 1

H54.1132 Blindness right eye category 3, low vision left eye category 2

✓7th H54.114 Blindness right eye category 4, low vision left eye

H54.1141 Blindness right eye category 4, low vision left eye category 1

H54.1142 Blindness right eye category 4, low vision left eye category 2

✓7th H54.115 Blindness right eye category 5, low vision left eye

H54.1151 Blindness right eye category 5, low vision left eye category 1

H54.1152 Blindness right eye category 5, low vision left eye category 2

✓6th H54.12 Blindness, left eye, low vision right eye

✓7th H54.121 Low vision right eye category 1, blindness left eye

H54.1213 Low vision right eye category 1, blindness left eye category 3

H54.1214 Low vision right eye category 1, blindness left eye category 4

H54.1215 Low vision right eye category 1, blindness left eye category 5

✓7th H54.122 Low vision right eye category 2, blindness left eye

H54.1223 Low vision right eye category 2, blindness left eye category 3

H54.1224 Low vision right eye category 2, blindness left eye category 4

H54.1225 Low vision right eye category 2, blindness left eye category 5

✓5th H54.2 Low vision, both eyes

Visual impairment categories 1 or 2 in both eyes.

✓6th H54.2X Low vision, both eyes, different category levels

✓7th H54.2X1 Low vision, right eye, category 1

H54.2X11 Low vision right eye category 1, low vision left eye category 1

H54.2X12 Low vision right eye category 1, low vision left eye category 2

✓7th H54.2X2 Low vision, right eye, category 2

H54.2X21 Low vision right eye category 2, low vision left eye category 1

H54.2X22 Low vision right eye category 2, low vision left eye category 2

H54.3 Unqualified visual loss, both eyes

Visual impairment category 9 in both eyes.

TIP: Assign only when both eyes are documented as affected by blindness or low vision but the visual impairment category is not documented.

✓5th H54.4 Blindness, one eye

Visual impairment categories 3, 4, 5 in one eye [normal vision in other eye]

H54.40 Blindness, one eye, unspecified eye

✓6th H54.41 Blindness, right eye, normal vision left eye

✓7th H54.413 Blindness, right eye, category 3

H54.413A Blindness right eye category 3, normal vision left eye

✓7th H54.414 Blindness, right eye, category 4

H54.414A Blindness right eye category 4, normal vision left eye

✓7th H54.415 Blindness, right eye, category 5

H54.415A Blindness right eye category 5, normal vision left eye

✓6th H54.42 Blindness, left eye, normal vision right eye

✓7th H54.42A Blindness, left eye, category 3-5

H54.42A3 Blindness left eye category 3, normal vision right eye

H54.42A4 Blindness left eye category 4, normal vision right eye

H54.42A5 Blindness left eye category 5, normal vision right eye

✓5th H54.5 Low vision, one eye

Visual impairment categories 1 or 2 in one eye [normal vision in other eye].

H54.50 Low vision, one eye, unspecified eye

✓6th H54.51 Low vision, right eye, normal vision left eye

✓7th H54.511 Low vision, right eye, category 1-2

H54.511A Low vision right eye category 1, normal vision left eye

H54.512A Low vision right eye category 2, normal vision left eye

✓7th H54.52A Low vision, left eye, category 1-2

H54.52A1 Low vision left eye category 1, normal vision right eye

H54.52A2 Low vision left eye category 2, normal vision right eye

✓5th H54.6 Unqualified visual loss, one eye

Visual impairment category 9 in one eye [normal vision in other eye].

TIP: Assign a code from this category only when one eye is documented as affected by blindness or low vision but the visual impairment category is not documented.

H54.60 Unqualified visual loss, one eye, unspecified

H54.61 Unqualified visual loss, right eye, normal vision left eye

H54.62 Unqualified visual loss, left eye, normal vision right eye

H54.7 Unspecified visual loss   UPD

Visual impairment category 9 NOS

TIP: Assign only when documentation specifies blindness, visual loss, or low vision but not whether one or both eyes are affected or the visual impairment category.

N Newborn: 0   P Pediatric: 0-17   M Maternity: 9-64   A Adult: 15-124   MCC Major Complication/Comorbidity   CC Complication/Comorbidity   SW Severe Wound Dx

628

ICD-10-CM 2022

H54.8   **Legal blindness,** as defined in USA
Blindness NOS according to USA definition

> **EXCLUDES 1**   *legal blindness with specification of impairment level (H54.0-H54.7)*

> **NOTE**   The table below gives a classification of severity of visual impairment recommended by a WHO Study Group on the Prevention of Blindness, Geneva, 6-10 November 1972.
>
> The term "low vision" in category H54 comprises categories 1 and 2 of the table, the term "blindness" categories 3, 4 and 5, and the term "unqualified visual loss" category 9.
>
> If the extent of the visual field is taken into account, patients with a field no greater than 10 but greater than 5 around central fixation should be placed in category 3 and patients with a field no greater than 5 around central fixation should be placed in category 4, even if the central acuity is not impaired.

Category of visual impairment	Visual acuity with best possible correction	
	Maximum less than:	**Minimum equal to or better than:**
1	6/18 3/10 (0.3) 20/70	6/60 1/10 (0.1) 20/200
2	6/60 1/10 (0.1) 20/200	3/60 1/20 (0.05) 20/400
3	3/60 1/200 (0.05) 20/400	1/60 (finger counting at one meter) 1/50 (0.02) 5/300 (20/1200)
4	1/60 (finger counting at one meter) 1/50 (0.02) 5/300	Light perception
5	No light perception	
9	Undetermined or unspecified	

Other disorders of eye and adnexa (H55-H57)

H55   **Nystagmus and other** irregular eye movements

   H55.0   **Nystagmus**
> **DEF:** Rapid, rhythmic, involuntary movements of the eyeball in vertical, horizontal, rotational, or mixed directions.

     H55.00   **Unspecified nystagmus**
     H55.01   **Congenital** nystagmus
     H55.02   **Latent** nystagmus
     H55.03   **Visual deprivation** nystagmus
     H55.04   **Dissociated** nystagmus
     H55.09   **Other forms of nystagmus**

   H55.8   **Other irregular eye movements**
> **AHA:** 2020,4Q,25

     H55.81   **Deficient saccadic** eye movements
     H55.82   **Deficient smooth pursuit** eye movements
     H55.89   **Other irregular eye movements**

H57   **Other disorders of eye and adnexa**

   H57.0   **Anomalies of pupillary function**
     H57.00   **Unspecified anomaly of pupillary function**
     H57.01   **Argyll Robertson pupil, atypical**
> **EXCLUDES 1**   *syphilitic Argyll Robertson pupil (A52.19)*

     H57.02   **Anisocoria**
     H57.03   **Miosis**
     H57.04   **Mydriasis**
     H57.05   **Tonic pupil**
       H57.051   **Tonic pupil, right** eye
       H57.052   **Tonic pupil, left** eye
       H57.053   **Tonic pupil, bilateral**
       H57.059   **Tonic pupil, unspecified eye**
     H57.09   **Other anomalies of pupillary function**

   H57.1   **Ocular pain**
     H57.10   **Ocular pain, unspecified eye**
     H57.11   **Ocular pain, right** eye
     H57.12   **Ocular pain, left** eye
     H57.13   **Ocular pain, bilateral**

   H57.8   **Other specified disorders of eye and adnexa**
> **AHA:** 2018,4Q,15-16

     H57.81   **Brow ptosis**
       H57.811   **Brow ptosis, right**
       H57.812   **Brow ptosis, left**
       H57.813   **Brow ptosis, bilateral**
       H57.819   **Brow ptosis, unspecified**
     H57.89   **Other specified disorders of eye and adnexa**

   H57.9   **Unspecified disorder of eye and adnexa**   **UPD**

Intraoperative and postprocedural complications and disorders of eye and adnexa, not elsewhere classified (H59)

H59   **Intraoperative and postprocedural complications and disorders of eye and adnexa, not elsewhere classified**

> **EXCLUDES 1**   *mechanical complication of intraocular lens (T85.2)*
> *mechanical complication of other ocular prosthetic devices, implants and grafts (T85.3)*
> *pseudophakia (Z96.1)*
> *secondary cataracts (H26.4-)*

   H59.0   **Disorders of the eye** following cataract surgery
     H59.01   **Keratopathy (bullous aphakic) following cataract surgery**
> Vitreal corneal syndrome
> Vitreous (touch) syndrome

       H59.011   **Keratopathy (bullous aphakic) following cataract surgery, right** eye   **CC**
       H59.012   **Keratopathy (bullous aphakic) following cataract surgery, left** eye   **CC**
       H59.013   **Keratopathy (bullous aphakic) following cataract surgery, bilateral**   **CC**
       H59.019   **Keratopathy (bullous aphakic) following cataract surgery, unspecified eye**   **CC**

     H59.02   **Cataract (lens) fragments in eye following cataract surgery**
       H59.021   **Cataract (lens) fragments in eye following cataract surgery, right** eye
       H59.022   **Cataract (lens) fragments in eye following cataract surgery, left** eye
       H59.023   **Cataract (lens) fragments in eye following cataract surgery, bilateral**
       H59.029   **Cataract (lens) fragments in eye following cataract surgery, unspecified eye**

     H59.03   **Cystoid macular edema following cataract surgery**
       H59.031   **Cystoid macular edema following cataract surgery, right** eye   **CC**
       H59.032   **Cystoid macular edema following cataract surgery, left** eye   **CC**
       H59.033   **Cystoid macular edema following cataract surgery, bilateral**   **CC**
       H59.039   **Cystoid macular edema following cataract surgery, unspecified eye**   **CC**

     H59.09   **Other disorders of the eye following cataract surgery**
       H59.091   **Other disorders of the right eye following cataract surgery**   **CC**
       H59.092   **Other disorders of the left eye following cataract surgery**   **CC**
       H59.093   **Other disorders of the eye following cataract surgery, bilateral**   **CC**
       H59.099   **Other disorders of unspecified eye following cataract surgery**   **CC**

   H59.1   **Intraoperative hemorrhage and hematoma** of eye and adnexa complicating a procedure
> **EXCLUDES 1**   *intraoperative hemorrhage and hematoma of eye and adnexa due to accidental puncture or laceration during a procedure (H59.2-)*

     H59.11   **Intraoperative hemorrhage and hematoma of eye and adnexa complicating an ophthalmic procedure**
       H59.111   **Intraoperative hemorrhage and hematoma of right eye and adnexa complicating an ophthalmic procedure**   **CC**

H59.112 Intraoperative hemorrhage and hematoma of left eye and adnexa complicating an ophthalmic procedure **CC**

H59.113 Intraoperative hemorrhage and hematoma of eye and adnexa complicating an ophthalmic procedure, bilateral **CC**

H59.119 Intraoperative hemorrhage and hematoma of unspecified eye and adnexa complicating an ophthalmic procedure **CC**

√6th H59.12 Intraoperative hemorrhage and hematoma of eye and adnexa complicating other procedure

H59.121 Intraoperative hemorrhage and hematoma of right eye and adnexa complicating other procedure **CC**

H59.122 Intraoperative hemorrhage and hematoma of left eye and adnexa complicating other procedure **CC**

H59.123 Intraoperative hemorrhage and hematoma of eye and adnexa complicating other procedure, bilateral **CC**

H59.129 Intraoperative hemorrhage and hematoma of unspecified eye and adnexa complicating other procedure **CC**

√5th H59.2 Accidental puncture and laceration of eye and adnexa during a procedure

√6th H59.21 Accidental puncture and laceration of eye and adnexa during an ophthalmic procedure

H59.211 Accidental puncture and laceration of right eye and adnexa during an ophthalmic procedure **CC**

H59.212 Accidental puncture and laceration of left eye and adnexa during an ophthalmic procedure **CC**

H59.213 Accidental puncture and laceration of eye and adnexa during an ophthalmic procedure, bilateral **CC**

H59.219 Accidental puncture and laceration of unspecified eye and adnexa during an ophthalmic procedure **CC**

√6th H59.22 Accidental puncture and laceration of eye and adnexa during other procedure

H59.221 Accidental puncture and laceration of right eye and adnexa during other procedure **CC**

H59.222 Accidental puncture and laceration of left eye and adnexa during other procedure **CC**

H59.223 Accidental puncture and laceration of eye and adnexa during other procedure, bilateral **CC**

H59.229 Accidental puncture and laceration of unspecified eye and adnexa during other procedure **CC**

√5th H59.3 Postprocedural hemorrhage, hematoma, and seroma of eye and adnexa following a procedure

AHA: 2016,4Q,9-10

√6th H59.31 Postprocedural hemorrhage of eye and adnexa following an ophthalmic procedure

H59.311 Postprocedural hemorrhage of right eye and adnexa following an ophthalmic procedure **CC**

H59.312 Postprocedural hemorrhage of left eye and adnexa following an ophthalmic procedure **CC**

H59.313 Postprocedural hemorrhage of eye and adnexa following an ophthalmic procedure, bilateral **CC**

H59.319 Postprocedural hemorrhage of unspecified eye and adnexa following an ophthalmic procedure **CC**

√6th H59.32 Postprocedural hemorrhage of eye and adnexa following other procedure

H59.321 Postprocedural hemorrhage of right eye and adnexa following other procedure **CC**

H59.322 Postprocedural hemorrhage of left eye and adnexa following other procedure **CC**

H59.323 Postprocedural hemorrhage of eye and adnexa following other procedure, bilateral **CC**

H59.329 Postprocedural hemorrhage of unspecified eye and adnexa following other procedure **CC**

√6th H59.33 Postprocedural hematoma of eye and adnexa following an ophthalmic procedure

H59.331 Postprocedural hematoma of right eye and adnexa following an ophthalmic procedure **CC**

H59.332 Postprocedural hematoma of left eye and adnexa following an ophthalmic procedure **CC**

H59.333 Postprocedural hematoma of eye and adnexa following an ophthalmic procedure, bilateral **CC**

H59.339 Postprocedural hematoma of unspecified eye and adnexa following an ophthalmic procedure **CC**

√6th H59.34 Postprocedural hematoma of eye and adnexa following other procedure

H59.341 Postprocedural hematoma of right eye and adnexa following other procedure **CC**

H59.342 Postprocedural hematoma of left eye and adnexa following other procedure **CC**

H59.343 Postprocedural hematoma of eye and adnexa following other procedure, bilateral **CC**

H59.349 Postprocedural hematoma of unspecified eye and adnexa following other procedure **CC**

√6th H59.35 Postprocedural seroma of eye and adnexa following an ophthalmic procedure

H59.351 Postprocedural seroma of right eye and adnexa following an ophthalmic procedure **CC**

H59.352 Postprocedural seroma of left eye and adnexa following an ophthalmic procedure **CC**

H59.353 Postprocedural seroma of eye and adnexa following an ophthalmic procedure, bilateral **CC**

H59.359 Postprocedural seroma of unspecified eye and adnexa following an ophthalmic procedure **CC**

√6th H59.36 Postprocedural seroma of eye and adnexa following other procedure

H59.361 Postprocedural seroma of right eye and adnexa following other procedure **CC**

H59.362 Postprocedural seroma of left eye and adnexa following other procedure **CC**

H59.363 Postprocedural seroma of eye and adnexa following other procedure, bilateral **CC**

H59.369 Postprocedural seroma of unspecified eye and adnexa following other procedure **CC**

√5th H59.4 Inflammation (infection) of postprocedural bleb

Postprocedural blebitis

EXCLUDES 1   filtering (vitreous) bleb after glaucoma surgery status (Z98.83)

H59.40 Inflammation (infection) of postprocedural bleb, unspecified

H59.41 Inflammation (infection) of postprocedural bleb, stage 1

H59.42 Inflammation (infection) of postprocedural bleb, stage 2

H59.43 Inflammation (infection) of postprocedural bleb, stage 3

Bleb endophthalmitis

√5th H59.8 Other intraoperative and postprocedural complications and disorders of eye and adnexa, not elsewhere classified

√6th H59.81 Chorioretinal scars after surgery for detachment

H59.811 Chorioretinal scars after surgery for detachment, right eye **CC**

H59.812 Chorioretinal scars after surgery for detachment, left eye **CC**

H59.813 Chorioretinal scars after surgery for detachment, bilateral **CC**

N Newborn: 0   P Pediatric: 0-17   M Maternity: 9-64   A Adult: 15-124   MCC Major Complication/Comorbidity   CC Complication/Comorbidity   SW Severe Wound Dx

630

ICD-10-CM 2022

    H59.819 Chorioretinal scars after surgery for detachment, unspecified eye   `CC`

H59.88 Other intraoperative complications of eye and adnexa, not elsewhere classified   `CC`

H59.89 Other postprocedural complications and disorders of eye and adnexa, not elsewhere classified   `CC`
    AHA: 2020,3Q,29

☑ Additional Character Required   ✓x 7ᵗʰ Placeholder   Questionable PDx   Manifestation   Unspecified Dx   **UPD** Unacceptable PDx   **H1 - H14** HAC   **HCC** CMS-HCC Dx   **HIV** HIV Dx

ICD-10-CM 2022   631

Chapter 7. Diseases of the Eye and Adnexa

H59.819–H59.89

Chapter 8. Diseases of the Ear and Mastoid Process (H60–H95)

Chapter-specific Guidelines with Coding Examples
Reserved for future guideline expansion.

Chapter 8. Diseases of the Ear and Mastoid Process (H60-H95)

NOTE Use an external cause code following the code for the ear condition, if applicable, to identify the cause of the ear condition

EXCLUDES 2   *certain conditions originating in the perinatal period (P04-P96)*
certain infectious and parasitic diseases (A00-B99)
complications of pregnancy, childbirth and the puerperium (O00-O9A)
congenital malformations, deformations and chromosomal abnormalities (Q00-Q99)
endocrine, nutritional and metabolic diseases (E00-E88)
injury, poisoning and certain other consequences of external causes (S00-T88)
neoplasms (C00-D49)
symptoms, signs and abnormal clinical and laboratory findings, not elsewhere classified (R00-R94)

This chapter contains the following blocks:

H60-H62   Diseases of external ear
H65-H75   Diseases of middle ear and mastoid
H80-H83   Diseases of inner ear
H90-H94   Other disorders of ear
H95   Intraoperative and postprocedural complications and disorders of ear and mastoid process, not elsewhere classified

Diseases of external ear (H60-H62)

✓4ᵗʰ **H60 Otitis externa**

TIP: When the specific infectious agent is identified, a code from Chapter 1 is assigned instead of a code from this category.

✓5ᵗʰ **H60.0 Abscess of external ear**

Boil of external ear
Carbuncle of auricle or external auditory canal
Furuncle of external ear

H60.00 Abscess of external ear, unspecified ear
H60.01 Abscess of right external ear
H60.02 Abscess of left external ear
H60.03 Abscess of external ear, bilateral

✓5ᵗʰ **H60.1 Cellulitis of external ear**

Cellulitis of auricle
Cellulitis of external auditory canal

H60.10 Cellulitis of external ear, unspecified ear
H60.11 Cellulitis of right external ear
H60.12 Cellulitis of left external ear
H60.13 Cellulitis of external ear, bilateral

✓5ᵗʰ **H60.2 Malignant otitis externa**

H60.20 Malignant otitis externa, unspecified ear   CC
H60.21 Malignant otitis externa, right ear   CC
H60.22 Malignant otitis externa, left ear   CC
H60.23 Malignant otitis externa, bilateral   CC

✓5ᵗʰ **H60.3 Other infective otitis externa**

✓6ᵗʰ **H60.31 Diffuse otitis externa**

H60.311 Diffuse otitis externa, right ear
H60.312 Diffuse otitis externa, left ear
H60.313 Diffuse otitis externa, bilateral
H60.319 Diffuse otitis externa, unspecified ear

✓6ᵗʰ **H60.32 Hemorrhagic otitis externa**

H60.321 Hemorrhagic otitis externa, right ear
H60.322 Hemorrhagic otitis externa, left ear
H60.323 Hemorrhagic otitis externa, bilateral
H60.329 Hemorrhagic otitis externa, unspecified ear

✓6ᵗʰ **H60.33 Swimmer's ear**

DEF: Commonly occurs when water gets trapped in the ear after swimming.

H60.331 Swimmer's ear, right ear
H60.332 Swimmer's ear, left ear
H60.333 Swimmer's ear, bilateral
H60.339 Swimmer's ear, unspecified ear

✓6ᵗʰ **H60.39 Other infective otitis externa**

H60.391 Other infective otitis externa, right ear
H60.392 Other infective otitis externa, left ear
H60.393 Other infective otitis externa, bilateral
H60.399 Other infective otitis externa, unspecified ear

✓5ᵗʰ **H60.4 Cholesteatoma of external ear**

Keratosis obturans of external ear (canal)

EXCLUDES 2   *cholesteatoma of middle ear (H71.-)*
recurrent cholesteatoma of postmastoidectomy cavity (H95.0-)

DEF: Cholesteatoma: Noncancerous cyst-like mass of cell debris, including cholesterol and epithelial cells resulting from trauma, repeated or improperly healed infections, and congenital enclosure of epidermal cells.

H60.40 Cholesteatoma of external ear, unspecified ear
H60.41 Cholesteatoma of right external ear
H60.42 Cholesteatoma of left external ear
H60.43 Cholesteatoma of external ear, bilateral

✓5ᵗʰ **H60.5 Acute noninfective otitis externa**

✓6ᵗʰ **H60.50 Unspecified acute noninfective otitis externa**

Acute otitis externa NOS

H60.501 Unspecified acute noninfective otitis externa, right ear
H60.502 Unspecified acute noninfective otitis externa, left ear
H60.503 Unspecified acute noninfective otitis externa, bilateral
H60.509 Unspecified acute noninfective otitis externa, unspecified ear

✓6ᵗʰ **H60.51 Acute actinic otitis externa**

H60.511 Acute actinic otitis externa, right ear
H60.512 Acute actinic otitis externa, left ear
H60.513 Acute actinic otitis externa, bilateral
H60.519 Acute actinic otitis externa, unspecified ear

✓6ᵗʰ **H60.52 Acute chemical otitis externa**

H60.521 Acute chemical otitis externa, right ear
H60.522 Acute chemical otitis externa, left ear
H60.523 Acute chemical otitis externa, bilateral
H60.529 Acute chemical otitis externa, unspecified ear

✓6ᵗʰ **H60.53 Acute contact otitis externa**

H60.531 Acute contact otitis externa, right ear
H60.532 Acute contact otitis externa, left ear
H60.533 Acute contact otitis externa, bilateral
H60.539 Acute contact otitis externa, unspecified ear

✓6ᵗʰ **H60.54 Acute eczematoid otitis externa**

H60.541 Acute eczematoid otitis externa, right ear
H60.542 Acute eczematoid otitis externa, left ear
H60.543 Acute eczematoid otitis externa, bilateral
H60.549 Acute eczematoid otitis externa, unspecified ear

✓6ᵗʰ **H60.55 Acute reactive otitis externa**

H60.551 Acute reactive otitis externa, right ear
H60.552 Acute reactive otitis externa, left ear
H60.553 Acute reactive otitis externa, bilateral
H60.559 Acute reactive otitis externa, unspecified ear

✓6ᵗʰ **H60.59 Other noninfective acute otitis externa**

H60.591 Other noninfective acute otitis externa, right ear
H60.592 Other noninfective acute otitis externa, left ear
H60.593 Other noninfective acute otitis externa, bilateral
H60.599 Other noninfective acute otitis externa, unspecified ear

✓5ᵗʰ **H60.6 Unspecified chronic otitis externa**

H60.60 Unspecified chronic otitis externa, unspecified ear
H60.61 Unspecified chronic otitis externa, right ear
H60.62 Unspecified chronic otitis externa, left ear
H60.63 Unspecified chronic otitis externa, bilateral

✓5ᵗʰ **H60.8 Other otitis externa**

✓6ᵗʰ **H60.8X Other otitis externa**

H60.8X1 Other otitis externa, right ear
H60.8X2 Other otitis externa, left ear
H60.8X3 Other otitis externa, bilateral
H60.8X9 Other otitis externa, unspecified ear

✓6ᵗʰ **H60.9 Unspecified otitis externa**

H60.90 Unspecified otitis externa, unspecified ear
H60.91 Unspecified otitis externa, right ear

H60.92 **Unspecified otitis externa,** left **ear**

H60.93 **Unspecified otitis externa,** bilateral

✓4ᵗʰ **H61 Other disorders of external ear**

✓5ᵗʰ **H61.0 Chondritis and perichondritis of external ear**

Chondrodermatitis nodularis chronica helicis
Perichondritis of auricle
Perichondritis of pinna

✓6ᵗʰ **H61.00 Unspecified** perichondritis **of external ear**

H61.001 **Unspecified perichondritis of** right **external ear**

H61.002 **Unspecified perichondritis of** left **external ear**

H61.003 **Unspecified perichondritis of external ear,** bilateral

H61.009 **Unspecified perichondritis of external ear, unspecified ear**

✓6ᵗʰ **H61.01** Acute perichondritis **of external ear**

H61.011 **Acute perichondritis of** right **external ear**

H61.012 **Acute perichondritis of** left **external ear**

H61.013 **Acute perichondritis of external ear,** bilateral

H61.019 **Acute perichondritis of external ear, unspecified ear**

✓6ᵗʰ **H61.02** Chronic perichondritis **of external ear**

H61.021 **Chronic perichondritis of** right **external ear**

H61.022 **Chronic perichondritis of** left **external ear**

H61.023 **Chronic perichondritis of external ear,** bilateral

H61.029 **Chronic perichondritis of external ear, unspecified ear**

✓6ᵗʰ **H61.03** Chondritis **of external ear**

Chondritis of auricle
Chondritis of pinna
AHA: 2015,1Q,18
DEF: Infection that has progressed into the cartilage and presents as indurated and edematous skin over the pinna. Vascular compromise occurs with tissue necrosis and deformity.

H61.031 **Chondritis of** right **external ear**

H61.032 **Chondritis of** left **external ear**

H61.033 **Chondritis of external ear,** bilateral

H61.039 **Chondritis of external ear, unspecified ear**

✓5ᵗʰ **H61.1 Noninfective disorders of pinna**

EXCLUDES 2 cauliflower ear (M95.1-)
gouty tophi of ear (M1A.-)

✓6ᵗʰ **H61.10 Unspecified noninfective disorders of pinna**

Disorder of pinna NOS

H61.101 **Unspecified noninfective disorders of pinna,** right **ear**

H61.102 **Unspecified noninfective disorders of pinna,** left **ear**

H61.103 **Unspecified noninfective disorders of pinna,** bilateral

H61.109 **Unspecified noninfective disorders of pinna, unspecified ear**

✓6ᵗʰ **H61.11 Acquired deformity of pinna**

Acquired deformity of auricle
EXCLUDES 2 cauliflower ear (M95.1-)

H61.111 **Acquired deformity of pinna,** right **ear**

H61.112 **Acquired deformity of pinna,** left **ear**

H61.113 **Acquired deformity of pinna,** bilateral

H61.119 **Acquired deformity of pinna, unspecified ear**

✓6ᵗʰ **H61.12 Hematoma of pinna**

Hematoma of auricle

H61.121 **Hematoma of pinna,** right **ear**

H61.122 **Hematoma of pinna,** left **ear**

H61.123 **Hematoma of pinna,** bilateral

H61.129 **Hematoma of pinna, unspecified ear**

✓6ᵗʰ **H61.19 Other noninfective disorders of pinna**

H61.191 **Noninfective disorders of pinna,** right **ear**

H61.192 **Noninfective disorders of pinna,** left **ear**

H61.193 **Noninfective disorders of pinna,** bilateral

H61.199 **Noninfective disorders of pinna, unspecified ear**

✓5ᵗʰ **H61.2 Impacted cerumen**

Wax in ear

H61.20 **Impacted cerumen, unspecified ear**

H61.21 **Impacted cerumen,** right **ear**

H61.22 **Impacted cerumen,** left **ear**

H61.23 **Impacted cerumen,** bilateral

✓5ᵗʰ **H61.3 Acquired stenosis of external ear canal**

Collapse of external ear canal
EXCLUDES 1 postprocedural stenosis of external ear canal (H95.81-)

✓6ᵗʰ **H61.30 Acquired stenosis of external ear canal, unspecified**

H61.301 **Acquired stenosis of** right **external ear canal, unspecified**

H61.302 **Acquired stenosis of** left **external ear canal, unspecified**

H61.303 **Acquired stenosis of external ear canal, unspecified,** bilateral

H61.309 **Acquired stenosis of external ear canal, unspecified, unspecified ear**

✓6ᵗʰ **H61.31 Acquired stenosis of external ear canal** secondary to trauma

H61.311 **Acquired stenosis of** right **external ear canal secondary to trauma**

H61.312 **Acquired stenosis of** left **external ear canal secondary to trauma**

H61.313 **Acquired stenosis of external ear canal secondary to trauma,** bilateral

H61.319 **Acquired stenosis of external ear canal secondary to trauma, unspecified ear**

✓6ᵗʰ **H61.32 Acquired stenosis of external ear canal** secondary to inflammation and infection

DEF: Narrowing of the external ear canal due to chronic inflammation or infection.

H61.321 **Acquired stenosis of** right **external ear canal secondary to inflammation and infection**

H61.322 **Acquired stenosis of** left **external ear canal secondary to inflammation and infection**

H61.323 **Acquired stenosis of external ear canal secondary to inflammation and infection,** bilateral

H61.329 **Acquired stenosis of external ear canal secondary to inflammation and infection, unspecified ear**

✓6ᵗʰ **H61.39 Other acquired stenosis of external ear canal**

H61.391 **Other acquired stenosis of** right **external ear canal**

H61.392 **Other acquired stenosis of** left **external ear canal**

H61.393 **Other acquired stenosis of external ear canal,** bilateral

H61.399 **Other acquired stenosis of external ear canal, unspecified ear**

✓5ᵗʰ **H61.8 Other specified disorders of external ear**

✓6ᵗʰ **H61.81 Exostosis of external canal**

H61.811 **Exostosis of** right **external canal**

H61.812 **Exostosis of** left **external canal**

H61.813 **Exostosis of external canal,** bilateral

H61.819 **Exostosis of external canal, unspecified ear**

✓6ᵗʰ **H61.89 Other specified disorders of external ear**

H61.891 **Other specified disorders of** right **external ear**

H61.892 **Other specified disorders of** left **external ear**

H61.893 **Other specified disorders of external ear,** bilateral

H61.899 **Other specified disorders of external ear, unspecified ear**

✓5ᵗʰ **H61.9 Disorder of external ear, unspecified**

H61.90 **Disorder of external ear, unspecified, unspecified ear**

H61.91 **Disorder of** right **external ear, unspecified**

H61.92 **Disorder of** left **external ear, unspecified**

H61.93 **Disorder of external ear, unspecified,** bilateral

✔ Additional Character Required   ✓x7ᵗʰ Placeholder   Questionable PDx   Manifestation   Unspecified Dx   UPD Unacceptable PDx   H1-H14 HAC   HCC CMS-HCC Dx   HIV HIV Dx

ICD-10-CM 2022   635

✓4ᵗʰ **H62** **Disorders of external ear in diseases classified elsewhere**

  ✓5ᵗʰ **H62.4** **Otitis externa in other diseases classified elsewhere**

    Code first underlying disease, such as:
      erysipelas (A46)
      impetigo (L01.0)
    EXCLUDES 1   *otitis externa (in):*
        candidiasis (B37.84)
        herpes viral [herpes simplex] (B00.1)
        herpes zoster (B02.8)

    H62.40 *Otitis externa in other diseases classified elsewhere, unspecified ear*

    H62.41 *Otitis externa in other diseases classified elsewhere, right ear*

    H62.42 *Otitis externa in other diseases classified elsewhere, left ear*

    H62.43 *Otitis externa in other diseases classified elsewhere, bilateral*

  ✓5ᵗʰ **H62.8** **Other disorders of external ear in diseases classified elsewhere**

    Code first underlying disease, such as:
      gout (M1A.-, M10.-)

    ✓6ᵗʰ **H62.8X** **Other disorders of external ear in diseases classified elsewhere**

      H62.8X1 *Other disorders of right external ear in diseases classified elsewhere*

      H62.8X2 *Other disorders of left external ear in diseases classified elsewhere*

      H62.8X3 *Other disorders of external ear in diseases classified elsewhere, bilateral*

      H62.8X9 *Other disorders of external ear in diseases classified elsewhere, unspecified ear*

Diseases of middle ear and mastoid (H65-H75)

✓4ᵗʰ **H65** **Nonsuppurative otitis media**

  INCLUDES   nonsuppurative otitis media with myringitis
  Use additional code for any associated perforated tympanic membrane (H72.-)
  Use additional code, if applicable, to identify:
    exposure to environmental tobacco smoke (Z77.22)
    exposure to tobacco smoke in the perinatal period (P96.81)
    history of tobacco dependence (Z87.891)
    infectious agent (B95-B97)
    occupational exposure to environmental tobacco smoke (Z57.31)
    tobacco dependence (F17.-)
    tobacco use (Z72.0)

  ✓5ᵗʰ **H65.0** **Acute serous otitis media**

    Acute and subacute secretory otitis

    H65.00 **Acute serous otitis media, unspecified ear**

    H65.01 **Acute serous otitis media, right ear**

    H65.02 **Acute serous otitis media, left ear**

    H65.03 **Acute serous otitis media, bilateral**

    H65.04 **Acute serous otitis media, recurrent, right ear**

    H65.05 **Acute serous otitis media, recurrent, left ear**

    H65.06 **Acute serous otitis media, recurrent, bilateral**

    H65.07 **Acute serous otitis media, recurrent, unspecified ear**

  ✓5ᵗʰ **H65.1** **Other acute nonsuppurative otitis media**

    EXCLUDES 1   *otitic barotrauma (T70.0)*
      otitis media (acute) NOS (H66.9)

    ✓6ᵗʰ **H65.11** **Acute and subacute allergic otitis media (mucoid) (sanguinous) (serous)**

      H65.111 **Acute and subacute allergic otitis media (mucoid) (sanguinous) (serous), right ear**

      H65.112 **Acute and subacute allergic otitis media (mucoid) (sanguinous) (serous), left ear**

      H65.113 **Acute and subacute allergic otitis media (mucoid) (sanguinous) (serous), bilateral**

      H65.114 **Acute and subacute allergic otitis media (mucoid) (sanguinous) (serous), recurrent, right ear**

      H65.115 **Acute and subacute allergic otitis media (mucoid) (sanguinous) (serous), recurrent, left ear**

      H65.116 **Acute and subacute allergic otitis media (mucoid) (sanguinous) (serous), recurrent, bilateral**

      H65.117 **Acute and subacute allergic otitis media (mucoid) (sanguinous) (serous), recurrent, unspecified ear**

      H65.119 **Acute and subacute allergic otitis media (mucoid) (sanguinous) (serous), unspecified ear**

    ✓6ᵗʰ **H65.19** **Other acute nonsuppurative otitis media**

      Acute and subacute mucoid otitis media
      Acute and subacute nonsuppurative otitis media NOS
      Acute and subacute sanguinous otitis media
      Acute and subacute seromucinous otitis media

      H65.191 **Other acute nonsuppurative otitis media, right ear**

      H65.192 **Other acute nonsuppurative otitis media, left ear**

      H65.193 **Other acute nonsuppurative otitis media, bilateral**

      H65.194 **Other acute nonsuppurative otitis media, recurrent, right ear**

      H65.195 **Other acute nonsuppurative otitis media, recurrent, left ear**

      H65.196 **Other acute nonsuppurative otitis media, recurrent, bilateral**

      H65.197 **Other acute nonsuppurative otitis media recurrent, unspecified ear**

      H65.199 **Other acute nonsuppurative otitis media, unspecified ear**

  ✓5ᵗʰ **H65.2** **Chronic serous otitis media**

    Chronic tubotympanal catarrh

    H65.20 **Chronic serous otitis media, unspecified ear**

    H65.21 **Chronic serous otitis media, right ear**

    H65.22 **Chronic serous otitis media, left ear**

    H65.23 **Chronic serous otitis media, bilateral**

  ✓5ᵗʰ **H65.3** **Chronic mucoid otitis media**

    Chronic mucinous otitis media
    Chronic secretory otitis media
    Chronic transudative otitis media
    Glue ear
    EXCLUDES 1   *adhesive middle ear disease (H74.1)*

    H65.30 **Chronic mucoid otitis media, unspecified ear**

    H65.31 **Chronic mucoid otitis media, right ear**

    H65.32 **Chronic mucoid otitis media, left ear**

    H65.33 **Chronic mucoid otitis media, bilateral**

  ✓5ᵗʰ **H65.4** **Other chronic nonsuppurative otitis media**

    ✓6ᵗʰ **H65.41** **Chronic allergic otitis media**

      H65.411 **Chronic allergic otitis media, right ear**

      H65.412 **Chronic allergic otitis media, left ear**

      H65.413 **Chronic allergic otitis media, bilateral**

      H65.419 **Chronic allergic otitis media, unspecified ear**

    ✓6ᵗʰ **H65.49** **Other chronic nonsuppurative otitis media**

      Chronic exudative otitis media
      Chronic nonsuppurative otitis media NOS
      Chronic otitis media with effusion (nonpurulent)
      Chronic seromucinous otitis media

      H65.491 **Other chronic nonsuppurative otitis media, right ear**

      H65.492 **Other chronic nonsuppurative otitis media, left ear**

      H65.493 **Other chronic nonsuppurative otitis media, bilateral**

      H65.499 **Other chronic nonsuppurative otitis media, unspecified ear**

  ✓5ᵗʰ **H65.9** **Unspecified nonsuppurative otitis media**

    Allergic otitis media NOS
    Catarrhal otitis media NOS
    Exudative otitis media NOS
    Mucoid otitis media NOS
    Otitis media with effusion (nonpurulent) NOS
    Secretory otitis media NOS
    Seromucinous otitis media NOS
    Serous otitis media NOS
    Transudative otitis media NOS

    H65.90 **Unspecified nonsuppurative otitis media, unspecified ear**

    H65.91 **Unspecified nonsuppurative otitis media, right ear**

    H65.92 **Unspecified nonsuppurative otitis media, left ear**

    H65.93 **Unspecified nonsuppurative otitis media, bilateral**

Ⓝ Newborn: 0   Ⓟ Pediatric: 0-17   Ⓜ Maternity: 9-64   Ⓐ Adult: 15-124   MCC Major Complication/Comorbidity   CC Complication/Comorbidity   SW Severe Wound Dx

636   ICD-10-CM 2022

☑4ᵗʰ **H66 Suppurative and unspecified otitis media**

> INCLUDES   suppurative and unspecified otitis media with myringitis
> Use additional code to identify:
>   exposure to environmental tobacco smoke (Z77.22)
>   exposure to tobacco smoke in the perinatal period (P96.81)
>   history of tobacco dependence (Z87.891)
>   occupational exposure to environmental tobacco smoke (Z57.31)
>   tobacco dependence (F17.-)
>   tobacco use (Z72.0)
> **AHA:** 2016,1Q,34

☑5ᵗʰ **H66.0 Acute suppurative otitis media**

   ☑6ᵗʰ **H66.00 Acute suppurative otitis media without spontaneous rupture of ear drum**

     H66.001 Acute suppurative otitis media without spontaneous rupture of ear drum, right ear

     H66.002 Acute suppurative otitis media without spontaneous rupture of ear drum, left ear

     H66.003 Acute suppurative otitis media without spontaneous rupture of ear drum, bilateral

     H66.004 Acute suppurative otitis media without spontaneous rupture of ear drum, recurrent, right ear

     H66.005 Acute suppurative otitis media without spontaneous rupture of ear drum, recurrent, left ear

     H66.006 Acute suppurative otitis media without spontaneous rupture of ear drum, recurrent, bilateral

     H66.007 Acute suppurative otitis media without spontaneous rupture of ear drum, recurrent, unspecified ear

     H66.009 Acute suppurative otitis media without spontaneous rupture of ear drum, unspecified ear

   ☑6ᵗʰ **H66.01 Acute suppurative otitis media with spontaneous rupture of ear drum**

> **DEF:** Sudden, severe inflammation of the middle ear, causing pressure that perforates the ear drum tissue.

     H66.011 Acute suppurative otitis media with spontaneous rupture of ear drum, right ear

     H66.012 Acute suppurative otitis media with spontaneous rupture of ear drum, left ear

     H66.013 Acute suppurative otitis media with spontaneous rupture of ear drum, bilateral

     H66.014 Acute suppurative otitis media with spontaneous rupture of ear drum, recurrent, right ear

     H66.015 Acute suppurative otitis media with spontaneous rupture of ear drum, recurrent, left ear

     H66.016 Acute suppurative otitis media with spontaneous rupture of ear drum, recurrent, bilateral

     H66.017 Acute suppurative otitis media with spontaneous rupture of ear drum, recurrent, unspecified ear

     H66.019 Acute suppurative otitis media with spontaneous rupture of ear drum, unspecified ear

☑5ᵗʰ **H66.1 Chronic tubotympanic suppurative otitis media**

> Benign chronic suppurative otitis media
> Chronic tubotympanic disease
> Use additional code for any associated perforated tympanic membrane (H72.-)

   H66.10 Chronic tubotympanic suppurative otitis media, unspecified

   H66.11 Chronic tubotympanic suppurative otitis media, right ear

   H66.12 Chronic tubotympanic suppurative otitis media, left ear

   H66.13 Chronic tubotympanic suppurative otitis media, bilateral

☑5ᵗʰ **H66.2 Chronic atticoantral suppurative otitis media**

> Chronic atticoantral disease
> Use additional code for any associated perforated tympanic membrane (H72.-)

   H66.20 Chronic atticoantral suppurative otitis media, unspecified ear

   H66.21 Chronic atticoantral suppurative otitis media, right ear

   H66.22 Chronic atticoantral suppurative otitis media, left ear

   H66.23 Chronic atticoantral suppurative otitis media, bilateral

☑5ᵗʰ **H66.3 Other chronic suppurative otitis media**

> Chronic suppurative otitis media NOS
> Use additional code for any associated perforated tympanic membrane (H72.-)
> EXCLUDES 1   *tuberculous otitis media (A18.6)*

   ☑6ᵗʰ **H66.3X Other chronic suppurative otitis media**

     H66.3X1 Other chronic suppurative otitis media, right ear

     H66.3X2 Other chronic suppurative otitis media, left ear

     H66.3X3 Other chronic suppurative otitis media, bilateral

     H66.3X9 Other chronic suppurative otitis media, unspecified ear

☑5ᵗʰ **H66.4 Suppurative otitis media, unspecified**

> Purulent otitis media NOS
> Use additional code for any associated perforated tympanic membrane (H72.-)

   H66.40 Suppurative otitis media, unspecified, unspecified ear

   H66.41 Suppurative otitis media, unspecified, right ear

   H66.42 Suppurative otitis media, unspecified, left ear

   H66.43 Suppurative otitis media, unspecified, bilateral

☑5ᵗʰ **H66.9 Otitis media, unspecified**

> Otitis media NOS
> Acute otitis media NOS
> Chronic otitis media NOS
> Use additional code for any associated perforated tympanic membrane (H72.-)

   H66.90 Otitis media, unspecified, unspecified ear

   H66.91 Otitis media, unspecified, right ear

   H66.92 Otitis media, unspecified, left ear

   H66.93 Otitis media, unspecified, bilateral

☑4ᵗʰ **H67 Otitis media in diseases classified elsewhere**

> Code first underlying disease, such as:
>   plasminogen deficiency (E88.02)
>   viral disease NEC (B00-B34)
> Use additional code for any associated perforated tympanic membrane (H72.-)
> EXCLUDES 1   *otitis media in:*
>   *influenza (J09.X9, J10.83, J11.83)*
>   *measles (B05.3)*
>   *scarlet fever (A38.0)*
>   *tuberculosis (A18.6)*

   H67.1 *Otitis media in diseases classified elsewhere, right ear*

   H67.2 *Otitis media in diseases classified elsewhere, left ear*

   H67.3 *Otitis media in diseases classified elsewhere, bilateral*

   H67.9 *Otitis media in diseases classified elsewhere, unspecified ear*

☑4ᵗʰ **H68 Eustachian salpingitis and obstruction**

> **DEF:** Eustachian tube: Internal channel between the tympanic cavity and the nasopharynx that equalizes internal pressure to the outside pressure and drains mucous production from the middle ear.

☑5ᵗʰ **H68.0 Eustachian salpingitis**

   ☑6ᵗʰ **H68.00 Unspecified Eustachian salpingitis**

     H68.001 Unspecified Eustachian salpingitis, right ear

     H68.002 Unspecified Eustachian salpingitis, left ear

     H68.003 Unspecified Eustachian salpingitis, bilateral

     H68.009 Unspecified Eustachian salpingitis, unspecified ear

   ☑6ᵗʰ **H68.01 Acute Eustachian salpingitis**

     H68.011 Acute Eustachian salpingitis, right ear

     H68.012 Acute Eustachian salpingitis, left ear

     H68.013 Acute Eustachian salpingitis, bilateral

     H68.019 Acute Eustachian salpingitis, unspecified ear

   ☑6ᵗʰ **H68.02 Chronic Eustachian salpingitis**

     H68.021 Chronic Eustachian salpingitis, right ear

     H68.022 Chronic Eustachian salpingitis, left ear

☑ Additional Character Required   ☑x7ᵗʰ Placeholder   Questionable PDx   Manifestation   Unspecified Dx   UPD Unacceptable PDx   H1-H14 HAC   HCC CMS-HCC Dx   HIV HIV Dx

H68.023 **Chronic Eustachian salpingitis,** bilateral
H68.029 **Chronic Eustachian salpingitis, unspecified ear**

√5ᵗʰ H68.1 **Obstruction** of Eustachian tube
  Stenosis of Eustachian tube
  Stricture of Eustachian tube

√6ᵗʰ H68.10 **Unspecified obstruction of Eustachian tube**
  H68.101 **Unspecified obstruction of Eustachian tube,** right **ear**
  H68.102 **Unspecified obstruction of Eustachian tube,** left **ear**
  H68.103 **Unspecified obstruction of Eustachian tube,** bilateral
  H68.109 **Unspecified obstruction of Eustachian tube, unspecified ear**

√6ᵗʰ H68.11 **Osseous** obstruction of Eustachian tube
  H68.111 **Osseous obstruction of Eustachian tube,** right **ear**
  H68.112 **Osseous obstruction of Eustachian tube,** left **ear**
  H68.113 **Osseous obstruction of Eustachian tube,** bilateral
  H68.119 **Osseous obstruction of Eustachian tube, unspecified ear**

√6ᵗʰ H68.12 **Intrinsic cartilagenous** obstruction of Eustachian **tube**
  H68.121 **Intrinsic cartilagenous obstruction of Eustachian tube,** right **ear**
  H68.122 **Intrinsic cartilagenous obstruction of Eustachian tube,** left **ear**
  H68.123 **Intrinsic cartilagenous obstruction of Eustachian tube,** bilateral
  H68.129 **Intrinsic cartilagenous obstruction of Eustachian tube, unspecified ear**

√6ᵗʰ H68.13 **Extrinsic cartilagenous** obstruction of Eustachian **tube**
  Compression of Eustachian tube
  H68.131 **Extrinsic cartilagenous obstruction of Eustachian tube,** right **ear**
  H68.132 **Extrinsic cartilagenous obstruction of Eustachian tube,** left **ear**
  H68.133 **Extrinsic cartilagenous obstruction of Eustachian tube,** bilateral
  H68.139 **Extrinsic cartilagenous obstruction of Eustachian tube, unspecified ear**

√4ᵗʰ H69 **Other and unspecified disorders of Eustachian tube**
  DEF: Eustachian tube: Internal channel between the tympanic cavity and the nasopharynx that equalizes internal pressure to the outside pressure and drains mucous production from the middle ear.

√5ᵗʰ H69.0 **Patulous** Eustachian tube
  H69.00 **Patulous Eustachian tube, unspecified ear**
  H69.01 **Patulous Eustachian tube,** right **ear**
  H69.02 **Patulous Eustachian tube,** left **ear**
  H69.03 **Patulous Eustachian tube,** bilateral

√5ᵗʰ H69.8 **Other specified disorders of Eustachian tube**
  H69.80 **Other specified disorders of Eustachian tube, unspecified ear**
  H69.81 **Other specified disorders of Eustachian tube,** right **ear**
  H69.82 **Other specified disorders of Eustachian tube,** left **ear**
  H69.83 **Other specified disorders of Eustachian tube,** bilateral

√5ᵗʰ H69.9 **Unspecified Eustachian tube disorder**
  H69.90 **Unspecified Eustachian tube disorder, unspecified ear**
  H69.91 **Unspecified Eustachian tube disorder,** right **ear**
  H69.92 **Unspecified Eustachian tube disorder,** left **ear**
  H69.93 **Unspecified Eustachian tube disorder,** bilateral

√4ᵗʰ H70 **Mastoiditis and related conditions**

√5ᵗʰ H70.0 **Acute** mastoiditis
  Abscess of mastoid
  Empyema of mastoid

√6ᵗʰ H70.00 **Acute mastoiditis** without complications
  H70.001 **Acute mastoiditis without complications,** right **ear** CC
  H70.002 **Acute mastoiditis without complications,** left **ear** CC

H70.003 **Acute mastoiditis without complications,** bilateral CC
H70.009 **Acute mastoiditis without complications, unspecified ear** CC

√6ᵗʰ H70.01 **Subperiosteal abscess of mastoid**
  H70.011 **Subperiosteal abscess of mastoid,** right **ear**
  H70.012 **Subperiosteal abscess of mastoid,** left **ear** CC
  H70.013 **Subperiosteal abscess of mastoid,** bilateral CC
  H70.019 **Subperiosteal abscess of mastoid, unspecified ear** CC

√6ᵗʰ H70.09 **Acute mastoiditis with other complications**
  H70.091 **Acute mastoiditis with other complications,** right **ear** CC
  H70.092 **Acute mastoiditis with other complications,** left **ear** CC
  H70.093 **Acute mastoiditis with other complications,** bilateral CC
  H70.099 **Acute mastoiditis with other complications, unspecified ear** CC

√5ᵗʰ H70.1 **Chronic** mastoiditis
  Caries of mastoid
  Fistula of mastoid
  EXCLUDES 1   tuberculous mastoiditis (A18.03)
  H70.10 **Chronic mastoiditis, unspecified ear**
  H70.11 **Chronic mastoiditis,** right **ear**
  H70.12 **Chronic mastoiditis,** left **ear**
  H70.13 **Chronic mastoiditis,** bilateral

√5ᵗʰ H70.2 **Petrositis**
  Inflammation of petrous bone
  √6ᵗʰ H70.20 **Unspecified petrositis**
  H70.201 **Unspecified petrositis,** right **ear**
  H70.202 **Unspecified petrositis,** left **ear**
  H70.203 **Unspecified petrositis,** bilateral
  H70.209 **Unspecified petrositis, unspecified ear**

√6ᵗʰ H70.21 **Acute petrositis**
  DEF: Sudden, severe inflammation of the petrous temporal bone behind the ear, associated with a middle ear infection.
  H70.211 **Acute petrositis,** right **ear**
  H70.212 **Acute petrositis,** left **ear**
  H70.213 **Acute petrositis,** bilateral
  H70.219 **Acute petrositis, unspecified ear**

√6ᵗʰ H70.22 **Chronic petrositis**
  H70.221 **Chronic petrositis,** right **ear**
  H70.222 **Chronic petrositis,** left **ear**
  H70.223 **Chronic petrositis,** bilateral
  H70.229 **Chronic petrositis, unspecified ear**

√5ᵗʰ H70.8 **Other mastoiditis and related conditions**
  EXCLUDES 1   preauricular sinus and cyst (Q18.1)
            sinus, fistula, and cyst of branchial cleft (Q18.0)

√6ᵗʰ H70.81 **Postauricular fistula**
  H70.811 **Postauricular fistula,** right **ear** SW
  H70.812 **Postauricular fistula,** left **ear** SW
  H70.813 **Postauricular fistula,** bilateral SW
  H70.819 **Postauricular fistula, unspecified ear** SW

√6ᵗʰ H70.89 **Other mastoiditis and related conditions**
  H70.891 **Other mastoiditis and related conditions,** right **ear**
  H70.892 **Other mastoiditis and related conditions,** left **ear**
  H70.893 **Other mastoiditis and related conditions,** bilateral
  H70.899 **Other mastoiditis and related conditions, unspecified ear**

√5ᵗʰ H70.9 **Unspecified mastoiditis**
  H70.90 **Unspecified mastoiditis, unspecified ear**
  H70.91 **Unspecified mastoiditis,** right **ear**
  H70.92 **Unspecified mastoiditis,** left **ear**
  H70.93 **Unspecified mastoiditis,** bilateral

✓4ᵗʰ **H71 Cholesteatoma of middle ear**

> EXCLUDES 2   cholesteatoma of external ear (H60.4-)
> recurrent cholesteatoma of postmastoidectomy cavity (H95.0-)

DEF: Cholesteatoma: Noncancerous cyst-like mass of cell debris, including cholesterol and epithelial cells resulting from trauma, repeated or improperly healed infections, and congenital enclosure of epidermal cells.

Cholesteatoma of Middle Ear

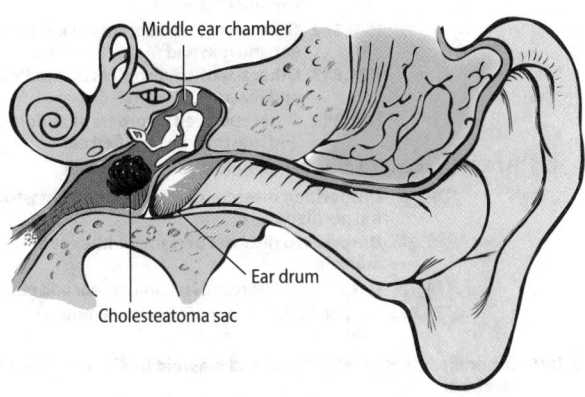

Middle ear chamber

Ear drum

Cholesteatoma sac

✓5ᵗʰ **H71.0 Cholesteatoma of attic**

   H71.00   Cholesteatoma of attic, unspecified ear
   H71.01   Cholesteatoma of attic, right ear
   H71.02   Cholesteatoma of attic, left ear
   H71.03   Cholesteatoma of attic, bilateral

✓5ᵗʰ **H71.1 Cholesteatoma of tympanum**

   H71.10   Cholesteatoma of tympanum, unspecified ear
   H71.11   Cholesteatoma of tympanum, right ear
   H71.12   Cholesteatoma of tympanum, left ear
   H71.13   Cholesteatoma of tympanum, bilateral

✓5ᵗʰ **H71.2 Cholesteatoma of mastoid**

   H71.20   Cholesteatoma of mastoid, unspecified ear
   H71.21   Cholesteatoma of mastoid, right ear
   H71.22   Cholesteatoma of mastoid, left ear
   H71.23   Cholesteatoma of mastoid, bilateral

✓5ᵗʰ **H71.3 Diffuse cholesteatosis**

   H71.30   Diffuse cholesteatosis, unspecified ear
   H71.31   Diffuse cholesteatosis, right ear
   H71.32   Diffuse cholesteatosis, left ear
   H71.33   Diffuse cholesteatosis, bilateral

✓5ᵗʰ **H71.9 Unspecified cholesteatoma**

   H71.90   Unspecified cholesteatoma, unspecified ear
   H71.91   Unspecified cholesteatoma, right ear
   H71.92   Unspecified cholesteatoma, left ear
   H71.93   Unspecified cholesteatoma, bilateral

✓4ᵗʰ **H72 Perforation of tympanic membrane**

> INCLUDES   persistent post-traumatic perforation of ear drum
> postinflammatory perforation of ear drum

Code first any associated otitis media (H65.-, H66.1-, H66.2-, H66.3-, H66.4-, H66.9-, H67.-)

> EXCLUDES 1   acute suppurative otitis media with rupture of the tympanic membrane (H66.01-)
> traumatic rupture of ear drum (S09.2-)

✓5ᵗʰ **H72.0 Central perforation of tympanic membrane**

   H72.00   Central perforation of tympanic membrane, unspecified ear
   H72.01   Central perforation of tympanic membrane, right ear
   H72.02   Central perforation of tympanic membrane, left ear
   H72.03   Central perforation of tympanic membrane, bilateral

✓5ᵗʰ **H72.1 Attic perforation of tympanic membrane**

   Perforation of pars flaccida

   H72.10   Attic perforation of tympanic membrane, unspecified ear
   H72.11   Attic perforation of tympanic membrane, right ear
   H72.12   Attic perforation of tympanic membrane, left ear
   H72.13   Attic perforation of tympanic membrane, bilateral

✓5ᵗʰ **H72.2 Other marginal perforations of tympanic membrane**

✓6ᵗʰ **H72.2X Other marginal perforations of tympanic membrane**

   H72.2X1   Other marginal perforations of tympanic membrane, right ear
   H72.2X2   Other marginal perforations of tympanic membrane, left ear
   H72.2X3   Other marginal perforations of tympanic membrane, bilateral
   H72.2X9   Other marginal perforations of tympanic membrane, unspecified ear

✓5ᵗʰ **H72.8 Other perforations of tympanic membrane**

✓6ᵗʰ **H72.81 Multiple perforations of tympanic membrane**

   H72.811   Multiple perforations of tympanic membrane, right ear
   H72.812   Multiple perforations of tympanic membrane, left ear
   H72.813   Multiple perforations of tympanic membrane, bilateral
   H72.819   Multiple perforations of tympanic membrane, unspecified ear

✓6ᵗʰ **H72.82 Total perforations of tympanic membrane**

   H72.821   Total perforations of tympanic membrane, right ear
   H72.822   Total perforations of tympanic membrane, left ear
   H72.823   Total perforations of tympanic membrane, bilateral
   H72.829   Total perforations of tympanic membrane, unspecified ear

✓5ᵗʰ **H72.9 Unspecified perforation of tympanic membrane**

   H72.90   Unspecified perforation of tympanic membrane, unspecified ear
   H72.91   Unspecified perforation of tympanic membrane, right ear
   H72.92   Unspecified perforation of tympanic membrane, left ear
   H72.93   Unspecified perforation of tympanic membrane, bilateral

✓4ᵗʰ **H73 Other disorders of tympanic membrane**

✓5ᵗʰ **H73.0 Acute myringitis**

> EXCLUDES 1   acute myringitis with otitis media (H65, H66)

✓6ᵗʰ **H73.00 Unspecified acute myringitis**

   Acute tympanitis NOS

   H73.001   Acute myringitis, right ear
   H73.002   Acute myringitis, left ear
   H73.003   Acute myringitis, bilateral
   H73.009   Acute myringitis, unspecified ear

✓6ᵗʰ **H73.01 Bullous myringitis**

   DEF: Bacterial or viral otitis media that is characterized by the appearance of serous or hemorrhagic blebs on the ear drum and sudden onset of severe pain in ear.

   H73.011   Bullous myringitis, right ear
   H73.012   Bullous myringitis, left ear
   H73.013   Bullous myringitis, bilateral
   H73.019   Bullous myringitis, unspecified ear

✓6ᵗʰ **H73.09 Other acute myringitis**

   H73.091   Other acute myringitis, right ear
   H73.092   Other acute myringitis, left ear
   H73.093   Other acute myringitis, bilateral
   H73.099   Other acute myringitis, unspecified ear

✓5ᵗʰ **H73.1 Chronic myringitis**

   Chronic tympanitis

> EXCLUDES 1   chronic myringitis with otitis media (H65, H66)

   H73.10   Chronic myringitis, unspecified ear
   H73.11   Chronic myringitis, right ear
   H73.12   Chronic myringitis, left ear
   H73.13   Chronic myringitis, bilateral

✓5ᵗʰ **H73.2 Unspecified myringitis**

   H73.20   Unspecified myringitis, unspecified ear
   H73.21   Unspecified myringitis, right ear
   H73.22   Unspecified myringitis, left ear
   H73.23   Unspecified myringitis, bilateral

✓5ᵗʰ **H73.8 Other specified disorders of tympanic membrane**

✓6ᵗʰ **H73.81 Atrophic flaccid tympanic membrane**

   H73.811   Atrophic flaccid tympanic membrane, right ear

✓ Additional Character Required   ✓x7ᵗʰ Placeholder   Questionable PDx   Manifestation   Unspecified Dx   UPD Unacceptable PDx   H1-H14 HAC   HCC CMS-HCC Dx   HIV HIV Dx

ICD-10-CM 2022   639

Chapter 8. Diseases of the Ear and Mastoid Process

H73.812 Atrophic flaccid tympanic membrane, left ear

H73.813 Atrophic flaccid tympanic membrane, bilateral

H73.819 Atrophic flaccid tympanic membrane, unspecified ear

☑6ᵗʰ **H73.82 Atrophic nonflaccid tympanic membrane**

H73.821 Atrophic nonflaccid tympanic membrane, right ear

H73.822 Atrophic nonflaccid tympanic membrane, left ear

H73.823 Atrophic nonflaccid tympanic membrane, bilateral

H73.829 Atrophic nonflaccid tympanic membrane, unspecified ear

☑6ᵗʰ **H73.89 Other specified disorders of tympanic membrane**

H73.891 Other specified disorders of tympanic membrane, right ear

H73.892 Other specified disorders of tympanic membrane, left ear

H73.893 Other specified disorders of tympanic membrane, bilateral

H73.899 Other specified disorders of tympanic membrane, unspecified ear

☑5ᵗʰ **H73.9 Unspecified disorder of tympanic membrane**

H73.90 Unspecified disorder of tympanic membrane, unspecified ear

H73.91 Unspecified disorder of tympanic membrane, right ear

H73.92 Unspecified disorder of tympanic membrane, left ear

H73.93 Unspecified disorder of tympanic membrane, bilateral

☑4ᵗʰ **H74 Other disorders of middle ear mastoid**

EXCLUDES 2   mastoiditis (H70.-)

☑5ᵗʰ **H74.0 Tympanosclerosis**

DEF: Calcification of tissue in the ear drum, middle ear bones, and middle ear canal.

H74.01 Tympanosclerosis, right ear

H74.02 Tympanosclerosis, left ear

H74.03 Tympanosclerosis, bilateral

H74.09 Tympanosclerosis, unspecified ear

☑5ᵗʰ **H74.1 Adhesive middle ear disease**

Adhesive otitis

EXCLUDES 1   glue ear (H65.3-)

H74.11 Adhesive right middle ear disease

H74.12 Adhesive left middle ear disease

H74.13 Adhesive middle ear disease, bilateral

H74.19 Adhesive middle ear disease, unspecified ear

☑5ᵗʰ **H74.2 Discontinuity and dislocation of ear ossicles**

H74.20 Discontinuity and dislocation of ear ossicles, unspecified ear

H74.21 Discontinuity and dislocation of right ear ossicles

H74.22 Discontinuity and dislocation of left ear ossicles

H74.23 Discontinuity and dislocation of ear ossicles, bilateral

☑5ᵗʰ **H74.3 Other acquired abnormalities of ear ossicles**

☑6ᵗʰ **H74.31 Ankylosis of ear ossicles**

H74.311 Ankylosis of ear ossicles, right ear

H74.312 Ankylosis of ear ossicles, left ear

H74.313 Ankylosis of ear ossicles, bilateral

H74.319 Ankylosis of ear ossicles, unspecified ear

☑6ᵗʰ **H74.32 Partial loss of ear ossicles**

H74.321 Partial loss of ear ossicles, right ear

H74.322 Partial loss of ear ossicles, left ear

H74.323 Partial loss of ear ossicles, bilateral

H74.329 Partial loss of ear ossicles, unspecified ear

☑6ᵗʰ **H74.39 Other acquired abnormalities of ear ossicles**

H74.391 Other acquired abnormalities of right ear ossicles

H74.392 Other acquired abnormalities of left ear ossicles

H74.393 Other acquired abnormalities of ear ossicles, bilateral

H74.399 Other acquired abnormalities of ear ossicles, unspecified ear

☑5ᵗʰ **H74.4 Polyp of middle ear**

H74.40 Polyp of middle ear, unspecified ear

H74.41 Polyp of right middle ear

H74.42 Polyp of left middle ear

H74.43 Polyp of middle ear, bilateral

☑5ᵗʰ **H74.8 Other specified disorders of middle ear and mastoid**

☑6ᵗʰ **H74.8X Other specified disorders of middle ear and mastoid**

H74.8X1 Other specified disorders of right middle ear and mastoid

H74.8X2 Other specified disorders of left middle ear and mastoid

H74.8X3 Other specified disorders of middle ear and mastoid, bilateral

H74.8X9 Other specified disorders of middle ear and mastoid, unspecified ear

☑5ᵗʰ **H74.9 Unspecified disorder of middle ear and mastoid**

H74.90 Unspecified disorder of middle ear and mastoid, unspecified ear

H74.91 Unspecified disorder of right middle ear and mastoid

H74.92 Unspecified disorder of left middle ear and mastoid

H74.93 Unspecified disorder of middle ear and mastoid, bilateral

☑4ᵗʰ **H75 Other disorders of middle ear and mastoid in diseases classified elsewhere**

Code first underlying disease

☑5ᵗʰ **H75.0 Mastoiditis in infectious and parasitic diseases classified elsewhere**

EXCLUDES 1   mastoiditis (in):

syphilis (A52.77)

tuberculosis (A18.03)

H75.00 Mastoiditis in infectious and parasitic diseases classified elsewhere, unspecified ear

H75.01 Mastoiditis in infectious and parasitic diseases classified elsewhere, right ear

H75.02 Mastoiditis in infectious and parasitic diseases classified elsewhere, left ear

H75.03 Mastoiditis in infectious and parasitic diseases classified elsewhere, bilateral

☑5ᵗʰ **H75.8 Other specified disorders of middle ear and mastoid in diseases classified elsewhere**

H75.80 Other specified disorders of middle ear and mastoid in diseases classified elsewhere, unspecified ear

H75.81 Other specified disorders of right middle ear and mastoid in diseases classified elsewhere

H75.82 Other specified disorders of left middle ear and mastoid in diseases classified elsewhere

H75.83 Other specified disorders of middle ear and mastoid in diseases classified elsewhere, bilateral

Diseases of inner ear (H80-H83)

☑4ᵗʰ **H80 Otosclerosis**

INCLUDES   otospongiosis

☑5ᵗʰ **H80.0 Otosclerosis involving oval window, nonobliterative**

H80.00 Otosclerosis involving oval window, nonobliterative, unspecified ear

H80.01 Otosclerosis involving oval window, nonobliterative, right ear

H80.02 Otosclerosis involving oval window, nonobliterative, left ear

H80.03 Otosclerosis involving oval window, nonobliterative, bilateral

☑5ᵗʰ **H80.1 Otosclerosis involving oval window, obliterative**

H80.10 Otosclerosis involving oval window, obliterative, unspecified ear

H80.11 Otosclerosis involving oval window, obliterative, right ear

H80.12 Otosclerosis involving oval window, obliterative, left ear

H80.13 Otosclerosis involving oval window, obliterative, bilateral

☑5ᵗʰ **H80.2 Cochlear otosclerosis**

Otosclerosis involving otic capsule

Otosclerosis involving round window

H80.20 Cochlear otosclerosis, unspecified ear

H80.21 Cochlear otosclerosis, right ear

H80.22 Cochlear otosclerosis, left ear

H80.23 Cochlear otosclerosis, bilateral

Ⓝ Newborn: 0   Ⓟ Pediatric: 0-17   Ⓜ Maternity: 9-64   Ⓐ Adult: 15-124   MCC Major Complication/Comorbidity   CC Complication/Comorbidity   SW Severe Wound Dx

640

ICD-10-CM 2022

☑5ᵗʰ H80.8 Other otosclerosis

     H80.80 Other otosclerosis, unspecified ear
     H80.81 Other otosclerosis, right ear
     H80.82 Other otosclerosis, left ear
     H80.83 Other otosclerosis, bilateral

☑5ᵗʰ H80.9 Unspecified otosclerosis

     H80.90 Unspecified otosclerosis, unspecified ear
     H80.91 Unspecified otosclerosis, right ear
     H80.92 Unspecified otosclerosis, left ear
     H80.93 Unspecified otosclerosis, bilateral

☑4ᵗʰ H81 Disorders of vestibular function

     EXCLUDES 1   epidemic vertigo (A88.1)
               vertigo NOS (R42)

☑5ᵗʰ H81.0 Ménière's disease

     Labyrinthine hydrops
     Ménière's syndrome or vertigo
     DEF: Distended membranous labyrinth of the middle ear from fluctuating pressure of fluid (hydrops) that causes vertigo, tinnitus, pressure, and hearing loss that may last on and off for several hours. Episodes may occur in clusters or may subside for weeks, months, or even years.

     H81.01 Ménière's disease, right ear
     H81.02 Ménière's disease, left ear
     H81.03 Ménière's disease, bilateral
     H81.09 Ménière's disease, unspecified ear

☑5ᵗʰ H81.1 Benign paroxysmal vertigo

     H81.10 Benign paroxysmal vertigo, unspecified ear
     H81.11 Benign paroxysmal vertigo, right ear
     H81.12 Benign paroxysmal vertigo, left ear
     H81.13 Benign paroxysmal vertigo, bilateral

☑5ᵗʰ H81.2 Vestibular neuronitis

     DEF: Transient benign vertigo caused by inflammation of the vestibular nerve. It is characterized by response to caloric stimulation on one side and nystagmus with rhythmic movement of the eyes. Normal auditory function is present.

     H81.20 Vestibular neuronitis, unspecified ear
     H81.21 Vestibular neuronitis, right ear
     H81.22 Vestibular neuronitis, left ear
     H81.23 Vestibular neuronitis, bilateral

☑5ᵗʰ H81.3 Other peripheral vertigo

     ☑6ᵗʰ H81.31 Aural vertigo

         H81.311 Aural vertigo, right ear
         H81.312 Aural vertigo, left ear
         H81.313 Aural vertigo, bilateral
         H81.319 Aural vertigo, unspecified ear

     ☑6ᵗʰ H81.39 Other peripheral vertigo

         Lermoyez' syndrome
         Otogenic vertigo
         Peripheral vertigo NOS
         H81.391 Other peripheral vertigo, right ear
         H81.392 Other peripheral vertigo, left ear
         H81.393 Other peripheral vertigo, bilateral
         H81.399 Other peripheral vertigo, unspecified ear

H81.4 Vertigo of central origin

     Central positional nystagmus

☑5ᵗʰ H81.8 Other disorders of vestibular function

     ☑6ᵗʰ H81.8X Other disorders of vestibular function

         H81.8X1 Other disorders of vestibular function, right ear
         H81.8X2 Other disorders of vestibular function, left ear
         H81.8X3 Other disorders of vestibular function, bilateral
         H81.8X9 Other disorders of vestibular function, unspecified ear

☑5ᵗʰ H81.9 Unspecified disorder of vestibular function

     Vertiginous syndrome NOS

     H81.90 Unspecified disorder of vestibular function, unspecified ear
     H81.91 Unspecified disorder of vestibular function, right ear
     H81.92 Unspecified disorder of vestibular function, left ear
     H81.93 Unspecified disorder of vestibular function, bilateral

☑4ᵗʰ H82 Vertiginous syndromes in diseases classified elsewhere

     Code first underlying disease
     EXCLUDES 1   epidemic vertigo (A88.1)

     H82.1 Vertiginous syndromes in diseases classified elsewhere, right ear
     H82.2 Vertiginous syndromes in diseases classified elsewhere, left ear
     H82.3 Vertiginous syndromes in diseases classified elsewhere, bilateral
     H82.9 Vertiginous syndromes in diseases classified elsewhere, unspecified ear

☑4ᵗʰ H83 Other diseases of inner ear

☑5ᵗʰ H83.0 Labyrinthitis

     DEF: Inflammation of the inner ear, or labyrinth, characterized by pus, vertigo, dizziness, nausea, and hearing loss.

     H83.01 Labyrinthitis, right ear
     H83.02 Labyrinthitis, left ear
     H83.03 Labyrinthitis, bilateral
     H83.09 Labyrinthitis, unspecified ear

☑5ᵗʰ H83.1 Labyrinthine fistula

     H83.11 Labyrinthine fistula, right ear
     H83.12 Labyrinthine fistula, left ear   SW
     H83.13 Labyrinthine fistula, bilateral   SW
     H83.19 Labyrinthine fistula, unspecified ear   SW

☑5ᵗʰ H83.2 Labyrinthine dysfunction

     Labyrinthine hypersensitivity
     Labyrinthine hypofunction
     Labyrinthine loss of function
     DEF: Decreased function of the labyrinth sensors.

     ☑6ᵗʰ H83.2X Labyrinthine dysfunction

         H83.2X1 Labyrinthine dysfunction, right ear
         H83.2X2 Labyrinthine dysfunction, left ear
         H83.2X3 Labyrinthine dysfunction, bilateral
         H83.2X9 Labyrinthine dysfunction, unspecified ear

☑5ᵗʰ H83.3 Noise effects on inner ear

     Acoustic trauma of inner ear
     Noise-induced hearing loss of inner ear

     ☑6ᵗʰ H83.3X Noise effects on inner ear

         H83.3X1 Noise effects on right inner ear
         H83.3X2 Noise effects on left inner ear
         H83.3X3 Noise effects on inner ear, bilateral
         H83.3X9 Noise effects on inner ear, unspecified ear

☑5ᵗʰ H83.8 Other specified diseases of inner ear

     ☑6ᵗʰ H83.8X Other specified diseases of inner ear

         H83.8X1 Other specified diseases of right inner ear
         H83.8X2 Other specified diseases of left inner ear
         H83.8X3 Other specified diseases of inner ear, bilateral
         H83.8X9 Other specified diseases of inner ear, unspecified ear

☑5ᵗʰ H83.9 Unspecified disease of inner ear

     H83.90 Unspecified disease of inner ear, unspecified ear
     H83.91 Unspecified disease of right inner ear
     H83.92 Unspecified disease of left inner ear
     H83.93 Unspecified disease of inner ear, bilateral

Other disorders of ear (H90-H94)

☑4ᵗʰ H90 Conductive and sensorineural hearing loss

     EXCLUDES 1   deaf nonspeaking NEC (H91.3)
               deafness NOS (H91.9-)
               hearing loss NOS (H91.9-)
               noise-induced hearing loss (H83.3-)
               ototoxic hearing loss (H91.0-)
               sudden (idiopathic) hearing loss (H91.2-)

     AHA: 2015,2Q,7
     DEF: Conductive hearing loss: Hearing loss due to the inability of soundwaves to move from the outer (external) ear to the inner ear.
     DEF: Sensorineural hearing loss: Hearing loss that occurs from damage to the hair cells of the inner ear or problems with the nerve pathways from the inner ear to the brain.

     H90.0 Conductive hearing loss, bilateral

☑ Additional Character Required   ☑x7ᵗʰ Placeholder   Questionable PDx   Manifestation   Unspecified Dx   UPD Unacceptable PDx   H1-H14 HAC   HCC CMS-HCC Dx   HIV HIV Dx

ICD-10-CM 2022   641

✓5ᵗʰ H90.1 Conductive hearing loss, unilateral with unrestricted hearing on the contralateral side

    H90.11 Conductive hearing loss, unilateral, right ear, with unrestricted hearing on the contralateral side

    H90.12 Conductive hearing loss, unilateral, left ear, with unrestricted hearing on the contralateral side

H90.2 Conductive hearing loss, unspecified

    Conductive deafness NOS

H90.3 Sensorineural hearing loss, bilateral

✓5ᵗʰ H90.4 Sensorineural hearing loss, unilateral with unrestricted hearing on the contralateral side

    H90.41 Sensorineural hearing loss, unilateral, right ear, with unrestricted hearing on the contralateral side

    H90.42 Sensorineural hearing loss, unilateral, left ear, with unrestricted hearing on the contralateral side

H90.5 Unspecified sensorineural hearing loss

    Central hearing loss NOS

    Congenital deafness NOS

    Neural hearing loss NOS

    Perceptive hearing loss NOS

    Sensorineural deafness NOS

    Sensory hearing loss NOS

    EXCLUDES 1   *abnormal auditory perception (H93.2-)*

                            psychogenic deafness (F44.6)

H90.6 Mixed conductive and sensorineural hearing loss, bilateral

    AHA: 2015,2Q,7

✓5ᵗʰ H90.7 Mixed conductive and sensorineural hearing loss, unilateral with unrestricted hearing on the contralateral side

    H90.71 Mixed conductive and sensorineural hearing loss, unilateral, right ear, with unrestricted hearing on the contralateral side

    H90.72 Mixed conductive and sensorineural hearing loss, unilateral, left ear, with unrestricted hearing on the contralateral side

H90.8 Mixed conductive and sensorineural hearing loss, unspecified

✓5ᵗʰ H90.A Conductive and sensorineural hearing loss with restricted hearing on the contralateral side

    AHA: 2016,4Q,23-25

    ✓6ᵗʰ H90.A1 Conductive hearing loss, unilateral, with restricted hearing on the contralateral side

        H90.A11 Conductive hearing loss, unilateral, right ear with restricted hearing on the contralateral side

        H90.A12 Conductive hearing loss, unilateral, left ear with restricted hearing on the contralateral side

    ✓6ᵗʰ H90.A2 Sensorineural hearing loss, unilateral, with restricted hearing on the contralateral side

        H90.A21 Sensorineural hearing loss, unilateral, right ear, with restricted hearing on the contralateral side

        H90.A22 Sensorineural hearing loss, unilateral, left ear, with restricted hearing on the contralateral side

    ✓6ᵗʰ H90.A3 Mixed conductive and sensorineural hearing loss, unilateral with restricted hearing on the contralateral side

        H90.A31 Mixed conductive and sensorineural hearing loss, unilateral, right ear with restricted hearing on the contralateral side

        H90.A32 Mixed conductive and sensorineural hearing, unilateral, left ear with restricted hearing on the contralateral side

✓4ᵗʰ H91 Other and unspecified hearing loss

    EXCLUDES 1   *abnormal auditory perception (H93.2-)*

                            hearing loss as classified in H90.-

                            impacted cerumen (H61.2-)

                            noise-induced hearing loss (H83.3-)

                            psychogenic deafness (F44.6)

                            transient ischemic deafness (H93.01-)

    ✓5ᵗʰ H91.0 Ototoxic hearing loss

        Code first poisoning due to drug or toxin, if applicable (T36-T65 with fifth or sixth character 1-4 or 6)

        Use additional code for adverse effect, if applicable, to identify drug (T36-T50 with fifth or sixth character 5)

        H91.01 Ototoxic hearing loss, right ear

        H91.02 Ototoxic hearing loss, left ear

        H91.03 Ototoxic hearing loss, bilateral

        H91.09 Ototoxic hearing loss, unspecified ear

✓5ᵗʰ H91.1 Presbycusis

    Presbyacusia

    H91.10 Presbycusis, unspecified ear

    H91.11 Presbycusis, right ear

    H91.12 Presbycusis, left ear

    H91.13 Presbycusis, bilateral

✓5ᵗʰ H91.2 Sudden idiopathic hearing loss

    Sudden hearing loss NOS

    H91.20 Sudden idiopathic hearing loss, unspecified ear

    H91.21 Sudden idiopathic hearing loss, right ear

    H91.22 Sudden idiopathic hearing loss, left ear

    H91.23 Sudden idiopathic hearing loss, bilateral

H91.3 Deaf nonspeaking, not elsewhere classified

✓5ᵗʰ H91.8 Other specified hearing loss

    ✓6ᵗʰ H91.8X Other specified hearing loss

        H91.8X1 Other specified hearing loss, right ear

        H91.8X2 Other specified hearing loss, left ear

        H91.8X3 Other specified hearing loss, bilateral

        H91.8X9 Other specified hearing loss, unspecified ear

✓5ᵗʰ H91.9 Unspecified hearing loss

    Deafness NOS

    High frequency deafness

    Low frequency deafness

    H91.90 Unspecified hearing loss, unspecified ear

    H91.91 Unspecified hearing loss, right ear

    H91.92 Unspecified hearing loss, left ear

    H91.93 Unspecified hearing loss, bilateral

✓4ᵗʰ H92 Otalgia and effusion of ear

    ✓5ᵗʰ H92.0 Otalgia

        H92.01 Otalgia, right ear

        H92.02 Otalgia, left ear

        H92.03 Otalgia, bilateral

        H92.09 Otalgia, unspecified ear

    ✓5ᵗʰ H92.1 Otorrhea

        EXCLUDES 1   *leakage of cerebrospinal fluid through ear (G96.0)*

        H92.10 Otorrhea, unspecified ear

        H92.11 Otorrhea, right ear

        H92.12 Otorrhea, left ear

        H92.13 Otorrhea, bilateral

    ✓5ᵗʰ H92.2 Otorrhagia

        EXCLUDES 1   *traumatic otorrhagia - code to injury*

        H92.20 Otorrhagia, unspecified ear

        H92.21 Otorrhagia, right ear

        H92.22 Otorrhagia, left ear

        H92.23 Otorrhagia, bilateral

✓4ᵗʰ H93 Other disorders of ear, not elsewhere classified

    ✓5ᵗʰ H93.0 Degenerative and vascular disorders of ear

        EXCLUDES 1   *presbycusis (H91.1)*

        ✓6ᵗʰ H93.01 Transient ischemic deafness

            H93.011 Transient ischemic deafness, right ear

            H93.012 Transient ischemic deafness, left ear

            H93.013 Transient ischemic deafness, bilateral

            H93.019 Transient ischemic deafness, unspecified ear

        ✓6ᵗʰ H93.09 Unspecified degenerative and vascular disorders of ear

            H93.091 Unspecified degenerative and vascular disorders of right ear

            H93.092 Unspecified degenerative and vascular disorders of left ear

            H93.093 Unspecified degenerative and vascular disorders of ear, bilateral

            H93.099 Unspecified degenerative and vascular disorders of unspecified ear

    ✓5ᵗʰ H93.1 Tinnitus

        H93.11 Tinnitus, right ear

        H93.12 Tinnitus, left ear

        H93.13 Tinnitus, bilateral

        H93.19 Tinnitus, unspecified ear

    ✓5ᵗʰ H93.A Pulsatile tinnitus

        AHA: 2016,4Q,25-26

        H93.A1 Pulsatile tinnitus, right ear

        H93.A2 Pulsatile tinnitus, left ear

        H93.A3 Pulsatile tinnitus, bilateral

N Newborn: 0   **P** Pediatric: 0-17   **M** Maternity: 9-64   **A** Adult: 15-124   **MCC** Major Complication/Comorbidity   **CC** Complication/Comorbidity   **SW** Severe Wound Dx

642   ICD-10-CM 2022

H93.A9   **Pulsatile tinnitus, unspecified ear**

√5ᵗʰ **H93.2**   **Other abnormal auditory perceptions**
- EXCLUDES 2   auditory hallucinations (R44.0)

√6ᵗʰ **H93.21**   **Auditory recruitment**
- H93.211   **Auditory recruitment, right ear**
- H93.212   **Auditory recruitment, left ear**
- H93.213   **Auditory recruitment, bilateral**
- H93.219   **Auditory recruitment, unspecified ear**

√6ᵗʰ **H93.22**   **Diplacusis**
- H93.221   **Diplacusis, right ear**
- H93.222   **Diplacusis, left ear**
- H93.223   **Diplacusis, bilateral**
- H93.229   **Diplacusis, unspecified ear**

√6ᵗʰ **H93.23**   **Hyperacusis**
- DEF: Exceptionally acute sense of hearing caused by such conditions as Bell's palsy. This term may also refer to painful sensitivity to sounds.
- H93.231   **Hyperacusis, right ear**
- H93.232   **Hyperacusis, left ear**
- H93.233   **Hyperacusis, bilateral**
- H93.239   **Hyperacusis, unspecified ear**

√6ᵗʰ **H93.24**   **Temporary auditory threshold shift**
- H93.241   **Temporary auditory threshold shift, right ear**
- H93.242   **Temporary auditory threshold shift, left ear**
- H93.243   **Temporary auditory threshold shift, bilateral**
- H93.249   **Temporary auditory threshold shift, unspecified ear**

H93.25   **Central auditory processing disorder**
- Congenital auditory imperception
- Word deafness
- EXCLUDES 1   mixed receptive-expressive language disorder (F80.2)

√6ᵗʰ **H93.29**   **Other abnormal auditory perceptions**
- H93.291   **Other abnormal auditory perceptions, right ear**
- H93.292   **Other abnormal auditory perceptions, left ear**
- H93.293   **Other abnormal auditory perceptions, bilateral**
- H93.299   **Other abnormal auditory perceptions, unspecified ear**

√5ᵗʰ **H93.3**   **Disorders of acoustic nerve**
- Disorder of 8th cranial nerve
- EXCLUDES 1   acoustic neuroma (D33.3)
-      syphilitic acoustic neuritis (A52.15)

√6ᵗʰ **H93.3X**   **Disorders of acoustic nerve**
- H93.3X1   **Disorders of right acoustic nerve**
- H93.3X2   **Disorders of left acoustic nerve**
- H93.3X3   **Disorders of bilateral acoustic nerves**
- H93.3X9   **Disorders of unspecified acoustic nerve**

√5ᵗʰ **H93.8**   **Other specified disorders of ear**

√6ᵗʰ **H93.8X**   **Other specified disorders of ear**
- H93.8X1   **Other specified disorders of right ear**
- H93.8X2   **Other specified disorders of left ear**
- H93.8X3   **Other specified disorders of ear, bilateral**
- H93.8X9   **Other specified disorders of ear, unspecified ear**

√5ᵗʰ **H93.9**   **Unspecified disorder of ear**
- H93.90   **Unspecified disorder of ear, unspecified ear**   UPD
- H93.91   **Unspecified disorder of right ear**   UPD
- H93.92   **Unspecified disorder of left ear**   UPD
- H93.93   **Unspecified disorder of ear, bilateral**   UPD

√4ᵗʰ **H94**   **Other disorders of ear in diseases classified elsewhere**

√5ᵗʰ **H94.0**   **Acoustic neuritis in infectious and parasitic diseases classified elsewhere**
- Code first underlying disease, such as:
-      parasitic disease (B65-B89)
- EXCLUDES 1   acoustic neuritis (in):
-      herpes zoster (B02.29)
-      syphilis (A52.15)
- H94.00   *Acoustic neuritis in infectious and parasitic diseases classified elsewhere, unspecified ear*

H94.01   *Acoustic neuritis in infectious and parasitic diseases classified elsewhere, right ear*

H94.02   *Acoustic neuritis in infectious and parasitic diseases classified elsewhere, left ear*

H94.03   *Acoustic neuritis in infectious and parasitic diseases classified elsewhere, bilateral*

√5ᵗʰ **H94.8**   **Other specified disorders of ear in diseases classified elsewhere**
- Code first underlying disease, such as:
-      congenital syphilis (A50.0)
- EXCLUDES 1   aural myiasis (B87.4)
-      syphilitic labyrinthitis (A52.79)
- H94.80   *Other specified disorders of ear in diseases classified elsewhere, unspecified ear*
- H94.81   *Other specified disorders of right ear in diseases classified elsewhere*
- H94.82   *Other specified disorders of left ear in diseases classified elsewhere*
- H94.83   *Other specified disorders of ear in diseases classified elsewhere, bilateral*

Intraoperative and postprocedural complications and disorders of ear and mastoid process, not elsewhere classified (H95)

√4ᵗʰ **H95**   **Intraoperative and postprocedural complications and disorders of ear and mastoid process, not elsewhere classified**
- AHA: 2016,4Q,9-10

√5ᵗʰ **H95.0**   **Recurrent cholesteatoma of postmastoidectomy cavity**
- H95.00   **Recurrent cholesteatoma of postmastoidectomy cavity, unspecified ear**
- H95.01   **Recurrent cholesteatoma of postmastoidectomy cavity, right ear**
- H95.02   **Recurrent cholesteatoma of postmastoidectomy cavity, left ear**
- H95.03   **Recurrent cholesteatoma of postmastoidectomy cavity, bilateral ears**

√5ᵗʰ **H95.1**   **Other disorders of ear and mastoid process following mastoidectomy**

√6ᵗʰ **H95.11**   **Chronic inflammation of postmastoidectomy cavity**
- H95.111   **Chronic inflammation of postmastoidectomy cavity, right ear**
- H95.112   **Chronic inflammation of postmastoidectomy cavity, left ear**
- H95.113   **Chronic inflammation of postmastoidectomy cavity, bilateral ears**
- H95.119   **Chronic inflammation of postmastoidectomy cavity, unspecified ear**

√6ᵗʰ **H95.12**   **Granulation of postmastoidectomy cavity**
- H95.121   **Granulation of postmastoidectomy cavity, right ear**
- H95.122   **Granulation of postmastoidectomy cavity, left ear**
- H95.123   **Granulation of postmastoidectomy cavity, bilateral ears**
- H95.129   **Granulation of postmastoidectomy cavity, unspecified ear**

√6ᵗʰ **H95.13**   **Mucosal cyst of postmastoidectomy cavity**
- H95.131   **Mucosal cyst of postmastoidectomy cavity, right ear**
- H95.132   **Mucosal cyst of postmastoidectomy cavity, left ear**
- H95.133   **Mucosal cyst of postmastoidectomy cavity, bilateral ears**
- H95.139   **Mucosal cyst of postmastoidectomy cavity, unspecified ear**

√6ᵗʰ **H95.19**   **Other disorders following mastoidectomy**
- H95.191   **Other disorders following mastoidectomy, right ear**
- H95.192   **Other disorders following mastoidectomy, left ear**
- H95.193   **Other disorders following mastoidectomy, bilateral ears**
- H95.199   **Other disorders following mastoidectomy, unspecified ear**

✓ Additional Character Required   √x7ᵗʰ Placeholder   Questionable PDx   Manifestation   Unspecified Dx   UPD Unacceptable PDx   H1-H14 HAC   HCC CMS-HCC Dx   HIV HIV Dx

ICD-10-CM 2022   643

✓5ᵗʰ **H95.2** Intraoperative hemorrhage and hematoma of ear and mastoid process complicating a procedure

> **EXCLUDES 1**   *intraoperative hemorrhage and hematoma of ear and mastoid process due to accidental puncture or laceration during a procedure (H95.3-)*

     H95.21 Intraoperative hemorrhage and hematoma of ear and mastoid process complicating a procedure on the ear and mastoid process   CC

     H95.22 Intraoperative hemorrhage and hematoma of ear and mastoid process complicating other procedure   CC

✓5ᵗʰ **H95.3** Accidental puncture and laceration of ear and mastoid process during a procedure

     H95.31 Accidental puncture and laceration of the ear and mastoid process during a procedure on the ear and mastoid process   CC

     H95.32 Accidental puncture and laceration of the ear and mastoid process during other procedure   CC

✓5ᵗʰ **H95.4** Postprocedural hemorrhage of ear and mastoid process following a procedure

     H95.41 Postprocedural hemorrhage of ear and mastoid process following a procedure on the ear and mastoid process   CC

     H95.42 Postprocedural hemorrhage of ear and mastoid process following other procedure   CC

✓5ᵗʰ **H95.5** Postprocedural hematoma and seroma of ear and mastoid process following a procedure

     H95.51 Postprocedural hematoma of ear and mastoid process following a procedure on the ear and mastoid process   CC

     H95.52 Postprocedural hematoma of ear and mastoid process following other procedure   CC

     H95.53 Postprocedural seroma of ear and mastoid process following a procedure on the ear and mastoid process   CC

     H95.54 Postprocedural seroma of ear and mastoid process following other procedure   CC

✓5ᵗʰ **H95.8** Other intraoperative and postprocedural complications and disorders of the ear and mastoid process, not elsewhere classified

> **EXCLUDES 2**   *postprocedural complications and disorders following mastoidectomy (H95.0-, H95.1-)*

     ✓6ᵗʰ **H95.81** Postprocedural stenosis of external ear canal

         H95.811 Postprocedural stenosis of right external ear canal   CC

         H95.812 Postprocedural stenosis of left external ear canal   CC

         H95.813 Postprocedural stenosis of external ear canal, bilateral   CC

         H95.819 Postprocedural stenosis of unspecified external ear canal   CC

     H95.88 Other intraoperative complications and disorders of the ear and mastoid process, not elsewhere classified   CC

> Use additional code, if applicable, to further specify disorder

     H95.89 Other postprocedural complications and disorders of the ear and mastoid process, not elsewhere classified   CC

> Use additional code, if applicable, to further specify disorder

N Newborn: 0   P Pediatric: 0-17   M Maternity: 9-64   A Adult: 15-124   MCC Major Complication/Comorbidity   CC Complication/Comorbidity   SW Severe Wound Dx

644   ICD-10-CM 2022

Chapter 9. Diseases of the Circulatory System (I00–I99)

Chapter-specific Guidelines with Coding Examples

The chapter-specific guidelines from the ICD-10-CM Official Guidelines for Coding and Reporting have been provided below. Along with these guidelines are coding examples, contained in the shaded boxes, that have been developed to help illustrate the coding and/or sequencing guidance found in these guidelines.

a. Hypertension

The classification presumes a causal relationship between hypertension and heart involvement and between hypertension and kidney involvement, as the two conditions are linked by the term "with" in the Alphabetic Index. These conditions should be coded as related even in the absence of provider documentation explicitly linking them, unless the documentation clearly states the conditions are unrelated.

For hypertension and conditions not specifically linked by relational terms such as "with," "associated with" or "due to" in the classification, provider documentation must link the conditions in order to code them as related.

1) Hypertension with heart disease

Hypertension with heart conditions classified to I50.- or I51.4-I51.7, I51.89, I51.9, are assigned to a code from category I11, Hypertensive heart disease. Use additional code(s) from category I50, Heart failure, to identify the type(s) of heart failure in those patients with heart failure.

The same heart conditions (I50.-, I51.4-I51.7, I51.89, I51.9) with hypertension are coded separately if the provider has documented they are unrelated to the hypertension. Sequence according to the circumstances of the admission/encounter.

> Patient is admitted in left heart failure. Patient also has a history of hypertension managed by medication.
>
> **I11.0**   **Hypertensive heart disease with heart failure**
>
> **I50.1**   **Left ventricular failure, unspecified**
>
> *Explanation*: Without a diagnostic statement to the contrary, hypertension and heart failure have an assumed causal relationship, and a combination code should be used. An additional code to identify the type of heart failure (I50.-) should also be provided.

2) Hypertensive chronic kidney disease

Assign codes from category I12, Hypertensive chronic kidney disease, when both hypertension and a condition classifiable to category N18, Chronic kidney disease (CKD), are present. CKD should not be coded as hypertensive if the provider indicates the CKD is not related to the hypertension.

The appropriate code from category N18 should be used as a secondary code with a code from category I12 to identify the stage of chronic kidney disease.

See Section I.C.14. Chronic kidney disease.

If a patient has hypertensive chronic kidney disease and acute renal failure, the acute renal failure should also be coded. Sequence according to the circumstances of the admission/encounter.

> Patient is admitted with stage IV chronic kidney disease (CKD) due to polycystic kidney disease. Patient also is on lisinopril for hypertension.
>
> **N18.4**   **Chronic kidney disease, stage 4 (severe)**
>
> **Q61.3**   **Polycystic kidney, unspecified**
>
> **I10**   **Essential (primary) hypertension**
>
> *Explanation*: A combination code describing a relationship between hypertension and CKD is not used because the physician documentation identifies the polycystic kidney disease as the cause for the CKD.

3) Hypertensive heart and chronic kidney disease

Assign codes from combination category I13, Hypertensive heart and chronic kidney disease, when there is hypertension with both heart and kidney involvement. If heart failure is present, assign an additional code from category I50 to identify the type of heart failure.

The appropriate code from category N18, Chronic kidney disease, should be used as a secondary code with a code from category I13 to identify the stage of chronic kidney disease.

See Section I.C.14. Chronic kidney disease.

The codes in category I13, Hypertensive heart and chronic kidney disease, are combination codes that include hypertension, heart disease and chronic kidney disease. The Includes note at I13 specifies that the conditions included at I11 and I12 are included together in I13. If a patient has hypertension, heart disease and chronic kidney disease, then a code from I13 should be used, not individual codes for hypertension, heart disease and chronic kidney disease, or codes from I11 or I12.

For patients with both acute renal failure and chronic kidney disease, the acute renal failure should also be coded. Sequence according to the circumstances of the admission/encounter.

> Patient admitted with acute tubular necrosis, history of hypertensive heart and kidney disease with congestive heart failure and stage 3a chronic kidney disease
>
> **N17.0**   **Acute kidney failure with tubular necrosis**
>
> **I13.0**   **Hypertensive heart and chronic kidney disease with heart failure and stage 1 through stage 4 chronic kidney disease, or unspecified chronic kidney disease**
>
> **I50.9**   **Heart failure, unspecified**
>
> **N18.31**   **Chronic kidney disease, stage 3a**
>
> *Explanation*: It is appropriate to report an acute kidney failure code and a chronic kidney failure code when both conditions are treated during an encounter. In this instance, the acute renal failure was the focus of treatment and therefore sequenced as principal diagnosis. Combination codes in category I13 are used to report conditions classifiable to *both* categories I11 and I12. Do not report conditions classifiable to I11 and I12 separately. Use additional codes to report the type of heart failure and stage of CKD.

4) Hypertensive cerebrovascular disease

For hypertensive cerebrovascular disease, first assign the appropriate code from categories I60-I69, followed by the appropriate hypertension code.

> Rupture of cerebral aneurysm caused by malignant hypertension
>
> **I60.7**   **Nontraumatic subarachnoid hemorrhage from unspecified intracranial artery**
>
> **I10**   **Essential (primary) hypertension**
>
> *Explanation*: Hypertensive cerebrovascular disease requires two codes: the appropriate I60–I69 code followed by the appropriate hypertension code.

5) Hypertensive retinopathy

Subcategory H35.0, Background retinopathy and retinal vascular changes, should be used **along** with a code from categor**ies** I10-I15, **in the** Hypertensive diseases **section,** to include the systemic hypertension. The sequencing is based on the reason for the encounter.

6) Hypertension, secondary

Secondary hypertension is due to an underlying condition. Two codes are required: one to identify the underlying etiology and one from category I15 to identify the hypertension. Sequencing of codes is determined by the reason for admission/encounter.

> Renovascular hypertension due to renal artery atherosclerosis
>
> **I15.0**   **Renovascular hypertension**
>
> **I70.1**   **Atherosclerosis of renal artery**
>
> *Explanation*: Secondary hypertension requires two codes: a code to identify the etiology and the appropriate I15 code.

7) Hypertension, transient

Assign code R03.0, Elevated blood pressure reading without diagnosis of hypertension, unless patient has an established diagnosis of hypertension. Assign code O13.-, Gestational [pregnancy-induced] hypertension without significant proteinuria, or O14.-, Pre-eclampsia, for transient hypertension of pregnancy.

8) Hypertension, controlled

This diagnostic statement usually refers to an existing state of hypertension under control by therapy. Assign the appropriate code from categories I10-I15, Hypertensive diseases.

9) Hypertension, uncontrolled

Uncontrolled hypertension may refer to untreated hypertension or hypertension not responding to current therapeutic regimen. In either case, assign the appropriate code from categories I10-I15, Hypertensive diseases.

10) Hypertensive crisis

Assign a code from category I16, Hypertensive crisis, for documented hypertensive urgency, hypertensive emergency or unspecified

Chapter 9. Diseases of the Circulatory System

hypertensive crisis. Code also any identified hypertensive disease (I10-I15). The sequencing is based on the reason for the encounter.

11) Pulmonary hypertension

Pulmonary hypertension is classified to category I27, Other pulmonary heart diseases. For secondary pulmonary hypertension (I27.1, I27.2-), code also any associated conditions or adverse effects of drugs or toxins. The sequencing is based on the reason for the encounter, except for adverse effects of drugs (See Section I.C.19.e.).

b. Atherosclerotic coronary artery disease and angina

ICD-10-CM has combination codes for atherosclerotic heart disease with angina pectoris. The subcategories for these codes are I25.11, Atherosclerotic heart disease of native coronary artery with angina pectoris and I25.7, Atherosclerosis of coronary artery bypass graft(s) and coronary artery of transplanted heart with angina pectoris.

When using one of these combination codes it is not necessary to use an additional code for angina pectoris. A causal relationship can be assumed in a patient with both atherosclerosis and angina pectoris, unless the documentation indicates the angina is due to something other than the atherosclerosis.

If a patient with coronary artery disease is admitted due to an acute myocardial infarction (AMI), the AMI should be sequenced before the coronary artery disease.

See Section I.C.9. Acute myocardial infarction (AMI)

c. Intraoperative and postprocedural cerebrovascular accident

Medical record documentation should clearly specify the cause- and- effect relationship between the medical intervention and the cerebrovascular accident in order to assign a code for intraoperative or postprocedural cerebrovascular accident.

Proper code assignment depends on whether it was an infarction or hemorrhage and whether it occurred intraoperatively or postoperatively. If it was a cerebral hemorrhage, code assignment depends on the type of procedure performed.

Embolic cerebral infarction of the right middle cerebral artery that occurred during hip replacement surgery. The surgeon documented as due to the surgery.

I97.811	**Intraoperative cerebrovascular infarction during other surgery**
I63.411	**Cerebral infarction due to embolism of right middle cerebral artery**

Explanation: Code assignment for intraoperative or postprocedural cerebrovascular accident is based on the provider's documentation of a cause-and-effect relationship between the condition and the procedure. Proper code assignment also depends on whether the cerebrovascular accident was an infarction or hemorrhage, occurred intraoperatively or postoperatively, and the type of procedure performed.

d. Sequelae of cerebrovascular disease

1) Category I69, Sequelae of cerebrovascular disease

Category I69 is used to indicate conditions classifiable to categories I60-I67 as the causes of sequela (neurologic deficits), themselves classified elsewhere. These "late effects" include neurologic deficits that persist after initial onset of conditions classifiable to categories I60-I67. The neurologic deficits caused by cerebrovascular disease may be present from the onset or may arise at any time after the onset of the condition classifiable to categories I60-I67.

Codes from category I69, Sequelae of cerebrovascular disease, that specify hemiplegia, hemiparesis and monoplegia identify whether the dominant or nondominant side is affected. Should the affected side be documented, but not specified as dominant or nondominant, and the classification system does not indicate a default, code selection is as follows:

- For ambidextrous patients, the default should be dominant.
- If the left side is affected, the default is non-dominant.
- If the right side is affected, the default is dominant.

2) Codes from category I69 with codes from I60–I67

Codes from category I69 may be assigned on a health care record with codes from I60-I67, if the patient has a current cerebrovascular disease and deficits from an old cerebrovascular disease.

3) Codes from category I69 and personal history of transient ischemic attack (TIA) and cerebral infarction (Z86.73)

Codes from category I69 should not be assigned if the patient does not have neurologic deficits.

See Section I.C.21. 4. History (of) for use of personal history codes

e. Acute myocardial infarction (AMI)

1) Type 1 ST elevation myocardial infarction (STEMI) and non ST elevation myocardial infarction (NSTEMI)

The ICD-10-CM codes for type 1 acute myocardial infarction (AMI) identify the site, such as anterolateral wall or true posterior wall. Subcategories I21.0-I21.2 and code I21.3 are used for type 1 ST elevation myocardial infarction (STEMI). Code I21.4, Non-ST elevation (NSTEMI) myocardial infarction, is used for type 1 non-ST elevation myocardial infarction (NSTEMI) and nontransmural MIs.

If a type 1 NSTEMI evolves to STEMI, assign the STEMI code. If a type 1 STEMI converts to NSTEMI due to thrombolytic therapy, it is still coded as STEMI.

For encounters occurring while the myocardial infarction is equal to, or less than, four weeks old, including transfers to another acute setting or a postacute setting, and the myocardial infarction meets the definition for "other diagnoses" (see Section III, Reporting Additional Diagnoses), codes from category I21 may continue to be reported. For encounters after the 4-week time frame and the patient is still receiving care related to the myocardial infarction, the appropriate aftercare code should be assigned, rather than a code from category I21. For old or healed myocardial infarctions not requiring further care, code I25.2, Old myocardial infarction, may be assigned.

2) Acute myocardial infarction, unspecified

Code I21.9, Acute myocardial infarction, unspecified, is the default for unspecified acute myocardial infarction or unspecified type. If only type 1 STEMI or transmural MI without the site is documented, assign code I21.3, ST elevation (STEMI) myocardial infarction of unspecified site.

3) AMI documented as nontransmural or subendocardial but site provided

If an AMI is documented as nontransmural or subendocardial, but the site is provided, it is still coded as a subendocardial AMI.

See Section I.C.21.3 for information on coding status post administration of tPA in a different facility within the last 24 hours.

4) Subsequent acute myocardial infarction

A code from category I22, Subsequent ST elevation (STEMI) and non-ST elevation (NSTEMI) myocardial infarction, is to be used when a patient who has suffered a type 1 or unspecified AMI has a new AMI within the 4-week time frame of the initial AMI. A code from category I22 must be used in conjunction with a code from category I21. The sequencing of the I22 and I21 codes depends on the circumstances of the encounter.

Do not assign code I22 for subsequent myocardial infarctions other than type 1 or unspecified. For subsequent type 2 AMI assign only code I21.A1. For subsequent type 4 or type 5 AMI, assign only code I21.A9.

If a subsequent myocardial infarction of one type occurs within 4 weeks of a myocardial infarction of a different type, assign the appropriate codes from category I21 to identify each type. Do not assign a code from I22. Codes from category I22 should only be assigned if both the initial and subsequent myocardial infarctions are type 1 or unspecified.

5) Other types of myocardial infarction

The ICD-10-CM provides codes for different types of myocardial infarction. Type 1 myocardial infarctions are assigned to codes I21.0-I21.4.

Type 2 myocardial infarction (myocardial infarction due to demand ischemia or secondary to ischemic imbalance) is assigned to code I21.A1, Myocardial infarction type 2 with the underlying cause coded first. Do not assign code I24.8, Other forms of acute ischemic heart disease, for the demand ischemia. If a type 2 AMI is described as NSTEMI or STEMI, only assign code I21.A1. Codes I21.01-I21.4 should only be assigned for type 1 AMIs.

Acute myocardial infarctions type 3, 4a, 4b, 4c and 5 are assigned to code I21.A9, Other myocardial infarction type.

The "Code also" and "Code first" notes should be followed related to complications, and for coding of postprocedural myocardial infarctions during or following cardiac surgery.

Myocardial infarction involving the left circumflex artery occurring during PTCA with stent insertion to treat coronary artery disease

I25.10	**Atherosclerotic heart disease of native coronary artery without angina pectoris**
I97.790	**Other intraoperative cardiac functional disturbances during cardiac surgery**
I21.A9	**Other myocardial infarction type**

Explanation: A myocardial infarction occurring during a revascularization procedure is not considered a type 1 myocardial infarction (MI) and should not be coded to a type 1 MI code (I21.0-, I21.1-, I21.2-, I21.3) even when the specific site of the MI is documented. According to the code first instruction at I21.A9, the complication code (I97.790) should be sequenced before code I21.A9.

Chapter 9. Diseases of the Circulatory System (I00-I99)

EXCLUDES 2
- certain conditions originating in the perinatal period (P04-P96)
- certain infectious and parasitic diseases (A00-B99)
- complications of pregnancy, childbirth and the puerperium (O00-O9A)
- congenital malformations, deformations, and chromosomal abnormalities (Q00-Q99)
- endocrine, nutritional and metabolic diseases (E00-E88)
- injury, poisoning and certain other consequences of external causes (S00-T88)
- neoplasms (C00-D49)
- symptoms, signs and abnormal clinical and laboratory findings, not elsewhere classified (R00-R94)
- systemic connective tissue disorders (M30-M36)
- transient cerebral ischemic attacks and related syndromes (G45.-)

This chapter contains the following blocks:

I00-I02	Acute rheumatic fever
I05-I09	Chronic rheumatic heart diseases
I10-I16	Hypertensive diseases
I20-I25	Ischemic heart diseases
I26-I28	Pulmonary heart disease and diseases of pulmonary circulation
▶I30-I5A◀	Other forms of heart disease
I60-I69	Cerebrovascular diseases
I70-I79	Diseases of arteries, arterioles and capillaries
I80-I89	Diseases of veins, lymphatic vessels and lymph nodes, not elsewhere classified
I95-I99	Other and unspecified disorders of the circulatory system

Acute rheumatic fever (I00-I02)

DEF: Rheumatic fever: Inflammatory disease that can follow a throat infection by group A *streptococci*. Complications can involve the joints (arthritis), subcutaneous tissue (nodules), skin (erythema marginatum), heart (carditis), or brain (chorea).

I00 Rheumatic fever without heart involvement
- INCLUDES   arthritis, rheumatic, acute or subacute
- EXCLUDES 1   rheumatic fever with heart involvement (I01.0-I01.9)

✓4ᵗʰ **I01 Rheumatic fever with heart involvement**
- EXCLUDES 1   chronic diseases of rheumatic origin (I05-I09) unless rheumatic fever is also present or there is evidence of reactivation or activity of the rheumatic process

- **I01.0 Acute rheumatic pericarditis**   CC
  - Any condition in I00 with pericarditis
  - Rheumatic pericarditis (acute)
  - EXCLUDES 1   acute pericarditis not specified as rheumatic (I30.-)

- **I01.1 Acute rheumatic endocarditis**   CC
  - Any condition in I00 with endocarditis or valvulitis
  - Acute rheumatic valvulitis

- **I01.2 Acute rheumatic myocarditis**   CC
  - Any condition in I00 with myocarditis

- **I01.8 Other acute rheumatic heart disease**   CC
  - Any condition in I00 with other or multiple types of heart involvement
  - Acute rheumatic pancarditis

- **I01.9 Acute rheumatic heart disease, unspecified**   CC
  - Any condition in I00 with unspecified type of heart involvement
  - Rheumatic carditis, acute
  - Rheumatic heart disease, active or acute

✓4ᵗʰ **I02 Rheumatic chorea**
- INCLUDES   Sydenham's chorea
- EXCLUDES 1   chorea NOS (G25.5)
  - Huntington's chorea (G10)

- **I02.0 Rheumatic chorea with heart involvement**   CC
  - Chorea NOS with heart involvement
  - Rheumatic chorea with heart involvement of any type classifiable under I01.-

- **I02.9 Rheumatic chorea without heart involvement**   CC
  - Rheumatic chorea NOS

Chronic rheumatic heart diseases (I05-I09)

✓4ᵗʰ **I05 Rheumatic mitral valve diseases**
- INCLUDES   conditions classifiable to both I05.0 and I05.2-I05.9, whether specified as rheumatic or not
- EXCLUDES 1   mitral valve disease specified as nonrheumatic (I34.-)
  - mitral valve disease with aortic and/or tricuspid valve involvement (I08.-)

- **I05.0 Rheumatic mitral stenosis**
  - Mitral (valve) obstruction (rheumatic)
  - **DEF:** Narrowing of the mitral valve between the left atrium and left ventricle due to rheumatic fever. Symptoms include shortness of breath during or after exercise, fatigue, palpitations, chest discomfort, and swelling of feet or legs.

- **I05.1 Rheumatic mitral insufficiency**
  - Rheumatic mitral incompetence
  - Rheumatic mitral regurgitation
  - EXCLUDES 1   mitral insufficiency not specified as rheumatic (I34.0)

- **I05.2 Rheumatic mitral stenosis with insufficiency**
  - Rheumatic mitral stenosis with incompetence or regurgitation

- **I05.8 Other rheumatic mitral valve diseases**
  - Rheumatic mitral (valve) failure

- **I05.9 Rheumatic mitral valve disease, unspecified**
  - Rheumatic mitral (valve) disorder (chronic) NOS

✓4ᵗʰ **I06 Rheumatic aortic valve diseases**
- EXCLUDES 1   aortic valve disease not specified as rheumatic (I35.-)
  - aortic valve disease with mitral and/or tricuspid valve involvement (I08.-)

- **I06.0 Rheumatic aortic stenosis**
  - Rheumatic aortic (valve) obstruction

- **I06.1 Rheumatic aortic insufficiency**
  - Rheumatic aortic incompetence
  - Rheumatic aortic regurgitation

- **I06.2 Rheumatic aortic stenosis with insufficiency**
  - Rheumatic aortic stenosis with incompetence or regurgitation

- **I06.8 Other rheumatic aortic valve diseases**

- **I06.9 Rheumatic aortic valve disease, unspecified**
  - Rheumatic aortic (valve) disease NOS

✓4ᵗʰ **I07 Rheumatic tricuspid valve diseases**
- INCLUDES   rheumatic tricuspid valve diseases specified as rheumatic or unspecified
- EXCLUDES 1   tricuspid valve disease specified as nonrheumatic (I36.-)
  - tricuspid valve disease with aortic and/or mitral valve involvement (I08.-)

- **I07.0 Rheumatic tricuspid stenosis**
  - Tricuspid (valve) stenosis (rheumatic)

- **I07.1 Rheumatic tricuspid insufficiency**
  - Tricuspid (valve) insufficiency (rheumatic)

- **I07.2 Rheumatic tricuspid stenosis and insufficiency**

- **I07.8 Other rheumatic tricuspid valve diseases**

- **I07.9 Rheumatic tricuspid valve disease, unspecified**
  - Rheumatic tricuspid valve disorder NOS

✓4ᵗʰ **I08 Multiple valve diseases**
- INCLUDES   multiple valve diseases specified as rheumatic or unspecified
- EXCLUDES 1   endocarditis, valve unspecified (I38)
  - multiple valve disease specified a nonrheumatic (I34.-, I35.-, I36.-, I37.-, I38.-, Q22.-, Q23.-, Q24.8-)
  - rheumatic valve disease NOS (I09.1)

- **I08.0 Rheumatic disorders of both mitral and aortic valves**
  - Involvement of both mitral and aortic valves specified as rheumatic or unspecified
  - **AHA:** 2019,2Q,5

- **I08.1 Rheumatic disorders of both mitral and tricuspid valves**

- **I08.2 Rheumatic disorders of both aortic and tricuspid valves**

- **I08.3 Combined rheumatic disorders of mitral, aortic and tricuspid valves**

- **I08.8 Other rheumatic multiple valve diseases**

- **I08.9 Rheumatic multiple valve disease, unspecified**

✓4ᵗʰ **I09 Other rheumatic heart diseases**

- **I09.0 Rheumatic myocarditis**   CC
  - EXCLUDES 1   myocarditis not specified as rheumatic (I51.4)

✔ Additional Character Required   ✓x7ᵗʰ Placeholder   Questionable PDx   Manifestation   Unspecified Dx   UPD Unacceptable PDx   H1-H14 HAC   HCC CMS-HCC Dx   HIV HIV Dx

ICD-10-CM 2022   647

Chapter 9. Diseases of the Circulatory System

I09.1   Rheumatic diseases of endocardium, valve unspecified
Rheumatic endocarditis (chronic)
Rheumatic valvulitis (chronic)
> EXCLUDES 1   *endocarditis, valve unspecified (I38)*

I09.2   Chronic rheumatic pericarditis   CC
Adherent pericardium, rheumatic
Chronic rheumatic mediastinopericarditis
Chronic rheumatic myopericarditis
> EXCLUDES 1   *chronic pericarditis not specified as rheumatic (I31.-)*

✓5th **I09.8   Other specified rheumatic heart diseases**

I09.81   Rheumatic heart failure   CC HCC
Use additional code to identify type of heart failure (I50.-)
DEF: Decreased cardiac output, edema, and hypertension due to rheumatic heart disease.

I09.89   Other specified rheumatic heart diseases
Rheumatic disease of pulmonary valve

I09.9   Rheumatic heart disease, unspecified
Rheumatic carditis
> EXCLUDES 1   *rheumatoid carditis (M05.31)*

Hypertensive diseases (I10-I16)

Use additional code to identify:
exposure to environmental tobacco smoke (Z77.22)
history of tobacco dependence (Z87.891)
occupational exposure to environmental tobacco smoke (Z57.31)
tobacco dependence (F17.-)
tobacco use (Z72.0)
> EXCLUDES 1   *neonatal hypertension (P29.2)*
> *primary pulmonary hypertension (I27.0)*
> EXCLUDES 2   *hypertensive disease complicating pregnancy, childbirth and the puerperium (O10-O11, O13-O16)*

I10   Essential (primary) hypertension
> INCLUDES   high blood pressure
> hypertension (arterial) (benign) (essential) (malignant) (primary) (systemic)
> EXCLUDES 1   *hypertensive disease complicating pregnancy, childbirth and the puerperium (O10-O11, O13-O16)*
> EXCLUDES 2   *essential (primary) hypertension involving vessels of brain (I60-I69)*
> *essential (primary) hypertension involving vessels of eye (H35.0-)*

AHA: 2020,1Q,12; 2018,2Q,9; 2016,4Q,27

✓4th **I11   Hypertensive heart disease**
> INCLUDES   any condition in I50.- or I51.4-I51.7, I51.89, I51.9 due to hypertension

AHA: 2018,2Q,9
TIP: Do not assign a code from this category when provider documentation indicates the heart disease is attributable to another cause.

I11.0   Hypertensive heart disease with heart failure   HCC
Hypertensive heart failure
Use additional code to identify type of heart failure (I50.-)
AHA: 2017,1Q,47

I11.9   Hypertensive heart disease without heart failure
Hypertensive heart disease NOS

✓4th **I12   Hypertensive chronic kidney disease**
> INCLUDES   any condition in N18 and N26 — due to hypertension
> arteriosclerosis of kidney
> arteriosclerotic nephritis (chronic) (interstitial)
> hypertensive nephropathy
> nephrosclerosis
> EXCLUDES 1   *hypertension due to kidney disease (I15.0, I15.1)*
> *renovascular hypertension (I15.0)*
> *secondary hypertension (I15.-)*
> EXCLUDES 2   *acute kidney failure (N17.-)*

AHA: 2019,3Q,3; 2018,4Q,88; 2016,3Q,22
TIP: Do not assign a code from this category when provider documentation indicates the chronic kidney disease (CKD) is attributable to another cause.

I12.0   Hypertensive chronic kidney disease with stage 5 chronic kidney disease or end stage renal disease   CC HCC
Use additional code to identify the stage of chronic kidney disease (N18.5, N18.6)

I12.9   Hypertensive chronic kidney disease with stage 1 through stage 4 chronic kidney disease, or unspecified chronic kidney disease
Hypertensive chronic kidney disease NOS
Hypertensive renal disease NOS
Use additional code to identify the stage of chronic kidney disease (N18.1-N18.4, N18.9)

✓4th **I13   Hypertensive heart and chronic kidney disease**
> INCLUDES   any condition in I11.- with any condition in I12.-
> cardiorenal disease
> cardiovascular renal disease

TIP: Do not assign a code from this category when provider documentation indicates the heart and/or chronic kidney disease is attributable to another cause.

I13.0   Hypertensive heart and chronic kidney disease with heart failure and stage 1 through stage 4 chronic kidney disease, or unspecified chronic kidney disease   CC HCC
Use additional code to identify type of heart failure (I50.-)
Use additional code to identify stage of chronic kidney disease (N18.1-N18.4, N18.9)

✓5th **I13.1   Hypertensive heart and chronic kidney disease without heart failure**

I13.10   Hypertensive heart and chronic kidney disease without heart failure, with stage 1 through stage 4 chronic kidney disease, or unspecified chronic kidney disease
Hypertensive heart disease and hypertensive chronic kidney disease NOS
Use additional code to identify the stage of chronic kidney disease (N18.1-N18.4, N18.9)

I13.11   Hypertensive heart and chronic kidney disease without heart failure, with stage 5 chronic kidney disease, or end stage renal disease   CC HCC
Use additional code to identify the stage of chronic kidney disease (N18.5, N18.6)

I13.2   Hypertensive heart and chronic kidney disease with heart failure and with stage 5 chronic kidney disease, or end stage renal disease   CC HCC
Use additional code to identify type of heart failure (I50.-)
Use additional code to identify the stage of chronic kidney disease (N18.5, N18.6)

✓4th **I15   Secondary hypertension**
Code also underlying condition
> EXCLUDES 1   *postprocedural hypertension (I97.3)*
> EXCLUDES 2   *secondary hypertension involving vessels of brain (I60-I69)*
> *secondary hypertension involving vessels of eye (H35.0-)*

I15.0   Renovascular hypertension
I15.1   Hypertension secondary to other renal disorders
> **AHA:** 2016,3Q,22
I15.2   Hypertension secondary to endocrine disorders
I15.8   Other secondary hypertension
I15.9   Secondary hypertension, unspecified

✓4th **I16   Hypertensive crisis**
Code also any identified hypertensive disease (I10-I15)
AHA: 2016,4Q,26-28
I16.0   Hypertensive urgency
I16.1   Hypertensive emergency   CC
I16.9   Hypertensive crisis, unspecified   CC

N Newborn: 0   P Pediatric: 0-17   M Maternity: 9-64   A Adult: 15-124   MCC Major Complication/Comorbidity   CC Complication/Comorbidity   SW Severe Wound Dx

Ischemic heart diseases (I20-I25)

▶Code also the presence of hypertension (I10-I16)◀
~~Use additional code to identify presence of hypertension (I10-I16)~~

✓4ᵗʰ I20 Angina pectoris

Use additional code to identify:
exposure to environmental tobacco smoke (Z77.22)
history of tobacco dependence (Z87.891)
occupational exposure to environmental tobacco smoke (Z57.31)
tobacco dependence (F17.-)
tobacco use (Z72.0)

EXCLUDES 1   *angina pectoris with atherosclerotic heart disease of native coronary arteries (I25.1-)*
atherosclerosis of coronary artery bypass graft(s) and coronary artery of transplanted heart with angina pectoris (I25.7-)
postinfarction angina (I23.7)

DEF: Chest pain due to reduced blood flow resulting in a lack of oxygen to the heart muscles.

I20.0 Unstable angina   CC HCC
Accelerated angina
Crescendo angina
De novo effort angina
Intermediate coronary syndrome
Preinfarction syndrome
Worsening effort angina
DEF: Condition representing an intermediate stage between angina of effort and acute myocardial infarction.

I20.1 Angina pectoris with documented spasm   CC HCC
Angiospastic angina
Prinzmetal angina
Spasm-induced angina
Variant angina

I20.8 Other forms of angina pectoris   HCC
Angina equivalent
Angina of effort
Coronary slow flow syndrome
Stable angina
Stenocardia
Use additional code(s) for symptoms associated with angina equivalent

I20.9 Angina pectoris, unspecified   HCC
Angina NOS
Anginal syndrome
Cardiac angina
Ischemic chest pain

✓4ᵗʰ I21 Acute myocardial infarction

INCLUDES   cardiac infarction
coronary (artery) embolism
coronary (artery) occlusion
coronary (artery) rupture
coronary (artery) thrombosis
infarction of heart, myocardium, or ventricle
myocardial infarction specified as acute or with a stated duration of 4 weeks (28 days) or less from onset

Use additional code, if applicable, to identify:
exposure to environmental tobacco smoke (Z77.22)
history of tobacco dependence (Z87.891)
occupational exposure to environmental tobacco smoke (Z57.31)
status post administration of tPA (rtPA) in a different facility within the last 24 hours prior to admission to current facility (Z92.82)
tobacco dependence (F17.-)
tobacco use (Z72.0)

EXCLUDES 2   *old myocardial infarction (I25.2)*
postmyocardial infarction syndrome (I24.1)
subsequent type 1 myocardial infarction (I22.-)

AHA: 2019,2Q,5; 2018,4Q,68; 2018,3Q,5; 2017,4Q,12-14; 2017,1Q,44-45; 2016,4Q,140; 2015,2Q,16; 2013,1Q,25; 2012,4Q,96,102-103

TIP: When chronic total occlusion and myocardial infarction are documented as being in different vessels, assign code I25.82 Chronic total occlusion of coronary artery, in addition to the myocardial infarction code.

✓5ᵗʰ I21.0 ST elevation (STEMI) myocardial infarction of anterior wall
Type 1 ST elevation myocardial infarction of anterior wall
DEF: ST elevation myocardial infarction: Complete obstruction of one or more coronary arteries causing decreased blood flow (ischemia) and necrosis of myocardial muscle cells.

I21.01 ST elevation (STEMI) myocardial infarction involving left main coronary artery   MCC HCC

I21.02 ST elevation (STEMI) myocardial infarction involving left anterior descending coronary artery   MCC HCC
ST elevation (STEMI) myocardial infarction involving diagonal coronary artery
AHA: 2013,1Q,25

I21.09 ST elevation (STEMI) myocardial infarction involving other coronary artery of anterior wall   MCC HCC
Acute transmural myocardial infarction of anterior wall
Anteroapical transmural (Q wave) infarction (acute)
Anterolateral transmural (Q wave) infarction (acute)
Anteroseptal transmural (Q wave) infarction (acute)
Transmural (Q wave) infarction (acute) (of) anterior (wall) NOS
AHA: 2012,4Q,102-103

✓5ᵗʰ I21.1 ST elevation (STEMI) myocardial infarction of inferior wall
Type 1 ST elevation myocardial infarction of inferior wall
DEF: ST elevation myocardial infarction: Complete obstruction of one or more coronary arteries causing decreased blood flow (ischemia) and necrosis of myocardial muscle cells.

I21.11 ST elevation (STEMI) myocardial infarction involving right coronary artery   MCC HCC
Inferoposterior transmural (Q wave) infarction (acute)

I21.19 ST elevation (STEMI) myocardial infarction involving other coronary artery of inferior wall   MCC HCC
Acute transmural myocardial infarction of inferior wall
Inferolateral transmural (Q wave) infarction (acute)
Transmural (Q wave) infarction (acute) (of) diaphragmatic wall
Transmural (Q wave) infarction (acute) (of) inferior (wall) NOS

EXCLUDES 2   *ST elevation (STEMI) myocardial infarction involving left circumflex coronary artery (I21.21)*

AHA: 2012,4Q,96

☑ ▶Additional Character Required   ✓x7ᵗʰ Placeholder   Questionable PDx   Manifestation   Unspecified Dx   UPD Unacceptable PDx   H1-H14 HAC   HCC CMS-HCC Dx   HIV HIV Dx

ICD-10-CM 2022   649

✓5ᵗʰ I21.2 ST elevation (STEMI) myocardial infarction of other sites

Type 1 ST elevation myocardial infarction of other sites
DEF: ST elevation myocardial infarction: Complete obstruction of one or more coronary arteries causing decreased blood flow (ischemia) and necrosis of myocardial muscle cells.

I21.21 ST elevation (STEMI) myocardial infarction involving left circumflex coronary artery MCC HCC

ST elevation (STEMI) myocardial infarction involving oblique marginal coronary artery

I21.29 ST elevation (STEMI) myocardial infarction involving other sites MCC HCC

Acute transmural myocardial infarction of other sites
Apical-lateral transmural (Q wave) infarction (acute)
Basal-lateral transmural (Q wave) infarction (acute)
High lateral transmural (Q wave) infarction (acute)
Lateral (wall) NOS transmural (Q wave) infarction (acute)
Posterior (true) transmural (Q wave) infarction (acute)
Posterobasal transmural (Q wave) infarction (acute)
Posterolateral transmural (Q wave) infarction (acute)
Posteroseptal transmural (Q wave) infarction (acute)
Septal transmural (Q wave) infarction (acute) NOS

I21.3 ST elevation (STEMI) myocardial infarction of unspecified site MCC HCC

Acute transmural myocardial infarction of unspecified site
Transmural (Q wave) myocardial infarction NOS
Type 1 ST elevation myocardial infarction of unspecified site
DEF: ST elevation myocardial infarction: Complete obstruction of one or more coronary arteries causing decreased blood flow (ischemia) and necrosis of myocardial muscle cells.

I21.4 Non-ST elevation (NSTEMI) myocardial infarction MCC HCC

Acute subendocardial myocardial infarction
Non-Q wave myocardial infarction NOS
Nontransmural myocardial infarction NOS
Type 1 non-ST elevation myocardial infarction
AHA: 2019,2Q,33; 2017,1Q,44-45
DEF: Partial obstruction of one or more coronary arteries that causes decreased blood flow (ischemia) and may cause partial thickness necrosis of myocardial muscle cells.

I21.9 Acute myocardial infarction, unspecified MCC HCC

Myocardial infarction (acute) NOS

✓6ᵗʰ I21.A Other type of myocardial infarction

AHA: 2019,2Q,5

I21.A1 Myocardial infarction type 2 MCC HCC

Myocardial infarction due to demand ischemia
Myocardial infarction secondary to ischemic imbalance
Code first the underlying cause, such as:
anemia (D50.0-D64.9)
chronic obstructive pulmonary disease (J44.-)
paroxysmal tachycardia (I47.0-I47.9)
shock (R57.0-R57.9)
AHA: 2019,4Q,53; 2017,4Q,13-14
DEF: Often referred to as due to demand ischemia, myocardial infarction (MI) type 2 refers to an MI due to ischemia and necrosis resulting from an oxygen imbalance to the heart. This mismatch between oxygen decreased supply and increased demand is caused by conditions other than coronary artery disease such as vasospasm, embolism, anemia, hypertension, hypotension, or arrhythmias.

I21.A9 Other myocardial infarction type MCC HCC

Myocardial infarction associated with revascularization procedure
Myocardial infarction type 3
Myocardial infarction type 4a
Myocardial infarction type 4b
Myocardial infarction type 4c
Myocardial infarction type 5
Code first, if applicable, postprocedural myocardial infarction following cardiac surgery (I97.190), or postprocedural myocardial infarction during cardiac surgery (I97.790)
Code also complication, if known and applicable, such as:
(acute) stent occlusion (T82.897-)
(acute) stent stenosis (T82.855-)
(acute) stent thrombosis (T82.867-)
cardiac arrest due to underlying cardiac condition (I46.2)
complication of percutaneous coronary intervention (PCI) (I97.89)
occlusion of coronary artery bypass graft (T82.218-)
AHA: 2019,2Q,33

✓4ᵗʰ I22 Subsequent ST elevation (STEMI) and non-ST elevation (NSTEMI) myocardial infarction

INCLUDES   acute myocardial infarction occurring within four weeks (28 days) of a previous acute myocardial infarction, regardless of site
cardiac infarction
coronary (artery) embolism
coronary (artery) occlusion
coronary (artery) rupture
coronary (artery) thrombosis
infarction of heart, myocardium, or ventricle
recurrent myocardial infarction
reinfarction of myocardium
rupture of heart, myocardium, or ventricle
subsequent type 1 myocardial infarction

Use additional code, if applicable, to identify:
exposure to environmental tobacco smoke (Z77.22)
history of tobacco dependence (Z87.891)
occupational exposure to environmental tobacco smoke (Z57.31)
status post administration of tPA (rtPA) in a different facility within the last 24 hours prior to admission to current facility (Z92.82)
tobacco dependence (F17.-)
tobacco use (Z72.0)

EXCLUDES 1   subsequent myocardial infarction, type 2 (I21.A1)
subsequent myocardial infarction of other type (type 3) (type 4) (type 5) (I21.A9)

AHA: 2018,4Q,68; 2018,3Q,5; 2017,4Q,12-13; 2017,2Q,11; 2013,1Q,25; 2012,4Q,97,102-103
DEF: Non-ST elevation myocardial infarction: Partial obstruction of one or more coronary arteries that causes decreased blood flow (ischemia) and may cause partial thickness necrosis of myocardial muscle cells.
DEF: ST elevation myocardial infarction: Complete obstruction of one or more coronary arteries causing decreased blood flow (ischemia) and necrosis of myocardial muscle cells.
TIP: When chronic total occlusion and myocardial infarction are documented as being in different vessels, assign code I25.82 Chronic total occlusion of coronary artery, in addition to the myocardial infarction code.

I22.0 Subsequent ST elevation (STEMI) myocardial infarction of anterior wall MCC HCC

Subsequent acute transmural myocardial infarction of anterior wall
Subsequent transmural (Q wave) infarction (acute)(of) anterior (wall) NOS
Subsequent anteroapical transmural (Q wave) infarction (acute)
Subsequent anterolateral transmural (Q wave) infarction (acute)
Subsequent anteroseptal transmural (Q wave) infarction (acute)

I22.1 **Subsequent ST elevation (STEMI) myocardial infarction of inferior wall** `MCC` `HCC`

Subsequent acute transmural myocardial infarction of inferior wall

Subsequent transmural (Q wave) infarction (acute)(of) diaphragmatic wall

Subsequent transmural (Q wave) infarction (acute)(of) inferior (wall) NOS

Subsequent inferolateral transmural (Q wave) infarction (acute)

Subsequent inferoposterior transmural (Q wave) infarction (acute)

AHA: 2012,4Q,102

I22.2 **Subsequent non-ST elevation (NSTEMI) myocardial infarction** `MCC` `HCC`

Subsequent acute subendocardial myocardial infarction

Subsequent non-Q wave myocardial infarction NOS

Subsequent nontransmural myocardial infarction NOS

I22.8 **Subsequent ST elevation (STEMI) myocardial infarction of other sites** `MCC` `HCC`

Subsequent acute transmural myocardial infarction of other sites

Subsequent apical-lateral transmural (Q wave) myocardial infarction (acute)

Subsequent basal-lateral transmural (Q wave) myocardial infarction (acute)

Subsequent high lateral transmural (Q wave) myocardial infarction (acute)

Subsequent transmural (Q wave) myocardial infarction (acute)(of) lateral (wall) NOS

Subsequent posterior (true) transmural (Q wave) myocardial infarction (acute)

Subsequent posterobasal transmural (Q wave) myocardial infarction (acute)

Subsequent posterolateral transmural (Q wave) myocardial infarction (acute)

Subsequent posteroseptal transmural (Q wave) myocardial infarction (acute)

Subsequent septal NOS transmural (Q wave) myocardial infarction (acute)

I22.9 **Subsequent ST elevation (STEMI) myocardial infarction of unspecified site** `MCC` `HCC`

Subsequent acute myocardial infarction of unspecified site

Subsequent myocardial infarction (acute) NOS

☑4ᵗʰ **I23** **Certain current complications following ST elevation (STEMI) and non-ST elevation (NSTEMI) myocardial infarction (within the 28 day period)**

AHA: 2017,2Q,11

DEF: ST elevation myocardial infarction: Complete obstruction of one or more coronary arteries causing decreased blood flow (ischemia) and necrosis of myocardial muscle cells.

DEF: Non-ST elevation myocardial infarction: Partial obstruction of one or more coronary arteries that causes decreased blood flow (ischemia) and may cause partial thickness necrosis of myocardial muscle cells.

I23.0 **Hemopericardium as current complication following acute myocardial infarction** `CC` `HCC` `A`

EXCLUDES 1   *hemopericardium not specified as current complication following acute myocardial infarction (I31.2)*

I23.1 **Atrial septal defect as current complication following acute myocardial infarction** `CC` `HCC` `A`

EXCLUDES 1   *acquired atrial septal defect not specified as current complication following acute myocardial infarction (I51.0)*

I23.2 **Ventricular septal defect as current complication following acute myocardial infarction** `CC` `HCC` `A`

EXCLUDES 1   *acquired ventricular septal defect not specified as current complication following acute myocardial infarction (I51.0)*

I23.3 **Rupture of cardiac wall without hemopericardium as current complication following acute myocardial infarction** `CC` `HCC` `A`

I23.4 **Rupture of chordae tendineae as current complication following acute myocardial infarction** `MCC` `HCC`

EXCLUDES 1   *rupture of chordae tendineae not specified as current complication following acute myocardial infarction (I51.1)*

I23.5 **Rupture of papillary muscle as current complication following acute myocardial infarction** `MCC` `HCC`

EXCLUDES 1   *rupture of papillary muscle not specified as current complication following acute myocardial infarction (I51.2)*

I23.6 **Thrombosis of atrium, auricular appendage, and ventricle as current complications following acute myocardial infarction** `CC` `HCC` `A`

EXCLUDES 1   *thrombosis of atrium, auricular appendage, and ventricle not specified as current complication following acute myocardial infarction (I51.3)*

I23.7 **Postinfarction angina** `CC` `HCC` `A`

AHA: 2015,2Q,16

TIP: When postinfarction angina occurs with atherosclerotic coronary artery disease, code both I23.7 and I25.118 for atherosclerotic disease with other forms of angina pectoris.

I23.8 **Other current complications following acute myocardial infarction** `CC` `HCC` `A`

☑4ᵗʰ **I24** **Other acute ischemic heart diseases**

EXCLUDES 1   *angina pectoris (I20.-)*

           transient myocardial ischemia in newborn (P29.4)

EXCLUDES 2   ►*non-ischemic myocardial injury (I5A)*◄

I24.0 **Acute coronary thrombosis not resulting in myocardial infarction** `CC` `HCC`

Acute coronary (artery) (vein) embolism not resulting in myocardial infarction

Acute coronary (artery) (vein) occlusion not resulting in myocardial infarction

Acute coronary (artery) (vein) thromboembolism not resulting in myocardial infarction

EXCLUDES 1   *atherosclerotic heart disease (I25.1-)*

AHA: 2013,1Q,24

I24.1 **Dressler's syndrome** `CC` `HCC`

Postmyocardial infarction syndrome

EXCLUDES 1   *postinfarction angina (I23.7)*

DEF: Fever, leukocytosis, chest pain, evidence of pericarditis, pleurisy, and pneumonia occurring days or weeks after a myocardial infarction.

I24.8 **Other forms of acute ischemic heart disease** `CC` `HCC`

EXCLUDES 1   *myocardial infarction due to demand ischemia (I21.A1)*

AHA: 2019,4Q,53; 2017,4Q,13

I24.9 **Acute ischemic heart disease, unspecified** `CC` `HCC`

EXCLUDES 1   *ischemic heart disease (chronic) NOS (I25.9)*

☑ Additional Character Required   √x7ᵗʰ Placeholder   Questionable PDx   Manifestation   Unspecified Dx   `UPD` Unacceptable PDx   `H1`-`H14` HAC   `HCC` CMS-HCC Dx   `HIV` HIV Dx

ICD-10-CM 2022   651

✓4th I25 Chronic ischemic heart disease
Use additional code to identify:
chronic total occlusion of coronary artery (I25.82)
exposure to environmental tobacco smoke (Z77.22)
history of tobacco dependence (Z87.891)
occupational exposure to environmental tobacco smoke (Z57.31)
tobacco dependence (F17.-)
tobacco use (Z72.0)
EXCLUDES 2 ▶non-ischemic myocardial injury (I5A)◀

✓5th I25.1 Atherosclerotic heart disease of native coronary artery
Atherosclerotic cardiovascular disease
Coronary (artery) atheroma
Coronary (artery) atherosclerosis
Coronary (artery) disease
Coronary (artery) sclerosis
Use additional code, if applicable, to identify:
coronary atherosclerosis due to calcified coronary lesion (I25.84)
coronary atherosclerosis due to lipid rich plaque (I25.83)
EXCLUDES 2 atheroembolism (I75.-)
atherosclerosis of coronary artery bypass graft(s) and transplanted heart (I25.7-)

Atheromas

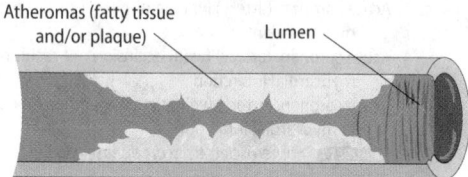

Atheromas (fatty tissue and/or plaque)
Lumen

I25.10 Atherosclerotic heart disease of native coronary artery without angina pectoris A
Atherosclerotic heart disease NOS
AHA: 2015,2Q,16; 2012,4Q,92

✓6th I25.11 Atherosclerotic heart disease of native coronary artery with angina pectoris

I25.110 Atherosclerotic heart disease of native coronary artery with unstable angina pectoris CC HCC A
EXCLUDES 1 unstable angina without atherosclerotic heart disease (I20.0)

I25.111 Atherosclerotic heart disease of native coronary artery with angina pectoris with documented spasm HCC A
EXCLUDES 1 angina pectoris with documented spasm without atherosclerotic heart disease (I20.1)

I25.118 Atherosclerotic heart disease of native coronary artery with other forms of angina pectoris HCC A
EXCLUDES 1 other forms of angina pectoris without atherosclerotic heart disease (I20.8)
AHA: 2015,2Q,16
TIP: When postinfarction angina occurs with atherosclerotic coronary artery disease, code both I23.7 and I25.118 for atherosclerotic disease with other forms of angina pectoris.

I25.119 Atherosclerotic heart disease of native coronary artery with unspecified angina pectoris HCC A
Atherosclerotic heart disease with angina NOS
Atherosclerotic heart disease with ischemic chest pain
EXCLUDES 1 unspecified angina pectoris without atherosclerotic heart disease (I20.9)

I25.2 Old myocardial infarction
Healed myocardial infarction
Past myocardial infarction diagnosed by ECG or other investigation, but currently presenting no symptoms

I25.3 Aneurysm of heart CC
Mural aneurysm
Ventricular aneurysm

✓5th I25.4 Coronary artery aneurysm and dissection

I25.41 Coronary artery aneurysm
Coronary arteriovenous fistula, acquired
EXCLUDES 1 congenital coronary (artery) aneurysm (Q24.5)

I25.42 Coronary artery dissection MCC
DEF: Tear in the intimal arterial wall of a coronary artery resulting in the sudden intrusion of blood within the layers of the wall.

I25.5 Ischemic cardiomyopathy
EXCLUDES 2 coronary atherosclerosis (I25.1-, I25.7-)

I25.6 Silent myocardial ischemia

✓5th I25.7 Atherosclerosis of coronary artery bypass graft(s) and coronary artery of transplanted heart with angina pectoris
Use additional code, if applicable, to identify:
coronary atherosclerosis due to calcified coronary lesion (I25.84)
coronary atherosclerosis due to lipid rich plaque (I25.83)
EXCLUDES 1 atherosclerosis of bypass graft(s) of transplanted heart without angina pectoris (I25.812)
atherosclerosis of coronary artery bypass graft(s) without angina pectoris (I25.810)
atherosclerosis of native coronary artery of transplanted heart without angina pectoris (I25.811)

✓6th I25.70 Atherosclerosis of coronary artery bypass graft(s), unspecified, with angina pectoris

I25.700 Atherosclerosis of coronary artery bypass graft(s), unspecified, with unstable angina pectoris CC HCC A
EXCLUDES 1 unstable angina pectoris without atherosclerosis of coronary artery bypass graft (I20.0)

I25.701 Atherosclerosis of coronary artery bypass graft(s), unspecified, with angina pectoris with documented spasm HCC A
EXCLUDES 1 angina pectoris with documented spasm without atherosclerosis of coronary artery bypass graft (I20.1)

I25.708 Atherosclerosis of coronary artery bypass graft(s), unspecified, with other forms of angina pectoris HCC A
EXCLUDES 1 other forms of angina pectoris without atherosclerosis of coronary artery bypass graft (I20.8)

I25.709 Atherosclerosis of coronary artery bypass graft(s), unspecified, with unspecified angina pectoris HCC A
EXCLUDES 1 unspecified angina pectoris without atherosclerosis of coronary artery bypass graft (I20.9)

✓6th I25.71 Atherosclerosis of autologous vein coronary artery bypass graft(s) with angina pectoris

I25.710 Atherosclerosis of autologous vein coronary artery bypass graft(s) with unstable angina pectoris CC HCC A
EXCLUDES 1 unstable angina without atherosclerosis of autologous vein coronary artery bypass graft(s) (I20.0)
EXCLUDES 2 embolism or thrombus of coronary artery bypass graft(s) (T82.8-)

I25.711　**Atherosclerosis of autologous vein coronary artery bypass graft(s) with angina pectoris with** documented spasm　`CC` `HCC` `A`
> **EXCLUDES 1**　*angina pectoris with documented spasm without atherosclerosis of autologous vein coronary artery bypass graft(s) (I20.1)*

I25.718　**Atherosclerosis of autologous vein coronary artery bypass graft(s) with other forms of angina pectoris**　`CC` `HCC` `A`
> **EXCLUDES 1**　*other forms of angina pectoris without atherosclerosis of autologous vein coronary artery bypass graft(s) (I20.8)*

I25.719　**Atherosclerosis of autologous vein coronary artery bypass graft(s) with unspecified angina pectoris**　`CC` `HCC` `A`
> **EXCLUDES 1**　*unspecified angina pectoris without atherosclerosis of autologous vein coronary artery bypass graft(s) (I20.9)*

✓6ᵗʰ　I25.72　**Atherosclerosis of** autologous artery **coronary artery bypass graft(s) with angina pectoris**
　　Atherosclerosis of internal mammary artery graft with angina pectoris

I25.720　**Atherosclerosis of autologous artery coronary artery bypass graft(s) with** unstable **angina pectoris**　`CC` `HCC` `A`
> **EXCLUDES 1**　*unstable angina without atherosclerosis of autologous artery coronary artery bypass graft(s) (I20.0)*

I25.721　**Atherosclerosis of autologous artery coronary artery bypass graft(s) with angina pectoris with** documented spasm　`CC` `HCC` `A`
> **EXCLUDES 1**　*angina pectoris with documented spasm without atherosclerosis of autologous artery coronary artery bypass graft(s) (I20.1)*

I25.728　**Atherosclerosis of autologous artery coronary artery bypass graft(s) with other forms of angina pectoris**　`CC` `HCC` `A`
> **EXCLUDES 1**　*other forms of angina pectoris without atherosclerosis of autologous artery coronary artery bypass graft(s) (I20.8)*

I25.729　**Atherosclerosis of autologous artery coronary artery bypass graft(s) with unspecified angina pectoris**　`CC` `HCC` `A`
> **EXCLUDES 1**　*unspecified angina pectoris without atherosclerosis of autologous artery coronary artery bypass graft(s) (I20.9)*

✓6ᵗʰ　I25.73　**Atherosclerosis of** nonautologous biological **coronary artery bypass graft(s) with angina pectoris**

I25.730　**Atherosclerosis of nonautologous biological coronary artery bypass graft(s) with** unstable **angina pectoris**　`CC` `HCC` `A`
> **EXCLUDES 1**　*unstable angina without atherosclerosis of nonautologous biological coronary artery bypass graft(s) (I20.0)*

I25.731　**Atherosclerosis of nonautologous biological coronary artery bypass graft(s) with angina pectoris with** documented spasm　`CC` `HCC` `A`
> **EXCLUDES 1**　*angina pectoris with documented spasm without atherosclerosis of nonautologous biological coronary artery bypass graft(s) (I20.1)*

I25.738　**Atherosclerosis of nonautologous biological coronary artery bypass graft(s) with other forms of angina pectoris**　`CC` `HCC` `A`
> **EXCLUDES 1**　*other forms of angina pectoris without atherosclerosis of nonautologous biological coronary artery bypass graft(s) (I20.8)*

I25.739　**Atherosclerosis of nonautologous biological coronary artery bypass graft(s) with unspecified angina pectoris**　`CC` `HCC` `A`
> **EXCLUDES 1**　*unspecified angina pectoris without atherosclerosis of nonautologous biological coronary artery bypass graft(s) (I20.9)*

✓6ᵗʰ　I25.75　**Atherosclerosis of** native **coronary artery of** transplanted heart **with angina pectoris**
> **EXCLUDES 1**　*atherosclerosis of native coronary artery of transplanted heart without angina pectoris (I25.811)*

I25.750　**Atherosclerosis of native coronary artery of transplanted heart with** unstable **angina**　`CC` `HCC`

I25.751　**Atherosclerosis of native coronary artery of transplanted heart with angina pectoris with** documented spasm　`CC` `HCC`

I25.758　**Atherosclerosis of native coronary artery of transplanted heart with other forms of angina pectoris**　`CC` `HCC`

I25.759　**Atherosclerosis of native coronary artery of transplanted heart with unspecified angina pectoris**　`CC` `HCC`

✓6ᵗʰ　I25.76　**Atherosclerosis of** bypass graft **of coronary artery of** transplanted heart **with angina pectoris**
> **EXCLUDES 1**　*atherosclerosis of bypass graft of coronary artery of transplanted heart without angina pectoris (I25.812)*

I25.760　**Atherosclerosis of bypass graft of coronary artery of transplanted heart with** unstable **angina**　`CC` `HCC` `A`

I25.761　**Atherosclerosis of bypass graft of coronary artery of transplanted heart with angina pectoris with** documented spasm　`CC` `HCC` `A`

I25.768　**Atherosclerosis of bypass graft of coronary artery of transplanted heart with other forms of angina pectoris**　`CC` `HCC` `A`

I25.769　**Atherosclerosis of bypass graft of coronary artery of transplanted heart with unspecified angina pectoris**　`CC` `HCC` `A`

✓6ᵗʰ　I25.79　**Atherosclerosis of other coronary artery bypass graft(s) with angina pectoris**

I25.790　**Atherosclerosis of other coronary artery bypass graft(s) with** unstable **angina pectoris**　`CC` `HCC` `A`
> **EXCLUDES 1**　*unstable angina without atherosclerosis of other coronary artery bypass graft(s) (I20.0)*

✓ Additional Character Required　✓x7ᵗʰ Placeholder　Questionable PDx　Manifestation　Unspecified Dx　`UPD` Unacceptable PDx　`H1`-`H14` HAC　`HCC` CMS-HCC Dx　`HIV` HIV Dx

ICD-10-CM 2022　　　　653

Chapter 9. Diseases of the Circulatory System

I25.791   **Atherosclerosis of other coronary artery bypass graft(s) with angina pectoris with documented spasm**   `CC` `HCC` `A`
> *EXCLUDES 1*   *angina pectoris with documented spasm without atherosclerosis of other coronary artery bypass graft(s) (I20.1)*

I25.798   **Atherosclerosis of other coronary artery bypass graft(s) with other forms of angina pectoris**   `CC` `HCC` `A`
> *EXCLUDES 1*   *other forms of angina pectoris without atherosclerosis of other coronary artery bypass graft(s) (I20.8)*

I25.799   **Atherosclerosis of other coronary artery bypass graft(s) with unspecified angina pectoris**   `CC` `HCC` `A`
> *EXCLUDES 1*   *unspecified angina pectoris without atherosclerosis of other coronary artery bypass graft(s) (I20.9)*

√5th **I25.8**   **Other forms of chronic ischemic heart disease**

√6th **I25.81**   **Atherosclerosis of other coronary vessels without angina pectoris**
Use additional code, if applicable, to identify:
coronary atherosclerosis due to calcified coronary lesion (I25.84)
coronary atherosclerosis due to lipid rich plaque (I25.83)
> *EXCLUDES 2*   *atherosclerotic heart disease of native coronary artery without angina pectoris (I25.10)*

I25.810   **Atherosclerosis of coronary artery bypass graft(s) without angina pectoris**   `CC` `A`
Atherosclerosis of coronary artery bypass graft NOS
> *EXCLUDES 1*   *atherosclerosis of coronary bypass graft(s) with angina pectoris (I25.70-I25.73-, I25.79-)*

I25.811   **Atherosclerosis of native coronary artery of transplanted heart without angina pectoris**   `CC`
Atherosclerosis of native coronary artery of transplanted heart NOS
> *EXCLUDES 1*   *atherosclerosis of native coronary artery of transplanted heart with angina pectoris (I25.75-)*

I25.812   **Atherosclerosis of bypass graft of coronary artery of transplanted heart without angina pectoris**   `CC` `A`
Atherosclerosis of bypass graft of transplanted heart NOS
> *EXCLUDES 1*   *atherosclerosis of bypass graft of transplanted heart with angina pectoris (I25.76)*

I25.82   **Chronic total occlusion of coronary artery**   `UPD`
Complete occlusion of coronary artery
Total occlusion of coronary artery
Code first coronary atherosclerosis (I25.1-, I25.7-, I25.81-)
> *EXCLUDES 1*   *acute coronary occlusion with myocardial infarction (I21.0-I21.9, I22.-)*
> *acute coronary occlusion without myocardial infarction (I24.0)*

AHA: 2018,3Q,5
DEF: Complete blockage of the coronary artery due to plaque accumulation over an extended period of time, resulting in substantial reduction of blood flow. Symptoms include angina or chest pain.
TIP: Report this code in addition to a code from category I21 or I22 when the chronic total occlusion and the myocardial infarction are documented as being in different vessels.

I25.83   **Coronary atherosclerosis due to lipid rich plaque**   `UPD` `A`
Code first coronary atherosclerosis (I25.1-, I25.7-, I25.81-)

I25.84   **Coronary atherosclerosis due to calcified coronary lesion**   `UPD`
Coronary atherosclerosis due to severely calcified coronary lesion
Code first coronary atherosclerosis (I25.1-, I25.7-, I25.81-)

I25.89   **Other forms of chronic ischemic heart disease**

I25.9   **Chronic ischemic heart disease, unspecified**
Ischemic heart disease (chronic) NOS

Pulmonary heart disease and diseases of pulmonary circulation (I26-I28)

√4th **I26**   **Pulmonary embolism**
> *INCLUDES*   pulmonary (acute)(artery)(vein) infarction
> pulmonary (acute) (artery)(vein) thromboembolism
> pulmonary (acute)(artery)(vein) thrombosis
> *EXCLUDES 2*   *chronic pulmonary embolism (I27.82)*
> *personal history of pulmonary embolism (Z86.711)*
> *pulmonary embolism complicating abortion, ectopic or molar pregnancy (O00-O07, O08.2)*
> *pulmonary embolism complicating pregnancy, childbirth and the puerperium (O88.-)*
> *pulmonary embolism due to trauma (T79.0, T79.1)*
> *pulmonary embolism due to complications of surgical and medical care (T80.0, T81.7-, T82.8-)*
> *septic (non-pulmonary) arterial embolism (I76)*

√5th **I26.0**   **Pulmonary embolism with acute cor pulmonale**
DEF: Cor pulmonale: Heart-lung disease appearing in identifiable forms as chronic or acute. The chronic form of this heart-lung disease is marked by dilation, hypertrophy and failure of the right ventricle due to a disease that has affected the function of the lungs, excluding congenital or left heart diseases and is also called chronic cardiopulmonary disease. The acute form is an overload of the right ventricle from a rapid onset of pulmonary hypertension, usually arising from a pulmonary embolism.

I26.01   **Septic pulmonary embolism with acute cor pulmonale**   `MCC` `UPD` `HCC`
Code first underlying infection

I26.02   **Saddle embolus of pulmonary artery with acute cor pulmonale**   `MCC` `H10` `HCC`

I26.09   **Other pulmonary embolism with acute cor pulmonale**   `MCC` `H10` `HCC`
Acute cor pulmonale NOS
AHA: 2014,4Q,21

√5th **I26.9**   **Pulmonary embolism without acute cor pulmonale**

I26.90   **Septic pulmonary embolism without acute cor pulmonale**   `MCC` `UPD` `HCC`
Code first underlying infection

I26.92   **Saddle embolus of pulmonary artery without acute cor pulmonale**   `MCC` `H10` `HCC`

I26.93   **Single subsegmental pulmonary embolism without acute cor pulmonale**   `MCC` `H10` `HCC`
Subsegmental pulmonary embolism NOS
AHA: 2021,2Q,9; 2019,4Q,6-7

I26.94   **Multiple subsegmental pulmonary emboli without acute cor pulmonale**   `MCC` `H10` `HCC`
AHA: 2021,2Q,9; 2019,4Q,6-7

I26.99   **Other pulmonary embolism without acute cor pulmonale**   `MCC` `H10` `HCC`
Acute pulmonary embolism NOS
Pulmonary embolism NOS
AHA: 2020,3Q,10-11; 2019,2Q,22

`N` Newborn: 0   `P` Pediatric: 0-17   `M` Maternity: 9-64   `A` Adult: 15-124   `MCC` Major Complication/Comorbidity   `CC` Complication/Comorbidity   `SW` Severe Wound Dx

654

ICD-10-CM 2022

I25.791–I26.99

✓4th I27 Other pulmonary heart diseases

I27.0 Primary pulmonary hypertension [CC] [HCC]
Heritable pulmonary arterial hypertension
Idiopathic pulmonary arterial hypertension
Primary group 1 pulmonary hypertension
Primary pulmonary arterial hypertension
> **EXCLUDES 1** persistent pulmonary hypertension of newborn
> (P29.30)
> pulmonary hypertension NOS (I27.20)
> secondary pulmonary arterial hypertension (I27.21)
> secondary pulmonary hypertension (I27.29)

DEF: Condition that occurs when pressure within the pulmonary artery is elevated and vascular resistance is observed in the lungs.

I27.1 Kyphoscoliotic heart disease [CC] [HCC]

✓5th I27.2 Other secondary pulmonary hypertension
Code also associated underlying condition
> **EXCLUDES 1** Eisenmenger's syndrome (I27.83)

AHA: 2017,4Q,14-15; 2014,4Q,21
DEF: Condition that occurs when pressure within the pulmonary artery is elevated and vascular resistance is observed in the lungs.

I27.20 Pulmonary hypertension, unspecified [HCC]
Pulmonary hypertension NOS

I27.21 Secondary pulmonary arterial hypertension [HCC]
(Associated) (drug-induced) (toxin-induced) pulmonary arterial hypertension NOS
(Associated) (drug-induced) (toxin-induced) (secondary) group 1 pulmonary hypertension
Code also associated conditions if applicable, or adverse effects of drugs or toxins, such as:
> adverse effect of appetite depressants (T50.5X5)
> congenital heart disease (Q20-Q28)
> human immunodeficiency virus [HIV] disease (B20)
> polymyositis (M33.2-)
> portal hypertension (K76.6)
> rheumatoid arthritis (M05.-)
> schistosomiasis (B65.-)
> Sjögren syndrome (M35.0-)
> systemic sclerosis (M34.-)

I27.22 Pulmonary hypertension due to left heart disease [HCC]
Group 2 pulmonary hypertension
Code also associated left heart disease, if known, such as:
> multiple valve disease (I08.-)
> rheumatic aortic valve diseases (I06.-)
> rheumatic mitral valve diseases (I05.-)

I27.23 Pulmonary hypertension due to lung diseases and hypoxia [HCC]
Group 3 pulmonary hypertension
Code also associated lung disease, if known, such as:
> bronchiectasis (J47.-)
> cystic fibrosis with pulmonary manifestations (E84.0)
> interstitial lung disease (J84.-)
> pleural effusion (J90)
> sleep apnea (G47.3-)

I27.24 Chronic thromboembolic pulmonary hypertension [HCC]
Group 4 pulmonary hypertension
Code also associated pulmonary embolism, if applicable (I26.-, I27.82)

I27.29 Other secondary pulmonary hypertension [HCC]
Group 5 pulmonary hypertension
Pulmonary hypertension with unclear multifactorial mechanisms
Pulmonary hypertension due to hematologic disorders
Pulmonary hypertension due to metabolic disorders
Pulmonary hypertension due to other systemic disorders
Code also other associated disorders, if known, such as:
> chronic myeloid leukemia (C92.10-C92.22)
> essential thrombocythemia (D47.3)
> Gaucher disease (E75.22)
> hypertensive chronic kidney disease with end stage renal disease (I12.0, I13.11, I13.2)
> hyperthyroidism (E05.-)
> hypothyroidism (E00-E03)
> polycythemia vera (D45)
> sarcoidosis (D86.-)

AHA: 2016,2Q,8

✓5th I27.8 Other specified pulmonary heart diseases

I27.81 Cor pulmonale (chronic) [HCC]
Cor pulmonale NOS
> **EXCLUDES 1** acute cor pulmonale (I26.0-)

AHA: 2014,4Q,21
DEF: Heart-lung disease appearing in identifiable forms as chronic or acute. The chronic form of this heart-lung disease is marked by dilation, hypertrophy and failure of the right ventricle due to a disease that has affected the function of the lungs, excluding congenital or left heart diseases and is also called chronic cardiopulmonary disease. The acute form is an overload of the right ventricle from a rapid onset of pulmonary hypertension, usually arising from a pulmonary embolism.

I27.82 Chronic pulmonary embolism [CC] [HCC]
Use additional code, if applicable, for associated long-term (current) use of anticoagulants (Z79.01)
> **EXCLUDES 1** personal history of pulmonary embolism (Z86.711)

AHA: 2021,2Q,9
DEF: Long-standing condition commonly associated with pulmonary hypertension in which small blood clots travel to the lungs repeatedly over many weeks, months, or years, requiring continuation of established anticoagulant or thrombolytic therapy.

I27.83 Eisenmenger's syndrome [HCC]
Eisenmenger's complex
(Irreversible) Eisenmenger's disease
Pulmonary hypertension with right to left shunt related to congenital heart disease
Code also underlying heart defect, if known, such as:
> atrial septal defect (Q21.1)
> Eisenmenger's defect (Q21.8)
> patent ductus arteriosus (Q25.0)
> ventricular septal defect (Q21.0)

DEF: Pulmonary hypertension with congenital communication between two circulations resulting in a right to left shunt. This causes reduced oxygen saturation in the arterial blood, leading to cyanosis and organ damage. Once it develops, this life-threating condition is irreversible.

I27.89 Other specified pulmonary heart diseases [HCC]

I27.9 Pulmonary heart disease, unspecified [HCC]
Chronic cardiopulmonary disease

✓4th I28 Other diseases of pulmonary vessels

I28.0 Arteriovenous fistula of pulmonary vessels [CC] [HCC]
> **EXCLUDES 1** congenital arteriovenous fistula (Q25.72)

I28.1 Aneurysm of pulmonary artery [CC] [HCC]
> **EXCLUDES 1** congenital aneurysm (Q25.79)
> congenital arteriovenous aneurysm (Q25.72)

I28.8 Other diseases of pulmonary vessels [HCC]
Pulmonary arteritis
Pulmonary endarteritis
Rupture of pulmonary vessels
Stenosis of pulmonary vessels
Stricture of pulmonary vessels

I28.9 Disease of pulmonary vessels, unspecified [HCC]

Other forms of heart disease ▶(I30-I5A)◀

✓4ᵗʰ **I30 Acute pericarditis**
   INCLUDES   acute mediastinopericarditis
          acute myopericarditis
          acute pericardial effusion
          acute pleuropericarditis
          acute pneumopericarditis
   EXCLUDES 1   *Dressler's syndrome (I24.1)*
          rheumatic pericarditis (acute) (I01.0)
          viral pericarditis due to Coxsakie virus (B33.23)
   DEF: Pericarditis: Inflammation affecting the pericardium, the fibroserous membrane that surrounds the heart.

I30.0 Acute nonspecific idiopathic pericarditis [CC]

I30.1 Infective pericarditis [CC]
Pneumococcal pericarditis
Pneumopyopericardium
Purulent pericarditis
Pyopericarditis
Pyopericardium
Pyopneumopericardium
Staphylococcal pericarditis
Streptococcal pericarditis
Suppurative pericarditis
Viral pericarditis
Use additional code (B95-B97) to identify infectious agent

I30.8 Other forms of acute pericarditis [CC]

I30.9 Acute pericarditis, unspecified [CC]

✓4ᵗʰ **I31 Other diseases of pericardium**
   EXCLUDES 1   *diseases of pericardium specified as rheumatic (I09.2)*
          postcardiotomy syndrome (I97.0)
          traumatic injury to pericardium (S26.-)

I31.0 Chronic adhesive pericarditis [CC]
Accretio cordis
Adherent pericardium
Adhesive mediastinopericarditis

I31.1 Chronic constrictive pericarditis [CC]
Concretio cordis
Pericardial calcification

I31.2 Hemopericardium, not elsewhere classified [CC]
   EXCLUDES 1   *hemopericardium as current complication following acute myocardial infarction (I23.0)*
   DEF: Presence of blood in the pericardial sac (pericardium). It can lead to potentially fatal cardiac tamponade if enough blood enters the pericardial cavity.

I31.3 Pericardial effusion (noninflammatory) [CC]
Chylopericardium
   EXCLUDES 1   *acute pericardial effusion (I30.9)*
   AHA: 2019,1Q,16
   TIP: Assign this code for documented malignant pericardial effusion. If the sole reason for admission is to treat the effusion with no treatment rendered for the associated malignancy, this code may be sequenced first.

I31.4 Cardiac tamponade [CC] [UPD]
Code first underlying cause
   DEF: Life-threatening condition in which fluid or blood accumulates in the space between the muscle of the heart (myocardium) and the outer sac that covers the heart (pericardium), resulting in compression of the heart.

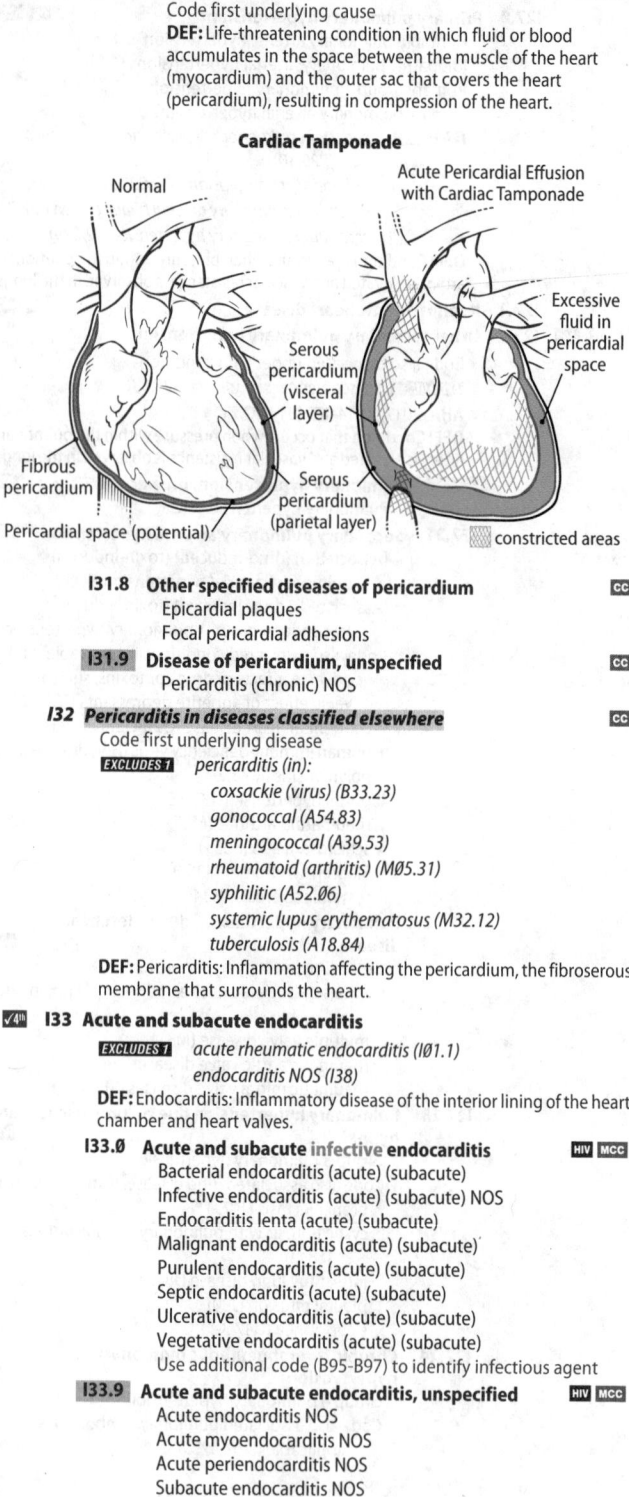

Cardiac Tamponade

Normal — Acute Pericardial Effusion with Cardiac Tamponade — Serous pericardium (visceral layer) — Excessive fluid in pericardial space — Fibrous pericardium — Serous pericardium (parietal layer) — Pericardial space (potential) — ▨ constricted areas

I31.8 Other specified diseases of pericardium [CC]
Epicardial plaques
Focal pericardial adhesions

I31.9 Disease of pericardium, unspecified [CC]
Pericarditis (chronic) NOS

I32 Pericarditis in diseases classified elsewhere [CC]
Code first underlying disease
   EXCLUDES 1   *pericarditis (in):*
          coxsackie (virus) (B33.23)
          gonococcal (A54.83)
          meningococcal (A39.53)
          rheumatoid (arthritis) (M05.31)
          syphilitic (A52.06)
          systemic lupus erythematosus (M32.12)
          tuberculosis (A18.84)
   DEF: Pericarditis: Inflammation affecting the pericardium, the fibroserous membrane that surrounds the heart.

✓4ᵗʰ **I33 Acute and subacute endocarditis**
   EXCLUDES 1   *acute rheumatic endocarditis (I01.1)*
          endocarditis NOS (I38)
   DEF: Endocarditis: Inflammatory disease of the interior lining of the heart chamber and heart valves.

I33.0 Acute and subacute infective endocarditis [HIV] [MCC]
Bacterial endocarditis (acute) (subacute)
Infective endocarditis (acute) (subacute) NOS
Endocarditis lenta (acute) (subacute)
Malignant endocarditis (acute) (subacute)
Purulent endocarditis (acute) (subacute)
Septic endocarditis (acute) (subacute)
Ulcerative endocarditis (acute) (subacute)
Vegetative endocarditis (acute) (subacute)
Use additional code (B95-B97) to identify infectious agent

I33.9 Acute and subacute endocarditis, unspecified [HIV] [MCC]
Acute endocarditis NOS
Acute myoendocarditis NOS
Acute periendocarditis NOS
Subacute endocarditis NOS
Subacute myoendocarditis NOS
Subacute periendocarditis NOS

✓4ᵗʰ **I34 Nonrheumatic mitral valve disorders**

> **EXCLUDES 1**   mitral valve disease (I05.9)
> mitral valve failure (I05.8)
> mitral valve stenosis (I05.0)
> mitral valve disorder of unspecified cause with diseases of aortic and/or tricuspid valve(s) (I08.-)
> mitral valve disorder of unspecified cause with mitral stenosis or obstruction (I05.0)
> mitral valve disorder specified as congenital (Q23.2, Q23.9)
> mitral valve disorder specified as rheumatic (I05.-)

I34.0 Nonrheumatic mitral (valve) insufficiency
Nonrheumatic mitral (valve) incompetence NOS
Nonrheumatic mitral (valve) regurgitation NOS

I34.1 Nonrheumatic mitral (valve) prolapse
Floppy nonrheumatic mitral valve syndrome
> **EXCLUDES 1**   Marfan's syndrome (Q87.4-)

I34.2 Nonrheumatic mitral (valve) stenosis

I34.8 Other nonrheumatic mitral valve disorders

I34.9 Nonrheumatic mitral valve disorder, unspecified

✓4ᵗʰ **I35 Nonrheumatic aortic valve disorders**

> **EXCLUDES 1**   aortic valve disorder of unspecified cause but with diseases of mitral and/or tricuspid valve(s) (I08.-)
> aortic valve disorder specified as congenital (Q23.0, Q23.1)
> aortic valve disorder specified as rheumatic (I06.-)
> hypertrophic subaortic stenosis (I42.1)

I35.0 Nonrheumatic aortic (valve) stenosis

I35.1 Nonrheumatic aortic (valve) insufficiency
Nonrheumatic aortic (valve) incompetence NOS
Nonrheumatic aortic (valve) regurgitation NOS

I35.2 Nonrheumatic aortic (valve) stenosis with insufficiency

I35.8 Other nonrheumatic aortic valve disorders

I35.9 Nonrheumatic aortic valve disorder, unspecified

✓4ᵗʰ **I36 Nonrheumatic tricuspid valve disorders**

> **EXCLUDES 1**   tricuspid valve disorders of unspecified cause (I07.-)
> tricuspid valve disorders specified as congenital (Q22.4, Q22.8, Q22.9)
> tricuspid valve disorders specified as rheumatic (I07.-)
> tricuspid valve disorders with aortic and/or mitral valve involvement (I08.-)

I36.0 Nonrheumatic tricuspid (valve) stenosis

I36.1 Nonrheumatic tricuspid (valve) insufficiency
Nonrheumatic tricuspid (valve) incompetence
Nonrheumatic tricuspid (valve) regurgitation

I36.2 Nonrheumatic tricuspid (valve) stenosis with insufficiency

I36.8 Other nonrheumatic tricuspid valve disorders

I36.9 Nonrheumatic tricuspid valve disorder, unspecified

✓4ᵗʰ **I37 Nonrheumatic pulmonary valve disorders**

> **EXCLUDES 1**   pulmonary valve disorder specified as congenital (Q22.1, Q22.2, Q22.3)
> pulmonary valve disorder specified as rheumatic (I09.89)

I37.0 Nonrheumatic pulmonary valve stenosis

I37.1 Nonrheumatic pulmonary valve insufficiency
Nonrheumatic pulmonary valve incompetence
Nonrheumatic pulmonary valve regurgitation

I37.2 Nonrheumatic pulmonary valve stenosis with insufficiency

I37.8 Other nonrheumatic pulmonary valve disorders

I37.9 Nonrheumatic pulmonary valve disorder, unspecified

I38 Endocarditis, valve unspecified   **CC**

> **INCLUDES**   endocarditis (chronic) NOS
> valvular incompetence NOS
> valvular insufficiency NOS
> valvular regurgitation NOS
> valvular stenosis NOS
> valvulitis (chronic) NOS

> **EXCLUDES 1**   congenital insufficiency of cardiac valve NOS (Q24.8)
> congenital stenosis of cardiac valve NOS (Q24.8)
> endocardial fibroelastosis (I42.4)
> endocarditis specified as rheumatic (I09.1)

DEF: Endocarditis: Inflammatory disease of the interior lining of the heart chamber and heart valves.

I39 Endocarditis and heart valve disorders in diseases classified elsewhere   **CC**

Code first underlying disease, such as:
Q fever (A78)

> **EXCLUDES 1**   endocardial involvement in:
> candidiasis (B37.6)
> gonococcal infection (A54.83)
> Libman-Sacks disease (M32.11)
> listerosis (A32.82)
> meningococcal infection (A39.51)
> rheumatoid arthritis (M05.31)
> syphilis (A52.03)
> tuberculosis (A18.84)
> typhoid fever (A01.02)

DEF: Endocarditis: Inflammatory disease of the interior lining of the heart chamber and heart valves.

✓4ᵗʰ **I40 Acute myocarditis**

> **INCLUDES**   subacute myocarditis
> **EXCLUDES 1**   acute rheumatic myocarditis (I01.2)

DEF: Myocarditis: Inflammation of the middle layer of the heart, which is composed of muscle tissue.

I40.0 Infective myocarditis   **HIV** **MCC**
Septic myocarditis
Use additional code (B95-B97) to identify infectious agent

I40.1 Isolated myocarditis   **HIV** **MCC**
Fiedler's myocarditis
Giant cell myocarditis
Idiopathic myocarditis

I40.8 Other acute myocarditis   **HIV** **MCC**

I40.9 Acute myocarditis, unspecified   **HIV** **MCC**

I41 Myocarditis in diseases classified elsewhere   **MCC**

Code first underlying disease, such as:
typhus (A75.0-A75.9)

> **EXCLUDES 1**   myocarditis (in):
> Chagas' disease (chronic) (B57.2)
> acute (B57.0)
> coxsackie (virus) infection (B33.22)
> diphtheritic (A36.81)
> gonococcal (A54.83)
> influenzal (J09.X9, J10.82, J11.82)
> meningococcal (A39.52)
> mumps (B26.82)
> rheumatoid arthritis (M05.31)
> sarcoid (D86.85)
> syphilis (A52.06)
> toxoplasmosis (B58.81)
> tuberculous (A18.84)

DEF: Myocarditis: Inflammation of the middle layer of the heart, which is composed of muscle tissue.

✓4ᵗʰ **I42 Cardiomyopathy**

> **INCLUDES**   myocardiopathy

Code first pre-existing cardiomyopathy complicating pregnancy and puerperium (O99.4)

> **EXCLUDES 2**   ischemic cardiomyopathy (I25.5)
> peripartum cardiomyopathy (O90.3)
> ventricular hypertrophy (I51.7)

I42.0 Dilated cardiomyopathy   **CC** **HCC**
Congestive cardiomyopathy

I42.1 Obstructive hypertrophic cardiomyopathy   **CC** **HCC**
Hypertrophic subaortic stenosis (idiopathic)
DEF: Cardiomyopathy marked by left ventricle hypertrophy and an enlarged septum that result in obstructed blood flow, arrhythmias, mitral regurgitation, and sudden cardiac death.
TIP: When this condition is described as inherited, assign code Q24.8.

I42.2 Other hypertrophic cardiomyopathy   **CC** **HCC**
Nonobstructive hypertrophic cardiomyopathy

I42.3 Endomyocardial (eosinophilic) disease   **CC** **HCC**
Endomyocardial (tropical) fibrosis
Löffler's endocarditis

I42.4 Endocardial fibroelastosis   **CC** **HCC**
Congenital cardiomyopathy
Elastomyofibrosis

✓ Additional Character Required   ✓x7ᵗʰ Placeholder   Questionable PDx   Manifestation   Unspecified Dx   **UPD** Unacceptable PDx   **H1**-**H14** HAC   **HCC** CMS-HCC Dx   **HIV** HIV Dx

ICD-10-CM 2022   657

I42.5 **Other restrictive cardiomyopathy** `CC` `HCC`
　　Constrictive cardiomyopathy NOS

I42.6 **Alcoholic cardiomyopathy** `CC` `HCC`
　　Code also presence of alcoholism (F10.-)

I42.7 **Cardiomyopathy due to drug and external agent** `CC` `HCC`
　　Code first poisoning due to drug or toxin, if applicable (T36-T65 with fifth or sixth character 1-4 or 6)
　　Use additional code for adverse effect, if applicable, to identify drug (T36-T50 with fifth or sixth character 5)

I42.8 **Other cardiomyopathies** `CC` `HCC`

I42.9 **Cardiomyopathy, unspecified** `CC` `HCC`
　　Cardiomyopathy (primary) (secondary) NOS

I43 *Cardiomyopathy in diseases classified elsewhere* `CC` `HCC`
　　Code first underlying disease, such as:
　　　amyloidosis (E85.-)
　　　glycogen storage disease (E74.0)
　　　gout (M10.0-)
　　　thyrotoxicosis (E05.0-E05.9-)
　　　EXCLUDES 1　cardiomyopathy (in):
　　　　　coxsackie (virus) (B33.24)
　　　　　diphtheria (A36.81)
　　　　　sarcoidosis (D86.85)
　　　　　tuberculosis (A18.84)

✓4ᵗʰ **I44 Atrioventricular and left bundle-branch block**

I44.0 **Atrioventricular block, first degree**

I44.1 **Atrioventricular block, second degree**
　　Atrioventricular block, type I and II
　　Möbitz block, type I and II
　　Second degree block, type I and II
　　Wenckebach's block

I44.2 **Atrioventricular block, complete** `CC` `HCC`
　　Complete heart block NOS
　　Third degree block
　　AHA: 2019,2Q,4

✓5ᵗʰ **I44.3** **Other and unspecified atrioventricular block**
　　Atrioventricular block NOS
　　　I44.30 **Unspecified atrioventricular block**
　　　I44.39 **Other atrioventricular block**

I44.4 **Left anterior fascicular block**

I44.5 **Left posterior fascicular block**

✓5ᵗʰ **I44.6** **Other and unspecified fascicular block**
　　　I44.60 **Unspecified fascicular block**
　　　　Left bundle-branch hemiblock NOS
　　　I44.69 **Other fascicular block**

I44.7 **Left bundle-branch block, unspecified**

Conduction Disorders

Sinoatrial node (pacemaker)
Internodal tracts:
　Anterior
　Middle
　Posterior
Atrioventricular node
Atrioventricular bundle (of His)
Atrioventricular block
Accessory bundle (of Kent)
Right bundle branch
Right bundle branch block
Moderator band
Bachmann's bundle
Left bundle branch block
Left bundle branch:
　Anterior fascicle
　Posterior fascicle
Left bundle branch hemiblock
Purkinje fibers

✓4ᵗʰ **I45 Other conduction disorders**

I45.0 **Right fascicular block**

✓5ᵗʰ **I45.1** **Other and unspecified right bundle-branch block**
　　　I45.10 **Unspecified right bundle-branch block**
　　　　Right bundle-branch block NOS
　　　I45.19 **Other right bundle-branch block**

I45.2 **Bifascicular block** `CC`

I45.3 **Trifascicular block** `CC`

I45.4 **Nonspecific intraventricular block**
　　Bundle-branch block NOS

I45.5 **Other specified heart block**
　　Sinoatrial block
　　Sinoauricular block
　　EXCLUDES 1　heart block NOS (I45.9)

I45.6 **Pre-excitation syndrome**
　　Accelerated atrioventricular conduction
　　Accessory atrioventricular conduction
　　Anomalous atrioventricular excitation
　　Lown-Ganong-Levine syndrome
　　Pre-excitation atrioventricular conduction
　　Wolff-Parkinson-White syndrome

✓5ᵗʰ **I45.8** **Other specified conduction disorders**
　　　I45.81 **Long QT syndrome**
　　　　DEF: Condition characterized by recurrent syncope, malignant arrhythmias, and sudden death. This syndrome has a characteristic prolonged Q-T interval on an electrocardiogram.
　　　I45.89 **Other specified conduction disorders** `CC`
　　　　Atrioventricular [AV] dissociation
　　　　Interference dissociation
　　　　Isorhythmic dissociation
　　　　Nonparoxysmal AV nodal tachycardia
　　　　AHA: 2013,2Q,31

I45.9 **Conduction disorder, unspecified**
　　Heart block NOS
　　Stokes-Adams syndrome

✓4ᵗʰ **I46 Cardiac arrest**
　　EXCLUDES 2　cardiogenic shock (R57.0)
　　AHA: 2019,2Q,4-5

I46.2 **Cardiac arrest due to underlying cardiac condition** `MCC` `UPD` `HCC`
　　Code first underlying cardiac condition

I46.8 **Cardiac arrest due to other underlying condition** `MCC` `UPD` `HCC`
　　Code first underlying condition

I46.9 **Cardiac arrest, cause unspecified** `MCC` `HCC`
　　AHA: 2020,3Q,26

✓4ᵗʰ **I47 Paroxysmal tachycardia**
　　Code first tachycardia complicating:
　　　abortion or ectopic or molar pregnancy (O00-O07, O08.8)
　　　obstetric surgery and procedures (O75.4)
　　EXCLUDES 1　tachycardia NOS (R00.0)
　　　　sinoauricular tachycardia NOS (R00.0)
　　　　sinus [sinusal] tachycardia NOS (R00.0)

I47.0 **Re-entry ventricular arrhythmia** `CC` `HCC`

I47.1 **Supraventricular tachycardia** `CC` `HCC`
　　Atrial (paroxysmal) tachycardia
　　Atrioventricular [AV] (paroxysmal) tachycardia
　　Atrioventricular re-entrant (nodal) tachycardia [AVNRT] [AVRT]
　　Junctional (paroxysmal) tachycardia
　　Nodal (paroxysmal) tachycardia

I47.2 **Ventricular tachycardia** `CC` `HCC`
　　AHA: 2013,3Q,23

I47.9 **Paroxysmal tachycardia, unspecified** `HCC`
　　Bouveret (-Hoffman) syndrome

✓4ᵗʰ **I48 Atrial fibrillation and flutter**

I48.0 **Paroxysmal atrial fibrillation** `HCC`
　　AHA: 2021,2Q,8; 2018,3Q,6

✓5ᵗʰ **I48.1** **Persistent atrial fibrillation**
　　EXCLUDES 1　permanent atrial fibrillation (I48.21)
　　AHA: 2021,2Q,8; 2019,4Q,7; 2019,2Q,3; 2018,3Q,6
　　　I48.11 **Longstanding persistent atrial fibrillation** `CC` `HCC`

`N` Newborn: 0　`P` Pediatric: 0-17　`M` Maternity: 9-64　`A` Adult: 15-124　`MCC` Major Complication/Comorbidity　`CC` Complication/Comorbidity　`SW` Severe Wound Dx

658　ICD-10-CM 2022

I48.19   **Other persistent** atrial fibrillation   `CC` `HCC`
Chronic persistent atrial fibrillation
Persistent atrial fibrillation, NOS
AHA: 2019,4Q,7

☑5ᵗʰ **I48.2**   **Chronic atrial fibrillation**
AHA: 2021,2Q,8; 2019,4Q,7; 2019,2Q,3; 2018,3Q,6

I48.20   **Chronic atrial fibrillation, unspecified**   `CC` `HCC`
EXCLUDES 1   *chronic persistent atrial fibrillation (I48.19)*

I48.21   **Permanent** atrial fibrillation   `CC` `HCC`

I48.3   **Typical** atrial flutter   `CC` `HCC`
Type I atrial flutter

I48.4   **Atypical** atrial flutter   `CC` `HCC`
Type II atrial flutter

☑5ᵗʰ **I48.9**   **Unspecified atrial fibrillation and atrial flutter**

I48.91   **Unspecified** atrial **fibrillation**   `HCC`

I48.92   **Unspecified** atrial **flutter**   `CC` `HCC`

☑4ᵗʰ **I49**   **Other cardiac arrhythmias**
Code first cardiac arrhythmia complicating:
   abortion or ectopic or molar pregnancy (O00-O07, O08.8)
   obstetric surgery and procedures (O75.4)
EXCLUDES 1   *neonatal dysrhythmia (P29.1-)*
            sinoatrial bradycardia (R00.1)
            sinus bradycardia (R00.1)
            vagal bradycardia (R00.1)
EXCLUDES 2   *bradycardia NOS (R00.1)*

☑5ᵗʰ **I49.0**   **Ventricular** fibrillation and flutter

I49.01   **Ventricular** fibrillation   `MCC` `HCC`

I49.02   **Ventricular** flutter   `MCC` `HCC`

I49.1   **Atrial premature** depolarization
Atrial premature beats

I49.2   **Junctional premature** depolarization   `CC` `HCC`

I49.3   **Ventricular premature** depolarization
AHA: 2020,2Q,23

☑6ᵗʰ **I49.4**   **Other and unspecified premature depolarization**

I49.40   **Unspecified premature depolarization**
Premature beats NOS

I49.49   **Other premature depolarization**
Ectopic beats
Extrasystoles
Extrasystolic arrhythmias
Premature contractions

I49.5   **Sick sinus syndrome**   `HCC`
Tachycardia-bradycardia syndrome
AHA: 2019,1Q,33
TIP: The presence of a pacemaker controls but does not cure sick sinus syndrome and therefore is considered a reportable chronic condition. When a pacemaker is evaluated by a provider, this code and code Z95.0 Presence of cardiac pacemaker, should be reported, even in the absence of any notable changes or management.

I49.8   **Other specified cardiac arrhythmias**
Brugada syndrome
Coronary sinus rhythm disorder
Ectopic rhythm disorder
Nodal rhythm disorder

I49.9   **Cardiac arrhythmia, unspecified**
Arrhythmia (cardiac) NOS

☑4ᵗʰ **I50**   **Heart failure**
Code first:
   heart failure complicating abortion or ectopic or molar pregnancy
     (O00-O07, O08.8)
   heart failure due to hypertension (I11.0)
   heart failure due to hypertension with chronic kidney disease (I13.-)
   heart failure following surgery (I97.13-)
   obstetric surgery and procedures (O75.4)
   rheumatic heart failure (I09.81)
EXCLUDES 1   ~~*neonatal cardiac failure (P29.0)*~~
EXCLUDES 2   *cardiac arrest (I46.-)*
        ►*neonatal cardiac failure (P29.0)*◄
AHA: 2018,4Q,67; 2018,2Q,9; 2017,1Q,47; 2014,1Q,25; 2013,2Q,33

I50.1   **Left ventricular** failure, unspecified   `CC` `HCC`
Cardiac asthma
Edema of lung with heart disease NOS
Edema of lung with heart failure
Left heart failure
Pulmonary edema with heart disease NOS
Pulmonary edema with heart failure
EXCLUDES 1   *edema of lung without heart disease or heart failure*
            (J81.-)
            pulmonary edema without heart disease or failure
            (J81.-)

☑5ᵗʰ **I50.2**   **Systolic (congestive) heart failure**
Heart failure with reduced ejection fraction [HFrEF]
Systolic left ventricular heart failure
Code also end stage heart failure, if applicable (I50.84)
EXCLUDES 1   *combined systolic (congestive) and diastolic*
            (congestive) heart failure (I50.4-)
AHA: 2020,3Q,32; 2017,1Q,46; 2016,1Q,10

I50.20   **Unspecified systolic (congestive) heart**
            failure   `CC` `HCC`

I50.21   **Acute systolic (congestive) heart failure**   `MCC` `HCC`

I50.22   **Chronic systolic (congestive) heart failure**   `CC` `HCC`

I50.23   **Acute on chronic systolic (congestive) heart**
            failure   `MCC` `HCC`

☑5ᵗʰ **I50.3**   **Diastolic (congestive) heart failure**
Diastolic left ventricular heart failure
Heart failure with normal ejection fraction
Heart failure with preserved ejection fraction [HFpEF]
Code also end stage heart failure, if applicable (I50.84)
EXCLUDES 1   *combined systolic (congestive) and diastolic*
            (congestive) heart failure (I50.4-)
AHA: 2020,3Q,32; 2017,1Q,46; 2016,1Q,10

I50.30   **Unspecified diastolic (congestive) heart**
            failure   `CC` `HCC`

I50.31   **Acute diastolic (congestive) heart**
            failure   `MCC` `HCC`

I50.32   **Chronic diastolic (congestive) heart**
            failure   `CC` `HCC`

I50.33   **Acute on chronic diastolic (congestive) heart**
            failure   `MCC` `HCC`

☑5ᵗʰ **I50.4**   **Combined systolic (congestive) and diastolic (congestive) heart failure**
Combined systolic and diastolic left ventricular heart failure
Heart failure with reduced ejection fraction and diastolic dysfunction
Code also end stage heart failure, if applicable (I50.84)
AHA: 2017,1Q,46; 2016,1Q,10

I50.40   **Unspecified combined systolic (congestive) and**
            diastolic (congestive) heart failure   `CC` `HCC`

I50.41   **Acute combined systolic (congestive) and diastolic**
            (congestive) heart failure   `MCC` `HCC`

I50.42   **Chronic combined systolic (congestive) and diastolic**
            (congestive) heart failure   `CC` `HCC`

I50.43   **Acute on chronic combined systolic (congestive)**
            and diastolic (congestive) heart failure   `MCC` `HCC`

☑5ᵗʰ **I50.8**   **Other heart failure**
AHA: 2017,4Q,15-16

☑6ᵗʰ **I50.81**   **Right heart failure**
Right ventricular failure

I50.810   **Right heart failure, unspecified**   `HCC`
Right heart failure without mention of left
     heart failure
Right ventricular failure NOS

Chapter 9. Diseases of the Circulatory System

I50.811–I5A

I50.811   **Acute right heart failure**   `HCC`
  Acute isolated right heart failure
  Acute (isolated) right ventricular failure

I50.812   **Chronic right heart failure**   `HCC`
  Chronic isolated right heart failure
  Chronic (isolated) right ventricular failure

I50.813   **Acute on chronic right heart failure**   `HCC`
  Acute on chronic isolated right heart failure
  Acute on chronic (isolated) right ventricular failure
  Acute decompensation of chronic (isolated) right ventricular failure
  Acute exacerbation of chronic (isolated) right ventricular failure

I50.814   **Right heart failure due to left heart failure**   `HCC`
  Right ventricular failure secondary to left ventricular failure
  Code also the type of left ventricular failure, if known (I50.2-I50.43)
  EXCLUDES 1   *right heart failure with but not due to left heart failure (I50.82)*

I50.82   **Biventricular heart failure**   `HCC`
  Code also the type of left ventricular failure as systolic, diastolic, or combined, if known (I50.2-I50.43)

I50.83   **High output heart failure**   `HCC`
  DEF: Occurs when the high demand for blood exceeds the capacity of a normally functioning heart to meet the demand.

I50.84   **End stage heart failure**   `HCC`
  Stage D heart failure
  Code also the type of heart failure as systolic, diastolic, or combined, if known (I50.2-I50.43)

I50.89   **Other heart failure**   `HCC`

I50.9   **Heart failure, unspecified**   `HCC`
  Cardiac, heart or myocardial failure NOS
  Congestive heart disease
  Congestive heart failure NOS
  EXCLUDES 2   *fluid overload unrelated to congestive heart failure (E87.70)*
  AHA: 2017,4Q,15-16; 2017,1Q,45-46; 2014,4Q,21; 2012,4Q,92

`√4ᵗʰ` **I51**   **Complications and ill-defined descriptions of heart disease**
  EXCLUDES 1   *any condition in I51.4-I51.9 due to hypertension (I11.-)*
         any condition in I51.4-I51.9 due to hypertension and chronic kidney disease (I13.-)
         heart disease specified as rheumatic (I00-I09)

I51.0   **Cardiac septal defect, acquired**   `CC` `A`
  Acquired septal atrial defect (old)
  Acquired septal auricular defect (old)
  Acquired septal ventricular defect (old)
  EXCLUDES 1   *cardiac septal defect as current complication following acute myocardial infarction (I23.1, I23.2)*
  DEF: Abnormal communication between opposite heart chambers due to a defect of the septum. It is not present at birth.

I51.1   **Rupture of chordae tendineae, not elsewhere classified**   `MCC` `HCC`
  EXCLUDES 1   *rupture of chordae tendineae as current complication following acute myocardial infarction (I23.4)*

I51.2   **Rupture of papillary muscle, not elsewhere classified**   `MCC` `HCC`
  EXCLUDES 1   *rupture of papillary muscle as current complication following acute myocardial infarction (I23.5)*

I51.3   **Intracardiac thrombosis, not elsewhere classified**
  Apical thrombosis (old)
  Atrial thrombosis (old)
  Auricular thrombosis (old)
  Mural thrombosis (old)
  Ventricular thrombosis (old)
  EXCLUDES 1   *intracardiac thrombosis as current complication following acute myocardial infarction (I23.6)*
  AHA: 2013,1Q,24

I51.4   **Myocarditis, unspecified**   `HCC`
  Chronic (interstitial) myocarditis
  Myocardial fibrosis
  Myocarditis NOS
  EXCLUDES 1   *acute or subacute myocarditis (I40.-)*
  AHA: 2018,4Q,67; 2018,2Q,9

I51.5   **Myocardial degeneration**   `HCC`
  Fatty degeneration of heart or myocardium
  Myocardial disease
  Senile degeneration of heart or myocardium
  AHA: 2018,4Q,67; 2018,2Q,9

I51.7   **Cardiomegaly**
  Cardiac dilatation
  Cardiac hypertrophy
  Ventricular dilatation
  AHA: 2018,4Q,67; 2018,2Q,9

`√5ᵗʰ` **I51.8**   **Other ill-defined heart diseases**
  AHA: 2018,2Q,9

I51.81   **Takotsubo syndrome**   `CC`
  Reversible left ventricular dysfunction following sudden emotional stress
  Stress induced cardiomyopathy
  Takotsubo cardiomyopathy
  Transient left ventricular apical ballooning syndrome
  DEF: Complex of symptoms mimicking myocardial infarct in absence of heart disease, with the majority of cases occurring in postmenopausal women. Heart muscles are temporarily weakened, and a sudden, massive surge of adrenalin stuns the heart, greatly reducing the ability to pump blood.

I51.89   **Other ill-defined heart diseases**
  Carditis (acute)(chronic)
  Pancarditis (acute)(chronic)
  AHA: 2019,2Q,5; 2018,4Q,67

I51.9   **Heart disease, unspecified**
  AHA: 2018,4Q,67; 2018,2Q,9

I52   ***Other heart disorders in diseases classified elsewhere***
  Code first underlying disease, such as:
     congenital syphilis (A50.5)
     mucopolysaccharidosis (E76.3)
     schistosomiasis (B65.0-B65.9)
  EXCLUDES 1   *heart disease (in):*
        gonococcal infection (A54.83)
        meningococcal infection (A39.50)
        rheumatoid arthritis (M05.31)
        syphilis (A52.06)

● **I5A**   **Non-ischemic myocardial injury (non-traumatic)**   `CC`
  Acute (non-ischemic) myocardial injury
  Chronic (non-ischemic) myocardial injury
  Unspecified (non-ischemic) myocardial injury
  Code first the underlying cause, if known and applicable, such as:
     acute kidney failure (N17.-)
     acute myocarditis (I40.-)
     cardiomyopathy (I42.-)
     chronic kidney disease (CKD) (N18.-)
     heart failure (I50.-)
     hypertensive urgency (I16.0)
     nonrheumatic aortic valve disorders (I35.-)
     paroxysmal tachycardia (I47.-)
     pulmonary embolism (I26.-)
     pulmonary hypertension (I27.0, I27.2-)
     sepsis (A41.-)
     takotsubo syndrome (I51.81)
  EXCLUDES 1   *acute myocardial infarction (I21.-)*
        injury of heart (S26.-)
  EXCLUDES 2   *other acute ischemic heart diseases (I24.-)*

Cerebrovascular diseases (I60-I69)

Use additional code to identify presence of:
 alcohol abuse and dependence (F10.-)
 exposure to environmental tobacco smoke (Z77.22)
 history of tobacco dependence (Z87.891)
 hypertension (I10-I16)
 occupational exposure to environmental tobacco smoke (Z57.31)
 tobacco dependence (F17.-)
 tobacco use (Z72.0)

EXCLUDES 1   *traumatic intracranial hemorrhage (S06.-)*
AHA: 2014,3Q,5; 2012,4Q,91-92

✓4ᵗʰ   I60   Nontraumatic subarachnoid hemorrhage

EXCLUDES 1   *syphilitic ruptured cerebral aneurysm (A52.05)*
EXCLUDES 2   *sequelae of subarachnoid hemorrhage (I69.0-)*

✓5ᵗʰ   **I60.0**   **Nontraumatic subarachnoid hemorrhage from** carotid siphon and bifurcation

     I60.00   Nontraumatic subarachnoid hemorrhage from unspecified carotid siphon and bifurcation   MCC HCC

     I60.01   Nontraumatic subarachnoid hemorrhage from right carotid siphon and bifurcation   MCC HCC

     I60.02   Nontraumatic subarachnoid hemorrhage from left carotid siphon and bifurcation   MCC HCC

✓5ᵗʰ   **I60.1**   **Nontraumatic subarachnoid hemorrhage from** middle cerebral artery

     I60.10   Nontraumatic subarachnoid hemorrhage from unspecified middle cerebral artery   MCC HCC

     I60.11   Nontraumatic subarachnoid hemorrhage from right middle cerebral artery   MCC HCC

     I60.12   Nontraumatic subarachnoid hemorrhage from left middle cerebral artery   MCC HCC

I60.2   **Nontraumatic subarachnoid hemorrhage from** anterior communicating artery   MCC HCC

✓5ᵗʰ   **I60.3**   **Nontraumatic subarachnoid hemorrhage from** posterior communicating artery

     I60.30   Nontraumatic subarachnoid hemorrhage from unspecified posterior communicating artery   MCC HCC

     I60.31   Nontraumatic subarachnoid hemorrhage from right posterior communicating artery   MCC HCC

     I60.32   Nontraumatic subarachnoid hemorrhage from left posterior communicating artery   MCC HCC

I60.4   **Nontraumatic subarachnoid hemorrhage from** basilar artery   MCC HCC

✓5ᵗʰ   **I60.5**   **Nontraumatic subarachnoid hemorrhage from** vertebral artery

     I60.50   Nontraumatic subarachnoid hemorrhage from unspecified vertebral artery   MCC HCC

     I60.51   Nontraumatic subarachnoid hemorrhage from right vertebral artery   MCC HCC

     I60.52   Nontraumatic subarachnoid hemorrhage from left vertebral artery   MCC HCC

I60.6   **Nontraumatic subarachnoid hemorrhage from other intracranial arteries**   MCC HCC

I60.7   **Nontraumatic subarachnoid hemorrhage from unspecified intracranial artery**   MCC HCC
Ruptured (congenital) berry aneurysm
Ruptured (congenital) cerebral aneurysm
Subarachnoid hemorrhage (nontraumatic) from cerebral artery NOS
Subarachnoid hemorrhage (nontraumatic) from communicating artery NOS

EXCLUDES 1   *berry aneurysm, nonruptured (I67.1)*

I60.8   **Other nontraumatic subarachnoid hemorrhage**   MCC HCC
Meningeal hemorrhage
Rupture of cerebral arteriovenous malformation

I60.9   **Nontraumatic subarachnoid hemorrhage, unspecified**   MCC HCC

✓4ᵗʰ   I61   Nontraumatic intracerebral hemorrhage

EXCLUDES 2   *sequelae of intracerebral hemorrhage (I69.1-)*
AHA: 2017,2Q,9-10

I61.0   **Nontraumatic intracerebral hemorrhage in** hemisphere, subcortical   MCC HCC
Deep intracerebral hemorrhage (nontraumatic)
AHA: 2016,4Q,27

I61.1   **Nontraumatic intracerebral hemorrhage in** hemisphere, cortical   MCC HCC
Cerebral lobe hemorrhage (nontraumatic)
Superficial intracerebral hemorrhage (nontraumatic)

I61.2   **Nontraumatic intracerebral hemorrhage in** hemisphere, unspecified   MCC HCC

I61.3   **Nontraumatic intracerebral hemorrhage in** brain stem   MCC HCC

I61.4   **Nontraumatic intracerebral hemorrhage in** cerebellum   MCC HCC

I61.5   **Nontraumatic intracerebral hemorrhage, intraventricular**   MCC HCC

I61.6   **Nontraumatic intracerebral hemorrhage, multiple localized**   MCC HCC

I61.8   **Other nontraumatic intracerebral hemorrhage**   MCC HCC

I61.9   **Nontraumatic intracerebral hemorrhage, unspecified**   MCC HCC

✓4ᵗʰ   I62   Other and unspecified nontraumatic intracranial hemorrhage

EXCLUDES 2   *sequelae of intracranial hemorrhage (I69.2)*

✓5ᵗʰ   **I62.0**   **Nontraumatic subdural hemorrhage**

     I62.00   Nontraumatic subdural hemorrhage, unspecified   MCC HCC

     I62.01   Nontraumatic acute subdural hemorrhage   MCC HCC

     I62.02   Nontraumatic subacute subdural hemorrhage   MCC HCC

     I62.03   Nontraumatic chronic subdural hemorrhage   MCC HCC

I62.1   **Nontraumatic extradural hemorrhage**   MCC HCC
Nontraumatic epidural hemorrhage

I62.9   **Nontraumatic intracranial hemorrhage, unspecified**   CC HCC

✓4ᵗʰ   I63   Cerebral infarction

INCLUDES   occlusion and stenosis of cerebral and precerebral arteries, resulting in cerebral infarction

Use additional code, if applicable, to identify status post administration of tPA (rtPA) in a different facility within the last 24 hours prior to admission to current facility (Z92.82)

Use additional code, if known, to indicate National Institutes of Health Stroke Scale (NIHSS) score (R29.7-)

EXCLUDES 1   *neonatal cerebral infarction (P91.82-)*
EXCLUDES 2   *sequelae of cerebral infarction (I69.3-)*

AHA: 2017,2Q,9-10; 2016,4Q,28,61-62; 2015,1Q,25; 2014,1Q,23
TIP: Weakness on one side of the body documented as secondary to stroke is synonymous with hemiparesis/hemiplegia (G81.-). Weakness of one limb documented as secondary to stroke is synonymous with monoplegia (G83.1-, G83.2-, G83.3-).

✓5ᵗʰ   **I63.0**   **Cerebral infarction due to** thrombosis of precerebral arteries

     I63.00   Cerebral infarction due to thrombosis of unspecified precerebral artery   MCC HCC

     ✓6ᵗʰ   **I63.01**   Cerebral infarction due to thrombosis of vertebral artery

       I63.011   Cerebral infarction due to thrombosis of right vertebral artery   MCC HCC

       I63.012   Cerebral infarction due to thrombosis of left vertebral artery   MCC HCC

       I63.013   Cerebral infarction due to thrombosis of bilateral vertebral arteries   MCC HCC

       I63.019   Cerebral infarction due to thrombosis of unspecified vertebral artery   MCC HCC

     I63.02   Cerebral infarction due to thrombosis of basilar artery   MCC HCC

     ✓6ᵗʰ   **I63.03**   Cerebral infarction due to thrombosis of carotid artery

       I63.031   Cerebral infarction due to thrombosis of right carotid artery   MCC HCC

       I63.032   Cerebral infarction due to thrombosis of left carotid artery   MCC HCC

       I63.033   Cerebral infarction due to thrombosis of bilateral carotid arteries   MCC HCC

       I63.039   Cerebral infarction due to thrombosis of unspecified carotid artery   MCC HCC

     I63.09   Cerebral infarction due to thrombosis of other precerebral artery   MCC HCC

✓5ᵗʰ   **I63.1**   **Cerebral infarction due to** embolism of precerebral arteries

     I63.10   Cerebral infarction due to embolism of unspecified precerebral artery   MCC HCC

☑ Additional Character Required   ✓x7ᵗʰ Placeholder   Questionable PDx   Manifestation   Unspecified Dx   UPD Unacceptable PDx   H1-H14 HAC   HCC CMS-HCC Dx   HIV HIV Dx

Chapter 9. Diseases of the Circulatory System

I63.11–I63.449

√6ᵗʰ **I63.11** Cerebral infarction due to embolism of vertebral artery

     I63.111 Cerebral infarction due to embolism of right vertebral artery `MCC` `HCC`

     I63.112 Cerebral infarction due to embolism of left vertebral artery `MCC` `HCC`

     I63.113 Cerebral infarction due to embolism of bilateral vertebral arteries `MCC` `HCC`

     I63.119 Cerebral infarction due to embolism of unspecified vertebral artery `MCC` `HCC`

I63.12 Cerebral infarction due to embolism of basilar artery `MCC` `HCC`

√6ᵗʰ **I63.13** Cerebral infarction due to embolism of carotid artery

     I63.131 Cerebral infarction due to embolism of right carotid artery `MCC` `HCC`

     I63.132 Cerebral infarction due to embolism of left carotid artery `MCC` `HCC`

     I63.133 Cerebral infarction due to embolism of bilateral carotid arteries `MCC` `HCC`

     I63.139 Cerebral infarction due to embolism of unspecified carotid artery `MCC` `HCC`

I63.19 Cerebral infarction due to embolism of other precerebral artery `MCC` `HCC`

√5ᵗʰ **I63.2** Cerebral infarction due to unspecified occlusion or stenosis of precerebral arteries

     AHA: 2020,3Q,27-28

     I63.20 Cerebral infarction due to unspecified occlusion or stenosis of unspecified precerebral arteries `MCC` `HCC`

√6ᵗʰ **I63.21** Cerebral infarction due to unspecified occlusion or stenosis of vertebral arteries

     I63.211 Cerebral infarction due to unspecified occlusion or stenosis of right vertebral artery `MCC` `HCC`

     I63.212 Cerebral infarction due to unspecified occlusion or stenosis of left vertebral artery `MCC` `HCC`

     I63.213 Cerebral infarction due to unspecified occlusion or stenosis of bilateral vertebral arteries `MCC` `HCC`

     I63.219 Cerebral infarction due to unspecified occlusion or stenosis of unspecified vertebral artery `MCC` `HCC`

I63.22 Cerebral infarction due to unspecified occlusion or stenosis of basilar artery `MCC` `HCC`

√6ᵗʰ **I63.23** Cerebral infarction due to unspecified occlusion or stenosis of carotid arteries

     I63.231 Cerebral infarction due to unspecified occlusion or stenosis of right carotid arteries `MCC` `HCC`

     I63.232 Cerebral infarction due to unspecified occlusion or stenosis of left carotid arteries `MCC` `HCC`

     I63.233 Cerebral infarction due to unspecified occlusion or stenosis of bilateral carotid arteries `MCC` `HCC`

     I63.239 Cerebral infarction due to unspecified occlusion or stenosis of unspecified carotid artery `MCC` `HCC`

I63.29 Cerebral infarction due to unspecified occlusion or stenosis of other precerebral arteries `MCC` `HCC`

√5ᵗʰ **I63.3** Cerebral infarction due to thrombosis of cerebral arteries

     I63.30 Cerebral infarction due to thrombosis of unspecified cerebral artery `MCC` `HCC`

√6ᵗʰ **I63.31** Cerebral infarction due to thrombosis of middle cerebral artery

     I63.311 Cerebral infarction due to thrombosis of right middle cerebral artery `MCC` `HCC`

     I63.312 Cerebral infarction due to thrombosis of left middle cerebral artery `MCC` `HCC`

     I63.313 Cerebral infarction due to thrombosis of bilateral middle cerebral arteries `MCC` `HCC`

     I63.319 Cerebral infarction due to thrombosis of unspecified middle cerebral artery `MCC` `HCC`

√6ᵗʰ **I63.32** Cerebral infarction due to thrombosis of anterior cerebral artery

     I63.321 Cerebral infarction due to thrombosis of right anterior cerebral artery `MCC` `HCC`

     I63.322 Cerebral infarction due to thrombosis of left anterior cerebral artery `MCC` `HCC`

     I63.323 Cerebral infarction due to thrombosis of bilateral anterior cerebral arteries `MCC` `HCC`

     I63.329 Cerebral infarction due to thrombosis of unspecified anterior cerebral artery `MCC` `HCC`

√6ᵗʰ **I63.33** Cerebral infarction due to thrombosis of posterior cerebral artery

     I63.331 Cerebral infarction due to thrombosis of right posterior cerebral artery `MCC` `HCC`

     I63.332 Cerebral infarction due to thrombosis of left posterior cerebral artery `MCC` `HCC`

     I63.333 Cerebral infarction due to thrombosis of bilateral posterior cerebral arteries `MCC` `HCC`

     I63.339 Cerebral infarction due to thrombosis of unspecified posterior cerebral artery `MCC` `HCC`

√6ᵗʰ **I63.34** Cerebral infarction due to thrombosis of cerebellar artery

     I63.341 Cerebral infarction due to thrombosis of right cerebellar artery `MCC` `HCC`

     I63.342 Cerebral infarction due to thrombosis of left cerebellar artery `MCC` `HCC`

     I63.343 Cerebral infarction due to thrombosis of bilateral cerebellar arteries `MCC` `HCC`

     I63.349 Cerebral infarction due to thrombosis of unspecified cerebellar artery `MCC` `HCC`

I63.39 Cerebral infarction due to thrombosis of other cerebral artery `MCC` `HCC`

√5ᵗʰ **I63.4** Cerebral infarction due to embolism of cerebral arteries

     I63.40 Cerebral infarction due to embolism of unspecified cerebral artery `MCC` `HCC`

√6ᵗʰ **I63.41** Cerebral infarction due to embolism of middle cerebral artery

     I63.411 Cerebral infarction due to embolism of right middle cerebral artery `MCC` `HCC`

     I63.412 Cerebral infarction due to embolism of left middle cerebral artery `MCC` `HCC`

     I63.413 Cerebral infarction due to embolism of bilateral middle cerebral arteries `MCC` `HCC`

     I63.419 Cerebral infarction due to embolism of unspecified middle cerebral artery `MCC` `HCC`

√6ᵗʰ **I63.42** Cerebral infarction due to embolism of anterior cerebral artery

     I63.421 Cerebral infarction due to embolism of right anterior cerebral artery `MCC` `HCC`

     I63.422 Cerebral infarction due to embolism of left anterior cerebral artery `MCC` `HCC`

     I63.423 Cerebral infarction due to embolism of bilateral anterior cerebral arteries `MCC` `HCC`

     I63.429 Cerebral infarction due to embolism of unspecified anterior cerebral artery `MCC` `HCC`

√6ᵗʰ **I63.43** Cerebral infarction due to embolism of posterior cerebral artery

     I63.431 Cerebral infarction due to embolism of right posterior cerebral artery `MCC` `HCC`

     I63.432 Cerebral infarction due to embolism of left posterior cerebral artery `MCC` `HCC`

     I63.433 Cerebral infarction due to embolism of bilateral posterior cerebral arteries `MCC` `HCC`

     I63.439 Cerebral infarction due to embolism of unspecified posterior cerebral artery `MCC` `HCC`

√6ᵗʰ **I63.44** Cerebral infarction due to embolism of cerebellar artery

     I63.441 Cerebral infarction due to embolism of right cerebellar artery `MCC` `HCC`

     I63.442 Cerebral infarction due to embolism of left cerebellar artery `MCC` `HCC`

     I63.443 Cerebral infarction due to embolism of bilateral cerebellar arteries `MCC` `HCC`

     I63.449 Cerebral infarction due to embolism of unspecified cerebellar artery `MCC` `HCC`

N Newborn: 0   P Pediatric: 0-17   M Maternity: 9-64   A Adult: 15-124   `MCC` Major Complication/Comorbidity   `CC` Complication/Comorbidity   `SW` Severe Wound Dx

662   ICD-10-CM 2022

I63.49   Cerebral infarction due to embolism of other cerebral artery   `MCC` `HCC`

√5ᵗʰ **I63.5**   **Cerebral infarction due to unspecified occlusion or stenosis of cerebral arteries**

    I63.50   Cerebral infarction due to unspecified occlusion or stenosis of unspecified cerebral artery   `MCC` `HCC`

    √6ᵗʰ **I63.51**   Cerebral infarction due to unspecified occlusion or stenosis of middle cerebral artery

       I63.511   Cerebral infarction due to unspecified occlusion or stenosis of right middle cerebral artery   `MCC` `HCC`

       I63.512   Cerebral infarction due to unspecified occlusion or stenosis of left middle cerebral artery   `MCC` `HCC`

       I63.513   Cerebral infarction due to unspecified occlusion or stenosis of bilateral middle cerebral arteries   `MCC` `HCC`

       I63.519   Cerebral infarction due to unspecified occlusion or stenosis of unspecified middle cerebral artery   `MCC` `HCC`

    √6ᵗʰ **I63.52**   Cerebral infarction due to unspecified occlusion or stenosis of anterior cerebral artery

       I63.521   Cerebral infarction due to unspecified occlusion or stenosis of right anterior cerebral artery   `MCC` `HCC`

       I63.522   Cerebral infarction due to unspecified occlusion or stenosis of left anterior cerebral artery   `MCC` `HCC`

       I63.523   Cerebral infarction due to unspecified occlusion or stenosis of bilateral anterior cerebral arteries   `MCC` `HCC`

       I63.529   Cerebral infarction due to unspecified occlusion or stenosis of unspecified anterior cerebral artery   `MCC` `HCC`

    √6ᵗʰ **I63.53**   Cerebral infarction due to unspecified occlusion or stenosis of posterior cerebral artery

       I63.531   Cerebral infarction due to unspecified occlusion or stenosis of right posterior cerebral artery   `MCC` `HCC`

       I63.532   Cerebral infarction due to unspecified occlusion or stenosis of left posterior cerebral artery   `MCC` `HCC`

       I63.533   Cerebral infarction due to unspecified occlusion or stenosis of bilateral posterior cerebral arteries   `MCC` `HCC`

       I63.539   Cerebral infarction due to unspecified occlusion or stenosis of unspecified posterior cerebral artery   `MCC` `HCC`

    √6ᵗʰ **I63.54**   Cerebral infarction due to unspecified occlusion or stenosis of cerebellar artery

       I63.541   Cerebral infarction due to unspecified occlusion or stenosis of right cerebellar artery   `MCC` `HCC`

       I63.542   Cerebral infarction due to unspecified occlusion or stenosis of left cerebellar artery   `MCC` `HCC`

       I63.543   Cerebral infarction due to unspecified occlusion or stenosis of bilateral cerebellar arteries   `MCC` `HCC`

       I63.549   Cerebral infarction due to unspecified occlusion or stenosis of unspecified cerebellar artery   `MCC` `HCC`

    I63.59   Cerebral infarction due to unspecified occlusion or stenosis of other cerebral artery   `MCC` `HCC`

I63.6   Cerebral infarction due to cerebral venous thrombosis, nonpyogenic   `MCC` `HCC`

√6ᵗʰ **I63.8**   **Other cerebral infarction**

    AHA: 2018,4Q,16

    I63.81   Other cerebral infarction due to occlusion or stenosis of small artery   `MCC` `HCC`
       Lacunar infarction
       AHA: 2020,3Q,27

    I63.89   Other cerebral infarction   `MCC` `HCC`

I63.9   **Cerebral infarction, unspecified**   `MCC` `HCC`
    Stroke NOS
    EXCLUDES 2   *transient cerebral ischemic attacks and related syndromes (G45.-)*

    AHA: 2020,2Q,29

    TIP: When provider documentation does not identify the location of an infarction, imaging reports can be used to pinpoint the location and lead to a more specific infarction code.

√4ᵗʰ **I65**   **Occlusion and stenosis of precerebral arteries, not resulting in cerebral infarction**

    INCLUDES   embolism of precerebral artery
           narrowing of precerebral artery
           obstruction (complete) (partial) of precerebral artery
           thrombosis of precerebral artery

    EXCLUDES 1   *insufficiency, NOS, of precerebral artery (G45.-)*
           insufficiency of precerebral arteries causing cerebral infarction (I63.0-I63.2)

    AHA: 2018,2Q,9

    √5ᵗʰ **I65.0**   **Occlusion and stenosis of vertebral artery**

       I65.01   Occlusion and stenosis of right vertebral artery

       I65.02   Occlusion and stenosis of left vertebral artery

       I65.03   Occlusion and stenosis of bilateral vertebral arteries

       I65.09   Occlusion and stenosis of unspecified vertebral artery

    I65.1   **Occlusion and stenosis of basilar artery**

    √5ᵗʰ **I65.2**   **Occlusion and stenosis of carotid artery**

       AHA: 2021,1Q,4; 2020,3Q,28

       I65.21   Occlusion and stenosis of right carotid artery

       I65.22   Occlusion and stenosis of left carotid artery

       I65.23   Occlusion and stenosis of bilateral carotid arteries

       I65.29   Occlusion and stenosis of unspecified carotid artery

    I65.8   **Occlusion and stenosis of other precerebral arteries**

    I65.9   **Occlusion and stenosis of unspecified precerebral artery**
       Occlusion and stenosis of precerebral artery NOS

√4ᵗʰ **I66**   **Occlusion and stenosis of cerebral arteries, not resulting in cerebral infarction**

    INCLUDES   embolism of cerebral artery
           narrowing of cerebral artery
           obstruction (complete) (partial) of cerebral artery
           thrombosis of cerebral artery

    EXCLUDES 1   *occlusion and stenosis of cerebral artery causing cerebral infarction (I63.3-I63.5)*

    √5ᵗʰ **I66.0**   **Occlusion and stenosis of middle cerebral artery**

       I66.01   Occlusion and stenosis of right middle cerebral artery

       I66.02   Occlusion and stenosis of left middle cerebral artery

       I66.03   Occlusion and stenosis of bilateral middle cerebral arteries

       I66.09   Occlusion and stenosis of unspecified middle cerebral artery

    √5ᵗʰ **I66.1**   **Occlusion and stenosis of anterior cerebral artery**

       I66.11   Occlusion and stenosis of right anterior cerebral artery

       I66.12   Occlusion and stenosis of left anterior cerebral artery

       I66.13   Occlusion and stenosis of bilateral anterior cerebral arteries

       I66.19   Occlusion and stenosis of unspecified anterior cerebral artery

    √5ᵗʰ **I66.2**   **Occlusion and stenosis of posterior cerebral artery**

       I66.21   Occlusion and stenosis of right posterior cerebral artery

       I66.22   Occlusion and stenosis of left posterior cerebral artery

       I66.23   Occlusion and stenosis of bilateral posterior cerebral arteries

       I66.29   Occlusion and stenosis of unspecified posterior cerebral artery

    I66.3   **Occlusion and stenosis of cerebellar arteries**

    I66.8   **Occlusion and stenosis of other cerebral arteries**
       Occlusion and stenosis of perforating arteries

    I66.9   **Occlusion and stenosis of unspecified cerebral artery**

√4ᵗʰ **I67**   **Other cerebrovascular diseases**

    EXCLUDES 2   *sequelae of the listed conditions (I69.8)*

    I67.0   **Dissection of cerebral arteries, nonruptured**   `MCC` `HCC`
       EXCLUDES 1   *ruptured cerebral arteries (I60.7)*

✔ Additional Character Required   √x7ᵗʰ Placeholder   Questionable PDx   Manifestation   Unspecified Dx   `UPD` Unacceptable PDx   `H1`-`H14` HAC   `HCC` CMS-HCC Dx   `HIV` HIV Dx

ICD-10-CM 2022   663

I67.1 Cerebral aneurysm, nonruptured
Cerebral aneurysm NOS
Cerebral arteriovenous fistula, acquired
Internal carotid artery aneurysm, intracranial portion
Internal carotid artery aneurysm, NOS
> **EXCLUDES 1**   congenital cerebral aneurysm, nonruptured (Q28.-)
>   ruptured cerebral aneurysm (I60.7)

Berry Aneurysm

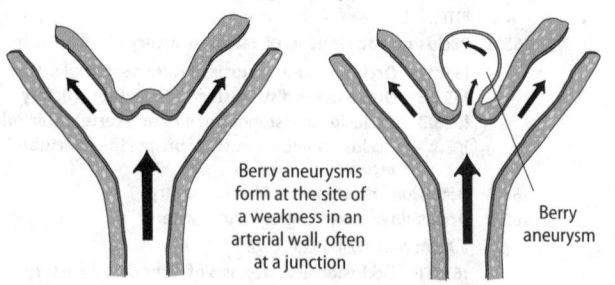

Berry aneurysms form at the site of a weakness in an arterial wall, often at a junction

Berry aneurysm

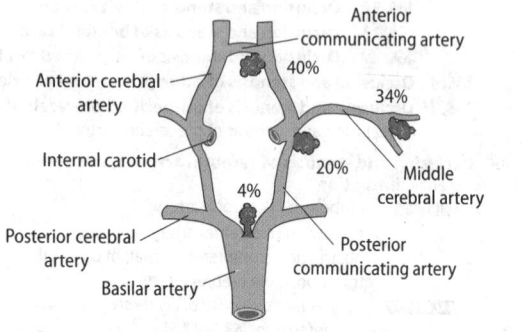

Common sites of berry aneurysms in the circle of Willis arteries

I67.2 Cerebral atherosclerosis   Ⓐ
Atheroma of cerebral and precerebral arteries

I67.3 Progressive vascular leukoencephalopathy   HIV CC HCC
Binswanger's disease

I67.4 Hypertensive encephalopathy   CC
> **EXCLUDES 2**   insufficiency, NOS, of precerebral arteries (G45.2)

I67.5 Moyamoya disease   CC
DEF: Cerebrovascular ischemia. Vessels occlude and rupture, causing tiny hemorrhages at the base of brain. It affects predominantly Japanese people.

I67.6 Nonpyogenic thrombosis of intracranial venous system   CC
Nonpyogenic thrombosis of cerebral vein
Nonpyogenic thrombosis of intracranial venous sinus
> **EXCLUDES 1**   nonpyogenic thrombosis of intracranial venous
>   system causing infarction (I63.6)

I67.7 Cerebral arteritis, not elsewhere classified   CC
Granulomatous angiitis of the nervous system
> **EXCLUDES 1**   allergic granulomatous angiitis (M30.1)

✓5ᵗʰ I67.8 Other specified cerebrovascular diseases

I67.81 Acute cerebrovascular insufficiency   CC
Acute cerebrovascular insufficiency unspecified as to location or reversibility

I67.82 Cerebral ischemia   CC
Chronic cerebral ischemia

I67.83 Posterior reversible encephalopathy syndrome   HIV MCC
PRES

✓6ᵗʰ I67.84 Cerebral vasospasm and vasoconstriction

I67.841 Reversible cerebrovascular vasoconstriction syndrome   CC
Call-Fleming syndrome
Code first underlying condition, if applicable, such as eclampsia (O15.00-O15.9)

I67.848 Other cerebrovascular vasospasm and vasoconstriction   CC

✓6ᵗʰ I67.85 Hereditary cerebrovascular diseases
AHA: 2018,4Q,17

I67.850 Cerebral autosomal dominant arteriopathy with subcortical infarcts and leukoencephalopathy   CC
CADASIL
Code also any associated diagnoses, such as:
epilepsy (G40.-)
stroke (I63.-)
vascular dementia (F01.-)

I67.858 Other hereditary cerebrovascular disease   CC

I67.89 Other cerebrovascular disease   CC

I67.9 Cerebrovascular disease, unspecified

✓4ᵗʰ I68 Cerebrovascular disorders in diseases classified elsewhere

I68.0 Cerebral amyloid angiopathy
Code first underlying amyloidosis (E85.-)

I68.2 Cerebral arteritis in other diseases classified elsewhere   CC
Code first underlying disease
> **EXCLUDES 1**   cerebral arteritis (in):
>   listerosis (A32.89)
>   syphilis (A52.04)
>   systemic lupus erythematosus (M32.19)
>   tuberculosis (A18.89)

I68.8 Other cerebrovascular disorders in diseases classified elsewhere
Code first underlying disease
> **EXCLUDES 1**   syphilitic cerebral aneurysm (A52.05)

✓4ᵗʰ I69 Sequelae of cerebrovascular disease

> **NOTE**   Category I69 is to be used to indicate conditions in I60-I67 as the cause of sequelae. The "sequelae" include conditions specified as such or as residuals which may occur at any time after the onset of the causal condition

> **EXCLUDES 1**   personal history of cerebral infarction without residual deficit (Z86.73)
>   personal history of prolonged reversible ischemic neurologic deficit (PRIND) (Z86.73)
>   personal history of reversible ischemic neurologcial deficit (RIND) (Z86.73)
>   sequelae of traumatic intracranial injury (S06.-)

AHA: 2020,2Q,29; 2017,1Q,47; 2016,4Q,28; 2015,1Q,25; 2012,4Q,106
TIP: Weakness on one side of the body (unilateral weakness) documented as secondary to old cerebrovascular disease is synonymous with hemiparesis/hemiplegia. Weakness of one limb documented as secondary to old cerebrovascular disease is synonymous with monoplegia.
TIP: For codes describing hemiplegia, hemiparesis, and monoplegia; if the documentation identifies the affected side but not whether it is the dominant or nondominant side, the default is as follows: for ambidextrous patients, the default is dominant; when the left side is affected, the default is nondominant; and when the right side is affected, the default is dominant.

✓5ᵗʰ I69.0 Sequelae of nontraumatic subarachnoid hemorrhage

I69.00 Unspecified sequelae of nontraumatic subarachnoid hemorrhage

✓6ᵗʰ I69.01 Cognitive deficits following nontraumatic subarachnoid hemorrhage

I69.010 Attention and concentration deficit following nontraumatic subarachnoid hemorrhage

I69.011 Memory deficit following nontraumatic subarachnoid hemorrhage

I69.012 Visuospatial deficit and spatial neglect following nontraumatic subarachnoid hemorrhage

I69.013 Psychomotor deficit following nontraumatic subarachnoid hemorrhage

I69.014 Frontal lobe and executive function deficit following nontraumatic subarachnoid hemorrhage

I69.015 Cognitive social or emotional deficit following nontraumatic subarachnoid hemorrhage

I69.018 Other symptoms and signs involving cognitive functions following nontraumatic subarachnoid hemorrhage

I69.019 Unspecified symptoms and signs involving cognitive functions following nontraumatic subarachnoid hemorrhage

Ⓝ Newborn: 0   Ⓟ Pediatric: 0-17   Ⓜ Maternity: 9-64   Ⓐ Adult: 15-124   MCC Major Complication/Comorbidity   CC Complication/Comorbidity   SW Severe Wound Dx

664

ICD-10-CM 2022

✓6ᵗʰ **I69.02　Speech and language deficits following nontraumatic subarachnoid hemorrhage**

I69.020　Aphasia following nontraumatic subarachnoid hemorrhage

I69.021　Dysphasia following nontraumatic subarachnoid hemorrhage

I69.022　Dysarthria following nontraumatic subarachnoid hemorrhage

I69.023　Fluency disorder following nontraumatic subarachnoid hemorrhage

　　　　Stuttering following nontraumatic subarachnoid hemorrhage

I69.028　Other speech and language deficits following nontraumatic subarachnoid hemorrhage

✓6ᵗʰ **I69.03　Monoplegia of upper limb following nontraumatic subarachnoid hemorrhage**

AHA: 2017,1Q,47

I69.031　Monoplegia of upper limb following nontraumatic subarachnoid hemorrhage affecting right dominant side HCC

I69.032　Monoplegia of upper limb following nontraumatic subarachnoid hemorrhage affecting left dominant side HCC

I69.033　Monoplegia of upper limb following nontraumatic subarachnoid hemorrhage affecting right non-dominant side HCC

I69.034　Monoplegia of upper limb following nontraumatic subarachnoid hemorrhage affecting left non-dominant side HCC

I69.039　Monoplegia of upper limb following nontraumatic subarachnoid hemorrhage affecting unspecified side HCC

✓6ᵗʰ **I69.04　Monoplegia of lower limb following nontraumatic subarachnoid hemorrhage**

AHA: 2017,1Q,47

I69.041　Monoplegia of lower limb following nontraumatic subarachnoid hemorrhage affecting right dominant side HCC

I69.042　Monoplegia of lower limb following nontraumatic subarachnoid hemorrhage affecting left dominant side HCC

I69.043　Monoplegia of lower limb following nontraumatic subarachnoid hemorrhage affecting right non-dominant side HCC

I69.044　Monoplegia of lower limb following nontraumatic subarachnoid hemorrhage affecting left non-dominant side HCC

I69.049　Monoplegia of lower limb following nontraumatic subarachnoid hemorrhage affecting unspecified side HCC

✓6ᵗʰ **I69.05　Hemiplegia and hemiparesis following nontraumatic subarachnoid hemorrhage**

AHA: 2015,1Q,25

I69.051　Hemiplegia and hemiparesis following nontraumatic subarachnoid hemorrhage affecting right dominant side CC HCC

I69.052　Hemiplegia and hemiparesis following nontraumatic subarachnoid hemorrhage affecting left dominant side CC HCC

I69.053　Hemiplegia and hemiparesis following nontraumatic subarachnoid hemorrhage affecting right non-dominant side CC HCC

I69.054　Hemiplegia and hemiparesis following nontraumatic subarachnoid hemorrhage affecting left non-dominant side CC HCC

I69.059　Hemiplegia and hemiparesis following nontraumatic subarachnoid hemorrhage affecting unspecified side CC HCC

✓6ᵗʰ **I69.06　Other paralytic syndrome following nontraumatic subarachnoid hemorrhage**

　　　Use additional code to identify type of paralytic syndrome, such as:
　　　　locked-in state (G83.5)
　　　　quadriplegia (G82.5-)

　　　EXCLUDES 1　*hemiplegia/hemiparesis following nontraumatic subarachnoid hemorrhage (I69.05-)*
　　　　monoplegia of lower limb following nontraumatic subarachnoid hemorrhage (I69.04-)
　　　　monoplegia of upper limb following nontraumatic subarachnoid hemorrhage (I69.03-)

I69.061　Other paralytic syndrome following nontraumatic subarachnoid hemorrhage affecting right dominant side HCC

I69.062　Other paralytic syndrome following nontraumatic subarachnoid hemorrhage affecting left dominant side HCC

I69.063　Other paralytic syndrome following nontraumatic subarachnoid hemorrhage affecting right non-dominant side HCC

I69.064　Other paralytic syndrome following nontraumatic subarachnoid hemorrhage affecting left non-dominant side HCC

I69.065　Other paralytic syndrome following nontraumatic subarachnoid hemorrhage, bilateral HCC

I69.069　Other paralytic syndrome following nontraumatic subarachnoid hemorrhage affecting unspecified side HCC

✓6ᵗʰ **I69.09　Other sequelae of nontraumatic subarachnoid hemorrhage**

I69.090　Apraxia following nontraumatic subarachnoid hemorrhage

I69.091　Dysphagia following nontraumatic subarachnoid hemorrhage

　　　Use additional code to identify the type of dysphagia, if known (R13.1-)

I69.092　Facial weakness following nontraumatic subarachnoid hemorrhage

　　　Facial droop following nontraumatic subarachnoid hemorrhage

I69.093　Ataxia following nontraumatic subarachnoid hemorrhage

I69.098　Other sequelae following nontraumatic subarachnoid hemorrhage

　　　Alterations of sensation following nontraumatic subarachnoid hemorrhage

　　　Disturbance of vision following nontraumatic subarachnoid hemorrhage

　　　Use additional code to identify the sequelae

✓5ᵗʰ **I69.1　Sequelae of nontraumatic intracerebral hemorrhage**

I69.10　Unspecified sequelae of nontraumatic intracerebral hemorrhage

✓6ᵗʰ **I69.11　Cognitive deficits following nontraumatic intracerebral hemorrhage**

I69.110　Attention and concentration deficit following nontraumatic intracerebral hemorrhage

I69.111　Memory deficit following nontraumatic intracerebral hemorrhage

I69.112　Visuospatial deficit and spatial neglect following nontraumatic intracerebral hemorrhage

I69.113　Psychomotor deficit following nontraumatic intracerebral hemorrhage

I69.114　Frontal lobe and executive function deficit following nontraumatic intracerebral hemorrhage

I69.115　Cognitive social or emotional deficit following nontraumatic intracerebral hemorrhage

I69.118　Other symptoms and signs involving cognitive functions following nontraumatic intracerebral hemorrhage

✓ Additional Character Required　✓x7ᵗʰ Placeholder　Questionable PDx　Manifestation　Unspecified Dx　UPD Unacceptable PDx　H1-H4 HAC　HCC CMS-HCC Dx　HIV HIV Dx

ICD-10-CM 2022　　　665

I69.119 Unspecified symptoms and signs involving cognitive functions following nontraumatic intracerebral hemorrhage

√6ᵗʰ **I69.12** **Speech and language deficits** following nontraumatic intracerebral hemorrhage

I69.120 **Aphasia** following nontraumatic intracerebral hemorrhage

I69.121 **Dysphasia** following nontraumatic intracerebral hemorrhage

I69.122 **Dysarthria** following nontraumatic intracerebral hemorrhage

I69.123 **Fluency disorder** following nontraumatic intracerebral hemorrhage

Stuttering following nontraumatic intracerebral hemorrhage

I69.128 Other speech and language deficits following nontraumatic intracerebral hemorrhage

√6ᵗʰ **I69.13** **Monoplegia of upper limb** following nontraumatic intracerebral hemorrhage

AHA: 2017,1Q,47

I69.131 Monoplegia of upper limb following nontraumatic intracerebral hemorrhage affecting **right dominant** side `HCC`

I69.132 Monoplegia of upper limb following nontraumatic intracerebral hemorrhage affecting **left dominant** side `HCC`

I69.133 Monoplegia of upper limb following nontraumatic intracerebral hemorrhage affecting **right non-dominant** side `HCC`

I69.134 Monoplegia of upper limb following nontraumatic intracerebral hemorrhage affecting **left non-dominant** side `HCC`

I69.139 Monoplegia of upper limb following nontraumatic intracerebral hemorrhage affecting unspecified side `HCC`

√6ᵗʰ **I69.14** **Monoplegia of lower limb** following nontraumatic intracerebral hemorrhage

AHA: 2017,1Q,47

I69.141 Monoplegia of lower limb following nontraumatic intracerebral hemorrhage affecting **right dominant** side `HCC`

I69.142 Monoplegia of lower limb following nontraumatic intracerebral hemorrhage affecting **left dominant** side `HCC`

I69.143 Monoplegia of lower limb following nontraumatic intracerebral hemorrhage affecting **right non-dominant** side `HCC`

I69.144 Monoplegia of lower limb following nontraumatic intracerebral hemorrhage affecting **left non-dominant** side `HCC`

I69.149 Monoplegia of lower limb following nontraumatic intracerebral hemorrhage affecting unspecified side `HCC`

√6ᵗʰ **I69.15** **Hemiplegia and hemiparesis** following nontraumatic intracerebral hemorrhage

AHA: 2015,1Q,25

I69.151 Hemiplegia and hemiparesis following nontraumatic intracerebral hemorrhage affecting **right dominant** side `CC` `HCC`

I69.152 Hemiplegia and hemiparesis following nontraumatic intracerebral hemorrhage affecting **left dominant** side `CC` `HCC`

I69.153 Hemiplegia and hemiparesis following nontraumatic intracerebral hemorrhage affecting **right non-dominant** side `CC` `HCC`

I69.154 Hemiplegia and hemiparesis following nontraumatic intracerebral hemorrhage affecting **left non-dominant** side `CC` `HCC`

I69.159 Hemiplegia and hemiparesis following nontraumatic intracerebral hemorrhage affecting unspecified side `CC` `HCC`

√6ᵗʰ **I69.16** Other **paralytic syndrome** following nontraumatic intracerebral hemorrhage

Use additional code to identify type of paralytic syndrome, such as:

locked-in state (G83.5)

quadriplegia (G82.5-)

EXCLUDES 1 *hemiplegia/hemiparesis following nontraumatic intracerebral hemorrhage (I69.15-)*

monoplegia of lower limb following nontraumatic intracerebral hemorrhage (I69.14-)

monoplegia of upper limb following nontraumatic intracerebral hemorrhage (I69.13-)

I69.161 Other paralytic syndrome following nontraumatic intracerebral hemorrhage affecting **right dominant** side `HCC`

I69.162 Other paralytic syndrome following nontraumatic intracerebral hemorrhage affecting **left dominant** side `HCC`

I69.163 Other paralytic syndrome following nontraumatic intracerebral hemorrhage affecting **right non-dominant** side `HCC`

I69.164 Other paralytic syndrome following nontraumatic intracerebral hemorrhage affecting **left non-dominant** side `HCC`

I69.165 Other paralytic syndrome following nontraumatic intracerebral hemorrhage, bilateral `HCC`

I69.169 Other paralytic syndrome following nontraumatic intracerebral hemorrhage affecting unspecified side `HCC`

√6ᵗʰ **I69.19** Other sequelae of nontraumatic intracerebral hemorrhage

I69.190 **Apraxia** following nontraumatic intracerebral hemorrhage

I69.191 **Dysphagia** following nontraumatic intracerebral hemorrhage

Use additional code to identify the type of dysphagia, if known (R13.1-)

I69.192 **Facial weakness** following nontraumatic intracerebral hemorrhage

Facial droop following nontraumatic intracerebral hemorrhage

I69.193 **Ataxia** following nontraumatic intracerebral hemorrhage

I69.198 Other sequelae of nontraumatic intracerebral hemorrhage

Alteration of sensations following nontraumatic intracerebral hemorrhage

Disturbance of vision following nontraumatic intracerebral hemorrhage

Use additional code to identify the sequelae

√5ᵗʰ **I69.2** **Sequelae of other nontraumatic intracranial hemorrhage**

I69.20 Unspecified sequelae of other nontraumatic intracranial hemorrhage

√6ᵗʰ **I69.21** **Cognitive deficits** following other nontraumatic intracranial hemorrhage

I69.210 **Attention and concentration** deficit following other nontraumatic intracranial hemorrhage

I69.211 **Memory** deficit following other nontraumatic intracranial hemorrhage

I69.212 **Visuospatial** deficit and **spatial neglect** following other nontraumatic intracranial hemorrhage

I69.213 **Psychomotor** deficit following other nontraumatic intracranial hemorrhage

I69.214 **Frontal lobe and executive function** deficit following other nontraumatic intracranial hemorrhage

I69.215 **Cognitive social or emotional** deficit following other nontraumatic intracranial hemorrhage

I69.218 Other symptoms and signs involving cognitive functions following other nontraumatic intracranial hemorrhage

`N` Newborn: 0   `P` Pediatric: 0-17   `M` Maternity: 9-64   `A` Adult: 15-124   `MCC` Major Complication/Comorbidity   `CC` Complication/Comorbidity   `SW` Severe Wound Dx

666

ICD-10-CM 2022

I69.219　Unspecified symptoms and signs involving cognitive functions following other nontraumatic intracranial hemorrhage

✓6th　**I69.22　Speech and language deficits following other nontraumatic intracranial hemorrhage**

I69.220　Aphasia following other nontraumatic intracranial hemorrhage

I69.221　Dysphasia following other nontraumatic intracranial hemorrhage

I69.222　Dysarthria following other nontraumatic intracranial hemorrhage

I69.223　Fluency disorder following other nontraumatic intracranial hemorrhage
Stuttering following other nontraumatic intracranial hemorrhage

I69.228　Other speech and language deficits following other nontraumatic intracranial hemorrhage

✓6th　**I69.23　Monoplegia of upper limb following other nontraumatic intracranial hemorrhage**
AHA: 2017,1Q,47

I69.231　Monoplegia of upper limb following other nontraumatic intracranial hemorrhage affecting right dominant side　HCC

I69.232　Monoplegia of upper limb following other nontraumatic intracranial hemorrhage affecting left dominant side　HCC

I69.233　Monoplegia of upper limb following other nontraumatic intracranial hemorrhage affecting right non-dominant side　HCC

I69.234　Monoplegia of upper limb following other nontraumatic intracranial hemorrhage affecting left non-dominant side　HCC

I69.239　Monoplegia of upper limb following other nontraumatic intracranial hemorrhage affecting unspecified side　HCC

✓6th　**I69.24　Monoplegia of lower limb following other nontraumatic intracranial hemorrhage**
AHA: 2017,1Q,47

I69.241　Monoplegia of lower limb following other nontraumatic intracranial hemorrhage affecting right dominant side　HCC

I69.242　Monoplegia of lower limb following other nontraumatic intracranial hemorrhage affecting left dominant side　HCC

I69.243　Monoplegia of lower limb following other nontraumatic intracranial hemorrhage affecting right non-dominant side　HCC

I69.244　Monoplegia of lower limb following other nontraumatic intracranial hemorrhage affecting left non-dominant side　HCC

I69.249　Monoplegia of lower limb following other nontraumatic intracranial hemorrhage affecting unspecified side　HCC

✓6th　**I69.25　Hemiplegia and hemiparesis following other nontraumatic intracranial hemorrhage**
AHA: 2015,1Q,25

I69.251　Hemiplegia and hemiparesis following other nontraumatic intracranial hemorrhage affecting right dominant side　CC　HCC

I69.252　Hemiplegia and hemiparesis following other nontraumatic intracranial hemorrhage affecting left dominant side　CC　HCC

I69.253　Hemiplegia and hemiparesis following other nontraumatic intracranial hemorrhage affecting right non-dominant side　CC　HCC

I69.254　Hemiplegia and hemiparesis following other nontraumatic intracranial hemorrhage affecting left non-dominant side　CC　HCC

I69.259　Hemiplegia and hemiparesis following other nontraumatic intracranial hemorrhage affecting unspecified side　CC　HCC

✓6th　**I69.26　Other paralytic syndrome following other nontraumatic intracranial hemorrhage**
Use additional code to identify type of paralytic syndrome, such as:
locked-in state (G83.5)
quadriplegia (G82.5-)

EXCLUDES 1　hemiplegia/hemiparesis following other nontraumatic intracranial hemorrhage (I69.25-)
monoplegia of lower limb following other nontraumatic intracranial hemorrhage (I69.24-)
monoplegia of upper limb following other nontraumatic intracranial hemorrhage (I69.23-)

I69.261　Other paralytic syndrome following other nontraumatic intracranial hemorrhage affecting right dominant side　HCC

I69.262　Other paralytic syndrome following other nontraumatic intracranial hemorrhage affecting left dominant side　HCC

I69.263　Other paralytic syndrome following other nontraumatic intracranial hemorrhage affecting right non-dominant side　HCC

I69.264　Other paralytic syndrome following other nontraumatic intracranial hemorrhage affecting left non-dominant side　HCC

I69.265　Other paralytic syndrome following other nontraumatic intracranial hemorrhage, bilateral　HCC

I69.269　Other paralytic syndrome following other nontraumatic intracranial hemorrhage affecting unspecified side　HCC

✓6th　**I69.29　Other sequelae of other nontraumatic intracranial hemorrhage**

I69.290　Apraxia following other nontraumatic intracranial hemorrhage

I69.291　Dysphagia following other nontraumatic intracranial hemorrhage
Use additional code to identify the type of dysphagia, if known (R13.1-)

I69.292　Facial weakness following other nontraumatic intracranial hemorrhage
Facial droop following other nontraumatic intracranial hemorrhage

I69.293　Ataxia following other nontraumatic intracranial hemorrhage

I69.298　Other sequelae of other nontraumatic intracranial hemorrhage
Alteration of sensation following other nontraumatic intracranial hemorrhage
Disturbance of vision following other nontraumatic intracranial hemorrhage
Use additional code to identify the sequelae

✓5th　**I69.3　Sequelae of cerebral infarction**
Sequelae of stroke NOS
AHA: 2013,4Q,127-128; 2012,4Q,92,94

I69.30　Unspecified sequelae of cerebral infarction

✓6th　**I69.31　Cognitive deficits following cerebral infarction**

I69.310　Attention and concentration deficit following cerebral infarction

I69.311　Memory deficit following cerebral infarction

I69.312　Visuospatial deficit and spatial neglect following cerebral infarction

I69.313　Psychomotor deficit following cerebral infarction

I69.314　Frontal lobe and executive function deficit following cerebral infarction

I69.315　Cognitive social or emotional deficit following cerebral infarction

I69.318　Other symptoms and signs involving cognitive functions following cerebral infarction

I69.319　Unspecified symptoms and signs involving cognitive functions following cerebral infarction

✓6ᵗʰ **169.32** Speech and language deficits following cerebral infarction

169.320 Aphasia following cerebral infarction

169.321 Dysphasia following cerebral infarction
AHA: 2012,4Q,91

169.322 Dysarthria following cerebral infarction
EXCLUDES 2   *transient ischemic attack (TIA) (G45.9)*

169.323 Fluency disorder following cerebral infarction
Stuttering following cerebral infarction

169.328 Other speech and language deficits following cerebral infarction

✓6ᵗʰ **169.33** Monoplegia of upper limb following cerebral infarction
AHA: 2017,1Q,47

169.331 Monoplegia of upper limb following cerebral infarction affecting right dominant side   HCC

169.332 Monoplegia of upper limb following cerebral infarction affecting left dominant side   HCC

169.333 Monoplegia of upper limb following cerebral infarction affecting right non-dominant side   HCC

169.334 Monoplegia of upper limb following cerebral infarction affecting left non-dominant side   HCC

169.339 Monoplegia of upper limb following cerebral infarction affecting unspecified side   HCC

✓6ᵗʰ **169.34** Monoplegia of lower limb following cerebral infarction
AHA: 2017,1Q,47

169.341 Monoplegia of lower limb following cerebral infarction affecting right dominant side   HCC

169.342 Monoplegia of lower limb following cerebral infarction affecting left dominant side   HCC

169.343 Monoplegia of lower limb following cerebral infarction affecting right non-dominant side   HCC

169.344 Monoplegia of lower limb following cerebral infarction affecting left non-dominant side   HCC

169.349 Monoplegia of lower limb following cerebral infarction affecting unspecified side   HCC

✓6ᵗʰ **169.35** Hemiplegia and hemiparesis following cerebral infarction
AHA: 2015,1Q,25

169.351 Hemiplegia and hemiparesis following cerebral infarction affecting right dominant side   CC HCC
EXCLUDES 2   *transient ischemic attack (TIA) (G45.9)*

169.352 Hemiplegia and hemiparesis following cerebral infarction affecting left dominant side   CC HCC

169.353 Hemiplegia and hemiparesis following cerebral infarction affecting right non-dominant side   CC HCC

169.354 Hemiplegia and hemiparesis following cerebral infarction affecting left non-dominant side   CC HCC
AHA: 2012,4Q,91

169.359 Hemiplegia and hemiparesis following cerebral infarction affecting unspecified side   CC HCC

✓6ᵗʰ **169.36** Other paralytic syndrome following cerebral infarction
Use additional code to identify type of paralytic syndrome, such as:
locked-in state (G83.5)
quadriplegia (G82.5-)
EXCLUDES 1   *hemiplegia/hemiparesis following cerebral infarction (169.35-)*
monoplegia of lower limb following cerebral infarction (169.34-)
monoplegia of upper limb following cerebral infarction (169.33-)

169.361 Other paralytic syndrome following cerebral infarction affecting right dominant side   HCC

169.362 Other paralytic syndrome following cerebral infarction affecting left dominant side   HCC

169.363 Other paralytic syndrome following cerebral infarction affecting right non-dominant side   HCC

169.364 Other paralytic syndrome following cerebral infarction affecting left non-dominant side   HCC

169.365 Other paralytic syndrome following cerebral infarction, bilateral   HCC

169.369 Other paralytic syndrome following cerebral infarction affecting unspecified side   HCC

✓6ᵗʰ **169.39** Other sequelae of cerebral infarction

169.390 Apraxia following cerebral infarction

169.391 Dysphagia following cerebral infarction
Use additional code to identify the type of dysphagia, if known (R13.1-)

169.392 Facial weakness following cerebral infarction
Facial droop following cerebral infarction

169.393 Ataxia following cerebral infarction

169.398 Other sequelae of cerebral infarction
Alteration of sensation following cerebral infarction
Disturbance of vision following cerebral infarction
Use additional code to identify the sequelae
AHA: 2020,2Q,29

✓5ᵗʰ **169.8** Sequelae of other cerebrovascular diseases
EXCLUDES 1   *sequelae of traumatic intracranial injury (S06.-)*

169.80 Unspecified sequelae of other cerebrovascular disease

✓6ᵗʰ **169.81** Cognitive deficits following other cerebrovascular disease

169.810 Attention and concentration deficit following other cerebrovascular disease

169.811 Memory deficit following other cerebrovascular disease

169.812 Visuospatial deficit and spatial neglect following other cerebrovascular disease

169.813 Psychomotor deficit following other cerebrovascular disease

169.814 Frontal lobe and executive function deficit following other cerebrovascular disease

169.815 Cognitive social or emotional deficit following other cerebrovascular disease

169.818 Other symptoms and signs involving cognitive functions following other cerebrovascular disease

169.819 Unspecified symptoms and signs involving cognitive functions following other cerebrovascular disease

✓6ᵗʰ **169.82** Speech and language deficits following other cerebrovascular disease

169.820 Aphasia following other cerebrovascular disease

169.821 Dysphasia following other cerebrovascular disease

169.822 Dysarthria following other cerebrovascular disease

I69.823 Fluency disorder following other cerebrovascular disease
Stuttering following other cerebrovascular disease

I69.828 Other speech and language deficits following other cerebrovascular disease
AHA: 2019,3Q,8

✓6ᵗʰ **I69.83 Monoplegia of upper limb following other cerebrovascular disease**
AHA: 2017,1Q,47

I69.831 Monoplegia of upper limb following other cerebrovascular disease affecting right dominant side HCC

I69.832 Monoplegia of upper limb following other cerebrovascular disease affecting left dominant side HCC

I69.833 Monoplegia of upper limb following other cerebrovascular disease affecting right non-dominant side HCC

I69.834 Monoplegia of upper limb following other cerebrovascular disease affecting left non-dominant side HCC

I69.839 Monoplegia of upper limb following other cerebrovascular disease affecting unspecified side HCC

✓6ᵗʰ **I69.84 Monoplegia of lower limb following other cerebrovascular disease**
AHA: 2017,1Q,47

I69.841 Monoplegia of lower limb following other cerebrovascular disease affecting right dominant side HCC

I69.842 Monoplegia of lower limb following other cerebrovascular disease affecting left dominant side HCC

I69.843 Monoplegia of lower limb following other cerebrovascular disease affecting right non-dominant side HCC

I69.844 Monoplegia of lower limb following other cerebrovascular disease affecting left non-dominant side HCC

I69.849 Monoplegia of lower limb following other cerebrovascular disease affecting unspecified side HCC

✓6ᵗʰ **I69.85 Hemiplegia and hemiparesis following other cerebrovascular disease**
AHA: 2015,1Q,25

I69.851 Hemiplegia and hemiparesis following other cerebrovascular disease affecting right dominant side CC HCC

I69.852 Hemiplegia and hemiparesis following other cerebrovascular disease affecting left dominant side CC HCC

I69.853 Hemiplegia and hemiparesis following other cerebrovascular disease affecting right non-dominant side CC HCC

I69.854 Hemiplegia and hemiparesis following other cerebrovascular disease affecting left non-dominant side CC HCC

I69.859 Hemiplegia and hemiparesis following other cerebrovascular disease affecting unspecified side CC HCC

✓6ᵗʰ **I69.86 Other paralytic syndrome following other cerebrovascular disease**
Use additional code to identify type of paralytic syndrome, such as:
locked-in state (G83.5)
quadriplegia (G82.5-)
EXCLUDES 1 hemiplegia/hemiparesis following other cerebrovascular disease (I69.85-)
monoplegia of lower limb following other cerebrovascular disease (I69.84-)
monoplegia of upper limb following other cerebrovascular disease (I69.83-)

I69.861 Other paralytic syndrome following other cerebrovascular disease affecting right dominant side HCC

I69.862 Other paralytic syndrome following other cerebrovascular disease affecting left dominant side HCC

I69.863 Other paralytic syndrome following other cerebrovascular disease affecting right non-dominant side HCC

I69.864 Other paralytic syndrome following other cerebrovascular disease affecting left non-dominant side HCC

I69.865 Other paralytic syndrome following other cerebrovascular disease, bilateral HCC

I69.869 Other paralytic syndrome following other cerebrovascular disease affecting unspecified side HCC

✓6ᵗʰ **I69.89 Other sequelae of other cerebrovascular disease**

I69.890 Apraxia following other cerebrovascular disease

I69.891 Dysphagia following other cerebrovascular disease
Use additional code to identify the type of dysphagia, if known (R13.1-)

I69.892 Facial weakness following other cerebrovascular disease
Facial droop following other cerebrovascular disease

I69.893 Ataxia following other cerebrovascular disease

I69.898 Other sequelae of other cerebrovascular disease
Alteration of sensation following other cerebrovascular disease
Disturbance of vision following other cerebrovascular disease
Use additional code to identify the sequelae

✓5ᵗʰ **I69.9 Sequelae of unspecified cerebrovascular diseases**
EXCLUDES 1 sequelae of stroke (I69.3)
sequelae of traumatic intracranial injury (S06.-)

I69.90 Unspecified sequelae of unspecified cerebrovascular disease

✓6ᵗʰ **I69.91 Cognitive deficits following unspecified cerebrovascular disease**

I69.910 Attention and concentration deficit following unspecified cerebrovascular disease

I69.911 Memory deficit following unspecified cerebrovascular disease

I69.912 Visuospatial deficit and spatial neglect following unspecified cerebrovascular disease

I69.913 Psychomotor deficit following unspecified cerebrovascular disease

I69.914 Frontal lobe and executive function deficit following unspecified cerebrovascular disease

I69.915 Cognitive social or emotional deficit following unspecified cerebrovascular disease

I69.918 Other symptoms and signs involving cognitive functions following unspecified cerebrovascular disease

I69.919 Unspecified symptoms and signs involving cognitive functions following unspecified cerebrovascular disease

✓6ᵗʰ **I69.92 Speech and language deficits following unspecified cerebrovascular disease**

I69.920 Aphasia following unspecified cerebrovascular disease

I69.921 Dysphasia following unspecified cerebrovascular disease

I69.922 Dysarthria following unspecified cerebrovascular disease

I69.923 Fluency disorder following unspecified cerebrovascular disease
Stuttering following unspecified cerebrovascular disease

I69.928 Other speech and language deficits following unspecified cerebrovascular disease

✓6ᵗʰ **I69.93 Monoplegia of upper limb following unspecified cerebrovascular disease**
AHA: 2017,1Q,47

I69.931 Monoplegia of upper limb following unspecified cerebrovascular disease affecting right dominant side HCC

I69.932 Monoplegia of upper limb following unspecified cerebrovascular disease affecting left dominant side HCC

Chapter 9. Diseases of the Circulatory System

I69.933   **Monoplegia of upper limb following unspecified cerebrovascular disease affecting right non-dominant side** `HCC`

I69.934   **Monoplegia of upper limb following unspecified cerebrovascular disease affecting left non-dominant side** `HCC`

I69.939   **Monoplegia of upper limb following unspecified cerebrovascular disease affecting unspecified side** `HCC`

✓6ᵗʰ **I69.94**   **Monoplegia of lower limb following unspecified cerebrovascular disease**
AHA: 2017,1Q,47

I69.941   **Monoplegia of lower limb following unspecified cerebrovascular disease affecting right dominant side** `HCC`

I69.942   **Monoplegia of lower limb following unspecified cerebrovascular disease affecting left dominant side** `HCC`

I69.943   **Monoplegia of lower limb following unspecified cerebrovascular disease affecting right non-dominant side** `HCC`

I69.944   **Monoplegia of lower limb following unspecified cerebrovascular disease affecting left non-dominant side** `HCC`

I69.949   **Monoplegia of lower limb following unspecified cerebrovascular disease affecting unspecified side** `HCC`

✓6ᵗʰ **I69.95**   **Hemiplegia and hemiparesis following unspecified cerebrovascular disease**
AHA: 2015,1Q,25

I69.951   **Hemiplegia and hemiparesis following unspecified cerebrovascular disease affecting right dominant side** `CC` `HCC`

I69.952   **Hemiplegia and hemiparesis following unspecified cerebrovascular disease affecting left dominant side** `CC` `HCC`

I69.953   **Hemiplegia and hemiparesis following unspecified cerebrovascular disease affecting right non-dominant side** `CC` `HCC`

I69.954   **Hemiplegia and hemiparesis following unspecified cerebrovascular disease affecting left non-dominant side** `CC` `HCC`

I69.959   **Hemiplegia and hemiparesis following unspecified cerebrovascular disease affecting unspecified side** `CC` `HCC`

✓6ᵗʰ **I69.96**   **Other paralytic syndrome following unspecified cerebrovascular disease**
Use additional code to identify type of paralytic syndrome, such as:
locked-in state (G83.5)
quadriplegia (G82.5-)
EXCLUDES 1   *hemiplegia/hemiparesis following unspecified cerebrovascular disease (I69.95-)*
monoplegia of lower limb following unspecified cerebrovascular disease (I69.94-)
monoplegia of upper limb following unspecified cerebrovascular disease (I69.93-)

I69.961   **Other paralytic syndrome following unspecified cerebrovascular disease affecting right dominant side** `HCC`

I69.962   **Other paralytic syndrome following unspecified cerebrovascular disease affecting left dominant side** `HCC`

I69.963   **Other paralytic syndrome following unspecified cerebrovascular disease affecting right non-dominant side** `HCC`

I69.964   **Other paralytic syndrome following unspecified cerebrovascular disease affecting left non-dominant side** `HCC`

I69.965   **Other paralytic syndrome following unspecified cerebrovascular disease, bilateral** `HCC`

I69.969   **Other paralytic syndrome following unspecified cerebrovascular disease affecting unspecified side** `HCC`

✓6ᵗʰ **I69.99**   **Other sequelae of unspecified cerebrovascular disease**

I69.990   **Apraxia following unspecified cerebrovascular disease**

I69.991   **Dysphagia following unspecified cerebrovascular disease**
Use additional code to identify the type of dysphagia, if known (R13.1-)

I69.992   **Facial weakness following unspecified cerebrovascular disease**
Facial droop following unspecified cerebrovascular disease

I69.993   **Ataxia following unspecified cerebrovascular disease**

I69.998   **Other sequelae following unspecified cerebrovascular disease**
Alteration in sensation following unspecified cerebrovascular disease
Disturbance of vision following unspecified cerebrovascular disease
Use additional code to identify the sequelae

Diseases of arteries, arterioles and capillaries (I70-I79)

✓4ᵗʰ **I70**   **Atherosclerosis**

`INCLUDES`   arterial degeneration
arteriolosclerosis
arteriosclerosis
arteriosclerotic vascular disease
arteriovascular degeneration
atheroma
endarteritis deformans or obliterans
senile arteritis
senile endarteritis
vascular degeneration
Use additional code to identify:
exposure to environmental tobacco smoke (Z77.22)
history of tobacco dependence (Z87.891)
occupational exposure to environmental tobacco smoke (Z57.31)
tobacco dependence (F17.-)
tobacco use (Z72.0)
EXCLUDES 2   *arteriosclerotic cardiovascular disease (I25.1-)*
arteriosclerotic heart disease (I25.1-)
atheroembolism (I75.-)
cerebral atherosclerosis (I67.2)
coronary atherosclerosis (I25.1-)
mesenteric atherosclerosis (K55.1)
precerebral atherosclerosis (I67.2)
primary pulmonary atherosclerosis (I27.0)

I70.0   **Atherosclerosis of aorta** `HCC` `A`

I70.1   **Atherosclerosis of renal artery** `HCC` `A`
Goldblatt's kidney
EXCLUDES 2   *atherosclerosis of renal arterioles (I12.-)*

✓5ᵗʰ **I70.2**   **Atherosclerosis of native arteries of the extremities**
Mönckeberg's (medial) sclerosis
Use additional code, if applicable, to identify chronic total occlusion of artery of extremity (I70.92)
EXCLUDES 2   *atherosclerosis of bypass graft of extremities (I70.30-I70.79)*
AHA: 2020,4Q,98; 2018,3Q,4; 2018,2Q,7

✓6ᵗʰ **I70.20**   **Unspecified atherosclerosis of native arteries of extremities**

I70.201   **Unspecified atherosclerosis of native arteries of extremities, right leg** `HCC` `A`

I70.202   **Unspecified atherosclerosis of native arteries of extremities, left leg** `HCC` `A`

I70.203   **Unspecified atherosclerosis of native arteries of extremities, bilateral legs** `HCC` `A`

I70.208   **Unspecified atherosclerosis of native arteries of extremities, other extremity** `HCC` `A`

I70.209   **Unspecified atherosclerosis of native arteries of extremities, unspecified extremity** `HCC` `A`

√6ᵗʰ I70.21 Atherosclerosis of native arteries of extremities with intermittent claudication

    I70.211 Atherosclerosis of native arteries of extremities with intermittent claudication, right leg   HCC A

    I70.212 Atherosclerosis of native arteries of extremities with intermittent claudication, left leg   HCC A

    I70.213 Atherosclerosis of native arteries of extremities with intermittent claudication, bilateral legs   HCC A

    I70.218 Atherosclerosis of native arteries of extremities with intermittent claudication, other extremity   HCC A

    I70.219 Atherosclerosis of native arteries of extremities with intermittent claudication, unspecified extremity   HCC A

√6ᵗʰ I70.22 Atherosclerosis of native arteries of extremities with rest pain

    INCLUDES   any condition classifiable to I70.21-

    chronic limb-threatening ischemia NOS of native arteries of extremities

    chronic limb-threatening ischemia of native arteries of extremities with rest pain

    critical limb ischemia NOS of native arteries of extremities

    critical limb ischemia of native arteries of extremities with rest pain

    I70.221 Atherosclerosis of native arteries of extremities with rest pain, right leg   HCC A

    I70.222 Atherosclerosis of native arteries of extremities with rest pain, left leg   HCC A

    I70.223 Atherosclerosis of native arteries of extremities with rest pain, bilateral legs   HCC A

    I70.228 Atherosclerosis of native arteries of extremities with rest pain, other extremity   HCC A

    I70.229 Atherosclerosis of native arteries of extremities with rest pain, unspecified extremity   HCC A

√6ᵗʰ I70.23 Atherosclerosis of native arteries of right leg with ulceration

    INCLUDES   any condition classifiable to I70.211 and I70.221

    chronic limb-threatening ischemia of native arteries of right leg with ulceration

    critical limb ischemia of native arteries of right leg with ulceration

    Use additional code to identify severity of ulcer (L97.-)

    I70.231 Atherosclerosis of native arteries of right leg with ulceration of thigh   HCC A

    I70.232 Atherosclerosis of native arteries of right leg with ulceration of calf   HCC A

    I70.233 Atherosclerosis of native arteries of right leg with ulceration of ankle   HCC A

    I70.234 Atherosclerosis of native arteries of right leg with ulceration of heel and midfoot   HCC A

    Atherosclerosis of native arteries of right leg with ulceration of plantar surface of midfoot

    I70.235 Atherosclerosis of native arteries of right leg with ulceration of other part of foot   HCC A

    Atherosclerosis of native arteries of right leg extremities with ulceration of toe

    I70.238 Atherosclerosis of native arteries of right leg with ulceration of other part of lower leg   HCC A

    I70.239 Atherosclerosis of native arteries of right leg with ulceration of unspecified site   HCC A

√6ᵗʰ I70.24 Atherosclerosis of native arteries of left leg with ulceration

    INCLUDES   any condition classifiable to I70.212 and I70.222

    chronic limb-threatening ischemia of native arteries of left leg with ulceration

    critical limb ischemia of native arteries of left leg with ulceration

    Use additional code to identify severity of ulcer (L97.-)

    I70.241 Atherosclerosis of native arteries of left leg with ulceration of thigh   HCC A

    I70.242 Atherosclerosis of native arteries of left leg with ulceration of calf   HCC A

    I70.243 Atherosclerosis of native arteries of left leg with ulceration of ankle   HCC A

    I70.244 Atherosclerosis of native arteries of left leg with ulceration of heel and midfoot   HCC A

    Atherosclerosis of native arteries of left leg with ulceration of plantar surface of midfoot

    I70.245 Atherosclerosis of native arteries of left leg with ulceration of other part of foot   HCC A

    Atherosclerosis of native arteries of left leg extremities with ulceration of toe

    I70.248 Atherosclerosis of native arteries of left leg with ulceration of other part of lower leg   HCC A

    I70.249 Atherosclerosis of native arteries of left leg with ulceration of unspecified site   HCC A

I70.25 Atherosclerosis of native arteries of other extremities with ulceration   HCC A

    INCLUDES   any condition classifiable to I70.218 and I70.228

    Use additional code to identify the severity of the ulcer (L98.49-)

√6ᵗʰ I70.26 Atherosclerosis of native arteries of extremities with gangrene

    INCLUDES   any condition classifiable to I70.21-, I70.22-, I70.23-, I70.24-, and I70.25-

    chronic limb-threatening ischemia of native arteries of extremities with gangrene

    critical limb ischemia of native arteries of extremities with gangrene

    Use additional code to identify the severity of any ulcer (L97.-, L98.49-), if applicable

    I70.261 Atherosclerosis of native arteries of extremities with gangrene, right leg   CC HCC A

    I70.262 Atherosclerosis of native arteries of extremities with gangrene, left leg   CC HCC A

    I70.263 Atherosclerosis of native arteries of extremities with gangrene, bilateral legs   CC HCC A

    I70.268 Atherosclerosis of native arteries of extremities with gangrene, other extremity   CC HCC A

    I70.269 Atherosclerosis of native arteries of extremities with gangrene, unspecified extremity   CC HCC A

√6ᵗʰ I70.29 Other atherosclerosis of native arteries of extremities

    I70.291 Other atherosclerosis of native arteries of extremities, right leg   HCC A

    I70.292 Other atherosclerosis of native arteries of extremities, left leg   HCC A

    I70.293 Other atherosclerosis of native arteries of extremities, bilateral legs   HCC A

    I70.298 Other atherosclerosis of native arteries of extremities, other extremity   HCC A

    I70.299 Other atherosclerosis of native arteries of extremities, unspecified extremity   HCC A

✔ Additional Character Required   √x7ᵗʰ Placeholder   Questionable PDx   Manifestation   Unspecified Dx   UPD Unacceptable PDx   H1-H14 HAC   HCC CMS-HCC Dx   HIV HIV Dx

ICD-10-CM 2022   671

Chapter 9. Diseases of the Circulatory System

I70.3–I70.348

✓5ᵗʰ **I70.3** **Atherosclerosis of** unspecified type of bypass graft(s) **of the extremities**

Use additional code, if applicable, to identify chronic total occlusion of artery of extremity (I70.92)

EXCLUDES 1   embolism or thrombus of bypass graft(s) of extremities (T82.8-)

AHA: 2020,4Q,98

✓6ᵗʰ **I70.30** **Unspecified atherosclerosis of unspecified type of bypass graft(s) of the extremities**

I70.301 **Unspecified atherosclerosis of unspecified type of bypass graft(s) of the extremities,** right leg   HCC A

I70.302 **Unspecified atherosclerosis of unspecified type of bypass graft(s) of the extremities,** left leg   HCC A

I70.303 **Unspecified atherosclerosis of unspecified type of bypass graft(s) of the extremities,** bilateral legs   HCC A

I70.308 **Unspecified atherosclerosis of unspecified type of bypass graft(s) of the extremities,** other extremity   HCC A

I70.309 **Unspecified atherosclerosis of unspecified type of bypass graft(s) of the extremities, unspecified extremity**   HCC A

✓6ᵗʰ **I70.31** **Atherosclerosis of unspecified type of bypass graft(s) of the extremities with** intermittent claudication

I70.311 **Atherosclerosis of unspecified type of bypass graft(s) of the extremities with intermittent claudication,** right leg   HCC A

I70.312 **Atherosclerosis of unspecified type of bypass graft(s) of the extremities with intermittent claudication,** left leg   HCC A

I70.313 **Atherosclerosis of unspecified type of bypass graft(s) of the extremities with intermittent claudication,** bilateral legs   HCC A

I70.318 **Atherosclerosis of unspecified type of bypass graft(s) of the extremities with intermittent claudication, other extremity**   HCC A

I70.319 **Atherosclerosis of unspecified type of bypass graft(s) of the extremities with intermittent claudication, unspecified extremity**   HCC A

✓6ᵗʰ **I70.32** **Atherosclerosis of unspecified type of bypass graft(s) of the extremities with** rest pain

INCLUDES   any condition classifiable to I70.31-

chronic limb-threatening ischemia NOS of unspecified type of bypass graft(s) of the extremities

chronic limb-threatening ischemia of unspecified type of bypass graft(s) of the extremities with rest pain, right leg

critical limb ischemia NOS of unspecified type of bypass graft(s) of the extremities

critical limb ischemia of unspecified type of bypass graft(s) of the extremities with rest pain

I70.321 **Atherosclerosis of unspecified type of bypass graft(s) of the extremities with rest pain,** right leg   HCC A

I70.322 **Atherosclerosis of unspecified type of bypass graft(s) of the extremities with rest pain,** left leg   HCC A

I70.323 **Atherosclerosis of unspecified type of bypass graft(s) of the extremities with rest pain,** bilateral legs   HCC A

I70.328 **Atherosclerosis of unspecified type of bypass graft(s) of the extremities with rest pain, other extremity**   HCC A

I70.329 **Atherosclerosis of unspecified type of bypass graft(s) of the extremities with rest pain, unspecified extremity**   HCC A

✓6ᵗʰ **I70.33** **Atherosclerosis of unspecified type of bypass graft(s) of the** right leg **with** ulceration

INCLUDES   any condition classifiable to I70.311 and I70.321

chronic limb-threatening ischemia of unspecified type of bypass graft(s) of the right leg with ulceration

critical limb ischemia of unspecified type of bypass graft(s) of the right leg with ulceration

Use additional code to identify severity of ulcer (L97.-)

I70.331 **Atherosclerosis of unspecified type of bypass graft(s) of the right leg with ulceration of** thigh   CC HCC A

I70.332 **Atherosclerosis of unspecified type of bypass graft(s) of the right leg with ulceration of** calf   CC HCC A

I70.333 **Atherosclerosis of unspecified type of bypass graft(s) of the right leg with ulceration of** ankle   CC HCC A

I70.334 **Atherosclerosis of unspecified type of bypass graft(s) of the right leg with ulceration of** heel and midfoot   CC HCC A

Atherosclerosis of unspecified type of bypass graft(s) of right leg with ulceration of plantar surface of midfoot

I70.335 **Atherosclerosis of unspecified type of bypass graft(s) of the right leg with ulceration of other part of foot**   HCC A

Atherosclerosis of unspecified type of bypass graft(s) of the right leg with ulceration of toe

I70.338 **Atherosclerosis of unspecified type of bypass graft(s) of the right leg with ulceration of other part of lower leg**   CC HCC A

I70.339 **Atherosclerosis of unspecified type of bypass graft(s) of the right leg with ulceration of unspecified site**   CC HCC A

✓6ᵗʰ **I70.34** **Atherosclerosis of unspecified type of bypass graft(s) of the** left leg **with** ulceration

INCLUDES   any condition classifiable to I70.312 and I70.322

chronic limb-threatening ischemia of unspecified type of bypass graft(s) of the left leg with ulceration

critical limb ischemia of unspecified type of bypass graft(s) of the left leg with ulceration

Use additional code to identify severity of ulcer (L97.-)

I70.341 **Atherosclerosis of unspecified type of bypass graft(s) of the left leg with ulceration of** thigh   CC HCC A

I70.342 **Atherosclerosis of unspecified type of bypass graft(s) of the left leg with ulceration of** calf   CC HCC A

I70.343 **Atherosclerosis of unspecified type of bypass graft(s) of the left leg with ulceration of** ankle   CC HCC A

I70.344 **Atherosclerosis of unspecified type of bypass graft(s) of the left leg with ulceration of** heel and midfoot   CC HCC A

Atherosclerosis of unspecified type of bypass graft(s) of left leg with ulceration of plantar surface of midfoot

I70.345 **Atherosclerosis of unspecified type of bypass graft(s) of the left leg with ulceration of other part of foot**   HCC A

Atherosclerosis of unspecified type of bypass graft(s) of the left leg with ulceration of toe

I70.348 **Atherosclerosis of unspecified type of bypass graft(s) of the left leg with ulceration of other part of lower leg**   CC HCC A

N Newborn: 0   P Pediatric: 0-17   M Maternity: 9-64   A Adult: 15-124   MCC Major Complication/Comorbidity   CC Complication/Comorbidity   SW Severe Wound Dx

672

ICD-10-CM 2022

I70.349 Atherosclerosis of unspecified type of bypass graft(s) of the left leg with ulceration of unspecified site　CC HCC A

I70.35 Atherosclerosis of unspecified type of bypass graft(s) of other extremity with ulceration　HCC A
> INCLUDES any condition classifiable to I70.318 and I70.328
> Use additional code to identify severity of ulcer (L98.49-)

I70.36 Atherosclerosis of unspecified type of bypass graft(s) of the extremities with gangrene
> INCLUDES any condition classifiable to I70.31-, I70.32-, I70.33-, I70.34-, I70.35
> chronic limb-threatening ischemia of unspecified type of bypass graft(s) of the extremities with gangrene
> critical limb ischemia of unspecified type of bypass graft(s) of the extremities with gangrene
> Use additional code to identify the severity of any ulcer (L97.-, L98.49-), if applicable

I70.361 Atherosclerosis of unspecified type of bypass graft(s) of the extremities with gangrene, right leg　CC HCC A

I70.362 Atherosclerosis of unspecified type of bypass graft(s) of the extremities with gangrene, left leg　CC HCC A

I70.363 Atherosclerosis of unspecified type of bypass graft(s) of the extremities with gangrene, bilateral legs　CC HCC A

I70.368 Atherosclerosis of unspecified type of bypass graft(s) of the extremities with gangrene, other extremity　CC HCC A

I70.369 Atherosclerosis of unspecified type of bypass graft(s) of the extremities with gangrene, unspecified extremity　CC HCC A

I70.39 Other atherosclerosis of unspecified type of bypass graft(s) of the extremities

I70.391 Other atherosclerosis of unspecified type of bypass graft(s) of the extremities, right leg　HCC A

I70.392 Other atherosclerosis of unspecified type of bypass graft(s) of the extremities, left leg　HCC A

I70.393 Other atherosclerosis of unspecified type of bypass graft(s) of the extremities, bilateral legs　HCC A

I70.398 Other atherosclerosis of unspecified type of bypass graft(s) of the extremities, other extremity　HCC A

I70.399 Other atherosclerosis of unspecified type of bypass graft(s) of the extremities, unspecified extremity　HCC A

I70.4 Atherosclerosis of autologous vein bypass graft(s) of the extremities
> Use additional code, if applicable, to identify chronic total occlusion of artery of extremity (I70.92)
> AHA: 2020,4Q,98

I70.40 Unspecified atherosclerosis of autologous vein bypass graft(s) of the extremities

I70.401 Unspecified atherosclerosis of autologous vein bypass graft(s) of the extremities, right leg　HCC A

I70.402 Unspecified atherosclerosis of autologous vein bypass graft(s) of the extremities, left leg　HCC A

I70.403 Unspecified atherosclerosis of autologous vein bypass graft(s) of the extremities, bilateral legs　HCC A

I70.408 Unspecified atherosclerosis of autologous vein bypass graft(s) of the extremities, other extremity　HCC A

I70.409 Unspecified atherosclerosis of autologous vein bypass graft(s) of the extremities, unspecified extremity　HCC A

I70.41 Atherosclerosis of autologous vein bypass graft(s) of the extremities with intermittent claudication

I70.411 Atherosclerosis of autologous vein bypass graft(s) of the extremities with intermittent claudication, right leg　HCC A

I70.412 Atherosclerosis of autologous vein bypass graft(s) of the extremities with intermittent claudication, left leg　HCC A

I70.413 Atherosclerosis of autologous vein bypass graft(s) of the extremities with intermittent claudication, bilateral legs　HCC A

I70.418 Atherosclerosis of autologous vein bypass graft(s) of the extremities with intermittent claudication, other extremity　HCC A

I70.419 Atherosclerosis of autologous vein bypass graft(s) of the extremities with intermittent claudication, unspecified extremity　HCC A

I70.42 Atherosclerosis of autologous vein bypass graft(s) of the extremities with rest pain
> INCLUDES any condition classifiable to I70.41-
> chronic limb-threatening ischemia NOS of autologous vein bypass graft(s) of the extremities
> chronic limb-threatening ischemia of autologous vein bypass graft(s) of the extremities with rest pain
> critical limb ischemia NOS of autologous vein bypass graft(s) of the extremities
> critical limb ischemia of autologous vein bypass graft(s) of the extremities with rest pain

I70.421 Atherosclerosis of autologous vein bypass graft(s) of the extremities with rest pain, right leg　HCC A

I70.422 Atherosclerosis of autologous vein bypass graft(s) of the extremities with rest pain, left leg　HCC A

I70.423 Atherosclerosis of autologous vein bypass graft(s) of the extremities with rest pain, bilateral legs　HCC A

I70.428 Atherosclerosis of autologous vein bypass graft(s) of the extremities with rest pain, other extremity　HCC A

I70.429 Atherosclerosis of autologous vein bypass graft(s) of the extremities with rest pain, unspecified extremity　HCC A

I70.43 Atherosclerosis of autologous vein bypass graft(s) of the right leg with ulceration
> INCLUDES any condition classifiable to I70.411 and I70.421
> chronic limb-threatening ischemia of autologous vein bypass graft(s) of the right leg with ulceration
> critical limb ischemia of autologous vein bypass graft(s) of the right leg with ulceration
> Use additional code to identify severity of ulcer (L97.-)

I70.431 Atherosclerosis of autologous vein bypass graft(s) of the right leg with ulceration of thigh　CC HCC A

I70.432 Atherosclerosis of autologous vein bypass graft(s) of the right leg with ulceration of calf　CC HCC A

I70.433 Atherosclerosis of autologous vein bypass graft(s) of the right leg with ulceration of ankle　CC HCC A

I70.434 Atherosclerosis of autologous vein bypass graft(s) of the right leg with ulceration of heel and midfoot　CC HCC A
> Atherosclerosis of autologous vein bypass graft(s) of right leg with ulceration of plantar surface of midfoot

Chapter 9. Diseases of the Circulatory System

I70.435–I70.519

I70.435 Atherosclerosis of autologous vein bypass graft(s) of the right leg with ulceration of other part of foot `HCC` `A`
    Atherosclerosis of autologous vein bypass graft(s) of right leg with ulceration of toe

I70.438 Atherosclerosis of autologous vein bypass graft(s) of the right leg with ulceration of other part of lower leg `CC` `HCC` `A`

I70.439 Atherosclerosis of autologous vein bypass graft(s) of the right leg with ulceration of unspecified site `CC` `HCC` `A`

√6ᵗʰ **I70.44** Atherosclerosis of autologous vein bypass graft(s) of the left leg with ulceration
    [INCLUDES] any condition classifiable to I70.412 and I70.422
    chronic limb-threatening ischemia of autologous vein bypass graft(s) of the left leg with ulceration
    critical limb ischemia of autologous vein bypass graft(s) of the left leg with ulceration
    Use additional code to identify severity of ulcer (L97.-)

I70.441 Atherosclerosis of autologous vein bypass graft(s) of the left leg with ulceration of thigh `CC` `HCC` `A`

I70.442 Atherosclerosis of autologous vein bypass graft(s) of the left leg with ulceration of calf `CC` `HCC` `A`

I70.443 Atherosclerosis of autologous vein bypass graft(s) of the left leg with ulceration of ankle `CC` `HCC` `A`

I70.444 Atherosclerosis of autologous vein bypass graft(s) of the left leg with ulceration of heel and midfoot `CC` `HCC` `A`
    Atherosclerosis of autologous vein bypass graft(s) of left leg with ulceration of plantar surface of midfoot

I70.445 Atherosclerosis of autologous vein bypass graft(s) of the left leg with ulceration of other part of foot `HCC` `A`
    Atherosclerosis of autologous vein bypass graft(s) of left leg with ulceration of toe

I70.448 Atherosclerosis of autologous vein bypass graft(s) of the left leg with ulceration of other part of lower leg `CC` `HCC` `A`

I70.449 Atherosclerosis of autologous vein bypass graft(s) of the left leg with ulceration of unspecified site `CC` `HCC` `A`

I70.45 Atherosclerosis of autologous vein bypass graft(s) of other extremity with ulceration `HCC` `A`
    [INCLUDES] any condition classifiable to I70.418, I70.428, and I70.438
    Use additional code to identify severity of ulcer (L98.49)

√6ᵗʰ **I70.46** Atherosclerosis of autologous vein bypass graft(s) of the extremities with gangrene
    [INCLUDES] any condition classifiable to I70.41-, I70.42-, and I70.43-, I70.44-, I70.45
    chronic limb-threatening ischemia of autologous vein bypass graft(s) of the extremities with gangrene
    critical limb ischemia of autologous vein bypass graft(s) of the extremities with gangrene
    Use additional code to identify the severity of any ulcer (L97.-, L98.49-), if applicable

I70.461 Atherosclerosis of autologous vein bypass graft(s) of the extremities with gangrene, right leg `CC` `HCC` `A`

I70.462 Atherosclerosis of autologous vein bypass graft(s) of the extremities with gangrene, left leg `CC` `HCC` `A`

I70.463 Atherosclerosis of autologous vein bypass graft(s) of the extremities with gangrene, bilateral legs `CC` `HCC` `A`

I70.468 Atherosclerosis of autologous vein bypass graft(s) of the extremities with gangrene, other extremity `CC` `HCC` `A`

I70.469 Atherosclerosis of autologous vein bypass graft(s) of the extremities with gangrene, unspecified extremity `CC` `HCC` `A`

√6ᵗʰ **I70.49** Other atherosclerosis of autologous vein bypass graft(s) of the extremities

I70.491 Other atherosclerosis of autologous vein bypass graft(s) of the extremities, right leg `HCC` `A`

I70.492 Other atherosclerosis of autologous vein bypass graft(s) of the extremities, left leg `HCC` `A`

I70.493 Other atherosclerosis of autologous vein bypass graft(s) of the extremities, bilateral legs `HCC` `A`

I70.498 Other atherosclerosis of autologous vein bypass graft(s) of the extremities, other extremity `HCC` `A`

I70.499 Other atherosclerosis of autologous vein bypass graft(s) of the extremities, unspecified extremity `HCC` `A`

√5ᵗʰ **I70.5** Atherosclerosis of nonautologous biological bypass graft(s) of the extremities
    Use additional code, if applicable, to identify chronic total occlusion of artery of extremity (I70.92)
    AHA: 2020,4Q,98

√6ᵗʰ **I70.50** Unspecified atherosclerosis of nonautologous biological bypass graft(s) of the extremities

I70.501 Unspecified atherosclerosis of nonautologous biological bypass graft(s) of the extremities, right leg `HCC` `A`

I70.502 Unspecified atherosclerosis of nonautologous biological bypass graft(s) of the extremities, left leg `HCC` `A`

I70.503 Unspecified atherosclerosis of nonautologous biological bypass graft(s) of the extremities, bilateral legs `HCC` `A`

I70.508 Unspecified atherosclerosis of nonautologous biological bypass graft(s) of the extremities, other extremity `HCC` `A`

I70.509 Unspecified atherosclerosis of nonautologous biological bypass graft(s) of the extremities, unspecified extremity `HCC` `A`

√6ᵗʰ **I70.51** Atherosclerosis of nonautologous biological bypass graft(s) of the extremities intermittent claudication

I70.511 Atherosclerosis of nonautologous biological bypass graft(s) of the extremities with intermittent claudication, right leg `HCC` `A`

I70.512 Atherosclerosis of nonautologous biological bypass graft(s) of the extremities with intermittent claudication, left leg `HCC` `A`

I70.513 Atherosclerosis of nonautologous biological bypass graft(s) of the extremities with intermittent claudication, bilateral legs `HCC` `A`

I70.518 Atherosclerosis of nonautologous biological bypass graft(s) of the extremities with intermittent claudication, other extremity `HCC` `A`

I70.519 Atherosclerosis of nonautologous biological bypass graft(s) of the extremities with intermittent claudication, unspecified extremity `HCC` `A`

✓6ᵗʰ **I70.52** **Atherosclerosis of nonautologous biological bypass graft(s) of the extremities with** rest pain

INCLUDES any condition classifiable to I70.51-

chronic limb-threatening ischemia NOS of nonautologous biological bypass graft(s) of the extremities

chronic limb-threatening ischemia of nonautologous biological bypass graft(s) of the extremities with rest pain

critical limb ischemia NOS of nonautologous biological bypass graft(s) of the extremities

critical limb ischemia of nonautologous biological bypass graft(s) of the extremities with rest pain

I70.521 **Atherosclerosis of nonautologous biological bypass graft(s) of the extremities with rest pain,** right leg HCC A

I70.522 **Atherosclerosis of nonautologous biological bypass graft(s) of the extremities with rest pain,** left leg HCC A

I70.523 **Atherosclerosis of nonautologous biological bypass graft(s) of the extremities with rest pain,** bilateral legs HCC A

I70.528 **Atherosclerosis of nonautologous biological bypass graft(s) of the extremities with rest pain, other extremity** HCC A

I70.529 **Atherosclerosis of nonautologous biological bypass graft(s) of the extremities with rest pain, unspecified extremity** HCC A

✓6ᵗʰ **I70.53** **Atherosclerosis of nonautologous biological bypass graft(s) of the** right leg **with** ulceration

INCLUDES any condition classifiable to I70.511 and I70.521

chronic limb-threatening ischemia of nonautologous biological bypass graft(s) of the right leg with ulceration

critical limb ischemia of nonautologous biological bypass graft(s) of the right leg with ulceration

Use additional code to identify severity of ulcer (L97.-)

I70.531 **Atherosclerosis of nonautologous biological bypass graft(s) of the right leg with ulceration of** thigh CC HCC A

I70.532 **Atherosclerosis of nonautologous biological bypass graft(s) of the right leg with ulceration of** calf CC HCC A

I70.533 **Atherosclerosis of nonautologous biological bypass graft(s) of the right leg with ulceration of** ankle CC HCC A

I70.534 **Atherosclerosis of nonautologous biological bypass graft(s) of the right leg with ulceration of** heel and midfoot CC HCC A

Atherosclerosis of nonautologous biological bypass graft(s) of right leg with ulceration of plantar surface of midfoot

I70.535 **Atherosclerosis of nonautologous biological bypass graft(s) of the right leg with ulceration of other part of foot** HCC A

Atherosclerosis of nonautologous biological bypass graft(s) of the right leg with ulceration of toe

I70.538 **Atherosclerosis of nonautologous biological bypass graft(s) of the right leg with ulceration of other part of lower leg** CC HCC A

I70.539 **Atherosclerosis of nonautologous biological bypass graft(s) of the right leg with ulceration of unspecified site** CC HCC A

✓6ᵗʰ **I70.54** **Atherosclerosis of nonautologous biological bypass graft(s) of the** left leg **with** ulceration

INCLUDES any condition classifiable to I70.512 and I70.522

chronic limb-threatening ischemia of nonautologous biological bypass graft(s) of the left leg with ulceration

critical limb ischemia of nonautologous biological bypass graft(s) of the left leg with ulceration

Use additional code to identify severity of ulcer (L97.-)

I70.541 **Atherosclerosis of nonautologous biological bypass graft(s) of the left leg with ulceration of** thigh CC HCC A

I70.542 **Atherosclerosis of nonautologous biological bypass graft(s) of the left leg with ulceration of** calf CC HCC A

I70.543 **Atherosclerosis of nonautologous biological bypass graft(s) of the left leg with ulceration of** ankle CC HCC A

I70.544 **Atherosclerosis of nonautologous biological bypass graft(s) of the left leg with ulceration of** heel and midfoot CC HCC A

Atherosclerosis of nonautologous biological bypass graft(s) of left leg with ulceration of plantar surface of midfoot

I70.545 **Atherosclerosis of nonautologous biological bypass graft(s) of the left leg with ulceration of other part of foot** HCC A

Atherosclerosis of nonautologous biological bypass graft(s) of the left leg with ulceration of toe

I70.548 **Atherosclerosis of nonautologous biological bypass graft(s) of the left leg with ulceration of other part of lower leg** CC HCC A

I70.549 **Atherosclerosis of nonautologous biological bypass graft(s) of the left leg with ulceration of unspecified site** CC HCC A

I70.55 **Atherosclerosis of nonautologous biological bypass graft(s) of other extremity with** ulceration HCC A

INCLUDES any condition classifiable to I70.518, I70.528, and I70.538

Use additional code to identify severity of ulcer (L98.49)

✓6ᵗʰ **I70.56** **Atherosclerosis of nonautologous biological bypass graft(s) of the extremities with** gangrene

INCLUDES any condition classifiable to I70.51-, I70.52-, and I70.53-, I70.54-, I70.55

chronic limb-threatening ischemia of nonautologous biological bypass graft(s) of the extremities with gangrene

critical limb ischemia of nonautologous biological bypass graft(s) of the extremities with gangrene

Use additional code to identify the severity of any ulcer (L97.-, L98.49-), if applicable

I70.561 **Atherosclerosis of nonautologous biological bypass graft(s) of the extremities with gangrene,** right leg CC HCC A

I70.562 **Atherosclerosis of nonautologous biological bypass graft(s) of the extremities with gangrene,** left leg CC HCC A

I70.563 **Atherosclerosis of nonautologous biological bypass graft(s) of the extremities with gangrene,** bilateral legs CC HCC A

I70.568 **Atherosclerosis of nonautologous biological bypass graft(s) of the extremities with gangrene, other extremity** CC HCC A

✓ Additional Character Required   ✓x7ᵗʰ Placeholder   Questionable PDx   ■ Manifestation   Unspecified Dx   UPD Unacceptable PDx   H1-H14 HAC   HCC CMS-HCC Dx   HIV HIV Dx

ICD-10-CM 2022   675

    I70.569   Atherosclerosis of nonautologous biological bypass graft(s) of the extremities with gangrene, unspecified extremity   `CC` `HCC` `A`

✓6ᵗʰ **I70.59**   Other atherosclerosis of nonautologous biological bypass graft(s) of the extremities

    I70.591   Other atherosclerosis of nonautologous biological bypass graft(s) of the extremities, right leg   `HCC` `A`

    I70.592   Other atherosclerosis of nonautologous biological bypass graft(s) of the extremities, left leg   `HCC` `A`

    I70.593   Other atherosclerosis of nonautologous biological bypass graft(s) of the extremities, bilateral legs   `HCC` `A`

    I70.598   Other atherosclerosis of nonautologous biological bypass graft(s) of the extremities, other extremity   `HCC` `A`

    I70.599   Other atherosclerosis of nonautologous biological bypass graft(s) of the extremities, unspecified extremity   `HCC` `A`

✓6ᵗʰ **I70.6**   Atherosclerosis of nonbiological bypass graft(s) of the extremities

Use additional code, if applicable, to identify chronic total occlusion of artery of extremity (I70.92)

AHA: 2020,4Q,98

✓6ᵗʰ **I70.60**   Unspecified atherosclerosis of nonbiological bypass graft(s) of the extremities

    I70.601   Unspecified atherosclerosis of nonbiological bypass graft(s) of the extremities, right leg   `HCC` `A`

    I70.602   Unspecified atherosclerosis of nonbiological bypass graft(s) of the extremities, left leg   `HCC` `A`

    I70.603   Unspecified atherosclerosis of nonbiological bypass graft(s) of the extremities, bilateral legs   `HCC` `A`

    I70.608   Unspecified atherosclerosis of nonbiological bypass graft(s) of the extremities, other extremity   `HCC` `A`

    I70.609   Unspecified atherosclerosis of nonbiological bypass graft(s) of the extremities, unspecified extremity   `HCC` `A`

✓6ᵗʰ **I70.61**   Atherosclerosis of nonbiological bypass graft(s) of the extremities with intermittent claudication

    I70.611   Atherosclerosis of nonbiological bypass graft(s) of the extremities with intermittent claudication, right leg   `HCC` `A`

    I70.612   Atherosclerosis of nonbiological bypass graft(s) of the extremities with intermittent claudication, left leg   `HCC` `A`

    I70.613   Atherosclerosis of nonbiological bypass graft(s) of the extremities with intermittent claudication, bilateral legs   `HCC` `A`

    I70.618   Atherosclerosis of nonbiological bypass graft(s) of the extremities with intermittent claudication, other extremity   `HCC` `A`

    I70.619   Atherosclerosis of nonbiological bypass graft(s) of the extremities with intermittent claudication, unspecified extremity   `HCC` `A`

✓6ᵗʰ **I70.62**   Atherosclerosis of nonbiological bypass graft(s) of the extremities with rest pain

INCLUDES   any condition classifiable to I70.61-

chronic limb-threatening ischemia NOS of nonbiological bypass graft(s) of the extremities

chronic limb-threatening ischemia of nonbiological bypass graft(s) of the extremities with rest pain

critical limb ischemia NOS of nonbiological bypass graft(s) of the extremities

critical limb ischemia of nonbiological bypass graft(s) of the extremities with rest pain

    I70.621   Atherosclerosis of nonbiological bypass graft(s) of the extremities with rest pain, right leg   `HCC` `A`

    I70.622   Atherosclerosis of nonbiological bypass graft(s) of the extremities with rest pain, left leg   `HCC` `A`

    I70.623   Atherosclerosis of nonbiological bypass graft(s) of the extremities with rest pain, bilateral legs   `HCC` `A`

    I70.628   Atherosclerosis of nonbiological bypass graft(s) of the extremities with rest pain, other extremity   `HCC` `A`

    I70.629   Atherosclerosis of nonbiological bypass graft(s) of the extremities with rest pain, unspecified extremity   `HCC` `A`

✓6ᵗʰ **I70.63**   Atherosclerosis of nonbiological bypass graft(s) of the right leg with ulceration

INCLUDES   any condition classifiable to I70.611 and I70.621

chronic limb-threatening ischemia of nonbiological bypass graft(s) of the right leg with ulceration

critical limb ischemia of nonbiological bypass graft(s) of the right leg with ulceration

Use additional code to identify severity of ulcer (L97.-)

    I70.631   Atherosclerosis of nonbiological bypass graft(s) of the right leg with ulceration of thigh   `CC` `HCC` `A`

    I70.632   Atherosclerosis of nonbiological bypass graft(s) of the right leg with ulceration of calf   `CC` `HCC` `A`

    I70.633   Atherosclerosis of nonbiological bypass graft(s) of the right leg with ulceration of ankle   `CC` `HCC` `A`

    I70.634   Atherosclerosis of nonbiological bypass graft(s) of the right leg with ulceration of heel and midfoot   `CC` `HCC` `A`

Atherosclerosis of nonbiological bypass graft(s) of right leg with ulceration of plantar surface of midfoot

    I70.635   Atherosclerosis of nonbiological bypass graft(s) of the right leg with ulceration of other part of foot   `HCC` `A`

Atherosclerosis of nonbiological bypass graft(s) of the right leg with ulceration of toe

    I70.638   Atherosclerosis of nonbiological bypass graft(s) of the right leg with ulceration of other part of lower leg   `CC` `HCC` `A`

    I70.639   Atherosclerosis of nonbiological bypass graft(s) of the right leg with ulceration of unspecified site   `CC` `HCC` `A`

N Newborn: 0   P Pediatric: 0-17   M Maternity: 9-64   A Adult: 15-124   MCC Major Complication/Comorbidity   CC Complication/Comorbidity   SW Severe Wound Dx

676   ICD-10-CM 2022

✓6th I70.64 **Atherosclerosis of nonbiological bypass graft(s) of the left leg with ulceration**

 INCLUDES any condition classifiable to I70.612 and I70.622

 chronic limb-threatening ischemia of nonbiological bypass graft(s) of the left leg with ulceration

 critical limb ischemia of nonbiological bypass graft(s) of the left leg with ulceration

 Use additional code to identify severity of ulcer (L97.-)

 I70.641 **Atherosclerosis of nonbiological bypass graft(s) of the left leg with ulceration of thigh** CC HCC A

 I70.642 **Atherosclerosis of nonbiological bypass graft(s) of the left leg with ulceration of calf** CC HCC A

 I70.643 **Atherosclerosis of nonbiological bypass graft(s) of the left leg with ulceration of ankle** CC HCC A

 I70.644 **Atherosclerosis of nonbiological bypass graft(s) of the left leg with ulceration of heel and midfoot** CC HCC A

 Atherosclerosis of nonbiological bypass graft(s) of left leg with ulceration of plantar surface of midfoot

 I70.645 **Atherosclerosis of nonbiological bypass graft(s) of the left leg with ulceration of other part of foot** HCC A

 Atherosclerosis of nonbiological bypass graft(s) of the left leg with ulceration of toe

 I70.648 **Atherosclerosis of nonbiological bypass graft(s) of the left leg with ulceration of other part of lower leg** CC HCC A

 I70.649 **Atherosclerosis of nonbiological bypass graft(s) of the left leg with ulceration of unspecified site** CC HCC A

 I70.65 **Atherosclerosis of nonbiological bypass graft(s) of other extremity with ulceration** HCC A

 INCLUDES any condition classifiable to I70.618 and I70.628

 Use additional code to identify severity of ulcer (L98.49)

✓6th I70.66 **Atherosclerosis of nonbiological bypass graft(s) of the extremities with gangrene**

 INCLUDES any condition classifiable to I70.61-, I70.62-, I70.63-, I70.64-, I70.65

 chronic limb-threatening ischemia of nonbiological bypass graft(s) of the extremities with gangrene

 critical limb ischemia of nonbiological bypass graft(s) of the extremities with gangrene

 Use additional code to identify the severity of any ulcer (L97.-, L98.49-), if applicable

 I70.661 **Atherosclerosis of nonbiological bypass graft(s) of the extremities with gangrene, right leg** CC HCC A

 I70.662 **Atherosclerosis of nonbiological bypass graft(s) of the extremities with gangrene, left leg** CC HCC A

 I70.663 **Atherosclerosis of nonbiological bypass graft(s) of the extremities with gangrene, bilateral legs** CC HCC A

 I70.668 **Atherosclerosis of nonbiological bypass graft(s) of the extremities with gangrene, other extremity** CC HCC A

 I70.669 **Atherosclerosis of nonbiological bypass graft(s) of the extremities with gangrene, unspecified extremity** CC HCC A

✓6th I70.69 **Other atherosclerosis of nonbiological bypass graft(s) of the extremities**

 I70.691 **Other atherosclerosis of nonbiological bypass graft(s) of the extremities, right leg** HCC A

 I70.692 **Other atherosclerosis of nonbiological bypass graft(s) of the extremities, left leg** HCC A

 I70.693 **Other atherosclerosis of nonbiological bypass graft(s) of the extremities, bilateral legs** HCC A

 I70.698 **Other atherosclerosis of nonbiological bypass graft(s) of the extremities, other extremity** HCC A

 I70.699 **Other atherosclerosis of nonbiological bypass graft(s) of the extremities, unspecified extremity** HCC A

✓5th I70.7 **Atherosclerosis of other type of bypass graft(s) of the extremities**

 Use additional code, if applicable, to identify chronic total occlusion of artery of extremity (I70.92)

 AHA: 2020,4Q,98

✓6th I70.70 **Unspecified atherosclerosis of other type of bypass graft(s) of the extremities**

 I70.701 **Unspecified atherosclerosis of other type of bypass graft(s) of the extremities, right leg** HCC A

 I70.702 **Unspecified atherosclerosis of other type of bypass graft(s) of the extremities, left leg** HCC A

 I70.703 **Unspecified atherosclerosis of other type of bypass graft(s) of the extremities, bilateral legs** HCC A

 I70.708 **Unspecified atherosclerosis of other type of bypass graft(s) of the extremities, other extremity** HCC A

 I70.709 **Unspecified atherosclerosis of other type of bypass graft(s) of the extremities, unspecified extremity** HCC A

✓6th I70.71 **Atherosclerosis of other type of bypass graft(s) of the extremities with intermittent claudication**

 I70.711 **Atherosclerosis of other type of bypass graft(s) of the extremities with intermittent claudication, right leg** HCC A

 I70.712 **Atherosclerosis of other type of bypass graft(s) of the extremities with intermittent claudication, left leg** HCC A

 I70.713 **Atherosclerosis of other type of bypass graft(s) of the extremities with intermittent claudication, bilateral legs** HCC A

 I70.718 **Atherosclerosis of other type of bypass graft(s) of the extremities with intermittent claudication, other extremity** HCC A

 I70.719 **Atherosclerosis of other type of bypass graft(s) of the extremities with intermittent claudication, unspecified extremity** HCC A

✓6th I70.72 **Atherosclerosis of other type of bypass graft(s) of the extremities with rest pain**

 INCLUDES any condition classifiable to I70.71-

 chronic limb-threatening ischemia NOS of other type of bypass graft(s) of the extremities

 chronic limb-threatening ischemia of other type of bypass graft(s) of the extremities with rest pain

 critical limb ischemia NOS of other type of bypass graft(s) of the extremities

 critical limb ischemia of other type of bypass graft(s) of the extremities with rest pain

 I70.721 **Atherosclerosis of other type of bypass graft(s) of the extremities with rest pain, right leg** HCC A

 I70.722 **Atherosclerosis of other type of bypass graft(s) of the extremities with rest pain, left leg** HCC A

 I70.723 **Atherosclerosis of other type of bypass graft(s) of the extremities with rest pain, bilateral legs** HCC A

 I70.728 **Atherosclerosis of other type of bypass graft(s) of the extremities with rest pain, other extremity** HCC A

 I70.729 **Atherosclerosis of other type of bypass graft(s) of the extremities with rest pain, unspecified extremity** HCC A

✔ Additional Character Required   ✓x7th Placeholder   Questionable PDx   Manifestation   Unspecified Dx   UPD Unacceptable PDx   H1-H14 HAC   HCC CMS-HCC Dx   HIV HIV Dx

ICD-10-CM 2022   677

Chapter 9. Diseases of the Circulatory System

✓6ᵗʰ **I70.73 Atherosclerosis of other type of bypass graft(s) of the right leg with ulceration**

> INCLUDES   any condition classifiable to I70.711 and I70.721
>
> chronic limb-threatening ischemia of other type of bypass graft(s) of the right leg with ulceration
>
> critical limb ischemia of other type of bypass graft(s) of the right leg with ulceration

Use additional code to identify severity of ulcer (L97.-)

I70.731 Atherosclerosis of other type of bypass graft(s) of the right leg with ulceration of thigh CC HCC A

I70.732 Atherosclerosis of other type of bypass graft(s) of the right leg with ulceration of calf CC HCC A

I70.733 Atherosclerosis of other type of bypass graft(s) of the right leg with ulceration of ankle CC HCC A

I70.734 Atherosclerosis of other type of bypass graft(s) of the right leg with ulceration of heel and midfoot CC HCC A

> Atherosclerosis of other type of bypass graft(s) of right leg with ulceration of plantar surface of midfoot

I70.735 Atherosclerosis of other type of bypass graft(s) of the right leg with ulceration of other part of foot HCC A

> Atherosclerosis of other type of bypass graft(s) of right leg with ulceration of toe

I70.738 Atherosclerosis of other type of bypass graft(s) of the right leg with ulceration of other part of lower leg CC HCC A

I70.739 Atherosclerosis of other type of bypass graft(s) of the right leg with ulceration of unspecified site CC HCC A

✓6ᵗʰ **I70.74 Atherosclerosis of other type of bypass graft(s) of the left leg with ulceration**

> INCLUDES   any condition classifiable to I70.712 and I70.722
>
> chronic limb-threatening ischemia of other type of bypass graft(s) of the left leg with ulceration
>
> critical limb ischemia of other type of bypass graft(s) of the left leg with ulceration

Use additional code to identify severity of ulcer (L97.-)

I70.741 Atherosclerosis of other type of bypass graft(s) of the left leg with ulceration of thigh CC HCC A

I70.742 Atherosclerosis of other type of bypass graft(s) of the left leg with ulceration of calf CC HCC A

I70.743 Atherosclerosis of other type of bypass graft(s) of the left leg with ulceration of ankle CC HCC A

I70.744 Atherosclerosis of other type of bypass graft(s) of the left leg with ulceration of heel and midfoot CC HCC A

> Atherosclerosis of other type of bypass graft(s) of left leg with ulceration of plantar surface of midfoot

I70.745 Atherosclerosis of other type of bypass graft(s) of the left leg with ulceration of other part of foot HCC A

> Atherosclerosis of other type of bypass graft(s) of left leg with ulceration of toe

I70.748 Atherosclerosis of other type of bypass graft(s) of the left leg with ulceration of other part of lower leg CC HCC A

I70.749 Atherosclerosis of other type of bypass graft(s) of the left leg with ulceration of unspecified site CC HCC A

✓6ᵗʰ **I70.75 Atherosclerosis of other type of bypass graft(s) of other extremity with ulceration** HCC A

> INCLUDES   any condition classifiable to I70.718 and I70.728

Use additional code to identify severity of ulcer (L98.49)

✓6ᵗʰ **I70.76 Atherosclerosis of other type of bypass graft(s) of the extremities with gangrene**

> INCLUDES   any condition classifiable to I70.71-, I70.72-, I70.73-, I70.74-, I70.75
>
> chronic limb-threatening ischemia of other type of bypass graft(s) of the extremities with gangrene
>
> critical limb ischemia of other type of bypass graft(s) of the extremities with gangrene

Use additional code to identify the severity of any ulcer (L97.-, L98.49-), if applicable

I70.761 Atherosclerosis of other type of bypass graft(s) of the extremities with gangrene, right leg CC HCC A

I70.762 Atherosclerosis of other type of bypass graft(s) of the extremities with gangrene, left leg CC HCC A

I70.763 Atherosclerosis of other type of bypass graft(s) of the extremities with gangrene, bilateral legs CC HCC A

I70.768 Atherosclerosis of other type of bypass graft(s) of the extremities with gangrene, other extremity CC HCC A

I70.769 Atherosclerosis of other type of bypass graft(s) of the extremities with gangrene, unspecified extremity CC HCC A

✓6ᵗʰ **I70.79 Other atherosclerosis of other type of bypass graft(s) of the extremities**

I70.791 Other atherosclerosis of other type of bypass graft(s) of the extremities, right leg HCC A

I70.792 Other atherosclerosis of other type of bypass graft(s) of the extremities, left leg HCC A

I70.793 Other atherosclerosis of other type of bypass graft(s) of the extremities, bilateral legs HCC A

I70.798 Other atherosclerosis of other type of bypass graft(s) of the extremities, other extremity HCC A

I70.799 Other atherosclerosis of other type of bypass graft(s) of the extremities, unspecified extremity HCC A

I70.8 Atherosclerosis of other arteries A

> **TIP:** Arteriosclerosis of the iliac arteries is coded here.

✓5ᵗʰ **I70.9 Other and unspecified atherosclerosis**

I70.90 Unspecified atherosclerosis A

I70.91 Generalized atherosclerosis A

I70.92 Chronic total occlusion of artery of the extremities CC UPD HCC A

> Complete occlusion of artery of the extremities
>
> Total occlusion of artery of the extremities
>
> Code first atherosclerosis of arteries of the extremities (I70.2-, I70.3-, I70.4-, I70.5-, I70.6-, I70.7-)

✓4ᵗʰ **I71 Aortic aneurysm and dissection**

> EXCLUDES 1   aortic ectasia (I77.81-)
>
> syphilitic aortic aneurysm (A52.01)
>
> traumatic aortic aneurysm (S25.09, S35.09)

✓5ᵗʰ **I71.0 Dissection of aorta**

I71.00 Dissection of unspecified site of aorta MCC HCC

I71.01 Dissection of thoracic aorta MCC HCC

I71.02 Dissection of abdominal aorta MCC HCC

I71.03 Dissection of thoracoabdominal aorta MCC HCC

I71.1 Thoracic aortic aneurysm, ruptured MCC HCC

I71.2 Thoracic aortic aneurysm, without rupture HCC

I71.3 Abdominal aortic aneurysm, ruptured MCC HCC

I71.4 Abdominal aortic aneurysm, without rupture HCC

I71.5 Thoracoabdominal aortic aneurysm, ruptured MCC HCC

I71.6 Thoracoabdominal aortic aneurysm, without rupture HCC

N Newborn: 0   P Pediatric: 0-17   M Maternity: 9-64   A Adult: 15-124   MCC Major Complication/Comorbidity   CC Complication/Comorbidity   SW Severe Wound Dx

678

ICD-10-CM 2022

I71.8   **Aortic aneurysm of unspecified site, ruptured**   `MCC` `HCC`
Rupture of aorta NOS

I71.9   **Aortic aneurysm of unspecified site, without rupture**   `HCC`
Aneurysm of aorta
Dilatation of aorta
Hyaline necrosis of aorta

✓4ᵗʰ I72   Other aneurysm

`INCLUDES`   aneurysm (cirsoid) (false) (ruptured)
`EXCLUDES 2`   acquired aneurysm (I77.Ø)
     aneurysm (of) aorta (I71.-)
     aneurysm (of) arteriovenous NOS (Q27.3-)
     carotid artery dissection (I77.71)
     cerebral (nonruptured) aneurysm (I67.1)
     coronary aneurysm (I25.4)
     coronary artery dissection (I25.42)
     dissection of artery NEC (I77.79)
     dissection of precerebral artery, congenital (nonruptured) (Q28.1)
     heart aneurysm (I25.3)
     iliac artery dissection (I77.72)
     precerebral artery, congential (nonruptured) (Q28.1)
     pulmonary artery aneurysm (I28.1)
     renal artery dissection (I77.73)
     retinal aneurysm (H35.Ø)
     ruptured cerebral aneurysm (I60.7)
     varicose aneurysm (I77.Ø)
     vertebral artery dissection (I77.74)
AHA: 2016,4Q,28-29

I72.Ø   **Aneurysm of carotid artery**   `HCC`
Aneurysm of common carotid artery
Aneurysm of external carotid artery
Aneurysm of internal carotid artery, extracranial portion
`EXCLUDES 1`   aneurysm of internal carotid artery, intracranial portion (I67.1)
     aneurysm of internal carotid artery NOS (I67.1)

I72.1   **Aneurysm of artery of upper extremity**   `HCC`

I72.2   **Aneurysm of renal artery**   `HCC`

I72.3   **Aneurysm of iliac artery**   `HCC`

I72.4   **Aneurysm of artery of lower extremity**   `HCC`
AHA: 2019,2Q,21

I72.5   **Aneurysm of other precerebral arteries**   `HCC`
Aneurysm of basilar artery (trunk)
`EXCLUDES 2`   aneurysm of carotid artery (I72.Ø)
     aneurysm of vertebral artery (I72.6)
     dissection of carotid artery (I77.71)
     dissection of other precerebral arteries (I77.75)
     dissection of vertebral artery (I77.74)

I72.6   **Aneurysm of vertebral artery**   `HCC`
`EXCLUDES 2`   dissection of vertebral artery (I77.74)

I72.8   **Aneurysm of other specified arteries**   `HCC`

I72.9   **Aneurysm of unspecified site**   `HCC`

Aneurysm

Outer layer
Layers of muscular and elastic tissue
Inner layer
Aneurysm

✓4ᵗʰ I73   Other peripheral vascular diseases

`EXCLUDES 2`   chilblains (T69.1)
     frostbite (T33-T34)
     immersion hand or foot (T69.Ø-)
     spasm of cerebral artery (G45.9)
AHA: 2018,4Q,87

✓5ᵗʰ I73.Ø   Raynaud's syndrome

Raynaud's disease
Raynaud's phenomenon (secondary)
DEF: Constriction of the arteries of the digits caused by cold or by nerve or arterial damage and can be prompted by stress or emotion. Blood cannot reach the skin and soft tissues and the skin turns white with blue mottling.

I73.ØØ   **Raynaud's syndrome without gangrene**

I73.Ø1   **Raynaud's syndrome with gangrene**   `CC` `HCC`

I73.1   **Thromboangiitis obliterans [Buerger's disease]**   `HCC`
DEF: Inflammatory disease of the extremity blood vessels, mainly the lower blood vessels. This disease is associated with heavy tobacco use. The arteries are more affected than veins. It occurs primarily in young men and leads to tissue ischemia and gangrene.

✓5ᵗʰ I73.8   Other specified peripheral vascular diseases

`EXCLUDES 1`   diabetic (peripheral) angiopathy (EØ8-E13 with .51-.52)

I73.81   **Erythromelalgia**   `HCC`

I73.89   **Other specified peripheral vascular diseases**   `HCC`
Acrocyanosis
Erythrocyanosis
Simple acroparesthesia [Schultze's type]
Vasomotor acroparesthesia [Nothnagel's type]

I73.9   **Peripheral vascular disease, unspecified**   `HCC`
Intermittent claudication
Peripheral angiopathy NOS
Spasm of artery
`EXCLUDES 1`   atherosclerosis of the extremities (I70.2-I70.7-)
AHA: 2018,2Q,7

✓4ᵗʰ I74   Arterial embolism and thrombosis

`INCLUDES`   embolic infarction
     embolic occlusion
     thrombotic infarction
     thrombotic occlusion
Code first:
     embolism and thrombosis complicating abortion or ectopic or molar pregnancy (OØØ-OØ7, OØ8.2)
     embolism and thrombosis complicating pregnancy, childbirth and the puerperium (O88.-)
`EXCLUDES 2`   atheroembolism (I75.-)
     basilar embolism and thrombosis (I63.Ø-I63.2, I65.1)
     carotid embolism and thrombosis (I63.Ø-I63.2, I65.2)
     cerebral embolism and thrombosis (I63.3-I63.5, I66.-)
     coronary embolism and thrombosis (I21-I25)
     mesenteric embolism and thrombosis (K55.Ø-)
     ophthalmic embolism and thrombosis (H34.-)
     precerebral embolism and thrombosis NOS (I63.Ø-I63.2, I65.9)
     pulmonary embolism and thrombosis (I26.-)
     renal embolism and thrombosis (N28.Ø)
     retinal embolism and thrombosis (H34.-)
     septic embolism and thrombosis (I76)
     vertebral embolism and thrombosis (I63.Ø-I63.2, I65.Ø)

✓5ᵗʰ I74.Ø   Embolism and thrombosis of abdominal aorta

I74.Ø1   **Saddle embolus of abdominal aorta**   `MCC` `HCC`

I74.Ø9   **Other arterial embolism and thrombosis of abdominal aorta**   `CC` `HCC`
Aortic bifurcation syndrome
Aortoiliac obstruction
Leriche's syndrome

✓5ᵗʰ I74.1   Embolism and thrombosis of other and unspecified parts of aorta

I74.1Ø   **Embolism and thrombosis of unspecified parts of aorta**   `CC` `HCC`

I74.11   **Embolism and thrombosis of thoracic aorta**   `CC` `HCC`

I74.19   **Embolism and thrombosis of other parts of aorta**   `CC` `HCC`

I74.2   **Embolism and thrombosis of arteries of the upper extremities**   `CC` `HCC`

✔ Additional Character Required   ✓x7ᵗʰ Placeholder   Questionable PDx   Manifestation   Unspecified Dx   `UPD` Unacceptable PDx   `H1`-`H14` HAC   `HCC` CMS-HCC Dx   `HIV` HIV Dx

ICD-10-CM 2022   679

Chapter 9. Diseases of the Circulatory System

I74.3   **Embolism and thrombosis of arteries of the** lower **extremities** `CC` `HCC`

I74.4   **Embolism and thrombosis of arteries of extremities, unspecified** `CC` `HCC`
Peripheral arterial embolism NOS

I74.5   **Embolism and thrombosis of** iliac **artery** `CC` `HCC`

I74.8   **Embolism and thrombosis of other arteries** `CC` `HCC`

I74.9   **Embolism and thrombosis of unspecified artery** `CC` `HCC`

✓4th **I75**   **Atheroembolism**
INCLUDES   atherothrombotic microembolism
      cholesterol embolism

✓5th **I75.0**   **Atheroembolism of** extremities

✓6th **I75.01**   **Atheroembolism of** upper **extremity**

I75.011   **Atheroembolism of** right **upper extremity** `CC` `HCC`

I75.012   **Atheroembolism of** left **upper extremity** `CC` `HCC`

I75.013   **Atheroembolism of** bilateral **upper extremities** `CC` `HCC`

I75.019   **Atheroembolism of unspecified upper extremity** `CC` `HCC`

✓6th **I75.02**   **Atheroembolism of** lower **extremity**

I75.021   **Atheroembolism of** right **lower extremity** `CC` `HCC`

I75.022   **Atheroembolism of** left **lower extremity** `CC` `HCC`

I75.023   **Atheroembolism of** bilateral **lower extremities** `CC` `HCC`

I75.029   **Atheroembolism of unspecified lower extremity** `CC` `HCC`

✓5th **I75.8**   **Atheroembolism of other sites**

I75.81   **Atheroembolism of** kidney `CC` `HCC`
Use additional code for any associated acute kidney failure and chronic kidney disease (N17.-, N18.-)

I75.89   **Atheroembolism of other site** `CC` `HCC`

I76   **Septic arterial embolism** `CC` `UPD` `HCC`
Code first underlying infection, such as:
     infective endocarditis (I33.0)
     lung abscess (J85.-)
Use additional code to identify the site of the embolism (I74.-)
EXCLUDES 2   septic pulmonary embolism (I26.01, I26.90)

✓4th **I77**   **Other disorders of arteries and arterioles**
EXCLUDES 2   collagen (vascular) diseases (M30-M36)
      hypersensitivity angiitis (M31.0)
      pulmonary artery (I28.-)

I77.0   **Arteriovenous fistula, acquired** `HCC`
Aneurysmal varix
Arteriovenous aneurysm, acquired
EXCLUDES 1   arteriovenous aneurysm NOS (Q27.3-)
      presence of arteriovenous shunt (fistula) for dialysis (Z99.2)
      traumatic - see injury of blood vessel by body region
EXCLUDES 2   cerebral (I67.1)
      coronary (I25.4)
DEF: Communication between an artery and vein caused by trauma or invasive procedures.

I77.1   **Stricture of artery** `HCC`
Narrowing of artery

I77.2   **Rupture of artery** `CC` `HCC`
Erosion of artery
Fistula of artery
Ulcer of artery
EXCLUDES 1   traumatic rupture of artery - see injury of blood vessel by body region

I77.3   **Arterial fibromuscular dysplasia** `HCC`
Fibromuscular hyperplasia (of) carotid artery
Fibromuscular hyperplasia (of) renal artery

I77.4   **Celiac artery compression syndrome** `CC` `HCC`

I77.5   **Necrosis of artery** `CC` `HCC`

I77.6   **Arteritis, unspecified** `HCC`
Aortitis NOS
Endarteritis NOS
EXCLUDES 1   arteritis or endarteritis:
      aortic arch (M31.4)
      cerebral NEC (I67.7)
      coronary (I25.89)
      deformans (I70.-)
      giant cell (M31.5, M31.6)
      obliterans (I70.-)
      senile (I70.-)

✓5th **I77.7**   **Other arterial dissection**
EXCLUDES 2   dissection of aorta (I71.0-)
      dissection of coronary artery (I25.42)
AHA: 2016,4Q,28-29

I77.70   **Dissection of unspecified artery** `MCC` `HCC`

I77.71   **Dissection of** carotid **artery** `MCC` `HCC`

I77.72   **Dissection of** iliac **artery** `MCC` `HCC`

I77.73   **Dissection of** renal **artery** `MCC` `HCC`

I77.74   **Dissection of** vertebral **artery** `MCC` `HCC`
EXCLUDES 2   aneurysm of vertebral artery (I72.6)

I77.75   **Dissection of other precerebral arteries** `MCC` `HCC`
Dissection of basilar artery (trunk)
EXCLUDES 2   aneurysm of carotid artery (I72.0)
      aneurysm of other precerebral arteries (I72.5)
      aneurysm of vertebral artery (I72.6)
      dissection of carotid artery (I77.71)
      dissection of vertebral artery (I77.74)

I77.76   **Dissection of artery of** upper extremity `MCC` `HCC`

I77.77   **Dissection of artery of** lower extremity `MCC` `HCC`

I77.79   **Dissection of other specified artery** `MCC` `HCC`

✓5th **I77.8**   **Other specified disorders of arteries and arterioles**

✓6th **I77.81**   **Aortic ectasia**
Ectasis aorta
EXCLUDES 1   aortic aneurysm and dissection (I71.0-)

I77.810   **Thoracic aortic ectasia** `HCC`

I77.811   **Abdominal aortic ectasia** `HCC`

I77.812   **Thoracoabdominal aortic ectasia** `HCC`

I77.819   **Aortic ectasia, unspecified site** `HCC`

I77.89   **Other specified disorders of arteries and arterioles** `HCC`
AHA: 2021,1Q,23

I77.9   **Disorder of arteries and arterioles, unspecified** `HCC`
AHA: 2021,1Q,4; 2018,2Q,7

✓4th **I78**   **Diseases of capillaries**

I78.0   **Hereditary hemorrhagic telangiectasia** `HCC`
Rendu-Osler-Weber disease

I78.1   **Nevus, non-neoplastic**
Araneus nevus
Senile nevus
Spider nevus
Stellar nevus
EXCLUDES 1   nevus NOS (D22.-)
      vascular NOS (Q82.5)
EXCLUDES 2   blue nevus (D22.-)
      flammeus nevus (Q82.5)
      hairy nevus (D22.-)
      melanocytic nevus (D22.-)
      pigmented nevus (D22.-)
      portwine nevus (Q82.5)
      sanguineous nevus (Q82.5)
      strawberry nevus (Q82.5)
      verrucous nevus (Q82.5)
AHA: 2019,1Q,21

I78.8   **Other diseases of capillaries**

I78.9   **Disease of capillaries, unspecified**

✓4th **I79**   **Disorders of arteries, arterioles and capillaries in diseases classified elsewhere**

I79.0   *Aneurysm of aorta in diseases classified elsewhere* `HCC`
Code first underlying disease
EXCLUDES 1   syphilitic aneurysm (A52.01)

N Newborn: 0   P Pediatric: 0-17   M Maternity: 9-64   A Adult: 15-124   MCC Major Complication/Comorbidity   CC Complication/Comorbidity   SW Severe Wound Dx

680   ICD-10-CM 2022

I79.1 Aortitis in diseases classified elsewhere   `HCC`
    Code first underlying disease
     EXCLUDES 1   syphilitic aortitis (A52.02)

I79.8 Other disorders of arteries, arterioles and capillaries in diseases classified elsewhere   `HCC`
    Code first underlying disease, such as:
     amyloidosis (E85.-)
     EXCLUDES 1   diabetic (peripheral) angiopathy (E08-E13 with .51-.52)
         syphilitic endarteritis (A52.09)
         tuberculous endarteritis (A18.89)

Diseases of veins, lymphatic vessels and lymph nodes, not elsewhere classified (I80-I89)

✓4ᵗʰ I80 Phlebitis and thrombophlebitis
     `INCLUDES`   endophlebitis
         inflammation, vein
         periphlebitis
         suppurative phlebitis
    Code first:
     phlebitis and thrombophlebitis complicating abortion, ectopic or molar pregnancy (O00-O07, O08.7)
     phlebitis and thrombophlebitis complicating pregnancy, childbirth and the puerperium (O22.-, O87.-)
     EXCLUDES 1   venous embolism and thrombosis of lower extremities (I82.4-, I82.5-, I82.81-)

✓5ᵗʰ I80.0 Phlebitis and thrombophlebitis of superficial vessels of lower extremities
     Phlebitis and thrombophlebitis of femoropopliteal vein
     I80.00 Phlebitis and thrombophlebitis of superficial vessels of unspecified lower extremity
     I80.01 Phlebitis and thrombophlebitis of superficial vessels of right lower extremity
     I80.02 Phlebitis and thrombophlebitis of superficial vessels of left lower extremity
     I80.03 Phlebitis and thrombophlebitis of superficial vessels of lower extremities, bilateral

✓5ᵗʰ I80.1 Phlebitis and thrombophlebitis of femoral vein
     Phlebitis and thrombophlebitis of common femoral vein
     Phlebitis and thrombophlebitis of deep femoral vein
     I80.10 Phlebitis and thrombophlebitis of unspecified femoral vein   `CC` `HCC`
     I80.11 Phlebitis and thrombophlebitis of right femoral vein   `CC` `HCC`
     I80.12 Phlebitis and thrombophlebitis of left femoral vein   `CC` `HCC`
     I80.13 Phlebitis and thrombophlebitis of femoral vein, bilateral   `CC` `HCC`

✓5ᵗʰ I80.2 Phlebitis and thrombophlebitis of other and unspecified deep vessels of lower extremities
     ✓6ᵗʰ I80.20 Phlebitis and thrombophlebitis of unspecified deep vessels of lower extremities
         I80.201 Phlebitis and thrombophlebitis of unspecified deep vessels of right lower extremity   `CC` `HCC`
         I80.202 Phlebitis and thrombophlebitis of unspecified deep vessels of left lower extremity   `CC` `HCC`
         I80.203 Phlebitis and thrombophlebitis of unspecified deep vessels of lower extremities, bilateral   `CC` `HCC`
         I80.209 Phlebitis and thrombophlebitis of unspecified deep vessels of unspecified lower extremity   `CC` `HCC`
     ✓6ᵗʰ I80.21 Phlebitis and thrombophlebitis of iliac vein
         Phlebitis and thrombophlebitis of common iliac vein
         Phlebitis and thrombophlebitis of external iliac vein
         Phlebitis and thrombophlebitis of internal iliac vein
         I80.211 Phlebitis and thrombophlebitis of right iliac vein   `CC` `HCC`
         I80.212 Phlebitis and thrombophlebitis of left iliac vein   `CC` `HCC`
         I80.213 Phlebitis and thrombophlebitis of iliac vein, bilateral   `CC` `HCC`
         I80.219 Phlebitis and thrombophlebitis of unspecified iliac vein   `CC` `HCC`
     ✓6ᵗʰ I80.22 Phlebitis and thrombophlebitis of popliteal vein
         I80.221 Phlebitis and thrombophlebitis of right popliteal vein   `CC` `HCC`
         I80.222 Phlebitis and thrombophlebitis of left popliteal vein   `CC` `HCC`
         I80.223 Phlebitis and thrombophlebitis of popliteal vein, bilateral   `CC` `HCC`
         I80.229 Phlebitis and thrombophlebitis of unspecified popliteal vein   `CC` `HCC`
     ✓6ᵗʰ I80.23 Phlebitis and thrombophlebitis of tibial vein
         Phlebitis and thrombophlebitis of anterior tibial vein
         Phlebitis and thrombophlebitis of posterior tibial vein
         I80.231 Phlebitis and thrombophlebitis of right tibial vein   `CC` `HCC`
         I80.232 Phlebitis and thrombophlebitis of left tibial vein   `CC` `HCC`
         I80.233 Phlebitis and thrombophlebitis of tibial vein, bilateral   `CC` `HCC`
         I80.239 Phlebitis and thrombophlebitis of unspecified tibial vein   `CC` `HCC`
     ✓6ᵗʰ I80.24 Phlebitis and thrombophlebitis of peroneal vein
         AHA: 2019,4Q,8
         I80.241 Phlebitis and thrombophlebitis of right peroneal vein   `CC` `HCC`
         I80.242 Phlebitis and thrombophlebitis of left peroneal vein   `CC` `HCC`
         I80.243 Phlebitis and thrombophlebitis of peroneal vein, bilateral   `CC` `HCC`
         I80.249 Phlebitis and thrombophlebitis of unspecified peroneal vein   `CC` `HCC`
     ✓6ᵗʰ I80.25 Phlebitis and thrombophlebitis of calf muscular vein
         Phlebitis and thrombophlebitis of calf muscular vein, NOS
         Phlebitis and thrombophlebitis of gastrocnemial vein
         Phlebitis and thrombophlebitis of soleal vein
         AHA: 2019,4Q,8
         I80.251 Phlebitis and thrombophlebitis of right calf muscular vein   `HCC`
         I80.252 Phlebitis and thrombophlebitis of left calf muscular vein   `HCC`
         I80.253 Phlebitis and thrombophlebitis of calf muscular vein, bilateral   `HCC`
         I80.259 Phlebitis and thrombophlebitis of unspecified calf muscular vein   `HCC`
     ✓6ᵗʰ I80.29 Phlebitis and thrombophlebitis of other deep vessels of lower extremities
         I80.291 Phlebitis and thrombophlebitis of other deep vessels of right lower extremity   `CC` `HCC`
         I80.292 Phlebitis and thrombophlebitis of other deep vessels of left lower extremity   `CC` `HCC`
         I80.293 Phlebitis and thrombophlebitis of other deep vessels of lower extremity, bilateral   `CC` `HCC`
         I80.299 Phlebitis and thrombophlebitis of other deep vessels of unspecified lower extremity   `CC` `HCC`

I80.3 Phlebitis and thrombophlebitis of lower extremities, unspecified

I80.8 Phlebitis and thrombophlebitis of other sites

I80.9 Phlebitis and thrombophlebitis of unspecified site

I81 Portal vein thrombosis   `MCC`
    Portal (vein) obstruction
     EXCLUDES 2   hepatic vein thrombosis (I82.0)
         phlebitis of portal vein (K75.1)
    AHA: 2019,4Q,68

✓4ᵗʰ I82 Other venous embolism and thrombosis

Code first venous embolism and thrombosis complicating:
abortion, ectopic or molar pregnancy (O00-O07, O08.7)
pregnancy, childbirth and the puerperium (O22.-, O87.-)

EXCLUDES 2   venous embolism and thrombosis (of):
cerebral (I63.6, I67.6)
coronary (I21-I25)
intracranial and intraspinal, septic or NOS (G08)
intracranial, nonpyogenic (I67.6)
intraspinal, nonpyogenic (G95.1)
mesenteric (K55.0-)
portal (I81)
pulmonary (I26.-)

I82.0 Budd-Chiari syndrome   MCC HCC
Hepatic vein thrombosis
DEF: Thrombosis or other obstruction of the hepatic veins. Symptoms include an enlarged liver, extensive collateral vessels, intractable ascites, and severe portal hypertension.

I82.1 Thrombophlebitis migrans   CC

✓5ᵗʰ I82.2 Embolism and thrombosis of vena cava and other thoracic veins

✓6ᵗʰ I82.21 Embolism and thrombosis of superior vena cava

I82.210 Acute embolism and thrombosis of superior vena cava   CC HCC
Embolism and thrombosis of superior vena cava NOS

I82.211 Chronic embolism and thrombosis of superior vena cava   CC HCC

✓6ᵗʰ I82.22 Embolism and thrombosis of inferior vena cava

I82.220 Acute embolism and thrombosis of inferior vena cava   MCC HCC
Embolism and thrombosis of inferior vena cava NOS

I82.221 Chronic embolism and thrombosis of inferior vena cava   MCC HCC

✓6ᵗʰ I82.29 Embolism and thrombosis of other thoracic veins
Embolism and thrombosis of brachiocephalic (innominate) vein

I82.290 Acute embolism and thrombosis of other thoracic veins   CC HCC

I82.291 Chronic embolism and thrombosis of other thoracic veins   CC HCC

I82.3 Embolism and thrombosis of renal vein   CC HCC

✓5ᵗʰ I82.4 Acute embolism and thrombosis of deep veins of lower extremity

✓6ᵗʰ I82.40 Acute embolism and thrombosis of unspecified deep veins of lower extremity
Deep vein thrombosis NOS
DVT NOS

EXCLUDES 1   acute embolism and thrombosis of unspecified deep veins of distal lower extremity (I82.4Z-)
acute embolism and thrombosis of unspecified deep veins of proximal lower extremity (I82.4Y-)

I82.401 Acute embolism and thrombosis of unspecified deep veins of right lower extremity   CC H10 HCC

I82.402 Acute embolism and thrombosis of unspecified deep veins of left lower extremity   CC H10 HCC

I82.403 Acute embolism and thrombosis of unspecified deep veins of lower extremity, bilateral   CC H10 HCC

I82.409 Acute embolism and thrombosis of unspecified deep veins of unspecified lower extremity   CC H10 HCC

✓6ᵗʰ I82.41 Acute embolism and thrombosis of femoral vein
Acute embolism and thrombosis of common femoral vein
Acute embolism and thrombosis of deep femoral vein

I82.411 Acute embolism and thrombosis of right femoral vein   CC H10 HCC

I82.412 Acute embolism and thrombosis of left femoral vein   CC H10 HCC

I82.413 Acute embolism and thrombosis of femoral vein, bilateral   CC H10 HCC

I82.419 Acute embolism and thrombosis of unspecified femoral vein   CC H10 HCC

✓6ᵗʰ I82.42 Acute embolism and thrombosis of iliac vein
Acute embolism and thrombosis of common iliac vein
Acute embolism and thrombosis of external iliac vein
Acute embolism and thrombosis of internal iliac vein

I82.421 Acute embolism and thrombosis of right iliac vein   CC H10 HCC

I82.422 Acute embolism and thrombosis of left iliac vein   CC H10 HCC

I82.423 Acute embolism and thrombosis of iliac vein, bilateral   CC H10 HCC

I82.429 Acute embolism and thrombosis of unspecified iliac vein   CC H10 HCC

✓6ᵗʰ I82.43 Acute embolism and thrombosis of popliteal vein

I82.431 Acute embolism and thrombosis of right popliteal vein   CC H10 HCC

I82.432 Acute embolism and thrombosis of left popliteal vein   CC H10 HCC

I82.433 Acute embolism and thrombosis of popliteal vein, bilateral   CC H10 HCC

I82.439 Acute embolism and thrombosis of unspecified popliteal vein   CC H10 HCC

✓6ᵗʰ I82.44 Acute embolism and thrombosis of tibial vein
Acute embolism and thrombosis of anterior tibial vein
Acute embolism and thrombosis of posterior tibial vein

I82.441 Acute embolism and thrombosis of right tibial vein   CC H10 HCC

I82.442 Acute embolism and thrombosis of left tibial vein   CC H10 HCC

I82.443 Acute embolism and thrombosis of tibial vein, bilateral   CC H10 HCC

I82.449 Acute embolism and thrombosis of unspecified tibial vein   CC H10 HCC

✓6ᵗʰ I82.45 Acute embolism and thrombosis of peroneal vein
AHA: 2019,4Q,8-10

I82.451 Acute embolism and thrombosis of right peroneal vein   CC H10 HCC

I82.452 Acute embolism and thrombosis of left peroneal vein   CC H10 HCC

I82.453 Acute embolism and thrombosis of peroneal vein, bilateral   CC H10 HCC

I82.459 Acute embolism and thrombosis of unspecified peroneal vein   CC H10 HCC

✓6ᵗʰ I82.46 Acute embolism and thrombosis of calf muscular vein
Acute embolism and thrombosis of calf muscular vein, NOS
Acute embolism and thrombosis of gastrocnemial vein
Acute embolism and thrombosis of soleal vein
AHA: 2019,4Q,8-10

I82.461 Acute embolism and thrombosis of right calf muscular vein   HCC

I82.462 Acute embolism and thrombosis of left calf muscular vein   HCC

I82.463 Acute embolism and thrombosis of calf muscular vein, bilateral   HCC

I82.469 Acute embolism and thrombosis of unspecified calf muscular vein   HCC

✓6ᵗʰ I82.49 Acute embolism and thrombosis of other specified deep vein of lower extremity

I82.491 Acute embolism and thrombosis of other specified deep vein of right lower extremity   CC H10 HCC

I82.492 Acute embolism and thrombosis of other specified deep vein of left lower extremity   CC H10 HCC

I82.493 Acute embolism and thrombosis of other specified deep vein of lower extremity, bilateral   CC H10 HCC

I82.499 Acute embolism and thrombosis of other specified deep vein of unspecified lower extremity   CC H10 HCC

√6ᵗʰ **I82.4Y** **Acute embolism and thrombosis of unspecified deep veins of proximal lower extremity**
Acute embolism and thrombosis of deep vein of thigh NOS
Acute embolism and thrombosis of deep vein of upper leg NOS

I82.4Y1 **Acute embolism and thrombosis of unspecified deep veins of right proximal lower extremity** `CC` `H10` `HCC`

I82.4Y2 **Acute embolism and thrombosis of unspecified deep veins of left proximal lower extremity** `CC` `H10` `HCC`

I82.4Y3 **Acute embolism and thrombosis of unspecified deep veins of proximal lower extremity, bilateral** `CC` `H10` `HCC`

I82.4Y9 **Acute embolism and thrombosis of unspecified deep veins of unspecified proximal lower extremity** `CC` `H10` `HCC`

√6ᵗʰ **I82.4Z** **Acute embolism and thrombosis of unspecified deep veins of distal lower extremity**
Acute embolism and thrombosis of deep vein of calf NOS
Acute embolism and thrombosis of deep vein of lower leg NOS

I82.4Z1 **Acute embolism and thrombosis of unspecified deep veins of right distal lower extremity** `CC` `H10` `HCC`

I82.4Z2 **Acute embolism and thrombosis of unspecified deep veins of left distal lower extremity** `CC` `H10` `HCC`

I82.4Z3 **Acute embolism and thrombosis of unspecified deep veins of distal lower extremity, bilateral** `CC` `H10` `HCC`

I82.4Z9 **Acute embolism and thrombosis of unspecified deep veins of unspecified distal lower extremity** `CC` `H10` `HCC`

√6ᵗʰ **I82.5** **Chronic embolism and thrombosis of deep veins of lower extremity**
Use additional code, if applicable, for associated long-term (current) use of anticoagulants (Z79.01)
EXCLUDES 1   *personal history of venous embolism and thrombosis (Z86.718)*

AHA: 2020,2Q,20

√6ᵗʰ **I82.50** **Chronic embolism and thrombosis of unspecified deep veins of lower extremity**
EXCLUDES 1   *chronic embolism and thrombosis of unspecified deep veins of distal lower extremity (I82.5Z-)*
chronic embolism and thrombosis of unspecified deep veins of proximal lower extremity (I82.5Y-)

I82.501 **Chronic embolism and thrombosis of unspecified deep veins of right lower extremity** `CC` `HCC`

I82.502 **Chronic embolism and thrombosis of unspecified deep veins of left lower extremity** `CC` `HCC`

I82.503 **Chronic embolism and thrombosis of unspecified deep veins of lower extremity, bilateral** `CC` `HCC`

I82.509 **Chronic embolism and thrombosis of unspecified deep veins of unspecified lower extremity** `CC` `HCC`

√6ᵗʰ **I82.51** **Chronic embolism and thrombosis of femoral vein**
Chronic embolism and thrombosis of common femoral vein
Chronic embolism and thrombosis of deep femoral vein

I82.511 **Chronic embolism and thrombosis of right femoral vein** `CC` `HCC`

I82.512 **Chronic embolism and thrombosis of left femoral vein** `CC` `HCC`

I82.513 **Chronic embolism and thrombosis of femoral vein, bilateral** `CC` `HCC`

I82.519 **Chronic embolism and thrombosis of unspecified femoral vein** `CC` `HCC`

√6ᵗʰ **I82.52** **Chronic embolism and thrombosis of iliac vein**
Chronic embolism and thrombosis of common iliac vein
Chronic embolism and thrombosis of external iliac vein
Chronic embolism and thrombosis of internal iliac vein

I82.521 **Chronic embolism and thrombosis of right iliac vein** `CC` `HCC`

I82.522 **Chronic embolism and thrombosis of left iliac vein** `CC` `HCC`

I82.523 **Chronic embolism and thrombosis of iliac vein, bilateral** `CC` `HCC`

I82.529 **Chronic embolism and thrombosis of unspecified iliac vein** `CC` `HCC`

√6ᵗʰ **I82.53** **Chronic embolism and thrombosis of popliteal vein**

I82.531 **Chronic embolism and thrombosis of right popliteal vein** `CC` `HCC`

I82.532 **Chronic embolism and thrombosis of left popliteal vein** `CC` `HCC`

I82.533 **Chronic embolism and thrombosis of popliteal vein, bilateral** `CC` `HCC`

I82.539 **Chronic embolism and thrombosis of unspecified popliteal vein** `CC` `HCC`

√6ᵗʰ **I82.54** **Chronic embolism and thrombosis of tibial vein**
Chronic embolism and thrombosis of anterior tibial vein
Chronic embolism and thrombosis of posterior tibial vein

I82.541 **Chronic embolism and thrombosis of right tibial vein** `CC` `HCC`

I82.542 **Chronic embolism and thrombosis of left tibial vein** `CC` `HCC`

I82.543 **Chronic embolism and thrombosis of tibial vein, bilateral** `CC` `HCC`

I82.549 **Chronic embolism and thrombosis of unspecified tibial vein** `CC` `HCC`

√6ᵗʰ **I82.55** **Chronic embolism and thrombosis of peroneal vein**
AHA: 2019,4Q,8-10

I82.551 **Chronic embolism and thrombosis of right peroneal vein** `CC` `HCC`

I82.552 **Chronic embolism and thrombosis of left peroneal vein** `CC` `HCC`

I82.553 **Chronic embolism and thrombosis of peroneal vein, bilateral** `CC` `HCC`

I82.559 **Chronic embolism and thrombosis of unspecified peroneal vein** `CC` `HCC`

√6ᵗʰ **I82.56** **Chronic embolism and thrombosis of calf muscular vein**
Chronic embolism and thrombosis of calf muscular vein NOS
Chronic embolism and thrombosis of gastrocnemial vein
Chronic embolism and thrombosis of soleal vein
AHA: 2019,4Q,8-10

I82.561 **Chronic embolism and thrombosis of right calf muscular vein** `HCC`

I82.562 **Chronic embolism and thrombosis of left calf muscular vein** `HCC`

I82.563 **Chronic embolism and thrombosis of calf muscular vein, bilateral** `HCC`

I82.569 **Chronic embolism and thrombosis of unspecified calf muscular vein** `HCC`

√6ᵗʰ **I82.59** **Chronic embolism and thrombosis of other specified deep vein of lower extremity**

I82.591 **Chronic embolism and thrombosis of other specified deep vein of right lower extremity** `CC` `HCC`

I82.592 **Chronic embolism and thrombosis of other specified deep vein of left lower extremity** `CC` `HCC`

I82.593 **Chronic embolism and thrombosis of other specified deep vein of lower extremity, bilateral** `CC` `HCC`

I82.599 **Chronic embolism and thrombosis of other specified deep vein of unspecified lower extremity** `CC` `HCC`

☑ Additional Character Required   √x7ᵗʰ Placeholder   Questionable PDx   Manifestation   Unspecified Dx   `UPD` Unacceptable PDx   `H1`-`H14` HAC   `HCC` CMS-HCC Dx   `HIV` HIV Dx

ICD-10-CM 2022   683

✓6ᵗʰ I82.5Y Chronic embolism and thrombosis of unspecified deep veins of proximal lower extremity
Chronic embolism and thrombosis of deep veins of thigh NOS
Chronic embolism and thrombosis of deep veins of upper leg NOS

I82.5Y1 Chronic embolism and thrombosis of unspecified deep veins of right proximal lower extremity CC HCC

I82.5Y2 Chronic embolism and thrombosis of unspecified deep veins of left proximal lower extremity CC HCC

I82.5Y3 Chronic embolism and thrombosis of unspecified deep veins of proximal lower extremity, bilateral CC HCC

I82.5Y9 Chronic embolism and thrombosis of unspecified deep veins of unspecified proximal lower extremity CC HCC

✓6ᵗʰ I82.5Z Chronic embolism and thrombosis of unspecified deep veins of distal lower extremity
Chronic embolism and thrombosis of deep veins of calf NOS
Chronic embolism and thrombosis of deep veins of lower leg NOS

I82.5Z1 Chronic embolism and thrombosis of unspecified deep veins of right distal lower extremity CC HCC

I82.5Z2 Chronic embolism and thrombosis of unspecified deep veins of left distal lower extremity CC HCC

I82.5Z3 Chronic embolism and thrombosis of unspecified deep veins of distal lower extremity, bilateral CC HCC

I82.5Z9 Chronic embolism and thrombosis of unspecified deep veins of unspecified distal lower extremity CC HCC

✓5ᵗʰ I82.6 Acute embolism and thrombosis of veins of upper extremity

✓6ᵗʰ I82.60 Acute embolism and thrombosis of unspecified veins of upper extremity

I82.601 Acute embolism and thrombosis of unspecified veins of right upper extremity CC

I82.602 Acute embolism and thrombosis of unspecified veins of left upper extremity CC

I82.603 Acute embolism and thrombosis of unspecified veins of upper extremity, bilateral CC

I82.609 Acute embolism and thrombosis of unspecified veins of unspecified upper extremity CC

✓6ᵗʰ I82.61 Acute embolism and thrombosis of superficial veins of upper extremity
Acute embolism and thrombosis of antecubital vein
Acute embolism and thrombosis of basilic vein
Acute embolism and thrombosis of cephalic vein

I82.611 Acute embolism and thrombosis of superficial veins of right upper extremity CC

I82.612 Acute embolism and thrombosis of superficial veins of left upper extremity CC

I82.613 Acute embolism and thrombosis of superficial veins of upper extremity, bilateral CC

I82.619 Acute embolism and thrombosis of superficial veins of unspecified upper extremity CC

✓6ᵗʰ I82.62 Acute embolism and thrombosis of deep veins of upper extremity
Acute embolism and thrombosis of brachial vein
Acute embolism and thrombosis of radial vein
Acute embolism and thrombosis of ulnar vein

I82.621 Acute embolism and thrombosis of deep veins of right upper extremity CC HCC

I82.622 Acute embolism and thrombosis of deep veins of left upper extremity CC HCC

I82.623 Acute embolism and thrombosis of deep veins of upper extremity, bilateral CC HCC

I82.629 Acute embolism and thrombosis of deep veins of unspecified upper extremity CC HCC

✓5ᵗʰ I82.7 Chronic embolism and thrombosis of veins of upper extremity
Use additional code, if applicable, for associated long-term (current) use of anticoagulants (Z79.01)
EXCLUDES 1   personal history of venous embolism and thrombosis (Z86.718)

✓6ᵗʰ I82.70 Chronic embolism and thrombosis of unspecified veins of upper extremity

I82.701 Chronic embolism and thrombosis of unspecified veins of right upper extremity CC

I82.702 Chronic embolism and thrombosis of unspecified veins of left upper extremity CC

I82.703 Chronic embolism and thrombosis of unspecified veins of upper extremity, bilateral CC

I82.709 Chronic embolism and thrombosis of unspecified veins of unspecified upper extremity CC

✓6ᵗʰ I82.71 Chronic embolism and thrombosis of superficial veins of upper extremity
Chronic embolism and thrombosis of antecubital vein
Chronic embolism and thrombosis of basilic vein
Chronic embolism and thrombosis of cephalic vein

I82.711 Chronic embolism and thrombosis of superficial veins of right upper extremity CC

I82.712 Chronic embolism and thrombosis of superficial veins of left upper extremity CC

I82.713 Chronic embolism and thrombosis of superficial veins of upper extremity, bilateral CC

I82.719 Chronic embolism and thrombosis of superficial veins of unspecified upper extremity CC

✓6ᵗʰ I82.72 Chronic embolism and thrombosis of deep veins of upper extremity
Chronic embolism and thrombosis of brachial vein
Chronic embolism and thrombosis of radial vein
Chronic embolism and thrombosis of ulnar vein

I82.721 Chronic embolism and thrombosis of deep veins of right upper extremity CC HCC

I82.722 Chronic embolism and thrombosis of deep veins of left upper extremity CC HCC

I82.723 Chronic embolism and thrombosis of deep veins of upper extremity, bilateral CC HCC

I82.729 Chronic embolism and thrombosis of deep veins of unspecified upper extremity CC HCC

✓5ᵗʰ I82.A Embolism and thrombosis of axillary vein

✓6ᵗʰ I82.A1 Acute embolism and thrombosis of axillary vein

I82.A11 Acute embolism and thrombosis of right axillary vein CC HCC

I82.A12 Acute embolism and thrombosis of left axillary vein CC HCC

I82.A13 Acute embolism and thrombosis of axillary vein, bilateral CC HCC

I82.A19 Acute embolism and thrombosis of unspecified axillary vein CC HCC

✓6ᵗʰ I82.A2 Chronic embolism and thrombosis of axillary vein

I82.A21 Chronic embolism and thrombosis of right axillary vein CC HCC

I82.A22 Chronic embolism and thrombosis of left axillary vein CC HCC

I82.A23 Chronic embolism and thrombosis of axillary vein, bilateral CC HCC

I82.A29 Chronic embolism and thrombosis of unspecified axillary vein CC HCC

✓5ᵗʰ I82.B Embolism and thrombosis of subclavian vein

✓6ᵗʰ I82.B1 Acute embolism and thrombosis of subclavian vein

I82.B11 Acute embolism and thrombosis of right subclavian vein CC HCC

N Newborn: 0   P Pediatric: 0-17   M Maternity: 9-64   A Adult: 15-124   MCC Major Complication/Comorbidity   CC Complication/Comorbidity   SW Severe Wound Dx

684   ICD-10-CM 2022

I82.B12 Acute embolism and thrombosis of left subclavian vein `CC` `HCC`

I82.B13 Acute embolism and thrombosis of subclavian vein, bilateral `CC` `HCC`

I82.B19 Acute embolism and thrombosis of unspecified subclavian vein `CC` `HCC`

✓6ᵗʰ **I82.B2** Chronic embolism and thrombosis of subclavian vein

I82.B21 Chronic embolism and thrombosis of right subclavian vein `CC` `HCC`

I82.B22 Chronic embolism and thrombosis of left subclavian vein `CC` `HCC`

I82.B23 Chronic embolism and thrombosis of subclavian vein, bilateral `CC` `HCC`

I82.B29 Chronic embolism and thrombosis of unspecified subclavian vein `CC` `HCC`

✓5ᵗʰ **I82.C** Embolism and thrombosis of internal jugular vein

✓6ᵗʰ **I82.C1** Acute embolism and thrombosis of internal jugular vein

I82.C11 Acute embolism and thrombosis of right internal jugular vein `CC` `HCC`

I82.C12 Acute embolism and thrombosis of left internal jugular vein `CC` `HCC`

I82.C13 Acute embolism and thrombosis of internal jugular vein, bilateral `CC` `HCC`

I82.C19 Acute embolism and thrombosis of unspecified internal jugular vein `CC` `HCC`

✓6ᵗʰ **I82.C2** Chronic embolism and thrombosis of internal jugular vein

I82.C21 Chronic embolism and thrombosis of right internal jugular vein `CC` `HCC`

I82.C22 Chronic embolism and thrombosis of left internal jugular vein `CC` `HCC`

I82.C23 Chronic embolism and thrombosis of internal jugular vein, bilateral `CC` `HCC`

I82.C29 Chronic embolism and thrombosis of unspecified internal jugular vein `CC` `HCC`

✓5ᵗʰ **I82.8** Embolism and thrombosis of other specified veins

Use additional code, if applicable, for associated long-term (current) use of anticoagulants (Z79.01)

✓6ᵗʰ **I82.81** Embolism and thrombosis of superficial veins of lower extremities

Embolism and thrombosis of saphenous vein (greater) (lesser)

I82.811 Embolism and thrombosis of superficial veins of right lower extremity `CC`

I82.812 Embolism and thrombosis of superficial veins of left lower extremity `CC`

I82.813 Embolism and thrombosis of superficial veins of lower extremities, bilateral `CC`

I82.819 Embolism and thrombosis of superficial veins of unspecified lower extremity `CC`

✓6ᵗʰ **I82.89** Embolism and thrombosis of other specified veins

I82.890 Acute embolism and thrombosis of other specified veins `CC`

I82.891 Chronic embolism and thrombosis of other specified veins `CC`

✓5ᵗʰ **I82.9** Embolism and thrombosis of unspecified vein

I82.90 Acute embolism and thrombosis of unspecified vein `CC`

Embolism of vein NOS
Thrombosis (vein) NOS

I82.91 Chronic embolism and thrombosis of unspecified vein `CC`

✓4ᵗʰ **I83** Varicose veins of lower extremities

EXCLUDES 1   *varicose veins complicating pregnancy (O22.0-)*
     varicose veins complicating the puerperium (O87.4)

EXCLUDES 2   ▶*varicose veins complicating pregnancy (O22.0-)*◀
     ▶*varicose veins complicating the puerperium (O87.4)*◀

✓5ᵗʰ **I83.0** Varicose veins of lower extremities with ulcer

Use additional code to identify severity of ulcer (L97.-)

✓6ᵗʰ **I83.00** Varicose veins of unspecified lower extremity with ulcer

I83.001 Varicose veins of unspecified lower extremity with ulcer of thigh `HCC` `A`

I83.002 Varicose veins of unspecified lower extremity with ulcer of calf `HCC` `A`

I83.003 Varicose veins of unspecified lower extremity with ulcer of ankle `HCC` `A`

I83.004 Varicose veins of unspecified lower extremity with ulcer of heel and midfoot `HCC` `A`

Varicose veins of unspecified lower extremity with ulcer of plantar surface of midfoot

I83.005 Varicose veins of unspecified lower extremity with ulcer other part of foot `HCC` `A`

Varicose veins of unspecified lower extremity with ulcer of toe

I83.008 Varicose veins of unspecified lower extremity with ulcer other part of lower leg `HCC` `A`

I83.009 Varicose veins of unspecified lower extremity with ulcer of unspecified site `HCC` `A`

✓6ᵗʰ **I83.01** Varicose veins of right lower extremity with ulcer

I83.011 Varicose veins of right lower extremity with ulcer of thigh `HCC` `A`

I83.012 Varicose veins of right lower extremity with ulcer of calf `HCC` `A`

I83.013 Varicose veins of right lower extremity with ulcer of ankle `HCC` `A`

I83.014 Varicose veins of right lower extremity with ulcer of heel and midfoot `HCC` `A`

Varicose veins of right lower extremity with ulcer of plantar surface of midfoot

I83.015 Varicose veins of right lower extremity with ulcer other part of foot `HCC` `A`

Varicose veins of right lower extremity with ulcer of toe

I83.018 Varicose veins of right lower extremity with ulcer other part of lower leg `HCC` `A`

I83.019 Varicose veins of right lower extremity with ulcer of unspecified site `HCC` `A`

✓6ᵗʰ **I83.02** Varicose veins of left lower extremity with ulcer

I83.021 Varicose veins of left lower extremity with ulcer of thigh `HCC` `A`

I83.022 Varicose veins of left lower extremity with ulcer of calf `HCC` `A`

I83.023 Varicose veins of left lower extremity with ulcer of ankle `HCC` `A`

I83.024 Varicose veins of left lower extremity with ulcer of heel and midfoot `HCC` `A`

Varicose veins of left lower extremity with ulcer of plantar surface of midfoot

I83.025 Varicose veins of left lower extremity with ulcer other part of foot `HCC` `A`

Varicose veins of left lower extremity with ulcer of toe

I83.028 Varicose veins of left lower extremity with ulcer other part of lower leg `HCC` `A`

I83.029 Varicose veins of left lower extremity with ulcer of unspecified site `HCC` `A`

✓5ᵗʰ **I83.1** Varicose veins of lower extremities with inflammation

I83.10 Varicose veins of unspecified lower extremity with inflammation `A`

I83.11 Varicose veins of right lower extremity with inflammation `A`

I83.12 Varicose veins of left lower extremity with inflammation `A`

✓5ᵗʰ **I83.2** Varicose veins of lower extremities with both ulcer and inflammation

Use additional code to identify severity of ulcer (L97.-)

✓6ᵗʰ **I83.20** Varicose veins of unspecified lower extremity with both ulcer and inflammation

I83.201 Varicose veins of unspecified lower extremity with both ulcer of thigh and inflammation `CC` `HCC` `A`

I83.202 Varicose veins of unspecified lower extremity with both ulcer of calf and inflammation `CC` `HCC` `A`

✓ Additional Character Required   ✓×7ᵗʰ Placeholder   Questionable PDx   Manifestation   Unspecified Dx   `UPD` Unacceptable PDx   `H1`-`H14` HAC   `HCC` CMS-HCC Dx   `HIV` HIV Dx

ICD-10-CM 2022   685

I83.203 Varicose veins of unspecified lower extremity with both ulcer of ankle and inflammation `CC` `HCC` `A`

I83.204 Varicose veins of unspecified lower extremity with both ulcer of heel and midfoot and inflammation `CC` `HCC` `A`
  Varicose veins of unspecified lower extremity with both ulcer of plantar surface of midfoot and inflammation

I83.205 Varicose veins of unspecified lower extremity with both ulcer of other part of foot and inflammation `CC` `HCC` `A`
  Varicose veins of unspecified lower extremity with both ulcer of toe and inflammation

I83.208 Varicose veins of unspecified lower extremity with both ulcer of other part of lower extremity and inflammation `CC` `HCC` `A`

I83.209 Varicose veins of unspecified lower extremity with both ulcer of unspecified site and inflammation `CC` `HCC` `A`

√6ᵗʰ **I83.21** Varicose veins of right lower extremity with both ulcer and inflammation

I83.211 Varicose veins of right lower extremity with both ulcer of thigh and inflammation `CC` `HCC` `A`

I83.212 Varicose veins of right lower extremity with both ulcer of calf and inflammation `CC` `HCC` `A`

I83.213 Varicose veins of right lower extremity with both ulcer of ankle and inflammation `CC` `HCC` `A`

I83.214 Varicose veins of right lower extremity with both ulcer of heel and midfoot and inflammation `CC` `HCC` `A`
  Varicose veins of right lower extremity with both ulcer of plantar surface of midfoot and inflammation

I83.215 Varicose veins of right lower extremity with both ulcer other part of foot and inflammation `CC` `HCC` `A`
  Varicose veins of right lower extremity with both ulcer of toe and inflammation

I83.218 Varicose veins of right lower extremity with both ulcer of other part of lower extremity and inflammation `CC` `HCC` `A`

I83.219 Varicose veins of right lower extremity with both ulcer of unspecified site and inflammation `CC` `HCC` `A`

√6ᵗʰ **I83.22** Varicose veins of left lower extremity with both ulcer and inflammation

I83.221 Varicose veins of left lower extremity with both ulcer of thigh and inflammation `CC` `HCC` `A`

I83.222 Varicose veins of left lower extremity with both ulcer of calf and inflammation `CC` `HCC` `A`

I83.223 Varicose veins of left lower extremity with both ulcer of ankle and inflammation `CC` `HCC` `A`

I83.224 Varicose veins of left lower extremity with both ulcer of heel and midfoot and inflammation `CC` `HCC` `A`
  Varicose veins of left lower extremity with both ulcer of plantar surface of midfoot and inflammation

I83.225 Varicose veins of left lower extremity with both ulcer other part of foot and inflammation `CC` `HCC` `A`
  Varicose veins of left lower extremity with both ulcer of toe and inflammation

I83.228 Varicose veins of left lower extremity with both ulcer of other part of lower extremity and inflammation `CC` `HCC` `A`

I83.229 Varicose veins of left lower extremity with both ulcer of unspecified site and inflammation `CC` `HCC` `A`

√5ᵗʰ **I83.8** Varicose veins of lower extremities with other complications

√6ᵗʰ **I83.81** Varicose veins of lower extremities with pain

I83.811 Varicose veins of right lower extremity with pain `A`

I83.812 Varicose veins of left lower extremity with pain `A`

I83.813 Varicose veins of bilateral lower extremities with pain `A`

I83.819 Varicose veins of unspecified lower extremity with pain `A`

√6ᵗʰ **I83.89** Varicose veins of lower extremities with other complications
  Varicose veins of lower extremities with edema
  Varicose veins of lower extremities with swelling

I83.891 Varicose veins of right lower extremity with other complications `A`

I83.892 Varicose veins of left lower extremity with other complications `A`

I83.893 Varicose veins of bilateral lower extremities with other complications `A`

I83.899 Varicose veins of unspecified lower extremity with other complications `A`

√5ᵗʰ **I83.9** Asymptomatic varicose veins of lower extremities
  Phlebectasia of lower extremities
  Varicose veins of lower extremities
  Varix of lower extremities

I83.90 Asymptomatic varicose veins of unspecified lower extremity `A`
  Varicose veins NOS

I83.91 Asymptomatic varicose veins of right lower extremity `A`

I83.92 Asymptomatic varicose veins of left lower extremity `A`

I83.93 Asymptomatic varicose veins of bilateral lower extremities `A`

√4ᵗʰ **I85** Esophageal varices
  Use additional code to identify:
  alcohol abuse and dependence (F10.-)

√5ᵗʰ **I85.0** Esophageal varices
  Idiopathic esophageal varices
  Primary esophageal varices

I85.00 Esophageal varices without bleeding `CC` `HCC`
  Esophageal varices NOS

I85.01 Esophageal varices with bleeding `MCC` `HCC`

√6ᵗʰ **I85.1** Secondary esophageal varices
  Esophageal varices secondary to alcoholic liver disease
  Esophageal varices secondary to cirrhosis of liver
  Esophageal varices secondary to schistosomiasis
  Esophageal varices secondary to toxic liver disease
  Code first underlying disease

I85.10 Secondary esophageal varices without bleeding `CC` `HCC`

I85.11 Secondary esophageal varices with bleeding `MCC` `HCC`

√4ᵗʰ **I86** Varicose veins of other sites
  EXCLUDES 1   varicose veins of unspecified site (I83.9-)
  EXCLUDES 2   retinal varices (H35.0-)

I86.0 Sublingual varices
  DEF: Distended, tortuous veins beneath the tongue.

I86.1 Scrotal varices ♂
  Varicocele

I86.2 Pelvic varices

I86.3 Vulval varices ♀
  EXCLUDES 1   vulval varices complicating childbirth and the puerperium (O87.8)
  vulval varices complicating pregnancy (O22.1-)

I86.4 Gastric varices

I86.8 Varicose veins of other specified sites `A`
  Varicose ulcer of nasal septum

√4ᵗʰ **I87** Other disorders of veins

√5ᵗʰ **I87.0** Postthrombotic syndrome
  Chronic venous hypertension due to deep vein thrombosis
  Postphlebitic syndrome
  EXCLUDES 1   chronic venous hypertension without deep vein thrombosis (I87.3-)

√6ᵗʰ **I87.00** Postthrombotic syndrome without complications
  Asymptomatic postthrombotic syndrome

I87.001 Postthrombotic syndrome without complications of right lower extremity

`N` Newborn: 0   `P` Pediatric: 0-17   `M` Maternity: 9-64   `A` Adult: 15-124   `MCC` Major Complication/Comorbidity   `CC` Complication/Comorbidity   `SW` Severe Wound Dx

686   ICD-10-CM 2022

I87.002 **Postthrombotic syndrome without complications of** left lower **extremity**

I87.003 **Postthrombotic syndrome without complications of** bilateral lower **extremity**

I87.009 **Postthrombotic syndrome without complications of unspecified extremity**
Postthrombotic syndrome NOS

✓6ᵗʰ   I87.01 **Postthrombotic syndrome with** ulcer
Use additional code to specify site and severity of ulcer (L97.-)

I87.011 **Postthrombotic syndrome with ulcer of** right lower **extremity** `CC` `HCC`

I87.012 **Postthrombotic syndrome with ulcer of** left lower **extremity** `CC` `HCC`

I87.013 **Postthrombotic syndrome with ulcer of** bilateral lower **extremity** `CC` `HCC`

I87.019 **Postthrombotic syndrome with ulcer of unspecified lower extremity** `CC` `HCC`

✓6ᵗʰ   I87.02 **Postthrombotic syndrome with** inflammation

I87.021 **Postthrombotic syndrome with inflammation of** right lower **extremity**

I87.022 **Postthrombotic syndrome with inflammation of** left lower **extremity**

I87.023 **Postthrombotic syndrome with inflammation of** bilateral lower **extremity**

I87.029 **Postthrombotic syndrome with inflammation of unspecified lower extremity**

✓6ᵗʰ   I87.03 **Postthrombotic syndrome with** ulcer and inflammation
Use additional code to specify site and severity of ulcer (L97.-)

I87.031 **Postthrombotic syndrome with ulcer and inflammation of** right lower **extremity** `CC` `HCC`

I87.032 **Postthrombotic syndrome with ulcer and inflammation of** left lower **extremity** `CC` `HCC`

I87.033 **Postthrombotic syndrome with ulcer and inflammation of** bilateral lower **extremity** `CC` `HCC`

I87.039 **Postthrombotic syndrome with ulcer and inflammation of unspecified lower extremity** `CC` `HCC`

✓6ᵗʰ   I87.09 **Postthrombotic syndrome with other complications**

I87.091 **Postthrombotic syndrome with other complications of** right lower **extremity**

I87.092 **Postthrombotic syndrome with other complications of** left lower **extremity**

I87.093 **Postthrombotic syndrome with other complications of** bilateral lower **extremity**

I87.099 **Postthrombotic syndrome with other complications of unspecified lower extremity**

I87.1 **Compression of vein** `CC`
Stricture of vein
Vena cava syndrome (inferior) (superior)
EXCLUDES 2   *compression of pulmonary vein (I28.8)*

I87.2 **Venous insufficiency (chronic) (peripheral)**
Stasis dermatitis
EXCLUDES 1   *stasis dermatitis with varicose veins of lower extremities (I83.1-, I83.2-)*
DEF: Insufficient drainage of venous blood in any part of the body that results in edema or dermatosis.

✓5ᵗʰ   I87.3 **Chronic venous hypertension (idiopathic)**
Stasis edema
EXCLUDES 1   *chronic venous hypertension due to deep vein thrombosis (I87.0-)*
varicose veins of lower extremities (I83.-)

✓6ᵗʰ   I87.30 **Chronic venous hypertension (idiopathic)** without complications
Asymptomatic chronic venous hypertension (idiopathic)

I87.301 **Chronic venous hypertension (idiopathic) without complications of** right lower **extremity**

I87.302 **Chronic venous hypertension (idiopathic) without complications of** left lower **extremity**

I87.303 **Chronic venous hypertension (idiopathic) without complications of** bilateral lower **extremity**

I87.309 **Chronic venous hypertension (idiopathic) without complications of unspecified lower extremity**
Chronic venous hypertension NOS

✓6ᵗʰ   I87.31 **Chronic venous hypertension (idiopathic) with** ulcer
Use additional code to specify site and severity of ulcer (L97.-)

I87.311 **Chronic venous hypertension (idiopathic) with ulcer of** right lower **extremity** `CC` `HCC`

I87.312 **Chronic venous hypertension (idiopathic) with ulcer of** left lower **extremity** `CC` `HCC`

I87.313 **Chronic venous hypertension (idiopathic) with ulcer of** bilateral lower **extremity** `CC` `HCC`

I87.319 **Chronic venous hypertension (idiopathic) with ulcer of unspecified lower extremity** `CC` `HCC`

✓6ᵗʰ   I87.32 **Chronic venous hypertension (idiopathic) with** inflammation

I87.321 **Chronic venous hypertension (idiopathic) with inflammation of** right lower **extremity**

I87.322 **Chronic venous hypertension (idiopathic) with inflammation of** left lower **extremity**

I87.323 **Chronic venous hypertension (idiopathic) with inflammation of** bilateral lower **extremity**

I87.329 **Chronic venous hypertension (idiopathic) with inflammation of unspecified lower extremity**

✓6ᵗʰ   I87.33 **Chronic venous hypertension (idiopathic) with** ulcer and inflammation
Use additional code to specify site and severity of ulcer (L97.-)

I87.331 **Chronic venous hypertension (idiopathic) with ulcer and inflammation of** right lower **extremity** `CC` `HCC`

I87.332 **Chronic venous hypertension (idiopathic) with ulcer and inflammation of** left lower **extremity** `CC` `HCC`

I87.333 **Chronic venous hypertension (idiopathic) with ulcer and inflammation of** bilateral lower **extremity** `CC` `HCC`

I87.339 **Chronic venous hypertension (idiopathic) with ulcer and inflammation of unspecified lower extremity** `CC` `HCC`

✓6ᵗʰ   I87.39 **Chronic venous hypertension (idiopathic) with other complications**

I87.391 **Chronic venous hypertension (idiopathic) with other complications of** right lower **extremity**

I87.392 **Chronic venous hypertension (idiopathic) with other complications of** left lower **extremity**

I87.393 **Chronic venous hypertension (idiopathic) with other complications of** bilateral lower **extremity**

I87.399 **Chronic venous hypertension (idiopathic) with other complications of unspecified lower extremity**

I87.8 **Other specified disorders of veins**
Phlebosclerosis
Venofibrosis

I87.9 **Disorder of vein, unspecified**

✓4ᵗʰ   I88 **Nonspecific lymphadenitis**
EXCLUDES 1   *acute lymphadenitis, except mesenteric (L04.-)*
enlarged lymph nodes NOS (R59.-)
human immunodeficiency virus [HIV] disease resulting in generalized lymphadenopathy (B20)

I88.0 **Nonspecific mesenteric lymphadenitis**
Mesenteric lymphadenitis (acute)(chronic)

I88.1 **Chronic lymphadenitis, except mesenteric**
Adenitis
Lymphadenitis

I88.8 **Other nonspecific lymphadenitis**

Chapter 9. Diseases of the Circulatory System

I88.9 Nonspecific lymphadenitis, unspecified
Lymphadenitis NOS

✓4ᵗʰ I89 Other noninfective disorders of lymphatic vessels and lymph nodes
    EXCLUDES 1   chylocele, tunica vaginalis (nonfilarial) NOS (N50.89)
           enlarged lymph nodes NOS (R59.-)
           filarial chylocele (B74.-)
           hereditary lymphedema (Q82.0)

I89.0 Lymphedema, not elsewhere classified
Elephantiasis (nonfilarial) NOS
Lymphangiectasis
Obliteration, lymphatic vessel
Praecox lymphedema
Secondary lymphedema
    EXCLUDES 1   postmastectomy lymphedema (I97.2)

I89.1 Lymphangitis
Chronic lymphangitis
Lymphangitis NOS
Subacute lymphangitis
    EXCLUDES 1   acute lymphangitis (L03.-)

I89.8 Other specified noninfective disorders of lymphatic vessels and lymph nodes
Chylocele (nonfilarial)
Chylous ascites
Chylous cyst
Lipomelanotic reticulosis
Lymph node or vessel fistula
Lymph node or vessel infarction
Lymph node or vessel rupture

I89.9 Noninfective disorder of lymphatic vessels and lymph nodes, unspecified
Disease of lymphatic vessels NOS

Other and unspecified disorders of the circulatory system (I95-I99)

✓4ᵗʰ I95 Hypotension
    EXCLUDES 1   cardiovascular collapse (R57.9) (~R57.9)
           maternal hypotension syndrome (O26.5-)
           nonspecific low blood pressure reading NOS (R03.1)

I95.0 Idiopathic hypotension

I95.1 Orthostatic hypotension
Hypotension, postural
    EXCLUDES 1   neurogenic orthostatic hypotension [Shy-Drager] (G90.3)
           orthostatic hypotension due to drugs (I95.2)

I95.2 Hypotension due to drugs
Orthostatic hypotension due to drugs
Use additional code for adverse effect, if applicable, to identify drug (T36-T50 with fifth or sixth character 5)

I95.3 Hypotension of hemodialysis
Intra-dialytic hypotension

✓5ᵗʰ I95.8 Other hypotension
I95.81 Postprocedural hypotension
I95.89 Other hypotension
Chronic hypotension

I95.9 Hypotension, unspecified

I96 Gangrene, not elsewhere classified   CC HCC
Gangrenous cellulitis
    EXCLUDES 1   gangrene in atherosclerosis of native arteries of the extremities (I70.26)
           gangrene in hernia (K40.1, K40.4, K41.1, K41.4, K42.1, K43.1-, K44.1, K45.1, K46.1)
           gangrene in other peripheral vascular diseases (I73.-)
           gangrene of certain specified sites - see Alphabetical Index
           gas gangrene (A48.0)
           pyoderma gangrenosum (L88)
    EXCLUDES 2   gangrene in diabetes mellitus (E08-E13 with .52)
    AHA: 2018,4Q,87; 2018,3Q,3; 2017,3Q,6; 2013,2Q,34

✓4ᵗʰ I97 Intraoperative and postprocedural complications and disorders of circulatory system, not elsewhere classified
    EXCLUDES 2   postprocedural shock (T81.1-)
    AHA: 2021,1Q,13; 2019,2Q,21

I97.0 Postcardiotomy syndrome

✓5ᵗʰ I97.1 Other postprocedural cardiac functional disturbances
    EXCLUDES 2   acute pulmonary insufficiency following thoracic surgery (J95.1)
           intraoperative cardiac functional disturbances (I97.7-)

✓6ᵗʰ I97.11 Postprocedural cardiac insufficiency
I97.110 Postprocedural cardiac insufficiency following cardiac surgery CC
I97.111 Postprocedural cardiac insufficiency following other surgery CC

✓6ᵗʰ I97.12 Postprocedural cardiac arrest
I97.120 Postprocedural cardiac arrest following cardiac surgery CC
I97.121 Postprocedural cardiac arrest following other surgery CC

✓6ᵗʰ I97.13 Postprocedural heart failure
Use additional code to identify the heart failure (I50.-)
I97.130 Postprocedural heart failure following cardiac surgery CC
I97.131 Postprocedural heart failure following other surgery CC

✓6ᵗʰ I97.19 Other postprocedural cardiac functional disturbances
Use additional code, if applicable, to further specify disorder
I97.190 Other postprocedural cardiac functional disturbances following cardiac surgery CC
Use additional code, if applicable, for type 4 or type 5 myocardial infarction, to further specify disorder
AHA: 2019,2Q,33
I97.191 Other postprocedural cardiac functional disturbances following other surgery CC

I97.2 Postmastectomy lymphedema syndrome A
Elephantiasis due to mastectomy
Obliteration of lymphatic vessels

I97.3 Postprocedural hypertension

✓5ᵗʰ I97.4 Intraoperative hemorrhage and hematoma of a circulatory system organ or structure complicating a procedure
    EXCLUDES 1   intraoperative hemorrhage and hematoma of a circulatory system organ or structure due to accidental puncture and laceration during a procedure (I97.5-)
    EXCLUDES 2   intraoperative cerebrovascular hemorrhage complicating a procedure (G97.3-)

✓6ᵗʰ I97.41 Intraoperative hemorrhage and hematoma of a circulatory system organ or structure complicating a circulatory system procedure
I97.410 Intraoperative hemorrhage and hematoma of a circulatory system organ or structure complicating a cardiac catheterization CC
I97.411 Intraoperative hemorrhage and hematoma of a circulatory system organ or structure complicating a cardiac bypass CC
I97.418 Intraoperative hemorrhage and hematoma of a circulatory system organ or structure complicating other circulatory system procedure CC

I97.42 Intraoperative hemorrhage and hematoma of a circulatory system organ or structure complicating other procedure CC
AHA: 2020,1Q,19

✓5ᵗʰ I97.5 Accidental puncture and laceration of a circulatory system organ or structure during a procedure
    EXCLUDES 2   accidental puncture and laceration of brain during a procedure (G97.4-)

I97.51 Accidental puncture and laceration of a circulatory system organ or structure during a circulatory system procedure CC
AHA: 2019,2Q,24

I97.52 Accidental puncture and laceration of a circulatory system organ or structure during other procedure CC

N Newborn: 0   P Pediatric: 0-17   M Maternity: 9-64   A Adult: 15-124   MCC Major Complication/Comorbidity   CC Complication/Comorbidity   SW Severe Wound Dx

688   ICD-10-CM 2022

✓5ᵗʰ **I97.6** Postprocedural hemorrhage, hematoma and seroma **of a circulatory system organ or structure following a procedure**

     EXCLUDES 2   *postprocedural cerebrovascular hemorrhage complicating a procedure (G97.5-)*

     AHA: 2016,4Q,9-10

   ✓6ᵗʰ **I97.61** Postprocedural hemorrhage **of a circulatory system organ or structure following a** circulatory system procedure

      I97.610 **Postprocedural hemorrhage of a circulatory system organ or structure following a** cardiac catheterization   **CC**

      I97.611 **Postprocedural hemorrhage of a circulatory system organ or structure following** cardiac bypass   **CC**

      I97.618 **Postprocedural hemorrhage of a circulatory system organ or structure following** other circulatory system procedure   **CC**

   ✓6ᵗʰ **I97.62** Postprocedural hemorrhage, hematoma and seroma **of a circulatory system organ or structure following** other procedure

      I97.620 **Postprocedural** hemorrhage **of a circulatory system organ or structure following other procedure**   **CC**

      I97.621 **Postprocedural** hematoma **of a circulatory system organ or structure following other procedure**   **CC**

      I97.622 **Postprocedural** seroma **of a circulatory system organ or structure following other procedure**   **CC**

   ✓6ᵗʰ **I97.63** Postprocedural hematoma **of a circulatory system organ or structure following a** circulatory system procedure

      I97.630 **Postprocedural hematoma of a circulatory system organ or structure following a** cardiac catheterization   **CC**

      I97.631 **Postprocedural hematoma of a circulatory system organ or structure following** cardiac bypass   **CC**

      I97.638 **Postprocedural hematoma of a circulatory system organ or structure following** other circulatory system procedure   **CC**

   ✓6ᵗʰ **I97.64** Postprocedural seroma **of a circulatory system organ or structure following a circulatory system procedure**

      I97.640 **Postprocedural seroma of a circulatory system organ or structure following a** cardiac catheterization   **CC**

      I97.641 **Postprocedural seroma of a circulatory system organ or structure following** cardiac bypass   **CC**

      I97.648 **Postprocedural seroma of a circulatory system organ or structure following other** circulatory system procedure   **CC**

✓5ᵗʰ **I97.7** Intraoperative **cardiac** functional disturbances

     EXCLUDES 2   *acute pulmonary insufficiency following thoracic surgery (J95.1)*

        postprocedural cardiac functional disturbances (I97.1-)

   ✓6ᵗʰ **I97.71** Intraoperative cardiac arrest

      I97.710 **Intraoperative cardiac arrest during** cardiac surgery   **CC**

      I97.711 **Intraoperative cardiac arrest during** other surgery   **CC**

   ✓6ᵗʰ **I97.79** **Other intraoperative cardiac functional disturbances**

      Use additional code, if applicable, to further specify disorder

      I97.790 **Other intraoperative cardiac functional disturbances during** cardiac surgery   **CC**

      I97.791 **Other intraoperative cardiac functional disturbances during** other surgery   **CC**

✓5ᵗʰ **I97.8** **Other intraoperative and postprocedural complications and disorders of the circulatory system, not elsewhere classified**

     Use additional code, if applicable, to further specify disorder

   ✓6ᵗʰ **I97.81** Intraoperative cerebrovascular infarction

      I97.810 **Intraoperative cerebrovascular infarction during** cardiac surgery   **CC HCC**

      I97.811 **Intraoperative cerebrovascular infarction during** other surgery   **CC HCC**

   ✓6ᵗʰ **I97.82** Postprocedural **cerebrovascular infarction**

      I97.820 **Postprocedural cerebrovascular infarction following** cardiac surgery   **CC HCC**

      I97.821 **Postprocedural cerebrovascular infarction following** other surgery   **CC HCC**

     I97.88 **Other intraoperative complications of the circulatory system, not elsewhere classified**   **CC**

     I97.89 **Other postprocedural complications and disorders of the circulatory system, not elsewhere classified**   **CC**

      AHA: 2020,3Q,3-8; 2019,2Q,33

✓4ᵗʰ **I99** **Other and unspecified disorders of circulatory system**

   I99.8 **Other disorder of circulatory system**

     AHA: 2020,4Q,98

   I99.9 **Unspecified disorder of circulatory system**

✅ Additional Character Required   ✓x7ᵗʰ Placeholder   Questionable PDx   Manifestation   Unspecified Dx   **UPD** Unacceptable PDx   **H1-H14** HAC   **HCC** CMS-HCC Dx   **HIV** HIV Dx

ICD-10-CM 2022   689

Chapter 10. Diseases of the Respiratory System (J00–J99)

Chapter-specific Guidelines with Coding Examples

The chapter-specific guidelines from the ICD-10-CM Official Guidelines for Coding and Reporting have been provided below. Along with these guidelines are coding examples, contained in the shaded boxes, that have been developed to help illustrate the coding and/or sequencing guidance found in these guidelines.

a. Chronic obstructive pulmonary disease [COPD] and asthma

1) Acute exacerbation of chronic obstructive bronchitis and asthma

The codes in categories J44 and J45 distinguish between uncomplicated cases and those in acute exacerbation. An acute exacerbation is a worsening or a decompensation of a chronic condition. An acute exacerbation is not equivalent to an infection superimposed on a chronic condition, though an exacerbation may be triggered by an infection.

Vancomycin IV was started to treat a patient with acute pneumonia due to *Streptococcus pneumoniae*. Patient also with acute exacerbation of COPD continued on home meds.

J13   **Pneumonia due to Streptococcus pneumoniae**

J44.0   **Chronic obstructive pulmonary disease with (acute) lower respiratory infection**

J44.1   **Chronic obstructive pulmonary disease with (acute) exacerbation**

Explanation: ICD-10-CM uses combination codes to create organism-specific classifications for acute pneumonia. Category J44 codes include combination codes with severity components, which differentiate between COPD with acute lower respiratory infection (acute pneumonia), COPD with acute exacerbation, and COPD without mention of a complication (unspecified).

An acute exacerbation is a worsening or a decompensation of a chronic condition. An acute exacerbation is not equivalent to an infection superimposed on a chronic condition, though an exacerbation may be triggered by an infection, as in this example. Treatment of the pneumonia necessitated the inpatient admission. Instructional notes at J44.0 say to "code also to identify the infection," which informs the coder that another code must be assigned if applicable. Sequencing of the pneumonia and COPD exacerbation are governed by the Section II, "Selection of Principal Diagnosis," guidelines. In this case it was the pneumonia that was "chiefly responsible for occasioning the admission" with the IV vancomycin treatment.

Exacerbation of moderate persistent asthma with status asthmaticus

J45.42   **Moderate persistent asthma with status asthmaticus**

Explanation: Category J45 Asthma includes severity-specific subcategories and fifth-character codes to distinguish between uncomplicated cases, those in acute exacerbation, and those with status asthmaticus.

---

b. Acute respiratory failure

1) Acute respiratory failure as principal diagnosis

A code from subcategory J96.0, Acute respiratory failure, or subcategory J96.2, Acute and chronic respiratory failure, may be assigned as a principal diagnosis when it is the condition established after study to be chiefly responsible for occasioning the admission to the hospital, and the selection is supported by the Alphabetic Index and Tabular List. However, chapter-specific coding guidelines (such as obstetrics, poisoning, HIV, newborn) that provide sequencing direction take precedence.

Acute hypoxic respiratory failure due to COPD exacerbation

J96.01   **Acute respiratory failure with hypoxia**

J44.1   **Chronic obstructive pulmonary disease with (acute) exacerbation**

Explanation: Category J96 classifies respiratory failure with combination codes that designate the severity and the presence of hypoxia and hypercapnia. Code J96.01 is sequenced as the first-listed diagnosis, as the reason for the admission. Respiratory failure may be assigned as a principal diagnosis when it is the condition established after study to be chiefly responsible for occasioning the admission to the hospital and the selection is supported by the Alphabetic Index and Tabular List.

---

2) Acute respiratory failure as secondary diagnosis

Respiratory failure may be listed as a secondary diagnosis if it occurs after admission, or if it is present on admission, but does not meet the definition of principal diagnosis.

Acute respiratory failure due to accidental oxycodone overdose

T40.2X1A   **Poisoning by other opioids, accidental (unintentional), initial encounter**

J96.00   **Acute respiratory failure, unspecified whether with hypoxia or hypercapnia**

Explanation: Respiratory failure may be assigned as a principal diagnosis when it is the condition established after study to be chiefly responsible for occasioning the admission to the hospital, and the selection is supported by the Alphabetic Index and Tabular List. However, chapter-specific coding guidelines, such as poisoning, that provide sequencing direction take precedence. When coding a poisoning or reaction to the improper use of a medication (e.g. overdose, wrong substance given or taken in error, wrong route of administration), first assign the appropriate code from categories T36–T50. Use additional code(s) for all manifestations of the poisoning. In this instance, the respiratory failure is a manifestation of the poisoning and is sequenced as a secondary diagnosis.

Acute pneumococcal pneumonia with subsequent development of acute respiratory failure

J13   **Pneumonia due to Streptococcus pneumoniae**

J96.00   **Acute respiratory failure, unspecified whether with hypoxia or hypercapnia**

Explanation: Acute respiratory failure may be listed as a secondary diagnosis if it occurs after admission, or if it is present on admission but does not meet the definition of principal diagnosis.

---

3) Sequencing of acute respiratory failure and another acute condition

When a patient is admitted with respiratory failure and another acute condition, (e.g., myocardial infarction, cerebrovascular accident, aspiration pneumonia), the principal diagnosis will not be the same in every situation. This applies whether the other acute condition is a respiratory or nonrespiratory condition. Selection of the principal diagnosis will be dependent on the circumstances of admission. If both the respiratory failure and the other acute condition are equally responsible for occasioning the admission to the hospital, and there are no chapter-specific sequencing rules, the guideline regarding two or more diagnoses that equally meet the definition for principal diagnosis (*Section II, C.*) may be applied in these situations.

If the documentation is not clear as to whether acute respiratory failure and another condition are equally responsible for occasioning the admission, query the provider for clarification.

Acute pneumococcal pneumonia and acute respiratory failure, both present on admission

J96.00   **Acute respiratory failure, unspecified whether with hypoxia or hypercapnia**

J13   **Pneumonia due to Streptococcus pneumoniae**

Explanation: When a patient is admitted with respiratory failure and another acute condition, such as a bacterial pneumonia, the principal diagnosis is not the same in every situation. This applies whether the other acute condition is a respiratory or nonrespiratory condition. The principal diagnosis depends on the circumstances of admission.

---

c. Influenza due to certain identified influenza viruses

Code only confirmed cases of influenza due to certain identified influenza viruses (category J09), and due to other identified influenza virus (category J10). This is an exception to the hospital inpatient guideline Section II, H. (Uncertain Diagnosis).

In this context, "confirmation" does not require documentation of positive laboratory testing specific for avian or other novel influenza A or other identified influenza virus. However, coding should be based on the provider's diagnostic statement that the patient has avian influenza, or other novel influenza A, for category J09, or has another particular identified strain of influenza, such as H1N1 or H3N2, but not identified as novel or variant, for category J10.

If the provider records "suspected" or "possible" or "probable" avian influenza, or novel influenza, or other identified influenza, then the appropriate influenza code from category J11, Influenza due to unidentified influenza virus, should be assigned. A code from category J09, Influenza due to certain identified influenza viruses, should not be assigned nor should a code from category J10, Influenza due to other identified influenza virus.

Influenza due to avian influenza virus with pneumonia

J09.X1	Influenza due to identified novel influenza A virus with pneumonia

Explanation: Codes in category J09 Influenza due to certain identified influenza viruses should be assigned only for confirmed cases. "Confirmation" does not require positive laboratory testing of a specific influenza virus but does need to be based on the provider's diagnostic statement, which should not include terms such as "possible," "probable," or "suspected."

---

d. Ventilator associated pneumonia

1) Documentation of ventilator associated pneumonia

As with all procedural or postprocedural complications, code assignment is based on the provider's documentation of the relationship between the condition and the procedure.

Code J95.851, Ventilator associated pneumonia, should be assigned only when the provider has documented ventilator associated pneumonia (VAP). An additional code to identify the organism (e.g., Pseudomonas aeruginosa, code B96.5) should also be assigned. Do not assign an additional code from categories J12-J18 to identify the type of pneumonia.

Code J95.851 should not be assigned for cases where the patient has pneumonia and is on a mechanical ventilator and the provider has not specifically stated that the pneumonia is ventilator-associated pneumonia. If the documentation is unclear as to whether the patient has a pneumonia that is a complication attributable to the mechanical ventilator, query the provider.

2) Ventilator associated pneumonia develops after admission

A patient may be admitted with one type of pneumonia (e.g., code J13, Pneumonia due to Streptococcus pneumonia) and subsequently develop VAP. In this instance, the principal diagnosis would be the appropriate code from categories J12-J18 for the pneumonia diagnosed at the time of admission. Code J95.851, Ventilator associated pneumonia, would be assigned as an additional diagnosis when the provider has also documented the presence of ventilator associated pneumonia.

Patient with pneumonia due to *Klebsiella pneumoniae* develops superimposed MRSA ventilator-associated pneumonia

J15.0	Pneumonia due to Klebsiella pneumoniae
J95.851	Ventilator associated pneumonia
B95.62	Methicillin resistant Staphylococcus aureus infection as the cause of diseases classified elsewhere

Explanation: Code assignment for ventilator-associated pneumonia is based on the provider's documentation of the relationship between the condition and the procedure and is reported only when the provider has documented ventilator-associated pneumonia (VAP).

A patient may be admitted with one type of pneumonia and subsequently develop VAP. In this example, the principal diagnosis code describes the pneumonia diagnosed at the time of admission, with code J95.851 Ventilator associated pneumonia, assigned as secondary.

---

e. Vaping-related disorders

For patients presenting with condition(s) related to vaping, assign code U07.0, Vaping-related disorder, as the principal diagnosis. For lung injury due to vaping, assign only code U07.0. Assign additional codes for other manifestations, such as acute respiratory failure (subcategory J96.0-) or pneumonitis (code J68.0).

Associated respiratory signs and symptoms due to vaping, such as cough, shortness of breath, etc., are not coded separately, when a definitive diagnosis has been established. However, it would be appropriate to code separately any gastrointestinal symptoms, such as diarrhea and abdominal pain.

See Section I.C.1.g.1.c.i. for Pneumonia confirmed as due to COVID-19

23-year-old patient with history of anxiety disorder admitted with fever, dyspnea and nonproductive cough. Patient's respiratory function continued to clinically worsen, requiring intubation for suspected ARDS and required OGT suction for coffee ground hematemesis. Following extubating, patient confirmed the use of THC vaping cartridge preceding development of symptoms. Discharge diagnosis is ARDS due to EVALI and anxiety disorder.

U07.0	Vaping related disorder
J80	Acute respiratory distress syndrome
K92.0	Hematemesis
F41.9	Anxiety disorder, unspecified

Explanation: Codes U07.0 and J80 represent the vaping-related disorder and its associated manifestation, the acute respiratory distress syndrome (ARDS). The symptoms that brought the patient in are not coded separately because these are integral to the vaping disorder and the ARDS, unlike the hematemesis (vomiting blood) a gastrointestinal symptom that is not integral to either of these conditions.

Chapter 10. Diseases of the Respiratory System (J00-J99)

NOTE   When a respiratory condition is described as occurring in more than one site and is not specifically indexed, it should be classified to the lower anatomic site (e.g., tracheobronchitis to bronchitis in J40).

Use additional code, where applicable, to identify:
exposure to environmental tobacco smoke (Z77.22)
exposure to tobacco smoke in the perinatal period (P96.81)
history of tobacco dependence (Z87.891)
occupational exposure to environmental tobacco smoke (Z57.31)
tobacco dependence (F17.-)
tobacco use (Z72.0)

EXCLUDES 2   certain conditions originating in the perinatal period (P04-P96)
certain infectious and parasitic diseases (A00-B99)
complications of pregnancy, childbirth and the puerperium (O00-O9A)
congenital malformations, deformations and chromosomal abnormalities (Q00-Q99)
endocrine, nutritional and metabolic diseases (E00-E88)
injury, poisoning and certain other consequences of external causes (S00-T88)
neoplasms (C00-D49)
smoke inhalation (T59.81-)
symptoms, signs and abnormal clinical and laboratory findings, not elsewhere classified (R00-R94)

This chapter contains the following blocks:
J00-J06   Acute upper respiratory infections
J09-J18   Influenza and pneumonia
J20-J22   Other acute lower respiratory infections
J30-J39   Other diseases of upper respiratory tract
J40-J47   Chronic lower respiratory diseases
J60-J70   Lung diseases due to external agents
J80-J84   Other respiratory diseases principally affecting the interstitium
J85-J86   Suppurative and necrotic conditions of the lower respiratory tract
J90-J94   Other diseases of the pleura
J95   Intraoperative and postprocedural complications and disorders of respiratory system, not elsewhere classified
J96-J99   Other diseases of the respiratory system

Acute upper respiratory infections (J00-J06)

EXCLUDES 1   chronic obstructive pulmonary disease with acute lower respiratory infection (J44.0)

J00   Acute nasopharyngitis [common cold]
Acute rhinitis
Coryza (acute)
Infective nasopharyngitis NOS
Infective rhinitis
Nasal catarrh, acute
Nasopharyngitis NOS
EXCLUDES 1   acute pharyngitis (J02.-)
acute sore throat NOS (J02.9)
influenza virus with other respiratory manifestations (J09.X2, J10.1, J11.1)
pharyngitis NOS (J02.9)
rhinitis NOS (J31.0)
sore throat NOS (J02.9)
EXCLUDES 2   allergic rhinitis (J30.1-J30.9)
chronic pharyngitis (J31.2)
chronic rhinitis (J31.0)
chronic sore throat (J31.2)
nasopharyngitis, chronic (J31.1)
vasomotor rhinitis (J30.0)
DEF: Acute inflammation of the mucous membranes that extends from the nares to the pharynx. It is characterized by nasal obstruction, sneezing, runny nose, and sore throat.

✓4ᵗʰ J01   Acute sinusitis
INCLUDES   acute abscess of sinus
acute empyema of sinus
acute infection of sinus
acute inflammation of sinus
acute suppuration of sinus
Use additional code (B95-B97) to identify infectious agent
EXCLUDES 1   sinusitis NOS (J32.9)
EXCLUDES 2   chronic sinusitis (J32.0-J32.8)

✓5ᵗʰ J01.0   Acute maxillary sinusitis
Acute antritis
J01.00   Acute maxillary sinusitis, unspecified
J01.01   Acute recurrent maxillary sinusitis

✓5ᵗʰ J01.1   Acute frontal sinusitis
J01.10   Acute frontal sinusitis, unspecified
J01.11   Acute recurrent frontal sinusitis
✓5ᵗʰ J01.2   Acute ethmoidal sinusitis
J01.20   Acute ethmoidal sinusitis, unspecified
J01.21   Acute recurrent ethmoidal sinusitis
✓5ᵗʰ J01.3   Acute sphenoidal sinusitis
J01.30   Acute sphenoidal sinusitis, unspecified
J01.31   Acute recurrent sphenoidal sinusitis
✓5ᵗʰ J01.4   Acute pansinusitis
J01.40   Acute pansinusitis, unspecified
J01.41   Acute recurrent pansinusitis
✓5ᵗʰ J01.8   Other acute sinusitis
J01.80   Other acute sinusitis
Acute sinusitis involving more than one sinus but not pansinusitis
J01.81   Other acute recurrent sinusitis
Acute recurrent sinusitis involving more than one sinus but not pansinusitis
✓5ᵗʰ J01.9   Acute sinusitis, unspecified
J01.90   Acute sinusitis, unspecified
J01.91   Acute recurrent sinusitis, unspecified

✓4ᵗʰ J02   Acute pharyngitis
INCLUDES   acute sore throat
EXCLUDES 1   acute laryngopharyngitis (J06.0)
peritonsillar abscess (J36)
pharyngeal abscess (J39.1)
retropharyngeal abscess (J39.0)
EXCLUDES 2   chronic pharyngitis (J31.2)

J02.0   Streptococcal pharyngitis
Septic pharyngitis
Streptococcal sore throat
EXCLUDES 2   scarlet fever (A38.-)

J02.8   Acute pharyngitis due to other specified organisms
Use additional code (B95-B97) to identify infectious agent
EXCLUDES 1   acute pharyngitis due to coxsackie virus (B08.5)
acute pharyngitis due to gonococcus (A54.5)
acute pharyngitis due to herpes [simplex] virus (B00.2)
acute pharyngitis due to infectious mononucleosis (B27.-)
enteroviral vesicular pharyngitis (B08.5)

J02.9   Acute pharyngitis, unspecified
Gangrenous pharyngitis (acute)
Infective pharyngitis (acute) NOS
Pharyngitis (acute) NOS
Sore throat (acute) NOS
Suppurative pharyngitis (acute)
Ulcerative pharyngitis (acute)
EXCLUDES 1   influenza virus with other respiratory manifestations (J09.X2, J10.1, J11.1)

✓4ᵗʰ J03   Acute tonsillitis
EXCLUDES 1   acute sore throat (J02.-)
hypertrophy of tonsils (J35.1)
peritonsillar abscess (J36)
sore throat NOS (J02.9)
streptococcal sore throat (J02.0)
EXCLUDES 2   chronic tonsillitis (J35.0)
✓5ᵗʰ J03.0   Streptococcal tonsillitis
J03.00   Acute streptococcal tonsillitis, unspecified
J03.01   Acute recurrent streptococcal tonsillitis
✓5ᵗʰ J03.8   Acute tonsillitis due to other specified organisms
Use additional code (B95-B97) to identify infectious agent
EXCLUDES 1   diphtheritic tonsillitis (A36.0)
herpesviral pharyngotonsillitis (B00.2)
streptococcal tonsillitis (J03.0)
tuberculous tonsillitis (A15.8)
Vincent's tonsillitis (A69.1)
J03.80   Acute tonsillitis due to other specified organisms
J03.81   Acute recurrent tonsillitis due to other specified organisms

✓5ᵗʰ **J03.9**   **Acute tonsillitis, unspecified**
     Follicular tonsillitis (acute)
     Gangrenous tonsillitis (acute)
     Infective tonsillitis (acute)
     Tonsillitis (acute) NOS
     Ulcerative tonsillitis (acute)
       EXCLUDES 1   *influenza virus with other respiratory manifestations (J09.X2, J10.1, J11.1)*

    J03.90   **Acute tonsillitis, unspecified**
    J03.91   **Acute recurrent tonsillitis, unspecified**

✓4ᵗʰ **J04**   **Acute laryngitis and tracheitis**
     Code also influenza, if present, such as:
     influenza due to identified novel influenza A virus with other respiratory manifestations (J09.X2)
     influenza due to other identified influenza virus with other respiratory manifestations (J10.1)
     influenza due to unidentified influenza virus with other respiratory manifestations (J11.1)
     Use additional code (B95-B97) to identify infectious agent
       EXCLUDES 1   *acute obstructive laryngitis [croup] and epiglottitis (J05.-)*
       EXCLUDES 2   *laryngismus (stridulus) (J38.5)*

    J04.0   **Acute laryngitis**
       Edematous laryngitis (acute)
       Laryngitis (acute) NOS
       Subglottic laryngitis (acute)
       Suppurative laryngitis (acute)
       Ulcerative laryngitis (acute)
         EXCLUDES 1   *acute obstructive laryngitis (J05.0)*
         EXCLUDES 2   *chronic laryngitis (J37.0)*

    ✓5ᵗʰ **J04.1**   **Acute tracheitis**
       Acute viral tracheitis
       Catarrhal tracheitis (acute)
       Tracheitis (acute) NOS
         EXCLUDES 2   *chronic tracheitis (J42)*
       J04.10   **Acute tracheitis without obstruction**
       J04.11   **Acute tracheitis with obstruction**   MCC

    J04.2   **Acute laryngotracheitis**
       Laryngotracheitis NOS
       Tracheitis (acute) with laryngitis (acute)
         EXCLUDES 1   *acute obstructive laryngotracheitis (J05.0)*
         EXCLUDES 2   *chronic laryngotracheitis (J37.1)*

    ✓5ᵗʰ **J04.3**   **Supraglottitis, unspecified**
       J04.30   **Supraglottitis, unspecified, without obstruction**
       J04.31   **Supraglottitis, unspecified, with obstruction**   MCC

✓4ᵗʰ **J05**   **Acute obstructive laryngitis [croup] and epiglottitis**
     ►Code also, influenza, if present, such as:◄
     influenza due to identified novel influenza A virus with other respiratory manifestations (J09.X2)
     influenza due to other identified influenza virus with other respiratory manifestations (J10.1)
     influenza due to unidentified influenza virus with other respiratory manifestations (J11.1)
     Use additional code (B95-B97) to identify infectious agent

    J05.0   **Acute obstructive laryngitis [croup]**
       Obstructive laryngitis (acute) NOS
       Obstructive laryngotracheitis NOS
       DEF: Acute laryngeal obstruction due to allergies, foreign bodies, or in the majority of cases a viral infection. Symptoms include a harsh, barking cough, hoarseness, and a persistent, high-pitched respiratory sound (stridor).

    ✓5ᵗʰ **J05.1**   **Acute epiglottitis**
         EXCLUDES 2   *epiglottitis, chronic (J37.0)*
       J05.10   **Acute epiglottitis without obstruction**   CC
         Epiglottitis NOS
       J05.11   **Acute epiglottitis with obstruction**   MCC

✓4ᵗʰ **J06**   **Acute upper respiratory infections of multiple and unspecified sites**
       EXCLUDES 1   *acute respiratory infection NOS (J22)*
           influenza virus with other respiratory manifestations (J09.X2, J10.1, J11.1)
           streptococcal pharyngitis (J02.0)

    J06.0   **Acute laryngopharyngitis**

J06.9   **Acute upper respiratory infection, unspecified**
     Upper respiratory disease, acute
     Upper respiratory infection NOS
     Use additional code (B95-B97) to identify infectious agent, if known, such as:
     respiratory syncytial virus (RSV) (B97.4)
     AHA: 2020,1Q,22

Influenza and pneumonia (J09-J18)

EXCLUDES 2   *allergic or eosinophilic pneumonia (J82)*
       aspiration pneumonia NOS (J69.0)
       meconium pneumonia (P24.01)
       neonatal aspiration pneumonia (P24.-)
       pneumonia due to solids and liquids (J69.-)
       congenital pneumonia (P23.9)
       lipid pneumonia (J69.1)
       rheumatic pneumonia (I00)
       ventilator associated pneumonia (J95.851)
AHA: 2017,4Q,96
TIP: Hemoptysis (R04.2) is not customarily associated with pneumonia and may be reported separately.

✓4ᵗʰ **J09**   **Influenza due to certain identified influenza viruses**
       EXCLUDES 1   *influenza A/H1N1 (J10.-)*
           influenza due to other identified influenza virus (J10.-)
           influenza due to unidentified influenza virus (J11.-)
           seasonal influenza due to other identified influenza virus (J10.-)
           seasonal influenza due to unidentified influenza virus (J11.-)

    ✓5ᵗʰ **J09.X**   **Influenza due to identified novel influenza A virus**
       Avian influenza
       Bird influenza
       Influenza A/H5N1
       Influenza of other animal origin, not bird or swine
       Swine influenza virus (viruses that normally cause infections in pigs)
       AHA: 2016,3Q,10

       J09.X1   **Influenza due to identified novel influenza A virus with pneumonia**   HIV MCC
         Code also, if applicable, associated:
         lung abscess (J85.1)
         other specified type of pneumonia

       J09.X2   **Influenza due to identified novel influenza A virus with other respiratory manifestations**
         Influenza due to identified novel influenza A virus NOS
         Influenza due to identified novel influenza A virus with laryngitis
         Influenza due to identified novel influenza A virus with pharyngitis
         Influenza due to identified novel influenza A virus with upper respiratory symptoms
         Use additional code, if applicable, for associated:
         pleural effusion (J91.8)
         sinusitis (J01.-)

       J09.X3   **Influenza due to identified novel influenza A virus with gastrointestinal manifestations**
         Influenza due to identified novel influenza A virus gastroenteritis
           EXCLUDES 1   *'intestinal flu' [viral gastroenteritis] (A08.-)*

       J09.X9   **Influenza due to identified novel influenza A virus with other manifestations**
         Influenza due to identified novel influenza A virus with encephalopathy
         Influenza due to identified novel influenza A virus with myocarditis
         Influenza due to identified novel influenza A virus with otitis media
         Use additional code to identify manifestation

N Newborn: 0   P Pediatric: 0-17   M Maternity: 9-64   A Adult: 15-124   MCC Major Complication/Comorbidity   CC Complication/Comorbidity   SW Severe Wound Dx

694   ICD-10-CM 2022

✓4th **J10 Influenza due to other identified influenza virus**

    INCLUDES   influenza A (non-novel)
                     influenza B
                     influenza C

    EXCLUDES 1   *influenza due to avian influenza virus (J09.X-)*
                 influenza due to swine flu (J09.X-)
                 influenza due to unidentifed influenza virus (J11.-)

✓5th **J10.0 Influenza due to other identified influenza virus with pneumonia**

     Code also associated lung abscess, if applicable (J85.1)

    J10.00 Influenza due to other identified influenza virus with unspecified type of pneumonia   MCC

    J10.01 Influenza due to other identified influenza virus with the same other identified influenza virus pneumonia   MCC

    J10.08 Influenza due to other identified influenza virus with other specified pneumonia   HIV MCC

         Code also other specified type of pneumonia

J10.1 Influenza due to other identified influenza virus with other respiratory manifestations

     Influenza due to other identified influenza virus NOS
     Influenza due to other identified influenza virus with laryngitis
     Influenza due to other identified influenza virus with pharyngitis
     Influenza due to other identified influenza virus with upper respiratory symptoms
     Use additional code for associated pleural effusion, if applicable (J91.8)
     Use additional code for associated sinusitis, if applicable (J01.-)
     AHA: 2016,3Q,10-11

J10.2 Influenza due to other identified influenza virus with gastrointestinal manifestations

     Influenza due to other identified influenza virus gastroenteritis
    EXCLUDES 1   *"intestinal flu" [viral gastroenteritis] (A08.-)*

✓5th **J10.8 Influenza due to other identified influenza virus with other manifestations**

    J10.81 Influenza due to other identified influenza virus with encephalopathy

    J10.82 Influenza due to other identified influenza virus with myocarditis

    J10.83 Influenza due to other identified influenza virus with otitis media

         Use additional code for any associated perforated tympanic membrane (H72.-)

    J10.89 Influenza due to other identified influenza virus with other manifestations

         Use additional codes to identify the manifestations

✓4th **J11 Influenza due to unidentified influenza virus**

✓5th **J11.0 Influenza due to unidentified influenza virus with pneumonia**

     Code also associated lung abscess, if applicable (J85.1)
     AHA: 2016,3Q,11

    J11.00 Influenza due to unidentified influenza virus with unspecified type of pneumonia   MCC
         Influenza with pneumonia NOS

    J11.08 Influenza due to unidentified influenza virus with specified pneumonia   MCC
         Code also other specified type of pneumonia

J11.1 Influenza due to unidentified influenza virus with other respiratory manifestations

     Influenza NOS
     Influenzal laryngitis NOS
     Influenzal pharyngitis NOS
     Influenza with upper respiratory symptoms NOS
     Use additional code for associated pleural effusion, if applicable (J91.8)
     Use additional code for associated sinusitis, if applicable (J01.-)

J11.2 Influenza due to unidentified influenza virus with gastrointestinal manifestations

     Influenza gastroenteritis NOS
    EXCLUDES 1   *"intestinal flu" [viral gastroenteritis] (A08.-)*

✓5th **J11.8 Influenza due to unidentified influenza virus with other manifestations**

    J11.81 Influenza due to unidentified influenza virus with encephalopathy
         Influenzal encephalopathy NOS

    J11.82 Influenza due to unidentified influenza virus with myocarditis
         Influenzal myocarditis NOS

    J11.83 Influenza due to unidentified influenza virus with otitis media
         Influenzal otitis media NOS
         Use additional code for any associated perforated tympanic membrane (H72.-)

    J11.89 Influenza due to unidentified influenza virus with other manifestations
         Use additional codes to identify the manifestations

✓4th **J12 Viral pneumonia, not elsewhere classified**

    INCLUDES   bronchopneumonia due to viruses other than influenza viruses

     Code first associated influenza, if applicable (J09.X1, J10.0-, J11.0-)
     Code also associated abscess, if applicable (J85.1)

    EXCLUDES 1   *aspiration pneumonia due to anesthesia during labor and delivery (O74.0)*
                 aspiration pneumonia due to anesthesia during pregnancy (O29)
                 aspiration pneumonia due to anesthesia during puerperium (O89.0)
                 aspiration pneumonia due to solids and liquids (J69.-)
                 aspiration pneumonia NOS (J69.0)
                 congenital pneumonia (P23.0)
                 congenital rubella pneumonitis (P35.0)
                 interstitial pneumonia NOS (J84.9)
                 lipid pneumonia (J69.1)
                 neonatal aspiration pneumonia (P24.-)

     AHA: 2020,2Q,28; 2019,1Q,35; 2018,3Q,24; 2016,3Q,15; 2013,4Q,118

J12.0 Adenoviral pneumonia   MCC

J12.1 Respiratory syncytial virus pneumonia   MCC
     RSV pneumonia

J12.2 Parainfluenza virus pneumonia   MCC

J12.3 Human metapneumovirus pneumonia   HIV MCC

✓5th **J12.8 Other viral pneumonia**

    J12.81 Pneumonia due to SARS-associated coronavirus   HIV MCC
         Severe acute respiratory syndrome NOS
         DEF: Inflammation of the lungs with consolidation, caused by the severe adult respiratory syndrome (SARS)-associated coronavirus or SARS-CoV. This pneumonia should not be confused with that caused by SARS-CoV-2 (COVID-19).

    J12.82 Pneumonia due to coronavirus disease 2019   HIV MCC UPD
         Pneumonia due to 2019 novel coronavirus (SARS-CoV-2)
         Pneumonia due to COVID-19
         Code first COVID-19 (U07.1)
         AHA: 2021,1Q,25-30,31-49

    J12.89 Other viral pneumonia   HIV MCC
         AHA: 2021,1Q,33-34; 2020,2Q,8,11; 2020,1Q,34-36

J12.9 Viral pneumonia, unspecified   HIV MCC

J13 Pneumonia due to Streptococcus pneumoniae   HIV MCC HCC

     Bronchopneumonia due to S. pneumoniae
     Code first associated influenza, if applicable (J09.X1, J10.0-, J11.0-)
     Code also associated abscess, if applicable (J85.1)
    EXCLUDES 1   *congenital pneumonia due to S. pneumoniae (P23.6)*
                 lobar pneumonia, unspecified organism (J18.1)
                 pneumonia due to other streptococci (J15.3-J15.4)
     AHA: 2020,2Q,28; 2019,1Q,35; 2018,3Q,24; 2016,3Q,15; 2013,4Q,118

J14 Pneumonia due to Hemophilus influenzae   HIV MCC HCC

     Bronchopneumonia due to H. influenzae
     Code first associated influenza, if applicable (J09.X1, J10.0-, J11.0-)
     Code also associated abscess, if applicable (J85.1)
    EXCLUDES 1   *congenital pneumonia due to H. influenzae (P23.6)*
     AHA: 2020,2Q,28; 2019,1Q,35; 2018,3Q,24; 2016,3Q,15; 2013,4Q,118

Chapter 10. Diseases of the Respiratory System

J15–J18.9

✓4ᵗʰ J15 Bacterial pneumonia, not elsewhere classified
> INCLUDES Bronchopneumonia due to bacteria other than S. pneumoniae and H. influenzae
>
> Code first associated influenza, if applicable (J09.X1, J10.0-, -J11.0-)
> Code also associated abscess, if applicable (J85.1)
>
> EXCLUDES 1 chlamydial pneumonia (J16.0)
> congenital pneumonia (P23.-)
> Legionnaires' disease (A48.1)
> spirochetal pneumonia (A69.8)
>
> AHA: 2020,2Q,28; 2019,1Q,35; 2018,3Q,24; 2016,3Q,15; 2013,4Q,118

J15.0 Pneumonia due to Klebsiella pneumoniae HIV MCC HCC
J15.1 Pneumonia due to Pseudomonas HIV MCC HCC
✓5ᵗʰ J15.2 Pneumonia due to staphylococcus
> **J15.20 Pneumonia due to staphylococcus, unspecified** HIV MCC HCC
> **✓6ᵗʰ J15.21 Pneumonia due to Staphylococcus aureus**
>> **J15.211 Pneumonia due to methicillin susceptible Staphylococcus aureus** HIV MCC HCC
>> MSSA pneumonia
>> Pneumonia due to Staphylococcus aureus NOS
>> **J15.212 Pneumonia due to methicillin resistant Staphylococcus aureus** HIV MCC HCC
> **J15.29 Pneumonia due to other staphylococcus** HIV MCC HCC

J15.3 Pneumonia due to streptococcus, group B HIV MCC HCC
J15.4 Pneumonia due to other streptococci HIV MCC HCC
> EXCLUDES 1 pneumonia due to streptococcus, group B (J15.3)
> pneumonia due to Streptococcus pneumoniae (J13)

J15.5 Pneumonia due to Escherichia coli HIV MCC HCC
J15.6 Pneumonia due to other Gram-negative bacteria HIV MCC HCC
> Pneumonia due to other aerobic Gram-negative bacteria
> Pneumonia due to Serratia marcescens
> AHA: 2020,2Q,28

J15.7 Pneumonia due to Mycoplasma pneumoniae MCC
J15.8 Pneumonia due to other specified bacteria HIV MCC HCC
J15.9 Unspecified bacterial pneumonia HIV MCC
> Pneumonia due to gram-positive bacteria

✓4ᵗʰ J16 Pneumonia due to other infectious organisms, not elsewhere classified
> Code first associated influenza, if applicable (J09.X1, J10.0-, J11.0-)
> Code also associated abscess, if applicable (J85.1)
>
> EXCLUDES 1 congenital pneumonia (P23.-)
> ornithosis (A70)
> pneumocystosis (B59)
> pneumonia NOS (J18.9)
>
> AHA: 2020,2Q,28; 2019,1Q,35; 2018,3Q,24; 2016,3Q,15; 2013,4Q,118

J16.0 Chlamydial pneumonia MCC
J16.8 Pneumonia due to other specified infectious organisms MCC

J17 Pneumonia in diseases classified elsewhere MCC
> Code first underlying disease, such as:
> Q fever (A78)
> rheumatic fever (I00)
> schistosomiasis (B65.0-B65.9)
>
> EXCLUDES 1 candidial pneumonia (B37.1)
> chlamydial pneumonia (J16.0)
> gonorrheal pneumonia (A54.84)
> histoplasmosis pneumonia (B39.0-B39.2)
> measles pneumonia (B05.2)
> nocardiosis pneumonia (A43.0)
> pneumocystosis (B59)
> pneumonia due to Pneumocystis carinii (B59)
> pneumonia due to Pneumocystis jiroveci (B59)
> pneumonia in actinomycosis (A42.0)
> pneumonia in anthrax (A22.1)
> pneumonia in ascariasis (B77.81)
> pneumonia in aspergillosis (B44.0-B44.1)
> pneumonia in coccidioidomycosis (B38.0-B38.2)
> pneumonia in cytomegalovirus disease (B25.0)
> pneumonia in toxoplasmosis (B58.3)
> rubella pneumonia (B06.81)
> salmonella pneumonia (A02.22)
> spirochetal infection NEC with pneumonia (A69.8)
> tularemia pneumonia (A21.2)
> typhoid fever with pneumonia (A01.03)
> varicella pneumonia (B01.2)
> whooping cough with pneumonia (A37 with fifth character 1)
>
> AHA: 2020,2Q,28; 2019,1Q,35; 2016,3Q,15; 2013,4Q,118

✓4ᵗʰ J18 Pneumonia, unspecified organism
> Code first associated influenza, if applicable (J09.X1, J10.0-, J11.0-)
>
> EXCLUDES 1 abscess of lung with pneumonia (J85.1)
> aspiration pneumonia due to anesthesia during labor and delivery (O74.0)
> aspiration pneumonia due to anesthesia during pregnancy (O29)
> aspiration pneumonia due to anesthesia during puerperium (O89.0)
> aspiration pneumonia due to solids and liquids (J69.-)
> aspiration pneumonia NOS (J69.0)
> congenital pneumonia (P23.0)
> drug-induced interstitial lung disorder (J70.2-J70.4)
> interstitial pneumonia NOS (J84.9)
> lipid pneumonia (J69.1)
> neonatal aspiration pneumonia (P24.-)
> pneumonitis due to external agents (J67-J70)
> pneumonitis due to fumes and vapors (J68.0)
> usual interstitial pneumonia (J84.178)
>
> AHA: 2020,2Q,28; 2019,1Q,35; 2016,3Q,15; 2013,4Q,118

J18.0 Bronchopneumonia, unspecified organism MCC
> EXCLUDES 1 hypostatic bronchopneumonia (J18.2)
> lipid pneumonia (J69.1)
> EXCLUDES 2 acute bronchiolitis (J21.-)
> chronic bronchiolitis (J44.9)

J18.1 Lobar pneumonia, unspecified organism HIV MCC HCC
> AHA: 2019,3Q,37; 2018,3Q,24
>
> TIP: Assign J18.1 only when the provider specifically documents "lobar pneumonia" without specifying a causal organism. Lobar pneumonia may not be assumed based on an imaging report that identifies pneumonia in a specific lobe.
>
> TIP: Use this code for documented lobar pneumonia or multilobar pneumonia when the causal organism is not identified. If the causal organism is identified, codes from categories J12-J16 should be used, depending on the organism that is present.

J18.2 Hypostatic pneumonia, unspecified organism CC
> Hypostatic bronchopneumonia
> Passive pneumonia

J18.8 Other pneumonia, unspecified organism HIV MCC
J18.9 Pneumonia, unspecified organism HIV MCC
> AHA: 2020,2Q,28; 2019,3Q,15; 2019,2Q,28; 2014,3Q,4; 2013,4Q,119; 2012,4Q,94

Other acute lower respiratory infections (J20-J22)

EXCLUDES 2   *chronic obstructive pulmonary disease with acute lower respiratory infection (J44.0)*

✓4ᵗʰ **J20   Acute bronchitis**

     INCLUDES   acute and subacute bronchitis (with) bronchospasm

                acute and subacute bronchitis (with) tracheitis

                acute and subacute bronchitis (with) tracheobronchitis, acute

                acute and subacute fibrinous bronchitis

                acute and subacute membranous bronchitis

                acute and subacute purulent bronchitis

                acute and subacute septic bronchitis

     EXCLUDES 1   *bronchitis NOS (J40)*

                tracheobronchitis NOS (J40)

     EXCLUDES 2   *acute bronchitis with bronchiectasis (J47.0)*

                acute bronchitis with chronic obstructive asthma (J44.0)

                acute bronchitis with chronic obstructive pulmonary disease (J44.0)

                allergic bronchitis NOS (J45.909-)

                bronchitis due to chemicals, fumes and vapors (J68.0)

                chronic bronchitis NOS (J42)

                chronic mucopurulent bronchitis (J41.1)

                chronic obstructive bronchitis (J44.-)

                chronic obstructive tracheobronchitis (J44.-)

                chronic simple bronchitis (J41.0)

                chronic tracheobronchitis (J42)

     AHA: 2019,1Q,35; 2016,3Q,10,16

     DEF: Acute inflammation of the main branches of the bronchial tree due to infectious or irritant agents. Symptoms include cough with a varied production of sputum, fever, substernal soreness, and lung rales. Bronchitis usually lasts three to 10 days.

     J20.0   Acute bronchitis due to Mycoplasma pneumoniae

     J20.1   Acute bronchitis due to Hemophilus influenzae

     J20.2   Acute bronchitis due to streptococcus

     J20.3   Acute bronchitis due to coxsackievirus

     J20.4   Acute bronchitis due to parainfluenza virus

     J20.5   Acute bronchitis due to respiratory syncytial virus

         Acute bronchitis due to RSV

     J20.6   Acute bronchitis due to rhinovirus

     J20.7   Acute bronchitis due to echovirus

     J20.8   Acute bronchitis due to other specified organisms

         AHA: 2020,1Q,34-36

         TIP: Assign as a secondary code for a patient with acute bronchitis confirmed as due to COVID-19; assign U07.1 as the principal or first-listed code.

     J20.9   Acute bronchitis, unspecified

✓4ᵗʰ **J21   Acute bronchiolitis**

     INCLUDES   acute bronchiolitis with bronchospasm

     EXCLUDES 2   *respiratory bronchiolitis interstitial lung disease (J84.115)*

     J21.0   Acute bronchiolitis due to respiratory syncytial virus   CC

         Acute bronchiolitis due to RSV

     J21.1   Acute bronchiolitis due to human metapneumovirus   CC

     J21.8   Acute bronchiolitis due to other specified organisms   CC

     J21.9   Acute bronchiolitis, unspecified   CC

         Bronchiolitis (acute)

         EXCLUDES 1   *chronic bronchiolitis (J44.-)*

J22   Unspecified acute lower respiratory infection

     Acute (lower) respiratory (tract) infection NOS

     EXCLUDES 1   *upper respiratory infection (acute) (J06.9)*

     AHA: 2020,1Q,22,34-36

     TIP: Assign as a secondary code for a patient with a respiratory infection specified as acute or lower that is documented as being associated with COVID-19; assign U07.1 as the principal or first-listed code. If the respiratory infection documentation does not specify acute or lower, assign J98.8.

Other diseases of upper respiratory tract (J30-J39)

✓4ᵗʰ **J30   Vasomotor and allergic rhinitis**

     INCLUDES   spasmodic rhinorrhea

     EXCLUDES 1   *allergic rhinitis with asthma (bronchial) (J45.909)*

                rhinitis NOS (J31.0)

     J30.0   Vasomotor rhinitis

         DEF: Noninfectious and nonallergic type of rhinitis for which the cause is often unknown. Symptoms often mimic those of allergic rhinitis with a diagnosis of vasomotor rhinitis typically made after ruling out allergens as the cause.

     J30.1   Allergic rhinitis due to pollen

         Allergy NOS due to pollen

         Hay fever

         Pollinosis

     J30.2   Other seasonal allergic rhinitis

     J30.5   Allergic rhinitis due to food

✓5ᵗʰ   **J30.8   Other allergic rhinitis**

     J30.81   Allergic rhinitis due to animal (cat) (dog) hair and dander

     J30.89   Other allergic rhinitis

         Perennial allergic rhinitis

     J30.9   Allergic rhinitis, unspecified

✓4ᵗʰ **J31   Chronic rhinitis, nasopharyngitis and pharyngitis**

     Use additional code to identify:

       exposure to environmental tobacco smoke (Z77.22)

       exposure to tobacco smoke in the perinatal period (P96.81)

       history of tobacco dependence (Z87.891)

       occupational exposure to environmental tobacco smoke (Z57.31)

       tobacco dependence (F17.-)

       tobacco use (Z72.0)

     J31.0   Chronic rhinitis

         Atrophic rhinitis (chronic)

         Granulomatous rhinitis (chronic)

         Hypertrophic rhinitis (chronic)

         Obstructive rhinitis (chronic)

         Ozena

         Purulent rhinitis (chronic)

         Rhinitis (chronic) NOS

         Ulcerative rhinitis (chronic)

         EXCLUDES 1   *allergic rhinitis (J30.1-J30.9)*

                vasomotor rhinitis (J30.0)

         DEF: Persistent inflammation of the mucous membranes of the nose, characterized by a postnasal drip.

     J31.1   Chronic nasopharyngitis

         EXCLUDES 2   *acute nasopharyngitis (J00)*

         DEF: Persistent inflammation of the mucous membranes extending from the nares to the pharynx. It is characterized by constant irritation in the nasopharynx and postnasal drip.

     J31.2   Chronic pharyngitis

         Atrophic pharyngitis (chronic)

         Chronic sore throat

         Granular pharyngitis (chronic)

         Hypertrophic pharyngitis (chronic)

         EXCLUDES 2   *acute pharyngitis (J02.9)*

✓4ᵗʰ **J32   Chronic sinusitis**

     INCLUDES   sinus abscess

                sinus empyema

                sinus infection

                sinus suppuration

     Use additional code to identify:

       exposure to environmental tobacco smoke (Z77.22)

       exposure to tobacco smoke in the perinatal period (P96.81)

       history of tobacco dependence (Z87.891)

       infectious agent (B95-B97)

       occupational exposure to environmental tobacco smoke (Z57.31)

       tobacco dependence (F17.-)

       tobacco use (Z72.0)

     EXCLUDES 2   *acute sinusitis (J01.-)*

     J32.0   Chronic maxillary sinusitis

         Antritis (chronic)

         Maxillary sinusitis NOS

     J32.1   Chronic frontal sinusitis

         Frontal sinusitis NOS

✔ Additional Character Required   ✓x7ᵗʰ Placeholder   Questionable PDx   Manifestation   Unspecified Dx   UPD Unacceptable PDx   H1-H14 HAC   HCC CMS-HCC Dx   HIV HIV Dx

ICD-10-CM 2022   **697**

Chapter 10. Diseases of the Respiratory System

J32.2   **Chronic ethmoidal sinusitis**
Ethmoidal sinusitis NOS
   EXCLUDES 1   *Woakes' ethmoiditis (J33.1)*

J32.3   **Chronic sphenoidal sinusitis**
Sphenoidal sinusitis NOS

J32.4   **Chronic pansinusitis**
Pansinusitis NOS

J32.8   **Other chronic sinusitis**
Sinusitis (chronic) involving more than one sinus but not pansinusitis

J32.9   **Chronic sinusitis, unspecified**
Sinusitis (chronic) NOS

✓4ᵗʰ **J33**   **Nasal polyp**
Use additional code to identify:
exposure to environmental tobacco smoke (Z77.22)
exposure to tobacco smoke in the perinatal period (P96.81)
history of tobacco dependence (Z87.891)
occupational exposure to environmental tobacco smoke (Z57.31)
tobacco dependence (F17.-)
tobacco use (Z72.0)
   EXCLUDES 1   *adenomatous polyps (D14.0)*

J33.0   **Polyp of nasal cavity**
Choanal polyp
Nasopharyngeal polyp

J33.1   **Polypoid sinus degeneration**
Woakes' syndrome or ethmoiditis

J33.8   **Other polyp of sinus**
Accessory polyp of sinus
Ethmoidal polyp of sinus
Maxillary polyp of sinus
Sphenoidal polyp of sinus

J33.9   **Nasal polyp, unspecified**

✓4ᵗʰ **J34**   **Other and unspecified disorders of nose and nasal sinuses**
   EXCLUDES 2   *varicose ulcer of nasal septum (I86.8)*

J34.0   **Abscess, furuncle and carbuncle of nose**
Cellulitis of nose
Necrosis of nose
Ulceration of nose

J34.1   **Cyst and mucocele of nose and nasal sinus**

J34.2   **Deviated nasal septum**
Deflection or deviation of septum (nasal) (acquired)
   EXCLUDES 1   *congenital deviated nasal septum (Q67.4)*
DEF: Condition in which the nasal septum, a thin wall composed of cartilage and bone that separates the two nostrils, is crooked or displaced from the midline.

J34.3   **Hypertrophy of nasal turbinates**
DEF: Overgrowth of bones within the nasal turbinate, which are ridges of bone and soft tissue that project from the sidewalls of the nasal passages. Hypertrophy can cause obstruction of the nasal passages.

✓5ᵗʰ **J34.8**   **Other specified disorders of nose and nasal sinuses**

J34.81   **Nasal mucositis (ulcerative)**
Code also type of associated therapy, such as:
antineoplastic and immunosuppressive drugs (T45.1X-)
radiological procedure and radiotherapy (Y84.2)
   EXCLUDES 2   *gastrointestinal mucositis (ulcerative) (K92.81)*
mucositis (ulcerative) of vagina and vulva (N76.81)
oral mucositis (ulcerative) (K12.3-)

J34.89   **Other specified disorders of nose and nasal sinuses**
Perforation of nasal septum NOS
Rhinolith

J34.9   **Unspecified disorder of nose and nasal sinuses**

✓4ᵗʰ **J35**   **Chronic diseases of tonsils and adenoids**
Use additional code to identify:
exposure to environmental tobacco smoke (Z77.22)
exposure to tobacco smoke in the perinatal period (P96.81)
history of tobacco dependence (Z87.891)
occupational exposure to environmental tobacco smoke (Z57.31)
tobacco dependence (F17.-)
tobacco use (Z72.0)

✓5ᵗʰ **J35.0**   **Chronic tonsillitis and adenoiditis**
   EXCLUDES 2   *acute tonsillitis (J03.-)*

J35.01   **Chronic tonsillitis**

J35.02   **Chronic adenoiditis**
J35.03   **Chronic tonsillitis and adenoiditis**

J35.1   **Hypertrophy of tonsils**
Enlargement of tonsils
   EXCLUDES 1   *hypertrophy of tonsils with tonsillitis (J35.0-)*

J35.2   **Hypertrophy of adenoids**
Enlargement of adenoids
   EXCLUDES 1   *hypertrophy of adenoids with adenoiditis (J35.0-)*

J35.3   **Hypertrophy of tonsils with hypertrophy of adenoids**
   EXCLUDES 1   *hypertrophy of tonsils and adenoids with tonsillitis and adenoiditis (J35.03)*

J35.8   **Other chronic diseases of tonsils and adenoids**
Adenoid vegetations
Amygdalolith
Calculus, tonsil
Cicatrix of tonsil (and adenoid)
Tonsillar tag
Ulcer of tonsil

J35.9   **Chronic disease of tonsils and adenoids, unspecified**
Disease (chronic) of tonsils and adenoids NOS

J36   **Peritonsillar abscess**   CC
   INCLUDES   abscess of tonsil
peritonsillar cellulitis
quinsy
Use additional code (B95-B97) to identify infectious agent
   EXCLUDES 1   *acute tonsillitis (J03.-)*
chronic tonsillitis (J35.0)
retropharyngeal abscess (J39.0)
tonsillitis NOS (J03.9-)

✓4ᵗʰ **J37**   **Chronic laryngitis and laryngotracheitis**
Use additional code to identify:
exposure to environmental tobacco smoke (Z77.22)
exposure to tobacco smoke in the perinatal period (P96.81)
history of tobacco dependence (Z87.891)
infectious agent (B95-B97)
occupational exposure to environmental tobacco smoke (Z57.31)
tobacco dependence (F17.-)
tobacco use (Z72.0)

J37.0   **Chronic laryngitis**
Catarrhal laryngitis
Hypertrophic laryngitis
Sicca laryngitis
   EXCLUDES 2   *acute laryngitis (J04.0)*
obstructive (acute) laryngitis (J05.0)

J37.1   **Chronic laryngotracheitis**
Laryngitis, chronic, with tracheitis (chronic)
Tracheitis, chronic, with laryngitis
   EXCLUDES 1   *chronic tracheitis (J42)*
   EXCLUDES 2   *acute laryngotracheitis (J04.2)*
acute tracheitis (J04.1)

✓4ᵗʰ **J38**   **Diseases of vocal cords and larynx, not elsewhere classified**
Use additional code to identify:
exposure to environmental tobacco smoke (Z77.22)
exposure to tobacco smoke in the perinatal period (P96.81)
history of tobacco dependence (Z87.891)
occupational exposure to environmental tobacco smoke (Z57.31)
tobacco dependence (F17.-)
tobacco use (Z72.0)
   EXCLUDES 1   *congenital laryngeal stridor (P28.89)*
obstructive laryngitis (acute) (J05.0)
postprocedural subglottic stenosis (J95.5)
stridor (R06.1)
ulcerative laryngitis (J04.0)

✓5ᵗʰ **J38.0**   **Paralysis of vocal cords and larynx**
Laryngoplegia
Paralysis of glottis

J38.00   **Paralysis of vocal cords and larynx, unspecified**
J38.01   **Paralysis of vocal cords and larynx, unilateral**
J38.02   **Paralysis of vocal cords and larynx, bilateral**

J38.1   **Polyp of vocal cord and larynx**
   EXCLUDES 1   *adenomatous polyps (D14.1)*

J38.2   Nodules **of vocal cords**
Chorditis (fibrinous)(nodosa)(tuberosa)
Singer's nodes
Teacher's nodes

J38.3   **Other diseases of vocal cords**
Abscess of vocal cords
Cellulitis of vocal cords
Granuloma of vocal cords
Leukokeratosis of vocal cords
Leukoplakia of vocal cords

J38.4   Edema **of larynx**
Edema (of) glottis
Subglottic edema
Supraglottic edema
    EXCLUDES 1   *acute obstructive laryngitis [croup] (J05.0)*
              edematous laryngitis (J04.0)

J38.5   **Laryngeal** spasm
Laryngismus (stridulus)

J38.6   Stenosis **of larynx**

J38.7   **Other diseases of larynx**
Abscess of larynx
Cellulitis of larynx
Disease of larynx NOS
Necrosis of larynx
Pachyderma of larynx
Perichondritis of larynx
Ulcer of larynx

✓4ᵗʰ **J39**   **Other diseases of upper respiratory tract**
    EXCLUDES 1   *acute respiratory infection NOS (J22)*
              acute upper respiratory infection (J06.9)
              upper respiratory inflammation due to chemicals, gases,
                 fumes or vapors (J68.2)

J39.0   **Retropharyngeal and parapharyngeal abscess**   `CC`
Peripharyngeal abscess
    EXCLUDES 1   *peritonsillar abscess (J36)*
    DEF: Purulent infection behind the pharynx and the front of the precerebral fascia, characterized by neck stiffness, cervical lymphadenopathy, sore throat, fever, and stridor.

J39.1   **Other** abscess **of pharynx**   `CC`
Cellulitis of pharynx
Nasopharyngeal abscess

J39.2   **Other diseases of pharynx**
Cyst of pharynx
Edema of pharynx
    EXCLUDES 2   *chronic pharyngitis (J31.2)*
              ulcerative pharyngitis (J02.9)

J39.3   **Upper respiratory tract hypersensitivity reaction, site unspecified**
    EXCLUDES 1   *hypersensitivity reaction of upper respiratory tract,*
              such as:
              extrinsic allergic alveolitis (J67.9)
              pneumoconiosis (J60-J67.9)

J39.8   **Other specified diseases of upper respiratory tract**

J39.9   **Disease of upper respiratory tract, unspecified**

Chronic lower respiratory diseases (J40-J47)

    EXCLUDES 1   *bronchitis due to chemicals, gases, fumes and vapors (J68.0)*
    EXCLUDES 2   *cystic fibrosis (E84.-)*

J40   **Bronchitis,** not specified as acute or chronic
Bronchitis NOS
Bronchitis with tracheitis NOS
Catarrhal bronchitis
Tracheobronchitis NOS
Use additional code to identify:
   exposure to environmental tobacco smoke (Z77.22)
   exposure to tobacco smoke in the perinatal period (P96.81)
   history of tobacco dependence (Z87.891)
   occupational exposure to environmental tobacco smoke (Z57.31)
   tobacco dependence (F17.-)
   tobacco use (Z72.0)
    EXCLUDES 1   *acute bronchitis (J20.-)*
              allergic bronchitis NOS (J45.909-)
              asthmatic bronchitis NOS (J45.9-)
              bronchitis due to chemicals, gases, fumes and vapors (J68.0)
AHA: 2020,1Q,34-36
TIP: Assign as a secondary code for a patient with bronchitis of unspecified acuity due to COVID-19; assign U07.1 as the principal or first-listed code.

✓4ᵗʰ **J41**   **Simple and mucopurulent chronic** bronchitis
Use additional code to identify:
   exposure to environmental tobacco smoke (Z77.22)
   exposure to tobacco smoke in the perinatal period (P96.81)
   history of tobacco dependence (Z87.891)
   occupational exposure to environmental tobacco smoke (Z57.31)
   tobacco dependence (F17.-)
   tobacco use (Z72.0)
    EXCLUDES 1   *chronic bronchitis NOS (J42)*
              chronic obstructive bronchitis (J44.-)

J41.0   **Simple chronic bronchitis**   `HCC`

J41.1   **Mucopurulent chronic bronchitis**   `HCC`

J41.8   **Mixed simple and mucopurulent chronic bronchitis**   `HCC`

J42   **Unspecified** chronic **bronchitis**   `HCC`
Chronic bronchitis NOS
Chronic tracheitis
Chronic tracheobronchitis
Use additional code to identify:
   exposure to environmental tobacco smoke (Z77.22)
   exposure to tobacco smoke in the perinatal period (P96.81)
   history of tobacco dependence (Z87.891)
   occupational exposure to environmental tobacco smoke (Z57.31)
   tobacco dependence (F17.-)
   tobacco use (Z72.0)
    EXCLUDES 1   *chronic asthmatic bronchitis (J44.-)*
              chronic bronchitis with airways obstruction (J44.-)
              chronic emphysematous bronchitis (J44.-)
              chronic obstructive pulmonary disease NOS (J44.9)
              simple and mucopurulent chronic bronchitis (J41.-)

Chapter 10. Diseases of the Respiratory System

J38.2–J42

Chapter 10. Diseases of the Respiratory System

✓4ᵗʰ J43 Emphysema

Use additional code to identify:
exposure to environmental tobacco smoke (Z77.22)
history of tobacco dependence (Z87.891)
occupational exposure to environmental tobacco smoke (Z57.31)
tobacco dependence (F17.-)
tobacco use (Z72.0)

EXCLUDES 1   *compensatory emphysema (J98.3)*
emphysema due to inhalation of chemicals, gases, fumes or vapors (J68.4)
emphysema with chronic (obstructive) bronchitis (J44.-)
emphysematous (obstructive) bronchitis (J44.-)
interstitial emphysema (J98.2)
mediastinal emphysema (J98.2)
neonatal interstitial emphysema (P25.0)
surgical (subcutaneous) emphysema (T81.82)

EXCLUDES 2   *traumatic subcutaneous emphysema (T79.7)*

DEF: Pathological condition in which there is destructive enlargement of the air sacs in the lungs resulting in damage and lack of elasticity to the alveolar walls, commonly seen in long-term smokers.

Emphysema

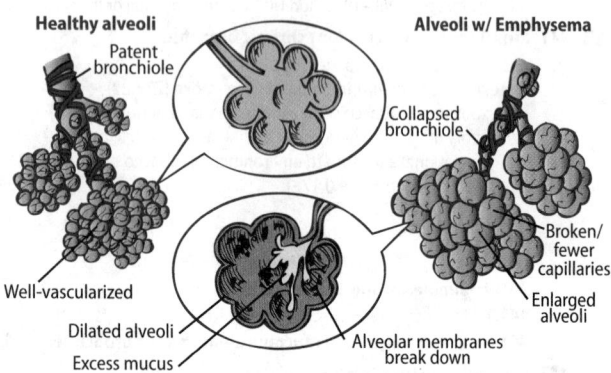

Healthy alveoli — Patent bronchiole — Well-vascularized — Dilated alveoli — Excess mucus
Alveoli w/ Emphysema — Collapsed bronchiole — Broken/fewer capillaries — Enlarged alveoli — Alveolar membranes break down

J43.0 Unilateral pulmonary emphysema [MacLeod's syndrome]   HCC
Swyer-James syndrome
Unilateral emphysema
Unilateral hyperlucent lung
Unilateral pulmonary artery functional hypoplasia
Unilateral transparency of lung

J43.1 Panlobular emphysema   HCC
Panacinar emphysema

J43.2 Centrilobular emphysema   HCC

J43.8 Other emphysema   HCC

J43.9 Emphysema, unspecified   HCC
Bullous emphysema (lung)(pulmonary)
Emphysema (lung)(pulmonary) NOS
Emphysematous bleb
Vesicular emphysema (lung)(pulmonary)
AHA: 2019,1Q,34-36; 2017,4Q,97-98

✓4ᵗʰ J44 Other chronic obstructive pulmonary disease

INCLUDES   asthma with chronic obstructive pulmonary disease
chronic asthmatic (obstructive) bronchitis
►chronic bronchitis with airway obstruction◄
chronic bronchitis with emphysema
chronic emphysematous bronchitis
chronic obstructive asthma
chronic obstructive bronchitis
chronic obstructive tracheobronchitis

Code also type of asthma, if applicable (J45.-)
Use additional code to identify:
exposure to environmental tobacco smoke (Z77.22)
history of tobacco dependence (Z87.891)
occupational exposure to environmental tobacco smoke (Z57.31)
tobacco dependence (F17.-)
tobacco use (Z72.0)

EXCLUDES 1   *bronchiectasis (J47.-)*
chronic bronchitis NOS (J42)
chronic simple and mucopurulent bronchitis (J41.-)
chronic tracheitis (J42)
chronic tracheobronchitis (J42)
emphysema without chronic bronchitis (J43.-)

AHA: 2019,1Q,34-36; 2017,4Q,97-98; 2017,1Q,25-26; 2016,3Q,15-16; 2013,4Q,109

J44.0 Chronic obstructive pulmonary disease with (acute) lower respiratory infection   CC HCC
Code also to identify the infection
AHA: 2019,1Q,35; 2017,4Q,96; 2017,1Q,24-25
TIP: Do not assign when only aspiration pneumonia is present. Aspiration pneumonia is not classified as a respiratory infection.

J44.1 Chronic obstructive pulmonary disease with (acute) exacerbation   CC HCC
Decompensated COPD
Decompensated COPD with (acute) exacerbation
EXCLUDES 2   *chronic obstructive pulmonary disease [COPD] with acute bronchitis (J44.0)*
lung diseases due to external agents (J60-J70)
AHA: 2019,1Q,34; 2017,4Q,96; 2017,1Q,26; 2016,1Q,36
TIP: Exacerbation of COPD should not be assumed based upon worsening of a concomitant respiratory disease or when COPD is described as end-stage.

J44.9 Chronic obstructive pulmonary disease, unspecified   HCC
Chronic obstructive airway disease NOS
Chronic obstructive lung disease NOS
EXCLUDES 2   *lung diseases due to external agents (J60-J70)*
AHA: 2019,1Q,36; 2017,4Q,96-97; 2016,1Q,36; 2014,4Q,21; 2013,4Q,109

✓4ᵗʰ **J45 Asthma**

INCLUDES   allergic (predominantly) asthma
allergic bronchitis NOS
allergic rhinitis with asthma
atopic asthma
extrinsic allergic asthma
hay fever with asthma
idiosyncratic asthma
intrinsic nonallergic asthma
nonallergic asthma

Use additional code to identify:
eosinophilic asthma (J82.83)
exposure to environmental tobacco smoke (Z77.22)
exposure to tobacco smoke in the perinatal period (P96.81)
history of tobacco dependence (Z87.891)
occupational exposure to environmental tobacco smoke (Z57.31)
tobacco dependence (F17.-)
tobacco use (Z72.0)

EXCLUDES 1   detergent asthma (J69.8)
eosinophilic asthma (J82)
miner's asthma (J60)
wheezing NOS (R06.2)
wood asthma (J67.8)

EXCLUDES 2   asthma with chronic obstructive pulmonary disease (J44.9)
chronic asthmatic (obstructive) bronchitis (J44.9)
chronic obstructive asthma (J44.9)

AHA: 2019,1Q,36; 2017,1Q,25-26; 2012,4Q,99

DEF: Status asthmaticus: Severe, intractable episode of asthma that is unresponsive to normal therapeutic measures.

Asthma

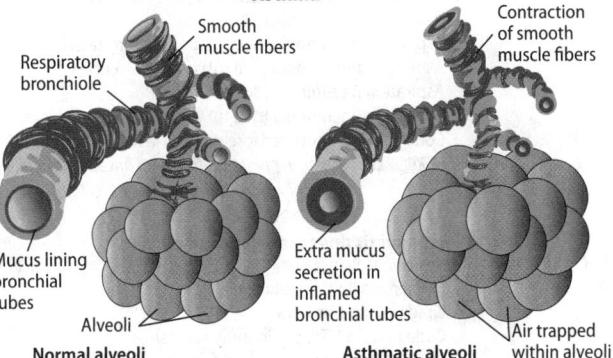

Respiratory bronchiole
Smooth muscle fibers
Contraction of smooth muscle fibers
Mucus lining bronchial tubes
Extra mucus secretion in inflamed bronchial tubes
Alveoli
Air trapped within alveoli
Normal alveoli   **Asthmatic alveoli**

✓5ᵗʰ **J45.2 Mild intermittent asthma**

   J45.20 Mild intermittent asthma, uncomplicated
Mild intermittent asthma NOS

   J45.21 Mild intermittent asthma with (acute) exacerbation CC

   J45.22 Mild intermittent asthma with status asthmaticus CC

✓5ᵗʰ **J45.3 Mild persistent asthma**

   J45.30 Mild persistent asthma, uncomplicated
Mild persistent asthma NOS

   J45.31 Mild persistent asthma with (acute) exacerbation CC
     AHA: 2016,1Q,35

   J45.32 Mild persistent asthma with status asthmaticus CC

✓5ᵗʰ **J45.4 Moderate persistent asthma**

   J45.40 Moderate persistent asthma, uncomplicated
Moderate persistent asthma NOS

   J45.41 Moderate persistent asthma with (acute) exacerbation CC
     AHA: 2017,1Q,26

   J45.42 Moderate persistent asthma with status asthmaticus CC

✓5ᵗʰ **J45.5 Severe persistent asthma**

   J45.50 Severe persistent asthma, uncomplicated
Severe persistent asthma NOS

   J45.51 Severe persistent asthma with (acute) exacerbation CC

   J45.52 Severe persistent asthma with status asthmaticus CC

✓5ᵗʰ **J45.9 Other and unspecified asthma**

✓6ᵗʰ **J45.90 Unspecified asthma**
Asthmatic bronchitis NOS
Childhood asthma NOS
Late onset asthma
AHA: 2017,4Q,96; 2017,1Q,25

   J45.901 Unspecified asthma with (acute) exacerbation CC

   J45.902 Unspecified asthma with status asthmaticus CC

   J45.909 Unspecified asthma, uncomplicated
Asthma NOS
     EXCLUDES 2   lung diseases due to external agents (J60-J70)
     AHA: 2017,1Q,25

✓6ᵗʰ **J45.99 Other asthma**

   J45.990 Exercise induced bronchospasm

   J45.991 Cough variant asthma

   J45.998 Other asthma

✓4ᵗʰ **J47 Bronchiectasis**

INCLUDES   bronchiolectasis

Use additional code to identify:
exposure to environmental tobacco smoke (Z77.22)
exposure to tobacco smoke in the perinatal period (P96.81)
history of tobacco dependence (Z87.891)
occupational exposure to environmental tobacco smoke (Z57.31)
tobacco dependence (F17.-)
tobacco use (Z72.0)

EXCLUDES 1   congenital bronchiectasis (Q33.4)
tuberculous bronchiectasis (current disease) (A15.0)

DEF: Dilation of the bronchi with mucus production and persistent cough due to infection or chronic conditions that causes diminished lung capacity and frequent infections of the lung.

   J47.0 Bronchiectasis with acute lower respiratory infection CC HCC
Bronchiectasis with acute bronchitis
►Code also to identify infection, if applicable◄
~~Use additional code to identify the infection~~

   J47.1 Bronchiectasis with (acute) exacerbation CC HCC
     AHA: 2021,1Q,23

   J47.9 Bronchiectasis, uncomplicated HCC
Bronchiectasis NOS

Lung diseases due to external agents (J60-J70)

EXCLUDES 2   asthma (J45.-)
malignant neoplasm of bronchus and lung (C34.-)

DEF: Pneumoconiosis: Condition caused by inhaling inorganic dust particles, typically associated with occupations that require regular exposure to mineral dusts. A form of interstitial lung disease that contributes to the inflammation of the air sacs, causing the lung tissue to harden.

   J60 Coalworker's pneumoconiosis HCC A
Anthracosilicosis
Anthracosis
Black lung disease
Coalworker's lung
     EXCLUDES 1   coalworker pneumoconiosis with tuberculosis, any type in A15 (J65)

   J61 Pneumoconiosis due to asbestos and other mineral fibers HCC A
Asbestosis
     EXCLUDES 1   pleural plaque with asbestosis (J92.0)
pneumoconiosis with tuberculosis, any type in A15 (J65)

✓4ᵗʰ **J62 Pneumoconiosis due to dust containing silica**
     INCLUDES   silicotic fibrosis (massive) of lung
     EXCLUDES 1   pneumoconiosis with tuberculosis, any type in A15 (J65)

   J62.0 Pneumoconiosis due to talc dust HCC

   J62.8 Pneumoconiosis due to other dust containing silica HCC
Silicosis NOS

✓4ᵗʰ **J63 Pneumoconiosis due to other inorganic dusts**
     EXCLUDES 1   pneumoconiosis with tuberculosis, any type in A15 (J65)

   J63.0 Aluminosis (of lung) HCC

   J63.1 Bauxite fibrosis (of lung) HCC

   J63.2 Berylliosis HCC

   J63.3 Graphite fibrosis (of lung) HCC

Chapter 10. Diseases of the Respiratory System

J63.4 **Siderosis** `HCC`
    AHA: 2019,3Q,8

J63.5 **Stannosis** `HCC`

J63.6 **Pneumoconiosis due to other specified inorganic dusts** `HCC`

J64 **Unspecified pneumoconiosis** `HCC`
    `EXCLUDES 1` *pneumonoconiosis with tuberculosis, any type in A15 (J65)*

J65 **Pneumoconiosis** associated with tuberculosis `HCC`
    Any condition in J60-J64 with tuberculosis, any type in A15
    Silicotuberculosis

✓4ᵗʰ **J66** **Airway disease due to specific** organic dust
    `EXCLUDES 2` *allergic alveolitis (J67.-)*
             asbestosis (J61)
             bagassosis (J67.1)
             farmer's lung (J67.0)
             hypersensitivity pneumonitis due to organic dust (J67.-)
             reactive airways dysfunction syndrome (J68.3)

J66.0 **Byssinosis** `HCC`
    Airway disease due to cotton dust

J66.1 **Flax-dressers' disease** `HCC`

J66.2 **Cannabinosis** `HCC`

J66.8 **Airway disease due to other specific organic dusts** `HCC`

✓4ᵗʰ **J67** **Hypersensitivity pneumonitis due to organic dust**
    `INCLUDES` allergic alveolitis and pneumonitis due to inhaled organic dust and particles of fungal, actinomycetic or other origin
    `EXCLUDES 1` *pneumonitis due to inhalation of chemicals, gases, fumes or vapors (J68.0)*

J67.0 **Farmer's lung** `HCC`
    Harvester's lung
    Haymaker's lung
    Moldy hay disease

J67.1 **Bagassosis** `HCC`
    Bagasse disease
    Bagasse pneumonitis

J67.2 **Bird fancier's lung** `HCC`
    Budgerigar fancier's disease or lung
    Pigeon fancier's disease or lung

J67.3 **Suberosis** `HCC`
    Corkhandler's disease or lung
    Corkworker's disease or lung

J67.4 **Maltworker's lung** `HCC`
    Alveolitis due to Aspergillus clavatus

J67.5 **Mushroom-worker's lung** `HCC`

J67.6 **Maple-bark-stripper's lung** `HCC`
    Alveolitis due to Cryptostroma corticale
    Cryptostromosis

J67.7 **Air conditioner and humidifier lung** `CC` `HCC`
    Allergic alveolitis due to fungal, thermophilic actinomycetes and other organisms growing in ventilation [air conditioning] systems

J67.8 **Hypersensitivity pneumonitis due to other organic dusts** `CC` `HCC`
    Cheese-washer's lung
    Coffee-worker's lung
    Fish-meal worker's lung
    Furrier's lung
    Sequoiosis

J67.9 **Hypersensitivity pneumonitis due to unspecified organic dust** `CC` `HCC`
    Allergic alveolitis (extrinsic) NOS
    Hypersensitivity pneumonitis NOS

✓4ᵗʰ **J68** **Respiratory conditions due to inhalation of chemicals, gases, fumes and vapors**
    Code first (T51-T65) to identify cause
    Use additional code to identify associated respiratory conditions, such as:
    acute respiratory failure (J96.0-)

J68.0 **Bronchitis and pneumonitis** due to chemicals, gases, fumes and vapors `CC` `HCC`
    Chemical bronchitis (acute)
    AHA: 2019,2Q,31

J68.1 **Pulmonary edema** due to chemicals, gases, fumes and vapors `MCC` `HCC`
    Chemical pulmonary edema (acute) (chronic)
    `EXCLUDES 1` *pulmonary edema (acute) (chronic) NOS (J81.-)*

J68.2 **Upper respiratory inflammation** due to chemicals, gases, fumes and vapors, not elsewhere classified `HCC`

J68.3 **Other** acute and subacute respiratory conditions due to chemicals, gases, fumes and vapors `HCC`
    Reactive airways dysfunction syndrome

J68.4 **Chronic respiratory conditions** due to chemicals, gases, fumes and vapors `HCC`
    Emphysema (diffuse) (chronic) due to inhalation of chemicals, gases, fumes and vapors
    Obliterative bronchiolitis (chronic) (subacute) due to inhalation of chemicals, gases, fumes and vapors
    Pulmonary fibrosis (chronic) due to inhalation of chemicals, gases, fumes and vapors
    `EXCLUDES 1` *chronic pulmonary edema due to chemicals, gases, fumes and vapors (J68.1)*

J68.8 **Other respiratory conditions due to chemicals, gases, fumes and vapors** `HCC`

J68.9 **Unspecified respiratory condition due to chemicals, gases, fumes and vapors** `HCC`

✓4ᵗʰ **J69** **Pneumonitis due to solids and liquids**
    `EXCLUDES 1` *neonatal aspiration syndromes (P24.-)*
             postprocedural pneumonitis (J95.4)
    AHA: 2017,1Q,24
    DEF: Pneumonitis: Noninfectious inflammation of the walls of the alveoli in the lung tissue due to inhalation of food, vomit, oils, essences, or other solids or liquids.

J69.0 **Pneumonitis due to** inhalation of food and vomit `MCC` `HCC`
    Aspiration pneumonia NOS
    Aspiration pneumonia (due to) food (regurgitated)
    Aspiration pneumonia (due to) gastric secretions
    Aspiration pneumonia (due to) milk
    Aspiration pneumonia (due to) vomit
    Code also any associated foreign body in respiratory tract (T17.-)
    `EXCLUDES 1` *chemical pneumonitis due to anesthesia (J95.4)*
             obstetric aspiration pneumonitis (O74.0)
    AHA: 2020,2Q,11,28; 2019,3Q,17; 2019,2Q,6,31

J69.1 **Pneumonitis due to** inhalation of oils and essences `MCC` `HCC`
    Exogenous lipoid pneumonia
    Lipid pneumonia NOS
    Code first (T51-T65) to identify substance
    `EXCLUDES 1` *endogenous lipoid pneumonia (J84.89)*

J69.8 **Pneumonitis due to inhalation of other solids and liquids** `MCC` `HCC`
    Pneumonitis due to aspiration of blood
    Pneumonitis due to aspiration of detergent
    Code first (T51-T65) to identify substance

✓4ᵗʰ **J70** **Respiratory conditions due to other external agents**

J70.0 **Acute pulmonary manifestations due to** radiation `CC` `HCC`
    Radiation pneumonitis
    Use additional code (W88-W90, X39.0-) to identify the external cause

J70.1 **Chronic** and other pulmonary manifestations due to radiation `CC` `HCC`
    Fibrosis of lung following radiation
    Use additional code (W88-W90, X39.0-) to identify the external cause

J70.2 **Acute drug-induced interstitial lung disorders** `HCC`
    Use additional code for adverse effect, if applicable, to identify drug (T36-T50 with fifth or sixth character 5)
    `EXCLUDES 1` *interstitial pneumonia NOS (J84.9)*
             lymphoid interstitial pneumonia (J84.2)
    AHA: 2019,2Q,28

J70.3 **Chronic drug-induced interstitial lung disorders** `HCC`
    Use additional code for adverse effect, if applicable, to identify drug (T36-T50 with fifth or sixth character 5)
    `EXCLUDES 1` *interstitial pneumonia NOS (J84.9)*
             lymphoid interstitial pneumonia (J84.2)

`N` Newborn: 0   `P` Pediatric: 0-17   `M` Maternity: 9-64   `A` Adult: 15-124   `MCC` Major Complication/Comorbidity   `CC` Complication/Comorbidity   `SW` Severe Wound Dx

702

ICD-10-CM 2022

J70.4 **Drug-induced interstitial lung disorders, unspecified** `HCC`
Use additional code for adverse effect, if applicable, to identify drug (T36-T50 with fifth or sixth character 5)
> _EXCLUDES 1_   _interstitial pneumonia NOS (J84.9)_
> _lymphoid interstitial pneumonia (J84.2)_

AHA: 2019,2Q,28

J70.5 **Respiratory conditions due to smoke inhalation** `HCC`
Code first smoke inhalation (T59.81-)
> _EXCLUDES 2_   _smoke inhalation due to chemicals, gases, fumes and vapors (J68.9)_

AHA: 2013,4Q,121

J70.8 **Respiratory conditions due to other specified external agents** `HCC`
Code first (T51-T65) to identify the external agent

J70.9 **Respiratory conditions due to unspecified external agent** `HCC`
Code first (T51-T65) to identify the external agent

Other respiratory diseases principally affecting the interstitium (J80-J84)

J80 **Acute respiratory distress syndrome** `MCC` `HCC`
Acute respiratory distress syndrome in adult or child
Adult hyaline membrane disease
> _EXCLUDES 1_   _respiratory distress syndrome in newborn (perinatal) (P22.0)_

AHA: 2021,1Q,23; 2020,4Q,96; 2020,1Q,34-36; 2017,1Q,26
DEF: Lung inflammation or injury resulting in a build-up of fluid in the air sacs, preventing the passage of oxygen from the air into the bloodstream.
TIP: Assign as a secondary code for a patient with acute respiratory distress syndrome (ARDS) due to COVID-19; assign code U07.1 as the principal or first-listed code.

J81 **Pulmonary edema**
Use additional code to identify:
exposure to environmental tobacco smoke (Z77.22)
history of tobacco dependence (Z87.891)
occupational exposure to environmental tobacco smoke (Z57.31)
tobacco dependence (F17.-)
tobacco use (Z72.0)
> _EXCLUDES 1_   _chemical (acute) pulmonary edema (J68.1)_
> _hypostatic pneumonia (J18.2)_
> _passive pneumonia (J18.2)_
> _pulmonary edema due to external agents (J60-J70)_
> _pulmonary edema with heart disease NOS (I50.1)_
> _pulmonary edema with heart failure (I50.1)_

DEF: Accumulation of fluid in the air sacs of the lungs, making it difficult to breathe.

J81.0 **Acute pulmonary edema** `MCC` `HCC`
Acute edema of lung
AHA: 2020,3Q,27

J81.1 **Chronic pulmonary edema** `CC`
Pulmonary congestion (chronic) (passive)
Pulmonary edema NOS

J82 **Pulmonary eosinophilia, not elsewhere classified**
> _EXCLUDES 2_   _pulmonary eosinophilia due to aspergillosis (B44.-)_
> _pulmonary eosinophilia due to drugs (J70.2-J70.4)_
> _pulmonary eosinophilia due to specified parasitic infection (B50-B83)_
> _pulmonary eosinophilia due to systemic connective tissue disorders (M30-M36)_
> _pulmonary infiltrate NOS (R91.8)_

DEF: Infiltration of eosinophils (white blood cells of the immune system) into the parenchyma of the lungs, resulting in cough, fever, and dyspnea.

J82.8 **Pulmonary eosinophilia, not elsewhere classified**
AHA: 2020,4Q,25-27

J82.81 **Chronic eosinophilic pneumonia** `CC` `HCC`
Eosinophilic pneumonia, NOS

J82.82 **Acute eosinophilic pneumonia** `CC`

J82.83 **Eosinophilic asthma** `CC`
Code first asthma, by type, such as:
mild intermittent asthma (J45.2-)
mild persistent asthma (J45.3-)
moderate persistent asthma (J45.4-)
severe persistent asthma (J45.5-)

J82.89 **Other pulmonary eosinophilia, not elsewhere classified** `CC` `HCC`
Allergic pneumonia
Löffler's pneumonia
Tropical (pulmonary) eosinophilia NOS

J84 **Other interstitial pulmonary diseases**
> _EXCLUDES 1_   _drug-induced interstitial lung disorders (J70.2-J70.4)_
> _interstitial emphysema (J98.2)_
> _EXCLUDES 2_   _lung diseases due to external agents (J60-J70)_

DEF: Interstitial: Within the small spaces or gaps occurring in tissue or organs.

J84.0 **Alveolar and parieto-alveolar conditions**

J84.01 **Alveolar proteinosis** `CC` `HCC`
DEF: Reduced ventilation due to proteinaceous deposits on alveoli. Symptoms include dyspnea, cough, chest pain, weakness, weight loss, and hemoptysis.

J84.02 **Pulmonary alveolar microlithiasis** `CC` `HCC`

J84.03 **Idiopathic pulmonary hemosiderosis** `CC` `HCC`
Essential brown induration of lung
Code first underlying disease, such as:
disorders of iron metabolism (E83.1-)
> _EXCLUDES 1_   _acute idiopathic pulmonary hemorrhage in infants [AIPHI] (R04.81)_

DEF: Fibrosis of the alveolar walls marked by abnormal accumulation of iron as hemosiderin in the lungs. It primarily affects children and symptoms include anemia, fluid in the lungs, and blood in the sputum. Etiology is unknown.

J84.09 **Other alveolar and parieto-alveolar conditions** `CC` `HCC`

J84.1 **Other interstitial pulmonary diseases with fibrosis**
> _EXCLUDES 1_   _pulmonary fibrosis (chronic) due to inhalation of chemicals, gases, fumes or vapors (J68.4)_
> _pulmonary fibrosis (chronic) following radiation (J70.1)_

J84.10 **Pulmonary fibrosis, unspecified** `HCC`
Capillary fibrosis of lung
Cirrhosis of lung (chronic) NOS
Fibrosis of lung (atrophic) (chronic) (confluent) (massive) (perialveolar) (peribronchial) NOS
Induration of lung (chronic) NOS
Postinflammatory pulmonary fibrosis

J84.11 **Idiopathic interstitial pneumonia**
> _EXCLUDES 1_   _lymphoid interstitial pneumonia (J84.2)_
> _pneumocystis pneumonia (B59)_

J84.111 **Idiopathic interstitial pneumonia, not otherwise specified** `HCC`

J84.112 **Idiopathic pulmonary fibrosis** `HCC`
Cryptogenic fibrosing alveolitis
Idiopathic fibrosing alveolitis

J84.113 **Idiopathic non-specific interstitial pneumonitis** `HCC`
> _EXCLUDES 1_   _non-specific interstitial pneumonia NOS, or due to known underlying cause (J84.89)_

J84.114 **Acute interstitial pneumonitis** `CC` `HCC`
Hamman-Rich syndrome
> _EXCLUDES 1_   _pneumocystis pneumonia (B59)_

J84.115 **Respiratory bronchiolitis interstitial lung disease** `HCC`

J84.116 **Cryptogenic organizing pneumonia** `CC` `HCC`
> _EXCLUDES 1_   _organizing pneumonia NOS, or due to known underlying cause (J84.89)_

J84.117 **Desquamative interstitial pneumonia** `CC` `HCC`

✓6ᵗʰ **J84.17** **Other interstitial pulmonary diseases with fibrosis in diseases classified elsewhere**
AHA: 2020,4Q,27-28

J84.17Ø *Interstitial lung disease with progressive fibrotic phenotype in diseases classified elsewhere* HCC
Progressive fibrotic interstitial lung disease
Code first underlying disease, such as:
lung diseases due to external agents (J6Ø-J7Ø)
rheumatoid arthritis (MØ5.ØØ-MØ6.9)
sarcoidosis (D86)
systemic connective tissue disorders (M3Ø-M36)

J84.178 *Other interstitial pulmonary diseases with fibrosis in diseases classified elsewhere* HCC
Interstitial pneumonia (nonspecific) (usual) due to collagen vascular disease
Interstitial pneumonia (nonspecific) (usual) in diseases classified elsewhere
Organizing pneumonia due to collagen vascular disease
Organizing pneumonia in diseases classified elsewhere
Code first underlying disease, such as:
progressive systemic sclerosis (M34.Ø)
rheumatoid arthritis (MØ5.ØØ-MØ6.9)
systemic lupus erythematosis (M32.Ø-M32.9)

J84.2 **Lymphoid interstitial pneumonia** CC HCC
Lymphoid interstitial pneumonitis

✓5ᵗʰ **J84.8** **Other specified interstitial pulmonary diseases**
EXCLUDES 1   *exogenous lipoid pneumonia (J69.1)*
unspecified lipoid pneumonia (J69.1)

J84.81 **Lymphangioleiomyomatosis** MCC HCC
Lymphangiomyomatosis

J84.82 **Adult pulmonary Langerhans cell histiocytosis** CC HCC A
Adult PLCH

J84.83 **Surfactant mutations of the lung** MCC HCC
DEF: Genetic disorder resulting in insufficient secretion of a complex mixture of phospholipids and proteins that reduce surface tension in the alveoli following the onset of breathing to facilitate lung expansion in the newborn. It is the leading indication for pediatric lung transplantation.

✓6ᵗʰ **J84.84** **Other interstitial lung diseases of childhood**
J84.841 **Neuroendocrine cell hyperplasia of infancy** MCC HCC
J84.842 **Pulmonary interstitial glycogenosis** MCC HCC
J84.843 **Alveolar capillary dysplasia with vein misalignment** MCC HCC
J84.848 **Other interstitial lung diseases of childhood** MCC HCC

J84.89 **Other specified interstitial pulmonary diseases** HCC
Endogenous lipoid pneumonia
Interstitial pneumonitis
Non-specific interstitial pneumonitis NOS
Organizing pneumonia NOS
Code first, if applicable:
poisoning due to drug or toxin (T51-T65 with fifth or sixth character to indicate intent), for toxic pneumonopathy
underlying cause of pneumonopathy, if known
Use additional code, for adverse effect, to identify drug (T36-T5Ø with fifth or sixth character 5), if drug-induced
EXCLUDES 1   *cryptogenic organizing pneumonia (J84.116)*
idiopathic non-specific interstitial pneumonitis (J84.113)
lymphoid interstitial pneumonia (J84.2)
lipoid pneumonia, exogenous or unspecified (J69.1)
AHA: 2021,1Q,48; 2019,2Q,28

J84.9 **Interstitial pulmonary disease, unspecified** CC HCC
Interstitial pneumonia NOS

Suppurative and necrotic conditions of the lower respiratory tract (J85-J86)

✓4ᵗʰ **J85** **Abscess of lung and mediastinum**
Use additional code (B95-B97) to identify infectious agent
J85.Ø **Gangrene and necrosis of lung** MCC HCC
J85.1 **Abscess of lung with pneumonia** MCC HCC
Code also the type of pneumonia
J85.2 **Abscess of lung without pneumonia** MCC HCC
Abscess of lung NOS
J85.3 **Abscess of mediastinum** MCC HCC

✓4ᵗʰ **J86** **Pyothorax**
Use additional code (B95-B97) to identify infectious agent
EXCLUDES 1   *abscess of lung (J85.-)*
pyothorax due to tuberculosis (A15.6)
DEF: Collection of pus in the pleural space that is commonly caused by an infection that spreads from the lung, such as bacterial pneumonia or a lung abscess.
J86.Ø **Pyothorax with fistula** MCC HCC SW
Bronchocutaneous fistula
Bronchopleural fistula
Hepatopleural fistula
Mediastinal fistula
Pleural fistula
Thoracic fistula
Any condition classifiable to J86.9 with fistula
DEF: Purulent infection of the respiratory cavity, with communication from a cavity to another structure.
J86.9 **Pyothorax without fistula** MCC HCC
Abscess of pleura
Abscess of thorax
Empyema (chest) (lung) (pleura)
Fibrinopurulent pleurisy
Purulent pleurisy
Pyopneumothorax
Septic pleurisy
Seropurulent pleurisy
Suppurative pleurisy

Other diseases of the pleura (J9Ø-J94)

J9Ø **Pleural effusion, not elsewhere classified** CC
Encysted pleurisy
Pleural effusion NOS
Pleurisy with effusion (exudative) (serous)
EXCLUDES 1   *chylous (pleural) effusion (J94.Ø)*
malignant pleural effusion (J91.Ø))
pleurisy NOS (RØ9.1)
tuberculous pleural effusion (A15.6)
DEF: Collection of lymph and other fluid within the pleural space.

✓4ᵗʰ **J91** **Pleural effusion in conditions classified elsewhere**
EXCLUDES 2   *pleural effusion in heart failure (I5Ø.-)*
pleural effusion in systemic lupus erythematosus (M32.13)
DEF: Collection of lymph and other fluid within the pleural space.
J91.Ø *Malignant pleural effusion* CC
Code first underlying neoplasm

J91.8 *Pleural effusion in other conditions classified elsewhere* `CC`
Code first underlying disease, such as:
filariasis (B74.0-B74.9)
influenza (J09.X2, J10.1, J11.1)
AHA: 2015,2Q,15
TIP: Assign this code as a secondary diagnosis to congestive heart failure (I50.-) only if pleural effusion is specifically evaluated or treated.

Pleural Effusion

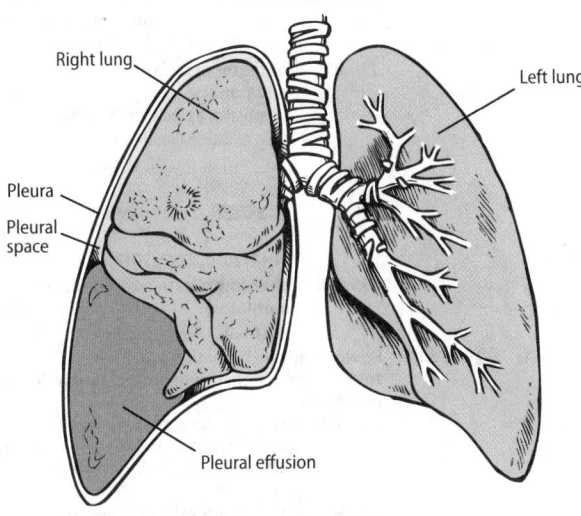

Right lung
Left lung
Pleura
Pleural space
Pleural effusion

✓4ᵗʰ **J92 Pleural plaque**
INCLUDES pleural thickening
DEF: Areas of fibrous thickening that form on the parietal or visceral pleura, the membranes that line the ribs and lungs.
J92.0 Pleural plaque with presence of asbestos
J92.9 Pleural plaque without asbestos
Pleural plaque NOS

✓4ᵗʰ **J93 Pneumothorax and air leak**
EXCLUDES 1 congenital or perinatal pneumothorax (P25.1)
postprocedural air leak (J95.812)
postprocedural pneumothorax (J95.811)
pyopneumothorax (J86.-)
traumatic pneumothorax (S27.0)
tuberculous (current disease) pneumothorax (A15.-)
DEF: Pneumothorax: Lung displacement due to abnormal leakage of air or gas that is trapped in the pleural space formed by the membrane that encloses the lungs and lines the thoracic cavity.
J93.0 Spontaneous tension pneumothorax `MCC`
DEF: Leaking air from the lung into the lining, causing collapse.
✓5ᵗʰ **J93.1 Other** spontaneous **pneumothorax**
J93.11 Primary spontaneous pneumothorax `CC`
J93.12 Secondary spontaneous pneumothorax `CC` `UPD`
Code first underlying condition, such as:
catamenial pneumothorax due to endometriosis (N80.8)
cystic fibrosis (E84.-)
eosinophilic pneumonia (J82)
lymphangioleiomyomatosis (J84.81)
malignant neoplasm of bronchus and lung (C34.-)
Marfan's syndrome (Q87.4)
pneumonia due to Pneumocystis carinii (B59)
secondary malignant neoplasm of lung (C78.0-)
spontaneous rupture of the esophagus (K22.3)
✓5ᵗʰ **J93.8 Other** pneumothorax and air leak
J93.81 Chronic pneumothorax `CC`
J93.82 Other air leak `CC`
Persistent air leak
J93.83 Other pneumothorax `CC`
Acute pneumothorax
Spontaneous pneumothorax NOS
AHA: 2020,3Q,9-10
J93.9 Pneumothorax, unspecified `CC`
Pneumothorax NOS

✓4ᵗʰ **J94 Other pleural conditions**
EXCLUDES 1 pleurisy NOS (R09.1)
traumatic hemopneumothorax (S27.2)
traumatic hemothorax (S27.1)
tuberculous pleural conditions (current disease) (A15.-)
J94.0 Chylous effusion `CC`
Chyliform effusion
DEF: Fluid within the pleural space due to the leaking of lymph contents into the space, usually as a result of thoracic duct damage or injury or mediastinal lymphoma.
J94.1 Fibrothorax
DEF: Fibrosis within the pleural lining of the lungs commonly seen as a stiff layer surrounding the lung typically attributed to traumatic hemothorax or pleural effusion.
J94.2 Hemothorax `CC`
Hemopneumothorax
J94.8 Other specified pleural conditions `CC`
Hydropneumothorax
Hydrothorax
AHA: 2021,1Q,48
J94.9 Pleural condition, unspecified

Intraoperative and postprocedural complications and disorders of respiratory system, not elsewhere classified (J95)

✓4ᵗʰ **J95 Intraoperative and postprocedural complications and disorders of respiratory system, not elsewhere classified**
EXCLUDES 2 aspiration pneumonia (J69.-)
emphysema (subcutaneous) resulting from a procedure (T81.82)
hypostatic pneumonia (J18.2)
pulmonary manifestations due to radiation (J70.0-J70.1)
✓5ᵗʰ **J95.0 Tracheostomy complications**
DEF: Tracheostomy: Formation of a tracheal opening on the neck surface with tube insertion to allow for respiration in cases of obstruction or decreased patency. A tracheostomy may be planned or performed on an emergency basis for temporary or long-term use.

Tracheostomy

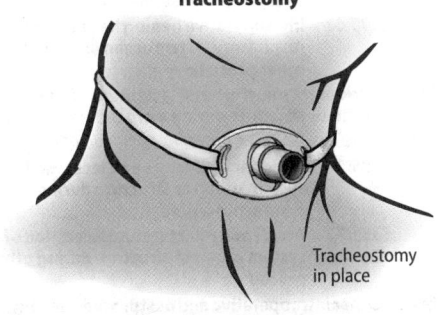

Tracheostomy in place

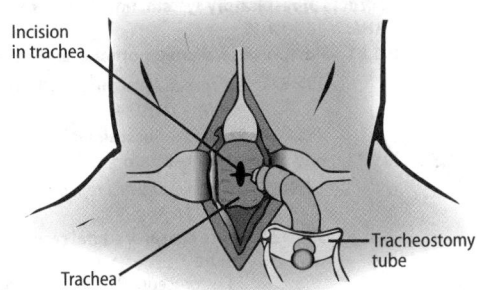

Incision in trachea
Trachea
Tracheostomy tube

J95.00 Unspecified tracheostomy complication `CC` `HCC`
J95.01 Hemorrhage from tracheostomy stoma `CC` `HCC`
J95.02 Infection of tracheostomy stoma `CC` `HCC`
Use additional code to identify type of infection, such as:
cellulitis of neck (L03.221)
sepsis (A40, A41.-)

J95.03 Malfunction of tracheostomy stoma CC HCC
Mechanical complication of tracheostomy stoma
Obstruction of tracheostomy airway
Tracheal stenosis due to tracheostomy

J95.04 Tracheo-esophageal fistula following tracheostomy CC HCC

J95.09 Other tracheostomy complication CC HCC

J95.1 Acute pulmonary insufficiency following thoracic surgery MCC HCC
> EXCLUDES 2   functional disturbances following cardiac surgery (I97.0, I97.1-)

J95.2 Acute pulmonary insufficiency following nonthoracic surgery MCC HCC
> EXCLUDES 2   functional disturbances following cardiac surgery (I97.0, I97.1-)

J95.3 Chronic pulmonary insufficiency following surgery MCC HCC
> EXCLUDES 2   functional disturbances following cardiac surgery (I97.0, I97.1-)

J95.4 Chemical pneumonitis due to anesthesia CC
Mendelson's syndrome
Postprocedural aspiration pneumonia
Use additional code for adverse effect, if applicable, to identify drug (T41.- with fifth or sixth character 5)
> EXCLUDES 1   aspiration pneumonitis due to anesthesia complicating labor and delivery (O74.0)
> aspiration pneumonitis due to anesthesia complicating pregnancy (O29)
> aspiration pneumonitis due to anesthesia complicating the puerperium (O89.01)

J95.5 Postprocedural subglottic stenosis CC

✓5ᵗʰ **J95.6 Intraoperative hemorrhage and hematoma of a respiratory system organ or structure complicating a procedure**
> EXCLUDES 1   intraoperative hemorrhage and hematoma of a respiratory system organ or structure due to accidental puncture and laceration during procedure (J95.7-)

J95.61 Intraoperative hemorrhage and hematoma of a respiratory system organ or structure complicating a respiratory system procedure CC

J95.62 Intraoperative hemorrhage and hematoma of a respiratory system organ or structure complicating other procedure CC

✓5ᵗʰ **J95.7 Accidental puncture and laceration of a respiratory system organ or structure during a procedure**
> EXCLUDES 2   postprocedural pneumothorax (J95.811)

J95.71 Accidental puncture and laceration of a respiratory system organ or structure during a respiratory system procedure CC

J95.72 Accidental puncture and laceration of a respiratory system organ or structure during other procedure CC

✓5ᵗʰ **J95.8 Other intraoperative and postprocedural complications and disorders of respiratory system, not elsewhere classified**
AHA: 2016,4Q,9-10

✓6ᵗʰ **J95.81 Postprocedural pneumothorax and air leak**

J95.811 Postprocedural pneumothorax CC H14
AHA: 2021,1Q,48

J95.812 Postprocedural air leak CC

✓6ᵗʰ **J95.82 Postprocedural respiratory failure**
> EXCLUDES 1   respiratory failure in other conditions (J96.-)

J95.821 Acute postprocedural respiratory failure MCC HCC
Postprocedural respiratory failure NOS

J95.822 Acute and chronic postprocedural respiratory failure MCC HCC

✓6ᵗʰ **J95.83 Postprocedural hemorrhage of a respiratory system organ or structure following a procedure**

J95.830 Postprocedural hemorrhage of a respiratory system organ or structure following a respiratory system procedure CC

J95.831 Postprocedural hemorrhage of a respiratory system organ or structure following other procedure CC

J95.84 Transfusion-related acute lung injury (TRALI) CC
DEF: Relatively rare, but serious, pulmonary complication of blood transfusion, with acute respiratory distress, noncardiogenic pulmonary edema, cyanosis, hypoxemia, hypotension, fever, and chills.

✓6ᵗʰ **J95.85 Complication of respirator [ventilator]**

J95.850 Mechanical complication of respirator CC HCC
> EXCLUDES 1   encounter for respirator [ventilator] dependence during power failure (Z99.12)

J95.851 Ventilator associated pneumonia CC HCC
Ventilator associated pneumonitis
Use additional code to identify the organism, if known (B95.-, B96.-, B97.-)
> EXCLUDES 1   ventilator lung in newborn (P27.8)
AHA: 2020,2Q,17; 2017,1Q,25

J95.859 Other complication of respirator [ventilator] CC HCC
AHA: 2021,1Q,48

✓6ᵗʰ **J95.86 Postprocedural hematoma and seroma of a respiratory system organ or structure following a procedure**

J95.860 Postprocedural hematoma of a respiratory system organ or structure following a respiratory system procedure CC

J95.861 Postprocedural hematoma of a respiratory system organ or structure following other procedure CC

J95.862 Postprocedural seroma of a respiratory system organ or structure following a respiratory system procedure CC

J95.863 Postprocedural seroma of a respiratory system organ or structure following other procedure CC

J95.88 Other intraoperative complications of respiratory system, not elsewhere classified CC

J95.89 Other postprocedural complications and disorders of respiratory system, not elsewhere classified CC
Use additional code to identify disorder, such as:
aspiration pneumonia (J69.-)
bacterial or viral pneumonia (J12-J18)
> EXCLUDES 2   acute pulmonary insufficiency following thoracic surgery (J95.1)
> postprocedural subglottic stenosis (J95.5)

Other diseases of the respiratory system (J96-J99)

✓4ᵗʰ **J96 Respiratory failure, not elsewhere classified**
> EXCLUDES 1   acute respiratory distress syndrome (J80)
> cardiorespiratory failure (R09.2)
> newborn respiratory distress syndrome (P22.0)
> postprocedural respiratory failure (J95.82-)
> respiratory arrest (R09.2)
> respiratory arrest of newborn (P28.81)
> respiratory failure of newborn (P28.5)
AHA: 2021,1Q,27,44-45; 2020,4Q,96

✓5ᵗʰ **J96.0 Acute respiratory failure**

J96.00 Acute respiratory failure, unspecified whether with hypoxia or hypercapnia MCC HCC
AHA: 2016,3Q,14; 2013,4Q,121

J96.01 Acute respiratory failure with hypoxia MCC HCC
AHA: 2020,3Q,12

J96.02 Acute respiratory failure with hypercapnia MCC HCC

✓5ᵗʰ **J96.1 Chronic respiratory failure**

J96.10 Chronic respiratory failure, unspecified whether with hypoxia or hypercapnia CC HCC
AHA: 2016,1Q,38; 2015,1Q,21

J96.11 Chronic respiratory failure with hypoxia CC HCC
AHA: 2013,4Q,129

J96.12 Chronic respiratory failure with hypercapnia CC HCC

√5ᵗʰ J96.2 Acute and chronic respiratory failure

Acute on chronic respiratory failure

    J96.20 Acute and chronic respiratory failure, unspecified whether with hypoxia or hypercapnia `MCC` `HCC`

    J96.21 Acute and chronic respiratory failure with hypoxia `MCC` `HCC`

    J96.22 Acute and chronic respiratory failure with hypercapnia `MCC` `HCC`

√5ᵗʰ J96.9 Respiratory failure, unspecified

    J96.90 Respiratory failure, unspecified, unspecified whether with hypoxia or hypercapnia `MCC` `HCC`

    J96.91 Respiratory failure, unspecified with hypoxia `MCC` `HCC`

    J96.92 Respiratory failure, unspecified with hypercapnia `MCC` `HCC`

√4ᵗʰ J98 Other respiratory disorders

Use additional code to identify:

exposure to environmental tobacco smoke (Z77.22)

exposure to tobacco smoke in the perinatal period (P96.81)

history of tobacco dependence (Z87.891)

occupational exposure to environmental tobacco smoke (Z57.31)

tobacco dependence (F17.-)

tobacco use (Z72.0)

    EXCLUDES 1   newborn apnea (P28.4)

               newborn sleep apnea (P28.3)

    EXCLUDES 2   apnea NOS (R06.81)

               sleep apnea (G47.3-)

√5ᵗʰ J98.0 Diseases of bronchus, not elsewhere classified

    J98.01 Acute bronchospasm

        EXCLUDES 1   acute bronchiolitis with bronchospasm (J21.-)

                    acute bronchitis with bronchospasm (J20.-)

                    asthma (J45.-)

                    exercise induced bronchospasm (J45.990)

    J98.09 Other diseases of bronchus, not elsewhere classified

         Broncholithiasis

         Calcification of bronchus

         Stenosis of bronchus

         Tracheobronchial collapse

         Tracheobronchial dyskinesia

         Ulcer of bronchus

√5ᵗʰ J98.1 Pulmonary collapse

    EXCLUDES 1   therapeutic collapse of lung status (Z98.3)

    J98.11 Atelectasis `CC`

        EXCLUDES 1   newborn atelectasis

                    tuberculous atelectasis (current disease) (A15)

        DEF: Collapse of lung tissue affecting part or all of one lung, preventing normal oxygen absorption to healthy tissues.

    J98.19 Other pulmonary collapse `CC`

J98.2 Interstitial emphysema `HCC`

Mediastinal emphysema

    EXCLUDES 1   emphysema NOS (J43.9)

               emphysema in newborn (P25.0)

               surgical emphysema (subcutaneous) (T81.82)

               traumatic subcutaneous emphysema (T79.7)

J98.3 Compensatory emphysema `HCC`

DEF: Distention of all or part of the lung caused by disease processes or surgical intervention that decreased volume in another part of the lung, causing an overcompensation reaction. Compensatory emphysema occurs in association with pneumonias, pleural effusions, atelectasis, empyema, and pneumothorax.

J98.4 Other disorders of lung

Calcification of lung

Cystic lung disease (acquired)

Lung disease NOS

Pulmolithiasis

    EXCLUDES 1   acute interstitial pneumonitis (J84.114)

              pulmonary insufficiency following surgery (J95.1-J95.2)

√5ᵗʰ J98.5 Diseases of mediastinum, not elsewhere classified

    EXCLUDES 2   abscess of mediastinum (J85.3)

    AHA: 2016,4Q,29

    J98.51 Mediastinitis `MCC` `H8`

         Code first underlying condition, if applicable, such as postoperative mediastinitis (T81.-)

    J98.59 Other diseases of mediastinum, not elsewhere classified `MCC` `H8`

         Fibrosis of mediastinum

         Hernia of mediastinum

         Retraction of mediastinum

J98.6 Disorders of diaphragm

Diaphragmatitis

Paralysis of diaphragm

Relaxation of diaphragm

    EXCLUDES 1   congenital malformation of diaphragm NEC (Q79.1)

              congenital diaphragmatic hernia (Q79.0)

    EXCLUDES 2   diaphragmatic hernia (K44.-)

J98.8 Other specified respiratory disorders

AHA: 2020,1Q,34-36

TIP: Assign as a secondary code for a patient with a respiratory infection that is not further specified but is documented as being associated with COVID-19; assign U07.1 as the principal or first-listed code. If the respiratory infection documentation specifies acute or lower respiratory infection (NOS), assign J22 instead.

J98.9 Respiratory disorder, unspecified

Respiratory disease (chronic) NOS

J99 Respiratory disorders in diseases classified elsewhere `HCC`

Code first underlying disease, such as:

amyloidosis (E85.-)

ankylosing spondylitis (M45)

congenital syphilis (A50.5)

cryoglobulinemia (D89.1)

early congenital syphilis (A50.0)

plasminogen deficiency (E88.02)

schistosomiasis (B65.0-B65.9)

    EXCLUDES 1   respiratory disorders in:

         amebiasis (A06.5)

         blastomycosis (B40.0-B40.2)

         candidiasis (B37.1)

         coccidioidomycosis (B38.0-B38.2)

         cystic fibrosis with pulmonary manifestations (E84.0)

         dermatomyositis (M33.01, M33.11)

         histoplasmosis (B39.0-B39.2)

         late syphilis (A52.72, A52.73)

         polymyositis (M33.21)

         ▶Sjögren syndrome◀ (M35.02)

         systemic lupus erythematosus (M32.13)

         systemic sclerosis (M34.81)

         Wegener's granulomatosis (M31.30-M31.31)

☑ Additional Character Required   √x7ᵗʰ Placeholder   Questionable PDx   Manifestation   Unspecified Dx   `UPD` Unacceptable PDx   `H1`-`H4` HAC   `HCC` CMS-HCC Dx   `HIV` HIV Dx

ICD-10-CM 2022   707

Chapter 11. Diseases of the Digestive System (KØØ–K95)

Chapter-specific Guidelines with Coding Examples
Reserved for future guideline expansion.

Chapter 11. Diseases of the Digestive System (K00-K95)

EXCLUDES 2   certain conditions originating in the perinatal period (P04-P96)
certain infectious and parasitic diseases (A00-B99)
complications of pregnancy, childbirth and the puerperium (O00-O9A)
congenital malformations, deformations and chromosomal abnormalities (Q00-Q99)
endocrine, nutritional and metabolic diseases (E00-E88)
injury, poisoning and certain other consequences of external causes (S00-T88)
neoplasms (C00-D49)
symptoms, signs and abnormal clinical and laboratory findings, not elsewhere classified (R00-R94)

This chapter contains the following blocks:

K00-K14	Diseases of oral cavity and salivary glands
K20-K31	Diseases of esophagus, stomach and duodenum
K35-K38	Diseases of appendix
K40-K46	Hernia
K50-K52	Noninfective enteritis and colitis
K55-K64	Other diseases of intestines
K65-K68	Diseases of peritoneum and retroperitoneum
K70-K77	Diseases of liver
K80-K87	Disorders of gallbladder, biliary tract and pancreas
K90-K95	Other diseases of the digestive system

Diseases of oral cavity and salivary glands (K00-K14)

✓4ᵗʰ K00 Disorders of tooth development and eruption

EXCLUDES 2   embedded and impacted teeth (K01.-)

K00.0 Anodontia
Hypodontia
Oligodontia
EXCLUDES 1   acquired absence of teeth (K08.1-)
DEF: Partial or complete absence of teeth due to a congenital defect involving the tooth bud.

K00.1 Supernumerary teeth
Distomolar
Fourth molar
Mesiodens
Paramolar
Supplementary teeth
EXCLUDES 2   supernumerary roots (K00.2)

K00.2 Abnormalities of size and form of teeth
Concrescence of teeth
Fusion of teeth
Gemination of teeth
Dens evaginatus
Dens in dente
Dens invaginatus
Enamel pearls
Macrodontia
Microdontia
Peg-shaped [conical] teeth
Supernumerary roots
Taurodontism
Tuberculum paramolare
EXCLUDES 1   abnormalities of teeth due to congenital syphilis (A50.5)
tuberculum Carabelli, which is regarded as a normal variation and should not be coded

K00.3 Mottled teeth
Dental fluorosis
Mottling of enamel
Nonfluoride enamel opacities
EXCLUDES 2   deposits [accretions] on teeth (K03.6)

K00.4 Disturbances in tooth formation
Aplasia and hypoplasia of cementum
Dilaceration of tooth
Enamel hypoplasia (neonatal) (postnatal) (prenatal)
Regional odontodysplasia
Turner's tooth
EXCLUDES 1   Hutchinson's teeth and mulberry molars in congenital syphilis (A50.5)
EXCLUDES 2   mottled teeth (K00.3)

K00.5 Hereditary disturbances in tooth structure, not elsewhere classified
Amelogenesis imperfecta
Dentinogenesis imperfecta
Odontogenesis imperfecta
Dentinal dysplasia
Shell teeth

K00.6 Disturbances in tooth eruption
Dentia praecox
Natal tooth
Neonatal tooth
Premature eruption of tooth
Premature shedding of primary [deciduous] tooth
Prenatal teeth
Retained [persistent] primary tooth
EXCLUDES 2   embedded and impacted teeth (K01.-)

K00.7 Teething syndrome

K00.8 Other disorders of tooth development
Color changes during tooth formation
Intrinsic staining of teeth NOS
EXCLUDES 2   posteruptive color changes (K03.7)

K00.9 Disorder of tooth development, unspecified
Disorder of odontogenesis NOS

✓4ᵗʰ K01 Embedded and impacted teeth
EXCLUDES 1   abnormal position of fully erupted teeth (M26.3-)

K01.0 Embedded teeth
K01.1 Impacted teeth

✓4ᵗʰ K02 Dental caries
INCLUDES   caries of dentine
dental cavities
early childhood caries
pre-eruptive caries
recurrent caries (dentino enamel junction) (enamel) (to the pulp)
tooth decay
DEF: Localized section of tooth decay that begins on the tooth surface with destruction of the calcified enamel, allowing bacterial destruction to continue and form cavities and may extend to the dentin and pulp.

Tooth Anatomy

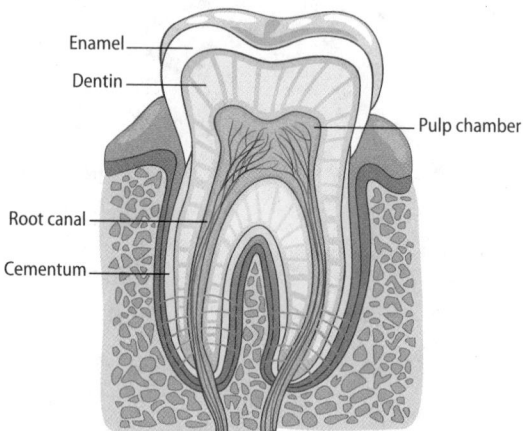

Enamel
Dentin
Pulp chamber
Root canal
Cementum

K02.3 Arrested dental caries
Arrested coronal and root caries

✓5ᵗʰ K02.5 Dental caries on pit and fissure surface
Dental caries on chewing surface of tooth

K02.51 Dental caries on pit and fissure surface limited to enamel
White spot lesions [initial caries] on pit and fissure surface of tooth

K02.52 Dental caries on pit and fissure surface penetrating into dentin
Primary dental caries, cervical origin

K02.53 Dental caries on pit and fissure surface penetrating into pulp

✓5ᵗʰ K02.6 Dental caries on smooth surface

K02.61 Dental caries on smooth surface limited to enamel
White spot lesions [initial caries] on smooth surface of tooth

K02.62   **Dental caries on smooth surface** penetrating into dentin

K02.63   **Dental caries on smooth surface** penetrating into pulp

K02.7   **Dental** root **caries**

K02.9   **Dental caries, unspecified**

✓4ᵗʰ **K03**   **Other diseases of hard tissues of teeth**

> **EXCLUDES 2**   bruxism (F45.8)
> dental caries (K02.-)
> teeth-grinding NOS (F45.8)

K03.0   **Excessive attrition of teeth**
Approximal wear of teeth
Occlusal wear of teeth
DEF: Attrition: In dentistry, wearing away or erosion of tooth surface from abrasive food or grinding teeth.

K03.1   **Abrasion of teeth**
Dentifrice abrasion of teeth
Habitual abrasion of teeth
Occupational abrasion of teeth
Ritual abrasion of teeth
Traditional abrasion of teeth
Wedge defect NOS

K03.2   **Erosion of teeth**
Erosion of teeth due to diet
Erosion of teeth due to drugs and medicaments
Erosion of teeth due to persistent vomiting
Erosion of teeth NOS
Idiopathic erosion of teeth
Occupational erosion of teeth

K03.3   **Pathological resorption of teeth**
Internal granuloma of pulp
Resorption of teeth (external)

K03.4   **Hypercementosis**
Cementation hyperplasia

K03.5   **Ankylosis of teeth**

K03.6   **Deposits [accretions] on teeth**
Betel deposits [accretions] on teeth
Black deposits [accretions] on teeth
Extrinsic staining of teeth NOS
Green deposits [accretions] on teeth
Materia alba deposits [accretions] on teeth
Orange deposits [accretions] on teeth
Staining of teeth NOS
Subgingival dental calculus
Supragingival dental calculus
Tobacco deposits [accretions] on teeth

K03.7   **Posteruptive color changes of dental hard tissues**
> **EXCLUDES 2**   deposits [accretions] on teeth (K03.6)

✓5ᵗʰ **K03.8**   **Other specified diseases of hard tissues of teeth**

K03.81   **Cracked tooth**
> **EXCLUDES 1**   asymptomatic craze lines in enamel - omit code
> broken or fractured tooth due to trauma (S02.5)

K03.89   **Other specified diseases of hard tissues of teeth**

K03.9   **Disease of hard tissues of teeth, unspecified**

✓4ᵗʰ **K04**   **Diseases of pulp and periapical tissues**
AHA: 2016,4Q,29-30

✓5ᵗʰ **K04.0**   **Pulpitis**
Acute pulpitis
Chronic (hyperplastic) (ulcerative) pulpitis

K04.01   Reversible **pulpitis**   CC

K04.02   Irreversible **pulpitis**   CC

K04.1   **Necrosis of pulp**
Pulpal gangrene

K04.2   **Pulp degeneration**
Denticles
Pulpal calcifications
Pulpal stones

K04.3   **Abnormal hard tissue formation in pulp**
Secondary or irregular dentine

K04.4   **Acute apical periodontitis of pulpal origin**   CC
Acute apical periodontitis NOS
> **EXCLUDES 1**   acute periodontitis (K05.2-)
DEF: Severe inflammation of the area surrounding the tip of a tooth's root that is often secondary to infection or trauma.

K04.5   **Chronic apical periodontitis**
Apical or periapical granuloma
Apical periodontitis NOS
> **EXCLUDES 1**   chronic periodontitis (K05.3-)

K04.6   **Periapical abscess with sinus**   SW
Dental abscess with sinus
Dentoalveolar abscess with sinus

K04.7   **Periapical abscess without sinus**
Dental abscess without sinus
Dentoalveolar abscess without sinus

K04.8   **Radicular cyst**
Apical (periodontal) cyst
Periapical cyst
Residual radicular cyst
> **EXCLUDES 2**   lateral periodontal cyst (K09.0)
DEF: Most common odontogenic cyst in tissue around the tooth apex due to chronic inflammation of dental pulp.

✓5ᵗʰ **K04.9**   **Other and unspecified diseases of pulp and periapical tissues**

K04.90   **Unspecified diseases of pulp and periapical tissues**

K04.99   **Other diseases of pulp and periapical tissues**

✓4ᵗʰ **K05**   **Gingivitis and periodontal diseases**
Use additional code to identify:
alcohol abuse and dependence (F10.-)
exposure to environmental tobacco smoke (Z77.22)
exposure to tobacco smoke in the perinatal period (P96.81)
history of tobacco dependence (Z87.891)
occupational exposure to environmental tobacco smoke (Z57.31)
tobacco dependence (F17.-)
tobacco use (Z72.0)
AHA: 2016,4Q,29-30

✓5ᵗʰ **K05.0**   **Acute gingivitis**
> **EXCLUDES 1**   acute necrotizing ulcerative gingivitis (A69.1)
> herpesviral [herpes simplex] gingivostomatitis (B00.2)

K05.00   **Acute gingivitis,** plaque induced
Acute gingivitis NOS
Plaque induced gingival disease

K05.01   **Acute gingivitis,** non-plaque induced

✓5ᵗʰ **K05.1**   **Chronic gingivitis**
Desquamative gingivitis (chronic)
Gingivitis (chronic) NOS
Hyperplastic gingivitis (chronic)
Pregnancy associated gingivitis
Simple marginal gingivitis (chronic)
Ulcerative gingivitis (chronic)
Code first, if applicable, diseases of the digestive system complicating pregnacy (O99.61-)

K05.10   **Chronic gingivitis,** plaque induced
Chronic gingivitis NOS
Gingivitis NOS

K05.11   **Chronic gingivitis,** non-plaque induced

✓5ᵗʰ **K05.2**   **Aggressive periodontitis**
Acute pericoronitis
> **EXCLUDES 1**   acute apical periodontitis (K04.4)
> periapical abscess (K04.7)
> periapical abscess with sinus (K04.6)

K05.20   **Aggressive periodontitis, unspecified**

✓6ᵗʰ **K05.21**   **Aggressive periodontitis,** localized
Periodontal abscess

K05.211   **Aggressive periodontitis, localized,** slight

K05.212   **Aggressive periodontitis, localized,** moderate

K05.213   **Aggressive periodontitis, localized,** severe

K05.219   **Aggressive periodontitis, localized, unspecified severity**

✓6ᵗʰ **K05.22**   **Aggressive periodontitis,** generalized

K05.221   **Aggressive periodontitis, generalized,** slight

K05.222   **Aggressive periodontitis, generalized,** moderate

K05.223   **Aggressive periodontitis, generalized,** severe

     K05.229 Aggressive periodontitis, generalized, unspecified severity

✓5ᵗʰ **K05.3 Chronic periodontitis**
- Chronic pericoronitis
- Complex periodontitis
- Periodontitis NOS
- Simplex periodontitis

   EXCLUDES 1   *chronic apical periodontitis (K04.5)*

   K05.30 Chronic periodontitis, unspecified

✓6ᵗʰ **K05.31** Chronic periodontitis, localized

    K05.311 Chronic periodontitis, localized, slight
    K05.312 Chronic periodontitis, localized, moderate
    K05.313 Chronic periodontitis, localized, severe
    K05.319 Chronic periodontitis, localized, unspecified severity

✓6ᵗʰ **K05.32** Chronic periodontitis, generalized

    K05.321 Chronic periodontitis, generalized, slight
    K05.322 Chronic periodontitis, generalized, moderate
    K05.323 Chronic periodontitis, generalized, severe
    K05.329 Chronic periodontitis, generalized, unspecified

K05.4 Periodontosis
- Juvenile periodontosis

K05.5 Other periodontal diseases
- Combined periodontic-endodontic lesion
- Narrow gingival width (of periodontal soft tissue)

   EXCLUDES 2   *leukoplakia of gingiva (K13.21)*

K05.6 Periodontal disease, unspecified

✓4ᵗʰ **K06 Other disorders of gingiva and edentulous alveolar ridge**

   EXCLUDES 2   *acute gingivitis (K05.0)*
       atrophy of edentulous alveolar ridge (K08.2)
       chronic gingivitis (K05.1)
       gingivitis NOS (K05.1)

AHA: 2016,4Q,29-30

✓5ᵗʰ **K06.0 Gingival recession**
- Gingival recession (postinfective) (postprocedural)

   AHA: 2017,4Q,16

✓6ᵗʰ **K06.01** Gingival recession, localized

    K06.010 Localized gingival recession, unspecified
      Localized gingival recession, NOS
    K06.011 Localized gingival recession, minimal
    K06.012 Localized gingival recession, moderate
    K06.013 Localized gingival recession, severe

✓6ᵗʰ **K06.02** Gingival recession, generalized

    K06.020 Generalized gingival recession, unspecified
      Generalized gingival recession, NOS
    K06.021 Generalized gingival recession, minimal
    K06.022 Generalized gingival recession, moderate
    K06.023 Generalized gingival recession, severe

K06.1 Gingival enlargement
- Gingival fibromatosis

K06.2 Gingival and edentulous alveolar ridge lesions associated with trauma
- Irritative hyperplasia of edentulous ridge [denture hyperplasia]
- Use additional code (Chapter 20) to identify external cause or denture status (Z97.2)

K06.3 Horizontal alveolar bone loss

K06.8 Other specified disorders of gingiva and edentulous alveolar ridge
- Fibrous epulis
- Flabby alveolar ridge
- Giant cell epulis
- Peripheral giant cell granuloma of gingiva
- Pyogenic granuloma of gingiva
- Vertical ridge deficiency

   EXCLUDES 2   *gingival cyst (K09.0)*

K06.9 Disorder of gingiva and edentulous alveolar ridge, unspecified

✓4ᵗʰ **K08 Other disorders of teeth and supporting structures**

   EXCLUDES 2   *dentofacial anomalies [including malocclusion] (M26.-)*
       disorders of jaw (M27.-)

AHA: 2016,4Q,29-30

K08.0 Exfoliation of teeth due to systemic causes
- Code also underlying systemic condition

✓5ᵗʰ **K08.1 Complete loss of teeth**
- Acquired loss of teeth, complete

   EXCLUDES 1   *congenital absence of teeth (K00.0)*
       exfoliation of teeth due to systemic causes (K08.0)
       partial loss of teeth (K08.4-)

   DEF: Loss of all teeth as a result of caries, trauma, extraction, periodontal disease, or other specified or unspecified causes.
   Synonym(s): complete edentulism

✓6ᵗʰ **K08.10** Complete loss of teeth, unspecified cause

    K08.101 Complete loss of teeth, unspecified cause, class I
    K08.102 Complete loss of teeth, unspecified cause, class II
    K08.103 Complete loss of teeth, unspecified cause, class III
    K08.104 Complete loss of teeth, unspecified cause, class IV
    K08.109 Complete loss of teeth, unspecified cause, unspecified class
      Edentulism NOS

✓6ᵗʰ **K08.11** Complete loss of teeth due to trauma

    K08.111 Complete loss of teeth due to trauma, class I
    K08.112 Complete loss of teeth due to trauma, class II
    K08.113 Complete loss of teeth due to trauma, class III
    K08.114 Complete loss of teeth due to trauma, class IV
    K08.119 Complete loss of teeth due to trauma, unspecified class

✓6ᵗʰ **K08.12** Complete loss of teeth due to periodontal diseases

    K08.121 Complete loss of teeth due to periodontal diseases, class I
    K08.122 Complete loss of teeth due to periodontal diseases, class II
    K08.123 Complete loss of teeth due to periodontal diseases, class III
    K08.124 Complete loss of teeth due to periodontal diseases, class IV
    K08.129 Complete loss of teeth due to periodontal diseases, unspecified class

✓6ᵗʰ **K08.13** Complete loss of teeth due to caries

    K08.131 Complete loss of teeth due to caries, class I
    K08.132 Complete loss of teeth due to caries, class II
    K08.133 Complete loss of teeth due to caries, class III
    K08.134 Complete loss of teeth due to caries, class IV
    K08.139 Complete loss of teeth due to caries, unspecified class

✓6ᵗʰ **K08.19** Complete loss of teeth due to other specified cause

    K08.191 Complete loss of teeth due to other specified cause, class I
    K08.192 Complete loss of teeth due to other specified cause, class II
    K08.193 Complete loss of teeth due to other specified cause, class III
    K08.194 Complete loss of teeth due to other specified cause, class IV
    K08.199 Complete loss of teeth due to other specified cause, unspecified class

✓5ᵗʰ **K08.2 Atrophy of edentulous alveolar ridge**

   K08.20 Unspecified atrophy of edentulous alveolar ridge
      Atrophy of the mandible NOS
      Atrophy of the maxilla NOS

   K08.21 Minimal atrophy of the mandible
      Minimal atrophy of the edentulous mandible

   K08.22 Moderate atrophy of the mandible
      Moderate atrophy of the edentulous mandible

N Newborn: 0   P Pediatric: 0-17   M Maternity: 9-64   A Adult: 15-124   MCC Major Complication/Comorbidity   CC Complication/Comorbidity   SW Severe Wound Dx

712   ICD-10-CM 2022

K08.23 Severe atrophy of the mandible
Severe atrophy of the edentulous mandible

K08.24 Minimal atrophy of maxilla
Minimal atrophy of the edentulous maxilla

K08.25 Moderate atrophy of the maxilla
Moderate atrophy of the edentulous maxilla

K08.26 Severe atrophy of the maxilla
Severe atrophy of the edentulous maxilla

K08.3 Retained dental root

√5th **K08.4 Partial loss of teeth**
Acquired loss of teeth, partial
EXCLUDES 1   complete loss of teeth (K08.1-)
     congenital absence of teeth (K00.0)
EXCLUDES 2   exfoliation of teeth due to systemic causes (K08.0)

√6th **K08.40 Partial loss of teeth, unspecified cause**

K08.401 Partial loss of teeth, unspecified cause, class I

K08.402 Partial loss of teeth, unspecified cause, class II

K08.403 Partial loss of teeth, unspecified cause, class III

K08.404 Partial loss of teeth, unspecified cause, class IV

K08.409 Partial loss of teeth, unspecified cause, unspecified class
Tooth extraction status NOS

√6th **K08.41 Partial loss of teeth due to trauma**

K08.411 Partial loss of teeth due to trauma, class I

K08.412 Partial loss of teeth due to trauma, class II

K08.413 Partial loss of teeth due to trauma, class III

K08.414 Partial loss of teeth due to trauma, class IV

K08.419 Partial loss of teeth due to trauma, unspecified class

√6th **K08.42 Partial loss of teeth due to periodontal diseases**

K08.421 Partial loss of teeth due to periodontal diseases, class I

K08.422 Partial loss of teeth due to periodontal diseases, class II

K08.423 Partial loss of teeth due to periodontal diseases, class III

K08.424 Partial loss of teeth due to periodontal diseases, class IV

K08.429 Partial loss of teeth due to periodontal diseases, unspecified class

√6th **K08.43 Partial loss of teeth due to caries**

K08.431 Partial loss of teeth due to caries, class I

K08.432 Partial loss of teeth due to caries, class II

K08.433 Partial loss of teeth due to caries, class III

K08.434 Partial loss of teeth due to caries, class IV

K08.439 Partial loss of teeth due to caries, unspecified class

√6th **K08.49 Partial loss of teeth due to other specified cause**

K08.491 Partial loss of teeth due to other specified cause, class I

K08.492 Partial loss of teeth due to other specified cause, class II

K08.493 Partial loss of teeth due to other specified cause, class III

K08.494 Partial loss of teeth due to other specified cause, class IV

K08.499 Partial loss of teeth due to other specified cause, unspecified class

√5th **K08.5 Unsatisfactory restoration of tooth**
Defective bridge, crown, filling
Defective dental restoration
EXCLUDES 1   dental restoration status (Z98.811)
EXCLUDES 2   endosseous dental implant failure (M27.6-)
     unsatisfactory endodontic treatment (M27.5-)

K08.50 Unsatisfactory restoration of tooth, unspecified
Defective dental restoration NOS

K08.51 Open restoration margins of tooth
Dental restoration failure of marginal integrity
Open margin on tooth restoration
Poor gingival margin to tooth restoration

K08.52 Unrepairable overhanging of dental restorative materials
Overhanging of tooth restoration

√6th **K08.53 Fractured dental restorative material**
EXCLUDES 1   cracked tooth (K03.81)
     traumatic fracture of tooth (S02.5)

K08.530 Fractured dental restorative material without loss of material

K08.531 Fractured dental restorative material with loss of material

K08.539 Fractured dental restorative material, unspecified

K08.54 Contour of existing restoration of tooth biologically incompatible with oral health
Dental restoration failure of periodontal anatomical integrity
Unacceptable contours of existing restoration of tooth
Unacceptable morphology of existing restoration of tooth

K08.55 Allergy to existing dental restorative material
Use additional code to identify the specific type of allergy

K08.56 Poor aesthetic of existing restoration of tooth
Dental restoration aesthetically inadequate or displeasing

K08.59 Other unsatisfactory restoration of tooth
Other defective dental restoration

√5th **K08.8 Other specified disorders of teeth and supporting structures**

K08.81 Primary occlusal trauma

K08.82 Secondary occlusal trauma

K08.89 Other specified disorders of teeth and supporting structures
Enlargement of alveolar ridge NOS
Insufficient anatomic crown height
Insufficient clinical crown length
Irregular alveolar process
Toothache NOS

K08.9 Disorder of teeth and supporting structures, unspecified

√4th **K09 Cysts of oral region, not elsewhere classified**
INCLUDES   lesions showing histological features both of aneurysmal cyst and of another fibro-osseous lesion
EXCLUDES 2   cysts of jaw (M27.0-, M27.4-)
     radicular cyst (K04.8)

K09.0 Developmental odontogenic cysts
Dentigerous cyst
Eruption cyst
Follicular cyst
Gingival cyst
Lateral periodontal cyst
Primordial cyst
EXCLUDES 2   keratocysts (D16.4, D16.5)
     odontogenic keratocystic tumors (D16.4, D16.5)

K09.1 Developmental (nonodontogenic) cysts of oral region
Cyst (of) incisive canal
Cyst (of) palatine of papilla
Globulomaxillary cyst
Median palatal cyst
Nasoalveolar cyst
Nasolabial cyst
Nasopalatine duct cyst

K09.8 Other cysts of oral region, not elsewhere classified
Dermoid cyst
Epidermoid cyst
Lymphoepithelial cyst
Epstein's pearl

K09.9 Cyst of oral region, unspecified

√4th **K11 Diseases of salivary glands**
Use additional code to identify:
alcohol abuse and dependence (F10.-)
exposure to environmental tobacco smoke (Z77.22)
exposure to tobacco smoke in the perinatal period (P96.81)
history of tobacco dependence (Z87.891)
occupational exposure to environmental tobacco smoke (Z57.31)
tobacco dependence (F17.-)
tobacco use (Z72.0)

K11.0 Atrophy of salivary gland

K11.1 **Hypertrophy** of salivary gland
> **DEF:** Overgrowth of or enlarged salivary gland tissue caused by infection, salivary duct blockage, autoimmune diseases, and benign and malignant tumors.

✓5ᵗʰ **K11.2** Sialoadenitis
> Parotitis
> **EXCLUDES 1**   epidemic parotitis (B26.-)
>   mumps (B26.-)
>   uveoparotid fever [Heerfordt] (D86.89)
> **DEF:** Inflammation of the salivary gland.

   K11.20 **Sialoadenitis, unspecified**
   K11.21 **Acute** sialoadenitis
>   **EXCLUDES 1**   acute recurrent sialoadenitis (K11.22)

   K11.22 **Acute recurrent** sialoadenitis
   K11.23 **Chronic** sialoadenitis

K11.3 **Abscess** of salivary gland   `CC`

K11.4 **Fistula** of salivary gland   `CC` `SW`
> **EXCLUDES 1**   congenital fistula of salivary gland (Q38.4)

K11.5 Sialolithiasis
> Calculus of salivary gland or duct
> Stone of salivary gland or duct

K11.6 **Mucocele** of salivary gland
> Mucous extravasation cyst of salivary gland
> Mucous retention cyst of salivary gland
> Ranula

K11.7 **Disturbances of salivary** secretion
> Hypoptyalism
> Ptyalism
> Xerostomia
> **EXCLUDES 2**   dry mouth NOS (R68.2)

K11.8 **Other diseases of salivary glands**
> Benign lymphoepithelial lesion of salivary gland
> Mikulicz' disease
> Necrotizing sialometaplasia
> Sialectasia
> Stenosis of salivary duct
> Stricture of salivary duct
> **EXCLUDES 1**   ▶Sjögren syndrome◀ (M35.0-)

K11.9 **Disease of salivary gland, unspecified**
> Sialoadenopathy NOS

✓4ᵗʰ **K12** **Stomatitis and related lesions**
> Use additional code to identify:
>   alcohol abuse and dependence (F10.-)
>   exposure to environmental tobacco smoke (Z77.22)
>   exposure to tobacco smoke in the perinatal period (P96.81)
>   history of tobacco dependence (Z87.891)
>   occupational exposure to environmental tobacco smoke (Z57.31)
>   tobacco dependence (F17.-)
>   tobacco use (Z72.0)
> **EXCLUDES 1**   cancrum oris (A69.0)
>   cheilitis (K13.0)
>   gangrenous stomatitis (A69.0)
>   herpesviral [herpes simplex] gingivostomatitis (B00.2)
>   noma (A69.0)

K12.0 **Recurrent oral aphthae**
> Aphthous stomatitis (major) (minor)
> Bednar's aphthae
> Periadenitis mucosa necrotica recurrens
> Recurrent aphthous ulcer
> Stomatitis herpetiformis
> **DEF:** Disorder of unknown etiology with small oval or round painful ulcers of the mouth marked by a grayish exudate and a red halo effect.

K12.1 **Other forms of stomatitis**
> Stomatitis NOS
> Denture stomatitis
> Ulcerative stomatitis
> Vesicular stomatitis
> **EXCLUDES 1**   acute necrotizing ulcerative stomatitis (A69.1)
>   Vincent's stomatitis (A69.1)

K12.2 **Cellulitis and abscess of mouth**   `CC`
> Cellulitis of mouth (floor)
> Submandibular abscess
> **EXCLUDES 2**   abscess of salivary gland (K11.3)
>   abscess of tongue (K14.0)
>   periapical abscess (K04.6-K04.7)
>   periodontal abscess (K05.21)
>   peritonsillar abscess (J36)

✓5ᵗʰ **K12.3** **Oral mucositis (ulcerative)**
> Mucositis (oral) (oropharyneal)
> **EXCLUDES 2**   gastrointestinal mucositis (ulcerative) (K92.81)
>   mucositis (ulcerative) of vagina and vulva (N76.81)
>   nasal mucositis (ulcerative) (J34.81)

   K12.30 **Oral mucositis (ulcerative), unspecified**
   K12.31 **Oral mucositis (ulcerative) due to** antineoplastic therapy
>   Use additional code for adverse effect, if applicable, to identify antineoplastic and immunosuppressive drugs (T45.1X5)
>   Use additional code for other antineoplastic therapy, such as:
>   radiological procedure and radiotherapy (Y84.2)

   K12.32 **Oral mucositis (ulcerative) due to other drugs**
>   Use additional code for adverse effect, if applicable, to identify drug (T36-T50 with fifth or sixth character 5)

   K12.33 **Oral mucositis (ulcerative) due to** radiation
>   Use additional external cause code (W88-W90, X39.0-) to identify cause

   K12.39 **Other oral mucositis (ulcerative)**
>   Viral oral mucositis (ulcerative)

✓4ᵗʰ **K13** **Other diseases of lip and oral mucosa**
> **INCLUDES**   epithelial disturbances of tongue
> Use additional code to identify:
>   alcohol abuse and dependence (F10.-)
>   exposure to environmental tobacco smoke (Z77.22)
>   exposure to tobacco smoke in the perinatal period (P96.81)
>   history of tobacco dependence (Z87.891)
>   occupational exposure to environmental tobacco smoke (Z57.31)
>   tobacco dependence (F17.-)
>   tobacco use (Z72.0)
> **EXCLUDES 2**   certain disorders of gingiva and edentulous alveolar ridge (K05-K06)
>   cysts of oral region (K09.-)
>   diseases of tongue (K14.-)
>   stomatitis and related lesions (K12.-)

K13.0 **Diseases of lips**
> Abscess of lips
> Angular cheilitis
> Cellulitis of lips
> Cheilitis NOS
> Cheilodynia
> Cheilosis
> Exfoliative cheilitis
> Fistula of lips
> Glandular cheilitis
> Hypertrophy of lips
> Perlèche NEC
> **EXCLUDES 1**   ariboflavinosis (E53.0)
>   cheilitis due to radiation-related disorders (L55-L59)
>   congenital fistula of lips (Q38.0)
>   congenital hypertrophy of lips (Q18.6)
>   perlèche due to candidiasis (B37.83)
>   perlèche due to riboflavin deficiency (E53.0)

K13.1 **Cheek and lip biting**

`N` Newborn: 0   `P` Pediatric: 0-17   `M` Maternity: 9-64   `A` Adult: 15-124   `MCC` Major Complication/Comorbidity   `CC` Complication/Comorbidity   `SW` Severe Wound Dx

714   ICD-10-CM 2022

✓5th **K13.2 Leukoplakia and other disturbances of oral epithelium, including tongue**

> EXCLUDES 1   *carcinoma in situ of oral epithelium (D00.0-)*
> *hairy leukoplakia (K13.3)*

> **DEF:** Leukoplakia: Thickened white patches or lesions appearing on a mucous membrane, such as oral mucosa or tongue.

    K13.21 Leukoplakia of oral mucosa, including tongue
> Leukokeratosis of oral mucosa
> Leukoplakia of gingiva, lips, tongue
> EXCLUDES 1   *hairy leukoplakia (K13.3)*
> *leukokeratosis nicotina palati (K13.24)*

    K13.22 Minimal keratinized residual ridge mucosa
> Minimal keratinization of alveolar ridge mucosa

    K13.23 Excessive keratinized residual ridge mucosa
> Excessive keratinization of alveolar ridge mucosa

    K13.24 Leukokeratosis nicotina palati
> Smoker's palate

    K13.29 Other disturbances of oral epithelium, including tongue
> Erythroplakia of mouth or tongue
> Focal epithelial hyperplasia of mouth or tongue
> Leukoedema of mouth or tongue
> Other oral epithelium disturbances

K13.3 Hairy leukoplakia

K13.4 Granuloma and granuloma-like lesions of oral mucosa
> Eosinophilic granuloma
> Granuloma pyogenicum
> Verrucous xanthoma

K13.5 Oral submucous fibrosis
> Submucous fibrosis of tongue

K13.6 Irritative hyperplasia of oral mucosa
> EXCLUDES 2   *irritative hyperplasia of edentulous ridge [denture hyperplasia] (K06.2)*

✓5th **K13.7 Other and unspecified lesions of oral mucosa**
    K13.70 Unspecified lesions of oral mucosa
    K13.79 Other lesions of oral mucosa
> Focal oral mucinosis

✓4th **K14 Diseases of tongue**
> Use additional code to identify:
> alcohol abuse and dependence (F10.-)
> exposure to environmental tobacco smoke (Z77.22)
> history of tobacco dependence (Z87.891)
> occupational exposure to environmental tobacco smoke (Z57.31)
> tobacco dependence (F17.-)
> tobacco use (Z72.0)
> EXCLUDES 2   *erythroplakia (K13.29)*
> *focal epithelial hyperplasia (K13.29)*
> *leukedema of tongue (K13.29)*
> *leukoplakia of tongue (K13.21)*
> *hairy leukoplakia (K13.3)*
> *macroglossia (congenital) (Q38.2)*
> *submucous fibrosis of tongue (K13.5)*

    K14.0 Glossitis
> Abscess of tongue
> Ulceration (traumatic) of tongue
> EXCLUDES 1   *atrophic glossitis (K14.4)*
> **DEF:** Inflammation and swelling of the tongue that may be associated with infection, adverse drug reactions, smoking, or injury.

    K14.1 Geographic tongue
> Benign migratory glossitis
> Glossitis areata exfoliativa

    K14.2 Median rhomboid glossitis

    K14.3 Hypertrophy of tongue papillae
> Black hairy tongue
> Coated tongue
> Hypertrophy of foliate papillae
> Lingua villosa nigra

    K14.4 Atrophy of tongue papillae
> Atrophic glossitis

    K14.5 Plicated tongue
> Fissured tongue
> Furrowed tongue
> Scrotal tongue
> EXCLUDES 1   *fissured tongue, congenital (Q38.3)*

    K14.6 Glossodynia
> Glossopyrosis
> Painful tongue

    K14.8 Other diseases of tongue
> Atrophy of tongue
> Crenated tongue
> Enlargement of tongue
> Glossocele
> Glossoptosis
> Hypertrophy of tongue

    K14.9 Disease of tongue, unspecified
> Glossopathy NOS

Diseases of esophagus, stomach and duodenum (K20-K31)

> EXCLUDES 2   *hiatus hernia (K44.-)*

✓4th **K20 Esophagitis**
> Use additional code to identify:
> alcohol abuse and dependence (F10.-)
> EXCLUDES 1   *erosion of esophagus (K22.1-)*
> *esophagitis with gastro-esophageal reflux disease (K21.0-)*
> *reflux esophagitis (K21.0-)*
> *ulcerative esophagitis (K22.1-)*
> EXCLUDES 2   *eosinophilic gastritis or gastroenteritis (K52.81)*

    K20.0 Eosinophilic esophagitis
> AHA: 2020,4Q,9

✓5th **K20.8 Other esophagitis**
> AHA: 2020,4Q,28-29
    K20.80 Other esophagitis without bleeding
> Abscess of esophagus
> Other esophagitis NOS
    K20.81 Other esophagitis with bleeding   MCC

✓5th **K20.9 Esophagitis, unspecified**
> AHA: 2020,4Q,28-29
    K20.90 Esophagitis, unspecified without bleeding
> Esophagitis NOS
    K20.91 Esophagitis, unspecified with bleeding   MCC

✓4th **K21 Gastro-esophageal reflux disease**
> EXCLUDES 1   *newborn esophageal reflux (P78.83)*

✓5th **K21.0 Gastro-esophageal reflux disease with esophagitis**
> AHA: 2020,4Q,28-29
    K21.00 Gastro-esophageal reflux disease with esophagitis, without bleeding
> Reflux esophagitis
    K21.01 Gastro-esophageal reflux disease with esophagitis, with bleeding   MCC
    K21.9 Gastro-esophageal reflux disease without esophagitis
> Esophageal reflux NOS
> AHA: 2016,1Q,18

✓4th **K22 Other diseases of esophagus**
> EXCLUDES 2   *esophageal varices (I85.-)*

    K22.0 Achalasia of cardia
> Achalasia NOS
> Cardiospasm
> EXCLUDES 1   *congenital cardiospasm (Q39.5)*
> **DEF:** Esophageal motility disorder that is caused by absence of the esophageal peristalsis and impaired relaxation of the lower esophageal sphincter. It is characterized by dysphagia, regurgitation, and heartburn.

✔ Additional Character Required   ✓x7th Placeholder   Questionable PDx   Manifestation   Unspecified Dx   UPD Unacceptable PDx   H1-H14 HAC   HCC CMS-HCC Dx   HIV HIV Dx

ICD-10-CM 2022   715

Chapter 11. Diseases of the Digestive System

✓5th **K22.1** **Ulcer** of esophagus

Barrett's ulcer
Erosion of esophagus
Fungal ulcer of esophagus
Peptic ulcer of esophagus
Ulcer of esophagus due to ingestion of chemicals
Ulcer of esophagus due to ingestion of drugs and medicaments
Ulcerative esophagitis
Code first poisoning due to drug or toxin, if applicable (T36-T65 with fifth or sixth character 1-4 or 6)
Use additional code for adverse effect, if applicable, to identify drug (T36-T50 with fifth or sixth character 5)

　EXCLUDES 1　Barrett's esophagus (K22.7-)

AHA: 2018,3Q,22; 2017,3Q,27

TIP: Assign a code for "with bleeding" when an esophageal ulcer and bleeding (hematemesis) are documented. The ICD-10-CM classification assumes the two are related without the provider linking the two conditions. Evidence of bleeding during a procedure is not required.

K22.10 **Ulcer of esophagus** without bleeding　　CC
Ulcer of esophagus NOS

K22.11 **Ulcer of esophagus** with bleeding　　MCC

　EXCLUDES 2　bleeding esophageal varices (I85.01, I85.11)

TIP: For bleeding esophageal ulcers resulting from anticoagulant therapy, assign this code, code D68.32 Hemorrhagic disorder due to extrinsic circulating anticoagulant, and adverse effect code T45.515- with the appropriate seventh character. Either code K22.11 or D68.32 may be sequenced first, depending on the circumstances of admission.

K22.2 **Esophageal** obstruction

Compression of esophagus
Constriction of esophagus
Stenosis of esophagus
Stricture of esophagus

　EXCLUDES 1　congenital stenosis or stricture of esophagus (Q39.3)

K22.3 **Perforation** of esophagus　　MCC

Rupture of esophagus

　EXCLUDES 1　traumatic perforation of (thoracic) esophagus (S27.8-)

K22.4 **Dyskinesia** of esophagus

Corkscrew esophagus
Diffuse esophageal spasm
Spasm of esophagus

　EXCLUDES 1　cardiospasm (K22.0)

K22.5 **Diverticulum** of esophagus, acquired

Esophageal pouch, acquired

　EXCLUDES 1　diverticulum of esophagus (congenital) (Q39.6)

K22.6 **Gastro-esophageal** laceration-hemorrhage **syndrome**　MCC
Mallory-Weiss syndrome

✓5th **K22.7** **Barrett's** esophagus

Barrett's disease
Barrett's syndrome

　EXCLUDES 1　Barrett's ulcer (K22.1)
　　　　　　malignant neoplasm of esophagus (C15.-)

DEF: Metaplastic disorder in which specialized columnar epithelial cells replace the normal squamous epithelial cells. Secondary to chronic gastroesophageal reflux damage to the mucosa, this disorder increases the risk of developing adenocarcinoma.

K22.70 **Barrett's esophagus** without dysplasia
Barrett's esophagus NOS

✓6th **K22.71** **Barrett's esophagus** with dysplasia

K22.710 **Barrett's esophagus with** low grade **dysplasia**

K22.711 **Barrett's esophagus with** high grade **dysplasia**

K22.719 **Barrett's esophagus with dysplasia, unspecified**

▲ ✓5th **K22.8** **Other specified diseases of esophagus**

~~Hemorrhage of esophagus NOS~~

　EXCLUDES 2　esophageal varices (I85.-)
　　　　　　Paterson-Kelly syndrome (D50.1)

AHA: 2020,1Q,16

● **K22.81** **Esophageal polyp**

　EXCLUDES 1　benign neoplasm of esophagus (D13.0)

● **K22.82** **Esophagogastric junction polyp**

　EXCLUDES 1　benign neoplasm of stomach (D13.1)

● **K22.89** **Other specified disease of esophagus**
Hemorrhage of esophagus NOS

K22.9 **Disease of esophagus, unspecified**

K23 *Disorders of esophagus in diseases classified elsewhere*

Code first underlying disease, such as:
congenital syphilis (A50.5)

　EXCLUDES 1　late syphilis (A52.79)
　　　　　　megaesophagus due to Chagas' disease (B57.31)
　　　　　　tuberculosis (A18.83)

✓4th **K25** **Gastric ulcer**

　INCLUDES　erosion (acute) of stomach
　　　　　pylorus ulcer (peptic)
　　　　　stomach ulcer (peptic)

Use additional code to identify:
alcohol abuse and dependence (F10.-)

　EXCLUDES 1　acute gastritis (K29.0-)
　　　　　　peptic ulcer NOS (K27.-)

AHA: 2021,1Q,9,11; 2017,3Q,27

TIP: Assign a code for "with hemorrhage" when a gastric ulcer and GI bleeding are documented. The ICD-10-CM classification assumes the two are related without the provider linking the two conditions. Evidence of bleeding during a procedure is not required.

TIP: For bleeding ulcers resulting from anticoagulant therapy, assign the appropriate "with hemorrhage" ulcer code from this category, code D68.32 Hemorrhagic disorder due to extrinsic circulating anticoagulant, and adverse effect code T45.515- with the appropriate seventh character. Either the bleeding ulcer code or code D68.32 may be sequenced first, depending on the circumstances of admission.

K25.0 **Acute gastric ulcer** with hemorrhage　　MCC

K25.1 **Acute gastric ulcer** with perforation　　MCC HCC

K25.2 **Acute gastric ulcer** with both hemorrhage and perforation　　MCC HCC

K25.3 **Acute gastric ulcer** without hemorrhage or perforation　　CC

K25.4 **Chronic or unspecified gastric ulcer** with hemorrhage　　MCC

K25.5 **Chronic or unspecified gastric ulcer** with perforation　　MCC HCC

K25.6 **Chronic or unspecified gastric ulcer** with both hemorrhage and perforation　　MCC HCC

K25.7 **Chronic gastric ulcer** without hemorrhage or perforation

K25.9 **Gastric ulcer, unspecified as acute or chronic, without hemorrhage or perforation**

Gastrointestinal Ulcers

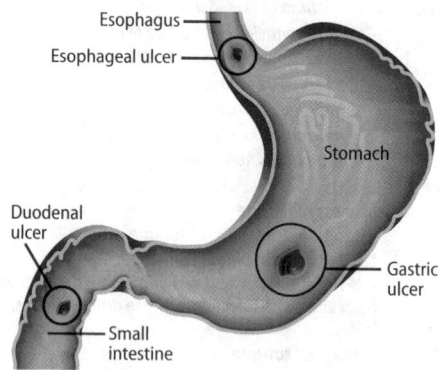

N Newborn: 0　**P** Pediatric: 0-17　**M** Maternity: 9-64　**A** Adult: 15-124　**MCC** Major Complication/Comorbidity　**CC** Complication/Comorbidity　**SW** Severe Wound Dx

☑4ᵗʰ **K26 Duodenal ulcer**

INCLUDES erosion (acute) of duodenum
duodenum ulcer (peptic)
postpyloric ulcer (peptic)

Use additional code to identify:
alcohol abuse and dependence (F10.-)

EXCLUDES 1 *peptic ulcer NOS (K27.-)*

AHA: 2017,3Q,27

TIP: Assign a code for "with hemorrhage" when a duodenal ulcer and GI bleeding are documented. The ICD-10-CM classification assumes the two are related without the provider linking the two conditions. Evidence of bleeding during a procedure is not required.

TIP: For bleeding ulcers resulting from anticoagulant therapy, assign the appropriate "with hemorrhage" ulcer code from this category, code D68.32 Hemorrhagic disorder due to extrinsic circulating anticoagulant, and adverse effect code T45.515- with the appropriate seventh character. Either the bleeding ulcer code or code D68.32 may be sequenced first, depending on the circumstances of admission.

K26.0   Acute **duodenal ulcer with hemorrhage**   MCC

K26.1   Acute **duodenal ulcer with perforation**   MCC HCC

K26.2   Acute **duodenal ulcer with both hemorrhage and perforation**   MCC HCC

K26.3   Acute **duodenal ulcer without hemorrhage or perforation**   CC

K26.4   Chronic **or unspecified duodenal ulcer with hemorrhage**   MCC
     AHA: 2016,1Q,14

K26.5   Chronic **or unspecified duodenal ulcer with perforation**   MCC HCC

K26.6   Chronic **or unspecified duodenal ulcer with both hemorrhage and perforation**   MCC HCC

K26.7   Chronic **duodenal ulcer without hemorrhage or perforation**

K26.9   **Duodenal ulcer, unspecified as acute or chronic, without hemorrhage or perforation**

☑4ᵗʰ **K27 Peptic ulcer, site unspecified**

INCLUDES gastroduodenal ulcer NOS
peptic ulcer NOS

Use additional code to identify:
alcohol abuse and dependence (F10.-)

EXCLUDES 1 *peptic ulcer of newborn (P78.82)*

AHA: 2017,3Q,27

TIP: Assign a code for "with hemorrhage" when a peptic ulcer and GI bleeding are documented. The ICD-10-CM classification assumes the two are related without the provider linking the two conditions. Evidence of bleeding during a procedure is not required.

TIP: For bleeding ulcers resulting from anticoagulant therapy, assign the appropriate "with hemorrhage" ulcer code from this category, code D68.32 Hemorrhagic disorder due to extrinsic circulating anticoagulant, and adverse effect code T45.515- with the appropriate seventh character. Either the bleeding ulcer code or code D68.32 may be sequenced first, depending on the circumstances of admission.

K27.0   Acute **peptic ulcer, site unspecified, with hemorrhage**   MCC

K27.1   Acute **peptic ulcer, site unspecified, with perforation**   MCC HCC

K27.2   Acute **peptic ulcer, site unspecified, with both hemorrhage and perforation**   MCC HCC

K27.3   Acute **peptic ulcer, site unspecified, without hemorrhage or perforation**   CC

K27.4   Chronic **or unspecified peptic ulcer, site unspecified, with hemorrhage**   MCC

K27.5   Chronic **or unspecified peptic ulcer, site unspecified, with perforation**   MCC HCC

K27.6   Chronic **or unspecified peptic ulcer, site unspecified, with both hemorrhage and perforation**   MCC HCC

K27.7   Chronic **peptic ulcer, site unspecified, without hemorrhage or perforation**

K27.9   **Peptic ulcer, site unspecified, unspecified as acute or chronic, without hemorrhage or perforation**

☑4ᵗʰ **K28 Gastrojejunal ulcer**

INCLUDES anastomotic ulcer (peptic) or erosion
gastrocolic ulcer (peptic) or erosion
gastrointestinal ulcer (peptic) or erosion
gastrojejunal ulcer (peptic) or erosion
jejunal ulcer (peptic) or erosion
marginal ulcer (peptic) or erosion
stomal ulcer (peptic) or erosion

Use additional code to identify:
alcohol abuse and dependence (F10.-)

EXCLUDES 1 *primary ulcer of small intestine (K63.3)*

AHA: 2017,3Q,27

TIP: Assign a code for "with hemorrhage" when a gastrojejunal ulcer and GI bleeding are documented. The ICD-10-CM classification assumes the two are related without the provider linking the two conditions. Evidence of bleeding during a procedure is not required.

TIP: For bleeding ulcers resulting from anticoagulant therapy, assign the appropriate "with hemorrhage" ulcer code from this category, code D68.32 Hemorrhagic disorder due to extrinsic circulating anticoagulant, and adverse effect code T45.515- with the appropriate seventh character. Either the bleeding ulcer code or code D68.32 may be sequenced first, depending on the circumstances of admission.

K28.0   Acute **gastrojejunal ulcer with hemorrhage**   MCC

K28.1   Acute **gastrojejunal ulcer with perforation**   MCC HCC

K28.2   Acute **gastrojejunal ulcer with both hemorrhage and perforation**   MCC HCC

K28.3   Acute **gastrojejunal ulcer without hemorrhage or perforation**   CC

K28.4   Chronic **or unspecified gastrojejunal ulcer with hemorrhage**   MCC

K28.5   Chronic **or unspecified gastrojejunal ulcer with perforation**   MCC HCC

K28.6   Chronic **or unspecified gastrojejunal ulcer with both hemorrhage and perforation**   MCC HCC

K28.7   Chronic **gastrojejunal ulcer without hemorrhage or perforation**

K28.9   **Gastrojejunal ulcer, unspecified as acute or chronic, without hemorrhage or perforation**

☑4ᵗʰ **K29 Gastritis and duodenitis**

EXCLUDES 1 *eosinophilic gastritis or gastroenteritis (K52.81)*
Zollinger-Ellison syndrome (E16.4)

AHA: 2018,3Q,22

TIP: Assign a code for "with bleeding" when gastritis or duodenitis and GI bleeding are documented. The ICD-10-CM classification assumes the two are related without the provider linking the two conditions. Evidence of bleeding during a procedure is not required.

TIP: For bleeding ulcers resulting from anticoagulant therapy, assign the appropriate "with hemorrhage" ulcer code from this category, code D68.32 Hemorrhagic disorder due to extrinsic circulating anticoagulant, and adverse effect code T45.515- with the appropriate seventh character. Either the bleeding ulcer code or code D68.32 may be sequenced first, depending on the circumstances of admission.

☑5ᵗʰ **K29.0**   Acute **gastritis**

Use additional code to identify:
alcohol abuse and dependence (F10.-)

EXCLUDES 1 *erosion (acute) of stomach (K25.-)*

   K29.00   Acute **gastritis without bleeding**

   K29.01   Acute **gastritis with bleeding**   MCC

☑5ᵗʰ **K29.2**   Alcoholic **gastritis**

Use additional code to identify:
alcohol abuse and dependence (F10.-)

   K29.20   Alcoholic **gastritis without bleeding**

   K29.21   Alcoholic **gastritis with bleeding**   MCC

☑5ᵗʰ **K29.3**   Chronic superficial **gastritis**

   K29.30   Chronic superficial **gastritis without bleeding**

   K29.31   Chronic superficial **gastritis with bleeding**   MCC

☑5ᵗʰ **K29.4**   Chronic atrophic **gastritis**

Gastric atrophy

   K29.40   Chronic atrophic **gastritis without bleeding**

   K29.41   Chronic atrophic **gastritis with bleeding**   MCC

☑5ᵗʰ **K29.5**   Unspecified chronic **gastritis**

Chronic antral gastritis
Chronic fundal gastritis

   K29.50   **Unspecified chronic gastritis without bleeding**

   K29.51   **Unspecified chronic gastritis with bleeding**   MCC

☑ Additional Character Required   √ₓ7ᵗʰ Placeholder   Questionable PDx   Manifestation   Unspecified Dx   UPD Unacceptable PDx   H1-H14 HAC   HCC CMS-HCC Dx   HIV HIV Dx

ICD-10-CM 2022   717

√5ᵗʰ **K29.6　Other gastritis**
Giant hypertrophic gastritis
Granulomatous gastritis
Ménétrier's disease
　　K29.60　Other gastritis without bleeding
　　K29.61　Other gastritis with bleeding　　MCC
√5ᵗʰ **K29.7　Gastritis, unspecified**
　　K29.70　Gastritis, unspecified, without bleeding
　　K29.71　Gastritis, unspecified, with bleeding　MCC
√5ᵗʰ **K29.8　Duodenitis**
　　K29.80　Duodenitis without bleeding
　　K29.81　Duodenitis with bleeding　　MCC
√5ᵗʰ **K29.9　Gastroduodenitis, unspecified**
　　K29.90　Gastroduodenitis, unspecified, without bleeding
　　K29.91　Gastroduodenitis, unspecified, with bleeding　MCC

K30　Functional dyspepsia
Indigestion
EXCLUDES 1　*dyspepsia NOS (R10.13)*
　　　　heartburn (R12)
　　　　nervous dyspepsia (F45.8)
　　　　neurotic dyspepsia (F45.8)
　　　　psychogenic dyspepsia (F45.8)

√4ᵗʰ **K31　Other diseases of stomach and duodenum**
INCLUDES　functional disorders of stomach
EXCLUDES 2　*diabetic gastroparesis (E08.43, E09.43, E10.43, E11.43, E13.43)*
　　　　diverticulum of duodenum (K57.00-K57.13)
K31.0　Acute dilatation of stomach　　CC
Acute distention of stomach
K31.1　Adult hypertrophic pyloric stenosis　　CC A
Pyloric stenosis NOS
　EXCLUDES 1　*congenital or infantile pyloric stenosis (Q40.0)*
K31.2　Hourglass stricture and stenosis of stomach
　EXCLUDES 1　*congenital hourglass stomach (Q40.2)*
　　　　hourglass contraction of stomach (K31.89)
K31.3　Pylorospasm, not elsewhere classified
　EXCLUDES 1　*congenital or infantile pylorospasm (Q40.0)*
　　　　neurotic pylorospasm (F45.8)
　　　　psychogenic pylorospasm (F45.8)
K31.4　Gastric diverticulum
　EXCLUDES 1　*congenital diverticulum of stomach (Q40.2)*
K31.5　Obstruction of duodenum　　CC
Constriction of duodenum
Duodenal ileus (chronic)
Stenosis of duodenum
Stricture of duodenum
Volvulus of duodenum
　EXCLUDES 1　*congenital stenosis of duodenum (Q41.0)*
K31.6　Fistula of stomach and duodenum　　CC SW
Gastrocolic fistula
Gastrojejunocolic fistula
K31.7　Polyp of stomach and duodenum
　EXCLUDES 1　*adenomatous polyp of stomach (D13.1)*
　AHA: 2020,1Q,16
√5ᵗʰ **K31.8　Other specified diseases of stomach and duodenum**
　√6ᵗʰ **K31.81　Angiodysplasia of stomach and duodenum**
　　　　TIP: Assign a code for "with bleeding" when angiodysplasia of the stomach or the duodenum and GI bleeding are documented. The ICD-10-CM classification assumes the two are related without the provider linking the two conditions. Evidence of bleeding during a procedure is not required.
　　　　K31.811　Angiodysplasia of stomach and duodenum with bleeding　MCC
　　　　K31.819　Angiodysplasia of stomach and duodenum without bleeding
　　　　　　Angiodysplasia of stomach and duodenum NOS

K31.82　Dieulafoy lesion (hemorrhagic) of stomach and duodenum　MCC
　EXCLUDES 2　*Dieulafoy lesion of intestine (K63.81)*
　DEF: Abnormally large submucosal artery protruding through a defect in the stomach mucosa or intestines that can cause massive and life-threatening hemorrhaging.
K31.83　Achlorhydria
　DEF: Absence of hydrochloric acid in gastric secretions due to gastric mucosa atrophy. Achlorhydria is unresponsive to histamines.
K31.84　Gastroparesis
Gastroparalysis
Code first underlying disease, if known, such as:
　anorexia nervosa (F50.0-)
　diabetes mellitus (E08.43, E09.43, E10.43, E11.43, E13.43)
　scleroderma (M34.-)
　AHA: 2013,4Q,114
K31.89　Other diseases of stomach and duodenum
　AHA: 2020,1Q,15; 2017,1Q,28
K31.9　Disease of stomach and duodenum, unspecified
● √5ᵗʰ **K31.A　Gastric intestinal metaplasia**
● 　**K31.A0　Gastric intestinal metaplasia, unspecified**
　　　Gastric intestinal metaplasia indefinite for dysplasia
　　　Gastric intestinal metaplasia NOS
● √6ᵗʰ **K31.A1　Gastric intestinal metaplasia without dysplasia**
● 　　**K31.A11　Gastric intestinal metaplasia without dysplasia, involving the antrum**
● 　　**K31.A12　Gastric intestinal metaplasia without dysplasia, involving the body (corpus)**
● 　　**K31.A13　Gastric intestinal metaplasia without dysplasia, involving the fundus**
● 　　**K31.A14　Gastric intestinal metaplasia without dysplasia, involving the cardia**
● 　　**K31.A15　Gastric intestinal metaplasia without dysplasia, involving multiple sites**
● 　　**K31.A19　Gastric intestinal metaplasia without dysplasia, unspecified site**
● √6ᵗʰ **K31.A2　Gastric intestinal metaplasia with dysplasia**
　　　K31.A21　Gastric intestinal metaplasia with low grade dysplasia
　　　K31.A22　Gastric intestinal metaplasia with high grade dysplasia
● 　　**K31.A29　Gastric intestinal metaplasia with dysplasia, unspecified**

Diseases of appendix (K35-K38)

√4ᵗʰ **K35　Acute appendicitis**
　AHA: 2018,4Q,17-18
√5ᵗʰ **K35.2　Acute appendicitis with generalized peritonitis**
Appendicitis (acute) with generalized (diffuse) peritonitis following rupture or perforation of appendix
K35.20　Acute appendicitis with generalized peritonitis, without abscess　　CC
　(Acute) appendicitis with generalized peritonitis NOS
K35.21　Acute appendicitis with generalized peritonitis, with abscess　　MCC
√5ᵗʰ **K35.3　Acute appendicitis with localized peritonitis**
K35.30　Acute appendicitis with localized peritonitis, without perforation or gangrene　CC
　Acute appendicitis with localized peritonitis NOS
K35.31　Acute appendicitis with localized peritonitis and gangrene, without perforation　CC
K35.32　Acute appendicitis with perforation and localized peritonitis, without abscess　MCC
　(Acute) appendicitis with perforation NOS
　Perforated appendix NOS
　Ruptured appendix (with localized peritonitis) NOS
　AHA: 2020,1Q,16
K35.33　Acute appendicitis with perforation and localized peritonitis, with abscess　MCC
　(Acute) appendicitis with (peritoneal) abscess NOS
　Ruptured appendix with localized peritonitis and abscess

✓5ᵗʰ **K35.8 Other and unspecified acute appendicitis**

    K35.80 Unspecified acute appendicitis `CC`
        Acute appendicitis NOS
        Acute appendicitis without (localized) (generalized) peritonitis

    ✓6ᵗʰ **K35.89 Other acute appendicitis**
        AHA: 2020,1Q,16

        K35.890 Other acute appendicitis without perforation or gangrene `CC`

        K35.891 Other acute appendicitis without perforation, with gangrene `CC`
            (Acute) appendicitis with gangrene NOS

K36 Other appendicitis
    Chronic appendicitis
    Recurrent appendicitis

K37 Unspecified appendicitis
    EXCLUDES 1   unspecified appendicitis with peritonitis (K35.2-, K35.3-)

✓4ᵗʰ **K38 Other diseases of appendix**

    K38.0 Hyperplasia of appendix

    K38.1 Appendicular concretions
        Fecalith of appendix
        Stercolith of appendix

    K38.2 Diverticulum of appendix

    K38.3 Fistula of appendix

    K38.8 Other specified diseases of appendix
        Intussusception of appendix

    K38.9 Disease of appendix, unspecified

Hernia (K40-K46)

NOTE   Hernia with both gangrene and obstruction is classified to hernia with gangrene.

INCLUDES   acquired hernia
             congenital [except diaphragmatic or hiatus] hernia
             recurrent hernia

✓4ᵗʰ **K40 Inguinal hernia**

    INCLUDES   bubonocele
          direct inguinal hernia
          double inguinal hernia
          indirect inguinal hernia
          inguinal hernia NOS
          oblique inguinal hernia
          scrotal hernia

    DEF: Within the groin region.

    ✓5ᵗʰ **K40.0 Bilateral inguinal hernia, with obstruction, without gangrene**
        Inguinal hernia (bilateral) causing obstruction without gangrene
        Incarcerated inguinal hernia (bilateral) without gangrene
        Irreducible inguinal hernia (bilateral) without gangrene
        Strangulated inguinal hernia (bilateral) without gangrene

        K40.00 Bilateral inguinal hernia, with obstruction, without gangrene, not specified as recurrent `CC`
            Bilateral inguinal hernia, with obstruction, without gangrene NOS

        K40.01 Bilateral inguinal hernia, with obstruction, without gangrene, recurrent `CC`

    ✓5ᵗʰ **K40.1 Bilateral inguinal hernia, with gangrene**

        K40.10 Bilateral inguinal hernia, with gangrene, not specified as recurrent `MCC`
            Bilateral inguinal hernia, with gangrene NOS

        K40.11 Bilateral inguinal hernia, with gangrene, recurrent `MCC`

    ✓5ᵗʰ **K40.2 Bilateral inguinal hernia, without obstruction or gangrene**

        K40.20 Bilateral inguinal hernia, without obstruction or gangrene, not specified as recurrent
            Bilateral inguinal hernia NOS

        K40.21 Bilateral inguinal hernia, without obstruction or gangrene, recurrent

✓5ᵗʰ **K40.3 Unilateral inguinal hernia, with obstruction, without gangrene**
    Inguinal hernia (unilateral) causing obstruction without gangrene
    Incarcerated inguinal hernia (unilateral) without gangrene
    Irreducible inguinal hernia (unilateral) without gangrene
    Strangulated inguinal hernia (unilateral) without gangrene

    K40.30 Unilateral inguinal hernia, with obstruction, without gangrene, not specified as recurrent `CC`
        Inguinal hernia, with obstruction NOS
        Unilateral inguinal hernia, with obstruction, without gangrene NOS

    K40.31 Unilateral inguinal hernia, with obstruction, without gangrene, recurrent `CC`

✓5ᵗʰ **K40.4 Unilateral inguinal hernia, with gangrene**

    K40.40 Unilateral inguinal hernia, with gangrene, not specified as recurrent `MCC`
        Inguinal hernia with gangrene NOS
        Unilateral inguinal hernia with gangrene NOS

    K40.41 Unilateral inguinal hernia, with gangrene, recurrent `MCC`

✓5ᵗʰ **K40.9 Unilateral inguinal hernia, without obstruction or gangrene**

    K40.90 Unilateral inguinal hernia, without obstruction or gangrene, not specified as recurrent
        Inguinal hernia NOS
        Unilateral inguinal hernia NOS

    K40.91 Unilateral inguinal hernia, without obstruction or gangrene, recurrent

Hernia Sites

✓4ᵗʰ **K41 Femoral hernia**

    ✓5ᵗʰ **K41.0 Bilateral femoral hernia, with obstruction, without gangrene**
        Femoral hernia (bilateral) causing obstruction, without gangrene
        Incarcerated femoral hernia (bilateral), without gangrene
        Irreducible femoral hernia (bilateral), without gangrene
        Strangulated femoral hernia (bilateral), without gangrene

        K41.00 Bilateral femoral hernia, with obstruction, without gangrene, not specified as recurrent `CC`
            Bilateral femoral hernia, with obstruction, without gangrene NOS

        K41.01 Bilateral femoral hernia, with obstruction, without gangrene, recurrent `CC`

    ✓5ᵗʰ **K41.1 Bilateral femoral hernia, with gangrene**

        K41.10 Bilateral femoral hernia, with gangrene, not specified as recurrent `MCC`
            Bilateral femoral hernia, with gangrene NOS

        K41.11 Bilateral femoral hernia, with gangrene, recurrent `MCC`

    ✓5ᵗʰ **K41.2 Bilateral femoral hernia, without obstruction or gangrene**

        K41.20 Bilateral femoral hernia, without obstruction or gangrene, not specified as recurrent
            Bilateral femoral hernia NOS

        K41.21 Bilateral femoral hernia, without obstruction or gangrene, recurrent

✓ Additional Character Required   ✓x7ᵗʰ Placeholder   Questionable PDx   Manifestation   Unspecified Dx   UPD Unacceptable PDx   H1-H14 HAC   HCC CMS-HCC Dx   HIV HIV Dx

ICD-10-CM 2022   719

✓5ᵗʰ **K41.3** Unilateral **femoral hernia, with obstruction, without gangrene**

    Femoral hernia (unilateral) causing obstruction, without gangrene

    Incarcerated femoral hernia (unilateral), without gangrene

    Irreducible femoral hernia (unilateral), without gangrene

    Strangulated femoral hernia (unilateral), without gangrene

    K41.30 Unilateral **femoral hernia, with obstruction, without gangrene,** not specified as recurrent   `CC`

        Femoral hernia, with obstruction NOS

        Unilateral femoral hernia, with obstruction NOS

    K41.31 Unilateral **femoral hernia, with obstruction, without gangrene,** recurrent   `CC`

✓5ᵗʰ **K41.4** Unilateral **femoral hernia, with gangrene**

    K41.40 Unilateral **femoral hernia, with gangrene,** not specified as recurrent   `MCC`

        Femoral hernia, with gangrene NOS

        Unilateral femoral hernia, with gangrene NOS

    K41.41 Unilateral **femoral hernia, with gangrene,** recurrent   `MCC`

✓5ᵗʰ **K41.9** Unilateral **femoral hernia, without obstruction or gangrene**

    K41.90 Unilateral **femoral hernia, without obstruction or gangrene,** not specified as recurrent

        Femoral hernia NOS

        Unilateral femoral hernia NOS

    K41.91 Unilateral **femoral hernia, without obstruction or gangrene,** recurrent

✓4ᵗʰ **K42** Umbilical **hernia**

    `INCLUDES`   paraumbilical hernia

    `EXCLUDES 1`   omphalocele (Q79.2)

    K42.0 Umbilical **hernia with obstruction, without gangrene**   `CC`

        Umbilical hernia causing obstruction, without gangrene

        Incarcerated umbilical hernia, without gangrene

        Irreducible umbilical hernia, without gangrene

        Strangulated umbilical hernia, without gangrene

    K42.1 Umbilical **hernia with gangrene**   `MCC`

        Gangrenous umbilical hernia

    K42.9 Umbilical **hernia without obstruction or gangrene**

        Umbilical hernia NOS

✓4ᵗʰ **K43** Ventral **hernia**

    DEF: Condition in which a loop of bowel protrudes through a weakness in the abdominal wall muscles that may occur as a birth defect, past surgical site (incisional), or form at a stomal site (parastomal).

    K43.0 Incisional **hernia with obstruction, without gangrene**   `CC`

        Incisional hernia causing obstruction, without gangrene

        Incarcerated incisional hernia, without gangrene

        Irreducible incisional hernia, without gangrene

        Strangulated incisional hernia, without gangrene

    K43.1 Incisional **hernia with gangrene**   `MCC`

        Gangrenous incisional hernia

        AHA: 2020,2Q,22

    K43.2 Incisional **hernia without obstruction or gangrene**

        Incisional hernia NOS

    K43.3 Parastomal **hernia with obstruction, without gangrene**   `CC`

        Incarcerated parastomal hernia, without gangrene

        Irreducible parastomal hernia, without gangrene

        Parastomal hernia causing obstruction, without gangrene

        Strangulated parastomal hernia, without gangrene

    K43.4 Parastomal **hernia with gangrene**   `MCC`

        Gangrenous parastomal hernia

    K43.5 Parastomal **hernia without obstruction or gangrene**

        Parastomal hernia NOS

K43.6 Other and unspecified ventral hernia with obstruction, without gangrene   `CC`

    Epigastric hernia causing obstruction, without gangrene

    Hypogastric hernia causing obstruction, without gangrene

    Incarcerated epigastric hernia without gangrene

    Incarcerated hypogastric hernia without gangrene

    Incarcerated midline hernia without gangrene

    Incarcerated spigelian hernia without gangrene

    Incarcerated subxiphoid hernia without gangrene

    Irreducible epigastric hernia without gangrene

    Irreducible hypogastric hernia without gangrene

    Irreducible midline hernia without gangrene

    Irreducible spigelian hernia without gangrene

    Irreducible subxiphoid hernia without gangrene

    Midline hernia causing obstruction, without gangrene

    Spigelian hernia causing obstruction, without gangrene

    Strangulated epigastric hernia without gangrene

    Strangulated hypogastric hernia without gangrene

    Strangulated midline hernia without gangrene

    Strangulated spigelian hernia without gangrene

    Strangulated subxiphoid hernia without gangrene

    Subxiphoid hernia causing obstruction, without gangrene

K43.7 Other and unspecified ventral hernia with gangrene   `MCC`

    Any condition listed under K43.6 specified as gangrenous

K43.9 Ventral hernia without obstruction or gangrene

    Epigastric hernia

    Ventral hernia NOS

✓4ᵗʰ **K44** Diaphragmatic **hernia**

    `INCLUDES`   hiatus hernia (esophageal) (sliding)

                 paraesophageal hernia

    `EXCLUDES 1`   congenital diaphragmatic hernia (Q79.0)

                  congenital hiatus hernia (Q40.1)

    DEF: Protrusion of an abdominal organ, usually the stomach, through the esophageal opening within the diaphragm and occurring in two types: the sliding hiatal hernia and the paraesophageal hernia.

Hiatal Hernia

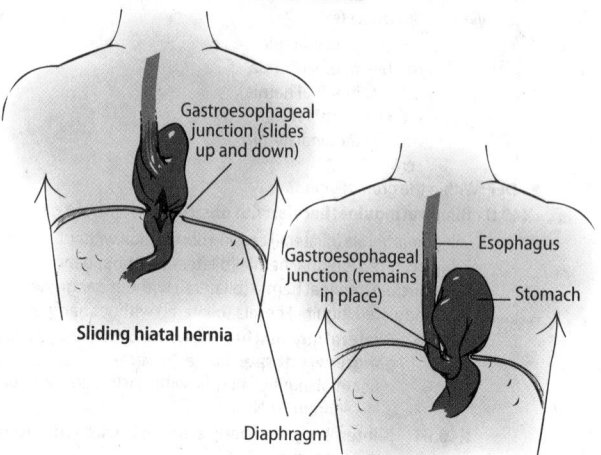

Gastroesophageal junction (slides up and down)

Sliding hiatal hernia

Gastroesophageal junction (remains in place)

Esophagus

Stomach

Diaphragm

Paraesophageal hiatal hernia

    K44.0 Diaphragmatic **hernia with obstruction, without gangrene**   `CC`

        Diaphragmatic hernia causing obstruction

        Incarcerated diaphragmatic hernia

        Irreducible diaphragmatic hernia

        Strangulated diaphragmatic hernia

    K44.1 Diaphragmatic **hernia with gangrene**   `MCC`

        Gangrenous diaphragmatic hernia

    K44.9 Diaphragmatic **hernia without obstruction or gangrene**

        Diaphragmatic hernia NOS

`N` Newborn: 0   `P` Pediatric: 0-17   `M` Maternity: 9-64   `A` Adult: 15-124   `MCC` Major Complication/Comorbidity   `CC` Complication/Comorbidity   `SW` Severe Wound Dx

720

ICD-10-CM 2022

√4ᵗʰ **K45 Other abdominal hernia**

     INCLUDES   abdominal hernia, specified site NEC
                lumbar hernia
                obturator hernia
                pudendal hernia
                retroperitoneal hernia
                sciatic hernia

   K45.0 Other specified abdominal hernia with obstruction, without gangrene   CC
      Other specified abdominal hernia causing obstruction
      Other specified incarcerated abdominal hernia
      Other specified irreducible abdominal hernia
      Other specified strangulated abdominal hernia

   K45.1 Other specified abdominal hernia with gangrene   MCC
      Any condition listed under K45 specified as gangrenous

   K45.8 Other specified abdominal hernia without obstruction or gangrene

√4ᵗʰ **K46 Unspecified abdominal hernia**

     INCLUDES   enterocele
                epiplocele
                hernia NOS
                interstitial hernia
                intestinal hernia
                intra-abdominal hernia
     EXCLUDES 1   *vaginal enterocele (N81.5)*

   K46.0 Unspecified abdominal hernia with obstruction, without gangrene   CC
      Unspecified abdominal hernia causing obstruction
      Unspecified incarcerated abdominal hernia
      Unspecified irreducible abdominal hernia
      Unspecified strangulated abdominal hernia

   K46.1 Unspecified abdominal hernia with gangrene   MCC
      Any condition listed under K46 specified as gangrenous

   K46.9 Unspecified abdominal hernia without obstruction or gangrene
      Abdominal hernia NOS

Noninfective enteritis and colitis (K50-K52)

   INCLUDES   noninfective inflammatory bowel disease
   EXCLUDES 1   *irritable bowel syndrome (K58.-)*
                  megacolon (K59.3-)

√4ᵗʰ **K50 Crohn's disease [regional enteritis]**

     INCLUDES   granulomatous enteritis
     Use additional code to identify manifestations, such as:
       pyoderma gangrenosum (L88)
     EXCLUDES 1   *ulcerative colitis (K51.-)*
     AHA: 2019,3Q,5; 2012,4Q,104
     DEF: Chronic inflammation of the gastrointestinal tract characterized by chronic granulomatous disease, most commonly affecting the intestines and the terminal ileum.

√5ᵗʰ   **K50.0 Crohn's disease of** small intestine
      Crohn's disease [regional enteritis] of duodenum
      Crohn's disease [regional enteritis] of ileum
      Crohn's disease [regional enteritis] of jejunum
      Regional ileitis
      Terminal ileitis
     EXCLUDES 1   *Crohn's disease of both small and large intestine (K50.8-)*

     K50.00 Crohn's disease of small intestine without complications   CC HCC

     √6ᵗʰ **K50.01 Crohn's disease of small intestine** with complications
        K50.011 Crohn's disease of small intestine with rectal bleeding   CC HCC
        K50.012 Crohn's disease of small intestine with intestinal obstruction   CC HCC
        K50.013 Crohn's disease of small intestine with fistula   CC HCC SW
        K50.014 Crohn's disease of small intestine with abscess   CC HCC
          AHA: 2012,4Q,104
        K50.018 Crohn's disease of small intestine with other complication   CC HCC
        K50.019 Crohn's disease of small intestine with unspecified complications   CC HCC

√5ᵗʰ   **K50.1 Crohn's disease of** large intestine
      Crohn's disease [regional enteritis] of colon
      Crohn's disease [regional enteritis] of large bowel
      Crohn's disease [regional enteritis] of rectum
      Granulomatous colitis
      Regional colitis
     EXCLUDES 1   *Crohn's disease of both small and large intestine (K50.8)*

     K50.10 Crohn's disease of large intestine without complications   CC HCC

     √6ᵗʰ **K50.11 Crohn's disease of large intestine** with complications
        K50.111 Crohn's disease of large intestine with rectal bleeding   CC HCC
        K50.112 Crohn's disease of large intestine with intestinal obstruction   CC HCC
        K50.113 Crohn's disease of large intestine with fistula   CC HCC SW
        K50.114 Crohn's disease of large intestine with abscess   CC HCC
        K50.118 Crohn's disease of large intestine with other complication   CC HCC
        K50.119 Crohn's disease of large intestine with unspecified complications   CC HCC

√5ᵗʰ   **K50.8 Crohn's disease of** both small and large intestine
     K50.80 Crohn's disease of both small and large intestine without complications   CC HCC

     √6ᵗʰ **K50.81 Crohn's disease of both small and large intestine** with complications
        K50.811 Crohn's disease of both small and large intestine with rectal bleeding   CC HCC
        K50.812 Crohn's disease of both small and large intestine with intestinal obstruction   CC HCC
        K50.813 Crohn's disease of both small and large intestine with fistula   CC HCC SW
        K50.814 Crohn's disease of both small and large intestine with abscess   CC HCC
        K50.818 Crohn's disease of both small and large intestine with other complication   CC HCC
        K50.819 Crohn's disease of both small and large intestine with unspecified complications   CC HCC

√5ᵗʰ   **K50.9 Crohn's disease, unspecified**
     K50.90 Crohn's disease, unspecified, without complications   CC HCC
      Crohn's disease NOS
      Regional enteritis NOS

     √6ᵗʰ **K50.91 Crohn's disease, unspecified,** with complications
        K50.911 Crohn's disease, unspecified, with rectal bleeding   CC HCC
        K50.912 Crohn's disease, unspecified, with intestinal obstruction   CC HCC
        K50.913 Crohn's disease, unspecified, with fistula   CC HCC SW
        K50.914 Crohn's disease, unspecified, with abscess   CC HCC
        K50.918 Crohn's disease, unspecified, with other complication   CC HCC
        K50.919 Crohn's disease, unspecified, with unspecified complications   CC HCC

√4ᵗʰ **K51 Ulcerative colitis**

     Use additional code to identify manifestations, such as:
       pyoderma gangrenosum (L88)
     EXCLUDES 1   *Crohn's disease [regional enteritis] (K50.-)*

√5ᵗʰ   **K51.0 Ulcerative (chronic)** pancolitis
      Backwash ileitis
     K51.00 Ulcerative (chronic) pancolitis without complications   CC HCC
      Ulcerative (chronic) pancolitis NOS

     √6ᵗʰ **K51.01 Ulcerative (chronic) pancolitis** with complications
        K51.011 Ulcerative (chronic) pancolitis with rectal bleeding   CC HCC
        K51.012 Ulcerative (chronic) pancolitis with intestinal obstruction   CC HCC
        K51.013 Ulcerative (chronic) pancolitis with fistula   CC HCC SW

K51.014   **Ulcerative (chronic) pancolitis with abscess** `CC` `HCC`

K51.018   **Ulcerative (chronic) pancolitis with other complication** `CC` `HCC`

K51.019   **Ulcerative (chronic) pancolitis with unspecified complications** `CC` `HCC`

√5ᵗʰ **K51.2**   **Ulcerative (chronic) proctitis**

     K51.20   **Ulcerative (chronic) proctitis without complications** `CC` `HCC`
         Ulcerative (chronic) proctitis NOS

     √6ᵗʰ **K51.21**   **Ulcerative (chronic) proctitis with complications**

         K51.211   **Ulcerative (chronic) proctitis with rectal bleeding** `CC` `HCC`

         K51.212   **Ulcerative (chronic) proctitis with intestinal obstruction** `CC` `HCC`

         K51.213   **Ulcerative (chronic) proctitis with fistula** `CC` `HCC` `SW`

         K51.214   **Ulcerative (chronic) proctitis with abscess** `CC` `HCC`

         K51.218   **Ulcerative (chronic) proctitis with other complication** `CC` `HCC`

         K51.219   **Ulcerative (chronic) proctitis with unspecified complications** `CC` `HCC`

√5ᵗʰ **K51.3**   **Ulcerative (chronic) rectosigmoiditis**

     K51.30   **Ulcerative (chronic) rectosigmoiditis without complications** `CC` `HCC`
         Ulcerative (chronic) rectosigmoiditis NOS

     √6ᵗʰ **K51.31**   **Ulcerative (chronic) rectosigmoiditis with complications**

         K51.311   **Ulcerative (chronic) rectosigmoiditis with rectal bleeding** `CC` `HCC`

         K51.312   **Ulcerative (chronic) rectosigmoiditis with intestinal obstruction** `CC` `HCC`

         K51.313   **Ulcerative (chronic) rectosigmoiditis with fistula** `CC` `HCC` `SW`

         K51.314   **Ulcerative (chronic) rectosigmoiditis with abscess** `CC` `HCC`

         K51.318   **Ulcerative (chronic) rectosigmoiditis with other complication** `CC` `HCC`

         K51.319   **Ulcerative (chronic) rectosigmoiditis with unspecified complications** `CC` `HCC`

√5ᵗʰ **K51.4**   **Inflammatory polyps of colon**

     `EXCLUDES 1`   adenomatous polyp of colon (D12.6)
         polyposis of colon (D12.6)
         polyps of colon NOS (K63.5)

     K51.40   **Inflammatory polyps of colon without complications** `CC` `HCC`
         Inflammatory polyps of colon NOS

     √6ᵗʰ **K51.41**   **Inflammatory polyps of colon with complications**

         K51.411   **Inflammatory polyps of colon with rectal bleeding** `CC` `HCC`

         K51.412   **Inflammatory polyps of colon with intestinal obstruction** `CC` `HCC`

         K51.413   **Inflammatory polyps of colon with fistula** `CC` `HCC` `SW`

         K51.414   **Inflammatory polyps of colon with abscess** `CC` `HCC`

         K51.418   **Inflammatory polyps of colon with other complication** `CC` `HCC`

         K51.419   **Inflammatory polyps of colon with unspecified complications** `CC` `HCC`

√5ᵗʰ **K51.5**   **Left sided colitis**
     Left hemicolitis

     K51.50   **Left sided colitis without complications** `CC` `HCC`
         Left sided colitis NOS

     √6ᵗʰ **K51.51**   **Left sided colitis with complications**

         K51.511   **Left sided colitis with rectal bleeding** `CC` `HCC`

         K51.512   **Left sided colitis with intestinal obstruction** `CC` `HCC`

         K51.513   **Left sided colitis with fistula** `CC` `HCC` `SW`

         K51.514   **Left sided colitis with abscess** `CC` `HCC`

         K51.518   **Left sided colitis with other complication** `CC` `HCC`

         K51.519   **Left sided colitis with unspecified complications** `CC` `HCC`

√5ᵗʰ **K51.8**   **Other ulcerative colitis**

     K51.80   **Other ulcerative colitis without complications** `CC` `HCC`

     √6ᵗʰ **K51.81**   **Other ulcerative colitis with complications**

         K51.811   **Other ulcerative colitis with rectal bleeding** `CC` `HCC`

         K51.812   **Other ulcerative colitis with intestinal obstruction** `CC` `HCC`

         K51.813   **Other ulcerative colitis with fistula** `CC` `HCC` `SW`

         K51.814   **Other ulcerative colitis with abscess** `CC` `HCC`

         K51.818   **Other ulcerative colitis with other complication** `CC` `HCC`

         K51.819   **Other ulcerative colitis with unspecified complications** `CC` `HCC`

√5ᵗʰ **K51.9**   **Ulcerative colitis, unspecified**

     K51.90   **Ulcerative colitis, unspecified, without complications** `CC` `HCC`

     √6ᵗʰ **K51.91**   **Ulcerative colitis, unspecified, with complications**

         K51.911   **Ulcerative colitis, unspecified with rectal bleeding** `CC` `HCC`

         K51.912   **Ulcerative colitis, unspecified with intestinal obstruction** `CC` `HCC`

         K51.913   **Ulcerative colitis, unspecified with fistula** `CC` `HCC` `SW`

         K51.914   **Ulcerative colitis, unspecified with abscess** `CC` `HCC`

         K51.918   **Ulcerative colitis, unspecified with other complication** `CC` `HCC`

         K51.919   **Ulcerative colitis, unspecified with unspecified complications** `CC` `HCC`

√4ᵗʰ **K52**   **Other and unspecified noninfective gastroenteritis and colitis**

     AHA: 2016,4Q,30-31

     K52.0   **Gastroenteritis and colitis due to radiation** `CC`

     K52.1   **Toxic gastroenteritis and colitis** `CC`
         Drug-induced gastroenteritis and colitis
         Code first (T51-T65) to identify toxic agent
         Use additional code for adverse effect, if applicable, to identify drug (T36-T50 with fifth or sixth character 5)
         AHA: 2019,1Q,17

     √5ᵗʰ **K52.2**   **Allergic and dietetic gastroenteritis and colitis**
         Food hypersensitivity gastroenteritis or colitis
         Use additional code to identify type of food allergy (Z91.01-, Z91.02-)

         `EXCLUDES 2`   allergic eosinophilic colitis (K52.82)
                 allergic eosinophilic esophagitis (K20.0)
                 allergic eosinophilic gastritis (K52.81)
                 allergic eosinophilic gastroenteritis (K52.81)
                 ~~food protein-induced proctocolitis (K52.82)~~

         DEF: True immunoglobulin E (IgE)-mediated allergic reaction of the lining of the stomach, intestines, or colon to food proteins. It causes nausea, vomiting, diarrhea, and abdominal cramping.

         K52.21   **Food protein-induced enterocolitis syndrome**
                 FPIES
                 Use additional code for hypovolemic shock, if present (R57.1)

         K52.22   **Food protein-induced enteropathy**

         K52.29   **Other allergic and dietetic gastroenteritis and colitis**
                 ►Allergic proctocolitis◄
                 Food hypersensitivity gastroenteritis or colitis
                 ►Food-induced eosinophilic proctocolitis◄
                 ►Food protein-induced proctocolitis◄
                 Immediate gastrointestinal hypersensitivity
                 ►Milk protein-induced proctocolitis◄

     K52.3   **Indeterminate colitis**
         Colonic inflammatory bowel disease unclassified (IBDU)
         `EXCLUDES 1`   unspecified colitis (K52.9)

N Newborn: 0   P Pediatric: 0-17   M Maternity: 9-64   A Adult: 15-124   MCC Major Complication/Comorbidity   CC Complication/Comorbidity   SW Severe Wound Dx

722   ICD-10-CM 2022

✓5ᵗʰ **K52.8 Other specified noninfective gastroenteritis and colitis**

   K52.81 Eosinophilic gastritis or gastroenteritis
     Eosinophilic enteritis
     EXCLUDES 2 *eosinophilic esophagitis (K20.0)*
     DEF: Disorder involving the accumulation of eosinophil in the lining of the stomach or multiple levels of the gastrointestinal tract, but without a known cause such as connective tissue disease, drug reaction, malignancy, or parasitic infection.

   K52.82 Eosinophilic colitis
     ~~Allergic proctocolitis~~
     ~~Food-induced eosinophilic proctocolitis~~
     ~~Food protein-induced proctocolitis~~
     ~~Milk protein-induced proctocolitis~~
     EXCLUDES 2 ▶*allergic proctocolitis (K52.29)*◀
        ▶*food-induced eosinophilic proctocolitis (K52.29)*◀
        ▶*food protein-induced enterocolitis syndrome (FPIES) (K52.21)*◀
        ▶*food protein-induced proctocolitis (K52.29)*◀
        ▶*milk protein-induced proctocolitis (K52.29)*◀
     DEF: Disorder involving the accumulation of eosinophil in the tissues lining the colon, but without a known cause such as connective tissue disease, drug reaction, malignancy, or parasitic infection. The resultant inflammation may cause extreme abdominal pain, diarrhea, or bloody stool.

  ✓6ᵗʰ **K52.83 Microscopic colitis**
     K52.831 Collagenous colitis
     K52.832 Lymphocytic colitis
     K52.838 Other microscopic colitis
     K52.839 Microscopic colitis, unspecified
   K52.89 Other specified noninfective gastroenteritis and colitis
     AHA: 2019,1Q,20

K52.9 Noninfective gastroenteritis and colitis, unspecified
    Colitis NOS
    Enteritis NOS
    Gastroenteritis NOS
    Ileitis NOS
    Jejunitis NOS
    Sigmoiditis NOS
    EXCLUDES 1 *diarrhea NOS (R19.7)*
        functional diarrhea (K59.1)
        infectious gastroenteritis and colitis NOS (A09)
        neonatal diarrhea (noninfective) (P78.3)
        psychogenic diarrhea (F45.8)

Other diseases of intestines (K55-K64)

✓4ᵗʰ **K55 Vascular disorders of intestine**
   EXCLUDES 1 *necrotizing enterocolitis of newborn (P77.-)*
   AHA: 2016,4Q,32

 ✓5ᵗʰ **K55.0 Acute vascular disorders of intestine**
    Infarction of appendices epiploicae
    Mesenteric (artery) (vein) embolism
    Mesenteric (artery) (vein) infarction
    Mesenteric (artery) (vein) thrombosis
    AHA: 2019,4Q,68

  ✓6ᵗʰ **K55.01 Acute (reversible) ischemia of small intestine**
     K55.011 Focal (segmental) acute (reversible) ischemia of small intestine MCC HCC
     K55.012 Diffuse acute (reversible) ischemia of small intestine MCC HCC
     K55.019 Acute (reversible) ischemia of small intestine, extent unspecified MCC HCC

  ✓6ᵗʰ **K55.02 Acute infarction of small intestine**
    Gangrene of small intestine
    Necrosis of small intestine
     K55.021 Focal (segmental) acute infarction of small intestine MCC HCC
     K55.022 Diffuse acute infarction of small intestine MCC HCC
     K55.029 Acute infarction of small intestine, extent unspecified MCC HCC

  ✓6ᵗʰ **K55.03 Acute (reversible) ischemia of large intestine**
    Acute fulminant ischemic colitis
    Subacute ischemic colitis
     K55.031 Focal (segmental) acute (reversible) ischemia of large intestine MCC HCC
     K55.032 Diffuse acute (reversible) ischemia of large intestine MCC HCC
     K55.039 Acute (reversible) ischemia of large intestine, extent unspecified MCC HCC
      AHA: 2019,4Q,68

  ✓6ᵗʰ **K55.04 Acute infarction of large intestine**
    Gangrene of large intestine
    Necrosis of large intestine
     K55.041 Focal (segmental) acute infarction of large intestine MCC HCC
     K55.042 Diffuse acute infarction of large intestine MCC HCC
     K55.049 Acute infarction of large intestine, extent unspecified MCC HCC

  ✓6ᵗʰ **K55.05 Acute (reversible) ischemia of intestine, part unspecified**
     K55.051 Focal (segmental) acute (reversible) ischemia of intestine, part unspecified MCC HCC
     K55.052 Diffuse acute (reversible) ischemia of intestine, part unspecified MCC HCC
     K55.059 Acute (reversible) ischemia of intestine, part and extent unspecified MCC HCC

  ✓6ᵗʰ **K55.06 Acute infarction of intestine, part unspecified**
    Acute intestinal infarction
    Gangrene of intestine
    Necrosis of intestine
     K55.061 Focal (segmental) acute infarction of intestine, part unspecified MCC HCC
     K55.062 Diffuse acute infarction of intestine, part unspecified MCC HCC
     K55.069 Acute infarction of intestine, part and extent unspecified MCC HCC

K55.1 Chronic vascular disorders of intestine CC HCC
    Chronic ischemic colitis
    Chronic ischemic enteritis
    Chronic ischemic enterocolitis
    Ischemic stricture of intestine
    Mesenteric atherosclerosis
    Mesenteric vascular insufficiency

 ✓5ᵗʰ **K55.2 Angiodysplasia of colon**
    AHA: 2018,3Q,21
    TIP: Assign a code for "with hemorrhage" when angiodysplasia and GI bleeding are documented. The ICD-10-CM classification assumes the two are related without the provider linking the two conditions. Evidence of bleeding during a procedure is not required.
   K55.20 Angiodysplasia of colon without hemorrhage
   K55.21 Angiodysplasia of colon with hemorrhage MCC
     DEF: Small vascular abnormalities due to fragile blood vessels in the colon, resulting in blood loss from the gastrointestinal (GI) tract.

 ✓5ᵗʰ **K55.3 Necrotizing enterocolitis**
   EXCLUDES 1 *necrotizing enterocolitis of newborn (P77.-)*
   EXCLUDES 2 *necrotizing enterocolitis due to Clostridium difficile (A04.7-)*
   K55.30 Necrotizing enterocolitis, unspecified MCC HCC
     Necrotizing enterocolitis, NOS
   K55.31 Stage 1 necrotizing enterocolitis MCC HCC
     Necrotizing enterocolitis without pneumatosis, without perforation
   K55.32 Stage 2 necrotizing enterocolitis MCC HCC
     Necrotizing enterocolitis with pneumatosis, without perforation
   K55.33 Stage 3 necrotizing enterocolitis MCC HCC
     Necrotizing enterocolitis with perforation
     Necrotizing enterocolitis with pneumatosis and perforation

K55.8 Other vascular disorders of intestine CC HCC

☑ Additional Character Required   ✓x7ᵗʰ Placeholder   Questionable PDx   Manifestation   Unspecified Dx   UPD Unacceptable PDx   H1-H16 HAC   HCC CMS-HCC Dx   HIV HIV Dx

ICD-10-CM 2022   723

K55.9 Vascular disorder of intestine, unspecified `CC` `HCC`
Ischemic colitis
Ischemic enteritis
Ischemic enterocolitis

✓4ᵗʰ K56 Paralytic ileus and intestinal obstruction without hernia
> *EXCLUDES 1* congenital stricture or stenosis of intestine (Q41-Q42)
> cystic fibrosis with meconium ileus (E84.11)
> ischemic stricture of intestine (K55.1)
> meconium ileus NOS (P76.0)
> neonatal intestinal obstructions classifiable to P76.-
> obstruction of duodenum (K31.5)
> postprocedural intestinal obstruction (K91.3-)
> *EXCLUDES 2* stenosis of anus or rectum (K62.4)

K56.0 Paralytic ileus `CC` `HCC`
Paralysis of bowel
Paralysis of colon
Paralysis of intestine
> *EXCLUDES 1* gallstone ileus (K56.3)
> ileus NOS (K56.7)
> obstructive ileus NOS (K56.69-)

DEF: Intestinal obstruction due to paralysis of bowel motility or peristalsis.

K56.1 Intussusception `CC` `HCC`
Intussusception or invagination of bowel
Intussusception or invagination of colon
Intussusception or invagination of intestine
Intussusception or invagination of rectum
> *EXCLUDES 2* intussusception of appendix (K38.8)

DEF: Intestinal obstruction due to prolapse of a bowel section into an adjacent section. It occurs primarily in children and symptoms include acute abdominal pain, vomiting, and passage of blood and mucus from the rectum.

K56.2 Volvulus `MCC` `HCC`
Strangulation of colon or intestine
Torsion of colon or intestine
Twist of colon or intestine
> *EXCLUDES 2* volvulus of duodenum (K31.5)

DEF: Twisting, knotting, or entanglement of the bowel on itself that may quickly compromise oxygen supply to the intestinal tissues. A volvulus usually occurs at the sigmoid and ileocecal areas of the intestines.

Volvulus

Knotted intestine (volvulus)

K56.3 Gallstone ileus `CC` `HCC`
Obstruction of intestine by gallstone

✓5ᵗʰ K56.4 Other impaction of intestine
> **K56.41 Fecal impaction** `HCC`
> > *EXCLUDES 1* constipation (K59.0-)
> > incomplete defecation (R15.0)
> **K56.49 Other impaction of intestine** `CC` `HCC`

✓5ᵗʰ K56.5 Intestinal adhesions [bands] with obstruction (postinfection)
Abdominal hernia due to adhesions with obstruction
Peritoneal adhesions [bands] with intestinal obstruction (postinfection)
AHA: 2017,4Q,16-17

> **K56.50 Intestinal adhesions [bands], unspecified as to partial versus complete obstruction** `CC` `HCC`
> Intestinal adhesions with obstruction NOS
> **K56.51 Intestinal adhesions [bands], with partial obstruction** `CC` `HCC`
> Intestinal adhesions with incomplete obstruction
> **K56.52 Intestinal adhesions [bands] with complete obstruction** `CC` `HCC`

✓5ᵗʰ K56.6 Other and unspecified intestinal obstruction
AHA: 2017,4Q,16-17; 2017,2Q,12

> **✓6ᵗʰ K56.60 Unspecified intestinal obstruction**
> > **K56.600 Partial intestinal obstruction, unspecified as to cause** `CC` `HCC`
> > Incomplete intestinal obstruction, NOS
> > **K56.601 Complete intestinal obstruction, unspecified as to cause** `CC` `HCC`
> > **K56.609 Unspecified intestinal obstruction, unspecified as to partial versus complete obstruction** `CC` `HCC`
> > Intestinal obstruction NOS

> **✓6ᵗʰ K56.69 Other intestinal obstruction**
> Enterostenosis NOS
> Obstructive ileus NOS
> Occlusion of colon or intestine NOS
> Stenosis of colon or intestine NOS
> Stricture of colon or intestine NOS
> > *EXCLUDES 1* intestinal obstruction due to specified condition - code to condition
> > **K56.690 Other partial intestinal obstruction** `CC` `HCC`
> > Other incomplete intestinal obstruction
> > **K56.691 Other complete intestinal obstruction** `CC` `HCC`
> > **K56.699 Other intestinal obstruction unspecified as to partial versus complete obstruction** `CC` `HCC`
> > Other intestinal obstruction, NEC

K56.7 Ileus, unspecified `CC` `HCC`
> *EXCLUDES 1* obstructive ileus (K56.69-)
> *EXCLUDES 2* intestinal obstruction with hernia (K40-K46)
> **AHA:** 2017,1Q,40

✓4ᵗʰ K57 Diverticular disease of intestine
Code also if applicable peritonitis K65.-
> *EXCLUDES 1* congenital diverticulum of intestine (Q43.8)
> Meckel's diverticulum (Q43.0)
> *EXCLUDES 2* diverticulum of appendix (K38.2)
AHA: 2021,1Q,9,11; 2018,3Q,21
TIP: Assign a code for "with bleeding" when diverticular disease of the intestine and GI bleeding are documented. The ICD-10-CM classification assumes the two are related without the provider linking the two conditions. Evidence of bleeding during a procedure is not required.

✓5ᵗʰ K57.0 Diverticulitis of small intestine with perforation and abscess
> *EXCLUDES 1* diverticulitis of both small and large intestine with perforation and abscess (K57.4-)
> **K57.00 Diverticulitis of small intestine with perforation and abscess without bleeding** `CC`
> **K57.01 Diverticulitis of small intestine with perforation and abscess with bleeding** `MCC`

✓5ᵗʰ K57.1 Diverticular disease of small intestine without perforation or abscess
> *EXCLUDES 1* diverticular disease of both small and large intestine without perforation or abscess (K57.5-)
> **K57.10 Diverticulosis of small intestine without perforation or abscess without bleeding**
> Diverticular disease of small intestine NOS
> **K57.11 Diverticulosis of small intestine without perforation or abscess with bleeding** `MCC`
> **K57.12 Diverticulitis of small intestine without perforation or abscess without bleeding** `CC`
> **K57.13 Diverticulitis of small intestine without perforation or abscess with bleeding** `MCC`

`N` Newborn: 0   `P` Pediatric: 0-17   `M` Maternity: 9-64   `A` Adult: 15-124   `MCC` Major Complication/Comorbidity   `CC` Complication/Comorbidity   `SW` Severe Wound Dx

724   ICD-10-CM 2022

√5ᵗʰ K57.2 Diverticulitis of large intestine with perforation and abscess

> **EXCLUDES 1**   *diverticulitis of both small and large intestine with perforation and abscess (K57.4-)*

    K57.20 Diverticulitis of large intestine with perforation and abscess without bleeding   `CC`

    K57.21 Diverticulitis of large intestine with perforation and abscess with bleeding   `MCC`

√5ᵗʰ K57.3 Diverticular disease of large intestine without perforation or abscess

> **EXCLUDES 1**   *diverticular disease of both small and large intestine without perforation or abscess (K57.5-)*

    K57.30 Diverticulosis of large intestine without perforation or abscess without bleeding
      Diverticular disease of colon NOS

    K57.31 Diverticulosis of large intestine without perforation or abscess with bleeding   `MCC`

    K57.32 Diverticulitis of large intestine without perforation or abscess without bleeding   `CC`

    K57.33 Diverticulitis of large intestine without perforation or abscess with bleeding   `MCC`

√5ᵗʰ K57.4 Diverticulitis of both small and large intestine with perforation and abscess

    K57.40 Diverticulitis of both small and large intestine with perforation and abscess without bleeding   `CC`

    K57.41 Diverticulitis of both small and large intestine with perforation and abscess with bleeding   `MCC`

√5ᵗʰ K57.5 Diverticular disease of both small and large intestine without perforation or abscess

    K57.50 Diverticulosis of both small and large intestine without perforation or abscess without bleeding
      Diverticular disease of both small and large intestine NOS

    K57.51 Diverticulosis of both small and large intestine without perforation or abscess with bleeding   `MCC`

    K57.52 Diverticulitis of both small and large intestine without perforation or abscess without bleeding   `CC`

    K57.53 Diverticulitis of both small and large intestine without perforation or abscess with bleeding   `MCC`

√5ᵗʰ K57.8 Diverticulitis of intestine, part unspecified, with perforation and abscess

    K57.80 Diverticulitis of intestine, part unspecified, with perforation and abscess without bleeding   `CC`

    K57.81 Diverticulitis of intestine, part unspecified, with perforation and abscess with bleeding   `MCC`

√5ᵗʰ K57.9 Diverticular disease of intestine, part unspecified, without perforation or abscess

    K57.90 Diverticulosis of intestine, part unspecified, without perforation or abscess without bleeding
      Diverticular disease of intestine NOS

    K57.91 Diverticulosis of intestine, part unspecified, without perforation or abscess with bleeding   `MCC`

    K57.92 Diverticulitis of intestine, part unspecified, without perforation or abscess without bleeding   `CC`

    K57.93 Diverticulitis of intestine, part unspecified, without perforation or abscess with bleeding   `MCC`

√4ᵗʰ K58 Irritable bowel syndrome

> **INCLUDES**   irritable colon
> spastic colon

AHA: 2016,4Q,32-33

    K58.0 Irritable bowel syndrome with diarrhea

    K58.1 Irritable bowel syndrome with constipation

    K58.2 Mixed irritable bowel syndrome

    K58.8 Other irritable bowel syndrome

    K58.9 Irritable bowel syndrome without diarrhea
      Irritable bowel syndrome NOS

√4ᵗʰ K59 Other functional intestinal disorders

> **EXCLUDES 1**   *change in bowel habit NOS (R19.4)*
> *intestinal malabsorption (K90.-)*
> *psychogenic intestinal disorders (F45.8)*
> **EXCLUDES 2**   *functional disorders of stomach (K31.-)*

√5ᵗʰ K59.0 Constipation

> **EXCLUDES 1**   *fecal impaction (K56.41)*
> *incomplete defecation (R15.0)*

AHA: 2016,4Q,33

    K59.00 Constipation, unspecified

    K59.01 Slow transit constipation
      DEF: Delay in the transit of fecal material through the colon secondary to smooth muscle dysfunction or decreased peristaltic contractions along the colon.

    K59.02 Outlet dysfunction constipation

    K59.03 Drug induced constipation
      Use additional code for adverse effect, if applicable, to identify drug (T36-T50 with fifth or sixth character 5)

    K59.04 Chronic idiopathic constipation
      Functional constipation

    K59.09 Other constipation
      Chronic constipation

K59.1 Functional diarrhea

> **EXCLUDES 1**   *diarrhea NOS (R19.7)*
> *irritable bowel syndrome with diarrhea (K58.0)*

K59.2 Neurogenic bowel, not elsewhere classified   `CC`
DEF: Disorder of bowel due to a spinal cord lesion because of injury or as a complication of conditions such as multiple sclerosis (MS) or spina bifida. Loss of bowel control is the primary symptom, manifested as constipation or bowel incontinence.

√5ᵗʰ K59.3 Megacolon, not elsewhere classified

    Dilatation of colon
    Code first, if applicable (T51-T65) to identify toxic agent

> **EXCLUDES 1**   *congenital megacolon (aganglionic) (Q43.1)*
> *megacolon (due to) (in) Chagas' disease (B57.32)*
> *megacolon (due to) (in) Clostridium difficile (A04.7-)*
> *megacolon (due to) (in) Hirschsprung's disease (Q43.1)*

AHA: 2016,4Q,33-34

    K59.31 Toxic megacolon   `CC` `HCC`

    K59.39 Other megacolon   `CC`
      Megacolon NOS

K59.4 Anal spasm
    Proctalgia fugax

√5ᵗʰ K59.8 Other specified functional intestinal disorders

AHA: 2020,4Q,29-30

    K59.81 Ogilvie syndrome
      Acute colonic pseudo-obstruction (ACPO)

    K59.89 Other specified functional intestinal disorders
      Atony of colon
      Pseudo-obstruction (acute) (chronic) of intestine

K59.9 Functional intestinal disorder, unspecified

√4ᵗʰ K60 Fissure and fistula of anal and rectal regions

> **EXCLUDES 1**   *fissure and fistula of anal and rectal regions with abscess or cellulitis (K61.-)*
> **EXCLUDES 2**   *anal sphincter tear (healed) (nontraumatic) (old) (K62.81)*

K60.0 Acute anal fissure

K60.1 Chronic anal fissure

K60.2 Anal fissure, unspecified

K60.3 Anal fistula   `SW`

K60.4 Rectal fistula   `SW`
    Fistula of rectum to skin

> **EXCLUDES 1**   *rectovaginal fistula (N82.3)*
> *vesicorectal fistual (N32.1)*

K60.5 Anorectal fistula   `SW`

√4ᵗʰ K61 Abscess of anal and rectal regions

> **INCLUDES**   abscess of anal and rectal regions
> cellulitis of anal and rectal regions

K61.0 Anal abscess   `CC`
    Perianal abscess

> **EXCLUDES 2**   *intrasphincteric abscess (K61.4)*

K61.1 Rectal abscess   `CC`
    Perirectal abscess

> **EXCLUDES 1**   *ischiorectal abscess (K61.39)*

AHA: 2012,4Q,104

K61.2 Anorectal abscess   `CC`

√5ᵗʰ K61.3 Ischiorectal abscess

AHA: 2018,4Q,19

    K61.31 Horseshoe abscess

    K61.39 Other ischiorectal abscess
      Abscess of ischiorectal fossa
      Ischiorectal abscess, NOS

☑ Additional Character Required   √ₓ7ᵗʰ Placeholder   Questionable PDx   Manifestation   Unspecified Dx   `UPD` Unacceptable PDx   `H1`-`H14` HAC   `HCC` CMS-HCC Dx   `HIV` HIV Dx

K61.4 Intrasphincteric abscess `CC`
Intersphincteric abscess

K61.5 Supralevator abscess
AHA: 2018,4Q,19

✓4ᵗʰ **K62 Other diseases of anus and rectum**
`INCLUDES` anal canal
`EXCLUDES 2` colostomy and enterostomy malfunction (K94.0-, K94.1-)
fecal incontinence (R15.-)
hemorrhoids (K64.-)

K62.0 Anal polyp

K62.1 Rectal polyp
`EXCLUDES 1` adenomatous polyp (D12.8)
AHA: 2018,1Q,6

K62.2 Anal prolapse
Prolapse of anal canal

K62.3 Rectal prolapse
Prolapse of rectal mucosa

K62.4 Stenosis of anus and rectum
Stricture of anus (sphincter)
AHA: 2019,2Q,13

K62.5 Hemorrhage of anus and rectum `CC`
`EXCLUDES 1` gastrointestinal bleeding NOS (K92.2)
melena (K92.1)
neonatal rectal hemorrhage (P54.2)
AHA: 2019,1Q,21

K62.6 Ulcer of anus and rectum `CC`
Solitary ulcer of anus and rectum
Stercoral ulcer of anus and rectum
`EXCLUDES 1` fissure and fistula of anus and rectum (K60.-)
ulcerative colitis (K51.-)

K62.7 Radiation proctitis
Use additional code to identify the type of radiation (W88.-) or radiation therapy (Y84.2)
AHA: 2019,1Q,21

✓5ᵗʰ **K62.8 Other specified diseases of anus and rectum**
`EXCLUDES 2` ulcerative proctitis (K51.2)

K62.81 Anal sphincter tear (healed) (nontraumatic) (old)
Tear of anus, nontraumatic
Use additional code for any associated fecal incontinence (R15.-)
`EXCLUDES 2` anal fissure (K60.-)
anal sphincter tear (healed) (old) complicating delivery (O34.7-)
traumatic tear of anal sphincter (S31.831)

K62.82 Dysplasia of anus
Anal intraepithelial neoplasia I and II (AIN I and II) (histologically confirmed)
Dysplasia of anus NOS
Mild and moderate dysplasia of anus (histologically confirmed)
`EXCLUDES 1` abnormal results from anal cytologic examination without histologic confirmation (R85.61-)
anal intraepithelial neoplasia III (D01.3)
carcinoma in situ of anus (D01.3)
HGSIL of anus (R85.613)
severe dysplasia of anus (D01.3)

K62.89 Other specified diseases of anus and rectum
Proctitis NOS
Use additional code for any associated fecal incontinence (R15.-)

K62.9 Disease of anus and rectum, unspecified

✓4ᵗʰ **K63 Other diseases of intestine**

K63.0 Abscess of intestine `CC`
`EXCLUDES 1` abscess of intestine with Crohn's disease (K50.014, K50.114, K50.814, K50.914)
abscess of intestine with diverticular disease (K57.0, K57.2, K57.4, K57.8)
abscess of intestine with ulcerative colitis (K51.014, K51.214, K51.314, K51.414, K51.514, K51.814, K51.914)
`EXCLUDES 2` abscess of anal and rectal regions (K61.-)
abscess of appendix (K35.3-)

K63.1 Perforation of intestine (nontraumatic) `MCC` `HCC`
Perforation (nontraumatic) of rectum
`EXCLUDES 1` perforation (nontraumatic) of duodenum (K26.-)
perforation (nontraumatic) of intestine with diverticular disease (K57.0, K57.2, K57.4, K57.8)
`EXCLUDES 2` perforation (nontraumatic) of appendix (K35.2-, K35.3-)
AHA: 2020,2Q,22

K63.2 Fistula of intestine `CC` `SW`
`EXCLUDES 1` fistula of duodenum (K31.6)
fistula of intestine with Crohn's disease (K50.013, K50.113, K50.813, K50.913)
fistula of intestine with ulcerative colitis (K51.013, K51.213, K51.313, K51.413, K51.513, K51.813, K51.913)
`EXCLUDES 2` fistula of anal and rectal regions (K60.-)
fistula of appendix (K38.3)
intestinal-genital fistula, female (N82.2-N82.4)
vesicointestinal fistula (N32.1)
AHA: 2017,3Q,4

K63.3 Ulcer of intestine `CC`
Primary ulcer of small intestine
`EXCLUDES 1` duodenal ulcer (K26.-)
gastrointestinal ulcer (K28.-)
gastrojejunal ulcer (K28.-)
jejunal ulcer (K28.-)
peptic ulcer, site unspecified (K27.-)
ulcer of intestine with perforation (K63.1)
ulcer of anus or rectum (K62.6)
ulcerative colitis (K51.-)

K63.4 Enteroptosis

K63.5 Polyp of colon
`EXCLUDES 1` adenomatous polyp of colon (D12.-)
inflammatory polyp of colon (K51.4-)
polyposis of colon (D12.6)
AHA: 2019,1Q,33; 2018,2Q,14; 2017,1Q,15; 2015,2Q,14
TIP: Assign this code when documentation states hyperplastic colon polyp regardless of the site in the colon. Slow-growing, hyperplastic polyps are not precancerous and are classified differently from benign or adenomatous polyps.

✓5ᵗʰ **K63.8 Other specified diseases of intestine**

K63.81 Dieulafoy lesion of intestine `MCC`
`EXCLUDES 2` Dieulafoy lesion of stomach and duodenum (K31.82)
DEF: Abnormally large submucosal artery protruding through a defect in the stomach mucosa or intestines that can cause massive and life-threatening hemorrhaging.

K63.89 Other specified diseases of intestine
AHA: 2013,2Q,31

K63.9 Disease of intestine, unspecified

N Newborn: 0 P Pediatric: 0-17 M Maternity: 9-64 A Adult: 15-124 `MCC` Major Complication/Comorbidity `CC` Complication/Comorbidity `SW` Severe Wound Dx

726
ICD-10-CM 2022

✓4ᵗʰ K64 Hemorrhoids and perianal venous thrombosis

    INCLUDES   piles

    EXCLUDES 1   *hemorrhoids complicating childbirth and the puerperium*
                 (O87.2)
                 hemorrhoids complicating pregnancy (O22.4)

Hemorrhoids

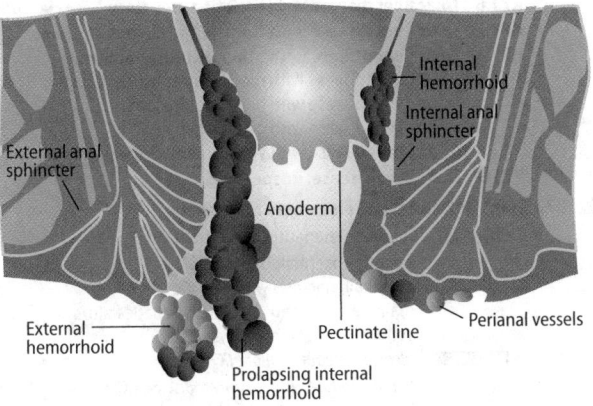

K64.0 First degree hemorrhoids
     Grade/stage I hemorrhoids
     Hemorrhoids (bleeding) without prolapse outside of anal canal

K64.1 Second degree hemorrhoids
     Grade/stage II hemorrhoids
     Hemorrhoids (bleeding) that prolapse with straining, but retract
         spontaneously

K64.2 Third degree hemorrhoids
     Grade/stage III hemorrhoids
     Hemorrhoids (bleeding) that prolapse with straining and require
         manual replacement back inside anal canal

K64.3 Fourth degree hemorrhoids
     Grade/stage IV hemorrhoids
     Hemorrhoids (bleeding) with prolapsed tissue that cannot be
         manually replaced

K64.4 Residual hemorrhoidal skin tags
     External hemorrhoids, NOS
     Skin tags of anus

K64.5 Perianal venous thrombosis
     External hemorrhoids with thrombosis
     Perianal hematoma
     Thrombosed hemorrhoids NOS

K64.8 Other hemorrhoids
     Internal hemorrhoids, without mention of degree
     Prolapsed hemorrhoids, degree not specified

K64.9 Unspecified hemorrhoids
     Hemorrhoids (bleeding) NOS
     Hemorrhoids (bleeding) without mention of degree

Diseases of peritoneum and retroperitoneum (K65-K68)

✓4ᵗʰ K65 Peritonitis

     Use additional code (B95-B97), to identify infectious agent, if known
     Code also if applicable diverticular disease of intestine (K57.-)

    EXCLUDES 1   *acute appendicitis with generalized peritonitis (K35.2-)*
                 aseptic peritonitis (T81.6)
                 benign paroxysmal peritonitis (E85.0)
                 chemical peritonitis (T81.6)
                 gonococcal peritonitis (A54.85)
                 neonatal peritonitis (P78.0-P78.1)
                 pelvic peritonitis, female (N73.3-N73.5)
                 periodic familial peritonitis (E85.0)
                 peritonitis due to talc or other foreign substance (T81.6)
                 peritonitis in chlamydia (A74.81)
                 peritonitis in diphtheria (A36.89)
                 peritonitis in syphilis (late) (A52.74)
                 peritonitis in tuberculosis (A18.31)
                 peritonitis with or following abortion or ectopic or molar
                     pregnancy (O00-O07, O08.0)
                 peritonitis with or following appendicitis (K35.-)
                 puerperal peritonitis (O85)
                 retroperitoneal infections (K68.-)

K65.0 Generalized (acute) peritonitis   `MCC` `HCC`
     Pelvic peritonitis (acute), male
     Subphrenic peritonitis (acute)
     Suppurative peritonitis (acute)

K65.1 Peritoneal abscess   `MCC` `HCC`
     Abdominopelvic abscess
     Abscess (of) omentum
     Abscess (of) peritoneum
     Mesenteric abscess
     Retrocecal abscess
     Subdiaphragmatic abscess
     Subhepatic abscess
     Subphrenic abscess
     AHA: 2019,1Q,15

K65.2 Spontaneous bacterial peritonitis   `MCC` `HCC`
    EXCLUDES 1   *bacterial peritonitis NOS (K65.9)*

K65.3 Choleperitonitis   `MCC` `HCC`
     Peritonitis due to bile
     DEF: Inflammation of the peritoneum due to leakage of bile into
     the peritoneal cavity resulting from rupture of the bile passages
     or gallbladder.

K65.4 Sclerosing mesenteritis   `CC` `HCC`
     Fat necrosis of peritoneum
     (Idiopathic) sclerosing mesenteric fibrosis
     Mesenteric lipodystrophy
     Mesenteric panniculitis
     Retractile mesenteritis

K65.8 Other peritonitis   `MCC` `HCC`
     Chronic proliferative peritonitis
     Peritonitis due to urine

K65.9 Peritonitis, unspecified   `MCC` `HCC`
     Bacterial peritonitis NOS
     AHA: 2013,2Q,31

✓4ᵗʰ K66 Other disorders of peritoneum

    EXCLUDES 2   *ascites (R18.-)*
                 peritoneal effusion (chronic) (R18.8)

K66.0 Peritoneal adhesions (postprocedural) (postinfection)
     Adhesions (of) abdominal (wall)
     Adhesions (of) diaphragm
     Adhesions (of) intestine
     Adhesions (of) male pelvis
     Adhesions (of) omentum
     Adhesions (of) stomach
     Adhesive bands
     Mesenteric adhesions
    EXCLUDES 1   *female pelvic adhesions [bands] (N73.6)*
                 peritoneal adhesions with intestinal obstruction
                     (K56.5-)

K66.1 Hemoperitoneum   `MCC`
    EXCLUDES 1   *traumatic hemoperitoneum (S36.8-)*

K66.8 Other specified disorders of peritoneum

K66.9 Disorder of peritoneum, unspecified

✔ Additional Character Required   ✓x7ᵗʰ Placeholder   Questionable PDx   Manifestation   Unspecified Dx   UPD Unacceptable PDx   H1 - H14 HAC   HCC CMS-HCC Dx   HIV HIV Dx

ICD-10-CM 2022   727

K67 Disorders of peritoneum in infectious diseases classified elsewhere `MCC` `HCC`

Code first underlying disease, such as:
   congenital syphilis (A50.0)
   helminthiasis (B65.0-B83.9)

EXCLUDES 1   peritonitis in chlamydia (A74.81)
        peritonitis in diphtheria (A36.89)
        peritonitis in gonococcal (A54.85)
        peritonitis in syphilis (late) (A52.74)
        peritonitis in tuberculosis (A18.31)

✓4th **K68 Disorders of retroperitoneum**

✓5th **K68.1 Retroperitoneal abscess**

     K68.11 Postprocedural retroperitoneal abscess `CC` `H11` `H12` `H13`

        EXCLUDES 2   infection following procedure (T81.4-)

     K68.12 Psoas muscle abscess `MCC` `HCC`

     K68.19 Other retroperitoneal abscess `MCC` `HCC`

        AHA: 2019,1Q,15

        TIP: This code should be used for a diagnosis of internal presacral abscess. If an intra-abdominal abscess is also present, code K65.1 can also be assigned; sequencing depends on the circumstances of admission.

     K68.9 Other disorders of retroperitoneum `MCC`

Diseases of liver (K70-K77)

EXCLUDES 1   jaundice NOS (R17)
EXCLUDES 2   hemochromatosis (E83.11-)
        Reye's syndrome (G93.7)
        viral hepatitis (B15-B19)
        Wilson's disease (E83.0)

✓4th **K70 Alcoholic liver disease**

Use additional code to identify:
     alcohol abuse and dependence (F10.-)

     K70.0 Alcoholic fatty liver `A`

✓5th **K70.1 Alcoholic hepatitis**

     K70.10 Alcoholic hepatitis without ascites `A`

     K70.11 Alcoholic hepatitis with ascites `A`

     K70.2 Alcoholic fibrosis and sclerosis of liver `A`

✓5th **K70.3 Alcoholic cirrhosis of liver**

     Alcoholic cirrhosis NOS

     K70.30 Alcoholic cirrhosis of liver without ascites `HCC` `A`

     K70.31 Alcoholic cirrhosis of liver with ascites `HCC` `A`

        AHA: 2018,1Q,4

✓5th **K70.4 Alcoholic hepatic failure**

     Acute alcoholic hepatic failure
     Alcoholic hepatic failure NOS
     Chronic alcoholic hepatic failure
     Subacute alcoholic hepatic failure

     K70.40 Alcoholic hepatic failure without coma `HCC` `A`

     K70.41 Alcoholic hepatic failure with coma `MCC` `HCC` `A`

     K70.9 Alcoholic liver disease, unspecified `HCC` `A`

✓4th **K71 Toxic liver disease**

INCLUDES   drug-induced idiosyncratic (unpredictable) liver disease
          drug-induced toxic (predictable) liver disease

Code first poisoning due to drug or toxin, if applicable (T36-T65 with fifth or sixth character 1-4 or 6)
Use additional code for adverse effect, if applicable, to identify drug (T36-T50 with fifth or sixth character 5)

EXCLUDES 2   alcoholic liver disease (K70.-)
        Budd-Chiari syndrome (I82.0)

     K71.0 Toxic liver disease with cholestasis

     Cholestasis with hepatocyte injury
     "Pure" cholestasis

✓5th **K71.1 Toxic liver disease with hepatic necrosis**

     Hepatic failure (acute) (chronic) due to drugs

     K71.10 Toxic liver disease with hepatic necrosis, without coma

     K71.11 Toxic liver disease with hepatic necrosis, with coma `MCC` `HCC`

     K71.2 Toxic liver disease with acute hepatitis

     K71.3 Toxic liver disease with chronic persistent hepatitis

     K71.4 Toxic liver disease with chronic lobular hepatitis

✓5th **K71.5 Toxic liver disease with chronic active hepatitis**

     Toxic liver disease with lupoid hepatitis

     K71.50 Toxic liver disease with chronic active hepatitis without ascites

     K71.51 Toxic liver disease with chronic active hepatitis with ascites

        AHA: 2018,1Q,4

     K71.6 Toxic liver disease with hepatitis, not elsewhere classified

     K71.7 Toxic liver disease with fibrosis and cirrhosis of liver

     K71.8 Toxic liver disease with other disorders of liver

     Toxic liver disease with focal nodular hyperplasia
     Toxic liver disease with hepatic granulomas
     Toxic liver disease with peliosis hepatis
     Toxic liver disease with veno-occlusive disease of liver

     K71.9 Toxic liver disease, unspecified

✓4th **K72 Hepatic failure, not elsewhere classified**

INCLUDES   fulminant hepatitis NEC, with hepatic failure
          hepatic encephalopathy NOS
          liver (cell) necrosis with hepatic failure
          malignant hepatitis NEC, with hepatic failure
          yellow liver atrophy or dystrophy

EXCLUDES 1   alcoholic hepatic failure (K70.4)
        hepatic failure with toxic liver disease (K71.1-)
        icterus of newborn (P55-P59)
        postprocedural hepatic failure (K91.82)

EXCLUDES 2   hepatic failure complicating abortion or ectopic or molar pregnancy (O00-O07, O08.8)
        hepatic failure complicating pregnancy, childbirth and the puerperium (O26.6-)
        viral hepatitis with hepatic coma (B15-B19)

     AHA: 2017,1Q,41

✓5th **K72.0 Acute and subacute hepatic failure**

     Acute non-viral hepatitis NOS
     AHA: 2015,2Q,17; 2014,2Q,13

     K72.00 Acute and subacute hepatic failure without coma `MCC`

        AHA: 2021,1Q,13

     K72.01 Acute and subacute hepatic failure with coma `MCC` `HCC`

✓5th **K72.1 Chronic hepatic failure**

     ▶End stage liver disease◀

     K72.10 Chronic hepatic failure without coma `HCC`

        AHA: 2021,1Q,13

     K72.11 Chronic hepatic failure with coma `MCC` `HCC`

✓5th **K72.9 Hepatic failure, unspecified**

     K72.90 Hepatic failure, unspecified without coma `HCC`

        AHA: 2018,4Q,20; 2016,2Q,35

     K72.91 Hepatic failure, unspecified with coma `MCC` `HCC`

     Hepatic coma NOS

✓4th **K73 Chronic hepatitis, not elsewhere classified**

EXCLUDES 1   alcoholic hepatitis (chronic) (K70.1-)
        drug-induced hepatitis (chronic) (K71.-)
        granulomatous hepatitis (chronic) NEC (K75.3)
        reactive, nonspecific hepatitis (chronic) (K75.2)
        viral hepatitis (chronic) (B15-B19)

     K73.0 Chronic persistent hepatitis, not elsewhere classified `HCC`

     K73.1 Chronic lobular hepatitis, not elsewhere classified `HCC`

     K73.2 Chronic active hepatitis, not elsewhere classified `HCC`

     K73.8 Other chronic hepatitis, not elsewhere classified `HCC`

     K73.9 Chronic hepatitis, unspecified `HCC`

✓4th **K74 Fibrosis and cirrhosis of liver**

Code also, if applicable, viral hepatitis (acute) (chronic) (B15-B19)

EXCLUDES 1   alcoholic cirrhosis (of liver) (K70.3)
        alcoholic fibrosis of liver (K70.2)
        cardiac sclerosis of liver (K76.1)
        cirrhosis (of liver) with toxic liver disease (K71.7)
        congenital cirrhosis (of liver) (P78.81)
        pigmentary cirrhosis (of liver) (E83.110)

✓5th **K74.0 Hepatic fibrosis**

     Code first underlying liver disease, such as:
        nonalcoholic steatohepatitis (NASH) (K75.81)
     AHA: 2020,4Q,30-31

     K74.00 Hepatic fibrosis, unspecified `UPD`

`N` Newborn: 0   `P` Pediatric: 0-17   `M` Maternity: 9-64   `A` Adult: 15-124   `MCC` Major Complication/Comorbidity   `CC` Complication/Comorbidity   `SW` Severe Wound Dx

728   ICD-10-CM 2022

K74.01 **Hepatic fibrosis, early fibrosis** `UPD`
Hepatic fibrosis, stage F1 or stage F2

K74.02 **Hepatic fibrosis, advanced fibrosis** `UPD`
Hepatic fibrosis, stage F3
`EXCLUDES 1` *cirrhosis of liver (K74.6-)*
hepatic fibrosis, stage F4 (K74.6-)

K74.1 **Hepatic sclerosis**

K74.2 **Hepatic fibrosis with hepatic sclerosis**

K74.3 **Primary biliary cirrhosis** `HCC`
Chronic nonsuppurative destructive cholangitis
Primary biliary cholangitis
`EXCLUDES 2` *primary sclerosing cholangitis (K83.01)*

K74.4 **Secondary biliary cirrhosis** `HCC`

K74.5 **Biliary cirrhosis, unspecified** `HCC`

✓5ᵗʰ K74.6 **Other and unspecified cirrhosis of liver**
AHA: 2020,4Q,30-31

K74.60 **Unspecified cirrhosis of liver** `HCC`
Cirrhosis (of liver) NOS
AHA: 2018,1Q,4

K74.69 **Other cirrhosis of liver** `HCC`
Cryptogenic cirrhosis (of liver)
Macronodular cirrhosis (of liver)
Micronodular cirrhosis (of liver)
Mixed type cirrhosis (of liver)
Portal cirrhosis (of liver)
Postnecrotic cirrhosis (of liver)

✓4ᵗʰ K75 **Other inflammatory liver diseases**
`EXCLUDES 2` *toxic liver disease (K71.-)*

K75.0 **Abscess of liver** `MCC`
Cholangitic hepatic abscess
Hematogenic hepatic abscess
Hepatic abscess NOS
Lymphogenic hepatic abscess
Pylephlebitic hepatic abscess
`EXCLUDES 1` *amebic liver abscess (A06.4)*
cholangitis without liver abscess (K83.09)
pylephlebitis without liver abscess (K75.1)
`EXCLUDES 2` *acute or subacute hepatitis NOS (B17.9)*
acute or subacute non-viral hepatitis (K72.0)
chronic hepatitis NEC (K73.8)

K75.1 **Phlebitis of portal vein** `MCC`
Pylephlebitis
`EXCLUDES 1` *pylephlebitic liver abscess (K75.0)*
DEF: Inflammation of the portal vein or branches due to diverticulitis, perforated appendicitis, or peritonitis. Symptoms include fever, chills, jaundice, sweating, and abscess in various body parts.

K75.2 **Nonspecific reactive hepatitis**
`EXCLUDES 1` *acute or subacute hepatitis (K72.0-)*
chronic hepatitis NEC (K73.-)
viral hepatitis (B15-B19)

K75.3 **Granulomatous hepatitis, not elsewhere classified**
`EXCLUDES 1` *acute or subacute hepatitis (K72.0-)*
chronic hepatitis NEC (K73.-)
viral hepatitis (B15-B19)

K75.4 **Autoimmune hepatitis** `HCC`
Lupoid hepatitis NEC

✓5ᵗʰ K75.8 **Other specified inflammatory liver diseases**

K75.81 **Nonalcoholic steatohepatitis (NASH)**
Use additional code, if applicable, hepatic fibrosis (K74.0-)

K75.89 **Other specified inflammatory liver diseases**

K75.9 **Inflammatory liver disease, unspecified**
Hepatitis NOS
`EXCLUDES 1` *acute or subacute hepatitis (K72.0-)*
chronic hepatitis NEC (K73.-)
viral hepatitis (B15-B19)
AHA: 2015,2Q,17

✓4ᵗʰ K76 **Other diseases of liver**
`EXCLUDES 2` *alcoholic liver disease (K70.-)*
amyloid degeneration of liver (E85.-)
cystic disease of liver (congenital) (Q44.6)
hepatic vein thrombosis (I82.0)
hepatomegaly NOS (R16.0)
pigmentary cirrhosis (of liver) (E83.110)
portal vein thrombosis (I81)
toxic liver disease (K71.-)

K76.0 **Fatty (change of) liver, not elsewhere classified**
Nonalcoholic fatty liver disease (NAFLD)
`EXCLUDES 1` *nonalcoholic steatohepatitis (NASH) (K75.81)*

K76.1 **Chronic passive congestion of liver**
Cardiac cirrhosis
Cardiac sclerosis

K76.2 **Central hemorrhagic necrosis of liver** `MCC`
`EXCLUDES 1` *liver necrosis with hepatic failure (K72.-)*

K76.3 **Infarction of liver** `MCC`

K76.4 **Peliosis hepatis**
Hepatic angiomatosis

K76.5 **Hepatic veno-occlusive disease**
`EXCLUDES 1` *Budd-Chiari syndrome (I82.0)*

K76.6 **Portal hypertension** `CC` `HCC`
Use additional code for any associated complications, such as:
portal hypertensive gastropathy (K31.89)
AHA: 2020,1Q,15

K76.7 **Hepatorenal syndrome** `MCC` `HCC`
`EXCLUDES 1` *hepatorenal syndrome following labor and delivery (O90.4)*
postprocedural hepatorenal syndrome (K91.83)

✓5ᵗʰ K76.8 **Other specified diseases of liver**

K76.81 **Hepatopulmonary syndrome** `UPD` `HCC`
Code first underlying liver disease, such as:
alcoholic cirrhosis of liver (K70.3-)
cirrhosis of liver without mention of alcohol (K74.6-)

K76.89 **Other specified diseases of liver**
Cyst (simple) of liver
Focal nodular hyperplasia of liver
Hepatoptosis

K76.9 **Liver disease, unspecified**

K77 *Liver disorders in diseases classified elsewhere* `CC`
Code first underlying disease, such as:
amyloidosis (E85.-)
congenital syphilis (A50.0, A50.5)
congenital toxoplasmosis (P37.1)
▶infectious mononucleosis with liver disease (B27.0-B27.9 with .9)◄
schistosomiasis (B65.0-B65.9)
`EXCLUDES 1` *alcoholic hepatitis (K70.1-)*
alcoholic liver disease (K70.-)
cytomegaloviral hepatitis (B25.1)
herpesviral [herpes simplex] hepatitis (B00.81)
~~infectious mononucleosis with liver disease (B27.0-B27.9 with .9)~~
mumps hepatitis (B26.81)
sarcoidosis with liver disease (D86.89)
secondary syphilis with liver disease (A51.45)
syphilis (late) with liver disease (A52.74)
toxoplasmosis (acquired) hepatitis (B58.1)
tuberculosis with liver disease (A18.83)

Disorders of gallbladder, biliary tract and pancreas (K80-K87)

☑4ᵗʰ **K80** **Cholelithiasis**

> **EXCLUDES 1**   *retained cholelithiasis following cholecystectomy (K91.86)*
> **AHA:** 2018,4Q,20
> **DEF:** Presence or formation of concretions (calculi or "gallstones") in the gallbladder. The stones contain cholesterol, calcium carbonate, or calcium bilirubinate in pure forms or in various combinations.

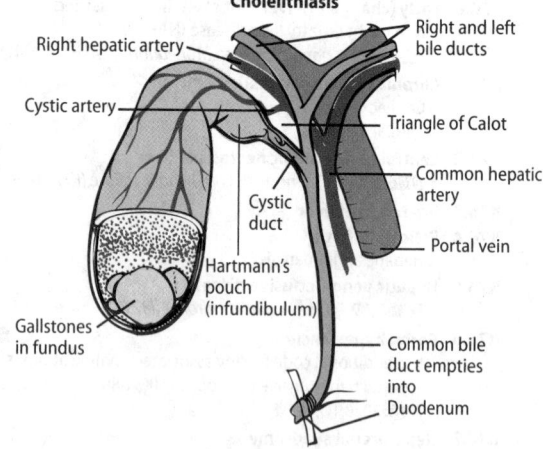

Cholelithiasis

☑5ᵗʰ **K80.0** **Calculus of** gallbladder with acute cholecystitis

> Any condition listed in K80.2 with acute cholecystitis
> Use additional code if applicable for associated gangrene of gallbladder (K82.A1), or perforation of gallbladder (K82.A2)

    K80.00   **Calculus of gallbladder with acute cholecystitis without obstruction**   cc

    K80.01   **Calculus of gallbladder with acute cholecystitis with obstruction**   cc

☑5ᵗʰ **K80.1** **Calculus of** gallbladder with other cholecystitis

> Use additional code if applicable for associated gangrene of gallbladder (K82.A1), or perforation of gallbladder (K82.A2)

    K80.10   **Calculus of gallbladder with** chronic **cholecystitis without obstruction**   cc
> Cholelithiasis with cholecystitis NOS

    K80.11   **Calculus of gallbladder with** chronic **cholecystitis with obstruction**   cc

    K80.12   **Calculus of gallbladder with** acute and chronic **cholecystitis without obstruction**   cc

    K80.13   **Calculus of gallbladder with** acute and chronic **cholecystitis with obstruction**   cc

    K80.18   **Calculus of gallbladder with other cholecystitis without obstruction**   cc

    K80.19   **Calculus of gallbladder with other cholecystitis with obstruction**   cc

☑5ᵗʰ **K80.2** **Calculus of** gallbladder without cholecystitis

> Cholecystolithiasis without cholecystitis
> Cholelithiasis (without cholecystitis)
> Colic (recurrent) of gallbladder (without cholecystitis)
> Gallstone (impacted) of cystic duct (without cholecystitis)
> Gallstone (impacted) of gallbladder (without cholecystitis)

    K80.20   **Calculus of gallbladder without cholecystitis without obstruction**

    K80.21   **Calculus of gallbladder without cholecystitis with obstruction**   cc

☑5ᵗʰ **K80.3** **Calculus of** bile duct with cholangitis

> Any condition listed in K80.5 with cholangitis
> **DEF:** Cholangitis: Inflammation of the bile ducts.

    K80.30   **Calculus of bile duct with cholangitis, unspecified, without obstruction**   cc

    K80.31   **Calculus of bile duct with cholangitis, unspecified, with obstruction**   cc

    K80.32   **Calculus of bile duct with** acute **cholangitis without obstruction**   cc

    K80.33   **Calculus of bile duct with** acute **cholangitis with obstruction**   cc

    K80.34   **Calculus of bile duct with** chronic **cholangitis without obstruction**   cc

    K80.35   **Calculus of bile duct with** chronic **cholangitis with obstruction**   cc

    K80.36   **Calculus of bile duct with** acute and chronic **cholangitis without obstruction**   cc

    K80.37   **Calculus of bile duct with** acute and chronic **cholangitis with obstruction**   cc

☑5ᵗʰ **K80.4** **Calculus of** bile duct with cholecystitis

> Any condition listed in K80.5 with cholecystitis (with cholangitis)
> Codes also fistula of bile duct (K83.3)
> Use additional code if applicable for associated gangrene of gallbladder (K82.A1), or perforation of gallbladder (K82.A2)
> **AHA:** 2019,1Q,17

    K80.40   **Calculus of bile duct with cholecystitis, unspecified, without obstruction**   cc

    K80.41   **Calculus of bile duct with cholecystitis, unspecified, with obstruction**   cc
> **AHA:** 2019,1Q,17

    K80.42   **Calculus of bile duct with** acute **cholecystitis without obstruction**   cc

    K80.43   **Calculus of bile duct with** acute **cholecystitis with obstruction**   cc

    K80.44   **Calculus of bile duct with** chronic **cholecystitis without obstruction**   cc

    K80.45   **Calculus of bile duct with** chronic **cholecystitis with obstruction**   cc

    K80.46   **Calculus of bile duct with** acute and chronic **cholecystitis without obstruction**   cc

    K80.47   **Calculus of bile duct with** acute and chronic **cholecystitis with obstruction**   cc

☑5ᵗʰ **K80.5** **Calculus of** bile duct without cholangitis or cholecystitis

> Choledocholithiasis (without cholangitis or cholecystitis)
> Gallstone (impacted) of bile duct NOS (without cholangitis or cholecystitis)
> Gallstone (impacted) of common duct (without cholangitis or cholecystitis)
> Gallstone (impacted) of hepatic duct (without cholangitis or cholecystitis)
> Hepatic cholelithiasis (without cholangitis or cholecystitis)
> Hepatic colic (recurrent) (without cholangitis or cholecystitis)
> **DEF:** Cholangitis: Inflammation of the bile ducts.

    K80.50   **Calculus of bile duct without cholangitis or cholecystitis without obstruction**

    K80.51   **Calculus of bile duct without cholangitis or cholecystitis with obstruction**   cc

☑5ᵗʰ **K80.6** **Calculus of** gallbladder and bile duct with cholecystitis

> Use additional code if applicable for associated gangrene of gallbladder (K82.A1), or perforation of gallbladder (K82.A2)

    K80.60   **Calculus of gallbladder and bile duct with cholecystitis, unspecified, without obstruction**   cc

    K80.61   **Calculus of gallbladder and bile duct with cholecystitis, unspecified, with obstruction**   cc

    K80.62   **Calculus of gallbladder and bile duct with** acute **cholecystitis without obstruction**   cc

    K80.63   **Calculus of gallbladder and bile duct with** acute **cholecystitis with obstruction**   cc

    K80.64   **Calculus of gallbladder and bile duct with** chronic **cholecystitis without obstruction**   cc

    K80.65   **Calculus of gallbladder and bile duct with** chronic **cholecystitis with obstruction**   cc

    K80.66   **Calculus of gallbladder and bile duct with** acute and chronic **cholecystitis without obstruction**   cc

    K80.67   **Calculus of gallbladder and bile duct with** acute and chronic **cholecystitis with obstruction**   MCC

☑5ᵗʰ **K80.7** **Calculus of** gallbladder and bile duct without cholecystitis

    K80.70   **Calculus of gallbladder and bile duct without cholecystitis without obstruction**

    K80.71   **Calculus of gallbladder and bile duct without cholecystitis with obstruction**   cc

☑5ᵗʰ **K80.8** **Other cholelithiasis**

    K80.80   **Other cholelithiasis without obstruction**

    K80.81   **Other cholelithiasis with obstruction**   cc

✓4ᵗʰ **K81** **Cholecystitis**
Use additional code if applicable for associated gangrene of gallbladder (K82.A1), or perforation of gallbladder (K82.A2)
EXCLUDES 1   *cholecystitis with cholelithiasis (K80.-)*
AHA: 2018,4Q,20

K81.0 **Acute cholecystitis**   `CC`
Abscess of gallbladder
Angiocholecystitis
Emphysematous (acute) cholecystitis
Empyema of gallbladder
Gangrene of gallbladder
Gangrenous cholecystitis
Suppurative cholecystitis

K81.1 **Chronic cholecystitis**

K81.2 **Acute cholecystitis with chronic cholecystitis**   `CC`

K81.9 **Cholecystitis, unspecified**

✓4ᵗʰ **K82** **Other diseases of gallbladder**
EXCLUDES 1   *nonvisualization of gallbladder (R93.2)*
postcholecystectomy syndrome (K91.5)

K82.0 **Obstruction of gallbladder**   `CC`
Occlusion of cystic duct or gallbladder without cholelithiasis
Stenosis of cystic duct or gallbladder without cholelithiasis
Stricture of cystic duct or gallbladder without cholelithiasis
EXCLUDES 1   *obstruction of gallbladder with cholelithiasis (K80.-)*

K82.1 **Hydrops of gallbladder**   `CC`
Mucocele of gallbladder

K82.2 **Perforation of gallbladder**   `MCC`
Rupture of cystic duct or gallbladder
EXCLUDES 1   *perforation of gallbladder in cholecystitis (K82.A2)*

K82.3 **Fistula of gallbladder**   `CC`
Cholecystocolic fistula
Cholecystoduodenal fistula

K82.4 **Cholesterolosis of gallbladder**
Strawberry gallbladder
EXCLUDES 1   *cholesterolosis of gallbladder with cholecystitis (K81.-)*
cholesterolosis of gallbladder with cholelithiasis (K80.-)

K82.8 **Other specified diseases of gallbladder**
Adhesions of cystic duct or gallbladder
Atrophy of cystic duct or gallbladder
Cyst of cystic duct or gallbladder
Dyskinesia of cystic duct or gallbladder
Hypertrophy of cystic duct or gallbladder
Nonfunctioning of cystic duct or gallbladder
Ulcer of cystic duct or gallbladder

K82.9 **Disease of gallbladder, unspecified**

✓5ᵗʰ **K82.A** **Disorders of gallbladder in diseases classified elsewhere**
Code first the type of cholecystitis (K81.-), or cholelithiasis with cholecystitis (K80.00-K80.19, K80.40-K80.47, K80.60-K80.67)
AHA: 2018,4Q,19-20
K82.A1 *Gangrene of gallbladder in cholecystitis*
K82.A2 *Perforation of gallbladder in cholecystitis*   `CC`

✓4ᵗʰ **K83** **Other diseases of biliary tract**
EXCLUDES 1   *postcholecystectomy syndrome (K91.5)*
EXCLUDES 2   *conditions involving the gallbladder (K81-K82)*
conditions involving the cystic duct (K81-K82)

✓5ᵗʰ **K83.0** **Cholangitis**
EXCLUDES 1   *cholangitic liver abscess (K75.0)*
cholangitis with choledocholithiasis (K80.3-, K80.4-)
EXCLUDES 2   *chronic nonsuppurative destructive cholangitis (K74.3)*
primary biliary cholangitis (K74.3)
primary biliary cirrhosis (K74.3)
AHA: 2018,4Q,20
K83.01 **Primary sclerosing cholangitis**   `CC`

K83.09 **Other cholangitis**   `CC`
Ascending cholangitis
Cholangitis NOS
Primary cholangitis
Recurrent cholangitis
Sclerosing cholangitis
Secondary cholangitis
Stenosing cholangitis
Suppurative cholangitis

K83.1 **Obstruction of bile duct**   `MCC`
Occlusion of bile duct without cholelithiasis
Stenosis of bile duct without cholelithiasis
Stricture of bile duct without cholelithiasis
EXCLUDES 1   *congenital obstruction of bile duct (Q44.3)*
obstruction of bile duct with cholelithiasis (K80.-)
AHA: 2016,1Q,18

K83.2 **Perforation of bile duct**   `MCC`
Rupture of bile duct

K83.3 **Fistula of bile duct**   `CC`
Choledochoduodenal fistula
AHA: 2019,1Q,17

K83.4 **Spasm of sphincter of Oddi**

K83.5 **Biliary cyst**

K83.8 **Other specified diseases of biliary tract**
Adhesions of biliary tract
Atrophy of biliary tract
Hypertrophy of biliary tract
Ulcer of biliary tract

K83.9 **Disease of biliary tract, unspecified**

✓4ᵗʰ **K85** **Acute pancreatitis**
INCLUDES   acute (recurrent) pancreatitis
subacute pancreatitis
AHA: 2016,4Q,34

✓5ᵗʰ **K85.0** **Idiopathic acute pancreatitis**
K85.00 **Idiopathic acute pancreatitis without necrosis or infection**   `MCC`
K85.01 **Idiopathic acute pancreatitis with uninfected necrosis**   `MCC`
K85.02 **Idiopathic acute pancreatitis with infected necrosis**   `MCC`

✓5ᵗʰ **K85.1** **Biliary acute pancreatitis**
Gallstone pancreatitis
K85.10 **Biliary acute pancreatitis without necrosis or infection**   `MCC`
K85.11 **Biliary acute pancreatitis with uninfected necrosis**   `MCC`
K85.12 **Biliary acute pancreatitis with infected necrosis**   `MCC`

✓5ᵗʰ **K85.2** **Alcohol induced acute pancreatitis**
EXCLUDES 2   *alcohol induced chronic pancreatitis (K86.0)*
K85.20 **Alcohol induced acute pancreatitis without necrosis or infection**   `MCC`
AHA: 2020,1Q,9
K85.21 **Alcohol induced acute pancreatitis with uninfected necrosis**   `MCC`
K85.22 **Alcohol induced acute pancreatitis with infected necrosis**   `MCC`

✓5ᵗʰ **K85.3** **Drug induced acute pancreatitis**
Use additional code for adverse effect, if applicable, to identify drug (T36-T50 with fifth or sixth character 5)
Use additional code to identify drug abuse and dependence (F11.- F17.-)
K85.30 **Drug induced acute pancreatitis without necrosis or infection**   `MCC`
K85.31 **Drug induced acute pancreatitis with uninfected necrosis**   `MCC`
K85.32 **Drug induced acute pancreatitis with infected necrosis**   `MCC`

✓5ᵗʰ **K85.8** **Other acute pancreatitis**
K85.80 **Other acute pancreatitis without necrosis or infection**   `MCC`
K85.81 **Other acute pancreatitis with uninfected necrosis**   `MCC`
K85.82 **Other acute pancreatitis with infected necrosis**   `MCC`

Chapter 11. Diseases of the Digestive System

✓5ᵗʰ **K85.9 Acute pancreatitis, unspecified**
Pancreatitis NOS

    K85.90 Acute pancreatitis without necrosis or infection, **unspecified** `MCC`

    K85.91 Acute pancreatitis with uninfected necrosis, **unspecified** `MCC`

    K85.92 Acute pancreatitis with infected necrosis, **unspecified** `MCC`

✓4ᵗʰ **K86 Other diseases of pancreas**
    EXCLUDES 2   fibrocystic disease of pancreas (E84.-)
           islet cell tumor (of pancreas) (D13.7)
           pancreatic steatorrhea (K90.3)

    K86.0 Alcohol-induced chronic pancreatitis `CC` `HCC`
Use additional code to identify:
    alcohol abuse and dependence (F10.-)
Code also exocrine pancreatic insufficiency (K86.81)
    EXCLUDES 2   alcohol induced acute pancreatitis (K85.2-)

    K86.1 Other chronic pancreatitis `CC` `HCC`
Chronic pancreatitis NOS
Infectious chronic pancreatitis
Recurrent chronic pancreatitis
Relapsing chronic pancreatitis
Code also exocrine pancreatic insufficiency (K86.81)

    K86.2 Cyst of pancreas `CC`
    K86.3 Pseudocyst of pancreas `CC`

✓5ᵗʰ **K86.8 Other specified diseases of pancreas**
    AHA: 2016,4Q,34-35

    K86.81 Exocrine pancreatic insufficiency

    K86.89 Other specified diseases of pancreas
Aseptic pancreatic necrosis, unrelated to acute pancreatitis
Atrophy of pancreas
Calculus of pancreas
Cirrhosis of pancreas
Fibrosis of pancreas
Pancreatic fat necrosis, unrelated to acute pancreatitis
Pancreatic infantilism
Pancreatic necrosis NOS, unrelated to acute pancreatitis

    K86.9 Disease of pancreas, unspecified

K87 Disorders of gallbladder, biliary tract and pancreas in diseases classified elsewhere
Code first underlying disease
    EXCLUDES 1   cytomegaloviral pancreatitis (B25.2)
           mumps pancreatitis (B26.3)
           syphilitic gallbladder (A52.74)
           syphilitic pancreas (A52.74)
           tuberculosis of gallbladder (A18.83)
           tuberculosis of pancreas (A18.83)

Other diseases of the digestive system (K90-K95)

✓4ᵗʰ **K90 Intestinal malabsorption**
    EXCLUDES 1   intestinal malabsorption following gastrointestinal surgery (K91.2)
    AHA: 2017,4Q,108

    K90.0 Celiac disease
Celiac disease with steatorrhea
Celiac gluten-sensitive enteropathy
Nontropical sprue
Use additional code for associated disorders including:
    dermatitis herpetiformis (L13.0)
    gluten ataxia (G32.81)
Code also exocrine pancreatic insufficiency (K86.81)
DEF: Malabsorption syndrome due to gluten consumption. Symptoms include fetid, bulky, frothy, oily stools; a distended abdomen; gas; asthenia; electrolyte depletion; and vitamin B, D, and K deficiency.

    K90.1 Tropical sprue `CC`
Sprue NOS
Tropical steatorrhea

    K90.2 Blind loop syndrome, not elsewhere classified `CC`
Blind loop syndrome NOS
    EXCLUDES 1   congenital blind loop syndrome (Q43.8)
           postsurgical blind loop syndrome (K91.2)

    K90.3 Pancreatic steatorrhea `CC`

✓5ᵗʰ **K90.4 Other malabsorption due to intolerance**
    EXCLUDES 2   celiac gluten-sensitive enteropathy (K90.0)
           lactose intolerance (E73.-)
    AHA: 2016,4Q,35-36

    K90.41 Non-celiac gluten sensitivity `CC`
Gluten sensitivity NOS
Non-celiac gluten sensitive enteropathy

    K90.49 Malabsorption due to intolerance, not elsewhere classified `CC`
Malabsorption due to intolerance to carbohydrate
Malabsorption due to intolerance to fat
Malabsorption due to intolerance to protein
Malabsorption due to intolerance to starch

✓5ᵗʰ **K90.8 Other intestinal malabsorption**

    K90.81 Whipple's disease `CC`
    K90.89 Other intestinal malabsorption `CC`

    K90.9 Intestinal malabsorption, unspecified `CC`

✓4ᵗʰ **K91 Intraoperative and postprocedural complications and disorders of digestive system, not elsewhere classified**
    EXCLUDES 2   complications of artificial opening of digestive system (K94.-)
           complications of bariatric procedures (K95.-)
           gastrojejunal ulcer (K28.-)
           postprocedural (radiation) retroperitoneal abscess (K68.11)
           radiation colitis (K52.0)
           radiation gastroenteritis (K52.0)
           radiation proctitis (K62.7)
    AHA: 2016,4Q,9-10

    K91.0 Vomiting following gastrointestinal surgery

    K91.1 Postgastric surgery syndromes
Dumping syndrome
Postgastrectomy syndrome
Postvagotomy syndrome

    K91.2 Postsurgical malabsorption, not elsewhere classified `CC`
Postsurgical blind loop syndrome
    EXCLUDES 1   malabsorption osteomalacia in adults (M83.2)
           malabsorption osteoporosis, postsurgical (M80.8-, M81.8)

✓5ᵗʰ **K91.3 Postprocedural** intestinal obstruction
    AHA: 2017,4Q,16-17; 2017,1Q,40

    K91.30 Postprocedural intestinal obstruction, unspecified as to partial versus complete `CC`
Postprocedural intestinal obstruction NOS

    K91.31 Postprocedural partial **intestinal obstruction** `CC`
Postprocedural incomplete intestinal obstruction

    K91.32 Postprocedural complete **intestinal obstruction** `CC`

    K91.5 Postcholecystectomy syndrome

✓5ᵗʰ **K91.6 Intraoperative hemorrhage and hematoma** of a digestive system organ or structure complicating a procedure
    EXCLUDES 1   intraoperative hemorrhage and hematoma of a digestive system organ or structure due to accidental puncture and laceration during a procedure (K91.7-)

    K91.61 Intraoperative hemorrhage and hematoma of a digestive system organ or structure complicating a digestive system procedure `CC`
    AHA: 2020,1Q,19

    K91.62 Intraoperative hemorrhage and hematoma of a digestive system organ or structure complicating other procedure `CC`

✓5ᵗʰ **K91.7 Accidental puncture and laceration** of a digestive system organ or structure during a procedure

    K91.71 Accidental puncture and laceration of a digestive system organ or structure during a digestive system procedure `CC`
    AHA: 2021,2Q,11

    K91.72 Accidental puncture and laceration of a digestive system organ or structure during other procedure `CC`
    AHA: 2019,2Q,23

✓5ᵗʰ **K91.8 Other intraoperative and postprocedural complications and disorders of digestive system**

    K91.81 Other intraoperative complications of digestive system `CC`

    K91.82 Postprocedural hepatic failure `CC`

    K91.83 Postprocedural hepatorenal syndrome `CC`

N Newborn: 0   **P** Pediatric: 0-17   **M** Maternity: 9-64   **A** Adult: 15-124   **MCC** Major Complication/Comorbidity   **CC** Complication/Comorbidity   **SW** Severe Wound Dx

732   ICD-10-CM 2022

✓6ᵗʰ	**K91.84**	**Postprocedural** hemorrhage **of a digestive system organ or structure** following a procedure

K91.840 Postprocedural hemorrhage of a digestive system organ or structure following a digestive system procedure `CC`
　　　　AHA: 2016,1Q,15

K91.841 Postprocedural hemorrhage of a digestive system organ or structure following other procedure `CC`

✓6ᵗʰ **K91.85** **Complications of** intestinal pouch

K91.850 **Pouchitis** `CC` `HCC`
　　　　Inflammation of internal ileoanal pouch
　　　　DEF: Inflammatory complication of an existing surgically created ileoanal pouch, resulting in multiple GI complaints, including diarrhea, abdominal pain, rectal bleeding, fecal urgency, or incontinence.

K91.858 **Other complications of intestinal pouch** `CC` `HCC`
　　　　AHA: 2019,2Q,13

K91.86 Retained cholelithiasis **following cholecystectomy** `CC`

✓6ᵗʰ **K91.87** Postprocedural hematoma and seroma **of a digestive system organ or structure following a procedure**

K91.870 Postprocedural hematoma **of a digestive system organ or structure following a** digestive system procedure `CC`

K91.871 Postprocedural hematoma **of a digestive system organ or structure following** other procedure `CC`

K91.872 Postprocedural seroma **of a digestive system organ or structure following a** digestive system procedure `CC`

K91.873 Postprocedural seroma **of a digestive system organ or structure following** other procedure `CC`

K91.89 **Other postprocedural complications and disorders of digestive system** `CC`
　　　　Use additional code, if applicable, to further specify disorder
　　　　EXCLUDES 2　postprocedural retroperitoneal abscess (K68.11)
　　　　AHA: 2020,2Q,22; 2017,1Q,40

✓4ᵗʰ **K92** **Other diseases of digestive system**
　　　EXCLUDES 1　neonatal gastrointestinal hemorrhage (P54.0-P54.3)

K92.0 **Hematemesis** `CC`

K92.1 **Melena** `CC`
　　　EXCLUDES 1　occult blood in feces (R19.5)

K92.2 **Gastrointestinal hemorrhage, unspecified** `CC`
　　　　Gastric hemorrhage NOS
　　　　Intestinal hemorrhage NOS
　　　EXCLUDES 1　acute hemorrhagic gastritis (K29.01)
　　　　　hemorrhage of anus and rectum (K62.5)
　　　　　angiodysplasia of stomach with hemorrhage (K31.811)
　　　　　diverticular disease with hemorrhage (K57.-)
　　　　　gastritis and duodenitis with hemorrhage (K29.-)
　　　　　peptic ulcer with hemorrhage (K25-K28)
　　　　AHA: 2021,1Q,11

✓5ᵗʰ **K92.8** **Other specified diseases of the digestive system**

K92.81 **Gastrointestinal mucositis (ulcerative)** `CC`
　　　　Code also type of associated therapy, such as:
　　　　　antineoplastic and immunosuppressive drugs (T45.1X-)
　　　　　radiological procedure and radiotherapy (Y84.2)
　　　EXCLUDES 2　mucositis (ulcerative) of vagina and vulva (N76.81)
　　　　　nasal mucositis (ulcerative) (J34.81)
　　　　　oral mucositis (ulcerative) (K12.3-)

K92.89 **Other specified diseases of the digestive system**

K92.9 **Disease of digestive system, unspecified**

✓4ᵗʰ **K94** **Complications of artificial openings of the digestive system**

✓5ᵗʰ **K94.0** Colostomy **complications**

K94.00 **Colostomy complication, unspecified** `HCC`
K94.01 **Colostomy** hemorrhage `CC` `HCC`

K94.02 **Colostomy** infection `CC` `HCC`
　　　　Use additional code to specify type of infection, such as:
　　　　　cellulitis of abdominal wall (L03.311)
　　　　　sepsis (A40.-, A41.-)

K94.03 **Colostomy** malfunction `CC` `HCC`
　　　　Mechanical complication of colostomy

K94.09 **Other complications of colostomy** `CC` `HCC`

✓5ᵗʰ **K94.1** Enterostomy **complications**

K94.10 **Enterostomy complication, unspecified** `HCC`
K94.11 **Enterostomy** hemorrhage `CC` `HCC`
K94.12 **Enterostomy** infection `CC` `HCC`
　　　　Use additional code to specify type of infection, such as:
　　　　　cellulitis of abdominal wall (L03.311)
　　　　　sepsis (A40.-, A41.-)

K94.13 **Enterostomy** malfunction `CC` `HCC`
　　　　Mechanical complication of enterostomy

K94.19 **Other complications of enterostomy** `CC` `HCC`

✓5ᵗʰ **K94.2** Gastrostomy **complications**

K94.20 **Gastrostomy complication, unspecified** `HCC`
K94.21 **Gastrostomy** hemorrhage `HCC`
K94.22 **Gastrostomy** infection `CC` `HCC`
　　　　Use additional code to specify type of infection, such as:
　　　　　cellulitis of abdominal wall (L03.311)
　　　　　sepsis (A40.-, A41.-)

K94.23 **Gastrostomy** malfunction `CC` `HCC`
　　　　Mechanical complication of gastrostomy
　　　　AHA: 2019,1Q,26

K94.29 **Other complications of gastrostomy** `HCC`

✓5ᵗʰ **K94.3** Esophagostomy **complications**

K94.30 **Esophagostomy complications, unspecified** `CC` `HCC`
K94.31 **Esophagostomy** hemorrhage `CC` `HCC`
K94.32 **Esophagostomy** infection `CC` `HCC`
　　　　Use additional code to identify the infection

K94.33 **Esophagostomy** malfunction `CC` `HCC`
　　　　Mechanical complication of esophagostomy

K94.39 **Other complications of esophagostomy** `CC` `HCC`

✓4ᵗʰ **K95** **Complications of bariatric procedures**

✓5ᵗʰ **K95.0** **Complications of** gastric band procedure

K95.01 Infection **due to gastric band procedure** `CC` `H11`
　　　　Use additional code to specify type of infection or organism, such as:
　　　　　bacterial and viral infectious agents (B95.-, B96.-)
　　　　　cellulitis of abdominal wall (L03.311)
　　　　　sepsis (A40.-, A41.-)

K95.09 **Other complications of gastric band procedure** `CC`
　　　　Use additional code, if applicable, to further specify complication

✓5ᵗʰ **K95.8** **Complications of other bariatric procedure**
　　　EXCLUDES 1　complications of gastric band surgery (K95.0-)

K95.81 Infection **due to other bariatric procedure** `CC` `H11`
　　　　Use additional code to specify type of infection or organism, such as:
　　　　　bacterial and viral infectious agents (B95.-, B96.-)
　　　　　cellulitis of abdominal wall (L03.311)
　　　　　sepsis (A40.-, A41.-)

K95.89 **Other complications of other bariatric procedure** `CC`
　　　　Use additional code, if applicable, to further specify complication

✓ Additional Character Required　　✓x7ᵗʰ Placeholder　　Questionable PDx　　Manifestation　　Unspecified Dx　　`UPD` Unacceptable PDx　　`H1`-`H14` HAC　　`HCC` CMS-HCC Dx　　`HIV` HIV Dx

ICD-10-CM 2022　　　　　　　　　　　　　　　　　　　　　　　　　　　　　　733

Chapter 12. Diseases of the Skin and Subcutaneous Tissue (L00–L99)

Chapter-specific Guidelines with Coding Examples

The chapter-specific guidelines from the ICD-10-CM Official Guidelines for Coding and Reporting have been provided below. Along with these guidelines are coding examples, contained in the shaded boxes, that have been developed to help illustrate the coding and/or sequencing guidance found in these guidelines.

a. Pressure ulcer stage codes

1) Pressure ulcer stages

Codes in category L89, Pressure ulcer, identify the site and stage of the pressure ulcer.

The ICD-10-CM classifies pressure ulcer stages based on severity, which is designated by stages 1-4, deep tissue pressure injury, unspecified stage, and unstageable.

Assign as many codes from category L89 as needed to identify all the pressure ulcers the patient has, if applicable.

See Section I.B.14 for pressure ulcer stage documentation by clinicians other than patient's provider

> Nursing notes: Dressings changed daily on stage 4 ulcer on heel and stage 2 ulcer on elbow
>
> Discharge summary: Pressure ulcers on right heel and left elbow
>
> **L89.614   Pressure ulcer of right heel, stage 4**
>
> **L89.022   Pressure ulcer of left elbow, stage 2**
>
> *Explanation:* Right heel and left elbow pressure ulcers were documented by the patient's provider in the discharge summary. Although the stage of these ulcers was not included in the provider's diagnostic statement, it is appropriate to code the stage from documentation from other clinicians involved in the patient's care, such as the nurse's notes, according to section I.B.14. Combination codes from category L89 Pressure ulcer, identify the site of the pressure ulcer as well as the stage. Assign as many codes from category L89 as needed to identify all the pressure ulcers the patient has.

2) Unstageable pressure ulcers

Assignment of the code for unstageable pressure ulcer (L89.--0) should be based on the clinical documentation. These codes are used for pressure ulcers whose stage cannot be clinically determined (e.g., the ulcer is covered by eschar or has been treated with a skin or muscle graft). This code should not be confused with the codes for unspecified stage (L89.--9). When there is no documentation regarding the stage of the pressure ulcer, assign the appropriate code for unspecified stage (L89.--9).

> Pressure ulcer of the right lower back documented as unstageable due to the presence of thick eschar covering the ulcer
>
> **L89.130   Pressure ulcer of right lower back, unstageable**
>
> *Explanation:* Codes for unstageable pressure ulcers are assigned when the stage cannot be clinically determined (e.g., the ulcer is covered by eschar or has been treated with a skin or muscle graft).

If during an encounter, the stage of an unstageable pressure ulcer is revealed after debridement, assign only the code for the stage revealed following debridement.

3) Documented pressure ulcer stage

Assignment of the pressure ulcer stage code should be guided by clinical documentation of the stage or documentation of the terms found in the Alphabetic Index. For clinical terms describing the stage that are not found in the Alphabetic Index, and there is no documentation of the stage, the provider should be queried.

> Left heel pressure ulcer with partial thickness skin loss involving the dermis
>
> **L89.622   Pressure ulcer of left heel, stage 2**
>
> *Explanation:* Code assignment for the pressure ulcer stage should be guided by either the clinical documentation of the stage or the documentation of terms found in the Alphabetic Index. The clinical documentation describing the left heel pressure ulcer "partial thickness skin loss involving the dermis" matches the ICD-10-CM index parenthetical description for stage 2 "(abrasion, blister, partial thickness skin loss involving epidermis and/or dermis)."

4) Patients admitted with pressure ulcers documented as healed

No code is assigned if the documentation states that the pressure ulcer is completely healed at the time of admission.

5) Pressure ulcers documented as healing

Pressure ulcers described as healing should be assigned the appropriate pressure ulcer stage code based on the documentation in the medical record. If the documentation does not provide information about the stage of the healing pressure ulcer, assign the appropriate code for unspecified stage.

If the documentation is unclear as to whether the patient has a current (new) pressure ulcer or if the patient is being treated for a healing pressure ulcer, query the provider.

For ulcers that were present on admission but healed at the time of discharge, assign the code for the site and stage of the pressure ulcer at the time of admission.

> H & P noted healing stage 2 sacral pressure ulcer. Resolved at time of discharge summary.
>
> **L89.152   Pressure ulcer of sacral region, stage 2**
>
> *Explanation:* Although completely healed upon discharge, the pressure ulcer required observation and/or treatment and should be coded based on the site and stage upon admission.

6) Patient admitted with pressure ulcer evolving into another stage during the admission

If a patient is admitted to an inpatient hospital with a pressure ulcer at one stage and it progresses to a higher stage, two separate codes should be assigned: one code for the site and stage of the ulcer on admission and a second code for the same ulcer site and the highest stage reported during the stay.

> Stage 3 right hip pressure ulcer worsened during admission to a stage 4
>
> **L89.213   Pressure ulcer of right hip, stage 3**
>
> **L89.214   Pressure ulcer of right hip, stage 4**
>
> *Explanation:* A pressure ulcer that progresses from a lower stage to a higher stage is assigned two codes, one for the documented stage upon admission and one for the documented stage at discharge.

7) Pressure-induced deep tissue damage

For pressure-induced deep tissue damage or deep tissue pressure injury, assign only the appropriate code for pressure-induced deep tissue damage (L89.--6).

b. Non-pressure chronic ulcers

1) Patients admitted with non-pressure ulcers documented as healed

No code is assigned if the documentation states that the non-pressure ulcer is completely healed at the time of admission.

2) Non-pressure ulcers documented as healing

Non-pressure ulcers described as healing should be assigned the appropriate non-pressure ulcer code based on the documentation in the medical record. If the documentation does not provide information about the severity of the healing non-pressure ulcer, assign the appropriate code for unspecified severity.

If the documentation is unclear as to whether the patient has a current (new) non-pressure ulcer or if the patient is being treated for a healing non-pressure ulcer, query the provider.

For ulcers that were present on admission but healed at the time of discharge, assign the code for the site and severity of the non-pressure ulcer at the time of admission.

> Admission diagnosis: Chronic ulcer, fat layer exposed, on left ankle
>
> Discharge diagnosis: Resolution of ulcer on the left ankle
>
> **L97.322   Non-pressure chronic ulcer of left ankle with fat layer exposed**
>
> *Explanation:* Although the ulcer was documented as resolved (healed) at discharge, a code representing the site and severity of the ulcer upon admission should be appended.

3) Patient admitted with non-pressure ulcer that progresses to another severity level during the admission

If a patient is admitted to an inpatient hospital with a non-pressure ulcer at one severity level and it progresses to a higher severity level, two separate codes should be assigned: one code for the site and severity level of the ulcer on admission and a second code for the same ulcer site and the highest severity level reported during the stay.

See Section I.B.14 for pressure ulcer stage documentation by clinicians other than patient's provider

Chapter 12. Diseases of the Skin and Subcutaneous Tissue (L00-L99)

EXCLUDES 2   *certain conditions originating in the perinatal period (P04-P96)*
certain infectious and parasitic diseases (A00-B99)
complications of pregnancy, childbirth and the puerperium (O00-O9A)
congenital malformations, deformations, and chromosomal abnormalities (Q00-Q99)
endocrine, nutritional and metabolic diseases (E00-E88)
lipomelanotic reticulosis (I89.8)
neoplasms (C00-D49)
symptoms, signs and abnormal clinical and laboratory findings, not elsewhere classified (R00-R94)
systemic connective tissue disorders (M30-M36)
viral warts (B07.-)

This chapter contains the following blocks:

L00-L08	Infections of the skin and subcutaneous tissue
L10-L14	Bullous disorders
L20-L30	Dermatitis and eczema
L40-L45	Papulosquamous disorders
L49-L54	Urticaria and erythema
L55-L59	Radiation-related disorders of the skin and subcutaneous tissue
L60-L75	Disorders of skin appendages
L76	Intraoperative and postprocedural complications of skin and subcutaneous tissue
L80-L99	Other disorders of the skin and subcutaneous tissue

Infections of the skin and subcutaneous tissue (L00-L08)

Use additional code (B95-B97) to identify infectious agent

EXCLUDES 2   *hordeolum (H00.0)*
infective dermatitis (L30.3)
local infections of skin classified in Chapter 1
lupus panniculitis (L93.2)
panniculitis NOS (M79.3)
panniculitis of neck and back (M54.0-)
perlèche NOS (K13.0)
perlèche due to candidiasis (B37.0)
perlèche due to riboflavin deficiency (E53.0)
pyogenic granuloma (L98.0)
relapsing panniculitis [Weber-Christian] (M35.6)
viral warts (B07.-)
zoster (B02.-)

L00   Staphylococcal scalded skin syndrome

Ritter's disease
Use additional code to identify percentage of skin exfoliation (L49.-)

EXCLUDES 1   *bullous impetigo (L01.03)*
pemphigus neonatorum (L01.03)
toxic epidermal necrolysis [Lyell] (L51.2)

DEF: Infectious skin disease of children younger than 5 years marked by eruptions ranging from a few localized blisters to widespread, easily ruptured, fine vesicles and bullae affecting almost the entire body. It results in exfoliation of large planes of skin and leaves raw areas.

✓4ᵗʰ L01   Impetigo

EXCLUDES 1   *impetigo herpetiformis (L40.1)*

DEF: Acute, superficial, highly contagious skin infection commonly occurring in children. Skin lesions usually appear on the face and consist of vesicles and bullae that burst and form yellow crusts.

✓5ᵗʰ L01.0   Impetigo

Impetigo contagiosa
Impetigo vulgaris

L01.00   Impetigo, unspecified
Impetigo NOS

L01.01   Non-bullous impetigo

L01.02   Bockhart's impetigo
Impetigo follicularis
Perifolliculitis NOS
Superficial pustular perifolliculitis
DEF: Superficial inflammation of the hair follicles commonly caused by *Staphylococcus aureus* that manifests as rounded, sphere-shaped, pustular eruptions in the areas of the scalp, beard, underarms, extremities, and buttocks.

L01.03   Bullous impetigo
Impetigo neonatorum
Pemphigus neonatorum

L01.09   Other impetigo
Ulcerative impetigo

L01.1   Impetiginization of other dermatoses

✓4ᵗʰ L02   Cutaneous abscess, furuncle and carbuncle

Use additional code to identify organism (B95-B96)

EXCLUDES 2   *abscess of anus and rectal regions (K61.-)*
abscess of female genital organs (external) (N76.4)
abscess of male genital organs (external) (N48.2, N49.-)

DEF: Carbuncle: Infection of the skin that arises from a collection of interconnected infected boils or furuncles, usually from hair follicles infected by *Staphylococcus*. This condition can produce pus and form drainage cavities.
DEF: Furuncle: Inflamed, painful abscess, cyst, or nodule on the skin caused by bacteria, often *Staphylococcus*, entering along the hair follicle.

✓5ᵗʰ L02.0   Cutaneous abscess, furuncle and carbuncle of face

EXCLUDES 2   *abscess of ear, external (H60.0)*
abscess of eyelid (H00.0)
abscess of head [any part, except face] (L02.8)
abscess of lacrimal gland (H04.0)
abscess of lacrimal passages (H04.3)
abscess of mouth (K12.2)
abscess of nose (J34.0)
abscess of orbit (H05.0)
submandibular abscess (K12.2)

L02.01   Cutaneous abscess of face   CC

L02.02   Furuncle of face
Boil of face
Folliculitis of face

L02.03   Carbuncle of face

✓5ᵗʰ L02.1   Cutaneous abscess, furuncle and carbuncle of neck

L02.11   Cutaneous abscess of neck   CC

L02.12   Furuncle of neck
Boil of neck
Folliculitis of neck

L02.13   Carbuncle of neck

✓5ᵗʰ L02.2   Cutaneous abscess, furuncle and carbuncle of trunk

EXCLUDES 1   *non-newborn omphalitis (L08.82)*
omphalitis of newborn (P38.-)

EXCLUDES 2   *abscess of breast (N61.1)*
abscess of buttocks (L02.3)
abscess of female external genital organs (N76.4)
abscess of hip (L02.4)
abscess of male external genital organs (N48.2, N49.-)

✓6ᵗʰ L02.21   Cutaneous abscess of trunk

L02.211   Cutaneous abscess of abdominal wall   CC
L02.212   Cutaneous abscess of back [any part, except buttock]   CC
L02.213   Cutaneous abscess of chest wall   CC
L02.214   Cutaneous abscess of groin   CC
L02.215   Cutaneous abscess of perineum   CC
L02.216   Cutaneous abscess of umbilicus   CC
L02.219   Cutaneous abscess of trunk, unspecified   CC

✓6ᵗʰ L02.22   Furuncle of trunk

Boil of trunk
Folliculitis of trunk
L02.221   Furuncle of abdominal wall
L02.222   Furuncle of back [any part, except buttock]
L02.223   Furuncle of chest wall
L02.224   Furuncle of groin
L02.225   Furuncle of perineum
L02.226   Furuncle of umbilicus
L02.229   Furuncle of trunk, unspecified

✓6ᵗʰ L02.23   Carbuncle of trunk

L02.231   Carbuncle of abdominal wall
L02.232   Carbuncle of back [any part, except buttock]
L02.233   Carbuncle of chest wall
L02.234   Carbuncle of groin
L02.235   Carbuncle of perineum
L02.236   Carbuncle of umbilicus
L02.239   Carbuncle of trunk, unspecified

✓5ᵗʰ L02.3   Cutaneous abscess, furuncle and carbuncle of buttock

EXCLUDES 1   *pilonidal cyst with abscess (L05.01)*

L02.31   Cutaneous abscess of buttock   CC
Cutaneous abscess of gluteal region

N Newborn: 0   P Pediatric: 0-17   M Maternity: 9-64   A Adult: 15-124   MCC Major Complication/Comorbidity   CC Complication/Comorbidity   SW Severe Wound Dx

736   ICD-10-CM 2022

L02.32 **Furuncle** of buttock
Boil of buttock
Folliculitis of buttock
Furuncle of gluteal region

L02.33 **Carbuncle** of buttock
Carbuncle of gluteal region

✓5ᵗʰ **L02.4** **Cutaneous abscess, furuncle and carbuncle of** limb

EXCLUDES 2   cutaneous abscess, furuncle and carbuncle of groin (L02.214, L02.224, L02.234)
cutaneous abscess, furuncle and carbuncle of hand (L02.5-)
cutaneous abscess, furuncle and carbuncle of foot (L02.6-)

✓6ᵗʰ **L02.41** **Cutaneous abscess** of limb

L02.411 **Cutaneous abscess of** right axilla   `CC`
L02.412 **Cutaneous abscess of** left axilla   `CC`
L02.413 **Cutaneous abscess of** right upper limb   `CC`
L02.414 **Cutaneous abscess of** left upper limb   `CC`
L02.415 **Cutaneous abscess of** right lower limb   `CC`
L02.416 **Cutaneous abscess of** left lower limb   `CC`
L02.419 **Cutaneous abscess of limb, unspecified**   `CC`

✓6ᵗʰ **L02.42** **Furuncle** of limb
Boil of limb
Folliculitis of limb

L02.421 **Furuncle of** right axilla
L02.422 **Furuncle of** left axilla
L02.423 **Furuncle of** right upper **limb**
L02.424 **Furuncle of** left upper **limb**
L02.425 **Furuncle of** right lower **limb**
L02.426 **Furuncle of** left lower **limb**
L02.429 **Furuncle of limb, unspecified**

✓6ᵗʰ **L02.43** **Carbuncle** of limb

L02.431 **Carbuncle of** right axilla
L02.432 **Carbuncle of** left axilla
L02.433 **Carbuncle of** right upper **limb**
L02.434 **Carbuncle of** left upper **limb**
L02.435 **Carbuncle of** right lower **limb**
L02.436 **Carbuncle of** left lower **limb**
L02.439 **Carbuncle of limb, unspecified**

✓5ᵗʰ **L02.5** **Cutaneous abscess, furuncle and carbuncle of** hand

✓6ᵗʰ **L02.51** **Cutaneous abscess** of hand

L02.511 **Cutaneous abscess of** right **hand**   `CC`
L02.512 **Cutaneous abscess of** left **hand**   `CC`
L02.519 **Cutaneous abscess of unspecified hand**   `CC`

✓6ᵗʰ **L02.52** **Furuncle** hand
Boil of hand
Folliculitis of hand

L02.521 **Furuncle** right **hand**
L02.522 **Furuncle** left **hand**
L02.529 **Furuncle unspecified hand**

✓6ᵗʰ **L02.53** **Carbuncle** of hand

L02.531 **Carbuncle of** right **hand**
L02.532 **Carbuncle of** left **hand**
L02.539 **Carbuncle of unspecified hand**

✓5ᵗʰ **L02.6** **Cutaneous abscess, furuncle and carbuncle of** foot

✓6ᵗʰ **L02.61** **Cutaneous abscess** of foot

L02.611 **Cutaneous abscess of** right **foot**   `CC`
L02.612 **Cutaneous abscess of** left **foot**   `CC`
L02.619 **Cutaneous abscess of unspecified foot**   `CC`

✓6ᵗʰ **L02.62** **Furuncle** of foot
Boil of foot
Folliculitis of foot

L02.621 **Furuncle of** right **foot**
L02.622 **Furuncle of** left **foot**
L02.629 **Furuncle of unspecified foot**

✓6ᵗʰ **L02.63** **Carbuncle** of foot

L02.631 **Carbuncle of** right **foot**
L02.632 **Carbuncle of** left **foot**
L02.639 **Carbuncle of unspecified foot**

✓5ᵗʰ **L02.8** **Cutaneous abscess, furuncle and carbuncle of other sites**

✓6ᵗʰ **L02.81** **Cutaneous abscess** of other sites

L02.811 **Cutaneous abscess of** head [any part, except face]   `CC`
L02.818 **Cutaneous abscess of other sites**   `CC`

✓6ᵗʰ **L02.82** **Furuncle** of other sites
Boil of other sites
Folliculitis of other sites

L02.821 **Furuncle of** head [any part, except face]
L02.828 **Furuncle of other sites**

✓6ᵗʰ **L02.83** **Carbuncle** of other sites

L02.831 **Carbuncle of** head [any part, except face]
L02.838 **Carbuncle of other sites**

✓5ᵗʰ **L02.9** **Cutaneous abscess, furuncle and carbuncle, unspecified**

L02.91 **Cutaneous abscess, unspecified**   `CC`
L02.92 **Furuncle, unspecified**
Boil NOS
Furunculosis NOS
L02.93 **Carbuncle, unspecified**

✓4ᵗʰ **L03** **Cellulitis and acute lymphangitis**

EXCLUDES 2   cellulitis of anal and rectal region (K61.-)
cellulitis of external auditory canal (H60.1)
cellulitis of eyelid (H00.0)
cellulitis of female external genital organs (N76.4)
cellulitis of lacrimal apparatus (H04.3)
cellulitis of male external genital organs (N48.2, N49.-)
cellulitis of mouth (K12.2)
cellulitis of nose (J34.0)
eosinophilic cellulitis [Wells] (L98.3)
febrile neutrophilic dermatosis [Sweet] (L98.2)
lymphangitis (chronic) (subacute) (I89.1)

AHA: 2017,4Q,100
DEF: Cellulitis: Infection of the skin and subcutaneous tissues, most often caused by *Staphylococcus* or *Streptococcus* bacteria secondary to a cutaneous lesion. Progression of the inflammation may lead to abscess and tissue death, or even systemic infection-like bacteremia.
DEF: Lymphangitis: Inflammation of the lymph channels most often caused by *Streptococcus*.

✓5ᵗʰ **L03.0** **Cellulitis and acute lymphangitis of** finger and toe
Infection of nail
Onychia
Paronychia
Perionychia

✓6ᵗʰ **L03.01** **Cellulitis** of finger
Felon
Whitlow
EXCLUDES 1   herpetic whitlow (B00.89)
DEF: Felon: Superficial bacterial skin infection at the tip of the finger.
L03.011 **Cellulitis of** right **finger**
L03.012 **Cellulitis of** left **finger**
L03.019 **Cellulitis of unspecified finger**

✓6ᵗʰ **L03.02** **Acute lymphangitis** of finger
Hangnail with lymphangitis of finger
L03.021 **Acute lymphangitis of** right **finger**
L03.022 **Acute lymphangitis of** left **finger**
L03.029 **Acute lymphangitis of unspecified finger**

✓6ᵗʰ **L03.03** **Cellulitis** of toe
L03.031 **Cellulitis of** right **toe**
L03.032 **Cellulitis of** left **toe**
L03.039 **Cellulitis of unspecified toe**

✓6ᵗʰ **L03.04** **Acute lymphangitis** of toe
Hangnail with lymphangitis of toe
L03.041 **Acute lymphangitis of** right **toe**
L03.042 **Acute lymphangitis of** left **toe**
L03.049 **Acute lymphangitis of unspecified toe**

✓5ᵗʰ **L03.1** **Cellulitis and acute lymphangitis of other parts of limb**

✓6ᵗʰ **L03.11** **Cellulitis** of other parts of limb
EXCLUDES 2   cellulitis of fingers (L03.01-)
cellulitis of toes (L03.03-)
groin (L03.314)
L03.111 **Cellulitis of** right axilla   `CC`
L03.112 **Cellulitis of** left axilla   `CC`
L03.113 **Cellulitis of** right upper **limb**   `CC`
L03.114 **Cellulitis of** left upper **limb**   `CC`

L03.115   Cellulitis of right lower limb   `CC`
L03.116   Cellulitis of left lower limb   `CC`
L03.119   Cellulitis of unspecified part of limb   `CC`

✓6ᵗʰ **L03.12**   Acute lymphangitis of other parts of limb
    EXCLUDES 2   *acute lymphangitis of fingers (L03.2-)*
           acute lymphangitis of groin (L03.324)
           acute lymphangitis of toes (L03.04-)
L03.121   Acute lymphangitis of right axilla   `CC`
L03.122   Acute lymphangitis of left axilla   `CC`
L03.123   Acute lymphangitis of right upper limb   `CC`
L03.124   Acute lymphangitis of left upper limb   `CC`
L03.125   Acute lymphangitis of right lower limb   `CC`
L03.126   Acute lymphangitis of left lower limb   `CC`
L03.129   Acute lymphangitis of unspecified part of limb   `CC`

✓5ᵗʰ **L03.2**   Cellulitis and acute lymphangitis of face and neck

✓6ᵗʰ **L03.21**   Cellulitis and acute lymphangitis of face
L03.211   Cellulitis of face   `CC`
    EXCLUDES 2   *abscess of orbit (H05.01-)*
           cellulitis of ear (H60.1-)
           cellulitis of eyelid (H00.0-)
           cellulitis of head (L03.81)
           cellulitis of lacrimal apparatus (H04.3)
           cellulitis of lip (K13.0)
           cellulitis of mouth (K12.2)
           cellulitis of nose (internal) (J34.0)
           cellulitis of orbit (H05.01-)
           cellulitis of scalp (L03.81)
    AHA: 2013,4Q,123
L03.212   Acute lymphangitis of face   `CC`
L03.213   Periorbital cellulitis   `CC`
    Preseptal cellulitis
    AHA: 2016,4Q,36

✓6ᵗʰ **L03.22**   Cellulitis and acute lymphangitis of neck
L03.221   Cellulitis of neck   `CC`
L03.222   Acute lymphangitis of neck   `CC`

✓5ᵗʰ **L03.3**   Cellulitis and acute lymphangitis of trunk

✓6ᵗʰ **L03.31**   Cellulitis of trunk
    EXCLUDES 2   *cellulitis of anal and rectal regions (K61.-)*
           cellulitis of breast NOS (N61.0)
           cellulitis of female external genital organs (N76.4)
           cellulitis of male external genital organs (N48.2, N49.-)
           omphalitis of newborn (P38.-)
           puerperal cellulitis of breast (O91.2)
L03.311   Cellulitis of abdominal wall   `CC`
    EXCLUDES 2   *cellulitis of umbilicus (L03.316)*
           cellulitis of groin (L03.314)
L03.312   Cellulitis of back [any part except buttock]   `CC`
L03.313   Cellulitis of chest wall   `CC`
L03.314   Cellulitis of groin   `CC`
L03.315   Cellulitis of perineum   `CC`
L03.316   Cellulitis of umbilicus   `CC`
L03.317   Cellulitis of buttock   `CC`
L03.319   Cellulitis of trunk, unspecified   `CC`

✓6ᵗʰ **L03.32**   Acute lymphangitis of trunk
L03.321   Acute lymphangitis of abdominal wall   `CC`
L03.322   Acute lymphangitis of back [any part except buttock]   `CC`
L03.323   Acute lymphangitis of chest wall   `CC`
L03.324   Acute lymphangitis of groin   `CC`
L03.325   Acute lymphangitis of perineum   `CC`
L03.326   Acute lymphangitis of umbilicus   `CC`
L03.327   Acute lymphangitis of buttock   `CC`

L03.329   Acute lymphangitis of trunk, unspecified   `CC`

✓5ᵗʰ **L03.8**   Cellulitis and acute lymphangitis of other sites

✓6ᵗʰ **L03.81**   Cellulitis of other sites
L03.811   Cellulitis of head [any part, except face]   `CC`
    Cellulitis of scalp
    EXCLUDES 2   *cellulitis of face (L03.211)*
L03.818   Cellulitis of other sites   `CC`

✓6ᵗʰ **L03.89**   Acute lymphangitis of other sites
L03.891   Acute lymphangitis of head [any part, except face]   `CC`
L03.898   Acute lymphangitis of other sites   `CC`

✓5ᵗʰ **L03.9**   Cellulitis and acute lymphangitis, unspecified
L03.90   Cellulitis, unspecified   `CC`
L03.91   Acute lymphangitis, unspecified   `CC`
    EXCLUDES 1   *lymphangitis NOS (I89.1)*

✓4ᵗʰ **L04**   **Acute lymphadenitis**
    INCLUDES   abscess (acute) of lymph nodes, except mesenteric
           acute lymphadenitis, except mesenteric
    EXCLUDES 1   *chronic or subacute lymphadenitis, except mesenteric (I88.1)*
           enlarged lymph nodes (R59.-)
           human immunodeficiency virus [HIV] disease resulting in generalized lymphadenopathy (B20)
           lymphadenitis NOS (I88.9)
           nonspecific mesenteric lymphadenitis (I88.0)
    DEF: Inflammation or enlargement of the lymph nodes.

L04.0   Acute lymphadenitis of face, head and neck
L04.1   Acute lymphadenitis of trunk
L04.2   Acute lymphadenitis of upper limb
    Acute lymphadenitis of axilla
    Acute lymphadenitis of shoulder
L04.3   Acute lymphadenitis of lower limb
    Acute lymphadenitis of hip
    EXCLUDES 2   *acute lymphadenitis of groin (L04.1)*
L04.8   Acute lymphadenitis of other sites
L04.9   Acute lymphadenitis, unspecified

✓4ᵗʰ **L05**   **Pilonidal cyst and sinus**
    DEF: Pilonidal cyst: Sac or sinus cavity of trapped epithelial tissues in the sacrococcygeal region, usually associated with ingrown hair.
    DEF: Pilonidal sinus: Fistula, tract, or channel that extends from an infected area of ingrown hair to another site within the skin or out to the skin surface.

Pilonidal Cyst

✓5ᵗʰ **L05.0**   Pilonidal cyst and sinus with abscess
L05.01   Pilonidal cyst with abscess   `CC` `SW`
    Pilonidal abscess
    Pilonidal dimple with abscess
    Postanal dimple with abscess
    EXCLUDES 2   *congenital sacral dimple (Q82.6)*
           parasacral dimple (Q82.6)
L05.02   Pilonidal sinus with abscess   `CC` `SW`
    Coccygeal fistula with abscess
    Coccygeal sinus with abscess
    Pilonidal fistula with abscess

N Newborn: 0   P Pediatric: 0-17   M Maternity: 9-64   A Adult: 15-124   MCC Major Complication/Comorbidity   CC Complication/Comorbidity   SW Severe Wound Dx

738   ICD-10-CM 2022

✓5th **L05.9** **Pilonidal cyst and sinus** without abscess

     L05.91 **Pilonidal** cyst **without abscess**
         Pilonidal dimple
         Postanal dimple
         Pilonidal cyst NOS
         EXCLUDES 2   *congenital sacral dimple (Q82.6)*
                   parasacral dimple (Q82.6)

     L05.92 **Pilonidal** sinus **without abscess**   `SW`
         Coccygeal fistula
         Coccygeal sinus without abscess
         Pilonidal fistula

✓4th **L08** **Other local infections of skin and subcutaneous tissue**

     L08.0 **Pyoderma**
         Dermatitis gangrenosa
         Purulent dermatitis
         Septic dermatitis
         Suppurative dermatitis
         EXCLUDES 1   *pyoderma gangrenosum (L88)*
                   pyoderma vegetans (L08.81)
         DEF: Any superficial skin disease commonly characterized by the discharging of pus not attributed to another condition.

     L08.1 **Erythrasma**   `HIV` `CC`
         DEF: Chronic, superficial skin infection of brown scaly patches, commonly found in skin folds most prevalent in the overweight or diabetic population.

✓5th **L08.8** **Other specified local infections of the skin and subcutaneous tissue**

     L08.81 **Pyoderma vegetans**
         EXCLUDES 1   *pyoderma gangrenosum (L88)*
                   pyoderma NOS (L08.0)

     L08.82 **Omphalitis not of newborn**
         EXCLUDES 1   *omphalitis of newborn (P38.-)*

     L08.89 **Other specified local infections of the skin and subcutaneous tissue**

     L08.9 **Local infection of the skin and subcutaneous tissue, unspecified**

Bullous disorders (L10-L14)

EXCLUDES 1   *benign familial pemphigus [Hailey-Hailey] (Q82.8)*
             staphylococcal scalded skin syndrome (L00)
             toxic epidermal necrolysis [Lyell] (L51.2)

✓4th **L10** **Pemphigus**

     EXCLUDES 1   *pemphigus neonatorum (L01.03)*

     L10.0 **Pemphigus** vulgaris   `CC`
     L10.1 **Pemphigus** vegetans   `CC`
     L10.2 **Pemphigus** foliaceous   `CC`
     L10.3 **Brazilian pemphigus [fogo selvagem]**   `CC`
     L10.4 **Pemphigus erythematosus**   `CC`
         Senear-Usher syndrome
     L10.5 **Drug-induced pemphigus**   `CC`
         Use additional code for adverse effect, if applicable, to identify drug (T36-T50 with fifth or sixth character 5)

✓5th **L10.8** **Other pemphigus**

     L10.81 **Paraneoplastic pemphigus**   `CC`
     L10.89 **Other pemphigus**   `CC`
     L10.9 **Pemphigus, unspecified**   `CC`

✓4th **L11** **Other acantholytic disorders**

     L11.0 **Acquired keratosis follicularis**
         EXCLUDES 1   *keratosis follicularis (congenital) [Darier-White]*
                   (Q82.8)
     L11.1 **Transient acantholytic dermatosis [Grover]**
     L11.8 **Other specified acantholytic disorders**
     L11.9 **Acantholytic disorder, unspecified**

✓4th **L12** **Pemphigoid**

     EXCLUDES 1   *herpes gestationis (O26.4-)*
                   impetigo herpetiformis (L40.1)

     L12.0 **Bullous pemphigoid**   `CC`
     L12.1 **Cicatricial pemphigoid**
         Benign mucous membrane pemphigoid
         DEF: Chronic autoimmune disease characterized by subepidermal blistering lesions of the mucosa, including the conjunctiva. It is seen predominantly in the elderly and produces adhesions and scarring.

     L12.2 **Chronic bullous disease of childhood**   `P`
         Juvenile dermatitis herpetiformis

✓5th **L12.3** **Acquired epidermolysis bullosa**

     EXCLUDES 1   *epidermolysis bullosa (congenital) (Q81.-)*

     L12.30 **Acquired epidermolysis bullosa, unspecified**   `CC` `HCC`
     L12.31 **Epidermolysis bullosa** due to drug   `CC` `HCC`
         Use additional code for adverse effect, if applicable, to identify drug (T36-T50 with fifth or sixth character 5)
     L12.35 **Other acquired epidermolysis bullosa**   `CC` `HCC`

     L12.8 **Other pemphigoid**   `CC`
     L12.9 **Pemphigoid, unspecified**   `CC`

✓4th **L13** **Other bullous disorders**

     L13.0 **Dermatitis herpetiformis**
         Duhring's disease
         Hydroa herpetiformis
         EXCLUDES 1   *juvenile dermatitis herpetiformis (L12.2)*
                   senile dermatitis herpetiformis (L12.0)
         DEF: Skin disease to which people are genetically predisposed resulting from an immunological response to gluten. Dermatitis herpetiformis is an extremely pruritic eruption of various lesions that frequently heal, leaving hyperpigmentation or hypopigmentation and occasionally scarring. It is usually associated with asymptomatic gluten-sensitive enteropathy.

     L13.1 **Subcorneal pustular dermatitis**
         Sneddon-Wilkinson disease
     L13.8 **Other specified bullous disorders**
     L13.9 **Bullous disorder, unspecified**

L14 *Bullous disorders in diseases classified elsewhere*
     Code first underlying disease

Dermatitis and eczema (L20-L30)

`NOTE`   In this block the terms dermatitis and eczema are used synonymously and interchangeably.

EXCLUDES 2   *chronic (childhood) granulomatous disease (D71)*
             dermatitis gangrenosa (L08.0)
             dermatitis herpetiformis (L13.0)
             dry skin dermatitis (L85.3)
             factitial dermatitis (L98.1)
             perioral dermatitis (L71.0)
             radiation-related disorders of the skin and subcutaneous tissue (L55-L59)
             stasis dermatitis (I87.2)

✓4th **L20** **Atopic dermatitis**

     L20.0 **Besnier's prurigo**

✓5th **L20.8** **Other atopic dermatitis**

     EXCLUDES 2   *circumscribed neurodermatitis (L28.0)*

     L20.81 **Atopic neurodermatitis**
         Diffuse neurodermatitis
     L20.82 **Flexural eczema**
     L20.83 **Infantile (acute) (chronic) eczema**   `P`
     L20.84 **Intrinsic (allergic) eczema**
     L20.89 **Other atopic dermatitis**
     L20.9 **Atopic dermatitis, unspecified**

✓4th **L21** **Seborrheic dermatitis**

     EXCLUDES 2   *infective dermatitis (L30.3)*
             seborrheic keratosis (L82.-)

     L21.0 **Seborrhea** capitis
         Cradle cap
         AHA: 2018,1Q,6
         TIP: Assign for dandruff in an adult patient.
     L21.1 **Seborrheic** infantile **dermatitis**   `P`
     L21.8 **Other seborrheic dermatitis**
     L21.9 **Seborrheic dermatitis, unspecified**
         Seborrhea NOS

     L22 **Diaper dermatitis**
         Diaper erythema
         Diaper rash
         Psoriasiform diaper rash

✔ Additional Character Required   ✓x7th Placeholder   Questionable PDx   Manifestation   Unspecified Dx   `UPD` Unacceptable PDx   `H1`-`H14` HAC   `HCC` CMS-HCC Dx   `HIV` HIV Dx

ICD-10-CM 2022   739

✓4ᵗʰ L23 Allergic contact dermatitis

EXCLUDES 1   *allergy NOS (T78.40)*
     contact dermatitis NOS (L25.9)
     dermatitis NOS (L30.9)

EXCLUDES 2   *dermatitis due to substances taken internally (L27.-)*
     dermatitis of eyelid (H01.1-)
     diaper dermatitis (L22)
     eczema of external ear (H60.5-)
     irritant contact dermatitis (L24.-)
     perioral dermatitis (L71.0)
     radiation-related disorders of the skin and subcutaneous tissue (L55-L59)

L23.0 Allergic contact dermatitis due to metals
   Allergic contact dermatitis due to chromium
   Allergic contact dermatitis due to nickel

L23.1 Allergic contact dermatitis due to adhesives

L23.2 Allergic contact dermatitis due to cosmetics

L23.3 Allergic contact dermatitis due to drugs in contact with skin
   Use additional code for adverse effect, if applicable, to identify drug (T36-T50 with fifth or sixth character 5)
     EXCLUDES 2   *dermatitis due to ingested drugs and medicaments (L27.0-L27.1)*

L23.4 Allergic contact dermatitis due to dyes

L23.5 Allergic contact dermatitis due to other chemical products
   Allergic contact dermatitis due to cement
   Allergic contact dermatitis due to insecticide
   Allergic contact dermatitis due to plastic
   Allergic contact dermatitis due to rubber

L23.6 Allergic contact dermatitis due to food in contact with the skin
     EXCLUDES 2   *dermatitis due to ingested food (L27.2)*

L23.7 Allergic contact dermatitis due to plants, except food
     EXCLUDES 2   *allergy NOS due to pollen (J30.1)*

✓5ᵗʰ L23.8 Allergic contact dermatitis due to other agents

   L23.81 Allergic contact dermatitis due to animal (cat) (dog) dander
     Allergic contact dermatitis due to animal (cat) (dog) hair

   L23.89 Allergic contact dermatitis due to other agents

L23.9 Allergic contact dermatitis, unspecified cause
   Allergic contact eczema NOS

✓4ᵗʰ L24 Irritant contact dermatitis

EXCLUDES 1   *allergy NOS (T78.40)*
     contact dermatitis NOS (L25.9)
     dermatitis NOS (L30.9)

EXCLUDES 2   *allergic contact dermatitis (L23.-)*
     dermatitis due to substances taken internally (L27.-)
     dermatitis of eyelid (H01.1-)
     diaper dermatitis (L22)
     eczema of external ear (H60.5-)
     perioral dermatitis (L71.0)
     radiation-related disorders of the skin and subcutaneous tissue (L55-L59)

L24.0 Irritant contact dermatitis due to detergents

L24.1 Irritant contact dermatitis due to oils and greases

L24.2 Irritant contact dermatitis due to solvents
   Irritant contact dermatitis due to chlorocompound
   Irritant contact dermatitis due to cyclohexane
   Irritant contact dermatitis due to ester
   Irritant contact dermatitis due to glycol
   Irritant contact dermatitis due to hydrocarbon
   Irritant contact dermatitis due to ketone

L24.3 Irritant contact dermatitis due to cosmetics

L24.4 Irritant contact dermatitis due to drugs in contact with skin
   Use additional code for adverse effect, if applicable, to identify drug (T36-T50 with fifth or sixth character 5)

L24.5 Irritant contact dermatitis due to other chemical products
   Irritant contact dermatitis due to cement
   Irritant contact dermatitis due to insecticide
   Irritant contact dermatitis due to plastic
   Irritant contact dermatitis due to rubber

L24.6 Irritant contact dermatitis due to food in contact with skin
     EXCLUDES 2   *dermatitis due to ingested food (L27.2)*

L24.7 Irritant contact dermatitis due to plants, except food
     EXCLUDES 2   *allergy NOS to pollen (J30.1)*

✓5ᵗʰ L24.8 Irritant contact dermatitis due to other agents

   L24.81 Irritant contact dermatitis due to metals
     Irritant contact dermatitis due to chromium
     Irritant contact dermatitis due to nickel

   L24.89 Irritant contact dermatitis due to other agents
     Irritant contact dermatitis due to dyes

L24.9 Irritant contact dermatitis, unspecified cause
   Irritant contact eczema NOS

● ✓5ᵗʰ L24.A Irritant contact dermatitis due to friction or contact with body fluids
     EXCLUDES 1   *irritant contact dermatitis related to stoma or fistula (L24.B-)*
     EXCLUDES 2   *erythema intertrigo (L30.4)*

   ● L24.A0 Irritant contact dermatitis due to friction or contact with body fluids, unspecified

   ● L24.A1 Irritant contact dermatitis due to saliva

   ● L24.A2 Irritant contact dermatitis due to fecal, urinary or dual incontinence
     EXCLUDES 1   *diaper dermatitis (L22)*

   ● L24.A9 Irritant contact dermatitis due friction or contact with other specified body fluids
     Irritant contact dermatitis related to endotracheal tube
     Wound fluids, exudate

● ✓5ᵗʰ L24.B Irritant contact dermatitis related to stoma or fistula
   Use additional code to identify any artificial opening status (Z93.-), if applicable, for contact dermatitis related to stoma secretions

   ● L24.B0 Irritant contact dermatitis related to unspecified stoma or fistula
     Irritant contact dermatitis related to fistula NOS
     Irritant contact dermatitis related to stoma NOS

   ● L24.B1 Irritant contact dermatitis related to digestive stoma or fistula
     Irritant contact dermatitis related to gastrostomy
     Irritant contact dermatitis related to jejunostomy
     Irritant contact dermatitis related to saliva or spit fistula

   ● L24.B2 Irritant contact dermatitis related to respiratory stoma or fistula
     Irritant contact dermatitis related to tracheostomy

   ● L24.B3 Irritant contact dermatitis related to fecal or urinary stoma or fistula
     Irritant contact dermatitis related to colostomy
     Irritant contact dermatitis related to enterocutaneous fistula
     Irritant contact dermatitis related to ileostomy

✓4ᵗʰ L25 Unspecified contact dermatitis

EXCLUDES 1   *allergic contact dermatitis (L23.-)*
     allergy NOS (T78.40)
     dermatitis NOS (L30.9)
     irritant contact dermatitis (L24.-)

EXCLUDES 2   *dermatitis due to ingested substances (L27.-)*
     dermatitis of eyelid (H01.1-)
     eczema of external ear (H60.5-)
     perioral dermatitis (L71.0)
     radiation-related disorders of the skin and subcutaneous tissue (L55-L59)

L25.0 Unspecified contact dermatitis due to cosmetics

L25.1 Unspecified contact dermatitis due to drugs in contact with skin
   Use additional code for adverse effect, if applicable, to identify drug (T36-T50 with fifth or sixth character 5)
     EXCLUDES 2   *dermatitis due to ingested drugs and medicaments (L27.0-L27.1)*

L25.2 Unspecified contact dermatitis due to dyes

L25.3 Unspecified contact dermatitis due to other chemical products
   Unspecified contact dermatitis due to cement
   Unspecified contact dermatitis due to insecticide

L25.4 Unspecified contact dermatitis due to food in contact with skin
     EXCLUDES 2   *dermatitis due to ingested food (L27.2)*

N Newborn: 0   P Pediatric: 0-17   M Maternity: 9-64   A Adult: 15-124   MCC Major Complication/Comorbidity   CC Complication/Comorbidity   SW Severe Wound Dx

740   ICD-10-CM 2022

L25.5 **Unspecified contact dermatitis due to** plants, except food
- EXCLUDES 1 nettle rash (L50.9)
- EXCLUDES 2 allergy NOS due to pollen (J30.1)

L25.8 **Unspecified contact dermatitis due to other agents**

L25.9 **Unspecified contact dermatitis, unspecified cause**
- Contact dermatitis (occupational) NOS
- Contact eczema (occupational) NOS

L26 Exfoliative dermatitis
- Hebra's pityriasis
- EXCLUDES 1 Ritter's disease (L00)

✓4ᵗʰ **L27 Dermatitis due to substances taken internally**
- EXCLUDES 1 allergy NOS (T78.40)
- EXCLUDES 2 adverse food reaction, except dermatitis (T78.0-T78.1)
  - contact dermatitis (L23-L25)
  - drug photoallergic response (L56.1)
  - drug phototoxic response (L56.0)
  - urticaria (L50.-)

L27.0 **Generalized skin eruption due to drugs and medicaments taken internally**
- Use additional code for adverse effect, if applicable, to identify drug (T36-T50 with fifth or sixth character 5)

L27.1 **Localized skin eruption due to drugs and medicaments taken internally**
- Use additional code for adverse effect, if applicable, to identify drug (T36-T50 with fifth or sixth character 5)

L27.2 **Dermatitis due to ingested food**
- EXCLUDES 2 dermatitis due to food in contact with skin (L23.6, L24.6, L25.4)

L27.8 **Dermatitis due to other substances taken internally**

L27.9 **Dermatitis due to unspecified substance taken internally**

✓4ᵗʰ **L28 Lichen simplex chronicus and prurigo**

L28.0 **Lichen simplex chronicus**
- Circumscribed neurodermatitis
- Lichen NOS

L28.1 **Prurigo nodularis**

L28.2 **Other prurigo**
- Prurigo NOS
- Prurigo Hebra
- Prurigo mitis
- Urticaria papulosa

✓4ᵗʰ **L29 Pruritus**
- EXCLUDES 1 neurotic excoriation (L98.1)
  - psychogenic pruritus (F45.8)

L29.0 **Pruritus ani**

L29.1 **Pruritus scroti**   ♂

L29.2 **Pruritus vulvae**   ♀

L29.3 **Anogenital pruritus, unspecified**

L29.8 **Other pruritus**

L29.9 **Pruritus, unspecified**
- Itch NOS

✓4ᵗʰ **L30 Other and unspecified dermatitis**
- EXCLUDES 2 contact dermatitis (L23-L25)
  - dry skin dermatitis (L85.3)
  - small plaque parapsoriasis (L41.3)
  - stasis dermatitis (I87.2)

L30.0 **Nummular dermatitis**

L30.1 **Dyshidrosis [pompholyx]**

L30.2 **Cutaneous autosensitization**
- Candidid [levurid]
- Dermatophytid
- Eczematid

L30.3 **Infective dermatitis**
- Infectious eczematoid dermatitis

L30.4 **Erythema intertrigo**

L30.5 **Pityriasis alba**
- AHA: 2018,1Q,6

L30.8 **Other specified dermatitis**

L30.9 **Dermatitis, unspecified**
- Eczema NOS

Papulosquamous disorders (L40-L45)

✓4ᵗʰ **L40 Psoriasis**
- **DEF:** Chronic autoimmune condition that speeds up skin cell growth, causing excessive immature skin cells to form raised, rounded erythematous lesions covered by dry, silvery scaling patches. Most commonly found on the scalp, elbows, knees, hands, feet, and genitals, it can also affect the joints with stiffness and swelling.

L40.0 **Psoriasis vulgaris**
- Nummular psoriasis
- Plaque psoriasis

L40.1 **Generalized pustular psoriasis**
- Impetigo herpetiformis
- Von Zumbusch's disease

L40.2 **Acrodermatitis continua**

L40.3 **Pustulosis palmaris et plantaris**

L40.4 **Guttate psoriasis**

✓5ᵗʰ **L40.5 Arthropathic psoriasis**
- L40.50 **Arthropathic psoriasis, unspecified**   HCC
- L40.51 **Distal interphalangeal psoriatic arthropathy**   HCC
- L40.52 **Psoriatic arthritis mutilans**   HCC
- L40.53 **Psoriatic spondylitis**   HCC
- L40.54 **Psoriatic juvenile arthropathy**   HCC
- L40.59 **Other psoriatic arthropathy**   HCC

L40.8 **Other psoriasis**
- Flexural psoriasis

L40.9 **Psoriasis, unspecified**

✓4ᵗʰ **L41 Parapsoriasis**
- EXCLUDES 1 poikiloderma vasculare atrophicans (L94.5)

L41.0 **Pityriasis lichenoides et varioliformis acuta**
- Mucha-Habermann disease

L41.1 **Pityriasis lichenoides chronica**

L41.3 **Small plaque parapsoriasis**

L41.4 **Large plaque parapsoriasis**

L41.5 **Retiform parapsoriasis**

L41.8 **Other parapsoriasis**

L41.9 **Parapsoriasis, unspecified**

L42 Pityriasis rosea

✓4ᵗʰ **L43 Lichen planus**
- EXCLUDES 1 lichen planopilaris (L66.1)

L43.0 **Hypertrophic lichen planus**

L43.1 **Bullous lichen planus**

L43.2 **Lichenoid drug reaction**
- Use additional code for adverse effect, if applicable, to identify drug (T36-T50 with fifth or sixth character 5)

L43.3 **Subacute (active) lichen planus**
- Lichen planus tropicus

L43.8 **Other lichen planus**

L43.9 **Lichen planus, unspecified**

✓4ᵗʰ **L44 Other papulosquamous disorders**

L44.0 **Pityriasis rubra pilaris**

L44.1 **Lichen nitidus**
- **DEF:** Chronic, inflammatory, asymptomatic skin disorder, characterized by numerous glistening, flat-topped, discrete, skin-colored micropapules, most often on the penis, lower abdomen, inner thighs, wrists, forearms, breasts, and buttocks.

L44.2 **Lichen striatus**

L44.3 **Lichen ruber moniliformis**

L44.4 **Infantile papular acrodermatitis [Gianotti-Crosti]**   P

L44.8 **Other specified papulosquamous disorders**

L44.9 **Papulosquamous disorder, unspecified**

L45 Papulosquamous disorders in diseases classified elsewhere
- Code first underlying disease

✔ Additional Character Required   ✓x7ᵗʰ Placeholder   Questionable PDx   Manifestation   Unspecified Dx   UPD Unacceptable PDx   H1 - H14 HAC   HCC CMS-HCC Dx   HIV HIV Dx

ICD-10-CM 2022   741

Chapter 12. Diseases of the Skin and Subcutaneous Tissue

L49–L55.9

Urticaria and erythema (L49-L54)

> EXCLUDES 1   Lyme disease (A69.2-)
> rosacea (L71.-)

✓4ᵗʰ **L49 Exfoliation due to erythematous conditions according to extent of body surface involved**

Code first erythematous condition causing exfoliation, such as:
Ritter's disease (L00)
(Staphylococcal) scalded skin syndrome (L00)
Stevens-Johnson syndrome (L51.1)
Stevens-Johnson syndrome-toxic epidermal necrolysis overlap syndrome (L51.3)
toxic epidermal necrolysis (L51.2)
DEF: Exfoliation: Falling or sloughing off skin in layers.

L49.0 Exfoliation due to erythematous condition involving less than 10 percent of body surface   UPD
Exfoliation due to erythematous condition NOS

L49.1 Exfoliation due to erythematous condition involving 10-19 percent of body surface   UPD

L49.2 Exfoliation due to erythematous condition involving 20-29 percent of body surface   UPD

L49.3 Exfoliation due to erythematous condition involving 30-39 percent of body surface   CC UPD

L49.4 Exfoliation due to erythematous condition involving 40-49 percent of body surface   CC UPD

L49.5 Exfoliation due to erythematous condition involving 50-59 percent of body surface   CC UPD

L49.6 Exfoliation due to erythematous condition involving 60-69 percent of body surface   CC UPD

L49.7 Exfoliation due to erythematous condition involving 70-79 percent of body surface   CC UPD

L49.8 Exfoliation due to erythematous condition involving 80-89 percent of body surface   CC UPD

L49.9 Exfoliation due to erythematous condition involving 90 or more percent of body surface   CC UPD

✓4ᵗʰ **L50 Urticaria**

> EXCLUDES 1   allergic contact dermatitis (L23.-)
> angioneurotic edema (T78.3)
> giant urticaria (T78.3)
> hereditary angio-edema (D84.1)
> Quincke's edema (T78.3)
> serum urticaria (T80.6-)
> solar urticaria (L56.3)
> urticaria neonatorum (P83.8)
> urticaria papulosa (L28.2)
> urticaria pigmentosa (D47.01)

DEF: Eruption of itching edema of the skin. **Synonym(s):** *hives.*

L50.0 Allergic urticaria

L50.1 Idiopathic urticaria

L50.2 Urticaria due to cold and heat
> EXCLUDES 2   familial cold urticaria (M04.2)

L50.3 Dermatographic urticaria

L50.4 Vibratory urticaria

L50.5 Cholinergic urticaria

L50.6 Contact urticaria

L50.8 Other urticaria
Chronic urticaria
Recurrent periodic urticaria

L50.9 Urticaria, unspecified

✓4ᵗʰ **L51 Erythema multiforme**

Use additional code for adverse effect, if applicable, to identify drug (T36-T50 with fifth or sixth character 5)
Use additional code to identify associated manifestations, such as:
arthropathy associated with dermatological disorders (M14.8-)
conjunctival edema (H11.42)
conjunctivitis (H10.22-)
corneal scars and opacities (H17.-)
corneal ulcer (H16.0-)
edema of eyelid (H02.84-)
inflammation of eyelid (H01.8)
keratoconjunctivitis sicca (H16.22-)
mechanical lagophthalmos (H02.22-)
stomatitis (K12.-)
symblepharon (H11.23-)
Use additional code to identify percentage of skin exfoliation (L49.-)

> EXCLUDES 1   staphylococcal scalded skin syndrome (L00)
> Ritter's disease (L00)

DEF: Acute complex of symptoms with a varied pattern of skin eruptions, such as macular, bullous, papular, nodose, or vesicular lesions on the neck, face, and legs. Erythema (redness of skin and mucous membranes) multiforme (multiple forms) is a hypersensitivity (allergic) reaction that can occur at any age but primarily affects children or young adults.

L51.0 Nonbullous erythema multiforme

L51.1 Stevens-Johnson syndrome   CC HCC

L51.2 Toxic epidermal necrolysis [Lyell]   CC HCC

L51.3 Stevens-Johnson syndrome-toxic epidermal necrolysis overlap syndrome   CC HCC
SJS-TEN overlap syndrome

L51.8 Other erythema multiforme

L51.9 Erythema multiforme, unspecified
Erythema iris
Erythema multiforme major NOS
Erythema multiforme minor NOS
Herpes iris

L52 Erythema nodosum

> EXCLUDES 1   tuberculous erythema nodosum (A18.4)

DEF: Form of panniculitis (inflammation of the fat layer beneath the skin) most often occurring in women. Commonly seen as a hypersensitivity reaction to infections, drugs, sarcoidosis, and specific enteropathies. The acute stage is associated with fever, malaise, and arthralgia. The lesions are pink to blue in color as tender nodules and are found on the front of the legs below the knees.

✓4ᵗʰ **L53 Other erythematous conditions**

> EXCLUDES 1   erythema ab igne (L59.0)
> erythema due to external agents in contact with skin (L23-L25)
> erythema intertrigo (L30.4)

L53.0 Toxic erythema   CC
Code first poisoning due to drug or toxin, if applicable (T36-T65 with fifth or sixth character 1-4 or 6)
Use additional code for adverse effect, if applicable, to identify drug (T36-T50 with fifth or sixth character 5)
> EXCLUDES 1   neonatal erythema toxicum (P83.1)

L53.1 Erythema annulare centrifugum   CC

L53.2 Erythema marginatum   CC

L53.3 Other chronic figurate erythema   CC

L53.8 Other specified erythematous conditions

L53.9 Erythematous condition, unspecified
Erythema NOS
Erythroderma NOS

L54 *Erythema in diseases classified elsewhere*
Code first underlying disease

Radiation-related disorders of the skin and subcutaneous tissue (L55-L59)

✓4ᵗʰ **L55 Sunburn**

L55.0 Sunburn of first degree

L55.1 Sunburn of second degree

L55.2 Sunburn of third degree

L55.9 Sunburn, unspecified

N Newborn: 0   P Pediatric: 0-17   M Maternity: 9-64   A Adult: 15-124   MCC Major Complication/Comorbidity   CC Complication/Comorbidity   SW Severe Wound Dx

742   ICD-10-CM 2022

✓4ᵗʰ L56　Other acute skin changes due to ultraviolet radiation

Use additional code to identify the source of the ultraviolet radiation (W89, X32)

L56.0　Drug phototoxic response

Use additional code for adverse effect, if applicable, to identify drug (T36-T50 with fifth or sixth character 5)

L56.1　Drug photoallergic response

Use additional code for adverse effect, if applicable, to identify drug (T36-T50 with fifth or sixth character 5)

L56.2　Photocontact dermatitis [berloque dermatitis]

L56.3　Solar urticaria

L56.4　Polymorphous light eruption

L56.5　Disseminated superficial actinic porokeratosis (DSAP)

DEF: Autosomal dominant skin condition occurring in sun-exposed areas of the skin (particularly the arms and legs), characterized by superficial annular, keratotic, brownish-red spots or thickenings with depressed centers and sharp, ridged borders. It may evolve into squamous cell carcinoma.

L56.8　Other specified acute skin changes due to ultraviolet radiation

L56.9　Acute skin change due to ultraviolet radiation, unspecified

✓4ᵗʰ L57　Skin changes due to chronic exposure to nonionizing radiation

Use additional code to identify the source of the ultraviolet radiation (W89), or other nonionizing radiation (W90)

L57.0　Actinic keratosis

Keratosis NOS
Senile keratosis
Solar keratosis

L57.1　Actinic reticuloid

L57.2　Cutis rhomboidalis nuchae

L57.3　Poikiloderma of Civatte

L57.4　Cutis laxa senilis

Elastosis senilis

L57.5　Actinic granuloma

L57.8　Other skin changes due to chronic exposure to nonionizing radiation

Farmer's skin
Sailor's skin
Solar dermatitis

L57.9　Skin changes due to chronic exposure to nonionizing radiation, unspecified

✓4ᵗʰ L58　Radiodermatitis

Use additional code to identify the source of the radiation (W88, W90)

L58.0　Acute radiodermatitis

L58.1　Chronic radiodermatitis

L58.9　Radiodermatitis, unspecified

✓4ᵗʰ L59　Other disorders of skin and subcutaneous tissue related to radiation

L59.0　Erythema ab igne [dermatitis ab igne]

L59.8　Other specified disorders of the skin and subcutaneous tissue related to radiation

AHA: 2017,1Q,33

L59.9　Disorder of the skin and subcutaneous tissue related to radiation, unspecified

Disorders of skin appendages (L60-L75)

EXCLUDES 1　congenital malformations of integument (Q84.-)

✓4ᵗʰ L60　Nail disorders

EXCLUDES 2　clubbing of nails (R68.3)
onychia and paronychia (L03.0-)

Nail Disorders

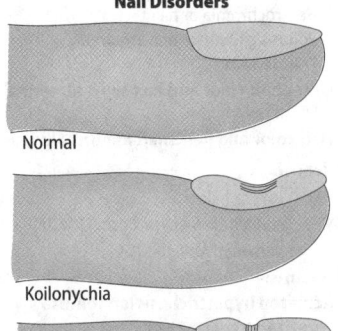

Normal

Koilonychia

Beau's Lines

L60.0　Ingrowing nail

L60.1　Onycholysis

L60.2　Onychogryphosis

L60.3　Nail dystrophy

L60.4　Beau's lines

L60.5　Yellow nail syndrome

L60.8　Other nail disorders

L60.9　Nail disorder, unspecified

L62　*Nail disorders in diseases classified elsewhere*

Code first underlying disease, such as:
pachydermoperiostosis (M89.4-)

✓4ᵗʰ L63　Alopecia areata

L63.0　Alopecia (capitis) totalis

L63.1　Alopecia universalis

L63.2　Ophiasis

L63.8　Other alopecia areata

L63.9　Alopecia areata, unspecified

✓4ᵗʰ L64　Androgenic alopecia

INCLUDES　male-pattern baldness

L64.0　Drug-induced androgenic alopecia

Use additional code for adverse effect, if applicable, to identify drug (T36-T50 with fifth or sixth character 5)

L64.8　Other androgenic alopecia

L64.9　Androgenic alopecia, unspecified

✓4ᵗʰ L65　Other nonscarring hair loss

Use additional code for adverse effect, if applicable, to identify drug (T36-T50 with fifth or sixth character 5)

EXCLUDES 1　trichotillomania (F63.3)

L65.0　Telogen effluvium

DEF: Form of nonscarring alopecia characterized by shedding of hair from premature telogen development in follicles due to stress, including shock, childbirth, surgery, drugs, or weight loss.

L65.1　Anagen effluvium

L65.2　Alopecia mucinosa

L65.8　Other specified nonscarring hair loss

L65.9　Nonscarring hair loss, unspecified

Alopecia NOS

✓4ᵗʰ L66　Cicatricial alopecia [scarring hair loss]

L66.0　Pseudopelade

L66.1　Lichen planopilaris

Follicular lichen planus

L66.2　Folliculitis decalvans

L66.3　Perifolliculitis capitis abscedens

L66.4　Folliculitis ulerythematosa reticulata

L66.8　Other cicatricial alopecia

AHA: 2015,1Q,19

L66.9　Cicatricial alopecia, unspecified

✓ Additional Character Required　　✓x7ᵗʰ Placeholder　　Questionable PDx　　Manifestation　　Unspecified Dx　　UPD Unacceptable PDx　　H1 - H14 HAC　　HCC CMS-HCC Dx　　HIV HIV Dx

ICD-10-CM 2022　　743

Chapter 12. Diseases of the Skin and Subcutaneous Tissue

L56–L66.9

Chapter 12. Diseases of the Skin and Subcutaneous Tissue

L67–L76.22

☑4ᵗʰ **L67 Hair color and hair shaft abnormalities**

     EXCLUDES 1   *monilethrix (Q84.1)*
                 pili annulati (Q84.1)
                 telogen effluvium (L65.0)

   L67.0 Trichorrhexis nodosa

   L67.1 Variations in hair color
         Canities
         Greyness, hair (premature)
         Heterochromia of hair
         Poliosis circumscripta, acquired
         Poliosis NOS

   L67.8 Other hair color and hair shaft abnormalities
         Fragilitas crinium

   L67.9 Hair color and hair shaft abnormality, unspecified

☑4ᵗʰ **L68 Hypertrichosis**

     INCLUDES   excess hair
     EXCLUDES 1   *congenital hypertrichosis (Q84.2)*
                 persistent lanugo (Q84.2)

   L68.0 Hirsutism
   L68.1 Acquired hypertrichosis lanuginosa
   L68.2 Localized hypertrichosis
   L68.3 Polytrichia
   L68.8 Other hypertrichosis
   L68.9 Hypertrichosis, unspecified

☑4ᵗʰ **L70 Acne**

     EXCLUDES 2   *acne keloid (L73.0)*

   L70.0 Acne vulgaris
   L70.1 Acne conglobata
   L70.2 Acne varioliformis
         Acne necrotica miliaris
         DEF: Rare form of acne characterized by development of persistent brown papulopustules followed by scar formation. This type of acne usually presents on the brow and temporoparietal part of the scalp.
   L70.3 Acne tropica
   L70.4 Infantile acne   P
   L70.5 Acné excoriée
         Acné excoriée des jeunes filles
         Picker's acne
   L70.8 Other acne
   L70.9 Acne, unspecified

☑4ᵗʰ **L71 Rosacea**

     Use additional code for adverse effect, if applicable, to identify drug (T36-T50 with fifth or sixth character 5)

   L71.0 Perioral dermatitis
   L71.1 Rhinophyma
   L71.8 Other rosacea
         AHA: 2018,4Q,15
   L71.9 Rosacea, unspecified

☑4ᵗʰ **L72 Follicular cysts of skin and subcutaneous tissue**

   L72.0 Epidermal cyst
   ☑5ᵗʰ **L72.1 Pilar and trichodermal cyst**
       L72.11 Pilar cyst
       L72.12 Trichodermal cyst
           Trichilemmal (proliferating) cyst
   L72.2 Steatocystoma multiplex
   L72.3 Sebaceous cyst
       EXCLUDES 2   *pilar cyst (L72.11)*
                  trichilemmal (proliferating) cyst (L72.12)
   L72.8 Other follicular cysts of the skin and subcutaneous tissue
   L72.9 Follicular cyst of the skin and subcutaneous tissue, unspecified

☑4ᵗʰ **L73 Other follicular disorders**

   L73.0 Acne keloid
   L73.1 Pseudofolliculitis barbae
   L73.2 Hidradenitis suppurativa
   L73.8 Other specified follicular disorders
         Sycosis barbae
   L73.9 Follicular disorder, unspecified

☑4ᵗʰ **L74 Eccrine sweat disorders**

     EXCLUDES 2   *generalized hyperhidrosis (R61)*
     DEF: Eccrine sweat glands: Glands found in the dermal and hypodermal layer of the skin throughout the body, particularly on the forehead, scalp, axillae, palms, and soles. These glands produce watery and neutral or slightly acidic sweat.

   L74.0 Miliaria rubra
   L74.1 Miliaria crystallina
   L74.2 Miliaria profunda
         Miliaria tropicalis
   L74.3 Miliaria, unspecified
   L74.4 Anhidrosis
         Hypohidrosis
         DEF: Inability to sweat normally. When the body can't cool itself through perspiration it can lead to heatstroke, a life-threatening condition.
   ☑5ᵗʰ **L74.5 Focal hyperhidrosis**
       ☑6ᵗʰ **L74.51 Primary focal hyperhidrosis**
           L74.510 Primary focal hyperhidrosis, axilla
           L74.511 Primary focal hyperhidrosis, face
           L74.512 Primary focal hyperhidrosis, palms
           L74.513 Primary focal hyperhidrosis, soles
           L74.519 Primary focal hyperhidrosis, unspecified
       L74.52 Secondary focal hyperhidrosis
           Frey's syndrome
   L74.8 Other eccrine sweat disorders
   L74.9 Eccrine sweat disorder, unspecified
         Sweat gland disorder NOS

☑4ᵗʰ **L75 Apocrine sweat disorders**

     EXCLUDES 1   *dyshidrosis (L30.1)*
                 hidradenitis suppurativa (L73.2)
     DEF: Apocrine sweat glands: Found in the axilla, areola, and circumanal region, these glands begin to function in puberty and produce viscid milky secretions in response to external stimuli.

   L75.0 Bromhidrosis
   L75.1 Chromhidrosis
   L75.2 Apocrine miliaria
         Fox-Fordyce disease
         DEF: Chronic, usually pruritic disease evidenced by small follicular papular eruptions, especially in the axillary and pubic areas. Apocrine miliaria develops from the closure and rupture of the affected apocrine glands' intraepidermal portion of the ducts.
   L75.8 Other apocrine sweat disorders
   L75.9 Apocrine sweat disorder, unspecified

Intraoperative and postprocedural complications of skin and subcutaneous tissue (L76)

☑4ᵗʰ **L76 Intraoperative and postprocedural complications of skin and subcutaneous tissue**

     AHA: 2016,4Q,9-10

   ☑5ᵗʰ **L76.0 Intraoperative hemorrhage and hematoma of skin and subcutaneous tissue complicating a procedure**
       EXCLUDES 1   *intraoperative hemorrhage and hematoma of skin and subcutaneous tissue due to accidental puncture and laceration during a procedure (L76.1-)*
       L76.01 Intraoperative hemorrhage and hematoma of skin and subcutaneous tissue complicating a dermatologic procedure   CC
       L76.02 Intraoperative hemorrhage and hematoma of skin and subcutaneous tissue complicating other procedure   CC
   ☑5ᵗʰ **L76.1 Accidental puncture and laceration of skin and subcutaneous tissue during a procedure**
       L76.11 Accidental puncture and laceration of skin and subcutaneous tissue during a dermatologic procedure   CC
       L76.12 Accidental puncture and laceration of skin and subcutaneous tissue during other procedure   CC
   ☑5ᵗʰ **L76.2 Postprocedural hemorrhage of skin and subcutaneous tissue following a procedure**
       L76.21 Postprocedural hemorrhage of skin and subcutaneous tissue following a dermatologic procedure   CC
       L76.22 Postprocedural hemorrhage of skin and subcutaneous tissue following other procedure   CC

N Newborn: 0   P Pediatric: 0-17   M Maternity: 9-64   A Adult: 15-124   MCC Major Complication/Comorbidity   CC Complication/Comorbidity   SW Severe Wound Dx

744   ICD-10-CM 2022

✓5ᵗʰ L76.3 Postprocedural hematoma and seroma of skin and subcutaneous tissue following a procedure

  L76.31 Postprocedural hematoma of skin and subcutaneous tissue following a dermatologic procedure   CC

  L76.32 Postprocedural hematoma of skin and subcutaneous tissue following other procedure   CC

  L76.33 Postprocedural seroma of skin and subcutaneous tissue following a dermatologic procedure   CC

  L76.34 Postprocedural seroma of skin and subcutaneous tissue following other procedure   CC

✓5ᵗʰ L76.8 Other intraoperative and postprocedural complications of skin and subcutaneous tissue

  Use additional code, if applicable, to further specify disorder

  L76.81 Other intraoperative complications of skin and subcutaneous tissue

  L76.82 Other postprocedural complications of skin and subcutaneous tissue

    AHA: 2017,3Q,6

Other disorders of the skin and subcutaneous tissue (L80-L99)

L80 Vitiligo

  EXCLUDES 2   vitiligo of eyelids (H02.73-)
           vitiligo of vulva (N90.89)

  DEF: Persistent, progressive development of nonpigmented white patches on otherwise normal skin.

✓4ᵗʰ L81 Other disorders of pigmentation

  EXCLUDES 1   birthmark NOS (Q82.5)
           Peutz-Jeghers syndrome (Q85.8)

  EXCLUDES 2   nevus - see Alphabetical Index

  L81.0 Postinflammatory hyperpigmentation

  L81.1 Chloasma

  L81.2 Freckles

  L81.3 Café au lait spots

  L81.4 Other melanin hyperpigmentation
    Lentigo

  L81.5 Leukoderma, not elsewhere classified

  L81.6 Other disorders of diminished melanin formation

  L81.7 Pigmented purpuric dermatosis
    Angioma serpiginosum

  L81.8 Other specified disorders of pigmentation
    Iron pigmentation
    Tattoo pigmentation

  L81.9 Disorder of pigmentation, unspecified

✓4ᵗʰ L82 Seborrheic keratosis

  INCLUDES   basal cell papilloma
           dermatosis papulosa nigra
           Leser-Trélat disease

  EXCLUDES 2   seborrheic dermatitis (L21.-)

  DEF: Common, benign, noninvasive, lightly pigmented, warty growth composed of basaloid cells that usually appear at middle age as soft, easily crumbling plaques on the face, trunk, and extremities.

  L82.0 Inflamed seborrheic keratosis

  L82.1 Other seborrheic keratosis
    Seborrheic keratosis NOS

L83 Acanthosis nigricans

  Confluent and reticulated papillomatosis

  DEF: Diffuse, velvety hyperplasia of the spinous skin layer of the axilla and other body folds marked by gray, brown, or black pigmentation. In adult form, it is often associated with malignant acanthosis nigricans in a benign, nevoid form relatively generalized.

L84 Corns and callosities
  Callus
  Clavus

✓4ᵗʰ L85 Other epidermal thickening

  EXCLUDES 2   hypertrophic disorders of the skin (L91.-)

  L85.0 Acquired ichthyosis
    EXCLUDES 1   congenital ichthyosis (Q80.-)

  L85.1 Acquired keratosis [keratoderma] palmaris et plantaris
    EXCLUDES 1   inherited keratosis palmaris et plantaris (Q82.8)

  L85.2 Keratosis punctata (palmaris et plantaris)

  L85.3 Xerosis cutis
    Dry skin dermatitis

  L85.8 Other specified epidermal thickening
    Cutaneous horn

  L85.9 Epidermal thickening, unspecified

L86 Keratoderma in diseases classified elsewhere

  Code first underlying disease, such as:
    Reiter's disease (M02.3-)

  EXCLUDES 1   gonococcal keratoderma (A54.89)
           gonococcal keratosis (A54.89)
           keratoderma due to vitamin A deficiency (E50.8)
           keratosis due to vitamin A deficiency (E50.8)
           xeroderma due to vitamin A deficiency (E50.8)

✓4ᵗʰ L87 Transepidermal elimination disorders

  EXCLUDES 1   granuloma annulare (perforating) (L92.0)

  L87.0 Keratosis follicularis et parafollicularis in cutem penetrans
    Hyperkeratosis follicularis penetrans
    Kyrle disease

  L87.1 Reactive perforating collagenosis

  L87.2 Elastosis perforans serpiginosa

  L87.8 Other transepidermal elimination disorders

  L87.9 Transepidermal elimination disorder, unspecified

L88 Pyoderma gangrenosum   CC
  Phagedenic pyoderma

  EXCLUDES 1   dermatitis gangrenosa (L08.0)

  DEF: Persistent debilitating skin disease characterized by irregular, boggy, blue-red ulcerations, with central healing and undermined edges.

✓4ᵗʰ L89 Pressure ulcer

  INCLUDES   bed sore
           decubitus ulcer
           plaster ulcer
           pressure area
           pressure sore

  Code first any associated gangrene (I96)

  EXCLUDES 2   decubitus (trophic) ulcer of cervix (uteri) (N86)
           diabetic ulcers (E08.621, E08.622, E09.621, E09.622, E10.621, E10.622, E11.621, E11.622, E13.621, E13.622)
           non-pressure chronic ulcer of skin (L97.-)
           skin infections (L00-L08)
           varicose ulcer (I83.0, I83.2)

  AHA: 2021,1Q,24; 2019,4Q,10-11,54; 2018,4Q,69; 2018,3Q,3; 2018,2Q,21; 2017,4Q,109; 2017,1Q,49; 2016,4Q,143

  TIP: The stage of a diagnosed pressure ulcer can be based on documentation from clinicians who are not the patient's provider.

Four Stages of Pressure Ulcer

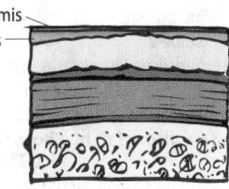
Epidermis
Dermis
Stage 1
Persistent focal edema

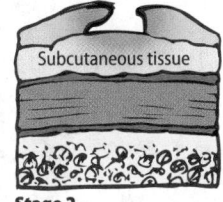
Subcutaneous tissue
Stage 2
Abrasion, blister, partial thickness skin loss involving epidermis and/or dermis

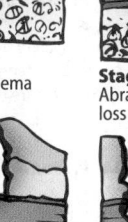
Superficial fascia
Muscle
Stage 3
Full thickness skin loss involving damage or necrosis of subcutaneous tissue

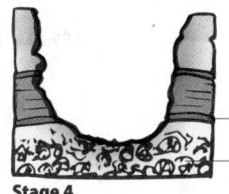
Deep fascia
Bone
Stage 4
Necrosis of soft tissues through to underlying muscle, tendon, or bone

  ✓5ᵗʰ L89.0 Pressure ulcer of elbow

    ✓6ᵗʰ L89.00 Pressure ulcer of unspecified elbow

      L89.000 Pressure ulcer of unspecified elbow, unstageable   HCC   SW

☑ Additional Character Required   ✓x7ᵗʰ Placeholder   Questionable PDx   Manifestation   Unspecified Dx   UPD Unacceptable PDx   H1 - H14 HAC   HCC CMS-HCC Dx   HIV HIV Dx

ICD-10-CM 2022   745

L89.001   **Pressure ulcer of unspecified elbow, stage 1**
> Healing pressure ulcer of unspecified elbow, stage 1
> Pressure pre-ulcer skin changes limited to persistent focal edema, unspecified elbow

L89.002   **Pressure ulcer of unspecified elbow, stage 2**   `HCC`
> Healing pressure ulcer of unspecified elbow, stage 2
> Pressure ulcer with abrasion, blister, partial thickness skin loss involving epidermis and/or dermis, unspecified elbow

L89.003   **Pressure ulcer of unspecified elbow, stage 3**   `MCC` `H4` `HCC` `SW`
> Healing pressure ulcer of unspecified elbow, stage 3
> Pressure ulcer with full thickness skin loss involving damage or necrosis of subcutaneous tissue, unspecified elbow

L89.004   **Pressure ulcer of unspecified elbow, stage 4**   `MCC` `H4` `HCC` `SW`
> Healing pressure ulcer of unspecified elbow, stage 4
> Pressure ulcer with necrosis of soft tissues through to underlying muscle, tendon, or bone, unspecified elbow

L89.006   **Pressure-induced deep tissue damage of unspecified elbow**

L89.009   **Pressure ulcer of unspecified elbow, unspecified stage**
> Healing pressure ulcer of elbow NOS
> Healing pressure ulcer of unspecified elbow, unspecified stage

√6ᵗʰ   **L89.01**   **Pressure ulcer of right elbow**

L89.010   **Pressure ulcer of right elbow, unstageable**   `HCC` `SW`

L89.011   **Pressure ulcer of right elbow, stage 1**
> Healing pressure ulcer of right elbow, stage 1
> Pressure pre-ulcer skin changes limited to persistent focal edema, right elbow

L89.012   **Pressure ulcer of right elbow, stage 2**   `HCC`
> Healing pressure ulcer of right elbow, stage 2
> Pressure ulcer with abrasion, blister, partial thickness skin loss involving epidermis and/or dermis, right elbow

L89.013   **Pressure ulcer of right elbow, stage 3**   `MCC` `H4` `HCC` `SW`
> Healing pressure ulcer of right elbow, stage 3
> Pressure ulcer with full thickness skin loss involving damage or necrosis of subcutaneous tissue, right elbow

L89.014   **Pressure ulcer of right elbow, stage 4**   `MCC` `H4` `HCC` `SW`
> Healing pressure ulcer of right elbow, stage 4
> Pressure ulcer with necrosis of soft tissues through to underlying muscle, tendon, or bone, right elbow

L89.016   **Pressure-induced deep tissue damage of right elbow**

L89.019   **Pressure ulcer of right elbow, unspecified stage**
> ►Healing pressure ulcer of right elbow NOS◄
> Healing pressure ulcer of right elbow, unspecified stage

√6ᵗʰ   **L89.02**   **Pressure ulcer of left elbow**

L89.020   **Pressure ulcer of left elbow, unstageable**   `HCC` `SW`

L89.021   **Pressure ulcer of left elbow, stage 1**
> Healing pressure ulcer of left elbow, stage 1
> Pressure pre-ulcer skin changes limited to persistent focal edema, left elbow

L89.022   **Pressure ulcer of left elbow, stage 2**   `HCC`
> Healing pressure ulcer of left elbow, stage 2
> Pressure ulcer with abrasion, blister, partial thickness skin loss involving epidermis and/or dermis, left elbow

L89.023   **Pressure ulcer of left elbow, stage 3**   `MCC` `H4` `HCC` `SW`
> Healing pressure ulcer of left elbow, stage 3
> Pressure ulcer with full thickness skin loss involving damage or necrosis of subcutaneous tissue, left elbow

L89.024   **Pressure ulcer of left elbow, stage 4**   `MCC` `H4` `HCC` `SW`
> Healing pressure ulcer of left elbow, stage 4
> Pressure ulcer with necrosis of soft tissues through to underlying muscle, tendon, or bone, left elbow

L89.026   **Pressure-induced deep tissue damage of left elbow**

L89.029   **Pressure ulcer of left elbow, unspecified stage**
> ►Healing pressure ulcer of left elbow NOS◄
> Healing pressure ulcer of left elbow, unspecified stage

√5ᵗʰ   **L89.1**   **Pressure ulcer of back**

√6ᵗʰ   **L89.10**   **Pressure ulcer of unspecified part of back**

L89.100   **Pressure ulcer of unspecified part of back, unstageable**   `HCC` `SW`

L89.101   **Pressure ulcer of unspecified part of back, stage 1**
> Healing pressure ulcer of unspecified part of back, stage 1
> Pressure pre-ulcer skin changes limited to persistent focal edema, unspecified part of back

L89.102   **Pressure ulcer of unspecified part of back, stage 2**   `HCC`
> Healing pressure ulcer of unspecified part of back, stage 2
> Pressure ulcer with abrasion, blister, partial thickness skin loss involving epidermis and/or dermis, unspecified part of back

L89.103   **Pressure ulcer of unspecified part of back, stage 3**   `MCC` `H4` `HCC` `SW`
> Healing pressure ulcer of unspecified part of back, stage 3
> Pressure ulcer with full thickness skin loss involving damage or necrosis of subcutaneous tissue, unspecified part of back

L89.104   **Pressure ulcer of unspecified part of back, stage 4**   `MCC` `H4` `HCC` `SW`
> Healing pressure ulcer of unspecified part of back, stage 4
> Pressure ulcer with necrosis of soft tissues through to underlying muscle, tendon, or bone, unspecified part of back

L89.106   **Pressure-induced deep tissue damage of unspecified part of back**

L89.109   **Pressure ulcer of unspecified part of back, unspecified stage**
> Healing pressure ulcer of unspecified part of back NOS
> Healing pressure ulcer of unspecified part of back, unspecified stage

√6ᵗʰ **L89.11**   **Pressure ulcer of right upper back**

Pressure ulcer of right shoulder blade

L89.110   **Pressure ulcer of right upper back, unstageable**   HCC SW

L89.111   **Pressure ulcer of right upper back, stage 1**

Healing pressure ulcer of right upper back, stage 1

Pressure pre-ulcer skin changes limited to persistent focal edema, right upper back

L89.112   **Pressure ulcer of right upper back, stage 2**   HCC

Healing pressure ulcer of right upper back, stage 2

Pressure ulcer with abrasion, blister, partial thickness skin loss involving epidermis and/or dermis, right upper back

L89.113   **Pressure ulcer of right upper back, stage 3**   MCC H4 HCC SW

Healing pressure ulcer of right upper back, stage 3

Pressure ulcer with full thickness skin loss involving damage or necrosis of subcutaneous tissue, right upper back

L89.114   **Pressure ulcer of right upper back, stage 4**   MCC H4 HCC SW

Healing pressure ulcer of right upper back, stage 4

Pressure ulcer with necrosis of soft tissues through to underlying muscle, tendon, or bone, right upper back

L89.116   **Pressure-induced deep tissue damage of right upper back**

L89.119   **Pressure ulcer of right upper back, unspecified stage**

Healing pressure ulcer of right upper back NOS

Healing pressure ulcer of right upper back, unspecified stage

√6ᵗʰ **L89.12**   **Pressure ulcer of left upper back**

Pressure ulcer of left shoulder blade

L89.120   **Pressure ulcer of left upper back, unstageable**   HCC SW

L89.121   **Pressure ulcer of left upper back, stage 1**

Healing pressure ulcer of left upper back, stage 1

Pressure pre-ulcer skin changes limited to persistent focal edema, left upper back

L89.122   **Pressure ulcer of left upper back, stage 2**   HCC

Healing pressure ulcer of left upper back, stage 2

Pressure ulcer with abrasion, blister, partial thickness skin loss involving epidermis and/or dermis, left upper back

L89.123   **Pressure ulcer of left upper back, stage 3**   MCC H4 HCC SW

Healing pressure ulcer of left upper back, stage 3

Pressure ulcer with full thickness skin loss involving damage or necrosis of subcutaneous tissue, left upper back

L89.124   **Pressure ulcer of left upper back, stage 4**   MCC H4 HCC SW

Healing pressure ulcer of left upper back, stage 4

Pressure ulcer with necrosis of soft tissues through to underlying muscle, tendon, or bone, left upper back

L89.126   **Pressure-induced deep tissue damage of left upper back**

L89.129   **Pressure ulcer of left upper back, unspecified stage**

Healing pressure ulcer of left upper back NOS

Healing pressure ulcer of left upper back, unspecified stage

√6ᵗʰ **L89.13**   **Pressure ulcer of right lower back**

L89.130   **Pressure ulcer of right lower back, unstageable**   HCC SW

L89.131   **Pressure ulcer of right lower back, stage 1**

Healing pressure ulcer of right lower back, stage 1

Pressure pre-ulcer skin changes limited to persistent focal edema, right lower back

L89.132   **Pressure ulcer of right lower back, stage 2**   HCC

Healing pressure ulcer of right lower back, stage 2

Pressure ulcer with abrasion, blister, partial thickness skin loss involving epidermis and/or dermis, right lower back

L89.133   **Pressure ulcer of right lower back, stage 3**   MCC H4 HCC SW

Healing pressure ulcer of right lower back, stage 3

Pressure ulcer with full thickness skin loss involving damage or necrosis of subcutaneous tissue, right lower back

L89.134   **Pressure ulcer of right lower back, stage 4**   MCC H4 HCC SW

Healing pressure ulcer of right lower back, stage 4

Pressure ulcer with necrosis of soft tissues through to underlying muscle, tendon, or bone, right lower back

L89.136   **Pressure-induced deep tissue damage of right lower back**

L89.139   **Pressure ulcer of right lower back, unspecified stage**

Healing pressure ulcer of right lower back NOS

Healing pressure ulcer of right lower back, unspecified stage

√6ᵗʰ **L89.14**   **Pressure ulcer of left lower back**

L89.140   **Pressure ulcer of left lower back, unstageable**   HCC SW

L89.141   **Pressure ulcer of left lower back, stage 1**

Healing pressure ulcer of left lower back, stage 1

Pressure pre-ulcer skin changes limited to persistent focal edema, left lower back

L89.142   **Pressure ulcer of left lower back, stage 2**   HCC

Healing pressure ulcer of left lower back, stage 2

Pressure ulcer with abrasion, blister, partial thickness skin loss involving epidermis and/or dermis, left lower back

L89.143   **Pressure ulcer of left lower back, stage 3**   MCC H4 HCC SW

Healing pressure ulcer of left lower back, stage 3

Pressure ulcer with full thickness skin loss involving damage or necrosis of subcutaneous tissue, left lower back

L89.144   **Pressure ulcer of left lower back, stage 4**   MCC H4 HCC SW

Healing pressure ulcer of left lower back, stage 4

Pressure ulcer with necrosis of soft tissues through to underlying muscle, tendon, or bone, left lower back

L89.146   **Pressure-induced deep tissue damage of left lower back**

✔ Additional Character Required   √x7ᵗʰ Placeholder   Questionable PDx   Manifestation   Unspecified Dx   UPD Unacceptable PDx   H1 -H14 HAC   HCC CMS-HCC Dx   HIV HIV Dx

ICD-10-CM 2022   747

Chapter 12. Diseases of the Skin and Subcutaneous Tissue

L89.149–L89.300

L89.149 Pressure ulcer of left lower back, unspecified stage
Healing pressure ulcer of left lower back NOS
Healing pressure ulcer of left lower back, unspecified stage

√6ᵗʰ **L89.15 Pressure ulcer of sacral region**
Pressure ulcer of coccyx
Pressure ulcer of tailbone

L89.150 Pressure ulcer of sacral region, unstageable HCC SW

L89.151 Pressure ulcer of sacral region, stage 1
Healing pressure ulcer of sacral region, stage 1
Pressure pre-ulcer skin changes limited to persistent focal edema, sacral region

L89.152 Pressure ulcer of sacral region, stage 2 HCC
Healing pressure ulcer of sacral region, stage 2
Pressure ulcer with abrasion, blister, partial thickness skin loss involving epidermis and/or dermis, sacral region

L89.153 Pressure ulcer of sacral region, stage 3 MCC H4 HCC SW
Healing pressure ulcer of sacral region, stage 3
Pressure ulcer with full thickness skin loss involving damage or necrosis of subcutaneous tissue, sacral region

L89.154 Pressure ulcer of sacral region, stage 4 MCC H4 HCC SW
Healing pressure ulcer of sacral region, stage 4
Pressure ulcer with necrosis of soft tissues through to underlying muscle, tendon, or bone, sacral region

L89.156 Pressure-induced deep tissue damage of sacral region

L89.159 Pressure ulcer of sacral region, unspecified stage
Healing pressure ulcer of sacral region NOS
Healing pressure ulcer of sacral region, unspecified stage

√5ᵗʰ **L89.2 Pressure ulcer of hip**

√6ᵗʰ **L89.20 Pressure ulcer of unspecified hip**

L89.200 Pressure ulcer of unspecified hip, unstageable HCC SW

L89.201 Pressure ulcer of unspecified hip, stage 1
Healing pressure ulcer of unspecified hip back, stage 1
Pressure pre-ulcer skin changes limited to persistent focal edema, unspecified hip

L89.202 Pressure ulcer of unspecified hip, stage 2 HCC
Healing pressure ulcer of unspecified hip, stage 2
Pressure ulcer with abrasion, blister, partial thickness skin loss involving epidermis and/or dermis, unspecified hip

L89.203 Pressure ulcer of unspecified hip, stage 3 MCC H4 HCC SW
Healing pressure ulcer of unspecified hip, stage 3
Pressure ulcer with full thickness skin loss involving damage or necrosis of subcutaneous tissue, unspecified hip

L89.204 Pressure ulcer of unspecified hip, stage 4 MCC H4 HCC SW
Healing pressure ulcer of unspecified hip, stage 4
Pressure ulcer with necrosis of soft tissues through to underlying muscle, tendon, or bone, unspecified hip

L89.206 Pressure-induced deep tissue damage of unspecified hip

L89.209 Pressure ulcer of unspecified hip, unspecified stage
Healing pressure ulcer of unspecified hip NOS
Healing pressure ulcer of unspecified hip, unspecified stage

√6ᵗʰ **L89.21 Pressure ulcer of right hip**

L89.210 Pressure ulcer of right hip, unstageable HCC SW

L89.211 Pressure ulcer of right hip, stage 1
Healing pressure ulcer of right hip back, stage 1
Pressure pre-ulcer skin changes limited to persistent focal edema, right hip

L89.212 Pressure ulcer of right hip, stage 2 HCC
Healing pressure ulcer of right hip, stage 2
Pressure ulcer with abrasion, blister, partial thickness skin loss involving epidermis and/or dermis, right hip

L89.213 Pressure ulcer of right hip, stage 3 MCC H4 HCC SW
Healing pressure ulcer of right hip, stage 3
Pressure ulcer with full thickness skin loss involving damage or necrosis of subcutaneous tissue, right hip

L89.214 Pressure ulcer of right hip, stage 4 MCC H4 HCC SW
Healing pressure ulcer of right hip, stage 4
Pressure ulcer with necrosis of soft tissues through to underlying muscle, tendon, or bone, right hip

L89.216 Pressure-induced deep tissue damage of right hip

L89.219 Pressure ulcer of right hip, unspecified stage
Healing pressure ulcer of right hip NOS
Healing pressure ulcer of right hip, unspecified stage

√6ᵗʰ **L89.22 Pressure ulcer of left hip**

L89.220 Pressure ulcer of left hip, unstageable HCC SW

L89.221 Pressure ulcer of left hip, stage 1
Healing pressure ulcer of left hip back, stage 1
Pressure pre-ulcer skin changes limited to persistent focal edema, left hip

L89.222 Pressure ulcer of left hip, stage 2 HCC
Healing pressure ulcer of left hip, stage 2
Pressure ulcer with abrasion, blister, partial thickness skin loss involving epidermis and/or dermis, left hip

L89.223 Pressure ulcer of left hip, stage 3 MCC H4 HCC SW
Healing pressure ulcer of left hip, stage 3
Pressure ulcer with full thickness skin loss involving damage or necrosis of subcutaneous tissue, left hip

L89.224 Pressure ulcer of left hip, stage 4 MCC H4 HCC SW
Healing pressure ulcer of left hip, stage 4
Pressure ulcer with necrosis of soft tissues through to underlying muscle, tendon, or bone, left hip

L89.226 Pressure-induced deep tissue damage of left hip

L89.229 Pressure ulcer of left hip, unspecified stage
Healing pressure ulcer of left hip NOS
Healing pressure ulcer of left hip, unspecified stage

√5ᵗʰ **L89.3 Pressure ulcer of buttock**

√6ᵗʰ **L89.30 Pressure ulcer of unspecified buttock**

L89.300 Pressure ulcer of unspecified buttock, unstageable HCC SW

L89.301 **Pressure ulcer of unspecified buttock, stage 1**
Healing pressure ulcer of unspecified buttock, stage 1
Pressure pre-ulcer skin changes limited to persistent focal edema, unspecified buttock

L89.302 **Pressure ulcer of unspecified buttock, stage 2** `HCC`
Healing pressure ulcer of unspecified buttock, stage 2
Pressure ulcer with abrasion, blister, partial thickness skin loss involving epidermis and/or dermis, unspecified buttock

L89.303 **Pressure ulcer of unspecified buttock, stage 3** `MCC` `H4` `HCC` `SW`
Healing pressure ulcer of unspecified buttock, stage 3
Pressure ulcer with full thickness skin loss involving damage or necrosis of subcutaneous tissue, unspecified buttock

L89.304 **Pressure ulcer of unspecified buttock, stage 4** `MCC` `H4` `HCC` `SW`
Healing pressure ulcer of unspecified buttock, stage 4
Pressure ulcer with necrosis of soft tissues through to underlying muscle, tendon, or bone, unspecified buttock

L89.306 **Pressure-induced deep tissue damage of unspecified buttock**

L89.309 **Pressure ulcer of unspecified buttock, unspecified stage**
Healing pressure ulcer of unspecified buttock NOS
Healing pressure ulcer of unspecified buttock, unspecified stage

√6ᵗʰ **L89.31** **Pressure ulcer of right buttock**

L89.310 **Pressure ulcer of right buttock, unstageable** `HCC` `SW`

L89.311 **Pressure ulcer of right buttock, stage 1**
Healing pressure ulcer of right buttock, stage 1
Pressure pre-ulcer skin changes limited to persistent focal edema, right buttock

L89.312 **Pressure ulcer of right buttock, stage 2** `HCC`
Healing pressure ulcer of right buttock, stage 2
Pressure ulcer with abrasion, blister, partial thickness skin loss involving epidermis and/or dermis, right buttock

L89.313 **Pressure ulcer of right buttock, stage 3** `MCC` `H4` `HCC` `SW`
Healing pressure ulcer of right buttock, stage 3
Pressure ulcer with full thickness skin loss involving damage or necrosis of subcutaneous tissue, right buttock

L89.314 **Pressure ulcer of right buttock, stage 4** `MCC` `H4` `HCC` `SW`
Healing pressure ulcer of right buttock, stage 4
Pressure ulcer with necrosis of soft tissues through to underlying muscle, tendon, or bone, right buttock

L89.316 **Pressure-induced deep tissue damage of right buttock**

L89.319 **Pressure ulcer of right buttock, unspecified stage**
Healing pressure ulcer of right buttock NOS
Healing pressure ulcer of right buttock, unspecified stage

√6ᵗʰ **L89.32** **Pressure ulcer of left buttock**

L89.320 **Pressure ulcer of left buttock, unstageable** `HCC` `SW`

L89.321 **Pressure ulcer of left buttock, stage 1**
Healing pressure ulcer of left buttock, stage 1
Pressure pre-ulcer skin changes limited to persistent focal edema, left buttock

L89.322 **Pressure ulcer of left buttock, stage 2** `HCC`
Healing pressure ulcer of left buttock, stage 2
Pressure ulcer with abrasion, blister, partial thickness skin loss involving epidermis and/or dermis, left buttock

L89.323 **Pressure ulcer of left buttock, stage 3** `MCC` `H4` `HCC` `SW`
Healing pressure ulcer of left buttock, stage 3
Pressure ulcer with full thickness skin loss involving damage or necrosis of subcutaneous tissue, left buttock

L89.324 **Pressure ulcer of left buttock, stage 4** `MCC` `H4` `HCC` `SW`
Healing pressure ulcer of left buttock, stage 4
Pressure ulcer with necrosis of soft tissues through to underlying muscle, tendon, or bone, left buttock

L89.326 **Pressure-induced deep tissue damage of left buttock**

L89.329 **Pressure ulcer of left buttock, unspecified stage**
Healing pressure ulcer of left buttock NOS
Healing pressure ulcer of left buttock, unspecified stage

√5ᵗʰ **L89.4** **Pressure ulcer of contiguous site of back, buttock and hip**

L89.40 **Pressure ulcer of contiguous site of back, buttock and hip, unspecified stage**
Healing pressure ulcer of contiguous site of back, buttock and hip NOS
Healing pressure ulcer of contiguous site of back, buttock and hip, unspecified stage

L89.41 **Pressure ulcer of contiguous site of back, buttock and hip, stage 1**
Healing pressure ulcer of contiguous site of back, buttock and hip, stage 1
Pressure pre-ulcer skin changes limited to persistent focal edema, contiguous site of back, buttock and hip

L89.42 **Pressure ulcer of contiguous site of back, buttock and hip, stage 2** `HCC`
Healing pressure ulcer of contiguous site of back, buttock and hip, stage 2
Pressure ulcer with abrasion, blister, partial thickness skin loss involving epidermis and/or dermis, contiguous site of back, buttock and hip

L89.43 **Pressure ulcer of contiguous site of back, buttock and hip, stage 3** `MCC` `H4` `HCC` `SW`
Healing pressure ulcer of contiguous site of back, buttock and hip, stage 3
Pressure ulcer with full thickness skin loss involving damage or necrosis of subcutaneous tissue, contiguous site of back, buttock and hip

L89.44 **Pressure ulcer of contiguous site of back, buttock and hip, stage 4** `MCC` `H4` `HCC` `SW`
Healing pressure ulcer of contiguous site of back, buttock and hip, stage 4
Pressure ulcer with necrosis of soft tissues through to underlying muscle, tendon, or bone, contiguous site of back, buttock and hip

L89.45 **Pressure ulcer of contiguous site of back, buttock and hip, unstageable** `HCC` `SW`

L89.46 **Pressure-induced deep tissue damage of contiguous site of back, buttock and hip**

√5ᵗʰ **L89.5** **Pressure ulcer of ankle**

√6ᵗʰ **L89.50** **Pressure ulcer of unspecified ankle**

L89.500 **Pressure ulcer of unspecified ankle, unstageable** `HCC` `SW`

☑ Additional Character Required   √x7ᵗʰ Placeholder   Questionable PDx   Manifestation   Unspecified Dx   UPD Unacceptable PDx   H1-H14 HAC   HCC CMS-HCC Dx   HIV HIV Dx

ICD-10-CM 2022   749

Chapter 12. Diseases of the Skin and Subcutaneous Tissue

L89.301–L89.500

Chapter 12. Diseases of the Skin and Subcutaneous Tissue

L89.501 **Pressure ulcer of unspecified ankle, stage 1**
Healing pressure ulcer of unspecified ankle, stage 1
Pressure pre-ulcer skin changes limited to persistent focal edema, unspecified ankle

L89.502 **Pressure ulcer of unspecified ankle, stage 2** `HCC`
Healing pressure ulcer of unspecified ankle, stage 2
Pressure ulcer with abrasion, blister, partial thickness skin loss involving epidermis and/or dermis, unspecified ankle

L89.503 **Pressure ulcer of unspecified ankle, stage 3** `MCC` `H4` `HCC` `SW`
Healing pressure ulcer of unspecified ankle, stage 3
Pressure ulcer with full thickness skin loss involving damage or necrosis of subcutaneous tissue, unspecified ankle

L89.504 **Pressure ulcer of unspecified ankle, stage 4** `MCC` `H4` `HCC` `SW`
Healing pressure ulcer of unspecified ankle, stage 4
Pressure ulcer with necrosis of soft tissues through to underlying muscle, tendon, or bone, unspecified ankle

L89.506 **Pressure-induced** deep tissue damage **of unspecified ankle**

L89.509 **Pressure ulcer of unspecified ankle, unspecified stage**
Healing pressure ulcer of unspecified ankle NOS
Healing pressure ulcer of unspecified ankle, unspecified stage

✓6ᵗʰ **L89.51** **Pressure ulcer of** right **ankle**

L89.510 **Pressure ulcer of right ankle, unstageable** `HCC` `SW`

L89.511 **Pressure ulcer of right ankle, stage 1**
Healing pressure ulcer of right ankle, stage 1
Pressure pre-ulcer skin changes limited to persistent focal edema, right ankle

L89.512 **Pressure ulcer of right ankle, stage 2** `HCC`
Healing pressure ulcer of right ankle, stage 2
Pressure ulcer with abrasion, blister, partial thickness skin loss involving epidermis and/or dermis, right ankle

L89.513 **Pressure ulcer of right ankle, stage 3** `MCC` `H4` `HCC` `SW`
Healing pressure ulcer of right ankle, stage 3
Pressure ulcer with full thickness skin loss involving damage or necrosis of subcutaneous tissue, right ankle

L89.514 **Pressure ulcer of right ankle, stage 4** `MCC` `H4` `HCC` `SW`
Healing pressure ulcer of right ankle, stage 4
Pressure ulcer with necrosis of soft tissues through to underlying muscle, tendon, or bone, right ankle

L89.516 **Pressure-induced** deep tissue damage **of right ankle**

L89.519 **Pressure ulcer of right ankle, unspecified stage**
Healing pressure ulcer of right ankle NOS
Healing pressure ulcer of right ankle, unspecified stage

✓6ᵗʰ **L89.52** **Pressure ulcer of** left **ankle**

L89.520 **Pressure ulcer of left ankle, unstageable** `HCC` `SW`

L89.521 **Pressure ulcer of left ankle, stage 1**
Healing pressure ulcer of left ankle, stage 1
Pressure pre-ulcer skin changes limited to persistent focal edema, left ankle

L89.522 **Pressure ulcer of left ankle, stage 2** `HCC`
Healing pressure ulcer of left ankle, stage 2
Pressure ulcer with abrasion, blister, partial thickness skin loss involving epidermis and/or dermis, left ankle

L89.523 **Pressure ulcer of left ankle, stage 3** `MCC` `H4` `HCC` `SW`
Healing pressure ulcer of left ankle, stage 3
Pressure ulcer with full thickness skin loss involving damage or necrosis of subcutaneous tissue, left ankle

L89.524 **Pressure ulcer of left ankle, stage 4** `MCC` `H4` `HCC` `SW`
Healing pressure ulcer of left ankle, stage 4
Pressure ulcer with necrosis of soft tissues through to underlying muscle, tendon, or bone, left ankle

L89.526 **Pressure-induced** deep tissue damage **of left ankle**

L89.529 **Pressure ulcer of left ankle, unspecified stage**
Healing pressure ulcer of left ankle NOS
Healing pressure ulcer of left ankle, unspecified stage

✓5ᵗʰ **L89.6** **Pressure ulcer of** heel

✓6ᵗʰ **L89.60** **Pressure ulcer of unspecified heel**

L89.600 **Pressure ulcer of unspecified heel, unstageable** `HCC` `SW`

L89.601 **Pressure ulcer of unspecified heel, stage 1**
Healing pressure ulcer of unspecified heel, stage 1
Pressure pre-ulcer skin changes limited to persistent focal edema, unspecified heel

L89.602 **Pressure ulcer of unspecified heel, stage 2** `HCC`
Healing pressure ulcer of unspecified heel, stage 2
Pressure ulcer with abrasion, blister, partial thickness skin loss involving epidermis and/or dermis, unspecified heel

L89.603 **Pressure ulcer of unspecified heel, stage 3** `MCC` `H4` `HCC` `SW`
Healing pressure ulcer of unspecified heel, stage 3
Pressure ulcer with full thickness skin loss involving damage or necrosis of subcutaneous tissue, unspecified heel

L89.604 **Pressure ulcer of unspecified heel, stage 4** `MCC` `H4` `HCC` `SW`
Healing pressure ulcer of unspecified heel, stage 4
Pressure ulcer with necrosis of soft tissues through to underlying muscle, tendon, or bone, unspecified heel

L89.606 **Pressure-induced** deep tissue damage **of unspecified heel**

L89.609 **Pressure ulcer of unspecified heel, unspecified stage**
Healing pressure ulcer of unspecified heel NOS
Healing pressure ulcer of unspecified heel, unspecified stage

✓6ᵗʰ **L89.61** **Pressure ulcer of** right **heel**

L89.610 **Pressure ulcer of right heel, unstageable** `HCC` `SW`

L89.611 **Pressure ulcer of right heel, stage 1**
Healing pressure ulcer of right heel, stage 1
Pressure pre-ulcer skin changes limited to persistent focal edema, right heel

L89.612 Pressure ulcer of right heel, stage 2 `HCC`
  Healing pressure ulcer of right heel, stage 2
  Pressure ulcer with abrasion, blister, partial thickness skin loss involving epidermis and/or dermis, right heel

L89.613 Pressure ulcer of right heel, stage 3 `MCC` `H4` `HCC` `SW`
  Healing pressure ulcer of right heel, stage 3
  Pressure ulcer with full thickness skin loss involving damage or necrosis of subcutaneous tissue, right heel

L89.614 Pressure ulcer of right heel, stage 4 `MCC` `H4` `HCC` `SW`
  Healing pressure ulcer of right heel, stage 4
  Pressure ulcer with necrosis of soft tissues through to underlying muscle, tendon, or bone, right heel

L89.616 Pressure-induced deep tissue damage of right heel

L89.619 Pressure ulcer of right heel, unspecified stage
  Healing pressure ulcer of right heel NOS
  Healing pressure ulcer of right heel, unspecified stage

✓6ᵗʰ **L89.62 Pressure ulcer of left heel**

L89.620 Pressure ulcer of left heel, unstageable `HCC` `SW`

L89.621 Pressure ulcer of left heel, stage 1
  Healing pressure ulcer of left heel, stage 1
  Pressure pre-ulcer skin changes limited to persistent focal edema, left heel

L89.622 Pressure ulcer of left heel, stage 2 `HCC`
  Healing pressure ulcer of left heel, stage 2
  Pressure ulcer with abrasion, blister, partial thickness skin loss involving epidermis and/or dermis, left heel

L89.623 Pressure ulcer of left heel, stage 3 `MCC` `H4` `HCC` `SW`
  Healing pressure ulcer of left heel, stage 3
  Pressure ulcer with full thickness skin loss involving damage or necrosis of subcutaneous tissue, left heel

L89.624 Pressure ulcer of left heel, stage 4 `MCC` `H4` `HCC` `SW`
  Healing pressure ulcer of left heel, stage 4
  Pressure ulcer with necrosis of soft tissues through to underlying muscle, tendon, or bone, left heel

L89.626 Pressure-induced deep tissue damage of left heel

L89.629 Pressure ulcer of left heel, unspecified stage
  Healing pressure ulcer of left heel NOS
  Healing pressure ulcer of left heel, unspecified stage

✓5ᵗʰ **L89.8 Pressure ulcer of other site**

✓6ᵗʰ **L89.81 Pressure ulcer of head**
  Pressure ulcer of face

L89.810 Pressure ulcer of head, unstageable `HCC` `SW`

L89.811 Pressure ulcer of head, stage 1
  Healing pressure ulcer of head, stage 1
  Pressure pre-ulcer skin changes limited to persistent focal edema, head

L89.812 Pressure ulcer of head, stage 2 `HCC`
  Healing pressure ulcer of head, stage 2
  Pressure ulcer with abrasion, blister, partial thickness skin loss involving epidermis and/or dermis, head

L89.813 Pressure ulcer of head, stage 3 `MCC` `H4` `HCC` `SW`
  Healing pressure ulcer of head, stage 3
  Pressure ulcer with full thickness skin loss involving damage or necrosis of subcutaneous tissue, head

L89.814 Pressure ulcer of head, stage 4 `MCC` `H4` `HCC` `SW`
  Healing pressure ulcer of head, stage 4
  Pressure ulcer with necrosis of soft tissues through to underlying muscle, tendon, or bone, head

L89.816 Pressure-induced deep tissue damage of head

L89.819 Pressure ulcer of head, unspecified stage
  Healing pressure ulcer of head NOS
  Healing pressure ulcer of head, unspecified stage

✓6ᵗʰ **L89.89 Pressure ulcer of other site**

L89.890 Pressure ulcer of other site, unstageable `HCC` `SW`

L89.891 Pressure ulcer of other site, stage 1
  Healing pressure ulcer of other site, stage 1
  Pressure pre-ulcer skin changes limited to persistent focal edema, other site

L89.892 Pressure ulcer of other site, stage 2 `HCC`
  Healing pressure ulcer of other site, stage 2
  Pressure ulcer with abrasion, blister, partial thickness skin loss involving epidermis and/or dermis, other site

L89.893 Pressure ulcer of other site, stage 3 `MCC` `H4` `HCC` `SW`
  Healing pressure ulcer of other site, stage 3
  Pressure ulcer with full thickness skin loss involving damage or necrosis of subcutaneous tissue, other site

L89.894 Pressure ulcer of other site, stage 4 `MCC` `H4` `HCC` `SW`
  Healing pressure ulcer of other site, stage 4
  Pressure ulcer with necrosis of soft tissues through to underlying muscle, tendon, or bone, other site

L89.896 Pressure-induced deep tissue damage of other site

L89.899 Pressure ulcer of other site, unspecified stage
  Healing pressure ulcer of other site NOS
  Healing pressure ulcer of other site, unspecified stage

✓5ᵗʰ **L89.9 Pressure ulcer of unspecified site**

L89.90 Pressure ulcer of unspecified site, unspecified stage
  Healing pressure ulcer of unspecified site NOS
  Healing pressure ulcer of unspecified site, unspecified stage

L89.91 Pressure ulcer of unspecified site, stage 1
  Healing pressure ulcer of unspecified site, stage 1
  Pressure pre-ulcer skin changes limited to persistent focal edema, unspecified site

L89.92 Pressure ulcer of unspecified site, stage 2 `HCC`
  Healing pressure ulcer of unspecified site, stage 2
  Pressure ulcer with abrasion, blister, partial thickness skin loss involving epidermis and/or dermis, unspecified site

L89.93 Pressure ulcer of unspecified site, stage 3 `MCC` `H4` `HCC` `SW`
  Healing pressure ulcer of unspecified site, stage 3
  Pressure ulcer with full thickness skin loss involving damage or necrosis of subcutaneous tissue, unspecified site

L89.94 Pressure ulcer of unspecified site, stage 4 `MCC` `H4` `HCC` `SW`
  Healing pressure ulcer of unspecified site, stage 4
  Pressure ulcer with necrosis of soft tissues through to underlying muscle, tendon, or bone, unspecified site

L89.95 Pressure ulcer of unspecified site, unstageable `HCC` `SW`

L89.96 Pressure-induced deep tissue damage of unspecified site

✔ Additional Character Required   ✓x7ᵗʰ Placeholder   Questionable PDx   Manifestation   Unspecified Dx   `UPD` Unacceptable PDx   `H1`-`H14` HAC   `HCC` CMS-HCC Dx   `HIV` HIV Dx

ICD-10-CM 2022   **751**

✓4ᵗʰ L90 Atrophic disorders of skin

L90.0 Lichen sclerosus et atrophicus
> EXCLUDES 2   lichen sclerosus of external female genital organs (N90.4)
> lichen sclerosus of external male genital organs (N48.0)

L90.1 Anetoderma of Schweninger-Buzzi

L90.2 Anetoderma of Jadassohn-Pellizzari

L90.3 Atrophoderma of Pasini and Pierini

L90.4 Acrodermatitis chronica atrophicans

L90.5 Scar conditions and fibrosis of skin
Adherent scar (skin)
Cicatrix
Disfigurement of skin due to scar
Fibrosis of skin NOS
Scar NOS
> EXCLUDES 2   hypertrophic scar (L91.0)
> keloid scar (L91.0)

AHA: 2016,2Q,5; 2015,1Q,19

L90.6 Striae atrophicae

L90.8 Other atrophic disorders of skin

L90.9 Atrophic disorder of skin, unspecified

✓4ᵗʰ L91 Hypertrophic disorders of skin

L91.0 Hypertrophic scar
Keloid
Keloid scar
> EXCLUDES 2   acne keloid (L73.0)
> scar NOS (L90.5)

DEF: Overgrowth of scar tissue due to excess amounts of collagen during connective tissue repair, occurring mainly on the upper trunk and face.

L91.8 Other hypertrophic disorders of the skin

L91.9 Hypertrophic disorder of the skin, unspecified

✓4ᵗʰ L92 Granulomatous disorders of skin and subcutaneous tissue
> EXCLUDES 2   actinic granuloma (L57.5)

L92.0 Granuloma annulare
Perforating granuloma annulare

L92.1 Necrobiosis lipoidica, not elsewhere classified
> EXCLUDES 1   necrobiosis lipoidica associated with diabetes mellitus (E08-E13 with .620)

L92.2 Granuloma faciale [eosinophilic granuloma of skin]

L92.3 Foreign body granuloma of the skin and subcutaneous tissue
Use additional code to identify the type of retained foreign body (Z18.-)

L92.8 Other granulomatous disorders of the skin and subcutaneous tissue

L92.9 Granulomatous disorder of the skin and subcutaneous tissue, unspecified
> EXCLUDES 2   umbilical granuloma (P83.81)

AHA: 2017,4Q,21-22

✓4ᵗʰ L93 Lupus erythematosus
Use additional code for adverse effect, if applicable, to identify drug (T36-T50 with fifth or sixth character 5)
> EXCLUDES 1   lupus exedens (A18.4)
> lupus vulgaris (A18.4)
> scleroderma (M34.-)
> systemic lupus erythematosus (M32.-)

DEF: Inflammatory, autoimmune skin condition in which the body's autoimmune system attacks healthy tissue of the integumentary system.

L93.0 Discoid lupus erythematosus
Lupus erythematosus NOS

L93.1 Subacute cutaneous lupus erythematosus

L93.2 Other local lupus erythematosus
Lupus erythematosus profundus
Lupus panniculitis

✓4ᵗʰ L94 Other localized connective tissue disorders
> EXCLUDES 1   systemic connective tissue disorders (M30-M36)

L94.0 Localized scleroderma [morphea]
Circumscribed scleroderma

L94.1 Linear scleroderma
En coup de sabre lesion

L94.2 Calcinosis cutis

L94.3 Sclerodactyly

L94.4 Gottron's papules

L94.5 Poikiloderma vasculare atrophicans

L94.6 Ainhum

L94.8 Other specified localized connective tissue disorders

L94.9 Localized connective tissue disorder, unspecified

✓4ᵗʰ L95 Vasculitis limited to skin, not elsewhere classified
> EXCLUDES 1   angioma serpiginosum (L81.7)
> Henoch(-Schönlein) purpura (D69.0)
> hypersensitivity angiitis (M31.0)
> lupus panniculitis (L93.2)
> panniculitis NOS (M79.3)
> panniculitis of neck and back (M54.0-)
> polyarteritis nodosa (M30.0)
> relapsing panniculitis (M35.6)
> rheumatoid vasculitis (M05.2)
> serum sickness (T80.6-)
> urticaria (L50.-)
> Wegener's granulomatosis (M31.3-)

L95.0 Livedoid vasculitis
Atrophie blanche (en plaque)

L95.1 Erythema elevatum diutinum

L95.8 Other vasculitis limited to the skin

L95.9 Vasculitis limited to the skin, unspecified

✓4ᵗʰ L97 Non-pressure chronic ulcer of lower limb, not elsewhere classified
> INCLUDES   chronic ulcer of skin of lower limb NOS
> non-healing ulcer of skin
> non-infected sinus of skin
> trophic ulcer NOS
> tropical ulcer NOS
> ulcer of skin of lower limb NOS

Code first any associated underlying condition, such as:
any associated gangrene (I96)
atherosclerosis of the lower extremities (I70.23-, I70.24-, I70.33-, I70.34-, I70.43-, I70.44-, I70.53-, I70.54-, I70.63-, I70.64-, I70.73-, I70.74-)
chronic venous hypertension (I87.31-, I87.33-)
diabetic ulcers (E08.621, E08.622, E09.621, E09.622, E10.621, E10.622, E11.621, E11.622, E13.621, E13.622)
postphlebitic syndrome (I87.01-, I87.03-)
postthrombotic syndrome (I87.01-, I87.03-)
varicose ulcer (I83.0-, I83.2-)
> EXCLUDES 2   pressure ulcer (pressure area) (L89.-)
> skin infections (L00-L08)
> specific infections classified to A00-B99

AHA: 2021,1Q,7; 2020,2Q,19; 2018,4Q,69; 2017,4Q,17

TIP: The depth and/or severity of a diagnosed nonpressure ulcer can be determined based on medical record documentation from clinicians who are not the patient's provider.

TIP: Assign a code from this category/subcategory for nonpressure ulcers documented as acute.

✓5ᵗʰ L97.1 Non-pressure chronic ulcer of thigh

✓6ᵗʰ L97.10 Non-pressure chronic ulcer of unspecified thigh

L97.101 Non-pressure chronic ulcer of unspecified thigh limited to breakdown of skin   CC HCC

L97.102 Non-pressure chronic ulcer of unspecified thigh with fat layer exposed   CC HCC SW

L97.103 Non-pressure chronic ulcer of unspecified thigh with necrosis of muscle   CC HCC SW

L97.104 Non-pressure chronic ulcer of unspecified thigh with necrosis of bone   CC HCC SW

L97.105 Non-pressure chronic ulcer of unspecified thigh with muscle involvement without evidence of necrosis   CC HCC

L97.106 Non-pressure chronic ulcer of unspecified thigh with bone involvement without evidence of necrosis   CC HCC

L97.108 Non-pressure chronic ulcer of unspecified thigh with other specified severity   CC HCC

L97.109 Non-pressure chronic ulcer of unspecified thigh with unspecified severity   CC HCC

✓6ᵗʰ L97.11 Non-pressure chronic ulcer of right thigh

L97.111 Non-pressure chronic ulcer of right thigh limited to breakdown of skin   CC HCC

L97.112 Non-pressure chronic ulcer of right thigh with fat layer exposed   CC HCC SW

L97.113   **Non-pressure chronic ulcer of right thigh with necrosis of muscle** `CC` `HCC` `SW`

L97.114   **Non-pressure chronic ulcer of right thigh with necrosis of bone** `CC` `HCC` `SW`

L97.115   **Non-pressure chronic ulcer of right thigh with muscle involvement without evidence of necrosis** `CC` `HCC`

L97.116   **Non-pressure chronic ulcer of right thigh with bone involvement without evidence of necrosis** `CC` `HCC`

L97.118   **Non-pressure chronic ulcer of right thigh with other specified severity** `CC` `HCC`

L97.119   **Non-pressure chronic ulcer of right thigh with unspecified severity** `CC` `HCC`

√6ᵗʰ   **L97.12**   **Non-pressure chronic ulcer of left thigh**

L97.121   **Non-pressure chronic ulcer of left thigh limited to breakdown of skin** `CC` `HCC`

L97.122   **Non-pressure chronic ulcer of left thigh with fat layer exposed** `CC` `HCC` `SW`

L97.123   **Non-pressure chronic ulcer of left thigh with necrosis of muscle** `CC` `HCC` `SW`

L97.124   **Non-pressure chronic ulcer of left thigh with necrosis of bone** `CC` `HCC` `SW`

L97.125   **Non-pressure chronic ulcer of left thigh with muscle involvement without evidence of necrosis** `CC` `HCC`

L97.126   **Non-pressure chronic ulcer of left thigh with bone involvement without evidence of necrosis** `CC` `HCC`

L97.128   **Non-pressure chronic ulcer of left thigh with other specified severity** `CC` `HCC`

L97.129   **Non-pressure chronic ulcer of left thigh with unspecified severity** `CC` `HCC`

√5ᵗʰ   **L97.2**   **Non-pressure chronic ulcer of calf**

√6ᵗʰ   **L97.20**   **Non-pressure chronic ulcer of unspecified calf**

L97.201   **Non-pressure chronic ulcer of unspecified calf limited to breakdown of skin** `CC` `HCC`

L97.202   **Non-pressure chronic ulcer of unspecified calf with fat layer exposed** `CC` `HCC` `SW`

L97.203   **Non-pressure chronic ulcer of unspecified calf with necrosis of muscle** `CC` `HCC` `SW`

L97.204   **Non-pressure chronic ulcer of unspecified calf with necrosis of bone** `CC` `HCC` `SW`

L97.205   **Non-pressure chronic ulcer of unspecified calf with muscle involvement without evidence of necrosis** `CC` `HCC`

L97.206   **Non-pressure chronic ulcer of unspecified calf with bone involvement without evidence of necrosis** `CC` `HCC`

L97.208   **Non-pressure chronic ulcer of unspecified calf with other specified severity** `CC` `HCC`

L97.209   **Non-pressure chronic ulcer of unspecified calf with unspecified severity** `CC` `HCC`

√6ᵗʰ   **L97.21**   **Non-pressure chronic ulcer of right calf**

L97.211   **Non-pressure chronic ulcer of right calf limited to breakdown of skin** `CC` `HCC`

L97.212   **Non-pressure chronic ulcer of right calf with fat layer exposed** `CC` `HCC` `SW`

L97.213   **Non-pressure chronic ulcer of right calf with necrosis of muscle** `CC` `HCC` `SW`

L97.214   **Non-pressure chronic ulcer of right calf with necrosis of bone** `CC` `HCC` `SW`

L97.215   **Non-pressure chronic ulcer of right calf with muscle involvement without evidence of necrosis** `CC` `HCC`

L97.216   **Non-pressure chronic ulcer of right calf with bone involvement without evidence of necrosis** `CC` `HCC`

L97.218   **Non-pressure chronic ulcer of right calf with other specified severity** `CC` `HCC`

L97.219   **Non-pressure chronic ulcer of right calf with unspecified severity** `CC` `HCC`

√6ᵗʰ   **L97.22**   **Non-pressure chronic ulcer of left calf**

L97.221   **Non-pressure chronic ulcer of left calf limited to breakdown of skin** `CC` `HCC`

L97.222   **Non-pressure chronic ulcer of left calf with fat layer exposed** `CC` `HCC` `SW`

L97.223   **Non-pressure chronic ulcer of left calf with necrosis of muscle** `CC` `HCC` `SW`

L97.224   **Non-pressure chronic ulcer of left calf with necrosis of bone** `CC` `HCC` `SW`

L97.225   **Non-pressure chronic ulcer of left calf with muscle involvement without evidence of necrosis** `CC` `HCC`

L97.226   **Non-pressure chronic ulcer of left calf with bone involvement without evidence of necrosis** `CC` `HCC`

L97.228   **Non-pressure chronic ulcer of left calf with other specified severity** `CC` `HCC`

L97.229   **Non-pressure chronic ulcer of left calf with unspecified severity** `CC` `HCC`

√5ᵗʰ   **L97.3**   **Non-pressure chronic ulcer of ankle**

√6ᵗʰ   **L97.30**   **Non-pressure chronic ulcer of unspecified ankle**

L97.301   **Non-pressure chronic ulcer of unspecified ankle limited to breakdown of skin** `CC` `HCC`

L97.302   **Non-pressure chronic ulcer of unspecified ankle with fat layer exposed** `CC` `HCC` `SW`

L97.303   **Non-pressure chronic ulcer of unspecified ankle with necrosis of muscle** `CC` `HCC` `SW`

L97.304   **Non-pressure chronic ulcer of unspecified ankle with necrosis of bone** `CC` `HCC` `SW`

L97.305   **Non-pressure chronic ulcer of unspecified ankle with muscle involvement without evidence of necrosis** `CC` `HCC`

L97.306   **Non-pressure chronic ulcer of unspecified ankle with bone involvement without evidence of necrosis** `CC` `HCC`

L97.308   **Non-pressure chronic ulcer of unspecified ankle with other specified severity** `CC` `HCC`

L97.309   **Non-pressure chronic ulcer of unspecified ankle with unspecified severity** `CC` `HCC`

√6ᵗʰ   **L97.31**   **Non-pressure chronic ulcer of right ankle**

L97.311   **Non-pressure chronic ulcer of right ankle limited to breakdown of skin** `CC` `HCC`

L97.312   **Non-pressure chronic ulcer of right ankle with fat layer exposed** `CC` `HCC` `SW`

L97.313   **Non-pressure chronic ulcer of right ankle with necrosis of muscle** `CC` `HCC` `SW`

L97.314   **Non-pressure chronic ulcer of right ankle with necrosis of bone** `CC` `HCC` `SW`

L97.315   **Non-pressure chronic ulcer of right ankle with muscle involvement without evidence of necrosis** `CC` `HCC`

L97.316   **Non-pressure chronic ulcer of right ankle with bone involvement without evidence of necrosis** `CC` `HCC`

L97.318   **Non-pressure chronic ulcer of right ankle with other specified severity** `CC` `HCC`

L97.319   **Non-pressure chronic ulcer of right ankle with unspecified severity** `CC` `HCC`

√6ᵗʰ   **L97.32**   **Non-pressure chronic ulcer of left ankle**

L97.321   **Non-pressure chronic ulcer of left ankle limited to breakdown of skin** `CC` `HCC`

L97.322   **Non-pressure chronic ulcer of left ankle with fat layer exposed** `CC` `HCC` `SW`

L97.323   **Non-pressure chronic ulcer of left ankle with necrosis of muscle** `CC` `HCC` `SW`

L97.324   **Non-pressure chronic ulcer of left ankle with necrosis of bone** `CC` `HCC` `SW`

L97.325   **Non-pressure chronic ulcer of left ankle with muscle involvement without evidence of necrosis** `CC` `HCC`

L97.326   **Non-pressure chronic ulcer of left ankle with bone involvement without evidence of necrosis** `CC` `HCC`

L97.328   **Non-pressure chronic ulcer of left ankle with other specified severity** `CC` `HCC`

L97.329   **Non-pressure chronic ulcer of left ankle with unspecified severity** `CC` `HCC`

✔ Additional Character Required   √x7ᵗʰ Placeholder   Questionable PDx   Manifestation   Unspecified Dx   UPD Unacceptable PDx   H1-H4 HAC   HCC CMS-HCC Dx   HIV HIV Dx

ICD-10-CM 2022   753

✓5ᵗʰ **L97.4　Non-pressure chronic ulcer of** heel and midfoot

　　　Non-pressure chronic ulcer of plantar surface of midfoot

✓6ᵗʰ **L97.40　Non-pressure chronic ulcer of unspecified heel and midfoot**

　　　L97.401　Non-pressure chronic ulcer of unspecified heel and midfoot limited to breakdown of skin　**CC HCC**

　　　L97.402　Non-pressure chronic ulcer of unspecified heel and midfoot with fat layer exposed　**CC HCC SW**

　　　L97.403　Non-pressure chronic ulcer of unspecified heel and midfoot with necrosis of muscle　**CC HCC SW**

　　　L97.404　Non-pressure chronic ulcer of unspecified heel and midfoot with necrosis of bone　**CC HCC SW**

　　　L97.405　Non-pressure chronic ulcer of unspecified heel and midfoot with muscle involvement without evidence of necrosis　**CC HCC**

　　　L97.406　Non-pressure chronic ulcer of unspecified heel and midfoot with bone involvement without evidence of necrosis　**CC HCC**

　　　L97.408　Non-pressure chronic ulcer of unspecified heel and midfoot with other specified severity　**CC HCC**

　　　L97.409　Non-pressure chronic ulcer of unspecified heel and midfoot with unspecified severity　**CC HCC**

✓6ᵗʰ **L97.41　Non-pressure chronic ulcer of** right heel and midfoot

　　　L97.411　Non-pressure chronic ulcer of right heel and midfoot limited to breakdown of skin　**CC HCC**

　　　L97.412　Non-pressure chronic ulcer of right heel and midfoot with fat layer exposed　**CC HCC SW**
　　　　　AHA: 2020,2Q,19

　　　L97.413　Non-pressure chronic ulcer of right heel and midfoot with necrosis of muscle　**CC HCC SW**

　　　L97.414　Non-pressure chronic ulcer of right heel and midfoot with necrosis of bone　**CC HCC SW**

　　　L97.415　Non-pressure chronic ulcer of right heel and midfoot with muscle involvement without evidence of necrosis　**CC HCC**

　　　L97.416　Non-pressure chronic ulcer of right heel and midfoot with bone involvement without evidence of necrosis　**CC HCC**

　　　L97.418　Non-pressure chronic ulcer of right heel and midfoot with other specified severity　**CC HCC**

　　　L97.419　Non-pressure chronic ulcer of right heel and midfoot with unspecified severity　**CC HCC**

✓6ᵗʰ **L97.42　Non-pressure chronic ulcer of** left heel and midfoot

　　　L97.421　Non-pressure chronic ulcer of left heel and midfoot limited to breakdown of skin　**CC HCC**
　　　　　AHA: 2016,1Q,12

　　　L97.422　Non-pressure chronic ulcer of left heel and midfoot with fat layer exposed　**CC HCC SW**
　　　　　AHA: 2020,2Q,19

　　　L97.423　Non-pressure chronic ulcer of left heel and midfoot with necrosis of muscle　**CC HCC SW**

　　　L97.424　Non-pressure chronic ulcer of left heel and midfoot with necrosis of bone　**CC HCC SW**

　　　L97.425　Non-pressure chronic ulcer of left heel and midfoot with muscle involvement without evidence of necrosis　**CC HCC**

　　　L97.426　Non-pressure chronic ulcer of left heel and midfoot with bone involvement without evidence of necrosis　**CC HCC**

　　　L97.428　Non-pressure chronic ulcer of left heel and midfoot with other specified severity　**CC HCC**

　　　L97.429　Non-pressure chronic ulcer of left heel and midfoot with unspecified severity　**CC HCC**

✓5ᵗʰ **L97.5　Non-pressure chronic ulcer of other part of** foot

　　　Non-pressure chronic ulcer of toe

✓6ᵗʰ **L97.50　Non-pressure chronic ulcer of other part of unspecified foot**

　　　L97.501　Non-pressure chronic ulcer of other part of unspecified foot limited to breakdown of skin　**HCC**

　　　L97.502　Non-pressure chronic ulcer of other part of unspecified foot with fat layer exposed　**HCC SW**

　　　L97.503　Non-pressure chronic ulcer of other part of unspecified foot with necrosis of muscle　**HCC SW**

　　　L97.504　Non-pressure chronic ulcer of other part of unspecified foot with necrosis of bone　**HCC SW**

　　　L97.505　Non-pressure chronic ulcer of other part of unspecified foot with muscle involvement without evidence of necrosis　**CC HCC**

　　　L97.506　Non-pressure chronic ulcer of other part of unspecified foot with bone involvement without evidence of necrosis　**CC HCC**

　　　L97.508　Non-pressure chronic ulcer of other part of unspecified foot with other specified severity　**CC HCC**

　　　L97.509　Non-pressure chronic ulcer of other part of unspecified foot with unspecified severity　**HCC**

✓6ᵗʰ **L97.51　Non-pressure chronic ulcer of other part of** right foot
　　　AHA: 2020,1Q,12

　　　L97.511　Non-pressure chronic ulcer of other part of right foot limited to breakdown of skin　**HCC**

　　　L97.512　Non-pressure chronic ulcer of other part of right foot with fat layer exposed　**HCC SW**
　　　　　AHA: 2020,2Q,19

　　　L97.513　Non-pressure chronic ulcer of other part of right foot with necrosis of muscle　**HCC SW**

　　　L97.514　Non-pressure chronic ulcer of other part of right foot with necrosis of bone　**HCC SW**

　　　L97.515　Non-pressure chronic ulcer of other part of right foot with muscle involvement without evidence of necrosis　**CC HCC**

　　　L97.516　Non-pressure chronic ulcer of other part of right foot with bone involvement without evidence of necrosis　**CC HCC**

　　　L97.518　Non-pressure chronic ulcer of other part of right foot with other specified severity　**CC HCC**

　　　L97.519　Non-pressure chronic ulcer of other part of right foot with unspecified severity　**HCC**

✓6ᵗʰ **L97.52　Non-pressure chronic ulcer of other part of** left foot
　　　AHA: 2020,1Q,12

　　　L97.521　Non-pressure chronic ulcer of other part of left foot limited to breakdown of skin　**HCC**

　　　L97.522　Non-pressure chronic ulcer of other part of left foot with fat layer exposed　**HCC SW**
　　　　　AHA: 2020,2Q,19

　　　L97.523　Non-pressure chronic ulcer of other part of left foot with necrosis of muscle　**HCC SW**

　　　L97.524　Non-pressure chronic ulcer of other part of left foot with necrosis of bone　**HCC SW**

　　　L97.525　Non-pressure chronic ulcer of other part of left foot with muscle involvement without evidence of necrosis　**CC HCC**

　　　L97.526　Non-pressure chronic ulcer of other part of left foot with bone involvement without evidence of necrosis　**CC HCC**

         L97.528   Non-pressure chronic ulcer of other part of left foot with other specified severity   `CC` `HCC`

         L97.529   Non-pressure chronic ulcer of other part of left foot with unspecified severity   `HCC`

☑️5ᵗʰ **L97.8**   Non-pressure chronic ulcer of other part of lower leg

    ☑️6ᵗʰ **L97.80**   Non-pressure chronic ulcer of other part of unspecified lower leg

         L97.801   Non-pressure chronic ulcer of other part of unspecified lower leg limited to breakdown of skin   `CC` `HCC`

         L97.802   Non-pressure chronic ulcer of other part of unspecified lower leg with fat layer exposed   `CC` `HCC` `SW`

         L97.803   Non-pressure chronic ulcer of other part of unspecified lower leg with necrosis of muscle   `CC` `HCC` `SW`

         L97.804   Non-pressure chronic ulcer of other part of unspecified lower leg with necrosis of bone   `CC` `HCC` `SW`

         L97.805   Non-pressure chronic ulcer of other part of unspecified lower leg with muscle involvement without evidence of necrosis   `CC` `HCC`

         L97.806   Non-pressure chronic ulcer of other part of unspecified lower leg with bone involvement without evidence of necrosis   `CC` `HCC`

         L97.808   Non-pressure chronic ulcer of other part of unspecified lower leg with other specified severity   `CC` `HCC`

         L97.809   Non-pressure chronic ulcer of other part of unspecified lower leg with unspecified severity   `CC` `HCC`

    ☑️6ᵗʰ **L97.81**   Non-pressure chronic ulcer of other part of right lower leg

         L97.811   Non-pressure chronic ulcer of other part of right lower leg limited to breakdown of skin   `CC` `HCC`

         L97.812   Non-pressure chronic ulcer of other part of right lower leg with fat layer exposed   `CC` `HCC` `SW`

         L97.813   Non-pressure chronic ulcer of other part of right lower leg with necrosis of muscle   `CC` `HCC` `SW`

         L97.814   Non-pressure chronic ulcer of other part of right lower leg with necrosis of bone   `CC` `HCC` `SW`

         L97.815   Non-pressure chronic ulcer of other part of right lower leg with muscle involvement without evidence of necrosis   `CC` `HCC`

         L97.816   Non-pressure chronic ulcer of other part of right lower leg with bone involvement without evidence of necrosis   `CC` `HCC`

         L97.818   Non-pressure chronic ulcer of other part of right lower leg with other specified severity   `CC` `HCC`

         L97.819   Non-pressure chronic ulcer of other part of right lower leg with unspecified severity   `CC` `HCC`

    ☑️6ᵗʰ **L97.82**   Non-pressure chronic ulcer of other part of left lower leg

         L97.821   Non-pressure chronic ulcer of other part of left lower leg limited to breakdown of skin   `CC` `HCC`

         L97.822   Non-pressure chronic ulcer of other part of left lower leg with fat layer exposed   `CC` `HCC` `SW`

         L97.823   Non-pressure chronic ulcer of other part of left lower leg with necrosis of muscle   `CC` `HCC` `SW`

         L97.824   Non-pressure chronic ulcer of other part of left lower leg with necrosis of bone   `CC` `HCC` `SW`

         L97.825   Non-pressure chronic ulcer of other part of left lower leg with muscle involvement without evidence of necrosis   `CC` `HCC`

         L97.826   Non-pressure chronic ulcer of other part of left lower leg with bone involvement without evidence of necrosis   `CC` `HCC`

         L97.828   Non-pressure chronic ulcer of other part of left lower leg with other specified severity   `CC` `HCC`

         L97.829   Non-pressure chronic ulcer of other part of left lower leg with unspecified severity   `CC` `HCC`

☑️5ᵗʰ **L97.9**   Non-pressure chronic ulcer of unspecified part of lower leg

    ☑️6ᵗʰ **L97.90**   Non-pressure chronic ulcer of unspecified part of unspecified lower leg

         L97.901   Non-pressure chronic ulcer of unspecified part of unspecified lower leg limited to breakdown of skin   `CC` `HCC`

         L97.902   Non-pressure chronic ulcer of unspecified part of unspecified lower leg with fat layer exposed   `CC` `HCC` `SW`

         L97.903   Non-pressure chronic ulcer of unspecified part of unspecified lower leg with necrosis of muscle   `CC` `HCC` `SW`

         L97.904   Non-pressure chronic ulcer of unspecified part of unspecified lower leg with necrosis of bone   `CC` `HCC` `SW`

         L97.905   Non-pressure chronic ulcer of unspecified part of unspecified lower leg with muscle involvement without evidence of necrosis   `CC` `HCC`

         L97.906   Non-pressure chronic ulcer of unspecified part of unspecified lower leg with bone involvement without evidence of necrosis   `CC` `HCC`

         L97.908   Non-pressure chronic ulcer of unspecified part of unspecified lower leg with other specified severity   `CC` `HCC`

         L97.909   Non-pressure chronic ulcer of unspecified part of unspecified lower leg with unspecified severity   `CC` `HCC`

    ☑️6ᵗʰ **L97.91**   Non-pressure chronic ulcer of unspecified part of right lower leg

         L97.911   Non-pressure chronic ulcer of unspecified part of right lower leg limited to breakdown of skin   `CC` `HCC`

         L97.912   Non-pressure chronic ulcer of unspecified part of right lower leg with fat layer exposed   `CC` `HCC` `SW`

         L97.913   Non-pressure chronic ulcer of unspecified part of right lower leg with necrosis of muscle   `CC` `HCC` `SW`

         L97.914   Non-pressure chronic ulcer of unspecified part of right lower leg with necrosis of bone   `CC` `HCC` `SW`

         L97.915   Non-pressure chronic ulcer of unspecified part of right lower leg with muscle involvement without evidence of necrosis   `CC` `HCC`

         L97.916   Non-pressure chronic ulcer of unspecified part of right lower leg with bone involvement without evidence of necrosis   `CC` `HCC`

         L97.918   Non-pressure chronic ulcer of unspecified part of right lower leg with other specified severity   `CC` `HCC`

         L97.919   Non-pressure chronic ulcer of unspecified part of right lower leg with unspecified severity   `CC` `HCC`

    ☑️6ᵗʰ **L97.92**   Non-pressure chronic ulcer of unspecified part of left lower leg

         L97.921   Non-pressure chronic ulcer of unspecified part of left lower leg limited to breakdown of skin   `CC` `HCC` `SW`

         L97.922   Non-pressure chronic ulcer of unspecified part of left lower leg with fat layer exposed   `CC` `HCC` `SW`

         L97.923   Non-pressure chronic ulcer of unspecified part of left lower leg with necrosis of muscle   `CC` `HCC` `SW`

         L97.924   Non-pressure chronic ulcer of unspecified part of left lower leg with necrosis of bone   `CC` `HCC` `SW`

         L97.925   Non-pressure chronic ulcer of unspecified part of left lower leg with muscle involvement without evidence of necrosis   `CC` `HCC`

☑️ Additional Character Required   ☑️x7ᵗʰ Placeholder   Questionable PDx   Manifestation   Unspecified Dx   `UPD` Unacceptable PDx   `H1`-`H14` HAC   `HCC` CMS-HCC Dx   `HIV` HIV Dx

         L97.926   Non-pressure chronic ulcer of unspecified part of left lower leg with bone involvement without evidence of necrosis   CC HCC

         L97.928   Non-pressure chronic ulcer of unspecified part of left lower leg with other specified severity   CC HCC

         L97.929   Non-pressure chronic ulcer of unspecified part of left lower leg with unspecified severity   CC HCC

✓4ᵗʰ **L98**   **Other disorders of skin and subcutaneous tissue, not elsewhere classified**

     L98.0   **Pyogenic granuloma**

         EXCLUDES 2   *pyogenic granuloma of gingiva (K06.8)*

                   pyogenic granuloma of maxillary alveolar ridge (K04.5)

                   pyogenic granuloma of oral mucosa (K13.4)

         DEF: Solitary polypoid capillary hemangioma often associated with local irritation, trauma, and superimposed inflammation. Located on the skin and gingival or oral mucosa, they bleed easily and may ulcerate and form crusted sores.

     L98.1   **Factitial dermatitis**

         Neurotic excoriation

         EXCLUDES 1   *excoriation (skin-picking) disorder (F42.4)*

         AHA: 2016,4Q,15

         DEF: Self-inflicted skin lesions to satisfy an unconscious psychological or emotional need. Methods used to injure the skin include deep excoriations with a sharp instrument, scarification with a knife, or the application of caustic chemicals and burning, sometimes with a cigarette.

     L98.2   **Febrile neutrophilic dermatosis [Sweet]**

     L98.3   **Eosinophilic cellulitis [Wells]**   CC

✓6ᵗʰ   **L98.4**   **Non-pressure chronic ulcer of skin, not elsewhere classified**

         Chronic ulcer of skin NOS

         Tropical ulcer NOS

         Ulcer of skin NOS

         EXCLUDES 2   *gangrene (I96)*

                   pressure ulcer (pressure area) (L89.-)

                   skin infections (L00-L08)

                   specific infections classified to A00-B99

                   ulcer of lower limb NEC (L97.-)

                   varicose ulcer (I83.0-I83.93)

         AHA: 2017,4Q,17

         TIP: The depth and/or severity of a diagnosed nonpressure ulcer can be determined based on medical record documentation from clinicians who are not the patient's provider.

         TIP: Assign a code from this category/subcategory for nonpressure ulcers documented as acute.

✓6ᵗʰ   **L98.41**   **Non-pressure chronic ulcer of buttock**

         L98.411   Non-pressure chronic ulcer of buttock limited to breakdown of skin   HCC

         L98.412   Non-pressure chronic ulcer of buttock with fat layer exposed   HCC SW

         L98.413   Non-pressure chronic ulcer of buttock with necrosis of muscle   HCC SW

         L98.414   Non-pressure chronic ulcer of buttock with necrosis of bone   HCC SW

         L98.415   Non-pressure chronic ulcer of buttock with muscle involvement without evidence of necrosis   CC HCC

         L98.416   Non-pressure chronic ulcer of buttock with bone involvement without evidence of necrosis   CC HCC

         L98.418   Non-pressure chronic ulcer of buttock with other specified severity   CC HCC

         L98.419   Non-pressure chronic ulcer of buttock with unspecified severity   HCC

✓6ᵗʰ   **L98.42**   **Non-pressure chronic ulcer of back**

         L98.421   Non-pressure chronic ulcer of back limited to breakdown of skin   HCC

         L98.422   Non-pressure chronic ulcer of back with fat layer exposed   HCC SW

         L98.423   Non-pressure chronic ulcer of back with necrosis of muscle   HCC SW

         L98.424   Non-pressure chronic ulcer of back with necrosis of bone   HCC SW

         L98.425   Non-pressure chronic ulcer of back with muscle involvement without evidence of necrosis   CC HCC

         L98.426   Non-pressure chronic ulcer of back with bone involvement without evidence of necrosis   CC HCC

         L98.428   Non-pressure chronic ulcer of back with other specified severity   CC HCC

         L98.429   Non-pressure chronic ulcer of back with unspecified severity   HCC

✓6ᵗʰ   **L98.49**   **Non-pressure chronic ulcer of skin of other sites**

         Non-pressure chronic ulcer of skin NOS

         L98.491   Non-pressure chronic ulcer of skin of other sites limited to breakdown of skin   HCC

         L98.492   Non-pressure chronic ulcer of skin of other sites with fat layer exposed   HCC SW

         L98.493   Non-pressure chronic ulcer of skin of other sites with necrosis of muscle   HCC SW

         L98.494   Non-pressure chronic ulcer of skin of other sites with necrosis of bone   HCC SW

         L98.495   Non-pressure chronic ulcer of skin of other sites with muscle involvement without evidence of necrosis   CC HCC

         L98.496   Non-pressure chronic ulcer of skin of other sites with bone involvement without evidence of necrosis   CC HCC

         L98.498   Non-pressure chronic ulcer of skin of other sites with other specified severity   CC HCC

         L98.499   Non-pressure chronic ulcer of skin of other sites with unspecified severity   HCC

     L98.5   **Mucinosis of the skin**

         Focal mucinosis

         Lichen myxedematosus

         Reticular erythematous mucinosis

         EXCLUDES 1   *focal oral mucinosis (K13.79)*

                   myxedema (E03.9)

     L98.6   **Other infiltrative disorders of the skin and subcutaneous tissue**

         EXCLUDES 1   *hyalinosis cutis et mucosae (E78.89)*

     L98.7   **Excessive and redundant skin and subcutaneous tissue**

         Loose or sagging skin, following bariatric surgery weight loss

         Loose or sagging skin following dietary weight loss

         Loose or sagging skin, NOS

         EXCLUDES 2   *acquired excess or redundant skin of eyelid (H02.3-)*

                   congenital excess or redundant skin of eyelid (Q10.3)

                   skin changes due to chronic exposure to nonionizing radiation (L57.-)

         AHA: 2016,4Q,36

     L98.8   **Other specified disorders of the skin and subcutaneous tissue**

         AHA: 2013,2Q,32

     L98.9   **Disorder of the skin and subcutaneous tissue, unspecified**

L99   *Other disorders of skin and subcutaneous tissue in diseases classified elsewhere*

         Code first underlying disease, such as:

            amyloidosis (E85.-)

         EXCLUDES 1   *skin disorders in diabetes ▶(E08-E13 with .62-)◀*

                   skin disorders in gonorrhea (A54.89)

                   skin disorders in syphilis (A51.31, A52.79)

         AHA: 2021,1Q,39

N Newborn: 0   P Pediatric: 0-17   M Maternity: 9-64   A Adult: 15-124   MCC Major Complication/Comorbidity   CC Complication/Comorbidity   SW Severe Wound Dx

756   ICD-10-CM 2022

Chapter 13. Diseases of the Musculoskeletal System and Connective Tissue (M00–M99)

Chapter-specific Guidelines with Coding Examples

The chapter-specific guidelines from the ICD-10-CM Official Guidelines for Coding and Reporting have been provided below. Along with these guidelines are coding examples, contained in the shaded boxes, that have been developed to help illustrate the coding and/or sequencing guidance found in these guidelines.

a. Site and laterality

Most of the codes within Chapter 13 have site and laterality designations. The site represents the bone, joint or the muscle involved. For some conditions where more than one bone, joint or muscle is usually involved, such as osteoarthritis, there is a "multiple sites" code available. For categories where no multiple site code is provided and more than one bone, joint or muscle is involved, multiple codes should be used to indicate the different sites involved.

> Rheumatoid arthritis of multiple sites without rheumatoid factor
>
> **M06.09**   **Rheumatoid arthritis without rheumatoid factor, multiple sites**
>
> *Explanation:* For some conditions where more than one bone, joint or muscle is usually involved, such as rheumatoid arthritis, there is a "multiple sites" code available.

> Osteomyelitis of the fourth thoracic and second lumbar vertebrae
>
> **M46.24**   **Osteomyelitis of vertebra, thoracic region**
>
> **M46.26**   **Osteomyelitis of vertebra, lumbar region**
>
> *Explanation:* For categories without a multiple site code and more than one bone, joint, or muscle is involved, multiple codes should be used to indicate the different sites involved.

1) Bone versus joint

For certain conditions, the bone may be affected at the upper or lower end, (e.g., avascular necrosis of bone, M87, Osteoporosis, M80, M81). Though the portion of the bone affected may be at the joint, the site designation will be the bone, not the joint.

> Idiopathic avascular necrosis of the femoral head of the left hip joint
>
> **M87.052**   **Idiopathic aseptic necrosis of left femur**
>
> *Explanation:* For certain conditions such as avascular necrosis, the bone may be affected at the joint, but the site designation is the bone, not the joint.

b. Acute traumatic versus chronic or recurrent musculoskeletal conditions

Many musculoskeletal conditions are a result of previous injury or trauma to a site, or are recurrent conditions. Bone, joint or muscle conditions that are the result of a healed injury are usually found in chapter 13. Recurrent bone, joint or muscle conditions are also usually found in chapter 13. Any current, acute injury should be coded to the appropriate injury code from chapter 19. Chronic or recurrent conditions should generally be coded with a code from chapter 13. If it is difficult to determine from the documentation in the record which code is best to describe a condition, query the provider.

> Acute traumatic bucket-handle tear of right medial meniscus
>
> **S83.211A**   **Bucket-handle tear of medial meniscus, current injury, right knee, initial encounter**
>
> *Explanation:* Any current, acute injury is not coded in chapter 13. It should instead be coded to the appropriate injury code from chapter 19.

> Old bucket-handle tear of right medial meniscus
>
> **M23.203**   **Derangement of unspecified medial meniscus due to old tear or injury, right knee**
>
> *Explanation:* Chronic or recurrent conditions should generally be coded with a code from chapter 13.

c. Coding of pathologic fractures

7th character A is for use as long as the patient is receiving active treatment for the fracture. Examples of active treatment are: surgical treatment, emergency department encounter, evaluation and continuing treatment by the same or a different physician. While the patient may be seen by a new or different provider over the course of treatment for a pathological fracture, assignment of the 7th character is based on whether the patient is undergoing active treatment and not whether the provider is seeing the patient for the first time.

> Patient admitted for repair of pathologic fracture of left foot, unknown cause. The surgery will be performed by his orthopedic specialist who he has been seeing for this fracture for the past month.
>
> **M84.475A**   **Pathological fracture, left foot, initial encounter for fracture**
>
> *Explanation:* Seventh character A is for use as long as the patient is receiving active treatment for a pathologic fracture. Examples of active treatment are surgical treatment, emergency department encounter, evaluation, and continuing treatment by the same or a different physician.
>
> The seventh character is based on whether the patient is undergoing active treatment such as surgery, and not whether the provider is seeing the patient for the first time.

7th character D is to be used for encounters after the patient has completed active treatment for the fracture and is receiving routine care for the fracture during the healing or recovery phase. The other 7th characters, listed under each subcategory in the Tabular List, are to be used for subsequent encounters for treatment of problems associated with the healing, such as malunions, nonunions, and sequelae.

Care for complications of surgical treatment for fracture repairs during the healing or recovery phase should be coded with the appropriate complication codes.

See Section I.C.19. Coding of traumatic fractures.

d. Osteoporosis

Osteoporosis is a systemic condition, meaning that all bones of the musculoskeletal system are affected. Therefore, site is not a component of the codes under category M81, Osteoporosis without current pathological fracture. The site codes under category M80, Osteoporosis with current pathological fracture, identify the site of the fracture, not the osteoporosis.

1) Osteoporosis without pathological fracture

Category M81, Osteoporosis without current pathological fracture, is for use for patients with osteoporosis who do not currently have a pathologic fracture due to the osteoporosis, even if they have had a fracture in the past. For patients with a history of osteoporosis fractures, status code Z87.310, Personal history of (healed) osteoporosis fracture, should follow the code from M81.

> Age-related osteoporosis with healed osteoporotic fracture of the lumbar vertebra
>
> **M81.0**   **Age-related osteoporosis without current pathological fracture**
>
> **Z87.310**   **Personal history of (healed) osteoporosis fracture**
>
> *Explanation:* Category M81 is used for patients with osteoporosis who do not currently have a pathologic fracture due to the osteoporosis. To report a previous (healed) fracture, status code Z87.310 Personal history of (healed) osteoporosis fracture, should follow the code from M81.

2) Osteoporosis with current pathological fracture

Category M80, Osteoporosis with current pathological fracture, is for patients who have a current pathologic fracture at the time of an encounter. The codes under M80 identify the site of the fracture. A code from category M80, not a traumatic fracture code, should be used for any patient with known osteoporosis who suffers a fracture, even if the patient had a minor fall or trauma, if that fall or trauma would not usually break a normal, healthy bone.

> Disuse osteoporosis with current fracture of right shoulder sustained lifting a grocery bag, initial encounter
>
> **M80.811A**   **Other osteoporosis with current pathological fracture, right shoulder, initial encounter for fracture**
>
> *Explanation:* A code from category M80, not a traumatic fracture code, should be used for any patient with known osteoporosis who suffers a fracture, even if the patient had a minor fall or trauma, if that fall or trauma would not usually break a normal, healthy bone.

e. Multisystem inflammatory syndrome

See Section I.C.1.g.1.l for Multisystem Inflammatory Syndrome

Muscle/Tendon Table

ICD-10-CM categorizes certain muscles and tendons in the upper and lower extremities by their action (e.g., extension, flexion), their anatomical location (e.g., posterior, anterior), and/or whether they are intrinsic or extrinsic to a certain anatomical area. The Muscle/Tendon Table is provided at the beginning of chapters 13 and 19 as a resource to help users when code selection depends on one or more of these characteristics. Please note that this table is not all-inclusive, and proper code assignment should be based on the provider's documentation.

Body Region	Muscle	Extensor Tendon	Flexor Tendon	Other Tendon
Shoulder				
	Deltoid	Posterior deltoid	Anterior deltoid	
	Rotator cuff			
	Infraspinatus			Infraspinatus
	Subscapularis			Subscapularis
	Supraspinatus			Supraspinatus
	Teres minor			Teres minor
	Teres major	Teres major		
Upper arm				
	Anterior muscles			
	Biceps brachii — long head		Biceps brachii — long head	
	Biceps brachii — short head		Biceps brachii — short head	
	Brachialis		Brachialis	
	Coracobrachialis		Coracobrachialis	
	Posterior muscles			
	Triceps brachii	Triceps brachii		
Forearm				
	Anterior muscles			
	Flexors			
	Deep			
	Flexor digitorum profundus		Flexor digitorum profundus	
	Flexor pollicis longus		Flexor pollicis longus	
	Intermediate			
	Flexor digitorum superficialis		Flexor digitorum superficialis	
	Superficial			
	Flexor carpi radialis		Flexor carpi radialis	
	Flexor carpi ulnaris		Flexor carpi ulnaris	
	Palmaris longus		Palmaris longus	
	Pronators			
	Pronator quadratus			Pronator quadratus
	Pronator teres			Pronator teres
	Posterior muscles			
	Extensors			
	Deep			
	Abductor pollicis longus			Abductor pollicis longus
	Extensor indicis	Extensor indicis		
	Extensor pollicis brevis	Extensor pollicis brevis		
	Extensor pollicis longus	Extensor pollicis longus		
	Superficial			
	Brachioradialis			Brachioradialis
	Extensor carpi radialis brevis	Extensor carpi radialis brevis		
	Extensor carpi radialis longus	Extensor carpi radialis longus		
	Extensor carpi ulnaris	Extensor carpi ulnaris		
	Extensor digiti minimi	Extensor digiti minimi		
	Extensor digitorum	Extensor digitorum		
	Anconeus	Anconeus		
	Supinator			Supinator

Body Region	Muscle	Extensor Tendon	Flexor Tendon	Other Tendon
Hand				
Extrinsic — attach to a site in the forearm as well as a site in the hand with action related to hand movement at the wrist				
	Extensor carpi radialis brevis	Extensor carpi radialis brevis		
	Extensor carpi radialis longus	Extensor carpi radialis longus		
	Extensor carpi ulnaris	Extensor carpi ulnaris		
	Flexor carpi radialis		Flexor carpi radialis	
	Flexor carpi ulnaris		Flexor carpi ulnaris	
	Flexor digitorum superficialis		Flexor digitorum superficialis	
	Palmaris longus		Palmaris longus	
Extrinsic — attach to a site in the forearm as well as a site in the hand with action in the hand related to finger movement				
	Adductor pollicis longus			Adductor pollicis longus
	Extensor digiti minimi	Extensor digiti minimi		
	Extensor digitorum	Extensor digitorum		
	Extensor indicis	Extensor indicis		
	Flexor digitorum profundus		Flexor digitorum profundus	
	Flexor digitorum superficialis		Flexor digitorum superficialis	
Extrinsic — attach to a site in the forearm as well as a site in the hand with action in the hand related to thumb movement				
	Extensor pollicis brevis	Extensor pollicis brevis		
	Extensor pollicis longus	Extensor pollicis longus		
	Flexor pollicis longus		Flexor pollicis longus	
Intrinsic — found within the hand only				
	Adductor pollicis			Adductor pollicis
	Dorsal interossei	Dorsal interossei	Dorsal interossei	
	Lumbricals	Lumbricals	Lumbricals	
	Palmaris brevis			Palmaris brevis
	Palmar interossei	Palmar interossei	Palmar interossei	
	Hypothenar muscles			
	Abductor digiti minimi			Abductor digiti minimi
	Flexor digiti minimi brevis		Flexor digiti minimi brevis	
	Opponens digiti minimi		Opponens digiti minimi	
	Thenar muscles			
	Abductor pollicis brevis			Abductor pollicis brevis
	Flexor pollicis brevis		Flexor pollicis brevis	
	Opponens pollicis		Opponens pollicis	
Thigh				
	Anterior muscles			
	Iliopsoas		Iliopsoas	
	Pectineus		Pectineus	
	Quadriceps	Quadriceps		
	Rectus femoris	Rectus femoris — Extends knee	Rectus femoris — Flexes hip	
	Vastus intermedius	Vastus intermedius		
	Vastus lateralis	Vastus lateralis		
	Vastus medialis	Vastus medialis		
	Sartorius		Sartorius	
	Medial muscles			
	Adductor brevis			Adductor brevis
	Adductor longus			Adductor longus
	Adductor magnus			Adductor magnus
	Gracilis			Gracilis
	Obturator externus			Obturator externus
	Posterior muscles			
	Hamstring	Hamstring — Extends hip	Hamstring — Flexes knee	
	Biceps femoris	Biceps femoris	Biceps femoris	
	Semimembranosus	Semimembranosus	Semimembranosus	
	Semitendinosus	Semitendinosus	Semitendinosus	

Chapter 13. Diseases of the Musculoskeletal System and Connective Tissue

Body Region	Muscle	Extensor Tendon	Flexor Tendon	Other Tendon
Lower leg				
	Anterior muscles			
	Extensor digitorum longus	Extensor digitorum longus		
	Extensor hallucis longus	Extensor hallucis longus		
	Fibularis (peroneus) tertius	Fibularis (peroneus) tertius		
	Tibialis anterior	Tibialis anterior		Tibialis anterior
	Lateral muscles			
	Fibularis (peroneus) brevis		Fibularis (peroneus) brevis	
	Fibularis (peroneus) longus		Fibularis (peroneus) longus	
	Posterior muscles			
	Deep			
	Flexor digitorum longus		Flexor digitorum longus	
	Flexor hallucis longus		Flexor hallucis longus	
	Popliteus		Popliteus	
	Tibialis posterior		Tibialis posterior	
	Superficial			
	Gastrocnemius		Gastrocnemius	
	Plantaris		Plantaris	
	Soleus		Soleus	
				Calcaneal (Achilles)
Ankle/Foot				
Extrinsic — attach to a site in the lower leg as well as a site in the foot with action related to foot movement at the ankle				
	Plantaris		Plantaris	
	Soleus		Soleus	
	Tibialis anterior	Tibialis anterior		
	Tibialis posterior		Tibialis posterior	
Extrinsic — attach to a site in the lower leg as well as a site in the foot with action in the foot related to toe movement				
	Extensor digitorum longus	Extensor digitorum longus		
	Extensor hallucis longus	Extensor hallucis longus		
	Flexor digitorum longus		Flexor digitorum longus	
	Flexor hallucis longus		Flexor hallucis longus	
Intrinsic — found within the ankle/foot only				
	Dorsal muscles			
	Extensor digitorum brevis	Extensor digitorum brevis		
	Extensor hallucis brevis	Extensor hallucis brevis		
	Plantar muscles			
	Abductor digiti minimi		Abductor digiti minimi	
	Abductor hallucis		Abductor hallucis	
	Dorsal interossei	Dorsal interossei	Dorsal interossei	
	Flexor digiti minimi brevis		Flexor digiti minimi brevis	
	Flexor digitorum brevis		Flexor digitorum brevis	
	Flexor hallucis brevis		Flexor hallucis brevis	
	Lumbricals	Lumbricals	Lumbricals	
	Quadratus plantae		Quadratus plantae	
	Plantar interossei	Plantar interossei	Plantar interossei	

Chapter 13. Diseases of the Musculoskeletal System and Connective Tissue (M00-M99)

NOTE Use an external cause code following the code for the musculoskeletal condition, if applicable, to identify the cause of the musculoskeletal condition

EXCLUDES 2 arthropathic psoriasis (L40.5-)
certain conditions originating in the perinatal period (P04-P96)
certain infectious and parasitic diseases (A00-B99)
compartment syndrome (traumatic) (T79.A-)
complications of pregnancy, childbirth and the puerperium (O00-O9A)
congenital malformations, deformations, and chromosomal abnormalities (Q00-Q99)
endocrine, nutritional and metabolic diseases (E00-E88)
injury, poisoning and certain other consequences of external causes (S00-T88)
neoplasms (C00-D49)
symptoms, signs and abnormal clinical and laboratory findings, not elsewhere classified (R00-R94)

This chapter contains the following blocks:

M00-M02   Infectious arthropathies
M04   Autoinflammatory syndromes
M05-M14   Inflammatory polyarthropathies
M15-M19   Osteoarthritis
M20-M25   Other joint disorders
M26-M27   Dentofacial anomalies [including malocclusion] and other disorders of jaw
M30-M36   Systemic connective tissue disorders
M40-M43   Deforming dorsopathies
M45-M49   Spondylopathies
M50-M54   Other dorsopathies
M60-M63   Disorders of muscles
M65-M67   Disorders of synovium and tendon
M70-M79   Other soft tissue disorders
M80-M85   Disorders of bone density and structure
M86-M90   Other osteopathies
M91-M94   Chondropathies
M95   Other disorders of the musculoskeletal system and connective tissue
M96   Intraprocedural and postprocedural complications and disorders of musculoskeletal system, not elsewhere classified
M97   Periprosthetic fracture around internal prosthetic joint
M99   Biomechanical lesions, not elsewhere classified

ARTHROPATHIES (M00-M25)

INCLUDES disorders affecting predominantly peripheral (limb) joints

Infectious arthropathies (M00-M02)

NOTE This block comprises arthropathies due to microbiological agents. Distinction is made between the following types of etiological relationship:

a) direct infection of joint, where organisms invade synovial tissue and microbial antigen is present in the joint;

b) indirect infection, which may be of two types: a reactive arthropathy, where microbial infection of the body is established but neither organisms nor antigens can be identified in the joint, and a postinfective arthropathy, where microbial antigen is present but recovery of an organism is inconstant and evidence of local multiplication is lacking.

AHA: 2019,3Q,16

☑4ᵗʰ **M00 Pyogenic arthritis**

EXCLUDES 2 infection and inflammatory reaction due to internal joint prosthesis (T84.5-)

DEF: Pyogenic: Relating to or involving pus production, often referred to as suppurative or purulent.

☑5ᵗʰ **M00.0 Staphylococcal arthritis and polyarthritis**

Use additional code (B95.61-B95.8) to identify bacterial agent

    M00.00 Staphylococcal arthritis, unspecified joint `CC` `HCC`

☑6ᵗʰ **M00.01 Staphylococcal arthritis, shoulder**

    M00.011 Staphylococcal arthritis, right shoulder `CC` `HCC`

    M00.012 Staphylococcal arthritis, left shoulder `CC` `HCC`

    M00.019 Staphylococcal arthritis, unspecified shoulder `CC` `HCC`

☑6ᵗʰ **M00.02 Staphylococcal arthritis, elbow**

    M00.021 Staphylococcal arthritis, right elbow `CC` `HCC`

    M00.022 Staphylococcal arthritis, left elbow `CC` `HCC`

    M00.029 Staphylococcal arthritis, unspecified elbow `CC` `HCC`

☑6ᵗʰ **M00.03 Staphylococcal arthritis, wrist**

Staphylococcal arthritis of carpal bones

    M00.031 Staphylococcal arthritis, right wrist `CC` `HCC`

    M00.032 Staphylococcal arthritis, left wrist `CC` `HCC`

    M00.039 Staphylococcal arthritis, unspecified wrist `CC` `HCC`

☑6ᵗʰ **M00.04 Staphylococcal arthritis, hand**

Staphylococcal arthritis of metacarpus and phalanges

    M00.041 Staphylococcal arthritis, right hand `CC` `HCC`

    M00.042 Staphylococcal arthritis, left hand `CC` `HCC`

    M00.049 Staphylococcal arthritis, unspecified hand `CC` `HCC`

☑6ᵗʰ **M00.05 Staphylococcal arthritis, hip**

    M00.051 Staphylococcal arthritis, right hip `CC` `HCC`

    M00.052 Staphylococcal arthritis, left hip `CC` `HCC`

    M00.059 Staphylococcal arthritis, unspecified hip `CC` `HCC`

☑6ᵗʰ **M00.06 Staphylococcal arthritis, knee**

    M00.061 Staphylococcal arthritis, right knee `CC` `HCC`

    M00.062 Staphylococcal arthritis, left knee `CC` `HCC`

    M00.069 Staphylococcal arthritis, unspecified knee `CC` `HCC`

☑6ᵗʰ **M00.07 Staphylococcal arthritis, ankle and foot**

Staphylococcal arthritis, tarsus, metatarsus and phalanges

    M00.071 Staphylococcal arthritis, right ankle and foot `CC` `HCC`

    M00.072 Staphylococcal arthritis, left ankle and foot `CC` `HCC`

    M00.079 Staphylococcal arthritis, unspecified ankle and foot `CC` `HCC`

    M00.08 Staphylococcal arthritis, vertebrae `CC` `HCC`

    M00.09 Staphylococcal polyarthritis `CC` `HCC`

☑5ᵗʰ **M00.1 Pneumococcal arthritis and polyarthritis**

    M00.10 Pneumococcal arthritis, unspecified joint `CC` `HCC`

☑6ᵗʰ **M00.11 Pneumococcal arthritis, shoulder**

    M00.111 Pneumococcal arthritis, right shoulder `CC` `HCC`

    M00.112 Pneumococcal arthritis, left shoulder `CC` `HCC`

    M00.119 Pneumococcal arthritis, unspecified shoulder `CC` `HCC`

☑6ᵗʰ **M00.12 Pneumococcal arthritis, elbow**

    M00.121 Pneumococcal arthritis, right elbow `CC` `HCC`

    M00.122 Pneumococcal arthritis, left elbow `CC` `HCC`

    M00.129 Pneumococcal arthritis, unspecified elbow `CC` `HCC`

☑6ᵗʰ **M00.13 Pneumococcal arthritis, wrist**

Pneumococcal arthritis of carpal bones

    M00.131 Pneumococcal arthritis, right wrist `CC` `HCC`

    M00.132 Pneumococcal arthritis, left wrist `CC` `HCC`

    M00.139 Pneumococcal arthritis, unspecified wrist `CC` `HCC`

☑6ᵗʰ **M00.14 Pneumococcal arthritis, hand**

Pneumococcal arthritis of metacarpus and phalanges

    M00.141 Pneumococcal arthritis, right hand `CC` `HCC`

    M00.142 Pneumococcal arthritis, left hand `CC` `HCC`

    M00.149 Pneumococcal arthritis, unspecified hand `CC` `HCC`

☑6ᵗʰ **M00.15 Pneumococcal arthritis, hip**

    M00.151 Pneumococcal arthritis, right hip `CC` `HCC`

M00.152 **Pneumococcal arthritis, left** hip   `CC` `HCC`

M00.159 **Pneumococcal arthritis, unspecified** hip   `CC` `HCC`

√6ᵗʰ M00.16 **Pneumococcal arthritis, knee**

  M00.161 **Pneumococcal arthritis, right** knee   `CC` `HCC`

  M00.162 **Pneumococcal arthritis, left** knee   `CC` `HCC`

  M00.169 **Pneumococcal arthritis, unspecified** knee   `CC` `HCC`

√6ᵗʰ M00.17 **Pneumococcal arthritis, ankle and foot**

Pneumococcal arthritis, tarsus, metatarsus and phalanges

  M00.171 **Pneumococcal arthritis, right ankle and** foot   `CC` `HCC`

  M00.172 **Pneumococcal arthritis, left ankle and** foot   `CC` `HCC`

  M00.179 **Pneumococcal arthritis, unspecified ankle and** foot   `CC` `HCC`

M00.18 **Pneumococcal arthritis, vertebrae**   `CC` `HCC`

M00.19 **Pneumococcal polyarthritis**   `CC` `HCC`

√5ᵗʰ M00.2 **Other streptococcal arthritis and polyarthritis**

Use additional code (B95.0-B95.2, B95.4-B95.5) to identify bacterial agent

  M00.20 **Other streptococcal arthritis, unspecified** joint   `CC` `HCC`

√6ᵗʰ M00.21 **Other streptococcal arthritis, shoulder**

  M00.211 **Other streptococcal arthritis, right** shoulder   `CC` `HCC`

  M00.212 **Other streptococcal arthritis, left** shoulder   `CC` `HCC`

  M00.219 **Other streptococcal arthritis, unspecified** shoulder   `CC` `HCC`

√6ᵗʰ M00.22 **Other streptococcal arthritis, elbow**

  M00.221 **Other streptococcal arthritis, right** elbow   `CC` `HCC`

  M00.222 **Other streptococcal arthritis, left** elbow   `CC` `HCC`

  M00.229 **Other streptococcal arthritis, unspecified** elbow   `CC` `HCC`

√6ᵗʰ M00.23 **Other streptococcal arthritis, wrist**

Other streptococcal arthritis of carpal bones

  M00.231 **Other streptococcal arthritis, right** wrist   `CC` `HCC`

  M00.232 **Other streptococcal arthritis, left** wrist   `CC` `HCC`

  M00.239 **Other streptococcal arthritis, unspecified** wrist   `CC` `HCC`

√6ᵗʰ M00.24 **Other streptococcal arthritis, hand**

Other streptococcal arthritis metacarpus and phalanges

  M00.241 **Other streptococcal arthritis, right** hand   `CC` `HCC`

  M00.242 **Other streptococcal arthritis, left** hand   `CC` `HCC`

  M00.249 **Other streptococcal arthritis, unspecified** hand   `CC` `HCC`

√6ᵗʰ M00.25 **Other streptococcal arthritis, hip**

  M00.251 **Other streptococcal arthritis, right** hip   `CC` `HCC`

  M00.252 **Other streptococcal arthritis, left** hip   `CC` `HCC`

  M00.259 **Other streptococcal arthritis, unspecified** hip   `CC` `HCC`

√6ᵗʰ M00.26 **Other streptococcal arthritis, knee**

  M00.261 **Other streptococcal arthritis, right** knee   `CC` `HCC`

  M00.262 **Other streptococcal arthritis, left** knee   `CC` `HCC`

  M00.269 **Other streptococcal arthritis, unspecified** knee   `CC` `HCC`

√6ᵗʰ M00.27 **Other streptococcal arthritis, ankle and foot**

Other streptococcal arthritis, tarsus, metatarsus and phalanges

  M00.271 **Other streptococcal arthritis, right ankle and foot**   `CC` `HCC`

  M00.272 **Other streptococcal arthritis, left ankle and foot**   `CC` `HCC`

  M00.279 **Other streptococcal arthritis, unspecified ankle and foot**   `CC` `HCC`

M00.28 **Other streptococcal arthritis, vertebrae**   `CC` `HCC`

M00.29 **Other streptococcal polyarthritis**   `CC` `HCC`

√5ᵗʰ M00.8 **Arthritis and polyarthritis due to other bacteria**

Use additional code (B96) to identify bacteria

  M00.80 **Arthritis due to other bacteria, unspecified** joint   `CC` `HCC`

√6ᵗʰ M00.81 **Arthritis due to other bacteria, shoulder**

  M00.811 **Arthritis due to other bacteria, right** shoulder   `CC` `HCC`

  M00.812 **Arthritis due to other bacteria, left** shoulder   `CC` `HCC`

  M00.819 **Arthritis due to other bacteria, unspecified shoulder**   `CC` `HCC`

√6ᵗʰ M00.82 **Arthritis due to other bacteria, elbow**

  M00.821 **Arthritis due to other bacteria, right** elbow   `CC` `HCC`

  M00.822 **Arthritis due to other bacteria, left** elbow   `CC` `HCC`

  M00.829 **Arthritis due to other bacteria, unspecified elbow**   `CC` `HCC`

√6ᵗʰ M00.83 **Arthritis due to other bacteria, wrist**

Arthritis due to other bacteria, carpal bones

  M00.831 **Arthritis due to other bacteria, right** wrist   `CC` `HCC`

  M00.832 **Arthritis due to other bacteria, left** wrist   `CC` `HCC`

  M00.839 **Arthritis due to other bacteria, unspecified wrist**   `CC` `HCC`

√6ᵗʰ M00.84 **Arthritis due to other bacteria, hand**

Arthritis due to other bacteria, metacarpus and phalanges

  M00.841 **Arthritis due to other bacteria, right** hand   `CC` `HCC`

  M00.842 **Arthritis due to other bacteria, left** hand   `CC` `HCC`

  M00.849 **Arthritis due to other bacteria, unspecified hand**   `CC` `HCC`

√6ᵗʰ M00.85 **Arthritis due to other bacteria, hip**

  M00.851 **Arthritis due to other bacteria, right** hip   `CC` `HCC`

  M00.852 **Arthritis due to other bacteria, left** hip   `CC` `HCC`

  M00.859 **Arthritis due to other bacteria, unspecified hip**   `CC` `HCC`

√6ᵗʰ M00.86 **Arthritis due to other bacteria, knee**

AHA: 2019,3Q,16

  M00.861 **Arthritis due to other bacteria, right** knee   `CC` `HCC`

  M00.862 **Arthritis due to other bacteria, left** knee   `CC` `HCC`

  M00.869 **Arthritis due to other bacteria, unspecified knee**   `CC` `HCC`

√6ᵗʰ M00.87 **Arthritis due to other bacteria, ankle and foot**

Arthritis due to other bacteria, tarsus, metatarsus, and phalanges

  M00.871 **Arthritis due to other bacteria, right ankle and foot**   `CC` `HCC`

  M00.872 **Arthritis due to other bacteria, left ankle and foot**   `CC` `HCC`

  M00.879 **Arthritis due to other bacteria, unspecified ankle and foot**   `CC` `HCC`

M00.88 **Arthritis due to other bacteria, vertebrae**   `CC` `HCC`

M00.89 **Polyarthritis due to other bacteria**   `CC` `HCC`

M00.9 **Pyogenic arthritis, unspecified**   `CC` `HCC`

Infective arthritis NOS

N Newborn: 0   P Pediatric: 0-17   M Maternity: 9-64   A Adult: 15-124   `MCC` Major Complication/Comorbidity   `CC` Complication/Comorbidity   `SW` Severe Wound Dx

762   ICD-10-CM 2022

✓4ᵗʰ **M01** **Direct infections of joint in infectious and parasitic diseases classified elsewhere**

Code first underlying disease, such as:
leprosy [Hansen's disease] (A3Ø.-)
mycoses (B35-B49)
O'nyong-nyong fever (A92.1)
paratyphoid fever (AØ1.1-AØ1.4)

EXCLUDES 1   *arthropathy in Lyme disease (A69.23)*
gonococcal arthritis (A54.42)
meningococcal arthritis (A39.83)
mumps arthritis (B26.85)
postinfective arthropathy (MØ2.-)
postmeningococcal arthritis (A39.84)
reactive arthritis (MØ2.3)
rubella arthritis (BØ6.82)
sarcoidosis arthritis (D86.86)
typhoid fever arthritis (AØ1.Ø4)
tuberculosis arthritis (A18.Ø1-A18.Ø2)

✓5ᵗʰ **M01.X** **Direct infection of joint in infectious and parasitic diseases classified elsewhere**

M01.XØ   *Direct infection of unspecified joint in infectious and parasitic diseases classified elsewhere*   CC   HCC

✓6ᵗʰ **M01.X1** **Direct infection of shoulder joint in infectious and parasitic diseases classified elsewhere**

M01.X11   *Direct infection of right shoulder in infectious and parasitic diseases classified elsewhere*   CC   HCC

M01.X12   *Direct infection of left shoulder in infectious and parasitic diseases classified elsewhere*   CC   HCC

M01.X19   *Direct infection of unspecified shoulder in infectious and parasitic diseases classified elsewhere*   CC   HCC

✓6ᵗʰ **M01.X2** **Direct infection of elbow in infectious and parasitic diseases classified elsewhere**

M01.X21   *Direct infection of right elbow in infectious and parasitic diseases classified elsewhere*   CC   HCC

M01.X22   *Direct infection of left elbow in infectious and parasitic diseases classified elsewhere*   CC   HCC

M01.X29   *Direct infection of unspecified elbow in infectious and parasitic diseases classified elsewhere*   CC   HCC

✓6ᵗʰ **M01.X3** **Direct infection of wrist in infectious and parasitic diseases classified elsewhere**

Direct infection of carpal bones in infectious and parasitic diseases classified elsewhere

M01.X31   *Direct infection of right wrist in infectious and parasitic diseases classified elsewhere*   CC   HCC

M01.X32   *Direct infection of left wrist in infectious and parasitic diseases classified elsewhere*   CC   HCC

M01.X39   *Direct infection of unspecified wrist in infectious and parasitic diseases classified elsewhere*   CC   HCC

✓6ᵗʰ **M01.X4** **Direct infection of hand in infectious and parasitic diseases classified elsewhere**

Direct infection of metacarpus and phalanges in infectious and parasitic diseases classified elsewhere

M01.X41   *Direct infection of right hand in infectious and parasitic diseases classified elsewhere*   CC   HCC

M01.X42   *Direct infection of left hand in infectious and parasitic diseases classified elsewhere*   CC   HCC

M01.X49   *Direct infection of unspecified hand in infectious and parasitic diseases classified elsewhere*   CC   HCC

✓6ᵗʰ **M01.X5** **Direct infection of hip in infectious and parasitic diseases classified elsewhere**

M01.X51   *Direct infection of right hip in infectious and parasitic diseases classified elsewhere*   CC   HCC

M01.X52   *Direct infection of left hip in infectious and parasitic diseases classified elsewhere*   CC   HCC

M01.X59   *Direct infection of unspecified hip in infectious and parasitic diseases classified elsewhere*   CC   HCC

✓6ᵗʰ **M01.X6** **Direct infection of knee in infectious and parasitic diseases classified elsewhere**

M01.X61   *Direct infection of right knee in infectious and parasitic diseases classified elsewhere*   CC   HCC

M01.X62   *Direct infection of left knee in infectious and parasitic diseases classified elsewhere*   CC   HCC

M01.X69   *Direct infection of unspecified knee in infectious and parasitic diseases classified elsewhere*   CC   HCC

✓6ᵗʰ **M01.X7** **Direct infection of ankle and foot in infectious and parasitic diseases classified elsewhere**

Direct infection of tarsus, metatarsus and phalanges in infectious and parasitic diseases classified elsewhere

M01.X71   *Direct infection of right ankle and foot in infectious and parasitic diseases classified elsewhere*   CC   HCC

M01.X72   *Direct infection of left ankle and foot in infectious and parasitic diseases classified elsewhere*   CC   HCC

M01.X79   *Direct infection of unspecified ankle and foot in infectious and parasitic diseases classified elsewhere*   CC   HCC

M01.X8   *Direct infection of vertebrae in infectious and parasitic diseases classified elsewhere*   CC   HCC

M01.X9   *Direct infection of multiple joints in infectious and parasitic diseases classified elsewhere*   CC   HCC

✓4ᵗʰ **M02** **Postinfective and reactive arthropathies**

Code first underlying disease, such as:
congenital syphilis [Clutton's joints] (A5Ø.5)
enteritis due to Yersinia enterocolitica (AØ4.6)
infective endocarditis (I33.Ø)
viral hepatitis (B15-B19)

EXCLUDES 1   *Behçet's disease (M35.2)*
direct infections of joint in infectious and parasitic diseases classified elsewhere (MØ1.-)
mumps arthritis (B26.85)
postmeningococcal arthritis (A39.84)
rheumatic fever (IØØ)
rubella arthritis (BØ6.82)
syphilis arthritis (late) (A52.77)
tabetic arthropathy [Charcôt's] (A52.16)

✓5ᵗʰ **M02.Ø** **Arthropathy following intestinal bypass**

M02.ØØ   **Arthropathy following intestinal bypass, unspecified site**

✓6ᵗʰ **M02.Ø1**   **Arthropathy following intestinal bypass, shoulder**

M02.Ø11   **Arthropathy following intestinal bypass, right shoulder**

M02.Ø12   **Arthropathy following intestinal bypass, left shoulder**

M02.Ø19   **Arthropathy following intestinal bypass, unspecified shoulder**

✓6ᵗʰ **M02.Ø2**   **Arthropathy following intestinal bypass, elbow**

M02.Ø21   **Arthropathy following intestinal bypass, right elbow**

M02.Ø22   **Arthropathy following intestinal bypass, left elbow**

M02.Ø29   **Arthropathy following intestinal bypass, unspecified elbow**

✓6ᵗʰ **M02.Ø3**   **Arthropathy following intestinal bypass, wrist**

Arthropathy following intestinal bypass, carpal bones

M02.Ø31   **Arthropathy following intestinal bypass, right wrist**

M02.Ø32   **Arthropathy following intestinal bypass, left wrist**

M02.Ø39   **Arthropathy following intestinal bypass, unspecified wrist**

✓6ᵗʰ **M02.Ø4**   **Arthropathy following intestinal bypass, hand**

Arthropathy following intestinal bypass, metacarpals and phalanges

M02.Ø41   **Arthropathy following intestinal bypass, right hand**

M02.Ø42   **Arthropathy following intestinal bypass, left hand**

✓ Additional Character Required   ✓x7ᵗʰ Placeholder   Questionable PDx   Manifestation   Unspecified Dx   UPD Unacceptable PDx   H1-H14 HAC   HCC CMS-HCC Dx   HIV HIV Dx

M02.049 Arthropathy following intestinal bypass, unspecified hand

✓6ᵗʰ **M02.05** Arthropathy following intestinal bypass, hip

M02.051 Arthropathy following intestinal bypass, right hip

M02.052 Arthropathy following intestinal bypass, left hip

M02.059 Arthropathy following intestinal bypass, unspecified hip

✓6ᵗʰ **M02.06** Arthropathy following intestinal bypass, knee

M02.061 Arthropathy following intestinal bypass, right knee

M02.062 Arthropathy following intestinal bypass, left knee

M02.069 Arthropathy following intestinal bypass, unspecified knee

✓6ᵗʰ **M02.07** Arthropathy following intestinal bypass, ankle and foot

Arthropathy following intestinal bypass, tarsus, metatarsus and phalanges

M02.071 Arthropathy following intestinal bypass, right ankle and foot

M02.072 Arthropathy following intestinal bypass, left ankle and foot

M02.079 Arthropathy following intestinal bypass, unspecified ankle and foot

M02.08 Arthropathy following intestinal bypass, vertebrae

M02.09 Arthropathy following intestinal bypass, multiple sites

✓5ᵗʰ **M02.1** Postdysenteric arthropathy

M02.10 Postdysenteric arthropathy, unspecified site **CC** **HCC**

✓6ᵗʰ **M02.11** Postdysenteric arthropathy, shoulder

M02.111 Postdysenteric arthropathy, right shoulder **CC** **HCC**

M02.112 Postdysenteric arthropathy, left shoulder **CC** **HCC**

M02.119 Postdysenteric arthropathy, unspecified shoulder **CC** **HCC**

✓6ᵗʰ **M02.12** Postdysenteric arthropathy, elbow

M02.121 Postdysenteric arthropathy, right elbow **CC** **HCC**

M02.122 Postdysenteric arthropathy, left elbow **CC** **HCC**

M02.129 Postdysenteric arthropathy, unspecified elbow **CC** **HCC**

✓6ᵗʰ **M02.13** Postdysenteric arthropathy, wrist

Postdysenteric arthropathy, carpal bones

M02.131 Postdysenteric arthropathy, right wrist **CC** **HCC**

M02.132 Postdysenteric arthropathy, left wrist **CC** **HCC**

M02.139 Postdysenteric arthropathy, unspecified wrist **CC** **HCC**

✓6ᵗʰ **M02.14** Postdysenteric arthropathy, hand

Postdysenteric arthropathy, metacarpus and phalanges

M02.141 Postdysenteric arthropathy, right hand **CC** **HCC**

M02.142 Postdysenteric arthropathy, left hand **CC** **HCC**

M02.149 Postdysenteric arthropathy, unspecified hand **CC** **HCC**

✓6ᵗʰ **M02.15** Postdysenteric arthropathy, hip

M02.151 Postdysenteric arthropathy, right hip **CC** **HCC**

M02.152 Postdysenteric arthropathy, left hip **CC** **HCC**

M02.159 Postdysenteric arthropathy, unspecified hip **CC** **HCC**

✓6ᵗʰ **M02.16** Postdysenteric arthropathy, knee

M02.161 Postdysenteric arthropathy, right knee **CC** **HCC**

M02.162 Postdysenteric arthropathy, left knee **CC** **HCC**

M02.169 Postdysenteric arthropathy, unspecified knee **CC** **HCC**

✓6ᵗʰ **M02.17** Postdysenteric arthropathy, ankle and foot

Postdysenteric arthropathy, tarsus, metatarsus and phalanges

M02.171 Postdysenteric arthropathy, right ankle and foot **CC** **HCC**

M02.172 Postdysenteric arthropathy, left ankle and foot **CC** **HCC**

M02.179 Postdysenteric arthropathy, unspecified ankle and foot **CC** **HCC**

M02.18 Postdysenteric arthropathy, vertebrae **CC** **HCC**

M02.19 Postdysenteric arthropathy, multiple sites **CC** **HCC**

✓5ᵗʰ **M02.2** Postimmunization arthropathy

M02.20 Postimmunization arthropathy, unspecified site

✓6ᵗʰ **M02.21** Postimmunization arthropathy, shoulder

M02.211 Postimmunization arthropathy, right shoulder

M02.212 Postimmunization arthropathy, left shoulder

M02.219 Postimmunization arthropathy, unspecified shoulder

✓6ᵗʰ **M02.22** Postimmunization arthropathy, elbow

M02.221 Postimmunization arthropathy, right elbow

M02.222 Postimmunization arthropathy, left elbow

M02.229 Postimmunization arthropathy, unspecified elbow

✓6ᵗʰ **M02.23** Postimmunization arthropathy, wrist

Postimmunization arthropathy, carpal bones

M02.231 Postimmunization arthropathy, right wrist

M02.232 Postimmunization arthropathy, left wrist

M02.239 Postimmunization arthropathy, unspecified wrist

✓6ᵗʰ **M02.24** Postimmunization arthropathy, hand

Postimmunization arthropathy, metacarpus and phalanges

M02.241 Postimmunization arthropathy, right hand

M02.242 Postimmunization arthropathy, left hand

M02.249 Postimmunization arthropathy, unspecified hand

✓6ᵗʰ **M02.25** Postimmunization arthropathy, hip

M02.251 Postimmunization arthropathy, right hip

M02.252 Postimmunization arthropathy, left hip

M02.259 Postimmunization arthropathy, unspecified hip

✓6ᵗʰ **M02.26** Postimmunization arthropathy, knee

M02.261 Postimmunization arthropathy, right knee

M02.262 Postimmunization arthropathy, left knee

M02.269 Postimmunization arthropathy, unspecified knee

✓6ᵗʰ **M02.27** Postimmunization arthropathy, ankle and foot

Postimmunization arthropathy, tarsus, metatarsus and phalanges

M02.271 Postimmunization arthropathy, right ankle and foot

M02.272 Postimmunization arthropathy, left ankle and foot

M02.279 Postimmunization arthropathy, unspecified ankle and foot

M02.28 Postimmunization arthropathy, vertebrae

M02.29 Postimmunization arthropathy, multiple sites

✓5ᵗʰ **M02.3** Reiter's disease

Reactive arthritis

DEF: Arthritis, iridocyclitis, and urethritis, sometimes with diarrhea. While symptoms may recur, arthritis is constant.

M02.30 Reiter's disease, unspecified site **CC** **HCC**

✓6ᵗʰ **M02.31** Reiter's disease, shoulder

M02.311 Reiter's disease, right shoulder **CC** **HCC**

M02.312 Reiter's disease, left shoulder **CC** **HCC**

M02.319 Reiter's disease, unspecified shoulder **CC** **HCC**

✓6ᵗʰ **M02.32** Reiter's disease, elbow

M02.321 Reiter's disease, right elbow **CC** **HCC**

M02.322 Reiter's disease, left elbow **CC** **HCC**

Ⓝ Newborn: 0   Ⓟ Pediatric: 0-17   Ⓜ Maternity: 9-64   Ⓐ Adult: 15-124   **MCC** Major Complication/Comorbidity   **CC** Complication/Comorbidity   **SW** Severe Wound Dx

764

ICD-10-CM 2022

M02.329   Reiter's disease, unspecified elbow   `CC` `HCC`

✓6ᵗʰ   **M02.33**   **Reiter's disease, wrist**

Reiter's disease, carpal bones

M02.331   Reiter's disease, **right** wrist   `CC` `HCC`

M02.332   Reiter's disease, **left** wrist   `CC` `HCC`

M02.339   Reiter's disease, unspecified wrist   `CC` `HCC`

✓6ᵗʰ   **M02.34**   **Reiter's disease, hand**

Reiter's disease, metacarpus and phalanges

M02.341   Reiter's disease, **right** hand   `CC` `HCC`

M02.342   Reiter's disease, **left** hand   `CC` `HCC`

M02.349   Reiter's disease, unspecified hand   `CC` `HCC`

✓6ᵗʰ   **M02.35**   **Reiter's disease, hip**

M02.351   Reiter's disease, **right** hip   `CC` `HCC`

M02.352   Reiter's disease, **left** hip   `CC` `HCC`

M02.359   Reiter's disease, unspecified hip   `CC` `HCC`

✓6ᵗʰ   **M02.36**   **Reiter's disease, knee**

M02.361   Reiter's disease, **right** knee   `CC` `HCC`

M02.362   Reiter's disease, **left** knee   `CC` `HCC`

M02.369   Reiter's disease, unspecified knee   `CC` `HCC`

✓6ᵗʰ   **M02.37**   **Reiter's disease, ankle and foot**

Reiter's disease, tarsus, metatarsus and phalanges

M02.371   Reiter's disease, **right** ankle and foot   `CC` `HCC`

M02.372   Reiter's disease, **left** ankle and foot   `CC` `HCC`

M02.379   Reiter's disease, unspecified ankle and foot   `CC` `HCC`

M02.38   Reiter's disease, vertebrae   `CC` `HCC`

M02.39   Reiter's disease, multiple sites   `CC` `HCC`

✓5ᵗʰ   **M02.8**   **Other reactive arthropathies**

M02.80   *Other reactive arthropathies, unspecified site*   `CC` `HCC`

✓6ᵗʰ   **M02.81**   **Other reactive arthropathies, shoulder**

M02.811   *Other reactive arthropathies, right shoulder*   `CC` `HCC`

M02.812   *Other reactive arthropathies, left shoulder*   `CC` `HCC`

M02.819   *Other reactive arthropathies, unspecified shoulder*   `CC` `HCC`

✓6ᵗʰ   **M02.82**   **Other reactive arthropathies, elbow**

M02.821   *Other reactive arthropathies, right elbow*   `CC` `HCC`

M02.822   *Other reactive arthropathies, left elbow*   `CC` `HCC`

M02.829   *Other reactive arthropathies, unspecified elbow*   `CC` `HCC`

✓6ᵗʰ   **M02.83**   **Other reactive arthropathies, wrist**

Other reactive arthropathies, carpal bones

M02.831   *Other reactive arthropathies, right wrist*   `CC` `HCC`

M02.832   *Other reactive arthropathies, left wrist*   `CC` `HCC`

M02.839   *Other reactive arthropathies, unspecified wrist*   `CC` `HCC`

✓6ᵗʰ   **M02.84**   **Other reactive arthropathies, hand**

Other reactive arthropathies, metacarpus and phalanges

M02.841   *Other reactive arthropathies, right hand*   `CC` `HCC`

M02.842   *Other reactive arthropathies, left hand*   `CC` `HCC`

M02.849   *Other reactive arthropathies, unspecified hand*   `CC` `HCC`

✓6ᵗʰ   **M02.85**   **Other reactive arthropathies, hip**

M02.851   *Other reactive arthropathies, right hip*   `CC` `HCC`

M02.852   *Other reactive arthropathies, left hip*   `CC` `HCC`

M02.859   *Other reactive arthropathies, unspecified hip*   `CC` `HCC`

✓6ᵗʰ   **M02.86**   **Other reactive arthropathies, knee**

M02.861   *Other reactive arthropathies, right knee*   `CC` `HCC`

M02.862   *Other reactive arthropathies, left knee*   `CC` `HCC`

M02.869   *Other reactive arthropathies, unspecified knee*   `CC` `HCC`

✓6ᵗʰ   **M02.87**   **Other reactive arthropathies, ankle and foot**

Other reactive arthropathies, tarsus, metatarsus and phalanges

M02.871   *Other reactive arthropathies, right ankle and foot*   `CC` `HCC`

M02.872   *Other reactive arthropathies, left ankle and foot*   `CC` `HCC`

M02.879   *Other reactive arthropathies, unspecified ankle and foot*   `CC` `HCC`

M02.88   *Other reactive arthropathies, vertebrae*   `CC` `HCC`

M02.89   *Other reactive arthropathies, multiple sites*   `CC` `HCC`

M02.9   **Reactive arthropathy, unspecified**   `HCC`

Autoinflammatory syndromes (M04)

✓4ᵗʰ   **M04**   **Autoinflammatory syndromes**

EXCLUDES 2   *Crohn's disease (K50.-)*

AHA: 2016,4Q,37

M04.1   **Periodic fever syndromes**   `HCC`

Familial Mediterranean fever

Hyperimmunoglobin D syndrome

Mevalonate kinase deficiency

Tumor necrosis factor receptor associated periodic syndrome [TRAPS]

M04.2   **Cryopyrin-associated periodic syndromes**   `HCC`

Chronic infantile neurological, cutaneous and articular syndrome [CINCA]

Familial cold autoinflammatory syndrome

Familial cold urticaria

Muckle-Wells syndrome

Neonatal onset multisystemic inflammatory disorder [NOMID]

M04.8   **Other autoinflammatory syndromes**   `HCC`

Blau syndrome

Deficiency of interleukin 1 receptor antagonist [DIRA]

Majeed syndrome

Periodic fever, aphthous stomatitis, pharyngitis, and adenopathy syndrome [PFAPA]

Pyogenic arthritis, pyoderma gangrenosum, and acne syndrome [PAPA]

M04.9   **Autoinflammatory syndrome, unspecified**   `HCC`

Inflammatory polyarthropathies (M05-M14)

✓4ᵗʰ   **M05**   **Rheumatoid arthritis with rheumatoid factor**

EXCLUDES 1   *rheumatic fever (I00)*

juvenile rheumatoid arthritis (M08.-)

rheumatoid arthritis of spine (M45.-)

AHA: 2020,4Q,31-32

DEF: Rheumatoid arthritis: Autoimmune systemic disease that causes chronic inflammation of the joints and other areas of the body, manifested by inflammatory changes in articular structures and synovial membranes, atrophy, and loss in bone density.

✓5ᵗʰ   **M05.0**   **Felty's syndrome**

Rheumatoid arthritis with splenoadenomegaly and leukopenia

M05.00   **Felty's syndrome, unspecified site**   `HCC`

✓6ᵗʰ   **M05.01**   **Felty's syndrome, shoulder**

M05.011   Felty's syndrome, **right** shoulder   `HCC`

M05.012   Felty's syndrome, **left** shoulder   `HCC`

M05.019   Felty's syndrome, unspecified shoulder   `HCC`

✓6ᵗʰ   **M05.02**   **Felty's syndrome, elbow**

M05.021   Felty's syndrome, **right** elbow   `HCC`

M05.022   Felty's syndrome, **left** elbow   `HCC`

M05.029   Felty's syndrome, unspecified elbow   `HCC`

✓6ᵗʰ   **M05.03**   **Felty's syndrome, wrist**

Felty's syndrome, carpal bones

M05.031   Felty's syndrome, **right** wrist   `HCC`

M05.032   Felty's syndrome, **left** wrist   `HCC`

✓ Additional Character Required   ✓7ᵗʰ Placeholder   Questionable PDx   Manifestation   Unspecified Dx   `UPD` Unacceptable PDx   `H1`-`H14` HAC   `HCC` CMS-HCC Dx   `HIV` HIV Dx

ICD-10-CM 2022   **765**

M05.039   Felty's syndrome, unspecified wrist   `HCC`

✓6ᵗʰ M05.04   Felty's syndrome, hand

   Felty's syndrome, metacarpus and phalanges

    M05.041   Felty's syndrome, right hand   `HCC`

    M05.042   Felty's syndrome, left hand   `HCC`

    M05.049   Felty's syndrome, unspecified hand   `HCC`

✓6ᵗʰ M05.05   Felty's syndrome, hip

    M05.051   Felty's syndrome, right hip   `HCC`

    M05.052   Felty's syndrome, left hip   `HCC`

    M05.059   Felty's syndrome, unspecified hip   `HCC`

✓6ᵗʰ M05.06   Felty's syndrome, knee

    M05.061   Felty's syndrome, right knee   `HCC`

    M05.062   Felty's syndrome, left knee   `HCC`

    M05.069   Felty's syndrome, unspecified knee   `HCC`

✓6ᵗʰ M05.07   Felty's syndrome, ankle and foot

   Felty's syndrome, tarsus, metatarsus and phalanges

    M05.071   Felty's syndrome, right ankle and foot   `HCC`

    M05.072   Felty's syndrome, left ankle and foot   `HCC`

    M05.079   Felty's syndrome, unspecified ankle and foot   `HCC`

   M05.09   Felty's syndrome, multiple sites   `HCC`

✓5ᵗʰ M05.1   Rheumatoid lung disease with rheumatoid arthritis

   DEF: Lung disorders associated with rheumatoid arthritis.

    M05.10   Rheumatoid lung disease with rheumatoid arthritis of unspecified site   `HCC`

✓6ᵗʰ M05.11   Rheumatoid lung disease with rheumatoid arthritis of shoulder

    M05.111   Rheumatoid lung disease with rheumatoid arthritis of right shoulder   `HCC`

    M05.112   Rheumatoid lung disease with rheumatoid arthritis of left shoulder   `HCC`

    M05.119   Rheumatoid lung disease with rheumatoid arthritis of unspecified shoulder   `HCC`

✓6ᵗʰ M05.12   Rheumatoid lung disease with rheumatoid arthritis of elbow

    M05.121   Rheumatoid lung disease with rheumatoid arthritis of right elbow   `HCC`

    M05.122   Rheumatoid lung disease with rheumatoid arthritis of left elbow   `HCC`

    M05.129   Rheumatoid lung disease with rheumatoid arthritis of unspecified elbow   `HCC`

✓6ᵗʰ M05.13   Rheumatoid lung disease with rheumatoid arthritis of wrist

   Rheumatoid lung disease with rheumatoid arthritis, carpal bones

    M05.131   Rheumatoid lung disease with rheumatoid arthritis of right wrist   `HCC`

    M05.132   Rheumatoid lung disease with rheumatoid arthritis of left wrist   `HCC`

    M05.139   Rheumatoid lung disease with rheumatoid arthritis of unspecified wrist   `HCC`

✓6ᵗʰ M05.14   Rheumatoid lung disease with rheumatoid arthritis of hand

   Rheumatoid lung disease with rheumatoid arthritis, metacarpus and phalanges

    M05.141   Rheumatoid lung disease with rheumatoid arthritis of right hand   `HCC`

    M05.142   Rheumatoid lung disease with rheumatoid arthritis of left hand   `HCC`

    M05.149   Rheumatoid lung disease with rheumatoid arthritis of unspecified hand   `HCC`

✓6ᵗʰ M05.15   Rheumatoid lung disease with rheumatoid arthritis of hip

    M05.151   Rheumatoid lung disease with rheumatoid arthritis of right hip   `HCC`

    M05.152   Rheumatoid lung disease with rheumatoid arthritis of left hip   `HCC`

    M05.159   Rheumatoid lung disease with rheumatoid arthritis of unspecified hip   `HCC`

✓6ᵗʰ M05.16   Rheumatoid lung disease with rheumatoid arthritis of knee

    M05.161   Rheumatoid lung disease with rheumatoid arthritis of right knee   `HCC`

    M05.162   Rheumatoid lung disease with rheumatoid arthritis of left knee   `HCC`

    M05.169   Rheumatoid lung disease with rheumatoid arthritis of unspecified knee   `HCC`

✓6ᵗʰ M05.17   Rheumatoid lung disease with rheumatoid arthritis of ankle and foot

   Rheumatoid lung disease with rheumatoid arthritis, tarsus, metatarsus and phalanges

    M05.171   Rheumatoid lung disease with rheumatoid arthritis of right ankle and foot   `HCC`

    M05.172   Rheumatoid lung disease with rheumatoid arthritis of left ankle and foot   `HCC`

    M05.179   Rheumatoid lung disease with rheumatoid arthritis of unspecified ankle and foot   `HCC`

   M05.19   Rheumatoid lung disease with rheumatoid arthritis of multiple sites   `HCC`

✓5ᵗʰ M05.2   Rheumatoid vasculitis with rheumatoid arthritis

    M05.20   Rheumatoid vasculitis with rheumatoid arthritis of unspecified site   `HCC`

✓6ᵗʰ M05.21   Rheumatoid vasculitis with rheumatoid arthritis of shoulder

    M05.211   Rheumatoid vasculitis with rheumatoid arthritis of right shoulder   `HCC`

    M05.212   Rheumatoid vasculitis with rheumatoid arthritis of left shoulder   `HCC`

    M05.219   Rheumatoid vasculitis with rheumatoid arthritis of unspecified shoulder   `HCC`

✓6ᵗʰ M05.22   Rheumatoid vasculitis with rheumatoid arthritis of elbow

    M05.221   Rheumatoid vasculitis with rheumatoid arthritis of right elbow   `HCC`

    M05.222   Rheumatoid vasculitis with rheumatoid arthritis of left elbow   `HCC`

    M05.229   Rheumatoid vasculitis with rheumatoid arthritis of unspecified elbow   `HCC`

✓6ᵗʰ M05.23   Rheumatoid vasculitis with rheumatoid arthritis of wrist

   Rheumatoid vasculitis with rheumatoid arthritis, carpal bones

    M05.231   Rheumatoid vasculitis with rheumatoid arthritis of right wrist   `HCC`

    M05.232   Rheumatoid vasculitis with rheumatoid arthritis of left wrist   `HCC`

    M05.239   Rheumatoid vasculitis with rheumatoid arthritis of unspecified wrist   `HCC`

✓6ᵗʰ M05.24   Rheumatoid vasculitis with rheumatoid arthritis of hand

   Rheumatoid vasculitis with rheumatoid arthritis, metacarpus and phalanges

    M05.241   Rheumatoid vasculitis with rheumatoid arthritis of right hand   `HCC`

    M05.242   Rheumatoid vasculitis with rheumatoid arthritis of left hand   `HCC`

    M05.249   Rheumatoid vasculitis with rheumatoid arthritis of unspecified hand   `HCC`

✓6ᵗʰ M05.25   Rheumatoid vasculitis with rheumatoid arthritis of hip

    M05.251   Rheumatoid vasculitis with rheumatoid arthritis of right hip   `HCC`

    M05.252   Rheumatoid vasculitis with rheumatoid arthritis of left hip   `HCC`

    M05.259   Rheumatoid vasculitis with rheumatoid arthritis of unspecified hip   `HCC`

✓6ᵗʰ M05.26   Rheumatoid vasculitis with rheumatoid arthritis of knee

    M05.261   Rheumatoid vasculitis with rheumatoid arthritis of right knee   `HCC`

    M05.262   Rheumatoid vasculitis with rheumatoid arthritis of left knee   `HCC`

Ⓝ Newborn: 0   Ⓟ Pediatric: 0-17   Ⓜ Maternity: 9-64   Ⓐ Adult: 15-124   `MCC` Major Complication/Comorbidity   `CC` Complication/Comorbidity   `SW` Severe Wound Dx

766   ICD-10-CM 2022

        M05.269 Rheumatoid vasculitis with rheumatoid arthritis of unspecified knee `HCC`

☑6ᵗʰ **M05.27** Rheumatoid vasculitis with rheumatoid arthritis of ankle and foot

        Rheumatoid vasculitis with rheumatoid arthritis, tarsus, metatarsus and phalanges

        M05.271 Rheumatoid vasculitis with rheumatoid arthritis of right ankle and foot `HCC`

        M05.272 Rheumatoid vasculitis with rheumatoid arthritis of left ankle and foot `HCC`

        M05.279 Rheumatoid vasculitis with rheumatoid arthritis of unspecified ankle and foot `HCC`

     M05.29 Rheumatoid vasculitis with rheumatoid arthritis of multiple sites `HCC`

☑5ᵗʰ **M05.3** Rheumatoid heart disease with rheumatoid arthritis

     Rheumatoid carditis
     Rheumatoid endocarditis
     Rheumatoid myocarditis
     Rheumatoid pericarditis

     M05.30 Rheumatoid heart disease with rheumatoid arthritis of unspecified site `HCC`

☑6ᵗʰ **M05.31** Rheumatoid heart disease with rheumatoid arthritis of shoulder

        M05.311 Rheumatoid heart disease with rheumatoid arthritis of right shoulder `HCC`

        M05.312 Rheumatoid heart disease with rheumatoid arthritis of left shoulder `HCC`

        M05.319 Rheumatoid heart disease with rheumatoid arthritis of unspecified shoulder `HCC`

☑6ᵗʰ **M05.32** Rheumatoid heart disease with rheumatoid arthritis of elbow

        M05.321 Rheumatoid heart disease with rheumatoid arthritis of right elbow `HCC`

        M05.322 Rheumatoid heart disease with rheumatoid arthritis of left elbow `HCC`

        M05.329 Rheumatoid heart disease with rheumatoid arthritis of unspecified elbow `HCC`

☑6ᵗʰ **M05.33** Rheumatoid heart disease with rheumatoid arthritis of wrist

        Rheumatoid heart disease with rheumatoid arthritis, carpal bones

        M05.331 Rheumatoid heart disease with rheumatoid arthritis of right wrist `HCC`

        M05.332 Rheumatoid heart disease with rheumatoid arthritis of left wrist `HCC`

        M05.339 Rheumatoid heart disease with rheumatoid arthritis of unspecified wrist `HCC`

☑6ᵗʰ **M05.34** Rheumatoid heart disease with rheumatoid arthritis of hand

        Rheumatoid heart disease with rheumatoid arthritis, metacarpus and phalanges

        M05.341 Rheumatoid heart disease with rheumatoid arthritis of right hand `HCC`

        M05.342 Rheumatoid heart disease with rheumatoid arthritis of left hand `HCC`

        M05.349 Rheumatoid heart disease with rheumatoid arthritis of unspecified hand `HCC`

☑6ᵗʰ **M05.35** Rheumatoid heart disease with rheumatoid arthritis of hip

        M05.351 Rheumatoid heart disease with rheumatoid arthritis of right hip `HCC`

        M05.352 Rheumatoid heart disease with rheumatoid arthritis of left hip `HCC`

        M05.359 Rheumatoid heart disease with rheumatoid arthritis of unspecified hip `HCC`

☑6ᵗʰ **M05.36** Rheumatoid heart disease with rheumatoid arthritis of knee

        M05.361 Rheumatoid heart disease with rheumatoid arthritis of right knee `HCC`

        M05.362 Rheumatoid heart disease with rheumatoid arthritis of left knee `HCC`

        M05.369 Rheumatoid heart disease with rheumatoid arthritis of unspecified knee `HCC`

☑6ᵗʰ **M05.37** Rheumatoid heart disease with rheumatoid arthritis of ankle and foot

        Rheumatoid heart disease with rheumatoid arthritis, tarsus, metatarsus and phalanges

        M05.371 Rheumatoid heart disease with rheumatoid arthritis of right ankle and foot `HCC`

        M05.372 Rheumatoid heart disease with rheumatoid arthritis of left ankle and foot `HCC`

        M05.379 Rheumatoid heart disease with rheumatoid arthritis of unspecified ankle and foot `HCC`

     M05.39 Rheumatoid heart disease with rheumatoid arthritis of multiple sites `HCC`

☑5ᵗʰ **M05.4** Rheumatoid myopathy with rheumatoid arthritis

     M05.40 Rheumatoid myopathy with rheumatoid arthritis of unspecified site `CC` `HCC`

☑6ᵗʰ **M05.41** Rheumatoid myopathy with rheumatoid arthritis of shoulder

        M05.411 Rheumatoid myopathy with rheumatoid arthritis of right shoulder `CC` `HCC`

        M05.412 Rheumatoid myopathy with rheumatoid arthritis of left shoulder `CC` `HCC`

        M05.419 Rheumatoid myopathy with rheumatoid arthritis of unspecified shoulder `CC` `HCC`

☑6ᵗʰ **M05.42** Rheumatoid myopathy with rheumatoid arthritis of elbow

        M05.421 Rheumatoid myopathy with rheumatoid arthritis of right elbow `CC` `HCC`

        M05.422 Rheumatoid myopathy with rheumatoid arthritis of left elbow `CC` `HCC`

        M05.429 Rheumatoid myopathy with rheumatoid arthritis of unspecified elbow `CC` `HCC`

☑6ᵗʰ **M05.43** Rheumatoid myopathy with rheumatoid arthritis of wrist

        Rheumatoid myopathy with rheumatoid arthritis, carpal bones

        M05.431 Rheumatoid myopathy with rheumatoid arthritis of right wrist `CC` `HCC`

        M05.432 Rheumatoid myopathy with rheumatoid arthritis of left wrist `CC` `HCC`

        M05.439 Rheumatoid myopathy with rheumatoid arthritis of unspecified wrist `CC` `HCC`

☑6ᵗʰ **M05.44** Rheumatoid myopathy with rheumatoid arthritis of hand

        Rheumatoid myopathy with rheumatoid arthritis, metacarpus and phalanges

        M05.441 Rheumatoid myopathy with rheumatoid arthritis of right hand `CC` `HCC`

        M05.442 Rheumatoid myopathy with rheumatoid arthritis of left hand `CC` `HCC`

        M05.449 Rheumatoid myopathy with rheumatoid arthritis of unspecified hand `CC` `HCC`

☑6ᵗʰ **M05.45** Rheumatoid myopathy with rheumatoid arthritis of hip

        M05.451 Rheumatoid myopathy with rheumatoid arthritis of right hip `CC` `HCC`

        M05.452 Rheumatoid myopathy with rheumatoid arthritis of left hip `CC` `HCC`

        M05.459 Rheumatoid myopathy with rheumatoid arthritis of unspecified hip `CC` `HCC`

☑6ᵗʰ **M05.46** Rheumatoid myopathy with rheumatoid arthritis of knee

        M05.461 Rheumatoid myopathy with rheumatoid arthritis of right knee `CC` `HCC`

        M05.462 Rheumatoid myopathy with rheumatoid arthritis of left knee `CC` `HCC`

        M05.469 Rheumatoid myopathy with rheumatoid arthritis of unspecified knee `CC` `HCC`

☑6ᵗʰ **M05.47** Rheumatoid myopathy with rheumatoid arthritis of ankle and foot

        Rheumatoid myopathy with rheumatoid arthritis, tarsus, metatarsus and phalanges

        M05.471 Rheumatoid myopathy with rheumatoid arthritis of right ankle and foot `CC` `HCC`

☑ Additional Character Required   ☑x7ᵗʰ Placeholder   Questionable PDx   Manifestation   Unspecified Dx   `UPD` Unacceptable PDx   `H1`-`H14` HAC   `HCC` CMS-HCC Dx   `HIV` HIV Dx

M05.472 **Rheumatoid myopathy with rheumatoid arthritis of left ankle and foot** `CC` `HCC`

M05.479 **Rheumatoid myopathy with rheumatoid arthritis of unspecified ankle and foot** `CC` `HCC`

M05.49 **Rheumatoid myopathy with rheumatoid arthritis of multiple sites** `CC` `HCC`

✓5ᵗʰ **M05.5 Rheumatoid polyneuropathy with rheumatoid arthritis**

M05.50 **Rheumatoid polyneuropathy with rheumatoid arthritis of unspecified site** `HCC`

✓6ᵗʰ M05.51 **Rheumatoid polyneuropathy with rheumatoid arthritis of shoulder**

M05.511 **Rheumatoid polyneuropathy with rheumatoid arthritis of right shoulder** `HCC`

M05.512 **Rheumatoid polyneuropathy with rheumatoid arthritis of left shoulder** `HCC`

M05.519 **Rheumatoid polyneuropathy with rheumatoid arthritis of unspecified shoulder** `HCC`

✓6ᵗʰ M05.52 **Rheumatoid polyneuropathy with rheumatoid arthritis of elbow**

M05.521 **Rheumatoid polyneuropathy with rheumatoid arthritis of right elbow** `HCC`

M05.522 **Rheumatoid polyneuropathy with rheumatoid arthritis of left elbow** `HCC`

M05.529 **Rheumatoid polyneuropathy with rheumatoid arthritis of unspecified elbow** `HCC`

✓6ᵗʰ M05.53 **Rheumatoid polyneuropathy with rheumatoid arthritis of wrist**

Rheumatoid polyneuropathy with rheumatoid arthritis, carpal bones

M05.531 **Rheumatoid polyneuropathy with rheumatoid arthritis of right wrist** `HCC`

M05.532 **Rheumatoid polyneuropathy with rheumatoid arthritis of left wrist** `HCC`

M05.539 **Rheumatoid polyneuropathy with rheumatoid arthritis of unspecified wrist** `HCC`

✓6ᵗʰ M05.54 **Rheumatoid polyneuropathy with rheumatoid arthritis of hand**

Rheumatoid polyneuropathy with rheumatoid arthritis, metacarpus and phalanges

M05.541 **Rheumatoid polyneuropathy with rheumatoid arthritis of right hand** `HCC`

M05.542 **Rheumatoid polyneuropathy with rheumatoid arthritis of left hand** `HCC`

M05.549 **Rheumatoid polyneuropathy with rheumatoid arthritis of unspecified hand** `HCC`

✓6ᵗʰ M05.55 **Rheumatoid polyneuropathy with rheumatoid arthritis of hip**

M05.551 **Rheumatoid polyneuropathy with rheumatoid arthritis of right hip** `HCC`

M05.552 **Rheumatoid polyneuropathy with rheumatoid arthritis of left hip** `HCC`

M05.559 **Rheumatoid polyneuropathy with rheumatoid arthritis of unspecified hip** `HCC`

✓6ᵗʰ M05.56 **Rheumatoid polyneuropathy with rheumatoid arthritis of knee**

M05.561 **Rheumatoid polyneuropathy with rheumatoid arthritis of right knee** `HCC`

M05.562 **Rheumatoid polyneuropathy with rheumatoid arthritis of left knee** `HCC`

M05.569 **Rheumatoid polyneuropathy with rheumatoid arthritis of unspecified knee** `HCC`

✓6ᵗʰ M05.57 **Rheumatoid polyneuropathy with rheumatoid arthritis of ankle and foot**

Rheumatoid polyneuropathy with rheumatoid arthritis, tarsus, metatarsus and phalanges

M05.571 **Rheumatoid polyneuropathy with rheumatoid arthritis of right ankle and foot** `HCC`

M05.572 **Rheumatoid polyneuropathy with rheumatoid arthritis of left ankle and foot** `HCC`

M05.579 **Rheumatoid polyneuropathy with rheumatoid arthritis of unspecified ankle and foot** `HCC`

M05.59 **Rheumatoid polyneuropathy with rheumatoid arthritis of multiple sites** `HCC`

✓5ᵗʰ **M05.6 Rheumatoid arthritis with involvement of other organs and systems**

M05.60 **Rheumatoid arthritis of unspecified site with involvement of other organs and systems** `HCC`

✓6ᵗʰ M05.61 **Rheumatoid arthritis of shoulder with involvement of other organs and systems**

M05.611 **Rheumatoid arthritis of right shoulder with involvement of other organs and systems** `HCC`

M05.612 **Rheumatoid arthritis of left shoulder with involvement of other organs and systems** `HCC`

M05.619 **Rheumatoid arthritis of unspecified shoulder with involvement of other organs and systems** `HCC`

✓6ᵗʰ M05.62 **Rheumatoid arthritis of elbow with involvement of other organs and systems**

M05.621 **Rheumatoid arthritis of right elbow with involvement of other organs and systems** `HCC`

M05.622 **Rheumatoid arthritis of left elbow with involvement of other organs and systems** `HCC`

M05.629 **Rheumatoid arthritis of unspecified elbow with involvement of other organs and systems** `HCC`

✓6ᵗʰ M05.63 **Rheumatoid arthritis of wrist with involvement of other organs and systems**

Rheumatoid arthritis of carpal bones with involvement of other organs and systems

M05.631 **Rheumatoid arthritis of right wrist with involvement of other organs and systems** `HCC`

M05.632 **Rheumatoid arthritis of left wrist with involvement of other organs and systems** `HCC`

M05.639 **Rheumatoid arthritis of unspecified wrist with involvement of other organs and systems** `HCC`

✓6ᵗʰ M05.64 **Rheumatoid arthritis of hand with involvement of other organs and systems**

Rheumatoid arthritis of metacarpus and phalanges with involvement of other organs and systems

M05.641 **Rheumatoid arthritis of right hand with involvement of other organs and systems** `HCC`

M05.642 **Rheumatoid arthritis of left hand with involvement of other organs and systems** `HCC`

M05.649 **Rheumatoid arthritis of unspecified hand with involvement of other organs and systems** `HCC`

✓6ᵗʰ M05.65 **Rheumatoid arthritis of hip with involvement of other organs and systems**

M05.651 **Rheumatoid arthritis of right hip with involvement of other organs and systems** `HCC`

M05.652 **Rheumatoid arthritis of left hip with involvement of other organs and systems** `HCC`

M05.659 **Rheumatoid arthritis of unspecified hip with involvement of other organs and systems** `HCC`

✓6ᵗʰ M05.66 **Rheumatoid arthritis of knee with involvement of other organs and systems**

M05.661 **Rheumatoid arthritis of right knee with involvement of other organs and systems** `HCC`

M05.662 **Rheumatoid arthritis of left knee with involvement of other organs and systems** `HCC`

M05.669 **Rheumatoid arthritis of unspecified knee with involvement of other organs and systems** `HCC`

N Newborn: 0   P Pediatric: 0-17   M Maternity: 9-64   A Adult: 15-124   `MCC` Major Complication/Comorbidity   `CC` Complication/Comorbidity   `SW` Severe Wound Dx

✓6ᵗʰ **M05.67 Rheumatoid arthritis of** ankle and foot **with involvement of other organs and systems**
Rheumatoid arthritis of tarsus, metatarsus and phalanges with involvement of other organs and systems

    M05.671 Rheumatoid arthritis of right **ankle and foot with involvement of other organs and systems** `HCC`

    M05.672 Rheumatoid arthritis of left **ankle and foot with involvement of other organs and systems** `HCC`

    M05.679 Rheumatoid arthritis of unspecified ankle and foot with involvement of other organs and systems `HCC`

  M05.69 Rheumatoid arthritis of multiple sites **with involvement of other organs and systems** `HCC`

✓5ᵗʰ **M05.7 Rheumatoid arthritis** with rheumatoid factor without organ or systems involvement

  M05.70 Rheumatoid arthritis with rheumatoid factor of unspecified site without organ or systems involvement `HCC`

✓6ᵗʰ **M05.71 Rheumatoid arthritis with rheumatoid factor of** shoulder **without organ or systems involvement**

    M05.711 Rheumatoid arthritis with rheumatoid factor of right **shoulder without organ or systems involvement** `HCC`

    M05.712 Rheumatoid arthritis with rheumatoid factor of left **shoulder without organ or systems involvement** `HCC`

    M05.719 Rheumatoid arthritis with rheumatoid factor of unspecified shoulder without organ or systems involvement `HCC`

✓6ᵗʰ **M05.72 Rheumatoid arthritis with rheumatoid factor of** elbow **without organ or systems involvement**

    M05.721 Rheumatoid arthritis with rheumatoid factor of right **elbow without organ or systems involvement** `HCC`

    M05.722 Rheumatoid arthritis with rheumatoid factor of left **elbow without organ or systems involvement** `HCC`

    M05.729 Rheumatoid arthritis with rheumatoid factor of unspecified elbow without organ or systems involvement `HCC`

✓6ᵗʰ **M05.73 Rheumatoid arthritis with rheumatoid factor of** wrist **without organ or systems involvement**

    M05.731 Rheumatoid arthritis with rheumatoid factor of right **wrist without organ or systems involvement** `HCC`

    M05.732 Rheumatoid arthritis with rheumatoid factor of left **wrist without organ or systems involvement** `HCC`

    M05.739 Rheumatoid arthritis with rheumatoid factor of unspecified wrist without organ or systems involvement `HCC`

✓6ᵗʰ **M05.74 Rheumatoid arthritis with rheumatoid factor of** hand **without organ or systems involvement**

    M05.741 Rheumatoid arthritis with rheumatoid factor of right **hand without organ or systems involvement** `HCC`

    M05.742 Rheumatoid arthritis with rheumatoid factor of left **hand without organ or systems involvement** `HCC`

    M05.749 Rheumatoid arthritis with rheumatoid factor of unspecified hand without organ or systems involvement `HCC`

✓6ᵗʰ **M05.75 Rheumatoid arthritis with rheumatoid factor of** hip **without organ or systems involvement**

    M05.751 Rheumatoid arthritis with rheumatoid factor of right **hip without organ or systems involvement** `HCC`

    M05.752 Rheumatoid arthritis with rheumatoid factor of left **hip without organ or systems involvement** `HCC`

    M05.759 Rheumatoid arthritis with rheumatoid factor of unspecified hip without organ or systems involvement `HCC`

✓6ᵗʰ **M05.76 Rheumatoid arthritis with rheumatoid factor of** knee **without organ or systems involvement**

    M05.761 Rheumatoid arthritis with rheumatoid factor of right **knee without organ or systems involvement** `HCC`

    M05.762 Rheumatoid arthritis with rheumatoid factor of left **knee without organ or systems involvement** `HCC`

    M05.769 Rheumatoid arthritis with rheumatoid factor of unspecified knee without organ or systems involvement `HCC`

✓6ᵗʰ **M05.77 Rheumatoid arthritis with rheumatoid factor of** ankle and foot **without organ or systems involvement**

    M05.771 Rheumatoid arthritis with rheumatoid factor of right **ankle and foot without organ or systems involvement** `HCC`

    M05.772 Rheumatoid arthritis with rheumatoid factor of left **ankle and foot without organ or systems involvement** `HCC`

    M05.779 Rheumatoid arthritis with rheumatoid factor of unspecified ankle and foot without organ or systems involvement `HCC`

  M05.79 Rheumatoid arthritis with rheumatoid factor of multiple sites **without organ or systems involvement** `HCC`

  M05.7A Rheumatoid arthritis with rheumatoid factor of other specified site without organ or systems involvement `HCC`

✓5ᵗʰ **M05.8 Other rheumatoid arthritis** with rheumatoid factor

  M05.80 Other rheumatoid arthritis with rheumatoid factor of unspecified site `HCC`

✓6ᵗʰ **M05.81 Other rheumatoid arthritis with rheumatoid factor of** shoulder

    M05.811 Other rheumatoid arthritis with rheumatoid factor of right **shoulder** `HCC`

    M05.812 Other rheumatoid arthritis with rheumatoid factor of left **shoulder** `HCC`

    M05.819 Other rheumatoid arthritis with rheumatoid factor of unspecified shoulder `HCC`

✓6ᵗʰ **M05.82 Other rheumatoid arthritis with rheumatoid factor of** elbow

    M05.821 Other rheumatoid arthritis with rheumatoid factor of right **elbow** `HCC`

    M05.822 Other rheumatoid arthritis with rheumatoid factor of left **elbow** `HCC`

    M05.829 Other rheumatoid arthritis with rheumatoid factor of unspecified elbow `HCC`

✓6ᵗʰ **M05.83 Other rheumatoid arthritis with rheumatoid factor of** wrist

    M05.831 Other rheumatoid arthritis with rheumatoid factor of right **wrist** `HCC`

    M05.832 Other rheumatoid arthritis with rheumatoid factor of left **wrist** `HCC`

    M05.839 Other rheumatoid arthritis with rheumatoid factor of unspecified wrist `HCC`

✓6ᵗʰ **M05.84 Other rheumatoid arthritis with rheumatoid factor of** hand

    M05.841 Other rheumatoid arthritis with rheumatoid factor of right **hand** `HCC`

    M05.842 Other rheumatoid arthritis with rheumatoid factor of left **hand** `HCC`

    M05.849 Other rheumatoid arthritis with rheumatoid factor of unspecified hand `HCC`

✓6ᵗʰ **M05.85 Other rheumatoid arthritis with rheumatoid factor of** hip

    M05.851 Other rheumatoid arthritis with rheumatoid factor of right **hip** `HCC`

    M05.852 Other rheumatoid arthritis with rheumatoid factor of left **hip** `HCC`

    M05.859 Other rheumatoid arthritis with rheumatoid factor of unspecified hip `HCC`

✓6ᵗʰ **M05.86 Other rheumatoid arthritis with rheumatoid factor of** knee

    M05.861 Other rheumatoid arthritis with rheumatoid factor of right **knee** `HCC`

    M05.862 Other rheumatoid arthritis with rheumatoid factor of left **knee** `HCC`

M05.869 **Other rheumatoid arthritis with rheumatoid factor of unspecified knee** HCC

✓6ᵗʰ M05.87 **Other rheumatoid arthritis with rheumatoid factor of** ankle and foot

M05.871 **Other rheumatoid arthritis with rheumatoid factor of** right **ankle and foot** HCC

M05.872 **Other rheumatoid arthritis with rheumatoid factor of** left **ankle and foot** HCC

M05.879 **Other rheumatoid arthritis with rheumatoid factor of unspecified ankle and foot** HCC

M05.89 **Other rheumatoid arthritis with rheumatoid factor of** multiple sites HCC

M05.8A **Other rheumatoid arthritis with rheumatoid factor of other specified site** HCC

M05.9 **Rheumatoid arthritis with rheumatoid factor, unspecified** HCC

✓4ᵗʰ **M06 Other rheumatoid arthritis**

AHA: 2020,4Q,31-32

DEF: Rheumatoid arthritis: Autoimmune systemic disease that causes chronic inflammation of the joints and other areas of the body, manifested by inflammatory changes in articular structures and synovial membranes, atrophy, and loss in bone density.

✓5ᵗʰ **M06.0 Rheumatoid arthritis** without rheumatoid factor

M06.00 **Rheumatoid arthritis without rheumatoid factor, unspecified site** HCC

✓6ᵗʰ M06.01 **Rheumatoid arthritis without rheumatoid factor,** shoulder

M06.011 **Rheumatoid arthritis without rheumatoid factor,** right **shoulder** HCC

M06.012 **Rheumatoid arthritis without rheumatoid factor,** left **shoulder** HCC

M06.019 **Rheumatoid arthritis without rheumatoid factor, unspecified shoulder** HCC

✓6ᵗʰ M06.02 **Rheumatoid arthritis without rheumatoid factor,** elbow

M06.021 **Rheumatoid arthritis without rheumatoid factor,** right **elbow** HCC

M06.022 **Rheumatoid arthritis without rheumatoid factor,** left **elbow** HCC

M06.029 **Rheumatoid arthritis without rheumatoid factor, unspecified elbow** HCC

✓6ᵗʰ M06.03 **Rheumatoid arthritis without rheumatoid factor,** wrist

M06.031 **Rheumatoid arthritis without rheumatoid factor,** right **wrist** HCC

M06.032 **Rheumatoid arthritis without rheumatoid factor,** left **wrist** HCC

M06.039 **Rheumatoid arthritis without rheumatoid factor, unspecified wrist** HCC

✓6ᵗʰ M06.04 **Rheumatoid arthritis without rheumatoid factor,** hand

M06.041 **Rheumatoid arthritis without rheumatoid factor,** right **hand** HCC

M06.042 **Rheumatoid arthritis without rheumatoid factor,** left **hand** HCC

M06.049 **Rheumatoid arthritis without rheumatoid factor, unspecified hand** HCC

✓6ᵗʰ M06.05 **Rheumatoid arthritis without rheumatoid factor,** hip

M06.051 **Rheumatoid arthritis without rheumatoid factor,** right **hip** HCC

M06.052 **Rheumatoid arthritis without rheumatoid factor,** left **hip** HCC

M06.059 **Rheumatoid arthritis without rheumatoid factor, unspecified hip** HCC

✓6ᵗʰ M06.06 **Rheumatoid arthritis without rheumatoid factor,** knee

M06.061 **Rheumatoid arthritis without rheumatoid factor,** right **knee** HCC

M06.062 **Rheumatoid arthritis without rheumatoid factor,** left **knee** HCC

M06.069 **Rheumatoid arthritis without rheumatoid factor, unspecified knee** HCC

✓6ᵗʰ M06.07 **Rheumatoid arthritis without rheumatoid factor,** ankle and foot

M06.071 **Rheumatoid arthritis without rheumatoid factor,** right **ankle and foot** HCC

M06.072 **Rheumatoid arthritis without rheumatoid factor,** left **ankle and foot** HCC

M06.079 **Rheumatoid arthritis without rheumatoid factor, unspecified ankle and foot** HCC

M06.08 **Rheumatoid arthritis without rheumatoid factor,** vertebrae HCC

M06.09 **Rheumatoid arthritis without rheumatoid factor,** multiple sites HCC

M06.0A **Rheumatoid arthritis without rheumatoid factor, other specified site** HCC

M06.1 **Adult-onset Still's disease** HCC A

EXCLUDES 1 Still's disease NOS (M08.2-)

DEF: Type of systemic arthritis characterized by a transient rash and spiking fevers. This condition may resolve or develop into a chronic condition and may affect internal organs, as well as joints.

Synonym(s): AOSD

✓5ᵗʰ **M06.2 Rheumatoid bursitis**

M06.20 **Rheumatoid bursitis, unspecified site** HCC

✓6ᵗʰ M06.21 **Rheumatoid bursitis,** shoulder

M06.211 **Rheumatoid bursitis,** right **shoulder** HCC

M06.212 **Rheumatoid bursitis, left shoulder** HCC

M06.219 **Rheumatoid bursitis, unspecified shoulder** HCC

✓6ᵗʰ M06.22 **Rheumatoid bursitis,** elbow

M06.221 **Rheumatoid bursitis, right elbow** HCC

M06.222 **Rheumatoid bursitis, left elbow** HCC

M06.229 **Rheumatoid bursitis, unspecified elbow** HCC

✓6ᵗʰ M06.23 **Rheumatoid bursitis,** wrist

M06.231 **Rheumatoid bursitis, right wrist** HCC

M06.232 **Rheumatoid bursitis, left wrist** HCC

M06.239 **Rheumatoid bursitis, unspecified wrist** HCC

✓6ᵗʰ M06.24 **Rheumatoid bursitis,** hand

M06.241 **Rheumatoid bursitis, right hand** HCC

M06.242 **Rheumatoid bursitis, left hand** HCC

M06.249 **Rheumatoid bursitis, unspecified hand** HCC

✓6ᵗʰ M06.25 **Rheumatoid bursitis,** hip

M06.251 **Rheumatoid bursitis,** right **hip** HCC

M06.252 **Rheumatoid bursitis,** left **hip** HCC

M06.259 **Rheumatoid bursitis, unspecified hip** HCC

✓6ᵗʰ M06.26 **Rheumatoid bursitis,** knee

M06.261 **Rheumatoid bursitis, right knee** HCC

M06.262 **Rheumatoid bursitis, left knee** HCC

M06.269 **Rheumatoid bursitis, unspecified knee** HCC

✓6ᵗʰ M06.27 **Rheumatoid bursitis,** ankle and foot

M06.271 **Rheumatoid bursitis,** right **ankle and foot** HCC

M06.272 **Rheumatoid bursitis,** left **ankle and foot** HCC

M06.279 **Rheumatoid bursitis, unspecified ankle and foot** HCC

M06.28 **Rheumatoid bursitis,** vertebrae HCC

M06.29 **Rheumatoid bursitis,** multiple sites HCC

✓5ᵗʰ **M06.3 Rheumatoid nodule**

M06.30 **Rheumatoid nodule, unspecified site** HCC

✓6ᵗʰ M06.31 **Rheumatoid nodule,** shoulder

M06.311 **Rheumatoid nodule,** right **shoulder** HCC

M06.312 **Rheumatoid nodule, left shoulder** HCC

M06.319 **Rheumatoid nodule, unspecified shoulder** HCC

✓6ᵗʰ M06.32 **Rheumatoid nodule,** elbow

M06.321 **Rheumatoid nodule, right elbow** HCC

M06.322 **Rheumatoid nodule, left elbow** HCC

M06.329 **Rheumatoid nodule, unspecified elbow** HCC

✓6ᵗʰ M06.33 **Rheumatoid nodule,** wrist

M06.331 **Rheumatoid nodule, right wrist** HCC

M06.332 **Rheumatoid nodule, left wrist** HCC

M06.339 **Rheumatoid nodule, unspecified wrist** HCC

✓6th **M06.34** **Rheumatoid nodule,** hand

    M06.341 **Rheumatoid nodule,** right **hand** `HCC`
    M06.342 **Rheumatoid nodule,** left **hand** `HCC`
    M06.349 **Rheumatoid nodule, unspecified hand** `HCC`

✓6th **M06.35** **Rheumatoid nodule,** hip

    M06.351 **Rheumatoid nodule,** right **hip** `HCC`
    M06.352 **Rheumatoid nodule,** left **hip** `HCC`
    M06.359 **Rheumatoid nodule, unspecified hip** `HCC`

✓6th **M06.36** **Rheumatoid nodule,** knee

    M06.361 **Rheumatoid nodule,** right **knee** `HCC`
    M06.362 **Rheumatoid nodule,** left **knee** `HCC`
    M06.369 **Rheumatoid nodule, unspecified knee** `HCC`

✓6th **M06.37** **Rheumatoid nodule,** ankle and foot

    M06.371 **Rheumatoid nodule,** right **ankle and foot** `HCC`
    M06.372 **Rheumatoid nodule,** left **ankle and foot** `HCC`
    M06.379 **Rheumatoid nodule, unspecified ankle and foot** `HCC`

    M06.38 **Rheumatoid nodule,** vertebrae `HCC`
    M06.39 **Rheumatoid nodule,** multiple sites `HCC`

M06.4 **Inflammatory polyarthropathy** `HCC`

    EXCLUDES 1   *polyarthritis NOS (M13.0)*

✓5th **M06.8** **Other specified rheumatoid arthritis**

    M06.80 **Other specified rheumatoid arthritis, unspecified site** `HCC`

✓6th **M06.81** **Other specified rheumatoid arthritis,** shoulder

    M06.811 **Other specified rheumatoid arthritis, right shoulder** `HCC`
    M06.812 **Other specified rheumatoid arthritis,** left **shoulder** `HCC`
    M06.819 **Other specified rheumatoid arthritis, unspecified shoulder** `HCC`

✓6th **M06.82** **Other specified rheumatoid arthritis,** elbow

    M06.821 **Other specified rheumatoid arthritis, right elbow** `HCC`
    M06.822 **Other specified rheumatoid arthritis,** left **elbow** `HCC`
    M06.829 **Other specified rheumatoid arthritis, unspecified elbow** `HCC`

✓6th **M06.83** **Other specified rheumatoid arthritis,** wrist

    M06.831 **Other specified rheumatoid arthritis, right wrist** `HCC`
    M06.832 **Other specified rheumatoid arthritis,** left **wrist** `HCC`
    M06.839 **Other specified rheumatoid arthritis, unspecified wrist** `HCC`

✓6th **M06.84** **Other specified rheumatoid arthritis,** hand

    M06.841 **Other specified rheumatoid arthritis, right hand** `HCC`
    M06.842 **Other specified rheumatoid arthritis,** left **hand** `HCC`
    M06.849 **Other specified rheumatoid arthritis, unspecified hand** `HCC`

✓6th **M06.85** **Other specified rheumatoid arthritis,** hip

    M06.851 **Other specified rheumatoid arthritis, right hip** `HCC`
    M06.852 **Other specified rheumatoid arthritis,** left **hip** `HCC`
    M06.859 **Other specified rheumatoid arthritis, unspecified hip** `HCC`

✓6th **M06.86** **Other specified rheumatoid arthritis,** knee

    M06.861 **Other specified rheumatoid arthritis, right knee** `HCC`
    M06.862 **Other specified rheumatoid arthritis,** left **knee** `HCC`
    M06.869 **Other specified rheumatoid arthritis, unspecified knee** `HCC`

✓6th **M06.87** **Other specified rheumatoid arthritis,** ankle and foot

    M06.871 **Other specified rheumatoid arthritis, right ankle and foot** `HCC`
    M06.872 **Other specified rheumatoid arthritis,** left **ankle and foot** `HCC`

    M06.879 **Other specified rheumatoid arthritis, unspecified ankle and foot** `HCC`

    M06.88 **Other specified rheumatoid arthritis,** vertebrae `HCC`

    M06.89 **Other specified rheumatoid arthritis,** multiple sites `HCC`

    M06.8A **Other specified rheumatoid arthritis, other specified site** `HCC`

    M06.9 **Rheumatoid arthritis, unspecified** `HCC`

✓4th **M07** **Enteropathic arthropathies**

    Code also associated enteropathy, such as:
       regional enteritis [Crohn's disease] (K50.-)
       ulcerative colitis (K51.-)
       EXCLUDES 1   *psoriatic arthropathies (L40.5-)*

✓5th **M07.6** **Enteropathic arthropathies**

    M07.60 **Enteropathic arthropathies, unspecified site**

✓6th **M07.61** **Enteropathic arthropathies,** shoulder

    M07.611 **Enteropathic arthropathies,** right **shoulder**
    M07.612 **Enteropathic arthropathies,** left **shoulder**
    M07.619 **Enteropathic arthropathies, unspecified shoulder**

✓6th **M07.62** **Enteropathic arthropathies,** elbow

    M07.621 **Enteropathic arthropathies,** right **elbow**
    M07.622 **Enteropathic arthropathies,** left **elbow**
    M07.629 **Enteropathic arthropathies, unspecified elbow**

✓6th **M07.63** **Enteropathic arthropathies,** wrist

    M07.631 **Enteropathic arthropathies,** right **wrist**
    M07.632 **Enteropathic arthropathies,** left **wrist**
    M07.639 **Enteropathic arthropathies, unspecified wrist**

✓6th **M07.64** **Enteropathic arthropathies,** hand

    M07.641 **Enteropathic arthropathies,** right **hand**
    M07.642 **Enteropathic arthropathies,** left **hand**
    M07.649 **Enteropathic arthropathies, unspecified hand**

✓6th **M07.65** **Enteropathic arthropathies,** hip

    M07.651 **Enteropathic arthropathies,** right **hip**
    M07.652 **Enteropathic arthropathies,** left **hip**
    M07.659 **Enteropathic arthropathies, unspecified hip**

✓6th **M07.66** **Enteropathic arthropathies,** knee

    M07.661 **Enteropathic arthropathies,** right **knee**
    M07.662 **Enteropathic arthropathies,** left **knee**
    M07.669 **Enteropathic arthropathies, unspecified knee**

✓6th **M07.67** **Enteropathic arthropathies,** ankle and foot

    M07.671 **Enteropathic arthropathies,** right **ankle and foot**
    M07.672 **Enteropathic arthropathies,** left **ankle and foot**
    M07.679 **Enteropathic arthropathies, unspecified ankle and foot**

    M07.68 **Enteropathic arthropathies,** vertebrae
    M07.69 **Enteropathic arthropathies,** multiple sites

✓4th **M08** **Juvenile arthritis**

    Code also any associated underlying condition, such as:
       regional enteritis [Crohn's disease] (K50.-)
       ulcerative colitis (K51.-)
       EXCLUDES 1   *arthropathy in Whipple's disease (M14.8)*
                 Felty's syndrome (M05.0)
                 juvenile dermatomyositis (M33.0-)
                 psoriatic juvenile arthropathy (L40.54)

    AHA: 2020,4Q,31-32

✓5th **M08.0** **Unspecified juvenile rheumatoid arthritis**

    Juvenile rheumatoid arthritis with or without rheumatoid factor

    M08.00 **Unspecified juvenile rheumatoid arthritis of unspecified site** `HCC`

✓6th **M08.01** **Unspecified juvenile rheumatoid arthritis,** shoulder

    M08.011 **Unspecified juvenile rheumatoid arthritis, right shoulder** `HCC`
    M08.012 **Unspecified juvenile rheumatoid arthritis,** left **shoulder** `HCC`
    M08.019 **Unspecified juvenile rheumatoid arthritis, unspecified shoulder** `HCC`

✓ Additional Character Required   ✓x7th Placeholder   Questionable PDx   Manifestation   Unspecified Dx   `UPD` Unacceptable PDx   `H1`-`H14` HAC   `HCC` CMS-HCC Dx   `HIV` HIV Dx

ICD-10-CM 2022   771

Chapter 13. Diseases of the Musculoskeletal System and Connective Tissue

✓6ᵗʰ M08.02 Unspecified juvenile rheumatoid arthritis of elbow

- M08.021 Unspecified juvenile rheumatoid arthritis, right elbow `HCC`
- M08.022 Unspecified juvenile rheumatoid arthritis, left elbow `HCC`
- M08.029 Unspecified juvenile rheumatoid arthritis, unspecified elbow `HCC`

✓6ᵗʰ M08.03 Unspecified juvenile rheumatoid arthritis, wrist

- M08.031 Unspecified juvenile rheumatoid arthritis, right wrist `HCC`
- M08.032 Unspecified juvenile rheumatoid arthritis, left wrist `HCC`
- M08.039 Unspecified juvenile rheumatoid arthritis, unspecified wrist `HCC`

✓6ᵗʰ M08.04 Unspecified juvenile rheumatoid arthritis, hand

- M08.041 Unspecified juvenile rheumatoid arthritis, right hand `HCC`
- M08.042 Unspecified juvenile rheumatoid arthritis, left hand `HCC`
- M08.049 Unspecified juvenile rheumatoid arthritis, unspecified hand `HCC`

✓6ᵗʰ M08.05 Unspecified juvenile rheumatoid arthritis, hip

- M08.051 Unspecified juvenile rheumatoid arthritis, right hip `HCC`
- M08.052 Unspecified juvenile rheumatoid arthritis, left hip `HCC`
- M08.059 Unspecified juvenile rheumatoid arthritis, unspecified hip `HCC`

✓6ᵗʰ M08.06 Unspecified juvenile rheumatoid arthritis, knee

- M08.061 Unspecified juvenile rheumatoid arthritis, right knee `HCC`
- M08.062 Unspecified juvenile rheumatoid arthritis, left knee `HCC`
- M08.069 Unspecified juvenile rheumatoid arthritis, unspecified knee `HCC`

✓6ᵗʰ M08.07 Unspecified juvenile rheumatoid arthritis, ankle and foot

- M08.071 Unspecified juvenile rheumatoid arthritis, right ankle and foot `HCC`
- M08.072 Unspecified juvenile rheumatoid arthritis, left ankle and foot `HCC`
- M08.079 Unspecified juvenile rheumatoid arthritis, unspecified ankle and foot `HCC`

M08.08 Unspecified juvenile rheumatoid arthritis, vertebrae `HCC`

M08.09 Unspecified juvenile rheumatoid arthritis, multiple sites `HCC`

M08.0A Unspecified juvenile rheumatoid arthritis, other specified site `HCC`

M08.1 Juvenile ankylosing spondylitis `HCC`

> EXCLUDES 1   ankylosing spondylitis in adults (M45.0-)

✓5ᵗʰ M08.2 Juvenile rheumatoid arthritis with systemic onset

Still's disease NOS

> EXCLUDES 1   adult-onset Still's disease (M06.1-)

DEF: Systemic juvenile rheumatoid arthritis characterized by a transient rash and spiking fevers that may affect internal organs, as well as joints.

M08.20 Juvenile rheumatoid arthritis with systemic onset, unspecified site `HCC`

✓6ᵗʰ M08.21 Juvenile rheumatoid arthritis with systemic onset, shoulder

- M08.211 Juvenile rheumatoid arthritis with systemic onset, right shoulder `HCC`
- M08.212 Juvenile rheumatoid arthritis with systemic onset, left shoulder `HCC`
- M08.219 Juvenile rheumatoid arthritis with systemic onset, unspecified shoulder `HCC`

✓6ᵗʰ M08.22 Juvenile rheumatoid arthritis with systemic onset, elbow

- M08.221 Juvenile rheumatoid arthritis with systemic onset, right elbow `HCC`
- M08.222 Juvenile rheumatoid arthritis with systemic onset, left elbow `HCC`
- M08.229 Juvenile rheumatoid arthritis with systemic onset, unspecified elbow `HCC`

✓6ᵗʰ M08.23 Juvenile rheumatoid arthritis with systemic onset, wrist

- M08.231 Juvenile rheumatoid arthritis with systemic onset, right wrist `HCC`
- M08.232 Juvenile rheumatoid arthritis with systemic onset, left wrist `HCC`
- M08.239 Juvenile rheumatoid arthritis with systemic onset, unspecified wrist `HCC`

✓6ᵗʰ M08.24 Juvenile rheumatoid arthritis with systemic onset, hand

- M08.241 Juvenile rheumatoid arthritis with systemic onset, right hand `HCC`
- M08.242 Juvenile rheumatoid arthritis with systemic onset, left hand `HCC`
- M08.249 Juvenile rheumatoid arthritis with systemic onset, unspecified hand `HCC`

✓6ᵗʰ M08.25 Juvenile rheumatoid arthritis with systemic onset, hip

- M08.251 Juvenile rheumatoid arthritis with systemic onset, right hip `HCC`
- M08.252 Juvenile rheumatoid arthritis with systemic onset, left hip `HCC`
- M08.259 Juvenile rheumatoid arthritis with systemic onset, unspecified hip `HCC`

✓6ᵗʰ M08.26 Juvenile rheumatoid arthritis with systemic onset, knee

- M08.261 Juvenile rheumatoid arthritis with systemic onset, right knee `HCC`
- M08.262 Juvenile rheumatoid arthritis with systemic onset, left knee `HCC`
- M08.269 Juvenile rheumatoid arthritis with systemic onset, unspecified knee `HCC`

✓6ᵗʰ M08.27 Juvenile rheumatoid arthritis with systemic onset, ankle and foot

- M08.271 Juvenile rheumatoid arthritis with systemic onset, right ankle and foot `HCC`
- M08.272 Juvenile rheumatoid arthritis with systemic onset, left ankle and foot `HCC`
- M08.279 Juvenile rheumatoid arthritis with systemic onset, unspecified ankle and foot `HCC`

M08.28 Juvenile rheumatoid arthritis with systemic onset, vertebrae `HCC`

M08.29 Juvenile rheumatoid arthritis with systemic onset, multiple sites `HCC`

M08.2A Juvenile rheumatoid arthritis with systemic onset, other specified site `HCC`

M08.3 Juvenile rheumatoid polyarthritis (seronegative) `HCC`

✓5ᵗʰ M08.4 Pauciarticular juvenile rheumatoid arthritis

M08.40 Pauciarticular juvenile rheumatoid arthritis, unspecified site `HCC`

✓6ᵗʰ M08.41 Pauciarticular juvenile rheumatoid arthritis, shoulder

- M08.411 Pauciarticular juvenile rheumatoid arthritis, right shoulder `HCC`
- M08.412 Pauciarticular juvenile rheumatoid arthritis, left shoulder `HCC`
- M08.419 Pauciarticular juvenile rheumatoid arthritis, unspecified shoulder `HCC`

✓6ᵗʰ M08.42 Pauciarticular juvenile rheumatoid arthritis, elbow

- M08.421 Pauciarticular juvenile rheumatoid arthritis, right elbow `HCC`
- M08.422 Pauciarticular juvenile rheumatoid arthritis, left elbow `HCC`
- M08.429 Pauciarticular juvenile rheumatoid arthritis, unspecified elbow `HCC`

✓6ᵗʰ M08.43 Pauciarticular juvenile rheumatoid arthritis, wrist

- M08.431 Pauciarticular juvenile rheumatoid arthritis, right wrist `HCC`
- M08.432 Pauciarticular juvenile rheumatoid arthritis, left wrist `HCC`
- M08.439 Pauciarticular juvenile rheumatoid arthritis, unspecified wrist `HCC`

✓6ᵗʰ M08.44 Pauciarticular juvenile rheumatoid arthritis, hand

- M08.441 Pauciarticular juvenile rheumatoid arthritis, right hand `HCC`
- M08.442 Pauciarticular juvenile rheumatoid arthritis, left hand `HCC`

N Newborn: 0   P Pediatric: 0-17   M Maternity: 9-64   A Adult: 15-124   MCC Major Complication/Comorbidity   CC Complication/Comorbidity   SW Severe Wound Dx

772   ICD-10-CM 2022

M08.449 Pauciarticular juvenile rheumatoid arthritis, unspecified hand `HCC`

√6ᵗʰ **M08.45 Pauciarticular juvenile rheumatoid arthritis, hip**

M08.451 Pauciarticular juvenile rheumatoid arthritis, right hip

M08.452 Pauciarticular juvenile rheumatoid arthritis, left hip `HCC`

M08.459 Pauciarticular juvenile rheumatoid arthritis, unspecified hip `HCC`

√6ᵗʰ **M08.46 Pauciarticular juvenile rheumatoid arthritis, knee**

M08.461 Pauciarticular juvenile rheumatoid arthritis, right knee `HCC`

M08.462 Pauciarticular juvenile rheumatoid arthritis, left knee `HCC`

M08.469 Pauciarticular juvenile rheumatoid arthritis, unspecified knee `HCC`

√6ᵗʰ **M08.47 Pauciarticular juvenile rheumatoid arthritis, ankle and foot**

M08.471 Pauciarticular juvenile rheumatoid arthritis, right ankle and foot `HCC`

M08.472 Pauciarticular juvenile rheumatoid arthritis, left ankle and foot `HCC`

M08.479 Pauciarticular juvenile rheumatoid arthritis, unspecified ankle and foot `HCC`

M08.48 Pauciarticular juvenile rheumatoid arthritis, vertebrae `HCC`

M08.4A Pauciarticular juvenile rheumatoid arthritis, other specified site `HCC`

√5ᵗʰ **M08.8 Other juvenile arthritis**

M08.80 Other juvenile arthritis, unspecified site `HCC`

√6ᵗʰ **M08.81 Other juvenile arthritis, shoulder**

M08.811 Other juvenile arthritis, right shoulder `HCC`

M08.812 Other juvenile arthritis, left shoulder `HCC`

M08.819 Other juvenile arthritis, unspecified shoulder `HCC`

√6ᵗʰ **M08.82 Other juvenile arthritis, elbow**

M08.821 Other juvenile arthritis, right elbow `HCC`

M08.822 Other juvenile arthritis, left elbow `HCC`

M08.829 Other juvenile arthritis, unspecified elbow `HCC`

√6ᵗʰ **M08.83 Other juvenile arthritis, wrist**

M08.831 Other juvenile arthritis, right wrist `HCC`

M08.832 Other juvenile arthritis, left wrist `HCC`

M08.839 Other juvenile arthritis, unspecified wrist `HCC`

√6ᵗʰ **M08.84 Other juvenile arthritis, hand**

M08.841 Other juvenile arthritis, right hand `HCC`

M08.842 Other juvenile arthritis, left hand `HCC`

M08.849 Other juvenile arthritis, unspecified hand `HCC`

√6ᵗʰ **M08.85 Other juvenile arthritis, hip**

M08.851 Other juvenile arthritis, right hip `HCC`

M08.852 Other juvenile arthritis, left hip `HCC`

M08.859 Other juvenile arthritis, unspecified hip `HCC`

√6ᵗʰ **M08.86 Other juvenile arthritis, knee**

M08.861 Other juvenile arthritis, right knee `HCC`

M08.862 Other juvenile arthritis, left knee `HCC`

M08.869 Other juvenile arthritis, unspecified knee `HCC`

√6ᵗʰ **M08.87 Other juvenile arthritis, ankle and foot**

M08.871 Other juvenile arthritis, right ankle and foot `HCC`

M08.872 Other juvenile arthritis, left ankle and foot `HCC`

M08.879 Other juvenile arthritis, unspecified ankle and foot `HCC`

M08.88 Other juvenile arthritis, other specified site `HCC`
Other juvenile arthritis, vertebrae

M08.89 Other juvenile arthritis, multiple sites `HCC`

√5ᵗʰ **M08.9 Juvenile arthritis, unspecified**

EXCLUDES 1   juvenile rheumatoid arthritis, unspecified (M08.0-)

M08.90 Juvenile arthritis, unspecified, unspecified site `HCC`

√6ᵗʰ **M08.91 Juvenile arthritis, unspecified, shoulder**

M08.911 Juvenile arthritis, unspecified, right shoulder `HCC`

M08.912 Juvenile arthritis, unspecified, left shoulder `HCC`

M08.919 Juvenile arthritis, unspecified, unspecified shoulder `HCC`

√6ᵗʰ **M08.92 Juvenile arthritis, unspecified, elbow**

M08.921 Juvenile arthritis, unspecified, right elbow `HCC`

M08.922 Juvenile arthritis, unspecified, left elbow `HCC`

M08.929 Juvenile arthritis, unspecified, unspecified elbow `HCC`

√6ᵗʰ **M08.93 Juvenile arthritis, unspecified, wrist**

M08.931 Juvenile arthritis, unspecified, right wrist `HCC`

M08.932 Juvenile arthritis, unspecified, left wrist `HCC`

M08.939 Juvenile arthritis, unspecified, unspecified wrist `HCC`

√6ᵗʰ **M08.94 Juvenile arthritis, unspecified, hand**

M08.941 Juvenile arthritis, unspecified, right hand `HCC`

M08.942 Juvenile arthritis, unspecified, left hand `HCC`

M08.949 Juvenile arthritis, unspecified, unspecified hand `HCC`

√6ᵗʰ **M08.95 Juvenile arthritis, unspecified, hip**

M08.951 Juvenile arthritis, unspecified, right hip `HCC`

M08.952 Juvenile arthritis, unspecified, left hip `HCC`

M08.959 Juvenile arthritis, unspecified, unspecified hip `HCC`

√6ᵗʰ **M08.96 Juvenile arthritis, unspecified, knee**

M08.961 Juvenile arthritis, unspecified, right knee `HCC`

M08.962 Juvenile arthritis, unspecified, left knee `HCC`

M08.969 Juvenile arthritis, unspecified, unspecified knee `HCC`

√6ᵗʰ **M08.97 Juvenile arthritis, unspecified, ankle and foot**

M08.971 Juvenile arthritis, unspecified, right ankle and foot `HCC`

M08.972 Juvenile arthritis, unspecified, left ankle and foot `HCC`

M08.979 Juvenile arthritis, unspecified, unspecified ankle and foot `HCC`

M08.98 Juvenile arthritis, unspecified, vertebrae `HCC`

M08.99 Juvenile arthritis, unspecified, multiple sites `HCC`

M08.9A Juvenile arthritis, unspecified, other specified site `HCC`

√4ᵗʰ **M1A Chronic gout**

Use additional code to identify:
autonomic neuropathy in diseases classified elsewhere (G99.0)
calculus of urinary tract in diseases classified elsewhere (N22)
cardiomyopathy in diseases classified elsewhere (I43)
disorders of external ear in diseases classified elsewhere (H61.1-, H62.8-)
disorders of iris and ciliary body in diseases classified elsewhere (H22)
glomerular disorders in diseases classified elsewhere (N08)

EXCLUDES 1   gout NOS (M10.-)

EXCLUDES 2   acute gout (M10.-)

The appropriate 7th character is to be added to each code from category M1A.
0   without tophus (tophi)
1   with tophus (tophi)

√5ᵗʰ **M1A.0 Idiopathic chronic gout**

Chronic gouty bursitis
Primary chronic gout

√x7ᵗʰ **M1A.00 Idiopathic chronic gout, unspecified site**

✔ Additional Character Required   √x7ᵗʰ Placeholder   Questionable PDx   Manifestation   Unspecified Dx   `UPD` Unacceptable PDx   `H1`-`H14` HAC   `HCC` CMS-HCC Dx   `HIV` HIV Dx

ICD-10-CM 2022   **773**

✓6ᵗʰ **M1A.Ø1** Idiopathic chronic gout, shoulder
    ✓7ᵗʰ **M1A.Ø11** Idiopathic chronic gout, right shoulder
    ✓7ᵗʰ **M1A.Ø12** Idiopathic chronic gout, left shoulder
    ✓7ᵗʰ **M1A.Ø19** Idiopathic chronic gout, unspecified shoulder

✓6ᵗʰ **M1A.Ø2** Idiopathic chronic gout, elbow
    ✓7ᵗʰ **M1A.Ø21** Idiopathic chronic gout, right elbow
    ✓7ᵗʰ **M1A.Ø22** Idiopathic chronic gout, left elbow
    ✓7ᵗʰ **M1A.Ø29** Idiopathic chronic gout, unspecified elbow

✓6ᵗʰ **M1A.Ø3** Idiopathic chronic gout, wrist
    ✓7ᵗʰ **M1A.Ø31** Idiopathic chronic gout, right wrist
    ✓7ᵗʰ **M1A.Ø32** Idiopathic chronic gout, left wrist
    ✓7ᵗʰ **M1A.Ø39** Idiopathic chronic gout, unspecified wrist

✓6ᵗʰ **M1A.Ø4** Idiopathic chronic gout, hand
    ✓7ᵗʰ **M1A.Ø41** Idiopathic chronic gout, right hand
    ✓7ᵗʰ **M1A.Ø42** Idiopathic chronic gout, left hand
    ✓7ᵗʰ **M1A.Ø49** Idiopathic chronic gout, unspecified hand

✓6ᵗʰ **M1A.Ø5** Idiopathic chronic gout, hip
    ✓7ᵗʰ **M1A.Ø51** Idiopathic chronic gout, right hip
    ✓7ᵗʰ **M1A.Ø52** Idiopathic chronic gout, left hip
    ✓7ᵗʰ **M1A.Ø59** Idiopathic chronic gout, unspecified hip

✓6ᵗʰ **M1A.Ø6** Idiopathic chronic gout, knee
    ✓7ᵗʰ **M1A.Ø61** Idiopathic chronic gout, right knee
    ✓7ᵗʰ **M1A.Ø62** Idiopathic chronic gout, left knee
    ✓7ᵗʰ **M1A.Ø69** Idiopathic chronic gout, unspecified knee

✓6ᵗʰ **M1A.Ø7** Idiopathic chronic gout, ankle and foot
    ✓7ᵗʰ **M1A.Ø71** Idiopathic chronic gout, right ankle and foot
    ✓7ᵗʰ **M1A.Ø72** Idiopathic chronic gout, left ankle and foot
    ✓7ᵗʰ **M1A.Ø79** Idiopathic chronic gout, unspecified ankle and foot

✓x7ᵗʰ **M1A.Ø8** Idiopathic chronic gout, vertebrae

✓x7ᵗʰ **M1A.Ø9** Idiopathic chronic gout, multiple sites

✓5ᵗʰ **M1A.1** Lead-induced chronic gout
    Code first toxic effects of lead and its compounds (T56.Ø-)

✓x7ᵗʰ **M1A.10** Lead-induced chronic gout, unspecified site

✓6ᵗʰ **M1A.11** Lead-induced chronic gout, shoulder
    ✓7ᵗʰ **M1A.111** Lead-induced chronic gout, right shoulder
    ✓7ᵗʰ **M1A.112** Lead-induced chronic gout, left shoulder
    ✓7ᵗʰ **M1A.119** Lead-induced chronic gout, unspecified shoulder

✓6ᵗʰ **M1A.12** Lead-induced chronic gout, elbow
    ✓7ᵗʰ **M1A.121** Lead-induced chronic gout, right elbow
    ✓7ᵗʰ **M1A.122** Lead-induced chronic gout, left elbow
    ✓7ᵗʰ **M1A.129** Lead-induced chronic gout, unspecified elbow

✓6ᵗʰ **M1A.13** Lead-induced chronic gout, wrist
    ✓7ᵗʰ **M1A.131** Lead-induced chronic gout, right wrist
    ✓7ᵗʰ **M1A.132** Lead-induced chronic gout, left wrist
    ✓7ᵗʰ **M1A.139** Lead-induced chronic gout, unspecified wrist

✓6ᵗʰ **M1A.14** Lead-induced chronic gout, hand
    ✓7ᵗʰ **M1A.141** Lead-induced chronic gout, right hand
    ✓7ᵗʰ **M1A.142** Lead-induced chronic gout, left hand
    ✓7ᵗʰ **M1A.149** Lead-induced chronic gout, unspecified hand

✓6ᵗʰ **M1A.15** Lead-induced chronic gout, hip
    ✓7ᵗʰ **M1A.151** Lead-induced chronic gout, right hip
    ✓7ᵗʰ **M1A.152** Lead-induced chronic gout, left hip
    ✓7ᵗʰ **M1A.159** Lead-induced chronic gout, unspecified hip

✓6ᵗʰ **M1A.16** Lead-induced chronic gout, knee
    ✓7ᵗʰ **M1A.161** Lead-induced chronic gout, right knee
    ✓7ᵗʰ **M1A.162** Lead-induced chronic gout, left knee
    ✓7ᵗʰ **M1A.169** Lead-induced chronic gout, unspecified knee

✓6ᵗʰ **M1A.17** Lead-induced chronic gout, ankle and foot
    ✓7ᵗʰ **M1A.171** Lead-induced chronic gout, right ankle and foot
    ✓7ᵗʰ **M1A.172** Lead-induced chronic gout, left ankle and foot
    ✓7ᵗʰ **M1A.179** Lead-induced chronic gout, unspecified ankle and foot

✓x7ᵗʰ **M1A.18** Lead-induced chronic gout, vertebrae

✓x7ᵗʰ **M1A.19** Lead-induced chronic gout, multiple sites

✓5ᵗʰ **M1A.2** Drug-induced chronic gout
    Use additional code for adverse effect, if applicable, to identify drug (T36-T5Ø with fifth or sixth character 5)

✓x7ᵗʰ **M1A.20** Drug-induced chronic gout, unspecified site

✓6ᵗʰ **M1A.21** Drug-induced chronic gout, shoulder
    ✓7ᵗʰ **M1A.211** Drug-induced chronic gout, right shoulder
    ✓7ᵗʰ **M1A.212** Drug-induced chronic gout, left shoulder
    ✓7ᵗʰ **M1A.219** Drug-induced chronic gout, unspecified shoulder

✓6ᵗʰ **M1A.22** Drug-induced chronic gout, elbow
    ✓7ᵗʰ **M1A.221** Drug-induced chronic gout, right elbow
    ✓7ᵗʰ **M1A.222** Drug-induced chronic gout, left elbow
    ✓7ᵗʰ **M1A.229** Drug-induced chronic gout, unspecified elbow

✓6ᵗʰ **M1A.23** Drug-induced chronic gout, wrist
    ✓7ᵗʰ **M1A.231** Drug-induced chronic gout, right wrist
    ✓7ᵗʰ **M1A.232** Drug-induced chronic gout, left wrist
    ✓7ᵗʰ **M1A.239** Drug-induced chronic gout, unspecified wrist

✓6ᵗʰ **M1A.24** Drug-induced chronic gout, hand
    ✓7ᵗʰ **M1A.241** Drug-induced chronic gout, right hand
    ✓7ᵗʰ **M1A.242** Drug-induced chronic gout, left hand
    ✓7ᵗʰ **M1A.249** Drug-induced chronic gout, unspecified hand

✓6ᵗʰ **M1A.25** Drug-induced chronic gout, hip
    ✓7ᵗʰ **M1A.251** Drug-induced chronic gout, right hip
    ✓7ᵗʰ **M1A.252** Drug-induced chronic gout, left hip
    ✓7ᵗʰ **M1A.259** Drug-induced chronic gout, unspecified hip

✓6ᵗʰ **M1A.26** Drug-induced chronic gout, knee
    ✓7ᵗʰ **M1A.261** Drug-induced chronic gout, right knee
    ✓7ᵗʰ **M1A.262** Drug-induced chronic gout, left knee
    ✓7ᵗʰ **M1A.269** Drug-induced chronic gout, unspecified knee

✓6ᵗʰ **M1A.27** Drug-induced chronic gout, ankle and foot
    ✓7ᵗʰ **M1A.271** Drug-induced chronic gout, right ankle and foot
    ✓7ᵗʰ **M1A.272** Drug-induced chronic gout, left ankle and foot
    ✓7ᵗʰ **M1A.279** Drug-induced chronic gout, unspecified ankle and foot

✓x7ᵗʰ **M1A.28** Drug-induced chronic gout, vertebrae

✓x7ᵗʰ **M1A.29** Drug-induced chronic gout, multiple sites

✓5ᵗʰ **M1A.3** Chronic gout due to renal impairment
    Code first associated renal disease

✓x7ᵗʰ **M1A.30** Chronic gout due to renal impairment, unspecified site

✓6ᵗʰ **M1A.31** Chronic gout due to renal impairment, shoulder
    ✓7ᵗʰ **M1A.311** Chronic gout due to renal impairment, right shoulder
    ✓7ᵗʰ **M1A.312** Chronic gout due to renal impairment, left shoulder
    ✓7ᵗʰ **M1A.319** Chronic gout due to renal impairment, unspecified shoulder

✓6ᵗʰ **M1A.32** Chronic gout due to renal impairment, elbow
    ✓7ᵗʰ **M1A.321** Chronic gout due to renal impairment, right elbow
    ✓7ᵗʰ **M1A.322** Chronic gout due to renal impairment, left elbow
    ✓7ᵗʰ **M1A.329** Chronic gout due to renal impairment, unspecified elbow

✓6ᵗʰ **M1A.33** Chronic gout due to renal impairment, wrist
    ✓7ᵗʰ **M1A.331** Chronic gout due to renal impairment, right wrist

Ⓝ Newborn: 0   Ⓟ Pediatric: 0-17   Ⓜ Maternity: 9-64   Ⓐ Adult: 15-124   MCC Major Complication/Comorbidity   CC Complication/Comorbidity   SW Severe Wound Dx

774

ICD-10-CM 2022

☑7ᵗʰ **M1A.332** Chronic gout due to renal impairment, left wrist

☑7ᵗʰ **M1A.339** Chronic gout due to renal impairment, unspecified wrist

☑6ᵗʰ **M1A.34** Chronic gout due to renal impairment, hand

  ☑7ᵗʰ **M1A.341** Chronic gout due to renal impairment, right hand

  ☑7ᵗʰ **M1A.342** Chronic gout due to renal impairment, left hand

  ☑7ᵗʰ **M1A.349** Chronic gout due to renal impairment, unspecified hand

☑6ᵗʰ **M1A.35** Chronic gout due to renal impairment, hip

  ☑7ᵗʰ **M1A.351** Chronic gout due to renal impairment, right hip

  ☑7ᵗʰ **M1A.352** Chronic gout due to renal impairment, left hip

  ☑7ᵗʰ **M1A.359** Chronic gout due to renal impairment, unspecified hip

☑6ᵗʰ **M1A.36** Chronic gout due to renal impairment, knee

  ☑7ᵗʰ **M1A.361** Chronic gout due to renal impairment, right knee

  ☑7ᵗʰ **M1A.362** Chronic gout due to renal impairment, left knee

  ☑7ᵗʰ **M1A.369** Chronic gout due to renal impairment, unspecified knee

☑6ᵗʰ **M1A.37** Chronic gout due to renal impairment, ankle and foot

  ☑7ᵗʰ **M1A.371** Chronic gout due to renal impairment, right ankle and foot

  ☑7ᵗʰ **M1A.372** Chronic gout due to renal impairment, left ankle and foot

  ☑7ᵗʰ **M1A.379** Chronic gout due to renal impairment, unspecified ankle and foot

☑✗7ᵗʰ **M1A.38** Chronic gout due to renal impairment, vertebrae

☑✗7ᵗʰ **M1A.39** Chronic gout due to renal impairment, multiple sites

☑5ᵗʰ **M1A.4** Other secondary chronic gout

  Code first associated condition

☑✗7ᵗʰ **M1A.40** Other secondary chronic gout, unspecified site

☑6ᵗʰ **M1A.41** Other secondary chronic gout, shoulder

  ☑7ᵗʰ **M1A.411** Other secondary chronic gout, right shoulder

  ☑7ᵗʰ **M1A.412** Other secondary chronic gout, left shoulder

  ☑7ᵗʰ **M1A.419** Other secondary chronic gout, unspecified shoulder

☑6ᵗʰ **M1A.42** Other secondary chronic gout, elbow

  ☑7ᵗʰ **M1A.421** Other secondary chronic gout, right elbow

  ☑7ᵗʰ **M1A.422** Other secondary chronic gout, left elbow

  ☑7ᵗʰ **M1A.429** Other secondary chronic gout, unspecified elbow

☑6ᵗʰ **M1A.43** Other secondary chronic gout, wrist

  ☑7ᵗʰ **M1A.431** Other secondary chronic gout, right wrist

  ☑7ᵗʰ **M1A.432** Other secondary chronic gout, left wrist

  ☑7ᵗʰ **M1A.439** Other secondary chronic gout, unspecified wrist

☑6ᵗʰ **M1A.44** Other secondary chronic gout, hand

  ☑7ᵗʰ **M1A.441** Other secondary chronic gout, right hand

  ☑7ᵗʰ **M1A.442** Other secondary chronic gout, left hand

  ☑7ᵗʰ **M1A.449** Other secondary chronic gout, unspecified hand

☑6ᵗʰ **M1A.45** Other secondary chronic gout, hip

  ☑7ᵗʰ **M1A.451** Other secondary chronic gout, right hip

  ☑7ᵗʰ **M1A.452** Other secondary chronic gout, left hip

  ☑7ᵗʰ **M1A.459** Other secondary chronic gout, unspecified hip

☑6ᵗʰ **M1A.46** Other secondary chronic gout, knee

  ☑7ᵗʰ **M1A.461** Other secondary chronic gout, right knee

  ☑7ᵗʰ **M1A.462** Other secondary chronic gout, left knee

  ☑7ᵗʰ **M1A.469** Other secondary chronic gout, unspecified knee

☑6ᵗʰ **M1A.47** Other secondary chronic gout, ankle and foot

  ☑7ᵗʰ **M1A.471** Other secondary chronic gout, right ankle and foot

  ☑7ᵗʰ **M1A.472** Other secondary chronic gout, left ankle and foot

☑7ᵗʰ **M1A.479** Other secondary chronic gout, unspecified ankle and foot

☑✗7ᵗʰ **M1A.48** Other secondary chronic gout, vertebrae

☑✗7ᵗʰ **M1A.49** Other secondary chronic gout, multiple sites

☑✗7ᵗʰ **M1A.9** Chronic gout, unspecified

☑4ᵗʰ **M10 Gout**

  Acute gout

  Gout attack

  Gout flare

  Podagra

  Use additional code to identify:

    autonomic neuropathy in diseases classified elsewhere (G99.0)

    calculus of urinary tract in diseases classified elsewhere (N22)

    cardiomyopathy in diseases classified elsewhere (I43)

    disorders of external ear in diseases classified elsewhere (H61.1-, H62.8-)

    disorders of iris and ciliary body in diseases classified elsewhere (H22)

    glomerular disorders in diseases classified elsewhere (N08)

  EXCLUDES 2   chronic gout (M1A.-)

  DEF: Purine and pyrimidine metabolic disorders, manifested by hyperuricemia and recurrent acute inflammatory arthritis. Monosodium urate or monohydrate crystals may be deposited in and around the joints, leading to joint destruction and severe crippling.

☑5ᵗʰ **M10.0** Idiopathic gout

  Gouty bursitis

  Primary gout

  M10.00 Idiopathic gout, unspecified site

☑6ᵗʰ **M10.01** Idiopathic gout, shoulder

  M10.011 Idiopathic gout, right shoulder

  M10.012 Idiopathic gout, left shoulder

  M10.019 Idiopathic gout, unspecified shoulder

☑6ᵗʰ **M10.02** Idiopathic gout, elbow

  M10.021 Idiopathic gout, right elbow

  M10.022 Idiopathic gout, left elbow

  M10.029 Idiopathic gout, unspecified elbow

☑6ᵗʰ **M10.03** Idiopathic gout, wrist

  M10.031 Idiopathic gout, right wrist

  M10.032 Idiopathic gout, left wrist

  M10.039 Idiopathic gout, unspecified wrist

☑6ᵗʰ **M10.04** Idiopathic gout, hand

  M10.041 Idiopathic gout, right hand

  M10.042 Idiopathic gout, left hand

  M10.049 Idiopathic gout, unspecified hand

☑6ᵗʰ **M10.05** Idiopathic gout, hip

  M10.051 Idiopathic gout, right hip

  M10.052 Idiopathic gout, left hip

  M10.059 Idiopathic gout, unspecified hip

☑6ᵗʰ **M10.06** Idiopathic gout, knee

  M10.061 Idiopathic gout, right knee

  M10.062 Idiopathic gout, left knee

  M10.069 Idiopathic gout, unspecified knee

☑6ᵗʰ **M10.07** Idiopathic gout, ankle and foot

  M10.071 Idiopathic gout, right ankle and foot

  M10.072 Idiopathic gout, left ankle and foot

  M10.079 Idiopathic gout, unspecified ankle and foot

  M10.08 Idiopathic gout, vertebrae

  M10.09 Idiopathic gout, multiple sites

☑5ᵗʰ **M10.1** Lead-induced gout

  Code first toxic effects of lead and its compounds (T56.0-)

  M10.10 Lead-induced gout, unspecified site

☑6ᵗʰ **M10.11** Lead-induced gout, shoulder

  M10.111 Lead-induced gout, right shoulder

  M10.112 Lead-induced gout, left shoulder

  M10.119 Lead-induced gout, unspecified shoulder

☑6ᵗʰ **M10.12** Lead-induced gout, elbow

  M10.121 Lead-induced gout, right elbow

  M10.122 Lead-induced gout, left elbow

  M10.129 Lead-induced gout, unspecified elbow

☑6ᵗʰ **M10.13** Lead-induced gout, wrist

  M10.131 Lead-induced gout, right wrist

  M10.132 Lead-induced gout, left wrist

  M10.139 Lead-induced gout, unspecified wrist

☑6ᵗʰ **M10.14** Lead-induced gout, hand

  M10.141 Lead-induced gout, right hand

☑ Additional Character Required   ☑✗7ᵗʰ Placeholder   Questionable PDx   Manifestation   Unspecified Dx   **UPD** Unacceptable PDx   **H1**-**H14** HAC   **HCC** CMS-HCC Dx   **HIV** HIV Dx

ICD-10-CM 2022   775

M10.142 Lead-induced gout, left hand
M10.149 Lead-induced gout, unspecified hand

✓6th M10.15 Lead-induced gout, hip

M10.151 Lead-induced gout, right hip
M10.152 Lead-induced gout, left hip
M10.159 Lead-induced gout, unspecified hip

✓6th M10.16 Lead-induced gout, knee

M10.161 Lead-induced gout, right knee
M10.162 Lead-induced gout, left knee
M10.169 Lead-induced gout, unspecified knee

✓6th M10.17 Lead-induced gout, ankle and foot

M10.171 Lead-induced gout, right ankle and foot
M10.172 Lead-induced gout, left ankle and foot
M10.179 Lead-induced gout, unspecified ankle and foot

M10.18 Lead-induced gout, vertebrae
M10.19 Lead-induced gout, multiple sites

✓5th M10.2 Drug-induced gout

Use additional code for adverse effect, if applicable, to identify drug (T36-T50 with fifth or sixth character 5)

M10.20 Drug-induced gout, unspecified site

✓6th M10.21 Drug-induced gout, shoulder

M10.211 Drug-induced gout, right shoulder
M10.212 Drug-induced gout, left shoulder
M10.219 Drug-induced gout, unspecified shoulder

✓6th M10.22 Drug-induced gout, elbow

M10.221 Drug-induced gout, right elbow
M10.222 Drug-induced gout, left elbow
M10.229 Drug-induced gout, unspecified elbow

✓6th M10.23 Drug-induced gout, wrist

M10.231 Drug-induced gout, right wrist
M10.232 Drug-induced gout, left wrist
M10.239 Drug-induced gout, unspecified wrist

✓6th M10.24 Drug-induced gout, hand

M10.241 Drug-induced gout, right hand
M10.242 Drug-induced gout, left hand
M10.249 Drug-induced gout, unspecified hand

✓6th M10.25 Drug-induced gout, hip

M10.251 Drug-induced gout, right hip
M10.252 Drug-induced gout, left hip
M10.259 Drug-induced gout, unspecified hip

✓6th M10.26 Drug-induced gout, knee

M10.261 Drug-induced gout, right knee
M10.262 Drug-induced gout, left knee
M10.269 Drug-induced gout, unspecified knee

✓6th M10.27 Drug-induced gout, ankle and foot

M10.271 Drug-induced gout, right ankle and foot
M10.272 Drug-induced gout, left ankle and foot
M10.279 Drug-induced gout, unspecified ankle and foot

M10.28 Drug-induced gout, vertebrae
M10.29 Drug-induced gout, multiple sites

✓5th M10.3 Gout due to renal impairment

Code first associated renal disease

M10.30 Gout due to renal impairment, unspecified site

✓6th M10.31 Gout due to renal impairment, shoulder

M10.311 Gout due to renal impairment, right shoulder
M10.312 Gout due to renal impairment, left shoulder
M10.319 Gout due to renal impairment, unspecified shoulder

✓6th M10.32 Gout due to renal impairment, elbow

M10.321 Gout due to renal impairment, right elbow
M10.322 Gout due to renal impairment, left elbow
M10.329 Gout due to renal impairment, unspecified elbow

✓6th M10.33 Gout due to renal impairment, wrist

M10.331 Gout due to renal impairment, right wrist
M10.332 Gout due to renal impairment, left wrist
M10.339 Gout due to renal impairment, unspecified wrist

✓6th M10.34 Gout due to renal impairment, hand

M10.341 Gout due to renal impairment, right hand
M10.342 Gout due to renal impairment, left hand

M10.349 Gout due to renal impairment, unspecified hand

✓6th M10.35 Gout due to renal impairment, hip

M10.351 Gout due to renal impairment, right hip
M10.352 Gout due to renal impairment, left hip
M10.359 Gout due to renal impairment, unspecified hip

✓6th M10.36 Gout due to renal impairment, knee

M10.361 Gout due to renal impairment, right knee
M10.362 Gout due to renal impairment, left knee
M10.369 Gout due to renal impairment, unspecified knee

✓6th M10.37 Gout due to renal impairment, ankle and foot

M10.371 Gout due to renal impairment, right ankle and foot
M10.372 Gout due to renal impairment, left ankle and foot
M10.379 Gout due to renal impairment, unspecified ankle and foot

M10.38 Gout due to renal impairment, vertebrae
M10.39 Gout due to renal impairment, multiple sites

✓5th M10.4 Other secondary gout

Code first associated condition

M10.40 Other secondary gout, unspecified site

✓6th M10.41 Other secondary gout, shoulder

M10.411 Other secondary gout, right shoulder
M10.412 Other secondary gout, left shoulder
M10.419 Other secondary gout, unspecified shoulder

✓6th M10.42 Other secondary gout, elbow

M10.421 Other secondary gout, right elbow
M10.422 Other secondary gout, left elbow
M10.429 Other secondary gout, unspecified elbow

✓6th M10.43 Other secondary gout, wrist

M10.431 Other secondary gout, right wrist
M10.432 Other secondary gout, left wrist
M10.439 Other secondary gout, unspecified wrist

✓6th M10.44 Other secondary gout, hand

M10.441 Other secondary gout, right hand
M10.442 Other secondary gout, left hand
M10.449 Other secondary gout, unspecified hand

✓6th M10.45 Other secondary gout, hip

M10.451 Other secondary gout, right hip
M10.452 Other secondary gout, left hip
M10.459 Other secondary gout, unspecified hip

✓6th M10.46 Other secondary gout, knee

M10.461 Other secondary gout, right knee
M10.462 Other secondary gout, left knee
M10.469 Other secondary gout, unspecified knee

✓6th M10.47 Other secondary gout, ankle and foot

M10.471 Other secondary gout, right ankle and foot
M10.472 Other secondary gout, left ankle and foot
M10.479 Other secondary gout, unspecified ankle and foot

M10.48 Other secondary gout, vertebrae
M10.49 Other secondary gout, multiple sites

M10.9 Gout, unspecified
Gout NOS

✓4th M11 Other crystal arthropathies

✓5th M11.0 Hydroxyapatite deposition disease

DEF: Disease caused by deposits of calcium phosphate crystals in the soft tissues close to the joint (especially tendons) or in the joints. These calcifications can be mono or polyarticular and can cause destruction of the joint involved.

M11.00 Hydroxyapatite deposition disease, unspecified site

✓6th M11.01 Hydroxyapatite deposition disease, shoulder

M11.011 Hydroxyapatite deposition disease, right shoulder
M11.012 Hydroxyapatite deposition disease, left shoulder
M11.019 Hydroxyapatite deposition disease, unspecified shoulder

✓6th M11.02 Hydroxyapatite deposition disease, elbow

M11.021 Hydroxyapatite deposition disease, right elbow

Ⓝ Newborn: 0   Ⓟ Pediatric: 0-17   Ⓜ Maternity: 9-64   Ⓐ Adult: 15-124   MCC Major Complication/Comorbidity   CC Complication/Comorbidity   SW Severe Wound Dx

776   ICD-10-CM 2022

M11.022 Hydroxyapatite deposition disease, left elbow

M11.029 Hydroxyapatite deposition disease, unspecified elbow

✓6ᵗʰ M11.03 Hydroxyapatite deposition disease, wrist

M11.031 Hydroxyapatite deposition disease, right wrist

M11.032 Hydroxyapatite deposition disease, left wrist

M11.039 Hydroxyapatite deposition disease, unspecified wrist

✓6ᵗʰ M11.04 Hydroxyapatite deposition disease, hand

M11.041 Hydroxyapatite deposition disease, right hand

M11.042 Hydroxyapatite deposition disease, left hand

M11.049 Hydroxyapatite deposition disease, unspecified hand

✓6ᵗʰ M11.05 Hydroxyapatite deposition disease, hip

M11.051 Hydroxyapatite deposition disease, right hip

M11.052 Hydroxyapatite deposition disease, left hip

M11.059 Hydroxyapatite deposition disease, unspecified hip

✓6ᵗʰ M11.06 Hydroxyapatite deposition disease, knee

M11.061 Hydroxyapatite deposition disease, right knee

M11.062 Hydroxyapatite deposition disease, left knee

M11.069 Hydroxyapatite deposition disease, unspecified knee

✓6ᵗʰ M11.07 Hydroxyapatite deposition disease, ankle and foot

M11.071 Hydroxyapatite deposition disease, right ankle and foot

M11.072 Hydroxyapatite deposition disease, left ankle and foot

M11.079 Hydroxyapatite deposition disease, unspecified ankle and foot

M11.08 Hydroxyapatite deposition disease, vertebrae

M11.09 Hydroxyapatite deposition disease, multiple sites

✓5ᵗʰ M11.1 Familial chondrocalcinosis

M11.10 Familial chondrocalcinosis, unspecified site

✓6ᵗʰ M11.11 Familial chondrocalcinosis, shoulder

M11.111 Familial chondrocalcinosis, right shoulder

M11.112 Familial chondrocalcinosis, left shoulder

M11.119 Familial chondrocalcinosis, unspecified shoulder

✓6ᵗʰ M11.12 Familial chondrocalcinosis, elbow

M11.121 Familial chondrocalcinosis, right elbow

M11.122 Familial chondrocalcinosis, left elbow

M11.129 Familial chondrocalcinosis, unspecified elbow

✓6ᵗʰ M11.13 Familial chondrocalcinosis, wrist

M11.131 Familial chondrocalcinosis, right wrist

M11.132 Familial chondrocalcinosis, left wrist

M11.139 Familial chondrocalcinosis, unspecified wrist

✓6ᵗʰ M11.14 Familial chondrocalcinosis, hand

M11.141 Familial chondrocalcinosis, right hand

M11.142 Familial chondrocalcinosis, left hand

M11.149 Familial chondrocalcinosis, unspecified hand

✓6ᵗʰ M11.15 Familial chondrocalcinosis, hip

M11.151 Familial chondrocalcinosis, right hip

M11.152 Familial chondrocalcinosis, left hip

M11.159 Familial chondrocalcinosis, unspecified hip

✓6ᵗʰ M11.16 Familial chondrocalcinosis, knee

M11.161 Familial chondrocalcinosis, right knee

M11.162 Familial chondrocalcinosis, left knee

M11.169 Familial chondrocalcinosis, unspecified knee

✓6ᵗʰ M11.17 Familial chondrocalcinosis, ankle and foot

M11.171 Familial chondrocalcinosis, right ankle and foot

M11.172 Familial chondrocalcinosis, left ankle and foot

M11.179 Familial chondrocalcinosis, unspecified ankle and foot

M11.18 Familial chondrocalcinosis, vertebrae

M11.19 Familial chondrocalcinosis, multiple sites

✓5ᵗʰ M11.2 Other chondrocalcinosis

Chondrocalcinosis NOS

AHA: 2018,3Q,20

TIP: Pseudogout is captured with codes in this subcategory.

M11.20 Other chondrocalcinosis, unspecified site

✓6ᵗʰ M11.21 Other chondrocalcinosis, shoulder

M11.211 Other chondrocalcinosis, right shoulder

M11.212 Other chondrocalcinosis, left shoulder

M11.219 Other chondrocalcinosis, unspecified shoulder

✓6ᵗʰ M11.22 Other chondrocalcinosis, elbow

M11.221 Other chondrocalcinosis, right elbow

M11.222 Other chondrocalcinosis, left elbow

M11.229 Other chondrocalcinosis, unspecified elbow

✓6ᵗʰ M11.23 Other chondrocalcinosis, wrist

M11.231 Other chondrocalcinosis, right wrist

M11.232 Other chondrocalcinosis, left wrist

M11.239 Other chondrocalcinosis, unspecified wrist

✓6ᵗʰ M11.24 Other chondrocalcinosis, hand

M11.241 Other chondrocalcinosis, right hand

M11.242 Other chondrocalcinosis, left hand

M11.249 Other chondrocalcinosis, unspecified hand

✓6ᵗʰ M11.25 Other chondrocalcinosis, hip

M11.251 Other chondrocalcinosis, right hip

M11.252 Other chondrocalcinosis, left hip

M11.259 Other chondrocalcinosis, unspecified hip

✓6ᵗʰ M11.26 Other chondrocalcinosis, knee

M11.261 Other chondrocalcinosis, right knee

M11.262 Other chondrocalcinosis, left knee

M11.269 Other chondrocalcinosis, unspecified knee

✓6ᵗʰ M11.27 Other chondrocalcinosis, ankle and foot

M11.271 Other chondrocalcinosis, right ankle and foot

M11.272 Other chondrocalcinosis, left ankle and foot

M11.279 Other chondrocalcinosis, unspecified ankle and foot

M11.28 Other chondrocalcinosis, vertebrae

M11.29 Other chondrocalcinosis, multiple sites

✓5ᵗʰ M11.8 Other specified crystal arthropathies

M11.80 Other specified crystal arthropathies, unspecified site

✓6ᵗʰ M11.81 Other specified crystal arthropathies, shoulder

M11.811 Other specified crystal arthropathies, right shoulder

M11.812 Other specified crystal arthropathies, left shoulder

M11.819 Other specified crystal arthropathies, unspecified shoulder

✓6ᵗʰ M11.82 Other specified crystal arthropathies, elbow

M11.821 Other specified crystal arthropathies, right elbow

M11.822 Other specified crystal arthropathies, left elbow

M11.829 Other specified crystal arthropathies, unspecified elbow

✓6ᵗʰ M11.83 Other specified crystal arthropathies, wrist

M11.831 Other specified crystal arthropathies, right wrist

M11.832 Other specified crystal arthropathies, left wrist

M11.839 Other specified crystal arthropathies, unspecified wrist

✓6ᵗʰ M11.84 Other specified crystal arthropathies, hand

M11.841 Other specified crystal arthropathies, right hand

M11.842 Other specified crystal arthropathies, left hand

M11.849 Other specified crystal arthropathies, unspecified hand

✓ Additional Character Required   ✓x7ᵗʰ Placeholder   Questionable PDx   Manifestation   Unspecified Dx   UPD Unacceptable PDx   H1-H14 HAC   HCC CMS-HCC Dx   HIV HIV Dx

ICD-10-CM 2022   777

✓6th **M11.85 Other specified crystal arthropathies, hip**

    M11.851 Other specified crystal arthropathies, right hip

    M11.852 Other specified crystal arthropathies, left hip

    M11.859 Other specified crystal arthropathies, unspecified hip

✓6th **M11.86 Other specified crystal arthropathies, knee**

    M11.861 Other specified crystal arthropathies, right knee

    M11.862 Other specified crystal arthropathies, left knee

    M11.869 Other specified crystal arthropathies, unspecified knee

✓6th **M11.87 Other specified crystal arthropathies, ankle and foot**

    M11.871 Other specified crystal arthropathies, right ankle and foot

    M11.872 Other specified crystal arthropathies, left ankle and foot

    M11.879 Other specified crystal arthropathies, unspecified ankle and foot

M11.88 Other specified crystal arthropathies, vertebrae

M11.89 Other specified crystal arthropathies, multiple sites

M11.9 Crystal arthropathy, unspecified

✓4th **M12 Other and unspecified arthropathy**

    EXCLUDES 1   *arthrosis (M15-M19)*

                 cricoarytenoid arthropathy (J38.7)

✓5th **M12.0 Chronic postrheumatic arthropathy [Jaccoud]**

    M12.00 Chronic postrheumatic arthropathy [Jaccoud], unspecified site HCC

✓6th **M12.01 Chronic postrheumatic arthropathy [Jaccoud], shoulder**

    M12.011 Chronic postrheumatic arthropathy [Jaccoud], right shoulder HCC

    M12.012 Chronic postrheumatic arthropathy [Jaccoud], left shoulder HCC

    M12.019 Chronic postrheumatic arthropathy [Jaccoud], unspecified shoulder HCC

✓6th **M12.02 Chronic postrheumatic arthropathy [Jaccoud], elbow**

    M12.021 Chronic postrheumatic arthropathy [Jaccoud], right elbow HCC

    M12.022 Chronic postrheumatic arthropathy [Jaccoud], left elbow HCC

    M12.029 Chronic postrheumatic arthropathy [Jaccoud], unspecified elbow HCC

✓6th **M12.03 Chronic postrheumatic arthropathy [Jaccoud], wrist**

    M12.031 Chronic postrheumatic arthropathy [Jaccoud], right wrist HCC

    M12.032 Chronic postrheumatic arthropathy [Jaccoud], left wrist HCC

    M12.039 Chronic postrheumatic arthropathy [Jaccoud], unspecified wrist HCC

✓6th **M12.04 Chronic postrheumatic arthropathy [Jaccoud], hand**

    M12.041 Chronic postrheumatic arthropathy [Jaccoud], right hand HCC

    M12.042 Chronic postrheumatic arthropathy [Jaccoud], left hand HCC

    M12.049 Chronic postrheumatic arthropathy [Jaccoud], unspecified hand HCC

✓6th **M12.05 Chronic postrheumatic arthropathy [Jaccoud], hip**

    M12.051 Chronic postrheumatic arthropathy [Jaccoud], right hip HCC

    M12.052 Chronic postrheumatic arthropathy [Jaccoud], left hip HCC

    M12.059 Chronic postrheumatic arthropathy [Jaccoud], unspecified hip HCC

✓6th **M12.06 Chronic postrheumatic arthropathy [Jaccoud], knee**

    M12.061 Chronic postrheumatic arthropathy [Jaccoud], right knee HCC

    M12.062 Chronic postrheumatic arthropathy [Jaccoud], left knee HCC

    M12.069 Chronic postrheumatic arthropathy [Jaccoud], unspecified knee HCC

✓6th **M12.07 Chronic postrheumatic arthropathy [Jaccoud], ankle and foot**

    M12.071 Chronic postrheumatic arthropathy [Jaccoud], right ankle and foot HCC

    M12.072 Chronic postrheumatic arthropathy [Jaccoud], left ankle and foot HCC

    M12.079 Chronic postrheumatic arthropathy [Jaccoud], unspecified ankle and foot HCC

M12.08 Chronic postrheumatic arthropathy [Jaccoud], other specified site HCC

    Chronic postrheumatic arthropathy [Jaccoud], vertebrae

M12.09 Chronic postrheumatic arthropathy [Jaccoud], multiple sites HCC

✓5th **M12.1 Kaschin-Beck disease**

    Osteochondroarthrosis deformans endemica

    M12.10 Kaschin-Beck disease, unspecified site

✓6th **M12.11 Kaschin-Beck disease, shoulder**

    M12.111 Kaschin-Beck disease, right shoulder

    M12.112 Kaschin-Beck disease, left shoulder

    M12.119 Kaschin-Beck disease, unspecified shoulder

✓6th **M12.12 Kaschin-Beck disease, elbow**

    M12.121 Kaschin-Beck disease, right elbow

    M12.122 Kaschin-Beck disease, left elbow

    M12.129 Kaschin-Beck disease, unspecified elbow

✓6th **M12.13 Kaschin-Beck disease, wrist**

    M12.131 Kaschin-Beck disease, right wrist

    M12.132 Kaschin-Beck disease, left wrist

    M12.139 Kaschin-Beck disease, unspecified wrist

✓6th **M12.14 Kaschin-Beck disease, hand**

    M12.141 Kaschin-Beck disease, right hand

    M12.142 Kaschin-Beck disease, left hand

    M12.149 Kaschin-Beck disease, unspecified hand

✓6th **M12.15 Kaschin-Beck disease, hip**

    M12.151 Kaschin-Beck disease, right hip

    M12.152 Kaschin-Beck disease, left hip

    M12.159 Kaschin-Beck disease, unspecified hip

✓6th **M12.16 Kaschin-Beck disease, knee**

    M12.161 Kaschin-Beck disease, right knee

    M12.162 Kaschin-Beck disease, left knee

    M12.169 Kaschin-Beck disease, unspecified knee

✓6th **M12.17 Kaschin-Beck disease, ankle and foot**

    M12.171 Kaschin-Beck disease, right ankle and foot

    M12.172 Kaschin-Beck disease, left ankle and foot

    M12.179 Kaschin-Beck disease, unspecified ankle and foot

M12.18 Kaschin-Beck disease, vertebrae

M12.19 Kaschin-Beck disease, multiple sites

✓5th **M12.2 Villonodular synovitis (pigmented)**

    M12.20 Villonodular synovitis (pigmented), unspecified site

✓6th **M12.21 Villonodular synovitis (pigmented), shoulder**

    M12.211 Villonodular synovitis (pigmented), right shoulder

    M12.212 Villonodular synovitis (pigmented), left shoulder

    M12.219 Villonodular synovitis (pigmented), unspecified shoulder

✓6th **M12.22 Villonodular synovitis (pigmented), elbow**

    M12.221 Villonodular synovitis (pigmented), right elbow

    M12.222 Villonodular synovitis (pigmented), left elbow

    M12.229 Villonodular synovitis (pigmented), unspecified elbow

✓6th **M12.23 Villonodular synovitis (pigmented), wrist**

    M12.231 Villonodular synovitis (pigmented), right wrist

    M12.232 Villonodular synovitis (pigmented), left wrist

    M12.239 Villonodular synovitis (pigmented), unspecified wrist

✓6th **M12.24 Villonodular synovitis (pigmented), hand**

    M12.241 Villonodular synovitis (pigmented), right hand

    M12.242 Villonodular synovitis (pigmented), left hand

    M12.249 Villonodular synovitis (pigmented), unspecified hand

N Newborn: 0   P Pediatric: 0-17   M Maternity: 9-64   A Adult: 15-124   MCC Major Complication/Comorbidity   CC Complication/Comorbidity   SW Severe Wound Dx

778   ICD-10-CM 2022

✓6th **M12.25 Villonodular synovitis (pigmented),** hip

     M12.251 Villonodular synovitis (pigmented), right hip

     M12.252 Villonodular synovitis (pigmented), left hip

     M12.259 Villonodular synovitis (pigmented), unspecified hip

✓6th **M12.26 Villonodular synovitis (pigmented),** knee

     M12.261 Villonodular synovitis (pigmented), right knee

     M12.262 Villonodular synovitis (pigmented), left knee

     M12.269 Villonodular synovitis (pigmented), unspecified knee

✓6th **M12.27 Villonodular synovitis (pigmented),** ankle and foot

     M12.271 Villonodular synovitis (pigmented), right ankle and foot

     M12.272 Villonodular synovitis (pigmented), left ankle and foot

     M12.279 Villonodular synovitis (pigmented), unspecified ankle and foot

M12.28 Villonodular synovitis (pigmented), other specified site

     Villonodular synovitis (pigmented), vertebrae

M12.29 Villonodular synovitis (pigmented), multiple sites

✓5th **M12.3 Palindromic rheumatism**

     DEF: Sudden and recurring attacks of moderate to severe joint pain and swelling generally occurring in the hands or feet of unknown etiology. After the attack subsides, the joints appear normal again.

     M12.30 Palindromic rheumatism, unspecified site

✓6th **M12.31 Palindromic rheumatism,** shoulder

     M12.311 Palindromic rheumatism, right shoulder

     M12.312 Palindromic rheumatism, left shoulder

     M12.319 Palindromic rheumatism, unspecified shoulder

✓6th **M12.32 Palindromic rheumatism,** elbow

     M12.321 Palindromic rheumatism, right elbow

     M12.322 Palindromic rheumatism, left elbow

     M12.329 Palindromic rheumatism, unspecified elbow

✓6th **M12.33 Palindromic rheumatism,** wrist

     M12.331 Palindromic rheumatism, right wrist

     M12.332 Palindromic rheumatism, left wrist

     M12.339 Palindromic rheumatism, unspecified wrist

✓6th **M12.34 Palindromic rheumatism,** hand

     M12.341 Palindromic rheumatism, right hand

     M12.342 Palindromic rheumatism, left hand

     M12.349 Palindromic rheumatism, unspecified hand

✓6th **M12.35 Palindromic rheumatism,** hip

     M12.351 Palindromic rheumatism, right hip

     M12.352 Palindromic rheumatism, left hip

     M12.359 Palindromic rheumatism, unspecified hip

✓6th **M12.36 Palindromic rheumatism,** knee

     M12.361 Palindromic rheumatism, right knee

     M12.362 Palindromic rheumatism, left knee

     M12.369 Palindromic rheumatism, unspecified knee

✓6th **M12.37 Palindromic rheumatism,** ankle and foot

     M12.371 Palindromic rheumatism, right ankle and foot

     M12.372 Palindromic rheumatism, left ankle and foot

     M12.379 Palindromic rheumatism, unspecified ankle and foot

M12.38 Palindromic rheumatism, other specified site

     Palindromic rheumatism, vertebrae

M12.39 Palindromic rheumatism, multiple sites

✓6th **M12.4 Intermittent hydrarthrosis**

     M12.40 Intermittent hydrarthrosis, unspecified site

✓6th **M12.41 Intermittent hydrarthrosis,** shoulder

     M12.411 Intermittent hydrarthrosis, right shoulder

     M12.412 Intermittent hydrarthrosis, left shoulder

     M12.419 Intermittent hydrarthrosis, unspecified shoulder

✓6th **M12.42 Intermittent hydrarthrosis,** elbow

     M12.421 Intermittent hydrarthrosis, right elbow

     M12.422 Intermittent hydrarthrosis, left elbow

     M12.429 Intermittent hydrarthrosis, unspecified elbow

✓6th **M12.43 Intermittent hydrarthrosis,** wrist

     M12.431 Intermittent hydrarthrosis, right wrist

     M12.432 Intermittent hydrarthrosis, left wrist

     M12.439 Intermittent hydrarthrosis, unspecified wrist

✓6th **M12.44 Intermittent hydrarthrosis,** hand

     M12.441 Intermittent hydrarthrosis, right hand

     M12.442 Intermittent hydrarthrosis, left hand

     M12.449 Intermittent hydrarthrosis, unspecified hand

✓6th **M12.45 Intermittent hydrarthrosis,** hip

     M12.451 Intermittent hydrarthrosis, right hip

     M12.452 Intermittent hydrarthrosis, left hip

     M12.459 Intermittent hydrarthrosis, unspecified hip

✓6th **M12.46 Intermittent hydrarthrosis,** knee

     M12.461 Intermittent hydrarthrosis, right knee

     M12.462 Intermittent hydrarthrosis, left knee

     M12.469 Intermittent hydrarthrosis, unspecified knee

✓6th **M12.47 Intermittent hydrarthrosis,** ankle and foot

     M12.471 Intermittent hydrarthrosis, right ankle and foot

     M12.472 Intermittent hydrarthrosis, left ankle and foot

     M12.479 Intermittent hydrarthrosis, unspecified ankle and foot

M12.48 Intermittent hydrarthrosis, other site

M12.49 Intermittent hydrarthrosis, multiple sites

✓5th **M12.5 Traumatic arthropathy**

     EXCLUDES 1   *current injury—see Alphabetic Index*

         post-traumatic osteoarthritis of first carpometacarpal joint (M18.2-M18.3)

         post-traumatic osteoarthritis of hip (M16.4-M16.5)

         post-traumatic osteoarthritis of knee (M17.2-M17.3)

         post-traumatic osteoarthritis NOS (M19.1-)

         post-traumatic osteoarthritis of other single joints (M19.1-)

     AHA: 2015,1Q,17

     M12.50 Traumatic arthropathy, unspecified site

✓6th **M12.51 Traumatic arthropathy,** shoulder

     M12.511 Traumatic arthropathy, right shoulder

     M12.512 Traumatic arthropathy, left shoulder

     M12.519 Traumatic arthropathy, unspecified shoulder

✓6th **M12.52 Traumatic arthropathy,** elbow

     M12.521 Traumatic arthropathy, right elbow

     M12.522 Traumatic arthropathy, left elbow

     M12.529 Traumatic arthropathy, unspecified elbow

✓6th **M12.53 Traumatic arthropathy,** wrist

     M12.531 Traumatic arthropathy, right wrist

     M12.532 Traumatic arthropathy, left wrist

     M12.539 Traumatic arthropathy, unspecified wrist

✓6th **M12.54 Traumatic arthropathy,** hand

     M12.541 Traumatic arthropathy, right hand

     M12.542 Traumatic arthropathy, left hand

     M12.549 Traumatic arthropathy, unspecified hand

✓6th **M12.55 Traumatic arthropathy,** hip

     M12.551 Traumatic arthropathy, right hip

     M12.552 Traumatic arthropathy, left hip

     M12.559 Traumatic arthropathy, unspecified hip

✓6th **M12.56 Traumatic arthropathy,** knee

     M12.561 Traumatic arthropathy, right knee

     M12.562 Traumatic arthropathy, left knee

     M12.569 Traumatic arthropathy, unspecified knee

✓6th **M12.57 Traumatic arthropathy,** ankle and foot

     M12.571 Traumatic arthropathy, right ankle and foot

     M12.572 Traumatic arthropathy, left ankle and foot

✓ Additional Character Required   ✓x7th Placeholder   Questionable PDx   Manifestation   Unspecified Dx   UPD Unacceptable PDx   H1-H14 HAC   HCC CMS-HCC Dx   HIV HIV Dx

ICD-10-CM 2022   **779**

M12.579   Traumatic arthropathy, unspecified ankle and foot

M12.58   Traumatic arthropathy, other specified site
Traumatic arthropathy, vertebrae

M12.59   Traumatic arthropathy, multiple sites

✓5ᵗʰ M12.8   Other specific arthropathies, not elsewhere classified
Transient arthropathy

M12.80   Other specific arthropathies, not elsewhere classified, unspecified site

✓6ᵗʰ M12.81   Other specific arthropathies, not elsewhere classified, shoulder

M12.811   Other specific arthropathies, not elsewhere classified, right shoulder

M12.812   Other specific arthropathies, not elsewhere classified, left shoulder

M12.819   Other specific arthropathies, not elsewhere classified, unspecified shoulder

✓6ᵗʰ M12.82   Other specific arthropathies, not elsewhere classified, elbow

M12.821   Other specific arthropathies, not elsewhere classified, right elbow

M12.822   Other specific arthropathies, not elsewhere classified, left elbow

M12.829   Other specific arthropathies, not elsewhere classified, unspecified elbow

✓6ᵗʰ M12.83   Other specific arthropathies, not elsewhere classified, wrist

M12.831   Other specific arthropathies, not elsewhere classified, right wrist

M12.832   Other specific arthropathies, not elsewhere classified, left wrist

M12.839   Other specific arthropathies, not elsewhere classified, unspecified wrist

✓6ᵗʰ M12.84   Other specific arthropathies, not elsewhere classified, hand

M12.841   Other specific arthropathies, not elsewhere classified, right hand

M12.842   Other specific arthropathies, not elsewhere classified, left hand

M12.849   Other specific arthropathies, not elsewhere classified, unspecified hand

✓6ᵗʰ M12.85   Other specific arthropathies, not elsewhere classified, hip

M12.851   Other specific arthropathies, not elsewhere classified, right hip

M12.852   Other specific arthropathies, not elsewhere classified, left hip

M12.859   Other specific arthropathies, not elsewhere classified, unspecified hip

✓6ᵗʰ M12.86   Other specific arthropathies, not elsewhere classified, knee

M12.861   Other specific arthropathies, not elsewhere classified, right knee

M12.862   Other specific arthropathies, not elsewhere classified, left knee

M12.869   Other specific arthropathies, not elsewhere classified, unspecified knee

✓6ᵗʰ M12.87   Other specific arthropathies, not elsewhere classified, ankle and foot

M12.871   Other specific arthropathies, not elsewhere classified, right ankle and foot

M12.872   Other specific arthropathies, not elsewhere classified, left ankle and foot

M12.879   Other specific arthropathies, not elsewhere classified, unspecified ankle and foot

M12.88   Other specific arthropathies, not elsewhere classified, other specified site
Other specific arthropathies, not elsewhere classified, vertebrae

M12.89   Other specific arthropathies, not elsewhere classified, multiple sites

M12.9   Arthropathy, unspecified

✓4ᵗʰ M13   Other arthritis

EXCLUDES 1   arthrosis (M15-M19)
osteoarthritis (M15-M19)

M13.0   Polyarthritis, unspecified

✓5ᵗʰ M13.1   Monoarthritis, not elsewhere classified

M13.10   Monoarthritis, not elsewhere classified, unspecified site

✓6ᵗʰ M13.11   Monoarthritis, not elsewhere classified, shoulder

M13.111   Monoarthritis, not elsewhere classified, right shoulder

M13.112   Monoarthritis, not elsewhere classified, left shoulder

M13.119   Monoarthritis, not elsewhere classified, unspecified shoulder

✓6ᵗʰ M13.12   Monoarthritis, not elsewhere classified, elbow

M13.121   Monoarthritis, not elsewhere classified, right elbow

M13.122   Monoarthritis, not elsewhere classified, left elbow

M13.129   Monoarthritis, not elsewhere classified, unspecified elbow

✓6ᵗʰ M13.13   Monoarthritis, not elsewhere classified, wrist

M13.131   Monoarthritis, not elsewhere classified, right wrist

M13.132   Monoarthritis, not elsewhere classified, left wrist

M13.139   Monoarthritis, not elsewhere classified, unspecified wrist

✓6ᵗʰ M13.14   Monoarthritis, not elsewhere classified, hand

M13.141   Monoarthritis, not elsewhere classified, right hand

M13.142   Monoarthritis, not elsewhere classified, left hand

M13.149   Monoarthritis, not elsewhere classified, unspecified hand

✓6ᵗʰ M13.15   Monoarthritis, not elsewhere classified, hip

M13.151   Monoarthritis, not elsewhere classified, right hip

M13.152   Monoarthritis, not elsewhere classified, left hip

M13.159   Monoarthritis, not elsewhere classified, unspecified hip

✓6ᵗʰ M13.16   Monoarthritis, not elsewhere classified, knee

M13.161   Monoarthritis, not elsewhere classified, right knee

M13.162   Monoarthritis, not elsewhere classified, left knee

M13.169   Monoarthritis, not elsewhere classified, unspecified knee

✓6ᵗʰ M13.17   Monoarthritis, not elsewhere classified, ankle and foot

M13.171   Monoarthritis, not elsewhere classified, right ankle and foot

M13.172   Monoarthritis, not elsewhere classified, left ankle and foot

M13.179   Monoarthritis, not elsewhere classified, unspecified ankle and foot

✓5ᵗʰ M13.8   Other specified arthritis
Allergic arthritis
EXCLUDES 1   osteoarthritis (M15-M19)

M13.80   Other specified arthritis, unspecified site

✓6ᵗʰ M13.81   Other specified arthritis, shoulder

M13.811   Other specified arthritis, right shoulder

M13.812   Other specified arthritis, left shoulder

M13.819   Other specified arthritis, unspecified shoulder

✓6ᵗʰ M13.82   Other specified arthritis, elbow

M13.821   Other specified arthritis, right elbow

M13.822   Other specified arthritis, left elbow

M13.829   Other specified arthritis, unspecified elbow

✓6ᵗʰ M13.83   Other specified arthritis, wrist

M13.831   Other specified arthritis, right wrist

M13.832   Other specified arthritis, left wrist

M13.839   Other specified arthritis, unspecified wrist

✓6ᵗʰ M13.84   Other specified arthritis, hand

M13.841   Other specified arthritis, right hand

M13.842   Other specified arthritis, left hand

M13.849   Other specified arthritis, unspecified hand

✓6ᵗʰ M13.85   Other specified arthritis, hip

M13.851   Other specified arthritis, right hip

M13.852   Other specified arthritis, left hip

M13.859   Other specified arthritis, unspecified hip

N Newborn: 0   P Pediatric: 0-17   M Maternity: 9-64   A Adult: 15-124   MCC Major Complication/Comorbidity   CC Complication/Comorbidity   SW Severe Wound Dx

780

ICD-10-CM 2022

✓6th **M13.86** **Other specified arthritis,** knee

    M13.861 **Other specified arthritis,** right **knee**

    M13.862 **Other specified arthritis,** left **knee**

    M13.869 **Other specified arthritis, unspecified knee**

✓6th **M13.87** **Other specified arthritis,** ankle and foot

    M13.871 **Other specified arthritis,** right **ankle and foot**

    M13.872 **Other specified arthritis,** left **ankle and foot**

    M13.879 **Other specified arthritis, unspecified ankle and foot**

M13.88 **Other specified arthritis, other site**

M13.89 **Other specified arthritis,** multiple sites

✓4th **M14** **Arthropathies in other diseases classified elsewhere**

    EXCLUDES 1   arthropathy in:

         diabetes mellitus (E08-E13 with .61-)

         hematological disorders (M36.2-M36.3)

         hypersensitivity reactions (M36.4)

         neoplastic disease (M36.1)

         neurosyphillis (A52.16)

         sarcoidosis (D86.86)

         enteropathic arthropathies (M07.-)

         juvenile psoriatic arthropathy (L40.54)

         lipoid dermatoarthritis (E78.81)

✓5th **M14.6** **Charcôt's joint**

    Neuropathic arthropathy

    EXCLUDES 1   Charcôt's joint in diabetes mellitus (E08-E13 with .610)

         Charcôt's joint in tabes dorsalis (A52.16)

    DEF: Progressive neurologic arthropathy in which chronic degeneration of joints in the weight-bearing areas with peripheral hypertrophy occurs as a complication of a neuropathy disorder. Supporting structures relax from a loss of sensation resulting in chronic joint instability.

M14.60 **Charcôt's joint, unspecified site**

✓6th **M14.61** **Charcôt's joint,** shoulder

    M14.611 **Charcôt's joint,** right **shoulder**

    M14.612 **Charcôt's joint,** left **shoulder**

    M14.619 **Charcôt's joint, unspecified shoulder**

✓6th **M14.62** **Charcôt's joint,** elbow

    M14.621 **Charcôt's joint,** right **elbow**

    M14.622 **Charcôt's joint,** left **elbow**

    M14.629 **Charcôt's joint, unspecified elbow**

✓6th **M14.63** **Charcôt's joint,** wrist

    M14.631 **Charcôt's joint,** right **wrist**

    M14.632 **Charcôt's joint,** left **wrist**

    M14.639 **Charcôt's joint, unspecified wrist**

✓6th **M14.64** **Charcôt's joint,** hand

    M14.641 **Charcôt's joint,** right **hand**

    M14.642 **Charcôt's joint,** left **hand**

    M14.649 **Charcôt's joint, unspecified hand**

✓6th **M14.65** **Charcôt's joint,** hip

    M14.651 **Charcôt's joint,** right **hip**

    M14.652 **Charcôt's joint,** left **hip**

    M14.659 **Charcôt's joint, unspecified hip**

✓6th **M14.66** **Charcôt's joint,** knee

    M14.661 **Charcôt's joint,** right **knee**

    M14.662 **Charcôt's joint,** left **knee**

    M14.669 **Charcôt's joint, unspecified knee**

✓6th **M14.67** **Charcôt's joint,** ankle and foot

    M14.671 **Charcôt's joint,** right **ankle and foot**

    M14.672 **Charcôt's joint,** left **ankle and foot**

    M14.679 **Charcôt's joint, unspecified ankle and foot**

M14.68 **Charcôt's joint,** vertebrae

M14.69 **Charcôt's joint,** multiple sites

✓5th **M14.8** **Arthropathies in other specified diseases classified elsewhere**

    Code first underlying disease, such as:

         amyloidosis (E85.-)

         erythema multiforme (L51.-)

         erythema nodosum (L52)

         hemochromatosis (E83.11-)

         hyperparathyroidism (E21.-)

         hypothyroidism (E00-E03)

         sickle-cell disorders (D57.-)

         thyrotoxicosis [hyperthyroidism] (E05.-)

         Whipple's disease (K90.81)

M14.80 **Arthropathies in other specified diseases classified elsewhere, unspecified site**

✓6th **M14.81** **Arthropathies in other specified diseases classified elsewhere,** shoulder

    M14.811 **Arthropathies in other specified diseases classified elsewhere,** right **shoulder**

    M14.812 **Arthropathies in other specified diseases classified elsewhere,** left **shoulder**

    M14.819 **Arthropathies in other specified diseases classified elsewhere, unspecified shoulder**

✓6th **M14.82** **Arthropathies in other specified diseases classified elsewhere,** elbow

    M14.821 **Arthropathies in other specified diseases classified elsewhere,** right **elbow**

    M14.822 **Arthropathies in other specified diseases classified elsewhere,** left **elbow**

    M14.829 **Arthropathies in other specified diseases classified elsewhere, unspecified elbow**

✓6th **M14.83** **Arthropathies in other specified diseases classified elsewhere,** wrist

    M14.831 **Arthropathies in other specified diseases classified elsewhere,** right **wrist**

    M14.832 **Arthropathies in other specified diseases classified elsewhere,** left **wrist**

    M14.839 **Arthropathies in other specified diseases classified elsewhere, unspecified wrist**

✓6th **M14.84** **Arthropathies in other specified diseases classified elsewhere,** hand

    M14.841 **Arthropathies in other specified diseases classified elsewhere,** right **hand**

    M14.842 **Arthropathies in other specified diseases classified elsewhere,** left **hand**

    M14.849 **Arthropathies in other specified diseases classified elsewhere, unspecified hand**

✓6th **M14.85** **Arthropathies in other specified diseases classified elsewhere,** hip

    M14.851 **Arthropathies in other specified diseases classified elsewhere,** right **hip**

    M14.852 **Arthropathies in other specified diseases classified elsewhere,** left **hip**

    M14.859 **Arthropathies in other specified diseases classified elsewhere, unspecified hip**

✓6th **M14.86** **Arthropathies in other specified diseases classified elsewhere,** knee

    M14.861 **Arthropathies in other specified diseases classified elsewhere,** right **knee**

    M14.862 **Arthropathies in other specified diseases classified elsewhere,** left **knee**

    M14.869 **Arthropathies in other specified diseases classified elsewhere, unspecified knee**

✓6th **M14.87** **Arthropathies in other specified diseases classified elsewhere,** ankle and foot

    M14.871 **Arthropathies in other specified diseases classified elsewhere,** right **ankle and foot**

    M14.872 **Arthropathies in other specified diseases classified elsewhere,** left **ankle and foot**

    M14.879 **Arthropathies in other specified diseases classified elsewhere, unspecified ankle and foot**

M14.88 **Arthropathies in other specified diseases classified elsewhere,** vertebrae

M14.89 **Arthropathies in other specified diseases classified elsewhere,** multiple sites

✔ Additional Character Required   ✓x7th Placeholder   Questionable PDx   Manifestation   Unspecified Dx   UPD Unacceptable PDx   H1-H14 HAC   HCC CMS-HCC Dx   HIV HIV Dx

ICD-10-CM 2022   781

Osteoarthritis (M15-M19)

EXCLUDES 2   *osteoarthritis of spine (M47.-)*

AHA: 2020,2Q,14; 2016,4Q,147

TIP: Assign a primary osteoarthritis code when the site of the osteoarthritis is documented but the type of osteoarthritis — primary, secondary, generalized, or post-traumatic — is not documented. Primary is considered the default.

✓4ᵗʰ **M15 Polyosteoarthritis**

     INCLUDES   arthritis of multiple sites

     EXCLUDES 1   *bilateral involvement of single joint (M16-M19)*

M15.0 Primary generalized (osteo)arthritis

M15.1 Heberden's nodes (with arthropathy)
     Interphalangeal distal osteoarthritis

M15.2 Bouchard's nodes (with arthropathy)
     Juxtaphalangeal distal osteoarthritis

M15.3 Secondary multiple arthritis
     Post-traumatic polyosteoarthritis

M15.4 Erosive (osteo)arthritis

M15.8 Other polyosteoarthritis

M15.9 Polyosteoarthritis, unspecified
     Generalized osteoarthritis NOS

✓4ᵗʰ **M16 Osteoarthritis of hip**

     AHA: 2016,4Q,146

M16.0 Bilateral primary osteoarthritis of hip
     AHA: 2018,2Q,15

✓5ᵗʰ **M16.1 Unilateral primary osteoarthritis of hip**
     Primary osteoarthritis of hip NOS
     AHA: 2018,2Q,15

     M16.10 Unilateral primary osteoarthritis, unspecified hip
     M16.11 Unilateral primary osteoarthritis, right hip
     M16.12 Unilateral primary osteoarthritis, left hip

M16.2 Bilateral osteoarthritis resulting from hip dysplasia

✓5ᵗʰ **M16.3 Unilateral osteoarthritis resulting from hip dysplasia**
     Dysplastic osteoarthritis of hip NOS

     M16.30 Unilateral osteoarthritis resulting from hip dysplasia, unspecified hip
     M16.31 Unilateral osteoarthritis resulting from hip dysplasia, right hip
     M16.32 Unilateral osteoarthritis resulting from hip dysplasia, left hip

M16.4 Bilateral post-traumatic osteoarthritis of hip

✓5ᵗʰ **M16.5 Unilateral post-traumatic osteoarthritis of hip**
     Post-traumatic osteoarthritis of hip NOS

     M16.50 Unilateral post-traumatic osteoarthritis, unspecified hip
     M16.51 Unilateral post-traumatic osteoarthritis, right hip
     M16.52 Unilateral post-traumatic osteoarthritis, left hip

M16.6 Other bilateral secondary osteoarthritis of hip

M16.7 Other unilateral secondary osteoarthritis of hip
     Secondary osteoarthritis of hip NOS

M16.9 Osteoarthritis of hip, unspecified

✓4ᵗʰ **M17 Osteoarthritis of knee**

     AHA: 2016,4Q,146-147

M17.0 Bilateral primary osteoarthritis of knee
     AHA: 2018,2Q,15

✓5ᵗʰ **M17.1 Unilateral primary osteoarthritis of knee**
     Primary osteoarthritis of knee NOS
     AHA: 2018,2Q,15

     M17.10 Unilateral primary osteoarthritis, unspecified knee
     M17.11 Unilateral primary osteoarthritis, right knee
     M17.12 Unilateral primary osteoarthritis, left knee

M17.2 Bilateral post-traumatic osteoarthritis of knee

✓5ᵗʰ **M17.3 Unilateral post-traumatic osteoarthritis of knee**
     Post-traumatic osteoarthritis of knee NOS

     M17.30 Unilateral post-traumatic osteoarthritis, unspecified knee
     M17.31 Unilateral post-traumatic osteoarthritis, right knee
     M17.32 Unilateral post-traumatic osteoarthritis, left knee

M17.4 Other bilateral secondary osteoarthritis of knee

M17.5 Other unilateral secondary osteoarthritis of knee
     Secondary osteoarthritis of knee NOS

M17.9 Osteoarthritis of knee, unspecified

✓4ᵗʰ **M18 Osteoarthritis of first carpometacarpal joint**

M18.0 Bilateral primary osteoarthritis of first carpometacarpal joints

✓5ᵗʰ **M18.1 Unilateral primary osteoarthritis of first carpometacarpal joint**
     Primary osteoarthritis of first carpometacarpal joint NOS

     M18.10 Unilateral primary osteoarthritis of first carpometacarpal joint, unspecified hand
     M18.11 Unilateral primary osteoarthritis of first carpometacarpal joint, right hand
     M18.12 Unilateral primary osteoarthritis of first carpometacarpal joint, left hand

M18.2 Bilateral post-traumatic osteoarthritis of first carpometacarpal joints

✓5ᵗʰ **M18.3 Unilateral post-traumatic osteoarthritis of first carpometacarpal joint**
     Post-traumatic osteoarthritis of first carpometacarpal joint NOS

     M18.30 Unilateral post-traumatic osteoarthritis of first carpometacarpal joint, unspecified hand
     M18.31 Unilateral post-traumatic osteoarthritis of first carpometacarpal joint, right hand
     M18.32 Unilateral post-traumatic osteoarthritis of first carpometacarpal joint, left hand

M18.4 Other bilateral secondary osteoarthritis of first carpometacarpal joints

✓5ᵗʰ **M18.5 Other unilateral secondary osteoarthritis of first carpometacarpal joint**
     Secondary osteoarthritis of first carpometacarpal joint NOS

     M18.50 Other unilateral secondary osteoarthritis of first carpometacarpal joint, unspecified hand
     M18.51 Other unilateral secondary osteoarthritis of first carpometacarpal joint, right hand
     M18.52 Other unilateral secondary osteoarthritis of first carpometacarpal joint, left hand

M18.9 Osteoarthritis of first carpometacarpal joint, unspecified

✓4ᵗʰ **M19 Other and unspecified osteoarthritis**

     EXCLUDES 1   *polyarthritis (M15.-)*

     EXCLUDES 2   *arthrosis of spine (M47.-)*
                 hallux rigidus (M20.2)
                 osteoarthritis of spine (M47.-)

     AHA: 2020,4Q,31-32

✓5ᵗʰ **M19.0 Primary osteoarthritis of other joints**
     AHA: 2018,2Q,15; 2016,4Q,145

     ✓6ᵗʰ **M19.01 Primary osteoarthritis, shoulder**

         M19.011 Primary osteoarthritis, right shoulder
         M19.012 Primary osteoarthritis, left shoulder
         M19.019 Primary osteoarthritis, unspecified shoulder

     ✓6ᵗʰ **M19.02 Primary osteoarthritis, elbow**

         M19.021 Primary osteoarthritis, right elbow
         M19.022 Primary osteoarthritis, left elbow
         M19.029 Primary osteoarthritis, unspecified elbow

     ✓6ᵗʰ **M19.03 Primary osteoarthritis, wrist**

         M19.031 Primary osteoarthritis, right wrist
         M19.032 Primary osteoarthritis, left wrist
         M19.039 Primary osteoarthritis, unspecified wrist

     ✓6ᵗʰ **M19.04 Primary osteoarthritis, hand**

         EXCLUDES 2   *primary osteoarthritis of first carpometacarpal joint (M18.0-, M18.1-)*

         M19.041 Primary osteoarthritis, right hand
         M19.042 Primary osteoarthritis, left hand
         M19.049 Primary osteoarthritis, unspecified hand

     ✓6ᵗʰ **M19.07 Primary osteoarthritis ankle and foot**

         M19.071 Primary osteoarthritis, right ankle and foot
         M19.072 Primary osteoarthritis, left ankle and foot
         M19.079 Primary osteoarthritis, unspecified ankle and foot

     M19.09 Primary osteoarthritis, other specified site

✓5ᵗʰ **M19.1 Post-traumatic osteoarthritis of other joints**

     ✓6ᵗʰ **M19.11 Post-traumatic osteoarthritis, shoulder**

         M19.111 Post-traumatic osteoarthritis, right shoulder
         M19.112 Post-traumatic osteoarthritis, left shoulder
         M19.119 Post-traumatic osteoarthritis, unspecified shoulder

     ✓6ᵗʰ **M19.12 Post-traumatic osteoarthritis, elbow**

         M19.121 Post-traumatic osteoarthritis, right elbow
         M19.122 Post-traumatic osteoarthritis, left elbow

N Newborn: 0   **P** Pediatric: 0-17   **M** Maternity: 9-64   **A** Adult: 15-124   **MCC** Major Complication/Comorbidity   **CC** Complication/Comorbidity   **SW** Severe Wound Dx

782   ICD-10-CM 2022

M19.129 Post-traumatic osteoarthritis, unspecified elbow

√6ᵗʰ **M19.13** Post-traumatic osteoarthritis, wrist

M19.131 Post-traumatic osteoarthritis, right wrist
M19.132 Post-traumatic osteoarthritis, left wrist
M19.139 Post-traumatic osteoarthritis, unspecified wrist

√6ᵗʰ **M19.14** Post-traumatic osteoarthritis, hand

EXCLUDES 2   post-traumatic osteoarthritis of first carpometacarpal joint (M18.2-, M18.3-)

M19.141 Post-traumatic osteoarthritis, right hand
M19.142 Post-traumatic osteoarthritis, left hand
M19.149 Post-traumatic osteoarthritis, unspecified hand

√6ᵗʰ **M19.17** Post-traumatic osteoarthritis, ankle and foot

M19.171 Post-traumatic osteoarthritis, right ankle and foot
M19.172 Post-traumatic osteoarthritis, left ankle and foot
M19.179 Post-traumatic osteoarthritis, unspecified ankle and foot

M19.19 Post-traumatic osteoarthritis, other specified site

√5ᵗʰ **M19.2** Secondary osteoarthritis of other joints

√6ᵗʰ **M19.21** Secondary osteoarthritis, shoulder

M19.211 Secondary osteoarthritis, right shoulder
M19.212 Secondary osteoarthritis, left shoulder
M19.219 Secondary osteoarthritis, unspecified shoulder

√6ᵗʰ **M19.22** Secondary osteoarthritis, elbow

M19.221 Secondary osteoarthritis, right elbow
M19.222 Secondary osteoarthritis, left elbow
M19.229 Secondary osteoarthritis, unspecified elbow

√6ᵗʰ **M19.23** Secondary osteoarthritis, wrist

M19.231 Secondary osteoarthritis, right wrist
M19.232 Secondary osteoarthritis, left wrist
M19.239 Secondary osteoarthritis, unspecified wrist

√6ᵗʰ **M19.24** Secondary osteoarthritis, hand

M19.241 Secondary osteoarthritis, right hand
M19.242 Secondary osteoarthritis, left hand
M19.249 Secondary osteoarthritis, unspecified hand

√6ᵗʰ **M19.27** Secondary osteoarthritis, ankle and foot

M19.271 Secondary osteoarthritis, right ankle and foot
M19.272 Secondary osteoarthritis, left ankle and foot
M19.279 Secondary osteoarthritis, unspecified ankle and foot

M19.29 Secondary osteoarthritis, other specified site

√5ᵗʰ **M19.9** Osteoarthritis, unspecified

TIP: Assign M19.90 when neither the site nor the type of osteoarthritis — primary, secondary, or post-traumatic — is documented.

M19.90 Unspecified osteoarthritis, unspecified site
Arthrosis NOS
Arthritis NOS
Osteoarthritis NOS
AHA: 2016,4Q,145-147

M19.91 Primary osteoarthritis, unspecified site
Primary osteoarthritis NOS

M19.92 Post-traumatic osteoarthritis, unspecified site
Post-traumatic osteoarthritis NOS

M19.93 Secondary osteoarthritis, unspecified site
Secondary osteoarthritis NOS

Other joint disorders (M20-M25)

EXCLUDES 2   joints of the spine (M40-M54)

√4ᵗʰ **M20** Acquired deformities of fingers and toes

EXCLUDES 1   acquired absence of fingers and toes (Z89.-)
congenital absence of fingers and toes (Q71.3-, Q72.3-)
congenital deformities and malformations of fingers and toes (Q66.-, Q68-Q70, Q74.-)

√5ᵗʰ **M20.0** Deformity of finger(s)

EXCLUDES 1   clubbing of fingers (R68.3)
palmar fascial fibromatosis [Dupuytren] (M72.0)
trigger finger (M65.3)

√6ᵗʰ **M20.00** Unspecified deformity of finger(s)

M20.001 Unspecified deformity of right finger(s)
M20.002 Unspecified deformity of left finger(s)
M20.009 Unspecified deformity of unspecified finger(s)

√6ᵗʰ **M20.01** Mallet finger

M20.011 Mallet finger of right finger(s)
M20.012 Mallet finger of left finger(s)
M20.019 Mallet finger of unspecified finger(s)

√6ᵗʰ **M20.02** Boutonnière deformity

DEF: Deformity of the finger caused by flexion of the proximal interphalangeal joint and hyperextension of the distal joint. The deformity results from rheumatoid arthritis, osteoarthritis, or injury.

M20.021 Boutonnière deformity of right finger(s)
M20.022 Boutonnière deformity of left finger(s)
M20.029 Boutonnière deformity of unspecified finger(s)

√6ᵗʰ **M20.03** Swan-neck deformity

DEF: Flexed distal and hyperextended proximal interphalangeal joint most commonly caused by rheumatoid arthritis.

M20.031 Swan-neck deformity of right finger(s)
M20.032 Swan-neck deformity of left finger(s)
M20.039 Swan-neck deformity of unspecified finger(s)

√6ᵗʰ **M20.09** Other deformity of finger(s)

M20.091 Other deformity of right finger(s)
M20.092 Other deformity of left finger(s)
M20.099 Other deformity of finger(s), unspecified

√5ᵗʰ **M20.1** Hallux valgus (acquired)

EXCLUDES 2   bunion (M21.6-)
AHA: 2016,4Q,38
DEF: Deformity in which the great toe deviates toward the other toes and may even be positioned over or under the second toe.

Hallux Valgus

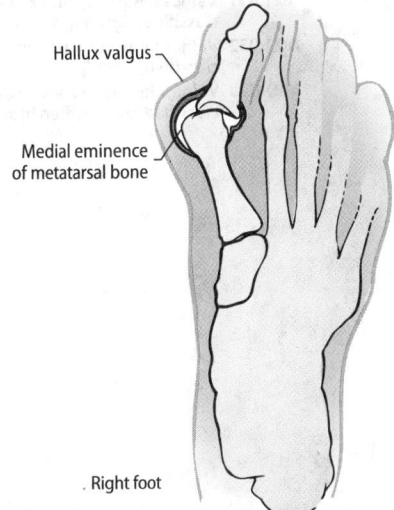

Hallux valgus

Medial eminence of metatarsal bone

Right foot

M20.10 Hallux valgus (acquired), unspecified foot
M20.11 Hallux valgus (acquired), right foot
M20.12 Hallux valgus (acquired), left foot

√5ᵗʰ **M20.2** Hallux rigidus

     M20.20 **Hallux rigidus, unspecified foot**

     M20.21 **Hallux rigidus, right foot**

     M20.22 **Hallux rigidus, left foot**

√5ᵗʰ **M20.3** Hallux varus (acquired)

     DEF: Deformity in which the great toe deviates away from the other toes.

     M20.30 **Hallux varus (acquired), unspecified foot**

     M20.31 **Hallux varus (acquired), right foot**

     M20.32 **Hallux varus (acquired), left foot**

√5ᵗʰ **M20.4** Other hammer toe(s) (acquired)

     M20.40 **Other hammer toe(s) (acquired), unspecified foot**

     M20.41 **Other hammer toe(s) (acquired), right foot**

     M20.42 **Other hammer toe(s) (acquired), left foot**

√5ᵗʰ **M20.5** Other deformities of toe(s) (acquired)

     √6ᵗʰ **M20.5X** **Other deformities of toe(s) (acquired)**

         M20.5X1 **Other deformities of toe(s) (acquired), right foot**

         M20.5X2 **Other deformities of toe(s) (acquired), left foot**

         M20.5X9 **Other deformities of toe(s) (acquired), unspecified foot**

√5ᵗʰ **M20.6** Acquired deformities of toe(s), unspecified

     M20.60 **Acquired deformities of toe(s), unspecified, unspecified foot**

     M20.61 **Acquired deformities of toe(s), unspecified, right foot**

     M20.62 **Acquired deformities of toe(s), unspecified, left foot**

√4ᵗʰ **M21** **Other acquired deformities of limbs**

     EXCLUDES 1   acquired absence of limb (Z89.-)

         congenital absence of limbs (Q71-Q73)

         congenital deformities and malformations of limbs (Q65-Q66, Q68-Q74)

     EXCLUDES 2   acquired deformities of fingers or toes (M20.-)

         coxa plana (M91.2)

√5ᵗʰ **M21.0** Valgus deformity, not elsewhere classified

     EXCLUDES 1   metatarsus valgus (Q66.6)

         talipes calcaneovalgus (Q66.4-)

     M21.00 **Valgus deformity, not elsewhere classified, unspecified site**

     √6ᵗʰ **M21.02** **Valgus deformity, not elsewhere classified, elbow**

         Cubitus valgus

         M21.021 **Valgus deformity, not elsewhere classified, right elbow**

         M21.022 **Valgus deformity, not elsewhere classified, left elbow**

         M21.029 **Valgus deformity, not elsewhere classified, unspecified elbow**

     √6ᵗʰ **M21.05** **Valgus deformity, not elsewhere classified, hip**

         M21.051 **Valgus deformity, not elsewhere classified, right hip**

         M21.052 **Valgus deformity, not elsewhere classified, left hip**

         M21.059 **Valgus deformity, not elsewhere classified, unspecified hip**

√6ᵗʰ **M21.06** **Valgus deformity, not elsewhere classified, knee**

     Genu valgum

     Knock knee

     DEF: Genu valga/valgum: Condition in which the thighs slant inward, causing the knees to be angled abnormally close together, leaving the space between the ankles wider than normal.

Genu Valga (knock-knee)

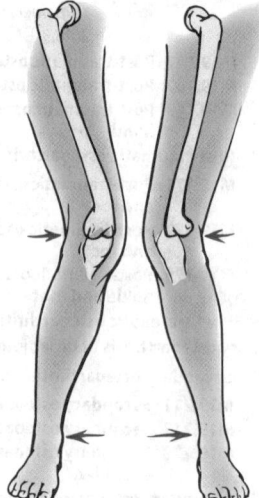

     M21.061 **Valgus deformity, not elsewhere classified, right knee**

     M21.062 **Valgus deformity, not elsewhere classified, left knee**

     M21.069 **Valgus deformity, not elsewhere classified, unspecified knee**

√6ᵗʰ **M21.07** **Valgus deformity, not elsewhere classified, ankle**

     M21.071 **Valgus deformity, not elsewhere classified, right ankle**

     M21.072 **Valgus deformity, not elsewhere classified, left ankle**

     M21.079 **Valgus deformity, not elsewhere classified, unspecified ankle**

√5ᵗʰ **M21.1** Varus deformity, not elsewhere classified

     EXCLUDES 1   metatarsus varus (Q66.22-)

         tibia vara (M92.51-)

     M21.10 **Varus deformity, not elsewhere classified, unspecified site**

     √6ᵗʰ **M21.12** **Varus deformity, not elsewhere classified, elbow**

         Cubitus varus, elbow

         M21.121 **Varus deformity, not elsewhere classified, right elbow**

         M21.122 **Varus deformity, not elsewhere classified, left elbow**

         M21.129 **Varus deformity, not elsewhere classified, unspecified elbow**

     √6ᵗʰ **M21.15** **Varus deformity, not elsewhere classified, hip**

         M21.151 **Varus deformity, not elsewhere classified, right hip**

         M21.152 **Varus deformity, not elsewhere classified, left hip**

         M21.159 **Varus deformity, not elsewhere classified, unspecified**

N Newborn: 0   P Pediatric: 0-17   M Maternity: 9-64   A Adult: 15-124   MCC Major Complication/Comorbidity   CC Complication/Comorbidity   SW Severe Wound Dx

784   ICD-10-CM 2022

☑6ᵗʰ **M21.16 Varus deformity, not elsewhere classified,** knee
Bow leg
Genu varum
DEF: Genu varus/varum: Condition in which the thighs and/or legs are bowed in an outward curve with an abnormally increased space between the knees.

Genu Varus (bowleg)

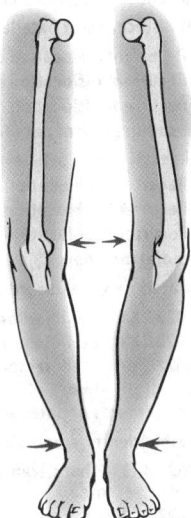

     M21.161 Varus deformity, not elsewhere classified, right knee
     M21.162 Varus deformity, not elsewhere classified, left knee
     M21.169 Varus deformity, not elsewhere classified, unspecified knee
☑6ᵗʰ **M21.17 Varus deformity, not elsewhere classified,** ankle
     M21.171 Varus deformity, not elsewhere classified, right ankle
     M21.172 Varus deformity, not elsewhere classified, left ankle
     M21.179 Varus deformity, not elsewhere classified, unspecified ankle
☑5ᵗʰ **M21.2 Flexion deformity**
     M21.20 Flexion deformity, unspecified site
☑6ᵗʰ **M21.21 Flexion deformity,** shoulder
     M21.211 Flexion deformity, right shoulder
     M21.212 Flexion deformity, left shoulder
     M21.219 Flexion deformity, unspecified shoulder
☑6ᵗʰ **M21.22 Flexion deformity,** elbow
     M21.221 Flexion deformity, right elbow
     M21.222 Flexion deformity, left elbow
     M21.229 Flexion deformity, unspecified elbow
☑6ᵗʰ **M21.23 Flexion deformity,** wrist
     M21.231 Flexion deformity, right wrist
     M21.232 Flexion deformity, left wrist
     M21.239 Flexion deformity, unspecified wrist
☑6ᵗʰ **M21.24 Flexion deformity,** finger joints
     M21.241 Flexion deformity, right finger joints
     M21.242 Flexion deformity, left finger joints
     M21.249 Flexion deformity, unspecified finger joints
☑6ᵗʰ **M21.25 Flexion deformity,** hip
     M21.251 Flexion deformity, right hip
     M21.252 Flexion deformity, left hip
     M21.259 Flexion deformity, unspecified hip
☑6ᵗʰ **M21.26 Flexion deformity,** knee
     M21.261 Flexion deformity, right knee
     M21.262 Flexion deformity, left knee
     M21.269 Flexion deformity, unspecified knee
☑6ᵗʰ **M21.27 Flexion deformity,** ankle and toes
     M21.271 Flexion deformity, right ankle and toes
     M21.272 Flexion deformity, left ankle and toes
     M21.279 Flexion deformity, unspecified ankle and toes

☑5ᵗʰ **M21.3 Wrist or foot drop (acquired)**
☑6ᵗʰ **M21.33 Wrist drop (acquired)**
     M21.331 Wrist drop, right wrist
     M21.332 Wrist drop, left wrist
     M21.339 Wrist drop, unspecified wrist
☑6ᵗʰ **M21.37 Foot drop (acquired)**
     M21.371 Foot drop, right foot
     M21.372 Foot drop, left foot
     M21.379 Foot drop, unspecified foot
☑5ᵗʰ **M21.4 Flat foot [pes planus] (acquired)**
    EXCLUDES 1   congenital pes planus (Q66.5-)
     M21.40 Flat foot [pes planus] (acquired), unspecified foot
     M21.41 Flat foot [pes planus] (acquired), right foot
     M21.42 Flat foot [pes planus] (acquired), left foot
☑5ᵗʰ **M21.5 Acquired** clawhand, clubhand, clawfoot and clubfoot
    EXCLUDES 1   clubfoot, not specified as acquired (Q66.89)
☑6ᵗʰ **M21.51 Acquired** clawhand
     M21.511 Acquired clawhand, right hand
     M21.512 Acquired clawhand, left hand
     M21.519 Acquired clawhand, unspecified hand
☑6ᵗʰ **M21.52 Acquired** clubhand
     M21.521 Acquired clubhand, right hand
     M21.522 Acquired clubhand, left hand
     M21.529 Acquired clubhand, unspecified hand
☑6ᵗʰ **M21.53 Acquired** clawfoot
    DEF: High foot arch with hyperextended toes at the metatarsophalangeal joint and flexed toes at the distal joints.
     M21.531 Acquired clawfoot, right foot
     M21.532 Acquired clawfoot, left foot
     M21.539 Acquired clawfoot, unspecified foot
☑6ᵗʰ **M21.54 Acquired** clubfoot
    DEF: Acquired anomaly of the foot with the heel elevated and rotated outward and the toes pointing inward.
     M21.541 Acquired clubfoot, right foot
     M21.542 Acquired clubfoot, left foot
     M21.549 Acquired clubfoot, unspecified foot
☑5ᵗʰ **M21.6 Other acquired deformities of foot**
    EXCLUDES 2   deformities of toe (acquired) (M20.1-M20.6-)
    AHA: 2016,4Q,38
☑6ᵗʰ **M21.61 Bunion**
     M21.611 Bunion of right foot
     M21.612 Bunion of left foot
     M21.619 Bunion of unspecified foot
☑6ᵗʰ **M21.62 Bunionette**
     M21.621 Bunionette of right foot
     M21.622 Bunionette of left foot
     M21.629 Bunionette of unspecified foot
☑6ᵗʰ **M21.6X Other acquired deformities of** foot
     M21.6X1 Other acquired deformities of right foot
     M21.6X2 Other acquired deformities of left foot
     M21.6X9 Other acquired deformities of unspecified foot
☑5ᵗʰ **M21.7 Unequal limb length (acquired)**
    NOTE   The site used should correspond to the shorter limb
     M21.70 Unequal limb length (acquired), unspecified site
☑6ᵗʰ **M21.72 Unequal limb length (acquired),** humerus
     M21.721 Unequal limb length (acquired), right humerus
     M21.722 Unequal limb length (acquired), left humerus
     M21.729 Unequal limb length (acquired), unspecified humerus
☑6ᵗʰ **M21.73 Unequal limb length (acquired),** ulna and radius
     M21.731 Unequal limb length (acquired), right ulna
     M21.732 Unequal limb length (acquired), left ulna
     M21.733 Unequal limb length (acquired), right radius
     M21.734 Unequal limb length (acquired), left radius
     M21.739 Unequal limb length (acquired), unspecified ulna and radius

✓6th **M21.75** Unequal limb length (acquired), femur

M21.751 Unequal limb length (acquired), right femur

M21.752 Unequal limb length (acquired), left femur

M21.759 Unequal limb length (acquired), unspecified femur

✓6th **M21.76** Unequal limb length (acquired), tibia and fibula

M21.761 Unequal limb length (acquired), right tibia

M21.762 Unequal limb length (acquired), left tibia

M21.763 Unequal limb length (acquired), right fibula

M21.764 Unequal limb length (acquired), left fibula

M21.769 Unequal limb length (acquired), unspecified tibia and fibula

✓5th **M21.8** Other specified acquired deformities of limbs

EXCLUDES 2   coxa plana (M91.2)

M21.80 Other specified acquired deformities of unspecified limb

✓6th **M21.82** Other specified acquired deformities of upper arm

M21.821 Other specified acquired deformities of right upper arm

M21.822 Other specified acquired deformities of left upper arm

M21.829 Other specified acquired deformities of unspecified upper arm

✓6th **M21.83** Other specified acquired deformities of forearm

M21.831 Other specified acquired deformities of right forearm

M21.832 Other specified acquired deformities of left forearm

M21.839 Other specified acquired deformities of unspecified forearm

✓6th **M21.85** Other specified acquired deformities of thigh

M21.851 Other specified acquired deformities of right thigh

M21.852 Other specified acquired deformities of left thigh

M21.859 Other specified acquired deformities of unspecified thigh

✓6th **M21.86** Other specified acquired deformities of lower leg

M21.861 Other specified acquired deformities of right lower leg

M21.862 Other specified acquired deformities of left lower leg

M21.869 Other specified acquired deformities of unspecified lower leg

✓5th **M21.9** Unspecified acquired deformity of limb and hand

M21.90 Unspecified acquired deformity of unspecified limb

✓6th **M21.92** Unspecified acquired deformity of upper arm

M21.921 Unspecified acquired deformity of right upper arm

M21.922 Unspecified acquired deformity of left upper arm

M21.929 Unspecified acquired deformity of unspecified upper arm

✓6th **M21.93** Unspecified acquired deformity of forearm

M21.931 Unspecified acquired deformity of right forearm

M21.932 Unspecified acquired deformity of left forearm

M21.939 Unspecified acquired deformity of unspecified forearm

✓6th **M21.94** Unspecified acquired deformity of hand

M21.941 Unspecified acquired deformity of hand, right hand

M21.942 Unspecified acquired deformity of hand, left hand

M21.949 Unspecified acquired deformity of hand, unspecified hand

✓6th **M21.95** Unspecified acquired deformity of thigh

M21.951 Unspecified acquired deformity of right thigh

M21.952 Unspecified acquired deformity of left thigh

M21.959 Unspecified acquired deformity of unspecified thigh

✓6th **M21.96** Unspecified acquired deformity of lower leg

M21.961 Unspecified acquired deformity of right lower leg

M21.962 Unspecified acquired deformity of left lower leg

M21.969 Unspecified acquired deformity of unspecified lower leg

✓4th **M22** Disorder of patella

EXCLUDES 2   traumatic dislocation of patella (S83.0-)

✓5th **M22.0** Recurrent dislocation of patella

M22.00 Recurrent dislocation of patella, unspecified knee

M22.01 Recurrent dislocation of patella, right knee

M22.02 Recurrent dislocation of patella, left knee

✓5th **M22.1** Recurrent subluxation of patella

Incomplete dislocation of patella

M22.10 Recurrent subluxation of patella, unspecified knee

M22.11 Recurrent subluxation of patella, right knee

M22.12 Recurrent subluxation of patella, left knee

✓5th **M22.2** Patellofemoral disorders

✓6th **M22.2X** Patellofemoral disorders

M22.2X1 Patellofemoral disorders, right knee

M22.2X2 Patellofemoral disorders, left knee

M22.2X9 Patellofemoral disorders, unspecified knee

✓5th **M22.3** Other derangements of patella

✓6th **M22.3X** Other derangements of patella

M22.3X1 Other derangements of patella, right knee

M22.3X2 Other derangements of patella, left knee

M22.3X9 Other derangements of patella, unspecified knee

✓5th **M22.4** Chondromalacia patellae

M22.40 Chondromalacia patellae, unspecified knee

M22.41 Chondromalacia patellae, right knee

M22.42 Chondromalacia patellae, left knee

✓5th **M22.8** Other disorders of patella

✓6th **M22.8X** Other disorders of patella

M22.8X1 Other disorders of patella, right knee

M22.8X2 Other disorders of patella, left knee

M22.8X9 Other disorders of patella, unspecified knee

✓5th **M22.9** Unspecified disorder of patella

M22.90 Unspecified disorder of patella, unspecified knee

M22.91 Unspecified disorder of patella, right knee

M22.92 Unspecified disorder of patella, left knee

✓4th **M23** Internal derangement of knee

EXCLUDES 1   ankylosis (M24.66)

deformity of knee (M21.-)

osteochondritis dissecans (M93.2)

EXCLUDES 2   current injury - see injury of knee and lower leg (S80-S89)

recurrent dislocation or subluxation of joints (M24.4)

recurrent dislocation or subluxation of patella (M22.0-M22.1)

✓5th **M23.0** Cystic meniscus

✓6th **M23.00** Cystic meniscus, unspecified meniscus

Cystic meniscus, unspecified lateral meniscus

Cystic meniscus, unspecified medial meniscus

M23.000 Cystic meniscus, unspecified lateral meniscus, right knee

M23.001 Cystic meniscus, unspecified lateral meniscus, left knee

M23.002 Cystic meniscus, unspecified lateral meniscus, unspecified knee

M23.003 Cystic meniscus, unspecified medial meniscus, right knee

M23.004 Cystic meniscus, unspecified medial meniscus, left knee

M23.005 Cystic meniscus, unspecified medial meniscus, unspecified knee

M23.006 Cystic meniscus, unspecified meniscus, right knee

M23.007 Cystic meniscus, unspecified meniscus, left knee

M23.009 Cystic meniscus, unspecified meniscus, unspecified knee

N Newborn: 0   P Pediatric: 0-17   M Maternity: 9-64   A Adult: 15-124   MCC Major Complication/Comorbidity   CC Complication/Comorbidity   SW Severe Wound Dx

786   ICD-10-CM 2022

✓6th **M23.01 Cystic meniscus, anterior horn of medial meniscus**
     M23.011 Cystic meniscus, anterior horn of medial meniscus, right knee
     M23.012 Cystic meniscus, anterior horn of medial meniscus, left knee
     M23.019 Cystic meniscus, anterior horn of medial meniscus, unspecified knee

✓6th **M23.02 Cystic meniscus, posterior horn of medial meniscus**
     M23.021 Cystic meniscus, posterior horn of medial meniscus, right knee
     M23.022 Cystic meniscus, posterior horn of medial meniscus, left knee
     M23.029 Cystic meniscus, posterior horn of medial meniscus, unspecified knee

✓6th **M23.03 Cystic meniscus, other medial meniscus**
     M23.031 Cystic meniscus, other medial meniscus, right knee
     M23.032 Cystic meniscus, other medial meniscus, left knee
     M23.039 Cystic meniscus, other medial meniscus, unspecified knee

✓6th **M23.04 Cystic meniscus, anterior horn of lateral meniscus**
     M23.041 Cystic meniscus, anterior horn of lateral meniscus, right knee
     M23.042 Cystic meniscus, anterior horn of lateral meniscus, left knee
     M23.049 Cystic meniscus, anterior horn of lateral meniscus, unspecified knee

✓6th **M23.05 Cystic meniscus, posterior horn of lateral meniscus**
     M23.051 Cystic meniscus, posterior horn of lateral meniscus, right knee
     M23.052 Cystic meniscus, posterior horn of lateral meniscus, left knee
     M23.059 Cystic meniscus, posterior horn of lateral meniscus, unspecified knee

✓6th **M23.06 Cystic meniscus, other lateral meniscus**
     M23.061 Cystic meniscus, other lateral meniscus, right knee
     M23.062 Cystic meniscus, other lateral meniscus, left knee
     M23.069 Cystic meniscus, other lateral meniscus, unspecified knee

✓5th **M23.2 Derangement of meniscus due to old tear or injury**
     Old bucket-handle tear
     AHA: 2019,2Q,26

Derangement of Meniscus

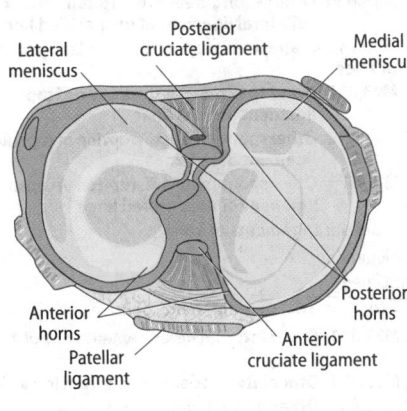

Overhead view of right knee

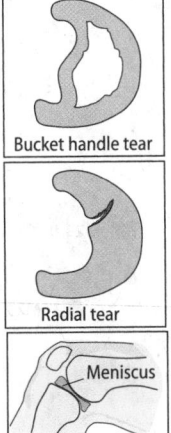

Bucket handle tear

Radial tear

Meniscus

✓6th **M23.20 Derangement of unspecified meniscus due to old tear or injury**
     Derangement of unspecified lateral meniscus due to old tear or injury
     Derangement of unspecified medial meniscus due to old tear or injury
     M23.200 Derangement of unspecified lateral meniscus due to old tear or injury, right knee
     M23.201 Derangement of unspecified lateral meniscus due to old tear or injury, left knee

M23.202 Derangement of unspecified lateral meniscus due to old tear or injury, unspecified knee
M23.203 Derangement of unspecified medial meniscus due to old tear or injury, right knee
M23.204 Derangement of unspecified medial meniscus due to old tear or injury, left knee
M23.205 Derangement of unspecified medial meniscus due to old tear or injury, unspecified knee
M23.206 Derangement of unspecified meniscus due to old tear or injury, right knee
M23.207 Derangement of unspecified meniscus due to old tear or injury, left knee
M23.209 Derangement of unspecified meniscus due to old tear or injury, unspecified knee

✓6th **M23.21 Derangement of anterior horn of medial meniscus due to old tear or injury**
     M23.211 Derangement of anterior horn of medial meniscus due to old tear or injury, right knee
     M23.212 Derangement of anterior horn of medial meniscus due to old tear or injury, left knee
     M23.219 Derangement of anterior horn of medial meniscus due to old tear or injury, unspecified knee

✓6th **M23.22 Derangement of posterior horn of medial meniscus due to old tear or injury**
     M23.221 Derangement of posterior horn of medial meniscus due to old tear or injury, right knee
     M23.222 Derangement of posterior horn of medial meniscus due to old tear or injury, left knee
     M23.229 Derangement of posterior horn of medial meniscus due to old tear or injury, unspecified knee

✓6th **M23.23 Derangement of other medial meniscus due to old tear or injury**
     M23.231 Derangement of other medial meniscus due to old tear or injury, right knee
     M23.232 Derangement of other medial meniscus due to old tear or injury, left knee
     M23.239 Derangement of other medial meniscus due to old tear or injury, unspecified knee

✓6th **M23.24 Derangement of anterior horn of lateral meniscus due to old tear or injury**
     M23.241 Derangement of anterior horn of lateral meniscus due to old tear or injury, right knee
     M23.242 Derangement of anterior horn of lateral meniscus due to old tear or injury, left knee
     M23.249 Derangement of anterior horn of lateral meniscus due to old tear or injury, unspecified knee

✓6th **M23.25 Derangement of posterior horn of lateral meniscus due to old tear or injury**
     M23.251 Derangement of posterior horn of lateral meniscus due to old tear or injury, right knee
     M23.252 Derangement of posterior horn of lateral meniscus due to old tear or injury, left knee
     M23.259 Derangement of posterior horn of lateral meniscus due to old tear or injury, unspecified knee

✓6th **M23.26 Derangement of other lateral meniscus due to old tear or injury**
     M23.261 Derangement of other lateral meniscus due to old tear or injury, right knee
     M23.262 Derangement of other lateral meniscus due to old tear or injury, left knee
     M23.269 Derangement of other lateral meniscus due to old tear or injury, unspecified knee

☑5ᵗʰ **M23.3** **Other meniscus derangements**
Degenerate meniscus
Detached meniscus
Retained meniscus

☑6ᵗʰ **M23.30** **Other meniscus derangements, unspecified meniscus**
Other meniscus derangements, unspecified lateral meniscus
Other meniscus derangements, unspecified medial meniscus

M23.300 **Other meniscus derangements, unspecified lateral meniscus, right knee**

M23.301 **Other meniscus derangements, unspecified lateral meniscus, left knee**

M23.302 **Other meniscus derangements, unspecified lateral meniscus, unspecified knee**

M23.303 **Other meniscus derangements, unspecified medial meniscus, right knee**

M23.304 **Other meniscus derangements, unspecified medial meniscus, left knee**

M23.305 **Other meniscus derangements, unspecified medial meniscus, unspecified knee**

M23.306 **Other meniscus derangements, unspecified meniscus, right knee**

M23.307 **Other meniscus derangements, unspecified meniscus, left knee**

M23.309 **Other meniscus derangements, unspecified meniscus, unspecified knee**

☑6ᵗʰ **M23.31** **Other meniscus derangements, anterior horn of medial meniscus**

M23.311 **Other meniscus derangements, anterior horn of medial meniscus, right knee**

M23.312 **Other meniscus derangements, anterior horn of medial meniscus, left knee**

M23.319 **Other meniscus derangements, anterior horn of medial meniscus, unspecified knee**

☑6ᵗʰ **M23.32** **Other meniscus derangements, posterior horn of medial meniscus**

M23.321 **Other meniscus derangements, posterior horn of medial meniscus, right knee**

M23.322 **Other meniscus derangements, posterior horn of medial meniscus, left knee**

M23.329 **Other meniscus derangements, posterior horn of medial meniscus, unspecified knee**

☑6ᵗʰ **M23.33** **Other meniscus derangements, other medial meniscus**

M23.331 **Other meniscus derangements, other medial meniscus, right knee**

M23.332 **Other meniscus derangements, other medial meniscus, left knee**

M23.339 **Other meniscus derangements, other medial meniscus, unspecified knee**

☑6ᵗʰ **M23.34** **Other meniscus derangements, anterior horn of lateral meniscus**

M23.341 **Other meniscus derangements, anterior horn of lateral meniscus, right knee**

M23.342 **Other meniscus derangements, anterior horn of lateral meniscus, left knee**

M23.349 **Other meniscus derangements, anterior horn of lateral meniscus, unspecified knee**

☑6ᵗʰ **M23.35** **Other meniscus derangements, posterior horn of lateral meniscus**

M23.351 **Other meniscus derangements, posterior horn of lateral meniscus, right knee**

M23.352 **Other meniscus derangements, posterior horn of lateral meniscus, left knee**

M23.359 **Other meniscus derangements, posterior horn of lateral meniscus, unspecified knee**

☑6ᵗʰ **M23.36** **Other meniscus derangements, other lateral meniscus**

M23.361 **Other meniscus derangements, other lateral meniscus, right knee**

M23.362 **Other meniscus derangements, other lateral meniscus, left knee**

M23.369 **Other meniscus derangements, other lateral meniscus, unspecified knee**

☑5ᵗʰ **M23.4** **Loose body in knee**

M23.40 **Loose body in knee, unspecified knee**

M23.41 **Loose body in knee, right knee**

M23.42 **Loose body in knee, left knee**

☑5ᵗʰ **M23.5** **Chronic instability of knee**

M23.50 **Chronic instability of knee, unspecified knee**

M23.51 **Chronic instability of knee, right knee**

M23.52 **Chronic instability of knee, left knee**

☑5ᵗʰ **M23.6** **Other spontaneous disruption of ligament(s) of knee**

☑6ᵗʰ **M23.60** **Other spontaneous disruption of unspecified ligament of knee**

M23.601 **Other spontaneous disruption of unspecified ligament of right knee**

M23.602 **Other spontaneous disruption of unspecified ligament of left knee**

M23.609 **Other spontaneous disruption of unspecified ligament of unspecified knee**

☑6ᵗʰ **M23.61** **Other spontaneous disruption of anterior cruciate ligament of knee**

M23.611 **Other spontaneous disruption of anterior cruciate ligament of right knee**

M23.612 **Other spontaneous disruption of anterior cruciate ligament of left knee**

M23.619 **Other spontaneous disruption of anterior cruciate ligament of unspecified knee**

☑6ᵗʰ **M23.62** **Other spontaneous disruption of posterior cruciate ligament of knee**

M23.621 **Other spontaneous disruption of posterior cruciate ligament of right knee**

M23.622 **Other spontaneous disruption of posterior cruciate ligament of left knee**

M23.629 **Other spontaneous disruption of posterior cruciate ligament of unspecified knee**

☑6ᵗʰ **M23.63** **Other spontaneous disruption of medial collateral ligament of knee**

M23.631 **Other spontaneous disruption of medial collateral ligament of right knee**

M23.632 **Other spontaneous disruption of medial collateral ligament of left knee**

M23.639 **Other spontaneous disruption of medial collateral ligament of unspecified knee**

☑6ᵗʰ **M23.64** **Other spontaneous disruption of lateral collateral ligament of knee**

M23.641 **Other spontaneous disruption of lateral collateral ligament of right knee**

M23.642 **Other spontaneous disruption of lateral collateral ligament of left knee**

M23.649 **Other spontaneous disruption of lateral collateral ligament of unspecified knee**

☑6ᵗʰ **M23.67** **Other spontaneous disruption of capsular ligament of knee**

M23.671 **Other spontaneous disruption of capsular ligament of right knee**

M23.672 **Other spontaneous disruption of capsular ligament of left knee**

M23.679 **Other spontaneous disruption of capsular ligament of unspecified knee**

☑5ᵗʰ **M23.8** **Other internal derangements of knee**
Laxity of ligament of knee
Snapping knee

☑6ᵗʰ **M23.8X** **Other internal derangements of knee**

M23.8X1 **Other internal derangements of right knee**

M23.8X2 **Other internal derangements of left knee**

M23.8X9 **Other internal derangements of unspecified knee**

☑5ᵗʰ **M23.9** **Unspecified internal derangement of knee**

M23.90 **Unspecified internal derangement of unspecified knee**

M23.91 **Unspecified internal derangement of right knee**

M23.92 **Unspecified internal derangement of left knee**

Ⓝ Newborn: 0   Ⓟ Pediatric: 0-17   Ⓜ Maternity: 9-64   Ⓐ Adult: 15-124   **MCC** Major Complication/Comorbidity   **CC** Complication/Comorbidity   **SW** Severe Wound Dx

788   ICD-10-CM 2022

✓4ᵗʰ **M24** **Other specific joint derangements**

     EXCLUDES 1   *current injury - see injury of joint by body region*

     EXCLUDES 2   *ganglion (M67.4)*

                 snapping knee (M23.8-)

                 temporomandibular joint disorders (M26.6-)

     AHA: 2020,4Q,31-32

✓5ᵗʰ **M24.0** **Loose body in joint**

         EXCLUDES 2   *loose body in knee (M23.4)*

     M24.00   Loose body in unspecified joint

     ✓6ᵗʰ **M24.01**   Loose body in shoulder

         M24.011   Loose body in right shoulder

         M24.012   Loose body in left shoulder

         M24.019   Loose body in unspecified shoulder

     ✓6ᵗʰ **M24.02**   Loose body in elbow

         M24.021   Loose body in right elbow

         M24.022   Loose body in left elbow

         M24.029   Loose body in unspecified elbow

     ✓6ᵗʰ **M24.03**   Loose body in wrist

         M24.031   Loose body in right wrist

         M24.032   Loose body in left wrist

         M24.039   Loose body in unspecified wrist

     ✓6ᵗʰ **M24.04**   Loose body in finger joints

         M24.041   Loose body in right finger joint(s)

         M24.042   Loose body in left finger joint(s)

         M24.049   Loose body in unspecified finger joint(s)

     ✓6ᵗʰ **M24.05**   Loose body in hip

         M24.051   Loose body in right hip

         M24.052   Loose body in left hip

         M24.059   Loose body in unspecified hip

     ✓6ᵗʰ **M24.07**   Loose body in ankle and toe joints

         M24.071   Loose body in right ankle

         M24.072   Loose body in left ankle

         M24.073   Loose body in unspecified ankle

         M24.074   Loose body in right toe joint(s)

         M24.075   Loose body in left toe joint(s)

         M24.076   Loose body in unspecified toe joints

     M24.08   Loose body, other site

✓5ᵗʰ **M24.1** **Other articular cartilage disorders**

         EXCLUDES 2   *chondrocalcinosis (M11.1, M11.2-)*

                 internal derangement of knee (M23.-)

                 metastatic calcification (E83.5)

                 ochronosis (E70.2)

     M24.10   Other articular cartilage disorders, unspecified site

     ✓6ᵗʰ **M24.11**   Other articular cartilage disorders, shoulder

         M24.111   Other articular cartilage disorders, right shoulder

         M24.112   Other articular cartilage disorders, left shoulder

         M24.119   Other articular cartilage disorders, unspecified shoulder

     ✓6ᵗʰ **M24.12**   Other articular cartilage disorders, elbow

         M24.121   Other articular cartilage disorders, right elbow

         M24.122   Other articular cartilage disorders, left elbow

         M24.129   Other articular cartilage disorders, unspecified elbow

     ✓6ᵗʰ **M24.13**   Other articular cartilage disorders, wrist

         M24.131   Other articular cartilage disorders, right wrist

         M24.132   Other articular cartilage disorders, left wrist

         M24.139   Other articular cartilage disorders, unspecified wrist

     ✓6ᵗʰ **M24.14**   Other articular cartilage disorders, hand

         M24.141   Other articular cartilage disorders, right hand

         M24.142   Other articular cartilage disorders, left hand

         M24.149   Other articular cartilage disorders, unspecified hand

     ✓6ᵗʰ **M24.15**   Other articular cartilage disorders, hip

         M24.151   Other articular cartilage disorders, right hip

         M24.152   Other articular cartilage disorders, left hip

         M24.159   Other articular cartilage disorders, unspecified hip

     ✓6ᵗʰ **M24.17**   Other articular cartilage disorders, ankle and foot

         M24.171   Other articular cartilage disorders, right ankle

         M24.172   Other articular cartilage disorders, left ankle

         M24.173   Other articular cartilage disorders, unspecified ankle

         M24.174   Other articular cartilage disorders, right foot

         M24.175   Other articular cartilage disorders, left foot

         M24.176   Other articular cartilage disorders, unspecified foot

     M24.19   Other articular cartilage disorders, other specified site

✓5ᵗʰ **M24.2** **Disorder of ligament**

     Instability secondary to old ligament injury

     Ligamentous laxity NOS

         EXCLUDES 1   *familial ligamentous laxity (M35.7)*

         EXCLUDES 2   *internal derangement of knee (M23.5-M23.8X9)*

     M24.20   Disorder of ligament, unspecified site

     ✓6ᵗʰ **M24.21**   Disorder of ligament, shoulder

         M24.211   Disorder of ligament, right shoulder

         M24.212   Disorder of ligament, left shoulder

         M24.219   Disorder of ligament, unspecified shoulder

     ✓6ᵗʰ **M24.22**   Disorder of ligament, elbow

         M24.221   Disorder of ligament, right elbow

         M24.222   Disorder of ligament, left elbow

         M24.229   Disorder of ligament, unspecified elbow

     ✓6ᵗʰ **M24.23**   Disorder of ligament, wrist

         M24.231   Disorder of ligament, right wrist

         M24.232   Disorder of ligament, left wrist

         M24.239   Disorder of ligament, unspecified wrist

     ✓6ᵗʰ **M24.24**   Disorder of ligament, hand

         M24.241   Disorder of ligament, right hand

         M24.242   Disorder of ligament, left hand

         M24.249   Disorder of ligament, unspecified hand

     ✓6ᵗʰ **M24.25**   Disorder of ligament, hip

         M24.251   Disorder of ligament, right hip

         M24.252   Disorder of ligament, left hip

         M24.259   Disorder of ligament, unspecified hip

     ✓6ᵗʰ **M24.27**   Disorder of ligament, ankle and foot

         M24.271   Disorder of ligament, right ankle

         M24.272   Disorder of ligament, left ankle

         M24.273   Disorder of ligament, unspecified ankle

         M24.274   Disorder of ligament, right foot

         M24.275   Disorder of ligament, left foot

         M24.276   Disorder of ligament, unspecified foot

     M24.28   Disorder of ligament, vertebrae

     M24.29   Disorder of ligament, other specified site

✓5ᵗʰ **M24.3** **Pathological dislocation of joint, not elsewhere classified**

         EXCLUDES 1   *congenital dislocation or displacement of joint - see congenital malformations and deformations of the musculoskeletal system (Q65-Q79)*

                 current injury - see injury of joints and ligaments by body region

                 recurrent dislocation of joint (M24.4-)

     M24.30   Pathological dislocation of unspecified joint, not elsewhere classified

     ✓6ᵗʰ **M24.31**   Pathological dislocation of shoulder, not elsewhere classified

         M24.311   Pathological dislocation of right shoulder, not elsewhere classified

         M24.312   Pathological dislocation of left shoulder, not elsewhere classified

         M24.319   Pathological dislocation of unspecified shoulder, not elsewhere classified

     ✓6ᵗʰ **M24.32**   Pathological dislocation of elbow, not elsewhere classified

         M24.321   Pathological dislocation of right elbow, not elsewhere classified

         M24.322   Pathological dislocation of left elbow, not elsewhere classified

         M24.329   Pathological dislocation of unspecified elbow, not elsewhere classified

✔ Additional Character Required   ✓x7ᵗʰ Placeholder   Questionable PDx   Manifestation   Unspecified Dx   UPD Unacceptable PDx   H1 - H14 HAC   HCC CMS-HCC Dx   HIV HIV Dx

ICD-10-CM 2022   789

✓6th **M24.33 Pathological dislocation of** wrist, not elsewhere classified
  M24.331 Pathological dislocation of right wrist, not elsewhere classified
  M24.332 Pathological dislocation of left wrist, not elsewhere classified
  M24.339 Pathological dislocation of unspecified wrist, not elsewhere classified

✓6th **M24.34 Pathological dislocation of** hand, not elsewhere classified
  M24.341 Pathological dislocation of right hand, not elsewhere classified
  M24.342 Pathological dislocation of left hand, not elsewhere classified
  M24.349 Pathological dislocation of unspecified hand, not elsewhere classified

✓6th **M24.35 Pathological dislocation of** hip, not elsewhere classified
  M24.351 Pathological dislocation of right hip, not elsewhere classified
  M24.352 Pathological dislocation of left hip, not elsewhere classified
  M24.359 Pathological dislocation of unspecified hip, not elsewhere classified

✓6th **M24.36 Pathological dislocation of** knee, not elsewhere classified
  M24.361 Pathological dislocation of right knee, not elsewhere classified
  M24.362 Pathological dislocation of left knee, not elsewhere classified
  M24.369 Pathological dislocation of unspecified knee, not elsewhere classified

✓6th **M24.37 Pathological dislocation of** ankle and foot, not elsewhere classified
  M24.371 Pathological dislocation of right ankle, not elsewhere classified
  M24.372 Pathological dislocation of left ankle, not elsewhere classified
  M24.373 Pathological dislocation of unspecified ankle, not elsewhere classified
  M24.374 Pathological dislocation of right foot, not elsewhere classified
  M24.375 Pathological dislocation of left foot, not elsewhere classified
  M24.376 Pathological dislocation of unspecified foot, not elsewhere classified

  M24.39 Pathological dislocation of other specified joint, not elsewhere classified

✓5th **M24.4 Recurrent dislocation of joint**
  Recurrent subluxation of joint
  EXCLUDES 2   recurrent dislocation of patella (M22.0-M22.1)
         recurrent vertebral dislocation (M43.3-, M43.4, M43.5-)

  M24.40 Recurrent dislocation, unspecified joint
✓6th **M24.41 Recurrent dislocation,** shoulder
  M24.411 Recurrent dislocation, right shoulder
  M24.412 Recurrent dislocation, left shoulder
  M24.419 Recurrent dislocation, unspecified shoulder
✓6th **M24.42 Recurrent dislocation,** elbow
  M24.421 Recurrent dislocation, right elbow
  M24.422 Recurrent dislocation, left elbow
  M24.429 Recurrent dislocation, unspecified elbow
✓6th **M24.43 Recurrent dislocation,** wrist
  M24.431 Recurrent dislocation, right wrist
  M24.432 Recurrent dislocation, left wrist
  M24.439 Recurrent dislocation, unspecified wrist
✓6th **M24.44 Recurrent dislocation,** hand and finger(s)
  M24.441 Recurrent dislocation, right hand
  M24.442 Recurrent dislocation, left hand
  M24.443 Recurrent dislocation, unspecified hand
  M24.444 Recurrent dislocation, right finger
  M24.445 Recurrent dislocation, left finger
  M24.446 Recurrent dislocation, unspecified finger
✓6th **M24.45 Recurrent dislocation,** hip
  M24.451 Recurrent dislocation, right hip
  M24.452 Recurrent dislocation, left hip
  M24.459 Recurrent dislocation, unspecified hip
✓6th **M24.46 Recurrent dislocation,** knee
  M24.461 Recurrent dislocation, right knee

  M24.462 Recurrent dislocation, left knee
  M24.469 Recurrent dislocation, unspecified knee
✓6th **M24.47 Recurrent dislocation,** ankle, foot and toes
  M24.471 Recurrent dislocation, right ankle
  M24.472 Recurrent dislocation, left ankle
  M24.473 Recurrent dislocation, unspecified ankle
  M24.474 Recurrent dislocation, right foot
  M24.475 Recurrent dislocation, left foot
  M24.476 Recurrent dislocation, unspecified foot
  M24.477 Recurrent dislocation, right toe(s)
  M24.478 Recurrent dislocation, left toe(s)
  M24.479 Recurrent dislocation, unspecified toe(s)
  M24.49 Recurrent dislocation, other specified joint

✓5th **M24.5 Contracture of joint**
  EXCLUDES 1   contracture of muscle without contracture of joint (M62.4-)
         contracture of tendon (sheath) without contracture of joint (M62.4-)
         Dupuytren's contracture (M72.0)
  EXCLUDES 2   acquired deformities of limbs (M20-M21)
  AHA: 2016,2Q,6

  M24.50 Contracture, unspecified joint
✓6th **M24.51 Contracture,** shoulder
  M24.511 Contracture, right shoulder
  M24.512 Contracture, left shoulder
  M24.519 Contracture, unspecified shoulder
✓6th **M24.52 Contracture,** elbow
  M24.521 Contracture, right elbow
  M24.522 Contracture, left elbow
  M24.529 Contracture, unspecified elbow
✓6th **M24.53 Contracture,** wrist
  M24.531 Contracture, right wrist
  M24.532 Contracture, left wrist
  M24.539 Contracture, unspecified wrist
✓6th **M24.54 Contracture,** hand
  M24.541 Contracture, right hand
  M24.542 Contracture, left hand
  M24.549 Contracture, unspecified hand
✓6th **M24.55 Contracture,** hip
  M24.551 Contracture, right hip
  M24.552 Contracture, left hip
  M24.559 Contracture, unspecified hip
✓6th **M24.56 Contracture,** knee
  M24.561 Contracture, right knee
  M24.562 Contracture, left knee
  M24.569 Contracture, unspecified knee
✓6th **M24.57 Contracture,** ankle and foot
  M24.571 Contracture, right ankle
  M24.572 Contracture, left ankle
  M24.573 Contracture, unspecified ankle
  M24.574 Contracture, right foot
  M24.575 Contracture, left foot
  M24.576 Contracture, unspecified foot
  M24.59 Contracture, other specified joint

✓5th **M24.6 Ankylosis of joint**
  EXCLUDES 1   stiffness of joint without ankylosis (M25.6-)
  EXCLUDES 2   spine (M43.2-)
  DEF: Ankylosis: Abnormal union or fusion of bones in a joint, which is normally moveable.

  M24.60 Ankylosis, unspecified joint
✓6th **M24.61 Ankylosis,** shoulder
  M24.611 Ankylosis, right shoulder
  M24.612 Ankylosis, left shoulder
  M24.619 Ankylosis, unspecified shoulder
✓6th **M24.62 Ankylosis,** elbow
  M24.621 Ankylosis, right elbow
  M24.622 Ankylosis, left elbow
  M24.629 Ankylosis, unspecified elbow
✓6th **M24.63 Ankylosis,** wrist
  M24.631 Ankylosis, right wrist
  M24.632 Ankylosis, left wrist
  M24.639 Ankylosis, unspecified wrist
✓6th **M24.64 Ankylosis,** hand
  M24.641 Ankylosis, right hand
  M24.642 Ankylosis, left hand

M24.649 Ankylosis, unspecified hand

✓6ᵗʰ **M24.65** Ankylosis, hip

    M24.651 Ankylosis, right hip
    M24.652 Ankylosis, left hip
    M24.659 Ankylosis, unspecified hip

✓6ᵗʰ **M24.66** Ankylosis, knee

    M24.661 Ankylosis, right knee
    M24.662 Ankylosis, left knee
    M24.669 Ankylosis, unspecified knee

✓6ᵗʰ **M24.67** Ankylosis, ankle and foot

    M24.671 Ankylosis, right ankle
    M24.672 Ankylosis, left ankle
    M24.673 Ankylosis, unspecified ankle
    M24.674 Ankylosis, right foot
    M24.675 Ankylosis, left foot
    M24.676 Ankylosis, unspecified foot

    M24.69 Ankylosis, other specified joint

M24.7 Protrusio acetabuli

    DEF: Intrapelvic protrusion of the acetabulum characterized by the sinking of the floor of the acetabulum, causing the femoral head to protrude. It limits hip movement and is of unknown etiology. *Synonym(s): Otto's pelvis.*

✓5ᵗʰ **M24.8** Other specific joint derangements, not elsewhere classified

    EXCLUDES 2   *iliotibial band syndrome (M76.3)*

    M24.80 Other specific joint derangements of unspecified joint, not elsewhere classified

✓6ᵗʰ **M24.81** Other specific joint derangements of shoulder, not elsewhere classified
    M24.811 Other specific joint derangements of right shoulder, not elsewhere classified
    M24.812 Other specific joint derangements of left shoulder, not elsewhere classified
    M24.819 Other specific joint derangements of unspecified shoulder, not elsewhere classified

✓6ᵗʰ **M24.82** Other specific joint derangements of elbow, not elsewhere classified
    M24.821 Other specific joint derangements of right elbow, not elsewhere classified
    M24.822 Other specific joint derangements of left elbow, not elsewhere classified
    M24.829 Other specific joint derangements of unspecified elbow, not elsewhere classified

✓6ᵗʰ **M24.83** Other specific joint derangements of wrist, not elsewhere classified
    M24.831 Other specific joint derangements of right wrist, not elsewhere classified
    M24.832 Other specific joint derangements of left wrist, not elsewhere classified
    M24.839 Other specific joint derangements of unspecified wrist, not elsewhere classified

✓6ᵗʰ **M24.84** Other specific joint derangements of hand, not elsewhere classified
    M24.841 Other specific joint derangements of right hand, not elsewhere classified
    M24.842 Other specific joint derangements of left hand, not elsewhere classified
    M24.849 Other specific joint derangements of unspecified hand, not elsewhere classified

✓6ᵗʰ **M24.85** Other specific joint derangements of hip, not elsewhere classified
    Irritable hip
    M24.851 Other specific joint derangements of right hip, not elsewhere classified
    M24.852 Other specific joint derangements of left hip, not elsewhere classified
    M24.859 Other specific joint derangements of unspecified hip, not elsewhere classified

✓6ᵗʰ **M24.87** Other specific joint derangements of ankle and foot, not elsewhere classified
    M24.871 Other specific joint derangements of right ankle, not elsewhere classified
    M24.872 Other specific joint derangements of left ankle, not elsewhere classified
    M24.873 Other specific joint derangements of unspecified ankle, not elsewhere classified

    M24.874 Other specific joint derangements of right foot, not elsewhere classified
    M24.875 Other specific joint derangements left foot, not elsewhere classified
    M24.876 Other specific joint derangements of unspecified foot, not elsewhere classified

    M24.89 Other specific joint derangement of other specified joint, not elsewhere classified

M24.9 Joint derangement, unspecified

✓4ᵗʰ **M25** Other joint disorder, not elsewhere classified

    EXCLUDES 2   *abnormality of gait and mobility (R26.-)*
      acquired deformities of limb (M20-M21)
      calcification of bursa (M71.4-)
      calcification of shoulder (joint) (M75.3)
      calcification of tendon (M65.2-)
      difficulty in walking (R26.2)
      temporomandibular joint disorder (M26.6-)

    AHA: 2020,4Q,31-32

✓5ᵗʰ **M25.0** Hemarthrosis

    EXCLUDES 1   *current injury - see injury of joint by body region*
      hemophilic arthropathy (M36.2)

    M25.00 Hemarthrosis, unspecified joint   CC

✓6ᵗʰ **M25.01** Hemarthrosis, shoulder
    M25.011 Hemarthrosis, right shoulder   CC
    M25.012 Hemarthrosis, left shoulder   CC
    M25.019 Hemarthrosis, unspecified shoulder   CC

✓6ᵗʰ **M25.02** Hemarthrosis, elbow
    M25.021 Hemarthrosis, right elbow   CC
    M25.022 Hemarthrosis, left elbow   CC
    M25.029 Hemarthrosis, unspecified elbow   CC

✓6ᵗʰ **M25.03** Hemarthrosis, wrist
    M25.031 Hemarthrosis, right wrist   CC
    M25.032 Hemarthrosis, left wrist   CC
    M25.039 Hemarthrosis, unspecified wrist   CC

✓6ᵗʰ **M25.04** Hemarthrosis, hand
    M25.041 Hemarthrosis, right hand   CC
    M25.042 Hemarthrosis, left hand   CC
    M25.049 Hemarthrosis, unspecified hand   CC

✓6ᵗʰ **M25.05** Hemarthrosis, hip
    M25.051 Hemarthrosis, right hip   CC
    M25.052 Hemarthrosis, left hip   CC
    M25.059 Hemarthrosis, unspecified hip   CC

✓6ᵗʰ **M25.06** Hemarthrosis, knee
    M25.061 Hemarthrosis, right knee   CC
    M25.062 Hemarthrosis, left knee   CC
    M25.069 Hemarthrosis, unspecified knee   CC

✓6ᵗʰ **M25.07** Hemarthrosis, ankle and foot
    M25.071 Hemarthrosis, right ankle   CC
    M25.072 Hemarthrosis, left ankle   CC
    M25.073 Hemarthrosis, unspecified ankle   CC
    M25.074 Hemarthrosis, right foot   CC
    M25.075 Hemarthrosis, left foot   CC
    M25.076 Hemarthrosis, unspecified foot   CC

    M25.08 Hemarthrosis, other specified site   CC
      Hemarthrosis, vertebrae

✓5ᵗʰ **M25.1** Fistula of joint

    M25.10 Fistula, unspecified joint   SW

✓6ᵗʰ **M25.11** Fistula, shoulder
    M25.111 Fistula, right shoulder   SW
    M25.112 Fistula, left shoulder   SW
    M25.119 Fistula, unspecified shoulder   SW

✓6ᵗʰ **M25.12** Fistula, elbow
    M25.121 Fistula, right elbow   SW
    M25.122 Fistula, left elbow   SW
    M25.129 Fistula, unspecified elbow   SW

✓6ᵗʰ **M25.13** Fistula, wrist
    M25.131 Fistula, right wrist   SW
    M25.132 Fistula, left wrist   SW
    M25.139 Fistula, unspecified wrist   SW

✓6ᵗʰ **M25.14** Fistula, hand
    M25.141 Fistula, right hand   SW
    M25.142 Fistula, left hand   SW

M25.149 Fistula, unspecified hand `SW`

✓6ᵗʰ M25.15 **Fistula**, hip

M25.151 **Fistula**, right hip `SW`
M25.152 **Fistula**, left hip `SW`
M25.159 Fistula, unspecified hip `SW`

✓6ᵗʰ M25.16 **Fistula**, knee

M25.161 **Fistula**, right knee `SW`
M25.162 **Fistula**, left knee `SW`
M25.169 Fistula, unspecified knee `SW`

✓6ᵗʰ M25.17 **Fistula**, ankle and foot

M25.171 **Fistula**, right ankle `SW`
M25.172 **Fistula**, left ankle `SW`
M25.173 Fistula, unspecified ankle `SW`
M25.174 **Fistula**, right foot `SW`
M25.175 **Fistula**, left foot `SW`
M25.176 Fistula, unspecified foot `SW`

M25.18 **Fistula, other specified site** `SW`
Fistula, vertebrae

✓5ᵗʰ M25.2 **Flail joint**

DEF: Hinged joint that exhibits an abnormal or excessive degree of range and mobility.

M25.20 **Flail joint, unspecified joint**

✓6ᵗʰ M25.21 **Flail joint**, shoulder

M25.211 **Flail joint**, right shoulder
M25.212 **Flail joint**, left shoulder
M25.219 Flail joint, unspecified shoulder

✓6ᵗʰ M25.22 **Flail joint**, elbow

M25.221 **Flail joint**, right elbow
M25.222 **Flail joint**, left elbow
M25.229 Flail joint, unspecified elbow

✓6ᵗʰ M25.23 **Flail joint**, wrist

M25.231 **Flail joint**, right wrist
M25.232 **Flail joint**, left wrist
M25.239 Flail joint, unspecified wrist

✓6ᵗʰ M25.24 **Flail joint**, hand

M25.241 **Flail joint**, right hand
M25.242 **Flail joint**, left hand
M25.249 Flail joint, unspecified hand

✓6ᵗʰ M25.25 **Flail joint**, hip

M25.251 **Flail joint**, right hip
M25.252 **Flail joint**, left hip
M25.259 Flail joint, unspecified hip

✓6ᵗʰ M25.26 **Flail joint**, knee

M25.261 **Flail joint**, right knee
M25.262 **Flail joint**, left knee
M25.269 Flail joint, unspecified knee

✓6ᵗʰ M25.27 **Flail joint**, ankle and foot

M25.271 **Flail joint**, right ankle and foot
M25.272 **Flail joint**, left ankle and foot
M25.279 Flail joint, unspecified ankle and foot

M25.28 **Flail joint, other site**

✓5ᵗʰ M25.3 **Other instability of joint**

EXCLUDES 1 instability of joint secondary to old ligament injury (M24.2-)
instability of joint secondary to removal of joint prosthesis (M96.8-)
EXCLUDES 2 spinal instabilities (M53.2-)

M25.30 **Other instability, unspecified joint**

✓6ᵗʰ M25.31 **Other instability**, shoulder

M25.311 **Other instability**, right shoulder
M25.312 **Other instability**, left shoulder
M25.319 Other instability, unspecified shoulder

✓6ᵗʰ M25.32 **Other instability**, elbow

M25.321 **Other instability**, right elbow
M25.322 **Other instability**, left elbow
M25.329 Other instability, unspecified elbow

✓6ᵗʰ M25.33 **Other instability**, wrist

M25.331 **Other instability**, right wrist
M25.332 **Other instability**, left wrist
M25.339 Other instability, unspecified wrist

✓6ᵗʰ M25.34 **Other instability**, hand

M25.341 **Other instability**, right hand
M25.342 **Other instability**, left hand
M25.349 Other instability, unspecified hand

✓6ᵗʰ M25.35 **Other instability**, hip

M25.351 **Other instability**, right hip
M25.352 **Other instability**, left hip
M25.359 Other instability, unspecified hip

✓6ᵗʰ M25.36 **Other instability**, knee

M25.361 **Other instability**, right knee
M25.362 **Other instability**, left knee
M25.369 Other instability, unspecified knee

✓6ᵗʰ M25.37 **Other instability**, ankle and foot

M25.371 **Other instability**, right ankle
M25.372 **Other instability**, left ankle
M25.373 Other instability, unspecified ankle
M25.374 **Other instability**, right foot
M25.375 **Other instability**, left foot
M25.376 Other instability, unspecified foot

M25.39 **Other instability, other specified joint**

✓5ᵗʰ M25.4 **Effusion of joint**

EXCLUDES 1 hydrarthrosis in yaws (A66.6)
intermittent hydrarthrosis (M12.4-)
other infective (teno)synovitis (M65.1-)

M25.40 **Effusion, unspecified joint**

✓6ᵗʰ M25.41 **Effusion**, shoulder

M25.411 **Effusion**, right shoulder
M25.412 **Effusion**, left shoulder
M25.419 Effusion, unspecified shoulder

✓6ᵗʰ M25.42 **Effusion**, elbow

M25.421 **Effusion**, right elbow
M25.422 **Effusion**, left elbow
M25.429 Effusion, unspecified elbow

✓6ᵗʰ M25.43 **Effusion**, wrist

M25.431 **Effusion**, right wrist
M25.432 **Effusion**, left wrist
M25.439 Effusion, unspecified wrist

✓6ᵗʰ M25.44 **Effusion**, hand

M25.441 **Effusion**, right hand
M25.442 **Effusion**, left hand
M25.449 Effusion, unspecified hand

✓6ᵗʰ M25.45 **Effusion**, hip

M25.451 **Effusion**, right hip
M25.452 **Effusion**, left hip
M25.459 Effusion, unspecified hip

✓6ᵗʰ M25.46 **Effusion**, knee

M25.461 **Effusion**, right knee
M25.462 **Effusion**, left knee
M25.469 Effusion, unspecified knee

✓6ᵗʰ M25.47 **Effusion**, ankle and foot

M25.471 **Effusion**, right ankle
M25.472 **Effusion**, left ankle
M25.473 Effusion, unspecified ankle
M25.474 **Effusion**, right foot
M25.475 **Effusion**, left foot
M25.476 Effusion, unspecified foot

M25.48 **Effusion, other site**

✓5ᵗʰ M25.5 **Pain in joint**

EXCLUDES 2 pain in hand (M79.64-)
pain in fingers (M79.64-)
pain in foot (M79.67-)
pain in limb (M79.6-)
pain in toes (M79.67-)

M25.50 **Pain in unspecified joint**

✓6ᵗʰ M25.51 **Pain in** shoulder

M25.511 **Pain in** right shoulder
M25.512 **Pain in** left shoulder
M25.519 Pain in unspecified shoulder

✓6ᵗʰ M25.52 **Pain in** elbow

M25.521 **Pain in** right elbow
M25.522 **Pain in** left elbow
M25.529 Pain in unspecified elbow

✓6ᵗʰ M25.53 **Pain in** wrist

M25.531 **Pain in** right wrist
M25.532 **Pain in** left wrist
M25.539 Pain in unspecified wrist

✓6ᵗʰ M25.54 **Pain in** joints of hand

AHA: 2016,4Q,38

M25.541 **Pain in joints of right hand**

N Newborn: 0   P Pediatric: 0-17   M Maternity: 9-64   A Adult: 15-124   MCC Major Complication/Comorbidity   CC Complication/Comorbidity   SW Severe Wound Dx

792

ICD-10-CM 2022

M25.542   Pain in joints of left hand
M25.549   Pain in joints of unspecified hand
       Pain in joints of hand NOS

√6ᵗʰ   **M25.55**   **Pain in hip**

M25.551   Pain in right hip
M25.552   Pain in left hip
M25.559   Pain in unspecified hip

√6ᵗʰ   **M25.56**   **Pain in knee**

M25.561   Pain in right knee
M25.562   Pain in left knee
M25.569   Pain in unspecified knee

√6ᵗʰ   **M25.57**   **Pain in ankle and joints of foot**

M25.571   Pain in right ankle and joints of right foot
M25.572   Pain in left ankle and joints of left foot
M25.579   Pain in unspecified ankle and joints of unspecified foot

M25.59   Pain in other specified joint

√5ᵗʰ   **M25.6**   **Stiffness of joint, not elsewhere classified**

> **EXCLUDES 1**   ankylosis of joint (M24.6-)
>   contracture of joint (M24.5-)

M25.60   Stiffness of unspecified joint, not elsewhere classified

√6ᵗʰ   **M25.61**   **Stiffness of shoulder, not elsewhere classified**

M25.611   Stiffness of right shoulder, not elsewhere classified
M25.612   Stiffness of left shoulder, not elsewhere classified
M25.619   Stiffness of unspecified shoulder, not elsewhere classified

√6ᵗʰ   **M25.62**   **Stiffness of elbow, not elsewhere classified**

M25.621   Stiffness of right elbow, not elsewhere classified
M25.622   Stiffness of left elbow, not elsewhere classified
M25.629   Stiffness of unspecified elbow, not elsewhere classified

√6ᵗʰ   **M25.63**   **Stiffness of wrist, not elsewhere classified**

M25.631   Stiffness of right wrist, not elsewhere classified
M25.632   Stiffness of left wrist, not elsewhere classified
M25.639   Stiffness of unspecified wrist, not elsewhere classified

√6ᵗʰ   **M25.64**   **Stiffness of hand, not elsewhere classified**

M25.641   Stiffness of right hand, not elsewhere classified
M25.642   Stiffness of left hand, not elsewhere classified
M25.649   Stiffness of unspecified hand, not elsewhere classified

√6ᵗʰ   **M25.65**   **Stiffness of hip, not elsewhere classified**

M25.651   Stiffness of right hip, not elsewhere classified
M25.652   Stiffness of left hip, not elsewhere classified
M25.659   Stiffness of unspecified hip, not elsewhere classified

√6ᵗʰ   **M25.66**   **Stiffness of knee, not elsewhere classified**

M25.661   Stiffness of right knee, not elsewhere classified
M25.662   Stiffness of left knee, not elsewhere classified
M25.669   Stiffness of unspecified knee, not elsewhere classified

√6ᵗʰ   **M25.67**   **Stiffness of ankle and foot, not elsewhere classified**

M25.671   Stiffness of right ankle, not elsewhere classified
M25.672   Stiffness of left ankle, not elsewhere classified
M25.673   Stiffness of unspecified ankle, not elsewhere classified
M25.674   Stiffness of right foot, not elsewhere classified
M25.675   Stiffness of left foot, not elsewhere classified
M25.676   Stiffness of unspecified foot, not elsewhere classified

M25.69   Stiffness of other specified joint, not elsewhere classified

√5ᵗʰ   **M25.7**   **Osteophyte**

M25.70   Osteophyte, unspecified joint

√6ᵗʰ   **M25.71**   **Osteophyte, shoulder**

M25.711   Osteophyte, right shoulder
M25.712   Osteophyte, left shoulder
M25.719   Osteophyte, unspecified shoulder

√6ᵗʰ   **M25.72**   **Osteophyte, elbow**

M25.721   Osteophyte, right elbow
M25.722   Osteophyte, left elbow
M25.729   Osteophyte, unspecified elbow

√6ᵗʰ   **M25.73**   **Osteophyte, wrist**

M25.731   Osteophyte, right wrist
M25.732   Osteophyte, left wrist
M25.739   Osteophyte, unspecified wrist

√6ᵗʰ   **M25.74**   **Osteophyte, hand**

M25.741   Osteophyte, right hand
M25.742   Osteophyte, left hand
M25.749   Osteophyte, unspecified hand

√6ᵗʰ   **M25.75**   **Osteophyte, hip**

M25.751   Osteophyte, right hip
M25.752   Osteophyte, left hip
M25.759   Osteophyte, unspecified hip

√6ᵗʰ   **M25.76**   **Osteophyte, knee**

M25.761   Osteophyte, right knee
M25.762   Osteophyte, left knee
M25.769   Osteophyte, unspecified knee

√6ᵗʰ   **M25.77**   **Osteophyte, ankle and foot**

M25.771   Osteophyte, right ankle
M25.772   Osteophyte, left ankle
M25.773   Osteophyte, unspecified ankle
M25.774   Osteophyte, right foot
M25.775   Osteophyte, left foot
M25.776   Osteophyte, unspecified foot

M25.78   Osteophyte, vertebrae

√5ᵗʰ   **M25.8**   **Other specified joint disorders**

M25.80   Other specified joint disorders, unspecified joint

√6ᵗʰ   **M25.81**   **Other specified joint disorders, shoulder**

M25.811   Other specified joint disorders, right shoulder
M25.812   Other specified joint disorders, left shoulder
M25.819   Other specified joint disorders, unspecified shoulder

√6ᵗʰ   **M25.82**   **Other specified joint disorders, elbow**

M25.821   Other specified joint disorders, right elbow
M25.822   Other specified joint disorders, left elbow
M25.829   Other specified joint disorders, unspecified elbow

√6ᵗʰ   **M25.83**   **Other specified joint disorders, wrist**

M25.831   Other specified joint disorders, right wrist
M25.832   Other specified joint disorders, left wrist
M25.839   Other specified joint disorders, unspecified wrist

√6ᵗʰ   **M25.84**   **Other specified joint disorders, hand**

M25.841   Other specified joint disorders, right hand
M25.842   Other specified joint disorders, left hand
M25.849   Other specified joint disorders, unspecified hand

√6ᵗʰ   **M25.85**   **Other specified joint disorders, hip**

     AHA: 2014,4Q,25

M25.851   Other specified joint disorders, right hip
M25.852   Other specified joint disorders, left hip
M25.859   Other specified joint disorders, unspecified hip

√6ᵗʰ   **M25.86**   **Other specified joint disorders, knee**

M25.861   Other specified joint disorders, right knee
M25.862   Other specified joint disorders, left knee
M25.869   Other specified joint disorders, unspecified knee

√6ᵗʰ   **M25.87**   **Other specified joint disorders, ankle and foot**

M25.871   Other specified joint disorders, right ankle and foot
M25.872   Other specified joint disorders, left ankle and foot
M25.879   Other specified joint disorders, unspecified ankle and foot

✔ Additional Character Required   √x7ᵗʰ Placeholder   Questionable PDx   Manifestation   Unspecified Dx   UPD Unacceptable PDx   H1-H14 HAC   HCC CMS-HCC Dx   HIV HIV Dx

ICD-10-CM 2022   793

M25.542–M25.879

M25.9   Joint disorder, unspecified

Dentofacial anomalies [including malocclusion] and other disorders of jaw (M26-M27)

EXCLUDES 1   *hemifacial atrophy or hypertrophy (Q67.4)*
unilateral condylar hyperplasia or hypoplasia (M27.8)

✓4ᵗʰ M26   **Dentofacial anomalies [including malocclusion]**

  ✓5ᵗʰ M26.0   **Major anomalies of jaw size**

    EXCLUDES 1   *acromegaly (E22.0)*
       Robin's syndrome (Q87.0)

    M26.00   **Unspecified anomaly of jaw size**
    M26.01   **Maxillary hyperplasia**
    M26.02   **Maxillary hypoplasia**
      AHA: 2014,3Q,23
    M26.03   **Mandibular hyperplasia**
    M26.04   **Mandibular hypoplasia**
    M26.05   **Macrogenia**
    M26.06   **Microgenia**
    M26.07   **Excessive tuberosity of jaw**
      Entire maxillary tuberosity
    M26.09   **Other specified anomalies of jaw size**

  ✓5ᵗʰ M26.1   **Anomalies of jaw-cranial base relationship**

    M26.10   **Unspecified anomaly of jaw-cranial base relationship**
    M26.11   **Maxillary asymmetry**
    M26.12   **Other jaw asymmetry**
    M26.19   **Other specified anomalies of jaw-cranial base relationship**
      AHA: 2020,1Q,21

  ✓5ᵗʰ M26.2   **Anomalies of dental arch relationship**

    M26.20   **Unspecified anomaly of dental arch relationship**
  ✓6ᵗʰ M26.21   **Malocclusion, Angle's class**
    M26.211   **Malocclusion, Angle's class I**
      Neutro-occlusion
    M26.212   **Malocclusion, Angle's class II**
      Disto-occlusion Division I
      Disto-occlusion Division II
    M26.213   **Malocclusion, Angle's class III**
      Mesio-occlusion
    M26.219   **Malocclusion, Angle's class, unspecified**
  ✓6ᵗʰ M26.22   **Open occlusal relationship**
    M26.220   **Open anterior occlusal relationship**
      Anterior open bite
    M26.221   **Open posterior occlusal relationship**
      Posterior open bite
    M26.23   **Excessive horizontal overlap**
      Excessive horizontal overjet
    M26.24   **Reverse articulation**
      Crossbite (anterior) (posterior)
    M26.25   **Anomalies of interarch distance**
    M26.29   **Other anomalies of dental arch relationship**
      Midline deviation of dental arch
      Overbite (excessive) deep
      Overbite (excessive) horizontal
      Overbite (excessive) vertical
      Posterior lingual occlusion of mandibular teeth

  ✓5ᵗʰ M26.3   **Anomalies of tooth position of fully erupted tooth or teeth**

    EXCLUDES 2   *embedded and impacted teeth (K01.-)*

    M26.30   **Unspecified anomaly of tooth position of fully erupted tooth or teeth**
      Abnormal spacing of fully erupted tooth or teeth NOS
      Displacement of fully erupted tooth or teeth NOS
      Transposition of fully erupted tooth or teeth NOS
    M26.31   **Crowding of fully erupted teeth**
    M26.32   **Excessive spacing of fully erupted teeth**
      Diastema of fully erupted tooth or teeth NOS
    M26.33   **Horizontal displacement of fully erupted tooth or teeth**
      Tipped tooth or teeth
      Tipping of fully erupted tooth
    M26.34   **Vertical displacement of fully erupted tooth or teeth**
      Extruded tooth
      Infraeruption of tooth or teeth
      Supraeruption of tooth or teeth
    M26.35   **Rotation of fully erupted tooth or teeth**

    M26.36   **Insufficient interocclusal distance of fully erupted teeth (ridge)**
      Lack of adequate intermaxillary vertical dimension of fully erupted teeth
    M26.37   **Excessive interocclusal distance of fully erupted teeth**
      Excessive intermaxillary vertical dimension of fully erupted teeth
      Loss of occlusal vertical dimension of fully erupted teeth
    M26.39   **Other anomalies of tooth position of fully erupted tooth or teeth**

  M26.4   **Malocclusion, unspecified**

  ✓5ᵗʰ M26.5   **Dentofacial functional abnormalities**

    EXCLUDES 1   *bruxism (F45.8)*
      teeth-grinding NOS (F45.8)

    M26.50   **Dentofacial functional abnormalities, unspecified**
    M26.51   **Abnormal jaw closure**
    M26.52   **Limited mandibular range of motion**
    M26.53   **Deviation in opening and closing of the mandible**
    M26.54   **Insufficient anterior guidance**
      Insufficient anterior occlusal guidance
    M26.55   **Centric occlusion maximum intercuspation discrepancy**
      EXCLUDES 1   *centric occlusion NOS (M26.59)*
    M26.56   **Non-working side interference**
      Balancing side interference
    M26.57   **Lack of posterior occlusal support**
    M26.59   **Other dentofacial functional abnormalities**
      Centric occlusion (of teeth) NOS
      Malocclusion due to abnormal swallowing
      Malocclusion due to mouth breathing
      Malocclusion due to tongue, lip or finger habits

  ✓5ᵗʰ M26.6   **Temporomandibular joint disorders**

    EXCLUDES 2   *current temporomandibular joint dislocation (S03.0)*
      current temporomandibular joint sprain (S03.4)

    AHA: 2016,4Q,38-39

Temporomandibular Joint

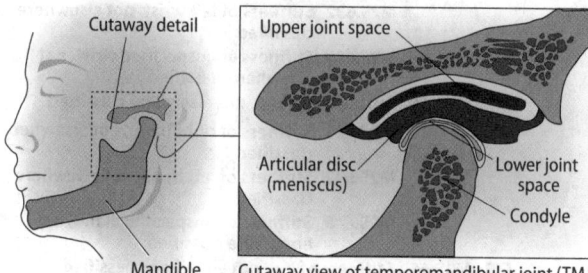

Cutaway detail — Upper joint space — Articular disc (meniscus) — Lower joint space — Condyle — Mandible

Cutaway view of temporomandibular joint (TMJ)

  ✓6ᵗʰ M26.60   **Temporomandibular joint disorder, unspecified**
    M26.601   **Right temporomandibular joint disorder, unspecified**
    M26.602   **Left temporomandibular joint disorder, unspecified**
    M26.603   **Bilateral temporomandibular joint disorder, unspecified**
    M26.609   **Unspecified temporomandibular joint disorder, unspecified side**
      Temporomandibular joint disorder NOS
  ✓6ᵗʰ M26.61   **Adhesions and ankylosis of temporomandibular joint**
    M26.611   **Adhesions and ankylosis of right temporomandibular joint**
    M26.612   **Adhesions and ankylosis of left temporomandibular joint**
    M26.613   **Adhesions and ankylosis of bilateral temporomandibular joint**
    M26.619   **Adhesions and ankylosis of temporomandibular joint, unspecified side**
  ✓6ᵗʰ M26.62   **Arthralgia of temporomandibular joint**
    M26.621   **Arthralgia of right temporomandibular joint**
    M26.622   **Arthralgia of left temporomandibular joint**
    M26.623   **Arthralgia of bilateral temporomandibular joint**

N Newborn: 0   **P** Pediatric: 0-17   **M** Maternity: 9-64   **A** Adult: 15-124   **MCC** Major Complication/Comorbidity   **CC** Complication/Comorbidity   **SW** Severe Wound Dx

794   ICD-10-CM 2022

     M26.629   **Arthralgia of temporomandibular joint, unspecified side**

☑6ᵗʰ   M26.63   Articular disc disorder of temporomandibular joint

     M26.631   **Articular disc disorder of right temporomandibular joint**

     M26.632   **Articular disc disorder of left temporomandibular joint**

     M26.633   **Articular disc disorder of bilateral temporomandibular joint**

     M26.639   **Articular disc disorder of temporomandibular joint, unspecified side**

☑6ᵗʰ   M26.64   Arthritis of temporomandibular joint

       AHA: 2020,4Q,32

     M26.641   **Arthritis of right temporomandibular joint**

     M26.642   **Arthritis of left temporomandibular joint**

     M26.643   **Arthritis of bilateral temporomandibular joint**

     M26.649   **Arthritis of unspecified temporomandibular joint**

☑6ᵗʰ   M26.65   Arthropathy of temporomandibular joint

       AHA: 2020,4Q,32

     M26.651   **Arthropathy of right temporomandibular joint**

     M26.652   **Arthropathy of left temporomandibular joint**

     M26.653   **Arthropathy of bilateral temporomandibular joint**

     M26.659   **Arthropathy of unspecified temporomandibular joint**

     M26.69   **Other specified disorders of temporomandibular joint**

☑5ᵗʰ   M26.7   **Dental alveolar anomalies**

     M26.70   **Unspecified alveolar anomaly**

     M26.71   **Alveolar maxillary hyperplasia**

     M26.72   **Alveolar mandibular hyperplasia**

     M26.73   **Alveolar maxillary hypoplasia**

     M26.74   **Alveolar mandibular hypoplasia**

     M26.79   **Other specified alveolar anomalies**

☑5ᵗʰ   M26.8   **Other dentofacial anomalies**

     M26.81   **Anterior soft tissue impingement**

       Anterior soft tissue impingement on teeth

     M26.82   **Posterior soft tissue impingement**

       Posterior soft tissue impingement on teeth

     M26.89   **Other dentofacial anomalies**

     M26.9   **Dentofacial anomaly, unspecified**

☑4ᵗʰ   **M27   Other diseases of jaws**

     M27.0   **Developmental disorders of jaws**

       Latent bone cyst of jaw

       Stafne's cyst

       Torus mandibularis

       Torus palatinus

     M27.1   **Giant cell granuloma, central**

       Giant cell granuloma NOS

       EXCLUDES 1   *peripheral giant cell granuloma (K06.8)*

     M27.2   **Inflammatory conditions of jaws**

       Osteitis of jaw(s)

       Osteomyelitis (neonatal) jaw(s)

       Osteoradionecrosis jaw(s)

       Periostitis jaw(s)

       Sequestrum of jaw bone

       Use additional code (W88-W90, X39.0) to identify radiation, if radiation-induced

       EXCLUDES 2   *osteonecrosis of jaw due to drug (M87.180)*

     M27.3   **Alveolitis of jaws**

       Alveolar osteitis

       Dry socket

☑5ᵗʰ   M27.4   **Other and unspecified cysts of jaw**

       EXCLUDES 1   *cysts of oral region (K09.-)*

               latent bone cyst of jaw (M27.0)

               Stafne's cyst (M27.0)

     M27.40   **Unspecified cyst of jaw**

       Cyst of jaw NOS

     M27.49   **Other cysts of jaw**

       Aneurysmal cyst of jaw

       Hemorrhagic cyst of jaw

       Traumatic cyst of jaw

☑5ᵗʰ   M27.5   **Periradicular pathology associated with previous endodontic treatment**

     M27.51   **Perforation of root canal space due to endodontic treatment**

     M27.52   **Endodontic overfill**

     M27.53   **Endodontic underfill**

     M27.59   **Other periradicular pathology associated with previous endodontic treatment**

☑5ᵗʰ   M27.6   **Endosseous dental implant failure**

     M27.61   Osseointegration failure of dental implant

       Hemorrhagic complications of dental implant placement

       Iatrogenic osseointegration failure of dental implant

       Osseointegration failure of dental implant due to complications of systemic disease

       Osseointegration failure of dental implant due to poor bone quality

       Pre-integration failure of dental implant NOS

       Pre-osseointegration failure of dental implant

     M27.62   Post-osseointegration biological failure of dental implant

       Failure of dental implant due to lack of attached gingiva

       Failure of dental implant due to occlusal trauma (caused by poor prosthetic design)

       Failure of dental implant due to parafunctional habits

       Failure of dental implant due to periodontal infection (peri-implantitis)

       Failure of dental implant due to poor oral hygiene

       Iatrogenic post-osseointegration failure of dental implant

       Post-osseointegration failure of dental implant due to complications of systemic disease

     M27.63   Post-osseointegration mechanical failure of dental implant

       Failure of dental prosthesis causing loss of dental implant

       Fracture of dental implant

       EXCLUDES 2   *cracked tooth (K03.81)*

               fractured dental restorative material with loss of material (K08.531)

               fractured dental restorative material without loss of material (K08.530)

               fractured tooth (S02.5)

     M27.69   **Other endosseous dental implant failure**

       Dental implant failure NOS

     M27.8   **Other specified diseases of jaws**

       Cherubism

       Exostosis

       Fibrous dysplasia

       Unilateral condylar hyperplasia

       Unilateral condylar hypoplasia

       EXCLUDES 1   *jaw pain (R68.84)*

     M27.9   **Disease of jaws, unspecified**

Systemic connective tissue disorders (M30-M36)

INCLUDES   autoimmune disease NOS

           collagen (vascular) disease NOS

           systemic autoimmune disease

           systemic collagen (vascular) disease

EXCLUDES 1   *autoimmune disease, single organ or single cell-type-code to relevant condition category*

☑4ᵗʰ   **M30   Polyarteritis nodosa and related conditions**

       EXCLUDES 1   *microscopic polyarteritis (M31.7)*

     M30.0   **Polyarteritis nodosa**   CC HCC

     M30.1   **Polyarteritis with lung involvement [Churg-Strauss]**   CC HCC

       Allergic granulomatous angiitis

       Eosinophilic granulomatosis with polyangiitis [EGPA]

       AHA: 2021,1Q,23

     M30.2   **Juvenile polyarteritis**   CC HCC

     M30.3   **Mucocutaneous lymph node syndrome [Kawasaki]**   CC HCC

☑ Additional Character Required   ✓x7ᵗʰ Placeholder   Questionable PDx   Manifestation   Unspecified Dx   UPD Unacceptable PDx   H1-H14 HAC   HCC CMS-HCC Dx   HIV HIV Dx

ICD-10-CM 2022   795

M30.8 Other conditions related to polyarteritis nodosa `CC` `HCC`
Polyangiitis overlap syndrome

✓4ᵗʰ **M31 Other necrotizing vasculopathies**

M31.0 Hypersensitivity angiitis `CC` `HCC`
Goodpasture's syndrome

▲ ✓5ᵗʰ **M31.1 Thrombotic microangiopathy**
~~Thrombotic thrombocytopenic purpura~~

● **M31.10 Thrombotic microangiopathy, unspecified** `MCC`

● **M31.11 Hematopoietic stem cell transplantation-associated thrombotic microangiopathy [HSCT-TMA]** `MCC`
Transplant-associated thrombotic microangiopathy [TA-TMA]
Code first if applicable:
complications of bone marrow transplant (T86.0-)
complications of stem cell transplant (T86.5)
Use additional code to identify specific organ dysfunction, such as:
acute kidney failure (N17.-)
acute respiratory distress syndrome (J80)
capillary leak syndrome (I78.8)
diffuse alveolar hemorrhage (R04.89)
encephalopathy (metabolic) (septic) (G93.41)
fluid overload, unspecified (E87.70)
graft versus host disease (D89.81-)
hemolytic uremic syndrome (D59.3)
hepatic failure (K72.-)
hepatic veno-occlusive disease (K76.5)
idiopathic interstitial pneumonia (J84.11-)
sinusoidal obstruction syndrome (K76.5)

● **M31.19 Other thrombotic microangiopathy** `MCC`
Thrombotic thrombocytopenic purpura

M31.2 Lethal midline granuloma `CC` `HCC`

✓5ᵗʰ **M31.3 Wegener's granulomatosis**
Granulomatosis with polyangiitis
Necrotizing respiratory granulomatosis
AHA: 2021,1Q,23

M31.30 Wegener's granulomatosis without renal involvement `CC` `HCC`
Wegener's granulomatosis NOS
AHA: 2021,2Q,10

M31.31 Wegener's granulomatosis with renal involvement `CC` `HCC`

M31.4 Aortic arch syndrome [Takayasu] `CC` `HCC`

M31.5 Giant cell arteritis with polymyalgia rheumatica `HCC`

M31.6 Other giant cell arteritis `HCC`

M31.7 Microscopic polyangiitis `CC` `HCC`
Microscopic polyarteritis
EXCLUDES 1 polyarteritis nodosa (M30.0)
AHA: 2021,1Q,23

M31.8 Other specified necrotizing vasculopathies `CC` `HCC`
Hypocomplementemic vasculitis
Septic vasculitis

M31.9 Necrotizing vasculopathy, unspecified `CC` `HCC`

✓4ᵗʰ **M32 Systemic lupus erythematosus (SLE)**
EXCLUDES 1 lupus erythematosus (discoid) (NOS) (L93.0)
AHA: 2020,4Q,11; 2018,3Q,14
TIP: There is no default code for "lupus NOS." Query the provider for the specific type of lupus in order to assign the appropriate code.

M32.0 Drug-induced systemic lupus erythematosus `HCC`
Use additional code for adverse effect, if applicable, to identify drug (T36-T50 with fifth or sixth character 5)

✓5ᵗʰ **M32.1 Systemic lupus erythematosus** with organ or system involvement

M32.10 Systemic lupus erythematosus, organ or system involvement unspecified `HCC`

M32.11 Endocarditis in systemic lupus erythematosus `CC` `HCC`
Libman-Sacks disease

M32.12 Pericarditis in systemic lupus erythematosus `CC` `HCC`
Lupus pericarditis

M32.13 Lung involvement in systemic lupus erythematosus `HCC`
Pleural effusion due to systemic lupus erythematosus

M32.14 Glomerular disease in systemic lupus erythematosus `HCC`
Lupus renal disease NOS
AHA: 2013,4Q,125

M32.15 Tubulo-interstitial nephropathy in systemic lupus erythematosus `HCC`

M32.19 Other organ or system involvement in systemic lupus erythematosus `HCC`

M32.8 Other forms of systemic lupus erythematosus `HCC`

M32.9 Systemic lupus erythematosus, unspecified `HCC`
SLE NOS
Systemic lupus erythematosus NOS
Systemic lupus erythematosus without organ involvement

✓4ᵗʰ **M33 Dermatopolymyositis**
AHA: 2017,4Q,18

✓5ᵗʰ **M33.0 Juvenile dermatomyositis**

M33.00 Juvenile dermatomyositis, organ involvement unspecified `CC` `HCC`

M33.01 Juvenile dermatomyositis with respiratory involvement `CC` `HCC`

M33.02 Juvenile dermatomyositis with myopathy `CC` `HCC`

M33.03 Juvenile dermatomyositis without myopathy `CC` `HCC`

M33.09 Juvenile dermatomyositis with other organ involvement `CC` `HCC`

✓5ᵗʰ **M33.1 Other dermatomyositis**
Adult dermatomyositis

M33.10 Other dermatomyositis, organ involvement unspecified `CC` `HCC`

M33.11 Other dermatomyositis with respiratory involvement `CC` `HCC`

M33.12 Other dermatomyositis with myopathy `CC` `HCC`

M33.13 Other dermatomyositis without myopathy `CC` `HCC`
Dermatomyositis NOS

M33.19 Other dermatomyositis with other organ involvement `CC` `HCC`

✓5ᵗʰ **M33.2 Polymyositis**

M33.20 Polymyositis, organ involvement unspecified `CC` `HCC`

M33.21 Polymyositis with respiratory involvement `CC` `HCC`

M33.22 Polymyositis with myopathy `CC` `HCC`

M33.29 Polymyositis with other organ involvement `CC` `HCC`

✓5ᵗʰ **M33.9 Dermatopolymyositis, unspecified**

M33.90 Dermatopolymyositis, unspecified, organ involvement unspecified `CC` `HCC`

M33.91 Dermatopolymyositis, unspecified with respiratory involvement `CC` `HCC`

M33.92 Dermatopolymyositis, unspecified with myopathy `CC` `HCC`

M33.93 Dermatopolymyositis, unspecified without myopathy `CC` `HCC`

M33.99 Dermatopolymyositis, unspecified with other organ involvement `CC` `HCC`

✓4ᵗʰ **M34 Systemic sclerosis [scleroderma]**
EXCLUDES 1 circumscribed scleroderma (L94.0)
neonatal scleroderma (P83.88)

M34.0 Progressive systemic sclerosis `HCC`

M34.1 CR(E)ST syndrome `HCC`
Combination of calcinosis, Raynaud's phenomenon, esophageal dysfunction, sclerodactyly, telangiectasia

M34.2 Systemic sclerosis induced by drug and chemical `HCC`
Code first poisoning due to drug or toxin, if applicable (T36-T65 with fifth or sixth character 1-4 or 6)
Use additional code for adverse effect, if applicable, to identify drug (T36-T50 with fifth or sixth character 5)

✓5ᵗʰ **M34.8 Other forms of systemic sclerosis**

M34.81 Systemic sclerosis with lung involvement `CC` `HCC`
▶Code also if applicable:◀
▶other interstitial pulmonary diseases (J84.89)◀
▶secondary pulmonary arterial hypertension (I27.21)◀

M34.82 Systemic sclerosis with myopathy `CC` `HCC`

M34.83 **Systemic sclerosis with** polyneuropathy `HCC`

M34.89 **Other systemic sclerosis** `HCC`

M34.9 **Systemic sclerosis, unspecified** `HCC`

✓4ᵗʰ **M35 Other systemic involvement of connective tissue**
  EXCLUDES 1   reactive perforating collagenosis (L87.1)

▲ ✓5ᵗʰ **M35.0 Sjögren syndrome**
  ▶Sicca syndrome◀
  ▶Use additional code to identify associated manifestations◀
    EXCLUDES 1 ▶dry mouth, unspecified (R68.2)◀
  DEF: Autoimmune disease associated with keratoconjunctivitis, laryngopharyngitis, rhinitis, dry mouth, enlarged parotid gland, and chronic polyarthritis.

▲ M35.00 **Sjögren syndrome, unspecified** `HCC`
▲ M35.01 **Sjögren syndrome with** keratoconjunctivitis `HCC`
▲ M35.02 **Sjögren syndrome with** lung involvement `HCC`
▲ M35.03 **Sjögren syndrome with** myopathy `CC` `HCC`
▲ M35.04 **Sjögren syndrome with** tubulo-interstitial nephropathy `HCC`
  Renal tubular acidosis in sicca syndrome
● M35.05 **Sjögren syndrome with** inflammatory arthritis
● M35.06 **Sjögren syndrome with** peripheral nervous system involvement
● M35.07 **Sjögren syndrome with** central nervous system involvement `CC`
● M35.08 **Sjögren syndrome with** gastrointestinal involvement
● M35.0A **Sjögren syndrome with** glomerular disease
● M35.0B **Sjögren syndrome with** vasculitis
● M35.0C **Sjögren syndrome with** dental involvement
▲ M35.09 **Sjögren syndrome with other organ involvement** `HCC`

M35.1 **Other overlap syndromes** `CC` `HCC`
  Mixed connective tissue disease
    EXCLUDES 1   polyangiitis overlap syndrome (M30.8)

M35.2 **Behçet's disease** `CC` `HCC`

M35.3 **Polymyalgia rheumatica** `HCC`
    EXCLUDES 1   polymyalgia rheumatica with giant cell arteritis (M31.5)

M35.4 **Diffuse (eosinophilic) fasciitis**

M35.5 **Multifocal fibrosclerosis** `CC` `HCC`

M35.6 **Relapsing panniculitis [Weber-Christian]**
    EXCLUDES 1   lupus panniculitis (L93.2)
                 panniculitis NOS (M79.3-)

M35.7 **Hypermobility syndrome**
  Familial ligamentous laxity
    EXCLUDES 1   Ehlers-Danlos syndromes (Q79.6-)
                 ligamentous laxity, NOS (M24.2-)
    EXCLUDES 2 ▶Ehlers-Danlos syndromes (Q79.6-)◀

✓5ᵗʰ **M35.8 Other specified systemic involvement of connective tissue**
  AHA: 2021,1Q,36; 2020,3Q,13-14

  M35.81 **Multisystem inflammatory syndrome** `CC` `HCC`
    MIS-A
    MIS-C
    Multisystem inflammatory syndrome in adults
    Multisystem inflammatory syndrome in children
    Pediatric inflammatory multisystem syndrome
    PIMS
    Code first, if applicable, COVID-19 (U07.1)
    Code also any associated complications such as:
      acute hepatic failure (K72.0-)
      acute kidney failure (N17.-)
      acute myocarditis (I40.-)
      acute respiratory distress syndrome (J80)
      cardiac arrhythmia (I47-I49.-)
      pneumonia due to COVID-19 (J12.82)
      severe sepsis (R65.2-)
      viral cardiomyopathy (B33.24)
      viral pericarditis (B33.23)
    Use additional code, if applicable, for:
      exposure to COVID-19 or SARS-CoV-2 infection (Z20.822)
      personal history of COVID-19 (Z86.16)
      ▶post COVID-19 condition (U09.9)◀
      sequelae of COVID-19 (B94.8)
    AHA: 2021,1Q,29,36,41
    DEF: Hyperinflammatory condition that seems to be largely associated with past or present coronavirus disease 2019 (COVID-19) infection. Predominantly occurring in children, with less frequent occurrences in adults, symptoms often include fever, laboratory evidence of inflammation, and evidence of clinically severe illness requiring hospitalization with multisystem (two or more) organ involvement. **Synonym(s):** MIS, MIS-C.

  M35.89 **Other specified systemic involvement of connective tissue** `CC` `HCC`

M35.9 **Systemic involvement of connective tissue, unspecified** `HCC`
  Autoimmune disease (systemic) NOS
  Collagen (vascular) disease NOS

✓4ᵗʰ **M36 Systemic disorders of connective tissue in diseases classified elsewhere**
    EXCLUDES 2   arthropathies in diseases classified elsewhere (M14.-)

M36.0 *Dermato(poly)myositis in neoplastic disease* `CC` `HCC`
  Code first underlying neoplasm (C00-D49)

M36.1 *Arthropathy in neoplastic disease*
  Code first underlying neoplasm, such as:
    leukemia (C91-C95)
    malignant histiocytosis (C96.A)
    multiple myeloma (C90.0)

M36.2 *Hemophilic arthropathy*
  Hemarthrosis in hemophilic arthropathy
  Code first underlying disease, such as:
    factor VIII deficiency (D66)
      with vascular defect (D68.0)
    factor IX deficiency (D67)
    hemophilia (classical) (D66)
    hemophilia B (D67)
    hemophilia C (D68.1)

M36.3 *Arthropathy in other blood disorders*

M36.4 *Arthropathy in hypersensitivity reactions classified elsewhere*
  Code first underlying disease, such as:
    Henoch (-Schönlein) purpura (D69.0)
    serum sickness (T80.6-)

M36.8 *Systemic disorders of connective tissue in other diseases classified elsewhere* `HCC`
  Code first underlying disease, such as:
    alkaptonuria (E70.2)
    hypogammaglobulinemia (D80.-)
    ochronosis (E70.2)

☑ Additional Character Required   ✓x7ᵗʰ Placeholder   Questionable PDx   Manifestation   Unspecified Dx   `UPD` Unacceptable PDx   `H1`-`H14` HAC   `HCC` CMS-HCC Dx   `HIV` HIV Dx

ICD-10-CM 2022   797

DORSOPATHIES (M40-M54)

Deforming dorsopathies (M40-M43)

✓4ᵗʰ **M40 Kyphosis and lordosis**
▶Code first underlying disease◀
EXCLUDES 1   congenital kyphosis and lordosis (Q76.4)
              kyphoscoliosis (M41.-)
              postprocedural kyphosis and lordosis (M96.-)

Kyphosis and Lordosis

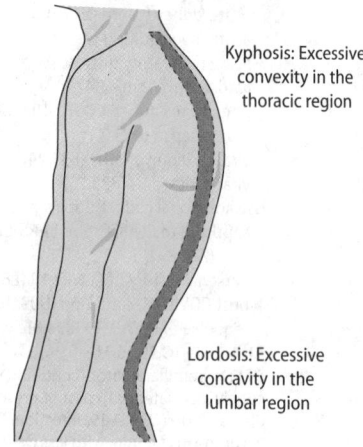

Kyphosis: Excessive convexity in the thoracic region

Lordosis: Excessive concavity in the lumbar region

✓5ᵗʰ **M40.0 Postural kyphosis**
EXCLUDES 1   osteochondrosis of spine (M42.-)
M40.00 Postural kyphosis, site unspecified
M40.03 Postural kyphosis, cervicothoracic region
M40.04 Postural kyphosis, thoracic region
M40.05 Postural kyphosis, thoracolumbar region

✓5ᵗʰ **M40.1 Other secondary kyphosis**
M40.10 Other secondary kyphosis, site unspecified
M40.12 Other secondary kyphosis, cervical region
M40.13 Other secondary kyphosis, cervicothoracic region
M40.14 Other secondary kyphosis, thoracic region
M40.15 Other secondary kyphosis, thoracolumbar region

✓5ᵗʰ **M40.2 Other and unspecified kyphosis**
✓6ᵗʰ **M40.20 Unspecified kyphosis**
M40.202 Unspecified kyphosis, cervical region
M40.203 Unspecified kyphosis, cervicothoracic region
M40.204 Unspecified kyphosis, thoracic region
M40.205 Unspecified kyphosis, thoracolumbar region
M40.209 Unspecified kyphosis, site unspecified
✓6ᵗʰ **M40.29 Other kyphosis**
M40.292 Other kyphosis, cervical region
M40.293 Other kyphosis, cervicothoracic region
M40.294 Other kyphosis, thoracic region
M40.295 Other kyphosis, thoracolumbar region
M40.299 Other kyphosis, site unspecified

✓5ᵗʰ **M40.3 Flatback syndrome**
M40.30 Flatback syndrome, site unspecified
M40.35 Flatback syndrome, thoracolumbar region
M40.36 Flatback syndrome, lumbar region
M40.37 Flatback syndrome, lumbosacral region

✓5ᵗʰ **M40.4 Postural lordosis**
Acquired lordosis
M40.40 Postural lordosis, site unspecified
M40.45 Postural lordosis, thoracolumbar region
M40.46 Postural lordosis, lumbar region
M40.47 Postural lordosis, lumbosacral region

✓5ᵗʰ **M40.5 Lordosis, unspecified**
M40.50 Lordosis, unspecified, site unspecified
M40.55 Lordosis, unspecified, thoracolumbar region
M40.56 Lordosis, unspecified, lumbar region
M40.57 Lordosis, unspecified, lumbosacral region

✓4ᵗʰ **M41 Scoliosis**
INCLUDES   kyphoscoliosis
EXCLUDES 1 congenital scoliosis due to bony malformation (Q76.3)
            congenital scoliosis NOS (Q67.5)
            kyphoscoliotic heart disease (I27.1)
            ~~postprocedural scoliosis (M96.-)~~
            postural congenital scoliosis (Q67.5)
EXCLUDES 2 ▶postprocedural scoliosis (M96.-)◀

Scoliosis

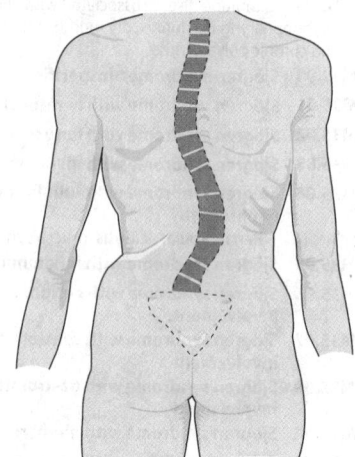

Lateral curvature of spine

✓5ᵗʰ **M41.0 Infantile idiopathic scoliosis**
AHA: 2014,4Q,26
M41.00 Infantile idiopathic scoliosis, site unspecified
M41.02 Infantile idiopathic scoliosis, cervical region
M41.03 Infantile idiopathic scoliosis, cervicothoracic region
M41.04 Infantile idiopathic scoliosis, thoracic region
M41.05 Infantile idiopathic scoliosis, thoracolumbar region
M41.06 Infantile idiopathic scoliosis, lumbar region
M41.07 Infantile idiopathic scoliosis, lumbosacral region
M41.08 Infantile idiopathic scoliosis, sacral and sacrococcygeal region

✓5ᵗʰ **M41.1 Juvenile and adolescent idiopathic scoliosis**
✓6ᵗʰ **M41.11 Juvenile idiopathic scoliosis**
AHA: 2014,4Q,28
M41.112 Juvenile idiopathic scoliosis, cervical region
M41.113 Juvenile idiopathic scoliosis, cervicothoracic region
M41.114 Juvenile idiopathic scoliosis, thoracic region
M41.115 Juvenile idiopathic scoliosis, thoracolumbar region
M41.116 Juvenile idiopathic scoliosis, lumbar region
M41.117 Juvenile idiopathic scoliosis, lumbosacral region
M41.119 Juvenile idiopathic scoliosis, site unspecified
✓6ᵗʰ **M41.12 Adolescent scoliosis**
M41.122 Adolescent idiopathic scoliosis, cervical region
M41.123 Adolescent idiopathic scoliosis, cervicothoracic region
M41.124 Adolescent idiopathic scoliosis, thoracic region
M41.125 Adolescent idiopathic scoliosis, thoracolumbar region
M41.126 Adolescent idiopathic scoliosis, lumbar region
M41.127 Adolescent idiopathic scoliosis, lumbosacral region
M41.129 Adolescent idiopathic scoliosis, site unspecified

✓5ᵗʰ **M41.2 Other idiopathic scoliosis**
M41.20 Other idiopathic scoliosis, site unspecified
M41.22 Other idiopathic scoliosis, cervical region
M41.23 Other idiopathic scoliosis, cervicothoracic region

M41.24   **Other idiopathic scoliosis, thoracic region**

M41.25   **Other idiopathic scoliosis, thoracolumbar region**

M41.26   **Other idiopathic scoliosis, lumbar region**

M41.27   **Other idiopathic scoliosis, lumbosacral region**

✓5ᵗʰ **M41.3 Thoracogenic scoliosis**

M41.30   **Thoracogenic scoliosis, site unspecified**

M41.34   **Thoracogenic scoliosis, thoracic region**

M41.35   **Thoracogenic scoliosis, thoracolumbar region**

✓5ᵗʰ **M41.4 Neuromuscular scoliosis**

Scoliosis secondary to cerebral palsy, Friedreich's ataxia, poliomyelitis and other neuromuscular disorders

Code also underlying condition

AHA: 2014,4Q,27

M41.40   **Neuromuscular scoliosis, site unspecified**

M41.41   **Neuromuscular scoliosis, occipito-atlanto-axial region**

M41.42   **Neuromuscular scoliosis, cervical region**

M41.43   **Neuromuscular scoliosis, cervicothoracic region**

M41.44   **Neuromuscular scoliosis, thoracic region**

M41.45   **Neuromuscular scoliosis, thoracolumbar region**

M41.46   **Neuromuscular scoliosis, lumbar region**

M41.47   **Neuromuscular scoliosis, lumbosacral region**

✓5ᵗʰ **M41.5 Other secondary scoliosis**

▶Code first underlying disease◀

AHA: 2019,1Q,19

M41.50   **Other secondary scoliosis, site unspecified**

M41.52   **Other secondary scoliosis, cervical region**

M41.53   **Other secondary scoliosis, cervicothoracic region**

M41.54   **Other secondary scoliosis, thoracic region**

M41.55   **Other secondary scoliosis, thoracolumbar region**

M41.56   **Other secondary scoliosis, lumbar region**

M41.57   **Other secondary scoliosis, lumbosacral region**

✓5ᵗʰ **M41.8 Other forms of scoliosis**

M41.80   **Other forms of scoliosis, site unspecified**

M41.82   **Other forms of scoliosis, cervical region**

M41.83   **Other forms of scoliosis, cervicothoracic region**

M41.84   **Other forms of scoliosis, thoracic region**

M41.85   **Other forms of scoliosis, thoracolumbar region**

M41.86   **Other forms of scoliosis, lumbar region**

M41.87   **Other forms of scoliosis, lumbosacral region**

M41.9   **Scoliosis, unspecified**

✓4ᵗʰ **M42 Spinal osteochondrosis**

✓5ᵗʰ **M42.0 Juvenile osteochondrosis of spine**

Calvé's disease

Scheuermann's disease

EXCLUDES 1   *postural kyphosis (M40.0)*

M42.00   **Juvenile osteochondrosis of spine, site unspecified**

M42.01   **Juvenile osteochondrosis of spine, occipito-atlanto-axial region**

M42.02   **Juvenile osteochondrosis of spine, cervical region**

M42.03   **Juvenile osteochondrosis of spine, cervicothoracic region**

M42.04   **Juvenile osteochondrosis of spine, thoracic region**

M42.05   **Juvenile osteochondrosis of spine, thoracolumbar region**

M42.06   **Juvenile osteochondrosis of spine, lumbar region**

M42.07   **Juvenile osteochondrosis of spine, lumbosacral region**

M42.08   **Juvenile osteochondrosis of spine, sacral and sacrococcygeal region**

M42.09   **Juvenile osteochondrosis of spine, multiple sites in spine**

✓5ᵗʰ **M42.1 Adult osteochondrosis of spine**

M42.10   **Adult osteochondrosis of spine, site unspecified**   Ⓐ

M42.11   **Adult osteochondrosis of spine, occipito-atlanto-axial region**   Ⓐ

M42.12   **Adult osteochondrosis of spine, cervical region**   Ⓐ

M42.13   **Adult osteochondrosis of spine, cervicothoracic region**   Ⓐ

M42.14   **Adult osteochondrosis of spine, thoracic region**   Ⓐ

M42.15   **Adult osteochondrosis of spine, thoracolumbar region**   Ⓐ

M42.16   **Adult osteochondrosis of spine, lumbar region**   Ⓐ

M42.17   **Adult osteochondrosis of spine, lumbosacral region**   Ⓐ

M42.18   **Adult osteochondrosis of spine, sacral and sacrococcygeal region**   Ⓐ

M42.19   **Adult osteochondrosis of spine, multiple sites in spine**   Ⓐ

M42.9   **Spinal osteochondrosis, unspecified**

✓4ᵗʰ **M43 Other deforming dorsopathies**

EXCLUDES 1   *congenital spondylolysis and spondylolisthesis (Q76.2)*

hemivertebra (Q76.3-Q76.4)

Klippel-Feil syndrome (Q76.1)

lumbarization and sacralization (Q76.4)

platyspondylisis (Q76.4)

spina bifida occulta (Q76.0)

spinal curvature in osteoporosis (M80.-)

spinal curvature in Paget's disease of bone [osteitis deformans] (M88.-)

✓5ᵗʰ **M43.0 Spondylolysis**

EXCLUDES 1   *congenital spondylolysis (Q76.2)*

spondylolisthesis (M43.1)

M43.00   **Spondylolysis, site unspecified**

M43.01   **Spondylolysis, occipito-atlanto-axial region**

M43.02   **Spondylolysis, cervical region**

M43.03   **Spondylolysis, cervicothoracic region**

M43.04   **Spondylolysis, thoracic region**

M43.05   **Spondylolysis, thoracolumbar region**

M43.06   **Spondylolysis, lumbar region**

M43.07   **Spondylolysis, lumbosacral region**

M43.08   **Spondylolysis, sacral and sacrococcygeal region**

M43.09   **Spondylolysis, multiple sites in spine**

✓5ᵗʰ **M43.1 Spondylolisthesis**

EXCLUDES 1   *acute traumatic of lumbosacral region (S33.1)*

acute traumatic of sites other than lumbosacral - code to Fracture, vertebra, by region

congenital spondylolisthesis (Q76.2)

AHA: 2020,2Q,21; 2018,3Q,18

TIP: Code also any associated radiculopathy (M54.1-) and/or myelopathy (G99.2).

M43.10   **Spondylolisthesis, site unspecified**

M43.11   **Spondylolisthesis, occipito-atlanto-axial region**

M43.12   **Spondylolisthesis, cervical region**

M43.13   **Spondylolisthesis, cervicothoracic region**

M43.14   **Spondylolisthesis, thoracic region**

M43.15   **Spondylolisthesis, thoracolumbar region**

M43.16   **Spondylolisthesis, lumbar region**

M43.17   **Spondylolisthesis, lumbosacral region**

M43.18   **Spondylolisthesis, sacral and sacrococcygeal region**

M43.19   **Spondylolisthesis, multiple sites in spine**

✓5ᵗʰ **M43.2 Fusion of spine**

Ankylosis of spinal joint

EXCLUDES 1   *ankylosing spondylitis (M45.0-)*

congenital fusion of spine (Q76.4)

EXCLUDES 2   *arthrodesis status (Z98.1)*

pseudoarthrosis after fusion or arthrodesis (M96.0)

M43.20   **Fusion of spine, site unspecified**

M43.21   **Fusion of spine, occipito-atlanto-axial region**

M43.22   **Fusion of spine, cervical region**

M43.23   **Fusion of spine, cervicothoracic region**

M43.24   **Fusion of spine, thoracic region**

M43.25   **Fusion of spine, thoracolumbar region**

M43.26   **Fusion of spine, lumbar region**

M43.27   **Fusion of spine, lumbosacral region**

M43.28   **Fusion of spine, sacral and sacrococcygeal region**

M43.3   **Recurrent atlantoaxial dislocation with myelopathy**

M43.4   **Other recurrent atlantoaxial dislocation**

✓5ᵗʰ **M43.5 Other recurrent vertebral dislocation**

EXCLUDES 1   *biomechanical lesions NEC (M99.-)*

✓6ᵗʰ **M43.5X Other recurrent vertebral dislocation**

M43.5X2   **Other recurrent vertebral dislocation, cervical region**

M43.5X3   **Other recurrent vertebral dislocation, cervicothoracic region**

M43.5X4   **Other recurrent vertebral dislocation, thoracic region**

M43.5X5   **Other recurrent vertebral dislocation, thoracolumbar region**

✓ Additional Character Required   ✓x7ᵗʰ Placeholder   Questionable PDx   Manifestation   Unspecified Dx   UPD Unacceptable PDx   H1-H14 HAC   HCC CMS-HCC Dx   HIV HIV Dx

ICD-10-CM 2022   799

        M43.5X6   **Other recurrent vertebral dislocation, lumbar region**

        M43.5X7   **Other recurrent vertebral dislocation, lumbosacral region**

        M43.5X8   **Other recurrent vertebral dislocation, sacral and sacrococcygeal region**

        M43.5X9   **Other recurrent vertebral dislocation, site unspecified**

M43.6   **Torticollis**
> EXCLUDES 1   congenital (sternomastoid) torticollis (Q68.0)
> current injury - see Injury, of spine, by body region
> ocular torticollis (R29.891)
> psychogenic torticollis (F45.8)
> spasmodic torticollis (G24.3)
> torticollis due to birth injury (P15.2)

DEF: Twisted, unnatural position of the neck due to contracted cervical muscles that pull the head to one side.

√5th M43.8   **Other specified deforming dorsopathies**
> EXCLUDES 2   kyphosis and lordosis (M40.-)
> scoliosis (M41.-)

√6th M43.8X   **Other specified deforming dorsopathies**

    M43.8X1   **Other specified deforming dorsopathies, occipito-atlanto-axial region**

    M43.8X2   **Other specified deforming dorsopathies, cervical region**

    M43.8X3   **Other specified deforming dorsopathies, cervicothoracic region**

    M43.8X4   **Other specified deforming dorsopathies, thoracic region**

    M43.8X5   **Other specified deforming dorsopathies, thoracolumbar region**

    M43.8X6   **Other specified deforming dorsopathies, lumbar region**

    M43.8X7   **Other specified deforming dorsopathies, lumbosacral region**

    M43.8X8   **Other specified deforming dorsopathies, sacral and sacrococcygeal region**

    M43.8X9   **Other specified deforming dorsopathies, site unspecified**

M43.9   **Deforming dorsopathy, unspecified**
Curvature of spine NOS

Spondylopathies (M45-M49)

√4th **M45 Ankylosing spondylitis**
Rheumatoid arthritis of spine
> EXCLUDES 1   arthropathy in Reiter's disease (M02.3-)
> juvenile (ankylosing) spondylitis (M08.1)
> EXCLUDES 2   Behçet's disease (M35.2)

M45.0   **Ankylosing spondylitis of multiple sites in spine**   HCC

M45.1   **Ankylosing spondylitis of occipito-atlanto-axial region**   HCC

M45.2   **Ankylosing spondylitis of cervical region**   HCC

M45.3   **Ankylosing spondylitis of cervicothoracic region**   HCC

M45.4   **Ankylosing spondylitis of thoracic region**   HCC

M45.5   **Ankylosing spondylitis of thoracolumbar region**   HCC

M45.6   **Ankylosing spondylitis lumbar region**   HCC

M45.7   **Ankylosing spondylitis of lumbosacral region**   HCC

M45.8   **Ankylosing spondylitis sacral and sacrococcygeal region**   HCC

M45.9   **Ankylosing spondylitis of unspecified sites in spine**   HCC

√5th M45.A   **Non-radiographic axial spondyloarthritis**

    M45.A0   **Non-radiographic axial spondyloarthritis of unspecified sites in spine**

    M45.A1   **Non-radiographic axial spondyloarthritis of occipito-atlanto-axial region**

    M45.A2   **Non-radiographic axial spondyloarthritis of cervical region**

    M45.A3   **Non-radiographic axial spondyloarthritis of cervicothoracic region**

    M45.A4   **Non-radiographic axial spondyloarthritis of thoracic region**

    M45.A5   **Non-radiographic axial spondyloarthritis of thoracolumbar region**

    M45.A6   **Non-radiographic axial spondyloarthritis of lumbar region**

    M45.A7   **Non-radiographic axial spondyloarthritis of lumbosacral region**

    M45.A8   **Non-radiographic axial spondyloarthritis of sacral and sacrococcygeal region**

    M45.AB   **Non-radiographic axial spondyloarthritis of multiple sites in spine**

√4th **M46 Other inflammatory spondylopathies**

√5th M46.0   **Spinal enthesopathy**
Disorder of ligamentous or muscular attachments of spine

    M46.00   **Spinal enthesopathy, site unspecified**   HCC

    M46.01   **Spinal enthesopathy, occipito-atlanto-axial region**   HCC

    M46.02   **Spinal enthesopathy, cervical region**   HCC

    M46.03   **Spinal enthesopathy, cervicothoracic region**   HCC

    M46.04   **Spinal enthesopathy, thoracic region**   HCC

    M46.05   **Spinal enthesopathy, thoracolumbar region**   HCC

    M46.06   **Spinal enthesopathy, lumbar region**   HCC

    M46.07   **Spinal enthesopathy, lumbosacral region**   HCC

    M46.08   **Spinal enthesopathy, sacral and sacrococcygeal region**   HCC

    M46.09   **Spinal enthesopathy, multiple sites in spine**   HCC

M46.1   **Sacroiliitis, not elsewhere classified**   HCC
AHA: 2020,2Q,14
DEF: Inflammation of the sacroiliac joint (situated at the juncture of the sacrum and hip). Symptoms include pain in the buttocks or lower back that can extend down one or both legs.

√5th M46.2   **Osteomyelitis of vertebra**

    M46.20   **Osteomyelitis of vertebra, site unspecified**   CC HCC

    M46.21   **Osteomyelitis of vertebra, occipito-atlanto-axial region**   CC HCC

    M46.22   **Osteomyelitis of vertebra, cervical region**   CC HCC

    M46.23   **Osteomyelitis of vertebra, cervicothoracic region**   CC HCC

    M46.24   **Osteomyelitis of vertebra, thoracic region**   CC HCC

    M46.25   **Osteomyelitis of vertebra, thoracolumbar region**   CC HCC

    M46.26   **Osteomyelitis of vertebra, lumbar region**   CC HCC

    M46.27   **Osteomyelitis of vertebra, lumbosacral region**   CC HCC

    M46.28   **Osteomyelitis of vertebra, sacral and sacrococcygeal region**   CC HCC

√5th M46.3   **Infection of intervertebral disc (pyogenic)**
Use additional code (B95-B97) to identify infectious agent

    M46.30   **Infection of intervertebral disc (pyogenic), site unspecified**   CC HCC

    M46.31   **Infection of intervertebral disc (pyogenic), occipito-atlanto-axial region**   CC HCC

    M46.32   **Infection of intervertebral disc (pyogenic), cervical region**   CC HCC

    M46.33   **Infection of intervertebral disc (pyogenic), cervicothoracic region**   CC HCC

    M46.34   **Infection of intervertebral disc (pyogenic), thoracic region**   CC HCC

    M46.35   **Infection of intervertebral disc (pyogenic), thoracolumbar region**   CC HCC

    M46.36   **Infection of intervertebral disc (pyogenic), lumbar region**   CC HCC

    M46.37   **Infection of intervertebral disc (pyogenic), lumbosacral region**   CC HCC

    M46.38   **Infection of intervertebral disc (pyogenic), sacral and sacrococcygeal region**   CC HCC

    M46.39   **Infection of intervertebral disc (pyogenic), multiple sites in spine**   CC HCC

√5th M46.4   **Discitis, unspecified**

    M46.40   **Discitis, unspecified, site unspecified**

    M46.41   **Discitis, unspecified, occipito-atlanto-axial region**

    M46.42   **Discitis, unspecified, cervical region**

    M46.43   **Discitis, unspecified, cervicothoracic region**

    M46.44   **Discitis, unspecified, thoracic region**

    M46.45   **Discitis, unspecified, thoracolumbar region**

    M46.46   **Discitis, unspecified, lumbar region**

    M46.47   **Discitis, unspecified, lumbosacral region**

    M46.48   **Discitis, unspecified, sacral and sacrococcygeal region**

    M46.49   **Discitis, unspecified, multiple sites in spine**

✓5ᵗʰ **M46.5 Other infective spondylopathies**

     M46.50   **Other infective spondylopathies, site unspecified**   HCC

     M46.51   **Other infective spondylopathies, occipito-atlanto-axial region**   HCC

     M46.52   **Other infective spondylopathies, cervical region**   HCC

     M46.53   **Other infective spondylopathies, cervicothoracic region**   HCC

     M46.54   **Other infective spondylopathies, thoracic region**   HCC

     M46.55   **Other infective spondylopathies, thoracolumbar region**   HCC

     M46.56   **Other infective spondylopathies, lumbar region**   HCC

     M46.57   **Other infective spondylopathies, lumbosacral region**   HCC

     M46.58   **Other infective spondylopathies, sacral and sacrococcygeal region**   HCC

     M46.59   **Other infective spondylopathies, multiple sites in spine**   HCC

✓5ᵗʰ **M46.8 Other specified inflammatory spondylopathies**

     M46.80   **Other specified inflammatory spondylopathies, site unspecified**   HCC

     M46.81   **Other specified inflammatory spondylopathies, occipito-atlanto-axial region**   HCC

     M46.82   **Other specified inflammatory spondylopathies, cervical region**   HCC

     M46.83   **Other specified inflammatory spondylopathies, cervicothoracic region**   HCC

     M46.84   **Other specified inflammatory spondylopathies, thoracic region**   HCC

     M46.85   **Other specified inflammatory spondylopathies, thoracolumbar region**   HCC

     M46.86   **Other specified inflammatory spondylopathies, lumbar region**   HCC

     M46.87   **Other specified inflammatory spondylopathies, lumbosacral region**   HCC

     M46.88   **Other specified inflammatory spondylopathies, sacral and sacrococcygeal region**   HCC

     M46.89   **Other specified inflammatory spondylopathies, multiple sites in spine**   HCC

✓5ᵗʰ **M46.9 Unspecified inflammatory spondylopathy**

     M46.90   **Unspecified inflammatory spondylopathy, site unspecified**   HCC

     M46.91   **Unspecified inflammatory spondylopathy, occipito-atlanto-axial region**   HCC

     M46.92   **Unspecified inflammatory spondylopathy, cervical region**   HCC
         AHA: 2019,3Q,10

     M46.93   **Unspecified inflammatory spondylopathy, cervicothoracic region**   HCC

     M46.94   **Unspecified inflammatory spondylopathy, thoracic region**   HCC

     M46.95   **Unspecified inflammatory spondylopathy, thoracolumbar region**   HCC

     M46.96   **Unspecified inflammatory spondylopathy, lumbar region**   HCC

     M46.97   **Unspecified inflammatory spondylopathy, lumbosacral region**   HCC

     M46.98   **Unspecified inflammatory spondylopathy, sacral and sacrococcygeal region**   HCC

     M46.99   **Unspecified inflammatory spondylopathy, multiple sites in spine**   HCC

✓4ᵗʰ **M47 Spondylosis**

     INCLUDES   arthrosis or osteoarthritis of spine
                degeneration of facet joints

     AHA: 2020,1Q,17; 2019,3Q,10-11; 2016,4Q,147

✓5ᵗʰ **M47.0 Anterior spinal and vertebral artery compression syndromes**

     ✓6ᵗʰ **M47.01**   **Anterior spinal artery compression syndromes**

         M47.011   **Anterior spinal artery compression syndromes, occipito-atlanto-axial region**   CC

         M47.012   **Anterior spinal artery compression syndromes, cervical region**   CC

         M47.013   **Anterior spinal artery compression syndromes, cervicothoracic region**   CC

         M47.014   **Anterior spinal artery compression syndromes, thoracic region**   CC

         M47.015   **Anterior spinal artery compression syndromes, thoracolumbar region**   CC

         M47.016   **Anterior spinal artery compression syndromes, lumbar region**   CC

         M47.019   **Anterior spinal artery compression syndromes, site unspecified**   CC

     ✓6ᵗʰ **M47.02**   **Vertebral artery compression syndromes**

         M47.021   **Vertebral artery compression syndromes, occipito-atlanto-axial region**   CC

         M47.022   **Vertebral artery compression syndromes, cervical region**   CC

         M47.029   **Vertebral artery compression syndromes, site unspecified**   CC

✓5ᵗʰ **M47.1 Other spondylosis with myelopathy**

     Spondylogenic compression of spinal cord

     EXCLUDES 1   vertebral subluxation (M43.3-M43.5X9)

     AHA: 2020,1Q,17

     M47.10   **Other spondylosis with myelopathy, site unspecified**   CC

     M47.11   **Other spondylosis with myelopathy, occipito-atlanto-axial region**   CC

     M47.12   **Other spondylosis with myelopathy, cervical region**   CC

     M47.13   **Other spondylosis with myelopathy, cervicothoracic region**   CC

     M47.14   **Other spondylosis with myelopathy, thoracic region**   CC

     M47.15   **Other spondylosis with myelopathy, thoracolumbar region**   CC

     M47.16   **Other spondylosis with myelopathy, lumbar region**   CC

✓5ᵗʰ **M47.2 Other spondylosis with radiculopathy**

     AHA: 2020,1Q,17

     M47.20   **Other spondylosis with radiculopathy, site unspecified**

     M47.21   **Other spondylosis with radiculopathy, occipito-atlanto-axial region**

     M47.22   **Other spondylosis with radiculopathy, cervical region**

     M47.23   **Other spondylosis with radiculopathy, cervicothoracic region**

     M47.24   **Other spondylosis with radiculopathy, thoracic region**

     M47.25   **Other spondylosis with radiculopathy, thoracolumbar region**

     M47.26   **Other spondylosis with radiculopathy, lumbar region**

     M47.27   **Other spondylosis with radiculopathy, lumbosacral region**

     M47.28   **Other spondylosis with radiculopathy, sacral and sacrococcygeal region**

✓5ᵗʰ **M47.8 Other spondylosis**

     ✓6ᵗʰ **M47.81**   **Spondylosis without myelopathy or radiculopathy**
         AHA: 2019,3Q,10-11; 2018,2Q,14

         M47.811   **Spondylosis without myelopathy or radiculopathy, occipito-atlanto-axial region**

         M47.812   **Spondylosis without myelopathy or radiculopathy, cervical region**

         M47.813   **Spondylosis without myelopathy or radiculopathy, cervicothoracic region**

         M47.814   **Spondylosis without myelopathy or radiculopathy, thoracic region**

         M47.815   **Spondylosis without myelopathy or radiculopathy, thoracolumbar region**

         M47.816   **Spondylosis without myelopathy or radiculopathy, lumbar region**

         M47.817   **Spondylosis without myelopathy or radiculopathy, lumbosacral region**

         M47.818   **Spondylosis without myelopathy or radiculopathy, sacral and sacrococcygeal region**

         M47.819   **Spondylosis without myelopathy or radiculopathy, site unspecified**

     ✓6ᵗʰ **M47.89**   **Other spondylosis**

         M47.891   **Other spondylosis, occipito-atlanto-axial region**

         M47.892   **Other spondylosis, cervical region**

✔ Additional Character Required   ✓x7ᵗʰ Placeholder   Questionable PDx   Manifestation   Unspecified Dx   UPD Unacceptable PDx   H1-H14 HAC   HCC CMS-HCC Dx   HIV HIV Dx

ICD-10-CM 2022   801

M47.893 Other spondylosis, cervicothoracic region
M47.894 Other spondylosis, thoracic region
M47.895 Other spondylosis, thoracolumbar region
M47.896 Other spondylosis, lumbar region
M47.897 Other spondylosis, lumbosacral region
M47.898 Other spondylosis, sacral and sacrococcygeal region
M47.899 Other spondylosis, site unspecified

M47.9 Spondylosis, unspecified

√4th **M48 Other spondylopathies**

√5th **M48.0 Spinal stenosis**

Caudal stenosis
AHA: 2020,1Q,17; 2018,3Q,18-19
TIP: Code also any associated radiculopathy (M54.1-) and/or myelopathy (G99.2).

M48.00 Spinal stenosis, site unspecified
M48.01 Spinal stenosis, occipito-atlanto-axial region
M48.02 Spinal stenosis, cervical region
M48.03 Spinal stenosis, cervicothoracic region
M48.04 Spinal stenosis, thoracic region
M48.05 Spinal stenosis, thoracolumbar region

√6th M48.06 Spinal stenosis, lumbar region

AHA: 2018,3Q,19; 2017,4Q,18-19
DEF: Spinal canal narrowing in the lumbar area with nerve root compression, causing muscle pain, fatigue, and weakness during extension of the lumbar spine. Pain is relieved by sitting or bending.

M48.061 Spinal stenosis, lumbar region without neurogenic claudication
Spinal stenosis, lumbar region NOS
M48.062 Spinal stenosis, lumbar region with neurogenic claudication

M48.07 Spinal stenosis, lumbosacral region
M48.08 Spinal stenosis, sacral and sacrococcygeal region

√5th **M48.1 Ankylosing hyperostosis [Forestier]**

Diffuse idiopathic skeletal hyperostosis [DISH]

M48.10 Ankylosing hyperostosis [Forestier], site unspecified
M48.11 Ankylosing hyperostosis [Forestier], occipito-atlanto-axial region
M48.12 Ankylosing hyperostosis [Forestier], cervical region
M48.13 Ankylosing hyperostosis [Forestier], cervicothoracic region
M48.14 Ankylosing hyperostosis [Forestier], thoracic region
M48.15 Ankylosing hyperostosis [Forestier], thoracolumbar region
M48.16 Ankylosing hyperostosis [Forestier], lumbar region
M48.17 Ankylosing hyperostosis [Forestier], lumbosacral region
M48.18 Ankylosing hyperostosis [Forestier], sacral and sacrococcygeal region
M48.19 Ankylosing hyperostosis [Forestier], multiple sites in spine

√5th **M48.2 Kissing spine**

M48.20 Kissing spine, site unspecified
M48.21 Kissing spine, occipito-atlanto-axial region
M48.22 Kissing spine, cervical region
M48.23 Kissing spine, cervicothoracic region
M48.24 Kissing spine, thoracic region
M48.25 Kissing spine, thoracolumbar region
M48.26 Kissing spine, lumbar region
M48.27 Kissing spine, lumbosacral region

√5th **M48.3 Traumatic spondylopathy**

M48.30 Traumatic spondylopathy, site unspecified ᴄᴄ
M48.31 Traumatic spondylopathy, occipito-atlanto-axial region ᴄᴄ
M48.32 Traumatic spondylopathy, cervical region ᴄᴄ
M48.33 Traumatic spondylopathy, cervicothoracic region ᴄᴄ
M48.34 Traumatic spondylopathy, thoracic region ᴄᴄ
M48.35 Traumatic spondylopathy, thoracolumbar region ᴄᴄ
M48.36 Traumatic spondylopathy, lumbar region ᴄᴄ
M48.37 Traumatic spondylopathy, lumbosacral region ᴄᴄ
M48.38 Traumatic spondylopathy, sacral and sacrococcygeal region ᴄᴄ

√5th **M48.4 Fatigue fracture of vertebra**

Stress fracture of vertebra
EXCLUDES 1 *pathological fracture NOS (M84.4-)*
pathological fracture of vertebra due to neoplasm (M84.58)
pathological fracture of vertebra due to osteoporosis (M80.-)
pathological fracture of vertebra due to other diagnosis (M84.68)
traumatic fracture of vertebrae (S12.0-S12.3-, S22.0-, S32.0-)

The appropriate 7th character is to be added to each code from subcategory M48.4.
A initial encounter for fracture
D subsequent encounter for fracture with routine healing
G subsequent encounter for fracture with delayed healing
S sequela of fracture

√x7th M48.40 Fatigue fracture of vertebra, site unspecified
√x7th M48.41 Fatigue fracture of vertebra, occipito-atlanto-axial region
√x7th M48.42 Fatigue fracture of vertebra, cervical region
√x7th M48.43 Fatigue fracture of vertebra, cervicothoracic region
√x7th M48.44 Fatigue fracture of vertebra, thoracic region
√x7th M48.45 Fatigue fracture of vertebra, thoracolumbar region
√x7th M48.46 Fatigue fracture of vertebra, lumbar region
√x7th M48.47 Fatigue fracture of vertebra, lumbosacral region
√x7th M48.48 Fatigue fracture of vertebra, sacral and sacrococcygeal region

√5th **M48.5 Collapsed vertebra, not elsewhere classified**

Collapsed vertebra NOS
Compression fracture of vertebra NOS
Wedging of vertebra NOS
EXCLUDES 1 *current injury - see Injury of spine, by body region*
fatigue fracture of vertebra (M48.4)
pathological fracture NOS (M84.4-)
pathological fracture of vertebra due to neoplasm (M84.58)
pathological fracture of vertebra due to osteoporosis (M80.-)
pathological fracture of vertebra due to other diagnosis (M84.68)
stress fracture of vertebra (M48.4-)
traumatic fracture of vertebra (S12.-, S22.-, S32.-)

The appropriate 7th character is to be added to each code from subcategory M48.5.
A initial encounter for fracture
D subsequent encounter for fracture with routine healing
G subsequent encounter for fracture with delayed healing
S sequela of fracture

6 √x7th M48.50 Collapsed vertebra, not elsewhere classified, site unspecified ᴄᴄ ʜᴄᴄ
6 √x7th M48.51 Collapsed vertebra, not elsewhere classified, occipito-atlanto-axial region ᴄᴄ ʜᴄᴄ
6 √x7th M48.52 Collapsed vertebra, not elsewhere classified, cervical region ᴄᴄ ʜᴄᴄ
6 √x7th M48.53 Collapsed vertebra, not elsewhere classified, cervicothoracic region ᴄᴄ ʜᴄᴄ
6 √x7th M48.54 Collapsed vertebra, not elsewhere classified, thoracic region ᴄᴄ ʜᴄᴄ
6 √x7th M48.55 Collapsed vertebra, not elsewhere classified, thoracolumbar region ᴄᴄ ʜᴄᴄ
6 √x7th M48.56 Collapsed vertebra, not elsewhere classified, lumbar region ᴄᴄ ʜᴄᴄ
6 √x7th M48.57 Collapsed vertebra, not elsewhere classified, lumbosacral region ᴄᴄ ʜᴄᴄ
6 √x7th M48.58 Collapsed vertebra, not elsewhere classified, sacral and sacrococcygeal region ᴄᴄ ʜᴄᴄ

√5th **M48.8 Other specified spondylopathies**

Ossification of posterior longitudinal ligament

√6th M48.8X Other specified spondylopathies

M48.8X1 Other specified spondylopathies, occipito-atlanto-axial region ʜᴄᴄ
M48.8X2 Other specified spondylopathies, cervical region ʜᴄᴄ

Ⓝ Newborn: 0 Ⓟ Pediatric: 0-17 Ⓜ Maternity: 9-64 Ⓐ Adult: 15-124 ᴍᴄᴄ Major Complication/Comorbidity ᴄᴄ Complication/Comorbidity ꜱᴡ Severe Wound Dx

802

ICD-10-CM 2022

M48.8X3   **Other specified spondylopathies, cervicothoracic region**   `HCC`

M48.8X4   **Other specified spondylopathies, thoracic region**   `HCC`

M48.8X5   **Other specified spondylopathies, thoracolumbar region**   `HCC`

M48.8X6   **Other specified spondylopathies, lumbar region**   `HCC`

M48.8X7   **Other specified spondylopathies, lumbosacral region**   `HCC`

M48.8X8   **Other specified spondylopathies, sacral and sacrococcygeal region**   `HCC`

M48.8X9   **Other specified spondylopathies, site unspecified**   `HCC`

M48.9   **Spondylopathy, unspecified**

✓4th **M49**   **Spondylopathies in diseases classified elsewhere**

> INCLUDES   curvature of spine in diseases classified elsewhere
> deformity of spine in diseases classified elsewhere
> kyphosis in diseases classified elsewhere
> scoliosis in diseases classified elsewhere
> spondylopathy in diseases classified elsewhere

Code first underlying disease, such as:
brucellosis (A23.-)
Charcôt-Marie-Tooth disease (G60.0)
enterobacterial infections (A01-A04)
osteitis fibrosa cystica (E21.0)

> EXCLUDES 1   curvature of spine in tuberculosis [Pott's] (A18.01)
> enteropathic arthropathies (M07.-)
> gonococcal spondylitis (A54.41)
> neuropathic spondylopathy in syringomyelia (G95.0)
> neuropathic spondylopathy in tabes dorsalis (A52.11)
> neuropathic [tabes dorsalis] spondylitis (A52.11)
> nonsyphilitic neuropathic spondylopathy NEC (G98.0)
> spondylitis in syphilis (acquired) (A52.77)
> tuberculous spondylitis (A18.01)
> typhoid fever spondylitis (A01.05)

✓5th **M49.8**   **Spondylopathy in diseases classified elsewhere**

M49.80   *Spondylopathy in diseases classified elsewhere, site unspecified*   `HCC`

M49.81   *Spondylopathy in diseases classified elsewhere, occipito-atlanto-axial region*   `HCC`

M49.82   *Spondylopathy in diseases classified elsewhere, cervical region*   `HCC`

M49.83   *Spondylopathy in diseases classified elsewhere, cervicothoracic region*   `HCC`

M49.84   *Spondylopathy in diseases classified elsewhere, thoracic region*   `HCC`

M49.85   *Spondylopathy in diseases classified elsewhere, thoracolumbar region*   `HCC`

M49.86   *Spondylopathy in diseases classified elsewhere, lumbar region*   `HCC`

M49.87   *Spondylopathy in diseases classified elsewhere, lumbosacral region*   `HCC`

M49.88   *Spondylopathy in diseases classified elsewhere, sacral and sacrococcygeal region*   `HCC`

M49.89   *Spondylopathy in diseases classified elsewhere, multiple sites in spine*   `HCC`

Other dorsopathies (M50-M54)

> EXCLUDES 1   current injury - see injury of spine by body region
> discitis NOS (M46.4-)

✓4th **M50**   **Cervical disc disorders**

> NOTE   Code to the most superior level of disorder
> INCLUDES   cervicothoracic disc disorders
> cervicothoracic disc disorders with cervicalgia

AHA: 2016,4Q,39-40; 2016,1Q,17

✓5th **M50.0**   **Cervical disc disorder with myelopathy**

AHA: 2018,3Q,19

M50.00   **Cervical disc disorder with myelopathy, unspecified cervical region**   `CC`

M50.01   **Cervical disc disorder with myelopathy, high cervical region**   `CC`
C2-C3 disc disorder with myelopathy
C3-C4 disc disorder with myelopathy

✓6th **M50.02**   **Cervical disc disorder with myelopathy, mid-cervical region**

M50.020   **Cervical disc disorder with myelopathy, mid-cervical region, unspecified level**   `CC`

M50.021   **Cervical disc disorder at C4-C5 level with myelopathy**   `CC`
C4-C5 disc disorder with myelopathy

M50.022   **Cervical disc disorder at C5-C6 level with myelopathy**   `CC`
C5-C6 disc disorder with myelopathy

M50.023   **Cervical disc disorder at C6-C7 level with myelopathy**   `CC`
C6-C7 disc disorder with myelopathy

M50.03   **Cervical disc disorder with myelopathy, cervicothoracic region**   `CC`
C7-T1 disc disorder with myelopathy

✓5th **M50.1**   **Cervical disc disorder with radiculopathy**

> EXCLUDES 2   brachial radiculitis NOS (M54.13)

AHA: 2018,3Q,19

M50.10   **Cervical disc disorder with radiculopathy, unspecified cervical region**

M50.11   **Cervical disc disorder with radiculopathy, high cervical region**
C2-C3 disc disorder with radiculopathy
C3 radiculopathy due to disc disorder
C3-C4 disc disorder with radiculopathy
C4 radiculopathy due to disc disorder

✓6th **M50.12**   **Cervical disc disorder with radiculopathy, mid-cervical region**

M50.120   **Mid-cervical disc disorder, unspecified level**

M50.121   **Cervical disc disorder at C4-C5 level with radiculopathy**
C4-C5 disc disorder with radiculopathy
C5 radiculopathy due to disc disorder

M50.122   **Cervical disc disorder at C5-C6 level with radiculopathy**
C5-C6 disc disorder with radiculopathy
C6 radiculopathy due to disc disorder

M50.123   **Cervical disc disorder at C6-C7 level with radiculopathy**
C6-C7 disc disorder with radiculopathy
C7 radiculopathy due to disc disorder

M50.13   **Cervical disc disorder with radiculopathy, cervicothoracic region**
C7-T1 disc disorder with radiculopathy
C8 radiculopathy due to disc disorder

✓5th **M50.2**   **Other cervical disc displacement**

M50.20   **Other cervical disc displacement, unspecified cervical region**

M50.21   **Other cervical disc displacement, high cervical region**
Other C2-C3 cervical disc displacement
Other C3-C4 cervical disc displacement

✓6th **M50.22**   **Other cervical disc displacement, mid-cervical region**

M50.220   **Other cervical disc displacement, mid-cervical region, unspecified level**

M50.221   **Other cervical disc displacement at C4-C5 level**
Other C4-C5 cervical disc displacement

M50.222   **Other cervical disc displacement at C5-C6 level**
Other C5-C6 cervical disc displacement

M50.223   **Other cervical disc displacement at C6-C7 level**
Other C6-C7 cervical disc displacement

M50.23   **Other cervical disc displacement, cervicothoracic region**
Other C7-T1 cervical disc displacement

✓5th **M50.3**   **Other cervical disc degeneration**

M50.30   **Other cervical disc degeneration, unspecified cervical region**

M50.31   **Other cervical disc degeneration, high cervical region**
Other C2-C3 cervical disc degeneration
Other C3-C4 cervical disc degeneration

✓ Additional Character Required   √x7th Placeholder   Questionable PDx   Manifestation   Unspecified Dx   UPD Unacceptable PDx   H1-H14 HAC   HCC CMS-HCC Dx   HIV HIV Dx

ICD-10-CM 2022   803

√6ᵗʰ **M50.32** **Other cervical disc degeneration, mid-cervical region**

     M50.320 **Other cervical disc degeneration, mid-cervical region, unspecified level**

     M50.321 **Other cervical disc degeneration at C4-C5 level**

         Other C4-C5 cervical disc degeneration

     M50.322 **Other cervical disc degeneration at C5-C6 level**

         Other C5-C6 cervical disc degeneration

     M50.323 **Other cervical disc degeneration at C6-C7 level**

         Other C6-C7 cervical disc degeneration

     M50.33 **Other cervical disc degeneration, cervicothoracic region**

         Other C7-T1 cervical disc degeneration

√5ᵗʰ **M50.8** **Other cervical disc disorders**

     M50.80 **Other cervical disc disorders, unspecified cervical region**

     M50.81 **Other cervical disc disorders, high cervical region**

         Other C2-C3 cervical disc disorders

         Other C3-C4 cervical disc disorders

√6ᵗʰ **M50.82** **Other cervical disc disorders, mid-cervical region**

     M50.820 **Other cervical disc disorders, mid-cervical region, unspecified level**

     M50.821 **Other cervical disc disorders at C4-C5 level**

         Other C4-C5 cervical disc disorders

     M50.822 **Other cervical disc disorders at C5-C6 level**

         Other C5-C6 cervical disc disorders

     M50.823 **Other cervical disc disorders at C6-C7 level**

         Other C6-C7 cervical disc disorders

     M50.83 **Other cervical disc disorders, cervicothoracic region**

         Other C7-T1 cervical disc disorders

√5ᵗʰ **M50.9** **Cervical disc disorder, unspecified**

     M50.90 **Cervical disc disorder, unspecified, unspecified cervical region**

     M50.91 **Cervical disc disorder, unspecified, high cervical region**

         C2-C3 cervical disc disorder, unspecified

         C3-C4 cervical disc disorder, unspecified

√6ᵗʰ **M50.92** **Cervical disc disorder, unspecified, mid-cervical region**

     M50.920 **Unspecified cervical disc disorder, mid-cervical region, unspecified level**

     M50.921 **Unspecified cervical disc disorder at C4-C5 level**

         Unspecified C4-C5 cervical disc disorder

     M50.922 **Unspecified cervical disc disorder at C5-C6 level**

         Unspecified C5-C6 cervical disc disorder

     M50.923 **Unspecified cervical disc disorder at C6-C7 level**

         Unspecified C6-C7 cervical disc disorder

     M50.93 **Cervical disc disorder, unspecified, cervicothoracic region**

         C7-T1 cervical disc disorder, unspecified

√4ᵗʰ **M51** **Thoracic, thoracolumbar, and lumbosacral intervertebral disc disorders**

     EXCLUDES 2   cervical and cervicothoracic disc disorders (M50.-)

                 sacral and sacrococcygeal disorders (M53.3)

√5ᵗʰ **M51.0** **Thoracic, thoracolumbar and lumbosacral intervertebral disc disorders with myelopathy**

     M51.04 **Intervertebral disc disorders with myelopathy, thoracic region** CC

     M51.05 **Intervertebral disc disorders with myelopathy, thoracolumbar region** CC

     M51.06 **Intervertebral disc disorders with myelopathy, lumbar region** CC

√5ᵗʰ **M51.1** **Thoracic, thoracolumbar and lumbosacral intervertebral disc disorders with radiculopathy**

     Sciatica due to intervertebral disc disorder

     EXCLUDES 1   lumbar radiculitis NOS (M54.16)

                 sciatica NOS (M54.3)

     AHA: 2018,3Q,18

     M51.14 **Intervertebral disc disorders with radiculopathy, thoracic region**

     M51.15 **Intervertebral disc disorders with radiculopathy, thoracolumbar region**

     M51.16 **Intervertebral disc disorders with radiculopathy, lumbar region**

     M51.17 **Intervertebral disc disorders with radiculopathy, lumbosacral region**

√5ᵗʰ **M51.2** **Other thoracic, thoracolumbar and lumbosacral intervertebral disc displacement**

     Lumbago due to displacement of intervertebral disc

Displacement Intervertebral Disc

Nucleus pulposus — Lamina — Ligamentum flavum — Spinal cord — Disc annulus — Herniates through annulus — Spinal nerve

Normal Top View   Herniated Top View

     M51.24 **Other intervertebral disc displacement, thoracic region**

     M51.25 **Other intervertebral disc displacement, thoracolumbar region**

     M51.26 **Other intervertebral disc displacement, lumbar region**

     M51.27 **Other intervertebral disc displacement, lumbosacral region**

√5ᵗʰ **M51.3** **Other thoracic, thoracolumbar and lumbosacral intervertebral disc degeneration**

     AHA: 2018,2Q,15; 2013,3Q,22

     M51.34 **Other intervertebral disc degeneration, thoracic region**

     M51.35 **Other intervertebral disc degeneration, thoracolumbar region**

     M51.36 **Other intervertebral disc degeneration, lumbar region**

     M51.37 **Other intervertebral disc degeneration, lumbosacral region**

√5ᵗʰ **M51.4** **Schmorl's nodes**

     DEF: Irregular bone defect in the margin of the vertebral body that causes herniation into the end plate of the vertebral body.

     M51.44 **Schmorl's nodes, thoracic region**

     M51.45 **Schmorl's nodes, thoracolumbar region**

     M51.46 **Schmorl's nodes, lumbar region**

     M51.47 **Schmorl's nodes, lumbosacral region**

√5ᵗʰ **M51.8** **Other thoracic, thoracolumbar and lumbosacral intervertebral disc disorders**

     M51.84 **Other intervertebral disc disorders, thoracic region**

     M51.85 **Other intervertebral disc disorders, thoracolumbar region**

     M51.86 **Other intervertebral disc disorders, lumbar region**

     M51.87 **Other intervertebral disc disorders, lumbosacral region**

     M51.9 **Unspecified thoracic, thoracolumbar and lumbosacral intervertebral disc disorder**

√4ᵗʰ **M53** **Other and unspecified dorsopathies, not elsewhere classified**

     M53.0 **Cervicocranial syndrome**

         Posterior cervical sympathetic syndrome

     M53.1 **Cervicobrachial syndrome**

         EXCLUDES 2   cervical disc disorder (M50.-)

                    thoracic outlet syndrome (G54.0)

√5ᵗʰ **M53.2** **Spinal instabilities**

     √6ᵗʰ **M53.2X** **Spinal instabilities**

         M53.2X1 **Spinal instabilities, occipito-atlanto-axial region**

         M53.2X2 **Spinal instabilities, cervical region**

         M53.2X3 **Spinal instabilities, cervicothoracic region**

         M53.2X4 **Spinal instabilities, thoracic region**

         M53.2X5 **Spinal instabilities, thoracolumbar region**

         M53.2X6 **Spinal instabilities, lumbar region**

         M53.2X7 **Spinal instabilities, lumbosacral region**

N Newborn: 0   P Pediatric: 0-17   M Maternity: 9-64   A Adult: 15-124   MCC Major Complication/Comorbidity   CC Complication/Comorbidity   SW Severe Wound Dx

804   ICD-10-CM 2022

M53.2X8 Spinal instabilities, sacral and sacrococcygeal region

M53.2X9 Spinal instabilities, site unspecified

M53.3 Sacrococcygeal disorders, not elsewhere classified
Coccygodynia

✓5ᵗʰ **M53.8** Other specified dorsopathies

    M53.80 Other specified dorsopathies, site unspecified

    M53.81 Other specified dorsopathies, occipito-atlanto-axial region

    M53.82 Other specified dorsopathies, cervical region

    M53.83 Other specified dorsopathies, cervicothoracic region

    M53.84 Other specified dorsopathies, thoracic region

    M53.85 Other specified dorsopathies, thoracolumbar region

    M53.86 Other specified dorsopathies, lumbar region

    M53.87 Other specified dorsopathies, lumbosacral region

    M53.88 Other specified dorsopathies, sacral and sacrococcygeal region

M53.9 Dorsopathy, unspecified

✓4ᵗʰ **M54** Dorsalgia

    EXCLUDES 1   psychogenic dorsalgia (F45.41)

✓5ᵗʰ **M54.0** Panniculitis affecting regions of neck and back

    EXCLUDES 1   lupus panniculitis (L93.2)
               panniculitis NOS (M79.3)
               relapsing [Weber-Christian] panniculitis (M35.6)

    M54.00 Panniculitis affecting regions of neck and back, site unspecified

    M54.01 Panniculitis affecting regions of neck and back, occipito-atlanto-axial region

    M54.02 Panniculitis affecting regions of neck and back, cervical region

    M54.03 Panniculitis affecting regions of neck and back, cervicothoracic region

    M54.04 Panniculitis affecting regions of neck and back, thoracic region

    M54.05 Panniculitis affecting regions of neck and back, thoracolumbar region

    M54.06 Panniculitis affecting regions of neck and back, lumbar region

    M54.07 Panniculitis affecting regions of neck and back, lumbosacral region

    M54.08 Panniculitis affecting regions of neck and back, sacral and sacrococcygeal region

    M54.09 Panniculitis affecting regions, neck and back, multiple sites in spine

✓5ᵗʰ **M54.1** Radiculopathy

    Brachial neuritis or radiculitis NOS
    Lumbar neuritis or radiculitis NOS
    Lumbosacral neuritis or radiculitis NOS
    Thoracic neuritis or radiculitis NOS
    Radiculitis NOS

    EXCLUDES 1   neuralgia and neuritis NOS (M79.2)
               radiculopathy with cervical disc disorder (M50.1)
               radiculopathy with lumbar and other intervertebral disc disorder (M51.1-)
               radiculopathy with spondylosis (M47.2-)

    AHA: 2018,3Q,18

    TIP: A code from this subcategory can be used in addition to a spondylolisthesis code (M43.1-) or a spinal stenosis code (M48.0-) when either condition is documented as the cause of the radiculopathy.

    M54.10 Radiculopathy, site unspecified

    M54.11 Radiculopathy, occipito-atlanto-axial region

    M54.12 Radiculopathy, cervical region

    M54.13 Radiculopathy, cervicothoracic region

    M54.14 Radiculopathy, thoracic region

    M54.15 Radiculopathy, thoracolumbar region

    M54.16 Radiculopathy, lumbar region

    M54.17 Radiculopathy, lumbosacral region

    M54.18 Radiculopathy, sacral and sacrococcygeal region

M54.2 Cervicalgia

    EXCLUDES 1   cervicalgia due to intervertebral cervical disc disorder (M50.-)

✓5ᵗʰ **M54.3** Sciatica

    EXCLUDES 1   lesion of sciatic nerve (G57.0)
               sciatica due to intervertebral disc disorder (M51.1-)
               sciatica with lumbago (M54.4-)

    M54.30 Sciatica, unspecified side

    M54.31 Sciatica, right side

    M54.32 Sciatica, left side

✓5ᵗʰ **M54.4** Lumbago with sciatica

    EXCLUDES 1   lumbago with sciatica due to intervertebral disc disorder (M51.1-)

    AHA: 2016,2Q,7

    M54.40 Lumbago with sciatica, unspecified side

    M54.41 Lumbago with sciatica, right side

    M54.42 Lumbago with sciatica, left side

▲ ✓5ᵗʰ **M54.5** Low back pain

    ~~Loin pain~~
    ~~Lumbago NOS~~

    EXCLUDES 1   low back strain (S39.012)
               lumbago due to intervertebral disc displacement (M51.2-)
               lumbago with sciatica (M54.4-)

●   **M54.50** Low back pain, unspecified
           Loin pain
           Lumbago NOS

●   **M54.51** Vertebrogenic low back pain
           Low back vertebral endplate pain

●   **M54.59** Other low back pain

M54.6 Pain in thoracic spine

    EXCLUDES 1   pain in thoracic spine due to intervertebral disc disorder (M51.-)

✓5ᵗʰ **M54.8** Other dorsalgia

    EXCLUDES 1   dorsalgia in thoracic region (M54.6)
               low back pain ▶(M54.5-)◀

    M54.81 Occipital neuralgia

    M54.89 Other dorsalgia

M54.9 Dorsalgia, unspecified
    Backache NOS
    Back pain NOS

SOFT TISSUE DISORDERS (M60-M79)

Disorders of muscles (M60-M63)

EXCLUDES 1   dermatopolymyositis (M33.-)
            muscular dystrophies and myopathies (G71-G72)
            myopathy in amyloidosis (E85.-)
            myopathy in polyarteritis nodosa (M30.0)
            myopathy in rheumatoid arthritis (M05.32)
            myopathy in scleroderma (M34.-)
            myopathy in Sjögren's syndrome (M35.03)
            myopathy in systemic lupus erythematosus (M32.-)

✓4ᵗʰ **M60** Myositis

    EXCLUDES 2   inclusion body myositis [IBM] (G72.41)

✓5ᵗʰ **M60.0** Infective myositis

    Tropical pyomyositis
    Use additional code (B95-B97) to identify infectious agent

    ✓6ᵗʰ **M60.00** Infective myositis, unspecified site

        M60.000 Infective myositis, unspecified right arm   `CC`
            Infective myositis, right upper limb NOS

        M60.001 Infective myositis, unspecified left arm   `CC`
            Infective myositis, left upper limb NOS

        M60.002 Infective myositis, unspecified arm   `CC`
            Infective myositis, upper limb NOS

        M60.003 Infective myositis, unspecified right leg   `CC`
            Infective myositis, right lower limb NOS

        M60.004 Infective myositis, unspecified left leg   `CC`
            Infective myositis, left lower limb NOS

        M60.005 Infective myositis, unspecified leg   `CC`
            Infective myositis, lower limb NOS

        M60.009 Infective myositis, unspecified site   `CC`

    ✓6ᵗʰ **M60.01** Infective myositis, shoulder

        M60.011 Infective myositis, right shoulder   `CC`

✓ Additional Character Required   ✓x7ᵗʰ Placeholder   Questionable PDx   Manifestation   Unspecified Dx   **UPD** Unacceptable PDx   **H1-H4** HAC   **HCC** CMS-HCC Dx   **HIV** HIV Dx

ICD-10-CM 2022   **805**

M60.012 Infective myositis, left shoulder   CC
M60.019 Infective myositis, unspecified shoulder   CC

✓6ᵗʰ M60.02 Infective myositis, upper arm

M60.021 Infective myositis, right upper arm   CC
M60.022 Infective myositis, left upper arm   CC
M60.029 Infective myositis, unspecified upper arm   CC

✓6ᵗʰ M60.03 Infective myositis, forearm

M60.031 Infective myositis, right forearm   CC
M60.032 Infective myositis, left forearm   CC
M60.039 Infective myositis, unspecified forearm   CC

✓6ᵗʰ M60.04 Infective myositis, hand and fingers

M60.041 Infective myositis, right hand   CC
M60.042 Infective myositis, left hand   CC
M60.043 Infective myositis, unspecified hand   CC
M60.044 Infective myositis, right finger(s)   CC
M60.045 Infective myositis, left finger(s)   CC
M60.046 Infective myositis, unspecified finger(s)   CC

✓6ᵗʰ M60.05 Infective myositis, thigh

M60.051 Infective myositis, right thigh   CC
M60.052 Infective myositis, left thigh   CC
M60.059 Infective myositis, unspecified thigh   CC

✓6ᵗʰ M60.06 Infective myositis, lower leg

M60.061 Infective myositis, right lower leg   CC
M60.062 Infective myositis, left lower leg   CC
M60.069 Infective myositis, unspecified lower leg   CC

✓6ᵗʰ M60.07 Infective myositis, ankle, foot and toes

M60.070 Infective myositis, right ankle   CC
M60.071 Infective myositis, left ankle   CC
M60.072 Infective myositis, unspecified ankle   CC
M60.073 Infective myositis, right foot   CC
M60.074 Infective myositis, left foot   CC
M60.075 Infective myositis, unspecified foot   CC
M60.076 Infective myositis, right toe(s)   CC
M60.077 Infective myositis, left toe(s)   CC
M60.078 Infective myositis, unspecified toe(s)   CC

M60.08 Infective myositis, other site   CC
M60.09 Infective myositis, multiple sites   CC

✓5ᵗʰ M60.1 Interstitial myositis

M60.10 Interstitial myositis of unspecified site

✓6ᵗʰ M60.11 Interstitial myositis, shoulder

M60.111 Interstitial myositis, right shoulder
M60.112 Interstitial myositis, left shoulder
M60.119 Interstitial myositis, unspecified shoulder

✓6ᵗʰ M60.12 Interstitial myositis, upper arm

M60.121 Interstitial myositis, right upper arm
M60.122 Interstitial myositis, left upper arm
M60.129 Interstitial myositis, unspecified upper arm

✓6ᵗʰ M60.13 Interstitial myositis, forearm

M60.131 Interstitial myositis, right forearm
M60.132 Interstitial myositis, left forearm
M60.139 Interstitial myositis, unspecified forearm

✓6ᵗʰ M60.14 Interstitial myositis, hand

M60.141 Interstitial myositis, right hand
M60.142 Interstitial myositis, left hand
M60.149 Interstitial myositis, unspecified hand

✓6ᵗʰ M60.15 Interstitial myositis, thigh

M60.151 Interstitial myositis, right thigh
M60.152 Interstitial myositis, left thigh
M60.159 Interstitial myositis, unspecified thigh

✓6ᵗʰ M60.16 Interstitial myositis, lower leg

M60.161 Interstitial myositis, right lower leg
M60.162 Interstitial myositis, left lower leg
M60.169 Interstitial myositis, unspecified lower leg

✓6ᵗʰ M60.17 Interstitial myositis, ankle and foot

M60.171 Interstitial myositis, right ankle and foot
M60.172 Interstitial myositis, left ankle and foot
M60.179 Interstitial myositis, unspecified ankle and foot

M60.18 Interstitial myositis, other site
M60.19 Interstitial myositis, multiple sites

✓5ᵗʰ M60.2 Foreign body granuloma of soft tissue, not elsewhere classified

Use additional code to identify the type of retained foreign body (Z18.-)

EXCLUDES 1   foreign body granuloma of skin and subcutaneous tissue (L92.3)

M60.20 Foreign body granuloma of soft tissue, not elsewhere classified, unspecified site

✓6ᵗʰ M60.21 Foreign body granuloma of soft tissue, not elsewhere classified, shoulder

M60.211 Foreign body granuloma of soft tissue, not elsewhere classified, right shoulder
M60.212 Foreign body granuloma of soft tissue, not elsewhere classified, left shoulder
M60.219 Foreign body granuloma of soft tissue, not elsewhere classified, unspecified shoulder

✓6ᵗʰ M60.22 Foreign body granuloma of soft tissue, not elsewhere classified, upper arm

M60.221 Foreign body granuloma of soft tissue, not elsewhere classified, right upper arm
M60.222 Foreign body granuloma of soft tissue, not elsewhere classified, left upper arm
M60.229 Foreign body granuloma of soft tissue, not elsewhere classified, unspecified upper arm

✓6ᵗʰ M60.23 Foreign body granuloma of soft tissue, not elsewhere classified, forearm

M60.231 Foreign body granuloma of soft tissue, not elsewhere classified, right forearm
M60.232 Foreign body granuloma of soft tissue, not elsewhere classified, left forearm
M60.239 Foreign body granuloma of soft tissue, not elsewhere classified, unspecified forearm

✓6ᵗʰ M60.24 Foreign body granuloma of soft tissue, not elsewhere classified, hand

M60.241 Foreign body granuloma of soft tissue, not elsewhere classified, right hand
M60.242 Foreign body granuloma of soft tissue, not elsewhere classified, left hand
M60.249 Foreign body granuloma of soft tissue, not elsewhere classified, unspecified hand

✓6ᵗʰ M60.25 Foreign body granuloma of soft tissue, not elsewhere classified, thigh

M60.251 Foreign body granuloma of soft tissue, not elsewhere classified, right thigh
M60.252 Foreign body granuloma of soft tissue, not elsewhere classified, left thigh
M60.259 Foreign body granuloma of soft tissue, not elsewhere classified, unspecified thigh

✓6ᵗʰ M60.26 Foreign body granuloma of soft tissue, not elsewhere classified, lower leg

M60.261 Foreign body granuloma of soft tissue, not elsewhere classified, right lower leg
M60.262 Foreign body granuloma of soft tissue, not elsewhere classified, left lower leg
M60.269 Foreign body granuloma of soft tissue, not elsewhere classified, unspecified lower leg

✓6ᵗʰ M60.27 Foreign body granuloma of soft tissue, not elsewhere classified, ankle and foot

M60.271 Foreign body granuloma of soft tissue, not elsewhere classified, right ankle and foot
M60.272 Foreign body granuloma of soft tissue, not elsewhere classified, left ankle and foot
M60.279 Foreign body granuloma of soft tissue, not elsewhere classified, unspecified ankle and foot

M60.28 Foreign body granuloma of soft tissue, not elsewhere classified, other site

N Newborn: 0   P Pediatric: 0-17   M Maternity: 9-64   A Adult: 15-124   MCC Major Complication/Comorbidity   CC Complication/Comorbidity   SW Severe Wound Dx

806

ICD-10-CM 2022

√5ᵗʰ **M60.8 Other myositis**

    M60.80 Other myositis, unspecified site

    √6ᵗʰ **M60.81** Other myositis shoulder

      M60.811 Other myositis, right shoulder
      M60.812 Other myositis, left shoulder
      M60.819 Other myositis, unspecified shoulder

    √6ᵗʰ **M60.82** Other myositis, upper arm

      M60.821 Other myositis, right upper arm
      M60.822 Other myositis, left upper arm
      M60.829 Other myositis, unspecified upper arm

    √6ᵗʰ **M60.83** Other myositis, forearm

      M60.831 Other myositis, right forearm
      M60.832 Other myositis, left forearm
      M60.839 Other myositis, unspecified forearm

    √6ᵗʰ **M60.84** Other myositis, hand

      M60.841 Other myositis, right hand
      M60.842 Other myositis, left hand
      M60.849 Other myositis, unspecified hand

    √6ᵗʰ **M60.85** Other myositis, thigh

      M60.851 Other myositis, right thigh
      M60.852 Other myositis, left thigh
      M60.859 Other myositis, unspecified thigh

    √6ᵗʰ **M60.86** Other myositis, lower leg

      M60.861 Other myositis, right lower leg
      M60.862 Other myositis, left lower leg
      M60.869 Other myositis, unspecified lower leg

    √6ᵗʰ **M60.87** Other myositis, ankle and foot

      M60.871 Other myositis, right ankle and foot
      M60.872 Other myositis, left ankle and foot
      M60.879 Other myositis, unspecified ankle and foot

    M60.88 Other myositis, other site
    M60.89 Other myositis, multiple sites ·

  M60.9 Myositis, unspecified

√4ᵗʰ **M61 Calcification and ossification of muscle**

   √5ᵗʰ **M61.0 Myositis ossificans traumatica**

     M61.00 Myositis ossificans traumatica, unspecified site

     √6ᵗʰ **M61.01** Myositis ossificans traumatica, shoulder

       M61.011 Myositis ossificans traumatica, right shoulder
       M61.012 Myositis ossificans traumatica, left shoulder
       M61.019 Myositis ossificans traumatica, unspecified shoulder

     √6ᵗʰ **M61.02** Myositis ossificans traumatica, upper arm

       M61.021 Myositis ossificans traumatica, right upper arm
       M61.022 Myositis ossificans traumatica, left upper arm
       M61.029 Myositis ossificans traumatica, unspecified upper arm

     √6ᵗʰ **M61.03** Myositis ossificans traumatica, forearm

       M61.031 Myositis ossificans traumatica, right forearm
       M61.032 Myositis ossificans traumatica, left forearm
       M61.039 Myositis ossificans traumatica, unspecified forearm

     √6ᵗʰ **M61.04** Myositis ossificans traumatica, hand

       M61.041 Myositis ossificans traumatica, right hand
       M61.042 Myositis ossificans traumatica, left hand
       M61.049 Myositis ossificans traumatica, unspecified hand

     √6ᵗʰ **M61.05** Myositis ossificans traumatica, thigh

       M61.051 Myositis ossificans traumatica, right thigh
       M61.052 Myositis ossificans traumatica, left thigh
       M61.059 Myositis ossificans traumatica, unspecified thigh

     √6ᵗʰ **M61.06** Myositis ossificans traumatica, lower leg

       M61.061 Myositis ossificans traumatica, right lower leg
       M61.062 Myositis ossificans traumatica, left lower leg
       M61.069 Myositis ossificans traumatica, unspecified lower leg

     √6ᵗʰ **M61.07** Myositis ossificans traumatica, ankle and foot

       M61.071 Myositis ossificans traumatica, right ankle and foot
       M61.072 Myositis ossificans traumatica, left ankle and foot
       M61.079 Myositis ossificans traumatica, unspecified ankle and foot

     M61.08 Myositis ossificans traumatica, other site
     M61.09 Myositis ossificans traumatica, multiple sites

   √5ᵗʰ **M61.1 Myositis ossificans progressiva**

     Fibrodysplasia ossificans progressiva

     M61.10 Myositis ossificans progressiva, unspecified site

     √6ᵗʰ **M61.11** Myositis ossificans progressiva, shoulder

       M61.111 Myositis ossificans progressiva, right shoulder
       M61.112 Myositis ossificans progressiva, left shoulder
       M61.119 Myositis ossificans progressiva, unspecified shoulder

     √6ᵗʰ **M61.12** Myositis ossificans progressiva, upper arm

       M61.121 Myositis ossificans progressiva, right upper arm
       M61.122 Myositis ossificans progressiva, left upper arm
       M61.129 Myositis ossificans progressiva, unspecified arm

     √6ᵗʰ **M61.13** Myositis ossificans progressiva, forearm

       M61.131 Myositis ossificans progressiva, right forearm
       M61.132 Myositis ossificans progressiva, left forearm
       M61.139 Myositis ossificans progressiva, unspecified forearm

     √6ᵗʰ **M61.14** Myositis ossificans progressiva, hand and finger(s)

       M61.141 Myositis ossificans progressiva, right hand
       M61.142 Myositis ossificans progressiva, left hand
       M61.143 Myositis ossificans progressiva, unspecified hand
       M61.144 Myositis ossificans progressiva, right finger(s)
       M61.145 Myositis ossificans progressiva, left finger(s)
       M61.146 Myositis ossificans progressiva, unspecified finger(s)

     √6ᵗʰ **M61.15** Myositis ossificans progressiva, thigh

       M61.151 Myositis ossificans progressiva, right thigh
       M61.152 Myositis ossificans progressiva, left thigh
       M61.159 Myositis ossificans progressiva, unspecified thigh

     √6ᵗʰ **M61.16** Myositis ossificans progressiva, lower leg

       M61.161 Myositis ossificans progressiva, right lower leg
       M61.162 Myositis ossificans progressiva, left lower leg
       M61.169 Myositis ossificans progressiva, unspecified lower leg

     √6ᵗʰ **M61.17** Myositis ossificans progressiva, ankle, foot and toe(s)

       M61.171 Myositis ossificans progressiva, right ankle
       M61.172 Myositis ossificans progressiva, left ankle
       M61.173 Myositis ossificans progressiva, unspecified ankle
       M61.174 Myositis ossificans progressiva, right foot
       M61.175 Myositis ossificans progressiva, left foot
       M61.176 Myositis ossificans progressiva, unspecified foot
       M61.177 Myositis ossificans progressiva, right toe(s)
       M61.178 Myositis ossificans progressiva, left toe(s)
       M61.179 Myositis ossificans progressiva, unspecified toe(s)

     M61.18 Myositis ossificans progressiva, other site
     M61.19 Myositis ossificans progressiva, multiple sites

   √5ᵗʰ **M61.2 Paralytic calcification and ossification of muscle**

     Myositis ossificans associated with quadriplegia or paraplegia

     M61.20 Paralytic calcification and ossification of muscle, unspecified site

✔ Additional Character Required   √x7ᵗʰ Placeholder   Questionable PDx   **Manifestation**   Unspecified Dx   UPD Unacceptable PDx   H1-H14 HAC   HCC CMS-HCC Dx   HIV HIV Dx

ICD-10-CM 2022   **807**

√6ᵗʰ **M61.21 Paralytic calcification and ossification of muscle, shoulder**
- M61.211 Paralytic calcification and ossification of muscle, right shoulder
- M61.212 Paralytic calcification and ossification of muscle, left shoulder
- M61.219 Paralytic calcification and ossification of muscle, unspecified shoulder

√6ᵗʰ **M61.22 Paralytic calcification and ossification of muscle, upper arm**
- M61.221 Paralytic calcification and ossification of muscle, right upper arm
- M61.222 Paralytic calcification and ossification of muscle, left upper arm
- M61.229 Paralytic calcification and ossification of muscle, unspecified upper arm

√6ᵗʰ **M61.23 Paralytic calcification and ossification of muscle, forearm**
- M61.231 Paralytic calcification and ossification of muscle, right forearm
- M61.232 Paralytic calcification and ossification of muscle, left forearm
- M61.239 Paralytic calcification and ossification of muscle, unspecified forearm

√6ᵗʰ **M61.24 Paralytic calcification and ossification of muscle, hand**
- M61.241 Paralytic calcification and ossification of muscle, right hand
- M61.242 Paralytic calcification and ossification of muscle, left hand
- M61.249 Paralytic calcification and ossification of muscle, unspecified hand

√6ᵗʰ **M61.25 Paralytic calcification and ossification of muscle, thigh**
- M61.251 Paralytic calcification and ossification of muscle, right thigh
- M61.252 Paralytic calcification and ossification of muscle, left thigh
- M61.259 Paralytic calcification and ossification of muscle, unspecified thigh

√6ᵗʰ **M61.26 Paralytic calcification and ossification of muscle, lower leg**
- M61.261 Paralytic calcification and ossification of muscle, right lower leg
- M61.262 Paralytic calcification and ossification of muscle, left lower leg
- M61.269 Paralytic calcification and ossification of muscle, unspecified lower leg

√6ᵗʰ **M61.27 Paralytic calcification and ossification of muscle, ankle and foot**
- M61.271 Paralytic calcification and ossification of muscle, right ankle and foot
- M61.272 Paralytic calcification and ossification of muscle, left ankle and foot
- M61.279 Paralytic calcification and ossification of muscle, unspecified ankle and foot

M61.28 Paralytic calcification and ossification of muscle, other site

M61.29 Paralytic calcification and ossification of muscle, multiple sites

√5ᵗʰ **M61.3 Calcification and ossification of muscles associated with burns**

     Myositis ossificans associated with burns

M61.30 Calcification and ossification of muscles associated with burns, unspecified site

√6ᵗʰ **M61.31 Calcification and ossification of muscles associated with burns, shoulder**
- M61.311 Calcification and ossification of muscles associated with burns, right shoulder
- M61.312 Calcification and ossification of muscles associated with burns, left shoulder
- M61.319 Calcification and ossification of muscles associated with burns, unspecified shoulder

√6ᵗʰ **M61.32 Calcification and ossification of muscles associated with burns, upper arm**
- M61.321 Calcification and ossification of muscles associated with burns, right upper arm
- M61.322 Calcification and ossification of muscles associated with burns, left upper arm
- M61.329 Calcification and ossification of muscles associated with burns, unspecified upper arm

√6ᵗʰ **M61.33 Calcification and ossification of muscles associated with burns, forearm**
- M61.331 Calcification and ossification of muscles associated with burns, right forearm
- M61.332 Calcification and ossification of muscles associated with burns, left forearm
- M61.339 Calcification and ossification of muscles associated with burns, unspecified forearm

√6ᵗʰ **M61.34 Calcification and ossification of muscles associated with burns, hand**
- M61.341 Calcification and ossification of muscles associated with burns, right hand
- M61.342 Calcification and ossification of muscles associated with burns, left hand
- M61.349 Calcification and ossification of muscles associated with burns, unspecified hand

√6ᵗʰ **M61.35 Calcification and ossification of muscles associated with burns, thigh**
- M61.351 Calcification and ossification of muscles associated with burns, right thigh
- M61.352 Calcification and ossification of muscles associated with burns, left thigh
- M61.359 Calcification and ossification of muscles associated with burns, unspecified thigh

√6ᵗʰ **M61.36 Calcification and ossification of muscles associated with burns, lower leg**
- M61.361 Calcification and ossification of muscles associated with burns, right lower leg
- M61.362 Calcification and ossification of muscles associated with burns, left lower leg
- M61.369 Calcification and ossification of muscles associated with burns, unspecified lower leg

√6ᵗʰ **M61.37 Calcification and ossification of muscles associated with burns, ankle and foot**
- M61.371 Calcification and ossification of muscles associated with burns, right ankle and foot
- M61.372 Calcification and ossification of muscles associated with burns, left ankle and foot
- M61.379 Calcification and ossification of muscles associated with burns, unspecified ankle and foot

M61.38 Calcification and ossification of muscles associated with burns, other site

M61.39 Calcification and ossification of muscles associated with burns, multiple sites

√5ᵗʰ **M61.4 Other calcification of muscle**

     EXCLUDES 1   calcific tendinitis NOS (M65.2-)
                 calcific tendinitis of shoulder (M75.3)

M61.40 Other calcification of muscle, unspecified site

√6ᵗʰ **M61.41 Other calcification of muscle, shoulder**
- M61.411 Other calcification of muscle, right shoulder
- M61.412 Other calcification of muscle, left shoulder
- M61.419 Other calcification of muscle, unspecified shoulder

√6ᵗʰ **M61.42 Other calcification of muscle, upper arm**
- M61.421 Other calcification of muscle, right upper arm
- M61.422 Other calcification of muscle, left upper arm
- M61.429 Other calcification of muscle, unspecified upper arm

√6ᵗʰ **M61.43 Other calcification of muscle, forearm**
- M61.431 Other calcification of muscle, right forearm
- M61.432 Other calcification of muscle, left forearm
- M61.439 Other calcification of muscle, unspecified forearm

√6ᵗʰ **M61.44 Other calcification of muscle, hand**
- M61.441 Other calcification of muscle, right hand
- M61.442 Other calcification of muscle, left hand
- M61.449 Other calcification of muscle, unspecified hand

√6ᵗʰ **M61.45 Other calcification of muscle, thigh**
- M61.451 Other calcification of muscle, right thigh
- M61.452 Other calcification of muscle, left thigh

N Newborn: 0   P Pediatric: 0-17   M Maternity: 9-64   A Adult: 15-124   MCC Major Complication/Comorbidity   CC Complication/Comorbidity   SW Severe Wound Dx

808

ICD-10-CM 2022

M61.459 Other calcification of muscle, unspecified thigh

√6ᵗʰ **M61.46** Other calcification of muscle, lower leg

M61.461 Other calcification of muscle, right lower leg

M61.462 Other calcification of muscle, left lower leg

M61.469 Other calcification of muscle, unspecified lower leg

√6ᵗʰ **M61.47** Other calcification of muscle, ankle and foot

M61.471 Other calcification of muscle, right ankle and foot

M61.472 Other calcification of muscle, left ankle and foot

M61.479 Other calcification of muscle, unspecified ankle and foot

M61.48 Other calcification of muscle, other site

M61.49 Other calcification of muscle, multiple sites

√5ᵗʰ **M61.5** Other ossification of muscle

M61.50 Other ossification of muscle, unspecified site

√6ᵗʰ **M61.51** Other ossification of muscle, shoulder

M61.511 Other ossification of muscle, right shoulder

M61.512 Other ossification of muscle, left shoulder

M61.519 Other ossification of muscle, unspecified shoulder

√6ᵗʰ **M61.52** Other ossification of muscle, upper arm

M61.521 Other ossification of muscle, right upper arm

M61.522 Other ossification of muscle, left upper arm

M61.529 Other ossification of muscle, unspecified upper arm

√6ᵗʰ **M61.53** Other ossification of muscle, forearm

M61.531 Other ossification of muscle, right forearm

M61.532 Other ossification of muscle, left forearm

M61.539 Other ossification of muscle, unspecified forearm

√6ᵗʰ **M61.54** Other ossification of muscle, hand

M61.541 Other ossification of muscle, right hand

M61.542 Other ossification of muscle, left hand

M61.549 Other ossification of muscle, unspecified hand

√6ᵗʰ **M61.55** Other ossification of muscle, thigh

M61.551 Other ossification of muscle, right thigh

M61.552 Other ossification of muscle, left thigh

M61.559 Other ossification of muscle, unspecified thigh

√6ᵗʰ **M61.56** Other ossification of muscle, lower leg

M61.561 Other ossification of muscle, right lower leg

M61.562 Other ossification of muscle, left lower leg

M61.569 Other ossification of muscle, unspecified lower leg

√6ᵗʰ **M61.57** Other ossification of muscle, ankle and foot

M61.571 Other ossification of muscle, right ankle and foot

M61.572 Other ossification of muscle, left ankle and foot

M61.579 Other ossification of muscle, unspecified ankle and foot

M61.58 Other ossification of muscle, other site

M61.59 Other ossification of muscle, multiple sites

M61.9 Calcification and ossification of muscle, unspecified

√4ᵗʰ **M62** Other disorders of muscle

EXCLUDES 1   *alcoholic myopathy (G72.1)*
cramp and spasm (R25.2)
drug-induced myopathy (G72.0)
myalgia (M79.1-)
stiff-man syndrome (G25.82)

EXCLUDES 2   *nontraumatic hematoma of muscle (M79.81)*

√5ᵗʰ **M62.0** Separation of muscle (nontraumatic)

Diastasis of muscle

EXCLUDES 1   *diastasis recti complicating pregnancy, labor and delivery (O71.8)*
traumatic separation of muscle - see strain of muscle by body region

M62.00 Separation of muscle (nontraumatic), unspecified site

√6ᵗʰ **M62.01** Separation of muscle (nontraumatic), shoulder

M62.011 Separation of muscle (nontraumatic), right shoulder

M62.012 Separation of muscle (nontraumatic), left shoulder

M62.019 Separation of muscle (nontraumatic), unspecified shoulder

√6ᵗʰ **M62.02** Separation of muscle (nontraumatic), upper arm

M62.021 Separation of muscle (nontraumatic), right upper arm

M62.022 Separation of muscle (nontraumatic), left upper arm

M62.029 Separation of muscle (nontraumatic), unspecified upper arm

√6ᵗʰ **M62.03** Separation of muscle (nontraumatic), forearm

M62.031 Separation of muscle (nontraumatic), right forearm

M62.032 Separation of muscle (nontraumatic), left forearm

M62.039 Separation of muscle (nontraumatic), unspecified forearm

√6ᵗʰ **M62.04** Separation of muscle (nontraumatic), hand

M62.041 Separation of muscle (nontraumatic), right hand

M62.042 Separation of muscle (nontraumatic), left hand

M62.049 Separation of muscle (nontraumatic), unspecified hand

√6ᵗʰ **M62.05** Separation of muscle (nontraumatic), thigh

M62.051 Separation of muscle (nontraumatic), right thigh

M62.052 Separation of muscle (nontraumatic), left thigh

M62.059 Separation of muscle (nontraumatic), unspecified thigh

√6ᵗʰ **M62.06** Separation of muscle (nontraumatic), lower leg

M62.061 Separation of muscle (nontraumatic), right lower leg

M62.062 Separation of muscle (nontraumatic), left lower leg

M62.069 Separation of muscle (nontraumatic), unspecified lower leg

√6ᵗʰ **M62.07** Separation of muscle (nontraumatic), ankle and foot

M62.071 Separation of muscle (nontraumatic), right ankle and foot

M62.072 Separation of muscle (nontraumatic), left ankle and foot

M62.079 Separation of muscle (nontraumatic), unspecified ankle and foot

M62.08 Separation of muscle (nontraumatic), other site

√5ᵗʰ **M62.1** Other rupture of muscle (nontraumatic)

EXCLUDES 1   *traumatic rupture of muscle - see strain of muscle by body region*

EXCLUDES 2   *rupture of tendon (M66.-)*

M62.10 Other rupture of muscle (nontraumatic), unspecified site

√6ᵗʰ **M62.11** Other rupture of muscle (nontraumatic), shoulder

M62.111 Other rupture of muscle (nontraumatic), right shoulder

M62.112 Other rupture of muscle (nontraumatic), left shoulder

M62.119 Other rupture of muscle (nontraumatic), unspecified shoulder

✔ Additional Character Required   √x7ᵗʰ Placeholder   Questionable PDx   Manifestation   Unspecified Dx   UPD Unacceptable PDx   H1-H14 HAC   HCC CMS-HCC Dx   HIV HIV Dx

ICD-10-CM 2022   809

✓6ᵗʰ **M62.12 Other rupture of muscle (nontraumatic), upper arm**

     M62.121 Other rupture of muscle (nontraumatic), right upper arm

     M62.122 Other rupture of muscle (nontraumatic), left upper arm

     M62.129 Other rupture of muscle (nontraumatic), unspecified upper arm

✓6ᵗʰ **M62.13 Other rupture of muscle (nontraumatic), forearm**

     M62.131 Other rupture of muscle (nontraumatic), right forearm

     M62.132 Other rupture of muscle (nontraumatic), left forearm

     M62.139 Other rupture of muscle (nontraumatic), unspecified forearm

✓6ᵗʰ **M62.14 Other rupture of muscle (nontraumatic), hand**

     M62.141 Other rupture of muscle (nontraumatic), right hand

     M62.142 Other rupture of muscle (nontraumatic), left hand

     M62.149 Other rupture of muscle (nontraumatic), unspecified hand

✓6ᵗʰ **M62.15 Other rupture of muscle (nontraumatic), thigh**

     M62.151 Other rupture of muscle (nontraumatic), right thigh

     M62.152 Other rupture of muscle (nontraumatic), left thigh

     M62.159 Other rupture of muscle (nontraumatic), unspecified thigh

✓6ᵗʰ **M62.16 Other rupture of muscle (nontraumatic), lower leg**

     M62.161 Other rupture of muscle (nontraumatic), right lower leg

     M62.162 Other rupture of muscle (nontraumatic), left lower leg

     M62.169 Other rupture of muscle (nontraumatic), unspecified lower leg

✓6ᵗʰ **M62.17 Other rupture of muscle (nontraumatic), ankle and foot**

     M62.171 Other rupture of muscle (nontraumatic), right ankle and foot

     M62.172 Other rupture of muscle (nontraumatic), left ankle and foot

     M62.179 Other rupture of muscle (nontraumatic), unspecified ankle and foot

     M62.18 Other rupture of muscle (nontraumatic), other site

✓5ᵗʰ **M62.2 Nontraumatic ischemic infarction of muscle**

     EXCLUDES 1   compartment syndrome (traumatic) (T79.A-)

          nontraumatic compartment syndrome (M79.A-)

          rhabdomyolysis (M62.82)

          traumatic ischemia of muscle (T79.6)

          Volkmann's ischemic contracture (T79.6)

     M62.20 Nontraumatic ischemic infarction of muscle, unspecified site

✓6ᵗʰ **M62.21 Nontraumatic ischemic infarction of muscle, shoulder**

     M62.211 Nontraumatic ischemic infarction of muscle, right shoulder

     M62.212 Nontraumatic ischemic infarction of muscle, left shoulder

     M62.219 Nontraumatic ischemic infarction of muscle, unspecified shoulder

✓6ᵗʰ **M62.22 Nontraumatic ischemic infarction of muscle, upper arm**

     M62.221 Nontraumatic ischemic infarction of muscle, right upper arm

     M62.222 Nontraumatic ischemic infarction of muscle, left upper arm

     M62.229 Nontraumatic ischemic infarction of muscle, unspecified upper arm

✓6ᵗʰ **M62.23 Nontraumatic ischemic infarction of muscle, forearm**

     M62.231 Nontraumatic ischemic infarction of muscle, right forearm

     M62.232 Nontraumatic ischemic infarction of muscle, left forearm

     M62.239 Nontraumatic ischemic infarction of muscle, unspecified forearm

✓6ᵗʰ **M62.24 Nontraumatic ischemic infarction of muscle, hand**

     M62.241 Nontraumatic ischemic infarction of muscle, right hand

     M62.242 Nontraumatic ischemic infarction of muscle, left hand

     M62.249 Nontraumatic ischemic infarction of muscle, unspecified hand

✓6ᵗʰ **M62.25 Nontraumatic ischemic infarction of muscle, thigh**

     M62.251 Nontraumatic ischemic infarction of muscle, right thigh

     M62.252 Nontraumatic ischemic infarction of muscle, left thigh

     M62.259 Nontraumatic ischemic infarction of muscle, unspecified thigh

✓6ᵗʰ **M62.26 Nontraumatic ischemic infarction of muscle, lower leg**

     M62.261 Nontraumatic ischemic infarction of muscle, right lower leg

     M62.262 Nontraumatic ischemic infarction of muscle, left lower leg

     M62.269 Nontraumatic ischemic infarction of muscle, unspecified lower leg

✓6ᵗʰ **M62.27 Nontraumatic ischemic infarction of muscle, ankle and foot**

     M62.271 Nontraumatic ischemic infarction of muscle, right ankle and foot

     M62.272 Nontraumatic ischemic infarction of muscle, left ankle and foot

     M62.279 Nontraumatic ischemic infarction of muscle, unspecified ankle and foot

     M62.28 Nontraumatic ischemic infarction of muscle, other site

     M62.3 Immobility syndrome (paraplegic)

✓5ᵗʰ **M62.4 Contracture of muscle**

     Contracture of tendon (sheath)

     EXCLUDES 1   contracture of joint (M24.5-)

     M62.40 Contracture of muscle, unspecified site

✓6ᵗʰ **M62.41 Contracture of muscle, shoulder**

     M62.411 Contracture of muscle, right shoulder

     M62.412 Contracture of muscle, left shoulder

     M62.419 Contracture of muscle, unspecified shoulder

✓6ᵗʰ **M62.42 Contracture of muscle, upper arm**

     M62.421 Contracture of muscle, right upper arm

     M62.422 Contracture of muscle, left upper arm

     M62.429 Contracture of muscle, unspecified upper arm

✓6ᵗʰ **M62.43 Contracture of muscle, forearm**

     M62.431 Contracture of muscle, right forearm

     M62.432 Contracture of muscle, left forearm

     M62.439 Contracture of muscle, unspecified forearm

✓6ᵗʰ **M62.44 Contracture of muscle, hand**

     M62.441 Contracture of muscle, right hand

     M62.442 Contracture of muscle, left hand

     M62.449 Contracture of muscle, unspecified hand

✓6ᵗʰ **M62.45 Contracture of muscle, thigh**

     M62.451 Contracture of muscle, right thigh

     M62.452 Contracture of muscle, left thigh

     M62.459 Contracture of muscle, unspecified thigh

✓6ᵗʰ **M62.46 Contracture of muscle, lower leg**

     M62.461 Contracture of muscle, right lower leg

     M62.462 Contracture of muscle, left lower leg

     M62.469 Contracture of muscle, unspecified lower leg

✓6ᵗʰ **M62.47 Contracture of muscle, ankle and foot**

     M62.471 Contracture of muscle, right ankle and foot

     M62.472 Contracture of muscle, left ankle and foot

     M62.479 Contracture of muscle, unspecified ankle and foot

     M62.48 Contracture of muscle, other site

     M62.49 Contracture of muscle, multiple sites

✓5ᵗʰ **M62.5 Muscle wasting and atrophy, not elsewhere classified**

     Disuse atrophy NEC

     EXCLUDES 1   neuralgic amyotrophy (G54.5)

          progressive muscular atrophy (G12.21)

          sarcopenia (M62.84)

     EXCLUDES 2   pelvic muscle wasting (N81.84)

     M62.50 Muscle wasting and atrophy, not elsewhere classified, unspecified site

N Newborn: 0   P Pediatric: 0-17   M Maternity: 9-64   A Adult: 15-124   MCC Major Complication/Comorbidity   CC Complication/Comorbidity   SW Severe Wound Dx

810   ICD-10-CM 2022

✓6ᵗʰ **M62.51 Muscle wasting and atrophy, not elsewhere classified, shoulder**
- **M62.511 Muscle wasting and atrophy, not elsewhere classified, right shoulder**
- **M62.512 Muscle wasting and atrophy, not elsewhere classified, left shoulder**
- **M62.519 Muscle wasting and atrophy, not elsewhere classified, unspecified shoulder**

✓6ᵗʰ **M62.52 Muscle wasting and atrophy, not elsewhere classified, upper arm**
- **M62.521 Muscle wasting and atrophy, not elsewhere classified, right upper arm**
- **M62.522 Muscle wasting and atrophy, not elsewhere classified, left upper arm**
- **M62.529 Muscle wasting and atrophy, not elsewhere classified, unspecified upper arm**

✓6ᵗʰ **M62.53 Muscle wasting and atrophy, not elsewhere classified, forearm**
- **M62.531 Muscle wasting and atrophy, not elsewhere classified, right forearm**
- **M62.532 Muscle wasting and atrophy, not elsewhere classified, left forearm**
- **M62.539 Muscle wasting and atrophy, not elsewhere classified, unspecified forearm**

✓6ᵗʰ **M62.54 Muscle wasting and atrophy, not elsewhere classified, hand**
- **M62.541 Muscle wasting and atrophy, not elsewhere classified, right hand**
- **M62.542 Muscle wasting and atrophy, not elsewhere classified, left hand**
- **M62.549 Muscle wasting and atrophy, not elsewhere classified, unspecified hand**

✓6ᵗʰ **M62.55 Muscle wasting and atrophy, not elsewhere classified, thigh**
- **M62.551 Muscle wasting and atrophy, not elsewhere classified, right thigh**
- **M62.552 Muscle wasting and atrophy, not elsewhere classified, left thigh**
- **M62.559 Muscle wasting and atrophy, not elsewhere classified, unspecified thigh**

✓6ᵗʰ **M62.56 Muscle wasting and atrophy, not elsewhere classified, lower leg**
- **M62.561 Muscle wasting and atrophy, not elsewhere classified, right lower leg**
- **M62.562 Muscle wasting and atrophy, not elsewhere classified, left lower leg**
- **M62.569 Muscle wasting and atrophy, not elsewhere classified, unspecified lower leg**

✓6ᵗʰ **M62.57 Muscle wasting and atrophy, not elsewhere classified, ankle and foot**
- **M62.571 Muscle wasting and atrophy, not elsewhere classified, right ankle and foot**
- **M62.572 Muscle wasting and atrophy, not elsewhere classified, left ankle and foot**
- **M62.579 Muscle wasting and atrophy, not elsewhere classified, unspecified ankle and foot**

M62.58 Muscle wasting and atrophy, not elsewhere classified, other site

M62.59 Muscle wasting and atrophy, not elsewhere classified, multiple sites

✓5ᵗʰ **M62.8 Other specified disorders of muscle**
> EXCLUDES 2   nontraumatic hematoma of muscle (M79.81)

M62.81 Muscle weakness (generalized)
> EXCLUDES 1   muscle weakness in sarcopenia (M62.84)

M62.82 Rhabdomyolysis   CC
> EXCLUDES 1   traumatic rhabdomyolysis (T79.6)

   AHA: 2019,2Q,12
   DEF: Rapid disintegration or destruction of skeletal muscle caused by direct or indirect injury, resulting in the excretion of muscle protein myoglobin into the urine.

✓6ᵗʰ **M62.83 Muscle spasm**
- **M62.830 Muscle spasm of back**
- **M62.831 Muscle spasm of calf**
  - Charley-horse
- **M62.838 Other muscle spasm**

M62.84 Sarcopenia
> Age-related sarcopenia
> Code first underlying disease, if applicable, such as:
>   disorders of myoneural junction and muscle disease in diseases classified elsewhere (G73.-)
>   other and unspecified myopathies (G72.-)
>   primary disorders of muscles (G71.-)
> **AHA:** 2016,4Q,41

M62.89 Other specified disorders of muscle
> Muscle (sheath) hernia

M62.9 Disorder of muscle, unspecified

✓4ᵗʰ **M63 Disorders of muscle in diseases classified elsewhere**
> Code first underlying disease, such as:
>   leprosy (A30.-)
>   neoplasm (C49.-, C79.89, D21.-, D48.1)
>   schistosomiasis (B65.-)
>   trichinellosis (B75)
> EXCLUDES 1   myopathy in cysticercosis (B69.81)
>   myopathy in endocrine diseases (G73.7)
>   myopathy in metabolic diseases (G73.7)
>   myopathy in sarcoidosis (D86.87)
>   myopathy in secondary syphilis (A51.49)
>   myopathy in syphilis (late) (A52.78)
>   myopathy in toxoplasmosis (B58.82)
>   myopathy in tuberculosis (A18.09)

✓5ᵗʰ **M63.8 Disorders of muscle in diseases classified elsewhere**

M63.80 *Disorders of muscle in diseases classified elsewhere, unspecified site*

✓6ᵗʰ **M63.81 Disorders of muscle in diseases classified elsewhere, shoulder**
- **M63.811 *Disorders of muscle in diseases classified elsewhere, right shoulder***
- **M63.812 *Disorders of muscle in diseases classified elsewhere, left shoulder***
- **M63.819 *Disorders of muscle in diseases classified elsewhere, unspecified shoulder***

✓6ᵗʰ **M63.82 Disorders of muscle in diseases classified elsewhere, upper arm**
- **M63.821 *Disorders of muscle in diseases classified elsewhere, right upper arm***
- **M63.822 *Disorders of muscle in diseases classified elsewhere, left upper arm***
- **M63.829 *Disorders of muscle in diseases classified elsewhere, unspecified upper arm***

✓6ᵗʰ **M63.83 Disorders of muscle in diseases classified elsewhere, forearm**
- **M63.831 *Disorders of muscle in diseases classified elsewhere, right forearm***
- **M63.832 *Disorders of muscle in diseases classified elsewhere, left forearm***
- **M63.839 *Disorders of muscle in diseases classified elsewhere, unspecified forearm***

✓6ᵗʰ **M63.84 Disorders of muscle in diseases classified elsewhere, hand**
- **M63.841 *Disorders of muscle in diseases classified elsewhere, right hand***
- **M63.842 *Disorders of muscle in diseases classified elsewhere, left hand***
- **M63.849 *Disorders of muscle in diseases classified elsewhere, unspecified hand***

✓6ᵗʰ **M63.85 Disorders of muscle in diseases classified elsewhere, thigh**
- **M63.851 *Disorders of muscle in diseases classified elsewhere, right thigh***
- **M63.852 *Disorders of muscle in diseases classified elsewhere, left thigh***
- **M63.859 *Disorders of muscle in diseases classified elsewhere, unspecified thigh***

✓6ᵗʰ **M63.86 Disorders of muscle in diseases classified elsewhere, lower leg**
- **M63.861 *Disorders of muscle in diseases classified elsewhere, right lower leg***
- **M63.862 *Disorders of muscle in diseases classified elsewhere, left lower leg***
- **M63.869 *Disorders of muscle in diseases classified elsewhere, unspecified lower leg***

✓6ᵗʰ **M63.87 Disorders of muscle in diseases classified elsewhere, ankle and foot**
- **M63.871 *Disorders of muscle in diseases classified elsewhere, right ankle and foot***

✔ Additional Character Required   ✓x7ᵗʰ Placeholder   Questionable PDx   Manifestation   Unspecified Dx   UPD Unacceptable PDx   H1–H14 HAC   HCC CMS-HCC Dx   HIV HIV Dx

ICD-10-CM 2022   811

       M63.872 *Disorders of muscle in diseases classified elsewhere, left ankle and foot*

       M63.879 *Disorders of muscle in diseases classified elsewhere, unspecified ankle and foot*

    M63.88 *Disorders of muscle in diseases classified elsewhere, other site*

    M63.89 *Disorders of muscle in diseases classified elsewhere, multiple sites*

Disorders of synovium and tendon (M65-M67)

✓4ᵗʰ **M65 Synovitis and tenosynovitis**

    EXCLUDES 1   *chronic crepitant synovitis of hand and wrist (M70.0-)*

        current injury - see injury of ligament or tendon by body region

        soft tissue disorders related to use, overuse and pressure (M70.-)

  ✓5ᵗʰ **M65.0 Abscess of tendon sheath**

    Use additional code (B95-B96) to identify bacterial agent.

    M65.00 Abscess of tendon sheath, unspecified site

    ✓6ᵗʰ **M65.01 Abscess of tendon sheath, shoulder**

       M65.011 Abscess of tendon sheath, right shoulder

       M65.012 Abscess of tendon sheath, left shoulder

       M65.019 Abscess of tendon sheath, unspecified shoulder

    ✓6ᵗʰ **M65.02 Abscess of tendon sheath, upper arm**

       M65.021 Abscess of tendon sheath, right upper arm

       M65.022 Abscess of tendon sheath, left upper arm

       M65.029 Abscess of tendon sheath, unspecified upper arm

    ✓6ᵗʰ **M65.03 Abscess of tendon sheath, forearm**

       M65.031 Abscess of tendon sheath, right forearm

       M65.032 Abscess of tendon sheath, left forearm

       M65.039 Abscess of tendon sheath, unspecified forearm

    ✓6ᵗʰ **M65.04 Abscess of tendon sheath, hand**

       M65.041 Abscess of tendon sheath, right hand

       M65.042 Abscess of tendon sheath, left hand

       M65.049 Abscess of tendon sheath, unspecified hand

    ✓6ᵗʰ **M65.05 Abscess of tendon sheath, thigh**

       M65.051 Abscess of tendon sheath, right thigh

       M65.052 Abscess of tendon sheath, left thigh

       M65.059 Abscess of tendon sheath, unspecified thigh

    ✓6ᵗʰ **M65.06 Abscess of tendon sheath, lower leg**

       M65.061 Abscess of tendon sheath, right lower leg

       M65.062 Abscess of tendon sheath, left lower leg

       M65.069 Abscess of tendon sheath, unspecified lower leg

    ✓6ᵗʰ **M65.07 Abscess of tendon sheath, ankle and foot**

       M65.071 Abscess of tendon sheath, right ankle and foot

       M65.072 Abscess of tendon sheath, left ankle and foot

       M65.079 Abscess of tendon sheath, unspecified ankle and foot

    M65.08 Abscess of tendon sheath, other site

  ✓5ᵗʰ **M65.1 Other infective (teno)synovitis**

    M65.10 Other infective (teno)synovitis, unspecified site

    ✓6ᵗʰ **M65.11 Other infective (teno)synovitis, shoulder**

       M65.111 Other infective (teno)synovitis, right shoulder

       M65.112 Other infective (teno)synovitis, left shoulder

       M65.119 Other infective (teno)synovitis, unspecified shoulder

    ✓6ᵗʰ **M65.12 Other infective (teno)synovitis, elbow**

       M65.121 Other infective (teno)synovitis, right elbow

       M65.122 Other infective (teno)synovitis, left elbow

       M65.129 Other infective (teno)synovitis, unspecified elbow

    ✓6ᵗʰ **M65.13 Other infective (teno)synovitis, wrist**

       M65.131 Other infective (teno)synovitis, right wrist

       M65.132 Other infective (teno)synovitis, left wrist

       M65.139 Other infective (teno)synovitis, unspecified wrist

    ✓6ᵗʰ **M65.14 Other infective (teno)synovitis, hand**

       M65.141 Other infective (teno)synovitis, right hand

       M65.142 Other infective (teno)synovitis, left hand

       M65.149 Other infective (teno)synovitis, unspecified hand

    ✓6ᵗʰ **M65.15 Other infective (teno)synovitis, hip**

       M65.151 Other infective (teno)synovitis, right hip

       M65.152 Other infective (teno)synovitis, left hip

       M65.159 Other infective (teno)synovitis, unspecified hip

    ✓6ᵗʰ **M65.16 Other infective (teno)synovitis, knee**

       M65.161 Other infective (teno)synovitis, right knee

       M65.162 Other infective (teno)synovitis, left knee

       M65.169 Other infective (teno)synovitis, unspecified knee

    ✓6ᵗʰ **M65.17 Other infective (teno)synovitis, ankle and foot**

       M65.171 Other infective (teno)synovitis, right ankle and foot

       M65.172 Other infective (teno)synovitis, left ankle and foot

       M65.179 Other infective (teno)synovitis, unspecified ankle and foot

    M65.18 Other infective (teno)synovitis, other site

    M65.19 Other infective (teno)synovitis, multiple sites

  ✓5ᵗʰ **M65.2 Calcific tendinitis**

    EXCLUDES 1   *tendinitis as classified in M75-M77*

        calcified tendinitis of shoulder (M75.3)

    M65.20 Calcific tendinitis, unspecified site

    ✓6ᵗʰ **M65.22 Calcific tendinitis, upper arm**

       M65.221 Calcific tendinitis, right upper arm

       M65.222 Calcific tendinitis, left upper arm

       M65.229 Calcific tendinitis, unspecified upper arm

    ✓6ᵗʰ **M65.23 Calcific tendinitis, forearm**

       M65.231 Calcific tendinitis, right forearm

       M65.232 Calcific tendinitis, left forearm

       M65.239 Calcific tendinitis, unspecified forearm

    ✓6ᵗʰ **M65.24 Calcific tendinitis, hand**

       M65.241 Calcific tendinitis, right hand

       M65.242 Calcific tendinitis, left hand

       M65.249 Calcific tendinitis, unspecified hand

    ✓6ᵗʰ **M65.25 Calcific tendinitis, thigh**

       M65.251 Calcific tendinitis, right thigh

       M65.252 Calcific tendinitis, left thigh

       M65.259 Calcific tendinitis, unspecified thigh

    ✓6ᵗʰ **M65.26 Calcific tendinitis, lower leg**

       M65.261 Calcific tendinitis, right lower leg

       M65.262 Calcific tendinitis, left lower leg

       M65.269 Calcific tendinitis, unspecified lower leg

    ✓6ᵗʰ **M65.27 Calcific tendinitis, ankle and foot**

       M65.271 Calcific tendinitis, right ankle and foot

       M65.272 Calcific tendinitis, left ankle and foot

       M65.279 Calcific tendinitis, unspecified ankle and foot

    M65.28 Calcific tendinitis, other site

    M65.29 Calcific tendinitis, multiple sites

  ✓5ᵗʰ **M65.3 Trigger finger**

    Nodular tendinous disease

    M65.30 Trigger finger, unspecified finger

    ✓6ᵗʰ **M65.31 Trigger thumb**

       M65.311 Trigger thumb, right thumb

       M65.312 Trigger thumb, left thumb

       M65.319 Trigger thumb, unspecified thumb

    ✓6ᵗʰ **M65.32 Trigger finger, index finger**

       M65.321 Trigger finger, right index finger

       M65.322 Trigger finger, left index finger

       M65.329 Trigger finger, unspecified index finger

    ✓6ᵗʰ **M65.33 Trigger finger, middle finger**

       M65.331 Trigger finger, right middle finger

       M65.332 Trigger finger, left middle finger

       M65.339 Trigger finger, unspecified middle finger

    ✓6ᵗʰ **M65.34 Trigger finger, ring finger**

       M65.341 Trigger finger, right ring finger

       M65.342 Trigger finger, left ring finger

       M65.349 Trigger finger, unspecified ring finger

N Newborn: 0   P Pediatric: 0-17   M Maternity: 9-64   A Adult: 15-124   MCC Major Complication/Comorbidity   CC Complication/Comorbidity   SW Severe Wound Dx

812
ICD-10-CM 2022

✓6ᵗʰ **M65.35 Trigger finger,** little finger

    M65.351 **Trigger finger,** right little finger
    M65.352 **Trigger finger,** left little finger
    M65.359 **Trigger finger, unspecified little finger**

M65.4 Radial styloid tenosynovitis [de Quervain]

✓5ᵗʰ **M65.8 Other synovitis and tenosynovitis**

    M65.80 **Other synovitis and tenosynovitis, unspecified site**

    ✓6ᵗʰ M65.81 **Other synovitis and tenosynovitis,** shoulder

        M65.811 **Other synovitis and tenosynovitis,** right shoulder
        M65.812 **Other synovitis and tenosynovitis,** left shoulder
        M65.819 **Other synovitis and tenosynovitis, unspecified shoulder**

    ✓6ᵗʰ M65.82 **Other synovitis and tenosynovitis,** upper arm

        M65.821 **Other synovitis and tenosynovitis,** right upper arm
        M65.822 **Other synovitis and tenosynovitis,** left upper arm
        M65.829 **Other synovitis and tenosynovitis, unspecified upper arm**

    ✓6ᵗʰ M65.83 **Other synovitis and tenosynovitis,** forearm

        M65.831 **Other synovitis and tenosynovitis,** right forearm
        M65.832 **Other synovitis and tenosynovitis,** left forearm
        M65.839 **Other synovitis and tenosynovitis, unspecified forearm**

    ✓6ᵗʰ M65.84 **Other synovitis and tenosynovitis,** hand

        M65.841 **Other synovitis and tenosynovitis,** right hand
        M65.842 **Other synovitis and tenosynovitis,** left hand
        M65.849 **Other synovitis and tenosynovitis, unspecified hand**

    ✓6ᵗʰ M65.85 **Other synovitis and tenosynovitis,** thigh

        M65.851 **Other synovitis and tenosynovitis,** right thigh
        M65.852 **Other synovitis and tenosynovitis,** left thigh
        M65.859 **Other synovitis and tenosynovitis, unspecified thigh**

    ✓6ᵗʰ M65.86 **Other synovitis and tenosynovitis,** lower leg

        M65.861 **Other synovitis and tenosynovitis,** right lower leg
        M65.862 **Other synovitis and tenosynovitis,** left lower leg
        M65.869 **Other synovitis and tenosynovitis, unspecified lower leg**

    ✓6ᵗʰ M65.87 **Other synovitis and tenosynovitis,** ankle and foot

        M65.871 **Other synovitis and tenosynovitis,** right ankle and foot
        M65.872 **Other synovitis and tenosynovitis,** left ankle and foot
        M65.879 **Other synovitis and tenosynovitis, unspecified ankle and foot**

    M65.88 **Other synovitis and tenosynovitis, other site**
    M65.89 **Other synovitis and tenosynovitis,** multiple sites

    M65.9 **Synovitis and tenosynovitis, unspecified**

✓4ᵗʰ **M66 Spontaneous rupture of synovium and tendon**

    INCLUDES rupture that occurs when a normal force is applied to tissues that are inferred to have less than normal strength

    EXCLUDES 2 *rotator cuff syndrome (M75.1-)*
        rupture where an abnormal force is applied to normal tissue - see injury of tendon by body region

M66.0 Rupture of popliteal cyst

✓5ᵗʰ **M66.1 Rupture of** synovium

    Rupture of synovial cyst
    EXCLUDES 2 *rupture of popliteal cyst (M66.0)*

    M66.10 **Rupture of synovium, unspecified joint**

    ✓6ᵗʰ M66.11 **Rupture of synovium,** shoulder

        M66.111 **Rupture of synovium,** right shoulder
        M66.112 **Rupture of synovium,** left shoulder
        M66.119 **Rupture of synovium, unspecified shoulder**

    ✓6ᵗʰ M66.12 **Rupture of synovium,** elbow

        M66.121 **Rupture of synovium,** right elbow

        M66.122 **Rupture of synovium,** left elbow
        M66.129 **Rupture of synovium, unspecified elbow**

✓6ᵗʰ M66.13 **Rupture of synovium,** wrist

    M66.131 **Rupture of synovium,** right wrist
    M66.132 **Rupture of synovium,** left wrist
    M66.139 **Rupture of synovium, unspecified wrist**

✓6ᵗʰ M66.14 **Rupture of synovium,** hand and fingers

    M66.141 **Rupture of synovium,** right hand
    M66.142 **Rupture of synovium,** left hand
    M66.143 **Rupture of synovium, unspecified hand**
    M66.144 **Rupture of synovium,** right finger(s)
    M66.145 **Rupture of synovium,** left finger(s)
    M66.146 **Rupture of synovium, unspecified finger(s)**

✓6ᵗʰ M66.15 **Rupture of synovium,** hip

    M66.151 **Rupture of synovium,** right hip
    M66.152 **Rupture of synovium,** left hip
    M66.159 **Rupture of synovium, unspecified hip**

✓6ᵗʰ M66.17 **Rupture of synovium,** ankle, foot and toes

    M66.171 **Rupture of synovium,** right ankle
    M66.172 **Rupture of synovium,** left ankle
    M66.173 **Rupture of synovium, unspecified ankle**
    M66.174 **Rupture of synovium,** right foot
    M66.175 **Rupture of synovium,** left foot
    M66.176 **Rupture of synovium, unspecified foot**
    M66.177 **Rupture of synovium,** right toe(s)
    M66.178 **Rupture of synovium,** left toe(s)
    M66.179 **Rupture of synovium, unspecified toe(s)**

    M66.18 **Rupture of synovium, other site**

✓5ᵗʰ **M66.2 Spontaneous rupture of** extensor tendons

    TIP: Refer to the Muscle/Tendon table at the beginning of this chapter.

    M66.20 **Spontaneous rupture of extensor tendons, unspecified site**

    ✓6ᵗʰ M66.21 **Spontaneous rupture of extensor tendons,** shoulder

        M66.211 **Spontaneous rupture of extensor tendons,** right shoulder
        M66.212 **Spontaneous rupture of extensor tendons,** left shoulder
        M66.219 **Spontaneous rupture of extensor tendons, unspecified shoulder**

    ✓6ᵗʰ M66.22 **Spontaneous rupture of extensor tendons,** upper arm

        M66.221 **Spontaneous rupture of extensor tendons,** right upper arm
        M66.222 **Spontaneous rupture of extensor tendons,** left upper arm
        M66.229 **Spontaneous rupture of extensor tendons, unspecified upper arm**

    ✓6ᵗʰ M66.23 **Spontaneous rupture of extensor tendons,** forearm

        M66.231 **Spontaneous rupture of extensor tendons,** right forearm
        M66.232 **Spontaneous rupture of extensor tendons,** left forearm
        M66.239 **Spontaneous rupture of extensor tendons, unspecified forearm**

    ✓6ᵗʰ M66.24 **Spontaneous rupture of extensor tendons,** hand

        M66.241 **Spontaneous rupture of extensor tendons,** right hand
        M66.242 **Spontaneous rupture of extensor tendons,** left hand
        M66.249 **Spontaneous rupture of extensor tendons, unspecified hand**

    ✓6ᵗʰ M66.25 **Spontaneous rupture of extensor tendons,** thigh

        M66.251 **Spontaneous rupture of extensor tendons,** right thigh
        M66.252 **Spontaneous rupture of extensor tendons,** left thigh
        M66.259 **Spontaneous rupture of extensor tendons, unspecified thigh**

    ✓6ᵗʰ M66.26 **Spontaneous rupture of extensor tendons,** lower leg

        M66.261 **Spontaneous rupture of extensor tendons,** right lower leg
        M66.262 **Spontaneous rupture of extensor tendons,** left lower leg
        M66.269 **Spontaneous rupture of extensor tendons, unspecified lower leg**

√6th **M66.27** **Spontaneous rupture of extensor tendons,** ankle and foot

    M66.271 **Spontaneous rupture of extensor tendons,** right **ankle and foot**

    M66.272 **Spontaneous rupture of extensor tendons,** left **ankle and foot**

    M66.279 **Spontaneous rupture of extensor tendons, unspecified ankle and foot**

M66.28 **Spontaneous rupture of extensor tendons, other site**

M66.29 **Spontaneous rupture of extensor tendons,** multiple sites

√5th **M66.3** **Spontaneous rupture of** flexor tendons

    TIP: Refer to the Muscle/Tendon table at the beginning of this chapter.

    M66.30 **Spontaneous rupture of flexor tendons, unspecified site**

√6th **M66.31** **Spontaneous rupture of flexor tendons,** shoulder

    M66.311 **Spontaneous rupture of flexor tendons,** right **shoulder**

    M66.312 **Spontaneous rupture of flexor tendons,** left **shoulder**

    M66.319 **Spontaneous rupture of flexor tendons, unspecified shoulder**

√6th **M66.32** **Spontaneous rupture of flexor tendons,** upper arm

    M66.321 **Spontaneous rupture of flexor tendons,** right **upper arm**

    M66.322 **Spontaneous rupture of flexor tendons,** left **upper arm**

    M66.329 **Spontaneous rupture of flexor tendons, unspecified upper arm**

√6th **M66.33** **Spontaneous rupture of flexor tendons,** forearm

    M66.331 **Spontaneous rupture of flexor tendons,** right **forearm**

    M66.332 **Spontaneous rupture of flexor tendons,** left **forearm**

    M66.339 **Spontaneous rupture of flexor tendons, unspecified forearm**

√6th **M66.34** **Spontaneous rupture of flexor tendons,** hand

    M66.341 **Spontaneous rupture of flexor tendons,** right **hand**

    M66.342 **Spontaneous rupture of flexor tendons,** left **hand**

    M66.349 **Spontaneous rupture of flexor tendons, unspecified hand**

√6th **M66.35** **Spontaneous rupture of flexor tendons,** thigh

    M66.351 **Spontaneous rupture of flexor tendons,** right **thigh**

    M66.352 **Spontaneous rupture of flexor tendons,** left **thigh**

    M66.359 **Spontaneous rupture of flexor tendons, unspecified thigh**

√6th **M66.36** **Spontaneous rupture of flexor tendons,** lower leg

    M66.361 **Spontaneous rupture of flexor tendons,** right **lower leg**

    M66.362 **Spontaneous rupture of flexor tendons,** left **lower leg**

    M66.369 **Spontaneous rupture of flexor tendons, unspecified lower leg**

√6th **M66.37** **Spontaneous rupture of flexor tendons,** ankle and foot

    M66.371 **Spontaneous rupture of flexor tendons,** right **ankle and foot**

    M66.372 **Spontaneous rupture of flexor tendons,** left **ankle and foot**

    M66.379 **Spontaneous rupture of flexor tendons, unspecified ankle and foot**

M66.38 **Spontaneous rupture of flexor tendons, other site**

M66.39 **Spontaneous rupture of flexor tendons,** multiple sites

√5th **M66.8** **Spontaneous rupture of** other tendons

    TIP: Refer to the Muscle/Tendon table at the beginning of this chapter.

    M66.80 **Spontaneous rupture of other tendons, unspecified site**

√6th **M66.81** **Spontaneous rupture of other tendons,** shoulder

    M66.811 **Spontaneous rupture of other tendons,** right **shoulder**

    M66.812 **Spontaneous rupture of other tendons,** left **shoulder**

    M66.819 **Spontaneous rupture of other tendons, unspecified shoulder**

√6th **M66.82** **Spontaneous rupture of other tendons,** upper arm

    M66.821 **Spontaneous rupture of other tendons,** right **upper arm**

    M66.822 **Spontaneous rupture of other tendons,** left **upper arm**

    M66.829 **Spontaneous rupture of other tendons, unspecified upper arm**

√6th **M66.83** **Spontaneous rupture of other tendons,** forearm

    M66.831 **Spontaneous rupture of other tendons,** right **forearm**

    M66.832 **Spontaneous rupture of other tendons,** left **forearm**

    M66.839 **Spontaneous rupture of other tendons, unspecified forearm**

√6th **M66.84** **Spontaneous rupture of other tendons,** hand

    M66.841 **Spontaneous rupture of other tendons,** right **hand**

    M66.842 **Spontaneous rupture of other tendons,** left **hand**

    M66.849 **Spontaneous rupture of other tendons, unspecified hand**

√6th **M66.85** **Spontaneous rupture of other tendons,** thigh

    M66.851 **Spontaneous rupture of other tendons,** right **thigh**

    M66.852 **Spontaneous rupture of other tendons,** left **thigh**

    M66.859 **Spontaneous rupture of other tendons, unspecified thigh**

√6th **M66.86** **Spontaneous rupture of other tendons,** lower leg

    M66.861 **Spontaneous rupture of other tendons,** right **lower leg**

    M66.862 **Spontaneous rupture of other tendons,** left **lower leg**

    M66.869 **Spontaneous rupture of other tendons, unspecified lower leg**

√6th **M66.87** **Spontaneous rupture of other tendons,** ankle and foot

    M66.871 **Spontaneous rupture of other tendons,** right **ankle and foot**

    M66.872 **Spontaneous rupture of other tendons,** left **ankle and foot**

    M66.879 **Spontaneous rupture of other tendons, unspecified ankle and foot**

M66.88 **Spontaneous rupture of other tendons, other sites**

M66.89 **Spontaneous rupture of other tendons,** multiple sites

M66.9 **Spontaneous rupture of unspecified tendon**

    Rupture at musculotendinous junction, nontraumatic

√4th **M67** **Other disorders of synovium and tendon**

    EXCLUDES 1   *palmar fascial fibromatosis [Dupuytren] (M72.0)*

          tendinitis NOS (M77.9-)

          xanthomatosis localized to tendons (E78.2)

√5th **M67.0** **Short Achilles tendon (acquired)**

    M67.00 **Short Achilles tendon (acquired), unspecified ankle**

    M67.01 **Short Achilles tendon (acquired),** right **ankle**

    M67.02 **Short Achilles tendon (acquired),** left **ankle**

√5th **M67.2** **Synovial hypertrophy, not elsewhere classified**

    EXCLUDES 1   *villonodular synovitis (pigmented) (M12.2-)*

    M67.20 **Synovial hypertrophy, not elsewhere classified, unspecified site**

√6th **M67.21** **Synovial hypertrophy, not elsewhere classified,** shoulder

    M67.211 **Synovial hypertrophy, not elsewhere classified,** right **shoulder**

    M67.212 **Synovial hypertrophy, not elsewhere classified,** left **shoulder**

    M67.219 **Synovial hypertrophy, not elsewhere classified, unspecified shoulder**

√6th **M67.22** **Synovial hypertrophy, not elsewhere classified,** upper arm

    M67.221 **Synovial hypertrophy, not elsewhere classified,** right **upper arm**

    M67.222 **Synovial hypertrophy, not elsewhere classified,** left **upper arm**

    M67.229 **Synovial hypertrophy, not elsewhere classified, unspecified upper arm**

N Newborn: 0   P Pediatric: 0-17   M Maternity: 9-64   A Adult: 15-124   MCC Major Complication/Comorbidity   CC Complication/Comorbidity   SW Severe Wound Dx

814   ICD-10-CM 2022

√6ᵗʰ **M67.23** **Synovial hypertrophy, not elsewhere classified, forearm**

    M67.231 Synovial hypertrophy, not elsewhere classified, right forearm

    M67.232 Synovial hypertrophy, not elsewhere classified, left forearm

    M67.239 Synovial hypertrophy, not elsewhere classified, unspecified forearm

√6ᵗʰ **M67.24** **Synovial hypertrophy, not elsewhere classified, hand**

    M67.241 Synovial hypertrophy, not elsewhere classified, right hand

    M67.242 Synovial hypertrophy, not elsewhere classified, left hand

    M67.249 Synovial hypertrophy, not elsewhere classified, unspecified hand

√6ᵗʰ **M67.25** **Synovial hypertrophy, not elsewhere classified, thigh**

    M67.251 Synovial hypertrophy, not elsewhere classified, right thigh

    M67.252 Synovial hypertrophy, not elsewhere classified, left thigh

    M67.259 Synovial hypertrophy, not elsewhere classified, unspecified thigh

√6ᵗʰ **M67.26** **Synovial hypertrophy, not elsewhere classified, lower leg**

    M67.261 Synovial hypertrophy, not elsewhere classified, right lower leg

    M67.262 Synovial hypertrophy, not elsewhere classified, left lower leg

    M67.269 Synovial hypertrophy, not elsewhere classified, unspecified lower leg

√6ᵗʰ **M67.27** **Synovial hypertrophy, not elsewhere classified, ankle and foot**

    M67.271 Synovial hypertrophy, not elsewhere classified, right ankle and foot

    M67.272 Synovial hypertrophy, not elsewhere classified, left ankle and foot

    M67.279 Synovial hypertrophy, not elsewhere classified, unspecified ankle and foot

M67.28 **Synovial hypertrophy, not elsewhere classified, other site**

M67.29 **Synovial hypertrophy, not elsewhere classified, multiple sites**

√5ᵗʰ **M67.3** **Transient synovitis**

    Toxic synovitis

    EXCLUDES 1 *palindromic rheumatism (M12.3-)*

    M67.30 Transient synovitis, unspecified site

√6ᵗʰ **M67.31** **Transient synovitis, shoulder**

    M67.311 Transient synovitis, right shoulder

    M67.312 Transient synovitis, left shoulder

    M67.319 Transient synovitis, unspecified shoulder

√6ᵗʰ **M67.32** **Transient synovitis, elbow**

    M67.321 Transient synovitis, right elbow

    M67.322 Transient synovitis, left elbow

    M67.329 Transient synovitis, unspecified elbow

√6ᵗʰ **M67.33** **Transient synovitis, wrist**

    M67.331 Transient synovitis, right wrist

    M67.332 Transient synovitis, left wrist

    M67.339 Transient synovitis, unspecified wrist

√6ᵗʰ **M67.34** **Transient synovitis, hand**

    M67.341 Transient synovitis, right hand

    M67.342 Transient synovitis, left hand

    M67.349 Transient synovitis, unspecified hand

√6ᵗʰ **M67.35** **Transient synovitis, hip**

    M67.351 Transient synovitis, right hip

    M67.352 Transient synovitis, left hip

    M67.359 Transient synovitis, unspecified hip

√6ᵗʰ **M67.36** **Transient synovitis, knee**

    M67.361 Transient synovitis, right knee

    M67.362 Transient synovitis, left knee

    M67.369 Transient synovitis, unspecified knee

√6ᵗʰ **M67.37** **Transient synovitis, ankle and foot**

    M67.371 Transient synovitis, right ankle and foot

    M67.372 Transient synovitis, left ankle and foot

    M67.379 Transient synovitis, unspecified ankle and foot

M67.38 **Transient synovitis, other site**

M67.39 **Transient synovitis, multiple sites**

√5ᵗʰ **M67.4** **Ganglion**

    Ganglion of joint or tendon (sheath)

    EXCLUDES 1 *ganglion in yaws (A66.6)*

    EXCLUDES 2 *cyst of bursa (M71.2-M71.3)*

        cyst of synovium (M71.2-M71.3)

    DEF: Fluid-filled, benign cyst appearing on a tendon sheath or aponeurosis, frequently connecting to an underlying joint.

    M67.40 Ganglion, unspecified site

√6ᵗʰ **M67.41** **Ganglion, shoulder**

    M67.411 Ganglion, right shoulder

    M67.412 Ganglion, left shoulder

    M67.419 Ganglion, unspecified shoulder

√6ᵗʰ **M67.42** **Ganglion, elbow**

    M67.421 Ganglion, right elbow

    M67.422 Ganglion, left elbow

    M67.429 Ganglion, unspecified elbow

√6ᵗʰ **M67.43** **Ganglion, wrist**

Ganglion of Wrist

Extensor tendon sheaths

Ganglion of wrist (fluid-filled sac)

    M67.431 Ganglion, right wrist

    M67.432 Ganglion, left wrist

    M67.439 Ganglion, unspecified wrist

√6ᵗʰ **M67.44** **Ganglion, hand**

    M67.441 Ganglion, right hand

    M67.442 Ganglion, left hand

    M67.449 Ganglion, unspecified hand

√6ᵗʰ **M67.45** **Ganglion, hip**

    M67.451 Ganglion, right hip

    M67.452 Ganglion, left hip

    M67.459 Ganglion, unspecified hip

√6ᵗʰ **M67.46** **Ganglion, knee**

    M67.461 Ganglion, right knee

    M67.462 Ganglion, left knee

    M67.469 Ganglion, unspecified knee

√6ᵗʰ **M67.47** **Ganglion, ankle and foot**

    M67.471 Ganglion, right ankle and foot

    M67.472 Ganglion, left ankle and foot

    M67.479 Ganglion, unspecified ankle and foot

M67.48 **Ganglion, other site**

M67.49 **Ganglion, multiple sites**

√5ᵗʰ **M67.5** **Plica syndrome**

    Plica knee

    M67.50 Plica syndrome, unspecified knee

    M67.51 Plica syndrome, right knee

    M67.52 Plica syndrome, left knee

√5ᵗʰ **M67.8** **Other specified disorders of synovium and tendon**

    M67.80 Other specified disorders of synovium and tendon, unspecified site

√6ᵗʰ **M67.81** **Other specified disorders of synovium and tendon, shoulder**

    M67.811 Other specified disorders of synovium, right shoulder

    M67.812 Other specified disorders of synovium, left shoulder

    M67.813 Other specified disorders of tendon, right shoulder

☑ Additional Character Required   √x7ᵗʰ Placeholder   Questionable PDx   Manifestation   Unspecified Dx   UPD Unacceptable PDx   H1-H14 HAC   HCC CMS-HCC Dx   HIV HIV Dx

ICD-10-CM 2022   815

Chapter 13. Diseases of the Musculoskeletal System and Connective Tissue

M67.814–M70.041

        M67.814   Other specified disorders of tendon, left shoulder

        M67.819   Other specified disorders of synovium and tendon, unspecified shoulder

✓6ᵗʰ   M67.82   Other specified disorders of synovium and tendon, elbow

        M67.821   Other specified disorders of synovium, right elbow

        M67.822   Other specified disorders of synovium, left elbow

        M67.823   Other specified disorders of tendon, right elbow

        M67.824   Other specified disorders of tendon, left elbow

        M67.829   Other specified disorders of synovium and tendon, unspecified elbow

✓6ᵗʰ   M67.83   Other specified disorders of synovium and tendon, wrist

        M67.831   Other specified disorders of synovium, right wrist

        M67.832   Other specified disorders of synovium, left wrist

        M67.833   Other specified disorders of tendon, right wrist

        M67.834   Other specified disorders of tendon, left wrist

        M67.839   Other specified disorders of synovium and tendon, unspecified wrist

✓6ᵗʰ   M67.84   Other specified disorders of synovium and tendon, hand

        M67.841   Other specified disorders of synovium, right hand

        M67.842   Other specified disorders of synovium, left hand

        M67.843   Other specified disorders of tendon, right hand

        M67.844   Other specified disorders of tendon, left hand

        M67.849   Other specified disorders of synovium and tendon, unspecified hand

✓6ᵗʰ   M67.85   Other specified disorders of synovium and tendon, hip

        M67.851   Other specified disorders of synovium, right hip

        M67.852   Other specified disorders of synovium, left hip

        M67.853   Other specified disorders of tendon, right hip

        M67.854   Other specified disorders of tendon, left hip

        M67.859   Other specified disorders of synovium and tendon, unspecified hip

✓6ᵗʰ   M67.86   Other specified disorders of synovium and tendon, knee

        M67.861   Other specified disorders of synovium, right knee

        M67.862   Other specified disorders of synovium, left knee

        M67.863   Other specified disorders of tendon, right knee

        M67.864   Other specified disorders of tendon, left knee

        M67.869   Other specified disorders of synovium and tendon, unspecified knee

✓6ᵗʰ   M67.87   Other specified disorders of synovium and tendon, ankle and foot

        M67.871   Other specified disorders of synovium, right ankle and foot

        M67.872   Other specified disorders of synovium, left ankle and foot

        M67.873   Other specified disorders of tendon, right ankle and foot

        M67.874   Other specified disorders of tendon, left ankle and foot

        M67.879   Other specified disorders of synovium and tendon, unspecified ankle and foot

     M67.88   Other specified disorders of synovium and tendon, other site

     M67.89   Other specified disorders of synovium and tendon, multiple sites

✓5ᵗʰ   M67.9   Unspecified disorder of synovium and tendon

     M67.90   Unspecified disorder of synovium and tendon, unspecified site

✓6ᵗʰ   M67.91   Unspecified disorder of synovium and tendon, shoulder

        M67.911   Unspecified disorder of synovium and tendon, right shoulder

        M67.912   Unspecified disorder of synovium and tendon, left shoulder

        M67.919   Unspecified disorder of synovium and tendon, unspecified shoulder

✓6ᵗʰ   M67.92   Unspecified disorder of synovium and tendon, upper arm

        M67.921   Unspecified disorder of synovium and tendon, right upper arm

        M67.922   Unspecified disorder of synovium and tendon, left upper arm

        M67.929   Unspecified disorder of synovium and tendon, unspecified upper arm

✓6ᵗʰ   M67.93   Unspecified disorder of synovium and tendon, forearm

        M67.931   Unspecified disorder of synovium and tendon, right forearm

        M67.932   Unspecified disorder of synovium and tendon, left forearm

        M67.939   Unspecified disorder of synovium and tendon, unspecified forearm

✓6ᵗʰ   M67.94   Unspecified disorder of synovium and tendon, hand

        M67.941   Unspecified disorder of synovium and tendon, right hand

        M67.942   Unspecified disorder of synovium and tendon, left hand

        M67.949   Unspecified disorder of synovium and tendon, unspecified hand

✓6ᵗʰ   M67.95   Unspecified disorder of synovium and tendon, thigh

        M67.951   Unspecified disorder of synovium and tendon, right thigh

        M67.952   Unspecified disorder of synovium and tendon, left thigh

        M67.959   Unspecified disorder of synovium and tendon, unspecified thigh

✓6ᵗʰ   M67.96   Unspecified disorder of synovium and tendon, lower leg

        M67.961   Unspecified disorder of synovium and tendon, right lower leg

        M67.962   Unspecified disorder of synovium and tendon, left lower leg

        M67.969   Unspecified disorder of synovium and tendon, unspecified lower leg

✓6ᵗʰ   M67.97   Unspecified disorder of synovium and tendon, ankle and foot

        M67.971   Unspecified disorder of synovium and tendon, right ankle and foot

        M67.972   Unspecified disorder of synovium and tendon, left ankle and foot

        M67.979   Unspecified disorder of synovium and tendon, unspecified ankle and foot

     M67.98   Unspecified disorder of synovium and tendon, other site

     M67.99   Unspecified disorder of synovium and tendon, multiple sites

Other soft tissue disorders (M70-M79)

✓4ᵗʰ   **M70**   Soft tissue disorders related to use, overuse and pressure

    INCLUDES   soft tissue disorders of occupational origin

    Use additional external cause code to identify activity causing disorder (Y93.-)

    EXCLUDES 1   bursitis NOS (M71.9-)

    EXCLUDES 2   bursitis of shoulder (M75.5)

               enthesopathies (M76-M77)

               pressure ulcer (pressure area) (L89.-)

✓5ᵗʰ   **M70.0**   Crepitant synovitis (acute) (chronic) of hand and wrist

✓6ᵗʰ   M70.03   Crepitant synovitis (acute) (chronic), wrist

        M70.031   Crepitant synovitis (acute) (chronic), right wrist

        M70.032   Crepitant synovitis (acute) (chronic), left wrist

        M70.039   Crepitant synovitis (acute) (chronic), unspecified wrist

✓6ᵗʰ   M70.04   Crepitant synovitis (acute) (chronic), hand

        M70.041   Crepitant synovitis (acute) (chronic), right hand

N Newborn: 0   P Pediatric: 0-17   M Maternity: 9-64   A Adult: 15-124   **MCC** Major Complication/Comorbidity   **CC** Complication/Comorbidity   **SW** Severe Wound Dx

816   ICD-10-CM 2022

M70.042 Crepitant synovitis (acute) (chronic), left hand

M70.049 Crepitant synovitis (acute) (chronic), unspecified hand

✓5ᵗʰ M70.1 Bursitis of hand

M70.10 Bursitis, unspecified hand

M70.11 Bursitis, right hand

M70.12 Bursitis, left hand

✓5ᵗʰ M70.2 Olecranon bursitis

M70.20 Olecranon bursitis, unspecified elbow

M70.21 Olecranon bursitis, right elbow

M70.22 Olecranon bursitis, left elbow

✓5ᵗʰ M70.3 Other bursitis of elbow

M70.30 Other bursitis of elbow, unspecified elbow

M70.31 Other bursitis of elbow, right elbow

M70.32 Other bursitis of elbow, left elbow

✓5ᵗʰ M70.4 Prepatellar bursitis

M70.40 Prepatellar bursitis, unspecified knee

M70.41 Prepatellar bursitis, right knee

M70.42 Prepatellar bursitis, left knee

Knee Bursae

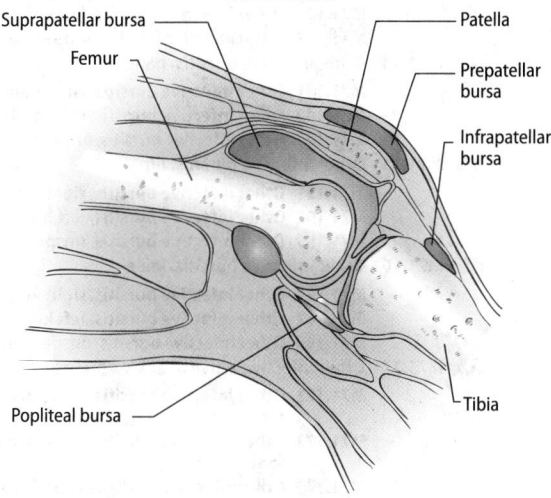

Suprapatellar bursa — Patella
Femur
Prepatellar bursa
Infrapatellar bursa
Popliteal bursa — Tibia

✓5ᵗʰ M70.5 Other bursitis of knee

M70.50 Other bursitis of knee, unspecified knee

M70.51 Other bursitis of knee, right knee

M70.52 Other bursitis of knee, left knee

✓5ᵗʰ M70.6 Trochanteric bursitis

Trochanteric tendinitis

M70.60 Trochanteric bursitis, unspecified hip

M70.61 Trochanteric bursitis, right hip

M70.62 Trochanteric bursitis, left hip

✓5ᵗʰ M70.7 Other bursitis of hip

Ischial bursitis

M70.70 Other bursitis of hip, unspecified hip

M70.71 Other bursitis of hip, right hip

M70.72 Other bursitis of hip, left hip

✓5ᵗʰ M70.8 Other soft tissue disorders related to use, overuse and pressure

M70.80 Other soft tissue disorders related to use, overuse and pressure of unspecified site

✓6ᵗʰ M70.81 Other soft tissue disorders related to use, overuse and pressure of shoulder

M70.811 Other soft tissue disorders related to use, overuse and pressure, right shoulder

M70.812 Other soft tissue disorders related to use, overuse and pressure, left shoulder

M70.819 Other soft tissue disorders related to use, overuse and pressure, unspecified shoulder

✓6ᵗʰ M70.82 Other soft tissue disorders related to use, overuse and pressure of upper arm

M70.821 Other soft tissue disorders related to use, overuse and pressure, right upper arm

M70.822 Other soft tissue diseases related to use, overuse and pressure, left upper arm

M70.829 Other soft tissue disorders related to use, overuse and pressure, unspecified upper arms

✓6ᵗʰ M70.83 Other soft tissue disorders related to use, overuse and pressure of forearm

M70.831 Other soft tissue disorders related to use, overuse and pressure, right forearm

M70.832 Other soft tissue disorders related to use, overuse and pressure, left forearm

M70.839 Other soft tissue disorders related to use, overuse and pressure, unspecified forearm

✓6ᵗʰ M70.84 Other soft tissue disorders related to use, overuse and pressure of hand

M70.841 Other soft tissue disorders related to use, overuse and pressure, right hand

M70.842 Other soft tissue disorders related to use, overuse and pressure, left hand

M70.849 Other soft tissue disorders related to use, overuse and pressure, unspecified hand

✓6ᵗʰ M70.85 Other soft tissue disorders related to use, overuse and pressure of thigh

M70.851 Other soft tissue disorders related to use, overuse and pressure, right thigh

M70.852 Other soft tissue disorders related to use, overuse and pressure, left thigh

M70.859 Other soft tissue disorders related to use, overuse and pressure, unspecified thigh

✓6ᵗʰ M70.86 Other soft tissue disorders related to use, overuse and pressure lower leg

M70.861 Other soft tissue disorders related to use, overuse and pressure, right lower leg

M70.862 Other soft tissue disorders related to use, overuse and pressure, left lower leg

M70.869 Other soft tissue disorders related to use, overuse and pressure, unspecified leg

✓6ᵗʰ M70.87 Other soft tissue disorders related to use, overuse and pressure of ankle and foot

M70.871 Other soft tissue disorders related to use, overuse and pressure, right ankle and foot

M70.872 Other soft tissue disorders related to use, overuse and pressure, left ankle and foot

M70.879 Other soft tissue disorders related to use, overuse and pressure, unspecified ankle and foot

M70.88 Other soft tissue disorders related to use, overuse and pressure other site

M70.89 Other soft tissue disorders related to use, overuse and pressure multiple sites

✓5ᵗʰ M70.9 Unspecified soft tissue disorder related to use, overuse and pressure

M70.90 Unspecified soft tissue disorder related to use, overuse and pressure of unspecified site

✓6ᵗʰ M70.91 Unspecified soft tissue disorder related to use, overuse and pressure of shoulder

M70.911 Unspecified soft tissue disorder related to use, overuse and pressure, right shoulder

M70.912 Unspecified soft tissue disorder related to use, overuse and pressure, left shoulder

M70.919 Unspecified soft tissue disorder related to use, overuse and pressure, unspecified shoulder

✓6ᵗʰ M70.92 Unspecified soft tissue disorder related to use, overuse and pressure of upper arm

M70.921 Unspecified soft tissue disorder related to use, overuse and pressure, right upper arm

M70.922 Unspecified soft tissue disorder related to use, overuse and pressure, left upper arm

M70.929 Unspecified soft tissue disorder related to use, overuse and pressure, unspecified upper arm

✓6ᵗʰ M70.93 Unspecified soft tissue disorder related to use, overuse and pressure of forearm

M70.931 Unspecified soft tissue disorder related to use, overuse and pressure, right forearm

M70.932 Unspecified soft tissue disorder related to use, overuse and pressure, left forearm

M70.939 Unspecified soft tissue disorder related to use, overuse and pressure, unspecified forearm

✓6ᵗʰ **M70.94** Unspecified soft tissue disorder related to use, overuse and pressure of hand

M70.941 Unspecified soft tissue disorder related to use, overuse and pressure, right hand

M70.942 Unspecified soft tissue disorder related to use, overuse and pressure, left hand

M70.949 Unspecified soft tissue disorder related to use, overuse and pressure, unspecified hand

✓6ᵗʰ **M70.95** Unspecified soft tissue disorder related to use, overuse and pressure of thigh

M70.951 Unspecified soft tissue disorder related to use, overuse and pressure, right thigh

M70.952 Unspecified soft tissue disorder related to use, overuse and pressure, left thigh

M70.959 Unspecified soft tissue disorder related to use, overuse and pressure, unspecified thigh

✓6ᵗʰ **M70.96** Unspecified soft tissue disorder related to use, overuse and pressure lower leg

M70.961 Unspecified soft tissue disorder related to use, overuse and pressure, right lower leg

M70.962 Unspecified soft tissue disorder related to use, overuse and pressure, left lower leg

M70.969 Unspecified soft tissue disorder related to use, overuse and pressure, unspecified lower leg

✓6ᵗʰ **M70.97** Unspecified soft tissue disorder related to use, overuse and pressure of ankle and foot

M70.971 Unspecified soft tissue disorder related to use, overuse and pressure, right ankle and foot

M70.972 Unspecified soft tissue disorder related to use, overuse and pressure, left ankle and foot

M70.979 Unspecified soft tissue disorder related to use, overuse and pressure, unspecified ankle and foot

M70.98 Unspecified soft tissue disorder related to use, overuse and pressure other

M70.99 Unspecified soft tissue disorder related to use, overuse and pressure multiple sites

✓4ᵗʰ **M71** **Other bursopathies**

> EXCLUDES 1   bunion (M20.1)
> bursitis related to use, overuse or pressure (M70.-)
> enthesopathies (M76-M77)

✓5ᵗʰ **M71.0** **Abscess of bursa**

> Use additional code (B95.-, B96.-) to identify causative organism

M71.00 Abscess of bursa, unspecified site

✓6ᵗʰ **M71.01** Abscess of bursa, shoulder

M71.011 Abscess of bursa, right shoulder

M71.012 Abscess of bursa, left shoulder

M71.019 Abscess of bursa, unspecified shoulder

✓6ᵗʰ **M71.02** Abscess of bursa, elbow

M71.021 Abscess of bursa, right elbow

M71.022 Abscess of bursa, left elbow

M71.029 Abscess of bursa, unspecified elbow

✓6ᵗʰ **M71.03** Abscess of bursa, wrist

M71.031 Abscess of bursa, right wrist

M71.032 Abscess of bursa, left wrist

M71.039 Abscess of bursa, unspecified wrist

✓6ᵗʰ **M71.04** Abscess of bursa, hand

M71.041 Abscess of bursa, right hand

M71.042 Abscess of bursa, left hand

M71.049 Abscess of bursa, unspecified hand

✓6ᵗʰ **M71.05** Abscess of bursa, hip

M71.051 Abscess of bursa, right hip

M71.052 Abscess of bursa, left hip

M71.059 Abscess of bursa, unspecified hip

✓6ᵗʰ **M71.06** Abscess of bursa, knee

M71.061 Abscess of bursa, right knee

M71.062 Abscess of bursa, left knee

M71.069 Abscess of bursa, unspecified knee

✓6ᵗʰ **M71.07** Abscess of bursa, ankle and foot

M71.071 Abscess of bursa, right ankle and foot

M71.072 Abscess of bursa, left ankle and foot

M71.079 Abscess of bursa, unspecified ankle and foot

M71.08 Abscess of bursa, other site

M71.09 Abscess of bursa, multiple sites

✓5ᵗʰ **M71.1** **Other infective bursitis**

> Use additional code (B95.-, B96.-) to identify causative organism

M71.10 Other infective bursitis, unspecified site

✓6ᵗʰ **M71.11** Other infective bursitis, shoulder

M71.111 Other infective bursitis, right shoulder

M71.112 Other infective bursitis, left shoulder

M71.119 Other infective bursitis, unspecified shoulder

✓6ᵗʰ **M71.12** Other infective bursitis, elbow

M71.121 Other infective bursitis, right elbow

M71.122 Other infective bursitis, left elbow

M71.129 Other infective bursitis, unspecified elbow

✓6ᵗʰ **M71.13** Other infective bursitis, wrist

M71.131 Other infective bursitis, right wrist

M71.132 Other infective bursitis, left wrist

M71.139 Other infective bursitis, unspecified wrist

✓6ᵗʰ **M71.14** Other infective bursitis, hand

M71.141 Other infective bursitis, right hand

M71.142 Other infective bursitis, left hand

M71.149 Other infective bursitis, unspecified hand

✓6ᵗʰ **M71.15** Other infective bursitis, hip

M71.151 Other infective bursitis, right hip

M71.152 Other infective bursitis, left hip

M71.159 Other infective bursitis, unspecified hip

✓6ᵗʰ **M71.16** Other infective bursitis, knee

M71.161 Other infective bursitis, right knee

M71.162 Other infective bursitis, left knee

M71.169 Other infective bursitis, unspecified knee

✓6ᵗʰ **M71.17** Other infective bursitis, ankle and foot

M71.171 Other infective bursitis, right ankle and foot

M71.172 Other infective bursitis, left ankle and foot

M71.179 Other infective bursitis, unspecified ankle and foot

M71.18 Other infective bursitis, other site

M71.19 Other infective bursitis, multiple sites

✓5ᵗʰ **M71.2** **Synovial cyst of popliteal space [Baker]**

> EXCLUDES 1   synovial cyst of popliteal space with rupture (M66.0)
> **DEF:** Sac filled with clear synovial fluid in adults, usually secondary to disease inside the joint, located on the back of the knee in the popliteal fossa area. In children, the cyst usually represents a ganglion of one of the tendons in the knee.

Baker's Cyst

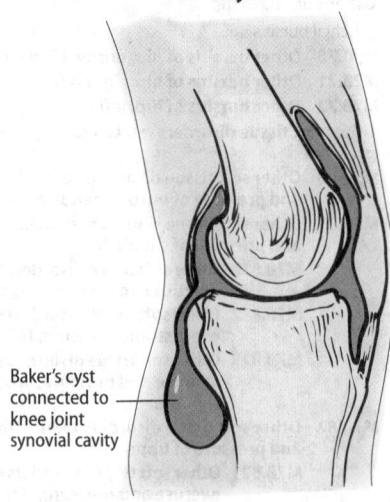

Baker's cyst connected to knee joint synovial cavity

M71.20 Synovial cyst of popliteal space [Baker], unspecified knee

M71.21 Synovial cyst of popliteal space [Baker], right knee

Ⓝ Newborn: 0   Ⓟ Pediatric: 0-17   Ⓜ Maternity: 9-64   Ⓐ Adult: 15-124   **MCC** Major Complication/Comorbidity   **CC** Complication/Comorbidity   **SW** Severe Wound Dx

818   ICD-10-CM 2022

M71.22   Synovial cyst of popliteal space [Baker], left knee

✓5ᵗʰ **M71.3   Other bursal cyst**

Synovial cyst NOS

EXCLUDES 1   *synovial cyst with rupture (M66.1-)*

M71.30   Other bursal cyst, unspecified site

✓6ᵗʰ **M71.31   Other bursal cyst, shoulder**

M71.311   Other bursal cyst, right shoulder
M71.312   Other bursal cyst, left shoulder
M71.319   Other bursal cyst, unspecified shoulder

✓6ᵗʰ **M71.32   Other bursal cyst, elbow**

M71.321   Other bursal cyst, right elbow
M71.322   Other bursal cyst, left elbow
M71.329   Other bursal cyst, unspecified elbow

✓6ᵗʰ **M71.33   Other bursal cyst, wrist**

M71.331   Other bursal cyst, right wrist
M71.332   Other bursal cyst, left wrist
M71.339   Other bursal cyst, unspecified wrist

✓6ᵗʰ **M71.34   Other bursal cyst, hand**

M71.341   Other bursal cyst, right hand
M71.342   Other bursal cyst, left hand
M71.349   Other bursal cyst, unspecified hand

✓6ᵗʰ **M71.35   Other bursal cyst, hip**

M71.351   Other bursal cyst, right hip
M71.352   Other bursal cyst, left hip
M71.359   Other bursal cyst, unspecified hip

✓6ᵗʰ **M71.37   Other bursal cyst, ankle and foot**

M71.371   Other bursal cyst, right ankle and foot
M71.372   Other bursal cyst, left ankle and foot
M71.379   Other bursal cyst, unspecified ankle and foot

M71.38   Other bursal cyst, other site

M71.39   Other bursal cyst, multiple sites

✓5ᵗʰ **M71.4   Calcium deposit in bursa**

EXCLUDES 2   *calcium deposit in bursa of shoulder (M75.3)*

M71.40   Calcium deposit in bursa, unspecified site

✓6ᵗʰ **M71.42   Calcium deposit in bursa, elbow**

M71.421   Calcium deposit in bursa, right elbow
M71.422   Calcium deposit in bursa, left elbow
M71.429   Calcium deposit in bursa, unspecified elbow

✓6ᵗʰ **M71.43   Calcium deposit in bursa, wrist**

M71.431   Calcium deposit in bursa, right wrist
M71.432   Calcium deposit in bursa, left wrist
M71.439   Calcium deposit in bursa, unspecified wrist

✓6ᵗʰ **M71.44   Calcium deposit in bursa, hand**

M71.441   Calcium deposit in bursa, right hand
M71.442   Calcium deposit in bursa, left hand
M71.449   Calcium deposit in bursa, unspecified hand

✓6ᵗʰ **M71.45   Calcium deposit in bursa, hip**

M71.451   Calcium deposit in bursa, right hip
M71.452   Calcium deposit in bursa, left hip
M71.459   Calcium deposit in bursa, unspecified hip

✓6ᵗʰ **M71.46   Calcium deposit in bursa, knee**

M71.461   Calcium deposit in bursa, right knee
M71.462   Calcium deposit in bursa, left knee
M71.469   Calcium deposit in bursa, unspecified knee

✓6ᵗʰ **M71.47   Calcium deposit in bursa, ankle and foot**

M71.471   Calcium deposit in bursa, right ankle and foot
M71.472   Calcium deposit in bursa, left ankle and foot
M71.479   Calcium deposit in bursa, unspecified ankle and foot

M71.48   Calcium deposit in bursa, other site

M71.49   Calcium deposit in bursa, multiple sites

✓5ᵗʰ **M71.5   Other bursitis, not elsewhere classified**

EXCLUDES 1   *bursitis NOS (M71.9-)*
EXCLUDES 2   *bursitis of shoulder (M75.5)*
        bursitis of tibial collateral [Pellegrini-Stieda] (M76.4-)

M71.50   Other bursitis, not elsewhere classified, unspecified site

✓6ᵗʰ **M71.52   Other bursitis, not elsewhere classified, elbow**

M71.521   Other bursitis, not elsewhere classified, right elbow
M71.522   Other bursitis, not elsewhere classified, left elbow
M71.529   Other bursitis, not elsewhere classified, unspecified elbow

✓6ᵗʰ **M71.53   Other bursitis, not elsewhere classified, wrist**

M71.531   Other bursitis, not elsewhere classified, right wrist
M71.532   Other bursitis, not elsewhere classified, left wrist
M71.539   Other bursitis, not elsewhere classified, unspecified wrist

✓6ᵗʰ **M71.54   Other bursitis, not elsewhere classified, hand**

M71.541   Other bursitis, not elsewhere classified, right hand
M71.542   Other bursitis, not elsewhere classified, left hand
M71.549   Other bursitis, not elsewhere classified, unspecified hand

✓6ᵗʰ **M71.55   Other bursitis, not elsewhere classified, hip**

M71.551   Other bursitis, not elsewhere classified, right hip
M71.552   Other bursitis, not elsewhere classified, left hip
M71.559   Other bursitis, not elsewhere classified, unspecified hip

✓6ᵗʰ **M71.56   Other bursitis, not elsewhere classified, knee**

M71.561   Other bursitis, not elsewhere classified, right knee
M71.562   Other bursitis, not elsewhere classified, left knee
M71.569   Other bursitis, not elsewhere classified, unspecified knee

✓6ᵗʰ **M71.57   Other bursitis, not elsewhere classified, ankle and foot**

M71.571   Other bursitis, not elsewhere classified, right ankle and foot
M71.572   Other bursitis, not elsewhere classified, left ankle and foot
M71.579   Other bursitis, not elsewhere classified, unspecified ankle and foot

M71.58   Other bursitis, not elsewhere classified, other site

✓5ᵗʰ **M71.8   Other specified bursopathies**

M71.80   Other specified bursopathies, unspecified site

✓6ᵗʰ **M71.81   Other specified bursopathies, shoulder**

M71.811   Other specified bursopathies, right shoulder
M71.812   Other specified bursopathies, left shoulder
M71.819   Other specified bursopathies, unspecified shoulder

✓6ᵗʰ **M71.82   Other specified bursopathies, elbow**

M71.821   Other specified bursopathies, right elbow
M71.822   Other specified bursopathies, left elbow
M71.829   Other specified bursopathies, unspecified elbow

✓6ᵗʰ **M71.83   Other specified bursopathies, wrist**

M71.831   Other specified bursopathies, right wrist
M71.832   Other specified bursopathies, left wrist
M71.839   Other specified bursopathies, unspecified wrist

✓6ᵗʰ **M71.84   Other specified bursopathies, hand**

M71.841   Other specified bursopathies, right hand
M71.842   Other specified bursopathies, left hand
M71.849   Other specified bursopathies, unspecified hand

✓6ᵗʰ **M71.85   Other specified bursopathies, hip**

M71.851   Other specified bursopathies, right hip
M71.852   Other specified bursopathies, left hip
M71.859   Other specified bursopathies, unspecified hip

✓6ᵗʰ **M71.86   Other specified bursopathies, knee**

M71.861   Other specified bursopathies, right knee
M71.862   Other specified bursopathies, left knee
M71.869   Other specified bursopathies, unspecified knee

✔ Additional Character Required   ✓x7ᵗʰ Placeholder   Questionable PDx   Manifestation   Unspecified Dx   UPD Unacceptable PDx   H1-H14 HAC   HCC CMS-HCC Dx   HIV HIV Dx

ICD-10-CM 2022   819

✓6th **M71.87** **Other specified bursopathies,** ankle and foot

    M71.871 **Other specified bursopathies,** right ankle and foot

    M71.872 **Other specified bursopathies,** left ankle and foot

    M71.879 **Other specified bursopathies,** unspecified ankle and foot

    M71.88 **Other specified bursopathies,** other site

    M71.89 **Other specified bursopathies,** multiple sites

M71.9 **Bursopathy, unspecified**

    Bursitis NOS

✓4th **M72** **Fibroblastic disorders**

    EXCLUDES 2   retroperitoneal fibromatosis (D48.3)

M72.0 **Palmar fascial fibromatosis [Dupuytren]** A

    DEF: Dupuytren's contracture: Flexion deformity of a finger, due to shortened, thickened fibrosing of palmar fascia. The cause is unknown, but it is associated with long-standing epilepsy.

M72.1 **Knuckle pads**

M72.2 **Plantar fascial fibromatosis**

    Plantar fasciitis

    DEF: Rapid-growing and multiplanar nodular swellings and pain in the foot that is not associated with contractures.

M72.4 **Pseudosarcomatous fibromatosis**

    Nodular fasciitis

M72.6 **Necrotizing fasciitis**   MCC   HCC

    Use additional code (B95.-, B96.-) to identify causative organism

M72.8 **Other fibroblastic disorders**

    Abscess of fascia

    Fasciitis NEC

    Other infective fasciitis

    Use additional code to (B95.-, B96.-) identify causative organism

    EXCLUDES 1   diffuse (eosinophilic) fasciitis (M35.4)

               necrotizing fasciitis (M72.6)

               nodular fasciitis (M72.4)

               perirenal fasciitis NOS (N13.5)

               perirenal fasciitis with infection (N13.6)

               plantar fasciitis (M72.2)

M72.9 **Fibroblastic disorder, unspecified**

    Fasciitis NOS

    Fibromatosis NOS

✓4th **M75** **Shoulder lesions**

    EXCLUDES 2   shoulder-hand syndrome (M89.0-)

✓5th **M75.0** **Adhesive capsulitis of shoulder**

    Frozen shoulder

    Periarthritis of shoulder

    AHA: 2015, 2Q, 23

    M75.00 **Adhesive capsulitis of unspecified shoulder**

    M75.01 **Adhesive capsulitis of** right **shoulder**

    M75.02 **Adhesive capsulitis of** left **shoulder**

✓5th **M75.1** **Rotator cuff tear or rupture, not specified as traumatic**

    Rotator cuff syndrome

    Supraspinatus syndrome

    Supraspinatus tear or rupture, not specified as traumatic

    EXCLUDES 1   tear of rotator cuff, traumatic (S46.01-)

✓6th   **M75.10** **Unspecified rotator cuff tear or rupture, not specified as traumatic**

    M75.100 **Unspecified rotator cuff tear or rupture of unspecified shoulder, not specified as traumatic**

    M75.101 **Unspecified rotator cuff tear or rupture of** right **shoulder, not specified as traumatic**

    M75.102 **Unspecified rotator cuff tear or rupture of** left **shoulder, not specified as traumatic**

✓6th   **M75.11** **Incomplete rotator cuff tear or rupture not specified as traumatic**

    M75.110 **Incomplete rotator cuff tear or rupture of unspecified shoulder, not specified as traumatic**

    M75.111 **Incomplete rotator cuff tear or rupture of** right **shoulder, not specified as traumatic**

    M75.112 **Incomplete rotator cuff tear or rupture of** left **shoulder, not specified as traumatic**

✓6th **M75.12** **Complete rotator cuff tear or rupture not specified as traumatic**

    M75.120 **Complete rotator cuff tear or rupture of unspecified shoulder, not specified as traumatic**

    M75.121 **Complete rotator cuff tear or rupture of** right **shoulder, not specified as traumatic**

    M75.122 **Complete rotator cuff tear or rupture of** left **shoulder, not specified as traumatic**

✓5th **M75.2** **Bicipital** tendinitis

    M75.20 **Bicipital tendinitis,** unspecified shoulder

    M75.21 **Bicipital tendinitis,** right shoulder

    M75.22 **Bicipital tendinitis,** left shoulder

✓5th **M75.3** **Calcific** tendinitis of shoulder

    Calcified bursa of shoulder

    M75.30 **Calcific tendinitis of unspecified shoulder**

    M75.31 **Calcific tendinitis of** right **shoulder**

    M75.32 **Calcific tendinitis of** left **shoulder**

✓5th **M75.4** **Impingement syndrome** of shoulder

    M75.40 **Impingement syndrome of unspecified shoulder**

    M75.41 **Impingement syndrome of** right **shoulder**

    M75.42 **Impingement syndrome of** left **shoulder**

✓5th **M75.5** **Bursitis** of shoulder

    M75.50 **Bursitis of unspecified shoulder**

    M75.51 **Bursitis of** right **shoulder**

    M75.52 **Bursitis of** left **shoulder**

✓5th **M75.8** **Other shoulder lesions**

    M75.80 **Other shoulder lesions,** unspecified shoulder

    M75.81 **Other shoulder lesions,** right **shoulder**

    M75.82 **Other shoulder lesions,** left **shoulder**

✓5th **M75.9** **Shoulder lesion, unspecified**

    M75.90 **Shoulder lesion, unspecified,** unspecified shoulder

    M75.91 **Shoulder lesion, unspecified,** right **shoulder**

    M75.92 **Shoulder lesion, unspecified,** left **shoulder**

✓4th **M76** **Enthesopathies, lower limb, excluding foot**

    EXCLUDES 2   bursitis due to use, overuse and pressure (M70.-)

               enthesopathies of ankle and foot (M77.5-)

✓5th **M76.0** **Gluteal** tendinitis

    M76.00 **Gluteal tendinitis,** unspecified hip

    M76.01 **Gluteal tendinitis,** right **hip**

    M76.02 **Gluteal tendinitis,** left **hip**

✓5th **M76.1** **Psoas** tendinitis

    M76.10 **Psoas tendinitis,** unspecified hip

    M76.11 **Psoas tendinitis,** right **hip**

    M76.12 **Psoas tendinitis,** left **hip**

✓5th **M76.2** **Iliac crest** spur

    M76.20 **Iliac crest spur,** unspecified hip

    M76.21 **Iliac crest spur,** right **hip**

    M76.22 **Iliac crest spur,** left **hip**

✓5th **M76.3** **Iliotibial band** syndrome

    M76.30 **Iliotibial band syndrome,** unspecified leg

    M76.31 **Iliotibial band syndrome,** right **leg**

    M76.32 **Iliotibial band syndrome,** left **leg**

✓5th **M76.4** **Tibial collateral bursitis [Pellegrini-Stieda]**

    M76.40 **Tibial collateral bursitis [Pellegrini-Stieda],** unspecified leg

    M76.41 **Tibial collateral bursitis [Pellegrini-Stieda],** right **leg**

    M76.42 **Tibial collateral bursitis [Pellegrini-Stieda],** left **leg**

✓5th **M76.5** **Patellar** tendinitis

    M76.50 **Patellar tendinitis,** unspecified knee

    M76.51 **Patellar tendinitis,** right **knee**

    M76.52 **Patellar tendinitis,** left **knee**

✓5th **M76.6** **Achilles** tendinitis

    Achilles bursitis

    M76.60 **Achilles tendinitis,** unspecified leg

    M76.61 **Achilles tendinitis,** right **leg**

    M76.62 **Achilles tendinitis,** left **leg**

✓5th **M76.7** **Peroneal** tendinitis

    M76.70 **Peroneal tendinitis,** unspecified leg

    M76.71 **Peroneal tendinitis,** right **leg**

    M76.72 **Peroneal tendinitis,** left **leg**

N Newborn: 0   P Pediatric: 0-17   M Maternity: 9-64   A Adult: 15-124   MCC Major Complication/Comorbidity   CC Complication/Comorbidity   SW Severe Wound Dx

820   ICD-10-CM 2022

✓5ᵗʰ **M76.8 Other specified enthesopathies of lower limb, excluding foot**

    ✓6ᵗʰ **M76.81 Anterior tibial syndrome**

        M76.811 Anterior tibial syndrome, right leg

        M76.812 Anterior tibial syndrome, left leg

        M76.819 Anterior tibial syndrome, unspecified leg

    ✓6ᵗʰ **M76.82 Posterior tibial tendinitis**

        M76.821 Posterior tibial tendinitis, right leg

        M76.822 Posterior tibial tendinitis, left leg

        M76.829 Posterior tibial tendinitis, unspecified leg

    ✓6ᵗʰ **M76.89 Other specified enthesopathies of lower limb, excluding foot**

        M76.891 Other specified enthesopathies of right lower limb, excluding foot

        M76.892 Other specified enthesopathies of left lower limb, excluding foot

        M76.899 Other specified enthesopathies of unspecified lower limb, excluding foot

    M76.9 Unspecified enthesopathy, lower limb, excluding foot

✓4ᵗʰ **M77 Other enthesopathies**

    EXCLUDES 1   bursitis NOS (M71.9-)

    EXCLUDES 2   bursitis due to use, overuse and pressure (M70.-)

                osteophyte (M25.7)

                spinal enthesopathy (M46.0-)

    ✓5ᵗʰ **M77.0 Medial epicondylitis**

        M77.00 Medial epicondylitis, unspecified elbow

        M77.01 Medial epicondylitis, right elbow

        M77.02 Medial epicondylitis, left elbow

    ✓5ᵗʰ **M77.1 Lateral epicondylitis**

        Tennis elbow

        M77.10 Lateral epicondylitis, unspecified elbow

        M77.11 Lateral epicondylitis, right elbow

        M77.12 Lateral epicondylitis, left elbow

    ✓5ᵗʰ **M77.2 Periarthritis of wrist**

        M77.20 Periarthritis, unspecified wrist

        M77.21 Periarthritis, right wrist

        M77.22 Periarthritis, left wrist

    ✓5ᵗʰ **M77.3 Calcaneal spur**

        DEF: Overgrowth of calcaneus bone on the underside of the heel that causes pain on walking. Calcaneal spur is due to a chronic avulsion injury of the plantar fascia from the calcaneus.

        M77.30 Calcaneal spur, unspecified foot

        M77.31 Calcaneal spur, right foot

        M77.32 Calcaneal spur, left foot

    ✓5ᵗʰ **M77.4 Metatarsalgia**

        EXCLUDES 1   Morton's metatarsalgia (G57.6)

        M77.40 Metatarsalgia, unspecified foot

        M77.41 Metatarsalgia, right foot

        M77.42 Metatarsalgia, left foot

    ✓5ᵗʰ **M77.5 Other enthesopathy of foot and ankle**

        M77.50 Other enthesopathy of unspecified foot and ankle

        M77.51 Other enthesopathy of right foot and ankle

        M77.52 Other enthesopathy of left foot and ankle

    M77.8 Other enthesopathies, not elsewhere classified

    M77.9 Enthesopathy, unspecified

        Bone spur NOS

        Capsulitis NOS

        Periarthritis NOS

        Tendinitis NOS

✓4ᵗʰ **M79 Other and unspecified soft tissue disorders, not elsewhere classified**

    EXCLUDES 1   psychogenic rheumatism (F45.8)

                soft tissue pain, psychogenic (F45.41)

    M79.0 Rheumatism, unspecified

        EXCLUDES 1   fibromyalgia (M79.7)

                palindromic rheumatism (M12.3-)

    ✓5ᵗʰ **M79.1 Myalgia**

        Myofascial pain syndrome

        EXCLUDES 1   fibromyalgia (M79.7)

                myositis (M60.-)

        AHA: 2018,4Q,21

        M79.10 Myalgia, unspecified site

        M79.11 Myalgia of mastication muscle

        M79.12 Myalgia of auxiliary muscles, head and neck

        M79.18 Myalgia, other site

M79.2 Neuralgia and neuritis, unspecified

    EXCLUDES 1   brachial radiculitis NOS (M54.1)

                lumbosacral radiculitis NOS (M54.1)

                mononeuropathies (G56-G58)

                radiculitis NOS (M54.1)

                sciatica (M54.3-M54.4)

    TIP: Assign for documented neuropathic pain.

M79.3 Panniculitis, unspecified

    EXCLUDES 1   lupus panniculitis (L93.2)

                neck and back panniculitis (M54.0-)

                relapsing [Weber-Christian] panniculitis (M35.6)

M79.4 Hypertrophy of (infrapatellar) fat pad

M79.5 Residual foreign body in soft tissue

    EXCLUDES 1   foreign body granuloma of skin and subcutaneous tissue (L92.3)

                foreign body granuloma of soft tissue (M60.2-)

✓5ᵗʰ **M79.6 Pain in limb, hand, foot, fingers and toes**

    EXCLUDES 2   pain in joint (M25.5-)

    ✓6ᵗʰ **M79.60 Pain in limb, unspecified**

        M79.601 Pain in right arm

            Pain in right upper limb NOS

        M79.602 Pain in left arm

            Pain in left upper limb NOS

        M79.603 Pain in arm, unspecified

            Pain in upper limb NOS

        M79.604 Pain in right leg

            Pain in right lower limb NOS

        M79.605 Pain in left leg

            Pain in left lower limb NOS

        M79.606 Pain in leg, unspecified

            Pain in lower limb NOS

        M79.609 Pain in unspecified limb

            Pain in limb NOS

    ✓6ᵗʰ **M79.62 Pain in upper arm**

        Pain in axillary region

        M79.621 Pain in right upper arm

        M79.622 Pain in left upper arm

        M79.629 Pain in unspecified upper arm

    ✓6ᵗʰ **M79.63 Pain in forearm**

        M79.631 Pain in right forearm

        M79.632 Pain in left forearm

        M79.639 Pain in unspecified forearm

    ✓6ᵗʰ **M79.64 Pain in hand and fingers**

        M79.641 Pain in right hand

        M79.642 Pain in left hand

        M79.643 Pain in unspecified hand

        M79.644 Pain in right finger(s)

        M79.645 Pain in left finger(s)

        M79.646 Pain in unspecified finger(s)

    ✓6ᵗʰ **M79.65 Pain in thigh**

        M79.651 Pain in right thigh

        M79.652 Pain in left thigh

        M79.659 Pain in unspecified thigh

    ✓6ᵗʰ **M79.66 Pain in lower leg**

        M79.661 Pain in right lower leg

        M79.662 Pain in left lower leg

        M79.669 Pain in unspecified lower leg

    ✓6ᵗʰ **M79.67 Pain in foot and toes**

        M79.671 Pain in right foot

        M79.672 Pain in left foot

        M79.673 Pain in unspecified foot

        M79.674 Pain in right toe(s)

        M79.675 Pain in left toe(s)

        M79.676 Pain in unspecified toe(s)

M79.7 Fibromyalgia

    Fibromyositis

    Fibrositis

    Myofibrositis

☑ Additional Character Required   ✓x7ᵗʰ Placeholder   Questionable PDx   Manifestation   Unspecified Dx   UPD Unacceptable PDx   H1-H14 HAC   HCC CMS-HCC Dx   HIV HIV Dx

ICD-10-CM 2022   821

✓5ᵗʰ **M79.A Nontraumatic compartment syndrome**

Code first, if applicable, associated postprocedural complication

EXCLUDES 1   *compartment syndrome NOS (T79.A-)*
fibromyalgia (M79.7)
nontraumatic ischemic infarction of muscle (M62.2-)
traumatic compartment syndrome (T79.A-)

✓6ᵗʰ **M79.A1 Nontraumatic compartment syndrome of** upper extremity

Nontraumatic compartment syndrome of shoulder, arm, forearm, wrist, hand, and fingers

M79.A11 Nontraumatic compartment syndrome of right **upper extremity**   CC

M79.A12 Nontraumatic compartment syndrome of left **upper extremity**   CC

M79.A19 Nontraumatic compartment syndrome of unspecified upper extremity   CC

✓6ᵗʰ **M79.A2 Nontraumatic compartment syndrome of** lower extremity

Nontraumatic compartment syndrome of hip, buttock, thigh, leg, foot, and toes

M79.A21 Nontraumatic compartment syndrome of right **lower extremity**   CC

M79.A22 Nontraumatic compartment syndrome of left **lower extremity**   CC

M79.A29 Nontraumatic compartment syndrome of unspecified lower extremity   CC

M79.A3 Nontraumatic compartment syndrome of abdomen   CC

M79.A9 Nontraumatic compartment syndrome of other sites   CC

✓5ᵗʰ **M79.8 Other specified soft tissue disorders**

M79.81 Nontraumatic hematoma of soft tissue
Nontraumatic hematoma of muscle
Nontraumatic seroma of muscle and soft tissue

M79.89 Other specified soft tissue disorders
Polyalgia

M79.9 Soft tissue disorder, unspecified

OSTEOPATHIES AND CHONDROPATHIES (M80-M94)

Disorders of bone density and structure (M80-M85)

✓4ᵗʰ **M80 Osteoporosis** with current pathological fracture

INCLUDES   osteoporosis with current fragility fracture

Use additional code to identify major osseous defect, if applicable (M89.7-)

EXCLUDES 1   *collapsed vertebra NOS (M48.5)*
pathological fracture NOS (M84.4)
wedging of vertebra NOS (M48.5)

EXCLUDES 2   *personal history of (healed) osteoporosis fracture (Z87.310)*

AHA: 2018,2Q,12

TIP: The site codes in this category identify the site of the fracture, not the site of the osteoporosis.

The appropriate 7th character is to be added to each code from category M80:
A   initial encounter for fracture
D   subsequent encounter for fracture with routine healing
G   subsequent encounter for fracture with delayed healing
K   subsequent encounter for fracture with nonunion
P   subsequent encounter for fracture with malunion
S   sequela

✓5ᵗʰ **M80.0 Age-related osteoporosis with current pathological fracture**
Involutional osteoporosis with current pathological fracture
Osteoporosis NOS with current pathological fracture
Postmenopausal osteoporosis with current pathological fracture
Senile osteoporosis with current pathological fracture

3 ✓x7ᵗʰ **M80.00 Age-related osteoporosis with current pathological fracture, unspecified site**   CC A

✓6ᵗʰ **M80.01 Age-related osteoporosis with current pathological fracture,** shoulder

3 ✓7ᵗʰ **M80.011 Age-related osteoporosis with current pathological fracture,** right **shoulder**   CC A

3 ✓7ᵗʰ **M80.012 Age-related osteoporosis with current pathological fracture,** left **shoulder**   CC A

3 ✓7ᵗʰ **M80.019 Age-related osteoporosis with current pathological fracture, unspecified shoulder**   CC A

✓6ᵗʰ **M80.02 Age-related osteoporosis with current pathological fracture,** humerus

3 ✓7ᵗʰ **M80.021 Age-related osteoporosis with current pathological fracture,** right **humerus**   CC A

3 ✓7ᵗʰ **M80.022 Age-related osteoporosis with current pathological fracture,** left **humerus**   CC A

3 ✓7ᵗʰ **M80.029 Age-related osteoporosis with current pathological fracture, unspecified humerus**   CC A

✓6ᵗʰ **M80.03 Age-related osteoporosis with current pathological fracture,** forearm
Age-related osteoporosis with current pathological fracture of wrist

3 ✓7ᵗʰ **M80.031 Age-related osteoporosis with current pathological fracture,** right **forearm**   CC A

3 ✓7ᵗʰ **M80.032 Age-related osteoporosis with current pathological fracture,** left **forearm**   CC A

3 ✓7ᵗʰ **M80.039 Age-related osteoporosis with current pathological fracture, unspecified forearm**   CC A

✓6ᵗʰ **M80.04 Age-related osteoporosis with current pathological fracture,** hand

3 ✓7ᵗʰ **M80.041 Age-related osteoporosis with current pathological fracture,** right **hand**   CC A

3 ✓7ᵗʰ **M80.042 Age-related osteoporosis with current pathological fracture,** left **hand**   CC A

3 ✓7ᵗʰ **M80.049 Age-related osteoporosis with current pathological fracture, unspecified hand**   CC A

✓6ᵗʰ **M80.05 Age-related osteoporosis with current pathological fracture,** femur
Age-related osteoporosis with current pathological fracture of hip

3,6 ✓7ᵗʰ **M80.051 Age-related osteoporosis with current pathological fracture,** right **femur**   CC HCC A

3,6 ✓7ᵗʰ **M80.052 Age-related osteoporosis with current pathological fracture,** left **femur**   CC HCC A

3,6 ✓7ᵗʰ **M80.059 Age-related osteoporosis with current pathological fracture, unspecified femur**   CC HCC A

✓6ᵗʰ **M80.06 Age-related osteoporosis with current pathological fracture,** lower leg

3 ✓7ᵗʰ **M80.061 Age-related osteoporosis with current pathological fracture,** right lower leg   CC A

3 ✓7ᵗʰ **M80.062 Age-related osteoporosis with current pathological fracture,** left lower leg   CC A

3 ✓7ᵗʰ **M80.069 Age-related osteoporosis with current pathological fracture, unspecified lower leg**   CC A

✓6ᵗʰ **M80.07 Age-related osteoporosis with current pathological fracture,** ankle and foot

3 ✓7ᵗʰ **M80.071 Age-related osteoporosis with current pathological fracture,** right ankle and foot   CC A

3 ✓7ᵗʰ **M80.072 Age-related osteoporosis with current pathological fracture,** left ankle and foot   CC A

3 ✓7ᵗʰ **M80.079 Age-related osteoporosis with current pathological fracture, unspecified ankle and foot**   CC A

3,6 ✓x7ᵗʰ **M80.08 Age-related osteoporosis with current pathological fracture,** vertebra(e)   CC HCC A

3 ✓x7ᵗʰ **M80.0A Age-related osteoporosis with current pathological fracture, other site**   CC A
AHA: 2020,4Q,32-33

☑5ᵗʰ **M80.8** **Other osteoporosis with current pathological fracture**

Drug-induced osteoporosis with current pathological fracture
Idiopathic osteoporosis with current pathological fracture
Osteoporosis of disuse with current pathological fracture
Postoophorectomy osteoporosis with current pathological fracture
Postsurgical malabsorption osteoporosis with current pathological fracture
Post-traumatic osteoporosis with current pathological fracture
Use additional code for adverse effect, if applicable, to identify drug (T36-T50 with fifth or sixth character 5)

3 ✓x7ᵗʰ **M80.80** **Other osteoporosis with current pathological fracture, unspecified site** `CC`

✓6ᵗʰ **M80.81** **Other osteoporosis with pathological fracture, shoulder**

     3 ✓7ᵗʰ **M80.811** **Other osteoporosis with current pathological fracture, right shoulder** `CC`

     3 ✓7ᵗʰ **M80.812** **Other osteoporosis with current pathological fracture, left shoulder** `CC`

     3 ✓7ᵗʰ **M80.819** **Other osteoporosis with current pathological fracture, unspecified shoulder** `CC`

✓6ᵗʰ **M80.82** **Other osteoporosis with current pathological fracture, humerus**

     3 ✓7ᵗʰ **M80.821** **Other osteoporosis with current pathological fracture, right humerus** `CC`

     3 ✓7ᵗʰ **M80.822** **Other osteoporosis with current pathological fracture, left humerus** `CC`

     3 ✓7ᵗʰ **M80.829** **Other osteoporosis with current pathological fracture, unspecified humerus** `CC`

✓6ᵗʰ **M80.83** **Other osteoporosis with current pathological fracture, forearm**

Other osteoporosis with current pathological fracture of wrist

     3 ✓7ᵗʰ **M80.831** **Other osteoporosis with current pathological fracture, right forearm** `CC`

     3 ✓7ᵗʰ **M80.832** **Other osteoporosis with current pathological fracture, left forearm** `CC`

     3 ✓7ᵗʰ **M80.839** **Other osteoporosis with current pathological fracture, unspecified forearm** `CC`

✓6ᵗʰ **M80.84** **Other osteoporosis with current pathological fracture, hand**

     3 ✓7ᵗʰ **M80.841** **Other osteoporosis with current pathological fracture, right hand** `CC`

     3 ✓7ᵗʰ **M80.842** **Other osteoporosis with current pathological fracture, left hand** `CC`

     3 ✓7ᵗʰ **M80.849** **Other osteoporosis with current pathological fracture, unspecified hand** `CC`

✓6ᵗʰ **M80.85** **Other osteoporosis with current pathological fracture, femur**

Other osteoporosis with current pathological fracture of hip

     3,6 ✓7ᵗʰ **M80.851** **Other osteoporosis with current pathological fracture, right femur** `CC` `HCC`

     3,6 ✓7ᵗʰ **M80.852** **Other osteoporosis with current pathological fracture, left femur** `CC` `HCC`

     3,6 ✓7ᵗʰ **M80.859** **Other osteoporosis with current pathological fracture, unspecified femur** `CC` `HCC`

✓6ᵗʰ **M80.86** **Other osteoporosis with current pathological fracture, lower leg**

     3 ✓7ᵗʰ **M80.861** **Other osteoporosis with current pathological fracture, right lower leg** `CC`

     3 ✓7ᵗʰ **M80.862** **Other osteoporosis with current pathological fracture, left lower leg** `CC`

     3 ✓7ᵗʰ **M80.869** **Other osteoporosis with current pathological fracture, unspecified lower leg** `CC`

✓6ᵗʰ **M80.87** **Other osteoporosis with current pathological fracture, ankle and foot**

     3 ✓7ᵗʰ **M80.871** **Other osteoporosis with current pathological fracture, right ankle and foot** `CC`

     3 ✓7ᵗʰ **M80.872** **Other osteoporosis with current pathological fracture, left ankle and foot** `CC`

     3 ✓7ᵗʰ **M80.879** **Other osteoporosis with current pathological fracture, unspecified ankle and foot** `CC`

3,6 ✓x7ᵗʰ **M80.88** **Other osteoporosis with current pathological fracture, vertebra(e)** `CC` `HCC`

3 ✓x7ᵗʰ **M80.8A** **Other osteoporosis with current pathological fracture, other site** `CC`

AHA: 2020,4Q,32

☑4ᵗʰ **M81** **Osteoporosis without current pathological fracture**

Use additional code to identify:
major osseous defect, if applicable (M89.7-)
personal history of (healed) osteoporosis fracture, if applicable (Z87.310)

EXCLUDES 1   *osteoporosis with current pathological fracture (M80.-)*
Sudeck's atrophy (M89.0)

M81.0 **Age-related osteoporosis without current pathological fracture** `A`

Involutional osteoporosis without current pathological fracture
Osteoporosis NOS
Postmenopausal osteoporosis without current pathological fracture
Senile osteoporosis without current pathological fracture

M81.6 **Localized osteoporosis [Lequesne]**
EXCLUDES 1   *Sudeck's atrophy (M89.0)*

M81.8 **Other osteoporosis without current pathological fracture**

Drug-induced osteoporosis without current pathological fracture
Idiopathic osteoporosis without current pathological fracture
Osteoporosis of disuse without current pathological fracture
Postoophorectomy osteoporosis without current pathological fracture
Postsurgical malabsorption osteoporosis without current pathological fracture
Post-traumatic osteoporosis without current pathological fracture
Use additional code for adverse effect, if applicable, to identify drug (T36-T50 with fifth or sixth character 5)

☑4ᵗʰ **M83** **Adult osteomalacia**

EXCLUDES 1   *infantile and juvenile osteomalacia (E55.0)*
renal osteodystrophy (N25.0)
rickets (active) (E55.0)
rickets (active) sequelae (E64.3)
vitamin D-resistant osteomalacia (E83.3)
vitamin D-resistant rickets (active) (E83.3)

M83.0 **Puerperal osteomalacia** `M` ♀

M83.1 **Senile osteomalacia** `A`

M83.2 **Adult osteomalacia due to malabsorption** `A`
Postsurgical malabsorption osteomalacia in adults

M83.3 **Adult osteomalacia due to malnutrition** `A`

M83.4 **Aluminum bone disease**

M83.5 **Other drug-induced osteomalacia in adults** `A`
Use additional code for adverse effect, if applicable, to identify drug (T36-T50 with fifth or sixth character 5)

M83.8 **Other adult osteomalacia** `A`

M83.9 **Adult osteomalacia, unspecified** `A`

☑ Additional Character Required   ✓x7ᵗʰ Placeholder   Questionable PDx   **Manifestation**   Unspecified Dx   `UPD` Unacceptable PDx   `H1`-`H14` HAC   `HCC` CMS-HCC Dx   `HIV` HIV Dx

√4th **M84 Disorder of continuity of bone**

> EXCLUDES 2   *traumatic fracture of bone-see fracture, by site*

√5th **M84.3 Stress fracture**

> Fatigue fracture
> March fracture
> Stress fracture NOS
> Stress reaction
> Use additional external cause code(s) to identify the cause of the stress fracture
>
> EXCLUDES 1   *pathological fracture due to osteoporosis (M80.-)*
> *pathological fracture NOS (M84.4.-)*
> *traumatic fracture (S12.-, S22.-, S32.-, S42.-, S52.-, S62.-, S72.-, S82.-, S92.-)*
>
> EXCLUDES 2   *personal history of (healed) stress (fatigue) fracture (Z87.312)*
> *stress fracture of vertebra (M48.4-)*

> The appropriate 7th character is to be added to each code from subcategory M84.3.
> A   initial encounter for fracture
> D   subsequent encounter for fracture with routine healing
> G   subsequent encounter for fracture with delayed healing
> K   subsequent encounter for fracture with nonunion
> P   subsequent encounter for fracture with malunion
> S   sequela

4 √x7th **M84.30** Stress fracture, unspecified site   CC

√6th **M84.31** Stress fracture, shoulder

   4 √7th **M84.311** Stress fracture, right shoulder   CC

   4 √7th **M84.312** Stress fracture, left shoulder   CC

   4 √7th **M84.319** Stress fracture, unspecified shoulder   CC

√6th **M84.32** Stress fracture, humerus

   4 √7th **M84.321** Stress fracture, right humerus   CC

   4 √7th **M84.322** Stress fracture, left humerus   CC

   4 √7th **M84.329** Stress fracture, unspecified humerus   CC

√6th **M84.33** Stress fracture, ulna and radius

   4 √7th **M84.331** Stress fracture, right ulna   CC

   4 √7th **M84.332** Stress fracture, left ulna   CC

   4 √7th **M84.333** Stress fracture, right radius   CC

   4 √7th **M84.334** Stress fracture, left radius   CC

   4 √7th **M84.339** Stress fracture, unspecified ulna and radius   CC

√6th **M84.34** Stress fracture, hand and fingers

   4 √7th **M84.341** Stress fracture, right hand   CC

   4 √7th **M84.342** Stress fracture, left hand   CC

   4 √7th **M84.343** Stress fracture, unspecified hand   CC

   4 √7th **M84.344** Stress fracture, right finger(s)   CC

   4 √7th **M84.345** Stress fracture, left finger(s)   CC

   4 √7th **M84.346** Stress fracture, unspecified finger(s)   CC

√6th **M84.35** Stress fracture, pelvis and femur

   Stress fracture, hip

   4 √7th **M84.350** Stress fracture, pelvis   CC

   4 √7th **M84.351** Stress fracture, right femur   CC

   4 √7th **M84.352** Stress fracture, left femur   CC

   4 √7th **M84.353** Stress fracture, unspecified femur   CC

   4 √7th **M84.359** Stress fracture, hip, unspecified   CC

√6th **M84.36** Stress fracture, tibia and fibula

   4 √7th **M84.361** Stress fracture, right tibia   CC

   4 √7th **M84.362** Stress fracture, left tibia   CC

   4 √7th **M84.363** Stress fracture, right fibula   CC

   4 √7th **M84.364** Stress fracture, left fibula   CC

   4 √7th **M84.369** Stress fracture, unspecified tibia and fibula   CC

√6th **M84.37** Stress fracture, ankle, foot and toes

   4 √7th **M84.371** Stress fracture, right ankle   CC

   4 √7th **M84.372** Stress fracture, left ankle   CC

   4 √7th **M84.373** Stress fracture, unspecified ankle   CC

   4 √7th **M84.374** Stress fracture, right foot   CC

   4 √7th **M84.375** Stress fracture, left foot   CC

   4 √7th **M84.376** Stress fracture, unspecified foot   CC

   4 √7th **M84.377** Stress fracture, right toe(s)   CC

   4 √7th **M84.378** Stress fracture, left toe(s)   CC

   4 √7th **M84.379** Stress fracture, unspecified toe(s)   CC

4 √x7th **M84.38** Stress fracture, other site   CC

> EXCLUDES 2   *stress fracture of vertebra (M48.4-)*

√5th **M84.4 Pathological fracture, not elsewhere classified**

> Chronic fracture
> Pathological fracture NOS
>
> EXCLUDES 1   *collapsed vertebra NEC (M48.5)*
> *pathological fracture in neoplastic disease (M84.5-)*
> *pathological fracture in osteoporosis (M80.-)*
> *pathological fracture in other disease (M84.6-)*
> *stress fracture (M84.3-)*
> *traumatic fracture (S12.-, S22.-, S32.-, S42.-, S52.-, S62.-, S72.-, S82.-, S92.-)*
>
> EXCLUDES 2   *personal history of (healed) pathological fracture (Z87.311)*

> The appropriate 7th character is to be added to each code from subcategory M84.4.
> A   initial encounter for fracture
> D   subsequent encounter for fracture with routine healing
> G   subsequent encounter for fracture with delayed healing
> K   subsequent encounter for fracture with nonunion
> P   subsequent encounter for fracture with malunion
> S   sequela

3 √x7th **M84.40** Pathological fracture, unspecified site   CC

√6th **M84.41** Pathological fracture, shoulder

   3 √7th **M84.411** Pathological fracture, right shoulder   CC

   3 √7th **M84.412** Pathological fracture, left shoulder   CC

   3 √7th **M84.419** Pathological fracture, unspecified shoulder   CC

√6th **M84.42** Pathological fracture, humerus

   3 √7th **M84.421** Pathological fracture, right humerus   CC

   3 √7th **M84.422** Pathological fracture, left humerus   CC

   3 √7th **M84.429** Pathological fracture, unspecified humerus   CC

√6th **M84.43** Pathological fracture, ulna and radius

   3 √7th **M84.431** Pathological fracture, right ulna   CC

   3 √7th **M84.432** Pathological fracture, left ulna   CC

   3 √7th **M84.433** Pathological fracture, right radius   CC

   3 √7th **M84.434** Pathological fracture, left radius   CC

   3 √7th **M84.439** Pathological fracture, unspecified ulna and radius   CC

√6th **M84.44** Pathological fracture, hand and fingers

   3 √7th **M84.441** Pathological fracture, right hand   CC

   3 √7th **M84.442** Pathological fracture, left hand   CC

   3 √7th **M84.443** Pathological fracture, unspecified hand   CC

   3 √7th **M84.444** Pathological fracture, right finger(s)   CC

   3 √7th **M84.445** Pathological fracture, left finger(s)

   3 √7th **M84.446** Pathological fracture, unspecified finger(s)   CC

√6th **M84.45** Pathological fracture, femur and pelvis

   AHA: 2016,4Q,43

   3,6 √7th **M84.451** Pathological fracture, right femur   CC HCC

   3,6 √7th **M84.452** Pathological fracture, left femur   CC HCC

   3,6 √7th **M84.453** Pathological fracture, unspecified femur   CC HCC

   3 √7th **M84.454** Pathological fracture, pelvis   CC

   3,6 √7th **M84.459** Pathological fracture, hip, unspecified   CC HCC

√6th **M84.46** Pathological fracture, tibia and fibula

   3 √7th **M84.461** Pathological fracture, right tibia   CC

   3 √7th **M84.462** Pathological fracture, left tibia   CC

   3 √7th **M84.463** Pathological fracture, right fibula   CC

   3 √7th **M84.464** Pathological fracture, left fibula   CC

N Newborn: 0   P Pediatric: 0-17   M Maternity: 9-64   A Adult: 15-124   MCC Major Complication/Comorbidity   CC Complication/Comorbidity   SW Severe Wound Dx

824   ICD-10-CM 2022

³ √7ᵗʰ **M84.469** Pathological fracture, unspecified tibia and fibula   CC

√6ᵗʰ **M84.47** Pathological fracture, ankle, foot and toes

    ³ √7ᵗʰ **M84.471** Pathological fracture, right ankle   CC

    ³ √7ᵗʰ **M84.472** Pathological fracture, left ankle   CC

    ³ √7ᵗʰ **M84.473** Pathological fracture, unspecified ankle   CC

    ³ √7ᵗʰ **M84.474** Pathological fracture, right foot   CC

    ³ √7ᵗʰ **M84.475** Pathological fracture, left foot   CC

    ³ √7ᵗʰ **M84.476** Pathological fracture, unspecified foot   CC

    ³ √7ᵗʰ **M84.477** Pathological fracture, right toe(s)   CC

    ³ √7ᵗʰ **M84.478** Pathological fracture, left toe(s)   CC

    ³ √7ᵗʰ **M84.479** Pathological fracture, unspecified toe(s)   CC

³ √x7ᵗʰ **M84.48** Pathological fracture, other site   CC

√5ᵗʰ **M84.5** Pathological fracture in neoplastic disease

    Code also underlying neoplasm

    The appropriate 7th character is to be added to each code from subcategory M84.5.
    A   initial encounter for fracture
    D   subsequent encounter for fracture with routine healing
    G   subsequent encounter for fracture with delayed healing
    K   subsequent encounter for fracture with nonunion
    P   subsequent encounter for fracture with malunion
    S   sequela

³ √x7ᵗʰ **M84.50** Pathological fracture in neoplastic disease, unspecified site   CC

√6ᵗʰ **M84.51** Pathological fracture in neoplastic disease, shoulder

    ³ √7ᵗʰ **M84.511** Pathological fracture in neoplastic disease, right shoulder   CC

    ³ √7ᵗʰ **M84.512** Pathological fracture in neoplastic disease, left shoulder   CC

    ³ √7ᵗʰ **M84.519** Pathological fracture in neoplastic disease, unspecified shoulder   CC

√6ᵗʰ **M84.52** Pathological fracture in neoplastic disease, humerus

    ³ √7ᵗʰ **M84.521** Pathological fracture in neoplastic disease, right humerus   CC

    ³ √7ᵗʰ **M84.522** Pathological fracture in neoplastic disease, left humerus   CC

    ³ √7ᵗʰ **M84.529** Pathological fracture in neoplastic disease, unspecified humerus   CC

√6ᵗʰ **M84.53** Pathological fracture in neoplastic disease, ulna and radius

    ³ √7ᵗʰ **M84.531** Pathological fracture in neoplastic disease, right ulna   CC

    ³ √7ᵗʰ **M84.532** Pathological fracture in neoplastic disease, left ulna   CC

    ³ √7ᵗʰ **M84.533** Pathological fracture in neoplastic disease, right radius   CC

    ³ √7ᵗʰ **M84.534** Pathological fracture in neoplastic disease, left radius   CC

    ³ √7ᵗʰ **M84.539** Pathological fracture in neoplastic disease, unspecified ulna and radius   CC

√6ᵗʰ **M84.54** Pathological fracture in neoplastic disease, hand

    ³ √7ᵗʰ **M84.541** Pathological fracture in neoplastic disease, right hand   CC

    ³ √7ᵗʰ **M84.542** Pathological fracture in neoplastic disease, left hand   CC

    ³ √7ᵗʰ **M84.549** Pathological fracture in neoplastic disease, unspecified hand   CC

√6ᵗʰ **M84.55** Pathological fracture in neoplastic disease, pelvis and femur

    ³ √7ᵗʰ **M84.550** Pathological fracture in neoplastic disease, pelvis   CC

    ³,⁶ √7ᵗʰ **M84.551** Pathological fracture in neoplastic disease, right femur   CC HCC

    ³,⁶ √7ᵗʰ **M84.552** Pathological fracture in neoplastic disease, left femur   CC HCC

    ³,⁶ √7ᵗʰ **M84.553** Pathological fracture in neoplastic disease, unspecified femur   CC HCC

    ³,⁶ √7ᵗʰ **M84.559** Pathological fracture in neoplastic disease, hip, unspecified   CC HCC

√6ᵗʰ **M84.56** Pathological fracture in neoplastic disease, tibia and fibula

    ³ √7ᵗʰ **M84.561** Pathological fracture in neoplastic disease, right tibia

    ³ √7ᵗʰ **M84.562** Pathological fracture in neoplastic disease, left tibia   CC

    ³ √7ᵗʰ **M84.563** Pathological fracture in neoplastic disease, right fibula

    ³ √7ᵗʰ **M84.564** Pathological fracture in neoplastic disease, left fibula

    ³ √7ᵗʰ **M84.569** Pathological fracture in neoplastic disease, unspecified tibia and fibula   CC

√6ᵗʰ **M84.57** Pathological fracture in neoplastic disease, ankle and foot

    ³ √7ᵗʰ **M84.571** Pathological fracture in neoplastic disease, right ankle   CC

    ³ √7ᵗʰ **M84.572** Pathological fracture in neoplastic disease, left ankle   CC

    ³ √7ᵗʰ **M84.573** Pathological fracture in neoplastic disease, unspecified ankle   CC

    ³ √7ᵗʰ **M84.574** Pathological fracture in neoplastic disease, right foot   CC

    ³ √7ᵗʰ **M84.575** Pathological fracture in neoplastic disease, left foot   CC

    ³ √7ᵗʰ **M84.576** Pathological fracture in neoplastic disease, unspecified foot   CC

³ √x7ᵗʰ **M84.58** Pathological fracture in neoplastic disease, other specified site   CC

      Pathological fracture in neoplastic disease, vertebrae

√5ᵗʰ **M84.6** Pathological fracture in other disease

    Code also underlying condition

    EXCLUDES 1   pathological fracture in osteoporosis (M80.-)

    The appropriate 7th character is to be added to each code from subcategory M84.6.
    A   initial encounter for fracture
    D   subsequent encounter for fracture with routine healing
    G   subsequent encounter for fracture with delayed healing
    K   subsequent encounter for fracture with nonunion
    P   subsequent encounter for fracture with malunion
    S   sequela

³ √x7ᵗʰ **M84.60** Pathological fracture in other disease, unspecified site   CC

√6ᵗʰ **M84.61** Pathological fracture in other disease, shoulder

    ³ √7ᵗʰ **M84.611** Pathological fracture in other disease, right shoulder   CC

    ³ √7ᵗʰ **M84.612** Pathological fracture in other disease, left shoulder   CC

    ³ √7ᵗʰ **M84.619** Pathological fracture in other disease, unspecified shoulder   CC

√6ᵗʰ **M84.62** Pathological fracture in other disease, humerus

    ³ √7ᵗʰ **M84.621** Pathological fracture in other disease, right humerus   CC

    ³ √7ᵗʰ **M84.622** Pathological fracture in other disease, left humerus   CC

    ³ √7ᵗʰ **M84.629** Pathological fracture in other disease, unspecified humerus   CC

√6ᵗʰ **M84.63** Pathological fracture in other disease, ulna and radius

    ³ √7ᵗʰ **M84.631** Pathological fracture in other disease, right ulna   CC

    ³ √7ᵗʰ **M84.632** Pathological fracture in other disease, left ulna   CC

    ³ √7ᵗʰ **M84.633** Pathological fracture in other disease, right radius   CC

    ³ √7ᵗʰ **M84.634** Pathological fracture in other disease, left radius   CC

    ³ √7ᵗʰ **M84.639** Pathological fracture in other disease, unspecified ulna and radius   CC

√6ᵗʰ **M84.64** Pathological fracture in other disease, hand

    ³ √7ᵗʰ **M84.641** Pathological fracture in other disease, right hand   CC

    ³ √7ᵗʰ **M84.642** Pathological fracture in other disease, left hand   CC

    ³ √7ᵗʰ **M84.649** Pathological fracture in other disease, unspecified hand   CC

☑ Additional Character Required   √x7ᵗʰ Placeholder   Questionable PDx   Manifestation   Unspecified Dx   UPD Unacceptable PDx   H1-H14 HAC   HCC CMS-HCC Dx   HIV HIV Dx

ICD-10-CM 2022   **825**

√6ᵗʰ **M84.65** **Pathological fracture in other disease,** pelvis and femur

³ √7ᵗʰ **M84.65Ø** **Pathological fracture in other disease,** pelvis `CC`

³,⁶ √7ᵗʰ **M84.651** **Pathological fracture in other disease,** right femur `CC` `HCC`

³,⁶ √7ᵗʰ **M84.652** **Pathological fracture in other disease,** left femur `CC` `HCC`

³,⁶ √7ᵗʰ **M84.653** **Pathological fracture in other disease,** unspecified femur `CC` `HCC`

³,⁶ √7ᵗʰ **M84.659** **Pathological fracture in other disease,** hip, unspecified `CC` `HCC`

√6ᵗʰ **M84.66** **Pathological fracture in other disease,** tibia and fibula

³ √7ᵗʰ **M84.661** **Pathological fracture in other disease,** right tibia `CC`

³ √7ᵗʰ **M84.662** **Pathological fracture in other disease,** left tibia `CC`

³ √7ᵗʰ **M84.663** **Pathological fracture in other disease,** right fibula `CC`

³ √7ᵗʰ **M84.664** **Pathological fracture in other disease,** left fibula `CC`

³ √7ᵗʰ **M84.669** **Pathological fracture in other disease,** unspecified tibia and fibula `CC`

√6ᵗʰ **M84.67** **Pathological fracture in other disease,** ankle and foot

³ √7ᵗʰ **M84.671** **Pathological fracture in other disease,** right ankle `CC`

³ √7ᵗʰ **M84.672** **Pathological fracture in other disease,** left ankle `CC`

³ √7ᵗʰ **M84.673** **Pathological fracture in other disease,** unspecified ankle `CC`

³ √7ᵗʰ **M84.674** **Pathological fracture in other disease,** right foot `CC`

³ √7ᵗʰ **M84.675** **Pathological fracture in other disease,** left foot `CC`

³ √7ᵗʰ **M84.676** **Pathological fracture in other disease,** unspecified foot `CC`

³ √x7ᵗʰ **M84.68** **Pathological fracture in other disease, other site** `CC`

√5ᵗʰ **M84.7** **Nontraumatic fracture, not elsewhere classified**

√6ᵗʰ **M84.75** **Atypical femoral fracture**

AHA: 2016,4Q,41-42

> The appropriate 7th character is to be added to each code from M84.75.
> A   initial encounter for fracture
> D   subsequent encounter for fracture with routine healing
> G   subsequent encounter for fracture with delayed healing
> K   subsequent encounter for fracture with nonunion
> P   subsequent encounter for fracture with malunion
> S   sequela

³ √7ᵗʰ **M84.75Ø** **Atypical femoral fracture, unspecified** `CC`

³ √7ᵗʰ **M84.751** **Incomplete atypical femoral fracture, right leg** `CC`

³ √7ᵗʰ **M84.752** **Incomplete atypical femoral fracture, left leg** `CC`

³ √7ᵗʰ **M84.753** **Incomplete atypical femoral fracture, unspecified leg** `CC`

³,⁶ √7ᵗʰ **M84.754** **Complete transverse atypical femoral fracture, right leg** `CC` `HCC`

³,⁶ √7ᵗʰ **M84.755** **Complete transverse atypical femoral fracture, left leg** `CC` `HCC`

³,⁶ √7ᵗʰ **M84.756** **Complete transverse atypical femoral fracture, unspecified leg** `CC` `HCC`

³,⁶ √7ᵗʰ **M84.757** **Complete oblique atypical femoral fracture, right leg** `CC` `HCC`

³,⁶ √7ᵗʰ **M84.758** **Complete oblique atypical femoral fracture, left leg** `CC` `HCC`

³,⁶ √7ᵗʰ **M84.759** **Complete oblique atypical femoral fracture, unspecified leg** `CC` `HCC`

√5ᵗʰ **M84.8** **Other disorders of continuity of bone**

M84.8Ø **Other disorders of continuity of bone, unspecified site**

√6ᵗʰ **M84.81** **Other disorders of continuity of bone,** shoulder

M84.811 **Other disorders of continuity of bone,** right shoulder

M84.812 **Other disorders of continuity of bone,** left shoulder

M84.819 **Other disorders of continuity of bone,** unspecified shoulder

√6ᵗʰ **M84.82** **Other disorders of continuity of bone,** humerus

M84.821 **Other disorders of continuity of bone,** right humerus

M84.822 **Other disorders of continuity of bone,** left humerus

M84.829 **Other disorders of continuity of bone,** unspecified humerus

√6ᵗʰ **M84.83** **Other disorders of continuity of bone,** ulna and radius

M84.831 **Other disorders of continuity of bone,** right ulna

M84.832 **Other disorders of continuity of bone,** left ulna

M84.833 **Other disorders of continuity of bone,** right radius

M84.834 **Other disorders of continuity of bone,** left radius

M84.839 **Other disorders of continuity of bone,** unspecified ulna and radius

√6ᵗʰ **M84.84** **Other disorders of continuity of bone,** hand

M84.841 **Other disorders of continuity of bone,** right hand

M84.842 **Other disorders of continuity of bone,** left hand

M84.849 **Other disorders of continuity of bone,** unspecified hand

√6ᵗʰ **M84.85** **Other disorders of continuity of bone,** pelvic region and thigh

M84.851 **Other disorders of continuity of bone,** right pelvic region and thigh

M84.852 **Other disorders of continuity of bone,** left pelvic region and thigh

M84.859 **Other disorders of continuity of bone,** unspecified pelvic region and thigh

√6ᵗʰ **M84.86** **Other disorders of continuity of bone,** tibia and fibula

M84.861 **Other disorders of continuity of bone,** right tibia

M84.862 **Other disorders of continuity of bone,** left tibia

M84.863 **Other disorders of continuity of bone,** right fibula

M84.864 **Other disorders of continuity of bone,** left fibula

M84.869 **Other disorders of continuity of bone,** unspecified tibia and fibula

√6ᵗʰ **M84.87** **Other disorders of continuity of bone,** ankle and foot

M84.871 **Other disorders of continuity of bone,** right ankle and foot

M84.872 **Other disorders of continuity of bone,** left ankle and foot

M84.879 **Other disorders of continuity of bone,** unspecified ankle and foot

M84.88 **Other disorders of continuity of bone, other site**

M84.9 **Disorder of continuity of bone, unspecified**

√4ᵗʰ **M85** **Other disorders of bone density and structure**

EXCLUDES 1   osteogenesis imperfecta (Q78.Ø)
osteopetrosis (Q78.2)
osteopoikilosis (Q78.8)
polyostotic fibrous dysplasia (Q78.1)

√5ᵗʰ **M85.Ø** **Fibrous dysplasia (monostotic)**

EXCLUDES 2   fibrous dysplasia of jaw (M27.8)

M85.ØØ **Fibrous dysplasia (monostotic), unspecified site**

√6ᵗʰ **M85.Ø1** **Fibrous dysplasia (monostotic),** shoulder

M85.Ø11 **Fibrous dysplasia (monostotic),** right shoulder

M85.Ø12 **Fibrous dysplasia (monostotic),** left shoulder

M85.Ø19 **Fibrous dysplasia (monostotic),** unspecified shoulder

N Newborn: 0   P Pediatric: 0-17   M Maternity: 9-64   A Adult: 15-124   MCC Major Complication/Comorbidity   CC Complication/Comorbidity   SW Severe Wound Dx

826   ICD-10-CM 2022

✓6ᵗʰ **M85.02** Fibrous dysplasia (monostotic), upper arm

     M85.021 Fibrous dysplasia (monostotic), right upper arm

     M85.022 Fibrous dysplasia (monostotic), left upper arm

     M85.029 Fibrous dysplasia (monostotic), unspecified upper arm

✓6ᵗʰ **M85.03** Fibrous dysplasia (monostotic), forearm

     M85.031 Fibrous dysplasia (monostotic), right forearm

     M85.032 Fibrous dysplasia (monostotic), left forearm

     M85.039 Fibrous dysplasia (monostotic), unspecified forearm

✓6ᵗʰ **M85.04** Fibrous dysplasia (monostotic), hand

     M85.041 Fibrous dysplasia (monostotic), right hand

     M85.042 Fibrous dysplasia (monostotic), left hand

     M85.049 Fibrous dysplasia (monostotic), unspecified hand

✓6ᵗʰ **M85.05** Fibrous dysplasia (monostotic), thigh

     M85.051 Fibrous dysplasia (monostotic), right thigh

     M85.052 Fibrous dysplasia (monostotic), left thigh

     M85.059 Fibrous dysplasia (monostotic), unspecified thigh

✓6ᵗʰ **M85.06** Fibrous dysplasia (monostotic), lower leg

     M85.061 Fibrous dysplasia (monostotic), right lower leg

     M85.062 Fibrous dysplasia (monostotic), left lower leg

     M85.069 Fibrous dysplasia (monostotic), unspecified lower leg

✓6ᵗʰ **M85.07** Fibrous dysplasia (monostotic), ankle and foot

     M85.071 Fibrous dysplasia (monostotic), right ankle and foot

     M85.072 Fibrous dysplasia (monostotic), left ankle and foot

     M85.079 Fibrous dysplasia (monostotic), unspecified ankle and foot

     M85.08 Fibrous dysplasia (monostotic), other site

     M85.09 Fibrous dysplasia (monostotic), multiple sites

✓5ᵗʰ **M85.1** Skeletal fluorosis

     M85.10 Skeletal fluorosis, unspecified site

✓6ᵗʰ **M85.11** Skeletal fluorosis, shoulder

     M85.111 Skeletal fluorosis, right shoulder

     M85.112 Skeletal fluorosis, left shoulder

     M85.119 Skeletal fluorosis, unspecified shoulder

✓6ᵗʰ **M85.12** Skeletal fluorosis, upper arm

     M85.121 Skeletal fluorosis, right upper arm

     M85.122 Skeletal fluorosis, left upper arm

     M85.129 Skeletal fluorosis, unspecified upper arm

✓6ᵗʰ **M85.13** Skeletal fluorosis, forearm

     M85.131 Skeletal fluorosis, right forearm

     M85.132 Skeletal fluorosis, left forearm

     M85.139 Skeletal fluorosis, unspecified forearm

✓6ᵗʰ **M85.14** Skeletal fluorosis, hand

     M85.141 Skeletal fluorosis, right hand

     M85.142 Skeletal fluorosis, left hand

     M85.149 Skeletal fluorosis, unspecified hand

✓6ᵗʰ **M85.15** Skeletal fluorosis, thigh

     M85.151 Skeletal fluorosis, right thigh

     M85.152 Skeletal fluorosis, left thigh

     M85.159 Skeletal fluorosis, unspecified thigh

✓6ᵗʰ **M85.16** Skeletal fluorosis, lower leg

     M85.161 Skeletal fluorosis, right lower leg

     M85.162 Skeletal fluorosis, left lower leg

     M85.169 Skeletal fluorosis, unspecified lower leg

✓6ᵗʰ **M85.17** Skeletal fluorosis, ankle and foot

     M85.171 Skeletal fluorosis, right ankle and foot

     M85.172 Skeletal fluorosis, left ankle and foot

     M85.179 Skeletal fluorosis, unspecified ankle and foot

     M85.18 Skeletal fluorosis, other site

     M85.19 Skeletal fluorosis, multiple sites

M85.2 Hyperostosis of skull

     DEF: Abnormal bone growth on the inner aspect of the cranial bones.

✓5ᵗʰ **M85.3** Osteitis condensans

     M85.30 Osteitis condensans, unspecified site

✓6ᵗʰ **M85.31** Osteitis condensans, shoulder

     M85.311 Osteitis condensans, right shoulder

     M85.312 Osteitis condensans, left shoulder

     M85.319 Osteitis condensans, unspecified shoulder

✓6ᵗʰ **M85.32** Osteitis condensans, upper arm

     M85.321 Osteitis condensans, right upper arm

     M85.322 Osteitis condensans, left upper arm

     M85.329 Osteitis condensans, unspecified upper arm

✓6ᵗʰ **M85.33** Osteitis condensans, forearm

     M85.331 Osteitis condensans, right forearm

     M85.332 Osteitis condensans, left forearm

     M85.339 Osteitis condensans, unspecified forearm

✓6ᵗʰ **M85.34** Osteitis condensans, hand

     M85.341 Osteitis condensans, right hand

     M85.342 Osteitis condensans, left hand

     M85.349 Osteitis condensans, unspecified hand

✓6ᵗʰ **M85.35** Osteitis condensans, thigh

     M85.351 Osteitis condensans, right thigh

     M85.352 Osteitis condensans, left thigh

     M85.359 Osteitis condensans, unspecified thigh

✓6ᵗʰ **M85.36** Osteitis condensans, lower leg

     M85.361 Osteitis condensans, right lower leg

     M85.362 Osteitis condensans, left lower leg

     M85.369 Osteitis condensans, unspecified lower leg

✓6ᵗʰ **M85.37** Osteitis condensans, ankle and foot

     M85.371 Osteitis condensans, right ankle and foot

     M85.372 Osteitis condensans, left ankle and foot

     M85.379 Osteitis condensans, unspecified ankle and foot

     M85.38 Osteitis condensans, other site

     M85.39 Osteitis condensans, multiple sites

✓5ᵗʰ **M85.4** Solitary bone cyst

     EXCLUDES 2   solitary cyst of jaw (M27.4)

     M85.40 Solitary bone cyst, unspecified site

✓6ᵗʰ **M85.41** Solitary bone cyst, shoulder

     M85.411 Solitary bone cyst, right shoulder

     M85.412 Solitary bone cyst, left shoulder

     M85.419 Solitary bone cyst, unspecified shoulder

✓6ᵗʰ **M85.42** Solitary bone cyst, humerus

     M85.421 Solitary bone cyst, right humerus

     M85.422 Solitary bone cyst, left humerus

     M85.429 Solitary bone cyst, unspecified humerus

✓6ᵗʰ **M85.43** Solitary bone cyst, ulna and radius

     M85.431 Solitary bone cyst, right ulna and radius

     M85.432 Solitary bone cyst, left ulna and radius

     M85.439 Solitary bone cyst, unspecified ulna and radius

✓6ᵗʰ **M85.44** Solitary bone cyst, hand

     M85.441 Solitary bone cyst, right hand

     M85.442 Solitary bone cyst, left hand

     M85.449 Solitary bone cyst, unspecified hand

✓6ᵗʰ **M85.45** Solitary bone cyst, pelvis

     M85.451 Solitary bone cyst, right pelvis

     M85.452 Solitary bone cyst, left pelvis

     M85.459 Solitary bone cyst, unspecified pelvis

✓6ᵗʰ **M85.46** Solitary bone cyst, tibia and fibula

     M85.461 Solitary bone cyst, right tibia and fibula

     M85.462 Solitary bone cyst, left tibia and fibula

     M85.469 Solitary bone cyst, unspecified tibia and fibula

✓6ᵗʰ **M85.47** Solitary bone cyst, ankle and foot

     M85.471 Solitary bone cyst, right ankle and foot

     M85.472 Solitary bone cyst, left ankle and foot

     M85.479 Solitary bone cyst, unspecified ankle and foot

     M85.48 Solitary bone cyst, other site

✔ Additional Character Required   ✓x7ᵗʰ Placeholder   Questionable PDx   Manifestation   Unspecified Dx   **UPD** Unacceptable PDx   **H1**-**H14** HAC   **HCC** CMS-HCC Dx   **HIV** HIV Dx

ICD-10-CM 2022   **827**

✓5ᵗʰ **M85.5 Aneurysmal bone cyst**

> EXCLUDES 2   *aneurysmal cyst of jaw (M27.4)*
> **DEF:** Solitary bone lesion that bulges into the periosteum and is marked by a calcified rim.

   M85.50 **Aneurysmal bone cyst, unspecified site**

✓6ᵗʰ   M85.51 **Aneurysmal bone cyst, shoulder**

    M85.511 **Aneurysmal bone cyst, right shoulder**
    M85.512 **Aneurysmal bone cyst, left shoulder**
    M85.519 **Aneurysmal bone cyst, unspecified shoulder**

✓6ᵗʰ   M85.52 **Aneurysmal bone cyst, upper arm**

    M85.521 **Aneurysmal bone cyst, right upper arm**
    M85.522 **Aneurysmal bone cyst, left upper arm**
    M85.529 **Aneurysmal bone cyst, unspecified upper arm**

✓6ᵗʰ   M85.53 **Aneurysmal bone cyst, forearm**

    M85.531 **Aneurysmal bone cyst, right forearm**
    M85.532 **Aneurysmal bone cyst, left forearm**
    M85.539 **Aneurysmal bone cyst, unspecified forearm**

✓6ᵗʰ   M85.54 **Aneurysmal bone cyst, hand**

    M85.541 **Aneurysmal bone cyst, right hand**
    M85.542 **Aneurysmal bone cyst, left hand**
    M85.549 **Aneurysmal bone cyst, unspecified hand**

✓6ᵗʰ   M85.55 **Aneurysmal bone cyst, thigh**

    M85.551 **Aneurysmal bone cyst, right thigh**
    M85.552 **Aneurysmal bone cyst, left thigh**
    M85.559 **Aneurysmal bone cyst, unspecified thigh**

✓6ᵗʰ   M85.56 **Aneurysmal bone cyst, lower leg**

    M85.561 **Aneurysmal bone cyst, right lower leg**
    M85.562 **Aneurysmal bone cyst, left lower leg**
    M85.569 **Aneurysmal bone cyst, unspecified lower leg**

✓6ᵗʰ   M85.57 **Aneurysmal bone cyst, ankle and foot**

    M85.571 **Aneurysmal bone cyst, right ankle and foot**
    M85.572 **Aneurysmal bone cyst, left ankle and foot**
    M85.579 **Aneurysmal bone cyst, unspecified ankle and foot**

   M85.58 **Aneurysmal bone cyst, other site**
   M85.59 **Aneurysmal bone cyst, multiple sites**

✓5ᵗʰ **M85.6 Other cyst of bone**

> EXCLUDES 1   *cyst of jaw NEC (M27.4)*
> *osteitis fibrosa cystica generalisata [von Recklinghausen's disease of bone] (E21.0)*

   M85.60 **Other cyst of bone, unspecified site**

✓6ᵗʰ   M85.61 **Other cyst of bone, shoulder**

    M85.611 **Other cyst of bone, right shoulder**
    M85.612 **Other cyst of bone, left shoulder**
    M85.619 **Other cyst of bone, unspecified shoulder**

✓6ᵗʰ   M85.62 **Other cyst of bone, upper arm**

    M85.621 **Other cyst of bone, right upper arm**
    M85.622 **Other cyst of bone, left upper arm**
    M85.629 **Other cyst of bone, unspecified upper arm**

✓6ᵗʰ   M85.63 **Other cyst of bone, forearm**

    M85.631 **Other cyst of bone, right forearm**
    M85.632 **Other cyst of bone, left forearm**
    M85.639 **Other cyst of bone, unspecified forearm**

✓6ᵗʰ   M85.64 **Other cyst of bone, hand**

    M85.641 **Other cyst of bone, right hand**
    M85.642 **Other cyst of bone, left hand**
    M85.649 **Other cyst of bone, unspecified hand**

✓6ᵗʰ   M85.65 **Other cyst of bone, thigh**

    M85.651 **Other cyst of bone, right thigh**
    M85.652 **Other cyst of bone, left thigh**
    M85.659 **Other cyst of bone, unspecified thigh**

✓6ᵗʰ   M85.66 **Other cyst of bone, lower leg**

    M85.661 **Other cyst of bone, right lower leg**
    M85.662 **Other cyst of bone, left lower leg**
    M85.669 **Other cyst of bone, unspecified lower leg**

✓6ᵗʰ   M85.67 **Other cyst of bone, ankle and foot**

    M85.671 **Other cyst of bone, right ankle and foot**
    M85.672 **Other cyst of bone, left ankle and foot**
    M85.679 **Other cyst of bone, unspecified ankle and foot**

   M85.68 **Other cyst of bone, other site**

   M85.69 **Other cyst of bone, multiple sites**

✓5ᵗʰ **M85.8 Other specified disorders of bone density and structure**

> Hyperostosis of bones, except skull
> Osteosclerosis, acquired
> EXCLUDES 1   *diffuse idiopathic skeletal hyperostosis [DISH] (M48.1)*
> *osteosclerosis congenita (Q77.4)*
> *osteosclerosis fragilitas (generalista) (Q78.2)*
> *osteosclerosis myelofibrosis (D75.81)*

   M85.80 **Other specified disorders of bone density and structure, unspecified site**

✓6ᵗʰ   M85.81 **Other specified disorders of bone density and structure, shoulder**

    M85.811 **Other specified disorders of bone density and structure, right shoulder**
    M85.812 **Other specified disorders of bone density and structure, left shoulder**
    M85.819 **Other specified disorders of bone density and structure, unspecified shoulder**

✓6ᵗʰ   M85.82 **Other specified disorders of bone density and structure, upper arm**

    M85.821 **Other specified disorders of bone density and structure, right upper arm**
    M85.822 **Other specified disorders of bone density and structure, left upper arm**
    M85.829 **Other specified disorders of bone density and structure, unspecified upper arm**

✓6ᵗʰ   M85.83 **Other specified disorders of bone density and structure, forearm**

    M85.831 **Other specified disorders of bone density and structure, right forearm**
    M85.832 **Other specified disorders of bone density and structure, left forearm**
    M85.839 **Other specified disorders of bone density and structure, unspecified forearm**

✓6ᵗʰ   M85.84 **Other specified disorders of bone density and structure, hand**

    M85.841 **Other specified disorders of bone density and structure, right hand**
    M85.842 **Other specified disorders of bone density and structure, left hand**
    M85.849 **Other specified disorders of bone density and structure, unspecified hand**

✓6ᵗʰ   M85.85 **Other specified disorders of bone density and structure, thigh**

    M85.851 **Other specified disorders of bone density and structure, right thigh**
    M85.852 **Other specified disorders of bone density and structure, left thigh**
    M85.859 **Other specified disorders of bone density and structure, unspecified thigh**

✓6ᵗʰ   M85.86 **Other specified disorders of bone density and structure, lower leg**

    M85.861 **Other specified disorders of bone density and structure, right lower leg**
    M85.862 **Other specified disorders of bone density and structure, left lower leg**
    M85.869 **Other specified disorders of bone density and structure, unspecified lower leg**

✓6ᵗʰ   M85.87 **Other specified disorders of bone density and structure, ankle and foot**

    M85.871 **Other specified disorders of bone density and structure, right ankle and foot**
    M85.872 **Other specified disorders of bone density and structure, left ankle and foot**
    M85.879 **Other specified disorders of bone density and structure, unspecified ankle and foot**

   M85.88 **Other specified disorders of bone density and structure, other site**

   M85.89 **Other specified disorders of bone density and structure, multiple sites**

   M85.9 **Disorder of bone density and structure, unspecified**

N Newborn: 0   P Pediatric: 0-17   M Maternity: 9-64   A Adult: 15-124   MCC Major Complication/Comorbidity   CC Complication/Comorbidity   SW Severe Wound Dx

828

ICD-10-CM 2022

Other osteopathies (M86-M90)

EXCLUDES 1   *postprocedural osteopathies (M96.-)*

✓4ᵗʰ **M86 Osteomyelitis**

Use additional code (B95-B97) to identify infectious agent
Use additional code to identify major osseous defect, if applicable (M89.7-)

     EXCLUDES 1   *osteomyelitis due to:*
       echinococcus (B67.2)
       gonococcus (A54.43)
       salmonella (A02.24)

     EXCLUDES 2   *osteomyelitis of:*
       orbit (H05.0-)
       petrous bone (H70.2-)
       vertebra (M46.2-)

✓5ᵗʰ **M86.0 Acute hematogenous osteomyelitis**

     M86.00 Acute hematogenous osteomyelitis, unspecified site   CC HCC

     ✓6ᵗʰ **M86.01 Acute hematogenous osteomyelitis, shoulder**

       M86.011 Acute hematogenous osteomyelitis, right shoulder   CC HCC
       M86.012 Acute hematogenous osteomyelitis, left shoulder   CC HCC
       M86.019 Acute hematogenous osteomyelitis, unspecified shoulder   CC HCC

     ✓6ᵗʰ **M86.02 Acute hematogenous osteomyelitis, humerus**

       M86.021 Acute hematogenous osteomyelitis, right humerus   CC HCC
       M86.022 Acute hematogenous osteomyelitis, left humerus   CC HCC
       M86.029 Acute hematogenous osteomyelitis, unspecified humerus   CC HCC

     ✓6ᵗʰ **M86.03 Acute hematogenous osteomyelitis, radius and ulna**

       M86.031 Acute hematogenous osteomyelitis, right radius and ulna   CC HCC
       M86.032 Acute hematogenous osteomyelitis, left radius and ulna   CC HCC
       M86.039 Acute hematogenous osteomyelitis, unspecified radius and ulna   CC HCC

     ✓6ᵗʰ **M86.04 Acute hematogenous osteomyelitis, hand**

       M86.041 Acute hematogenous osteomyelitis, right hand   CC HCC
       M86.042 Acute hematogenous osteomyelitis, left hand   CC HCC
       M86.049 Acute hematogenous osteomyelitis, unspecified hand   CC HCC

     ✓6ᵗʰ **M86.05 Acute hematogenous osteomyelitis, femur**

       M86.051 Acute hematogenous osteomyelitis, right femur   CC HCC
       M86.052 Acute hematogenous osteomyelitis, left femur   CC HCC
       M86.059 Acute hematogenous osteomyelitis, unspecified femur   CC HCC

     ✓6ᵗʰ **M86.06 Acute hematogenous osteomyelitis, tibia and fibula**

       M86.061 Acute hematogenous osteomyelitis, right tibia and fibula   CC HCC
       M86.062 Acute hematogenous osteomyelitis, left tibia and fibula   CC HCC
       M86.069 Acute hematogenous osteomyelitis, unspecified tibia and fibula   CC HCC

     ✓6ᵗʰ **M86.07 Acute hematogenous osteomyelitis, ankle and foot**

       M86.071 Acute hematogenous osteomyelitis, right ankle and foot   CC HCC
       M86.072 Acute hematogenous osteomyelitis, left ankle and foot   CC HCC
       M86.079 Acute hematogenous osteomyelitis, unspecified ankle and foot   CC HCC

     M86.08 Acute hematogenous osteomyelitis, other sites   CC HCC

     M86.09 Acute hematogenous osteomyelitis, multiple sites   CC HCC

✓5ᵗʰ **M86.1 Other acute osteomyelitis**

     M86.10 Other acute osteomyelitis, unspecified site   CC HCC

✓6ᵗʰ **M86.11 Other acute osteomyelitis, shoulder**

     M86.111 Other acute osteomyelitis, right shoulder   CC HCC
     M86.112 Other acute osteomyelitis, left shoulder   CC HCC
     M86.119 Other acute osteomyelitis, unspecified shoulder   CC HCC

✓6ᵗʰ **M86.12 Other acute osteomyelitis, humerus**

     M86.121 Other acute osteomyelitis, right humerus   CC HCC
     M86.122 Other acute osteomyelitis, left humerus   CC HCC
     M86.129 Other acute osteomyelitis, unspecified humerus   CC HCC

✓6ᵗʰ **M86.13 Other acute osteomyelitis, radius and ulna**

     M86.131 Other acute osteomyelitis, right radius and ulna   CC HCC
     M86.132 Other acute osteomyelitis, left radius and ulna   CC HCC
     M86.139 Other acute osteomyelitis, unspecified radius and ulna   CC HCC

✓6ᵗʰ **M86.14 Other acute osteomyelitis, hand**

     M86.141 Other acute osteomyelitis, right hand   CC HCC
     M86.142 Other acute osteomyelitis, left hand   CC HCC
     M86.149 Other acute osteomyelitis, unspecified hand   CC HCC

✓6ᵗʰ **M86.15 Other acute osteomyelitis, femur**

     M86.151 Other acute osteomyelitis, right femur   CC HCC
     M86.152 Other acute osteomyelitis, left femur   CC HCC
     M86.159 Other acute osteomyelitis, unspecified femur   CC HCC

✓6ᵗʰ **M86.16 Other acute osteomyelitis, tibia and fibula**

     M86.161 Other acute osteomyelitis, right tibia and fibula   CC HCC
     M86.162 Other acute osteomyelitis, left tibia and fibula   CC HCC
     M86.169 Other acute osteomyelitis, unspecified tibia and fibula   CC HCC

✓6ᵗʰ **M86.17 Other acute osteomyelitis, ankle and foot**

     AHA: 2020,1Q,12

     M86.171 Other acute osteomyelitis, right ankle and foot   CC HCC
     M86.172 Other acute osteomyelitis, left ankle and foot   CC HCC
     M86.179 Other acute osteomyelitis, unspecified ankle and foot   CC HCC

     M86.18 Other acute osteomyelitis, other site   CC HCC

     M86.19 Other acute osteomyelitis, multiple sites   CC HCC

✓5ᵗʰ **M86.2 Subacute osteomyelitis**

     M86.20 Subacute osteomyelitis, unspecified site   CC HCC

     ✓6ᵗʰ **M86.21 Subacute osteomyelitis, shoulder**

       M86.211 Subacute osteomyelitis, right shoulder   CC HCC
       M86.212 Subacute osteomyelitis, left shoulder   CC HCC
       M86.219 Subacute osteomyelitis, unspecified shoulder   CC HCC

     ✓6ᵗʰ **M86.22 Subacute osteomyelitis, humerus**

       M86.221 Subacute osteomyelitis, right humerus   CC HCC
       M86.222 Subacute osteomyelitis, left humerus   CC HCC
       M86.229 Subacute osteomyelitis, unspecified humerus   CC HCC

     ✓6ᵗʰ **M86.23 Subacute osteomyelitis, radius and ulna**

       M86.231 Subacute osteomyelitis, right radius and ulna   CC HCC
       M86.232 Subacute osteomyelitis, left radius and ulna   CC HCC
       M86.239 Subacute osteomyelitis, unspecified radius and ulna   CC HCC

     ✓6ᵗʰ **M86.24 Subacute osteomyelitis, hand**

       M86.241 Subacute osteomyelitis, right hand   CC HCC

✔ Additional Character Required   ✓x7ᵗʰ Placeholder   Questionable PDx   Manifestation   Unspecified Dx   UPD Unacceptable PDx   H1-H14 HAC   HCC CMS-HCC Dx   HIV HIV Dx

ICD-10-CM 2022   829

M86.242 Subacute osteomyelitis, left hand `CC` `HCC`

M86.249 Subacute osteomyelitis, unspecified hand `CC` `HCC`

✓6ᵗʰ M86.25 Subacute osteomyelitis, femur

    M86.251 Subacute osteomyelitis, right femur `CC` `HCC`

    M86.252 Subacute osteomyelitis, left femur `CC` `HCC`

    M86.259 Subacute osteomyelitis, unspecified femur `CC` `HCC`

✓6ᵗʰ M86.26 Subacute osteomyelitis, tibia and fibula

    M86.261 Subacute osteomyelitis, right tibia and fibula `CC` `HCC`

    M86.262 Subacute osteomyelitis, left tibia and fibula `CC` `HCC`

    M86.269 Subacute osteomyelitis, unspecified tibia and fibula `CC` `HCC`

✓6ᵗʰ M86.27 Subacute osteomyelitis, ankle and foot

    M86.271 Subacute osteomyelitis, right ankle and foot `CC` `HCC`

    M86.272 Subacute osteomyelitis, left ankle and foot `CC` `HCC`

    M86.279 Subacute osteomyelitis, unspecified ankle and foot `CC` `HCC`

M86.28 Subacute osteomyelitis, other site `CC` `HCC`

M86.29 Subacute osteomyelitis, multiple sites `CC` `HCC`

✓5ᵗʰ M86.3 Chronic multifocal osteomyelitis

    M86.30 Chronic multifocal osteomyelitis, unspecified site `CC` `HCC`

✓6ᵗʰ M86.31 Chronic multifocal osteomyelitis, shoulder

    M86.311 Chronic multifocal osteomyelitis, right shoulder `CC` `HCC`

    M86.312 Chronic multifocal osteomyelitis, left shoulder `CC` `HCC`

    M86.319 Chronic multifocal osteomyelitis, unspecified shoulder `CC` `HCC`

✓6ᵗʰ M86.32 Chronic multifocal osteomyelitis, humerus

    M86.321 Chronic multifocal osteomyelitis, right humerus `CC` `HCC`

    M86.322 Chronic multifocal osteomyelitis, left humerus `CC` `HCC`

    M86.329 Chronic multifocal osteomyelitis, unspecified humerus `CC` `HCC`

✓6ᵗʰ M86.33 Chronic multifocal osteomyelitis, radius and ulna

    M86.331 Chronic multifocal osteomyelitis, right radius and ulna `CC` `HCC`

    M86.332 Chronic multifocal osteomyelitis, left radius and ulna `CC` `HCC`

    M86.339 Chronic multifocal osteomyelitis, unspecified radius and ulna `CC` `HCC`

✓6ᵗʰ M86.34 Chronic multifocal osteomyelitis, hand

    M86.341 Chronic multifocal osteomyelitis, right hand `CC` `HCC`

    M86.342 Chronic multifocal osteomyelitis, left hand `CC` `HCC`

    M86.349 Chronic multifocal osteomyelitis, unspecified hand `CC` `HCC`

✓6ᵗʰ M86.35 Chronic multifocal osteomyelitis, femur

    M86.351 Chronic multifocal osteomyelitis, right femur `CC` `HCC`

    M86.352 Chronic multifocal osteomyelitis, left femur `CC` `HCC`

    M86.359 Chronic multifocal osteomyelitis, unspecified femur `CC` `HCC`

✓6ᵗʰ M86.36 Chronic multifocal osteomyelitis, tibia and fibula

    M86.361 Chronic multifocal osteomyelitis, right tibia and fibula `CC` `HCC`

    M86.362 Chronic multifocal osteomyelitis, left tibia and fibula `CC` `HCC`

    M86.369 Chronic multifocal osteomyelitis, unspecified tibia and fibula `CC` `HCC`

✓6ᵗʰ M86.37 Chronic multifocal osteomyelitis, ankle and foot

    M86.371 Chronic multifocal osteomyelitis, right ankle and foot `CC` `HCC`

    M86.372 Chronic multifocal osteomyelitis, left ankle and foot `CC` `HCC`

    M86.379 Chronic multifocal osteomyelitis, unspecified ankle and foot `CC` `HCC`

M86.38 Chronic multifocal osteomyelitis, other site `CC` `HCC`

M86.39 Chronic multifocal osteomyelitis, multiple sites `CC` `HCC`

✓5ᵗʰ M86.4 Chronic osteomyelitis with draining sinus

    M86.40 Chronic osteomyelitis with draining sinus, unspecified site `CC` `HCC`

✓6ᵗʰ M86.41 Chronic osteomyelitis with draining sinus, shoulder

    M86.411 Chronic osteomyelitis with draining sinus, right shoulder `CC` `HCC`

    M86.412 Chronic osteomyelitis with draining sinus, left shoulder `CC` `HCC`

    M86.419 Chronic osteomyelitis with draining sinus, unspecified shoulder `CC` `HCC`

✓6ᵗʰ M86.42 Chronic osteomyelitis with draining sinus, humerus

    M86.421 Chronic osteomyelitis with draining sinus, right humerus `CC` `HCC`

    M86.422 Chronic osteomyelitis with draining sinus, left humerus `CC` `HCC`

    M86.429 Chronic osteomyelitis with draining sinus, unspecified humerus `CC` `HCC`

✓6ᵗʰ M86.43 Chronic osteomyelitis with draining sinus, radius and ulna

    M86.431 Chronic osteomyelitis with draining sinus, right radius and ulna `CC` `HCC`

    M86.432 Chronic osteomyelitis with draining sinus, left radius and ulna `CC` `HCC`

    M86.439 Chronic osteomyelitis with draining sinus, unspecified radius and ulna `CC` `HCC`

✓6ᵗʰ M86.44 Chronic osteomyelitis with draining sinus, hand

    M86.441 Chronic osteomyelitis with draining sinus, right hand `CC` `HCC`

    M86.442 Chronic osteomyelitis with draining sinus, left hand `CC` `HCC`

    M86.449 Chronic osteomyelitis with draining sinus, unspecified hand `CC` `HCC`

✓6ᵗʰ M86.45 Chronic osteomyelitis with draining sinus, femur

    M86.451 Chronic osteomyelitis with draining sinus, right femur `CC` `HCC`

    M86.452 Chronic osteomyelitis with draining sinus, left femur `CC` `HCC`

    M86.459 Chronic osteomyelitis with draining sinus, unspecified femur `CC` `HCC`

✓6ᵗʰ M86.46 Chronic osteomyelitis with draining sinus, tibia and fibula

    M86.461 Chronic osteomyelitis with draining sinus, right tibia and fibula `CC` `HCC`

    M86.462 Chronic osteomyelitis with draining sinus, left tibia and fibula `CC` `HCC`

    M86.469 Chronic osteomyelitis with draining sinus, unspecified tibia and fibula `CC` `HCC`

✓6ᵗʰ M86.47 Chronic osteomyelitis with draining sinus, ankle and foot

    M86.471 Chronic osteomyelitis with draining sinus, right ankle and foot `CC` `HCC`

    M86.472 Chronic osteomyelitis with draining sinus, left ankle and foot `CC` `HCC`

    M86.479 Chronic osteomyelitis with draining sinus, unspecified ankle and foot `CC` `HCC`

M86.48 Chronic osteomyelitis with draining sinus, other site `CC` `HCC`

M86.49 Chronic osteomyelitis with draining sinus, multiple sites `CC` `HCC`

✓5ᵗʰ M86.5 Other chronic hematogenous osteomyelitis

    M86.50 Other chronic hematogenous osteomyelitis, unspecified site `CC` `HCC`

✓6ᵗʰ M86.51 Other chronic hematogenous osteomyelitis, shoulder

    M86.511 Other chronic hematogenous osteomyelitis, right shoulder `CC` `HCC`

    M86.512 Other chronic hematogenous osteomyelitis, left shoulder `CC` `HCC`

    M86.519 Other chronic hematogenous osteomyelitis, unspecified shoulder `CC` `HCC`

Ⓝ Newborn: 0   Ⓟ Pediatric: 0-17   Ⓜ Maternity: 9-64   Ⓐ Adult: 15-124   `MCC` Major Complication/Comorbidity   `CC` Complication/Comorbidity   `SW` Severe Wound Dx

✓6ᵗʰ **M86.52** **Other chronic hematogenous osteomyelitis, humerus**

     M86.521 Other chronic hematogenous osteomyelitis, right humerus   `CC` `HCC`

     M86.522 Other chronic hematogenous osteomyelitis, left humerus   `CC` `HCC`

     M86.529 Other chronic hematogenous osteomyelitis, unspecified humerus

✓6ᵗʰ **M86.53** **Other chronic hematogenous osteomyelitis, radius and ulna**

     M86.531 Other chronic hematogenous osteomyelitis, right radius and ulna   `CC` `HCC`

     M86.532 Other chronic hematogenous osteomyelitis, left radius and ulna   `CC` `HCC`

     M86.539 Other chronic hematogenous osteomyelitis, unspecified radius and ulna   `CC` `HCC`

✓6ᵗʰ **M86.54** **Other chronic hematogenous osteomyelitis, hand**

     M86.541 Other chronic hematogenous osteomyelitis, right hand   `CC` `HCC`

     M86.542 Other chronic hematogenous osteomyelitis, left hand   `CC` `HCC`

     M86.549 Other chronic hematogenous osteomyelitis, unspecified hand   `CC` `HCC`

✓6ᵗʰ **M86.55** **Other chronic hematogenous osteomyelitis, femur**

     M86.551 Other chronic hematogenous osteomyelitis, right femur   `CC` `HCC`

     M86.552 Other chronic hematogenous osteomyelitis, left femur   `CC` `HCC`

     M86.559 Other chronic hematogenous osteomyelitis, unspecified femur   `CC` `HCC`

✓6ᵗʰ **M86.56** **Other chronic hematogenous osteomyelitis, tibia and fibula**

     M86.561 Other chronic hematogenous osteomyelitis, right tibia and fibula   `CC` `HCC`

     M86.562 Other chronic hematogenous osteomyelitis, left tibia and fibula   `CC` `HCC`

     M86.569 Other chronic hematogenous osteomyelitis, unspecified tibia and fibula   `CC` `HCC`

✓6ᵗʰ **M86.57** **Other chronic hematogenous osteomyelitis, ankle and foot**

     M86.571 Other chronic hematogenous osteomyelitis, right ankle and foot   `CC` `HCC`

     M86.572 Other chronic hematogenous osteomyelitis, left ankle and foot   `CC` `HCC`

     M86.579 Other chronic hematogenous osteomyelitis, unspecified ankle and foot   `CC` `HCC`

   M86.58 Other chronic hematogenous osteomyelitis, other site   `CC` `HCC`

   M86.59 Other chronic hematogenous osteomyelitis, multiple sites   `CC` `HCC`

✓5ᵗʰ **M86.6** **Other chronic osteomyelitis**

     M86.60 Other chronic osteomyelitis, unspecified site   `CC` `HCC`

✓6ᵗʰ **M86.61** **Other chronic osteomyelitis, shoulder**

     M86.611 Other chronic osteomyelitis, right shoulder   `CC` `HCC`

     M86.612 Other chronic osteomyelitis, left shoulder   `CC` `HCC`

     M86.619 Other chronic osteomyelitis, unspecified shoulder   `CC` `HCC`

✓6ᵗʰ **M86.62** **Other chronic osteomyelitis, humerus**

     M86.621 Other chronic osteomyelitis, right humerus   `CC` `HCC`

     M86.622 Other chronic osteomyelitis, left humerus   `CC` `HCC`

     M86.629 Other chronic osteomyelitis, unspecified humerus   `CC` `HCC`

✓6ᵗʰ **M86.63** **Other chronic osteomyelitis, radius and ulna**

     M86.631 Other chronic osteomyelitis, right radius and ulna   `CC` `HCC`

     M86.632 Other chronic osteomyelitis, left radius and ulna   `CC` `HCC`

     M86.639 Other chronic osteomyelitis, unspecified radius and ulna

✓6ᵗʰ **M86.64** **Other chronic osteomyelitis, hand**

     M86.641 Other chronic osteomyelitis, right hand   `CC` `HCC`

     M86.642 Other chronic osteomyelitis, left hand   `CC` `HCC`

     M86.649 Other chronic osteomyelitis, unspecified hand   `CC` `HCC`

✓6ᵗʰ **M86.65** **Other chronic osteomyelitis, thigh**

     M86.651 Other chronic osteomyelitis, right thigh   `CC` `HCC`

     M86.652 Other chronic osteomyelitis, left thigh   `CC` `HCC`

     M86.659 Other chronic osteomyelitis, unspecified thigh   `CC` `HCC`

✓6ᵗʰ **M86.66** **Other chronic osteomyelitis, tibia and fibula**

     M86.661 Other chronic osteomyelitis, right tibia and fibula   `CC` `HCC`

     M86.662 Other chronic osteomyelitis, left tibia and fibula   `CC` `HCC`

     M86.669 Other chronic osteomyelitis, unspecified tibia and fibula   `CC` `HCC`

✓6ᵗʰ **M86.67** **Other chronic osteomyelitis, ankle and foot**

     M86.671 Other chronic osteomyelitis, right ankle and foot   `CC` `HCC`

       AHA: 2016,1Q,13

     M86.672 Other chronic osteomyelitis, left ankle and foot   `CC` `HCC`

     M86.679 Other chronic osteomyelitis, unspecified ankle and foot   `CC` `HCC`

   M86.68 Other chronic osteomyelitis, other site   `CC` `HCC`

   M86.69 Other chronic osteomyelitis, multiple sites   `CC` `HCC`

✓5ᵗʰ **M86.8** **Other osteomyelitis**

     Brodie's abscess

✓6ᵗʰ **M86.8X** **Other osteomyelitis**

     M86.8X0 Other osteomyelitis, multiple sites   `CC` `HCC`

     M86.8X1 Other osteomyelitis, shoulder   `CC` `HCC`

     M86.8X2 Other osteomyelitis, upper arm   `CC` `HCC`

     M86.8X3 Other osteomyelitis, forearm   `CC` `HCC`

     M86.8X4 Other osteomyelitis, hand   `CC` `HCC`

     M86.8X5 Other osteomyelitis, thigh   `CC` `HCC`

     M86.8X6 Other osteomyelitis, lower leg   `CC` `HCC`

     M86.8X7 Other osteomyelitis, ankle and foot   `CC` `HCC`

     M86.8X8 Other osteomyelitis, other site   `CC` `HCC`

     M86.8X9 Other osteomyelitis, unspecified sites   `CC` `HCC`

   M86.9 **Osteomyelitis, unspecified**   `CC` `HCC`

     Infection of bone NOS

     Periostitis without osteomyelitis

✓4ᵗʰ **M87** **Osteonecrosis**

   `INCLUDES`   avascular necrosis of bone

   Use additional code to identify major osseous defect, if applicable (M89.7-)

   `EXCLUDES 1`   *juvenile osteonecrosis (M91-M92)*
         osteochondropathies (M90-M93)

✓5ᵗʰ **M87.0** **Idiopathic aseptic necrosis of bone**

     M87.00 Idiopathic aseptic necrosis of unspecified bone   `CC` `HCC`

✓6ᵗʰ **M87.01** **Idiopathic aseptic necrosis of shoulder**

     Idiopathic aseptic necrosis of clavicle and scapula

     M87.011 Idiopathic aseptic necrosis of right shoulder   `CC` `HCC`

     M87.012 Idiopathic aseptic necrosis of left shoulder   `CC` `HCC`

     M87.019 Idiopathic aseptic necrosis of unspecified shoulder   `CC` `HCC`

☑ Additional Character Required   ✓x7ᵗʰ Placeholder   Questionable PDx   *Manifestation*   Unspecified Dx   `UPD` Unacceptable PDx   `H1`-`H14` HAC   `HCC` CMS-HCC Dx   `HIV` HIV Dx

ICD-10-CM 2022   831

✓6ᵗʰ **M87.02 Idiopathic aseptic necrosis of humerus**

     M87.021 Idiopathic aseptic necrosis of right humerus `CC` `HCC`

     M87.022 Idiopathic aseptic necrosis of left humerus `CC` `HCC`

     M87.029 Idiopathic aseptic necrosis of unspecified humerus `CC` `HCC`

✓6ᵗʰ **M87.03 Idiopathic aseptic necrosis of radius, ulna and carpus**

     M87.031 Idiopathic aseptic necrosis of right radius `CC` `HCC`

     M87.032 Idiopathic aseptic necrosis of left radius `CC` `HCC`

     M87.033 Idiopathic aseptic necrosis of unspecified radius `CC` `HCC`

     M87.034 Idiopathic aseptic necrosis of right ulna `CC` `HCC`

     M87.035 Idiopathic aseptic necrosis of left ulna `CC` `HCC`

     M87.036 Idiopathic aseptic necrosis of unspecified ulna `CC` `HCC`

     M87.037 Idiopathic aseptic necrosis of right carpus `CC` `HCC`

     M87.038 Idiopathic aseptic necrosis of left carpus `CC` `HCC`

     M87.039 Idiopathic aseptic necrosis of unspecified carpus `CC` `HCC`

✓6ᵗʰ **M87.04 Idiopathic aseptic necrosis of hand and fingers**

     Idiopathic aseptic necrosis of metacarpals and phalanges of hands

     M87.041 Idiopathic aseptic necrosis of right hand `CC` `HCC`

     M87.042 Idiopathic aseptic necrosis of left hand `CC` `HCC`

     M87.043 Idiopathic aseptic necrosis of unspecified hand `CC` `HCC`

     M87.044 Idiopathic aseptic necrosis of right finger(s) `CC` `HCC`

     M87.045 Idiopathic aseptic necrosis of left finger(s) `CC` `HCC`

     M87.046 Idiopathic aseptic necrosis of unspecified finger(s) `CC` `HCC`

✓6ᵗʰ **M87.05 Idiopathic aseptic necrosis of pelvis and femur**

     M87.050 Idiopathic aseptic necrosis of pelvis `CC` `HCC`

     M87.051 Idiopathic aseptic necrosis of right femur `CC` `HCC`

     M87.052 Idiopathic aseptic necrosis of left femur `CC` `HCC`

     M87.059 Idiopathic aseptic necrosis of unspecified femur `CC` `HCC`

✓6ᵗʰ **M87.06 Idiopathic aseptic necrosis of tibia and fibula**

     M87.061 Idiopathic aseptic necrosis of right tibia `CC` `HCC`

     M87.062 Idiopathic aseptic necrosis of left tibia `CC` `HCC`

     M87.063 Idiopathic aseptic necrosis of unspecified tibia `CC` `HCC`

     M87.064 Idiopathic aseptic necrosis of right fibula `CC` `HCC`

     M87.065 Idiopathic aseptic necrosis of left fibula `CC` `HCC`

     M87.066 Idiopathic aseptic necrosis of unspecified fibula `CC` `HCC`

✓6ᵗʰ **M87.07 Idiopathic aseptic necrosis of ankle, foot and toes**

     Idiopathic aseptic necrosis of metatarsus, tarsus, and phalanges of toes

     M87.071 Idiopathic aseptic necrosis of right ankle `CC` `HCC`

     M87.072 Idiopathic aseptic necrosis of left ankle `CC` `HCC`

     M87.073 Idiopathic aseptic necrosis of unspecified ankle `CC` `HCC`

     M87.074 Idiopathic aseptic necrosis of right foot `CC` `HCC`

     M87.075 Idiopathic aseptic necrosis of left foot `CC` `HCC`

     M87.076 Idiopathic aseptic necrosis of unspecified foot `CC` `HCC`

     M87.077 Idiopathic aseptic necrosis of right toe(s) `CC` `HCC`

     M87.078 Idiopathic aseptic necrosis of left toe(s) `CC` `HCC`

     M87.079 Idiopathic aseptic necrosis of unspecified toe(s) `CC` `HCC`

     M87.08 Idiopathic aseptic necrosis of bone, other site `CC` `HCC`

     M87.09 Idiopathic aseptic necrosis of bone, multiple sites `CC` `HCC`

✓5ᵗʰ **M87.1 Osteonecrosis due to drugs**

     Use additional code for adverse effect, if applicable, to identify drug (T36-T50 with fifth or sixth character 5)

     M87.10 Osteonecrosis due to drugs, unspecified bone `CC` `HCC`

✓6ᵗʰ **M87.11 Osteonecrosis due to drugs, shoulder**

     M87.111 Osteonecrosis due to drugs, right shoulder `CC` `HCC`

     M87.112 Osteonecrosis due to drugs, left shoulder `CC` `HCC`

     M87.119 Osteonecrosis due to drugs, unspecified shoulder `CC` `HCC`

✓6ᵗʰ **M87.12 Osteonecrosis due to drugs, humerus**

     M87.121 Osteonecrosis due to drugs, right humerus `CC` `HCC`

     M87.122 Osteonecrosis due to drugs, left humerus `CC` `HCC`

     M87.129 Osteonecrosis due to drugs, unspecified humerus `CC` `HCC`

✓6ᵗʰ **M87.13 Osteonecrosis due to drugs of radius, ulna and carpus**

     M87.131 Osteonecrosis due to drugs of right radius `CC` `HCC`

     M87.132 Osteonecrosis due to drugs of left radius `CC` `HCC`

     M87.133 Osteonecrosis due to drugs of unspecified radius `CC` `HCC`

     M87.134 Osteonecrosis due to drugs of right ulna `CC` `HCC`

     M87.135 Osteonecrosis due to drugs of left ulna `CC` `HCC`

     M87.136 Osteonecrosis due to drugs of unspecified ulna `CC` `HCC`

     M87.137 Osteonecrosis due to drugs of right carpus `CC` `HCC`

     M87.138 Osteonecrosis due to drugs of left carpus `CC` `HCC`

     M87.139 Osteonecrosis due to drugs of unspecified carpus `CC` `HCC`

✓6ᵗʰ **M87.14 Osteonecrosis due to drugs, hand and fingers**

     M87.141 Osteonecrosis due to drugs, right hand `CC` `HCC`

     M87.142 Osteonecrosis due to drugs, left hand `CC` `HCC`

     M87.143 Osteonecrosis due to drugs, unspecified hand `CC` `HCC`

     M87.144 Osteonecrosis due to drugs, right finger(s) `CC` `HCC`

     M87.145 Osteonecrosis due to drugs, left finger(s) `CC` `HCC`

     M87.146 Osteonecrosis due to drugs, unspecified finger(s) `CC` `HCC`

✓6ᵗʰ **M87.15 Osteonecrosis due to drugs, pelvis and femur**

     M87.150 Osteonecrosis due to drugs, pelvis `CC` `HCC`

     M87.151 Osteonecrosis due to drugs, right femur `CC` `HCC`

     M87.152 Osteonecrosis due to drugs, left femur `CC` `HCC`

     M87.159 Osteonecrosis due to drugs, unspecified femur `CC` `HCC`

✓6ᵗʰ **M87.16 Osteonecrosis due to drugs, tibia and fibula**

     M87.161 Osteonecrosis due to drugs, right tibia `CC` `HCC`

     M87.162 Osteonecrosis due to drugs, left tibia `CC` `HCC`

     M87.163 Osteonecrosis due to drugs, unspecified tibia `CC` `HCC`

Ⓝ Newborn: 0   Ⓟ Pediatric: 0-17   Ⓜ Maternity: 9-64   Ⓐ Adult: 15-124   `MCC` Major Complication/Comorbidity   `CC` Complication/Comorbidity   `SW` Severe Wound Dx

832   ICD-10-CM 2022

M87.164 Osteonecrosis due to drugs, right fibula `CC` `HCC`

M87.165 Osteonecrosis due to drugs, left fibula `CC` `HCC`

M87.166 Osteonecrosis due to drugs, unspecified fibula

✓6ᵗʰ M87.17 Osteonecrosis due to drugs, ankle, foot and toes

M87.171 Osteonecrosis due to drugs, right ankle `CC` `HCC`

M87.172 Osteonecrosis due to drugs, left ankle `CC` `HCC`

M87.173 Osteonecrosis due to drugs, unspecified ankle

M87.174 Osteonecrosis due to drugs, right foot `CC` `HCC`

M87.175 Osteonecrosis due to drugs, left foot `CC` `HCC`

M87.176 Osteonecrosis due to drugs, unspecified foot

M87.177 Osteonecrosis due to drugs, right toe(s) `CC` `HCC`

M87.178 Osteonecrosis due to drugs, left toe(s) `CC` `HCC`

M87.179 Osteonecrosis due to drugs, unspecified toe(s) `CC` `HCC`

✓6ᵗʰ M87.18 Osteonecrosis due to drugs, other site

M87.180 Osteonecrosis due to drugs, jaw `CC` `HCC`

M87.188 Osteonecrosis due to drugs, other site `CC` `HCC`

M87.19 Osteonecrosis due to drugs, multiple sites `CC` `HCC`

✓5ᵗʰ M87.2 Osteonecrosis due to previous trauma

M87.20 Osteonecrosis due to previous trauma, unspecified bone `CC` `HCC`

✓6ᵗʰ M87.21 Osteonecrosis due to previous trauma, shoulder

M87.211 Osteonecrosis due to previous trauma, right shoulder `CC` `HCC`

M87.212 Osteonecrosis due to previous trauma, left shoulder `CC` `HCC`

M87.219 Osteonecrosis due to previous trauma, unspecified shoulder `CC` `HCC`

✓6ᵗʰ M87.22 Osteonecrosis due to previous trauma, humerus

M87.221 Osteonecrosis due to previous trauma, right humerus `CC` `HCC`

M87.222 Osteonecrosis due to previous trauma, left humerus `CC` `HCC`

M87.229 Osteonecrosis due to previous trauma, unspecified humerus `CC` `HCC`

✓6ᵗʰ M87.23 Osteonecrosis due to previous trauma of radius, ulna and carpus

M87.231 Osteonecrosis due to previous trauma of right radius `CC` `HCC`

M87.232 Osteonecrosis due to previous trauma of left radius `CC` `HCC`

M87.233 Osteonecrosis due to previous trauma of unspecified radius `CC` `HCC`

M87.234 Osteonecrosis due to previous trauma of right ulna `CC` `HCC`

M87.235 Osteonecrosis due to previous trauma of left ulna `CC` `HCC`

M87.236 Osteonecrosis due to previous trauma of unspecified ulna `CC` `HCC`

M87.237 Osteonecrosis due to previous trauma of right carpus `CC` `HCC`

M87.238 Osteonecrosis due to previous trauma of left carpus `CC` `HCC`

M87.239 Osteonecrosis due to previous trauma of unspecified carpus `CC` `HCC`

✓6ᵗʰ M87.24 Osteonecrosis due to previous trauma, hand and fingers

M87.241 Osteonecrosis due to previous trauma, right hand `CC` `HCC`

M87.242 Osteonecrosis due to previous trauma, left hand `CC` `HCC`

M87.243 Osteonecrosis due to previous trauma, unspecified hand `CC` `HCC`

M87.244 Osteonecrosis due to previous trauma, right finger(s) `CC` `HCC`

M87.245 Osteonecrosis due to previous trauma, left finger(s) `CC` `HCC`

M87.246 Osteonecrosis due to previous trauma, unspecified finger(s) `CC` `HCC`

✓6ᵗʰ M87.25 Osteonecrosis due to previous trauma, pelvis and femur

M87.250 Osteonecrosis due to previous trauma, pelvis `CC` `HCC`

M87.251 Osteonecrosis due to previous trauma, right femur `CC` `HCC`

M87.252 Osteonecrosis due to previous trauma, left femur `CC` `HCC`

M87.256 Osteonecrosis due to previous trauma, unspecified femur `CC` `HCC`

✓6ᵗʰ M87.26 Osteonecrosis due to previous trauma, tibia and fibula

M87.261 Osteonecrosis due to previous trauma, right tibia `CC` `HCC`

M87.262 Osteonecrosis due to previous trauma, left tibia `CC` `HCC`

M87.263 Osteonecrosis due to previous trauma, unspecified tibia `CC` `HCC`

M87.264 Osteonecrosis due to previous trauma, right fibula `CC` `HCC`

M87.265 Osteonecrosis due to previous trauma, left fibula `CC` `HCC`

M87.266 Osteonecrosis due to previous trauma, unspecified fibula `CC` `HCC`

✓6ᵗʰ M87.27 Osteonecrosis due to previous trauma, ankle, foot and toes

M87.271 Osteonecrosis due to previous trauma, right ankle `CC` `HCC`

M87.272 Osteonecrosis due to previous trauma, left ankle `CC` `HCC`

M87.273 Osteonecrosis due to previous trauma, unspecified ankle `CC` `HCC`

M87.274 Osteonecrosis due to previous trauma, right foot `CC` `HCC`

M87.275 Osteonecrosis due to previous trauma, left foot `CC` `HCC`

M87.276 Osteonecrosis due to previous trauma, unspecified foot `CC` `HCC`

M87.277 Osteonecrosis due to previous trauma, right toe(s) `CC` `HCC`

M87.278 Osteonecrosis due to previous trauma, left toe(s) `CC` `HCC`

M87.279 Osteonecrosis due to previous trauma, unspecified toe(s) `CC` `HCC`

M87.28 Osteonecrosis due to previous trauma, other site `CC` `HCC`

M87.29 Osteonecrosis due to previous trauma, multiple sites `CC` `HCC`

✓5ᵗʰ M87.3 Other secondary osteonecrosis

M87.30 Other secondary osteonecrosis, unspecified bone `CC` `HCC`

✓6ᵗʰ M87.31 Other secondary osteonecrosis, shoulder

M87.311 Other secondary osteonecrosis, right shoulder `CC` `HCC`

M87.312 Other secondary osteonecrosis, left shoulder `CC` `HCC`

M87.319 Other secondary osteonecrosis, unspecified shoulder `CC` `HCC`

✓6ᵗʰ M87.32 Other secondary osteonecrosis, humerus

M87.321 Other secondary osteonecrosis, right humerus `CC` `HCC`

M87.322 Other secondary osteonecrosis, left humerus `CC` `HCC`

M87.329 Other secondary osteonecrosis, unspecified humerus `CC` `HCC`

✓6ᵗʰ M87.33 Other secondary osteonecrosis of radius, ulna and carpus

M87.331 Other secondary osteonecrosis of right radius `CC` `HCC`

M87.332 Other secondary osteonecrosis of left radius `CC` `HCC`

M87.333 Other secondary osteonecrosis of unspecified radius `CC` `HCC`

M87.334 Other secondary osteonecrosis of right ulna `CC` `HCC`

☑ Additional Character Required   ✓x7ᵗʰ Placeholder   Questionable PDx   Manifestation   Unspecified Dx   UPD Unacceptable PDx   H1-H14 HAC   HCC CMS-HCC Dx   HIV HIV Dx

ICD-10-CM 2022

833

M87.335 Other secondary osteonecrosis of left ulna `CC` `HCC`

M87.336 Other secondary osteonecrosis of unspecified ulna `CC` `HCC`

M87.337 Other secondary osteonecrosis of right carpus `CC` `HCC`

M87.338 Other secondary osteonecrosis of left carpus `CC` `HCC`

M87.339 Other secondary osteonecrosis of unspecified carpus `CC` `HCC`

√6ᵗʰ **M87.34 Other secondary osteonecrosis, hand and fingers**

M87.341 Other secondary osteonecrosis, right hand `CC` `HCC`

M87.342 Other secondary osteonecrosis, left hand `CC` `HCC`

M87.343 Other secondary osteonecrosis, unspecified hand `CC` `HCC`

M87.344 Other secondary osteonecrosis, right finger(s) `CC` `HCC`

M87.345 Other secondary osteonecrosis, left finger(s) `CC` `HCC`

M87.346 Other secondary osteonecrosis, unspecified finger(s) `CC` `HCC`

√6ᵗʰ **M87.35 Other secondary osteonecrosis, pelvis and femur**

M87.350 Other secondary osteonecrosis, pelvis `CC` `HCC`

M87.351 Other secondary osteonecrosis, right femur `CC` `HCC`

M87.352 Other secondary osteonecrosis, left femur `CC` `HCC`

M87.353 Other secondary osteonecrosis, unspecified femur `CC` `HCC`

√6ᵗʰ **M87.36 Other secondary osteonecrosis, tibia and fibula**

M87.361 Other secondary osteonecrosis, right tibia `CC` `HCC`

M87.362 Other secondary osteonecrosis, left tibia `CC` `HCC`

M87.363 Other secondary osteonecrosis, unspecified tibia `CC` `HCC`

M87.364 Other secondary osteonecrosis, right fibula `CC` `HCC`

M87.365 Other secondary osteonecrosis, left fibula `CC` `HCC`

M87.366 Other secondary osteonecrosis, unspecified fibula `CC` `HCC`

√6ᵗʰ **M87.37 Other secondary osteonecrosis, ankle and foot**

M87.371 Other secondary osteonecrosis, right ankle `CC` `HCC`

M87.372 Other secondary osteonecrosis, left ankle `CC` `HCC`

M87.373 Other secondary osteonecrosis, unspecified ankle `CC` `HCC`

M87.374 Other secondary osteonecrosis, right foot `CC` `HCC`

M87.375 Other secondary osteonecrosis, left foot `CC` `HCC`

M87.376 Other secondary osteonecrosis, unspecified foot `CC` `HCC`

M87.377 Other secondary osteonecrosis, right toe(s) `CC` `HCC`

M87.378 Other secondary osteonecrosis, left toe(s) `CC` `HCC`

M87.379 Other secondary osteonecrosis, unspecified toe(s) `CC` `HCC`

M87.38 Other secondary osteonecrosis, other site `CC` `HCC`

M87.39 Other secondary osteonecrosis, multiple sites `CC` `HCC`

√5ᵗʰ **M87.8 Other osteonecrosis**

M87.80 Other osteonecrosis, unspecified bone `CC` `HCC`

√6ᵗʰ **M87.81 Other osteonecrosis, shoulder**

M87.811 Other osteonecrosis, right shoulder `CC` `HCC`

M87.812 Other osteonecrosis, left shoulder `CC` `HCC`

M87.819 Other osteonecrosis, unspecified shoulder `CC` `HCC`

√6ᵗʰ **M87.82 Other osteonecrosis, humerus**

M87.821 Other osteonecrosis, right humerus `CC` `HCC`

M87.822 Other osteonecrosis, left humerus `CC` `HCC`

M87.829 Other osteonecrosis, unspecified humerus `CC` `HCC`

√6ᵗʰ **M87.83 Other osteonecrosis of radius, ulna and carpus**

M87.831 Other osteonecrosis of right radius `CC` `HCC`

M87.832 Other osteonecrosis of left radius `CC` `HCC`

M87.833 Other osteonecrosis of unspecified radius `CC` `HCC`

M87.834 Other osteonecrosis of right ulna `CC` `HCC`

M87.835 Other osteonecrosis of left ulna `CC` `HCC`

M87.836 Other osteonecrosis of unspecified ulna `CC` `HCC`

M87.837 Other osteonecrosis of right carpus `CC` `HCC`

M87.838 Other osteonecrosis of left carpus `CC` `HCC`

M87.839 Other osteonecrosis of unspecified carpus `CC` `HCC`

√6ᵗʰ **M87.84 Other osteonecrosis, hand and fingers**

M87.841 Other osteonecrosis, right hand `CC` `HCC`

M87.842 Other osteonecrosis, left hand `CC` `HCC`

M87.843 Other osteonecrosis, unspecified hand `CC` `HCC`

M87.844 Other osteonecrosis, right finger(s) `CC` `HCC`

M87.845 Other osteonecrosis, left finger(s) `CC` `HCC`

M87.849 Other osteonecrosis, unspecified finger(s) `CC` `HCC`

√6ᵗʰ **M87.85 Other osteonecrosis, pelvis and femur**

M87.850 Other osteonecrosis, pelvis `CC` `HCC`

M87.851 Other osteonecrosis, right femur `CC` `HCC`

M87.852 Other osteonecrosis, left femur `CC` `HCC`

M87.859 Other osteonecrosis, unspecified femur `CC` `HCC`

√6ᵗʰ **M87.86 Other osteonecrosis, tibia and fibula**

M87.861 Other osteonecrosis, right tibia `CC` `HCC`

M87.862 Other osteonecrosis, left tibia `CC` `HCC`

M87.863 Other osteonecrosis, unspecified tibia `CC` `HCC`

M87.864 Other osteonecrosis, right fibula `CC` `HCC`

M87.865 Other osteonecrosis, left fibula `CC` `HCC`

M87.869 Other osteonecrosis, unspecified fibula `CC` `HCC`

√6ᵗʰ **M87.87 Other osteonecrosis, ankle, foot and toes**

M87.871 Other osteonecrosis, right ankle `CC` `HCC`

M87.872 Other osteonecrosis, left ankle `CC` `HCC`

M87.873 Other osteonecrosis, unspecified ankle `CC` `HCC`

M87.874 Other osteonecrosis, right foot `CC` `HCC`

M87.875 Other osteonecrosis, left foot `CC` `HCC`

M87.876 Other osteonecrosis, unspecified foot `CC` `HCC`

M87.877 Other osteonecrosis, right toe(s) `CC` `HCC`

M87.878 Other osteonecrosis, left toe(s) `CC` `HCC`

M87.879 Other osteonecrosis, unspecified toe(s) `CC` `HCC`

M87.88 Other osteonecrosis, other site `CC` `HCC`

M87.89 Other osteonecrosis, multiple sites `CC` `HCC`

M87.9 Osteonecrosis, unspecified `CC` `HCC`

Necrosis of bone NOS

√4ᵗʰ **M88 Osteitis deformans [Paget's disease of bone]**

> *EXCLUDES 1*   *osteitis deformans in neoplastic disease (M90.6)*

DEF: Bone disease characterized by numerous cycles of bone resorption by the body. Resorption is followed by accelerated repair attempts, causing bone deformities and bowing, with associated fractures and pain.

M88.0 Osteitis deformans of skull

M88.1 Osteitis deformans of vertebrae

Ⓝ Newborn: 0   Ⓟ Pediatric: 0-17   Ⓜ Maternity: 9-64   Ⓐ Adult: 15-124   `MCC` Major Complication/Comorbidity   `CC` Complication/Comorbidity   `SW` Severe Wound Dx

834

ICD-10-CM 2022

☑5ᵗʰ **M88.8 Osteitis deformans of other bones**

  ☑6ᵗʰ **M88.81 Osteitis deformans of** shoulder

    M88.811 Osteitis deformans of right shoulder
    M88.812 Osteitis deformans of left shoulder
    M88.819 Osteitis deformans of unspecified shoulder

  ☑6ᵗʰ **M88.82 Osteitis deformans of** upper arm

    M88.821 Osteitis deformans of right upper arm
    M88.822 Osteitis deformans of left upper arm
    M88.829 Osteitis deformans of unspecified upper arm

  ☑6ᵗʰ **M88.83 Osteitis deformans of** forearm

    M88.831 Osteitis deformans of right forearm
    M88.832 Osteitis deformans of left forearm
    M88.839 Osteitis deformans of unspecified forearm

  ☑6ᵗʰ **M88.84 Osteitis deformans of** hand

    M88.841 Osteitis deformans of right hand
    M88.842 Osteitis deformans of left hand
    M88.849 Osteitis deformans of unspecified hand

  ☑6ᵗʰ **M88.85 Osteitis deformans of** thigh

    M88.851 Osteitis deformans of right thigh
    M88.852 Osteitis deformans of left thigh
    M88.859 Osteitis deformans of unspecified thigh

  ☑6ᵗʰ **M88.86 Osteitis deformans of** lower leg

    M88.861 Osteitis deformans of right lower leg
    M88.862 Osteitis deformans of left lower leg
    M88.869 Osteitis deformans of unspecified lower leg

  ☑6ᵗʰ **M88.87 Osteitis deformans of** ankle and foot

    M88.871 Osteitis deformans of right ankle and foot
    M88.872 Osteitis deformans of left ankle and foot
    M88.879 Osteitis deformans of unspecified ankle and foot

  M88.88 Osteitis deformans of other bones

    EXCLUDES 2   osteitis deformans of skull (M88.0)
               osteitis deformans of vertebrae (M88.1)

  M88.89 Osteitis deformans of multiple sites

M88.9 Osteitis deformans of unspecified bone

☑4ᵗʰ **M89 Other disorders of bone**

  ☑5ᵗʰ **M89.0 Algoneurodystrophy**

    Shoulder-hand syndrome
    Sudeck's atrophy

    EXCLUDES 1   causalgia, lower limb (G57.7-)
               causalgia, upper limb (G56.4-)
               complex regional pain syndrome II, lower limb (G57.7-)
               complex regional pain syndrome II, upper limb (G56.4-)
               reflex sympathetic dystrophy (G90.5-)

    M89.00 Algoneurodystrophy, unspecified site

  ☑6ᵗʰ **M89.01 Algoneurodystrophy,** shoulder

    M89.011 Algoneurodystrophy, right shoulder
    M89.012 Algoneurodystrophy, left shoulder
    M89.019 Algoneurodystrophy, unspecified shoulder

  ☑6ᵗʰ **M89.02 Algoneurodystrophy,** upper arm

    M89.021 Algoneurodystrophy, right upper arm
    M89.022 Algoneurodystrophy, left upper arm
    M89.029 Algoneurodystrophy, unspecified upper arm

  ☑6ᵗʰ **M89.03 Algoneurodystrophy,** forearm

    M89.031 Algoneurodystrophy, right forearm
    M89.032 Algoneurodystrophy, left forearm
    M89.039 Algoneurodystrophy, unspecified forearm

  ☑6ᵗʰ **M89.04 Algoneurodystrophy,** hand

    M89.041 Algoneurodystrophy, right hand
    M89.042 Algoneurodystrophy, left hand
    M89.049 Algoneurodystrophy, unspecified hand

  ☑6ᵗʰ **M89.05 Algoneurodystrophy,** thigh

    M89.051 Algoneurodystrophy, right thigh
    M89.052 Algoneurodystrophy, left thigh
    M89.059 Algoneurodystrophy, unspecified thigh

  ☑6ᵗʰ **M89.06 Algoneurodystrophy,** lower leg

    M89.061 Algoneurodystrophy, right lower leg
    M89.062 Algoneurodystrophy, left lower leg
    M89.069 Algoneurodystrophy, unspecified lower leg

  ☑6ᵗʰ **M89.07 Algoneurodystrophy,** ankle and foot

    M89.071 Algoneurodystrophy, right ankle and foot
    M89.072 Algoneurodystrophy, left ankle and foot
    M89.079 Algoneurodystrophy, unspecified ankle and foot

  M89.08 Algoneurodystrophy, other site

  M89.09 Algoneurodystrophy, multiple sites

  ☑5ᵗʰ **M89.1 Physeal arrest**

    Arrest of growth plate
    Epiphyseal arrest
    Growth plate arrest

  ☑6ᵗʰ **M89.12 Physeal arrest, humerus**

    M89.121 Complete physeal arrest, right proximal humerus
    M89.122 Complete physeal arrest, left proximal humerus
    M89.123 Partial physeal arrest, right proximal humerus
    M89.124 Partial physeal arrest, left proximal humerus
    M89.125 Complete physeal arrest, right distal humerus
    M89.126 Complete physeal arrest, left distal humerus
    M89.127 Partial physeal arrest, right distal humerus
    M89.128 Partial physeal arrest, left distal humerus
    M89.129 Physeal arrest, humerus, unspecified

  ☑6ᵗʰ **M89.13 Physeal arrest,** forearm

    M89.131 Complete physeal arrest, right distal radius
    M89.132 Complete physeal arrest, left distal radius
    M89.133 Partial physeal arrest, right distal radius
    M89.134 Partial physeal arrest, left distal radius
    M89.138 Other physeal arrest of forearm
    M89.139 Physeal arrest, forearm, unspecified

  ☑6ᵗʰ **M89.15 Physeal arrest,** femur

    M89.151 Complete physeal arrest, right proximal femur
    M89.152 Complete physeal arrest, left proximal femur
    M89.153 Partial physeal arrest, right proximal femur
    M89.154 Partial physeal arrest, left proximal femur
    M89.155 Complete physeal arrest, right distal femur
    M89.156 Complete physeal arrest, left distal femur
    M89.157 Partial physeal arrest, right distal femur
    M89.158 Partial physeal arrest, left distal femur
    M89.159 Physeal arrest, femur, unspecified

  ☑6ᵗʰ **M89.16 Physeal arrest,** lower leg

    M89.160 Complete physeal arrest, right proximal tibia
    M89.161 Complete physeal arrest, left proximal tibia
    M89.162 Partial physeal arrest, right proximal tibia
    M89.163 Partial physeal arrest, left proximal tibia
    M89.164 Complete physeal arrest, right distal tibia
    M89.165 Complete physeal arrest, left distal tibia
    M89.166 Partial physeal arrest, right distal tibia
    M89.167 Partial physeal arrest, left distal tibia
    M89.168 Other physeal arrest of lower leg
    M89.169 Physeal arrest, lower leg, unspecified

  M89.18 Physeal arrest, other site

  ☑5ᵗʰ **M89.2 Other disorders of bone development and growth**

    M89.20 Other disorders of bone development and growth, unspecified site

  ☑6ᵗʰ **M89.21 Other disorders of bone development and growth,** shoulder

    M89.211 Other disorders of bone development and growth, right shoulder
    M89.212 Other disorders of bone development and growth, left shoulder

☑ Additional Character Required   ☑x7ᵗʰ Placeholder   Questionable PDx   Manifestation   Unspecified Dx   UPD Unacceptable PDx   H1 - H14 HAC   HCC CMS-HCC Dx   HIV HIV Dx

ICD-10-CM 2022   835

M89.219 Other disorders of bone development and growth, unspecified shoulder

√6ᵗʰ M89.22 Other disorders of bone development and growth, humerus

M89.221 Other disorders of bone development and growth, right humerus

M89.222 Other disorders of bone development and growth, left humerus

M89.229 Other disorders of bone development and growth, unspecified humerus

√6ᵗʰ M89.23 Other disorders of bone development and growth, ulna and radius

M89.231 Other disorders of bone development and growth, right ulna

M89.232 Other disorders of bone development and growth, left ulna

M89.233 Other disorders of bone development and growth, right radius

M89.234 Other disorders of bone development and growth, left radius

M89.239 Other disorders of bone development and growth, unspecified ulna and radius

√6ᵗʰ M89.24 Other disorders of bone development and growth, hand

M89.241 Other disorders of bone development and growth, right hand

M89.242 Other disorders of bone development and growth, left hand

M89.249 Other disorders of bone development and growth, unspecified hand

√6ᵗʰ M89.25 Other disorders of bone development and growth, femur

M89.251 Other disorders of bone development and growth, right femur

M89.252 Other disorders of bone development and growth, left femur

M89.259 Other disorders of bone development and growth, unspecified femur

√6ᵗʰ M89.26 Other disorders of bone development and growth, tibia and fibula

M89.261 Other disorders of bone development and growth, right tibia

M89.262 Other disorders of bone development and growth, left tibia

M89.263 Other disorders of bone development and growth, right fibula

M89.264 Other disorders of bone development and growth, left fibula

M89.269 Other disorders of bone development and growth, unspecified lower leg

√6ᵗʰ M89.27 Other disorders of bone development and growth, ankle and foot

M89.271 Other disorders of bone development and growth, right ankle and foot

M89.272 Other disorders of bone development and growth, left ankle and foot

M89.279 Other disorders of bone development and growth, unspecified ankle and foot

M89.28 Other disorders of bone development and growth, other site

M89.29 Other disorders of bone development and growth, multiple sites

√5ᵗʰ M89.3 Hypertrophy of bone

M89.30 Hypertrophy of bone, unspecified site

√6ᵗʰ M89.31 Hypertrophy of bone, shoulder

M89.311 Hypertrophy of bone, right shoulder

M89.312 Hypertrophy of bone, left shoulder

M89.319 Hypertrophy of bone, unspecified shoulder

√6ᵗʰ M89.32 Hypertrophy of bone, humerus

M89.321 Hypertrophy of bone, right humerus

M89.322 Hypertrophy of bone, left humerus

M89.329 Hypertrophy of bone, unspecified humerus

√6ᵗʰ M89.33 Hypertrophy of bone, ulna and radius

M89.331 Hypertrophy of bone, right ulna

M89.332 Hypertrophy of bone, left ulna

M89.333 Hypertrophy of bone, right radius

M89.334 Hypertrophy of bone, left radius

M89.339 Hypertrophy of bone, unspecified ulna and radius

√6ᵗʰ M89.34 Hypertrophy of bone, hand

M89.341 Hypertrophy of bone, right hand

M89.342 Hypertrophy of bone, left hand

M89.349 Hypertrophy of bone, unspecified hand

√6ᵗʰ M89.35 Hypertrophy of bone, femur

M89.351 Hypertrophy of bone, right femur

M89.352 Hypertrophy of bone, left femur

M89.359 Hypertrophy of bone, unspecified femur

√6ᵗʰ M89.36 Hypertrophy of bone, tibia and fibula

M89.361 Hypertrophy of bone, right tibia

M89.362 Hypertrophy of bone, left tibia

M89.363 Hypertrophy of bone, right fibula

M89.364 Hypertrophy of bone, left fibula

M89.369 Hypertrophy of bone, unspecified tibia and fibula

√6ᵗʰ M89.37 Hypertrophy of bone, ankle and foot

M89.371 Hypertrophy of bone, right ankle and foot

M89.372 Hypertrophy of bone, left ankle and foot

M89.379 Hypertrophy of bone, unspecified ankle and foot

M89.38 Hypertrophy of bone, other site

M89.39 Hypertrophy of bone, multiple sites

√5ᵗʰ M89.4 Other hypertrophic osteoarthropathy

Marie-Bamberger disease
Pachydermoperiostosis

M89.40 Other hypertrophic osteoarthropathy, unspecified site

√6ᵗʰ M89.41 Other hypertrophic osteoarthropathy, shoulder

M89.411 Other hypertrophic osteoarthropathy, right shoulder

M89.412 Other hypertrophic osteoarthropathy, left shoulder

M89.419 Other hypertrophic osteoarthropathy, unspecified shoulder

√6ᵗʰ M89.42 Other hypertrophic osteoarthropathy, upper arm

M89.421 Other hypertrophic osteoarthropathy, right upper arm

M89.422 Other hypertrophic osteoarthropathy, left upper arm

M89.429 Other hypertrophic osteoarthropathy, unspecified upper arm

√6ᵗʰ M89.43 Other hypertrophic osteoarthropathy, forearm

M89.431 Other hypertrophic osteoarthropathy, right forearm

M89.432 Other hypertrophic osteoarthropathy, left forearm

M89.439 Other hypertrophic osteoarthropathy, unspecified forearm

√6ᵗʰ M89.44 Other hypertrophic osteoarthropathy, hand

M89.441 Other hypertrophic osteoarthropathy, right hand

M89.442 Other hypertrophic osteoarthropathy, left hand

M89.449 Other hypertrophic osteoarthropathy, unspecified hand

√6ᵗʰ M89.45 Other hypertrophic osteoarthropathy, thigh

M89.451 Other hypertrophic osteoarthropathy, right thigh

M89.452 Other hypertrophic osteoarthropathy, left thigh

M89.459 Other hypertrophic osteoarthropathy, unspecified thigh

√6ᵗʰ M89.46 Other hypertrophic osteoarthropathy, lower leg

M89.461 Other hypertrophic osteoarthropathy, right lower leg

M89.462 Other hypertrophic osteoarthropathy, left lower leg

M89.469 Other hypertrophic osteoarthropathy, unspecified lower leg

√6ᵗʰ M89.47 Other hypertrophic osteoarthropathy, ankle and foot

M89.471 Other hypertrophic osteoarthropathy, right ankle and foot

M89.472 Other hypertrophic osteoarthropathy, left ankle and foot

M89.479 Other hypertrophic osteoarthropathy, unspecified ankle and foot

M89.48 Other hypertrophic osteoarthropathy, other site

Ⓝ Newborn: 0   Ⓟ Pediatric: 0-17   Ⓜ Maternity: 9-64   Ⓐ Adult: 15-124   ᴹᶜᶜ Major Complication/Comorbidity   ᶜᶜ Complication/Comorbidity   ˢʷ Severe Wound Dx

836

ICD-10-CM 2022

M89.49　Other hypertrophic osteoarthropathy, multiple sites

✓5ᵗʰ **M89.5**　Osteolysis

Use additional code to identify major osseous defect, if applicable (M89.7-)

EXCLUDES 2　periprosthetic osteolysis of internal prosthetic joint (T84.05-)

M89.50　Osteolysis, unspecified site

✓6ᵗʰ **M89.51**　Osteolysis, shoulder

　　M89.511　Osteolysis, right shoulder
　　M89.512　Osteolysis, left shoulder
　　M89.519　Osteolysis, unspecified shoulder

✓6ᵗʰ **M89.52**　Osteolysis, upper arm

　　M89.521　Osteolysis, right upper arm
　　M89.522　Osteolysis, left upper arm
　　M89.529　Osteolysis, unspecified upper arm

✓6ᵗʰ **M89.53**　Osteolysis, forearm

　　M89.531　Osteolysis, right forearm
　　M89.532　Osteolysis, left forearm
　　M89.539　Osteolysis, unspecified forearm

✓6ᵗʰ **M89.54**　Osteolysis, hand

　　M89.541　Osteolysis, right hand
　　M89.542　Osteolysis, left hand
　　M89.549　Osteolysis, unspecified hand

✓6ᵗʰ **M89.55**　Osteolysis, thigh

　　M89.551　Osteolysis, right thigh
　　M89.552　Osteolysis, left thigh
　　M89.559　Osteolysis, unspecified thigh

✓6ᵗʰ **M89.56**　Osteolysis, lower leg

　　M89.561　Osteolysis, right lower leg
　　M89.562　Osteolysis, left lower leg
　　M89.569　Osteolysis, unspecified lower leg

✓6ᵗʰ **M89.57**　Osteolysis, ankle and foot

　　M89.571　Osteolysis, right ankle and foot
　　M89.572　Osteolysis, left ankle and foot
　　M89.579　Osteolysis, unspecified ankle and foot

M89.58　Osteolysis, other site
M89.59　Osteolysis, multiple sites

✓5ᵗʰ **M89.6**　Osteopathy after poliomyelitis

Use additional code (B91) to identify previous poliomyelitis

EXCLUDES 1　postpolio syndrome (G14)

M89.60　Osteopathy after poliomyelitis, unspecified site　HCC

✓6ᵗʰ **M89.61**　Osteopathy after poliomyelitis, shoulder

　　M89.611　Osteopathy after poliomyelitis, right shoulder　HCC
　　M89.612　Osteopathy after poliomyelitis, left shoulder　HCC
　　M89.619　Osteopathy after poliomyelitis, unspecified shoulder　HCC

✓6ᵗʰ **M89.62**　Osteopathy after poliomyelitis, upper arm

　　M89.621　Osteopathy after poliomyelitis, right upper arm　HCC
　　M89.622　Osteopathy after poliomyelitis, left upper arm　HCC
　　M89.629　Osteopathy after poliomyelitis, unspecified upper arm　HCC

✓6ᵗʰ **M89.63**　Osteopathy after poliomyelitis, forearm

　　M89.631　Osteopathy after poliomyelitis, right forearm　HCC
　　M89.632　Osteopathy after poliomyelitis, left forearm　HCC
　　M89.639　Osteopathy after poliomyelitis, unspecified forearm　HCC

✓6ᵗʰ **M89.64**　Osteopathy after poliomyelitis, hand

　　M89.641　Osteopathy after poliomyelitis, right hand　HCC
　　M89.642　Osteopathy after poliomyelitis, left hand　HCC
　　M89.649　Osteopathy after poliomyelitis, unspecified hand　HCC

✓6ᵗʰ **M89.65**　Osteopathy after poliomyelitis, thigh

　　M89.651　Osteopathy after poliomyelitis, right thigh　HCC
　　M89.652　Osteopathy after poliomyelitis, left thigh　HCC

M89.659　Osteopathy after poliomyelitis, unspecified thigh　HCC

✓6ᵗʰ **M89.66**　Osteopathy after poliomyelitis, lower leg

　　M89.661　Osteopathy after poliomyelitis, right lower leg　HCC
　　M89.662　Osteopathy after poliomyelitis, left lower leg　HCC
　　M89.669　Osteopathy after poliomyelitis, unspecified lower leg　HCC

✓6ᵗʰ **M89.67**　Osteopathy after poliomyelitis, ankle and foot

　　M89.671　Osteopathy after poliomyelitis, right ankle and foot　HCC
　　M89.672　Osteopathy after poliomyelitis, left ankle and foot　HCC
　　M89.679　Osteopathy after poliomyelitis, unspecified ankle and foot　HCC

M89.68　Osteopathy after poliomyelitis, other site　HCC
M89.69　Osteopathy after poliomyelitis, multiple sites　HCC

✓5ᵗʰ **M89.7**　Major osseous defect

Code first underlying disease, if known, such as:
　aseptic necrosis of bone (M87.-)
　malignant neoplasm of bone (C40.-)
　osteolysis (M89.5)
　osteomyelitis (M86.-)
　osteonecrosis (M87.-)
　osteoporosis (M80.-, M81.-)
　periprosthetic osteolysis (T84.05-)

M89.70　Major osseous defect, unspecified site

✓6ᵗʰ **M89.71**　Major osseous defect, shoulder region

　　Major osseous defect clavicle or scapula

　　M89.711　Major osseous defect, right shoulder region
　　M89.712　Major osseous defect, left shoulder region
　　M89.719　Major osseous defect, unspecified shoulder region

✓6ᵗʰ **M89.72**　Major osseous defect, humerus

　　M89.721　Major osseous defect, right humerus
　　M89.722　Major osseous defect, left humerus
　　M89.729　Major osseous defect, unspecified humerus

✓6ᵗʰ **M89.73**　Major osseous defect, forearm

　　Major osseous defect of radius and ulna

　　M89.731　Major osseous defect, right forearm
　　M89.732　Major osseous defect, left forearm
　　M89.739　Major osseous defect, unspecified forearm

✓6ᵗʰ **M89.74**　Major osseous defect, hand

　　Major osseous defect of carpus, fingers, metacarpus

　　M89.741　Major osseous defect, right hand
　　M89.742　Major osseous defect, left hand
　　M89.749　Major osseous defect, unspecified hand

✓6ᵗʰ **M89.75**　Major osseous defect, pelvic region and thigh

　　Major osseous defect of femur and pelvis

　　M89.751　Major osseous defect, right pelvic region and thigh
　　M89.752　Major osseous defect, left pelvic region and thigh
　　M89.759　Major osseous defect, unspecified pelvic region and thigh

✓6ᵗʰ **M89.76**　Major osseous defect, lower leg

　　Major osseous defect of fibula and tibia

　　M89.761　Major osseous defect, right lower leg
　　M89.762　Major osseous defect, left lower leg
　　M89.769　Major osseous defect, unspecified lower leg

✓6ᵗʰ **M89.77**　Major osseous defect, ankle and foot

　　Major osseous defect of metatarsus, tarsus, toes

　　M89.771　Major osseous defect, right ankle and foot
　　M89.772　Major osseous defect, left ankle and foot
　　M89.779　Major osseous defect, unspecified ankle and foot

M89.78　Major osseous defect, other site
M89.79　Major osseous defect, multiple sites

☑ Additional Character Required　✓x7ᵗʰ Placeholder　Questionable PDx　Manifestation　Unspecified Dx　UPD Unacceptable PDx　H1-H14 HAC　HCC CMS-HCC Dx　HIV HIV Dx

ICD-10-CM 2022　　　837

√5ᵗʰ **M89.8** **Other specified disorders of bone**
     Infantile cortical hyperostoses
     Post-traumatic subperiosteal ossification
     √6ᵗʰ **M89.8X** **Other specified disorders of bone**
         M89.8X0 **Other specified disorders of bone,** multiple sites
         M89.8X1 **Other specified disorders of bone,** shoulder
         M89.8X2 **Other specified disorders of bone,** upper arm
         M89.8X3 **Other specified disorders of bone,** forearm
             AHA: 2019,3Q,9
         M89.8X4 **Other specified disorders of bone,** hand
         M89.8X5 **Other specified disorders of bone,** thigh
         M89.8X6 **Other specified disorders of bone,** lower leg
         M89.8X7 **Other specified disorders of bone,** ankle and foot
         M89.8X8 **Other specified disorders of bone, other** site
         M89.8X9 **Other specified disorders of bone,** unspecified site

M89.9 **Disorder of bone, unspecified**

√4ᵗʰ **M90** **Osteopathies in diseases classified elsewhere**
     EXCLUDES 1   osteochondritis, osteomyelitis, and osteopathy (in):
         cryptococcosis (B45.3)
         diabetes mellitus (E08-E13 with .69-)
         gonococcal (A54.43)
         neurogenic syphilis (A52.11)
         renal osteodystrophy (N25.0)
         salmonellosis (A02.24)
         secondary syphilis (A51.46)
         syphilis (late) (A52.77)

√5ᵗʰ **M90.5** **Osteonecrosis in diseases classified elsewhere**
     Code first underlying disease, such as:
         caisson disease (T70.3)
         hemoglobinopathy (D50-D64)
     M90.50 *Osteonecrosis in diseases classified elsewhere,* unspecified site   CC HCC
     √6ᵗʰ **M90.51** **Osteonecrosis in diseases classified elsewhere,** shoulder
         M90.511 *Osteonecrosis in diseases classified elsewhere, right shoulder*   CC HCC
         M90.512 *Osteonecrosis in diseases classified elsewhere, left shoulder*   CC HCC
         M90.519 *Osteonecrosis in diseases classified elsewhere, unspecified shoulder*   CC HCC
     √6ᵗʰ **M90.52** **Osteonecrosis in diseases classified elsewhere,** upper arm
         M90.521 *Osteonecrosis in diseases classified elsewhere, right upper arm*   CC HCC
         M90.522 *Osteonecrosis in diseases classified elsewhere, left upper arm*   CC HCC
         M90.529 *Osteonecrosis in diseases classified elsewhere, unspecified upper arm*   CC HCC
     √6ᵗʰ **M90.53** **Osteonecrosis in diseases classified elsewhere,** forearm
         M90.531 *Osteonecrosis in diseases classified elsewhere, right forearm*   CC HCC
         M90.532 *Osteonecrosis in diseases classified elsewhere, left forearm*   CC HCC
         M90.539 *Osteonecrosis in diseases classified elsewhere, unspecified forearm*   CC HCC
     √6ᵗʰ **M90.54** **Osteonecrosis in diseases classified elsewhere,** hand
         M90.541 *Osteonecrosis in diseases classified elsewhere, right hand*   CC HCC
         M90.542 *Osteonecrosis in diseases classified elsewhere, left hand*   CC HCC
         M90.549 *Osteonecrosis in diseases classified elsewhere, unspecified hand*   CC HCC
     √6ᵗʰ **M90.55** **Osteonecrosis in diseases classified elsewhere,** thigh
         M90.551 *Osteonecrosis in diseases classified elsewhere, right thigh*   CC HCC
         M90.552 *Osteonecrosis in diseases classified elsewhere, left thigh*   CC HCC

         M90.559 *Osteonecrosis in diseases classified elsewhere, unspecified thigh*   CC HCC
     √6ᵗʰ **M90.56** **Osteonecrosis in diseases classified elsewhere,** lower leg
         M90.561 *Osteonecrosis in diseases classified elsewhere, right lower leg*   CC HCC
         M90.562 *Osteonecrosis in diseases classified elsewhere, left lower leg*   CC HCC
         M90.569 *Osteonecrosis in diseases classified elsewhere, unspecified lower leg*   CC HCC
     √6ᵗʰ **M90.57** **Osteonecrosis in diseases classified elsewhere,** ankle and foot
         M90.571 *Osteonecrosis in diseases classified elsewhere, right ankle and foot*   CC HCC
         M90.572 *Osteonecrosis in diseases classified elsewhere, left ankle and foot*   CC HCC
         M90.579 *Osteonecrosis in diseases classified elsewhere, unspecified ankle and foot*   CC HCC
     M90.58 *Osteonecrosis in diseases classified elsewhere, other site*   CC HCC
     M90.59 *Osteonecrosis in diseases classified elsewhere, multiple sites*   CC HCC

√5ᵗʰ **M90.6** **Osteitis deformans in neoplastic diseases**
     Osteitis deformans in malignant neoplasm of bone
     Code first the neoplasm (C40.-, C41.-)
     EXCLUDES 1   osteitis deformans [Paget's disease of bone] (M88.-)
     M90.60 *Osteitis deformans in neoplastic diseases, unspecified site*
     √6ᵗʰ **M90.61** **Osteitis deformans in neoplastic diseases,** shoulder
         M90.611 *Osteitis deformans in neoplastic diseases, right shoulder*
         M90.612 *Osteitis deformans in neoplastic diseases, left shoulder*
         M90.619 *Osteitis deformans in neoplastic diseases, unspecified shoulder*
     √6ᵗʰ **M90.62** **Osteitis deformans in neoplastic diseases,** upper arm
         M90.621 *Osteitis deformans in neoplastic diseases, right upper arm*
         M90.622 *Osteitis deformans in neoplastic diseases, left upper arm*
         M90.629 *Osteitis deformans in neoplastic diseases, unspecified upper arm*
     √6ᵗʰ **M90.63** **Osteitis deformans in neoplastic diseases,** forearm
         M90.631 *Osteitis deformans in neoplastic diseases, right forearm*
         M90.632 *Osteitis deformans in neoplastic diseases, left forearm*
         M90.639 *Osteitis deformans in neoplastic diseases, unspecified forearm*
     √6ᵗʰ **M90.64** **Osteitis deformans in neoplastic diseases,** hand
         M90.641 *Osteitis deformans in neoplastic diseases, right hand*
         M90.642 *Osteitis deformans in neoplastic diseases, left hand*
         M90.649 *Osteitis deformans in neoplastic diseases, unspecified hand*
     √6ᵗʰ **M90.65** **Osteitis deformans in neoplastic diseases,** thigh
         M90.651 *Osteitis deformans in neoplastic diseases, right thigh*
         M90.652 *Osteitis deformans in neoplastic diseases, left thigh*
         M90.659 *Osteitis deformans in neoplastic diseases, unspecified thigh*
     √6ᵗʰ **M90.66** **Osteitis deformans in neoplastic diseases,** lower leg
         M90.661 *Osteitis deformans in neoplastic diseases, right lower leg*
         M90.662 *Osteitis deformans in neoplastic diseases, left lower leg*
         M90.669 *Osteitis deformans in neoplastic diseases, unspecified lower leg*
     √6ᵗʰ **M90.67** **Osteitis deformans in neoplastic diseases,** ankle and foot
         M90.671 *Osteitis deformans in neoplastic diseases, right ankle and foot*
         M90.672 *Osteitis deformans in neoplastic diseases, left ankle and foot*
         M90.679 *Osteitis deformans in neoplastic diseases, unspecified ankle and foot*

M90.68   *Osteitis deformans in neoplastic diseases, other site*

M90.69   *Osteitis deformans in neoplastic diseases, multiple sites*

✓5ᵗʰ **M90.8**   **Osteopathy in diseases classified elsewhere**

Code first underlying disease, such as:
   rickets (E55.0)
   vitamin-D-resistant rickets (E83.3)

M90.80   *Osteopathy in diseases classified elsewhere, unspecified site*

✓6ᵗʰ **M90.81**   **Osteopathy in diseases classified elsewhere, shoulder**

M90.811   *Osteopathy in diseases classified elsewhere, right shoulder*

M90.812   *Osteopathy in diseases classified elsewhere, left shoulder*

M90.819   *Osteopathy in diseases classified elsewhere, unspecified shoulder*

✓6ᵗʰ **M90.82**   **Osteopathy in diseases classified elsewhere, upper arm**

M90.821   *Osteopathy in diseases classified elsewhere, right upper arm*

M90.822   *Osteopathy in diseases classified elsewhere, left upper arm*

M90.829   *Osteopathy in diseases classified elsewhere, unspecified upper arm*

✓6ᵗʰ **M90.83**   **Osteopathy in diseases classified elsewhere, forearm**

M90.831   *Osteopathy in diseases classified elsewhere, right forearm*

M90.832   *Osteopathy in diseases classified elsewhere, left forearm*

M90.839   *Osteopathy in diseases classified elsewhere, unspecified forearm*

✓6ᵗʰ **M90.84**   **Osteopathy in diseases classified elsewhere, hand**

M90.841   *Osteopathy in diseases classified elsewhere, right hand*

M90.842   *Osteopathy in diseases classified elsewhere, left hand*

M90.849   *Osteopathy in diseases classified elsewhere, unspecified hand*

✓6ᵗʰ **M90.85**   **Osteopathy in diseases classified elsewhere, thigh**

M90.851   *Osteopathy in diseases classified elsewhere, right thigh*

M90.852   *Osteopathy in diseases classified elsewhere, left thigh*

M90.859   *Osteopathy in diseases classified elsewhere, unspecified thigh*

✓6ᵗʰ **M90.86**   **Osteopathy in diseases classified elsewhere, lower leg**

M90.861   *Osteopathy in diseases classified elsewhere, right lower leg*

M90.862   *Osteopathy in diseases classified elsewhere, left lower leg*

M90.869   *Osteopathy in diseases classified elsewhere, unspecified lower leg*

✓6ᵗʰ **M90.87**   **Osteopathy in diseases classified elsewhere, ankle and foot**

M90.871   *Osteopathy in diseases classified elsewhere, right ankle and foot*

M90.872   *Osteopathy in diseases classified elsewhere, left ankle and foot*

M90.879   *Osteopathy in diseases classified elsewhere, unspecified ankle and foot*

M90.88   *Osteopathy in diseases classified elsewhere, other site*

M90.89   *Osteopathy in diseases classified elsewhere, multiple sites*

Chondropathies (M91-M94)

EXCLUDES 1   *postprocedural chondropathies (M96.-)*

✓4ᵗʰ **M91**   **Juvenile osteochondrosis of hip and pelvis**

EXCLUDES 1   *slipped upper femoral epiphysis (nontraumatic) (M93.0)*

M91.0   **Juvenile osteochondrosis of pelvis**

Osteochondrosis (juvenile) of acetabulum
Osteochondrosis (juvenile) of iliac crest [Buchanan]
Osteochondrosis (juvenile) of ischiopubic synchondrosis [van Neck]
Osteochondrosis (juvenile) of symphysis pubis [Pierson]

✓6ᵗʰ **M91.1**   **Juvenile osteochondrosis of head of femur [Legg-Calvé-Perthes]**

M91.10   Juvenile osteochondrosis of head of femur [Legg-Calvé-Perthes], unspecified leg

M91.11   Juvenile osteochondrosis of head of femur [Legg-Calvé-Perthes], right leg

M91.12   Juvenile osteochondrosis of head of femur [Legg-Calvé-Perthes], left leg

✓5ᵗʰ **M91.2**   **Coxa plana**

Hip deformity due to previous juvenile osteochondrosis

M91.20   Coxa plana, unspecified hip

M91.21   Coxa plana, right hip

M91.22   Coxa plana, left hip

✓5ᵗʰ **M91.3**   **Pseudocoxalgia**

M91.30   Pseudocoxalgia, unspecified hip

M91.31   Pseudocoxalgia, right hip

M91.32   Pseudocoxalgia, left hip

✓5ᵗʰ **M91.4**   **Coxa magna**

M91.40   Coxa magna, unspecified hip

M91.41   Coxa magna, right hip

M91.42   Coxa magna, left hip

✓5ᵗʰ **M91.8**   **Other juvenile osteochondrosis of hip and pelvis**

Juvenile osteochondrosis after reduction of congenital dislocation of hip

M91.80   Other juvenile osteochondrosis of hip and pelvis, unspecified leg

M91.81   Other juvenile osteochondrosis of hip and pelvis, right leg

M91.82   Other juvenile osteochondrosis of hip and pelvis, left leg

✓5ᵗʰ **M91.9**   **Juvenile osteochondrosis of hip and pelvis, unspecified**

M91.90   Juvenile osteochondrosis of hip and pelvis, unspecified, unspecified leg

M91.91   Juvenile osteochondrosis of hip and pelvis, unspecified, right leg

M91.92   Juvenile osteochondrosis of hip and pelvis, unspecified, left leg

✓4ᵗʰ **M92**   **Other juvenile osteochondrosis**

✓5ᵗʰ **M92.0**   **Juvenile osteochondrosis of humerus**

Osteochondrosis (juvenile) of capitulum of humerus [Panner]
Osteochondrosis (juvenile) of head of humerus [Haas]

M92.00   Juvenile osteochondrosis of humerus, unspecified arm

M92.01   Juvenile osteochondrosis of humerus, right arm

M92.02   Juvenile osteochondrosis of humerus, left arm

✓5ᵗʰ **M92.1**   **Juvenile osteochondrosis of radius and ulna**

Osteochondrosis (juvenile) of lower ulna [Burns]
Osteochondrosis (juvenile) of radial head [Brailsford]

M92.10   Juvenile osteochondrosis of radius and ulna, unspecified arm

M92.11   Juvenile osteochondrosis of radius and ulna, right arm

M92.12   Juvenile osteochondrosis of radius and ulna, left arm

✓5ᵗʰ **M92.2**   **Juvenile osteochondrosis, hand**

✓6ᵗʰ **M92.20**   **Unspecified juvenile osteochondrosis, hand**

M92.201   Unspecified juvenile osteochondrosis, right hand

M92.202   Unspecified juvenile osteochondrosis, left hand

M92.209   Unspecified juvenile osteochondrosis, unspecified hand

✓6ᵗʰ **M92.21**   **Osteochondrosis (juvenile) of carpal lunate [Kienböck]**

M92.211   Osteochondrosis (juvenile) of carpal lunate [Kienböck], right hand

M92.212   Osteochondrosis (juvenile) of carpal lunate [Kienböck], left hand

M92.219   Osteochondrosis (juvenile) of carpal lunate [Kienböck], unspecified hand

✓6ᵗʰ **M92.22**   **Osteochondrosis (juvenile) of metacarpal heads [Mauclaire]**

M92.221   Osteochondrosis (juvenile) of metacarpal heads [Mauclaire], right hand

M92.222   Osteochondrosis (juvenile) of metacarpal heads [Mauclaire], left hand

M92.229   Osteochondrosis (juvenile) of metacarpal heads [Mauclaire], unspecified hand

✓ Additional Character Required   ✓x7ᵗʰ Placeholder   Questionable PDx   Manifestation   Unspecified Dx   UPD Unacceptable PDx   H1-H4 HAC   HCC CMS-HCC Dx   HIV HIV Dx

ICD-10-CM 2022   839

☑6ᵗʰ **M92.29** Other juvenile osteochondrosis, hand

     M92.291 Other juvenile osteochondrosis, right hand

     M92.292 Other juvenile osteochondrosis, left hand

     M92.299 Other juvenile osteochondrosis, unspecified hand

☑5ᵗʰ **M92.3** Other juvenile osteochondrosis, upper limb

     M92.30 Other juvenile osteochondrosis, unspecified upper limb

     M92.31 Other juvenile osteochondrosis, right upper limb

     M92.32 Other juvenile osteochondrosis, left upper limb

☑5ᵗʰ **M92.4** Juvenile osteochondrosis of patella

     Osteochondrosis (juvenile) of primary patellar center [Köhler]

     Osteochondrosis (juvenile) of secondary patellar centre [Sinding Larsen]

     M92.40 Juvenile osteochondrosis of patella, unspecified knee

     M92.41 Juvenile osteochondrosis of patella, right knee

     M92.42 Juvenile osteochondrosis of patella, left knee

☑5ᵗʰ **M92.5** Juvenile osteochondrosis of tibia and fibula

     AHA: 2020,4Q,33-34

     ☑6ᵗʰ **M92.50** Unspecified juvenile osteochondrosis of tibia and fibula

         M92.501 Unspecified juvenile osteochondrosis, right leg

         M92.502 Unspecified juvenile osteochondrosis, left leg

         M92.503 Unspecified juvenile osteochondrosis, bilateral leg

         M92.509 Unspecified juvenile osteochondrosis, unspecified leg

     ☑6ᵗʰ **M92.51** Juvenile osteochondrosis of proximal tibia

         Blount disease

         Tibia vara

         M92.511 Juvenile osteochondrosis of proximal tibia, right leg

         M92.512 Juvenile osteochondrosis of proximal tibia, left leg

         M92.513 Juvenile osteochondrosis of proximal tibia, bilateral

         M92.519 Juvenile osteochondrosis of proximal tibia, unspecified leg

     ☑6ᵗʰ **M92.52** Juvenile osteochondrosis of tibia tubercle

         Osgood-Schlatter disease

         M92.521 Juvenile osteochondrosis of tibia tubercle, right leg

         M92.522 Juvenile osteochondrosis of tibia tubercle, left leg

         M92.523 Juvenile osteochondrosis of tibia tubercle, bilateral

         M92.529 Juvenile osteochondrosis of tibia tubercle, unspecified leg

     ☑6ᵗʰ **M92.59** Other juvenile osteochondrosis of tibia and fibula

         M92.591 Other juvenile osteochondrosis of tibia and fibula, right leg

         M92.592 Other juvenile osteochondrosis of tibia and fibula, left leg

         M92.593 Other juvenile osteochondrosis of tibia and fibula, bilateral

         M92.599 Other juvenile osteochondrosis of tibia and fibula, unspecified leg

☑5ᵗʰ **M92.6** Juvenile osteochondrosis of tarsus

     Osteochondrosis (juvenile) of calcaneum [Sever]

     Osteochondrosis (juvenile) of os tibiale externum [Haglund]

     Osteochondrosis (juvenile) of talus [Diaz]

     Osteochondrosis (juvenile) of tarsal navicular [Köhler]

     M92.60 Juvenile osteochondrosis of tarsus, unspecified ankle

     M92.61 Juvenile osteochondrosis of tarsus, right ankle

     M92.62 Juvenile osteochondrosis of tarsus, left ankle

☑5ᵗʰ **M92.7** Juvenile osteochondrosis of metatarsus

     Osteochondrosis (juvenile) of fifth metatarsus [Iselin]

     Osteochondrosis (juvenile) of second metatarsus [Freiberg]

     M92.70 Juvenile osteochondrosis of metatarsus, unspecified foot

     M92.71 Juvenile osteochondrosis of metatarsus, right foot

     M92.72 Juvenile osteochondrosis of metatarsus, left foot

M92.8 Other specified juvenile osteochondrosis

     Calcaneal apophysitis

     DEF: Calcaneal apophysitis: Inflammation of the calcaneus at the point of Achilles tendon insertion usually occurring in boys ages 8 to 14. Pain, tenderness, and localized swelling are present.

M92.9 Juvenile osteochondrosis, unspecified

     Juvenile apophysitis NOS

     Juvenile epiphysitis NOS

     Juvenile osteochondritis NOS

     Juvenile osteochondrosis NOS

☑4ᵗʰ **M93** Other osteochondropathies

     EXCLUDES 2   osteochondrosis of spine (M42.-)

☑5ᵗʰ **M93.0** Slipped upper femoral epiphysis (nontraumatic)

     Use additional code for associated chondrolysis (M94.3)

     ☑6ᵗʰ **M93.00** Unspecified slipped upper femoral epiphysis (nontraumatic)

         M93.001 Unspecified slipped upper femoral epiphysis (nontraumatic), right hip

         M93.002 Unspecified slipped upper femoral epiphysis (nontraumatic), left hip

         M93.003 Unspecified slipped upper femoral epiphysis (nontraumatic), unspecified hip

     ☑6ᵗʰ **M93.01** Acute slipped upper femoral epiphysis (nontraumatic)

         M93.011 Acute slipped upper femoral epiphysis (nontraumatic), right hip

         M93.012 Acute slipped upper femoral epiphysis (nontraumatic), left hip

         M93.013 Acute slipped upper femoral epiphysis (nontraumatic), unspecified hip

     ☑6ᵗʰ **M93.02** Chronic slipped upper femoral epiphysis (nontraumatic)

         M93.021 Chronic slipped upper femoral epiphysis (nontraumatic), right hip

         M93.022 Chronic slipped upper femoral epiphysis (nontraumatic), left hip

         M93.023 Chronic slipped upper femoral epiphysis (nontraumatic), unspecified hip

     ☑6ᵗʰ **M93.03** Acute on chronic slipped upper femoral epiphysis (nontraumatic)

         M93.031 Acute on chronic slipped upper femoral epiphysis (nontraumatic), right hip

         M93.032 Acute on chronic slipped upper femoral epiphysis (nontraumatic), left hip

         M93.033 Acute on chronic slipped upper femoral epiphysis (nontraumatic), unspecified hip

M93.1 Kienböck's disease of adults   Ⓐ

     Adult osteochondrosis of carpal lunates

☑5ᵗʰ **M93.2** Osteochondritis dissecans

     DEF: Avascular necrosis caused by lack of blood flow to the bone and cartilage of a joint causing the bone to die. This can result in splinters or pieces of cartilage breaking off in the joint.

     M93.20 Osteochondritis dissecans of unspecified site

     ☑6ᵗʰ **M93.21** Osteochondritis dissecans of shoulder

         M93.211 Osteochondritis dissecans, right shoulder

         M93.212 Osteochondritis dissecans, left shoulder

         M93.219 Osteochondritis dissecans, unspecified shoulder

     ☑6ᵗʰ **M93.22** Osteochondritis dissecans of elbow

         M93.221 Osteochondritis dissecans, right elbow

         M93.222 Osteochondritis dissecans, left elbow

         M93.229 Osteochondritis dissecans, unspecified elbow

     ☑6ᵗʰ **M93.23** Osteochondritis dissecans of wrist

         M93.231 Osteochondritis dissecans, right wrist

         M93.232 Osteochondritis dissecans, left wrist

         M93.239 Osteochondritis dissecans, unspecified wrist

     ☑6ᵗʰ **M93.24** Osteochondritis dissecans of joints of hand

         M93.241 Osteochondritis dissecans, joints of right hand

         M93.242 Osteochondritis dissecans, joints of left hand

         M93.249 Osteochondritis dissecans, joints of unspecified hand

     ☑6ᵗʰ **M93.25** Osteochondritis dissecans of hip

         M93.251 Osteochondritis dissecans, right hip

         M93.252 Osteochondritis dissecans, left hip

Ⓝ Newborn: 0   Ⓟ Pediatric: 0-17   Ⓜ Maternity: 9-64   Ⓐ Adult: 15-124   **MCC** Major Complication/Comorbidity   **CC** Complication/Comorbidity   **SW** Severe Wound Dx

840   ICD-10-CM 2022

M93.259 Osteochondritis dissecans, unspecified hip

✓6ᵗʰ M93.26 Osteochondritis dissecans knee

     M93.261 Osteochondritis dissecans, right knee

     M93.262 Osteochondritis dissecans, left knee

     M93.269 Osteochondritis dissecans, unspecified knee

✓6ᵗʰ M93.27 Osteochondritis dissecans of ankle and joints of foot

     M93.271 Osteochondritis dissecans, right ankle and joints of right foot

     M93.272 Osteochondritis dissecans, left ankle and joints of left foot

     M93.279 Osteochondritis dissecans, unspecified ankle and joints of foot

M93.28 Osteochondritis dissecans other site

M93.29 Osteochondritis dissecans multiple sites

✓5ᵗʰ M93.8 Other specified osteochondropathies

     M93.80 Other specified osteochondropathies of unspecified site

✓6ᵗʰ M93.81 Other specified osteochondropathies of shoulder

     M93.811 Other specified osteochondropathies, right shoulder

     M93.812 Other specified osteochondropathies, left shoulder

     M93.819 Other specified osteochondropathies, unspecified shoulder

✓6ᵗʰ M93.82 Other specified osteochondropathies of upper arm

     M93.821 Other specified osteochondropathies, right upper arm

     M93.822 Other specified osteochondropathies, left upper arm

     M93.829 Other specified osteochondropathies, unspecified upper arm

✓6ᵗʰ M93.83 Other specified osteochondropathies of forearm

     M93.831 Other specified osteochondropathies, right forearm

     M93.832 Other specified osteochondropathies, left forearm

     M93.839 Other specified osteochondropathies, unspecified forearm

✓6ᵗʰ M93.84 Other specified osteochondropathies of hand

     M93.841 Other specified osteochondropathies, right hand

     M93.842 Other specified osteochondropathies, left hand

     M93.849 Other specified osteochondropathies, unspecified hand

✓6ᵗʰ M93.85 Other specified osteochondropathies of thigh

     M93.851 Other specified osteochondropathies, right thigh

     M93.852 Other specified osteochondropathies, left thigh

     M93.859 Other specified osteochondropathies, unspecified thigh

✓6ᵗʰ M93.86 Other specified osteochondropathies lower leg

     M93.861 Other specified osteochondropathies, right lower leg

     M93.862 Other specified osteochondropathies, left lower leg

     M93.869 Other specified osteochondropathies, unspecified lower leg

✓6ᵗʰ M93.87 Other specified osteochondropathies of ankle and foot

     M93.871 Other specified osteochondropathies, right ankle and foot

     M93.872 Other specified osteochondropathies, left ankle and foot

     M93.879 Other specified osteochondropathies, unspecified ankle and foot

M93.88 Other specified osteochondropathies other site

M93.89 Other specified osteochondropathies multiple sites

✓5ᵗʰ M93.9 Osteochondropathy, unspecified

     Apophysitis NOS

     Epiphysitis NOS

     Osteochondritis NOS

     Osteochondrosis NOS

     M93.90 Osteochondropathy, unspecified of unspecified site

✓6ᵗʰ M93.91 Osteochondropathy, unspecified of shoulder

     M93.911 Osteochondropathy, unspecified, right shoulder

     M93.912 Osteochondropathy, unspecified, left shoulder

     M93.919 Osteochondropathy, unspecified, unspecified shoulder

✓6ᵗʰ M93.92 Osteochondropathy, unspecified of upper arm

     M93.921 Osteochondropathy, unspecified, right upper arm

     M93.922 Osteochondropathy, unspecified, left upper arm

     M93.929 Osteochondropathy, unspecified, unspecified upper arm

✓6ᵗʰ M93.93 Osteochondropathy, unspecified of forearm

     M93.931 Osteochondropathy, unspecified, right forearm

     M93.932 Osteochondropathy, unspecified, left forearm

     M93.939 Osteochondropathy, unspecified, unspecified forearm

✓6ᵗʰ M93.94 Osteochondropathy, unspecified of hand

     M93.941 Osteochondropathy, unspecified, right hand

     M93.942 Osteochondropathy, unspecified, left hand

     M93.949 Osteochondropathy, unspecified, unspecified hand

✓6ᵗʰ M93.95 Osteochondropathy, unspecified of thigh

     M93.951 Osteochondropathy, unspecified, right thigh

     M93.952 Osteochondropathy, unspecified, left thigh

     M93.959 Osteochondropathy, unspecified, unspecified thigh

✓6ᵗʰ M93.96 Osteochondropathy, unspecified lower leg

     M93.961 Osteochondropathy, unspecified, right lower leg

     M93.962 Osteochondropathy, unspecified, left lower leg

     M93.969 Osteochondropathy, unspecified, unspecified lower leg

✓6ᵗʰ M93.97 Osteochondropathy, unspecified of ankle and foot

     M93.971 Osteochondropathy, unspecified, right ankle and foot

     M93.972 Osteochondropathy, unspecified, left ankle and foot

     M93.979 Osteochondropathy, unspecified, unspecified ankle and foot

M93.98 Osteochondropathy, unspecified other site

M93.99 Osteochondropathy, unspecified multiple sites

✓4ᵗʰ **M94 Other disorders of cartilage**

M94.0 Chondrocostal junction syndrome [Tietze]

     Costochondritis

M94.1 Relapsing polychondritis

✓5ᵗʰ M94.2 Chondromalacia

     EXCLUDES 1   chondromalacia patellae (M22.4)

     M94.20 Chondromalacia, unspecified site

✓6ᵗʰ M94.21 Chondromalacia, shoulder

     M94.211 Chondromalacia, right shoulder

     M94.212 Chondromalacia, left shoulder

     M94.219 Chondromalacia, unspecified shoulder

✓6ᵗʰ M94.22 Chondromalacia, elbow

     M94.221 Chondromalacia, right elbow

     M94.222 Chondromalacia, left elbow

     M94.229 Chondromalacia, unspecified elbow

✓6ᵗʰ M94.23 Chondromalacia, wrist

     M94.231 Chondromalacia, right wrist

     M94.232 Chondromalacia, left wrist

     M94.239 Chondromalacia, unspecified wrist

✓6ᵗʰ M94.24 Chondromalacia, joints of hand

     M94.241 Chondromalacia, joints of right hand

     M94.242 Chondromalacia, joints of left hand

     M94.249 Chondromalacia, joints of unspecified hand

✓6ᵗʰ M94.25 Chondromalacia, hip

     M94.251 Chondromalacia, right hip

     M94.252 Chondromalacia, left hip

☑ Additional Character Required   ✓x7ᵗʰ Placeholder   Questionable PDx   Manifestation   Unspecified Dx   UPD Unacceptable PDx   H1-H4 HAC   HCC CMS-HCC Dx   HIV HIV Dx

ICD-10-CM 2022   841

         M94.259   Chondromalacia, unspecified hip

✓6ᵗʰ   M94.26   Chondromalacia, knee

     M94.261   Chondromalacia, right knee

     M94.262   Chondromalacia, left knee

     M94.269   Chondromalacia, unspecified knee

✓6ᵗʰ   M94.27   Chondromalacia, ankle and joints of foot

     M94.271   Chondromalacia, right ankle and joints of right foot

     M94.272   Chondromalacia, left ankle and joints of left foot

     M94.279   Chondromalacia, unspecified ankle and joints of foot

     M94.28   Chondromalacia, other site

     M94.29   Chondromalacia, multiple sites

✓5ᵗʰ   M94.3   Chondrolysis

     Code first any associated slipped upper femoral epiphysis (nontraumatic) (M93.0-)

✓6ᵗʰ   M94.35   Chondrolysis, hip

     M94.351   Chondrolysis, right hip

     M94.352   Chondrolysis, left hip

     M94.359   Chondrolysis, unspecified hip

✓5ᵗʰ   M94.8   Other specified disorders of cartilage

✓6ᵗʰ   M94.8X   Other specified disorders of cartilage

     M94.8X0   Other specified disorders of cartilage, multiple sites

     M94.8X1   Other specified disorders of cartilage, shoulder

     M94.8X2   Other specified disorders of cartilage, upper arm

     M94.8X3   Other specified disorders of cartilage, forearm

     M94.8X4   Other specified disorders of cartilage, hand

     M94.8X5   Other specified disorders of cartilage, thigh

     M94.8X6   Other specified disorders of cartilage, lower leg

     M94.8X7   Other specified disorders of cartilage, ankle and foot

     M94.8X8   Other specified disorders of cartilage, other site

     M94.8X9   Other specified disorders of cartilage, unspecified sites

     M94.9   Disorder of cartilage, unspecified

Other disorders of the musculoskeletal system and connective tissue (M95)

✓4ᵗʰ   M95   Other acquired deformities of musculoskeletal system and connective tissue

EXCLUDES 2   acquired absence of limbs and organs (Z89-Z90)

     acquired deformities of limbs (M20-M21)

     congenital malformations and deformations of the musculoskeletal system (Q65-Q79)

     deforming dorsopathies (M40-M43)

     dentofacial anomalies [including malocclusion] (M26.-)

     postprocedural musculoskeletal disorders (M96.-)

     M95.0   Acquired deformity of nose

     EXCLUDES 2   deviated nasal septum (J34.2)

✓5ᵗʰ   M95.1   Cauliflower ear

     EXCLUDES 2   other acquired deformities of ear (H61.1)

     DEF: Acquired deformity of the external ear due to injury or subsequent perichondritis.

     M95.10   Cauliflower ear, unspecified ear

     M95.11   Cauliflower ear, right ear

     M95.12   Cauliflower ear, left ear

     M95.2   Other acquired deformity of head

     M95.3   Acquired deformity of neck

     M95.4   Acquired deformity of chest and rib

     AHA: 2014,4Q,26-27

     M95.5   Acquired deformity of pelvis

     EXCLUDES 1   maternal care for known or suspected disproportion (O33.-)

     M95.8   Other specified acquired deformities of musculoskeletal system

     M95.9   Acquired deformity of musculoskeletal system, unspecified

Intraoperative and postprocedural complications and disorders of musculoskeletal system, not elsewhere classified (M96)

✓4ᵗʰ   M96   Intraoperative and postprocedural complications and disorders of musculoskeletal system, not elsewhere classified

EXCLUDES 2   arthropathy following intestinal bypass (M02.0-)

     complications of internal orthopedic prosthetic devices, implants and grafts (T84.-)

     disorders associated with osteoporosis (M80)

     periprosthetic fracture around internal prosthetic joint (M97.-)

     presence of functional implants and other devices (Z96-Z97)

     M96.0   Pseudarthrosis after fusion or arthrodesis   CC

     M96.1   Postlaminectomy syndrome, not elsewhere classified

     M96.2   Postradiation kyphosis

     M96.3   Postlaminectomy kyphosis

     M96.4   Postsurgical lordosis

     M96.5   Postradiation scoliosis

✓5ᵗʰ   M96.6   Fracture of bone following insertion of orthopedic implant, joint prosthesis, or bone plate

     Intraoperative fracture of bone during insertion of orthopedic implant, joint prosthesis, or bone plate

     EXCLUDES 2   complication of internal orthopedic devices, implants or grafts (T84.-)

✓6ᵗʰ   M96.62   Fracture of humerus following insertion of orthopedic implant, joint prosthesis, or bone plate

     M96.621   Fracture of humerus following insertion of orthopedic implant, joint prosthesis, or bone plate, right arm   CC HCC

     M96.622   Fracture of humerus following insertion of orthopedic implant, joint prosthesis, or bone plate, left arm   CC HCC

     M96.629   Fracture of humerus following insertion of orthopedic implant, joint prosthesis, or bone plate, unspecified arm   CC HCC

✓6ᵗʰ   M96.63   Fracture of radius or ulna following insertion of orthopedic implant, joint prosthesis, or bone plate

     M96.631   Fracture of radius or ulna following insertion of orthopedic implant, joint prosthesis, or bone plate, right arm   CC HCC

     M96.632   Fracture of radius or ulna following insertion of orthopedic implant, joint prosthesis, or bone plate, left arm   CC HCC

     M96.639   Fracture of radius or ulna following insertion of orthopedic implant, joint prosthesis, or bone plate, unspecified arm   CC HCC

     M96.65   Fracture of pelvis following insertion of orthopedic implant, joint prosthesis, or bone plate   CC HCC

✓6ᵗʰ   M96.66   Fracture of femur following insertion of orthopedic implant, joint prosthesis, or bone plate

     M96.661   Fracture of femur following insertion of orthopedic implant, joint prosthesis, or bone plate, right leg   CC HCC

     M96.662   Fracture of femur following insertion of orthopedic implant, joint prosthesis, or bone plate, left leg   CC HCC

     M96.669   Fracture of femur following insertion of orthopedic implant, joint prosthesis, or bone plate, unspecified leg   CC HCC

✓6ᵗʰ   M96.67   Fracture of tibia or fibula following insertion of orthopedic implant, joint prosthesis, or bone plate

     M96.671   Fracture of tibia or fibula following insertion of orthopedic implant, joint prosthesis, or bone plate, right leg   CC HCC

     M96.672   Fracture of tibia or fibula following insertion of orthopedic implant, joint prosthesis, or bone plate, left leg   CC HCC

     M96.679   Fracture of tibia or fibula following insertion of orthopedic implant, joint prosthesis, or bone plate, unspecified leg   CC HCC

     M96.69   Fracture of other bone following insertion of orthopedic implant, joint prosthesis, or bone plate   CC HCC

N Newborn: 0   P Pediatric: 0-17   M Maternity: 9-64   A Adult: 15-124   MCC Major Complication/Comorbidity   CC Complication/Comorbidity   SW Severe Wound Dx

842

ICD-10-CM 2022

✓5ᵗʰ **M96.8** **Other intraoperative and postprocedural complications and disorders of musculoskeletal system, not elsewhere classified**
AHA: 2016,4Q,9-10

    ✓6ᵗʰ **M96.81** Intraoperative hemorrhage and hematoma of a musculoskeletal structure complicating a procedure
       EXCLUDES 1   intraoperative hemorrhage and hematoma of a musculoskeletal structure due to accidental puncture and laceration during a procedure (M96.82-)

       M96.810 Intraoperative hemorrhage and hematoma of a musculoskeletal structure complicating a musculoskeletal system procedure CC
       M96.811 Intraoperative hemorrhage and hematoma of a musculoskeletal structure complicating other procedure CC

    ✓6ᵗʰ **M96.82** Accidental puncture and laceration of a musculoskeletal structure during a procedure
       M96.820 Accidental puncture and laceration of a musculoskeletal structure during a musculoskeletal system procedure CC
       M96.821 Accidental puncture and laceration of a musculoskeletal structure during other procedure CC

    ✓6ᵗʰ **M96.83** Postprocedural hemorrhage of a musculoskeletal structure following a procedure
       M96.830 Postprocedural hemorrhage of a musculoskeletal structure following a musculoskeletal system procedure CC
       M96.831 Postprocedural hemorrhage of a musculoskeletal structure following other procedure CC

    ✓6ᵗʰ **M96.84** Postprocedural hematoma and seroma of a musculoskeletal structure following a procedure
       M96.840 Postprocedural hematoma of a musculoskeletal structure following a musculoskeletal system procedure CC
       M96.841 Postprocedural hematoma of a musculoskeletal structure following other procedure CC
         AHA: 2016,4Q,10
       M96.842 Postprocedural seroma of a musculoskeletal structure following a musculoskeletal system procedure CC
       M96.843 Postprocedural seroma of a musculoskeletal structure following other procedure CC
         AHA: 2018,3Q,6

    M96.89 Other intraoperative and postprocedural complications and disorders of the musculoskeletal system CC
       Instability of joint secondary to removal of joint prosthesis
       Use additional code, if applicable, to further specify disorder
         AHA: 2021,1Q,5

Periprosthetic fractures around internal prosthetic joint (M97)

✓4ᵗʰ **M97** **Periprosthetic fracture around internal prosthetic joint**
    EXCLUDES 2   breakage (fracture) of prosthetic joint (T84.01-)
       fracture of bone following insertion of orthopedic implant, joint prosthesis or bone plate (M96.6-)

AHA: 2016,4Q,42-43

The appropriate 7th character is to be added to each code from category M97.
A   initial encounter
D   subsequent encounter
S   sequela

    ✓5ᵗʰ **M97.0** **Periprosthetic fracture around internal prosthetic hip joint**
         AHA: 2018,1Q,21; 2016,4Q,42
      ✓x7ᵗʰ **M97.01** Periprosthetic fracture around internal prosthetic right hip joint CC HCC
      ✓x7ᵗʰ **M97.02** Periprosthetic fracture around internal prosthetic left hip joint CC HCC

    ✓5ᵗʰ **M97.1** **Periprosthetic fracture around internal prosthetic knee joint**
      ✓x7ᵗʰ **M97.11** Periprosthetic fracture around internal prosthetic right knee joint CC

      ✓x7ᵗʰ **M97.12** Periprosthetic fracture around internal prosthetic left knee joint CC

    ✓5ᵗʰ **M97.2** **Periprosthetic fracture around internal prosthetic ankle joint**
      ✓x7ᵗʰ **M97.21** Periprosthetic fracture around internal prosthetic right ankle joint CC
      ✓x7ᵗʰ **M97.22** Periprosthetic fracture around internal prosthetic left ankle joint CC

    ✓5ᵗʰ **M97.3** **Periprosthetic fracture around internal prosthetic shoulder joint**
      ✓x7ᵗʰ **M97.31** Periprosthetic fracture around internal prosthetic right shoulder joint CC
      ✓x7ᵗʰ **M97.32** Periprosthetic fracture around internal prosthetic left shoulder joint CC

    ✓5ᵗʰ **M97.4** **Periprosthetic fracture around internal prosthetic elbow joint**
      ✓x7ᵗʰ **M97.41** Periprosthetic fracture around internal prosthetic right elbow joint CC
      ✓x7ᵗʰ **M97.42** Periprosthetic fracture around internal prosthetic left elbow joint CC

    ✓x7ᵗʰ **M97.8** **Periprosthetic fracture around other internal prosthetic joint** CC
       Periprosthetic fracture around internal prosthetic finger joint
       Periprosthetic fracture around internal prosthetic spinal joint
       Periprosthetic fracture around internal prosthetic toe joint
       Periprosthetic fracture around internal prosthetic wrist joint
       Use additional code to identify the joint (Z96.6-)

    ✓x7ᵗʰ **M97.9** **Periprosthetic fracture around unspecified internal prosthetic joint** CC

Biomechanical lesions, not elsewhere classified (M99)

✓4ᵗʰ **M99** **Biomechanical lesions, not elsewhere classified**
    NOTE   This category should not be used if the condition can be classified elsewhere.
    DEF: Biomechanical lesion: Term used by osteopathic and chiropractic physicians to describe musculoskeletal conditions treated that are not more appropriately classified elsewhere.

    ✓5ᵗʰ **M99.0** **Segmental and somatic dysfunction**
       M99.00 Segmental and somatic dysfunction of head region
       M99.01 Segmental and somatic dysfunction of cervical region
       M99.02 Segmental and somatic dysfunction of thoracic region
       M99.03 Segmental and somatic dysfunction of lumbar region
       M99.04 Segmental and somatic dysfunction of sacral region
       M99.05 Segmental and somatic dysfunction of pelvic region
       M99.06 Segmental and somatic dysfunction of lower extremity
       M99.07 Segmental and somatic dysfunction of upper extremity
       M99.08 Segmental and somatic dysfunction of rib cage
       M99.09 Segmental and somatic dysfunction of abdomen and other regions

    ✓5ᵗʰ **M99.1** **Subluxation complex (vertebral)**
       M99.10 Subluxation complex (vertebral) of head region CC H5
       M99.11 Subluxation complex (vertebral) of cervical region CC H5
       M99.12 Subluxation complex (vertebral) of thoracic region
       M99.13 Subluxation complex (vertebral) of lumbar region
       M99.14 Subluxation complex (vertebral) of sacral region
       M99.15 Subluxation complex (vertebral) of pelvic region
       M99.16 Subluxation complex (vertebral) of lower extremity
       M99.17 Subluxation complex (vertebral) of upper extremity
       M99.18 Subluxation complex (vertebral) of rib cage CC H5
       M99.19 Subluxation complex (vertebral) of abdomen and other regions

    ✓5ᵗʰ **M99.2** **Subluxation stenosis of neural canal**
       M99.20 Subluxation stenosis of neural canal of head region
       M99.21 Subluxation stenosis of neural canal of cervical region
       M99.22 Subluxation stenosis of neural canal of thoracic region
       M99.23 Subluxation stenosis of neural canal of lumbar region
       M99.24 Subluxation stenosis of neural canal of sacral region
       M99.25 Subluxation stenosis of neural canal of pelvic region

M99.26   **Subluxation stenosis of neural canal of** lower extremity

M99.27   **Subluxation stenosis of neural canal of** upper extremity

M99.28   **Subluxation stenosis of neural canal of** rib cage

M99.29   **Subluxation stenosis of neural canal of** abdomen and other **regions**

✓5ᵗʰ **M99.3   Osseous stenosis of neural canal**

M99.30   **Osseous stenosis of neural canal of** head **region**

M99.31   **Osseous stenosis of neural canal of** cervical **region**

M99.32   **Osseous stenosis of neural canal of** thoracic **region**

M99.33   **Osseous stenosis of neural canal of** lumbar **region**

M99.34   **Osseous stenosis of neural canal of** sacral **region**

M99.35   **Osseous stenosis of neural canal of** pelvic **region**

M99.36   **Osseous stenosis of neural canal of** lower extremity

M99.37   **Osseous stenosis of neural canal of** upper extremity

M99.38   **Osseous stenosis of neural canal of** rib cage

M99.39   **Osseous stenosis of neural canal of** abdomen and other **regions**

✓5ᵗʰ **M99.4   Connective tissue stenosis of neural canal**

M99.40   **Connective tissue stenosis of neural canal of** head region

M99.41   **Connective tissue stenosis of neural canal of** cervical region

M99.42   **Connective tissue stenosis of neural canal of** thoracic **region**

M99.43   **Connective tissue stenosis of neural canal of** lumbar region

M99.44   **Connective tissue stenosis of neural canal of** sacral region

M99.45   **Connective tissue stenosis of neural canal of** pelvic region

M99.46   **Connective tissue stenosis of neural canal of** lower extremity

M99.47   **Connective tissue stenosis of neural canal of** upper extremity

M99.48   **Connective tissue stenosis of neural canal of** rib cage

M99.49   **Connective tissue stenosis of neural canal of** abdomen and other **regions**

✓5ᵗʰ **M99.5   Intervertebral disc stenosis of neural canal**

M99.50   **Intervertebral disc stenosis of neural canal of** head region

M99.51   **Intervertebral disc stenosis of neural canal of** cervical **region**

M99.52   **Intervertebral disc stenosis of neural canal of** thoracic **region**

M99.53   **Intervertebral disc stenosis of neural canal of** lumbar **region**

M99.54   **Intervertebral disc stenosis of neural canal of** sacral region

M99.55   **Intervertebral disc stenosis of neural canal of** pelvic region

M99.56   **Intervertebral disc stenosis of neural canal of** lower extremity

M99.57   **Intervertebral disc stenosis of neural canal of** upper extremity

M99.58   **Intervertebral disc stenosis of neural canal of** rib cage

M99.59   **Intervertebral disc stenosis of neural canal of** abdomen and other **regions**

✓5ᵗʰ **M99.6   Osseous and subluxation stenosis of intervertebral foramina**

M99.60   **Osseous and subluxation stenosis of intervertebral foramina of** head region

M99.61   **Osseous and subluxation stenosis of intervertebral foramina of** cervical **region**

M99.62   **Osseous and subluxation stenosis of intervertebral foramina of** thoracic **region**

M99.63   **Osseous and subluxation stenosis of intervertebral foramina of** lumbar **region**

M99.64   **Osseous and subluxation stenosis of intervertebral foramina of** sacral **region**

M99.65   **Osseous and subluxation stenosis of intervertebral foramina of** pelvic region

M99.66   **Osseous and subluxation stenosis of intervertebral foramina of** lower extremity

M99.67   **Osseous and subluxation stenosis of intervertebral foramina of** upper extremity

M99.68   **Osseous and subluxation stenosis of intervertebral foramina of** rib cage

M99.69   **Osseous and subluxation stenosis of intervertebral foramina of** abdomen and other **regions**

✓5ᵗʰ **M99.7   Connective tissue and disc stenosis of intervertebral foramina**

M99.70   **Connective tissue and disc stenosis of intervertebral foramina of** head region

M99.71   **Connective tissue and disc stenosis of intervertebral foramina of** cervical region

M99.72   **Connective tissue and disc stenosis of intervertebral foramina of** thoracic **region**

M99.73   **Connective tissue and disc stenosis of intervertebral foramina of** lumbar **region**

M99.74   **Connective tissue and disc stenosis of intervertebral foramina of** sacral region

M99.75   **Connective tissue and disc stenosis of intervertebral foramina of** pelvic region

M99.76   **Connective tissue and disc stenosis of intervertebral foramina of** lower extremity

M99.77   **Connective tissue and disc stenosis of intervertebral foramina of** upper extremity

M99.78   **Connective tissue and disc stenosis of intervertebral foramina of** rib cage

M99.79   **Connective tissue and disc stenosis of intervertebral foramina of** abdomen and other **regions**

✓5ᵗʰ **M99.8   Other biomechanical lesions**

M99.80   **Other biomechanical lesions of** head **region**

M99.81   **Other biomechanical lesions of** cervical **region**

M99.82   **Other biomechanical lesions of** thoracic **region**

M99.83   **Other biomechanical lesions of** lumbar **region**

M99.84   **Other biomechanical lesions of** sacral **region**

M99.85   **Other biomechanical lesions of** pelvic **region**

M99.86   **Other biomechanical lesions of** lower extremity

M99.87   **Other biomechanical lesions of** upper extremity

M99.88   **Other biomechanical lesions of** rib cage

M99.89   **Other biomechanical lesions of** abdomen and other **regions**

M99.9   Biomechanical lesion, unspecified

Ⓝ Newborn: 0   Ⓟ Pediatric: 0-17   Ⓜ Maternity: 9-64   Ⓐ Adult: 15-124   MCC Major Complication/Comorbidity   CC Complication/Comorbidity   SW Severe Wound Dx

844   ICD-10-CM 2022

Chapter 14. Diseases of Genitourinary System (NØØ–N99)

Chapter-specific Guidelines with Coding Examples

The chapter-specific guidelines from the ICD-10-CM Official Guidelines for Coding and Reporting have been provided below. Along with these guidelines are coding examples, contained in the shaded boxes, that have been developed to help illustrate the coding and/or sequencing guidance found in these guidelines.

a. Chronic kidney disease

1) Stages of chronic kidney disease (CKD)

The ICD-10-CM classifies CKD based on severity. The severity of CKD is designated by stages 1-5. Stage 2, code N18.2, equates to mild CKD; stage 3, codes N18.3Ø-N18.32, equate to moderate CKD; and stage 4, code N18.4, equates to severe CKD. Code N18.6, End stage renal disease (ESRD), is assigned when the provider has documented end-stage renal disease (ESRD).

If both a stage of CKD and ESRD are documented, assign code N18.6 only.

> Stage 5 chronic kidney disease with ESRD requiring chronic dialysis
>
> **N18.6**   **End stage renal disease**
>
> **Z99.2**   **Dependence on renal dialysis**
>
> *Explanation:* The diagnostic statement indicates the patient has chronic kidney disease, documented both as stage 5 and as ESRD requiring chronic dialysis. Code N18.6 End stage renal disease (ESRD), is assigned when the provider has documented end-stage-renal disease (ESRD). If both a stage of CKD and ESRD are documented, assign code N18.6 only.

2) Chronic kidney disease and kidney transplant status

Patients who have undergone kidney transplant may still have some form of chronic kidney disease (CKD) because the kidney transplant may not fully restore kidney function. Therefore, the presence of CKD alone does not constitute a transplant complication. Assign the appropriate N18 code for the patient's stage of CKD and code Z94.Ø, Kidney transplant status. If a transplant complication such as failure or rejection or other transplant complication is documented, see section I.C.19.g for information on coding complications of a kidney transplant. If the documentation is unclear as to whether the patient has a complication of the transplant, query the provider.

> Patient with residual chronic kidney disease stage 1 after kidney transplant
>
> **N18.1**   **Chronic kidney disease, stage 1**
>
> **Z94.Ø**   **Kidney transplant status**
>
> *Explanation:* Patients who have undergone kidney transplant may still have some form of chronic kidney disease (CKD) because the kidney transplant may not fully restore kidney function. The presence of CKD alone does not constitute a transplant complication. Assign the appropriate N18 code for the patient's stage of CKD and code Z94.Ø Kidney transplant status.

3) Chronic kidney disease with other conditions

Patients with CKD may also suffer from other serious conditions, most commonly diabetes mellitus and hypertension. The sequencing of the CKD code in relationship to codes for other contributing conditions is based on the conventions in the Tabular List.

See I.C.9. Hypertensive chronic kidney disease.

See I.C.19. Chronic kidney disease and kidney transplant complications.

> Type 1 diabetic chronic kidney disease, stage 2
>
> **E1Ø.22**   **Type 1 diabetes mellitus with diabetic chronic kidney disease**
>
> **N18.2**   **Chronic kidney disease, stage 2 (mild)**
>
> *Explanation:* Patients with CKD may also suffer from other serious conditions such as diabetes mellitus. The sequencing of the CKD code in relationship to codes for other contributing conditions is based on the conventions in the Tabular List. Diabetic CKD code E1Ø.22 includes an instructional note to "Use additional code to identify stage of chronic kidney disease (N18.1–N18.6)," thus providing sequencing direction.

Chapter 14. Diseases of the Genitourinary System (N00-N99)

EXCLUDES 2   certain conditions originating in the perinatal period (P04-P96)
certain infectious and parasitic diseases (A00-B99)
complications of pregnancy, childbirth and the puerperium (O00-O9A)
congenital malformations, deformations and chromosomal abnormalities (Q00-Q99)
endocrine, nutritional and metabolic diseases (E00-E88)
injury, poisoning and certain other consequences of external causes (S00-T88)
neoplasms (C00-D49)
symptoms, signs and abnormal clinical and laboratory findings, not elsewhere classified (R00-R94)

This chapter contains the following blocks:

N00-N08   Glomerular diseases
N10-N16   Renal tubulo-interstitial diseases
N17-N19   Acute kidney failure and chronic kidney disease
N20-N23   Urolithiasis
N25-N29   Other disorders of kidney and ureter
N30-N39   Other diseases of the urinary system
N40-N53   Diseases of male genital organs
N60-N65   Disorders of breast
N70-N77   Inflammatory diseases of female pelvic organs
N80-N98   Noninflammatory disorders of female genital tract
N99   Intraoperative and postprocedural complications and disorders of genitourinary system, not elsewhere classified

Glomerular diseases (N00-N08)

Code also any associated kidney failure (N17-N19).
EXCLUDES 1   hypertensive chronic kidney disease (I12.-)
AHA: 2020,4Q,34-35
DEF: Glomeruli: Clusters of microscopic blood vessels located within the kidneys containing small pores through which waste products are filtered from the blood and urine is formed.
DEF: Glomerulonephritis: Disease of the kidney with diffuse inflammation of the capillary loops of the glomeruli.

✓4th **N00**   Acute **nephritic syndrome**

INCLUDES   acute glomerular disease
acute glomerulonephritis
acute nephritis
EXCLUDES 1   acute tubulo-interstitial nephritis (N10)
nephritic syndrome NOS (N05.-)

AHA: 2021,1Q,23

N00.0   **Acute nephritic syndrome with** minor glomerular abnormality   MCC
Acute nephritic syndrome with minimal change lesion

N00.1   **Acute nephritic syndrome with** focal and segmental glomerular lesions   MCC
Acute nephritic syndrome with focal and segmental hyalinosis
Acute nephritic syndrome with focal and segmental sclerosis
Acute nephritic syndrome with focal glomerulonephritis

N00.2   **Acute nephritic syndrome with** diffuse membranous glomerulonephritis   MCC

N00.3   **Acute nephritic syndrome with** diffuse mesangial proliferative glomerulonephritis   MCC

N00.4   **Acute nephritic syndrome with** diffuse endocapillary proliferative glomerulonephritis   MCC

N00.5   **Acute nephritic syndrome with** diffuse mesangiocapillary glomerulonephritis   MCC
Acute nephritic syndrome with membranoproliferative glomerulonephritis, types 1 and 3, or NOS
EXCLUDES 1   acute nephritic syndrome with C3 glomerulonephritis (N00.A)
acute nephritic syndrome with C3 glomerulopathy (N00.A)

N00.6   **Acute nephritic syndrome with** dense deposit disease   MCC
Acute nephritic syndrome with C3 glomerulopathy with dense deposit disease
Acute nephritic syndrome with membranoproliferative glomerulonephritis, type 2

N00.7   **Acute nephritic syndrome with** diffuse crescentic glomerulonephritis   MCC
Acute nephritic syndrome with extracapillary glomerulonephritis

N00.8   **Acute nephritic syndrome with other morphologic changes**   MCC
Acute nephritic syndrome with proliferative glomerulonephritis NOS

N00.9   **Acute nephritic syndrome with unspecified morphologic changes**   MCC

N00.A   **Acute nephritic syndrome with** C3 glomerulonephritis   MCC
Acute nephritic syndrome with C3 glomerulopathy, NOS
EXCLUDES 1   acute nephritic syndrome (with C3 glomerulopathy) with dense deposit disease (N00.6)

✓4th **N01**   Rapidly progressive **nephritic syndrome**

INCLUDES   rapidly progressive glomerular disease
rapidly progressive glomerulonephritis
rapidly progressive nephritis
EXCLUDES 1   nephritic syndrome NOS (N05.-)

AHA: 2021,1Q,23

N01.0   **Rapidly progressive nephritic syndrome with** minor glomerular abnormality   MCC
Rapidly progressive nephritic syndrome with minimal change lesion

N01.1   **Rapidly progressive nephritic syndrome with** focal and segmental glomerular lesions   MCC
Rapidly progressive nephritic syndrome with focal and segmental hyalinosis
Rapidly progressive nephritic syndrome with focal and segmental sclerosis
Rapidly progressive nephritic syndrome with focal glomerulonephritis

N01.2   **Rapidly progressive nephritic syndrome with** diffuse membranous glomerulonephritis   MCC

N01.3   **Rapidly progressive nephritic syndrome with** diffuse mesangial proliferative glomerulonephritis   MCC

N01.4   **Rapidly progressive nephritic syndrome with** diffuse endocapillary proliferative glomerulonephritis   MCC

N01.5   **Rapidly progressive nephritic syndrome with** diffuse mesangiocapillary glomerulonephritis   MCC
Rapidly progressive nephritic syndrome with membranoproliferative glomerulonephritis, types 1 and 3, or NOS
EXCLUDES 1   rapidly progressive nephritic syndrome with C3 glomerulonephritis (N01.A)
rapidly progressive nephritic syndrome with C3 glomerulopathy (N01.A)

N01.6   **Rapidly progressive nephritic syndrome with** dense deposit disease   MCC
Rapidly progressive nephritic syndrome with C3 glomerulopathy with dense deposit disease
Rapidly progressive nephritic syndrome with membranoproliferative glomerulonephritis, type 2

N01.7   **Rapidly progressive nephritic syndrome with** diffuse crescentic glomerulonephritis   MCC
Rapidly progressive nephritic syndrome with extracapillary glomerulonephritis

N01.8   **Rapidly progressive nephritic syndrome with other morphologic changes**   MCC
Rapidly progressive nephritic syndrome with proliferative glomerulonephritis NOS

N01.9   **Rapidly progressive nephritic syndrome with unspecified morphologic changes**   MCC

N01.A   **Rapidly progressive nephritic syndrome with** C3 glomerulonephritis   MCC
Rapidly progressive nephritic syndrome with C3 glomerulopathy, NOS
EXCLUDES 1   rapidly progressive nephritic syndrome (with C3 glomerulopathy) with dense deposit disease (N01.6)

✓4th **N02**   Recurrent and persistent hematuria

EXCLUDES 1   acute cystitis with hematuria (N30.01)
hematuria NOS (R31.9)
hematuria not associated with specified morphologic lesions (R31.-)

N02.0   **Recurrent and persistent hematuria with** minor glomerular abnormality   CC
Recurrent and persistent hematuria with minimal change lesion

N02.1 **Recurrent and persistent hematuria with** focal and segmental glomerular lesions   `CC`
  Recurrent and persistent hematuria with focal and segmental hyalinosis
  Recurrent and persistent hematuria with focal and segmental sclerosis
  Recurrent and persistent hematuria with focal glomerulonephritis

N02.2 **Recurrent and persistent hematuria with** diffuse membranous glomerulonephritis   `CC`

N02.3 **Recurrent and persistent hematuria with** diffuse mesangial proliferative glomerulonephritis   `CC`

N02.4 **Recurrent and persistent hematuria with** diffuse endocapillary proliferative glomerulonephritis   `CC`

N02.5 **Recurrent and persistent hematuria with** diffuse mesangiocapillary glomerulonephritis   `CC`
  Recurrent and persistent hematuria with membranoproliferative glomerulonephritis, types 1 and 3, or NOS
  `EXCLUDES 1`   *recurrent and persistent hematuria with C3 glomerulonephritis (N02.A)*
      recurrent and persistent hematuria with C3 glomerulopathy (N02.A)

N02.6 **Recurrent and persistent hematuria with** dense deposit disease   `CC`
  Recurrent and persistent hematuria with C3 glomerulopathy with dense deposit disease
  Recurrent and persistent hematuria with membranoproliferative glomerulonephritis, type 2

N02.7 **Recurrent and persistent hematuria with** diffuse crescentic glomerulonephritis   `CC`
  Recurrent and persistent hematuria with extracapillary glomerulonephritis

N02.8 **Recurrent and persistent hematuria with** other morphologic changes   `CC`
  Recurrent and persistent hematuria with proliferative glomerulonephritis NOS

N02.9 **Recurrent and persistent hematuria with** unspecified morphologic changes   `CC`
  AHA: 2017,2Q,5

N02.A **Recurrent and persistent hematuria with** C3 glomerulonephritis   `CC`
  Recurrent and persistent hematuria with C3 glomerulopathy
  `EXCLUDES 1`   *recurrent and persistent hematuria (with C3 glomerulopathy) with dense deposit disease (N02.6)*

`✓4ᵗʰ` **N03** **Chronic** nephritic syndrome

  `INCLUDES`   chronic glomerular disease
      chronic glomerulonephritis
      chronic nephritis
  `EXCLUDES 1`   *chronic tubulo-interstitial nephritis (N11.-)*
      diffuse sclerosing glomerulonephritis (N05.8-)
      nephritic syndrome NOS (N05.-)

  AHA: 2021,1Q,23
  DEF: Slow, progressive type of nephritis characterized by inflammation of the capillary loops in the glomeruli of the kidney, which leads to renal failure.

N03.0 **Chronic nephritic syndrome with** minor glomerular abnormality   `CC`
  Chronic nephritic syndrome with minimal change lesion

N03.1 **Chronic nephritic syndrome with** focal and segmental glomerular lesions   `CC`
  Chronic nephritic syndrome with focal and segmental hyalinosis
  Chronic nephritic syndrome with focal and segmental sclerosis
  Chronic nephritic syndrome with focal glomerulonephritis

N03.2 **Chronic nephritic syndrome with** diffuse membranous glomerulonephritis   `CC`

N03.3 **Chronic nephritic syndrome with** diffuse mesangial proliferative glomerulonephritis   `CC`

N03.4 **Chronic nephritic syndrome with** diffuse endocapillary proliferative glomerulonephritis   `CC`

N03.5 **Chronic nephritic syndrome with** diffuse mesangiocapillary glomerulonephritis   `CC`
  Chronic nephritic syndrome with membranoproliferative glomerulonephritis, types 1 and 3, or NOS
  `EXCLUDES 1`   *chronic nephritic syndrome with C3 glomerulonephritis (N03.A)*
      chronic nephritic syndrome with C3 glomerulopathy (N03.A)

N03.6 **Chronic nephritic syndrome with** dense deposit disease   `CC`
  Chronic nephritic syndrome with C3 glomerulopathy with dense deposit disease
  Chronic nephritic syndrome with membranoproliferative glomerulonephritis, type 2

N03.7 **Chronic nephritic syndrome with** diffuse crescentic glomerulonephritis   `CC`
  Chronic nephritic syndrome with extracapillary glomerulonephritis

N03.8 **Chronic nephritic syndrome with** other morphologic changes   `CC`
  Chronic nephritic syndrome with proliferative glomerulonephritis NOS

N03.9 **Chronic nephritic syndrome with** unspecified morphologic changes   `CC`

N03.A **Chronic nephritic syndrome with** C3 glomerulonephritis   `CC`
  Chronic nephritic syndrome with C3 glomerulopathy
  `EXCLUDES 1`   *chronic nephritic syndrome (with C3 glomerulopathy) with dense deposit disease (N03.6)*

`✓4ᵗʰ` **N04** **Nephrotic syndrome**

  `INCLUDES`   congenital nephrotic syndrome
      lipoid nephrosis

N04.0 **Nephrotic syndrome with** minor glomerular abnormality   `CC`
  Nephrotic syndrome with minimal change lesion

N04.1 **Nephrotic syndrome with** focal and segmental glomerular lesions   `CC`
  Nephrotic syndrome with focal and segmental hyalinosis
  Nephrotic syndrome with focal and segmental sclerosis
  Nephrotic syndrome with focal glomerulonephritis

N04.2 **Nephrotic syndrome with** diffuse membranous glomerulonephritis   `CC`

N04.3 **Nephrotic syndrome with** diffuse mesangial proliferative glomerulonephritis   `CC`

N04.4 **Nephrotic syndrome with** diffuse endocapillary proliferative glomerulonephritis   `CC`

N04.5 **Nephrotic syndrome with** diffuse mesangiocapillary glomerulonephritis   `CC`
  Nephrotic syndrome with membranoproliferative glomerulonephritis, types 1 and 3, or NOS
  `EXCLUDES 1`   *nephrotic syndrome with C3 glomerulonephritis (N04.A)*
      nephrotic syndrome with C3 glomerulopathy (N04.A)

N04.6 **Nephrotic syndrome with** dense deposit disease   `CC`
  Nephrotic syndrome with C3 glomerulopathy with dense deposit disease
  Nephrotic syndrome with membranoproliferative glomerulonephritis, type 2

N04.7 **Nephrotic syndrome with** diffuse crescentic glomerulonephritis   `CC`
  Nephrotic syndrome with extracapillary glomerulonephritis

N04.8 **Nephrotic syndrome with** other morphologic changes   `CC`
  Nephrotic syndrome with proliferative glomerulonephritis NOS

N04.9 **Nephrotic syndrome with** unspecified morphologic changes   `CC`

N04.A **Nephrotic syndrome with** C3 glomerulonephritis   `CC`
  Nephrotic syndrome with C3 glomerulopathy
  `EXCLUDES 1`   *nephrotic syndrome (with C3 glomerulopathy) with dense deposit disease (N04.6)*

Chapter 14. Diseases of the Genitourinary System

✓4ᵗʰ **N05 Unspecified nephritic syndrome**

INCLUDES   glomerular disease NOS
glomerulonephritis NOS
nephritis NOS
nephropathy NOS and renal disease NOS with morphological lesion specified in .0-.8

EXCLUDES 1   *nephropathy NOS with no stated morphological lesion (N28.9)*
renal disease NOS with no stated morphological lesion (N28.9)
tubulo-interstitial nephritis NOS (N12)

N05.0 Unspecified nephritic syndrome with minor glomerular abnormality
Unspecified nephritic syndrome with minimal change lesion

N05.1 Unspecified nephritic syndrome with focal and segmental glomerular lesions
Unspecified nephritic syndrome with focal and segmental hyalinosis
Unspecified nephritic syndrome with focal and segmental sclerosis
Unspecified nephritic syndrome with focal glomerulonephritis

N05.2 Unspecified nephritic syndrome with diffuse membranous glomerulonephritis CC

N05.3 Unspecified nephritic syndrome with diffuse mesangial proliferative glomerulonephritis CC

N05.4 Unspecified nephritic syndrome with diffuse endocapillary proliferative glomerulonephritis CC

N05.5 Unspecified nephritic syndrome with diffuse mesangiocapillary glomerulonephritis CC
Unspecified nephritic syndrome with membranoproliferative glomerulonephritis, types 1 and 3, or NOS
EXCLUDES 1   *unspecified nephritic syndrome with C3 glomerulonephritis (N05.A)*
unspecified nephritic syndrome with C3 glomerulopathy (N05.A)

N05.6 Unspecified nephritic syndrome with dense deposit disease
Unspecified nephritic syndrome with C3 glomerulopathy with dense deposit disease
Unspecified nephritic syndrome with membranoproliferative glomerulonephritis, type 2

N05.7 Unspecified nephritic syndrome with diffuse crescentic glomerulonephritis
Unspecified nephritic syndrome with extracapillary glomerulonephritis

N05.8 Unspecified nephritic syndrome with other morphologic changes
Unspecified nephritic syndrome with proliferative glomerulonephritis NOS

N05.9 Unspecified nephritic syndrome with unspecified morphologic changes

N05.A Unspecified nephritic syndrome with C3 glomerulonephritis CC
Unspecified nephritic syndrome with C3 glomerulopathy
EXCLUDES 1   *unspecified nephritic syndrome (with C3 glomerulopathy) with dense deposit disease (N05.6)*

✓4ᵗʰ **N06 Isolated proteinuria with specified morphological lesion**
EXCLUDES 1   *proteinuria not associated with specific morphologic lesions (R80.0)*

N06.0 Isolated proteinuria with minor glomerular abnormality
Isolated proteinuria with minimal change lesion

N06.1 Isolated proteinuria with focal and segmental glomerular lesions
Isolated proteinuria with focal and segmental hyalinosis
Isolated proteinuria with focal and segmental sclerosis
Isolated proteinuria with focal glomerulonephritis

N06.2 Isolated proteinuria with diffuse membranous glomerulonephritis CC

N06.3 Isolated proteinuria with diffuse mesangial proliferative glomerulonephritis CC

N06.4 Isolated proteinuria with diffuse endocapillary proliferative glomerulonephritis CC

N06.5 Isolated proteinuria with diffuse mesangiocapillary glomerulonephritis CC
Isolated proteinuria with membranoproliferative glomerulonephritis, types 1 and 3, or NOS
EXCLUDES 1   *isolated proteinuria with C3 glomerulonephritis (N06.A)*
isolated proteinuria with C3 glomerulopathy (N06.A)

N06.6 Isolated proteinuria with dense deposit disease
Isolated proteinuria with C3 glomerulopathy with dense deposit disease
Isolated proteinuria with membranoproliferative glomerulonephritis, type 2

N06.7 Isolated proteinuria with diffuse crescentic glomerulonephritis
Isolated proteinuria with extracapillary glomerulonephritis

N06.8 Isolated proteinuria with other morphologic lesion
Isolated proteinuria with proliferative glomerulonephritis NOS

N06.9 Isolated proteinuria with unspecified morphologic lesion

N06.A Isolated proteinuria with C3 glomerulonephritis CC
Isolated proteinuria with C3 glomerulopathy
EXCLUDES 1   *isolated proteinuria (with C3 glomerulopathy) with dense deposit disease (N06.6)*

✓4ᵗʰ **N07 Hereditary nephropathy, not elsewhere classified**
EXCLUDES 2   *Alport's syndrome (Q87.81-)*
hereditary amyloid nephropathy (E85.-)
nail patella syndrome (Q87.2)
non-neuropathic heredofamilial amyloidosis (E85.-)

N07.0 Hereditary nephropathy, not elsewhere classified with minor glomerular abnormality
Hereditary nephropathy, not elsewhere classified with minimal change lesion

N07.1 Hereditary nephropathy, not elsewhere classified with focal and segmental glomerular lesions
Hereditary nephropathy, not elsewhere classified with focal and segmental hyalinosis
Hereditary nephropathy, not elsewhere classified with focal and segmental sclerosis
Hereditary nephropathy, not elsewhere classified with focal glomerulonephritis

N07.2 Hereditary nephropathy, not elsewhere classified with diffuse membranous glomerulonephritis CC

N07.3 Hereditary nephropathy, not elsewhere classified with diffuse mesangial proliferative glomerulonephritis CC

N07.4 Hereditary nephropathy, not elsewhere classified with diffuse endocapillary proliferative glomerulonephritis CC

N07.5 Hereditary nephropathy, not elsewhere classified with diffuse mesangiocapillary glomerulonephritis CC
Hereditary nephropathy, not elsewhere classified with membranoproliferative glomerulonephritis, types 1 and 3, or NOS
EXCLUDES 1   *hereditary nephropathy, not elsewhere classified with C3 glomerulonephritis (N07.A)*
hereditary nephropathy, not elsewhere classified with C3 glomerulopathy (N07.A)

N07.6 Hereditary nephropathy, not elsewhere classified with dense deposit disease
Hereditary nephropathy, not elsewhere classified with C3 glomerulopathy with dense deposit disease
Hereditary nephropathy, not elsewhere classified with membranoproliferative glomerulonephritis, type 2

N07.7 Hereditary nephropathy, not elsewhere classified with diffuse crescentic glomerulonephritis
Hereditary nephropathy, not elsewhere classified with extracapillary glomerulonephritis

N07.8 Hereditary nephropathy, not elsewhere classified with other morphologic lesions
Hereditary nephropathy, not elsewhere classified with proliferative glomerulonephritis NOS

N07.9 Hereditary nephropathy, not elsewhere classified with unspecified morphologic lesions

N07.A Hereditary nephropathy, not elsewhere classified with C3 glomerulonephritis CC
Hereditary nephropathy, not elsewhere classified with C3 glomerulopathy
EXCLUDES 1   *hereditary nephropathy, not elsewhere classified (with C3 glomerulopathy) with dense deposit disease (N07.6)*

N Newborn: 0   P Pediatric: 0-17   M Maternity: 9-64   A Adult: 15-124   MCC Major Complication/Comorbidity   CC Complication/Comorbidity   SW Severe Wound Dx

848   ICD-10-CM 2022

N08   *Glomerular disorders in diseases classified elsewhere*

Glomerulonephritis
Nephritis
Nephropathy
Code first underlying disease, such as:
   amyloidosis (E85.-)
   congenital syphilis (A50.5)
   cryoglobulinemia (D89.1)
   disseminated intravascular coagulation (D65)
   gout (M1A.-, M10.-)
   microscopic polyangiitis (M31.7)
   multiple myeloma (C90.0-)
   sepsis (A40.0-A41.9)
   sickle-cell disease (D57.0-D57.8)

> **EXCLUDES 1**   *glomerulonephritis, nephritis and nephropathy (in):*
>   *antiglomerular basement membrane disease (M31.0)*
>   *diabetes (E08-E13 with .21)*
>   *gonococcal (A54.21)*
>   *Goodpasture's syndrome (M31.0)*
>   *hemolytic-uremic syndrome (D59.3)*
>   *lupus (M32.14)*
>   *mumps (B26.83)*
>   *syphilis (A52.75)*
>   *systemic lupus erythematosus (M32.14)*
>   *Wegener's granulomatosis (M31.31)*
> *pyelonephritis in diseases classified elsewhere (N16)*
> *renal tubulo-interstitial disorders classified elsewhere (N16)*

Renal tubulo-interstitial diseases (N10-N16)

> **INCLUDES**   pyelonephritis
> **EXCLUDES 1**   *pyeloureteritis cystica (N28.85)*

N10   Acute pyelonephritis   `CC` `H6`

Acute infectious interstitial nephritis
Acute pyelitis
Acute tubulo-interstitial nephritis
Hemoglobin nephrosis
Myoglobin nephrosis
Use additional code (B95-B97), to identify infectious agent
AHA: 2020,3Q,25; 2019,3Q,13

✓4ᵗʰ N11   Chronic tubulo-interstitial nephritis

> **INCLUDES**   chronic infectious interstitial nephritis
>   chronic pyelitis
>   chronic pyelonephritis

Use additional code (B95-B97), to identify infectious agent

N11.0   Nonobstructive reflux-associated chronic pyelonephritis
Pyelonephritis (chronic) associated with (vesicoureteral) reflux
> **EXCLUDES 1**   *vesicoureteral reflux NOS (N13.70)*

N11.1   Chronic obstructive pyelonephritis   `CC`
Pyelonephritis (chronic) associated with anomaly of pelviureteric junction
Pyelonephritis (chronic) associated with anomaly of pyeloureteric junction
Pyelonephritis (chronic) associated with crossing of vessel
Pyelonephritis (chronic) associated with kinking of ureter
Pyelonephritis (chronic) associated with obstruction of ureter
Pyelonephritis (chronic) associated with stricture of pelviureteric junction
Pyelonephritis (chronic) associated with stricture of ureter
> **EXCLUDES 1**   *calculous pyelonephritis (N20.9)*
>   *obstructive uropathy (N13.-)*

N11.8   Other chronic tubulo-interstitial nephritis   `CC`
Nonobstructive chronic pyelonephritis NOS

N11.9   Chronic tubulo-interstitial nephritis, unspecified   `CC` `H6`
Chronic interstitial nephritis NOS
Chronic pyelitis NOS
Chronic pyelonephritis NOS

N12   Tubulo-interstitial nephritis, not specified as acute or chronic   `CC` `H6`

Interstitial nephritis NOS
Pyelitis NOS
Pyelonephritis NOS
> **EXCLUDES 1**   *calculous pyelonephritis (N20.9)*

✓4ᵗʰ N13   Obstructive and reflux uropathy

> **EXCLUDES 2**   *calculus of kidney and ureter without hydronephrosis (N20.-)*
> *congenital obstructive defects of renal pelvis and ureter (Q62.0-Q62.3)*
> *hydronephrosis with ureteropelvic junction obstruction (Q62.11)*
> *obstructive pyelonephritis (N11.1)*

DEF: Hydronephrosis: Distension of the kidney caused by an accumulation of urine that cannot flow out due to an obstruction that may be caused by conditions such as kidney stones or vesicoureteral reflux.

N13.0   Hydronephrosis with ureteropelvic junction obstruction   `CC`
Hydronephrosis due to acquired occlusion of ureteropelvic junction
> **EXCLUDES 2**   *hydronephrosis with ureteropelvic junction obstruction due to calculus (N13.2)*

AHA: 2016,4Q,43

Hydronephrosis/UPJ Obstruction

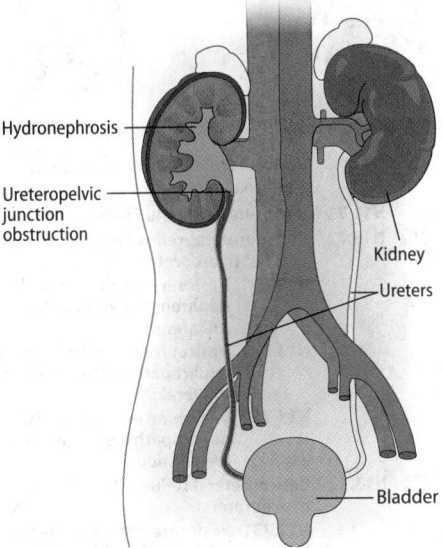

Hydronephrosis
Ureteropelvic junction obstruction
Kidney
Ureters
Bladder

N13.1   Hydronephrosis with ureteral stricture, not elsewhere classified   `CC`
> **EXCLUDES 1**   *hydronephrosis with ureteral stricture with infection (N13.6)*

N13.2   Hydronephrosis with renal and ureteral calculous obstruction   `CC`
> **EXCLUDES 1**   *hydronephrosis with renal and ureteral calculous obstruction with infection (N13.6)*

✓5ᵗʰ N13.3   Other and unspecified hydronephrosis
> **EXCLUDES 1**   *hydronephrosis with infection (N13.6)*

   N13.30   Unspecified hydronephrosis   `CC`
   N13.39   Other hydronephrosis   `CC`

N13.4   Hydroureter   `CC`
> **EXCLUDES 1**   *congenital hydroureter (Q62.3-)*
> *hydroureter with infection (N13.6)*
> *vesicoureteral-reflux with hydroureter (N13.73-)*

DEF: Abnormal enlargement or distension of the ureter with water or urine caused by an obstruction.

N13.5   Crossing vessel and stricture of ureter without hydronephrosis
Kinking and stricture of ureter without hydronephrosis
> **EXCLUDES 1**   *crossing vessel and stricture of ureter without hydronephrosis with infection (N13.6)*

N13.6   Pyonephrosis   `CC` `H6`
Conditions in N13.0-N13.5 with infection
Obstructive uropathy with infection
Use additional code (B95-B97), to identify infectious agent
AHA: 2018,2Q,21

Chapter 14. Diseases of the Genitourinary System

✓5ᵗʰ **N13.7 Vesicoureteral-reflux**

> EXCLUDES 1   reflux-associated pyelonephritis (N11.0)

> **DEF:** Urine passage from the bladder flows backward up into the ureter and kidneys that can lead to bacterial infection and an increase in hydrostatic pressure, causing kidney damage.

Vesicoureteral Reflux

Kidneys

Ureters

Bladder

Normal flow of urine   Urine flowing the wrong way (VUR)

N13.70 Vesicoureteral-reflux, unspecified
Vesicoureteral-reflux NOS

N13.71 Vesicoureteral-reflux without reflux nephropathy

✓6ᵗʰ **N13.72 Vesicoureteral-reflux** with reflux nephropathy without hydroureter

     N13.721 Vesicoureteral-reflux with reflux nephropathy without hydroureter, unilateral

     N13.722 Vesicoureteral-reflux with reflux nephropathy without hydroureter, bilateral

     N13.729 Vesicoureteral-reflux with reflux nephropathy without hydroureter, unspecified

✓6ᵗʰ **N13.73 Vesicoureteral-reflux** with reflux nephropathy with hydroureter

     N13.731 Vesicoureteral-reflux with reflux nephropathy with hydroureter, unilateral

     N13.732 Vesicoureteral-reflux with reflux nephropathy with hydroureter, bilateral

     N13.739 Vesicoureteral-reflux with reflux nephropathy with hydroureter, unspecified

N13.8 Other obstructive and reflux uropathy   CC
Urinary tract obstruction due to specified cause
Code first, if applicable, any causal condition, such as:
     enlarged prostate (N40.1)

N13.9 Obstructive and reflux uropathy, unspecified
Urinary tract obstruction NOS

✓4ᵗʰ **N14 Drug- and heavy-metal-induced tubulo-interstitial and tubular conditions**

Code first poisoning due to drug or toxin, if applicable (T36-T65 with fifth or sixth character 1-4 or 6)
Use additional code for adverse effect, if applicable, to identify drug (T36-T50 with fifth or sixth character 5)

N14.0 Analgesic nephropathy

N14.1 Nephropathy induced by other drugs, medicaments and biological substances

N14.2 Nephropathy induced by unspecified drug, medicament or biological substance

N14.3 Nephropathy induced by heavy metals

N14.4 Toxic nephropathy, not elsewhere classified

✓4ᵗʰ **N15 Other renal tubulo-interstitial diseases**

N15.0 Balkan nephropathy
Balkan endemic nephropathy

N15.1 Renal and perinephric abscess   MCC H6

N15.8 Other specified renal tubulo-interstitial diseases

N15.9 Renal tubulo-interstitial disease, unspecified
Infection of kidney NOS

> EXCLUDES 1   urinary tract infection NOS (N39.0)

N16 Renal tubulo-interstitial disorders in diseases classified elsewhere

Pyelonephritis
Tubulo-interstitial nephritis
Code first underlying disease, such as:
     brucellosis (A23.0-A23.9)
     cryoglobulinemia (D89.1)
     glycogen storage disease (E74.0)
     leukemia (C91-C95)
     lymphoma (C81.0-C85.9, C96.0-C96.9)
     multiple myeloma (C90.0-)
     sepsis (A40.0-A41.9)
     Wilson's disease (E83.0)

> EXCLUDES 1   diphtheritic pyelonephritis and tubulo-interstitial nephritis (A36.84)
> pyelonephritis and tubulo-interstitial nephritis in candidiasis (B37.49)
> pyelonephritis and tubulo-interstitial nephritis in cystinosis (E72.04)
> pyelonephritis and tubulo-interstitial nephritis in salmonella infection (A02.25)
> pyelonephritis and tubulo-interstitial nephritis in sarcoidosis (D86.84)
> ▶pyelonephritis and tubulo-interstitial nephritis in Sjögren syndrome◀ (M35.04)
> pyelonephritis and tubulo-interstitial nephritis in systemic lupus erythematosus (M32.15)
> pyelonephritis and tubulo-interstitial nephritis in toxoplasmosis (B58.83)
> renal tubular degeneration in diabetes (E08-E13 with .29)
> syphilitic pyelonephritis and tubulo-interstitial nephritis (A52.75)

Acute kidney failure and chronic kidney disease (N17-N19)

> EXCLUDES 2   congenital renal failure (P96.0)
> drug- and heavy-metal-induced tubulo-interstitial and tubular conditions (N14.-)
> extrarenal uremia (R39.2)
> hemolytic-uremic syndrome (D59.3)
> hepatorenal syndrome (K76.7)
> postpartum hepatorenal syndrome (O90.4)
> posttraumatic renal failure (T79.5)
> prerenal uremia (R39.2)
> renal failure complicating abortion or ectopic or molar pregnancy (O00-O07, O08.4)
> renal failure following labor and delivery (O90.4)
> renal failure postprocedural (N99.0)

✓4ᵗʰ **N17 Acute kidney failure**

Code also associated underlying condition

> EXCLUDES 1   posttraumatic renal failure (T79.5)

AHA: 2020,3Q,22; 2019,2Q,7; 2019,1Q,12; 2013,4Q,124

N17.0 Acute kidney failure with tubular necrosis   MCC HCC
Acute tubular necrosis
Renal tubular necrosis
Tubular necrosis NOS

N17.1 Acute kidney failure with acute cortical necrosis   MCC HCC
Acute cortical necrosis
Cortical necrosis NOS
Renal cortical necrosis

N17.2 Acute kidney failure with medullary necrosis   MCC HCC
Medullary [papillary] necrosis NOS
Acute medullary [papillary] necrosis
Renal medullary [papillary] necrosis

N17.8 Other acute kidney failure   CC HCC

N17.9 Acute kidney failure, unspecified   CC HCC
Acute kidney injury (nontraumatic)

> EXCLUDES 2   traumatic kidney injury (S37.0-)

✓4ᵗʰ **N18 Chronic kidney disease (CKD)**

Code first any associated:
     diabetic chronic kidney disease (E08.22, E09.22, E10.22, E11.22, E13.22)
     hypertensive chronic kidney disease (I12.-, I13.-)
Use additional code to identify kidney transplant status, if applicable, (Z94.0)

AHA: 2019,3Q,3; 2018,4Q,88; 2013,1Q,24

N18.1 Chronic kidney disease, stage 1

N18.2 Chronic kidney disease, stage 2 (mild)

N Newborn: 0   P Pediatric: 0-17   M Maternity: 9-64   A Adult: 15-124   MCC Major Complication/Comorbidity   CC Complication/Comorbidity   SW Severe Wound Dx

850

ICD-10-CM 2022

Chapter 14. Diseases of the Genitourinary System

✓5ᵗʰ **N18.3** **Chronic kidney disease, stage 3 (moderate)**
    AHA: 2020,4Q,35
    N18.30 **Chronic kidney disease, stage 3 unspecified** HCC
    N18.31 **Chronic kidney disease, stage 3a** HCC
    N18.32 **Chronic kidney disease, stage 3b** HCC

N18.4 **Chronic kidney disease, stage 4 (severe)** CC HCC

N18.5 **Chronic kidney disease, stage 5** CC HCC
    EXCLUDES 1   *chronic kidney disease, stage 5 requiring chronic dialysis (N18.6)*
    DEF: End-stage renal disease (ESRD) with a GFR value of 15 ml/min or less not yet requiring chronic dialysis.
    TIP: When both ESRD and CKD 5 are documented, code only for ESRD.

N18.6 **End stage renal disease** MCC HCC
    Chronic kidney disease requiring chronic dialysis
    Use additional code to identify dialysis status (Z99.2)
    AHA: 2016,3Q,22; 2016,1Q,12; 2013,4Q,124-125
    TIP: When both ESRD and CKD 5 are documented, code only for ESRD.

N18.9 **Chronic kidney disease, unspecified**
    Chronic renal disease
    Chronic renal failure NOS
    Chronic renal insufficiency
    Chronic uremia NOS
    Diffuse sclerosing glomerulonephritis NOS

N19 **Unspecified kidney failure**
    Uremia NOS
    EXCLUDES 1   *acute kidney failure (N17.-)*
        chronic kidney disease (N18.-)
        chronic uremia (N18.9)
        extrarenal uremia (R39.2)
        prerenal uremia (R39.2)
        renal insufficiency (acute) (N28.9)
        uremia of newborn (P96.0)

Urolithiasis (N20-N23)

AHA: 2017,1Q,5; 2015,2Q,8
TIP: Codes from this code block can be assigned based on the diagnosis listed in a radiology report when authenticated by a radiologist and available at the time of code assignment.

✓4ᵗʰ **N20** **Calculus of kidney and ureter**
    Calculous pyelonephritis
    EXCLUDES 1   *nephrocalcinosis (E83.5)*
        that with hydronephrosis (N13.2)
    AHA: 2019,3Q,13

N20.0 **Calculus of kidney**
    Nephrolithiasis NOS
    Renal calculus
    Renal stone
    Staghorn calculus
    Stone in kidney
    AHA: 2019,3Q,13

N20.1 **Calculus of ureter** CC
    Calculus of the ureteropelvic junction
    Ureteric stone
    AHA: 2016,3Q,22

N20.2 **Calculus of kidney with calculus of ureter** CC

N20.9 **Urinary calculus, unspecified**

✓4ᵗʰ **N21** **Calculus of lower urinary tract**
    INCLUDES   calculus of lower urinary tract with cystitis and urethritis

N21.0 **Calculus in bladder**
    Calculus in diverticulum of bladder
    Urinary bladder stone
    EXCLUDES 2   *staghorn calculus (N20.0)*

N21.1 **Calculus in urethra**
    EXCLUDES 2   *calculus of prostate (N42.0)*

N21.8 **Other lower urinary tract calculus**

N21.9 **Calculus of lower urinary tract, unspecified**
    EXCLUDES 1   *calculus of urinary tract NOS (N20.9)*

N22 *Calculus of urinary tract in diseases classified elsewhere*
    Code first underlying disease, such as:
        gout (M1A.-, M10.-)
        schistosomiasis (B65.0-B65.9)

N23 **Unspecified renal colic**

Other disorders of kidney and ureter (N25-N29)

EXCLUDES 2   *disorders of kidney and ureter with urolithiasis (N20-N23)*

✓4ᵗʰ **N25** **Disorders resulting from impaired renal tubular function**

N25.0 **Renal osteodystrophy**
    Azotemic osteodystrophy
    Phosphate-losing tubular disorders
    Renal rickets
    Renal short stature
    EXCLUDES 2   *metabolic disorders classifiable to E70-E88*
    DEF: Various bone diseases occurring when kidney function is impaired or fails. Abnormal levels of phosphorous and calcium can lead to osteomalacia, osteoporosis, or osteosclerosis.

N25.1 **Nephrogenic diabetes insipidus** CC HCC
    EXCLUDES 1   *diabetes insipidus NOS (E23.2)*
    DEF: Type of diabetes due to the inability of renal tubules to reabsorb water back into the body. It is not responsive to vasopressin (antidiuretic hormone) and it is characterized by excessive thirst and excessive urine production. It may develop into chronic renal insufficiency.

✓5ᵗʰ **N25.8** **Other disorders resulting from impaired renal tubular function**

N25.81 **Secondary hyperparathyroidism of renal origin** CC HCC
    EXCLUDES 1   *secondary hyperparathyroidism, non-renal (E21.1)*
    EXCLUDES 2   *metabolic disorders classifiable to E70-E88*
    DEF: Parathyroid dysfunction caused by chronic renal failure. Phosphate clearance and vitamin D production is impaired resulting in lowered calcium blood levels and an excessive production of parathyroid hormone.

N25.89 **Other disorders resulting from impaired renal tubular function**
    Hypokalemic nephropathy
    Lightwood-Albright syndrome
    Renal tubular acidosis NOS

N25.9 **Disorder resulting from impaired renal tubular function, unspecified**

✓4ᵗʰ **N26** **Unspecified contracted kidney**
    EXCLUDES 1   *contracted kidney due to hypertension (I12.-)*
        diffuse sclerosing glomerulonephritis (N05.8.-)
        hypertensive nephrosclerosis (arteriolar) (arteriosclerotic) (I12.-)
        small kidney of unknown cause (N27.-)

N26.1 **Atrophy of kidney (terminal)**
N26.2 **Page kidney**
N26.9 **Renal sclerosis, unspecified**

✓4ᵗʰ **N27** **Small kidney of unknown cause**
    INCLUDES   oligonephronia

N27.0 **Small kidney, unilateral**
N27.1 **Small kidney, bilateral**
N27.9 **Small kidney, unspecified**

✓4ᵗʰ **N28** **Other disorders of kidney and ureter, not elsewhere classified**

N28.0 **Ischemia and infarction of kidney** CC HCC
    Renal artery embolism
    Renal artery obstruction
    Renal artery occlusion
    Renal artery thrombosis
    Renal infarct
    EXCLUDES 1   *atherosclerosis of renal artery (extrarenal part) (I70.1)*
        congenital stenosis of renal artery (Q27.1)
        Goldblatt's kidney (I70.1)

N28.1 **Cyst of kidney, acquired**
    Cyst (multiple) (solitary) of kidney (acquired)
    EXCLUDES 1   *cystic kidney disease (congenital) (Q61.-)*

✓5ᵗʰ **N28.8** **Other specified disorders of kidney and ureter**
    EXCLUDES 1   *hydroureter (N13.4)*
        ureteric stricture with hydronephrosis (N13.1)
        ureteric stricture without hydronephrosis (N13.5)

N28.81 **Hypertrophy of kidney**
N28.82 **Megaloureter**
N28.83 **Nephroptosis**
N28.84 **Pyelitis cystica** CC H6
N28.85 **Pyeloureteritis cystica** CC H6
N28.86 **Ureteritis cystica** CC H6

✔ Additional Character Required   ✓x7ᵗʰ Placeholder   Questionable PDx   Manifestation   Unspecified Dx   UPD Unacceptable PDx   H1-H14 HAC   HCC CMS-HCC Dx   HIV HIV Dx

ICD-10-CM 2022   851

Chapter 14. Diseases of the Genitourinary System

N18.3–N28.86

N28.89   Other specified disorders of kidney and ureter

N28.9   Disorder of kidney and ureter, unspecified
Nephropathy NOS
Renal disease (acute) NOS
Renal insufficiency (acute)
EXCLUDES 1   *chronic renal insufficiency (N18.9)*
unspecified nephritic syndrome (N05.-)
AHA: 2016,1Q,13

N29   Other disorders of kidney and ureter in diseases classified elsewhere
Code first underlying disease, such as:
amyloidosis (E85.-)
nephrocalcinosis (E83.5)
schistosomiasis (B65.0-B65.9)
EXCLUDES 1   *disorders of kidney and ureter in:*
cystinosis (E72.0)
gonorrhea (A54.21)
syphilis (A52.75)
tuberculosis (A18.11)

Other diseases of the urinary system (N30-N39)

EXCLUDES 1   *urinary infection (complicating):*
abortion or ectopic or molar pregnancy (O00-O07, O08.8)
pregnancy, childbirth and the puerperium (O23.-, O75.3, O86.2-)
EXCLUDES 2   ►*urinary infection (complicating):*◄
►*abortion or ectopic or molar pregnancy (O00-O07, O08.8)*◄
►*pregnancy, childbirth and the puerperium (O23.-, O75.3, O86.2-)*◄

N30   Cystitis
Use additional code to identify infectious agent (B95-B97)
EXCLUDES 1   *prostatocystitis (N41.3)*
AHA: 2017,1Q,6
DEF: Inflammation of the urinary bladder. Symptoms include dysuria, frequency of urination, urgency, and hematuria.

N30.0   Acute cystitis
EXCLUDES 1   *irradiation cystitis (N30.4-)*
trigonitis (N30.3-)
N30.00   Acute cystitis without hematuria   CC H6
N30.01   Acute cystitis with hematuria   CC H6

N30.1   Interstitial cystitis (chronic)
N30.10   Interstitial cystitis (chronic) without hematuria
N30.11   Interstitial cystitis (chronic) with hematuria

N30.2   Other chronic cystitis
N30.20   Other chronic cystitis without hematuria
N30.21   Other chronic cystitis with hematuria

N30.3   Trigonitis
Urethrotrigonitis
N30.30   Trigonitis without hematuria
N30.31   Trigonitis with hematuria

N30.4   Irradiation cystitis
N30.40   Irradiation cystitis without hematuria   CC
N30.41   Irradiation cystitis with hematuria   CC

N30.8   Other cystitis
Abscess of bladder
N30.80   Other cystitis without hematuria
N30.81   Other cystitis with hematuria

N30.9   Cystitis, unspecified
N30.90   Cystitis, unspecified without hematuria
N30.91   Cystitis, unspecified with hematuria

N31   Neuromuscular dysfunction of bladder, not elsewhere classified
Use additional code to identify any associated urinary incontinence (N39.3-N39.4-)
EXCLUDES 1   *cord bladder NOS (G95.89)*
neurogenic bladder due to cauda equina syndrome (G83.4)
neuromuscular dysfunction due to spinal cord lesion (G95.89)
N31.0   Uninhibited neuropathic bladder, not elsewhere classified
N31.1   Reflex neuropathic bladder, not elsewhere classified
N31.2   Flaccid neuropathic bladder, not elsewhere classified
Atonic (motor) (sensory) neuropathic bladder
Autonomous neuropathic bladder
Nonreflex neuropathic bladder
N31.8   Other neuromuscular dysfunction of bladder
N31.9   Neuromuscular dysfunction of bladder, unspecified
Neurogenic bladder dysfunction NOS

N32   Other disorders of bladder
EXCLUDES 2   *calculus of bladder (N21.0)*
cystocele (N81.1-)
hernia or prolapse of bladder, female (N81.1-)

N32.0   Bladder-neck obstruction
Bladder-neck stenosis (acquired)
EXCLUDES 1   *congenital bladder-neck obstruction (Q64.3-)*
DEF: Bladder outlet and vesicourethral obstruction that occurs as a consequence of benign prostatic hypertrophy or prostatic cancer. It may also occur in either sex due to strictures, radiation, cystoscopy, catheterization, injury, infection, blood clots, bladder cancer, impaction, or other disease that compresses the bladder neck.

N32.1   Vesicointestinal fistula   CC
Vesicorectal fistula

N32.2   Vesical fistula, not elsewhere classified   CC
EXCLUDES 1   *fistula between bladder and female genital tract (N82.0-N82.1)*

N32.3   Diverticulum of bladder
EXCLUDES 1   *congenital diverticulum of bladder (Q64.6)*
diverticulitis of bladder (N30.8-)

N32.8   Other specified disorders of bladder
N32.81   Overactive bladder
Detrusor muscle hyperactivity
EXCLUDES 1   *frequent urination due to specified bladder condition — code to condition*
DEF: Sudden involuntary contractions of the muscular wall of the bladder that results in a sudden, strong urge to urinate.
N32.89   Other specified disorders of bladder
Bladder hemorrhage
Bladder hypertrophy
Calcified bladder
Contracted bladder

N32.9   Bladder disorder, unspecified

N33   Bladder disorders in diseases classified elsewhere
Code first underlying disease, such as:
schistosomiasis (B65.0-B65.9)
EXCLUDES 1   *bladder disorder in syphilis (A52.76)*
bladder disorder in tuberculosis (A18.12)
candidal cystitis (B37.41)
chlamydial cystitis (A56.01)
cystitis in gonorrhea (A54.01)
cystitis in neurogenic bladder (N31.-)
diphtheritic cystitis (A36.85)
neurogenic bladder (N31.-)
syphilitic cystitis (A52.76)
trichomonal cystitis (A59.03)

N34   Urethritis and urethral syndrome
Use additional code (B95-B97), to identify infectious agent
EXCLUDES 2   *Reiter's disease (M02.3-)*
urethritis in diseases with a predominantly sexual mode of transmission (A50-A64)
urethrotrigonitis (N30.3-)
AHA: 2017,1Q,6

N34.0   Urethral abscess   CC H6
Abscess (of) Cowper's gland
Abscess (of) Littré's gland
Abscess (of) urethral (gland)
Periurethral abscess
EXCLUDES 1   *urethral caruncle (N36.2)*

N34.1   Nonspecific urethritis
Nongonococcal urethritis
Nonvenereal urethritis

N34.2   Other urethritis
Meatitis, urethral
Postmenopausal urethritis
Ulcer of urethra (meatus)
Urethritis NOS

N34.3   Urethral syndrome, unspecified

N Newborn: 0   P Pediatric: 0-17   M Maternity: 9-64   A Adult: 15-124   MCC Major Complication/Comorbidity   CC Complication/Comorbidity   SW Severe Wound Dx

852

ICD-10-CM 2022

☑4ᵗʰ **N35**   **Urethral stricture**
> *EXCLUDES 1*   congenital urethral stricture (Q64.3-)
>   postprocedural urethral stricture (N99.1-)

AHA: 2018,4Q,21-22

☑5ᵗʰ **N35.0**   **Post-traumatic urethral stricture**
> Urethral stricture due to injury
> *EXCLUDES 1*   postprocedural urethral stricture (N99.1-)

     ☑6ᵗʰ **N35.01**   **Post-traumatic urethral stricture, male**

         N35.010   **Post-traumatic urethral stricture, male, meatal** ♂

         N35.011   **Post-traumatic bulbous urethral stricture** ♂

         N35.012   **Post-traumatic membranous urethral stricture** ♂

         N35.013   **Post-traumatic anterior urethral stricture** ♂

         N35.014   **Post-traumatic urethral stricture, male, unspecified** ♂

         N35.016   **Post-traumatic urethral stricture, male, overlapping sites** ♂

     ☑6ᵗʰ **N35.02**   **Post-traumatic urethral stricture, female**

         N35.021   **Urethral stricture due to childbirth** ♀

         N35.028   **Other post-traumatic urethral stricture, female** ♀

☑5ᵗʰ **N35.1**   **Postinfective urethral stricture, not elsewhere classified**
> *EXCLUDES 1*   gonococcal urethral stricture (A54.01)
>   syphilitic urethral stricture (A52.76)
>   urethral stricture associated with schistosomiasis (B65.-, N29)

     ☑6ᵗʰ **N35.11**   **Postinfective urethral stricture, not elsewhere classified, male**

         N35.111   **Postinfective urethral stricture, not elsewhere classified, male, meatal** ♂

         N35.112   **Postinfective bulbous urethral stricture, not elsewhere classified, male** ♂

         N35.113   **Postinfective membranous urethral stricture, not elsewhere classified, male** ♂

         N35.114   **Postinfective anterior urethral stricture, not elsewhere classified, male** ♂

         N35.116   **Postinfective urethral stricture, not elsewhere classified, male, overlapping sites** ♂

         N35.119   **Postinfective urethral stricture, not elsewhere classified, male, unspecified** ♂

     N35.12   **Postinfective urethral stricture, not elsewhere classified, female** ♀

☑5ᵗʰ **N35.8**   **Other urethral stricture**
> *EXCLUDES 1*   postprocedural urethral stricture (N99.1-)

     ☑6ᵗʰ **N35.81**   **Other urethral stricture, male**

         N35.811   **Other urethral stricture, male, meatal** ♂

         N35.812   **Other urethral bulbous stricture, male** ♂

         N35.813   **Other membranous urethral stricture, male** ♂

         N35.814   **Other anterior urethral stricture, male** ♂

         N35.816   **Other urethral stricture, male, overlapping sites** ♂

         N35.819   **Other urethral stricture, male, unspecified site** ♂

     N35.82   **Other urethral stricture, female** ♀

☑5ᵗʰ **N35.9**   **Urethral stricture, unspecified**

     ☑6ᵗʰ **N35.91**   **Urethral stricture, unspecified, male**

         N35.911   **Unspecified urethral stricture, male, meatal** ♂

         N35.912   **Unspecified bulbous urethral stricture, male** ♂

         N35.913   **Unspecified membranous urethral stricture, male** ♂

         N35.914   **Unspecified anterior urethral stricture, male** ♂

         N35.916   **Unspecified urethral stricture, male, overlapping sites** ♂

         N35.919   **Unspecified urethral stricture, male, unspecified site** ♂
> Pinhole meatus NOS
> Urethral stricture NOS

     N35.92   **Unspecified urethral stricture, female** ♀

☑4ᵗʰ **N36**   **Other disorders of urethra**

     N36.0   **Urethral fistula**   cc
> Urethroperineal fistula
> Urethrorectal fistula
> Urinary fistula NOS
> *EXCLUDES 1*   urethroscrotal fistula (N50.89)
>   urethrovaginal fistula (N82.1)
>   urethrovesicovaginal fistula (N82.1)

     N36.1   **Urethral diverticulum**

     N36.2   **Urethral caruncle**

     ☑5ᵗʰ **N36.4**   **Urethral functional and muscular disorders**
> Use additional code to identify associated urinary stress incontinence (N39.3)

         N36.41   **Hypermobility of urethra**

         N36.42   **Intrinsic sphincter deficiency (ISD)**

         N36.43   **Combined hypermobility of urethra and intrinsic sphincter deficiency**

         N36.44   **Muscular disorders of urethra**
> Bladder sphincter dyssynergy

     N36.5   **Urethral false passage**

     N36.8   **Other specified disorders of urethra**
> *EXCLUDES 1*   congenital urethrocele (Q64.7)
>   female urethrocele (N81.0)

     N36.9   **Urethral disorder, unspecified**

N37   *Urethral disorders in diseases classified elsewhere*
> Code first underlying disease
> *EXCLUDES 1*   urethritis (in):
>   candidal infection (B37.41)
>   chlamydial (A56.01)
>   gonorrhea (A54.01)
>   syphilis (A52.76)
>   trichomonal infection (A59.03)
>   tuberculosis (A18.13)

☑4ᵗʰ **N39**   **Other disorders of urinary system**
> *EXCLUDES 2*   hematuria NOS (R31.-)
>   recurrent or persistent hematuria (N02.-)
>   recurrent or persistent hematuria with specified morphological lesion (N02.-)
>   proteinuria NOS (R80.-)

     N39.0   **Urinary tract infection, site not specified**   cc H6
> Use additional code (B95-B97), to identify infectious agent
> *EXCLUDES 1*   candidiasis of urinary tract (B37.4-)
>   neonatal urinary tract infection (P39.3)
>   pyuria (R82.81)
>   urinary tract infection of specified site, such as:
>   cystitis (N30.-)
>   urethritis (N34.-)

       AHA: 2019,3Q,17; 2018,2Q,21,22; 2018,1Q,16; 2017,1Q,6; 2012,4Q,94

     N39.3   **Stress incontinence (female) (male)**
> Code also any associated overactive bladder (N32.81)
> *EXCLUDES 1*   mixed incontinence (N39.46)

     ☑5ᵗʰ **N39.4**   **Other specified urinary incontinence**
> Code also any associated overactive bladder (N32.81)
> *EXCLUDES 1*   enuresis NOS (R32)
>   functional urinary incontinence (R39.81)
>   urinary incontinence associated with cognitive impairment (R39.81)
>   urinary incontinence NOS (R32)
>   urinary incontinence of nonorganic origin (F98.0)

         N39.41   **Urge incontinence**
> *EXCLUDES 1*   mixed incontinence (N39.46)

         N39.42   **Incontinence without sensory awareness**
> Insensible (urinary) incontinence

         N39.43   **Post-void dribbling**

         N39.44   **Nocturnal enuresis**
> *EXCLUDES 2*   ►nocturnal polyuria (R35.81)◄

         N39.45   **Continuous leakage**

☑ Additional Character Required   ☑x7ᵗʰ Placeholder   Questionable PDx   Manifestation   Unspecified Dx   UPD Unacceptable PDx   H1 - H14 HAC   HCC CMS-HCC Dx   HIV HIV Dx

ICD-10-CM 2022   853

N39.46 **Mixed incontinence**
Urge and stress incontinence

✓6th **N39.49** **Other specified urinary incontinence**
AHA: 2016,4Q,44

N39.490 **Overflow incontinence**
N39.491 **Coital incontinence**
N39.492 **Postural (urinary) incontinence**
N39.498 **Other specified urinary incontinence**
Reflex incontinence
Total incontinence

N39.8 **Other specified disorders of urinary system**
N39.9 **Disorder of urinary system, unspecified**

Diseases of male genital organs (N40-N53)

✓4th **N4Ø** **Benign prostatic hyperplasia**
[INCLUDES] adenofibromatous hypertrophy of prostate
benign hypertrophy of the prostate
benign prostatic hypertrophy
BPH
enlarged prostate
nodular prostate
polyp of prostate
[EXCLUDES 1] benign neoplasms of prostate (adenoma, benign)
(fibroadenoma) (fibroma) (myoma) (D29.1)
[EXCLUDES 2] malignant neoplasm of prostate (C61)
DEF: Enlargement of the prostate gland due to an abnormal proliferation of fibrostromal tissue in the paraurethral glands. This condition causes impingement of the urethra resulting in obstructed urinary flow.

N4Ø.Ø **Benign prostatic hyperplasia** without lower urinary tract symptoms   A ♂
Enlarged prostate NOS
Enlarged prostate without LUTS

N4Ø.1 **Benign prostatic hyperplasia** with lower urinary tract symptoms   A ♂
Enlarged prostate with LUTS
Use additional code for associated symptoms, when specified:
incomplete bladder emptying (R39.14)
nocturia (R35.1)
straining on urination (R39.16)
urinary frequency (R35.Ø)
urinary hesitancy (R39.11)
urinary incontinence (N39.4-)
urinary obstruction (N13.8)
urinary retention (R33.8)
urinary urgency (R39.15)
weak urinary stream (R39.12)
AHA: 2018,4Q,55

N4Ø.2 **Nodular prostate** without lower urinary tract symptoms   A ♂
Nodular prostate without LUTS

N4Ø.3 **Nodular prostate** with lower urinary tract symptoms   A ♂
Use additional code for associated symptoms, when specified:
incomplete bladder emptying (R39.14)
nocturia (R35.1)
straining on urination (R39.16)
urinary frequency (R35.Ø)
urinary hesitancy (R39.11)
urinary incontinence (N39.4-)
urinary obstruction (N13.8)
urinary retention (R33.8)
urinary urgency (R39.15)
weak urinary stream (R39.12)

✓4th **N41** **Inflammatory diseases of prostate**
Use additional code (B95-B97), to identify infectious agent
N41.Ø **Acute prostatitis**   CC A ♂
N41.1 **Chronic prostatitis**   A ♂
N41.2 **Abscess of prostate**   CC A ♂
N41.3 **Prostatocystitis**   A ♂
N41.4 **Granulomatous prostatitis**   A ♂
N41.8 **Other inflammatory diseases of prostate**   A ♂
N41.9 **Inflammatory disease of prostate, unspecified**   A ♂
Prostatitis NOS

✓4th **N42** **Other and unspecified disorders of prostate**
N42.Ø **Calculus of prostate**   A ♂
Prostatic stone
DEF: Formation of a small, solid stone often composed of calcium carbonate or calcium phosphate in the prostate gland.

N42.1 **Congestion and hemorrhage of prostate**   A ♂
[EXCLUDES 1] enlarged prostate (N4Ø.-)
hematuria (R31.-)
hyperplasia of prostate (N4Ø.-)
inflammatory diseases of prostate (N41.-)

✓5th **N42.3** **Dysplasia of prostate**
AHA: 2016,4Q,44
N42.30 **Unspecified dysplasia of prostate**   ♂
N42.31 **Prostatic intraepithelial neoplasia**   ♂
PIN
Prostatic intraepithelial neoplasia I (PIN I)
Prostatic intraepithelial neoplasia II (PIN II)
[EXCLUDES 1] prostatic intraepithelial neoplasia III (PIN III) (DØ7.5)
DEF: Abnormality of shape and size of the intraepithelial tissues of the prostate. It is a premalignant condition characterized by stalks and absence of a basilar cell layer.
N42.32 **Atypical small acinar proliferation of prostate**   ♂
N42.39 **Other dysplasia of prostate**   ♂

✓5th **N42.8** **Other specified disorders of prostate**
N42.81 **Prostatodynia syndrome**   A ♂
Painful prostate syndrome
N42.82 **Prostatosis syndrome**   A ♂
N42.83 **Cyst of prostate**   A ♂
N42.89 **Other specified disorders of prostate**   A ♂
N42.9 **Disorder of prostate, unspecified**   A ♂

✓4th **N43** **Hydrocele and spermatocele**
[INCLUDES] hydrocele of spermatic cord, testis or tunica vaginalis
[EXCLUDES 1] congenital hydrocele (P83.5)
DEF: Hydrocele: Serous fluid that collects in the tunica vaginalis of the scrotum along the spermatic cord in males.
N43.Ø **Encysted hydrocele**   ♂
N43.1 **Infected hydrocele**   CC ♂
Use additional code (B95-B97), to identify infectious agent
N43.2 **Other hydrocele**   ♂

Hydrocele

Normal | Noncommunicating hydrocele | Communicating hydrocele | Hydrocele of the cord

Testicle
Scrotum

N43.3 **Hydrocele, unspecified**   ♂
✓5th **N43.4** **Spermatocele of epididymis**
Spermatic cyst
DEF: Spermatocele: Noncancerous accumulation of fluid and dead sperm cells normally located at the head of the epididymis that exhibits itself as a hard, smooth scrotal mass and do not normally require treatment unless they become enlarged or cause pain.
N43.40 **Spermatocele of epididymis, unspecified**   ♂
N43.41 **Spermatocele of epididymis, single**   ♂
N43.42 **Spermatocele of epididymis, multiple**   ♂

✓4th **N44** **Noninflammatory disorders of testis**
✓5th **N44.Ø** **Torsion of testis**
N44.00 **Torsion of testis, unspecified**   CC ♂
N44.01 **Extravaginal torsion of spermatic cord**   CC ♂
DEF: Torsion of the spermatic cord just below the tunica vaginalis attachments.

    N44.02   Intravaginal **torsion of spermatic cord**   cc ♂
          Torsion of spermatic cord NOS

    N44.03   **Torsion of** appendix testis   cc ♂

    N44.04   **Torsion of** appendix epididymis   cc ♂

  N44.1   **Cyst of tunica albuginea testis**   ♂

  N44.2   **Benign cyst of testis**   ♂

  N44.8   **Other noninflammatory disorders of the testis**   ♂

✓4ᵗʰ N45   Orchitis and epididymitis

     Use additional code (B95-B97), to identify infectious agent

  N45.1   **Epididymitis**   ♂

  N45.2   **Orchitis**   ♂

  N45.3   **Epididymo-orchitis**   ♂

  N45.4   **Abscess of epididymis or testis**   cc ♂

✓4ᵗʰ N46   Male infertility

     EXCLUDES 1   vasectomy status (Z98.52)

  ✓5ᵗʰ **N46.0**   **Azoospermia**

       Absolute male infertility
       Male infertility due to germinal (cell) aplasia
       Male infertility due to spermatogenic arrest (complete)
       DEF: Failure of the development of sperm or the absence of sperm in semen.

    N46.01   Organic **azoospermia**   A ♂
         Azoospermia NOS

    ✓6ᵗʰ **N46.02**   **Azoospermia due to** extratesticular causes

         Code also associated cause

        N46.021   **Azoospermia due to** drug
               therapy   A ♂

        N46.022   **Azoospermia due to** infection   A ♂

        N46.023   **Azoospermia due to** obstruction of
               efferent ducts   A ♂

        N46.024   **Azoospermia due to** radiation   A ♂

        N46.025   **Azoospermia due to** systemic
               disease   A ♂

        N46.029   **Azoospermia due to other** extratesticular
               causes   A ♂

  ✓5ᵗʰ **N46.1**   **Oligospermia**

       Male infertility due to germinal cell desquamation
       Male infertility due to hypospermatogenesis
       Male infertility due to incomplete spermatogenic arrest
       DEF: Insufficient production of sperm in semen.

    N46.11   Organic **oligospermia**   A ♂
         Oligospermia NOS

    ✓6ᵗʰ **N46.12**   **Oligospermia due to** extratesticular causes

         Code also associated cause

        N46.121   **Oligospermia due to** drug
               therapy   A ♂

        N46.122   **Oligospermia due to** infection   A ♂

        N46.123   **Oligospermia due to** obstruction of
               efferent ducts   A ♂

        N46.124   **Oligospermia due to** radiation   A ♂

        N46.125   **Oligospermia due to** systemic
               disease   A ♂

        N46.129   **Oligospermia due to other extratesticular**
               causes   A ♂

  N46.8   **Other male infertility**   A ♂

  N46.9   **Male infertility, unspecified**   A ♂

✓4ᵗʰ N47   Disorders of prepuce

  N47.0   **Adherent prepuce, newborn**   N ♂

  N47.1   **Phimosis**   ♂
       DEF: Condition in which the foreskin is contracted and cannot be drawn back behind the glans penis.

  N47.2   **Paraphimosis**   ♂

  N47.3   **Deficient foreskin**   ♂

  N47.4   **Benign cyst of prepuce**   ♂

  N47.5   **Adhesions of prepuce and glans penis**   ♂

  N47.6   **Balanoposthitis**
       Use additional code (B95-B97), to identify infectious agent
       EXCLUDES 1   balanitis (N48.1)

  N47.7   **Other inflammatory diseases of prepuce**   ♂
       Use additional code (B95-B97), to identify infectious agent

  N47.8   **Other disorders of prepuce**   ♂

✓4ᵗʰ N48   Other disorders of penis

  N48.0   **Leukoplakia of penis**   ♂
       Balanitis xerotica obliterans
       Kraurosis of penis
       Lichen sclerosus of external male genital organs
       EXCLUDES 1   carcinoma in situ of penis (D07.4)

  N48.1   **Balanitis**   ♂
       Use additional code (B95-B97), to identify infectious agent
       EXCLUDES 1   amebic balanitis (A06.8)
              balanitis xerotica obliterans (N48.0)
              candidal balanitis (B37.42)
              gonococcal balanitis (A54.23)
              herpesviral [herpes simplex] balanitis (A60.01)
       DEF: Inflammation of the glans penis, most often affecting uncircumcised males.

  ✓5ᵗʰ **N48.2**   **Other inflammatory disorders of penis**
       Use additional code (B95-B97), to identify infectious agent
       EXCLUDES 1   balanitis (N48.1)
              balanitis xerotica obliterans (N48.0)
              balanoposthitis (N47.6)

    N48.21   **Abscess of corpus cavernosum and penis**   ♂

    N48.22   **Cellulitis of corpus cavernosum and penis**   ♂

    N48.29   **Other inflammatory disorders of penis**   ♂

  ✓6ᵗʰ **N48.3**   **Priapism**
       Painful erection
       Code first underlying cause

    N48.30   **Priapism, unspecified**   cc ♂

    N48.31   **Priapism** due to trauma   cc ♂

    N48.32   *Priapism due to disease classified elsewhere*   cc ♂

    N48.33   **Priapism,** drug-induced   cc ♂

    N48.39   **Other priapism**   cc ♂

  N48.5   **Ulcer of penis**   ♂

  N48.6   **Induration penis plastica**   ♂
       Peyronie's disease
       Plastic induration of penis

  ✓5ᵗʰ **N48.8**   **Other specified disorders of penis**

    N48.81   **Thrombosis of superficial vein of penis**   ♂

    N48.82   **Acquired torsion of penis**   ♂
         Acquired torsion of penis NOS
         EXCLUDES 1   congenital torsion of penis (Q55.63)

    N48.83   **Acquired buried penis**   ♂
         EXCLUDES 1   congenital hidden penis (Q55.64)

    N48.89   **Other specified disorders of penis**   ♂

  N48.9   **Disorder of penis, unspecified**   ♂

✓4ᵗʰ N49   Inflammatory disorders of male genital organs, not elsewhere classified

     Use additional code (B95-B97), to identify infectious agent
     EXCLUDES 1   inflammation of penis (N48.1, N48.2-)
             orchitis and epididymitis (N45.-)

  N49.0   **Inflammatory disorders of** seminal vesicle   ♂
       Vesiculitis NOS

  N49.1   **Inflammatory disorders of** spermatic cord, tunica vaginalis and vas deferens   ♂
       Vasitis

  N49.2   **Inflammatory disorders of** scrotum   ♂

  N49.3   Fournier gangrene   ♂
       AHA: 2020, 2Q, 18

  N49.8   **Inflammatory disorders of other specified male genital organs**   ♂
       Inflammation of multiple sites in male genital organs

  N49.9   **Inflammatory disorder of unspecified male genital organ**   ♂
       Abscess of unspecified male genital organ
       Boil of unspecified male genital organ
       Carbuncle of unspecified male genital organ
       Cellulitis of unspecified male genital organ

✓4ᵗʰ N50   Other and unspecified disorders of male genital organs

     EXCLUDES 2   torsion of testis (N44.0-)

  N50.0   **Atrophy of testis**   ♂

  N50.1   **Vascular disorders of male genital organs**   ♂
       Hematocele, NOS, of male genital organs
       Hemorrhage of male genital organs
       Thrombosis of male genital organs

  N50.3   **Cyst of epididymis**   ♂

✓ Additional Character Required   ✓x7ᵗʰ Placeholder   Questionable PDx   Manifestation   Unspecified Dx   UPD Unacceptable PDx   H1-H14 HAC   HCC CMS-HCC Dx   HIV HIV Dx

ICD-10-CM 2022   855

✓5th **N50.8 Other specified disorders of male genital organs**
> AHA: 2016,4Q,45

  ✓6th **N50.81 Testicular** pain

    N50.811 Right testicular pain ♂

    N50.812 Left testicular pain ♂

    N50.819 Testicular pain, unspecified ♂

  N50.82 Scrotal pain ♂

  N50.89 Other specified disorders of the male genital organs ♂

> Atrophy of scrotum, seminal vesicle, spermatic cord, tunica vaginalis and vas deferens
> Chylocele, tunica vaginalis (nonfilarial) NOS
> Edema of scrotum, seminal vesicle, spermatic cord, tunica vaginalis and vas deferens
> Hypertrophy of scrotum, seminal vesicle, spermatic cord, tunica vaginalis and vas deferens
> Stricture of spermatic cord, tunica vaginalis, and vas deferens
> Ulcer of scrotum, seminal vesicle, spermatic cord, testis, tunica vaginalis and vas deferens
> Urethroscrotal fistula

N50.9 Disorder of male genital organs, unspecified ♂

N51 Disorders of male genital organs in diseases classified elsewhere ♂

> Code first underlying disease, such as:
> filariasis (B74.0-B74.9)

  EXCLUDES 1 *amebic balanitis (A06.8)*
> *candidal balanitis (B37.42)*
> *gonococcal balanitis (A54.23)*
> *gonococcal prostatitis (A54.22)*
> *herpesviral [herpes simplex] balanitis (A60.01)*
> *trichomonal prostatitis (A59.02)*
> *tuberculous prostatitis (A18.14)*

✓4th **N52 Male erectile dysfunction**

  EXCLUDES 1 *psychogenic impotence (F52.21)*

  ✓5th **N52.0 Vasculogenic erectile dysfunction**

    N52.01 Erectile dysfunction due to arterial insufficiency A ♂

    N52.02 Corporo-venous occlusive erectile dysfunction A ♂

    N52.03 Combined arterial insufficiency and corporo-venous occlusive erectile dysfunction A ♂

  N52.1 Erectile dysfunction due to diseases classified elsewhere A ♂

> Code first underlying disease

  N52.2 Drug-induced erectile dysfunction A ♂

  ✓5th **N52.3 Postprocedural erectile dysfunction**

> AHA: 2016,4Q,45

    N52.31 Erectile dysfunction following radical prostatectomy A ♂

    N52.32 Erectile dysfunction following radical cystectomy A ♂

    N52.33 Erectile dysfunction following urethral surgery A ♂

    N52.34 Erectile dysfunction following simple prostatectomy A ♂

    N52.35 Erectile dysfunction following radiation therapy A ♂

    N52.36 Erectile dysfunction following interstitial seed therapy A ♂

    N52.37 Erectile dysfunction following prostate ablative therapy A ♂

> Erectile dysfunction following cryotherapy
> Erectile dysfunction following other prostate ablative therapies
> Erectile dysfunction following ultrasound ablative therapies

    N52.39 Other and unspecified postprocedural erectile dysfunction A ♂

  N52.8 Other male erectile dysfunction A ♂

  N52.9 Male erectile dysfunction, unspecified A ♂

> Impotence NOS

✓4th **N53 Other male sexual dysfunction**

  EXCLUDES 1 *psychogenic sexual dysfunction (F52.-)*

  ✓5th **N53.1 Ejaculatory dysfunction**

    EXCLUDES 1 *premature ejaculation (F52.4)*

    N53.11 Retarded ejaculation ♂

    N53.12 Painful ejaculation ♂

    N53.13 Anejaculatory orgasm ♂

    N53.14 Retrograde ejaculation ♂

> **DEF:** Form of male sexual dysfunction in which the semen enters the bladder instead of going out through the urethra during ejaculation.

    N53.19 Other ejaculatory dysfunction ♂

> Ejaculatory dysfunction NOS

  N53.8 Other male sexual dysfunction ♂

  N53.9 Unspecified male sexual dysfunction ♂

Disorders of breast (N60-N65)

EXCLUDES 1 *disorders of breast associated with childbirth (O91-O92)*

✓4th **N60 Benign mammary dysplasia**

  INCLUDES fibrocystic mastopathy

  ✓5th **N60.0 Solitary cyst of breast**

> Cyst of breast

    N60.01 Solitary cyst of right breast

    N60.02 Solitary cyst of left breast

    N60.09 Solitary cyst of unspecified breast

  ✓5th **N60.1 Diffuse cystic mastopathy**

> Cystic breast
> Fibrocystic disease of breast

    EXCLUDES 1 *diffuse cystic mastopathy with epithelial proliferation (N60.3-)*

    N60.11 Diffuse cystic mastopathy of right breast A

    N60.12 Diffuse cystic mastopathy of left breast A

    N60.19 Diffuse cystic mastopathy of unspecified breast A

  ✓5th **N60.2 Fibroadenosis of breast**

> Adenofibrosis of breast

    EXCLUDES 2 *fibroadenoma of breast (D24.-)*

    N60.21 Fibroadenosis of right breast

    N60.22 Fibroadenosis of left breast

    N60.29 Fibroadenosis of unspecified breast

  ✓5th **N60.3 Fibrosclerosis of breast**

> Cystic mastopathy with epithelial proliferation

    N60.31 Fibrosclerosis of right breast

    N60.32 Fibrosclerosis of left breast

    N60.39 Fibrosclerosis of unspecified breast

  ✓5th **N60.4 Mammary duct ectasia**

    N60.41 Mammary duct ectasia of right breast

    N60.42 Mammary duct ectasia of left breast

    N60.49 Mammary duct ectasia of unspecified breast

  ✓5th **N60.8 Other benign mammary dysplasias**

    N60.81 Other benign mammary dysplasias of right breast

    N60.82 Other benign mammary dysplasias of left breast

    N60.89 Other benign mammary dysplasias of unspecified breast

  ✓5th **N60.9 Unspecified benign mammary dysplasia**

    N60.91 Unspecified benign mammary dysplasia of right breast

    N60.92 Unspecified benign mammary dysplasia of left breast

    N60.99 Unspecified benign mammary dysplasia of unspecified breast

✓4th **N61 Inflammatory disorders of breast**

  EXCLUDES 1 *inflammatory carcinoma of breast (C50.9)*
> *inflammatory disorder of breast associated with childbirth (O91.-)*
> *neonatal infective mastitis (P39.0)*
> *thrombophlebitis of breast [Mondor's disease] (I80.8)*

  N61.0 Mastitis without abscess

> Infective mastitis (acute) (nonpuerperal) (subacute)
> Mastitis (acute) (nonpuerperal) (subacute) NOS
> Cellulitis (acute) (nonpuerperal) (subacute) of breast NOS
> Cellulitis (acute) (nonpuerperal) (subacute) of nipple NOS

N Newborn: 0 P Pediatric: 0-17 M Maternity: 9-64 A Adult: 15-124 MCC Major Complication/Comorbidity CC Complication/Comorbidity SW Severe Wound Dx

856   ICD-10-CM 2022

N61.1 Abscess of the breast and nipple
Abscess (acute) (chronic) (nonpuerperal) of areola
Abscess (acute) (chronic) (nonpuerperal) of breast
Carbuncle of breast
Mastitis with abscess

✓5ᵗʰ **N61.2 Granulomatous mastitis**
AHA: 2020,4Q,35

     N61.20 Granulomatous mastitis, **unspecified breast**
     N61.21 Granulomatous mastitis, **right breast**
     N61.22 Granulomatous mastitis, **left breast**
     N61.23 Granulomatous mastitis, **bilateral breast**

N62 Hypertrophy of breast
Gynecomastia
Hypertrophy of breast NOS
Massive pubertal hypertrophy of breast
     EXCLUDES 1   breast engorgement of newborn (P83.4)
                 disproportion of reconstructed breast (N65.1)

✓4ᵗʰ **N63 Unspecified lump in breast**
Nodule(s) NOS in breast
AHA: 2019,4Q,12; 2017,4Q,19

     N63.0 Unspecified lump in unspecified breast
✓5ᵗʰ **N63.1** Unspecified lump in the **right breast**
     N63.10 Unspecified lump in the right breast, unspecified quadrant
     N63.11 Unspecified lump in the right breast, **upper outer quadrant**
     N63.12 Unspecified lump in the right breast, **upper inner quadrant**
     N63.13 Unspecified lump in the right breast, **lower outer quadrant**
     N63.14 Unspecified lump in the right breast, **lower inner quadrant**
     N63.15 Unspecified lump in the right breast, **overlapping quadrants**

✓5ᵗʰ **N63.2** Unspecified lump in the **left breast**
     N63.20 Unspecified lump in the left breast, unspecified quadrant
     N63.21 Unspecified lump in the left breast, **upper outer quadrant**
     N63.22 Unspecified lump in the left breast, **upper inner quadrant**
     N63.23 Unspecified lump in the left breast, **lower outer quadrant**
     N63.24 Unspecified lump in the left breast, **lower inner quadrant**
     N63.25 Unspecified lump in the left breast, **overlapping quadrants**

✓5ᵗʰ **N63.3** Unspecified lump in **axillary tail**
     N63.31 Unspecified lump in axillary tail of the **right breast**
     N63.32 Unspecified lump in axillary tail of the **left breast**

✓5ᵗʰ **N63.4** Unspecified lump in breast, **subareolar**
     N63.41 Unspecified lump in **right breast, subareolar**
     N63.42 Unspecified lump in **left breast, subareolar**

✓4ᵗʰ **N64 Other disorders of breast**
     EXCLUDES 2   mechanical complication of breast prosthesis and implant (T85.4-)

     N64.0 Fissure and fistula of nipple
     N64.1 Fat necrosis of breast   UPD
         Fat necrosis (segmental) of breast
         Code first breast necrosis due to breast graft (T85.898)
     N64.2 Atrophy of breast
     N64.3 Galactorrhea not associated with childbirth
     N64.4 Mastodynia
✓5ᵗʰ **N64.5** Other signs and symptoms in breast
         EXCLUDES 2   abnormal findings on diagnostic imaging of breast (R92.-)
     N64.51 Induration of breast
     N64.52 Nipple discharge
         EXCLUDES 1   abnormal findings in nipple discharge (R89.-)
     N64.53 Retraction of nipple
     N64.59 Other signs and symptoms in breast

✓5ᵗʰ **N64.8 Other specified disorders of breast**
     N64.81 Ptosis of breast   A
         EXCLUDES 1   ptosis of native breast in relation to reconstructed breast (N65.1)
     N64.82 Hypoplasia of breast   A
         Micromastia
         EXCLUDES 1   congenital absence of breast (Q83.0)
                 hypoplasia of native breast in relation to reconstructed breast (N65.1)
     N64.89 Other specified disorders of breast
         Galactocele
         Subinvolution of breast (postlactational)
         AHA: 2019,1Q,32; 2018,1Q,3
     N64.9 Disorder of breast, unspecified

✓4ᵗʰ **N65 Deformity and disproportion of reconstructed breast**
     N65.0 Deformity of reconstructed breast   A
         Contour irregularity in reconstructed breast
         Excess tissue in reconstructed breast
         Misshapen reconstructed breast
     N65.1 Disproportion of reconstructed breast   A
         Breast asymmetry between native breast and reconstructed breast
         Disproportion between native breast and reconstructed breast

Inflammatory diseases of female pelvic organs (N70-N77)

     EXCLUDES 1   inflammatory diseases of female pelvic organs complicating:
             abortion or ectopic or molar pregnancy (O00-O07, O08.0)
             pregnancy, childbirth and the puerperium (O23.-, O75.3, O85, O86.-)

✓4ᵗʰ **N70 Salpingitis and oophoritis**
     INCLUDES   abscess (of) fallopian tube
             abscess (of) ovary
             pyosalpinx
             salpingo-oophoritis
             tubo-ovarian abscess
             tubo-ovarian inflammatory disease
     Use additional code (B95-B97), to identify infectious agent
     EXCLUDES 1   gonococcal infection (A54.24)
             tuberculous infection (A18.17)

✓5ᵗʰ **N70.0** Acute salpingitis and oophoritis
     N70.01 Acute salpingitis   CC ♀
     N70.02 Acute oophoritis   CC ♀
     N70.03 Acute salpingitis and oophoritis   CC ♀
✓5ᵗʰ **N70.1** Chronic salpingitis and oophoritis
     Hydrosalpinx
     N70.11 Chronic salpingitis   ♀
     N70.12 Chronic oophoritis   ♀
     N70.13 Chronic salpingitis and oophoritis   ♀
✓5ᵗʰ **N70.9** Salpingitis and oophoritis, unspecified
     N70.91 Salpingitis, unspecified   ♀
     N70.92 Oophoritis, unspecified   ♀
     N70.93 Salpingitis and oophoritis, unspecified   ♀

✓4ᵗʰ **N71 Inflammatory disease of uterus, except cervix**
     INCLUDES   endo (myo) metritis
             metritis
             myometritis
             pyometra
             uterine abscess
     Use additional code (B95-B97), to identify infectious agent
     EXCLUDES 1   hyperplastic endometritis (N85.0-)
             infection of uterus following delivery (O85, O86.-)
     N71.0 Acute inflammatory disease of uterus   CC ♀
     N71.1 Chronic inflammatory disease of uterus   ♀
     N71.9 Inflammatory disease of uterus, unspecified   ♀

N72 Inflammatory disease of cervix uteri   ♀
     INCLUDES   cervicitis (with or without erosion or ectropion)
             endocervicitis (with or without erosion or ectropion)
             exocervicitis (with or without erosion or ectropion)
     Use additional code (B95-B97), to identify infectious agent
     EXCLUDES 1   erosion and ectropion of cervix without cervicitis (N86)

Chapter 14. Diseases of the Genitourinary System *(side tab)*

✓4ᵗʰ **N73 Other female pelvic inflammatory diseases**

Use additional code (B95-B97), to identify infectious agent

N73.0 Acute parametritis and pelvic cellulitis   CC ♀

Abscess of broad ligament

Abscess of parametrium

Pelvic cellulitis, female

DEF: Parametritis: Inflammation of the parametrium.

N73.1 Chronic parametritis and pelvic cellulitis   ♀

Any condition in N73.0 specified as chronic

EXCLUDES 1   *tuberculous parametritis and pelvic cellultis (A18.17)*

N73.2 Unspecified parametritis and pelvic cellulitis   ♀

Any condition in N73.0 unspecified whether acute or chronic

N73.3 Female acute pelvic peritonitis   MCC ♀

N73.4 Female chronic pelvic peritonitis   CC ♀

EXCLUDES 1   *tuberculous pelvic (female) peritonitis (A18.17)*

N73.5 Female pelvic peritonitis, unspecified   ♀

N73.6 Female pelvic peritoneal adhesions (postinfective)   ♀

EXCLUDES 2   *postprocedural pelvic peritoneal adhesions (N99.4)*

AHA: 2014,1Q,6

N73.8 Other specified female pelvic inflammatory diseases   ♀

N73.9 Female pelvic inflammatory disease, unspecified   ♀

Female pelvic infection or inflammation NOS

N74 Female pelvic inflammatory disorders in diseases classified elsewhere   ♀

Code first underlying disease

EXCLUDES 1   *chlamydial cervicitis (A56.02)*

chlamydial pelvic inflammatory disease (A56.11)

gonococcal cervicitis (A54.03)

gonococcal pelvic inflammatory disease (A54.24)

herpesviral [herpes simplex] cervicitis (A60.03)

herpesviral [herpes simplex] pelvic inflammatory disease (A60.09)

syphilitic cervicitis (A52.76)

syphilitic pelvic inflammatory disease (A52.76)

trichomonal cervicitis (A59.09)

tuberculous cervicitis (A18.16)

tuberculous pelvic inflammatory disease (A18.17)

✓4ᵗʰ **N75 Diseases of Bartholin's gland**

DEF: Bartholin's gland: Mucous-producing gland found in the vestibular bulbs on either side of the vaginal orifice and connected to the mucosal membrane at the opening by a duct.

N75.0 Cyst of Bartholin's gland   ♀

N75.1 Abscess of Bartholin's gland   CC ♀

N75.8 Other diseases of Bartholin's gland   ♀

Bartholinitis

N75.9 Disease of Bartholin's gland, unspecified   ♀

✓4ᵗʰ **N76 Other inflammation of vagina and vulva**

Use additional code (B95-B97), to identify infectious agent

EXCLUDES 2   *senile (atrophic) vaginitis (N95.2)*

vulvar vestibulitis (N94.810)

N76.0 Acute vaginitis   ♀

Acute vulvovaginitis

Vaginitis NOS

Vulvovaginitis NOS

N76.1 Subacute and chronic vaginitis   ♀

Chronic vulvovaginitis

Subacute vulvovaginitis

N76.2 Acute vulvitis   ♀

Vulvitis NOS

N76.3 Subacute and chronic vulvitis   ♀

N76.4 Abscess of vulva   CC ♀

Furuncle of vulva

N76.5 Ulceration of vagina   ♀

N76.6 Ulceration of vulva   ♀

✓5ᵗʰ **N76.8 Other specified inflammation of vagina and vulva**

N76.81 Mucositis (ulcerative) of vagina and vulva   CC ♀

Code also type of associated therapy, such as:

antineoplastic and immunosuppressive drugs (T45.1X-)

radiological procedure and radiotherapy (Y84.2)

EXCLUDES 2   *gastrointestinal mucositis (ulcerative) (K92.81)*

nasal mucositis (ulcerative) (J34.81)

oral mucositis (ulcerative) (K12.3-)

N76.89 Other specified inflammation of vagina and vulva   ♀

✓4ᵗʰ **N77 Vulvovaginal ulceration and inflammation in diseases classified elsewhere**

N77.0 Ulceration of vulva in diseases classified elsewhere   ♀

Code first underlying disease, such as:

Behçet's disease (M35.2)

EXCLUDES 1   *ulceration of vulva in gonococcal infection (A54.02)*

ulceration of vulva in herpesviral [herpes simplex] infection (A60.04)

ulceration of vulva in syphilis (A51.0)

ulceration of vulva in tuberculosis (A18.18)

N77.1 Vaginitis, vulvitis and vulvovaginitis in diseases classified elsewhere   ♀

Code first underlying disease, such as:

pinworm (B80)

EXCLUDES 1   *candidal vulvovaginitis (B37.3)*

chlamydial vulvovaginitis (A56.02)

gonococcal vulvovaginitis (A54.02)

herpesviral [herpes simplex] vulvovaginitis (A60.04)

trichomonal vulvovaginitis (A59.01)

tuberculous vulvovaginitis (A18.18)

vulvovaginitis in early syphilis (A51.0)

vulvovaginitis in late syphilis (A52.76)

Noninflammatory disorders of female genital tract (N80-N98)

✓4ᵗʰ **N80 Endometriosis**

DEF: Aberrant uterine mucosal tissue appearing in areas of the pelvic cavity outside of its normal location, lining the uterus, and inflaming surrounding tissues often resulting in infertility or spontaneous abortion.

N80.0 Endometriosis of uterus   ♀

Adenomyosis

EXCLUDES 1   *stromal endometriosis (D39.0)*

N80.1 Endometriosis of ovary   ♀

N80.2 Endometriosis of fallopian tube   ♀

N80.3 Endometriosis of pelvic peritoneum   ♀

N80.4 Endometriosis of rectovaginal septum and vagina   ♀

N80.5 Endometriosis of intestine   ♀

N80.6 Endometriosis in cutaneous scar   ♀

N80.8 Other endometriosis   ♀

Endometriosis of thorax

N80.9 Endometriosis, unspecified   ♀

Ⓝ Newborn: 0   Ⓟ Pediatric: 0-17   Ⓜ Maternity: 9-64   Ⓐ Adult: 15-124   MCC Major Complication/Comorbidity   CC Complication/Comorbidity   SW Severe Wound Dx

858   ICD-10-CM 2022

N73–N80.9 *(side tab)*

☑️4ᵗʰ **N81 Female genital prolapse**

> EXCLUDES 1   genital prolapse complicating pregnancy, labor or delivery (O34.5-)
> prolapse and hernia of ovary and fallopian tube (N83.4-)
> prolapse of vaginal vault after hysterectomy (N99.3)

Types of Pelvic Organ Prolapse

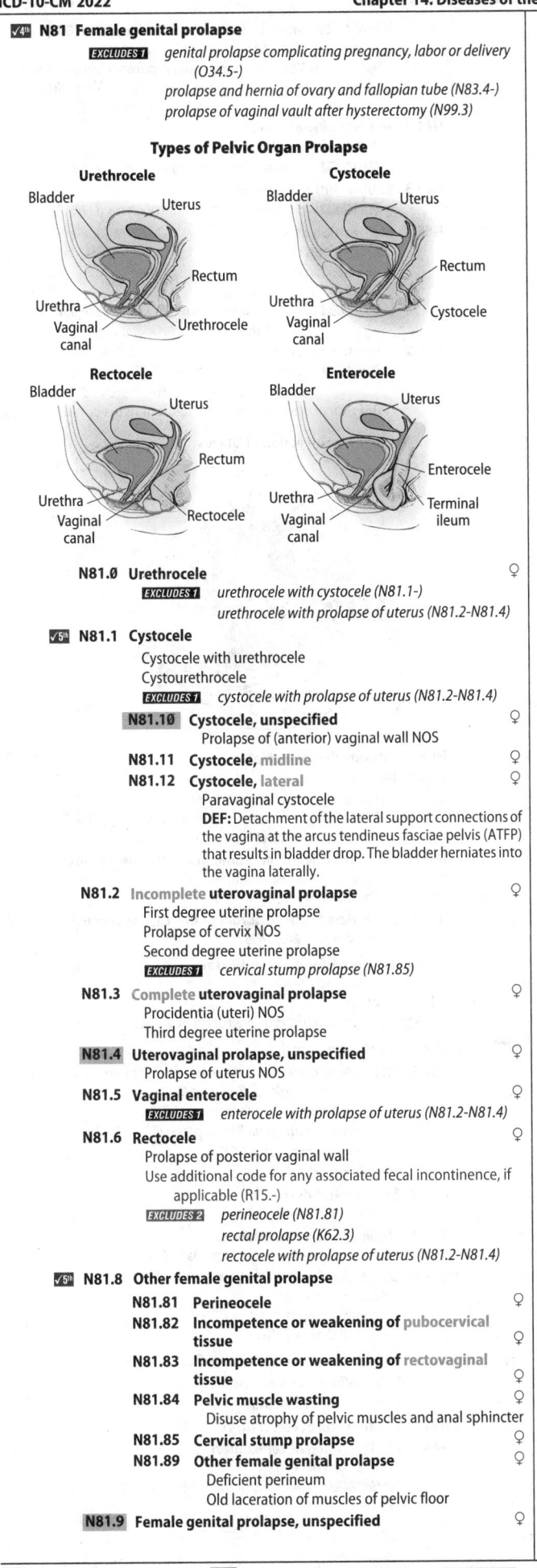

N81.0 Urethrocele ♀
> EXCLUDES 1   urethrocele with cystocele (N81.1-)
> urethrocele with prolapse of uterus (N81.2-N81.4)

☑️5ᵗʰ **N81.1 Cystocele**
Cystocele with urethrocele
Cystourethrocele
> EXCLUDES 1   cystocele with prolapse of uterus (N81.2-N81.4)

   N81.10 Cystocele, unspecified ♀
Prolapse of (anterior) vaginal wall NOS

   N81.11 Cystocele, midline ♀

   N81.12 Cystocele, lateral ♀
Paravaginal cystocele
DEF: Detachment of the lateral support connections of the vagina at the arcus tendineus fasciae pelvis (ATFP) that results in bladder drop. The bladder herniates into the vagina laterally.

N81.2 Incomplete uterovaginal prolapse ♀
First degree uterine prolapse
Prolapse of cervix NOS
Second degree uterine prolapse
> EXCLUDES 1   cervical stump prolapse (N81.85)

N81.3 Complete uterovaginal prolapse ♀
Procidentia (uteri) NOS
Third degree uterine prolapse

N81.4 Uterovaginal prolapse, unspecified ♀
Prolapse of uterus NOS

N81.5 Vaginal enterocele ♀
> EXCLUDES 1   enterocele with prolapse of uterus (N81.2-N81.4)

N81.6 Rectocele ♀
Prolapse of posterior vaginal wall
Use additional code for any associated fecal incontinence, if applicable (R15.-)
> EXCLUDES 2   perineocele (N81.81)
> rectal prolapse (K62.3)
> rectocele with prolapse of uterus (N81.2-N81.4)

☑️5ᵗʰ **N81.8 Other female genital prolapse**
   N81.81 Perineocele ♀
   N81.82 Incompetence or weakening of pubocervical tissue ♀
   N81.83 Incompetence or weakening of rectovaginal tissue ♀
   N81.84 Pelvic muscle wasting ♀
Disuse atrophy of pelvic muscles and anal sphincter
   N81.85 Cervical stump prolapse ♀
   N81.89 Other female genital prolapse ♀
Deficient perineum
Old laceration of muscles of pelvic floor

   N81.9 Female genital prolapse, unspecified ♀

☑️4ᵗʰ **N82 Fistulae involving female genital tract**
> EXCLUDES 1   vesicointestinal fistulae (N32.1)

N82.0 Vesicovaginal fistula CC SW ♀

N82.1 Other female urinary-genital tract fistulae CC ♀
Cervicovesical fistula
Ureterovaginal fistula
Urethrovaginal fistula
Uteroureteric fistula
Uterovesical fistula
AHA: 2017,3Q,3

N82.2 Fistula of vagina to small intestine CC SW ♀

N82.3 Fistula of vagina to large intestine CC SW ♀
Rectovaginal fistula

N82.4 Other female intestinal-genital tract fistulae CC SW ♀
Intestinouterine fistula

N82.5 Female genital tract-skin fistulae CC SW ♀
Uterus to abdominal wall fistula
Vaginoperineal fistula

N82.8 Other female genital tract fistulae CC ♀

N82.9 Female genital tract fistula, unspecified CC ♀

☑️4ᵗʰ **N83 Noninflammatory disorders of ovary, fallopian tube and broad ligament**
> EXCLUDES 2   hydrosalpinx (N70.1-)

AHA: 2016,4Q,46

☑️5ᵗʰ **N83.0 Follicular cyst of ovary**
Cyst of graafian follicle
Hemorrhagic follicular cyst (of ovary)
   N83.00 Follicular cyst of ovary, unspecified side ♀
   N83.01 Follicular cyst of right ovary ♀
   N83.02 Follicular cyst of left ovary ♀

☑️5ᵗʰ **N83.1 Corpus luteum cyst**
Hemorrhagic corpus luteum cyst
   N83.10 Corpus luteum cyst of ovary, unspecified side ♀
   N83.11 Corpus luteum cyst of right ovary ♀
   N83.12 Corpus luteum cyst of left ovary ♀

☑️5ᵗʰ **N83.2 Other and unspecified ovarian cysts**
> EXCLUDES 1   developmental ovarian cyst (Q50.1)
> neoplastic ovarian cyst (D27.-)
> polycystic ovarian syndrome (E28.2)
> Stein-Leventhal syndrome (E28.2)

   ☑️6ᵗʰ **N83.20 Unspecified ovarian cysts**
     N83.201 Unspecified ovarian cyst, right side ♀
     N83.202 Unspecified ovarian cyst, left side ♀
     N83.209 Unspecified ovarian cyst, unspecified side ♀
Ovarian cyst, NOS

   ☑️6ᵗʰ **N83.29 Other ovarian cysts**
Retention cyst of ovary
Simple cyst of ovary
     N83.291 Other ovarian cyst, right side ♀
     N83.292 Other ovarian cyst, left side ♀
     N83.299 Other ovarian cyst, unspecified side ♀

☑️5ᵗʰ **N83.3 Acquired atrophy of ovary and fallopian tube**
   ☑️6ᵗʰ **N83.31 Acquired atrophy of ovary**
     N83.311 Acquired atrophy of right ovary ♀
     N83.312 Acquired atrophy of left ovary ♀
     N83.319 Acquired atrophy of ovary, unspecified side ♀
Acquired atrophy of ovary, NOS

   ☑️6ᵗʰ **N83.32 Acquired atrophy of fallopian tube**
     N83.321 Acquired atrophy of right fallopian tube ♀
     N83.322 Acquired atrophy of left fallopian tube ♀
     N83.329 Acquired atrophy of fallopian tube, unspecified side ♀
Acquired atrophy of fallopian tube, NOS

   ☑️6ᵗʰ **N83.33 Acquired atrophy of ovary and fallopian tube**
     N83.331 Acquired atrophy of right ovary and fallopian tube ♀
     N83.332 Acquired atrophy of left ovary and fallopian tube ♀

☑️ Additional Character Required   ☑️x7ᵗʰ Placeholder   Questionable PDx   Manifestation   Unspecified Dx   UPD Unacceptable PDx   H1-H14 HAC   HCC CMS-HCC Dx   HIV HIV Dx

ICD-10-CM 2022   **859**

N83.339 **Acquired atrophy of ovary and fallopian tube, unspecified side** ♀
Acquired atrophy of ovary and fallopian tube, NOS

✓6ᵗʰ N83.4 **Prolapse and hernia of ovary and fallopian tube**

N83.40 **Prolapse and hernia of ovary and fallopian tube, unspecified side** ♀
Prolapse and hernia of ovary and fallopian tube, NOS

N83.41 **Prolapse and hernia of right ovary and fallopian tube** ♀

N83.42 **Prolapse and hernia of left ovary and fallopian tube** ♀

✓6ᵗʰ N83.5 **Torsion of ovary, ovarian pedicle and fallopian tube**
Torsion of accessory tube

✓6ᵗʰ N83.51 **Torsion of ovary and ovarian pedicle**

N83.511 **Torsion of right ovary and ovarian pedicle** CC ♀

N83.512 **Torsion of left ovary and ovarian pedicle** CC ♀

N83.519 **Torsion of ovary and ovarian pedicle, unspecified side** CC ♀
Torsion of ovary and ovarian pedicle, NOS

✓6ᵗʰ N83.52 **Torsion of fallopian tube**
Torsion of hydatid of Morgagni

N83.521 **Torsion of right fallopian tube** CC ♀

N83.522 **Torsion of left fallopian tube** CC ♀

N83.529 **Torsion of fallopian tube, unspecified side** CC ♀
Torsion of fallopian tube, NOS

N83.53 **Torsion of ovary, ovarian pedicle and fallopian tube** CC ♀

N83.6 **Hematosalpinx** ♀
EXCLUDES 1   *hematosalpinx (with) (in):*
hematocolpos (N89.7)
hematometra (N85.7)
tubal pregnancy (O00.1-)

N83.7 **Hematoma of broad ligament** ♀

N83.8 **Other noninflammatory disorders of ovary, fallopian tube and broad ligament** ♀
Broad ligament laceration syndrome [Allen-Masters]

N83.9 **Noninflammatory disorder of ovary, fallopian tube and broad ligament, unspecified** ♀

✓4ᵗʰ **N84 Polyp of female genital tract**
EXCLUDES 1   *adenomatous polyp (D28.-)*
placental polyp (O90.89)

N84.0 **Polyp of corpus uteri** ♀
Polyp of endometrium
Polyp of uterus NOS
EXCLUDES 1   *polypoid endometrial hyperplasia (N85.0-)*

N84.1 **Polyp of cervix uteri** ♀
Mucous polyp of cervix

N84.2 **Polyp of vagina** ♀

N84.3 **Polyp of vulva** ♀
Polyp of labia

N84.8 **Polyp of other parts of female genital tract** ♀

N84.9 **Polyp of female genital tract, unspecified** ♀

✓4ᵗʰ **N85 Other noninflammatory disorders of uterus, except cervix**
EXCLUDES 1   *endometriosis (N80.-)*
inflammatory diseases of uterus (N71.-)
noninflammatory disorders of cervix, except malposition (N86-N88)
polyp of corpus uteri (N84.0)
uterine prolapse (N81.-)

✓5ᵗʰ N85.0 **Endometrial hyperplasia**

N85.00 **Endometrial hyperplasia, unspecified** ♀
Hyperplasia (adenomatous) (cystic) (glandular) of endometrium
Hyperplastic endometritis

N85.01 **Benign endometrial hyperplasia** ♀
Endometrial hyperplasia (complex) (simple) without atypia

N85.02 **Endometrial intraepithelial neoplasia [EIN]** ♀
Endometrial hyperplasia with atypia
EXCLUDES 1   *malignant neoplasm of endometrium (with endometrial intraepithelial neoplasia [EIN]) (C54.1)*

N85.2 **Hypertrophy of uterus** ♀
Bulky or enlarged uterus
EXCLUDES 1   *puerperal hypertrophy of uterus (O90.89)*

N85.3 **Subinvolution of uterus** ♀
EXCLUDES 1   *puerperal subinvolution of uterus (O90.89)*

N85.4 **Malposition of uterus** ♀
Anteversion of uterus
Retroflexion of uterus
Retroversion of uterus
EXCLUDES 1   *malposition of uterus complicating pregnancy, labor or delivery (O34.5-, O65.5)*

N85.5 **Inversion of uterus** ♀
EXCLUDES 1   *current obstetric trauma (O71.2)*
postpartum inversion of uterus (O71.2)
DEF: Abnormality in which the uterus turns inside out.

Inversion of Uterus

Uterus

N85.6 **Intrauterine synechiae** ♀

N85.7 **Hematometra** ♀
Hematosalpinx with hematometra
EXCLUDES 1   *hematometra with hematocolpos (N89.7)*
DEF: Accumulation of blood within the uterus.

N85.8 **Other specified noninflammatory disorders of uterus** ♀
Atrophy of uterus, acquired
Fibrosis of uterus NOS

N85.9 **Noninflammatory disorder of uterus, unspecified** ♀
Disorder of uterus NOS

N86 Erosion and ectropion of cervix uteri ♀
Decubitus (trophic) ulcer of cervix
Eversion of cervix
EXCLUDES 1   *erosion and ectropion of cervix with cervicitis (N72)*

✓4ᵗʰ **N87 Dysplasia of cervix uteri**
EXCLUDES 1   *abnormal results from cervical cytologic examination without histologic confirmation (R87.61-)*
carcinoma in situ of cervix uteri (D06.-)
cervical intraepithelial neoplasia III [CIN III] (D06.-)
HGSIL of cervix (R87.613)
severe dysplasia of cervix uteri (D06.-)

N87.0 **Mild cervical dysplasia** ♀
Cervical intraepithelial neoplasia I [CIN I]

N87.1 **Moderate cervical dysplasia** ♀
Cervical intraepithelial neoplasia II [CIN II]

N87.9 **Dysplasia of cervix uteri, unspecified** ♀
Anaplasia of cervix
Cervical atypism
Cervical dysplasia NOS

✓4ᵗʰ **N88 Other noninflammatory disorders of cervix uteri**
EXCLUDES 2   *inflammatory disease of cervix (N72)*
polyp of cervix (N84.1)

N88.0 **Leukoplakia of cervix uteri** ♀

N88.1 **Old laceration of cervix uteri** ♀
Adhesions of cervix
EXCLUDES 1   *current obstetric trauma (O71.3)*

N88.2   **Stricture and stenosis of cervix uteri** ♀
> EXCLUDES 1   *stricture and stenosis of cervix uteri complicating labor (O65.5)*

N88.3   **Incompetence of cervix uteri** ♀
Investigation and management of (suspected) cervical incompetence in a nonpregnant woman
> EXCLUDES 1   *cervical incompetence complicating pregnancy (O34.3-)*

DEF: Inadequate functioning of the cervix marked by abnormal widening during pregnancy and causing premature birth or miscarriage.

N88.4   **Hypertrophic elongation of cervix uteri** ♀
N88.8   **Other specified noninflammatory disorders of cervix uteri** ♀
> EXCLUDES 1   *current obstetric trauma (O71.3)*

N88.9   **Noninflammatory disorder of cervix uteri, unspecified** ♀

✓4ᵗʰ **N89**   **Other noninflammatory disorders of vagina**
> EXCLUDES 1   *abnormal results from vaginal cytologic examination without histologic confirmation (R87.62-)*
> *carcinoma in situ of vagina (D07.2)*
> *HGSIL of vagina (R87.623)*
> *inflammation of vagina (N76.-)*
> *senile (atrophic) vaginitis (N95.2)*
> *severe dysplasia of vagina (D07.2)*
> *trichomonal leukorrhea (A59.00)*
> *vaginal intraepithelial neoplasia [VAIN], grade III (D07.2)*

N89.0   **Mild vaginal dysplasia** ♀
Vaginal intraepithelial neoplasia [VAIN], grade I

N89.1   **Moderate vaginal dysplasia** ♀
Vaginal intraepithelial neoplasia [VAIN], grade II

N89.3   **Dysplasia of vagina, unspecified** ♀
N89.4   **Leukoplakia of vagina** ♀
N89.5   **Stricture and atresia of vagina** ♀
Vaginal adhesions
Vaginal stenosis
> EXCLUDES 1   *congenital atresia or stricture (Q52.4)*
> *postprocedural adhesions of vagina (N99.2)*

N89.6   **Tight hymenal ring** ♀
Rigid hymen
Tight introitus
> EXCLUDES 1   *imperforate hymen (Q52.3)*

N89.7   **Hematocolpos** ♀
Hematocolpos with hematometra or hematosalpinx
AHA: 2016,4Q,58

N89.8   **Other specified noninflammatory disorders of vagina** ♀
Leukorrhea NOS
Old vaginal laceration
Pessary ulcer of vagina
> EXCLUDES 1   *current obstetric trauma (O70.-, O71.4, O71.7-O71.8)*
> *old laceration involving muscles of pelvic floor (N81.8)*

N89.9   **Noninflammatory disorder of vagina, unspecified** ♀

✓4ᵗʰ **N90**   **Other noninflammatory disorders of vulva and perineum**
> EXCLUDES 1   *anogenital (venereal) warts (A63.0)*
> *carcinoma in situ of vulva (D07.1)*
> *condyloma acuminatum (A63.0)*
> *current obstetric trauma (O70.-, O71.7-O71.8)*
> *inflammation of vulva (N76.-)*
> *severe dysplasia of vulva (D07.1)*
> *vulvar intraepithelial neoplasm III [VIN III] (D07.1)*

N90.0   **Mild vulvar dysplasia** ♀
Vulvar intraepithelial neoplasia [VIN], grade I

N90.1   **Moderate vulvar dysplasia** ♀
Vulvar intraepithelial neoplasia [VIN], grade II

N90.3   **Dysplasia of vulva, unspecified** ♀
N90.4   **Leukoplakia of vulva** ♀
Dystrophy of vulva
Kraurosis of vulva
Lichen sclerosus of external female genital organs

N90.5   **Atrophy of vulva** ♀
Stenosis of vulva

✓5ᵗʰ **N90.6**   **Hypertrophy of vulva**
AHA: 2016,4Q,46

N90.60   **Unspecified hypertrophy of vulva** ♀
Unspecified hypertrophy of labia

N90.61   **Childhood asymmetric labium majus enlargement** ♀
CALME

N90.69   **Other specified hypertrophy of vulva** ♀
Other specified hypertrophy of labia

N90.7   **Vulvar cyst** ♀

✓5ᵗʰ **N90.8**   **Other specified noninflammatory disorders of vulva and perineum**

✓6ᵗʰ **N90.81**   **Female genital mutilation status**
Female genital cutting status

N90.810   **Female genital mutilation status, unspecified** ♀
Female genital cutting status, unspecified
Female genital mutilation status NOS

N90.811   **Female genital mutilation Type I status** ♀
Clitorectomy status
Female genital cutting Type I status

N90.812   **Female genital mutilation Type II status** ♀
Clitorectomy with excision of labia minora status
Female genital cutting Type II status

N90.813   **Female genital mutilation Type III status** ♀
Female genital cutting Type III status
Infibulation status

N90.818   **Other female genital mutilation status** ♀
Female genital cutting Type IV status
Female genital mutilation Type IV status
Other female genital cutting status

N90.89   **Other specified noninflammatory disorders of vulva and perineum** ♀
Adhesions of vulva
Hypertrophy of clitoris

N90.9   **Noninflammatory disorder of vulva and perineum, unspecified** ♀

✓4ᵗʰ **N91**   **Absent, scanty and rare menstruation**
> EXCLUDES 1   *ovarian dysfunction (E28.-)*

N91.0   **Primary amenorrhea** ♀
N91.1   **Secondary amenorrhea** ♀
N91.2   **Amenorrhea, unspecified** ♀
N91.3   **Primary oligomenorrhea** ♀
N91.4   **Secondary oligomenorrhea** ♀
N91.5   **Oligomenorrhea, unspecified** ♀
Hypomenorrhea NOS

✓4ᵗʰ **N92**   **Excessive, frequent and irregular menstruation**
> EXCLUDES 1   *postmenopausal bleeding (N95.0)*
> *precocious puberty (menstruation) (E30.1)*

N92.0   **Excessive and frequent menstruation with regular cycle** ♀
Heavy periods NOS
Menorrhagia NOS
Polymenorrhea

N92.1   **Excessive and frequent menstruation with irregular cycle** ♀
Irregular intermenstrual bleeding
Irregular, shortened intervals between menstrual bleeding
Menometrorrhagia
Metrorrhagia

N92.2   **Excessive menstruation at puberty** P ♀
Excessive bleeding associated with onset of menstrual periods
Pubertal menorrhagia
Puberty bleeding

N92.3   **Ovulation bleeding** ♀
Regular intermenstrual bleeding

N92.4 Excessive bleeding in the premenopausal period ♀
Climacteric menorrhagia or metrorrhagia
Menopausal menorrhagia or metrorrhagia
Perimenopausal bleeding
Perimenopausal menorrhagia or metrorrhagia
Preclimacteric menorrhagia or metrorrhagia
Premenopausal menorrhagia or metrorrhagia

N92.5 Other specified irregular menstruation ♀

N92.6 Irregular menstruation, unspecified ♀
Irregular bleeding NOS
Irregular periods NOS
> EXCLUDES 1   *irregular menstruation with:*
>   *lengthened intervals or scanty bleeding*
>   *(N91.3-N91.5)*
>   *shortened intervals or excessive bleeding (N92.1)*

☑4ᵗʰ **N93 Other abnormal uterine and vaginal bleeding**
> EXCLUDES 1   *neonatal vaginal hemorrhage (P54.6)*
>   *precocious puberty (menstruation) (E3Ø.1)*
>   *pseudomenses (P54.6)*

N93.Ø Postcoital and contact bleeding ♀

N93.1 Pre-pubertal vaginal bleeding ♀
AHA: 2016,4Q,47

N93.8 Other specified abnormal uterine and vaginal bleeding ♀
Dysfunctional or functional uterine or vaginal bleeding NOS

N93.9 Abnormal uterine and vaginal bleeding, unspecified ♀

☑4ᵗʰ **N94 Pain and other conditions associated with female genital organs and menstrual cycle**

N94.Ø Mittelschmerz ♀
DEF: One-sided, lower abdominal pain occurring between menstrual periods that is associated with ovulation.

☑5ᵗʰ **N94.1 Dyspareunia**
> EXCLUDES 1   *psychogenic dyspareunia (F52.6)*
AHA: 2016,4Q,47

    N94.1Ø Unspecified dyspareunia ♀
    N94.11 Superficial (introital) dyspareunia ♀
    N94.12 Deep dyspareunia ♀
    N94.19 Other specified dyspareunia ♀

N94.2 Vaginismus ♀
> EXCLUDES 1   *psychogenic vaginismus (F52.5)*
DEF: Spontaneous contractions of the muscles surrounding the vagina, causing it to constrict or close.

N94.3 Premenstrual tension syndrome ♀
Code also associated menstrual migraine (G43.82-, G43.83-)
> EXCLUDES 1   *premenstrual dysphoric disorder (F32.81)*

N94.4 Primary dysmenorrhea ♀
N94.5 Secondary dysmenorrhea ♀
N94.6 Dysmenorrhea, unspecified ♀
> EXCLUDES 1   *psychogenic dysmenorrhea (F45.8)*

☑5ᵗʰ **N94.8 Other specified conditions associated with female genital organs and menstrual cycle**

   ☑6ᵗʰ **N94.81 Vulvodynia**
     N94.81Ø Vulvar vestibulitis ♀
     N94.818 Other vulvodynia ♀
     N94.819 Vulvodynia, unspecified ♀
      Vulvodynia NOS

   N94.89 Other specified conditions associated with female genital organs and menstrual cycle ♀
     DEF: Hydrocele: Serous fluid that collects in the canal of Nuck in females.

N94.9 Unspecified condition associated with female genital organs and menstrual cycle ♀

☑4ᵗʰ **N95 Menopausal and other perimenopausal disorders**
Menopausal and other perimenopausal disorders due to naturally occurring (age-related) menopause and perimenopause
> EXCLUDES 1   *excessive bleeding in the premenopausal period (N92.4)*
>   *menopausal and perimenopausal disorders due to artificial or premature menopause (E89.4-, E28.31-)*
>   *premature menopause (E28.31-)*
> EXCLUDES 2   *postmenopausal osteoporosis (M81.Ø-)*
>   *postmenopausal osteoporosis with current pathological fracture (M80.Ø-)*
>   *postmenopausal urethritis (N34.2)*

N95.Ø Postmenopausal bleeding ♀

N95.1 Menopausal and female climacteric states ♀
Symptoms such as flushing, sleeplessness, headache, lack of concentration, associated with natural (age-related) menopause
Use additional code for associated symptoms
> EXCLUDES 1   *asymptomatic menopausal state (Z78.Ø)*
>   *symptoms associated with artificial menopause (E89.41)*
>   *symptoms associated with premature menopause (E28.31Ø)*

N95.2 Postmenopausal atrophic vaginitis ♀
Senile (atrophic) vaginitis

N95.8 Other specified menopausal and perimenopausal disorders ♀

N95.9 Unspecified menopausal and perimenopausal disorder ♀

N96 Recurrent pregnancy loss ♀
Investigation or care in a nonpregnant woman with history of recurrent pregnancy loss
> EXCLUDES 1   *recurrent pregnancy loss with current pregnancy (O26.2-)*

☑4ᵗʰ **N97 Female infertility**
> INCLUDES   inability to achieve a pregnancy
>   sterility, female NOS
> EXCLUDES 1   *female infertility associated with:*
>   *hypopituitarism (E23.Ø)*
>   *Stein-Leventhal syndrome (E28.2)*
> EXCLUDES 2   ▸*female infertility associated with:*◂
>   ▸*hypopituitarism (E23.Ø)*◂
>   ▸*Stein-Leventhal syndrome (E28.2)*◂
>   *incompetence of cervix uteri (N88.3)*

DEF: Infertility: Inability to conceive for at least one year with regular intercourse.
DEF: Primary infertility: Infertility occurring in patients who have never conceived.
DEF: Secondary infertility: Infertility occurring in patients who have previously conceived.

N97.Ø Female infertility associated with anovulation ♀
N97.1 Female infertility of tubal origin ♀
Female infertility associated with congenital anomaly of tube
Female infertility due to tubal block
Female infertility due to tubal occlusion
Female infertility due to tubal stenosis

N97.2 Female infertility of uterine origin ♀
Female infertility associated with congenital anomaly of uterus
Female infertility due to nonimplantation of ovum

N97.8 Female infertility of other origin ♀
N97.9 Female infertility, unspecified ♀

☑4ᵗʰ **N98 Complications associated with artificial fertilization**

N98.Ø Infection associated with artificial insemination CC ♀
N98.1 Hyperstimulation of ovaries CC ♀
Hyperstimulation of ovaries NOS
Hyperstimulation of ovaries associated with induced ovulation

N98.2 Complications of attempted introduction of fertilized ovum following in vitro fertilization ♀

N98.3 Complications of attempted introduction of embryo in embryo transfer CC ♀

N98.8 Other complications associated with artificial fertilization CC ♀

N98.9 Complication associated with artificial fertilization, unspecified CC ♀

Intraoperative and postprocedural complications and disorders of genitourinary system, not elsewhere classified (N99)

☑4ᵗʰ **N99 Intraoperative and postprocedural complications and disorders of genitourinary system, not elsewhere classified**
> EXCLUDES 2   *irradiation cystitis (N3Ø.4-)*
>   *postoophorectomy osteoporosis with current pathological fracture (M8Ø.8-)*
>   *postoophorectomy osteoporosis without current pathological fracture (M81.8)*

N99.Ø Postprocedural (acute) (chronic) kidney failure
Use additional code to type of kidney disease

N Newborn: 0   P Pediatric: 0-17   M Maternity: 9-64   A Adult: 15-124   MCC Major Complication/Comorbidity   CC Complication/Comorbidity   SW Severe Wound Dx

862

ICD-10-CM 2022

✓5th **N99.1** **Postprocedural** urethral stricture
     Postcatheterization urethral stricture
   ✓6th **N99.11** **Postprocedural urethral stricture,** male
      AHA: 2016,4Q,47-48
     N99.110 **Postprocedural urethral stricture, male,** meatal ♂
     N99.111 **Postprocedural** bulbous **urethral stricture, male** ♂
     N99.112 **Postprocedural** membranous **urethral stricture, male** ♂
     N99.113 **Postprocedural** anterior bulbous **urethral stricture, male** ♂
     N99.114 **Postprocedural urethral stricture, male, unspecified** ♂
     N99.115 **Postprocedural** fossa navicularis **urethral stricture** ♂
     N99.116 **Postprocedural urethral stricture, male, overlapping** sites ♂
   N99.12 **Postprocedural urethral stricture, female** ♀
  N99.2 **Postprocedural** adhesions of vagina ♀
  N99.3 Prolapse of vaginal vault **after hysterectomy** ♀
  N99.4 **Postprocedural** pelvic peritoneal adhesions
    EXCLUDES 2   pelvic peritoneal adhesions NOS (N73.6)
          postinfective pelvic peritoneal adhesions (N73.6)
✓5th **N99.5** **Complications of stoma of urinary tract**
    EXCLUDES 2   mechanical complication of urinary catheter (T83.0-)
    AHA: 2016,4Q,48
   ✓6th **N99.51** **Complication of** cystostomy
     N99.510 **Cystostomy** hemorrhage   CC HCC
     N99.511 **Cystostomy** infection   CC HCC
     N99.512 **Cystostomy** malfunction   CC HCC
     N99.518 **Other cystostomy complication**   CC HCC
   ✓6th **N99.52** **Complication of** incontinent external stoma **of urinary tract**
     N99.520 Hemorrhage **of incontinent external stoma of urinary tract**   HCC
     N99.521 Infection **of incontinent external stoma of urinary tract**   HCC
     N99.522 Malfunction **of incontinent external stoma of urinary tract**   HCC
     N99.523 Herniation **of incontinent stoma of urinary tract**   HCC
     N99.524 Stenosis **of incontinent stoma of urinary tract**   HCC
     N99.528 **Other complication of incontinent external stoma of urinary tract**   HCC
   ✓6th **N99.53** **Complication of** continent stoma **of urinary tract**
     N99.530 Hemorrhage **of continent stoma of urinary tract**   HCC
     N99.531 Infection **of continent stoma of urinary tract**   HCC
     N99.532 Malfunction **of continent stoma of urinary tract**   HCC
     N99.533 Herniation **of continent stoma of urinary tract**   HCC
     N99.534 Stenosis **of continent stoma of urinary tract**   HCC
     N99.538 **Other complication of continent stoma of urinary tract**   HCC
✓5th **N99.6** Intraoperative hemorrhage and hematoma **of a genitourinary system organ or structure complicating a procedure**
    EXCLUDES 1   intraoperative hemorrhage and hematoma of a genitourinary system organ or structure due to accidental puncture or laceration during a procedure (N99.7-)
   N99.61 **Intraoperative hemorrhage and hematoma of a genitourinary system organ or structure complicating a** genitourinary system procedure   CC
   N99.62 **Intraoperative hemorrhage and hematoma of a genitourinary system organ or structure complicating** other procedure   CC
✓5th **N99.7** Accidental puncture and laceration **of a genitourinary system organ or structure during a procedure**
   N99.71 **Accidental puncture and laceration of a genitourinary system organ or structure during a** genitourinary system procedure   CC

   N99.72 **Accidental puncture and laceration of a genitourinary system organ or structure during** other procedure   CC
✓5th **N99.8** **Other intraoperative and postprocedural complications and disorders of genitourinary system**
    AHA: 2016,4Q,9-10
   N99.81 **Other** intraoperative complications **of genitourinary system**
   ✓6th **N99.82** Postprocedural hemorrhage **of a genitourinary system organ or structure following a procedure**
     N99.820 **Postprocedural hemorrhage of a genitourinary system organ or structure following a** genitourinary system procedure   CC
     N99.821 **Postprocedural hemorrhage of a genitourinary system organ or structure following** other procedure   CC
   N99.83 Residual ovary syndrome ♀
   ✓6th **N99.84** Postprocedural hematoma and seroma **of a genitourinary system organ or structure following a procedure**
     N99.840 **Postprocedural** hematoma **of a genitourinary system organ or structure following a** genitourinary system procedure   CC
     N99.841 **Postprocedural** hematoma **of a genitourinary system organ or structure following** other procedure   CC
     N99.842 **Postprocedural** seroma **of a genitourinary system organ or structure following a** genitourinary system procedure   CC
     N99.843 **Postprocedural** seroma **of a genitourinary system organ or structure following** other procedure   CC
   N99.85 Post endometrial ablation syndrome ♀
     AHA: 2019,4Q,12
   N99.89 **Other postprocedural complications and disorders of genitourinary system**

✔ Additional Character Required   ✓x7th Placeholder   Questionable PDx   Manifestation   Unspecified Dx   UPD Unacceptable PDx   H1-H14 HAC   HCC CMS-HCC Dx   HIV HIV Dx

ICD-10-CM 2022   863

Chapter 15. Pregnancy, Childbirth and the Puerperium (O00–O9A)

Chapter-specific Guidelines with Coding Examples

The chapter-specific guidelines from the ICD-10-CM Official Guidelines for Coding and Reporting have been provided below. Along with these guidelines are coding examples, contained in the shaded boxes, that have been developed to help illustrate the coding and/or sequencing guidance found in these guidelines.

a. General rules for obstetric cases

1) Codes from Chapter 15 and sequencing priority

Obstetric cases require codes from chapter 15, codes in the range O00-O9A, Pregnancy, Childbirth, and the Puerperium. Chapter 15 codes have sequencing priority over codes from other chapters. Additional codes from other chapters may be used in conjunction with chapter 15 codes to further specify conditions. Should the provider document that the pregnancy is incidental to the encounter, then code Z33.1, Pregnant state, incidental, should be used in place of any chapter 15 codes. It is the provider's responsibility to state that the condition being treated is not affecting the pregnancy.

Pregnant patient at 25 weeks' gestation admitted for bladder abscess	
O23.12	Infections of bladder in pregnancy, second trimester
N30.80	Other cystitis without hematuria
Z3A.25	25 weeks gestation of pregnancy

Explanation: The documentation does not indicate that the pregnancy is incidental or in any way unaffected by the bladder abscess; therefore, an obstetrics code should be sequenced first. An additional code was provided to identify the specific bladder condition as this information is not called out specifically in the obstetrics code.

2) Chapter 15 codes used only on the maternal record

Chapter 15 codes are to be used only on the maternal record, never on the record of the newborn.

3) Final character for trimester

The majority of codes in Chapter 15 have a final character indicating the trimester of pregnancy. The timeframes for the trimesters are indicated at the beginning of the chapter. If trimester is not a component of a code, it is because the condition always occurs in a specific trimester, or the concept of trimester of pregnancy is not applicable. Certain codes have characters for only certain trimesters because the condition does not occur in all trimesters, but it may occur in more than just one.

Assignment of the final character for trimester should be based on the provider's documentation of the trimester (or number of weeks) for the current admission/encounter. This applies to the assignment of trimester for pre-existing conditions as well as those that develop during or are due to the pregnancy. The provider's documentation of the number of weeks may be used to assign the appropriate code identifying the trimester.

Whenever delivery occurs during the current admission, and there is an "in childbirth" option for the obstetric complication being coded, the "in childbirth" code should be assigned. **When the classification does not provide an obstetric code with an "in childbirth" option, it is appropriate to assign a code describing the current trimester.**

Pregnant patient at 21 weeks' gestation admitted with excessive vomiting	
O21.2	Late vomiting of pregnancy
Z3A.21	21 weeks gestation of pregnancy

Explanation: Category O21 classifies vomiting in pregnancy. Although code selection is based on whether the vomiting is before or after 20 completed weeks, these codes are not further classified by trimester. If vomiting only in the second trimester was documented, the provider should be queried for the specific week of gestation, as this will affect code selection.

4) Selection of trimester for inpatient admissions that encompass more than one trimester

In instances when a patient is admitted to a hospital for complications of pregnancy during one trimester and remains in the hospital into a subsequent trimester, the trimester character for the antepartum complication code should be assigned on the basis of the trimester when the complication developed, not the trimester of the discharge. If the condition developed prior to the current admission/encounter or represents a pre-existing condition, the trimester character for the trimester at the time of the admission/encounter should be assigned.

Patient admitted at 27 6/7 weeks' gestation for hemorrhaging from partial placenta previa; three days after admission at 28 1/7 weeks' gestation, she developed gestational hypertension	
O44.32	Partial placenta previa with hemorrhage, second trimester
O13.3	Gestational [pregnancy-induced] hypertension without significant proteinuria, third trimester
Z3A.27	27 weeks gestation of pregnancy

Explanation: The patient presented with hemorrhaging from partial placenta previa while still in her 27th week, which falls within the second trimester. The gestational hypertension did not occur until three days after admission, putting the patient in her 28th week of pregnancy or what is considered to be the third trimester. The weeks of gestation captured by a code from category Z3A should represent only the gestational weeks upon admission.

5) Unspecified trimester

Each category that includes codes for trimester has a code for "unspecified trimester." The "unspecified trimester" code should rarely be used, such as when the documentation in the record is insufficient to determine the trimester and it is not possible to obtain clarification.

6) 7th character for fetus identification

Where applicable, a 7th character is to be assigned for certain categories (O31, O32, O33.3 - O33.6, O35, O36, O40, O41, O60.1, O60.2, O64, and O69) to identify the fetus for which the complication code applies.

Assign 7th character "0":

- For single gestations
- When the documentation in the record is insufficient to determine the fetus affected and it is not possible to obtain clarification.
- When it is not possible to clinically determine which fetus is affected.

b. Selection of OB principal or first-listed diagnosis

1) Routine outpatient prenatal visits

For routine outpatient prenatal visits when no complications are present, a code from category Z34, Encounter for supervision of normal pregnancy, should be used as the first-listed diagnosis. These codes should not be used in conjunction with chapter 15 codes.

2) Supervision of high-risk pregnancy

Codes from category O09, Supervision of high-risk pregnancy, are intended for use only during the prenatal period. For complications during the labor or delivery episode as a result of a high-risk pregnancy, assign the applicable complication codes from Chapter 15. If there are no complications during the labor or delivery episode, assign code O80, Encounter for full-term uncomplicated delivery.

For routine prenatal outpatient visits for patients with high-risk pregnancies, a code from category O09, Supervision of high-risk pregnancy, should be used as the first-listed diagnosis. Secondary chapter 15 codes may be used in conjunction with these codes if appropriate.

36-year-old with history of preterm labor admitted in labor with second child at 39 weeks' gestation, delivered healthy baby without complications	
O80	Encounter for full-term uncomplicated delivery
Z3A.39	39 weeks gestation of pregnancy
Z37.0	Single live birth

Explanation: Although this patient is over 35 and having her second child (elderly multigravida) and has a history of preterm labor with her first child, no codes from category O09.- should be appended. In the absence of any other complications noted during the encounter, code O80 is the most appropriate code to describe the principal diagnosis.

3) Episodes when no delivery occurs

In episodes when no delivery occurs, the principal diagnosis should correspond to the principal complication of the pregnancy which necessitated the encounter. Should more than one complication exist, all of which are treated or monitored, any of the complication codes may be sequenced first.

Chapter 15. Pregnancy, Childbirth and the Puerperium

4) When a delivery occurs

When an obstetric patient is admitted and delivers during that admission, the condition that prompted the admission should be sequenced as the principal diagnosis. If multiple conditions prompted the admission, sequence the one most related to the delivery as the principal diagnosis. A code for any complication of the delivery should be assigned as an additional diagnosis. In cases of cesarean delivery, if the patient was admitted with a condition that resulted in the performance of a cesarean procedure, that condition should be selected as the principal diagnosis. If the reason for the admission was unrelated to the condition resulting in the cesarean delivery, the condition related to the reason for the admission should be selected as the principal diagnosis.

Maternal patient with diet-controlled gestational diabetes was admitted at 38 weeks' gestation in obstructed labor due to footling presentation; cesarean performed for the malpresentation

O64.8XX0	**Obstructed labor due to other malposition and malpresentation, not applicable or unspecified**
O24.420	**Gestational diabetes mellitus in childbirth, diet controlled**
Z3A.38	**38 weeks gestation of pregnancy**
Z37.0	**Single live birth**

Explanation: The obstructed labor necessitated the cesarean procedure.

At 39 weeks' gestation, a maternal patient presents with hemorrhage with coagulation defect; the next day the patient goes into labor and eventually delivers via cesarean section due to arrested active phase of labor

O46.003	**Antepartum hemorrhage with coagulation defect, unspecified, third trimester**
O62.1	**Secondary uterine inertia**
Z3A.39	**39 weeks gestation of pregnancy**
Z37.0	**Single live birth**

Explanation: The patient was admitted because of the antepartum hemorrhage with coagulation defect. The arrested active phase, although the reason for the cesarean delivery, did not develop until later into the stay.

---

5) Outcome of delivery

A code from category Z37, Outcome of delivery, should be included on every maternal record when a delivery has occurred. These codes are not to be used on subsequent records or on the newborn record.

c. Pre-existing conditions versus conditions due to the pregnancy

Certain categories in Chapter 15 distinguish between conditions of the mother that existed prior to pregnancy (pre-existing) and those that are a direct result of pregnancy. When assigning codes from Chapter 15, it is important to assess if a condition was pre-existing prior to pregnancy or developed during or due to the pregnancy in order to assign the correct code.

Categories that do not distinguish between pre-existing and pregnancy-related conditions may be used for either. It is acceptable to use codes specifically for the puerperium with codes complicating pregnancy and childbirth if a condition arises postpartum during the delivery encounter.

d. Pre-existing hypertension in pregnancy

Category O10, Pre-existing hypertension complicating pregnancy, childbirth and the puerperium, includes codes for hypertensive heart and hypertensive chronic kidney disease. When assigning one of the O10 codes that includes hypertensive heart disease or hypertensive chronic kidney disease, it is necessary to add a secondary code from the appropriate hypertension category to specify the type of heart failure or chronic kidney disease.

See Section I.C.9. Hypertension.

e. Fetal conditions affecting the management of the mother

1) Codes from categories O35 and O36

Codes from categories O35, Maternal care for known or suspected fetal abnormality and damage, and O36, Maternal care for other fetal problems, are assigned only when the fetal condition is actually responsible for modifying the management of the mother, i.e., by requiring diagnostic studies, additional observation, special care, or

---

termination of pregnancy. The fact that the fetal condition exists does not justify assigning a code from this series to the mother's record.

A patient is seen in ED for spotting 15 weeks into her pregnancy; the doctors also suspect fetal hydrocephalus.

O26.852	**Spotting complicating pregnancy, second trimester**
Z3A.15	**15 weeks gestation of pregnancy**

Explanation: Whether the fetal hydrocephalus was suspected or confirmed, an additional code is not warranted for this condition as the documentation does not indicate that this fetal condition is in any way altering the management of the mother or complicating her pregnancy.

---

2) In utero surgery

In cases when surgery is performed on the fetus, a diagnosis code from category O35, Maternal care for known or suspected fetal abnormality and damage, should be assigned identifying the fetal condition. Assign the appropriate procedure code for the procedure performed.

No code from Chapter 16, the perinatal codes, should be used on the mother's record to identify fetal conditions. Surgery performed in utero on a fetus is still to be coded as an obstetric encounter.

f. HIV infection in pregnancy, childbirth and the puerperium

During pregnancy, childbirth or the puerperium, a patient admitted because of an HIV-related illness should receive a principal diagnosis from subcategory O98.7-, Human immunodeficiency [HIV] disease complicating pregnancy, childbirth and the puerperium, followed by the code(s) for the HIV-related illness(es).

Patients with asymptomatic HIV infection status admitted during pregnancy, childbirth, or the puerperium should receive codes of O98.7- and Z21, Asymptomatic human immunodeficiency virus [HIV] infection status.

A previously asymptomatic HIV patient who is 13 weeks pregnant is admitted with oral thrush.

O98.711	**Human immunodeficiency virus [HIV] disease complicating pregnancy, first trimester**
B20	**Human immunodeficiency virus [HIV] disease**
B37.0	**Candidal stomatitis**
Z3A.13	**13 weeks gestation of pregnancy**

Explanation: Because oral thrush is an HIV-related condition, this patient is now considered to have HIV disease. An obstetrics code indicating that HIV is complicating the pregnancy is coded first, followed by B20 for HIV disease as well as a code for the oral thrush.

---

g. Diabetes mellitus in pregnancy

Diabetes mellitus is a significant complicating factor in pregnancy. Pregnant **patients** who are diabetic should be assigned a code from category O24, Diabetes mellitus in pregnancy, childbirth, and the puerperium, first, followed by the appropriate diabetes code(s) (E08-E13) from Chapter 4.

h. Long term use of insulin and oral hypoglycemics

See section I.C.4.a.3 for information on the long-term use of insulin and oral hypoglycemics.

i. Gestational (pregnancy induced) diabetes

Gestational (pregnancy induced) diabetes can occur during the second and third trimester of pregnancy in **patients** who were not diabetic prior to pregnancy. Gestational diabetes can cause complications in the pregnancy similar to those of pre-existing diabetes mellitus. It also puts the **patient** at greater risk of developing diabetes after the pregnancy.

Codes for gestational diabetes are in subcategory O24.4, Gestational diabetes mellitus. No other code from category O24, Diabetes mellitus in pregnancy, childbirth, and the puerperium, should be used with a code from O24.4.

The codes under subcategory O24.4 include diet controlled, insulin controlled, and controlled by oral hypoglycemic drugs. If a patient with gestational diabetes is treated with both diet and insulin, only the code for insulin-controlled is required. If a patient with gestational diabetes is treated with both diet and oral hypoglycemic medications, only the code for "controlled by oral hypoglycemic drugs" is required. Code Z79.4, Long-term (current) use of insulin or code Z79.84, Long-term (current) use of oral hypoglycemic drugs, should not be assigned with codes from subcategory O24.4.

An abnormal glucose tolerance in pregnancy is assigned a code from subcategory O99.81, Abnormal glucose complicating pregnancy, childbirth, and the puerperium.

> Patient at 39 weeks term pregnancy with gestational diabetes was admitted in labor and delivered a healthy newborn. Patient is on a diabetic diet with daily metformin.
>
> **O24.425**   **Gestational diabetes mellitus in childbirth, controlled by oral hypoglycemic drugs**
>
> **Z3A.39**   **39 weeks gestation of pregnancy**
>
> **Z37.0**   **Single live birth**
>
> *Explanation:* When the patient is admitted for delivery and the patient's gestational diabetes is controlled by both diet and oral hypoglycemic medications, only the combination code in subcategory O24.4- Gestational diabetes mellitus, is reported. No code is added for diet controlled diabetes, and no Z code for long-term use of oral hypoglycemics is reported with the O24.4 combination codes.

j. Sepsis and septic shock complicating abortion, pregnancy, childbirth and the puerperium

When assigning a chapter 15 code for sepsis complicating abortion, pregnancy, childbirth, and the puerperium, a code for the specific type of infection should be assigned as an additional diagnosis. If severe sepsis is present, a code from subcategory R65.2, Severe sepsis, and code(s) for associated organ dysfunction(s) should also be assigned as additional diagnoses.

> Patient is seen several days after a miscarriage with sepsis; cultures return MSSA
>
> **O03.87**   **Sepsis following complete or unspecified spontaneous abortion**
>
> **B95.61**   **Methicillin susceptible Staphylococcus aureus infection as the cause of diseases classified elsewhere**
>
> *Explanation:* The type of infection that caused this patient to become septic was methicillin susceptible *Staphylococcus aureus* (MSSA), which as a secondary code helps capture all aspects related to this patient's septic condition.

k. Puerperal sepsis

Code O85, Puerperal sepsis, should be assigned with a secondary code to identify the causal organism (e.g., for a bacterial infection, assign a code from category B95-B96, Bacterial infections in conditions classified elsewhere). A code from category A40, Streptococcal sepsis, or A41, Other sepsis, should not be used for puerperal sepsis. If applicable, use additional codes to identify severe sepsis (R65.2-) and any associated acute organ dysfunction.

Code O85 should not be assigned for sepsis following an obstetrical procedure (See Section I.C.1.d.5.b., Sepsis due to a postprocedural infection).

l. Alcohol, tobacco and drug use during pregnancy, childbirth and the puerperium

1) Alcohol use during pregnancy, childbirth and the puerperium

Codes under subcategory O99.31, Alcohol use complicating pregnancy, childbirth, and the puerperium, should be assigned for any pregnancy case when a **patient** uses alcohol during the pregnancy or postpartum. A secondary code from category F10, Alcohol related disorders, should also be assigned to identify manifestations of the alcohol use.

2) Tobacco use during pregnancy, childbirth and the puerperium

Codes under subcategory O99.33, Smoking (tobacco) complicating pregnancy, childbirth, and the puerperium, should be assigned for any pregnancy case when a **patient** uses any type of tobacco product during the pregnancy or postpartum.

A secondary code from category F17, Nicotine dependence, should also be assigned to identify the type of nicotine dependence.

3) Drug use during pregnancy, childbirth and the puerperium

Codes under subcategory O99.32, Drug use complicating pregnancy, childbirth, and the puerperium, should be assigned for any pregnancy case when a **patient** uses drugs during the pregnancy or postpartum. This can involve illegal drugs, or inappropriate use or abuse of prescription drugs. Secondary code(s) from categories F11-F16 and F18-F19 should also be assigned to identify manifestations of the drug use.

m. Poisoning, toxic effects, adverse effects and underdosing in a pregnant patient

A code from subcategory O9A.2, Injury, poisoning and certain other consequences of external causes complicating pregnancy, childbirth, and the puerperium, should be sequenced first, followed by the appropriate injury, poisoning, toxic effect, adverse effect or underdosing code, and then the additional code(s) that specifies the condition caused by the poisoning, toxic effect, adverse effect or underdosing.

See Section I.C.19. Adverse effects, poisoning, underdosing and toxic effects.

> Patient admitted with accidental carbon monoxide poisoning from a gas heating implement; the patient is 18 weeks' pregnant
>
> **O9A.212**   **Injury, poisoning and certain other consequences of external causes complicating pregnancy, second trimester**
>
> **T58.11XA**   **Toxic effect of carbon monoxide from utility gas, accidental (unintentional), initial encounter**
>
> **Z3A.18**   **18 weeks gestation of pregnancy**
>
> *Explanation:* Although the carbon monoxide poisoning is the reason the patient was admitted, a code from the obstetrics chapter must be sequenced first. Chapter 15 codes have sequencing priority over codes from other chapters.

n. Normal delivery, code O80

1) Encounter for full term uncomplicated delivery

Code O80 should be assigned when a **patient** is admitted for a full-term normal delivery and delivers a single, healthy infant without any complications antepartum, during the delivery, or postpartum during the delivery episode. Code O80 is always a principal diagnosis. It is not to be used if any other code from chapter 15 is needed to describe a current complication of the antenatal, delivery, or postnatal period. Additional codes from other chapters may be used with code O80 if they are not related to or are in any way complicating the pregnancy.

2) Uncomplicated delivery with resolved antepartum complication

Code O80 may be used if the patient had a complication at some point during the pregnancy, but the complication is not present at the time of the admission for delivery.

> Patient presents in labor at 39 weeks' gestation and delivers a healthy newborn; patient had abnormal glucose levels in her first trimester, which have since resolved
>
> **O80**   **Encounter for full-term uncomplicated delivery**
>
> **Z37.0**   **Single live birth**
>
> *Explanation:* The abnormal glucose levels during the first trimester cannot be coded if they are not affecting the patient's current trimester. Without additional complications associated with the pregnancy, fetus, or mother, code O80 is appropriate.

3) Outcome of delivery for O80

Z37.0, Single live birth, is the only outcome of delivery code appropriate for use with O80.

o. The peripartum and postpartum periods

1) Peripartum and postpartum periods

The postpartum period begins immediately after delivery and continues for six weeks following delivery. The peripartum period is defined as the last month of pregnancy to five months postpartum.

2) Peripartum and postpartum complication

A postpartum complication is any complication occurring within the six-week period.

3) Pregnancy-related complications after 6-week period

Chapter 15 codes may also be used to describe pregnancy-related complications after the peripartum or postpartum period if the provider documents that a condition is pregnancy related.

Chapter 15. Pregnancy, Childbirth and the Puerperium

Patient admitted for varicose veins. She had a baby boy three months ago; the varicose veins started to appear one month ago. The doctor attributes the patient's pregnancy as the cause of the varicose veins, which continue to be painful and bother the patient. She is seeking surgical relief.

O87.4   Varicose veins of the lower extremity in the puerperium

Explanation: Although the varicose veins occurred several months after the delivery of the newborn, the doctor attributed the varicose veins to pregnancy and therefore a code from chapter 15 is appropriate.

4) Admission for routine postpartum care following delivery outside hospital

When the mother delivers outside the hospital prior to admission and is admitted for routine postpartum care and no complications are noted, code Z39.0, Encounter for care and examination of mother immediately after delivery, should be assigned as the principal diagnosis.

5) Pregnancy associated cardiomyopathy

Pregnancy associated cardiomyopathy, code O90.3, is unique in that it may be diagnosed in the third trimester of pregnancy but may continue to progress months after delivery. For this reason, it is referred to as peripartum cardiomyopathy. Code O90.3 is only for use when the cardiomyopathy develops as a result of pregnancy in a **patient** who did not have pre-existing heart disease.

p. Code O94, Sequelae of complication of pregnancy, childbirth, and the puerperium

1) Code O94

Code O94, Sequelae of complication of pregnancy, childbirth, and the puerperium, is for use in those cases when an initial complication of a pregnancy develops a **sequela or** sequelae requiring care or treatment at a future date.

2) After the initial postpartum period

This code may be used at any time after the initial postpartum period.

3) Sequencing of code O94

This code, like all sequela codes, is to be sequenced following the code describing the sequelae of the complication.

q. Termination of pregnancy and spontaneous abortions

1) Abortion with liveborn fetus

When an attempted termination of pregnancy results in a liveborn fetus, assign code Z33.2, Encounter for elective termination of pregnancy and a code from category Z37, Outcome of Delivery.

2) Retained products of conception following an abortion

Subsequent encounters for retained products of conception following a spontaneous abortion or elective termination of pregnancy, without complications are assigned O03.4, Incomplete spontaneous, abortion without complication, or code O07.4, Failed attempted termination of pregnancy without complication. This advice is appropriate even when the patient was discharged previously with a discharge diagnosis of complete abortion. If the patient has a specific complication associated with the spontaneous abortion or elective termination of pregnancy in addition to retained products of conception, assign the appropriate complication code (e.g., O03.-, O04.-, O07.-) instead of code O03.4 or O07.4.

Patient was seen two days ago for complete spontaneous abortion but returns today for urinary tract infection (UTI) with ultrasound showing retained products of conception

O03.38   Urinary tract infection following incomplete spontaneous abortion

Explanation: Although the diagnosis from the patient's previous stay indicated that the patient had a complete abortion, it is now determined that there were actually retained products of conception (POC). An abortion with retained POC is considered incomplete and in this case resulted in the patient developing a UTI.

3) Complications leading to abortion

Codes from Chapter 15 may be used as additional codes to identify any documented complications of the pregnancy in conjunction with codes in categories in O04, O07 and O08.

r. Abuse in a pregnant patient

For suspected or confirmed cases of abuse of a pregnant patient, a code(s) from subcategories O9A.3, Physical abuse complicating pregnancy, childbirth, and the puerperium, O9A.4, Sexual abuse complicating pregnancy, childbirth, and the puerperium, and O9A.5, Psychological abuse complicating pregnancy, childbirth, and the puerperium, should be sequenced first, followed by the appropriate codes (if applicable) to identify any associated current injury due to physical abuse, sexual abuse, and the perpetrator of abuse.

See Section I.C.19. Adult and child abuse, neglect and other maltreatment.

s. COVID-19 infection in pregnancy, childbirth, and the puerperium

During pregnancy, childbirth or the puerperium, when COVID-19 is the reason for admission/encounter , code O98.5-, Other viral diseases complicating pregnancy, childbirth and the puerperium, should be sequenced as the principal/first-listed diagnosis, and code U07.1, COVID-19, and the appropriate codes for associated manifestation(s) should be assigned as additional diagnoses. Codes from Chapter 15 always take sequencing priority.

If the reason for admission/encounter is unrelated to COVID-19 but the patient tests positive for COVID-19 during the admission/encounter, the appropriate code for the reason for admission/encounter should be sequenced as the principal/first-listed diagnosis, and codes O98.5- and U07.1, as well as the appropriate codes for associated COVID-19 manifestations, should be assigned as additional diagnoses.

Patient admitted in labor at 39 weeks' gestation and delivered a healthy newborn. Prenatal care consisted of some hyperemesis early in the pregnancy that has since resolved. No complications encountered during or following delivery. As per hospital protocol, during the pandemic, all patients are to be screened for COVID-19, and the patient tested positive. She remains asymptomatic, will be sent home to quarantine for 14 days.

O98.52   Other viral diseases complicating childbirth

U07.1   COVID-19

Z3A.39   39 weeks gestation of pregnancy

Z37.0   Single live birth

Explanation: No code is assigned for the hyperemesis as it resolved prior to this admission. Per guideline I.C.1.g.1.f, a screening code is generally not appropriate during the pandemic phase of COVID-19. Most hospitals screen their patients upon admission to the hospital to ensure proper protocols are in place for monitoring and treating those patients who do test positive for the disease. A positive test result alone is confirmation of the disease, according to guideline I.C.1.g.1.a, and code U07.1 should be assigned. A claim for any patient admitted during pregnancy, childbirth, or the puerperium and who tests positive or is treated for COVID-19 should have a code from subcategory O98.5- sequenced first, followed by code U07.1. As the patient was asymptomatic, no additional codes are assigned to represent any manifestation of the COVID-19 infection.

Chapter 15. Pregnancy, Childbirth and the Puerperium (O00-O9A)

NOTE CODES FROM THIS CHAPTER ARE FOR USE ONLY ON MATERNAL RECORDS, NEVER ON NEWBORN RECORDS

Codes from this chapter are for use for conditions related to or aggravated by the pregnancy, childbirth, or by the puerperium (maternal causes or obstetrical causes)

NOTE Trimesters are counted from the first day of the last menstrual period. They are defined as follows:

1st trimester- less than 14 weeks 0 days

2nd trimester- 14 weeks 0 days to less than 28 weeks 0 days

3rd trimester- 28 weeks 0 days until delivery

Use additional code from category Z3A, Weeks of gestation, to identify the specific week of the pregnancy, if known.

EXCLUDES 1 *supervision of normal pregnancy (Z34.-)*

EXCLUDES 2 *mental and behavioral disorders associated with the puerperium (F53.-)*
obstetrical tetanus (A34)
postpartum necrosis of pituitary gland (E23.0)
puerperal osteomalacia (M83.0)

AHA: 2016,1Q,3-5; 2014,3Q,17

This chapter contains the following blocks:

O00-O08   Pregnancy with abortive outcome
O09   Supervision of high risk pregnancy
O10-O16   Edema, proteinuria and hypertensive disorders in pregnancy, childbirth and the puerperium
O20-O29   Other maternal disorders predominantly related to pregnancy
O30-O48   Maternal care related to the fetus and amniotic cavity and possible delivery problems
O60-O77   Complications of labor and delivery
O80-O82   Encounter for delivery
O85-O92   Complications predominantly related to the puerperium
O94-O9A   Other obstetric conditions, not elsewhere classified

Pregnancy with abortive outcome (O00-O08)

EXCLUDES 1 *continuing pregnancy in multiple gestation after abortion of one fetus or more (O31.1-, O31.3-)*

TIP: Do not assign a code from category Z3A with codes in this code block.

✓4ᵗʰ O00 Ectopic pregnancy

INCLUDES ruptured ectopic pregnancy

Use additional code from category O08 to identify any associated complication

AHA: 2016,4Q,48-50; 2014,3Q,17

DEF: Implantation of a fertilized egg outside the uterus, usually in the fallopian tube or abdomen that requires emergency treatment.

Ectopic Pregnancy

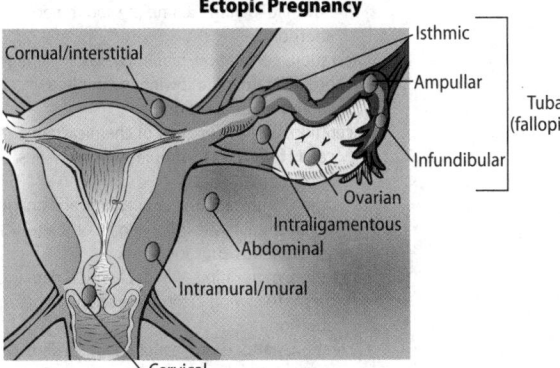

✓5ᵗʰ O00.0 Abdominal pregnancy

EXCLUDES 1 *maternal care for viable fetus in abdominal pregnancy (O36.7-)*

O00.00 Abdominal pregnancy without intrauterine **pregnancy**   CC M ♀
Abdominal pregnancy NOS

O00.01 Abdominal pregnancy with intrauterine **pregnancy**   CC M ♀

✓5ᵗʰ O00.1 Tubal pregnancy

Fallopian pregnancy
Rupture of (fallopian) tube due to pregnancy
Tubal abortion

AHA: 2017,4Q,20

✓6ᵗʰ O00.10 Tubal pregnancy without intrauterine pregnancy

Tubal pregnancy NOS

O00.101 Right tubal pregnancy without intrauterine pregnancy   CC M ♀

O00.102 Left tubal pregnancy without intrauterine pregnancy   CC M ♀

O00.109 Unspecified tubal pregnancy without intrauterine pregnancy   CC M ♀

✓6ᵗʰ O00.11 Tubal pregnancy with intrauterine pregnancy

O00.111 Right tubal pregnancy with intrauterine pregnancy   CC M ♀

O00.112 Left tubal pregnancy with intrauterine pregnancy   CC M ♀

O00.119 Unspecified tubal pregnancy with intrauterine pregnancy   CC M ♀

✓5ᵗʰ O00.2 Ovarian pregnancy

AHA: 2017,4Q,20

✓6ᵗʰ O00.20 Ovarian pregnancy without intrauterine pregnancy

Ovarian pregnancy NOS

O00.201 Right ovarian pregnancy without intrauterine pregnancy   CC M ♀

O00.202 Left ovarian pregnancy without intrauterine pregnancy   CC M ♀

O00.209 Unspecified ovarian pregnancy without intrauterine pregnancy   CC M ♀

✓6ᵗʰ O00.21 Ovarian pregnancy with intrauterine pregnancy

O00.211 Right ovarian pregnancy with intrauterine pregnancy   CC M ♀

O00.212 Left ovarian pregnancy with intrauterine pregnancy   CC M ♀

O00.219 Unspecified ovarian pregnancy with intrauterine pregnancy   CC M ♀

✓5ᵗʰ O00.8 Other ectopic pregnancy

Cervical pregnancy
Cornual pregnancy
Intraligamentous pregnancy
Mural pregnancy

O00.80 Other ectopic pregnancy without intrauterine **pregnancy**   CC M ♀
Other ectopic pregnancy NOS

O00.81 Other ectopic pregnancy with intrauterine **pregnancy**   CC M ♀

✓5ᵗʰ O00.9 Ectopic pregnancy, unspecified

O00.90 Unspecified ectopic pregnancy without intrauterine **pregnancy**   CC M ♀
Ectopic pregnancy NOS

O00.91 Unspecified ectopic pregnancy with intrauterine **pregnancy**   CC M ♀

✓4ᵗʰ O01 Hydatidiform mole

Use additional code from category O08 to identify any associated complication

EXCLUDES 1 *chorioadenoma (destruens) (D39.2)*
malignant hydatidiform mole (D39.2)

AHA: 2014,3Q,17

DEF: Abnormal product of pregnancy, marked by a mass of cysts resembling a bunch of grapes due to chorionic villi proliferation and dissolution. It must be surgically removed.

O01.0 Classical hydatidiform mole   M ♀
Complete hydatidiform mole

O01.1 Incomplete and partial hydatidiform mole   M ♀

O01.9 Hydatidiform mole, unspecified   M ♀
Trophoblastic disease NOS
Vesicular mole NOS

☑ Additional Character Required   ✓x7ᵗʰ Placeholder   Questionable PDx   ■ Manifestation   Unspecified Dx   UPD Unacceptable PDx   H1 - H14 HAC   HCC CMS-HCC Dx   HIV HIV Dx

ICD-10-CM 2022   869

✓4ᵗʰ **O02 Other abnormal products of conception**

Use additional code from category O08 to identify any associated complication

EXCLUDES 1   *papyraceous fetus (O31.0-)*

AHA: 2014,3Q,17

O02.0 Blighted ovum and nonhydatidiform mole   M♀

Carneous mole
Fleshy mole
Intrauterine mole NOS
Molar pregnancy NEC
Pathological ovum

O02.1 Missed abortion   M♀

Early fetal death, before completion of 20 weeks of gestation, with retention of dead fetus

EXCLUDES 1   *failed induced abortion (O07.-)*
         fetal death (intrauterine) (late) (O36.4)
         missed abortion with blighted ovum (O02.0)
         missed abortion with hydatidiform mole (O01.-)
         missed abortion with nonhydatidiform (O02.0)
         missed abortion with other abnormal products of conception (O02.8-)
         missed delivery (O36.4)
         stillbirth (P95)

AHA: 2019,3Q,11

✓5ᵗʰ **O02.8 Other specified abnormal products of conception**

EXCLUDES 1   *abnormal products of conception with blighted ovum (O02.0)*
         abnormal products of conception with hydatidiform mole (O01.-)
         abnormal products of conception with nonhydatidiform mole (O02.0)

O02.81 Inappropriate change in quantitative human chorionic gonadotropin (hCG) in early pregnancy   M♀

Biochemical pregnancy
Chemical pregnancy
Inappropriate level of quantitative human chorionic gonadotropin (hCG) for gestational age in early pregnancy

O02.89 Other abnormal products of conception   M♀

O02.9 Abnormal product of conception, unspecified   M♀

✓4ᵗʰ **O03 Spontaneous abortion**

NOTE   Incomplete abortion includes retained products of conception following spontaneous abortion

INCLUDES   miscarriage

O03.0 Genital tract and pelvic infection following incomplete spontaneous abortion   CC M♀

Endometritis following incomplete spontaneous abortion
Oophoritis following incomplete spontaneous abortion
Parametritis following incomplete spontaneous abortion
Pelvic peritonitis following incomplete spontaneous abortion
Salpingitis following incomplete spontaneous abortion
Salpingo-oophoritis following incomplete spontaneous abortion

EXCLUDES 1   *sepsis following incomplete spontaneous abortion (O03.37)*
         urinary tract infection following incomplete spontaneous abortion (O03.38)

O03.1 Delayed or excessive hemorrhage following incomplete spontaneous abortion   M♀

Afibrinogenemia following incomplete spontaneous abortion
Defibrination syndrome following incomplete spontaneous abortion
Hemolysis following incomplete spontaneous abortion
Intravascular coagulation following incomplete spontaneous abortion

O03.2 Embolism following incomplete spontaneous abortion   MCC M♀

Air embolism following incomplete spontaneous abortion
Amniotic fluid embolism following incomplete spontaneous abortion
Blood-clot embolism following incomplete spontaneous abortion
Embolism NOS following incomplete spontaneous abortion
Fat embolism following incomplete spontaneous abortion
Pulmonary embolism following incomplete spontaneous abortion
Pyemic embolism following incomplete spontaneous abortion
Septic or septicopyemic embolism following incomplete spontaneous abortion
Soap embolism following incomplete spontaneous abortion

✓5ᵗʰ **O03.3 Other and unspecified complications following incomplete spontaneous abortion**

O03.30 Unspecified complication following incomplete spontaneous abortion   CC M♀

O03.31 Shock following incomplete spontaneous abortion   MCC M♀

Circulatory collapse following incomplete spontaneous abortion
Shock (postprocedural) following incomplete spontaneous abortion

EXCLUDES 1   *shock due to infection following incomplete spontaneous abortion (O03.37)*

O03.32 Renal failure following incomplete spontaneous abortion   MCC M♀

Kidney failure (acute) following incomplete spontaneous abortion
Oliguria following incomplete spontaneous abortion
Renal shutdown following incomplete spontaneous abortion
Renal tubular necrosis following incomplete spontaneous abortion
Uremia following incomplete spontaneous abortion

O03.33 Metabolic disorder following incomplete spontaneous abortion   CC M♀

O03.34 Damage to pelvic organs following incomplete spontaneous abortion   CC M♀

Laceration, perforation, tear or chemical damage of bladder following incomplete spontaneous abortion
Laceration, perforation, tear or chemical damage of bowel following incomplete spontaneous abortion
Laceration, perforation, tear or chemical damage of broad ligament following incomplete spontaneous abortion
Laceration, perforation, tear or chemical damage of cervix following incomplete spontaneous abortion
Laceration, perforation, tear or chemical damage of periurethral tissue following incomplete spontaneous abortion
Laceration, perforation, tear or chemical damage of uterus following incomplete spontaneous abortion
Laceration, perforation, tear or chemical damage of vagina following incomplete spontaneous abortion

O03.35 Other venous complications following incomplete spontaneous abortion   CC♀

O03.36 Cardiac arrest following incomplete spontaneous abortion   CC M♀

O03.37 Sepsis following incomplete spontaneous abortion   CC M♀

Use additional code to identify infectious agent (B95-B97)
Use additional code to identify severe sepsis, if applicable (R65.2-)

EXCLUDES 1   *septic or septicopyemic embolism following incomplete spontaneous abortion (O03.2)*

O03.38   Urinary tract infection **following** incomplete **spontaneous abortion**   `CC` `M` ♀
> Cystitis following incomplete spontaneous abortion

O03.39   **Incomplete spontaneous abortion with other complications**   `CC` `M` ♀

O03.4   Incomplete **spontaneous abortion** without complication   `M` ♀

O03.5   Genital tract and pelvic infection **following** complete or unspecified **spontaneous abortion**   `CC` `M` ♀
> Endometritis following complete or unspecified spontaneous abortion
> Oophoritis following complete or unspecified spontaneous abortion
> Parametritis following complete or unspecified spontaneous abortion
> Pelvic peritonitis following complete or unspecified spontaneous abortion
> Salpingitis following complete or unspecified spontaneous abortion
> Salpingo-oophoritis following complete or unspecified spontaneous abortion
>> **EXCLUDES 1**   *sepsis following complete or unspecified spontaneous abortion (O03.87)*
>> *urinary tract infection following complete or unspecified spontaneous abortion (O03.88)*

O03.6   Delayed or excessive hemorrhage **following** complete or unspecified **spontaneous abortion**   `M` ♀
> Afibrinogenemia following complete or unspecified spontaneous abortion
> Defibrination syndrome following complete or unspecified spontaneous abortion
> Hemolysis following complete or unspecified spontaneous abortion
> Intravascular coagulation following complete or unspecified spontaneous abortion

O03.7   Embolism **following** complete or unspecified **spontaneous abortion**   `CC` `M` ♀
> Air embolism following complete or unspecified spontaneous abortion
> Amniotic fluid embolism following complete or unspecified spontaneous abortion
> Blood-clot embolism following complete or unspecified spontaneous abortion
> Embolism NOS following complete or unspecified spontaneous abortion
> Fat embolism following complete or unspecified spontaneous abortion
> Pulmonary embolism following complete or unspecified spontaneous abortion
> Pyemic embolism following complete or unspecified spontaneous abortion
> Septic or septicopyemic embolism following complete or unspecified spontaneous abortion
> Soap embolism following complete or unspecified spontaneous abortion

`✓5ᵗʰ` **O03.8**   **Other and unspecified complications following complete or unspecified spontaneous abortion**

     O03.80   Unspecified complication following complete or unspecified **spontaneous abortion**   `CC` `M` ♀

     O03.81   Shock **following** complete or unspecified **spontaneous abortion**   `MCC` `M` ♀
>> Circulatory collapse following complete or unspecified spontaneous abortion
>> Shock (postprocedural) following complete or unspecified spontaneous abortion
>>> **EXCLUDES 1**   *shock due to infection following complete or unspecified spontaneous abortion (O03.87)*

O03.82   Renal failure **following** complete or unspecified **spontaneous abortion**   `MCC` `M` ♀
> Kidney failure (acute) following complete or unspecified spontaneous abortion
> Oliguria following complete or unspecified spontaneous abortion
> Renal shutdown following complete or unspecified spontaneous abortion
> Renal tubular necrosis following complete or unspecified spontaneous abortion
> Uremia following complete or unspecified spontaneous abortion

O03.83   Metabolic **disorder following** complete or unspecified **spontaneous abortion**   `CC` `M` ♀

O03.84   Damage to pelvic organs **following** complete or unspecified **spontaneous abortion**   `CC` `M` ♀
> Laceration, perforation, tear or chemical damage of bladder following complete or unspecified spontaneous abortion
> Laceration, perforation, tear or chemical damage of bowel following complete or unspecified spontaneous abortion
> Laceration, perforation, tear or chemical damage of broad ligament following complete or unspecified spontaneous abortion
> Laceration, perforation, tear or chemical damage of cervix following complete or unspecified spontaneous abortion
> Laceration, perforation, tear or chemical damage of periurethral tissue following complete or unspecified spontaneous abortion
> Laceration, perforation, tear or chemical damage of uterus following complete or unspecified spontaneous abortion
> Laceration, perforation, tear or chemical damage of vagina following complete or unspecified spontaneous abortion

O03.85   Other venous complications following complete or unspecified **spontaneous abortion**   `CC` `M` ♀

O03.86   Cardiac arrest **following** complete or unspecified **spontaneous abortion**   `CC` `M` ♀

O03.87   Sepsis **following** complete or unspecified **spontaneous abortion**   `CC` `M` ♀
> Use additional code to identify infectious agent (B95-B97)
> Use additional code to identify severe sepsis, if applicable (R65.2-)
>> **EXCLUDES 1**   *septic or septicopyemic embolism following complete or unspecified spontaneous abortion (O03.7)*

O03.88   Urinary tract infection **following** complete or unspecified **spontaneous abortion**   `CC` `M` ♀
> Cystitis following complete or unspecified spontaneous abortion

O03.89   Complete or unspecified **spontaneous abortion with other complications**   `CC` `M` ♀

O03.9   Complete or unspecified **spontaneous abortion** without complication   `M` ♀
> Miscarriage NOS
> Spontaneous abortion NOS

✔ Additional Character Required   `✓x7ᵗʰ` Placeholder   Questionable PDx   Manifestation   Unspecified Dx   `UPD` Unacceptable PDx   `H1`-`H14` HAC   `HCC` CMS-HCC Dx   `HIV` HIV Dx

ICD-10-CM 2022   **871**

✓4ᵗʰ O04　Complications following (induced) termination of pregnancy

> INCLUDES　complications following (induced) termination of pregnancy
>
> EXCLUDES 1　*encounter for elective termination of pregnancy, uncomplicated (Z33.2)*
> *failed attempted termination of pregnancy (O07.-)*

O04.5　Genital tract and pelvic infection following (induced) termination of pregnancy　CC M ♀
> Endometritis following (induced) termination of pregnancy
> Oophoritis following (induced) termination of pregnancy
> Parametritis following (induced) termination of pregnancy
> Pelvic peritonitis following (induced) termination of pregnancy
> Salpingitis following (induced) termination of pregnancy
> Salpingo-oophoritis following (induced) termination of pregnancy
>> EXCLUDES 1　*sepsis following (induced) termination of pregnancy (O04.87)*
>> *urinary tract infection following (induced) termination of pregnancy (O04.88)*

O04.6　Delayed or excessive hemorrhage following (induced) termination of pregnancy　M ♀
> Afibrinogenemia following (induced) termination of pregnancy
> Defibrination syndrome following (induced) termination of pregnancy
> Hemolysis following (induced) termination of pregnancy
> Intravascular coagulation following (induced) termination of pregnancy
> **AHA:** 2019,3Q,11

O04.7　Embolism following (induced) termination of pregnancy　MCC M ♀
> Air embolism following (induced) termination of pregnancy
> Amniotic fluid embolism following (induced) termination of pregnancy
> Blood-clot embolism following (induced) termination of pregnancy
> Embolism NOS following (induced) termination of pregnancy
> Fat embolism following (induced) termination of pregnancy
> Pulmonary embolism following (induced) termination of pregnancy
> Pyemic embolism following (induced) termination of pregnancy
> Septic or septicopyemic embolism following (induced) termination of pregnancy
> Soap embolism following (induced) termination of pregnancy

✓5ᵗʰ O04.8　(Induced) termination of pregnancy with other and unspecified complications

O04.80　(Induced) termination of pregnancy with unspecified complications　CC M ♀

O04.81　Shock following (induced) termination of pregnancy　MCC M ♀
> Circulatory collapse following (induced) termination of pregnancy
> Shock (postprocedural) following (induced) termination of pregnancy
>> EXCLUDES 1　*shock due to infection following (induced) termination of pregnancy (O04.87)*

O04.82　Renal failure following (induced) termination of pregnancy　MCC M ♀
> Kidney failure (acute) following (induced) termination of pregnancy
> Oliguria following (induced) termination of pregnancy
> Renal shutdown following (induced) termination of pregnancy
> Renal tubular necrosis following (induced) termination of pregnancy
> Uremia following (induced) termination of pregnancy

O04.83　Metabolic disorder following (induced) termination of pregnancy　CC M ♀

O04.84　Damage to pelvic organs following (induced) termination of pregnancy　CC M ♀
> Laceration, perforation, tear or chemical damage of bladder following (induced) termination of pregnancy
> Laceration, perforation, tear or chemical damage of bowel following (induced) termination of pregnancy
> Laceration, perforation, tear or chemical damage of broad ligament following (induced) termination of pregnancy
> Laceration, perforation, tear or chemical damage of cervix following (induced) termination of pregnancy
> Laceration, perforation, tear or chemical damage of periurethral tissue following (induced) termination of pregnancy
> Laceration, perforation, tear or chemical damage of uterus following (induced) termination of pregnancy
> Laceration, perforation, tear or chemical damage of vagina following (induced) termination of pregnancy

O04.85　Other venous complications following (induced) termination of pregnancy　CC M ♀

O04.86　Cardiac arrest following (induced) termination of pregnancy　CC M ♀

O04.87　Sepsis following (induced) termination of pregnancy　CC M ♀
> Use additional code to identify infectious agent (B95-B97)
> Use additional code to identify severe sepsis, if applicable (R65.2-)
>> EXCLUDES 1　*septic or septicopyemic embolism following (induced) termination of pregnancy (O04.7)*

O04.88　Urinary tract infection following (induced) termination of pregnancy　CC M ♀
> Cystitis following (induced) termination of pregnancy

O04.89　(Induced) termination of pregnancy with other complications　CC M ♀

✓4ᵗʰ O07　Failed attempted termination of pregnancy

> INCLUDES　failure of attempted induction of termination of pregnancy
> incomplete elective abortion
>
> EXCLUDES 1　*incomplete spontaneous abortion (O03.0-)*

O07.0　Genital tract and pelvic infection following failed attempted termination of pregnancy　CC M ♀
> Endometritis following failed attempted termination of pregnancy
> Oophoritis following failed attempted termination of pregnancy
> Parametritis following failed attempted termination of pregnancy
> Pelvic peritonitis following failed attempted termination of pregnancy
> Salpingitis following failed attempted termination of pregnancy
> Salpingo-oophoritis following failed attempted termination of pregnancy
>> EXCLUDES 1　*sepsis following failed attempted termination of pregnancy (O07.37)*
>> *urinary tract infection following failed attempted termination of pregnancy (O07.38)*

O07.1　Delayed or excessive hemorrhage following failed attempted termination of pregnancy　CC M ♀
> Afibrinogenemia following failed attempted termination of pregnancy
> Defibrination syndrome following failed attempted termination of pregnancy
> Hemolysis following failed attempted termination of pregnancy
> Intravascular coagulation following failed attempted termination of pregnancy

N Newborn: 0　P Pediatric: 0-17　M Maternity: 9-64　A Adult: 15-124　MCC Major Complication/Comorbidity　CC Complication/Comorbidity　SW Severe Wound Dx

872

ICD-10-CM 2022

O07.2   **Embolism following failed attempted termination of pregnancy**   MCC M ♀
>Air embolism following failed attempted termination of pregnancy
>Amniotic fluid embolism following failed attempted termination of pregnancy
>Blood-clot embolism following failed attempted termination of pregnancy
>Embolism NOS following failed attempted termination of pregnancy
>Fat embolism following failed attempted termination of pregnancy
>Pulmonary embolism following failed attempted termination of pregnancy
>Pyemic embolism following failed attempted termination of pregnancy
>Septic or septicopyemic embolism following failed attempted termination of pregnancy
>Soap embolism following failed attempted termination of pregnancy

✓6ᵗʰ **O07.3**   **Failed attempted termination of pregnancy with other and unspecified complications**

O07.30   **Failed attempted termination of pregnancy with unspecified complications**   CC M ♀

O07.31   **Shock following failed attempted termination of pregnancy**   MCC M ♀
>Circulatory collapse following failed attempted termination of pregnancy
>Shock (postprocedural) following failed attempted termination of pregnancy
>*EXCLUDES 1*   *shock due to infection following failed attempted termination of pregnancy (O07.37)*

O07.32   **Renal failure following failed attempted termination of pregnancy**   MCC M ♀
>Kidney failure (acute) following failed attempted termination of pregnancy
>Oliguria following failed attempted termination of pregnancy
>Renal shutdown following failed attempted termination of pregnancy
>Renal tubular necrosis following failed attempted termination of pregnancy
>Uremia following failed attempted termination of pregnancy

O07.33   **Metabolic disorder following failed attempted termination of pregnancy**   CC M ♀

O07.34   **Damage to pelvic organs following failed attempted termination of pregnancy**   CC M ♀
>Laceration, perforation, tear or chemical damage of bladder following failed attempted termination of pregnancy
>Laceration, perforation, tear or chemical damage of bowel following failed attempted termination of pregnancy
>Laceration, perforation, tear or chemical damage of broad ligament following failed attempted termination of pregnancy
>Laceration, perforation, tear or chemical damage of cervix following failed attempted termination of pregnancy
>Laceration, perforation, tear or chemical damage of periurethral tissue following failed attempted termination of pregnancy
>Laceration, perforation, tear or chemical damage of uterus following failed attempted termination of pregnancy
>Laceration, perforation, tear or chemical damage of vagina following failed attempted termination of pregnancy

O07.35   **Other venous complications following failed attempted termination of pregnancy**   CC M ♀

O07.36   **Cardiac arrest following failed attempted termination of pregnancy**   CC M ♀

O07.37   **Sepsis following failed attempted termination of pregnancy**   CC M ♀
>Use additional code (B95-B97), to identify infectious agent
>Use additional code (R65.2-) to identify severe sepsis, if applicable
>*EXCLUDES 1*   *septic or septicopyemic embolism following failed attempted termination of pregnancy (O07.2)*

O07.38   **Urinary tract infection following failed attempted termination of pregnancy**   CC M ♀
>Cystitis following failed attempted termination of pregnancy

O07.39   **Failed attempted termination of pregnancy with other complications**   CC M ♀

O07.4   **Failed attempted termination of pregnancy without complication**   M ♀

✓4ᵗʰ **O08**   **Complications following ectopic and molar pregnancy**
>This category is for use with categories O00-O02 to identify any associated complications

O08.0   **Genital tract and pelvic infection following ectopic and molar pregnancy**   CC M ♀
>Endometritis following ectopic and molar pregnancy
>Oophoritis following ectopic and molar pregnancy
>Parametritis following ectopic and molar pregnancy
>Pelvic peritonitis following ectopic and molar pregnancy
>Salpingitis following ectopic and molar pregnancy
>Salpingo-oophoritis following ectopic and molar pregnancy
>*EXCLUDES 1*   *sepsis following ectopic and molar pregnancy (O08.82)*
>*urinary tract infection (O08.83)*

O08.1   **Delayed or excessive hemorrhage following ectopic and molar pregnancy**   CC M ♀
>Afibrinogenemia following ectopic and molar pregnancy
>Defibrination syndrome following ectopic and molar pregnancy
>Hemolysis following ectopic and molar pregnancy
>Intravascular coagulation following ectopic and molar pregnancy
>*EXCLUDES 1*   *delayed or excessive hemorrhage due to incomplete abortion (O03.1)*

O08.2   **Embolism following ectopic and molar pregnancy**   MCC M ♀
>Air embolism following ectopic and molar pregnancy
>Amniotic fluid embolism following ectopic and molar pregnancy
>Blood-clot embolism following ectopic and molar pregnancy
>Embolism NOS following ectopic and molar pregnancy
>Fat embolism following ectopic and molar pregnancy
>Pulmonary embolism following ectopic and molar pregnancy
>Pyemic embolism following ectopic and molar pregnancy
>Septic or septicopyemic embolism following ectopic and molar pregnancy
>Soap embolism following ectopic and molar pregnancy

O08.3   **Shock following ectopic and molar pregnancy**   MCC M ♀
>Circulatory collapse following ectopic and molar pregnancy
>Shock (postprocedural) following ectopic and molar pregnancy
>*EXCLUDES 1*   *shock due to infection following ectopic and molar pregnancy (O08.82)*

O08.4   **Renal failure following ectopic and molar pregnancy**   MCC M ♀
>Kidney failure (acute) following ectopic and molar pregnancy
>Oliguria following ectopic and molar pregnancy
>Renal shutdown following ectopic and molar pregnancy
>Renal tubular necrosis following ectopic and molar pregnancy
>Uremia following ectopic and molar pregnancy

O08.5   **Metabolic disorders following an ectopic and molar pregnancy**   CC M ♀

✔ Additional Character Required   ✓ₓ7ᵗʰ Placeholder   Questionable PDx   Manifestation   Unspecified Dx   UPD Unacceptable PDx   H1-H14 HAC   HCC CMS-HCC Dx   HIV HIV Dx

ICD-10-CM 2022   873

O08.6 **Damage to pelvic organs and tissues** **following an ectopic and molar pregnancy** CC M ♀
Laceration, perforation, tear or chemical damage of bladder following an ectopic and molar pregnancy
Laceration, perforation, tear or chemical damage of bowel following an ectopic and molar pregnancy
Laceration, perforation, tear or chemical damage of broad ligament following an ectopic and molar pregnancy
Laceration, perforation, tear or chemical damage of cervix following an ectopic and molar pregnancy
Laceration, perforation, tear or chemical damage of periurethral tissue following an ectopic and molar pregnancy
Laceration, perforation, tear or chemical damage of uterus following an ectopic and molar pregnancy
Laceration, perforation, tear or chemical damage of vagina following an ectopic and molar pregnancy

O08.7 **Other venous complications following an ectopic and molar pregnancy** CC M ♀

√5ᵗʰ **O08.8** **Other complications following an ectopic and molar pregnancy**

O08.81 **Cardiac arrest following an ectopic and molar pregnancy** CC M ♀

O08.82 **Sepsis following ectopic and molar pregnancy** CC M ♀
Use additional code (B95-B97), to identify infectious agent
Use additional code (R65.2-) to identify severe sepsis, if applicable
EXCLUDES 1 *septic or septicopyemic embolism following ectopic and molar pregnancy (O08.2)*

O08.83 **Urinary tract infection following an ectopic and molar pregnancy** CC M ♀
Cystitis following an ectopic and molar pregnancy

O08.89 **Other complications following an ectopic and molar pregnancy**

O08.9 **Unspecified complication following an ectopic and molar pregnancy** CC M ♀

Supervision of high risk pregnancy (O09)

√4ᵗʰ **O09** **Supervision of high risk pregnancy**
AHA: 2019,3Q,5; 2016,4Q,48-50,150

√6ᵗʰ **O09.0** **Supervision of pregnancy with history of infertility**
DEF: Infertility: Inability to conceive for at least one year with regular intercourse.

O09.00 **Supervision of pregnancy with history of infertility, unspecified trimester** UPD M ♀

O09.01 **Supervision of pregnancy with history of infertility, first trimester** UPD M ♀

O09.02 **Supervision of pregnancy with history of infertility, second trimester** UPD M ♀

O09.03 **Supervision of pregnancy with history of infertility, third trimester** UPD M ♀

√5ᵗʰ **O09.1** **Supervision of pregnancy with history of ectopic pregnancy**
DEF: Ectopic pregnancy: Implantation of a fertilized egg outside the uterus, usually in the fallopian tube or abdomen that requires emergency treatment.

O09.10 **Supervision of pregnancy with history of ectopic pregnancy, unspecified trimester** UPD M ♀

O09.11 **Supervision of pregnancy with history of ectopic pregnancy, first trimester** UPD M ♀

O09.12 **Supervision of pregnancy with history of ectopic pregnancy, second trimester** UPD M ♀

O09.13 **Supervision of pregnancy with history of ectopic pregnancy, third trimester** UPD M ♀

√5ᵗʰ **O09.A** **Supervision of pregnancy with history of molar pregnancy**
DEF: Molar pregnancy: Trophoblastic neoplasm that mimics pregnancy by proliferating from a pathologic ovum and resulting only in a mass of cysts resembling grapes, 80 percent of which are benign, but require surgical removal.

O09.A0 **Supervision of pregnancy with history of molar pregnancy, unspecified trimester** UPD M ♀

O09.A1 **Supervision of pregnancy with history of molar pregnancy, first trimester** UPD M ♀

O09.A2 **Supervision of pregnancy with history of molar pregnancy, second trimester** UPD M ♀

O09.A3 **Supervision of pregnancy with history of molar pregnancy, third trimester** UPD M ♀

√5ᵗʰ **O09.2** **Supervision of pregnancy with other poor reproductive or obstetric history**
EXCLUDES 2 *pregnancy care for patient with history of recurrent pregnancy loss (O26.2-)*

√6ᵗʰ **O09.21** **Supervision of pregnancy with history of pre-term labor**

O09.211 **Supervision of pregnancy with history of pre-term labor, first trimester** UPD M ♀

O09.212 **Supervision of pregnancy with history of pre-term labor, second trimester** UPD M ♀

O09.213 **Supervision of pregnancy with history of pre-term labor, third trimester** UPD M ♀

O09.219 **Supervision of pregnancy with history of pre-term labor, unspecified trimester** UPD M ♀

√6ᵗʰ **O09.29** **Supervision of pregnancy with other poor reproductive or obstetric history**
Supervision of pregnancy with history of neonatal death
Supervision of pregnancy with history of stillbirth

O09.291 **Supervision of pregnancy with other poor reproductive or obstetric history, first trimester** UPD M ♀

O09.292 **Supervision of pregnancy with other poor reproductive or obstetric history, second trimester** UPD M ♀

O09.293 **Supervision of pregnancy with other poor reproductive or obstetric history, third trimester** UPD M ♀

O09.299 **Supervision of pregnancy with other poor reproductive or obstetric history, unspecified trimester** UPD M ♀

√5ᵗʰ **O09.3** **Supervision of pregnancy with insufficient antenatal care**
Supervision of concealed pregnancy
Supervision of hidden pregnancy

O09.30 **Supervision of pregnancy with insufficient antenatal care, unspecified trimester** UPD M ♀

O09.31 **Supervision of pregnancy with insufficient antenatal care, first trimester** UPD M ♀

O09.32 **Supervision of pregnancy with insufficient antenatal care, second trimester** UPD M ♀

O09.33 **Supervision of pregnancy with insufficient antenatal care, third trimester** UPD M ♀

√5ᵗʰ **O09.4** **Supervision of pregnancy with grand multiparity**

O09.40 **Supervision of pregnancy with grand multiparity, unspecified trimester** UPD M ♀

O09.41 **Supervision of pregnancy with grand multiparity, first trimester** UPD M ♀

O09.42 **Supervision of pregnancy with grand multiparity, second trimester** UPD M ♀

O09.43 **Supervision of pregnancy with grand multiparity, third trimester** UPD M ♀

√5ᵗʰ **O09.5** **Supervision of elderly primigravida and multigravida**
Pregnancy for a female 35 years and older at expected date of delivery

√6ᵗʰ **O09.51** **Supervision of elderly primigravida**

O09.511 **Supervision of elderly primigravida, first trimester** UPD M ♀

O09.512 **Supervision of elderly primigravida, second trimester** UPD M ♀

O09.513 **Supervision of elderly primigravida, third trimester** UPD M ♀

O09.519 **Supervision of elderly primigravida, unspecified trimester** UPD M ♀

√6ᵗʰ **O09.52** **Supervision of elderly multigravida**

O09.521 **Supervision of elderly multigravida, first trimester** UPD M ♀

O09.522 **Supervision of elderly multigravida, second trimester** UPD M ♀

O09.523 **Supervision of elderly multigravida, third trimester** UPD M ♀

O09.529 **Supervision of elderly multigravida, unspecified trimester** M ♀

☑5ᵗʰ O09.6 Supervision of young primigravida and multigravida
Supervision of pregnancy for a female less than 16 years old at expected date of delivery

  ☑6ᵗʰ O09.61 Supervision of young primigravida

    O09.611 **Supervision of young primigravida, first trimester** UPD M ♀

    O09.612 **Supervision of young primigravida, second trimester** UPD M ♀

    O09.613 **Supervision of young primigravida, third trimester** UPD M ♀

    O09.619 **Supervision of young primigravida, unspecified trimester** UPD M ♀

  ☑6ᵗʰ O09.62 Supervision of young multigravida

    O09.621 **Supervision of young multigravida, first trimester** UPD M ♀

    O09.622 **Supervision of young multigravida, second trimester** UPD M ♀

    O09.623 **Supervision of young multigravida, third trimester** UPD M ♀

    O09.629 **Supervision of young multigravida, unspecified trimester** UPD M ♀

☑5ᵗʰ O09.7 Supervision of high risk pregnancy due to social problems

    O09.70 **Supervision of high risk pregnancy due to social problems, unspecified trimester** UPD M ♀

    O09.71 **Supervision of high risk pregnancy due to social problems, first trimester** UPD M ♀

    O09.72 **Supervision of high risk pregnancy due to social problems, second trimester** UPD M ♀

    O09.73 **Supervision of high risk pregnancy due to social problems, third trimester** UPD M ♀

☑5ᵗʰ O09.8 Supervision of other high risk pregnancies

  ☑6ᵗʰ O09.81 Supervision of pregnancy resulting from assisted reproductive technology
Supervision of pregnancy resulting from in-vitro fertilization

    EXCLUDES 2   *gestational carrier status (Z33.3)*

    O09.811 **Supervision of pregnancy resulting from assisted reproductive technology, first trimester** UPD M ♀

    O09.812 **Supervision of pregnancy resulting from assisted reproductive technology, second trimester** UPD M ♀

    O09.813 **Supervision of pregnancy resulting from assisted reproductive technology, third trimester** UPD M ♀

    O09.819 **Supervision of pregnancy resulting from assisted reproductive technology, unspecified trimester** UPD M ♀

  ☑6ᵗʰ O09.82 Supervision of pregnancy with history of in utero procedure during previous pregnancy

    O09.821 **Supervision of pregnancy with history of in utero procedure during previous pregnancy, first trimester** UPD M ♀

    O09.822 **Supervision of pregnancy with history of in utero procedure during previous pregnancy, second trimester** UPD M ♀

    O09.823 **Supervision of pregnancy with history of in utero procedure during previous pregnancy, third trimester** UPD M ♀

    O09.829 **Supervision of pregnancy with history of in utero procedure during previous pregnancy, unspecified trimester** UPD M ♀

      EXCLUDES 1   *supervision of pregnancy affected by in utero procedure during current pregnancy (O35.7)*

  ☑6ᵗʰ O09.89 Supervision of other high risk pregnancies

    O09.891 **Supervision of other high risk pregnancies, first trimester** UPD M ♀

    O09.892 **Supervision of other high risk pregnancies, second trimester** UPD M ♀

    O09.893 **Supervision of other high risk pregnancies, third trimester** UPD M ♀

    O09.899 **Supervision of other high risk pregnancies, unspecified trimester** UPD M ♀

☑5ᵗʰ O09.9 Supervision of high risk pregnancy, unspecified

    O09.90 **Supervision of high risk pregnancy, unspecified, unspecified trimester** UPD M ♀

    O09.91 **Supervision of high risk pregnancy, unspecified, first trimester** UPD M ♀

    O09.92 **Supervision of high risk pregnancy, unspecified, second trimester** UPD M ♀

    O09.93 **Supervision of high risk pregnancy, unspecified, third trimester** UPD M ♀

Edema, proteinuria and hypertensive disorders in pregnancy, childbirth and the puerperium (O10-O16)

AHA: 2016,4Q,50

☑4ᵗʰ O10 Pre-existing hypertension complicating pregnancy, childbirth and the puerperium

  INCLUDES   pre-existing hypertension with pre-existing proteinuria complicating pregnancy, childbirth and the puerperium

  EXCLUDES 2   *pre-existing hypertension with superimposed pre-eclampsia complicating pregnancy, childbirth and the puerperium (O11.-)*

☑5ᵗʰ O10.0 Pre-existing essential hypertension complicating pregnancy, childbirth and the puerperium
Any condition in I10 specified as a reason for obstetric care during pregnancy, childbirth or the puerperium

  ☑6ᵗʰ O10.01 Pre-existing essential hypertension complicating pregnancy

    O10.011 **Pre-existing essential hypertension complicating pregnancy, first trimester** CC M ♀

    O10.012 **Pre-existing essential hypertension complicating pregnancy, second trimester** CC M ♀

    O10.013 **Pre-existing essential hypertension complicating pregnancy, third trimester** CC ♀

    O10.019 **Pre-existing essential hypertension complicating pregnancy, unspecified trimester** M ♀

    O10.02 **Pre-existing essential hypertension complicating childbirth** CC ♀

    O10.03 **Pre-existing essential hypertension complicating the puerperium** M ♀

☑5ᵗʰ O10.1 Pre-existing hypertensive heart disease complicating pregnancy, childbirth and the puerperium
Any condition in I11 specified as a reason for obstetric care during pregnancy, childbirth or the puerperium
Use additional code from I11 to identify the type of hypertensive heart disease

  ☑6ᵗʰ O10.11 Pre-existing hypertensive heart disease complicating pregnancy

    O10.111 **Pre-existing hypertensive heart disease complicating pregnancy, first trimester** M ♀

    O10.112 **Pre-existing hypertensive heart disease complicating pregnancy, second trimester** M ♀

    O10.113 **Pre-existing hypertensive heart disease complicating pregnancy, third trimester** M ♀

    O10.119 **Pre-existing hypertensive heart disease complicating pregnancy, unspecified trimester** M ♀

    O10.12 **Pre-existing hypertensive heart disease complicating childbirth** M ♀

    O10.13 **Pre-existing hypertensive heart disease complicating the puerperium** M ♀

☑5ᵗʰ O10.2 Pre-existing hypertensive chronic kidney disease complicating pregnancy, childbirth and the puerperium
Any condition in I12 specified as a reason for obstetric care during pregnancy, childbirth or the puerperium
Use additional code from I12 to identify the type of hypertensive chronic kidney disease

  ☑6ᵗʰ O10.21 Pre-existing hypertensive chronic kidney disease complicating pregnancy

    O10.211 **Pre-existing hypertensive chronic kidney disease complicating pregnancy, first trimester** M ♀

    O10.212 **Pre-existing hypertensive chronic kidney disease complicating pregnancy, second trimester** M ♀

Chapter 15. Pregnancy, Childbirth and the Puerperium

O10.213–O13.9

O10.213 Pre-existing hypertensive chronic kidney disease complicating pregnancy, **third trimester** Ⓜ♀

O10.219 Pre-existing hypertensive chronic kidney disease complicating pregnancy, **unspecified trimester** Ⓜ♀

O10.22 Pre-existing hypertensive chronic kidney disease complicating **childbirth** Ⓜ♀

O10.23 Pre-existing hypertensive chronic kidney disease complicating the **puerperium** Ⓜ♀

✓5ᵗʰ **O10.3** Pre-existing hypertensive heart and chronic kidney disease complicating pregnancy, childbirth and the puerperium
Any condition in I13 specified as a reason for obstetric care during pregnancy, childbirth or the puerperium
Use additional code from I13 to identify the type of hypertensive heart and chronic kidney disease

✓6ᵗʰ **O10.31** Pre-existing hypertensive heart and chronic kidney disease complicating **pregnancy**

O10.311 Pre-existing hypertensive heart and chronic kidney disease complicating pregnancy, **first trimester** Ⓜ♀

O10.312 Pre-existing hypertensive heart and chronic kidney disease complicating pregnancy, **second trimester** Ⓜ♀

O10.313 Pre-existing hypertensive heart and chronic kidney disease complicating pregnancy, **third trimester** Ⓜ♀

O10.319 Pre-existing hypertensive heart and chronic kidney disease complicating pregnancy, **unspecified trimester** Ⓜ♀

O10.32 Pre-existing hypertensive heart and chronic kidney disease complicating **childbirth** Ⓜ♀

O10.33 Pre-existing hypertensive heart and chronic kidney disease complicating the **puerperium** Ⓜ♀

✓5ᵗʰ **O10.4** Pre-existing **secondary** hypertension complicating pregnancy, childbirth and the puerperium
Any condition in I15 specified as a reason for obstetric care during pregnancy, childbirth or the puerperium
Use additional code from I15 to identify the type of secondary hypertension

✓6ᵗʰ **O10.41** Pre-existing secondary hypertension complicating **pregnancy**

O10.411 Pre-existing secondary hypertension complicating pregnancy, **first trimester** CC Ⓜ♀

O10.412 Pre-existing secondary hypertension complicating pregnancy, **second trimester** CC Ⓜ♀

O10.413 Pre-existing secondary hypertension complicating pregnancy, **third trimester** CC Ⓜ♀

O10.419 Pre-existing secondary hypertension complicating pregnancy, **unspecified trimester** Ⓜ♀

O10.42 Pre-existing secondary hypertension complicating **childbirth** MCC Ⓜ♀

O10.43 Pre-existing secondary hypertension complicating the **puerperium** CC Ⓜ♀

✓5ᵗʰ **O10.9** Unspecified pre-existing hypertension complicating pregnancy, childbirth and the puerperium

✓6ᵗʰ **O10.91** Unspecified pre-existing hypertension complicating **pregnancy**

O10.911 Unspecified pre-existing hypertension complicating pregnancy, **first trimester** CC Ⓜ♀

O10.912 Unspecified pre-existing hypertension complicating pregnancy, **second trimester** CC Ⓜ♀

O10.913 Unspecified pre-existing hypertension complicating pregnancy, **third trimester** CC Ⓜ♀

O10.919 Unspecified pre-existing hypertension complicating pregnancy, **unspecified trimester** Ⓜ♀

O10.92 Unspecified pre-existing hypertension complicating **childbirth** CC Ⓜ♀

O10.93 Unspecified pre-existing hypertension complicating the **puerperium** Ⓜ♀

✓4ᵗʰ **O11** Pre-existing **hypertension with pre-eclampsia**
INCLUDES conditions in O10 complicated by pre-eclampsia
pre-eclampsia superimposed pre-existing in hypertension
Use additional code from O10 to identify the type of hypertension
DEF: Complication of pregnancy manifesting in the development of borderline hypertension, protein in the urine, and unresponsive swelling between the 20th week of pregnancy and the end of the first week following birth in mild to moderate cases. Severe preeclampsia presents with hypertension, associated with marked swelling, proteinuria, abdominal pain, and/or visual changes.

O11.1 Pre-existing hypertension with pre-eclampsia, **first trimester** MCC Ⓜ♀

O11.2 Pre-existing hypertension with pre-eclampsia, **second trimester** MCC Ⓜ♀

O11.3 Pre-existing hypertension with pre-eclampsia, **third trimester** MCC Ⓜ♀

O11.4 Pre-existing hypertension with pre-eclampsia, complicating **childbirth** Ⓜ♀

O11.5 Pre-existing hypertension with pre-eclampsia, complicating the **puerperium** Ⓜ♀

O11.9 Pre-existing hypertension with pre-eclampsia, **unspecified trimester** Ⓜ♀

✓4ᵗʰ **O12** Gestational **[pregnancy-induced] edema and proteinuria** without **hypertension**

✓5ᵗʰ **O12.0** Gestational **edema**

O12.00 Gestational edema, unspecified trimester Ⓜ♀

O12.01 Gestational edema, **first trimester** Ⓜ♀

O12.02 Gestational edema, **second trimester** Ⓜ♀

O12.03 Gestational edema, **third trimester** Ⓜ♀

O12.04 Gestational edema, complicating **childbirth** Ⓜ♀

O12.05 Gestational edema, complicating the **puerperium** Ⓜ♀

✓5ᵗʰ **O12.1** Gestational **proteinuria**

O12.10 Gestational proteinuria, unspecified trimester Ⓜ♀

O12.11 Gestational proteinuria, **first trimester** CC Ⓜ♀

O12.12 Gestational proteinuria, **second trimester** CC Ⓜ♀

O12.13 Gestational proteinuria, **third trimester** CC Ⓜ♀

O12.14 Gestational proteinuria, complicating **childbirth** Ⓜ♀

O12.15 Gestational proteinuria, complicating the **puerperium** Ⓜ♀

✓5ᵗʰ **O12.2** Gestational **edema with proteinuria**

O12.20 Gestational edema with proteinuria, unspecified trimester Ⓜ♀

O12.21 Gestational edema with proteinuria, **first trimester** CC Ⓜ♀

O12.22 Gestational edema with proteinuria, **second trimester** CC Ⓜ♀

O12.23 Gestational edema with proteinuria, **third trimester** CC Ⓜ♀

O12.24 Gestational edema with proteinuria, complicating **childbirth** Ⓜ♀

O12.25 Gestational edema with proteinuria, complicating the **puerperium** Ⓜ♀

✓4ᵗʰ **O13** Gestational **[pregnancy-induced] hypertension without significant proteinuria**
INCLUDES gestational hypertension NOS
transient hypertension of pregnancy
AHA: 2016,1Q,5

O13.1 Gestational [pregnancy-induced] hypertension without significant proteinuria, **first trimester** Ⓜ♀

O13.2 Gestational [pregnancy-induced] hypertension without significant proteinuria, **second trimester** Ⓜ♀

O13.3 Gestational [pregnancy-induced] hypertension without significant proteinuria, **third trimester** Ⓜ♀

O13.4 Gestational [pregnancy-induced] hypertension without significant proteinuria, complicating **childbirth** Ⓜ♀

O13.5 Gestational [pregnancy-induced] hypertension without significant proteinuria, complicating the **puerperium** Ⓜ♀

O13.9 Gestational [pregnancy-induced] hypertension without significant proteinuria, **unspecified trimester** Ⓜ♀

Ⓝ Newborn: 0   Ⓟ Pediatric: 0-17   Ⓜ Maternity: 9-64   Ⓐ Adult: 15-124   MCC Major Complication/Comorbidity   CC Complication/Comorbidity   SW Severe Wound Dx

876   ICD-10-CM 2022

✓4ᵗʰ O14 Pre-eclampsia

> **EXCLUDES 1**   *pre-existing hypertension with pre-eclampsia (O11)*
>
> **DEF:** Complication of pregnancy manifesting in the development of borderline hypertension, protein in the urine, and unresponsive swelling between the 20th week of pregnancy and the end of the first week following birth in mild to moderate cases. Severe preeclampsia presents with hypertension, associated with marked swelling, proteinuria, abdominal pain, and/or visual changes.

✓5ᵗʰ O14.0 Mild to moderate pre-eclampsia

> **AHA:** 2019,3Q,12; 2019,2Q,8

- **O14.00** Mild to moderate pre-eclampsia, unspecified trimester   Ⓜ ♀
- **O14.02** Mild to moderate pre-eclampsia, second trimester   CC Ⓜ ♀
- **O14.03** Mild to moderate pre-eclampsia, third trimester   CC Ⓜ ♀
- **O14.04** Mild to moderate pre-eclampsia, complicating childbirth   Ⓜ ♀
  - **AHA:** 2019,2Q,8
- **O14.05** Mild to moderate pre-eclampsia, complicating the puerperium   Ⓜ ♀

✓5ᵗʰ O14.1 Severe pre-eclampsia

> **EXCLUDES 1**   *HELLP syndrome (O14.2-)*
>
> **AHA:** 2019,3Q,12

- **O14.10** Severe pre-eclampsia, unspecified trimester   Ⓜ ♀
- **O14.12** Severe pre-eclampsia, second trimester   MCC Ⓜ ♀
- **O14.13** Severe pre-eclampsia, third trimester   MCC Ⓜ ♀
- **O14.14** Severe pre-eclampsia complicating childbirth   Ⓜ ♀
- **O14.15** Severe pre-eclampsia, complicating the puerperium   Ⓜ ♀

✓6ᵗʰ O14.2 HELLP syndrome

> Severe pre-eclampsia with hemolysis, elevated liver enzymes and low platelet count (HELLP)
>
> **AHA:** 2019,3Q,12

- **O14.20** HELLP syndrome (HELLP), unspecified trimester   Ⓜ ♀
- **O14.22** HELLP syndrome (HELLP), second trimester   MCC Ⓜ ♀
- **O14.23** HELLP syndrome (HELLP), third trimester   MCC Ⓜ ♀
- **O14.24** HELLP syndrome, complicating childbirth   Ⓜ ♀
- **O14.25** HELLP syndrome, complicating the puerperium   Ⓜ ♀

✓5ᵗʰ O14.9 Unspecified pre-eclampsia

- **O14.90** Unspecified pre-eclampsia, unspecified trimester   Ⓜ ♀
- **O14.92** Unspecified pre-eclampsia, second trimester   CC Ⓜ ♀
- **O14.93** Unspecified pre-eclampsia, third trimester   CC Ⓜ ♀
- **O14.94** Unspecified pre-eclampsia, complicating childbirth   Ⓜ ♀
- **O14.95** Unspecified pre-eclampsia, complicating the puerperium   Ⓜ ♀

✓4ᵗʰ O15 Eclampsia

> **INCLUDES**   convulsions following conditions in O10-O14 and O16
>
> **DEF:** Tetany and toxemia producing seizure activity or coma in a pregnant patient who most often has presented with prior preeclampsia (i.e., hypertension, albuminuria, and edema).

✓5ᵗʰ O15.0 Eclampsia complicating pregnancy

- **O15.00** Eclampsia complicating pregnancy, unspecified trimester   Ⓜ ♀
- **O15.02** Eclampsia complicating pregnancy, second trimester   MCC Ⓜ ♀
- **O15.03** Eclampsia complicating pregnancy, third trimester   MCC Ⓜ ♀
- **O15.1** Eclampsia complicating labor   MCC Ⓜ ♀
- **O15.2** Eclampsia complicating the puerperium   MCC Ⓜ ♀
- **O15.9** Eclampsia, unspecified as to time period   Ⓜ ♀
  - Eclampsia NOS

✓4ᵗʰ O16 Unspecified maternal hypertension

- **O16.1** Unspecified maternal hypertension, first trimester   CC Ⓜ ♀
- **O16.2** Unspecified maternal hypertension, second trimester   CC Ⓜ ♀
- **O16.3** Unspecified maternal hypertension, third trimester   CC Ⓜ ♀
- **O16.4** Unspecified maternal hypertension, complicating childbirth   Ⓜ ♀
- **O16.5** Unspecified maternal hypertension, complicating the puerperium   Ⓜ ♀
- **O16.9** Unspecified maternal hypertension, unspecified trimester   Ⓜ ♀

Other maternal disorders predominantly related to pregnancy (O20-O29)

> **EXCLUDES 2**   *maternal care related to the fetus and amniotic cavity and possible delivery problems (O30-O48)*
> *maternal diseases classifiable elsewhere but complicating pregnancy, labor and delivery, and the puerperium (O98-O99)*

✓4ᵗʰ O20 Hemorrhage in early pregnancy

> **INCLUDES**   hemorrhage before completion of 20 weeks gestation
> **EXCLUDES 1**   *pregnancy with abortive outcome (O00-O08)*

- **O20.0** Threatened abortion   CC Ⓜ ♀
  - Hemorrhage specified as due to threatened abortion
  - **DEF:** Bloody discharge during pregnancy. The cervix may be dilated and pregnancy threatened, but the pregnancy is not terminated.
- **O20.8** Other hemorrhage in early pregnancy   Ⓜ ♀
- **O20.9** Hemorrhage in early pregnancy, unspecified   CC Ⓜ ♀

✓4ᵗʰ O21 Excessive vomiting in pregnancy

- **O21.0** Mild hyperemesis gravidarum   Ⓜ ♀
  - Hyperemesis gravidarum, mild or unspecified, starting before the end of the 20th week of gestation
- **O21.1** Hyperemesis gravidarum with metabolic disturbance   Ⓜ ♀
  - Hyperemesis gravidarum, starting before the end of the 20th week of gestation, with metabolic disturbance such as carbohydrate depletion
  - Hyperemesis gravidarum, starting before the end of the 20th week of gestation, with metabolic disturbance such as dehydration
  - Hyperemesis gravidarum, starting before the end of the 20th week of gestation, with metabolic disturbance such as electrolyte imbalance
- **O21.2** Late vomiting of pregnancy   Ⓜ ♀
  - Excessive vomiting starting after 20 completed weeks of gestation
- **O21.8** Other vomiting complicating pregnancy   Ⓜ ♀
  - Vomiting due to diseases classified elsewhere, complicating pregnancy
  - Use additional code, to identify cause
- **O21.9** Vomiting of pregnancy, unspecified   Ⓜ ♀

✓4ᵗʰ O22 Venous complications and hemorrhoids in pregnancy

> **EXCLUDES 1**   *venous complications of:*
> *abortion NOS (O03.9)*
> *ectopic or molar pregnancy (O08.7)*
> *failed attempted abortion (O07.35)*
> *induced abortion (O04.85)*
> *spontaneous abortion (O03.89)*
> **EXCLUDES 2**   *obstetric pulmonary embolism (O88.-)*
> *venous complications and hemorrhoids of childbirth and the puerperium (O87.-)*

✓5ᵗʰ O22.0 Varicose veins of lower extremity in pregnancy

> Varicose veins NOS in pregnancy
> **DEF:** Distended, tortuous veins of the lower extremities associated with pregnancy.

- **O22.00** Varicose veins of lower extremity in pregnancy, unspecified trimester   Ⓜ ♀
- **O22.01** Varicose veins of lower extremity in pregnancy, first trimester   Ⓜ ♀
- **O22.02** Varicose veins of lower extremity in pregnancy, second trimester   Ⓜ ♀
- **O22.03** Varicose veins of lower extremity in pregnancy, third trimester   Ⓜ ♀

✓5ᵗʰ O22.1 Genital varices in pregnancy

> Perineal varices in pregnancy
> Vaginal varices in pregnancy
> Vulval varices in pregnancy

- **O22.10** Genital varices in pregnancy, unspecified trimester   Ⓜ ♀
- **O22.11** Genital varices in pregnancy, first trimester   Ⓜ ♀
- **O22.12** Genital varices in pregnancy, second trimester   Ⓜ ♀

✔ Additional Character Required   ✓x7ᵗʰ Placeholder   Questionable PDx   Manifestation   Unspecified Dx   UPD Unacceptable PDx   H1-H14 HAC   HCC CMS-HCC Dx   HIV HIV Dx

ICD-10-CM 2022   877

Chapter 15. Pregnancy, Childbirth and the Puerperium

O14–O22.12

Chapter 15. Pregnancy, Childbirth and the Puerperium

O22.13 Genital varices in pregnancy, third trimester M ♀

✓5ᵗʰ O22.2 Superficial thrombophlebitis in pregnancy
Phlebitis in pregnancy NOS
Thrombophlebitis of legs in pregnancy
Thrombosis in pregnancy NOS
Use additional code to identify the superficial thrombophlebitis (I80.0-)

O22.20 Superficial thrombophlebitis in pregnancy, unspecified trimester cc M ♀

O22.21 Superficial thrombophlebitis in pregnancy, first trimester cc M ♀

O22.22 Superficial thrombophlebitis in pregnancy, second trimester cc M ♀

O22.23 Superficial thrombophlebitis in pregnancy, third trimester cc M ♀

✓6ᵗʰ O22.3 Deep phlebothrombosis in pregnancy
Deep vein thrombosis, antepartum
Use additional code to identify the deep vein thrombosis
▶(I82.4-, I82.5-, I82.62-, I82.72-)◀
Use additional code, if applicable, for associated long-term (current) use of anticoagulants (Z79.01)

O22.30 Deep phlebothrombosis in pregnancy, unspecified trimester cc M ♀

O22.31 Deep phlebothrombosis in pregnancy, first trimester MCC M ♀

O22.32 Deep phlebothrombosis in pregnancy, second trimester MCC M ♀

O22.33 Deep phlebothrombosis in pregnancy, third trimester MCC M ♀

✓5ᵗʰ O22.4 Hemorrhoids in pregnancy

O22.40 Hemorrhoids in pregnancy, unspecified trimester cc M ♀

O22.41 Hemorrhoids in pregnancy, first trimester cc M ♀

O22.42 Hemorrhoids in pregnancy, second trimester cc M ♀

O22.43 Hemorrhoids in pregnancy, third trimester cc M ♀

✓5ᵗʰ O22.5 Cerebral venous thrombosis in pregnancy
Cerebrovenous sinus thrombosis in pregnancy

O22.50 Cerebral venous thrombosis in pregnancy, unspecified trimester cc M ♀

O22.51 Cerebral venous thrombosis in pregnancy, first trimester cc M ♀

O22.52 Cerebral venous thrombosis in pregnancy, second trimester cc M ♀

O22.53 Cerebral venous thrombosis in pregnancy, third trimester cc M ♀

✓5ᵗʰ O22.8 Other venous complications in pregnancy

✓6ᵗʰ O22.8X Other venous complications in pregnancy

O22.8X1 Other venous complications in pregnancy, first trimester cc M ♀

O22.8X2 Other venous complications in pregnancy, second trimester cc M ♀

O22.8X3 Other venous complications in pregnancy, third trimester cc M ♀

O22.8X9 Other venous complications in pregnancy, unspecified trimester cc M ♀

✓5ᵗʰ O22.9 Venous complication in pregnancy, unspecified
Gestational phlebitis NOS
Gestational phlebopathy NOS
Gestational thrombosis NOS

O22.90 Venous complication in pregnancy, unspecified, unspecified trimester cc M ♀

O22.91 Venous complication in pregnancy, unspecified, first trimester M ♀

O22.92 Venous complication in pregnancy, unspecified, second trimester M ♀

O22.93 Venous complication in pregnancy, unspecified, third trimester M ♀

✓4ᵗʰ O23 Infections of genitourinary tract in pregnancy
Use additional code to identify organism (B95.-, B96.-)
EXCLUDES 2   gonococcal infections complicating pregnancy, childbirth and the puerperium (O98.2)
infections with a predominantly sexual mode of transmission NOS complicating pregnancy, childbirth and the puerperium (O98.3)
syphilis complicating pregnancy, childbirth and the puerperium (O98.1)
tuberculosis of genitourinary system complicating pregnancy, childbirth and the puerperium (O98.0)
venereal disease NOS complicating pregnancy, childbirth and the puerperium (O98.3)

AHA: 2018,2Q,20

✓5ᵗʰ O23.0 Infections of kidney in pregnancy
Pyelonephritis in pregnancy

O23.00 Infections of kidney in pregnancy, unspecified trimester M ♀

O23.01 Infections of kidney in pregnancy, first trimester cc M ♀

O23.02 Infections of kidney in pregnancy, second trimester cc M ♀

O23.03 Infections of kidney in pregnancy, third trimester cc M ♀

✓5ᵗʰ O23.1 Infections of bladder in pregnancy

O23.10 Infections of bladder in pregnancy, unspecified trimester M ♀

O23.11 Infections of bladder in pregnancy, first trimester cc M ♀

O23.12 Infections of bladder in pregnancy, second trimester cc M ♀

O23.13 Infections of bladder in pregnancy, third trimester cc M ♀

✓5ᵗʰ O23.2 Infections of urethra in pregnancy

O23.20 Infections of urethra in pregnancy, unspecified trimester M ♀

O23.21 Infections of urethra in pregnancy, first trimester cc M ♀

O23.22 Infections of urethra in pregnancy, second trimester cc M ♀

O23.23 Infections of urethra in pregnancy, third trimester cc M ♀

✓5ᵗʰ O23.3 Infections of other parts of urinary tract in pregnancy

O23.30 Infections of other parts of urinary tract in pregnancy, unspecified trimester M ♀

O23.31 Infections of other parts of urinary tract in pregnancy, first trimester cc M ♀

O23.32 Infections of other parts of urinary tract in pregnancy, second trimester cc M ♀

O23.33 Infections of other parts of urinary tract in pregnancy, third trimester cc M ♀

✓5ᵗʰ O23.4 Unspecified infection of urinary tract in pregnancy

O23.40 Unspecified infection of urinary tract in pregnancy, unspecified trimester M ♀

O23.41 Unspecified infection of urinary tract in pregnancy, first trimester cc M ♀

O23.42 Unspecified infection of urinary tract in pregnancy, second trimester cc M ♀

O23.43 Unspecified infection of urinary tract in pregnancy, third trimester cc M ♀

✓5ᵗʰ O23.5 Infections of the genital tract in pregnancy

✓6ᵗʰ O23.51 Infection of cervix in pregnancy

O23.511 Infections of cervix in pregnancy, first trimester cc M ♀

O23.512 Infections of cervix in pregnancy, second trimester cc ♀

O23.513 Infections of cervix in pregnancy, third trimester cc M ♀

O23.519 Infections of cervix in pregnancy, unspecified trimester M ♀

✓6ᵗʰ O23.52 Salpingo-oophoritis in pregnancy
Oophoritis in pregnancy
Salpingitis in pregnancy

O23.521 Salpingo-oophoritis in pregnancy, first trimester cc M ♀

O23.522 Salpingo-oophoritis in pregnancy, second trimester cc M ♀

      O23.523 **Salpingo-oophoritis in pregnancy, third trimester** cc M ♀

      O23.529 **Salpingo-oophoritis in pregnancy, unspecified trimester** M ♀

    ✓6ᵗʰ **O23.59** **Infection of other part of genital tract in pregnancy**

      O23.591 **Infection of other part of genital tract in pregnancy, first trimester** cc M ♀

      O23.592 **Infection of other part of genital tract in pregnancy, second trimester** cc M ♀

      O23.593 **Infection of other part of genital tract in pregnancy, third trimester** cc M ♀

      O23.599 **Infection of other part of genital tract in pregnancy, unspecified trimester** M ♀

  ✓5ᵗʰ **O23.9** **Unspecified genitourinary tract infection in pregnancy**

    Genitourinary tract infection in pregnancy NOS

    O23.90 **Unspecified genitourinary tract infection in pregnancy, unspecified trimester** M ♀

    O23.91 **Unspecified genitourinary tract infection in pregnancy, first trimester** cc M ♀

    O23.92 **Unspecified genitourinary tract infection in pregnancy, second trimester** cc M ♀

    O23.93 **Unspecified genitourinary tract infection in pregnancy, third trimester** cc M ♀

✓4ᵗʰ **O24** **Diabetes mellitus in pregnancy, childbirth and the puerperium**

  ✓5ᵗʰ **O24.0** **Pre-existing type 1 diabetes mellitus, in pregnancy, childbirth and the puerperium**

    Juvenile onset diabetes mellitus, in pregnancy, childbirth and the puerperium

    Ketosis-prone diabetes mellitus in pregnancy, childbirth and the puerperium

    Use additional code from category E10 to further identify any manifestations

    ✓6ᵗʰ **O24.01** **Pre-existing type 1 diabetes mellitus, in pregnancy**

      O24.011 **Pre-existing type 1 diabetes mellitus, in pregnancy, first trimester** cc M ♀

      O24.012 **Pre-existing type 1 diabetes mellitus, in pregnancy, second trimester** cc M ♀

      O24.013 **Pre-existing type 1 diabetes mellitus, in pregnancy, third trimester** cc M ♀

      O24.019 **Pre-existing type 1 diabetes mellitus, in pregnancy, unspecified trimester** cc M ♀

    O24.02 **Pre-existing type 1 diabetes mellitus, in childbirth** MCC M ♀

    O24.03 **Pre-existing type 1 diabetes mellitus, in the puerperium** cc M ♀

  ✓5ᵗʰ **O24.1** **Pre-existing type 2 diabetes mellitus, in pregnancy, childbirth and the puerperium**

    Insulin-resistant diabetes mellitus in pregnancy, childbirth and the puerperium

    Use additional code (for):

      from category E11 to further identify any manifestations

      long-term (current) use of insulin (Z79.4)

    ✓6ᵗʰ **O24.11** **Pre-existing type 2 diabetes mellitus, in pregnancy**

      O24.111 **Pre-existing type 2 diabetes mellitus, in pregnancy, first trimester** cc M ♀

      O24.112 **Pre-existing type 2 diabetes mellitus, in pregnancy, second trimester** cc M ♀

      O24.113 **Pre-existing type 2 diabetes mellitus, in pregnancy, third trimester** cc M ♀

      O24.119 **Pre-existing type 2 diabetes mellitus, in pregnancy, unspecified trimester** cc M ♀

    O24.12 **Pre-existing type 2 diabetes mellitus, in childbirth** MCC M ♀

    O24.13 **Pre-existing type 2 diabetes mellitus, in the puerperium** cc M ♀

  ✓5ᵗʰ **O24.3** **Unspecified pre-existing diabetes mellitus in pregnancy, childbirth and the puerperium**

    Use additional code (for):

      from category E11 to further identify any manifestation

      long-term (current) use of insulin (Z79.4)

    ✓6ᵗʰ **O24.31** **Unspecified pre-existing diabetes mellitus in pregnancy**

      O24.311 **Unspecified pre-existing diabetes mellitus in pregnancy, first trimester** cc M ♀

      O24.312 **Unspecified pre-existing diabetes mellitus in pregnancy, second trimester** cc M ♀

      O24.313 **Unspecified pre-existing diabetes mellitus in pregnancy, third trimester** cc M ♀

      O24.319 **Unspecified pre-existing diabetes mellitus in pregnancy, unspecified trimester** cc M ♀

    O24.32 **Unspecified pre-existing diabetes mellitus in childbirth** MCC M ♀

    O24.33 **Unspecified pre-existing diabetes mellitus in the puerperium** cc M ♀

  ✓5ᵗʰ **O24.4** **Gestational diabetes mellitus**

    Diabetes mellitus arising in pregnancy

    Gestational diabetes mellitus NOS

    AHA: 2020,3Q,30; 2016,4Q,50; 2015,4Q,34

    ✓6ᵗʰ **O24.41** **Gestational diabetes mellitus in pregnancy**

      O24.410 **Gestational diabetes mellitus in pregnancy, diet controlled** M ♀

      O24.414 **Gestational diabetes mellitus in pregnancy, insulin controlled** M ♀

      O24.415 **Gestational diabetes mellitus in pregnancy, controlled by oral hypoglycemic drugs** M ♀

        Gestational diabetes mellitus in pregnancy, controlled by oral antidiabetic drugs

      O24.419 **Gestational diabetes mellitus in pregnancy, unspecified control** M ♀

    ✓6ᵗʰ **O24.42** **Gestational diabetes mellitus in childbirth**

      AHA: 2016,1Q,5

      O24.420 **Gestational diabetes mellitus in childbirth, diet controlled** M ♀

      O24.424 **Gestational diabetes mellitus in childbirth, insulin controlled** M ♀

      O24.425 **Gestational diabetes mellitus in childbirth, controlled by oral hypoglycemic drugs** M ♀

        Gestational diabetes mellitus in childbirth, controlled by oral antidiabetic drugs

      O24.429 **Gestational diabetes mellitus in childbirth, unspecified control** M ♀

    ✓6ᵗʰ **O24.43** **Gestational diabetes mellitus in the puerperium**

      O24.430 **Gestational diabetes mellitus in the puerperium, diet controlled** M ♀

      O24.434 **Gestational diabetes mellitus in the puerperium, insulin controlled** M ♀

      O24.435 **Gestational diabetes mellitus in puerperium, controlled by oral hypoglycemic drugs** M ♀

        Gestational diabetes mellitus in puerperium, controlled by oral antidiabetic drugs

      O24.439 **Gestational diabetes mellitus in the puerperium, unspecified control** M ♀

  ✓5ᵗʰ **O24.8** **Other pre-existing diabetes mellitus in pregnancy, childbirth, and the puerperium**

    Use additional code (for):

      from categories E08, E09 and E13 to further identify any manifestation

      long-term (current) use of insulin (Z79.4)

    ✓6ᵗʰ **O24.81** **Other pre-existing diabetes mellitus in pregnancy**

      O24.811 **Other pre-existing diabetes mellitus in pregnancy, first trimester** cc M ♀

      O24.812 **Other pre-existing diabetes mellitus in pregnancy, second trimester** cc M ♀

      O24.813 **Other pre-existing diabetes mellitus in pregnancy, third trimester** cc M ♀

      O24.819 **Other pre-existing diabetes mellitus in pregnancy, unspecified trimester** cc M ♀

    O24.82 **Other pre-existing diabetes mellitus in childbirth** MCC M ♀

    O24.83 **Other pre-existing diabetes mellitus in the puerperium** cc M ♀

✔ Additional Character Required   ✓x7ᵗʰ Placeholder   Questionable PDx   Manifestation   Unspecified Dx   UPD Unacceptable PDx   H1-H14 HAC   HCC CMS-HCC Dx   HIV HIV Dx

ICD-10-CM 2022   879

Chapter 15. Pregnancy, Childbirth and the Puerperium

O24.9–O26.842

√5ᵗʰ **O24.9** **Unspecified diabetes mellitus in pregnancy, childbirth and the puerperium**
Use additional code for long-term (current) use of insulin (Z79.4)

√6ᵗʰ **O24.91** **Unspecified diabetes mellitus in** pregnancy

O24.911 **Unspecified diabetes mellitus in pregnancy,** first trimester   cc M ♀

O24.912 **Unspecified diabetes mellitus in pregnancy,** second trimester   cc M ♀

O24.913 **Unspecified diabetes mellitus in pregnancy,** third trimester   cc M ♀

O24.919 **Unspecified diabetes mellitus in pregnancy, unspecified trimester**   cc M ♀

O24.92 **Unspecified diabetes mellitus in** childbirth   M ♀

O24.93 **Unspecified diabetes mellitus in the** puerperium   cc M ♀

√4ᵗʰ **O25** **Malnutrition in pregnancy, childbirth and the puerperium**

√5ᵗʰ **O25.1** **Malnutrition in** pregnancy

O25.10 **Malnutrition in pregnancy, unspecified trimester**   M ♀

O25.11 **Malnutrition in pregnancy,** first trimester   M ♀

O25.12 **Malnutrition in pregnancy,** second trimester   M ♀

O25.13 **Malnutrition in pregnancy,** third trimester   M ♀

O25.2 **Malnutrition in** childbirth   M ♀

O25.3 **Malnutrition in the** puerperium   M ♀

√4ᵗʰ **O26** **Maternal care for other conditions predominantly related to pregnancy**

√5ᵗʰ **O26.0** **Excessive weight gain in pregnancy**
EXCLUDES 2   gestational edema (O12.0, O12.2)

O26.00 **Excessive weight gain in pregnancy, unspecified trimester**   M ♀

O26.01 **Excessive weight gain in pregnancy,** first trimester   M ♀

O26.02 **Excessive weight gain in pregnancy,** second trimester   M ♀

O26.03 **Excessive weight gain in pregnancy,** third trimester   M ♀

√5ᵗʰ **O26.1** **Low weight gain in pregnancy**

O26.10 **Low weight gain in pregnancy, unspecified trimester**   M ♀

O26.11 **Low weight gain in pregnancy,** first trimester   M ♀

O26.12 **Low weight gain in pregnancy,** second trimester   M ♀

O26.13 **Low weight gain in pregnancy,** third trimester   M ♀

√5ᵗʰ **O26.2** **Pregnancy care for patient with recurrent pregnancy loss**

O26.20 **Pregnancy care for patient with recurrent pregnancy loss, unspecified trimester**   M ♀

O26.21 **Pregnancy care for patient with recurrent pregnancy loss,** first trimester   M ♀

O26.22 **Pregnancy care for patient with recurrent pregnancy loss,** second trimester   M ♀

O26.23 **Pregnancy care for patient with recurrent pregnancy loss,** third trimester   M ♀

√5ᵗʰ **O26.3** **Retained intrauterine contraceptive device in pregnancy**

O26.30 **Retained intrauterine contraceptive device in pregnancy, unspecified trimester**   M ♀

O26.31 **Retained intrauterine contraceptive device in pregnancy,** first trimester   M ♀

O26.32 **Retained intrauterine contraceptive device in pregnancy,** second trimester   M ♀

O26.33 **Retained intrauterine contraceptive device in pregnancy,** third trimester   M ♀

√5ᵗʰ **O26.4** **Herpes gestationis**
DEF: Rare skin disorder of unknown origin that appears on the abdomen in the second and third trimester as intensely itchy blisters that spread to other sites.

O26.40 **Herpes gestationis, unspecified trimester**   M ♀

O26.41 **Herpes gestationis,** first trimester   M ♀

O26.42 **Herpes gestationis,** second trimester   M ♀

O26.43 **Herpes gestationis,** third trimester   M ♀

√5ᵗʰ **O26.5** **Maternal hypotension syndrome**
Supine hypotensive syndrome

O26.50 **Maternal hypotension syndrome, unspecified trimester**   M ♀

O26.51 **Maternal hypotension syndrome,** first trimester   M ♀

O26.52 **Maternal hypotension syndrome,** second trimester   M ♀

O26.53 **Maternal hypotension syndrome,** third trimester   M ♀

√5ᵗʰ **O26.6** **Liver and biliary tract disorders in pregnancy, childbirth and the puerperium**
Use additional code to identify the specific disorder
EXCLUDES 2   hepatorenal syndrome following labor and delivery (O90.4)

√6ᵗʰ **O26.61** **Liver and biliary tract disorders in** pregnancy

O26.611 **Liver and biliary tract disorders in pregnancy,** first trimester   cc M ♀

O26.612 **Liver and biliary tract disorders in pregnancy,** second trimester   cc M ♀

O26.613 **Liver and biliary tract disorders in pregnancy,** third trimester   cc M ♀

O26.619 **Liver and biliary tract disorders in pregnancy, unspecified trimester**   M ♀

O26.62 **Liver and biliary tract disorders in** childbirth   cc M ♀

O26.63 **Liver and biliary tract disorders in the** puerperium   M ♀

√5ᵗʰ **O26.7** **Subluxation of symphysis (pubis) in pregnancy, childbirth and the puerperium**
EXCLUDES 1   traumatic separation of symphysis (pubis) during childbirth (O71.6)

√6ᵗʰ **O26.71** **Subluxation of symphysis (pubis) in** pregnancy

O26.711 **Subluxation of symphysis (pubis) in pregnancy,** first trimester   M ♀

O26.712 **Subluxation of symphysis (pubis) in pregnancy,** second trimester   M ♀

O26.713 **Subluxation of symphysis (pubis) in pregnancy,** third trimester   M ♀

O26.719 **Subluxation of symphysis (pubis) in pregnancy, unspecified trimester**   M ♀

O26.72 **Subluxation of symphysis (pubis) in** childbirth   M ♀

O26.73 **Subluxation of symphysis (pubis) in the** puerperium   M ♀

√5ᵗʰ **O26.8** **Other specified pregnancy related conditions**

√6ᵗʰ **O26.81** **Pregnancy related exhaustion and fatigue**

O26.811 **Pregnancy related exhaustion and fatigue,** first trimester   M ♀

O26.812 **Pregnancy related exhaustion and fatigue,** second trimester   M ♀

O26.813 **Pregnancy related exhaustion and fatigue,** third trimester   M ♀

O26.819 **Pregnancy related exhaustion and fatigue, unspecified trimester**   M ♀

√6ᵗʰ **O26.82** **Pregnancy related peripheral neuritis**

O26.821 **Pregnancy related peripheral neuritis,** first trimester   M ♀

O26.822 **Pregnancy related peripheral neuritis,** second trimester   M ♀

O26.823 **Pregnancy related peripheral neuritis,** third trimester   M ♀

O26.829 **Pregnancy related peripheral neuritis, unspecified trimester**   M ♀

√6ᵗʰ **O26.83** **Pregnancy related renal disease**
Use additional code to identify the specific disorder

O26.831 **Pregnancy related renal disease,** first trimester   cc M ♀

O26.832 **Pregnancy related renal disease,** second trimester   cc M ♀

O26.833 **Pregnancy related renal disease,** third trimester   cc M ♀

O26.839 **Pregnancy related renal disease, unspecified trimester**   M ♀

√6ᵗʰ **O26.84** **Uterine size-date discrepancy complicating pregnancy**
EXCLUDES 1   encounter for suspected problem with fetal growth ruled out (Z03.74)

O26.841 **Uterine size-date discrepancy,** first trimester   M ♀

O26.842 **Uterine size-date discrepancy,** second trimester   M ♀

N Newborn: 0   P Pediatric: 0-17   M Maternity: 9-64   A Adult: 15-124   MCC Major Complication/Comorbidity   CC Complication/Comorbidity   SW Severe Wound Dx

880   ICD-10-CM 2022

O26.843 Uterine size-date discrepancy, third trimester   M ♀

O26.849 Uterine size-date discrepancy, unspecified trimester   M ♀

√6ᵗʰ **O26.85** Spotting complicating pregnancy

O26.851 Spotting complicating pregnancy, first trimester   M ♀

O26.852 Spotting complicating pregnancy, second trimester   M ♀

O26.853 Spotting complicating pregnancy, third trimester   M ♀

O26.859 Spotting complicating pregnancy, unspecified trimester   M ♀

O26.86 Pruritic urticarial papules and plaques of pregnancy (PUPPP)   M ♀

Polymorphic eruption of pregnancy

√6ᵗʰ **O26.87** Cervical shortening

EXCLUDES 1   *encounter for suspected cervical shortening ruled out (Z03.75)*

DEF: Cervix that has shortened to less than 25 mm before the 24th week of pregnancy. A shortened cervix is a warning sign for impending premature delivery and is treated by cervical cerclage placement or progesterone.

O26.872 Cervical shortening, second trimester   CC M ♀

O26.873 Cervical shortening, third trimester   CC M ♀

O26.879 Cervical shortening, unspecified trimester   CC M ♀

√6ᵗʰ **O26.89** Other specified pregnancy related conditions

AHA: 2015,3Q,40

O26.891 Other specified pregnancy related conditions, first trimester   M ♀

O26.892 Other specified pregnancy related conditions, second trimester   M ♀

O26.893 Other specified pregnancy related conditions, third trimester   M ♀

O26.899 Other specified pregnancy related conditions, unspecified trimester   M ♀

√5ᵗʰ **O26.9** Pregnancy related conditions, unspecified

O26.90 Pregnancy related conditions, unspecified, unspecified trimester   M ♀

O26.91 Pregnancy related conditions, unspecified, first trimester   M ♀

O26.92 Pregnancy related conditions, unspecified, second trimester   M ♀

O26.93 Pregnancy related conditions, unspecified, third trimester   M ♀

√4ᵗʰ **O28** Abnormal findings on antenatal screening of mother

EXCLUDES 1   *diagnostic findings classified elsewhere - see Alphabetical Index*

O28.0 Abnormal hematological finding on antenatal screening of mother   M ♀

O28.1 Abnormal biochemical finding on antenatal screening of mother   M ♀

O28.2 Abnormal cytological finding on antenatal screening of mother   M ♀

O28.3 Abnormal ultrasonic finding on antenatal screening of mother   M ♀

O28.4 Abnormal radiological finding on antenatal screening of mother   M ♀

O28.5 Abnormal chromosomal and genetic finding on antenatal screening of mother   M ♀

O28.8 Other abnormal findings on antenatal screening of mother   M ♀

O28.9 Unspecified abnormal findings on antenatal screening of mother   M ♀

√4ᵗʰ **O29** Complications of anesthesia during pregnancy

INCLUDES   maternal complications arising from the administration of a general, regional or local anesthetic, analgesic or other sedation during pregnancy

Use additional code, if necessary, to identify the complication

EXCLUDES 2   *complications of anesthesia during labor and delivery (O74.-)*
complications of anesthesia during the puerperium (O89.-)

√5ᵗʰ **O29.0** Pulmonary complications of anesthesia during pregnancy

√6ᵗʰ **O29.01** Aspiration pneumonitis due to anesthesia during pregnancy

Inhalation of stomach contents or secretions NOS due to anesthesia during pregnancy

Mendelson's syndrome due to anesthesia during pregnancy

O29.011 Aspiration pneumonitis due to anesthesia during pregnancy, first trimester   M ♀

O29.012 Aspiration pneumonitis due to anesthesia during pregnancy, second trimester   M ♀

O29.013 Aspiration pneumonitis due to anesthesia during pregnancy, third trimester   M ♀

O29.019 Aspiration pneumonitis due to anesthesia during pregnancy, unspecified trimester   M ♀

√6ᵗʰ **O29.02** Pressure collapse of lung due to anesthesia during pregnancy

O29.021 Pressure collapse of lung due to anesthesia during pregnancy, first trimester   M ♀

O29.022 Pressure collapse of lung due to anesthesia during pregnancy, second trimester   M ♀

O29.023 Pressure collapse of lung due to anesthesia during pregnancy, third trimester   M ♀

O29.029 Pressure collapse of lung due to anesthesia during pregnancy, unspecified trimester   M ♀

√6ᵗʰ **O29.09** Other pulmonary complications of anesthesia during pregnancy

O29.091 Other pulmonary complications of anesthesia during pregnancy, first trimester   M ♀

O29.092 Other pulmonary complications of anesthesia during pregnancy, second trimester   M ♀

O29.093 Other pulmonary complications of anesthesia during pregnancy, third trimester   M ♀

O29.099 Other pulmonary complications of anesthesia during pregnancy, unspecified trimester   M ♀

√5ᵗʰ **O29.1** Cardiac complications of anesthesia during pregnancy

√6ᵗʰ **O29.11** Cardiac arrest due to anesthesia during pregnancy

O29.111 Cardiac arrest due to anesthesia during pregnancy, first trimester   M ♀

O29.112 Cardiac arrest due to anesthesia during pregnancy, second trimester   M ♀

O29.113 Cardiac arrest due to anesthesia during pregnancy, third trimester   M ♀

O29.119 Cardiac arrest due to anesthesia during pregnancy, unspecified trimester   M ♀

√6ᵗʰ **O29.12** Cardiac failure due to anesthesia during pregnancy

O29.121 Cardiac failure due to anesthesia during pregnancy, first trimester   M ♀

O29.122 Cardiac failure due to anesthesia during pregnancy, second trimester   M ♀

O29.123 Cardiac failure due to anesthesia during pregnancy, third trimester   M ♀

O29.129 Cardiac failure due to anesthesia during pregnancy, unspecified trimester   M ♀

√6ᵗʰ **O29.19** Other cardiac complications of anesthesia during pregnancy

O29.191 Other cardiac complications of anesthesia during pregnancy, first trimester   M ♀

O29.192 Other cardiac complications of anesthesia during pregnancy, second trimester   M ♀

O29.193 Other cardiac complications of anesthesia during pregnancy, third trimester   M ♀

☑ Additional Character Required   ✓ₓ7ᵗʰ Placeholder   Questionable PDx   Manifestation   Unspecified Dx   UPD Unacceptable PDx   H1-H16 HAC   HCC CMS-HCC Dx   HIV HIV Dx

ICD-10-CM 2022   881

Chapter 15. Pregnancy, Childbirth and the Puerperium

029.199–030.029

O29.199   Other cardiac complications of anesthesia during pregnancy, unspecified trimester   M ♀

√5th   O29.2   Central nervous system complications of anesthesia during pregnancy

    √6th   O29.21   Cerebral anoxia due to anesthesia during pregnancy

       O29.211   Cerebral anoxia due to anesthesia during pregnancy, first trimester   M ♀

       O29.212   Cerebral anoxia due to anesthesia during pregnancy, second trimester   M ♀

       O29.213   Cerebral anoxia due to anesthesia during pregnancy, third trimester   M ♀

       O29.219   Cerebral anoxia due to anesthesia during pregnancy, unspecified trimester   M ♀

    √6th   O29.29   Other central nervous system complications of anesthesia during pregnancy

       O29.291   Other central nervous system complications of anesthesia during pregnancy, first trimester   M ♀

       O29.292   Other central nervous system complications of anesthesia during pregnancy, second trimester   M ♀

       O29.293   Other central nervous system complications of anesthesia during pregnancy, third trimester   M ♀

       O29.299   Other central nervous system complications of anesthesia during pregnancy, unspecified trimester   M ♀

√5th   O29.3   Toxic reaction to local anesthesia during pregnancy

    √6th   O29.3X   Toxic reaction to local anesthesia during pregnancy

       O29.3X1   Toxic reaction to local anesthesia during pregnancy, first trimester   M ♀

       O29.3X2   Toxic reaction to local anesthesia during pregnancy, second trimester   M ♀

       O29.3X3   Toxic reaction to local anesthesia during pregnancy, third trimester   M ♀

       O29.3X9   Toxic reaction to local anesthesia during pregnancy, unspecified trimester   M ♀

√5th   O29.4   Spinal and epidural anesthesia induced headache during pregnancy

    O29.40   Spinal and epidural anesthesia induced headache during pregnancy, unspecified trimester   M ♀

    O29.41   Spinal and epidural anesthesia induced headache during pregnancy, first trimester   M ♀

    O29.42   Spinal and epidural anesthesia induced headache during pregnancy, second trimester   M ♀

    O29.43   Spinal and epidural anesthesia induced headache during pregnancy, third trimester   M ♀

√5th   O29.5   Other complications of spinal and epidural anesthesia during pregnancy

    √6th   O29.5X   Other complications of spinal and epidural anesthesia during pregnancy

       O29.5X1   Other complications of spinal and epidural anesthesia during pregnancy, first trimester   M ♀

       O29.5X2   Other complications of spinal and epidural anesthesia during pregnancy, second trimester   M ♀

       O29.5X3   Other complications of spinal and epidural anesthesia during pregnancy, third trimester   M ♀

       O29.5X9   Other complications of spinal and epidural anesthesia during pregnancy, unspecified trimester   M ♀

√5th   O29.6   Failed or difficult intubation for anesthesia during pregnancy

    O29.60   Failed or difficult intubation for anesthesia during pregnancy, unspecified trimester   M ♀

    O29.61   Failed or difficult intubation for anesthesia during pregnancy, first trimester   M ♀

    O29.62   Failed or difficult intubation for anesthesia during pregnancy, second trimester   M ♀

    O29.63   Failed or difficult intubation for anesthesia during pregnancy, third trimester   M ♀

√5th   O29.8   Other complications of anesthesia during pregnancy

    √6th   O29.8X   Other complications of anesthesia during pregnancy

       O29.8X1   Other complications of anesthesia during pregnancy, first trimester   M ♀

       O29.8X2   Other complications of anesthesia during pregnancy, second trimester   M ♀

       O29.8X3   Other complications of anesthesia during pregnancy, third trimester   M ♀

       O29.8X9   Other complications of anesthesia during pregnancy, unspecified trimester   M ♀

√5th   O29.9   Unspecified complication of anesthesia during pregnancy

    O29.90   Unspecified complication of anesthesia during pregnancy, unspecified trimester   M ♀

    O29.91   Unspecified complication of anesthesia during pregnancy, first trimester   M ♀

    O29.92   Unspecified complication of anesthesia during pregnancy, second trimester   M ♀

    O29.93   Unspecified complication of anesthesia during pregnancy, third trimester   M ♀

Maternal care related to the fetus and amniotic cavity and possible delivery problems (O30-O48)

√4th   **O30**   **Multiple gestation**

    Code also any complications specific to multiple gestation

    AHA: 2016,4Q,51

    √5th   O30.0   Twin pregnancy

      √6th   O30.00   Twin pregnancy, unspecified number of placenta and unspecified number of amniotic sacs

        O30.001   Twin pregnancy, unspecified number of placenta and unspecified number of amniotic sacs, first trimester   M ♀

        O30.002   Twin pregnancy, unspecified number of placenta and unspecified number of amniotic sacs, second trimester   M ♀

        O30.003   Twin pregnancy, unspecified number of placenta and unspecified number of amniotic sacs, third trimester   M ♀

        O30.009   Twin pregnancy, unspecified number of placenta and unspecified number of amniotic sacs, unspecified trimester   M ♀

      √6th   O30.01   Twin pregnancy, monochorionic/monoamniotic

        Twin pregnancy, one placenta, one amniotic sac

        EXCLUDES 1   conjoined twins (O30.02-)

Twin Gestation – Monochorionic/Monoamniotic

- 1 Chorionic sac
- 1 Amniotic sac
- 2 Fetuses
- 2 Umbilical cords
- 1 Placenta

        O30.011   Twin pregnancy, monochorionic/monoamniotic, first trimester   M ♀

        O30.012   Twin pregnancy, monochorionic/monoamniotic, second trimester   M ♀

        O30.013   Twin pregnancy, monochorionic/monoamniotic, third trimester   M ♀

        O30.019   Twin pregnancy, monochorionic/monoamniotic, unspecified trimester   M ♀

      √6th   O30.02   Conjoined twin pregnancy

        O30.021   Conjoined twin pregnancy, first trimester   M ♀

        O30.022   Conjoined twin pregnancy, second trimester   M ♀

        O30.023   Conjoined twin pregnancy, third trimester   M ♀

        O30.029   Conjoined twin pregnancy, unspecified trimester   M ♀

N Newborn: 0   P Pediatric: 0-17   M Maternity: 9-64   A Adult: 15-124   MCC Major Complication/Comorbidity   CC Complication/Comorbidity   SW Severe Wound Dx

882   ICD-10-CM 2022

✓6th **O30.03**   **Twin pregnancy,** monochorionic/diamniotic
Twin pregnancy, one placenta, two amniotic sacs

Twin Gestation – Monochorionic/Diamniotic

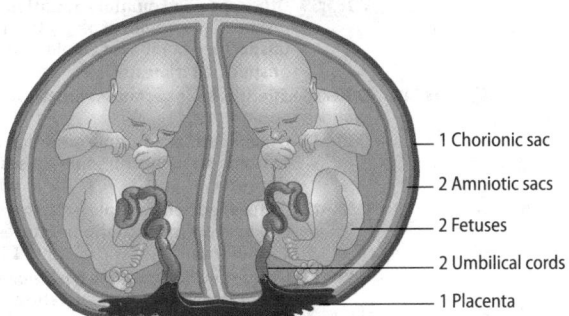

— 1 Chorionic sac
— 2 Amniotic sacs
— 2 Fetuses
— 2 Umbilical cords
— 1 Placenta

O30.031   Twin pregnancy, monochorionic/diamniotic, first trimester   M ♀

O30.032   Twin pregnancy, monochorionic/diamniotic, second trimester   M ♀

O30.033   Twin pregnancy, monochorionic/diamniotic, third trimester   M ♀

O30.039   Twin pregnancy, monochorionic/diamniotic, unspecified trimester   M ♀

✓6th **O30.04**   **Twin pregnancy,** dichorionic/diamniotic
Twin pregnancy, two placentae, two amniotic sacs

Twin Gestation – Dichorionic/Diamniotic

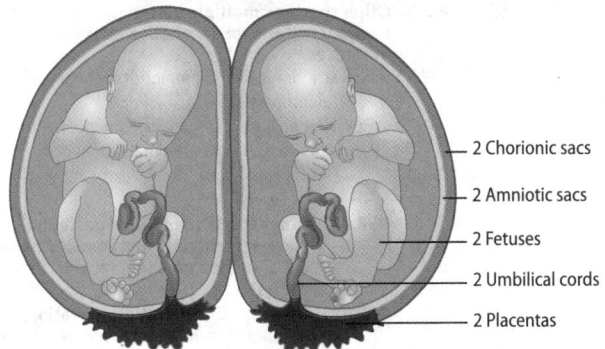

— 2 Chorionic sacs
— 2 Amniotic sacs
— 2 Fetuses
— 2 Umbilical cords
— 2 Placentas

O30.041   Twin pregnancy, dichorionic/diamniotic, first trimester   M ♀

O30.042   Twin pregnancy, dichorionic/diamniotic, second trimester   M ♀

O30.043   Twin pregnancy, dichorionic/diamniotic, third trimester   M ♀

O30.049   Twin pregnancy, dichorionic/diamniotic, unspecified trimester   M ♀

✓6th **O30.09**   **Twin pregnancy,** unable to determine number of placenta and number of amniotic sacs

O30.091   Twin pregnancy, unable to determine number of placenta and number of amniotic sacs, first trimester   M ♀

O30.092   Twin pregnancy, unable to determine number of placenta and number of amniotic sacs, second trimester   M ♀

O30.093   Twin pregnancy, unable to determine number of placenta and number of amniotic sacs, third trimester   M ♀

O30.099   Twin pregnancy, unable to determine number of placenta and number of amniotic sacs, unspecified trimester   M ♀

✓5th **O30.1**   **Triplet** pregnancy

✓6th **O30.10**   **Triplet pregnancy, unspecified number of placenta and unspecified number of amniotic sacs**
AHA: 2016,2Q,8

O30.101   Triplet pregnancy, unspecified number of placenta and unspecified number of amniotic sacs, first trimester   CC M ♀

O30.102   Triplet pregnancy, unspecified number of placenta and unspecified number of amniotic sacs, second trimester   CC M ♀

O30.103   Triplet pregnancy, unspecified number of placenta and unspecified number of amniotic sacs, third trimester   CC M ♀

O30.109   Triplet pregnancy, unspecified number of placenta and unspecified number of amniotic sacs, unspecified trimester   M ♀

✓6th **O30.11**   **Triplet pregnancy with** two or more monochorionic fetuses

O30.111   Triplet pregnancy with two or more monochorionic fetuses, first trimester   CC M ♀

O30.112   Triplet pregnancy with two or more monochorionic fetuses, second trimester   CC M ♀

O30.113   Triplet pregnancy with two or more monochorionic fetuses, third trimester   CC M ♀

O30.119   Triplet pregnancy with two or more monochorionic fetuses, unspecified trimester   M ♀

✓6th **O30.12**   **Triplet pregnancy with** two or more monoamniotic fetuses

O30.121   Triplet pregnancy with two or more monoamniotic fetuses, first trimester   CC M ♀

O30.122   Triplet pregnancy with two or more monoamniotic fetuses, second trimester   CC M ♀

O30.123   Triplet pregnancy with two or more monoamniotic fetuses, third trimester   CC M ♀

O30.129   Triplet pregnancy with two or more monoamniotic fetuses, unspecified trimester   M ♀

✓6th **O30.13**   **Triplet pregnancy,** trichorionic/triamniotic
AHA: 2018,4Q,22

O30.131   Triplet pregnancy, trichorionic/triamniotic, first trimester   CC M ♀

O30.132   Triplet pregnancy, trichorionic/triamniotic, second trimester   CC M ♀

O30.133   Triplet pregnancy, trichorionic/triamniotic, third trimester   CC M ♀

O30.139   Triplet pregnancy, trichorionic/triamniotic, unspecified trimester   M ♀

✓6th **O30.19**   **Triplet pregnancy,** unable to determine number of placenta and number of amniotic sacs

O30.191   Triplet pregnancy, unable to determine number of placenta and number of amniotic sacs, first trimester   CC M ♀

O30.192   Triplet pregnancy, unable to determine number of placenta and number of amniotic sacs, second trimester   CC M ♀

O30.193   Triplet pregnancy, unable to determine number of placenta and number of amniotic sacs, third trimester   CC M ♀

O30.199   Triplet pregnancy, unable to determine number of placenta and number of amniotic sacs, unspecified trimester   M ♀

✓5th **O30.2**   **Quadruplet** pregnancy

✓6th **O30.20**   **Quadruplet pregnancy, unspecified number of placenta and unspecified number of amniotic sacs**

O30.201   Quadruplet pregnancy, unspecified number of placenta and unspecified number of amniotic sacs, first trimester   CC M ♀

O30.202   Quadruplet pregnancy, unspecified number of placenta and unspecified number of amniotic sacs, second trimester   CC M ♀

✓ Additional Character Required   ✓x7th Placeholder   Questionable PDx   Manifestation   Unspecified Dx   UPD Unacceptable PDx   H1-H14 HAC   HCC CMS-HCC Dx   HIV HIV Dx

ICD-10-CM 2022   **883**

Chapter 15. Pregnancy, Childbirth and the Puerperium

O30.203–O30.899

- **O30.203** Quadruplet pregnancy, unspecified number of placenta and unspecified number of amniotic sacs, **third trimester** `CC` `M` ♀
- **O30.209** Quadruplet pregnancy, unspecified number of placenta and unspecified number of amniotic sacs, unspecified trimester `M` ♀

✓6ᵗʰ **O30.21** Quadruplet pregnancy with two or more monochorionic fetuses
- **O30.211** Quadruplet pregnancy with two or more monochorionic fetuses, **first trimester** `CC` `M` ♀
- **O30.212** Quadruplet pregnancy with two or more monochorionic fetuses, **second trimester** `CC` `M` ♀
- **O30.213** Quadruplet pregnancy with two or more monochorionic fetuses, **third trimester** `CC` `M` ♀
- **O30.219** Quadruplet pregnancy with two or more monochorionic fetuses, unspecified trimester `M` ♀

✓6ᵗʰ **O30.22** Quadruplet pregnancy with two or more monoamniotic fetuses
- **O30.221** Quadruplet pregnancy with two or more monoamniotic fetuses, **first trimester** `CC` `M` ♀
- **O30.222** Quadruplet pregnancy with two or more monoamniotic fetuses, **second trimester** `CC` `M` ♀
- **O30.223** Quadruplet pregnancy with two or more monoamniotic fetuses, **third trimester** `CC` `M` ♀
- **O30.229** Quadruplet pregnancy with two or more monoamniotic fetuses, unspecified trimester `M` ♀

✓6ᵗʰ **O30.23** Quadruplet pregnancy, quadrachorionic/quadra-amniotic
    AHA: 2018,4Q,22
- **O30.231** Quadruplet pregnancy, quadrachorionic/quadra-amniotic, **first trimester** `CC` `M` ♀
- **O30.232** Quadruplet pregnancy, quadrachorionic/quadra-amniotic, **second trimester** `CC` `M` ♀
- **O30.233** Quadruplet pregnancy, quadrachorionic/quadra-amniotic, **third trimester** `CC` `M` ♀
- **O30.239** Quadruplet pregnancy, quadrachorionic/quadra-amniotic, unspecified trimester `M` ♀

✓6ᵗʰ **O30.29** Quadruplet pregnancy, unable to determine number of placenta and number of amniotic sacs
- **O30.291** Quadruplet pregnancy, unable to determine number of placenta and number of amniotic sacs, **first trimester** `CC` `M` ♀
- **O30.292** Quadruplet pregnancy, unable to determine number of placenta and number of amniotic sacs, **second trimester** `CC` `M` ♀
- **O30.293** Quadruplet pregnancy, unable to determine number of placenta and number of amniotic sacs, **third trimester** `CC` `M` ♀
- **O30.299** Quadruplet pregnancy, unable to determine number of placenta and number of amniotic sacs, unspecified trimester `M` ♀

✓5ᵗʰ **O30.8** Other specified multiple gestation
    Multiple gestation pregnancy greater then quadruplets

✓6ᵗʰ **O30.80** Other specified multiple gestation, unspecified number of placenta and unspecified number of amniotic sacs
- **O30.801** Other specified multiple gestation, unspecified number of placenta and unspecified number of amniotic sacs, **first trimester** `CC` `M` ♀
- **O30.802** Other specified multiple gestation, unspecified number of placenta and unspecified number of amniotic sacs, **second trimester** `CC` `M` ♀
- **O30.803** Other specified multiple gestation, unspecified number of placenta and unspecified number of amniotic sacs, **third trimester** `CC` `M` ♀
- **O30.809** Other specified multiple gestation, unspecified number of placenta and unspecified number of amniotic sacs, unspecified trimester `M` ♀

✓6ᵗʰ **O30.81** Other specified multiple gestation with two or more monochorionic fetuses
- **O30.811** Other specified multiple gestation with two or more monochorionic fetuses, **first trimester** `CC` `M` ♀
- **O30.812** Other specified multiple gestation with two or more monochorionic fetuses, **second trimester** `CC` `M` ♀
- **O30.813** Other specified multiple gestation with two or more monochorionic fetuses, **third trimester** `CC` `M` ♀
- **O30.819** Other specified multiple gestation with two or more monochorionic fetuses, unspecified trimester `M` ♀

✓6ᵗʰ **O30.82** Other specified multiple gestation with two or more monoamniotic fetuses
- **O30.821** Other specified multiple gestation with two or more monoamniotic fetuses, **first trimester** `CC` `M` ♀
- **O30.822** Other specified multiple gestation with two or more monoamniotic fetuses, **second trimester** `CC` `M` ♀
- **O30.823** Other specified multiple gestation with two or more monoamniotic fetuses, **third trimester** `CC` `M` ♀
- **O30.829** Other specified multiple gestation with two or more monoamniotic fetuses, unspecified trimester `M` ♀

✓6ᵗʰ **O30.83** Other specified multiple gestation, number of chorions and amnions are both equal to the number of fetuses
    Pentachorionic, penta-amniotic pregnancy (quintuplets)
    Hexachorionic, hexa-amniotic pregnancy (sextuplets)
    Heptachorionic, hepta-amniotic pregnancy (septuplets)
    AHA: 2018,4Q,22
- **O30.831** Other specified multiple gestation, number of chorions and amnions are both equal to the number of fetuses, **first trimester** `CC` `M` ♀
- **O30.832** Other specified multiple gestation, number of chorions and amnions are both equal to the number of fetuses, **second trimester** `CC` `M` ♀
- **O30.833** Other specified multiple gestation, number of chorions and amnions are both equal to the number of fetuses, **third trimester** `CC` `M` ♀
- **O30.839** Other specified multiple gestation, number of chorions and amnions are both equal to the number of fetuses, unspecified trimester `M` ♀

✓6ᵗʰ **O30.89** Other specified multiple gestation, unable to determine number of placenta and number of amniotic sacs
- **O30.891** Other specified multiple gestation, unable to determine number of placenta and number of amniotic sacs, **first trimester** `CC` `M` ♀
- **O30.892** Other specified multiple gestation, unable to determine number of placenta and number of amniotic sacs, **second trimester** `CC` `M` ♀
- **O30.893** Other specified multiple gestation, unable to determine number of placenta and number of amniotic sacs, **third trimester** `CC` `M` ♀
- **O30.899** Other specified multiple gestation, unable to determine number of placenta and number of amniotic sacs, unspecified trimester `M` ♀

`N` Newborn: 0   `P` Pediatric: 0-17   `M` Maternity: 9-64   `A` Adult: 15-124   `MCC` Major Complication/Comorbidity   `CC` Complication/Comorbidity   `SW` Severe Wound Dx

884   ICD-10-CM 2022

√5ᵗʰ **O30.9 Multiple gestation, unspecified**

    Multiple pregnancy NOS

    O30.90 Multiple gestation, unspecified, unspecified trimester Ⓜ♀

    O30.91 Multiple gestation, unspecified, first trimester Ⓜ♀

    O30.92 Multiple gestation, unspecified, second trimester Ⓜ♀

    O30.93 Multiple gestation, unspecified, third trimester Ⓜ♀

√4ᵗʰ **O31 Complications specific to multiple gestation**

    EXCLUDES 2   delayed delivery of second twin, triplet, etc. (O63.2)

         malpresentation of one fetus or more (O32.9)

         placental transfusion syndromes (O43.0-)

    AHA: 2012,4Q,107

> One of the following 7th characters is to be assigned to each code under category O31. 7th character Ø is for single gestations and multiple gestations where the fetus is unspecified. 7th characters 1 through 9 are for cases of multiple gestations to identify the fetus for which the code applies. The appropriate code from category O30, Multiple gestation, must also be assigned when assigning a code from category O31 that has a 7th character of 1 through 9.
>
> Ø   not applicable or unspecified
> 1   fetus 1
> 2   fetus 2
> 3   fetus 3
> 4   fetus 4
> 5   fetus 5
> 9   other fetus

√5ᵗʰ **O31.Ø Papyraceous fetus**

    Fetus compressus

    DEF: Fetus that has died, but remains in utero for weeks before delivery, becoming compacted and mummified in appearance, with skin resembling parchment. Occurs most commonly in multigestational pregnancies. *Synonym(s): paper doll fetus.*

    √x7ᵗʰ **O31.ØØ Papyraceous fetus, unspecified trimester** Ⓜ♀

    √x7ᵗʰ **O31.Ø1 Papyraceous fetus, first trimester** Ⓜ♀

    √x7ᵗʰ **O31.Ø2 Papyraceous fetus, second trimester** Ⓜ♀

    √x7ᵗʰ **O31.Ø3 Papyraceous fetus, third trimester** Ⓜ♀

√5ᵗʰ **O31.1 Continuing pregnancy after spontaneous abortion of one fetus or more**

    √x7ᵗʰ **O31.10 Continuing pregnancy after spontaneous abortion of one fetus or more, unspecified trimester** Ⓜ♀

    √x7ᵗʰ **O31.11 Continuing pregnancy after spontaneous abortion of one fetus or more, first trimester** Ⓜ♀

    √x7ᵗʰ **O31.12 Continuing pregnancy after spontaneous abortion of one fetus or more, second trimester** Ⓜ♀

    √x7ᵗʰ **O31.13 Continuing pregnancy after spontaneous abortion of one fetus or more, third trimester** Ⓜ♀

√5ᵗʰ **O31.2 Continuing pregnancy after intrauterine death of one fetus or more**

    √x7ᵗʰ **O31.20 Continuing pregnancy after intrauterine death of one fetus or more, unspecified trimester** Ⓜ♀

    √x7ᵗʰ **O31.21 Continuing pregnancy after intrauterine death of one fetus or more, first trimester** Ⓜ♀

    √x7ᵗʰ **O31.22 Continuing pregnancy after intrauterine death of one fetus or more, second trimester** Ⓜ♀

    √x7ᵗʰ **O31.23 Continuing pregnancy after intrauterine death of one fetus or more, third trimester** Ⓜ♀

√5ᵗʰ **O31.3 Continuing pregnancy after elective fetal reduction of one fetus or more**

    Continuing pregnancy after selective termination of one fetus or more

    √x7ᵗʰ **O31.30 Continuing pregnancy after elective fetal reduction of one fetus or more, unspecified trimester** Ⓜ♀

    √x7ᵗʰ **O31.31 Continuing pregnancy after elective fetal reduction of one fetus or more, first trimester** Ⓜ♀

    √x7ᵗʰ **O31.32 Continuing pregnancy after elective fetal reduction of one fetus or more, second trimester** Ⓜ♀

    √x7ᵗʰ **O31.33 Continuing pregnancy after elective fetal reduction of one fetus or more, third trimester** Ⓜ♀

√5ᵗʰ **O31.8 Other complications specific to multiple gestation**

    √6ᵗʰ **O31.8X Other complications specific to multiple gestation**

       √7ᵗʰ **O31.8X1 Other complications specific to multiple gestation, first trimester** cc Ⓜ♀

       √7ᵗʰ **O31.8X2 Other complications specific to multiple gestation, second trimester** cc Ⓜ♀

       √7ᵗʰ **O31.8X3 Other complications specific to multiple gestation, third trimester** cc Ⓜ♀

       √7ᵗʰ **O31.8X9 Other complications specific to multiple gestation, unspecified trimester** cc Ⓜ♀

√4ᵗʰ **O32 Maternal care for malpresentation of fetus**

    INCLUDES   the listed conditions as a reason for observation, hospitalization or other obstetric care of the mother, or for cesarean delivery before onset of labor

    EXCLUDES 1   malpresentation of fetus with obstructed labor (O64.-)

    AHA: 2012,4Q,107

> One of the following 7th characters is to be assigned to each code under category O32. 7th character Ø is for single gestations and multiple gestations where the fetus is unspecified. 7th characters 1 through 9 are for cases of multiple gestations to identify the fetus for which the code applies. The appropriate code from category O30, Multiple gestation, must also be assigned when assigning a code from category O32 that has a 7th character of 1 through 9.
>
> Ø   not applicable or unspecified
> 1   fetus 1
> 2   fetus 2
> 3   fetus 3
> 4   fetus 4
> 5   fetus 5
> 9   other fetus

Fetal Malpresentation

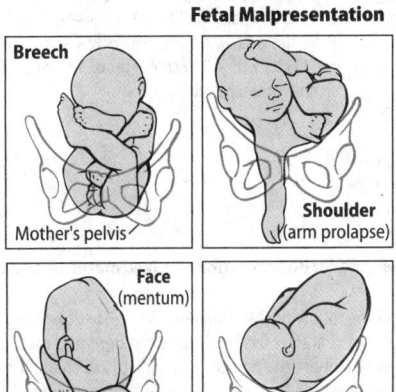
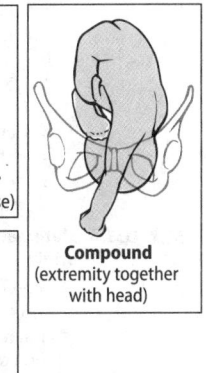

Breech — Mother's pelvis

Shoulder (arm prolapse)

Compound (extremity together with head)

Face (mentum)

Oblique

    √x7ᵗʰ **O32.Ø Maternal care for unstable lie** Ⓜ♀

    √x7ᵗʰ **O32.1 Maternal care for breech presentation** Ⓜ♀

        Maternal care for buttocks presentation

        Maternal care for complete breech

        Maternal care for frank breech

        EXCLUDES 1   footling presentation (O32.8)

             incomplete breech (O32.8)

        DEF: Fetus presentation in a longitudinal lie with the buttocks or feet closest to birth canal that may require external cephalic version or cesarean delivery.

    √x7ᵗʰ **O32.2 Maternal care for transverse and oblique lie** Ⓜ♀

        Maternal care for oblique presentation

        Maternal care for transverse presentation

    √x7ᵗʰ **O32.3 Maternal care for face, brow and chin presentation** Ⓜ♀

    √x7ᵗʰ **O32.4 Maternal care for high head at term** Ⓜ♀

        Maternal care for failure of head to enter pelvic brim

    √x7ᵗʰ **O32.6 Maternal care for compound presentation** Ⓜ♀

    √x7ᵗʰ **O32.8 Maternal care for other malpresentation of fetus** Ⓜ♀

        Maternal care for footling presentation

        Maternal care for incomplete breech

    √x7ᵗʰ **O32.9 Maternal care for malpresentation of fetus, unspecified** Ⓜ♀

✔ Additional Character Required   √x7ᵗʰ Placeholder   Questionable PDx   Manifestation   Unspecified Dx   UPD Unacceptable PDx   H1-H14 HAC   HCC CMS-HCC Dx   HIV HIV Dx

ICD-10-CM 2022   885

Chapter 15. Pregnancy, Childbirth and the Puerperium

O33–O34.13

✓4ᵗʰ **O33 Maternal care for disproportion**

> INCLUDES   the listed conditions as a reason for observation, hospitalization or other obstetric care of the mother, or for cesarean delivery before onset of labor
>
> EXCLUDES 1   *disproportion with obstructed labor (O65-O66)*

O33.0 Maternal care for disproportion due to deformity of maternal pelvic bones   CC M ♀

> Maternal care for disproportion due to pelvic deformity causing disproportion NOS

O33.1 Maternal care for disproportion due to generally contracted pelvis   M ♀

> Maternal care for disproportion due to contracted pelvis NOS causing disproportion

O33.2 Maternal care for disproportion due to inlet contraction of pelvis   M ♀

> Maternal care for disproportion due to inlet contraction (pelvis) causing disproportion

✓x7ᵗʰ **O33.3 Maternal care for disproportion due to outlet contraction of pelvis**   M ♀

> Maternal care for disproportion due to mid-cavity contraction (pelvis)
>
> Maternal care for disproportion due to outlet contraction (pelvis)
>
> One of the following 7th characters is to be assigned to code O33.3. 7th character 0 is for single gestations and multiple gestations where the fetus is unspecified. 7th characters 1 through 9 are for cases of multiple gestations to identify the fetus for which the code applies. The appropriate code from category O30, Multiple gestation, must also be assigned when assigning code O33.3 with a 7th character of 1 through 9.
>
> 0   not applicable or unspecified
> 1   fetus 1
> 2   fetus 2
> 3   fetus 3
> 4   fetus 4
> 5   fetus 5
> 9   other fetus

✓x7ᵗʰ **O33.4 Maternal care for disproportion of mixed maternal and fetal origin**   M ♀

> One of the following 7th characters is to be assigned to code O33.4. 7th character 0 is for single gestations and multiple gestations where the fetus is unspecified. 7th characters 1 through 9 are for cases of multiple gestations to identify the fetus for which the code applies. The appropriate code from category O30, Multiple gestation, must also be assigned when assigning code O33.4 with a 7th character of 1 through 9.
>
> 0   not applicable or unspecified
> 1   fetus 1
> 2   fetus 2
> 3   fetus 3
> 4   fetus 4
> 5   fetus 5
> 9   other fetus

✓x7ᵗʰ **O33.5 Maternal care for disproportion due to unusually large fetus**   M ♀

> Maternal care for disproportion due to disproportion of fetal origin with normally formed fetus
>
> Maternal care for disproportion due to fetal disproportion NOS
>
> One of the following 7th characters is to be assigned to code O33.5. 7th character 0 is for single gestations and multiple gestations where the fetus is unspecified. 7th characters 1 through 9 are for cases of multiple gestations to identify the fetus for which the code applies. The appropriate code from category O30, Multiple gestation, must also be assigned when assigning code O33.5 with a 7th character of 1 through 9.
>
> 0   not applicable or unspecified
> 1   fetus 1
> 2   fetus 2
> 3   fetus 3
> 4   fetus 4
> 5   fetus 5
> 9   other fetus

✓x7ᵗʰ **O33.6 Maternal care for disproportion due to hydrocephalic fetus**   M ♀

> One of the following 7th characters is to be assigned to code O33.6. 7th character 0 is for single gestations and multiple gestations where the fetus is unspecified. 7th characters 1 through 9 are for cases of multiple gestations to identify the fetus for which the code applies. The appropriate code from category O30, Multiple gestation, must also be assigned when assigning code O33.6 with a 7th character of 1 through 9.
>
> 0   not applicable or unspecified
> 1   fetus 1
> 2   fetus 2
> 3   fetus 3
> 4   fetus 4
> 5   fetus 5
> 9   other fetus

✓x7ᵗʰ **O33.7 Maternal care for disproportion due to other fetal deformities**   M ♀

> Maternal care for disproportion due to fetal ascites
> Maternal care for disproportion due to fetal hydrops
> Maternal care for disproportion due to fetal meningomyelocele
> Maternal care for disproportion due to fetal sacral teratoma
> Maternal care for disproportion due to fetal tumor
>
> EXCLUDES 1   *obstructed labor due to other fetal deformities (O66.3)*
>
> **AHA:** 2016,4Q,51
>
> One of the following 7th characters is to be assigned to code O33.7. 7th character 0 is for single gestations and multiple gestations where the fetus is unspecified. 7th characters 1 through 9 are for cases of multiple gestations to identify the fetus for which the code applies. The appropriate code from category O30, Multiple gestation, must also be assigned when assigning code O33.7 with a 7th character of 1 through 9.
>
> 0   not applicable or unspecified
> 1   fetus 1
> 2   fetus 2
> 3   fetus 3
> 4   fetus 4
> 5   fetus 5
> 9   other fetus

O33.8 Maternal care for disproportion of other origin   M ♀

O33.9 Maternal care for disproportion, unspecified   M ♀

> Maternal care for disproportion due to cephalopelvic disproportion NOS
>
> Maternal care for disproportion due to fetopelvic disproportion NOS

✓4ᵗʰ **O34 Maternal care for abnormality of pelvic organs**

> INCLUDES   the listed conditions as a reason for hospitalization or other obstetric care of the mother, or for cesarean delivery before onset of labor
>
> Code first any associated obstructed labor (O65.5)
> Use additional code for specific condition

✓5ᵗʰ **O34.0 Maternal care for congenital malformation of uterus**

> Maternal care for double uterus
> Maternal care for uterus bicornis

O34.00 Maternal care for unspecified congenital malformation of uterus, unspecified trimester   M ♀

O34.01 Maternal care for unspecified congenital malformation of uterus, first trimester   M ♀

O34.02 Maternal care for unspecified congenital malformation of uterus, second trimester   M ♀

O34.03 Maternal care for unspecified congenital malformation of uterus, third trimester   M ♀

✓5ᵗʰ **O34.1 Maternal care for benign tumor of corpus uteri**

> EXCLUDES 2   *maternal care for benign tumor of cervix (O34.4-)*
> *maternal care for malignant neoplasm of uterus (O9A.1-)*

O34.10 Maternal care for benign tumor of corpus uteri, unspecified trimester   M ♀

O34.11 Maternal care for benign tumor of corpus uteri, first trimester   M ♀

O34.12 Maternal care for benign tumor of corpus uteri, second trimester   M ♀

O34.13 Maternal care for benign tumor of corpus uteri, third trimester   M ♀

N Newborn: 0   P Pediatric: 0-17   M Maternity: 9-64   A Adult: 15-124   MCC Major Complication/Comorbidity   CC Complication/Comorbidity   SW Severe Wound Dx

886   ICD-10-CM 2022

☑5ᵗʰ **O34.2** **Maternal care due to** uterine scar from previous surgery
    AHA: 2020,4Q,36; 2016,4Q,76

    ☑6ᵗʰ **O34.21** **Maternal care for scar** from previous cesarean delivery
       AHA: 2018,3Q,23; 2016,4Q,51-52

       O34.211 **Maternal care for** low transverse **scar from previous cesarean delivery** Ⓜ♀

       O34.212 **Maternal care for** vertical **scar from previous cesarean delivery** Ⓜ♀
          Maternal care for classical scar from previous cesarean delivery

       O34.218 **Maternal care for other type scar from previous cesarean delivery** Ⓜ♀
          Mid-transverse T incision

       O34.219 **Maternal care for unspecified type scar from previous cesarean delivery** Ⓜ♀

    O34.22 **Maternal care for** cesarean scar defect **(isthmocele)** Ⓜ♀

    O34.29 **Maternal care due to** uterine scar from other previous surgery Ⓜ♀
       Maternal care due to uterine scar from other transmural uterine incision

☑5ᵗʰ **O34.3** **Maternal care for** cervical incompetence
    Maternal care for cerclage with or without cervical incompetence
    Maternal care for Shirodkar suture with or without cervical incompetence
    DEF: Inadequate functioning of the cervix marked by abnormal widening during pregnancy and causing premature birth or miscarriage.

    O34.30 **Maternal care for cervical incompetence, unspecified trimester** Ⓜ♀

    O34.31 **Maternal care for cervical incompetence,** first trimester ᴹᶜᶜ Ⓜ♀

    O34.32 **Maternal care for cervical incompetence,** second trimester ᴹᶜᶜ Ⓜ♀

    O34.33 **Maternal care for cervical incompetence,** third trimester ᴹᶜᶜ Ⓜ♀

☑5ᵗʰ **O34.4** **Maternal care for** other abnormalities of cervix

    O34.40 **Maternal care for other abnormalities of cervix, unspecified trimester** Ⓜ♀

    O34.41 **Maternal care for other abnormalities of cervix,** first trimester Ⓜ♀

    O34.42 **Maternal care for other abnormalities of cervix,** second trimester Ⓜ♀

    O34.43 **Maternal care for other abnormalities of cervix,** third trimester Ⓜ♀

☑5ᵗʰ **O34.5** **Maternal care for** other abnormalities of gravid uterus

    ☑6ᵗʰ **O34.51** **Maternal care for** incarceration **of gravid uterus**

       O34.511 **Maternal care for incarceration of gravid uterus,** first trimester Ⓜ♀

       O34.512 **Maternal care for incarceration of gravid uterus,** second trimester Ⓜ♀

       O34.513 **Maternal care for incarceration of gravid uterus,** third trimester Ⓜ♀

       O34.519 **Maternal care for incarceration of gravid uterus, unspecified trimester** Ⓜ♀

    ☑6ᵗʰ **O34.52** **Maternal care for** prolapse **of gravid uterus**

       O34.521 **Maternal care for prolapse of gravid uterus,** first trimester Ⓜ♀

       O34.522 **Maternal care for prolapse of gravid uterus,** second trimester Ⓜ♀

       O34.523 **Maternal care for prolapse of gravid uterus,** third trimester Ⓜ♀

       O34.529 **Maternal care for prolapse of gravid uterus, unspecified trimester** Ⓜ♀

    ☑6ᵗʰ **O34.53** **Maternal care for** retroversion **of gravid uterus**

       O34.531 **Maternal care for retroversion of gravid uterus,** first trimester Ⓜ♀

       O34.532 **Maternal care for retroversion of gravid uterus,** second trimester Ⓜ♀

       O34.533 **Maternal care for retroversion of gravid uterus,** third trimester Ⓜ♀

       O34.539 **Maternal care for retroversion of gravid uterus, unspecified trimester** Ⓜ♀

    ☑6ᵗʰ **O34.59** **Maternal care for other abnormalities of gravid uterus**

       O34.591 **Maternal care for other abnormalities of gravid uterus, first trimester** Ⓜ♀

       O34.592 **Maternal care for other abnormalities of gravid uterus,** second trimester Ⓜ♀

       O34.593 **Maternal care for other abnormalities of gravid uterus,** third trimester Ⓜ♀

       O34.599 **Maternal care for other abnormalities of gravid uterus, unspecified trimester** Ⓜ♀

☑5ᵗʰ **O34.6** **Maternal care for** abnormality of vagina
    EXCLUDES 2   maternal care for vaginal varices in pregnancy (O22.1-)

    O34.60 **Maternal care for abnormality of vagina, unspecified trimester** Ⓜ♀

    O34.61 **Maternal care for abnormality of vagina,** first trimester Ⓜ♀

    O34.62 **Maternal care for abnormality of vagina,** second trimester Ⓜ♀

    O34.63 **Maternal care for abnormality of vagina,** third trimester Ⓜ♀

☑5ᵗʰ **O34.7** **Maternal care for** abnormality of vulva and perineum
    EXCLUDES 2   maternal care for perineal and vulval varices in pregnancy (O22.1-)

    O34.70 **Maternal care for abnormality of vulva and perineum, unspecified trimester** Ⓜ♀

    O34.71 **Maternal care for abnormality of vulva and perineum,** first trimester Ⓜ♀

    O34.72 **Maternal care for abnormality of vulva and perineum,** second trimester Ⓜ♀

    O34.73 **Maternal care for abnormality of vulva and perineum,** third trimester Ⓜ♀

☑5ᵗʰ **O34.8** **Maternal care for** other abnormalities of pelvic organs

    O34.80 **Maternal care for other abnormalities of pelvic organs, unspecified trimester** Ⓜ♀

    O34.81 **Maternal care for other abnormalities of pelvic organs,** first trimester Ⓜ♀

    O34.82 **Maternal care for other abnormalities of pelvic organs,** second trimester Ⓜ♀

    O34.83 **Maternal care for other abnormalities of pelvic organs,** third trimester Ⓜ♀

☑5ᵗʰ **O34.9** **Maternal care for** abnormality of pelvic organ, unspecified

    O34.90 **Maternal care for abnormality of pelvic organ, unspecified, unspecified trimester** Ⓜ♀

    O34.91 **Maternal care for abnormality of pelvic organ, unspecified,** first trimester Ⓜ♀

    O34.92 **Maternal care for abnormality of pelvic organ, unspecified,** second trimester Ⓜ♀

    O34.93 **Maternal care for abnormality of pelvic organ, unspecified,** third trimester Ⓜ♀

☑4ᵗʰ **O35** **Maternal care for known or suspected fetal abnormality and damage**
    INCLUDES   the listed conditions in the fetus as a reason for hospitalization or other obstetric care to the mother, or for termination of pregnancy
    Code also any associated maternal condition
    EXCLUDES 1   encounter for suspected maternal and fetal conditions ruled out (Z03.7-)

    One of the following 7th characters is to be assigned to each code under category O35. 7th character Ø is for single gestations and multiple gestations where the fetus is unspecified. 7th characters 1 through 9 are for cases of multiple gestations to identify the fetus for which the code applies. The appropriate code from category O30, Multiple gestation, must also be assigned when assigning a code from category O35 that has a 7th character of 1 through 9.
    Ø   not applicable or unspecified
    1   fetus 1
    2   fetus 2
    3   fetus 3
    4   fetus 4
    5   fetus 5
    9   other fetus

☑ₓ7ᵗʰ **O35.0** **Maternal care for (suspected)** central nervous system malformation in fetus Ⓜ♀
    Maternal care for fetal anencephaly
    Maternal care for fetal hydrocephalus
    Maternal care for fetal spina bifida
    EXCLUDES 2   chromosomal abnormality in fetus (O35.1)

☑ₓ7ᵗʰ **O35.1** **Maternal care for (suspected)** chromosomal abnormality in fetus Ⓜ♀

√x7th **O35.2** **Maternal care for (suspected)** hereditary disease in fetus Ⓜ♀
> EXCLUDES 2   *chromosomal abnormality in fetus (O35.1)*

√x7th **O35.3** **Maternal care for (suspected)** damage to fetus from viral disease in mother Ⓜ♀
> Maternal care for damage to fetus from maternal cytomegalovirus infection
> Maternal care for damage to fetus from maternal rubella

√x7th **O35.4** **Maternal care for (suspected)** damage to fetus from alcohol Ⓜ♀

√x7th **O35.5** **Maternal care for (suspected)** damage to fetus by drugs Ⓜ♀
> Maternal care for damage to fetus from drug addiction

√x7th **O35.6** **Maternal care for (suspected)** damage to fetus by radiation Ⓜ♀

√x7th **O35.7** **Maternal care for (suspected)** damage to fetus by other medical procedures Ⓜ♀
> Maternal care for damage to fetus by amniocentesis
> Maternal care for damage to fetus by biopsy procedures
> Maternal care for damage to fetus by hematological investigation
> Maternal care for damage to fetus by intrauterine contraceptive device
> Maternal care for damage to fetus by intrauterine surgery

√x7th **O35.8** **Maternal care for other (suspected)** fetal abnormality and damage Ⓜ♀
> Maternal care for damage to fetus from maternal listeriosis
> Maternal care for damage to fetus from maternal toxoplasmosis

√x7th **O35.9** **Maternal care for (suspected)** fetal abnormality and damage, unspecified Ⓜ♀

√4th **O36** **Maternal care for other fetal problems**
> INCLUDES   the listed conditions in the fetus as a reason for hospitalization or other obstetric care of the mother, or for termination of pregnancy
> EXCLUDES 1   *encounter for suspected maternal and fetal conditions ruled out (Z03.7-)*
> *placental transfusion syndromes (O43.0-)*
> EXCLUDES 2   *labor and delivery complicated by fetal stress (O77.-)*
> **AHA:** 2015,3Q,40

One of the following 7th characters is to be assigned to each code under category O36. 7th character Ø is for single gestations and multiple gestations where the fetus is unspecified. 7th characters 1 through 9 are for cases of multiple gestations to identify the fetus for which the code applies. The appropriate code from category O30, Multiple gestation, must also be assigned when assigning a code from category O36 that has a 7th character of 1 through 9.
Ø   not applicable or unspecified
1   fetus 1
2   fetus 2
3   fetus 3
4   fetus 4
5   fetus 5
9   other fetus

√5th **O36.0** **Maternal care for rhesus isoimmunization**
> Maternal care for Rh incompatibility (with hydrops fetalis)
> √6th **O36.01** **Maternal care for** anti-D [Rh] antibodies
> > **AHA:** 2014,4Q,17
> > √7th **O36.011** **Maternal care for anti-D [Rh] antibodies,** first trimester ᴄᴄ Ⓜ♀
> > √7th **O36.012** **Maternal care for anti-D [Rh] antibodies,** second trimester ᴄᴄ Ⓜ♀
> > √7th **O36.013** **Maternal care for anti-D [Rh] antibodies,** third trimester ᴄᴄ Ⓜ♀
> > √7th **O36.019** **Maternal care for anti-D [Rh] antibodies,** unspecified trimester Ⓜ♀
> √6th **O36.09** **Maternal care for other rhesus isoimmunization**
> > √7th **O36.091** **Maternal care for other rhesus isoimmunization,** first trimester ᴄᴄ Ⓜ♀
> > √7th **O36.092** **Maternal care for other rhesus isoimmunization,** second trimester ᴄᴄ Ⓜ♀
> > √7th **O36.093** **Maternal care for other rhesus isoimmunization,** third trimester ᴄᴄ Ⓜ♀
> > √7th **O36.099** **Maternal care for other rhesus isoimmunization,** unspecified trimester Ⓜ♀

√5th **O36.1** **Maternal care for other isoimmunization**
> Maternal care for ABO isoimmunization
> √6th **O36.11** **Maternal care for** Anti-A sensitization
> > Maternal care for isoimmunization NOS (with hydrops fetalis)
> > √7th **O36.111** **Maternal care for Anti-A sensitization,** first trimester Ⓜ♀
> > √7th **O36.112** **Maternal care for Anti-A sensitization,** second trimester Ⓜ♀
> > √7th **O36.113** **Maternal care for Anti-A sensitization,** third trimester Ⓜ♀
> > √7th **O36.119** **Maternal care for Anti-A sensitization,** unspecified trimester Ⓜ♀
> √6th **O36.19** **Maternal care for other isoimmunization**
> > Maternal care for Anti-B sensitization
> > √7th **O36.191** **Maternal care for other isoimmunization,** first trimester Ⓜ♀
> > √7th **O36.192** **Maternal care for other isoimmunization,** second trimester Ⓜ♀
> > √7th **O36.193** **Maternal care for other isoimmunization,** third trimester Ⓜ♀
> > √7th **O36.199** **Maternal care for other isoimmunization,** unspecified trimester Ⓜ♀

√5th **O36.2** **Maternal care for hydrops fetalis**
> Maternal care for hydrops fetalis NOS
> Maternal care for hydrops fetalis not associated with isoimmunization
> EXCLUDES 1   *hydrops fetalis associated with ABO isoimmunization (O36.1-)*
> *hydrops fetalis associated with rhesus isoimmunization (O36.0-)*
> **DEF:** Hydrops fetalis: Abnormal fluid buildup in at least two of the following fetal organ spaces: the skin (edema), abdomen (ascites), around the heart (pericardia effusion), and around the lung (pleural effusion). Fluid accumulation may also occur in the mother as polyhydramnios and edema of the placenta.
> √x7th **O36.20** **Maternal care for hydrops fetalis, unspecified trimester** Ⓜ♀
> √x7th **O36.21** **Maternal care for hydrops fetalis,** first trimester Ⓜ♀
> √x7th **O36.22** **Maternal care for hydrops fetalis,** second trimester Ⓜ♀
> √x7th **O36.23** **Maternal care for hydrops fetalis,** third trimester Ⓜ♀

√x7th **O36.4** **Maternal care for intrauterine death** ᴄᴄ Ⓜ♀
> Maternal care for intrauterine fetal death NOS
> Maternal care for intrauterine fetal death after completion of 20 weeks of gestation
> Maternal care for late fetal death
> Maternal care for missed delivery
> EXCLUDES 1   *missed abortion (O02.1)*
> *stillbirth (P95)*

√5th **O36.5** **Maternal care for known or suspected poor fetal growth**
> √6th **O36.51** **Maternal care for known or suspected placental insufficiency**
> > √7th **O36.511** **Maternal care for known or suspected placental insufficiency,** first trimester Ⓜ♀
> > √7th **O36.512** **Maternal care for known or suspected placental insufficiency,** second trimester Ⓜ♀
> > √7th **O36.513** **Maternal care for known or suspected placental insufficiency,** third trimester Ⓜ♀
> > √7th **O36.519** **Maternal care for known or suspected placental insufficiency, unspecified trimester** Ⓜ♀
> √6th **O36.59** **Maternal care for other known or suspected poor fetal growth**
> > Maternal care for known or suspected light-for-dates NOS
> > Maternal care for known or suspected small-for-dates NOS
> > √7th **O36.591** **Maternal care for other known or suspected poor fetal growth,** first trimester Ⓜ♀
> > √7th **O36.592** **Maternal care for other known or suspected poor fetal growth,** second trimester Ⓜ♀

Ⓝ Newborn: 0   Ⓟ Pediatric: 0-17   Ⓜ Maternity: 9-64   Ⓐ Adult: 15-124   ᴹᶜᶜ Major Complication/Comorbidity   ᴄᴄ Complication/Comorbidity   ˢʷ Severe Wound Dx

888

ICD-10-CM 2022

√7ᵗʰ **O36.593** **Maternal care for other known or suspected poor fetal growth, third trimester** Ⓜ ♀

√7ᵗʰ **O36.599** **Maternal care for other known or suspected poor fetal growth, unspecified trimester** Ⓜ ♀

√5ᵗʰ **O36.6** **Maternal care for excessive fetal growth**

Maternal care for known or suspected large-for-dates

√x7ᵗʰ **O36.60** **Maternal care for excessive fetal growth, unspecified trimester** Ⓜ ♀

√x7ᵗʰ **O36.61** **Maternal care for excessive fetal growth,** first **trimester** Ⓜ ♀

√x7ᵗʰ **O36.62** **Maternal care for excessive fetal growth,** second **trimester** Ⓜ ♀

√x7ᵗʰ **O36.63** **Maternal care for excessive fetal growth,** third **trimester** Ⓜ ♀

√5ᵗʰ **O36.7** **Maternal care for viable fetus in abdominal pregnancy**

√x7ᵗʰ **O36.70** **Maternal care for viable fetus in abdominal pregnancy, unspecified trimester** Ⓜ ♀

√x7ᵗʰ **O36.71** **Maternal care for viable fetus in abdominal pregnancy,** first trimester Ⓜ ♀

√x7ᵗʰ **O36.72** **Maternal care for viable fetus in abdominal pregnancy,** second trimester Ⓜ ♀

√x7ᵗʰ **O36.73** **Maternal care for viable fetus in abdominal pregnancy,** third trimester Ⓜ ♀

√5ᵗʰ **O36.8** **Maternal care for other specified fetal problems**

√x7ᵗʰ **O36.80** **Pregnancy with inconclusive fetal viability** ᵁᴾᴰ Ⓜ ♀

Encounter to determine fetal viability of pregnancy

AHA: 2019,2Q,29

√6ᵗʰ **O36.81** **Decreased fetal movements**

√7ᵗʰ **O36.812** **Decreased fetal movements,** second trimester Ⓜ ♀

√7ᵗʰ **O36.813** **Decreased fetal movements,** third trimester Ⓜ ♀

√7ᵗʰ **O36.819** **Decreased fetal movements, unspecified trimester** Ⓜ ♀

√6ᵗʰ **O36.82** **Fetal anemia and thrombocytopenia**

√7ᵗʰ **O36.821** **Fetal anemia and thrombocytopenia,** first trimester Ⓜ ♀

√7ᵗʰ **O36.822** **Fetal anemia and thrombocytopenia,** second trimester Ⓜ ♀

√7ᵗʰ **O36.823** **Fetal anemia and thrombocytopenia,** third trimester Ⓜ ♀

√7ᵗʰ **O36.829** **Fetal anemia and thrombocytopenia, unspecified trimester** Ⓜ ♀

√6ᵗʰ **O36.83** **Maternal care for abnormalities of the fetal heart rate or rhythm**

Maternal care for depressed fetal heart rate tones

Maternal care for fetal bradycardia

Maternal care for fetal heart rate abnormal variability

Maternal care for fetal heart rate decelerations

Maternal care for fetal heart rate irregularity

Maternal care for fetal tachycardia

Maternal care for non-reassuring fetal heart rate or rhythm

AHA: 2017,4Q,20

TIP: Assign for documented fetal tachycardia, bradycardia, decelerations, or loss of variability detected during antenatal testing.

√7ᵗʰ **O36.831** **Maternal care for abnormalities of the fetal heart rate or rhythm,** first trimester Ⓜ ♀

√7ᵗʰ **O36.832** **Maternal care for abnormalities of the fetal heart rate or rhythm,** second trimester Ⓜ ♀

√7ᵗʰ **O36.833** **Maternal care for abnormalities of the fetal heart rate or rhythm,** third trimester Ⓜ ♀

√7ᵗʰ **O36.839** **Maternal care for abnormalities of the fetal heart rate or rhythm, unspecified trimester** Ⓜ ♀

√6ᵗʰ **O36.89** **Maternal care for other specified fetal problems**

√7ᵗʰ **O36.891** **Maternal care for other specified fetal problems,** first trimester Ⓜ ♀

√7ᵗʰ **O36.892** **Maternal care for other specified fetal problems,** second trimester Ⓜ ♀

√7ᵗʰ **O36.893** **Maternal care for other specified fetal problems,** third trimester Ⓜ ♀

√7ᵗʰ **O36.899** **Maternal care for other specified fetal problems, unspecified trimester** Ⓜ ♀

√5ᵗʰ **O36.9** **Maternal care for fetal problem, unspecified**

√x7ᵗʰ **O36.90** **Maternal care for fetal problem, unspecified, unspecified trimester** Ⓜ ♀

√x7ᵗʰ **O36.91** **Maternal care for fetal problem, unspecified,** first trimester Ⓜ ♀

√x7ᵗʰ **O36.92** **Maternal care for fetal problem, unspecified,** second trimester Ⓜ ♀

√x7ᵗʰ **O36.93** **Maternal care for fetal problem, unspecified,** third trimester Ⓜ ♀

√4ᵗʰ **O40** **Polyhydramnios**

INCLUDES   hydramnios

EXCLUDES 1   encounter for suspected maternal and fetal conditions ruled out (Z03.7-)

AHA: 2016,1Q,4

DEF: Excess amniotic fluid surrounding the fetus, typically defined as a total fluid volume of greater than 24 cm.

One of the following 7th characters is to be assigned to each code under category O40. 7th character 0 is for single gestations and multiple gestations where the fetus is unspecified. 7th characters 1 through 9 are for cases of multiple gestations to identify the fetus for which the code applies. The appropriate code from category O30, Multiple gestation, must also be assigned when assigning a code from category O40 that has a 7th character of 1 through 9.

0   not applicable or unspecified
1   fetus 1
2   fetus 2
3   fetus 3
4   fetus 4
5   fetus 5
9   other fetus

√x7ᵗʰ **O40.1** **Polyhydramnios,** first trimester Ⓜ ♀

√x7ᵗʰ **O40.2** **Polyhydramnios,** second trimester Ⓜ ♀

√x7ᵗʰ **O40.3** **Polyhydramnios,** third trimester Ⓜ ♀

√x7ᵗʰ **O40.9** **Polyhydramnios, unspecified trimester** Ⓜ ♀

√4ᵗʰ **O41** **Other disorders of amniotic fluid and membranes**

EXCLUDES 1   encounter for suspected maternal and fetal conditions ruled out (Z03.7-)

One of the following 7th characters is to be assigned to each code under category O41. 7th character 0 is for single gestations and multiple gestations where the fetus is unspecified. 7th characters 1 through 9 are for cases of multiple gestations to identify the fetus for which the code applies. The appropriate code from category O30, Multiple gestation, must also be assigned when assigning a code from category O41 that has a 7th character of 1 through 9.

0   not applicable or unspecified
1   fetus 1
2   fetus 2
3   fetus 3
4   fetus 4
5   fetus 5
9   other fetus

√5ᵗʰ **O41.0** **Oligohydramnios**

Oligohydramnios without rupture of membranes

DEF: Low amniotic fluid, occurring most frequently in the last trimester.

√x7ᵗʰ **O41.00** **Oligohydramnios, unspecified trimester** Ⓜ ♀

√x7ᵗʰ **O41.01** **Oligohydramnios,** first trimester ᶜᶜ Ⓜ ♀

√x7ᵗʰ **O41.02** **Oligohydramnios,** second trimester ᶜᶜ Ⓜ ♀

√x7ᵗʰ **O41.03** **Oligohydramnios,** third trimester ᶜᶜ Ⓜ ♀

√6ᵗʰ **O41.1** **Infection of amniotic sac and membranes**

√6ᵗʰ **O41.10** **Infection of amniotic sac and membranes, unspecified**

√7ᵗʰ **O41.101** **Infection of amniotic sac and membranes, unspecified,** first trimester ᴹᶜᶜ Ⓜ ♀

√7ᵗʰ **O41.102** **Infection of amniotic sac and membranes, unspecified,** second trimester ᴹᶜᶜ Ⓜ ♀

√7ᵗʰ **O41.103** **Infection of amniotic sac and membranes, unspecified,** third trimester ᴹᶜᶜ Ⓜ ♀

√7ᵗʰ **O41.109** **Infection of amniotic sac and membranes, unspecified, unspecified trimester** Ⓜ ♀

✔ Additional Character Required   √x7ᵗʰ Placeholder   Questionable PDx   Manifestation   Unspecified Dx   ᵁᴾᴰ Unacceptable PDx   ᴴ¹-ᴴ¹⁴ HAC   ᴴᶜᶜ CMS-HCC Dx   ᴴᴵⱽ HIV Dx

ICD-10-CM 2022   889

  ✓6ᵗʰ **O41.12** **Chorioamnionitis**
      AHA: 2019,2Q,34
      ✓7ᵗʰ **O41.121** **Chorioamnionitis,** first trimester   MCC Ⓜ ♀
      ✓7ᵗʰ **O41.122** **Chorioamnionitis,** second trimester   MCC Ⓜ ♀
      ✓7ᵗʰ **O41.123** **Chorioamnionitis,** third trimester   MCC Ⓜ ♀
      ✓7ᵗʰ **O41.129** **Chorioamnionitis, unspecified trimester**   Ⓜ ♀

  ✓6ᵗʰ **O41.14** **Placentitis**
      ✓7ᵗʰ **O41.141** **Placentitis,** first trimester   MCC Ⓜ ♀
      ✓7ᵗʰ **O41.142** **Placentitis,** second trimester   MCC Ⓜ ♀
      ✓7ᵗʰ **O41.143** **Placentitis,** third trimester   MCC Ⓜ ♀
      ✓7ᵗʰ **O41.149** **Placentitis, unspecified trimester**   Ⓜ ♀

 ✓5ᵗʰ **O41.8** **Other specified disorders of amniotic fluid and membranes**
  ✓6ᵗʰ **O41.8X** **Other specified disorders of amniotic fluid and membranes**
      ✓7ᵗʰ **O41.8X1** **Other specified disorders of amniotic fluid and membranes,** first trimester   Ⓜ ♀
      ✓7ᵗʰ **O41.8X2** **Other specified disorders of amniotic fluid and membranes,** second trimester   Ⓜ ♀
      ✓7ᵗʰ **O41.8X3** **Other specified disorders of amniotic fluid and membranes,** third trimester   Ⓜ ♀
      ✓7ᵗʰ **O41.8X9** **Other specified disorders of amniotic fluid and membranes, unspecified trimester**   Ⓜ ♀

 ✓5ᵗʰ **O41.9** **Disorder of amniotic fluid and membranes, unspecified**
  ✓x7ᵗʰ **O41.90** **Disorder of amniotic fluid and membranes, unspecified, unspecified trimester**   Ⓜ ♀
  ✓x7ᵗʰ **O41.91** **Disorder of amniotic fluid and membranes, unspecified,** first trimester   Ⓜ ♀
  ✓x7ᵗʰ **O41.92** **Disorder of amniotic fluid and membranes, unspecified,** second trimester   Ⓜ ♀
  ✓x7ᵗʰ **O41.93** **Disorder of amniotic fluid and membranes, unspecified,** third trimester   Ⓜ ♀

✓4ᵗʰ **O42** **Premature rupture of membranes**
  AHA: 2016,1Q,3

 ✓5ᵗʰ **O42.0** **Premature rupture of membranes,** onset of labor within 24 hours of rupture
  O42.00 **Premature rupture of membranes, onset of labor within 24 hours of rupture, unspecified weeks of gestation**   Ⓜ ♀
  ✓6ᵗʰ **O42.01** Preterm **premature rupture of membranes, onset of labor within 24 hours of rupture**
    Premature rupture of membranes before 37 completed weeks of gestation
    O42.011 **Preterm premature rupture of membranes, onset of labor within 24 hours of rupture,** first trimester   Ⓜ ♀
    O42.012 **Preterm premature rupture of membranes, onset of labor within 24 hours of rupture,** second trimester   Ⓜ ♀
    O42.013 **Preterm premature rupture of membranes, onset of labor within 24 hours of rupture,** third trimester   Ⓜ ♀
    O42.019 **Preterm premature rupture of membranes, onset of labor within 24 hours of rupture, unspecified trimester**   Ⓜ ♀
  O42.02 Full-term **premature rupture of membranes, onset of labor within 24 hours of rupture**   Ⓜ ♀
    Premature rupture of membranes at or after 37 completed weeks of gestation, onset of labor within 24 hours of rupture

 ✓5ᵗʰ **O42.1** **Premature rupture of membranes,** onset of labor more than 24 hours following rupture
  AHA: 2016,1Q,5
  O42.10 **Premature rupture of membranes, onset of labor more than 24 hours following rupture, unspecified weeks of gestation**   Ⓜ ♀

  ✓6ᵗʰ **O42.11** Preterm **premature rupture of membranes, onset of labor more than 24 hours following rupture**
    Premature rupture of membranes before 37 completed weeks of gestation
    O42.111 **Preterm premature rupture of membranes, onset of labor more than 24 hours following rupture,** first trimester   Ⓜ ♀
    O42.112 **Preterm premature rupture of membranes, onset of labor more than 24 hours following rupture,** second trimester   Ⓜ ♀
    O42.113 **Preterm premature rupture of membranes, onset of labor more than 24 hours following rupture,** third trimester   Ⓜ ♀
    O42.119 **Preterm premature rupture of membranes, onset of labor more than 24 hours following rupture, unspecified trimester**   Ⓜ ♀
  O42.12 Full-term **premature rupture of membranes, onset of labor more than 24 hours following rupture**   Ⓜ ♀
    Premature rupture of membranes at or after 37 completed weeks of gestation, onset of labor more than 24 hours following rupture

 ✓5ᵗʰ **O42.9** **Premature rupture of membranes,** unspecified as to length of time between rupture and onset of labor
  O42.90 **Premature rupture of membranes, unspecified as to length of time between rupture and onset of labor, unspecified weeks of gestation**   Ⓜ ♀
  ✓6ᵗʰ **O42.91** Preterm **premature rupture of membranes, unspecified as to length of time between rupture and onset of labor**
    Premature rupture of membranes before 37 completed weeks of gestation
    O42.911 **Preterm premature rupture of membranes, unspecified as to length of time between rupture and onset of labor, first trimester**   Ⓜ ♀
    O42.912 **Preterm premature rupture of membranes, unspecified as to length of time between rupture and onset of labor,** second trimester   Ⓜ ♀
    O42.913 **Preterm premature rupture of membranes, unspecified as to length of time between rupture and onset of labor,** third trimester   Ⓜ ♀
    O42.919 **Preterm premature rupture of membranes, unspecified as to length of time between rupture and onset of labor, unspecified trimester**   Ⓜ ♀
  O42.92 Full-term **premature rupture of membranes, unspecified as to length of time between rupture and onset of labor**   Ⓜ ♀
    Premature rupture of membranes at or after 37 completed weeks of gestation, unspecified as to length of time between rupture and onset of labor

✓4ᵗʰ **O43** **Placental disorders**
  EXCLUDES 2   *maternal care for poor fetal growth due to placental insufficiency (O36.5-)*
    placenta previa (O44.-)
    placental polyp (O90.89)
    placentitis (O41.14-)
    premature separation of placenta [abruptio placentae] (O45.-)

 ✓5ᵗʰ **O43.0** **Placental transfusion syndromes**
  ✓6ᵗʰ **O43.01** Fetomaternal **placental transfusion syndrome**
    Maternofetal placental transfusion syndrome
    O43.011 **Fetomaternal placental transfusion syndrome,** first trimester   Ⓜ ♀
    O43.012 **Fetomaternal placental transfusion syndrome,** second trimester   Ⓜ ♀
    O43.013 **Fetomaternal placental transfusion syndrome,** third trimester   Ⓜ ♀
    O43.019 **Fetomaternal placental transfusion syndrome, unspecified trimester**   Ⓜ ♀

Ⓝ Newborn: 0   Ⓟ Pediatric: 0-17   Ⓜ Maternity: 9-64   Ⓐ Adult: 15-124   MCC Major Complication/Comorbidity   CC Complication/Comorbidity   SW Severe Wound Dx

✓6ᵗʰ **O43.02 Fetus-to-fetus placental transfusion syndrome**

DEF: Condition in which an imbalance in amniotic fluid occurs due to uneven blood flow between twins sharing a placenta.

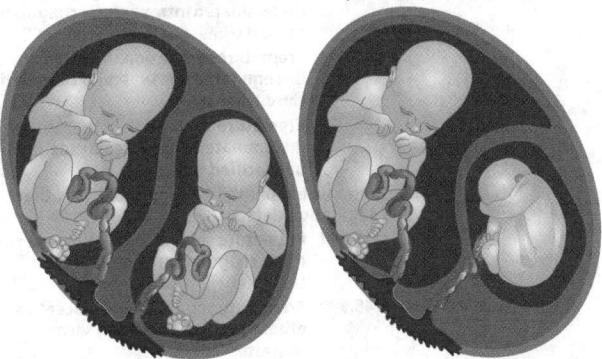

Twin to Twin Transfusion Syndrome (TTTS)

Healthy twins   Twins with TTTS

O43.021 Fetus-to-fetus placental transfusion syndrome, first trimester Ⓜ♀

O43.022 Fetus-to-fetus placental transfusion syndrome, second trimester Ⓜ♀

O43.023 Fetus-to-fetus placental transfusion syndrome, third trimester Ⓜ♀

O43.029 Fetus-to-fetus placental transfusion syndrome, unspecified trimester Ⓜ♀

✓5ᵗʰ **O43.1 Malformation of placenta**

✓6ᵗʰ **O43.10 Malformation of placenta, unspecified**

Abnormal placenta NOS

O43.101 Malformation of placenta, unspecified, first trimester Ⓜ♀

O43.102 Malformation of placenta, unspecified, second trimester Ⓜ♀

O43.103 Malformation of placenta, unspecified, third trimester Ⓜ♀

O43.109 Malformation of placenta, unspecified, unspecified trimester Ⓜ♀

✓6ᵗʰ **O43.11 Circumvallate placenta**

O43.111 Circumvallate placenta, first trimester Ⓜ♀

O43.112 Circumvallate placenta, second trimester Ⓜ♀

O43.113 Circumvallate placenta, third trimester Ⓜ♀

O43.119 Circumvallate placenta, unspecified trimester Ⓜ♀

✓6ᵗʰ **O43.12 Velamentous insertion of umbilical cord**

O43.121 Velamentous insertion of umbilical cord, first trimester Ⓜ♀

O43.122 Velamentous insertion of umbilical cord, second trimester Ⓜ♀

O43.123 Velamentous insertion of umbilical cord, third trimester Ⓜ♀

O43.129 Velamentous insertion of umbilical cord, unspecified trimester Ⓜ♀

✓6ᵗʰ **O43.19 Other malformation of placenta**

O43.191 Other malformation of placenta, first trimester Ⓜ♀

O43.192 Other malformation of placenta, second trimester Ⓜ♀

O43.193 Other malformation of placenta, third trimester Ⓜ♀

O43.199 Other malformation of placenta, unspecified trimester Ⓜ♀

✓5ᵗʰ **O43.2 Morbidly adherent placenta**

Code also associated third stage postpartum hemorrhage, if applicable (O72.0)

EXCLUDES 1 retained placenta (O73.-)

✓6ᵗʰ **O43.21 Placenta accreta**

DEF: Condition where the placenta adheres too deeply to the uterine wall; often associated with placenta previa.

O43.211 Placenta accreta, first trimester Ⓜ♀

O43.212 Placenta accreta, second trimester Ⓜ♀

O43.213 Placenta accreta, third trimester Ⓜ♀

O43.219 Placenta accreta, unspecified trimester Ⓜ♀

✓6ᵗʰ **O43.22 Placenta increta**

DEF: Condition where the placenta adheres too deeply to the uterine wall and penetrates the muscle; often associated with placenta previa.

O43.221 Placenta increta, first trimester Ⓜ♀

O43.222 Placenta increta, second trimester Ⓜ♀

O43.223 Placenta increta, third trimester Ⓜ♀

O43.229 Placenta increta, unspecified trimester Ⓜ♀

✓6ᵗʰ **O43.23 Placenta percreta**

DEF: Condition where the placenta attaches through the uterine muscle and may invade other organs, resulting in antenatal complications, premature delivery, retention of all or a portion of the placenta, or postpartum bleeding.

O43.231 Placenta percreta, first trimester Ⓜ♀

O43.232 Placenta percreta, second trimester Ⓜ♀

O43.233 Placenta percreta, third trimester Ⓜ♀

O43.239 Placenta percreta, unspecified trimester Ⓜ♀

✓5ᵗʰ **O43.8 Other placental disorders**

✓6ᵗʰ **O43.81 Placental infarction**

O43.811 Placental infarction, first trimester Ⓜ♀

O43.812 Placental infarction, second trimester Ⓜ♀

O43.813 Placental infarction, third trimester Ⓜ♀

O43.819 Placental infarction, unspecified trimester Ⓜ♀

✓6ᵗʰ **O43.89 Other placental disorders**

Placental dysfunction

O43.891 Other placental disorders, first trimester Ⓜ♀

O43.892 Other placental disorders, second trimester Ⓜ♀

O43.893 Other placental disorders, third trimester Ⓜ♀

O43.899 Other placental disorders, unspecified trimester Ⓜ♀

✓5ᵗʰ **O43.9 Unspecified placental disorder**

O43.90 Unspecified placental disorder, unspecified trimester Ⓜ♀

O43.91 Unspecified placental disorder, first trimester Ⓜ♀

O43.92 Unspecified placental disorder, second trimester Ⓜ♀

O43.93 Unspecified placental disorder, third trimester Ⓜ♀

✓4ᵗʰ **O44 Placenta previa**

AHA: 2016,4Q,52-53

DEF: Placenta implanted in the lower segment of the uterus, which commonly causes hemorrhage in the last trimester of pregnancy.

✓5ᵗʰ **O44.0 Complete placenta previa NOS or without hemorrhage**

Placenta previa NOS

O44.00 Complete placenta previa NOS or without hemorrhage, unspecified trimester Ⓜ♀

O44.01 Complete placenta previa NOS or without hemorrhage, first trimester CC Ⓜ♀

O44.02 Complete placenta previa NOS or without hemorrhage, second trimester CC Ⓜ♀

O44.03 Complete placenta previa NOS or without hemorrhage, third trimester CC Ⓜ♀

✓5ᵗʰ **O44.1 Complete placenta previa with hemorrhage**

EXCLUDES 1 labor and delivery complicated by hemorrhage from vasa previa (O69.4)

O44.10 Complete placenta previa with hemorrhage, unspecified trimester Ⓜ♀

O44.11 Complete placenta previa with hemorrhage, first trimester MCC Ⓜ♀

✔ Additional Character Required   ✓x7ᵗʰ Placeholder   Questionable PDx   Manifestation   Unspecified Dx   UPD Unacceptable PDx   H1-H14 HAC   HCC CMS-HCC Dx   HIV HIV Dx

ICD-10-CM 2022   891

O44.12   **Complete placenta previa with hemorrhage,** second **trimester**   MCC M ♀

O44.13   **Complete placenta previa with hemorrhage,** third **trimester**   MCC M ♀

√5ᵗʰ **O44.2** Partial **placenta previa** without hemorrhage

   Marginal placenta previa, NOS or without hemorrhage

O44.20   **Partial placenta previa NOS or without hemorrhage, unspecified trimester**   M ♀

O44.21   **Partial placenta previa NOS or without hemorrhage,** first **trimester**   CC M ♀

O44.22   **Partial placenta previa NOS or without hemorrhage,** second **trimester**   CC M ♀

O44.23   **Partial placenta previa NOS or without hemorrhage,** third **trimester**   CC M ♀

√5ᵗʰ **O44.3** Partial **placenta previa** with hemorrhage

   Marginal placenta previa with hemorrhage

O44.30   **Partial placenta previa with hemorrhage, unspecified trimester**   M ♀

O44.31   **Partial placenta previa with hemorrhage,** first **trimester**   MCC M ♀

O44.32   **Partial placenta previa with hemorrhage,** second **trimester**   MCC M ♀

O44.33   **Partial placenta previa with hemorrhage,** third **trimester**   MCC M ♀

√5ᵗʰ **O44.4** Low lying **placenta NOS or** without hemorrhage

   Low implantation of placenta NOS or without hemorrhage

O44.40   **Low lying placenta NOS or without hemorrhage, unspecified trimester**   M ♀

O44.41   **Low lying placenta NOS or without hemorrhage,** first **trimester**   CC M ♀

O44.42   **Low lying placenta NOS or without hemorrhage,** second **trimester**   CC M ♀

O44.43   **Low lying placenta NOS or without hemorrhage,** third **trimester**   CC M ♀

√5ᵗʰ **O44.5** Low lying **placenta** with hemorrhage

   Low implantation of placenta with hemorrhage

O44.50   **Low lying placenta with hemorrhage, unspecified trimester**   M ♀

O44.51   **Low lying placenta with hemorrhage,** first **trimester**   MCC M ♀

O44.52   **Low lying placenta with hemorrhage,** second **trimester**   MCC M ♀

O44.53   **Low lying placenta with hemorrhage,** third **trimester**   MCC M ♀

√4ᵗʰ **O45 Premature separation of placenta [abruptio placentae]**

√5ᵗʰ **O45.0** **Premature separation of placenta** with coagulation defect

√6ᵗʰ O45.00   **Premature separation of placenta with coagulation defect, unspecified**

O45.001   **Premature separation of placenta with coagulation defect, unspecified,** first **trimester**   MCC M ♀

O45.002   **Premature separation of placenta with coagulation defect, unspecified,** second **trimester**   MCC M ♀

O45.003   **Premature separation of placenta with coagulation defect, unspecified,** third **trimester**   MCC M ♀

O45.009   **Premature separation of placenta with coagulation defect, unspecified, unspecified trimester**   M ♀

√6ᵗʰ O45.01   **Premature separation of placenta with afibrinogenemia**

   Premature separation of placenta with hypofibrinogenemia

O45.011   **Premature separation of placenta with afibrinogenemia,** first **trimester**   MCC M ♀

O45.012   **Premature separation of placenta with afibrinogenemia,** second **trimester**   MCC M ♀

O45.013   **Premature separation of placenta with afibrinogenemia,** third **trimester**   MCC M ♀

O45.019   **Premature separation of placenta with afibrinogenemia, unspecified trimester**   M ♀

√6ᵗʰ O45.02   **Premature separation of placenta** with disseminated intravascular coagulation

O45.021   **Premature separation of placenta with disseminated intravascular coagulation,** first **trimester**   MCC M ♀

O45.022   **Premature separation of placenta with disseminated intravascular coagulation,** second **trimester**   MCC M ♀

O45.023   **Premature separation of placenta with disseminated intravascular coagulation,** third **trimester**   MCC M ♀

O45.029   **Premature separation of placenta with disseminated intravascular coagulation, unspecified trimester**   M ♀

√6ᵗʰ O45.09   **Premature separation of placenta with other coagulation defect**

O45.091   **Premature separation of placenta with other coagulation defect,** first **trimester**   MCC M ♀

O45.092   **Premature separation of placenta with other coagulation defect,** second **trimester**   MCC M ♀

O45.093   **Premature separation of placenta with other coagulation defect,** third **trimester**   MCC M ♀

O45.099   **Premature separation of placenta with other coagulation defect, unspecified trimester**   M ♀

√5ᵗʰ **O45.8** **Other premature separation of placenta**

√6ᵗʰ O45.8X   **Other premature separation of placenta**

O45.8X1   **Other premature separation of placenta,** first **trimester**   MCC M ♀

O45.8X2   **Other premature separation of placenta,** second **trimester**   MCC M ♀

O45.8X3   **Other premature separation of placenta,** third **trimester**   MCC M ♀

O45.8X9   **Other premature separation of placenta, unspecified trimester**   M ♀

√5ᵗʰ **O45.9** **Premature separation of placenta, unspecified**

   Abruptio placentae NOS

O45.90   **Premature separation of placenta, unspecified, unspecified trimester**   M ♀

O45.91   **Premature separation of placenta, unspecified,** first **trimester**   MCC M ♀

O45.92   **Premature separation of placenta, unspecified,** second **trimester**   MCC M ♀

O45.93   **Premature separation of placenta, unspecified,** third **trimester**   MCC M ♀

√4ᵗʰ **O46 Antepartum hemorrhage, not elsewhere classified**

EXCLUDES 1   *hemorrhage in early pregnancy (O20.-)*
          intrapartum hemorrhage NEC (O67.-)
          placenta previa (O44.-)
          premature separation of placenta [abruptio placentae] (O45.-)

DEF: Uterine hemorrhage prior to delivery that is not related to placenta previa or abruptio placentae.

√5ᵗʰ **O46.0** **Antepartum hemorrhage** with coagulation defect

√6ᵗʰ O46.00   **Antepartum hemorrhage with coagulation defect, unspecified**

O46.001   **Antepartum hemorrhage with coagulation defect, unspecified,** first **trimester**   MCC M ♀

O46.002   **Antepartum hemorrhage with coagulation defect, unspecified,** second **trimester**   MCC M ♀

O46.003   **Antepartum hemorrhage with coagulation defect, unspecified,** third **trimester**   MCC M ♀

O46.009   **Antepartum hemorrhage with coagulation defect, unspecified, unspecified trimester**   M ♀

√6ᵗʰ O46.01   **Antepartum hemorrhage** with afibrinogenemia

   Antepartum hemorrhage with hypofibrinogenemia

O46.011   **Antepartum hemorrhage with afibrinogenemia,** first **trimester**   MCC M ♀

O46.012   **Antepartum hemorrhage with afibrinogenemia,** second **trimester**   MCC M ♀

N Newborn: 0   P Pediatric: 0-17   M Maternity: 9-64   A Adult: 15-124   MCC Major Complication/Comorbidity   CC Complication/Comorbidity   SW Severe Wound Dx

892   ICD-10-CM 2022

O46.013 **Antepartum hemorrhage with afibrinogenemia**, third trimester `MCC` Ⓜ ♀

O46.019 **Antepartum hemorrhage with afibrinogenemia**, unspecified trimester Ⓜ ♀

√6ᵗʰ O46.02 **Antepartum hemorrhage** with disseminated intravascular coagulation

O46.021 **Antepartum hemorrhage with disseminated intravascular coagulation**, first trimester `MCC` Ⓜ ♀

O46.022 **Antepartum hemorrhage with disseminated intravascular coagulation**, second trimester `MCC` Ⓜ ♀

O46.023 **Antepartum hemorrhage with disseminated intravascular coagulation**, third trimester `MCC` Ⓜ ♀

O46.029 **Antepartum hemorrhage with disseminated intravascular coagulation**, unspecified trimester Ⓜ ♀

√6ᵗʰ O46.09 **Antepartum hemorrhage with** other **coagulation defect**

O46.091 **Antepartum hemorrhage with other coagulation defect**, first trimester `MCC` Ⓜ ♀

O46.092 **Antepartum hemorrhage with other coagulation defect**, second trimester `MCC` Ⓜ ♀

O46.093 **Antepartum hemorrhage with other coagulation defect**, third trimester `MCC` Ⓜ ♀

O46.099 **Antepartum hemorrhage with other coagulation defect**, unspecified trimester Ⓜ ♀

√6ᵗʰ O46.8 **Other antepartum hemorrhage**

√6ᵗʰ O46.8X **Other antepartum hemorrhage**

O46.8X1 **Other antepartum hemorrhage**, first trimester Ⓜ ♀

O46.8X2 **Other antepartum hemorrhage**, second trimester Ⓜ ♀

O46.8X3 **Other antepartum hemorrhage**, third trimester Ⓜ ♀

O46.8X9 **Other antepartum hemorrhage**, unspecified trimester Ⓜ ♀

√5ᵗʰ O46.9 **Antepartum hemorrhage, unspecified**

O46.90 **Antepartum hemorrhage, unspecified, unspecified trimester** Ⓜ ♀

O46.91 **Antepartum hemorrhage, unspecified,** first trimester Ⓜ ♀

O46.92 **Antepartum hemorrhage, unspecified,** second trimester Ⓜ ♀

O46.93 **Antepartum hemorrhage, unspecified,** third trimester Ⓜ ♀

√4ᵗʰ **O47 False labor**

INCLUDES   Braxton Hicks contractions

threatened labor

EXCLUDES 1   *preterm labor (O60.-)*

AHA: 2021,1Q,10

√5ᵗʰ O47.0 **False labor** before 37 completed weeks of gestation

O47.00 **False labor before 37 completed weeks of gestation, unspecified trimester** Ⓜ ♀

O47.02 **False labor before 37 completed weeks of gestation,** second trimester `CC` Ⓜ ♀

O47.03 **False labor before 37 completed weeks of gestation,** third trimester `CC` Ⓜ ♀

O47.1 **False labor** at or after 37 completed weeks of gestation `CC` Ⓜ ♀

O47.9 **False labor, unspecified** Ⓜ ♀

√4ᵗʰ **O48 Late pregnancy**

O48.0 **Post-term pregnancy** Ⓜ ♀
Pregnancy over 40 completed weeks to 42 completed weeks gestation

O48.1 **Prolonged pregnancy** Ⓜ ♀
Pregnancy which has advanced beyond 42 completed weeks gestation
AHA: 2016,1Q,5

Complications of labor and delivery (O60-O77)

√4ᵗʰ **O60 Preterm labor**

INCLUDES   onset (spontaneous) of labor before 37 completed weeks of gestation

EXCLUDES 1   *false labor (O47.0-)*

threatened labor NOS (O47.0-)

√5ᵗʰ O60.0 **Preterm labor** without delivery

O60.00 **Preterm labor without delivery, unspecified trimester** Ⓜ ♀

O60.02 **Preterm labor without delivery,** second trimester `MCC` Ⓜ ♀

O60.03 **Preterm labor without delivery,** third trimester `MCC` Ⓜ ♀

√5ᵗʰ O60.1 **Preterm labor** with preterm delivery

AHA: 2016,2Q,10

One of the following 7th characters is to be assigned to each code under subcategory O60.1. 7th character 0 is for single gestations and multiple gestations where the fetus is unspecified. 7th characters 1 through 9 are for cases of multiple gestations to identify the fetus for which the code applies. The appropriate code from category O30, Multiple gestation, must also be assigned when assigning a code from subcategory O60.1 that has a 7th character of 1 through 9.

0   not applicable or unspecified
1   fetus 1
2   fetus 2
3   fetus 3
4   fetus 4
5   fetus 5
9   other fetus

√x7ᵗʰ O60.10 **Preterm labor with preterm delivery, unspecified trimester** `CC` Ⓜ ♀
Preterm labor with delivery NOS

√x7ᵗʰ O60.12 **Preterm labor** second trimester **with preterm delivery** second trimester `MCC` Ⓜ ♀

√x7ᵗʰ O60.13 **Preterm labor** second trimester **with preterm delivery** third trimester `MCC` Ⓜ ♀

√x7ᵗʰ O60.14 **Preterm labor** third trimester **with preterm delivery** third trimester `MCC` Ⓜ ♀

√5ᵗʰ O60.2 **Term delivery with preterm labor**

One of the following 7th characters is to be assigned to each code under subcategory O60.2. 7th character 0 is for single gestations and multiple gestations where the fetus is unspecified. 7th characters 1 through 9 are for cases of multiple gestations to identify the fetus for which the code applies. The appropriate code from category O30, Multiple gestation, must also be assigned when assigning a code from subcategory O60.2 that has a 7th character of 1 through 9.

0   not applicable or unspecified
1   fetus 1
2   fetus 2
3   fetus 3
4   fetus 4
5   fetus 5
9   other fetus

√x7ᵗʰ O60.20 **Term delivery with preterm labor, unspecified trimester** `CC` Ⓜ ♀

√x7ᵗʰ O60.22 **Term delivery with preterm labor,** second trimester `MCC` Ⓜ ♀

√x7ᵗʰ O60.23 **Term delivery with preterm labor,** third trimester `MCC` Ⓜ ♀

√4ᵗʰ **O61 Failed induction of labor**

O61.0 **Failed** medical **induction of labor** Ⓜ ♀
Failed induction (of labor) by oxytocin
Failed induction (of labor) by prostaglandins

O61.1 **Failed** instrumental **induction of labor** Ⓜ ♀
Failed mechanical induction (of labor)
Failed surgical induction (of labor)

O61.8 **Other failed induction of labor** Ⓜ ♀

O61.9 **Failed induction of labor, unspecified** Ⓜ ♀

☑ Additional Character Required   √x7ᵗʰ Placeholder   Questionable PDx   Manifestation   Unspecified Dx   UPD Unacceptable PDx   H1-H14 HAC   HCC CMS-HCC Dx   HIV HIV Dx

ICD-10-CM 2022   893

✓4th **062** **Abnormalities of forces of labor**

> **DEF:** Uterine inertia: Weak or poorly coordinated contractions of the uterus during labor.

062.0 **Primary inadequate contractions**   M ♀
> Failure of cervical dilatation
> Primary hypotonic uterine dysfunction
> Uterine inertia during latent phase of labor

062.1 **Secondary uterine inertia**   M ♀
> Arrested active phase of labor
> Secondary hypotonic uterine dysfunction

062.2 **Other uterine inertia**   M ♀
> Atony of uterus without hemorrhage
> Atony of uterus NOS
> Desultory labor
> Hypotonic uterine dysfunction NOS
> Irregular labor
> Poor contractions
> Slow slope active phase of labor
> Uterine inertia NOS
>> **EXCLUDES 1**   atony of uterus with hemorrhage (postpartum) (072.1)
>> postpartum atony of uterus without hemorrhage (075.89)
>
> **DEF:** Uterine atony: Failure of the uterine muscles to contract after the fetus and placenta are delivered.

062.3 **Precipitate labor**   M ♀
> **DEF:** Rapid labor with delivery occurring in three hours or less from the onset of contractions.

062.4 **Hypertonic, incoordinate, and prolonged uterine contractions**   M ♀
> Cervical spasm
> Contraction ring dystocia
> Dyscoordinate labor
> Hour-glass contraction of uterus
> Hypertonic uterine dysfunction
> Incoordinate uterine action
> Tetanic contractions
> Uterine dystocia NOS
> Uterine spasm
>> **EXCLUDES 1**   dystocia (fetal) (maternal) NOS (066.9)

062.8 **Other abnormalities of forces of labor**   M ♀
062.9 **Abnormality of forces of labor, unspecified**   M ♀

✓4th **063** **Long labor**

063.0 **Prolonged first stage (of labor)**   M ♀
063.1 **Prolonged second stage (of labor)**   M ♀
063.2 **Delayed delivery of second twin, triplet, etc.**   M ♀
063.9 **Long labor, unspecified**   CC M ♀
> Prolonged labor NOS

✓4th **064** **Obstructed labor due to malposition and malpresentation of fetus**

> One of the following 7th characters is to be assigned to each code under category 064. 7th character Ø is for single gestations and multiple gestations where the fetus is unspecified. 7th characters 1 through 9 are for cases of multiple gestations to identify the fetus for which the code applies. The appropriate code from category O3Ø, Multiple gestation, must also be assigned when assigning a code from category 064 that has a 7th character of 1 through 9.
> Ø   not applicable or unspecified
> 1   fetus 1
> 2   fetus 2
> 3   fetus 3
> 4   fetus 4
> 5   fetus 5
> 9   other fetus

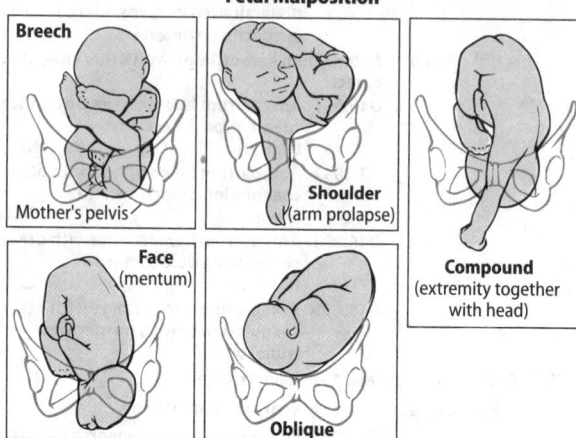

Fetal Malposition

Breech — Mother's pelvis

Shoulder (arm prolapse)

Face (mentum)

Compound (extremity together with head)

Oblique

✓x7th **064.0** **Obstructed labor due to incomplete rotation of fetal head**   M ♀
> Deep transverse arrest
> Obstructed labor due to persistent occipitoiliac (position)
> Obstructed labor due to persistent occipitoposterior (position)
> Obstructed labor due to persistent occipitosacral (position)
> Obstructed labor due to persistent occipitotransverse (position)

✓x7th **064.1** **Obstructed labor due to breech presentation**   M ♀
> Obstructed labor due to buttocks presentation
> Obstructed labor due to complete breech presentation
> Obstructed labor due to frank breech presentation

✓x7th **064.2** **Obstructed labor due to face presentation**   M ♀
> Obstructed labor due to chin presentation

✓x7th **064.3** **Obstructed labor due to brow presentation**   M ♀

✓x7th **064.4** **Obstructed labor due to shoulder presentation**   M ♀
> Prolapsed arm
>> **EXCLUDES 1**   impacted shoulders (066.0)
>> shoulder dystocia (066.0)

✓x7th **064.5** **Obstructed labor due to compound presentation**   M ♀

✓x7th **064.8** **Obstructed labor due to other malposition and malpresentation**   M ♀
> Obstructed labor due to footling presentation
> Obstructed labor due to incomplete breech presentation

✓x7th **064.9** **Obstructed labor due to malposition and malpresentation, unspecified**   M ♀

✓4th **065** **Obstructed labor due to maternal pelvic abnormality**

065.0 **Obstructed labor due to deformed pelvis**   M ♀
065.1 **Obstructed labor due to generally contracted pelvis**   M ♀
065.2 **Obstructed labor due to pelvic inlet contraction**   M ♀
065.3 **Obstructed labor due to pelvic outlet and mid-cavity contraction**   M ♀
065.4 **Obstructed labor due to fetopelvic disproportion, unspecified**   M ♀
>> **EXCLUDES 1**   dystocia due to abnormality of fetus (066.2-066.3)
065.5 **Obstructed labor due to abnormality of maternal pelvic organs**   M ♀
> Obstructed labor due to conditions listed in O34.-
> Use additional code to identify abnormality of pelvic organs O34.-

O65.8   **Obstructed labor due to other maternal pelvic abnormalities**   M ♀

O65.9   **Obstructed labor due to maternal pelvic abnormality, unspecified**   M ♀

✓4th **O66**   **Other obstructed labor**

O66.0   **Obstructed labor due to shoulder dystocia**   M ♀
Impacted shoulders
DEF: Obstructed labor due to impacted fetal shoulders. It is an emergency condition that may require cesarean section, forceps delivery, vacuum extraction, or symphysiotomy.

O66.1   **Obstructed labor due to locked twins**   M ♀

O66.2   **Obstructed labor due to unusually large fetus**   M ♀

O66.3   **Obstructed labor due to other abnormalities of fetus**   M ♀
Dystocia due to fetal ascites
Dystocia due to fetal hydrops
Dystocia due to fetal meningomyelocele
Dystocia due to fetal sacral teratoma
Dystocia due to fetal tumor
Dystocia due to hydrocephalic fetus
Use additional code to identify cause of obstruction

✓5th **O66.4**   **Failed trial of labor**

O66.40   **Failed trial of labor, unspecified**   M ♀

O66.41   **Failed attempted vaginal birth after previous cesarean delivery**   M ♀
Code first rupture of uterus, if applicable (O71.0-, O71.1)

O66.5   **Attempted application of vacuum extractor and forceps**   M ♀
Attempted application of vacuum or forceps, with subsequent delivery by forceps or cesarean delivery

O66.6   **Obstructed labor due to other multiple fetuses**   M ♀

O66.8   **Other specified obstructed labor**   M ♀
Use additional code to identify cause of obstruction

O66.9   **Obstructed labor, unspecified**   M ♀
Dystocia NOS
Fetal dystocia NOS
Maternal dystocia NOS

✓4th **O67**   **Labor and delivery complicated by intrapartum hemorrhage, not elsewhere classified**
EXCLUDES 1   antepartum hemorrhage NEC (O46.-)
placenta previa (O44.-)
premature separation of placenta [abruptio placentae] (O45.-)
EXCLUDES 2   postpartum hemorrhage (O72.-)

O67.0   **Intrapartum hemorrhage with coagulation defect**   MCC M ♀
Intrapartum hemorrhage (excessive) associated with afibrinogenemia
Intrapartum hemorrhage (excessive) associated with disseminated intravascular coagulation
Intrapartum hemorrhage (excessive) associated with hyperfibrinolysis
Intrapartum hemorrhage (excessive) associated with hypofibrinogenemia

O67.8   **Other intrapartum hemorrhage**   M ♀
Excessive intrapartum hemorrhage

O67.9   **Intrapartum hemorrhage, unspecified**   M ♀

O68   **Labor and delivery complicated by abnormality of fetal acid-base balance**   CC M ♀
Fetal acidemia complicating labor and delivery
Fetal acidosis complicating labor and delivery
Fetal alkalosis complicating labor and delivery
Fetal metabolic acidemia complicating labor and delivery
EXCLUDES 1   fetal stress NOS (O77.9)
labor and delivery complicated by electrocardiographic evidence of fetal stress (O77.8)
labor and delivery complicated by ultrasonic evidence of fetal stress (O77.8)
EXCLUDES 2   abnormality in fetal heart rate or rhythm (O76)
labor and delivery complicated by meconium in amniotic fluid (O77.0)

✓4th **O69**   **Labor and delivery complicated by umbilical cord complications**
AHA: 2016,1Q,5

One of the following 7th characters is to be assigned to each code under category O69. 7th character Ø is for single gestations and multiple gestations where the fetus is unspecified. 7th characters 1 through 9 are for cases of multiple gestations to identify the fetus for which the code applies. The appropriate code from category O30, Multiple gestation, must also be assigned when assigning a code from category O69 that has a 7th character of 1 through 9.
Ø   not applicable or unspecified
1   fetus 1
2   fetus 2
3   fetus 3
4   fetus 4
5   fetus 5
9   other fetus

✓x7th **O69.0**   **Labor and delivery complicated by prolapse of cord**   M ♀
DEF: Abnormal presentation of the fetus marked by a protruding umbilical cord during labor. It can cause fetal death.

✓x7th **O69.1**   **Labor and delivery complicated by cord around neck, with compression**   M ♀
EXCLUDES 1   labor and delivery complicated by cord around neck, without compression (O69.81)

✓x7th **O69.2**   **Labor and delivery complicated by other cord entanglement, with compression**   M ♀
Labor and delivery complicated by compression of cord NOS
Labor and delivery complicated by entanglement of cords of twins in monoamniotic sac
Labor and delivery complicated by knot in cord
EXCLUDES 1   labor and delivery complicated by other cord entanglement, without compression (O69.82)

✓x7th **O69.3**   **Labor and delivery complicated by short cord**   M ♀

✓x7th **O69.4**   **Labor and delivery complicated by vasa previa**   M ♀
Labor and delivery complicated by hemorrhage from vasa previa

✓x7th **O69.5**   **Labor and delivery complicated by vascular lesion of cord**   M ♀
Labor and delivery complicated by cord bruising
Labor and delivery complicated by cord hematoma
Labor and delivery complicated by thrombosis of umbilical vessels

✓5th **O69.8**   **Labor and delivery complicated by other cord complications**

✓x7th **O69.81**   **Labor and delivery complicated by cord around neck, without compression**   M ♀
AHA: 2016,1Q,5

✓x7th **O69.82**   **Labor and delivery complicated by other cord entanglement, without compression**   M ♀

✓x7th **O69.89**   **Labor and delivery complicated by other cord complications**   M ♀

✓x7th **O69.9**   **Labor and delivery complicated by cord complication, unspecified**   M ♀

✓4th **O70**   **Perineal laceration during delivery**
INCLUDES   episiotomy extended by laceration
EXCLUDES 1   obstetric high vaginal laceration alone (O71.4)
AHA: 2016,2Q,34; 2016,1Q,3-4,5

O70.0   **First degree perineal laceration during delivery**   M ♀
Perineal laceration, rupture or tear involving fourchette during delivery
Perineal laceration, rupture or tear involving labia during delivery
Perineal laceration, rupture or tear involving skin during delivery
Perineal laceration, rupture or tear involving vagina during delivery
Perineal laceration, rupture or tear involving vulva during delivery
Slight perineal laceration, rupture or tear during delivery

O70.1   **Second degree perineal laceration during delivery**   M ♀
Perineal laceration, rupture or tear during delivery as in O70.0, also involving pelvic floor
Perineal laceration, rupture or tear during delivery as in O70.0, also involving perineal muscles
Perineal laceration, rupture or tear during delivery as in O70.0, also involving vaginal muscles
EXCLUDES 1   perineal laceration involving anal sphincter (O70.2)

✔ Additional Character Required   ✓x7th Placeholder   Questionable PDx   Manifestation   Unspecified Dx   UPD Unacceptable PDx   H1-H14 HAC   HCC CMS-HCC Dx   HIV HIV Dx

ICD-10-CM 2022   895

✓5ᵗʰ O70.2 Third degree perineal laceration during delivery

Perineal laceration, rupture or tear during delivery as in O70.1, also involving anal sphincter

Perineal laceration, rupture or tear during delivery as in O70.1, also involving rectovaginal septum

Perineal laceration, rupture or tear during delivery as in O70.1, also involving sphincter NOS

> **EXCLUDES 1**   anal sphincter tear during delivery without third degree perineal laceration (O70.4)
>
> perineal laceration involving anal or rectal mucosa (O70.3)

AHA: 2016,4Q,53-54

O70.20 Third degree perineal laceration during delivery, unspecified   cc M ♀

O70.21 Third degree perineal laceration during delivery, IIIa   cc M ♀

Third degree perineal laceration during delivery with less than 50% of external anal sphincter (EAS) thickness torn

O70.22 Third degree perineal laceration during delivery, IIIb   cc M ♀

Third degree perineal laceration during delivery with more than 50% external anal sphincter (EAS) thickness torn

O70.23 Third degree perineal laceration during delivery, IIIc   cc M ♀

Third degree perineal laceration during delivery with both external anal sphincter (EAS) and internal anal sphincter (IAS) torn

O70.3 Fourth degree perineal laceration during delivery   cc M ♀

Perineal laceration, rupture or tear during delivery as in O70.2, also involving anal mucosa

Perineal laceration, rupture or tear during delivery as in O70.2, also involving rectal mucosa

O70.4 Anal sphincter tear complicating delivery, not associated with third degree laceration   cc M ♀

> **EXCLUDES 1**   anal sphincter tear with third degree perineal laceration (O70.2)

O70.9 Perineal laceration during delivery, unspecified   M ♀

✓4ᵗʰ O71 Other obstetric trauma

> **INCLUDES**   obstetric damage from instruments

✓5ᵗʰ O71.0 Rupture of uterus (spontaneous) before onset of labor

> **EXCLUDES 1**   disruption of (current) cesarean delivery wound (O90.0)
>
> laceration of uterus, NEC (O71.81)

O71.00 Rupture of uterus before onset of labor, unspecified trimester   M ♀

O71.02 Rupture of uterus before onset of labor, second trimester   MCC M ♀

O71.03 Rupture of uterus before onset of labor, third trimester   MCC M ♀

O71.1 Rupture of uterus during labor   MCC M ♀

Rupture of uterus not stated as occurring before onset of labor

> **EXCLUDES 1**   disruption of cesarean delivery wound (O90.0)
>
> laceration of uterus, NEC (O71.81)

O71.2 Postpartum inversion of uterus   cc M ♀

O71.3 Obstetric laceration of cervix   cc M ♀

Annular detachment of cervix

O71.4 Obstetric high vaginal laceration alone   cc M ♀

Laceration of vaginal wall without perineal laceration

> **EXCLUDES 1**   obstetric high vaginal laceration with perineal laceration (O70.-)

AHA: 2016,1Q,5

O71.5 Other obstetric injury to pelvic organs   cc M ♀

Obstetric injury to bladder

Obstetric injury to urethra

> **EXCLUDES 2**   obstetric periurethral trauma (O71.82)

AHA: 2014,4Q,18

O71.6 Obstetric damage to pelvic joints and ligaments   cc M ♀

Obstetric avulsion of inner symphyseal cartilage

Obstetric damage to coccyx

Obstetric traumatic separation of symphysis (pubis)

O71.7 Obstetric hematoma of pelvis   cc M ♀

Obstetric hematoma of perineum

Obstetric hematoma of vagina

Obstetric hematoma of vulva

✓5ᵗʰ O71.8 Other specified obstetric trauma

O71.81 Laceration of uterus, not elsewhere classified   M ♀

O71.82 Other specified trauma to perineum and vulva   M ♀

Obstetric periurethral trauma

AHA: 2016,1Q,4; 2014,4Q,18

O71.89 Other specified obstetric trauma   M ♀

O71.9 Obstetric trauma, unspecified   M ♀

✓4ᵗʰ O72 Postpartum hemorrhage

> **INCLUDES**   hemorrhage after delivery of fetus or infant

O72.0 Third-stage hemorrhage   cc M ♀

Hemorrhage associated with retained, trapped or adherent placenta

Retained placenta NOS

Code also type of adherent placenta (O43.2-)

AHA: 2019,3Q,11

O72.1 Other immediate postpartum hemorrhage   cc M ♀

Hemorrhage following delivery of placenta

Postpartum hemorrhage (atonic) NOS

Uterine atony with hemorrhage

> **EXCLUDES 1**   uterine atony NOS (O62.2)
>
> uterine atony without hemorrhage (O62.2)
>
> postpartum atony of uterus without hemorrhage (O75.89)

AHA: 2016,1Q,4

DEF: Uterine atony: Failure of the uterine muscles to contract after the fetus and placenta are delivered.

O72.2 Delayed and secondary postpartum hemorrhage   cc M ♀

Hemorrhage associated with retained portions of placenta or membranes after the first 24 hours following delivery of placenta

Retained products of conception NOS, following delivery

O72.3 Postpartum coagulation defects   M ♀

Postpartum afibrinogenemia

Postpartum fibrinolysis

✓4ᵗʰ O73 Retained placenta and membranes, without hemorrhage

> **EXCLUDES 1**   placenta accreta (O43.21-)
>
> placenta increta (O43.22-)
>
> placenta percreta (O43.23-)

DEF: Postpartum condition resulting from failure to expel placental membrane tissues due to failed contractions of the uterine wall.

O73.0 Retained placenta without hemorrhage   M ♀

Adherent placenta, without hemorrhage

Trapped placenta without hemorrhage

O73.1 Retained portions of placenta and membranes, without hemorrhage   M ♀

Retained products of conception following delivery, without hemorrhage

✓4ᵗʰ O74 Complications of anesthesia during labor and delivery

> **INCLUDES**   maternal complications arising from the administration of a general, regional or local anesthetic, analgesic or other sedation during labor and delivery

Use additional code, if applicable, to identify specific complication

O74.0 Aspiration pneumonitis due to anesthesia during labor and delivery   M ♀

Inhalation of stomach contents or secretions NOS due to anesthesia during labor and delivery

Mendelson's syndrome due to anesthesia during labor and delivery

O74.1 Other pulmonary complications of anesthesia during labor and delivery   M ♀

O74.2 Cardiac complications of anesthesia during labor and delivery   M ♀

O74.3 Central nervous system complications of anesthesia during labor and delivery   M ♀

O74.4 Toxic reaction to local anesthesia during labor and delivery   M ♀

O74.5 Spinal and epidural anesthesia-induced headache during labor and delivery   M ♀

O74.6 Other complications of spinal and epidural anesthesia during labor and delivery   M ♀

N Newborn: 0   P Pediatric: 0-17   M Maternity: 9-64   A Adult: 15-124   MCC Major Complication/Comorbidity   CC Complication/Comorbidity   SW Severe Wound Dx

896

ICD-10-CM 2022

O74.7 Failed or difficult intubation for anesthesia during labor and delivery   Ⓜ ♀

O74.8 Other complications of anesthesia during labor and delivery   Ⓜ ♀

O74.9 Complication of anesthesia during labor and delivery, unspecified   Ⓜ ♀

✓4ᵗʰ **O75** Other complications of labor and delivery, not elsewhere classified

     EXCLUDES 2   *puerperal (postpartum) infection (O86.-)*
            puerperal (postpartum) sepsis (O85)

O75.0 Maternal distress during labor and delivery   Ⓜ ♀

O75.1 Shock during or following labor and delivery   ᴹᶜᶜ Ⓜ ♀
     Obstetric shock following labor and delivery

O75.2 Pyrexia during labor, not elsewhere classified   ᶜᶜ Ⓜ ♀

O75.3 Other infection during labor   ᴹᶜᶜ Ⓜ ♀
     Sepsis during labor
     Use additional code (B95-B97), to identify infectious agent

O75.4 Other complications of obstetric surgery and procedures   Ⓜ ♀
     Cardiac arrest following obstetric surgery or procedures
     Cardiac failure following obstetric surgery or procedures
     Cerebral anoxia following obstetric surgery or procedures
     Pulmonary edema following obstetric surgery or procedures
     Use additional code to identify specific complication
     EXCLUDES 2   *complications of anesthesia during labor and delivery (O74.-)*
            disruption of obstetrical (surgical) wound (O90.0-O90.1)
            hematoma of obstetrical (surgical) wound (O90.2)
            infection of obstetrical (surgical) wound (O86.0-)

O75.5 Delayed delivery after artificial rupture of membranes   Ⓜ ♀

✓5ᵗʰ **O75.8** Other specified complications of labor and delivery

     O75.81 Maternal exhaustion complicating labor and delivery   Ⓜ ♀

     O75.82 Onset (spontaneous) of labor after 37 completed weeks of gestation but before 39 completed weeks gestation, with delivery by (planned) cesarean section   Ⓜ ♀
         Delivery by (planned) cesarean section occurring after 37 completed weeks of gestation but before 39 completed weeks gestation due to (spontaneous) onset of labor
         Code first to specify reason for planned cesarean section such as:
            cephalopelvic disproportion (normally formed fetus) (O33.9)
            previous cesarean delivery (O34.21)

     O75.89 Other specified complications of labor and delivery   Ⓜ ♀

O75.9 Complication of labor and delivery, unspecified   Ⓜ ♀

O76 Abnormality in fetal heart rate and rhythm complicating labor and delivery   Ⓜ ♀
     Depressed fetal heart rate tones complicating labor and delivery
     Fetal bradycardia complicating labor and delivery
     Fetal heart rate decelerations complicating labor and delivery
     Fetal heart rate irregularity complicating labor and delivery
     Fetal heart rate abnormal variability complicating labor and delivery
     Fetal tachycardia complicating labor and delivery
     Non-reassuring fetal heart rate or rhythm complicating labor and delivery
     EXCLUDES 1   *fetal stress NOS (O77.9)*
            labor and delivery complicated by electrocardiographic evidence of fetal stress (O77.8)
            labor and delivery complicated by ultrasonic evidence of fetal stress (O77.8)
     EXCLUDES 2   *fetal metabolic acidemia (O68)*
            other fetal stress (O77.0-O77.1)
     AHA: 2013,4Q,118

✓4ᵗʰ **O77** Other fetal stress complicating labor and delivery

     O77.0 Labor and delivery complicated by meconium in amniotic fluid   Ⓜ ♀
         AHA: 2013,4Q,117-118

     O77.1 Fetal stress in labor or delivery due to drug administration   Ⓜ ♀

O77.8 Labor and delivery complicated by other evidence of fetal stress   Ⓜ ♀
     Labor and delivery complicated by electrocardiographic evidence of fetal stress
     Labor and delivery complicated by ultrasonic evidence of fetal stress
     EXCLUDES 1   *abnormality of fetal acid-base balance (O68)*
            abnormality in fetal heart rate or rhythm (O76)
            fetal metabolic acidemia (O68)

O77.9 Labor and delivery complicated by fetal stress, unspecified   Ⓜ ♀
     EXCLUDES 1   *abnormality of fetal acid-base balance (O68)*
            abnormality in fetal heart rate or rhythm (O76)
            fetal metabolic acidemia (O68)

Encounter for delivery (O80-O82)

O80 Encounter for full-term uncomplicated delivery   Ⓜ ♀
     NOTE   Delivery requiring minimal or no assistance, with or without episiotomy, without fetal manipulation [e.g., rotation version] or instrumentation [forceps] of a spontaneous, cephalic, vaginal, full-term, single, live-born infant. This code is for use as a single diagnosis code and is not to be used with any other code from chapter 15.
     Use additional code to indicate outcome of delivery (Z37.0)
     AHA: 2016,4Q,150; 2014,2Q,9

O82 Encounter for cesarean delivery without indication   Ⓜ ♀
     Use additional code to indicate outcome of delivery (Z37.0)

Complications predominantly related to the puerperium (O85-O92)

     EXCLUDES 2   *mental and behavioral disorders associated with the puerperium (F53.-)*
            obstetrical tetanus (A34)
            puerperal osteomalacia (M83.0)

O85 Puerperal sepsis   ᴹᶜᶜ Ⓜ ♀
     Postpartum sepsis
     Puerperal peritonitis
     Puerperal pyemia
     Use additional code (B95-B97), to identify infectious agent
     Use additional code (R65.2-) to identify severe sepsis, if applicable
     EXCLUDES 1   *fever of unknown origin following delivery (O86.4)*
            genital tract infection following delivery (O86.1-)
            obstetric pyemic and septic embolism (O88.3-)
            puerperal septic thrombophlebitis (O86.81)
            urinary tract infection following delivery (O86.2-)
     EXCLUDES 2   *sepsis during labor (O75.3)*
     AHA: 2020,2Q,32; 2019,2Q,39; 2018,4Q,23

✓4ᵗʰ **O86** Other puerperal infections
     Use additional code (B95-B97), to identify infectious agent
     EXCLUDES 2   *infection during labor (O75.3)*
            obstetrical tetanus (A34)

✓5ᵗʰ **O86.0** Infection of obstetric surgical wound
     Infected cesarean delivery wound following delivery
     Infected perineal repair following delivery
     EXCLUDES 1   *complications of procedures, not elsewhere classified (T81.4-)*
            postprocedural fever NOS (R50.82)
            postprocedural retroperitoneal abscess (K68.11)
     AHA: 2020,2Q,32; 2018,4Q,22-23,62

     O86.00 Infection of obstetric surgical wound, unspecified   Ⓜ ♀

     O86.01 Infection of obstetric surgical wound, superficial incisional site   Ⓜ ♀
         Subcutaneous abscess following an obstetrical procedure
         Stitch abscess following an obstetrical procedure

     O86.02 Infection of obstetric surgical wound, deep incisional site   Ⓜ ♀
         Intramuscular abscess following an obstetrical procedure
         Sub-fascial abscess following an obstetrical procedure
         AHA: 2020,2Q,32

    O86.03   **Infection of obstetric surgical wound,** organ and space site   M ♀
         Intraabdominal abscess following an obstetrical procedure
         Subphrenic abscess following an obstetrical procedure

    O86.04   **Sepsis** following an obstetrical procedure   MCC M ♀
         Use additional code to identify the sepsis
         AHA: 2020,2Q,32; 2019,2Q,39

    O86.09   **Infection of obstetric surgical wound, other surgical site**   M ♀

✓5ᵗʰ **O86.1**   **Other infection of** genital tract **following delivery**

    O86.11   **Cervicitis following delivery**   CC M ♀
    O86.12   **Endometritis following delivery**   CC M ♀
    O86.13   **Vaginitis following delivery**   CC M ♀
    O86.19   **Other infection of genital tract following delivery**   CC M ♀

✓5ᵗʰ **O86.2**   **Urinary tract infection following delivery**

    O86.20   **Urinary tract infection following delivery, unspecified**   CC M ♀
         Puerperal urinary tract infection NOS
    O86.21   **Infection of kidney following delivery**   CC M ♀
    O86.22   **Infection of bladder following delivery**   CC M ♀
         Infection of urethra following delivery
    O86.29   **Other urinary tract infection following delivery**   CC M ♀

O86.4   **Pyrexia of unknown origin following delivery**   CC M ♀
     Puerperal infection NOS following delivery
     Puerperal pyrexia NOS following delivery
     EXCLUDES 2   pyrexia during labor (O75.2)
     DEF: Fever of unknown origin experienced by the mother after childbirth.

✓5ᵗʰ **O86.8**   **Other specified puerperal infections**

    O86.81   **Puerperal** septic thrombophlebitis   MCC M ♀
    O86.89   **Other specified puerperal infections**   MCC M ♀

✓4ᵗʰ **O87**   **Venous complications and hemorrhoids in the puerperium**
     INCLUDES   venous complications in labor, delivery and the puerperium
     EXCLUDES 2   obstetric embolism (O88.-)
         puerperal septic thrombophlebitis (O86.81)
         venous complications in pregnancy (O22.-)

O87.0   **Superficial thrombophlebitis in the puerperium**   CC M ♀
     Puerperal phlebitis NOS
     Puerperal thrombosis NOS

O87.1   **Deep phlebothrombosis in the puerperium**   MCC M ♀
     Deep vein thrombosis, postpartum
     Pelvic thrombophlebitis, postpartum
     Use additional code to identify the deep vein thrombosis
         ▶(I82.4-, I82.5-, I82.62-, I82.72-)◀
     Use additional code, if applicable, for associated long-term (current) use of anticoagulants (Z79.01)

O87.2   **Hemorrhoids in the puerperium**   CC M ♀
O87.3   **Cerebral venous thrombosis in the puerperium**   CC M ♀
     Cerebrovenous sinus thrombosis in the puerperium
O87.4   **Varicose veins of lower extremity in the puerperium**   M ♀
O87.8   **Other venous complications in the puerperium**   CC M ♀
     Genital varices in the puerperium
O87.9   **Venous complication in the puerperium, unspecified**   M ♀
     Puerperal phlebopathy NOS

✓4ᵗʰ **O88**   **Obstetric embolism**
     EXCLUDES 1   embolism complicating abortion NOS (O03.2)
         embolism complicating ectopic or molar pregnancy (O08.2)
         embolism complicating failed attempted abortion (O07.2)
         embolism complicating induced abortion (O04.7)
         embolism complicating spontaneous abortion (O03.2, O03.7)

✓5ᵗʰ **O88.0**   **Obstetric** air embolism
     DEF: Sudden blocking of the pulmonary artery or right ventricle with air or nitrogen bubbles.

  ✓6ᵗʰ **O88.01**   **Obstetric air embolism in** pregnancy
    O88.011   **Air embolism in pregnancy,** first trimester   MCC M ♀
    O88.012   **Air embolism in pregnancy,** second trimester   MCC M ♀
    O88.013   **Air embolism in pregnancy,** third trimester   MCC M ♀

    O88.019   **Air embolism in pregnancy, unspecified trimester**   M ♀
    O88.02   **Air embolism in** childbirth   MCC M ♀
    O88.03   **Air embolism in the** puerperium   MCC M ♀

✓5ᵗʰ **O88.1**   **Amniotic fluid embolism**
     Anaphylactoid syndrome in pregnancy

  ✓6ᵗʰ **O88.11**   **Amniotic fluid embolism in** pregnancy
    O88.111   **Amniotic fluid embolism in pregnancy,** first trimester   MCC M ♀
    O88.112   **Amniotic fluid embolism in pregnancy,** second trimester   MCC M ♀
    O88.113   **Amniotic fluid embolism in pregnancy,** third trimester   MCC M ♀
    O88.119   **Amniotic fluid embolism in pregnancy, unspecified trimester**   M ♀
    O88.12   **Amniotic fluid embolism in** childbirth   MCC M ♀
    O88.13   **Amniotic fluid embolism in the** puerperium   MCC M ♀

✓5ᵗʰ **O88.2**   **Obstetric** thromboembolism

  ✓6ᵗʰ **O88.21**   **Thromboembolism in** pregnancy
     Obstetric (pulmonary) embolism NOS
    O88.211   **Thromboembolism in pregnancy,** first trimester   MCC M ♀
    O88.212   **Thromboembolism in pregnancy,** second trimester   MCC M ♀
    O88.213   **Thromboembolism in pregnancy,** third trimester   MCC M ♀
    O88.219   **Thromboembolism in pregnancy, unspecified trimester**   M ♀
    O88.22   **Thromboembolism in** childbirth   MCC M ♀
    O88.23   **Thromboembolism in the** puerperium   MCC M ♀
         Puerperal (pulmonary) embolism NOS

✓5ᵗʰ **O88.3**   **Obstetric** pyemic and septic embolism

  ✓6ᵗʰ **O88.31**   **Pyemic and septic embolism in** pregnancy
    O88.311   **Pyemic and septic embolism in pregnancy,** first trimester   MCC M ♀
    O88.312   **Pyemic and septic embolism in pregnancy,** second trimester   MCC M ♀
    O88.313   **Pyemic and septic embolism in pregnancy,** third trimester   MCC M ♀
    O88.319   **Pyemic and septic embolism in pregnancy, unspecified trimester**   CC M ♀
    O88.32   **Pyemic and septic embolism in** childbirth   MCC M ♀
    O88.33   **Pyemic and septic embolism in the** puerperium   MCC M ♀

✓5ᵗʰ **O88.8**   **Other obstetric embolism**
     Obstetric fat embolism

  ✓6ᵗʰ **O88.81**   **Other embolism in** pregnancy
    O88.811   **Other embolism in pregnancy,** first trimester   M ♀
    O88.812   **Other embolism in pregnancy,** second trimester   MCC M ♀
    O88.813   **Other embolism in pregnancy,** third trimester   MCC M ♀
    O88.819   **Other embolism in pregnancy, unspecified trimester**   M ♀
    O88.82   **Other embolism in** childbirth   MCC M ♀
    O88.83   **Other embolism in the** puerperium   MCC M ♀

✓4ᵗʰ **O89**   **Complications of anesthesia during the puerperium**
     INCLUDES   maternal complications arising from the administration of a general, regional or local anesthetic, analgesic or other sedation during the puerperium
     Use additional code, if applicable, to identify specific complication

✓5ᵗʰ **O89.0**   **Pulmonary complications of anesthesia during the puerperium**
    O89.01   **Aspiration pneumonitis due to anesthesia during the puerperium**   M ♀
         Inhalation of stomach contents or secretions NOS due to anesthesia during the puerperium
         Mendelson's syndrome due to anesthesia during the puerperium
    O89.09   **Other pulmonary complications of anesthesia during the puerperium**   M ♀

O89.1   **Cardiac complications of anesthesia during the puerperium**   M ♀

N Newborn: 0   P Pediatric: 0-17   M Maternity: 9-64   A Adult: 15-124   MCC Major Complication/Comorbidity   CC Complication/Comorbidity   SW Severe Wound Dx

898   ICD-10-CM 2022

O89.2   Central nervous system **complications of anesthesia during the puerperium**   M ♀

O89.3   Toxic reaction **to local anesthesia during the puerperium**   M ♀

O89.4   Spinal and epidural anesthesia-induced headache **during the puerperium**   M ♀

O89.5   Other complications of spinal and epidural anesthesia **during the puerperium**   M ♀

O89.6   Failed or difficult intubation **for anesthesia during the puerperium**   M ♀

O89.8   Other complications of anesthesia during the **puerperium**   M ♀

O89.9   Complication of anesthesia during the puerperium, **unspecified**   M ♀

✔4ᵗʰ **O90**   **Complications of the puerperium, not elsewhere classified**

   O90.0   **Disruption of cesarean delivery wound**   M ♀
     Dehiscence of cesarean delivery wound
     EXCLUDES 1   *rupture of uterus (spontaneous) before onset of labor (O71.0-)*
         rupture of uterus during labor (O71.1)

   O90.1   **Disruption of perineal obstetric wound**   M ♀
     Disruption of wound of episiotomy
     Disruption of wound of perineal laceration
     Secondary perineal tear

   O90.2   **Hematoma of obstetric wound**   M ♀

   O90.3   **Peripartum cardiomyopathy**   MCC M ♀
     Conditions in I42- arising during pregnancy and the puerperium
     EXCLUDES 1   *pre-existing heart disease complicating pregnancy and the puerperium (O99.4-)*
     DEF: Any structural or functional abnormality of the ventricular myocardium. It is a noninflammatory disease of obscure or unknown etiology with onset during the postpartum period.

   O90.4   **Postpartum acute kidney failure**   MCC M ♀
     Hepatorenal syndrome following labor and delivery

   O90.5   **Postpartum thyroiditis**   M ♀

   O90.6   **Postpartum mood disturbance**   M ♀
     Postpartum blues
     Postpartum dysphoria
     Postpartum sadness
     EXCLUDES 1   *postpartum depression (F53.0)*
         puerperal psychosis (F53.1)

✔5ᵗʰ **O90.8**   **Other complications of the puerperium, not elsewhere classified**

     O90.81   **Anemia of the puerperium**   M ♀
       Postpartum anemia NOS
       EXCLUDES 1   *pre-existing anemia complicating the puerperium (O99.03)*
       AHA: 2019,3Q,11

     O90.89   **Other complications of the puerperium, not elsewhere classified**   M ♀
       Placental polyp

   O90.9   **Complication of the puerperium, unspecified**   M ♀

✔4ᵗʰ **O91**   **Infections of breast associated with pregnancy, the puerperium and lactation**
     Use additional code to identify infection

✔5ᵗʰ **O91.0**   **Infection of nipple associated with pregnancy, the puerperium and lactation**

     ✔6ᵗʰ **O91.01**   **Infection of nipple associated with** pregnancy
       Gestational abscess of nipple

       O91.011   **Infection of nipple associated with pregnancy,** first trimester   M ♀

       O91.012   **Infection of nipple associated with pregnancy,** second trimester   M ♀

       O91.013   **Infection of nipple associated with pregnancy,** third trimester   M ♀

       O91.019   **Infection of nipple associated with pregnancy,** unspecified trimester   M ♀

     O91.02   **Infection of nipple associated with the** puerperium   M ♀
       Puerperal abscess of nipple

     O91.03   **Infection of nipple associated with** lactation   M ♀
       Abscess of nipple associated with lactation

✔5ᵗʰ **O91.1**   **Abscess of breast associated with pregnancy, the puerperium and lactation**

     ✔6ᵗʰ **O91.11**   **Abscess of breast associated with** pregnancy
       Gestational mammary abscess
       Gestational purulent mastitis
       Gestational subareolar abscess

       O91.111   **Abscess of breast associated with pregnancy,** first trimester   M ♀

       O91.112   **Abscess of breast associated with pregnancy,** second trimester   M ♀

       O91.113   **Abscess of breast associated with pregnancy,** third trimester   M ♀

       O91.119   **Abscess of breast associated with pregnancy,** unspecified trimester   M ♀

     O91.12   **Abscess of breast associated with the** puerperium   M ♀
       Puerperal mammary abscess
       Puerperal purulent mastitis
       Puerperal subareolar abscess

     O91.13   **Abscess of breast associated with** lactation   M ♀
       Mammary abscess associated with lactation
       Purulent mastitis associated with lactation
       Subareolar abscess associated with lactation

✔5ᵗʰ **O91.2**   **Nonpurulent mastitis associated with pregnancy, the puerperium and lactation**

     ✔6ᵗʰ **O91.21**   **Nonpurulent mastitis associated with** pregnancy
       Gestational interstitial mastitis
       Gestational lymphangitis of breast
       Gestational mastitis NOS
       Gestational parenchymatous mastitis

       O91.211   **Nonpurulent mastitis associated with pregnancy,** first trimester   M ♀

       O91.212   **Nonpurulent mastitis associated with pregnancy,** second trimester   M ♀

       O91.213   **Nonpurulent mastitis associated with pregnancy,** third trimester   M ♀

       O91.219   **Nonpurulent mastitis associated with pregnancy,** unspecified trimester   M ♀

     O91.22   **Nonpurulent mastitis associated with the** puerperium   M ♀
       Puerperal interstitial mastitis
       Puerperal lymphangitis of breast
       Puerperal mastitis NOS
       Puerperal parenchymatous mastitis

     O91.23   **Nonpurulent mastitis associated with** lactation   M ♀
       Interstitial mastitis associated with lactation
       Lymphangitis of breast associated with lactation
       Mastitis NOS associated with lactation
       Parenchymatous mastitis associated with lactation

✔4ᵗʰ **O92**   **Other disorders of breast and disorders of lactation associated with pregnancy and the puerperium**

✔5ᵗʰ **O92.0**   **Retracted nipple associated with pregnancy, the puerperium, and lactation**

     ✔6ᵗʰ **O92.01**   **Retracted nipple associated with** pregnancy

       O92.011   **Retracted nipple associated with pregnancy,** first trimester   M ♀

       O92.012   **Retracted nipple associated with pregnancy,** second trimester   M ♀

       O92.013   **Retracted nipple associated with pregnancy,** third trimester   M ♀

       O92.019   **Retracted nipple associated with pregnancy,** unspecified trimester   M ♀

     O92.02   **Retracted nipple associated with the** puerperium   M ♀

     O92.03   **Retracted nipple associated with** lactation   M ♀

✔5ᵗʰ **O92.1**   **Cracked nipple associated with pregnancy, the puerperium, and lactation**
     Fissure of nipple, gestational or puerperal

     ✔6ᵗʰ **O92.11**   **Cracked nipple associated with** pregnancy

       O92.111   **Cracked nipple associated with pregnancy,** first trimester   M ♀

       O92.112   **Cracked nipple associated with pregnancy,** second trimester   M ♀

       O92.113   **Cracked nipple associated with pregnancy,** third trimester   M ♀

       O92.119   **Cracked nipple associated with pregnancy,** unspecified trimester   M ♀

O92.12 **Cracked nipple associated with the puerperium** M ♀

O92.13 **Cracked nipple associated with** lactation M ♀

✓5ᵗʰ **O92.2** **Other and unspecified disorders of breast associated with pregnancy and the puerperium**

O92.20 **Unspecified disorder of breast associated with pregnancy and the puerperium** M ♀

O92.29 **Other disorders of breast associated with pregnancy and the puerperium** M ♀

O92.3 **Agalactia** M ♀
Primary agalactia
EXCLUDES 1   *elective agalactia (O92.5)*
secondary agalactia (O92.5)
therapeutic agalactia (O92.5)
DEF: Absence of milk secretion in a female after delivery.

O92.4 **Hypogalactia** M ♀

O92.5 **Suppressed lactation** M ♀
Elective agalactia
Secondary agalactia
Therapeutic agalactia
EXCLUDES 1   *primary agalactia (O92.3)*

O92.6 **Galactorrhea** M ♀
DEF: Excessive or persistent milk secretion by the breast that may occur in the absence of nursing.

✓5ᵗʰ **O92.7** **Other and unspecified disorders of lactation**

O92.70 **Unspecified disorders of lactation** M ♀

O92.79 **Other disorders of lactation** M ♀
Puerperal galactocele

Other obstetric conditions, not elsewhere classified (O94-O9A)

O94 **Sequelae of complication of pregnancy, childbirth, and the puerperium** UPD M ♀

NOTE   This category is to be used to indicate conditions in O00-O77.-, O85-O94 and O98-O9A.- as the cause of late effects. The sequelae include conditions specified as such, or as late effects, which may occur at any time after the puerperium
Code first condition resulting from (sequela) of complication of pregnancy, childbirth, and the puerperium

✓4ᵗʰ **O98** **Maternal infectious and parasitic diseases classifiable elsewhere but complicating pregnancy, childbirth and the puerperium**
INCLUDES   the listed conditions when complicating the pregnant state, when aggravated by the pregnancy, or as a reason for obstetric care
Use additional code (Chapter 1), to identify specific infectious or parasitic disease
EXCLUDES 2   *herpes gestationis (O26.4-)*
infectious carrier state (O99.82-, O99.83-)
obstetrical tetanus (A34)
puerperal infection (O86.-)
puerperal sepsis (O85)
when the reason for maternal care is that the disease is known or suspected to have affected the fetus (O35-O36)

✓5ᵗʰ **O98.0** **Tuberculosis complicating pregnancy, childbirth and the puerperium**
Conditions in A15-A19

✓6ᵗʰ **O98.01** **Tuberculosis complicating** pregnancy

O98.011 **Tuberculosis complicating pregnancy, first trimester** cc M ♀

O98.012 **Tuberculosis complicating pregnancy, second trimester** cc M ♀

O98.013 **Tuberculosis complicating pregnancy, third trimester** cc M ♀

O98.019 **Tuberculosis complicating pregnancy, unspecified trimester** M ♀

O98.02 **Tuberculosis complicating** childbirth cc M ♀

O98.03 **Tuberculosis complicating the puerperium** cc M ♀

✓5ᵗʰ **O98.1** **Syphilis complicating pregnancy, childbirth and the puerperium**
Conditions in A50-A53

✓6ᵗʰ **O98.11** **Syphilis complicating** pregnancy

O98.111 **Syphilis complicating pregnancy, first trimester** cc M ♀

O98.112 **Syphilis complicating pregnancy,** second trimester cc M ♀

O98.113 **Syphilis complicating pregnancy,** third trimester cc M ♀

O98.119 **Syphilis complicating pregnancy, unspecified trimester** M ♀

O98.12 **Syphilis complicating** childbirth cc M ♀

O98.13 **Syphilis complicating the** puerperium cc M ♀

✓5ᵗʰ **O98.2** **Gonorrhea complicating pregnancy, childbirth and the puerperium**
Conditions in A54.-

✓6ᵗʰ **O98.21** **Gonorrhea complicating** pregnancy

O98.211 **Gonorrhea complicating pregnancy,** first trimester cc M ♀

O98.212 **Gonorrhea complicating pregnancy, second trimester** cc M ♀

O98.213 **Gonorrhea complicating pregnancy,** third trimester cc M ♀

O98.219 **Gonorrhea complicating pregnancy, unspecified trimester** M ♀

O98.22 **Gonorrhea complicating** childbirth cc M ♀

O98.23 **Gonorrhea complicating the** puerperium cc M ♀

✓5ᵗʰ **O98.3** **Other infections with a predominantly sexual mode of transmission complicating pregnancy, childbirth and the puerperium**
Conditions in A55-A64
AHA: 2020,1Q,20

✓6ᵗʰ **O98.31** **Other infections with a predominantly sexual mode of transmission complicating** pregnancy

O98.311 **Other infections with a predominantly sexual mode of transmission complicating pregnancy,** first trimester cc M ♀

O98.312 **Other infections with a predominantly sexual mode of transmission complicating pregnancy,** second trimester cc M ♀

O98.313 **Other infections with a predominantly sexual mode of transmission complicating pregnancy,** third trimester cc M ♀

O98.319 **Other infections with a predominantly sexual mode of transmission complicating pregnancy, unspecified trimester** M ♀

O98.32 **Other infections with a predominantly sexual mode of transmission complicating** childbirth cc M ♀

O98.33 **Other infections with a predominantly sexual mode of transmission complicating the** puerperium cc M ♀

✓5ᵗʰ **O98.4** **Viral hepatitis complicating pregnancy, childbirth and the puerperium**
Conditions in B15-B19

✓6ᵗʰ **O98.41** **Viral hepatitis complicating** pregnancy

O98.411 **Viral hepatitis complicating pregnancy, first trimester** cc M ♀

O98.412 **Viral hepatitis complicating pregnancy, second trimester** cc M ♀

O98.413 **Viral hepatitis complicating pregnancy, third trimester** cc M ♀

O98.419 **Viral hepatitis complicating pregnancy, unspecified trimester** M ♀

O98.42 **Viral hepatitis complicating** childbirth cc M ♀

O98.43 **Viral hepatitis complicating the** puerperium cc M ♀

✓5ᵗʰ **O98.5** **Other viral diseases complicating pregnancy, childbirth and the puerperium**
Conditions in A80-B09, B25-B34, R87.81-, R87.82-
EXCLUDES 1   *human immunodeficiency virus [HIV] disease complicating pregnancy, childbirth and the puerperium (O98.7-)*
TIP: Assign a code from this subcategory as the principal or first-listed diagnosis for a patient admitted/presenting during pregnancy, childbirth, or the puerperium because of COVID-19; assign U07.1 and codes for associated manifestations as secondary codes.

✓6ᵗʰ **O98.51** **Other viral diseases complicating** pregnancy

O98.511 **Other viral diseases complicating pregnancy,** first trimester cc M ♀

O98.512 **Other viral diseases complicating pregnancy,** second trimester cc M ♀

O98.513 **Other viral diseases complicating pregnancy,** third trimester cc M ♀

O98.519 Other viral diseases complicating pregnancy, unspecified trimester   M ♀

O98.52 Other viral diseases complicating childbirth   CC M ♀

O98.53 Other viral diseases complicating the puerperium   CC M ♀

✓5ᵗʰ **O98.6** Protozoal diseases complicating pregnancy, childbirth and the puerperium
Conditions in B50-B64

✓6ᵗʰ **O98.61** Protozoal diseases complicating pregnancy

O98.611 Protozoal diseases complicating pregnancy, first trimester   CC M ♀

O98.612 Protozoal diseases complicating pregnancy, second trimester   CC M ♀

O98.613 Protozoal diseases complicating pregnancy, third trimester   CC M ♀

O98.619 Protozoal diseases complicating pregnancy, unspecified trimester   M ♀

O98.62 Protozoal diseases complicating childbirth   CC M ♀

O98.63 Protozoal diseases complicating the puerperium   CC M ♀

✓5ᵗʰ **O98.7** Human immunodeficiency virus [HIV] disease complicating pregnancy, childbirth and the puerperium
Use additional code to identify the type of HIV disease:
acquired immune deficiency syndrome (AIDS) (B20)
asymptomatic HIV status (Z21)
HIV positive NOS (Z21)
symptomatic HIV disease (B20)

✓6ᵗʰ **O98.71** Human immunodeficiency virus [HIV] disease complicating pregnancy

O98.711 Human immunodeficiency virus [HIV] disease complicating pregnancy, first trimester   CC M ♀

O98.712 Human immunodeficiency virus [HIV] disease complicating pregnancy, second trimester   CC M ♀

O98.713 Human immunodeficiency virus [HIV] disease complicating pregnancy, third trimester   CC M ♀

O98.719 Human immunodeficiency virus [HIV] disease complicating pregnancy, unspecified trimester   M ♀

O98.72 Human immunodeficiency virus [HIV] disease complicating childbirth   CC M ♀

O98.73 Human immunodeficiency virus [HIV] disease complicating the puerperium   CC M ♀

✓5ᵗʰ **O98.8** Other maternal infectious and parasitic diseases complicating pregnancy, childbirth and the puerperium
AHA: 2020,1Q,10

✓6ᵗʰ **O98.81** Other maternal infectious and parasitic diseases complicating pregnancy

O98.811 Other maternal infectious and parasitic diseases complicating pregnancy, first trimester   CC M ♀

O98.812 Other maternal infectious and parasitic diseases complicating pregnancy, second trimester   CC M ♀

O98.813 Other maternal infectious and parasitic diseases complicating pregnancy, third trimester   CC M ♀

O98.819 Other maternal infectious and parasitic diseases complicating pregnancy, unspecified trimester   M ♀

O98.82 Other maternal infectious and parasitic diseases complicating childbirth   CC M ♀

O98.83 Other maternal infectious and parasitic diseases complicating the puerperium   CC M ♀

✓5ᵗʰ **O98.9** Unspecified maternal infectious and parasitic disease complicating pregnancy, childbirth and the puerperium

✓6ᵗʰ **O98.91** Unspecified maternal infectious and parasitic disease complicating pregnancy

O98.911 Unspecified maternal infectious and parasitic disease complicating pregnancy, first trimester   CC M ♀

O98.912 Unspecified maternal infectious and parasitic disease complicating pregnancy, second trimester   CC M ♀

O98.913 Unspecified maternal infectious and parasitic disease complicating pregnancy, third trimester   CC M ♀

O98.919 Unspecified maternal infectious and parasitic disease complicating pregnancy, unspecified trimester   M ♀

O98.92 Unspecified maternal infectious and parasitic disease complicating childbirth   CC M ♀

O98.93 Unspecified maternal infectious and parasitic disease complicating the puerperium   CC M ♀

✓4ᵗʰ **O99** Other maternal diseases classifiable elsewhere but complicating pregnancy, childbirth and the puerperium

INCLUDES   conditions which complicate the pregnant state, are aggravated by the pregnancy or are a main reason for obstetric care

Use additional code to identify specific condition

EXCLUDES 2   when the reason for maternal care is that the condition is known or suspected to have affected the fetus (O35-O36)

✓5ᵗʰ **O99.0** Anemia complicating pregnancy, childbirth and the puerperium
Conditions in D50-D64

EXCLUDES 1   anemia arising in the puerperium (O90.81)
postpartum anemia NOS (O90.81)

AHA: 2019,3Q,11

✓6ᵗʰ **O99.01** Anemia complicating pregnancy
AHA: 2016,1Q,4

O99.011 Anemia complicating pregnancy, first trimester   M ♀

O99.012 Anemia complicating pregnancy, second trimester   M ♀

O99.013 Anemia complicating pregnancy, third trimester   M ♀

O99.019 Anemia complicating pregnancy, unspecified trimester   M ♀

O99.02 Anemia complicating childbirth   M ♀

O99.03 Anemia complicating the puerperium   M ♀

EXCLUDES 1   postpartum anemia not pre-existing prior to delivery (O90.81)

✓5ᵗʰ **O99.1** Other diseases of the blood and blood-forming organs and certain disorders involving the immune mechanism complicating pregnancy, childbirth and the puerperium
Conditions in D65-D89

EXCLUDES 1   hemorrhage with coagulation defects (O45.-, O46.0-, O67.0, O72.3)

✓6ᵗʰ **O99.11** Other diseases of the blood and blood-forming organs and certain disorders involving the immune mechanism complicating pregnancy

O99.111 Other diseases of the blood and blood-forming organs and certain disorders involving the immune mechanism complicating pregnancy, first trimester   CC M ♀

O99.112 Other diseases of the blood and blood-forming organs and certain disorders involving the immune mechanism complicating pregnancy, second trimester   CC M ♀

O99.113 Other diseases of the blood and blood-forming organs and certain disorders involving the immune mechanism complicating pregnancy, third trimester   CC M ♀

O99.119 Other diseases of the blood and blood-forming organs and certain disorders involving the immune mechanism complicating pregnancy, unspecified trimester   CC M ♀

O99.12 Other diseases of the blood and blood-forming organs and certain disorders involving the immune mechanism complicating childbirth   CC M ♀

O99.13 Other diseases of the blood and blood-forming organs and certain disorders involving the immune mechanism complicating the puerperium   CC M ♀

☑ Additional Character Required   ✓x7ᵗʰ Placeholder   Questionable PDx   Manifestation   Unspecified Dx   UPD Unacceptable PDx   H1-H14 HAC   HCC CMS-HCC Dx   HIV HIV Dx

ICD-10-CM 2022   **901**

✓5th **O99.2** **Endocrine, nutritional and metabolic diseases** complicating **pregnancy, childbirth and the puerperium**
Conditions in E00-E89
EXCLUDES 2   *diabetes mellitus (O24.-)*
malnutrition (O25.-)
postpartum thyroiditis (O90.5)

✓6th **O99.21** **Obesity** complicating pregnancy, childbirth, and the puerperium
Use additional code to identify the type of obesity (E66.-)
AHA: 2021,2Q,10; 2018,4Q,80
TIP: Do not assign a BMI code (Z68.-) for obese or overweight patients who are pregnant.

O99.210 **Obesity complicating pregnancy, unspecified trimester** Ⓜ♀
O99.211 **Obesity complicating pregnancy, first** trimester Ⓜ♀
O99.212 **Obesity complicating pregnancy, second** trimester Ⓜ♀
O99.213 **Obesity complicating pregnancy, third** trimester Ⓜ♀
O99.214 **Obesity complicating** childbirth Ⓜ♀
O99.215 **Obesity complicating the** puerperium Ⓜ♀

✓6th **O99.28** **Other endocrine, nutritional and metabolic diseases** complicating pregnancy, childbirth and the puerperium
AHA: 2021,1Q,8

O99.280 **Endocrine, nutritional and metabolic diseases complicating pregnancy, unspecified trimester** Ⓜ♀
O99.281 **Endocrine, nutritional and metabolic diseases complicating pregnancy, first** trimester Ⓜ♀
O99.282 **Endocrine, nutritional and metabolic diseases complicating pregnancy, second** trimester Ⓜ♀
O99.283 **Endocrine, nutritional and metabolic diseases complicating pregnancy, third** trimester Ⓜ♀
O99.284 **Endocrine, nutritional and metabolic diseases complicating** childbirth Ⓜ♀
O99.285 **Endocrine, nutritional and metabolic diseases complicating the** puerperium Ⓜ♀

✓5th **O99.3** **Mental disorders** and diseases of the **nervous system** complicating pregnancy, childbirth and the puerperium

✓6th **O99.31** **Alcohol use** complicating pregnancy, childbirth, and the puerperium
Use additional code(s) from F10 to identify manifestations of the alcohol use

O99.310 **Alcohol use complicating pregnancy, unspecified trimester** Ⓜ♀
O99.311 **Alcohol use complicating pregnancy, first** trimester Ⓜ♀
O99.312 **Alcohol use complicating pregnancy, second trimester** Ⓜ♀
O99.313 **Alcohol use complicating pregnancy, third trimester** Ⓜ♀
O99.314 **Alcohol use complicating childbirth** Ⓜ♀
O99.315 **Alcohol use complicating the** puerperium Ⓜ♀

✓6th **O99.32** **Drug use** complicating pregnancy, childbirth, and the puerperium
Use additional code(s) from F11-F16 and F18-F19 to identify manifestations of the drug use
AHA: 2018,4Q,69-70; 2018,2Q,10
TIP: When drug use is documented during pregnancy, assign first a code from this subcategory followed by an additional code from F11-F16 and F18-F19 identifying the specific drug use even if not documented as associated with a physical, mental, or behavioral disorder. According to chapter 15 guidelines, it is the provider's responsibility to state that the condition being treated is *not* affecting the pregnancy.

O99.320 **Drug use complicating pregnancy, unspecified trimester** Ⓜ♀
O99.321 **Drug use complicating pregnancy, first** trimester Ⓒⓒ Ⓜ♀
O99.322 **Drug use complicating pregnancy, second** trimester Ⓒⓒ Ⓜ♀

O99.323 **Drug use complicating pregnancy, third** trimester Ⓒⓒ Ⓜ♀
O99.324 **Drug use complicating childbirth** Ⓒⓒ Ⓜ♀
O99.325 **Drug use complicating the** puerperium Ⓒⓒ Ⓜ♀

✓6th **O99.33** **Tobacco use disorder** complicating pregnancy, childbirth, and the puerperium
Smoking complicating pregnancy, childbirth, and the puerperium
Use additional code from category F17 to identify type of tobacco nicotine dependence

O99.330 **Smoking (tobacco) complicating pregnancy, unspecified trimester** Ⓜ♀
O99.331 **Smoking (tobacco) complicating pregnancy, first trimester** Ⓜ♀
O99.332 **Smoking (tobacco) complicating pregnancy, second trimester** Ⓜ♀
O99.333 **Smoking (tobacco) complicating pregnancy, third trimester** Ⓜ♀
O99.334 **Smoking (tobacco) complicating childbirth** Ⓜ♀
O99.335 **Smoking (tobacco) complicating the puerperium** Ⓜ♀

✓6th **O99.34** **Other mental disorders complicating pregnancy, childbirth, and the puerperium**
Conditions in F01-F09, F20-F52 and F54-F99
EXCLUDES 2   *postpartum mood disturbance (O90.6)*
postnatal psychosis (F53.1)
puerperal psychosis (F53.1)

O99.340 **Other mental disorders complicating pregnancy, unspecified trimester** Ⓜ♀
O99.341 **Other mental disorders complicating pregnancy, first trimester** Ⓜ♀
O99.342 **Other mental disorders complicating pregnancy, second trimester** Ⓜ♀
O99.343 **Other mental disorders complicating pregnancy, third trimester** Ⓜ♀
O99.344 **Other mental disorders complicating childbirth** Ⓜ♀
O99.345 **Other mental disorders complicating the puerperium** Ⓜ♀
AHA: 2018,4Q,8

✓6th **O99.35** **Diseases of the nervous system** complicating pregnancy, childbirth, and the puerperium
Conditions in G00-G99
EXCLUDES 2   *pregnancy related peripheral neuritis (O26.8-)*

O99.350 **Diseases of the nervous system complicating pregnancy, unspecified trimester** Ⓜ♀
O99.351 **Diseases of the nervous system complicating pregnancy, first trimester** Ⓜ♀
O99.352 **Diseases of the nervous system complicating pregnancy, second trimester** Ⓜ♀
O99.353 **Diseases of the nervous system complicating pregnancy, third trimester** Ⓜ♀
O99.354 **Diseases of the nervous system complicating childbirth** Ⓒⓒ Ⓜ♀
O99.355 **Diseases of the nervous system complicating the puerperium** Ⓒⓒ Ⓜ♀

✓5ᵗʰ O99.4 Diseases of the circulatory system complicating pregnancy, childbirth and the puerperium
Conditions in I00-I99
EXCLUDES 1   peripartum cardiomyopathy (O90.3)
EXCLUDES 2   hypertensive disorders (O10-O16)
    obstetric embolism (O88.-)
    venous complications and cerebrovenous sinus thrombosis in labor, childbirth and the puerperium (O87.-)
    venous complications and cerebrovenous sinus thrombosis in pregnancy (O22.-)

AHA: 2016,2Q,8

✓6ᵗʰ O99.41 Diseases of the circulatory system complicating pregnancy
    O99.411 Diseases of the circulatory system complicating pregnancy, first trimester cc M ♀
    O99.412 Diseases of the circulatory system complicating pregnancy, second trimester cc M ♀
    O99.413 Diseases of the circulatory system complicating pregnancy, third trimester cc M ♀
    O99.419 Diseases of the circulatory system complicating pregnancy, unspecified trimester M ♀

O99.42 Diseases of the circulatory system complicating childbirth MCC M ♀

O99.43 Diseases of the circulatory system complicating the puerperium cc M ♀

✓5ᵗʰ O99.5 Diseases of the respiratory system complicating pregnancy, childbirth and the puerperium
Conditions in J00-J99
✓6ᵗʰ O99.51 Diseases of the respiratory system complicating pregnancy
    O99.511 Diseases of the respiratory system complicating pregnancy, first trimester M ♀
    O99.512 Diseases of the respiratory system complicating pregnancy, second trimester M ♀
    O99.513 Diseases of the respiratory system complicating pregnancy, third trimester M ♀
    O99.519 Diseases of the respiratory system complicating pregnancy, unspecified trimester M ♀

O99.52 Diseases of the respiratory system complicating childbirth M ♀

O99.53 Diseases of the respiratory system complicating the puerperium M ♀

✓5ᵗʰ O99.6 Diseases of the digestive system complicating pregnancy, childbirth and the puerperium
Conditions in K00-K93
EXCLUDES 2   hemorrhoids in pregnancy (O22.4-)
    liver and biliary tract disorders in pregnancy, childbirth and the puerperium (O26.6-)

✓6ᵗʰ O99.61 Diseases of the digestive system complicating pregnancy
AHA: 2016,1Q,4
    O99.611 Diseases of the digestive system complicating pregnancy, first trimester M ♀
    O99.612 Diseases of the digestive system complicating pregnancy, second trimester M ♀
    O99.613 Diseases of the digestive system complicating pregnancy, third trimester M ♀
    O99.619 Diseases of the digestive system complicating pregnancy, unspecified trimester M ♀

O99.62 Diseases of the digestive system complicating childbirth M ♀

O99.63 Diseases of the digestive system complicating the puerperium M ♀

✓5ᵗʰ O99.7 Diseases of the skin and subcutaneous tissue complicating pregnancy, childbirth and the puerperium
Conditions in L00-L99
EXCLUDES 2   herpes gestationis (O26.4)
    pruritic urticarial papules and plaques of pregnancy (PUPPP) (O26.86)

✓6ᵗʰ O99.71 Diseases of the skin and subcutaneous tissue complicating pregnancy
    O99.711 Diseases of the skin and subcutaneous tissue complicating pregnancy, first trimester M ♀
    O99.712 Diseases of the skin and subcutaneous tissue complicating pregnancy, second trimester M ♀
    O99.713 Diseases of the skin and subcutaneous tissue complicating pregnancy, third trimester M ♀
    O99.719 Diseases of the skin and subcutaneous tissue complicating pregnancy, unspecified trimester M ♀

O99.72 Diseases of the skin and subcutaneous tissue complicating childbirth M ♀

O99.73 Diseases of the skin and subcutaneous tissue complicating the puerperium M ♀

✓5ᵗʰ O99.8 Other specified diseases and conditions complicating pregnancy, childbirth and the puerperium
Conditions in D00-D48, H00-H95, M00-N99, and Q00-Q99
Use additional code to identify condition
EXCLUDES 2   genitourinary infections in pregnancy (O23.-)
    infection of genitourinary tract following delivery (O86.1-O86.4)
    malignant neoplasm complicating pregnancy, childbirth and the puerperium (O9A.1-)
    maternal care for known or suspected abnormality of maternal pelvic organs (O34.-)
    postpartum acute kidney failure (O90.4)
    traumatic injuries in pregnancy (O9A.2-)

✓6ᵗʰ O99.81 Abnormal glucose complicating pregnancy, childbirth and the puerperium
EXCLUDES 1   gestational diabetes (O24.4-)
    O99.810 Abnormal glucose complicating pregnancy M ♀
    O99.814 Abnormal glucose complicating childbirth M ♀
    O99.815 Abnormal glucose complicating the puerperium M ♀

✓6ᵗʰ O99.82 Streptococcus B carrier state complicating pregnancy, childbirth and the puerperium
EXCLUDES 1   carrier of streptococcus group B (GBS) in a nonpregnant woman (Z22.330)
DEF: *Streptococcus* group B colonization: Bacteria normally found in the vagina or lower intestine of many healthy adult women that may infect the fetus during childbirth, causing mental or physical handicaps or death. Women who test positive for *Streptococcus* group B during pregnancy are considered a "colonized" status and are treated with IV antibiotics at the time of delivery and may also be treated with oral antibiotics during the pregnancy.
    O99.820 Streptococcus B carrier state complicating pregnancy UPD M ♀
    O99.824 Streptococcus B carrier state complicating childbirth M ♀
       AHA: 2019,2Q,8
    O99.825 Streptococcus B carrier state complicating the puerperium UPD M ♀

✓6ᵗʰ O99.83 Other infection carrier state complicating pregnancy, childbirth and the puerperium
Use additional code to identify the carrier state (Z22.-)
    O99.830 Other infection carrier state complicating pregnancy cc M ♀
    O99.834 Other infection carrier state complicating childbirth cc M ♀
    O99.835 Other infection carrier state complicating the puerperium cc M ♀

✓6ᵗʰ **O99.84** Bariatric surgery status **complicating pregnancy, childbirth and the puerperium**
Gastric banding status complicating pregnancy, childbirth and the puerperium
Gastric bypass status for obesity complicating pregnancy, childbirth and the puerperium
Obesity surgery status complicating pregnancy, childbirth and the puerperium

    O99.840 **Bariatric surgery status complicating pregnancy, unspecified trimester** Ⓜ ♀

    O99.841 **Bariatric surgery status complicating pregnancy, first trimester** Ⓜ ♀

    O99.842 **Bariatric surgery status complicating pregnancy, second trimester** Ⓜ ♀

    O99.843 **Bariatric surgery status complicating pregnancy, third trimester** Ⓜ ♀

    O99.844 **Bariatric surgery status complicating childbirth** Ⓜ ♀

    O99.845 **Bariatric surgery status complicating the puerperium** Ⓜ ♀

✓6ᵗʰ **O99.89** **Other specified diseases and conditions complicating pregnancy, childbirth and the puerperium**
AHA: 2020,4Q,36-37

    O99.891 **Other specified diseases and conditions complicating pregnancy** Ⓜ ♀

    O99.892 **Other specified diseases and conditions complicating childbirth** Ⓜ ♀

    O99.893 **Other specified diseases and conditions complicating puerperium** Ⓜ ♀

✓4ᵗʰ **O9A** **Maternal malignant neoplasms, traumatic injuries and abuse classifiable elsewhere but complicating pregnancy, childbirth and the puerperium**

✓5ᵗʰ **O9A.1** Malignant neoplasm **complicating pregnancy, childbirth and the puerperium**
Conditions in C00-C96
Use additional code to identify neoplasm
    EXCLUDES 2   *maternal care for benign tumor of corpus uteri (O34.1-)*
       maternal care for benign tumor of cervix (O34.4-)
AHA: 2015,3Q,19

✓6ᵗʰ **O9A.11** **Malignant neoplasm complicating pregnancy**

    O9A.111 **Malignant neoplasm complicating pregnancy, first trimester** Ⓜ ♀

    O9A.112 **Malignant neoplasm complicating pregnancy, second trimester** Ⓜ ♀

    O9A.113 **Malignant neoplasm complicating pregnancy, third trimester** Ⓜ ♀

    O9A.119 **Malignant neoplasm complicating pregnancy, unspecified trimester** Ⓜ ♀

    O9A.12 **Malignant neoplasm complicating childbirth** Ⓜ ♀

    O9A.13 **Malignant neoplasm complicating the puerperium** Ⓜ ♀

✓5ᵗʰ **O9A.2** Injury, poisoning and **certain other consequences of** external causes **complicating pregnancy, childbirth and the puerperium**
Conditions in S00-T88, except T74 and T76
Use additional code(s) to identify the injury or poisoning
    EXCLUDES 2   *physical, sexual and psychological abuse complicating pregnancy, childbirth and the puerperium (O9A.3-, O9A.4-, O9A.5-)*

✓6ᵗʰ **O9A.21** **Injury, poisoning and certain other consequences of external causes complicating pregnancy**

    O9A.211 **Injury, poisoning and certain other consequences of external causes complicating pregnancy, first trimester** Ⓜ ♀

    O9A.212 **Injury, poisoning and certain other consequences of external causes complicating pregnancy, second trimester** Ⓜ ♀

    O9A.213 **Injury, poisoning and certain other consequences of external causes complicating pregnancy, third trimester** Ⓜ ♀

    O9A.219 **Injury, poisoning and certain other consequences of external causes complicating pregnancy, unspecified trimester** Ⓜ ♀

    O9A.22 **Injury, poisoning and certain other consequences of external causes complicating childbirth** Ⓜ ♀

    O9A.23 **Injury, poisoning and certain other consequences of external causes complicating the puerperium** Ⓜ ♀

✓5ᵗʰ **O9A.3** Physical abuse **complicating pregnancy, childbirth and the puerperium**
Conditions in T74.11 or T76.11
Use additional code (if applicable):
    to identify any associated current injury due to physical abuse
    to identify the perpetrator of abuse (Y07.-)
    EXCLUDES 2   *sexual abuse complicating pregnancy, childbirth and the puerperium (O9A.4)*

✓6ᵗʰ **O9A.31** **Physical abuse complicating pregnancy**

    O9A.311 **Physical abuse complicating pregnancy, first trimester** Ⓜ ♀

    O9A.312 **Physical abuse complicating pregnancy, second trimester** Ⓜ ♀

    O9A.313 **Physical abuse complicating pregnancy, third trimester** Ⓜ ♀

    O9A.319 **Physical abuse complicating pregnancy, unspecified trimester** Ⓜ ♀

    O9A.32 **Physical abuse complicating childbirth** Ⓜ ♀

    O9A.33 **Physical abuse complicating the puerperium** Ⓜ ♀

✓5ᵗʰ **O9A.4** Sexual abuse **complicating pregnancy, childbirth and the puerperium**
Conditions in T74.21 or T76.21
Use additional code (if applicable):
    to identify any associated current injury due to sexual abuse
    to identify the perpetrator of abuse (Y07.-)

✓6ᵗʰ **O9A.41** **Sexual abuse complicating pregnancy**

    O9A.411 **Sexual abuse complicating pregnancy, first trimester** Ⓜ ♀

    O9A.412 **Sexual abuse complicating pregnancy, second trimester** Ⓜ ♀

    O9A.413 **Sexual abuse complicating pregnancy, third trimester** Ⓜ ♀

    O9A.419 **Sexual abuse complicating pregnancy, unspecified trimester** Ⓜ ♀

    O9A.42 **Sexual abuse complicating childbirth** Ⓜ ♀

    O9A.43 **Sexual abuse complicating the puerperium** Ⓜ ♀

✓5ᵗʰ **O9A.5** Psychological abuse **complicating pregnancy, childbirth and the puerperium**
Conditions in T74.31 or T76.31
Use additional code to identify the perpetrator of abuse (Y07.-)

✓6ᵗʰ **O9A.51** **Psychological abuse complicating pregnancy**

    O9A.511 **Psychological abuse complicating pregnancy, first trimester** Ⓜ ♀

    O9A.512 **Psychological abuse complicating pregnancy, second trimester** Ⓜ ♀

    O9A.513 **Psychological abuse complicating pregnancy, third trimester** Ⓜ ♀

    O9A.519 **Psychological abuse complicating pregnancy, unspecified trimester** Ⓜ ♀

    O9A.52 **Psychological abuse complicating childbirth** Ⓜ ♀

    O9A.53 **Psychological abuse complicating the puerperium** Ⓜ ♀

Chapter 16. Certain Conditions Originating in the Perinatal Period (PØØ–P96)

Chapter-specific Guidelines with Coding Examples

The chapter-specific guidelines from the ICD-10-CM Official Guidelines for Coding and Reporting have been provided below. Along with these guidelines are coding examples, contained in the shaded boxes, that have been developed to help illustrate the coding and/or sequencing guidance found in these guidelines.

For coding and reporting purposes the perinatal period is defined as before birth through the 28th day following birth. The following guidelines are provided for reporting purposes

a. General perinatal rules

1) Use of Chapter 16 codes

Codes in this chapter are <u>never</u> for use on the maternal record. Codes from Chapter 15, the obstetric chapter, are never permitted on the newborn record. Chapter 16 codes may be used throughout the life of the patient if the condition is still present.

2) Principal diagnosis for birth record

When coding the birth episode in a newborn record, assign a code from category Z38, Liveborn infants according to place of birth and type of delivery, as the principal diagnosis. A code from category Z38 is assigned only once, to a newborn at the time of birth. If a newborn is transferred to another institution, a code from category Z38 should not be used at the receiving hospital.

A code from category Z38 is used only on the newborn record, not on the mother's record.

> Newborn delivered via vaginal delivery in Rural Hospital A, experienced meconium aspiration resulting in pneumonia. Rural Hospital A is not equipped to handle the extensive respiratory therapy this baby needs and transfers the patient to Metropolis Hospital B, where the pneumonia resolves and the newborn is eventually discharged.
>
> *Rural Hospital A*
>
> **Z38.ØØ**   **Single liveborn infant, delivered vaginally**
>
> **P24.Ø1**   **Meconium aspiration with respiratory symptoms**
>
> *Metropolis Hospital B*
>
> **P24.Ø1**   **Meconium aspiration with respiratory symptoms**
>
> *Explanation:* A code from category Z38 is a one-time use only code. The hospital that actually delivered the newborn, in this case Rural Hospital A, can append a code from category Z38 but for the delivery admission only. Once the patient is transferred or discharged, the Z38 category no longer applies for that patient.
>
> The reason for the transfer to Metropolis Hospital B was for the respiratory symptoms (pneumonia) the newborn was exhibiting secondary to aspirating meconium.

3) Use of codes from other chapters with codes from Chapter 16

Codes from other chapters may be used with codes from chapter 16 if the codes from the other chapters provide more specific detail. Codes for signs and symptoms may be assigned when a definitive diagnosis has not been established. If the reason for the encounter is a perinatal condition, the code from chapter 16 should be sequenced first.

4) Use of Chapter 16 codes after the perinatal period

Should a condition originate in the perinatal period, and continue throughout the life of the patient, the perinatal code should continue to be used regardless of the patient's age.

> A 7-year-old patient with history of birth injury that resulted in Erb's palsy is seen for subscapularis release
>
> **P14.Ø**   **Erb's paralysis due to birth injury**
>
> *Explanation:* Although in this instance Erb's palsy is specifically related to a birth injury, it has not resolved and continues to be a health concern. A perinatal code is appropriate even though this patient is beyond the perinatal period.

5) Birth process or community acquired conditions

If a newborn has a condition that may be either due to the birth process or community acquired and the documentation does not indicate which it is, the default is due to the birth process and the code from Chapter 16 should be used. If the condition is community-acquired, a code from Chapter 16 should not be assigned.

For COVID-19 infection in a newborn, see guideline I.C.16.h.

6) Code all clinically significant conditions

All clinically significant conditions noted on routine newborn examination should be coded. A condition is clinically significant if it requires:

clinical evaluation; or

therapeutic treatment; or

diagnostic procedures; or

extended length of hospital stay; or

increased nursing care and/or monitoring; or

has implications for future health care needs

Note: The perinatal guidelines listed above are the same as the general coding guidelines for "additional diagnoses", except for the final point regarding implications for future health care needs. Codes should be assigned for conditions that have been specified by the provider as having implications for future health care needs.

b. Observation and evaluation of newborns for suspected conditions not found

1) Use of Z05 codes

Assign a code from category Z05, Observation and evaluation of newborns and infants for suspected conditions ruled out, to identify those instances when a healthy newborn is evaluated for a suspected condition that is determined after study not to be present. Do not use a code from category Z05 when the patient has identified signs or symptoms of a suspected problem; in such cases code the sign or symptom.

2) Z05 on other than the birth record

A code from category Z05 may also be assigned as a principal or first-listed code for readmissions or encounters when the code from category Z38 code no longer applies. Codes from category Z05 are for use only for healthy newborns and infants for which no condition after study is found to be present.

3) Z05 on a birth record

A code from category Z05 is to be used as a secondary code after the code from category Z38, Liveborn infants according to place of birth and type of delivery.

> Newborn delivered via vaginal delivery; previous ultrasounds showed what appeared to be an abnormality of the right kidney. Kidney function tests were performed and ultrasounds taken and any genitourinary conditions ruled out.
>
> **Z38.ØØ**   **Single liveborn infant, delivered vaginally**
>
> **Z05.6**   **Observation and evaluation of newborn for suspected genitourinary condition ruled out**
>
> Explanation: The newborn had no signs or symptoms of kidney or other genitourinary condition but was evaluated after delivery due to the abnormal prenatal ultrasound findings. A Z code describing the type and place of birth should be coded first, followed by a Z05 category code for the work performed to rule out a suspected genitourinary condition.

c. Coding additional perinatal diagnoses

1) Assigning codes for conditions that require treatment

Assign codes for conditions that require treatment or further investigation, prolong the length of stay, or require resource utilization.

Chapter 16. Certain Conditions Originating in the Perinatal Period

2) **Codes for conditions specified as having implications for future health care needs**

Assign codes for conditions that have been specified by the provider as having implications for future health care needs.

Note: This guideline should not be used for adult patients.

> An abnormal noise was heard in the left hip of a post-term newborn during a physical examination. The pediatrician would like to follow the patient after discharge as a hip click can be an early sign of hip dysplasia. The newborn was delivered via cesarean at 41 weeks.
>
> **Z38.01**   **Single liveborn infant, delivered by cesarean**
>
> **P08.21**   **Post-term newborn**
>
> **R29.4**   **Clicking hip**
>
> *Explanation:* The abnormal hip noise or click is appended as a secondary diagnosis not only because it is an abnormal finding upon examination, but also due to its potential to be part of a bigger health issue. The hip dysplasia has not yet been diagnosed and does not warrant a code at this time.

d. **Prematurity and fetal growth retardation**

Providers utilize different criteria in determining prematurity. A code for prematurity should not be assigned unless it is documented. Assignment of codes in categories P05, Disorders of newborn related to slow fetal growth and fetal malnutrition, and P07, Disorders of newborn related to short gestation and low birth weight, not elsewhere classified, should be based on the recorded birth weight and estimated gestational age.

When both birth weight and gestational age are available, two codes from category P07 should be assigned, with the code for birth weight sequenced before the code for gestational age.

e. **Low birth weight and immaturity status**

Codes from category P07, Disorders of newborn related to short gestation and low birth weight, not elsewhere classified, are for use for a child or adult who was premature or had a low birth weight as a newborn and this is affecting the patient's current health status.

See Section I.C.21. Factors influencing health status and contact with health services, Status.

> A 35-year-old patient, who weighed 659 grams at birth, is seen for heart disease documented as being a consequence of the low birth weight
>
> **I51.9**   **Heart disease, unspecified**
>
> **P07.02**   **Extremely low birth weight newborn, 500–749 grams**
>
> *Explanation:* A code from subcategories P07.0- and P07.1- is appropriate, regardless of the age of the patient, as long as the documentation provides a clear link between the patient's current illness and the low birth weight.

f. **Bacterial sepsis of newborn**

Category P36, Bacterial sepsis of newborn, includes congenital sepsis. If a perinate is documented as having sepsis without documentation of congenital or community acquired, the default is congenital and a code from category P36 should be assigned. If the P36 code includes the causal organism, an additional code from category B95, Streptococcus, Staphylococcus, and Enterococcus as the cause of diseases classified elsewhere, or B96, Other bacterial agents as the cause of diseases classified elsewhere, should not be assigned. If the P36 code does not include the causal organism, assign an additional code from category B96. If applicable, use additional codes to identify severe sepsis (R65.2-) and any associated acute organ dysfunction.

> A full-term infant develops severe sepsis 24 hours after discharge from the hospital and is readmitted; cultures identified *E. coli* as the infective agent
>
> **P36.4**   **Sepsis of newborn due to Escherichia coli**
>
> **R65.20**   **Severe sepsis without septic shock**
>
> *Explanation:* Even though this newborn was discharged and could have acquired *E. coli* from his/her external environment, due to the lack of documentation specifying specifically how this pathogen was acquired, the default is to code the *E. coli* sepsis as congenital. A code from chapter 1, "Certain Infectious and Parasitic Diseases," is not required because the perinatal sepsis code identifies both the sepsis and the bacteria causing the sepsis.

g. **Stillbirth**

Code P95, Stillbirth, is only for use in institutions that maintain separate records for stillbirths. No other code should be used with P95. Code P95 should not be used on the mother's record.

h. **COVID-19 infection in newborn**

For a newborn that tests positive for COVID-19, assign code U07.1, COVID-19, and the appropriate codes for associated manifestation(s) in neonates/newborns in the absence of documentation indicating a specific type of transmission. For a newborn that tests positive for COVID-19 and the provider documents the condition was contracted in utero or during the birth process, assign codes P35.8, Other congenital viral diseases, and U07.1, COVID-19. When coding the birth episode in a newborn record, the appropriate code from category Z38, Liveborn infants according to place of birth and type of delivery, should be assigned as the principal diagnosis.

Chapter 16. Certain Conditions Originating in the Perinatal Period (P00-P96)

NOTE   Codes from this chapter are for use on newborn records only, never on maternal records

INCLUDES   conditions that have their origin in the fetal or perinatal period (before birth through the first 28 days after birth) even if morbidity occurs later

EXCLUDES 2   congenital malformations, deformations and chromosomal abnormalities (Q00-Q99)

endocrine, nutritional and metabolic diseases (E00-E88)

injury, poisoning and certain other consequences of external causes (S00-T88)

neoplasms (C00-D49)

tetanus neonatorum (A33)

This chapter contains the following blocks:

P00-P04   Newborn affected by maternal factors and by complications of pregnancy, labor, and delivery
P05-P08   Disorders of newborn related to length of gestation and fetal growth
P09   Abnormal findings on neonatal screening
P10-P15   Birth trauma
P19-P29   Respiratory and cardiovascular disorders specific to the perinatal period
P35-P39   Infections specific to the perinatal period
P50-P61   Hemorrhagic and hematological disorders of newborn
P70-P74   Transitory endocrine and metabolic disorders specific to newborn
P76-P78   Digestive system disorders of newborn
P80-P83   Conditions involving the integument and temperature regulation of newborn
P84   Other problems with newborn
P90-P96   Other disorders originating in the perinatal period

Newborn affected by maternal factors and by complications of pregnancy, labor, and delivery (P00-P04)

NOTE   These codes are for use when the listed maternal conditions are specified as the cause of confirmed morbidity or potential morbidity which have their origin in the perinatal period (before birth through the first 28 days after birth).

AHA: 2016,4Q,54-55

✓4ᵗʰ P00 Newborn affected by maternal conditions that may be unrelated to present pregnancy

Code first any current condition in newborn

EXCLUDES 2   encounter for observation of newborn for suspected diseases and conditions ruled out (Z05.-)

newborn affected by maternal complications of pregnancy (P01.-)

newborn affected by maternal endocrine and metabolic disorders (P70-P74)

newborn affected by noxious substances transmitted via placenta or breast milk (P04.-)

P00.0 Newborn affected by maternal hypertensive disorders
Newborn affected by maternal conditions classifiable to O10-O11, O13-O16

P00.1 Newborn affected by maternal renal and urinary tract diseases
Newborn affected by maternal conditions classifiable to N00-N39

P00.2 Newborn affected by maternal infectious and parasitic diseases
Newborn affected by maternal infectious disease classifiable to A00-B99, J09 and J10

EXCLUDES 1   maternal genital tract or other localized infections (P00.8)

EXCLUDES 2   infections specific to the perinatal period (P35-P39)
▶newborn affected by (positive) maternal group B streptococcus (GBS) colonization (P00.82)◄

AHA: 2019,2Q,10; 2015,3Q,20

P00.3 Newborn affected by other maternal circulatory and respiratory diseases
Newborn affected by maternal conditions classifiable to I00-I99, J00-J99, Q20-Q34 and not included in P00.0, P00.2

P00.4 Newborn affected by maternal nutritional disorders
Newborn affected by maternal disorders classifiable to E40-E64
Maternal malnutrition NOS

P00.5 Newborn affected by maternal injury
Newborn affected by maternal conditions classifiable to O9A.2-

P00.6 Newborn affected by surgical procedure on mother
Newborn affected by amniocentesis

EXCLUDES 1   Cesarean delivery for present delivery (P03.4)
damage to placenta from amniocentesis, Cesarean delivery or surgical induction (P02.1)
previous surgery to uterus or pelvic organs (P03.89)

EXCLUDES 2   newborn affected by complication of (fetal) intrauterine procedure (P96.5)

P00.7 Newborn affected by other medical procedures on mother, not elsewhere classified
Newborn affected by radiation to mother

EXCLUDES 1   damage to placenta from amniocentesis, cesarean delivery or surgical induction (P02.1)
newborn affected by other complications of labor and delivery (P03.-)

✓5ᵗʰ P00.8 Newborn affected by other maternal conditions

P00.81 Newborn affected by periodontal disease in mother

P00.82 Newborn affected by (positive) maternal group B streptococcus (GBS) colonization
Contact with positive maternal group B streptococcus

P00.89 Newborn affected by other maternal conditions
Newborn affected by conditions classifiable to T80-T88
Newborn affected by maternal genital tract or other localized infections
Newborn affected by maternal systemic lupus erythematosus
Use additional code to identify infectious agent, if known

EXCLUDES 2   ▶newborn affected by positive maternal group B streptococcus (GBS) colonization (P00.82)◄

AHA: 2019,2Q,9

P00.9 Newborn affected by unspecified maternal condition

✓4ᵗʰ P01 Newborn affected by maternal complications of pregnancy

Code first any current condition in newborn

EXCLUDES 2   encounter for observation of newborn for suspected diseases and conditions ruled out (Z05.-)

P01.0 Newborn affected by incompetent cervix

P01.1 Newborn affected by premature rupture of membranes

P01.2 Newborn affected by oligohydramnios

EXCLUDES 1   oligohydramnios due to premature rupture of membranes (P01.1)

DEF: Oligohydramnios: Low amniotic fluid level, resulting in underdeveloped organs in the fetus.

P01.3 Newborn affected by polyhydramnios
Newborn affected by hydramnios
DEF: Excess amniotic fluid surrounding the fetus, typically defined as a total fluid volume of greater than 24 cm.

P01.4 Newborn affected by ectopic pregnancy
Newborn affected by abdominal pregnancy

P01.5 Newborn affected by multiple pregnancy
Newborn affected by triplet (pregnancy)
Newborn affected by twin (pregnancy)

P01.6 Newborn affected by maternal death

P01.7 Newborn affected by malpresentation before labor
Newborn affected by breech presentation before labor
Newborn affected by external version before labor
Newborn affected by face presentation before labor
Newborn affected by transverse lie before labor
Newborn affected by unstable lie before labor

P01.8 Newborn affected by other maternal complications of pregnancy

P01.9 Newborn affected by maternal complication of pregnancy, unspecified

✓4ᵗʰ P02 Newborn affected by complications of placenta, cord and membranes

Code first any current condition in newborn

EXCLUDES 2   encounter for observation of newborn for suspected diseases and conditions ruled out (Z05.-)

P02.0 Newborn affected by placenta previa
DEF: Placenta developed in the lower segment of the uterus that can cause hemorrhaging leading to preterm delivery.

✓ Additional Character Required   **√x7ᵗʰ** Placeholder   Questionable PDx   Manifestation   Unspecified Dx   **UPD** Unacceptable PDx   **H1-H14** HAC   **HCC** CMS-HCC Dx   **HIV** HIV Dx

ICD-10-CM 2022   907

Chapter 16. Certain Conditions Originating in the Perinatal Period

P02.1   **Newborn affected by other forms of placental** separation and hemorrhage
    Newborn affected by abruptio placenta
    Newborn affected by accidental hemorrhage
    Newborn affected by antepartum hemorrhage
    Newborn affected by damage to placenta from amniocentesis, cesarean delivery or surgical induction
    Newborn affected by maternal blood loss
    Newborn affected by premature separation of placenta

✓5ᵗʰ **P02.2**   **Newborn affected by other and unspecified** morphological and functional abnormalities of placenta

    P02.20   **Newborn affected by unspecified morphological and functional abnormalities of placenta**

    P02.29   **Newborn affected by other morphological and functional abnormalities of placenta**
       Newborn affected by placental dysfunction
       Newborn affected by placental infarction
       Newborn affected by placental insufficiency

P02.3   **Newborn affected by** placental transfusion syndromes
    Newborn affected by placental and cord abnormalities resulting in twin-to-twin or other transplacental transfusion

P02.4   **Newborn affected by** prolapsed cord

P02.5   **Newborn affected by other compression of umbilical cord**
    Newborn affected by umbilical cord (tightly) around neck
    Newborn affected by entanglement of umbilical cord
    Newborn affected by knot in umbilical cord

✓5ᵗʰ **P02.6**   **Newborn affected by other and unspecified** conditions of umbilical cord

    P02.60   **Newborn affected by unspecified conditions of umbilical cord**

    P02.69   **Newborn affected by other conditions of umbilical cord**
       Newborn affected by short umbilical cord
       Newborn affected by vasa previa
       EXCLUDES 1   newborn affected by single umbilical artery (Q27.0)

✓5ᵗʰ **P02.7**   **Newborn affected by** chorioamnionitis

    AHA: 2018,4Q,23-24
    DEF: Inflammation of the fetal membranes due to maternal infection characterized by fetal tachycardia, respiratory distress, apnea, weak cries, and poor sucking.

    P02.70   **Newborn affected by** fetal inflammatory response syndrome   **HCC**
       Newborn affected by FIRS

    P02.78   **Newborn affected by other conditions from chorioamnionitis**
       Newborn affected by amnionitis
       Newborn affected by membranitis
       Newborn affected by placentitis

P02.8   **Newborn affected by other abnormalities of membranes**

P02.9   **Newborn affected by abnormality of membranes, unspecified**

✓4ᵗʰ **P03**   **Newborn affected by other complications of** labor and delivery

    Code first any current condition in newborn
    EXCLUDES 2   encounter for observation of newborn for suspected diseases and conditions ruled out (Z05.-)

P03.0   **Newborn affected by** breech delivery and extraction

P03.1   **Newborn affected by other** malpresentation, malposition and disproportion **during labor and delivery**
    Newborn affected by contracted pelvis
    Newborn affected by conditions classifiable to O64-O66
    Newborn affected by persistent occipitoposterior
    Newborn affected by transverse lie

P03.2   **Newborn affected by** forceps delivery

Forceps Assisted Birth

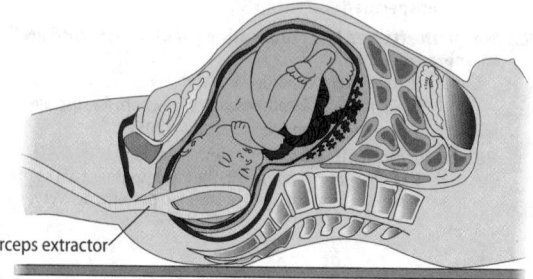

Forceps extractor

P03.3   **Newborn affected by delivery by** vacuum extractor [ventouse]

Vacuum Assisted Birth

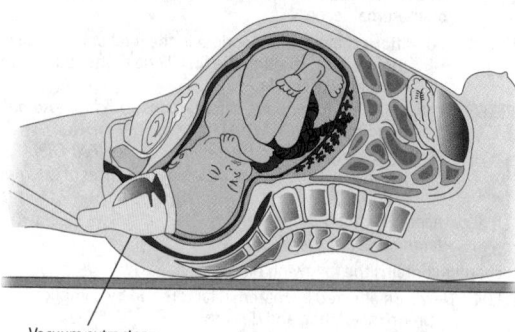

Vacuum extractor

P03.4   **Newborn affected by** Cesarean delivery

P03.5   **Newborn affected by** precipitate delivery
    Newborn affected by rapid second stage

P03.6   **Newborn affected by** abnormal uterine contractions
    Newborn affected by conditions classifiable to O62.-, except O62.3
    Newborn affected by hypertonic labor
    Newborn affected by uterine inertia

✓5ᵗʰ **P03.8**   **Newborn affected by other specified complications of labor and delivery**

    ✓6ᵗʰ **P03.81**   **Newborn affected by** abnormality in fetal (intrauterine) heart rate or rhythm
       EXCLUDES 1   neonatal cardiac dysrhythmia (P29.1-)

       P03.810   **Newborn affected by abnormality in fetal (intrauterine) heart rate or rhythm** before the onset of labor

       P03.811   **Newborn affected by abnormality in fetal (intrauterine) heart rate or rhythm** during labor

       P03.819   **Newborn affected by abnormality in fetal (intrauterine) heart rate or rhythm, unspecified as to time of onset**

    P03.82   Meconium passage **during delivery**
       EXCLUDES 1   meconium aspiration (P24.00, P24.01)
          meconium staining (P96.83)
       DEF: Fetal intestinal activity that increases in response to a fetomaternal distressed state during delivery. The anal sphincter relaxes and meconium is passed into the amniotic fluid.

    P03.89   **Newborn affected by other specified complications of labor and delivery**
       Newborn affected by abnormality of maternal soft tissues
       Newborn affected by conditions classifiable to O60-O75 and by procedures used in labor and delivery not included in P02.- and P03.0-P03.6
       Newborn affected by induction of labor

P03.9   **Newborn affected by complication of labor and delivery, unspecified**

✓4ᵗʰ **P04**   **Newborn affected by** noxious substances transmitted via placenta or breast milk

    INCLUDES   nonteratogenic effects of substances transmitted via placenta

    ►Code first any current condition in newborn, if applicable◄
    EXCLUDES 2   congenital malformations (Q00-Q99)
       encounter for observation of newborn for suspected diseases and conditions ruled out (Z05.-)
       neonatal jaundice from excessive hemolysis due to drugs or toxins transmitted from mother (P58.4)
       newborn in contact with and (suspected) exposures hazardous to health not transmitted via placenta or breast milk (Z77.-)

P04.0   **Newborn affected by maternal** anesthesia and analgesia **in pregnancy, labor and delivery**
    Newborn affected by reactions and intoxications from maternal opiates and tranquilizers administered for procedures during pregnancy or labor and delivery
    EXCLUDES 2   newborn affected by other maternal medication (P04.1-)

N Newborn: 0   **P** Pediatric: 0-17   **M** Maternity: 9-64   **A** Adult: 15-124   **MCC** Major Complication/Comorbidity   **CC** Complication/Comorbidity   **SW** Severe Wound Dx

908   ICD-10-CM 2022

✓5ᵗʰ **P04.1 Newborn affected by other maternal medication**

Code first withdrawal symptoms from maternal use of drugs of addiction, if applicable (P96.1)

EXCLUDES 1   *dysmorphism due to warfarin (Q86.2)*
fetal hydantoin syndrome (Q86.1)

EXCLUDES 2   *maternal anesthesia and analgesia in pregnancy, labor and delivery (P04.0)*
maternal use of drugs of addiction (P04.4-)

AHA: 2018,4Q,24-25

P04.11 Newborn affected by maternal antineoplastic chemotherapy

P04.12 Newborn affected by maternal cytotoxic drugs

P04.13 Newborn affected by maternal use of anticonvulsants

P04.14 Newborn affected by maternal use of opiates

P04.15 Newborn affected by maternal use of antidepressants

P04.16 Newborn affected by maternal use of amphetamines

P04.17 Newborn affected by maternal use of sedative-hypnotics

P04.1A Newborn affected by maternal use of anxiolytics

P04.18 Newborn affected by other maternal medication

P04.19 Newborn affected by maternal use of unspecified medication

P04.2 Newborn affected by maternal use of tobacco

Newborn affected by exposure in utero to tobacco smoke

EXCLUDES 2   *newborn exposure to environmental tobacco smoke (P96.81)*

P04.3 Newborn affected by maternal use of alcohol

EXCLUDES 1   *fetal alcohol syndrome (Q86.0)*

✓5ᵗʰ **P04.4 Newborn affected by maternal use of** drugs of addiction

AHA: 2018,4Q,25

P04.40 Newborn affected by maternal use of unspecified drugs of addiction

P04.41 Newborn affected by maternal use of cocaine

P04.42 Newborn affected by maternal use of hallucinogens

EXCLUDES 2   *newborn affected by other maternal medication (P04.1-)*

P04.49 Newborn affected by maternal use of other drugs of addiction

EXCLUDES 2   *newborn affected by maternal anesthesia and analgesia (P04.0)*
withdrawal symptoms from maternal use of drugs of addiction (P96.1)

P04.5 Newborn affected by maternal use of nutritional chemical substances

P04.6 Newborn affected by maternal exposure to environmental chemical substances

✓5ᵗʰ **P04.8 Newborn affected by other maternal** noxious substances

AHA: 2018,4Q,25

P04.81 Newborn affected by maternal use of cannabis

P04.89 Newborn affected by other maternal noxious substances

P04.9 Newborn affected by maternal noxious substance, unspecified

Disorders of newborn related to length of gestation and fetal growth (P05-P08)

✓4ᵗʰ **P05 Disorders of newborn related to slow fetal growth and fetal malnutrition**

AHA: 2016,4Q,55-56

✓5ᵗʰ **P05.0 Newborn light for gestational age**

Newborn light-for-dates
Weight below but length above 10th percentile for gestational age

P05.00 Newborn light for gestational age, unspecified weight

P05.01 Newborn light for gestational age, less than 500 grams

P05.02 Newborn light for gestational age, 500-749 grams

P05.03 Newborn light for gestational age, 750-999 grams

P05.04 Newborn light for gestational age, 1000-1249 grams

P05.05 Newborn light for gestational age, 1250-1499 grams

P05.06 Newborn light for gestational age, 1500-1749 grams

P05.07 Newborn light for gestational age, 1750-1999 grams

P05.08 Newborn light for gestational age, 2000-2499 grams

P05.09 Newborn light for gestational age, 2500 grams and over

Newborn light for gestational age, other

✓5ᵗʰ **P05.1 Newborn small for gestational age**

Newborn small-and-light-for-dates
Newborn small-for-dates
Weight and length below 10th percentile for gestational age

P05.10 Newborn small for gestational age, unspecified weight

P05.11 Newborn small for gestational age, less than 500 grams

P05.12 Newborn small for gestational age, 500-749 grams

P05.13 Newborn small for gestational age, 750-999 grams

P05.14 Newborn small for gestational age, 1000-1249 grams

P05.15 Newborn small for gestational age, 1250-1499 grams

P05.16 Newborn small for gestational age, 1500-1749 grams

P05.17 Newborn small for gestational age, 1750-1999 grams

P05.18 Newborn small for gestational age, 2000-2499 grams

P05.19 Newborn small for gestational age, other

Newborn small for gestational age, 2500 grams and over

P05.2 Newborn affected by fetal (intrauterine) malnutrition **not light or small for gestational age**

Infant, not light or small for gestational age, showing signs of fetal malnutrition, such as dry, peeling skin and loss of subcutaneous tissue

EXCLUDES 1   *newborn affected by fetal malnutrition with light for gestational age (P05.0-)*
newborn affected by fetal malnutrition with small for gestational age (P05.1-)

P05.9 Newborn affected by slow intrauterine growth, unspecified

Newborn affected by fetal growth retardation NOS

✓4ᵗʰ **P07 Disorders of newborn related to short gestation and low birth weight, not elsewhere classified**

NOTE   When both birth weight and gestational age of the newborn are available, both should be coded with birth weight sequenced before gestational age

INCLUDES   the listed conditions, without further specification, as the cause of morbidity or additional care, in newborn

✓5ᵗʰ **P07.0 Extremely low birth weight newborn**

Newborn birth weight 999 g. or less

EXCLUDES 1   *low birth weight due to slow fetal growth and fetal malnutrition (P05.-)*

P07.00 Extremely low birth weight newborn, unspecified weight

P07.01 Extremely low birth weight newborn, less than 500 grams

P07.02 Extremely low birth weight newborn, 500-749 grams

P07.03 Extremely low birth weight newborn, 750-999 grams

✓5ᵗʰ **P07.1 Other low birth weight newborn**

Newborn birth weight 1000-2499 g.

EXCLUDES 1   *low birth weight due to slow fetal growth and fetal malnutrition (P05.-)*

P07.10 Other low birth weight newborn, unspecified weight

P07.14 Other low birth weight newborn, 1000-1249 grams

P07.15 Other low birth weight newborn, 1250-1499 grams

P07.16 Other low birth weight newborn, 1500-1749 grams

P07.17 Other low birth weight newborn, 1750-1999 grams

P07.18 Other low birth weight newborn, 2000-2499 grams

✓5ᵗʰ **P07.2 Extreme immaturity of newborn**

Less than 28 completed weeks (less than 196 completed days) of gestation.

P07.20 Extreme immaturity of newborn, unspecified weeks of gestation

Gestational age less than 28 completed weeks NOS

☑ Additional Character Required   ✓x7ᵗʰ Placeholder   Questionable PDx   Manifestation   Unspecified Dx   UPD Unacceptable PDx   H1-H14 HAC   HCC CMS-HCC Dx   HIV HIV Dx

ICD-10-CM 2022   909

P07.21 **Extreme immaturity of newborn, gestational age** less than 23 completed weeks

Extreme immaturity of newborn, gestational age less than 23 weeks, 0 days

P07.22 **Extreme immaturity of newborn, gestational age** 23 completed weeks

Extreme immaturity of newborn, gestational age 23 weeks, 0 days through 23 weeks, 6 days

P07.23 **Extreme immaturity of newborn, gestational age** 24 completed weeks

Extreme immaturity of newborn, gestational age 24 weeks, 0 days through 24 weeks, 6 days

P07.24 **Extreme immaturity of newborn, gestational age** 25 completed weeks

Extreme immaturity of newborn, gestational age 25 weeks, 0 days through 25 weeks, 6 days

P07.25 **Extreme immaturity of newborn, gestational age** 26 completed weeks

Extreme immaturity of newborn, gestational age 26 weeks, 0 days through 26 weeks, 6 days

P07.26 **Extreme immaturity of newborn, gestational age** 27 completed weeks

Extreme immaturity of newborn, gestational age 27 weeks, 0 days through 27 weeks, 6 days

√5ᵗʰ **P07.3 Preterm [premature] newborn [other]**

28 completed weeks or more but less than 37 completed weeks (196 completed days but less than 259 completed days) of gestation

Prematurity NOS

AHA: 2017,3Q,26

P07.30 **Preterm newborn, unspecified weeks of gestation**

P07.31 **Preterm newborn, gestational age** 28 completed weeks

Preterm newborn, gestational age 28 weeks, 0 days through 28 weeks, 6 days

P07.32 **Preterm newborn, gestational age** 29 completed weeks

Preterm newborn, gestational age 29 weeks, 0 days through 29 weeks, 6 days

P07.33 **Preterm newborn, gestational age** 30 completed weeks

Preterm newborn, gestational age 30 weeks, 0 days through 30 weeks, 6 days

P07.34 **Preterm newborn, gestational age** 31 completed weeks

Preterm newborn, gestational age 31 weeks, 0 days through 31 weeks, 6 days

P07.35 **Preterm newborn, gestational age** 32 completed weeks

Preterm newborn, gestational age 32 weeks, 0 days through 32 weeks, 6 days

P07.36 **Preterm newborn, gestational age** 33 completed weeks

Preterm newborn, gestational age 33 weeks, 0 days through 33 weeks, 6 days

P07.37 **Preterm newborn, gestational age** 34 completed weeks

Preterm newborn, gestational age 34 weeks, 0 days through 34 weeks, 6 days

P07.38 **Preterm newborn, gestational age** 35 completed weeks

Preterm newborn, gestational age 35 weeks, 0 days through 35 weeks, 6 days

P07.39 **Preterm newborn, gestational age** 36 completed weeks

Preterm newborn, gestational age 36 weeks, 0 days through 36 weeks, 6 days

√4ᵗʰ **P08 Disorders of newborn related to long gestation and high birth weight**

NOTE When both birth weight and gestational age of the newborn are available, priority of assignment should be given to birth weight

INCLUDES the listed conditions, without further specification, as causes of morbidity or additional care, in newborn

P08.0 **Exceptionally large newborn baby**

Usually implies a birth weight of 4500 g. or more

EXCLUDES 1 *syndrome of infant of diabetic mother (P70.1)*

syndrome of infant of mother with gestational diabetes (P70.0)

P08.1 **Other heavy for gestational age newborn**

Other newborn heavy- or large-for-dates regardless of period of gestation

Usually implies a birth weight of 4000 g. to 4499 g.

EXCLUDES 1 *newborn with a birth weight of 4500 or more (P08.0)*

syndrome of infant of diabetic mother (P70.1)

▶*syndrome of infant of mother with gestational diabetes (P70.0)*◀

√5ᵗʰ **P08.2 Late newborn, not heavy for gestational age**

AHA: 2014,1Q,14

P08.21 **Post-term newborn**

Newborn with gestation period over 40 completed weeks to 42 completed weeks

P08.22 **Prolonged gestation of newborn**

Newborn with gestation period over 42 completed weeks (294 days or more), not heavy- or large-for-dates.

Postmaturity NOS

Abnormal findings on neonatal screening (P09)

▲√4ᵗʰ **P09 Abnormal findings on neonatal screening**

INCLUDES ▶Abnormal findings on state mandated newborn screens◀

▶Failed newborn screening◀

~~Use additional code to identify signs, symptoms and conditions associated with the screening~~

EXCLUDES 2 *nonspecific serologic evidence of human immunodeficiency virus [HIV] (R75)*

● P09.1 **Abnormal findings on neonatal screening for** inborn errors of metabolism

● P09.2 **Abnormal findings on neonatal screening for** congenital endocrine disease

Abnormal findings on neonatal screening for congenital adrenal hyperplasia

Abnormal findings on neonatal screening for hypothyroidism screen

● P09.3 **Abnormal findings on neonatal screening for** congenital hematologic disorders

Abnormal findings for hemoglobinothies screen

Abnormal findings on red cell membrane defects screen

Abnormal findings on sickle cell screen

● P09.4 **Abnormal findings on neonatal screening for** cystic fibrosis

● P09.5 **Abnormal findings on neonatal screening for** critical congenital heart disease

Neonatal congenital heart disease screening failure

● P09.6 **Abnormal findings on neonatal screening for** neonatal hearing loss

EXCLUDES 2 *encounter for hearing examination following failed hearing screening (Z01.110)*

● P09.8 **Other abnormal findings on neonatal screening**

● P09.9 **Abnormal findings on neonatal screening, unspecified**

Birth trauma (P10-P15)

√4ᵗʰ **P10 Intracranial laceration and hemorrhage due to birth injury**

EXCLUDES 1 *intracranial hemorrhage of newborn NOS (P52.9)*

intracranial hemorrhage of newborn due to anoxia or hypoxia (P52.-)

nontraumatic intracranial hemorrhage of newborn (P52.-)

P10.0 **Subdural hemorrhage due to birth injury** **MCC**

Subdural hematoma (localized) due to birth injury

EXCLUDES 1 *subdural hemorrhage accompanying tentorial tear (P10.4)*

P10.1 **Cerebral hemorrhage due to birth injury** **MCC**

P10.2 **Intraventricular hemorrhage due to birth injury** **CC**

N Newborn: 0   **P** Pediatric: 0-17   **M** Maternity: 9-64   **A** Adult: 15-124   **MCC** Major Complication/Comorbidity   **CC** Complication/Comorbidity   **SW** Severe Wound Dx

910   ICD-10-CM 2022

P10.3 Subarachnoid hemorrhage due to birth injury   `MCC`

P10.4 Tentorial tear due to birth injury   `MCC`

P10.8 Other intracranial lacerations and hemorrhages due to birth injury   `MCC`

P10.9 Unspecified intracranial laceration and hemorrhage due to birth injury   `MCC`

✓4ᵗʰ **P11** Other birth injuries to central nervous system

P11.0 Cerebral edema due to birth injury   `MCC`

P11.1 Other specified brain damage due to birth injury

P11.2 Unspecified brain damage due to birth injury   `MCC`

P11.3 Birth injury to facial nerve
Facial palsy due to birth injury

P11.4 Birth injury to other cranial nerves

P11.5 Birth injury to spine and spinal cord
Fracture of spine due to birth injury

P11.9 Birth injury to central nervous system, unspecified   `MCC`

✓4ᵗʰ **P12** Birth injury to scalp

Birth Injuries to Scalp

P12.0 Cephalhematoma due to birth injury
DEF: Condition that occurs in a neonate when blood vessels between the skull and periosteum rupture and blood collects in the subperiosteal space (below the periosteum). It is typically caused by prolonged labor or trauma due to instrument-assisted delivery (e.g., forceps, vacuum extraction), although in rare circumstances, it may indicate a linear skull fracture with intracranial hemorrhage.

P12.1 Chignon (from vacuum extraction) due to birth injury
DEF: Artificial swelling of the scalp that occurs when a collection of interstitial fluid and blood forms in the area of the scalp where the suction cup was applied during a vacuum-assisted delivery.

P12.2 Epicranial subaponeurotic hemorrhage due to birth injury   `CC`
Subgaleal hemorrhage

P12.3 Bruising of scalp due to birth injury

P12.4 Injury of scalp of newborn due to monitoring equipment
Sampling incision of scalp of newborn
Scalp clip (electrode) injury of newborn

✓5ᵗʰ **P12.8** Other birth injuries to scalp

P12.81 Caput succedaneum
DEF: Swelling of the scalp as a result of pressure being exerted on the head from the vaginal walls, uterus, or instrumentation used in assisting a delivery (e.g., vacuum).

P12.89 Other birth injuries to scalp

P12.9 Birth injury to scalp, unspecified

✓4ᵗʰ **P13** Birth injury to skeleton
`EXCLUDES 2` birth injury to spine (P11.5)

P13.0 Fracture of skull due to birth injury

P13.1 Other birth injuries to skull
`EXCLUDES 1` cephalhematoma (P12.0)

P13.2 Birth injury to femur

P13.3 Birth injury to other long bones

P13.4 Fracture of clavicle due to birth injury

P13.8 Birth injuries to other parts of skeleton

P13.9 Birth injury to skeleton, unspecified

✓4ᵗʰ **P14** Birth injury to peripheral nervous system

P14.0 Erb's paralysis due to birth injury
DEF: Erb's paralysis: Most common type of brachial plexus (peripheral nerve) injury in a neonate that involves nerve damage at the level of C5-C6. *Synonym(s): Erb's palsy*

P14.1 Klumpke's paralysis due to birth injury

P14.2 Phrenic nerve paralysis due to birth injury

P14.3 Other brachial plexus birth injuries

P14.8 Birth injuries to other parts of peripheral nervous system

P14.9 Birth injury to peripheral nervous system, unspecified

✓4ᵗʰ **P15** Other birth injuries

P15.0 Birth injury to liver
Rupture of liver due to birth injury

P15.1 Birth injury to spleen
Rupture of spleen due to birth injury

P15.2 Sternomastoid injury due to birth injury

P15.3 Birth injury to eye
Subconjunctival hemorrhage due to birth injury
Traumatic glaucoma due to birth injury

P15.4 Birth injury to face
Facial congestion due to birth injury

P15.5 Birth injury to external genitalia

P15.6 Subcutaneous fat necrosis due to birth injury

P15.8 Other specified birth injuries

P15.9 Birth injury, unspecified

Respiratory and cardiovascular disorders specific to the perinatal period (P19-P29)

✓4ᵗʰ **P19** Metabolic acidemia in newborn
`INCLUDES` metabolic acidemia in newborn

P19.0 Metabolic acidemia in newborn first noted before onset of labor

P19.1 Metabolic acidemia in newborn first noted during labor

P19.2 Metabolic acidemia noted at birth

P19.9 Metabolic acidemia, unspecified

✓4ᵗʰ **P22** Respiratory distress of newborn
AHA: 2019,2Q,29

P22.0 Respiratory distress syndrome of newborn   `MCC`
Cardiorespiratory distress syndrome of newborn
Hyaline membrane disease
Idiopathic respiratory distress syndrome [IRDS or RDS] of newborn
Pulmonary hypoperfusion syndrome
Respiratory distress syndrome, type I
`EXCLUDES 2` respiratory arrest of newborn (P28.81)
respiratory failure of newborn NOS (P28.5)

AHA: 2019,2Q,29
DEF: Severe chest contractions upon air intake and expiratory grunting. The infant appears blue due to oxygen deficiency and has a rapid respiratory rate, formerly called hyaline membrane disease.

P22.1 Transient tachypnea of newborn
Idiopathic tachypnea of newborn
Respiratory distress syndrome, type II
Wet lung syndrome
DEF: Rapid, labored breathing of a newborn. It is a short-term problem that begins after birth and lasts about three days.

P22.8 Other respiratory distress of newborn
`EXCLUDES 1` respiratory arrest of newborn (P28.81)
respiratory failure of newborn NOS (P28.5)

P22.9 Respiratory distress of newborn, unspecified
`EXCLUDES 1` respiratory arrest of newborn (P28.81)
respiratory failure of newborn NOS (P28.5)

✓4ᵗʰ **P23** Congenital pneumonia
`INCLUDES` infective pneumonia acquired in utero or during birth
`EXCLUDES 1` neonatal pneumonia resulting from aspiration (P24.-)

P23.0 Congenital pneumonia due to viral agent   `MCC`
Use additional code (B97) to identify organism
`EXCLUDES 1` congenital rubella pneumonitis (P35.0)

P23.1 Congenital pneumonia due to Chlamydia   `MCC`

P23.2 Congenital pneumonia due to staphylococcus   `MCC`

P23.3 Congenital pneumonia due to streptococcus, group B   `MCC`

P23.4 Congenital pneumonia due to Escherichia coli   `MCC`

P23.5 Congenital pneumonia due to Pseudomonas   `MCC`

Chapter 16. Certain Conditions Originating in the Perinatal Period

P23.6   Congenital pneumonia due to other bacterial agents `MCC`
Congenital pneumonia due to Hemophilus influenzae
Congenital pneumonia due to Klebsiella pneumoniae
Congenital pneumonia due to Mycoplasma
Congenital pneumonia due to Streptococcus, except group B
Use additional code (B95-B96) to identify organism

P23.8   Congenital pneumonia due to other organisms `MCC`

P23.9   Congenital pneumonia, unspecified `MCC`

✓4ᵗʰ **P24   Neonatal aspiration**
`INCLUDES`   aspiration in utero and during delivery

  ✓5ᵗʰ **P24.0   Meconium aspiration**
    `EXCLUDES 1`   meconium passage (without aspiration) during delivery (P03.82)
       meconium staining (P96.83)
    DEF: Meconium in the trachea or seen on chest x-ray after birth.

    P24.00   Meconium aspiration without respiratory symptoms
       Meconium aspiration NOS

    P24.01   Meconium aspiration with respiratory symptoms `MCC`
       Meconium aspiration pneumonia
       Meconium aspiration pneumonitis
       Meconium aspiration syndrome NOS
       Use additional code to identify any secondary pulmonary hypertension, if applicable (I27.2-)
      DEF: Aspiration of fetal intestinal material during or prior to delivery. It is usually a complication of placental insufficiency, causing pneumonitis and bronchial obstruction (inflammatory reaction of lungs).

  ✓5ᵗʰ **P24.1   Neonatal aspiration of (clear) amniotic fluid and mucus**
     Neonatal aspiration of liquor (amnii)

    P24.10   Neonatal aspiration of (clear) amniotic fluid and mucus without respiratory symptoms
       Neonatal aspiration of amniotic fluid and mucus NOS

    P24.11   Neonatal aspiration of (clear) amniotic fluid and mucus with respiratory symptoms `MCC`
       Neonatal aspiration of amniotic fluid and mucus with pneumonia
       Neonatal aspiration of amniotic fluid and mucus with pneumonitis
       Use additional code to identify any secondary pulmonary hypertension, if applicable (I27.2-)

  ✓5ᵗʰ **P24.2   Neonatal aspiration of blood**

    P24.20   Neonatal aspiration of blood without respiratory symptoms
       Neonatal aspiration of blood NOS

    P24.21   Neonatal aspiration of blood with respiratory symptoms `MCC`
       Neonatal aspiration of blood with pneumonia
       Neonatal aspiration of blood with pneumonitis
       Use additional code to identify any secondary pulmonary hypertension, if applicable (I27.2-)

  ✓5ᵗʰ **P24.3   Neonatal aspiration of milk and regurgitated food**
     Neonatal aspiration of stomach contents

    P24.30   Neonatal aspiration of milk and regurgitated food without respiratory symptoms
       Neonatal aspiration of milk and regurgitated food NOS

    P24.31   Neonatal aspiration of milk and regurgitated food with respiratory symptoms `MCC`
       Neonatal aspiration of milk and regurgitated food with pneumonia
       Neonatal aspiration of milk and regurgitated food with pneumonitis
       Use additional code to identify any secondary pulmonary hypertension, if applicable (I27.2-)

  ✓5ᵗʰ **P24.8   Other neonatal aspiration**

    P24.80   Other neonatal aspiration without respiratory symptoms
       Neonatal aspiration NEC

P24.81   Other neonatal aspiration with respiratory symptoms `MCC`
Neonatal aspiration pneumonia NEC
Neonatal aspiration with pneumonitis NEC
Neonatal aspiration with pneumonia NOS
Neonatal aspiration with pneumonitis NOS
Use additional code to identify any secondary pulmonary hypertension, if applicable (I27.2-)

P24.9   Neonatal aspiration, unspecified

✓4ᵗʰ **P25   Interstitial emphysema and related conditions originating in the perinatal period**

  P25.0   Interstitial emphysema originating in the perinatal period `MCC`

  P25.1   Pneumothorax originating in the perinatal period `MCC`

  P25.2   Pneumomediastinum originating in the perinatal period `MCC`

  P25.3   Pneumopericardium originating in the perinatal period `MCC`

  P25.8   Other conditions related to interstitial emphysema originating in the perinatal period `MCC`

✓4ᵗʰ **P26   Pulmonary hemorrhage originating in the perinatal period**
  `EXCLUDES 1`   acute idiopathic hemorrhage in infants over 28 days old (R04.81)

  P26.0   Tracheobronchial hemorrhage originating in the perinatal period `MCC`

  P26.1   Massive pulmonary hemorrhage originating in the perinatal period `MCC`

  P26.8   Other pulmonary hemorrhages originating in the perinatal period `MCC`

  P26.9   Unspecified pulmonary hemorrhage originating in the perinatal period `MCC`

✓4ᵗʰ **P27   Chronic respiratory disease originating in the perinatal period**
  `EXCLUDES 2`   respiratory distress of newborn (P22.0-P22.9)

  P27.0   Wilson-Mikity syndrome `MCC`
     Pulmonary dysmaturity
    DEF: Pulmonary insufficiency in newborn babies, especially those with low birth weight. Rapid onset of hypercapnia and cyanosis occur during the first month of life frequently resulting in death.

  P27.1   Bronchopulmonary dysplasia originating in the perinatal period `MCC`

  P27.8   Other chronic respiratory diseases originating in the perinatal period `MCC`
     Congenital pulmonary fibrosis
     Ventilator lung in newborn

  P27.9   Unspecified chronic respiratory disease originating in the perinatal period `MCC`

✓4ᵗʰ **P28   Other respiratory conditions originating in the perinatal period**
  `EXCLUDES 1`   congenital malformations of the respiratory system (Q30-Q34)

  P28.0   Primary atelectasis of newborn `CC`
     Primary failure to expand terminal respiratory units
     Pulmonary hypoplasia associated with short gestation
     Pulmonary immaturity NOS

  ✓5ᵗʰ **P28.1   Other and unspecified atelectasis of newborn**

    P28.10   Unspecified atelectasis of newborn `CC`
       Atelectasis of newborn NOS

    P28.11   Resorption atelectasis without respiratory distress syndrome `CC`
      `EXCLUDES 1`   resorption atelectasis with respiratory distress syndrome (P22.0)

    P28.19   Other atelectasis of newborn `CC`
       Partial atelectasis of newborn
       Secondary atelectasis of newborn

  P28.2   Cyanotic attacks of newborn `CC`
    `EXCLUDES 1`   apnea of newborn (P28.3-P28.4)

  P28.3   Primary sleep apnea of newborn `CC`
     Central sleep apnea of newborn
     Obstructive sleep apnea of newborn
     Sleep apnea of newborn NOS
    DEF: Unexplained cessation of breathing when a neonate makes no respiratory effort for 20 seconds or longer or when a neonate's breathing cessation is accompanied by cyanosis, bradycardia, or hypotonia.

P23.6–P28.3

N Newborn: 0   P Pediatric: 0-17   M Maternity: 9-64   A Adult: 15-124   `MCC` Major Complication/Comorbidity   `CC` Complication/Comorbidity   `SW` Severe Wound Dx

912   ICD-10-CM 2022

P28.4 Other apnea of newborn `CC`
Apnea of prematurity
Obstructive apnea of newborn
EXCLUDES 1   *obstructive sleep apnea of newborn (P28.3)*

P28.5 Respiratory failure of newborn `MCC`
EXCLUDES 1   *respiratory arrest of newborn (P28.81)*
respiratory distress of newborn (P22.0-)
AHA: 2019,2Q,29

✓5ᵗʰ **P28.8 Other specified respiratory conditions of newborn**
P28.81   Respiratory arrest of newborn `MCC`
P28.89   Other specified respiratory conditions of newborn
Congenital laryngeal stridor
Sniffles in newborn
Snuffles in newborn
EXCLUDES 1   *early congenital syphilitic rhinitis (A50.05)*

P28.9 Respiratory condition of newborn, unspecified
Respiratory depression in newborn

✓4ᵗʰ **P29 Cardiovascular disorders originating in the perinatal period**
EXCLUDES 1   *congenital malformations of the circulatory system (Q20-Q28)*
EXCLUDES 2   ▶*congenital malformations of the circulatory system (Q20-Q28)*◀

P29.0 Neonatal cardiac failure
✓5ᵗʰ **P29.1 Neonatal cardiac dysrhythmia**
P29.11   Neonatal tachycardia
P29.12   Neonatal bradycardia
P29.2 Neonatal hypertension
✓5ᵗʰ **P29.3 Persistent fetal circulation**
AHA: 2017,4Q,20-21
P29.30   Pulmonary hypertension of newborn `MCC`
Persistent pulmonary hypertension of newborn
DEF: Condition that occurs when pressure within the pulmonary artery is elevated and vascular resistance is observed in the lungs.
P29.38   Other persistent fetal circulation `MCC`
Delayed closure of ductus arteriosus
P29.4 Transient myocardial ischemia in newborn
✓5ᵗʰ **P29.8 Other cardiovascular disorders originating in the perinatal period**
P29.81   Cardiac arrest of newborn `MCC`
P29.89   Other cardiovascular disorders originating in the perinatal period
AHA: 2014,4Q,23
P29.9 Cardiovascular disorder originating in the perinatal period, unspecified

Infections specific to the perinatal period (P35-P39)

Infections acquired in utero, during birth via the umbilicus, or during the first 28 days after birth
EXCLUDES 2   *asymptomatic human immunodeficiency virus [HIV] infection status (Z21)*
congenital gonococcal infection (A54.-)
congenital pneumonia (P23.-)
congenital syphilis (A50.-)
human immunodeficiency virus [HIV] disease (B20)
infant botulism (A48.51)
infectious diseases not specific to the perinatal period (A00-B99, J09, J10.-)
intestinal infectious disease (A00-A09)
laboratory evidence of human immunodeficiency virus [HIV] (R75)
tetanus neonatorum (A33)

✓4ᵗʰ **P35 Congenital viral diseases**
INCLUDES   infections acquired in utero or during birth
P35.0 Congenital rubella syndrome `CC`
Congenital rubella pneumonitis
P35.1 Congenital cytomegalovirus infection `MCC`
P35.2 Congenital herpesviral [herpes simplex] infection `MCC`
P35.3 Congenital viral hepatitis `MCC`
P35.4 Congenital Zika virus disease `MCC`
Use additional code to identify manifestations of congenital Zika virus disease
AHA: 2018,4Q,25-26
P35.8 Other congenital viral diseases `MCC`
Congenital varicella [chickenpox]
AHA: 2020,2Q,13
P35.9 Congenital viral disease, unspecified `MCC`

✓4ᵗʰ **P36 Bacterial sepsis of newborn**
INCLUDES   congenital sepsis
Use additional code(s), if applicable, to identify severe sepsis (R65.2-) and associated acute organ dysfunction(s)
P36.0 Sepsis of newborn due to streptococcus, group B `MCC` `HCC`
✓5ᵗʰ **P36.1 Sepsis of newborn due to other and unspecified streptococci**
P36.10   Sepsis of newborn due to unspecified streptococci `MCC` `HCC`
P36.19   Sepsis of newborn due to other streptococci `MCC` `HCC`
P36.2 Sepsis of newborn due to Staphylococcus aureus `MCC` `HCC`
✓5ᵗʰ **P36.3 Sepsis of newborn due to other and unspecified staphylococci**
P36.30   Sepsis of newborn due to unspecified staphylococci `MCC` `HCC`
P36.39   Sepsis of newborn due to other staphylococci `MCC` `HCC`
P36.4 Sepsis of newborn due to Escherichia coli `MCC` `HCC`
P36.5 Sepsis of newborn due to anaerobes `MCC` `HCC`
P36.8 Other bacterial sepsis of newborn `MCC` `HCC`
Use additional code from category B96 to identify organism
P36.9 Bacterial sepsis of newborn, unspecified `MCC` `HCC`

✓4ᵗʰ **P37 Other congenital infectious and parasitic diseases**
EXCLUDES 2   *congenital syphilis (A50.-)*
infectious neonatal diarrhea (A00-A09)
necrotizing enterocolitis in newborn (P77.-)
noninfectious neonatal diarrhea (P78.3)
ophthalmia neonatorum due to gonococcus (A54.31)
tetanus neonatorum (A33)
P37.0 Congenital tuberculosis `MCC`
P37.1 Congenital toxoplasmosis `MCC`
Hydrocephalus due to congenital toxoplasmosis
P37.2 Neonatal (disseminated) listeriosis `MCC`
P37.3 Congenital falciparum malaria `MCC`
P37.4 Other congenital malaria
P37.5 Neonatal candidiasis
P37.8 Other specified congenital infectious and parasitic diseases `MCC`
P37.9 Congenital infectious or parasitic disease, unspecified `MCC`

✓4ᵗʰ **P38 Omphalitis of newborn**
EXCLUDES 1   *omphalitis not of newborn (L08.82)*
tetanus omphalitis (A33)
umbilical hemorrhage of newborn (P51.-)
DEF: Omphalitis: Infection and inflammation of the umbilical stump, often due to bacteria that can spread beyond the umbilical stump to the fascia, muscle, or even the umbilical vessels.
P38.1 Omphalitis with mild hemorrhage `CC`
P38.9 Omphalitis without hemorrhage `CC`
Omphalitis of newborn NOS

✓4ᵗʰ **P39 Other infections specific to the perinatal period**
Use additional code to identify organism or specific infection
P39.0 Neonatal infective mastitis `CC`
EXCLUDES 1   *breast engorgement of newborn (P83.4)*
noninfective mastitis of newborn (P83.4)
P39.1 Neonatal conjunctivitis and dacryocystitis
Neonatal chlamydial conjunctivitis
Ophthalmia neonatorum NOS
EXCLUDES 1   *gonococcal conjunctivitis (A54.31)*
P39.2 Intra-amniotic infection affecting newborn, not elsewhere classified `CC`
P39.3 Neonatal urinary tract infection `CC`
P39.4 Neonatal skin infection `CC`
Neonatal pyoderma
EXCLUDES 1   *pemphigus neonatorum (L00)*
staphylococcal scalded skin syndrome (L00)
P39.8 Other specified infections specific to the perinatal period `CC`
P39.9 Infection specific to the perinatal period, unspecified `CC`

Hemorrhagic and hematological disorders of newborn (P50-P61)

EXCLUDES 1   congenital stenosis and stricture of bile ducts (Q44.3)
Crigler-Najjar syndrome (E80.5)
Dubin-Johnson syndrome (E80.6)
Gilbert syndrome (E80.4)
hereditary hemolytic anemias (D55-D58)

✓4th P50 Newborn affected by intrauterine (fetal) blood loss

EXCLUDES 1   congenital anemia from intrauterine (fetal) blood loss (P61.3)

P50.0 Newborn affected by intrauterine (fetal) blood loss from vasa previa

P50.1 Newborn affected by intrauterine (fetal) blood loss from ruptured cord

P50.2 Newborn affected by intrauterine (fetal) blood loss from placenta

P50.3 Newborn affected by hemorrhage into co-twin

P50.4 Newborn affected by hemorrhage into maternal circulation

P50.5 Newborn affected by intrauterine (fetal) blood loss from cut end of co-twin's cord

P50.8 Newborn affected by other intrauterine (fetal) blood loss

P50.9 Newborn affected by intrauterine (fetal) blood loss, unspecified
Newborn affected by fetal hemorrhage NOS

✓4th P51 Umbilical hemorrhage of newborn

EXCLUDES 1   omphalitis with mild hemorrhage (P38.1)
umbilical hemorrhage from cut end of co-twins cord (P50.5)

P51.0 Massive umbilical hemorrhage of newborn

P51.8 Other umbilical hemorrhages of newborn
Slipped umbilical ligature NOS

P51.9 Umbilical hemorrhage of newborn, unspecified

✓4th P52 Intracranial nontraumatic hemorrhage of newborn

INCLUDES   intracranial hemorrhage due to anoxia or hypoxia

EXCLUDES 1   intracranial hemorrhage due to birth injury (P10.-)
intracranial hemorrhage due to other injury (S06.-)

P52.0 Intraventricular (nontraumatic) hemorrhage, grade 1, of newborn CC
Subependymal hemorrhage (without intraventricular extension)
Bleeding into germinal matrix

P52.1 Intraventricular (nontraumatic) hemorrhage, grade 2, of newborn CC
Subependymal hemorrhage with intraventricular extension
Bleeding into ventricle

✓5th P52.2 Intraventricular (nontraumatic) hemorrhage, grade 3 and grade 4, of newborn

P52.21 Intraventricular (nontraumatic) hemorrhage, grade 3, of newborn MCC
Subependymal hemorrhage with intraventricular extension with enlargement of ventricle

P52.22 Intraventricular (nontraumatic) hemorrhage, grade 4, of newborn MCC
Bleeding into cerebral cortex
Subependymal hemorrhage with intracerebral extension

P52.3 Unspecified intraventricular (nontraumatic) hemorrhage of newborn CC

P52.4 Intracerebral (nontraumatic) hemorrhage of newborn MCC

P52.5 Subarachnoid (nontraumatic) hemorrhage of newborn MCC

P52.6 Cerebellar (nontraumatic) and posterior fossa hemorrhage of newborn MCC

P52.8 Other intracranial (nontraumatic) hemorrhages of newborn MCC

P52.9 Intracranial (nontraumatic) hemorrhage of newborn, unspecified MCC

P53 Hemorrhagic disease of newborn CC
Vitamin K deficiency of newborn

✓4th P54 Other neonatal hemorrhages

EXCLUDES 1   newborn affected by (intrauterine) blood loss (P50.-)
pulmonary hemorrhage originating in the perinatal period (P26.-)

P54.0 Neonatal hematemesis

EXCLUDES 1   neonatal hematemesis due to swallowed maternal blood (P78.2)

P54.1 Neonatal melena MCC

EXCLUDES 1   neonatal melena due to swallowed maternal blood (P78.2)

P54.2 Neonatal rectal hemorrhage MCC

P54.3 Other neonatal gastrointestinal hemorrhage MCC

P54.4 Neonatal adrenal hemorrhage CC

P54.5 Neonatal cutaneous hemorrhage
Neonatal bruising
Neonatal ecchymoses
Neonatal petechiae
Neonatal superficial hematomata

EXCLUDES 2   bruising of scalp due to birth injury (P12.3)
cephalhematoma due to birth injury (P12.0)

P54.6 Neonatal vaginal hemorrhage ♀
Neonatal pseudomenses

P54.8 Other specified neonatal hemorrhages

P54.9 Neonatal hemorrhage, unspecified

✓4th P55 Hemolytic disease of newborn

P55.0 Rh isoimmunization of newborn
DEF: Incompatible Rh fetal-maternal blood grouping that prematurely destroys red blood cells. Symptoms include jaundice, asphyxia, pulmonary hypertension, edema, respiratory distress, kernicterus, and coagulopathies. It is detected by a Coombs test.
TIP: A positive Coombs test without documentation of associated Rh isoimmunization should be coded to R79.89 Other specified abnormal findings of blood chemistry.

P55.1 ABO isoimmunization of newborn
AHA: 2015,3Q,20

P55.8 Other hemolytic diseases of newborn
AHA: 2018,3Q,24

P55.9 Hemolytic disease of newborn, unspecified

✓4th P56 Hydrops fetalis due to hemolytic disease

EXCLUDES 1   hydrops fetalis NOS (P83.2)

P56.0 Hydrops fetalis due to isoimmunization MCC

✓5th P56.9 Hydrops fetalis due to other and unspecified hemolytic disease

P56.90 Hydrops fetalis due to unspecified hemolytic disease MCC

P56.99 Hydrops fetalis due to other hemolytic disease MCC

✓4th P57 Kernicterus

P57.0 Kernicterus due to isoimmunization MCC
DEF: Complication of erythroblastosis fetalis associated with severe neural symptoms, high blood bilirubin levels, and nerve cell destruction. It results in bilirubin-pigmented gray matter of the central nervous system.

P57.8 Other specified kernicterus MCC

EXCLUDES 1   Crigler-Najjar syndrome (E80.5)

P57.9 Kernicterus, unspecified MCC

✓4th P58 Neonatal jaundice due to other excessive hemolysis

EXCLUDES 1   jaundice due to isoimmunization (P55-P57)

P58.0 Neonatal jaundice due to bruising

P58.1 Neonatal jaundice due to bleeding

P58.2 Neonatal jaundice due to infection

P58.3 Neonatal jaundice due to polycythemia

✓5th P58.4 Neonatal jaundice due to drugs or toxins transmitted from mother or given to newborn
Code first poisoning due to drug or toxin, if applicable (T36-T65 with fifth or sixth character 1-4 or 6)
Use additional code for adverse effect, if applicable, to identify drug (T36-T50 with fifth or sixth character 5)

P58.41 Neonatal jaundice due to drugs or toxins transmitted from mother

P58.42 Neonatal jaundice due to drugs or toxins given to newborn

P58.5 Neonatal jaundice due to swallowed maternal blood

P58.8 Neonatal jaundice due to other specified excessive hemolysis

P58.9 Neonatal jaundice due to excessive hemolysis, unspecified

☑4ᵗʰ **P59 Neonatal jaundice from other and unspecified causes**

> *EXCLUDES 1*   *jaundice due to inborn errors of metabolism (E70-E88)*
> *kernicterus (P57.-)*

P59.0 Neonatal jaundice associated with preterm delivery
Hyperbilirubinemia of prematurity
Jaundice due to delayed conjugation associated with preterm delivery

P59.1 Inspissated bile syndrome   `MCC`
DEF: Biliary obstruction in newborn resulting from obstruction of outflow tract.

☑5ᵗʰ **P59.2 Neonatal jaundice from other and unspecified hepatocellular damage**

> *EXCLUDES 1*   *congenital viral hepatitis (P35.3)*

P59.20 Neonatal jaundice from unspecified hepatocellular damage   `MCC`

P59.29 Neonatal jaundice from other hepatocellular damage   `MCC`
Neonatal giant cell hepatitis
Neonatal (idiopathic) hepatitis

P59.3 Neonatal jaundice from breast milk inhibitor

P59.8 Neonatal jaundice from other specified causes

P59.9 Neonatal jaundice, unspecified
Neonatal physiological jaundice (intense)(prolonged) NOS
AHA: 2015,3Q,20

P60 Disseminated intravascular coagulation of newborn   `MCC`
Defibrination syndrome of newborn

☑4ᵗʰ **P61 Other perinatal hematological disorders**

> *EXCLUDES 1*   *transient hypogammaglobulinemia of infancy (D80.7)*

P61.0 Transient neonatal thrombocytopenia   `MCC`
Neonatal thrombocytopenia due to exchange transfusion
Neonatal thrombocytopenia due to idiopathic maternal thrombocytopenia
Neonatal thrombocytopenia due to isoimmunization
DEF: Temporary decrease in blood platelets of a newborn that is secondary to placental insufficiency.

P61.1 Polycythemia neonatorum
DEF: Abnormal increase of total red blood cells of a newborn that results in hyperviscosity, which slows the flow of blood through small blood vessels.

P61.2 Anemia of prematurity   `CC`

P61.3 Congenital anemia from fetal blood loss   `CC`

P61.4 Other congenital anemias, not elsewhere classified   `CC`
Congenital anemia NOS

P61.5 Transient neonatal neutropenia   `MCC`

> *EXCLUDES 1*   *congenital neutropenia (nontransient) (D70.0)*

DEF: Low blood neutrophil counts of newborn that occurs due to maternal hypertension, sepsis, twin-twin transfusion, alloimmunization, and hemolytic disease.

P61.6 Other transient neonatal disorders of coagulation   `CC`

P61.8 Other specified perinatal hematological disorders

P61.9 Perinatal hematological disorder, unspecified

Transitory endocrine and metabolic disorders specific to newborn (P70-P74)

> `INCLUDES`   transitory endocrine and metabolic disturbances caused by the infant's response to maternal endocrine and metabolic factors, or its adjustment to extrauterine environment

AHA: 2018,2Q,6

☑4ᵗʰ **P70 Transitory disorders of carbohydrate metabolism specific to newborn**

P70.0 Syndrome of infant of mother with gestational diabetes
Newborn (with hypoglycemia) affected by maternal gestational diabetes

> *EXCLUDES 1*   *newborn (with hypoglycemia) affected by maternal (pre-existing) diabetes mellitus (P70.1)*
> *syndrome of infant of a diabetic mother (P70.1)*

P70.1 Syndrome of infant of a diabetic mother
Newborn (with hypoglycemia) affected by maternal (pre-existing) diabetes mellitus

> *EXCLUDES 1*   *newborn (with hypoglycemia) affected by maternal gestational diabetes (P70.0)*
> *syndrome of infant of mother with gestational diabetes (P70.0)*

P70.2 Neonatal diabetes mellitus   `CC`

P70.3 Iatrogenic neonatal hypoglycemia

P70.4 Other neonatal hypoglycemia
Transitory neonatal hypoglycemia

P70.8 Other transitory disorders of carbohydrate metabolism of newborn   `CC`

P70.9 Transitory disorder of carbohydrate metabolism of newborn, unspecified

☑4ᵗʰ **P71 Transitory neonatal disorders of calcium and magnesium metabolism**

P71.0 Cow's milk hypocalcemia in newborn   `CC`

P71.1 Other neonatal hypocalcemia   `CC`

> *EXCLUDES 1*   *neonatal hypoparathyroidism (P71.4)*

P71.2 Neonatal hypomagnesemia

P71.3 Neonatal tetany without calcium or magnesium deficiency   `CC`
Neonatal tetany NOS

P71.4 Transitory neonatal hypoparathyroidism

P71.8 Other transitory neonatal disorders of calcium and magnesium metabolism   `CC`
AHA: 2016,4Q,54

P71.9 Transitory neonatal disorder of calcium and magnesium metabolism, unspecified   `CC`

☑4ᵗʰ **P72 Other transitory neonatal endocrine disorders**

> *EXCLUDES 1*   *congenital hypothyroidism with or without goiter (E03.0-E03.1)*
> *dyshormogenetic goiter (E07.1)*
> *Pendred's syndrome (E07.1)*

P72.0 Neonatal goiter, not elsewhere classified   `CC`
Transitory congenital goiter with normal functioning

P72.1 Transitory neonatal hyperthyroidism
Neonatal thyrotoxicosis

P72.2 Other transitory neonatal disorders of thyroid function, not elsewhere classified   `CC`
Transitory neonatal hypothyroidism

P72.8 Other specified transitory neonatal endocrine disorders   `CC`

P72.9 Transitory neonatal endocrine disorder, unspecified

☑4ᵗʰ **P74 Other transitory neonatal electrolyte and metabolic disturbances**
AHA: 2018,4Q,26-27

P74.0 Late metabolic acidosis of newborn   `MCC`

> *EXCLUDES 1*   *(fetal) metabolic acidosis of newborn (P19)*

P74.1 Dehydration of newborn

☑5ᵗʰ **P74.2 Disturbances of sodium balance of newborn**

P74.21 Hypernatremia of newborn

P74.22 Hyponatremia of newborn

☑5ᵗʰ **P74.3 Disturbances of potassium balance of newborn**

P74.31 Hyperkalemia of newborn

P74.32 Hypokalemia of newborn

☑5ᵗʰ **P74.4 Other transitory electrolyte disturbances of newborn**

P74.41 Alkalosis of newborn   `CC`
Hyperbicarbonatemia

☑6ᵗʰ **P74.42 Disturbances of chlorine balance of newborn**

P74.421 Hyperchloremia of newborn
Hyperchloremic metabolic acidosis

> *EXCLUDES 2*   *late metabolic acidosis of the newborn (P74.0)*

P74.422 Hypochloremia of newborn

P74.49 Other transitory electrolyte disturbance of newborn

P74.5 Transitory tyrosinemia of newborn   `CC`

P74.6 Transitory hyperammonemia of newborn   `CC`

P74.8 Other transitory metabolic disturbances of newborn   `CC`
Amino-acid metabolic disorders described as transitory

P74.9 Transitory metabolic disturbance of newborn, unspecified

Digestive system disorders of newborn (P76-P78)

☑4ᵗʰ **P76 Other intestinal obstruction of newborn**

P76.0 Meconium plug syndrome
Meconium ileus NOS

> *EXCLUDES 1*   *meconium ileus in cystic fibrosis (E84.11)*

DEF: Meconium obstruction of a newborn's intestines, resulting from unusually thick or hard meconium.

P76.1 Transitory ileus of newborn   `CC`

> *EXCLUDES 1*   *Hirschsprung's disease (Q43.1)*

P76.2 Intestinal obstruction due to inspissated milk

P76.8 **Other specified intestinal obstruction of newborn**
> EXCLUDES 1   *intestinal obstruction classifiable to K56.-*

P76.9 **Intestinal obstruction of newborn, unspecified**

☑4ᵗʰ **P77** **Necrotizing enterocolitis of newborn**
> **DEF:** Serious intestinal infection and inflammation in preterm infants. Severity is measured by stages and may progress to life-threatening perforation or peritonitis. Resection surgical treatment may be necessary.

P77.1 **Stage 1 necrotizing enterocolitis in newborn**   MCC
> Necrotizing enterocolitis without pneumatosis, without perforation
> **DEF:** Broad-spectrum symptoms with nonspecific signs, including feeding intolerance, abdominal distention, bradycardia, and metabolic abnormalities.

P77.2 **Stage 2 necrotizing enterocolitis in newborn**   MCC
> Necrotizing enterocolitis with pneumatosis, without perforation
> **DEF:** Radiographic confirmation of necrotizing enterocolitis showing intestinal dilatation, fixed loops of bowels, pneumatosis intestinalis, metabolic acidosis, and thrombocytopenia.

P77.3 **Stage 3 necrotizing enterocolitis in newborn**   MCC
> Necrotizing enterocolitis with perforation
> Necrotizing enterocolitis with pneumatosis and perforation
> **DEF:** Advanced stage in which an infant demonstrates signs of bowel perforation, septic shock, metabolic acidosis, ascites, disseminated intravascular coagulopathy, and neutropenia.

P77.9 **Necrotizing enterocolitis in newborn, unspecified**   MCC
> Necrotizing enterocolitis in newborn, NOS

☑4ᵗʰ **P78** **Other perinatal digestive system disorders**
> EXCLUDES 1   *cystic fibrosis (E84.0-E84.9)*
> *neonatal gastrointestinal hemorrhages (P54.0-P54.3)*

P78.0 **Perinatal intestinal perforation**   MCC
> Meconium peritonitis

P78.1 **Other neonatal peritonitis**
> Neonatal peritonitis NOS

P78.2 **Neonatal hematemesis and melena due to swallowed maternal blood**

P78.3 **Noninfective neonatal diarrhea**
> Neonatal diarrhea NOS

☑5ᵗʰ **P78.8** **Other specified perinatal digestive system disorders**

P78.81 **Congenital cirrhosis (of liver)**

P78.82 **Peptic ulcer of newborn**

P78.83 **Newborn esophageal reflux**
> Neonatal esophageal reflux

P78.84 **Gestational alloimmune liver disease**
> GALD
> Neonatal hemochromatosis
> EXCLUDES 1   *hemochromatosis (E83.11-)*
> **AHA:** 2017,4Q,21
> **DEF:** Severe hepatic injury with onset during fetal development with manifestations beginning during fetal life. It is due to maternal antibodies to fetal hepatic cells (hepatocytes) that cross the placenta into the fetal circulation, causing hepatic cell necrosis.

P78.89 **Other specified perinatal digestive system disorders**

P78.9 **Perinatal digestive system disorder, unspecified**

Conditions involving the integument and temperature regulation of newborn (P80-P83)

☑4ᵗʰ **P80** **Hypothermia of newborn**
> **DEF:** Decrease in newborn body temperature due to their larger ratio of surface area to body weight, thin skin with blood vessels close to the surface, and a limited amount of subcutaneous fat.

P80.0 **Cold injury syndrome**
> Severe and usually chronic hypothermia associated with a pink flushed appearance, edema and neurological and biochemical abnormalities.
> EXCLUDES 1   *mild hypothermia of newborn (P80.8)*

P80.8 **Other hypothermia of newborn**
> Mild hypothermia of newborn

P80.9 **Hypothermia of newborn, unspecified**

☑4ᵗʰ **P81** **Other disturbances of temperature regulation of newborn**

P81.0 **Environmental hyperthermia of newborn**

P81.8 **Other specified disturbances of temperature regulation of newborn**

P81.9 **Disturbance of temperature regulation of newborn, unspecified**
> Fever of newborn NOS

☑4ᵗʰ **P83** **Other conditions of integument specific to newborn**
> EXCLUDES 1   *congenital malformations of skin and integument (Q80-Q84)*
> *hydrops fetalis due to hemolytic disease (P56.-)*
> *neonatal skin infection (P39.4)*
> *staphylococcal scalded skin syndrome (L00)*
> EXCLUDES 2   *cradle cap (L21.0)*
> *diaper [napkin] dermatitis (L22)*

P83.0 **Sclerema neonatorum**   CC
> **DEF:** Diffuse, rapidly progressing white, waxy, nonpitting hardening of tissue, usually of legs and feet that is life-threatening. It is found in preterm or debilitated infants. Etiology is unknown.

P83.1 **Neonatal erythema toxicum**

P83.2 **Hydrops fetalis not due to hemolytic disease**   MCC
> Hydrops fetalis NOS
> **DEF:** Severe, life-threatening problem of a newborn characterized by severe edema of the entire body. It is unrelated to immune response.

☑5ᵗʰ **P83.3** **Other and unspecified edema specific to newborn**

P83.30 **Unspecified edema specific to newborn**   CC

P83.39 **Other edema specific to newborn**   CC

P83.4 **Breast engorgement of newborn**
> Noninfective mastitis of newborn

P83.5 **Congenital hydrocele**   ♂
> **DEF:** Hydrocele: Serous fluid that collects in the tunica vaginalis of the scrotum along the spermatic cord in males.

P83.6 **Umbilical polyp of newborn**

☑5ᵗʰ **P83.8** **Other specified conditions of integument specific to newborn**
> **AHA:** 2017,4Q,21-22

P83.81 **Umbilical granuloma**
> EXCLUDES 2   *granulomatous disorder of the skin and subcutaneous tissue, unspecified (L92.9)*

P83.88 **Other specified conditions of integument specific to newborn**
> Bronze baby syndrome
> Neonatal scleroderma
> Urticaria neonatorum

P83.9 **Condition of the integument specific to newborn, unspecified**

Other problems with newborn (P84)

P84 **Other problems with newborn**
> Acidemia of newborn
> Acidosis of newborn
> Anoxia of newborn NOS
> Asphyxia of newborn NOS
> Hypercapnia of newborn
> Hypoxemia of newborn
> Hypoxia of newborn NOS
> Mixed metabolic and respiratory acidosis of newborn
> EXCLUDES 1   *intracranial hemorrhage due to anoxia or hypoxia (P52.-)*
> *hypoxic ischemic encephalopathy [HIE] (P91.6-)*
> *late metabolic acidosis of newborn (P74.0)*

Other disorders originating in the perinatal period (P90-P96)

P90 **Convulsions of newborn**   MCC
> EXCLUDES 1   *benign myoclonic epilepsy in infancy (G40.3-)*
> *benign neonatal convulsions (familial) (G40.3-)*

☑4ᵗʰ **P91** **Other disturbances of cerebral status of newborn**

P91.0 **Neonatal cerebral ischemia**   MCC
> EXCLUDES 1   *neonatal cerebral infarction (P91.82-)*

P91.1 **Acquired periventricular cysts of newborn**   MCC

P91.2 **Neonatal cerebral leukomalacia**   MCC
> Periventricular leukomalacia

P91.3 **Neonatal cerebral irritability**   MCC

P91.4 **Neonatal cerebral depression**   MCC

P91.5 **Neonatal coma**   MCC

√5ᵗʰ P91.6 Hypoxic ischemic encephalopathy [HIE]

EXCLUDES 1   *neonatal cerebral depression (P91.4)*
neonatal cerebral irritability (P91.3)
neonatal coma (P91.5)

AHA: 2017,4Q,22

P91.60 Hypoxic ischemic encephalopathy [HIE], unspecified   CC

P91.61 Mild hypoxic ischemic encephalopathy [HIE]   CC

P91.62 Moderate hypoxic ischemic encephalopathy [HIE]   CC

P91.63 Severe hypoxic ischemic encephalopathy [HIE]   MCC

√5ᵗʰ P91.8 Other specified disturbances of cerebral status of newborn

AHA: 2017,4Q,22

√6ᵗʰ P91.81 Neonatal encephalopathy

P91.811 Neonatal encephalopathy in diseases classified elsewhere
Code first underlying condition, if known, such as:
congenital cirrhosis (of liver) (P78.81)
intracranial nontraumatic hemorrhage of newborn (P52.-)
kernicterus (P57.-)

P91.819 Neonatal encephalopathy, unspecified

√6ᵗʰ P91.82 Neonatal cerebral infarction

Neonatal stroke
Perinatal arterial ischemic stroke
Perinatal cerebral infarction

EXCLUDES 1   *cerebral infarction (I63.-)*

EXCLUDES 2   *intracranial hemorrhage of newborn (P52.-)*

AHA: 2020,4Q,37-38

P91.821 Neonatal cerebral infarction, right side of brain   MCC HCC

P91.822 Neonatal cerebral infarction, left side of brain   MCC HCC

P91.823 Neonatal cerebral infarction, bilateral   MCC HCC

P91.829 Neonatal cerebral infarction, unspecified side   MCC HCC

P91.88 Other specified disturbances of cerebral status of newborn

P91.9 Disturbance of cerebral status of newborn, unspecified

√4ᵗʰ P92 Feeding problems of newborn

EXCLUDES 1   *eating disorders (F50.-)*
~~feeding problems in child over 28 days old (R63.3)~~

EXCLUDES 2   ▶*feeding problems in child over 28 days old (R63.3)*◀

AHA: 2016,3Q,19

√5ᵗʰ P92.0 Vomiting of newborn

EXCLUDES 1   *vomiting of child over 28 days old (R11.-)*

P92.01 Bilious vomiting of newborn   MCC

EXCLUDES 1   *bilious vomiting in child over 28 days old (R11.14)*

P92.09 Other vomiting of newborn

EXCLUDES 1   *regurgitation of food in newborn (P92.1)*

P92.1 Regurgitation and rumination of newborn

P92.2 Slow feeding of newborn

P92.3 Underfeeding of newborn

P92.4 Overfeeding of newborn

P92.5 Neonatal difficulty in feeding at breast

AHA: 2017,1Q,28

P92.6 Failure to thrive in newborn

EXCLUDES 1   *failure to thrive in child over 28 days old (R62.51)*

P92.8 Other feeding problems of newborn

P92.9 Feeding problem of newborn, unspecified

√4ᵗʰ P93 Reactions and intoxications due to drugs administered to newborn

INCLUDES   reactions and intoxications due to drugs administered to fetus affecting newborn

EXCLUDES 1   *jaundice due to drugs or toxins transmitted from mother or given to newborn (P58.4-)*
reactions and intoxications from maternal opiates, tranquilizers and other medication (P04.0-P04.1, P04.4-)
withdrawal symptoms from maternal use of drugs of addiction (P96.1)
withdrawal symptoms from therapeutic use of drugs in newborn (P96.2)

P93.0 Grey baby syndrome   CC
Grey syndrome from chloramphenicol administration in newborn

P93.8 Other reactions and intoxications due to drugs administered to newborn   CC
Use additional code for adverse effect, if applicable, to identify drug (T36-T50 with fifth or sixth character 5)

√4ᵗʰ P94 Disorders of muscle tone of newborn

P94.0 Transient neonatal myasthenia gravis   CC

EXCLUDES 1   *myasthenia gravis (G70.0)*

P94.1 Congenital hypertonia

P94.2 Congenital hypotonia
Floppy baby syndrome, unspecified

P94.8 Other disorders of muscle tone of newborn

P94.9 Disorder of muscle tone of newborn, unspecified

P95 Stillbirth
Deadborn fetus NOS
Fetal death of unspecified cause
Stillbirth NOS

EXCLUDES 1   *maternal care for intrauterine death (O36.4)*
missed abortion (O02.1)
outcome of delivery, stillbirth (Z37.1, Z37.3, Z37.4, Z37.7)

√4ᵗʰ P96 Other conditions originating in the perinatal period

P96.0 Congenital renal failure
Uremia of newborn

P96.1 Neonatal withdrawal symptoms from maternal use of drugs of addiction   CC
Drug withdrawal syndrome in infant of dependent mother
Neonatal abstinence syndrome

EXCLUDES 1   *reactions and intoxications from maternal opiates and tranquilizers administered during labor and delivery (P04.0)*

AHA: 2018,4Q,24-25

P96.2 Withdrawal symptoms from therapeutic use of drugs in newborn   CC

P96.3 Wide cranial sutures of newborn
Neonatal craniotabes

P96.5 Complication to newborn due to (fetal) intrauterine procedure

EXCLUDES 2   *newborn affected by amniocentesis (P00.6)*

√5ᵗʰ P96.8 Other specified conditions originating in the perinatal period

P96.81 Exposure to (parental) (environmental) tobacco smoke in the perinatal period

EXCLUDES 2   *newborn affected by in utero exposure to tobacco (P04.2)*
exposure to environmental tobacco smoke after the perinatal period (Z77.22)

P96.82 Delayed separation of umbilical cord

P96.83 Meconium staining

EXCLUDES 1   *meconium aspiration (P24.00, P24.01)*
meconium passage during delivery (P03.82)

DEF: Meconium passed in utero causing discoloration on the fetal skin and nails or on the umbilicus. This staining may be incidental or may be an indicator of significant fetal stress that could affect outcomes.

P96.89 Other specified conditions originating in the perinatal period
Use additional code to specify condition

P96.9 Condition originating in the perinatal period, unspecified
Congenital debility NOS

✔ Additional Character Required   √x7ᵗʰ Placeholder   Questionable PDx   Manifestation   Unspecified Dx   UPD Unacceptable PDx   H1-H14 HAC   HCC CMS-HCC Dx   HIV HIV Dx

ICD-10-CM 2022   917

Chapter 17. Congenital Malformations, Deformations and Chromosomal Abnormalities (Q00–Q99)

Chapter-specific Guidelines with Coding Examples

The chapter-specific guidelines from the ICD-10-CM Official Guidelines for Coding and Reporting have been provided below. Along with these guidelines are coding examples, contained in the shaded boxes, that have been developed to help illustrate the coding and/or sequencing guidance found in these guidelines.

Assign an appropriate code(s) from categories Q00-Q99, Congenital malformations, deformations, and chromosomal abnormalities when a malformation/deformation or chromosomal abnormality is documented. A malformation/deformation/or chromosomal abnormality may be the principal/first-listed diagnosis on a record or a secondary diagnosis.

When a malformation/deformation/or chromosomal abnormality does not have a unique code assignment, assign additional code(s) for any manifestations that may be present.

When the code assignment specifically identifies the malformation/deformation/or chromosomal abnormality, manifestations that are an inherent component of the anomaly should not be coded separately. Additional codes should be assigned for manifestations that are not an inherent component.

8-day-old infant with tetralogy of Fallot and pulmonary stenosis

Q21.3   **Tetralogy of Fallot**

Explanation: Pulmonary stenosis is inherent in the disease process of tetralogy of Fallot. When the code assignment specifically identifies the malformation/deformation/or chromosomal abnormality, manifestations that are inherent components of the anomaly should not be coded separately.

7-month-old infant with Down syndrome and common atrioventricular canal

Q90.9   **Down syndrome, unspecified**

Q21.2   **Atrioventricular septal defect**

Explanation: While a common atrioventricular canal is often associated with patients with Down syndrome, this manifestation is not an inherent component and may be reported separately. When the code assignment specifically identifies the anomaly, manifestations that are inherent components of the condition should not be coded separately. Additional codes should be assigned for manifestations that are not inherent components.

Codes from Chapter 17 may be used throughout the life of the patient. If a congenital malformation or deformity has been corrected, a personal history code should be used to identify the history of the malformation or deformity. Although present at birth, a malformation/deformation/or chromosomal abnormality may not be identified until later in life. Whenever the condition is diagnosed by the provider, it is appropriate to assign a code from codes Q00-Q99. For the birth admission, the appropriate code from category Z38, Liveborn infants, according to place of birth and type of delivery, should be sequenced as the principal diagnosis, followed by any congenital anomaly codes, Q00- Q99.

Three-year-old with history of corrected ventricular septal defect

Z87.74   **Personal history of (corrected) congenital malformations of heart and circulatory system**

Explanation: If a congenital malformation or deformity has been corrected, a personal history code should be used to identify the history of the malformation or deformity.

Forty-year-old man with headaches diagnosed with congenital arteriovenous malformation of cerebral vessels by brain scan

Q28.2   **Arteriovenous malformation of cerebral vessels**

Explanation: Although present at birth, malformations may not be identified until later in life. Whenever a congenital condition is diagnosed by the physician, it is appropriate to assign a code from the range Q00–Q99.

Newborn with anencephaly delivered vaginally in hospital

Z38.00   **Single liveborn infant, delivered vaginally**

Q00.0   **Anencephaly**

Explanation: For the birth admission, the appropriate code from category Z38 Liveborn infants, according to place of birth and type of delivery, should be sequenced as the principal diagnosis, followed by any congenital anomaly codes, Q00–Q99.

Chapter 17. Congenital Malformations, Deformations and Chromosomal Abnormalities (Q00-Q99)

NOTE   Codes from this chapter are not for use on maternal records

EXCLUDES 2   *inborn errors of metabolism (E70-E88)*

This chapter contains the following blocks:

Q00-Q07   Congenital malformations of the nervous system
Q10-Q18   Congenital malformations of eye, ear, face and neck
Q20-Q28   Congenital malformations of the circulatory system
Q30-Q34   Congenital malformations of the respiratory system
Q35-Q37   Cleft lip and cleft palate
Q38-Q45   Other congenital malformations of the digestive system
Q50-Q56   Congenital malformations of genital organs
Q60-Q64   Congenital malformations of the urinary system
Q65-Q79   Congenital malformations and deformations of the musculoskeletal system
Q80-Q89   Other congenital malformations
Q90-Q99   Chromosomal abnormalities, not elsewhere classified

Congenital malformations of the nervous system (Q00-Q07)

✓4ᵗʰ Q00 Anencephaly and similar malformations

    Q00.0 Anencephaly   `MCC` `HCC`
       Acephaly
       Acrania
       Amyelencephaly
       Hemianencephaly
       Hemicephaly

    Q00.1 Craniorachischisis   `MCC` `HCC`
    Q00.2 Iniencephaly   `MCC` `HCC`

✓4ᵗʰ Q01 Encephalocele

    INCLUDES   Arnold-Chiari syndrome, type III
           encephalocystocele
           encephalomyelocele
           hydroencephalocele
           hydromeningocele, cranial
           meningocele, cerebral
           meningoencephalocele

    EXCLUDES 1   *Meckel-Gruber syndrome (Q61.9)*

    DEF: Congenital protrusion of brain tissue through a defect in the skull.

    Q01.0 Frontal encephalocele   `CC` `HCC`
    Q01.1 Nasofrontal encephalocele   `CC` `HCC`
    Q01.2 Occipital encephalocele   `CC` `HCC`
    Q01.8 Encephalocele of other sites   `CC` `HCC`
    Q01.9 Encephalocele, unspecified   `CC` `HCC`

Q02 Microcephaly   `HCC`

    INCLUDES   hydromicrocephaly
           micrencephalon

    Code first, if applicable, congenital Zika virus disease

    EXCLUDES 1   *Meckel-Gruber syndrome (Q61.9)*

    AHA: 2018,4Q,26

    DEF: Congenital disorder in which the head circumference is more than two standard deviations below the mean for age, sex, race, and gestation and associated with a decreased life expectancy.

✓4ᵗʰ Q03 Congenital hydrocephalus

    INCLUDES   hydrocephalus in newborn

    EXCLUDES 1   *Arnold-Chiari syndrome, type II (Q07.0-)*
           acquired hydrocephalus (G91.-)
           hydrocephalus due to congenital toxoplasmosis (P37.1)
           hydrocephalus with spina bifida (Q05.0-Q05.4)

    DEF: Hydrocephalus: Abnormal buildup of cerebrospinal fluid in the brain causing dilation of the ventricles.

Congenital Hydrocephalus

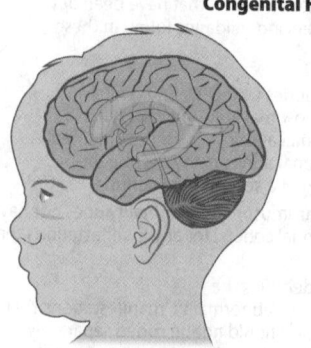
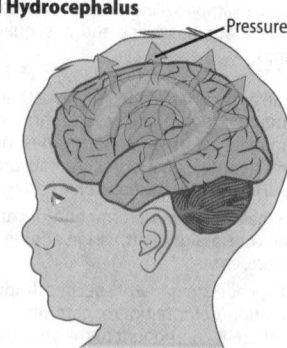

Pressure

Normal ventricles   Hydrocephalic ventricles

    Q03.0 Malformations of aqueduct of Sylvius   `HCC`
       Anomaly of aqueduct of Sylvius
       Obstruction of aqueduct of Sylvius, congenital
       Stenosis of aqueduct of Sylvius

    Q03.1 Atresia of foramina of Magendie and Luschka   `HCC`
       Dandy-Walker syndrome

    Q03.8 Other congenital hydrocephalus   `HCC`
    Q03.9 Congenital hydrocephalus, unspecified   `HCC`

✓4ᵗʰ Q04 Other congenital malformations of brain

    EXCLUDES 1   *cyclopia (Q87.0)*
           macrocephaly (Q75.3)

    Q04.0 Congenital malformations of corpus callosum   `MCC` `HCC`
       Agenesis of corpus callosum

    Q04.1 Arhinencephaly   `MCC` `HCC`
    Q04.2 Holoprosencephaly   `MCC` `HCC`
    Q04.3 Other reduction deformities of brain   `MCC` `HCC`
       Absence of part of brain
       Agenesis of part of brain
       Agyria
       Aplasia of part of brain
       Hydranencephaly
       Hypoplasia of part of brain
       Lissencephaly
       Microgyria
       Pachygyria
    EXCLUDES 1   *congenital malformations of corpus callosum (Q04.0)*

    Q04.4 Septo-optic dysplasia of brain   `CC` `HCC`
    Q04.5 Megalencephaly   `CC` `HCC`
    Q04.6 Congenital cerebral cysts   `CC` `HCC`
       Porencephaly
       Schizencephaly
    EXCLUDES 1   *acquired porencephalic cyst (G93.0)*

    Q04.8 Other specified congenital malformations of brain   `CC` `HCC`
       Arnold-Chiari syndrome, type IV
       Macrogyria

    Q04.9 Congenital malformation of brain, unspecified   `HCC`
       Congenital anomaly NOS of brain
       Congenital deformity NOS of brain
       Congenital disease or lesion NOS of brain
       Multiple anomalies NOS of brain, congenital

N Newborn: 0   **P** Pediatric: 0-17   **M** Maternity: 9-64   **A** Adult: 15-124   `MCC` Major Complication/Comorbidity   `CC` Complication/Comorbidity   `SW` Severe Wound Dx

920   ICD-10-CM 2022

☑4ᵗʰ **Q05 Spina bifida**

> [INCLUDES]   hydromeningocele (spinal)
> meningocele (spinal)
> meningomyelocele
> myelocele
> myelomeningocele
> rachischisis
> spina bifida (aperta)(cystica)
> syringomyelocele

Use additional code for any associated paraplegia (paraparesis) (G82.2-)

> [EXCLUDES 1]   *Arnold-Chiari syndrome, type II (Q07.0-)*
> *spina bifida occulta (Q76.0)*

DEF: Lack of closure in the vertebral column with protrusion of the spinal cord through the defect, often in the lumbosacral area. This condition can be recognized by the presence of alpha-fetoproteins in the amniotic fluid.

Spina Bifida

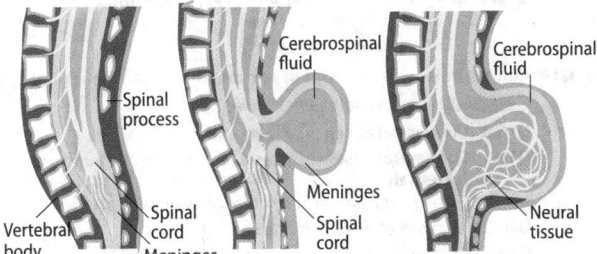

Spina bifida occulta   Meningocele   Myelomeningocele

Q05.0	Cervical **spina bifida with hydrocephalus**	CC HCC
Q05.1	Thoracic **spina bifida with hydrocephalus**	CC HCC
	Dorsal spina bifida with hydrocephalus	
	Thoracolumbar spina bifida with hydrocephalus	
Q05.2	Lumbar **spina bifida with hydrocephalus**	CC HCC
	Lumbosacral spina bifida with hydrocephalus	
Q05.3	Sacral **spina bifida with hydrocephalus**	CC HCC
Q05.4	**Unspecified spina bifida with hydrocephalus**	CC HCC
Q05.5	Cervical **spina bifida without hydrocephalus**	HCC
Q05.6	Thoracic **spina bifida without hydrocephalus**	HCC
	Dorsal spina bifida NOS	
	Thoracolumbar spina bifida NOS	
Q05.7	Lumbar **spina bifida without hydrocephalus**	HCC
	Lumbosacral spina bifida NOS	
Q05.8	Sacral **spina bifida without hydrocephalus**	HCC
Q05.9	**Spina bifida, unspecified**	HCC

☑4ᵗʰ **Q06 Other congenital malformations of spinal cord**

Q06.0	**Amyelia**	HCC
Q06.1	**Hypoplasia and dysplasia of spinal cord**	HCC
	Atelomyelia	
	Myelatelia	
	Myelodysplasia of spinal cord	
Q06.2	**Diastematomyelia**	HCC

> **DEF:** Rare congenital anomaly often associated with spina bifida. The spinal cord is separated into longitudinal halves by a bony, cartilaginous or fibrous septum, each half surrounded by a dural sac.

Q06.3	**Other congenital cauda equina malformations**	HCC
Q06.4	**Hydromyelia**	HCC
	Hydrorachis	
Q06.8	**Other specified congenital malformations of spinal cord**	HCC
Q06.9	**Congenital malformation of spinal cord, unspecified**	HCC
	Congenital anomaly NOS of spinal cord	
	Congenital deformity NOS of spinal cord	
	Congenital disease or lesion NOS of spinal cord	

☑4ᵗʰ **Q07 Other congenital malformations of nervous system**

> [EXCLUDES 2]   *congenital central alveolar hypoventilation syndrome (G47.35)*
> *familial dysautonomia [Riley-Day] (G90.1)*
> *neurofibromatosis (nonmalignant) (Q85.0-)*

☑5ᵗʰ **Q07.0 Arnold-Chiari syndrome**

> Arnold-Chiari syndrome, type II
>
> [EXCLUDES 1]   *Arnold-Chiari syndrome, type III (Q01.-)*
> *Arnold-Chiari syndrome, type IV (Q04.8)*
>
> **DEF:** Congenital malformation of the brain in which the cerebellum protrudes through the foramen magnum into the spinal canal.

Q07.00	**Arnold-Chiari syndrome** without spina bifida or hydrocephalus	HCC
Q07.01	**Arnold-Chiari syndrome** with spina bifida	HCC
Q07.02	**Arnold-Chiari syndrome** with hydrocephalus	CC HCC
Q07.03	**Arnold-Chiari syndrome** with spina bifida and hydrocephalus	CC HCC
Q07.8	**Other specified congenital malformations of nervous system**	HCC
	Agenesis of nerve	
	Displacement of brachial plexus	
	Jaw-winking syndrome	
	Marcus Gunn's syndrome	
Q07.9	**Congenital malformation of nervous system, unspecified**	HCC
	Congenital anomaly NOS of nervous system	
	Congenital deformity NOS of nervous system	
	Congenital disease or lesion NOS of nervous system	

Congenital malformations of eye, ear, face and neck (Q10-Q18)

> [EXCLUDES 2]   *cleft lip and cleft palate (Q35-Q37)*
> *congenital malformation of cervical spine (Q05.0, Q05.5, Q67.5, Q76.0-Q76.4)*
> *congenital malformation of larynx (Q31.-)*
> *congenital malformation of lip NEC (Q38.0)*
> *congenital malformation of nose (Q30.-)*
> *congenital malformation of parathyroid gland (Q89.2)*
> *congenital malformation of thyroid gland (Q89.2)*

☑4ᵗʰ **Q10 Congenital malformations of eyelid, lacrimal apparatus and orbit**

> [EXCLUDES 1]   *cryptophthalmos NOS (Q11.2)*
> *cryptophthalmos syndrome (Q87.0)*

Q10.0 Congenital ptosis

> **DEF:** Congenital drooping of the eyelid. Ptosis is mostly idiopathic, but may occur genetically.

Q10.1 Congenital ectropion

Q10.2 Congenital entropion

Q10.3 Other congenital malformations of eyelid

> Ablepharon
> Blepharophimosis, congenital
> Coloboma of eyelid
> Congenital absence or agenesis of cilia
> Congenital absence or agenesis of eyelid
> Congenital accessory eyelid
> Congenital accessory eye muscle
> Congenital malformation of eyelid NOS

Q10.4 Absence and agenesis of lacrimal apparatus

> Congenital absence of punctum lacrimale

Q10.5 Congenital stenosis and stricture of lacrimal duct

Q10.6 Other congenital malformations of lacrimal apparatus

> Congenital malformation of lacrimal apparatus NOS

Q10.7 Congenital malformation of orbit

☑4ᵗʰ **Q11 Anophthalmos, microphthalmos and macrophthalmos**

Q11.0 Cystic eyeball

Q11.1 Other anophthalmos

> Anophthalmos NOS
> Agenesis of eye
> Aplasia of eye

Q11.2 Microphthalmos

> Cryptophthalmos NOS
> Dysplasia of eye
> Hypoplasia of eye
> Rudimentary eye
>
> [EXCLUDES 1]   *cryptophthalmos syndrome (Q87.0)*

Q11.3 Macrophthalmos
> EXCLUDES 1   *macrophthalmos in congenital glaucoma (Q15.0)*

✓4ᵗʰ Q12 Congenital lens malformations

Q12.0 Congenital cataract
Q12.1 Congenital displaced lens
Q12.2 Coloboma of lens

Coloboma of Lens

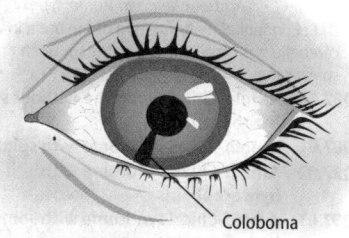

Coloboma

Q12.3 Congenital aphakia
Q12.4 Spherophakia
Q12.8 Other congenital lens malformations
> Microphakia

Q12.9 Congenital lens malformation, unspecified

✓4ᵗʰ Q13 Congenital malformations of anterior segment of eye

Q13.0 Coloboma of iris
> Coloboma NOS
> **DEF:** Defective or absent section of ocular tissue that may present as mild cupping or a small pit in the ocular disc due to extensive defects in the iris, ciliary body, choroids, and retina.

Q13.1 Absence of iris
> Aniridia
> Use additional code for associated glaucoma (H42)
> **DEF:** Incompletely formed or absent iris. It affects both eyes and is a dominant trait.

Q13.2 Other congenital malformations of iris
> Anisocoria, congenital
> Atresia of pupil
> Congenital malformation of iris NOS
> Corectopia

Q13.3 Congenital corneal opacity
Q13.4 Other congenital corneal malformations
> Congenital malformation of cornea NOS
> Microcornea
> Peter's anomaly

Q13.5 Blue sclera

✓5ᵗʰ Q13.8 Other congenital malformations of anterior segment of eye

Q13.81 Rieger's anomaly
> Use additional code for associated glaucoma (H42)

Q13.89 Other congenital malformations of anterior segment of eye

Q13.9 Congenital malformation of anterior segment of eye, unspecified

✓4ᵗʰ Q14 Congenital malformations of posterior segment of eye
> EXCLUDES 2   *optic nerve hypoplasia (H47.03-)*

Q14.0 Congenital malformation of vitreous humor
> Congenital vitreous opacity

Q14.1 Congenital malformation of retina
> Congenital retinal aneurysm

Q14.2 Congenital malformation of optic disc
> Coloboma of optic disc

Q14.3 Congenital malformation of choroid
Q14.8 Other congenital malformations of posterior segment of eye
> Coloboma of the fundus

Q14.9 Congenital malformation of posterior segment of eye, unspecified

✓4ᵗʰ Q15 Other congenital malformations of eye
> EXCLUDES 1   *congenital nystagmus (H55.01)*
>   *ocular albinism (E70.31-)*
>   *optic nerve hypoplasia (H47.03-)*
>   *retinitis pigmentosa (H35.52)*

Q15.0 Congenital glaucoma
> Axenfeld's anomaly
> Buphthalmos
> Glaucoma of childhood
> Glaucoma of newborn
> Hydrophthalmos
> Keratoglobus, congenital, with glaucoma
> Macrocornea with glaucoma
> Macrophthalmos in congenital glaucoma
> Megalocornea with glaucoma

Q15.8 Other specified congenital malformations of eye
Q15.9 Congenital malformation of eye, unspecified
> Congenital anomaly of eye
> Congenital deformity of eye

✓4ᵗʰ Q16 Congenital malformations of ear causing impairment of hearing
> EXCLUDES 1   *congenital deafness (H90.-)*

Q16.0 Congenital absence of (ear) auricle
Q16.1 Congenital absence, atresia and stricture of auditory canal (external)
> Congenital atresia or stricture of osseous meatus

Q16.2 Absence of eustachian tube
Q16.3 Congenital malformation of ear ossicles
> Congenital fusion of ear ossicles

Q16.4 Other congenital malformations of middle ear
> Congenital malformation of middle ear NOS

Q16.5 Congenital malformation of inner ear
> Congenital anomaly of membranous labyrinth
> Congenital anomaly of organ of Corti

Q16.9 Congenital malformation of ear causing impairment of hearing, unspecified
> Congenital absence of ear NOS

✓4ᵗʰ Q17 Other congenital malformations of ear
> EXCLUDES 1   *congenital malformations of ear with impairment of hearing (Q16.0-Q16.9)*
>   *preauricular sinus (Q18.1)*

Q17.0 Accessory auricle
> Accessory tragus
> Polyotia
> Preauricular appendage or tag
> Supernumerary ear
> Supernumerary lobule

Q17.1 Macrotia
> **DEF:** Birth defect characterized by abnormal enlargement of the pinna of the ear.

Q17.2 Microtia
Q17.3 Other misshapen ear
> Pointed ear

Q17.4 Misplaced ear
> Low-set ears
> EXCLUDES 1   *cervical auricle (Q18.2)*

Q17.5 Prominent ear
> Bat ear

Q17.8 Other specified congenital malformations of ear
> Congenital absence of lobe of ear

Q17.9 Congenital malformation of ear, unspecified
> Congenital anomaly of ear NOS

✓4ᵗʰ Q18 Other congenital malformations of face and neck
> EXCLUDES 1   *cleft lip and cleft palate (Q35-Q37)*
>   *conditions classified to Q67.0-Q67.4*
>   *congenital malformations of skull and face bones (Q75.-)*
>   *cyclopia (Q87.0)*
>   *dentofacial anomalies [including malocclusion] (M26.-)*
>   *malformation syndromes affecting facial appearance (Q87.0)*
>   *persistent thyroglossal duct (Q89.2)*

Q18.0 Sinus, fistula and cyst of branchial cleft
> Branchial vestige

Q18.1 Preauricular sinus and cyst   [SW]
> Fistula of auricle, congenital
> Cervicoaural fistula

N Newborn: 0   P Pediatric: 0-17   M Maternity: 9-64   A Adult: 15-124   MCC Major Complication/Comorbidity   CC Complication/Comorbidity   SW Severe Wound Dx

922

ICD-10-CM 2022

Q18.2   **Other branchial cleft malformations**
Branchial cleft malformation NOS
Cervical auricle
Otocephaly

Q18.3   **Webbing of neck**
Pterygium colli
DEF: Congenital malformation characterized by a thick, triangular skinfold that stretches from the lateral side of the neck across the shoulder. It is associated with genetic conditions such as Turner's and Noonan's syndromes.

Q18.4   **Macrostomia**
DEF: Rare congenital craniofacial bilateral or unilateral anomaly of the mouth due to malformed maxillary and mandibular processes. It results in an abnormally large mouth extending toward the ear.

Q18.5   **Microstomia**

Q18.6   **Macrocheilia**
Hypertrophy of lip, congenital

Q18.7   **Microcheilia**

Q18.8   **Other specified congenital malformations of face and neck**
Medial cyst of face and neck
Medial fistula of face and neck
Medial sinus of face and neck

Q18.9   **Congenital malformation of face and neck, unspecified**
Congenital anomaly NOS of face and neck

Congenital malformations of the circulatory system (Q20-Q28)

✓4ᵗʰ Q20   **Congenital malformations of cardiac chambers and connections**
    EXCLUDES 1   *dextrocardia with situs inversus (Q89.3)*
       mirror-image atrial arrangement with situs inversus (Q89.3)

Q20.0   **Common arterial trunk**   `MCC`
Persistent truncus arteriosus
    EXCLUDES 1   *aortic septal defect (Q21.4)*

Q20.1   **Double outlet right ventricle**   `MCC`
Taussig-Bing syndrome

Q20.2   **Double outlet left ventricle**   `MCC`

Q20.3   **Discordant ventriculoarterial connection**   `MCC`
Dextrotransposition of aorta
Transposition of great vessels (complete)

Q20.4   **Double inlet ventricle**   `MCC`
Common ventricle
Cor triloculare biatriatum
Single ventricle

Q20.5   **Discordant atrioventricular connection**   `CC`
Corrected transposition
Levotransposition
Ventricular inversion

Q20.6   **Isomerism of atrial appendages**
Isomerism of atrial appendages with asplenia or polysplenia

Q20.8   **Other congenital malformations of cardiac chambers and connections**
Cor binoculare

Q20.9   **Congenital malformation of cardiac chambers and connections, unspecified**

✓4ᵗʰ Q21   **Congenital malformations of cardiac septa**
    EXCLUDES 1   *acquired cardiac septal defect (I51.0)*

Q21.0   **Ventricular septal defect**   `CC`
Roger's disease

Ventricular Septal Defect

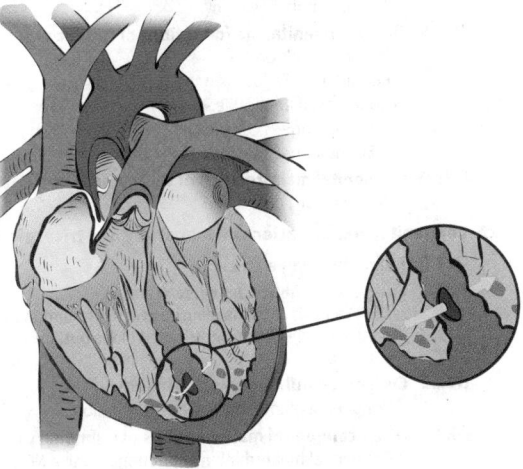

Q21.1   **Atrial septal defect**   `CC`
Coronary sinus defect
Patent or persistent foramen ovale
Patent or persistent ostium secundum defect (type II)
Patent or persistent sinus venosus defect

Atrial Septal Defect

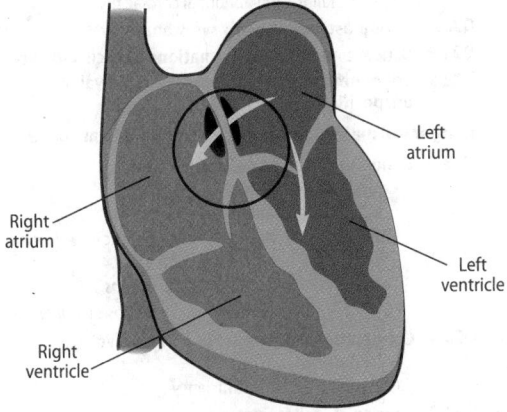

Right atrium — Left atrium — Left ventricle — Right ventricle

Q21.2   **Atrioventricular septal defect**   `CC`
Common atrioventricular canal
Endocardial cushion defect
Ostium primum atrial septal defect (type I)

Atrioventricular Septal Defect

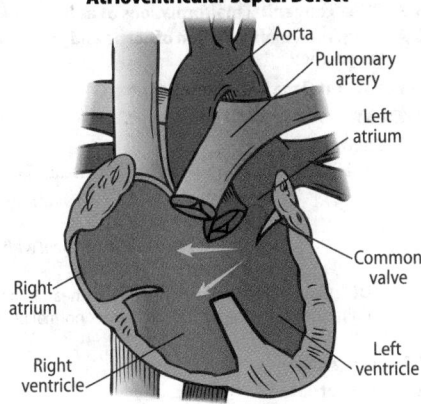

Aorta — Pulmonary artery — Left atrium — Common valve — Left ventricle — Right ventricle — Right atrium

Q21.3   **Tetralogy of Fallot**   `MCC`
Ventricular septal defect with pulmonary stenosis or atresia, dextroposition of aorta and hypertrophy of right ventricle.
AHA: 2014,3Q,16

Q21.4   **Aortopulmonary septal defect**
Aortic septal defect
Aortopulmonary window

Q21.8   **Other congenital malformations of cardiac septa**
Eisenmenger's defect
Pentalogy of Fallot
▶Code also, if applicable:◄
   Eisenmenger's complex (I27.83)
   Eisenmenger's syndrome (I27.83)

Q21.9   **Congenital malformation of cardiac septum, unspecified**
Septal (heart) defect NOS

✓4ᵗʰ **Q22**   **Congenital malformations of pulmonary and tricuspid valves**

Q22.0   **Pulmonary valve atresia**   `MCC`

Q22.1   **Congenital pulmonary valve stenosis**   `CC`
DEF: Stenosis of the opening between the pulmonary artery and right ventricle, causing obstructed blood outflow from the right ventricle.

Q22.2   **Congenital pulmonary valve insufficiency**   `CC`
Congenital pulmonary valve regurgitation

Q22.3   **Other congenital malformations of pulmonary valve**   `CC`
Congenital malformation of pulmonary valve NOS
Supernumerary cusps of pulmonary valve

Q22.4   **Congenital tricuspid stenosis**   `MCC`
Congenital tricuspid atresia

Q22.5   **Ebstein's anomaly**   `MCC`
DEF: Malformation of the tricuspid valve characterized by septal and posterior leaflets attaching to the wall of the right ventricle. Ebstein's anomaly causes the right ventricle to fuse with the atrium into a large right atrium and a small ventricle and leads to heart failure and abnormal cardiac rhythm.

Q22.6   **Hypoplastic right heart syndrome**   `MCC`

Q22.8   **Other congenital malformations of tricuspid valve**   `MCC`

Q22.9   **Congenital malformation of tricuspid valve, unspecified**   `MCC`

✓4ᵗʰ **Q23**   **Congenital malformations of aortic and mitral valves**

Q23.0   **Congenital stenosis of aortic valve**   `CC`
Congenital aortic atresia
Congenital aortic stenosis NOS
EXCLUDES 1   congenital stenosis of aortic valve in hypoplastic left heart syndrome (Q23.4)
    congenital subaortic stenosis (Q24.4)
    supravalvular aortic stenosis (congenital) (Q25.3)

Q23.1   **Congenital insufficiency of aortic valve**   `CC`
Bicuspid aortic valve
Congenital aortic insufficiency

Q23.2   **Congenital mitral stenosis**   `CC`
Congenital mitral atresia
DEF: Congenital stenosis of the mitral valve orifice between the left atrium and ventricle, at the supravalvular, valvular, or subvalvular levels, causing obstruction to left ventricular filling.

Q23.3   **Congenital mitral insufficiency**   `CC`

Q23.4   **Hypoplastic left heart syndrome**   `MCC`

Q23.8   **Other congenital malformations of aortic and mitral valves**

Q23.9   **Congenital malformation of aortic and mitral valves, unspecified**

✓4ᵗʰ **Q24**   **Other congenital malformations of heart**
EXCLUDES 1   endocardial fibroelastosis (I42.4)

Q24.0   **Dextrocardia**   `CC`
EXCLUDES 1   dextrocardia with situs inversus (Q89.3)
    isomerism of atrial appendages (with asplenia or polysplenia) (Q20.6)
    mirror-image atrial arrangement with situs inversus (Q89.3)
DEF: Congenital condition in which the heart is located on the right side of the chest rather than in its normal position on the left.

Q24.1   **Levocardia**   `CC`

Q24.2   **Cor triatriatum**   `MCC`

Q24.3   **Pulmonary infundibular stenosis**   `CC`
Subvalvular pulmonic stenosis

Q24.4   **Congenital subaortic stenosis**   `MCC`
DEF: Congenital heart defect characterized by stenosis of the left ventricular outflow tract due to a fibrous tissue ring or septal hypertrophy below the aortic valve.

Q24.5   **Malformation of coronary vessels**   `CC`
Congenital coronary (artery) aneurysm

Q24.6   **Congenital heart block**   `MCC`

Q24.8   **Other specified congenital malformations of heart**
Congenital diverticulum of left ventricle
Congenital malformation of myocardium
Congenital malformation of pericardium
Malposition of heart
Uhl's disease

Q24.9   **Congenital malformation of heart, unspecified**
Congenital anomaly of heart
Congenital disease of heart

✓4ᵗʰ **Q25**   **Congenital malformations of great arteries**

Q25.0   **Patent ductus arteriosus**   `CC`
Patent ductus Botallo
Persistent ductus arteriosus
DEF: Condition in which the normal channel between the pulmonary artery and the aorta fails to close at birth, causing arterial blood to recirculate in the lungs and inhibiting the blood supply to the aorta. *Synonym(s):* PDA.

Patent Ductus Arteriosus

Patent ductus arteriosus
Aorta
Pulmonary artery
Superior vena cava
Patent foramen ovale
Right atrium
Left atrium
Atria
Septum
Schematic showing foramen ovale

Q25.1   **Coarctation of aorta**   `CC`
Coarctation of aorta (preductal) (postductal)
Stenosis of aorta
AHA: 2016,4Q,56-57

✓5ᵗʰ **Q25.2**   **Atresia of aorta**
AHA: 2016,4Q,56-57

Q25.21   **Interruption of aortic arch**   `CC`
Atresia of aortic arch

Q25.29   **Other atresia of aorta**   `CC`
Atresia of aorta

Q25.3   **Supravalvular aortic stenosis**   `CC`
EXCLUDES 1   congenital aortic stenosis NOS (Q23.0)
    congenital stenosis of aortic valve (Q23.0)

✓5ᵗʰ **Q25.4**   **Other congenital malformations of aorta**
EXCLUDES 1   hypoplasia of aorta in hypoplastic left heart syndrome (Q23.4)
AHA: 2016,4Q,57

Q25.40   **Congenital malformation of aorta unspecified**   `CC`

Q25.41   **Absence and aplasia of aorta**   `CC`

Q25.42   **Hypoplasia of aorta**   `CC`

Q25.43   **Congenital aneurysm of aorta**   `CC`
Congenital aneurysm of aortic root
Congenital aneurysm of aortic sinus

Q25.44   **Congenital dilation of aorta**   `CC`

Q25.45 Double aortic arch `CC`
Vascular ring of aorta

Aortic Arch Anomalies

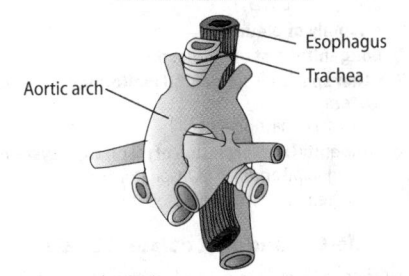

Normal aortic arch

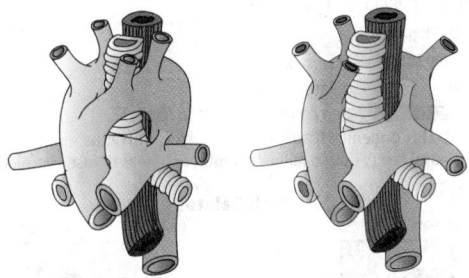

Double aortic arch   Right aortic arch

Q25.46 Tortuous aortic arch `CC`
Persistent convolutions of aortic arch

Q25.47 Right aortic arch `CC`
Persistent right aortic arch

Q25.48 Anomalous origin of subclavian artery `CC`

Q25.49 Other congenital malformations of aorta `CC`
Aortic arch
Bovine arch

Q25.5 Atresia of pulmonary artery `MCC`

Q25.6 Stenosis of pulmonary artery `MCC`
Supravalvular pulmonary stenosis

√5ᵗʰ **Q25.7 Other congenital malformations of pulmonary artery**

Q25.71 Coarctation of pulmonary artery `MCC`

Q25.72 Congenital pulmonary arteriovenous malformation `MCC`
Congenital pulmonary arteriovenous aneurysm

Q25.79 Other congenital malformations of pulmonary artery `MCC`
Aberrant pulmonary artery
Agenesis of pulmonary artery
Congenital aneurysm of pulmonary artery
Congenital anomaly of pulmonary artery
Hypoplasia of pulmonary artery

Q25.8 Other congenital malformations of other great arteries `CC`

Q25.9 Congenital malformation of great arteries, unspecified `CC`

√4ᵗʰ **Q26 Congenital malformations of great veins**

Q26.0 Congenital stenosis of vena cava `CC`
Congenital stenosis of vena cava (inferior)(superior)

Q26.1 Persistent left superior vena cava `CC`

Q26.2 Total anomalous pulmonary venous connection `CC`
Total anomalous pulmonary venous return [TAPVR], subdiaphragmatic
Total anomalous pulmonary venous return [TAPVR], supradiaphragmatic

Q26.3 Partial anomalous pulmonary venous connection `CC`
Partial anomalous pulmonary venous return

Q26.4 Anomalous pulmonary venous connection, unspecified `CC`

Q26.5 Anomalous portal venous connection

Q26.6 Portal vein-hepatic artery fistula

Q26.8 Other congenital malformations of great veins `CC`
Absence of vena cava (inferior) (superior)
Azygos continuation of inferior vena cava
Persistent left posterior cardinal vein
Scimitar syndrome

Q26.9 Congenital malformation of great vein, unspecified `CC`
Congenital anomaly of vena cava (inferior) (superior) NOS

√4ᵗʰ **Q27 Other congenital malformations of peripheral vascular system**
EXCLUDES 2 anomalies of cerebral and precerebral vessels (Q28.0-Q28.3)
anomalies of coronary vessels (Q24.5)
anomalies of pulmonary artery (Q25.5-Q25.7)
congenital retinal aneurysm (Q14.1)
hemangioma and lymphangioma (D18.-)

Q27.0 Congenital absence and hypoplasia of umbilical artery
Single umbilical artery

Q27.1 Congenital renal artery stenosis

Q27.2 Other congenital malformations of renal artery
Congenital malformation of renal artery NOS
Multiple renal arteries

√5ᵗʰ **Q27.3 Arteriovenous malformation (peripheral)**
Arteriovenous aneurysm
EXCLUDES 1 acquired arteriovenous aneurysm (I77.0)
EXCLUDES 2 arteriovenous malformation of cerebral vessels (Q28.2)
arteriovenous malformation of precerebral vessels (Q28.0)
DEF: Arteriovenous malformation: Connecting passage between an artery and a vein.

Q27.30 Arteriovenous malformation, site unspecified `CC`

Q27.31 Arteriovenous malformation of vessel of upper limb

Q27.32 Arteriovenous malformation of vessel of lower limb

Q27.33 Arteriovenous malformation of digestive system vessel
AHA: 2018,3Q,21

Q27.34 Arteriovenous malformation of renal vessel

Q27.39 Arteriovenous malformation, other site

Q27.4 Congenital phlebectasia `CC`

Q27.8 Other specified congenital malformations of peripheral vascular system
Absence of peripheral vascular system
Atresia of peripheral vascular system
Congenital aneurysm (peripheral)
Congenital stricture, artery
Congenital varix
EXCLUDES 1 arteriovenous malformation (Q27.3-)

Q27.9 Congenital malformation of peripheral vascular system, unspecified
Anomaly of artery or vein NOS

√4ᵗʰ **Q28 Other congenital malformations of circulatory system**
EXCLUDES 1 congenital aneurysm NOS (Q27.8)
congenital coronary aneurysm (Q24.5)
ruptured cerebral arteriovenous malformation (I60.8)
ruptured malformation of precerebral vessels (I72.0)
EXCLUDES 2 congenital peripheral aneurysm (Q27.8)
congenital pulmonary aneurysm (Q25.79)
congenital retinal aneurysm (Q14.1)

Q28.0 Arteriovenous malformation of precerebral vessels `CC`
Congenital arteriovenous precerebral aneurysm (nonruptured)

Q28.1 Other malformations of precerebral vessels `CC`
Congenital malformation of precerebral vessels NOS
Congenital precerebral aneurysm (nonruptured)

Q28.2 Arteriovenous malformation of cerebral vessels `MCC`
Arteriovenous malformation of brain NOS
Congenital arteriovenous cerebral aneurysm (nonruptured)

Q28.3 Other malformations of cerebral vessels `MCC`
Congenital cerebral aneurysm (nonruptured)
Congenital malformation of cerebral vessels NOS
Developmental venous anomaly

Q28.8 Other specified congenital malformations of circulatory system `CC`
Congenital aneurysm, specified site NEC
Spinal vessel anomaly

Q28.9 Congenital malformation of circulatory system, unspecified `CC`

Congenital malformations of the respiratory system (Q30-Q34)

✓4ᵗʰ Q30 Congenital malformations of nose

> **EXCLUDES 1**   congenital deviation of nasal septum (Q67.4)

Q30.0 Choanal atresia
Atresia of nares (anterior) (posterior)
Congenital stenosis of nares (anterior) (posterior)

Q30.1 Agenesis and underdevelopment of nose
Congenital absent of nose

Q30.2 Fissured, notched and cleft nose

Q30.3 Congenital perforated nasal septum

Q30.8 Other congenital malformations of nose
Accessory nose
Congenital anomaly of nasal sinus wall

Q30.9 Congenital malformation of nose, unspecified

✓4ᵗʰ Q31 Congenital malformations of larynx

> **EXCLUDES 1**   congenital laryngeal stridor NOS (P28.89)

Q31.0 Web of larynx
Glottic web of larynx
Subglottic web of larynx
Web of larynx NOS
DEF: Congenital malformation of the larynx marked by thin, translucent, or thick fibrotic membrane-like structure between the vocal folds. It is characterized by shortness of breath and stridor.

Q31.1 Congenital subglottic stenosis   `CC`

Q31.2 Laryngeal hypoplasia   `CC`

Q31.3 Laryngocele   `CC`

Q31.5 Congenital laryngomalacia   `CC`

Q31.8 Other congenital malformations of larynx   `CC`
Absence of larynx
Agenesis of larynx
Atresia of larynx
Congenital cleft thyroid cartilage
Congenital fissure of epiglottis
Congenital stenosis of larynx NEC
Posterior cleft of cricoid cartilage

Q31.9 Congenital malformation of larynx, unspecified   `CC`

✓4ᵗʰ Q32 Congenital malformations of trachea and bronchus

> **EXCLUDES 1**   congenital bronchiectasis (Q33.4)

Q32.0 Congenital tracheomalacia   `CC`

Q32.1 Other congenital malformations of trachea   `CC`
Atresia of trachea
Congenital anomaly of tracheal cartilage
Congenital dilatation of trachea
Congenital malformation of trachea
Congenital stenosis of trachea
Congenital tracheocele

Q32.2 Congenital bronchomalacia   `CC`

Q32.3 Congenital stenosis of bronchus   `CC`

Q32.4 Other congenital malformations of bronchus   `CC`
Absence of bronchus
Agenesis of bronchus
Atresia of bronchus
Congenital diverticulum of bronchus
Congenital malformation of bronchus NOS

✓4ᵗʰ Q33 Congenital malformations of lung

Q33.0 Congenital cystic lung   `CC`
Congenital cystic lung disease
Congenital honeycomb lung
Congenital polycystic lung disease
> **EXCLUDES 1**   cystic fibrosis (E84.0)
>   cystic lung disease, acquired or unspecified (J98.4)

Q33.1 Accessory lobe of lung
Azygos lobe (fissured), lung

Q33.2 Sequestration of lung   `MCC`

Q33.3 Agenesis of lung   `MCC`
Congenital absence of lung (lobe)

Q33.4 Congenital bronchiectasis   `CC`

Q33.5 Ectopic tissue in lung

Q33.6 Congenital hypoplasia and dysplasia of lung   `MCC`
> **EXCLUDES 1**   pulmonary hypoplasia associated with short gestation (P28.0)

Q33.8 Other congenital malformations of lung

Q33.9 Congenital malformation of lung, unspecified

✓4ᵗʰ Q34 Other congenital malformations of respiratory system

> **EXCLUDES 2**   congenital central alveolar hypoventilation syndrome (G47.35)

Q34.0 Anomaly of pleura

Q34.1 Congenital cyst of mediastinum

Q34.8 Other specified congenital malformations of respiratory system
Atresia of nasopharynx

Q34.9 Congenital malformation of respiratory system, unspecified
Congenital absence of respiratory system
Congenital anomaly of respiratory system NOS

Cleft lip and cleft palate (Q35-Q37)

Use additional code to identify associated malformation of the nose (Q30.2)
> **EXCLUDES 2**   Robin's syndrome (Q87.0)

✓4ᵗʰ Q35 Cleft palate

> **INCLUDES**   fissure of palate
>   palatoschisis
> **EXCLUDES 1**   cleft palate with cleft lip (Q37.-)

DEF: Congenital fissure or defect of the roof of the mouth opening to the nasal cavity due to failure of embryonic cells to fuse completely.

Cleft Palate

Cleft in soft palate — Hard palate — Soft palate — Cleft

Cleft in hard and soft palate — Cleft

Q35.1 Cleft hard palate

Q35.3 Cleft soft palate

Q35.5 Cleft hard palate with cleft soft palate

Q35.7 Cleft uvula

Q35.9 Cleft palate, unspecified
Cleft palate NOS

✓4ᵗʰ Q36 Cleft lip

> **INCLUDES**   cheiloschisis
>   congenital fissure of lip
>   harelip
>   labium leporinum
> **EXCLUDES 1**   cleft lip with cleft palate (Q37.-)

DEF: Congenital fissure or opening in the upper lip due to failure of embryonic cells to fuse completely.

Cleft Lip

Unilateral incomplete   Unilateral complete   Bilateral complete

Q36.0 Cleft lip, bilateral

Q36.1 Cleft lip, median

Q36.9 Cleft lip, unilateral
Cleft lip NOS

✓4ᵗʰ Q37 Cleft palate with cleft lip

> **INCLUDES**   cheilopalatoschisis

Q37.0 Cleft hard palate with bilateral cleft lip

Q37.1 Cleft hard palate with unilateral cleft lip
Cleft hard palate with cleft lip NOS

Q37.2 Cleft soft palate with bilateral cleft lip

Q37.3 Cleft soft palate with unilateral cleft lip
Cleft soft palate with cleft lip NOS

Q37.4 Cleft hard and soft palate with bilateral cleft lip

N Newborn: 0   P Pediatric: 0-17   M Maternity: 9-64   A Adult: 15-124   `MCC` Major Complication/Comorbidity   `CC` Complication/Comorbidity   `SW` Severe Wound Dx

926   ICD-10-CM 2022

Q37.5 **Cleft** hard and soft **palate with** unilateral **cleft lip**
Cleft hard and soft palate with cleft lip NOS

Q37.8 **Unspecified cleft palate with bilateral cleft lip**

Q37.9 **Unspecified cleft palate with unilateral cleft lip**
Cleft palate with cleft lip NOS

Other congenital malformations of the digestive system (Q38-Q45)

☑4ᵗʰ **Q38** **Other congenital malformations of** tongue, mouth and pharynx

> *EXCLUDES 1*   *dentofacial anomalies (M26.-)*
> *macrostomia (Q18.4)*
> *microstomia (Q18.5)*

Q38.0 **Congenital malformations of** lips, **not elsewhere classified**
Congenital fistula of lip
Congenital malformation of lip NOS
Van der Woude's syndrome

> *EXCLUDES 1*   *cleft lip (Q36.-)*
> *cleft lip with cleft palate (Q37.-)*
> *macrocheilia (Q18.6)*
> *microcheilia (Q18.7)*

Q38.1 **Ankyloglossia**
Tongue tie

Q38.2 **Macroglossia**
Congenital hypertrophy of tongue

Q38.3 **Other congenital malformations of tongue**
Aglossia
Bifid tongue
Congenital adhesion of tongue
Congenital fissure of tongue
Congenital malformation of tongue NOS
Double tongue
Hypoglossia
Hypoplasia of tongue
Microglossia

Q38.4 **Congenital malformations of** salivary glands and ducts
Atresia of salivary glands and ducts
Congenital absence of salivary glands and ducts
Congenital accessory salivary glands and ducts
Congenital fistula of salivary gland

Q38.5 **Congenital malformations of** palate, **not elsewhere classified**
Congenital absence of uvula
Congenital malformation of palate NOS
Congenital high arched palate

> *EXCLUDES 1*   *cleft palate (Q35.-)*
> *cleft palate with cleft lip (Q37.-)*

Q38.6 **Other congenital malformations of mouth**
Congenital malformation of mouth NOS

Q38.7 **Congenital** pharyngeal pouch
Congenital diverticulum of pharynx

> *EXCLUDES 1*   *pharyngeal pouch syndrome (D82.1)*

Q38.8 **Other congenital malformations of pharynx**
Congenital malformation of pharynx NOS
Imperforate pharynx

☑4ᵗʰ **Q39** **Congenital malformations of** esophagus

Q39.0 **Atresia of esophagus without fistula**   `MCC`
Atresia of esophagus NOS

Q39.1 **Atresia of esophagus with tracheo-esophageal fistula**   `MCC`
Atresia of esophagus with broncho-esophageal fistula

Q39.2 **Congenital** tracheo-esophageal fistula without atresia   `MCC`
Congenital tracheo-esophageal fistula NOS

Q39.3 **Congenital** stenosis and stricture of esophagus   `MCC`

Q39.4 **Esophageal** web   `MCC`

Q39.5 **Congenital** dilatation of esophagus   `CC`
Congenital cardiospasm

Q39.6 **Congenital** diverticulum of esophagus   `CC`
Congenital esophageal pouch

Q39.8 **Other congenital malformations of esophagus**   `CC`
Congenital absence of esophagus
Congenital displacement of esophagus
Congenital duplication of esophagus

Q39.9 **Congenital malformation of esophagus, unspecified**   `CC`

☑4ᵗʰ **Q40** **Other congenital malformations of** upper alimentary tract

Q40.0 **Congenital** hypertrophic pyloric stenosis
Congenital or infantile constriction
Congenital or infantile hypertrophy
Congenital or infantile spasm
Congenital or infantile stenosis
Congenital or infantile stricture

Q40.1 **Congenital** hiatus hernia
Congenital displacement of cardia through esophageal hiatus

> *EXCLUDES 1*   *congenital diaphragmatic hernia (Q79.0)*

Q40.2 **Other specified congenital malformations of stomach**
Congenital displacement of stomach
Congenital diverticulum of stomach
Congenital hourglass stomach
Congenital duplication of stomach
Megalogastria
Microgastria

Q40.3 **Congenital malformation of stomach, unspecified**

Q40.8 **Other specified congenital malformations of upper alimentary tract**

Q40.9 **Congenital malformation of upper alimentary tract, unspecified**
Congenital anomaly of upper alimentary tract
Congenital deformity of upper alimentary tract

☑4ᵗʰ **Q41** **Congenital absence, atresia and stenosis of** small intestine

> *INCLUDES*   congenital obstruction, occlusion or stricture of small intestine or intestine NOS
> *EXCLUDES 1*   *cystic fibrosis with intestinal manifestation (E84.11)*
> *meconium ileus NOS (without cystic fibrosis) (P76.0)*

Q41.0 **Congenital absence, atresia and stenosis of** duodenum   `CC`

Q41.1 **Congenital absence, atresia and stenosis of** jejunum   `CC`
Apple peel syndrome
Imperforate jejunum

Q41.2 **Congenital absence, atresia and stenosis of** ileum   `CC`

Q41.8 **Congenital absence, atresia and stenosis of other specified parts of small intestine**   `CC`

Q41.9 **Congenital absence, atresia and stenosis of small intestine, part unspecified**   `CC`
Congenital absence, atresia and stenosis of intestine NOS

☑4ᵗʰ **Q42** **Congenital absence, atresia and stenosis of** large intestine

> *INCLUDES*   congenital obstruction, occlusion and stricture of large intestine

Q42.0 **Congenital absence, atresia and stenosis of** rectum with fistula   `CC`

Q42.1 **Congenital absence, atresia and stenosis of** rectum without fistula   `CC`
Imperforate rectum

Q42.2 **Congenital absence, atresia and stenosis of** anus with fistula   `CC`

Q42.3 **Congenital absence, atresia and stenosis of** anus without fistula   `CC`
Imperforate anus

Q42.8 **Congenital absence, atresia and stenosis of other parts of large intestine**   `CC`

Q42.9 **Congenital absence, atresia and stenosis of large intestine, part unspecified**   `CC`

☑4ᵗʰ **Q43** **Other congenital malformations of** intestine

Q43.0 **Meckel's diverticulum (displaced) (hypertrophic)**
Persistent omphalomesenteric duct
Persistent vitelline duct
DEF: Congenital, abnormal remnant of embryonic digestive system development that leaves a sacculation or outpouching from the wall of the small intestine near the terminal part of the ileum made of acid-secreting tissue as in the stomach.

Q43.1 **Hirschsprung's disease**   `CC`
Aganglionosis
Congenital (aganglionic) megacolon
DEF: Congenital enlargement or dilation of the colon, with the absence of nerve cells in a segment of colon distally that causes the inability to defecate.

Q43.2 **Other congenital functional disorders of colon**   `CC`
Congenital dilatation of colon

☑ Additional Character Required   √x7ᵗʰ Placeholder   Questionable PDx   Manifestation   Unspecified Dx   `UPD` Unacceptable PDx   `H1`-`H14` HAC   `HCC` CMS-HCC Dx   `HIV` HIV Dx

ICD-10-CM 2022   927

Q43.3 **Congenital malformations of intestinal fixation** `CC`
Congenital omental, anomalous adhesions [bands]
Congenital peritoneal adhesions [bands]
Incomplete rotation of cecum and colon
Insufficient rotation of cecum and colon
Jackson's membrane
Malrotation of colon
Rotation failure of cecum and colon
Universal mesentery

Q43.4 **Duplication of intestine** `CC`

Q43.5 **Ectopic anus** `CC`

Q43.6 **Congenital fistula of rectum and anus** `CC`
EXCLUDES 1   congenital fistula of anus with absence, atresia and stenosis (Q42.2)
congenital fistula of rectum with absence, atresia and stenosis (Q42.0)
congenital rectovaginal fistula (Q52.2)
congenital urethrorectal fistula (Q64.73)
pilonidal fistula or sinus (L05.-)

Q43.7 **Persistent cloaca** `CC`
Cloaca NOS

Q43.8 **Other specified congenital malformations of intestine** `CC`
Congenital blind loop syndrome
Congenital diverticulitis, colon
Congenital diverticulum, intestine
Dolichocolon
Megaloappendix
Megaloduodenum
Microcolon
Transposition of appendix
Transposition of colon
Transposition of intestine
AHA: 2013,2Q,31

Q43.9 **Congenital malformation of intestine, unspecified** `CC`

✓4ᵗʰ Q44 **Congenital malformations of gallbladder, bile ducts and liver**

Q44.0 **Agenesis, aplasia and hypoplasia of gallbladder** `CC`
Congenital absence of gallbladder

Q44.1 **Other congenital malformations of gallbladder** `CC`
Congenital malformation of gallbladder NOS
Intrahepatic gallbladder

Q44.2 **Atresia of bile ducts** `MCC`

Q44.3 **Congenital stenosis and stricture of bile ducts** `MCC`

Q44.4 **Choledochal cyst** `CC`

Q44.5 **Other congenital malformations of bile ducts** `CC`
Accessory hepatic duct
Biliary duct duplication
Congenital malformation of bile duct NOS
Cystic duct duplication

Q44.6 **Cystic disease of liver** `CC`
Fibrocystic disease of liver

Q44.7 **Other congenital malformations of liver** `CC`
Accessory liver
Alagille's syndrome
Congenital absence of liver
Congenital hepatomegaly
Congenital malformation of liver NOS

✓4ᵗʰ Q45 **Other congenital malformations of digestive system**
EXCLUDES 2   congenital diaphragmatic hernia (Q79.0)
congenital hiatus hernia (Q40.1)

Q45.0 **Agenesis, aplasia and hypoplasia of pancreas** `CC`
Congenital absence of pancreas

Q45.1 **Annular pancreas** `CC`

Q45.2 **Congenital pancreatic cyst** `CC`

Q45.3 **Other congenital malformations of pancreas and pancreatic duct** `CC`
Accessory pancreas
Congenital malformation of pancreas or pancreatic duct NOS
EXCLUDES 1   congenital diabetes mellitus (E10.-)
cystic fibrosis (E84.0-E84.9)
fibrocystic disease of pancreas (E84.-)
neonatal diabetes mellitus (P70.2)

Q45.8 **Other specified congenital malformations of digestive system**
Absence (complete) (partial) of alimentary tract NOS
Duplication of digestive system
Malposition, congenital of digestive system

Q45.9 **Congenital malformation of digestive system, unspecified**
Congenital anomaly of digestive system
Congenital deformity of digestive system

Congenital malformations of genital organs (Q50-Q56)

EXCLUDES 1   androgen insensitivity syndrome (E34.5-)
syndromes associated with anomalies in the number and form of chromosomes (Q90-Q99)

✓4ᵗʰ Q50 **Congenital malformations of ovaries, fallopian tubes and broad ligaments**

✓5ᵗʰ Q50.0 **Congenital absence of ovary**
EXCLUDES 1   Turner's syndrome (Q96.-)

Q50.01 **Congenital absence of ovary, unilateral** ♀

Q50.02 **Congenital absence of ovary, bilateral** ♀

Q50.1 **Developmental ovarian cyst** ♀

Q50.2 **Congenital torsion of ovary** ♀

✓5ᵗʰ Q50.3 **Other congenital malformations of ovary**

Q50.31 **Accessory ovary** ♀

Q50.32 **Ovarian streak** ♀
46, XX with streak gonads

Q50.39 **Other congenital malformation of ovary** ♀
Congenital malformation of ovary NOS

Q50.4 **Embryonic cyst of fallopian tube** ♀
Fimbrial cyst

Q50.5 **Embryonic cyst of broad ligament** ♀
Epoophoron cyst
Parovarian cyst

Q50.6 **Other congenital malformations of fallopian tube and broad ligament** ♀
Absence of fallopian tube and broad ligament
Accessory fallopian tube and broad ligament
Atresia of fallopian tube and broad ligament
Congenital malformation of fallopian tube or broad ligament NOS

✓4ᵗʰ Q51 **Congenital malformations of uterus and cervix**

Q51.0 **Agenesis and aplasia of uterus** ♀
Congenital absence of uterus

✓5ᵗʰ Q51.1 **Doubling of uterus with doubling of cervix and vagina**

Q51.10 **Doubling of uterus with doubling of cervix and vagina without obstruction** ♀
Doubling of uterus with doubling of cervix and vagina NOS

Q51.11 **Doubling of uterus with doubling of cervix and vagina with obstruction** ♀

✓5ᵗʰ Q51.2 **Other doubling of uterus**
Doubling of uterus NOS
Septate uterus
AHA: 2018,4Q,27

Q51.21 **Complete doubling of uterus** ♀
Complete septate uterus

Q51.22 **Partial doubling of uterus** ♀
Partial septate uterus

Q51.28 **Other and unspecified doubling of uterus** ♀
Septate uterus NOS

Q51.3 **Bicornate uterus** ♀
Bicornate uterus, complete or partial

Q51.4 **Unicornate uterus** ♀
Unicornate uterus with or without a separate uterine horn
Uterus with only one functioning horn

Q51.5 **Agenesis and aplasia of cervix** ♀
Congenital absence of cervix

Q51.6 **Embryonic cyst of cervix** ♀

Q51.7 **Congenital fistulae between uterus and digestive and urinary tracts** ♀

✓5ᵗʰ Q51.8 **Other congenital malformations of uterus and cervix**

✓6ᵗʰ Q51.81 **Other congenital malformations of uterus**

Q51.810 **Arcuate uterus** ♀
Arcuatus uterus

Q51.811 **Hypoplasia of uterus** ♀

Q51.818 **Other congenital malformations of uterus** ♀
Müllerian anomaly of uterus NEC

√6ᵗʰ Q51.82 **Other congenital malformations of cervix**

Q51.820 **Cervical duplication** ♀
Q51.821 **Hypoplasia of cervix** ♀
Q51.828 **Other congenital malformations of cervix** ♀

Q51.9 **Congenital malformation of uterus and cervix, unspecified** ♀

√4ᵗʰ **Q52 Other congenital malformations of female genitalia**

Q52.0 **Congenital absence of vagina** ♀
Vaginal agenesis, total or partial

√5ᵗʰ Q52.1 **Doubling of vagina**
EXCLUDES 1   *doubling of vagina with doubling of uterus and cervix (Q51.1-)*

Q52.10 **Doubling of vagina, unspecified** ♀
Septate vagina NOS
Q52.11 **Transverse vaginal septum** ♀
√6ᵗʰ Q52.12 **Longitudinal vaginal septum**
AHA: 2016,4Q,58-59

Q52.120 **Longitudinal vaginal septum, nonobstructing** ♀
Q52.121 **Longitudinal vaginal septum, obstructing, right side** ♀
Q52.122 **Longitudinal vaginal septum, obstructing, left side** ♀
Q52.123 **Longitudinal vaginal septum, microperforate, right side** ♀
Q52.124 **Longitudinal vaginal septum, microperforate, left side** ♀
Q52.129 **Other and unspecified longitudinal vaginal septum** ♀

Q52.2 **Congenital rectovaginal fistula** ♀
EXCLUDES 1   *cloaca (Q43.7)*

Q52.3 **Imperforate hymen** ♀
DEF: Obstructive anomaly of vagina, characterized by complete closure of the membranous fold around the external opening of the vagina, obstructing the vaginal introitus.

Q52.4 **Other congenital malformations of vagina** ♀
Canal of Nuck cyst, congenital
Congenital malformation of vagina NOS
Embryonic vaginal cyst
Gartner's duct cyst

Q52.5 **Fusion of labia** ♀
Q52.6 **Congenital malformation of clitoris** ♀
√5ᵗʰ Q52.7 **Other and unspecified congenital malformations of vulva**

Q52.70 **Unspecified congenital malformations of vulva** ♀
Congenital malformation of vulva NOS
Q52.71 **Congenital absence of vulva** ♀
Q52.79 **Other congenital malformations of vulva** ♀
Congenital cyst of vulva

Q52.8 **Other specified congenital malformations of female genitalia** ♀
Q52.9 **Congenital malformation of female genitalia, unspecified** ♀

√4ᵗʰ **Q53 Undescended and ectopic testicle**

√5ᵗʰ Q53.0 **Ectopic testis**

Q53.00 **Ectopic testis, unspecified** ♂
Q53.01 **Ectopic testis, unilateral** ♂
Q53.02 **Ectopic testes, bilateral** ♂

√5ᵗʰ Q53.1 **Undescended testicle, unilateral**
AHA: 2017,4Q,22-23

Q53.10 **Unspecified undescended testicle, unilateral** ♂
√6ᵗʰ Q53.11 **Abdominal testis, unilateral**

Q53.111 **Unilateral intraabdominal testis** ♂
Q53.112 **Unilateral inguinal testis** ♂
Q53.12 **Ectopic perineal testis, unilateral** ♂
Q53.13 **Unilateral high scrotal testis** ♂

√5ᵗʰ Q53.2 **Undescended testicle, bilateral**
AHA: 2017,4Q,22-23

Q53.20 **Undescended testicle, unspecified, bilateral** ♂

√6ᵗʰ Q53.21 **Abdominal testis, bilateral**

Q53.211 **Bilateral intraabdominal testes** ♂
Q53.212 **Bilateral inguinal testes** ♂
Q53.22 **Ectopic perineal testis, bilateral** ♂
Q53.23 **Bilateral high scrotal testes** ♂
Q53.9 **Undescended testicle, unspecified** ♂
Cryptorchism NOS

√4ᵗʰ **Q54 Hypospadias**
EXCLUDES 1   *epispadias (Q64.0)*
DEF: Abnormal opening of the urethra on the ventral (underside) surface of the penis.

Hypospadias

- Balanic (glanular, coronal) hypospadias
- Subcoronal hypospadias
- Penile hypospadias
- Scrotal hypospadias
- Scrotum
Penile raphe
Penoscrotal hypospadias
Scrotal raphe
Perineal hypospadias   **Hypospadias (ventral view)**

Q54.0 **Hypospadias, balanic** ♂
Hypospadias, coronal
Hypospadias, glandular
Q54.1 **Hypospadias, penile** ♂
Q54.2 **Hypospadias, penoscrotal** ♂
Q54.3 **Hypospadias, perineal** ♂
Q54.4 **Congenital chordee** ♂
Chordee without hypospadias
Q54.8 **Other hypospadias** ♂
Hypospadias with intersex state
Q54.9 **Hypospadias, unspecified** ♂

√4ᵗʰ **Q55 Other congenital malformations of male genital organs**
EXCLUDES 1   *congenital hydrocele (P83.5)*
    hypospadias (Q54.-)

Q55.0 **Absence and aplasia of testis** ♂
Monorchism
Q55.1 **Hypoplasia of testis and scrotum** ♂
Fusion of testes
√5ᵗʰ Q55.2 **Other and unspecified congenital malformations of testis and scrotum**

Q55.20 **Unspecified congenital malformations of testis and scrotum** ♂
Congenital malformation of testis or scrotum NOS
Q55.21 **Polyorchism** ♂
DEF: Congenital anomaly in which there are more than two testes.
Q55.22 **Retractile testis** ♂
Q55.23 **Scrotal transposition** ♂
Q55.29 **Other congenital malformations of testis and scrotum** ♂

Q55.3 **Atresia of vas deferens** ♂
Code first any associated cystic fibrosis (E84.-)
Q55.4 **Other congenital malformations of vas deferens, epididymis, seminal vesicles and prostate** ♂
Absence or aplasia of prostate
Absence or aplasia of spermatic cord
Congenital malformation of vas deferens, epididymis, seminal vesicles or prostate NOS

Q55.5 **Congenital absence and aplasia of penis** ♂
√5ᵗʰ Q55.6 **Other congenital malformations of penis**

Q55.61 **Curvature of penis (lateral)** ♂
Q55.62 **Hypoplasia of penis** ♂
Micropenis
Q55.63 **Congenital torsion of penis** ♂
EXCLUDES 1   *acquired torsion of penis (N48.82)*

Q55.64 **Hidden penis** ♂
Buried penis
Concealed penis
EXCLUDES 1 *acquired buried penis (N48.83)*

Q55.69 **Other congenital malformation of penis** ♂
Congenital malformation of penis NOS

Q55.7 **Congenital vasocutaneous fistula** ♂

Q55.8 **Other specified congenital malformations of male genital organs** ♂

Q55.9 **Congenital malformation of male genital organ, unspecified** ♂
Congenital anomaly of male genital organ
Congenital deformity of male genital organ

✓4ᵗʰ **Q56** **Indeterminate sex and pseudohermaphroditism**
EXCLUDES 1 *46, XX true hermaphrodite (Q99.1)*
androgen insensitivity syndrome (E34.5-)
chimera 46, XX/46, XY true hermaphrodite (Q99.0)
female pseudohermaphroditism with adrenocortical disorder (E25.-)
pseudohermaphroditism with specified chromosomal anomaly (Q96-Q99)
pure gonadal dysgenesis (Q99.1)
DEF: Indeterminate sex: External genitalia that is nondescript, lacking the physical appearance specific to either sex.
DEF: Pseudohermaphroditism: Presence of gonads of one sex and external genitalia of another sex.

Q56.0 **Hermaphroditism, not elsewhere classified**
Ovotestis

Q56.1 **Male pseudohermaphroditism, not elsewhere classified** ♂
46, XY with streak gonads
Male pseudohermaphroditism NOS

Q56.2 **Female pseudohermaphroditism, not elsewhere classified** ♀
Female pseudohermaphroditism NOS

Q56.3 **Pseudohermaphroditism, unspecified**

Q56.4 **Indeterminate sex, unspecified**
Ambiguous genitalia

Congenital malformations of the urinary system (Q60-Q64)

✓4ᵗʰ **Q60** **Renal agenesis and other reduction defects of kidney**
INCLUDES congenital absence of kidney
congenital atrophy of kidney
infantile atrophy of kidney

Q60.0 **Renal agenesis, unilateral** CC

Q60.1 **Renal agenesis, bilateral** CC

Q60.2 **Renal agenesis, unspecified** CC

Q60.3 **Renal hypoplasia, unilateral** CC

Q60.4 **Renal hypoplasia, bilateral** CC

Q60.5 **Renal hypoplasia, unspecified** CC

Q60.6 **Potter's syndrome** CC

✓4ᵗʰ **Q61** **Cystic kidney disease**
EXCLUDES 1 *acquired cyst of kidney (N28.1)*
Potter's syndrome (Q60.6)

✓5ᵗʰ **Q61.0** **Congenital renal cyst**

Q61.00 **Congenital renal cyst, unspecified** CC
Cyst of kidney NOS (congenital)

Q61.01 **Congenital single renal cyst** CC

Q61.02 **Congenital multiple renal cysts** CC

✓5ᵗʰ **Q61.1** **Polycystic kidney, infantile type**
Polycystic kidney, autosomal recessive

Q61.11 **Cystic dilatation of collecting ducts** CC

Q61.19 **Other polycystic kidney, infantile type** CC

Q61.2 **Polycystic kidney, adult type**
Polycystic kidney, autosomal dominant

Q61.3 **Polycystic kidney, unspecified** CC
AHA: 2016,3Q,22

Q61.4 **Renal dysplasia** CC
Multicystic dysplastic kidney
Multicystic kidney (development)
Multicystic kidney disease
Multicystic renal dysplasia
EXCLUDES 1 *polycystic kidney disease (Q61.11-Q61.3)*

Q61.5 **Medullary cystic kidney** CC
►Nephronophthisis◄
Sponge kidney NOS
DEF: Sponge kidney: Dilated collecting tubules that are usually asymptomatic. Calcinosis in tubules may cause renal insufficiency.

Q61.8 **Other cystic kidney diseases** CC
Fibrocystic kidney
Fibrocystic renal degeneration or disease

Q61.9 **Cystic kidney disease, unspecified** CC
Meckel-Gruber syndrome

✓4ᵗʰ **Q62** **Congenital obstructive defects of renal pelvis and congenital malformations of ureter**

Q62.0 **Congenital hydronephrosis** CC

✓5ᵗʰ **Q62.1** **Congenital occlusion of ureter**
Atresia and stenosis of ureter

Q62.10 **Congenital occlusion of ureter, unspecified** CC

Q62.11 **Congenital occlusion of ureteropelvic junction** CC

Q62.12 **Congenital occlusion of ureterovesical orifice** CC

Q62.2 **Congenital megaureter** CC
Congenital dilatation of ureter

✓5ᵗʰ **Q62.3** **Other obstructive defects of renal pelvis and ureter**

Q62.31 **Congenital ureterocele, orthotopic** CC

Q62.32 **Cecoureterocele** CC
Ectopic ureterocele

Q62.39 **Other obstructive defects of renal pelvis and ureter** CC
Ureteropelvic junction obstruction NOS

Q62.4 **Agenesis of ureter**
Congenital absence ureter

Q62.5 **Duplication of ureter**
Accessory ureter
Double ureter

✓5ᵗʰ **Q62.6** **Malposition of ureter**

Q62.60 **Malposition of ureter, unspecified**

Q62.61 **Deviation of ureter**

Q62.62 **Displacement of ureter**

Q62.63 **Anomalous implantation of ureter**
Ectopia of ureter
Ectopic ureter

Q62.69 **Other malposition of ureter**

Q62.7 **Congenital vesico-uretero-renal reflux**

Q62.8 **Other congenital malformations of ureter**
Anomaly of ureter NOS

✓4ᵗʰ **Q63** **Other congenital malformations of kidney**
EXCLUDES 1 *congenital nephrotic syndrome (N04.-)*

Q63.0 **Accessory kidney**

Q63.1 **Lobulated, fused and horseshoe kidney**

Q63.2 **Ectopic kidney**
Congenital displaced kidney
Malrotation of kidney

Q63.3 **Hyperplastic and giant kidney**
Compensatory hypertrophy of kidney

Q63.8 **Other specified congenital malformations of kidney**
Congenital renal calculi

Q63.9 **Congenital malformation of kidney, unspecified**

✓4ᵗʰ **Q64** **Other congenital malformations of urinary system**

Q64.0 **Epispadias**
EXCLUDES 1 *hypospadias (Q54.-)*

Epispadias

Normal external urethral orifice
Glans penis
Foreskin (retracted)
Epispadias

Epispadias (dorsal view)

✓5ᵗʰ **Q64.1 Exstrophy of** urinary bladder

     Q64.10 Exstrophy of urinary bladder, unspecified cc
         Ectopia vesicae

     Q64.11 Supravesical fissure of urinary bladder cc

     Q64.12 Cloacal exstrophy of urinary bladder cc

     Q64.19 Other exstrophy of urinary bladder cc
         Extroversion of bladder

Q64.2 Congenital posterior urethral valves cc

✓5ᵗʰ **Q64.3 Other atresia and stenosis of urethra and bladder neck**

     Q64.31 Congenital bladder neck obstruction cc
         Congenital obstruction of vesicourethral orifice

     Q64.32 Congenital stricture of urethra cc

     Q64.33 Congenital stricture of urinary meatus cc

     Q64.39 Other atresia and stenosis of urethra and bladder neck cc
         Atresia and stenosis of urethra and bladder neck NOS

Q64.4 Malformation of urachus
     Cyst of urachus
     Patent urachus
     Prolapse of urachus

Q64.5 Congenital absence of bladder and urethra

Q64.6 Congenital diverticulum of bladder

✓5ᵗʰ **Q64.7 Other and unspecified congenital malformations of bladder and urethra**
     EXCLUDES 1 *congenital prolapse of bladder (mucosa) (Q79.4)*

     Q64.70 Unspecified congenital malformation of bladder and urethra
         Malformation of bladder or urethra NOS

     Q64.71 Congenital prolapse of urethra

     Q64.72 Congenital prolapse of urinary meatus

     Q64.73 Congenital urethrorectal fistula

     Q64.74 Double urethra

     Q64.75 Double urinary meatus

     Q64.79 Other congenital malformations of bladder and urethra

Q64.8 Other specified congenital malformations of urinary system

Q64.9 Congenital malformation of urinary system, unspecified
     Congenital anomaly NOS of urinary system
     Congenital deformity NOS of urinary system

Congenital malformations and deformations of the musculoskeletal system (Q65-Q79)

✓4ᵗʰ **Q65 Congenital deformities of hip**
     EXCLUDES 1 *clicking hip (R29.4)*

✓5ᵗʰ **Q65.0 Congenital dislocation of hip, unilateral**

     Q65.00 Congenital dislocation of unspecified hip, unilateral
     Q65.01 Congenital dislocation of right hip, unilateral
     Q65.02 Congenital dislocation of left hip, unilateral

Q65.1 Congenital dislocation of hip, bilateral

Q65.2 Congenital dislocation of hip, unspecified

✓5ᵗʰ **Q65.3 Congenital partial dislocation of hip, unilateral**

     Q65.30 Congenital partial dislocation of unspecified hip, unilateral
     Q65.31 Congenital partial dislocation of right hip, unilateral
     Q65.32 Congenital partial dislocation of left hip, unilateral

Q65.4 Congenital partial dislocation of hip, bilateral

Q65.5 Congenital partial dislocation of hip, unspecified

Q65.6 Congenital unstable hip
     Congenital dislocatable hip

✓5ᵗʰ **Q65.8 Other congenital deformities of hip**

     Q65.81 Congenital coxa valga
     Q65.82 Congenital coxa vara
     Q65.89 Other specified congenital deformities of hip
         Anteversion of femoral neck
         Congenital acetabular dysplasia

Q65.9 Congenital deformity of hip, unspecified

✓4ᵗʰ **Q66 Congenital deformities of feet**
     EXCLUDES 1 *reduction defects of feet (Q72.-)*
         valgus deformities (acquired) (M21.0-)
         varus deformities (acquired) (M21.1-)
     AHA: 2019,4Q,13

✓5ᵗʰ **Q66.0 Congenital talipes equinovarus**

     Q66.00 Congenital talipes equinovarus, unspecified foot

     Q66.01 Congenital talipes equinovarus, right foot
     Q66.02 Congenital talipes equinovarus, left foot

✓5ᵗʰ **Q66.1 Congenital talipes calcaneovarus**

     Q66.10 Congenital talipes calcaneovarus, unspecified foot
     Q66.11 Congenital talipes calcaneovarus, right foot
     Q66.12 Congenital talipes calcaneovarus, left foot

✓5ᵗʰ **Q66.2 Congenital metatarsus (primus) varus**
     AHA: 2016,4Q,59

     ✓6ᵗʰ **Q66.21 Congenital metatarsus primus varus**

         Q66.211 Congenital metatarsus primus varus, right foot
         Q66.212 Congenital metatarsus primus varus, left foot
         Q66.219 Congenital metatarsus primus varus, unspecified foot

     ✓6ᵗʰ **Q66.22 Congenital metatarsus adductus**
         Congenital metatarsus varus

         Q66.221 Congenital metatarsus adductus, right foot
         Q66.222 Congenital metatarsus adductus, left foot
         Q66.229 Congenital metatarsus adductus, unspecified foot

✓5ᵗʰ **Q66.3 Other congenital varus deformities of feet**
     Hallux varus, congenital

     Q66.30 Other congenital varus deformities of feet, unspecified foot
     Q66.31 Other congenital varus deformities of feet, right foot
     Q66.32 Other congenital varus deformities of feet, left foot

✓5ᵗʰ **Q66.4 Congenital talipes calcaneovalgus**

     Q66.40 Congenital talipes calcaneovalgus, unspecified foot
     Q66.41 Congenital talipes calcaneovalgus, right foot
     Q66.42 Congenital talipes calcaneovalgus, left foot

✓5ᵗʰ **Q66.5 Congenital pes planus**
     Congenital flat foot
     Congenital rigid flat foot
     Congenital spastic (everted) flat foot
     EXCLUDES 1 *pes planus, acquired (M21.4)*

     Q66.50 Congenital pes planus, unspecified foot
     Q66.51 Congenital pes planus, right foot
     Q66.52 Congenital pes planus, left foot

Q66.6 Other congenital valgus deformities of feet
     Congenital metatarsus valgus

✓5ᵗʰ **Q66.7 Congenital pes cavus**

     Q66.70 Congenital pes cavus, unspecified foot
     Q66.71 Congenital pes cavus, right foot
     Q66.72 Congenital pes cavus, left foot

✓5ᵗʰ **Q66.8 Other congenital deformities of feet**

     Q66.80 Congenital vertical talus deformity, unspecified foot

     Q66.81 Congenital vertical talus deformity, right foot

     Q66.82 Congenital vertical talus deformity, left foot

     Q66.89 Other specified congenital deformities of feet
         Congenital asymmetric talipes
         Congenital clubfoot NOS
         Congenital talipes NOS
         Congenital tarsal coalition
         Hammer toe, congenital
         DEF: Clubfoot: Congenital anomaly of the foot with the heel elevated and rotated outward and the toes pointing inward.

✓5ᵗʰ **Q66.9 Congenital deformity of feet, unspecified**

     Q66.90 Congenital deformity of feet, unspecified, unspecified foot

     Q66.91 Congenital deformity of feet, unspecified, right foot

     Q66.92 Congenital deformity of feet, unspecified, left foot

✓4ᵗʰ **Q67 Congenital musculoskeletal deformities of head, face, spine and chest**
     EXCLUDES 1 *congenital malformation syndromes classified to Q87.-*
         Potter's syndrome (Q60.6)

Q67.0 Congenital facial asymmetry

Q67.1 Congenital compression facies

Q67.2 Dolichocephaly

Q67.3 Plagiocephaly

✓ Additional Character Required   ✓x7ᵗʰ Placeholder   Questionable PDx   Manifestation   Unspecified Dx   UPD Unacceptable PDx   H1-H4 HAC   HCC CMS-HCC Dx   HIV HIV Dx

ICD-10-CM 2022   931

Q67.4 Other congenital deformities of skull, face and jaw
Congenital depressions in skull
Congenital hemifacial atrophy or hypertrophy
Deviation of nasal septum, congenital
Squashed or bent nose, congenital
EXCLUDES 1 *dentofacial anomalies [including malocclusion] (M26.-)*
syphilitic saddle nose (A50.5)
DEF: Deviated septum: Condition in which the nasal septum, a thin wall composed of cartilage and bone that separates the two nostrils, is crooked or displaced from the midline.

Q67.5 Congenital deformity of spine   CC
Congenital postural scoliosis
Congenital scoliosis NOS
EXCLUDES 1 *infantile idiopathic scoliosis (M41.0)*
scoliosis due to congenital bony malformation (Q76.3)
AHA: 2014,4Q,26

Q67.6 Pectus excavatum
Congenital funnel chest

Q67.7 Pectus carinatum
Congenital pigeon chest

Q67.8 Other congenital deformities of chest   CC
Congenital deformity of chest wall NOS

✓4ᵗʰ **Q68 Other congenital musculoskeletal deformities**
EXCLUDES 1 *reduction defects of limb(s) (Q71-Q73)*
EXCLUDES 2 *congenital myotonic chondrodystrophy (G71.13)*

Q68.0 Congenital deformity of sternocleidomastoid muscle
Congenital contracture of sternocleidomastoid (muscle)
Congenital (sternomastoid) torticollis
Sternomastoid tumor (congenital)

Q68.1 Congenital deformity of finger(s) and hand   CC
Congenital clubfinger
Spade-like hand (congenital)

Q68.2 Congenital deformity of knee
Congenital dislocation of knee
Congenital genu recurvatum

Q68.3 Congenital bowing of femur
EXCLUDES 1 *anteversion of femur (neck) (Q65.89)*

Q68.4 Congenital bowing of tibia and fibula

Q68.5 Congenital bowing of long bones of leg, unspecified

Q68.6 Discoid meniscus

Q68.8 Other specified congenital musculoskeletal deformities
Congenital deformity of clavicle
Congenital deformity of elbow
Congenital deformity of forearm
Congenital deformity of scapula
Congenital deformity of wrist
Congenital dislocation of elbow
Congenital dislocation of shoulder
Congenital dislocation of wrist

✓4ᵗʰ **Q69 Polydactyly**

Q69.0 Accessory finger(s)

Q69.1 Accessory thumb(s)

Q69.2 Accessory toe(s)
Accessory hallux

Q69.9 Polydactyly, unspecified
Supernumerary digit(s) NOS

✓4ᵗʰ **Q70 Syndactyly**

✓5ᵗʰ **Q70.0 Fused fingers**
Complex syndactyly of fingers with synostosis
Q70.00 Fused fingers, unspecified hand
Q70.01 Fused fingers, right **hand**
Q70.02 Fused fingers, left **hand**
Q70.03 Fused fingers, bilateral

✓5ᵗʰ **Q70.1 Webbed fingers**
Simple syndactyly of fingers without synostosis
Q70.10 Webbed fingers, unspecified hand
Q70.11 Webbed fingers, right **hand**
Q70.12 Webbed fingers, left **hand**
Q70.13 Webbed fingers, bilateral

✓5ᵗʰ **Q70.2 Fused toes**
Complex syndactyly of toes with synostosis
Q70.20 Fused toes, unspecified foot
Q70.21 Fused toes, right **foot**

Q70.22 Fused toes, left **foot**
Q70.23 Fused toes, bilateral

✓5ᵗʰ **Q70.3 Webbed toes**
Simple syndactyly of toes without synostosis
Q70.30 Webbed toes, unspecified foot
Q70.31 Webbed toes, right **foot**
Q70.32 Webbed toes, left **foot**
Q70.33 Webbed toes, bilateral

Q70.4 Polysyndactyly, unspecified
EXCLUDES 1 *specified syndactyly of hand and feet - code to specified conditions (Q70.0-Q70.3-)*

Q70.9 Syndactyly, unspecified
Symphalangy NOS

✓4ᵗʰ **Q71 Reduction defects of** upper limb

✓5ᵗʰ **Q71.0 Congenital** complete absence **of upper limb**
Q71.00 Congenital complete absence of unspecified upper limb
Q71.01 Congenital complete absence of right **upper limb**
Q71.02 Congenital complete absence of left **upper limb**
Q71.03 Congenital complete absence of upper limb, bilateral

✓5ᵗʰ **Q71.1 Congenital** absence of upper arm and forearm with hand present
Q71.10 Congenital absence of unspecified upper arm and forearm with hand present
Q71.11 Congenital absence of right **upper arm and forearm with hand present**
Q71.12 Congenital absence of left **upper arm and forearm with hand present**
Q71.13 Congenital absence of upper arm and forearm with hand present, bilateral

✓5ᵗʰ **Q71.2 Congenital** absence of both forearm and hand
Q71.20 Congenital absence of both forearm and hand, unspecified upper limb
Q71.21 Congenital absence of both forearm and hand, right **upper limb**
Q71.22 Congenital absence of both forearm and hand, left **upper limb**
Q71.23 Congenital absence of both forearm and hand, bilateral

✓5ᵗʰ **Q71.3 Congenital** absence of hand and finger
Q71.30 Congenital absence of unspecified hand and finger
Q71.31 Congenital absence of right **hand and finger**
Q71.32 Congenital absence of left **hand and finger**
Q71.33 Congenital absence of hand and finger, bilateral

✓5ᵗʰ **Q71.4 Longitudinal reduction defect of** radius
Clubhand (congenital)
Radial clubhand
Q71.40 Longitudinal reduction defect of unspecified radius
Q71.41 Longitudinal reduction defect of right **radius**
Q71.42 Longitudinal reduction defect of left **radius**
Q71.43 Longitudinal reduction defect of radius, bilateral

✓5ᵗʰ **Q71.5 Longitudinal reduction defect of** ulna
Q71.50 Longitudinal reduction defect of unspecified ulna
Q71.51 Longitudinal reduction defect of right **ulna**
Q71.52 Longitudinal reduction defect of left **ulna**
Q71.53 Longitudinal reduction defect of ulna, bilateral

✓5ᵗʰ **Q71.6 Lobster-claw hand**
Q71.60 Lobster-claw hand, unspecified hand
Q71.61 Lobster-claw right **hand**
Q71.62 Lobster-claw left **hand**
Q71.63 Lobster-claw hand, bilateral

✓5ᵗʰ **Q71.8 Other reduction defects of** upper limb
✓6ᵗʰ **Q71.81 Congenital** shortening **of upper limb**
Q71.811 Congenital shortening of right **upper limb**
Q71.812 Congenital shortening of left **upper limb**
Q71.813 Congenital shortening of upper limb, bilateral
Q71.819 Congenital shortening of unspecified upper limb
✓6ᵗʰ **Q71.89 Other reduction defects of upper limb**
Q71.891 Other reduction defects of right **upper limb**
Q71.892 Other reduction defects of left **upper limb**
Q71.893 Other reduction defects of upper limb, bilateral

Q71.899 Other reduction defects of unspecified upper limb

√5ᵗʰ **Q71.9** Unspecified reduction defect of upper limb

Q71.90 Unspecified reduction defect of unspecified upper limb

Q71.91 Unspecified reduction defect of right upper limb

Q71.92 Unspecified reduction defect of left upper limb

Q71.93 Unspecified reduction defect of upper limb, bilateral

√4ᵗʰ **Q72** Reduction defects of lower limb

√5ᵗʰ **Q72.0** Congenital complete absence of lower limb

Q72.00 Congenital complete absence of unspecified lower limb

Q72.01 Congenital complete absence of right lower limb

Q72.02 Congenital complete absence of left lower limb

Q72.03 Congenital complete absence of lower limb, bilateral

√5ᵗʰ **Q72.1** Congenital absence of thigh and lower leg with foot present

Q72.10 Congenital absence of unspecified thigh and lower leg with foot present

Q72.11 Congenital absence of right thigh and lower leg with foot present

Q72.12 Congenital absence of left thigh and lower leg with foot present

Q72.13 Congenital absence of thigh and lower leg with foot present, bilateral

√5ᵗʰ **Q72.2** Congenital absence of both lower leg and foot

Q72.20 Congenital absence of both lower leg and foot, unspecified lower limb

Q72.21 Congenital absence of both lower leg and foot, right lower limb

Q72.22 Congenital absence of both lower leg and foot, left lower limb

Q72.23 Congenital absence of both lower leg and foot, bilateral

√5ᵗʰ **Q72.3** Congenital absence of foot and toe(s)

Q72.30 Congenital absence of unspecified foot and toe(s)

Q72.31 Congenital absence of right foot and toe(s)

Q72.32 Congenital absence of left foot and toe(s)

Q72.33 Congenital absence of foot and toe(s), bilateral

√5ᵗʰ **Q72.4** Longitudinal reduction defect of femur

Proximal femoral focal deficiency

Q72.40 Longitudinal reduction defect of unspecified femur

Q72.41 Longitudinal reduction defect of right femur

Q72.42 Longitudinal reduction defect of left femur

Q72.43 Longitudinal reduction defect of femur, bilateral

√5ᵗʰ **Q72.5** Longitudinal reduction defect of tibia

Q72.50 Longitudinal reduction defect of unspecified tibia

Q72.51 Longitudinal reduction defect of right tibia

Q72.52 Longitudinal reduction defect of left tibia

Q72.53 Longitudinal reduction defect of tibia, bilateral

√5ᵗʰ **Q72.6** Longitudinal reduction defect of fibula

Q72.60 Longitudinal reduction defect of unspecified fibula

Q72.61 Longitudinal reduction defect of right fibula

Q72.62 Longitudinal reduction defect of left fibula

Q72.63 Longitudinal reduction defect of fibula, bilateral

√5ᵗʰ **Q72.7** Split foot

Q72.70 Split foot, unspecified lower limb

Q72.71 Split foot, right lower limb

Q72.72 Split foot, left lower limb

Q72.73 Split foot, bilateral

√5ᵗʰ **Q72.8** Other reduction defects of lower limb

√6ᵗʰ **Q72.81** Congenital shortening of lower limb

Q72.811 Congenital shortening of right lower limb

Q72.812 Congenital shortening of left lower limb

Q72.813 Congenital shortening of lower limb, bilateral

Q72.819 Congenital shortening of unspecified lower limb

√6ᵗʰ **Q72.89** Other reduction defects of lower limb

Q72.891 Other reduction defects of right lower limb

Q72.892 Other reduction defects of left lower limb

Q72.893 Other reduction defects of lower limb, bilateral

Q72.899 Other reduction defects of unspecified lower limb

√5ᵗʰ **Q72.9** Unspecified reduction defect of lower limb

Q72.90 Unspecified reduction defect of unspecified lower limb

Q72.91 Unspecified reduction defect of right lower limb

Q72.92 Unspecified reduction defect of left lower limb

Q72.93 Unspecified reduction defect of lower limb, bilateral

√4ᵗʰ **Q73** Reduction defects of unspecified limb

Q73.0 Congenital absence of unspecified limb(s)

Amelia NOS

Q73.1 Phocomelia, unspecified limb(s)

Phocomelia NOS

Q73.8 Other reduction defects of unspecified limb(s)

Longitudinal reduction deformity of unspecified limb(s)

Ectromelia of limb NOS

Hemimelia of limb NOS

Reduction defect of limb NOS

√4ᵗʰ **Q74** Other congenital malformations of limb(s)

EXCLUDES 1   polydactyly (Q69.-)

reduction defect of limb (Q71-Q73)

syndactyly (Q70.-)

Q74.0 Other congenital malformations of upper limb(s), including shoulder girdle

Accessory carpal bones

Cleidocranial dysostosis

Congenital pseudarthrosis of clavicle

Macrodactylia (fingers)

Madelung's deformity

Radioulnar synostosis

Sprengel's deformity

Triphalangeal thumb

Q74.1 Congenital malformation of knee

Congenital absence of patella

Congenital dislocation of patella

Congenital genu valgum

Congenital genu varum

Rudimentary patella

EXCLUDES 1   congenital dislocation of knee (Q68.2)

congenital genu recurvatum (Q68.2)

nail patella syndrome (Q87.2)

Q74.2 Other congenital malformations of lower limb(s), including pelvic girdle

Congenital fusion of sacroiliac joint

Congenital malformation of ankle joint

Congenital malformation of sacroiliac joint

EXCLUDES 1   anteversion of femur (neck) (Q65.89)

Q74.3 Arthrogryposis multiplex congenita   CC

Q74.8 Other specified congenital malformations of limb(s)

Q74.9 Unspecified congenital malformation of limb(s)

Congenital anomaly of limb(s) NOS

√4ᵗʰ **Q75** Other congenital malformations of skull and face bones

EXCLUDES 1   congenital malformation of face NOS (Q18.-)

congenital malformation syndromes classified to Q87.-

dentofacial anomalies [including malocclusion] (M26.-)

musculoskeletal deformities of head and face (Q67.0-Q67.4)

skull defects associated with congenital anomalies of brain

such as:

anencephaly (Q00.0)

encephalocele (Q01.-)

hydrocephalus (Q03.-)

microcephaly (Q02)

Q75.0 Craniosynostosis

Acrocephaly

Imperfect fusion of skull

Oxycephaly

Trigonocephaly

DEF: Congenital condition in which one or more of the cranial sutures fuse prematurely, creating a deformed or aberrant head shape.

Q75.1 Craniofacial dysostosis

Crouzon's disease

Q75.2 Hypertelorism

Q75.3 Macrocephaly

Q75.4 Mandibulofacial dysostosis
Francheschetti syndrome
Treacher Collins syndrome

Q75.5 Oculomandibular dysostosis

Q75.8 Other specified congenital malformations of skull and face bones
Absence of skull bone, congenital
Congenital deformity of forehead
Platybasia

Q75.9 Congenital malformation of skull and face bones, unspecified
Congenital anomaly of face bones NOS
Congenital anomaly of skull NOS

✓4ᵗʰ **Q76 Congenital malformations of spine and bony thorax**
> EXCLUDES 1   congenital musculoskeletal deformities of spine and chest (Q67.5-Q67.8)

Q76.0 Spina bifida occulta
> EXCLUDES 1   meningocele (spinal) (Q05.-)
>   spina bifida (aperta) (cystica) (Q05.-)

Q76.1 Klippel-Feil syndrome
Cervical fusion syndrome

Q76.2 Congenital spondylolisthesis
Congenital spondylolysis
> EXCLUDES 1   spondylolisthesis (acquired) (M43.1-)
>   spondylolysis (acquired) (M43.0-)

Q76.3 Congenital scoliosis due to congenital bony malformation   CC
Hemivertebra fusion or failure of segmentation with scoliosis

✓5ᵗʰ **Q76.4 Other congenital malformations of spine, not associated with scoliosis**
    ✓6ᵗʰ **Q76.41 Congenital kyphosis**
       Q76.411 Congenital kyphosis, occipito-atlanto-axial region
       Q76.412 Congenital kyphosis, cervical region
       Q76.413 Congenital kyphosis, cervicothoracic region
       Q76.414 Congenital kyphosis, thoracic region
       Q76.415 Congenital kyphosis, thoracolumbar region
       Q76.419 Congenital kyphosis, unspecified region
    ✓6ᵗʰ **Q76.42 Congenital lordosis**
       Q76.425 Congenital lordosis, thoracolumbar region   CC
       Q76.426 Congenital lordosis, lumbar region   CC
       Q76.427 Congenital lordosis, lumbosacral region   CC
       Q76.428 Congenital lordosis, sacral and sacrococcygeal region   CC
       Q76.429 Congenital lordosis, unspecified region   CC
    Q76.49 Other congenital malformations of spine, not associated with scoliosis
      Congenital absence of vertebra NOS
      Congenital fusion of spine NOS
      Congenital malformation of lumbosacral (joint) (region) NOS
      Congenital malformation of spine NOS
      Hemivertebra NOS
      Malformation of spine NOS
      Platyspondylisis NOS
      Supernumerary vertebra NOS

Q76.5 Cervical rib
Supernumerary rib in cervical region

Q76.6 Other congenital malformations of ribs   CC
Accessory rib
Congenital absence of rib
Congenital fusion of ribs
Congenital malformation of ribs NOS
> EXCLUDES 1   short rib syndrome (Q77.2)

Q76.7 Congenital malformation of sternum   CC
Congenital absence of sternum
Sternum bifidum

Q76.8 Other congenital malformations of bony thorax   CC

Q76.9 Congenital malformation of bony thorax, unspecified   CC

✓4ᵗʰ **Q77 Osteochondrodysplasia with defects of growth of tubular bones and spine**
> EXCLUDES 1   mucopolysaccharidosis (E76.0-E76.3)
> EXCLUDES 2   congenital myotonic chondrodystrophy (G71.13)

Q77.0 Achondrogenesis
Hypochondrogenesis

Q77.1 Thanatophoric short stature

Q77.2 Short rib syndrome   CC
Asphyxiating thoracic dysplasia [Jeune]

Q77.3 Chondrodysplasia punctata
> EXCLUDES 1   Rhizomelic chondrodysplasia punctata (E71.43)

Q77.4 Achondroplasia
Hypochondroplasia
Osteosclerosis congenita

Q77.5 Diastrophic dysplasia

Q77.6 Chondroectodermal dysplasia
Ellis-van Creveld syndrome

Q77.7 Spondyloepiphyseal dysplasia

Q77.8 Other osteochondrodysplasia with defects of growth of tubular bones and spine

Q77.9 Osteochondrodysplasia with defects of growth of tubular bones and spine, unspecified

✓4ᵗʰ **Q78 Other osteochondrodysplasias**
> EXCLUDES 2   congenital myotonic chondrodystrophy (G71.13)

Q78.0 Osteogenesis imperfecta   CC
Fragilitas ossium
Osteopsathyrosis

Q78.1 Polyostotic fibrous dysplasia
Albright(-McCune)(-Sternberg) syndrome

Q78.2 Osteopetrosis   CC
Albers-Schönberg syndrome
Osteosclerosis NOS
DEF: Rare congenital condition in which the bones are excessively dense, resulting from a discrepancy in the formation and breakdown of bone.

Q78.3 Progressive diaphyseal dysplasia
Camurati-Engelmann syndrome

Q78.4 Enchondromatosis
Maffucci's syndrome
Ollier's disease

Q78.5 Metaphyseal dysplasia
Pyle's syndrome

Q78.6 Multiple congenital exostoses
Diaphyseal aclasis

Q78.8 Other specified osteochondrodysplasias
Osteopoikilosis

Q78.9 Osteochondrodysplasia, unspecified
Chondrodystrophy NOS
Osteodystrophy NOS

✓4ᵗʰ **Q79 Congenital malformations of musculoskeletal system, not elsewhere classified**
> EXCLUDES 2   congenital (sternomastoid) torticollis (Q68.0)

Q79.0 Congenital diaphragmatic hernia   MCC
> EXCLUDES 1   congenital hiatus hernia (Q40.1)

Q79.1 Other congenital malformations of diaphragm   MCC
Absence of diaphragm
Congenital malformation of diaphragm NOS
Eventration of diaphragm

Q79.2 Exomphalos   MCC
Omphalocele
> EXCLUDES 1   umbilical hernia (K42.-)

N Newborn: 0   P Pediatric: 0-17   M Maternity: 9-64   A Adult: 15-124   MCC Major Complication/Comorbidity   CC Complication/Comorbidity   SW Severe Wound Dx

934   **ICD-10-CM 2022**

Q79.3   Gastroschisis   `MCC`

Gastroschisis

Herniated small bowel (gastroschisis)

Rectus abdominus m.

Umbilicus

skin

distal

proximal

Defect

Q79.4   Prune belly syndrome   `MCC`
Congenital prolapse of bladder mucosa
Eagle-Barrett syndrome

✓5th **Q79.5   Other congenital malformations of abdominal wall**
   EXCLUDES 1   umbilical hernia (K42.-)

   Q79.51   Congenital hernia of bladder   `MCC`

   Q79.59   Other congenital malformations of abdominal wall   `MCC`

✓5th **Q79.6   Ehlers-Danlos syndromes**
   AHA: 2019,4Q,13-14
   DEF: Connective tissue disorder that causes hyperextended skin and joints and results in fragile blood vessels with bleeding, poor wound healing, and subcutaneous pseudotumors.

   Q79.60   Ehlers-Danlos syndrome, unspecified   `CC`

   Q79.61   Classical Ehlers-Danlos syndrome   `CC`
     Classical EDS (cEDS)

   Q79.62   Hypermobile Ehlers-Danlos syndrome   `CC`
     Hypermobile EDS (hEDS)

   Q79.63   Vascular Ehlers-Danlos syndrome   `CC`
     Vascular EDS (vEDS)

   Q79.69   Other Ehlers-Danlos syndromes   `CC`

Q79.8   Other congenital malformations of musculoskeletal system
Absence of muscle
Absence of tendon
Accessory muscle
Amyotrophia congenita
Congenital constricting bands
Congenital shortening of tendon
Poland syndrome

Q79.9   Congenital malformation of musculoskeletal system, unspecified
Congenital anomaly of musculoskeletal system NOS
Congenital deformity of musculoskeletal system NOS

Other congenital malformations (Q80-Q89)

✓4th **Q80   Congenital ichthyosis**
   EXCLUDES 1   Refsum's disease (G60.1)
   DEF: Excessive production of skin cells resulting in red, dry, scaly skin.

   Q80.0   Ichthyosis vulgaris

   Q80.1   X-linked ichthyosis

   Q80.2   Lamellar ichthyosis
     Collodion baby

   Q80.3   Congenital bullous ichthyosiform erythroderma

   Q80.4   Harlequin fetus

   Q80.8   Other congenital ichthyosis

   Q80.9   Congenital ichthyosis, unspecified

✓4th **Q81   Epidermolysis bullosa**

   Q81.0   Epidermolysis bullosa simplex
     EXCLUDES 1   Cockayne's syndrome (Q87.19)

   Q81.1   Epidermolysis bullosa letalis
     Herlitz' syndrome

   Q81.2   Epidermolysis bullosa dystrophica

   Q81.8   Other epidermolysis bullosa

   Q81.9   Epidermolysis bullosa, unspecified

✓4th **Q82   Other congenital malformations of skin**
   EXCLUDES 1   acrodermatitis enteropathica (E83.2)
     congenital erythropoietic porphyria (E80.0)
     pilonidal cyst or sinus (L05.-)
     Sturge-Weber (-Dimitri) syndrome (Q85.8)

   Q82.0   Hereditary lymphedema

   Q82.1   Xeroderma pigmentosum

   Q82.2   Congenital cutaneous mastocytosis
     Congenital diffuse cutaneous mastocytosis
     Congenital maculopapular cutaneous mastocytosis
     Congenital urticaria pigmentosa
     EXCLUDES 1   cutaneous mastocytosis NOS (D47.01)
       diffuse cutaneous mastocytosis (with onset after newborn period) (D47.01)
       malignant mastocytosis (C96.2-)
       systemic mastocytosis (D47.02)
       urticaria pigmentosa (non-congenital) (with onset after newborn period) (D47.01)
     AHA: 2017,4Q,5

   Q82.3   Incontinentia pigmenti

   Q82.4   Ectodermal dysplasia (anhidrotic)
     EXCLUDES 1   Ellis-van Creveld syndrome (Q77.6)

   Q82.5   Congenital non-neoplastic nevus
     Birthmark NOS
     Flammeus Nevus
     Portwine Nevus
     Sanguineous Nevus
     Strawberry Nevus
     Vascular Nevus NOS
     Verrucous Nevus
     EXCLUDES 2   araneus nevus (I78.1)
       Café au lait spots (L81.3)
       lentigo (L81.4)
       melanocytic nevus (D22.-)
       nevus NOS (D22.-)
       pigmented nevus (D22.-)
       spider nevus (I78.1)
       stellar nevus (I78.1)

   Q82.6   Congenital sacral dimple
     Parasacral dimple
     EXCLUDES 2   pilonidal cyst with abscess (L05.01)
       pilonidal cyst without abscess (L05.91)
     AHA: 2016,4Q,60

   Q82.8   Other specified congenital malformations of skin
     Abnormal palmar creases
     Accessory skin tags
     Benign familial pemphigus [Hailey-Hailey]
     Congenital poikiloderma
     Cutis laxa (hyperelastica)
     Dermatoglyphic anomalies
     Inherited keratosis palmaris et plantaris
     Keratosis follicularis [Darier-White]
     EXCLUDES 1   Ehlers-Danlos syndromes (Q79.6-)
     AHA: 2016,1Q,17

   Q82.9   Congenital malformation of skin, unspecified

✓4th **Q83   Congenital malformations of breast**
   EXCLUDES 2   absence of pectoral muscle (Q79.8)
     hypoplasia of breast (N64.82)
     micromastia (N64.82)

   Q83.0   Congenital absence of breast with absent nipple

   Q83.1   Accessory breast
     Supernumerary breast

   Q83.2   Absent nipple

   Q83.3   Accessory nipple
     Supernumerary nipple

   Q83.8   Other congenital malformations of breast

   Q83.9   Congenital malformation of breast, unspecified

✓4th **Q84   Other congenital malformations of integument**

   Q84.0   Congenital alopecia
     Congenital atrichosis

✓ Additional Character Required   ✓x7th Placeholder   Questionable PDx   Manifestation   Unspecified Dx   `UPD` Unacceptable PDx   `H1`-`H14` HAC   `HCC` CMS-HCC Dx   `HIV` HIV Dx

ICD-10-CM 2022   935

Chapter 17. Congenital Malformations, Deformations and Chromosomal Abnormalities

Q84.1–Q89.01

Q84.1 Congenital morphological disturbances of hair, not elsewhere classified
Beaded hair
Monilethrix
Pili annulati
> **EXCLUDES 1** *Menkes' kinky hair syndrome (E83.0)*

Q84.2 Other congenital malformations of hair
Congenital hypertrichosis
Congenital malformation of hair NOS
Persistent lanugo

Q84.3 Anonychia
> **EXCLUDES 1** *nail patella syndrome (Q87.2)*

Q84.4 Congenital leukonychia

Q84.5 Enlarged and hypertrophic nails
Congenital onychauxis
Pachyonychia

Q84.6 Other congenital malformations of nails
Congenital clubnail
Congenital koilonychia
Congenital malformation of nail NOS

Q84.8 Other specified congenital malformations of integument
Aplasia cutis congenita

Q84.9 Congenital malformation of integument, unspecified
Congenital anomaly of integument NOS
Congenital deformity of integument NOS

✓4ᵗʰ Q85 Phakomatoses, not elsewhere classified
> **EXCLUDES 1** *ataxia telangiectasia [Louis-Bar] (G11.3)*
> *familial dysautonomia [Riley-Day] (G90.1)*

✓5ᵗʰ Q85.0 Neurofibromatosis (nonmalignant)

Q85.00 Neurofibromatosis, unspecified   HCC

Q85.01 Neurofibromatosis, type 1   HCC
Von Recklinghausen disease

Q85.02 Neurofibromatosis, type 2   HCC
Acoustic neurofibromatosis
DEF: Inherited condition with cutaneous lesions, benign tumors of peripheral nerves, and bilateral 8th nerve masses.

Q85.03 Schwannomatosis   HCC
DEF: Genetic mutation (SMARCB1/INI1) causing multiple benign tumors along the nerve pathways, except on the 8th cranial (vestibular) nerve.

Q85.09 Other neurofibromatosis   HCC

Q85.1 Tuberous sclerosis   CC HCC
Bourneville's disease
Epiloia

Q85.8 Other phakomatoses, not elsewhere classified   CC HCC
Peutz-Jeghers Syndrome
Sturge-Weber(-Dimitri) syndrome
von Hippel-Lindau syndrome
> **EXCLUDES 1** *Meckel-Gruber syndrome (Q61.9)*

Q85.9 Phakomatosis, unspecified   CC HCC
Hamartosis NOS

✓4ᵗʰ Q86 Congenital malformation syndromes due to known exogenous causes, not elsewhere classified
> **EXCLUDES 2** *iodine-deficiency-related hypothyroidism (E00-E02)*
> *nonteratogenic effects of substances transmitted via placenta or breast milk (P04.-)*

Q86.0 Fetal alcohol syndrome (dysmorphic)

Q86.1 Fetal hydantoin syndrome
Meadow's syndrome

Q86.2 Dysmorphism due to warfarin

Q86.8 Other congenital malformation syndromes due to known exogenous causes

✓4ᵗʰ Q87 Other specified congenital malformation syndromes affecting multiple systems
Use additional code(s) to identify all associated manifestations

Q87.0 Congenital malformation syndromes predominantly affecting facial appearance
Acrocephalopolysyndactyly
Acrocephalosyndactyly [Apert]
Cryptophthalmos syndrome
Cyclopia
Goldenhar syndrome
Moebius syndrome
Oro-facial-digital syndrome
Robin syndrome
Whistling face

✓5ᵗʰ Q87.1 Congenital malformation syndromes predominantly associated with short stature
> **EXCLUDES 1** *Ellis-van Creveld syndrome (Q77.6)*
> *Smith-Lemli-Opitz syndrome (E78.72)*

AHA: 2019,4Q,14-15

Q87.11 Prader-Willi syndrome   CC

Q87.19 Other congenital malformation syndromes predominantly associated with short stature   CC
Aarskog syndrome
Cockayne syndrome
De Lange syndrome
Dubowitz syndrome
Noonan syndrome
Robinow-Silverman-Smith syndrome
Russell-Silver syndrome
Seckel syndrome

Q87.2 Congenital malformation syndromes predominantly involving limbs   CC
Holt-Oram syndrome
Klippel-Trenaunay-Weber syndrome
Nail patella syndrome
Rubinstein-Taybi syndrome
Sirenomelia syndrome
Thrombocytopenia with absent radius [TAR] syndrome
VATER syndrome

Q87.3 Congenital malformation syndromes involving early overgrowth   CC
Beckwith-Wiedemann syndrome
Sotos syndrome
Weaver syndrome

✓5ᵗʰ Q87.4 Marfan's syndrome
DEF: Disorder that affects the connective tissue of multiple systems, including disproportionally long or abnormal bone structure and eye and cardiovascular complications.

Q87.40 Marfan's syndrome, unspecified   CC

✓6ᵗʰ Q87.41 Marfan's syndrome with cardiovascular manifestations

Q87.410 Marfan's syndrome with aortic dilation   CC

Q87.418 Marfan's syndrome with other cardiovascular manifestations   CC

Q87.42 Marfan's syndrome with ocular manifestations   CC

Q87.43 Marfan's syndrome with skeletal manifestation   CC

Q87.5 Other congenital malformation syndromes with other skeletal changes   CC

✓5ᵗʰ Q87.8 Other specified congenital malformation syndromes, not elsewhere classified
> **EXCLUDES 1** *Zellweger syndrome (E71.510)*

Q87.81 Alport syndrome   CC
Use additional code to identify stage of chronic kidney disease (N18.1-N18.6)

Q87.82 Arterial tortuosity syndrome   CC
AHA: 2016,4Q,60-61

Q87.89 Other specified congenital malformation syndromes, not elsewhere classified   CC
Laurence-Moon (-Bardet)-Biedl syndrome

✓4ᵗʰ Q89 Other congenital malformations, not elsewhere classified

✓5ᵗʰ Q89.0 Congenital absence and malformations of spleen
> **EXCLUDES 1** *isomerism of atrial appendages (with asplenia or polysplenia) (Q20.6)*

Q89.01 Asplenia (congenital)   CC

N Newborn: 0   **P** Pediatric: 0-17   **M** Maternity: 9-64   **A** Adult: 15-124   **MCC** Major Complication/Comorbidity   **CC** Complication/Comorbidity   **SW** Severe Wound Dx

936

ICD-10-CM 2022

       Q89.09   **Congenital malformations of spleen**   `CC`
            Congenital splenomegaly

  Q89.1   **Congenital malformations of adrenal gland**
        `EXCLUDES 1`   *adrenogenital disorders (E25.-)*
                congenital adrenal hyperplasia (E25.0)

  Q89.2   **Congenital malformations of other endocrine glands**
        Congenital malformation of parathyroid or thyroid gland
        Persistent thyroglossal duct
        Thyroglossal cyst
        `EXCLUDES 1`   *congenital goiter (E03.0)*
                congenital hypothyroidism (E03.1)

  Q89.3   **Situs inversus**   `CC`
        Dextrocardia with situs inversus
        Mirror-image atrial arrangement with situs inversus
        Situs inversus or transversus abdominalis
        Situs inversus or transversus thoracis
        Transposition of abdominal viscera
        Transposition of thoracic viscera
        `EXCLUDES 1`   *dextrocardia NOS (Q24.0)*
        DEF: Congenital anomaly in which the internal thoracic and abdominal organs are transposed laterally and found on the opposite side from the normal position.

  Q89.4   **Conjoined twins**   `MCC`
        Craniopagus
        Dicephaly
        Pygopagus
        Thoracopagus

  Q89.7   **Multiple congenital malformations, not elsewhere classified**   `CC`
        Multiple congenital anomalies NOS
        Multiple congenital deformities NOS
        `EXCLUDES 1`   *congenital malformation syndromes affecting multiple systems (Q87.-)*

  Q89.8   **Other specified congenital malformations**   `CC`
        Use additional code(s) to identify all associated manifestations

  Q89.9   **Congenital malformation, unspecified**
        Congenital anomaly NOS
        Congenital deformity NOS

Chromosomal abnormalities, not elsewhere classified (Q90-Q99)

       `EXCLUDES 2`   *mitochondrial metabolic disorders (E88.4-)*

`√4th` **Q90**   **Down syndrome**
        Use additional code(s) to identify any associated physical conditions and degree of intellectual disabilities (F70-F79)

  Q90.0   **Trisomy 21, nonmosaicism (meiotic nondisjunction)**
  Q90.1   **Trisomy 21, mosaicism (mitotic nondisjunction)**
  Q90.2   **Trisomy 21, translocation**
  Q90.9   **Down syndrome, unspecified**
        Trisomy 21 NOS

`√4th` **Q91**   **Trisomy 18 and Trisomy 13**

  Q91.0   **Trisomy 18, nonmosaicism (meiotic nondisjunction)**   `CC`
  Q91.1   **Trisomy 18, mosaicism (mitotic nondisjunction)**   `CC`
  Q91.2   **Trisomy 18, translocation**   `CC`
  Q91.3   **Trisomy 18, unspecified**   `CC`
  Q91.4   **Trisomy 13, nonmosaicism (meiotic nondisjunction)**   `CC`
  Q91.5   **Trisomy 13, mosaicism (mitotic nondisjunction)**   `CC`
  Q91.6   **Trisomy 13, translocation**   `CC`
  Q91.7   **Trisomy 13, unspecified**   `CC`

`√4th` **Q92**   **Other trisomies and partial trisomies of the autosomes, not elsewhere classified**
       `INCLUDES`   unbalanced translocations and insertions
       `EXCLUDES 1`   *trisomies of chromosomes 13, 18, 21 (Q90-Q91)*

  Q92.0   **Whole chromosome trisomy, nonmosaicism (meiotic nondisjunction)**
  Q92.1   **Whole chromosome trisomy, mosaicism (mitotic nondisjunction)**
  Q92.2   **Partial trisomy**
        Less than whole arm duplicated
        Whole arm or more duplicated
        `EXCLUDES 1`   *partial trisomy due to unbalanced translocation (Q92.5)*

  Q92.5   **Duplications with other complex rearrangements**
        Partial trisomy due to unbalanced translocations
        Code also any associated deletions due to unbalanced translocations, inversions and insertions (Q93.7)

`√5th` **Q92.6**   **Marker chromosomes**
        Trisomies due to dicentrics
        Trisomies due to extra rings
        Trisomies due to isochromosomes
        Individual with marker heterochromatin
       Q92.61   **Marker chromosomes in normal individual**
       Q92.62   **Marker chromosomes in abnormal individual**

  Q92.7   **Triploidy and polyploidy**
  Q92.8   **Other specified trisomies and partial trisomies of autosomes**
        Duplications identified by fluorescence in situ hybridization (FISH)
        Duplications identified by in situ hybridization (ISH)
        Duplications seen only at prometaphase
  Q92.9   **Trisomy and partial trisomy of autosomes, unspecified**

`√4th` **Q93**   **Monosomies and deletions from the autosomes, not elsewhere classified**

  Q93.0   **Whole chromosome monosomy, nonmosaicism (meiotic nondisjunction)**
  Q93.1   **Whole chromosome monosomy, mosaicism (mitotic nondisjunction)**
  Q93.2   **Chromosome replaced with ring, dicentric or isochromosome**
  Q93.3   **Deletion of short arm of chromosome 4**   `CC`
        Wolff-Hirschorn syndrome
  Q93.4   **Deletion of short arm of chromosome 5**   `CC`
        Cri-du-chat syndrome

`√5th` **Q93.5**   **Other deletions of part of a chromosome**
        AHA: 2018,4Q,28
       Q93.51   **Angelman syndrome**   `CC`
       Q93.59   **Other deletions of part of a chromosome**   `CC`

  Q93.7   **Deletions with other complex rearrangements**   `CC`
        Deletions due to unbalanced translocations, inversions and insertions
        Code also any associated duplications due to unbalanced translocations, inversions and insertions (Q92.5)

`√5th` **Q93.8**   **Other deletions from the autosomes**

       Q93.81   **Velo-cardio-facial syndrome**   `MCC`
           Deletion 22q11.2
           AHA: 2019,3Q,14
           DEF: Microdeletion syndrome affecting multiple organs characterized by a cleft palate, heart defects, an elongated face with almond-shaped eyes, wide nose, small ears, weak immune system, weak musculature, hypothyroidism, short stature, and scoliosis. The deletion occurs at q11.2 on the long arm of the chromosome 22.

       Q93.82   **Williams syndrome**   `CC`
           AHA: 2018,4Q,28-29

       Q93.88   **Other microdeletions**   `CC`
           Miller-Dieker syndrome
           Smith-Magenis syndrome

       Q93.89   **Other deletions from the autosomes**   `CC`
           Deletions identified by fluorescence in situ hybridization (FISH)
           Deletions identified by in situ hybridization (ISH)
           Deletions seen only at prometaphase

  Q93.9   **Deletion from autosomes, unspecified**   `CC`

`√4th` **Q95**   **Balanced rearrangements and structural markers, not elsewhere classified**
       `INCLUDES`   Robertsonian and balanced reciprocal translocations and insertions

  Q95.0   **Balanced translocation and insertion in normal individual**
  Q95.1   **Chromosome inversion in normal individual**
  Q95.2   **Balanced autosomal rearrangement in abnormal individual**
  Q95.3   **Balanced sex/autosomal rearrangement in abnormal individual**
  Q95.5   **Individual with autosomal fragile site**
  Q95.8   **Other balanced rearrangements and structural markers**
  Q95.9   **Balanced rearrangement and structural marker, unspecified**

`√4th` **Q96**   **Turner's syndrome**
       `EXCLUDES 1`   *Noonan syndrome (Q87.19)*

  Q96.0   **Karyotype 45, X**   ♀

✔ Additional Character Required   `√x7th` Placeholder   Questionable PDx   Manifestation   Unspecified Dx   `UPD` Unacceptable PDx   `H1`-`H14` HAC   `HCC` CMS-HCC Dx   `HIV` HIV Dx

ICD-10-CM 2022   937

Q96.1 Karyotype 46, X iso (Xq) ♀
Karyotype 46, isochromosome Xq

Q96.2 Karyotype 46, X with abnormal sex chromosome, except iso (Xq) ♀
Karyotype 46, X with abnormal sex chromosome, except isochromosome Xq

Q96.3 Mosaicism, 45, X/46, XX or XY ♀

Q96.4 Mosaicism, 45, X/other cell line(s) with abnormal sex chromosome ♀

Q96.8 Other variants of Turner's syndrome ♀

Q96.9 Turner's syndrome, unspecified ♀

✓4ᵗʰ **Q97 Other sex chromosome abnormalities, female phenotype, not elsewhere classified**
> EXCLUDES 1   Turner's syndrome (Q96.-)

Q97.0 Karyotype 47, XXX ♀

Q97.1 Female with more than three X chromosomes ♀

Q97.2 Mosaicism, lines with various numbers of X chromosomes ♀

Q97.3 Female with 46, XY karyotype ♀

Q97.8 Other specified sex chromosome abnormalities, female phenotype ♀

Q97.9 Sex chromosome abnormality, female phenotype, unspecified ♀

✓4ᵗʰ **Q98 Other sex chromosome abnormalities, male phenotype, not elsewhere classified**

Q98.0 Klinefelter syndrome karyotype 47, XXY ♂

Q98.1 Klinefelter syndrome, male with more than two X chromosomes ♂

Q98.3 Other male with 46, XX karyotype ♂

Q98.4 Klinefelter syndrome, unspecified ♂

Q98.5 Karyotype 47, XYY

Q98.6 Male with structurally abnormal sex chromosome ♂

Q98.7 Male with sex chromosome mosaicism ♂

Q98.8 Other specified sex chromosome abnormalities, male phenotype ♂

Q98.9 Sex chromosome abnormality, male phenotype, unspecified ♂

✓4ᵗʰ **Q99 Other chromosome abnormalities, not elsewhere classified**

Q99.0 Chimera 46, XX/46, XY
Chimera 46, XX/46, XY true hermaphrodite

Q99.1 46, XX true hermaphrodite
46, XX with streak gonads
46, XY with streak gonads
Pure gonadal dysgenesis

Q99.2 Fragile X chromosome
Fragile X syndrome

Q99.8 Other specified chromosome abnormalities

Q99.9 Chromosomal abnormality, unspecified

Chapter 18. Symptoms, Signs and Abnormal Clinical and Laboratory Findings (R00–R99)

Chapter-specific Guidelines with Coding Examples

The chapter-specific guidelines from the ICD-10-CM Official Guidelines for Coding and Reporting have been provided below. Along with these guidelines are coding examples, contained in the shaded boxes, that have been developed to help illustrate the coding and/or sequencing guidance found in these guidelines.

Chapter 18 includes symptoms, signs, abnormal results of clinical or other investigative procedures, and ill-defined conditions regarding which no diagnosis classifiable elsewhere is recorded. Signs and symptoms that point to a specific diagnosis have been assigned to a category in other chapters of the classification.

a. Use of symptom codes

Codes that describe symptoms and signs are acceptable for reporting purposes when a related definitive diagnosis has not been established (confirmed) by the provider.

> Chest pain of unknown origin
>
> **R07.9   Chest pain, unspecified**
>
> *Explanation:* Codes that describe symptoms such as chest pain are acceptable for reporting purposes when the provider has not established (confirmed) a related definitive diagnosis.

b. Use of a symptom code with a definitive diagnosis code

Codes for signs and symptoms may be reported in addition to a related definitive diagnosis when the sign or symptom is not routinely associated with that diagnosis, such as the various signs and symptoms associated with complex syndromes. The definitive diagnosis code should be sequenced before the symptom code.

Signs or symptoms that are associated routinely with a disease process should not be assigned as additional codes, unless otherwise instructed by the classification.

> Pneumonia with hemoptysis
>
> **J18.9   Pneumonia, unspecified organism**
>
> **R04.2   Hemoptysis**
>
> *Explanation:* Codes for signs and symptoms may be reported in addition to a related definitive diagnosis when the sign or symptom is not routinely associated with that diagnosis.

> Abdominal pain due to acute appendicitis
>
> **K35.80   Unspecified acute appendicitis**
>
> *Explanation:* Codes for signs or symptoms routinely associated with a disease process should not be assigned unless the classification instructs otherwise.

c. Combination codes that include symptoms

ICD-10-CM contains a number of combination codes that identify both the definitive diagnosis and common symptoms of that diagnosis. When using one of these combination codes, an additional code should not be assigned for the symptom.

> Acute gastritis with hemorrhage
>
> **K29.01   Acute gastritis with bleeding**
>
> *Explanation:* When a combination code identifies both the definitive diagnosis and the symptom, an additional code should not be assigned for the symptom.

d. Repeated falls

Code R29.6, Repeated falls, is for use for encounters when a patient has recently fallen and the reason for the fall is being investigated.

Code Z91.81, History of falling, is for use when a patient has fallen in the past and is at risk for future falls. When appropriate, both codes R29.6 and Z91.81 may be assigned together.

e. Coma

Code R40.20, Unspecified coma, may be assigned in conjunction with codes for any medical condition.

Do not report codes for **unspecified coma**, individual or total Glasgow coma scale scores for a patient with a medically induced coma or a sedated patient.

1) Coma scale

The coma scale codes (R40.21- **to R40.24-**) can be used in conjunction with traumatic brain injury codes. These codes are primarily for use by trauma registries, but they may be used in any setting where this information is collected. The coma scale codes should be sequenced after the diagnosis code(s).

These codes, one from each subcategory, are needed to complete the scale. The 7th character indicates when the scale was recorded. The 7th character should match for all three codes.

At a minimum, report the initial score documented on presentation at your facility. This may be a score from the emergency medicine technician (EMT) or in the emergency department. If desired, a facility may choose to capture multiple coma scale scores.

Assign code R40.24-, Glasgow coma scale, total score, when only the total score is documented in the medical record and not the individual score(s).

If multiple coma scores are captured within the first 24 hours after hospital admission, assign only the code for the score at the time of admission. ICD-10-CM does not classify coma scores that are reported after admission but less than 24 hours later.

See Section I.B.14 for coma scale documentation by clinicians other than patient's provider

> 23-year-old man found down after unknown injury with skull fracture and with concussion and loss of consciousness of unknown duration. EMS evaluated the patient in the field and reported the individual Glasgow coma scores:
>
> Eye opening response—3: eyes open to speech
>
> Verbal response—4: confused but coherent speech
>
> Motor response—6: obeys commands fully
>
> **S02.0XXA   Fracture of vault of skull, initial encounter for closed fracture**
>
> **S06.0X9A   Concussion with loss of consciousness of unspecified duration, initial encounter**
>
> **R40.2131   Coma scale, eyes open, to sound, in the field [EMT or ambulance]**
>
> **R40.2241   Coma scale, best verbal response, confused conversation, in the field [EMT or ambulance]**
>
> **R40.2361   Coma scale, best motor response, obeys commands, in the field [EMT or ambulance]**
>
> *Explanation:* When individual scores for the Glasgow coma scale are documented, one code from each category is needed to complete the scale. The seventh character indicates when the scale was recorded and should match for all three codes. Assign a code from subcategory R40.24- Glasgow coma scale, total score, when only the total and not the individual score(s) is documented.

f. Functional quadriplegia

GUIDELINE HAS BEEN DELETED EFFECTIVE OCTOBER 1, 2017

g. SIRS due to non-infectious process

The systemic inflammatory response syndrome (SIRS) can develop as a result of certain non-infectious disease processes, such as trauma, malignant neoplasm, or pancreatitis. When SIRS is documented with a noninfectious condition, and no subsequent infection is documented, the code for the underlying condition, such as an injury, should be assigned, followed by code R65.10, Systemic inflammatory response syndrome (SIRS) of non-infectious origin without acute organ dysfunction, or code R65.11, Systemic inflammatory response syndrome (SIRS) of non-infectious origin with acute organ dysfunction. If an associated acute organ dysfunction is documented, the appropriate code(s) for the specific type of organ dysfunction(s) should be assigned in addition to code R65.11. If acute organ dysfunction is documented, but it cannot be determined if the acute organ dysfunction is associated with SIRS or due to another condition (e.g., directly due to the trauma), the provider should be queried.

Systemic inflammatory response syndrome (SIRS) due to acute gallstone pancreatitis

K85.1Ø	**Biliary acute pancreatitis without necrosis or infection**
R65.1Ø	**Systemic inflammatory response syndrome [SIRS] of non-infectious origin without acute organ dysfunction**

Explanation: When SIRS is documented with a non-infectious condition without subsequent infection documented, the code for the underlying condition such as pancreatitis should be assigned followed by the appropriate code for SIRS of noninfectious origin, either with or without associated organ dysfunction.

h. Death NOS

Code R99, Ill-defined and unknown cause of mortality, is only for use in the very limited circumstance when a patient who has already died is brought into an emergency department or other healthcare facility and is pronounced dead upon arrival. It does not represent the discharge disposition of death.

i. NIHSS stroke scale

The NIH stroke scale (NIHSS) codes (R29.7- -) can be used in conjunction with acute stroke codes (I63) to identify the patient's neurological status and the severity of the stroke. The stroke scale codes should be sequenced after the acute stroke diagnosis code(s).

At a minimum, report the initial score documented. If desired, a facility may choose to capture multiple stroke scale scores.

See Section I.B.14 for NIHSS stroke scale documentation by clinicians other than patient's provider

Patient admitted with CVA seen by neurology consult who documents moderate to severe stroke, 17 on NIHSS stroke scale.

I63.9	**Cerebral infarction, unspecified**
R29.717	**NIHSS score 17**

Explanation: Unspecified cerebral vascular accident (CVA) is sequenced before the NIHSS stroke scale score code. The stroke scale is an assessment tool to help measure stroke-related neurological deficits. Fifteen items are evaluated by trained observers and include such conditions as levels of consciousness, language, dysarthria, ataxia, and sensory loss. A facility may report multiple stroke scale scores if it wants to.

Chapter 18. Symptoms, Signs and Abnormal Clinical and Laboratory Findings, Not Elsewhere Classified (R00-R99)

NOTE This chapter includes symptoms, signs, abnormal results of clinical or other investigative procedures, and ill-defined conditions regarding which no diagnosis classifiable elsewhere is recorded.

Signs and symptoms that point rather definitely to a given diagnosis have been assigned to a category in other chapters of the classification. In general, categories in this chapter include the less well-defined conditions and symptoms that, without the necessary study of the case to establish a final diagnosis, point perhaps equally to two or more diseases or to two or more systems of the body. Practically all categories in the chapter could be designated 'not otherwise specified', 'unknown etiology' or 'transient'. The Alphabetical Index should be consulted to determine which symptoms and signs are to be allocated here and which to other chapters. The residual subcategories, numbered .8, are generally provided for other relevant symptoms that cannot be allocated elsewhere in the classification.

The conditions and signs or symptoms included in categories R00-R94 consist of:

(a) cases for which no more specific diagnosis can be made even after all the facts bearing on the case have been investigated;

(b) signs or symptoms existing at the time of initial encounter that proved to be transient and whose causes could not be determined;

(c) provisional diagnosis in a patient who failed to return for further investigation or care;

(d) cases referred elsewhere for investigation or treatment before the diagnosis was made;

(e) cases in which a more precise diagnosis was not available for any other reason;

(f) certain symptoms, for which supplementary information is provided, that represent important problems in medical care in their own right.

EXCLUDES 2   *abnormal findings on antenatal screening of mother (O28.-)*
certain conditions originating in the perinatal period (P04-P96)
signs and symptoms classified in the body system chapters
signs and symptoms of breast (N63, N64.5)

AHA: 2017,1Q,6,7

This chapter contains the following blocks:

R00-R09   Symptoms and signs involving the circulatory and respiratory systems
R10-R19   Symptoms and signs involving the digestive system and abdomen
R20-R23   Symptoms and signs involving the skin and subcutaneous tissue
R25-R29   Symptoms and signs involving the nervous and musculoskeletal systems
R30-R39   Symptoms and signs involving the genitourinary system
R40-R46   Symptoms and signs involving cognition, perception, emotional state and behavior
R47-R49   Symptoms and signs involving speech and voice
R50-R69   General symptoms and signs
R70-R79   Abnormal findings on examination of blood, without diagnosis
R80-R82   Abnormal findings on examination of urine, without diagnosis
R83-R89   Abnormal findings on examination of other body fluids, substances and tissues, without diagnosis
R90-R94   Abnormal findings on diagnostic imaging and in function studies, without diagnosis
R97   Abnormal tumor markers
R99   Ill-defined and unknown cause of mortality

Symptoms and signs involving the circulatory and respiratory systems (R00-R09)

R00   **Abnormalities of heart beat**

> *EXCLUDES 1*   *abnormalities originating in the perinatal period (P29.1-)*
> *EXCLUDES 2*   *specified arrhythmias (I47-I49)*

R00.0   **Tachycardia, unspecified**
Rapid heart beat
Sinoauricular tachycardia NOS
Sinus [sinusal] tachycardia NOS
> *EXCLUDES 1*   *neonatal tachycardia (P29.11)*
> *paroxysmal tachycardia (I47.-)*

DEF: Excessively rapid heart rate of more than 100 beats per minute.

R00.1   **Bradycardia, unspecified**
Sinoatrial bradycardia
Sinus bradycardia
Slow heart beat
Vagal bradycardia
Use additional code for adverse effect, if applicable, to identify drug (T36-T50 with fifth or sixth character 5)
> *EXCLUDES 1*   *neonatal bradycardia (P29.12)*

AHA: 2020,2Q,23
DEF: Slowed heartbeat, usually defined as a rate fewer than 60 beats per minute. Heart rhythm may be slow as a result of a congenital defect or an acquired problem.

R00.2   **Palpitations**
Awareness of heart beat

R00.8   **Other abnormalities of heart beat**

R00.9   **Unspecified abnormalities of heart beat**

R01   **Cardiac murmurs and other cardiac sounds**

> *EXCLUDES 1*   *cardiac murmurs and sounds originating in the perinatal period (P29.8)*

R01.0   **Benign and innocent cardiac murmurs**
Functional cardiac murmur

R01.1   **Cardiac murmur, unspecified**
Cardiac bruit NOS
Heart murmur NOS
Systolic murmur NOS

R01.2   **Other cardiac sounds**
Cardiac dullness, increased or decreased
Precordial friction

R03   **Abnormal blood-pressure reading, without diagnosis**

R03.0   **Elevated blood-pressure reading, without diagnosis of hypertension**
> **NOTE** This category is to be used to record an episode of elevated blood pressure in a patient in whom no formal diagnosis of hypertension has been made, or as an isolated incidental finding.

R03.1   **Nonspecific low blood-pressure reading**
> *EXCLUDES 1*   *hypotension (I95.-)*
> *maternal hypotension syndrome (O26.5-)*
> *neurogenic orthostatic hypotension (G90.3)*

R04   **Hemorrhage from respiratory passages**

R04.0   **Epistaxis**
Hemorrhage from nose
Nosebleed

R04.1   **Hemorrhage from throat**
> *EXCLUDES 2*   *hemoptysis (R04.2)*

R04.2   **Hemoptysis**   **CC**
Blood-stained sputum
Cough with hemorrhage
AHA: 2013,4Q,118

R04.8   **Hemorrhage from other sites in respiratory passages**

> **R04.81**   **Acute idiopathic pulmonary hemorrhage in infants**   **CC P**
> AIPHI
> Acute idiopathic hemorrhage in infants over 28 days old
> > *EXCLUDES 1*   *perinatal pulmonary hemorrhage (P26.-)*
> > *von Willebrand's disease (D68.0)*

> **R04.89**   **Hemorrhage from other sites in respiratory passages**   **CC**
> Pulmonary hemorrhage NOS

R04.9   **Hemorrhage from respiratory passages, unspecified**   **CC**

R05   **Cough**

> *EXCLUDES 1*   *cough with hemorrhage (R04.2)*
> ▶*paroxysmal cough due to Bordetella pertussis (A37.0-)*◄
> *smoker's cough (J41.0)*
> *EXCLUDES 2*   ▶*cough with hemorrhage (R04.2)*◄
AHA: 2016,2Q,33

● **R05.1**   **Acute cough**

● **R05.2**   **Subacute cough**

● **R05.3**   **Chronic cough**
Persistent cough
Refractory cough
Unexplained cough

Chapter 18. Symptoms, Signs and Abnormal Clinical and Laboratory Findings

R05.4–R09.89

● **R05.4** **Cough** syncope
> Code first syncope and collapse (R55)

● **R05.8** **Other specified cough**

● **R05.9** **Cough, unspecified**

✓4ᵗʰ **R06** **Abnormalities of breathing**
> EXCLUDES 1 acute respiratory distress syndrome (J80)
> respiratory arrest (R09.2)
> respiratory arrest of newborn (P28.81)
> respiratory distress syndrome of newborn (P22.-)
> respiratory failure (J96.-)
> respiratory failure of newborn (P28.5)

✓5ᵗʰ **R06.0** **Dyspnea**
> EXCLUDES 1 tachypnea NOS (R06.82)
> transient tachypnea of newborn (P22.1)

R06.00 **Dyspnea, unspecified**
> AHA: 2017,1Q,26

R06.01 **Orthopnea**

R06.02 **Shortness of breath**

R06.03 **Acute respiratory distress**
> AHA: 2017,4Q,23

R06.09 **Other forms of dyspnea**

R06.1 **Stridor**
> EXCLUDES 1 congenital laryngeal stridor (P28.89)
> laryngismus (stridulus) (J38.5)
> **DEF:** Certain type of wheezing described as a loud, constant, musical sound produced when breathing with an obstructed airway, like the inspiratory sound heard when laryngeal or esophageal obstruction is present.

R06.2 **Wheezing**
> EXCLUDES 1 asthma (J45.-)
> **AHA:** 2016,2Q,33
> **DEF:** High-pitched whistling sound during breathing due to stenosis of the respiratory passageway. Wheezing is associated with asthma, sleep apnea, bronchiectasis, bronchiolitis, COPD, and pleural effusion.

R06.3 **Periodic breathing** CC
> Cheyne-Stokes breathing

R06.4 **Hyperventilation**
> EXCLUDES 1 psychogenic hyperventilation (F45.8)

R06.5 **Mouth breathing**
> EXCLUDES 2 dry mouth NOS (R68.2)

R06.6 **Hiccough**
> EXCLUDES 1 psychogenic hiccough (F45.8)

R06.7 **Sneezing**

✓5ᵗʰ **R06.8** **Other abnormalities of breathing**

R06.81 **Apnea, not elsewhere classified**
> Apnea NOS
> EXCLUDES 1 apnea (of) newborn (P28.4)
> sleep apnea (G47.3-)
> sleep apnea of newborn (primary) (P28.3)

R06.82 **Tachypnea, not elsewhere classified**
> Tachypnea NOS
> EXCLUDES 1 transitory tachypnea of newborn (P22.1)

R06.83 **Snoring**

R06.89 **Other abnormalities of breathing**
> Breath-holding (spells)
> Sighing

R06.9 **Unspecified abnormalities of breathing**

✓4ᵗʰ **R07** **Pain in throat and chest**
> EXCLUDES 1 epidemic myalgia (B33.0)
> EXCLUDES 2 jaw pain R68.84
> pain in breast (N64.4)

R07.0 **Pain in** throat
> EXCLUDES 1 chronic sore throat (J31.2)
> sore throat (acute) NOS (J02.9)
> EXCLUDES 2 dysphagia (R13.1-)
> pain in neck (M54.2)

R07.1 **Chest pain on breathing**
> Painful respiration

R07.2 **Precordial pain**
> **DEF:** Pain felt in the anterior (front) chest wall over the region of the heart. This type of pain is generally felt slightly to the left of the sternum, but may also extend into the surrounding chest wall region.

✓5ᵗʰ **R07.8** **Other chest pain**

R07.81 **Pleurodynia**
> Pleurodynia NOS
> EXCLUDES 1 epidemic pleurodynia (B33.0)

R07.82 **Intercostal pain**

R07.89 **Other chest pain**
> Anterior chest-wall pain NOS
> **AHA:** 2021,1Q,42

R07.9 **Chest pain, unspecified**

✓4ᵗʰ **R09** **Other symptoms and signs involving the circulatory and respiratory system**
> EXCLUDES 1 acute respiratory distress syndrome (J80)
> respiratory arrest of newborn (P28.81)
> respiratory distress syndrome of newborn (P22.0)
> respiratory failure (J96.-)
> respiratory failure of newborn (P28.5)

✓5ᵗʰ **R09.0** **Asphyxia and hypoxemia**
> EXCLUDES 1 asphyxia due to carbon monoxide (T58.-)
> asphyxia due to foreign body in respiratory tract (T17.-)
> birth (intrauterine) asphyxia (P84)
> hyperventilation (R06.4)
> traumatic asphyxia (T71.-)
> EXCLUDES 2 hypercapnia (R06.89)

R09.01 **Asphyxia** CC
> **DEF:** Interference of oxygen intake due to obstruction or injury of airways resulting in a lack of oxygen perfusion to the tissues or excessive carbon dioxide in the blood. Can cause unconsciousness or death.

R09.02 **Hypoxemia**
> **AHA:** 2019,3Q,15
> **DEF:** Insufficient oxygen in the arterial blood resulting in inadequate delivery of oxygen to the body tissues.

R09.1 **Pleurisy**
> EXCLUDES 1 pleurisy with effusion (J90)

1 **R09.2** **Respiratory arrest** MCC HCC
> Cardiorespiratory failure
> EXCLUDES 1 cardiac arrest (I46.-)
> respiratory arrest of newborn (P28.81)
> respiratory distress of newborn (P22.0)
> respiratory failure (J96.-)
> respiratory failure of newborn (P28.5)
> respiratory insufficiency (R06.89)
> respiratory insufficiency of newborn (P28.5)

R09.3 **Abnormal sputum**
> Abnormal amount of sputum
> Abnormal color of sputum
> Abnormal odor of sputum
> Excessive sputum
> EXCLUDES 1 blood-stained sputum (R04.2)

✓5ᵗʰ **R09.8** **Other specified symptoms and signs involving the circulatory and respiratory systems**

R09.81 **Nasal congestion**

R09.82 **Postnasal drip**

R09.89 **Other specified symptoms and signs involving the circulatory and respiratory systems**
> Abnormal chest percussion
> Bruit (arterial)
> Chest tympany
> Choking sensation
> Feeling of foreign body in throat
> Friction sounds in chest
> Rales
> Weak pulse
> EXCLUDES 2 foreign body in throat (T17.2-)
> wheezing (R06.2)
> **AHA:** 2021,1Q,42

N Newborn: 0   P Pediatric: 0-17   M Maternity: 9-64   A Adult: 15-124   MCC Major Complication/Comorbidity   CC Complication/Comorbidity   SW Severe Wound Dx

942

ICD-10-CM 2022

Symptoms and signs involving the digestive system and abdomen (R10-R19)

EXCLUDES 2   congenital or infantile pylorospasm (Q40.0)
gastrointestinal hemorrhage (K92.0-K92.2)
intestinal obstruction (K56.-)
newborn gastrointestinal hemorrhage (P54.0-P54.3)
newborn intestinal obstruction (P76.-)
pylorospasm (K31.3)
signs and symptoms involving the urinary system (R30-R39)
symptoms referable to female genital organs (N94.-)
symptoms referable to male genital organs (N48-N50)

✓4th **R10   Abdominal and pelvic pain**
    EXCLUDES 1   *renal colic (N23)*
    EXCLUDES 2   *dorsalgia (M54.-)*
             flatulence and related conditions (R14.-)

   R10.0   Acute abdomen
      Severe abdominal pain (generalized) (with abdominal rigidity)
      EXCLUDES 1   *abdominal rigidity NOS (R19.3)*
              generalized abdominal pain NOS (R10.84)
              localized abdominal pain (R10.1-R10.3-)

✓5th **R10.1   Pain localized to upper abdomen**
     R10.10   Upper abdominal pain, unspecified
     R10.11   Right upper quadrant pain
     R10.12   Left upper quadrant pain
     R10.13   Epigastric pain
         Dyspepsia
         EXCLUDES 1   *functional dyspepsia (K30)*

Abdominal Pain

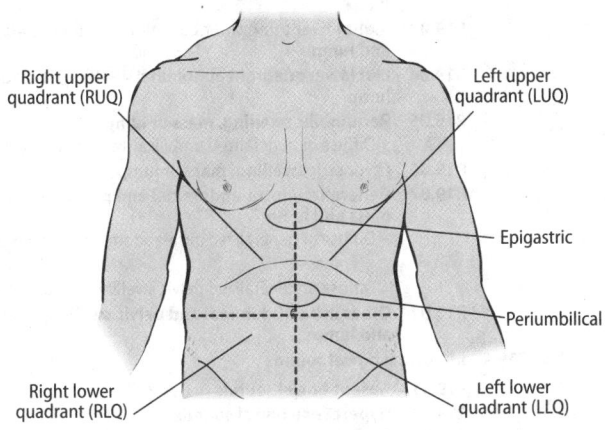

Right upper quadrant (RUQ)   Left upper quadrant (LUQ)
Epigastric
Periumbilical
Right lower quadrant (RLQ)   Left lower quadrant (LLQ)

   R10.2   Pelvic and perineal pain
      EXCLUDES 1   *vulvodynia (N94.81)*
✓5th **R10.3   Pain localized to other parts of lower abdomen**
     R10.30   Lower abdominal pain, unspecified
     R10.31   Right lower quadrant pain
     R10.32   Left lower quadrant pain
     R10.33   Periumbilical pain
✓5th **R10.8   Other abdominal pain**
    ✓6th **R10.81   Abdominal tenderness**
       Abdominal tenderness NOS
       R10.811   Right upper quadrant abdominal tenderness
       R10.812   Left upper quadrant abdominal tenderness
       R10.813   Right lower quadrant abdominal tenderness
       R10.814   Left lower quadrant abdominal tenderness
       R10.815   Periumbilic abdominal tenderness
       R10.816   Epigastric abdominal tenderness
       R10.817   Generalized abdominal tenderness
       R10.819   Abdominal tenderness, unspecified site
    ✓6th **R10.82   Rebound abdominal tenderness**
       R10.821   Right upper quadrant rebound abdominal tenderness
       R10.822   Left upper quadrant rebound abdominal tenderness
       R10.823   Right lower quadrant rebound abdominal tenderness

       R10.824   Left lower quadrant rebound abdominal tenderness
       R10.825   Periumbilic rebound abdominal tenderness
       R10.826   Epigastric rebound abdominal tenderness
       R10.827   Generalized rebound abdominal tenderness
       R10.829   Rebound abdominal tenderness, unspecified site
   R10.83   Colic   P
      Colic NOS
      Infantile colic
      EXCLUDES 1   *colic in adult and child over 12 months old (R10.84)*
      DEF: Inconsolable crying in an otherwise well-fed and healthy infant for more than three hours a day, three days a week, for more than three weeks.
   R10.84   Generalized abdominal pain
      EXCLUDES 1   *generalized abdominal pain associated with acute abdomen (R10.0)*
   R10.9   Unspecified abdominal pain

✓4th **R11   Nausea and vomiting**
    EXCLUDES 1   *cyclical vomiting associated with migraine (G43.A-)*
              excessive vomiting in pregnancy (O21.-)
              hematemesis (K92.0)
              neonatal hematemesis (P54.0)
              newborn vomiting (P92.0-)
              psychogenic vomiting (F50.89)
              vomiting associated with bulimia nervosa (F50.2)
              vomiting following gastrointestinal surgery (K91.0)
    AHA: 2017,1Q,28
   R11.0   Nausea
      Nausea NOS
      Nausea without vomiting
    ✓5th **R11.1   Vomiting**
     R11.10   Vomiting, unspecified
        Vomiting NOS
     R11.11   Vomiting without nausea
     R11.12   Projectile vomiting
     R11.13   Vomiting of fecal matter
     R11.14   Bilious vomiting
        Bilious emesis
     R11.15   Cyclical vomiting syndrome unrelated to migraine
        Cyclic vomiting syndrome NOS
        Persistent vomiting
        EXCLUDES 1   *cyclical vomiting in migraine (G43.A-)*
        EXCLUDES 2   *bulimia nervosa (F50.2)*
                diabetes mellitus due to underlying condition (E08.-)
        AHA: 2019,4Q,15
   R11.2   Nausea with vomiting, unspecified
      Persistent nausea with vomiting NOS
      AHA: 2020,1Q,8

   R12   Heartburn
      EXCLUDES 1   *dyspepsia NOS (R10.13)*
             functional dyspepsia (K30)

✓4th **R13   Aphagia and dysphagia**
   R13.0   Aphagia
      Inability to swallow
      EXCLUDES 1   *psychogenic aphagia (F50.9)*

✓5ᵗʰ **R13.1 Dysphagia**

Code first, if applicable, dysphagia following cerebrovascular disease (I69. with final characters -91)

EXCLUDES 1   *psychogenic dysphagia (F45.8)*

Swallowing Function

Oral phase

Oropharyngeal phase

Pharyngeal phase

Pharyngoesophageal phase

R13.10 Dysphagia, unspecified
Difficulty in swallowing NOS

R13.11 Dysphagia, oral phase

R13.12 Dysphagia, oropharyngeal phase

R13.13 Dysphagia, pharyngeal phase

R13.14 Dysphagia, pharyngoesophageal phase

R13.19 Other dysphagia
Cervical dysphagia
Neurogenic dysphagia

✓4ᵗʰ **R14 Flatulence and related conditions**

EXCLUDES 1   *psychogenic aerophagy (F45.8)*

R14.0 Abdominal distension (gaseous)
Bloating
Tympanites (abdominal) (intestinal)

R14.1 Gas pain

R14.2 Eructation

R14.3 Flatulence

✓4ᵗʰ **R15 Fecal incontinence**

INCLUDES   encopresis NOS

EXCLUDES 1   *fecal incontinence of nonorganic origin (F98.1)*

R15.0 Incomplete defecation

EXCLUDES 1   *constipation (K59.0-)*
fecal impaction (K56.41)

R15.1 Fecal smearing
Fecal soiling

R15.2 Fecal urgency

R15.9 Full incontinence of feces
Fecal incontinence NOS

✓4ᵗʰ **R16 Hepatomegaly and splenomegaly, not elsewhere classified**

R16.0 Hepatomegaly, not elsewhere classified
Hepatomegaly NOS

R16.1 Splenomegaly, not elsewhere classified
Splenomegaly NOS

R16.2 Hepatomegaly with splenomegaly, not elsewhere classified
Hepatosplenomegaly NOS

R17 Unspecified jaundice   CC

EXCLUDES 1   *neonatal jaundice (P55, P57-P59)*

✓4ᵗʰ **R18 Ascites**

INCLUDES   fluid in peritoneal cavity

EXCLUDES 1   *ascites in alcoholic cirrhosis (K70.31)*
ascites in alcoholic hepatitis (K70.11)
ascites in toxic liver disease with chronic active hepatitis (K71.51)

DEF: Abnormal accumulation of free fluid in the abdominal cavity, causing distention and tightness in addition to shortness of breath as the fluid accumulates. Ascites is usually an underlying disorder and can be a manifestation of any number of diseases.

R18.0 Malignant ascites   CC UPD

Code first malignancy, such as:
malignant neoplasm of ovary (C56.-)
secondary malignant neoplasm of retroperitoneum and peritoneum (C78.6)

R18.8 Other ascites   CC

Ascites NOS
Peritoneal effusion (chronic)
AHA: 2018,1Q,4

✓4ᵗʰ **R19 Other symptoms and signs involving the digestive system and abdomen**

EXCLUDES 1   *acute abdomen (R10.0)*

✓5ᵗʰ **R19.0 Intra-abdominal and pelvic swelling, mass and lump**

EXCLUDES 1   *abdominal distension (gaseous) (R14.-)*
ascites (R18.-)

R19.00 Intra-abdominal and pelvic swelling, mass and lump, unspecified site

R19.01 Right upper quadrant abdominal swelling, mass and lump

R19.02 Left upper quadrant abdominal swelling, mass and lump

R19.03 Right lower quadrant abdominal swelling, mass and lump

R19.04 Left lower quadrant abdominal swelling, mass and lump

R19.05 Periumbilic swelling, mass or lump
Diffuse or generalized umbilical swelling or mass

R19.06 Epigastric swelling, mass or lump

R19.07 Generalized intra-abdominal and pelvic swelling, mass and lump
Diffuse or generalized intra-abdominal swelling or mass NOS
Diffuse or generalized pelvic swelling or mass NOS

R19.09 Other intra-abdominal and pelvic swelling, mass and lump

✓5ᵗʰ **R19.1 Abnormal bowel sounds**

R19.11 Absent bowel sounds

R19.12 Hyperactive bowel sounds

R19.15 Other abnormal bowel sounds
Abnormal bowel sounds NOS

R19.2 Visible peristalsis
Hyperperistalsis
DEF: Visible movements of muscular attempts to move food through the digestive tract due to pyloric obstruction, stomach obstruction, or intestinal obstruction.

✓5ᵗʰ **R19.3 Abdominal rigidity**

EXCLUDES 1   *abdominal rigidity with severe abdominal pain (R10.0)*

R19.30 Abdominal rigidity, unspecified site

R19.31 Right upper quadrant abdominal rigidity

R19.32 Left upper quadrant abdominal rigidity

R19.33 Right lower quadrant abdominal rigidity

R19.34 Left lower quadrant abdominal rigidity

R19.35 Periumbilic abdominal rigidity

R19.36 Epigastric abdominal rigidity

R19.37 Generalized abdominal rigidity

R19.4 Change in bowel habit

EXCLUDES 1   *constipation (K59.0-)*
functional diarrhea (K59.1)

N Newborn: 0   P Pediatric: 0-17   M Maternity: 9-64   A Adult: 15-124   MCC Major Complication/Comorbidity   CC Complication/Comorbidity   SW Severe Wound Dx

944   ICD-10-CM 2022

R19.5 Other fecal abnormalities
Abnormal stool color
Bulky stools
Mucus in stools
Occult blood in feces
Occult blood in stools
    EXCLUDES 1   *melena (K92.1)*
                neonatal melena (P54.1)
    AHA: 2021,1Q,9; 2019,1Q,32

R19.6 Halitosis

R19.7 Diarrhea, unspecified
Diarrhea NOS
    EXCLUDES 1   *functional diarrhea (K59.1)*
                neonatal diarrhea (P78.3)
                psychogenic diarrhea (F45.8)

R19.8 Other specified symptoms and signs involving the digestive system and abdomen

Symptoms and signs involving the skin and subcutaneous tissue (R20-R23)

    EXCLUDES 2   *symptoms relating to breast (N64.4-N64.5)*

✓4ᵗʰ R20 Disturbances of skin sensation
    EXCLUDES 1   *dissociative anesthesia and sensory loss (F44.6)*
                psychogenic disturbances (F45.8)

R20.0 Anesthesia of skin

R20.1 Hypoesthesia of skin

R20.2 Paresthesia of skin
Formication
Pins and needles
Tingling skin
    EXCLUDES 1   *acroparesthesia (I73.8)*

R20.3 Hyperesthesia

R20.8 Other disturbances of skin sensation

R20.9 Unspecified disturbances of skin sensation

R21 Rash and other nonspecific skin eruption
    INCLUDES   rash NOS
    EXCLUDES 1   *specified type of rash - code to condition*
                vesicular eruption (R23.8)

✓4ᵗʰ R22 Localized swelling, mass and lump of skin and subcutaneous tissue
    INCLUDES   subcutaneous nodules (localized)(superficial)
    EXCLUDES 1   *abnormal findings on diagnostic imaging (R90-R93)*
                edema (R60.-)
                enlarged lymph nodes (R59.-)
                localized adiposity (E65)
                swelling of joint (M25.4-)

R22.0 Localized swelling, mass and lump, head

R22.1 Localized swelling, mass and lump, neck

R22.2 Localized swelling, mass and lump, trunk
    EXCLUDES 1   *intra-abdominal or pelvic mass and lump (R19.0-)*
                intra-abdominal or pelvic swelling (R19.0-)
    EXCLUDES 2   *breast mass and lump (N63)*

✓5ᵗʰ R22.3 Localized swelling, mass and lump, upper limb

    R22.30 Localized swelling, mass and lump, unspecified upper limb

    R22.31 Localized swelling, mass and lump, right upper limb

    R22.32 Localized swelling, mass and lump, left upper limb

    R22.33 Localized swelling, mass and lump, upper limb, bilateral

✓5ᵗʰ R22.4 Localized swelling, mass and lump, lower limb

    R22.40 Localized swelling, mass and lump, unspecified lower limb

    R22.41 Localized swelling, mass and lump, right lower limb

    R22.42 Localized swelling, mass and lump, left lower limb

    R22.43 Localized swelling, mass and lump, lower limb, bilateral

R22.9 Localized swelling, mass and lump, unspecified

✓4ᵗʰ R23 Other skin changes

R23.0 Cyanosis
    EXCLUDES 1   *acrocyanosis (I73.8)*
                cyanotic attacks of newborn (P28.2)
    DEF: Bluish or purplish discoloration of the skin due to an inadequate oxygen blood level.

R23.1 Pallor
Clammy skin

R23.2 Flushing
Excessive blushing
Code first, if applicable, menopausal and female climacteric states (N95.1)

R23.3 Spontaneous ecchymoses
Petechiae
    EXCLUDES 1   *ecchymoses of newborn (P54.5)*
                purpura (D69.-)

R23.4 Changes in skin texture
Desquamation of skin
Induration of skin
Scaling of skin
    EXCLUDES 1   *epidermal thickening NOS (L85.9)*

R23.8 Other skin changes

R23.9 Unspecified skin changes

Symptoms and signs involving the nervous and musculoskeletal systems (R25-R29)

✓4ᵗʰ R25 Abnormal involuntary movements
    EXCLUDES 1   *specific movement disorders (G20-G26)*
                stereotyped movement disorders (F98.4)
                tic disorders (F95.-)

R25.0 Abnormal head movements

R25.1 Tremor, unspecified
    EXCLUDES 1   *chorea NOS (G25.5)*
                essential tremor (G25.0)
                hysterical tremor (F44.4)
                intention tremor (G25.2)

R25.2 Cramp and spasm
    EXCLUDES 2   *carpopedal spasm (R29.0)*
                charley-horse (M62.831)
                infantile spasms (G40.4-)
                muscle spasm of back (M62.830)
                muscle spasm of calf (M62.831)

R25.3 Fasciculation
Twitching NOS

R25.8 Other abnormal involuntary movements

R25.9 Unspecified abnormal involuntary movements

✓4ᵗʰ R26 Abnormalities of gait and mobility
    EXCLUDES 1   *ataxia NOS (R27.0)*
                hereditary ataxia (G11.-)
                locomotor (syphilitic) ataxia (A52.11)
                immobility syndrome (paraplegic) (M62.3)

R26.0 Ataxic gait
Staggering gait

R26.1 Paralytic gait
Spastic gait

R26.2 Difficulty in walking, not elsewhere classified
    EXCLUDES 1   *falling (R29.6)*
                unsteadiness on feet (R26.81)
    AHA: 2016,2Q,7

✓5ᵗʰ R26.8 Other abnormalities of gait and mobility

    R26.81 Unsteadiness on feet

    R26.89 Other abnormalities of gait and mobility
        AHA: 2020,2Q,29

R26.9 Unspecified abnormalities of gait and mobility

✓4ᵗʰ R27 Other lack of coordination
    EXCLUDES 1   *ataxic gait (R26.0)*
                hereditary ataxia (G11.-)
                vertigo NOS (R42)

R27.0 Ataxia, unspecified
    EXCLUDES 1   *ataxia following cerebrovascular disease (I69. with final characters -93)*

R27.8 Other lack of coordination

R27.9 Unspecified lack of coordination

☑ Additional Character Required   ✓x7ᵗʰ Placeholder   Questionable PDx   Manifestation   Unspecified Dx   UPD Unacceptable PDx   H1-H14 HAC   HCC CMS-HCC Dx   HIV HIV Dx

ICD-10-CM 2022   945

✓4ᵗʰ **R29 Other symptoms and signs involving the nervous and musculoskeletal systems**

R29.0 Tetany CC
Carpopedal spasm
EXCLUDES 1 *hysterical tetany (F44.5)*
neonatal tetany (P71.3)
parathyroid tetany (E20.9)
post-thyroidectomy tetany (E89.2)
DEF: Calcium or other mineral imbalance causing voluntary muscles such as hands, feet, or larynx to spasm rhythmically.

R29.1 Meningismus CC

R29.2 Abnormal reflex
EXCLUDES 2 *abnormal pupillary reflex (H57.0)*
hyperactive gag reflex (J39.2)
vasovagal reaction or syncope (R55)

R29.3 Abnormal posture

R29.4 Clicking hip
EXCLUDES 1 *congenital deformities of hip (Q65.-)*

R29.5 Transient paralysis CC
Code first any associated spinal cord injury (S14.0, S14.1-, S24.0, S24.1-, S34.0-, S34.1-)
EXCLUDES 1 *transient ischemic attack (G45.9)*

R29.6 Repeated falls
Falling
Tendency to fall
EXCLUDES 2 *at risk for falling (Z91.81)*
history of falling (Z91.81)
AHA: 2016,2Q,6
TIP: Code in addition to Parkinson's disease (G20), when documented.

✓5ᵗʰ **R29.7 National Institutes of Health Stroke Scale (NIHSS) score**
Code first the type of cerebral infarction (I63.-)
AHA: 2016,4Q,61-62
TIP: Codes from this subcategory may be assigned based on medical record documentation from clinicians who are not the patient's provider.

✓6ᵗʰ **R29.70 NIHSS score 0-9**
R29.700 NIHSS score 0 UPD
R29.701 NIHSS score 1 UPD
R29.702 NIHSS score 2 UPD
R29.703 NIHSS score 3 UPD
R29.704 NIHSS score 4 UPD
R29.705 NIHSS score 5 UPD
R29.706 NIHSS score 6 UPD
R29.707 NIHSS score 7 UPD
R29.708 NIHSS score 8 UPD
R29.709 NIHSS score 9 UPD

✓6ᵗʰ **R29.71 NIHSS score 10-19**
R29.710 NIHSS score 10 UPD
R29.711 NIHSS score 11 UPD
R29.712 NIHSS score 12 UPD
R29.713 NIHSS score 13 UPD
R29.714 NIHSS score 14 UPD
R29.715 NIHSS score 15 UPD
R29.716 NIHSS score 16 UPD
R29.717 NIHSS score 17 UPD
R29.718 NIHSS score 18 UPD
R29.719 NIHSS score 19 UPD

✓6ᵗʰ **R29.72 NIHSS score 20-29**
R29.720 NIHSS score 20 UPD
R29.721 NIHSS score 21 UPD
R29.722 NIHSS score 22 UPD
R29.723 NIHSS score 23 UPD
R29.724 NIHSS score 24 UPD
R29.725 NIHSS score 25 UPD
R29.726 NIHSS score 26 UPD
R29.727 NIHSS score 27 UPD
R29.728 NIHSS score 28 UPD
R29.729 NIHSS score 29 UPD

✓6ᵗʰ **R29.73 NIHSS score 30-39**
R29.730 NIHSS score 30 UPD
R29.731 NIHSS score 31 UPD
R29.732 NIHSS score 32 UPD
R29.733 NIHSS score 33 UPD
R29.734 NIHSS score 34 UPD
R29.735 NIHSS score 35 UPD
R29.736 NIHSS score 36 UPD
R29.737 NIHSS score 37 UPD
R29.738 NIHSS score 38 UPD
R29.739 NIHSS score 39 UPD

✓6ᵗʰ **R29.74 NIHSS score 40-42**
R29.740 NIHSS score 40 UPD
R29.741 NIHSS score 41 UPD
R29.742 NIHSS score 42 UPD

✓5ᵗʰ **R29.8 Other symptoms and signs involving the nervous and musculoskeletal systems**

✓6ᵗʰ **R29.81 Other symptoms and signs involving the nervous system**
R29.810 Facial weakness
Facial droop
EXCLUDES 1 *Bell's palsy (G51.0)*
facial weakness following cerebrovascular disease (I69. with final characters -92)
R29.818 Other symptoms and signs involving the nervous system

✓6ᵗʰ **R29.89 Other symptoms and signs involving the musculoskeletal system**
EXCLUDES 2 *pain in limb (M79.6-)*
R29.890 Loss of height
EXCLUDES 1 *osteoporosis (M80-M81)*
R29.891 Ocular torticollis
EXCLUDES 1 *congenital (sternomastoid) torticollis Q68.0*
psychogenic torticollis (F45.8)
spasmodic torticollis (G24.3)
torticollis due to birth injury (P15.8)
torticollis NOS M43.6
DEF: Abnormal head posture as a result of a contracted state of cervical muscles to correct a visual disturbance, either double vision or a visual field defect.
R29.898 Other symptoms and signs involving the musculoskeletal system

✓5ᵗʰ **R29.9 Unspecified symptoms and signs involving the nervous and musculoskeletal systems**
R29.90 Unspecified symptoms and signs involving the nervous system
R29.91 Unspecified symptoms and signs involving the musculoskeletal system

Symptoms and signs involving the genitourinary system (R30-R39)

✓4ᵗʰ **R30 Pain associated with micturition**
EXCLUDES 1 *psychogenic pain associated with micturition (F45.8)*
R30.0 Dysuria
Strangury
R30.1 Vesical tenesmus
DEF: Feeling of a full bladder even when there is little or no urine in the bladder.
R30.9 Painful micturition, unspecified
Painful urination NOS

✓4ᵗʰ **R31 Hematuria**
EXCLUDES 1 *hematuria included with underlying conditions, such as:*
acute cystitis with hematuria (N30.01)
recurrent and persistent hematuria in glomerular diseases (N02.-)
AHA: 2017,1Q,17
R31.0 Gross hematuria
R31.1 Benign essential microscopic hematuria
✓5ᵗʰ **R31.2 Other microscopic hematuria**
AHA: 2016,4Q,62
R31.21 Asymptomatic microscopic hematuria
AMH
R31.29 Other microscopic hematuria
R31.9 Hematuria, unspecified

R32 Unspecified urinary incontinence
Enuresis NOS
> EXCLUDES 1   functional urinary incontinence (R39.81)
> nonorganic enuresis (F98.0)
> stress incontinence and other specified urinary incontinence (N39.3-N39.4-)
> urinary incontinence associated with cognitive impairment (R39.81)

✓4ᵗʰ **R33 Retention of urine**
> EXCLUDES 1   psychogenic retention of urine (F45.8)

R33.0 Drug induced retention of urine
Use additional code for adverse effect, if applicable, to identify drug (T36-T50 with fifth or sixth character 5)

R33.8 Other retention of urine
Code first, if applicable, any causal condition, such as:
enlarged prostate (N40.1)
AHA: 2018,4Q,55

R33.9 Retention of urine, unspecified

R34 Anuria and oliguria
> EXCLUDES 1   anuria and oliguria complicating abortion or ectopic or molar pregnancy (O00-O07, O08.4)
> anuria and oliguria complicating pregnancy (O26.83-)
> anuria and oliguria complicating the puerperium (O90.4)

✓4ᵗʰ **R35 Polyuria**
Code first, if applicable, any causal condition, such as:
enlarged prostate (N40.1)
> EXCLUDES 1   psychogenic polyuria (F45.8)

R35.0 Frequency of micturition
R35.1 Nocturia
▲ ✓6ᵗʰ **R35.8 Other polyuria**
Polyuria NOS
● **R35.81 Nocturnal polyuria**
> EXCLUDES 2   nocturnal enuresis (N39.44)
● **R35.89 Other polyuria**
Polyuria NOS

✓4ᵗʰ **R36 Urethral discharge**
R36.0 Urethral discharge without blood
R36.1 Hematospermia   ♂
R36.9 Urethral discharge, unspecified
Penile discharge NOS
Urethrorrhea

R37 Sexual dysfunction, unspecified

✓4ᵗʰ **R39 Other and unspecified symptoms and signs involving the genitourinary system**
R39.0 Extravasation of urine   CC
✓6ᵗʰ **R39.1 Other difficulties with micturition**
Code first, if applicable, any causal condition, such as:
enlarged prostate (N40.1)
R39.11 Hesitancy of micturition
R39.12 Poor urinary stream
Weak urinary steam
R39.13 Splitting of urinary stream
R39.14 Feeling of incomplete bladder emptying
R39.15 Urgency of urination
> EXCLUDES 1   urge incontinence (N39.41, N39.46)
R39.16 Straining to void
✓6ᵗʰ **R39.19 Other difficulties with micturition**
AHA: 2016,4Q,63
R39.191 Need to immediately re-void
R39.192 Position dependent micturition
R39.198 Other difficulties with micturition
R39.2 Extrarenal uremia
Prerenal uremia
> EXCLUDES 1   uremia NOS (N19)
✓5ᵗʰ **R39.8 Other symptoms and signs involving the genitourinary system**
AHA: 2017,4Q,22-23
R39.81 Functional urinary incontinence
Urinary incontinence due to cognitive impairment, or severe physical disability or immobility
> EXCLUDES 1   stress incontinence and other specified urinary incontinence (N39.3-N39.4-)
> urinary incontinence NOS (R32)

R39.82 Chronic bladder pain
AHA: 2016,4Q,64
R39.83 Unilateral non-palpable testicle   ♂
R39.84 Bilateral non-palpable testicles   ♂
R39.89 Other symptoms and signs involving the genitourinary system
R39.9 Unspecified symptoms and signs involving the genitourinary system

Symptoms and signs involving cognition, perception, emotional state and behavior (R40-R46)

> EXCLUDES 2   symptoms and signs constituting part of a pattern of mental disorder (F01-F99)

✓4ᵗʰ **R40 Somnolence, stupor and coma**
> EXCLUDES 1   neonatal coma (P91.5)
> somnolence, stupor and coma in diabetes (E08-E13)
> somnolence, stupor and coma in hepatic failure (K72.-)
> somnolence, stupor and coma in hypoglycemia (nondiabetic) (E15)

R40.0 Somnolence
Drowsiness
> EXCLUDES 1   coma (R40.2-)

R40.1 Stupor
Catatonic stupor
Semicoma
> EXCLUDES 1   catatonic schizophrenia (F20.2)
> coma (R40.2-)
> depressive stupor (F31-F33)
> dissociative stupor (F44.2)
> manic stupor (F30.2)

✓5ᵗʰ **R40.2 Coma**
Code first any associated:
fracture of skull (S02.-)
intracranial injury (S06.-)
> NOTE   One code from each subcategory, R40.21-R40.23, is required to complete the coma scale

AHA: 2020,3Q,46; 2019,2Q,12; 2018,4Q,70; 2017,4Q,23-25,95; 2015,2Q,17; 2014,1Q,19
TIP: The codes for individual (R40.21-, R40.22-, R40.23-) or total (R40.24-) coma scale scores are only assigned as secondary diagnoses with traumatic brain injury (TBI) codes (S06.2X-, S06.30-, S06.9X-). While individual or total coma scale scores may be useful to providers in their clinical decision making when trying to establish a diagnosis, the codes reflecting these scores may not be assigned in conjunction with conditions other than TBIs.
TIP: Codes for individual (R40.21-, R40.22-, R40.23-) or total (R40.24-) coma scale scores may be assigned based on medical record documentation from clinicians who are not the patient's provider.
TIP: It is not appropriate to assign individual (R40.21-, R40.22-, R40.23-) or total (R40.24-) coma scale score codes for patients who are sedated or in medically induced comas.

R40.20 Unspecified coma   MCC HCC
Coma NOS
Unconsciousness NOS
AHA: 2021,2Q,5
✓6ᵗʰ **R40.21 Coma scale, eyes open**

> The following appropriate 7th character is to be added to subcategory R40.21-, R40.22-, R40.23-, and R40.24-.
> 0   unspecified time
> 1   in the field [EMT or ambulance]
> 2   at arrival to emergency department
> 3   at hospital admission
> 4   24 hours or more after hospital admission

✓7ᵗʰ **R40.211 Coma scale, eyes open, never**   MCC UPD HCC
Coma scale eye opening score of 1
✓7ᵗʰ **R40.212 Coma scale, eyes open, to pain**   MCC UPD HCC
Coma scale eye opening score of 2
✓7ᵗʰ **R40.213 Coma scale, eyes open, to sound**   UPD
Coma scale eye opening score of 3
✓7ᵗʰ **R40.214 Coma scale, eyes open, spontaneous**   UPD
Coma scale eye opening score of 4

Chapter 18. Symptoms, Signs and Abnormal Clinical and Laboratory Findings

R40.22–R43.1

✓6ᵗʰ **R40.22 Coma scale, best verbal response**

✓7ᵗʰ **R40.221 Coma scale, best verbal response, none** `MCC` `UPD` `HCC`
Coma scale verbal score of 1

✓7ᵗʰ **R40.222 Coma scale, best verbal response, incomprehensible words** `MCC` `UPD` `HCC`
Coma scale verbal score of 2
Incomprehensible sounds (2-5 years of age)
Moans/grunts to pain; restless (< 2 years old)

✓7ᵗʰ **R40.223 Coma scale, best verbal response, inappropriate words** `UPD`
Coma scale verbal score of 3
Inappropriate crying or screaming (< 2 years of age)
Screaming (2-5 years of age)

✓7ᵗʰ **R40.224 Coma scale, best verbal response, confused conversation** `UPD`
Coma scale verbal score of 4
Inappropriate words (2-5 years of age)
Irritable cries (< 2 years of age)

✓7ᵗʰ **R40.225 Coma scale, best verbal response, oriented** `UPD`
Coma scale verbal score of 5
Cooing or babbling or crying appropriately (< 2 years of age)
Uses appropriate words (2-5 years of age)

✓6ᵗʰ **R40.23 Coma scale, best motor response**

✓7ᵗʰ **R40.231 Coma scale, best motor response, none** `MCC` `UPD` `HCC`
Coma scale motor score of 1

✓7ᵗʰ **R40.232 Coma scale, best motor response, extension** `MCC` `UPD` `HCC`
Abnormal extensor posturing to pain or noxious stimuli (< 2 years of age)
Coma scale motor score of 2
Extensor posturing to pain or noxious stimuli (2-5 years of age)

✓7ᵗʰ **R40.233 Coma scale, best motor response, abnormal flexion** `UPD`
Abnormal flexure posturing to pain or noxious stimuli (2-5 years of age)
Coma scale motor score of 3
Flexion/decorticate posturing (< 2 years of age)

✓7ᵗʰ **R40.234 Coma scale, best motor response, flexion withdrawal** `MCC` `UPD` `HCC`
Coma scale motor score of 4
Withdraws from pain or noxious stimuli (2-5 years of age)

✓7ᵗʰ **R40.235 Coma scale, best motor response, localizes pain** `UPD`
Coma scale motor score of 5
Localizes pain (2-5 years of age)
Withdraws to touch (< 2 years of age)

✓7ᵗʰ **R40.236 Coma scale, best motor response, obeys commands** `UPD`
Coma scale motor score of 6
Normal or spontaneous movement (< 2 years of age)
Obeys commands (2-5 years of age)

✓6ᵗʰ **R40.24 Glasgow coma scale, total score**

`NOTE` Assign a code from subcategory R40.24, when only the total coma score is documented

AHA: 2021,2Q,4; 2016,4Q,64-65

✓7ᵗʰ **R40.241 Glasgow coma scale score 13-15** `UPD`

✓7ᵗʰ **R40.242 Glasgow coma scale score 9-12** `UPD`

✓7ᵗʰ **R40.243 Glasgow coma scale score 3-8** `UPD` `HCC`

✓7ᵗʰ **R40.244 Other coma, without documented Glasgow coma scale score, or with partial score reported** `UPD` `HCC`

R40.3 Persistent vegetative state `CC` `HCC`
DEF: Persistent wakefulness without consciousness due to a nonfunctioning cerebral cortex.

R40.4 Transient alteration of awareness
AHA: 2020,2Q,24

✓4ᵗʰ **R41 Other symptoms and signs involving cognitive functions and awareness**

`EXCLUDES 1` dissociative [conversion] disorders (F44.-)
mild cognitive impairment, so stated (G31.84)

R41.0 Disorientation, unspecified
Confusion NOS
Delirium NOS
AHA: 2019,2Q,34

R41.1 Anterograde amnesia

R41.2 Retrograde amnesia

R41.3 Other amnesia
Amnesia NOS
Memory loss NOS
`EXCLUDES 1` amnestic disorder due to known physiologic condition (F04)
amnestic syndrome due to psychoactive substance use (F10-F19 with 5th character .6)
mild memory disturbance due to known physiological condition (F06.8)
transient global amnesia (G45.4)

R41.4 Neurologic neglect syndrome `CC`
Asomatognosia
Hemi-akinesia
Hemi-inattention
Hemispatial neglect
Left-sided neglect
Sensory neglect
Visuospatial neglect
`EXCLUDES 1` visuospatial deficit (R41.842)

✓5ᵗʰ **R41.8 Other symptoms and signs involving cognitive functions and awareness**

R41.81 Age-related cognitive decline `A`
Senility NOS

R41.82 Altered mental status, unspecified
Change in mental status NOS
`EXCLUDES 1` altered level of consciousness (R40.-)
altered mental status due to known condition - code to condition
delirium NOS (R41.0)
AHA: 2012,4Q,97

R41.83 Borderline intellectual functioning `UPD`
IQ level 71 to 84
`EXCLUDES 1` intellectual disabilities (F70-F79)

✓6ᵗʰ **R41.84 Other specified cognitive deficit**
`EXCLUDES 1` cognitive deficits as sequelae of cerebrovascular disease (I69.01-, I69.11-, I69.21-, I69.31-, I69.81-, I69.91-)

R41.840 Attention and concentration deficit
`EXCLUDES 1` attention-deficit hyperactivity disorders (F90.-)

R41.841 Cognitive communication deficit

R41.842 Visuospatial deficit

R41.843 Psychomotor deficit

R41.844 Frontal lobe and executive function deficit

R41.89 Other symptoms and signs involving cognitive functions and awareness
Anosognosia

R41.9 Unspecified symptoms and signs involving cognitive functions and awareness
Unspecified neurocognitive disorder

R42 Dizziness and giddiness
Light-headedness
Vertigo NOS
`EXCLUDES 1` vertiginous syndromes (H81.-)
vertigo from infrasound (T75.23)

✓4ᵗʰ **R43 Disturbances of smell and taste**

R43.0 Anosmia
DEF: Permanent or transient absence of smell that may be congenital or acquired.

R43.1 Parosmia
DEF: Abnormal perception of smell usually triggered by environmental odors.

`N` Newborn: 0   `P` Pediatric: 0-17   `M` Maternity: 9-64   `A` Adult: 15-124   `MCC` Major Complication/Comorbidity   `CC` Complication/Comorbidity   `SW` Severe Wound Dx

948

ICD-10-CM 2022

R43.2 Parageusia
    DEF: Abnormal perception of taste.

R43.8 Other disturbances of smell and taste
    Mixed disturbance of smell and taste

R43.9 Unspecified disturbances of smell and taste

✓4ᵗʰ **R44 Other symptoms and signs involving general sensations and perceptions**
    EXCLUDES 1   *alcoholic hallucinations (F10.151, F10.251, F10.951)*
       hallucinations in drug psychosis (F11-F19 with fifth to sixth characters 51)
       hallucinations in mood disorders with psychotic symptoms (F30.2, F31.5, F32.3, F33.3)
       hallucinations in schizophrenia, schizotypal and delusional disorders (F20-F29)
    EXCLUDES 2   *disturbances of skin sensation (R20.-)*

R44.0 Auditory hallucinations   `CC`

R44.1 Visual hallucinations

R44.2 Other hallucinations   `CC`

R44.3 Hallucinations, unspecified   `CC`

R44.8 Other symptoms and signs involving general sensations and perceptions

R44.9 Unspecified symptoms and signs involving general sensations and perceptions

✓4ᵗʰ **R45 Symptoms and signs involving emotional state**

R45.0 Nervousness
    Nervous tension

R45.1 Restlessness and agitation

R45.2 Unhappiness

R45.3 Demoralization and apathy
    EXCLUDES 1   *anhedonia (R45.84)*

R45.4 Irritability and anger

R45.5 Hostility

R45.6 Violent behavior

R45.7 State of emotional shock and stress, unspecified

✓5ᵗʰ **R45.8 Other symptoms and signs involving emotional state**

    R45.81 Low self-esteem

    R45.82 Worries

    R45.83 Excessive crying of child, adolescent or adult
       EXCLUDES 1   *excessive crying of infant (baby) R68.11*

    R45.84 Anhedonia

    ✓6ᵗʰ **R45.85 Homicidal and suicidal ideations**
       EXCLUDES 1   *suicide attempt (T14.91)*

       R45.850 Homicidal ideations   `UPD`

       R45.851 Suicidal ideations   `CC`
          DEF: Thoughts of committing suicide but no actual attempt of suicide has been made.

    R45.86 Emotional lability

    R45.87 Impulsiveness

    R45.88 Nonsuicidal self-harm
       Nonsuicidal self-injury
       Nonsuicidal self-mutilation
       Self-inflicted injury without suicidal intent
       Code also injury, if known

    R45.89 Other symptoms and signs involving emotional state

✓4ᵗʰ **R46 Symptoms and signs involving appearance and behavior**
    EXCLUDES 1   *appearance and behavior in schizophrenia, schizotypal and delusional disorders (F20-F29)*
       mental and behavioral disorders (F01-F99)

R46.0 Very low level of personal hygiene

R46.1 Bizarre personal appearance

R46.2 Strange and inexplicable behavior

R46.3 Overactivity

R46.4 Slowness and poor responsiveness
    EXCLUDES 1   *stupor (R40.1)*

R46.5 Suspiciousness and marked evasiveness

R46.6 Undue concern and preoccupation with stressful events

R46.7 Verbosity and circumstantial detail obscuring reason for contact

✓5ᵗʰ **R46.8 Other symptoms and signs involving appearance and behavior**

    R46.81 Obsessive-compulsive behavior   `UPD`
       EXCLUDES 1   *obsessive-compulsive disorder (F42.-)*

    R46.89 Other symptoms and signs involving appearance and behavior   `UPD`

Symptoms and signs involving speech and voice (R47-R49)

✓4ᵗʰ **R47 Speech disturbances, not elsewhere classified**
    EXCLUDES 1   *autism (F84.0)*
       cluttering (F80.81)
       specific developmental disorders of speech and language (F80.-)
       stuttering (F80.81)

✓5ᵗʰ **R47.0 Dysphasia and aphasia**

    R47.01 Aphasia   `CC`
       EXCLUDES 1   *aphasia following cerebrovascular disease (I69. with final characters -20)*
         progressive isolated aphasia (G31.01)

    R47.02 Dysphasia
       EXCLUDES 1   *dysphasia following cerebrovascular disease (I69. with final characters -21)*

R47.1 Dysarthria and anarthria
    EXCLUDES 1   *dysarthria following cerebrovascular disease (I69. with final characters -22)*

✓5ᵗʰ **R47.8 Other speech disturbances**
    EXCLUDES 1   *dysarthria following cerebrovascular disease (I69. with final characters -28)*

    R47.81 Slurred speech

    R47.82 *Fluency disorder in conditions classified elsewhere*
       Stuttering in conditions classified elsewhere
       Code first underlying disease or condition, such as:
       Parkinson's disease (G20)
       EXCLUDES 1   *adult onset fluency disorder (F98.5)*
         childhood onset fluency disorder (F80.81)
         fluency disorder (stuttering) following cerebrovascular disease (I69. with final characters -23)

    R47.89 Other speech disturbances

R47.9 Unspecified speech disturbances

✓4ᵗʰ **R48 Dyslexia and other symbolic dysfunctions, not elsewhere classified**
    EXCLUDES 1   *specific developmental disorders of scholastic skills (F81.-)*

R48.0 Dyslexia and alexia

R48.1 Agnosia
    Astereognosia (astereognosis)
    Autotopagnosia
    EXCLUDES 1   *visual object agnosia (R48.3)*
    DEF: Inability to recognize common things such as faces, objects, smells, or voices.

R48.2 Apraxia
    EXCLUDES 1   *apraxia following cerebrovascular disease (I69. with final characters -90)*

R48.3 Visual agnosia
    Prosopagnosia
    Simultanagnosia (asimultagnosia)

R48.8 Other symbolic dysfunctions
    Acalculia
    Agraphia
    AHA: 2017,1Q,27

R48.9 Unspecified symbolic dysfunctions

✓4ᵗʰ **R49 Voice and resonance disorders**
    EXCLUDES 1   *psychogenic voice and resonance disorders (F44.4)*

R49.0 Dysphonia
    Hoarseness

R49.1 Aphonia
    Loss of voice

✓5ᵗʰ **R49.2 Hypernasality and hyponasality**

    R49.21 Hypernasality

    R49.22 Hyponasality

R49.8 Other voice and resonance disorders

R49.9 Unspecified voice and resonance disorder
    Change in voice NOS
    Resonance disorder NOS

✓ Additional Character Required   ✓x7ᵗʰ Placeholder   Questionable PDx   Manifestation   Unspecified Dx   `UPD` Unacceptable PDx   H1-H14 HAC   HCC CMS-HCC Dx   HIV HIV Dx

ICD-10-CM 2022   949

Chapter 18. Symptoms, Signs and Abnormal Clinical and Laboratory Findings

General symptoms and signs (R50-R69)

✓4ᵗʰ **R50 Fever of other and unknown origin**

> EXCLUDES 1   *chills without fever (R68.83)*
> *febrile convulsions (R56.0-)*
> *fever of unknown origin during labor (O75.2)*
> *fever of unknown origin in newborn (P81.9)*
> *hypothermia due to illness (R68.0)*
> *malignant hyperthermia due to anesthesia (T88.3)*
> *puerperal pyrexia NOS (O86.4)*

  R50.2 Drug induced fever
> Use additional code for adverse effect, if applicable, to identify drug (T36-T50 with fifth or sixth character 5)
> EXCLUDES 1   *postvaccination (postimmunization) fever (R50.83)*

✓5ᵗʰ **R50.8 Other specified fever**

    R50.81   ***Fever presenting with conditions classified elsewhere***
> Code first underlying condition when associated fever is present, such as with:
> leukemia (C91-C95)
> neutropenia (D70.-)
> sickle-cell disease (D57.-)
> **AHA:** 2020,3Q,22; 2014,4Q,22

    R50.82 Postprocedural fever
> EXCLUDES 1   *postprocedural infection (T81.4-)*
> *posttransfusion fever (R50.84)*
> *postvaccination (postimmunization) fever (R50.83)*

    R50.83 Postvaccination fever
> Postimmunization fever

    R50.84 Febrile nonhemolytic transfusion reaction
> FNHTR
> Posttransfusion fever

  R50.9 Fever, unspecified
> Fever NOS
> Fever of unknown origin [FUO]
> Fever with chills
> Fever with rigors
> Hyperpyrexia NOS
> Persistent fever
> Pyrexia NOS

✓4ᵗʰ **R51 Headache**

> EXCLUDES 2   *atypical face pain (G50.1)*
> *migraine and other headache syndromes (G43-G44)*
> *trigeminal neuralgia (G50.0)*
> **AHA:** 2020,4Q,38-39

  R51.0 Headache with orthostatic component, not elsewhere classified
> Headache with positional component, not elsewhere classified

  R51.9 Headache, unspecified
> Facial pain NOS

R52 Pain, unspecified
> Acute pain NOS
> Generalized pain NOS
> Pain NOS
> EXCLUDES 1   *acute and chronic pain, not elsewhere classified (G89.-)*
> *localized pain, unspecified type - code to pain by site, such as:*
>   *abdomen pain (R10.-)*
>   *back pain (M54.9)*
>   *breast pain (N64.4)*
>   *chest pain (R07.1-R07.9)*
>   *ear pain (H92.0-)*
>   *eye pain (H57.1)*
>   *headache (R51.9)*
>   *joint pain (M25.5-)*
>   *limb pain (M79.6-)*
>   *lumbar region pain ▶(M54.5-)◀*
>   *pelvic and perineal pain (R10.2)*
>   *renal colic (N23)*
>   *shoulder pain (M25.51-)*
>   *spine pain (M54.-)*
>   *throat pain (R07.0)*
>   *tongue pain (K14.6)*
>   *tooth pain (K08.8)*
> *pain disorders exclusively related to psychological factors (F45.41)*

✓4ᵗʰ **R53 Malaise and fatigue**

  R53.0 Neoplastic (malignant) related fatigue
> Code first associated neoplasm

  R53.1 Weakness
> Asthenia NOS
> EXCLUDES 1   *age-related weakness (R54)*
> *muscle weakness (generalized) (M62.81)*
> *sarcopenia (M62.84)*
> *senile asthenia (R54)*
> **AHA:** 2017,1Q,7; 2015,1Q,25

  R53.2 Functional quadriplegia   MCC   HCC
> Complete immobility due to severe physical disability or frailty
> EXCLUDES 1   *frailty NOS (R54)*
> *hysterical paralysis (F44.4)*
> *immobility syndrome (M62.3)*
> *neurologic quadriplegia (G82.5-)*
> *quadriplegia (G82.50)*
> **AHA:** 2016,2Q,6
> **DEF:** Inability to move due to a nonphysiological condition, such as dementia. The patient has no mental ability to move independently.

✓5ᵗʰ **R53.8 Other malaise and fatigue**
> EXCLUDES 1   *combat exhaustion and fatigue (F43.0)*
> *congenital debility (P96.9)*
> *exhaustion and fatigue due to excessive exertion (T73.3)*
> *exhaustion and fatigue due to exposure (T73.2)*
> *exhaustion and fatigue due to heat (T67.-)*
> *exhaustion and fatigue due to pregnancy (O26.8-)*
> *exhaustion and fatigue due to recurrent depressive episode (F33)*
> *exhaustion and fatigue due to senile debility (R54)*

    R53.81 Other malaise
> Chronic debility
> Debility NOS
> General physical deterioration
> Malaise NOS
> Nervous debility
> EXCLUDES 1   *age-related physical debility (R54)*
> **AHA:** 2021,1Q,43

    R53.82 Chronic fatigue, unspecified
> Chronic fatigue syndrome NOS
> EXCLUDES 1   *postviral fatigue syndrome (G93.3)*

N Newborn: 0   P Pediatric: 0-17   M Maternity: 9-64   A Adult: 15-124   MCC Major Complication/Comorbidity   CC Complication/Comorbidity   SW Severe Wound Dx
950
ICD-10-CM 2022

R50–R53.82

R53.83   **Other fatigue**
Fatigue NOS
Lack of energy
Lethargy
Tiredness
EXCLUDES 2   exhaustion and fatigue due to depressive episode (F32.-)

R54   **Age-related physical debility**   Ⓐ
Frailty
Old age
Senescence
Senile asthenia
Senile debility
EXCLUDES 1   age-related cognitive decline (R41.81)
sarcopenia (M62.84)
senile psychosis (F03)
senility NOS (R41.81)

R55   **Syncope and collapse**
Blackout
Fainting
Vasovagal attack
EXCLUDES 1   cardiogenic shock (R57.0)
carotid sinus syncope (G90.01)
heat syncope (T67.1)
neurocirculatory asthenia (F45.8)
neurogenic orthostatic hypotension (G90.3)
orthostatic hypotension (I95.1)
postprocedural shock (T81.1-)
psychogenic syncope (F48.8)
shock NOS (R57.9)
shock complicating or following abortion or ectopic or molar pregnancy (O00-O07, O08.3)
shock complicating or following labor and delivery (O75.1)
Stokes-Adams attack (I45.9)
unconsciousness NOS (R40.2-)

✓4ᵗʰ **R56**   **Convulsions, not elsewhere classified**
EXCLUDES 1   dissociative convulsions and seizures (F44.5)
epileptic convulsions and seizures (G40.-)
newborn convulsions and seizures (P90)

✓5ᵗʰ **R56.0**   **Febrile convulsions**

R56.00   **Simple febrile convulsions**   CC HCC
Febrile convulsion NOS
Febrile seizure NOS

R56.01   **Complex febrile convulsions**   CC HCC
Atypical febrile seizure
Complex febrile seizure
Complicated febrile seizure
EXCLUDES 1   status epilepticus (G40.901)

R56.1   **Post traumatic seizures**   CC HCC
EXCLUDES 1   post traumatic epilepsy (G40.-)

R56.9   **Unspecified convulsions**   HCC
Convulsion disorder
Fit NOS
Recurrent convulsions
Seizure(s) (convulsive) NOS
AHA: 2021,1Q,3; 2019,1Q,19

✓4ᵗʰ **R57**   **Shock, not elsewhere classified**
EXCLUDES 1   anaphylactic shock NOS (T78.2)
anaphylactic reaction or shock due to adverse food reaction (T78.0-)
anaphylactic shock due to adverse effect of correct drug or medicament properly administered (T88.6)
anaphylactic shock due to serum (T80.5-)
anesthetic shock (T88.3)
electric shock (T75.4)
obstetric shock (O75.1)
postprocedural shock (T81.1-)
psychic shock (F43.0)
shock complicating or following ectopic or molar pregnancy (O00-O07, O08.3)
▶shock due to anesthesia (T88.2)◀
shock due to lightning (T75.01)
toxic shock syndrome (A48.3)
traumatic shock (T79.4)

¹ **R57.0**   **Cardiogenic shock**   MCC HCC
EXCLUDES 2   septic shock (R65.21)
AHA: 2020,3Q,26
DEF: Associated with myocardial infarction, cardiac tamponade, and massive pulmonary embolism. Symptoms include mental confusion, reduced blood pressure, tachycardia, pallor, and cold, clammy skin.

¹ **R57.1**   **Hypovolemic shock**   MCC HCC
AHA: 2019,2Q,7

¹ **R57.8**   **Other shock**   MCC HCC

R57.9   **Shock, unspecified**   CC HCC
Failure of peripheral circulation NOS

R58   **Hemorrhage, not elsewhere classified**
Hemorrhage NOS
EXCLUDES 1   hemorrhage included with underlying conditions, such as:
acute duodenal ulcer with hemorrhage (K26.0)
acute gastritis with bleeding (K29.01)
ulcerative enterocolitis with rectal bleeding (K51.01)

✓4ᵗʰ **R59**   **Enlarged lymph nodes**
INCLUDES   swollen glands
EXCLUDES 1   acute lymphadenitis (L04.-)
chronic lymphadenitis (I88.1)
lymphadenitis NOS (I88.9)
mesenteric (acute) (chronic) lymphadenitis (I88.0)

R59.0   **Localized enlarged lymph nodes**

R59.1   **Generalized enlarged lymph nodes**
Lymphadenopathy NOS

R59.9   **Enlarged lymph nodes, unspecified**

✓4ᵗʰ **R60**   **Edema, not elsewhere classified**
EXCLUDES 1   angioneurotic edema (T78.3)
ascites (R18.-)
cerebral edema (G93.6)
cerebral edema due to birth injury (P11.0)
edema of larynx (J38.4)
edema of nasopharynx (J39.2)
edema of pharynx (J39.2)
gestational edema (O12.0-)
hereditary edema (Q82.0)
hydrops fetalis NOS (P83.2)
hydrothorax (J94.8)
newborn edema (P83.3)
pulmonary edema (J81.-)

R60.0   **Localized edema**

R60.1   **Generalized edema**
EXCLUDES 2   nutritional edema (E40-E46)

R60.9   **Edema, unspecified**
Fluid retention NOS

R61   Generalized hyperhidrosis
Excessive sweating
Night sweats
Secondary hyperhidrosis
Code first, if applicable, menopausal and female climacteric states (N95.1)
> EXCLUDES 1   *focal (primary) (secondary) hyperhidrosis (L74.5-)*
> *Frey's syndrome (L74.52)*
> *localized (primary) (secondary) hyperhidrosis (L74.5-)*

✓4ᵗʰ **R62   Lack of expected normal physiological development in childhood and adults**
> EXCLUDES 1   *delayed puberty (E30.0)*
> *gonadal dysgenesis (Q99.1)*
> *hypopituitarism (E23.0)*

R62.0   Delayed milestone in childhood   P
Delayed attainment of expected physiological developmental stage
Late talker
Late walker

✓5ᵗʰ **R62.5   Other and unspecified lack of expected normal physiological development in childhood**
> EXCLUDES 1   *HIV disease resulting in failure to thrive (B20)*
> *physical retardation due to malnutrition (E45)*

   R62.50   Unspecified lack of expected normal physiological development in childhood
Infantilism NOS

   R62.51   Failure to thrive (child)   P
Failure to gain weight
> EXCLUDES 1   *failure to thrive in child under 28 days old (P92.6)*

AHA: 2018,4Q,82
DEF: Organic failure to thrive (FTT): Acute or chronic illness that interferes with nutritional intake, absorption, metabolism excretion, and energy requirements.
DEF: Nonorganic failure to thrive (FTT): Symptom of neglect or abuse.

   R62.52   Short stature (child)
Lack of growth
Physical retardation
Short stature NOS
> EXCLUDES 1   *short stature due to endocrine disorder (E34.3)*

   R62.59   Other lack of expected normal physiological development in childhood

R62.7   Adult failure to thrive   A

✓4ᵗʰ **R63   Symptoms and signs concerning food and fluid intake**
> EXCLUDES 1   *bulimia NOS (F50.2)*

R63.0   Anorexia
Loss of appetite
> EXCLUDES 1   *anorexia nervosa (F50.0-)*
> *loss of appetite of nonorganic origin (F50.89)*

AHA: 2018,4Q,82
TIP: Assign an additional code from category Z68 when BMI is documented. BMI can be based on documentation from clinicians who are not the patient's provider.

R63.1   Polydipsia
Excessive thirst

R63.2   Polyphagia
Excessive eating
Hyperalimentation NOS

▲   ✓5ᵗʰ **R63.3   Feeding difficulties**
~~Feeding problem (elderly) (infant) NOS~~
~~Picky eater~~
> EXCLUDES 1   *~~eating disorders (F50.-)~~*
> *~~feeding problems of newborn (P92.-)~~*
> *~~infant feeding disorder of nonorganic origin (F98.2-)~~*
> EXCLUDES 2   ▶*eating disorders (F50.-)*◀
> ▶*feeding problems of newborn (P92.-)*◀
> ▶*infant feeding disorder of nonorganic origin (F98.2-)*◀

AHA: 2017,1Q,28; 2016,3Q,19

   R63.30   Feeding difficulties, unspecified

● **R63.31   Pediatric feeding disorder, acute**
Pediatric feeding dysfunction, acute
Code also, if applicable, associated conditions such as:
   aspiration pneumonia (J69.0)
   dysphagia (R13.1-)
   gastro-esophageal reflux disease (K21.-)
   malnutrition (E40-E46)

● **R63.32   Pediatric feeding disorder, chronic**
Pediatric feeding dysfunction, chronic
Code also, if applicable, associated conditions such as:
   aspiration pneumonia (J69.0)
   dysphagia (R13.1-)
   gastro-esophageal reflux disease (K21.-)
   malnutrition (E40-E46)

● **R63.39   Other feeding difficulties**
Feeding problem (elderly) (infant) NOS
Picky eater

R63.4   Abnormal weight loss
AHA: 2018,4Q,82
TIP: Assign an additional code from category Z68 when BMI is documented. BMI can be based on documentation from clinicians who are not the patient's provider.

R63.5   Abnormal weight gain
> EXCLUDES 1   *excessive weight gain in pregnancy (O26.0-)*
> *obesity (E66.-)*

AHA: 2018,4Q,82
TIP: Assign an additional code from category Z68 when BMI is documented. BMI can be based on documentation from clinicians who are not the patient's provider.

R63.6   Underweight
Use additional code to identify body mass index (BMI), if known (Z68.-)
> EXCLUDES 1   *abnormal weight loss (R63.4)*
> *anorexia nervosa (F50.0-)*
> *malnutrition (E40-E46)*

AHA: 2018,4Q,82

R63.8   Other symptoms and signs concerning food and fluid intake

R64   Cachexia   CC   HCC
Wasting syndrome
Code first underlying condition, if known
> EXCLUDES 1   *abnormal weight loss (R63.4)*
> *nutritional marasmus (E41)*

AHA: 2018,4Q,82; 2017,3Q,24
TIP: Assign code E43 when emaciated or emaciation is documented in relation to malnutrition.

✓4ᵗʰ **R65   Symptoms and signs specifically associated with systemic inflammation and infection**
AHA: 2019,2Q,38
TIP: When documentation states SIRS with an infection, assign only a code for the infection. ICD-10-CM does not offer a code for SIRS due to infectious process. If sepsis is suspected, query the provider.

✓5ᵗʰ **R65.1   Systemic inflammatory response syndrome [SIRS] of non-infectious origin**
Code first underlying condition, such as:
   heatstroke (T67.0-)
   injury and trauma (S00-T88)
> EXCLUDES 1   *sepsis - code to infection*
> *severe sepsis (R65.2)*

   R65.10   Systemic inflammatory response syndrome [SIRS] of non-infectious origin without acute organ dysfunction   CC   UPD   HCC
Systemic inflammatory response syndrome (SIRS) NOS
AHA: 2019,2Q,24

N Newborn: 0   P Pediatric: 0-17   M Maternity: 9-64   A Adult: 15-124   MCC Major Complication/Comorbidity   CC Complication/Comorbidity   SW Severe Wound Dx

952   ICD-10-CM 2022

R65.11 **Systemic inflammatory response syndrome [SIRS] of non-infectious origin** with acute organ dysfunction `MCC` `UPD` `HCC`

Use additional code to identify specific acute organ dysfunction, such as:

acute kidney failure (N17.-)
acute respiratory failure (J96.0-)
critical illness myopathy (G72.81)
critical illness polyneuropathy (G62.81)
disseminated intravascular coagulopathy [DIC] (D65)
encephalopathy (metabolic) (septic) (G93.41)
hepatic failure (K72.0-)

✓5ᵗʰ **R65.2** **Severe sepsis**

Infection with associated acute organ dysfunction
Sepsis with acute organ dysfunction
Sepsis with multiple organ dysfunction
Systemic inflammatory response syndrome due to infectious process with acute organ dysfunction

Code first underlying infection, such as:

infection following a procedure (T81.4-)
infections following infusion, transfusion and therapeutic injection (T80.2-)
puerperal sepsis (O85)
sepsis following complete or unspecified spontaneous abortion (O03.87)
sepsis following ectopic and molar pregnancy (O08.82)
sepsis following incomplete spontaneous abortion (O03.37)
sepsis following (induced) termination of pregnancy (O04.87)
sepsis NOS (A41.9)

Use additional code to identify specific acute organ dysfunction, such as:

acute kidney failure (N17.-)
acute respiratory failure (J96.0-)
critical illness myopathy (G72.81)
critical illness polyneuropathy (G62.81)
disseminated intravascular coagulopathy [DIC] (D65)
encephalopathy (metabolic) (septic) (G93.41)
hepatic failure (K72.0-)

AHA: 2020,2Q,17; 2018,4Q,62-63; 2017,4Q,98-99; 2016,3Q,8

R65.20 **Severe sepsis** without septic shock `MCC` `UPD` `HCC`
Severe sepsis NOS
AHA: 2020,2Q,17; 2016,3Q,14; 2013,4Q,119

R65.21 **Severe sepsis** with septic shock `MCC` `UPD` `HCC`
AHA: 2018,4Q,63

✓4ᵗʰ **R68** **Other general symptoms and signs**

R68.0 **Hypothermia, not associated with low environmental temperature**
EXCLUDES 1   hypothermia NOS (accidental) (T68)
hypothermia due to anesthesia (T88.51)
hypothermia due to low environmental temperature (T68)
newborn hypothermia (P80.-)

✓5ᵗʰ **R68.1** **Nonspecific symptoms peculiar to infancy**
EXCLUDES 1   colic, infantile (R10.83)
neonatal cerebral irritability (P91.3)
teething syndrome (K00.7)

R68.11 **Excessive crying of infant (baby)** `P`
EXCLUDES 1   excessive crying of child, adolescent, or adult (R45.83)

R68.12 **Fussy infant (baby)** `P`
Irritable infant

R68.13 **Apparent life threatening event in infant (ALTE)** `P`
Apparent life threatening event in newborn
Brief resolved unexplained event (BRUE)
Code first confirmed diagnosis, if known
Use additional code(s) for associated signs and symptoms if no confirmed diagnosis established, or if signs and symptoms are not associated routinely with confirmed diagnosis, or provide additional information for cause of ALTE

R68.19 **Other nonspecific symptoms peculiar to infancy** `P`

R68.2 **Dry mouth, unspecified**
EXCLUDES 1   dry mouth due to dehydration (E86.0)
▶dry mouth due to Sjögren syndrome◀ (M35.0-)
salivary gland hyposecretion (K11.7)

R68.3 **Clubbing of fingers**
Clubbing of nails
EXCLUDES 1   congenital clubfinger (Q68.1)
DEF: Enlarged soft tissue of the distal fingers that usually occurs in heart and lung diseases.

✓5ᵗʰ **R68.8** **Other general symptoms and signs**

R68.81 **Early satiety**
DEF: Premature feeling of being full after eating only a small amount of food. The mechanism of satiety is multifactorial.

R68.82 **Decreased libido** `A`
Decreased sexual desire

R68.83 **Chills (without fever)**
Chills NOS
EXCLUDES 1   chills with fever (R50.9)

R68.84 **Jaw pain**
Mandibular pain
Maxilla pain
EXCLUDES 1   temporomandibular joint arthralgia (M26.62-)

R68.89 **Other general symptoms and signs**

`R69` **Illness, unspecified**
Unknown and unspecified cases of morbidity

Abnormal findings on examination of blood, without diagnosis (R70-R79)

EXCLUDES 2   abnormal findings on antenatal screening of mother (O28.-)
abnormalities of lipids (E78.-)
abnormalities of platelets and thrombocytes (D69.-)
abnormalities of white blood cells classified elsewhere (D70-D72)
coagulation hemorrhagic disorders (D65-D68)
diagnostic abnormal findings classified elsewhere - see Alphabetical Index
hemorrhagic and hematological disorders of newborn (P50-P61)

✓4ᵗʰ **R70** **Elevated erythrocyte sedimentation rate and abnormality of plasma viscosity**
R70.0 **Elevated erythrocyte sedimentation rate**
R70.1 **Abnormal plasma viscosity**

✓4ᵗʰ **R71** **Abnormality of red blood cells**
EXCLUDES 1   anemias (D50-D64)
anemia of premature infant (P61.2)
benign (familial) polycythemia (D75.0)
congenital anemias (P61.2-P61.4)
newborn anemia due to isoimmunization (P55.-)
polycythemia neonatorum (P61.1)
polycythemia NOS (D75.1)
polycythemia vera (D45)
secondary polycythemia (D75.1)

R71.0 **Precipitous drop in hematocrit** `cc`
Drop (precipitous) in hemoglobin
Drop in hematocrit

R71.8 **Other abnormality of red blood cells**
Abnormal red-cell morphology NOS
Abnormal red-cell volume NOS
Anisocytosis
Poikilocytosis

Chapter 18. Symptoms, Signs and Abnormal Clinical and Laboratory Findings

R73–R79.82

✓4th **R73 Elevated blood glucose level**

EXCLUDES 1   *diabetes mellitus (E08-E13)*

diabetes mellitus in pregnancy, childbirth and the puerperium (O24.-)

neonatal disorders (P70.0-P70.2)

postsurgical hypoinsulinemia (E89.1)

✓5th **R73.0 Abnormal glucose**

EXCLUDES 1   *abnormal glucose in pregnancy (O99.81-)*

diabetes mellitus (E08-E13)

dysmetabolic syndrome X (E88.81)

gestational diabetes (O24.4-)

glycosuria (R81)

hypoglycemia (E16.2)

R73.01 Impaired fasting glucose

Elevated fasting glucose

R73.02 Impaired glucose tolerance (oral)

Elevated glucose tolerance

R73.03 Prediabetes

Latent diabetes

AHA: 2016,4Q,65

R73.09 Other abnormal glucose

Abnormal glucose NOS

Abnormal non-fasting glucose tolerance

R73.9 Hyperglycemia, unspecified

✓4th **R74 Abnormal serum enzyme levels**

✓5th **R74.0 Nonspecific elevation of levels of transaminase and lactic acid dehydrogenase [LDH]**

AHA: 2020,4Q,39

R74.01 Elevation of levels of liver transaminase levels

Elevation of levels of alanine transaminase (ALT)

Elevation of levels of aspartate transaminase (AST)

R74.02 Elevation of levels of lactic acid dehydrogenase [LDH]

R74.8 Abnormal levels of other serum enzymes

Abnormal level of acid phosphatase

Abnormal level of alkaline phosphatase

Abnormal level of amylase

Abnormal level of lipase [triacylglycerol lipase]

AHA: 2019,2Q,6

R74.9 Abnormal serum enzyme level, unspecified

R75 Inconclusive laboratory evidence of human immunodeficiency virus [HIV]

Nonconclusive HIV-test finding in infants

EXCLUDES 1   *asymptomatic human immunodeficiency virus [HIV] infection status (Z21)*

human immunodeficiency virus [HIV] disease (B20)

✓4th **R76 Other abnormal immunological findings in serum**

R76.0 Raised antibody titer

EXCLUDES 1   *isoimmunization in pregnancy (O36.0-O36.1)*

isoimmunization affecting newborn (P55.-)

AHA: 2021,1Q,6

✓5th **R76.1 Nonspecific reaction to test for tuberculosis**

R76.11 Nonspecific reaction to tuberculin skin test without active tuberculosis

Abnormal result of Mantoux test

PPD positive

Tuberculin (skin test) positive

Tuberculin (skin test) reactor

EXCLUDES 1   *nonspecific reaction to cell mediated immunity measurement of gamma interferon antigen response without active tuberculosis (R76.12)*

R76.12 Nonspecific reaction to cell mediated immunity measurement of gamma interferon antigen response without active tuberculosis

Nonspecific reaction to QuantiFERON-TB test (QFT) without active tuberculosis

EXCLUDES 1   *nonspecific reaction to tuberculin skin test without active tuberculosis (R76.11)*

positive tuberculin skin test (R76.11)

R76.8 Other specified abnormal immunological findings in serum

Raised level of immunoglobulins NOS

AHA: 2021,1Q,6

R76.9 Abnormal immunological finding in serum, unspecified

✓4th **R77 Other abnormalities of plasma proteins**

EXCLUDES 1   *disorders of plasma-protein metabolism (E88.0-)*

R77.0 Abnormality of albumin

R77.1 Abnormality of globulin

Hyperglobulinemia NOS

R77.2 Abnormality of alphafetoprotein

R77.8 Other specified abnormalities of plasma proteins

R77.9 Abnormality of plasma protein, unspecified

AHA: 2019,2Q,6

✓4th **R78 Findings of drugs and other substances, not normally found in blood**

Use additional code to identify the any retained foreign body, if applicable (Z18.-)

EXCLUDES 1   *mental or behavioral disorders due to psychoactive substance use (F10-F19)*

R78.0 Finding of alcohol in blood

Use additional external cause code (Y90.-), for detail regarding alcohol level

R78.1 Finding of opiate drug in blood

R78.2 Finding of cocaine in blood

R78.3 Finding of hallucinogen in blood

R78.4 Finding of other drugs of addictive potential in blood

R78.5 Finding of other psychotropic drug in blood

R78.6 Finding of steroid agent in blood

✓5th **R78.7 Finding of abnormal level of heavy metals in blood**

R78.71 Abnormal lead level in blood

EXCLUDES 1   *lead poisoning (T56.0-)*

R78.79 Finding of abnormal level of heavy metals in blood

✓5th **R78.8 Finding of other specified substances, not normally found in blood**

R78.81 Bacteremia   CC

EXCLUDES 1   *sepsis — code to specified infection*

DEF: Laboratory finding of bacteria in the blood in the absence of two or more signs of sepsis. Transient in nature, it can progress to septicemia with a severe infectious process.

R78.89 Finding of other specified substances, not normally found in blood

Finding of abnormal level of lithium in blood

R78.9 Finding of unspecified substance, not normally found in blood

✓4th **R79 Other abnormal findings of blood chemistry**

Use additional code to identify any retained foreign body, if applicable (Z18.-)

EXCLUDES 1   *asymptomatic hyperuricemia (E79.0)*

hyperglycemia NOS (R73.9)

hypoglycemia NOS (E16.2)

neonatal hypoglycemia (P70.3-P70.4)

specific findings indicating disorder of amino-acid metabolism (E70-E72)

specific findings indicating disorder of carbohydrate metabolism (E73-E74)

specific findings indicating disorder of lipid metabolism (E75.-)

R79.0 Abnormal level of blood mineral

Abnormal blood level of cobalt

Abnormal blood level of copper

Abnormal blood level of iron

Abnormal blood level of magnesium

Abnormal blood level of mineral NEC

Abnormal blood level of zinc

EXCLUDES 1   *abnormal level of lithium (R78.89)*

disorders of mineral metabolism (E83.-)

neonatal hypomagnesemia (P71.2)

nutritional mineral deficiency (E58-E61)

R79.1 Abnormal coagulation profile

Abnormal or prolonged bleeding time

Abnormal or prolonged coagulation time

Abnormal or prolonged partial thromboplastin time [PTT]

Abnormal or prolonged prothrombin time [PT]

EXCLUDES 1   *coagulation defects (D68.-)*

EXCLUDES 2   *abnormality of fluid, electrolyte or acid-base balance (E86-E87)*

✓6th **R79.8 Other specified abnormal findings of blood chemistry**

R79.81 Abnormal blood-gas level

R79.82 Elevated C-reactive protein [CRP]

N Newborn: 0   P Pediatric: 0-17   M Maternity: 9-64   A Adult: 15-124   MCC Major Complication/Comorbidity   CC Complication/Comorbidity   SW Severe Wound Dx

954   ICD-10-CM 2022

- **R79.83** **Abnormal findings of blood amino-acid level**
  Homocysteinemia
  EXCLUDES 1   *disorders of amino-acid metabolism (E70-E72)*

R79.89 **Other specified abnormal findings of blood chemistry**
    AHA: 2019,2Q,6
    TIP: Assign for positive Coombs test when not further clarified in the documentation.

R79.9 **Abnormal finding of blood chemistry, unspecified**

Abnormal findings on examination of urine, without diagnosis (R80-R82)

EXCLUDES 1   *abnormal findings on antenatal screening of mother (O28.-)*
diagnostic abnormal findings classified elsewhere - see Alphabetical Index
specific findings indicating disorder of amino-acid metabolism (E70-E72)
specific findings indicating disorder of carbohydrate metabolism (E73-E74)

☑4ᵗʰ R80 Proteinuria
    EXCLUDES 1   *gestational proteinuria (O12.1-)*

R80.0 **Isolated proteinuria**
    Idiopathic proteinuria
    EXCLUDES 1   *isolated proteinuria with specific morphological lesion (N06.-)*

R80.1 **Persistent proteinuria, unspecified**

R80.2 **Orthostatic proteinuria, unspecified**
    Postural proteinuria

R80.3 **Bence Jones proteinuria**

R80.8 **Other proteinuria**

R80.9 **Proteinuria, unspecified**
    Albuminuria NOS

R81 Glycosuria
    EXCLUDES 1   *renal glycosuria (E74.818)*

☑4ᵗʰ R82 Other and unspecified abnormal findings in urine
    INCLUDES   chromoabnormalities in urine
    Use additional code to identify any retained foreign body, if applicable (Z18.-)
    EXCLUDES 2   *hematuria (R31.-)*

R82.0 **Chyluria**   CC
    EXCLUDES 1   *filarial chyluria (B74.-)*

R82.1 **Myoglobinuria**   CC

R82.2 **Biliuria**

R82.3 **Hemoglobinuria**
    EXCLUDES 1   *hemoglobinuria due to hemolysis from external causes NEC (D59.6)*
        hemoglobinuria due to paroxysmal nocturnal [Marchiafava-Micheli] (D59.5)
    DEF: Free hemoglobin in blood due to rapid hemolysis of red blood cells. Causes include burns, crushed injury, sickle cell anemia, thalassemia, parasitic infections, or kidney infections.

R82.4 **Acetonuria**
    Ketonuria
    DEF: Excessive excretion of acetone in urine that commonly occurs in diabetic acidosis.

R82.5 **Elevated urine levels of drugs, medicaments and biological substances**
    Elevated urine levels of catecholamines
    Elevated urine levels of indoleacetic acid
    Elevated urine levels of 17-ketosteroids
    Elevated urine levels of steroids

R82.6 **Abnormal urine levels of substances chiefly nonmedicinal as to source**
    Abnormal urine level of heavy metals

☑5ᵗʰ R82.7 **Abnormal findings on microbiological examination of urine**
    EXCLUDES 1   *colonization status (Z22.-)*
    AHA: 2016,4Q,65

R82.71 **Bacteriuria**

R82.79 **Other abnormal findings on microbiological examination of urine**
    Positive culture findings of urine

☑5ᵗʰ R82.8 **Abnormal findings on cytological and histological examination of urine**
    AHA: 2019,4Q,16

R82.81 **Pyuria**
    Sterile pyuria

R82.89 **Other abnormal findings on cytological and histological examination of urine**

☑5ᵗʰ R82.9 **Other and unspecified abnormal findings in urine**

R82.90 **Unspecified abnormal findings in urine**

R82.91 **Other chromoabnormalities of urine**
    Chromoconversion (dipstick)
    Idiopathic dipstick converts positive for blood with no cellular forms in sediment
    EXCLUDES 1   *hemoglobinuria (R82.3)*
        myoglobinuria (R82.1)

☑6ᵗʰ R82.99 **Other abnormal findings in urine**
    AHA: 2018,4Q,29-30

R82.991 **Hypocitraturia**

R82.992 **Hyperoxaluria**
    EXCLUDES 1   *primary hyperoxaluria (E72.53)*

R82.993 **Hyperuricosuria**

R82.994 **Hypercalciuria**
    Idiopathic hypercalciuria

R82.998 **Other abnormal findings in urine**
    Cells and casts in urine
    Crystalluria
    Melanuria

Abnormal findings on examination of other body fluids, substances and tissues, without diagnosis (R83-R89)

EXCLUDES 1   *abnormal findings on antenatal screening of mother (O28.-)*
diagnostic abnormal findings classified elsewhere - see Alphabetical Index

EXCLUDES 2   *abnormal findings on examination of blood, without diagnosis (R70-R79)*
abnormal findings on examination of urine, without diagnosis (R80-R82)
abnormal tumor markers (R97.-)

☑4ᵗʰ R83 Abnormal findings in cerebrospinal fluid

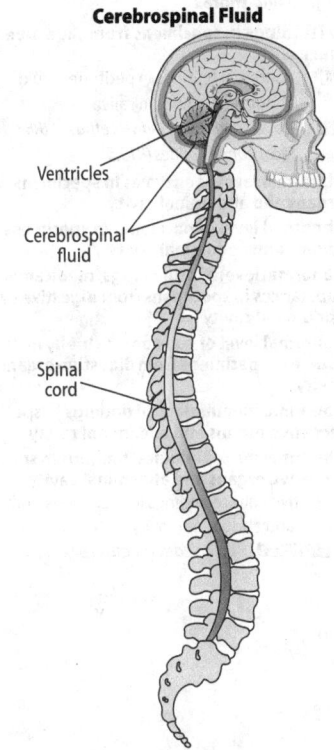

Cerebrospinal Fluid

Ventricles

Cerebrospinal fluid

Spinal cord

R83.0 **Abnormal level of enzymes in cerebrospinal fluid**

R83.1 **Abnormal level of hormones in cerebrospinal fluid**

R83.2 **Abnormal level of other drugs, medicaments and biological substances in cerebrospinal fluid**

R83.3 **Abnormal level of substances chiefly nonmedicinal as to source in cerebrospinal fluid**

✓ Additional Character Required   ✓x7ᵗʰ Placeholder   Questionable PDx   Manifestation   Unspecified Dx   UPD Unacceptable PDx   H1-H14 HAC   HCC CMS-HCC Dx   HIV HIV Dx

ICD-10-CM 2022   955

R83.4 **Abnormal immunological findings in cerebrospinal fluid**

R83.5 **Abnormal microbiological findings in cerebrospinal fluid**

Positive culture findings in cerebrospinal fluid

EXCLUDES 1   *colonization status (Z22.-)*

R83.6 **Abnormal cytological findings in cerebrospinal fluid**

R83.8 **Other abnormal findings in cerebrospinal fluid**

Abnormal chromosomal findings in cerebrospinal fluid

R83.9 **Unspecified abnormal finding in cerebrospinal fluid**

√4ᵗʰ **R84** **Abnormal findings in specimens from respiratory organs and thorax**

INCLUDES   abnormal findings in bronchial washings

abnormal findings in nasal secretions

abnormal findings in pleural fluid

abnormal findings in sputum

abnormal findings in throat scrapings

EXCLUDES 1   *blood-stained sputum (R04.2)*

R84.0 **Abnormal level of enzymes in specimens from respiratory organs and thorax**

R84.1 **Abnormal level of hormones in specimens from respiratory organs and thorax**

R84.2 **Abnormal level of other drugs, medicaments and biological substances in specimens from respiratory organs and thorax**

R84.3 **Abnormal level of substances chiefly nonmedicinal as to source in specimens from respiratory organs and thorax**

R84.4 **Abnormal immunological findings in specimens from respiratory organs and thorax**

R84.5 **Abnormal microbiological findings in specimens from respiratory organs and thorax**

Positive culture findings in specimens from respiratory organs and thorax

EXCLUDES 1   *colonization status (Z22.-)*

R84.6 **Abnormal cytological findings in specimens from respiratory organs and thorax**

R84.7 **Abnormal histological findings in specimens from respiratory organs and thorax**

R84.8 **Other abnormal findings in specimens from respiratory organs and thorax**

Abnormal chromosomal findings in specimens from respiratory organs and thorax

R84.9 **Unspecified abnormal finding in specimens from respiratory organs and thorax**

√4ᵗʰ **R85** **Abnormal findings in specimens from digestive organs and abdominal cavity**

INCLUDES   abnormal findings in peritoneal fluid

abnormal findings in saliva

EXCLUDES 1   *cloudy peritoneal dialysis effluent (R88.0)*

fecal abnormalities (R19.5)

R85.0 **Abnormal level of enzymes in specimens from digestive organs and abdominal cavity**

R85.1 **Abnormal level of hormones in specimens from digestive organs and abdominal cavity**

R85.2 **Abnormal level of other drugs, medicaments and biological substances in specimens from digestive organs and abdominal cavity**

R85.3 **Abnormal level of substances chiefly nonmedicinal as to source in specimens from digestive organs and abdominal cavity**

R85.4 **Abnormal immunological findings in specimens from digestive organs and abdominal cavity**

R85.5 **Abnormal microbiological findings in specimens from digestive organs and abdominal cavity**

Positive culture findings in specimens from digestive organs and abdominal cavity

EXCLUDES 1   *colonization status (Z22.-)*

√5ᵗʰ **R85.6** **Abnormal cytological findings in specimens from digestive organs and abdominal cavity**

√6ᵗʰ **R85.61** **Abnormal cytologic smear of anus**

EXCLUDES 1   *abnormal cytological findings in specimens from other digestive organs and abdominal cavity (R85.69)*

anal intraepithelial neoplasia I [AIN I] (K62.82)

anal intraepithelial neoplasia II [AIN II] (K62.82)

anal intraepithelial neoplasia III [AIN III] (D01.3)

carcinoma in situ of anus (histologically confirmed) (D01.3)

dysplasia (mild) (moderate) of anus (histologically confirmed) (K62.82)

severe dysplasia of anus (histologically confirmed) (D01.3)

EXCLUDES 2   *anal high risk human papillomavirus (HPV) DNA test positive (R85.81)*

anal low risk human papillomavirus (HPV) DNA test positive (R85.82)

R85.610 **Atypical squamous cells of undetermined significance on cytologic smear of anus [ASC-US]**

R85.611 **Atypical squamous cells cannot exclude high grade squamous intraepithelial lesion on cytologic smear of anus [ASC-H]**

R85.612 **Low grade squamous intraepithelial lesion on cytologic smear of anus [LGSIL]**

R85.613 **High grade squamous intraepithelial lesion on cytologic smear of anus [HGSIL]**

R85.614 **Cytologic evidence of malignancy on smear of anus**

R85.615 **Unsatisfactory cytologic smear of anus**

Inadequate sample of cytologic smear of anus

R85.616 **Satisfactory anal smear but lacking transformation zone**

R85.618 **Other abnormal cytological findings on specimens from anus**

R85.619 **Unspecified abnormal cytological findings in specimens from anus**

Abnormal anal cytology NOS

Atypical glandular cells of anus NOS

R85.69 **Abnormal cytological findings in specimens from other digestive organs and abdominal cavity**

R85.7 **Abnormal histological findings in specimens from digestive organs and abdominal cavity**

√5ᵗʰ **R85.8** **Other abnormal findings in specimens from digestive organs and abdominal cavity**

R85.81 **Anal high risk human papillomavirus [HPV] DNA test positive**

EXCLUDES 1   *anogenital warts due to human papillomavirus (HPV) (A63.0)*

condyloma acuminatum (A63.0)

R85.82 **Anal low risk human papillomavirus [HPV] DNA test positive**

Use additional code for associated human papillomavirus (B97.7)

R85.89 **Other abnormal findings in specimens from digestive organs and abdominal cavity**

Abnormal chromosomal findings in specimens from digestive organs and abdominal cavity

R85.9 **Unspecified abnormal finding in specimens from digestive organs and abdominal cavity**

√4ᵗʰ **R86** **Abnormal findings in specimens from male genital organs**

INCLUDES   abnormal findings in prostatic secretions

abnormal findings in semen, seminal fluid

abnormal spermatozoa

EXCLUDES 1   *azoospermia (N46.0-)*

oligospermia (N46.1-)

R86.0 **Abnormal level of enzymes in specimens from male genital organs** ♂

R86.1 **Abnormal level of hormones in specimens from male genital organs** ♂

R86.2 **Abnormal level of other drugs, medicaments and biological substances in specimens from male genital organs** ♂

R86.3 Abnormal level of substances chiefly nonmedicinal as to source in specimens from male genital organs   ♂

R86.4 Abnormal immunological findings in specimens from male genital organs   ♂

R86.5 Abnormal microbiological findings in specimens from male genital organs   ♂

Positive culture findings in specimens from male genital organs

EXCLUDES 1   colonization status (Z22.-)

R86.6 Abnormal cytological findings in specimens from male genital organs   ♂

R86.7 Abnormal histological findings in specimens from male genital organs   ♂

R86.8 Other abnormal findings in specimens from male genital organs   ♂

Abnormal chromosomal findings in specimens from male genital organs

R86.9 Unspecified abnormal finding in specimens from male genital organs   ♂

✓4ᵗʰ **R87** Abnormal findings in specimens from female genital organs

INCLUDES   abnormal findings in secretion and smears from cervix uteri
abnormal findings in secretion and smears from vagina
abnormal findings in secretion and smears from vulva

R87.0 Abnormal level of enzymes in specimens from female genital organs   ♀

R87.1 Abnormal level of hormones in specimens from female genital organs   ♀

R87.2 Abnormal level of other drugs, medicaments and biological substances in specimens from female genital organs   ♀

R87.3 Abnormal level of substances chiefly nonmedicinal as to source in specimens from female genital organs   ♀

R87.4 Abnormal immunological findings in specimens from female genital organs   ♀

R87.5 Abnormal microbiological findings in specimens from female genital organs   ♀

Positive culture findings in specimens from female genital organs

EXCLUDES 1   colonization status (Z22.-)

✓5ᵗʰ **R87.6** Abnormal cytological findings in specimens from female genital organs

✓6ᵗʰ **R87.61** Abnormal cytological findings in specimens from cervix uteri

EXCLUDES 1   abnormal cytological findings in specimens from other female genital organs (R87.69)
abnormal cytological findings in specimens from vagina (R87.62-)
carcinoma in situ of cervix uteri (histologically confirmed) (D06.-)
cervical intraepithelial neoplasia I [CIN I] (N87.0)
cervical intraepithelial neoplasia II [CIN II] (N87.1)
cervical intraepithelial neoplasia III [CIN III] (D06.-)
dysplasia (mild) (moderate) of cervix uteri (histologically confirmed) (N87.-)
severe dysplasia of cervix uteri (histologically confirmed) (D06.-)

EXCLUDES 2   cervical high risk human papillomavirus (HPV) DNA test positive (R87.810)
cervical low risk human papillomavirus (HPV) DNA test positive (R87.820)

R87.610 Atypical squamous cells of undetermined significance on cytologic smear of cervix [ASC-US]   ♀

R87.611 Atypical squamous cells cannot exclude high grade squamous intraepithelial lesion on cytologic smear of cervix [ASC-H]   ♀

R87.612 Low grade squamous intraepithelial lesion on cytologic smear of cervix [LGSIL]   ♀

R87.613 High grade squamous intraepithelial lesion on cytologic smear of cervix [HGSIL]   ♀

R87.614 Cytologic evidence of malignancy on smear of cervix   ♀

R87.615 Unsatisfactory cytologic smear of cervix   ♀

Inadequate sample of cytologic smear of cervix

R87.616 Satisfactory cervical smear but lacking transformation zone   ♀

R87.618 Other abnormal cytological findings on specimens from cervix uteri   ♀

R87.619 Unspecified abnormal cytological findings in specimens from cervix uteri   ♀

Abnormal cervical cytology NOS
Abnormal Papanicolaou smear of cervix NOS
Abnormal thin preparation smear of cervix NOS
Atypical endocervical cells of cervix NOS
Atypical endometrial cells of cervix NOS
Atypical glandular cells of cervix NOS

✓6ᵗʰ **R87.62** Abnormal cytological findings in specimens from vagina

Use additional code to identify acquired absence of uterus and cervix, if applicable (Z90.71-)

EXCLUDES 1   abnormal cytological findings in specimens from cervix uteri (R87.61-)
abnormal cytological findings in specimens from other female genital organs (R87.69)
carcinoma in situ of vagina (histologically confirmed) (D07.2)
dysplasia (mild) (moderate) of vagina (histologically confirmed) (N89.-)
severe dysplasia of vagina (histologically confirmed) (D07.2)
vaginal intraepithelial neoplasia I [VAIN I] (N89.0)
vaginal intraepithelial neoplasia II [VAIN II] (N89.1)
vaginal intraepithelial neoplasia III [VAIN III] (D07.2)

EXCLUDES 2   vaginal high risk human papillomavirus (HPV) DNA test positive (R87.811)
vaginal low risk human papillomavirus (HPV) DNA test positive (R87.821)

R87.620 Atypical squamous cells of undetermined significance on cytologic smear of vagina [ASC-US]   ♀

R87.621 Atypical squamous cells cannot exclude high grade squamous intraepithelial lesion on cytologic smear of vagina [ASC-H]   ♀

R87.622 Low grade squamous intraepithelial lesion on cytologic smear of vagina [LGSIL]   ♀

R87.623 High grade squamous intraepithelial lesion on cytologic smear of vagina [HGSIL]   ♀

R87.624 Cytologic evidence of malignancy on smear of vagina   ♀

R87.625 Unsatisfactory cytologic smear of vagina   ♀

Inadequate sample of cytologic smear of vagina

R87.628 Other abnormal cytological findings on specimens from vagina   ♀

R87.629 Unspecified abnormal cytological findings in specimens from vagina   ♀

Abnormal Papanicolaou smear of vagina NOS
Abnormal thin preparation smear of vagina NOS
Abnormal vaginal cytology NOS
Atypical endocervical cells of vagina NOS
Atypical endometrial cells of vagina NOS
Atypical glandular cells of vagina NOS

✓ Additional Character Required   ✓x7ᵗʰ Placeholder   Questionable PDx   Manifestation   Unspecified Dx   UPD Unacceptable PDx   H1-H14 HAC   HCC CMS-HCC Dx   .HIV HIV Dx

ICD-10-CM 2022   957

R87.69 **Abnormal cytological findings in specimens from other female genital organs** ♀
Abnormal cytological findings in specimens from female genital organs NOS
EXCLUDES 1   *dysplasia of vulva (histologically confirmed) (N90.0-N90.3)*

R87.7 **Abnormal histological findings in specimens from female genital organs** ♀
EXCLUDES 1   *carcinoma in situ (histologically confirmed) of female genital organs (D06-D07.3)*
cervical intraepithelial neoplasia I [CIN I] (N87.0)
cervical intraepithelial neoplasia II [CIN II] (N87.1)
cervical intraepithelial neoplasia III [CIN III] (D06.-)
dysplasia (mild) (moderate) of cervix uteri (histologically confirmed) (N87.-)
dysplasia (mild) (moderate) of vagina (histologically confirmed) (N89.-)
severe dysplasia of cervix uteri (histologically confirmed) (D06.-)
severe dysplasia of vagina (histologically confirmed) (D07.2)
vaginal intraepithelial neoplasia I [VAIN I] (N89.0)
vaginal intraepithelial neoplasia II [VAIN II] (N89.1)
vaginal intraepithelial neoplasia III [VAIN III] (D07.2)

✓5ᵗʰ R87.8 **Other abnormal findings in specimens from female genital organs**

✓6ᵗʰ R87.81 **High risk human papillomavirus [HPV] DNA test positive from female genital organs**
EXCLUDES 1   *anogenital warts due to human papillomavirus (HPV) (A63.0)*
condyloma acuminatum (A63.0)
R87.810 **Cervical high risk human papillomavirus [HPV] DNA test positive** ♀
R87.811 **Vaginal high risk human papillomavirus [HPV] DNA test positive** ♀

✓6ᵗʰ R87.82 **Low risk human papillomavirus [HPV] DNA test positive from female genital organs**
Use additional code for associated human papillomavirus (B97.7)
R87.820 **Cervical low risk human papillomavirus [HPV] DNA test positive** ♀
R87.821 **Vaginal low risk human papillomavirus [HPV] DNA test positive** ♀
R87.89 **Other abnormal findings in specimens from female genital organs** ♀
Abnormal chromosomal findings in specimens from female genital organs

R87.9 **Unspecified abnormal finding in specimens from female genital organs** ♀

✓4ᵗʰ R88 **Abnormal findings in other body fluids and substances**
R88.0 **Cloudy (hemodialysis) (peritoneal) dialysis effluent**
R88.8 **Abnormal findings in other body fluids and substances**

✓4ᵗʰ R89 **Abnormal findings in specimens from other organs, systems and tissues**
INCLUDES   abnormal findings in nipple discharge
abnormal findings in synovial fluid
abnormal findings in wound secretions
R89.0 **Abnormal level of enzymes in specimens from other organs, systems and tissues**
R89.1 **Abnormal level of hormones in specimens from other organs, systems and tissues**
R89.2 **Abnormal level of other drugs, medicaments and biological substances in specimens from other organs, systems and tissues**
R89.3 **Abnormal level of substances chiefly nonmedicinal as to source in specimens from other organs, systems and tissues**
R89.4 **Abnormal immunological findings in specimens from other organs, systems and tissues**
R89.5 **Abnormal microbiological findings in specimens from other organs, systems and tissues**
Positive culture findings in specimens from other organs, systems and tissues
EXCLUDES 1   *colonization status (Z22.-)*
R89.6 **Abnormal cytological findings in specimens from other organs, systems and tissues**
R89.7 **Abnormal histological findings in specimens from other organs, systems and tissues**

R89.8 **Other abnormal findings in specimens from other organs, systems and tissues**
Abnormal chromosomal findings in specimens from other organs, systems and tissues
R89.9 **Unspecified abnormal finding in specimens from other organs, systems and tissues**

Abnormal findings on diagnostic imaging and in function studies, without diagnosis (R90-R94)

INCLUDES   nonspecific abnormal findings on diagnostic imaging by computerized axial tomography [CAT scan]
nonspecific abnormal findings on diagnostic imaging by magnetic resonance imaging [MRI][NMR]
nonspecific abnormal findings on diagnostic imaging by positron emission tomography [PET scan]
nonspecific abnormal findings on diagnostic imaging by thermography
nonspecific abnormal findings on diagnostic imaging by ultrasound [echogram]
nonspecific abnormal findings on diagnostic imaging by X-ray examination
EXCLUDES 1   *abnormal findings on antenatal screening of mother (O28.-)*
diagnostic abnormal findings classified elsewhere - see Alphabetical Index

✓4ᵗʰ R90 **Abnormal findings on diagnostic imaging of central nervous system**
R90.0 **Intracranial space-occupying lesion found on diagnostic imaging of central nervous system**
✓5ᵗʰ R90.8 **Other abnormal findings on diagnostic imaging of central nervous system**
R90.81 **Abnormal echoencephalogram**
R90.82 **White matter disease, unspecified**
R90.89 **Other abnormal findings on diagnostic imaging of central nervous system**
Other cerebrovascular abnormality found on diagnostic imaging of central nervous system

✓4ᵗʰ R91 **Abnormal findings on diagnostic imaging of lung**
R91.1 **Solitary pulmonary nodule**
Coin lesion lung
Solitary pulmonary nodule, subsegmental branch of the bronchial tree
R91.8 **Other nonspecific abnormal finding of lung field**
Lung mass NOS found on diagnostic imaging of lung
Pulmonary infiltrate NOS
Shadow, lung

✓4ᵗʰ R92 **Abnormal and inconclusive findings on diagnostic imaging of breast**
R92.0 **Mammographic microcalcification found on diagnostic imaging of breast**
EXCLUDES 2   *mammographic calcification (calculus) found on diagnostic imaging of breast (R92.1)*
DEF: Calcium and cellular debris deposits in the breast that cannot be felt but can be detected on a mammogram. The deposits can be a sign of cancer, benign conditions, or changes in the breast tissue as a result of inflammation, injury, or an obstructed duct.
R92.1 **Mammographic calcification found on diagnostic imaging of breast**
Mammographic calculus found on diagnostic imaging of breast
R92.2 **Inconclusive mammogram**
Dense breasts NOS
Inconclusive mammogram NEC
Inconclusive mammography due to dense breasts
Inconclusive mammography NEC
AHA: 2015,1Q,24
R92.8 **Other abnormal and inconclusive findings on diagnostic imaging of breast**

✓4ᵗʰ R93 **Abnormal findings on diagnostic imaging of other body structures**
R93.0 **Abnormal findings on diagnostic imaging of skull and head, not elsewhere classified**
EXCLUDES 1   *intracranial space-occupying lesion found on diagnostic imaging (R90.0)*
R93.1 **Abnormal findings on diagnostic imaging of heart and coronary circulation**
Abnormal echocardiogram NOS
Abnormal heart shadow
R93.2 **Abnormal findings on diagnostic imaging of liver and biliary tract**
Nonvisualization of gallbladder

R93.3 **Abnormal findings on diagnostic imaging of other parts of digestive tract**

☑5ᵗʰ **R93.4** **Abnormal findings on diagnostic imaging of** urinary organs

     EXCLUDES 2   *hypertrophy of kidney (N28.81)*

     AHA: 2016,4Q,66

     R93.41 **Abnormal radiologic findings on diagnostic imaging of** renal pelvis, ureter, or bladder

         Filling defect of bladder found on diagnostic imaging

         Filling defect of renal pelvis found on diagnostic imaging

         Filling defect of ureter found on diagnostic imaging

     ☑6ᵗʰ **R93.42** **Abnormal radiologic findings on diagnostic imaging of kidney**

         R93.421 **Abnormal radiologic findings on diagnostic imaging of** right **kidney**

         R93.422 **Abnormal radiologic findings on diagnostic imaging of** left **kidney**

         R93.429 **Abnormal radiologic findings on diagnostic imaging of unspecified kidney**

     R93.49 **Abnormal radiologic findings on diagnostic imaging of other urinary organs**

R93.5 **Abnormal findings on diagnostic imaging of other abdominal regions, including retroperitoneum**

R93.6 **Abnormal findings on diagnostic imaging of** limbs

     EXCLUDES 2   *abnormal finding in skin and subcutaneous tissue (R93.8-)*

     AHA: 2020,1Q,14

R93.7 **Abnormal findings on diagnostic imaging of other parts of musculoskeletal system**

     EXCLUDES 2   *abnormal findings on diagnostic imaging of skull (R93.0)*

☑5ᵗʰ **R93.8** **Abnormal findings on diagnostic imaging of other specified body structures**

     AHA: 2018,4Q,30

     ☑6ᵗʰ **R93.81** **Abnormal radiologic findings on diagnostic imaging of** testis

         R93.811 **Abnormal radiologic findings on diagnostic imaging of** right **testicle**   ♂

         R93.812 **Abnormal radiologic findings on diagnostic imaging of** left **testicle**   ♂

         R93.813 **Abnormal radiologic findings on diagnostic imaging of testicles, bilateral**   ♂

         R93.819 **Abnormal radiologic findings on diagnostic imaging of unspecified testicle**   ♂

     R93.89 **Abnormal findings on diagnostic imaging of other specified body structures**

         Abnormal finding by radioisotope localization of placenta

         Abnormal radiological finding in skin and subcutaneous tissue

         Mediastinal shift

R93.9 **Diagnostic imaging inconclusive due to** excess body fat of patient

☑4ᵗʰ **R94** **Abnormal results of function studies**

     INCLUDES   abnormal results of radionuclide [radioisotope] uptake studies

             abnormal results of scintigraphy

☑5ᵗʰ **R94.0** **Abnormal results of function studies of** central nervous system

     R94.01 **Abnormal** electroencephalogram [EEG]

     R94.02 **Abnormal** brain scan

     R94.09 **Abnormal results of other function studies of central nervous system**

☑5ᵗʰ **R94.1** **Abnormal results of function studies of** peripheral nervous system and special senses

     ☑6ᵗʰ **R94.11** **Abnormal results of function studies of** eye

         R94.110 **Abnormal** electro-oculogram [EOG]

         R94.111 **Abnormal** electroretinogram [ERG]

             Abnormal retinal function study

         R94.112 **Abnormal** visually evoked potential [VEP]

         R94.113 **Abnormal** oculomotor study

         R94.118 **Abnormal results of other function studies of eye**

     ☑6ᵗʰ **R94.12** **Abnormal results of function studies of** ear and other special senses

         AHA: 2016,3Q,17

         R94.120 **Abnormal** auditory function study

         R94.121 **Abnormal** vestibular function study

         R94.128 **Abnormal results of other function studies of ear and other special senses**

     ☑6ᵗʰ **R94.13** **Abnormal results of function studies of** peripheral nervous system

         R94.130 **Abnormal response to nerve stimulation, unspecified**

         R94.131 **Abnormal** electromyogram [EMG]

             EXCLUDES 1   *electromyogram of eye (R94.113)*

         R94.138 **Abnormal results of other function studies of peripheral nervous system**

R94.2 **Abnormal results of** pulmonary function **studies**

     Reduced ventilatory capacity

     Reduced vital capacity

☑5ᵗʰ **R94.3** **Abnormal results of** cardiovascular function **studies**

     R94.30 **Abnormal result of cardiovascular function study, unspecified**

     R94.31 **Abnormal** electrocardiogram [ECG] [EKG]

         EXCLUDES 1   *long QT syndrome (I45.81)*

     R94.39 **Abnormal result of other cardiovascular function study**

         Abnormal electrophysiological intracardiac studies

         Abnormal phonocardiogram

         Abnormal vectorcardiogram

R94.4 **Abnormal results of** kidney function **studies**

     Abnormal renal function test

R94.5 **Abnormal results of** liver function **studies**

R94.6 **Abnormal results of** thyroid function **studies**

R94.7 **Abnormal results of other endocrine function studies**

     EXCLUDES 2   *abnormal glucose (R73.0-)*

R94.8 **Abnormal results of function studies of other organs and systems**

     Abnormal basal metabolic rate [BMR]

     Abnormal bladder function test

     Abnormal splenic function test

Abnormal tumor markers (R97)

☑4ᵗʰ **R97** **Abnormal tumor markers**

     Elevated tumor associated antigens [TAA]

     Elevated tumor specific antigens [TSA]

R97.0 **Elevated carcinoembryonic antigen [CEA]**

R97.1 **Elevated cancer antigen 125 [CA 125]**

☑5ᵗʰ **R97.2** **Elevated prostate specific antigen [PSA]**

     AHA: 2016,4Q,66

     R97.20 **Elevated prostate specific antigen [PSA]**   Ⓐ ♂

     R97.21 **Rising PSA following treatment for malignant neoplasm of prostate**   Ⓐ ♂

R97.8 **Other abnormal tumor markers**

Ill-defined and unknown cause of mortality (R99)

R99 **Ill-defined and unknown cause of mortality**

     Death (unexplained) NOS

     Unspecified cause of mortality

☑ Additional Character Required   ☑x7ᵗʰ Placeholder   Questionable PDx   Manifestation   Unspecified Dx   UPD Unacceptable PDx   H1 - H14 HAC   HCC CMS-HCC Dx   HIV HIV Dx

ICD-10-CM 2022   959

Chapter 19. Injury, Poisoning and Certain Other Consequences of External Causes (S00–T88)

Chapter-specific Guidelines with Coding Examples

The chapter-specific guidelines from the ICD-10-CM Official Guidelines for Coding and Reporting have been provided below. Along with these guidelines are coding examples, contained in the shaded boxes, that have been developed to help illustrate the coding and/or sequencing guidance found in these guidelines.

a. Application of 7th characters in Chapter 19

Most categories in chapter 19 have a 7th character requirement for each applicable code. Most categories in this chapter have three 7th character values (with the exception of fractures): A, initial encounter, D, subsequent encounter and S, sequela. Categories for traumatic fractures have additional 7th character values. While the patient may be seen by a new or different provider over the course of treatment for an injury, assignment of the 7th character is based on whether the patient is undergoing active treatment and not whether the provider is seeing the patient for the first time.

For complication codes, active treatment refers to treatment for the condition described by the code, even though it may be related to an earlier precipitating problem. For example, code T84.50XA, Infection and inflammatory reaction due to unspecified internal joint prosthesis, initial encounter, is used when active treatment is provided for the infection, even though the condition relates to the prosthetic device, implant or graft that was placed at a previous encounter.

7th character "A", initial encounter is used for each encounter where the patient is receiving active treatment for the condition.

> Patient admitted after fall from a skateboard onto the sidewalk, x-rays identify a nondisplaced fracture to the distal pole of the right scaphoid bone. The patient is placed in a cast.
>
> **S62.014A**   **Nondisplaced fracture of distal pole of navicular [scaphoid] bone of right wrist, initial encounter for closed fracture**
>
> **V00.131A**   **Fall from skateboard, initial encounter**
>
> **Y92.480**   **Sidewalk as the place of occurrence of the external cause**
>
> **Y93.51**   **Activity, roller skating (inline) and skateboarding**
>
> **Y99.8**   **Other external cause status**
>
> *Explanation:* This fracture would be coded with a seventh character A for initial encounter because the patient received x-rays to identify the site of the fracture and treatment was rendered; this would be considered active treatment.

7th character "D" subsequent encounter is used for encounters after the patient has completed active treatment of the condition and is receiving routine care for the condition during the healing or recovery phase.

> Patient admitted after fall from a skateboard onto the sidewalk resulted in casting of the right arm. X-rays are taken to evaluate how well the nondisplaced fracture to the distal pole of the right scaphoid bone is healing. The physician feels the fracture is healing appropriately; no adjustments to the cast are made.
>
> **S62.014D**   **Nondisplaced fracture of distal pole of navicular [scaphoid] bone of right wrist, subsequent encounter for fracture with routine healing**
>
> **V00.131D**   **Fall from skateboard, subsequent encounter**
>
> *Explanation:* This fracture would be coded with a seventh character D for subsequent encounter, whether the same physician who provided the initial cast application or a different physician is now seeing the patient. Although the patient received x-rays, the intent of the x-rays was to assess how the fracture was healing. There was no active treatment rendered and the visit is therefore considered a subsequent encounter.

The aftercare Z codes should not be used for aftercare for conditions such as injuries or poisonings, where 7th characters are provided to identify subsequent care. For example, for aftercare of an injury, assign the acute injury code with the 7th character "D" (subsequent encounter).

7th character "S", sequela, is for use for complications or conditions that arise as a direct result of a condition, such as scar formation after a burn. The scars are sequelae of the burn. When using 7th character "S", it is necessary to use both the injury code that precipitated the sequela and the code for the sequela itself. The "S" is added only to the injury code, not the sequela code. The 7th character "S" identifies the injury responsible for the sequela. The specific type of sequela (e.g. scar) is sequenced first, followed by the injury code.

See Section I.B.10 Sequelae, (Late Effects)

> Patient with a history of a nondisplaced fracture to the distal pole of the right scaphoid bone due to a fall from a skateboard is admitted for evaluation of arthritis to the right wrist that has developed as a consequence of the traumatic fracture.
>
> **M12.531**   **Traumatic arthropathy, right wrist**
>
> **S62.014S**   **Nondisplaced fracture of distal pole of navicular [scaphoid] bone of right wrist, sequela**
>
> **V00.131S**   **Fall from skateboard, sequela**
>
> *Explanation:* The code identifying the specific sequela condition (traumatic arthritis) should be coded first followed by the injury that instigated the development of the sequela (fracture). The scaphoid fracture injury code is given a 7th character S for sequela to represent its role as the inciting injury. The fracture has healed and is not being managed or treated on this admit and therefore is not applicable as a first listed or principal diagnosis. However, it is directly related to the development of the arthritis and should be appended as a secondary code to signify this cause and effect relationship.

b. Coding of injuries

When coding injuries, assign separate codes for each injury unless a combination code is provided, in which case the combination code is assigned. Codes from category T07, Unspecified multiple injuries should not be assigned in the inpatient setting unless information for a more specific code is not available. Traumatic injury codes (S00-T14.9) are not to be used for normal, healing surgical wounds or to identify complications of surgical wounds.

The code for the most serious injury, as determined by the provider and the focus of treatment, is sequenced first.

1) Superficial injuries

Superficial injuries such as abrasions or contusions are not coded when associated with more severe injuries of the same site.

2) Primary injury with damage to nerves/blood vessels

When a primary injury results in minor damage to peripheral nerves or blood vessels, the primary injury is sequenced first with additional code(s) for injuries to nerves and spinal cord (such as category S04), and/or injury to blood vessels (such as category S15). When the primary injury is to the blood vessels or nerves, that injury should be sequenced first.

3) Iatrogenic injuries

Injury codes from Chapter 19 should not be assigned for injuries that occur during, or as a result of, a medical intervention. Assign the appropriate complication code(s).

c. Coding of traumatic fractures

The principles of multiple coding of injuries should be followed in coding fractures. Fractures of specified sites are coded individually by site in accordance with both the provisions within categories S02, S12, S22, S32, S42, S49, S52, S59, S62, S72, S79, S82, S89, S92 and the level of detail furnished by medical record content.

A fracture not indicated as open or closed should be coded to closed. A fracture not indicated whether displaced or not displaced should be coded to displaced.

More specific guidelines are as follows:

1) Initial vs. subsequent encounter for fractures

Traumatic fractures are coded using the appropriate 7th character for initial encounter (A, B, C) for each encounter where the patient is receiving active treatment for the fracture. The appropriate 7th character for initial encounter should also be assigned for a patient who delayed seeking treatment for the fracture or nonunion.

Fractures are coded using the appropriate 7th character for subsequent care for encounters after the patient has completed active treatment of the fracture and is receiving routine care for the fracture during the healing or recovery phase.

Care for complications of surgical treatment for fracture repairs during the healing or recovery phase should be coded with the appropriate complication codes.

Care of complications of fractures, such as malunion and nonunion, should be reported with the appropriate 7th character for subsequent care with nonunion (K, M, N,) or subsequent care with malunion (P, Q, R).

Malunion/nonunion: The appropriate 7th character for initial encounter should also be assigned for a patient who delayed seeking treatment for the fracture or nonunion.

Female patient fell during a forest hiking excursion almost six months ago and until recently did not feel she needed to seek medical attention for her left ankle pain; x-rays show nonunion of lateral malleolus and surgery has been scheduled

S82.62XA	**Displaced fracture of lateral malleolus of left fibula, initial encounter for closed fracture**
W01.0XXA	**Fall on same level from slipping, tripping and stumbling without subsequent striking against object, initial encounter**
Y92.821	**Forest as place of occurrence of the external cause**
Y93.01	**Activity, walking, marching and hiking**
Y99.8	**Other external cause status**

Explanation: A seventh character of A is used for the lateral malleolus nonunion fracture to signify that the fracture is receiving active treatment. The delayed care for the fracture has resulted in a nonunion, but capturing the nonunion in the seventh character is trumped by the provision of active care.

The open fracture designations in the assignment of the 7th character for fractures of the forearm, femur and lower leg, including ankle are based on the Gustilo open fracture classification. When the Gustilo classification type is not specified for an open fracture, the 7th character for open fracture type I or II should be assigned (B, E, H, M, Q).

A 17-year-old arrives at the trauma center with open, displaced right forearm fracture with extensive soft tissue damage. He fell while being tackled playing football for his high school team. On-call orthopaedic specialist documents segmental type IIIA fracture of radial shaft with no need for plastic consult.

S52.361C	**Displaced segmental fracture of shaft of radius, right arm, initial encounter for open fracture type IIIA, IIIB, or IIIC**
W03.XXXA	**Other fall on same level due to collision with another person, initial encounter**
Y92.321	**Football field as the place of occurrence of the external cause**
Y93.61	**Activity, American tackle football**

Explanation: The seventh character for forearm fractures capture the type of encounter and whether the fracture is open or closed; open fractures are broken down further by the type of fracture based on the Gustilo classification. The Gustilo classification describes the severity of open fracture and soft tissue injury. Type IIIA describes an open fracture with extensive soft tissue injury but adequate soft tissue remaining for wound coverage. A segmental fracture means that the bone is broken in two places, leaving at least one segment unattached to the bone. There is no need to report an additional code for the soft tissue injury as it is captured in the fracture code.

A code from category M80, not a traumatic fracture code, should be used for any patient with known osteoporosis who suffers a fracture, even if the patient had a minor fall or trauma, if that fall or trauma would not usually break a normal, healthy bone.

See Section I.C.13. Osteoporosis.

The aftercare Z codes should not be used for aftercare for traumatic fractures. For aftercare of a traumatic fracture, assign the acute fracture code with the appropriate 7th character.

2) Multiple fractures sequencing

Multiple fractures are sequenced in accordance with the severity of the fracture.

3) Physeal fractures

For physeal fractures, assign only the code identifying the type of physeal fracture. Do not assign a separate code to identify the specific bone that is fractured.

d. Coding of burns and corrosions

The ICD-10-CM makes a distinction between burns and corrosions. The burn codes are for thermal burns, except sunburns, that come from a heat source, such as a fire or hot appliance. The burn codes are also for burns resulting from electricity and radiation. Corrosions are burns due to chemicals. The guidelines are the same for burns and corrosions.

Current burns (T20-T25) are classified by depth, extent and by agent (X code). Burns are classified by depth as first degree (erythema), second degree (blistering), and third degree (full-thickness involvement). Burns of the eye and internal organs (T26-T28) are classified by site, but not by degree.

1) Sequencing of burn and related condition codes

Sequence first the code that reflects the highest degree of burn when more than one burn is present.

a. When the reason for the admission or encounter is for treatment of external multiple burns, sequence first the code that reflects the burn of the highest degree.

b. When a patient has both internal and external burns, the circumstances of admission govern the selection of the principal diagnosis or first-listed diagnosis.

c. When a patient is admitted for burn injuries and other related conditions such as smoke inhalation and/or respiratory failure, the circumstances of admission govern the selection of the principal or first-listed diagnosis.

Patient admitted with minor first-degree burns to multiple sites of her right and left hands as well as severe smoke inhalation. While she was sleeping at home, a candle on her dresser lit the bedroom curtains on fire.

T59.811A	**Toxic effect of smoke, accidental (unintentional), initial encounter**
J70.5	**Respiratory conditions due to smoke inhalation**
T23.191A	**Burn of first degree of multiple sites of right wrist and hand, initial encounter**
T23.192A	**Burn of first degree of multiple sites of left wrist and hand, initial encounter**
X08.8XXA	**Exposure to other specified smoke, fire and flames, initial encounter**
Y92.003	**Bedroom of unspecified non-institutional (private) residence as the place of occurrence of the external cause**
Y93.84	**Activity, sleeping**

Explanation: Based on the documentation, the inhalation injury is more severe than the first-degree burns and is sequenced first. The burns to the hands are appended as secondary diagnoses.

---

2) Burns of the same anatomic site

Classify burns of the same anatomic site and on the same side but of different degrees to the subcategory identifying the highest degree recorded in the diagnosis (e.g., for second and third degree burns of right thigh, assign only code T24.311-).

3) Non-healing burns

Non-healing burns are coded as acute burns.

Necrosis of burned skin should be coded as a non-healed burn.

4) Infected burn

For any documented infected burn site, use an additional code for the infection.

5) Assign separate codes for each burn site

When coding burns, assign separate codes for each burn site. Category T30, Burn and corrosion, body region unspecified is extremely vague and should rarely be used.

Codes for burns of "multiple sites" should only be assigned when the medical record documentation does not specify the individual sites.

Patient is admitted with third-degree burns of the scalp as well as second-degree burns to the back of the right hand

T20.35XA	**Burn of third degree of scalp [any part], initial encounter**
T23.261A	**Burn of second degree of back of right hand, initial encounter**

Explanation: Two codes may be reported as the hand and face represent distinct burn sites.

---

6) Burns and corrosions classified according to extent of body surface involved

Assign codes from category T31, Burns classified according to extent of body surface involved, or T32, Corrosions classified according to extent of body surface involved, **for acute burns or corrosions** when the site of the burn **or corrosion** is not specified or when there is a need for additional data. It is advisable to use category T31 as additional coding when needed to provide data for evaluating burn mortality, such as that needed by burn units. It is also advisable to use category T31 as an additional code for reporting purposes when there is mention of a third-degree burn involving 20 percent or more of the body surface. **Codes from categories T31 and T32 should not be used for sequelae of burns or corrosions.**

Categories T31 and T32 are based on the classic "rule of nines" in estimating body surface involved: head and neck are assigned nine percent, each arm nine percent, each leg 18 percent, the anterior trunk 18 percent, posterior trunk 18 percent, and genitalia one percent. Providers may change these percentage assignments where necessary to accommodate infants and children who have proportionately larger heads than adults, and patients who have large buttocks, thighs, or abdomen that involve burns.

Patient seen in burn unit for dressing change after he accidentally spilled acetic acid on himself two days ago. The second-degree burns to his right thigh, covering about 3 percent of his body surface, are healing appropriately.

T54.2X1D	**Toxic effect of corrosive acids and acid-like substances, accidental (unintentional), subsequent encounter**
T24.611D	**Corrosion of second degree of right thigh, subsequent encounter**
T32.0	**Corrosions involving less than 10% of body surface**

Explanation: Code T32.0 provides additional information as to how much of the patient's body was affected by the corrosive substance.

---

7) **Encounters for treatment of sequela of burns**

Encounters for the treatment of the late effects of burns or corrosions (i.e., scars or joint contractures) should be coded with a burn or corrosion code with the 7th character "S" for sequela.

8) **Sequelae with a late effect code and current burn**

When appropriate, both a code for a current burn or corrosion with 7th character "A" or "D" and a burn or corrosion code with 7th character "S" may be assigned on the same record (when both a current burn and sequelae of an old burn exist). Burns and corrosions do not heal at the same rate and a current healing wound may still exist with sequela of a healed burn or corrosion.

See Section I.B.10 Sequela (Late Effects)

Female patient seen in ED for second-degree burn to the left ear; she also has significant scarring on her left elbow from a third-degree burn from childhood

T20.212A	**Burn of second degree of left ear [any part, except ear drum], initial encounter**
L90.5	**Scar conditions and fibrosis of skin**
T22.322S	**Burn of third degree of left elbow, sequela**

Explanation: The patient is being seen for management of a current second-degree burn, which is reflected in the code by appending the seventh character of A, indicating active treatment or management of this burn. The elbow scarring is a sequela of a previous third-degree burn. The sequela condition precedes the original burn injury, which is appended with a seventh character of S.

---

9) **Use of an external cause code with burns and corrosions**

An external cause code should be used with burns and corrosions to identify the source and intent of the burn, as well as the place where it occurred.

e. **Adverse effects, poisoning, underdosing and toxic effects**

Codes in categories T36-T65 are combination codes that include the substance that was taken as well as the intent. No additional external cause code is required for poisonings, toxic effects, adverse effects and underdosing codes.

1) **Do not code directly from the Table of Drugs**

Do not code directly from the Table of Drugs and Chemicals. Always refer back to the Tabular List.

2) **Use as many codes as necessary to describe**

Use as many codes as necessary to describe completely all drugs, medicinal or biological substances.

3) **If the same code would describe the causative agent**

If the same code would describe the causative agent for more than one adverse reaction, poisoning, toxic effect or underdosing, assign the code only once.

4) **If two or more drugs, medicinal or biological substances**

If two or more drugs, medicinal or biological substances are taken, code each individually unless a combination code is listed in the Table of Drugs and Chemicals.

If multiple unspecified drugs, medicinal or biological substances were taken, assign the appropriate code from subcategory T50.91, Poisoning by, adverse effect of and underdosing of multiple unspecified drugs, medicaments and biological substances.

5) **The occurrence of drug toxicity is classified in ICD-10-CM as follows:**

(a) **Adverse effect**

When coding an adverse effect of a drug that has been correctly prescribed and properly administered, assign the appropriate code for the nature of the adverse effect followed by the appropriate code for the adverse effect of the drug (T36-T50). The code for the drug should have a 5th or 6th character "5" (for example T36.0X5-) Examples of the nature of an adverse effect are tachycardia, delirium, gastrointestinal hemorrhaging, vomiting, hypokalemia, hepatitis, renal failure, or respiratory failure.

Patient admitted for stomach pain and jaundice, indicated by physician as possible side-effects of Inderal, recently started for hypertension. Inderal was discontinued and the patient switched to Atenolol instead.

R10.9	**Unspecified abdominal pain**
R17	**Unspecified jaundice**
T44.7X5A	**Adverse effect of beta-adrenoreceptor antagonists, initial encounter**
I10	**Essential (primary) hypertension**

Explanation: The side-effects caused by the drug are listed first, followed by the code for the adverse effect of the drug to capture the specific drug that was used.

(b) **Poisoning**

When coding a poisoning or reaction to the improper use of a medication (e.g., overdose, wrong substance given or taken in error, wrong route of administration), first assign the appropriate code from categories T36-T50. The poisoning codes have an associated intent as their 5th or 6th character (accidental, intentional self-harm, assault and undetermined). If the intent of the poisoning is unknown or unspecified, code the intent as accidental intent. The undetermined intent is only for use if the documentation in the record specifies that the intent cannot be determined. Use additional code(s) for all manifestations of poisonings.

A 55-year-old female status post recent left knee replacement is admitted due to confusion, dizziness, and nausea. Her spouse brought in her prescribed Xanax, Ambien, and Percocet bottles but has no idea how many she took. It is suspected that her symptoms are due to an overdose of these medications.

T42.4X1A	**Poisoning by benzodiazepines, accidental (unintentional), initial encounter**
T42.6X1A	**Poisoning by other antiepileptic and sedative-hypnotic drugs, accidental (unintentional), initial encounter**
T40.2X1A	**Poisoning by other opioids, accidental (unintentional), initial encounter**
R41.0	**Disorientation, unspecified**
R42	**Dizziness and giddiness**
R11.0	**Nausea**

Explanation: It was not documented whether the overdose of the drugs was accidental or intentional; therefore the correct reporting of the poisoning codes is accidental intent. The poisoning codes are sequenced first, followed by manifestations of the poisoning.

If there is also a diagnosis of abuse or dependence of the substance, the abuse or dependence is assigned as an additional code.

Examples of poisoning include:

(i) Error was made in drug prescription

Errors made in drug prescription or in the administration of the drug by provider, nurse, patient, or other person.

(ii) Overdose of a drug intentionally taken

If an overdose of a drug was intentionally taken or administered and resulted in drug toxicity, it would be coded as a poisoning.

(iii) Nonprescribed drug taken with correctly prescribed and properly administered drug

If a nonprescribed drug or medicinal agent was taken in combination with a correctly prescribed and properly administered drug, any drug toxicity or other reaction resulting from the interaction of the two drugs would be classified as a poisoning.

(iv) Interaction of drug(s) and alcohol

When a reaction results from the interaction of a drug(s) and alcohol, this would be classified as poisoning.

See Section I.C.4. if poisoning is the result of insulin pump malfunctions.

(c) Underdosing

Underdosing refers to taking less of a medication than is prescribed by a provider or a manufacturer's instruction. Discontinuing the use of a prescribed medication on the patient's own initiative (not directed by the patient's provider) is also classified as an underdosing. For underdosing, assign the code from categories T36-T50 (fifth or sixth character "6").

Codes for underdosing should never be assigned as principal or first-listed codes. If a patient has a relapse or exacerbation of the medical condition for which the drug is prescribed because of the reduction in dose, then the medical condition itself should be coded.

Noncompliance (Z91.12-, Z91.13- and Z91.14-) or complication of care (Y63.6-Y63.9) codes are to be used with an underdosing code to indicate intent, if known.

> Patient admitted for atrial fibrillation with history of chronic atrial fibrillation for which she is prescribed amiodarone. Financial concerns have left the patient unable to pay for her prescriptions and she has been skipping her amiodarone dose every other day to offset the cost.
>
> | I48.20 | Chronic atrial fibrillation, unspecified |
> | T46.2X6A | Underdosing of other antidysrhythmic drugs, initial encounter |
> | Z91.120 | Patient's intentional underdosing of medication regimen due to financial hardship |
>
> *Explanation:* By skipping her amiodarone pill every other day, the patient's atrial fibrillation returned. The condition for which the drug was being taken is reported first, followed by an underdosing code to show that the patient was not adhering to her prescription regimen. The Z code helps elaborate on the patient's social and/or economic circumstances that led to the patient taking less then what she was prescribed.

(d) Toxic effects

When a harmful substance is ingested or comes in contact with a person, this is classified as a toxic effect. The toxic effect codes are in categories T51-T65.

Toxic effect codes have an associated intent: accidental, intentional self-harm, assault and undetermined.

f. Adult and child abuse, neglect and other maltreatment

Sequence first the appropriate code from categories T74.- (Adult and child abuse, neglect and other maltreatment, confirmed) or T76.- (Adult and child abuse, neglect and other maltreatment, suspected) for abuse, neglect and other maltreatment, followed by any accompanying mental health or injury code(s).

If the documentation in the medical record states abuse or neglect it is coded as confirmed (T74.-). It is coded as suspected if it is documented as suspected (T76.-).

For cases of confirmed abuse or neglect an external cause code from the assault section (X92-Y09) should be added to identify the cause of any physical injuries. A perpetrator code (Y07) should be added when the perpetrator of the abuse is known. For suspected cases of abuse or neglect, do not report external cause or perpetrator code.

If a suspected case of abuse, neglect or mistreatment is ruled out during an encounter code Z04.71, Encounter for examination and observation following alleged physical adult abuse, ruled out, or code Z04.72, Encounter for examination and observation following alleged child physical abuse, ruled out, should be used, not a code from T76.

If a suspected case of alleged rape or sexual abuse is ruled out during an encounter code Z04.41, Encounter for examination and observation following alleged adult rape or code Z04.42, Encounter for examination and observation following alleged child rape, should be used, not a code from T76.

If a suspected case of forced sexual exploitation or forced labor exploitation is ruled out during an encounter, code Z04.81, Encounter for examination and observation of victim following forced sexual exploitation, or code Z04.82, Encounter for examination and observation of victim following forced labor exploitation, should be used, not a code from T76.

See Section I.C.15. Abuse in a pregnant patient.

g. Complications of care

1) General guidelines for complications of care

(a) Documentation of complications of care

See Section I.B.16. for information on documentation of complications of care.

2) Pain due to medical devices

Pain associated with devices, implants or grafts left in a surgical site (for example painful hip prosthesis) is assigned to the appropriate code(s) found in Chapter 19, Injury, poisoning, and certain other consequences of external causes. Specific codes for pain due to medical devices are found in the T code section of the ICD-10-CM. Use additional code(s) from category G89 to identify acute or chronic pain due to presence of the device, implant or graft (G89.18 or G89.28).

3) Transplant complications

(a) Transplant complications other than kidney

Codes under category T86, Complications of transplanted organs and tissues, are for use for both complications and rejection of transplanted organs. A transplant complication code is only assigned if the complication affects the function of the transplanted organ. Two codes are required to fully describe a transplant complication: the appropriate code from category T86 and a secondary code that identifies the complication.

Pre-existing conditions or conditions that develop after the transplant are not coded as complications unless they affect the function of the transplanted organs.

See I.C.21. for transplant organ removal status

See I.C.2. for malignant neoplasm associated with transplanted organ.

(b) Kidney transplant complications

Patients who have undergone kidney transplant may still have some form of chronic kidney disease (CKD) because the kidney transplant may not fully restore kidney function. Code T86.1- should be assigned for documented complications of a kidney transplant, such as transplant failure or rejection or other transplant complication. Code T86.1- should not be assigned for post kidney transplant patients who have chronic kidney (CKD) unless a transplant complication such as transplant failure or rejection is documented. If the documentation is unclear as to whether the patient has a complication of the transplant, query the provider.

Conditions that affect the function of the transplanted kidney, other than CKD, should be assigned a code from subcategory T86.1, Complications of transplanted organ, Kidney, and a secondary code that identifies the complication.

For patients with CKD following a kidney transplant, but who do not have a complication such as failure or rejection, *see section I.C.14. Chronic kidney disease and kidney transplant status.*

> Patient with chronic kidney disease stage 2; history of successful kidney transplant with no complications identified
>
> | N18.2 | Chronic kidney disease, stage 2 (mild) |
> | Z94.0 | Kidney transplant status |
>
> *Explanation:* This patient's stage 2 CKD is not indicated as being due to the transplanted kidney but instead is just the residual disease the patient had prior to the transplant.

4) Complication codes that include the external cause

As with certain other T codes, some of the complications of care codes have the external cause included in the code. The code includes the nature of the complication as well as the type of procedure that caused the complication. No external cause code indicating the type of procedure is necessary for these codes.

5) Complications of care codes within the body system chapters

Intraoperative and postprocedural complication codes are found within the body system chapters with codes specific to the organs and structures of that body system. These codes should be sequenced first, followed by a code(s) for the specific complication, if applicable.

Complication codes from the body system chapters should be assigned for intraoperative and postprocedural complications (e.g., the appropriate complication code from chapter 9 would be assigned for a vascular intraoperative or postprocedural complication) unless the complication is specifically indexed to a T code in chapter 19.

> During a spinal fusion procedure, the surgeon inadvertently punctured the dura. The midline durotomy was repaired, and the fusion procedure was completed.
>
> | G97.41 | Accidental puncture or laceration of dura during a procedure |
>
> *Explanation:* The accidental durotomy is not coded to an injury code in chapter 19 but instead is categorized to the nervous system chapter.

Muscle/Tendon Table

ICD-10-CM categorizes certain muscles and tendons in the upper and lower extremities by their action (e.g., extension, flexion), their anatomical location (e.g., posterior, anterior), and/or whether they are intrinsic or extrinsic to a certain anatomical area. The Muscle/Tendon Table is provided at the beginning of chapters 13 and 19 as a resource to help users when code selection depends on one or more of these characteristics. Please note that this table is not all-inclusive, and proper code assignment should be based on the provider's documentation.

Body Region	Muscle	Extensor Tendon	Flexor Tendon	Other Tendon
Shoulder				
	Deltoid	Posterior deltoid	Anterior deltoid	
	Rotator cuff			
	Infraspinatus			Infraspinatus
	Subscapularis			Subscapularis
	Supraspinatus			Supraspinatus
	Teres minor			Teres minor
	Teres major	Teres major		
Upper arm				
	Anterior muscles			
	Biceps brachii — long head		Biceps brachii — long head	
	Biceps brachii — short head		Biceps brachii — short head	
	Brachialis		Brachialis	
	Coracobrachialis		Coracobrachialis	
	Posterior muscles			
	Triceps brachii	Triceps brachii		
Forearm				
	Anterior muscles			
	Flexors			
	Deep			
	Flexor digitorum profundus		Flexor digitorum profundus	
	Flexor pollicis longus		Flexor pollicis longus	
	Intermediate			
	Flexor digitorum superficialis		Flexor digitorum superficialis	
	Superficial			
	Flexor carpi radialis		Flexor carpi radialis	
	Flexor carpi ulnaris		Flexor carpi ulnaris	
	Palmaris longus		Palmaris longus	
	Pronators			
	Pronator quadratus			Pronator quadratus
	Pronator teres			Pronator teres
	Posterior muscles			
	Extensors			
	Deep			
	Abductor pollicis longus			Abductor pollicis longus
	Extensor indicis	Extensor indicis		
	Extensor pollicis brevis	Extensor pollicis brevis		
	Extensor pollicis longus	Extensor pollicis longus		
	Superficial			
	Brachioradialis			Brachioradialis
	Extensor carpi radialis brevis	Extensor carpi radialis brevis		
	Extensor carpi radialis longus	Extensor carpi radialis longus		
	Extensor carpi ulnaris	Extensor carpi ulnaris		
	Extensor digiti minimi	Extensor digiti minimi		
	Extensor digitorum	Extensor digitorum		
	Anconeus	Anconeus		
	Supinator			Supinator

Chapter 19. Injury, Poisoning and Certain Other Consequences of External Causes

Body Region	Muscle	Extensor Tendon	Flexor Tendon	Other Tendon
Hand				
Extrinsic — attach to a site in the forearm as well as a site in the hand with action related to hand movement at the wrist				
	Extensor carpi radialis brevis	Extensor carpi radialis brevis		
	Extensor carpi radialis longus	Extensor carpi radialis longus		
	Extensor carpi ulnaris	Extensor carpi ulnaris		
	Flexor carpi radialis		Flexor carpi radialis	
	Flexor carpi ulnaris		Flexor carpi ulnaris	
	Flexor digitorum superficialis		Flexor digitorum superficialis	
	Palmaris longus		Palmaris longus	
Extrinsic — attach to a site in the forearm as well as a site in the hand with action in the hand related to finger movement				
	Adductor pollicis longus			Adductor pollicis longus
	Extensor digiti minimi	Extensor digiti minimi		
	Extensor digitorum	Extensor digitorum		
	Extensor indicis	Extensor indicis		
	Flexor digitorum profundus		Flexor digitorum profundus	
	Flexor digitorum superficialis		Flexor digitorum superficialis	
Extrinsic — attach to a site in the forearm as well as a site in the hand with action in the hand related to thumb movement				
	Extensor pollicis brevis	Extensor pollicis brevis		
	Extensor pollicis longus	Extensor pollicis longus		
	Flexor pollicis longus		Flexor pollicis longus	
Intrinsic — found within the hand only				
	Adductor pollicis			Adductor pollicis
	Dorsal interossei	Dorsal interossei	Dorsal interossei	
	Lumbricals	Lumbricals	Lumbricals	
	Palmaris brevis			Palmaris brevis
	Palmar interossei	Palmar interossei	Palmar interossei	
	Hypothenar muscles			
	Abductor digiti minimi			Abductor digiti minimi
	Flexor digiti minimi brevis		Flexor digiti minimi brevis	
	Opponens digiti minimi		Opponens digiti minimi	
	Thenar muscles			
	Abductor pollicis brevis			Abductor pollicis brevis
	Flexor pollicis brevis		Flexor pollicis brevis	
	Opponens pollicis		Opponens pollicis	
Thigh				
	Anterior muscles			
	Iliopsoas		Iliopsoas	
	Pectineus		Pectineus	
	Quadriceps	Quadriceps		
	Rectus femoris	Rectus femoris — Extends knee	Rectus femoris — Flexes hip	
	Vastus intermedius	Vastus intermedius		
	Vastus lateralis	Vastus lateralis		
	Vastus medialis	Vastus medialis		
	Sartorius		Sartorius	
	Medial muscles			
	Adductor brevis			Adductor brevis
	Adductor longus			Adductor longus
	Adductor magnus			Adductor magnus
	Gracilis			Gracilis
	Obturator externus			Obturator externus
	Posterior muscles			
	Hamstring	Hamstring — Extends hip	Hamstring — Flexes knee	
	Biceps femoris	Biceps femoris	Biceps femoris	
	Semimembranosus	Semimembranosus	Semimembranosus	
	Semitendinosus	Semitendinosus	Semitendinosus	

Body Region	Muscle	Extensor Tendon	Flexor Tendon	Other Tendon
Lower leg				
	Anterior muscles			
	Extensor digitorum longus	Extensor digitorum longus		
	Extensor hallucis longus	Extensor hallucis longus		
	Fibularis (peroneus) tertius	Fibularis (peroneus) tertius		
	Tibialis anterior	Tibialis anterior		Tibialis anterior
	Lateral muscles			
	Fibularis (peroneus) brevis		Fibularis (peroneus) brevis	
	Fibularis (peroneus) longus		Fibularis (peroneus) longus	
	Posterior muscles			
	Deep			
	Flexor digitorum longus		Flexor digitorum longus	
	Flexor hallucis longus		Flexor hallucis longus	
	Popliteus		Popliteus	
	Tibialis posterior		Tibialis posterior	
	Superficial			
	Gastrocnemius		Gastrocnemius	
	Plantaris		Plantaris	
	Soleus		Soleus	
				Calcaneal (Achilles)
Ankle/Foot				
Extrinsic — attach to a site in the lower leg as well as a site in the foot with action related to foot movement at the ankle				
	Plantaris		Plantaris	
	Soleus		Soleus	
	Tibialis anterior	Tibialis anterior		
	Tibialis posterior		Tibialis posterior	
Extrinsic — attach to a site in the lower leg as well as a site in the foot with action in the foot related to toe movement				
	Extensor digitorum longus	Extensor digitorum longus		
	Extensor hallucis longus	Extensor hallucis longus		
	Flexor digitorum longus		Flexor digitorum longus	
	Flexor hallucis longus		Flexor hallucis longus	
Intrinsic — found within the ankle/foot only				
	Dorsal muscles			
	Extensor digitorum brevis	Extensor digitorum brevis		
	Extensor hallucis brevis	Extensor hallucis brevis		
	Plantar muscles			
	Abductor digiti minimi		Abductor digiti minimi	
	Abductor hallucis		Abductor hallucis	
	Dorsal interossei	Dorsal interossei	Dorsal interossei	
	Flexor digiti minimi brevis		Flexor digiti minimi brevis	
	Flexor digitorum brevis		Flexor digitorum brevis	
	Flexor hallucis brevis		Flexor hallucis brevis	
	Lumbricals	Lumbricals	Lumbricals	
	Quadratus plantae		Quadratus plantae	
	Plantar interossei	Plantar interossei	Plantar interossei	

Chapter 19. Injury, Poisoning and Certain Other Consequences of External Causes (S00-T88)

NOTE   Use secondary code(s) from Chapter 20, External causes of morbidity, to indicate cause of injury. Codes within the T section that include the external cause do not require an additional external cause code.

Use additional code to identify any retained foreign body, if applicable (Z18.-)

EXCLUDES 1   birth trauma (P10-P15)
     obstetric trauma (O70-O71)

NOTE   The chapter uses the S-section for coding different types of injuries related to single body regions and the T-section to cover injuries to unspecified body regions as well as poisoning and certain other consequences of external causes.

AHA: 2016,2Q,3-7; 2015,4Q,35-38; 2015,3Q,37-39,40; 2015,2Q,6; 2015,1Q,3-21

TIP: The specific site of an injury can be determined from the radiology report when authenticated by a radiologist and available at the time of code assignment.

This chapter contains the following blocks:

S00-S09	Injuries to the head
S10-S19	Injuries to the neck
S20-S29	Injuries to the thorax
S30-S39	Injuries to the abdomen, lower back, lumbar spine, pelvis and external genitals
S40-S49	Injuries to the shoulder and upper arm
S50-S59	Injuries to the elbow and forearm
S60-S69	Injuries to the wrist, hand and fingers
S70-S79	Injuries to the hip and thigh
S80-S89	Injuries to the knee and lower leg
S90-S99	Injuries to the ankle and foot
T07	Injuries involving multiple body regions
T14	Injury of unspecified body region
T15-T19	Effects of foreign body entering through natural orifice
T20-T25	Burns and corrosions of external body surface, specified by site
T26-T28	Burns and corrosions confined to eye and internal organs
T30-T32	Burns and corrosions of multiple and unspecified body regions
T33-T34	Frostbite
T36-T50	Poisoning by, adverse effect of and underdosing of drugs, medicaments and biological substances
T51-T65	Toxic effects of substances chiefly nonmedicinal as to source
T66-T78	Other and unspecified effects of external causes
T79	Certain early complications of trauma
T80-T88	Complications of surgical and medical care, not elsewhere classified

Injuries to the head (S00-S09)

INCLUDES   injuries of ear
     injuries of eye
     injuries of face [any part]
     injuries of gum
     injuries of jaw
     injuries of oral cavity
     injuries of palate
     injuries of periocular area
     injuries of scalp
     injuries of temporomandibular joint area
     injuries of tongue
     injuries of tooth

Code also for any associated infection

EXCLUDES 2   burns and corrosions (T20-T32)
     effects of foreign body in ear (T16)
     effects of foreign body in larynx (T17.3)
     effects of foreign body in mouth NOS (T18.0)
     effects of foreign body in nose (T17.0-T17.1)
     effects of foreign body in pharynx (T17.2)
     effects of foreign body on external eye (T15.-)
     frostbite (T33-T34)
     insect bite or sting, venomous (T63.4)

✓4ᵗʰ S00   **Superficial injury of head**

EXCLUDES 1   diffuse cerebral contusion (S06.2-)
     focal cerebral contusion (S06.3-)
     injury of eye and orbit (S05.-)
     open wound of head (S01.-)

> The appropriate 7th character is to be added to each code from category S00.
> A   initial encounter
> D   subsequent encounter
> S   sequela

✓5ᵗʰ S00.0   **Superficial injury of scalp**

   ✓x7ᵗʰ S00.00   Unspecified superficial injury of scalp

   ✓x7ᵗʰ S00.01   Abrasion of scalp

   ✓x7ᵗʰ S00.02   Blister (nonthermal) of scalp

   ✓x7ᵗʰ S00.03   **Contusion of scalp**
       Bruise of scalp
       Hematoma of scalp

   ✓x7ᵗʰ S00.04   **External constriction** of part of scalp

   ✓x7ᵗʰ S00.05   **Superficial foreign body** of scalp
       Splinter in the scalp

   ✓x7ᵗʰ S00.06   **Insect bite** (nonvenomous) of scalp

   ✓x7ᵗʰ S00.07   **Other superficial** bite of scalp
       EXCLUDES 1   open bite of scalp (S01.05)

✓5ᵗʰ S00.1   **Contusion of** eyelid and periocular area
     Black eye
     EXCLUDES 2   contusion of eyeball and orbital tissues ▶(S05.1-)◀

   ✓x7ᵗʰ S00.10   Contusion of unspecified eyelid and periocular area

   ✓x7ᵗʰ S00.11   Contusion of right eyelid and periocular area

   ✓x7ᵗʰ S00.12   Contusion of left eyelid and periocular area

✓5ᵗʰ S00.2   **Other and unspecified superficial injuries of eyelid and periocular area**
     EXCLUDES 2   superficial injury of conjunctiva and cornea (S05.0-)

   ✓6ᵗʰ S00.20   **Unspecified superficial injury of eyelid and periocular area**

     ✓7ᵗʰ S00.201   Unspecified superficial injury of right eyelid and periocular area

     ✓7ᵗʰ S00.202   Unspecified superficial injury of left eyelid and periocular area

     ✓7ᵗʰ S00.209   Unspecified superficial injury of unspecified eyelid and periocular area

   ✓6ᵗʰ S00.21   **Abrasion** of eyelid and periocular area

     ✓7ᵗʰ S00.211   Abrasion of right eyelid and periocular area

     ✓7ᵗʰ S00.212   Abrasion of left eyelid and periocular area

     ✓7ᵗʰ S00.219   Abrasion of unspecified eyelid and periocular area

   ✓6ᵗʰ S00.22   **Blister (nonthermal)** of eyelid and periocular area

     ✓7ᵗʰ S00.221   Blister (nonthermal) of right eyelid and periocular area

     ✓7ᵗʰ S00.222   Blister (nonthermal) of left eyelid and periocular area

     ✓7ᵗʰ S00.229   Blister (nonthermal) of unspecified eyelid and periocular area

   ✓6ᵗʰ S00.24   **External constriction** of eyelid and periocular area

     ✓7ᵗʰ S00.241   External constriction of right eyelid and periocular area

     ✓7ᵗʰ S00.242   External constriction of left eyelid and periocular area

     ✓7ᵗʰ S00.249   External constriction of unspecified eyelid and periocular area

   ✓6ᵗʰ S00.25   **Superficial foreign body** of eyelid and periocular area
       Splinter of eyelid and periocular area
       EXCLUDES 2   retained foreign body in eyelid (H02.81-)

     ✓7ᵗʰ S00.251   Superficial foreign body of right eyelid and periocular area

     ✓7ᵗʰ S00.252   Superficial foreign body of left eyelid and periocular area

     ✓7ᵗʰ S00.259   Superficial foreign body of unspecified eyelid and periocular area

   ✓6ᵗʰ S00.26   **Insect bite** (nonvenomous) of eyelid and periocular area

     ✓7ᵗʰ S00.261   Insect bite (nonvenomous) of right eyelid and periocular area

     ✓7ᵗʰ S00.262   Insect bite (nonvenomous) of left eyelid and periocular area

     ✓7ᵗʰ S00.269   Insect bite (nonvenomous) of unspecified eyelid and periocular area

   ✓6ᵗʰ S00.27   **Other superficial** bite of eyelid and periocular area
       EXCLUDES 1   open bite of eyelid and periocular area (S01.15)

     ✓7ᵗʰ S00.271   Other superficial bite of right eyelid and periocular area

     ✓7ᵗʰ S00.272   Other superficial bite of left eyelid and periocular area

     ✓7ᵗʰ S00.279   Other superficial bite of unspecified eyelid and periocular area

✓5ᵗʰ S00.3   **Superficial injury of** nose

   ✓x7ᵗʰ S00.30   Unspecified superficial injury of nose

   ✓x7ᵗʰ S00.31   Abrasion of nose

   ✓x7ᵗʰ S00.32   Blister (nonthermal) of nose

N Newborn: 0   **P** Pediatric: 0-17   **M** Maternity: 9-64   **A** Adult: 15-124   **MCC** Major Complication/Comorbidity   **CC** Complication/Comorbidity   **SW** Severe Wound Dx

968   ICD-10-CM 2022

√x7ᵗʰ **S00.33** **Contusion** of nose
    Bruise of nose
    Hematoma of nose

√x7ᵗʰ **S00.34** **External constriction** of nose

√x7ᵗʰ **S00.35** **Superficial** foreign body of nose
    Splinter in the nose

√x7ᵗʰ **S00.36** Insect bite (nonvenomous) of nose

√x7ᵗʰ **S00.37** **Other superficial** bite of nose
    EXCLUDES 1   open bite of nose (S01.25)

√5ᵗʰ **S00.4** **Superficial injury of** ear

√6ᵗʰ **S00.40** **Unspecified superficial injury of ear**
    √7ᵗʰ **S00.401** Unspecified superficial injury of **right** ear
    √7ᵗʰ **S00.402** Unspecified superficial injury of **left** ear
    √7ᵗʰ **S00.409** Unspecified superficial injury of **unspecified** ear

√6ᵗʰ **S00.41** **Abrasion** of ear
    √7ᵗʰ **S00.411** **Abrasion** of **right** ear
    √7ᵗʰ **S00.412** **Abrasion** of **left** ear
    √7ᵗʰ **S00.419** **Abrasion** of unspecified ear

√6ᵗʰ **S00.42** **Blister (nonthermal)** of ear
    √7ᵗʰ **S00.421** **Blister (nonthermal)** of **right** ear
    √7ᵗʰ **S00.422** **Blister (nonthermal)** of **left** ear
    √7ᵗʰ **S00.429** **Blister (nonthermal)** of **unspecified** ear

√6ᵗʰ **S00.43** **Contusion** of ear
    Bruise of ear
    Hematoma of ear
    √7ᵗʰ **S00.431** **Contusion** of **right** ear
    √7ᵗʰ **S00.432** **Contusion** of **left** ear
    √7ᵗʰ **S00.439** **Contusion** of **unspecified** ear

√6ᵗʰ **S00.44** **External constriction** of ear
    √7ᵗʰ **S00.441** **External constriction** of **right** ear
    √7ᵗʰ **S00.442** **External constriction** of **left** ear
    √7ᵗʰ **S00.449** **External constriction** of **unspecified** ear

√6ᵗʰ **S00.45** **Superficial** foreign body of ear
    Splinter in the ear
    √7ᵗʰ **S00.451** **Superficial foreign body** of **right** ear
    √7ᵗʰ **S00.452** **Superficial foreign body** of **left** ear
    √7ᵗʰ **S00.459** **Superficial foreign body** of **unspecified** ear

√6ᵗʰ **S00.46** Insect bite (nonvenomous) of ear
    √7ᵗʰ **S00.461** Insect bite (nonvenomous) of **right** ear
    √7ᵗʰ **S00.462** Insect bite (nonvenomous) of **left** ear
    √7ᵗʰ **S00.469** Insect bite (nonvenomous) of **unspecified** ear

√6ᵗʰ **S00.47** **Other superficial** bite of ear
    EXCLUDES 1   open bite of ear (S01.35)
    √7ᵗʰ **S00.471** **Other superficial bite** of **right** ear
    √7ᵗʰ **S00.472** **Other superficial bite** of **left** ear
    √7ᵗʰ **S00.479** **Other superficial bite** of **unspecified** ear

√5ᵗʰ **S00.5** **Superficial injury of** lip and oral cavity

√6ᵗʰ **S00.50** **Unspecified superficial injury of lip and oral cavity**
    √7ᵗʰ **S00.501** Unspecified superficial injury of **lip**
    √7ᵗʰ **S00.502** Unspecified superficial injury of **oral cavity**

√6ᵗʰ **S00.51** **Abrasion** of lip and oral cavity
    √7ᵗʰ **S00.511** **Abrasion** of **lip**
    √7ᵗʰ **S00.512** **Abrasion** of **oral cavity**

√6ᵗʰ **S00.52** **Blister (nonthermal)** of lip and oral cavity
    √7ᵗʰ **S00.521** **Blister (nonthermal)** of **lip**
    √7ᵗʰ **S00.522** **Blister (nonthermal)** of **oral cavity**

√6ᵗʰ **S00.53** **Contusion** of lip and oral cavity
    √7ᵗʰ **S00.531** **Contusion** of **lip**
       Bruise of lip
       Hematoma of lip
    √7ᵗʰ **S00.532** **Contusion** of **oral cavity**
       Bruise of oral cavity
       Hematoma of oral cavity

√6ᵗʰ **S00.54** **External constriction** of lip and oral cavity
    √7ᵗʰ **S00.541** **External constriction** of **lip**

√7ᵗʰ **S00.542** **External constriction** of **oral cavity**

√6ᵗʰ **S00.55** **Superficial** foreign body of lip and oral cavity
    √7ᵗʰ **S00.551** **Superficial foreign body of lip**
       Splinter of lip and oral cavity
    √7ᵗʰ **S00.552** **Superficial foreign body of** oral cavity
       Splinter of lip and oral cavity

√6ᵗʰ **S00.56** Insect bite (nonvenomous) of lip and oral cavity
    √7ᵗʰ **S00.561** Insect bite (nonvenomous) of **lip**
    √7ᵗʰ **S00.562** Insect bite (nonvenomous) of **oral cavity**

√6ᵗʰ **S00.57** **Other superficial** bite of lip and oral cavity
    √7ᵗʰ **S00.571** **Other superficial bite of lip**
    EXCLUDES 1   open bite of lip (S01.551)
    √7ᵗʰ **S00.572** **Other superficial bite of** oral cavity
    EXCLUDES 1   open bite of oral cavity (S01.552)

√5ᵗʰ **S00.8** **Superficial injury of other parts of head**
    Superficial injuries of face [any part]

√x7ᵗʰ **S00.80** **Unspecified superficial injury of other part of head**

√x7ᵗʰ **S00.81** **Abrasion** of other part of head

√x7ᵗʰ **S00.82** **Blister (nonthermal)** of other part of head

√x7ᵗʰ **S00.83** **Contusion** of other part of head
    Bruise of other part of head
    Hematoma of other part of head

√x7ᵗʰ **S00.84** **External constriction** of other part of head

√x7ᵗʰ **S00.85** **Superficial** foreign body of other part of head
    Splinter in other part of head

√x7ᵗʰ **S00.86** Insect bite (nonvenomous) of other part of head

√x7ᵗʰ **S00.87** **Other superficial** bite of other part of head
    EXCLUDES 1   open bite of other part of head (S01.85)

√5ᵗʰ **S00.9** **Superficial injury of unspecified part of head**

√x7ᵗʰ **S00.90** **Unspecified superficial injury of unspecified part of head**

√x7ᵗʰ **S00.91** **Abrasion** of unspecified part of head

√x7ᵗʰ **S00.92** **Blister (nonthermal)** of unspecified part of head

√x7ᵗʰ **S00.93** **Contusion** of unspecified part of head
    Bruise of head
    Hematoma of head

√x7ᵗʰ **S00.94** **External constriction** of unspecified part of head

√x7ᵗʰ **S00.95** **Superficial** foreign body of unspecified part of head
    Splinter of head

√x7ᵗʰ **S00.96** Insect bite (nonvenomous) of unspecified part of head

√x7ᵗʰ **S00.97** **Other superficial** bite of unspecified part of head
    EXCLUDES 1   open bite of head (S01.95)

√4ᵗʰ **S01** **Open wound of head**
    Code also any associated:
      injury of cranial nerve (S04.-)
      injury of muscle and tendon of head (S09.1-)
      intracranial injury (S06.-)
      wound infection
    EXCLUDES 1   open skull fracture (S02.- with 7th character B)
    EXCLUDES 2   injury of eye and orbit (S05.-)
               traumatic amputation of part of head (S08.-)

> The appropriate 7th character is to be added to each code from category S01.
> A   initial encounter
> D   subsequent encounter
> S   sequela

√5ᵗʰ **S01.0** **Open wound of scalp**
    EXCLUDES 1   avulsion of scalp ▶(S08.0-)◀
    √x7ᵗʰ **S01.00** **Unspecified open wound of scalp**
    √x7ᵗʰ **S01.01** **Laceration without foreign body** of scalp
    √x7ᵗʰ **S01.02** **Laceration with foreign body** of scalp
    √x7ᵗʰ **S01.03** **Puncture wound without foreign body** of scalp
    √x7ᵗʰ **S01.04** **Puncture wound with foreign body** of scalp
    √x7ᵗʰ **S01.05** **Open bite** of scalp
       Bite of scalp NOS
       EXCLUDES 1   superficial bite of scalp (S00.06, S00.07-)

✓5ᵗʰ **S01.1** **Open wound of eyelid and periocular area**

Open wound of eyelid and periocular area with or without involvement of lacrimal passages

✓6ᵗʰ **S01.10** **Unspecified open wound of eyelid and periocular area**

✓7ᵗʰ **S01.101** Unspecified open wound of right eyelid and periocular area **cc**

✓7ᵗʰ **S01.102** Unspecified open wound of left eyelid and periocular area **cc**

✓7ᵗʰ **S01.109** Unspecified open wound of unspecified eyelid and periocular area **cc**

✓6ᵗʰ **S01.11** Laceration without foreign body of eyelid and periocular area

✓7ᵗʰ **S01.111** Laceration without foreign body of right eyelid and periocular area

✓7ᵗʰ **S01.112** Laceration without foreign body of left eyelid and periocular area

✓7ᵗʰ **S01.119** Laceration without foreign body of unspecified eyelid and periocular area

✓6ᵗʰ **S01.12** Laceration with foreign body of eyelid and periocular area

✓7ᵗʰ **S01.121** Laceration with foreign body of right eyelid and periocular area

✓7ᵗʰ **S01.122** Laceration with foreign body of left eyelid and periocular area

✓7ᵗʰ **S01.129** Laceration with foreign body of unspecified eyelid and periocular area

✓6ᵗʰ **S01.13** Puncture wound without foreign body of eyelid and periocular area

✓7ᵗʰ **S01.131** Puncture wound without foreign body of right eyelid and periocular area

✓7ᵗʰ **S01.132** Puncture wound without foreign body of left eyelid and periocular area

✓7ᵗʰ **S01.139** Puncture wound without foreign body of unspecified eyelid and periocular area

✓6ᵗʰ **S01.14** Puncture wound with foreign body of eyelid and periocular area

✓7ᵗʰ **S01.141** Puncture wound with foreign body of right eyelid and periocular area

✓7ᵗʰ **S01.142** Puncture wound with foreign body of left eyelid and periocular area

✓7ᵗʰ **S01.149** Puncture wound with foreign body of unspecified eyelid and periocular area

✓6ᵗʰ **S01.15** Open bite of eyelid and periocular area

Bite of eyelid and periocular area NOS

EXCLUDES 1 *superficial bite of eyelid and periocular area (S00.26, S00.27)*

✓7ᵗʰ **S01.151** Open bite of right eyelid and periocular area

✓7ᵗʰ **S01.152** Open bite of left eyelid and periocular area

✓7ᵗʰ **S01.159** Open bite of unspecified eyelid and periocular area

✓5ᵗʰ **S01.2** **Open wound of nose**

✓x7ᵗʰ **S01.20** **Unspecified open wound of nose**

✓x7ᵗʰ **S01.21** Laceration without foreign body of nose

✓x7ᵗʰ **S01.22** Laceration with foreign body of nose

✓x7ᵗʰ **S01.23** Puncture wound without foreign body of nose

✓x7ᵗʰ **S01.24** Puncture wound with foreign body of nose

✓x7ᵗʰ **S01.25** Open bite of nose

Bite of nose NOS

EXCLUDES 1 *superficial bite of nose (S00.36, S00.37)*

✓5ᵗʰ **S01.3** **Open wound of ear**

✓6ᵗʰ **S01.30** **Unspecified open wound of ear**

✓7ᵗʰ **S01.301** Unspecified open wound of right ear

✓7ᵗʰ **S01.302** Unspecified open wound of left ear

✓7ᵗʰ **S01.309** Unspecified open wound of unspecified ear

✓6ᵗʰ **S01.31** Laceration without foreign body of ear

✓7ᵗʰ **S01.311** Laceration without foreign body of right ear

✓7ᵗʰ **S01.312** Laceration without foreign body of left ear

✓7ᵗʰ **S01.319** Laceration without foreign body of unspecified ear

✓6ᵗʰ **S01.32** Laceration with foreign body of ear

✓7ᵗʰ **S01.321** Laceration with foreign body of right ear

✓7ᵗʰ **S01.322** Laceration with foreign body of left ear

✓7ᵗʰ **S01.329** Laceration with foreign body of unspecified ear

✓6ᵗʰ **S01.33** Puncture wound without foreign body of ear

✓7ᵗʰ **S01.331** Puncture wound without foreign body of right ear

✓7ᵗʰ **S01.332** Puncture wound without foreign body of left ear

✓7ᵗʰ **S01.339** Puncture wound without foreign body of unspecified ear

✓6ᵗʰ **S01.34** Puncture wound with foreign body of ear

✓7ᵗʰ **S01.341** Puncture wound with foreign body of right ear

✓7ᵗʰ **S01.342** Puncture wound with foreign body of left ear

✓7ᵗʰ **S01.349** Puncture wound with foreign body of unspecified ear

✓6ᵗʰ **S01.35** Open bite of ear

Bite of ear NOS

EXCLUDES 1 *superficial bite of ear (S00.46, S00.47)*

✓7ᵗʰ **S01.351** Open bite of right ear

✓7ᵗʰ **S01.352** Open bite of left ear

✓7ᵗʰ **S01.359** Open bite of unspecified ear

✓5ᵗʰ **S01.4** **Open wound of cheek and temporomandibular area**

✓6ᵗʰ **S01.40** **Unspecified open wound of cheek and temporomandibular area**

✓7ᵗʰ **S01.401** Unspecified open wound of right cheek and temporomandibular area

✓7ᵗʰ **S01.402** Unspecified open wound of left cheek and temporomandibular area

✓7ᵗʰ **S01.409** Unspecified open wound of unspecified cheek and temporomandibular area

✓6ᵗʰ **S01.41** Laceration without foreign body of cheek and temporomandibular area

✓7ᵗʰ **S01.411** Laceration without foreign body of right cheek and temporomandibular area

✓7ᵗʰ **S01.412** Laceration without foreign body of left cheek and temporomandibular area

✓7ᵗʰ **S01.419** Laceration without foreign body of unspecified cheek and temporomandibular area

✓6ᵗʰ **S01.42** Laceration with foreign body of cheek and temporomandibular area

✓7ᵗʰ **S01.421** Laceration with foreign body of right cheek and temporomandibular area

✓7ᵗʰ **S01.422** Laceration with foreign body of left cheek and temporomandibular area

✓7ᵗʰ **S01.429** Laceration with foreign body of unspecified cheek and temporomandibular area

✓6ᵗʰ **S01.43** Puncture wound without foreign body of cheek and temporomandibular area

✓7ᵗʰ **S01.431** Puncture wound without foreign body of right cheek and temporomandibular area

✓7ᵗʰ **S01.432** Puncture wound without foreign body of left cheek and temporomandibular area

✓7ᵗʰ **S01.439** Puncture wound without foreign body of unspecified cheek and temporomandibular area

✓6ᵗʰ **S01.44** Puncture wound with foreign body of cheek and temporomandibular area

✓7ᵗʰ **S01.441** Puncture wound with foreign body of right cheek and temporomandibular area

✓7ᵗʰ **S01.442** Puncture wound with foreign body of left cheek and temporomandibular area

✓7ᵗʰ **S01.449** Puncture wound with foreign body of unspecified cheek and temporomandibular area

✓6ᵗʰ **S01.45** Open bite of cheek and temporomandibular area

Bite of cheek and temporomandibular area NOS

EXCLUDES 2 *superficial bite of cheek and temporomandibular area (S00.86, S00.87)*

✓7ᵗʰ **S01.451** Open bite of right cheek and temporomandibular area

✓7ᵗʰ **S01.452** Open bite of left cheek and temporomandibular area

✓7ᵗʰ **S01.459** Open bite of unspecified cheek and temporomandibular area

Ⓝ Newborn: 0　Ⓟ Pediatric: 0-17　Ⓜ Maternity: 9-64　Ⓐ Adult: 15-124　**MCC** Major Complication/Comorbidity　**CC** Complication/Comorbidity　**SW** Severe Wound Dx

970

ICD-10-CM 2022

✓5ᵗʰ **S01.5** **Open wound of lip and oral cavity**
> EXCLUDES 2   tooth dislocation (S03.2)
>   tooth fracture (S02.5)

   ✓6ᵗʰ **S01.50** **Unspecified open wound of lip and oral cavity**

      ✓7ᵗʰ **S01.501** Unspecified open wound of **lip**

      ✓7ᵗʰ **S01.502** Unspecified open wound of **oral cavity**

   ✓6ᵗʰ **S01.51** **Laceration of lip and oral cavity without foreign body**

      ✓7ᵗʰ **S01.511** Laceration without foreign body of **lip**

      ✓7ᵗʰ **S01.512** Laceration without foreign body of **oral cavity**

   ✓6ᵗʰ **S01.52** **Laceration of lip and oral cavity with foreign body**

      ✓7ᵗʰ **S01.521** Laceration with foreign body of **lip**

      ✓7ᵗʰ **S01.522** Laceration with foreign body of **oral cavity**

   ✓6ᵗʰ **S01.53** **Puncture wound of lip and oral cavity without foreign body**

      ✓7ᵗʰ **S01.531** Puncture wound without foreign body of **lip**

      ✓7ᵗʰ **S01.532** Puncture wound without foreign body of **oral cavity**

   ✓6ᵗʰ **S01.54** **Puncture wound of lip and oral cavity with foreign body**

      ✓7ᵗʰ **S01.541** Puncture wound with foreign body of **lip**

      ✓7ᵗʰ **S01.542** Puncture wound with foreign body of **oral cavity**

   ✓6ᵗʰ **S01.55** **Open bite of lip and oral cavity**

      ✓7ᵗʰ **S01.551** Open bite of **lip**
>   Bite of lip NOS
>   EXCLUDES 1   superficial bite of lip (S00.571)

      ✓7ᵗʰ **S01.552** Open bite of **oral cavity**
>   Bite of oral cavity NOS
>   EXCLUDES 1   superficial bite of oral cavity (S00.572)

✓5ᵗʰ **S01.8** **Open wound of other parts of head**

   ✓x7ᵗʰ **S01.80** Unspecified open wound of other part of head

   ✓x7ᵗʰ **S01.81** Laceration without foreign body of other part of head

   ✓x7ᵗʰ **S01.82** Laceration with foreign body of other part of head

   ✓x7ᵗʰ **S01.83** Puncture wound without foreign body of other part of head

   ✓x7ᵗʰ **S01.84** Puncture wound with foreign body of other part of head

   ✓x7ᵗʰ **S01.85** Open bite of other part of head
>   Bite of other part of head NOS
>   EXCLUDES 1   superficial bite of other part of head (S00.87)

✓5ᵗʰ **S01.9** **Open wound of unspecified part of head**

   ✓x7ᵗʰ **S01.90** Unspecified open wound of unspecified part of head

   ✓x7ᵗʰ **S01.91** Laceration without foreign body of unspecified part of head

   ✓x7ᵗʰ **S01.92** Laceration with foreign body of unspecified part of head

   ✓x7ᵗʰ **S01.93** Puncture wound without foreign body of unspecified part of head

   ✓x7ᵗʰ **S01.94** Puncture wound with foreign body of unspecified part of head

   ✓x7ᵗʰ **S01.95** Open bite of unspecified part of head
>   Bite of head NOS
>   EXCLUDES 1   superficial bite of head NOS (S00.97)

✓4ᵗʰ **S02** **Fracture of skull and facial bones**

> NOTE   A fracture not indicated as open or closed should be coded to closed.

Code also any associated intracranial injury (S06.-)
AHA: 2021,1Q,6; 2017,1Q,42; 2016,4Q,66-67

> The appropriate 7th character is to be added to each code from category S02.
> A   initial encounter for closed fracture
> B   initial encounter for open fracture
> D   subsequent encounter for fracture with routine healing
> G   subsequent encounter for fracture with delayed healing
> K   subsequent encounter for fracture with nonunion
> S   sequela

2,3,7 ✓x7ᵗʰ **S02.0** **Fracture of vault of skull**   MCC CC H5 HCC
> Fracture of frontal bone
> Fracture of parietal bone

✓5ᵗʰ **S02.1** **Fracture of base of skull**
> EXCLUDES 2   lateral orbital wall (S02.84-)
>   medial orbital wall (S02.83-)
>   orbital floor (S02.3-)

     AHA: 2019,4Q,16-17

   ✓6ᵗʰ **S02.10** **Unspecified fracture of base of skull**

      2,3,7 ✓7ᵗʰ **S02.101** Fracture of base of skull, **right side**   MCC CC H5 HCC

      2,3,7 ✓7ᵗʰ **S02.102** Fracture of base of skull, **left side**   MCC CC H5 HCC

      2,3,7 ✓7ᵗʰ **S02.109** Fracture of base of skull, unspecified side   MCC CC H5 HCC

   ✓6ᵗʰ **S02.11** **Fracture of occiput**

      2,3,7 ✓7ᵗʰ **S02.110** Type I occipital condyle fracture, unspecified side   MCC CC H5 HCC

      2,3,7 ✓7ᵗʰ **S02.111** Type II occipital condyle fracture, unspecified side   MCC CC H5 HCC

      2,3,7 ✓7ᵗʰ **S02.112** Type III occipital condyle fracture, unspecified side   MCC CC H5 HCC

      2,3,7 ✓7ᵗʰ **S02.113** Unspecified occipital condyle fracture   MCC CC H5 HCC

      2,3,7 ✓7ᵗʰ **S02.118** Other fracture of occiput, unspecified side   MCC CC H5 HCC

      2,3,7 ✓7ᵗʰ **S02.119** Unspecified fracture of occiput   MCC CC H5 HCC

      2,3,7 ✓7ᵗʰ **S02.11A** Type I occipital condyle fracture, **right side**   MCC CC H5 HCC

      2,3,7 ✓7ᵗʰ **S02.11B** Type I occipital condyle fracture, **left side**   MCC CC H5 HCC

      2,3,7 ✓7ᵗʰ **S02.11C** Type II occipital condyle fracture, **right side**   MCC CC H5 HCC

      2,3,7 ✓7ᵗʰ **S02.11D** Type II occipital condyle fracture, **left side**   MCC CC H5 HCC

      2,3,7 ✓7ᵗʰ **S02.11E** Type III occipital condyle fracture, **right side**   MCC CC H5 HCC

      2,3,7 ✓7ᵗʰ **S02.11F** Type III occipital condyle fracture, **left side**   MCC CC H5 HCC

      2,3,7 ✓7ᵗʰ **S02.11G** Other fracture of occiput, **right side**   MCC CC H5 HCC

      2,3,7 ✓7ᵗʰ **S02.11H** Other fracture of occiput, **left side**   MCC CC H5 HCC

   ✓6ᵗʰ **S02.12** **Fracture of orbital roof**
      AHA: 2019,4Q,16-17

      2,3,7 ✓7ᵗʰ **S02.121** Fracture of orbital roof, **right side**   MCC CC H5 HCC

      2,3,7 ✓7ᵗʰ **S02.122** Fracture of orbital roof, **left side**   MCC CC H5 HCC

      2,3,7 ✓7ᵗʰ **S02.129** Fracture of orbital roof, unspecified side   MCC CC H5 HCC

    2,3,7 ✓x7ᵗʰ **S02.19** **Other fracture of base of skull**   MCC CC H5 HCC
> Fracture of anterior fossa of base of skull
> Fracture of ethmoid sinus
> Fracture of frontal sinus
> Fracture of middle fossa of base of skull
> Fracture of posterior fossa of base of skull
> Fracture of sphenoid
> Fracture of temporal bone

3 ✓x7ᵗʰ **S02.2** **Fracture of nasal bones**   CC H5

✓ Additional Character Required   ✓x7ᵗʰ Placeholder   Questionable PDx   Manifestation   Unspecified Dx   UPD Unacceptable PDx   H1-H14 HAC   HCC CMS-HCC Dx   HIV HIV Dx

√5ᵗʰ **S02.3** **Fracture of orbital floor**
Fracture of inferior orbital wall
EXCLUDES 1   orbit NOS (S02.85)
EXCLUDES 2   lateral orbital wall (S02.84-)
    medial orbital wall (S02.83-)
    orbital roof (S02.1-)

3,7 √x7ᵗʰ **S02.30** **Fracture of orbital floor, unspecified side** `CC` `H5` `HCC`

3,7 √x7ᵗʰ **S02.31** **Fracture of orbital floor, right side** `CC` `H5` `HCC`

3,7 √x7ᵗʰ **S02.32** **Fracture of orbital floor, left side** `CC` `H5` `HCC`

√5ᵗʰ **S02.4** **Fracture of malar, maxillary and zygoma bones**
Fracture of superior maxilla
Fracture of upper jaw (bone)
Fracture of zygomatic process of temporal bone

√6ᵗʰ **S02.40** **Fracture of malar, maxillary and zygoma bones, unspecified**

3,7 √7ᵗʰ **S02.400** **Malar fracture, unspecified side** `CC` `H5` `HCC`

3,7 √7ᵗʰ **S02.401** **Maxillary fracture, unspecified side** `CC` `H5` `HCC`

3,7 √7ᵗʰ **S02.402** **Zygomatic fracture, unspecified side** `CC` `H5` `HCC`

3,7 √7ᵗʰ **S02.40A** **Malar fracture, right side** `CC` `H5` `HCC`

3,7 √7ᵗʰ **S02.40B** **Malar fracture, left side** `CC` `H5` `HCC`

3,7 √7ᵗʰ **S02.40C** **Maxillary fracture, right side** `CC` `H5` `HCC`

3,7 √7ᵗʰ **S02.40D** **Maxillary fracture, left side** `CC` `H5` `HCC`

3,7 √7ᵗʰ **S02.40E** **Zygomatic fracture, right side** `CC` `H5` `HCC`

3,7 √7ᵗʰ **S02.40F** **Zygomatic fracture, left side** `CC` `H5` `HCC`

√6ᵗʰ **S02.41** **LeFort fracture**

DEF: Named for Rene Le Fort, these fractures describe different combinations of multiple fractures that occur from significant force to the midface. A common denominator in all three types of LeFort fractures is fracture of the pterygoid processes, which are two bony plates resembling wings that extend downward from the sphenoid bone.

LeFort Fracture Types

Frontal bone
Type III
Nasal bone
Orbital floor
Type II
Type I
Maxilla
Zygomatic bone (malar) and arch

3,7 √7ᵗʰ **S02.411** **LeFort I fracture** `CC` `H5` `HCC`

3,7 √7ᵗʰ **S02.412** **LeFort II fracture** `CC` `H5` `HCC`

3,7 √7ᵗʰ **S02.413** **LeFort III fracture** `CC` `H5` `HCC`

3,7 √x7ᵗʰ **S02.42** **Fracture of alveolus of maxilla** `CC` `H5` `HCC`

4 √x7ᵗʰ **S02.5** **Fracture of tooth (traumatic)** `CC`
Broken tooth
EXCLUDES 1   cracked tooth (nontraumatic) (K03.81)

√5ᵗʰ **S02.6** **Fracture of mandible**
Fracture of lower jaw (bone)

√6ᵗʰ **S02.60** **Fracture of mandible, unspecified**

3,7 √7ᵗʰ **S02.600** **Fracture of unspecified part of body of mandible, unspecified side** `CC` `H5` `HCC`

3,7 √7ᵗʰ **S02.601** **Fracture of unspecified part of body of right mandible**

3,7 √7ᵗʰ **S02.602** **Fracture of unspecified part of body of left mandible** `CC` `H5` `HCC`

3,7 √7ᵗʰ **S02.609** **Fracture of mandible, unspecified** `CC` `H5` `HCC`

√6ᵗʰ **S02.61** **Fracture of condylar process of mandible**

3,7 √7ᵗʰ **S02.610** **Fracture of condylar process of mandible, unspecified side** `CC` `H5` `HCC`

3,7 √7ᵗʰ **S02.611** **Fracture of condylar process of right mandible** `CC` `H5` `HCC`

3,7 √7ᵗʰ **S02.612** **Fracture of condylar process of left mandible** `CC` `H5` `HCC`

√6ᵗʰ **S02.62** **Fracture of subcondylar process of mandible**

3,7 √7ᵗʰ **S02.620** **Fracture of subcondylar process of mandible, unspecified side** `CC` `H5` `HCC`

3,7 √7ᵗʰ **S02.621** **Fracture of subcondylar process of right mandible** `CC` `H5` `HCC`

3,7 √7ᵗʰ **S02.622** **Fracture of subcondylar process of left mandible** `CC` `H5` `HCC`

√6ᵗʰ **S02.63** **Fracture of coronoid process of mandible**

3,7 √7ᵗʰ **S02.630** **Fracture of coronoid process of mandible, unspecified side** `CC` `H5` `HCC`

3,7 √7ᵗʰ **S02.631** **Fracture of coronoid process of right mandible** `CC` `H5` `HCC`

3,7 √7ᵗʰ **S02.632** **Fracture of coronoid process of left mandible** `CC` `H5` `HCC`

√6ᵗʰ **S02.64** **Fracture of ramus of mandible**

3,7 √7ᵗʰ **S02.640** **Fracture of ramus of mandible, unspecified side** `CC` `H5` `HCC`

3,7 √7ᵗʰ **S02.641** **Fracture of ramus of right mandible** `CC` `H5` `HCC`

3,7 √7ᵗʰ **S02.642** **Fracture of ramus of left mandible** `CC` `H5` `HCC`

√6ᵗʰ **S02.65** **Fracture of angle of mandible**

3,7 √7ᵗʰ **S02.650** **Fracture of angle of mandible, unspecified side** `CC` `H5` `HCC`

3,7 √7ᵗʰ **S02.651** **Fracture of angle of right mandible** `CC` `H5` `HCC`

3,7 √7ᵗʰ **S02.652** **Fracture of angle of left mandible** `CC` `H5` `HCC`

3,7 √x7ᵗʰ **S02.66** **Fracture of symphysis of mandible** `CC` `H5` `HCC`

√6ᵗʰ **S02.67** **Fracture of alveolus of mandible**

3,7 √7ᵗʰ **S02.670** **Fracture of alveolus of mandible, unspecified side** `CC` `H5` `HCC`

3,7 √7ᵗʰ **S02.671** **Fracture of alveolus of right mandible** `CC` `H5` `HCC`

3,7 √7ᵗʰ **S02.672** **Fracture of alveolus of left mandible** `CC` `H5` `HCC`

3,7 √x7ᵗʰ **S02.69** **Fracture of mandible of other specified site** `CC` `H5` `HCC`

√5ᵗʰ **S02.8** **Fractures of other specified skull and facial bones**
Fracture of palate
EXCLUDES 2   fracture of orbital floor (S02.3-)
    fracture of orbital roof (S02.12-)

3,7 √x7ᵗʰ **S02.80** **Fracture of other specified skull and facial bones, unspecified side** `CC` `H5` `HCC`

3,7 √x7ᵗʰ **S02.81** **Fracture of other specified skull and facial bones, right side** `CC` `H5` `HCC`

3,7 √x7ᵗʰ **S02.82** **Fracture of other specified skull and facial bones, left side** `CC` `H5` `HCC`

√6ᵗʰ **S02.83** **Fracture of medial orbital wall**
EXCLUDES 2   orbital floor (S02.3-)
    orbital roof (S02.12-)
AHA: 2019,4Q,16-17

3,7 √7ᵗʰ **S02.831** **Fracture of medial orbital wall, right side** `CC` `H5` `HCC`

3,7 √7ᵗʰ **S02.832** **Fracture of medial orbital wall, left side** `CC` `H5` `HCC`

3,7 √7ᵗʰ **S02.839** **Fracture of medial orbital wall, unspecified side** `CC` `H5` `HCC`

√6ᵗʰ **S02.84** **Fracture of lateral orbital wall**
EXCLUDES 2   orbital floor (S02.3-)
    orbital roof (S02.12-)
AHA: 2019,4Q,16-17

3,7 √7ᵗʰ **S02.841** **Fracture of lateral orbital wall, right side** `CC` `H5` `HCC`

3,7 √7ᵗʰ **S02.842** **Fracture of lateral orbital wall, left side** `CC` `H5` `HCC`

`N` Newborn: 0   `P` Pediatric: 0-17   `M` Maternity: 9-64   `A` Adult: 15-124   `MCC` Major Complication/Comorbidity   `CC` Complication/Comorbidity   `SW` Severe Wound Dx

972

ICD-10-CM 2022

3,7 ✓7ᵗʰ **S02.849** **Fracture of lateral orbital wall, unspecified side** CC H5 HCC

3,7 ✓x7ᵗʰ **S02.85** **Fracture of orbit, unspecified** CC H5 HCC
Fracture of orbit NOS
Fracture of orbit wall NOS
EXCLUDES 1 *lateral orbital wall (S02.84-)*
medial orbital wall (S02.83-)
orbital floor (S02.3-)
orbital roof (S02.12-)

✓5ᵗʰ **S02.9** **Fracture of unspecified skull and facial bones**

2,3,7 ✓x7ᵗʰ **S02.91** **Unspecified fracture of skull** MCC CC H5 HCC
AHA: 2020,2Q,24

3,7 ✓x7ᵗʰ **S02.92** **Unspecified fracture of facial bones** CC H5 HCC

✓4ᵗʰ **S03** **Dislocation and sprain of joints and ligaments of head**
INCLUDES avulsion of joint (capsule) or ligament of head
laceration of cartilage, joint (capsule) or ligament of head
sprain of cartilage, joint (capsule) or ligament of head
traumatic hemarthrosis of joint or ligament of head
traumatic rupture of joint or ligament of head
traumatic subluxation of joint or ligament of head
traumatic tear of joint or ligament of head
Code also any associated open wound
EXCLUDES 2 *strain of muscle or tendon of head (S09.1)*

The appropriate 7th character is to be added to each code from category S03.
A   initial encounter
D   subsequent encounter
S   sequela

✓5ᵗʰ **S03.0** **Dislocation of jaw**
Dislocation of jaw (cartilage) (meniscus)
Dislocation of mandible
Dislocation of temporomandibular (joint)
AHA: 2016,4Q,67

✓7ᵗʰ **S03.00** **Dislocation of jaw, unspecified side**

✓7ᵗʰ **S03.01** **Dislocation of jaw, right side**

✓7ᵗʰ **S03.02** **Dislocation of jaw, left side**

✓7ᵗʰ **S03.03** **Dislocation of jaw, bilateral**

✓x7ᵗʰ **S03.1** **Dislocation of septal cartilage of nose**

✓x7ᵗʰ **S03.2** **Dislocation of tooth**

✓5ᵗʰ **S03.4** **Sprain of jaw**
Sprain of temporomandibular (joint) (ligament)
AHA: 2016,4Q,67

✓7ᵗʰ **S03.40** **Sprain of jaw, unspecified side**

✓7ᵗʰ **S03.41** **Sprain of jaw, right side**

✓7ᵗʰ **S03.42** **Sprain of jaw, left side**

✓7ᵗʰ **S03.43** **Sprain of jaw, bilateral**

✓x7ᵗʰ **S03.8** **Sprain of joints and ligaments of other parts of head**

✓x7ᵗʰ **S03.9** **Sprain of joints and ligaments of unspecified parts of head**

✓4ᵗʰ **S04** **Injury of cranial nerve**
The selection of side should be based on the side of the body being affected
Code first any associated intracranial injury (S06.-)
Code also any associated:
open wound of head (S01.-)
skull fracture (S02.-)

The appropriate 7th character is to be added to each code from category S04.
A   initial encounter
D   subsequent encounter
S   sequela

✓5ᵗʰ **S04.0** **Injury of optic nerve and pathways**
Use additional code to identify any visual field defect or blindness (H53.4-, H54.-)

✓6ᵗʰ **S04.01** **Injury of optic nerve**
Injury of 2nd cranial nerve

✓7ᵗʰ **S04.011** **Injury of optic nerve, right eye** CC

✓7ᵗʰ **S04.012** **Injury of optic nerve, left eye** CC

✓7ᵗʰ **S04.019** **Injury of optic nerve, unspecified eye** CC
Injury of optic nerve NOS

✓x7ᵗʰ **S04.02** **Injury of optic chiasm** CC

✓6ᵗʰ **S04.03** **Injury of optic tract and pathways**
Injury of optic radiation

✓7ᵗʰ **S04.031** **Injury of optic tract and pathways, right side** CC

✓7ᵗʰ **S04.032** **Injury of optic tract and pathways, left side** CC

✓7ᵗʰ **S04.039** **Injury of optic tract and pathways, unspecified side** CC
Injury of optic tract and pathways NOS

✓6ᵗʰ **S04.04** **Injury of visual cortex**

✓7ᵗʰ **S04.041** **Injury of visual cortex, right side** CC

✓7ᵗʰ **S04.042** **Injury of visual cortex, left side** CC

✓7ᵗʰ **S04.049** **Injury of visual cortex, unspecified side** CC
Injury of visual cortex NOS

✓5ᵗʰ **S04.1** **Injury of oculomotor nerve**
Injury of 3rd cranial nerve

✓x7ᵗʰ **S04.10** **Injury of oculomotor nerve, unspecified side** CC

✓x7ᵗʰ **S04.11** **Injury of oculomotor nerve, right side** CC

✓x7ᵗʰ **S04.12** **Injury of oculomotor nerve, left side** CC

✓5ᵗʰ **S04.2** **Injury of trochlear nerve**
Injury of 4th cranial nerve

✓x7ᵗʰ **S04.20** **Injury of trochlear nerve, unspecified side** CC

✓x7ᵗʰ **S04.21** **Injury of trochlear nerve, right side** CC

✓x7ᵗʰ **S04.22** **Injury of trochlear nerve, left side** CC

✓5ᵗʰ **S04.3** **Injury of trigeminal nerve**
Injury of 5th cranial nerve

✓x7ᵗʰ **S04.30** **Injury of trigeminal nerve, unspecified side** CC

✓x7ᵗʰ **S04.31** **Injury of trigeminal nerve, right side** CC

✓x7ᵗʰ **S04.32** **Injury of trigeminal nerve, left side** CC

✓5ᵗʰ **S04.4** **Injury of abducent nerve**
Injury of 6th cranial nerve

✓x7ᵗʰ **S04.40** **Injury of abducent nerve, unspecified side** CC

✓x7ᵗʰ **S04.41** **Injury of abducent nerve, right side** CC

✓x7ᵗʰ **S04.42** **Injury of abducent nerve, left side** CC

✓5ᵗʰ **S04.5** **Injury of facial nerve**
Injury of 7th cranial nerve

✓x7ᵗʰ **S04.50** **Injury of facial nerve, unspecified side** CC

✓x7ᵗʰ **S04.51** **Injury of facial nerve, right side** CC

✓x7ᵗʰ **S04.52** **Injury of facial nerve, left side** CC

✓5ᵗʰ **S04.6** **Injury of acoustic nerve**
Injury of auditory nerve
Injury of 8th cranial nerve

✓x7ᵗʰ **S04.60** **Injury of acoustic nerve, unspecified side** CC

✓x7ᵗʰ **S04.61** **Injury of acoustic nerve, right side** CC

✓x7ᵗʰ **S04.62** **Injury of acoustic nerve, left side** CC

✓5ᵗʰ **S04.7** **Injury of accessory nerve**
Injury of 11th cranial nerve

✓x7ᵗʰ **S04.70** **Injury of accessory nerve, unspecified side** CC

✓x7ᵗʰ **S04.71** **Injury of accessory nerve, right side** CC

✓x7ᵗʰ **S04.72** **Injury of accessory nerve, left side** CC

✓6ᵗʰ **S04.8** **Injury of other cranial nerves**

✓6ᵗʰ **S04.81** **Injury of olfactory [1st] nerve**

✓7ᵗʰ **S04.811** **Injury of olfactory [1st] nerve, right side** CC

✓7ᵗʰ **S04.812** **Injury of olfactory [1st] nerve, left side** CC

✓7ᵗʰ **S04.819** **Injury of olfactory [1st] nerve, unspecified side** CC

✓6ᵗʰ **S04.89** **Injury of other cranial nerves**
Injury of vagus [10th] nerve

✓7ᵗʰ **S04.891** **Injury of other cranial nerves, right side** CC

✓7ᵗʰ **S04.892** **Injury of other cranial nerves, left side** CC

✓7ᵗʰ **S04.899** **Injury of other cranial nerves, unspecified side** CC

✓x7ᵗʰ **S04.9** **Injury of unspecified cranial nerve** CC

✓ Additional Character Required   ✓x7ᵗʰ Placeholder   Questionable PDx   Manifestation   Unspecified Dx   UPD Unacceptable PDx   H1-H14 HAC   HCC CMS-HCC Dx   HIV HIV Dx

ICD-10-CM 2022   973

✓4ᵗʰ S05 Injury of eye and orbit

     INCLUDES   open wound of eye and orbit

     EXCLUDES 2   2nd cranial [optic] nerve injury (S04.0-)

                  3rd cranial [oculomotor] nerve injury (S04.1-)

                  open wound of eyelid and periocular area (S01.1-)

                  orbital bone fracture (S02.1-, S02.3-, S02.8-)

                  superficial injury of eyelid (S00.1-S00.2)

> The appropriate 7th character is to be added to each code from category S05.
> A   initial encounter
> D   subsequent encounter
> S   sequela

✓5ᵗʰ S05.0 Injury of conjunctiva and corneal abrasion without foreign body

     EXCLUDES 1   foreign body in conjunctival sac (T15.1)

                  foreign body in cornea (T15.0)

   ✓x7ᵗʰ **S05.00 Injury of conjunctiva and corneal abrasion without foreign body, unspecified eye**

   ✓x7ᵗʰ **S05.01 Injury of conjunctiva and corneal abrasion without foreign body, right eye**

   ✓x7ᵗʰ **S05.02 Injury of conjunctiva and corneal abrasion without foreign body, left eye**

✓5ᵗʰ S05.1 Contusion of eyeball and orbital tissues

     Traumatic hyphema

     EXCLUDES 2   black eye NOS (S00.1)

                  contusion of eyelid and periocular area (S00.1)

   ✓x7ᵗʰ **S05.10 Contusion of eyeball and orbital tissues, unspecified eye**

   ✓x7ᵗʰ **S05.11 Contusion of eyeball and orbital tissues, right eye**

   ✓x7ᵗʰ **S05.12 Contusion of eyeball and orbital tissues, left eye**

✓5ᵗʰ S05.2 Ocular laceration and rupture with prolapse or loss of intraocular tissue

   ✓x7ᵗʰ **S05.20 Ocular laceration and rupture with prolapse or loss of intraocular tissue, unspecified eye** `CC`

   ✓x7ᵗʰ **S05.21 Ocular laceration and rupture with prolapse or loss of intraocular tissue, right eye** `CC`

   ✓x7ᵗʰ **S05.22 Ocular laceration and rupture with prolapse or loss of intraocular tissue, left eye** `CC`

✓5ᵗʰ S05.3 Ocular laceration without prolapse or loss of intraocular tissue

     Laceration of eye NOS

     DEF: Tear in ocular tissue without displacing structures that is due to blunt trauma. It is characterized by pain, redness, and decreased vision.

   ✓x7ᵗʰ **S05.30 Ocular laceration without prolapse or loss of intraocular tissue, unspecified eye** `CC`

   ✓x7ᵗʰ **S05.31 Ocular laceration without prolapse or loss of intraocular tissue, right eye** `CC`

   ✓x7ᵗʰ **S05.32 Ocular laceration without prolapse or loss of intraocular tissue, left eye** `CC`

✓5ᵗʰ S05.4 Penetrating wound of orbit with or without foreign body

     EXCLUDES 2   retained (old) foreign body following penetrating wound in orbit (H05.5-)

   ✓x7ᵗʰ **S05.40 Penetrating wound of orbit with or without foreign body, unspecified eye** `CC`

   ✓x7ᵗʰ **S05.41 Penetrating wound of orbit with or without foreign body, right eye** `CC`

   ✓x7ᵗʰ **S05.42 Penetrating wound of orbit with or without foreign body, left eye** `CC`

✓5ᵗʰ S05.5 Penetrating wound with foreign body of eyeball

     EXCLUDES 2   retained (old) intraocular foreign body (H44.6-, H44.7)

   ✓x7ᵗʰ **S05.50 Penetrating wound with foreign body of unspecified eyeball** `CC`

   ✓x7ᵗʰ **S05.51 Penetrating wound with foreign body of right eyeball**

   ✓x7ᵗʰ **S05.52 Penetrating wound with foreign body of left eyeball** `CC`

✓5ᵗʰ S05.6 Penetrating wound without foreign body of eyeball

     Ocular penetration NOS

   ✓x7ᵗʰ **S05.60 Penetrating wound without foreign body of unspecified eyeball**

   ✓x7ᵗʰ **S05.61 Penetrating wound without foreign body of right eyeball**

   ✓x7ᵗʰ **S05.62 Penetrating wound without foreign body of left eyeball**

✓5ᵗʰ S05.7 Avulsion of eye

     Traumatic enucleation

   ✓x7ᵗʰ **S05.70 Avulsion of unspecified eye** `CC`

   ✓x7ᵗʰ **S05.71 Avulsion of right eye** `CC`

   ✓x7ᵗʰ **S05.72 Avulsion of left eye** `CC`

✓5ᵗʰ S05.8 Other injuries of eye and orbit

     Lacrimal duct injury

   ✓6ᵗʰ **S05.8X Other injuries of eye and orbit**

     ✓7ᵗʰ **S05.8X1 Other injuries of right eye and orbit** `CC`

     ✓7ᵗʰ **S05.8X2 Other injuries of left eye and orbit** `CC`

     ✓7ᵗʰ **S05.8X9 Other injuries of unspecified eye and orbit** `CC`

✓5ᵗʰ S05.9 Unspecified injury of eye and orbit

     Injury of eye NOS

   ✓x7ᵗʰ **S05.90 Unspecified injury of unspecified eye and orbit**

   ✓x7ᵗʰ **S05.91 Unspecified injury of right eye and orbit** `CC`

   ✓x7ᵗʰ **S05.92 Unspecified injury of left eye and orbit** `CC`

✓4ᵗʰ S06 Intracranial injury

     NOTE   7th characters D and S do not apply to codes in category S06 with 6th character 7 – death due to brain injury prior to regaining consciousness, or 8 – death due to other cause prior to regaining consciousness.

     INCLUDES   traumatic brain injury

     Code also any associated:

       open wound of head (S01.-)

       skull fracture (S02.-)

     EXCLUDES 1   head injury NOS (S09.90)

     AHA: 2017,4Q,25; 2017,1Q,42; 2015,3Q,37

     TIP: Do not assign Z87.820 Personal history of traumatic brain injury, when residual conditions persist after an intracranial injury. The codes for the residual conditions should be first listed, followed by a code from category S06 using seventh character S to identify sequelae.

> The appropriate 7th character is to be added to each code from category S06.
> A   initial encounter
> D   subsequent encounter
> S   sequela

✓5ᵗʰ S06.0 Concussion

     Commotio cerebri

     EXCLUDES 1   concussion with other intracranial injuries classified in subcategories S06.1- to S06.6- , S06.81- and S06.82- - code to specified intracranial injury

     AHA: 2016,4Q,67-68

   ✓6ᵗʰ **S06.0X Concussion**

     8 ✓7ᵗʰ **S06.0X0 Concussion** without loss of consciousness `CC` `HCC`

     8 ✓7ᵗʰ **S06.0X1 Concussion with loss of consciousness of 30 minutes or less** `CC` `H5` `HCC`

     8 ✓7ᵗʰ **S06.0X9 Concussion with loss of consciousness of unspecified duration** `CC` `H5` `HCC`

       Concussion NOS

✓5ᵗʰ S06.1 Traumatic cerebral edema

     Diffuse traumatic cerebral edema

     Focal traumatic cerebral edema

     AHA: 2019,3Q,35; 2015,1Q,12-13

   ✓6ᵗʰ **S06.1X Traumatic cerebral edema**

     7 ✓7ᵗʰ **S06.1X0 Traumatic cerebral edema** without loss of consciousness `MCC` `HCC`

     7 ✓7ᵗʰ **S06.1X1 Traumatic cerebral edema with loss of consciousness of 30 minutes or less** `MCC` `H5` `HCC`

     7 ✓7ᵗʰ **S06.1X2 Traumatic cerebral edema with loss of consciousness of 31 minutes to 59 minutes** `MCC` `H5` `HCC`

     7 ✓7ᵗʰ **S06.1X3 Traumatic cerebral edema with loss of consciousness of 1 hour to 5 hours 59 minutes** `MCC` `H5` `HCC`

     7 ✓7ᵗʰ **S06.1X4 Traumatic cerebral edema with loss of consciousness of 6 hours to 24 hours** `MCC` `H5` `HCC`

     7 ✓7ᵗʰ **S06.1X5 Traumatic cerebral edema with loss of consciousness greater than 24 hours with return to pre-existing conscious level** `MCC` `H5` `HCC`

N Newborn: 0   **P** Pediatric: 0-17   **M** Maternity: 9-64   **A** Adult: 15-124   **MCC** Major Complication/Comorbidity   **CC** Complication/Comorbidity   **SW** Severe Wound Dx

974   ICD-10-CM 2022

7 √7ᵗʰ **S06.1X6 Traumatic cerebral edema with loss of consciousness** greater than 24 hours without return to pre-existing conscious level with patient surviving   `MCC` `H5` `HCC`

√7ᵗʰ **S06.1X7 Traumatic cerebral edema with loss of consciousness of** any duration with death due to brain injury prior to regaining consciousness   `MCC` `H5`

√7ᵗʰ **S06.1X8 Traumatic cerebral edema with loss of consciousness of** any duration with death due to **other** cause prior to regaining consciousness   `MCC` `H5`

7 √7ᵗʰ **S06.1X9 Traumatic cerebral edema with loss of consciousness of unspecified duration**   `MCC` `H5` `HCC`
    Traumatic cerebral edema NOS

√5ᵗʰ **S06.2 Diffuse traumatic brain injury**

Diffuse axonal brain injury

▶Use additional code, if applicable, for traumatic brain compression or herniation (S06.A-)◀

EXCLUDES 1   *traumatic diffuse cerebral edema (S06.1X-)*

AHA: 2020,3Q,46

TIP: Assign additional code(s) for individual (R40.21-, R40.22-, R40.23-) or total (R40.24-) coma scale scores. It is appropriate to code the coma scale scores based on documentation provided by clinicians who are not the patient's provider (such as emergency medical technician).

√6ᵗʰ **S06.2X Diffuse traumatic brain injury**

7 √7ᵗʰ **S06.2X0 Diffuse traumatic brain injury** without loss of consciousness   `HCC`

7 √7ᵗʰ **S06.2X1 Diffuse traumatic brain injury with loss of consciousness of** 30 minutes or less   `CC` `H5` `HCC`

7 √7ᵗʰ **S06.2X2 Diffuse traumatic brain injury with loss of consciousness of** 31 minutes to 59 minutes   `CC` `H5` `HCC`

7 √7ᵗʰ **S06.2X3 Diffuse traumatic brain injury with loss of consciousness of** 1 hour to 5 hours 59 minutes   `CC` `H5` `HCC`

7 √7ᵗʰ **S06.2X4 Diffuse traumatic brain injury with loss of consciousness of** 6 hours to 24 hours   `CC` `H5` `HCC`

7 √7ᵗʰ **S06.2X5 Diffuse traumatic brain injury with loss of consciousness** greater than 24 hours with return to pre-existing conscious levels   `CC` `H5` `HCC`

7 √7ᵗʰ **S06.2X6 Diffuse traumatic brain injury with loss of consciousness** greater than 24 hours without return to pre-existing conscious level with patient surviving   `MCC` `H5` `HCC`

√7ᵗʰ **S06.2X7 Diffuse traumatic brain injury with loss of consciousness of** any duration with death due to brain injury prior to regaining consciousness   `MCC` `H5`

√7ᵗʰ **S06.2X8 Diffuse traumatic brain injury with loss of consciousness of** any duration with death due to **other** cause prior to regaining consciousness   `MCC` `H5`

7 √7ᵗʰ **S06.2X9 Diffuse traumatic brain injury with loss of consciousness of unspecified duration**   `CC` `H5` `HCC`
    Diffuse traumatic brain injury NOS

√5ᵗʰ **S06.3 Focal traumatic brain injury**

▶Use additional code, if applicable, for traumatic brain compression or herniation (S06.A-)◀

EXCLUDES 1   *any condition classifiable to S06.4-S06.6*

EXCLUDES 2   *focal cerebral edema (S06.1)*

AHA: 2020,3Q,46; 2019,3Q,35; 2015,1Q,12-13

TIP: Assign additional code(s) for individual (R40.21-, R40.22-, R40.23-) or total (R40.24-) coma scale scores. It is appropriate to code the coma scale scores based on documentation provided by clinicians who are not the patient's provider (such as emergency medical technician).

√6ᵗʰ **S06.30 Unspecified focal traumatic brain injury**

7 √7ᵗʰ **S06.300 Unspecified focal traumatic brain injury** without loss of consciousness   `HCC`

7 √7ᵗʰ **S06.301 Unspecified focal traumatic brain injury with loss of consciousness of** 30 minutes or less   `CC` `H5` `HCC`

7 √7ᵗʰ **S06.302 Unspecified focal traumatic brain injury with loss of consciousness of** 31 minutes to 59 minutes   `CC` `H5` `HCC`

7 √7ᵗʰ **S06.303 Unspecified focal traumatic brain injury with loss of consciousness of** 1 hour to 5 hours 59 minutes   `CC` `H5` `HCC`

7 √7ᵗʰ **S06.304 Unspecified focal traumatic brain injury with loss of consciousness of** 6 hours to 24 hours   `CC` `H5` `HCC`

7 √7ᵗʰ **S06.305 Unspecified focal traumatic brain injury with loss of consciousness** greater than 24 hours with return to pre-existing conscious level   `CC` `H5` `HCC`

7 √7ᵗʰ **S06.306 Unspecified focal traumatic brain injury with loss of consciousness** greater than 24 hours without return to pre-existing conscious level with patient surviving   `MCC` `H5` `HCC`

√7ᵗʰ **S06.307 Unspecified focal traumatic brain injury with loss of consciousness of** any duration with death due to brain injury prior to regaining consciousness   `MCC` `H5`

√7ᵗʰ **S06.308 Unspecified focal traumatic brain injury with loss of consciousness of** any duration with death due to **other** cause prior to regaining consciousness   `MCC` `H5`

7 √7ᵗʰ **S06.309 Unspecified focal traumatic brain injury with loss of consciousness of unspecified duration**   `CC` `H5` `HCC`
    Unspecified focal traumatic brain injury NOS

√6ᵗʰ **S06.31 Contusion and laceration of** right cerebrum

7 √7ᵗʰ **S06.310 Contusion and laceration of right cerebrum** without loss of consciousness   `MCC` `H5` `HCC`

7 √7ᵗʰ **S06.311 Contusion and laceration of right cerebrum with loss of consciousness of** 30 minutes or less   `MCC` `H5` `HCC`

7 √7ᵗʰ **S06.312 Contusion and laceration of right cerebrum with loss of consciousness of** 31 minutes to 59 minutes   `MCC` `H5` `HCC`

7 √7ᵗʰ **S06.313 Contusion and laceration of right cerebrum with loss of consciousness of** 1 hour to 5 hours 59 minutes   `MCC` `H5` `HCC`

7 √7ᵗʰ **S06.314 Contusion and laceration of right cerebrum with loss of consciousness of** 6 hours to 24 hours   `MCC` `H5` `HCC`

7 √7ᵗʰ **S06.315 Contusion and laceration of right cerebrum with loss of consciousness** greater than 24 hours with return to pre-existing conscious level   `MCC` `H5` `HCC`

7 √7ᵗʰ **S06.316 Contusion and laceration of right cerebrum with loss of consciousness** greater than 24 hours without return to pre-existing conscious level with patient surviving   `MCC` `H5` `HCC`

√7ᵗʰ **S06.317 Contusion and laceration of right cerebrum with loss of consciousness of** any duration with death due to brain injury prior to regaining consciousness   `MCC` `H5`

√7ᵗʰ **S06.318 Contusion and laceration of right cerebrum with loss of consciousness of** any duration with death due to **other** cause prior to regaining consciousness   `MCC` `H5`

7 √7ᵗʰ **S06.319 Contusion and laceration of right cerebrum with loss of consciousness of unspecified duration**   `MCC` `H5` `HCC`
    Contusion and laceration of right cerebrum NOS

√6ᵗʰ **S06.32 Contusion and laceration of** left cerebrum

7 √7ᵗʰ **S06.320 Contusion and laceration of left cerebrum** without loss of consciousness   `MCC` `H5` `HCC`

7 √7ᵗʰ **S06.321 Contusion and laceration of left cerebrum with loss of consciousness of** 30 minutes or less   `MCC` `H5` `HCC`

7 √7ᵗʰ **S06.322 Contusion and laceration of left cerebrum with loss of consciousness of** 31 minutes to 59 minutes   `MCC` `H5` `HCC`

7 √7th **S06.323** **Contusion and laceration of left cerebrum with loss of consciousness of** 1 hour to 5 hours 59 minutes `MCC` `H5` `HCC`

7 √7th **S06.324** **Contusion and laceration of left cerebrum with loss of consciousness of** 6 hours to 24 hours `MCC` `H5` `HCC`

7 √7th **S06.325** **Contusion and laceration of left cerebrum with loss of consciousness** greater than 24 hours with return to pre-existing conscious level `MCC` `H5` `HCC`

7 √7th **S06.326** **Contusion and laceration of left cerebrum with loss of consciousness** greater than 24 hours without return to pre-existing conscious level with patient surviving `MCC` `H5` `HCC`

√7th **S06.327** **Contusion and laceration of left cerebrum with loss of consciousness of** any duration with death due to brain injury prior to regaining consciousness `MCC` `H5`

√7th **S06.328** **Contusion and laceration of left cerebrum with loss of consciousness of** any duration with death due to **other** cause prior to regaining consciousness `MCC` `H5`

7 √7th **S06.329** **Contusion and laceration of left cerebrum with loss of consciousness of unspecified duration** `MCC` `H5` `HCC`
Contusion and laceration of left cerebrum NOS

√6th **S06.33** **Contusion and laceration of cerebrum, unspecified**

7 √7th **S06.330** **Contusion and laceration of cerebrum, unspecified,** without loss of consciousness `MCC` `H5` `HCC`

7 √7th **S06.331** **Contusion and laceration of cerebrum, unspecified, with loss of consciousness of** 30 minutes or less `MCC` `H5` `HCC`

7 √7th **S06.332** **Contusion and laceration of cerebrum, unspecified, with loss of consciousness of** 31 minutes to 59 minutes `MCC` `H5` `HCC`

7 √7th **S06.333** **Contusion and laceration of cerebrum, unspecified, with loss of consciousness of** 1 hour to 5 hours 59 minutes `MCC` `H5` `HCC`

7 √7th **S06.334** **Contusion and laceration of cerebrum, unspecified, with loss of consciousness of** 6 hours to 24 hours `MCC` `H5` `HCC`

7 √7th **S06.335** **Contusion and laceration of cerebrum, unspecified, with loss of consciousness** greater than 24 hours with return to pre-existing conscious level `MCC` `H5` `HCC`

7 √7th **S06.336** **Contusion and laceration of cerebrum, unspecified, with loss of consciousness** greater than 24 hours without return to pre-existing conscious level with patient surviving `MCC` `H5` `HCC`

√7th **S06.337** **Contusion and laceration of cerebrum, unspecified, with loss of consciousness of** any duration with death due to brain injury prior to regaining consciousness `MCC` `H5`

√7th **S06.338** **Contusion and laceration of cerebrum, unspecified, with loss of consciousness of** any duration with death due to **other** cause prior to regaining consciousness `MCC` `H5`

7 √7th **S06.339** **Contusion and laceration of cerebrum, unspecified, with loss of consciousness of unspecified duration** `MCC` `H5` `HCC`
Contusion and laceration of cerebrum NOS

√6th **S06.34** **Traumatic hemorrhage of** right cerebrum
Traumatic intracerebral hemorrhage and hematoma of right cerebrum

7 √7th **S06.340** **Traumatic hemorrhage of right cerebrum** without loss of consciousness `MCC` `H5` `HCC`

7 √7th **S06.341** **Traumatic hemorrhage of right cerebrum with loss of consciousness of** 30 minutes or less `MCC` `H5` `HCC`

7 √7th **S06.342** **Traumatic hemorrhage of right cerebrum with loss of consciousness of** 31 minutes to 59 minutes `MCC` `H5` `HCC`

7 √7th **S06.343** **Traumatic hemorrhage of right cerebrum with loss of consciousness of** 1 hours to 5 hours 59 minutes `MCC` `H5` `HCC`

7 √7th **S06.344** **Traumatic hemorrhage of right cerebrum with loss of consciousness of** 6 hours to 24 hours `MCC` `H5` `HCC`

7 √7th **S06.345** **Traumatic hemorrhage of right cerebrum with loss of consciousness** greater than 24 hours with return to pre-existing conscious level `MCC` `H5` `HCC`

7 √7th **S06.346** **Traumatic hemorrhage of right cerebrum with loss of consciousness** greater than 24 hours without return to pre-existing conscious level with patient surviving `MCC` `H5` `HCC`

√7th **S06.347** **Traumatic hemorrhage of right cerebrum with loss of consciousness of** any duration with death due to brain injury prior to regaining consciousness `MCC` `H5`

√7th **S06.348** **Traumatic hemorrhage of right cerebrum with loss of consciousness of** any duration with death due to **other** cause prior to regaining consciousness `MCC` `H5`

7 √7th **S06.349** **Traumatic hemorrhage of right cerebrum with loss of consciousness of unspecified duration** `MCC` `H5` `HCC`
Traumatic hemorrhage of right cerebrum NOS

√6th **S06.35** **Traumatic hemorrhage of** left cerebrum
Traumatic intracerebral hemorrhage and hematoma of left cerebrum

7 √7th **S06.350** **Traumatic hemorrhage of left cerebrum** without loss of consciousness `MCC` `H5` `HCC`

7 √7th **S06.351** **Traumatic hemorrhage of left cerebrum with loss of consciousness of** 30 minutes or less `MCC` `H5` `HCC`

7 √7th **S06.352** **Traumatic hemorrhage of left cerebrum with loss of consciousness of** 31 minutes to 59 minutes `MCC` `H5` `HCC`

7 √7th **S06.353** **Traumatic hemorrhage of left cerebrum with loss of consciousness of** 1 hours to 5 hours 59 minutes `MCC` `H5` `HCC`

7 √7th **S06.354** **Traumatic hemorrhage of left cerebrum with loss of consciousness of** 6 hours to 24 hours `MCC` `H5` `HCC`

7 √7th **S06.355** **Traumatic hemorrhage of left cerebrum with loss of consciousness** greater than 24 hours with return to pre-existing conscious level `MCC` `H5` `HCC`

7 √7th **S06.356** **Traumatic hemorrhage of left cerebrum with loss of consciousness** greater than 24 hours without return to pre-existing conscious level with patient surviving `MCC` `H5` `HCC`

√7th **S06.357** **Traumatic hemorrhage of left cerebrum with loss of consciousness of** any duration with death due to brain injury prior to regaining consciousness `MCC` `H5`

√7th **S06.358** **Traumatic hemorrhage of left cerebrum with loss of consciousness of** any duration with death due to **other** cause prior to regaining consciousness `MCC` `H5`

7 √7th **S06.359** **Traumatic hemorrhage of left cerebrum with loss of consciousness of unspecified duration** `MCC` `H5` `HCC`
Traumatic hemorrhage of left cerebrum NOS

√6th **S06.36** **Traumatic hemorrhage of cerebrum, unspecified**
Traumatic intracerebral hemorrhage and hematoma, unspecified

7 √7th **S06.360** **Traumatic hemorrhage of cerebrum, unspecified,** without loss of consciousness `MCC` `H5` `HCC`

7 √7th **S06.361** **Traumatic hemorrhage of cerebrum, unspecified, with loss of consciousness of** 30 minutes or less `MCC` `H5` `HCC`

7 √7th **S06.362** **Traumatic hemorrhage of cerebrum, unspecified, with loss of consciousness of** 31 minutes to 59 minutes `MCC` `H5` `HCC`

7 √7ᵗʰ **S06.363** **Traumatic hemorrhage of cerebrum, unspecified, with loss of consciousness of** 1 hours to 5 hours 59 minutes   `MCC` `H5` `HCC`

7 √7ᵗʰ **S06.364** **Traumatic hemorrhage of cerebrum, unspecified, with loss of consciousness of** 6 hours to 24 hours   `MCC` `H5` `HCC`

7 √7ᵗʰ **S06.365** **Traumatic hemorrhage of cerebrum, unspecified, with loss of consciousness** greater than 24 hours with return to pre-existing conscious level   `MCC` `H5` `HCC`

7 √7ᵗʰ **S06.366** **Traumatic hemorrhage of cerebrum, unspecified, with loss of consciousness** greater than 24 hours without return to pre-existing conscious level with patient surviving   `MCC` `H5` `HCC`

√7ᵗʰ **S06.367** **Traumatic hemorrhage of cerebrum, unspecified, with loss of consciousness of** any duration with death due to brain injury prior to regaining consciousness   `MCC` `H5`

√7ᵗʰ **S06.368** **Traumatic hemorrhage of cerebrum, unspecified, with loss of consciousness of** any duration with death due to **other** cause prior to regaining consciousness   `MCC` `H5`

7 √7ᵗʰ **S06.369** **Traumatic hemorrhage of cerebrum, unspecified, with loss of consciousness of unspecified duration**   `MCC` `H5` `HCC`
     Traumatic hemorrhage of cerebrum NOS

√6ᵗʰ **S06.37** **Contusion, laceration, and hemorrhage of cerebellum**

7 √7ᵗʰ **S06.370** **Contusion, laceration, and hemorrhage of cerebellum** without loss of consciousness   `MCC` `H5` `HCC`

7 √7ᵗʰ **S06.371** **Contusion, laceration, and hemorrhage of cerebellum with loss of consciousness of** 30 minutes or less   `CC` `H5` `HCC`

7 √7ᵗʰ **S06.372** **Contusion, laceration, and hemorrhage of cerebellum with loss of consciousness of** 31 minutes to 59 minutes   `CC` `H5` `HCC`

7 √7ᵗʰ **S06.373** **Contusion, laceration, and hemorrhage of cerebellum with loss of consciousness of** 1 hour to 5 hours 59 minutes   `CC` `H5` `HCC`

7 √7ᵗʰ **S06.374** **Contusion, laceration, and hemorrhage of cerebellum with loss of consciousness of** 6 hours to 24 hours   `CC` `H5` `HCC`

7 √7ᵗʰ **S06.375** **Contusion, laceration, and hemorrhage of cerebellum with loss of consciousness** greater than 24 hours with return to pre-existing conscious level   `CC` `H5` `HCC`

7 √7ᵗʰ **S06.376** **Contusion, laceration, and hemorrhage of cerebellum with loss of consciousness** greater than 24 hours without return to pre-existing conscious level with patient surviving   `MCC` `H5` `HCC`

√7ᵗʰ **S06.377** **Contusion, laceration, and hemorrhage of cerebellum with loss of consciousness of** any duration with death due to brain injury prior to regaining consciousness   `MCC` `H5`

√7ᵗʰ **S06.378** **Contusion, laceration, and hemorrhage of cerebellum with loss of consciousness of** any duration with death due to **other** cause prior to regaining consciousness   `MCC` `H5`

7 √7ᵗʰ **S06.379** **Contusion, laceration, and hemorrhage of cerebellum with loss of consciousness of unspecified duration**   `CC` `H5` `HCC`
     Contusion, laceration, and hemorrhage of cerebellum NOS

√6ᵗʰ **S06.38** **Contusion, laceration, and hemorrhage of brainstem**

7 √7ᵗʰ **S06.380** **Contusion, laceration, and hemorrhage of brainstem** without loss of consciousness   `MCC` `H5` `HCC`

7 √7ᵗʰ **S06.381** **Contusion, laceration, and hemorrhage of brainstem with loss of consciousness of** 30 minutes or less   `CC` `H5` `HCC`

7 √7ᵗʰ **S06.382** **Contusion, laceration, and hemorrhage of brainstem with loss of consciousness of** 31 minutes to 59 minutes   `CC` `H5` `HCC`

7 √7ᵗʰ **S06.383** **Contusion, laceration, and hemorrhage of brainstem with loss of consciousness of** 1 hour to 5 hours 59 minutes   `CC` `H5` `HCC`

7 √7ᵗʰ **S06.384** **Contusion, laceration, and hemorrhage of brainstem with loss of consciousness of** 6 hours to 24 hours   `CC` `H5` `HCC`

7 √7ᵗʰ **S06.385** **Contusion, laceration, and hemorrhage of brainstem with loss of consciousness** greater than 24 hours with return to pre-existing conscious level   `CC` `H5` `HCC`

7 √7ᵗʰ **S06.386** **Contusion, laceration, and hemorrhage of brainstem with loss of consciousness** greater than 24 hours without return to pre-existing conscious level with patient surviving   `MCC` `H5` `HCC`

√7ᵗʰ **S06.387** **Contusion, laceration, and hemorrhage of brainstem with loss of consciousness of** any duration with death due to brain injury prior to regaining consciousness   `MCC` `H5`

√7ᵗʰ **S06.388** **Contusion, laceration, and hemorrhage of brainstem with loss of consciousness of** any duration with death due to **other** cause prior to regaining consciousness   `MCC` `H5`

7 √7ᵗʰ **S06.389** **Contusion, laceration, and hemorrhage of brainstem with loss of consciousness of unspecified duration**   `CC` `H5` `HCC`
     Contusion, laceration, and hemorrhage of brainstem NOS

√5ᵗʰ **S06.4** **Epidural hemorrhage**
     Extradural hemorrhage NOS
     Extradural hemorrhage (traumatic)
     DEF: Epidural space: Space between the endosteum of the cranium (skull) and the dura mater, the outermost layer of a three-layer membrane that covers the brain.

√6ᵗʰ **S06.4X** **Epidural hemorrhage**

7 √7ᵗʰ **S06.4X0** **Epidural hemorrhage** without loss of consciousness   `MCC` `H5` `HCC`

7 √7ᵗʰ **S06.4X1** **Epidural hemorrhage with loss of consciousness of** 30 minutes or less   `MCC` `H5` `HCC`

7 √7ᵗʰ **S06.4X2** **Epidural hemorrhage with loss of consciousness of** 31 minutes to 59 minutes   `MCC` `H5` `HCC`

7 √7ᵗʰ **S06.4X3** **Epidural hemorrhage with loss of consciousness of** 1 hour to 5 hours 59 minutes   `MCC` `H5` `HCC`

7 √7ᵗʰ **S06.4X4** **Epidural hemorrhage with loss of consciousness of** 6 hours to 24 hours   `MCC` `H5` `HCC`

7 √7ᵗʰ **S06.4X5** **Epidural hemorrhage with loss of consciousness** greater than 24 hours with return to pre-existing conscious level   `MCC` `H5` `HCC`

7 √7ᵗʰ **S06.4X6** **Epidural hemorrhage with loss of consciousness** greater than 24 hours without return to pre-existing conscious level with patient surviving   `MCC` `H5` `HCC`

√7ᵗʰ **S06.4X7** **Epidural hemorrhage with loss of consciousness of** any duration with death due to brain injury prior to regaining consciousness   `MCC` `H5`

√7ᵗʰ **S06.4X8** **Epidural hemorrhage with loss of consciousness of** any duration with death due to **other** causes prior to regaining consciousness   `MCC` `H5`

7 √7ᵗʰ **S06.4X9** **Epidural hemorrhage with loss of consciousness of unspecified duration**   `MCC` `H5` `HCC`
     Epidural hemorrhage NOS

√5ᵗʰ **S06.5** **Traumatic subdural hemorrhage**
     ▶Use additional code, if applicable, for traumatic brain compression or herniation (S06.A-)◀
     AHA: 2021,2Q,5; 2021,1Q,4
     DEF: Subdural: Potential space between the dura mater and arachnoid membrane around the brain.

√6ᵗʰ **S06.5X** **Traumatic subdural hemorrhage**

7 √7ᵗʰ **S06.5X0** **Traumatic subdural hemorrhage** without loss of consciousness   `MCC` `H5` `HCC`

7 ✓7ᵗʰ **S06.5X1** Traumatic subdural hemorrhage with loss of consciousness of 30 minutes or less `MCC` `H5` `HCC`

7 ✓7ᵗʰ **S06.5X2** Traumatic subdural hemorrhage with loss of consciousness of 31 minutes to 59 minutes `MCC` `H5` `HCC`

7 ✓7ᵗʰ **S06.5X3** Traumatic subdural hemorrhage with loss of consciousness of 1 hour to 5 hours 59 minutes `MCC` `H5` `HCC`

7 ✓7ᵗʰ **S06.5X4** Traumatic subdural hemorrhage with loss of consciousness of 6 hours to 24 hours `MCC` `H5` `HCC`

7 ✓7ᵗʰ **S06.5X5** Traumatic subdural hemorrhage with loss of consciousness greater than 24 hours with return to pre-existing conscious level `MCC` `H5` `HCC`

7 ✓7ᵗʰ **S06.5X6** Traumatic subdural hemorrhage with loss of consciousness greater than 24 hours without return to pre-existing conscious level with patient surviving `MCC` `H5` `HCC`

✓7ᵗʰ **S06.5X7** Traumatic subdural hemorrhage with loss of consciousness of any duration with death due to brain injury before regaining consciousness `MCC` `H5`

✓7ᵗʰ **S06.5X8** Traumatic subdural hemorrhage with loss of consciousness of any duration with death due to other cause before regaining consciousness `MCC` `H5`

7 ✓7ᵗʰ **S06.5X9** Traumatic subdural hemorrhage with loss of consciousness of unspecified duration `MCC` `H5` `HCC`
> Traumatic subdural hemorrhage NOS

✓5ᵗʰ **S06.6** **Traumatic subarachnoid hemorrhage**
▶ Use additional code, if applicable, for traumatic brain compression or herniation (S06.A-)◀
AHA: 2021,2Q,5; 2021,1Q,4
DEF: Subarachnoid: Space located between the arachnoid membrane and the pia mater that contains cerebrospinal fluid.

✓6ᵗʰ **S06.6X** **Traumatic subarachnoid hemorrhage**

7 ✓7ᵗʰ **S06.6X0** Traumatic subarachnoid hemorrhage without loss of consciousness `MCC` `H5` `HCC`

7 ✓7ᵗʰ **S06.6X1** Traumatic subarachnoid hemorrhage with loss of consciousness of 30 minutes or less `MCC` `H5` `HCC`

7 ✓7ᵗʰ **S06.6X2** Traumatic subarachnoid hemorrhage with loss of consciousness of 31 minutes to 59 minutes `MCC` `H5` `HCC`

7 ✓7ᵗʰ **S06.6X3** Traumatic subarachnoid hemorrhage with loss of consciousness of 1 hour to 5 hours 59 minutes `MCC` `H5` `HCC`

7 ✓7ᵗʰ **S06.6X4** Traumatic subarachnoid hemorrhage with loss of consciousness of 6 hours to 24 hours `MCC` `H5` `HCC`

7 ✓7ᵗʰ **S06.6X5** Traumatic subarachnoid hemorrhage with loss of consciousness greater than 24 hours with return to pre-existing conscious level `MCC` `H5` `HCC`

✓7ᵗʰ **S06.6X6** Traumatic subarachnoid hemorrhage with loss of consciousness greater than 24 hours without return to pre-existing conscious level with patient surviving `MCC` `H5` `HCC`

✓7ᵗʰ **S06.6X7** Traumatic subarachnoid hemorrhage with loss of consciousness of any duration with death due to brain injury prior to regaining consciousness `MCC` `H5`

✓7ᵗʰ **S06.6X8** Traumatic subarachnoid hemorrhage with loss of consciousness of any duration with death due to other cause prior to regaining consciousness `MCC` `H5`

7 ✓7ᵗʰ **S06.6X9** Traumatic subarachnoid hemorrhage with loss of consciousness of unspecified duration `MCC` `H5` `HCC`
> Traumatic subarachnoid hemorrhage NOS

✓5ᵗʰ **S06.8** **Other specified intracranial injuries**

✓6ᵗʰ **S06.81** Injury of right internal carotid artery, intracranial portion, not elsewhere classified

7 ✓7ᵗʰ **S06.810** Injury of right internal carotid artery, intracranial portion, not elsewhere classified without loss of consciousness `HCC`

7 ✓7ᵗʰ **S06.811** Injury of right internal carotid artery, intracranial portion, not elsewhere classified with loss of consciousness of 30 minutes or less `CC` `H5` `HCC`

7 ✓7ᵗʰ **S06.812** Injury of right internal carotid artery, intracranial portion, not elsewhere classified with loss of consciousness of 31 minutes to 59 minutes `CC` `H5` `HCC`

7 ✓7ᵗʰ **S06.813** Injury of right internal carotid artery, intracranial portion, not elsewhere classified with loss of consciousness of 1 hour to 5 hours 59 minutes `CC` `H5` `HCC`

7 ✓7ᵗʰ **S06.814** Injury of right internal carotid artery, intracranial portion, not elsewhere classified with loss of consciousness of 6 hours to 24 hours `CC` `H5` `HCC`

7 ✓7ᵗʰ **S06.815** Injury of right internal carotid artery, intracranial portion, not elsewhere classified with loss of consciousness greater than 24 hours with return to pre-existing conscious level `CC` `H5` `HCC`

7 ✓7ᵗʰ **S06.816** Injury of right internal carotid artery, intracranial portion, not elsewhere classified with loss of consciousness greater than 24 hours without return to pre-existing conscious level with patient surviving `MCC` `H5` `HCC`

✓7ᵗʰ **S06.817** Injury of right internal carotid artery, intracranial portion, not elsewhere classified with loss of consciousness of any duration with death due to brain injury prior to regaining consciousness `MCC` `H5`

✓7ᵗʰ **S06.818** Injury of right internal carotid artery, intracranial portion, not elsewhere classified with loss of consciousness of any duration with death due to other cause prior to regaining consciousness `MCC` `H5`

7 ✓7ᵗʰ **S06.819** Injury of right internal carotid artery, intracranial portion, not elsewhere classified with loss of consciousness of unspecified duration `CC` `H5` `HCC`
> Injury of right internal carotid artery, intracranial portion, not elsewhere classified NOS

✓6ᵗʰ **S06.82** Injury of left internal carotid artery, intracranial portion, not elsewhere classified

7 ✓7ᵗʰ **S06.820** Injury of left internal carotid artery, intracranial portion, not elsewhere classified without loss of consciousness `HCC`

7 ✓7ᵗʰ **S06.821** Injury of left internal carotid artery, intracranial portion, not elsewhere classified with loss of consciousness of 30 minutes or less `CC` `H5` `HCC`

7 ✓7ᵗʰ **S06.822** Injury of left internal carotid artery, intracranial portion, not elsewhere classified with loss of consciousness of 31 minutes to 59 minutes `CC` `H5` `HCC`

7 ✓7ᵗʰ **S06.823** Injury of left internal carotid artery, intracranial portion, not elsewhere classified with loss of consciousness of 1 hour to 5 hours 59 minutes `CC` `H5` `HCC`

7 ✓7ᵗʰ **S06.824** Injury of left internal carotid artery, intracranial portion, not elsewhere classified with loss of consciousness of 6 hours to 24 hours `CC` `H5` `HCC`

7 ✓7ᵗʰ **S06.825** Injury of left internal carotid artery, intracranial portion, not elsewhere classified with loss of consciousness greater than 24 hours with return to pre-existing conscious level `CC` `H5` `HCC`

Ⓝ Newborn: 0   Ⓟ Pediatric: 0-17   Ⓜ Maternity: 9-64   Ⓐ Adult: 15-124   `MCC` Major Complication/Comorbidity   `CC` Complication/Comorbidity   `SW` Severe Wound Dx

978   ICD-10-CM 2022

7 √7ᵗʰ **S06.826 Injury of left internal carotid artery, intracranial portion, not elsewhere classified with loss of consciousness** greater than 24 hours without return to pre-existing conscious level with patient surviving   MCC H5 HCC

√7ᵗʰ **S06.827 Injury of left internal carotid artery, intracranial portion, not elsewhere classified with loss of consciousness of** any duration with death due to brain injury prior to regaining consciousness   MCC H5

√7ᵗʰ **S06.828 Injury of left internal carotid artery, intracranial portion, not elsewhere classified with loss of consciousness of** any duration with death due to other cause prior to regaining consciousness   MCC H5

7 √7ᵗʰ **S06.829 Injury of left internal carotid artery, intracranial portion, not elsewhere classified with loss of consciousness of unspecified duration**   CC H5 HCC

Injury of left internal carotid artery, intracranial portion, not elsewhere classified NOS

√6ᵗʰ **S06.89 Other specified intracranial injury**
EXCLUDES 1   concussion (S06.0X-)

7 √7ᵗʰ **S06.890 Other specified intracranial injury** without loss of consciousness   HCC

7 √7ᵗʰ **S06.891 Other specified intracranial injury with loss of consciousness of** 30 minutes or less   CC H5 HCC

7 √7ᵗʰ **S06.892 Other specified intracranial injury with loss of consciousness of** 31 minutes to 59 minutes   CC H5 HCC

7 √7ᵗʰ **S06.893 Other specified intracranial injury with loss of consciousness of** 1 hour to 5 hours 59 minutes   CC H5 HCC

7 √7ᵗʰ **S06.894 Other specified intracranial injury with loss of consciousness of** 6 hours to 24 hours   CC H5 HCC

7 √7ᵗʰ **S06.895 Other specified intracranial injury with loss of consciousness** greater than 24 hours with return to pre-existing conscious level   CC H5 HCC

7 √7ᵗʰ **S06.896 Other specified intracranial injury with loss of consciousness** greater than 24 hours without return to pre-existing conscious level with patient surviving   MCC H5 HCC

√7ᵗʰ **S06.897 Other specified intracranial injury with loss of consciousness of** any duration with death due to brain injury prior to regaining consciousness   MCC H5

√7ᵗʰ **S06.898 Other specified intracranial injury with loss of consciousness of** any duration with death due to other cause prior to regaining consciousness   MCC H5

7 √7ᵗʰ **S06.899 Other specified intracranial injury with loss of consciousness of unspecified duration**   CC H5 HCC

√5ᵗʰ **S06.9 Unspecified intracranial injury**
Brain injury NOS
Head injury NOS with loss of consciousness
Traumatic brain injury NOS
EXCLUDES 1   conditions classifiable to S06.0- to S06.8- code to specified intracranial injury
head injury NOS (S09.90)
AHA: 2020,3Q,46; 2020,2Q,31
TIP: Assign additional code(s) for individual (R40.21-, R40.22-, R40.23-) or total (R40.24-) coma scale scores. It is appropriate to code the coma scale scores based on documentation provided by clinicians who are not the patient's provider (such as emergency medical technician).

√6ᵗʰ **S06.9X Unspecified intracranial injury**

7 √7ᵗʰ **S06.9X0 Unspecified intracranial injury** without loss of consciousness   HCC

7 √7ᵗʰ **S06.9X1 Unspecified intracranial injury with loss of consciousness of** 30 minutes or less   CC H5 HCC

7 √7ᵗʰ **S06.9X2 Unspecified intracranial injury with loss of consciousness of** 31 minutes to 59 minutes   CC H5 HCC

7 √7ᵗʰ **S06.9X3 Unspecified intracranial injury with loss of consciousness of** 1 hour to 5 hours 59 minutes   CC H5 HCC

7 √7ᵗʰ **S06.9X4 Unspecified intracranial injury with loss of consciousness of** 6 hours to 24 hours   CC H5 HCC

7 √7ᵗʰ **S06.9X5 Unspecified intracranial injury with loss of consciousness** greater than 24 hours with return to pre-existing conscious level   CC H5 HCC

7 √7ᵗʰ **S06.9X6 Unspecified intracranial injury with loss of consciousness** greater than 24 hours without return to pre-existing conscious level with patient surviving   MCC H5 HCC

√7ᵗʰ **S06.9X7 Unspecified intracranial injury with loss of consciousness of** any duration with death due to brain injury prior to regaining consciousness   MCC H5

√7ᵗʰ **S06.9X8 Unspecified intracranial injury with loss of consciousness of** any duration with death due to other cause prior to regaining consciousness   MCC H5

7 √7ᵗʰ **S06.9X9 Unspecified intracranial injury with loss of consciousness of unspecified duration**   CC H5 HCC

● √5ᵗʰ **S06.A Traumatic brain compression and herniation**
Traumatic cerebral compression
Code first the underlying traumatic brain injury, such as:
diffuse traumatic brain injury (S06.2-)
focal traumatic brain injury (S06.3-)
traumatic subdural hemorrhage (S06.5-)
traumatic subarachnoid hemorrhage (S06.6-)

● √x7ᵗʰ **S06.A0 Traumatic brain compression without herniation**   MCC
Traumatic brain compression NOS
Traumatic cerebral compression NOS

● √x7ᵗʰ **S06.A1 Traumatic brain compression with herniation**   MCC
Traumatic brain herniation
Traumatic brainstem compression with herniation
Traumatic cerebellar compression with herniation
Traumatic cerebral compression with herniation

√4ᵗʰ **S07 Crushing injury of head**
Use additional code for all associated injuries, such as:
intracranial injuries (S06.-)
skull fractures (S02.-)

> The appropriate 7th character is to be added to each code from category S07.
> A   initial encounter
> D   subsequent encounter
> S   sequela

√x7ᵗʰ **S07.0 Crushing injury of face**   CC H5

√x7ᵗʰ **S07.1 Crushing injury of skull**   CC H5

√x7ᵗʰ **S07.8 Crushing injury of other parts of head**   CC H5

√x7ᵗʰ **S07.9 Crushing injury of head, part unspecified**   CC H5

√4ᵗʰ **S08 Avulsion and traumatic amputation of part of head**
An amputation not identified as partial or complete should be coded to complete

> The appropriate 7th character is to be added to each code from category S08.
> A   initial encounter
> D   subsequent encounter
> S   sequela

√x7ᵗʰ **S08.0 Avulsion of scalp**

√5ᵗʰ **S08.1 Traumatic amputation of ear**

√6ᵗʰ **S08.11 Complete traumatic amputation of ear**

√7ᵗʰ **S08.111 Complete traumatic amputation of right ear**

√7ᵗʰ **S08.112 Complete traumatic amputation of left ear**

√7ᵗʰ **S08.119 Complete traumatic amputation of unspecified ear**

√6ᵗʰ S08.12 Partial traumatic amputation of ear
- **√7ᵗʰ S08.121 Partial traumatic amputation of right ear**
- **√7ᵗʰ S08.122 Partial traumatic amputation of left ear**
- **√7ᵗʰ S08.129 Partial traumatic amputation of unspecified ear**

√5ᵗʰ S08.8 Traumatic amputation of other parts of head
- **√6ᵗʰ S08.81 Traumatic amputation of nose**
  - **√7ᵗʰ S08.811 Complete traumatic amputation of nose**
  - **√7ᵗʰ S08.812 Partial traumatic amputation of nose**
- **√x7ᵗʰ S08.89 Traumatic amputation of other parts of head**

√4ᵗʰ S09 Other and unspecified injuries of head

The appropriate 7th character is to be added to each code from category S09.
A initial encounter
D subsequent encounter
S sequela

√x7ᵗʰ S09.0 Injury of blood vessels of head, not elsewhere classified cc
- EXCLUDES 1   *injury of cerebral blood vessels (S06.-)*
-          *injury of precerebral blood vessels (S15.-)*

√5ᵗʰ S09.1 Injury of muscle and tendon of head
- Code also any associated open wound (S01.-)
- EXCLUDES 2   *sprain to joints and ligament of head (S03.9)*
- **√x7ᵗʰ S09.10 Unspecified injury of muscle and tendon of head**
  - Injury of muscle and tendon of head NOS
- **√x7ᵗʰ S09.11 Strain of muscle and tendon of head**
- **√x7ᵗʰ S09.12 Laceration of muscle and tendon of head**
- **√x7ᵗʰ S09.19 Other specified injury of muscle and tendon of head**

√5ᵗʰ S09.2 Traumatic rupture of ear drum
- EXCLUDES 1   *traumatic rupture of ear drum due to blast injury (S09.31-)*
- **√x7ᵗʰ S09.20 Traumatic rupture of unspecified ear drum** cc
- **√x7ᵗʰ S09.21 Traumatic rupture of right ear drum** cc
- **√x7ᵗʰ S09.22 Traumatic rupture of left ear drum** cc

√5ᵗʰ S09.3 Other specified and unspecified injury of middle and inner ear
- EXCLUDES 1   *injury to ear NOS (S09.91-)*
- EXCLUDES 2   *injury to external ear (S00.4-, S01.3-, S08.1-)*
- **√6ᵗʰ S09.30 Unspecified injury of middle and inner ear**
  - **√7ᵗʰ S09.301 Unspecified injury of right middle and inner ear** cc
  - **√7ᵗʰ S09.302 Unspecified injury of left middle and inner ear** cc
  - **√7ᵗʰ S09.309 Unspecified injury of unspecified middle and inner ear** cc
- **√6ᵗʰ S09.31 Primary blast injury of ear**
  - Blast injury of ear NOS
  - **√7ᵗʰ S09.311 Primary blast injury of right ear** cc
  - **√7ᵗʰ S09.312 Primary blast injury of left ear** cc
  - **√7ᵗʰ S09.313 Primary blast injury of ear, bilateral** cc
  - **√7ᵗʰ S09.319 Primary blast injury of unspecified ear** cc
- **√6ᵗʰ S09.39 Other specified injury of middle and inner ear**
  - Secondary blast injury to ear
  - **√7ᵗʰ S09.391 Other specified injury of right middle and inner ear** cc
  - **√7ᵗʰ S09.392 Other specified injury of left middle and inner ear** cc
  - **√7ᵗʰ S09.399 Other specified injury of unspecified middle and inner ear** cc

√x7ᵗʰ S09.8 Other specified injuries of head

√6ᵗʰ S09.9 Unspecified injury of face and head
- **√x7ᵗʰ S09.90 Unspecified injury of head**
  - Head injury NOS
  - EXCLUDES 1   *brain injury NOS (S06.9-)*
  -          *head injury NOS with loss of consciousness (S06.9-)*
  -          *intracranial injury NOS (S06.9-)*
- **√x7ᵗʰ S09.91 Unspecified injury of ear**
  - Injury of ear NOS

√x7ᵗʰ S09.92 Unspecified injury of nose
- Injury of nose NOS
√x7ᵗʰ S09.93 Unspecified injury of face
- Injury of face NOS
- AHA: 2019,2Q,23

Injuries to the neck (S10-S19)

INCLUDES   injuries of nape
         injuries of supraclavicular region
         injuries of throat
EXCLUDES 2   *burns and corrosions (T20-T32)*
         effects of foreign body in esophagus (T18.1)
         effects of foreign body in larynx (T17.3)
         effects of foreign body in pharynx (T17.2)
         effects of foreign body in trachea (T17.4)
         frostbite (T33-T34)
         insect bite or sting, venomous (T63.4)

√4ᵗʰ S10 Superficial injury of neck

The appropriate 7th character is to be added to each code from category S10.
A initial encounter
D subsequent encounter
S sequela

√x7ᵗʰ S10.0 Contusion of throat
- Contusion of cervical esophagus
- Contusion of larynx
- Contusion of pharynx
- Contusion of trachea

√5ᵗʰ S10.1 Other and unspecified superficial injuries of throat
- **√x7ᵗʰ S10.10 Unspecified superficial injuries of throat**
- **√x7ᵗʰ S10.11 Abrasion of throat**
- **√x7ᵗʰ S10.12 Blister (nonthermal) of throat**
- **√x7ᵗʰ S10.14 External constriction of part of throat**
- **√x7ᵗʰ S10.15 Superficial foreign body of throat**
  - Splinter in the throat
- **√x7ᵗʰ S10.16 Insect bite (nonvenomous) of throat**
- **√x7ᵗʰ S10.17 Other superficial bite of throat**
  - EXCLUDES 1   *open bite of throat (S11.85)*

√5ᵗʰ S10.8 Superficial injury of other specified parts of neck
- **√x7ᵗʰ S10.80 Unspecified superficial injury of other specified part of neck**
- **√x7ᵗʰ S10.81 Abrasion of other specified part of neck**
- **√x7ᵗʰ S10.82 Blister (nonthermal) of other specified part of neck**
- **√x7ᵗʰ S10.83 Contusion of other specified part of neck**
- **√x7ᵗʰ S10.84 External constriction of other specified part of neck**
- **√x7ᵗʰ S10.85 Superficial foreign body of other specified part of neck**
  - Splinter in other specified part of neck
- **√x7ᵗʰ S10.86 Insect bite of other specified part of neck**
- **√x7ᵗʰ S10.87 Other superficial bite of other specified part of neck**
  - EXCLUDES 1   *open bite of other specified parts of neck (S11.85)*

√5ᵗʰ S10.9 Superficial injury of unspecified part of neck
- **√x7ᵗʰ S10.90 Unspecified superficial injury of unspecified part of neck**
- **√x7ᵗʰ S10.91 Abrasion of unspecified part of neck**
- **√x7ᵗʰ S10.92 Blister (nonthermal) of unspecified part of neck**
- **√x7ᵗʰ S10.93 Contusion of unspecified part of neck**
- **√x7ᵗʰ S10.94 External constriction of unspecified part of neck**
- **√x7ᵗʰ S10.95 Superficial foreign body of unspecified part of neck**
- **√x7ᵗʰ S10.96 Insect bite of unspecified part of neck**
- **√x7ᵗʰ S10.97 Other superficial bite of unspecified part of neck**

√4ᵗʰ **S11 Open wound of neck**

Code also any associated:
spinal cord injury (S14.0, S14.1-)
wound infection

EXCLUDES 2   *open fracture of vertebra (S12.- with 7th character B)*

The appropriate 7th character is to be added to each code from category S11.
A   initial encounter
D   subsequent encounter
S   sequela

√5ᵗʰ **S11.0 Open wound of larynx and trachea**

√6ᵗʰ **S11.01 Open wound of larynx**

EXCLUDES 2   *open wound of vocal cord (S11.03)*

√7ᵗʰ   **S11.011 Laceration without foreign body of larynx**   MCC

√7ᵗʰ   **S11.012 Laceration with foreign body of larynx**   MCC

√7ᵗʰ   **S11.013 Puncture wound without foreign body of larynx**   MCC

√7ᵗʰ   **S11.014 Puncture wound with foreign body of larynx**   MCC

√7ᵗʰ   **S11.015 Open bite of larynx**   MCC

Bite of larynx NOS

√7ᵗʰ   **S11.019 Unspecified open wound of larynx**   MCC

√6ᵗʰ **S11.02 Open wound of trachea**

Open wound of cervical trachea
Open wound of trachea NOS

EXCLUDES 2   *open wound of thoracic trachea (S27.5-)*

√7ᵗʰ   **S11.021 Laceration without foreign body of trachea**   MCC

√7ᵗʰ   **S11.022 Laceration with foreign body of trachea**   MCC

√7ᵗʰ   **S11.023 Puncture wound without foreign body of trachea**   MCC

√7ᵗʰ   **S11.024 Puncture wound with foreign body of trachea**   MCC

√7ᵗʰ   **S11.025 Open bite of trachea**   MCC

Bite of trachea NOS

√7ᵗʰ   **S11.029 Unspecified open wound of trachea**   MCC

√6ᵗʰ **S11.03 Open wound of vocal cord**

√7ᵗʰ   **S11.031 Laceration without foreign body of vocal cord**   MCC

√7ᵗʰ   **S11.032 Laceration with foreign body of vocal cord**   MCC

√7ᵗʰ   **S11.033 Puncture wound without foreign body of vocal cord**   MCC

√7ᵗʰ   **S11.034 Puncture wound with foreign body of vocal cord**   MCC

√7ᵗʰ   **S11.035 Open bite of vocal cord**   MCC

Bite of vocal cord NOS

√7ᵗʰ   **S11.039 Unspecified open wound of vocal cord**   MCC

√5ᵗʰ **S11.1 Open wound of thyroid gland**

√x7ᵗʰ   **S11.10 Unspecified open wound of thyroid gland**   CC

√x7ᵗʰ   **S11.11 Laceration without foreign body of thyroid gland**   CC

√x7ᵗʰ   **S11.12 Laceration with foreign body of thyroid gland**   CC

√x7ᵗʰ   **S11.13 Puncture wound without foreign body of thyroid gland**   CC

√x7ᵗʰ   **S11.14 Puncture wound with foreign body of thyroid gland**   CC

√x7ᵗʰ   **S11.15 Open bite of thyroid gland**   CC

Bite of thyroid gland NOS

√5ᵗʰ **S11.2 Open wound of pharynx and cervical esophagus**

EXCLUDES 1   *open wound of esophagus NOS (S27.8-)*

√x7ᵗʰ   **S11.20 Unspecified open wound of pharynx and cervical esophagus**   CC

√x7ᵗʰ   **S11.21 Laceration without foreign body of pharynx and cervical esophagus**   CC

√x7ᵗʰ   **S11.22 Laceration with foreign body of pharynx and cervical esophagus**   CC

√x7ᵗʰ   **S11.23 Puncture wound without foreign body of pharynx and cervical esophagus**   CC

√x7ᵗʰ   **S11.24 Puncture wound with foreign body of pharynx and cervical esophagus**   CC

√x7ᵗʰ   **S11.25 Open bite of pharynx and cervical esophagus**   CC

Bite of pharynx and cervical esophagus NOS

√5ᵗʰ **S11.8 Open wound of other specified parts of neck**

√x7ᵗʰ   **S11.80 Unspecified open wound of other specified part of neck**

√x7ᵗʰ   **S11.81 Laceration without foreign body of other specified part of neck**

√x7ᵗʰ   **S11.82 Laceration with foreign body of other specified part of neck**

√x7ᵗʰ   **S11.83 Puncture wound without foreign body of other specified part of neck**

√x7ᵗʰ   **S11.84 Puncture wound with foreign body of other specified part of neck**

√x7ᵗʰ   **S11.85 Open bite of other specified part of neck**

Bite of other specified part of neck NOS

EXCLUDES 1   *superficial bite of other specified part of neck (S10.87)*

√x7ᵗʰ   **S11.89 Other open wound of other specified part of neck**

√5ᵗʰ **S11.9 Open wound of unspecified part of neck**

√x7ᵗʰ   **S11.90 Unspecified open wound of unspecified part of neck**

√x7ᵗʰ   **S11.91 Laceration without foreign body of unspecified part of neck**

√x7ᵗʰ   **S11.92 Laceration with foreign body of unspecified part of neck**

√x7ᵗʰ   **S11.93 Puncture wound without foreign body of unspecified part of neck**

√x7ᵗʰ   **S11.94 Puncture wound with foreign body of unspecified part of neck**

√x7ᵗʰ   **S11.95 Open bite of unspecified part of neck**

Bite of neck NOS

EXCLUDES 1   *superficial bite of neck (S10.97)*

√4ᵗʰ **S12 Fracture of cervical vertebra and other parts of neck**

NOTE   A fracture not indicated as displaced or nondisplaced should be coded to displaced.

A fracture not indicated as open or closed should be coded to closed.

INCLUDES   fracture of cervical neural arch
fracture of cervical spine
fracture of cervical spinous process
fracture of cervical transverse process
fracture of cervical vertebral arch
fracture of neck

Code first any associated cervical spinal cord injury (S14.0, S14.1-)

AHA: 2021,1Q,6; 2018,2Q,12; 2015,3Q,37-39

The appropriate 7th character is to be added to all codes from subcategories S12.0-S12.6.
A   initial encounter for closed fracture
B   initial encounter for open fracture
D   subsequent encounter for fracture with routine healing
G   subsequent encounter for fracture with delayed healing
K   subsequent encounter for fracture with nonunion
S   sequela

√5ᵗʰ **S12.0 Fracture of first cervical vertebra**

Atlas

√6ᵗʰ **S12.00 Unspecified fracture of first cervical vertebra**

2,3,6 √7ᵗʰ   **S12.000 Unspecified displaced fracture of first cervical vertebra**   MCC CC H5 HCC

2,3,6 √7ᵗʰ   **S12.001 Unspecified nondisplaced fracture of first cervical vertebra**   MCC CC H5 HCC

2,3,6 √7ᵗʰ   **S12.01 Stable burst fracture of first cervical vertebra**   MCC CC H5 HCC

2,3,6 √7ᵗʰ   **S12.02 Unstable burst fracture of first cervical vertebra**   MCC CC H5 HCC

√6ᵗʰ **S12.03 Posterior arch fracture of first cervical vertebra**

2,3,6 √7ᵗʰ   **S12.030 Displaced posterior arch fracture of first cervical vertebra**   MCC CC H5 HCC

2,3,6 √7ᵗʰ   **S12.031 Nondisplaced posterior arch fracture of first cervical vertebra**   MCC CC H5 HCC

√6ᵗʰ **S12.04 Lateral mass fracture of first cervical vertebra**

2,3,6 √7ᵗʰ   **S12.040 Displaced lateral mass fracture of first cervical vertebra**   MCC CC H5 HCC

2,3,6 √7ᵗʰ   **S12.041 Nondisplaced lateral mass fracture of first cervical vertebra**   MCC CC H5 HCC

☑ Additional Character Required   √x7ᵗʰ Placeholder   Questionable PDx   Manifestation   Unspecified Dx   UPD Unacceptable PDx   H1 - H14 HAC   HCC CMS-HCC Dx   HIV HIV Dx

ICD-10-CM 2022   981

√6ᵗʰ **S12.09**   Other fracture of first cervical vertebra
- 2,3,6 √7ᵗʰ **S12.090**   Other displaced fracture of first cervical vertebra   `MCC` `CC` `H5` `HCC`
- 2,3,6 √7ᵗʰ **S12.091**   Other nondisplaced fracture of first cervical vertebra   `MCC` `CC` `H5` `HCC`

√5ᵗʰ **S12.1**   Fracture of second cervical vertebra
    Axis

√6ᵗʰ **S12.10**   Unspecified fracture of second cervical vertebra
- 2,3,6 √7ᵗʰ **S12.100**   Unspecified displaced fracture of second cervical vertebra   `MCC` `CC` `H5` `HCC`
- 2,3,6 √7ᵗʰ **S12.101**   Unspecified nondisplaced fracture of second cervical vertebra   `MCC` `CC` `H5` `HCC`

√6ᵗʰ **S12.11**   Type II dens fracture
- 2,3,6 √7ᵗʰ **S12.110**   Anterior displaced Type II dens fracture   `MCC` `CC` `H5` `HCC`
- 2,3,6 √7ᵗʰ **S12.111**   Posterior displaced Type II dens fracture   `MCC` `CC` `H5` `HCC`
- 2,3,6 √7ᵗʰ **S12.112**   Nondisplaced Type II dens fracture   `MCC` `CC` `H5` `HCC`

√6ᵗʰ **S12.12**   Other dens fracture
- 2,3,6 √7ᵗʰ **S12.120**   Other displaced dens fracture   `MCC` `CC` `H5` `HCC`
- 2,3,6 √7ᵗʰ **S12.121**   Other nondisplaced dens fracture   `MCC` `CC` `H5` `HCC`

√6ᵗʰ **S12.13**   Unspecified traumatic spondylolisthesis of second cervical vertebra
- 2,3,6 √7ᵗʰ **S12.130**   Unspecified traumatic displaced spondylolisthesis of second cervical vertebra   `MCC` `CC` `H5` `HCC`
- 2,3,6 √7ᵗʰ **S12.131**   Unspecified traumatic nondisplaced spondylolisthesis of second cervical vertebra   `MCC` `CC` `H5` `HCC`

2,3,6 √x7ᵗʰ **S12.14**   Type III traumatic spondylolisthesis of second cervical vertebra   `MCC` `CC` `H5` `HCC`

√6ᵗʰ **S12.15**   Other traumatic spondylolisthesis of second cervical vertebra
- 2,3,6 √7ᵗʰ **S12.150**   Other traumatic displaced spondylolisthesis of second cervical vertebra   `MCC` `CC` `H5` `HCC`
- 2,3,6 √7ᵗʰ **S12.151**   Other traumatic nondisplaced spondylolisthesis of second cervical vertebra   `MCC` `CC` `H5` `HCC`

√6ᵗʰ **S12.19**   Other fracture of second cervical vertebra
- 2,3,6 √7ᵗʰ **S12.190**   Other displaced fracture of second cervical vertebra   `MCC` `CC` `H5` `HCC`
- 2,3,6 √7ᵗʰ **S12.191**   Other nondisplaced fracture of second cervical vertebra   `MCC` `CC` `H5` `HCC`

√5ᵗʰ **S12.2**   Fracture of third cervical vertebra

√6ᵗʰ **S12.20**   Unspecified fracture of third cervical vertebra
- 2,3,6 √7ᵗʰ **S12.200**   Unspecified displaced fracture of third cervical vertebra   `MCC` `CC` `H5` `HCC`
- 2,3,6 √7ᵗʰ **S12.201**   Unspecified nondisplaced fracture of third cervical vertebra   `MCC` `CC` `H5` `HCC`

√6ᵗʰ **S12.23**   Unspecified traumatic spondylolisthesis of third cervical vertebra
- 2,3,6 √7ᵗʰ **S12.230**   Unspecified traumatic displaced spondylolisthesis of third cervical vertebra   `MCC` `CC` `H5` `HCC`
- 2,3,6 √7ᵗʰ **S12.231**   Unspecified traumatic nondisplaced spondylolisthesis of third cervical vertebra   `MCC` `CC` `H5` `HCC`

2,3,6 √x7ᵗʰ **S12.24**   Type III traumatic spondylolisthesis of third cervical vertebra   `MCC` `CC` `H5` `HCC`

√6ᵗʰ **S12.25**   Other traumatic spondylolisthesis of third cervical vertebra
- 2,3,6 √7ᵗʰ **S12.250**   Other traumatic displaced spondylolisthesis of third cervical vertebra   `MCC` `CC` `H5` `HCC`
- 2,3,6 √7ᵗʰ **S12.251**   Other traumatic nondisplaced spondylolisthesis of third cervical vertebra   `MCC` `CC` `H5` `HCC`

√6ᵗʰ **S12.29**   Other fracture of third cervical vertebra
- 2,3,6 √7ᵗʰ **S12.290**   Other displaced fracture of third cervical vertebra   `MCC` `CC` `H5` `HCC`
- 2,3,6 √7ᵗʰ **S12.291**   Other nondisplaced fracture of third cervical vertebra   `MCC` `CC` `H5` `HCC`

√5ᵗʰ **S12.3**   Fracture of fourth cervical vertebra

√6ᵗʰ **S12.30**   Unspecified fracture of fourth cervical vertebra
- 2,3,6 √7ᵗʰ **S12.300**   Unspecified displaced fracture of fourth cervical vertebra   `MCC` `CC` `H5` `HCC`
- 2,3,6 √7ᵗʰ **S12.301**   Unspecified nondisplaced fracture of fourth cervical vertebra   `MCC` `CC` `H5` `HCC`

√6ᵗʰ **S12.33**   Unspecified traumatic spondylolisthesis of fourth cervical vertebra
- 2,3,6 √7ᵗʰ **S12.330**   Unspecified traumatic displaced spondylolisthesis of fourth cervical vertebra   `MCC` `CC` `H5` `HCC`
- 2,3,6 √7ᵗʰ **S12.331**   Unspecified traumatic nondisplaced spondylolisthesis of fourth cervical vertebra   `MCC` `CC` `H5` `HCC`

2,3,6 √x7ᵗʰ **S12.34**   Type III traumatic spondylolisthesis of fourth cervical vertebra   `MCC` `CC` `H5` `HCC`

√6ᵗʰ **S12.35**   Other traumatic spondylolisthesis of fourth cervical vertebra
- 2,3,6 √7ᵗʰ **S12.350**   Other traumatic displaced spondylolisthesis of fourth cervical vertebra   `MCC` `CC` `H5` `HCC`
- 2,3,6 √7ᵗʰ **S12.351**   Other traumatic nondisplaced spondylolisthesis of fourth cervical vertebra   `MCC` `CC` `H5` `HCC`

√6ᵗʰ **S12.39**   Other fracture of fourth cervical vertebra
- 2,3,6 √7ᵗʰ **S12.390**   Other displaced fracture of fourth cervical vertebra   `MCC` `CC` `H5` `HCC`
- 2,3,6 √7ᵗʰ **S12.391**   Other nondisplaced fracture of fourth cervical vertebra   `MCC` `CC` `H5` `HCC`

√5ᵗʰ **S12.4**   Fracture of fifth cervical vertebra

√6ᵗʰ **S12.40**   Unspecified fracture of fifth cervical vertebra
- 2,3,6 √7ᵗʰ **S12.400**   Unspecified displaced fracture of fifth cervical vertebra   `MCC` `CC` `H5` `HCC`
- 2,3,6 √7ᵗʰ **S12.401**   Unspecified nondisplaced fracture of fifth cervical vertebra   `MCC` `CC` `H5` `HCC`

√6ᵗʰ **S12.43**   Unspecified traumatic spondylolisthesis of fifth cervical vertebra
- 2,3,6 √7ᵗʰ **S12.430**   Unspecified traumatic displaced spondylolisthesis of fifth cervical vertebra   `MCC` `CC` `H5` `HCC`
- 2,3,6 √7ᵗʰ **S12.431**   Unspecified traumatic nondisplaced spondylolisthesis of fifth cervical vertebra   `MCC` `CC` `H5` `HCC`

2,3,6 √x7ᵗʰ **S12.44**   Type III traumatic spondylolisthesis of fifth cervical vertebra   `MCC` `CC` `H5` `HCC`

√6ᵗʰ **S12.45**   Other traumatic spondylolisthesis of fifth cervical vertebra
- 2,3,6 √7ᵗʰ **S12.450**   Other traumatic displaced spondylolisthesis of fifth cervical vertebra   `MCC` `CC` `H5` `HCC`
- 2,3,6 √7ᵗʰ **S12.451**   Other traumatic nondisplaced spondylolisthesis of fifth cervical vertebra   `MCC` `CC` `H5` `HCC`

√6ᵗʰ **S12.49**   Other fracture of fifth cervical vertebra
- 2,3,6 √7ᵗʰ **S12.490**   Other displaced fracture of fifth cervical vertebra   `MCC` `CC` `H5` `HCC`
- 2,3,6 √7ᵗʰ **S12.491**   Other nondisplaced fracture of fifth cervical vertebra   `MCC` `CC` `H5` `HCC`

√5ᵗʰ **S12.5**   Fracture of sixth cervical vertebra

√6ᵗʰ **S12.50**   Unspecified fracture of sixth cervical vertebra
- 2,3,6 √7ᵗʰ **S12.500**   Unspecified displaced fracture of sixth cervical vertebra   `MCC` `CC` `H5` `HCC`
- 2,3,6 √7ᵗʰ **S12.501**   Unspecified nondisplaced fracture of sixth cervical vertebra   `MCC` `CC` `H5` `HCC`

√6ᵗʰ **S12.53**   Unspecified traumatic spondylolisthesis of sixth cervical vertebra
- 2,3,6 √7ᵗʰ **S12.530**   Unspecified traumatic displaced spondylolisthesis of sixth cervical vertebra   `MCC` `CC` `H5` `HCC`
- 2,3,6 √7ᵗʰ **S12.531**   Unspecified traumatic nondisplaced spondylolisthesis of sixth cervical vertebra   `MCC` `CC` `H5` `HCC`

2,3,6 √x7ᵗʰ **S12.54**   Type III traumatic spondylolisthesis of sixth cervical vertebra   `MCC` `CC` `H5` `HCC`

√6ᵗʰ **S12.55**   Other traumatic spondylolisthesis of sixth cervical vertebra
- 2,3,6 √7ᵗʰ **S12.550**   Other traumatic displaced spondylolisthesis of sixth cervical vertebra   `MCC` `CC` `H5` `HCC`

N Newborn: 0   P Pediatric: 0-17   M Maternity: 9-64   A Adult: 15-124   `MCC` Major Complication/Comorbidity   `CC` Complication/Comorbidity   `SW` Severe Wound Dx

982   ICD-10-CM 2022

2,3,6 √7ᵗʰ **S12.551** Other traumatic nondisplaced spondylolisthesis of sixth cervical vertebra `MCC` `CC` `H5` `HCC`

√6ᵗʰ **S12.59** Other fracture of sixth cervical vertebra

2,3,6 √7ᵗʰ **S12.590** Other displaced fracture of sixth cervical vertebra `MCC` `CC` `H5` `HCC`

2,3,6 √7ᵗʰ **S12.591** Other nondisplaced fracture of sixth cervical vertebra `MCC` `CC` `H5` `HCC`

√5ᵗʰ **S12.6** Fracture of seventh cervical vertebra

√6ᵗʰ **S12.60** Unspecified fracture of seventh cervical vertebra

2,3,6 √7ᵗʰ **S12.600** Unspecified displaced fracture of seventh cervical vertebra `MCC` `CC` `H5` `HCC`

2,3,6 √7ᵗʰ **S12.601** Unspecified nondisplaced fracture of seventh cervical vertebra `MCC` `CC` `H5` `HCC`

√6ᵗʰ **S12.63** Unspecified traumatic spondylolisthesis of seventh cervical vertebra

2,3,6 √7ᵗʰ **S12.630** Unspecified traumatic displaced spondylolisthesis of seventh cervical vertebra `MCC` `CC` `H5` `HCC`

2,3,6 √7ᵗʰ **S12.631** Unspecified traumatic nondisplaced spondylolisthesis of seventh cervical vertebra `MCC` `CC` `H5` `HCC`

2,3,6 √x7ᵗʰ **S12.64** Type III traumatic spondylolisthesis of seventh cervical vertebra `MCC` `CC` `H5` `HCC`

√6ᵗʰ **S12.65** Other traumatic spondylolisthesis of seventh cervical vertebra

2,3,6 √7ᵗʰ **S12.650** Other traumatic displaced spondylolisthesis of seventh cervical vertebra `MCC` `CC` `H5` `HCC`

2,3,6 √7ᵗʰ **S12.651** Other traumatic nondisplaced spondylolisthesis of seventh cervical vertebra `MCC` `CC` `H5` `HCC`

√6ᵗʰ **S12.69** Other fracture of seventh cervical vertebra

2,3,6 √7ᵗʰ **S12.690** Other displaced fracture of seventh cervical vertebra `MCC` `CC` `H5` `HCC`

2,3,6 √7ᵗʰ **S12.691** Other nondisplaced fracture of seventh cervical vertebra `MCC` `CC` `H5` `HCC`

6 √x7ᵗʰ **S12.8** Fracture of other parts of neck `MCC` `H5` `HCC`

Hyoid bone
Larynx
Thyroid cartilage
Trachea

> The appropriate 7th character is to be added to code S12.8.
> A   initial encounter
> D   subsequent encounter
> S   sequela

6 √x7ᵗʰ **S12.9** Fracture of neck, unspecified `CC` `H5` `HCC`

Fracture of neck NOS
Fracture of cervical spine NOS
Fracture of cervical vertebra NOS

> The appropriate 7th character is to be added to code S12.9.
> A   initial encounter
> D   subsequent encounter
> S   sequela

√4ᵗʰ **S13** Dislocation and sprain of joints and ligaments at neck level

`INCLUDES`   avulsion of joint or ligament at neck level
laceration of cartilage, joint or ligament at neck level
sprain of cartilage, joint or ligament at neck level
traumatic hemarthrosis of joint or ligament at neck level
traumatic rupture of joint or ligament at neck level
traumatic subluxation of joint or ligament at neck level
traumatic tear of joint or ligament at neck level

Code also any associated open wound

EXCLUDES 2   strain of muscle or tendon at neck level (S16.1)

> The appropriate 7th character is to be added to each code from category S13.
> A   initial encounter
> D   subsequent encounter
> S   sequela

√x7ᵗʰ **S13.0** Traumatic rupture of cervical intervertebral disc `CC` `H5`

EXCLUDES 1   rupture or displacement (nontraumatic) of cervical intervertebral disc NOS (M50.-)

√5ᵗʰ **S13.1** Subluxation and dislocation of cervical vertebrae

Code also any associated:
open wound of neck (S11.-)
spinal cord injury (S14.1-)

EXCLUDES 2   fracture of cervical vertebrae (S12.0-S12.3-)

√6ᵗʰ **S13.10** Subluxation and dislocation of unspecified cervical vertebrae

√7ᵗʰ **S13.100** Subluxation of unspecified cervical vertebrae `CC` `H5`

√7ᵗʰ **S13.101** Dislocation of unspecified cervical vertebrae `CC` `H5`

√6ᵗʰ **S13.11** Subluxation and dislocation of C0/C1 cervical vertebrae

Subluxation and dislocation of atlantooccipital joint
Subluxation and dislocation of atloidooccipital joint
Subluxation and dislocation of occipitoatloid joint

√7ᵗʰ **S13.110** Subluxation of C0/C1 cervical vertebrae

√7ᵗʰ **S13.111** Dislocation of C0/C1 cervical vertebrae `CC` `H5`

√6ᵗʰ **S13.12** Subluxation and dislocation of C1/C2 cervical vertebrae

Subluxation and dislocation of atlantoaxial joint

√7ᵗʰ **S13.120** Subluxation of C1/C2 cervical vertebrae `CC` `H5`

√7ᵗʰ **S13.121** Dislocation of C1/C2 cervical vertebrae `CC` `H5`

√6ᵗʰ **S13.13** Subluxation and dislocation of C2/C3 cervical vertebrae

√7ᵗʰ **S13.130** Subluxation of C2/C3 cervical vertebrae `CC` `H5`

√7ᵗʰ **S13.131** Dislocation of C2/C3 cervical vertebrae `CC` `H5`

√6ᵗʰ **S13.14** Subluxation and dislocation of C3/C4 cervical vertebrae

√7ᵗʰ **S13.140** Subluxation of C3/C4 cervical vertebrae `CC` `H5`

√7ᵗʰ **S13.141** Dislocation of C3/C4 cervical vertebrae `CC` `H5`

√6ᵗʰ **S13.15** Subluxation and dislocation of C4/C5 cervical vertebrae

√7ᵗʰ **S13.150** Subluxation of C4/C5 cervical vertebrae `CC` `H5`

√7ᵗʰ **S13.151** Dislocation of C4/C5 cervical vertebrae `CC` `H5`

√6ᵗʰ **S13.16** Subluxation and dislocation of C5/C6 cervical vertebrae

√7ᵗʰ **S13.160** Subluxation of C5/C6 cervical vertebrae

√7ᵗʰ **S13.161** Dislocation of C5/C6 cervical vertebrae `CC` `H5`

√6ᵗʰ **S13.17** Subluxation and dislocation of C6/C7 cervical vertebrae

√7ᵗʰ **S13.170** Subluxation of C6/C7 cervical vertebrae

√7ᵗʰ **S13.171** Dislocation of C6/C7 cervical vertebrae `CC` `H5`

√6ᵗʰ **S13.18** Subluxation and dislocation of C7/T1 cervical vertebrae

√7ᵗʰ **S13.180** Subluxation of C7/T1 cervical vertebrae

√7ᵗʰ **S13.181** Dislocation of C7/T1 cervical vertebrae `CC` `H5`

√5ᵗʰ **S13.2** Dislocation of other and unspecified parts of neck

√x7ᵗʰ **S13.20** Dislocation of unspecified parts of neck `CC` `H5`

√x7ᵗʰ **S13.29** Dislocation of other parts of neck `CC` `H5`

√x7ᵗʰ **S13.4** Sprain of ligaments of cervical spine

Sprain of anterior longitudinal (ligament), cervical
Sprain of atlanto-axial (joints)
Sprain of atlanto-occipital (joints)
Whiplash injury of cervical spine

√x7ᵗʰ **S13.5** Sprain of thyroid region

Sprain of cricoarytenoid (joint) (ligament)
Sprain of cricothyroid (joint) (ligament)
Sprain of thyroid cartilage

√x7ᵗʰ **S13.8** Sprain of joints and ligaments of other parts of neck

√x7ᵗʰ **S13.9** Sprain of joints and ligaments of unspecified parts of neck

✓4th S14 Injury of nerves and spinal cord at neck level

> **NOTE** Code to highest level of cervical cord injury

Code also any associated:
  fracture of cervical vertebra (S12.0- — S12.6.-)
  open wound of neck (S11.-)
  transient paralysis (R29.5)

> The appropriate 7th character is to be added to each code from category S14.
> A initial encounter
> D subsequent encounter
> S sequela

✓x7th S14.0 Concussion and edema of cervical spinal cord `MCC` `HCC`

✓5th S14.1 Other and unspecified injuries of cervical spinal cord

  ✓6th S14.10 Unspecified injury of cervical spinal cord

    ✓7th S14.101 Unspecified injury at C1 level of cervical spinal cord `MCC` `H5` `HCC`

    ✓7th S14.102 Unspecified injury at C2 level of cervical spinal cord `MCC` `H5` `HCC`

    ✓7th S14.103 Unspecified injury at C3 level of cervical spinal cord `MCC` `H5` `HCC`

    ✓7th S14.104 Unspecified injury at C4 level of cervical spinal cord `MCC` `H5` `HCC`

    ✓7th S14.105 Unspecified injury at C5 level of cervical spinal cord `MCC` `H5` `HCC`

    ✓7th S14.106 Unspecified injury at C6 level of cervical spinal cord `MCC` `H5` `HCC`

    ✓7th S14.107 Unspecified injury at C7 level of cervical spinal cord `MCC` `H5` `HCC`

    ✓7th S14.108 Unspecified injury at C8 level of cervical spinal cord `MCC` `HCC`

    ✓7th S14.109 Unspecified injury at unspecified level of cervical spinal cord `HCC`
      Injury of cervical spinal cord NOS

  ✓6th S14.11 Complete lesion of cervical spinal cord

    ✓7th S14.111 Complete lesion at C1 level of cervical spinal cord `MCC` `H5` `HCC`

    ✓7th S14.112 Complete lesion at C2 level of cervical spinal cord `MCC` `H5` `HCC`

    ✓7th S14.113 Complete lesion at C3 level of cervical spinal cord `MCC` `H5` `HCC`

    ✓7th S14.114 Complete lesion at C4 level of cervical spinal cord `MCC` `H5` `HCC`

    ✓7th S14.115 Complete lesion at C5 level of cervical spinal cord `MCC` `H5` `HCC`

    ✓7th S14.116 Complete lesion at C6 level of cervical spinal cord `MCC` `H5` `HCC`

    ✓7th S14.117 Complete lesion at C7 level of cervical spinal cord `MCC` `H5` `HCC`

    ✓7th S14.118 Complete lesion at C8 level of cervical spinal cord `MCC` `HCC`

    ✓7th S14.119 Complete lesion at unspecified level of cervical spinal cord `HCC`

  ✓6th S14.12 Central cord syndrome of cervical spinal cord

    ✓7th S14.121 Central cord syndrome at C1 level of cervical spinal cord `MCC` `H5` `HCC`

    ✓7th S14.122 Central cord syndrome at C2 level of cervical spinal cord `MCC` `H5` `HCC`

    ✓7th S14.123 Central cord syndrome at C3 level of cervical spinal cord `MCC` `H5` `HCC`

    ✓7th S14.124 Central cord syndrome at C4 level of cervical spinal cord `MCC` `H5` `HCC`

    ✓7th S14.125 Central cord syndrome at C5 level of cervical spinal cord `MCC` `H5` `HCC`

    ✓7th S14.126 Central cord syndrome at C6 level of cervical spinal cord `MCC` `H5` `HCC`

    ✓7th S14.127 Central cord syndrome at C7 level of cervical spinal cord `MCC` `H5` `HCC`

    ✓7th S14.128 Central cord syndrome at C8 level of cervical spinal cord `MCC` `HCC`

    ✓7th S14.129 Central cord syndrome at unspecified level of cervical spinal cord `HCC`

  ✓6th S14.13 Anterior cord syndrome of cervical spinal cord

    ✓7th S14.131 Anterior cord syndrome at C1 level of cervical spinal cord `MCC` `H5` `HCC`

    ✓7th S14.132 Anterior cord syndrome at C2 level of cervical spinal cord `MCC` `H5` `HCC`

    ✓7th S14.133 Anterior cord syndrome at C3 level of cervical spinal cord `MCC` `H5` `HCC`

    ✓7th S14.134 Anterior cord syndrome at C4 level of cervical spinal cord `MCC` `H5` `HCC`

    ✓7th S14.135 Anterior cord syndrome at C5 level of cervical spinal cord `MCC` `H5` `HCC`

    ✓7th S14.136 Anterior cord syndrome at C6 level of cervical spinal cord `MCC` `H5` `HCC`

    ✓7th S14.137 Anterior cord syndrome at C7 level of cervical spinal cord `MCC` `H5` `HCC`

    ✓7th S14.138 Anterior cord syndrome at C8 level of cervical spinal cord `MCC` `HCC`

    ✓7th S14.139 Anterior cord syndrome at unspecified level of cervical spinal cord `HCC`

  ✓6th S14.14 Brown-Séquard syndrome of cervical spinal cord

    ✓7th S14.141 Brown-Séquard syndrome at C1 level of cervical spinal cord `MCC` `HCC`

    ✓7th S14.142 Brown-Séquard syndrome at C2 level of cervical spinal cord `MCC` `HCC`

    ✓7th S14.143 Brown-Séquard syndrome at C3 level of cervical spinal cord `MCC` `HCC`

    ✓7th S14.144 Brown-Séquard syndrome at C4 level of cervical spinal cord `MCC` `HCC`

    ✓7th S14.145 Brown-Séquard syndrome at C5 level of cervical spinal cord `MCC` `HCC`

    ✓7th S14.146 Brown-Séquard syndrome at C6 level of cervical spinal cord `MCC` `HCC`

    ✓7th S14.147 Brown-Séquard syndrome at C7 level of cervical spinal cord `MCC` `HCC`

    ✓7th S14.148 Brown-Séquard syndrome at C8 level of cervical spinal cord `MCC` `HCC`

    ✓7th S14.149 Brown-Séquard syndrome at unspecified level of cervical spinal cord `HCC`

  ✓6th S14.15 Other incomplete lesions of cervical spinal cord
    Incomplete lesion of cervical spinal cord NOS
    Posterior cord syndrome of cervical spinal cord

    ✓7th S14.151 Other incomplete lesion at C1 level of cervical spinal cord `MCC` `H5` `HCC`

    ✓7th S14.152 Other incomplete lesion at C2 level of cervical spinal cord `MCC` `H5` `HCC`

    ✓7th S14.153 Other incomplete lesion at C3 level of cervical spinal cord `MCC` `H5` `HCC`

    ✓7th S14.154 Other incomplete lesion at C4 level of cervical spinal cord `MCC` `H5` `HCC`

    ✓7th S14.155 Other incomplete lesion at C5 level of cervical spinal cord `MCC` `H5` `HCC`

    ✓7th S14.156 Other incomplete lesion at C6 level of cervical spinal cord `MCC` `H5` `HCC`

    ✓7th S14.157 Other incomplete lesion at C7 level of cervical spinal cord `MCC` `H5` `HCC`

    ✓7th S14.158 Other incomplete lesion at C8 level of cervical spinal cord `MCC` `HCC`

    ✓7th S14.159 Other incomplete lesion at unspecified level of cervical spinal cord `HCC`

✓x7th S14.2 Injury of nerve root of cervical spine

✓x7th S14.3 Injury of brachial plexus

✓x7th S14.4 Injury of peripheral nerves of neck

✓x7th S14.5 Injury of cervical sympathetic nerves

✓x7th S14.8 Injury of other specified nerves of neck

✓x7th S14.9 Injury of unspecified nerves of neck

✓4th S15 Injury of blood vessels at neck level

Code also any associated open wound (S11.-)

> The appropriate 7th character is to be added to each code from category S15.
> A initial encounter
> D subsequent encounter
> S sequela

✓5th S15.0 Injury of carotid artery of neck

Injury of carotid artery (common) (external) (internal, extracranial portion)
Injury of carotid artery NOS

> **EXCLUDES 1**   injury of internal carotid artery, intracranial portion (S06.8)

  ✓6th S15.00 Unspecified injury of carotid artery

    ✓7th S15.001 Unspecified injury of right carotid artery `CC`

N Newborn: 0   **P** Pediatric: 0-17   **M** Maternity: 9-64   **A** Adult: 15-124   `MCC` Major Complication/Comorbidity   `CC` Complication/Comorbidity   `SW` Severe Wound Dx

984   ICD-10-CM 2022

√7ᵗʰ **S15.002** Unspecified injury of left carotid artery `CC`

√7ᵗʰ **S15.009** Unspecified injury of unspecified carotid artery `CC`

√6ᵗʰ **S15.01** Minor laceration of carotid artery

Incomplete transection of carotid artery
Laceration of carotid artery NOS
Superficial laceration of carotid artery

√7ᵗʰ **S15.011** Minor laceration of right carotid artery `CC`

√7ᵗʰ **S15.012** Minor laceration of left carotid artery `CC`

√7ᵗʰ **S15.019** Minor laceration of unspecified carotid artery `CC`

√6ᵗʰ **S15.02** Major laceration of carotid artery

Complete transection of carotid artery
Traumatic rupture of carotid artery

√7ᵗʰ **S15.021** Major laceration of right carotid artery `CC`

√7ᵗʰ **S15.022** Major laceration of left carotid artery `CC`

√7ᵗʰ **S15.029** Major laceration of unspecified carotid artery `CC`

√6ᵗʰ **S15.09** Other specified injury of carotid artery

√7ᵗʰ **S15.091** Other specified injury of right carotid artery `CC`

√7ᵗʰ **S15.092** Other specified injury of left carotid artery `CC`

√7ᵗʰ **S15.099** Other specified injury of unspecified carotid artery `CC`

√5ᵗʰ **S15.1** Injury of vertebral artery

√6ᵗʰ **S15.10** Unspecified injury of vertebral artery

√7ᵗʰ **S15.101** Unspecified injury of right vertebral artery `CC`

√7ᵗʰ **S15.102** Unspecified injury of left vertebral artery `CC`

√7ᵗʰ **S15.109** Unspecified injury of unspecified vertebral artery `CC`

√6ᵗʰ **S15.11** Minor laceration of vertebral artery

Incomplete transection of vertebral artery
Laceration of vertebral artery NOS
Superficial laceration of vertebral artery

√7ᵗʰ **S15.111** Minor laceration of right vertebral artery `CC`

√7ᵗʰ **S15.112** Minor laceration of left vertebral artery `CC`

√7ᵗʰ **S15.119** Minor laceration of unspecified vertebral artery `CC`

√6ᵗʰ **S15.12** Major laceration of vertebral artery

Complete transection of vertebral artery
Traumatic rupture of vertebral artery

√7ᵗʰ **S15.121** Major laceration of right vertebral artery `CC`

√7ᵗʰ **S15.122** Major laceration of left vertebral artery `CC`

√7ᵗʰ **S15.129** Major laceration of unspecified vertebral artery `CC`

√6ᵗʰ **S15.19** Other specified injury of vertebral artery

√7ᵗʰ **S15.191** Other specified injury of right vertebral artery `CC`

√7ᵗʰ **S15.192** Other specified injury of left vertebral artery `CC`

√7ᵗʰ **S15.199** Other specified injury of unspecified vertebral artery `CC`

√5ᵗʰ **S15.2** Injury of external jugular vein

√6ᵗʰ **S15.20** Unspecified injury of external jugular vein

√7ᵗʰ **S15.201** Unspecified injury of right external jugular vein `CC`

√7ᵗʰ **S15.202** Unspecified injury of left external jugular vein `CC`

√7ᵗʰ **S15.209** Unspecified injury of unspecified external jugular vein `CC`

√6ᵗʰ **S15.21** Minor laceration of external jugular vein

Incomplete transection of external jugular vein
Laceration of external jugular vein NOS
Superficial laceration of external jugular vein

√7ᵗʰ **S15.211** Minor laceration of right external jugular vein `CC`

√7ᵗʰ **S15.212** Minor laceration of left external jugular vein `CC`

√7ᵗʰ **S15.219** Minor laceration of unspecified external jugular vein `CC`

√6ᵗʰ **S15.22** Major laceration of external jugular vein

Complete transection of external jugular vein
Traumatic rupture of external jugular vein

√7ᵗʰ **S15.221** Major laceration of right external jugular vein `CC`

√7ᵗʰ **S15.222** Major laceration of left external jugular vein `CC`

√7ᵗʰ **S15.229** Major laceration of unspecified external jugular vein `CC`

√6ᵗʰ **S15.29** Other specified injury of external jugular vein

√7ᵗʰ **S15.291** Other specified injury of right external jugular vein `CC`

√7ᵗʰ **S15.292** Other specified injury of left external jugular vein `CC`

√7ᵗʰ **S15.299** Other specified injury of unspecified external jugular vein `CC`

√5ᵗʰ **S15.3** Injury of internal jugular vein

√6ᵗʰ **S15.30** Unspecified injury of internal jugular vein

√7ᵗʰ **S15.301** Unspecified injury of right internal jugular vein `CC`

√7ᵗʰ **S15.302** Unspecified injury of left internal jugular vein `CC`

√7ᵗʰ **S15.309** Unspecified injury of unspecified internal jugular vein `CC`

√6ᵗʰ **S15.31** Minor laceration of internal jugular vein

Incomplete transection of internal jugular vein
Laceration of internal jugular vein NOS
Superficial laceration of internal jugular vein

√7ᵗʰ **S15.311** Minor laceration of right internal jugular vein `CC`

√7ᵗʰ **S15.312** Minor laceration of left internal jugular vein `CC`

√7ᵗʰ **S15.319** Minor laceration of unspecified internal jugular vein `CC`

√6ᵗʰ **S15.32** Major laceration of internal jugular vein

Complete transection of internal jugular vein
Traumatic rupture of internal jugular vein

√7ᵗʰ **S15.321** Major laceration of right internal jugular vein `CC`

√7ᵗʰ **S15.322** Major laceration of left internal jugular vein `CC`

√7ᵗʰ **S15.329** Major laceration of unspecified internal jugular vein `CC`

√6ᵗʰ **S15.39** Other specified injury of internal jugular vein

√7ᵗʰ **S15.391** Other specified injury of right internal jugular vein `CC`

√7ᵗʰ **S15.392** Other specified injury of left internal jugular vein `CC`

√7ᵗʰ **S15.399** Other specified injury of unspecified internal jugular vein `CC`

√x7ᵗʰ **S15.8** Injury of other specified blood vessels at neck level `CC`

√x7ᵗʰ **S15.9** Injury of unspecified blood vessel at neck level `CC`

√4ᵗʰ **S16** Injury of muscle, fascia and tendon at neck level

Code also any associated open wound (S11.-)

EXCLUDES 2   sprain of joint or ligament at neck level (S13.9)

The appropriate 7th character is to be added to each code from category S16.
A   initial encounter
D   subsequent encounter
S   sequela

√x7ᵗʰ **S16.1** Strain of muscle, fascia and tendon at neck level

√x7ᵗʰ **S16.2** Laceration of muscle, fascia and tendon at neck level

√x7ᵗʰ **S16.8** Other specified injury of muscle, fascia and tendon at neck level

√x7ᵗʰ **S16.9** Unspecified injury of muscle, fascia and tendon at neck level

☑ Additional Character Required   √x7ᵗʰ Placeholder   Questionable PDx   Manifestation   Unspecified Dx   **UPD** Unacceptable PDx   **H1-H14** HAC   **HCC** CMS-HCC Dx   **HIV** HIV Dx

ICD-10-CM 2022   985

✓4ᵗʰ **S17 Crushing injury of neck**

     Use additional code for all associated injuries, such as:
       injury of blood vessels (S15.-)
       open wound of neck (S11.-)
       spinal cord injury (S14.0, S14.1-)
       vertebral fracture (S12.0- — S12.3-)

> The appropriate 7th character is to be added to each code from category S17.
> A   initial encounter
> D   subsequent encounter
> S   sequela

   ✓x7ᵗʰ **S17.0 Crushing injury of larynx and trachea**   `CC` `H5`

   ✓x7ᵗʰ **S17.8 Crushing injury of other specified parts of neck**   `CC` `H5`

   ✓x7ᵗʰ **S17.9 Crushing injury of neck, part unspecified**   `CC` `H5`

✓4ᵗʰ **S19 Other specified and unspecified injuries of neck**

> The appropriate 7th character is to be added to each code from category S19.
> A   initial encounter
> D   subsequent encounter
> S   sequela

   ✓5ᵗʰ **S19.8 Other specified injuries of neck**

     ✓x7ᵗʰ **S19.80 Other specified injuries of unspecified part of neck**

     ✓x7ᵗʰ **S19.81 Other specified injuries of larynx**

     ✓x7ᵗʰ **S19.82 Other specified injuries of cervical trachea**

       EXCLUDES 2   *other specified injury of thoracic trachea (S27.5-)*

     ✓x7ᵗʰ **S19.83 Other specified injuries of vocal cord**

     ✓x7ᵗʰ **S19.84 Other specified injuries of thyroid gland**

     ✓x7ᵗʰ **S19.85 Other specified injuries of pharynx and cervical esophagus**

     ✓x7ᵗʰ **S19.89 Other specified injuries of other specified part of neck**

   ✓x7ᵗʰ **S19.9 Unspecified injury of neck**

Injuries to the thorax (S20-S29)

INCLUDES   injuries of breast
       injuries of chest (wall)
       injuries of interscapular area

EXCLUDES 2   *burns and corrosions (T20-T32)*
       effects of foreign body in bronchus (T17.5)
       effects of foreign body in esophagus (T18.1)
       effects of foreign body in lung (T17.8)
       effects of foreign body in trachea (T17.4)
       frostbite (T33-T34)
       injuries of axilla
       injuries of clavicle
       injuries of scapular region
       injuries of shoulder
       insect bite or sting, venomous (T63.4)

✓4ᵗʰ **S20 Superficial injury of thorax**

     AHA: 2020,4Q,39

> The appropriate 7th character is to be added to each code from category S20.
> A   initial encounter
> D   subsequent encounter
> S   sequela

   ✓5ᵗʰ **S20.0 Contusion of breast**

     ✓x7ᵗʰ **S20.00 Contusion of breast, unspecified breast**

     ✓x7ᵗʰ **S20.01 Contusion of right breast**

     ✓x7ᵗʰ **S20.02 Contusion of left breast**

   ✓5ᵗʰ **S20.1 Other and unspecified superficial injuries of breast**

     ✓6ᵗʰ **S20.10 Unspecified superficial injuries of breast**

       ✓7ᵗʰ **S20.101 Unspecified superficial injuries of breast, right breast**

       ✓7ᵗʰ **S20.102 Unspecified superficial injuries of breast, left breast**

       ✓7ᵗʰ **S20.109 Unspecified superficial injuries of breast, unspecified breast**

     ✓6ᵗʰ **S20.11 Abrasion of breast**

       ✓7ᵗʰ **S20.111 Abrasion of breast, right breast**

       ✓7ᵗʰ **S20.112 Abrasion of breast, left breast**

       ✓7ᵗʰ **S20.119 Abrasion of breast, unspecified breast**

     ✓6ᵗʰ **S20.12 Blister (nonthermal) of breast**

       ✓7ᵗʰ **S20.121 Blister (nonthermal) of breast, right breast**

       ✓7ᵗʰ **S20.122 Blister (nonthermal) of breast, left breast**

       ✓7ᵗʰ **S20.129 Blister (nonthermal) of breast, unspecified breast**

     ✓6ᵗʰ **S20.14 External constriction of part of breast**

       ✓7ᵗʰ **S20.141 External constriction of part of breast, right breast**

       ✓7ᵗʰ **S20.142 External constriction of part of breast, left breast**

       ✓7ᵗʰ **S20.149 External constriction of part of breast, unspecified breast**

     ✓6ᵗʰ **S20.15 Superficial foreign body of breast**

       Splinter in the breast

       ✓7ᵗʰ **S20.151 Superficial foreign body of breast, right breast**

       ✓7ᵗʰ **S20.152 Superficial foreign body of breast, left breast**

       ✓7ᵗʰ **S20.159 Superficial foreign body of breast, unspecified breast**

     ✓6ᵗʰ **S20.16 Insect bite (nonvenomous) of breast**

       ✓7ᵗʰ **S20.161 Insect bite (nonvenomous) of breast, right breast**

       ✓7ᵗʰ **S20.162 Insect bite (nonvenomous) of breast, left breast**

       ✓7ᵗʰ **S20.169 Insect bite (nonvenomous) of breast, unspecified breast**

     ✓6ᵗʰ **S20.17 Other superficial bite of breast**

       EXCLUDES 1   *open bite of breast (S21.05-)*

       ✓7ᵗʰ **S20.171 Other superficial bite of breast, right breast**

       ✓7ᵗʰ **S20.172 Other superficial bite of breast, left breast**

       ✓7ᵗʰ **S20.179 Other superficial bite of breast, unspecified breast**

   ✓5ᵗʰ **S20.2 Contusion of thorax**

     ✓x7ᵗʰ **S20.20 Contusion of thorax, unspecified**

     ✓6ᵗʰ **S20.21 Contusion of front wall of thorax**

       ✓7ᵗʰ **S20.211 Contusion of right front wall of thorax**

       ✓7ᵗʰ **S20.212 Contusion of left front wall of thorax**

       ✓7ᵗʰ **S20.213 Contusion of bilateral front wall of thorax**

       ✓7ᵗʰ **S20.214 Contusion of middle front wall of thorax**

       ✓7ᵗʰ **S20.219 Contusion of unspecified front wall of thorax**

     ✓6ᵗʰ **S20.22 Contusion of back wall of thorax**

       ✓7ᵗʰ **S20.221 Contusion of right back wall of thorax**

       ✓7ᵗʰ **S20.222 Contusion of left back wall of thorax**

       ✓7ᵗʰ **S20.223 Contusion of bilateral back wall of thorax**

       ✓7ᵗʰ **S20.224 Contusion of middle back wall of thorax**

       ✓7ᵗʰ **S20.229 Contusion of unspecified back wall of thorax**

   ✓5ᵗʰ **S20.3 Other and unspecified superficial injuries of front wall of thorax**

     ✓6ᵗʰ **S20.30 Unspecified superficial injuries of front wall of thorax**

       ✓7ᵗʰ **S20.301 Unspecified superficial injuries of right front wall of thorax**

       ✓7ᵗʰ **S20.302 Unspecified superficial injuries of left front wall of thorax**

       ✓7ᵗʰ **S20.303 Unspecified superficial injuries of bilateral front wall of thorax**

       ✓7ᵗʰ **S20.304 Unspecified superficial injuries of middle front wall of thorax**

       ✓7ᵗʰ **S20.309 Unspecified superficial injuries of unspecified front wall of thorax**

     ✓6ᵗʰ **S20.31 Abrasion of front wall of thorax**

       ✓7ᵗʰ **S20.311 Abrasion of right front wall of thorax**

       ✓7ᵗʰ **S20.312 Abrasion of left front wall of thorax**

       ✓7ᵗʰ **S20.313 Abrasion of bilateral front wall of thorax**

       ✓7ᵗʰ **S20.314 Abrasion of middle front wall of thorax**

       ✓7ᵗʰ **S20.319 Abrasion of unspecified front wall of thorax**

     ✓6ᵗʰ **S20.32 Blister (nonthermal) of front wall of thorax**

       ✓7ᵗʰ **S20.321 Blister (nonthermal) of right front wall of thorax**

Ⓝ Newborn: 0   Ⓟ Pediatric: 0-17   Ⓜ Maternity: 9-64   Ⓐ Adult: 15-124   **MCC** Major Complication/Comorbidity   **CC** Complication/Comorbidity   **SW** Severe Wound Dx

986   ICD-10-CM 2022

√7ᵗʰ **S20.322** Blister (nonthermal) of left front wall of thorax

√7ᵗʰ **S20.323** Blister (nonthermal) of bilateral front wall of thorax

√7ᵗʰ **S20.324** Blister (nonthermal) of middle front wall of thorax

√7ᵗʰ **S20.329** Blister (nonthermal) of unspecified front wall of thorax

√6ᵗʰ **S20.34** External constriction of front wall of thorax

√7ᵗʰ **S20.341** External constriction of right front wall of thorax

√7ᵗʰ **S20.342** External constriction of left front wall of thorax

√7ᵗʰ **S20.343** External constriction of bilateral front wall of thorax

√7ᵗʰ **S20.344** External constriction of middle front wall of thorax

√7ᵗʰ **S20.349** External constriction of unspecified front wall of thorax

√6ᵗʰ **S20.35** Superficial foreign body of front wall of thorax

Splinter in front wall of thorax

√7ᵗʰ **S20.351** Superficial foreign body of right front wall of thorax

√7ᵗʰ **S20.352** Superficial foreign body of left front wall of thorax

√7ᵗʰ **S20.353** Superficial foreign body of bilateral front wall of thorax

√7ᵗʰ **S20.354** Superficial foreign body of middle front wall of thorax

√7ᵗʰ **S20.359** Superficial foreign body of unspecified front wall of thorax

√6ᵗʰ **S20.36** Insect bite (nonvenomous) of front wall of thorax

√7ᵗʰ **S20.361** Insect bite (nonvenomous) of right front wall of thorax

√7ᵗʰ **S20.362** Insect bite (nonvenomous) of left front wall of thorax

√7ᵗʰ **S20.363** Insect bite (nonvenomous) of bilateral front wall of thorax

√7ᵗʰ **S20.364** Insect bite (nonvenomous) of middle front wall of thorax

√7ᵗʰ **S20.369** Insect bite (nonvenomous) of unspecified front wall of thorax

√6ᵗʰ **S20.37** Other superficial bite of front wall of thorax

EXCLUDES 1   open bite of front wall of thorax (S21.15)

√7ᵗʰ **S20.371** Other superficial bite of right front wall of thorax

√7ᵗʰ **S20.372** Other superficial bite of left front wall of thorax

√7ᵗʰ **S20.373** Other superficial bite of bilateral front wall of thorax

√7ᵗʰ **S20.374** Other superficial bite of middle front wall of thorax

√7ᵗʰ **S20.379** Other superficial bite of unspecified front wall of thorax

√5ᵗʰ **S20.4** Other and unspecified superficial injuries of back wall of thorax

√6ᵗʰ **S20.40** Unspecified superficial injuries of back wall of thorax

√7ᵗʰ **S20.401** Unspecified superficial injuries of right back wall of thorax

√7ᵗʰ **S20.402** Unspecified superficial injuries of left back wall of thorax

√7ᵗʰ **S20.409** Unspecified superficial injuries of unspecified back wall of thorax

√6ᵗʰ **S20.41** Abrasion of back wall of thorax

√7ᵗʰ **S20.411** Abrasion of right back wall of thorax

√7ᵗʰ **S20.412** Abrasion of left back wall of thorax

√7ᵗʰ **S20.419** Abrasion of unspecified back wall of thorax

√6ᵗʰ **S20.42** Blister (nonthermal) of back wall of thorax

√7ᵗʰ **S20.421** Blister (nonthermal) of right back wall of thorax

√7ᵗʰ **S20.422** Blister (nonthermal) of left back wall of thorax

√7ᵗʰ **S20.429** Blister (nonthermal) of unspecified back wall of thorax

√6ᵗʰ **S20.44** External constriction of back wall of thorax

√7ᵗʰ **S20.441** External constriction of right back wall of thorax

√7ᵗʰ **S20.442** External constriction of left back wall of thorax

√7ᵗʰ **S20.449** External constriction of unspecified back wall of thorax

√6ᵗʰ **S20.45** Superficial foreign body of back wall of thorax

Splinter of back wall of thorax

√7ᵗʰ **S20.451** Superficial foreign body of right back wall of thorax

√7ᵗʰ **S20.452** Superficial foreign body of left back wall of thorax

√7ᵗʰ **S20.459** Superficial foreign body of unspecified back wall of thorax

√6ᵗʰ **S20.46** Insect bite (nonvenomous) of back wall of thorax

√7ᵗʰ **S20.461** Insect bite (nonvenomous) of right back wall of thorax

√7ᵗʰ **S20.462** Insect bite (nonvenomous) of left back wall of thorax

√7ᵗʰ **S20.469** Insect bite (nonvenomous) of unspecified back wall of thorax

√6ᵗʰ **S20.47** Other superficial bite of back wall of thorax

EXCLUDES 1   open bite of back wall of thorax (S21.25)

√7ᵗʰ **S20.471** Other superficial bite of right back wall of thorax

√7ᵗʰ **S20.472** Other superficial bite of left back wall of thorax

√7ᵗʰ **S20.479** Other superficial bite of unspecified back wall of thorax

√5ᵗʰ **S20.9** Superficial injury of unspecified parts of thorax

EXCLUDES 1   contusion of thorax NOS (S20.20)

√x7ᵗʰ **S20.90** Unspecified superficial injury of unspecified parts of thorax

Superficial injury of thoracic wall NOS

√x7ᵗʰ **S20.91** Abrasion of unspecified parts of thorax

√x7ᵗʰ **S20.92** Blister (nonthermal) of unspecified parts of thorax

√x7ᵗʰ **S20.94** External constriction of unspecified parts of thorax

√x7ᵗʰ **S20.95** Superficial foreign body of unspecified parts of thorax

Splinter in thorax NOS

√x7ᵗʰ **S20.96** Insect bite (nonvenomous) of unspecified parts of thorax

√x7ᵗʰ **S20.97** Other superficial bite of unspecified parts of thorax

EXCLUDES 1   open bite of thorax NOS (S21.95)

√4ᵗʰ **S21** Open wound of thorax

Code also any associated injury, such as:
injury of heart (S26.-)
injury of intrathoracic organs (S27.-)
rib fracture (S22.3-, S22.4-)
spinal cord injury (S24.0-, S24.1-)
traumatic hemopneumothorax (S27.3)
traumatic hemothorax (S27.1)
traumatic pneumothorax (S27.0)
wound infection

EXCLUDES 1   traumatic amputation (partial) of thorax (S28.1)

The appropriate 7th character is to be added to each code from category S21.
A   initial encounter
D   subsequent encounter
S   sequela

√5ᵗʰ **S21.0** Open wound of breast

√6ᵗʰ **S21.00** Unspecified open wound of breast

√7ᵗʰ **S21.001** Unspecified open wound of right breast

√7ᵗʰ **S21.002** Unspecified open wound of left breast

√7ᵗʰ **S21.009** Unspecified open wound of unspecified breast

√6ᵗʰ **S21.01** Laceration without foreign body of breast

√7ᵗʰ **S21.011** Laceration without foreign body of right breast

√7ᵗʰ **S21.012** Laceration without foreign body of left breast

√7ᵗʰ **S21.019** Laceration without foreign body of unspecified breast

√6ᵗʰ **S21.02** Laceration with foreign body of breast

√7ᵗʰ **S21.021** Laceration with foreign body of right breast

√7ᵗʰ **S21.022** Laceration with foreign body of left breast

√7ᵗʰ **S21.029** Laceration with foreign body of unspecified breast

☑ Additional Character Required   √x7ᵗʰ Placeholder   Questionable PDx   Manifestation   Unspecified Dx   UPD Unacceptable PDx   H1-H14 HAC   HCC CMS-HCC Dx   HIV HIV Dx

ICD-10-CM 2022   987

✓6ᵗʰ **S21.03** Puncture wound without foreign body of breast
- ✓7ᵗʰ **S21.031** Puncture wound without foreign body of right breast
- ✓7ᵗʰ **S21.032** Puncture wound without foreign body of left breast
- ✓7ᵗʰ **S21.039** Puncture wound without foreign body of unspecified breast

✓6ᵗʰ **S21.04** Puncture wound with foreign body of breast
- ✓7ᵗʰ **S21.041** Puncture wound with foreign body of right breast
- ✓7ᵗʰ **S21.042** Puncture wound with foreign body of left breast
- ✓7ᵗʰ **S21.049** Puncture wound with foreign body of unspecified breast

✓6ᵗʰ **S21.05** Open bite of breast
  Bite of breast NOS
  EXCLUDES 1 superficial bite of breast (S20.17)
- ✓7ᵗʰ **S21.051** Open bite of right breast
- ✓7ᵗʰ **S21.052** Open bite of left breast
- ✓7ᵗʰ **S21.059** Open bite of unspecified breast

✓5ᵗʰ **S21.1** Open wound of front wall of thorax without penetration into thoracic cavity
  Open wound of chest without penetration into thoracic cavity

✓6ᵗʰ **S21.10** Unspecified open wound of front wall of thorax without penetration into thoracic cavity
- ✓7ᵗʰ **S21.101** Unspecified open wound of right front wall of thorax without penetration into thoracic cavity **cc**
- ✓7ᵗʰ **S21.102** Unspecified open wound of left front wall of thorax without penetration into thoracic cavity **cc**
- ✓7ᵗʰ **S21.109** Unspecified open wound of unspecified front wall of thorax without penetration into thoracic cavity **cc**

✓6ᵗʰ **S21.11** Laceration without foreign body of front wall of thorax without penetration into thoracic cavity
- ✓7ᵗʰ **S21.111** Laceration without foreign body of right front wall of thorax without penetration into thoracic cavity **cc**
- ✓7ᵗʰ **S21.112** Laceration without foreign body of left front wall of thorax without penetration into thoracic cavity **cc**
- ✓7ᵗʰ **S21.119** Laceration without foreign body of unspecified front wall of thorax without penetration into thoracic cavity **cc**

✓6ᵗʰ **S21.12** Laceration with foreign body of front wall of thorax without penetration into thoracic cavity
- ✓7ᵗʰ **S21.121** Laceration with foreign body of right front wall of thorax without penetration into thoracic cavity **cc**
- ✓7ᵗʰ **S21.122** Laceration with foreign body of left front wall of thorax without penetration into thoracic cavity **cc**
- ✓7ᵗʰ **S21.129** Laceration with foreign body of unspecified front wall of thorax without penetration into thoracic cavity **cc**

✓6ᵗʰ **S21.13** Puncture wound without foreign body of front wall of thorax without penetration into thoracic cavity
- ✓7ᵗʰ **S21.131** Puncture wound without foreign body of right front wall of thorax without penetration into thoracic cavity **cc**
- ✓7ᵗʰ **S21.132** Puncture wound without foreign body of left front wall of thorax without penetration into thoracic cavity **cc**
- ✓7ᵗʰ **S21.139** Puncture wound without foreign body of unspecified front wall of thorax without penetration into thoracic cavity **cc**

✓6ᵗʰ **S21.14** Puncture wound with foreign body of front wall of thorax without penetration into thoracic cavity
- ✓7ᵗʰ **S21.141** Puncture wound with foreign body of right front wall of thorax without penetration into thoracic cavity **cc**
- ✓7ᵗʰ **S21.142** Puncture wound with foreign body of left front wall of thorax without penetration into thoracic cavity **cc**
- ✓7ᵗʰ **S21.149** Puncture wound with foreign body of unspecified front wall of thorax without penetration into thoracic cavity **cc**

✓6ᵗʰ **S21.15** Open bite of front wall of thorax without penetration into thoracic cavity
  Bite of front wall of thorax NOS
  EXCLUDES 1 superficial bite of front wall of thorax (S20.37)
- ✓7ᵗʰ **S21.151** Open bite of right front wall of thorax without penetration into thoracic cavity **cc**
- ✓7ᵗʰ **S21.152** Open bite of left front wall of thorax without penetration into thoracic cavity **cc**
- ✓7ᵗʰ **S21.159** Open bite of unspecified front wall of thorax without penetration into thoracic cavity **cc**

✓5ᵗʰ **S21.2** Open wound of back wall of thorax without penetration into thoracic cavity

✓6ᵗʰ **S21.20** Unspecified open wound of back wall of thorax without penetration into thoracic cavity
- ✓7ᵗʰ **S21.201** Unspecified open wound of right back wall of thorax without penetration into thoracic cavity
- ✓7ᵗʰ **S21.202** Unspecified open wound of left back wall of thorax without penetration into thoracic cavity
- ✓7ᵗʰ **S21.209** Unspecified open wound of unspecified back wall of thorax without penetration into thoracic cavity

✓6ᵗʰ **S21.21** Laceration without foreign body of back wall of thorax without penetration into thoracic cavity
- ✓7ᵗʰ **S21.211** Laceration without foreign body of right back wall of thorax without penetration into thoracic cavity
- ✓7ᵗʰ **S21.212** Laceration without foreign body of left back wall of thorax without penetration into thoracic cavity
- ✓7ᵗʰ **S21.219** Laceration without foreign body of unspecified back wall of thorax without penetration into thoracic cavity

✓6ᵗʰ **S21.22** Laceration with foreign body of back wall of thorax without penetration into thoracic cavity
- ✓7ᵗʰ **S21.221** Laceration with foreign body of right back wall of thorax without penetration into thoracic cavity
- ✓7ᵗʰ **S21.222** Laceration with foreign body of left back wall of thorax without penetration into thoracic cavity
- ✓7ᵗʰ **S21.229** Laceration with foreign body of unspecified back wall of thorax without penetration into thoracic cavity

✓6ᵗʰ **S21.23** Puncture wound without foreign body of back wall of thorax without penetration into thoracic cavity
- ✓7ᵗʰ **S21.231** Puncture wound without foreign body of right back wall of thorax without penetration into thoracic cavity
- ✓7ᵗʰ **S21.232** Puncture wound without foreign body of left back wall of thorax without penetration into thoracic cavity
- ✓7ᵗʰ **S21.239** Puncture wound without foreign body of unspecified back wall of thorax without penetration into thoracic cavity

✓6ᵗʰ **S21.24** Puncture wound with foreign body of back wall of thorax without penetration into thoracic cavity
- ✓7ᵗʰ **S21.241** Puncture wound with foreign body of right back wall of thorax without penetration into thoracic cavity
- ✓7ᵗʰ **S21.242** Puncture wound with foreign body of left back wall of thorax without penetration into thoracic cavity
- ✓7ᵗʰ **S21.249** Puncture wound with foreign body of unspecified back wall of thorax without penetration into thoracic cavity

✓6ᵗʰ **S21.25** Open bite of back wall of thorax without penetration into thoracic cavity
  Bite of back wall of thorax NOS
  EXCLUDES 1 superficial bite of back wall of thorax (S20.47)
- ✓7ᵗʰ **S21.251** Open bite of right back wall of thorax without penetration into thoracic cavity
- ✓7ᵗʰ **S21.252** Open bite of left back wall of thorax without penetration into thoracic cavity
- ✓7ᵗʰ **S21.259** Open bite of unspecified back wall of thorax without penetration into thoracic cavity

✓5th **S21.3 Open wound of** front wall of thorax with penetration **into thoracic cavity**

Open wound of chest with penetration into thoracic cavity

✓6th **S21.30 Unspecified open wound of front wall of thorax with penetration into thoracic cavity**

✓7th **S21.301 Unspecified open wound of** right **front wall of thorax with penetration into thoracic cavity** MCC

✓7th **S21.302 Unspecified open wound of** left **front wall of thorax with penetration into thoracic cavity** MCC

✓7th **S21.309 Unspecified open wound of unspecified front wall of thorax with penetration into thoracic cavity** MCC

✓6th **S21.31** Laceration without foreign body **of front wall of thorax with penetration into thoracic cavity**

✓7th **S21.311 Laceration without foreign body of** right **front wall of thorax with penetration into thoracic cavity** MCC

✓7th **S21.312 Laceration without foreign body of** left **front wall of thorax with penetration into thoracic cavity** MCC

✓7th **S21.319 Laceration without foreign body of unspecified front wall of thorax with penetration into thoracic cavity** MCC

✓6th **S21.32** Laceration with foreign body **of front wall of thorax with penetration into thoracic cavity**

✓7th **S21.321 Laceration with foreign body of** right **front wall of thorax with penetration into thoracic cavity** MCC

✓7th **S21.322 Laceration with foreign body of** left **front wall of thorax with penetration into thoracic cavity** MCC

✓7th **S21.329 Laceration with foreign body of unspecified front wall of thorax with penetration into thoracic cavity** MCC

✓6th **S21.33** Puncture wound without foreign body **of front wall of thorax with penetration into thoracic cavity**

✓7th **S21.331 Puncture wound without foreign body of** right **front wall of thorax with penetration into thoracic cavity** MCC

✓7th **S21.332 Puncture wound without foreign body of** left **front wall of thorax with penetration into thoracic cavity** MCC

✓7th **S21.339 Puncture wound without foreign body of unspecified front wall of thorax with penetration into thoracic cavity** MCC

✓6th **S21.34** Puncture wound with foreign body **of front wall of thorax with penetration into thoracic cavity**

✓7th **S21.341 Puncture wound with foreign body of** right **front wall of thorax with penetration into thoracic cavity** MCC

✓7th **S21.342 Puncture wound with foreign body of** left **front wall of thorax with penetration into thoracic cavity** MCC

✓7th **S21.349 Puncture wound with foreign body of unspecified front wall of thorax with penetration into thoracic cavity** MCC

✓6th **S21.35** Open bite **of front wall of thorax with penetration into thoracic cavity**

EXCLUDES 1   *superficial bite of front wall of thorax (S20.37)*

✓7th **S21.351 Open bite of** right **front wall of thorax with penetration into thoracic cavity** MCC

✓7th **S21.352 Open bite of** left **front wall of thorax with penetration into thoracic cavity** MCC

✓7th **S21.359 Open bite of unspecified front wall of thorax with penetration into thoracic cavity** MCC

✓5th **S21.4 Open wound of** back wall of thorax with penetration **into thoracic cavity**

✓6th **S21.40 Unspecified open wound of back wall of thorax with penetration into thoracic cavity**

✓7th **S21.401 Unspecified open wound of** right **back wall of thorax with penetration into thoracic cavity** MCC

✓7th **S21.402 Unspecified open wound of** left **back wall of thorax with penetration into thoracic cavity** MCC

✓7th **S21.409 Unspecified open wound of unspecified back wall of thorax with penetration into thoracic cavity** MCC

✓6th **S21.41** Laceration without foreign body **of back wall of thorax with penetration into thoracic cavity**

✓7th **S21.411 Laceration without foreign body of** right **back wall of thorax with penetration into thoracic cavity** MCC

✓7th **S21.412 Laceration without foreign body of** left **back wall of thorax with penetration into thoracic cavity** MCC

✓7th **S21.419 Laceration without foreign body of unspecified back wall of thorax with penetration into thoracic cavity** MCC

✓6th **S21.42** Laceration with foreign body **of back wall of thorax with penetration into thoracic cavity**

✓7th **S21.421 Laceration with foreign body of** right **back wall of thorax with penetration into thoracic cavity** MCC

✓7th **S21.422 Laceration with foreign body of** left **back wall of thorax with penetration into thoracic cavity** MCC

✓7th **S21.429 Laceration with foreign body of unspecified back wall of thorax with penetration into thoracic cavity** MCC

✓6th **S21.43** Puncture wound without foreign body **of back wall of thorax with penetration into thoracic cavity**

✓7th **S21.431 Puncture wound without foreign body of** right **back wall of thorax with penetration into thoracic cavity** MCC

✓7th **S21.432 Puncture wound without foreign body of** left **back wall of thorax with penetration into thoracic cavity** MCC

✓7th **S21.439 Puncture wound without foreign body of unspecified back wall of thorax with penetration into thoracic cavity** MCC

✓6th **S21.44** Puncture wound with foreign body **of back wall of thorax with penetration into thoracic cavity**

✓7th **S21.441 Puncture wound with foreign body of** right **back wall of thorax with penetration into thoracic cavity** MCC

✓7th **S21.442 Puncture wound with foreign body of** left **back wall of thorax with penetration into thoracic cavity** MCC

✓7th **S21.449 Puncture wound with foreign body of unspecified back wall of thorax with penetration into thoracic cavity** MCC

✓6th **S21.45** Open bite **of back wall of thorax with penetration into thoracic cavity**

Bite of back wall of thorax NOS

EXCLUDES 1   *superficial bite of back wall of thorax (S20.47)*

✓7th **S21.451 Open bite of** right **back wall of thorax with penetration into thoracic cavity** MCC

✓7th **S21.452 Open bite of** left **back wall of thorax with penetration into thoracic cavity** MCC

✓7th **S21.459 Open bite of unspecified back wall of thorax with penetration into thoracic cavity** MCC

✓5th **S21.9 Open wound of unspecified part of thorax**

Open wound of thoracic wall NOS

✓x7th **S21.90 Unspecified open wound of unspecified part of thorax** CC

✓x7th **S21.91 Laceration without foreign body of unspecified part of thorax** CC

✓x7th **S21.92 Laceration with foreign body of unspecified part of thorax** CC

✓x7th **S21.93 Puncture wound without foreign body of unspecified part of thorax** CC

✓x7th **S21.94 Puncture wound with foreign body of unspecified part of thorax** CC

✓x7th **S21.95 Open bite of unspecified part of thorax** CC

EXCLUDES 1   *superficial bite of thorax (S20.97)*

√4ᵗʰ **S22 Fracture of rib(s), sternum and thoracic spine**

> **NOTE**   A fracture not indicated as displaced or nondisplaced should be coded to displaced
>
>   A fracture not indicated as open or closed should be coded to closed

INCLUDES   fracture of thoracic neural arch
fracture of thoracic spinous process
fracture of thoracic transverse process
fracture of thoracic vertebra
fracture of thoracic vertebral arch

Code first any associated:
   injury of intrathoracic organ (S27.-)
   spinal cord injury (S24.0-, S24.1-)

EXCLUDES 1   *transection of thorax (S28.1)*

EXCLUDES 2   *fracture of clavicle (S42.0-)*
         fracture of scapula (S42.1-)

AHA: 2021,1Q,6; 2018,2Q,12; 2015,3Q,37-39

> The appropriate 7th character is to be added to each code from category S22.
> A   initial encounter for closed fracture
> B   initial encounter for open fracture
> D   subsequent encounter for fracture with routine healing
> G   subsequent encounter for fracture with delayed healing
> K   subsequent encounter for fracture with nonunion
> S   sequela

√5ᵗʰ **S22.0 Fracture of thoracic vertebra**

   √6ᵗʰ **S22.00 Fracture of unspecified thoracic vertebra**

     2,3,6 √7ᵗʰ **S22.000 Wedge compression fracture of unspecified thoracic vertebra** MCC CC H5 HCC

     2,3,6 √7ᵗʰ **S22.001 Stable burst fracture of unspecified thoracic vertebra** MCC CC H5 HCC

     2,3,6 √7ᵗʰ **S22.002 Unstable burst fracture of unspecified thoracic vertebra** MCC CC H5 HCC

     2,3,6 √7ᵗʰ **S22.008 Other fracture of unspecified thoracic vertebra** MCC CC H5 HCC

     2,3,6 √7ᵗʰ **S22.009 Unspecified fracture of unspecified thoracic vertebra** MCC CC H5 HCC

   √6ᵗʰ **S22.01 Fracture of first thoracic vertebra**

     2,3,6 √7ᵗʰ **S22.010 Wedge compression fracture of first thoracic vertebra** MCC CC H5 HCC

     2,3,6 √7ᵗʰ **S22.011 Stable burst fracture of first thoracic vertebra** MCC CC H5 HCC

     2,3,6 √7ᵗʰ **S22.012 Unstable burst fracture of first thoracic vertebra** MCC CC H5 HCC

     2,3,6 √7ᵗʰ **S22.018 Other fracture of first thoracic vertebra** MCC CC H5 HCC

     2,3,6 √7ᵗʰ **S22.019 Unspecified fracture of first thoracic vertebra** MCC CC H5 HCC

   √6ᵗʰ **S22.02 Fracture of second thoracic vertebra**

     2,3,6 √7ᵗʰ **S22.020 Wedge compression fracture of second thoracic vertebra** MCC CC H5 HCC

     2,3,6 √7ᵗʰ **S22.021 Stable burst fracture of second thoracic vertebra** MCC CC H5 HCC

     2,3,6 √7ᵗʰ **S22.022 Unstable burst fracture of second thoracic vertebra** MCC CC H5 HCC

     2,3,6 √7ᵗʰ **S22.028 Other fracture of second thoracic vertebra** MCC CC H5 HCC

     2,3,6 √7ᵗʰ **S22.029 Unspecified fracture of second thoracic vertebra** MCC CC H5 HCC

   √6ᵗʰ **S22.03 Fracture of third thoracic vertebra**

     2,3,6 √7ᵗʰ **S22.030 Wedge compression fracture of third thoracic vertebra** MCC CC H5 HCC

     2,3,6 √7ᵗʰ **S22.031 Stable burst fracture of third thoracic vertebra** MCC CC H5 HCC

     2,3,6 √7ᵗʰ **S22.032 Unstable burst fracture of third thoracic vertebra** MCC CC H5 HCC

     2,3,6 √7ᵗʰ **S22.038 Other fracture of third thoracic vertebra** MCC CC H5 HCC

     2,3,6 √7ᵗʰ **S22.039 Unspecified fracture of third thoracic vertebra** MCC CC H5 HCC

   √6ᵗʰ **S22.04 Fracture of fourth thoracic vertebra**

     2,3,6 √7ᵗʰ **S22.040 Wedge compression fracture of fourth thoracic vertebra** MCC CC H5 HCC

     2,3,6 √7ᵗʰ **S22.041 Stable burst fracture of fourth thoracic vertebra** MCC CC H5 HCC

     2,3,6 √7ᵗʰ **S22.042 Unstable burst fracture of fourth thoracic vertebra** MCC CC H5 HCC

     2,3,6 √7ᵗʰ **S22.048 Other fracture of fourth thoracic vertebra** MCC CC H5 HCC

     2,3,6 √7ᵗʰ **S22.049 Unspecified fracture of fourth thoracic vertebra** MCC CC H5 HCC

   √6ᵗʰ **S22.05 Fracture of T5-T6 vertebra**

     2,3,6 √7ᵗʰ **S22.050 Wedge compression fracture of T5-T6 vertebra** MCC CC H5 HCC

     2,3,6 √7ᵗʰ **S22.051 Stable burst fracture of T5-T6 vertebra** MCC CC H5 HCC

     2,3,6 √7ᵗʰ **S22.052 Unstable burst fracture of T5-T6 vertebra** MCC CC H5 HCC

     2,3,6 √7ᵗʰ **S22.058 Other fracture of T5-T6 vertebra** MCC CC H5 HCC

     2,3,6 √7ᵗʰ **S22.059 Unspecified fracture of T5-T6 vertebra** MCC CC H5 HCC

   √6ᵗʰ **S22.06 Fracture of T7-T8 vertebra**

     2,3,6 √7ᵗʰ **S22.060 Wedge compression fracture of T7-T8 vertebra** MCC CC H5 HCC

     2,3,6 √7ᵗʰ **S22.061 Stable burst fracture of T7-T8 vertebra** MCC CC H5 HCC

     2,3,6 √7ᵗʰ **S22.062 Unstable burst fracture of T7-T8 vertebra** MCC CC H5 HCC

     2,3,6 √7ᵗʰ **S22.068 Other fracture of T7-T8 thoracic vertebra** MCC CC H5 HCC

     2,3,6 √7ᵗʰ **S22.069 Unspecified fracture of T7-T8 vertebra** MCC CC H5 HCC

   √6ᵗʰ **S22.07 Fracture of T9-T10 vertebra**

     2,3,6 √7ᵗʰ **S22.070 Wedge compression fracture of T9-T10 vertebra** MCC CC H5 HCC

     2,3,6 √7ᵗʰ **S22.071 Stable burst fracture of T9-T10 vertebra** MCC CC H5 HCC

     2,3,6 √7ᵗʰ **S22.072 Unstable burst fracture of T9-T10 vertebra** MCC CC H5 HCC

     2,3,6 √7ᵗʰ **S22.078 Other fracture of T9-T10 vertebra** MCC CC H5 HCC

     2,3,6 √7ᵗʰ **S22.079 Unspecified fracture of T9-T10 vertebra** MCC CC H5 HCC

   √6ᵗʰ **S22.08 Fracture of T11-T12 vertebra**

     2,3,6 √7ᵗʰ **S22.080 Wedge compression fracture of T11-T12 vertebra** MCC CC H5 HCC

     2,3,6 √7ᵗʰ **S22.081 Stable burst fracture of T11-T12 vertebra** MCC CC H5 HCC

     2,3,6 √7ᵗʰ **S22.082 Unstable burst fracture of T11-T12 vertebra** MCC CC H5 HCC

     2,3,6 √7ᵗʰ **S22.088 Other fracture of T11-T12 vertebra** MCC CC H5 HCC

     2,3,6 √7ᵗʰ **S22.089 Unspecified fracture of T11-T12 vertebra** MCC CC H5 HCC

√5ᵗʰ **S22.2 Fracture of sternum**

> **DEF:** Break in flat bone (breast bone) in the anterior thorax caused by blunt trauma to the anterior chest.

   2,3 √x7ᵗʰ **S22.20 Unspecified fracture of sternum** MCC CC H5

   2,3 √x7ᵗʰ **S22.21 Fracture of manubrium** MCC CC H5

   2,3 √x7ᵗʰ **S22.22 Fracture of body of sternum** MCC CC H5

   2,3 √x7ᵗʰ **S22.23 Sternal manubrial dissociation** MCC CC H5

   2,3 √x7ᵗʰ **S22.24 Fracture of xiphoid process** MCC CC H5

√5ᵗʰ **S22.3 Fracture of one rib**

   AHA: 2021,1Q,5

   2,3 √x7ᵗʰ **S22.31 Fracture of one rib, right side** MCC CC H5

   2,3 √x7ᵗʰ **S22.32 Fracture of one rib, left side** MCC CC H5

   2,3 √x7ᵗʰ **S22.39 Fracture of one rib, unspecified side** MCC CC H5

√5ᵗʰ **S22.4 Multiple fractures of ribs**

   Fractures of two or more ribs

   EXCLUDES 1   *flail chest (S22.5-)*

   AHA: 2021,1Q,5

   2,3 √x7ᵗʰ **S22.41 Multiple fractures of ribs, right side** MCC CC H5

   2,3 √x7ᵗʰ **S22.42 Multiple fractures of ribs, left side** MCC CC H5

   2,3 √x7ᵗʰ **S22.43 Multiple fractures of ribs, bilateral** MCC CC H5

   2,3 √x7ᵗʰ **S22.49 Multiple fractures of ribs, unspecified side** MCC CC H5

4 √x7ᵗʰ **S22.5 Flail chest** MCC CC H5

2,3 √x7ᵗʰ **S22.9 Fracture of bony thorax, part unspecified** MCC CC H5

N Newborn: 0   P Pediatric: 0-17   M Maternity: 9-64   A Adult: 15-124   MCC Major Complication/Comorbidity   CC Complication/Comorbidity   SW Severe Wound Dx

990   ICD-10-CM 2022

☑4ᵗʰ **S23 Dislocation and sprain of joints and ligaments of thorax**

INCLUDES   avulsion of joint or ligament of thorax
laceration of cartilage, joint or ligament of thorax
sprain of cartilage, joint or ligament of thorax
traumatic hemarthrosis of joint or ligament of thorax
traumatic rupture of joint or ligament of thorax
traumatic subluxation of joint or ligament of thorax
traumatic tear of joint or ligament of thorax

Code also any associated open wound

EXCLUDES 2   dislocation, sprain of sternoclavicular joint (S43.2, S43.6)
strain of muscle or tendon of thorax (S29.01-)

The appropriate 7th character is to be added to each code from category S23.
A   initial encounter
D   subsequent encounter
S   sequela

☑x7ᵗʰ **S23.0 Traumatic rupture of thoracic intervertebral disc**

EXCLUDES 1   rupture or displacement (nontraumatic) of thoracic intervertebral disc NOS (M51.- with fifth character 4)

☑5ᵗʰ **S23.1 Subluxation and dislocation of thoracic vertebra**

▶Code also any associated:◀
open wound of thorax (S21.-)
spinal cord injury (S24.0-, S24.1-)

EXCLUDES 2   fracture of thoracic vertebrae (S22.0-)

☑6ᵗʰ **S23.10 Subluxation and dislocation of unspecified thoracic vertebra**

☑7ᵗʰ **S23.100 Subluxation** of unspecified thoracic vertebra

☑7ᵗʰ **S23.101 Dislocation** of unspecified thoracic vertebra

☑6ᵗʰ **S23.11 Subluxation and dislocation of** T1/T2 **thoracic vertebra**

☑7ᵗʰ **S23.110 Subluxation** of T1/T2 thoracic vertebra

☑7ᵗʰ **S23.111 Dislocation** of T1/T2 thoracic vertebra

☑6ᵗʰ **S23.12 Subluxation and dislocation of** T2/T3-T3/T4 **thoracic vertebra**

☑7ᵗʰ **S23.120 Subluxation** of T2/T3 thoracic vertebra

☑7ᵗʰ **S23.121 Dislocation** of T2/T3 thoracic vertebra

☑7ᵗʰ **S23.122 Subluxation** of T3/T4 thoracic vertebra

☑7ᵗʰ **S23.123 Dislocation** of T3/T4 thoracic vertebra

☑6ᵗʰ **S23.13 Subluxation and dislocation of** T4/T5-T5/T6 **thoracic vertebra**

☑7ᵗʰ **S23.130 Subluxation** of T4/T5 thoracic vertebra

☑7ᵗʰ **S23.131 Dislocation** of T4/T5 thoracic vertebra

☑7ᵗʰ **S23.132 Subluxation** of T5/T6 thoracic vertebra

☑7ᵗʰ **S23.133 Dislocation** of T5/T6 thoracic vertebra

☑6ᵗʰ **S23.14 Subluxation and dislocation of** T6/T7-T7/T8 **thoracic vertebra**

☑7ᵗʰ **S23.140 Subluxation** of T6/T7 thoracic vertebra

☑7ᵗʰ **S23.141 Dislocation** of T6/T7 thoracic vertebra

☑7ᵗʰ **S23.142 Subluxation** of T7/T8 thoracic vertebra

☑7ᵗʰ **S23.143 Dislocation** of T7/T8 thoracic vertebra

☑6ᵗʰ **S23.15 Subluxation and dislocation of** T8/T9-T9/T10 **thoracic vertebra**

☑7ᵗʰ **S23.150 Subluxation** of T8/T9 thoracic vertebra

☑7ᵗʰ **S23.151 Dislocation** of T8/T9 thoracic vertebra

☑7ᵗʰ **S23.152 Subluxation** of T9/T10 thoracic vertebra

☑7ᵗʰ **S23.153 Dislocation** of T9/T10 thoracic vertebra

☑6ᵗʰ **S23.16 Subluxation and dislocation of** T10/T11-T11/T12 **thoracic vertebra**

☑7ᵗʰ **S23.160 Subluxation** of T10/T11 thoracic vertebra

☑7ᵗʰ **S23.161 Dislocation** of T10/T11 thoracic vertebra

☑7ᵗʰ **S23.162 Subluxation** of T11/T12 thoracic vertebra

☑7ᵗʰ **S23.163 Dislocation** of T11/T12 thoracic vertebra

☑6ᵗʰ **S23.17 Subluxation and dislocation of** T12/L1 **thoracic vertebra**

☑7ᵗʰ **S23.170 Subluxation** of T12/L1 thoracic vertebra

☑7ᵗʰ **S23.171 Dislocation** of T12/L1 thoracic vertebra

☑5ᵗʰ **S23.2 Dislocation of other and unspecified parts of thorax**

☑x7ᵗʰ **S23.20 Dislocation of unspecified part of thorax**

☑x7ᵗʰ **S23.29 Dislocation of other parts of thorax**

☑x7ᵗʰ **S23.3 Sprain of ligaments of thoracic spine**

☑5ᵗʰ **S23.4 Sprain of ribs and sternum**

☑x7ᵗʰ **S23.41 Sprain of ribs**

☑6ᵗʰ **S23.42 Sprain of sternum**

☑7ᵗʰ **S23.420 Sprain of sternoclavicular (joint) (ligament)**

☑7ᵗʰ **S23.421 Sprain of chondrosternal joint**

☑7ᵗʰ **S23.428 Other sprain of sternum**

☑7ᵗʰ **S23.429 Unspecified sprain of sternum**

☑x7ᵗʰ **S23.8 Sprain of other specified parts of thorax**

☑x7ᵗʰ **S23.9 Sprain of unspecified parts of thorax**

☑4ᵗʰ **S24 Injury of nerves and spinal cord at thorax level**

NOTE   Code to highest level of thoracic spinal cord injury.
Injuries to the spinal cord (S24.0 and S24.1) refer to the cord level and not bone level injury, and can affect nerve roots at and below the level given.

Code also any associated:
fracture of thoracic vertebra (S22.0-)
open wound of thorax (S21.-)
transient paralysis (R29.5)

EXCLUDES 2   injury of brachial plexus (S14.3)

The appropriate 7th character is to be added to each code from category S24.
A   initial encounter
D   subsequent encounter
S   sequela

☑x7ᵗʰ **S24.0 Concussion and edema of thoracic spinal cord**   MCC HCC

☑5ᵗʰ **S24.1 Other and unspecified injuries of thoracic spinal cord**

☑6ᵗʰ **S24.10 Unspecified injury of thoracic spinal cord**

☑7ᵗʰ **S24.101 Unspecified injury at** T1 **level of thoracic spinal cord**   MCC H5 HCC

☑7ᵗʰ **S24.102 Unspecified injury at** T2-T6 **level of thoracic spinal cord**   MCC H5 HCC

☑7ᵗʰ **S24.103 Unspecified injury at** T7-T10 **level of thoracic spinal cord**   MCC H5 HCC

☑7ᵗʰ **S24.104 Unspecified injury at** T11-T12 **level of thoracic spinal cord**   MCC H5 HCC

☑7ᵗʰ **S24.109 Unspecified injury at unspecified level of thoracic spinal cord**   HCC
Injury of thoracic spinal cord NOS

☑6ᵗʰ **S24.11 Complete lesion of thoracic spinal cord**

☑7ᵗʰ **S24.111 Complete lesion at** T1 **level of thoracic spinal cord**   MCC H5 HCC

☑7ᵗʰ **S24.112 Complete lesion at** T2-T6 **level of thoracic spinal cord**   MCC H5 HCC

☑7ᵗʰ **S24.113 Complete lesion at** T7-T10 **level of thoracic spinal cord**   MCC H5 HCC

☑7ᵗʰ **S24.114 Complete lesion at** T11-T12 **level of thoracic spinal cord**   MCC H5 HCC

☑7ᵗʰ **S24.119 Complete lesion at unspecified level of thoracic spinal cord**   HCC

☑6ᵗʰ **S24.13 Anterior cord syndrome of thoracic spinal cord**

☑7ᵗʰ **S24.131 Anterior cord syndrome at** T1 **level of thoracic spinal cord**   MCC H5 HCC

☑7ᵗʰ **S24.132 Anterior cord syndrome at** T2-T6 **level of thoracic spinal cord**   MCC H5 HCC

☑7ᵗʰ **S24.133 Anterior cord syndrome at** T7-T10 **level of thoracic spinal cord**   MCC H5 HCC

☑7ᵗʰ **S24.134 Anterior cord syndrome at** T11-T12 **level of thoracic spinal cord**   MCC H5 HCC

☑7ᵗʰ **S24.139 Anterior cord syndrome at unspecified level of thoracic spinal cord**   HCC

☑6ᵗʰ **S24.14 Brown-Séquard syndrome of thoracic spinal cord**

☑7ᵗʰ **S24.141 Brown-Séquard syndrome at** T1 **level of thoracic spinal cord**   MCC HCC

☑7ᵗʰ **S24.142 Brown-Séquard syndrome at** T2-T6 **level of thoracic spinal cord**   MCC HCC

☑7ᵗʰ **S24.143 Brown-Séquard syndrome at** T7-T10 **level of thoracic spinal cord**   MCC HCC

☑7ᵗʰ **S24.144 Brown-Séquard syndrome at** T11-T12 **level of thoracic spinal cord**   MCC HCC

☑7ᵗʰ **S24.149 Brown-Séquard syndrome at unspecified level of thoracic spinal cord**   HCC

√6ᵗʰ **S24.15** Other incomplete lesions of thoracic spinal cord
- Incomplete lesion of thoracic spinal cord NOS
- Posterior cord syndrome of thoracic spinal cord

√7ᵗʰ **S24.151** Other incomplete lesion at **T1 level of thoracic spinal cord** `MCC` `H5` `HCC`

√7ᵗʰ **S24.152** Other incomplete lesion at **T2-T6 level of thoracic spinal cord** `MCC` `H5` `HCC`

√7ᵗʰ **S24.153** Other incomplete lesion at **T7-T10 level of thoracic spinal cord** `MCC` `H5` `HCC`

√7ᵗʰ **S24.154** Other incomplete lesion at **T11-T12 level of thoracic spinal cord** `MCC` `H5` `HCC`

√7ᵗʰ **S24.159** Other incomplete lesion at **unspecified level of thoracic spinal cord** `HCC`

√x7ᵗʰ **S24.2** Injury of nerve root of thoracic spine

√x7ᵗʰ **S24.3** Injury of peripheral nerves of thorax

√x7ᵗʰ **S24.4** Injury of thoracic sympathetic nervous system
- Injury of cardiac plexus
- Injury of esophageal plexus
- Injury of pulmonary plexus
- Injury of stellate ganglion
- Injury of thoracic sympathetic ganglion

√x7ᵗʰ **S24.8** Injury of other specified nerves of thorax

√x7ᵗʰ **S24.9** Injury of unspecified nerve of thorax

√4ᵗʰ **S25** Injury of blood vessels of thorax

Code also any associated open wound (S21.-)

The appropriate 7th character is to be added to each code from category S25.
- A initial encounter
- D subsequent encounter
- S sequela

√5ᵗʰ **S25.0** Injury of **thoracic aorta**

Injury of aorta NOS

√x7ᵗʰ **S25.00** Unspecified injury of thoracic aorta `MCC`

√x7ᵗʰ **S25.01** Minor laceration of thoracic aorta `MCC`
- Incomplete transection of thoracic aorta
- Laceration of thoracic aorta NOS
- Superficial laceration of thoracic aorta

√x7ᵗʰ **S25.02** Major laceration of thoracic aorta `MCC`
- Complete transection of thoracic aorta
- Traumatic rupture of thoracic aorta

√x7ᵗʰ **S25.09** Other specified injury of thoracic aorta `MCC`

√5ᵗʰ **S25.1** Injury of **innominate or subclavian artery**

√6ᵗʰ **S25.10** Unspecified injury of innominate or subclavian artery

√7ᵗʰ **S25.101** Unspecified injury of **right innominate or subclavian artery** `MCC`

√7ᵗʰ **S25.102** Unspecified injury of **left innominate or subclavian artery** `MCC`

√7ᵗʰ **S25.109** Unspecified injury of **unspecified innominate or subclavian artery** `MCC`

√6ᵗʰ **S25.11** Minor laceration of innominate or subclavian artery
- Incomplete transection of innominate or subclavian artery
- Laceration of innominate or subclavian artery NOS
- Superficial laceration of innominate or subclavian artery

√7ᵗʰ **S25.111** Minor laceration of **right innominate or subclavian artery** `MCC`

√7ᵗʰ **S25.112** Minor laceration of **left innominate or subclavian artery** `MCC`

√7ᵗʰ **S25.119** Minor laceration of **unspecified innominate or subclavian artery** `MCC`

√6ᵗʰ **S25.12** Major laceration of innominate or subclavian artery
- Complete transection of innominate or subclavian artery
- Traumatic rupture of innominate or subclavian artery

√7ᵗʰ **S25.121** Major laceration of **right innominate or subclavian artery** `MCC`

√7ᵗʰ **S25.122** Major laceration of **left innominate or subclavian artery** `MCC`

√7ᵗʰ **S25.129** Major laceration of **unspecified innominate or subclavian artery** `MCC`

√6ᵗʰ **S25.19** Other specified injury of innominate or subclavian artery

√7ᵗʰ **S25.191** Other specified injury of **right innominate or subclavian artery** `MCC`

√7ᵗʰ **S25.192** Other specified injury of **left innominate or subclavian artery** `MCC`

√7ᵗʰ **S25.199** Other specified injury of **unspecified innominate or subclavian artery** `MCC`

√5ᵗʰ **S25.2** Injury of **superior vena cava**

Injury of vena cava NOS

√x7ᵗʰ **S25.20** Unspecified injury of superior vena cava `MCC`

√x7ᵗʰ **S25.21** Minor laceration of superior vena cava `MCC`
- Incomplete transection of superior vena cava
- Laceration of superior vena cava NOS
- Superficial laceration of superior vena cava

√x7ᵗʰ **S25.22** Major laceration of superior vena cava `MCC`
- Complete transection of superior vena cava
- Traumatic rupture of superior vena cava

√x7ᵗʰ **S25.29** Other specified injury of superior vena cava `MCC`

√5ᵗʰ **S25.3** Injury of **innominate or subclavian vein**

√6ᵗʰ **S25.30** Unspecified injury of innominate or subclavian vein

√7ᵗʰ **S25.301** Unspecified injury of **right innominate or subclavian vein**

√7ᵗʰ **S25.302** Unspecified injury of **left innominate or subclavian vein** `MCC`

√7ᵗʰ **S25.309** Unspecified injury of **unspecified innominate or subclavian vein** `MCC`

√6ᵗʰ **S25.31** Minor laceration of innominate or subclavian vein
- Incomplete transection of innominate or subclavian vein
- Laceration of innominate or subclavian vein NOS
- Superficial laceration of innominate or subclavian vein

√7ᵗʰ **S25.311** Minor laceration of **right innominate or subclavian vein** `MCC`

√7ᵗʰ **S25.312** Minor laceration of **left innominate or subclavian vein** `MCC`

√7ᵗʰ **S25.319** Minor laceration of **unspecified innominate or subclavian vein** `MCC`

√6ᵗʰ **S25.32** Major laceration of innominate or subclavian vein
- Complete transection of innominate or subclavian vein
- Traumatic rupture of innominate or subclavian vein

√7ᵗʰ **S25.321** Major laceration of **right innominate or subclavian vein** `MCC`

√7ᵗʰ **S25.322** Major laceration of **left innominate or subclavian vein** `MCC`

√7ᵗʰ **S25.329** Major laceration of **unspecified innominate or subclavian vein** `MCC`

√6ᵗʰ **S25.39** Other specified injury of innominate or subclavian vein

√7ᵗʰ **S25.391** Other specified injury of **right innominate or subclavian vein** `MCC`

√7ᵗʰ **S25.392** Other specified injury of **left innominate or subclavian vein** `MCC`

√7ᵗʰ **S25.399** Other specified injury of **unspecified innominate or subclavian vein** `MCC`

√5ᵗʰ **S25.4** Injury of **pulmonary blood vessels**

√6ᵗʰ **S25.40** Unspecified injury of pulmonary blood vessels

√7ᵗʰ **S25.401** Unspecified injury of **right pulmonary blood vessels** `MCC`

√7ᵗʰ **S25.402** Unspecified injury of **left pulmonary blood vessels** `MCC`

√7ᵗʰ **S25.409** Unspecified injury of **unspecified pulmonary blood vessels** `MCC`

√6ᵗʰ **S25.41** Minor laceration of pulmonary blood vessels
- Incomplete transection of pulmonary blood vessels
- Laceration of pulmonary blood vessels NOS
- Superficial laceration of pulmonary blood vessels

√7ᵗʰ **S25.411** Minor laceration of **right pulmonary blood vessels** `MCC`

√7ᵗʰ **S25.412** Minor laceration of **left pulmonary blood vessels** `MCC`

√7ᵗʰ **S25.419** Minor laceration of **unspecified pulmonary blood vessels** `MCC`

Ⓝ Newborn: 0   Ⓟ Pediatric: 0-17   Ⓜ Maternity: 9-64   Ⓐ Adult: 15-124   `MCC` Major Complication/Comorbidity   `CC` Complication/Comorbidity   `SW` Severe Wound Dx

992

ICD-10-CM 2022

√6ᵗʰ **S25.42** Major laceration of pulmonary blood vessels
         Complete transection of pulmonary blood vessels
         Traumatic rupture of pulmonary blood vessels

√7ᵗʰ **S25.421** Major laceration of right pulmonary blood vessels   MCC

√7ᵗʰ **S25.422** Major laceration of left pulmonary blood vessels   MCC

√7ᵗʰ **S25.429** Major laceration of unspecified pulmonary blood vessels   MCC

√6ᵗʰ **S25.49** Other specified injury of pulmonary blood vessels

√7ᵗʰ **S25.491** Other specified injury of right pulmonary blood vessels   MCC

√7ᵗʰ **S25.492** Other specified injury of left pulmonary blood vessels   MCC

√7ᵗʰ **S25.499** Other specified injury of unspecified pulmonary blood vessels   MCC

√5ᵗʰ **S25.5** Injury of intercostal blood vessels

√6ᵗʰ **S25.50** Unspecified injury of intercostal blood vessels

√7ᵗʰ **S25.501** Unspecified injury of intercostal blood vessels, right side   CC

√7ᵗʰ **S25.502** Unspecified injury of intercostal blood vessels, left side   CC

√7ᵗʰ **S25.509** Unspecified injury of intercostal blood vessels, unspecified side   CC

√6ᵗʰ **S25.51** Laceration of intercostal blood vessels

√7ᵗʰ **S25.511** Laceration of intercostal blood vessels, right side   CC

√7ᵗʰ **S25.512** Laceration of intercostal blood vessels, left side   CC

√7ᵗʰ **S25.519** Laceration of intercostal blood vessels, unspecified side   CC

√6ᵗʰ **S25.59** Other specified injury of intercostal blood vessels

√7ᵗʰ **S25.591** Other specified injury of intercostal blood vessels, right side   CC

√7ᵗʰ **S25.592** Other specified injury of intercostal blood vessels, left side   CC

√7ᵗʰ **S25.599** Other specified injury of intercostal blood vessels, unspecified side   CC

√5ᵗʰ **S25.8** Injury of other blood vessels of thorax
         Injury of azygos vein
         Injury of mammary artery or vein

√6ᵗʰ **S25.80** Unspecified injury of other blood vessels of thorax

√7ᵗʰ **S25.801** Unspecified injury of other blood vessels of thorax, right side   CC

√7ᵗʰ **S25.802** Unspecified injury of other blood vessels of thorax, left side   CC

√7ᵗʰ **S25.809** Unspecified injury of other blood vessels of thorax, unspecified side   CC

√6ᵗʰ **S25.81** Laceration of other blood vessels of thorax

√7ᵗʰ **S25.811** Laceration of other blood vessels of thorax, right side   CC

√7ᵗʰ **S25.812** Laceration of other blood vessels of thorax, left side   CC

√7ᵗʰ **S25.819** Laceration of other blood vessels of thorax, unspecified side   CC

√6ᵗʰ **S25.89** Other specified injury of other blood vessels of thorax

√7ᵗʰ **S25.891** Other specified injury of other blood vessels of thorax, right side   CC

√7ᵗʰ **S25.892** Other specified injury of other blood vessels of thorax, left side   CC

√7ᵗʰ **S25.899** Other specified injury of other blood vessels of thorax, unspecified side   CC

√5ᵗʰ **S25.9** Injury of unspecified blood vessel of thorax

√x7ᵗʰ **S25.90** Unspecified injury of unspecified blood vessel of thorax   CC

√x7ᵗʰ **S25.91** Laceration of unspecified blood vessel of thorax   CC

√x7ᵗʰ **S25.99** Other specified injury of unspecified blood vessel of thorax   CC

√4ᵗʰ **S26** Injury of heart
     Code also any associated:
         open wound of thorax (S21.-)
         traumatic hemopneumothorax (S27.2)
         traumatic hemothorax (S27.1)
         traumatic pneumothorax (S27.0)

> The appropriate 7th character is to be added to each code from category S26.
> A   initial encounter
> D   subsequent encounter
> S   sequela

√5ᵗʰ **S26.0** Injury of heart with hemopericardium

√x7ᵗʰ **S26.00** Unspecified injury of heart with hemopericardium   CC

√x7ᵗʰ **S26.01** Contusion of heart with hemopericardium   CC

√6ᵗʰ **S26.02** Laceration of heart with hemopericardium

√7ᵗʰ **S26.020** Mild laceration of heart with hemopericardium   MCC
         Laceration of heart without penetration of heart chamber

√7ᵗʰ **S26.021** Moderate laceration of heart with hemopericardium   MCC
         Laceration of heart with penetration of heart chamber

√7ᵗʰ **S26.022** Major laceration of heart with hemopericardium   MCC
         Laceration of heart with penetration of multiple heart chambers

√x7ᵗʰ **S26.09** Other injury of heart with hemopericardium   CC

√5ᵗʰ **S26.1** Injury of heart without hemopericardium

√x7ᵗʰ **S26.10** Unspecified injury of heart without hemopericardium   CC

√x7ᵗʰ **S26.11** Contusion of heart without hemopericardium   CC

√x7ᵗʰ **S26.12** Laceration of heart without hemopericardium   MCC

√x7ᵗʰ **S26.19** Other injury of heart without hemopericardium   CC

√5ᵗʰ **S26.9** Injury of heart, unspecified with or without hemopericardium

√x7ᵗʰ **S26.90** Unspecified injury of heart, unspecified with or without hemopericardium   CC

√x7ᵗʰ **S26.91** Contusion of heart, unspecified with or without hemopericardium   CC
         DEF: Bruising within the heart muscle, with no mention of an open wound, usually caused by blunt chest trauma in motor vehicle accidents, falling from great heights, or receiving CPR.

√x7ᵗʰ **S26.92** Laceration of heart, unspecified with or without hemopericardium   MCC
         Laceration of heart NOS
         AHA: 2019,2Q,24

√x7ᵗʰ **S26.99** Other injury of heart, unspecified with or without hemopericardium   CC

√4ᵗʰ **S27** Injury of other and unspecified intrathoracic organs
     Code also any associated open wound of thorax (S21.-)
     EXCLUDES 2   injury of cervical esophagus (S10-S19)
                    injury of trachea (cervical) (S10-S19)

> The appropriate 7th character is to be added to each code from category S27.
> A   initial encounter
> D   subsequent encounter
> S   sequela

√x7ᵗʰ **S27.0** Traumatic pneumothorax   CC
     EXCLUDES 1   spontaneous pneumothorax (J93.-)

√x7ᵗʰ **S27.1** Traumatic hemothorax   MCC

√x7ᵗʰ **S27.2** Traumatic hemopneumothorax   MCC

√5ᵗʰ **S27.3** Other and unspecified injuries of lung

√6ᵗʰ **S27.30** Unspecified injury of lung

√7ᵗʰ **S27.301** Unspecified injury of lung, unilateral   CC

√7ᵗʰ **S27.302** Unspecified injury of lung, bilateral   CC

√7ᵗʰ **S27.309** Unspecified injury of lung, unspecified   CC

✔ Additional Character Required   √x7ᵗʰ Placeholder   Questionable PDx   Manifestation   Unspecified Dx   UPD Unacceptable PDx   H1-H14 HAC   HCC CMS-HCC Dx   HIV HIV Dx

ICD-10-CM 2022   993

Chapter 19. Injury, Poisoning and Certain Other Consequences of External Causes (left margin)

S27.31–S29.019 (left margin)

√6ᵗʰ **S27.31** Primary blast **injury of lung**
    Blast injury of lung NOS
    √7ᵗʰ **S27.311** **Primary blast injury of lung, unilateral**   CC
    √7ᵗʰ **S27.312** **Primary blast injury of lung, bilateral**   CC
    √7ᵗʰ **S27.319** **Primary blast injury of lung, unspecified**   CC

√6ᵗʰ **S27.32** Contusion **of lung**
    DEF: Bruising of the lung without mention of an open wound.
    √7ᵗʰ **S27.321** **Contusion of lung, unilateral**   CC
    √7ᵗʰ **S27.322** **Contusion of lung, bilateral**   CC
    √7ᵗʰ **S27.329** **Contusion of lung, unspecified**   CC

√6ᵗʰ **S27.33** Laceration **of lung**
    √7ᵗʰ **S27.331** **Laceration of lung, unilateral**   MCC
    √7ᵗʰ **S27.332** **Laceration of lung, bilateral**   MCC
    √7ᵗʰ **S27.339** **Laceration of lung, unspecified**   MCC

√6ᵗʰ **S27.39** Other injuries **of lung**
    Secondary blast injury of lung
    √7ᵗʰ **S27.391** **Other injuries of lung, unilateral**   CC
    √7ᵗʰ **S27.392** **Other injuries of lung, bilateral**   CC
    √7ᵗʰ **S27.399** **Other injuries of lung, unspecified**   CC

√5ᵗʰ **S27.4** Injury of **bronchus**
√6ᵗʰ **S27.40** **Unspecified injury of bronchus**
    √7ᵗʰ **S27.401** **Unspecified injury of bronchus, unilateral**   MCC
    √7ᵗʰ **S27.402** **Unspecified injury of bronchus, bilateral**   MCC
    √7ᵗʰ **S27.409** **Unspecified injury of bronchus, unspecified**   MCC

√6ᵗʰ **S27.41** Primary blast **injury of bronchus**
    Blast injury of bronchus NOS
    √7ᵗʰ **S27.411** **Primary blast injury of bronchus, unilateral**   MCC
    √7ᵗʰ **S27.412** **Primary blast injury of bronchus, bilateral**   MCC
    √7ᵗʰ **S27.419** **Primary blast injury of bronchus, unspecified**   MCC

√6ᵗʰ **S27.42** Contusion **of bronchus**
    √7ᵗʰ **S27.421** **Contusion of bronchus, unilateral**   MCC
    √7ᵗʰ **S27.422** **Contusion of bronchus, bilateral**   MCC
    √7ᵗʰ **S27.429** **Contusion of bronchus, unspecified**   MCC

√6ᵗʰ **S27.43** Laceration **of bronchus**
    √7ᵗʰ **S27.431** **Laceration of bronchus, unilateral**   MCC
    √7ᵗʰ **S27.432** **Laceration of bronchus, bilateral**   MCC
    √7ᵗʰ **S27.439** **Laceration of bronchus, unspecified**   MCC

√6ᵗʰ **S27.49** Other injury **of bronchus**
    Secondary blast injury of bronchus
    √7ᵗʰ **S27.491** **Other injury of bronchus, unilateral**   MCC
    √7ᵗʰ **S27.492** **Other injury of bronchus, bilateral**   MCC
    √7ᵗʰ **S27.499** **Other injury of bronchus, unspecified**   MCC

√5ᵗʰ **S27.5** Injury of **thoracic trachea**
√x7ᵗʰ **S27.50** **Unspecified injury of thoracic trachea**   CC
√x7ᵗʰ **S27.51** Primary blast **injury of thoracic trachea**   CC
    Blast injury of thoracic trachea NOS
√x7ᵗʰ **S27.52** Contusion **of thoracic trachea**   CC
√x7ᵗʰ **S27.53** Laceration **of thoracic trachea**   CC
√x7ᵗʰ **S27.59** Other injury **of thoracic trachea**   CC
    Secondary blast injury of thoracic trachea

√5ᵗʰ **S27.6** Injury of **pleura**
√x7ᵗʰ **S27.60** **Unspecified injury of pleura**   CC
√x7ᵗʰ **S27.63** Laceration **of pleura**   CC
√x7ᵗʰ **S27.69** Other injury **of pleura**   CC

√5ᵗʰ **S27.8** Injury of other specified intrathoracic organs
√6ᵗʰ **S27.80** **Injury of diaphragm**
    √7ᵗʰ **S27.802** **Contusion of diaphragm**   CC

√7ᵗʰ **S27.803** Laceration **of diaphragm**   CC
√7ᵗʰ **S27.808** Other injury **of diaphragm**   CC
√7ᵗʰ **S27.809** Unspecified injury of diaphragm   CC

√6ᵗʰ **S27.81** Injury of **esophagus (thoracic part)**
    √7ᵗʰ **S27.812** **Contusion of esophagus (thoracic part)**   MCC
    √7ᵗʰ **S27.813** **Laceration of esophagus (thoracic part)**   MCC
    √7ᵗʰ **S27.818** **Other injury of esophagus (thoracic part)**   MCC
    √7ᵗʰ **S27.819** **Unspecified injury of esophagus (thoracic part)**   MCC

√6ᵗʰ **S27.89** Injury of other specified intrathoracic organs
    Injury of lymphatic thoracic duct
    Injury of thymus gland
    √7ᵗʰ **S27.892** **Contusion of other specified intrathoracic organs**   CC
    √7ᵗʰ **S27.893** **Laceration of other specified intrathoracic organs**   CC
    √7ᵗʰ **S27.898** **Other injury of other specified intrathoracic organs**   CC
    √7ᵗʰ **S27.899** **Unspecified injury of other specified intrathoracic organs**   CC

√x7ᵗʰ **S27.9** **Injury of unspecified intrathoracic organ**   CC

√4ᵗʰ **S28** **Crushing injury of thorax, and traumatic amputation of part of thorax**

> The appropriate 7th character is to be added to each code from category S28.
> A   initial encounter
> D   subsequent encounter
> S   sequela

√x7ᵗʰ **S28.0** **Crushed chest**
    Use additional code for all associated injuries
    EXCLUDES 1   *flail chest (S22.5)*

√x7ᵗʰ **S28.1** **Traumatic amputation (partial) of** part of thorax, except breast   CC

√5ᵗʰ **S28.2** **Traumatic amputation of** breast
√6ᵗʰ **S28.21** Complete **traumatic amputation of breast**
    Traumatic amputation of breast NOS
    √7ᵗʰ **S28.211** **Complete traumatic amputation of** right breast
    √7ᵗʰ **S28.212** **Complete traumatic amputation of** left breast
    √7ᵗʰ **S28.219** **Complete traumatic amputation of unspecified breast**

√6ᵗʰ **S28.22** Partial **traumatic amputation of breast**
    √7ᵗʰ **S28.221** **Partial traumatic amputation of** right breast
    √7ᵗʰ **S28.222** **Partial traumatic amputation of** left breast
    √7ᵗʰ **S28.229** **Partial traumatic amputation of unspecified breast**

√4ᵗʰ **S29** **Other and unspecified injuries of thorax**
    Code also any associated open wound (S21.-)

> The appropriate 7th character is to be added to each code from category S29.
> A   initial encounter
> D   subsequent encounter
> S   sequela

√5ᵗʰ **S29.0** **Injury of muscle and tendon at thorax level**
√6ᵗʰ **S29.00** **Unspecified injury of muscle and tendon of thorax**
    √7ᵗʰ **S29.001** **Unspecified injury of muscle and tendon of** front wall of thorax
    √7ᵗʰ **S29.002** **Unspecified injury of muscle and tendon of** back wall of thorax
    √7ᵗʰ **S29.009** **Unspecified injury of muscle and tendon of unspecified wall of thorax**

√6ᵗʰ **S29.01** Strain **of muscle and tendon of thorax**
    √7ᵗʰ **S29.011** **Strain of muscle and tendon of** front wall of thorax
    √7ᵗʰ **S29.012** **Strain of muscle and tendon of** back wall of thorax
    √7ᵗʰ **S29.019** **Strain of muscle and tendon of unspecified wall of thorax**

N Newborn: 0   **P** Pediatric: 0-17   **M** Maternity: 9-64   **A** Adult: 15-124   **MCC** Major Complication/Comorbidity   **CC** Complication/Comorbidity   **SW** Severe Wound Dx

994   ICD-10-CM 2022

✓6ᵗʰ   **S29.02**   Laceration of muscle and tendon of thorax
- ✓7ᵗʰ   **S29.021**   **Laceration of muscle and tendon of front wall of thorax**   CC
- ✓7ᵗʰ   **S29.022**   **Laceration of muscle and tendon of back wall of thorax**
- ✓7ᵗʰ   **S29.029**   **Laceration of muscle and tendon of unspecified wall of thorax**   CC

✓6ᵗʰ   **S29.09**   Other injury of muscle and tendon of thorax
- ✓7ᵗʰ   **S29.091**   **Other injury of muscle and tendon of front wall of thorax**
- ✓7ᵗʰ   **S29.092**   **Other injury of muscle and tendon of back wall of thorax**
- ✓7ᵗʰ   **S29.099**   **Other injury of muscle and tendon of unspecified wall of thorax**

✓x7ᵗʰ   **S29.8**   **Other specified injuries of thorax**

✓x7ᵗʰ   **S29.9**   **Unspecified injury of thorax**

Injuries to the abdomen, lower back, lumbar spine, pelvis and external genitals (S30-S39)

INCLUDES   injuries to the abdominal wall
injuries to the anus
injuries to the buttock
injuries to the external genitalia
injuries to the flank
injuries to the groin

EXCLUDES 2   *burns and corrosions (T20-T32)*
effects of foreign body in anus and rectum (T18.5)
effects of foreign body in genitourinary tract (T19.-)
effects of foreign body in stomach, small intestine and colon (T18.2-T18.4)
frostbite (T33-T34)
insect bite or sting, venomous (T63.4)

✓4ᵗʰ   **S30**   **Superficial injury of abdomen, lower back, pelvis and external genitals**

     EXCLUDES 2   *superficial injury of hip (S70.-)*

     The appropriate 7th character is to be added to each code from category S30.
     A   initial encounter
     D   subsequent encounter
     S   sequela

✓x7ᵗʰ   **S30.0**   **Contusion of lower back and pelvis**
     Contusion of buttock

✓x7ᵗʰ   **S30.1**   **Contusion of abdominal wall**
     Contusion of flank
     Contusion of groin

✓5ᵗʰ   **S30.2**   **Contusion of external genital organs**
- ✓6ᵗʰ   **S30.20**   **Contusion of unspecified external genital organ**
  - ✓7ᵗʰ   **S30.201**   **Contusion of unspecified external genital organ, male**   ♂
  - ✓7ᵗʰ   **S30.202**   **Contusion of unspecified external genital organ, female**   ♀
- ✓x7ᵗʰ   **S30.21**   **Contusion of penis**   ♂
- ✓x7ᵗʰ   **S30.22**   **Contusion of scrotum and testes**   ♂
- ✓x7ᵗʰ   **S30.23**   **Contusion of vagina and vulva**   ♀

✓x7ᵗʰ   **S30.3**   **Contusion of anus**

✓5ᵗʰ   **S30.8**   **Other superficial injuries of abdomen, lower back, pelvis and external genitals**
- ✓6ᵗʰ   **S30.81**   Abrasion of abdomen, lower back, pelvis and external genitals
  - ✓7ᵗʰ   **S30.810**   **Abrasion of lower back and pelvis**
  - ✓7ᵗʰ   **S30.811**   **Abrasion of abdominal wall**
  - ✓7ᵗʰ   **S30.812**   **Abrasion of penis**   ♂
  - ✓7ᵗʰ   **S30.813**   **Abrasion of scrotum and testes**   ♂
  - ✓7ᵗʰ   **S30.814**   **Abrasion of vagina and vulva**   ♀
  - ✓7ᵗʰ   **S30.815**   **Abrasion of unspecified external genital organs, male**   ♂
  - ✓7ᵗʰ   **S30.816**   **Abrasion of unspecified external genital organs, female**   ♀
  - ✓7ᵗʰ   **S30.817**   **Abrasion of anus**
- ✓6ᵗʰ   **S30.82**   Blister (nonthermal) of abdomen, lower back, pelvis and external genitals
  - ✓7ᵗʰ   **S30.820**   **Blister (nonthermal) of lower back and pelvis**
  - ✓7ᵗʰ   **S30.821**   **Blister (nonthermal) of abdominal wall**
  - ✓7ᵗʰ   **S30.822**   **Blister (nonthermal) of penis**   ♂

- ✓7ᵗʰ   **S30.823**   **Blister (nonthermal) of scrotum and testes**   ♂
- ✓7ᵗʰ   **S30.824**   **Blister (nonthermal) of vagina and vulva**   ♀
- ✓7ᵗʰ   **S30.825**   **Blister (nonthermal) of unspecified external genital organs, male**   ♂
- ✓7ᵗʰ   **S30.826**   **Blister (nonthermal) of unspecified external genital organs, female**   ♀
- ✓7ᵗʰ   **S30.827**   **Blister (nonthermal) of anus**

✓6ᵗʰ   **S30.84**   External constriction of abdomen, lower back, pelvis and external genitals
- ✓7ᵗʰ   **S30.840**   **External constriction of lower back and pelvis**
- ✓7ᵗʰ   **S30.841**   **External constriction of abdominal wall**
- ✓7ᵗʰ   **S30.842**   **External constriction of penis**   ♂
  - Hair tourniquet syndrome of penis
  - Use additional cause code to identify the constricting item (W49.0-)
- ✓7ᵗʰ   **S30.843**   **External constriction of scrotum and testes**   ♂
- ✓7ᵗʰ   **S30.844**   **External constriction of vagina and vulva**   ♀
- ✓7ᵗʰ   **S30.845**   **External constriction of unspecified external genital organs, male**   ♂
- ✓7ᵗʰ   **S30.846**   **External constriction of unspecified external genital organs, female**   ♀

✓6ᵗʰ   **S30.85**   Superficial foreign body of abdomen, lower back, pelvis and external genitals
     Splinter in the abdomen, lower back, pelvis and external genitals
- ✓7ᵗʰ   **S30.850**   **Superficial foreign body of lower back and pelvis**
- ✓7ᵗʰ   **S30.851**   **Superficial foreign body of abdominal wall**
- ✓7ᵗʰ   **S30.852**   **Superficial foreign body of penis**   ♂
- ✓7ᵗʰ   **S30.853**   **Superficial foreign body of scrotum and testes**   ♂
- ✓7ᵗʰ   **S30.854**   **Superficial foreign body of vagina and vulva**   ♀
- ✓7ᵗʰ   **S30.855**   **Superficial foreign body of unspecified external genital organs, male**   ♂
- ✓7ᵗʰ   **S30.856**   **Superficial foreign body of unspecified external genital organs, female**   ♀
- ✓7ᵗʰ   **S30.857**   **Superficial foreign body of anus**

✓6ᵗʰ   **S30.86**   Insect bite (nonvenomous) of abdomen, lower back, pelvis and external genitals
- ✓7ᵗʰ   **S30.860**   **Insect bite (nonvenomous) of lower back and pelvis**
- ✓7ᵗʰ   **S30.861**   **Insect bite (nonvenomous) of abdominal wall**
- ✓7ᵗʰ   **S30.862**   **Insect bite (nonvenomous) of penis**   ♂
- ✓7ᵗʰ   **S30.863**   **Insect bite (nonvenomous) of scrotum and testes**   ♂
- ✓7ᵗʰ   **S30.864**   **Insect bite (nonvenomous) of vagina and vulva**   ♀
- ✓7ᵗʰ   **S30.865**   **Insect bite (nonvenomous) of unspecified external genital organs, male**   ♂
- ✓7ᵗʰ   **S30.866**   **Insect bite (nonvenomous) of unspecified external genital organs, female**   ♀
- ✓7ᵗʰ   **S30.867**   **Insect bite (nonvenomous) of anus**

✓6ᵗʰ   **S30.87**   Other superficial bite of abdomen, lower back, pelvis and external genitals
     EXCLUDES 1   *open bite of abdomen, lower back, pelvis and external genitals (S31.05, S31.15, S31.25, S31.35, S31.45, S31.55)*
- ✓7ᵗʰ   **S30.870**   **Other superficial bite of lower back and pelvis**
- ✓7ᵗʰ   **S30.871**   **Other superficial bite of abdominal wall**
- ✓7ᵗʰ   **S30.872**   **Other superficial bite of penis**   ♂
- ✓7ᵗʰ   **S30.873**   **Other superficial bite of scrotum and testes**   ♂
- ✓7ᵗʰ   **S30.874**   **Other superficial bite of vagina and vulva**   ♀
- ✓7ᵗʰ   **S30.875**   **Other superficial bite of unspecified external genital organs, male**   ♂
- ✓7ᵗʰ   **S30.876**   **Other superficial bite of unspecified external genital organs, female**   ♀
- ✓7ᵗʰ   **S30.877**   **Other superficial bite of anus**

✅ Additional Character Required   ✓x7ᵗʰ Placeholder   Questionable PDx   Manifestation   Unspecified Dx   **UPD** Unacceptable PDx   **H1-H14** HAC   **HCC** CMS-HCC Dx   **HIV** HIV Dx

√5ᵗʰ **S30.9 Unspecified superficial injury of abdomen, lower back, pelvis and external genitals**

√x7ᵗʰ **S30.91 Unspecified superficial injury of** lower back and pelvis

√x7ᵗʰ **S30.92 Unspecified superficial injury of** abdominal wall

√x7ᵗʰ **S30.93 Unspecified superficial injury of** penis ♂

√x7ᵗʰ **S30.94 Unspecified superficial injury of** scrotum and testes ♂

√x7ᵗʰ **S30.95 Unspecified superficial injury of** vagina and vulva ♀

√x7ᵗʰ **S30.96 Unspecified superficial injury of unspecified external genital organs, male** ♂

√x7ᵗʰ **S30.97 Unspecified superficial injury of unspecified external genital organs, female** ♀

√x7ᵗʰ **S30.98 Unspecified superficial injury of** anus

√4ᵗʰ **S31 Open wound of abdomen, lower back, pelvis and external genitals**

Code also any associated:
spinal cord injury (S24.0, S24.1-, S34.0-, S34.1-)
wound infection

EXCLUDES 1   *traumatic amputation of part of abdomen, lower back and pelvis (S38.2-, S38.3)*

EXCLUDES 2   *open wound of hip (S71.00-S71.02)*
open fracture of pelvis (S32.1- - S32.9 with 7th character B)

The appropriate 7th character is to be added to each code from category S31.
A   initial encounter
D   subsequent encounter
S   sequela

√5ᵗʰ **S31.0 Open wound of** lower back and pelvis

√6ᵗʰ **S31.00 Unspecified open wound of lower back and pelvis**

√7ᵗʰ **S31.000 Unspecified open wound of lower back and pelvis** without penetration into retroperitoneum
Unspecified open wound of lower back and pelvis NOS

√7ᵗʰ **S31.001 Unspecified open wound of lower back and pelvis** with penetration into retroperitoneum MCC

√6ᵗʰ **S31.01 Laceration without foreign body of lower back and pelvis**

√7ᵗʰ **S31.010 Laceration without foreign body of lower back and pelvis** without penetration into retroperitoneum
Laceration without foreign body of lower back and pelvis NOS

√7ᵗʰ **S31.011 Laceration without foreign body of lower back and pelvis** with penetration into retroperitoneum MCC

√6ᵗʰ **S31.02 Laceration with foreign body of lower back and pelvis**

√7ᵗʰ **S31.020 Laceration with foreign body of lower back and pelvis** without penetration into retroperitoneum
Laceration with foreign body of lower back and pelvis NOS

√7ᵗʰ **S31.021 Laceration with foreign body of lower back and pelvis** with penetration into retroperitoneum MCC

√6ᵗʰ **S31.03 Puncture wound without foreign body of lower back and pelvis**

√7ᵗʰ **S31.030 Puncture wound without foreign body of lower back and pelvis** without penetration into retroperitoneum
Puncture wound without foreign body of lower back and pelvis NOS

√7ᵗʰ **S31.031 Puncture wound without foreign body of lower back and pelvis** with penetration into retroperitoneum MCC

√6ᵗʰ **S31.04 Puncture wound with foreign body of lower back and pelvis**

√7ᵗʰ **S31.040 Puncture wound with foreign body of lower back and pelvis** without penetration into retroperitoneum
Puncture wound with foreign body of lower back and pelvis NOS

√7ᵗʰ **S31.041 Puncture wound with foreign body of lower back and pelvis** with penetration into retroperitoneum MCC

√6ᵗʰ **S31.05 Open bite of lower back and pelvis**
Bite of lower back and pelvis NOS

EXCLUDES 1   *superficial bite of lower back and pelvis (S30.860, S30.870)*

√7ᵗʰ **S31.050 Open bite of lower back and pelvis** without penetration into retroperitoneum
Open bite of lower back and pelvis NOS

√7ᵗʰ **S31.051 Open bite of lower back and pelvis** with penetration into retroperitoneum MCC

√5ᵗʰ **S31.1 Open wound of** abdominal wall without penetration into peritoneal cavity
Open wound of abdominal wall NOS

EXCLUDES 2   *open wound of abdominal wall with penetration into peritoneal cavity (S31.6-)*

√6ᵗʰ **S31.10 Unspecified open wound of abdominal wall without penetration into peritoneal cavity**

√7ᵗʰ **S31.100 Unspecified open wound of abdominal wall,** right upper quadrant without penetration into peritoneal cavity

√7ᵗʰ **S31.101 Unspecified open wound of abdominal wall,** left upper quadrant without penetration into peritoneal cavity

√7ᵗʰ **S31.102 Unspecified open wound of abdominal wall,** epigastric region without penetration into peritoneal cavity

√7ᵗʰ **S31.103 Unspecified open wound of abdominal wall,** right lower quadrant without penetration into peritoneal cavity

√7ᵗʰ **S31.104 Unspecified open wound of abdominal wall,** left lower quadrant without penetration into peritoneal cavity

√7ᵗʰ **S31.105 Unspecified open wound of abdominal wall,** periumbilic region without penetration into peritoneal cavity

√7ᵗʰ **S31.109 Unspecified open wound of abdominal wall, unspecified quadrant without penetration into peritoneal cavity**
Unspecified open wound of abdominal wall NOS

√6ᵗʰ **S31.11 Laceration without foreign body of abdominal wall without penetration into peritoneal cavity**

√7ᵗʰ **S31.110 Laceration without foreign body of abdominal wall,** right upper quadrant without penetration into peritoneal cavity

√7ᵗʰ **S31.111 Laceration without foreign body of abdominal wall,** left upper quadrant without penetration into peritoneal cavity

√7ᵗʰ **S31.112 Laceration without foreign body of abdominal wall,** epigastric region without penetration into peritoneal cavity

√7ᵗʰ **S31.113 Laceration without foreign body of abdominal wall,** right lower quadrant without penetration into peritoneal cavity

√7ᵗʰ **S31.114 Laceration without foreign body of abdominal wall,** left lower quadrant without penetration into peritoneal cavity

√7ᵗʰ **S31.115 Laceration without foreign body of abdominal wall,** periumbilic region without penetration into peritoneal cavity

√7ᵗʰ **S31.119 Laceration without foreign body of abdominal wall, unspecified quadrant without penetration into peritoneal cavity**

√6ᵗʰ **S31.12 Laceration with foreign body of abdominal wall without penetration into peritoneal cavity**

√7ᵗʰ **S31.120 Laceration of abdominal wall with foreign body,** right upper quadrant without penetration into peritoneal cavity

√7ᵗʰ **S31.121 Laceration of abdominal wall with foreign body,** left upper quadrant without penetration into peritoneal cavity

√7ᵗʰ **S31.122 Laceration of abdominal wall with foreign body,** epigastric region without penetration into peritoneal cavity

√7ᵗʰ **S31.123 Laceration of abdominal wall with foreign body,** right lower quadrant without penetration into peritoneal cavity

N Newborn: 0   P Pediatric: 0-17   M Maternity: 9-64   A Adult: 15-124   MCC Major Complication/Comorbidity   CC Complication/Comorbidity   SW Severe Wound Dx

996
ICD-10-CM 2022

√7th **S31.124** Laceration of abdominal wall with foreign body, left lower quadrant without penetration into peritoneal cavity

√7th **S31.125** Laceration of abdominal wall with foreign body, periumbilic region without penetration into peritoneal cavity

√7th **S31.129** Laceration of abdominal wall with foreign body, unspecified quadrant without penetration into peritoneal cavity

√6th **S31.13** Puncture wound of abdominal wall without foreign body without penetration into peritoneal cavity

√7th **S31.130** Puncture wound of abdominal wall without foreign body, right upper quadrant without penetration into peritoneal cavity

√7th **S31.131** Puncture wound of abdominal wall without foreign body, left upper quadrant without penetration into peritoneal cavity

√7th **S31.132** Puncture wound of abdominal wall without foreign body, epigastric region without penetration into peritoneal cavity

√7th **S31.133** Puncture wound of abdominal wall without foreign body, right lower quadrant without penetration into peritoneal cavity

√7th **S31.134** Puncture wound of abdominal wall without foreign body, left lower quadrant without penetration into peritoneal cavity

√7th **S31.135** Puncture wound of abdominal wall without foreign body, periumbilic region without penetration into peritoneal cavity

√7th **S31.139** Puncture wound of abdominal wall without foreign body, unspecified quadrant without penetration into peritoneal cavity

√6th **S31.14** Puncture wound of abdominal wall with foreign body without penetration into peritoneal cavity

√7th **S31.140** Puncture wound of abdominal wall with foreign body, right upper quadrant without penetration into peritoneal cavity

√7th **S31.141** Puncture wound of abdominal wall with foreign body, left upper quadrant without penetration into peritoneal cavity

√7th **S31.142** Puncture wound of abdominal wall with foreign body, epigastric region without penetration into peritoneal cavity

√7th **S31.143** Puncture wound of abdominal wall with foreign body, right lower quadrant without penetration into peritoneal cavity

√7th **S31.144** Puncture wound of abdominal wall with foreign body, left lower quadrant without penetration into peritoneal cavity

√7th **S31.145** Puncture wound of abdominal wall with foreign body, periumbilic region without penetration into peritoneal cavity

√7th **S31.149** Puncture wound of abdominal wall with foreign body, unspecified quadrant without penetration into peritoneal cavity

√6th **S31.15** Open bite of abdominal wall without penetration into peritoneal cavity

Bite of abdominal wall NOS

EXCLUDES 1   superficial bite of abdominal wall (S30.871)

√7th **S31.150** Open bite of abdominal wall, right upper quadrant without penetration into peritoneal cavity

√7th **S31.151** Open bite of abdominal wall, left upper quadrant without penetration into peritoneal cavity

√7th **S31.152** Open bite of abdominal wall, epigastric region without penetration into peritoneal cavity

√7th **S31.153** Open bite of abdominal wall, right lower quadrant without penetration into peritoneal cavity

√7th **S31.154** Open bite of abdominal wall, left lower quadrant without penetration into peritoneal cavity

√7th **S31.155** Open bite of abdominal wall, periumbilic region without penetration into peritoneal cavity

√7th **S31.159** Open bite of abdominal wall, unspecified quadrant without penetration into peritoneal cavity

√5th **S31.2** Open wound of penis

√x7th **S31.20** Unspecified open wound of penis ♂

√x7th **S31.21** Laceration without foreign body of penis ♂

√x7th **S31.22** Laceration with foreign body of penis ♂

√x7th **S31.23** Puncture wound without foreign body of penis ♂

√x7th **S31.24** Puncture wound with foreign body of penis ♂

√x7th **S31.25** Open bite of penis ♂

Bite of penis NOS

EXCLUDES 1   superficial bite of penis (S30.862, S30.872)

√5th **S31.3** Open wound of scrotum and testes

√x7th **S31.30** Unspecified open wound of scrotum and testes ♂

√x7th **S31.31** Laceration without foreign body of scrotum and testes ♂

√x7th **S31.32** Laceration with foreign body of scrotum and testes ♂

√x7th **S31.33** Puncture wound without foreign body of scrotum and testes ♂

√x7th **S31.34** Puncture wound with foreign body of scrotum and testes ♂

√x7th **S31.35** Open bite of scrotum and testes ♂

Bite of scrotum and testes NOS

EXCLUDES 1   superficial bite of scrotum and testes (S30.863, S30.873)

√5th **S31.4** Open wound of vagina and vulva

EXCLUDES 1   injury to vagina and vulva during delivery (O70.-, O71.4)

√x7th **S31.40** Unspecified open wound of vagina and vulva ♀

√x7th **S31.41** Laceration without foreign body of vagina and vulva ♀

√x7th **S31.42** Laceration with foreign body of vagina and vulva ♀

√x7th **S31.43** Puncture wound without foreign body of vagina and vulva ♀

√x7th **S31.44** Puncture wound with foreign body of vagina and vulva ♀

√x7th **S31.45** Open bite of vagina and vulva ♀

Bite of vagina and vulva NOS

EXCLUDES 1   superficial bite of vagina and vulva (S30.864, S30.874)

√5th **S31.5** Open wound of unspecified external genital organs

EXCLUDES 1   traumatic amputation of external genital organs (S38.21, S38.22)

√6th **S31.50** Unspecified open wound of unspecified external genital organs

√7th **S31.501** Unspecified open wound of unspecified external genital organs, male ♂

√7th **S31.502** Unspecified open wound of unspecified external genital organs, female ♀

√6th **S31.51** Laceration without foreign body of unspecified external genital organs

√7th **S31.511** Laceration without foreign body of unspecified external genital organs, male ♂

√7th **S31.512** Laceration without foreign body of unspecified external genital organs, female ♀

√6th **S31.52** Laceration with foreign body of unspecified external genital organs

√7th **S31.521** Laceration with foreign body of unspecified external genital organs, male ♂

√7th **S31.522** Laceration with foreign body of unspecified external genital organs, female ♀

✔ Additional Character Required   √x7th Placeholder   Questionable PDx   Manifestation   Unspecified Dx   UPD Unacceptable PDx   H1-H14 HAC   HCC CMS-HCC Dx   HIV HIV Dx

ICD-10-CM 2022   997

√6th **S31.53** Puncture wound without foreign body of unspecified external genital organs

√7th **S31.531** Puncture wound without foreign body of unspecified external genital organs, male ♂

√7th **S31.532** Puncture wound without foreign body of unspecified external genital organs, female ♀

√6th **S31.54** Puncture wound with foreign body of unspecified external genital organs

√7th **S31.541** Puncture wound with foreign body of unspecified external genital organs, male ♂

√7th **S31.542** Puncture wound with foreign body of unspecified external genital organs, female ♀

√6th **S31.55** Open bite of unspecified external genital organs

Bite of unspecified external genital organs NOS

EXCLUDES 1 superficial bite of unspecified external genital organs (S30.865, S30.866, S30.875, S30.876)

√7th **S31.551** Open bite of unspecified external genital organs, male ♂

√7th **S31.552** Open bite of unspecified external genital organs, female ♀

√5th **S31.6** Open wound of abdominal wall with penetration into peritoneal cavity

√6th **S31.60** Unspecified open wound of abdominal wall with penetration into peritoneal cavity

√7th **S31.600** Unspecified open wound of abdominal wall, right upper quadrant with penetration into peritoneal cavity MCC

√7th **S31.601** Unspecified open wound of abdominal wall, left upper quadrant with penetration into peritoneal cavity MCC

√7th **S31.602** Unspecified open wound of abdominal wall, epigastric region with penetration into peritoneal cavity MCC

√7th **S31.603** Unspecified open wound of abdominal wall, right lower quadrant with penetration into peritoneal cavity MCC

√7th **S31.604** Unspecified open wound of abdominal wall, left lower quadrant with penetration into peritoneal cavity MCC

√7th **S31.605** Unspecified open wound of abdominal wall, periumbilic region with penetration into peritoneal cavity MCC

√7th **S31.609** Unspecified open wound of abdominal wall, unspecified quadrant with penetration into peritoneal cavity MCC

√6th **S31.61** Laceration without foreign body of abdominal wall with penetration into peritoneal cavity

√7th **S31.610** Laceration without foreign body of abdominal wall, right upper quadrant with penetration into peritoneal cavity MCC

√7th **S31.611** Laceration without foreign body of abdominal wall, left upper quadrant with penetration into peritoneal cavity MCC

√7th **S31.612** Laceration without foreign body of abdominal wall, epigastric region with penetration into peritoneal cavity MCC

√7th **S31.613** Laceration without foreign body of abdominal wall, right lower quadrant with penetration into peritoneal cavity MCC

√7th **S31.614** Laceration without foreign body of abdominal wall, left lower quadrant with penetration into peritoneal cavity MCC

√7th **S31.615** Laceration without foreign body of abdominal wall, periumbilic region with penetration into peritoneal cavity MCC

√7th **S31.619** Laceration without foreign body of abdominal wall, unspecified quadrant with penetration into peritoneal cavity MCC

√6th **S31.62** Laceration with foreign body of abdominal wall with penetration into peritoneal cavity

√7th **S31.620** Laceration with foreign body of abdominal wall, right upper quadrant with penetration into peritoneal cavity MCC

√7th **S31.621** Laceration with foreign body of abdominal wall, left upper quadrant with penetration into peritoneal cavity MCC

√7th **S31.622** Laceration with foreign body of abdominal wall, epigastric region with penetration into peritoneal cavity MCC

√7th **S31.623** Laceration with foreign body of abdominal wall, right lower quadrant with penetration into peritoneal cavity MCC

√7th **S31.624** Laceration with foreign body of abdominal wall, left lower quadrant with penetration into peritoneal cavity MCC

√7th **S31.625** Laceration with foreign body of abdominal wall, periumbilic region with penetration into peritoneal cavity MCC

√7th **S31.629** Laceration with foreign body of abdominal wall, unspecified quadrant with penetration into peritoneal cavity MCC

√6th **S31.63** Puncture wound without foreign body of abdominal wall with penetration into peritoneal cavity

√7th **S31.630** Puncture wound without foreign body of abdominal wall, right upper quadrant with penetration into peritoneal cavity MCC

√7th **S31.631** Puncture wound without foreign body of abdominal wall, left upper quadrant with penetration into peritoneal cavity MCC

√7th **S31.632** Puncture wound without foreign body of abdominal wall, epigastric region with penetration into peritoneal cavity MCC

√7th **S31.633** Puncture wound without foreign body of abdominal wall, right lower quadrant with penetration into peritoneal cavity MCC

√7th **S31.634** Puncture wound without foreign body of abdominal wall, left lower quadrant with penetration into peritoneal cavity MCC

√7th **S31.635** Puncture wound without foreign body of abdominal wall, periumbilic region with penetration into peritoneal cavity MCC

√7th **S31.639** Puncture wound without foreign body of abdominal wall, unspecified quadrant with penetration into peritoneal cavity MCC

√6th **S31.64** Puncture wound with foreign body of abdominal wall with penetration into peritoneal cavity

√7th **S31.640** Puncture wound with foreign body of abdominal wall, right upper quadrant with penetration into peritoneal cavity MCC

√7th **S31.641** Puncture wound with foreign body of abdominal wall, left upper quadrant with penetration into peritoneal cavity MCC

√7th **S31.642** Puncture wound with foreign body of abdominal wall, epigastric region with penetration into peritoneal cavity MCC

√7th **S31.643** Puncture wound with foreign body of abdominal wall, right lower quadrant with penetration into peritoneal cavity MCC

√7th **S31.644** Puncture wound with foreign body of abdominal wall, left lower quadrant with penetration into peritoneal cavity MCC

√7th **S31.645** Puncture wound with foreign body of abdominal wall, periumbilic region with penetration into peritoneal cavity MCC

√7th **S31.649** Puncture wound with foreign body of abdominal wall, unspecified quadrant with penetration into peritoneal cavity MCC

√6th **S31.65** Open bite of abdominal wall with penetration into peritoneal cavity

EXCLUDES 1 superficial bite of abdominal wall (S30.861, S30.871)

√7th **S31.650** Open bite of abdominal wall, right upper quadrant with penetration into peritoneal cavity MCC

√7th **S31.651** Open bite of abdominal wall, left upper quadrant with penetration into peritoneal cavity MCC

☑7ᵗʰ **S31.652** Open bite of abdominal wall, epigastric region with penetration into peritoneal cavity   MCC

☑7ᵗʰ **S31.653** Open bite of abdominal wall, right lower quadrant with penetration into peritoneal cavity   MCC

☑7ᵗʰ **S31.654** Open bite of abdominal wall, left lower quadrant with penetration into peritoneal cavity   MCC

☑7ᵗʰ **S31.655** Open bite of abdominal wall, periumbilic region with penetration into peritoneal cavity   MCC

☑7ᵗʰ **S31.659** Open bite of abdominal wall, unspecified quadrant with penetration into peritoneal cavity   MCC

☑5ᵗʰ **S31.8** **Open wound of other parts of abdomen, lower back and pelvis**

  ☑6ᵗʰ **S31.80** **Open wound of unspecified buttock**

    ☑7ᵗʰ **S31.801** Laceration without foreign body of unspecified buttock

    ☑7ᵗʰ **S31.802** Laceration with foreign body of unspecified buttock

    ☑7ᵗʰ **S31.803** Puncture wound without foreign body of unspecified buttock

    ☑7ᵗʰ **S31.804** Puncture wound with foreign body of unspecified buttock

    ☑7ᵗʰ **S31.805** Open bite of unspecified buttock

         Bite of buttock NOS

         EXCLUDES 1   superficial bite of buttock (S30.870)

    ☑7ᵗʰ **S31.809** Unspecified open wound of unspecified buttock

  ☑6ᵗʰ **S31.81** **Open wound of right buttock**

    ☑7ᵗʰ **S31.811** Laceration without foreign body of right buttock

    ☑7ᵗʰ **S31.812** Laceration with foreign body of right buttock

    ☑7ᵗʰ **S31.813** Puncture wound without foreign body of right buttock

    ☑7ᵗʰ **S31.814** Puncture wound with foreign body of right buttock

    ☑7ᵗʰ **S31.815** Open bite of right buttock

         Bite of right buttock NOS

         EXCLUDES 1   superficial bite of buttock (S30.870)

    ☑7ᵗʰ **S31.819** Unspecified open wound of right buttock

  ☑6ᵗʰ **S31.82** **Open wound of left buttock**

    ☑7ᵗʰ **S31.821** Laceration without foreign body of left buttock

    ☑7ᵗʰ **S31.822** Laceration with foreign body of left buttock

    ☑7ᵗʰ **S31.823** Puncture wound without foreign body of left buttock

    ☑7ᵗʰ **S31.824** Puncture wound with foreign body of left buttock

    ☑7ᵗʰ **S31.825** Open bite of left buttock

         Bite of left buttock NOS

         EXCLUDES 1   superficial bite of buttock (S30.870)

    ☑7ᵗʰ **S31.829** Unspecified open wound of left buttock

  ☑6ᵗʰ **S31.83** **Open wound of anus**

    ☑7ᵗʰ **S31.831** Laceration without foreign body of anus

    ☑7ᵗʰ **S31.832** Laceration with foreign body of anus

    ☑7ᵗʰ **S31.833** Puncture wound without foreign body of anus

    ☑7ᵗʰ **S31.834** Puncture wound with foreign body of anus

    ☑7ᵗʰ **S31.835** Open bite of anus

         Bite of anus NOS

         EXCLUDES 1   superficial bite of anus (S30.877)

    ☑7ᵗʰ **S31.839** Unspecified open wound of anus

☑4ᵗʰ **S32** **Fracture of lumbar spine and pelvis**

  NOTE   A fracture not indicated as displaced or nondisplaced should be coded to displaced.

       A fracture not indicated as opened or closed should be coded to closed.

  INCLUDES   fracture of lumbosacral neural arch

       fracture of lumbosacral spinous process

       fracture of lumbosacral transverse process

       fracture of lumbosacral vertebra

       fracture of lumbosacral vertebral arch

Code first any associated spinal cord and spinal nerve injury (S34.-)

  EXCLUDES 1   transection of abdomen (S38.3)

  EXCLUDES 2   fracture of hip NOS (S72.0-)

AHA: 2021,1Q,6; 2018,2Q,12; 2015,3Q,37-39; 2012,4Q,93

The appropriate 7th character is to be added to each code from category S32.
A   initial encounter for closed fracture
B   initial encounter for open fracture
D   subsequent encounter for fracture with routine healing
G   subsequent encounter for fracture with delayed healing
K   subsequent encounter for fracture with nonunion
S   sequela

☑5ᵗʰ **S32.0** **Fracture of lumbar vertebra**

     Fracture of lumbar spine NOS

  ☑6ᵗʰ **S32.00** **Fracture of unspecified lumbar vertebra**

    2,3,6 ☑7ᵗʰ **S32.000** Wedge compression fracture of unspecified lumbar vertebra   MCC CC H5 HCC

    2,3,6 ☑7ᵗʰ **S32.001** Stable burst fracture of unspecified lumbar vertebra   MCC CC H5 HCC

    2,3,6 ☑7ᵗʰ **S32.002** Unstable burst fracture of unspecified lumbar vertebra   MCC CC H5 HCC

    2,3,6 ☑7ᵗʰ **S32.008** Other fracture of unspecified lumbar vertebra   MCC CC H5 HCC

    2,3,6 ☑7ᵗʰ **S32.009** Unspecified fracture of unspecified lumbar vertebra   MCC CC H5 HCC

  ☑6ᵗʰ **S32.01** **Fracture of first lumbar vertebra**

    2,3,6 ☑7ᵗʰ **S32.010** Wedge compression fracture of first lumbar vertebra   MCC CC H5 HCC

    2,3,6 ☑7ᵗʰ **S32.011** Stable burst fracture of first lumbar vertebra   MCC CC H5 HCC

    2,3,6 ☑7ᵗʰ **S32.012** Unstable burst fracture of first lumbar vertebra   MCC CC H5 HCC

    2,3,6 ☑7ᵗʰ **S32.018** Other fracture of first lumbar vertebra   MCC CC H5 HCC

    2,3,6 ☑7ᵗʰ **S32.019** Unspecified fracture of first lumbar vertebra   MCC CC H5 HCC

  ☑6ᵗʰ **S32.02** **Fracture of second lumbar vertebra**

    2,3,6 ☑7ᵗʰ **S32.020** Wedge compression fracture of second lumbar vertebra   MCC CC H5 HCC

    2,3,6 ☑7ᵗʰ **S32.021** Stable burst fracture of second lumbar vertebra   MCC CC H5 HCC

    2,3,6 ☑7ᵗʰ **S32.022** Unstable burst fracture of second lumbar vertebra   MCC CC H5 HCC

    2,3,6 ☑7ᵗʰ **S32.028** Other fracture of second lumbar vertebra   MCC CC H5 HCC

    2,3,6 ☑7ᵗʰ **S32.029** Unspecified fracture of second lumbar vertebra   MCC CC H5 HCC

  ☑6ᵗʰ **S32.03** **Fracture of third lumbar vertebra**

    2,3,6 ☑7ᵗʰ **S32.030** Wedge compression fracture of third lumbar vertebra   MCC CC H5 HCC

    2,3,6 ☑7ᵗʰ **S32.031** Stable burst fracture of third lumbar vertebra   MCC CC H5 HCC

    2,3,6 ☑7ᵗʰ **S32.032** Unstable burst fracture of third lumbar vertebra   MCC CC H5 HCC

    2,3,6 ☑7ᵗʰ **S32.038** Other fracture of third lumbar vertebra   MCC CC H5 HCC

    2,3,6 ☑7ᵗʰ **S32.039** Unspecified fracture of third lumbar vertebra   MCC CC H5 HCC

  ☑6ᵗʰ **S32.04** **Fracture of fourth lumbar vertebra**

    2,3,6 ☑7ᵗʰ **S32.040** Wedge compression fracture of fourth lumbar vertebra   MCC CC H5 HCC

    2,3,6 ☑7ᵗʰ **S32.041** Stable burst fracture of fourth lumbar vertebra   MCC CC H5 HCC

    2,3,6 ☑7ᵗʰ **S32.042** Unstable burst fracture of fourth lumbar vertebra   MCC CC H5 HCC

☑ Additional Character Required   ☑x7ᵗʰ Placeholder   Questionable PDx   Manifestation   Unspecified Dx   UPD Unacceptable PDx   H1-H4 HAC   HCC CMS-HCC Dx   HIV HIV Dx

ICD-10-CM 2022   999

Chapter 19. Injury, Poisoning and Certain Other Consequences of External Causes   S31.652–S32.042

2,3,6 √7ᵗʰ **S32.Ø48** Other fracture of fourth lumbar vertebra `MCC` `CC` `H5` `HCC`

2,3,6 √7ᵗʰ **S32.Ø49** Unspecified fracture of fourth lumbar vertebra `MCC` `CC` `H5` `HCC`

√6ᵗʰ **S32.Ø5** **Fracture of fifth lumbar vertebra**

2,3,6 √7ᵗʰ **S32.Ø5Ø** Wedge compression fracture of fifth lumbar vertebra `MCC` `CC` `H5` `HCC`

2,3,6 √7ᵗʰ **S32.Ø51** Stable burst fracture of fifth lumbar vertebra `MCC` `CC` `H5` `HCC`

2,3,6 √7ᵗʰ **S32.Ø52** Unstable burst fracture of fifth lumbar vertebra `MCC` `CC` `H5` `HCC`

2,3,6 √7ᵗʰ **S32.Ø58** Other fracture of fifth lumbar vertebra `MCC` `CC` `H5` `HCC`

2,3,6 √7ᵗʰ **S32.Ø59** Unspecified fracture of fifth lumbar vertebra `MCC` `CC` `H5` `HCC`

√5ᵗʰ **S32.1** **Fracture of sacrum**

> **NOTE** For vertical fractures, code to most medial fracture extension
>
> Use two codes if both a vertical and transverse fracture are present

Code also any associated fracture of pelvic ring (S32.8-)

2,3,6 √x7ᵗʰ **S32.1Ø** **Unspecified fracture of sacrum** `MCC` `CC` `H5` `HCC`

√6ᵗʰ **S32.11** **Zone I fracture of sacrum**

Vertical sacral ala fracture of sacrum

Vertical Sacral Fracture Zones

2,3,6 √7ᵗʰ **S32.11Ø** Nondisplaced Zone I fracture of sacrum `MCC` `CC` `H5` `HCC`

2,3,6 √7ᵗʰ **S32.111** Minimally displaced Zone I fracture of sacrum `MCC` `CC` `H5` `HCC`

2,3,6 √7ᵗʰ **S32.112** Severely displaced Zone I fracture of sacrum `MCC` `CC` `H5` `HCC`

2,3,6 √7ᵗʰ **S32.119** Unspecified Zone I fracture of sacrum `MCC` `CC` `H5` `HCC`

√6ᵗʰ **S32.12** **Zone II fracture of sacrum**

Vertical foraminal region fracture of sacrum

2,3,6 √7ᵗʰ **S32.12Ø** Nondisplaced Zone II fracture of sacrum `MCC` `CC` `H5` `HCC`

2,3,6 √7ᵗʰ **S32.121** Minimally displaced Zone II fracture of sacrum `MCC` `CC` `H5` `HCC`

2,3,6 √7ᵗʰ **S32.122** Severely displaced Zone II fracture of sacrum `MCC` `CC` `H5` `HCC`

2,3,6 √7ᵗʰ **S32.129** Unspecified Zone II fracture of sacrum `MCC` `CC` `H5` `HCC`

√6ᵗʰ **S32.13** **Zone III fracture of sacrum**

Vertical fracture into spinal canal region of sacrum

2,3,6 √7ᵗʰ **S32.13Ø** Nondisplaced Zone III fracture of sacrum `MCC` `CC` `H5` `HCC`

2,3,6 √7ᵗʰ **S32.131** Minimally displaced Zone III fracture of sacrum `MCC` `CC` `H5` `HCC`

2,3,6 √7ᵗʰ **S32.132** Severely displaced Zone III fracture of sacrum `MCC` `CC` `H5` `HCC`

2,3,6 √7ᵗʰ **S32.139** Unspecified Zone III fracture of sacrum `MCC` `CC` `H5` `HCC`

Transverse Sacral Fracture Types

Type 1   Type 2   Type 3   Type 4

2,3,6 √x7ᵗʰ **S32.14** Type 1 fracture of sacrum `MCC` `CC` `H5` `HCC`

Transverse flexion fracture of sacrum without displacement

2,3,6 √x7ᵗʰ **S32.15** Type 2 fracture of sacrum `MCC` `CC` `H5` `HCC`

Transverse flexion fracture of sacrum with posterior displacement

2,3,6 √x7ᵗʰ **S32.16** Type 3 fracture of sacrum `MCC` `CC` `H5` `HCC`

Transverse extension fracture of sacrum with anterior displacement

2,3,6 √x7ᵗʰ **S32.17** Type 4 fracture of sacrum `MCC` `CC` `H5` `HCC`

Transverse segmental comminution of upper sacrum

2,3,6 √x7ᵗʰ **S32.19** Other fracture of sacrum `MCC` `CC` `H5` `HCC`

2,3,6 √x7ᵗʰ **S32.2** **Fracture of coccyx** `MCC` `CC` `H5` `HCC`

√5ᵗʰ **S32.3** **Fracture of ilium**

> **EXCLUDES 1** fracture of ilium with associated disruption of pelvic ring (S32.8-)

√6ᵗʰ **S32.3Ø** **Unspecified fracture of ilium**

2,3,6 √7ᵗʰ **S32.3Ø1** Unspecified fracture of right ilium `MCC` `CC` `H5` `HCC`

2,3,6 √7ᵗʰ **S32.3Ø2** Unspecified fracture of left ilium `MCC` `CC` `H5` `HCC`

2,3,6 √7ᵗʰ **S32.3Ø9** Unspecified fracture of unspecified ilium `MCC` `CC` `H5` `HCC`

√6ᵗʰ **S32.31** **Avulsion fracture of ilium**

2,3,6 √7ᵗʰ **S32.311** Displaced avulsion fracture of right ilium `MCC` `CC` `H5` `HCC`

2,3,6 √7ᵗʰ **S32.312** Displaced avulsion fracture of left ilium `MCC` `CC` `H5` `HCC`

2,3,6 √7ᵗʰ **S32.313** Displaced avulsion fracture of unspecified ilium `MCC` `CC` `H5` `HCC`

2,3,6 √7ᵗʰ **S32.314** Nondisplaced avulsion fracture of right ilium `MCC` `CC` `H5` `HCC`

2,3,6 √7ᵗʰ **S32.315** Nondisplaced avulsion fracture of left ilium `MCC` `CC` `H5` `HCC`

2,3,6 √7ᵗʰ **S32.316** Nondisplaced avulsion fracture of unspecified ilium `MCC` `CC` `H5` `HCC`

√6ᵗʰ **S32.39** **Other fracture of ilium**

2,3,6 √7ᵗʰ **S32.391** Other fracture of right ilium `MCC` `CC` `H5` `HCC`

2,3,6 √7ᵗʰ **S32.392** Other fracture of left ilium `MCC` `CC` `H5` `HCC`

2,3,6 √7ᵗʰ **S32.399** Other fracture of unspecified ilium `MCC` `CC` `H5` `HCC`

√5ᵗʰ **S32.4** **Fracture of acetabulum**

Code also any associated fracture of pelvic ring (S32.8-)
AHA: 2016,3Q,16

√6ᵗʰ **S32.4Ø** **Unspecified fracture of acetabulum**

4,6 √7ᵗʰ **S32.4Ø1** Unspecified fracture of right acetabulum `MCC` `CC` `H5` `HCC`

4,6 √7ᵗʰ **S32.4Ø2** Unspecified fracture of left acetabulum `MCC` `CC` `H5` `HCC`

4,6 √7ᵗʰ **S32.4Ø9** Unspecified fracture of unspecified acetabulum `MCC` `CC` `H5` `HCC`

√6ᵗʰ **S32.41** **Fracture of anterior wall of acetabulum**

4,6 √7ᵗʰ **S32.411** Displaced fracture of anterior wall of right acetabulum `MCC` `CC` `H5` `HCC`

4,6 √7ᵗʰ **S32.412** Displaced fracture of anterior wall of left acetabulum `MCC` `CC` `H5` `HCC`

`N` Newborn: 0   `P` Pediatric: 0-17   `M` Maternity: 9-64   `A` Adult: 15-124   `MCC` Major Complication/Comorbidity   `CC` Complication/Comorbidity   `SW` Severe Wound Dx

1000 ICD-10-CM 2022

4,6 √7th **S32.413** Displaced fracture of anterior wall of unspecified acetabulum `MCC` `CC` `H5` `HCC`

4,6 √7th **S32.414** Nondisplaced fracture of anterior wall of right acetabulum `MCC` `CC` `H5` `HCC`

4,6 √7th **S32.415** Nondisplaced fracture of anterior wall of left acetabulum `MCC` `CC` `H5` `HCC`

4,6 √7th **S32.416** Nondisplaced fracture of anterior wall of unspecified acetabulum `MCC` `CC` `H5` `HCC`

√6th **S32.42** Fracture of posterior wall of acetabulum

4,6 √7th **S32.421** Displaced fracture of posterior wall of right acetabulum `MCC` `CC` `H5` `HCC`

4,6 √7th **S32.422** Displaced fracture of posterior wall of left acetabulum `MCC` `CC` `H5` `HCC`

4,6 √7th **S32.423** Displaced fracture of posterior wall of unspecified acetabulum `MCC` `CC` `H5` `HCC`

4,6 √7th **S32.424** Nondisplaced fracture of posterior wall of right acetabulum `MCC` `CC` `H5` `HCC`

4,6 √7th **S32.425** Nondisplaced fracture of posterior wall of left acetabulum `MCC` `CC` `H5` `HCC`

4,6 √7th **S32.426** Nondisplaced fracture of posterior wall of unspecified acetabulum `MCC` `CC` `H5` `HCC`

√6th **S32.43** Fracture of anterior column [iliopubic] of acetabulum

4,6 √7th **S32.431** Displaced fracture of anterior column [iliopubic] of right acetabulum `MCC` `CC` `H5` `HCC`

4,6 √7th **S32.432** Displaced fracture of anterior column [iliopubic] of left acetabulum `MCC` `CC` `H5` `HCC`

4,6 √7th **S32.433** Displaced fracture of anterior column [iliopubic] of unspecified acetabulum `MCC` `CC` `H5` `HCC`

4,6 √7th **S32.434** Nondisplaced fracture of anterior column [iliopubic] of right acetabulum `MCC` `CC` `H5` `HCC`

4,6 √7th **S32.435** Nondisplaced fracture of anterior column [iliopubic] of left acetabulum `MCC` `CC` `H5` `HCC`

4,6 √7th **S32.436** Nondisplaced fracture of anterior column [iliopubic] of unspecified acetabulum `MCC` `CC` `H5` `HCC`

√6th **S32.44** Fracture of posterior column [ilioischial] of acetabulum

4,6 √7th **S32.441** Displaced fracture of posterior column [ilioischial] of right acetabulum `MCC` `CC` `H5` `HCC`

4,6 √7th **S32.442** Displaced fracture of posterior column [ilioischial] of left acetabulum `MCC` `CC` `H5` `HCC`

4,6 √7th **S32.443** Displaced fracture of posterior column [ilioischial] of unspecified acetabulum `MCC` `CC` `H5` `HCC`

4,6 √7th **S32.444** Nondisplaced fracture of posterior column [ilioischial] of right acetabulum `MCC` `CC` `H5` `HCC`

4,6 √7th **S32.445** Nondisplaced fracture of posterior column [ilioischial] of left acetabulum `MCC` `CC` `H5` `HCC`

4,6 √7th **S32.446** Nondisplaced fracture of posterior column [ilioischial] of unspecified acetabulum `MCC` `CC` `H5` `HCC`

√6th **S32.45** Transverse fracture of acetabulum

4,6 √7th **S32.451** Displaced transverse fracture of right acetabulum `MCC` `CC` `H5` `HCC`

4,6 √7th **S32.452** Displaced transverse fracture of left acetabulum `MCC` `CC` `H5` `HCC`

4,6 √7th **S32.453** Displaced transverse fracture of unspecified acetabulum `MCC` `CC` `H5` `HCC`

4,6 √7th **S32.454** Nondisplaced transverse fracture of right acetabulum `MCC` `CC` `H5` `HCC`

4,6 √7th **S32.455** Nondisplaced transverse fracture of left acetabulum `MCC` `CC` `H5` `HCC`

4,6 √7th **S32.456** Nondisplaced transverse fracture of unspecified acetabulum `MCC` `CC` `H5` `HCC`

√6th **S32.46** Associated transverse-posterior fracture of acetabulum

4,6 √7th **S32.461** Displaced associated transverse-posterior fracture of right acetabulum `MCC` `CC` `H5` `HCC`

4,6 √7th **S32.462** Displaced associated transverse-posterior fracture of left acetabulum `MCC` `CC` `H5` `HCC`

4,6 √7th **S32.463** Displaced associated transverse-posterior fracture of unspecified acetabulum `MCC` `CC` `H5` `HCC`

4,6 √7th **S32.464** Nondisplaced associated transverse-posterior fracture of right acetabulum `MCC` `CC` `H5` `HCC`

4,6 √7th **S32.465** Nondisplaced associated transverse-posterior fracture of left acetabulum `MCC` `CC` `H5` `HCC`

4,6 √7th **S32.466** Nondisplaced associated transverse-posterior fracture of unspecified acetabulum `MCC` `CC` `H5` `HCC`

√6th **S32.47** Fracture of medial wall of acetabulum

4,6 √7th **S32.471** Displaced fracture of medial wall of right acetabulum `MCC` `CC` `H5` `HCC`

4,6 √7th **S32.472** Displaced fracture of medial wall of left acetabulum `MCC` `CC` `H5` `HCC`

4,6 √7th **S32.473** Displaced fracture of medial wall of unspecified acetabulum `MCC` `CC` `H5` `HCC`

4,6 √7th **S32.474** Nondisplaced fracture of medial wall of right acetabulum `MCC` `CC` `H5` `HCC`

4,6 √7th **S32.475** Nondisplaced fracture of medial wall of left acetabulum `MCC` `CC` `H5` `HCC`

4,6 √7th **S32.476** Nondisplaced fracture of medial wall of unspecified acetabulum `MCC` `CC` `H5` `HCC`

√6th **S32.48** Dome fracture of acetabulum

4,6 √7th **S32.481** Displaced dome fracture of right acetabulum `MCC` `CC` `H5` `HCC`

4,6 √7th **S32.482** Displaced dome fracture of left acetabulum `MCC` `CC` `H5` `HCC`

4,6 √7th **S32.483** Displaced dome fracture of unspecified acetabulum `MCC` `CC` `H5` `HCC`

4,6 √7th **S32.484** Nondisplaced dome fracture of right acetabulum `MCC` `CC` `H5` `HCC`

4,6 √7th **S32.485** Nondisplaced dome fracture of left acetabulum `MCC` `CC` `H5` `HCC`

4,6 √7th **S32.486** Nondisplaced dome fracture of unspecified acetabulum `MCC` `CC` `H5` `HCC`

√6th **S32.49** Other specified fracture of acetabulum

4,6 √7th **S32.491** Other specified fracture of right acetabulum `MCC` `CC` `H5` `HCC`

4,6 √7th **S32.492** Other specified fracture of left acetabulum `MCC` `CC` `H5` `HCC`

4,6 √7th **S32.499** Other specified fracture of unspecified acetabulum `MCC` `CC` `H5` `HCC`

√5th **S32.5** Fracture of pubis

> EXCLUDES 1   fracture of pubis with associated disruption of pelvic ring (S32.8-)

√6th **S32.50** Unspecified fracture of pubis

2,3,6 √7th **S32.501** Unspecified fracture of right pubis `MCC` `CC` `H5` `HCC`

2,3,6 √7th **S32.502** Unspecified fracture of left pubis `MCC` `CC` `H5` `HCC`

2,3,6 √7th **S32.509** Unspecified fracture of unspecified pubis `MCC` `CC` `H5` `HCC`

√6th **S32.51** Fracture of superior rim of pubis

2,3,6 √7th **S32.511** Fracture of superior rim of right pubis `MCC` `CC` `H5` `HCC`

2,3,6 √7th **S32.512** Fracture of superior rim of left pubis `MCC` `CC` `H5` `HCC`

2,3,6 √7th **S32.519** Fracture of superior rim of unspecified pubis `MCC` `CC` `H5` `HCC`

√6th **S32.59** Other specified fracture of pubis

2,3,6 √7th **S32.591** Other specified fracture of right pubis `MCC` `CC` `H5` `HCC`

2,3,6 √7th **S32.592** Other specified fracture of left pubis

2,3,6 ✓7th **S32.599** Other specified fracture of unspecified pubis   MCC CC H5 HCC

✓5th **S32.6** **Fracture of** ischium

   EXCLUDES 1   *fracture of ischium with associated disruption of pelvic ring (S32.8-)*

✓6th **S32.60** **Unspecified fracture of ischium**

2,3,6 ✓7th **S32.601** Unspecified fracture of right ischium   MCC CC H5 HCC

2,3,6 ✓7th **S32.602** Unspecified fracture of left ischium   MCC CC H5 HCC

2,3,6 ✓7th **S32.609** Unspecified fracture of unspecified ischium   MCC CC H5 HCC

✓6th **S32.61** **Avulsion fracture of ischium**

2,3,6 ✓7th **S32.611** Displaced avulsion fracture of right ischium   MCC CC H5 HCC

2,3,6 ✓7th **S32.612** Displaced avulsion fracture of left ischium   MCC CC H5 HCC

2,3,6 ✓7th **S32.613** Displaced avulsion fracture of unspecified ischium   MCC CC H5 HCC

2,3,6 ✓7th **S32.614** Nondisplaced avulsion fracture of right ischium   MCC CC H5 HCC

2,3,6 ✓7th **S32.615** Nondisplaced avulsion fracture of left ischium   MCC CC H5 HCC

2,3,6 ✓7th **S32.616** Nondisplaced avulsion fracture of unspecified ischium   MCC CC H5 HCC

✓6th **S32.69** **Other specified fracture of ischium**

2,3,6 ✓7th **S32.691** Other specified fracture of right ischium   MCC CC H5 HCC

2,3,6 ✓7th **S32.692** Other specified fracture of left ischium   MCC CC H5 HCC

2,3,6 ✓7th **S32.699** Other specified fracture of unspecified ischium   MCC CC H5 HCC

✓5th **S32.8** **Fracture of other parts of pelvis**

   Code also any associated:
     fracture of acetabulum (S32.4-)
     sacral fracture (S32.1-)

Fractures Disrupting Pelvic Circle

2,3,6 ✓6th **S32.81** **Multiple fractures of pelvis** with disruption of pelvic ring

   Multiple pelvic fractures with disruption of pelvic circle

2,3,6 ✓7th **S32.810** Multiple fractures of pelvis with stable disruption of pelvic ring   MCC CC H5 HCC

2,3,6 ✓7th **S32.811** Multiple fractures of pelvis with unstable disruption of pelvic ring   MCC CC H5 HCC

2,3,6 ✓x7th **S32.82** **Multiple fractures of pelvis** without disruption of pelvic ring   MCC CC H5 HCC

   Multiple pelvic fractures without disruption of pelvic circle

2,3,6 ✓x7th **S32.89** **Fracture of other parts of pelvis**   MCC CC H5 HCC

2,3,6 ✓x7th **S32.9** **Fracture of unspecified parts of lumbosacral spine and pelvis**   MCC CC H5 HCC

   Fracture of lumbosacral spine NOS
   Fracture of pelvis NOS
   AHA: 2012,4Q,93

✓4th **S33** **Dislocation and sprain of joints and ligaments of lumbar spine and pelvis**

   INCLUDES   avulsion of joint or ligament of lumbar spine and pelvis

     laceration of cartilage, joint or ligament of lumbar spine and pelvis

     sprain of cartilage, joint or ligament of lumbar spine and pelvis

     traumatic hemarthrosis of joint or ligament of lumbar spine and pelvis

     traumatic rupture of joint or ligament of lumbar spine and pelvis

     traumatic subluxation of joint or ligament of lumbar spine and pelvis

     traumatic tear of joint or ligament of lumbar spine and pelvis

   Code also any associated open wound

   EXCLUDES 1   *nontraumatic rupture or displacement of lumbar intervertebral disc NOS (M51.-)*

     obstetric damage to pelvic joints and ligaments (O71.6)

   EXCLUDES 2   *dislocation and sprain of joints and ligaments of hip (S73.-)*

     strain of muscle of lower back and pelvis (S39.01-)

   The appropriate 7th character is to be added to each code from category S33.
     A   initial encounter
     D   subsequent encounter
     S   sequela

✓x7th **S33.0** **Traumatic rupture of lumbar intervertebral disc**

   EXCLUDES 1   *rupture or displacement (nontraumatic) of lumbar intervertebral disc NOS (M51.- with fifth character 6)*

✓5th **S33.1** **Subluxation and dislocation of** lumbar vertebra

   Code also any associated:
     open wound of abdomen, lower back and pelvis (S31)
     spinal cord injury (S24.0, S24.1-, S34.0-, S34.1-)

   EXCLUDES 2   *fracture of lumbar vertebrae (S32.0-)*

✓6th **S33.10** **Subluxation and dislocation of unspecified lumbar vertebra**

✓7th **S33.100** Subluxation of unspecified lumbar vertebra

✓7th **S33.101** Dislocation of unspecified lumbar vertebra

✓6th **S33.11** **Subluxation and dislocation of** L1/L2 **lumbar vertebra**

✓7th **S33.110** Subluxation of L1/L2 lumbar vertebra

✓7th **S33.111** Dislocation of L1/L2 lumbar vertebra

✓6th **S33.12** **Subluxation and dislocation of** L2/L3 **lumbar vertebra**

✓7th **S33.120** Subluxation of L2/L3 lumbar vertebra

✓7th **S33.121** Dislocation of L2/L3 lumbar vertebra

✓6th **S33.13** **Subluxation and dislocation of** L3/L4 **lumbar vertebra**

✓7th **S33.130** Subluxation of L3/L4 lumbar vertebra

✓7th **S33.131** Dislocation of L3/L4 lumbar vertebra

✓6th **S33.14** **Subluxation and dislocation of** L4/L5 **lumbar vertebra**

✓7th **S33.140** Subluxation of L4/L5 lumbar vertebra

✓7th **S33.141** Dislocation of L4/L5 lumbar vertebra

✓x7th **S33.2** **Dislocation of** sacroiliac and sacrococcygeal **joint**

✓5th **S33.3** **Dislocation of other and unspecified parts of lumbar spine and pelvis**

✓x7th **S33.30** **Dislocation of unspecified parts of lumbar spine and pelvis**

✓x7th **S33.39** **Dislocation of other parts of lumbar spine and pelvis**

✓x7th **S33.4** **Traumatic rupture of** symphysis pubis

✓x7th **S33.5** **Sprain of ligaments of** lumbar spine

✓x7th **S33.6** **Sprain of** sacroiliac joint

✓x7th **S33.8** **Sprain of other parts of lumbar spine and pelvis**

✓x7th **S33.9** **Sprain of unspecified parts of lumbar spine and pelvis**

N Newborn: 0   P Pediatric: 0-17   M Maternity: 9-64   A Adult: 15-124   MCC Major Complication/Comorbidity   CC Complication/Comorbidity   SW Severe Wound Dx

1002   ICD-10-CM 2022

☑4ᵗʰ **S34 Injury of lumbar and sacral spinal cord and nerves at abdomen, lower back and pelvis level**

> **NOTE**   Code to highest level of lumbar cord injury.
>
> Injuries to the spinal cord (S34.0 and S34.1) refer to the cord level and not bone level injury, and can affect nerve roots at and below the level given.

Code also any associated:
> fracture of vertebra (S22.0-, S32.0-)
> open wound of abdomen, lower back and pelvis (S31.-)
> transient paralysis (R29.5)

> The appropriate 7th character is to be added to each code from category S34.
> A   initial encounter
> D   subsequent encounter
> S   sequela

☑5ᵗʰ **S34.0 Concussion and edema** of lumbar and sacral spinal cord

  ☑x7ᵗʰ **S34.01 Concussion and edema of** lumbar **spinal cord**   MCC HCC

  ☑x7ᵗʰ **S34.02 Concussion and edema of** sacral **spinal cord**   MCC HCC
       Concussion and edema of conus medullaris

☑5ᵗʰ **S34.1 Other and unspecified injury of lumbar and sacral spinal cord**

  ☑6ᵗʰ **S34.10 Unspecified injury to lumbar spinal cord**

    ☑7ᵗʰ **S34.101 Unspecified injury to** L1 **level of lumbar spinal cord**   MCC H5 HCC
        Unspecified injury to lumbar spinal cord level 1

    ☑7ᵗʰ **S34.102 Unspecified injury to** L2 **level of lumbar spinal cord**   MCC H5 HCC
        Unspecified injury to lumbar spinal cord level 2

    ☑7ᵗʰ **S34.103 Unspecified injury to** L3 **level of lumbar spinal cord**   MCC H5 HCC
        Unspecified injury to lumbar spinal cord level 3

    ☑7ᵗʰ **S34.104 Unspecified injury to** L4 **level of lumbar spinal cord**   MCC H5 HCC
        Unspecified injury to lumbar spinal cord level 4

    ☑7ᵗʰ **S34.105 Unspecified injury to** L5 **level of lumbar spinal cord**   MCC H5 HCC
        Unspecified injury to lumbar spinal cord level 5

    ☑7ᵗʰ **S34.109 Unspecified injury to unspecified level of lumbar spinal cord**   MCC H5 HCC

  ☑6ᵗʰ **S34.11 Complete lesion** of lumbar spinal cord

    ☑7ᵗʰ **S34.111 Complete lesion of** L1 **level of lumbar spinal cord**   MCC H5 HCC
        Complete lesion of lumbar spinal cord level 1

    ☑7ᵗʰ **S34.112 Complete lesion of** L2 **level of lumbar spinal cord**   MCC H5 HCC
        Complete lesion of lumbar spinal cord level 2

    ☑7ᵗʰ **S34.113 Complete lesion of** L3 **level of lumbar spinal cord**   MCC H5 HCC
        Complete lesion of lumbar spinal cord level 3

    ☑7ᵗʰ **S34.114 Complete lesion of** L4 **level of lumbar spinal cord**   MCC H5 HCC
        Complete lesion of lumbar spinal cord level 4

    ☑7ᵗʰ **S34.115 Complete lesion of** L5 **level of lumbar spinal cord**   MCC H5 HCC
        Complete lesion of lumbar spinal cord level 5

    ☑7ᵗʰ **S34.119 Complete lesion of unspecified level of lumbar spinal cord**   MCC H5 HCC

  ☑6ᵗʰ **S34.12 Incomplete lesion** of lumbar spinal cord

    ☑7ᵗʰ **S34.121 Incomplete lesion of** L1 **level of lumbar spinal cord**   MCC H5 HCC
        Incomplete lesion of lumbar spinal cord level 1

    ☑7ᵗʰ **S34.122 Incomplete lesion of** L2 **level of lumbar spinal cord**   MCC H5 HCC
        Incomplete lesion of lumbar spinal cord level 2

    ☑7ᵗʰ **S34.123 Incomplete lesion of** L3 **level of lumbar spinal cord**   MCC H5 HCC
        Incomplete lesion of lumbar spinal cord level 3

    ☑7ᵗʰ **S34.124 Incomplete lesion of** L4 **level of lumbar spinal cord**   MCC H5 HCC
        Incomplete lesion of lumbar spinal cord level 4

    ☑7ᵗʰ **S34.125 Incomplete lesion of** L5 **level of lumbar spinal cord**   MCC H5 HCC
        Incomplete lesion of lumbar spinal cord level 5

    ☑7ᵗʰ **S34.129 Incomplete lesion of unspecified level of lumbar spinal cord**   MCC H5 HCC

  ☑6ᵗʰ **S34.13 Other and unspecified injury to sacral spinal cord**
      Other injury to conus medullaris

    ☑7ᵗʰ **S34.131 Complete lesion of** sacral **spinal cord**   MCC H5 HCC
        Complete lesion of conus medullaris

    ☑7ᵗʰ **S34.132 Incomplete lesion of** sacral **spinal cord**   MCC H5 HCC
        Incomplete lesion of conus medullaris

    ☑7ᵗʰ **S34.139 Unspecified injury to sacral spinal cord**   MCC H5 HCC
        Unspecified injury of conus medullaris

☑5ᵗʰ **S34.2 Injury of nerve root of lumbar and sacral spine**

  ☑x7ᵗʰ **S34.21 Injury of nerve root of** lumbar **spine**

  ☑x7ᵗʰ **S34.22 Injury of nerve root of** sacral **spine**

6 ☑x7ᵗʰ **S34.3 Injury of cauda equina**   MCC H5 HCC

☑x7ᵗʰ **S34.4 Injury of lumbosacral plexus**

☑x7ᵗʰ **S34.5 Injury of lumbar, sacral and pelvic sympathetic nerves**
    Injury of celiac ganglion or plexus
    Injury of hypogastric plexus
    Injury of mesenteric plexus (inferior) (superior)
    Injury of splanchnic nerve

☑x7ᵗʰ **S34.6 Injury of peripheral nerve(s) at abdomen, lower back and pelvis level**

☑x7ᵗʰ **S34.8 Injury of other nerves at abdomen, lower back and pelvis level**

☑x7ᵗʰ **S34.9 Injury of unspecified nerves at abdomen, lower back and pelvis level**

☑4ᵗʰ **S35 Injury of blood vessels at abdomen, lower back and pelvis level**

> Code also any associated open wound (S31.-)

> The appropriate 7th character is to be added to each code from category S35.
> A   initial encounter
> D   subsequent encounter
> S   sequela

☑5ᵗʰ **S35.0 Injury of** abdominal aorta

  EXCLUDES 1   injury of aorta NOS (S25.0)

  ☑x7ᵗʰ **S35.00 Unspecified injury of abdominal aorta**   MCC

  ☑x7ᵗʰ **S35.01 Minor laceration of abdominal aorta**   MCC
      Incomplete transection of abdominal aorta
      Laceration of abdominal aorta NOS
      Superficial laceration of abdominal aorta

  ☑x7ᵗʰ **S35.02 Major laceration of abdominal aorta**   MCC
      Complete transection of abdominal aorta
      Traumatic rupture of abdominal aorta

  ☑x7ᵗʰ **S35.09 Other injury of abdominal aorta**   MCC

☑5ᵗʰ **S35.1 Injury of** inferior vena cava

  Injury of hepatic vein
  EXCLUDES 1   injury of vena cava NOS (S25.2)

  ☑x7ᵗʰ **S35.10 Unspecified injury of inferior vena cava**   MCC

  ☑x7ᵗʰ **S35.11 Minor laceration of inferior vena cava**   MCC
      Incomplete transection of inferior vena cava
      Laceration of inferior vena cava NOS
      Superficial laceration of inferior vena cava

√x7ᵗʰ **S35.12** Major laceration of inferior vena cava MCC
  Complete transection of inferior vena cava
  Traumatic rupture of inferior vena cava

√x7ᵗʰ **S35.19** Other injury of inferior vena cava MCC

√5ᵗʰ **S35.2** Injury of celiac or mesenteric artery and branches

√6ᵗʰ **S35.21** Injury of celiac artery

√7ᵗʰ **S35.211** Minor laceration of celiac artery MCC
  Incomplete transection of celiac artery
  Laceration of celiac artery NOS
  Superficial laceration of celiac artery

√7ᵗʰ **S35.212** Major laceration of celiac artery MCC
  Complete transection of celiac artery
  Traumatic rupture of celiac artery

√7ᵗʰ **S35.218** Other injury of celiac artery MCC

√7ᵗʰ **S35.219** Unspecified injury of celiac artery MCC

√6ᵗʰ **S35.22** Injury of superior mesenteric artery

√7ᵗʰ **S35.221** Minor laceration of superior mesenteric artery MCC
  Incomplete transection of superior mesenteric artery
  Laceration of superior mesenteric artery NOS
  Superficial laceration of superior mesenteric artery

√7ᵗʰ **S35.222** Major laceration of superior mesenteric artery MCC
  Complete transection of superior mesenteric artery
  Traumatic rupture of superior mesenteric artery

√7ᵗʰ **S35.228** Other injury of superior mesenteric artery MCC

√7ᵗʰ **S35.229** Unspecified injury of superior mesenteric artery MCC

√6ᵗʰ **S35.23** Injury of inferior mesenteric artery

√7ᵗʰ **S35.231** Minor laceration of inferior mesenteric artery MCC
  Incomplete transection of inferior mesenteric artery
  Laceration of inferior mesenteric artery NOS
  Superficial laceration of inferior mesenteric artery

√7ᵗʰ **S35.232** Major laceration of inferior mesenteric artery MCC
  Complete transection of inferior mesenteric artery
  Traumatic rupture of inferior mesenteric artery

√7ᵗʰ **S35.238** Other injury of inferior mesenteric artery MCC

√7ᵗʰ **S35.239** Unspecified injury of inferior mesenteric artery MCC

√6ᵗʰ **S35.29** Injury of branches of celiac and mesenteric artery
  Injury of gastric artery
  Injury of gastroduodenal artery
  Injury of hepatic artery
  Injury of splenic artery

√7ᵗʰ **S35.291** Minor laceration of branches of celiac and mesenteric artery MCC
  Incomplete transection of branches of celiac and mesenteric artery
  Laceration of branches of celiac and mesenteric artery NOS
  Superficial laceration of branches of celiac and mesenteric artery

√7ᵗʰ **S35.292** Major laceration of branches of celiac and mesenteric artery MCC
  Complete transection of branches of celiac and mesenteric artery
  Traumatic rupture of branches of celiac and mesenteric artery

√7ᵗʰ **S35.298** Other injury of branches of celiac and mesenteric artery MCC

√7ᵗʰ **S35.299** Unspecified injury of branches of celiac and mesenteric artery MCC

√5ᵗʰ **S35.3** Injury of portal or splenic vein and branches

√6ᵗʰ **S35.31** Injury of portal vein

√7ᵗʰ **S35.311** Laceration of portal vein MCC

√7ᵗʰ **S35.318** Other specified injury of portal vein MCC

√7ᵗʰ **S35.319** Unspecified injury of portal vein MCC

√6ᵗʰ **S35.32** Injury of splenic vein

√7ᵗʰ **S35.321** Laceration of splenic vein MCC

√7ᵗʰ **S35.328** Other specified injury of splenic vein MCC

√7ᵗʰ **S35.329** Unspecified injury of splenic vein MCC

√6ᵗʰ **S35.33** Injury of superior mesenteric vein

√7ᵗʰ **S35.331** Laceration of superior mesenteric vein MCC

√7ᵗʰ **S35.338** Other specified injury of superior mesenteric vein MCC

√7ᵗʰ **S35.339** Unspecified injury of superior mesenteric vein MCC

√6ᵗʰ **S35.34** Injury of inferior mesenteric vein

√7ᵗʰ **S35.341** Laceration of inferior mesenteric vein MCC

√7ᵗʰ **S35.348** Other specified injury of inferior mesenteric vein MCC

√7ᵗʰ **S35.349** Unspecified injury of inferior mesenteric vein MCC

√5ᵗʰ **S35.4** Injury of renal blood vessels

√6ᵗʰ **S35.40** Unspecified injury of renal blood vessel

√7ᵗʰ **S35.401** Unspecified injury of right renal artery MCC

√7ᵗʰ **S35.402** Unspecified injury of left renal artery MCC

√7ᵗʰ **S35.403** Unspecified injury of unspecified renal artery MCC

√7ᵗʰ **S35.404** Unspecified injury of right renal vein MCC

√7ᵗʰ **S35.405** Unspecified injury of left renal vein MCC

√7ᵗʰ **S35.406** Unspecified injury of unspecified renal vein MCC

√6ᵗʰ **S35.41** Laceration of renal blood vessel

√7ᵗʰ **S35.411** Laceration of right renal artery MCC

√7ᵗʰ **S35.412** Laceration of left renal artery MCC

√7ᵗʰ **S35.413** Laceration of unspecified renal artery MCC

√7ᵗʰ **S35.414** Laceration of right renal vein MCC

√7ᵗʰ **S35.415** Laceration of left renal vein MCC

√7ᵗʰ **S35.416** Laceration of unspecified renal vein MCC

√6ᵗʰ **S35.49** Other specified injury of renal blood vessel

√7ᵗʰ **S35.491** Other specified injury of right renal artery MCC

√7ᵗʰ **S35.492** Other specified injury of left renal artery MCC

√7ᵗʰ **S35.493** Other specified injury of unspecified renal artery MCC

√7ᵗʰ **S35.494** Other specified injury of right renal vein MCC

√7ᵗʰ **S35.495** Other specified injury of left renal vein MCC

√7ᵗʰ **S35.496** Other specified injury of unspecified renal vein MCC

√5ᵗʰ **S35.5** Injury of iliac blood vessels

√x7ᵗʰ **S35.50** Injury of unspecified iliac blood vessel(s) MCC

√6ᵗʰ **S35.51** Injury of iliac artery or vein
  Injury of hypogastric artery or vein

√7ᵗʰ **S35.511** Injury of right iliac artery MCC

√7ᵗʰ **S35.512** Injury of left iliac artery MCC

√7ᵗʰ **S35.513** Injury of unspecified iliac artery MCC

√7ᵗʰ **S35.514** Injury of right iliac vein MCC

√7ᵗʰ **S35.515** Injury of left iliac vein MCC

√7ᵗʰ **S35.516** Injury of unspecified iliac vein MCC

√6ᵗʰ **S35.53** Injury of uterine artery or vein

√7ᵗʰ **S35.531** Injury of right uterine artery CC ♀

√7ᵗʰ **S35.532** Injury of left uterine artery CC ♀

N Newborn: 0 P Pediatric: 0-17 M Maternity: 9-64 A Adult: 15-124 MCC Major Complication/Comorbidity CC Complication/Comorbidity SW Severe Wound Dx

1004 ICD-10-CM 2022

√7ᵗʰ **S35.533** Injury of unspecified uterine artery   CC ♀

√7ᵗʰ **S35.534** Injury of right uterine vein   CC ♀

√7ᵗʰ **S35.535** Injury of left uterine vein   CC ♀

√7ᵗʰ **S35.536** Injury of unspecified uterine vein   CC ♀

√x7ᵗʰ **S35.59** Injury of other iliac blood vessels   MCC

√5ᵗʰ **S35.8** Injury of other blood vessels at abdomen, lower back and pelvis level

Injury of ovarian artery or vein

√6ᵗʰ **S35.8X** Injury of other blood vessels at abdomen, lower back and pelvis level

√7ᵗʰ **S35.8X1** Laceration of other blood vessels at abdomen, lower back and pelvis level   CC

√7ᵗʰ **S35.8X8** Other specified injury of other blood vessels at abdomen, lower back and pelvis level   CC

√7ᵗʰ **S35.8X9** Unspecified injury of other blood vessels at abdomen, lower back and pelvis level   CC

√5ᵗʰ **S35.9** Injury of unspecified blood vessel at abdomen, lower back and pelvis level

√x7ᵗʰ **S35.90** Unspecified injury of unspecified blood vessel at abdomen, lower back and pelvis level   CC

√x7ᵗʰ **S35.91** Laceration of unspecified blood vessel at abdomen, lower back and pelvis level   CC

√x7ᵗʰ **S35.99** Other specified injury of unspecified blood vessel at abdomen, lower back and pelvis level   CC

√4ᵗʰ **S36 Injury of intra-abdominal organs**

Code also any associated open wound (S31.-)

The appropriate 7th character is to be added to each code from category S36.
A   initial encounter
D   subsequent encounter
S   sequela

√5ᵗʰ **S36.0** Injury of spleen

AHA: 2015,2Q,36; 2015,1Q,10

√x7ᵗʰ **S36.00** Unspecified injury of spleen   CC

√6ᵗʰ **S36.02** Contusion of spleen

TIP: When both traumatic splenic laceration and contusion are documented in the same encounter, code only the laceration, as contusions are not coded when they occur with a more severe injury in the same body site.

√7ᵗʰ **S36.020** Minor contusion of spleen   CC

Contusion of spleen less than 2 cm

√7ᵗʰ **S36.021** Major contusion of spleen   CC

Contusion of spleen greater than 2 cm

√7ᵗʰ **S36.029** Unspecified contusion of spleen   CC

√6ᵗʰ **S36.03** Laceration of spleen

TIP: When both traumatic splenic laceration and contusion are documented in the same encounter, code only the laceration, as contusions are not coded when they occur with a more severe injury in the same body site.

√7ᵗʰ **S36.030** Superficial (capsular) laceration of spleen   CC

Laceration of spleen less than 1 cm
Minor laceration of spleen

√7ᵗʰ **S36.031** Moderate laceration of spleen   MCC

Laceration of spleen 1 to 3 cm

√7ᵗʰ **S36.032** Major laceration of spleen   MCC

Avulsion of spleen
Laceration of spleen greater than 3 cm
Massive laceration of spleen
Multiple moderate lacerations of spleen
Stellate laceration of spleen

√7ᵗʰ **S36.039** Unspecified laceration of spleen   CC

√x7ᵗʰ **S36.09** Other injury of spleen   CC

√5ᵗʰ **S36.1** Injury of liver and gallbladder and bile duct

√6ᵗʰ **S36.11** Injury of liver

√7ᵗʰ **S36.112** Contusion of liver   CC

√7ᵗʰ **S36.113** Laceration of liver, unspecified degree   CC

√7ᵗʰ **S36.114** Minor laceration of liver   CC

Laceration involving capsule only, or, without significant involvement of hepatic parenchyma [i.e., less than 1 cm deep]

√7ᵗʰ **S36.115** Moderate laceration of liver   MCC

Laceration involving parenchyma but without major disruption of parenchyma [i.e., less than 10 cm long and less than 3 cm deep]

√7ᵗʰ **S36.116** Major laceration of liver   MCC

Laceration with significant disruption of hepatic parenchyma [i.e., greater than 10 cm long and 3 cm deep]
Multiple moderate lacerations, with or without hematoma
Stellate laceration of liver

√7ᵗʰ **S36.118** Other injury of liver   CC

√7ᵗʰ **S36.119** Unspecified injury of liver   CC

√6ᵗʰ **S36.12** Injury of gallbladder

√7ᵗʰ **S36.122** Contusion of gallbladder   CC

√7ᵗʰ **S36.123** Laceration of gallbladder   CC

√7ᵗʰ **S36.128** Other injury of gallbladder   CC

√7ᵗʰ **S36.129** Unspecified injury of gallbladder   CC

√x7ᵗʰ **S36.13** Injury of bile duct   CC

√5ᵗʰ **S36.2** Injury of pancreas

√6ᵗʰ **S36.20** Unspecified injury of pancreas

√7ᵗʰ **S36.200** Unspecified injury of head of pancreas   CC

√7ᵗʰ **S36.201** Unspecified injury of body of pancreas   CC

√7ᵗʰ **S36.202** Unspecified injury of tail of pancreas   CC

√7ᵗʰ **S36.209** Unspecified injury of unspecified part of pancreas   CC

√6ᵗʰ **S36.22** Contusion of pancreas

√7ᵗʰ **S36.220** Contusion of head of pancreas   CC

√7ᵗʰ **S36.221** Contusion of body of pancreas   CC

√7ᵗʰ **S36.222** Contusion of tail of pancreas   CC

√7ᵗʰ **S36.229** Contusion of unspecified part of pancreas   CC

√6ᵗʰ **S36.23** Laceration of pancreas, unspecified degree

√7ᵗʰ **S36.230** Laceration of head of pancreas, unspecified degree   CC

√7ᵗʰ **S36.231** Laceration of body of pancreas, unspecified degree   CC

√7ᵗʰ **S36.232** Laceration of tail of pancreas, unspecified degree   CC

√7ᵗʰ **S36.239** Laceration of unspecified part of pancreas, unspecified degree   CC

√6ᵗʰ **S36.24** Minor laceration of pancreas

√7ᵗʰ **S36.240** Minor laceration of head of pancreas   CC

√7ᵗʰ **S36.241** Minor laceration of body of pancreas   CC

√7ᵗʰ **S36.242** Minor laceration of tail of pancreas   CC

√7ᵗʰ **S36.249** Minor laceration of unspecified part of pancreas   CC

√6ᵗʰ **S36.25** Moderate laceration of pancreas

√7ᵗʰ **S36.250** Moderate laceration of head of pancreas   CC

√7ᵗʰ **S36.251** Moderate laceration of body of pancreas   CC

√7ᵗʰ **S36.252** Moderate laceration of tail of pancreas   CC

√7ᵗʰ **S36.259** Moderate laceration of unspecified part of pancreas   CC

√6ᵗʰ **S36.26** Major laceration of pancreas

√7ᵗʰ **S36.260** Major laceration of head of pancreas   CC

√7ᵗʰ **S36.261** Major laceration of body of pancreas   CC

√7ᵗʰ **S36.262** Major laceration of tail of pancreas   CC

√7ᵗʰ **S36.269** Major laceration of unspecified part of pancreas   CC

☑ Additional Character Required   √x7ᵗʰ Placeholder   Questionable PDx   Manifestation   Unspecified Dx   UPD Unacceptable PDx   H1-H14 HAC   HCC CMS-HCC Dx   HIV HIV Dx

ICD-10-CM 2022   1005

√6ᵗʰ **S36.29** Other injury of pancreas
　　√7ᵗʰ **S36.290** Other injury of head of pancreas　CC
　　√7ᵗʰ **S36.291** Other injury of body of pancreas　CC
　　√7ᵗʰ **S36.292** Other injury of tail of pancreas　CC
　　√7ᵗʰ **S36.299** Other injury of unspecified part of pancreas　CC

√5ᵗʰ **S36.3** Injury of stomach
　√x7ᵗʰ **S36.30** Unspecified injury of stomach　CC
　√x7ᵗʰ **S36.32** Contusion of stomach　CC
　√x7ᵗʰ **S36.33** Laceration of stomach　CC
　√x7ᵗʰ **S36.39** Other injury of stomach　CC

√5ᵗʰ **S36.4** Injury of small intestine
　√6ᵗʰ **S36.40** Unspecified injury of small intestine
　　√7ᵗʰ **S36.400** Unspecified injury of duodenum　CC
　　√7ᵗʰ **S36.408** Unspecified injury of other part of small intestine　CC
　　√7ᵗʰ **S36.409** Unspecified injury of unspecified part of small intestine　CC
　√6ᵗʰ **S36.41** Primary blast injury of small intestine
　　　Blast injury of small intestine NOS
　　√7ᵗʰ **S36.410** Primary blast injury of duodenum　CC
　　√7ᵗʰ **S36.418** Primary blast injury of other part of small intestine　CC
　　√7ᵗʰ **S36.419** Primary blast injury of unspecified part of small intestine　CC
　√6ᵗʰ **S36.42** Contusion of small intestine
　　√7ᵗʰ **S36.420** Contusion of duodenum　CC
　　√7ᵗʰ **S36.428** Contusion of other part of small intestine　CC
　　√7ᵗʰ **S36.429** Contusion of unspecified part of small intestine　CC
　√6ᵗʰ **S36.43** Laceration of small intestine
　　√7ᵗʰ **S36.430** Laceration of duodenum　CC
　　√7ᵗʰ **S36.438** Laceration of other part of small intestine　CC
　　√7ᵗʰ **S36.439** Laceration of unspecified part of small intestine　CC
　√6ᵗʰ **S36.49** Other injury of small intestine
　　√7ᵗʰ **S36.490** Other injury of duodenum　CC
　　√7ᵗʰ **S36.498** Other injury of other part of small intestine　CC
　　√7ᵗʰ **S36.499** Other injury of unspecified part of small intestine　CC

√6ᵗʰ **S36.5** Injury of colon
　　EXCLUDES 2　injury of rectum (S36.6-)
　√6ᵗʰ **S36.50** Unspecified injury of colon
　　√7ᵗʰ **S36.500** Unspecified injury of ascending [right] colon　CC
　　√7ᵗʰ **S36.501** Unspecified injury of transverse colon　CC
　　√7ᵗʰ **S36.502** Unspecified injury of descending [left] colon　CC
　　√7ᵗʰ **S36.503** Unspecified injury of sigmoid colon　CC
　　√7ᵗʰ **S36.508** Unspecified injury of other part of colon　CC
　　√7ᵗʰ **S36.509** Unspecified injury of unspecified part of colon　CC
　√6ᵗʰ **S36.51** Primary blast injury of colon
　　　Blast injury of colon NOS
　　√7ᵗʰ **S36.510** Primary blast injury of ascending [right] colon　CC
　　√7ᵗʰ **S36.511** Primary blast injury of transverse colon　CC
　　√7ᵗʰ **S36.512** Primary blast injury of descending [left] colon　CC
　　√7ᵗʰ **S36.513** Primary blast injury of sigmoid colon　CC
　　√7ᵗʰ **S36.518** Primary blast injury of other part of colon　CC
　　√7ᵗʰ **S36.519** Primary blast injury of unspecified part of colon　CC
　√6ᵗʰ **S36.52** Contusion of colon
　　√7ᵗʰ **S36.520** Contusion of ascending [right] colon　CC

　　√7ᵗʰ **S36.521** Contusion of transverse colon　CC
　　√7ᵗʰ **S36.522** Contusion of descending [left] colon　CC
　　√7ᵗʰ **S36.523** Contusion of sigmoid colon　CC
　　√7ᵗʰ **S36.528** Contusion of other part of colon　CC
　　√7ᵗʰ **S36.529** Contusion of unspecified part of colon　CC
　√6ᵗʰ **S36.53** Laceration of colon
　　√7ᵗʰ **S36.530** Laceration of ascending [right] colon　CC
　　√7ᵗʰ **S36.531** Laceration of transverse colon　CC
　　√7ᵗʰ **S36.532** Laceration of descending [left] colon　CC
　　√7ᵗʰ **S36.533** Laceration of sigmoid colon　CC
　　√7ᵗʰ **S36.538** Laceration of other part of colon　CC
　　√7ᵗʰ **S36.539** Laceration of unspecified part of colon　CC
　√6ᵗʰ **S36.59** Other injury of colon
　　　Secondary blast injury of colon
　　√7ᵗʰ **S36.590** Other injury of ascending [right] colon　CC
　　√7ᵗʰ **S36.591** Other injury of transverse colon　CC
　　√7ᵗʰ **S36.592** Other injury of descending [left] colon　CC
　　√7ᵗʰ **S36.593** Other injury of sigmoid colon　CC
　　√7ᵗʰ **S36.598** Other injury of other part of colon　CC
　　√7ᵗʰ **S36.599** Other injury of unspecified part of colon　CC

√5ᵗʰ **S36.6** Injury of rectum
　√x7ᵗʰ **S36.60** Unspecified injury of rectum　CC
　√x7ᵗʰ **S36.61** Primary blast injury of rectum　CC
　　　Blast injury of rectum NOS
　√x7ᵗʰ **S36.62** Contusion of rectum　CC
　√x7ᵗʰ **S36.63** Laceration of rectum　CC
　√x7ᵗʰ **S36.69** Other injury of rectum　CC
　　　Secondary blast injury of rectum

√5ᵗʰ **S36.8** Injury of other intra-abdominal organs
　√x7ᵗʰ **S36.81** Injury of peritoneum　CC
　√6ᵗʰ **S36.89** Injury of other intra-abdominal organs
　　　Injury of retroperitoneum
　　√7ᵗʰ **S36.892** Contusion of other intra-abdominal organs　CC
　　√7ᵗʰ **S36.893** Laceration of other intra-abdominal organs　CC
　　√7ᵗʰ **S36.898** Other injury of other intra-abdominal organs　CC
　　√7ᵗʰ **S36.899** Unspecified injury of other intra-abdominal organs　CC

√5ᵗʰ **S36.9** Injury of unspecified intra-abdominal organ
　√x7ᵗʰ **S36.90** Unspecified injury of unspecified intra-abdominal organ　CC
　√x7ᵗʰ **S36.92** Contusion of unspecified intra-abdominal organ　CC
　√x7ᵗʰ **S36.93** Laceration of unspecified intra-abdominal organ　CC
　√x7ᵗʰ **S36.99** Other injury of unspecified intra-abdominal organ　CC

√4ᵗʰ **S37** Injury of urinary and pelvic organs
　　Code also any associated open wound (S31.-)
　　EXCLUDES 1　obstetric trauma to pelvic organs (O71.-)
　　EXCLUDES 2　injury of peritoneum (S36.81)
　　　　　　　injury of retroperitoneum (S36.89-)

　　The appropriate 7th character is to be added to each code from category S37.
　　A　initial encounter
　　D　subsequent encounter
　　S　sequela

√5ᵗʰ **S37.0** Injury of kidney
　　EXCLUDES 2　acute kidney injury (nontraumatic) (N17.9)
　√6ᵗʰ **S37.00** Unspecified injury of kidney
　　√7ᵗʰ **S37.001** Unspecified injury of right kidney　CC
　　√7ᵗʰ **S37.002** Unspecified injury of left kidney　CC

    √7ᵗʰ **S37.009** Unspecified injury of unspecified kidney   CC

√6ᵗʰ **S37.01** Minor contusion of kidney
    Contusion of kidney less than 2 cm
    Contusion of kidney NOS
    √7ᵗʰ **S37.011** Minor contusion of right kidney   CC
    √7ᵗʰ **S37.012** Minor contusion of left kidney   CC
    √7ᵗʰ **S37.019** Minor contusion of unspecified kidney   CC

√6ᵗʰ **S37.02** Major contusion of kidney
    Contusion of kidney greater than 2 cm
    √7ᵗʰ **S37.021** Major contusion of right kidney   CC
    √7ᵗʰ **S37.022** Major contusion of left kidney   CC
    √7ᵗʰ **S37.029** Major contusion of unspecified kidney   CC

√6ᵗʰ **S37.03** Laceration of kidney, unspecified degree
    √7ᵗʰ **S37.031** Laceration of right kidney, unspecified degree   CC
    √7ᵗʰ **S37.032** Laceration of left kidney, unspecified degree   CC
    √7ᵗʰ **S37.039** Laceration of unspecified kidney, unspecified degree   CC

√6ᵗʰ **S37.04** Minor laceration of kidney
    Laceration of kidney less than 1 cm
    √7ᵗʰ **S37.041** Minor laceration of right kidney   CC
    √7ᵗʰ **S37.042** Minor laceration of left kidney   CC
    √7ᵗʰ **S37.049** Minor laceration of unspecified kidney   CC

√6ᵗʰ **S37.05** Moderate laceration of kidney
    Laceration of kidney 1 to 3 cm
    √7ᵗʰ **S37.051** Moderate laceration of right kidney   CC
    √7ᵗʰ **S37.052** Moderate laceration of left kidney   CC
    √7ᵗʰ **S37.059** Moderate laceration of unspecified kidney   CC

√6ᵗʰ **S37.06** Major laceration of kidney
    Avulsion of kidney
    Laceration of kidney greater than 3 cm
    Massive laceration of kidney
    Multiple moderate lacerations of kidney
    Stellate laceration of kidney
    √7ᵗʰ **S37.061** Major laceration of right kidney   MCC
    √7ᵗʰ **S37.062** Major laceration of left kidney   MCC
    √7ᵗʰ **S37.069** Major laceration of unspecified kidney   MCC

√6ᵗʰ **S37.09** Other injury of kidney
    √7ᵗʰ **S37.091** Other injury of right kidney   MCC
    √7ᵗʰ **S37.092** Other injury of left kidney   MCC
    √7ᵗʰ **S37.099** Other injury of unspecified kidney   MCC

√5ᵗʰ **S37.1** Injury of ureter
    √×7ᵗʰ **S37.10** Unspecified injury of ureter   CC
    √×7ᵗʰ **S37.12** Contusion of ureter   CC
    √×7ᵗʰ **S37.13** Laceration of ureter   CC
    √×7ᵗʰ **S37.19** Other injury of ureter   CC

√5ᵗʰ **S37.2** Injury of bladder
    √×7ᵗʰ **S37.20** Unspecified injury of bladder   CC
    √×7ᵗʰ **S37.22** Contusion of bladder   CC
    √×7ᵗʰ **S37.23** Laceration of bladder   CC
    √×7ᵗʰ **S37.29** Other injury of bladder   CC

√5ᵗʰ **S37.3** Injury of urethra
    √×7ᵗʰ **S37.30** Unspecified injury of urethra   CC
    √×7ᵗʰ **S37.32** Contusion of urethra   CC
    √×7ᵗʰ **S37.33** Laceration of urethra   CC
    √×7ᵗʰ **S37.39** Other injury of urethra   CC

√5ᵗʰ **S37.4** Injury of ovary
    √6ᵗʰ **S37.40** Unspecified injury of ovary
        √7ᵗʰ **S37.401** Unspecified injury of ovary, unilateral   ♀
        √7ᵗʰ **S37.402** Unspecified injury of ovary, bilateral   ♀

        √7ᵗʰ **S37.409** Unspecified injury of ovary, unspecified   ♀

√6ᵗʰ **S37.42** Contusion of ovary
    √7ᵗʰ **S37.421** Contusion of ovary, unilateral   ♀
    √7ᵗʰ **S37.422** Contusion of ovary, bilateral   ♀
    √7ᵗʰ **S37.429** Contusion of ovary, unspecified   ♀

√6ᵗʰ **S37.43** Laceration of ovary
    √7ᵗʰ **S37.431** Laceration of ovary, unilateral   ♀
    √7ᵗʰ **S37.432** Laceration of ovary, bilateral   ♀
    √7ᵗʰ **S37.439** Laceration of ovary, unspecified   ♀

√6ᵗʰ **S37.49** Other injury of ovary
    √7ᵗʰ **S37.491** Other injury of ovary, unilateral   ♀
    √7ᵗʰ **S37.492** Other injury of ovary, bilateral   ♀
    √7ᵗʰ **S37.499** Other injury of ovary, unspecified   ♀

√5ᵗʰ **S37.5** Injury of fallopian tube
    √6ᵗʰ **S37.50** Unspecified injury of fallopian tube
        √7ᵗʰ **S37.501** Unspecified injury of fallopian tube, unilateral   ♀
        √7ᵗʰ **S37.502** Unspecified injury of fallopian tube, bilateral   ♀
        √7ᵗʰ **S37.509** Unspecified injury of fallopian tube, unspecified   ♀

    √6ᵗʰ **S37.51** Primary blast injury of fallopian tube
        Blast injury of fallopian tube NOS
        √7ᵗʰ **S37.511** Primary blast injury of fallopian tube, unilateral   ♀
        √7ᵗʰ **S37.512** Primary blast injury of fallopian tube, bilateral   ♀
        √7ᵗʰ **S37.519** Primary blast injury of fallopian tube, unspecified   ♀

    √6ᵗʰ **S37.52** Contusion of fallopian tube
        √7ᵗʰ **S37.521** Contusion of fallopian tube, unilateral   ♀
        √7ᵗʰ **S37.522** Contusion of fallopian tube, bilateral   ♀
        √7ᵗʰ **S37.529** Contusion of fallopian tube, unspecified   ♀

    √6ᵗʰ **S37.53** Laceration of fallopian tube
        √7ᵗʰ **S37.531** Laceration of fallopian tube, unilateral   ♀
        √7ᵗʰ **S37.532** Laceration of fallopian tube, bilateral   ♀
        √7ᵗʰ **S37.539** Laceration of fallopian tube, unspecified   ♀

    √6ᵗʰ **S37.59** Other injury of fallopian tube
        Secondary blast injury of fallopian tube
        √7ᵗʰ **S37.591** Other injury of fallopian tube, unilateral   ♀
        √7ᵗʰ **S37.592** Other injury of fallopian tube, bilateral   ♀
        √7ᵗʰ **S37.599** Other injury of fallopian tube, unspecified   ♀

√5ᵗʰ **S37.6** Injury of uterus
    EXCLUDES 1   injury to gravid uterus (O9A.2-)
                       injury to uterus during delivery (O71.-)
    √×7ᵗʰ **S37.60** Unspecified injury of uterus   CC ♀
    √×7ᵗʰ **S37.62** Contusion of uterus   CC ♀
    √×7ᵗʰ **S37.63** Laceration of uterus   CC ♀
    √×7ᵗʰ **S37.69** Other injury of uterus   CC ♀

√5ᵗʰ **S37.8** Injury of other urinary and pelvic organs
    √6ᵗʰ **S37.81** Injury of adrenal gland
        √7ᵗʰ **S37.812** Contusion of adrenal gland   CC
        √7ᵗʰ **S37.813** Laceration of adrenal gland   CC
        √7ᵗʰ **S37.818** Other injury of adrenal gland   CC
        √7ᵗʰ **S37.819** Unspecified injury of adrenal gland   CC

    √6ᵗʰ **S37.82** Injury of prostate
        √7ᵗʰ **S37.822** Contusion of prostate   ♂
        √7ᵗʰ **S37.823** Laceration of prostate   ♂
        √7ᵗʰ **S37.828** Other injury of prostate   ♂
        √7ᵗʰ **S37.829** Unspecified injury of prostate   ♂

Chapter 19. Injury, Poisoning and Certain Other Consequences of External Causes

✓6ᵗʰ **S37.89** Injury of other urinary and pelvic organ

✓7ᵗʰ **S37.892** Contususion of other urinary and pelvic organ **cc**

✓7ᵗʰ **S37.893** Laceration of other urinary and pelvic organ **cc**

✓7ᵗʰ **S37.898** Other injury of other urinary and pelvic organ **cc**

✓7ᵗʰ **S37.899** Unspecified injury of other urinary and pelvic organ **cc**

✓5ᵗʰ **S37.9** Injury of unspecified urinary and pelvic organ

✓x7ᵗʰ **S37.90** Unspecified injury of unspecified urinary and pelvic organ **cc**

✓x7ᵗʰ **S37.92** Contusion of unspecified urinary and pelvic organ **cc**

✓x7ᵗʰ **S37.93** Laceration of unspecified urinary and pelvic organ **cc**

✓x7ᵗʰ **S37.99** Other injury of unspecified urinary and pelvic organ **cc**

✓4ᵗʰ **S38** Crushing injury and traumatic amputation of abdomen, lower back, pelvis and external genitals

> **NOTE** An amputation not identified as partial or complete should be coded to complete

> The appropriate 7th character is to be added to each code from category S38.
> A initial encounter
> D subsequent encounter
> S sequela

✓5ᵗʰ **S38.0** Crushing injury of external genital organs

Use additional code for any associated injuries

✓6ᵗʰ **S38.00** Crushing injury of unspecified external genital organs

✓7ᵗʰ **S38.001** Crushing injury of unspecified external genital organs, male ♂

✓7ᵗʰ **S38.002** Crushing injury of unspecified external genital organs, female ♀

✓x7ᵗʰ **S38.01** Crushing injury of penis ♂

✓x7ᵗʰ **S38.02** Crushing injury of scrotum and testis ♂

✓x7ᵗʰ **S38.03** Crushing injury of vulva ♀

✓x7ᵗʰ **S38.1** Crushing injury of abdomen, lower back, and pelvis

Use additional code for all associated injuries, such as:
fracture of thoracic or lumbar spine and pelvis (S22.0-, S32.-)
injury to intra-abdominal organs (S36.-)
injury to urinary and pelvic organs (S37.-)
open wound of abdominal wall (S31.-)
spinal cord injury (S34.0, S34.1-)

> **EXCLUDES 2** crushing injury of external genital organs (S38.0-)

✓5ᵗʰ **S38.2** Traumatic amputation of external genital organs

✓6ᵗʰ **S38.21** Traumatic amputation of female external genital organs

Traumatic amputation of clitoris
Traumatic amputation of labium (majus) (minus)
Traumatic amputation of vulva

✓7ᵗʰ **S38.211** Complete traumatic amputation of female external genital organs ♀

✓7ᵗʰ **S38.212** Partial traumatic amputation of female external genital organs ♀

✓6ᵗʰ **S38.22** Traumatic amputation of penis

✓7ᵗʰ **S38.221** Complete traumatic amputation of penis ♂

✓7ᵗʰ **S38.222** Partial traumatic amputation of penis ♂

✓6ᵗʰ **S38.23** Traumatic amputation of scrotum and testis

✓7ᵗʰ **S38.231** Complete traumatic amputation of scrotum and testis ♂

✓7ᵗʰ **S38.232** Partial traumatic amputation of scrotum and testis ♂

✓x7ᵗʰ **S38.3** Transection (partial) of abdomen

✓4ᵗʰ **S39** Other and unspecified injuries of abdomen, lower back, pelvis and external genitals

Code also any associated open wound (S31.-)

> **EXCLUDES 2** sprain of joints and ligaments of lumbar spine and pelvis (S33.-)

> The appropriate 7th character is to be added to each code from category S39.
> A initial encounter
> D subsequent encounter
> S sequela

✓5ᵗʰ **S39.0** Injury of muscle, fascia and tendon of abdomen, lower back and pelvis

✓6ᵗʰ **S39.00** Unspecified injury of muscle, fascia and tendon of abdomen, lower back and pelvis

✓7ᵗʰ **S39.001** Unspecified injury of muscle, fascia and tendon of abdomen

✓7ᵗʰ **S39.002** Unspecified injury of muscle, fascia and tendon of lower back

✓7ᵗʰ **S39.003** Unspecified injury of muscle, fascia and tendon of pelvis

✓6ᵗʰ **S39.01** Strain of muscle, fascia and tendon of abdomen, lower back and pelvis

✓7ᵗʰ **S39.011** Strain of muscle, fascia and tendon of abdomen

✓7ᵗʰ **S39.012** Strain of muscle, fascia and tendon of lower back

✓7ᵗʰ **S39.013** Strain of muscle, fascia and tendon of pelvis

✓6ᵗʰ **S39.02** Laceration of muscle, fascia and tendon of abdomen, lower back and pelvis

✓7ᵗʰ **S39.021** Laceration of muscle, fascia and tendon of abdomen

✓7ᵗʰ **S39.022** Laceration of muscle, fascia and tendon of lower back

✓7ᵗʰ **S39.023** Laceration of muscle, fascia and tendon of pelvis

✓6ᵗʰ **S39.09** Other injury of muscle, fascia and tendon of abdomen, lower back and pelvis

✓7ᵗʰ **S39.091** Other injury of muscle, fascia and tendon of abdomen

✓7ᵗʰ **S39.092** Other injury of muscle, fascia and tendon of lower back

✓7ᵗʰ **S39.093** Other injury of muscle, fascia and tendon of pelvis

✓5ᵗʰ **S39.8** Other specified injuries of abdomen, lower back, pelvis and external genitals

✓x7ᵗʰ **S39.81** Other specified injuries of abdomen

✓x7ᵗʰ **S39.82** Other specified injuries of lower back

✓x7ᵗʰ **S39.83** Other specified injuries of pelvis

✓6ᵗʰ **S39.84** Other specified injuries of external genitals

✓7ᵗʰ **S39.840** Fracture of corpus cavernosum penis ♂

✓7ᵗʰ **S39.848** Other specified injuries of external genitals

✓5ᵗʰ **S39.9** Unspecified injury of abdomen, lower back, pelvis and external genitals

✓x7ᵗʰ **S39.91** Unspecified injury of abdomen

✓x7ᵗʰ **S39.92** Unspecified injury of lower back

✓x7ᵗʰ **S39.93** Unspecified injury of pelvis

✓x7ᵗʰ **S39.94** Unspecified injury of external genitals

Injuries to the shoulder and upper arm (S40-S49)

> **INCLUDES** injuries of axilla
> injuries of scapular region
> **EXCLUDES 2** burns and corrosions (T20-T32)
> frostbite (T33-T34)
> injuries of elbow (S50-S59)
> insect bite or sting, venomous (T63.4)

✓4ᵗʰ **S40** Superficial injury of shoulder and upper arm

> The appropriate 7th character is to be added to each code from category S40.
> A initial encounter
> D subsequent encounter
> S sequela

✓5ᵗʰ **S40.0** Contusion of shoulder and upper arm

✓6ᵗʰ **S40.01** Contusion of shoulder

✓7ᵗʰ **S40.011** Contusion of right shoulder

N Newborn: 0 **P** Pediatric: 0-17 **M** Maternity: 9-64 **A** Adult: 15-124 **MCC** Major Complication/Comorbidity **CC** Complication/Comorbidity **SW** Severe Wound Dx

1008

ICD-10-CM 2022

√7ᵗʰ **S40.012 Contusion of** left **shoulder**

√7ᵗʰ **S40.019 Contusion of unspecified shoulder**

√6ᵗʰ **S40.02 Contusion of** upper arm

√7ᵗʰ **S40.021 Contusion of** right **upper arm**

√7ᵗʰ **S40.022 Contusion of** left **upper arm**

√7ᵗʰ **S40.029 Contusion of unspecified upper arm**

√5ᵗʰ **S40.2 Other superficial injuries of** shoulder

√6ᵗʰ **S40.21 Abrasion of shoulder**

√7ᵗʰ **S40.211 Abrasion of** right **shoulder**

√7ᵗʰ **S40.212 Abrasion of** left **shoulder**

√7ᵗʰ **S40.219 Abrasion of unspecified shoulder**

√6ᵗʰ **S40.22 Blister (nonthermal) of shoulder**

√7ᵗʰ **S40.221 Blister (nonthermal) of** right **shoulder**

√7ᵗʰ **S40.222 Blister (nonthermal) of** left **shoulder**

√7ᵗʰ **S40.229 Blister (nonthermal) of unspecified shoulder**

√6ᵗʰ **S40.24 External constriction of shoulder**

√7ᵗʰ **S40.241 External constriction of** right **shoulder**

√7ᵗʰ **S40.242 External constriction of** left **shoulder**

√7ᵗʰ **S40.249 External constriction of unspecified shoulder**

√6ᵗʰ **S40.25 Superficial** foreign body **of shoulder**

Splinter in the shoulder

√7ᵗʰ **S40.251 Superficial foreign body of** right **shoulder**

√7ᵗʰ **S40.252 Superficial foreign body of** left **shoulder**

√7ᵗʰ **S40.259 Superficial foreign body of unspecified shoulder**

√6ᵗʰ **S40.26 Insect bite (nonvenomous) of shoulder**

√7ᵗʰ **S40.261 Insect bite (nonvenomous) of** right **shoulder**

√7ᵗʰ **S40.262 Insect bite (nonvenomous) of** left **shoulder**

√7ᵗʰ **S40.269 Insect bite (nonvenomous) of unspecified shoulder**

√6ᵗʰ **S40.27 Other superficial** bite **of shoulder**

EXCLUDES 1   *open bite of shoulder (S41.05)*

√7ᵗʰ **S40.271 Other superficial bite of** right **shoulder**

√7ᵗʰ **S40.272 Other superficial bite of** left **shoulder**

√7ᵗʰ **S40.279 Other superficial bite of unspecified shoulder**

√5ᵗʰ **S40.8 Other superficial injuries of** upper arm

√6ᵗʰ **S40.81 Abrasion of upper arm**

√7ᵗʰ **S40.811 Abrasion of** right **upper arm**

√7ᵗʰ **S40.812 Abrasion of** left **upper arm**

√7ᵗʰ **S40.819 Abrasion of unspecified upper arm**

√6ᵗʰ **S40.82 Blister (nonthermal) of upper arm**

√7ᵗʰ **S40.821 Blister (nonthermal) of** right **upper arm**

√7ᵗʰ **S40.822 Blister (nonthermal) of** left **upper arm**

√7ᵗʰ **S40.829 Blister (nonthermal) of unspecified upper arm**

√6ᵗʰ **S40.84 External constriction of upper arm**

√7ᵗʰ **S40.841 External constriction of** right **upper arm**

√7ᵗʰ **S40.842 External constriction of** left **upper arm**

√7ᵗʰ **S40.849 External constriction of unspecified upper arm**

√6ᵗʰ **S40.85 Superficial** foreign body **of upper arm**

Splinter in the upper arm

√7ᵗʰ **S40.851 Superficial foreign body of** right **upper arm**

√7ᵗʰ **S40.852 Superficial foreign body of** left **upper arm**

√7ᵗʰ **S40.859 Superficial foreign body of unspecified upper arm**

√6ᵗʰ **S40.86 Insect bite (nonvenomous) of upper arm**

√7ᵗʰ **S40.861 Insect bite (nonvenomous) of** right **upper arm**

√7ᵗʰ **S40.862 Insect bite (nonvenomous) of** left **upper arm**

√7ᵗʰ **S40.869 Insect bite (nonvenomous) of unspecified upper arm**

√6ᵗʰ **S40.87 Other superficial** bite **of upper arm**

EXCLUDES 1   *open bite of upper arm (S41.14)*

EXCLUDES 2   *other superficial bite of shoulder (S40.27-)*

√7ᵗʰ **S40.871 Other superficial bite of** right **upper arm**

√7ᵗʰ **S40.872 Other superficial bite of** left **upper arm**

√7ᵗʰ **S40.879 Other superficial bite of unspecified upper arm**

√5ᵗʰ **S40.9 Unspecified superficial injury of shoulder and upper arm**

√6ᵗʰ **S40.91 Unspecified superficial injury of** shoulder

√7ᵗʰ **S40.911 Unspecified superficial injury of** right **shoulder**

√7ᵗʰ **S40.912 Unspecified superficial injury of** left **shoulder**

√7ᵗʰ **S40.919 Unspecified superficial injury of unspecified shoulder**

√6ᵗʰ **S40.92 Unspecified superficial injury of** upper arm

√7ᵗʰ **S40.921 Unspecified superficial injury of** right **upper arm**

√7ᵗʰ **S40.922 Unspecified superficial injury of** left **upper arm**

√7ᵗʰ **S40.929 Unspecified superficial injury of unspecified upper arm**

√4ᵗʰ **S41 Open wound of shoulder and upper arm**

Code also any associated wound infection

EXCLUDES 1   *traumatic amputation of shoulder and upper arm (S48.-)*

EXCLUDES 2   *open fracture of shoulder and upper arm (S42.- with 7th character B or C)*

The appropriate 7th character is to be added to each code from category S41.
A   initial encounter
D   subsequent encounter
S   sequela

√5ᵗʰ **S41.0 Open wound of** shoulder

√6ᵗʰ **S41.00 Unspecified open wound of shoulder**

√7ᵗʰ **S41.001 Unspecified open wound of** right **shoulder**

√7ᵗʰ **S41.002 Unspecified open wound of** left **shoulder**

√7ᵗʰ **S41.009 Unspecified open wound of unspecified shoulder**

√6ᵗʰ **S41.01 Laceration without foreign body of shoulder**

√7ᵗʰ **S41.011 Laceration without foreign body of** right **shoulder**

√7ᵗʰ **S41.012 Laceration without foreign body of** left **shoulder**

√7ᵗʰ **S41.019 Laceration without foreign body of unspecified shoulder**

√6ᵗʰ **S41.02 Laceration with foreign body of shoulder**

√7ᵗʰ **S41.021 Laceration with foreign body of** right **shoulder**

√7ᵗʰ **S41.022 Laceration with foreign body of** left **shoulder**

√7ᵗʰ **S41.029 Laceration with foreign body of unspecified shoulder**

√6ᵗʰ **S41.03 Puncture wound without foreign body of shoulder**

√7ᵗʰ **S41.031 Puncture wound without foreign body of** right **shoulder**

√7ᵗʰ **S41.032 Puncture wound without foreign body of** left **shoulder**

√7ᵗʰ **S41.039 Puncture wound without foreign body of unspecified shoulder**

√6ᵗʰ **S41.04 Puncture wound with foreign body of shoulder**

√7ᵗʰ **S41.041 Puncture wound with foreign body of** right **shoulder**

√7ᵗʰ **S41.042 Puncture wound with foreign body of** left **shoulder**

√7ᵗʰ **S41.049 Puncture wound with foreign body of unspecified shoulder**

√6ᵗʰ **S41.05 Open bite of shoulder**

Bite of shoulder NOS

EXCLUDES 1   *superficial bite of shoulder (S40.27)*

√7ᵗʰ **S41.051 Open bite of** right **shoulder**

√7ᵗʰ **S41.052 Open bite of** left **shoulder**

√7ᵗʰ **S41.059 Open bite of unspecified shoulder**

√5ᵗʰ S41.1   Open wound of upper arm

    √6ᵗʰ S41.10   Unspecified open wound of upper arm

       AHA: 2016,3Q,24

       √7ᵗʰ S41.101   Unspecified open wound of right **upper arm**

       √7ᵗʰ S41.102   Unspecified open wound of left **upper arm**

       √7ᵗʰ S41.109   Unspecified open wound of unspecified upper arm

    √6ᵗʰ S41.11   Laceration without foreign body of upper arm

       √7ᵗʰ S41.111   Laceration without foreign body of right **upper arm**

       √7ᵗʰ S41.112   Laceration without foreign body of left **upper arm**

       √7ᵗʰ S41.119   Laceration without foreign body of unspecified upper arm

    √6ᵗʰ S41.12   Laceration with foreign body of upper arm

       √7ᵗʰ S41.121   Laceration with foreign body of right **upper arm**

       √7ᵗʰ S41.122   Laceration with foreign body of left **upper arm**

       √7ᵗʰ S41.129   Laceration with foreign body of unspecified upper arm

    √6ᵗʰ S41.13   Puncture wound without foreign body of upper arm

       AHA: 2016,3Q,24

       √7ᵗʰ S41.131   Puncture wound without foreign body of right upper arm

       √7ᵗʰ S41.132   Puncture wound without foreign body of left upper arm

       √7ᵗʰ S41.139   Puncture wound without foreign body of unspecified upper arm

    √6ᵗʰ S41.14   Puncture wound with foreign body of upper arm

       AHA: 2016,3Q,24

       √7ᵗʰ S41.141   Puncture wound with foreign body of right upper arm

       √7ᵗʰ S41.142   Puncture wound with foreign body of left **upper arm**

       √7ᵗʰ S41.149   Puncture wound with foreign body of unspecified upper arm

    √6ᵗʰ S41.15   Open bite of upper arm

       Bite of upper arm NOS

       EXCLUDES 1   *superficial bite of upper arm (S40.87)*

       √7ᵗʰ S41.151   Open bite of right **upper arm**

       √7ᵗʰ S41.152   Open bite of left **upper arm**

       √7ᵗʰ S41.159   Open bite of unspecified upper arm

√4ᵗʰ S42   Fracture of shoulder and upper arm

    NOTE   A fracture not indicated as displaced or nondisplaced should be coded to displaced

       A fracture not indicated as open or closed should be coded to closed

    EXCLUDES 1   *traumatic amputation of shoulder and upper arm (S48.-)*

    AHA: 2018,2Q,12; 2015,3Q,37-39

    DEF: Diaphysis: Central shaft of a long bone.

    DEF: Epiphysis: Proximal and distal rounded ends of a long bone, communicates with the joint.

    DEF: Metaphysis: Section of a long bone located between the epiphysis and diaphysis at the proximal and distal ends.

    DEF: Physis (growth plate): Narrow zone of cartilaginous tissue between the epiphysis and metaphysis at each end of a long bone. In childhood, proliferation of cells in this zone lengthens the bone. As the bone matures, this area thins, ossification eventually fusing into solid bone and growth stops. *Synonym(s):* Epiphyseal plate.

> The appropriate 7th character is to be added to all codes from category S42 [unless otherwise indicated].
> A   initial encounter for closed fracture
> B   initial encounter for open fracture
> D   subsequent encounter for fracture with routine healing
> G   subsequent encounter for fracture with delayed healing
> K   subsequent encounter for fracture with nonunion
> P   subsequent encounter for fracture with malunion
> S   sequela

    √5ᵗʰ S42.0   Fracture of clavicle

       √6ᵗʰ S42.00   Fracture of unspecified part of clavicle

          ³ **√7ᵗʰ S42.001   Fracture of unspecified part of** right **clavicle** CC H5

          ³ **√7ᵗʰ S42.002   Fracture of unspecified part of** left **clavicle** CC H5

          ³ **√7ᵗʰ S42.009   Fracture of unspecified part of unspecified clavicle** CC H5

             AHA: 2012,4Q,93

       √6ᵗʰ S42.01   Fracture of sternal end of clavicle

          ³ **√7ᵗʰ S42.011   Anterior displaced fracture of sternal end of** right **clavicle** CC H5

          ³ **√7ᵗʰ S42.012   Anterior displaced fracture of sternal end of** left **clavicle** CC H5

          ³ **√7ᵗʰ S42.013   Anterior displaced fracture of sternal end of unspecified clavicle** CC H5

             Displaced fracture of sternal end of clavicle NOS

          ³ **√7ᵗʰ S42.014   Posterior displaced fracture of sternal end of** right **clavicle** CC H5

          ³ **√7ᵗʰ S42.015   Posterior displaced fracture of sternal end of** left **clavicle** CC H5

          ³ **√7ᵗʰ S42.016   Posterior displaced fracture of sternal end of unspecified clavicle** CC H5

          ³ **√7ᵗʰ S42.017   Nondisplaced fracture of sternal end of** right **clavicle** CC H5

          ³ **√7ᵗʰ S42.018   Nondisplaced fracture of sternal end of** left **clavicle** CC H5

          ³ **√7ᵗʰ S42.019   Nondisplaced fracture of sternal end of unspecified clavicle** CC H5

       √6ᵗʰ S42.02   Fracture of shaft of clavicle

          ³ **√7ᵗʰ S42.021   Displaced fracture of shaft of** right **clavicle** CC H5

          ³ **√7ᵗʰ S42.022   Displaced fracture of shaft of** left **clavicle** CC H5

          ³ **√7ᵗʰ S42.023   Displaced fracture of shaft of unspecified clavicle** CC H5

          ³ **√7ᵗʰ S42.024   Nondisplaced fracture of shaft of** right **clavicle** CC H5

          ³ **√7ᵗʰ S42.025   Nondisplaced fracture of shaft of** left **clavicle** CC H5

          ³ **√7ᵗʰ S42.026   Nondisplaced fracture of shaft of unspecified clavicle** CC H5

       √6ᵗʰ S42.03   Fracture of lateral end of clavicle

          Fracture of acromial end of clavicle

          ³ **√7ᵗʰ S42.031   Displaced fracture of lateral end of** right **clavicle** CC H5

          ³ **√7ᵗʰ S42.032   Displaced fracture of lateral end of** left **clavicle** CC H5

          ³ **√7ᵗʰ S42.033   Displaced fracture of lateral end of unspecified clavicle** CC H5

          ³ **√7ᵗʰ S42.034   Nondisplaced fracture of lateral end of** right **clavicle** CC H5

          ³ **√7ᵗʰ S42.035   Nondisplaced fracture of lateral end of** left **clavicle** CC H5

          ³ **√7ᵗʰ S42.036   Nondisplaced fracture of lateral end of unspecified clavicle** CC H5

    √5ᵗʰ S42.1   Fracture of scapula

       √6ᵗʰ S42.10   Fracture of unspecified part of scapula

          ³ **√7ᵗʰ S42.101   Fracture of unspecified part of scapula, right shoulder** CC H5

          ³ **√7ᵗʰ S42.102   Fracture of unspecified part of scapula, left shoulder** CC H5

          ³ **√7ᵗʰ S42.109   Fracture of unspecified part of scapula, unspecified shoulder** CC H5

       √6ᵗʰ S42.11   Fracture of body of scapula

          ³ **√7ᵗʰ S42.111   Displaced fracture of body of scapula, right shoulder** CC H5

          ³ **√7ᵗʰ S42.112   Displaced fracture of body of scapula,** left **shoulder** CC H5

          ³ **√7ᵗʰ S42.113   Displaced fracture of body of scapula, unspecified shoulder** CC H5

          ³ **√7ᵗʰ S42.114   Nondisplaced fracture of body of scapula, right shoulder** CC H5

          ³ **√7ᵗʰ S42.115   Nondisplaced fracture of body of scapula, left shoulder** CC H5

          ³ **√7ᵗʰ S42.116   Nondisplaced fracture of body of scapula, unspecified shoulder** CC H5

       √6ᵗʰ S42.12   Fracture of acromial process

          ³ **√7ᵗʰ S42.121   Displaced fracture of acromial process, right shoulder** CC H5

N Newborn: 0   P Pediatric: 0-17   M Maternity: 9-64   A Adult: 15-124   MCC Major Complication/Comorbidity   CC Complication/Comorbidity   SW Severe Wound Dx

1010   ICD-10-CM 2022

³ √7ᵗʰ **S42.122** Displaced fracture of acromial process, left shoulder `CC` `H5`

³ √7ᵗʰ **S42.123** Displaced fracture of acromial process, unspecified shoulder `CC` `H5`

³ √7ᵗʰ **S42.124** Nondisplaced fracture of acromial process, right shoulder `CC` `H5`

³ √7ᵗʰ **S42.125** Nondisplaced fracture of acromial process, left shoulder `CC` `H5`

³ √7ᵗʰ **S42.126** Nondisplaced fracture of acromial process, unspecified shoulder `CC` `H5`

√6ᵗʰ **S42.13** Fracture of coracoid process

³ √7ᵗʰ **S42.131** Displaced fracture of coracoid process, right shoulder `CC` `H5`

³ √7ᵗʰ **S42.132** Displaced fracture of coracoid process, left shoulder `CC` `H5`

³ √7ᵗʰ **S42.133** Displaced fracture of coracoid process, unspecified shoulder `CC` `H5`

³ √7ᵗʰ **S42.134** Nondisplaced fracture of coracoid process, right shoulder `CC` `H5`

³ √7ᵗʰ **S42.135** Nondisplaced fracture of coracoid process, left shoulder `CC` `H5`

³ √7ᵗʰ **S42.136** Nondisplaced fracture of coracoid process, unspecified shoulder `CC` `H5`

√6ᵗʰ **S42.14** Fracture of glenoid cavity of scapula

³ √7ᵗʰ **S42.141** Displaced fracture of glenoid cavity of scapula, right shoulder `CC` `H5`

³ √7ᵗʰ **S42.142** Displaced fracture of glenoid cavity of scapula, left shoulder `CC` `H5`

³ √7ᵗʰ **S42.143** Displaced fracture of glenoid cavity of scapula, unspecified shoulder `CC` `H5`

³ √7ᵗʰ **S42.144** Nondisplaced fracture of glenoid cavity of scapula, right shoulder `CC` `H5`

³ √7ᵗʰ **S42.145** Nondisplaced fracture of glenoid cavity of scapula, left shoulder `CC` `H5`

³ √7ᵗʰ **S42.146** Nondisplaced fracture of glenoid cavity of scapula, unspecified shoulder `CC` `H5`

√6ᵗʰ **S42.15** Fracture of neck of scapula

³ √7ᵗʰ **S42.151** Displaced fracture of neck of scapula, right shoulder `CC` `H5`

³ √7ᵗʰ **S42.152** Displaced fracture of neck of scapula, left shoulder `CC` `H5`

³ √7ᵗʰ **S42.153** Displaced fracture of neck of scapula, unspecified shoulder `CC` `H5`

³ √7ᵗʰ **S42.154** Nondisplaced fracture of neck of scapula, right shoulder `CC` `H5`

³ √7ᵗʰ **S42.155** Nondisplaced fracture of neck of scapula, left shoulder `CC` `H5`

³ √7ᵗʰ **S42.156** Nondisplaced fracture of neck of scapula, unspecified shoulder `CC` `H5`

√6ᵗʰ **S42.19** Fracture of other part of scapula

³ √7ᵗʰ **S42.191** Fracture of other part of scapula, right shoulder `CC` `H5`

³ √7ᵗʰ **S42.192** Fracture of other part of scapula, left shoulder `CC` `H5`

³ √7ᵗʰ **S42.199** Fracture of other part of scapula, unspecified shoulder `CC` `H5`

√5ᵗʰ **S42.2** Fracture of upper end of humerus

Fracture of proximal end of humerus

EXCLUDES 2 *fracture of shaft of humerus (S42.3-)*
physeal fracture of upper end of humerus (S49.0-)

√6ᵗʰ **S42.20** Unspecified fracture of upper end of humerus

²,³ √7ᵗʰ **S42.201** Unspecified fracture of upper end of right humerus `MCC` `CC` `H5`

²,³ √7ᵗʰ **S42.202** Unspecified fracture of upper end of left humerus `MCC` `CC` `H5`

²,³ √7ᵗʰ **S42.209** Unspecified fracture of upper end of unspecified humerus `MCC` `CC` `H5`

√6ᵗʰ **S42.21** Unspecified fracture of surgical neck of humerus

Fracture of neck of humerus NOS

²,³ √7ᵗʰ **S42.211** Unspecified displaced fracture of surgical neck of right humerus `MCC` `CC` `H5`

²,³ √7ᵗʰ **S42.212** Unspecified displaced fracture of surgical neck of left humerus `MCC` `CC` `H5`

²,³ √7ᵗʰ **S42.213** Unspecified displaced fracture of surgical neck of unspecified humerus `MCC` `CC` `H5`

²,³ √7ᵗʰ **S42.214** Unspecified nondisplaced fracture of surgical neck of right humerus `MCC` `CC` `H5`

²,³ √7ᵗʰ **S42.215** Unspecified nondisplaced fracture of surgical neck of left humerus `MCC` `CC` `H5`

²,³ √7ᵗʰ **S42.216** Unspecified nondisplaced fracture of surgical neck of unspecified humerus `MCC` `CC` `H5`

√6ᵗʰ **S42.22** 2-part fracture of surgical neck of humerus

²,³ √7ᵗʰ **S42.221** 2-part displaced fracture of surgical neck of right humerus `MCC` `CC` `H5`

²,³ √7ᵗʰ **S42.222** 2-part displaced fracture of surgical neck of left humerus `MCC` `CC` `H5`

²,³ √7ᵗʰ **S42.223** 2-part displaced fracture of surgical neck of unspecified humerus `MCC` `CC` `H5`

²,³ √7ᵗʰ **S42.224** 2-part nondisplaced fracture of surgical neck of right humerus `MCC` `CC` `H5`

²,³ √7ᵗʰ **S42.225** 2-part nondisplaced fracture of surgical neck of left humerus `MCC` `CC` `H5`

²,³ √7ᵗʰ **S42.226** 2-part nondisplaced fracture of surgical neck of unspecified humerus `MCC` `CC` `H5`

√6ᵗʰ **S42.23** 3-part fracture of surgical neck of humerus

²,³ √7ᵗʰ **S42.231** 3-part fracture of surgical neck of right humerus `MCC` `CC` `H5`

²,³ √7ᵗʰ **S42.232** 3-part fracture of surgical neck of left humerus `MCC` `CC` `H5`

²,³ √7ᵗʰ **S42.239** 3-part fracture of surgical neck of unspecified humerus `MCC` `CC` `H5`

√6ᵗʰ **S42.24** 4-part fracture of surgical neck of humerus

²,³ √7ᵗʰ **S42.241** 4-part fracture of surgical neck of right humerus `MCC` `CC` `H5`

²,³ √7ᵗʰ **S42.242** 4-part fracture of surgical neck of left humerus `MCC` `CC` `H5`

²,³ √7ᵗʰ **S42.249** 4-part fracture of surgical neck of unspecified humerus `MCC` `CC` `H5`

√6ᵗʰ **S42.25** Fracture of greater tuberosity of humerus

²,³ √7ᵗʰ **S42.251** Displaced fracture of greater tuberosity of right humerus `MCC` `CC` `H5`

²,³ √7ᵗʰ **S42.252** Displaced fracture of greater tuberosity of left humerus `MCC` `CC` `H5`

²,³ √7ᵗʰ **S42.253** Displaced fracture of greater tuberosity of unspecified humerus `MCC` `CC` `H5`

²,³ √7ᵗʰ **S42.254** Nondisplaced fracture of greater tuberosity of right humerus `MCC` `CC` `H5`

²,³ √7ᵗʰ **S42.255** Nondisplaced fracture of greater tuberosity of left humerus `MCC` `CC` `H5`

²,³ √7ᵗʰ **S42.256** Nondisplaced fracture of greater tuberosity of unspecified humerus `MCC` `CC` `H5`

√6ᵗʰ **S42.26** Fracture of lesser tuberosity of humerus

²,³ √7ᵗʰ **S42.261** Displaced fracture of lesser tuberosity of right humerus `MCC` `CC` `H5`

²,³ √7ᵗʰ **S42.262** Displaced fracture of lesser tuberosity of left humerus `MCC` `CC` `H5`

²,³ √7ᵗʰ **S42.263** Displaced fracture of lesser tuberosity of unspecified humerus `MCC` `CC` `H5`

²,³ √7ᵗʰ **S42.264** Nondisplaced fracture of lesser tuberosity of right humerus `MCC` `CC` `H5`

²,³ √7ᵗʰ **S42.265** Nondisplaced fracture of lesser tuberosity of left humerus `MCC` `CC` `H5`

²,³ √7ᵗʰ **S42.266** Nondisplaced fracture of lesser tuberosity of unspecified humerus `MCC` `CC` `H5`

√6ᵗʰ **S42.27**   **Torus** fracture of upper end of humerus

> The appropriate 7th character is to be added to all codes in subcategory S42.27
> A   initial encounter for closed fracture
> D   subsequent encounter for fracture with routine healing
> G   subsequent encounter for fracture with delayed healing
> K   subsequent encounter for fracture with nonunion
> P   subsequent encounter for fracture with malunion
> S   sequela

³ √7ᵗʰ **S42.271**   **Torus** fracture of upper end of right humerus   CC H5

³ √7ᵗʰ **S42.272**   **Torus** fracture of upper end of left humerus   CC H5

³ √7ᵗʰ **S42.279**   **Torus** fracture of upper end of unspecified humerus   CC H5

√6ᵗʰ **S42.29**   **Other** fracture of upper end of humerus

Fracture of anatomical neck of humerus
Fracture of articular head of humerus
AHA: 2019,1Q,18

²,³ √7ᵗʰ **S42.291**   Other **displaced** fracture of upper end of **right** humerus   MCC CC H5

²,³ √7ᵗʰ **S42.292**   Other **displaced** fracture of upper end of **left** humerus   MCC CC H5

²,³ √7ᵗʰ **S42.293**   Other **displaced** fracture of upper end of **unspecified** humerus   MCC CC H5

²,³ √7ᵗʰ **S42.294**   Other **nondisplaced** fracture of upper end of **right** humerus   MCC CC H5

²,³ √7ᵗʰ **S42.295**   Other **nondisplaced** fracture of upper end of **left** humerus   MCC CC H5

²,³ √7ᵗʰ **S42.296**   Other **nondisplaced** fracture of upper end of unspecified humerus   MCC CC H5

√5ᵗʰ **S42.3**   **Fracture of shaft of humerus**

Fracture of humerus NOS
Fracture of upper arm NOS
EXCLUDES 2   physeal fractures of upper end of humerus (S49.0-)
    physeal fractures of lower end of humerus (S49.1-)

√6ᵗʰ **S42.30**   **Unspecified** fracture of shaft of humerus

²,³ √7ᵗʰ **S42.301**   **Unspecified** fracture of shaft of humerus, **right** arm   MCC CC H5

²,³ √7ᵗʰ **S42.302**   **Unspecified** fracture of shaft of humerus, **left** arm   MCC CC H5

²,³ √7ᵗʰ **S42.309**   **Unspecified** fracture of shaft of humerus, **unspecified** arm   MCC CC H5

√6ᵗʰ **S42.31**   **Greenstick** fracture of shaft of humerus

> The appropriate 7th character is to be added to all codes in subcategory S42.31
> A   initial encounter for closed fracture
> D   subsequent encounter for fracture with routine healing
> G   subsequent encounter for fracture with delayed healing
> K   subsequent encounter for fracture with nonunion
> P   subsequent encounter for fracture with malunion
> S   sequela

³ √7ᵗʰ **S42.311**   **Greenstick** fracture of shaft of humerus, **right** arm   CC H5

³ √7ᵗʰ **S42.312**   **Greenstick** fracture of shaft of humerus, **left** arm   CC H5

³ √7ᵗʰ **S42.319**   **Greenstick** fracture of shaft of humerus, **unspecified** arm   CC H5

√6ᵗʰ **S42.32**   **Transverse** fracture of shaft of humerus

²,³ √7ᵗʰ **S42.321**   **Displaced transverse** fracture of shaft of humerus, **right** arm   MCC CC H5

²,³ √7ᵗʰ **S42.322**   **Displaced transverse** fracture of shaft of humerus, **left** arm   MCC CC H5

²,³ √7ᵗʰ **S42.323**   **Displaced transverse** fracture of shaft of humerus, **unspecified** arm   MCC CC H5

²,³ √7ᵗʰ **S42.324**   **Nondisplaced transverse** fracture of shaft of humerus, **right** arm   MCC CC H5

²,³ √7ᵗʰ **S42.325**   **Nondisplaced transverse** fracture of shaft of humerus, **left** arm   MCC CC H5

²,³ √7ᵗʰ **S42.326**   **Nondisplaced transverse** fracture of shaft of humerus, unspecified arm   MCC CC H5

√6ᵗʰ **S42.33**   **Oblique** fracture of shaft of humerus

²,³ √7ᵗʰ **S42.331**   **Displaced oblique** fracture of shaft of humerus, **right arm**   MCC CC H5

²,³ √7ᵗʰ **S42.332**   **Displaced oblique** fracture of shaft of humerus, **left arm**   MCC CC H5

²,³ √7ᵗʰ **S42.333**   **Displaced oblique** fracture of shaft of humerus, **unspecified arm**   MCC CC H5

²,³ √7ᵗʰ **S42.334**   **Nondisplaced oblique** fracture of shaft of humerus, **right arm**   MCC CC H5

²,³ √7ᵗʰ **S42.335**   **Nondisplaced oblique** fracture of shaft of humerus, **left arm**   MCC CC H5

²,³ √7ᵗʰ **S42.336**   **Nondisplaced oblique** fracture of shaft of humerus, **unspecified arm**   MCC CC H5

√6ᵗʰ **S42.34**   **Spiral** fracture of shaft of humerus

²,³ √7ᵗʰ **S42.341**   **Displaced spiral** fracture of shaft of humerus, **right arm**   MCC CC H5

²,³ √7ᵗʰ **S42.342**   **Displaced spiral** fracture of shaft of humerus, **left arm**   MCC CC H5

²,³ √7ᵗʰ **S42.343**   **Displaced spiral** fracture of shaft of humerus, **unspecified arm**   MCC CC H5

²,³ √7ᵗʰ **S42.344**   **Nondisplaced spiral** fracture of shaft of humerus, **right arm**   MCC CC H5

²,³ √7ᵗʰ **S42.345**   **Nondisplaced spiral** fracture of shaft of humerus, **left arm**   MCC CC H5

²,³ √7ᵗʰ **S42.346**   **Nondisplaced spiral** fracture of shaft of humerus, **unspecified arm**   MCC CC H5

√6ᵗʰ **S42.35**   **Comminuted** fracture of shaft of humerus

²,³ √7ᵗʰ **S42.351**   **Displaced comminuted** fracture of shaft of humerus, **right arm**   MCC CC H5

²,³ √7ᵗʰ **S42.352**   **Displaced comminuted** fracture of shaft of humerus, **left arm**   MCC CC H5

²,³ √7ᵗʰ **S42.353**   **Displaced comminuted** fracture of shaft of humerus, unspecified arm   MCC CC H5

²,³ √7ᵗʰ **S42.354**   **Nondisplaced comminuted** fracture of shaft of humerus, **right arm**   MCC CC H5

²,³ √7ᵗʰ **S42.355**   **Nondisplaced comminuted** fracture of shaft of humerus, **left arm**   MCC CC H5

²,³ √7ᵗʰ **S42.356**   **Nondisplaced comminuted** fracture of shaft of humerus, unspecified arm   MCC CC H5

√6ᵗʰ **S42.36**   **Segmental** fracture of shaft of humerus

²,³ √7ᵗʰ **S42.361**   **Displaced segmental** fracture of shaft of humerus, **right arm**   MCC CC H5

²,³ √7ᵗʰ **S42.362**   **Displaced segmental** fracture of shaft of humerus, **left arm**   MCC CC H5

²,³ √7ᵗʰ **S42.363**   **Displaced segmental** fracture of shaft of humerus, **unspecified arm**   MCC CC H5

²,³ √7ᵗʰ **S42.364**   **Nondisplaced segmental** fracture of shaft of humerus, **right arm**   MCC CC H5

²,³ √7ᵗʰ **S42.365**   **Nondisplaced segmental** fracture of shaft of humerus, **left arm**   MCC CC H5

²,³ √7ᵗʰ **S42.366**   **Nondisplaced segmental** fracture of shaft of humerus, unspecified arm   MCC CC H5

√6ᵗʰ **S42.39**   **Other** fracture of shaft of humerus

²,³ √7ᵗʰ **S42.391**   **Other** fracture of shaft of **right** humerus   MCC CC H5

²,³ √7ᵗʰ **S42.392**   **Other** fracture of shaft of **left** humerus   MCC CC H5

²,³ √7ᵗʰ **S42.399**   **Other** fracture of shaft of unspecified humerus   MCC CC H5

√5ᵗʰ **S42.4**   **Fracture of lower end of humerus**

Fracture of distal end of humerus
EXCLUDES 2   fracture of shaft of humerus (S42.3-)
    physeal fracture of lower end of humerus (S49.1-)

√6ᵗʰ **S42.40**   **Unspecified** fracture of lower end of humerus

Fracture of elbow NOS

²,³ √7ᵗʰ **S42.401**   **Unspecified** fracture of lower end of **right** humerus   MCC CC H5

²,³ √7ᵗʰ **S42.402**   **Unspecified** fracture of lower end of **left** humerus   MCC CC H5

²,³ √7ᵗʰ **S42.409**   **Unspecified** fracture of lower end of unspecified humerus   MCC CC H5

N Newborn: 0   P Pediatric: 0-17   M Maternity: 9-64   A Adult: 15-124   MCC Major Complication/Comorbidity   CC Complication/Comorbidity   SW Severe Wound Dx

1012   ICD-10-CM 2022

√6ᵗʰ **S42.41** Simple supracondylar fracture without intercondylar fracture of humerus

    2,3 √7ᵗʰ **S42.411** Displaced simple supracondylar fracture without intercondylar fracture of right humerus   `MCC` `CC` `H5`

    2,3 √7ᵗʰ **S42.412** Displaced simple supracondylar fracture without intercondylar fracture of left humerus   `MCC` `CC` `H5`

    2,3 √7ᵗʰ **S42.413** Displaced simple supracondylar fracture without intercondylar fracture of unspecified humerus   `MCC` `CC` `H5`

    2,3 √7ᵗʰ **S42.414** Nondisplaced simple supracondylar fracture without intercondylar fracture of right humerus   `MCC` `CC` `H5`

    2,3 √7ᵗʰ **S42.415** Nondisplaced simple supracondylar fracture without intercondylar fracture of left humerus   `MCC` `CC` `H5`

    2,3 √7ᵗʰ **S42.416** Nondisplaced simple supracondylar fracture without intercondylar fracture of unspecified humerus   `MCC` `CC` `H5`

√6ᵗʰ **S42.42** Comminuted supracondylar fracture without intercondylar fracture of humerus

    2,3 √7ᵗʰ **S42.421** Displaced comminuted supracondylar fracture without intercondylar fracture of right humerus   `MCC` `CC` `H5`

    2,3 √7ᵗʰ **S42.422** Displaced comminuted supracondylar fracture without intercondylar fracture of left humerus   `MCC` `CC` `H5`

    2,3 √7ᵗʰ **S42.423** Displaced comminuted supracondylar fracture without intercondylar fracture of unspecified humerus   `MCC` `CC` `H5`

    2,3 √7ᵗʰ **S42.424** Nondisplaced comminuted supracondylar fracture without intercondylar fracture of right humerus   `MCC` `CC` `H5`

    2,3 √7ᵗʰ **S42.425** Nondisplaced comminuted supracondylar fracture without intercondylar fracture of left humerus   `MCC` `CC` `H5`

    2,3 √7ᵗʰ **S42.426** Nondisplaced comminuted supracondylar fracture without intercondylar fracture of unspecified humerus   `MCC` `CC` `H5`

√6ᵗʰ **S42.43** Fracture (avulsion) of lateral epicondyle of humerus

    2,3 √7ᵗʰ **S42.431** Displaced fracture (avulsion) of lateral epicondyle of right humerus   `MCC` `CC` `H5`

    2,3 √7ᵗʰ **S42.432** Displaced fracture (avulsion) of lateral epicondyle of left humerus   `MCC` `CC` `H5`

    2,3 √7ᵗʰ **S42.433** Displaced fracture (avulsion) of lateral epicondyle of unspecified humerus   `MCC` `CC` `H5`

    2,3 √7ᵗʰ **S42.434** Nondisplaced fracture (avulsion) of lateral epicondyle of right humerus   `MCC` `CC` `H5`

    2,3 √7ᵗʰ **S42.435** Nondisplaced fracture (avulsion) of lateral epicondyle of left humerus   `MCC` `CC` `H5`

    2,3 √7ᵗʰ **S42.436** Nondisplaced fracture (avulsion) of lateral epicondyle of unspecified humerus   `MCC` `CC` `H5`

√6ᵗʰ **S42.44** Fracture (avulsion) of medial epicondyle of humerus

    2,3 √7ᵗʰ **S42.441** Displaced fracture (avulsion) of medial epicondyle of right humerus   `MCC` `CC` `H5`

    2,3 √7ᵗʰ **S42.442** Displaced fracture (avulsion) of medial epicondyle of left humerus   `MCC` `CC` `H5`

    2,3 √7ᵗʰ **S42.443** Displaced fracture (avulsion) of medial epicondyle of unspecified humerus   `MCC` `CC` `H5`

    2,3 √7ᵗʰ **S42.444** Nondisplaced fracture (avulsion) of medial epicondyle of right humerus   `MCC` `CC` `H5`

    2,3 √7ᵗʰ **S42.445** Nondisplaced fracture (avulsion) of medial epicondyle of left humerus   `MCC` `CC` `H5`

    2,3 √7ᵗʰ **S42.446** Nondisplaced fracture (avulsion) of medial epicondyle of unspecified humerus   `MCC` `CC` `H5`

    2,3 √7ᵗʰ **S42.447** Incarcerated fracture (avulsion) of medial epicondyle of right humerus   `MCC` `CC` `H5`

    2,3 √7ᵗʰ **S42.448** Incarcerated fracture (avulsion) of medial epicondyle of left humerus   `MCC` `CC` `H5`

    2,3 √7ᵗʰ **S42.449** Incarcerated fracture (avulsion) of medial epicondyle of unspecified humerus   `MCC` `CC` `H5`

√6ᵗʰ **S42.45** Fracture of lateral condyle of humerus

    Fracture of capitellum of humerus

    2,3 √7ᵗʰ **S42.451** Displaced fracture of lateral condyle of right humerus   `MCC` `CC` `H5`

    2,3 √7ᵗʰ **S42.452** Displaced fracture of lateral condyle of left humerus   `MCC` `CC` `H5`

    2,3 √7ᵗʰ **S42.453** Displaced fracture of lateral condyle of unspecified humerus   `MCC` `CC` `H5`

    2,3 √7ᵗʰ **S42.454** Nondisplaced fracture of lateral condyle of right humerus   `MCC` `CC` `H5`

    2,3 √7ᵗʰ **S42.455** Nondisplaced fracture of lateral condyle of left humerus   `MCC` `CC` `H5`

    2,3 √7ᵗʰ **S42.456** Nondisplaced fracture of lateral condyle of unspecified humerus   `MCC` `CC` `H5`

√6ᵗʰ **S42.46** Fracture of medial condyle of humerus

    Trochlea fracture of humerus

    2,3 √7ᵗʰ **S42.461** Displaced fracture of medial condyle of right humerus   `MCC` `CC` `H5`

    2,3 √7ᵗʰ **S42.462** Displaced fracture of medial condyle of left humerus   `MCC` `CC` `H5`

    2,3 √7ᵗʰ **S42.463** Displaced fracture of medial condyle of unspecified humerus   `MCC` `CC` `H5`

    2,3 √7ᵗʰ **S42.464** Nondisplaced fracture of medial condyle of right humerus   `MCC` `CC` `H5`

    2,3 √7ᵗʰ **S42.465** Nondisplaced fracture of medial condyle of left humerus   `MCC` `CC` `H5`

    2,3 √7ᵗʰ **S42.466** Nondisplaced fracture of medial condyle of unspecified humerus   `MCC` `CC` `H5`

√6ᵗʰ **S42.47** Transcondylar fracture of humerus

    2,3 √7ᵗʰ **S42.471** Displaced transcondylar fracture of right humerus   `MCC` `CC` `H5`

    2,3 √7ᵗʰ **S42.472** Displaced transcondylar fracture of left humerus   `MCC` `CC` `H5`

    2,3 √7ᵗʰ **S42.473** Displaced transcondylar fracture of unspecified humerus   `MCC` `CC` `H5`

    2,3 √7ᵗʰ **S42.474** Nondisplaced transcondylar fracture of right humerus   `MCC` `CC` `H5`

    2,3 √7ᵗʰ **S42.475** Nondisplaced transcondylar fracture of left humerus   `MCC` `CC` `H5`

    2,3 √7ᵗʰ **S42.476** Nondisplaced transcondylar fracture of unspecified humerus   `MCC` `CC` `H5`

√6ᵗʰ **S42.48** Torus fracture of lower end of humerus

> The appropriate 7th character is to be added to all codes in subcategory S42.48.
> A   initial encounter for closed fracture
> D   subsequent encounter for fracture with routine healing
> G   subsequent encounter for fracture with delayed healing
> K   subsequent encounter for fracture with nonunion
> P   subsequent encounter for fracture with malunion
> S   sequela

    3 √7ᵗʰ **S42.481** Torus fracture of lower end of right humerus   `CC` `H5`

    3 √7ᵗʰ **S42.482** Torus fracture of lower end of left humerus   `CC` `H5`

    3 √7ᵗʰ **S42.489** Torus fracture of lower end of unspecified humerus   `CC` `H5`

√6ᵗʰ **S42.49** Other fracture of lower end of humerus

    2,3 √7ᵗʰ **S42.491** Other displaced fracture of lower end of right humerus   `MCC` `CC` `H5`

    2,3 √7ᵗʰ **S42.492** Other displaced fracture of lower end of left humerus   `MCC` `CC` `H5`

    2,3 √7ᵗʰ **S42.493** Other displaced fracture of lower end of unspecified humerus   `MCC` `CC` `H5`

    2,3 √7ᵗʰ **S42.494** Other nondisplaced fracture of lower end of right humerus   `MCC` `CC` `H5`

    2,3 √7ᵗʰ **S42.495** Other nondisplaced fracture of lower end of left humerus   `MCC` `CC` `H5`

    2,3 √7ᵗʰ **S42.496** Other nondisplaced fracture of lower end of unspecified humerus   `MCC` `CC` `H5`

☑ Additional Character Required   √x7ᵗʰ Placeholder   Questionable PDx   Manifestation   Unspecified Dx   `UPD` Unacceptable PDx   `H1`-`H14` HAC   `HCC` CMS-HCC Dx   `HIV` HIV Dx

ICD-10-CM 2022   1013

√5ᵗʰ **S42.9** **Fracture of shoulder girdle, part unspecified**
    Fracture of shoulder NOS

2,3 √x7ᵗʰ **S42.90** **Fracture of unspecified shoulder girdle, part unspecified** `MCC` `CC` `H5`

2,3 √x7ᵗʰ **S42.91** **Fracture of right shoulder girdle, part unspecified** `MCC` `CC` `H5`

2,3 √x7ᵗʰ **S42.92** **Fracture of left shoulder girdle, part unspecified** `MCC` `CC` `H5`

√4ᵗʰ **S43** **Dislocation and sprain of joints and ligaments of shoulder girdle**

`INCLUDES`
    avulsion of joint or ligament of shoulder girdle
    laceration of cartilage, joint or ligament of shoulder girdle
    sprain of cartilage, joint or ligament of shoulder girdle
    traumatic hemarthrosis of joint or ligament of shoulder girdle
    traumatic rupture of joint or ligament of shoulder girdle
    traumatic subluxation of joint or ligament of shoulder girdle
    traumatic tear of joint or ligament of shoulder girdle

Code also any associated open wound

`EXCLUDES 2`   *strain of muscle, fascia and tendon of shoulder and upper arm (S46.-)*

The appropriate 7th character is to be added to each code from category S43.
  A   initial encounter
  D   subsequent encounter
  S   sequela

√5ᵗʰ **S43.0** **Subluxation and dislocation of shoulder joint**
    Dislocation of glenohumeral joint
    Subluxation of glenohumeral joint

√6ᵗʰ **S43.00** **Unspecified subluxation and dislocation of shoulder joint**
    Dislocation of humerus NOS
    Subluxation of humerus NOS

√7ᵗʰ **S43.001** **Unspecified subluxation of right shoulder joint**

√7ᵗʰ **S43.002** **Unspecified subluxation of left shoulder joint**

√7ᵗʰ **S43.003** **Unspecified subluxation of unspecified shoulder joint**

√7ᵗʰ **S43.004** **Unspecified dislocation of right shoulder joint**

√7ᵗʰ **S43.005** **Unspecified dislocation of left shoulder joint**

√7ᵗʰ **S43.006** **Unspecified dislocation of unspecified shoulder joint**

√6ᵗʰ **S43.01** **Anterior subluxation and dislocation of humerus**

√7ᵗʰ **S43.011** **Anterior subluxation of right humerus**

√7ᵗʰ **S43.012** **Anterior subluxation of left humerus**

√7ᵗʰ **S43.013** **Anterior subluxation of unspecified humerus**

√7ᵗʰ **S43.014** **Anterior dislocation of right humerus**

√7ᵗʰ **S43.015** **Anterior dislocation of left humerus**

√7ᵗʰ **S43.016** **Anterior dislocation of unspecified humerus**

√6ᵗʰ **S43.02** **Posterior subluxation and dislocation of humerus**

√7ᵗʰ **S43.021** **Posterior subluxation of right humerus**

√7ᵗʰ **S43.022** **Posterior subluxation of left humerus**

√7ᵗʰ **S43.023** **Posterior subluxation of unspecified humerus**

√7ᵗʰ **S43.024** **Posterior dislocation of right humerus**

√7ᵗʰ **S43.025** **Posterior dislocation of left humerus**

√7ᵗʰ **S43.026** **Posterior dislocation of unspecified humerus**

√6ᵗʰ **S43.03** **Inferior subluxation and dislocation of humerus**

√7ᵗʰ **S43.031** **Inferior subluxation of right humerus**

√7ᵗʰ **S43.032** **Inferior subluxation of left humerus**

√7ᵗʰ **S43.033** **Inferior subluxation of unspecified humerus**

√7ᵗʰ **S43.034** **Inferior dislocation of right humerus**

√7ᵗʰ **S43.035** **Inferior dislocation of left humerus**

√7ᵗʰ **S43.036** **Inferior dislocation of unspecified humerus**

√6ᵗʰ **S43.08** **Other subluxation and dislocation of shoulder joint**

√7ᵗʰ **S43.081** **Other subluxation of right shoulder joint**

√7ᵗʰ **S43.082** **Other subluxation of left shoulder joint**

√7ᵗʰ **S43.083** **Other subluxation of unspecified shoulder joint**

√7ᵗʰ **S43.084** **Other dislocation of right shoulder joint**

√7ᵗʰ **S43.085** **Other dislocation of left shoulder joint**

√7ᵗʰ **S43.086** **Other dislocation of unspecified shoulder joint**

√5ᵗʰ **S43.1** **Subluxation and dislocation of acromioclavicular joint**

√6ᵗʰ **S43.10** **Unspecified dislocation of acromioclavicular joint**

√7ᵗʰ **S43.101** **Unspecified dislocation of right acromioclavicular joint**

√7ᵗʰ **S43.102** **Unspecified dislocation of left acromioclavicular joint**

√7ᵗʰ **S43.109** **Unspecified dislocation of unspecified acromioclavicular joint**

√6ᵗʰ **S43.11** **Subluxation of acromioclavicular joint**

√7ᵗʰ **S43.111** **Subluxation of right acromioclavicular joint**

√7ᵗʰ **S43.112** **Subluxation of left acromioclavicular joint**

√7ᵗʰ **S43.119** **Subluxation of unspecified acromioclavicular joint**

√6ᵗʰ **S43.12** **Dislocation of acromioclavicular joint, 100%-200% displacement**

√7ᵗʰ **S43.121** **Dislocation of right acromioclavicular joint, 100%-200% displacement**

√7ᵗʰ **S43.122** **Dislocation of left acromioclavicular joint, 100%-200% displacement**

√7ᵗʰ **S43.129** **Dislocation of unspecified acromioclavicular joint, 100%-200% displacement**

√6ᵗʰ **S43.13** **Dislocation of acromioclavicular joint, greater than 200% displacement**

√7ᵗʰ **S43.131** **Dislocation of right acromioclavicular joint, greater than 200% displacement**

√7ᵗʰ **S43.132** **Dislocation of left acromioclavicular joint, greater than 200% displacement**

√7ᵗʰ **S43.139** **Dislocation of unspecified acromioclavicular joint, greater than 200% displacement**

√6ᵗʰ **S43.14** **Inferior dislocation of acromioclavicular joint**

√7ᵗʰ **S43.141** **Inferior dislocation of right acromioclavicular joint**

√7ᵗʰ **S43.142** **Inferior dislocation of left acromioclavicular joint**

√7ᵗʰ **S43.149** **Inferior dislocation of unspecified acromioclavicular joint**

√6ᵗʰ **S43.15** **Posterior dislocation of acromioclavicular joint**

√7ᵗʰ **S43.151** **Posterior dislocation of right acromioclavicular joint**

√7ᵗʰ **S43.152** **Posterior dislocation of left acromioclavicular joint**

√7ᵗʰ **S43.159** **Posterior dislocation of unspecified acromioclavicular joint**

√5ᵗʰ **S43.2** **Subluxation and dislocation of sternoclavicular joint**

√6ᵗʰ **S43.20** **Unspecified subluxation and dislocation of sternoclavicular joint**

√7ᵗʰ **S43.201** **Unspecified subluxation of right sternoclavicular joint** `CC` `H5`

√7ᵗʰ **S43.202** **Unspecified subluxation of left sternoclavicular joint** `CC` `H5`

√7ᵗʰ **S43.203** **Unspecified subluxation of unspecified sternoclavicular joint** `CC` `H5`

√7ᵗʰ **S43.204** **Unspecified dislocation of right sternoclavicular joint** `CC` `H5`

√7ᵗʰ **S43.205** **Unspecified dislocation of left sternoclavicular joint** `CC` `H5`

√7ᵗʰ **S43.206** **Unspecified dislocation of unspecified sternoclavicular joint** `CC` `H5`

√6ᵗʰ **S43.21** **Anterior subluxation and dislocation of sternoclavicular joint**

√7ᵗʰ **S43.211** **Anterior subluxation of right sternoclavicular joint** `CC` `H5`

√7ᵗʰ **S43.212** **Anterior subluxation of left sternoclavicular joint** `CC` `H5`

√7ᵗʰ **S43.213** **Anterior subluxation of unspecified sternoclavicular joint** `CC` `H5`

√7ᵗʰ **S43.214** **Anterior dislocation of right sternoclavicular joint** `CC` `H5`

√7ᵗʰ **S43.215** **Anterior dislocation of left sternoclavicular joint** `CC` `H5`

`N` Newborn: 0   `P` Pediatric: 0-17   `M` Maternity: 9-64   `A` Adult: 15-124   `MCC` Major Complication/Comorbidity   `CC` Complication/Comorbidity   `SW` Severe Wound Dx

1014   ICD-10-CM 2022

√6ᵗʰ **S43.216** Anterior dislocation of unspecified sternoclavicular joint   CC H5

√6ᵗʰ **S43.22** Posterior subluxation and dislocation of sternoclavicular joint

√7ᵗʰ **S43.221** Posterior subluxation of right sternoclavicular joint   CC H5

√7ᵗʰ **S43.222** Posterior subluxation of left sternoclavicular joint   CC H5

√7ᵗʰ **S43.223** Posterior subluxation of unspecified sternoclavicular joint   CC H5

√7ᵗʰ **S43.224** Posterior dislocation of right sternoclavicular joint   CC H5

√7ᵗʰ **S43.225** Posterior dislocation of left sternoclavicular joint   CC H5

√7ᵗʰ **S43.226** Posterior dislocation of unspecified sternoclavicular joint   CC H5

√5ᵗʰ **S43.3** Subluxation and dislocation of other and unspecified parts of shoulder girdle

√6ᵗʰ **S43.30** Subluxation and dislocation of unspecified parts of shoulder girdle

Dislocation of shoulder girdle NOS
Subluxation of shoulder girdle NOS

√7ᵗʰ **S43.301** Subluxation of unspecified parts of right shoulder girdle

√7ᵗʰ **S43.302** Subluxation of unspecified parts of left shoulder girdle

√7ᵗʰ **S43.303** Subluxation of unspecified parts of unspecified shoulder girdle

√7ᵗʰ **S43.304** Dislocation of unspecified parts of right shoulder girdle

√7ᵗʰ **S43.305** Dislocation of unspecified parts of left shoulder girdle

√7ᵗʰ **S43.306** Dislocation of unspecified parts of unspecified shoulder girdle

√6ᵗʰ **S43.31** Subluxation and dislocation of scapula

√7ᵗʰ **S43.311** Subluxation of right scapula

√7ᵗʰ **S43.312** Subluxation of left scapula

√7ᵗʰ **S43.313** Subluxation of unspecified scapula

√7ᵗʰ **S43.314** Dislocation of right scapula

√7ᵗʰ **S43.315** Dislocation of left scapula

√7ᵗʰ **S43.316** Dislocation of unspecified scapula

√6ᵗʰ **S43.39** Subluxation and dislocation of other parts of shoulder girdle

√7ᵗʰ **S43.391** Subluxation of other parts of right shoulder girdle

√7ᵗʰ **S43.392** Subluxation of other parts of left shoulder girdle

√7ᵗʰ **S43.393** Subluxation of other parts of unspecified shoulder girdle

√7ᵗʰ **S43.394** Dislocation of other parts of right shoulder girdle

√7ᵗʰ **S43.395** Dislocation of other parts of left shoulder girdle

√7ᵗʰ **S43.396** Dislocation of other parts of unspecified shoulder girdle

√5ᵗʰ **S43.4** Sprain of shoulder joint

√6ᵗʰ **S43.40** Unspecified sprain of shoulder joint

√7ᵗʰ **S43.401** Unspecified sprain of right shoulder joint

√7ᵗʰ **S43.402** Unspecified sprain of left shoulder joint

√7ᵗʰ **S43.409** Unspecified sprain of unspecified shoulder joint

√6ᵗʰ **S43.41** Sprain of coracohumeral (ligament)

√7ᵗʰ **S43.411** Sprain of right coracohumeral (ligament)

√7ᵗʰ **S43.412** Sprain of left coracohumeral (ligament)

√7ᵗʰ **S43.419** Sprain of unspecified coracohumeral (ligament)

√6ᵗʰ **S43.42** Sprain of rotator cuff capsule

EXCLUDES 1   rotator cuff syndrome (complete) (incomplete), not specified as traumatic (M75.1-)

EXCLUDES 2   injury of tendon of rotator cuff (S46.0-)

√7ᵗʰ **S43.421** Sprain of right rotator cuff capsule

√7ᵗʰ **S43.422** Sprain of left rotator cuff capsule

√7ᵗʰ **S43.429** Sprain of unspecified rotator cuff capsule

√6ᵗʰ **S43.43** Superior glenoid labrum lesion

SLAP lesion
AHA: 2019,2Q,26
DEF: Detachment injury of the superior aspect of the glenoid labrum, which is the ring of fibrocartilage attached to the rim of the glenoid cavity of the scapula.

√7ᵗʰ **S43.431** Superior glenoid labrum lesion of right shoulder

√7ᵗʰ **S43.432** Superior glenoid labrum lesion of left shoulder

√7ᵗʰ **S43.439** Superior glenoid labrum lesion of unspecified shoulder

√6ᵗʰ **S43.49** Other sprain of shoulder joint

√7ᵗʰ **S43.491** Other sprain of right shoulder joint

√7ᵗʰ **S43.492** Other sprain of left shoulder joint

√7ᵗʰ **S43.499** Other sprain of unspecified shoulder joint

√5ᵗʰ **S43.5** Sprain of acromioclavicular joint

Sprain of acromioclavicular ligament

√x7ᵗʰ **S43.50** Sprain of unspecified acromioclavicular joint

√x7ᵗʰ **S43.51** Sprain of right acromioclavicular joint

√x7ᵗʰ **S43.52** Sprain of left acromioclavicular joint

√5ᵗʰ **S43.6** Sprain of sternoclavicular joint

√x7ᵗʰ **S43.60** Sprain of unspecified sternoclavicular joint

√x7ᵗʰ **S43.61** Sprain of right sternoclavicular joint

√x7ᵗʰ **S43.62** Sprain of left sternoclavicular joint

√5ᵗʰ **S43.8** Sprain of other specified parts of shoulder girdle

√x7ᵗʰ **S43.80** Sprain of other specified parts of unspecified shoulder girdle

√x7ᵗʰ **S43.81** Sprain of other specified parts of right shoulder girdle

√x7ᵗʰ **S43.82** Sprain of other specified parts of left shoulder girdle

√5ᵗʰ **S43.9** Sprain of unspecified parts of shoulder girdle

√x7ᵗʰ **S43.90** Sprain of unspecified parts of unspecified shoulder girdle

Sprain of shoulder girdle NOS

√x7ᵗʰ **S43.91** Sprain of unspecified parts of right shoulder girdle

√x7ᵗʰ **S43.92** Sprain of unspecified parts of left shoulder girdle

√4ᵗʰ **S44** Injury of nerves at shoulder and upper arm level

Code also any associated open wound (S41.-)
EXCLUDES 2   injury of brachial plexus (S14.3-)

The appropriate 7th character is to be added to each code from category S44.
A   initial encounter
D   subsequent encounter
S   sequela

√5ᵗʰ **S44.0** Injury of ulnar nerve at upper arm level

EXCLUDES 1   ulnar nerve NOS (S54.0)

√x7ᵗʰ **S44.00** Injury of ulnar nerve at upper arm level, unspecified arm

√x7ᵗʰ **S44.01** Injury of ulnar nerve at upper arm level, right arm

√x7ᵗʰ **S44.02** Injury of ulnar nerve at upper arm level, left arm

√5ᵗʰ **S44.1** Injury of median nerve at upper arm level

EXCLUDES 1   median nerve NOS (S54.1)

√x7ᵗʰ **S44.10** Injury of median nerve at upper arm level, unspecified arm

√x7ᵗʰ **S44.11** Injury of median nerve at upper arm level, right arm

√x7ᵗʰ **S44.12** Injury of median nerve at upper arm level, left arm

√5ᵗʰ **S44.2** Injury of radial nerve at upper arm level

EXCLUDES 1   radial nerve NOS (S54.2)

√x7ᵗʰ **S44.20** Injury of radial nerve at upper arm level, unspecified arm

√x7ᵗʰ **S44.21** Injury of radial nerve at upper arm level, right arm

√x7ᵗʰ **S44.22** Injury of radial nerve at upper arm level, left arm

√5ᵗʰ **S44.3** Injury of axillary nerve

√x7ᵗʰ **S44.30** Injury of axillary nerve, unspecified arm

√x7ᵗʰ **S44.31** Injury of axillary nerve, right arm

√x7ᵗʰ **S44.32** Injury of axillary nerve, left arm

√5ᵗʰ **S44.4** Injury of musculocutaneous nerve

√x7ᵗʰ **S44.40** Injury of musculocutaneous nerve, unspecified arm

☑ Additional Character Required   √x7ᵗʰ Placeholder   Questionable PDx   Manifestation   Unspecified Dx   UPD Unacceptable PDx   H1-H14 HAC   HCC CMS-HCC Dx   HIV HIV Dx

ICD-10-CM 2022   1015

Chapter 19. Injury, Poisoning and Certain Other Consequences of External Causes

✓x7ᵗʰ **S44.41** Injury of musculocutaneous nerve, **right** arm

✓x7ᵗʰ **S44.42** Injury of musculocutaneous nerve, **left** arm

✓5ᵗʰ **S44.5** Injury of cutaneous sensory nerve at shoulder and upper arm level

     ✓x7ᵗʰ **S44.50** Injury of cutaneous sensory nerve at shoulder and upper arm level, unspecified arm

     ✓x7ᵗʰ **S44.51** Injury of cutaneous sensory nerve at shoulder and upper arm level, **right** arm

     ✓x7ᵗʰ **S44.52** Injury of cutaneous sensory nerve at shoulder and upper arm level, **left** arm

✓5ᵗʰ **S44.8** Injury of other nerves at shoulder and upper arm level

     ✓6ᵗʰ **S44.8X** Injury of other nerves at shoulder and upper arm level

         ✓7ᵗʰ **S44.8X1** Injury of other nerves at shoulder and upper arm level, **right** arm

         ✓7ᵗʰ **S44.8X2** Injury of other nerves at shoulder and upper arm level, **left** arm

         ✓7ᵗʰ **S44.8X9** Injury of other nerves at shoulder and upper arm level, unspecified arm

✓5ᵗʰ **S44.9** Injury of unspecified nerve at shoulder and upper arm level

     ✓x7ᵗʰ **S44.90** Injury of unspecified nerve at shoulder and upper arm level, unspecified arm

     ✓x7ᵗʰ **S44.91** Injury of unspecified nerve at shoulder and upper arm level, **right** arm

     ✓x7ᵗʰ **S44.92** Injury of unspecified nerve at shoulder and upper arm level, **left** arm

✓4ᵗʰ **S45** **Injury of blood vessels at shoulder and upper arm level**

     Code also any associated open wound (S41.-)

     EXCLUDES 2   injury of subclavian artery (S25.1)

                 injury of subclavian vein (S25.3)

     The appropriate 7th character is to be added to each code from category S45.
     A   initial encounter
     D   subsequent encounter
     S   sequela

✓5ᵗʰ **S45.0** Injury of axillary artery

     ✓6ᵗʰ **S45.00** Unspecified injury of axillary artery

         ✓7ᵗʰ **S45.001** Unspecified injury of axillary artery, **right** side   `MCC`

         ✓7ᵗʰ **S45.002** Unspecified injury of axillary artery, **left** side   `MCC`

         ✓7ᵗʰ **S45.009** Unspecified injury of axillary artery, unspecified side   `MCC`

     ✓6ᵗʰ **S45.01** Laceration of axillary artery

         ✓7ᵗʰ **S45.011** Laceration of axillary artery, **right** side   `MCC`

         ✓7ᵗʰ **S45.012** Laceration of axillary artery, **left** side   `MCC`

         ✓7ᵗʰ **S45.019** Laceration of axillary artery, unspecified side   `MCC`

     ✓6ᵗʰ **S45.09** Other specified injury of axillary artery

         ✓7ᵗʰ **S45.091** Other specified injury of axillary artery, **right** side   `MCC`

         ✓7ᵗʰ **S45.092** Other specified injury of axillary artery, **left** side   `MCC`

         ✓7ᵗʰ **S45.099** Other specified injury of axillary artery, unspecified side   `MCC`

✓5ᵗʰ **S45.1** Injury of brachial artery

     ✓6ᵗʰ **S45.10** Unspecified injury of brachial artery

         ✓7ᵗʰ **S45.101** Unspecified injury of brachial artery, **right** side   `CC`

         ✓7ᵗʰ **S45.102** Unspecified injury of brachial artery, **left** side   `CC`

         ✓7ᵗʰ **S45.109** Unspecified injury of brachial artery, unspecified side   `CC`

     ✓6ᵗʰ **S45.11** Laceration of brachial artery

         ✓7ᵗʰ **S45.111** Laceration of brachial artery, **right** side   `CC`

         ✓7ᵗʰ **S45.112** Laceration of brachial artery, **left** side   `CC`

         ✓7ᵗʰ **S45.119** Laceration of brachial artery, unspecified side   `CC`

     ✓6ᵗʰ **S45.19** Other specified injury of brachial artery

         ✓7ᵗʰ **S45.191** Other specified injury of brachial artery, **right** side   `CC`

         ✓7ᵗʰ **S45.192** Other specified injury of brachial artery, **left** side   `CC`

         ✓7ᵗʰ **S45.199** Other specified injury of brachial artery, unspecified side   `CC`

✓5ᵗʰ **S45.2** Injury of axillary or brachial vein

     ✓6ᵗʰ **S45.20** Unspecified injury of axillary or brachial vein

         ✓7ᵗʰ **S45.201** Unspecified injury of axillary or brachial vein, **right** side   `CC`

         ✓7ᵗʰ **S45.202** Unspecified injury of axillary or brachial vein, **left** side   `CC`

         ✓7ᵗʰ **S45.209** Unspecified injury of axillary or brachial vein, unspecified side   `CC`

     ✓6ᵗʰ **S45.21** Laceration of axillary or brachial vein

         ✓7ᵗʰ **S45.211** Laceration of axillary or brachial vein, **right** side   `CC`

         ✓7ᵗʰ **S45.212** Laceration of axillary or brachial vein, **left** side   `CC`

         ✓7ᵗʰ **S45.219** Laceration of axillary or brachial vein, unspecified side   `CC`

     ✓6ᵗʰ **S45.29** Other specified injury of axillary or brachial vein

         ✓7ᵗʰ **S45.291** Other specified injury of axillary or brachial vein, **right** side   `CC`

         ✓7ᵗʰ **S45.292** Other specified injury of axillary or brachial vein, **left** side   `CC`

         ✓7ᵗʰ **S45.299** Other specified injury of axillary or brachial vein, unspecified side   `CC`

✓5ᵗʰ **S45.3** Injury of superficial vein at shoulder and upper arm level

     ✓6ᵗʰ **S45.30** Unspecified injury of superficial vein at shoulder and upper arm level

         ✓7ᵗʰ **S45.301** Unspecified injury of superficial vein at shoulder and upper arm level, **right** arm   `CC`

         ✓7ᵗʰ **S45.302** Unspecified injury of superficial vein at shoulder and upper arm level, **left** arm   `CC`

         ✓7ᵗʰ **S45.309** Unspecified injury of superficial vein at shoulder and upper arm level, unspecified arm   `CC`

     ✓6ᵗʰ **S45.31** Laceration of superficial vein at shoulder and upper arm level

         ✓7ᵗʰ **S45.311** Laceration of superficial vein at shoulder and upper arm level, **right** arm   `CC`

         ✓7ᵗʰ **S45.312** Laceration of superficial vein at shoulder and upper arm level, **left** arm   `CC`

         ✓7ᵗʰ **S45.319** Laceration of superficial vein at shoulder and upper arm level, unspecified arm   `CC`

     ✓6ᵗʰ **S45.39** Other specified injury of superficial vein at shoulder and upper arm level

         ✓7ᵗʰ **S45.391** Other specified injury of superficial vein at shoulder and upper arm level, **right** arm   `CC`

         ✓7ᵗʰ **S45.392** Other specified injury of superficial vein at shoulder and upper arm level, **left** arm   `CC`

         ✓7ᵗʰ **S45.399** Other specified injury of superficial vein at shoulder and upper arm level, unspecified arm   `CC`

✓5ᵗʰ **S45.8** Injury of other specified blood vessels at shoulder and upper arm level

     ✓6ᵗʰ **S45.80** Unspecified injury of other specified blood vessels at shoulder and upper arm level

         ✓7ᵗʰ **S45.801** Unspecified injury of other specified blood vessels at shoulder and upper arm level, **right** arm   `CC`

         ✓7ᵗʰ **S45.802** Unspecified injury of other specified blood vessels at shoulder and upper arm level, **left** arm   `CC`

         ✓7ᵗʰ **S45.809** Unspecified injury of other specified blood vessels at shoulder and upper arm level, unspecified arm   `CC`

     ✓6ᵗʰ **S45.81** Laceration of other specified blood vessels at shoulder and upper arm level

         ✓7ᵗʰ **S45.811** Laceration of other specified blood vessels at shoulder and upper arm level, **right** arm   `CC`

         ✓7ᵗʰ **S45.812** Laceration of other specified blood vessels at shoulder and upper arm level, **left** arm   `CC`

         ✓7ᵗʰ **S45.819** Laceration of other specified blood vessels at shoulder and upper arm level, unspecified arm   `CC`

Ⓝ Newborn: 0   Ⓟ Pediatric: 0-17   Ⓜ Maternity: 9-64   Ⓐ Adult: 15-124   `MCC` Major Complication/Comorbidity   `CC` Complication/Comorbidity   `SW` Severe Wound Dx

1016   ICD-10-CM 2022

√6ᵗʰ **S45.89** **Other specified injury of other specified blood vessels at shoulder and upper arm level**

    √7ᵗʰ **S45.891** **Other specified injury of other specified blood vessels at shoulder and upper arm level, right arm** CC

    √7ᵗʰ **S45.892** **Other specified injury of other specified blood vessels at shoulder and upper arm level, left arm** CC

    √7ᵗʰ **S45.899** **Other specified injury of other specified blood vessels at shoulder and upper arm level, unspecified arm** CC

√5ᵗʰ **S45.9** **Injury of unspecified blood vessel at shoulder and upper arm level**

  √6ᵗʰ **S45.90** **Unspecified injury of unspecified blood vessel at shoulder and upper arm level**

    √7ᵗʰ **S45.901** **Unspecified injury of unspecified blood vessel at shoulder and upper arm level, right arm** CC

    √7ᵗʰ **S45.902** **Unspecified injury of unspecified blood vessel at shoulder and upper arm level, left arm** CC

    √7ᵗʰ **S45.909** **Unspecified injury of unspecified blood vessel at shoulder and upper arm level, unspecified arm** CC

  √6ᵗʰ **S45.91** **Laceration of unspecified blood vessel at shoulder and upper arm level**

    √7ᵗʰ **S45.911** **Laceration of unspecified blood vessel at shoulder and upper arm level, right arm** CC

    √7ᵗʰ **S45.912** **Laceration of unspecified blood vessel at shoulder and upper arm level, left arm** CC

    √7ᵗʰ **S45.919** **Laceration of unspecified blood vessel at shoulder and upper arm level, unspecified arm** CC

  √6ᵗʰ **S45.99** **Other specified injury of unspecified blood vessel at shoulder and upper arm level**

    √7ᵗʰ **S45.991** **Other specified injury of unspecified blood vessel at shoulder and upper arm level, right arm** CC

    √7ᵗʰ **S45.992** **Other specified injury of unspecified blood vessel at shoulder and upper arm level, left arm** CC

    √7ᵗʰ **S45.999** **Other specified injury of unspecified blood vessel at shoulder and upper arm level, unspecified arm** CC

√4ᵗʰ **S46** **Injury of muscle, fascia and tendon at shoulder and upper arm level**

Code also any associated open wound (S41.-)

EXCLUDES 2   *injury of muscle, fascia and tendon at elbow (S56.-)*

        sprain of joints and ligaments of shoulder girdle (S43.9)

TIP: Refer to the Muscle/Tendon table at the beginning of this chapter.

The appropriate 7th character is to be added to each code from category S46.
A   initial encounter
D   subsequent encounter
S   sequela

√5ᵗʰ **S46.0** **Injury of muscle(s) and tendon(s) of the rotator cuff of shoulder**

  √6ᵗʰ **S46.00** **Unspecified injury of muscle(s) and tendon(s) of the rotator cuff of shoulder**

    √7ᵗʰ **S46.001** **Unspecified injury of muscle(s) and tendon(s) of the rotator cuff of right shoulder**

    √7ᵗʰ **S46.002** **Unspecified injury of muscle(s) and tendon(s) of the rotator cuff of left shoulder**

    √7ᵗʰ **S46.009** **Unspecified injury of muscle(s) and tendon(s) of the rotator cuff of unspecified shoulder**

  √6ᵗʰ **S46.01** **Strain of muscle(s) and tendon(s) of the rotator cuff of shoulder**

    √7ᵗʰ **S46.011** **Strain of muscle(s) and tendon(s) of the rotator cuff of right shoulder**

    √7ᵗʰ **S46.012** **Strain of muscle(s) and tendon(s) of the rotator cuff of left shoulder**

    √7ᵗʰ **S46.019** **Strain of muscle(s) and tendon(s) of the rotator cuff of unspecified shoulder**

  √6ᵗʰ **S46.02** **Laceration of muscle(s) and tendon(s) of the rotator cuff of shoulder**

    √7ᵗʰ **S46.021** **Laceration of muscle(s) and tendon(s) of the rotator cuff of right shoulder** CC

    √7ᵗʰ **S46.022** **Laceration of muscle(s) and tendon(s) of the rotator cuff of left shoulder** CC

    √7ᵗʰ **S46.029** **Laceration of muscle(s) and tendon(s) of the rotator cuff of unspecified shoulder** CC

  √6ᵗʰ **S46.09** **Other injury of muscle(s) and tendon(s) of the rotator cuff of shoulder**

    √7ᵗʰ **S46.091** **Other injury of muscle(s) and tendon(s) of the rotator cuff of right shoulder**

    √7ᵗʰ **S46.092** **Other injury of muscle(s) and tendon(s) of the rotator cuff of left shoulder**

    √7ᵗʰ **S46.099** **Other injury of muscle(s) and tendon(s) of the rotator cuff of unspecified shoulder**

√5ᵗʰ **S46.1** **Injury of muscle, fascia and tendon of long head of biceps**

  √6ᵗʰ **S46.10** **Unspecified injury of muscle, fascia and tendon of long head of biceps**

    √7ᵗʰ **S46.101** **Unspecified injury of muscle, fascia and tendon of long head of biceps, right arm**

    √7ᵗʰ **S46.102** **Unspecified injury of muscle, fascia and tendon of long head of biceps, left arm**

    √7ᵗʰ **S46.109** **Unspecified injury of muscle, fascia and tendon of long head of biceps, unspecified arm**

  √6ᵗʰ **S46.11** **Strain of muscle, fascia and tendon of long head of biceps**

      AHA: 2020,1Q,38; 2019,2Q,27

    √7ᵗʰ **S46.111** **Strain of muscle, fascia and tendon of long head of biceps, right arm**

    √7ᵗʰ **S46.112** **Strain of muscle, fascia and tendon of long head of biceps, left arm**

    √7ᵗʰ **S46.119** **Strain of muscle, fascia and tendon of long head of biceps, unspecified arm**

  √6ᵗʰ **S46.12** **Laceration of muscle, fascia and tendon of long head of biceps**

    √7ᵗʰ **S46.121** **Laceration of muscle, fascia and tendon of long head of biceps, right arm** CC

    √7ᵗʰ **S46.122** **Laceration of muscle, fascia and tendon of long head of biceps, left arm** CC

    √7ᵗʰ **S46.129** **Laceration of muscle, fascia and tendon of long head of biceps, unspecified arm** CC

  √6ᵗʰ **S46.19** **Other injury of muscle, fascia and tendon of long head of biceps**

    √7ᵗʰ **S46.191** **Other injury of muscle, fascia and tendon of long head of biceps, right arm**

    √7ᵗʰ **S46.192** **Other injury of muscle, fascia and tendon of long head of biceps, left arm**

    √7ᵗʰ **S46.199** **Other injury of muscle, fascia and tendon of long head of biceps, unspecified arm**

√5ᵗʰ **S46.2** **Injury of muscle, fascia and tendon of other parts of biceps**

  √6ᵗʰ **S46.20** **Unspecified injury of muscle, fascia and tendon of other parts of biceps**

    √7ᵗʰ **S46.201** **Unspecified injury of muscle, fascia and tendon of other parts of biceps, right arm**

    √7ᵗʰ **S46.202** **Unspecified injury of muscle, fascia and tendon of other parts of biceps, left arm**

    √7ᵗʰ **S46.209** **Unspecified injury of muscle, fascia and tendon of other parts of biceps, unspecified arm**

  √6ᵗʰ **S46.21** **Strain of muscle, fascia and tendon of other parts of biceps**

    √7ᵗʰ **S46.211** **Strain of muscle, fascia and tendon of other parts of biceps, right arm**

    √7ᵗʰ **S46.212** **Strain of muscle, fascia and tendon of other parts of biceps, left arm**

    √7ᵗʰ **S46.219** **Strain of muscle, fascia and tendon of other parts of biceps, unspecified arm**

  √6ᵗʰ **S46.22** **Laceration of muscle, fascia and tendon of other parts of biceps**

    √7ᵗʰ **S46.221** **Laceration of muscle, fascia and tendon of other parts of biceps, right arm** CC

    √7ᵗʰ **S46.222** **Laceration of muscle, fascia and tendon of other parts of biceps, left arm** CC

    √7ᵗʰ **S46.229** **Laceration of muscle, fascia and tendon of other parts of biceps, unspecified arm** CC

  √6ᵗʰ **S46.29** **Other injury of muscle, fascia and tendon of other parts of biceps**

    √7ᵗʰ **S46.291** **Other injury of muscle, fascia and tendon of other parts of biceps, right arm**

    √7ᵗʰ **S46.292** **Other injury of muscle, fascia and tendon of other parts of biceps, left arm**

☑ Additional Character Required   √xᵗʰ Placeholder   Questionable PDx   Manifestation   Unspecified Dx   UPD Unacceptable PDx   H1-H4 HAC   HCC CMS-HCC Dx   HIV HIV Dx

ICD-10-CM 2022   1017

√7ᵗʰ **S46.299** Other injury of muscle, fascia and tendon of other parts of biceps, unspecified arm

√5ᵗʰ **S46.3** Injury of muscle, fascia and tendon of triceps

√6ᵗʰ **S46.30** Unspecified injury of muscle, fascia and tendon of triceps

√7ᵗʰ **S46.301** Unspecified injury of muscle, fascia and tendon of triceps, right arm

√7ᵗʰ **S46.302** Unspecified injury of muscle, fascia and tendon of triceps, left arm

√7ᵗʰ **S46.309** Unspecified injury of muscle, fascia and tendon of triceps, unspecified arm

√6ᵗʰ **S46.31** Strain of muscle, fascia and tendon of triceps

√7ᵗʰ **S46.311** Strain of muscle, fascia and tendon of triceps, right arm

√7ᵗʰ **S46.312** Strain of muscle, fascia and tendon of triceps, left arm

√7ᵗʰ **S46.319** Strain of muscle, fascia and tendon of triceps, unspecified arm

√6ᵗʰ **S46.32** Laceration of muscle, fascia and tendon of triceps

√7ᵗʰ **S46.321** Laceration of muscle, fascia and tendon of triceps, right arm　**CC**

√7ᵗʰ **S46.322** Laceration of muscle, fascia and tendon of triceps, left arm　**CC**

√7ᵗʰ **S46.329** Laceration of muscle, fascia and tendon of triceps, unspecified arm　**CC**

√6ᵗʰ **S46.39** Other injury of muscle, fascia and tendon of triceps

√7ᵗʰ **S46.391** Other injury of muscle, fascia and tendon of triceps, right arm

√7ᵗʰ **S46.392** Other injury of muscle, fascia and tendon of triceps, left arm

√7ᵗʰ **S46.399** Other injury of muscle, fascia and tendon of triceps, unspecified arm

√5ᵗʰ **S46.8** Injury of other muscles, fascia and tendons at shoulder and upper arm level

√6ᵗʰ **S46.80** Unspecified injury of other muscles, fascia and tendons at shoulder and upper arm level

√7ᵗʰ **S46.801** Unspecified injury of other muscles, fascia and tendons at shoulder and upper arm level, right arm

√7ᵗʰ **S46.802** Unspecified injury of other muscles, fascia and tendons at shoulder and upper arm level, left arm

√7ᵗʰ **S46.809** Unspecified injury of other muscles, fascia and tendons at shoulder and upper arm level, unspecified arm

√6ᵗʰ **S46.81** Strain of other muscles, fascia and tendons at shoulder and upper arm level

√7ᵗʰ **S46.811** Strain of other muscles, fascia and tendons at shoulder and upper arm level, right arm

√7ᵗʰ **S46.812** Strain of other muscles, fascia and tendons at shoulder and upper arm level, left arm

√7ᵗʰ **S46.819** Strain of other muscles, fascia and tendons at shoulder and upper arm level, unspecified arm

√6ᵗʰ **S46.82** Laceration of other muscles, fascia and tendons at shoulder and upper arm level

√7ᵗʰ **S46.821** Laceration of other muscles, fascia and tendons at shoulder and upper arm level, right arm　**CC**

√7ᵗʰ **S46.822** Laceration of other muscles, fascia and tendons at shoulder and upper arm level, left arm　**CC**

√7ᵗʰ **S46.829** Laceration of other muscles, fascia and tendons at shoulder and upper arm level, unspecified arm　**CC**

√6ᵗʰ **S46.89** Other injury of other muscles, fascia and tendons at shoulder and upper arm level

√7ᵗʰ **S46.891** Other injury of other muscles, fascia and tendons at shoulder and upper arm level, right arm

√7ᵗʰ **S46.892** Other injury of other muscles, fascia and tendons at shoulder and upper arm level, left arm

√7ᵗʰ **S46.899** Other injury of other muscles, fascia and tendons at shoulder and upper arm level, unspecified arm

√5ᵗʰ **S46.9** Injury of unspecified muscle, fascia and tendon at shoulder and upper arm level

√6ᵗʰ **S46.90** Unspecified injury of unspecified muscle, fascia and tendon at shoulder and upper arm level

√7ᵗʰ **S46.901** Unspecified injury of unspecified muscle, fascia and tendon at shoulder and upper arm level, right arm

√7ᵗʰ **S46.902** Unspecified injury of unspecified muscle, fascia and tendon at shoulder and upper arm level, left arm

√7ᵗʰ **S46.909** Unspecified injury of unspecified muscle, fascia and tendon at shoulder and upper arm level, unspecified arm

√6ᵗʰ **S46.91** Strain of unspecified muscle, fascia and tendon at shoulder and upper arm level

√7ᵗʰ **S46.911** Strain of unspecified muscle, fascia and tendon at shoulder and upper arm level, right arm

√7ᵗʰ **S46.912** Strain of unspecified muscle, fascia and tendon at shoulder and upper arm level, left arm

√7ᵗʰ **S46.919** Strain of unspecified muscle, fascia and tendon at shoulder and upper arm level, unspecified arm

√6ᵗʰ **S46.92** Laceration of unspecified muscle, fascia and tendon at shoulder and upper arm level

√7ᵗʰ **S46.921** Laceration of unspecified muscle, fascia and tendon at shoulder and upper arm level, right arm　**CC**

√7ᵗʰ **S46.922** Laceration of unspecified muscle, fascia and tendon at shoulder and upper arm level, left arm　**CC**

√7ᵗʰ **S46.929** Laceration of unspecified muscle, fascia and tendon at shoulder and upper arm level, unspecified arm　**CC**

√6ᵗʰ **S46.99** Other injury of unspecified muscle, fascia and tendon at shoulder and upper arm level

√7ᵗʰ **S46.991** Other injury of unspecified muscle, fascia and tendon at shoulder and upper arm level, right arm

√7ᵗʰ **S46.992** Other injury of unspecified muscle, fascia and tendon at shoulder and upper arm level, left arm

√7ᵗʰ **S46.999** Other injury of unspecified muscle, fascia and tendon at shoulder and upper arm level, unspecified arm

√4ᵗʰ **S47** Crushing injury of shoulder and upper arm

Use additional code for all associated injuries

EXCLUDES 2　crushing injury of elbow (S57.0-)

The appropriate 7th character is to be added to each code from category S47.
A　initial encounter
D　subsequent encounter
S　sequela

√x7ᵗʰ **S47.1** Crushing injury of right shoulder and upper arm

√x7ᵗʰ **S47.2** Crushing injury of left shoulder and upper arm

√x7ᵗʰ **S47.9** Crushing injury of shoulder and upper arm, unspecified arm

√4ᵗʰ **S48** Traumatic amputation of shoulder and upper arm

An amputation not identified as partial or complete should be coded to complete

EXCLUDES 1　traumatic amputation at elbow level (S58.0)

The appropriate 7th character is to be added to each code from category S48.
A　initial encounter
D　subsequent encounter
S　sequela

√5ᵗʰ **S48.0** Traumatic amputation at shoulder joint

√6ᵗʰ **S48.01** Complete traumatic amputation at shoulder joint

⁷ √7ᵗʰ **S48.011** Complete traumatic amputation at right shoulder joint　**CC** **HCC**

⁷ √7ᵗʰ **S48.012** Complete traumatic amputation at left shoulder joint　**CC** **HCC**

⁷ √7ᵗʰ **S48.019** Complete traumatic amputation at unspecified shoulder joint　**CC** **HCC**

√6ᵗʰ **S48.02** Partial traumatic amputation at shoulder joint

⁷ √7ᵗʰ **S48.021** Partial traumatic amputation at right shoulder joint　**CC** **HCC**

⁷ √7ᵗʰ **S48.022** Partial traumatic amputation at left shoulder joint　**CC** **HCC**

7 √7ᵗʰ **S48.029** Partial traumatic amputation at unspecified shoulder joint   CC HCC

√5ᵗʰ **S48.1** Traumatic amputation at level between shoulder and elbow

  √6ᵗʰ **S48.11** Complete traumatic amputation at level between shoulder and elbow

    7 √7ᵗʰ **S48.111** Complete traumatic amputation at level between right shoulder and elbow   CC HCC

    7 √7ᵗʰ **S48.112** Complete traumatic amputation at level between left shoulder and elbow   CC HCC

    7 √7ᵗʰ **S48.119** Complete traumatic amputation at level between unspecified shoulder and elbow   CC HCC

  √6ᵗʰ **S48.12** Partial traumatic amputation at level between shoulder and elbow

    7 √7ᵗʰ **S48.121** Partial traumatic amputation at level between right shoulder and elbow   CC HCC

    7 √7ᵗʰ **S48.122** Partial traumatic amputation at level between left shoulder and elbow   CC HCC

    7 √7ᵗʰ **S48.129** Partial traumatic amputation at level between unspecified shoulder and elbow   CC HCC

√5ᵗʰ **S48.9** Traumatic amputation of shoulder and upper arm, level unspecified

  √6ᵗʰ **S48.91** Complete traumatic amputation of shoulder and upper arm, level unspecified

    7 √7ᵗʰ **S48.911** Complete traumatic amputation of right shoulder and upper arm, level unspecified   CC HCC

    7 √7ᵗʰ **S48.912** Complete traumatic amputation of left shoulder and upper arm, level unspecified   CC HCC

    7 √7ᵗʰ **S48.919** Complete traumatic amputation of unspecified shoulder and upper arm, level unspecified   CC HCC

  √6ᵗʰ **S48.92** Partial traumatic amputation of shoulder and upper arm, level unspecified

    7 √7ᵗʰ **S48.921** Partial traumatic amputation of right shoulder and upper arm, level unspecified   CC HCC

    7 √7ᵗʰ **S48.922** Partial traumatic amputation of left shoulder and upper arm, level unspecified   CC HCC

    7 √7ᵗʰ **S48.929** Partial traumatic amputation of unspecified shoulder and upper arm, level unspecified   CC HCC

√4ᵗʰ **S49** Other and unspecified injuries of shoulder and upper arm

  AHA: 2018,2Q,12; 2018,1Q,3

> The appropriate 7th character is to be added to each code from subcategories S49.0 and S49.1.
> A   initial encounter for closed fracture
> D   subsequent encounter for fracture with routine healing
> G   subsequent encounter for fracture with delayed healing
> K   subsequent encounter for fracture with nonunion
> P   subsequent encounter for fracture with malunion
> S   sequela

√5ᵗʰ **S49.0** Physeal fracture of upper end of humerus

  AHA: 2019,4Q,56

  √6ᵗʰ **S49.00** Unspecified physeal fracture of upper end of humerus

    3 √7ᵗʰ **S49.001** Unspecified physeal fracture of upper end of humerus, right arm   CC H5

    3 √7ᵗʰ **S49.002** Unspecified physeal fracture of upper end of humerus, left arm   CC H5

    3 √7ᵗʰ **S49.009** Unspecified physeal fracture of upper end of humerus, unspecified arm   CC H5

  √6ᵗʰ **S49.01** Salter-Harris Type I physeal fracture of upper end of humerus

    3 √7ᵗʰ **S49.011** Salter-Harris Type I physeal fracture of upper end of humerus, right arm   CC H5

    3 √7ᵗʰ **S49.012** Salter-Harris Type I physeal fracture of upper end of humerus, left arm   CC H5

    3 √7ᵗʰ **S49.019** Salter-Harris Type I physeal fracture of upper end of humerus, unspecified arm   CC H5

  √6ᵗʰ **S49.02** Salter-Harris Type II physeal fracture of upper end of humerus

    3 √7ᵗʰ **S49.021** Salter-Harris Type II physeal fracture of upper end of humerus, right arm   CC H5

    3 √7ᵗʰ **S49.022** Salter-Harris Type II physeal fracture of upper end of humerus, left arm   CC H5

    3 √7ᵗʰ **S49.029** Salter-Harris Type II physeal fracture of upper end of humerus, unspecified arm   CC H5

  √6ᵗʰ **S49.03** Salter-Harris Type III physeal fracture of upper end of humerus

    3 √7ᵗʰ **S49.031** Salter-Harris Type III physeal fracture of upper end of humerus, right arm   CC H5

    3 √7ᵗʰ **S49.032** Salter-Harris Type III physeal fracture of upper end of humerus, left arm   CC H5

    3 √7ᵗʰ **S49.039** Salter-Harris Type III physeal fracture of upper end of humerus, unspecified arm   CC H5

  √6ᵗʰ **S49.04** Salter-Harris Type IV physeal fracture of upper end of humerus

    3 √7ᵗʰ **S49.041** Salter-Harris Type IV physeal fracture of upper end of humerus, right arm   CC H5

    3 √7ᵗʰ **S49.042** Salter-Harris Type IV physeal fracture of upper end of humerus, left arm   CC H5

    3 √7ᵗʰ **S49.049** Salter-Harris Type IV physeal fracture of upper end of humerus, unspecified arm   CC H5

  √6ᵗʰ **S49.09** Other physeal fracture of upper end of humerus

    3 √7ᵗʰ **S49.091** Other physeal fracture of upper end of humerus, right arm   CC H5

    3 √7ᵗʰ **S49.092** Other physeal fracture of upper end of humerus, left arm   CC H5

    3 √7ᵗʰ **S49.099** Other physeal fracture of upper end of humerus, unspecified arm   CC H5

√5ᵗʰ **S49.1** Physeal fracture of lower end of humerus

  AHA: 2019,4Q,56

  √6ᵗʰ **S49.10** Unspecified physeal fracture of lower end of humerus

    3 √7ᵗʰ **S49.101** Unspecified physeal fracture of lower end of humerus, right arm   CC H5

    3 √7ᵗʰ **S49.102** Unspecified physeal fracture of lower end of humerus, left arm   CC H5

    3 √7ᵗʰ **S49.109** Unspecified physeal fracture of lower end of humerus, unspecified arm   CC H5

  √6ᵗʰ **S49.11** Salter-Harris Type I physeal fracture of lower end of humerus

    3 √7ᵗʰ **S49.111** Salter-Harris Type I physeal fracture of lower end of humerus, right arm   CC H5

    3 √7ᵗʰ **S49.112** Salter-Harris Type I physeal fracture of lower end of humerus, left arm   CC H5

    3 √7ᵗʰ **S49.119** Salter-Harris Type I physeal fracture of lower end of humerus, unspecified arm   CC H5

  √6ᵗʰ **S49.12** Salter-Harris Type II physeal fracture of lower end of humerus

    3 √7ᵗʰ **S49.121** Salter-Harris Type II physeal fracture of lower end of humerus, right arm   CC H5

    3 √7ᵗʰ **S49.122** Salter-Harris Type II physeal fracture of lower end of humerus, left arm   CC H5

    3 √7ᵗʰ **S49.129** Salter-Harris Type II physeal fracture of lower end of humerus, unspecified arm   CC H5

  √6ᵗʰ **S49.13** Salter-Harris Type III physeal fracture of lower end of humerus

    3 √7ᵗʰ **S49.131** Salter-Harris Type III physeal fracture of lower end of humerus, right arm   CC H5

    3 √7ᵗʰ **S49.132** Salter-Harris Type III physeal fracture of lower end of humerus, left arm   CC H5

    3 √7ᵗʰ **S49.139** Salter-Harris Type III physeal fracture of lower end of humerus, unspecified arm   CC H5

☑ Additional Character Required   √x7ᵗʰ Placeholder   Questionable PDx   Manifestation   Unspecified Dx   UPD Unacceptable PDx   H1-H14 HAC   HCC CMS-HCC Dx   HIV HIV Dx

ICD-10-CM 2022   1019

Chapter 19. Injury, Poisoning and Certain Other Consequences of External Causes

S49.14–S50.919

✓6ᵗʰ **S49.14 Salter-Harris Type IV** physeal fracture of lower end of humerus

  ³ ✓7ᵗʰ **S49.141** Salter-Harris Type IV physeal fracture of lower end of humerus, right arm   CC H5

  ³ ✓7ᵗʰ **S49.142** Salter-Harris Type IV physeal fracture of lower end of humerus, left arm   CC H5

  ³ ✓7ᵗʰ **S49.149** Salter-Harris Type IV physeal fracture of lower end of humerus, unspecified arm   CC H5

✓6ᵗʰ **S49.19 Other** physeal fracture of lower end of humerus

  ³ ✓7ᵗʰ **S49.191** Other physeal fracture of lower end of humerus, right arm   CC H5

  ³ ✓7ᵗʰ **S49.192** Other physeal fracture of lower end of humerus, left arm   CC H5

  ³ ✓7ᵗʰ **S49.199** Other physeal fracture of lower end of humerus, unspecified arm   CC H5

✓5ᵗʰ **S49.8 Other specified injuries of shoulder and upper arm**

The appropriate 7th character is to be added to each code in subcategory S49.8.
A   initial encounter
D   subsequent encounter
S   sequela

✓✗7ᵗʰ **S49.80** Other specified injuries of shoulder and upper arm, unspecified arm

✓✗7ᵗʰ **S49.81** Other specified injuries of right shoulder and upper arm

✓✗7ᵗʰ **S49.82** Other specified injuries of left shoulder and upper arm

✓6ᵗʰ **S49.9 Unspecified injury of shoulder and upper arm**

The appropriate 7th character is to be added to each code in subcategory S49.9.
A   initial encounter
D   subsequent encounter
S   sequela

✓✗7ᵗʰ **S49.90** Unspecified injury of shoulder and upper arm, unspecified arm

✓✗7ᵗʰ **S49.91** Unspecified injury of right shoulder and upper arm

✓✗7ᵗʰ **S49.92** Unspecified injury of left shoulder and upper arm

Injuries to the elbow and forearm (S50-S59)

EXCLUDES 2   burns and corrosions (T20-T32)
     frostbite (T33-T34)
     injuries of wrist and hand (S60-S69)
     insect bite or sting, venomous (T63.4)

✓4ᵗʰ **S50 Superficial injury of elbow and forearm**

EXCLUDES 2   superficial injury of wrist and hand (S60.-)

The appropriate 7th character is to be added to each code from category S50.
A   initial encounter
D   subsequent encounter
S   sequela

✓5ᵗʰ **S50.0 Contusion of elbow**

  ✓✗7ᵗʰ **S50.00** Contusion of unspecified elbow

  ✓✗7ᵗʰ **S50.01** Contusion of right elbow

  ✓✗7ᵗʰ **S50.02** Contusion of left elbow

✓5ᵗʰ **S50.1 Contusion of forearm**

  ✓✗7ᵗʰ **S50.10** Contusion of unspecified forearm

  ✓✗7ᵗʰ **S50.11** Contusion of right forearm

  ✓✗7ᵗʰ **S50.12** Contusion of left forearm

✓5ᵗʰ **S50.3 Other superficial injuries of elbow**

  ✓6ᵗʰ **S50.31 Abrasion of elbow**

    ✓7ᵗʰ **S50.311** Abrasion of right elbow

    ✓7ᵗʰ **S50.312** Abrasion of left elbow

    ✓7ᵗʰ **S50.319** Abrasion of unspecified elbow

  ✓6ᵗʰ **S50.32 Blister (nonthermal) of elbow**

    ✓7ᵗʰ **S50.321** Blister (nonthermal) of right elbow

    ✓7ᵗʰ **S50.322** Blister (nonthermal) of left elbow

    ✓7ᵗʰ **S50.329** Blister (nonthermal) of unspecified elbow

  ✓6ᵗʰ **S50.34 External constriction of elbow**

    ✓7ᵗʰ **S50.341** External constriction of right elbow

    ✓7ᵗʰ **S50.342** External constriction of left elbow

    ✓7ᵗʰ **S50.349** External constriction of unspecified elbow

  ✓6ᵗʰ **S50.35 Superficial foreign body of elbow**

Splinter in the elbow

    ✓7ᵗʰ **S50.351** Superficial foreign body of right elbow

    ✓7ᵗʰ **S50.352** Superficial foreign body of left elbow

    ✓7ᵗʰ **S50.359** Superficial foreign body of unspecified elbow

  ✓6ᵗʰ **S50.36 Insect bite (nonvenomous) of elbow**

    ✓7ᵗʰ **S50.361** Insect bite (nonvenomous) of right elbow

    ✓7ᵗʰ **S50.362** Insect bite (nonvenomous) of left elbow

    ✓7ᵗʰ **S50.369** Insect bite (nonvenomous) of unspecified elbow

  ✓6ᵗʰ **S50.37 Other superficial bite of elbow**

    EXCLUDES 1   open bite of elbow (S51.05)

    ✓7ᵗʰ **S50.371** Other superficial bite of right elbow

    ✓7ᵗʰ **S50.372** Other superficial bite of left elbow

    ✓7ᵗʰ **S50.379** Other superficial bite of unspecified elbow

✓5ᵗʰ **S50.8 Other superficial injuries of forearm**

  ✓6ᵗʰ **S50.81 Abrasion of forearm**

    ✓7ᵗʰ **S50.811** Abrasion of right forearm

    ✓7ᵗʰ **S50.812** Abrasion of left forearm

    ✓7ᵗʰ **S50.819** Abrasion of unspecified forearm

  ✓6ᵗʰ **S50.82 Blister (nonthermal) of forearm**

    ✓7ᵗʰ **S50.821** Blister (nonthermal) of right forearm

    ✓7ᵗʰ **S50.822** Blister (nonthermal) of left forearm

    ✓7ᵗʰ **S50.829** Blister (nonthermal) of unspecified forearm

  ✓6ᵗʰ **S50.84 External constriction of forearm**

    ✓7ᵗʰ **S50.841** External constriction of right forearm

    ✓7ᵗʰ **S50.842** External constriction of left forearm

    ✓7ᵗʰ **S50.849** External constriction of unspecified forearm

  ✓6ᵗʰ **S50.85 Superficial foreign body of forearm**

Splinter in the forearm

    ✓7ᵗʰ **S50.851** Superficial foreign body of right forearm

    ✓7ᵗʰ **S50.852** Superficial foreign body of left forearm

    ✓7ᵗʰ **S50.859** Superficial foreign body of unspecified forearm

  ✓6ᵗʰ **S50.86 Insect bite (nonvenomous) of forearm**

    ✓7ᵗʰ **S50.861** Insect bite (nonvenomous) of right forearm

    ✓7ᵗʰ **S50.862** Insect bite (nonvenomous) of left forearm

    ✓7ᵗʰ **S50.869** Insect bite (nonvenomous) of unspecified forearm

  ✓6ᵗʰ **S50.87 Other superficial bite of forearm**

    EXCLUDES 1   open bite of forearm (S51.85)

    ✓7ᵗʰ **S50.871** Other superficial bite of right forearm

    ✓7ᵗʰ **S50.872** Other superficial bite of left forearm

    ✓7ᵗʰ **S50.879** Other superficial bite of unspecified forearm

✓5ᵗʰ **S50.9 Unspecified superficial injury of elbow and forearm**

  ✓6ᵗʰ **S50.90 Unspecified superficial injury of elbow**

    ✓7ᵗʰ **S50.901** Unspecified superficial injury of right elbow

    ✓7ᵗʰ **S50.902** Unspecified superficial injury of left elbow

    ✓7ᵗʰ **S50.909** Unspecified superficial injury of unspecified elbow

  ✓6ᵗʰ **S50.91 Unspecified superficial injury of forearm**

    ✓7ᵗʰ **S50.911** Unspecified superficial injury of right forearm

    ✓7ᵗʰ **S50.912** Unspecified superficial injury of left forearm

    ✓7ᵗʰ **S50.919** Unspecified superficial injury of unspecified forearm

☑4ᵗʰ S51 Open wound of elbow and forearm

Code also any associated wound infection

EXCLUDES 1   open fracture of elbow and forearm (S52.- with open fracture 7th character)

traumatic amputation of elbow and forearm (S58.-)

EXCLUDES 2   open wound of wrist and hand (S61.-)

The appropriate 7th character is to be added to each code from category S51.

A   initial encounter
D   subsequent encounter
S   sequela

☑5ᵗʰ S51.0 Open wound of elbow

   ☑6ᵗʰ S51.00 Unspecified open wound of elbow

      ☑7ᵗʰ S51.001 Unspecified open wound of right elbow

         AHA: 2012,4Q,108

      ☑7ᵗʰ S51.002 Unspecified open wound of left elbow

      ☑7ᵗʰ S51.009 Unspecified open wound of unspecified elbow

         Open wound of elbow NOS

   ☑6ᵗʰ S51.01 Laceration without foreign body of elbow

      ☑7ᵗʰ S51.011 Laceration without foreign body of right elbow

      ☑7ᵗʰ S51.012 Laceration without foreign body of left elbow

      ☑7ᵗʰ S51.019 Laceration without foreign body of unspecified elbow

   ☑6ᵗʰ S51.02 Laceration with foreign body of elbow

      ☑7ᵗʰ S51.021 Laceration with foreign body of right elbow

      ☑7ᵗʰ S51.022 Laceration with foreign body of left elbow

      ☑7ᵗʰ S51.029 Laceration with foreign body of unspecified elbow

   ☑6ᵗʰ S51.03 Puncture wound without foreign body of elbow

      ☑7ᵗʰ S51.031 Puncture wound without foreign body of right elbow

      ☑7ᵗʰ S51.032 Puncture wound without foreign body of left elbow

      ☑7ᵗʰ S51.039 Puncture wound without foreign body of unspecified elbow

   ☑6ᵗʰ S51.04 Puncture wound with foreign body of elbow

      ☑7ᵗʰ S51.041 Puncture wound with foreign body of right elbow

      ☑7ᵗʰ S51.042 Puncture wound with foreign body of left elbow

      ☑7ᵗʰ S51.049 Puncture wound with foreign body of unspecified elbow

   ☑6ᵗʰ S51.05 Open bite of elbow

      Bite of elbow NOS

      EXCLUDES 1   superficial bite of elbow (S50.36, S50.37)

      ☑7ᵗʰ S51.051 Open bite, right elbow

      ☑7ᵗʰ S51.052 Open bite, left elbow

      ☑7ᵗʰ S51.059 Open bite, unspecified elbow

☑5ᵗʰ S51.8 Open wound of forearm

   EXCLUDES 2   open wound of elbow (S51.0-)

   ☑6ᵗʰ S51.80 Unspecified open wound of forearm

      AHA: 2016,3Q,24

      ☑7ᵗʰ S51.801 Unspecified open wound of right forearm

      ☑7ᵗʰ S51.802 Unspecified open wound of left forearm

      ☑7ᵗʰ S51.809 Unspecified open wound of unspecified forearm

         Open wound of forearm NOS

   ☑6ᵗʰ S51.81 Laceration without foreign body of forearm

      ☑7ᵗʰ S51.811 Laceration without foreign body of right forearm

      ☑7ᵗʰ S51.812 Laceration without foreign body of left forearm

      ☑7ᵗʰ S51.819 Laceration without foreign body of unspecified forearm

   ☑6ᵗʰ S51.82 Laceration with foreign body of forearm

      ☑7ᵗʰ S51.821 Laceration with foreign body of right forearm

      ☑7ᵗʰ S51.822 Laceration with foreign body of left forearm

      ☑7ᵗʰ S51.829 Laceration with foreign body of unspecified forearm

   ☑6ᵗʰ S51.83 Puncture wound without foreign body of forearm

      AHA: 2016,3Q,24

      ☑7ᵗʰ S51.831 Puncture wound without foreign body of right forearm

      ☑7ᵗʰ S51.832 Puncture wound without foreign body of left forearm

      ☑7ᵗʰ S51.839 Puncture wound without foreign body of unspecified forearm

   ☑6ᵗʰ S51.84 Puncture wound with foreign body of forearm

      AHA: 2016,3Q,24

      ☑7ᵗʰ S51.841 Puncture wound with foreign body of right forearm

      ☑7ᵗʰ S51.842 Puncture wound with foreign body of left forearm

      ☑7ᵗʰ S51.849 Puncture wound with foreign body of unspecified forearm

   ☑6ᵗʰ S51.85 Open bite of forearm

      Bite of forearm NOS

      EXCLUDES 1   superficial bite of forearm (S50.86, S50.87)

      ☑7ᵗʰ S51.851 Open bite of right forearm

      ☑7ᵗʰ S51.852 Open bite of left forearm

      ☑7ᵗʰ S51.859 Open bite of unspecified forearm

☑4ᵗʰ S52 Fracture of forearm

   NOTE   A fracture not indicated as displaced or nondisplaced should be coded to displaced.

      A fracture not indicated as open or closed should be coded to closed.

      The open fracture designations are based on the Gustilo open fracture classification.

   EXCLUDES 1   traumatic amputation of forearm (S58.-)

   EXCLUDES 2   fracture at wrist and hand level (S62.-)

   AHA: 2018,2Q,12; 2016,1Q,33; 2015,3Q,37-39

   DEF: Diaphysis: Central shaft of a long bone.

   DEF: Epiphysis: Proximal and distal rounded ends of a long bone, communicates with the joint.

   DEF: Metaphysis: Section of a long bone located between the epiphysis and diaphysis at the proximal and distal ends.

   DEF: Physis (growth plate): Narrow zone of cartilaginous tissue between the epiphysis and metaphysis at each end of a long bone. In childhood, proliferation of cells in this zone lengthens the bone. As the bone matures, this area thins, ossification eventually fusing into solid bone and growth stops. **Synonym(s):** Epiphyseal plate.

The appropriate 7th character is to be added to all codes from category S52 [unless otherwise indicated].

A   initial encounter for closed fracture
B   initial encounter for open fracture type I or II
    initial encounter for open fracture NOS
C   initial encounter for open fracture type IIIA, IIIB, or IIIC
D   subsequent encounter for closed fracture with routine healing
E   subsequent encounter for open fracture type I or II with routine healing
F   subsequent encounter for open fracture type IIIA, IIIB, or IIIC with routine healing
G   subsequent encounter for closed fracture with delayed healing
H   subsequent encounter for open fracture type I or II with delayed healing
J   subsequent encounter for open fracture type IIIA, IIIB, or IIIC with delayed healing
K   subsequent encounter for closed fracture with nonunion
M   subsequent encounter for open fracture type I or II with nonunion
N   subsequent encounter for open fracture type IIIA, IIIB, or IIIC with nonunion
P   subsequent encounter for closed fracture with malunion
Q   subsequent encounter for open fracture type I or II with malunion
R   subsequent encounter for open fracture type IIIA, IIIB, or IIIC with malunion
S   sequela

☑5ᵗʰ S52.0 Fracture of upper end of ulna

   Fracture of proximal end of ulna

   EXCLUDES 2   fracture of elbow NOS (S42.40-)

            fractures of shaft of ulna (S52.2-)

   ☑6ᵗʰ S52.00 Unspecified fracture of upper end of ulna

      2,4 **☑7ᵗʰ S52.001 Unspecified fracture of upper end of right ulna**   MCC CC H5

      2,4 **☑7ᵗʰ S52.002 Unspecified fracture of upper end of left ulna**   MCC CC H5

☑ Additional Character Required   ☑7ᵗʰ Placeholder   Questionable PDx   Manifestation   Unspecified Dx   UPD Unacceptable PDx   H1-H14 HAC   HCC CMS-HCC Dx   HIV HIV Dx

ICD-10-CM 2022   1021

2,4 √7th **S52.009** Unspecified fracture of upper end of unspecified ulna MCC CC H5

√6th **S52.01** Torus fracture of upper end of ulna

> The appropriate 7th character is to be added to all codes in subcategory S52.01
> A   initial encounter for closed fracture
> D   subsequent encounter for fracture with routine healing
> G   subsequent encounter for fracture with delayed healing
> K   subsequent encounter for fracture with nonunion
> P   subsequent encounter for fracture with malunion
> S   sequela

3 √7th **S52.011** Torus fracture of upper end of right ulna CC H5

3 √7th **S52.012** Torus fracture of upper end of left ulna CC H5

3 √7th **S52.019** Torus fracture of upper end of unspecified ulna CC H5

√6th **S52.02** Fracture of olecranon process without intraarticular extension of ulna

2,4 √7th **S52.021** Displaced fracture of olecranon process without intraarticular extension of right ulna MCC CC H5

2,4 √7th **S52.022** Displaced fracture of olecranon process without intraarticular extension of left ulna MCC CC H5

2,4 √7th **S52.023** Displaced fracture of olecranon process without intraarticular extension of unspecified ulna MCC CC H5

2,4 √7th **S52.024** Nondisplaced fracture of olecranon process without intraarticular extension of right ulna MCC CC H5

2,4 √7th **S52.025** Nondisplaced fracture of olecranon process without intraarticular extension of left ulna MCC CC H5

2,4 √7th **S52.026** Nondisplaced fracture of olecranon process without intraarticular extension of unspecified ulna MCC CC H5

√6th **S52.03** Fracture of olecranon process with intraarticular extension of ulna

2,4 √7th **S52.031** Displaced fracture of olecranon process with intraarticular extension of right ulna MCC CC H5

2,4 √7th **S52.032** Displaced fracture of olecranon process with intraarticular extension of left ulna MCC CC H5

2,4 √7th **S52.033** Displaced fracture of olecranon process with intraarticular extension of unspecified ulna MCC CC H5

2,4 √7th **S52.034** Nondisplaced fracture of olecranon process with intraarticular extension of right ulna MCC CC H5

2,4 √7th **S52.035** Nondisplaced fracture of olecranon process with intraarticular extension of left ulna MCC CC H5

2,4 √7th **S52.036** Nondisplaced fracture of olecranon process with intraarticular extension of unspecified ulna MCC CC H5

√6th **S52.04** Fracture of coronoid process of ulna

2,4 √7th **S52.041** Displaced fracture of coronoid process of right ulna MCC CC H5

2,4 √7th **S52.042** Displaced fracture of coronoid process of left ulna MCC CC H5

2,4 √7th **S52.043** Displaced fracture of coronoid process of unspecified ulna MCC CC H5

2,4 √7th **S52.044** Nondisplaced fracture of coronoid process of right ulna MCC CC H5

2,4 √7th **S52.045** Nondisplaced fracture of coronoid process of left ulna MCC CC H5

2,4 √7th **S52.046** Nondisplaced fracture of coronoid process of unspecified ulna MCC CC H5

√6th **S52.09** Other fracture of upper end of ulna

2,4 √7th **S52.091** Other fracture of upper end of right ulna MCC CC H5

2,4 √7th **S52.092** Other fracture of upper end of left ulna MCC CC H5

2,4 √7th **S52.099** Other fracture of upper end of unspecified ulna MCC CC H5

√5th **S52.1** Fracture of upper end of radius

Fracture of proximal end of radius

EXCLUDES 2   physeal fractures of upper end of radius (S59.2-)
fracture of shaft of radius (S52.3-)

√6th **S52.10** Unspecified fracture of upper end of radius

2,4 √7th **S52.101** Unspecified fracture of upper end of right radius MCC CC H5

2,4 √7th **S52.102** Unspecified fracture of upper end of left radius MCC CC H5

2,4 √7th **S52.109** Unspecified fracture of upper end of unspecified radius MCC CC H5

√6th **S52.11** Torus fracture of upper end of radius

> The appropriate 7th character is to be added to all codes in subcategory S52.11
> A   initial encounter for closed fracture
> D   subsequent encounter for fracture with routine healing
> G   subsequent encounter for fracture with delayed healing
> K   subsequent encounter for fracture with nonunion
> P   subsequent encounter for fracture with malunion
> S   sequela

3 √7th **S52.111** Torus fracture of upper end of right radius CC H5

3 √7th **S52.112** Torus fracture of upper end of left radius CC H5

3 √7th **S52.119** Torus fracture of upper end of unspecified radius CC H5

√6th **S52.12** Fracture of head of radius

2,4 √7th **S52.121** Displaced fracture of head of right radius MCC CC H5

2,4 √7th **S52.122** Displaced fracture of head of left radius MCC CC H5

2,4 √7th **S52.123** Displaced fracture of head of unspecified radius MCC CC H5

2,4 √7th **S52.124** Nondisplaced fracture of head of right radius MCC CC H5

2,4 √7th **S52.125** Nondisplaced fracture of head of left radius MCC CC H5

2,4 √7th **S52.126** Nondisplaced fracture of head of unspecified radius MCC CC H5

√6th **S52.13** Fracture of neck of radius

2,4 √7th **S52.131** Displaced fracture of neck of right radius MCC CC H5

2,4 √7th **S52.132** Displaced fracture of neck of left radius MCC CC H5

2,4 √7th **S52.133** Displaced fracture of neck of unspecified radius MCC CC H5

2,4 √7th **S52.134** Nondisplaced fracture of neck of right radius MCC CC H5

2,4 √7th **S52.135** Nondisplaced fracture of neck of left radius MCC CC H5

2,4 √7th **S52.136** Nondisplaced fracture of neck of unspecified radius MCC CC H5

√6th **S52.18** Other fracture of upper end of radius

2,4 √7th **S52.181** Other fracture of upper end of right radius MCC CC H5

2,4 √7th **S52.182** Other fracture of upper end of left radius MCC CC H5

2,4 √7th **S52.189** Other fracture of upper end of unspecified radius MCC CC H5

√5th **S52.2** Fracture of shaft of ulna

√6th **S52.20** Unspecified fracture of shaft of ulna

Fracture of ulna NOS

2,3 √7th **S52.201** Unspecified fracture of shaft of right ulna MCC CC H5

2,3 √7th **S52.202** Unspecified fracture of shaft of left ulna MCC CC H5

2,3 √7th **S52.209** Unspecified fracture of shaft of unspecified ulna MCC CC H5

N Newborn: 0   P Pediatric: 0-17   M Maternity: 9-64   A Adult: 15-124   MCC Major Complication/Comorbidity   CC Complication/Comorbidity   SW Severe Wound Dx

1022   ICD-10-CM 2022

√6ᵗʰ **S52.21** Greenstick **fracture of shaft of ulna**

> The appropriate 7th character is to be added to all codes in subcategory S52.21
> A   initial encounter for closed fracture
> D   subsequent encounter for fracture with routine healing
> G   subsequent encounter for fracture with delayed healing
> K   subsequent encounter for fracture with nonunion
> P   subsequent encounter for fracture with malunion
> S   sequela

3 √7ᵗʰ **S52.211** Greenstick fracture of shaft of right ulna   CC H5

3 √7ᵗʰ **S52.212** Greenstick fracture of shaft of left ulna   CC H5

3 √7ᵗʰ **S52.219** Greenstick fracture of shaft of unspecified ulna   CC H5

√6ᵗʰ **S52.22** Transverse **fracture of shaft of ulna**

2,3 √7ᵗʰ **S52.221** Displaced transverse fracture of shaft of right ulna   MCC CC H5

2,3 √7ᵗʰ **S52.222** Displaced transverse fracture of shaft of left ulna   MCC CC H5

2,3 √7ᵗʰ **S52.223** Displaced transverse fracture of shaft of unspecified ulna   MCC CC H5

2,3 √7ᵗʰ **S52.224** Nondisplaced transverse fracture of shaft of right ulna   MCC CC H5

2,3 √7ᵗʰ **S52.225** Nondisplaced transverse fracture of shaft of left ulna   MCC CC H5

2,3 √7ᵗʰ **S52.226** Nondisplaced transverse fracture of shaft of unspecified ulna   MCC CC H5

√6ᵗʰ **S52.23** Oblique **fracture of shaft of ulna**

2,3 √7ᵗʰ **S52.231** Displaced oblique fracture of shaft of right ulna   MCC CC H5

2,3 √7ᵗʰ **S52.232** Displaced oblique fracture of shaft of left ulna   MCC CC H5

2,3 √7ᵗʰ **S52.233** Displaced oblique fracture of shaft of unspecified ulna   MCC CC H5

2,3 √7ᵗʰ **S52.234** Nondisplaced oblique fracture of shaft of right ulna   MCC CC H5

2,3 √7ᵗʰ **S52.235** Nondisplaced oblique fracture of shaft of left ulna   MCC CC H5

2,3 √7ᵗʰ **S52.236** Nondisplaced oblique fracture of shaft of unspecified ulna   MCC CC H5

√6ᵗʰ **S52.24** Spiral **fracture of shaft of ulna**

2,3 √7ᵗʰ **S52.241** Displaced spiral fracture of shaft of ulna, right arm   MCC CC H5

2,3 √7ᵗʰ **S52.242** Displaced spiral fracture of shaft of ulna, left arm   MCC CC H5

2,3 √7ᵗʰ **S52.243** Displaced spiral fracture of shaft of ulna, unspecified arm   MCC CC H5

2,3 √7ᵗʰ **S52.244** Nondisplaced spiral fracture of shaft of ulna, right arm   MCC CC H5

2,3 √7ᵗʰ **S52.245** Nondisplaced spiral fracture of shaft of ulna, left arm   MCC CC H5

2,3 √7ᵗʰ **S52.246** Nondisplaced spiral fracture of shaft of ulna, unspecified arm   MCC CC H5

√6ᵗʰ **S52.25** Comminuted **fracture of shaft of ulna**

2,3 √7ᵗʰ **S52.251** Displaced comminuted fracture of shaft of ulna, right arm   MCC CC H5

2,3 √7ᵗʰ **S52.252** Displaced comminuted fracture of shaft of ulna, left arm   MCC CC H5

2,3 √7ᵗʰ **S52.253** Displaced comminuted fracture of shaft of ulna, unspecified arm   MCC CC H5

2,3 √7ᵗʰ **S52.254** Nondisplaced comminuted fracture of shaft of ulna, right arm   MCC CC H5

2,3 √7ᵗʰ **S52.255** Nondisplaced comminuted fracture of shaft of ulna, left arm   MCC CC H5

2,3 √7ᵗʰ **S52.256** Nondisplaced comminuted fracture of shaft of ulna, unspecified arm   MCC CC H5

√6ᵗʰ **S52.26** Segmental **fracture of shaft of ulna**

2,3 √7ᵗʰ **S52.261** Displaced segmental fracture of shaft of ulna, right arm   MCC CC H5

2,3 √7ᵗʰ **S52.262** Displaced segmental fracture of shaft of ulna, left arm   MCC CC H5

2,3 √7ᵗʰ **S52.263** Displaced segmental fracture of shaft of ulna, unspecified arm   MCC CC H5

2,3 √7ᵗʰ **S52.264** Nondisplaced segmental fracture of shaft of ulna, right arm   MCC CC H5

2,3 √7ᵗʰ **S52.265** Nondisplaced segmental fracture of shaft of ulna, left arm   MCC CC H5

2,3 √7ᵗʰ **S52.266** Nondisplaced segmental fracture of shaft of ulna, unspecified arm   MCC CC H5

√6ᵗʰ **S52.27** Monteggia's **fracture of ulna**

> Fracture of upper shaft of ulna with dislocation of radial head

2,4 √7ᵗʰ **S52.271** Monteggia's fracture of right ulna   MCC CC H5

2,4 √7ᵗʰ **S52.272** Monteggia's fracture of left ulna   MCC CC H5

2,4 √7ᵗʰ **S52.279** Monteggia's fracture of unspecified ulna   MCC CC H5

√6ᵗʰ **S52.28** Bent bone **of ulna**

2,3 √7ᵗʰ **S52.281** Bent bone of right ulna   MCC CC H5

2,3 √7ᵗʰ **S52.282** Bent bone of left ulna   MCC CC H5

2,3 √7ᵗʰ **S52.283** Bent bone of unspecified ulna   MCC CC H5

√6ᵗʰ **S52.29** Other **fracture of shaft of ulna**

2,3 √7ᵗʰ **S52.291** Other fracture of shaft of right ulna   MCC CC H5

2,3 √7ᵗʰ **S52.292** Other fracture of shaft of left ulna   MCC CC H5

2,3 √7ᵗʰ **S52.299** Other fracture of shaft of unspecified ulna   MCC CC H5

√5ᵗʰ **S52.3** Fracture of **shaft of radius**

√6ᵗʰ **S52.30** Unspecified **fracture of shaft of radius**

2,3 √7ᵗʰ **S52.301** Unspecified fracture of shaft of right radius   MCC CC H5

2,3 √7ᵗʰ **S52.302** Unspecified fracture of shaft of left radius   MCC CC H5

2,3 √7ᵗʰ **S52.309** Unspecified fracture of shaft of unspecified radius   MCC CC H5

√6ᵗʰ **S52.31** Greenstick **fracture of shaft of radius**

> The appropriate 7th character is to be added to all codes in subcategory S52.31.
> A   initial encounter for closed fracture
> D   subsequent encounter for fracture with routine healing
> G   subsequent encounter for fracture with delayed healing
> K   subsequent encounter for fracture with nonunion
> P   subsequent encounter for fracture with malunion
> S   sequela

3 √7ᵗʰ **S52.311** Greenstick fracture of shaft of radius, right arm   CC H5

3 √7ᵗʰ **S52.312** Greenstick fracture of shaft of radius, left arm   CC H5

3 √7ᵗʰ **S52.319** Greenstick fracture of shaft of radius, unspecified arm   CC H5

√6ᵗʰ **S52.32** Transverse **fracture of shaft of radius**

2,3 √7ᵗʰ **S52.321** Displaced transverse fracture of shaft of right radius   MCC CC H5

2,3 √7ᵗʰ **S52.322** Displaced transverse fracture of shaft of left radius   MCC CC H5

2,3 √7ᵗʰ **S52.323** Displaced transverse fracture of shaft of unspecified radius   MCC CC H5

2,3 √7ᵗʰ **S52.324** Nondisplaced transverse fracture of shaft of right radius   MCC CC H5

2,3 √7ᵗʰ **S52.325** Nondisplaced transverse fracture of shaft of left radius   MCC CC H5

2,3 √7ᵗʰ **S52.326** Nondisplaced transverse fracture of shaft of unspecified radius   MCC CC H5

√6ᵗʰ **S52.33** Oblique **fracture of shaft of radius**

2,3 √7ᵗʰ **S52.331** Displaced oblique fracture of shaft of right radius   MCC CC H5

2,3 √7ᵗʰ **S52.332** Displaced oblique fracture of shaft of left radius   MCC CC H5

2,3 √7ᵗʰ **S52.333** Displaced oblique fracture of shaft of unspecified radius   MCC CC H5

☑ Additional Character Required   √×7ᵗʰ Placeholder   Questionable PDx   Manifestation   Unspecified Dx   UPD Unacceptable PDx   H1-H14 HAC   HCC CMS-HCC Dx   HIV HIV Dx

ICD-10-CM 2022   1023

2,3 √7ᵗʰ **S52.334** Nondisplaced oblique fracture of shaft of right radius   MCC CC H5

2,3 √7ᵗʰ **S52.335** Nondisplaced oblique fracture of shaft of left radius   MCC CC H5

2,3 √7ᵗʰ **S52.336** Nondisplaced oblique fracture of shaft of unspecified radius   MCC CC H5

√6ᵗʰ **S52.34** Spiral fracture of shaft of radius

2,3 √7ᵗʰ **S52.341** Displaced spiral fracture of shaft of radius, right arm   MCC CC H5

2,3 √7ᵗʰ **S52.342** Displaced spiral fracture of shaft of radius, left arm   MCC CC H5

2,3 √7ᵗʰ **S52.343** Displaced spiral fracture of shaft of radius, unspecified arm   MCC CC H5

2,3 √7ᵗʰ **S52.344** Nondisplaced spiral fracture of shaft of radius, right arm   MCC CC H5

2,3 √7ᵗʰ **S52.345** Nondisplaced spiral fracture of shaft of radius, left arm   MCC CC H5

2,3 √7ᵗʰ **S52.346** Nondisplaced spiral fracture of shaft of radius, unspecified arm   MCC CC H5

√6ᵗʰ **S52.35** Comminuted fracture of shaft of radius

2,3 √7ᵗʰ **S52.351** Displaced comminuted fracture of shaft of radius, right arm   MCC CC H5

2,3 √7ᵗʰ **S52.352** Displaced comminuted fracture of shaft of radius, left arm   MCC CC H5

2,3 √7ᵗʰ **S52.353** Displaced comminuted fracture of shaft of radius, unspecified arm   MCC CC H5

2,3 √7ᵗʰ **S52.354** Nondisplaced comminuted fracture of shaft of radius, right arm   MCC CC H5

2,3 √7ᵗʰ **S52.355** Nondisplaced comminuted fracture of shaft of radius, left arm   MCC CC H5

2,3 √7ᵗʰ **S52.356** Nondisplaced comminuted fracture of shaft of radius, unspecified arm   MCC CC H5

√6ᵗʰ **S52.36** Segmental fracture of shaft of radius

2,3 √7ᵗʰ **S52.361** Displaced segmental fracture of shaft of radius, right arm   MCC CC H5

2,3 √7ᵗʰ **S52.362** Displaced segmental fracture of shaft of radius, left arm   MCC CC H5

2,3 √7ᵗʰ **S52.363** Displaced segmental fracture of shaft of radius, unspecified arm   MCC CC H5

2,3 √7ᵗʰ **S52.364** Nondisplaced segmental fracture of shaft of radius, right arm   MCC CC H5

2,3 √7ᵗʰ **S52.365** Nondisplaced segmental fracture of shaft of radius, left arm   MCC CC H5

2,3 √7ᵗʰ **S52.366** Nondisplaced segmental fracture of shaft of radius, unspecified arm   MCC CC H5

√6ᵗʰ **S52.37** Galeazzi's fracture

Fracture of lower shaft of radius with radioulnar joint dislocation

2,3 √7ᵗʰ **S52.371** Galeazzi's fracture of right radius   MCC CC H5

2,3 √7ᵗʰ **S52.372** Galeazzi's fracture of left radius   MCC CC H5

2,3 √7ᵗʰ **S52.379** Galeazzi's fracture of unspecified radius   MCC CC H5

√6ᵗʰ **S52.38** Bent bone of radius

2,3 √7ᵗʰ **S52.381** Bent bone of right radius   MCC CC H5

2,3 √7ᵗʰ **S52.382** Bent bone of left radius   MCC CC H5

2,3 √7ᵗʰ **S52.389** Bent bone of unspecified radius   MCC CC H5

√6ᵗʰ **S52.39** Other fracture of shaft of radius

2,3 √7ᵗʰ **S52.391** Other fracture of shaft of radius, right arm   MCC CC H5

2,3 √7ᵗʰ **S52.392** Other fracture of shaft of radius, left arm   MCC CC H5

2,3 √7ᵗʰ **S52.399** Other fracture of shaft of radius, unspecified arm   MCC CC H5

√5ᵗʰ **S52.5** Fracture of lower end of radius

Fracture of distal end of radius

EXCLUDES 2   physeal fractures of lower end of radius (S59.2-)

DEF: Fracture of the distal end of the radius above the wrist, most commonly caused by a fall onto an outstretched hand.

√6ᵗʰ **S52.50** Unspecified fracture of the lower end of radius

2,3 √7ᵗʰ **S52.501** Unspecified fracture of the lower end of right radius   MCC CC H5

2,3 √7ᵗʰ **S52.502** Unspecified fracture of the lower end of left radius   MCC CC H5

2,3 √7ᵗʰ **S52.509** Unspecified fracture of the lower end of unspecified radius   MCC CC H5

√6ᵗʰ **S52.51** Fracture of radial styloid process

2,3 √7ᵗʰ **S52.511** Displaced fracture of right radial styloid process   MCC CC H5

2,3 √7ᵗʰ **S52.512** Displaced fracture of left radial styloid process   MCC CC H5

2,3 √7ᵗʰ **S52.513** Displaced fracture of unspecified radial styloid process   MCC CC H5

2,3 √7ᵗʰ **S52.514** Nondisplaced fracture of right radial styloid process   MCC CC H5

2,3 √7ᵗʰ **S52.515** Nondisplaced fracture of left radial styloid process   MCC CC H5

2,3 √7ᵗʰ **S52.516** Nondisplaced fracture of unspecified radial styloid process   MCC CC H5

√6ᵗʰ **S52.52** Torus fracture of lower end of radius

> The appropriate 7th character is to be added to all codes in subcategory S52.52.
> A   initial encounter for closed fracture
> D   subsequent encounter for fracture with routine healing
> G   subsequent encounter for fracture with delayed healing
> K   subsequent encounter for fracture with nonunion
> P   subsequent encounter for fracture with malunion
> S   sequela

3 √7ᵗʰ **S52.521** Torus fracture of lower end of right radius   CC H5

3 √7ᵗʰ **S52.522** Torus fracture of lower end of left radius   CC H5

3 √7ᵗʰ **S52.529** Torus fracture of lower end of unspecified radius   CC H5

√6ᵗʰ **S52.53** Colles' fracture

AHA: 2016,2Q,4

DEF: Fracture of the radius at the wrist in which the distal fragment is pushed posteriorly. The dorsal angulation of the fragment results in the wrist cocking up.

2,3 √7ᵗʰ **S52.531** Colles' fracture of right radius   MCC CC H5

2,3 √7ᵗʰ **S52.532** Colles' fracture of left radius   MCC CC H5

2,3 √7ᵗʰ **S52.539** Colles' fracture of unspecified radius   MCC CC H5

√6ᵗʰ **S52.54** Smith's fracture

2,3 √7ᵗʰ **S52.541** Smith's fracture of right radius   MCC CC H5

2,3 √7ᵗʰ **S52.542** Smith's fracture of left radius   MCC CC H5

2,3 √7ᵗʰ **S52.549** Smith's fracture of unspecified radius   MCC CC H5

√6ᵗʰ **S52.55** Other extraarticular fracture of lower end of radius

2,3 √7ᵗʰ **S52.551** Other extraarticular fracture of lower end of right radius   MCC CC H5

2,3 √7ᵗʰ **S52.552** Other extraarticular fracture of lower end of left radius   MCC CC H5

2,3 √7ᵗʰ **S52.559** Other extraarticular fracture of lower end of unspecified radius   MCC CC H5

√6ᵗʰ **S52.56** Barton's fracture

2,3 √7ᵗʰ **S52.561** Barton's fracture of right radius   MCC CC H5

2,3 √7ᵗʰ **S52.562** Barton's fracture of left radius   MCC CC H5

2,3 √7ᵗʰ **S52.569** Barton's fracture of unspecified radius   MCC CC H5

√6ᵗʰ **S52.57** Other intraarticular fracture of lower end of radius

2,3 √7ᵗʰ **S52.571** Other intraarticular fracture of lower end of right radius   MCC CC H5

2,3 √7ᵗʰ **S52.572** Other intraarticular fracture of lower end of left radius   MCC CC H5

2,3 √7ᵗʰ **S52.579** Other intraarticular fracture of lower end of unspecified radius   MCC CC H5

√6ᵗʰ **S52.59** Other fractures of lower end of radius

AHA: 2019,3Q,9

2,3 √7ᵗʰ **S52.591** Other fractures of lower end of right radius   MCC CC H5

2,3 √7th **S52.592 Other fractures of lower end of left radius** `MCC` `CC` `H5`

2,3 √7th **S52.599 Other fractures of lower end of unspecified radius** `MCC` `CC` `H5`

√6th **S52.6 Fracture of lower end of ulna**

√6th **S52.60 Unspecified fracture of lower end of ulna**

2,3 √7th **S52.601 Unspecified fracture of lower end of right ulna** `MCC` `CC` `H5`

2,3 √7th **S52.602 Unspecified fracture of lower end of left ulna** `MCC` `CC` `H5`

2,3 √7th **S52.609 Unspecified fracture of lower end of unspecified ulna** `MCC` `CC` `H5`

√6th **S52.61 Fracture of ulna styloid process**

2,3 √7th **S52.611 Displaced fracture of right ulna styloid process** `MCC` `CC` `H5`

2,3 √7th **S52.612 Displaced fracture of left ulna styloid process** `MCC` `CC` `H5`

2,3 √7th **S52.613 Displaced fracture of unspecified ulna styloid process** `MCC` `CC` `H5`

2,3 √7th **S52.614 Nondisplaced fracture of right ulna styloid process** `MCC` `CC` `H5`

2,3 √7th **S52.615 Nondisplaced fracture of left ulna styloid process** `MCC` `CC` `H5`

2,3 √7th **S52.616 Nondisplaced fracture of unspecified ulna styloid process** `MCC` `CC` `H5`

√6th **S52.62 Torus fracture of lower end of ulna**

> The appropriate 7th character is to be added to all codes in subcategory S52.62.
> A   initial encounter for closed fracture
> D   subsequent encounter for fracture with routine healing
> G   subsequent encounter for fracture with delayed healing
> K   subsequent encounter for fracture with nonunion
> P   subsequent encounter for fracture with malunion
> S   sequela

3 √7th **S52.621 Torus fracture of lower end of right ulna** `CC` `H5`

3 √7th **S52.622 Torus fracture of lower end of left ulna** `CC` `H5`

3 √7th **S52.629 Torus fracture of lower end of unspecified ulna** `CC` `H5`

√6th **S52.69 Other fracture of lower end of ulna**

AHA: 2019,3Q,9

2,3 √7th **S52.691 Other fracture of lower end of right ulna** `MCC` `CC` `H5`

2,3 √7th **S52.692 Other fracture of lower end of left ulna** `MCC` `CC` `H5`

2,3 √7th **S52.699 Other fracture of lower end of unspecified ulna** `MCC` `CC` `H5`

√5th **S52.9 Unspecified fracture of forearm**

2,3 √x7th **S52.90 Unspecified fracture of unspecified forearm** `MCC` `CC` `H5`

2,3 √x7th **S52.91 Unspecified fracture of right forearm** `MCC` `CC` `H5`

2,3 √x7th **S52.92 Unspecified fracture of left forearm** `MCC` `CC` `H5`

√4th **S53 Dislocation and sprain of joints and ligaments of elbow**

`INCLUDES`   avulsion of joint or ligament of elbow
laceration of cartilage, joint or ligament of elbow
sprain of cartilage, joint or ligament of elbow
traumatic hemarthrosis of joint or ligament of elbow
traumatic rupture of joint or ligament of elbow
traumatic subluxation of joint or ligament of elbow
traumatic tear of joint or ligament of elbow

Code also any associated open wound

`EXCLUDES 2`   *strain of muscle, fascia and tendon at forearm level (S56.-)*

> The appropriate 7th character is to be added to each code from category S53.
> A   initial encounter
> D   subsequent encounter
> S   sequela

√5th **S53.0 Subluxation and dislocation of radial head**

Dislocation of radiohumeral joint
Subluxation of radiohumeral joint

`EXCLUDES 1`   *Monteggia's fracture-dislocation (S52.27-)*

√6th **S53.00 Unspecified subluxation and dislocation of radial head**

√7th **S53.001 Unspecified subluxation of right radial head**

√7th **S53.002 Unspecified subluxation of left radial head**

√7th **S53.003 Unspecified subluxation of unspecified radial head**

√7th **S53.004 Unspecified dislocation of right radial head**

√7th **S53.005 Unspecified dislocation of left radial head**

√7th **S53.006 Unspecified dislocation of unspecified radial head**

√6th **S53.01 Anterior subluxation and dislocation of radial head**

Anteriomedial subluxation and dislocation of radial head

√7th **S53.011 Anterior subluxation of right radial head**

√7th **S53.012 Anterior subluxation of left radial head**

√7th **S53.013 Anterior subluxation of unspecified radial head**

√7th **S53.014 Anterior dislocation of right radial head**

√7th **S53.015 Anterior dislocation of left radial head**

√7th **S53.016 Anterior dislocation of unspecified radial head**

√6th **S53.02 Posterior subluxation and dislocation of radial head**

Posteriolateral subluxation and dislocation of radial head

√7th **S53.021 Posterior subluxation of right radial head**

√7th **S53.022 Posterior subluxation of left radial head**

√7th **S53.023 Posterior subluxation of unspecified radial head**

√7th **S53.024 Posterior dislocation of right radial head**

√7th **S53.025 Posterior dislocation of left radial head**

√7th **S53.026 Posterior dislocation of unspecified radial head**

√6th **S53.03 Nursemaid's elbow**

√7th **S53.031 Nursemaid's elbow, right elbow**

√7th **S53.032 Nursemaid's elbow, left elbow**

√7th **S53.033 Nursemaid's elbow, unspecified elbow**

√6th **S53.09 Other subluxation and dislocation of radial head**

√7th **S53.091 Other subluxation of right radial head**

√7th **S53.092 Other subluxation of left radial head**

√7th **S53.093 Other subluxation of unspecified radial head**

√7th **S53.094 Other dislocation of right radial head**

√7th **S53.095 Other dislocation of left radial head**

√7th **S53.096 Other dislocation of unspecified radial head**

√6th **S53.1 Subluxation and dislocation of ulnohumeral joint**

Subluxation and dislocation of elbow NOS

`EXCLUDES 1`   *dislocation of radial head alone (S53.0-)*

√6th **S53.10 Unspecified subluxation and dislocation of ulnohumeral joint**

√7th **S53.101 Unspecified subluxation of right ulnohumeral joint**

✔ Additional Character Required   √x7th Placeholder   Questionable PDx   Manifestation   Unspecified Dx   `UPD` Unacceptable PDx   `H1`-`H14` HAC   `HCC` CMS-HCC Dx   `HIV` HIV Dx

ICD-10-CM 2022   **1025**

√7ᵗʰ **S53.102** Unspecified subluxation of left ulnohumeral joint

√7ᵗʰ **S53.103** Unspecified subluxation of unspecified ulnohumeral joint

√7ᵗʰ **S53.104** Unspecified dislocation of right ulnohumeral joint

√7ᵗʰ **S53.105** Unspecified dislocation of left ulnohumeral joint

√7ᵗʰ **S53.106** Unspecified dislocation of unspecified ulnohumeral joint

√6ᵗʰ **S53.11** Anterior subluxation and dislocation of ulnohumeral joint

√7ᵗʰ **S53.111** Anterior subluxation of right ulnohumeral joint

√7ᵗʰ **S53.112** Anterior subluxation of left ulnohumeral joint

√7ᵗʰ **S53.113** Anterior subluxation of unspecified ulnohumeral joint

√7ᵗʰ **S53.114** Anterior dislocation of right ulnohumeral joint

AHA: 2012,4Q,108

√7ᵗʰ **S53.115** Anterior dislocation of left ulnohumeral joint

√7ᵗʰ **S53.116** Anterior dislocation of unspecified ulnohumeral joint

√6ᵗʰ **S53.12** Posterior subluxation and dislocation of ulnohumeral joint

√7ᵗʰ **S53.121** Posterior subluxation of right ulnohumeral joint

√7ᵗʰ **S53.122** Posterior subluxation of left ulnohumeral joint

√7ᵗʰ **S53.123** Posterior subluxation of unspecified ulnohumeral joint

√7ᵗʰ **S53.124** Posterior dislocation of right ulnohumeral joint

√7ᵗʰ **S53.125** Posterior dislocation of left ulnohumeral joint

√7ᵗʰ **S53.126** Posterior dislocation of unspecified ulnohumeral joint

√6ᵗʰ **S53.13** Medial subluxation and dislocation of ulnohumeral joint

√7ᵗʰ **S53.131** Medial subluxation of right ulnohumeral joint

√7ᵗʰ **S53.132** Medial subluxation of left ulnohumeral joint

√7ᵗʰ **S53.133** Medial subluxation of unspecified ulnohumeral joint

√7ᵗʰ **S53.134** Medial dislocation of right ulnohumeral joint

√7ᵗʰ **S53.135** Medial dislocation of left ulnohumeral joint

√7ᵗʰ **S53.136** Medial dislocation of unspecified ulnohumeral joint

√6ᵗʰ **S53.14** Lateral subluxation and dislocation of ulnohumeral joint

√7ᵗʰ **S53.141** Lateral subluxation of right ulnohumeral joint

√7ᵗʰ **S53.142** Lateral subluxation of left ulnohumeral joint

√7ᵗʰ **S53.143** Lateral subluxation of unspecified ulnohumeral joint

√7ᵗʰ **S53.144** Lateral dislocation of right ulnohumeral joint

√7ᵗʰ **S53.145** Lateral dislocation of left ulnohumeral joint

√7ᵗʰ **S53.146** Lateral dislocation of unspecified ulnohumeral joint

√6ᵗʰ **S53.19** Other subluxation and dislocation of ulnohumeral joint

√7ᵗʰ **S53.191** Other subluxation of right ulnohumeral joint

√7ᵗʰ **S53.192** Other subluxation of left ulnohumeral joint

√7ᵗʰ **S53.193** Other subluxation of unspecified ulnohumeral joint

√7ᵗʰ **S53.194** Other dislocation of right ulnohumeral joint

√7ᵗʰ **S53.195** Other dislocation of left ulnohumeral joint

√7ᵗʰ **S53.196** Other dislocation of unspecified ulnohumeral joint

√5ᵗʰ **S53.2** Traumatic rupture of radial collateral ligament

> EXCLUDES 1   sprain of radial collateral ligament NOS (S53.43-)

√x7ᵗʰ **S53.20** Traumatic rupture of unspecified radial collateral ligament

√x7ᵗʰ **S53.21** Traumatic rupture of right radial collateral ligament

√x7ᵗʰ **S53.22** Traumatic rupture of left radial collateral ligament

√5ᵗʰ **S53.3** Traumatic rupture of ulnar collateral ligament

> EXCLUDES 1   sprain of ulnar collateral ligament (S53.44-)

√x7ᵗʰ **S53.30** Traumatic rupture of unspecified ulnar collateral ligament

√x7ᵗʰ **S53.31** Traumatic rupture of right ulnar collateral ligament

√x7ᵗʰ **S53.32** Traumatic rupture of left ulnar collateral ligament

√5ᵗʰ **S53.4** Sprain of elbow

> EXCLUDES 2   traumatic rupture of radial collateral ligament (S53.2-)
>
>   traumatic rupture of ulnar collateral ligament (S53.3-)

√6ᵗʰ **S53.40** Unspecified sprain of elbow

√7ᵗʰ **S53.401** Unspecified sprain of right elbow

√7ᵗʰ **S53.402** Unspecified sprain of left elbow

√7ᵗʰ **S53.409** Unspecified sprain of unspecified elbow

Sprain of elbow NOS

√6ᵗʰ **S53.41** Radiohumeral (joint) sprain

√7ᵗʰ **S53.411** Radiohumeral (joint) sprain of right elbow

√7ᵗʰ **S53.412** Radiohumeral (joint) sprain of left elbow

√7ᵗʰ **S53.419** Radiohumeral (joint) sprain of unspecified elbow

√6ᵗʰ **S53.42** Ulnohumeral (joint) sprain

√7ᵗʰ **S53.421** Ulnohumeral (joint) sprain of right elbow

√7ᵗʰ **S53.422** Ulnohumeral (joint) sprain of left elbow

√7ᵗʰ **S53.429** Ulnohumeral (joint) sprain of unspecified elbow

√6ᵗʰ **S53.43** Radial collateral ligament sprain

√7ᵗʰ **S53.431** Radial collateral ligament sprain of right elbow

√7ᵗʰ **S53.432** Radial collateral ligament sprain of left elbow

√7ᵗʰ **S53.439** Radial collateral ligament sprain of unspecified elbow

√6ᵗʰ **S53.44** Ulnar collateral ligament sprain

√7ᵗʰ **S53.441** Ulnar collateral ligament sprain of right elbow

√7ᵗʰ **S53.442** Ulnar collateral ligament sprain of left elbow

√7ᵗʰ **S53.449** Ulnar collateral ligament sprain of unspecified elbow

√6ᵗʰ **S53.49** Other sprain of elbow

√7ᵗʰ **S53.491** Other sprain of right elbow

√7ᵗʰ **S53.492** Other sprain of left elbow

√7ᵗʰ **S53.499** Other sprain of unspecified elbow

√4ᵗʰ **S54** Injury of nerves at forearm level

Code also any associated open wound (S51.-)

> EXCLUDES 2   injury of nerves at wrist and hand level (S64.-)

The appropriate 7th character is to be added to each code from category S54.
A   initial encounter
D   subsequent encounter
S   sequela

√5ᵗʰ **S54.0** Injury of ulnar nerve at forearm level

Injury of ulnar nerve NOS

√x7ᵗʰ **S54.00** Injury of ulnar nerve at forearm level, unspecified arm

√x7ᵗʰ **S54.01** Injury of ulnar nerve at forearm level, right arm

√x7ᵗʰ **S54.02** Injury of ulnar nerve at forearm level, left arm

√5ᵗʰ **S54.1** Injury of median nerve at forearm level

Injury of median nerve NOS

√x7ᵗʰ **S54.10** Injury of median nerve at forearm level, unspecified arm

√x7ᵗʰ **S54.11** Injury of median nerve at forearm level, right arm

√x7ᵗʰ **S54.12** Injury of median nerve at forearm level, left arm

---

N Newborn: 0   P Pediatric: 0-17   M Maternity: 9-64   A Adult: 15-124   MCC Major Complication/Comorbidity   CC Complication/Comorbidity   SW Severe Wound Dx

1026   ICD-10-CM 2022

√5ᵗʰ **S54.2 Injury of radial nerve at forearm level**
    Injury of radial nerve NOS

  √x7ᵗʰ **S54.20** Injury of radial nerve at forearm level, unspecified arm

  √x7ᵗʰ **S54.21** Injury of radial nerve at forearm level, right arm

  √x7ᵗʰ **S54.22** Injury of radial nerve at forearm level, left arm

√5ᵗʰ **S54.3 Injury of cutaneous sensory nerve at forearm level**

  √x7ᵗʰ **S54.30** Injury of cutaneous sensory nerve at forearm level, unspecified arm

  √x7ᵗʰ **S54.31** Injury of cutaneous sensory nerve at forearm level, right arm

  √x7ᵗʰ **S54.32** Injury of cutaneous sensory nerve at forearm level, left arm

√5ᵗʰ **S54.8 Injury of other nerves at forearm level**

  √6ᵗʰ **S54.8X** Injury of other nerves at forearm level

    √7ᵗʰ **S54.8X1** Injury of other nerves at forearm level, right arm

    √7ᵗʰ **S54.8X2** Injury of other nerves at forearm level, left arm

    √7ᵗʰ **S54.8X9** Injury of other nerves at forearm level, unspecified arm

√5ᵗʰ **S54.9 Injury of unspecified nerve at forearm level**

  √x7ᵗʰ **S54.90** Injury of unspecified nerve at forearm level, unspecified arm

  √x7ᵗʰ **S54.91** Injury of unspecified nerve at forearm level, right arm

  √x7ᵗʰ **S54.92** Injury of unspecified nerve at forearm level, left arm

√4ᵗʰ **S55 Injury of blood vessels at forearm level**

  Code also any associated open wound (S51.-)

  EXCLUDES 2   *injury of blood vessels at wrist and hand level (S65.-)*
         injury of brachial vessels (S45.1-S45.2)

  The appropriate 7th character is to be added to each code from category S55.
  A   initial encounter
  D   subsequent encounter
  S   sequela

√5ᵗʰ **S55.0 Injury of ulnar artery at forearm level**

  √6ᵗʰ **S55.00** Unspecified injury of ulnar artery at forearm level

    √7ᵗʰ **S55.001** Unspecified injury of ulnar artery at forearm level, right arm   CC

    √7ᵗʰ **S55.002** Unspecified injury of ulnar artery at forearm level, left arm   CC

    √7ᵗʰ **S55.009** Unspecified injury of ulnar artery at forearm level, unspecified arm   CC

  √6ᵗʰ **S55.01** Laceration of ulnar artery at forearm level

    √7ᵗʰ **S55.011** Laceration of ulnar artery at forearm level, right arm   CC

    √7ᵗʰ **S55.012** Laceration of ulnar artery at forearm level, left arm   CC

    √7ᵗʰ **S55.019** Laceration of ulnar artery at forearm level, unspecified arm   CC

  √6ᵗʰ **S55.09** Other specified injury of ulnar artery at forearm level

    √7ᵗʰ **S55.091** Other specified injury of ulnar artery at forearm level, right arm   CC

    √7ᵗʰ **S55.092** Other specified injury of ulnar artery at forearm level, left arm   CC

    √7ᵗʰ **S55.099** Other specified injury of ulnar artery at forearm level, unspecified arm   CC

√5ᵗʰ **S55.1 Injury of radial artery at forearm level**

  √6ᵗʰ **S55.10** Unspecified injury of radial artery at forearm level

    √7ᵗʰ **S55.101** Unspecified injury of radial artery at forearm level, right arm   CC

    √7ᵗʰ **S55.102** Unspecified injury of radial artery at forearm level, left arm   CC

    √7ᵗʰ **S55.109** Unspecified injury of radial artery at forearm level, unspecified arm   CC

  √6ᵗʰ **S55.11** Laceration of radial artery at forearm level

    √7ᵗʰ **S55.111** Laceration of radial artery at forearm level, right arm   CC

    √7ᵗʰ **S55.112** Laceration of radial artery at forearm level, left arm   CC

    √7ᵗʰ **S55.119** Laceration of radial artery at forearm level, unspecified arm   CC

  √6ᵗʰ **S55.19** Other specified injury of radial artery at forearm level

    √7ᵗʰ **S55.191** Other specified injury of radial artery at forearm level, right arm   CC

    √7ᵗʰ **S55.192** Other specified injury of radial artery at forearm level, left arm   CC

    √7ᵗʰ **S55.199** Other specified injury of radial artery at forearm level, unspecified arm   CC

√5ᵗʰ **S55.2 Injury of vein at forearm level**

  √6ᵗʰ **S55.20** Unspecified injury of vein at forearm level

    √7ᵗʰ **S55.201** Unspecified injury of vein at forearm level, right arm   CC

    √7ᵗʰ **S55.202** Unspecified injury of vein at forearm level, left arm   CC

    √7ᵗʰ **S55.209** Unspecified injury of vein at forearm level, unspecified arm   CC

  √6ᵗʰ **S55.21** Laceration of vein at forearm level

    √7ᵗʰ **S55.211** Laceration of vein at forearm level, right arm   CC

    √7ᵗʰ **S55.212** Laceration of vein at forearm level, left arm   CC

    √7ᵗʰ **S55.219** Laceration of vein at forearm level, unspecified arm   CC

  √6ᵗʰ **S55.29** Other specified injury of vein at forearm level

    √7ᵗʰ **S55.291** Other specified injury of vein at forearm level, right arm   CC

    √7ᵗʰ **S55.292** Other specified injury of vein at forearm level, left arm   CC

    √7ᵗʰ **S55.299** Other specified injury of vein at forearm level, unspecified arm   CC

√5ᵗʰ **S55.8 Injury of other blood vessels at forearm level**

  √6ᵗʰ **S55.80** Unspecified injury of other blood vessels at forearm level

    √7ᵗʰ **S55.801** Unspecified injury of other blood vessels at forearm level, right arm   CC

    √7ᵗʰ **S55.802** Unspecified injury of other blood vessels at forearm level, left arm   CC

    √7ᵗʰ **S55.809** Unspecified injury of other blood vessels at forearm level, unspecified arm   CC

  √6ᵗʰ **S55.81** Laceration of other blood vessels at forearm level

    √7ᵗʰ **S55.811** Laceration of other blood vessels at forearm level, right arm   CC

    √7ᵗʰ **S55.812** Laceration of other blood vessels at forearm level, left arm   CC

    √7ᵗʰ **S55.819** Laceration of other blood vessels at forearm level, unspecified arm   CC

  √6ᵗʰ **S55.89** Other specified injury of other blood vessels at forearm level

    √7ᵗʰ **S55.891** Other specified injury of other blood vessels at forearm level, right arm   CC

    √7ᵗʰ **S55.892** Other specified injury of other blood vessels at forearm level, left arm   CC

    √7ᵗʰ **S55.899** Other specified injury of other blood vessels at forearm level, unspecified arm   CC

√5ᵗʰ **S55.9 Injury of unspecified blood vessel at forearm level**

  √6ᵗʰ **S55.90** Unspecified injury of unspecified blood vessel at forearm level

    √7ᵗʰ **S55.901** Unspecified injury of unspecified blood vessel at forearm level, right arm   CC

    √7ᵗʰ **S55.902** Unspecified injury of unspecified blood vessel at forearm level, left arm   CC

    √7ᵗʰ **S55.909** Unspecified injury of unspecified blood vessel at forearm level, unspecified arm   CC

  √6ᵗʰ **S55.91** Laceration of unspecified blood vessel at forearm level

    √7ᵗʰ **S55.911** Laceration of unspecified blood vessel at forearm level, right arm   CC

    √7ᵗʰ **S55.912** Laceration of unspecified blood vessel at forearm level, left arm   CC

    √7ᵗʰ **S55.919** Laceration of unspecified blood vessel at forearm level, unspecified arm   CC

  √6ᵗʰ **S55.99** Other specified injury of unspecified blood vessel at forearm level

    √7ᵗʰ **S55.991** Other specified injury of unspecified blood vessel at forearm level, right arm   CC

✔ Additional Character Required   √x7ᵗʰ Placeholder   Questionable PDx   Manifestation   Unspecified Dx   UPD Unacceptable PDx   H1-H14 HAC   HCC CMS-HCC Dx   HIV HIV Dx

☑7ᵗʰ **S55.992** Other specified injury of unspecified blood vessel at forearm level, left arm   cc

☑7ᵗʰ **S55.999** Other specified injury of unspecified blood vessel at forearm level, unspecified arm   cc

☑4ᵗʰ **S56** Injury of muscle, fascia and tendon at forearm level

Code also any associated open wound (S51.-)

EXCLUDES 2   injury of muscle, fascia and tendon at or below wrist (S66.-)
sprain of joints and ligaments of elbow (S53.4-)

TIP: Refer to the Muscle/Tendon table at the beginning of this chapter

The appropriate 7th character is to be added to each code from category S56.
A   initial encounter
D   subsequent encounter
S   sequela

☑5ᵗʰ **S56.0** Injury of flexor muscle, fascia and tendon of thumb at forearm level

☑6ᵗʰ **S56.00** Unspecified injury of flexor muscle, fascia and tendon of thumb at forearm level

☑7ᵗʰ **S56.001** Unspecified injury of flexor muscle, fascia and tendon of right thumb at forearm level

☑7ᵗʰ **S56.002** Unspecified injury of flexor muscle, fascia and tendon of left thumb at forearm level

☑7ᵗʰ **S56.009** Unspecified injury of flexor muscle, fascia and tendon of unspecified thumb at forearm level

☑6ᵗʰ **S56.01** Strain of flexor muscle, fascia and tendon of thumb at forearm level

☑7ᵗʰ **S56.011** Strain of flexor muscle, fascia and tendon of right thumb at forearm level

☑7ᵗʰ **S56.012** Strain of flexor muscle, fascia and tendon of left thumb at forearm level

☑7ᵗʰ **S56.019** Strain of flexor muscle, fascia and tendon of unspecified thumb at forearm level

☑6ᵗʰ **S56.02** Laceration of flexor muscle, fascia and tendon of thumb at forearm level

☑7ᵗʰ **S56.021** Laceration of flexor muscle, fascia and tendon of right thumb at forearm level   cc

☑7ᵗʰ **S56.022** Laceration of flexor muscle, fascia and tendon of left thumb at forearm level   cc

☑7ᵗʰ **S56.029** Laceration of flexor muscle, fascia and tendon of unspecified thumb at forearm level   cc

☑6ᵗʰ **S56.09** Other injury of flexor muscle, fascia and tendon of thumb at forearm level

☑7ᵗʰ **S56.091** Other injury of flexor muscle, fascia and tendon of right thumb at forearm level

☑7ᵗʰ **S56.092** Other injury of flexor muscle, fascia and tendon of left thumb at forearm level

☑7ᵗʰ **S56.099** Other injury of flexor muscle, fascia and tendon of unspecified thumb at forearm level

☑5ᵗʰ **S56.1** Injury of flexor muscle, fascia and tendon of other and unspecified finger at forearm level

☑6ᵗʰ **S56.10** Unspecified injury of flexor muscle, fascia and tendon of other and unspecified finger at forearm level

☑7ᵗʰ **S56.101** Unspecified injury of flexor muscle, fascia and tendon of right index finger at forearm level

☑7ᵗʰ **S56.102** Unspecified injury of flexor muscle, fascia and tendon of left index finger at forearm level

☑7ᵗʰ **S56.103** Unspecified injury of flexor muscle, fascia and tendon of right middle finger at forearm level

☑7ᵗʰ **S56.104** Unspecified injury of flexor muscle, fascia and tendon of left middle finger at forearm level

☑7ᵗʰ **S56.105** Unspecified injury of flexor muscle, fascia and tendon of right ring finger at forearm level

☑7ᵗʰ **S56.106** Unspecified injury of flexor muscle, fascia and tendon of left ring finger at forearm level

☑7ᵗʰ **S56.107** Unspecified injury of flexor muscle, fascia and tendon of right little finger at forearm level

☑7ᵗʰ **S56.108** Unspecified injury of flexor muscle, fascia and tendon of left little finger at forearm level

☑7ᵗʰ **S56.109** Unspecified injury of flexor muscle, fascia and tendon of unspecified finger at forearm level

☑6ᵗʰ **S56.11** Strain of flexor muscle, fascia and tendon of other and unspecified finger at forearm level

☑7ᵗʰ **S56.111** Strain of flexor muscle, fascia and tendon of right index finger at forearm level

☑7ᵗʰ **S56.112** Strain of flexor muscle, fascia and tendon of left index finger at forearm level

☑7ᵗʰ **S56.113** Strain of flexor muscle, fascia and tendon of right middle finger at forearm level

☑7ᵗʰ **S56.114** Strain of flexor muscle, fascia and tendon of left middle finger at forearm level

☑7ᵗʰ **S56.115** Strain of flexor muscle, fascia and tendon of right ring finger at forearm level

☑7ᵗʰ **S56.116** Strain of flexor muscle, fascia and tendon of left ring finger at forearm level

☑7ᵗʰ **S56.117** Strain of flexor muscle, fascia and tendon of right little finger at forearm level

☑7ᵗʰ **S56.118** Strain of flexor muscle, fascia and tendon of left little finger at forearm level

☑7ᵗʰ **S56.119** Strain of flexor muscle, fascia and tendon of finger of unspecified finger at forearm level

☑6ᵗʰ **S56.12** Laceration of flexor muscle, fascia and tendon of other and unspecified finger at forearm level

☑7ᵗʰ **S56.121** Laceration of flexor muscle, fascia and tendon of right index finger at forearm level   cc

☑7ᵗʰ **S56.122** Laceration of flexor muscle, fascia and tendon of left index finger at forearm level   cc

☑7ᵗʰ **S56.123** Laceration of flexor muscle, fascia and tendon of right middle finger at forearm level   cc

☑7ᵗʰ **S56.124** Laceration of flexor muscle, fascia and tendon of left middle finger at forearm level   cc

☑7ᵗʰ **S56.125** Laceration of flexor muscle, fascia and tendon of right ring finger at forearm level   cc

☑7ᵗʰ **S56.126** Laceration of flexor muscle, fascia and tendon of left ring finger at forearm level   cc

☑7ᵗʰ **S56.127** Laceration of flexor muscle, fascia and tendon of right little finger at forearm level   cc

☑7ᵗʰ **S56.128** Laceration of flexor muscle, fascia and tendon of left little finger at forearm level   cc

☑7ᵗʰ **S56.129** Laceration of flexor muscle, fascia and tendon of unspecified finger at forearm level   cc

☑6ᵗʰ **S56.19** Other injury of flexor muscle, fascia and tendon of other and unspecified finger at forearm level

☑7ᵗʰ **S56.191** Other injury of flexor muscle, fascia and tendon of right index finger at forearm level

☑7ᵗʰ **S56.192** Other injury of flexor muscle, fascia and tendon of left index finger at forearm level

☑7ᵗʰ **S56.193** Other injury of flexor muscle, fascia and tendon of right middle finger at forearm level

☑7ᵗʰ **S56.194** Other injury of flexor muscle, fascia and tendon of left middle finger at forearm level

☑7ᵗʰ **S56.195** Other injury of flexor muscle, fascia and tendon of right ring finger at forearm level

☑7ᵗʰ **S56.196** Other injury of flexor muscle, fascia and tendon of left ring finger at forearm level

☑7ᵗʰ **S56.197** Other injury of flexor muscle, fascia and tendon of right little finger at forearm level

☑7ᵗʰ **S56.198** Other injury of flexor muscle, fascia and tendon of left little finger at forearm level

☑7ᵗʰ **S56.199** Other injury of flexor muscle, fascia and tendon of unspecified finger at forearm level

Ⓝ Newborn: 0   Ⓟ Pediatric: 0-17   Ⓜ Maternity: 9-64   Ⓐ Adult: 15-124   ᴹᶜᶜ Major Complication/Comorbidity   cc Complication/Comorbidity   ˢʷ Severe Wound Dx

1028

ICD-10-CM 2022

√5ᵗʰ **S56.2** **Injury of other flexor muscle, fascia and tendon at forearm level**

√6ᵗʰ **S56.20** **Unspecified injury of other flexor muscle, fascia and tendon at forearm level**

√7ᵗʰ **S56.201** Unspecified injury of other flexor muscle, fascia and tendon at forearm level, right arm

√7ᵗʰ **S56.202** Unspecified injury of other flexor muscle, fascia and tendon at forearm level, left arm

√7ᵗʰ **S56.209** Unspecified injury of other flexor muscle, fascia and tendon at forearm level, unspecified arm

√6ᵗʰ **S56.21** Strain of other flexor muscle, fascia and tendon at forearm level

√7ᵗʰ **S56.211** Strain of other flexor muscle, fascia and tendon at forearm level, right arm

√7ᵗʰ **S56.212** Strain of other flexor muscle, fascia and tendon at forearm level, left arm

√7ᵗʰ **S56.219** Strain of other flexor muscle, fascia and tendon at forearm level, unspecified arm

√6ᵗʰ **S56.22** Laceration of other flexor muscle, fascia and tendon at forearm level

√7ᵗʰ **S56.221** Laceration of other flexor muscle, fascia and tendon at forearm level, right arm   CC

√7ᵗʰ **S56.222** Laceration of other flexor muscle, fascia and tendon at forearm level, left arm   CC

√7ᵗʰ **S56.229** Laceration of other flexor muscle, fascia and tendon at forearm level, unspecified arm   CC

√6ᵗʰ **S56.29** Other injury of other flexor muscle, fascia and tendon at forearm level

√7ᵗʰ **S56.291** Other injury of other flexor muscle, fascia and tendon at forearm level, right arm

√7ᵗʰ **S56.292** Other injury of other flexor muscle, fascia and tendon at forearm level, left arm

√7ᵗʰ **S56.299** Other injury of other flexor muscle, fascia and tendon at forearm level, unspecified arm

√5ᵗʰ **S56.3** **Injury of extensor or abductor muscles, fascia and tendons of thumb at forearm level**

√6ᵗʰ **S56.30** **Unspecified injury of extensor or abductor muscles, fascia and tendons of thumb at forearm level**

√7ᵗʰ **S56.301** Unspecified injury of extensor or abductor muscles, fascia and tendons of right thumb at forearm level

√7ᵗʰ **S56.302** Unspecified injury of extensor or abductor muscles, fascia and tendons of left thumb at forearm level

√7ᵗʰ **S56.309** Unspecified injury of extensor or abductor muscles, fascia and tendons of unspecified thumb at forearm level

√6ᵗʰ **S56.31** Strain of extensor or abductor muscles, fascia and tendons of thumb at forearm level

√7ᵗʰ **S56.311** Strain of extensor or abductor muscles, fascia and tendons of right thumb at forearm level

√7ᵗʰ **S56.312** Strain of extensor or abductor muscles, fascia and tendons of left thumb at forearm level

√7ᵗʰ **S56.319** Strain of extensor or abductor muscles, fascia and tendons of unspecified thumb at forearm level

√6ᵗʰ **S56.32** Laceration of extensor or abductor muscles, fascia and tendons of thumb at forearm level

√7ᵗʰ **S56.321** Laceration of extensor or abductor muscles, fascia and tendons of right thumb at forearm level   CC

√7ᵗʰ **S56.322** Laceration of extensor or abductor muscles, fascia and tendons of left thumb at forearm level   CC

√7ᵗʰ **S56.329** Laceration of extensor or abductor muscles, fascia and tendons of unspecified thumb at forearm level   CC

√6ᵗʰ **S56.39** Other injury of extensor or abductor muscles, fascia and tendons of thumb at forearm level

√7ᵗʰ **S56.391** Other injury of extensor or abductor muscles, fascia and tendons of right thumb at forearm level

√7ᵗʰ **S56.392** Other injury of extensor or abductor muscles, fascia and tendons of left thumb at forearm level

√7ᵗʰ **S56.399** Other injury of extensor or abductor muscles, fascia and tendons of unspecified thumb at forearm level

√5ᵗʰ **S56.4** **Injury of extensor muscle, fascia and tendon of other and unspecified finger at forearm level**

√6ᵗʰ **S56.40** **Unspecified injury of extensor muscle, fascia and tendon of other and unspecified finger at forearm level**

√7ᵗʰ **S56.401** Unspecified injury of extensor muscle, fascia and tendon of right index finger at forearm level

√7ᵗʰ **S56.402** Unspecified injury of extensor muscle, fascia and tendon of left index finger at forearm level

√7ᵗʰ **S56.403** Unspecified injury of extensor muscle, fascia and tendon of right middle finger at forearm level

√7ᵗʰ **S56.404** Unspecified injury of extensor muscle, fascia and tendon of left middle finger at forearm level

√7ᵗʰ **S56.405** Unspecified injury of extensor muscle, fascia and tendon of right ring finger at forearm level

√7ᵗʰ **S56.406** Unspecified injury of extensor muscle, fascia and tendon of left ring finger at forearm level

√7ᵗʰ **S56.407** Unspecified injury of extensor muscle, fascia and tendon of right little finger at forearm level

√7ᵗʰ **S56.408** Unspecified injury of extensor muscle, fascia and tendon of left little finger at forearm level

√7ᵗʰ **S56.409** Unspecified injury of extensor muscle, fascia and tendon of unspecified finger at forearm level

√6ᵗʰ **S56.41** Strain of extensor muscle, fascia and tendon of other and unspecified finger at forearm level

√7ᵗʰ **S56.411** Strain of extensor muscle, fascia and tendon of right index finger at forearm level

√7ᵗʰ **S56.412** Strain of extensor muscle, fascia and tendon of left index finger at forearm level

√7ᵗʰ **S56.413** Strain of extensor muscle, fascia and tendon of right middle finger at forearm level

√7ᵗʰ **S56.414** Strain of extensor muscle, fascia and tendon of left middle finger at forearm level

√7ᵗʰ **S56.415** Strain of extensor muscle, fascia and tendon of right ring finger at forearm level

√7ᵗʰ **S56.416** Strain of extensor muscle, fascia and tendon of left ring finger at forearm level

√7ᵗʰ **S56.417** Strain of extensor muscle, fascia and tendon of right little finger at forearm level

√7ᵗʰ **S56.418** Strain of extensor muscle, fascia and tendon of left little finger at forearm level

√7ᵗʰ **S56.419** Strain of extensor muscle, fascia and tendon of finger, unspecified finger at forearm level

√6ᵗʰ **S56.42** Laceration of extensor muscle, fascia and tendon of other and unspecified finger at forearm level

√7ᵗʰ **S56.421** Laceration of extensor muscle, fascia and tendon of right index finger at forearm level   CC

√7ᵗʰ **S56.422** Laceration of extensor muscle, fascia and tendon of left index finger at forearm level   CC

√7ᵗʰ **S56.423** Laceration of extensor muscle, fascia and tendon of right middle finger at forearm level   CC

√7ᵗʰ **S56.424** Laceration of extensor muscle, fascia and tendon of left middle finger at forearm level   CC

√7ᵗʰ **S56.425** Laceration of extensor muscle, fascia and tendon of right ring finger at forearm level   CC

√7ᵗʰ **S56.426** Laceration of extensor muscle, fascia and tendon of left ring finger at forearm level   CC

√7ᵗʰ **S56.427** Laceration of extensor muscle, fascia and tendon of right little finger at forearm level   cc

√7ᵗʰ **S56.428** Laceration of extensor muscle, fascia and tendon of left little finger at forearm level   cc

√7ᵗʰ **S56.429** Laceration of extensor muscle, fascia and tendon of unspecified finger at forearm level   cc

√6ᵗʰ **S56.49** Other injury of extensor muscle, fascia and tendon of other and unspecified finger at forearm level

√7ᵗʰ **S56.491** Other injury of extensor muscle, fascia and tendon of right index finger at forearm level

√7ᵗʰ **S56.492** Other injury of extensor muscle, fascia and tendon of left index finger at forearm level

√7ᵗʰ **S56.493** Other injury of extensor muscle, fascia and tendon of right middle finger at forearm level

√7ᵗʰ **S56.494** Other injury of extensor muscle, fascia and tendon of left middle finger at forearm level

√7ᵗʰ **S56.495** Other injury of extensor muscle, fascia and tendon of right ring finger at forearm level

√7ᵗʰ **S56.496** Other injury of extensor muscle, fascia and tendon of left ring finger at forearm level

√7ᵗʰ **S56.497** Other injury of extensor muscle, fascia and tendon of right little finger at forearm level

√7ᵗʰ **S56.498** Other injury of extensor muscle, fascia and tendon of left little finger at forearm level

√7ᵗʰ **S56.499** Other injury of extensor muscle, fascia and tendon of unspecified finger at forearm level

√6ᵗʰ **S56.5** Injury of other extensor muscle, fascia and tendon at forearm level

√6ᵗʰ **S56.50** Unspecified injury of other extensor muscle, fascia and tendon at forearm level

√7ᵗʰ **S56.501** Unspecified injury of other extensor muscle, fascia and tendon at forearm level, right arm

√7ᵗʰ **S56.502** Unspecified injury of other extensor muscle, fascia and tendon at forearm level, left arm

√7ᵗʰ **S56.509** Unspecified injury of other extensor muscle, fascia and tendon at forearm level, unspecified arm

√6ᵗʰ **S56.51** Strain of other extensor muscle, fascia and tendon at forearm level

√7ᵗʰ **S56.511** Strain of other extensor muscle, fascia and tendon at forearm level, right arm

√7ᵗʰ **S56.512** Strain of other extensor muscle, fascia and tendon at forearm level, left arm

√7ᵗʰ **S56.519** Strain of other extensor muscle, fascia and tendon at forearm level, unspecified arm

√6ᵗʰ **S56.52** Laceration of other extensor muscle, fascia and tendon at forearm level

√7ᵗʰ **S56.521** Laceration of other extensor muscle, fascia and tendon at forearm level, right arm   cc

√7ᵗʰ **S56.522** Laceration of other extensor muscle, fascia and tendon at forearm level, left arm   cc

√7ᵗʰ **S56.529** Laceration of other extensor muscle, fascia and tendon at forearm level, unspecified arm   cc

√6ᵗʰ **S56.59** Other injury of other extensor muscle, fascia and tendon at forearm level

√7ᵗʰ **S56.591** Other injury of other extensor muscle, fascia and tendon at forearm level, right arm

√7ᵗʰ **S56.592** Other injury of other extensor muscle, fascia and tendon at forearm level, left arm

√7ᵗʰ **S56.599** Other injury of other extensor muscle, fascia and tendon at forearm level, unspecified arm

√5ᵗʰ **S56.8** Injury of other muscles, fascia and tendons at forearm level

√6ᵗʰ **S56.80** Unspecified injury of other muscles, fascia and tendons at forearm level

√7ᵗʰ **S56.801** Unspecified injury of other muscles, fascia and tendons at forearm level, right arm

√7ᵗʰ **S56.802** Unspecified injury of other muscles, fascia and tendons at forearm level, left arm

√7ᵗʰ **S56.809** Unspecified injury of other muscles, fascia and tendons at forearm level, unspecified arm

√6ᵗʰ **S56.81** Strain of other muscles, fascia and tendons at forearm level

√7ᵗʰ **S56.811** Strain of other muscles, fascia and tendons at forearm level, right arm

√7ᵗʰ **S56.812** Strain of other muscles, fascia and tendons at forearm level, left arm

√7ᵗʰ **S56.819** Strain of other muscles, fascia and tendons at forearm level, unspecified arm

√6ᵗʰ **S56.82** Laceration of other muscles, fascia and tendons at forearm level

√7ᵗʰ **S56.821** Laceration of other muscles, fascia and tendons at forearm level, right arm   cc

√7ᵗʰ **S56.822** Laceration of other muscles, fascia and tendons at forearm level, left arm   cc

√7ᵗʰ **S56.829** Laceration of other muscles, fascia and tendons at forearm level, unspecified arm   cc

√6ᵗʰ **S56.89** Other injury of other muscles, fascia and tendons at forearm level

√7ᵗʰ **S56.891** Other injury of other muscles, fascia and tendons at forearm level, right arm

√7ᵗʰ **S56.892** Other injury of other muscles, fascia and tendons at forearm level, left arm

√7ᵗʰ **S56.899** Other injury of other muscles, fascia and tendons at forearm level, unspecified arm

√5ᵗʰ **S56.9** Injury of unspecified muscles, fascia and tendons at forearm level

√6ᵗʰ **S56.90** Unspecified injury of unspecified muscles, fascia and tendons at forearm level

√7ᵗʰ **S56.901** Unspecified injury of unspecified muscles, fascia and tendons at forearm level, right arm

√7ᵗʰ **S56.902** Unspecified injury of unspecified muscles, fascia and tendons at forearm level, left arm

√7ᵗʰ **S56.909** Unspecified injury of unspecified muscles, fascia and tendons at forearm level, unspecified arm

√6ᵗʰ **S56.91** Strain of unspecified muscles, fascia and tendons at forearm level

√7ᵗʰ **S56.911** Strain of unspecified muscles, fascia and tendons at forearm level, right arm

√7ᵗʰ **S56.912** Strain of unspecified muscles, fascia and tendons at forearm level, left arm

√7ᵗʰ **S56.919** Strain of unspecified muscles, fascia and tendons at forearm level, unspecified arm

√6ᵗʰ **S56.92** Laceration of unspecified muscles, fascia and tendons at forearm level

√7ᵗʰ **S56.921** Laceration of unspecified muscles, fascia and tendons at forearm level, right arm   cc

√7ᵗʰ **S56.922** Laceration of unspecified muscles, fascia and tendons at forearm level, left arm   cc

√7ᵗʰ **S56.929** Laceration of unspecified muscles, fascia and tendons at forearm level, unspecified arm   cc

√6ᵗʰ **S56.99** Other injury of unspecified muscles, fascia and tendons at forearm level

√7ᵗʰ **S56.991** Other injury of unspecified muscles, fascia and tendons at forearm level, right arm

√7ᵗʰ **S56.992** Other injury of unspecified muscles, fascia and tendons at forearm level, left arm

√7ᵗʰ **S56.999** Other injury of unspecified muscles, fascia and tendons at forearm level, unspecified arm

N Newborn: 0   P Pediatric: 0-17   M Maternity: 9-64   A Adult: 15-124   MCC Major Complication/Comorbidity   CC Complication/Comorbidity   SW Severe Wound Dx

1030   ICD-10-CM 2022

√4ᵗʰ **S57 Crushing injury** of elbow and forearm

    Use additional code(s) for all associated injuries

    EXCLUDES 2   crushing injury of wrist and hand (S67.-)

    The appropriate 7th character is to be added to each code from category S57.
    A   initial encounter
    D   subsequent encounter
    S   sequela

  √5ᵗʰ **S57.0 Crushing injury** of elbow

    √x7ᵗʰ **S57.00** Crushing injury of unspecified elbow

    √x7ᵗʰ **S57.01** Crushing injury of right elbow

    √x7ᵗʰ **S57.02** Crushing injury of left elbow

  √5ᵗʰ **S57.8 Crushing injury** of forearm

    √x7ᵗʰ **S57.80** Crushing injury of unspecified forearm

    √x7ᵗʰ **S57.81** Crushing injury of right forearm

    √x7ᵗʰ **S57.82** Crushing injury of left forearm

√4ᵗʰ **S58 Traumatic amputation** of elbow and forearm

    An amputation not identified as partial or complete should be coded to complete

    EXCLUDES 1   traumatic amputation of wrist and hand (S68.-)

    The appropriate 7th character is to be added to each code from category S58.
    A   initial encounter
    D   subsequent encounter
    S   sequela

  √5ᵗʰ **S58.0 Traumatic amputation** at elbow level

    √6ᵗʰ **S58.01 Complete** traumatic amputation at elbow level

      7 √7ᵗʰ **S58.011** Complete traumatic amputation at elbow level, right arm   CC HCC

      7 √7ᵗʰ **S58.012** Complete traumatic amputation at elbow level, left arm   CC HCC

      7 √7ᵗʰ **S58.019** Complete traumatic amputation at elbow level, unspecified arm   CC HCC

    √6ᵗʰ **S58.02 Partial** traumatic amputation at elbow level

      7 √7ᵗʰ **S58.021** Partial traumatic amputation at elbow level, right arm   CC HCC

      7 √7ᵗʰ **S58.022** Partial traumatic amputation at elbow level, left arm   CC HCC

      7 √7ᵗʰ **S58.029** Partial traumatic amputation at elbow level, unspecified arm   CC HCC

  √5ᵗʰ **S58.1 Traumatic amputation** at level between elbow and wrist

    √6ᵗʰ **S58.11 Complete** traumatic amputation at level between elbow and wrist

      7 √7ᵗʰ **S58.111** Complete traumatic amputation at level between elbow and wrist, right arm   CC HCC

      7 √7ᵗʰ **S58.112** Complete traumatic amputation at level between elbow and wrist, left arm   CC HCC

      7 √7ᵗʰ **S58.119** Complete traumatic amputation at level between elbow and wrist, unspecified arm   CC HCC

    √6ᵗʰ **S58.12 Partial** traumatic amputation at level between elbow and wrist

      7 √7ᵗʰ **S58.121** Partial traumatic amputation at level between elbow and wrist, right arm   CC HCC

      7 √7ᵗʰ **S58.122** Partial traumatic amputation at level between elbow and wrist, left arm   CC HCC

      7 √7ᵗʰ **S58.129** Partial traumatic amputation at level between elbow and wrist, unspecified arm   CC HCC

  √5ᵗʰ **S58.9 Traumatic amputation** of forearm, level unspecified

    EXCLUDES 1   traumatic amputation of wrist (S68.-)

    √6ᵗʰ **S58.91 Complete** traumatic amputation of forearm, level unspecified

      7 √7ᵗʰ **S58.911** Complete traumatic amputation of right forearm, level unspecified   CC HCC

      7 √7ᵗʰ **S58.912** Complete traumatic amputation of left forearm, level unspecified   CC HCC

      7 √7ᵗʰ **S58.919** Complete traumatic amputation of unspecified forearm, level unspecified   CC HCC

    √6ᵗʰ **S58.92 Partial** traumatic amputation of forearm, level unspecified

      7 √7ᵗʰ **S58.921** Partial traumatic amputation of right forearm, level unspecified   CC HCC

      7 √7ᵗʰ **S58.922** Partial traumatic amputation of left forearm, level unspecified   CC HCC

      7 √7ᵗʰ **S58.929** Partial traumatic amputation of unspecified forearm, level unspecified   CC HCC

√4ᵗʰ **S59 Other and unspecified injuries** of elbow and forearm

    EXCLUDES 2   other and unspecified injuries of wrist and hand (S69.-)

    AHA: 2018,2Q,12; 2018,1Q,3; 2015,3Q,37-39

    The appropriate 7th character is to be added to each code from subcategories S59.0, S59.1, and S59.2.
    A   initial encounter for closed fracture
    D   subsequent encounter for fracture with routine healing
    G   subsequent encounter for fracture with delayed healing
    K   subsequent encounter for fracture with nonunion
    P   subsequent encounter for fracture with malunion
    S   sequela

  √5ᵗʰ **S59.0 Physeal fracture** of lower end of ulna

    AHA: 2019,4Q,56

    √6ᵗʰ **S59.00 Unspecified** physeal fracture of lower end of ulna

      3 √7ᵗʰ **S59.001** Unspecified physeal fracture of lower end of ulna, right arm   CC H5

      3 √7ᵗʰ **S59.002** Unspecified physeal fracture of lower end of ulna, left arm   CC H5

      3 √7ᵗʰ **S59.009** Unspecified physeal fracture of lower end of ulna, unspecified arm   CC H5

    √6ᵗʰ **S59.01 Salter-Harris Type I** physeal fracture of lower end of ulna

      3 √7ᵗʰ **S59.011** Salter-Harris Type I physeal fracture of lower end of ulna, right arm   CC H5

      3 √7ᵗʰ **S59.012** Salter-Harris Type I physeal fracture of lower end of ulna, left arm   CC H5

      3 √7ᵗʰ **S59.019** Salter-Harris Type I physeal fracture of lower end of ulna, unspecified arm   CC H5

    √6ᵗʰ **S59.02 Salter-Harris Type II** physeal fracture of lower end of ulna

      3 √7ᵗʰ **S59.021** Salter-Harris Type II physeal fracture of lower end of ulna, right arm   CC H5

      3 √7ᵗʰ **S59.022** Salter-Harris Type II physeal fracture of lower end of ulna, left arm   CC H5

      3 √7ᵗʰ **S59.029** Salter-Harris Type II physeal fracture of lower end of ulna, unspecified arm   CC H5

    √6ᵗʰ **S59.03 Salter-Harris Type III** physeal fracture of lower end of ulna

      3 √7ᵗʰ **S59.031** Salter-Harris Type III physeal fracture of lower end of ulna, right arm   CC H5

      3 √7ᵗʰ **S59.032** Salter-Harris Type III physeal fracture of lower end of ulna, left arm   CC H5

      3 √7ᵗʰ **S59.039** Salter-Harris Type III physeal fracture of lower end of ulna, unspecified arm   CC H5

    √6ᵗʰ **S59.04 Salter-Harris Type IV** physeal fracture of lower end of ulna

      3 √7ᵗʰ **S59.041** Salter-Harris Type IV physeal fracture of lower end of ulna, right arm   CC H5

      3 √7ᵗʰ **S59.042** Salter-Harris Type IV physeal fracture of lower end of ulna, left arm   CC H5

      3 √7ᵗʰ **S59.049** Salter-Harris Type IV physeal fracture of lower end of ulna, unspecified arm   CC H5

    √6ᵗʰ **S59.09 Other** physeal fracture of lower end of ulna

      3 √7ᵗʰ **S59.091** Other physeal fracture of lower end of ulna, right arm   CC H5

      3 √7ᵗʰ **S59.092** Other physeal fracture of lower end of ulna, left arm   CC H5

      3 √7ᵗʰ **S59.099** Other physeal fracture of lower end of ulna, unspecified arm   CC H5

  √5ᵗʰ **S59.1 Physeal fracture** of upper end of radius

    AHA: 2019,4Q,56

    √6ᵗʰ **S59.10 Unspecified** physeal fracture of upper end of radius

      4 √7ᵗʰ **S59.101** Unspecified physeal fracture of upper end of radius, right arm   CC

✔ Additional Character Required   √x7ᵗʰ Placeholder   Questionable PDx   Manifestation   Unspecified Dx   UPD Unacceptable PDx   H1-H4 HAC   HCC CMS-HCC Dx   HIV HIV Dx

ICD-10-CM 2022   1031

4 √7th **S59.102** Unspecified physeal fracture of upper end of radius, **left** arm `CC`

4 √7th **S59.109** Unspecified physeal fracture of upper end of radius, **unspecified** arm `CC`

√6th **S59.11** Salter-Harris Type I physeal fracture of upper end of radius

4 √7th **S59.111** Salter-Harris Type I physeal fracture of upper end of radius, **right** arm `CC`

4 √7th **S59.112** Salter-Harris Type I physeal fracture of upper end of radius, **left** arm `CC`

4 √7th **S59.119** Salter-Harris Type I physeal fracture of upper end of radius, **unspecified** arm `CC`

√6th **S59.12** Salter-Harris Type II physeal fracture of upper end of radius

4 √7th **S59.121** Salter-Harris Type II physeal fracture of upper end of radius, **right** arm `CC`

4 √7th **S59.122** Salter-Harris Type II physeal fracture of upper end of radius, **left** arm `CC`

4 √7th **S59.129** Salter-Harris Type II physeal fracture of upper end of radius, **unspecified** arm `CC`

√6th **S59.13** Salter-Harris Type III physeal fracture of upper end of radius

4 √7th **S59.131** Salter-Harris Type III physeal fracture of upper end of radius, **right** arm `CC`

4 √7th **S59.132** Salter-Harris Type III physeal fracture of upper end of radius, **left** arm `CC`

4 √7th **S59.139** Salter-Harris Type III physeal fracture of upper end of radius, **unspecified** arm `CC`

√6th **S59.14** Salter-Harris Type IV physeal fracture of upper end of radius

4 √7th **S59.141** Salter-Harris Type IV physeal fracture of upper end of radius, **right** arm `CC`

4 √7th **S59.142** Salter-Harris Type IV physeal fracture of upper end of radius, **left** arm `CC`

4 √7th **S59.149** Salter-Harris Type IV physeal fracture of upper end of radius, **unspecified** arm `CC`

√6th **S59.19** Other physeal fracture of upper end of radius

4 √7th **S59.191** Other physeal fracture of upper end of radius, **right** arm `CC`

4 √7th **S59.192** Other physeal fracture of upper end of radius, **left** arm `CC`

4 √7th **S59.199** Other physeal fracture of upper end of radius, **unspecified** arm `CC`

√5th **S59.2** Physeal fracture of lower end of radius

AHA: 2019,4Q,56

√6th **S59.20** Unspecified physeal fracture of lower end of radius

3 √7th **S59.201** Unspecified physeal fracture of lower end of radius, **right** arm `CC` `H5`

3 √7th **S59.202** Unspecified physeal fracture of lower end of radius, **left** arm `CC` `H5`

3 √7th **S59.209** Unspecified physeal fracture of lower end of radius, **unspecified** arm `CC` `H5`

√6th **S59.21** Salter-Harris Type I physeal fracture of lower end of radius

3 √7th **S59.211** Salter-Harris Type I physeal fracture of lower end of radius, **right** arm `CC` `H5`

3 √7th **S59.212** Salter-Harris Type I physeal fracture of lower end of radius, **left** arm `CC` `H5`

3 √7th **S59.219** Salter-Harris Type I physeal fracture of lower end of radius, **unspecified** arm `CC` `H5`

√6th **S59.22** Salter-Harris Type II physeal fracture of lower end of radius

3 √7th **S59.221** Salter-Harris Type II physeal fracture of lower end of radius, **right** arm `CC` `H5`

3 √7th **S59.222** Salter-Harris Type II physeal fracture of lower end of radius, **left** arm `CC` `H5`

3 √7th **S59.229** Salter-Harris Type II physeal fracture of lower end of radius, **unspecified** arm `CC` `H5`

√6th **S59.23** Salter-Harris Type III physeal fracture of lower end of radius

3 √7th **S59.231** Salter-Harris Type III physeal fracture of lower end of radius, **right** arm `CC` `H5`

3 √7th **S59.232** Salter-Harris Type III physeal fracture of lower end of radius, **left** arm `CC` `H5`

3 √7th **S59.239** Salter-Harris Type III physeal fracture of lower end of radius, **unspecified** arm `CC` `H5`

√6th **S59.24** Salter-Harris Type IV physeal fracture of lower end of radius

3 √7th **S59.241** Salter-Harris Type IV physeal fracture of lower end of radius, **right** arm `CC` `H5`

3 √7th **S59.242** Salter-Harris Type IV physeal fracture of lower end of radius, **left** arm `CC` `H5`

3 √7th **S59.249** Salter-Harris Type IV physeal fracture of lower end of radius, **unspecified** arm `CC` `H5`

√6th **S59.29** Other physeal fracture of lower end of radius

3 √7th **S59.291** Other physeal fracture of lower end of radius, **right** arm `CC` `H5`

3 √7th **S59.292** Other physeal fracture of lower end of radius, **left** arm `CC` `H5`

3 √7th **S59.299** Other physeal fracture of lower end of radius, **unspecified** arm `CC` `H5`

√5th **S59.8** Other specified injuries of elbow and forearm

The appropriate 7th character is to be added to each code in subcategory S59.8.
A   initial encounter
D   subsequent encounter
S   sequela

√6th **S59.80** Other specified injuries of elbow

√7th **S59.801** Other specified injuries of **right** elbow

√7th **S59.802** Other specified injuries of **left** elbow

√7th **S59.809** Other specified injuries of **unspecified** elbow

√6th **S59.81** Other specified injuries of forearm

√7th **S59.811** Other specified injuries **right** forearm

√7th **S59.812** Other specified injuries **left** forearm

√7th **S59.819** Other specified injuries **unspecified** forearm

√5th **S59.9** Unspecified injury of elbow and forearm

The appropriate 7th character is to be added to each code in subcategory S59.9.
A   initial encounter
D   subsequent encounter
S   sequela

√6th **S59.90** Unspecified injury of elbow

√7th **S59.901** Unspecified injury of **right** elbow

√7th **S59.902** Unspecified injury of **left** elbow

√7th **S59.909** Unspecified injury of **unspecified** elbow

√6th **S59.91** Unspecified injury of forearm

√7th **S59.911** Unspecified injury of **right** forearm

√7th **S59.912** Unspecified injury of **left** forearm

√7th **S59.919** Unspecified injury of **unspecified** forearm

Injuries to the wrist, hand and fingers (S60-S69)

`EXCLUDES 2`   burns and corrosions (T20-T32)
frostbite (T33-T34)
insect bite or sting, venomous (T63.4)

√4th **S60** Superficial injury of wrist, hand and fingers

The appropriate 7th character is to be added to each code from category S60.
A   initial encounter
D   subsequent encounter
S   sequela

√5th **S60.0** Contusion of finger without damage to nail

`EXCLUDES 1`   contusion involving nail (matrix) (S60.1)

√x7th **S60.00** Contusion of unspecified finger without damage to nail

Contusion of finger(s) NOS

√6th **S60.01** Contusion of thumb without damage to nail

√7th **S60.011** Contusion of **right** thumb without damage to nail

√7th **S60.012** Contusion of **left** thumb without damage to nail

√7th **S60.019** Contusion of unspecified thumb without damage to nail

√6ᵗʰ **S60.02** Contusion of index finger without damage to nail
     √7ᵗʰ **S60.021** Contusion of right index finger without damage to nail
     √7ᵗʰ **S60.022** Contusion of left index finger without damage to nail
     √7ᵗʰ **S60.029** Contusion of unspecified index finger without damage to nail

√6ᵗʰ **S60.03** Contusion of middle finger without damage to nail
     √7ᵗʰ **S60.031** Contusion of right middle finger without damage to nail
     √7ᵗʰ **S60.032** Contusion of left middle finger without damage to nail
     √7ᵗʰ **S60.039** Contusion of unspecified middle finger without damage to nail

√6ᵗʰ **S60.04** Contusion of ring finger without damage to nail
     √7ᵗʰ **S60.041** Contusion of right ring finger without damage to nail
     √7ᵗʰ **S60.042** Contusion of left ring finger without damage to nail
     √7ᵗʰ **S60.049** Contusion of unspecified ring finger without damage to nail

√6ᵗʰ **S60.05** Contusion of little finger without damage to nail
     √7ᵗʰ **S60.051** Contusion of right little finger without damage to nail
     √7ᵗʰ **S60.052** Contusion of left little finger without damage to nail
     √7ᵗʰ **S60.059** Contusion of unspecified little finger without damage to nail

√5ᵗʰ **S60.1** Contusion of finger with damage to nail
   √x7ᵗʰ **S60.10** Contusion of unspecified finger with damage to nail

√6ᵗʰ **S60.11** Contusion of thumb with damage to nail
     √7ᵗʰ **S60.111** Contusion of right thumb with damage to nail
     √7ᵗʰ **S60.112** Contusion of left thumb with damage to nail
     √7ᵗʰ **S60.119** Contusion of unspecified thumb with damage to nail

√6ᵗʰ **S60.12** Contusion of index finger with damage to nail
     √7ᵗʰ **S60.121** Contusion of right index finger with damage to nail
     √7ᵗʰ **S60.122** Contusion of left index finger with damage to nail
     √7ᵗʰ **S60.129** Contusion of unspecified index finger with damage to nail

√6ᵗʰ **S60.13** Contusion of middle finger with damage to nail
     √7ᵗʰ **S60.131** Contusion of right middle finger with damage to nail
     √7ᵗʰ **S60.132** Contusion of left middle finger with damage to nail
     √7ᵗʰ **S60.139** Contusion of unspecified middle finger with damage to nail

√6ᵗʰ **S60.14** Contusion of ring finger with damage to nail
     √7ᵗʰ **S60.141** Contusion of right ring finger with damage to nail
     √7ᵗʰ **S60.142** Contusion of left ring finger with damage to nail
     √7ᵗʰ **S60.149** Contusion of unspecified ring finger with damage to nail

√6ᵗʰ **S60.15** Contusion of little finger with damage to nail
     √7ᵗʰ **S60.151** Contusion of right little finger with damage to nail
     √7ᵗʰ **S60.152** Contusion of left little finger with damage to nail
     √7ᵗʰ **S60.159** Contusion of unspecified little finger with damage to nail

√5ᵗʰ **S60.2** Contusion of wrist and hand
    EXCLUDES 2   contusion of fingers (S60.0-, S60.1-)

√6ᵗʰ **S60.21** Contusion of wrist
     √7ᵗʰ **S60.211** Contusion of right wrist
     √7ᵗʰ **S60.212** Contusion of left wrist
     √7ᵗʰ **S60.219** Contusion of unspecified wrist

√6ᵗʰ **S60.22** Contusion of hand
     √7ᵗʰ **S60.221** Contusion of right hand
     √7ᵗʰ **S60.222** Contusion of left hand
     √7ᵗʰ **S60.229** Contusion of unspecified hand

√5ᵗʰ **S60.3** Other superficial injuries of thumb

√6ᵗʰ **S60.31** Abrasion of thumb
     √7ᵗʰ **S60.311** Abrasion of right thumb
     √7ᵗʰ **S60.312** Abrasion of left thumb
     √7ᵗʰ **S60.319** Abrasion of unspecified thumb

√6ᵗʰ **S60.32** Blister (nonthermal) of thumb
     √7ᵗʰ **S60.321** Blister (nonthermal) of right thumb
     √7ᵗʰ **S60.322** Blister (nonthermal) of left thumb
     √7ᵗʰ **S60.329** Blister (nonthermal) of unspecified thumb

√6ᵗʰ **S60.34** External constriction of thumb
     Hair tourniquet syndrome of thumb
     Use additional cause code to identify the constricting item (W49.0-)
     √7ᵗʰ **S60.341** External constriction of right thumb
     √7ᵗʰ **S60.342** External constriction of left thumb
     √7ᵗʰ **S60.349** External constriction of unspecified thumb

√6ᵗʰ **S60.35** Superficial foreign body of thumb
     Splinter in the thumb
     √7ᵗʰ **S60.351** Superficial foreign body of right thumb
     √7ᵗʰ **S60.352** Superficial foreign body of left thumb
     √7ᵗʰ **S60.359** Superficial foreign body of unspecified thumb

√6ᵗʰ **S60.36** Insect bite (nonvenomous) of thumb
     √7ᵗʰ **S60.361** Insect bite (nonvenomous) of right thumb
     √7ᵗʰ **S60.362** Insect bite (nonvenomous) of left thumb
     √7ᵗʰ **S60.369** Insect bite (nonvenomous) of unspecified thumb

√6ᵗʰ **S60.37** Other superficial bite of thumb
     EXCLUDES 1   open bite of thumb (S61.05-, S61.15-)
     √7ᵗʰ **S60.371** Other superficial bite of right thumb
     √7ᵗʰ **S60.372** Other superficial bite of left thumb
     √7ᵗʰ **S60.379** Other superficial bite of unspecified thumb

√6ᵗʰ **S60.39** Other superficial injuries of thumb
     √7ᵗʰ **S60.391** Other superficial injuries of right thumb
     √7ᵗʰ **S60.392** Other superficial injuries of left thumb
     √7ᵗʰ **S60.399** Other superficial injuries of unspecified thumb

√5ᵗʰ **S60.4** Other superficial injuries of other fingers

√6ᵗʰ **S60.41** Abrasion of fingers
     √7ᵗʰ **S60.410** Abrasion of right index finger
     √7ᵗʰ **S60.411** Abrasion of left index finger
     √7ᵗʰ **S60.412** Abrasion of right middle finger
     √7ᵗʰ **S60.413** Abrasion of left middle finger
     √7ᵗʰ **S60.414** Abrasion of right ring finger
     √7ᵗʰ **S60.415** Abrasion of left ring finger
     √7ᵗʰ **S60.416** Abrasion of right little finger
     √7ᵗʰ **S60.417** Abrasion of left little finger
     √7ᵗʰ **S60.418** Abrasion of other finger
       Abrasion of specified finger with unspecified laterality
     √7ᵗʰ **S60.419** Abrasion of unspecified finger

√6ᵗʰ **S60.42** Blister (nonthermal) of fingers
     √7ᵗʰ **S60.420** Blister (nonthermal) of right index finger
     √7ᵗʰ **S60.421** Blister (nonthermal) of left index finger
     √7ᵗʰ **S60.422** Blister (nonthermal) of right middle finger
     √7ᵗʰ **S60.423** Blister (nonthermal) of left middle finger
     √7ᵗʰ **S60.424** Blister (nonthermal) of right ring finger
     √7ᵗʰ **S60.425** Blister (nonthermal) of left ring finger
     √7ᵗʰ **S60.426** Blister (nonthermal) of right little finger
     √7ᵗʰ **S60.427** Blister (nonthermal) of left little finger
     √7ᵗʰ **S60.428** Blister (nonthermal) of other finger
       Blister (nonthermal) of specified finger with unspecified laterality
     √7ᵗʰ **S60.429** Blister (nonthermal) of unspecified finger

Chapter 19. Injury, Poisoning and Certain Other Consequences of External Causes

S60.44–S60.919

√6ᵗʰ **S60.44** **External constriction** of fingers

Hair tourniquet syndrome of finger

Use additional cause code to identify the constricting item (W49.0-)

√7ᵗʰ **S60.440** External constriction of **right index** finger

√7ᵗʰ **S60.441** External constriction of **left index** finger

√7ᵗʰ **S60.442** External constriction of **right middle** finger

√7ᵗʰ **S60.443** External constriction of **left middle** finger

√7ᵗʰ **S60.444** External constriction of **right ring** finger

√7ᵗʰ **S60.445** External constriction of **left ring** finger

√7ᵗʰ **S60.446** External constriction of **right little** finger

√7ᵗʰ **S60.447** External constriction of **left little** finger

√7ᵗʰ **S60.448** External constriction of other finger

External constriction of specified finger with unspecified laterality

√7ᵗʰ **S60.449** External constriction of unspecified finger

√6ᵗʰ **S60.45** Superficial **foreign body** of fingers

Splinter in the finger(s)

√7ᵗʰ **S60.450** Superficial foreign body of **right index** finger

√7ᵗʰ **S60.451** Superficial foreign body of **left index** finger

√7ᵗʰ **S60.452** Superficial foreign body of **right middle** finger

√7ᵗʰ **S60.453** Superficial foreign body of **left middle** finger

√7ᵗʰ **S60.454** Superficial foreign body of **right ring** finger

√7ᵗʰ **S60.455** Superficial foreign body of **left ring** finger

√7ᵗʰ **S60.456** Superficial foreign body of **right little** finger

√7ᵗʰ **S60.457** Superficial foreign body of **left little** finger

√7ᵗʰ **S60.458** Superficial foreign body of other finger

Superficial foreign body of specified finger with unspecified laterality

√7ᵗʰ **S60.459** Superficial foreign body of unspecified finger

√6ᵗʰ **S60.46** Insect bite (nonvenomous) of fingers

√7ᵗʰ **S60.460** Insect bite (nonvenomous) of **right index** finger

√7ᵗʰ **S60.461** Insect bite (nonvenomous) of **left index** finger

√7ᵗʰ **S60.462** Insect bite (nonvenomous) of **right middle** finger

√7ᵗʰ **S60.463** Insect bite (nonvenomous) of **left middle** finger

√7ᵗʰ **S60.464** Insect bite (nonvenomous) of **right ring** finger

√7ᵗʰ **S60.465** Insect bite (nonvenomous) of **left ring** finger

√7ᵗʰ **S60.466** Insect bite (nonvenomous) of **right little** finger

√7ᵗʰ **S60.467** Insect bite (nonvenomous) of **left little** finger

√7ᵗʰ **S60.468** Insect bite (nonvenomous) of other finger

Insect bite (nonvenomous) of specified finger with unspecified laterality

√7ᵗʰ **S60.469** Insect bite (nonvenomous) of unspecified finger

√6ᵗʰ **S60.47** Other superficial **bite** of fingers

> EXCLUDES 1   *open bite of fingers (S61.25-, S61.35-)*

√7ᵗʰ **S60.470** Other superficial bite of **right index** finger

√7ᵗʰ **S60.471** Other superficial bite of **left index** finger

√7ᵗʰ **S60.472** Other superficial bite of **right middle** finger

√7ᵗʰ **S60.473** Other superficial bite of **left middle** finger

√7ᵗʰ **S60.474** Other superficial bite of **right ring** finger

√7ᵗʰ **S60.475** Other superficial bite of **left ring** finger

√7ᵗʰ **S60.476** Other superficial bite of **right little** finger

√7ᵗʰ **S60.477** Other superficial bite of **left little** finger

√7ᵗʰ **S60.478** Other superficial bite of other finger

Other superficial bite of specified finger with unspecified laterality

√7ᵗʰ **S60.479** Other superficial bite of unspecified finger

√5ᵗʰ **S60.5** Other superficial injuries of **hand**

> EXCLUDES 2   *superficial injuries of fingers (S60.3-, S60.4-)*

√6ᵗʰ **S60.51** **Abrasion** of hand

√7ᵗʰ **S60.511** Abrasion of **right** hand

√7ᵗʰ **S60.512** Abrasion of **left** hand

√7ᵗʰ **S60.519** Abrasion of unspecified hand

√6ᵗʰ **S60.52** **Blister** (nonthermal) of hand

√7ᵗʰ **S60.521** Blister (nonthermal) of **right** hand

√7ᵗʰ **S60.522** Blister (nonthermal) of **left** hand

√7ᵗʰ **S60.529** Blister (nonthermal) of unspecified hand

√6ᵗʰ **S60.54** **External constriction** of hand

√7ᵗʰ **S60.541** External constriction of **right** hand

√7ᵗʰ **S60.542** External constriction of **left** hand

√7ᵗʰ **S60.549** External constriction of unspecified hand

√6ᵗʰ **S60.55** Superficial **foreign body** of hand

Splinter in the hand

√7ᵗʰ **S60.551** Superficial foreign body of **right** hand

√7ᵗʰ **S60.552** Superficial foreign body of **left** hand

√7ᵗʰ **S60.559** Superficial foreign body of unspecified hand

√6ᵗʰ **S60.56** Insect bite (nonvenomous) of hand

√7ᵗʰ **S60.561** Insect bite (nonvenomous) of **right** hand

√7ᵗʰ **S60.562** Insect bite (nonvenomous) of **left** hand

√7ᵗʰ **S60.569** Insect bite (nonvenomous) of unspecified hand

√6ᵗʰ **S60.57** Other superficial **bite** of hand

> EXCLUDES 1   *open bite of hand (S61.45-)*

√7ᵗʰ **S60.571** Other superficial bite of hand of **right** hand

√7ᵗʰ **S60.572** Other superficial bite of hand of **left** hand

√7ᵗʰ **S60.579** Other superficial bite of hand of unspecified hand

√5ᵗʰ **S60.8** Other superficial injuries of **wrist**

√6ᵗʰ **S60.81** **Abrasion** of wrist

√7ᵗʰ **S60.811** Abrasion of **right** wrist

√7ᵗʰ **S60.812** Abrasion of **left** wrist

√7ᵗʰ **S60.819** Abrasion of unspecified wrist

√6ᵗʰ **S60.82** **Blister** (nonthermal) of wrist

√7ᵗʰ **S60.821** Blister (nonthermal) of **right** wrist

√7ᵗʰ **S60.822** Blister (nonthermal) of **left** wrist

√7ᵗʰ **S60.829** Blister (nonthermal) of unspecified wrist

√6ᵗʰ **S60.84** **External constriction** of wrist

√7ᵗʰ **S60.841** External constriction of **right** wrist

√7ᵗʰ **S60.842** External constriction of **left** wrist

√7ᵗʰ **S60.849** External constriction of unspecified wrist

√6ᵗʰ **S60.85** Superficial **foreign body** of wrist

Splinter in the wrist

√7ᵗʰ **S60.851** Superficial foreign body of **right** wrist

√7ᵗʰ **S60.852** Superficial foreign body of **left** wrist

√7ᵗʰ **S60.859** Superficial foreign body of unspecified wrist

√6ᵗʰ **S60.86** Insect bite (nonvenomous) of wrist

√7ᵗʰ **S60.861** Insect bite (nonvenomous) of **right** wrist

√7ᵗʰ **S60.862** Insect bite (nonvenomous) of **left** wrist

√7ᵗʰ **S60.869** Insect bite (nonvenomous) of unspecified wrist

√6ᵗʰ **S60.87** Other superficial **bite** of wrist

> EXCLUDES 1   *open bite of wrist (S61.55)*

√7ᵗʰ **S60.871** Other superficial bite of **right** wrist

√7ᵗʰ **S60.872** Other superficial bite of **left** wrist

√7ᵗʰ **S60.879** Other superficial bite of unspecified wrist

√5ᵗʰ **S60.9** Unspecified superficial injury of wrist, hand and fingers

√6ᵗʰ **S60.91** Unspecified superficial injury of **wrist**

√7ᵗʰ **S60.911** Unspecified superficial injury of **right** wrist

√7ᵗʰ **S60.912** Unspecified superficial injury of **left** wrist

√7ᵗʰ **S60.919** Unspecified superficial injury of unspecified wrist

N Newborn: 0   **P** Pediatric: 0-17   **M** Maternity: 9-64   **A** Adult: 15-124   **MCC** Major Complication/Comorbidity   **CC** Complication/Comorbidity   **SW** Severe Wound Dx

1034   ICD-10-CM 2022

✓6ᵗʰ **S60.92**   **Unspecified superficial injury of** hand

    ✓7ᵗʰ **S60.921**   **Unspecified superficial injury of** right hand

    ✓7ᵗʰ **S60.922**   **Unspecified superficial injury of** left hand

    ✓7ᵗʰ **S60.929**   **Unspecified superficial injury of unspecified hand**

✓6ᵗʰ **S60.93**   **Unspecified superficial injury of** thumb

    ✓7ᵗʰ **S60.931**   **Unspecified superficial injury of** right thumb

    ✓7ᵗʰ **S60.932**   **Unspecified superficial injury of** left thumb

    ✓7ᵗʰ **S60.939**   **Unspecified superficial injury of unspecified thumb**

✓6ᵗʰ **S60.94**   **Unspecified superficial injury of other** fingers

    ✓7ᵗʰ **S60.940**   **Unspecified superficial injury of** right index **finger**

    ✓7ᵗʰ **S60.941**   **Unspecified superficial injury of** left index finger

    ✓7ᵗʰ **S60.942**   **Unspecified superficial injury of** right middle **finger**

    ✓7ᵗʰ **S60.943**   **Unspecified superficial injury of** left middle **finger**

    ✓7ᵗʰ **S60.944**   **Unspecified superficial injury of** right ring finger

    ✓7ᵗʰ **S60.945**   **Unspecified superficial injury of** left ring finger

    ✓7ᵗʰ **S60.946**   **Unspecified superficial injury of** right little **finger**

    ✓7ᵗʰ **S60.947**   **Unspecified superficial injury of** left little finger

    ✓7ᵗʰ **S60.948**   **Unspecified superficial injury of other finger**

      Unspecified superficial injury of specified finger with unspecified laterality

    ✓7ᵗʰ **S60.949**   **Unspecified superficial injury of unspecified finger**

✓4ᵗʰ **S61**   **Open wound of wrist, hand and fingers**

    Code also any associated wound infection

    EXCLUDES 1   *open fracture of wrist, hand and finger (S62.- with 7th character B)*

           traumatic amputation of wrist and hand (S68.-)

    The appropriate 7th character is to be added to each code from category S61.
    A   initial encounter
    D   subsequent encounter
    S   sequela

✓5ᵗʰ **S61.0**   **Open wound of** thumb without damage to nail

    EXCLUDES 1   *open wound of thumb with damage to nail (S61.1-)*

    ✓6ᵗʰ **S61.00**   **Unspecified open wound of thumb without damage to nail**

      ✓7ᵗʰ **S61.001**   **Unspecified open wound of** right **thumb without damage to nail**

      ✓7ᵗʰ **S61.002**   **Unspecified open wound of** left **thumb without damage to nail**

      ✓7ᵗʰ **S61.009**   **Unspecified open wound of unspecified thumb without damage to nail**

    ✓6ᵗʰ **S61.01**   **Laceration** without foreign body **of thumb without damage to nail**

      ✓7ᵗʰ **S61.011**   **Laceration without foreign body of** right **thumb without damage to nail**

      ✓7ᵗʰ **S61.012**   **Laceration without foreign body of** left **thumb without damage to nail**

      ✓7ᵗʰ **S61.019**   **Laceration without foreign body of unspecified thumb without damage to nail**

    ✓6ᵗʰ **S61.02**   **Laceration** with foreign body **of thumb without damage to nail**

      ✓7ᵗʰ **S61.021**   **Laceration with foreign body of** right **thumb without damage to nail**

      ✓7ᵗʰ **S61.022**   **Laceration with foreign body of** left **thumb without damage to nail**

      ✓7ᵗʰ **S61.029**   **Laceration with foreign body of unspecified thumb without damage to nail**

    ✓6ᵗʰ **S61.03**   **Puncture wound** without foreign body **of thumb without damage to nail**

      ✓7ᵗʰ **S61.031**   **Puncture wound without foreign body of** right **thumb without damage to nail**

      ✓7ᵗʰ **S61.032**   **Puncture wound without foreign body of** left **thumb without damage to nail**

      ✓7ᵗʰ **S61.039**   **Puncture wound without foreign body of unspecified thumb without damage to nail**

    ✓6ᵗʰ **S61.04**   **Puncture wound** with foreign body **of thumb without damage to nail**

      ✓7ᵗʰ **S61.041**   **Puncture wound with foreign body of** right **thumb without damage to nail**

      ✓7ᵗʰ **S61.042**   **Puncture wound with foreign body of** left **thumb without damage to nail**

      ✓7ᵗʰ **S61.049**   **Puncture wound with foreign body of unspecified thumb without damage to nail**

    ✓6ᵗʰ **S61.05**   **Open bite** of thumb without damage to nail

      Bite of thumb NOS

      EXCLUDES 1   *superficial bite of thumb (S60.36-, S60.37-)*

      ✓7ᵗʰ **S61.051**   **Open bite of** right **thumb without damage to nail**

      ✓7ᵗʰ **S61.052**   **Open bite of** left **thumb without damage to nail**

      ✓7ᵗʰ **S61.059**   **Open bite of unspecified thumb without damage to nail**

✓5ᵗʰ **S61.1**   **Open wound of** thumb with damage to nail

    ✓6ᵗʰ **S61.10**   **Unspecified open wound of thumb with damage to nail**

      ✓7ᵗʰ **S61.101**   **Unspecified open wound of** right **thumb with damage to nail**

      ✓7ᵗʰ **S61.102**   **Unspecified open wound of** left **thumb with damage to nail**

      ✓7ᵗʰ **S61.109**   **Unspecified open wound of unspecified thumb with damage to nail**

    ✓6ᵗʰ **S61.11**   **Laceration** without foreign body **of thumb with damage to nail**

      ✓7ᵗʰ **S61.111**   **Laceration without foreign body of** right **thumb with damage to nail**

      ✓7ᵗʰ **S61.112**   **Laceration without foreign body of** left **thumb with damage to nail**

      ✓7ᵗʰ **S61.119**   **Laceration without foreign body of unspecified thumb with damage to nail**

    ✓6ᵗʰ **S61.12**   **Laceration** with foreign body **of thumb with damage to nail**

      ✓7ᵗʰ **S61.121**   **Laceration with foreign body of** right **thumb with damage to nail**

      ✓7ᵗʰ **S61.122**   **Laceration with foreign body of** left **thumb with damage to nail**

      ✓7ᵗʰ **S61.129**   **Laceration with foreign body of unspecified thumb with damage to nail**

    ✓6ᵗʰ **S61.13**   **Puncture wound** without foreign body **of thumb with damage to nail**

      ✓7ᵗʰ **S61.131**   **Puncture wound without foreign body of** right **thumb with damage to nail**

      ✓7ᵗʰ **S61.132**   **Puncture wound without foreign body of** left **thumb with damage to nail**

      ✓7ᵗʰ **S61.139**   **Puncture wound without foreign body of unspecified thumb with damage to nail**

    ✓6ᵗʰ **S61.14**   **Puncture wound** with foreign body **of thumb with damage to nail**

      ✓7ᵗʰ **S61.141**   **Puncture wound with foreign body of** right **thumb with damage to nail**

      ✓7ᵗʰ **S61.142**   **Puncture wound with foreign body of** left **thumb with damage to nail**

      ✓7ᵗʰ **S61.149**   **Puncture wound with foreign body of unspecified thumb with damage to nail**

    ✓6ᵗʰ **S61.15**   **Open bite** of thumb with damage to nail

      Bite of thumb with damage to nail NOS

      EXCLUDES 1   *superficial bite of thumb (S60.36-, S60.37-)*

      ✓7ᵗʰ **S61.151**   **Open bite of** right **thumb with damage to nail**

      ✓7ᵗʰ **S61.152**   **Open bite of** left **thumb with damage to nail**

      ✓7ᵗʰ **S61.159**   **Open bite of unspecified thumb with damage to nail**

✓5ᵗʰ **S61.2**   **Open wound of other** finger without damage to nail

    EXCLUDES 1   *open wound of finger involving nail (matrix) (S61.3-)*

    EXCLUDES 2   *open wound of thumb without damage to nail (S61.0-)*

    ✓6ᵗʰ **S61.20**   **Unspecified open wound of other finger without damage to nail**

      ✓7ᵗʰ **S61.200**   **Unspecified open wound of** right index **finger without damage to nail**

      ✓7ᵗʰ **S61.201**   **Unspecified open wound of** left index **finger without damage to nail**

✓ Additional Character Required   ✓x7ᵗʰ Placeholder   Questionable PDx   Manifestation   Unspecified Dx   UPD Unacceptable PDx   H1–H14 HAC   HCC CMS-HCC Dx   HIV HIV Dx

ICD-10-CM 2022   1035

√7ᵗʰ S61.202 Unspecified open wound of right middle **finger without damage to nail**

√7ᵗʰ S61.203 Unspecified open wound of left middle **finger without damage to nail**

√7ᵗʰ S61.204 Unspecified open wound of right ring **finger without damage to nail**

√7ᵗʰ S61.205 Unspecified open wound of left ring **finger without damage to nail**

√7ᵗʰ S61.206 Unspecified open wound of right little **finger without damage to nail**

√7ᵗʰ S61.207 Unspecified open wound of left little **finger without damage to nail**

√7ᵗʰ S61.208 Unspecified open wound of other finger without damage to nail
Unspecified open wound of specified finger with unspecified laterality without damage to nail

√7ᵗʰ S61.209 Unspecified open wound of unspecified finger without damage to nail

√6ᵗʰ S61.21 Laceration without foreign body of finger without damage to nail

√7ᵗʰ S61.210 Laceration without foreign body of right index **finger without damage to nail**

√7ᵗʰ S61.211 Laceration without foreign body of left index **finger without damage to nail**

√7ᵗʰ S61.212 Laceration without foreign body of right middle **finger without damage to nail**

√7ᵗʰ S61.213 Laceration without foreign body of left middle **finger without damage to nail**

√7ᵗʰ S61.214 Laceration without foreign body of right ring **finger without damage to nail**

√7ᵗʰ S61.215 Laceration without foreign body of left ring **finger without damage to nail**

√7ᵗʰ S61.216 Laceration without foreign body of right little **finger without damage to nail**

√7ᵗʰ S61.217 Laceration without foreign body of left little **finger without damage to nail**

√7ᵗʰ S61.218 Laceration without foreign body of other finger without damage to nail
Laceration without foreign body of specified finger with unspecified laterality without damage to nail

√7ᵗʰ S61.219 Laceration without foreign body of unspecified finger without damage to nail

√6ᵗʰ S61.22 Laceration with foreign body of finger without damage to nail

√7ᵗʰ S61.220 Laceration with foreign body of right index **finger without damage to nail**

√7ᵗʰ S61.221 Laceration with foreign body of left index **finger without damage to nail**

√7ᵗʰ S61.222 Laceration with foreign body of right middle **finger without damage to nail**

√7ᵗʰ S61.223 Laceration with foreign body of left middle **finger without damage to nail**

√7ᵗʰ S61.224 Laceration with foreign body of right ring **finger without damage to nail**

√7ᵗʰ S61.225 Laceration with foreign body of left ring **finger without damage to nail**

√7ᵗʰ S61.226 Laceration with foreign body of right little **finger without damage to nail**

√7ᵗʰ S61.227 Laceration with foreign body of left little **finger without damage to nail**

√7ᵗʰ S61.228 Laceration with foreign body of other finger without damage to nail
Laceration with foreign body of specified finger with unspecified laterality without damage to nail

√7ᵗʰ S61.229 Laceration with foreign body of unspecified finger without damage to nail

√6ᵗʰ S61.23 Puncture wound without foreign body of finger without damage to nail

√7ᵗʰ S61.230 Puncture wound without foreign body of right index **finger without damage to nail**

√7ᵗʰ S61.231 Puncture wound without foreign body of left index **finger without damage to nail**

√7ᵗʰ S61.232 Puncture wound without foreign body of right middle **finger without damage to nail**

√7ᵗʰ S61.233 Puncture wound without foreign body of left middle **finger without damage to nail**

√7ᵗʰ S61.234 Puncture wound without foreign body of right ring **finger without damage to nail**

√7ᵗʰ S61.235 Puncture wound without foreign body of left ring **finger without damage to nail**

√7ᵗʰ S61.236 Puncture wound without foreign body of right little **finger without damage to nail**

√7ᵗʰ S61.237 Puncture wound without foreign body of left little **finger without damage to nail**

√7ᵗʰ S61.238 Puncture wound without foreign body of other finger without damage to nail
Puncture wound without foreign body of specified finger with unspecified laterality without damage to nail

√7ᵗʰ S61.239 Puncture wound without foreign body of unspecified finger without damage to nail

√6ᵗʰ S61.24 Puncture wound with foreign body of finger without damage to nail

√7ᵗʰ S61.240 Puncture wound with foreign body of right index **finger without damage to nail**

√7ᵗʰ S61.241 Puncture wound with foreign body of left index **finger without damage to nail**

√7ᵗʰ S61.242 Puncture wound with foreign body of right middle **finger without damage to nail**

√7ᵗʰ S61.243 Puncture wound with foreign body of left middle **finger without damage to nail**

√7ᵗʰ S61.244 Puncture wound with foreign body of right ring **finger without damage to nail**

√7ᵗʰ S61.245 Puncture wound with foreign body of left ring **finger without damage to nail**

√7ᵗʰ S61.246 Puncture wound with foreign body of right little **finger without damage to nail**

√7ᵗʰ S61.247 Puncture wound with foreign body of left little **finger without damage to nail**

√7ᵗʰ S61.248 Puncture wound with foreign body of other finger without damage to nail
Puncture wound with foreign body of specified finger with unspecified laterality without damage to nail

√7ᵗʰ S61.249 Puncture wound with foreign body of unspecified finger without damage to nail

√6ᵗʰ S61.25 Open bite of finger without damage to nail
Bite of finger without damage to nail NOS
EXCLUDES 1 *superficial bite of finger (S60.46-, S60.47-)*

√7ᵗʰ S61.250 Open bite of right index **finger without damage to nail**

√7ᵗʰ S61.251 Open bite of left index **finger without damage to nail**

√7ᵗʰ S61.252 Open bite of right middle **finger without damage to nail**

√7ᵗʰ S61.253 Open bite of left middle **finger without damage to nail**

√7ᵗʰ S61.254 Open bite of right ring **finger without damage to nail**

√7ᵗʰ S61.255 Open bite of left ring **finger without damage to nail**

√7ᵗʰ S61.256 Open bite of right little **finger without damage to nail**

√7ᵗʰ S61.257 Open bite of left little **finger without damage to nail**

√7ᵗʰ S61.258 Open bite of other finger without damage to nail
Open bite of specified finger with unspecified laterality without damage to nail

√7ᵗʰ S61.259 Open bite of unspecified finger without damage to nail

√5ᵗʰ S61.3 Open wound of other finger with damage to nail

√6ᵗʰ S61.30 Unspecified open wound of finger with damage to nail

√7ᵗʰ S61.300 Unspecified open wound of right index **finger with damage to nail**

√7ᵗʰ S61.301 Unspecified open wound of left index **finger with damage to nail**

√7ᵗʰ S61.302 Unspecified open wound of right middle **finger with damage to nail**

√7ᵗʰ S61.303 Unspecified open wound of left middle **finger with damage to nail**

√7ᵗʰ S61.304 Unspecified open wound of right ring **finger with damage to nail**

N Newborn: 0   **P** Pediatric: 0-17   **M** Maternity: 9-64   **A** Adult: 15-124   **MCC** Major Complication/Comorbidity   **CC** Complication/Comorbidity   **SW** Severe Wound Dx

1036
ICD-10-CM 2022

√7ᵗʰ **S61.305** Unspecified open wound of left ring finger with damage to nail

√7ᵗʰ **S61.306** Unspecified open wound of right little finger with damage to nail

√7ᵗʰ **S61.307** Unspecified open wound of left little finger with damage to nail

√7ᵗʰ **S61.308** Unspecified open wound of other finger with damage to nail

Unspecified open wound of specified finger with unspecified laterality with damage to nail

√7ᵗʰ **S61.309** Unspecified open wound of unspecified finger with damage to nail

√6ᵗʰ **S61.31** Laceration without foreign body of finger with damage to nail

√7ᵗʰ **S61.310** Laceration without foreign body of right index finger with damage to nail

√7ᵗʰ **S61.311** Laceration without foreign body of left index finger with damage to nail

√7ᵗʰ **S61.312** Laceration without foreign body of right middle finger with damage to nail

√7ᵗʰ **S61.313** Laceration without foreign body of left middle finger with damage to nail

√7ᵗʰ **S61.314** Laceration without foreign body of right ring finger with damage to nail

√7ᵗʰ **S61.315** Laceration without foreign body of left ring finger with damage to nail

√7ᵗʰ **S61.316** Laceration without foreign body of right little finger with damage to nail

√7ᵗʰ **S61.317** Laceration without foreign body of left little finger with damage to nail

√7ᵗʰ **S61.318** Laceration without foreign body of other finger with damage to nail

Laceration without foreign body of specified finger with unspecified laterality with damage to nail

√7ᵗʰ **S61.319** Laceration without foreign body of unspecified finger with damage to nail

√6ᵗʰ **S61.32** Laceration with foreign body of finger with damage to nail

√7ᵗʰ **S61.320** Laceration with foreign body of right index finger with damage to nail

√7ᵗʰ **S61.321** Laceration with foreign body of left index finger with damage to nail

√7ᵗʰ **S61.322** Laceration with foreign body of right middle finger with damage to nail

√7ᵗʰ **S61.323** Laceration with foreign body of left middle finger with damage to nail

√7ᵗʰ **S61.324** Laceration with foreign body of right ring finger with damage to nail

√7ᵗʰ **S61.325** Laceration with foreign body of left ring finger with damage to nail

√7ᵗʰ **S61.326** Laceration with foreign body of right little finger with damage to nail

√7ᵗʰ **S61.327** Laceration with foreign body of left little finger with damage to nail

√7ᵗʰ **S61.328** Laceration with foreign body of other finger with damage to nail

Laceration with foreign body of specified finger with unspecified laterality with damage to nail

√7ᵗʰ **S61.329** Laceration with foreign body of unspecified finger with damage to nail

√6ᵗʰ **S61.33** Puncture wound without foreign body of finger with damage to nail

√7ᵗʰ **S61.330** Puncture wound without foreign body of right index finger with damage to nail

√7ᵗʰ **S61.331** Puncture wound without foreign body of left index finger with damage to nail

√7ᵗʰ **S61.332** Puncture wound without foreign body of right middle finger with damage to nail

√7ᵗʰ **S61.333** Puncture wound without foreign body of left middle finger with damage to nail

√7ᵗʰ **S61.334** Puncture wound without foreign body of right ring finger with damage to nail

√7ᵗʰ **S61.335** Puncture wound without foreign body of left ring finger with damage to nail

√7ᵗʰ **S61.336** Puncture wound without foreign body of right little finger with damage to nail

√7ᵗʰ **S61.337** Puncture wound without foreign body of left little finger with damage to nail

√7ᵗʰ **S61.338** Puncture wound without foreign body of other finger with damage to nail

Puncture wound without foreign body of specified finger with unspecified laterality with damage to nail

√7ᵗʰ **S61.339** Puncture wound without foreign body of unspecified finger with damage to nail

√6ᵗʰ **S61.34** Puncture wound with foreign body of finger with damage to nail

√7ᵗʰ **S61.340** Puncture wound with foreign body of right index finger with damage to nail

√7ᵗʰ **S61.341** Puncture wound with foreign body of left index finger with damage to nail

√7ᵗʰ **S61.342** Puncture wound with foreign body of right middle finger with damage to nail

√7ᵗʰ **S61.343** Puncture wound with foreign body of left middle finger with damage to nail

√7ᵗʰ **S61.344** Puncture wound with foreign body of right ring finger with damage to nail

√7ᵗʰ **S61.345** Puncture wound with foreign body of left ring finger with damage to nail

√7ᵗʰ **S61.346** Puncture wound with foreign body of right little finger with damage to nail

√7ᵗʰ **S61.347** Puncture wound with foreign body of left little finger with damage to nail

√7ᵗʰ **S61.348** Puncture wound with foreign body of other finger with damage to nail

Puncture wound with foreign body of specified finger with unspecified laterality with damage to nail

√7ᵗʰ **S61.349** Puncture wound with foreign body of unspecified finger with damage to nail

√6ᵗʰ **S61.35** Open bite of finger with damage to nail

Bite of finger with damage to nail NOS

EXCLUDES 1   superficial bite of finger (S60.46-, S60.47-)

√7ᵗʰ **S61.350** Open bite of right index finger with damage to nail

√7ᵗʰ **S61.351** Open bite of left index finger with damage to nail

√7ᵗʰ **S61.352** Open bite of right middle finger with damage to nail

√7ᵗʰ **S61.353** Open bite of left middle finger with damage to nail

√7ᵗʰ **S61.354** Open bite of right ring finger with damage to nail

√7ᵗʰ **S61.355** Open bite of left ring finger with damage to nail

√7ᵗʰ **S61.356** Open bite of right little finger with damage to nail

√7ᵗʰ **S61.357** Open bite of left little finger with damage to nail

√7ᵗʰ **S61.358** Open bite of other finger with damage to nail

Open bite of specified finger with unspecified laterality with damage to nail

√7ᵗʰ **S61.359** Open bite of unspecified finger with damage to nail

√5ᵗʰ **S61.4** Open wound of hand

√6ᵗʰ **S61.40** Unspecified open wound of hand

√7ᵗʰ **S61.401** Unspecified open wound of right hand

√7ᵗʰ **S61.402** Unspecified open wound of left hand

√7ᵗʰ **S61.409** Unspecified open wound of unspecified hand

√6ᵗʰ **S61.41** Laceration without foreign body of hand

√7ᵗʰ **S61.411** Laceration without foreign body of right hand

√7ᵗʰ **S61.412** Laceration without foreign body of left hand

√7ᵗʰ **S61.419** Laceration without foreign body of unspecified hand

√6ᵗʰ **S61.42** Laceration with foreign body of hand

√7ᵗʰ **S61.421** Laceration with foreign body of right hand

√7ᵗʰ **S61.422** Laceration with foreign body of left hand

√7ᵗʰ **S61.429** Laceration with foreign body of unspecified hand

√6ᵗʰ **S61.43** Puncture wound without foreign body of hand

√7ᵗʰ **S61.431** Puncture wound without foreign body of right hand

☑ Additional Character Required   √x7ᵗʰ Placeholder   Questionable PDx   Manifestation   Unspecified Dx   **UPD** Unacceptable PDx   **H1-H14** HAC   **HCC** CMS-HCC Dx   **HIV** HIV Dx

ICD-10-CM 2022   **1037**

√7ᵗʰ **S61.432** Puncture wound without foreign body of **left** hand

√7ᵗʰ **S61.439** Puncture wound without foreign body of **unspecified** hand

√6ᵗʰ **S61.44** Puncture wound with foreign body of hand

√7ᵗʰ **S61.441** Puncture wound with foreign body of **right** hand

√7ᵗʰ **S61.442** Puncture wound with foreign body of **left** hand

√7ᵗʰ **S61.449** Puncture wound with foreign body of **unspecified** hand

√6ᵗʰ **S61.45** Open bite of hand

Bite of hand NOS

EXCLUDES 1   *superficial bite of hand (S60.56-, S60.57-)*

√7ᵗʰ **S61.451** Open bite of **right** hand

√7ᵗʰ **S61.452** Open bite of **left** hand

√7ᵗʰ **S61.459** Open bite of unspecified hand

√5ᵗʰ **S61.5** Open wound of **wrist**

√6ᵗʰ **S61.50** Unspecified open wound of wrist

√7ᵗʰ **S61.501** Unspecified open wound of **right** wrist

√7ᵗʰ **S61.502** Unspecified open wound of **left** wrist

√7ᵗʰ **S61.509** Unspecified open wound of unspecified wrist

√6ᵗʰ **S61.51** Laceration without foreign body of wrist

√7ᵗʰ **S61.511** Laceration without foreign body of **right** wrist

√7ᵗʰ **S61.512** Laceration without foreign body of **left** wrist

√7ᵗʰ **S61.519** Laceration without foreign body of unspecified wrist

√6ᵗʰ **S61.52** Laceration with foreign body of wrist

√7ᵗʰ **S61.521** Laceration with foreign body of **right** wrist

√7ᵗʰ **S61.522** Laceration with foreign body of **left** wrist

√7ᵗʰ **S61.529** Laceration with foreign body of unspecified wrist

√6ᵗʰ **S61.53** Puncture wound without foreign body of wrist

√7ᵗʰ **S61.531** Puncture wound without foreign body of **right** wrist

√7ᵗʰ **S61.532** Puncture wound without foreign body of **left** wrist

√7ᵗʰ **S61.539** Puncture wound without foreign body of **unspecified** wrist

√6ᵗʰ **S61.54** Puncture wound with foreign body of wrist

√7ᵗʰ **S61.541** Puncture wound with foreign body of **right** wrist

√7ᵗʰ **S61.542** Puncture wound with foreign body of **left** wrist

√7ᵗʰ **S61.549** Puncture wound with foreign body of **unspecified** wrist

√6ᵗʰ **S61.55** Open bite of wrist

Bite of wrist NOS

EXCLUDES 1   *superficial bite of wrist (S60.86-, S60.87-)*

√7ᵗʰ **S61.551** Open bite of **right** wrist

√7ᵗʰ **S61.552** Open bite of **left** wrist

√7ᵗʰ **S61.559** Open bite of unspecified wrist

√4ᵗʰ **S62 Fracture at wrist and hand level**

NOTE   A fracture not indicated as displaced or nondisplaced should be coded to displaced

A fracture not indicated as open or closed should be coded to closed

EXCLUDES 1   *traumatic amputation of wrist and hand (S68.-)*

EXCLUDES 2   *fracture of distal parts of ulna and radius (S52.-)*

AHA: 2018,2Q,12; 2015,3Q,37-39

The appropriate 7th character is to be added to each code from category S62.
A   initial encounter for closed fracture
B   initial encounter for open fracture
D   subsequent encounter for fracture with routine healing
G   subsequent encounter for fracture with delayed healing
K   subsequent encounter for fracture with nonunion
P   subsequent encounter for fracture with malunion
S   sequela

√5ᵗʰ **S62.0** Fracture of **navicular [scaphoid] bone of wrist**

√6ᵗʰ **S62.00** Unspecified fracture of navicular [scaphoid] bone of wrist

³ √7ᵗʰ **S62.001** Unspecified fracture of navicular [scaphoid] bone of **right** wrist   CC H5

³ √7ᵗʰ **S62.002** Unspecified fracture of navicular [scaphoid] bone of **left** wrist   CC H5

       AHA: 2012,4Q,106

³ √7ᵗʰ **S62.009** Unspecified fracture of navicular [scaphoid] bone of unspecified wrist   CC H5

√6ᵗʰ **S62.01** Fracture of **distal pole of navicular [scaphoid] bone of wrist**

Fracture of volar tuberosity of navicular [scaphoid] bone of wrist

³ √7ᵗʰ **S62.011** Displaced fracture of distal pole of navicular [scaphoid] bone of **right** wrist   CC H5

³ √7ᵗʰ **S62.012** Displaced fracture of distal pole of navicular [scaphoid] bone of **left** wrist   CC H5

³ √7ᵗʰ **S62.013** Displaced fracture of distal pole of navicular [scaphoid] bone of unspecified wrist   CC H5

³ √7ᵗʰ **S62.014** Nondisplaced fracture of distal pole of navicular [scaphoid] bone of **right** wrist   CC H5

³ √7ᵗʰ **S62.015** Nondisplaced fracture of distal pole of navicular [scaphoid] bone of **left** wrist   CC H5

³ √7ᵗʰ **S62.016** Nondisplaced fracture of distal pole of navicular [scaphoid] bone of unspecified wrist   CC H5

√6ᵗʰ **S62.02** Fracture of **middle third of navicular [scaphoid] bone of wrist**

³ √7ᵗʰ **S62.021** Displaced fracture of middle third of navicular [scaphoid] bone of **right** wrist   CC H5

³ √7ᵗʰ **S62.022** Displaced fracture of middle third of navicular [scaphoid] bone of **left** wrist   CC H5

³ √7ᵗʰ **S62.023** Displaced fracture of middle third of navicular [scaphoid] bone of unspecified wrist   CC H5

³ √7ᵗʰ **S62.024** Nondisplaced fracture of middle third of navicular [scaphoid] bone of **right** wrist   CC H5

³ √7ᵗʰ **S62.025** Nondisplaced fracture of middle third of navicular [scaphoid] bone of **left** wrist   CC H5

³ √7ᵗʰ **S62.026** Nondisplaced fracture of middle third of navicular [scaphoid] bone of unspecified wrist   CC H5

√6ᵗʰ **S62.03** Fracture of **proximal third of navicular [scaphoid] bone of wrist**

³ √7ᵗʰ **S62.031** Displaced fracture of proximal third of navicular [scaphoid] bone of **right** wrist   CC H5

³ √7ᵗʰ **S62.032** Displaced fracture of proximal third of navicular [scaphoid] bone of **left** wrist   CC H5

3 √7ᵗʰ **S62.033** Displaced **fracture of proximal third of navicular [scaphoid] bone of unspecified wrist** `CC` `H5`

3 √7ᵗʰ **S62.034** Nondisplaced **fracture of proximal third of navicular [scaphoid] bone of right wrist** `CC` `H5`

3 √7ᵗʰ **S62.035** Nondisplaced **fracture of proximal third of navicular [scaphoid] bone of left wrist** `CC` `H5`

3 √7ᵗʰ **S62.036** Nondisplaced **fracture of proximal third of navicular [scaphoid] bone of unspecified wrist** `CC` `H5`

√5ᵗʰ **S62.1 Fracture of other and unspecified carpal bone(s)**

> EXCLUDES 2   *fracture of scaphoid of wrist (S62.0-)*

√6ᵗʰ **S62.10 Fracture of unspecified carpal bone**

Fracture of wrist NOS

3 √7ᵗʰ **S62.101** **Fracture of unspecified carpal bone, right wrist** `CC` `H5`

3 √7ᵗʰ **S62.102** **Fracture of unspecified carpal bone, left wrist** `CC` `H5`

AHA: 2012,4Q,95

3 √7ᵗʰ **S62.109** **Fracture of unspecified carpal bone, unspecified wrist** `CC` `H5`

√6ᵗʰ **S62.11 Fracture of triquetrum [cuneiform] bone of wrist**

3 √7ᵗʰ **S62.111** Displaced **fracture of triquetrum [cuneiform] bone, right wrist** `CC` `H5`

3 √7ᵗʰ **S62.112** Displaced **fracture of triquetrum [cuneiform] bone, left wrist** `CC` `H5`

3 √7ᵗʰ **S62.113** Displaced **fracture of triquetrum [cuneiform] bone, unspecified wrist** `CC` `H5`

3 √7ᵗʰ **S62.114** Nondisplaced **fracture of triquetrum [cuneiform] bone, right wrist** `CC` `H5`

3 √7ᵗʰ **S62.115** Nondisplaced **fracture of triquetrum [cuneiform] bone, left wrist** `CC` `H5`

3 √7ᵗʰ **S62.116** Nondisplaced **fracture of triquetrum [cuneiform] bone, unspecified wrist** `CC` `H5`

√6ᵗʰ **S62.12 Fracture of lunate [semilunar]**

3 √7ᵗʰ **S62.121** Displaced **fracture of lunate [semilunar], right wrist** `CC` `H5`

3 √7ᵗʰ **S62.122** Displaced **fracture of lunate [semilunar], left wrist** `CC` `H5`

3 √7ᵗʰ **S62.123** Displaced **fracture of lunate [semilunar], unspecified wrist** `CC` `H5`

3 √7ᵗʰ **S62.124** Nondisplaced **fracture of lunate [semilunar], right wrist** `CC` `H5`

3 √7ᵗʰ **S62.125** Nondisplaced **fracture of lunate [semilunar], left wrist** `CC` `H5`

3 √7ᵗʰ **S62.126** Nondisplaced **fracture of lunate [semilunar], unspecified wrist** `CC` `H5`

√6ᵗʰ **S62.13 Fracture of capitate [os magnum] bone**

3 √7ᵗʰ **S62.131** Displaced **fracture of capitate [os magnum] bone, right wrist** `CC` `H5`

3 √7ᵗʰ **S62.132** Displaced **fracture of capitate [os magnum] bone, left wrist** `CC` `H5`

3 √7ᵗʰ **S62.133** Displaced **fracture of capitate [os magnum] bone, unspecified wrist** `CC` `H5`

3 √7ᵗʰ **S62.134** Nondisplaced **fracture of capitate [os magnum] bone, right wrist** `CC` `H5`

3 √7ᵗʰ **S62.135** Nondisplaced **fracture of capitate [os magnum] bone, left wrist** `CC` `H5`

3 √7ᵗʰ **S62.136** Nondisplaced **fracture of capitate [os magnum] bone, unspecified wrist** `CC` `H5`

√6ᵗʰ **S62.14 Fracture of body of hamate [unciform] bone**

Fracture of hamate [unciform] bone NOS

3 √7ᵗʰ **S62.141** Displaced **fracture of body of hamate [unciform] bone, right wrist** `CC` `H5`

3 √7ᵗʰ **S62.142** Displaced **fracture of body of hamate [unciform] bone, left wrist** `CC` `H5`

3 √7ᵗʰ **S62.143** Displaced **fracture of body of hamate [unciform] bone, unspecified wrist** `CC` `H5`

3 √7ᵗʰ **S62.144** Nondisplaced **fracture of body of hamate [unciform] bone, right wrist** `CC` `H5`

3 √7ᵗʰ **S62.145** Nondisplaced **fracture of body of hamate [unciform] bone, left wrist** `CC` `H5`

3 √7ᵗʰ **S62.146** Nondisplaced **fracture of body of hamate [unciform] bone, unspecified wrist** `CC` `H5`

√6ᵗʰ **S62.15 Fracture of hook process of hamate [unciform] bone**

Fracture of unciform process of hamate [unciform] bone

3 √7ᵗʰ **S62.151** Displaced **fracture of hook process of hamate [unciform] bone, right wrist** `CC` `H5`

3 √7ᵗʰ **S62.152** Displaced **fracture of hook process of hamate [unciform] bone, left wrist** `CC` `H5`

3 √7ᵗʰ **S62.153** Displaced **fracture of hook process of hamate [unciform] bone, unspecified wrist** `CC` `H5`

3 √7ᵗʰ **S62.154** Nondisplaced **fracture of hook process of hamate [unciform] bone, right wrist** `CC` `H5`

3 √7ᵗʰ **S62.155** Nondisplaced **fracture of hook process of hamate [unciform] bone, left wrist** `CC` `H5`

3 √7ᵗʰ **S62.156** Nondisplaced **fracture of hook process of hamate [unciform] bone, unspecified wrist** `CC` `H5`

√6ᵗʰ **S62.16 Fracture of pisiform**

3 √7ᵗʰ **S62.161** Displaced **fracture of pisiform, right wrist** `CC` `H5`

3 √7ᵗʰ **S62.162** Displaced **fracture of pisiform, left wrist** `CC` `H5`

3 √7ᵗʰ **S62.163** Displaced **fracture of pisiform, unspecified wrist** `CC` `H5`

3 √7ᵗʰ **S62.164** Nondisplaced **fracture of pisiform, right wrist** `CC` `H5`

3 √7ᵗʰ **S62.165** Nondisplaced **fracture of pisiform, left wrist** `CC` `H5`

3 √7ᵗʰ **S62.166** Nondisplaced **fracture of pisiform, unspecified wrist** `CC` `H5`

√6ᵗʰ **S62.17 Fracture of trapezium [larger multangular]**

3 √7ᵗʰ **S62.171** Displaced **fracture of trapezium [larger multangular], right wrist** `CC` `H5`

3 √7ᵗʰ **S62.172** Displaced **fracture of trapezium [larger multangular], left wrist** `CC` `H5`

3 √7ᵗʰ **S62.173** Displaced **fracture of trapezium [larger multangular], unspecified wrist** `CC` `H5`

3 √7ᵗʰ **S62.174** Nondisplaced **fracture of trapezium [larger multangular], right wrist** `CC` `H5`

3 √7ᵗʰ **S62.175** Nondisplaced **fracture of trapezium [larger multangular], left wrist** `CC` `H5`

3 √7ᵗʰ **S62.176** Nondisplaced **fracture of trapezium [larger multangular], unspecified wrist** `CC` `H5`

√6ᵗʰ **S62.18 Fracture of trapezoid [smaller multangular]**

3 √7ᵗʰ **S62.181** Displaced **fracture of trapezoid [smaller multangular], right wrist** `CC` `H5`

3 √7ᵗʰ **S62.182** Displaced **fracture of trapezoid [smaller multangular], left wrist** `CC` `H5`

3 √7ᵗʰ **S62.183** Displaced **fracture of trapezoid [smaller multangular], unspecified wrist** `CC` `H5`

3 √7ᵗʰ **S62.184** Nondisplaced **fracture of trapezoid [smaller multangular], right wrist** `CC` `H5`

3 √7ᵗʰ **S62.185** Nondisplaced **fracture of trapezoid [smaller multangular], left wrist** `CC` `H5`

3 √7ᵗʰ **S62.186** Nondisplaced **fracture of trapezoid [smaller multangular], unspecified wrist** `CC` `H5`

√5ᵗʰ **S62.2 Fracture of first metacarpal bone**

√6ᵗʰ **S62.20 Unspecified fracture of first metacarpal bone**

3 √7ᵗʰ **S62.201** **Unspecified fracture of first metacarpal bone, right hand** `CC` `H5`

3 √7ᵗʰ **S62.202** **Unspecified fracture of first metacarpal bone, left hand** `CC` `H5`

3 √7ᵗʰ **S62.209** **Unspecified fracture of first metacarpal bone, unspecified hand** `CC` `H5`

☑ Additional Character Required   √x7ᵗʰ Placeholder   Questionable PDx   Manifestation   Unspecified Dx   `UPD` Unacceptable PDx   `H1`-`H14` HAC   `HCC` CMS-HCC Dx   `HIV` HIV Dx

ICD-10-CM 2022   1039

√6ᵗʰ **S62.21**   Bennett's fracture

DEF: Intra-articular, two-part fracture at the base of the first metacarpal bone (thumb) on the ulnar side at the carpometacarpal (CMC) joint.

³ √7ᵗʰ **S62.211**   Bennett's fracture, **right hand**   CC H5

³ √7ᵗʰ **S62.212**   Bennett's fracture, **left hand**   CC H5

³ √7ᵗʰ **S62.213**   Bennett's fracture, **unspecified hand**   CC H5

√6ᵗʰ **S62.22**   Rolando's fracture

DEF: Comminuted, three part intra-articular fracture at the base of the thumb metacarpal.

³ √7ᵗʰ **S62.221**   Displaced Rolando's fracture, **right hand**   CC H5

³ √7ᵗʰ **S62.222**   Displaced Rolando's fracture, **left hand**   CC H5

³ √7ᵗʰ **S62.223**   Displaced Rolando's fracture, **unspecified hand**   CC H5

³ √7ᵗʰ **S62.224**   Nondisplaced Rolando's fracture, **right hand**   CC H5

³ √7ᵗʰ **S62.225**   Nondisplaced Rolando's fracture, **left hand**   CC H5

³ √7ᵗʰ **S62.226**   Nondisplaced Rolando's fracture, **unspecified hand**   CC H5

√6ᵗʰ **S62.23**   Other fracture of base of first metacarpal bone

³ √7ᵗʰ **S62.231**   Other displaced fracture of base of first metacarpal bone, **right hand**   CC H5

³ √7ᵗʰ **S62.232**   Other displaced fracture of base of first metacarpal bone, **left hand**   CC H5

³ √7ᵗʰ **S62.233**   Other displaced fracture of base of first metacarpal bone, **unspecified hand**   CC H5

³ √7ᵗʰ **S62.234**   Other nondisplaced fracture of base of first metacarpal bone, **right hand**   CC H5

³ √7ᵗʰ **S62.235**   Other nondisplaced fracture of base of first metacarpal bone, **left hand**   CC H5

³ √7ᵗʰ **S62.236**   Other nondisplaced fracture of base of first metacarpal bone, **unspecified hand**   CC H5

√6ᵗʰ **S62.24**   Fracture of shaft of first metacarpal bone

³ √7ᵗʰ **S62.241**   Displaced fracture of shaft of first metacarpal bone, **right hand**   CC H5

³ √7ᵗʰ **S62.242**   Displaced fracture of shaft of first metacarpal bone, **left hand**   CC H5

³ √7ᵗʰ **S62.243**   Displaced fracture of shaft of first metacarpal bone, **unspecified hand**   CC H5

³ √7ᵗʰ **S62.244**   Nondisplaced fracture of shaft of first metacarpal bone, **right hand**   CC H5

³ √7ᵗʰ **S62.245**   Nondisplaced fracture of shaft of first metacarpal bone, **left hand**   CC H5

³ √7ᵗʰ **S62.246**   Nondisplaced fracture of shaft of first metacarpal bone, **unspecified hand**   CC H5

√6ᵗʰ **S62.25**   Fracture of neck of first metacarpal bone

³ √7ᵗʰ **S62.251**   Displaced fracture of neck of first metacarpal bone, **right hand**   CC H5

³ √7ᵗʰ **S62.252**   Displaced fracture of neck of first metacarpal bone, **left hand**   CC H5

³ √7ᵗʰ **S62.253**   Displaced fracture of neck of first metacarpal bone, **unspecified hand**   CC H5

³ √7ᵗʰ **S62.254**   Nondisplaced fracture of neck of first metacarpal bone, **right hand**   CC H5

³ √7ᵗʰ **S62.255**   Nondisplaced fracture of neck of first metacarpal bone, **left hand**   CC H5

³ √7ᵗʰ **S62.256**   Nondisplaced fracture of neck of first metacarpal bone, **unspecified hand**   CC H5

√6ᵗʰ **S62.29**   Other fracture of first metacarpal bone

³ √7ᵗʰ **S62.291**   Other fracture of first metacarpal bone, **right hand**   CC H5

³ √7ᵗʰ **S62.292**   Other fracture of first metacarpal bone, **left hand**   CC H5

³ √7ᵗʰ **S62.299**   Other fracture of first metacarpal bone, **unspecified hand**   CC H5

√5ᵗʰ **S62.3**   Fracture of other and unspecified metacarpal bone

EXCLUDES 2   fracture of first metacarpal bone (S62.2-)

√6ᵗʰ **S62.30**   Unspecified fracture of other metacarpal bone

³ √7ᵗʰ **S62.300**   Unspecified fracture of second metacarpal bone, **right hand**   CC H5

³ √7ᵗʰ **S62.301**   Unspecified fracture of second metacarpal bone, **left hand**   CC H5

³ √7ᵗʰ **S62.302**   Unspecified fracture of third metacarpal bone, **right hand**   CC H5

³ √7ᵗʰ **S62.303**   Unspecified fracture of third metacarpal bone, **left hand**   CC H5

³ √7ᵗʰ **S62.304**   Unspecified fracture of fourth metacarpal bone, **right hand**   CC H5

³ √7ᵗʰ **S62.305**   Unspecified fracture of fourth metacarpal bone, **left hand**   CC H5

³ √7ᵗʰ **S62.306**   Unspecified fracture of fifth metacarpal bone, **right hand**   CC H5

³ √7ᵗʰ **S62.307**   Unspecified fracture of fifth metacarpal bone, **left hand**   CC H5

³ √7ᵗʰ **S62.308**   Unspecified fracture of other metacarpal bone   CC H5

Unspecified fracture of specified metacarpal bone with unspecified laterality

³ √7ᵗʰ **S62.309**   Unspecified fracture of unspecified metacarpal bone   CC H5

√6ᵗʰ **S62.31**   Displaced fracture of base of other metacarpal bone

³ √7ᵗʰ **S62.310**   Displaced fracture of base of second metacarpal bone, **right hand**   CC H5

³ √7ᵗʰ **S62.311**   Displaced fracture of base of second metacarpal bone, **left hand**   CC H5

³ √7ᵗʰ **S62.312**   Displaced fracture of base of third metacarpal bone, **right hand**   CC H5

³ √7ᵗʰ **S62.313**   Displaced fracture of base of third metacarpal bone, **left hand**   CC H5

³ √7ᵗʰ **S62.314**   Displaced fracture of base of fourth metacarpal bone, **right hand**   CC H5

³ √7ᵗʰ **S62.315**   Displaced fracture of base of fourth metacarpal bone, **left hand**   CC H5

³ √7ᵗʰ **S62.316**   Displaced fracture of base of fifth metacarpal bone, **right hand**   CC H5

³ √7ᵗʰ **S62.317**   Displaced fracture of base of fifth metacarpal bone, **left hand**   CC H5

³ √7ᵗʰ **S62.318**   Displaced fracture of base of other metacarpal bone   CC H5

Displaced fracture of base of specified metacarpal bone with unspecified laterality

³ √7ᵗʰ **S62.319**   Displaced fracture of base of unspecified metacarpal bone   CC H5

√6ᵗʰ **S62.32**   Displaced fracture of shaft of other metacarpal bone

³ √7ᵗʰ **S62.320**   Displaced fracture of shaft of second metacarpal bone, **right hand**   CC H5

³ √7ᵗʰ **S62.321**   Displaced fracture of shaft of second metacarpal bone, **left hand**   CC H5

³ √7ᵗʰ **S62.322**   Displaced fracture of shaft of third metacarpal bone, **right hand**   CC H5

³ √7ᵗʰ **S62.323**   Displaced fracture of shaft of third metacarpal bone, **left hand**   CC H5

³ √7ᵗʰ **S62.324**   Displaced fracture of shaft of fourth metacarpal bone, **right hand**   CC H5

³ √7ᵗʰ **S62.325**   Displaced fracture of shaft of fourth metacarpal bone, **left hand**   CC H5

³ √7ᵗʰ **S62.326**   Displaced fracture of shaft of fifth metacarpal bone, **right hand**   CC H5

³ √7ᵗʰ **S62.327**   Displaced fracture of shaft of fifth metacarpal bone, **left hand**   CC H5

³ √7ᵗʰ **S62.328**   Displaced fracture of shaft of other metacarpal bone   CC H5

Displaced fracture of shaft of specified metacarpal bone with unspecified laterality

³ √7ᵗʰ **S62.329**   Displaced fracture of shaft of unspecified metacarpal bone   CC H5

√6ᵗʰ **S62.33**   Displaced fracture of neck of other metacarpal bone

³ √7ᵗʰ **S62.330**   Displaced fracture of neck of second metacarpal bone, **right hand**   CC H5

N Newborn: 0   P Pediatric: 0-17   M Maternity: 9-64   A Adult: 15-124   MCC Major Complication/Comorbidity   CC Complication/Comorbidity   SW Severe Wound Dx

1040   ICD-10-CM 2022

³ √7ᵗʰ **S62.331** **Displaced fracture of neck of second metacarpal bone, left hand** CC H5

³ √7ᵗʰ **S62.332** **Displaced fracture of neck of third metacarpal bone, right hand** CC H5

³ √7ᵗʰ **S62.333** **Displaced fracture of neck of third metacarpal bone, left hand** CC H5

³ √7ᵗʰ **S62.334** **Displaced fracture of neck of fourth metacarpal bone, right hand** CC H5

³ √7ᵗʰ **S62.335** **Displaced fracture of neck of fourth metacarpal bone, left hand** CC H5

³ √7ᵗʰ **S62.336** **Displaced fracture of neck of fifth metacarpal bone, right hand** CC H5

³ √7ᵗʰ **S62.337** **Displaced fracture of neck of fifth metacarpal bone, left hand** CC H5

³ √7ᵗʰ **S62.338** **Displaced fracture of neck of other metacarpal bone** CC H5

Displaced fracture of neck of specified metacarpal bone with unspecified laterality

³ √7ᵗʰ **S62.339** **Displaced fracture of neck of unspecified metacarpal bone** CC H5

√6ᵗʰ **S62.34** **Nondisplaced fracture of base of other metacarpal bone**

³ √7ᵗʰ **S62.340** **Nondisplaced fracture of base of second metacarpal bone, right hand** CC H5

³ √7ᵗʰ **S62.341** **Nondisplaced fracture of base of second metacarpal bone, left hand** CC H5

³ √7ᵗʰ **S62.342** **Nondisplaced fracture of base of third metacarpal bone, right hand** CC H5

³ √7ᵗʰ **S62.343** **Nondisplaced fracture of base of third metacarpal bone, left hand** CC H5

³ √7ᵗʰ **S62.344** **Nondisplaced fracture of base of fourth metacarpal bone, right hand** CC H5

³ √7ᵗʰ **S62.345** **Nondisplaced fracture of base of fourth metacarpal bone, left hand** CC H5

³ √7ᵗʰ **S62.346** **Nondisplaced fracture of base of fifth metacarpal bone, right hand** CC H5

³ √7ᵗʰ **S62.347** **Nondisplaced fracture of base of fifth metacarpal bone, left hand** CC H5

³ √7ᵗʰ **S62.348** **Nondisplaced fracture of base of other metacarpal bone** CC H5

Nondisplaced fracture of base of specified metacarpal bone with unspecified laterality

³ √7ᵗʰ **S62.349** **Nondisplaced fracture of base of unspecified metacarpal bone** CC H5

√6ᵗʰ **S62.35** **Nondisplaced fracture of shaft of other metacarpal bone**

³ √7ᵗʰ **S62.350** **Nondisplaced fracture of shaft of second metacarpal bone, right hand** CC H5

³ √7ᵗʰ **S62.351** **Nondisplaced fracture of shaft of second metacarpal bone, left hand** CC H5

³ √7ᵗʰ **S62.352** **Nondisplaced fracture of shaft of third metacarpal bone, right hand** CC H5

³ √7ᵗʰ **S62.353** **Nondisplaced fracture of shaft of third metacarpal bone, left hand** CC H5

³ √7ᵗʰ **S62.354** **Nondisplaced fracture of shaft of fourth metacarpal bone, right hand** CC H5

³ √7ᵗʰ **S62.355** **Nondisplaced fracture of shaft of fourth metacarpal bone, left hand** CC H5

³ √7ᵗʰ **S62.356** **Nondisplaced fracture of shaft of fifth metacarpal bone, right hand** CC H5

³ √7ᵗʰ **S62.357** **Nondisplaced fracture of shaft of fifth metacarpal bone, left hand** CC H5

³ √7ᵗʰ **S62.358** **Nondisplaced fracture of shaft of other metacarpal bone** CC H5

Nondisplaced fracture of shaft of specified metacarpal bone with unspecified laterality

³ √7ᵗʰ **S62.359** **Nondisplaced fracture of shaft of unspecified metacarpal bone** CC H5

√6ᵗʰ **S62.36** **Nondisplaced fracture of neck of other metacarpal bone**

³ √7ᵗʰ **S62.360** **Nondisplaced fracture of neck of second metacarpal bone, right hand** CC H5

³ √7ᵗʰ **S62.361** **Nondisplaced fracture of neck of second metacarpal bone, left hand** CC H5

³ √7ᵗʰ **S62.362** **Nondisplaced fracture of neck of third metacarpal bone, right hand** CC H5

³ √7ᵗʰ **S62.363** **Nondisplaced fracture of neck of third metacarpal bone, left hand** CC H5

³ √7ᵗʰ **S62.364** **Nondisplaced fracture of neck of fourth metacarpal bone, right hand** CC H5

³ √7ᵗʰ **S62.365** **Nondisplaced fracture of neck of fourth metacarpal bone, left hand** CC H5

³ √7ᵗʰ **S62.366** **Nondisplaced fracture of neck of fifth metacarpal bone, right hand** CC H5

³ √7ᵗʰ **S62.367** **Nondisplaced fracture of neck of fifth metacarpal bone, left hand** CC H5

³ √7ᵗʰ **S62.368** **Nondisplaced fracture of neck of other metacarpal bone** CC H5

Nondisplaced fracture of neck of specified metacarpal bone with unspecified laterality

³ √7ᵗʰ **S62.369** **Nondisplaced fracture of neck of unspecified metacarpal bone** CC H5

√6ᵗʰ **S62.39** **Other fracture of other metacarpal bone**

³ √7ᵗʰ **S62.390** **Other fracture of second metacarpal bone, right hand** CC H5

³ √7ᵗʰ **S62.391** **Other fracture of second metacarpal bone, left hand** CC H5

³ √7ᵗʰ **S62.392** **Other fracture of third metacarpal bone, right hand** CC H5

³ √7ᵗʰ **S62.393** **Other fracture of third metacarpal bone, left hand** CC H5

³ √7ᵗʰ **S62.394** **Other fracture of fourth metacarpal bone, right hand** CC H5

³ √7ᵗʰ **S62.395** **Other fracture of fourth metacarpal bone, left hand** CC H5

³ √7ᵗʰ **S62.396** **Other fracture of fifth metacarpal bone, right hand** CC H5

³ √7ᵗʰ **S62.397** **Other fracture of fifth metacarpal bone, left hand** CC H5

³ √7ᵗʰ **S62.398** **Other fracture of other metacarpal bone** CC H5

Other fracture of specified metacarpal bone with unspecified laterality

³ √7ᵗʰ **S62.399** **Other fracture of unspecified metacarpal bone** CC H5

√5ᵗʰ **S62.5** **Fracture of thumb**

√6ᵗʰ **S62.50** **Fracture of unspecified phalanx of thumb**

³ √7ᵗʰ **S62.501** **Fracture of unspecified phalanx of right thumb** CC H5

³ √7ᵗʰ **S62.502** **Fracture of unspecified phalanx of left thumb** CC H5

³ √7ᵗʰ **S62.509** **Fracture of unspecified phalanx of unspecified thumb** CC H5

√6ᵗʰ **S62.51** **Fracture of proximal phalanx of thumb**

³ √7ᵗʰ **S62.511** **Displaced fracture of proximal phalanx of right thumb** CC H5

³ √7ᵗʰ **S62.512** **Displaced fracture of proximal phalanx of left thumb** CC H5

³ √7ᵗʰ **S62.513** **Displaced fracture of proximal phalanx of unspecified thumb** CC H5

³ √7ᵗʰ **S62.514** **Nondisplaced fracture of proximal phalanx of right thumb** CC H5

³ √7ᵗʰ **S62.515** **Nondisplaced fracture of proximal phalanx of left thumb** CC H5

³ √7ᵗʰ **S62.516** **Nondisplaced fracture of proximal phalanx of unspecified thumb** CC H5

√6ᵗʰ **S62.52** **Fracture of distal phalanx of thumb**

³ √7ᵗʰ **S62.521** **Displaced fracture of distal phalanx of right thumb** CC H5

³ √7ᵗʰ **S62.522** **Displaced fracture of distal phalanx of left thumb** CC H5

³ √7ᵗʰ **S62.523** **Displaced fracture of distal phalanx of unspecified thumb** CC H5

³ √7ᵗʰ **S62.524** **Nondisplaced fracture of distal phalanx of right thumb** CC H5

³ √7ᵗʰ **S62.525** **Nondisplaced fracture of distal phalanx of left thumb** CC H5

³ √7ᵗʰ **S62.526** **Nondisplaced fracture of distal phalanx of unspecified thumb** CC H5

☑ Additional Character Required   √x7ᵗʰ Placeholder   Questionable PDx   Manifestation   Unspecified Dx   UPD Unacceptable PDx   H1–H14 HAC   HCC CMS-HCC Dx   HIV HIV Dx

ICD-10-CM 2022

1041

✓5th **S62.6** **Fracture of other and unspecified** finger(s)

> EXCLUDES 2   *fracture of thumb (S62.5-)*

✓6th **S62.60** **Fracture of unspecified phalanx of finger**

3 ✓7th **S62.600** Fracture of unspecified phalanx of right index finger   CC H5

3 ✓7th **S62.601** Fracture of unspecified phalanx of left index finger   CC H5

3 ✓7th **S62.602** Fracture of unspecified phalanx of right middle finger   CC H5

3 ✓7th **S62.603** Fracture of unspecified phalanx of left middle finger   CC H5

3 ✓7th **S62.604** Fracture of unspecified phalanx of right ring finger   CC H5

3 ✓7th **S62.605** Fracture of unspecified phalanx of left ring finger   CC H5

3 ✓7th **S62.606** Fracture of unspecified phalanx of right little finger   CC H5

3 ✓7th **S62.607** Fracture of unspecified phalanx of left little finger   CC H5

3 ✓7th **S62.608** Fracture of unspecified phalanx of other finger   CC H5
> Fracture of unspecified phalanx of specified finger with unspecified laterality

3 ✓7th **S62.609** Fracture of unspecified phalanx of unspecified finger   CC H5

✓6th **S62.61** **Displaced** fracture of proximal phalanx of finger

3 ✓7th **S62.610** Displaced fracture of proximal phalanx of right index finger   CC H5

3 ✓7th **S62.611** Displaced fracture of proximal phalanx of left index finger   CC H5

3 ✓7th **S62.612** Displaced fracture of proximal phalanx of right middle finger   CC H5

3 ✓7th **S62.613** Displaced fracture of proximal phalanx of left middle finger   CC H5

3 ✓7th **S62.614** Displaced fracture of proximal phalanx of right ring finger   CC H5

3 ✓7th **S62.615** Displaced fracture of proximal phalanx of left ring finger   CC H5

3 ✓7th **S62.616** Displaced fracture of proximal phalanx of right little finger   CC H5

3 ✓7th **S62.617** Displaced fracture of proximal phalanx of left little finger   CC H5

3 ✓7th **S62.618** Displaced fracture of proximal phalanx of other finger   CC H5
> Displaced fracture of proximal phalanx of specified finger with unspecified laterality

3 ✓7th **S62.619** Displaced fracture of proximal phalanx of unspecified finger   CC H5

✓6th **S62.62** **Displaced** fracture of middle phalanx of finger

3 ✓7th **S62.620** Displaced fracture of middle phalanx of right index finger   CC H5

3 ✓7th **S62.621** Displaced fracture of middle phalanx of left index finger   CC H5

3 ✓7th **S62.622** Displaced fracture of middle phalanx of right middle finger   CC H5

3 ✓7th **S62.623** Displaced fracture of middle phalanx of left middle finger   CC H5

3 ✓7th **S62.624** Displaced fracture of middle phalanx of right ring finger   CC H5

3 ✓7th **S62.625** Displaced fracture of middle phalanx of left ring finger   CC H5

3 ✓7th **S62.626** Displaced fracture of middle phalanx of right little finger   CC H5

3 ✓7th **S62.627** Displaced fracture of middle phalanx of left little finger   CC H5

3 ✓7th **S62.628** Displaced fracture of middle phalanx of other finger   CC H5
> Displaced fracture of middle phalanx of specified finger with unspecified laterality

3 ✓7th **S62.629** Displaced fracture of middle phalanx of unspecified finger   CC H5

✓6th **S62.63** **Displaced** fracture of distal phalanx of finger

3 ✓7th **S62.630** Displaced fracture of distal phalanx of right index finger   CC H5

3 ✓7th **S62.631** Displaced fracture of distal phalanx of left index finger   CC H5

3 ✓7th **S62.632** Displaced fracture of distal phalanx of right middle finger   CC H5

3 ✓7th **S62.633** Displaced fracture of distal phalanx of left middle finger   CC H5

3 ✓7th **S62.634** Displaced fracture of distal phalanx of right ring finger   CC H5

3 ✓7th **S62.635** Displaced fracture of distal phalanx of left ring finger   CC H5

3 ✓7th **S62.636** Displaced fracture of distal phalanx of right little finger   CC H5

3 ✓7th **S62.637** Displaced fracture of distal phalanx of left little finger   CC H5

3 ✓7th **S62.638** Displaced fracture of distal phalanx of other finger   CC H5
> Displaced fracture of distal phalanx of specified finger with unspecified laterality

3 ✓7th **S62.639** Displaced fracture of distal phalanx of unspecified finger   CC H5

✓6th **S62.64** **Nondisplaced** fracture of proximal phalanx of finger

3 ✓7th **S62.640** Nondisplaced fracture of proximal phalanx of right index finger   CC H5

3 ✓7th **S62.641** Nondisplaced fracture of proximal phalanx of left index finger   CC H5

3 ✓7th **S62.642** Nondisplaced fracture of proximal phalanx of right middle finger   CC H5

3 ✓7th **S62.643** Nondisplaced fracture of proximal phalanx of left middle finger   CC H5

3 ✓7th **S62.644** Nondisplaced fracture of proximal phalanx of right ring finger   CC H5

3 ✓7th **S62.645** Nondisplaced fracture of proximal phalanx of left ring finger   CC H5

3 ✓7th **S62.646** Nondisplaced fracture of proximal phalanx of right little finger   CC H5

3 ✓7th **S62.647** Nondisplaced fracture of proximal phalanx of left little finger   CC H5

3 ✓7th **S62.648** Nondisplaced fracture of proximal phalanx of other finger   CC H5
> Nondisplaced fracture of proximal phalanx of specified finger with unspecified laterality

3 ✓7th **S62.649** Nondisplaced fracture of proximal phalanx of unspecified finger   CC H5

✓6th **S62.65** **Nondisplaced** fracture of middle phalanx of finger

3 ✓7th **S62.650** Nondisplaced fracture of middle phalanx of right index finger   CC H5

3 ✓7th **S62.651** Nondisplaced fracture of middle phalanx of left index finger   CC H5

3 ✓7th **S62.652** Nondisplaced fracture of middle phalanx of right middle finger   CC H5

3 ✓7th **S62.653** Nondisplaced fracture of middle phalanx of left middle finger   CC H5

3 ✓7th **S62.654** Nondisplaced fracture of middle phalanx of right ring finger   CC H5

3 ✓7th **S62.655** Nondisplaced fracture of middle phalanx of left ring finger   CC H5

3 ✓7th **S62.656** Nondisplaced fracture of middle phalanx of right little finger   CC H5

3 ✓7th **S62.657** Nondisplaced fracture of middle phalanx of left little finger   CC H5

3 ✓7th **S62.658** Nondisplaced fracture of middle phalanx of other finger   CC H5
> Nondisplaced fracture of middle phalanx of specified finger with unspecified laterality

3 ✓7th **S62.659** Nondisplaced fracture of middle phalanx of unspecified finger   CC H5

✓6th **S62.66** **Nondisplaced** fracture of distal phalanx of finger

3 ✓7th **S62.660** Nondisplaced fracture of distal phalanx of right index finger   CC H5

3 ✓7th **S62.661** Nondisplaced fracture of distal phalanx of left index finger   CC H5

3 ✓7th **S62.662** Nondisplaced fracture of distal phalanx of right middle finger   CC H5

3 ✓7th **S62.663** Nondisplaced fracture of distal phalanx of left middle finger   CC H5

3 ✓7th **S62.664** Nondisplaced fracture of distal phalanx of right ring finger   CC H5

N Newborn: 0   P Pediatric: 0-17   M Maternity: 9-64   A Adult: 15-124   MCC Major Complication/Comorbidity   CC Complication/Comorbidity   SW Severe Wound Dx

1042   ICD-10-CM 2022

3 √7ᵗʰ **S62.665** **Nondisplaced fracture of distal phalanx of left ring finger** `CC` `H5`

3 √7ᵗʰ **S62.666** **Nondisplaced fracture of distal phalanx of right little finger** `CC` `H5`

3 √7ᵗʰ **S62.667** **Nondisplaced fracture of distal phalanx of left little finger** `CC` `H5`

3 √7ᵗʰ **S62.668** **Nondisplaced fracture of distal phalanx of other finger** `CC` `H5`

     Nondisplaced fracture of distal phalanx of specified finger with unspecified laterality

3 √7ᵗʰ **S62.669** **Nondisplaced fracture of distal phalanx of unspecified finger** `CC` `H5`

√5ᵗʰ **S62.9** **Unspecified fracture of wrist and hand**

3 √x7ᵗʰ **S62.90** **Unspecified fracture of unspecified wrist and hand** `CC` `H5`

3 √x7ᵗʰ **S62.91** **Unspecified fracture of right wrist and hand** `CC` `H5`

3 √x7ᵗʰ **S62.92** **Unspecified fracture of left wrist and hand** `CC` `H5`

√4ᵗʰ **S63** **Dislocation and sprain of joints and ligaments at wrist and hand level**

`INCLUDES`   avulsion of joint or ligament at wrist and hand level

     laceration of cartilage, joint or ligament at wrist and hand level

     sprain of cartilage, joint or ligament at wrist and hand level

     traumatic hemarthrosis of joint or ligament at wrist and hand level

     traumatic rupture of joint or ligament at wrist and hand level

     traumatic subluxation of joint or ligament at wrist and hand level

     traumatic tear of joint or ligament at wrist and hand level

Code also any associated open wound

`EXCLUDES 2`   *strain of muscle, fascia and tendon of wrist and hand (S66.-)*

The appropriate 7th character is to be added to each code from category S63.
A   initial encounter
D   subsequent encounter
S   sequela

√5ᵗʰ **S63.0** **Subluxation and dislocation of wrist and hand joints**

√6ᵗʰ **S63.00** **Unspecified subluxation and dislocation of wrist and hand**

     Dislocation of carpal bone NOS
     Dislocation of distal end of radius NOS
     Subluxation of carpal bone NOS
     Subluxation of distal end of radius NOS

√7ᵗʰ **S63.001** **Unspecified subluxation of right wrist and hand**

√7ᵗʰ **S63.002** **Unspecified subluxation of left wrist and hand**

√7ᵗʰ **S63.003** **Unspecified subluxation of unspecified wrist and hand**

√7ᵗʰ **S63.004** **Unspecified dislocation of right wrist and hand**

√7ᵗʰ **S63.005** **Unspecified dislocation of left wrist and hand**

√7ᵗʰ **S63.006** **Unspecified dislocation of unspecified wrist and hand**

√6ᵗʰ **S63.01** **Subluxation and dislocation of distal radioulnar joint**

√7ᵗʰ **S63.011** **Subluxation of distal radioulnar joint of right wrist**

√7ᵗʰ **S63.012** **Subluxation of distal radioulnar joint of left wrist**

√7ᵗʰ **S63.013** **Subluxation of distal radioulnar joint of unspecified wrist**

√7ᵗʰ **S63.014** **Dislocation of distal radioulnar joint of right wrist**

√7ᵗʰ **S63.015** **Dislocation of distal radioulnar joint of left wrist**

√7ᵗʰ **S63.016** **Dislocation of distal radioulnar joint of unspecified wrist**

√6ᵗʰ **S63.02** **Subluxation and dislocation of radiocarpal joint**

√7ᵗʰ **S63.021** **Subluxation of radiocarpal joint of right wrist**

√7ᵗʰ **S63.022** **Subluxation of radiocarpal joint of left wrist**

√7ᵗʰ **S63.023** **Subluxation of radiocarpal joint of unspecified wrist**

√7ᵗʰ **S63.024** **Dislocation of radiocarpal joint of right wrist**

√7ᵗʰ **S63.025** **Dislocation of radiocarpal joint of left wrist**

√7ᵗʰ **S63.026** **Dislocation of radiocarpal joint of unspecified wrist**

√6ᵗʰ **S63.03** **Subluxation and dislocation of midcarpal joint**

√7ᵗʰ **S63.031** **Subluxation of midcarpal joint of right wrist**

√7ᵗʰ **S63.032** **Subluxation of midcarpal joint of left wrist**

√7ᵗʰ **S63.033** **Subluxation of midcarpal joint of unspecified wrist**

√7ᵗʰ **S63.034** **Dislocation of midcarpal joint of right wrist**

√7ᵗʰ **S63.035** **Dislocation of midcarpal joint of left wrist**

√7ᵗʰ **S63.036** **Dislocation of midcarpal joint of unspecified wrist**

√6ᵗʰ **S63.04** **Subluxation and dislocation of carpometacarpal joint of thumb**

`EXCLUDES 2`   *interphalangeal subluxation and dislocation of thumb (S63.1-)*

√7ᵗʰ **S63.041** **Subluxation of carpometacarpal joint of right thumb**

√7ᵗʰ **S63.042** **Subluxation of carpometacarpal joint of left thumb**

√7ᵗʰ **S63.043** **Subluxation of carpometacarpal joint of unspecified thumb**

√7ᵗʰ **S63.044** **Dislocation of carpometacarpal joint of right thumb**

√7ᵗʰ **S63.045** **Dislocation of carpometacarpal joint of left thumb**

√7ᵗʰ **S63.046** **Dislocation of carpometacarpal joint of unspecified thumb**

√6ᵗʰ **S63.05** **Subluxation and dislocation of other carpometacarpal joint**

`EXCLUDES 2`   *subluxation and dislocation of carpometacarpal joint of thumb (S63.04-)*

√7ᵗʰ **S63.051** **Subluxation of other carpometacarpal joint of right hand**

√7ᵗʰ **S63.052** **Subluxation of other carpometacarpal joint of left hand**

√7ᵗʰ **S63.053** **Subluxation of other carpometacarpal joint of unspecified hand**

√7ᵗʰ **S63.054** **Dislocation of other carpometacarpal joint of right hand**

√7ᵗʰ **S63.055** **Dislocation of other carpometacarpal joint of left hand**

√7ᵗʰ **S63.056** **Dislocation of other carpometacarpal joint of unspecified hand**

√6ᵗʰ **S63.06** **Subluxation and dislocation of metacarpal (bone), proximal end**

√7ᵗʰ **S63.061** **Subluxation of metacarpal (bone), proximal end of right hand**

√7ᵗʰ **S63.062** **Subluxation of metacarpal (bone), proximal end of left hand**

√7ᵗʰ **S63.063** **Subluxation of metacarpal (bone), proximal end of unspecified hand**

√7ᵗʰ **S63.064** **Dislocation of metacarpal (bone), proximal end of right hand**

√7ᵗʰ **S63.065** **Dislocation of metacarpal (bone), proximal end of left hand**

√7ᵗʰ **S63.066** **Dislocation of metacarpal (bone), proximal end of unspecified hand**

√6ᵗʰ **S63.07** **Subluxation and dislocation of distal end of ulna**

√7ᵗʰ **S63.071** **Subluxation of distal end of right ulna**

√7ᵗʰ **S63.072** **Subluxation of distal end of left ulna**

√7ᵗʰ **S63.073** **Subluxation of distal end of unspecified ulna**

√7ᵗʰ **S63.074** **Dislocation of distal end of right ulna**

√7ᵗʰ **S63.075** **Dislocation of distal end of left ulna**

√7ᵗʰ **S63.076** **Dislocation of distal end of unspecified ulna**

√6ᵗʰ **S63.09** **Other subluxation and dislocation of wrist and hand**

√7ᵗʰ **S63.091** **Other subluxation of right wrist and hand**

√7ᵗʰ **S63.092** **Other subluxation of left wrist and hand**

√7ᵗʰ **S63.093** Other subluxation of unspecified wrist and hand

√7ᵗʰ **S63.094** Other dislocation of right wrist and hand

√7ᵗʰ **S63.095** Other dislocation of left wrist and hand

√7ᵗʰ **S63.096** Other dislocation of unspecified wrist and hand

√5ᵗʰ **S63.1 Subluxation and dislocation of thumb**

√6ᵗʰ **S63.10 Unspecified subluxation and dislocation of thumb**

√7ᵗʰ **S63.101** Unspecified subluxation of right thumb

√7ᵗʰ **S63.102** Unspecified subluxation of left thumb

√7ᵗʰ **S63.103** Unspecified subluxation of unspecified thumb

√7ᵗʰ **S63.104** Unspecified dislocation of right thumb

√7ᵗʰ **S63.105** Unspecified dislocation of left thumb

√7ᵗʰ **S63.106** Unspecified dislocation of unspecified thumb

√6ᵗʰ **S63.11 Subluxation and dislocation of metacarpophalangeal joint of thumb**

√7ᵗʰ **S63.111** Subluxation of metacarpophalangeal joint of right thumb

√7ᵗʰ **S63.112** Subluxation of metacarpophalangeal joint of left thumb

√7ᵗʰ **S63.113** Subluxation of metacarpophalangeal joint of unspecified thumb

√7ᵗʰ **S63.114** Dislocation of metacarpophalangeal joint of right thumb

√7ᵗʰ **S63.115** Dislocation of metacarpophalangeal joint of left thumb

√7ᵗʰ **S63.116** Dislocation of metacarpophalangeal joint of unspecified thumb

√6ᵗʰ **S63.12 Subluxation and dislocation of interphalangeal joint of thumb**

√7ᵗʰ **S63.121** Subluxation of interphalangeal joint of right thumb

√7ᵗʰ **S63.122** Subluxation of interphalangeal joint of left thumb

√7ᵗʰ **S63.123** Subluxation of interphalangeal joint of unspecified thumb

√7ᵗʰ **S63.124** Dislocation of interphalangeal joint of right thumb

√7ᵗʰ **S63.125** Dislocation of interphalangeal joint of left thumb

√7ᵗʰ **S63.126** Dislocation of interphalangeal joint of unspecified thumb

√5ᵗʰ **S63.2 Subluxation and dislocation of other finger(s)**

EXCLUDES 2   subluxation and dislocation of thumb (S63.1-)

√6ᵗʰ **S63.20 Unspecified subluxation of other finger**

√7ᵗʰ **S63.200** Unspecified subluxation of right index finger

√7ᵗʰ **S63.201** Unspecified subluxation of left index finger

√7ᵗʰ **S63.202** Unspecified subluxation of right middle finger

√7ᵗʰ **S63.203** Unspecified subluxation of left middle finger

√7ᵗʰ **S63.204** Unspecified subluxation of right ring finger

√7ᵗʰ **S63.205** Unspecified subluxation of left ring finger

√7ᵗʰ **S63.206** Unspecified subluxation of right little finger

√7ᵗʰ **S63.207** Unspecified subluxation of left little finger

√7ᵗʰ **S63.208** Unspecified subluxation of other finger

Unspecified subluxation of specified finger with unspecified laterality

√7ᵗʰ **S63.209** Unspecified subluxation of unspecified finger

√6ᵗʰ **S63.21 Subluxation of metacarpophalangeal joint of finger**

√7ᵗʰ **S63.210** Subluxation of metacarpophalangeal joint of right index finger

√7ᵗʰ **S63.211** Subluxation of metacarpophalangeal joint of left index finger

√7ᵗʰ **S63.212** Subluxation of metacarpophalangeal joint of right middle finger

√7ᵗʰ **S63.213** Subluxation of metacarpophalangeal joint of left middle finger

√7ᵗʰ **S63.214** Subluxation of metacarpophalangeal joint of right ring finger

√7ᵗʰ **S63.215** Subluxation of metacarpophalangeal joint of left ring finger

√7ᵗʰ **S63.216** Subluxation of metacarpophalangeal joint of right little finger

√7ᵗʰ **S63.217** Subluxation of metacarpophalangeal joint of left little finger

√7ᵗʰ **S63.218** Subluxation of metacarpophalangeal joint of other finger

Subluxation of metacarpophalangeal joint of specified finger with unspecified laterality

√7ᵗʰ **S63.219** Subluxation of metacarpophalangeal joint of unspecified finger

√6ᵗʰ **S63.22 Subluxation of unspecified interphalangeal joint of finger**

√7ᵗʰ **S63.220** Subluxation of unspecified interphalangeal joint of right index finger

√7ᵗʰ **S63.221** Subluxation of unspecified interphalangeal joint of left index finger

√7ᵗʰ **S63.222** Subluxation of unspecified interphalangeal joint of right middle finger

√7ᵗʰ **S63.223** Subluxation of unspecified interphalangeal joint of left middle finger

√7ᵗʰ **S63.224** Subluxation of unspecified interphalangeal joint of right ring finger

√7ᵗʰ **S63.225** Subluxation of unspecified interphalangeal joint of left ring finger

√7ᵗʰ **S63.226** Subluxation of unspecified interphalangeal joint of right little finger

√7ᵗʰ **S63.227** Subluxation of unspecified interphalangeal joint of left little finger

√7ᵗʰ **S63.228** Subluxation of unspecified interphalangeal joint of other finger

Subluxation of unspecified interphalangeal joint of specified finger with unspecified laterality

√7ᵗʰ **S63.229** Subluxation of unspecified interphalangeal joint of unspecified finger

√6ᵗʰ **S63.23 Subluxation of proximal interphalangeal joint of finger**

√7ᵗʰ **S63.230** Subluxation of proximal interphalangeal joint of right index finger

√7ᵗʰ **S63.231** Subluxation of proximal interphalangeal joint of left index finger

√7ᵗʰ **S63.232** Subluxation of proximal interphalangeal joint of right middle finger

√7ᵗʰ **S63.233** Subluxation of proximal interphalangeal joint of left middle finger

√7ᵗʰ **S63.234** Subluxation of proximal interphalangeal joint of right ring finger

√7ᵗʰ **S63.235** Subluxation of proximal interphalangeal joint of left ring finger

√7ᵗʰ **S63.236** Subluxation of proximal interphalangeal joint of right little finger

√7ᵗʰ **S63.237** Subluxation of proximal interphalangeal joint of left little finger

√7ᵗʰ **S63.238** Subluxation of proximal interphalangeal joint of other finger

Subluxation of proximal interphalangeal joint of specified finger with unspecified laterality

√7ᵗʰ **S63.239** Subluxation of proximal interphalangeal joint of unspecified finger

√6ᵗʰ **S63.24 Subluxation of distal interphalangeal joint of finger**

√7ᵗʰ **S63.240** Subluxation of distal interphalangeal joint of right index finger

√7ᵗʰ **S63.241** Subluxation of distal interphalangeal joint of left index finger

√7ᵗʰ **S63.242** Subluxation of distal interphalangeal joint of right middle finger

√7ᵗʰ **S63.243** Subluxation of distal interphalangeal joint of left middle finger

√7ᵗʰ **S63.244** Subluxation of distal interphalangeal joint of right ring finger

√7ᵗʰ **S63.245** Subluxation of distal interphalangeal joint of left ring finger

√7ᵗʰ **S63.246** Subluxation of distal interphalangeal joint of right little finger

√7ᵗʰ **S63.247** Subluxation of distal interphalangeal joint of left little finger

Ⓝ Newborn: 0   Ⓟ Pediatric: 0-17   Ⓜ Maternity: 9-64   Ⓐ Adult: 15-124   MCC Major Complication/Comorbidity   CC Complication/Comorbidity   SW Severe Wound Dx

1044   ICD-10-CM 2022

√7ᵗʰ **S63.248** Subluxation of distal interphalangeal joint of other finger
  Subluxation of distal interphalangeal joint of specified finger with unspecified laterality

√7ᵗʰ **S63.249** Subluxation of distal interphalangeal joint of unspecified finger

√6ᵗʰ **S63.25** Unspecified dislocation of other finger

√7ᵗʰ **S63.250** Unspecified dislocation of right index finger

√7ᵗʰ **S63.251** Unspecified dislocation of left index finger

√7ᵗʰ **S63.252** Unspecified dislocation of right middle finger

√7ᵗʰ **S63.253** Unspecified dislocation of left middle finger

√7ᵗʰ **S63.254** Unspecified dislocation of right ring finger

√7ᵗʰ **S63.255** Unspecified dislocation of left ring finger

√7ᵗʰ **S63.256** Unspecified dislocation of right little finger

√7ᵗʰ **S63.257** Unspecified dislocation of left little finger

√7ᵗʰ **S63.258** Unspecified dislocation of other finger
  Unspecified dislocation of specified finger with unspecified laterality

√7ᵗʰ **S63.259** Unspecified dislocation of unspecified finger
  Unspecified dislocation of unspecified finger with unspecified laterality

√6ᵗʰ **S63.26** Dislocation of metacarpophalangeal joint of finger

√7ᵗʰ **S63.260** Dislocation of metacarpophalangeal joint of right index finger

√7ᵗʰ **S63.261** Dislocation of metacarpophalangeal joint of left index finger

√7ᵗʰ **S63.262** Dislocation of metacarpophalangeal joint of right middle finger

√7ᵗʰ **S63.263** Dislocation of metacarpophalangeal joint of left middle finger

√7ᵗʰ **S63.264** Dislocation of metacarpophalangeal joint of right ring finger

√7ᵗʰ **S63.265** Dislocation of metacarpophalangeal joint of left ring finger

√7ᵗʰ **S63.266** Dislocation of metacarpophalangeal joint of right little finger

√7ᵗʰ **S63.267** Dislocation of metacarpophalangeal joint of left little finger

√7ᵗʰ **S63.268** Dislocation of metacarpophalangeal joint of other finger
  Dislocation of metacarpophalangeal joint of specified finger with unspecified laterality

√7ᵗʰ **S63.269** Dislocation of metacarpophalangeal joint of unspecified finger

√6ᵗʰ **S63.27** Dislocation of unspecified interphalangeal joint of finger

√7ᵗʰ **S63.270** Dislocation of unspecified interphalangeal joint of right index finger

√7ᵗʰ **S63.271** Dislocation of unspecified interphalangeal joint of left index finger

√7ᵗʰ **S63.272** Dislocation of unspecified interphalangeal joint of right middle finger

√7ᵗʰ **S63.273** Dislocation of unspecified interphalangeal joint of left middle finger

√7ᵗʰ **S63.274** Dislocation of unspecified interphalangeal joint of right ring finger

√7ᵗʰ **S63.275** Dislocation of unspecified interphalangeal joint of left ring finger

√7ᵗʰ **S63.276** Dislocation of unspecified interphalangeal joint of right little finger

√7ᵗʰ **S63.277** Dislocation of unspecified interphalangeal joint of left little finger

√7ᵗʰ **S63.278** Dislocation of unspecified interphalangeal joint of other finger
  Dislocation of unspecified interphalangeal joint of specified finger with unspecified laterality

√7ᵗʰ **S63.279** Dislocation of unspecified interphalangeal joint of unspecified finger
  Dislocation of unspecified interphalangeal joint of unspecified finger without specified laterality

√6ᵗʰ **S63.28** Dislocation of proximal interphalangeal joint of finger

√7ᵗʰ **S63.280** Dislocation of proximal interphalangeal joint of right index finger

√7ᵗʰ **S63.281** Dislocation of proximal interphalangeal joint of left index finger

√7ᵗʰ **S63.282** Dislocation of proximal interphalangeal joint of right middle finger

√7ᵗʰ **S63.283** Dislocation of proximal interphalangeal joint of left middle finger

√7ᵗʰ **S63.284** Dislocation of proximal interphalangeal joint of right ring finger

√7ᵗʰ **S63.285** Dislocation of proximal interphalangeal joint of left ring finger

√7ᵗʰ **S63.286** Dislocation of proximal interphalangeal joint of right little finger

√7ᵗʰ **S63.287** Dislocation of proximal interphalangeal joint of left little finger

√7ᵗʰ **S63.288** Dislocation of proximal interphalangeal joint of other finger
  Dislocation of proximal interphalangeal joint of specified finger with unspecified laterality

√7ᵗʰ **S63.289** Dislocation of proximal interphalangeal joint of unspecified finger

√6ᵗʰ **S63.29** Dislocation of distal interphalangeal joint of finger

√7ᵗʰ **S63.290** Dislocation of distal interphalangeal joint of right index finger

√7ᵗʰ **S63.291** Dislocation of distal interphalangeal joint of left index finger

√7ᵗʰ **S63.292** Dislocation of distal interphalangeal joint of right middle finger

√7ᵗʰ **S63.293** Dislocation of distal interphalangeal joint of left middle finger

√7ᵗʰ **S63.294** Dislocation of distal interphalangeal joint of right ring finger

√7ᵗʰ **S63.295** Dislocation of distal interphalangeal joint of left ring finger

√7ᵗʰ **S63.296** Dislocation of distal interphalangeal joint of right little finger

√7ᵗʰ **S63.297** Dislocation of distal interphalangeal joint of left little finger

√7ᵗʰ **S63.298** Dislocation of distal interphalangeal joint of other finger
  Dislocation of distal interphalangeal joint of specified finger with unspecified laterality

√7ᵗʰ **S63.299** Dislocation of distal interphalangeal joint of unspecified finger

√5ᵗʰ **S63.3** Traumatic rupture of ligament of wrist

√6ᵗʰ **S63.30** Traumatic rupture of unspecified ligament of wrist

√7ᵗʰ **S63.301** Traumatic rupture of unspecified ligament of right wrist

√7ᵗʰ **S63.302** Traumatic rupture of unspecified ligament of left wrist

√7ᵗʰ **S63.309** Traumatic rupture of unspecified ligament of unspecified wrist

√6ᵗʰ **S63.31** Traumatic rupture of collateral ligament of wrist

√7ᵗʰ **S63.311** Traumatic rupture of collateral ligament of right wrist

√7ᵗʰ **S63.312** Traumatic rupture of collateral ligament of left wrist

√7ᵗʰ **S63.319** Traumatic rupture of collateral ligament of unspecified wrist

√6ᵗʰ **S63.32** Traumatic rupture of radiocarpal ligament

√7ᵗʰ **S63.321** Traumatic rupture of right radiocarpal ligament

√7ᵗʰ **S63.322** Traumatic rupture of left radiocarpal ligament

√7ᵗʰ **S63.329** Traumatic rupture of unspecified radiocarpal ligament

√6ᵗʰ **S63.33** Traumatic rupture of ulnocarpal (palmar) ligament

√7ᵗʰ **S63.331** Traumatic rupture of right ulnocarpal (palmar) ligament

✓7th **S63.332** Traumatic rupture of left ulnocarpal (palmar) ligament

✓7th **S63.339** Traumatic rupture of unspecified ulnocarpal (palmar) ligament

✓6th **S63.39** Traumatic rupture of other ligament of wrist

  ✓7th **S63.391** Traumatic rupture of other ligament of right wrist

  ✓7th **S63.392** Traumatic rupture of other ligament of left wrist

  ✓7th **S63.399** Traumatic rupture of other ligament of unspecified wrist

✓5th **S63.4** Traumatic rupture of ligament of finger at metacarpophalangeal and interphalangeal joint(s)

  ✓6th **S63.40** Traumatic rupture of unspecified ligament of finger at metacarpophalangeal and interphalangeal joint

    ✓7th **S63.400** Traumatic rupture of unspecified ligament of right index finger at metacarpophalangeal and interphalangeal joint

    ✓7th **S63.401** Traumatic rupture of unspecified ligament of left index finger at metacarpophalangeal and interphalangeal joint

    ✓7th **S63.402** Traumatic rupture of unspecified ligament of right middle finger at metacarpophalangeal and interphalangeal joint

    ✓7th **S63.403** Traumatic rupture of unspecified ligament of left middle finger at metacarpophalangeal and interphalangeal joint

    ✓7th **S63.404** Traumatic rupture of unspecified ligament of right ring finger at metacarpophalangeal and interphalangeal joint

    ✓7th **S63.405** Traumatic rupture of unspecified ligament of left ring finger at metacarpophalangeal and interphalangeal joint

    ✓7th **S63.406** Traumatic rupture of unspecified ligament of right little finger at metacarpophalangeal and interphalangeal joint

    ✓7th **S63.407** Traumatic rupture of unspecified ligament of left little finger at metacarpophalangeal and interphalangeal joint

    ✓7th **S63.408** Traumatic rupture of unspecified ligament of other finger at metacarpophalangeal and interphalangeal joint

       Traumatic rupture of unspecified ligament of specified finger with unspecified laterality at metacarpophalangeal and interphalangeal joint

    ✓7th **S63.409** Traumatic rupture of unspecified ligament of unspecified finger at metacarpophalangeal and interphalangeal joint

  ✓6th **S63.41** Traumatic rupture of collateral ligament of finger at metacarpophalangeal and interphalangeal joint

    ✓7th **S63.410** Traumatic rupture of collateral ligament of right index finger at metacarpophalangeal and interphalangeal joint

    ✓7th **S63.411** Traumatic rupture of collateral ligament of left index finger at metacarpophalangeal and interphalangeal joint

    ✓7th **S63.412** Traumatic rupture of collateral ligament of right middle finger at metacarpophalangeal and interphalangeal joint

    ✓7th **S63.413** Traumatic rupture of collateral ligament of left middle finger at metacarpophalangeal and interphalangeal joint

    ✓7th **S63.414** Traumatic rupture of collateral ligament of right ring finger at metacarpophalangeal and interphalangeal joint

    ✓7th **S63.415** Traumatic rupture of collateral ligament of left ring finger at metacarpophalangeal and interphalangeal joint

    ✓7th **S63.416** Traumatic rupture of collateral ligament of right little finger at metacarpophalangeal and interphalangeal joint

    ✓7th **S63.417** Traumatic rupture of collateral ligament of left little finger at metacarpophalangeal and interphalangeal joint

    ✓7th **S63.418** Traumatic rupture of collateral ligament of other finger at metacarpophalangeal and interphalangeal joint

       Traumatic rupture of collateral ligament of specified finger with unspecified laterality at metacarpophalangeal and interphalangeal joint

    ✓7th **S63.419** Traumatic rupture of collateral ligament of unspecified finger at metacarpophalangeal and interphalangeal joint

  ✓6th **S63.42** Traumatic rupture of palmar ligament of finger at metacarpophalangeal and interphalangeal joint

    ✓7th **S63.420** Traumatic rupture of palmar ligament of right index finger at metacarpophalangeal and interphalangeal joint

    ✓7th **S63.421** Traumatic rupture of palmar ligament of left index finger at metacarpophalangeal and interphalangeal joint

    ✓7th **S63.422** Traumatic rupture of palmar ligament of right middle finger at metacarpophalangeal and interphalangeal joint

    ✓7th **S63.423** Traumatic rupture of palmar ligament of left middle finger at metacarpophalangeal and interphalangeal joint

    ✓7th **S63.424** Traumatic rupture of palmar ligament of right ring finger at metacarpophalangeal and interphalangeal joint

    ✓7th **S63.425** Traumatic rupture of palmar ligament of left ring finger at metacarpophalangeal and interphalangeal joint

    ✓7th **S63.426** Traumatic rupture of palmar ligament of right little finger at metacarpophalangeal and interphalangeal joint

    ✓7th **S63.427** Traumatic rupture of palmar ligament of left little finger at metacarpophalangeal and interphalangeal joint

    ✓7th **S63.428** Traumatic rupture of palmar ligament of other finger at metacarpophalangeal and interphalangeal joint

       Traumatic rupture of palmar ligament of specified finger with unspecified laterality at metacarpophalangeal and interphalangeal joint

    ✓7th **S63.429** Traumatic rupture of palmar ligament of unspecified finger at metacarpophalangeal and interphalangeal joint

  ✓6th **S63.43** Traumatic rupture of volar plate of finger at metacarpophalangeal and interphalangeal joint

    ✓7th **S63.430** Traumatic rupture of volar plate of right index finger at metacarpophalangeal and interphalangeal joint

    ✓7th **S63.431** Traumatic rupture of volar plate of left index finger at metacarpophalangeal and interphalangeal joint

    ✓7th **S63.432** Traumatic rupture of volar plate of right middle finger at metacarpophalangeal and interphalangeal joint

    ✓7th **S63.433** Traumatic rupture of volar plate of left middle finger at metacarpophalangeal and interphalangeal joint

    ✓7th **S63.434** Traumatic rupture of volar plate of right ring finger at metacarpophalangeal and interphalangeal joint

    ✓7th **S63.435** Traumatic rupture of volar plate of left ring finger at metacarpophalangeal and interphalangeal joint

    ✓7th **S63.436** Traumatic rupture of volar plate of right little finger at metacarpophalangeal and interphalangeal joint

    ✓7th **S63.437** Traumatic rupture of volar plate of left little finger at metacarpophalangeal and interphalangeal joint

N Newborn: 0   P Pediatric: 0-17   M Maternity: 9-64   A Adult: 15-124   MCC Major Complication/Comorbidity   CC Complication/Comorbidity   SW Severe Wound Dx

1046   ICD-10-CM 2022

√7ᵗʰ **S63.438 Traumatic rupture of volar plate of other finger at metacarpophalangeal and interphalangeal joint**

Traumatic rupture of volar plate of specified finger with unspecified laterality at metacarpophalangeal and interphalangeal joint

√7ᵗʰ **S63.439 Traumatic rupture of volar plate of unspecified finger at metacarpophalangeal and interphalangeal joint**

√6ᵗʰ **S63.49 Traumatic rupture of other ligament of finger at metacarpophalangeal and interphalangeal joint**

√7ᵗʰ **S63.490 Traumatic rupture of other ligament of right index finger at metacarpophalangeal and interphalangeal joint**

√7ᵗʰ **S63.491 Traumatic rupture of other ligament of left index finger at metacarpophalangeal and interphalangeal joint**

√7ᵗʰ **S63.492 Traumatic rupture of other ligament of right middle finger at metacarpophalangeal and interphalangeal joint**

√7ᵗʰ **S63.493 Traumatic rupture of other ligament of left middle finger at metacarpophalangeal and interphalangeal joint**

√7ᵗʰ **S63.494 Traumatic rupture of other ligament of right ring finger at metacarpophalangeal and interphalangeal joint**

√7ᵗʰ **S63.495 Traumatic rupture of other ligament of left ring finger at metacarpophalangeal and interphalangeal joint**

√7ᵗʰ **S63.496 Traumatic rupture of other ligament of right little finger at metacarpophalangeal and interphalangeal joint**

√7ᵗʰ **S63.497 Traumatic rupture of other ligament of left little finger at metacarpophalangeal and interphalangeal joint**

√7ᵗʰ **S63.498 Traumatic rupture of other ligament of other finger at metacarpophalangeal and interphalangeal joint**

Traumatic rupture of ligament of specified finger with unspecified laterality at metacarpophalangeal and interphalangeal joint

√7ᵗʰ **S63.499 Traumatic rupture of other ligament of unspecified finger at metacarpophalangeal and interphalangeal joint**

√5ᵗʰ **S63.5 Other and unspecified sprain of wrist**

√6ᵗʰ **S63.50 Unspecified sprain of wrist**

√7ᵗʰ **S63.501 Unspecified sprain of right wrist**

√7ᵗʰ **S63.502 Unspecified sprain of left wrist**

√7ᵗʰ **S63.509 Unspecified sprain of unspecified wrist**

√6ᵗʰ **S63.51 Sprain of carpal (joint)**

√7ᵗʰ **S63.511 Sprain of carpal joint of right wrist**

√7ᵗʰ **S63.512 Sprain of carpal joint of left wrist**

√7ᵗʰ **S63.519 Sprain of carpal joint of unspecified wrist**

√6ᵗʰ **S63.52 Sprain of radiocarpal joint**

EXCLUDES 1   traumatic rupture of radiocarpal ligament (S63.32-)

√7ᵗʰ **S63.521 Sprain of radiocarpal joint of right wrist**

√7ᵗʰ **S63.522 Sprain of radiocarpal joint of left wrist**

√7ᵗʰ **S63.529 Sprain of radiocarpal joint of unspecified wrist**

√6ᵗʰ **S63.59 Other specified sprain of wrist**

√7ᵗʰ **S63.591 Other specified sprain of right wrist**

√7ᵗʰ **S63.592 Other specified sprain of left wrist**

√7ᵗʰ **S63.599 Other specified sprain of unspecified wrist**

√5ᵗʰ **S63.6 Other and unspecified sprain of finger(s)**

EXCLUDES 1   traumatic rupture of ligament of finger at metacarpophalangeal and interphalangeal joint(s) (S63.4-)

√6ᵗʰ **S63.60 Unspecified sprain of thumb**

√7ᵗʰ **S63.601 Unspecified sprain of right thumb**

√7ᵗʰ **S63.602 Unspecified sprain of left thumb**

√7ᵗʰ **S63.609 Unspecified sprain of unspecified thumb**

√6ᵗʰ **S63.61 Unspecified sprain of other and unspecified finger(s)**

√7ᵗʰ **S63.610 Unspecified sprain of right index finger**

√7ᵗʰ **S63.611 Unspecified sprain of left index finger**

√7ᵗʰ **S63.612 Unspecified sprain of right middle finger**

√7ᵗʰ **S63.613 Unspecified sprain of left middle finger**

√7ᵗʰ **S63.614 Unspecified sprain of right ring finger**

√7ᵗʰ **S63.615 Unspecified sprain of left ring finger**

√7ᵗʰ **S63.616 Unspecified sprain of right little finger**

√7ᵗʰ **S63.617 Unspecified sprain of left little finger**

√7ᵗʰ **S63.618 Unspecified sprain of other finger**

Unspecified sprain of specified finger with unspecified laterality

√7ᵗʰ **S63.619 Unspecified sprain of unspecified finger**

√6ᵗʰ **S63.62 Sprain of interphalangeal joint of thumb**

√7ᵗʰ **S63.621 Sprain of interphalangeal joint of right thumb**

√7ᵗʰ **S63.622 Sprain of interphalangeal joint of left thumb**

√7ᵗʰ **S63.629 Sprain of interphalangeal joint of unspecified thumb**

√6ᵗʰ **S63.63 Sprain of interphalangeal joint of other and unspecified finger(s)**

√7ᵗʰ **S63.630 Sprain of interphalangeal joint of right index finger**

√7ᵗʰ **S63.631 Sprain of interphalangeal joint of left index finger**

√7ᵗʰ **S63.632 Sprain of interphalangeal joint of right middle finger**

√7ᵗʰ **S63.633 Sprain of interphalangeal joint of left middle finger**

√7ᵗʰ **S63.634 Sprain of interphalangeal joint of right ring finger**

√7ᵗʰ **S63.635 Sprain of interphalangeal joint of left ring finger**

√7ᵗʰ **S63.636 Sprain of interphalangeal joint of right little finger**

√7ᵗʰ **S63.637 Sprain of interphalangeal joint of left little finger**

√7ᵗʰ **S63.638 Sprain of interphalangeal joint of other finger**

√7ᵗʰ **S63.639 Sprain of interphalangeal joint of unspecified finger**

√6ᵗʰ **S63.64 Sprain of metacarpophalangeal joint of thumb**

√7ᵗʰ **S63.641 Sprain of metacarpophalangeal joint of right thumb**

√7ᵗʰ **S63.642 Sprain of metacarpophalangeal joint of left thumb**

√7ᵗʰ **S63.649 Sprain of metacarpophalangeal joint of unspecified thumb**

√6ᵗʰ **S63.65 Sprain of metacarpophalangeal joint of other and unspecified finger(s)**

√7ᵗʰ **S63.650 Sprain of metacarpophalangeal joint of right index finger**

√7ᵗʰ **S63.651 Sprain of metacarpophalangeal joint of left index finger**

√7ᵗʰ **S63.652 Sprain of metacarpophalangeal joint of right middle finger**

√7ᵗʰ **S63.653 Sprain of metacarpophalangeal joint of left middle finger**

√7ᵗʰ **S63.654 Sprain of metacarpophalangeal joint of right ring finger**

√7ᵗʰ **S63.655 Sprain of metacarpophalangeal joint of left ring finger**

√7ᵗʰ **S63.656 Sprain of metacarpophalangeal joint of right little finger**

√7ᵗʰ **S63.657 Sprain of metacarpophalangeal joint of left little finger**

√7ᵗʰ **S63.658 Sprain of metacarpophalangeal joint of other finger**

Sprain of metacarpophalangeal joint of specified finger with unspecified laterality

√7ᵗʰ **S63.659 Sprain of metacarpophalangeal joint of unspecified finger**

√6ᵗʰ **S63.68 Other sprain of thumb**

√7ᵗʰ **S63.681 Other sprain of right thumb**

☑ Additional Character Required   √X7ᵗʰ Placeholder   Questionable PDx   Manifestation   Unspecified Dx   UPD Unacceptable PDx   H1 - H14 HAC   HCC CMS-HCC Dx   HIV HIV Dx

ICD-10-CM 2022   1047

√7ᵗʰ **S63.682** Other sprain of left thumb

√7ᵗʰ **S63.689** Other sprain of unspecified thumb

√6ᵗʰ **S63.69** Other sprain of other and unspecified finger(s)

  √7ᵗʰ **S63.690** Other sprain of right index finger

  √7ᵗʰ **S63.691** Other sprain of left index finger

  √7ᵗʰ **S63.692** Other sprain of right middle finger

  √7ᵗʰ **S63.693** Other sprain of left middle finger

  √7ᵗʰ **S63.694** Other sprain of right ring finger

  √7ᵗʰ **S63.695** Other sprain of left ring finger

  √7ᵗʰ **S63.696** Other sprain of right little finger

  √7ᵗʰ **S63.697** Other sprain of left little finger

  √7ᵗʰ **S63.698** Other sprain of other finger

    Other sprain of specified finger with unspecified laterality

  √7ᵗʰ **S63.699** Other sprain of unspecified finger

√5ᵗʰ **S63.8** Sprain of other part of wrist and hand

  √6ᵗʰ **S63.8X** Sprain of other part of wrist and hand

    √7ᵗʰ **S63.8X1** Sprain of other part of right wrist and hand

    √7ᵗʰ **S63.8X2** Sprain of other part of left wrist and hand

    √7ᵗʰ **S63.8X9** Sprain of other part of unspecified wrist and hand

√5ᵗʰ **S63.9** Sprain of unspecified part of wrist and hand

  √x7ᵗʰ **S63.90** Sprain of unspecified part of unspecified wrist and hand

  √x7ᵗʰ **S63.91** Sprain of unspecified part of right wrist and hand

  √x7ᵗʰ **S63.92** Sprain of unspecified part of left wrist and hand

√4ᵗʰ **S64** Injury of nerves at wrist and hand level

Code also any associated open wound (S61.-)

The appropriate 7th character is to be added to each code from category S64.
A   initial encounter
D   subsequent encounter
S   sequela

√5ᵗʰ **S64.0** Injury of ulnar nerve at wrist and hand level

  √x7ᵗʰ **S64.00** Injury of ulnar nerve at wrist and hand level of unspecified arm

  √x7ᵗʰ **S64.01** Injury of ulnar nerve at wrist and hand level of right arm

  √x7ᵗʰ **S64.02** Injury of ulnar nerve at wrist and hand level of left arm

√5ᵗʰ **S64.1** Injury of median nerve at wrist and hand level

  √x7ᵗʰ **S64.10** Injury of median nerve at wrist and hand level of unspecified arm

  √x7ᵗʰ **S64.11** Injury of median nerve at wrist and hand level of right arm

  √x7ᵗʰ **S64.12** Injury of median nerve at wrist and hand level of left arm

√5ᵗʰ **S64.2** Injury of radial nerve at wrist and hand level

  √x7ᵗʰ **S64.20** Injury of radial nerve at wrist and hand level of unspecified arm

  √x7ᵗʰ **S64.21** Injury of radial nerve at wrist and hand level of right arm

  √x7ᵗʰ **S64.22** Injury of radial nerve at wrist and hand level of left arm

√5ᵗʰ **S64.3** Injury of digital nerve of thumb

  √x7ᵗʰ **S64.30** Injury of digital nerve of unspecified thumb

  √x7ᵗʰ **S64.31** Injury of digital nerve of right thumb

  √x7ᵗʰ **S64.32** Injury of digital nerve of left thumb

√5ᵗʰ **S64.4** Injury of digital nerve of other and unspecified finger

  √x7ᵗʰ **S64.40** Injury of digital nerve of unspecified finger

  √6ᵗʰ **S64.49** Injury of digital nerve of other finger

    √7ᵗʰ **S64.490** Injury of digital nerve of right index finger

    √7ᵗʰ **S64.491** Injury of digital nerve of left index finger

    √7ᵗʰ **S64.492** Injury of digital nerve of right middle finger

    √7ᵗʰ **S64.493** Injury of digital nerve of left middle finger

    √7ᵗʰ **S64.494** Injury of digital nerve of right ring finger

    √7ᵗʰ **S64.495** Injury of digital nerve of left ring finger

    √7ᵗʰ **S64.496** Injury of digital nerve of right little finger

    √7ᵗʰ **S64.497** Injury of digital nerve of left little finger

    √7ᵗʰ **S64.498** Injury of digital nerve of other finger

    Injury of digital nerve of specified finger with unspecified laterality

√5ᵗʰ **S64.8** Injury of other nerves at wrist and hand level

  √6ᵗʰ **S64.8X** Injury of other nerves at wrist and hand level

    √7ᵗʰ **S64.8X1** Injury of other nerves at wrist and hand level of right arm

    √7ᵗʰ **S64.8X2** Injury of other nerves at wrist and hand level of left arm

    √7ᵗʰ **S64.8X9** Injury of other nerves at wrist and hand level of unspecified arm

√5ᵗʰ **S64.9** Injury of unspecified nerve at wrist and hand level

  √x7ᵗʰ **S64.90** Injury of unspecified nerve at wrist and hand level of unspecified arm

  √x7ᵗʰ **S64.91** Injury of unspecified nerve at wrist and hand level of right arm

  √x7ᵗʰ **S64.92** Injury of unspecified nerve at wrist and hand level of left arm

√4ᵗʰ **S65** Injury of blood vessels at wrist and hand level

Code also any associated open wound (S61.-)

The appropriate 7th character is to be added to each code from category S65.
A   initial encounter
D   subsequent encounter
S   sequela

√5ᵗʰ **S65.0** Injury of ulnar artery at wrist and hand level

  √6ᵗʰ **S65.00** Unspecified injury of ulnar artery at wrist and hand level

    √7ᵗʰ **S65.001** Unspecified injury of ulnar artery at wrist and hand level of right arm CC

    √7ᵗʰ **S65.002** Unspecified injury of ulnar artery at wrist and hand level of left arm CC

    √7ᵗʰ **S65.009** Unspecified injury of ulnar artery at wrist and hand level of unspecified arm CC

  √6ᵗʰ **S65.01** Laceration of ulnar artery at wrist and hand level

    √7ᵗʰ **S65.011** Laceration of ulnar artery at wrist and hand level of right arm CC

    √7ᵗʰ **S65.012** Laceration of ulnar artery at wrist and hand level of left arm CC

    √7ᵗʰ **S65.019** Laceration of ulnar artery at wrist and hand level of unspecified arm CC

  √6ᵗʰ **S65.09** Other specified injury of ulnar artery at wrist and hand level

    √7ᵗʰ **S65.091** Other specified injury of ulnar artery at wrist and hand level of right arm CC

    √7ᵗʰ **S65.092** Other specified injury of ulnar artery at wrist and hand level of left arm CC

    √7ᵗʰ **S65.099** Other specified injury of ulnar artery at wrist and hand level of unspecified arm CC

√5ᵗʰ **S65.1** Injury of radial artery at wrist and hand level

  √6ᵗʰ **S65.10** Unspecified injury of radial artery at wrist and hand level

    √7ᵗʰ **S65.101** Unspecified injury of radial artery at wrist and hand level of right arm CC

    √7ᵗʰ **S65.102** Unspecified injury of radial artery at wrist and hand level of left arm CC

    √7ᵗʰ **S65.109** Unspecified injury of radial artery at wrist and hand level of unspecified arm CC

  √6ᵗʰ **S65.11** Laceration of radial artery at wrist and hand level

    √7ᵗʰ **S65.111** Laceration of radial artery at wrist and hand level of right arm CC

    √7ᵗʰ **S65.112** Laceration of radial artery at wrist and hand level of left arm CC

    √7ᵗʰ **S65.119** Laceration of radial artery at wrist and hand level of unspecified arm CC

  √6ᵗʰ **S65.19** Other specified injury of radial artery at wrist and hand level

    √7ᵗʰ **S65.191** Other specified injury of radial artery at wrist and hand level of right arm CC

    √7ᵗʰ **S65.192** Other specified injury of radial artery at wrist and hand level of left arm CC

    √7ᵗʰ **S65.199** Other specified injury of radial artery at wrist and hand level of unspecified arm CC

√5ᵗʰ **S65.2 Injury of** superficial palmar arch

  √6ᵗʰ **S65.20 Unspecified injury of superficial palmar arch**

    √7ᵗʰ **S65.201 Unspecified injury of superficial palmar arch of** right **hand** CC

    √7ᵗʰ **S65.202 Unspecified injury of superficial palmar arch of** left **hand** CC

    √7ᵗʰ **S65.209 Unspecified injury of superficial palmar arch of unspecified hand** CC

  √6ᵗʰ **S65.21 Laceration of superficial palmar arch**

    √7ᵗʰ **S65.211 Laceration of superficial palmar arch of** right **hand** CC

    √7ᵗʰ **S65.212 Laceration of superficial palmar arch of** left **hand** CC

    √7ᵗʰ **S65.219 Laceration of superficial palmar arch of unspecified hand** CC

  √6ᵗʰ **S65.29 Other specified injury of superficial palmar arch**

    √7ᵗʰ **S65.291 Other specified injury of superficial palmar arch of** right **hand** CC

    √7ᵗʰ **S65.292 Other specified injury of superficial palmar arch of** left **hand** CC

    √7ᵗʰ **S65.299 Other specified injury of superficial palmar arch of unspecified hand** CC

√5ᵗʰ **S65.3 Injury of** deep palmar arch

  √6ᵗʰ **S65.30 Unspecified injury of deep palmar arch**

    √7ᵗʰ **S65.301 Unspecified injury of deep palmar arch of** right **hand** CC

    √7ᵗʰ **S65.302 Unspecified injury of deep palmar arch of** left **hand** CC

    √7ᵗʰ **S65.309 Unspecified injury of deep palmar arch of unspecified hand** CC

  √6ᵗʰ **S65.31 Laceration of deep palmar arch**

    √7ᵗʰ **S65.311 Laceration of deep palmar arch of** right **hand** CC

    √7ᵗʰ **S65.312 Laceration of deep palmar arch of** left **hand** CC

    √7ᵗʰ **S65.319 Laceration of deep palmar arch of unspecified hand** CC

  √6ᵗʰ **S65.39 Other specified injury of deep palmar arch**

    √7ᵗʰ **S65.391 Other specified injury of deep palmar arch of** right **hand** CC

    √7ᵗʰ **S65.392 Other specified injury of deep palmar arch of** left **hand** CC

    √7ᵗʰ **S65.399 Other specified injury of deep palmar arch of unspecified hand** CC

√5ᵗʰ **S65.4 Injury of blood vessel of** thumb

  √6ᵗʰ **S65.40 Unspecified injury of blood vessel of thumb**

    √7ᵗʰ **S65.401 Unspecified injury of blood vessel of** right **thumb** CC

    √7ᵗʰ **S65.402 Unspecified injury of blood vessel of** left **thumb** CC

    √7ᵗʰ **S65.409 Unspecified injury of blood vessel of unspecified thumb** CC

  √6ᵗʰ **S65.41 Laceration of blood vessel of thumb**

    √7ᵗʰ **S65.411 Laceration of blood vessel of** right **thumb** CC

    √7ᵗʰ **S65.412 Laceration of blood vessel of** left **thumb** CC

    √7ᵗʰ **S65.419 Laceration of blood vessel of unspecified thumb** CC

  √6ᵗʰ **S65.49 Other specified injury of blood vessel of thumb**

    √7ᵗʰ **S65.491 Other specified injury of blood vessel of** right **thumb** CC

    √7ᵗʰ **S65.492 Other specified injury of blood vessel of** left **thumb** CC

    √7ᵗʰ **S65.499 Other specified injury of blood vessel of unspecified thumb** CC

√5ᵗʰ **S65.5 Injury of blood vessel of other and unspecified** finger

  √6ᵗʰ **S65.50 Unspecified injury of blood vessel of other and unspecified finger**

    √7ᵗʰ **S65.500 Unspecified injury of blood vessel of** right **index finger** CC

    √7ᵗʰ **S65.501 Unspecified injury of blood vessel of** left **index finger** CC

    √7ᵗʰ **S65.502 Unspecified injury of blood vessel of** right **middle finger** CC

    √7ᵗʰ **S65.503 Unspecified injury of blood vessel of** left **middle finger** CC

    √7ᵗʰ **S65.504 Unspecified injury of blood vessel of** right **ring finger** CC

    √7ᵗʰ **S65.505 Unspecified injury of blood vessel of** left **ring finger** CC

    √7ᵗʰ **S65.506 Unspecified injury of blood vessel of** right **little finger** CC

    √7ᵗʰ **S65.507 Unspecified injury of blood vessel of** left **little finger** CC

    √7ᵗʰ **S65.508 Unspecified injury of blood vessel of other finger** CC
         Unspecified injury of blood vessel of specified finger with unspecified laterality

    √7ᵗʰ **S65.509 Unspecified injury of blood vessel of unspecified finger** CC

  √6ᵗʰ **S65.51 Laceration of blood vessel of other and unspecified finger**

    √7ᵗʰ **S65.510 Laceration of blood vessel of** right index **finger** CC

    √7ᵗʰ **S65.511 Laceration of blood vessel of** left index **finger** CC

    √7ᵗʰ **S65.512 Laceration of blood vessel of** right middle **finger** CC

    √7ᵗʰ **S65.513 Laceration of blood vessel of** left middle **finger** CC

    √7ᵗʰ **S65.514 Laceration of blood vessel of** right ring **finger** CC

    √7ᵗʰ **S65.515 Laceration of blood vessel of** left ring **finger** CC

    √7ᵗʰ **S65.516 Laceration of blood vessel of** right little **finger** CC

    √7ᵗʰ **S65.517 Laceration of blood vessel of** left little **finger** CC

    √7ᵗʰ **S65.518 Laceration of blood vessel of other finger** CC
         Laceration of blood vessel of specified finger with unspecified laterality

    √7ᵗʰ **S65.519 Laceration of blood vessel of unspecified finger** CC

  √6ᵗʰ **S65.59 Other specified injury of blood vessel of other and unspecified finger**

    √7ᵗʰ **S65.590 Other specified injury of blood vessel of** right index **finger** CC

    √7ᵗʰ **S65.591 Other specified injury of blood vessel of** left index **finger** CC

    √7ᵗʰ **S65.592 Other specified injury of blood vessel of** right middle **finger** CC

    √7ᵗʰ **S65.593 Other specified injury of blood vessel of** left middle **finger** CC

    √7ᵗʰ **S65.594 Other specified injury of blood vessel of** right ring **finger** CC

    √7ᵗʰ **S65.595 Other specified injury of blood vessel of** left ring **finger** CC

    √7ᵗʰ **S65.596 Other specified injury of blood vessel of** right little **finger** CC

    √7ᵗʰ **S65.597 Other specified injury of blood vessel of** left little **finger** CC

    √7ᵗʰ **S65.598 Other specified injury of blood vessel of other finger** CC
         Other specified injury of blood vessel of specified finger with unspecified laterality

    √7ᵗʰ **S65.599 Other specified injury of blood vessel of unspecified finger** CC

√5ᵗʰ **S65.8 Injury of other blood vessels at** wrist and hand level

  √6ᵗʰ **S65.80 Unspecified injury of other blood vessels at wrist and hand level**

    √7ᵗʰ **S65.801 Unspecified injury of other blood vessels at wrist and hand level of right arm** CC

    √7ᵗʰ **S65.802 Unspecified injury of other blood vessels at wrist and hand level of left arm** CC

    √7ᵗʰ **S65.809 Unspecified injury of other blood vessels at wrist and hand level of unspecified arm** CC

  √6ᵗʰ **S65.81 Laceration of other blood vessels at wrist and hand level**

    √7ᵗʰ **S65.811 Laceration of other blood vessels at wrist and hand level of** right **arm** CC

    √7ᵗʰ **S65.812 Laceration of other blood vessels at wrist and hand level of** left **arm** CC

✔ Additional Character Required   √x7ᵗʰ Placeholder   Questionable PDx   Manifestation   Unspecified Dx   UPD Unacceptable PDx   H1-H14 HAC   HCC CMS-HCC Dx   HIV HIV Dx

ICD-10-CM 2022   **1049**

√7ᵗʰ **S65.819** Laceration of other blood vessels at wrist and hand level of unspecified arm **cc**

√6ᵗʰ **S65.89** Other specified injury of other blood vessels at wrist and hand level

    √7ᵗʰ **S65.891** Other specified injury of other blood vessels at wrist and hand level of right arm **cc**

    √7ᵗʰ **S65.892** Other specified injury of other blood vessels at wrist and hand level of left arm **cc**

    √7ᵗʰ **S65.899** Other specified injury of other blood vessels at wrist and hand level of unspecified arm **cc**

√5ᵗʰ **S65.9** Injury of unspecified blood vessel at wrist and hand level

    √6ᵗʰ **S65.90** Unspecified injury of unspecified blood vessel at wrist and hand level

       √7ᵗʰ **S65.901** Unspecified injury of unspecified blood vessel at wrist and hand level of right arm **cc**

       √7ᵗʰ **S65.902** Unspecified injury of unspecified blood vessel at wrist and hand level of left arm **cc**

       √7ᵗʰ **S65.909** Unspecified injury of unspecified blood vessel at wrist and hand level of unspecified arm **cc**

    √6ᵗʰ **S65.91** Laceration of unspecified blood vessel at wrist and hand level

       √7ᵗʰ **S65.911** Laceration of unspecified blood vessel at wrist and hand level of right arm **cc**

       √7ᵗʰ **S65.912** Laceration of unspecified blood vessel at wrist and hand level of left arm **cc**

       √7ᵗʰ **S65.919** Laceration of unspecified blood vessel at wrist and hand level of unspecified arm **cc**

    √6ᵗʰ **S65.99** Other specified injury of unspecified blood vessel at wrist and hand level

       √7ᵗʰ **S65.991** Other specified injury of unspecified blood vessel at wrist and hand of right arm **cc**

       √7ᵗʰ **S65.992** Other specified injury of unspecified blood vessel at wrist and hand of left arm **cc**

       √7ᵗʰ **S65.999** Other specified injury of unspecified blood vessel at wrist and hand of unspecified arm **cc**

√4ᵗʰ **S66 Injury of muscle, fascia and tendon at wrist and hand level**

Code also any associated open wound (S61.-)

EXCLUDES 2   sprain of joints and ligaments of wrist and hand (S63.-)

TIP: Refer to the Muscle/Tendon table at the beginning of this chapter.

> The appropriate 7th character is to be added to each code from category S66.
> A   initial encounter
> D   subsequent encounter
> S   sequela

√5ᵗʰ **S66.0** Injury of long flexor muscle, fascia and tendon of thumb at wrist and hand level

    √6ᵗʰ **S66.00** Unspecified injury of long flexor muscle, fascia and tendon of thumb at wrist and hand level

       √7ᵗʰ **S66.001** Unspecified injury of long flexor muscle, fascia and tendon of right thumb at wrist and hand level

       √7ᵗʰ **S66.002** Unspecified injury of long flexor muscle, fascia and tendon of left thumb at wrist and hand level

       √7ᵗʰ **S66.009** Unspecified injury of long flexor muscle, fascia and tendon of unspecified thumb at wrist and hand level

    √6ᵗʰ **S66.01** Strain of long flexor muscle, fascia and tendon of thumb at wrist and hand level

       √7ᵗʰ **S66.011** Strain of long flexor muscle, fascia and tendon of right thumb at wrist and hand level

       √7ᵗʰ **S66.012** Strain of long flexor muscle, fascia and tendon of left thumb at wrist and hand level

       √7ᵗʰ **S66.019** Strain of long flexor muscle, fascia and tendon of unspecified thumb at wrist and hand level

    √6ᵗʰ **S66.02** Laceration of long flexor muscle, fascia and tendon of thumb at wrist and hand level

       √7ᵗʰ **S66.021** Laceration of long flexor muscle, fascia and tendon of right thumb at wrist and hand level **cc**

       √7ᵗʰ **S66.022** Laceration of long flexor muscle, fascia and tendon of left thumb at wrist and hand level **cc**

       √7ᵗʰ **S66.029** Laceration of long flexor muscle, fascia and tendon of unspecified thumb at wrist and hand level **cc**

    √6ᵗʰ **S66.09** Other specified injury of long flexor muscle, fascia and tendon of thumb at wrist and hand level

       √7ᵗʰ **S66.091** Other specified injury of long flexor muscle, fascia and tendon of right thumb at wrist and hand level

       √7ᵗʰ **S66.092** Other specified injury of long flexor muscle, fascia and tendon of left thumb at wrist and hand level

       √7ᵗʰ **S66.099** Other specified injury of long flexor muscle, fascia and tendon of unspecified thumb at wrist and hand level

√5ᵗʰ **S66.1** Injury of flexor muscle, fascia and tendon of other and unspecified finger at wrist and hand level

    EXCLUDES 2   injury of long flexor muscle, fascia and tendon of thumb at wrist and hand level (S66.0-)

    √6ᵗʰ **S66.10** Unspecified injury of flexor muscle, fascia and tendon of other and unspecified finger at wrist and hand level

       √7ᵗʰ **S66.100** Unspecified injury of flexor muscle, fascia and tendon of right index finger at wrist and hand level

       √7ᵗʰ **S66.101** Unspecified injury of flexor muscle, fascia and tendon of left index finger at wrist and hand level

       √7ᵗʰ **S66.102** Unspecified injury of flexor muscle, fascia and tendon of right middle finger at wrist and hand level

       √7ᵗʰ **S66.103** Unspecified injury of flexor muscle, fascia and tendon of left middle finger at wrist and hand level

       √7ᵗʰ **S66.104** Unspecified injury of flexor muscle, fascia and tendon of right ring finger at wrist and hand level

       √7ᵗʰ **S66.105** Unspecified injury of flexor muscle, fascia and tendon of left ring finger at wrist and hand level

       √7ᵗʰ **S66.106** Unspecified injury of flexor muscle, fascia and tendon of right little finger at wrist and hand level

       √7ᵗʰ **S66.107** Unspecified injury of flexor muscle, fascia and tendon of left little finger at wrist and hand level

       √7ᵗʰ **S66.108** Unspecified injury of flexor muscle, fascia and tendon of other finger at wrist and hand level

          Unspecified injury of flexor muscle, fascia and tendon of specified finger with unspecified laterality at wrist and hand level

       √7ᵗʰ **S66.109** Unspecified injury of flexor muscle, fascia and tendon of unspecified finger at wrist and hand level

    √6ᵗʰ **S66.11** Strain of flexor muscle, fascia and tendon of other and unspecified finger at wrist and hand level

       √7ᵗʰ **S66.110** Strain of flexor muscle, fascia and tendon of right index finger at wrist and hand level

       √7ᵗʰ **S66.111** Strain of flexor muscle, fascia and tendon of left index finger at wrist and hand level

       √7ᵗʰ **S66.112** Strain of flexor muscle, fascia and tendon of right middle finger at wrist and hand level

       √7ᵗʰ **S66.113** Strain of flexor muscle, fascia and tendon of left middle finger at wrist and hand level

       √7ᵗʰ **S66.114** Strain of flexor muscle, fascia and tendon of right ring finger at wrist and hand level

       √7ᵗʰ **S66.115** Strain of flexor muscle, fascia and tendon of left ring finger at wrist and hand level

       √7ᵗʰ **S66.116** Strain of flexor muscle, fascia and tendon of right little finger at wrist and hand level

N Newborn: 0   **P** Pediatric: 0-17   **M** Maternity: 9-64   **A** Adult: 15-124   **MCC** Major Complication/Comorbidity   **CC** Complication/Comorbidity   **SW** Severe Wound Dx

1050   ICD-10-CM 2022

√7ᵗʰ **S66.117** Strain of flexor muscle, fascia and tendon of **left little** finger at wrist and hand level

√7ᵗʰ **S66.118** Strain of flexor muscle, fascia and tendon of **other finger** at wrist and hand level
Strain of flexor muscle, fascia and tendon of specified finger with unspecified laterality at wrist and hand level

√7ᵗʰ **S66.119** Strain of flexor muscle, fascia and tendon of unspecified finger at wrist and hand level

√6ᵗʰ **S66.12** Laceration of flexor muscle, fascia and tendon of other and unspecified finger at wrist and hand level

√7ᵗʰ **S66.120** Laceration of flexor muscle, fascia and tendon of **right index** finger at wrist and hand level   cc

√7ᵗʰ **S66.121** Laceration of flexor muscle, fascia and tendon of **left index** finger at wrist and hand level   cc

√7ᵗʰ **S66.122** Laceration of flexor muscle, fascia and tendon of **right middle** finger at wrist and hand level   cc

√7ᵗʰ **S66.123** Laceration of flexor muscle, fascia and tendon of **left middle** finger at wrist and hand level   cc

√7ᵗʰ **S66.124** Laceration of flexor muscle, fascia and tendon of **right ring** finger at wrist and hand level   cc

√7ᵗʰ **S66.125** Laceration of flexor muscle, fascia and tendon of **left ring** finger at wrist and hand level   cc

√7ᵗʰ **S66.126** Laceration of flexor muscle, fascia and tendon of **right little** finger at wrist and hand level   cc

√7ᵗʰ **S66.127** Laceration of flexor muscle, fascia and tendon of **left little** finger at wrist and hand level   cc

√7ᵗʰ **S66.128** Laceration of flexor muscle, fascia and tendon of **other finger** at wrist and hand level   cc
Laceration of flexor muscle, fascia and tendon of specified finger with unspecified laterality at wrist and hand level

√7ᵗʰ **S66.129** Laceration of flexor muscle, fascia and tendon of unspecified finger at wrist and hand level   cc

√6ᵗʰ **S66.19** Other injury of flexor muscle, fascia and tendon of other and unspecified finger at wrist and hand level

√7ᵗʰ **S66.190** Other injury of flexor muscle, fascia and tendon of **right index** finger at wrist and hand level

√7ᵗʰ **S66.191** Other injury of flexor muscle, fascia and tendon of **left index** finger at wrist and hand level

√7ᵗʰ **S66.192** Other injury of flexor muscle, fascia and tendon of **right middle** finger at wrist and hand level

√7ᵗʰ **S66.193** Other injury of flexor muscle, fascia and tendon of **left middle** finger at wrist and hand level

√7ᵗʰ **S66.194** Other injury of flexor muscle, fascia and tendon of **right ring** finger at wrist and hand level

√7ᵗʰ **S66.195** Other injury of flexor muscle, fascia and tendon of **left ring** finger at wrist and hand level

√7ᵗʰ **S66.196** Other injury of flexor muscle, fascia and tendon of **right little** finger at wrist and hand level

√7ᵗʰ **S66.197** Other injury of flexor muscle, fascia and tendon of **left little** finger at wrist and hand level

√7ᵗʰ **S66.198** Other injury of flexor muscle, fascia and tendon of **other finger** at wrist and hand level
Other injury of flexor muscle, fascia and tendon of specified finger with unspecified laterality at wrist and hand level

√7ᵗʰ **S66.199** Other injury of flexor muscle, fascia and tendon of unspecified finger at wrist and hand level

√5ᵗʰ **S66.2** Injury of extensor muscle, fascia and tendon of thumb at wrist and hand level

√6ᵗʰ **S66.20** Unspecified injury of extensor muscle, fascia and tendon of thumb at wrist and hand level

√7ᵗʰ **S66.201** Unspecified injury of extensor muscle, fascia and tendon of **right** thumb at wrist and hand level

√7ᵗʰ **S66.202** Unspecified injury of extensor muscle, fascia and tendon of **left** thumb at wrist and hand level

√7ᵗʰ **S66.209** Unspecified injury of extensor muscle, fascia and tendon of unspecified thumb at wrist and hand level

√6ᵗʰ **S66.21** Strain of extensor muscle, fascia and tendon of thumb at wrist and hand level

√7ᵗʰ **S66.211** Strain of extensor muscle, fascia and tendon of **right** thumb at wrist and hand level

√7ᵗʰ **S66.212** Strain of extensor muscle, fascia and tendon of **left** thumb at wrist and hand level

√7ᵗʰ **S66.219** Strain of extensor muscle, fascia and tendon of unspecified thumb at wrist and hand level

√6ᵗʰ **S66.22** Laceration of extensor muscle, fascia and tendon of thumb at wrist and hand level

√7ᵗʰ **S66.221** Laceration of extensor muscle, fascia and tendon of **right** thumb at wrist and hand level   cc

√7ᵗʰ **S66.222** Laceration of extensor muscle, fascia and tendon of **left** thumb at wrist and hand level   cc

√7ᵗʰ **S66.229** Laceration of extensor muscle, fascia and tendon of unspecified thumb at wrist and hand level   cc

√6ᵗʰ **S66.29** Other specified injury of extensor muscle, fascia and tendon of thumb at wrist and hand level

√7ᵗʰ **S66.291** Other specified injury of extensor muscle, fascia and tendon of **right** thumb at wrist and hand level

√7ᵗʰ **S66.292** Other specified injury of extensor muscle, fascia and tendon of **left** thumb at wrist and hand level

√7ᵗʰ **S66.299** Other specified injury of extensor muscle, fascia and tendon of unspecified thumb at wrist and hand level

√5ᵗʰ **S66.3** Injury of extensor muscle, fascia and tendon of other and unspecified finger at wrist and hand level
EXCLUDES 2   injury of extensor muscle, fascia and tendon of thumb at wrist and hand level (S66.2-)

√6ᵗʰ **S66.30** Unspecified injury of extensor muscle, fascia and tendon of other and unspecified finger at wrist and hand level

√7ᵗʰ **S66.300** Unspecified injury of extensor muscle, fascia and tendon of **right index** finger at wrist and hand level

√7ᵗʰ **S66.301** Unspecified injury of extensor muscle, fascia and tendon of **left index** finger at wrist and hand level

√7ᵗʰ **S66.302** Unspecified injury of extensor muscle, fascia and tendon of **right middle** finger at wrist and hand level

√7ᵗʰ **S66.303** Unspecified injury of extensor muscle, fascia and tendon of **left middle** finger at wrist and hand level

√7ᵗʰ **S66.304** Unspecified injury of extensor muscle, fascia and tendon of **right ring** finger at wrist and hand level

√7ᵗʰ **S66.305** Unspecified injury of extensor muscle, fascia and tendon of **left ring** finger at wrist and hand level

√7ᵗʰ **S66.306** Unspecified injury of extensor muscle, fascia and tendon of **right little** finger at wrist and hand level

√7ᵗʰ **S66.307** Unspecified injury of extensor muscle, fascia and tendon of **left little** finger at wrist and hand level

✔ Additional Character Required   √x7ᵗʰ Placeholder   Questionable PDx   Manifestation   Unspecified Dx   UPD Unacceptable PDx   H1-H14 HAC   HCC CMS-HCC Dx   HIV HIV Dx

ICD-10-CM 2022   1051

√7ᵗʰ **S66.308 Unspecified injury of extensor muscle, fascia and tendon of other finger at wrist and hand level**

Unspecified injury of extensor muscle, fascia and tendon of specified finger with unspecified laterality at wrist and hand level

√7ᵗʰ **S66.309 Unspecified injury of extensor muscle, fascia and tendon of unspecified finger at wrist and hand level**

√6ᵗʰ S66.31 Strain of extensor muscle, fascia and tendon of other and unspecified finger at wrist and hand level

√7ᵗʰ S66.310 Strain of extensor muscle, fascia and tendon of right index finger at wrist and hand level

√7ᵗʰ S66.311 Strain of extensor muscle, fascia and tendon of left index finger at wrist and hand level

√7ᵗʰ S66.312 Strain of extensor muscle, fascia and tendon of right middle finger at wrist and hand level

√7ᵗʰ S66.313 Strain of extensor muscle, fascia and tendon of left middle finger at wrist and hand level

√7ᵗʰ S66.314 Strain of extensor muscle, fascia and tendon of right ring finger at wrist and hand level

√7ᵗʰ S66.315 Strain of extensor muscle, fascia and tendon of left ring finger at wrist and hand level

√7ᵗʰ S66.316 Strain of extensor muscle, fascia and tendon of right little finger at wrist and hand level

√7ᵗʰ S66.317 Strain of extensor muscle, fascia and tendon of left little finger at wrist and hand level

√7ᵗʰ S66.318 Strain of extensor muscle, fascia and tendon of other finger at wrist and hand level

Strain of extensor muscle, fascia and tendon of specified finger with unspecified laterality at wrist and hand level

√7ᵗʰ **S66.319 Strain of extensor muscle, fascia and tendon of unspecified finger at wrist and hand level**

√6ᵗʰ S66.32 Laceration of extensor muscle, fascia and tendon of other and unspecified finger at wrist and hand level

√7ᵗʰ S66.320 Laceration of extensor muscle, fascia and tendon of right index finger at wrist and hand level　ᴄᴄ

√7ᵗʰ S66.321 Laceration of extensor muscle, fascia and tendon of left index finger at wrist and hand level　ᴄᴄ

√7ᵗʰ S66.322 Laceration of extensor muscle, fascia and tendon of right middle finger at wrist and hand level　ᴄᴄ

√7ᵗʰ S66.323 Laceration of extensor muscle, fascia and tendon of left middle finger at wrist and hand level　ᴄᴄ

√7ᵗʰ S66.324 Laceration of extensor muscle, fascia and tendon of right ring finger at wrist and hand level　ᴄᴄ

√7ᵗʰ S66.325 Laceration of extensor muscle, fascia and tendon of left ring finger at wrist and hand level　ᴄᴄ

√7ᵗʰ S66.326 Laceration of extensor muscle, fascia and tendon of right little finger at wrist and hand level　ᴄᴄ

√7ᵗʰ S66.327 Laceration of extensor muscle, fascia and tendon of left little finger at wrist and hand level　ᴄᴄ

√7ᵗʰ S66.328 Laceration of extensor muscle, fascia and tendon of other finger at wrist and hand level　ᴄᴄ

Laceration of extensor muscle, fascia and tendon of specified finger with unspecified laterality at wrist and hand level

√7ᵗʰ **S66.329 Laceration of extensor muscle, fascia and tendon of unspecified finger at wrist and hand level**　ᴄᴄ

√6ᵗʰ **S66.39 Other injury of extensor muscle, fascia and tendon of other and unspecified finger at wrist and hand level**

√7ᵗʰ S66.390 Other injury of extensor muscle, fascia and tendon of right index finger at wrist and hand level

√7ᵗʰ S66.391 Other injury of extensor muscle, fascia and tendon of left index finger at wrist and hand level

√7ᵗʰ S66.392 Other injury of extensor muscle, fascia and tendon of right middle finger at wrist and hand level

√7ᵗʰ S66.393 Other injury of extensor muscle, fascia and tendon of left middle finger at wrist and hand level

√7ᵗʰ S66.394 Other injury of extensor muscle, fascia and tendon of right ring finger at wrist and hand level

√7ᵗʰ S66.395 Other injury of extensor muscle, fascia and tendon of left ring finger at wrist and hand level

√7ᵗʰ S66.396 Other injury of extensor muscle, fascia and tendon of right little finger at wrist and hand level

√7ᵗʰ S66.397 Other injury of extensor muscle, fascia and tendon of left little finger at wrist and hand level

√7ᵗʰ S66.398 Other injury of extensor muscle, fascia and tendon of other finger at wrist and hand level

Other injury of extensor muscle, fascia and tendon of specified finger with unspecified laterality at wrist and hand level

√7ᵗʰ **S66.399 Other injury of extensor muscle, fascia and tendon of unspecified finger at wrist and hand level**

√5ᵗʰ S66.4 **Injury of intrinsic muscle, fascia and tendon of thumb at wrist and hand level**

√6ᵗʰ **S66.40 Unspecified injury of intrinsic muscle, fascia and tendon of thumb at wrist and hand level**

√7ᵗʰ **S66.401 Unspecified injury of intrinsic muscle, fascia and tendon of right thumb at wrist and hand level**

√7ᵗʰ **S66.402 Unspecified injury of intrinsic muscle, fascia and tendon of left thumb at wrist and hand level**

√7ᵗʰ **S66.409 Unspecified injury of intrinsic muscle, fascia and tendon of unspecified thumb at wrist and hand level**

√6ᵗʰ S66.41 Strain of intrinsic muscle, fascia and tendon of thumb at wrist and hand level

√7ᵗʰ S66.411 Strain of intrinsic muscle, fascia and tendon of right thumb at wrist and hand level

√7ᵗʰ S66.412 Strain of intrinsic muscle, fascia and tendon of left thumb at wrist and hand level

√7ᵗʰ **S66.419 Strain of intrinsic muscle, fascia and tendon of unspecified thumb at wrist and hand level**

√6ᵗʰ S66.42 Laceration of intrinsic muscle, fascia and tendon of thumb at wrist and hand level

√7ᵗʰ S66.421 Laceration of intrinsic muscle, fascia and tendon of right thumb at wrist and hand level　ᴄᴄ

√7ᵗʰ S66.422 Laceration of intrinsic muscle, fascia and tendon of left thumb at wrist and hand level　ᴄᴄ

√7ᵗʰ **S66.429 Laceration of intrinsic muscle, fascia and tendon of unspecified thumb at wrist and hand level**　ᴄᴄ

√6ᵗʰ S66.49 Other specified injury of intrinsic muscle, fascia and tendon of thumb at wrist and hand level

√7ᵗʰ S66.491 Other specified injury of intrinsic muscle, fascia and tendon of right thumb at wrist and hand level

√7ᵗʰ S66.492 Other specified injury of intrinsic muscle, fascia and tendon of left thumb at wrist and hand level

√7ᵗʰ **S66.499 Other specified injury of intrinsic muscle, fascia and tendon of unspecified thumb at wrist and hand level**

√5ᵗʰ **S66.5**　**Injury of** intrinsic **muscle, fascia and tendon of other and unspecified** finger **at wrist and hand level**

> **EXCLUDES 2**　injury of intrinsic muscle, fascia and tendon of thumb at wrist and hand level (S66.4-)

√6ᵗʰ **S66.50**　Unspecified injury of intrinsic muscle, fascia and tendon of other and unspecified finger at wrist and hand level

√7ᵗʰ **S66.500**　Unspecified injury of intrinsic muscle, fascia and tendon of right index finger at wrist and hand level

√7ᵗʰ **S66.501**　Unspecified injury of intrinsic muscle, fascia and tendon of left index finger at wrist and hand level

√7ᵗʰ **S66.502**　Unspecified injury of intrinsic muscle, fascia and tendon of right middle finger at wrist and hand level

√7ᵗʰ **S66.503**　Unspecified injury of intrinsic muscle, fascia and tendon of left middle finger at wrist and hand level

√7ᵗʰ **S66.504**　Unspecified injury of intrinsic muscle, fascia and tendon of right ring finger at wrist and hand level

√7ᵗʰ **S66.505**　Unspecified injury of intrinsic muscle, fascia and tendon of left ring finger at wrist and hand level

√7ᵗʰ **S66.506**　Unspecified injury of intrinsic muscle, fascia and tendon of right little finger at wrist and hand level

√7ᵗʰ **S66.507**　Unspecified injury of intrinsic muscle, fascia and tendon of left little finger at wrist and hand level

√7ᵗʰ **S66.508**　Unspecified injury of intrinsic muscle, fascia and tendon of other finger at wrist and hand level

> Unspecified injury of intrinsic muscle, fascia and tendon of specified finger with unspecified laterality at wrist and hand level

√7ᵗʰ **S66.509**　Unspecified injury of intrinsic muscle, fascia and tendon of unspecified finger at wrist and hand level

√6ᵗʰ **S66.51**　Strain **of intrinsic muscle, fascia and tendon of other and unspecified finger at wrist and hand level**

√7ᵗʰ **S66.510**　Strain of intrinsic muscle, fascia and tendon of right index finger at wrist and hand level

√7ᵗʰ **S66.511**　Strain of intrinsic muscle, fascia and tendon of left index finger at wrist and hand level

√7ᵗʰ **S66.512**　Strain of intrinsic muscle, fascia and tendon of right middle finger at wrist and hand level

√7ᵗʰ **S66.513**　Strain of intrinsic muscle, fascia and tendon of left middle finger at wrist and hand level

√7ᵗʰ **S66.514**　Strain of intrinsic muscle, fascia and tendon of right ring finger at wrist and hand level

√7ᵗʰ **S66.515**　Strain of intrinsic muscle, fascia and tendon of left ring finger at wrist and hand level

√7ᵗʰ **S66.516**　Strain of intrinsic muscle, fascia and tendon of right little finger at wrist and hand level

√7ᵗʰ **S66.517**　Strain of intrinsic muscle, fascia and tendon of left little finger at wrist and hand level

√7ᵗʰ **S66.518**　Strain of intrinsic muscle, fascia and tendon of other finger at wrist and hand level

> Strain of intrinsic muscle, fascia and tendon of specified finger with unspecified laterality at wrist and hand level

√7ᵗʰ **S66.519**　Strain of intrinsic muscle, fascia and tendon of unspecified finger at wrist and hand level

√6ᵗʰ **S66.52**　Laceration **of intrinsic muscle, fascia and tendon of other and unspecified finger at wrist and hand level**

√7ᵗʰ **S66.520**　Laceration of intrinsic muscle, fascia and tendon of right index finger at wrist and hand level　**CC**

√7ᵗʰ **S66.521**　Laceration of intrinsic muscle, fascia and tendon of left index finger at wrist and hand level　**CC**

√7ᵗʰ **S66.522**　Laceration of intrinsic muscle, fascia and tendon of right middle finger at wrist and hand level　**CC**

√7ᵗʰ **S66.523**　Laceration of intrinsic muscle, fascia and tendon of left middle finger at wrist and hand level　**CC**

√7ᵗʰ **S66.524**　Laceration of intrinsic muscle, fascia and tendon of right ring finger at wrist and hand level　**CC**

√7ᵗʰ **S66.525**　Laceration of intrinsic muscle, fascia and tendon of left ring finger at wrist and hand level　**CC**

√7ᵗʰ **S66.526**　Laceration of intrinsic muscle, fascia and tendon of right little finger at wrist and hand level　**CC**

√7ᵗʰ **S66.527**　Laceration of intrinsic muscle, fascia and tendon of left little finger at wrist and hand level　**CC**

√7ᵗʰ **S66.528**　Laceration of intrinsic muscle, fascia and tendon of other finger at wrist and hand level　**CC**

> Laceration of intrinsic muscle, fascia and tendon of specified finger with unspecified laterality at wrist and hand level

√7ᵗʰ **S66.529**　Laceration of intrinsic muscle, fascia and tendon of unspecified finger at wrist and hand level　**CC**

√6ᵗʰ **S66.59**　Other injury of intrinsic muscle, fascia and tendon of other and unspecified finger at wrist and hand level

√7ᵗʰ **S66.590**　Other injury of intrinsic muscle, fascia and tendon of right index finger at wrist and hand level

√7ᵗʰ **S66.591**　Other injury of intrinsic muscle, fascia and tendon of left index finger at wrist and hand level

√7ᵗʰ **S66.592**　Other injury of intrinsic muscle, fascia and tendon of right middle finger at wrist and hand level

√7ᵗʰ **S66.593**　Other injury of intrinsic muscle, fascia and tendon of left middle finger at wrist and hand level

√7ᵗʰ **S66.594**　Other injury of intrinsic muscle, fascia and tendon of right ring finger at wrist and hand level

√7ᵗʰ **S66.595**　Other injury of intrinsic muscle, fascia and tendon of left ring finger at wrist and hand level

√7ᵗʰ **S66.596**　Other injury of intrinsic muscle, fascia and tendon of right little finger at wrist and hand level

√7ᵗʰ **S66.597**　Other injury of intrinsic muscle, fascia and tendon of left little finger at wrist and hand level

√7ᵗʰ **S66.598**　Other injury of intrinsic muscle, fascia and tendon of other finger at wrist and hand level

> Other injury of intrinsic muscle, fascia and tendon of specified finger with unspecified laterality at wrist and hand level

√7ᵗʰ **S66.599**　Other injury of intrinsic muscle, fascia and tendon of unspecified finger at wrist and hand level

√5ᵗʰ **S66.8**　**Injury of other specified muscles, fascia and tendons at wrist and hand level**

√6ᵗʰ **S66.80**　Unspecified injury of other specified muscles, fascia and tendons at wrist and hand level

√7ᵗʰ **S66.801**　Unspecified injury of other specified muscles, fascia and tendons at wrist and hand level, right hand

√7ᵗʰ **S66.802**　Unspecified injury of other specified muscles, fascia and tendons at wrist and hand level, left hand

√7ᵗʰ **S66.809**　Unspecified injury of other specified muscles, fascia and tendons at wrist and hand level, unspecified hand

√6ᵗʰ **S66.81**　Strain **of other specified muscles, fascia and tendons at wrist and hand level**

√7ᵗʰ **S66.811**　Strain of other specified muscles, fascia and tendons at wrist and hand level, right hand

✔ Additional Character Required　√x7ᵗʰ Placeholder　Questionable PDx　Manifestation　Unspecified Dx　**UPD** Unacceptable PDx　**H1**-**H14** HAC　**HCC** CMS-HCC Dx　**HIV** HIV Dx

ICD-10-CM 2022　　　**1053**

√7ᵗʰ **S66.812** Strain of other specified muscles, fascia and tendons at wrist and hand level, left hand

√7ᵗʰ **S66.819** Strain of other specified muscles, fascia and tendons at wrist and hand level, unspecified hand

√6ᵗʰ **S66.82** Laceration of other specified muscles, fascia and tendons at wrist and hand level

√7ᵗʰ **S66.821** Laceration of other specified muscles, fascia and tendons at wrist and hand level, right hand   **CC**

√7ᵗʰ **S66.822** Laceration of other specified muscles, fascia and tendons at wrist and hand level, left hand   **CC**

√7ᵗʰ **S66.829** Laceration of other specified muscles, fascia and tendons at wrist and hand level, unspecified hand   **CC**

√6ᵗʰ **S66.89** Other injury of other specified muscles, fascia and tendons at wrist and hand level

√7ᵗʰ **S66.891** Other injury of other specified muscles, fascia and tendons at wrist and hand level, right hand

√7ᵗʰ **S66.892** Other injury of other specified muscles, fascia and tendons at wrist and hand level, left hand

√7ᵗʰ **S66.899** Other injury of other specified muscles, fascia and tendons at wrist and hand level, unspecified hand

√5ᵗʰ **S66.9** Injury of unspecified muscle, fascia and tendon at wrist and hand level

√6ᵗʰ **S66.90** Unspecified injury of unspecified muscle, fascia and tendon at wrist and hand level

√7ᵗʰ **S66.901** Unspecified injury of unspecified muscle, fascia and tendon at wrist and hand level, right hand

√7ᵗʰ **S66.902** Unspecified injury of unspecified muscle, fascia and tendon at wrist and hand level, left hand

√7ᵗʰ **S66.909** Unspecified injury of unspecified muscle, fascia and tendon at wrist and hand level, unspecified hand

√6ᵗʰ **S66.91** Strain of unspecified muscle, fascia and tendon at wrist and hand level

√7ᵗʰ **S66.911** Strain of unspecified muscle, fascia and tendon at wrist and hand level, right hand

√7ᵗʰ **S66.912** Strain of unspecified muscle, fascia and tendon at wrist and hand level, left hand

√7ᵗʰ **S66.919** Strain of unspecified muscle, fascia and tendon at wrist and hand level, unspecified hand

√6ᵗʰ **S66.92** Laceration of unspecified muscle, fascia and tendon at wrist and hand level

√7ᵗʰ **S66.921** Laceration of unspecified muscle, fascia and tendon at wrist and hand level, right hand   **CC**

√7ᵗʰ **S66.922** Laceration of unspecified muscle, fascia and tendon at wrist and hand level, left hand   **CC**

√7ᵗʰ **S66.929** Laceration of unspecified muscle, fascia and tendon at wrist and hand level, unspecified hand   **CC**

√6ᵗʰ **S66.99** Other injury of unspecified muscle, fascia and tendon at wrist and hand level

√7ᵗʰ **S66.991** Other injury of unspecified muscle, fascia and tendon at wrist and hand level, right hand

√7ᵗʰ **S66.992** Other injury of unspecified muscle, fascia and tendon at wrist and hand level, left hand

√7ᵗʰ **S66.999** Other injury of unspecified muscle, fascia and tendon at wrist and hand level, unspecified hand

√4ᵗʰ **S67** Crushing injury of wrist, hand and fingers

Use additional code for all associated injuries, such as:
fracture of wrist and hand (S62.-)
open wound of wrist and hand (S61.-)

The appropriate 7th character is to be added to each code from category S67.
A   initial encounter
D   subsequent encounter
S   sequela

√5ᵗʰ **S67.0** Crushing injury of thumb

√x7ᵗʰ **S67.00** Crushing injury of unspecified thumb

√x7ᵗʰ **S67.01** Crushing injury of right thumb

√x7ᵗʰ **S67.02** Crushing injury of left thumb

√5ᵗʰ **S67.1** Crushing injury of other and unspecified finger(s)

EXCLUDES 2   crushing injury of thumb (S67.0-)

√x7ᵗʰ **S67.10** Crushing injury of unspecified finger(s)

√6ᵗʰ **S67.19** Crushing injury of other finger(s)

√7ᵗʰ **S67.190** Crushing injury of right index finger

√7ᵗʰ **S67.191** Crushing injury of left index finger

√7ᵗʰ **S67.192** Crushing injury of right middle finger

√7ᵗʰ **S67.193** Crushing injury of left middle finger

√7ᵗʰ **S67.194** Crushing injury of right ring finger

√7ᵗʰ **S67.195** Crushing injury of left ring finger

√7ᵗʰ **S67.196** Crushing injury of right little finger

√7ᵗʰ **S67.197** Crushing injury of left little finger

√7ᵗʰ **S67.198** Crushing injury of other finger

Crushing injury of specified finger with unspecified laterality

√5ᵗʰ **S67.2** Crushing injury of hand

EXCLUDES 2   crushing injury of fingers (S67.1-)
crushing injury of thumb (S67.0-)

√x7ᵗʰ **S67.20** Crushing injury of unspecified hand

√x7ᵗʰ **S67.21** Crushing injury of right hand

√x7ᵗʰ **S67.22** Crushing injury of left hand

√5ᵗʰ **S67.3** Crushing injury of wrist

√x7ᵗʰ **S67.30** Crushing injury of unspecified wrist

√x7ᵗʰ **S67.31** Crushing injury of right wrist

√x7ᵗʰ **S67.32** Crushing injury of left wrist

√5ᵗʰ **S67.4** Crushing injury of wrist and hand

EXCLUDES 1   crushing injury of hand alone (S67.2-)
crushing injury of wrist alone (S67.3-)

EXCLUDES 2   crushing injury of fingers (S67.1-)
crushing injury of thumb (S67.0-)

√x7ᵗʰ **S67.40** Crushing injury of unspecified wrist and hand

√x7ᵗʰ **S67.41** Crushing injury of right wrist and hand

√x7ᵗʰ **S67.42** Crushing injury of left wrist and hand

√5ᵗʰ **S67.9** Crushing injury of unspecified part(s) of wrist, hand and fingers

√x7ᵗʰ **S67.90** Crushing injury of unspecified part(s) of unspecified wrist, hand and fingers

√x7ᵗʰ **S67.91** Crushing injury of unspecified part(s) of right wrist, hand and fingers

√x7ᵗʰ **S67.92** Crushing injury of unspecified part(s) of left wrist, hand and fingers

√4ᵗʰ **S68** Traumatic amputation of wrist, hand and fingers

An amputation not identified as partial or complete should be coded to complete.

The appropriate 7th character is to be added to each code from category S68.
A   initial encounter
D   subsequent encounter
S   sequela

√5ᵗʰ **S68.0** Traumatic metacarpophalangeal amputation of thumb

Traumatic amputation of thumb NOS

√6ᵗʰ **S68.01** Complete traumatic metacarpophalangeal amputation of thumb

8 √7ᵗʰ **S68.011** Complete traumatic metacarpophalangeal amputation of right thumb   **HCC**

N Newborn: 0   P Pediatric: 0-17   M Maternity: 9-64   A Adult: 15-124   MCC Major Complication/Comorbidity   CC Complication/Comorbidity   SW Severe Wound Dx

1054   ICD-10-CM 2022

8 √7th **S68.012** **Complete traumatic metacarpophalangeal amputation of** left **thumb** HCC

8 √7th **S68.019** **Complete traumatic metacarpophalangeal amputation of unspecified thumb** HCC

√6th **S68.02** Partial **traumatic metacarpophalangeal amputation of thumb**

8 √7th **S68.021** **Partial traumatic metacarpophalangeal amputation of** right **thumb** HCC

8 √7th **S68.022** **Partial traumatic metacarpophalangeal amputation of** left **thumb** HCC

8 √7th **S68.029** **Partial traumatic metacarpophalangeal amputation of unspecified thumb** HCC

√5th **S68.1** **Traumatic** metacarpophalangeal **amputation of other and unspecified** finger

Traumatic amputation of finger NOS

> EXCLUDES 2   traumatic metacarpophalangeal amputation of thumb (S68.0-)

√6th **S68.11** Complete **traumatic metacarpophalangeal amputation of other and unspecified finger**

8 √7th **S68.110** **Complete traumatic metacarpophalangeal amputation of** right index **finger** HCC

8 √7th **S68.111** **Complete traumatic metacarpophalangeal amputation of** left index **finger** HCC

8 √7th **S68.112** **Complete traumatic metacarpophalangeal amputation of** right middle **finger** HCC

8 √7th **S68.113** **Complete traumatic metacarpophalangeal amputation of** left middle **finger** HCC

8 √7th **S68.114** **Complete traumatic metacarpophalangeal amputation of** right ring **finger** HCC

8 √7th **S68.115** **Complete traumatic metacarpophalangeal amputation of** left ring **finger** HCC

8 √7th **S68.116** **Complete traumatic metacarpophalangeal amputation of** right little **finger** HCC

8 √7th **S68.117** **Complete traumatic metacarpophalangeal amputation of** left little **finger** HCC

8 √7th **S68.118** **Complete traumatic metacarpophalangeal amputation of other finger** HCC

> Complete traumatic metacarpophalangeal amputation of specified finger with unspecified laterality

8 √7th **S68.119** **Complete traumatic metacarpophalangeal amputation of unspecified finger** HCC

√6th **S68.12** Partial **traumatic metacarpophalangeal amputation of other and unspecified finger**

8 √7th **S68.120** **Partial traumatic metacarpophalangeal amputation of** right index **finger** HCC

8 √7th **S68.121** **Partial traumatic metacarpophalangeal amputation of** left index **finger** HCC

8 √7th **S68.122** **Partial traumatic metacarpophalangeal amputation of** right middle **finger** HCC

8 √7th **S68.123** **Partial traumatic metacarpophalangeal amputation of** left middle **finger** HCC

8 √7th **S68.124** **Partial traumatic metacarpophalangeal amputation of** right ring **finger** HCC

8 √7th **S68.125** **Partial traumatic metacarpophalangeal amputation of** left ring **finger** HCC

8 √7th **S68.126** **Partial traumatic metacarpophalangeal amputation of** right little **finger** HCC

8 √7th **S68.127** **Partial traumatic metacarpophalangeal amputation of** left little **finger** HCC

8 √7th **S68.128** **Partial traumatic metacarpophalangeal amputation of other finger** HCC

> Partial traumatic metacarpophalangeal amputation of specified finger with unspecified laterality

8 √7th **S68.129** **Partial traumatic metacarpophalangeal amputation of unspecified finger** HCC

√5th **S68.4** **Traumatic amputation of** hand at wrist level

Traumatic amputation of hand NOS
Traumatic amputation of wrist

√6th **S68.41** Complete **traumatic amputation of hand at wrist level**

7 √7th **S68.411** **Complete traumatic amputation of** right **hand at wrist level** CC HCC

7 √7th **S68.412** **Complete traumatic amputation of** left **hand at wrist level** CC HCC

7 √7th **S68.419** **Complete traumatic amputation of unspecified hand at wrist level** CC HCC

√6th **S68.42** Partial **traumatic amputation of hand at wrist level**

7 √7th **S68.421** **Partial traumatic amputation of** right **hand at wrist level** CC HCC

7 √7th **S68.422** **Partial traumatic amputation of** left **hand at wrist level** CC HCC

7 √7th **S68.429** **Partial traumatic amputation of unspecified hand at wrist level** CC HCC

√5th **S68.5** **Traumatic** transphalangeal **amputation of** thumb

Traumatic interphalangeal joint amputation of thumb

√6th **S68.51** Complete **traumatic transphalangeal amputation of thumb**

8 √7th **S68.511** **Complete traumatic transphalangeal amputation of** right **thumb** HCC

8 √7th **S68.512** **Complete traumatic transphalangeal amputation of** left **thumb** HCC

8 √7th **S68.519** **Complete traumatic transphalangeal amputation of unspecified thumb** HCC

√6th **S68.52** Partial **traumatic transphalangeal amputation of thumb**

8 √7th **S68.521** **Partial traumatic transphalangeal amputation of** right **thumb** HCC

8 √7th **S68.522** **Partial traumatic transphalangeal amputation of** left **thumb** HCC

8 √7th **S68.529** **Partial traumatic transphalangeal amputation of unspecified thumb** HCC

√5th **S68.6** **Traumatic** transphalangeal **amputation of other and unspecified** finger

√6th **S68.61** Complete **traumatic transphalangeal amputation of other and unspecified finger(s)**

8 √7th **S68.610** **Complete traumatic transphalangeal amputation of** right index **finger** HCC

8 √7th **S68.611** **Complete traumatic transphalangeal amputation of** left index **finger** HCC

8 √7th **S68.612** **Complete traumatic transphalangeal amputation of** right middle **finger** HCC

8 √7th **S68.613** **Complete traumatic transphalangeal amputation of** left middle **finger** HCC

8 √7th **S68.614** **Complete traumatic transphalangeal amputation of** right ring **finger** HCC

8 √7th **S68.615** **Complete traumatic transphalangeal amputation of** left ring **finger** HCC

8 √7th **S68.616** **Complete traumatic transphalangeal amputation of** right little **finger** HCC

8 √7th **S68.617** **Complete traumatic transphalangeal amputation of** left little **finger** HCC

8 √7th **S68.618** **Complete traumatic transphalangeal amputation of other finger** HCC

> Complete traumatic transphalangeal amputation of specified finger with unspecified laterality

8 √7th **S68.619** **Complete traumatic transphalangeal amputation of unspecified finger** HCC

√6th **S68.62** Partial **traumatic transphalangeal amputation of other and unspecified finger**

8 √7th **S68.620** **Partial traumatic transphalangeal amputation of** right index **finger** HCC

8 √7th **S68.621** **Partial traumatic transphalangeal amputation of** left index **finger** HCC

8 √7th **S68.622** **Partial traumatic transphalangeal amputation of** right middle **finger** HCC

8 √7th **S68.623** **Partial traumatic transphalangeal amputation of** left middle **finger** HCC

8 √7th **S68.624** **Partial traumatic transphalangeal amputation of** right ring **finger** HCC

8 √7th **S68.625** **Partial traumatic transphalangeal amputation of** left ring **finger** HCC

8 √7th **S68.626** **Partial traumatic transphalangeal amputation of** right little **finger** HCC

✔ Additional Character Required √x7th Placeholder Questionable PDx Manifestation Unspecified Dx UPD Unacceptable PDx H1-H14 HAC HCC CMS-HCC Dx HIV HIV Dx

ICD-10-CM 2022   1055

Chapter 19. Injury, Poisoning and Certain Other Consequences of External Causes

8   √7ᵗʰ   **S68.627**   **Partial traumatic transphalangeal amputation of left little finger**   HCC

8   √7ᵗʰ   **S68.628**   **Partial traumatic transphalangeal amputation of other finger**   HCC
    Partial traumatic transphalangeal amputation of specified finger with unspecified laterality

8   √7ᵗʰ   **S68.629**   **Partial traumatic transphalangeal amputation of unspecified finger**   HCC

√5ᵗʰ   **S68.7**   **Traumatic transmetacarpal amputation of hand**

    √6ᵗʰ   **S68.71**   **Complete traumatic transmetacarpal amputation of hand**

      7   √7ᵗʰ   **S68.711**   **Complete traumatic transmetacarpal amputation of right hand**   CC HCC

      7   √7ᵗʰ   **S68.712**   **Complete traumatic transmetacarpal amputation of left hand**   CC HCC

      7   √7ᵗʰ   **S68.719**   **Complete traumatic transmetacarpal amputation of unspecified hand**   CC HCC

    √6ᵗʰ   **S68.72**   **Partial traumatic transmetacarpal amputation of hand**

      7   √7ᵗʰ   **S68.721**   **Partial traumatic transmetacarpal amputation of right hand**   CC HCC

      7   √7ᵗʰ   **S68.722**   **Partial traumatic transmetacarpal amputation of left hand**   CC HCC

      7   √7ᵗʰ   **S68.729**   **Partial traumatic transmetacarpal amputation of unspecified hand**   CC HCC

√4ᵗʰ   **S69**   **Other and unspecified injuries of wrist, hand and finger(s)**

> The appropriate 7th character is to be added to each code from category S69.
> A   initial encounter
> D   subsequent encounter
> S   sequela

√5ᵗʰ   **S69.8**   **Other specified injuries of wrist, hand and finger(s)**

    √x7ᵗʰ   **S69.80**   **Other specified injuries of unspecified wrist, hand and finger(s)**

    √x7ᵗʰ   **S69.81**   **Other specified injuries of right wrist, hand and finger(s)**

    √x7ᵗʰ   **S69.82**   **Other specified injuries of left wrist, hand and finger(s)**

√5ᵗʰ   **S69.9**   **Unspecified injury of wrist, hand and finger(s)**

    √x7ᵗʰ   **S69.90**   **Unspecified injury of unspecified wrist, hand and finger(s)**

    √x7ᵗʰ   **S69.91**   **Unspecified injury of right wrist, hand and finger(s)**

    √x7ᵗʰ   **S69.92**   **Unspecified injury of left wrist, hand and finger(s)**

Injuries to the hip and thigh (S70-S79)

EXCLUDES 2   *burns and corrosions (T20-T32)*
               frostbite (T33-T34)
               snake bite (T63.0-)
               venomous insect bite or sting (T63.4-)

√4ᵗʰ   **S70**   **Superficial injury of hip and thigh**

> The appropriate 7th character is to be added to each code from category S70.
> A   initial encounter
> D   subsequent encounter
> S   sequela

√5ᵗʰ   **S70.0**   **Contusion of hip**

    √x7ᵗʰ   **S70.00**   **Contusion of unspecified hip**

    √x7ᵗʰ   **S70.01**   **Contusion of right hip**

    √x7ᵗʰ   **S70.02**   **Contusion of left hip**

√5ᵗʰ   **S70.1**   **Contusion of thigh**

    √x7ᵗʰ   **S70.10**   **Contusion of unspecified thigh**

    √x7ᵗʰ   **S70.11**   **Contusion of right thigh**

    √x7ᵗʰ   **S70.12**   **Contusion of left thigh**

√5ᵗʰ   **S70.2**   **Other superficial injuries of hip**

    √6ᵗʰ   **S70.21**   **Abrasion of hip**

      √7ᵗʰ   **S70.211**   **Abrasion, right hip**

      √7ᵗʰ   **S70.212**   **Abrasion, left hip**

      √7ᵗʰ   **S70.219**   **Abrasion, unspecified hip**

    √6ᵗʰ   **S70.22**   **Blister (nonthermal) of hip**

      √7ᵗʰ   **S70.221**   **Blister (nonthermal), right hip**

      √7ᵗʰ   **S70.222**   **Blister (nonthermal), left hip**

      √7ᵗʰ   **S70.229**   **Blister (nonthermal), unspecified hip**

    √6ᵗʰ   **S70.24**   **External constriction of hip**

      √7ᵗʰ   **S70.241**   **External constriction, right hip**

      √7ᵗʰ   **S70.242**   **External constriction, left hip**

      √7ᵗʰ   **S70.249**   **External constriction, unspecified hip**

    √6ᵗʰ   **S70.25**   **Superficial foreign body of hip**
      Splinter in the hip

      √7ᵗʰ   **S70.251**   **Superficial foreign body, right hip**

      √7ᵗʰ   **S70.252**   **Superficial foreign body, left hip**

      √7ᵗʰ   **S70.259**   **Superficial foreign body, unspecified hip**

    √6ᵗʰ   **S70.26**   **Insect bite (nonvenomous) of hip**

      √7ᵗʰ   **S70.261**   **Insect bite (nonvenomous), right hip**

      √7ᵗʰ   **S70.262**   **Insect bite (nonvenomous), left hip**

      √7ᵗʰ   **S70.269**   **Insect bite (nonvenomous), unspecified hip**

    √6ᵗʰ   **S70.27**   **Other superficial bite of hip**
      EXCLUDES 1   *open bite of hip (S71.05-)*

      √7ᵗʰ   **S70.271**   **Other superficial bite of hip, right hip**

      √7ᵗʰ   **S70.272**   **Other superficial bite of hip, left hip**

      √7ᵗʰ   **S70.279**   **Other superficial bite of hip, unspecified hip**

√5ᵗʰ   **S70.3**   **Other superficial injuries of thigh**

    √6ᵗʰ   **S70.31**   **Abrasion of thigh**

      √7ᵗʰ   **S70.311**   **Abrasion, right thigh**

      √7ᵗʰ   **S70.312**   **Abrasion, left thigh**

      √7ᵗʰ   **S70.319**   **Abrasion, unspecified thigh**

    √6ᵗʰ   **S70.32**   **Blister (nonthermal) of thigh**

      √7ᵗʰ   **S70.321**   **Blister (nonthermal), right thigh**

      √7ᵗʰ   **S70.322**   **Blister (nonthermal), left thigh**

      √7ᵗʰ   **S70.329**   **Blister (nonthermal), unspecified thigh**

    √6ᵗʰ   **S70.34**   **External constriction of thigh**

      √7ᵗʰ   **S70.341**   **External constriction, right thigh**

      √7ᵗʰ   **S70.342**   **External constriction, left thigh**

      √7ᵗʰ   **S70.349**   **External constriction, unspecified thigh**

    √6ᵗʰ   **S70.35**   **Superficial foreign body of thigh**
      Splinter in the thigh

      √7ᵗʰ   **S70.351**   **Superficial foreign body, right thigh**

      √7ᵗʰ   **S70.352**   **Superficial foreign body, left thigh**

      √7ᵗʰ   **S70.359**   **Superficial foreign body, unspecified thigh**

    √6ᵗʰ   **S70.36**   **Insect bite (nonvenomous) of thigh**

      √7ᵗʰ   **S70.361**   **Insect bite (nonvenomous), right thigh**

      √7ᵗʰ   **S70.362**   **Insect bite (nonvenomous), left thigh**

      √7ᵗʰ   **S70.369**   **Insect bite (nonvenomous), unspecified thigh**

    √6ᵗʰ   **S70.37**   **Other superficial bite of thigh**
      EXCLUDES 1   *open bite of thigh (S71.15)*

      √7ᵗʰ   **S70.371**   **Other superficial bite of right thigh**

      √7ᵗʰ   **S70.372**   **Other superficial bite of left thigh**

      √7ᵗʰ   **S70.379**   **Other superficial bite of unspecified thigh**

√5ᵗʰ   **S70.9**   **Unspecified superficial injury of hip and thigh**

    √6ᵗʰ   **S70.91**   **Unspecified superficial injury of hip**

      √7ᵗʰ   **S70.911**   **Unspecified superficial injury of right hip**

      √7ᵗʰ   **S70.912**   **Unspecified superficial injury of left hip**

      √7ᵗʰ   **S70.919**   **Unspecified superficial injury of unspecified hip**

    √6ᵗʰ   **S70.92**   **Unspecified superficial injury of thigh**

      √7ᵗʰ   **S70.921**   **Unspecified superficial injury of right thigh**

      √7ᵗʰ   **S70.922**   **Unspecified superficial injury of left thigh**

      √7ᵗʰ   **S70.929**   **Unspecified superficial injury of unspecified thigh**

N Newborn: 0   P Pediatric: 0-17   M Maternity: 9-64   A Adult: 15-124   MCC Major Complication/Comorbidity   CC Complication/Comorbidity   SW Severe Wound Dx

1056   ICD-10-CM 2022

√4ᵗʰ **S71 Open wound** of hip and thigh

Code also any associated wound infection

EXCLUDES 1   open fracture of hip and thigh (S72.-)

traumatic amputation of hip and thigh (S78.-)

EXCLUDES 2   bite of venomous animal (T63.-)

open wound of ankle, foot and toes (S91.-)

open wound of knee and lower leg (S81.-)

The appropriate 7th character is to be added to each code from category S71.
A   initial encounter
D   subsequent encounter
S   sequela

√5ᵗʰ **S71.0 Open wound** of hip

√6ᵗʰ **S71.00 Unspecified open wound** of hip

√7ᵗʰ **S71.001 Unspecified open wound, right** hip

√7ᵗʰ **S71.002 Unspecified open wound, left** hip

√7ᵗʰ **S71.009 Unspecified open wound, unspecified** hip

√6ᵗʰ **S71.01 Laceration without foreign body** of hip

√7ᵗʰ **S71.011 Laceration without foreign body, right** hip

√7ᵗʰ **S71.012 Laceration without foreign body, left** hip

√7ᵗʰ **S71.019 Laceration without foreign body, unspecified** hip

√6ᵗʰ **S71.02 Laceration with foreign body** of hip

√7ᵗʰ **S71.021 Laceration with foreign body, right** hip

√7ᵗʰ **S71.022 Laceration with foreign body, left** hip

√7ᵗʰ **S71.029 Laceration with foreign body, unspecified** hip

√6ᵗʰ **S71.03 Puncture wound without foreign body** of hip

√7ᵗʰ **S71.031 Puncture wound without foreign body, right** hip

√7ᵗʰ **S71.032 Puncture wound without foreign body, left** hip

√7ᵗʰ **S71.039 Puncture wound without foreign body, unspecified** hip

√6ᵗʰ **S71.04 Puncture wound with foreign body** of hip

√7ᵗʰ **S71.041 Puncture wound with foreign body, right** hip

√7ᵗʰ **S71.042 Puncture wound with foreign body, left** hip

√7ᵗʰ **S71.049 Puncture wound with foreign body, unspecified** hip

√6ᵗʰ **S71.05 Open bite** of hip

Bite of hip NOS

EXCLUDES 1   superficial bite of hip (S70.26, S70.27)

√7ᵗʰ **S71.051 Open bite, right** hip

√7ᵗʰ **S71.052 Open bite, left** hip

√7ᵗʰ **S71.059 Open bite, unspecified** hip

√5ᵗʰ **S71.1 Open wound** of thigh

√6ᵗʰ **S71.10 Unspecified open wound of thigh**

AHA: 2016,3Q,24

√7ᵗʰ **S71.101 Unspecified open wound, right** thigh

√7ᵗʰ **S71.102 Unspecified open wound, left** thigh

√7ᵗʰ **S71.109 Unspecified open wound, unspecified** thigh

√6ᵗʰ **S71.11 Laceration without foreign body** of thigh

√7ᵗʰ **S71.111 Laceration without foreign body, right** thigh

√7ᵗʰ **S71.112 Laceration without foreign body, left** thigh

√7ᵗʰ **S71.119 Laceration without foreign body, unspecified** thigh

√6ᵗʰ **S71.12 Laceration with foreign body** of thigh

√7ᵗʰ **S71.121 Laceration with foreign body, right** thigh

√7ᵗʰ **S71.122 Laceration with foreign body, left** thigh

√7ᵗʰ **S71.129 Laceration with foreign body, unspecified** thigh

√6ᵗʰ **S71.13 Puncture wound without foreign body** of thigh

AHA: 2016,3Q,24

√7ᵗʰ **S71.131 Puncture wound without foreign body, right** thigh

√7ᵗʰ **S71.132 Puncture wound without foreign body, left** thigh

√7ᵗʰ **S71.139 Puncture wound without foreign body, unspecified** thigh

√6ᵗʰ **S71.14 Puncture wound with foreign body** of thigh

AHA: 2016,3Q,24

√7ᵗʰ **S71.141 Puncture wound with foreign body, right** thigh

√7ᵗʰ **S71.142 Puncture wound with foreign body, left** thigh

√7ᵗʰ **S71.149 Puncture wound with foreign body, unspecified** thigh

√6ᵗʰ **S71.15 Open bite** of thigh

Bite of thigh NOS

EXCLUDES 1   superficial bite of thigh (S70.37-)

√7ᵗʰ **S71.151 Open bite, right** thigh

√7ᵗʰ **S71.152 Open bite, left** thigh

√7ᵗʰ **S71.159 Open bite, unspecified** thigh

√4ᵗʰ **S72 Fracture of femur**

NOTE   A fracture not indicated as displaced or nondisplaced should be coded to displaced.

A fracture not indicated as open or closed should be coded to closed.

The open fracture designations are based on the Gustilo open fracture classification.

EXCLUDES 1   traumatic amputation of hip and thigh (S78.-)

EXCLUDES 2   fracture of lower leg and ankle (S82.-)

fracture of foot (S92.-)

periprosthetic fracture of prosthetic implant of hip (M97.0-)

AHA: 2018,2Q,12; 2016,1Q,33; 2015,3Q,37-39; 2015,1Q,17; 2013,4Q,128

DEF: Diaphysis: Central shaft of a long bone.

DEF: Epiphysis: Proximal and distal rounded ends of a long bone communicates with the joint.

DEF: Metaphysis: Section of a long bone located between the epiphysis and diaphysis at the proximal and distal ends.

DEF: Physis (growth plate): Narrow zone of cartilaginous tissue between the epiphysis and metaphysis at each end of a long bone. In childhood, proliferation of cells in this zone lengthens the bone. As the bone matures, this area thins, ossification eventually fusing into solid bone and growth stops. **Synonym(s):** Epiphyseal plate.

The appropriate 7th character is to be added to all codes from category S72 [unless otherwise indicated].
A   initial encounter for closed fracture
B   initial encounter for open fracture type I or II
     initial encounter for open fracture NOS
C   initial encounter for open fracture type IIIA, IIIB, or IIIC
D   subsequent encounter for closed fracture with routine healing
E   subsequent encounter for open fracture type I or II with routine healing
F   subsequent encounter for open fracture type IIIA, IIIB, or IIIC with routine healing
G   subsequent encounter for closed fracture with delayed healing
H   subsequent encounter for open fracture type I or II with delayed healing
J   subsequent encounter for open fracture type IIIA, IIIB, or IIIC with delayed healing
K   subsequent encounter for closed fracture with nonunion
M   subsequent encounter for open fracture type I or II with nonunion
N   subsequent encounter for open fracture type IIIA, IIIB, or IIIC with nonunion
P   subsequent encounter for closed fracture with malunion
Q   subsequent encounter for open fracture type I or II with malunion
R   subsequent encounter for open fracture type IIIA, IIIB, or IIIC with malunion
S   sequela

√5ᵗʰ **S72.0 Fracture of head and neck** of femur

EXCLUDES 2   physeal fracture of upper end of femur (S79.0-)

AHA: 2016,3Q,16

√6ᵗʰ **S72.00 Fracture of unspecified part of neck of femur**

Fracture of hip NOS

Fracture of neck of femur NOS

4,6 √7ᵗʰ **S72.001 Fracture of unspecified part of neck of right femur**   MCC CC H5 HCC

4,6 √7ᵗʰ **S72.002 Fracture of unspecified part of neck of left femur**   MCC CC H5 HCC

4,6 √7ᵗʰ **S72.009 Fracture of unspecified part of neck of unspecified femur**   MCC CC H5 HCC

☑ Additional Character Required   √x7ᵗʰ Placeholder   Questionable PDx   Manifestation   Unspecified Dx   UPD Unacceptable PDx   H1 - H14 HAC   HCC CMS-HCC Dx   HIV HIV Dx

ICD-10-CM 2022   1057

√6th **S72.01** **Unspecified intracapsular fracture of femur**

Subcapital fracture of femur

4,6 √7th **S72.011** **Unspecified intracapsular fracture of right femur** MCC CC H5 HCC

4,6 √7th **S72.012** **Unspecified intracapsular fracture of left femur** MCC CC H5 HCC

4,6 √7th **S72.019** **Unspecified intracapsular fracture of unspecified femur** MCC CC H5 HCC

√6th **S72.02** **Fracture of epiphysis (separation) (upper) of femur**

Transepiphyseal fracture of femur

EXCLUDES 1   capital femoral epiphyseal fracture (pediatric) of femur (S79.01-)

Salter-Harris Type I physeal fracture of upper end of femur (S79.01-)

4,6 √7th **S72.021** **Displaced fracture of epiphysis (separation) (upper) of right femur** MCC CC H5 HCC

4,6 √7th **S72.022** **Displaced fracture of epiphysis (separation) (upper) of left femur** MCC CC H5 HCC

4,6 √7th **S72.023** **Displaced fracture of epiphysis (separation) (upper) of unspecified femur** MCC CC H5 HCC

4,6 √7th **S72.024** **Nondisplaced fracture of epiphysis (separation) (upper) of right femur** MCC CC H5 HCC

4,6 √7th **S72.025** **Nondisplaced fracture of epiphysis (separation) (upper) of left femur** MCC CC H5 HCC

4,6 √7th **S72.026** **Nondisplaced fracture of epiphysis (separation) (upper) of unspecified femur** MCC CC H5 HCC

√6th **S72.03** **Midcervical fracture of femur**

Transcervical fracture of femur NOS

4,6 √7th **S72.031** **Displaced midcervical fracture of right femur** MCC CC H5 HCC

4,6 √7th **S72.032** **Displaced midcervical fracture of left femur** MCC CC H5 HCC

4,6 √7th **S72.033** **Displaced midcervical fracture of unspecified femur** MCC CC H5 HCC

4,6 √7th **S72.034** **Nondisplaced midcervical fracture of right femur** MCC CC H5 HCC

4,6 √7th **S72.035** **Nondisplaced midcervical fracture of left femur** MCC CC H5 HCC

4,6 √7th **S72.036** **Nondisplaced midcervical fracture of unspecified femur** MCC CC H5 HCC

√6th **S72.04** **Fracture of base of neck of femur**

Cervicotrochanteric fracture of femur

4,6 √7th **S72.041** **Displaced fracture of base of neck of right femur** MCC CC H5 HCC

4,6 √7th **S72.042** **Displaced fracture of base of neck of left femur** MCC CC H5 HCC

4,6 √7th **S72.043** **Displaced fracture of base of neck of unspecified femur** MCC CC H5 HCC

4,6 √7th **S72.044** **Nondisplaced fracture of base of neck of right femur** MCC CC H5 HCC

4,6 √7th **S72.045** **Nondisplaced fracture of base of neck of left femur** MCC CC H5 HCC

4,6 √7th **S72.046** **Nondisplaced fracture of base of neck of unspecified femur** MCC CC H5 HCC

√6th **S72.05** **Unspecified fracture of head of femur**

Fracture of head of femur NOS

4,6 √7th **S72.051** **Unspecified fracture of head of right femur** MCC CC H5 HCC

4,6 √7th **S72.052** **Unspecified fracture of head of left femur** MCC CC H5 HCC

4,6 √7th **S72.059** **Unspecified fracture of head of unspecified femur** MCC CC H5 HCC

√6th **S72.06** **Articular fracture of head of femur**

4,6 √7th **S72.061** **Displaced articular fracture of head of right femur** MCC CC H5 HCC

4,6 √7th **S72.062** **Displaced articular fracture of head of left femur** MCC CC H5 HCC

4,6 √7th **S72.063** **Displaced articular fracture of head of unspecified femur** MCC CC H5 HCC

4,6 √7th **S72.064** **Nondisplaced articular fracture of head of right femur** MCC CC H5 HCC

4,6 √7th **S72.065** **Nondisplaced articular fracture of head of left femur** MCC CC H5 HCC

4,6 √7th **S72.066** **Nondisplaced articular fracture of head of unspecified femur** MCC CC H5 HCC

√6th **S72.09** **Other fracture of head and neck of femur**

4,6 √7th **S72.091** **Other fracture of head and neck of right femur** MCC CC H5 HCC

4,6 √7th **S72.092** **Other fracture of head and neck of left femur** MCC CC H5 HCC

4,6 √7th **S72.099** **Other fracture of head and neck of unspecified femur** MCC CC H5 HCC

√5th **S72.1** **Pertrochanteric fracture**

AHA: 2016,3Q,16

√6th **S72.10** **Unspecified trochanteric fracture of femur**

Fracture of trochanter NOS

4,6 √7th **S72.101** **Unspecified trochanteric fracture of right femur** MCC CC H5 HCC

4,6 √7th **S72.102** **Unspecified trochanteric fracture of left femur** MCC CC H5 HCC

4,6 √7th **S72.109** **Unspecified trochanteric fracture of unspecified femur** MCC CC H5 HCC

√6th **S72.11** **Fracture of greater trochanter of femur**

4,6 √7th **S72.111** **Displaced fracture of greater trochanter of right femur** MCC CC H5 HCC

4,6 √7th **S72.112** **Displaced fracture of greater trochanter of left femur** MCC CC H5 HCC

4,6 √7th **S72.113** **Displaced fracture of greater trochanter of unspecified femur** MCC CC H5 HCC

4,6 √7th **S72.114** **Nondisplaced fracture of greater trochanter of right femur** MCC CC H5 HCC

4,6 √7th **S72.115** **Nondisplaced fracture of greater trochanter of left femur** MCC CC H5 HCC

4,6 √7th **S72.116** **Nondisplaced fracture of greater trochanter of unspecified femur** MCC CC H5 HCC

√6th **S72.12** **Fracture of lesser trochanter of femur**

4,6 √7th **S72.121** **Displaced fracture of lesser trochanter of right femur** MCC CC H5 HCC

4,6 √7th **S72.122** **Displaced fracture of lesser trochanter of left femur** MCC CC H5 HCC

4,6 √7th **S72.123** **Displaced fracture of lesser trochanter of unspecified femur** MCC CC H5 HCC

4,6 √7th **S72.124** **Nondisplaced fracture of lesser trochanter of right femur** MCC CC H5 HCC

4,6 √7th **S72.125** **Nondisplaced fracture of lesser trochanter of left femur** MCC CC H5 HCC

4,6 √7th **S72.126** **Nondisplaced fracture of lesser trochanter of unspecified femur** MCC CC H5 HCC

√6th **S72.13** **Apophyseal fracture of femur**

EXCLUDES 1   chronic (nontraumatic) slipped upper femoral epiphysis (M93.0-)

4,6 √7th **S72.131** **Displaced apophyseal fracture of right femur** MCC CC H5 HCC

4,6 √7th **S72.132** **Displaced apophyseal fracture of left femur** MCC CC H5 HCC

4,6 √7th **S72.133** **Displaced apophyseal fracture of unspecified femur** MCC CC H5 HCC

4,6 √7th **S72.134** **Nondisplaced apophyseal fracture of right femur** MCC CC H5 HCC

4,6 √7th **S72.135** **Nondisplaced apophyseal fracture of left femur** MCC CC H5 HCC

4,6 √7th **S72.136** **Nondisplaced apophyseal fracture of unspecified femur** MCC CC H5 HCC

√6th **S72.14** **Intertrochanteric fracture of femur**

4,6 √7th **S72.141** **Displaced intertrochanteric fracture of right femur** MCC CC H5 HCC

4,6 √7th **S72.142** **Displaced intertrochanteric fracture of left femur** MCC CC H5 HCC

4,6 √7th **S72.143** **Displaced intertrochanteric fracture of unspecified femur** MCC CC H5 HCC

4,6 √7th **S72.144** **Nondisplaced intertrochanteric fracture of right femur** MCC CC H5 HCC

4,6 √7th **S72.145** **Nondisplaced intertrochanteric fracture of left femur** MCC CC H5 HCC

4,6 √7th **S72.146** **Nondisplaced intertrochanteric fracture of unspecified femur** MCC CC H5 HCC

√5th **S72.2** Subtrochanteric **fracture of femur**

4,6 √x7th **S72.21** Displaced subtrochanteric fracture of right femur   MCC CC H5 HCC

4,6 √x7th **S72.22** Displaced subtrochanteric fracture of left femur   MCC CC H5 HCC

4,6 √x7th **S72.23** Displaced subtrochanteric fracture of unspecified femur   MCC CC H5 HCC

4,6 √x7th **S72.24** Nondisplaced subtrochanteric fracture of right femur   MCC CC H5 HCC

4,6 √x7th **S72.25** Nondisplaced subtrochanteric fracture of left femur   MCC CC H5 HCC

4,6 √x7th **S72.26** Nondisplaced subtrochanteric fracture of unspecified femur   MCC CC H5 HCC

√5th **S72.3** Fracture of shaft of femur

√6th **S72.30** Unspecified fracture of shaft of femur

4,6 √7th **S72.301** Unspecified fracture of shaft of right femur   MCC CC H5 HCC

4,6 √7th **S72.302** Unspecified fracture of shaft of left femur   MCC CC H5 HCC

4,6 √7th **S72.309** Unspecified fracture of shaft of unspecified femur   MCC CC H5 HCC

√6th **S72.32** Transverse fracture of shaft of femur

4,6 √7th **S72.321** Displaced transverse fracture of shaft of right femur   MCC CC H5 HCC

4,6 √7th **S72.322** Displaced transverse fracture of shaft of left femur   MCC CC H5 HCC

4,6 √7th **S72.323** Displaced transverse fracture of shaft of unspecified femur   MCC CC H5 HCC

4,6 √7th **S72.324** Nondisplaced transverse fracture of shaft of right femur   MCC CC H5 HCC

4,6 √7th **S72.325** Nondisplaced transverse fracture of shaft of left femur   MCC CC H5 HCC

4,6 √7th **S72.326** Nondisplaced transverse fracture of shaft of unspecified femur   MCC CC H5 HCC

√6th **S72.33** Oblique fracture of shaft of femur

4,6 √7th **S72.331** Displaced oblique fracture of shaft of right femur   MCC CC H5 HCC

4,6 √7th **S72.332** Displaced oblique fracture of shaft of left femur   MCC CC H5 HCC

4,6 √7th **S72.333** Displaced oblique fracture of shaft of unspecified femur   MCC CC H5 HCC

4,6 √7th **S72.334** Nondisplaced oblique fracture of shaft of right femur   MCC CC H5 HCC

4,6 √7th **S72.335** Nondisplaced oblique fracture of shaft of left femur   MCC CC H5 HCC

4,6 √7th **S72.336** Nondisplaced oblique fracture of shaft of unspecified femur   MCC CC H5 HCC

√6th **S72.34** Spiral fracture of shaft of femur

4,6 √7th **S72.341** Displaced spiral fracture of shaft of right femur   MCC CC H5 HCC

4,6 √7th **S72.342** Displaced spiral fracture of shaft of left femur   MCC CC H5 HCC

4,6 √7th **S72.343** Displaced spiral fracture of shaft of unspecified femur   MCC CC H5 HCC

4,6 √7th **S72.344** Nondisplaced spiral fracture of shaft of right femur   MCC CC H5 HCC

4,6 √7th **S72.345** Nondisplaced spiral fracture of shaft of left femur   MCC CC H5 HCC

4,6 √7th **S72.346** Nondisplaced spiral fracture of shaft of unspecified femur   MCC CC H5 HCC

√6th **S72.35** Comminuted fracture of shaft of femur

4,6 √7th **S72.351** Displaced comminuted fracture of shaft of right femur   MCC CC H5 HCC

4,6 √7th **S72.352** Displaced comminuted fracture of shaft of left femur   MCC CC H5 HCC

4,6 √7th **S72.353** Displaced comminuted fracture of shaft of unspecified femur   MCC CC H5 HCC

4,6 √7th **S72.354** Nondisplaced comminuted fracture of shaft of right femur   MCC CC H5 HCC

4,6 √7th **S72.355** Nondisplaced comminuted fracture of shaft of left femur   MCC CC H5 HCC

4,6 √7th **S72.356** Nondisplaced comminuted fracture of shaft of unspecified femur   MCC CC H5 HCC

√6th **S72.36** Segmental fracture of shaft of femur

4,6 √7th **S72.361** Displaced segmental fracture of shaft of right femur   MCC CC H5 HCC

4,6 √7th **S72.362** Displaced segmental fracture of shaft of left femur   MCC CC H5 HCC

4,6 √7th **S72.363** Displaced segmental fracture of shaft of unspecified femur   MCC CC H5 HCC

4,6 √7th **S72.364** Nondisplaced segmental fracture of shaft of right femur   MCC CC H5 HCC

4,6 √7th **S72.365** Nondisplaced segmental fracture of shaft of left femur   MCC CC H5 HCC

4,6 √7th **S72.366** Nondisplaced segmental fracture of shaft of unspecified femur   MCC CC H5 HCC

√6th **S72.39** Other fracture of shaft of femur

4,6 √7th **S72.391** Other fracture of shaft of right femur   MCC CC H5 HCC

4,6 √7th **S72.392** Other fracture of shaft of left femur   MCC CC H5 HCC

4,6 √7th **S72.399** Other fracture of shaft of unspecified femur   MCC CC H5 HCC

√5th **S72.4** Fracture of lower end of femur

Fracture of distal end of femur

EXCLUDES 2   fracture of shaft of femur (S72.3-)

physeal fracture of lower end of femur (S79.1-)

AHA: 2016,4Q,42

√6th **S72.40** Unspecified fracture of lower end of femur

AHA: 2018,1Q,21; 2016,4Q,42

2,3,6 √7th **S72.401** Unspecified fracture of lower end of right femur   MCC CC H5 HCC

2,3,6 √7th **S72.402** Unspecified fracture of lower end of left femur   MCC CC H5 HCC

2,3,6 √7th **S72.409** Unspecified fracture of lower end of unspecified femur   MCC CC H5 HCC

√6th **S72.41** Unspecified condyle fracture of lower end of femur

Condyle fracture of femur NOS

2,3,6 √7th **S72.411** Displaced unspecified condyle fracture of lower end of right femur   MCC CC H5 HCC

2,3,6 √7th **S72.412** Displaced unspecified condyle fracture of lower end of left femur   MCC CC H5 HCC

2,3,6 √7th **S72.413** Displaced unspecified condyle fracture of lower end of unspecified femur   MCC CC H5 HCC

2,3,6 √7th **S72.414** Nondisplaced unspecified condyle fracture of lower end of right femur   MCC CC H5 HCC

2,3,6 √7th **S72.415** Nondisplaced unspecified condyle fracture of lower end of left femur   MCC CC H5 HCC

2,3,6 √7th **S72.416** Nondisplaced unspecified condyle fracture of lower end of unspecified femur   MCC CC H5 HCC

√6th **S72.42** Fracture of lateral condyle of femur

2,3,6 √7th **S72.421** Displaced fracture of lateral condyle of right femur   MCC CC H5 HCC

2,3,6 √7th **S72.422** Displaced fracture of lateral condyle of left femur   MCC CC H5 HCC

2,3,6 √7th **S72.423** Displaced fracture of lateral condyle of unspecified femur   MCC CC H5 HCC

2,3,6 √7th **S72.424** Nondisplaced fracture of lateral condyle of right femur   MCC CC H5 HCC

2,3,6 √7th **S72.425** Nondisplaced fracture of lateral condyle of left femur   MCC CC H5 HCC

2,3,6 √7th **S72.426** Nondisplaced fracture of lateral condyle of unspecified femur   MCC CC H5 HCC

√6th **S72.43** Fracture of medial condyle of femur

2,3,6 √7th **S72.431** Displaced fracture of medial condyle of right femur   MCC CC H5 HCC

2,3,6 √7th **S72.432** Displaced fracture of medial condyle of left femur   MCC CC H5 HCC

2,3,6 √7th **S72.433** Displaced fracture of medial condyle of unspecified femur   MCC CC H5 HCC

2,3,6 √7th **S72.434** Nondisplaced fracture of medial condyle of right femur   MCC CC H5 HCC

2,3,6 √7th **S72.435** Nondisplaced fracture of medial condyle of left femur   MCC CC H5 HCC

2,3,6 √7th **S72.436** Nondisplaced fracture of medial condyle of unspecified femur   MCC CC H5 HCC

✔ Additional Character Required   √x7th Placeholder   Questionable PDx   Manifestation   Unspecified Dx   UPD Unacceptable PDx   H1-H14 HAC   HCC CMS-HCC Dx   HIV HIV Dx

ICD-10-CM 2022   1059

√6th **S72.44** **Fracture of** lower epiphysis (separation) of femur

    EXCLUDES 1   *Salter-Harris Type I physeal fracture of lower end of femur (S79.11-)*

2,3,6 √7th **S72.441** Displaced **fracture of lower epiphysis (separation) of** right **femur** `MCC` `CC` `H5` `HCC`

2,3,6 √7th **S72.442** Displaced **fracture of lower epiphysis (separation) of** left **femur** `MCC` `CC` `H5` `HCC`

2,3,6 √7th **S72.443** Displaced **fracture of lower epiphysis (separation) of unspecified femur** `MCC` `CC` `H5` `HCC`

2,3,6 √7th **S72.444** Nondisplaced **fracture of lower epiphysis (separation) of** right **femur** `MCC` `CC` `H5` `HCC`

2,3,6 √7th **S72.445** Nondisplaced **fracture of lower epiphysis (separation) of** left **femur** `MCC` `CC` `H5` `HCC`

2,3,6 √7th **S72.446** Nondisplaced **fracture of lower epiphysis (separation) of unspecified femur** `MCC` `CC` `H5` `HCC`

√6th **S72.45** Supracondylar **fracture** without intracondylar extension of lower end of femur

    Supracondylar fracture of lower end of femur NOS

    EXCLUDES 1   *supracondylar fracture with intracondylar extension of lower end of femur (S72.46-)*

2,3,6 √7th **S72.451** Displaced **supracondylar fracture without intracondylar extension of lower end of** right **femur** `MCC` `CC` `H5` `HCC`

2,3,6 √7th **S72.452** Displaced **supracondylar fracture without intracondylar extension of lower end of** left **femur** `MCC` `CC` `H5` `HCC`

2,3,6 √7th **S72.453** Displaced **supracondylar fracture without intracondylar extension of lower end of unspecified femur** `MCC` `CC` `H5` `HCC`

2,3,6 √7th **S72.454** Nondisplaced **supracondylar fracture without intracondylar extension of lower end of** right **femur** `MCC` `CC` `H5` `HCC`

2,3,6 √7th **S72.455** Nondisplaced **supracondylar fracture without intracondylar extension of lower end of** left **femur** `MCC` `CC` `H5` `HCC`

2,3,6 √7th **S72.456** Nondisplaced **supracondylar fracture without intracondylar extension of lower end of unspecified femur** `MCC` `CC` `H5` `HCC`

√6th **S72.46** Supracondylar **fracture** with intracondylar extension of lower end of femur

    EXCLUDES 1   *supracondylar fracture without intracondylar extension of lower end of femur (S72.45-)*

2,3,6 √7th **S72.461** Displaced **supracondylar fracture with intracondylar extension of lower end of** right **femur** `MCC` `CC` `H5` `HCC`

2,3,6 √7th **S72.462** Displaced **supracondylar fracture with intracondylar extension of lower end of** left **femur** `MCC` `CC` `H5` `HCC`

2,3,6 √7th **S72.463** Displaced **supracondylar fracture with intracondylar extension of lower end of unspecified femur** `MCC` `CC` `H5` `HCC`

2,3,6 √7th **S72.464** Nondisplaced **supracondylar fracture with intracondylar extension of lower end of** right **femur** `MCC` `CC` `H5` `HCC`

2,3,6 √7th **S72.465** Nondisplaced **supracondylar fracture with intracondylar extension of lower end of** left **femur** `MCC` `CC` `H5` `HCC`

2,3,6 √7th **S72.466** Nondisplaced **supracondylar fracture with intracondylar extension of lower end of unspecified femur** `MCC` `CC` `H5` `HCC`

√6th **S72.47** Torus **fracture of lower end of femur**

The appropriate 7th character is to be added to all codes in subcategory S72.47.
A   initial encounter for closed fracture
D   subsequent encounter for fracture with routine healing
G   subsequent encounter for fracture with delayed healing
K   subsequent encounter for fracture with nonunion
P   subsequent encounter for fracture with malunion
S   sequela

3,6 √7th **S72.471** **Torus fracture of lower end of** right **femur** `CC` `H5` `HCC`

3,6 √7th **S72.472** **Torus fracture of lower end of** left **femur** `CC` `H5` `HCC`

3,6 √7th **S72.479** **Torus fracture of lower end of unspecified femur** `CC` `H5` `HCC`

√6th **S72.49** Other **fracture of lower end of femur**

2,3,6 √7th **S72.491** **Other fracture of lower end of** right **femur** `MCC` `CC` `H5` `HCC`

2,3,6 √7th **S72.492** **Other fracture of lower end of** left **femur** `MCC` `CC` `H5` `HCC`

2,3,6 √7th **S72.499** **Other fracture of lower end of unspecified femur** `MCC` `CC` `H5` `HCC`

√5th **S72.8** Other fracture of femur

√6th **S72.8X** Other **fracture of femur**

4,6 √7th **S72.8X1** **Other fracture of** right **femur** `MCC` `CC` `H5` `HCC`

4,6 √7th **S72.8X2** **Other fracture of** left **femur** `MCC` `CC` `H5` `HCC`

4,6 √7th **S72.8X9** **Other fracture of unspecified femur** `MCC` `CC` `H5` `HCC`

√5th **S72.9** **Unspecified fracture of femur**

    Fracture of thigh NOS
    Fracture of upper leg NOS

    EXCLUDES 1   *fracture of hip NOS (S72.00-, S72.01-)*

4,6 √x7th **S72.90** **Unspecified fracture of unspecified femur** `MCC` `CC` `H5` `HCC`

    AHA: 2012,4Q,93

4,6 √x7th **S72.91** **Unspecified fracture of** right **femur** `MCC` `CC` `H5` `HCC`

4,6 √x7th **S72.92** **Unspecified fracture of** left **femur** `MCC` `CC` `H5` `HCC`

√4th **S73** **Dislocation and sprain of joint and ligaments of hip**

    `INCLUDES`   avulsion of joint or ligament of hip
    laceration of cartilage, joint or ligament of hip
    sprain of cartilage, joint or ligament of hip
    traumatic hemarthrosis of joint or ligament of hip
    traumatic rupture of joint or ligament of hip
    traumatic subluxation of joint or ligament of hip
    traumatic tear of joint or ligament of hip

Code also any associated open wound

    EXCLUDES 2   *strain of muscle, fascia and tendon of hip and thigh (S76.-)*

The appropriate 7th character is to be added to each code from category S73.
A   initial encounter
D   subsequent encounter
S   sequela

√5th **S73.0** **Subluxation and dislocation of** hip

    EXCLUDES 2   *dislocation and subluxation of hip prosthesis (T84.020, T84.021)*

√6th **S73.00** **Unspecified subluxation and dislocation of hip**

    Dislocation of hip NOS
    Subluxation of hip NOS

6 √7th **S73.001** Unspecified **subluxation of** right **hip** `CC` `H5` `HCC`

6 √7th **S73.002** Unspecified **subluxation of** left **hip** `CC` `H5` `HCC`

6 √7th **S73.003** Unspecified **subluxation of unspecified hip** `CC` `H5` `HCC`

6 √7th **S73.004** Unspecified **dislocation of** right **hip** `CC` `H5` `HCC`

6 √7th **S73.005** Unspecified **dislocation of** left **hip** `CC` `H5` `HCC`

6 ✓7th **S73.006** Unspecified dislocation of unspecified hip   CC H5 HCC

✓6th **S73.01** Posterior subluxation and dislocation of hip

    6 ✓7th **S73.011** Posterior subluxation of right hip   CC H5 HCC

    6 ✓7th **S73.012** Posterior subluxation of left hip   CC H5 HCC

    6 ✓7th **S73.013** Posterior subluxation of unspecified hip   CC H5 HCC

    6 ✓7th **S73.014** Posterior dislocation of right hip   CC H5 HCC

    6 ✓7th **S73.015** Posterior dislocation of left hip   CC H5 HCC

    6 ✓7th **S73.016** Posterior dislocation of unspecified hip   CC H5 HCC

✓6th **S73.02** Obturator subluxation and dislocation of hip

    6 ✓7th **S73.021** Obturator subluxation of right hip   CC H5 HCC

    6 ✓7th **S73.022** Obturator subluxation of left hip   CC H5 HCC

    6 ✓7th **S73.023** Obturator subluxation of unspecified hip   CC H5 HCC

    6 ✓7th **S73.024** Obturator dislocation of right hip   CC H5 HCC

    6 ✓7th **S73.025** Obturator dislocation of left hip   CC H5 HCC

    6 ✓7th **S73.026** Obturator dislocation of unspecified hip   CC H5 HCC

✓6th **S73.03** Other anterior subluxation and dislocation of hip

    6 ✓7th **S73.031** Other anterior subluxation of right hip   CC H5 HCC

    6 ✓7th **S73.032** Other anterior subluxation of left hip   CC H5 HCC

    6 ✓7th **S73.033** Other anterior subluxation of unspecified hip   CC H5 HCC

    6 ✓7th **S73.034** Other anterior dislocation of right hip   CC H5 HCC

    6 ✓7th **S73.035** Other anterior dislocation of left hip   CC H5 HCC

    6 ✓7th **S73.036** Other anterior dislocation of unspecified hip   CC H5 HCC

✓6th **S73.04** Central subluxation and dislocation of hip

    6 ✓7th **S73.041** Central subluxation of right hip   CC H5 HCC

    6 ✓7th **S73.042** Central subluxation of left hip   CC H5 HCC

    6 ✓7th **S73.043** Central subluxation of unspecified hip   CC H5 HCC

    6 ✓7th **S73.044** Central dislocation of right hip   CC H5 HCC

    6 ✓7th **S73.045** Central dislocation of left hip   CC H5 HCC

    6 ✓7th **S73.046** Central dislocation of unspecified hip   CC H5 HCC

✓5th **S73.1** Sprain of hip

    AHA: 2014,4Q,25

    ✓6th **S73.10** Unspecified sprain of hip

       ✓7th **S73.101** Unspecified sprain of right hip

       ✓7th **S73.102** Unspecified sprain of left hip

       ✓7th **S73.109** Unspecified sprain of unspecified hip

    ✓6th **S73.11** Iliofemoral ligament sprain of hip

       ✓7th **S73.111** Iliofemoral ligament sprain of right hip

       ✓7th **S73.112** Iliofemoral ligament sprain of left hip

       ✓7th **S73.119** Iliofemoral ligament sprain of unspecified hip

    ✓6th **S73.12** Ischiocapsular (ligament) sprain of hip

       ✓7th **S73.121** Ischiocapsular ligament sprain of right hip

       ✓7th **S73.122** Ischiocapsular ligament sprain of left hip

       ✓7th **S73.129** Ischiocapsular ligament sprain of unspecified hip

    ✓6th **S73.19** Other sprain of hip

       ✓7th **S73.191** Other sprain of right hip

       ✓7th **S73.192** Other sprain of left hip

       ✓7th **S73.199** Other sprain of unspecified hip

✓4th **S74** Injury of nerves at hip and thigh level

Code also any associated open wound (S71.-)

EXCLUDES 2   *injury of nerves at ankle and foot level (S94.-)*

           injury of nerves at lower leg level (S84.-)

> The appropriate 7th character is to be added to each code from category S74.
> A   initial encounter
> D   subsequent encounter
> S   sequela

✓5th **S74.0** Injury of sciatic nerve at hip and thigh level

    ✓x7th **S74.00** Injury of sciatic nerve at hip and thigh level, unspecified leg

    ✓x7th **S74.01** Injury of sciatic nerve at hip and thigh level, right leg

    ✓x7th **S74.02** Injury of sciatic nerve at hip and thigh level, left leg

✓5th **S74.1** Injury of femoral nerve at hip and thigh level

    ✓x7th **S74.10** Injury of femoral nerve at hip and thigh level, unspecified leg

    ✓x7th **S74.11** Injury of femoral nerve at hip and thigh level, right leg

    ✓x7th **S74.12** Injury of femoral nerve at hip and thigh level, left leg

✓5th **S74.2** Injury of cutaneous sensory nerve at hip and thigh level

    ✓x7th **S74.20** Injury of cutaneous sensory nerve at hip and thigh level, unspecified leg

    ✓x7th **S74.21** Injury of cutaneous sensory nerve at hip and high level, right leg

    ✓x7th **S74.22** Injury of cutaneous sensory nerve at hip and thigh level, left leg

✓5th **S74.8** Injury of other nerves at hip and thigh level

    ✓6th **S74.8X** Injury of other nerves at hip and thigh level

       ✓7th **S74.8X1** Injury of other nerves at hip and thigh level, right leg

       ✓7th **S74.8X2** Injury of other nerves at hip and thigh level, left leg

       ✓7th **S74.8X9** Injury of other nerves at hip and thigh level, unspecified leg

✓5th **S74.9** Injury of unspecified nerve at hip and thigh level

    ✓x7th **S74.90** Injury of unspecified nerve at hip and thigh level, unspecified leg

    ✓x7th **S74.91** Injury of unspecified nerve at hip and thigh level, right leg

    ✓x7th **S74.92** Injury of unspecified nerve at hip and thigh level, left leg

✓4th **S75** Injury of blood vessels at hip and thigh level

Code also any associated open wound (S71.-)

EXCLUDES 2   *injury of blood vessels at lower leg level (S85.-)*

           injury of popliteal artery (S85.0)

> The appropriate 7th character is to be added to each code from category S75.
> A   initial encounter
> D   subsequent encounter
> S   sequela

✓5th **S75.0** Injury of femoral artery

    ✓6th **S75.00** Unspecified injury of femoral artery

       ✓7th **S75.001** Unspecified injury of femoral artery, right leg   MCC

       ✓7th **S75.002** Unspecified injury of femoral artery, left leg   MCC

       ✓7th **S75.009** Unspecified injury of femoral artery, unspecified leg   MCC

    ✓6th **S75.01** Minor laceration of femoral artery

       Incomplete transection of femoral artery

       Laceration of femoral artery NOS

       Superficial laceration of femoral artery

       ✓7th **S75.011** Minor laceration of femoral artery, right leg   MCC

       ✓7th **S75.012** Minor laceration of femoral artery, left leg   MCC

       ✓7th **S75.019** Minor laceration of femoral artery, unspecified leg   MCC

    ✓6th **S75.02** Major laceration of femoral artery

       Complete transection of femoral artery

       Traumatic rupture of femoral artery

       ✓7th **S75.021** Major laceration of femoral artery, right leg   MCC

✓ Additional Character Required   ✓x7th Placeholder   Questionable PDx   Manifestation   Unspecified Dx   UPD Unacceptable PDx   H1 - H14 HAC   HCC CMS-HCC Dx   HIV HIV Dx

ICD-10-CM 2022   **1061**

✓7ᵗʰ **S75.022** Major laceration of femoral artery, left leg   `MCC`

✓7ᵗʰ **S75.029** Major laceration of femoral artery, unspecified leg   `MCC`

✓6ᵗʰ **S75.09** Other specified injury of femoral artery

     ✓7ᵗʰ **S75.091** Other specified injury of femoral artery, right leg   `MCC`

     ✓7ᵗʰ **S75.092** Other specified injury of femoral artery, left leg   `MCC`

     ✓7ᵗʰ **S75.099** Other specified injury of femoral artery, unspecified leg   `MCC`

✓5ᵗʰ **S75.1** Injury of femoral vein at hip and thigh level

   ✓6ᵗʰ **S75.10** Unspecified injury of femoral vein at hip and thigh level

     ✓7ᵗʰ **S75.101** Unspecified injury of femoral vein at hip and thigh level, right leg   `MCC`

     ✓7ᵗʰ **S75.102** Unspecified injury of femoral vein at hip and thigh level, left leg   `MCC`

     ✓7ᵗʰ **S75.109** Unspecified injury of femoral vein at hip and thigh level, unspecified leg   `MCC`

   ✓6ᵗʰ **S75.11** Minor laceration of femoral vein at hip and thigh level

     Incomplete transection of femoral vein at hip and thigh level
     Laceration of femoral vein at hip and thigh level NOS
     Superficial laceration of femoral vein at hip and thigh level

     ✓7ᵗʰ **S75.111** Minor laceration of femoral vein at hip and thigh level, right leg   `MCC`

     ✓7ᵗʰ **S75.112** Minor laceration of femoral vein at hip and thigh level, left leg   `MCC`

     ✓7ᵗʰ **S75.119** Minor laceration of femoral vein at hip and thigh level, unspecified leg   `MCC`

   ✓6ᵗʰ **S75.12** Major laceration of femoral vein at hip and thigh level

     Complete transection of femoral vein at hip and thigh level
     Traumatic rupture of femoral vein at hip and thigh level

     ✓7ᵗʰ **S75.121** Major laceration of femoral vein at hip and thigh level, right leg   `MCC`

     ✓7ᵗʰ **S75.122** Major laceration of femoral vein at hip and thigh level, left leg   `MCC`

     ✓7ᵗʰ **S75.129** Major laceration of femoral vein at hip and thigh level, unspecified leg   `MCC`

   ✓6ᵗʰ **S75.19** Other specified injury of femoral vein at hip and thigh level

     ✓7ᵗʰ **S75.191** Other specified injury of femoral vein at hip and thigh level, right leg   `MCC`

     ✓7ᵗʰ **S75.192** Other specified injury of femoral vein at hip and thigh level, left leg   `MCC`

     ✓7ᵗʰ **S75.199** Other specified injury of femoral vein at hip and thigh level, unspecified leg   `MCC`

✓5ᵗʰ **S75.2** Injury of greater saphenous vein at hip and thigh level

   `EXCLUDES 1`   greater saphenous vein NOS (S85.3)

   ✓6ᵗʰ **S75.20** Unspecified injury of greater saphenous vein at hip and thigh level

     ✓7ᵗʰ **S75.201** Unspecified injury of greater saphenous vein at hip and thigh level, right leg   `CC`

     ✓7ᵗʰ **S75.202** Unspecified injury of greater saphenous vein at hip and thigh level, left leg   `CC`

     ✓7ᵗʰ **S75.209** Unspecified injury of greater saphenous vein at hip and thigh level, unspecified leg   `CC`

   ✓6ᵗʰ **S75.21** Minor laceration of greater saphenous vein at hip and thigh level

     Incomplete transection of greater saphenous vein at hip and thigh level
     Laceration of greater saphenous vein at hip and thigh level NOS
     Superficial laceration of greater saphenous vein at hip and thigh level

     ✓7ᵗʰ **S75.211** Minor laceration of greater saphenous vein at hip and thigh level, right leg   `CC`

     ✓7ᵗʰ **S75.212** Minor laceration of greater saphenous vein at hip and thigh level, left leg   `CC`

     ✓7ᵗʰ **S75.219** Minor laceration of greater saphenous vein at hip and thigh level, unspecified leg   `CC`

   ✓6ᵗʰ **S75.22** Major laceration of greater saphenous vein at hip and thigh level

     Complete transection of greater saphenous vein at hip and thigh level
     Traumatic rupture of greater saphenous vein at hip and thigh level

     ✓7ᵗʰ **S75.221** Major laceration of greater saphenous vein at hip and thigh level, right leg   `CC`

     ✓7ᵗʰ **S75.222** Major laceration of greater saphenous vein at hip and thigh level, left leg   `CC`

     ✓7ᵗʰ **S75.229** Major laceration of greater saphenous vein at hip and thigh level, unspecified leg   `CC`

   ✓6ᵗʰ **S75.29** Other specified injury of greater saphenous vein at hip and thigh level

     ✓7ᵗʰ **S75.291** Other specified injury of greater saphenous vein at hip and thigh level, right leg   `CC`

     ✓7ᵗʰ **S75.292** Other specified injury of greater saphenous vein at hip and thigh level, left leg   `CC`

     ✓7ᵗʰ **S75.299** Other specified injury of greater saphenous vein at hip and thigh level, unspecified leg   `CC`

✓5ᵗʰ **S75.8** Injury of other blood vessels at hip and thigh level

   ✓6ᵗʰ **S75.80** Unspecified injury of other blood vessels at hip and thigh level

     ✓7ᵗʰ **S75.801** Unspecified injury of other blood vessels at hip and thigh level, right leg   `CC`

     ✓7ᵗʰ **S75.802** Unspecified injury of other blood vessels at hip and thigh level, left leg   `CC`

     ✓7ᵗʰ **S75.809** Unspecified injury of other blood vessels at hip and thigh level, unspecified leg   `CC`

   ✓6ᵗʰ **S75.81** Laceration of other blood vessels at hip and thigh level

     ✓7ᵗʰ **S75.811** Laceration of other blood vessels at hip and thigh level, right leg   `CC`

     ✓7ᵗʰ **S75.812** Laceration of other blood vessels at hip and thigh level, left leg   `CC`

     ✓7ᵗʰ **S75.819** Laceration of other blood vessels at hip and thigh level, unspecified leg   `CC`

   ✓6ᵗʰ **S75.89** Other specified injury of other blood vessels at hip and thigh level

     ✓7ᵗʰ **S75.891** Other specified injury of other blood vessels at hip and thigh level, right leg   `CC`

     ✓7ᵗʰ **S75.892** Other specified injury of other blood vessels at hip and thigh level, left leg   `CC`

     ✓7ᵗʰ **S75.899** Other specified injury of other blood vessels at hip and thigh level, unspecified leg   `CC`

✓5ᵗʰ **S75.9** Injury of unspecified blood vessel at hip and thigh level

   ✓6ᵗʰ **S75.90** Unspecified injury of unspecified blood vessel at hip and thigh level

     ✓7ᵗʰ **S75.901** Unspecified injury of unspecified blood vessel at hip and thigh level, right leg   `CC`

     ✓7ᵗʰ **S75.902** Unspecified injury of unspecified blood vessel at hip and thigh level, left leg   `CC`

     ✓7ᵗʰ **S75.909** Unspecified injury of unspecified blood vessel at hip and thigh level, unspecified leg   `CC`

   ✓6ᵗʰ **S75.91** Laceration of unspecified blood vessel at hip and thigh level

     ✓7ᵗʰ **S75.911** Laceration of unspecified blood vessel at hip and thigh level, right leg   `CC`

     ✓7ᵗʰ **S75.912** Laceration of unspecified blood vessel at hip and thigh level, left leg   `CC`

     ✓7ᵗʰ **S75.919** Laceration of unspecified blood vessel at hip and thigh level, unspecified leg   `CC`

   ✓6ᵗʰ **S75.99** Other specified injury of unspecified blood vessel at hip and thigh level

     ✓7ᵗʰ **S75.991** Other specified injury of unspecified blood vessel at hip and thigh level, right leg   `CC`

`N` Newborn: 0   `P` Pediatric: 0-17   `M` Maternity: 9-64   `A` Adult: 15-124   `MCC` Major Complication/Comorbidity   `CC` Complication/Comorbidity   `SW` Severe Wound Dx

1062   ICD-10-CM 2022

   ☑7ᵗʰ **S75.992** **Other specified injury of unspecified blood vessel at hip and thigh level, left leg** `CC`

   ☑7ᵗʰ **S75.999** **Other specified injury of unspecified blood vessel at hip and thigh level, unspecified leg** `CC`

☑4ᵗʰ **S76** **Injury of muscle, fascia and tendon at hip and thigh level**

Code also any associated open wound (S71.-)

EXCLUDES 2   *injury of muscle, fascia and tendon at lower leg level (S86)*
           sprain of joint and ligament of hip (S73.1)

TIP: Refer to the Muscle/Tendon table at the beginning of this chapter.

The appropriate 7th character is to be added to each code from category S76.
A   initial encounter
D   subsequent encounter
S   sequela

☑5ᵗʰ **S76.0** **Injury of muscle, fascia and tendon of hip**

  ☑6ᵗʰ **S76.00** **Unspecified injury of muscle, fascia and tendon of hip**

    ☑7ᵗʰ **S76.001** **Unspecified injury of muscle, fascia and tendon of right hip**

    ☑7ᵗʰ **S76.002** **Unspecified injury of muscle, fascia and tendon of left hip**

    ☑7ᵗʰ **S76.009** **Unspecified injury of muscle, fascia and tendon of unspecified hip**

  ☑6ᵗʰ **S76.01** Strain of muscle, fascia and tendon of hip

    ☑7ᵗʰ **S76.011** **Strain of muscle, fascia and tendon of right hip**

    ☑7ᵗʰ **S76.012** **Strain of muscle, fascia and tendon of left hip**

    ☑7ᵗʰ **S76.019** **Strain of muscle, fascia and tendon of unspecified hip**

  ☑6ᵗʰ **S76.02** Laceration of muscle, fascia and tendon of hip

    ☑7ᵗʰ **S76.021** **Laceration of muscle, fascia and tendon of right hip** `CC`

    ☑7ᵗʰ **S76.022** **Laceration of muscle, fascia and tendon of left hip** `CC`

    ☑7ᵗʰ **S76.029** **Laceration of muscle, fascia and tendon of unspecified hip** `CC`

  ☑6ᵗʰ **S76.09** **Other specified injury of muscle, fascia and tendon of hip**

    ☑7ᵗʰ **S76.091** **Other specified injury of muscle, fascia and tendon of right hip**

    ☑7ᵗʰ **S76.092** **Other specified injury of muscle, fascia and tendon of left hip**

    ☑7ᵗʰ **S76.099** **Other specified injury of muscle, fascia and tendon of unspecified hip**

☑5ᵗʰ **S76.1** **Injury of quadriceps muscle, fascia and tendon**

Injury of patellar ligament (tendon)

  ☑6ᵗʰ **S76.10** **Unspecified injury of quadriceps muscle, fascia and tendon**

    ☑7ᵗʰ **S76.101** **Unspecified injury of right quadriceps muscle, fascia and tendon**

    ☑7ᵗʰ **S76.102** **Unspecified injury of left quadriceps muscle, fascia and tendon**

    ☑7ᵗʰ **S76.109** **Unspecified injury of unspecified quadriceps muscle, fascia and tendon**

  ☑6ᵗʰ **S76.11** Strain of quadriceps muscle, fascia and tendon

    ☑7ᵗʰ **S76.111** **Strain of right quadriceps muscle, fascia and tendon**

    ☑7ᵗʰ **S76.112** **Strain of left quadriceps muscle, fascia and tendon**

    ☑7ᵗʰ **S76.119** **Strain of unspecified quadriceps muscle, fascia and tendon**

  ☑6ᵗʰ **S76.12** Laceration of quadriceps muscle, fascia and tendon

    ☑7ᵗʰ **S76.121** **Laceration of right quadriceps muscle, fascia and tendon** `CC`

    ☑7ᵗʰ **S76.122** **Laceration of left quadriceps muscle, fascia and tendon** `CC`

    ☑7ᵗʰ **S76.129** **Laceration of unspecified quadriceps muscle, fascia and tendon** `CC`

  ☑6ᵗʰ **S76.19** **Other specified injury of quadriceps muscle, fascia and tendon**

    ☑7ᵗʰ **S76.191** **Other specified injury of right quadriceps muscle, fascia and tendon**

    ☑7ᵗʰ **S76.192** **Other specified injury of left quadriceps muscle, fascia and tendon**

    ☑7ᵗʰ **S76.199** **Other specified injury of unspecified quadriceps muscle, fascia and tendon**

☑5ᵗʰ **S76.2** **Injury of adductor muscle, fascia and tendon of thigh**

  ☑6ᵗʰ **S76.20** **Unspecified injury of adductor muscle, fascia and tendon of thigh**

    ☑7ᵗʰ **S76.201** **Unspecified injury of adductor muscle, fascia and tendon of right thigh**

    ☑7ᵗʰ **S76.202** **Unspecified injury of adductor muscle, fascia and tendon of left thigh**

    ☑7ᵗʰ **S76.209** **Unspecified injury of adductor muscle, fascia and tendon of unspecified thigh**

  ☑6ᵗʰ **S76.21** Strain of adductor muscle, fascia and tendon of thigh

    ☑7ᵗʰ **S76.211** **Strain of adductor muscle, fascia and tendon of right thigh**

    ☑7ᵗʰ **S76.212** **Strain of adductor muscle, fascia and tendon of left thigh**

    ☑7ᵗʰ **S76.219** **Strain of adductor muscle, fascia and tendon of unspecified thigh**

  ☑6ᵗʰ **S76.22** Laceration of adductor muscle, fascia and tendon of thigh

    ☑7ᵗʰ **S76.221** **Laceration of adductor muscle, fascia and tendon of right thigh** `CC`

    ☑7ᵗʰ **S76.222** **Laceration of adductor muscle, fascia and tendon of left thigh** `CC`

    ☑7ᵗʰ **S76.229** **Laceration of adductor muscle, fascia and tendon of unspecified thigh** `CC`

  ☑6ᵗʰ **S76.29** **Other injury of adductor muscle, fascia and tendon of thigh**

    ☑7ᵗʰ **S76.291** **Other injury of adductor muscle, fascia and tendon of right thigh**

    ☑7ᵗʰ **S76.292** **Other injury of adductor muscle, fascia and tendon of left thigh**

    ☑7ᵗʰ **S76.299** **Other injury of adductor muscle, fascia and tendon of unspecified thigh**

☑5ᵗʰ **S76.3** **Injury of muscle, fascia and tendon of the posterior muscle group at thigh level**

  ☑6ᵗʰ **S76.30** **Unspecified injury of muscle, fascia and tendon of the posterior muscle group at thigh level**

    ☑7ᵗʰ **S76.301** **Unspecified injury of muscle, fascia and tendon of the posterior muscle group at thigh level, right thigh**

    ☑7ᵗʰ **S76.302** **Unspecified injury of muscle, fascia and tendon of the posterior muscle group at thigh level, left thigh**

    ☑7ᵗʰ **S76.309** **Unspecified injury of muscle, fascia and tendon of the posterior muscle group at thigh level, unspecified thigh**

  ☑6ᵗʰ **S76.31** Strain of muscle, fascia and tendon of the posterior muscle group at thigh level

    ☑7ᵗʰ **S76.311** **Strain of muscle, fascia and tendon of the posterior muscle group at thigh level, right thigh**

    ☑7ᵗʰ **S76.312** **Strain of muscle, fascia and tendon of the posterior muscle group at thigh level, left thigh**

    ☑7ᵗʰ **S76.319** **Strain of muscle, fascia and tendon of the posterior muscle group at thigh level, unspecified thigh**

  ☑6ᵗʰ **S76.32** Laceration of muscle, fascia and tendon of the posterior muscle group at thigh level

    ☑7ᵗʰ **S76.321** **Laceration of muscle, fascia and tendon of the posterior muscle group at thigh level, right thigh** `CC`

    ☑7ᵗʰ **S76.322** **Laceration of muscle, fascia and tendon of the posterior muscle group at thigh level, left thigh** `CC`

    ☑7ᵗʰ **S76.329** **Laceration of muscle, fascia and tendon of the posterior muscle group at thigh level, unspecified thigh** `CC`

  ☑6ᵗʰ **S76.39** **Other specified injury of muscle, fascia and tendon of the posterior muscle group at thigh level**

    ☑7ᵗʰ **S76.391** **Other specified injury of muscle, fascia and tendon of the posterior muscle group at thigh level, right thigh**

    ☑7ᵗʰ **S76.392** **Other specified injury of muscle, fascia and tendon of the posterior muscle group at thigh level, left thigh**

    ☑7ᵗʰ **S76.399** **Other specified injury of muscle, fascia and tendon of the posterior muscle group at thigh level, unspecified thigh**

☑ Additional Character Required   ☑x7ᵗʰ Placeholder   Questionable PDx   Manifestation   Unspecified Dx   UPD Unacceptable PDx   H1-H14 HAC   HCC CMS-HCC Dx   HIV HIV Dx

ICD-10-CM 2022   1063

☑5ᵗʰ **S76.8** **Injury of other specified muscles, fascia and tendons at** thigh level

  ☑6ᵗʰ **S76.80** Unspecified injury of other specified muscles, fascia and tendons at thigh level

    ☑7ᵗʰ **S76.801** Unspecified injury of other specified muscles, fascia and tendons at thigh level, right thigh

    ☑7ᵗʰ **S76.802** Unspecified injury of other specified muscles, fascia and tendons at thigh level, left thigh

    ☑7ᵗʰ **S76.809** Unspecified injury of other specified muscles, fascia and tendons at thigh level, unspecified thigh

  ☑6ᵗʰ **S76.81** Strain of other specified muscles, fascia and tendons at thigh level

    ☑7ᵗʰ **S76.811** Strain of other specified muscles, fascia and tendons at thigh level, right thigh

    ☑7ᵗʰ **S76.812** Strain of other specified muscles, fascia and tendons at thigh level, left thigh

    ☑7ᵗʰ **S76.819** Strain of other specified muscles, fascia and tendons at thigh level, unspecified thigh

  ☑6ᵗʰ **S76.82** Laceration of other specified muscles, fascia and tendons at thigh level

    ☑7ᵗʰ **S76.821** Laceration of other specified muscles, fascia and tendons at thigh level, right thigh `CC`

    ☑7ᵗʰ **S76.822** Laceration of other specified muscles, fascia and tendons at thigh level, left thigh `CC`

    ☑7ᵗʰ **S76.829** Laceration of other specified muscles, fascia and tendons at thigh level, unspecified thigh `CC`

  ☑6ᵗʰ **S76.89** Other injury of other specified muscles, fascia and tendons at thigh level

    ☑7ᵗʰ **S76.891** Other injury of other specified muscles, fascia and tendons at thigh level, right thigh

    ☑7ᵗʰ **S76.892** Other injury of other specified muscles, fascia and tendons at thigh level, left thigh

    ☑7ᵗʰ **S76.899** Other injury of other specified muscles, fascia and tendons at thigh level, unspecified thigh

☑5ᵗʰ **S76.9** **Injury of unspecified muscles, fascia and tendons at** thigh level

  ☑6ᵗʰ **S76.90** Unspecified injury of unspecified muscles, fascia and tendons at thigh level

    ☑7ᵗʰ **S76.901** Unspecified injury of unspecified muscles, fascia and tendons at thigh level, right thigh

    ☑7ᵗʰ **S76.902** Unspecified injury of unspecified muscles, fascia and tendons at thigh level, left thigh

    ☑7ᵗʰ **S76.909** Unspecified injury of unspecified muscles, fascia and tendons at thigh level, unspecified thigh

  ☑6ᵗʰ **S76.91** Strain of unspecified muscles, fascia and tendons at thigh level

    ☑7ᵗʰ **S76.911** Strain of unspecified muscles, fascia and tendons at thigh level, right thigh

    ☑7ᵗʰ **S76.912** Strain of unspecified muscles, fascia and tendons at thigh level, left thigh

    ☑7ᵗʰ **S76.919** Strain of unspecified muscles, fascia and tendons at thigh level, unspecified thigh

  ☑6ᵗʰ **S76.92** Laceration of unspecified muscles, fascia and tendons at thigh level

    ☑7ᵗʰ **S76.921** Laceration of unspecified muscles, fascia and tendons at thigh level, right thigh `CC`

    ☑7ᵗʰ **S76.922** Laceration of unspecified muscles, fascia and tendons at thigh level, left thigh `CC`

    ☑7ᵗʰ **S76.929** Laceration of unspecified muscles, fascia and tendons at thigh level, unspecified thigh `CC`

  ☑6ᵗʰ **S76.99** Other specified injury of unspecified muscles, fascia and tendons at thigh level

    ☑7ᵗʰ **S76.991** Other specified injury of unspecified muscles, fascia and tendons at thigh level, right thigh

    ☑7ᵗʰ **S76.992** Other specified injury of unspecified muscles, fascia and tendons at thigh level, left thigh

    ☑7ᵗʰ **S76.999** Other specified injury of unspecified muscles, fascia and tendons at thigh level, unspecified thigh

☑4ᵗʰ **S77** **Crushing injury** of hip and thigh

  Use additional code(s) for all associated injuries

  EXCLUDES 2   *crushing injury of ankle and foot (S97.-)*
                crushing injury of lower leg (S87.-)

  The appropriate 7th character is to be added to each code from category S77.
  A   initial encounter
  D   subsequent encounter
  S   sequela

  ☑5ᵗʰ **S77.0** Crushing injury of hip

    ☑x7ᵗʰ **S77.00** Crushing injury of unspecified hip `CC` `H5`

    ☑x7ᵗʰ **S77.01** Crushing injury of right hip `CC` `H5`

    ☑x7ᵗʰ **S77.02** Crushing injury of left hip `CC` `H5`

  ☑5ᵗʰ **S77.1** Crushing injury of thigh

    ☑x7ᵗʰ **S77.10** Crushing injury of unspecified thigh `CC` `H5`

    ☑x7ᵗʰ **S77.11** Crushing injury of right thigh `CC` `H5`

    ☑x7ᵗʰ **S77.12** Crushing injury of left thigh `CC` `H5`

  ☑5ᵗʰ **S77.2** Crushing injury of hip with thigh

    ☑x7ᵗʰ **S77.20** Crushing injury of unspecified hip with thigh

    ☑x7ᵗʰ **S77.21** Crushing injury of right hip with thigh

    ☑x7ᵗʰ **S77.22** Crushing injury of left hip with thigh

☑4ᵗʰ **S78** **Traumatic amputation of hip and thigh**

  An amputation not identified as partial or complete should be coded to complete

  EXCLUDES 1   *traumatic amputation of knee (S88.0-)*

  The appropriate 7th character is to be added to each code from category S78.
  A   initial encounter
  D   subsequent encounter
  S   sequela

  ☑5ᵗʰ **S78.0** Traumatic amputation at hip joint

    ☑6ᵗʰ **S78.01** Complete traumatic amputation at hip joint

      ☑7ᵗʰ **S78.011** Complete traumatic amputation at right hip joint `CC` `MCC`

      ☑7ᵗʰ **S78.012** Complete traumatic amputation at left hip joint `CC` `MCC`

      ☑7ᵗʰ **S78.019** Complete traumatic amputation at unspecified hip joint `CC` `MCC`

    ☑6ᵗʰ **S78.02** Partial traumatic amputation at hip joint

      ☑7ᵗʰ **S78.021** Partial traumatic amputation at right hip joint `CC` `MCC`

      ☑7ᵗʰ **S78.022** Partial traumatic amputation at left hip joint `CC` `MCC`

      ☑7ᵗʰ **S78.029** Partial traumatic amputation at unspecified hip joint `CC` `MCC`

  ☑5ᵗʰ **S78.1** Traumatic amputation at level between hip and knee

    EXCLUDES 1   *traumatic amputation of knee (S88.0-)*

    ☑6ᵗʰ **S78.11** Complete traumatic amputation at level between hip and knee

      ☑7ᵗʰ **S78.111** Complete traumatic amputation at level between right hip and knee `CC` `MCC`

      ☑7ᵗʰ **S78.112** Complete traumatic amputation at level between left hip and knee `CC` `MCC`

      ☑7ᵗʰ **S78.119** Complete traumatic amputation at level between unspecified hip and knee `CC` `MCC`

    ☑6ᵗʰ **S78.12** Partial traumatic amputation at level between hip and knee

      ☑7ᵗʰ **S78.121** Partial traumatic amputation at level between right hip and knee `CC` `MCC`

      ☑7ᵗʰ **S78.122** Partial traumatic amputation at level between left hip and knee `CC` `MCC`

      ☑7ᵗʰ **S78.129** Partial traumatic amputation at level between unspecified hip and knee `CC` `MCC`

  ☑5ᵗʰ **S78.9** Traumatic amputation of hip and thigh, level unspecified

    ☑6ᵗʰ **S78.91** Complete traumatic amputation of hip and thigh, level unspecified

      ☑7ᵗʰ **S78.911** Complete traumatic amputation of right hip and thigh, level unspecified `CC` `MCC`

`N` Newborn: 0   `P` Pediatric: 0-17   `M` Maternity: 9-64   `A` Adult: 15-124   `MCC` Major Complication/Comorbidity   `CC` Complication/Comorbidity   `SW` Severe Wound Dx

1064   ICD-10-CM 2022

√7ᵗʰ **S78.912** Complete traumatic amputation of left hip and thigh, level unspecified `CC` `HCC`

√7ᵗʰ **S78.919** Complete traumatic amputation of unspecified hip and thigh, level unspecified `CC` `HCC`

√6ᵗʰ **S78.92** Partial traumatic amputation of hip and thigh, level unspecified

√7ᵗʰ **S78.921** Partial traumatic amputation of right hip and thigh, level unspecified `CC` `HCC`

√7ᵗʰ **S78.922** Partial traumatic amputation of left hip and thigh, level unspecified `CC` `HCC`

√7ᵗʰ **S78.929** Partial traumatic amputation of unspecified hip and thigh, level unspecified `CC` `HCC`

√4ᵗʰ **S79** Other and unspecified injuries of hip and thigh

> **NOTE** A fracture not indicated as open or closed should be coded to closed

AHA: 2018,2Q,12; 2018,1Q,3; 2015,3Q,37-39

The appropriate 7th character is to be added to each code from subcategories S79.0 and S79.1.
A   initial encounter for closed fracture
D   subsequent encounter for fracture with routine healing
G   subsequent encounter for fracture with delayed healing
K   subsequent encounter for fracture with nonunion
P   subsequent encounter for fracture with malunion
S   sequela

√5ᵗʰ **S79.0** Physeal fracture of upper end of femur

> **EXCLUDES 1** apophyseal fracture of upper end of femur (S72.13-)
> nontraumatic slipped upper femoral epiphysis (M93.0-)

AHA: 2019,4Q,56

√6ᵗʰ **S79.00** Unspecified physeal fracture of upper end of femur

4,6 √7ᵗʰ **S79.001** Unspecified physeal fracture of upper end of right femur `MCC` `CC` `H5` `HCC`

4,6 √7ᵗʰ **S79.002** Unspecified physeal fracture of upper end of left femur `MCC` `CC` `H5` `HCC`

4,6 √7ᵗʰ **S79.009** Unspecified physeal fracture of upper end of unspecified femur `MCC` `CC` `H5` `HCC`

√6ᵗʰ **S79.01** Salter-Harris Type I physeal fracture of upper end of femur

> Acute on chronic slipped capital femoral epiphysis (traumatic)
> Acute slipped capital femoral epiphysis (traumatic)
> Capital femoral epiphyseal fracture
> **EXCLUDES 1** chronic slipped upper femoral epiphysis (nontraumatic) (M93.02-)

4,6 √7ᵗʰ **S79.011** Salter-Harris Type I physeal fracture of upper end of right femur `MCC` `CC` `H5` `HCC`

4,6 √7ᵗʰ **S79.012** Salter-Harris Type I physeal fracture of upper end of left femur `MCC` `CC` `H5` `HCC`

4,6 √7ᵗʰ **S79.019** Salter-Harris Type I physeal fracture of upper end of unspecified femur `MCC` `CC` `H5` `HCC`

√6ᵗʰ **S79.09** Other physeal fracture of upper end of femur

4,6 √7ᵗʰ **S79.091** Other physeal fracture of upper end of right femur `MCC` `CC` `H5` `HCC`

4,6 √7ᵗʰ **S79.092** Other physeal fracture of upper end of left femur `MCC` `CC` `H5` `HCC`

4,6 √7ᵗʰ **S79.099** Other physeal fracture of upper end of unspecified femur `MCC` `CC` `H5` `HCC`

√5ᵗʰ **S79.1** Physeal fracture of lower end of femur

AHA: 2019,4Q,56

√6ᵗʰ **S79.10** Unspecified physeal fracture of lower end of femur

3,6 √7ᵗʰ **S79.101** Unspecified physeal fracture of lower end of right femur `CC` `H5` `HCC`

3,6 √7ᵗʰ **S79.102** Unspecified physeal fracture of lower end of left femur `CC` `H5` `HCC`

3,6 √7ᵗʰ **S79.109** Unspecified physeal fracture of lower end of unspecified femur `CC` `H5` `HCC`

√6ᵗʰ **S79.11** Salter-Harris Type I physeal fracture of lower end of femur

3,6 √7ᵗʰ **S79.111** Salter-Harris Type I physeal fracture of lower end of right femur `CC` `H5` `HCC`

3,6 √7ᵗʰ **S79.112** Salter-Harris Type I physeal fracture of lower end of left femur `CC` `H5` `HCC`

3,6 √7ᵗʰ **S79.119** Salter-Harris Type I physeal fracture of lower end of unspecified femur `CC` `H5` `HCC`

√6ᵗʰ **S79.12** Salter-Harris Type II physeal fracture of lower end of femur

3,6 √7ᵗʰ **S79.121** Salter-Harris Type II physeal fracture of lower end of right femur `CC` `H5` `HCC`

3,6 √7ᵗʰ **S79.122** Salter-Harris Type II physeal fracture of lower end of left femur `CC` `H5` `HCC`

3,6 √7ᵗʰ **S79.129** Salter-Harris Type II physeal fracture of lower end of unspecified femur `CC` `H5` `HCC`

√6ᵗʰ **S79.13** Salter-Harris Type III physeal fracture of lower end of femur

3,6 √7ᵗʰ **S79.131** Salter-Harris Type III physeal fracture of lower end of right femur `CC` `H5` `HCC`

3,6 √7ᵗʰ **S79.132** Salter-Harris Type III physeal fracture of lower end of left femur `CC` `H5` `HCC`

3,6 √7ᵗʰ **S79.139** Salter-Harris Type III physeal fracture of lower end of unspecified femur `CC` `H5` `HCC`

√6ᵗʰ **S79.14** Salter-Harris Type IV physeal fracture of lower end of femur

3,6 √7ᵗʰ **S79.141** Salter-Harris Type IV physeal fracture of lower end of right femur `CC` `H5` `HCC`

3,6 √7ᵗʰ **S79.142** Salter-Harris Type IV physeal fracture of lower end of left femur `CC` `H5` `HCC`

3,6 √7ᵗʰ **S79.149** Salter-Harris Type IV physeal fracture of lower end of unspecified femur `CC` `H5` `HCC`

√6ᵗʰ **S79.19** Other physeal fracture of lower end of femur

3,6 √7ᵗʰ **S79.191** Other physeal fracture of lower end of right femur `CC` `H5` `HCC`

3,6 √7ᵗʰ **S79.192** Other physeal fracture of lower end of left femur `CC` `H5` `HCC`

3,6 √7ᵗʰ **S79.199** Other physeal fracture of lower end of unspecified femur `CC` `H5` `HCC`

√5ᵗʰ **S79.8** Other specified injuries of hip and thigh

The appropriate 7th character is to be added to each code in subcategory S79.8.
A   initial encounter
D   subsequent encounter
S   sequela

√6ᵗʰ **S79.81** Other specified injuries of hip

√7ᵗʰ **S79.811** Other specified injuries of right hip

√7ᵗʰ **S79.812** Other specified injuries of left hip

√7ᵗʰ **S79.819** Other specified injuries of unspecified hip

√6ᵗʰ **S79.82** Other specified injuries of thigh

√7ᵗʰ **S79.821** Other specified injuries of right thigh

√7ᵗʰ **S79.822** Other specified injuries of left thigh

√7ᵗʰ **S79.829** Other specified injuries of unspecified thigh

√5ᵗʰ **S79.9** Unspecified injury of hip and thigh

The appropriate 7th character is to be added to each code in subcategory S79.9.
A   initial encounter
D   subsequent encounter
S   sequela

√6ᵗʰ **S79.91** Unspecified injury of hip

√7ᵗʰ **S79.911** Unspecified injury of right hip

√7ᵗʰ **S79.912** Unspecified injury of left hip

√7ᵗʰ **S79.919** Unspecified injury of unspecified hip

√6ᵗʰ **S79.92** Unspecified injury of thigh

√7ᵗʰ **S79.921** Unspecified injury of right thigh

√7ᵗʰ **S79.922** Unspecified injury of left thigh

√7ᵗʰ **S79.929** Unspecified injury of unspecified thigh

Injuries to the knee and lower leg (S80-S89)

EXCLUDES 2   burns and corrosions (T20-T32)
frostbite (T33-T34)
injuries of ankle and foot, except fracture of ankle and malleolus (S90-S99)
insect bite or sting, venomous (T63.4)

√4ᵗʰ **S80 Superficial injury of knee and lower leg**

  EXCLUDES 2   superficial injury of ankle and foot (S90.-)

The appropriate 7th character is to be added to each code from category S80.
A   initial encounter
D   subsequent encounter
S   sequela

√5ᵗʰ **S80.0 Contusion of** knee
   √x7ᵗʰ **S80.00 Contusion of unspecified knee**
   √x7ᵗʰ **S80.01 Contusion of right knee**
   √x7ᵗʰ **S80.02 Contusion of left knee**

√5ᵗʰ **S80.1 Contusion of** lower leg
   √x7ᵗʰ **S80.10 Contusion of unspecified lower leg**
   √x7ᵗʰ **S80.11 Contusion of right lower leg**
   √x7ᵗʰ **S80.12 Contusion of left lower leg**

√5ᵗʰ **S80.2 Other superficial injuries of** knee
   √6ᵗʰ **S80.21 Abrasion of knee**
     √7ᵗʰ **S80.211 Abrasion, right knee**
     √7ᵗʰ **S80.212 Abrasion, left knee**
     √7ᵗʰ **S80.219 Abrasion, unspecified knee**
   √6ᵗʰ **S80.22 Blister (nonthermal) of knee**
     √7ᵗʰ **S80.221 Blister (nonthermal), right knee**
     √7ᵗʰ **S80.222 Blister (nonthermal), left knee**
     √7ᵗʰ **S80.229 Blister (nonthermal), unspecified knee**
   √6ᵗʰ **S80.24 External constriction of knee**
     √7ᵗʰ **S80.241 External constriction, right knee**
     √7ᵗʰ **S80.242 External constriction, left knee**
     √7ᵗʰ **S80.249 External constriction, unspecified knee**
   √6ᵗʰ **S80.25 Superficial foreign body of knee**
     Splinter in the knee
     √7ᵗʰ **S80.251 Superficial foreign body, right knee**
     √7ᵗʰ **S80.252 Superficial foreign body, left knee**
     √7ᵗʰ **S80.259 Superficial foreign body, unspecified knee**
   √6ᵗʰ **S80.26 Insect bite (nonvenomous) of knee**
     √7ᵗʰ **S80.261 Insect bite (nonvenomous), right knee**
     √7ᵗʰ **S80.262 Insect bite (nonvenomous), left knee**
     √7ᵗʰ **S80.269 Insect bite (nonvenomous), unspecified knee**
   √6ᵗʰ **S80.27 Other superficial bite of knee**
     EXCLUDES 1 open bite of knee (S81.05-)
     √7ᵗʰ **S80.271 Other superficial bite of right knee**
     √7ᵗʰ **S80.272 Other superficial bite of left knee**
     √7ᵗʰ **S80.279 Other superficial bite of unspecified knee**

√5ᵗʰ **S80.8 Other superficial injuries of** lower leg
   √6ᵗʰ **S80.81 Abrasion of lower leg**
     √7ᵗʰ **S80.811 Abrasion, right lower leg**
     √7ᵗʰ **S80.812 Abrasion, left lower leg**
     √7ᵗʰ **S80.819 Abrasion, unspecified lower leg**
   √6ᵗʰ **S80.82 Blister (nonthermal) of lower leg**
     √7ᵗʰ **S80.821 Blister (nonthermal), right lower leg**
     √7ᵗʰ **S80.822 Blister (nonthermal), left lower leg**
     √7ᵗʰ **S80.829 Blister (nonthermal), unspecified lower leg**
   √6ᵗʰ **S80.84 External constriction of lower leg**
     √7ᵗʰ **S80.841 External constriction, right lower leg**
     √7ᵗʰ **S80.842 External constriction, left lower leg**
     √7ᵗʰ **S80.849 External constriction, unspecified lower leg**
   √6ᵗʰ **S80.85 Superficial foreign body of lower leg**
     Splinter in the lower leg
     √7ᵗʰ **S80.851 Superficial foreign body, right lower leg**

     √7ᵗʰ **S80.852 Superficial foreign body, left lower leg**
     √7ᵗʰ **S80.859 Superficial foreign body, unspecified lower leg**
   √6ᵗʰ **S80.86 Insect bite (nonvenomous) of lower leg**
     √7ᵗʰ **S80.861 Insect bite (nonvenomous), right lower leg**
     √7ᵗʰ **S80.862 Insect bite (nonvenomous), left lower leg**
     √7ᵗʰ **S80.869 Insect bite (nonvenomous), unspecified lower leg**
   √6ᵗʰ **S80.87 Other superficial bite of lower leg**
     EXCLUDES 1 open bite of lower leg (S81.85-)
     √7ᵗʰ **S80.871 Other superficial bite, right lower leg**
     √7ᵗʰ **S80.872 Other superficial bite, left lower leg**
     √7ᵗʰ **S80.879 Other superficial bite, unspecified lower leg**

√5ᵗʰ **S80.9 Unspecified superficial injury of knee and lower leg**
   √6ᵗʰ **S80.91 Unspecified superficial injury of** knee
     √7ᵗʰ **S80.911 Unspecified superficial injury of right knee**
     √7ᵗʰ **S80.912 Unspecified superficial injury of left knee**
     √7ᵗʰ **S80.919 Unspecified superficial injury of unspecified knee**
   √6ᵗʰ **S80.92 Unspecified superficial injury of** lower leg
     √7ᵗʰ **S80.921 Unspecified superficial injury of right lower leg**
     √7ᵗʰ **S80.922 Unspecified superficial injury of left lower leg**
     √7ᵗʰ **S80.929 Unspecified superficial injury of unspecified lower leg**

√4ᵗʰ **S81 Open wound of knee and lower leg**

Code also any associated wound infection
  EXCLUDES 1 open fracture of knee and lower leg (S82.-)
     traumatic amputation of lower leg (S88.-)
  EXCLUDES 2 open wound of ankle and foot (S91.-)

The appropriate 7th character is to be added to each code from category S81.
A   initial encounter
D   subsequent encounter
S   sequela

√5ᵗʰ **S81.0 Open wound of** knee
   √6ᵗʰ **S81.00 Unspecified open wound of knee**
     √7ᵗʰ **S81.001 Unspecified open wound, right knee**
     √7ᵗʰ **S81.002 Unspecified open wound, left knee**
     √7ᵗʰ **S81.009 Unspecified open wound, unspecified knee**
   √6ᵗʰ **S81.01 Laceration without foreign body of knee**
     √7ᵗʰ **S81.011 Laceration without foreign body, right knee**
     √7ᵗʰ **S81.012 Laceration without foreign body, left knee**
     √7ᵗʰ **S81.019 Laceration without foreign body, unspecified knee**
   √6ᵗʰ **S81.02 Laceration with foreign body of knee**
     √7ᵗʰ **S81.021 Laceration with foreign body, right knee**
     √7ᵗʰ **S81.022 Laceration with foreign body, left knee**
     √7ᵗʰ **S81.029 Laceration with foreign body, unspecified knee**
   √6ᵗʰ **S81.03 Puncture wound without foreign body of knee**
     √7ᵗʰ **S81.031 Puncture wound without foreign body, right knee**
     √7ᵗʰ **S81.032 Puncture wound without foreign body, left knee**
     √7ᵗʰ **S81.039 Puncture wound without foreign body, unspecified knee**
   √6ᵗʰ **S81.04 Puncture wound with foreign body of knee**
     √7ᵗʰ **S81.041 Puncture wound with foreign body, right knee**
     √7ᵗʰ **S81.042 Puncture wound with foreign body, left knee**
     √7ᵗʰ **S81.049 Puncture wound with foreign body, unspecified knee**
   √6ᵗʰ **S81.05 Open bite of knee**
     Bite of knee NOS
     EXCLUDES 1 superficial bite of knee (S80.27-)
     √7ᵗʰ **S81.051 Open bite, right knee**

     ✓7ᵗʰ **S81.052**   Open bite, left knee

     ✓7ᵗʰ **S81.059**   Open bite, unspecified knee

✓5ᵗʰ **S81.8**   **Open wound of** lower leg

   ✓6ᵗʰ **S81.80**   **Unspecified open wound of lower leg**

     AHA: 2016,3Q,24

     ✓7ᵗʰ **S81.801**   Unspecified open wound, right lower leg

     ✓7ᵗʰ **S81.802**   Unspecified open wound, left lower leg

     ✓7ᵗʰ **S81.809**   Unspecified open wound, unspecified lower leg

   ✓6ᵗʰ **S81.81**   **Laceration without foreign body of lower leg**

     ✓7ᵗʰ **S81.811**   Laceration without foreign body, right lower leg

     ✓7ᵗʰ **S81.812**   Laceration without foreign body, left lower leg

     ✓7ᵗʰ **S81.819**   Laceration without foreign body, unspecified lower leg

   ✓6ᵗʰ **S81.82**   **Laceration with foreign body of lower leg**

     ✓7ᵗʰ **S81.821**   Laceration with foreign body, right lower leg

     ✓7ᵗʰ **S81.822**   Laceration with foreign body, left lower leg

     ✓7ᵗʰ **S81.829**   Laceration with foreign body, unspecified lower leg

   ✓6ᵗʰ **S81.83**   **Puncture wound without foreign body of lower leg**

     AHA: 2016,3Q,24

     ✓7ᵗʰ **S81.831**   Puncture wound without foreign body, right lower leg

     ✓7ᵗʰ **S81.832**   Puncture wound without foreign body, left lower leg

     ✓7ᵗʰ **S81.839**   Puncture wound without foreign body, unspecified lower leg

   ✓6ᵗʰ **S81.84**   **Puncture wound with foreign body of lower leg**

     AHA: 2016,3Q,24

     ✓7ᵗʰ **S81.841**   Puncture wound with foreign body, right lower leg

     ✓7ᵗʰ **S81.842**   Puncture wound with foreign body, left lower leg

     ✓7ᵗʰ **S81.849**   Puncture wound with foreign body, unspecified lower leg

   ✓6ᵗʰ **S81.85**   **Open bite** of lower leg

     Bite of lower leg NOS

     EXCLUDES 1   *superficial bite of lower leg (S80.86-, S80.87-)*

     ✓7ᵗʰ **S81.851**   Open bite, right lower leg

     ✓7ᵗʰ **S81.852**   Open bite, left lower leg

     ✓7ᵗʰ **S81.859**   Open bite, unspecified lower leg

✓4ᵗʰ **S82**   **Fracture of lower leg, including ankle**

   NOTE   A fracture not indicated as displaced or nondisplaced should be coded to displaced

     A fracture not indicated as open or closed should be coded to closed

     The open fracture designations are based on the Gustilo open fracture classification.

   INCLUDES   fracture of malleolus

   EXCLUDES 1   *traumatic amputation of lower leg (S88.-)*

   EXCLUDES 2   *fracture of foot, except ankle (S92.-)*

     ▶*periprosthetic fracture around internal prosthetic implant of knee joint (M97.1-)*◀

AHA: 2018,2Q,12; 2016,1Q,33; 2015,3Q,37-39

DEF: Diaphysis: Central shaft of a long bone.

DEF: Epiphysis: Proximal and distal rounded ends of a long bone, communicates with the joint.

DEF: Metaphysis: Section of a long bone located between the epiphysis and diaphysis at the proximal and distal ends.

DEF: Physis (growth plate): Narrow zone of cartilaginous tissue between the epiphysis and metaphysis at each end of a long bone. In childhood, proliferation of cells in this zone lengthens the bone. As the bone matures, this area thins, ossification eventually fusing into solid bone and growth stops. ***Synonym(s):*** *Epiphyseal plate.*

The appropriate 7th character is to be added to all codes from category S82 [unless otherwise indicated].
A   initial encounter for closed fracture
B   initial encounter for open fracture type I or II
    initial encounter for open fracture NOS
C   initial encounter for open fracture type IIIA, IIIB, or IIIC
D   subsequent encounter for closed fracture with routine healing
E   subsequent encounter for open fracture type I or II with routine healing
F   subsequent encounter for open fracture type IIIA, IIIB, or IIIC with routine healing
G   subsequent encounter for closed fracture with delayed healing
H   subsequent encounter for open fracture type I or II with delayed healing
J   subsequent encounter for open fracture type IIIA, IIIB, or IIIC with delayed healing
K   subsequent encounter for closed fracture with nonunion
M   subsequent encounter for open fracture type I or II with nonunion
N   subsequent encounter for open fracture type IIIA, IIIB, or IIIC with nonunion
P   subsequent encounter for closed fracture with malunion
Q   subsequent encounter for open fracture type I or II with malunion
R   subsequent encounter for open fracture type IIIA, IIIB, or IIIC with malunion
S   sequela

   ✓5ᵗʰ **S82.0**   **Fracture of** patella

     Knee cap

     ✓6ᵗʰ **S82.00**   **Unspecified fracture of patella**

      ³ ✓7ᵗʰ **S82.001**   Unspecified fracture of right patella   **CC** **H5**

      ³ ✓7ᵗʰ **S82.002**   Unspecified fracture of left patella   **CC** **H5**

      ³ ✓7ᵗʰ **S82.009**   Unspecified fracture of unspecified patella   **CC** **H5**

     ✓6ᵗʰ **S82.01**   **Osteochondral fracture of patella**

      ³ ✓7ᵗʰ **S82.011**   Displaced osteochondral fracture of right patella   **CC** **H5**

      ³ ✓7ᵗʰ **S82.012**   Displaced osteochondral fracture of left patella   **CC** **H5**

      ³ ✓7ᵗʰ **S82.013**   Displaced osteochondral fracture of unspecified patella   **CC** **H5**

      ³ ✓7ᵗʰ **S82.014**   Nondisplaced osteochondral fracture of right patella   **CC** **H5**

      ³ ✓7ᵗʰ **S82.015**   Nondisplaced osteochondral fracture of left patella   **CC** **H5**

      ³ ✓7ᵗʰ **S82.016**   Nondisplaced osteochondral fracture of unspecified patella   **CC** **H5**

     ✓6ᵗʰ **S82.02**   **Longitudinal fracture of patella**

      ³ ✓7ᵗʰ **S82.021**   Displaced longitudinal fracture of right patella   **CC** **H5**

      ³ ✓7ᵗʰ **S82.022**   Displaced longitudinal fracture of left patella   **CC** **H5**

      ³ ✓7ᵗʰ **S82.023**   Displaced longitudinal fracture of unspecified patella   **CC** **H5**

✔ Additional Character Required   ✓x7ᵗʰ Placeholder   Questionable PDx   Manifestation   Unspecified Dx   **UPD** Unacceptable PDx   **H1**-**H14** HAC   **HCC** CMS-HCC Dx   **HIV** HIV Dx

ICD-10-CM 2022   **1067**

³ √7ᵗʰ **S82.024** Nondisplaced longitudinal fracture of right patella `CC` `H5`

³ √7ᵗʰ **S82.025** Nondisplaced longitudinal fracture of left patella `CC` `H5`

³ √7ᵗʰ **S82.026** Nondisplaced longitudinal fracture of unspecified patella `CC` `H5`

√6ᵗʰ **S82.03** Transverse fracture of patella

³ √7ᵗʰ **S82.031** Displaced transverse fracture of right patella `CC` `H5`

³ √7ᵗʰ **S82.032** Displaced transverse fracture of left patella `CC` `H5`

³ √7ᵗʰ **S82.033** Displaced transverse fracture of unspecified patella `CC` `H5`

³ √7ᵗʰ **S82.034** Nondisplaced transverse fracture of right patella `CC` `H5`

³ √7ᵗʰ **S82.035** Nondisplaced transverse fracture of left patella `CC` `H5`

³ √7ᵗʰ **S82.036** Nondisplaced transverse fracture of unspecified patella `CC` `H5`

√6ᵗʰ **S82.04** Comminuted fracture of patella

³ √7ᵗʰ **S82.041** Displaced comminuted fracture of right patella `CC` `H5`

³ √7ᵗʰ **S82.042** Displaced comminuted fracture of left patella `CC` `H5`

³ √7ᵗʰ **S82.043** Displaced comminuted fracture of unspecified patella `CC` `H5`

³ √7ᵗʰ **S82.044** Nondisplaced comminuted fracture of right patella `CC` `H5`

³ √7ᵗʰ **S82.045** Nondisplaced comminuted fracture of left patella `CC` `H5`

³ √7ᵗʰ **S82.046** Nondisplaced comminuted fracture of unspecified patella `CC` `H5`

√6ᵗʰ **S82.09** Other fracture of patella

³ √7ᵗʰ **S82.091** Other fracture of right patella `CC` `H5`

³ √7ᵗʰ **S82.092** Other fracture of left patella `CC` `H5`

³ √7ᵗʰ **S82.099** Other fracture of unspecified patella `CC` `H5`

√5ᵗʰ **S82.1** Fracture of upper end of tibia

Fracture of proximal end of tibia

EXCLUDES 2   *fracture of shaft of tibia (S82.2-)*
physeal fracture of upper end of tibia (S89.0-)

√6ᵗʰ **S82.10** Unspecified fracture of upper end of tibia

²,³ √7ᵗʰ **S82.101** Unspecified fracture of upper end of right tibia `MCC` `CC` `H5`

²,³ √7ᵗʰ **S82.102** Unspecified fracture of upper end of left tibia `MCC` `CC` `H5`

²,³ √7ᵗʰ **S82.109** Unspecified fracture of upper end of unspecified tibia `MCC` `CC` `H5`

√6ᵗʰ **S82.11** Fracture of tibial spine

²,³ √7ᵗʰ **S82.111** Displaced fracture of right tibial spine `MCC` `CC` `H5`

²,³ √7ᵗʰ **S82.112** Displaced fracture of left tibial spine `MCC` `CC` `H5`

²,³ √7ᵗʰ **S82.113** Displaced fracture of unspecified tibial spine `MCC` `CC` `H5`

²,³ √7ᵗʰ **S82.114** Nondisplaced fracture of right tibial spine `MCC` `CC` `H5`

²,³ √7ᵗʰ **S82.115** Nondisplaced fracture of left tibial spine `MCC` `CC` `H5`

²,³ √7ᵗʰ **S82.116** Nondisplaced fracture of unspecified tibial spine `MCC` `CC` `H5`

√6ᵗʰ **S82.12** Fracture of lateral condyle of tibia

²,³ √7ᵗʰ **S82.121** Displaced fracture of lateral condyle of right tibia `MCC` `CC` `H5`

²,³ √7ᵗʰ **S82.122** Displaced fracture of lateral condyle of left tibia `MCC` `CC` `H5`

²,³ √7ᵗʰ **S82.123** Displaced fracture of lateral condyle of unspecified tibia `MCC` `CC` `H5`

²,³ √7ᵗʰ **S82.124** Nondisplaced fracture of lateral condyle of right tibia `MCC` `CC` `H5`

²,³ √7ᵗʰ **S82.125** Nondisplaced fracture of lateral condyle of left tibia `MCC` `CC` `H5`

²,³ √7ᵗʰ **S82.126** Nondisplaced fracture of lateral condyle of unspecified tibia `MCC` `CC` `H5`

√6ᵗʰ **S82.13** Fracture of medial condyle of tibia

²,³ √7ᵗʰ **S82.131** Displaced fracture of medial condyle of right tibia `MCC` `CC` `H5`

²,³ √7ᵗʰ **S82.132** Displaced fracture of medial condyle of left tibia `MCC` `CC` `H5`

²,³ √7ᵗʰ **S82.133** Displaced fracture of medial condyle of unspecified tibia `MCC` `CC` `H5`

²,³ √7ᵗʰ **S82.134** Nondisplaced fracture of medial condyle of right tibia `MCC` `CC` `H5`

²,³ √7ᵗʰ **S82.135** Nondisplaced fracture of medial condyle of left tibia `MCC` `CC` `H5`

²,³ √7ᵗʰ **S82.136** Nondisplaced fracture of medial condyle of unspecified tibia `MCC` `CC` `H5`

√6ᵗʰ **S82.14** Bicondylar fracture of tibia

Fracture of tibial plateau NOS

²,³ √7ᵗʰ **S82.141** Displaced bicondylar fracture of right tibia `MCC` `CC` `H5`

²,³ √7ᵗʰ **S82.142** Displaced bicondylar fracture of left tibia `MCC` `CC` `H5`

²,³ √7ᵗʰ **S82.143** Displaced bicondylar fracture of unspecified tibia `MCC` `CC` `H5`

²,³ √7ᵗʰ **S82.144** Nondisplaced bicondylar fracture of right tibia `MCC` `CC` `H5`

²,³ √7ᵗʰ **S82.145** Nondisplaced bicondylar fracture of left tibia `MCC` `CC` `H5`

²,³ √7ᵗʰ **S82.146** Nondisplaced bicondylar fracture of unspecified tibia `MCC` `CC` `H5`

√6ᵗʰ **S82.15** Fracture of tibial tuberosity

²,³ √7ᵗʰ **S82.151** Displaced fracture of right tibial tuberosity `MCC` `CC` `H5`

²,³ √7ᵗʰ **S82.152** Displaced fracture of left tibial tuberosity `MCC` `CC` `H5`

²,³ √7ᵗʰ **S82.153** Displaced fracture of unspecified tibial tuberosity `MCC` `CC` `H5`

²,³ √7ᵗʰ **S82.154** Nondisplaced fracture of right tibial tuberosity `MCC` `CC` `H5`

²,³ √7ᵗʰ **S82.155** Nondisplaced fracture of left tibial tuberosity `MCC` `CC` `H5`

²,³ √7ᵗʰ **S82.156** Nondisplaced fracture of unspecified tibial tuberosity `MCC` `CC` `H5`

√6ᵗʰ **S82.16** Torus fracture of upper end of tibia

The appropriate 7th character is to be added to all codes in subcategory S82.16.
A   initial encounter for closed fracture
D   subsequent encounter for fracture with routine healing
G   subsequent encounter for fracture with delayed healing
K   subsequent encounter for fracture with nonunion
P   subsequent encounter for fracture with malunion
S   sequela

³ √7ᵗʰ **S82.161** Torus fracture of upper end of right tibia `CC` `H5`

³ √7ᵗʰ **S82.162** Torus fracture of upper end of left tibia `CC` `H5`

³ √7ᵗʰ **S82.169** Torus fracture of upper end of unspecified tibia `CC` `H5`

√6ᵗʰ **S82.19** Other fracture of upper end of tibia

²,³ √7ᵗʰ **S82.191** Other fracture of upper end of right tibia `MCC` `CC` `H5`

²,³ √7ᵗʰ **S82.192** Other fracture of upper end of left tibia `MCC` `CC` `H5`

²,³ √7ᵗʰ **S82.199** Other fracture of upper end of unspecified tibia `MCC` `CC` `H5`

√5ᵗʰ **S82.2** Fracture of shaft of tibia

√6ᵗʰ **S82.20** Unspecified fracture of shaft of tibia

Fracture of tibia NOS

²,³ √7ᵗʰ **S82.201** Unspecified fracture of shaft of right tibia `MCC` `CC` `H5`

²,³ √7ᵗʰ **S82.202** Unspecified fracture of shaft of left tibia `MCC` `CC` `H5`

²,³ √7ᵗʰ **S82.209** Unspecified fracture of shaft of unspecified tibia `MCC` `CC` `H5`

√6ᵗʰ **S82.22** Transverse fracture of shaft of tibia

²,³ √7ᵗʰ **S82.221** Displaced transverse fracture of shaft of right tibia `MCC` `CC` `H5`

²,³ √7ᵗʰ **S82.222** Displaced transverse fracture of shaft of left tibia `MCC` `CC` `H5`

Ⓝ Newborn: 0   Ⓟ Pediatric: 0-17   Ⓜ Maternity: 9-64   Ⓐ Adult: 15-124   `MCC` Major Complication/Comorbidity   `CC` Complication/Comorbidity   `SW` Severe Wound Dx

1068   ICD-10-CM 2022

2,3 √7ᵗʰ **S82.223** Displaced **transverse fracture of shaft of unspecified tibia** `MCC` `CC` `H5`

2,3 √7ᵗʰ **S82.224** Nondisplaced **transverse fracture of shaft of right tibia** `MCC` `CC` `H5`

2,3 √7ᵗʰ **S82.225** Nondisplaced **transverse fracture of shaft of left tibia** `MCC` `CC` `H5`

2,3 √7ᵗʰ **S82.226** Nondisplaced **transverse fracture of shaft of unspecified tibia** `MCC` `CC` `H5`

√6ᵗʰ **S82.23** Oblique **fracture of shaft of tibia**

2,3 √7ᵗʰ **S82.231** Displaced **oblique fracture of shaft of right tibia** `MCC` `CC` `H5`

2,3 √7ᵗʰ **S82.232** Displaced **oblique fracture of shaft of left tibia** `MCC` `CC` `H5`

2,3 √7ᵗʰ **S82.233** Displaced **oblique fracture of shaft of unspecified tibia** `MCC` `CC` `H5`

2,3 √7ᵗʰ **S82.234** Nondisplaced **oblique fracture of shaft of right tibia** `MCC` `CC` `H5`

2,3 √7ᵗʰ **S82.235** Nondisplaced **oblique fracture of shaft of left tibia** `MCC` `CC` `H5`

2,3 √7ᵗʰ **S82.236** Nondisplaced **oblique fracture of shaft of unspecified tibia** `MCC` `CC` `H5`

√6ᵗʰ **S82.24** Spiral **fracture of shaft of tibia**
    Toddler fracture

2,3 √7ᵗʰ **S82.241** Displaced **spiral fracture of shaft of right tibia** `MCC` `CC` `H5`

2,3 √7ᵗʰ **S82.242** Displaced **spiral fracture of shaft of left tibia** `MCC` `CC` `H5`

2,3 √7ᵗʰ **S82.243** Displaced **spiral fracture of shaft of unspecified tibia** `MCC` `CC` `H5`

2,3 √7ᵗʰ **S82.244** Nondisplaced **spiral fracture of shaft of right tibia** `MCC` `CC` `H5`

2,3 √7ᵗʰ **S82.245** Nondisplaced **spiral fracture of shaft of left tibia** `MCC` `CC` `H5`

2,3 √7ᵗʰ **S82.246** Nondisplaced **spiral fracture of shaft of unspecified tibia** `MCC` `CC` `H5`

√6ᵗʰ **S82.25** Comminuted **fracture of shaft of tibia**

2,3 √7ᵗʰ **S82.251** Displaced **comminuted fracture of shaft of right tibia** `MCC` `CC` `H5`

2,3 √7ᵗʰ **S82.252** Displaced **comminuted fracture of shaft of left tibia** `MCC` `CC` `H5`

2,3 √7ᵗʰ **S82.253** Displaced **comminuted fracture of shaft of unspecified tibia** `MCC` `CC` `H5`

2,3 √7ᵗʰ **S82.254** Nondisplaced **comminuted fracture of shaft of right tibia** `MCC` `CC` `H5`

2,3 √7ᵗʰ **S82.255** Nondisplaced **comminuted fracture of shaft of left tibia** `MCC` `CC` `H5`

2,3 √7ᵗʰ **S82.256** Nondisplaced **comminuted fracture of shaft of unspecified tibia** `MCC` `CC` `H5`

√6ᵗʰ **S82.26** Segmental **fracture of shaft of tibia**

2,3 √7ᵗʰ **S82.261** Displaced **segmental fracture of shaft of right tibia** `MCC` `CC` `H5`

2,3 √7ᵗʰ **S82.262** Displaced **segmental fracture of shaft of left tibia** `MCC` `CC` `H5`

2,3 √7ᵗʰ **S82.263** Displaced **segmental fracture of shaft of unspecified tibia** `MCC` `CC` `H5`

2,3 √7ᵗʰ **S82.264** Nondisplaced **segmental fracture of shaft of right tibia** `MCC` `CC` `H5`

2,3 √7ᵗʰ **S82.265** Nondisplaced **segmental fracture of shaft of left tibia** `MCC` `CC` `H5`

2,3 √7ᵗʰ **S82.266** Nondisplaced **segmental fracture of shaft of unspecified tibia** `MCC` `CC` `H5`

√6ᵗʰ **S82.29** Other **fracture of shaft of tibia**

2,3 √7ᵗʰ **S82.291** Other **fracture of shaft of right tibia** `MCC` `CC` `H5`

2,3 √7ᵗʰ **S82.292** Other **fracture of shaft of left tibia** `MCC` `CC` `H5`

2,3 √7ᵗʰ **S82.299** Other **fracture of shaft of unspecified tibia** `MCC` `CC` `H5`

√5ᵗʰ **S82.3** Fracture of lower end of tibia

EXCLUDES 1   bimalleolar fracture of lower leg (S82.84-)
    fracture of medial malleolus alone (S82.5-)
    Maisonneuve's fracture (S82.86-)
    pilon fracture of distal tibia (S82.87-)
    trimalleolar fractures of lower leg (S82.85-)

√6ᵗʰ **S82.30** Unspecified **fracture of lower end of tibia**

3 √7ᵗʰ **S82.301** Unspecified **fracture of lower end of right tibia** `CC` `H5`

3 √7ᵗʰ **S82.302** Unspecified **fracture of lower end of left tibia** `CC` `H5`

3 √7ᵗʰ **S82.309** Unspecified **fracture of lower end of unspecified tibia** `CC` `H5`

√6ᵗʰ **S82.31** Torus **fracture of lower end of tibia**

The appropriate 7th character is to be added to all codes in subcategory S82.31.
A   initial encounter for closed fracture
D   subsequent encounter for fracture with routine healing
G   subsequent encounter for fracture with delayed healing
K   subsequent encounter for fracture with nonunion
P   subsequent encounter for fracture with malunion
S   sequela

3 √7ᵗʰ **S82.311** Torus **fracture of lower end of right tibia** `CC` `H5`

3 √7ᵗʰ **S82.312** Torus **fracture of lower end of left tibia** `CC` `H5`

3 √7ᵗʰ **S82.319** Torus **fracture of lower end of unspecified tibia** `CC` `H5`

√6ᵗʰ **S82.39** Other **fracture of lower end of tibia**
    AHA: 2015,1Q,25

3 √7ᵗʰ **S82.391** Other **fracture of lower end of right tibia** `CC` `H5`

3 √7ᵗʰ **S82.392** Other **fracture of lower end of left tibia** `CC` `H5`

3 √7ᵗʰ **S82.399** Other **fracture of lower end of unspecified tibia** `CC` `H5`

√5ᵗʰ **S82.4** Fracture of shaft of fibula

EXCLUDES 2   fracture of lateral malleolus alone (S82.6-)

√6ᵗʰ **S82.40** Unspecified **fracture of shaft of fibula**

2,4 √7ᵗʰ **S82.401** Unspecified **fracture of shaft of right fibula** `MCC` `CC` `H5`

2,4 √7ᵗʰ **S82.402** Unspecified **fracture of shaft of left fibula** `MCC` `CC` `H5`

2,4 √7ᵗʰ **S82.409** Unspecified **fracture of shaft of unspecified fibula** `MCC` `CC` `H5`

√6ᵗʰ **S82.42** Transverse **fracture of shaft of fibula**

2,4 √7ᵗʰ **S82.421** Displaced **transverse fracture of shaft of right fibula** `MCC` `CC` `H5`

2,4 √7ᵗʰ **S82.422** Displaced **transverse fracture of shaft of left fibula** `MCC` `CC` `H5`

2,4 √7ᵗʰ **S82.423** Displaced **transverse fracture of shaft of unspecified fibula** `MCC` `CC` `H5`

2,4 √7ᵗʰ **S82.424** Nondisplaced **transverse fracture of shaft of right fibula** `MCC` `CC` `H5`

2,4 √7ᵗʰ **S82.425** Nondisplaced **transverse fracture of shaft of left fibula** `MCC` `CC` `H5`

2,4 √7ᵗʰ **S82.426** Nondisplaced **transverse fracture of shaft of unspecified fibula** `MCC` `CC` `H5`

√6ᵗʰ **S82.43** Oblique **fracture of shaft of fibula**

2,4 √7ᵗʰ **S82.431** Displaced **oblique fracture of shaft of right fibula** `MCC` `CC` `H5`

2,4 √7ᵗʰ **S82.432** Displaced **oblique fracture of shaft of left fibula** `MCC` `CC` `H5`

2,4 √7ᵗʰ **S82.433** Displaced **oblique fracture of shaft of unspecified fibula** `MCC` `CC` `H5`

2,4 √7ᵗʰ **S82.434** Nondisplaced **oblique fracture of shaft of right fibula** `MCC` `CC` `H5`

2,4 √7ᵗʰ **S82.435** Nondisplaced **oblique fracture of shaft of left fibula** `MCC` `CC` `H5`

2,4 √7ᵗʰ **S82.436** Nondisplaced **oblique fracture of shaft of unspecified fibula** `MCC` `CC` `H5`

√6ᵗʰ **S82.44** Spiral **fracture of shaft of fibula**

2,4 √7ᵗʰ **S82.441** Displaced **spiral fracture of shaft of right fibula** `MCC` `CC` `H5`

2,4 √7ᵗʰ **S82.442** Displaced **spiral fracture of shaft of left fibula** `MCC` `CC` `H5`

2,4 √7ᵗʰ **S82.443** Displaced **spiral fracture of shaft of unspecified fibula** `MCC` `CC` `H5`

2,4 √7ᵗʰ **S82.444** Nondisplaced **spiral fracture of shaft of right fibula** `MCC` `CC` `H5`

2,4 √7ᵗʰ **S82.445** Nondisplaced **spiral fracture of shaft of left fibula** `MCC` `CC` `H5`

2,4 ✓7ᵗʰ **S82.446** Nondisplaced spiral fracture of shaft of unspecified fibula   MCC CC H5

✓6ᵗʰ **S82.45** Comminuted fracture of shaft of fibula

   2,4 ✓7ᵗʰ **S82.451** Displaced comminuted fracture of shaft of right fibula   MCC CC H5

   2,4 ✓7ᵗʰ **S82.452** Displaced comminuted fracture of shaft of left fibula   MCC CC H5

   2,4 ✓7ᵗʰ **S82.453** Displaced comminuted fracture of shaft of unspecified fibula   MCC CC H5

   2,4 ✓7ᵗʰ **S82.454** Nondisplaced comminuted fracture of shaft of right fibula   MCC CC H5

   2,4 ✓7ᵗʰ **S82.455** Nondisplaced comminuted fracture of shaft of left fibula   MCC CC H5

   2,4 ✓7ᵗʰ **S82.456** Nondisplaced comminuted fracture of shaft of unspecified fibula   MCC CC H5

✓6ᵗʰ **S82.46** Segmental fracture of shaft of fibula

   2,4 ✓7ᵗʰ **S82.461** Displaced segmental fracture of shaft of right fibula   MCC CC H5

   2,4 ✓7ᵗʰ **S82.462** Displaced segmental fracture of shaft of left fibula   MCC CC H5

   2,4 ✓7ᵗʰ **S82.463** Displaced segmental fracture of shaft of unspecified fibula   MCC CC H5

   2,4 ✓7ᵗʰ **S82.464** Nondisplaced segmental fracture of shaft of right fibula   MCC CC H5

   2,4 ✓7ᵗʰ **S82.465** Nondisplaced segmental fracture of shaft of left fibula   MCC CC H5

   2,4 ✓7ᵗʰ **S82.466** Nondisplaced segmental fracture of shaft of unspecified fibula   MCC CC H5

✓6ᵗʰ **S82.49** Other fracture of shaft of fibula

   2,4 ✓7ᵗʰ **S82.491** Other fracture of shaft of right fibula   MCC CC H5

   2,4 ✓7ᵗʰ **S82.492** Other fracture of shaft of left fibula   MCC CC H5

   2,4 ✓7ᵗʰ **S82.499** Other fracture of shaft of unspecified fibula   MCC CC H5

✓5ᵗʰ **S82.5** Fracture of medial malleolus

   EXCLUDES 1   *pilon fracture of distal tibia (S82.87-)*
        Salter-Harris type III of lower end of tibia (S89.13-)
        Salter-Harris type IV of lower end of tibia (S89.14-)

   3 ✓x7ᵗʰ **S82.51** Displaced fracture of medial malleolus of right tibia   CC H5

   3 ✓x7ᵗʰ **S82.52** Displaced fracture of medial malleolus of left tibia   CC H5

   3 ✓x7ᵗʰ **S82.53** Displaced fracture of medial malleolus of unspecified tibia   CC H5

   3 ✓x7ᵗʰ **S82.54** Nondisplaced fracture of medial malleolus of right tibia   CC H5

   3 ✓x7ᵗʰ **S82.55** Nondisplaced fracture of medial malleolus of left tibia   CC H5

   3 ✓x7ᵗʰ **S82.56** Nondisplaced fracture of medial malleolus of unspecified tibia   CC H5

✓5ᵗʰ **S82.6** Fracture of lateral malleolus

   EXCLUDES 1   *pilon fracture of distal tibia (S82.87-)*

   3 ✓x7ᵗʰ **S82.61** Displaced fracture of lateral malleolus of right fibula   CC H5

   3 ✓x7ᵗʰ **S82.62** Displaced fracture of lateral malleolus of left fibula   CC H5

   3 ✓x7ᵗʰ **S82.63** Displaced fracture of lateral malleolus of unspecified fibula   CC H5

   3 ✓x7ᵗʰ **S82.64** Nondisplaced fracture of lateral malleolus of right fibula   CC H5

   3 ✓x7ᵗʰ **S82.65** Nondisplaced fracture of lateral malleolus of left fibula   CC H5

   3 ✓x7ᵗʰ **S82.66** Nondisplaced fracture of lateral malleolus of unspecified fibula   CC H5

✓5ᵗʰ **S82.8** Other fractures of lower leg

✓6ᵗʰ **S82.81** Torus fracture of upper end of fibula

> The appropriate 7th character is to be added to all codes in subcategory S82.81
> A   initial encounter for closed fracture
> D   subsequent encounter for fracture with routine healing
> G   subsequent encounter for fracture with delayed healing
> K   subsequent encounter for fracture with nonunion
> P   subsequent encounter for fracture with malunion
> S   sequela

   4 ✓7ᵗʰ **S82.811** Torus fracture of upper end of right fibula   CC

   4 ✓7ᵗʰ **S82.812** Torus fracture of upper end of left fibula   CC

   4 ✓7ᵗʰ **S82.819** Torus fracture of upper end of unspecified fibula   CC

✓6ᵗʰ **S82.82** Torus fracture of lower end of fibula

> The appropriate 7th character is to be added to all codes in subcategory S82.82.
> A   initial encounter for closed fracture
> D   subsequent encounter for fracture with routine healing
> G   subsequent encounter for fracture with delayed healing
> K   subsequent encounter for fracture with nonunion
> P   subsequent encounter for fracture with malunion
> S   sequela

   4 ✓7ᵗʰ **S82.821** Torus fracture of lower end of right fibula   CC

   4 ✓7ᵗʰ **S82.822** Torus fracture of lower end of left fibula   CC

   4 ✓7ᵗʰ **S82.829** Torus fracture of lower end of unspecified fibula   CC

✓6ᵗʰ **S82.83** Other fracture of upper and lower end of fibula

   AHA: 2015,1Q,25

   2,4 ✓7ᵗʰ **S82.831** Other fracture of upper and lower end of right fibula   MCC CC H5

   2,4 ✓7ᵗʰ **S82.832** Other fracture of upper and lower end of left fibula   MCC CC H5

   2,4 ✓7ᵗʰ **S82.839** Other fracture of upper and lower end of unspecified fibula   MCC CC H5

✓6ᵗʰ **S82.84** Bimalleolar fracture of lower leg

Right Bimalleolar Fracture

- Patella
- Tibial plateau
- Tibial tubercle
- Fibula
- Tibia
- Medial (tibial) malleolus
- Lateral (fibular) malleolus
- Fracture medial malleolus
- Talus
- Fracture lateral malleolus

   3 ✓7ᵗʰ **S82.841** Displaced bimalleolar fracture of right lower leg   CC H5

N Newborn: 0   P Pediatric: 0-17   M Maternity: 9-64   A Adult: 15-124   MCC Major Complication/Comorbidity   CC Complication/Comorbidity   SW Severe Wound Dx

1070   ICD-10-CM 2022

³ √7ᵗʰ **S82.842** Displaced **bimalleolar** fracture of left lower leg   CC H5

³ √7ᵗʰ **S82.843** Displaced **bimalleolar** fracture of unspecified lower leg   CC H5

³ √7ᵗʰ **S82.844** Nondisplaced **bimalleolar** fracture of right lower leg   CC H5

³ √7ᵗʰ **S82.845** Nondisplaced **bimalleolar** fracture of left lower leg   CC H5

³ √7ᵗʰ **S82.846** Nondisplaced **bimalleolar** fracture of unspecified lower leg   CC H5

√6ᵗʰ **S82.85** **Trimalleolar** fracture of lower leg

³ √7ᵗʰ **S82.851** Displaced **trimalleolar** fracture of right lower leg   CC H5

³ √7ᵗʰ **S82.852** Displaced **trimalleolar** fracture of left lower leg   CC H5

³ √7ᵗʰ **S82.853** Displaced **trimalleolar** fracture of unspecified lower leg   CC H5

³ √7ᵗʰ **S82.854** Nondisplaced **trimalleolar** fracture of right lower leg   CC H5

³ √7ᵗʰ **S82.855** Nondisplaced **trimalleolar** fracture of left lower leg   CC H5

³ √7ᵗʰ **S82.856** Nondisplaced **trimalleolar** fracture of unspecified lower leg   CC H5

√6ᵗʰ **S82.86** **Maisonneuve's** fracture

²,⁴ √7ᵗʰ **S82.861** Displaced **Maisonneuve's** fracture of right leg   MCC CC H5

²,⁴ √7ᵗʰ **S82.862** Displaced **Maisonneuve's** fracture of left leg   MCC CC H5

²,⁴ √7ᵗʰ **S82.863** Displaced **Maisonneuve's** fracture of unspecified leg   MCC CC H5

²,⁴ √7ᵗʰ **S82.864** Nondisplaced **Maisonneuve's** fracture of right leg   MCC CC H5

²,⁴ √7ᵗʰ **S82.865** Nondisplaced **Maisonneuve's** fracture of left leg   MCC CC H5

²,⁴ √7ᵗʰ **S82.866** Nondisplaced **Maisonneuve's** fracture of unspecified leg   MCC CC H5

√6ᵗʰ **S82.87** **Pilon** fracture of tibia

³ √7ᵗʰ **S82.871** Displaced **pilon** fracture of right tibia   CC H5

³ √7ᵗʰ **S82.872** Displaced **pilon** fracture of left tibia   CC H5

³ √7ᵗʰ **S82.873** Displaced **pilon** fracture of unspecified tibia   CC H5

³ √7ᵗʰ **S82.874** Nondisplaced **pilon** fracture of right tibia   CC H5

³ √7ᵗʰ **S82.875** Nondisplaced **pilon** fracture of left tibia   CC H5

³ √7ᵗʰ **S82.876** Nondisplaced **pilon** fracture of unspecified tibia   CC H5

√6ᵗʰ **S82.89** **Other fractures of lower leg**

Fracture of ankle NOS

³ √7ᵗʰ **S82.891** Other fracture of right lower leg   CC H5

³ √7ᵗʰ **S82.892** Other fracture of left lower leg   CC H5

³ √7ᵗʰ **S82.899** Other fracture of unspecified lower leg   CC H5

√5ᵗʰ **S82.9** **Unspecified fracture of lower leg**

³ √x7ᵗʰ **S82.90** Unspecified fracture of unspecified lower leg   CC H5

³ √x7ᵗʰ **S82.91** Unspecified fracture of right lower leg   CC H5

³ √x7ᵗʰ **S82.92** Unspecified fracture of left lower leg   CC H5

√4ᵗʰ **S83** **Dislocation and sprain of joints and ligaments of knee**

INCLUDES   avulsion of joint or ligament of knee
laceration of cartilage, joint or ligament of knee
sprain of cartilage, joint or ligament of knee
traumatic hemarthrosis of joint or ligament of knee
traumatic rupture of joint or ligament of knee
traumatic subluxation of joint or ligament of knee
traumatic tear of joint or ligament of knee

Code also any associated open wound

EXCLUDES 2   *derangement of patella (M22.0-M22.3)*
injury of patellar ligament (tendon) (S76.1-)
internal derangement of knee (M23.-)
old dislocation of knee (M24.36)
pathological dislocation of knee (M24.36)
recurrent dislocation of knee (M22.0)
strain of muscle, fascia and tendon of lower leg (S86.-)

The appropriate 7th character is to be added to each code from category S83.
A   initial encounter
D   subsequent encounter
S   sequela

√5ᵗʰ **S83.0** **Subluxation and dislocation of patella**

√6ᵗʰ **S83.00** Unspecified subluxation and dislocation of patella

√7ᵗʰ **S83.001** Unspecified **subluxation** of right patella

√7ᵗʰ **S83.002** Unspecified **subluxation** of left patella

√7ᵗʰ **S83.003** Unspecified **subluxation** of unspecified patella

√7ᵗʰ **S83.004** Unspecified **dislocation** of right patella

√7ᵗʰ **S83.005** Unspecified **dislocation** of left patella

√7ᵗʰ **S83.006** Unspecified **dislocation** of unspecified patella

√6ᵗʰ **S83.01** Lateral subluxation and dislocation of patella

√7ᵗʰ **S83.011** Lateral **subluxation** of right patella

√7ᵗʰ **S83.012** Lateral **subluxation** of left patella

√7ᵗʰ **S83.013** Lateral **subluxation** of unspecified patella

√7ᵗʰ **S83.014** Lateral **dislocation** of right patella

√7ᵗʰ **S83.015** Lateral **dislocation** of left patella

√7ᵗʰ **S83.016** Lateral **dislocation** of unspecified patella

√6ᵗʰ **S83.09** Other subluxation and dislocation of patella

√7ᵗʰ **S83.091** Other **subluxation** of right patella

√7ᵗʰ **S83.092** Other **subluxation** of left patella

√7ᵗʰ **S83.093** Other **subluxation** of unspecified patella

√7ᵗʰ **S83.094** Other **dislocation** of right patella

√7ᵗʰ **S83.095** Other **dislocation** of left patella

√7ᵗʰ **S83.096** Other **dislocation** of unspecified patella

√5ᵗʰ **S83.1** **Subluxation and dislocation of knee**

EXCLUDES 2   *instability of knee prosthesis (T84.022, T84.023)*

√6ᵗʰ **S83.10** Unspecified subluxation and dislocation of knee

√7ᵗʰ **S83.101** Unspecified **subluxation** of right knee

√7ᵗʰ **S83.102** Unspecified **subluxation** of left knee

√7ᵗʰ **S83.103** Unspecified **subluxation** of unspecified knee

√7ᵗʰ **S83.104** Unspecified **dislocation** of right knee

√7ᵗʰ **S83.105** Unspecified **dislocation** of left knee

√7ᵗʰ **S83.106** Unspecified **dislocation** of unspecified knee

√6ᵗʰ **S83.11** **Anterior** subluxation and dislocation of proximal end of tibia

Posterior subluxation and dislocation of distal end of femur

√7ᵗʰ **S83.111** Anterior **subluxation** of proximal end of tibia, right knee

√7ᵗʰ **S83.112** Anterior **subluxation** of proximal end of tibia, left knee

√7ᵗʰ **S83.113** Anterior **subluxation** of proximal end of tibia, unspecified knee

√7ᵗʰ **S83.114** Anterior **dislocation** of proximal end of tibia, right knee

√7ᵗʰ **S83.115** Anterior **dislocation** of proximal end of tibia, left knee

√7ᵗʰ **S83.116** Anterior **dislocation** of proximal end of tibia, unspecified knee

√6ᵗʰ **S83.12** **Posterior** subluxation and dislocation of proximal end of tibia
Anterior dislocation of distal end of femur

    √7ᵗʰ **S83.121** Posterior **subluxation** of proximal end of tibia, **right** knee

    √7ᵗʰ **S83.122** Posterior **subluxation** of proximal end of tibia, **left** knee

    √7ᵗʰ **S83.123** Posterior **subluxation** of proximal end of tibia, unspecified knee

    √7ᵗʰ **S83.124** Posterior **dislocation** of proximal end of tibia, **right** knee

    √7ᵗʰ **S83.125** Posterior **dislocation** of proximal end of tibia, **left** knee

    √7ᵗʰ **S83.126** Posterior **dislocation** of proximal end of tibia, unspecified knee

√6ᵗʰ **S83.13** **Medial** subluxation and dislocation of proximal end of tibia

    √7ᵗʰ **S83.131** Medial **subluxation** of proximal end of tibia, **right** knee

    √7ᵗʰ **S83.132** Medial **subluxation** of proximal end of tibia, **left** knee

    √7ᵗʰ **S83.133** Medial **subluxation** of proximal end of tibia, unspecified knee

    √7ᵗʰ **S83.134** Medial **dislocation** of proximal end of tibia, **right** knee

    √7ᵗʰ **S83.135** Medial **dislocation** of proximal end of tibia, **left** knee

    √7ᵗʰ **S83.136** Medial **dislocation** of proximal end of tibia, unspecified knee

√6ᵗʰ **S83.14** **Lateral** subluxation and dislocation of proximal end of tibia

    √7ᵗʰ **S83.141** Lateral **subluxation** of proximal end of tibia, **right** knee

    √7ᵗʰ **S83.142** Lateral **subluxation** of proximal end of tibia, **left** knee

    √7ᵗʰ **S83.143** Lateral **subluxation** of proximal end of tibia, unspecified knee

    √7ᵗʰ **S83.144** Lateral **dislocation** of proximal end of tibia, **right** knee

    √7ᵗʰ **S83.145** Lateral **dislocation** of proximal end of tibia, **left** knee

    √7ᵗʰ **S83.146** Lateral **dislocation** of proximal end of tibia, unspecified knee

√6ᵗʰ **S83.19** Other subluxation and dislocation of knee

    √7ᵗʰ **S83.191** Other **subluxation** of **right** knee

    √7ᵗʰ **S83.192** Other **subluxation** of **left** knee

    √7ᵗʰ **S83.193** Other **subluxation** of unspecified knee

    √7ᵗʰ **S83.194** Other **dislocation** of **right** knee

    √7ᵗʰ **S83.195** Other **dislocation** of **left** knee

    √7ᵗʰ **S83.196** Other **dislocation** of unspecified knee

√5ᵗʰ **S83.2** **Tear of meniscus, current injury**

    EXCLUDES 1   old bucket-handle tear (M23.2)

    AHA: 2019,2Q,26

    √6ᵗʰ **S83.20** **Tear of unspecified meniscus, current injury**
Tear of meniscus of knee NOS

      √7ᵗʰ **S83.200** **Bucket-handle** tear of unspecified meniscus, current injury, **right** knee

      √7ᵗʰ **S83.201** **Bucket-handle** tear of unspecified meniscus, current injury, **left** knee

      √7ᵗʰ **S83.202** **Bucket-handle** tear of unspecified meniscus, current injury, unspecified knee

      √7ᵗʰ **S83.203** Other tear of unspecified meniscus, current injury, **right** knee

      √7ᵗʰ **S83.204** Other tear of unspecified meniscus, current injury, **left** knee

      √7ᵗʰ **S83.205** Other tear of unspecified meniscus, current injury, unspecified knee

      √7ᵗʰ **S83.206** Unspecified tear of unspecified meniscus, current injury, **right** knee

      √7ᵗʰ **S83.207** Unspecified tear of unspecified meniscus, current injury, **left** knee

      √7ᵗʰ **S83.209** Unspecified tear of unspecified meniscus, current injury, unspecified knee

    √6ᵗʰ **S83.21** **Bucket-handle** tear of **medial** meniscus, current injury

      √7ᵗʰ **S83.211** Bucket-handle tear of medial meniscus, current injury, **right** knee

      √7ᵗʰ **S83.212** Bucket-handle tear of medial meniscus, current injury, **left** knee

      √7ᵗʰ **S83.219** Bucket-handle tear of medial meniscus, current injury, unspecified knee

    √6ᵗʰ **S83.22** **Peripheral** tear of **medial** meniscus, current injury

      √7ᵗʰ **S83.221** Peripheral tear of medial meniscus, current injury, **right** knee

      √7ᵗʰ **S83.222** Peripheral tear of medial meniscus, current injury, **left** knee

      √7ᵗʰ **S83.229** Peripheral tear of medial meniscus, current injury, unspecified knee

    √6ᵗʰ **S83.23** **Complex** tear of **medial** meniscus, current injury

      √7ᵗʰ **S83.231** Complex tear of medial meniscus, current injury, **right** knee

      √7ᵗʰ **S83.232** Complex tear of medial meniscus, current injury, **left** knee

      √7ᵗʰ **S83.239** Complex tear of medial meniscus, current injury, unspecified knee

    √6ᵗʰ **S83.24** **Other tear** of **medial** meniscus, current injury

      √7ᵗʰ **S83.241** Other tear of medial meniscus, current injury, **right** knee

      √7ᵗʰ **S83.242** Other tear of medial meniscus, current injury, **left** knee

      √7ᵗʰ **S83.249** Other tear of medial meniscus, current injury, unspecified knee

    √6ᵗʰ **S83.25** **Bucket-handle** tear of **lateral** meniscus, current injury

      √7ᵗʰ **S83.251** Bucket-handle tear of lateral meniscus, current injury, **right** knee

      √7ᵗʰ **S83.252** Bucket-handle tear of lateral meniscus, current injury, **left** knee

      √7ᵗʰ **S83.259** Bucket-handle tear of lateral meniscus, current injury, unspecified knee

    √6ᵗʰ **S83.26** **Peripheral** tear of **lateral** meniscus, current injury

      √7ᵗʰ **S83.261** Peripheral tear of lateral meniscus, current injury, **right** knee

      √7ᵗʰ **S83.262** Peripheral tear of lateral meniscus, current injury, **left** knee

      √7ᵗʰ **S83.269** Peripheral tear of lateral meniscus, current injury, unspecified knee

    √6ᵗʰ **S83.27** **Complex** tear of **lateral** meniscus, current injury

      √7ᵗʰ **S83.271** Complex tear of lateral meniscus, current injury, **right** knee

      √7ᵗʰ **S83.272** Complex tear of lateral meniscus, current injury, **left** knee

      √7ᵗʰ **S83.279** Complex tear of lateral meniscus, current injury, unspecified knee

    √6ᵗʰ **S83.28** **Other tear** of **lateral** meniscus, current injury

      √7ᵗʰ **S83.281** Other tear of lateral meniscus, current injury, **right** knee

      √7ᵗʰ **S83.282** Other tear of lateral meniscus, current injury, **left** knee

      √7ᵗʰ **S83.289** Other tear of lateral meniscus, current injury, unspecified knee

√5ᵗʰ **S83.3** **Tear of articular cartilage of knee, current**

    √x7ᵗʰ **S83.30** Tear of articular cartilage of unspecified knee, current

    √x7ᵗʰ **S83.31** Tear of articular cartilage of **right** knee, current

    √x7ᵗʰ **S83.32** Tear of articular cartilage of **left** knee, current

√5ᵗʰ **S83.4** **Sprain of collateral ligament of knee**

    √6ᵗʰ **S83.40** Sprain of unspecified collateral ligament of knee

      √7ᵗʰ **S83.401** Sprain of unspecified collateral ligament of **right** knee

      √7ᵗʰ **S83.402** Sprain of unspecified collateral ligament of **left** knee

      √7ᵗʰ **S83.409** Sprain of unspecified collateral ligament of unspecified knee

    √6ᵗʰ **S83.41** Sprain of **medial** collateral ligament of knee
Sprain of tibial collateral ligament

      √7ᵗʰ **S83.411** Sprain of medial collateral ligament of **right** knee

      √7ᵗʰ **S83.412** Sprain of medial collateral ligament of **left** knee

      √7ᵗʰ **S83.419** Sprain of medial collateral ligament of unspecified knee

    √6ᵗʰ **S83.42** Sprain of **lateral** collateral ligament of knee
Sprain of fibular collateral ligament

      √7ᵗʰ **S83.421** Sprain of lateral collateral ligament of **right** knee

      √7ᵗʰ **S83.422** Sprain of lateral collateral ligament of **left** knee

Ⓝ Newborn: 0   Ⓟ Pediatric: 0-17   Ⓜ Maternity: 9-64   Ⓐ Adult: 15-124   **MCC** Major Complication/Comorbidity   **CC** Complication/Comorbidity   **SW** Severe Wound Dx

1072   ICD-10-CM 2022

     √7ᵗʰ **S83.429** Sprain of lateral collateral ligament of unspecified knee

✓5ᵗʰ **S83.5** Sprain of cruciate ligament of knee

     AHA: 2016,2Q,3

     ✓6ᵗʰ **S83.50** Sprain of unspecified cruciate ligament of knee

         √7ᵗʰ **S83.501** Sprain of unspecified cruciate ligament of right knee

         √7ᵗʰ **S83.502** Sprain of unspecified cruciate ligament of left knee

         √7ᵗʰ **S83.509** Sprain of unspecified cruciate ligament of unspecified knee

     ✓6ᵗʰ **S83.51** Sprain of anterior cruciate ligament of knee

         √7ᵗʰ **S83.511** Sprain of anterior cruciate ligament of right knee

         √7ᵗʰ **S83.512** Sprain of anterior cruciate ligament of left knee

         √7ᵗʰ **S83.519** Sprain of anterior cruciate ligament of unspecified knee

     ✓6ᵗʰ **S83.52** Sprain of posterior cruciate ligament of knee

         √7ᵗʰ **S83.521** Sprain of posterior cruciate ligament of right knee

         √7ᵗʰ **S83.522** Sprain of posterior cruciate ligament of left knee

         √7ᵗʰ **S83.529** Sprain of posterior cruciate ligament of unspecified knee

✓5ᵗʰ **S83.6** Sprain of the superior tibiofibular joint and ligament

     √x7ᵗʰ **S83.60** Sprain of the superior tibiofibular joint and ligament, unspecified knee

     √x7ᵗʰ **S83.61** Sprain of the superior tibiofibular joint and ligament, right knee

     √x7ᵗʰ **S83.62** Sprain of the superior tibiofibular joint and ligament, left knee

✓5ᵗʰ **S83.8** Sprain of other specified parts of knee

     ✓6ᵗʰ **S83.8X** Sprain of other specified parts of knee

         √7ᵗʰ **S83.8X1** Sprain of other specified parts of right knee

         √7ᵗʰ **S83.8X2** Sprain of other specified parts of left knee

         √7ᵗʰ **S83.8X9** Sprain of other specified parts of unspecified knee

✓5ᵗʰ **S83.9** Sprain of unspecified site of knee

     √x7ᵗʰ **S83.90** Sprain of unspecified site of unspecified knee

     √x7ᵗʰ **S83.91** Sprain of unspecified site of right knee

     √x7ᵗʰ **S83.92** Sprain of unspecified site of left knee

✓4ᵗʰ **S84** Injury of nerves at lower leg level

     Code also any associated open wound (S81.-)

     EXCLUDES 2 injury of nerves at ankle and foot level (S94.-)

     The appropriate 7th character is to be added to each code from category S84.
     A   initial encounter
     D   subsequent encounter
     S   sequela

     ✓5ᵗʰ **S84.0** Injury of tibial nerve at lower leg level

         √x7ᵗʰ **S84.00** Injury of tibial nerve at lower leg level, unspecified leg

         √x7ᵗʰ **S84.01** Injury of tibial nerve at lower leg level, right leg

         √x7ᵗʰ **S84.02** Injury of tibial nerve at lower leg level, left leg

     ✓5ᵗʰ **S84.1** Injury of peroneal nerve at lower leg level

         √x7ᵗʰ **S84.10** Injury of peroneal nerve at lower leg level, unspecified leg

         √x7ᵗʰ **S84.11** Injury of peroneal nerve at lower leg level, right leg

         √x7ᵗʰ **S84.12** Injury of peroneal nerve at lower leg level, left leg

     ✓5ᵗʰ **S84.2** Injury of cutaneous sensory nerve at lower leg level

         √x7ᵗʰ **S84.20** Injury of cutaneous sensory nerve at lower leg level, unspecified leg

         √x7ᵗʰ **S84.21** Injury of cutaneous sensory nerve at lower leg level, right leg

         √x7ᵗʰ **S84.22** Injury of cutaneous sensory nerve at lower leg level, left leg

     ✓5ᵗʰ **S84.8** Injury of other nerves at lower leg level

         ✓6ᵗʰ **S84.80** Injury of other nerves at lower leg level

             √7ᵗʰ **S84.801** Injury of other nerves at lower leg level, right leg

             √7ᵗʰ **S84.802** Injury of other nerves at lower leg level, left leg

             √7ᵗʰ **S84.809** Injury of other nerves at lower leg level, unspecified leg

     ✓5ᵗʰ **S84.9** Injury of unspecified nerve at lower leg level

         √x7ᵗʰ **S84.90** Injury of unspecified nerve at lower leg level, unspecified leg

         √x7ᵗʰ **S84.91** Injury of unspecified nerve at lower leg level, right leg

         √x7ᵗʰ **S84.92** Injury of unspecified nerve at lower leg level, left leg

✓4ᵗʰ **S85** Injury of blood vessels at lower leg level

     Code also any associated open wound (S81.-)

     EXCLUDES 2 injury of blood vessels at ankle and foot level (S95.-)

     The appropriate 7th character is to be added to each code from category S85.
     A   initial encounter
     D   subsequent encounter
     S   sequela

     ✓5ᵗʰ **S85.0** Injury of popliteal artery

         ✓6ᵗʰ **S85.00** Unspecified injury of popliteal artery

             √7ᵗʰ **S85.001** Unspecified injury of popliteal artery, right leg   MCC

             √7ᵗʰ **S85.002** Unspecified injury of popliteal artery, left leg   MCC

             √7ᵗʰ **S85.009** Unspecified injury of popliteal artery, unspecified leg   MCC

         ✓6ᵗʰ **S85.01** Laceration of popliteal artery

             √7ᵗʰ **S85.011** Laceration of popliteal artery, right leg   MCC

             √7ᵗʰ **S85.012** Laceration of popliteal artery, left leg   MCC

             √7ᵗʰ **S85.019** Laceration of popliteal artery, unspecified leg   MCC

         ✓6ᵗʰ **S85.09** Other specified injury of popliteal artery

             √7ᵗʰ **S85.091** Other specified injury of popliteal artery, right leg   MCC

             √7ᵗʰ **S85.092** Other specified injury of popliteal artery, left leg   MCC

             √7ᵗʰ **S85.099** Other specified injury of popliteal artery, unspecified leg   MCC

     ✓5ᵗʰ **S85.1** Injury of tibial artery

         ✓6ᵗʰ **S85.10** Unspecified injury of unspecified tibial artery

             Injury of tibial artery NOS

             √7ᵗʰ **S85.101** Unspecified injury of unspecified tibial artery, right leg   CC

             √7ᵗʰ **S85.102** Unspecified injury of unspecified tibial artery, left leg   CC

             √7ᵗʰ **S85.109** Unspecified injury of unspecified tibial artery, unspecified leg   CC

         ✓6ᵗʰ **S85.11** Laceration of unspecified tibial artery

             √7ᵗʰ **S85.111** Laceration of unspecified tibial artery, right leg   CC

             √7ᵗʰ **S85.112** Laceration of unspecified tibial artery, left leg   CC

             √7ᵗʰ **S85.119** Laceration of unspecified tibial artery, unspecified leg   CC

         ✓6ᵗʰ **S85.12** Other specified injury of unspecified tibial artery

             √7ᵗʰ **S85.121** Other specified injury of unspecified tibial artery, right leg   CC

             √7ᵗʰ **S85.122** Other specified injury of unspecified tibial artery, left leg   CC

             √7ᵗʰ **S85.129** Other specified injury of unspecified tibial artery, unspecified leg   CC

         ✓6ᵗʰ **S85.13** Unspecified injury of anterior tibial artery

             √7ᵗʰ **S85.131** Unspecified injury of anterior tibial artery, right leg   CC

             √7ᵗʰ **S85.132** Unspecified injury of anterior tibial artery, left leg   CC

             √7ᵗʰ **S85.139** Unspecified injury of anterior tibial artery, unspecified leg   CC

         ✓6ᵗʰ **S85.14** Laceration of anterior tibial artery

             √7ᵗʰ **S85.141** Laceration of anterior tibial artery, right leg   CC

             √7ᵗʰ **S85.142** Laceration of anterior tibial artery, left leg   CC

             √7ᵗʰ **S85.149** Laceration of anterior tibial artery, unspecified leg   CC

✔ Additional Character Required   √x7ᵗʰ Placeholder   Questionable PDx   Manifestation   Unspecified Dx   **UPD** Unacceptable PDx   **H1-H14** HAC   **HCC** CMS-HCC Dx   **HIV** HIV Dx

√6ᵗʰ **S85.15** Other specified injury of anterior tibial artery

- √7ᵗʰ **S85.151** Other specified injury of anterior tibial artery, right leg   CC
- √7ᵗʰ **S85.152** Other specified injury of anterior tibial artery, left leg   CC
- √7ᵗʰ **S85.159** Other specified injury of anterior tibial artery, unspecified leg   CC

√6ᵗʰ **S85.16** Unspecified injury of posterior tibial artery

- √7ᵗʰ **S85.161** Unspecified injury of posterior tibial artery, right leg   CC
- √7ᵗʰ **S85.162** Unspecified injury of posterior tibial artery, left leg   CC
- √7ᵗʰ **S85.169** Unspecified injury of posterior tibial artery, unspecified leg   CC

√6ᵗʰ **S85.17** Laceration of posterior tibial artery

- √7ᵗʰ **S85.171** Laceration of posterior tibial artery, right leg   CC
- √7ᵗʰ **S85.172** Laceration of posterior tibial artery, left leg   CC
- √7ᵗʰ **S85.179** Laceration of posterior tibial artery, unspecified leg   CC

√6ᵗʰ **S85.18** Other specified injury of posterior tibial artery

- √7ᵗʰ **S85.181** Other specified injury of posterior tibial artery, right leg   CC
- √7ᵗʰ **S85.182** Other specified injury of posterior tibial artery, left leg   CC
- √7ᵗʰ **S85.189** Other specified injury of posterior tibial artery, unspecified leg   CC

√5ᵗʰ **S85.2** Injury of peroneal artery

√6ᵗʰ **S85.20** Unspecified injury of peroneal artery

- √7ᵗʰ **S85.201** Unspecified injury of peroneal artery, right leg   CC
- √7ᵗʰ **S85.202** Unspecified injury of peroneal artery, left leg   CC
- √7ᵗʰ **S85.209** Unspecified injury of peroneal artery, unspecified leg   CC

√6ᵗʰ **S85.21** Laceration of peroneal artery

- √7ᵗʰ **S85.211** Laceration of peroneal artery, right leg   CC
- √7ᵗʰ **S85.212** Laceration of peroneal artery, left leg   CC
- √7ᵗʰ **S85.219** Laceration of peroneal artery, unspecified leg   CC

√6ᵗʰ **S85.29** Other specified injury of peroneal artery

- √7ᵗʰ **S85.291** Other specified injury of peroneal artery, right leg   CC
- √7ᵗʰ **S85.292** Other specified injury of peroneal artery, left leg   CC
- √7ᵗʰ **S85.299** Other specified injury of peroneal artery, unspecified leg   CC

√5ᵗʰ **S85.3** Injury of greater saphenous vein at lower leg level

Injury of greater saphenous vein NOS
Injury of saphenous vein NOS

√6ᵗʰ **S85.30** Unspecified injury of greater saphenous vein at lower leg level

- √7ᵗʰ **S85.301** Unspecified injury of greater saphenous vein at lower leg level, right leg   CC
- √7ᵗʰ **S85.302** Unspecified injury of greater saphenous vein at lower leg level, left leg   CC
- √7ᵗʰ **S85.309** Unspecified injury of greater saphenous vein at lower leg level, unspecified leg   CC

√6ᵗʰ **S85.31** Laceration of greater saphenous vein at lower leg level

- √7ᵗʰ **S85.311** Laceration of greater saphenous vein at lower leg level, right leg   CC
- √7ᵗʰ **S85.312** Laceration of greater saphenous vein at lower leg level, left leg   CC
- √7ᵗʰ **S85.319** Laceration of greater saphenous vein at lower leg level, unspecified leg   CC

√6ᵗʰ **S85.39** Other specified injury of greater saphenous vein at lower leg level

- √7ᵗʰ **S85.391** Other specified injury of greater saphenous vein at lower leg level, right leg   CC
- √7ᵗʰ **S85.392** Other specified injury of greater saphenous vein at lower leg level, left leg   CC

- √7ᵗʰ **S85.399** Other specified injury of greater saphenous vein at lower leg level, unspecified leg   CC

√5ᵗʰ **S85.4** Injury of lesser saphenous vein at lower leg level

√6ᵗʰ **S85.40** Unspecified injury of lesser saphenous vein at lower leg level

- √7ᵗʰ **S85.401** Unspecified injury of lesser saphenous vein at lower leg level, right leg   CC
- √7ᵗʰ **S85.402** Unspecified injury of lesser saphenous vein at lower leg level, left leg   CC
- √7ᵗʰ **S85.409** Unspecified injury of lesser saphenous vein at lower leg level, unspecified leg   CC

√6ᵗʰ **S85.41** Laceration of lesser saphenous vein at lower leg level

- √7ᵗʰ **S85.411** Laceration of lesser saphenous vein at lower leg level, right leg   CC
- √7ᵗʰ **S85.412** Laceration of lesser saphenous vein at lower leg level, left leg   CC
- √7ᵗʰ **S85.419** Laceration of lesser saphenous vein at lower leg level, unspecified leg   CC

√6ᵗʰ **S85.49** Other specified injury of lesser saphenous vein at lower leg level

- √7ᵗʰ **S85.491** Other specified injury of lesser saphenous vein at lower leg level, right leg   CC
- √7ᵗʰ **S85.492** Other specified injury of lesser saphenous vein at lower leg level, left leg   CC
- √7ᵗʰ **S85.499** Other specified injury of lesser saphenous vein at lower leg level, unspecified leg   CC

√5ᵗʰ **S85.5** Injury of popliteal vein

√6ᵗʰ **S85.50** Unspecified injury of popliteal vein

- √7ᵗʰ **S85.501** Unspecified injury of popliteal vein, right leg   MCC
- √7ᵗʰ **S85.502** Unspecified injury of popliteal vein, left leg   MCC
- √7ᵗʰ **S85.509** Unspecified injury of popliteal vein, unspecified leg   MCC

√6ᵗʰ **S85.51** Laceration of popliteal vein

- √7ᵗʰ **S85.511** Laceration of popliteal vein, right leg   MCC
- √7ᵗʰ **S85.512** Laceration of popliteal vein, left leg   MCC
- √7ᵗʰ **S85.519** Laceration of popliteal vein, unspecified leg   MCC

√6ᵗʰ **S85.59** Other specified injury of popliteal vein

- √7ᵗʰ **S85.591** Other specified injury of popliteal vein, right leg   MCC
- √7ᵗʰ **S85.592** Other specified injury of popliteal vein, left leg   MCC
- √7ᵗʰ **S85.599** Other specified injury of popliteal vein, unspecified leg   MCC

√5ᵗʰ **S85.8** Injury of other blood vessels at lower leg level

√6ᵗʰ **S85.80** Unspecified injury of other blood vessels at lower leg level

- √7ᵗʰ **S85.801** Unspecified injury of other blood vessels at lower leg level, right leg   CC
- √7ᵗʰ **S85.802** Unspecified injury of other blood vessels at lower leg level, left leg   CC
- √7ᵗʰ **S85.809** Unspecified injury of other blood vessels at lower leg level, unspecified leg   CC

√6ᵗʰ **S85.81** Laceration of other blood vessels at lower leg level

- √7ᵗʰ **S85.811** Laceration of other blood vessels at lower leg level, right leg   CC
- √7ᵗʰ **S85.812** Laceration of other blood vessels at lower leg level, left leg   CC
- √7ᵗʰ **S85.819** Laceration of other blood vessels at lower leg level, unspecified leg   CC

√6ᵗʰ **S85.89** Other specified injury of other blood vessels at lower leg level

- √7ᵗʰ **S85.891** Other specified injury of other blood vessels at lower leg level, right leg   CC
- √7ᵗʰ **S85.892** Other specified injury of other blood vessels at lower leg level, left leg   CC
- √7ᵗʰ **S85.899** Other specified injury of other blood vessels at lower leg level, unspecified leg   CC

Ⓝ Newborn: 0   Ⓟ Pediatric: 0-17   Ⓜ Maternity: 9-64   Ⓐ Adult: 15-124   MCC Major Complication/Comorbidity   CC Complication/Comorbidity   SW Severe Wound Dx

1074

ICD-10-CM 2022

√5ᵗʰ **S85.9** Injury of unspecified blood vessel at lower leg level

  √6ᵗʰ **S85.90** Unspecified injury of unspecified blood vessel at lower leg level

    √7ᵗʰ **S85.901** Unspecified injury of unspecified blood vessel at lower leg level, **right leg** `cc`

    √7ᵗʰ **S85.902** Unspecified injury of unspecified blood vessel at lower leg level, **left leg** `cc`

    √7ᵗʰ **S85.909** Unspecified injury of unspecified blood vessel at lower leg level, unspecified leg `cc`

  √6ᵗʰ **S85.91** Laceration of unspecified blood vessel at lower leg level

    √7ᵗʰ **S85.911** Laceration of unspecified blood vessel at lower leg level, **right leg** `cc`

    √7ᵗʰ **S85.912** Laceration of unspecified blood vessel at lower leg level, **left leg** `cc`

    √7ᵗʰ **S85.919** Laceration of unspecified blood vessel at lower leg level, unspecified leg `cc`

  √6ᵗʰ **S85.99** Other specified injury of unspecified blood vessel at lower leg level

    √7ᵗʰ **S85.991** Other specified injury of unspecified blood vessel at lower leg level, **right leg** `cc`

    √7ᵗʰ **S85.992** Other specified injury of unspecified blood vessel at lower leg level, **left leg** `cc`

    √7ᵗʰ **S85.999** Other specified injury of unspecified blood vessel at lower leg level, unspecified leg `cc`

√4ᵗʰ **S86** **Injury of muscle, fascia and tendon at lower leg level**

  Code also any associated open wound (S81.-)

  EXCLUDES 2   injury of muscle, fascia and tendon at ankle (S96.-)

         injury of patellar ligament (tendon) (S76.1-)

         sprain of joints and ligaments of knee (S83.-)

  TIP: Refer to the Muscle/Tendon table at the beginning of this chapter.

  The appropriate 7th character is to be added to each code from category S86.

  A   initial encounter

  D   subsequent encounter

  S   sequela

√5ᵗʰ **S86.0** Injury of **Achilles tendon**

  √6ᵗʰ **S86.00** **Unspecified injury of Achilles tendon**

    √7ᵗʰ **S86.001** Unspecified injury of **right** Achilles tendon

    √7ᵗʰ **S86.002** Unspecified injury of **left** Achilles tendon

    √7ᵗʰ **S86.009** Unspecified injury of unspecified Achilles tendon

  √6ᵗʰ **S86.01** **Strain of Achilles tendon**

    √7ᵗʰ **S86.011** Strain of **right** Achilles tendon

    √7ᵗʰ **S86.012** Strain of **left** Achilles tendon

    √7ᵗʰ **S86.019** Strain of unspecified Achilles tendon

  √6ᵗʰ **S86.02** **Laceration of Achilles tendon**

    √7ᵗʰ **S86.021** Laceration of **right** Achilles tendon `cc`

    √7ᵗʰ **S86.022** Laceration of **left** Achilles tendon `cc`

    √7ᵗʰ **S86.029** Laceration of unspecified Achilles tendon `cc`

  √6ᵗʰ **S86.09** **Other specified injury of Achilles tendon**

    √7ᵗʰ **S86.091** Other specified injury of **right** Achilles tendon

    √7ᵗʰ **S86.092** Other specified injury of **left** Achilles tendon

    √7ᵗʰ **S86.099** Other specified injury of unspecified Achilles tendon

√5ᵗʰ **S86.1** Injury of other muscle(s) and tendon(s) of **posterior muscle group** at lower leg level

  √6ᵗʰ **S86.10** Unspecified injury of other muscle(s) and tendon(s) of posterior muscle group at lower leg level

    √7ᵗʰ **S86.101** Unspecified injury of other muscle(s) and tendon(s) of posterior muscle group at lower leg level, **right leg**

    √7ᵗʰ **S86.102** Unspecified injury of other muscle(s) and tendon(s) of posterior muscle group at lower leg level, **left leg**

    √7ᵗʰ **S86.109** Unspecified injury of other muscle(s) and tendon(s) of posterior muscle group at lower leg level, unspecified leg

√6ᵗʰ **S86.11** **Strain** of other muscle(s) and tendon(s) of posterior muscle group at lower leg level

  √7ᵗʰ **S86.111** Strain of other muscle(s) and tendon(s) of posterior muscle group at lower leg level, **right leg**

  √7ᵗʰ **S86.112** Strain of other muscle(s) and tendon(s) of posterior muscle group at lower leg level, **left leg**

  √7ᵗʰ **S86.119** Strain of other muscle(s) and tendon(s) of posterior muscle group at lower leg level, unspecified leg

√6ᵗʰ **S86.12** **Laceration** of other muscle(s) and tendon(s) of posterior muscle group at lower leg level

  √7ᵗʰ **S86.121** Laceration of other muscle(s) and tendon(s) of posterior muscle group at lower leg level, **right leg** `cc`

  √7ᵗʰ **S86.122** Laceration of other muscle(s) and tendon(s) of posterior muscle group at lower leg level, **left leg** `cc`

  √7ᵗʰ **S86.129** Laceration of other muscle(s) and tendon(s) of posterior muscle group at lower leg level, unspecified leg `cc`

√6ᵗʰ **S86.19** **Other injury of other muscle(s) and tendon(s) of posterior muscle group at lower leg level**

  √7ᵗʰ **S86.191** Other injury of other muscle(s) and tendon(s) of posterior muscle group at lower leg level, **right leg**

  √7ᵗʰ **S86.192** Other injury of other muscle(s) and tendon(s) of posterior muscle group at lower leg level, **left leg**

  √7ᵗʰ **S86.199** Other injury of other muscle(s) and tendon(s) of posterior muscle group at lower leg level, unspecified leg

√5ᵗʰ **S86.2** Injury of muscle(s) and tendon(s) of **anterior muscle group** at lower leg level

  √6ᵗʰ **S86.20** Unspecified injury of muscle(s) and tendon(s) of anterior muscle group at lower leg level

    √7ᵗʰ **S86.201** Unspecified injury of muscle(s) and tendon(s) of anterior muscle group at lower leg level, **right leg**

    √7ᵗʰ **S86.202** Unspecified injury of muscle(s) and tendon(s) of anterior muscle group at lower leg level, **left leg**

    √7ᵗʰ **S86.209** Unspecified injury of muscle(s) and tendon(s) of anterior muscle group at lower leg level, unspecified leg

√6ᵗʰ **S86.21** **Strain** of muscle(s) and tendon(s) of anterior muscle group at lower leg level

  √7ᵗʰ **S86.211** Strain of muscle(s) and tendon(s) of anterior muscle group at lower leg level, **right leg**

  √7ᵗʰ **S86.212** Strain of muscle(s) and tendon(s) of anterior muscle group at lower leg level, **left leg**

  √7ᵗʰ **S86.219** Strain of muscle(s) and tendon(s) of anterior muscle group at lower leg level, unspecified leg

√6ᵗʰ **S86.22** **Laceration** of muscle(s) and tendon(s) of anterior muscle group at lower leg level

  √7ᵗʰ **S86.221** Laceration of muscle(s) and tendon(s) of anterior muscle group at lower leg level, **right leg** `cc`

  √7ᵗʰ **S86.222** Laceration of muscle(s) and tendon(s) of anterior muscle group at lower leg level, **left leg** `cc`

  √7ᵗʰ **S86.229** Laceration of muscle(s) and tendon(s) of anterior muscle group at lower leg level, unspecified leg `cc`

√6ᵗʰ **S86.29** **Other injury of muscle(s) and tendon(s) of anterior muscle group at lower leg level**

  √7ᵗʰ **S86.291** Other injury of muscle(s) and tendon(s) of anterior muscle group at lower leg level, **right leg**

  √7ᵗʰ **S86.292** Other injury of muscle(s) and tendon(s) of anterior muscle group at lower leg level, **left leg**

  √7ᵗʰ **S86.299** Other injury of muscle(s) and tendon(s) of anterior muscle group at lower leg level, unspecified leg

✔ Additional Character Required   √x7ᵗʰ Placeholder   Questionable PDx   Manifestation   Unspecified Dx   UPD Unacceptable PDx   H1-H14 HAC   HCC CMS-HCC Dx   HIV HIV Dx

ICD-10-CM 2022   1075

✓5ᵗʰ S86.3 Injury of muscle(s) and tendon(s) of peroneal muscle group at lower leg level

  ✓6ᵗʰ S86.30 Unspecified injury of muscle(s) and tendon(s) of peroneal muscle group at lower leg level

    ✓7ᵗʰ S86.301 Unspecified injury of muscle(s) and tendon(s) of peroneal muscle group at lower leg level, right leg

    ✓7ᵗʰ S86.302 Unspecified injury of muscle(s) and tendon(s) of peroneal muscle group at lower leg level, left leg

    ✓7ᵗʰ S86.309 Unspecified injury of muscle(s) and tendon(s) of peroneal muscle group at lower leg level, unspecified leg

  ✓6ᵗʰ S86.31 Strain of muscle(s) and tendon(s) of peroneal muscle group at lower leg level

    ✓7ᵗʰ S86.311 Strain of muscle(s) and tendon(s) of peroneal muscle group at lower leg level, right leg

    ✓7ᵗʰ S86.312 Strain of muscle(s) and tendon(s) of peroneal muscle group at lower leg level, left leg

    ✓7ᵗʰ S86.319 Strain of muscle(s) and tendon(s) of peroneal muscle group at lower leg level, unspecified leg

  ✓6ᵗʰ S86.32 Laceration of muscle(s) and tendon(s) of peroneal muscle group at lower leg level

    ✓7ᵗʰ S86.321 Laceration of muscle(s) and tendon(s) of peroneal muscle group at lower leg level, right leg CC

    ✓7ᵗʰ S86.322 Laceration of muscle(s) and tendon(s) of peroneal muscle group at lower leg level, left leg CC

    ✓7ᵗʰ S86.329 Laceration of muscle(s) and tendon(s) of peroneal muscle group at lower leg level, unspecified leg CC

  ✓6ᵗʰ S86.39 Other injury of muscle(s) and tendon(s) of peroneal muscle group at lower leg level

    ✓7ᵗʰ S86.391 Other injury of muscle(s) and tendon(s) of peroneal muscle group at lower leg level, right leg

    ✓7ᵗʰ S86.392 Other injury of muscle(s) and tendon(s) of peroneal muscle group at lower leg level, left leg

    ✓7ᵗʰ S86.399 Other injury of muscle(s) and tendon(s) of peroneal muscle group at lower leg level, unspecified leg

✓5ᵗʰ S86.8 Injury of other muscles and tendons at lower leg level

  ✓6ᵗʰ S86.80 Unspecified injury of other muscles and tendons at lower leg level

    ✓7ᵗʰ S86.801 Unspecified injury of other muscle(s) and tendon(s) at lower leg level, right leg

    ✓7ᵗʰ S86.802 Unspecified injury of other muscle(s) and tendon(s) at lower leg level, left leg

    ✓7ᵗʰ S86.809 Unspecified injury of other muscle(s) and tendon(s) at lower leg level, unspecified leg

  ✓6ᵗʰ S86.81 Strain of other muscles and tendons at lower leg level

    ✓7ᵗʰ S86.811 Strain of other muscle(s) and tendon(s) at lower leg level, right leg

    ✓7ᵗʰ S86.812 Strain of other muscle(s) and tendon(s) at lower leg level, left leg

    ✓7ᵗʰ S86.819 Strain of other muscle(s) and tendon(s) at lower leg level, unspecified leg

  ✓6ᵗʰ S86.82 Laceration of other muscles and tendons at lower leg level

    ✓7ᵗʰ S86.821 Laceration of other muscle(s) and tendon(s) at lower leg level, right leg CC

    ✓7ᵗʰ S86.822 Laceration of other muscle(s) and tendon(s) at lower leg level, left leg CC

    ✓7ᵗʰ S86.829 Laceration of other muscle(s) and tendon(s) at lower leg level, unspecified leg CC

  ✓6ᵗʰ S86.89 Other injury of other muscles and tendons at lower leg level

    ✓7ᵗʰ S86.891 Other injury of other muscle(s) and tendon(s) at lower leg level, right leg

    ✓7ᵗʰ S86.892 Other injury of other muscle(s) and tendon(s) at lower leg level, left leg

    ✓7ᵗʰ S86.899 Other injury of other muscle(s) and tendon(s) at lower leg level, unspecified leg

✓5ᵗʰ S86.9 Injury of unspecified muscle and tendon at lower leg level

  ✓6ᵗʰ S86.90 Unspecified injury of unspecified muscle and tendon at lower leg level

    ✓7ᵗʰ S86.901 Unspecified injury of unspecified muscle(s) and tendon(s) at lower leg level, right leg

    ✓7ᵗʰ S86.902 Unspecified injury of unspecified muscle(s) and tendon(s) at lower leg level, left leg

    ✓7ᵗʰ S86.909 Unspecified injury of unspecified muscle(s) and tendon(s) at lower leg level, unspecified leg

  ✓6ᵗʰ S86.91 Strain of unspecified muscle and tendon at lower leg level

    ✓7ᵗʰ S86.911 Strain of unspecified muscle(s) and tendon(s) at lower leg level, right leg

    ✓7ᵗʰ S86.912 Strain of unspecified muscle(s) and tendon(s) at lower leg level, left leg

    ✓7ᵗʰ S86.919 Strain of unspecified muscle(s) and tendon(s) at lower leg level, unspecified leg

  ✓6ᵗʰ S86.92 Laceration of unspecified muscle and tendon at lower leg level

    ✓7ᵗʰ S86.921 Laceration of unspecified muscle(s) and tendon(s) at lower leg level, right leg CC

    ✓7ᵗʰ S86.922 Laceration of unspecified muscle(s) and tendon(s) at lower leg level, left leg CC

    ✓7ᵗʰ S86.929 Laceration of unspecified muscle(s) and tendon(s) at lower leg level, unspecified leg CC

  ✓6ᵗʰ S86.99 Other injury of unspecified muscle and tendon at lower leg level

    ✓7ᵗʰ S86.991 Other injury of unspecified muscle(s) and tendon(s) at lower leg level, right leg

    ✓7ᵗʰ S86.992 Other injury of unspecified muscle(s) and tendon(s) at lower leg level, left leg

    ✓7ᵗʰ S86.999 Other injury of unspecified muscle(s) and tendon(s) at lower leg level, unspecified leg

✓4ᵗʰ S87 Crushing injury of lower leg

  Use additional code(s) for all associated injuries

  EXCLUDES 2   crushing injury of ankle and foot (S97.-)

  The appropriate 7th character is to be added to each code from category S87.
  A   initial encounter
  D   subsequent encounter
  S   sequela

  ✓5ᵗʰ S87.0 Crushing injury of knee

    ✓x7ᵗʰ S87.00 Crushing injury of unspecified knee

    ✓x7ᵗʰ S87.01 Crushing injury of right knee

    ✓x7ᵗʰ S87.02 Crushing injury of left knee

  ✓5ᵗʰ S87.8 Crushing injury of lower leg

    ✓x7ᵗʰ S87.80 Crushing injury of unspecified lower leg

    ✓x7ᵗʰ S87.81 Crushing injury of right lower leg

    ✓x7ᵗʰ S87.82 Crushing injury of left lower leg

✓4ᵗʰ S88 Traumatic amputation of lower leg

  An amputation not identified as partial or complete should be coded to complete

  EXCLUDES 1   traumatic amputation of ankle and foot (S98.-)

  The appropriate 7th character is to be added to each code from category S88.
  A   initial encounter
  D   subsequent encounter
  S   sequela

  ✓5ᵗʰ S88.0 Traumatic amputation at knee level

    ✓6ᵗʰ S88.01 Complete traumatic amputation at knee level

      ✓7ᵗʰ S88.011 Complete traumatic amputation at knee level, right lower leg CC HCC

      ✓7ᵗʰ S88.012 Complete traumatic amputation at knee level, left lower leg CC HCC

      ✓7ᵗʰ S88.019 Complete traumatic amputation at knee level, unspecified lower leg CC HCC

    ✓6ᵗʰ S88.02 Partial traumatic amputation at knee level

      ✓7ᵗʰ S88.021 Partial traumatic amputation at knee level, right lower leg CC HCC

N Newborn: 0   P Pediatric: 0-17   M Maternity: 9-64   A Adult: 15-124   MCC Major Complication/Comorbidity   CC Complication/Comorbidity   SW Severe Wound Dx

√7ᵗʰ **S88.022** Partial traumatic amputation at knee level, left lower leg   CC HCC

√7ᵗʰ **S88.029** Partial traumatic amputation at knee level, unspecified lower leg   CC

√5ᵗʰ **S88.1** Traumatic amputation at level between knee and ankle

√6ᵗʰ **S88.11** Complete traumatic amputation at level between knee and ankle

√7ᵗʰ **S88.111** Complete traumatic amputation at level between knee and ankle, right lower leg   CC HCC

√7ᵗʰ **S88.112** Complete traumatic amputation at level between knee and ankle, left lower leg   CC HCC

√7ᵗʰ **S88.119** Complete traumatic amputation at level between knee and ankle, unspecified lower leg   CC HCC

√6ᵗʰ **S88.12** Partial traumatic amputation at level between knee and ankle

√7ᵗʰ **S88.121** Partial traumatic amputation at level between knee and ankle, right lower leg   CC HCC

√7ᵗʰ **S88.122** Partial traumatic amputation at level between knee and ankle, left lower leg   CC HCC

√7ᵗʰ **S88.129** Partial traumatic amputation at level between knee and ankle, unspecified lower leg   CC HCC

√5ᵗʰ **S88.9** Traumatic amputation of lower leg, level unspecified

√6ᵗʰ **S88.91** Complete traumatic amputation of lower leg, level unspecified

√7ᵗʰ **S88.911** Complete traumatic amputation of right lower leg, level unspecified   CC HCC

√7ᵗʰ **S88.912** Complete traumatic amputation of left lower leg, level unspecified   CC HCC

√7ᵗʰ **S88.919** Complete traumatic amputation of unspecified lower leg, level unspecified   CC HCC

√6ᵗʰ **S88.92** Partial traumatic amputation of lower leg, level unspecified

√7ᵗʰ **S88.921** Partial traumatic amputation of right lower leg, level unspecified   CC HCC

√7ᵗʰ **S88.922** Partial traumatic amputation of left lower leg, level unspecified   CC HCC

√7ᵗʰ **S88.929** Partial traumatic amputation of unspecified lower leg, level unspecified   CC HCC

√4ᵗʰ **S89 Other and unspecified injuries of lower leg**

NOTE A fracture not indicated as open or closed should be coded to closed.

EXCLUDES 2   *other and unspecified injuries of ankle and foot (S99.-)*

AHA: 2018,2Q,12; 2018,1Q,3; 2015,3Q,37-39

The appropriate 7th character is to be added to each code from subcategories S89.0, S89.1, S89.2, and S89.3.
A   initial encounter for closed fracture
D   subsequent encounter for fracture with routine healing
G   subsequent encounter for fracture with delayed healing
K   subsequent encounter for fracture with nonunion
P   subsequent encounter for fracture with malunion
S   sequela

√5ᵗʰ **S89.0** Physeal fracture of upper end of tibia

AHA: 2019,4Q,56

√6ᵗʰ **S89.00** Unspecified physeal fracture of upper end of tibia

³ √7ᵗʰ **S89.001** Unspecified physeal fracture of upper end of right tibia   CC H5

³ √7ᵗʰ **S89.002** Unspecified physeal fracture of upper end of left tibia   CC H5

³ √7ᵗʰ **S89.009** Unspecified physeal fracture of upper end of unspecified tibia   CC H5

√6ᵗʰ **S89.01** Salter-Harris Type I physeal fracture of upper end of tibia

³ √7ᵗʰ **S89.011** Salter-Harris Type I physeal fracture of upper end of right tibia   CC H5

³ √7ᵗʰ **S89.012** Salter-Harris Type I physeal fracture of upper end of left tibia   CC H5

³ √7ᵗʰ **S89.019** Salter-Harris Type I physeal fracture of upper end of unspecified tibia   CC H5

√6ᵗʰ **S89.02** Salter-Harris Type II physeal fracture of upper end of tibia

³ √7ᵗʰ **S89.021** Salter-Harris Type II physeal fracture of upper end of right tibia   CC H5

³ √7ᵗʰ **S89.022** Salter-Harris Type II physeal fracture of upper end of left tibia   CC H5

³ √7ᵗʰ **S89.029** Salter-Harris Type II physeal fracture of upper end of unspecified tibia   CC H5

√6ᵗʰ **S89.03** Salter-Harris Type III physeal fracture of upper end of tibia

³ √7ᵗʰ **S89.031** Salter-Harris Type III physeal fracture of upper end of right tibia   CC H5

³ √7ᵗʰ **S89.032** Salter-Harris Type III physeal fracture of upper end of left tibia   CC H5

³ √7ᵗʰ **S89.039** Salter-Harris Type III physeal fracture of upper end of unspecified tibia   CC H5

√6ᵗʰ **S89.04** Salter-Harris Type IV physeal fracture of upper end of tibia

³ √7ᵗʰ **S89.041** Salter-Harris Type IV physeal fracture of upper end of right tibia   CC H5

³ √7ᵗʰ **S89.042** Salter-Harris Type IV physeal fracture of upper end of left tibia   CC H5

³ √7ᵗʰ **S89.049** Salter-Harris Type IV physeal fracture of upper end of unspecified tibia   CC H5

√6ᵗʰ **S89.09** Other physeal fracture of upper end of tibia

³ √7ᵗʰ **S89.091** Other physeal fracture of upper end of right tibia   CC H5

³ √7ᵗʰ **S89.092** Other physeal fracture of upper end of left tibia   CC H5

³ √7ᵗʰ **S89.099** Other physeal fracture of upper end of unspecified tibia   CC H5

√5ᵗʰ **S89.1** Physeal fracture of lower end of tibia

AHA: 2019,4Q,56

√6ᵗʰ **S89.10** Unspecified physeal fracture of lower end of tibia

⁴ √7ᵗʰ **S89.101** Unspecified physeal fracture of lower end of right tibia   CC

⁴ √7ᵗʰ **S89.102** Unspecified physeal fracture of lower end of left tibia   CC

⁴ √7ᵗʰ **S89.109** Unspecified physeal fracture of lower end of unspecified tibia   CC

√6ᵗʰ **S89.11** Salter-Harris Type I physeal fracture of lower end of tibia

⁴ √7ᵗʰ **S89.111** Salter-Harris Type I physeal fracture of lower end of right tibia   CC

⁴ √7ᵗʰ **S89.112** Salter-Harris Type I physeal fracture of lower end of left tibia   CC

⁴ √7ᵗʰ **S89.119** Salter-Harris Type I physeal fracture of lower end of unspecified tibia   CC

√6ᵗʰ **S89.12** Salter-Harris Type II physeal fracture of lower end of tibia

⁴ √7ᵗʰ **S89.121** Salter-Harris Type II physeal fracture of lower end of right tibia   CC

⁴ √7ᵗʰ **S89.122** Salter-Harris Type II physeal fracture of lower end of left tibia   CC

⁴ √7ᵗʰ **S89.129** Salter-Harris Type II physeal fracture of lower end of unspecified tibia   CC

√6ᵗʰ **S89.13** Salter-Harris Type III physeal fracture of lower end of tibia

EXCLUDES 1   *fracture of medial malleolus (adult) (S82.5-)*

⁴ √7ᵗʰ **S89.131** Salter-Harris Type III physeal fracture of lower end of right tibia   CC

⁴ √7ᵗʰ **S89.132** Salter-Harris Type III physeal fracture of lower end of left tibia   CC

⁴ √7ᵗʰ **S89.139** Salter-Harris Type III physeal fracture of lower end of unspecified tibia   CC

√6ᵗʰ **S89.14** Salter-Harris Type IV physeal fracture of lower end of tibia

EXCLUDES 1   *fracture of medial malleolus (adult) (S82.5-)*

⁴ √7ᵗʰ **S89.141** Salter-Harris Type IV physeal fracture of lower end of right tibia   CC

⁴ √7ᵗʰ **S89.142** Salter-Harris Type IV physeal fracture of lower end of left tibia   CC

⁴ √7ᵗʰ **S89.149** Salter-Harris Type IV physeal fracture of lower end of unspecified tibia   CC

√6ᵗʰ **S89.19** Other physeal fracture of lower end of tibia

⁴ √7ᵗʰ **S89.191** Other physeal fracture of lower end of right tibia   CC

✔ Additional Character Required   √x7ᵗʰ Placeholder   Questionable PDx   Manifestation   Unspecified Dx   UPD Unacceptable PDx   H1-H14 HAC   HCC CMS-HCC Dx   HIV HIV Dx

ICD-10-CM 2022   1077

4 √7ᵗʰ   **S89.192**   Other physeal fracture of lower end of left tibia   **CC**

4 √7ᵗʰ   **S89.199**   Other physeal fracture of lower end of unspecified tibia   **MCC**

√5ᵗʰ   **S89.2**   **Physeal fracture of** upper end of fibula

     AHA: 2019,4Q,56

   √6ᵗʰ   **S89.20**   Unspecified physeal fracture of upper end of fibula

     4 √7ᵗʰ   **S89.201**   Unspecified physeal fracture of upper end of right fibula   **CC**

     4 √7ᵗʰ   **S89.202**   Unspecified physeal fracture of upper end of left fibula   **CC**

     4 √7ᵗʰ   **S89.209**   Unspecified physeal fracture of upper end of unspecified fibula   **CC**

   √6ᵗʰ   **S89.21**   Salter-Harris Type I physeal fracture of upper end of fibula

     4 √7ᵗʰ   **S89.211**   Salter-Harris Type I physeal fracture of upper end of right fibula   **CC**

     4 √7ᵗʰ   **S89.212**   Salter-Harris Type I physeal fracture of upper end of left fibula   **CC**

     4 √7ᵗʰ   **S89.219**   Salter-Harris Type I physeal fracture of upper end of unspecified fibula   **CC**

   √6ᵗʰ   **S89.22**   Salter-Harris Type II physeal fracture of upper end of fibula

     4 √7ᵗʰ   **S89.221**   Salter-Harris Type II physeal fracture of upper end of right fibula   **CC**

     4 √7ᵗʰ   **S89.222**   Salter-Harris Type II physeal fracture of upper end of left fibula   **CC**

     4 √7ᵗʰ   **S89.229**   Salter-Harris Type II physeal fracture of upper end of unspecified fibula   **CC**

   √6ᵗʰ   **S89.29**   Other physeal fracture of upper end of fibula

     4 √7ᵗʰ   **S89.291**   Other physeal fracture of upper end of right fibula   **CC**

     4 √7ᵗʰ   **S89.292**   Other physeal fracture of upper end of left fibula   **CC**

     4 √7ᵗʰ   **S89.299**   Other physeal fracture of upper end of unspecified fibula   **CC**

√5ᵗʰ   **S89.3**   **Physeal fracture of** lower end of fibula

     AHA: 2019,4Q,56

   √6ᵗʰ   **S89.30**   Unspecified physeal fracture of lower end of fibula

     4 √7ᵗʰ   **S89.301**   Unspecified physeal fracture of lower end of right fibula   **CC**

     4 √7ᵗʰ   **S89.302**   Unspecified physeal fracture of lower end of left fibula   **CC**

     4 √7ᵗʰ   **S89.309**   Unspecified physeal fracture of lower end of unspecified fibula   **CC**

   √6ᵗʰ   **S89.31**   Salter-Harris Type I physeal fracture of lower end of fibula

     4 √7ᵗʰ   **S89.311**   Salter-Harris Type I physeal fracture of lower end of right fibula   **CC**

     4 √7ᵗʰ   **S89.312**   Salter-Harris Type I physeal fracture of lower end of left fibula   **CC**

     4 √7ᵗʰ   **S89.319**   Salter-Harris Type I physeal fracture of lower end of unspecified fibula   **CC**

   √6ᵗʰ   **S89.32**   Salter-Harris Type II physeal fracture of lower end of fibula

     4 √7ᵗʰ   **S89.321**   Salter-Harris Type II physeal fracture of lower end of right fibula   **CC**

     4 √7ᵗʰ   **S89.322**   Salter-Harris Type II physeal fracture of lower end of left fibula   **CC**

     4 √7ᵗʰ   **S89.329**   Salter-Harris Type II physeal fracture of lower end of unspecified fibula   **CC**

   √6ᵗʰ   **S89.39**   Other physeal fracture of lower end of fibula

     4 √7ᵗʰ   **S89.391**   Other physeal fracture of lower end of right fibula   **CC**

     4 √7ᵗʰ   **S89.392**   Other physeal fracture of lower end of left fibula   **CC**

     4 √7ᵗʰ   **S89.399**   Other physeal fracture of lower end of unspecified fibula   **CC**

√5ᵗʰ   **S89.8**   **Other specified injuries of lower leg**

> The appropriate 7th character is to be added to each code in subcategory S89.8.
> A   initial encounter
> D   subsequent encounter
> S   sequela

   √x7ᵗʰ   **S89.80**   Other specified injuries of unspecified lower leg

   √x7ᵗʰ   **S89.81**   Other specified injuries of right lower leg

   √x7ᵗʰ   **S89.82**   Other specified injuries of left lower leg

---

   √5ᵗʰ   **S89.9**   **Unspecified injury of lower leg**

> The appropriate 7th character is to be added to each code in subcategory S89.9.
> A   initial encounter
> D   subsequent encounter
> S   sequela

   √x7ᵗʰ   **S89.90**   Unspecified injury of unspecified lower leg

   √x7ᵗʰ   **S89.91**   Unspecified injury of right lower leg

   √x7ᵗʰ   **S89.92**   Unspecified injury of left lower leg

Injuries to the ankle and foot (S90-S99)

EXCLUDES 2   burns and corrosions (T20-T32)
     fracture of ankle and malleolus (S82.-)
     frostbite (T33-T34)
     insect bite or sting, venomous (T63.4)

√4ᵗʰ   **S90**   **Superficial injury of ankle, foot and toes**

> The appropriate 7th character is to be added to each code from category S90.
> A   initial encounter
> D   subsequent encounter
> S   sequela

   √5ᵗʰ   **S90.0**   **Contusion of** ankle

     √x7ᵗʰ   **S90.00**   Contusion of unspecified ankle

     √x7ᵗʰ   **S90.01**   Contusion of right ankle

     √x7ᵗʰ   **S90.02**   Contusion of left ankle

   √5ᵗʰ   **S90.1**   **Contusion of** toe without damage to nail

     √6ᵗʰ   **S90.11**   Contusion of great toe without damage to nail

       √7ᵗʰ   **S90.111**   Contusion of right great toe without damage to nail

       √7ᵗʰ   **S90.112**   Contusion of left great toe without damage to nail

       √7ᵗʰ   **S90.119**   Contusion of unspecified great toe without damage to nail

     √6ᵗʰ   **S90.12**   Contusion of lesser toe without damage to nail

       √7ᵗʰ   **S90.121**   Contusion of right lesser toe(s) without damage to nail

       √7ᵗʰ   **S90.122**   Contusion of left lesser toe(s) without damage to nail

       √7ᵗʰ   **S90.129**   Contusion of unspecified lesser toe(s) without damage to nail
          Contusion of toe NOS

   √5ᵗʰ   **S90.2**   **Contusion of** toe with damage to nail

     √6ᵗʰ   **S90.21**   Contusion of great toe with damage to nail

       √7ᵗʰ   **S90.211**   Contusion of right great toe with damage to nail

       √7ᵗʰ   **S90.212**   Contusion of left great toe with damage to nail

       √7ᵗʰ   **S90.219**   Contusion of unspecified great toe with damage to nail

     √6ᵗʰ   **S90.22**   Contusion of lesser toe with damage to nail

       √7ᵗʰ   **S90.221**   Contusion of right lesser toe(s) with damage to nail

       √7ᵗʰ   **S90.222**   Contusion of left lesser toe(s) with damage to nail

       √7ᵗʰ   **S90.229**   Contusion of unspecified lesser toe(s) with damage to nail

   √5ᵗʰ   **S90.3**   **Contusion of** foot

     EXCLUDES 2   contusion of toes (S90.1-, S90.2-)

     √x7ᵗʰ   **S90.30**   Contusion of unspecified foot
          Contusion of foot NOS

     √x7ᵗʰ   **S90.31**   Contusion of right foot

     √x7ᵗʰ   **S90.32**   Contusion of left foot

   √5ᵗʰ   **S90.4**   **Other superficial injuries of** toe

     √6ᵗʰ   **S90.41**   Abrasion of toe

       √7ᵗʰ   **S90.411**   Abrasion, right great toe

       √7ᵗʰ   **S90.412**   Abrasion, left great toe

       √7ᵗʰ   **S90.413**   Abrasion, unspecified great toe

       √7ᵗʰ   **S90.414**   Abrasion, right lesser toe(s)

       √7ᵗʰ   **S90.415**   Abrasion, left lesser toe(s)

       √7ᵗʰ   **S90.416**   Abrasion, unspecified lesser toe(s)

     √6ᵗʰ   **S90.42**   Blister (nonthermal) of toe

       √7ᵗʰ   **S90.421**   Blister (nonthermal), right great toe

---

N Newborn: 0   **P** Pediatric: 0-17   **M** Maternity: 9-64   **A** Adult: 15-124   **MCC** Major Complication/Comorbidity   **CC** Complication/Comorbidity   **SW** Severe Wound Dx

1078   ICD-10-CM 2022

√7ᵗʰ **S90.422** Blister (nonthermal), left great toe

√7ᵗʰ **S90.423** Blister (nonthermal), unspecified great toe

√7ᵗʰ **S90.424** Blister (nonthermal), right lesser toe(s)

√7ᵗʰ **S90.425** Blister (nonthermal), left lesser toe(s)

√7ᵗʰ **S90.426** Blister (nonthermal), unspecified lesser toe(s)

√6ᵗʰ **S90.44** External constriction of toe

    Hair tourniquet syndrome of toe

√7ᵗʰ **S90.441** External constriction, right great toe

√7ᵗʰ **S90.442** External constriction, left great toe

√7ᵗʰ **S90.443** External constriction, unspecified great toe

√7ᵗʰ **S90.444** External constriction, right lesser toe(s)

√7ᵗʰ **S90.445** External constriction, left lesser toe(s)

√7ᵗʰ **S90.446** External constriction, unspecified lesser toe(s)

√6ᵗʰ **S90.45** Superficial foreign body of toe

    Splinter in the toe

√7ᵗʰ **S90.451** Superficial foreign body, right great toe

√7ᵗʰ **S90.452** Superficial foreign body, left great toe

√7ᵗʰ **S90.453** Superficial foreign body, unspecified great toe

√7ᵗʰ **S90.454** Superficial foreign body, right lesser toe(s)

√7ᵗʰ **S90.455** Superficial foreign body, left lesser toe(s)

√7ᵗʰ **S90.456** Superficial foreign body, unspecified lesser toe(s)

√6ᵗʰ **S90.46** Insect bite (nonvenomous) of toe

√7ᵗʰ **S90.461** Insect bite (nonvenomous), right great toe

√7ᵗʰ **S90.462** Insect bite (nonvenomous), left great toe

√7ᵗʰ **S90.463** Insect bite (nonvenomous), unspecified great toe

√7ᵗʰ **S90.464** Insect bite (nonvenomous), right lesser toe(s)

√7ᵗʰ **S90.465** Insect bite (nonvenomous), left lesser toe(s)

√7ᵗʰ **S90.466** Insect bite (nonvenomous), unspecified lesser toe(s)

√6ᵗʰ **S90.47** Other superficial bite of toe

    EXCLUDES 1 *open bite of toe (S91.15-, S91.25-)*

√7ᵗʰ **S90.471** Other superficial bite of right great toe

√7ᵗʰ **S90.472** Other superficial bite of left great toe

√7ᵗʰ **S90.473** Other superficial bite of unspecified great toe

√7ᵗʰ **S90.474** Other superficial bite of right lesser toe(s)

√7ᵗʰ **S90.475** Other superficial bite of left lesser toe(s)

√7ᵗʰ **S90.476** Other superficial bite of unspecified lesser toe(s)

√5ᵗʰ **S90.5** Other superficial injuries of ankle

√6ᵗʰ **S90.51** Abrasion of ankle

√7ᵗʰ **S90.511** Abrasion, right ankle

√7ᵗʰ **S90.512** Abrasion, left ankle

√7ᵗʰ **S90.519** Abrasion, unspecified ankle

√6ᵗʰ **S90.52** Blister (nonthermal) of ankle

√7ᵗʰ **S90.521** Blister (nonthermal), right ankle

√7ᵗʰ **S90.522** Blister (nonthermal), left ankle

√7ᵗʰ **S90.529** Blister (nonthermal), unspecified ankle

√6ᵗʰ **S90.54** External constriction of ankle

√7ᵗʰ **S90.541** External constriction, right ankle

√7ᵗʰ **S90.542** External constriction, left ankle

√7ᵗʰ **S90.549** External constriction, unspecified ankle

√6ᵗʰ **S90.55** Superficial foreign body of ankle

    Splinter in the ankle

√7ᵗʰ **S90.551** Superficial foreign body, right ankle

√7ᵗʰ **S90.552** Superficial foreign body, left ankle

√7ᵗʰ **S90.559** Superficial foreign body, unspecified ankle

√6ᵗʰ **S90.56** Insect bite (nonvenomous) of ankle

√7ᵗʰ **S90.561** Insect bite (nonvenomous), right ankle

√7ᵗʰ **S90.562** Insect bite (nonvenomous), left ankle

√7ᵗʰ **S90.569** Insect bite (nonvenomous), unspecified ankle

√6ᵗʰ **S90.57** Other superficial bite of ankle

    EXCLUDES 1 *open bite of ankle (S91.05-)*

√7ᵗʰ **S90.571** Other superficial bite of ankle, right ankle

√7ᵗʰ **S90.572** Other superficial bite of ankle, left ankle

√7ᵗʰ **S90.579** Other superficial bite of ankle, unspecified ankle

√5ᵗʰ **S90.8** Other superficial injuries of foot

√6ᵗʰ **S90.81** Abrasion of foot

√7ᵗʰ **S90.811** Abrasion, right foot

√7ᵗʰ **S90.812** Abrasion, left foot

√7ᵗʰ **S90.819** Abrasion, unspecified foot

√6ᵗʰ **S90.82** Blister (nonthermal) of foot

√7ᵗʰ **S90.821** Blister (nonthermal), right foot

√7ᵗʰ **S90.822** Blister (nonthermal), left foot

√7ᵗʰ **S90.829** Blister (nonthermal), unspecified foot

√6ᵗʰ **S90.84** External constriction of foot

√7ᵗʰ **S90.841** External constriction, right foot

√7ᵗʰ **S90.842** External constriction, left foot

√7ᵗʰ **S90.849** External constriction, unspecified foot

√6ᵗʰ **S90.85** Superficial foreign body of foot

    Splinter in the foot

√7ᵗʰ **S90.851** Superficial foreign body, right foot

√7ᵗʰ **S90.852** Superficial foreign body, left foot

√7ᵗʰ **S90.859** Superficial foreign body, unspecified foot

√6ᵗʰ **S90.86** Insect bite (nonvenomous) of foot

√7ᵗʰ **S90.861** Insect bite (nonvenomous), right foot

√7ᵗʰ **S90.862** Insect bite (nonvenomous), left foot

√7ᵗʰ **S90.869** Insect bite (nonvenomous), unspecified foot

√6ᵗʰ **S90.87** Other superficial bite of foot

    EXCLUDES 1 *open bite of foot (S91.35-)*

√7ᵗʰ **S90.871** Other superficial bite of right foot

√7ᵗʰ **S90.872** Other superficial bite of left foot

√7ᵗʰ **S90.879** Other superficial bite of unspecified foot

√5ᵗʰ **S90.9** Unspecified superficial injury of ankle, foot and toe

√6ᵗʰ **S90.91** Unspecified superficial injury of ankle

√7ᵗʰ **S90.911** Unspecified superficial injury of right ankle

√7ᵗʰ **S90.912** Unspecified superficial injury of left ankle

√7ᵗʰ **S90.919** Unspecified superficial injury of unspecified ankle

√6ᵗʰ **S90.92** Unspecified superficial injury of foot

√7ᵗʰ **S90.921** Unspecified superficial injury of right foot

√7ᵗʰ **S90.922** Unspecified superficial injury of left foot

√7ᵗʰ **S90.929** Unspecified superficial injury of unspecified foot

√6ᵗʰ **S90.93** Unspecified superficial injury of toes

√7ᵗʰ **S90.931** Unspecified superficial injury of right great toe

√7ᵗʰ **S90.932** Unspecified superficial injury of left great toe

√7ᵗʰ **S90.933** Unspecified superficial injury of unspecified great toe

√7ᵗʰ **S90.934** Unspecified superficial injury of right lesser toe(s)

√7ᵗʰ **S90.935** Unspecified superficial injury of left lesser toe(s)

√7ᵗʰ **S90.936** Unspecified superficial injury of unspecified lesser toe(s)

✔ Additional Character Required   √ₓ7ᵗʰ Placeholder   Questionable PDx   Manifestation   Unspecified Dx   **UPD** Unacceptable PDx   **H1**-**H14** HAC   **HCC** CMS-HCC Dx   **HIV** HIV Dx

ICD-10-CM 2022   1079

✓4th S91 Open wound of ankle, foot and toes

Code also any associated wound infection

> **EXCLUDES 1**   open fracture of ankle, foot and toes (S92.- with 7th character B)
>
> traumatic amputation of ankle and foot (S98.-)

AHA: 2021,1Q,7

The appropriate 7th character is to be added to each code from category S91.
A   initial encounter
D   subsequent encounter
S   sequela

✓5th S91.0   Open wound of ankle

   ✓6th S91.00   Unspecified open wound of ankle

     ✓7th S91.001   Unspecified open wound, right ankle

     ✓7th S91.002   Unspecified open wound, left ankle

     ✓7th S91.009   Unspecified open wound, unspecified ankle

   ✓6th S91.01   Laceration without foreign body of ankle

     ✓7th S91.011   Laceration without foreign body, right ankle

     ✓7th S91.012   Laceration without foreign body, left ankle

     ✓7th S91.019   Laceration without foreign body, unspecified ankle

   ✓6th S91.02   Laceration with foreign body of ankle

     ✓7th S91.021   Laceration with foreign body, right ankle

     ✓7th S91.022   Laceration with foreign body, left ankle

     ✓7th S91.029   Laceration with foreign body, unspecified ankle

   ✓6th S91.03   Puncture wound without foreign body of ankle

     ✓7th S91.031   Puncture wound without foreign body, right ankle

     ✓7th S91.032   Puncture wound without foreign body, left ankle

     ✓7th S91.039   Puncture wound without foreign body, unspecified ankle

   ✓6th S91.04   Puncture wound with foreign body of ankle

     ✓7th S91.041   Puncture wound with foreign body, right ankle

     ✓7th S91.042   Puncture wound with foreign body, left ankle

     ✓7th S91.049   Puncture wound with foreign body, unspecified ankle

   ✓6th S91.05   Open bite of ankle

> **EXCLUDES 1**   superficial bite of ankle (S90.56-, S90.57-)

     ✓7th S91.051   Open bite, right ankle

     ✓7th S91.052   Open bite, left ankle

     ✓7th S91.059   Open bite, unspecified ankle

✓5th S91.1   Open wound of toe without damage to nail

   ✓6th S91.10   Unspecified open wound of toe without damage to nail

     ✓7th S91.101   Unspecified open wound of right great toe without damage to nail

     ✓7th S91.102   Unspecified open wound of left great toe without damage to nail

     ✓7th S91.103   Unspecified open wound of unspecified great toe without damage to nail

     ✓7th S91.104   Unspecified open wound of right lesser toe(s) without damage to nail

     ✓7th S91.105   Unspecified open wound of left lesser toe(s) without damage to nail

     ✓7th S91.106   Unspecified open wound of unspecified lesser toe(s) without damage to nail

     ✓7th S91.109   Unspecified open wound of unspecified toe(s) without damage to nail

   ✓6th S91.11   Laceration without foreign body of toe without damage to nail

     ✓7th S91.111   Laceration without foreign body of right great toe without damage to nail

     ✓7th S91.112   Laceration without foreign body of left great toe without damage to nail

     ✓7th S91.113   Laceration without foreign body of unspecified great toe without damage to nail

     ✓7th S91.114   Laceration without foreign body of right lesser toe(s) without damage to nail

     ✓7th S91.115   Laceration without foreign body of left lesser toe(s) without damage to nail

     ✓7th S91.116   Laceration without foreign body of unspecified lesser toe(s) without damage to nail

     ✓7th S91.119   Laceration without foreign body of unspecified toe without damage to nail

   ✓6th S91.12   Laceration with foreign body of toe without damage to nail

     ✓7th S91.121   Laceration with foreign body of right great toe without damage to nail

     ✓7th S91.122   Laceration with foreign body of left great toe without damage to nail

     ✓7th S91.123   Laceration with foreign body of unspecified great toe without damage to nail

     ✓7th S91.124   Laceration with foreign body of right lesser toe(s) without damage to nail

     ✓7th S91.125   Laceration with foreign body of left lesser toe(s) without damage to nail

     ✓7th S91.126   Laceration with foreign body of unspecified lesser toe(s) without damage to nail

     ✓7th S91.129   Laceration with foreign body of unspecified toe(s) without damage to nail

   ✓6th S91.13   Puncture wound without foreign body of toe without damage to nail

     ✓7th S91.131   Puncture wound without foreign body of right great toe without damage to nail

     ✓7th S91.132   Puncture wound without foreign body of left great toe without damage to nail

     ✓7th S91.133   Puncture wound without foreign body of unspecified great toe without damage to nail

     ✓7th S91.134   Puncture wound without foreign body of right lesser toe(s) without damage to nail

     ✓7th S91.135   Puncture wound without foreign body of left lesser toe(s) without damage to nail

     ✓7th S91.136   Puncture wound without foreign body of unspecified lesser toe(s) without damage to nail

     ✓7th S91.139   Puncture wound without foreign body of unspecified toe(s) without damage to nail

   ✓6th S91.14   Puncture wound with foreign body of toe without damage to nail

     ✓7th S91.141   Puncture wound with foreign body of right great toe without damage to nail

     ✓7th S91.142   Puncture wound with foreign body of left great toe without damage to nail

     ✓7th S91.143   Puncture wound with foreign body of unspecified great toe without damage to nail

     ✓7th S91.144   Puncture wound with foreign body of right lesser toe(s) without damage to nail

     ✓7th S91.145   Puncture wound with foreign body of left lesser toe(s) without damage to nail

     ✓7th S91.146   Puncture wound with foreign body of unspecified lesser toe(s) without damage to nail

     ✓7th S91.149   Puncture wound with foreign body of unspecified toe(s) without damage to nail

   ✓6th S91.15   Open bite of toe without damage to nail

Bite of toe NOS

> **EXCLUDES 1**   superficial bite of toe (S90.46-, S90.47-)

     ✓7th S91.151   Open bite of right great toe without damage to nail

     ✓7th S91.152   Open bite of left great toe without damage to nail

     ✓7th S91.153   Open bite of unspecified great toe without damage to nail

     ✓7th S91.154   Open bite of right lesser toe(s) without damage to nail

     ✓7th S91.155   Open bite of left lesser toe(s) without damage to nail

     ✓7th S91.156   Open bite of unspecified lesser toe(s) without damage to nail

     ✓7th S91.159   Open bite of unspecified toe(s) without damage to nail

✓5th S91.2   Open wound of toe with damage to nail

   ✓6th S91.20   Unspecified open wound of toe with damage to nail

     ✓7th S91.201   Unspecified open wound of right great toe with damage to nail

     ✓7th S91.202   Unspecified open wound of left great toe with damage to nail

N Newborn: 0   **P** Pediatric: 0-17   **M** Maternity: 9-64   **A** Adult: 15-124   **MCC** Major Complication/Comorbidity   **CC** Complication/Comorbidity   **SW** Severe Wound Dx

1080   ICD-10-CM 2022

√7ᵗʰ **S91.203** Unspecified open wound of unspecified great toe with damage to nail

√7ᵗʰ **S91.204** Unspecified open wound of right lesser toe(s) with damage to nail

√7ᵗʰ **S91.205** Unspecified open wound of left lesser toe(s) with damage to nail

√7ᵗʰ **S91.206** Unspecified open wound of unspecified lesser toe(s) with damage to nail

√7ᵗʰ **S91.209** Unspecified open wound of unspecified toe(s) with damage to nail

√6ᵗʰ **S91.21** Laceration without foreign body of toe with damage to nail

√7ᵗʰ **S91.211** Laceration without foreign body of right great toe with damage to nail

√7ᵗʰ **S91.212** Laceration without foreign body of left great toe with damage to nail

√7ᵗʰ **S91.213** Laceration without foreign body of unspecified great toe with damage to nail

√7ᵗʰ **S91.214** Laceration without foreign body of right lesser toe(s) with damage to nail

√7ᵗʰ **S91.215** Laceration without foreign body of left lesser toe(s) with damage to nail

√7ᵗʰ **S91.216** Laceration without foreign body of unspecified lesser toe(s) with damage to nail

√7ᵗʰ **S91.219** Laceration without foreign body of unspecified toe(s) with damage to nail

√6ᵗʰ **S91.22** Laceration with foreign body of toe with damage to nail

√7ᵗʰ **S91.221** Laceration with foreign body of right great toe with damage to nail

√7ᵗʰ **S91.222** Laceration with foreign body of left great toe with damage to nail

√7ᵗʰ **S91.223** Laceration with foreign body of unspecified great toe with damage to nail

√7ᵗʰ **S91.224** Laceration with foreign body of right lesser toe(s) with damage to nail

√7ᵗʰ **S91.225** Laceration with foreign body of left lesser toe(s) with damage to nail

√7ᵗʰ **S91.226** Laceration with foreign body of unspecified lesser toe(s) with damage to nail

√7ᵗʰ **S91.229** Laceration with foreign body of unspecified toe(s) with damage to nail

√6ᵗʰ **S91.23** Puncture wound without foreign body of toe with damage to nail

√7ᵗʰ **S91.231** Puncture wound without foreign body of right great toe with damage to nail

√7ᵗʰ **S91.232** Puncture wound without foreign body of left great toe with damage to nail

√7ᵗʰ **S91.233** Puncture wound without foreign body of unspecified great toe with damage to nail

√7ᵗʰ **S91.234** Puncture wound without foreign body of right lesser toe(s) with damage to nail

√7ᵗʰ **S91.235** Puncture wound without foreign body of left lesser toe(s) with damage to nail

√7ᵗʰ **S91.236** Puncture wound without foreign body of unspecified lesser toe(s) with damage to nail

√7ᵗʰ **S91.239** Puncture wound without foreign body of unspecified toe(s) with damage to nail

√6ᵗʰ **S91.24** Puncture wound with foreign body of toe with damage to nail

√7ᵗʰ **S91.241** Puncture wound with foreign body of right great toe with damage to nail

√7ᵗʰ **S91.242** Puncture wound with foreign body of left great toe with damage to nail

√7ᵗʰ **S91.243** Puncture wound with foreign body of unspecified great toe with damage to nail

√7ᵗʰ **S91.244** Puncture wound with foreign body of right lesser toe(s) with damage to nail

√7ᵗʰ **S91.245** Puncture wound with foreign body of left lesser toe(s) with damage to nail

√7ᵗʰ **S91.246** Puncture wound with foreign body of unspecified lesser toe(s) with damage to nail

√7ᵗʰ **S91.249** Puncture wound with foreign body of unspecified toe(s) with damage to nail

√6ᵗʰ **S91.25** Open bite of toe with damage to nail

Bite of toe with damage to nail NOS

EXCLUDES 1   superficial bite of toe (S90.46-, S90.47-)

√7ᵗʰ **S91.251** Open bite of right great toe with damage to nail

√7ᵗʰ **S91.252** Open bite of left great toe with damage to nail

√7ᵗʰ **S91.253** Open bite of unspecified great toe with damage to nail

√7ᵗʰ **S91.254** Open bite of right lesser toe(s) with damage to nail

√7ᵗʰ **S91.255** Open bite of left lesser toe(s) with damage to nail

√7ᵗʰ **S91.256** Open bite of unspecified lesser toe(s) with damage to nail

√7ᵗʰ **S91.259** Open bite of unspecified toe(s) with damage to nail

√5ᵗʰ **S91.3** Open wound of foot

√6ᵗʰ **S91.30** Unspecified open wound of foot

√7ᵗʰ **S91.301** Unspecified open wound, right foot

√7ᵗʰ **S91.302** Unspecified open wound, left foot

√7ᵗʰ **S91.309** Unspecified open wound, unspecified foot

√6ᵗʰ **S91.31** Laceration without foreign body of foot

√7ᵗʰ **S91.311** Laceration without foreign body, right foot

√7ᵗʰ **S91.312** Laceration without foreign body, left foot

√7ᵗʰ **S91.319** Laceration without foreign body, unspecified foot

√6ᵗʰ **S91.32** Laceration with foreign body of foot

√7ᵗʰ **S91.321** Laceration with foreign body, right foot

√7ᵗʰ **S91.322** Laceration with foreign body, left foot

√7ᵗʰ **S91.329** Laceration with foreign body, unspecified foot

√6ᵗʰ **S91.33** Puncture wound without foreign body of foot

√7ᵗʰ **S91.331** Puncture wound without foreign body, right foot

√7ᵗʰ **S91.332** Puncture wound without foreign body, left foot

√7ᵗʰ **S91.339** Puncture wound without foreign body, unspecified foot

√6ᵗʰ **S91.34** Puncture wound with foreign body of foot

√7ᵗʰ **S91.341** Puncture wound with foreign body, right foot

√7ᵗʰ **S91.342** Puncture wound with foreign body, left foot

√7ᵗʰ **S91.349** Puncture wound with foreign body, unspecified foot

√6ᵗʰ **S91.35** Open bite of foot

EXCLUDES 1   superficial bite of foot (S90.86-, S90.87-)

√7ᵗʰ **S91.351** Open bite, right foot

√7ᵗʰ **S91.352** Open bite, left foot

√7ᵗʰ **S91.359** Open bite, unspecified foot

√4ᵗʰ **S92 Fracture of foot and toe, except ankle**

NOTE   A fracture not indicated as displaced or nondisplaced should be coded to displaced

A fracture not indicated as open or closed should be coded to closed.

EXCLUDES 1   ~~traumatic amputation of ankle and foot (S98.-)~~

EXCLUDES 2   fracture of ankle (S82.-)

fracture of malleolus (S82.-)

▶traumatic amputation of ankle and foot (S98.-)◀

AHA: 2018,2Q,12; 2015,3Q,37-39

The appropriate 7th character is to be added to each code from category S92.

A   initial encounter for closed fracture

B   initial encounter for open fracture

D   subsequent encounter for fracture with routine healing

G   subsequent encounter for fracture with delayed healing

K   subsequent encounter for fracture with nonunion

P   subsequent encounter for fracture with malunion

S   sequela

√5ᵗʰ **S92.0 Fracture of calcaneus**

Heel bone

Os calcis

EXCLUDES 2   physeal fracture of calcaneus (S99.0-)

√6ᵗʰ **S92.00** Unspecified fracture of calcaneus

³ √7ᵗʰ **S92.001** Unspecified fracture of right calcaneus   CC   H5

✔ Additional Character Required   √x7ᵗʰ Placeholder   Questionable PDx   Manifestation   Unspecified Dx   UPD Unacceptable PDx   H1-H14 HAC   HCC CMS-HCC Dx   HIV HIV Dx

ICD-10-CM 2022   1081

³ √7ᵗʰ **S92.002** Unspecified fracture of left calcaneus   CC H5

³ √7ᵗʰ **S92.009** Unspecified fracture of unspecified calcaneus   CC H5

√6ᵗʰ **S92.01** Fracture of body of calcaneus

³ √7ᵗʰ **S92.011** Displaced fracture of body of right calcaneus   CC H5

³ √7ᵗʰ **S92.012** Displaced fracture of body of left calcaneus   CC H5

³ √7ᵗʰ **S92.013** Displaced fracture of body of unspecified calcaneus   CC H5

³ √7ᵗʰ **S92.014** Nondisplaced fracture of body of right calcaneus   CC H5

³ √7ᵗʰ **S92.015** Nondisplaced fracture of body of left calcaneus   CC H5

³ √7ᵗʰ **S92.016** Nondisplaced fracture of body of unspecified calcaneus   CC H5

√6ᵗʰ **S92.02** Fracture of anterior process of calcaneus

³ √7ᵗʰ **S92.021** Displaced fracture of anterior process of right calcaneus   CC H5

³ √7ᵗʰ **S92.022** Displaced fracture of anterior process of left calcaneus   CC H5

³ √7ᵗʰ **S92.023** Displaced fracture of anterior process of unspecified calcaneus   CC H5

³ √7ᵗʰ **S92.024** Nondisplaced fracture of anterior process of right calcaneus   CC H5

³ √7ᵗʰ **S92.025** Nondisplaced fracture of anterior process of left calcaneus   CC H5

³ √7ᵗʰ **S92.026** Nondisplaced fracture of anterior process of unspecified calcaneus   CC H5

√6ᵗʰ **S92.03** Avulsion fracture of tuberosity of calcaneus

³ √7ᵗʰ **S92.031** Displaced avulsion fracture of tuberosity of right calcaneus   CC H5

³ √7ᵗʰ **S92.032** Displaced avulsion fracture of tuberosity of left calcaneus   CC H5

³ √7ᵗʰ **S92.033** Displaced avulsion fracture of tuberosity of unspecified calcaneus   CC H5

³ √7ᵗʰ **S92.034** Nondisplaced avulsion fracture of tuberosity of right calcaneus   CC H5

³ √7ᵗʰ **S92.035** Nondisplaced avulsion fracture of tuberosity of left calcaneus   CC H5

³ √7ᵗʰ **S92.036** Nondisplaced avulsion fracture of tuberosity of unspecified calcaneus   CC H5

√6ᵗʰ **S92.04** Other fracture of tuberosity of calcaneus

³ √7ᵗʰ **S92.041** Displaced other fracture of tuberosity of right calcaneus   CC H5

³ √7ᵗʰ **S92.042** Displaced other fracture of tuberosity of left calcaneus   CC H5

³ √7ᵗʰ **S92.043** Displaced other fracture of tuberosity of unspecified calcaneus   CC H5

³ √7ᵗʰ **S92.044** Nondisplaced other fracture of tuberosity of right calcaneus   CC H5

³ √7ᵗʰ **S92.045** Nondisplaced other fracture of tuberosity of left calcaneus   CC H5

³ √7ᵗʰ **S92.046** Nondisplaced other fracture of tuberosity of unspecified calcaneus   CC H5

√6ᵗʰ **S92.05** Other extraarticular fracture of calcaneus

³ √7ᵗʰ **S92.051** Displaced other extraarticular fracture of right calcaneus   CC H5

³ √7ᵗʰ **S92.052** Displaced other extraarticular fracture of left calcaneus   CC H5

³ √7ᵗʰ **S92.053** Displaced other extraarticular fracture of unspecified calcaneus   CC H5

³ √7ᵗʰ **S92.054** Nondisplaced other extraarticular fracture of right calcaneus   CC H5

³ √7ᵗʰ **S92.055** Nondisplaced other extraarticular fracture of left calcaneus   CC H5

³ √7ᵗʰ **S92.056** Nondisplaced other extraarticular fracture of unspecified calcaneus   CC H5

√6ᵗʰ **S92.06** Intraarticular fracture of calcaneus

³ √7ᵗʰ **S92.061** Displaced intraarticular fracture of right calcaneus   CC H5

³ √7ᵗʰ **S92.062** Displaced intraarticular fracture of left calcaneus   CC H5

³ √7ᵗʰ **S92.063** Displaced intraarticular fracture of unspecified calcaneus   CC H5

³ √7ᵗʰ **S92.064** Nondisplaced intraarticular fracture of right calcaneus   CC H5

³ √7ᵗʰ **S92.065** Nondisplaced intraarticular fracture of left calcaneus   CC H5

³ √7ᵗʰ **S92.066** Nondisplaced intraarticular fracture of unspecified calcaneus   CC H5

√5ᵗʰ **S92.1** Fracture of talus

Astragalus

√6ᵗʰ **S92.10** Unspecified fracture of talus

³ √7ᵗʰ **S92.101** Unspecified fracture of right talus   CC H5

³ √7ᵗʰ **S92.102** Unspecified fracture of left talus   CC H5

³ √7ᵗʰ **S92.109** Unspecified fracture of unspecified talus   CC H5

√6ᵗʰ **S92.11** Fracture of neck of talus

³ √7ᵗʰ **S92.111** Displaced fracture of neck of right talus   CC H5

³ √7ᵗʰ **S92.112** Displaced fracture of neck of left talus   CC H5

³ √7ᵗʰ **S92.113** Displaced fracture of neck of unspecified talus   CC H5

³ √7ᵗʰ **S92.114** Nondisplaced fracture of neck of right talus   CC H5

³ √7ᵗʰ **S92.115** Nondisplaced fracture of neck of left talus   CC H5

³ √7ᵗʰ **S92.116** Nondisplaced fracture of neck of unspecified talus   CC H5

√6ᵗʰ **S92.12** Fracture of body of talus

³ √7ᵗʰ **S92.121** Displaced fracture of body of right talus   CC H5

³ √7ᵗʰ **S92.122** Displaced fracture of body of left talus   CC H5

³ √7ᵗʰ **S92.123** Displaced fracture of body of unspecified talus   CC H5

³ √7ᵗʰ **S92.124** Nondisplaced fracture of body of right talus   CC H5

³ √7ᵗʰ **S92.125** Nondisplaced fracture of body of left talus   CC H5

³ √7ᵗʰ **S92.126** Nondisplaced fracture of body of unspecified talus   CC H5

√6ᵗʰ **S92.13** Fracture of posterior process of talus

³ √7ᵗʰ **S92.131** Displaced fracture of posterior process of right talus   CC H5

³ √7ᵗʰ **S92.132** Displaced fracture of posterior process of left talus   CC H5

³ √7ᵗʰ **S92.133** Displaced fracture of posterior process of unspecified talus   CC H5

³ √7ᵗʰ **S92.134** Nondisplaced fracture of posterior process of right talus   CC H5

³ √7ᵗʰ **S92.135** Nondisplaced fracture of posterior process of left talus   CC H5

³ √7ᵗʰ **S92.136** Nondisplaced fracture of posterior process of unspecified talus   CC H5

√6ᵗʰ **S92.14** Dome fracture of talus

EXCLUDES 1   osteochondritis dissecans (M93.2)

³ √7ᵗʰ **S92.141** Displaced dome fracture of right talus   CC H5

³ √7ᵗʰ **S92.142** Displaced dome fracture of left talus   CC H5

³ √7ᵗʰ **S92.143** Displaced dome fracture of unspecified talus   CC H5

³ √7ᵗʰ **S92.144** Nondisplaced dome fracture of right talus   CC H5

³ √7ᵗʰ **S92.145** Nondisplaced dome fracture of left talus   CC H5

³ √7ᵗʰ **S92.146** Nondisplaced dome fracture of unspecified talus   CC H5

√6ᵗʰ **S92.15** Avulsion fracture (chip fracture) of talus

³ √7ᵗʰ **S92.151** Displaced avulsion fracture (chip fracture) of right talus   CC H5

³ √7ᵗʰ **S92.152** Displaced avulsion fracture (chip fracture) of left talus   CC H5

³ √7ᵗʰ **S92.153** Displaced avulsion fracture (chip fracture) of unspecified talus   CC H5

³ √7ᵗʰ **S92.154** Nondisplaced avulsion fracture (chip fracture) of right talus   CC H5

N Newborn: 0   P Pediatric: 0-17   M Maternity: 9-64   A Adult: 15-124   MCC Major Complication/Comorbidity   CC Complication/Comorbidity   SW Severe Wound Dx

1082   ICD-10-CM 2022

3 √7ᵗʰ **S92.155** Nondisplaced avulsion fracture (chip fracture) of left talus   CC H5

3 √7ᵗʰ **S92.156** Nondisplaced avulsion fracture (chip fracture) of unspecified talus   CC H5

√6ᵗʰ **S92.19** Other fracture of talus

    3 √7ᵗʰ **S92.191** Other fracture of right talus   CC H5

    3 √7ᵗʰ **S92.192** Other fracture of left talus   CC H5

    3 √7ᵗʰ **S92.199** Other fracture of unspecified talus   CC H5

√5ᵗʰ **S92.2** Fracture of other and unspecified tarsal bone(s)

√6ᵗʰ **S92.20** Fracture of unspecified tarsal bone(s)

    3 √7ᵗʰ **S92.201** Fracture of unspecified tarsal bone(s) of right foot   CC H5

    3 √7ᵗʰ **S92.202** Fracture of unspecified tarsal bone(s) of left foot   CC H5

    3 √7ᵗʰ **S92.209** Fracture of unspecified tarsal bone(s) of unspecified foot   CC H5

√6ᵗʰ **S92.21** Fracture of cuboid bone

    3 √7ᵗʰ **S92.211** Displaced fracture of cuboid bone of right foot   CC H5

    3 √7ᵗʰ **S92.212** Displaced fracture of cuboid bone of left foot   CC H5

    3 √7ᵗʰ **S92.213** Displaced fracture of cuboid bone of unspecified foot   CC H5

    3 √7ᵗʰ **S92.214** Nondisplaced fracture of cuboid bone of right foot   CC H5

    3 √7ᵗʰ **S92.215** Nondisplaced fracture of cuboid bone of left foot   CC H5

    3 √7ᵗʰ **S92.216** Nondisplaced fracture of cuboid bone of unspecified foot   CC H5

√6ᵗʰ **S92.22** Fracture of lateral cuneiform

    3 √7ᵗʰ **S92.221** Displaced fracture of lateral cuneiform of right foot   CC H5

    3 √7ᵗʰ **S92.222** Displaced fracture of lateral cuneiform of left foot   CC H5

    3 √7ᵗʰ **S92.223** Displaced fracture of lateral cuneiform of unspecified foot   CC H5

    3 √7ᵗʰ **S92.224** Nondisplaced fracture of lateral cuneiform of right foot   CC H5

    3 √7ᵗʰ **S92.225** Nondisplaced fracture of lateral cuneiform of left foot   CC H5

    3 √7ᵗʰ **S92.226** Nondisplaced fracture of lateral cuneiform of unspecified foot   CC H5

√6ᵗʰ **S92.23** Fracture of intermediate cuneiform

    3 √7ᵗʰ **S92.231** Displaced fracture of intermediate cuneiform of right foot   CC H5

    3 √7ᵗʰ **S92.232** Displaced fracture of intermediate cuneiform of left foot   CC H5

    3 √7ᵗʰ **S92.233** Displaced fracture of intermediate cuneiform of unspecified foot   CC H5

    3 √7ᵗʰ **S92.234** Nondisplaced fracture of intermediate cuneiform of right foot   CC H5

    3 √7ᵗʰ **S92.235** Nondisplaced fracture of intermediate cuneiform of left foot   CC H5

    3 √7ᵗʰ **S92.236** Nondisplaced fracture of intermediate cuneiform of unspecified foot   CC H5

√6ᵗʰ **S92.24** Fracture of medial cuneiform

    3 √7ᵗʰ **S92.241** Displaced fracture of medial cuneiform of right foot   CC H5

    3 √7ᵗʰ **S92.242** Displaced fracture of medial cuneiform of left foot   CC H5

    3 √7ᵗʰ **S92.243** Displaced fracture of medial cuneiform of unspecified foot   CC H5

    3 √7ᵗʰ **S92.244** Nondisplaced fracture of medial cuneiform of right foot   CC H5

    3 √7ᵗʰ **S92.245** Nondisplaced fracture of medial cuneiform of left foot   CC H5

    3 √7ᵗʰ **S92.246** Nondisplaced fracture of medial cuneiform of unspecified foot   CC H5

√6ᵗʰ **S92.25** Fracture of navicular [scaphoid] of foot

    3 √7ᵗʰ **S92.251** Displaced fracture of navicular [scaphoid] of right foot   CC H5

    3 √7ᵗʰ **S92.252** Displaced fracture of navicular [scaphoid] of left foot   CC H5

    3 √7ᵗʰ **S92.253** Displaced fracture of navicular [scaphoid] of unspecified foot   CC H5

    3 √7ᵗʰ **S92.254** Nondisplaced fracture of navicular [scaphoid] of right foot   CC H5

3 √7ᵗʰ **S92.255** Nondisplaced fracture of navicular [scaphoid] of left foot   CC H5

3 √7ᵗʰ **S92.256** Nondisplaced fracture of navicular [scaphoid] of unspecified foot   CC H5

√5ᵗʰ **S92.3** Fracture of metatarsal bone(s)

    EXCLUDES 2   physeal fracture of metatarsal (S99.1-)

    • **AHA:** 2018,1Q,3

√6ᵗʰ **S92.30** Fracture of unspecified metatarsal bone(s)

    3 √7ᵗʰ **S92.301** Fracture of unspecified metatarsal bone(s), right foot   CC H5

    3 √7ᵗʰ **S92.302** Fracture of unspecified metatarsal bone(s), left foot   CC H5

    3 √7ᵗʰ **S92.309** Fracture of unspecified metatarsal bone(s), unspecified foot   CC H5

√6ᵗʰ **S92.31** Fracture of first metatarsal bone

    3 √7ᵗʰ **S92.311** Displaced fracture of first metatarsal bone, right foot   CC H5

    3 √7ᵗʰ **S92.312** Displaced fracture of first metatarsal bone, left foot   CC H5

    3 √7ᵗʰ **S92.313** Displaced fracture of first metatarsal bone, unspecified foot   CC H5

    3 √7ᵗʰ **S92.314** Nondisplaced fracture of first metatarsal bone, right foot   CC H5

    3 √7ᵗʰ **S92.315** Nondisplaced fracture of first metatarsal bone, left foot   CC H5

    3 √7ᵗʰ **S92.316** Nondisplaced fracture of first metatarsal bone, unspecified foot   CC H5

√6ᵗʰ **S92.32** Fracture of second metatarsal bone

    3 √7ᵗʰ **S92.321** Displaced fracture of second metatarsal bone, right foot   CC H5

    3 √7ᵗʰ **S92.322** Displaced fracture of second metatarsal bone, left foot   CC H5

    3 √7ᵗʰ **S92.323** Displaced fracture of second metatarsal bone, unspecified foot   CC H5

    3 √7ᵗʰ **S92.324** Nondisplaced fracture of second metatarsal bone, right foot   CC H5

    3 √7ᵗʰ **S92.325** Nondisplaced fracture of second metatarsal bone, left foot   CC H5

    3 √7ᵗʰ **S92.326** Nondisplaced fracture of second metatarsal bone, unspecified foot   CC H5

√6ᵗʰ **S92.33** Fracture of third metatarsal bone

    3 √7ᵗʰ **S92.331** Displaced fracture of third metatarsal bone, right foot   CC H5

    3 √7ᵗʰ **S92.332** Displaced fracture of third metatarsal bone, left foot   CC H5

    3 √7ᵗʰ **S92.333** Displaced fracture of third metatarsal bone, unspecified foot   CC H5

    3 √7ᵗʰ **S92.334** Nondisplaced fracture of third metatarsal bone, right foot   CC H5

    3 √7ᵗʰ **S92.335** Nondisplaced fracture of third metatarsal bone, left foot   CC H5

    3 √7ᵗʰ **S92.336** Nondisplaced fracture of third metatarsal bone, unspecified foot   CC H5

√6ᵗʰ **S92.34** Fracture of fourth metatarsal bone

    3 √7ᵗʰ **S92.341** Displaced fracture of fourth metatarsal bone, right foot   CC H5

    3 √7ᵗʰ **S92.342** Displaced fracture of fourth metatarsal bone, left foot   CC H5

    3 √7ᵗʰ **S92.343** Displaced fracture of fourth metatarsal bone, unspecified foot   CC H5

    3 √7ᵗʰ **S92.344** Nondisplaced fracture of fourth metatarsal bone, right foot   CC H5

    3 √7ᵗʰ **S92.345** Nondisplaced fracture of fourth metatarsal bone, left foot   CC H5

    3 √7ᵗʰ **S92.346** Nondisplaced fracture of fourth metatarsal bone, unspecified foot   CC H5

√6ᵗʰ **S92.35** Fracture of fifth metatarsal bone

    3 √7ᵗʰ **S92.351** Displaced fracture of fifth metatarsal bone, right foot   CC H5

    3 √7ᵗʰ **S92.352** Displaced fracture of fifth metatarsal bone, left foot   CC H5

    3 √7ᵗʰ **S92.353** Displaced fracture of fifth metatarsal bone, unspecified foot   CC H5

    3 √7ᵗʰ **S92.354** Nondisplaced fracture of fifth metatarsal bone, right foot

☑ Additional Character Required   √x7ᵗʰ Placeholder   Questionable PDx   Manifestation   Unspecified Dx   UPD Unacceptable PDx   H1-H14 HAC   HCC CMS-HCC Dx   HIV HIV Dx

ICD-10-CM 2022   1083

³ √7ᵗʰ **S92.355** Nondisplaced fracture of fifth metatarsal bone, left foot `CC` `H5`

³ √7ᵗʰ **S92.356** Nondisplaced fracture of fifth metatarsal bone, unspecified foot `CC` `H5`

√5ᵗʰ **S92.4** Fracture of great toe

> EXCLUDES 2 *physeal fracture of phalanx of toe (S99.2-)*

√6ᵗʰ **S92.40** Unspecified fracture of great toe

4 √7ᵗʰ **S92.401** Displaced unspecified fracture of right great toe `CC`

4 √7ᵗʰ **S92.402** Displaced unspecified fracture of left great toe `CC`

4 √7ᵗʰ **S92.403** Displaced unspecified fracture of unspecified great toe `CC`

4 √7ᵗʰ **S92.404** Nondisplaced unspecified fracture of right great toe `CC`

4 √7ᵗʰ **S92.405** Nondisplaced unspecified fracture of left great toe `CC`

4 √7ᵗʰ **S92.406** Nondisplaced unspecified fracture of unspecified great toe `CC`

√6ᵗʰ **S92.41** Fracture of proximal phalanx of great toe

4 √7ᵗʰ **S92.411** Displaced fracture of proximal phalanx of right great toe `CC`

4 √7ᵗʰ **S92.412** Displaced fracture of proximal phalanx of left great toe `CC`

4 √7ᵗʰ **S92.413** Displaced fracture of proximal phalanx of unspecified great toe `CC`

4 √7ᵗʰ **S92.414** Nondisplaced fracture of proximal phalanx of right great toe `CC`

4 √7ᵗʰ **S92.415** Nondisplaced fracture of proximal phalanx of left great toe `CC`

4 √7ᵗʰ **S92.416** Nondisplaced fracture of proximal phalanx of unspecified great toe `CC`

√6ᵗʰ **S92.42** Fracture of distal phalanx of great toe

4 √7ᵗʰ **S92.421** Displaced fracture of distal phalanx of right great toe `CC`

4 √7ᵗʰ **S92.422** Displaced fracture of distal phalanx of left great toe `CC`

4 √7ᵗʰ **S92.423** Displaced fracture of distal phalanx of unspecified great toe `CC`

4 √7ᵗʰ **S92.424** Nondisplaced fracture of distal phalanx of right great toe `CC`

4 √7ᵗʰ **S92.425** Nondisplaced fracture of distal phalanx of left great toe `CC`

4 √7ᵗʰ **S92.426** Nondisplaced fracture of distal phalanx of unspecified great toe `CC`

√6ᵗʰ **S92.49** Other fracture of great toe

4 √7ᵗʰ **S92.491** Other fracture of right great toe `CC`

4 √7ᵗʰ **S92.492** Other fracture of left great toe `CC`

4 √7ᵗʰ **S92.499** Other fracture of unspecified great toe `CC`

√5ᵗʰ **S92.5** Fracture of lesser toe(s)

> EXCLUDES 2 *physeal fracture of phalanx of toe (S99.2-)*

√6ᵗʰ **S92.50** Unspecified fracture of lesser toe(s)

4 √7ᵗʰ **S92.501** Displaced unspecified fracture of right lesser toe(s) `CC`

4 √7ᵗʰ **S92.502** Displaced unspecified fracture of left lesser toe(s) `CC`

4 √7ᵗʰ **S92.503** Displaced unspecified fracture of unspecified lesser toe(s) `CC`

4 √7ᵗʰ **S92.504** Nondisplaced unspecified fracture of right lesser toe(s) `CC`

4 √7ᵗʰ **S92.505** Nondisplaced unspecified fracture of left lesser toe(s) `CC`

4 √7ᵗʰ **S92.506** Nondisplaced unspecified fracture of unspecified lesser toe(s) `CC`

√6ᵗʰ **S92.51** Fracture of proximal phalanx of lesser toe(s)

4 √7ᵗʰ **S92.511** Displaced fracture of proximal phalanx of right lesser toe(s) `CC`

4 √7ᵗʰ **S92.512** Displaced fracture of proximal phalanx of left lesser toe(s) `CC`

4 √7ᵗʰ **S92.513** Displaced fracture of proximal phalanx of unspecified lesser toe(s) `CC`

4 √7ᵗʰ **S92.514** Nondisplaced fracture of proximal phalanx of right lesser toe(s) `CC`

4 √7ᵗʰ **S92.515** Nondisplaced fracture of proximal phalanx of left lesser toe(s)) `CC`

4 √7ᵗʰ **S92.516** Nondisplaced fracture of proximal phalanx of unspecified lesser toe(s) `CC`

√6ᵗʰ **S92.52** Fracture of middle phalanx of lesser toe(s)

4 √7ᵗʰ **S92.521** Displaced fracture of middle phalanx of right lesser toe(s) `CC`

4 √7ᵗʰ **S92.522** Displaced fracture of middle phalanx of left lesser toe(s) `CC`

4 √7ᵗʰ **S92.523** Displaced fracture of middle phalanx of unspecified lesser toe(s) `CC`

4 √7ᵗʰ **S92.524** Nondisplaced fracture of middle phalanx of right lesser toe(s) `CC`

4 √7ᵗʰ **S92.525** Nondisplaced fracture of middle phalanx of left lesser toe(s) `CC`

4 √7ᵗʰ **S92.526** Nondisplaced fracture of middle phalanx of unspecified lesser toe(s) `CC`

√6ᵗʰ **S92.53** Fracture of distal phalanx of lesser toe(s)

4 √7ᵗʰ **S92.531** Displaced fracture of distal phalanx of right lesser toe(s) `CC`

4 √7ᵗʰ **S92.532** Displaced fracture of distal phalanx of left lesser toe(s) `CC`

4 √7ᵗʰ **S92.533** Displaced fracture of distal phalanx of unspecified lesser toe(s) `CC`

4 √7ᵗʰ **S92.534** Nondisplaced fracture of distal phalanx of right lesser toe(s) `CC`

4 √7ᵗʰ **S92.535** Nondisplaced fracture of distal phalanx of left lesser toe(s) `CC`

4 √7ᵗʰ **S92.536** Nondisplaced fracture of distal phalanx of unspecified lesser toe(s) `CC`

√6ᵗʰ **S92.59** Other fracture of lesser toe(s)

4 √7ᵗʰ **S92.591** Other fracture of right lesser toe(s) `CC`

4 √7ᵗʰ **S92.592** Other fracture of left lesser toe(s) `CC`

4 √7ᵗʰ **S92.599** Other fracture of unspecified lesser toe(s) `CC`

√5ᵗʰ **S92.8** Other fracture of foot, except ankle

√6ᵗʰ **S92.81** Other fracture of foot

> Sesamoid fracture of foot
> **AHA:** 2016,4Q,68

³ √7ᵗʰ **S92.811** Other fracture of right foot `CC` `H5`

³ √7ᵗʰ **S92.812** Other fracture of left foot `CC` `H5`

³ √7ᵗʰ **S92.819** Other fracture of unspecified foot `CC` `H5`

√5ᵗʰ **S92.9** Unspecified fracture of foot and toe

√6ᵗʰ **S92.90** Unspecified fracture of foot

³ √7ᵗʰ **S92.901** Unspecified fracture of right foot `CC` `H5`

³ √7ᵗʰ **S92.902** Unspecified fracture of left foot `CC` `H5`

³ √7ᵗʰ **S92.909** Unspecified fracture of unspecified foot `CC` `H5`

√6ᵗʰ **S92.91** Unspecified fracture of toe

4 √7ᵗʰ **S92.911** Unspecified fracture of right toe(s) `CC`

4 √7ᵗʰ **S92.912** Unspecified fracture of left toe(s) `CC`

4 √7ᵗʰ **S92.919** Unspecified fracture of unspecified toe(s) `CC`

✓4ᵗʰ **S93** **Dislocation and sprain of joints and ligaments at ankle, foot and toe level**

    INCLUDES   avulsion of joint or ligament of ankle, foot and toe

             laceration of cartilage, joint or ligament of ankle, foot and toe

             sprain of cartilage, joint or ligament of ankle, foot and toe

             traumatic hemarthrosis of joint or ligament of ankle, foot and toe

             traumatic rupture of joint or ligament of ankle, foot and toe

             traumatic subluxation of joint or ligament of ankle, foot and toe

             traumatic tear of joint or ligament of ankle, foot and toe

    Code also any associated open wound

    EXCLUDES 2   *strain of muscle and tendon of ankle and foot (S96.-)*

> The appropriate 7th character is to be added to each code from category S93.
> A   initial encounter
> D   subsequent encounter
> S   sequela

✓5ᵗʰ **S93.0** **Subluxation and dislocation of** ankle joint

    Subluxation and dislocation of astragalus
    Subluxation and dislocation of fibula, lower end
    Subluxation and dislocation of talus
    Subluxation and dislocation of tibia, lower end

   ✓x7ᵗʰ   **S93.01**   Subluxation of right ankle joint

   ✓x7ᵗʰ   **S93.02**   Subluxation of left ankle joint

   ✓x7ᵗʰ   **S93.03**   Subluxation of unspecified ankle joint

   ✓x7ᵗʰ   **S93.04**   Dislocation of right ankle joint

   ✓x7ᵗʰ   **S93.05**   Dislocation of left ankle joint

   ✓x7ᵗʰ   **S93.06**   Dislocation of unspecified ankle joint

✓5ᵗʰ **S93.1** **Subluxation and dislocation of** toe

   ✓6ᵗʰ   **S93.10**   **Unspecified subluxation and dislocation of toe**

          Dislocation of toe NOS
          Subluxation of toe NOS

     ✓7ᵗʰ   **S93.101**   Unspecified subluxation of right toe(s)

     ✓7ᵗʰ   **S93.102**   Unspecified subluxation of left toe(s)

     ✓7ᵗʰ   **S93.103**   Unspecified subluxation of unspecified toe(s)

     ✓7ᵗʰ   **S93.104**   Unspecified dislocation of right toe(s)

     ✓7ᵗʰ   **S93.105**   Unspecified dislocation of left toe(s)

     ✓7ᵗʰ   **S93.106**   Unspecified dislocation of unspecified toe(s)

   ✓6ᵗʰ   **S93.11**   **Dislocation of** interphalangeal joint

     ✓7ᵗʰ   **S93.111**   Dislocation of interphalangeal joint of right great toe

     ✓7ᵗʰ   **S93.112**   Dislocation of interphalangeal joint of left great toe

     ✓7ᵗʰ   **S93.113**   Dislocation of interphalangeal joint of unspecified great toe

     ✓7ᵗʰ   **S93.114**   Dislocation of interphalangeal joint of right lesser toe(s)

     ✓7ᵗʰ   **S93.115**   Dislocation of interphalangeal joint of left lesser toe(s)

     ✓7ᵗʰ   **S93.116**   Dislocation of interphalangeal joint of unspecified lesser toe(s)

     ✓7ᵗʰ   **S93.119**   Dislocation of interphalangeal joint of unspecified toe(s)

   ✓6ᵗʰ   **S93.12**   **Dislocation of** metatarsophalangeal joint

     ✓7ᵗʰ   **S93.121**   Dislocation of metatarsophalangeal joint of right great toe

     ✓7ᵗʰ   **S93.122**   Dislocation of metatarsophalangeal joint of left great toe

     ✓7ᵗʰ   **S93.123**   Dislocation of metatarsophalangeal joint of unspecified great toe

     ✓7ᵗʰ   **S93.124**   Dislocation of metatarsophalangeal joint of right lesser toe(s)

     ✓7ᵗʰ   **S93.125**   Dislocation of metatarsophalangeal joint of left lesser toe(s)

     ✓7ᵗʰ   **S93.126**   Dislocation of metatarsophalangeal joint of unspecified lesser toe(s)

     ✓7ᵗʰ   **S93.129**   Dislocation of metatarsophalangeal joint of unspecified toe(s)

   ✓6ᵗʰ   **S93.13**   **Subluxation of** interphalangeal joint

     ✓7ᵗʰ   **S93.131**   Subluxation of interphalangeal joint of right great toe

     ✓7ᵗʰ   **S93.132**   Subluxation of interphalangeal joint of left great toe

     ✓7ᵗʰ   **S93.133**   Subluxation of interphalangeal joint of unspecified great toe

     ✓7ᵗʰ   **S93.134**   Subluxation of interphalangeal joint of right lesser toe(s)

     ✓7ᵗʰ   **S93.135**   Subluxation of interphalangeal joint of left lesser toe(s)

     ✓7ᵗʰ   **S93.136**   Subluxation of interphalangeal joint of unspecified lesser toe(s)

     ✓7ᵗʰ   **S93.139**   Subluxation of interphalangeal joint of unspecified toe(s)

   ✓6ᵗʰ   **S93.14**   **Subluxation of** metatarsophalangeal joint

     ✓7ᵗʰ   **S93.141**   Subluxation of metatarsophalangeal joint of right great toe

     ✓7ᵗʰ   **S93.142**   Subluxation of metatarsophalangeal joint of left great toe

     ✓7ᵗʰ   **S93.143**   Subluxation of metatarsophalangeal joint of unspecified great toe

     ✓7ᵗʰ   **S93.144**   Subluxation of metatarsophalangeal joint of right lesser toe(s)

     ✓7ᵗʰ   **S93.145**   Subluxation of metatarsophalangeal joint of left lesser toe(s)

     ✓7ᵗʰ   **S93.146**   Subluxation of metatarsophalangeal joint of unspecified lesser toe(s)

     ✓7ᵗʰ   **S93.149**   Subluxation of metatarsophalangeal joint of unspecified toe(s)

✓5ᵗʰ **S93.3** **Subluxation and dislocation of** foot

    EXCLUDES 2   *dislocation of toe (S93.1-)*

   ✓6ᵗʰ   **S93.30**   **Unspecified subluxation and dislocation of foot**

          Dislocation of foot NOS
          Subluxation of foot NOS

     ✓7ᵗʰ   **S93.301**   Unspecified subluxation of right foot

     ✓7ᵗʰ   **S93.302**   Unspecified subluxation of left foot

     ✓7ᵗʰ   **S93.303**   Unspecified subluxation of unspecified foot

     ✓7ᵗʰ   **S93.304**   Unspecified dislocation of right foot

     ✓7ᵗʰ   **S93.305**   Unspecified dislocation of left foot

     ✓7ᵗʰ   **S93.306**   Unspecified dislocation of unspecified foot

   ✓6ᵗʰ   **S93.31**   **Subluxation and dislocation of** tarsal joint

     ✓7ᵗʰ   **S93.311**   Subluxation of tarsal joint of right foot

     ✓7ᵗʰ   **S93.312**   Subluxation of tarsal joint of left foot

     ✓7ᵗʰ   **S93.313**   Subluxation of tarsal joint of unspecified foot

     ✓7ᵗʰ   **S93.314**   Dislocation of tarsal joint of right foot

     ✓7ᵗʰ   **S93.315**   Dislocation of tarsal joint of left foot

     ✓7ᵗʰ   **S93.316**   Dislocation of tarsal joint of unspecified foot

   ✓6ᵗʰ   **S93.32**   **Subluxation and dislocation of** tarsometatarsal joint

     ✓7ᵗʰ   **S93.321**   Subluxation of tarsometatarsal joint of right foot

     ✓7ᵗʰ   **S93.322**   Subluxation of tarsometatarsal joint of left foot

     ✓7ᵗʰ   **S93.323**   Subluxation of tarsometatarsal joint of unspecified foot

     ✓7ᵗʰ   **S93.324**   Dislocation of tarsometatarsal joint of right foot

     ✓7ᵗʰ   **S93.325**   Dislocation of tarsometatarsal joint of left foot

     ✓7ᵗʰ   **S93.326**   Dislocation of tarsometatarsal joint of unspecified foot

   ✓6ᵗʰ   **S93.33**   **Other subluxation and dislocation of foot**

     ✓7ᵗʰ   **S93.331**   Other subluxation of right foot

     ✓7ᵗʰ   **S93.332**   Other subluxation of left foot

     ✓7ᵗʰ   **S93.333**   Other subluxation of unspecified foot

     ✓7ᵗʰ   **S93.334**   Other dislocation of right foot

     ✓7ᵗʰ   **S93.335**   Other dislocation of left foot

     ✓7ᵗʰ   **S93.336**   Other dislocation of unspecified foot

✓5ᵗʰ **S93.4** **Sprain of** ankle

    EXCLUDES 2   *injury of Achilles tendon (S86.0-)*

   ✓6ᵗʰ   **S93.40**   **Sprain of unspecified ligament of ankle**

          Sprain of ankle NOS
          Sprained ankle NOS

     ✓7ᵗʰ   **S93.401**   Sprain of unspecified ligament of right ankle

✔ Additional Character Required   ✓x7ᵗʰ Placeholder   Questionable PDx   Manifestation   Unspecified Dx   UPD Unacceptable PDx   H1-H14 HAC   HCC CMS-HCC Dx   HIV HIV Dx

ICD-10-CM 2022   1085

√7ᵗʰ **S93.402** Sprain of unspecified ligament of left ankle

√7ᵗʰ **S93.409** Sprain of unspecified ligament of unspecified ankle

√6ᵗʰ **S93.41** Sprain of calcaneofibular ligament

√7ᵗʰ **S93.411** Sprain of calcaneofibular ligament of right ankle

√7ᵗʰ **S93.412** Sprain of calcaneofibular ligament of left ankle

√7ᵗʰ **S93.419** Sprain of calcaneofibular ligament of unspecified ankle

√6ᵗʰ **S93.42** Sprain of deltoid ligament

√7ᵗʰ **S93.421** Sprain of deltoid ligament of right ankle

√7ᵗʰ **S93.422** Sprain of deltoid ligament of left ankle

√7ᵗʰ **S93.429** Sprain of deltoid ligament of unspecified ankle

√6ᵗʰ **S93.43** Sprain of tibiofibular ligament

√7ᵗʰ **S93.431** Sprain of tibiofibular ligament of right ankle

√7ᵗʰ **S93.432** Sprain of tibiofibular ligament of left ankle

√7ᵗʰ **S93.439** Sprain of tibiofibular ligament of unspecified ankle

√6ᵗʰ **S93.49** Sprain of other ligament of ankle

Sprain of internal collateral ligament
Sprain of talofibular ligament

√7ᵗʰ **S93.491** Sprain of other ligament of right ankle

√7ᵗʰ **S93.492** Sprain of other ligament of left ankle

√7ᵗʰ **S93.499** Sprain of other ligament of unspecified ankle

√5ᵗʰ **S93.5** Sprain of toe

√6ᵗʰ **S93.50** Unspecified sprain of toe

S93.501 Unspecified sprain of right great toe

S93.502 Unspecified sprain of left great toe

S93.503 Unspecified sprain of unspecified great toe

√7ᵗʰ **S93.504** Unspecified sprain of right lesser toe(s)

√7ᵗʰ **S93.505** Unspecified sprain of left lesser toe(s)

√7ᵗʰ **S93.506** Unspecified sprain of unspecified lesser toe(s)

√7ᵗʰ **S93.509** Unspecified sprain of unspecified toe(s)

√6ᵗʰ **S93.51** Sprain of interphalangeal joint of toe

√7ᵗʰ **S93.511** Sprain of interphalangeal joint of right great toe

√7ᵗʰ **S93.512** Sprain of interphalangeal joint of left great toe

√7ᵗʰ **S93.513** Sprain of interphalangeal joint of unspecified great toe

√7ᵗʰ **S93.514** Sprain of interphalangeal joint of right lesser toe(s)

√7ᵗʰ **S93.515** Sprain of interphalangeal joint of left lesser toe(s)

√7ᵗʰ **S93.516** Sprain of interphalangeal joint of unspecified lesser toe(s)

√7ᵗʰ **S93.519** Sprain of interphalangeal joint of unspecified toe(s)

√6ᵗʰ **S93.52** Sprain of metatarsophalangeal joint of toe

√7ᵗʰ **S93.521** Sprain of metatarsophalangeal joint of right great toe

√7ᵗʰ **S93.522** Sprain of metatarsophalangeal joint of left great toe

√7ᵗʰ **S93.523** Sprain of metatarsophalangeal joint of unspecified great toe

√7ᵗʰ **S93.524** Sprain of metatarsophalangeal joint of right lesser toe(s)

√7ᵗʰ **S93.525** Sprain of metatarsophalangeal joint of left lesser toe(s)

√7ᵗʰ **S93.526** Sprain of metatarsophalangeal joint of unspecified lesser toe(s)

√7ᵗʰ **S93.529** Sprain of metatarsophalangeal joint of unspecified toe(s)

√5ᵗʰ **S93.6** Sprain of foot

EXCLUDES 2   sprain of metatarsophalangeal joint of toe (S93.52-)
sprain of toe (S93.5-)

√6ᵗʰ **S93.60** Unspecified sprain of foot

√7ᵗʰ **S93.601** Unspecified sprain of right foot

√7ᵗʰ **S93.602** Unspecified sprain of left foot

√7ᵗʰ **S93.609** Unspecified sprain of unspecified foot

√6ᵗʰ **S93.61** Sprain of tarsal ligament of foot

√7ᵗʰ **S93.611** Sprain of tarsal ligament of right foot

√7ᵗʰ **S93.612** Sprain of tarsal ligament of left foot

√7ᵗʰ **S93.619** Sprain of tarsal ligament of unspecified foot

√6ᵗʰ **S93.62** Sprain of tarsometatarsal ligament of foot

√7ᵗʰ **S93.621** Sprain of tarsometatarsal ligament of right foot

√7ᵗʰ **S93.622** Sprain of tarsometatarsal ligament of left foot

√7ᵗʰ **S93.629** Sprain of tarsometatarsal ligament of unspecified foot

√6ᵗʰ **S93.69** Other sprain of foot

√7ᵗʰ **S93.691** Other sprain of right foot

√7ᵗʰ **S93.692** Other sprain of left foot

√7ᵗʰ **S93.699** Other sprain of unspecified foot

√4ᵗʰ **S94** Injury of nerves at ankle and foot level

Code also any associated open wound (S91.-)

The appropriate 7th character is to be added to each code from category S94.
A   initial encounter
D   subsequent encounter
S   sequela

√5ᵗʰ **S94.0** Injury of lateral plantar nerve

√x7ᵗʰ **S94.00** Injury of lateral plantar nerve, unspecified leg

√x7ᵗʰ **S94.01** Injury of lateral plantar nerve, right leg

√x7ᵗʰ **S94.02** Injury of lateral plantar nerve, left leg

√5ᵗʰ **S94.1** Injury of medial plantar nerve

√x7ᵗʰ **S94.10** Injury of medial plantar nerve, unspecified leg

√x7ᵗʰ **S94.11** Injury of medial plantar nerve, right leg

√x7ᵗʰ **S94.12** Injury of medial plantar nerve, left leg

√5ᵗʰ **S94.2** Injury of deep peroneal nerve at ankle and foot level

Injury of terminal, lateral branch of deep peroneal nerve

√x7ᵗʰ **S94.20** Injury of deep peroneal nerve at ankle and foot level, unspecified leg

√x7ᵗʰ **S94.21** Injury of deep peroneal nerve at ankle and foot level, right leg

√x7ᵗʰ **S94.22** Injury of deep peroneal nerve at ankle and foot level, left leg

√5ᵗʰ **S94.3** Injury of cutaneous sensory nerve at ankle and foot level

√x7ᵗʰ **S94.30** Injury of cutaneous sensory nerve at ankle and foot level, unspecified leg

√x7ᵗʰ **S94.31** Injury of cutaneous sensory nerve at ankle and foot level, right leg

√x7ᵗʰ **S94.32** Injury of cutaneous sensory nerve at ankle and foot level, left leg

√5ᵗʰ **S94.8** Injury of other nerves at ankle and foot level

√6ᵗʰ **S94.8X** Injury of other nerves at ankle and foot level

√7ᵗʰ **S94.8X1** Injury of other nerves at ankle and foot level, right leg

√7ᵗʰ **S94.8X2** Injury of other nerves at ankle and foot level, left leg

√7ᵗʰ **S94.8X9** Injury of other nerves at ankle and foot level, unspecified leg

√5ᵗʰ **S94.9** Injury of unspecified nerve at ankle and foot level

√x7ᵗʰ **S94.90** Injury of unspecified nerve at ankle and foot level, unspecified leg

√x7ᵗʰ **S94.91** Injury of unspecified nerve at ankle and foot level, right leg

√x7ᵗʰ **S94.92** Injury of unspecified nerve at ankle and foot level, left leg

Ⓝ Newborn: 0   Ⓟ Pediatric: 0-17   Ⓜ Maternity: 9-64   Ⓐ Adult: 15-124   MCC Major Complication/Comorbidity   CC Complication/Comorbidity   SW Severe Wound Dx

1086   ICD-10-CM 2022

✓4th **S95 Injury of blood vessels at ankle and foot level**

Code also any associated open wound (S91.-)

EXCLUDES 2   *injury of posterior tibial artery and vein (S85.1-, S85.8-)*

The appropriate 7th character is to be added to each code from category S95.
A   initial encounter
D   subsequent encounter
S   sequela

✓5th **S95.0 Injury of dorsal artery of foot**

    ✓6th **S95.00 Unspecified injury of dorsal artery of foot**

       ✓7th **S95.001** Unspecified injury of dorsal artery of right foot   CC

       ✓7th **S95.002** Unspecified injury of dorsal artery of left foot   CC

       ✓7th **S95.009** Unspecified injury of dorsal artery of unspecified foot   CC

    ✓6th **S95.01 Laceration of dorsal artery of foot**

       ✓7th **S95.011** Laceration of dorsal artery of right foot   CC

       ✓7th **S95.012** Laceration of dorsal artery of left foot   CC

       ✓7th **S95.019** Laceration of dorsal artery of unspecified foot   CC

    ✓6th **S95.09 Other specified injury of dorsal artery of foot**

       ✓7th **S95.091** Other specified injury of dorsal artery of right foot   CC

       ✓7th **S95.092** Other specified injury of dorsal artery of left foot   CC

       ✓7th **S95.099** Other specified injury of dorsal artery of unspecified foot   CC

✓5th **S95.1 Injury of plantar artery of foot**

    ✓6th **S95.10 Unspecified injury of plantar artery of foot**

       ✓7th **S95.101** Unspecified injury of plantar artery of right foot   CC

       ✓7th **S95.102** Unspecified injury of plantar artery of left foot   CC

       ✓7th **S95.109** Unspecified injury of plantar artery of unspecified foot   CC

    ✓6th **S95.11 Laceration of plantar artery of foot**

       ✓7th **S95.111** Laceration of plantar artery of right foot   CC

       ✓7th **S95.112** Laceration of plantar artery of left foot   CC

       ✓7th **S95.119** Laceration of plantar artery of unspecified foot   CC

    ✓6th **S95.19 Other specified injury of plantar artery of foot**

       ✓7th **S95.191** Other specified injury of plantar artery of right foot   CC

       ✓7th **S95.192** Other specified injury of plantar artery of left foot   CC

       ✓7th **S95.199** Other specified injury of plantar artery of unspecified foot   CC

✓5th **S95.2 Injury of dorsal vein of foot**

    ✓6th **S95.20 Unspecified injury of dorsal vein of foot**

       ✓7th **S95.201** Unspecified injury of dorsal vein of right foot   CC

       ✓7th **S95.202** Unspecified injury of dorsal vein of left foot   CC

       ✓7th **S95.209** Unspecified injury of dorsal vein of unspecified foot   CC

    ✓6th **S95.21 Laceration of dorsal vein of foot**

       ✓7th **S95.211** Laceration of dorsal vein of right foot   CC

       ✓7th **S95.212** Laceration of dorsal vein of left foot   CC

       ✓7th **S95.219** Laceration of dorsal vein of unspecified foot   CC

    ✓6th **S95.29 Other specified injury of dorsal vein of foot**

       ✓7th **S95.291** Other specified injury of dorsal vein of right foot   CC

       ✓7th **S95.292** Other specified injury of dorsal vein of left foot   CC

       ✓7th **S95.299** Other specified injury of dorsal vein of unspecified foot   CC

✓5th **S95.8 Injury of other blood vessels at ankle and foot level**

    ✓6th **S95.80 Unspecified injury of other blood vessels at ankle and foot level**

       ✓7th **S95.801** Unspecified injury of other blood vessels at ankle and foot level, right leg   CC

       ✓7th **S95.802** Unspecified injury of other blood vessels at ankle and foot level, left leg   CC

       ✓7th **S95.809** Unspecified injury of other blood vessels at ankle and foot level, unspecified leg   CC

    ✓6th **S95.81 Laceration of other blood vessels at ankle and foot level**

       ✓7th **S95.811** Laceration of other blood vessels at ankle and foot level, right leg   CC

       ✓7th **S95.812** Laceration of other blood vessels at ankle and foot level, left leg   CC

       ✓7th **S95.819** Laceration of other blood vessels at ankle and foot level, unspecified leg   CC

    ✓6th **S95.89 Other specified injury of other blood vessels at ankle and foot level**

       ✓7th **S95.891** Other specified injury of other blood vessels at ankle and foot level, right leg   CC

       ✓7th **S95.892** Other specified injury of other blood vessels at ankle and foot level, left leg   CC

       ✓7th **S95.899** Other specified injury of other blood vessels at ankle and foot level, unspecified leg   CC

✓5th **S95.9 Injury of unspecified blood vessel at ankle and foot level**

    ✓6th **S95.90 Unspecified injury of unspecified blood vessel at ankle and foot level**

       ✓7th **S95.901** Unspecified injury of unspecified blood vessel at ankle and foot level, right leg   CC

       ✓7th **S95.902** Unspecified injury of unspecified blood vessel at ankle and foot level, left leg   CC

       ✓7th **S95.909** Unspecified injury of unspecified blood vessel at ankle and foot level, unspecified leg   CC

    ✓6th **S95.91 Laceration of unspecified blood vessel at ankle and foot level**

       ✓7th **S95.911** Laceration of unspecified blood vessel at ankle and foot level, right leg   CC

       ✓7th **S95.912** Laceration of unspecified blood vessel at ankle and foot level, left leg   CC

       ✓7th **S95.919** Laceration of unspecified blood vessel at ankle and foot level, unspecified leg   CC

    ✓6th **S95.99 Other specified injury of unspecified blood vessel at ankle and foot level**

       ✓7th **S95.991** Other specified injury of unspecified blood vessel at ankle and foot level, right leg   CC

       ✓7th **S95.992** Other specified injury of unspecified blood vessel at ankle and foot level, left leg   CC

       ✓7th **S95.999** Other specified injury of unspecified blood vessel at ankle and foot level, unspecified leg   CC

✓4th **S96 Injury of muscle and tendon at ankle and foot level**

Code also any associated open wound (S91.-)

EXCLUDES 2   *injury of Achilles tendon (S86.0-)*
         sprain of joints and ligaments of ankle and foot (S93.-)

TIP: Refer to the Muscle/Tendon table at the beginning of this chapter,

The appropriate 7th character is to be added to each code from category S96.
A   initial encounter
D   subsequent encounter
S   sequela

✓5th **S96.0 Injury of muscle and tendon of long flexor muscle of toe at ankle and foot level**

    ✓6th **S96.00 Unspecified injury of muscle and tendon of long flexor muscle of toe at ankle and foot level**

       ✓7th **S96.001** Unspecified injury of muscle and tendon of long flexor muscle of toe at ankle and foot level, right foot

       ✓7th **S96.002** Unspecified injury of muscle and tendon of long flexor muscle of toe at ankle and foot level, left foot

✓ Additional Character Required   ✓x7th Placeholder   Questionable PDx   Manifestation   Unspecified Dx   UPD Unacceptable PDx   H1-H14 HAC   HCC CMS-HCC Dx   HIV HIV Dx

ICD-10-CM 2022   1087

✓7th **S96.009** Unspecified injury of muscle and tendon of long flexor muscle of toe at ankle and foot level, unspecified foot

✓6th **S96.01** Strain of muscle and tendon of long flexor muscle of toe at ankle and foot level

    ✓7th S96.011 Strain of muscle and tendon of long flexor muscle of toe at ankle and foot level, right foot

    ✓7th S96.012 Strain of muscle and tendon of long flexor muscle of toe at ankle and foot level, left foot

    ✓7th **S96.019** Strain of muscle and tendon of long flexor muscle of toe at ankle and foot level, unspecified foot

✓6th **S96.02** Laceration of muscle and tendon of long flexor muscle of toe at ankle and foot level

    ✓7th S96.021 Laceration of muscle and tendon of long flexor muscle of toe at ankle and foot level, right foot   CC

    ✓7th S96.022 Laceration of muscle and tendon of long flexor muscle of toe at ankle and foot level, left foot   CC

    ✓7th **S96.029** Laceration of muscle and tendon of long flexor muscle of toe at ankle and foot level, unspecified foot   CC

✓6th **S96.09** Other injury of muscle and tendon of long flexor muscle of toe at ankle and foot level

    ✓7th S96.091 Other injury of muscle and tendon of long flexor muscle of toe at ankle and foot level, right foot

    ✓7th S96.092 Other injury of muscle and tendon of long flexor muscle of toe at ankle and foot level, left foot

    ✓7th **S96.099** Other injury of muscle and tendon of long flexor muscle of toe at ankle and foot level, unspecified foot

✓5th **S96.1** Injury of muscle and tendon of long extensor muscle of toe at ankle and foot level

✓6th **S96.10** Unspecified injury of muscle and tendon of long extensor muscle of toe at ankle and foot level

    ✓7th **S96.101** Unspecified injury of muscle and tendon of long extensor muscle of toe at ankle and foot level, right foot

    ✓7th **S96.102** Unspecified injury of muscle and tendon of long extensor muscle of toe at ankle and foot level, left foot

    ✓7th **S96.109** Unspecified injury of muscle and tendon of long extensor muscle of toe at ankle and foot level, unspecified foot

✓6th **S96.11** Strain of muscle and tendon of long extensor muscle of toe at ankle and foot level

    ✓7th S96.111 Strain of muscle and tendon of long extensor muscle of toe at ankle and foot level, right foot

    ✓7th S96.112 Strain of muscle and tendon of long extensor muscle of toe at ankle and foot level, left foot

    ✓7th **S96.119** Strain of muscle and tendon of long extensor muscle of toe at ankle and foot level, unspecified foot

✓6th **S96.12** Laceration of muscle and tendon of long extensor muscle of toe at ankle and foot level

    ✓7th S96.121 Laceration of muscle and tendon of long extensor muscle of toe at ankle and foot level, right foot   CC

    ✓7th S96.122 Laceration of muscle and tendon of long extensor muscle of toe at ankle and foot level, left foot   CC

    ✓7th **S96.129** Laceration of muscle and tendon of long extensor muscle of toe at ankle and foot level, unspecified foot   CC

✓6th **S96.19** Other specified injury of muscle and tendon of long extensor muscle of toe at ankle and foot level

    ✓7th S96.191 Other specified injury of muscle and tendon of long extensor muscle of toe at ankle and foot level, right foot

    ✓7th S96.192 Other specified injury of muscle and tendon of long extensor muscle of toe at ankle and foot level, left foot

    ✓7th **S96.199** Other specified injury of muscle and tendon of long extensor muscle of toe at ankle and foot level, unspecified foot

✓5th **S96.2** Injury of intrinsic muscle and tendon at ankle and foot level

✓6th **S96.20** Unspecified injury of intrinsic muscle and tendon at ankle and foot level

    ✓7th **S96.201** Unspecified injury of intrinsic muscle and tendon at ankle and foot level, right foot

    ✓7th **S96.202** Unspecified injury of intrinsic muscle and tendon at ankle and foot level, left foot

    ✓7th **S96.209** Unspecified injury of intrinsic muscle and tendon at ankle and foot level, unspecified foot

✓6th **S96.21** Strain of intrinsic muscle and tendon at ankle and foot level

    ✓7th S96.211 Strain of intrinsic muscle and tendon at ankle and foot level, right foot

    ✓7th S96.212 Strain of intrinsic muscle and tendon at ankle and foot level, left foot

    ✓7th **S96.219** Strain of intrinsic muscle and tendon at ankle and foot level, unspecified foot

✓6th **S96.22** Laceration of intrinsic muscle and tendon at ankle and foot level

    ✓7th S96.221 Laceration of intrinsic muscle and tendon at ankle and foot level, right foot   CC

    ✓7th S96.222 Laceration of intrinsic muscle and tendon at ankle and foot level, left foot   CC

    ✓7th **S96.229** Laceration of intrinsic muscle and tendon at ankle and foot level, unspecified foot   CC

✓6th **S96.29** Other specified injury of intrinsic muscle and tendon at ankle and foot level

    ✓7th S96.291 Other specified injury of intrinsic muscle and tendon at ankle and foot level, right foot

    ✓7th S96.292 Other specified injury of intrinsic muscle and tendon at ankle and foot level, left foot

    ✓7th **S96.299** Other specified injury of intrinsic muscle and tendon at ankle and foot level, unspecified foot

✓5th **S96.8** Injury of other specified muscles and tendons at ankle and foot level

✓6th **S96.80** Unspecified injury of other specified muscles and tendons at ankle and foot level

    ✓7th **S96.801** Unspecified injury of other specified muscles and tendons at ankle and foot level, right foot

    ✓7th **S96.802** Unspecified injury of other specified muscles and tendons at ankle and foot level, left foot

    ✓7th **S96.809** Unspecified injury of other specified muscles and tendons at ankle and foot level, unspecified foot

✓6th **S96.81** Strain of other specified muscles and tendons at ankle and foot level

    ✓7th S96.811 Strain of other specified muscles and tendons at ankle and foot level, right foot

    ✓7th S96.812 Strain of other specified muscles and tendons at ankle and foot level, left foot

    ✓7th **S96.819** Strain of other specified muscles and tendons at ankle and foot level, unspecified foot

✓6th **S96.82** Laceration of other specified muscles and tendons at ankle and foot level

    ✓7th S96.821 Laceration of other specified muscles and tendons at ankle and foot level, right foot   CC

    ✓7th S96.822 Laceration of other specified muscles and tendons at ankle and foot level, left foot   CC

    ✓7th **S96.829** Laceration of other specified muscles and tendons at ankle and foot level, unspecified foot   CC

✓6th **S96.89** Other specified injury of other specified muscles and tendons at ankle and foot level

    ✓7th S96.891 Other specified injury of other specified muscles and tendons at ankle and foot level, right foot

    ✓7th S96.892 Other specified injury of other specified muscles and tendons at ankle and foot level, left foot

    ✓7th **S96.899** Other specified injury of other specified muscles and tendons at ankle and foot level, unspecified foot

N Newborn: 0   P Pediatric: 0-17   M Maternity: 9-64   A Adult: 15-124   MCC Major Complication/Comorbidity   CC Complication/Comorbidity   SW Severe Wound Dx

1088   ICD-10-CM 2022

√5ᵗʰ **S96.9 Injury of unspecified muscle and tendon at ankle and foot level**

  √6ᵗʰ **S96.90 Unspecified injury of unspecified muscle and tendon at ankle and foot level**

    √7ᵗʰ **S96.901** Unspecified injury of unspecified muscle and tendon at ankle and foot level, right foot

    √7ᵗʰ **S96.902** Unspecified injury of unspecified muscle and tendon at ankle and foot level, left foot

    √7ᵗʰ **S96.909** Unspecified injury of unspecified muscle and tendon at ankle and foot level, unspecified foot

  √6ᵗʰ **S96.91 Strain of unspecified muscle and tendon at ankle and foot level**

    √7ᵗʰ **S96.911** Strain of unspecified muscle and tendon at ankle and foot level, right foot

    √7ᵗʰ **S96.912** Strain of unspecified muscle and tendon at ankle and foot level, left foot

    √7ᵗʰ **S96.919** Strain of unspecified muscle and tendon at ankle and foot level, unspecified foot

  √6ᵗʰ **S96.92 Laceration of unspecified muscle and tendon at ankle and foot level**

    √7ᵗʰ **S96.921** Laceration of unspecified muscle and tendon at ankle and foot level, right foot `CC`

    √7ᵗʰ **S96.922** Laceration of unspecified muscle and tendon at ankle and foot level, left foot `CC`

    √7ᵗʰ **S96.929** Laceration of unspecified muscle and tendon at ankle and foot level, unspecified foot `CC`

  √6ᵗʰ **S96.99 Other specified injury of unspecified muscle and tendon at ankle and foot level**

    √7ᵗʰ **S96.991** Other specified injury of unspecified muscle and tendon at ankle and foot level, right foot

    √7ᵗʰ **S96.992** Other specified injury of unspecified muscle and tendon at ankle and foot level, left foot

    √7ᵗʰ **S96.999** Other specified injury of unspecified muscle and tendon at ankle and foot level, unspecified foot

√4ᵗʰ **S97 Crushing injury of ankle and foot**

  Use additional code(s) for all associated injuries

  The appropriate 7th character is to be added to each code from category S97.
  A   initial encounter
  D   subsequent encounter
  S   sequela

  √5ᵗʰ **S97.0 Crushing injury of ankle**

    √×7ᵗʰ **S97.00** Crushing injury of unspecified ankle

    √×7ᵗʰ **S97.01** Crushing injury of right ankle

    √×7ᵗʰ **S97.02** Crushing injury of left ankle

  √5ᵗʰ **S97.1 Crushing injury of toe**

    √6ᵗʰ **S97.10 Crushing injury of unspecified toe(s)**

      √7ᵗʰ **S97.101** Crushing injury of unspecified right toe(s)

      √7ᵗʰ **S97.102** Crushing injury of unspecified left toe(s)

      √7ᵗʰ **S97.109** Crushing injury of unspecified toe(s)
        Crushing injury of toe NOS

    √6ᵗʰ **S97.11 Crushing injury of great toe**

      √7ᵗʰ **S97.111** Crushing injury of right great toe

      √7ᵗʰ **S97.112** Crushing injury of left great toe

      √7ᵗʰ **S97.119** Crushing injury of unspecified great toe

    √6ᵗʰ **S97.12 Crushing injury of lesser toe(s)**

      √7ᵗʰ **S97.121** Crushing injury of right lesser toe(s)

      √7ᵗʰ **S97.122** Crushing injury of left lesser toe(s)

      √7ᵗʰ **S97.129** Crushing injury of unspecified lesser toe(s)

  √5ᵗʰ **S97.8 Crushing injury of foot**

    √×7ᵗʰ **S97.80** Crushing injury of unspecified foot
      Crushing injury of foot NOS

    √×7ᵗʰ **S97.81** Crushing injury of right foot

    √×7ᵗʰ **S97.82** Crushing injury of left foot

√4ᵗʰ **S98 Traumatic amputation of ankle and foot**

  An amputation not identified as partial or complete should be coded to complete

  The appropriate 7th character is to be added to each code from category S98.
  A   initial encounter
  D   subsequent encounter
  S   sequela

  √5ᵗʰ **S98.0 Traumatic amputation of foot at ankle level**

    √6ᵗʰ **S98.01 Complete traumatic amputation of foot at ankle level**

      √7ᵗʰ **S98.011** Complete traumatic amputation of right foot at ankle level `CC` `HCC`

      √7ᵗʰ **S98.012** Complete traumatic amputation of left foot at ankle level `CC` `HCC`

      √7ᵗʰ **S98.019** Complete traumatic amputation of unspecified foot at ankle level `CC` `HCC`

    √6ᵗʰ **S98.02 Partial traumatic amputation of foot at ankle level**

      √7ᵗʰ **S98.021** Partial traumatic amputation of right foot at ankle level `CC` `HCC`

      √7ᵗʰ **S98.022** Partial traumatic amputation of left foot at ankle level `CC` `HCC`

      √7ᵗʰ **S98.029** Partial traumatic amputation of unspecified foot at ankle level `CC` `HCC`

  √5ᵗʰ **S98.1 Traumatic amputation of one toe**

    √6ᵗʰ **S98.11 Complete traumatic amputation of great toe**

      √7ᵗʰ **S98.111** Complete traumatic amputation of right great toe `HCC`

      √7ᵗʰ **S98.112** Complete traumatic amputation of left great toe `HCC`

      √7ᵗʰ **S98.119** Complete traumatic amputation of unspecified great toe `HCC`

    √6ᵗʰ **S98.12 Partial traumatic amputation of great toe**

      √7ᵗʰ **S98.121** Partial traumatic amputation of right great toe `HCC`

      √7ᵗʰ **S98.122** Partial traumatic amputation of left great toe `HCC`

      √7ᵗʰ **S98.129** Partial traumatic amputation of unspecified great toe `HCC`

    √6ᵗʰ **S98.13 Complete traumatic amputation of one lesser toe**
      Traumatic amputation of toe NOS

      √7ᵗʰ **S98.131** Complete traumatic amputation of one right lesser toe `HCC`

      √7ᵗʰ **S98.132** Complete traumatic amputation of one left lesser toe `HCC`

      √7ᵗʰ **S98.139** Complete traumatic amputation of one unspecified lesser toe `HCC`

    √6ᵗʰ **S98.14 Partial traumatic amputation of one lesser toe**

      √7ᵗʰ **S98.141** Partial traumatic amputation of one right lesser toe `HCC`

      √7ᵗʰ **S98.142** Partial traumatic amputation of one left lesser toe `HCC`

      √7ᵗʰ **S98.149** Partial traumatic amputation of one unspecified lesser toe `HCC`

  √5ᵗʰ **S98.2 Traumatic amputation of two or more lesser toes**

    √6ᵗʰ **S98.21 Complete traumatic amputation of two or more lesser toes**

      √7ᵗʰ **S98.211** Complete traumatic amputation of two or more right lesser toes `HCC`

      √7ᵗʰ **S98.212** Complete traumatic amputation of two or more left lesser toes `HCC`

      √7ᵗʰ **S98.219** Complete traumatic amputation of two or more unspecified lesser toes `HCC`

    √6ᵗʰ **S98.22 Partial traumatic amputation of two or more lesser toes**

      √7ᵗʰ **S98.221** Partial traumatic amputation of two or more right lesser toes

      √7ᵗʰ **S98.222** Partial traumatic amputation of two or more left lesser toes `HCC`

      √7ᵗʰ **S98.229** Partial traumatic amputation of two or more unspecified lesser toes `HCC`

  √5ᵗʰ **S98.3 Traumatic amputation of midfoot**

    √6ᵗʰ **S98.31 Complete traumatic amputation of midfoot**

      √7ᵗʰ **S98.311** Complete traumatic amputation of right midfoot `CC` `HCC`

      √7ᵗʰ **S98.312** Complete traumatic amputation of left midfoot `CC` `HCC`

✔ Additional Character Required   √×7ᵗʰ Placeholder   Questionable PDx   Manifestation   Unspecified Dx   `UPD` Unacceptable PDx   `H1`-`H14` HAC   `HCC` CMS-HCC Dx   `HIV` HIV Dx

ICD-10-CM 2022   1089

√7th **S98.319** Complete traumatic amputation of unspecified midfoot `CC` `HCC`

√6th **S98.32** Partial traumatic amputation of midfoot

√7th **S98.321** Partial traumatic amputation of right midfoot `CC` `HCC`

√7th **S98.322** Partial traumatic amputation of left midfoot `CC` `HCC`

√7th **S98.329** Partial traumatic amputation of unspecified midfoot `CC` `HCC`

√5th **S98.9** Traumatic amputation of foot, level unspecified

√6th **S98.91** Complete traumatic amputation of foot, level unspecified

√7th **S98.911** Complete traumatic amputation of right foot, level unspecified `CC` `HCC`

√7th **S98.912** Complete traumatic amputation of left foot, level unspecified `CC` `HCC`

√7th **S98.919** Complete traumatic amputation of unspecified foot, level unspecified `CC` `HCC`

√6th **S98.92** Partial traumatic amputation of foot, level unspecified

√7th **S98.921** Partial traumatic amputation of right foot, level unspecified `CC` `HCC`

√7th **S98.922** Partial traumatic amputation of left foot, level unspecified `CC` `HCC`

√7th **S98.929** Partial traumatic amputation of unspecified foot, level unspecified `CC` `HCC`

√4th **S99 Other and unspecified injuries of ankle and foot**

AHA: 2018,2Q,12; 2018,1Q,3; 2016,4Q,68-69

√5th **S99.0** Physeal fracture of calcaneus

AHA: 2019,4Q,56

The appropriate 7th character is to be added to each code from subcategory S99.0.
A   initial encounter for closed fracture
B   initial encounter for open fracture
D   subsequent encounter for fracture with routine healing
G   subsequent encounter for fracture with delayed healing
K   subsequent encounter for fracture with nonunion
P   subsequent encounter for fracture with malunion
S   sequela

√6th **S99.00** Unspecified physeal fracture of calcaneus

√7th **S99.001** Unspecified physeal fracture of right calcaneus

√7th **S99.002** Unspecified physeal fracture of left calcaneus

√7th **S99.009** Unspecified physeal fracture of unspecified calcaneus

√6th **S99.01** Salter-Harris Type I physeal fracture of calcaneus

√7th **S99.011** Salter-Harris Type I physeal fracture of right calcaneus

√7th **S99.012** Salter-Harris Type I physeal fracture of left calcaneus

√7th **S99.019** Salter-Harris Type I physeal fracture of unspecified calcaneus

√6th **S99.02** Salter-Harris Type II physeal fracture of calcaneus

√7th **S99.021** Salter-Harris Type II physeal fracture of right calcaneus

√7th **S99.022** Salter-Harris Type II physeal fracture of left calcaneus

√7th **S99.029** Salter-Harris Type II physeal fracture of unspecified calcaneus

√6th **S99.03** Salter-Harris Type III physeal fracture of calcaneus

√7th **S99.031** Salter-Harris Type III physeal fracture of right calcaneus

√7th **S99.032** Salter-Harris Type III physeal fracture of left calcaneus

√7th **S99.039** Salter-Harris Type III physeal fracture of unspecified calcaneus

√6th **S99.04** Salter-Harris Type IV physeal fracture of calcaneus

√7th **S99.041** Salter-Harris Type IV physeal fracture of right calcaneus

√7th **S99.042** Salter-Harris Type IV physeal fracture of left calcaneus

√7th **S99.049** Salter-Harris Type IV physeal fracture of unspecified calcaneus

√6th **S99.09** Other physeal fracture of calcaneus

√7th **S99.091** Other physeal fracture of right calcaneus

√7th **S99.092** Other physeal fracture of left calcaneus

√7th **S99.099** Other physeal fracture of unspecified calcaneus

√5th **S99.1** Physeal fracture of metatarsal

AHA: 2019,4Q,56

The appropriate 7th character is to be added to each code from subcategory S99.1
A   initial encounter for closed fracture
B   initial encounter for open fracture
D   subsequent encounter for fracture with routine healing
G   subsequent encounter for fracture with delayed healing
K   subsequent encounter for fracture with nonunion
P   subsequent encounter for fracture with malunion
S   sequela

√6th **S99.10** Unspecified physeal fracture of metatarsal

√7th **S99.101** Unspecified physeal fracture of right metatarsal

√7th **S99.102** Unspecified physeal fracture of left metatarsal

√7th **S99.109** Unspecified physeal fracture of unspecified metatarsal

√6th **S99.11** Salter-Harris Type I physeal fracture of metatarsal

√7th **S99.111** Salter-Harris Type I physeal fracture of right metatarsal

√7th **S99.112** Salter-Harris Type I physeal fracture of left metatarsal

√7th **S99.119** Salter-Harris Type I physeal fracture of unspecified metatarsal

√6th **S99.12** Salter-Harris Type II physeal fracture of metatarsal

√7th **S99.121** Salter-Harris Type II physeal fracture of right metatarsal

√7th **S99.122** Salter-Harris Type II physeal fracture of left metatarsal

√7th **S99.129** Salter-Harris Type II physeal fracture of unspecified metatarsal

√6th **S99.13** Salter-Harris Type III physeal fracture of metatarsal

√7th **S99.131** Salter-Harris Type III physeal fracture of right metatarsal

√7th **S99.132** Salter-Harris Type III physeal fracture of left metatarsal

√7th **S99.139** Salter-Harris Type III physeal fracture of unspecified metatarsal

√6th **S99.14** Salter-Harris Type IV physeal fracture of metatarsal

√7th **S99.141** Salter-Harris Type IV physeal fracture of right metatarsal

√7th **S99.142** Salter-Harris Type IV physeal fracture of left metatarsal

√7th **S99.149** Salter-Harris Type IV physeal fracture of unspecified metatarsal

√6th **S99.19** Other physeal fracture of metatarsal

√7th **S99.191** Other physeal fracture of right metatarsal

√7th **S99.192** Other physeal fracture of left metatarsal

√7th **S99.199** Other physeal fracture of unspecified metatarsal

√5th **S99.2** Physeal fracture of phalanx of toe

AHA: 2019,4Q,56

The appropriate 7th character is to be added to each code from subcategories S99.2.
A   initial encounter for closed fracture
B   initial encounter for open fracture
D   subsequent encounter for fracture with routine healing
G   subsequent encounter for fracture with delayed healing
K   subsequent encounter for fracture with nonunion
P   subsequent encounter for fracture with malunion
S   sequela

√6th **S99.20** Unspecified physeal fracture of phalanx of toe

√7th **S99.201** Unspecified physeal fracture of phalanx of right toe

√7th **S99.202** Unspecified physeal fracture of phalanx of left toe

√7th **S99.209** Unspecified physeal fracture of phalanx of unspecified toe

√6th **S99.21** Salter-Harris Type I physeal fracture of phalanx of toe

√7th **S99.211** Salter-Harris Type I physeal fracture of phalanx of right toe

√7th **S99.212** Salter-Harris Type I physeal fracture of phalanx of left toe

√7ᵗʰ **S99.219** Salter-Harris Type I physeal fracture of phalanx of unspecified toe

√6ᵗʰ **S99.22** Salter-Harris Type II physeal fracture of phalanx of toe

    √7ᵗʰ **S99.221** Salter-Harris Type II physeal fracture of phalanx of right toe

    √7ᵗʰ **S99.222** Salter-Harris Type II physeal fracture of phalanx of left toe

    √7ᵗʰ **S99.229** Salter-Harris Type II physeal fracture of phalanx of unspecified toe

√6ᵗʰ **S99.23** Salter-Harris Type III physeal fracture of phalanx of toe

    √7ᵗʰ **S99.231** Salter-Harris Type III physeal fracture of phalanx of right toe

    √7ᵗʰ **S99.232** Salter-Harris Type III physeal fracture of phalanx of left toe

    √7ᵗʰ **S99.239** Salter-Harris Type III physeal fracture of phalanx of unspecified toe

√6ᵗʰ **S99.24** Salter-Harris Type IV physeal fracture of phalanx of toe

    √7ᵗʰ **S99.241** Salter-Harris Type IV physeal fracture of phalanx of right toe

    √7ᵗʰ **S99.242** Salter-Harris Type IV physeal fracture of phalanx of left toe

    √7ᵗʰ **S99.249** Salter-Harris Type IV physeal fracture of phalanx of unspecified toe

√6ᵗʰ **S99.29** Other physeal fracture of phalanx of toe

    √7ᵗʰ **S99.291** Other physeal fracture of phalanx of right toe

    √7ᵗʰ **S99.292** Other physeal fracture of phalanx of left toe

    √7ᵗʰ **S99.299** Other physeal fracture of phalanx of unspecified toe

√5ᵗʰ **S99.8** Other specified injuries of ankle and foot

> The appropriate 7th character is to be added to each code from subcategory S99.8.
> A   initial encounter
> D   subsequent encounter
> S   sequela

√6ᵗʰ **S99.81** Other specified injuries of ankle

    √7ᵗʰ **S99.811** Other specified injuries of right ankle

    √7ᵗʰ **S99.812** Other specified injuries of left ankle

    √7ᵗʰ **S99.819** Other specified injuries of unspecified ankle

√6ᵗʰ **S99.82** Other specified injuries of foot

    √7ᵗʰ **S99.821** Other specified injuries of right foot

    √7ᵗʰ **S99.822** Other specified injuries of left foot

    √7ᵗʰ **S99.829** Other specified injuries of unspecified foot

√5ᵗʰ **S99.9** Unspecified injury of ankle and foot

> The appropriate 7th character is to be added to each code from subcategory S99.9.
> A   initial encounter
> D   subsequent encounter
> S   sequela

√6ᵗʰ **S99.91** Unspecified injury of ankle

    √7ᵗʰ **S99.911** Unspecified injury of right ankle

    √7ᵗʰ **S99.912** Unspecified injury of left ankle

    √7ᵗʰ **S99.919** Unspecified injury of unspecified ankle

√6ᵗʰ **S99.92** Unspecified injury of foot

    √7ᵗʰ **S99.921** Unspecified injury of right foot

    √7ᵗʰ **S99.922** Unspecified injury of left foot

    √7ᵗʰ **S99.929** Unspecified injury of unspecified foot

INJURY, POISONING AND CERTAIN OTHER CONSEQUENCES OF EXTERNAL CAUSES (T07-T88)

Injuries involving multiple body regions (T07)

EXCLUDES 1   *burns and corrosions (T20-T32)*
               frostbite (T33-T34)
               insect bite or sting, venomous (T63.4)
               sunburn (L55.-)

√x7ᵗʰ **T07** Unspecified multiple injuries

    EXCLUDES 1   *injury NOS (T14.90)*

    AHA: 2017,4Q,26

> The appropriate 7th character is to be added to code T07.
> A   initial encounter
> D   subsequent encounter
> S   sequela

Injury of unspecified body region (T14)

√4ᵗʰ **T14** Injury of unspecified body region

    EXCLUDES 1   *multiple unspecified injuries (T07)*

    AHA: 2017,4Q,26

> The appropriate 7th character is to be added to each code from category T14.
> A   initial encounter
> D   subsequent encounter
> S   sequela

√x7ᵗʰ **T14.8** Other injury of unspecified body region

    Abrasion NOS
    Contusion NOS
    Crush injury NOS
    Fracture NOS
    Skin injury NOS
    Vascular injury NOS
    Wound NOS

√5ᵗʰ **T14.9** Unspecified injury

    √x7ᵗʰ **T14.90** Injury, unspecified

        Injury NOS

    √x7ᵗʰ **T14.91** Suicide attempt   HCC

        Attempted suicide NOS

Effects of foreign body entering through natural orifice (T15-T19)

EXCLUDES 2   *foreign body accidentally left in operation wound (T81.5-)*
               foreign body in penetrating wound - see open wound by body region
               residual foreign body in soft tissue (M79.5)
               splinter, without open wound - see superficial injury by body region

√4ᵗʰ **T15** Foreign body on external eye

    EXCLUDES 2   *foreign body in penetrating wound of orbit and eye ball (S05.4-, S05.5-)*
               open wound of eyelid and periocular area (S01.1-)
               retained foreign body in eyelid (H02.8-)
               retained (old) foreign body in penetrating wound of orbit and eye ball (H05.5-, H44.6-, H44.7-)
               superficial foreign body of eyelid and periocular area (S00.25-)

> The appropriate 7th character is to be added to each code from category T15.
> A   initial encounter
> D   subsequent encounter
> S   sequela

√5ᵗʰ **T15.0** Foreign body in cornea

    √x7ᵗʰ **T15.00** Foreign body in cornea, unspecified eye

    √x7ᵗʰ **T15.01** Foreign body in cornea, right eye

    √x7ᵗʰ **T15.02** Foreign body in cornea, left eye

√5ᵗʰ **T15.1** Foreign body in conjunctival sac

    √x7ᵗʰ **T15.10** Foreign body in conjunctival sac, unspecified eye

    √x7ᵗʰ **T15.11** Foreign body in conjunctival sac, right eye

    √x7ᵗʰ **T15.12** Foreign body in conjunctival sac, left eye

√5ᵗʰ **T15.8** Foreign body in other and multiple parts of external eye

    Foreign body in lacrimal punctum

    √x7ᵗʰ **T15.80** Foreign body in other and multiple parts of external eye, unspecified eye

☑ Additional Character Required √x7ᵗʰ Placeholder Questionable PDx Manifestation Unspecified Dx UPD Unacceptable PDx H1-H4 HAC HCC CMS-HCC Dx HIV HIV Dx

ICD-10-CM 2022   1091

√x7ᵗʰ **T15.81** Foreign body in other and multiple parts of external eye, right eye

√x7ᵗʰ **T15.82** Foreign body in other and multiple parts of external eye, left eye

√5ᵗʰ **T15.9** Foreign body on external eye, part unspecified

√x7ᵗʰ **T15.90** Foreign body on external eye, part unspecified, unspecified eye

√x7ᵗʰ **T15.91** Foreign body on external eye, part unspecified, right eye

√x7ᵗʰ **T15.92** Foreign body on external eye, part unspecified, left eye

√4ᵗʰ **T16** Foreign body in ear

INCLUDES   foreign body in auditory canal

The appropriate 7th character is to be added to each code from category T16.
A   initial encounter
D   subsequent encounter
S   sequela

√x7ᵗʰ **T16.1** Foreign body in right ear

√x7ᵗʰ **T16.2** Foreign body in left ear

√x7ᵗʰ **T16.9** Foreign body in ear, unspecified ear

√4ᵗʰ **T17** Foreign body in respiratory tract

The appropriate 7th character is to be added to each code from category T17.
A   initial encounter
D   subsequent encounter
S   sequela

√x7ᵗʰ **T17.0** Foreign body in nasal sinus

√x7ᵗʰ **T17.1** Foreign body in nostril
Foreign body in nose NOS

√5ᵗʰ **T17.2** Foreign body in pharynx
Foreign body in nasopharynx
Foreign body in throat NOS

√6ᵗʰ **T17.20** Unspecified foreign body in pharynx

√7ᵗʰ **T17.200** Unspecified foreign body in pharynx causing asphyxiation

√7ᵗʰ **T17.208** Unspecified foreign body in pharynx causing other injury

√6ᵗʰ **T17.21** Gastric contents in pharynx
Aspiration of gastric contents into pharynx
Vomitus in pharynx

√7ᵗʰ **T17.210** Gastric contents in pharynx causing asphyxiation

√7ᵗʰ **T17.218** Gastric contents in pharynx causing other injury

√6ᵗʰ **T17.22** Food in pharynx
Bones in pharynx
Seeds in pharynx

√7ᵗʰ **T17.220** Food in pharynx causing asphyxiation

√7ᵗʰ **T17.228** Food in pharynx causing other injury

√6ᵗʰ **T17.29** Other foreign object in pharynx

√7ᵗʰ **T17.290** Other foreign object in pharynx causing asphyxiation

√7ᵗʰ **T17.298** Other foreign object in pharynx causing other injury

√5ᵗʰ **T17.3** Foreign body in larynx

√6ᵗʰ **T17.30** Unspecified foreign body in larynx

√7ᵗʰ **T17.300** Unspecified foreign body in larynx causing asphyxiation

√7ᵗʰ **T17.308** Unspecified foreign body in larynx causing other injury

√6ᵗʰ **T17.31** Gastric contents in larynx
Aspiration of gastric contents into larynx
Vomitus in larynx

√7ᵗʰ **T17.310** Gastric contents in larynx causing asphyxiation

√7ᵗʰ **T17.318** Gastric contents in larynx causing other injury

√6ᵗʰ **T17.32** Food in larynx
Bones in larynx
Seeds in larynx

√7ᵗʰ **T17.320** Food in larynx causing asphyxiation

√7ᵗʰ **T17.328** Food in larynx causing other injury

√6ᵗʰ **T17.39** Other foreign object in larynx

√7ᵗʰ **T17.390** Other foreign object in larynx causing asphyxiation

√7ᵗʰ **T17.398** Other foreign object in larynx causing other injury

√5ᵗʰ **T17.4** Foreign body in trachea

√6ᵗʰ **T17.40** Unspecified foreign body in trachea

√7ᵗʰ **T17.400** Unspecified foreign body in trachea causing asphyxiation   CC

√7ᵗʰ **T17.408** Unspecified foreign body in trachea causing other injury   CC

√6ᵗʰ **T17.41** Gastric contents in trachea
Aspiration of gastric contents into trachea
Vomitus in trachea

√7ᵗʰ **T17.410** Gastric contents in trachea causing asphyxiation   CC

√7ᵗʰ **T17.418** Gastric contents in trachea causing other injury   CC

√6ᵗʰ **T17.42** Food in trachea
Bones in trachea
Seeds in trachea

√7ᵗʰ **T17.420** Food in trachea causing asphyxiation   CC

√7ᵗʰ **T17.428** Food in trachea causing other injury   CC

√6ᵗʰ **T17.49** Other foreign object in trachea

√7ᵗʰ **T17.490** Other foreign object in trachea causing asphyxiation   CC

√7ᵗʰ **T17.498** Other foreign object in trachea causing other injury   CC

√5ᵗʰ **T17.5** Foreign body in bronchus

√6ᵗʰ **T17.50** Unspecified foreign body in bronchus

√7ᵗʰ **T17.500** Unspecified foreign body in bronchus causing asphyxiation   CC

√7ᵗʰ **T17.508** Unspecified foreign body in bronchus causing other injury   CC

√6ᵗʰ **T17.51** Gastric contents in bronchus
Aspiration of gastric contents into bronchus
Vomitus in bronchus

√7ᵗʰ **T17.510** Gastric contents in bronchus causing asphyxiation   CC

√7ᵗʰ **T17.518** Gastric contents in bronchus causing other injury   CC

√6ᵗʰ **T17.52** Food in bronchus
Bones in bronchus
Seeds in bronchus

√7ᵗʰ **T17.520** Food in bronchus causing asphyxiation   CC

√7ᵗʰ **T17.528** Food in bronchus causing other injury   CC

√6ᵗʰ **T17.59** Other foreign object in bronchus

√7ᵗʰ **T17.590** Other foreign object in bronchus causing asphyxiation   CC

√7ᵗʰ **T17.598** Other foreign object in bronchus causing other injury   CC

√5ᵗʰ **T17.8** Foreign body in other parts of respiratory tract
Foreign body in bronchioles
Foreign body in lung

√6ᵗʰ **T17.80** Unspecified foreign body in other parts of respiratory tract

√7ᵗʰ **T17.800** Unspecified foreign body in other parts of respiratory tract causing asphyxiation   CC

√7ᵗʰ **T17.808** Unspecified foreign body in other parts of respiratory tract causing other injury   CC

√6ᵗʰ **T17.81** Gastric contents in other parts of respiratory tract
Aspiration of gastric contents into other parts of respiratory tract
Vomitus in other parts of respiratory tract

√7ᵗʰ **T17.810** Gastric contents in other parts of respiratory tract causing asphyxiation   CC

√7ᵗʰ **T17.818** Gastric contents in other parts of respiratory tract causing other injury   CC

N Newborn: 0   P Pediatric: 0-17   M Maternity: 9-64   A Adult: 15-124   MCC Major Complication/Comorbidity   CC Complication/Comorbidity   SW Severe Wound Dx

1092   ICD-10-CM 2022

√6ᵗʰ **T17.82** **Food** in other parts of respiratory tract
    Bones in other parts of respiratory tract
    Seeds in other parts of respiratory tract

    √7ᵗʰ **T17.820** **Food in other parts of respiratory tract** causing asphyxiation   **cc**

    √7ᵗʰ **T17.828** **Food in other parts of respiratory tract** causing other injury   **cc**

√6ᵗʰ **T17.89** **Other foreign object** in other parts of respiratory tract

    √7ᵗʰ **T17.890** **Other foreign object in other parts of respiratory tract** causing asphyxiation   **cc**

    √7ᵗʰ **T17.898** **Other foreign object in other parts of respiratory tract** causing other injury   **cc**

√5ᵗʰ **T17.9** **Foreign body** in respiratory tract, part unspecified

  √6ᵗʰ **T17.90** **Unspecified foreign body** in respiratory tract, part unspecified

    √7ᵗʰ **T17.900** **Unspecified foreign body in respiratory tract, part unspecified** causing asphyxiation

    √7ᵗʰ **T17.908** **Unspecified foreign body in respiratory tract, part unspecified** causing other injury

  √6ᵗʰ **T17.91** **Gastric contents** in respiratory tract, part unspecified
    Aspiration of gastric contents into respiratory tract, part unspecified
    Vomitus in trachea respiratory tract, part unspecified

    √7ᵗʰ **T17.910** **Gastric contents in respiratory tract, part unspecified** causing asphyxiation

    √7ᵗʰ **T17.918** **Gastric contents in respiratory tract, part unspecified** causing other injury

  √6ᵗʰ **T17.92** **Food** in respiratory tract, part unspecified
    Bones in respiratory tract, part unspecified
    Seeds in respiratory tract, part unspecified

    √7ᵗʰ **T17.920** **Food in respiratory tract, part unspecified** causing asphyxiation

    √7ᵗʰ **T17.928** **Food in respiratory tract, part unspecified** causing other injury

  √6ᵗʰ **T17.99** **Other foreign object** in respiratory tract, part unspecified

    √7ᵗʰ **T17.990** **Other foreign object in respiratory tract, part unspecified in** causing asphyxiation
        AHA: 2019,3Q,15

    √7ᵗʰ **T17.998** **Other foreign object in respiratory tract, part unspecified** causing other injury

√4ᵗʰ **T18** **Foreign body in alimentary tract**
  EXCLUDES 2 *foreign body in pharynx (T17.2-)*

The appropriate 7th character is to be added to each code from category T18.
A initial encounter
D subsequent encounter
S sequela

√x7ᵗʰ **T18.0** **Foreign body in mouth**

√5ᵗʰ **T18.1** **Foreign body in esophagus**
  EXCLUDES 2 *foreign body in respiratory tract (T17.-)*

  √6ᵗʰ **T18.10** **Unspecified foreign body in esophagus**

    √7ᵗʰ **T18.100** **Unspecified foreign body in esophagus** causing compression of trachea
        Unspecified foreign body in esophagus causing obstruction of respiration

    √7ᵗʰ **T18.108** **Unspecified foreign body in esophagus** causing other injury

  √6ᵗʰ **T18.11** **Gastric contents in esophagus**
    Vomitus in esophagus

    √7ᵗʰ **T18.110** **Gastric contents in esophagus** causing compression of trachea
        Gastric contents in esophagus causing obstruction of respiration

    √7ᵗʰ **T18.118** **Gastric contents in esophagus** causing other injury

---

√6ᵗʰ **T18.12** **Food in esophagus**
    Bones in esophagus
    Seeds in esophagus

    √7ᵗʰ **T18.120** **Food in esophagus** causing compression of trachea
        Food in esophagus causing obstruction of respiration

    √7ᵗʰ **T18.128** **Food in esophagus** causing other injury

√6ᵗʰ **T18.19** **Other foreign object in esophagus**
    AHA: 2015,1Q,23

    √7ᵗʰ **T18.190** **Other foreign object in esophagus** causing compression of trachea
        Other foreign body in esophagus causing obstruction of respiration
        TIP: Any foreign object lodged in the esophagus requires immediate treatment and is considered an injury. Assign this code when there is respiratory compromise or compression. If no respiratory compromise or compression is documented, assign code T18.198-.

    √7ᵗʰ **T18.198** **Other foreign object in esophagus** causing other injury
        TIP: Any foreign object lodged in the esophagus requires immediate treatment and is considered an injury. Assign this code when there is no respiratory compromise or compression. If respiratory compromise or compression is documented, assign code T18.190-.

√x7ᵗʰ **T18.2** **Foreign body in stomach**

√x7ᵗʰ **T18.3** **Foreign body in small intestine**

√x7ᵗʰ **T18.4** **Foreign body in colon**

√x7ᵗʰ **T18.5** **Foreign body in anus and rectum**
    Foreign body in rectosigmoid (junction)

√x7ᵗʰ **T18.8** **Foreign body in other parts of alimentary tract**

√x7ᵗʰ **T18.9** **Foreign body of alimentary tract, part unspecified**
    Foreign body in digestive system NOS
    Swallowed foreign body NOS

√4ᵗʰ **T19** **Foreign body in genitourinary tract**
  EXCLUDES 2 *complications due to implanted mesh (T83.7-)*
    mechanical complications of contraceptive device (intrauterine) (vaginal) (T83.3-)
    presence of contraceptive device (intrauterine) (vaginal) (Z97.5)

The appropriate 7th character is to be added to each code from category T19.
A initial encounter
D subsequent encounter
S sequela

√x7ᵗʰ **T19.0** **Foreign body in urethra**

√x7ᵗʰ **T19.1** **Foreign body in bladder**

√x7ᵗʰ **T19.2** **Foreign body in vulva and vagina**   ♀

√x7ᵗʰ **T19.3** **Foreign body in uterus**   ♀

√x7ᵗʰ **T19.4** **Foreign body in penis**   ♂

√x7ᵗʰ **T19.8** **Foreign body in other parts of genitourinary tract**

√x7ᵗʰ **T19.9** **Foreign body in genitourinary tract, part unspecified**

BURNS AND CORROSIONS (T20-T32)

INCLUDES　burns (thermal) from electrical heating appliances
burns (thermal) from electricity
burns (thermal) from flame
burns (thermal) from friction
burns (thermal) from hot air and hot gases
burns (thermal) from hot objects
burns (thermal) from lightning
burns (thermal) from radiation
chemical burn [corrosion] (external) (internal)
scalds

EXCLUDES 2　erythema [dermatitis] ab igne (L59.Ø)
radiation-related disorders of the skin and subcutaneous tissue
(L55-L59)
sunburn (L55.-)

AHA: 2016,2Q,4

Burns and corrosions of external body surface, specified by site (T20-T25)

INCLUDES　burns and corrosions of first degree [erythema]
burns and corrosions of second degree [blisters] [epidermal loss]
burns and corrosions of third degree [deep necrosis of underlying
tissue] [full-thickness skin loss]

Use additional code from category T31 or T32 to identify extent of body surface
involved

✓4ᵗʰ **T20　Burn and corrosion of head, face, and neck**

EXCLUDES 2　burn and corrosion of ear drum (T28.41, T28.91)
burn and corrosion of eye and adnexa (T26.-)
burn and corrosion of mouth and pharynx (T28.Ø)

AHA: 2015,1Q,18-19

The appropriate 7th character is to be added to each code from
category T20.
A　initial encounter
D　subsequent encounter
S　sequela

✓5ᵗʰ **T20.Ø　Burn of unspecified degree of head, face, and neck**

Use additional external cause code to identify the source, place
and intent of the burn (XØØ-X19, X75-X77, X96-X98, Y92)

✓x7ᵗʰ **T20.ØØ**　Burn of unspecified degree of head, face, and neck,
unspecified site

✓6ᵗʰ **T20.Ø1**　Burn of unspecified degree of ear [any part, except
ear drum]

EXCLUDES 2　burn of ear drum (T28.41-)

✓7ᵗʰ **T20.Ø11**　Burn of unspecified degree of right ear
[any part, except ear drum]

✓7ᵗʰ **T20.Ø12**　Burn of unspecified degree of left ear [any
part, except ear drum]

✓7ᵗʰ **T20.Ø19**　Burn of unspecified degree of unspecified
ear [any part, except ear drum]

✓x7ᵗʰ **T20.Ø2**　Burn of unspecified degree of lip(s)

✓x7ᵗʰ **T20.Ø3**　Burn of unspecified degree of chin

✓x7ᵗʰ **T20.Ø4**　Burn of unspecified degree of nose (septum)

✓x7ᵗʰ **T20.Ø5**　Burn of unspecified degree of scalp [any part]

✓x7ᵗʰ **T20.Ø6**　Burn of unspecified degree of forehead and cheek

✓x7ᵗʰ **T20.Ø7**　Burn of unspecified degree of neck

✓x7ᵗʰ **T20.Ø9**　Burn of unspecified degree of multiple sites of head,
face, and neck

✓5ᵗʰ **T20.1　Burn of first degree of head, face, and neck**

Use additional external cause code to identify the source, place
and intent of the burn (XØØ-X19, X75-X77, X96-X98, Y92)

✓x7ᵗʰ **T20.1Ø**　Burn of first degree of head, face, and neck,
unspecified site

✓6ᵗʰ **T20.11**　Burn of first degree of ear [any part, except ear
drum]

EXCLUDES 2　burn of ear drum (T28.41-)

✓7ᵗʰ **T20.111**　Burn of first degree of right ear [any part,
except ear drum]

✓7ᵗʰ **T20.112**　Burn of first degree of left ear [any part,
except ear drum]

✓7ᵗʰ **T20.119**　Burn of first degree of unspecified ear
[any part, except ear drum]

✓x7ᵗʰ **T20.12**　Burn of first degree of lip(s)

✓x7ᵗʰ **T20.13**　Burn of first degree of chin

✓x7ᵗʰ **T20.14**　Burn of first degree of nose (septum)

✓x7ᵗʰ **T20.15**　Burn of first degree of scalp [any part]

✓x7ᵗʰ **T20.16**　Burn of first degree of forehead and cheek

✓x7ᵗʰ **T20.17**　Burn of first degree of neck

✓x7ᵗʰ **T20.19**　Burn of first degree of multiple sites of head, face,
and neck

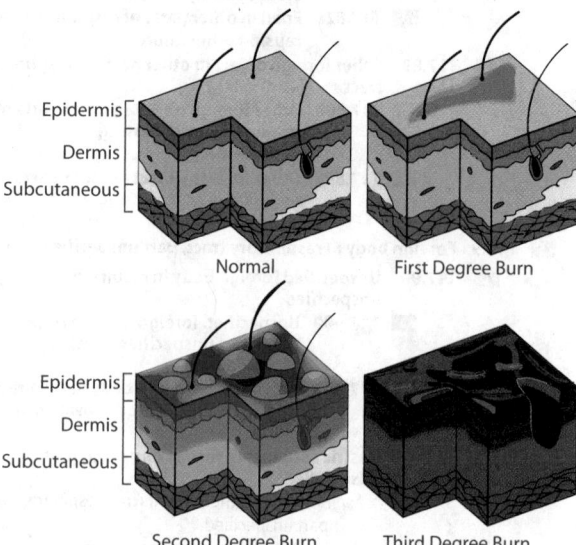

Degree of Burns

Epidermis
Dermis
Subcutaneous

Normal　　　　First Degree Burn

Epidermis
Dermis
Subcutaneous

Second Degree Burn　　　　Third Degree Burn

✓5ᵗʰ **T20.2　Burn of second degree of head, face, and neck**

Use additional external cause code to identify the source, place
and intent of the burn (XØØ-X19, X75-X77, X96-X98, Y92)

✓x7ᵗʰ **T20.2Ø**　Burn of second degree of head, face, and neck,
unspecified site

✓6ᵗʰ **T20.21**　Burn of second degree of ear [any part, except ear
drum]

EXCLUDES 2　burn of ear drum (T28.41-)

✓7ᵗʰ **T20.211**　Burn of second degree of right ear [any
part, except ear drum]

✓7ᵗʰ **T20.212**　Burn of second degree of left ear [any
part, except ear drum]

✓7ᵗʰ **T20.219**　Burn of second degree of unspecified ear
[any part, except ear drum]

✓x7ᵗʰ **T20.22**　Burn of second degree of lip(s)

✓x7ᵗʰ **T20.23**　Burn of second degree of chin

✓x7ᵗʰ **T20.24**　Burn of second degree of nose (septum)

✓x7ᵗʰ **T20.25**　Burn of second degree of scalp [any part]

✓x7ᵗʰ **T20.26**　Burn of second degree of forehead and cheek

✓x7ᵗʰ **T20.27**　Burn of second degree of neck

✓x7ᵗʰ **T20.29**　Burn of second degree of multiple sites of head,
face, and neck

✓5ᵗʰ **T20.3　Burn of third degree of head, face, and neck**

Use additional external cause code to identify the source, place
and intent of the burn (XØØ-X19, X75-X77, X96-X98, Y92)

✓x7ᵗʰ **T20.3Ø**　Burn of third degree of head, face, and neck,
unspecified site　　　CC H5 SW

✓6ᵗʰ **T20.31**　Burn of third degree of ear [any part, except ear
drum]

EXCLUDES 2　burn of ear drum (T28.41-)

AHA: 2015,1Q,18

✓7ᵗʰ **T20.311**　Burn of third degree of right ear [any
part, except ear drum]　　CC H5 SW

✓7ᵗʰ **T20.312**　Burn of third degree of left ear [any part,
except ear drum]　　CC H5 SW

✓7ᵗʰ **T20.319**　Burn of third degree of unspecified ear
[any part, except ear drum]　　CC H5 SW

✓x7ᵗʰ **T20.32**　Burn of third degree of lip(s)　　CC H5 SW

✓x7ᵗʰ **T20.33**　Burn of third degree of chin　　CC H5 SW

✓x7ᵗʰ **T20.34**　Burn of third degree of nose (septum)　　CC H5 SW

✓x7ᵗʰ **T20.35**　Burn of third degree of scalp [any part]　　CC H5 SW

✓x7ᵗʰ **T20.36**　Burn of third degree of forehead and
cheek　　CC H5 SW

✓x7ᵗʰ **T20.37**　Burn of third degree of neck　　CC H5 SW

✓x7ᵗʰ **T20.39**　Burn of third degree of multiple sites of head, face,
and neck　　CC H5 SW

√5ᵗʰ **T20.4** **Corrosion of unspecified degree of head, face, and neck**

Code first (T51-T65) to identify chemical and intent
Use additional external cause code to identify place (Y92)

√x7ᵗʰ **T20.40** **Corrosion of unspecified degree of head, face, and neck, unspecified site**

√6ᵗʰ **T20.41** **Corrosion of unspecified degree of ear [any part, except ear drum]**

EXCLUDES 2   *corrosion of ear drum (T28.91-)*

√7ᵗʰ **T20.411** **Corrosion of unspecified degree of right ear [any part, except ear drum]**

√7ᵗʰ **T20.412** **Corrosion of unspecified degree of left ear [any part, except ear drum]**

√7ᵗʰ **T20.419** **Corrosion of unspecified degree of unspecified ear [any part, except ear drum]**

√x7ᵗʰ **T20.42** **Corrosion of unspecified degree of lip(s)**

√x7ᵗʰ **T20.43** **Corrosion of unspecified degree of chin**

√x7ᵗʰ **T20.44** **Corrosion of unspecified degree of nose (septum)**

√x7ᵗʰ **T20.45** **Corrosion of unspecified degree of scalp [any part]**

√x7ᵗʰ **T20.46** **Corrosion of unspecified degree of forehead and cheek**

√x7ᵗʰ **T20.47** **Corrosion of unspecified degree of neck**

√x7ᵗʰ **T20.49** **Corrosion of unspecified degree of multiple sites of head, face, and neck**

√5ᵗʰ **T20.5** **Corrosion of first degree of head, face, and neck**

Code first (T51-T65) to identify chemical and intent
Use additional external cause code to identify place (Y92)

√x7ᵗʰ **T20.50** **Corrosion of first degree of head, face, and neck, unspecified site**

√6ᵗʰ **T20.51** **Corrosion of first degree of ear [any part, except ear drum]**

EXCLUDES 2   *corrosion of ear drum (T28.91-)*

√7ᵗʰ **T20.511** **Corrosion of first degree of right ear [any part, except ear drum]**

√7ᵗʰ **T20.512** **Corrosion of first degree of left ear [any part, except ear drum]**

√7ᵗʰ **T20.519** **Corrosion of first degree of unspecified ear [any part, except ear drum]**

√x7ᵗʰ **T20.52** **Corrosion of first degree of lip(s)**

√x7ᵗʰ **T20.53** **Corrosion of first degree of chin**

√x7ᵗʰ **T20.54** **Corrosion of first degree of nose (septum)**

√x7ᵗʰ **T20.55** **Corrosion of first degree of scalp [any part]**

√x7ᵗʰ **T20.56** **Corrosion of first degree of forehead and cheek**

√x7ᵗʰ **T20.57** **Corrosion of first degree of neck**

√x7ᵗʰ **T20.59** **Corrosion of first degree of multiple sites of head, face, and neck**

√5ᵗʰ **T20.6** **Corrosion of second degree of head, face, and neck**

Code first (T51-T65) to identify chemical and intent
Use additional external cause code to identify place (Y92)

√x7ᵗʰ **T20.60** **Corrosion of second degree of head, face, and neck, unspecified site**

√6ᵗʰ **T20.61** **Corrosion of second degree of ear [any part, except ear drum]**

EXCLUDES 2   *corrosion of ear drum (T28.91-)*

√7ᵗʰ **T20.611** **Corrosion of second degree of right ear [any part, except ear drum]**

√7ᵗʰ **T20.612** **Corrosion of second degree of left ear [any part, except ear drum]**

√7ᵗʰ **T20.619** **Corrosion of second degree of unspecified ear [any part, except ear drum]**

√x7ᵗʰ **T20.62** **Corrosion of second degree of lip(s)**

√x7ᵗʰ **T20.63** **Corrosion of second degree of chin**

√x7ᵗʰ **T20.64** **Corrosion of second degree of nose (septum)**

√x7ᵗʰ **T20.65** **Corrosion of second degree of scalp [any part]**

√x7ᵗʰ **T20.66** **Corrosion of second degree of forehead and cheek**

√x7ᵗʰ **T20.67** **Corrosion of second degree of neck**

√x7ᵗʰ **T20.69** **Corrosion of second degree of multiple sites of head, face, and neck**

√5ᵗʰ **T20.7** **Corrosion of third degree of head, face, and neck**

Code first (T51-T65) to identify chemical and intent
Use additional external cause code to identify place (Y92)

√x7ᵗʰ **T20.70** **Corrosion of third degree of head, face, and neck, unspecified site**   CC H5 SW

√6ᵗʰ **T20.71** **Corrosion of third degree of ear [any part, except ear drum]**

EXCLUDES 2   *corrosion of ear drum (T28.91-)*

√7ᵗʰ **T20.711** **Corrosion of third degree of right ear [any part, except ear drum]**   CC H5 SW

√7ᵗʰ **T20.712** **Corrosion of third degree of left ear [any part, except ear drum]**   CC H5 SW

√7ᵗʰ **T20.719** **Corrosion of third degree of unspecified ear [any part, except ear drum]**   CC H5 SW

√x7ᵗʰ **T20.72** **Corrosion of third degree of lip(s)**   CC H5 SW

√x7ᵗʰ **T20.73** **Corrosion of third degree of chin**   CC H5 SW

√x7ᵗʰ **T20.74** **Corrosion of third degree of nose (septum)**

√x7ᵗʰ **T20.75** **Corrosion of third degree of scalp [any part]**   CC H5 SW

√x7ᵗʰ **T20.76** **Corrosion of third degree of forehead and cheek**   CC H5 SW

√x7ᵗʰ **T20.77** **Corrosion of third degree of neck**   CC H5 SW

√x7ᵗʰ **T20.79** **Corrosion of third degree of multiple sites of head, face, and neck**   CC H5 SW

√4ᵗʰ **T21** **Burn and corrosion of trunk**

INCLUDES   burns and corrosion of hip region

EXCLUDES 2   *burns and corrosion of axilla (T22.- with fifth character 4)*

burns and corrosion of scapular region (T22.- with fifth character 6)

burns and corrosion of shoulder (T22.- with fifth character 5)

The appropriate 7th character is to be added to each code from category T21.

A   initial encounter
D   subsequent encounter
S   sequela

√5ᵗʰ **T21.0** **Burn of unspecified degree of trunk**

Use additional external cause code to identify the source, place and intent of the burn (X00-X19, X75-X77, X96-X98, Y92)

√x7ᵗʰ **T21.00** **Burn of unspecified degree of trunk, unspecified site**

√x7ᵗʰ **T21.01** **Burn of unspecified degree of chest wall**

Burn of unspecified degree of breast

√x7ᵗʰ **T21.02** **Burn of unspecified degree of abdominal wall**

Burn of unspecified degree of flank
Burn of unspecified degree of groin

√x7ᵗʰ **T21.03** **Burn of unspecified degree of upper back**

Burn of unspecified degree of interscapular region

√x7ᵗʰ **T21.04** **Burn of unspecified degree of lower back**

√x7ᵗʰ **T21.05** **Burn of unspecified degree of buttock**

Burn of unspecified degree of anus

√x7ᵗʰ **T21.06** **Burn of unspecified degree of male genital region**   ♂

Burn of unspecified degree of penis
Burn of unspecified degree of scrotum
Burn of unspecified degree of testis

√x7ᵗʰ **T21.07** **Burn of unspecified degree of female genital region**   ♀

Burn of unspecified degree of labium (majus) (minus)
Burn of unspecified degree of perineum
Burn of unspecified degree of vulva

EXCLUDES 2   *burn of vagina (T28.3)*

√x7ᵗʰ **T21.09** **Burn of unspecified degree of other site of trunk**

√5ᵗʰ **T21.1** **Burn of first degree of trunk**

Use additional external cause code to identify the source, place and intent of the burn (X00-X19, X75-X77, X96-X98, Y92)

√x7ᵗʰ **T21.10** **Burn of first degree of trunk, unspecified site**

√x7ᵗʰ **T21.11** **Burn of first degree of chest wall**

Burn of first degree of breast

√x7ᵗʰ **T21.12** **Burn of first degree of abdominal wall**

Burn of first degree of flank
Burn of first degree of groin

√x7ᵗʰ **T21.13** **Burn of first degree of upper back**

Burn of first degree of interscapular region

√x7ᵗʰ **T21.14** **Burn of first degree of lower back**

√x7ᵗʰ **T21.15** **Burn of first degree of buttock**

Burn of first degree of anus

✔ Additional Character Required   √x7ᵗʰ Placeholder   Questionable PDx   Manifestation   Unspecified Dx   UPD Unacceptable PDx   H1-H14 HAC   HCC CMS-HCC Dx   HIV HIV Dx

ICD-10-CM 2022   1095

Chapter 19. Injury, Poisoning and Certain Other Consequences of External Causes

√x7ᵗʰ **T21.16 Burn of first degree of male genital region** ♂
- Burn of first degree of penis
- Burn of first degree of scrotum
- Burn of first degree of testis

√x7ᵗʰ **T21.17 Burn of first degree of female genital region** ♀
- Burn of first degree of labium (majus) (minus)
- Burn of first degree of perineum
- Burn of first degree of vulva
- EXCLUDES 2   burn of vagina (T28.3)

√x7ᵗʰ **T21.19 Burn of first degree of other site of trunk**

√5ᵗʰ **T21.2 Burn of second degree of trunk**
- Use additional external cause code to identify the source, place and intent of the burn (X00-X19, X75-X77, X96-X98, Y92)

√x7ᵗʰ **T21.20 Burn of second degree of trunk, unspecified site**

√x7ᵗʰ **T21.21 Burn of second degree of chest wall**
- Burn of second degree of breast

√x7ᵗʰ **T21.22 Burn of second degree of abdominal wall**
- Burn of second degree of flank
- Burn of second degree of groin

√x7ᵗʰ **T21.23 Burn of second degree of upper back**
- Burn of second degree of interscapular region

√x7ᵗʰ **T21.24 Burn of second degree of lower back**

√x7ᵗʰ **T21.25 Burn of second degree of buttock**
- Burn of second degree of anus

√x7ᵗʰ **T21.26 Burn of second degree of male genital region** ♂
- Burn of second degree of penis
- Burn of second degree of scrotum
- Burn of second degree of testis

√x7ᵗʰ **T21.27 Burn of second degree of female genital region** ♀
- Burn of second degree of labium (majus) (minus)
- Burn of second degree of perineum
- Burn of second degree of vulva
- EXCLUDES 2   burn of vagina (T28.3)

√x7ᵗʰ **T21.29 Burn of second degree of other site of trunk**

√5ᵗʰ **T21.3 Burn of third degree of trunk**
- Use additional external cause code to identify the source, place and intent of the burn (X00-X19, X75-X77, X96-X98, Y92)

√x7ᵗʰ **T21.30 Burn of third degree of trunk, unspecified site** CC H5 SW

√x7ᵗʰ **T21.31 Burn of third degree of chest wall** CC H5 SW
- Burn of third degree of breast
- AHA: 2016,2Q,5

√x7ᵗʰ **T21.32 Burn of third degree of abdominal wall** CC H5 SW
- Burn of third degree of flank
- Burn of third degree of groin

√x7ᵗʰ **T21.33 Burn of third degree of upper back** CC H5 SW
- Burn of third degree of interscapular region

√x7ᵗʰ **T21.34 Burn of third degree of lower back** CC H5 SW

√x7ᵗʰ **T21.35 Burn of third degree of buttock** CC H5 SW
- Burn of third degree of anus

√x7ᵗʰ **T21.36 Burn of third degree of male genital region** CC H5 SW ♂
- Burn of third degree of penis
- Burn of third degree of scrotum
- Burn of third degree of testis

√x7ᵗʰ **T21.37 Burn of third degree of female genital region** CC H5 SW ♀
- Burn of third degree of labium (majus) (minus)
- Burn of third degree of perineum
- Burn of third degree of vulva
- EXCLUDES 2   burn of vagina (T28.3)

√x7ᵗʰ **T21.39 Burn of third degree of other site of trunk** CC H5 SW

√5ᵗʰ **T21.4 Corrosion of unspecified degree of trunk**
- Code first (T51-T65) to identify chemical and intent
- Use additional external cause code to identify place (Y92)

√x7ᵗʰ **T21.40 Corrosion of unspecified degree of trunk, unspecified site**

√x7ᵗʰ **T21.41 Corrosion of unspecified degree of chest wall**
- Corrosion of unspecified degree of breast

√x7ᵗʰ **T21.42 Corrosion of unspecified degree of abdominal wall**
- Corrosion of unspecified degree of flank
- Corrosion of unspecified degree of groin

√x7ᵗʰ **T21.43 Corrosion of unspecified degree of upper back**
- Corrosion of unspecified degree of interscapular region

√x7ᵗʰ **T21.44 Corrosion of unspecified degree of lower back**

√x7ᵗʰ **T21.45 Corrosion of unspecified degree of buttock**
- Corrosion of unspecified degree of anus

√x7ᵗʰ **T21.46 Corrosion of unspecified degree of male genital region** ♂
- Corrosion of unspecified degree of penis
- Corrosion of unspecified degree of scrotum
- Corrosion of unspecified degree of testis

√x7ᵗʰ **T21.47 Corrosion of unspecified degree of female genital region** ♀
- Corrosion of unspecified degree of labium (majus) (minus)
- Corrosion of unspecified degree of perineum
- Corrosion of unspecified degree of vulva
- EXCLUDES 2   corrosion of vagina (T28.8)

√x7ᵗʰ **T21.49 Corrosion of unspecified degree of other site of trunk**

√5ᵗʰ **T21.5 Corrosion of first degree of trunk**
- Code first (T51-T65) to identify chemical and intent
- Use additional external cause code to identify place (Y92)

√x7ᵗʰ **T21.50 Corrosion of first degree of trunk, unspecified site**

√x7ᵗʰ **T21.51 Corrosion of first degree of chest wall**
- Corrosion of first degree of breast

√x7ᵗʰ **T21.52 Corrosion of first degree of abdominal wall**
- Corrosion of first degree of flank
- Corrosion of first degree of groin

√x7ᵗʰ **T21.53 Corrosion of first degree of upper back**
- Corrosion of first degree of interscapular region

√x7ᵗʰ **T21.54 Corrosion of first degree of lower back**

√x7ᵗʰ **T21.55 Corrosion of first degree of buttock**
- Corrosion of first degree of anus

√x7ᵗʰ **T21.56 Corrosion of first degree of male genital region** ♂
- Corrosion of first degree of penis
- Corrosion of first degree of scrotum
- Corrosion of first degree of testis

√x7ᵗʰ **T21.57 Corrosion of first degree of female genital region** ♀
- Corrosion of first degree of labium (majus) (minus)
- Corrosion of first degree of perineum
- Corrosion of first degree of vulva
- EXCLUDES 2   corrosion of vagina (T28.8)

√x7ᵗʰ **T21.59 Corrosion of first degree of other site of trunk**

√5ᵗʰ **T21.6 Corrosion of second degree of trunk**
- Code first (T51-T65) to identify chemical and intent
- Use additional external cause code to identify place (Y92)

√x7ᵗʰ **T21.60 Corrosion of second degree of trunk, unspecified site**

√x7ᵗʰ **T21.61 Corrosion of second degree of chest wall**
- Corrosion of second degree of breast

√x7ᵗʰ **T21.62 Corrosion of second degree of abdominal wall**
- Corrosion of second degree of flank
- Corrosion of second degree of groin

√x7ᵗʰ **T21.63 Corrosion of second degree of upper back**
- Corrosion of second degree of interscapular region

√x7ᵗʰ **T21.64 Corrosion of second degree of lower back**

√x7ᵗʰ **T21.65 Corrosion of second degree of buttock**
- Corrosion of second degree of anus

√x7ᵗʰ **T21.66 Corrosion of second degree of male genital region** ♂
- Corrosion of second degree of penis
- Corrosion of second degree of scrotum
- Corrosion of second degree of testis

√x7ᵗʰ **T21.67 Corrosion of second degree of** female genital region   ♀

Corrosion of second degree of labium (majus) (minus)
Corrosion of second degree of perineum
Corrosion of second degree of vulva
EXCLUDES 2   corrosion of vagina (T28.8)

√x7ᵗʰ **T21.69 Corrosion of second degree of other site of trunk**

√5ᵗʰ **T21.7 Corrosion of** third degree **of trunk**

Code first (T51-T65) to identify chemical and intent
Use additional external cause code to identify place (Y92)

√x7ᵗʰ **T21.70 Corrosion of third degree of trunk, unspecified site**   CC H5 SW

√x7ᵗʰ **T21.71 Corrosion of third degree of** chest wall   CC H5 SW

Corrosion of third degree of breast

√x7ᵗʰ **T21.72 Corrosion of third degree of** abdominal wall   CC H5 SW

Corrosion of third degree of flank
Corrosion of third degree of groin

√x7ᵗʰ **T21.73 Corrosion of third degree of** upper back   CC H5 SW

Corrosion of third degree of interscapular region

√x7ᵗʰ **T21.74 Corrosion of third degree of** lower back   CC H5 SW

√x7ᵗʰ **T21.75 Corrosion of third degree of** buttock   CC H5 SW

Corrosion of third degree of anus

√x7ᵗʰ **T21.76 Corrosion of third degree of** male genital region   CC H5 SW ♂

Corrosion of third degree of penis
Corrosion of third degree of scrotum
Corrosion of third degree of testis

√x7ᵗʰ **T21.77 Corrosion of third degree of** female genital region   CC H5 SW ♀

Corrosion of third degree of labium (majus) (minus)
Corrosion of third degree of perineum
Corrosion of third degree of vulva
EXCLUDES 2   corrosion of vagina (T28.8)

√x7ᵗʰ **T21.79 Corrosion of third degree of other site of trunk**   CC H5 SW

√4ᵗʰ **T22 Burn and corrosion of shoulder and upper limb, except wrist and hand**

EXCLUDES 2   burn and corrosion of interscapular region (T21.-)
burn and corrosion of wrist and hand (T23.-)

The appropriate 7th character is to be added to each code from category T22.
A   initial encounter
D   subsequent encounter
S   sequela

√5ᵗʰ **T22.0 Burn of unspecified degree of shoulder and upper limb, except wrist and hand**

Use additional external cause code to identify the source, place and intent of the burn (X00-X19, X75-X77, X96-X98, Y92)

√x7ᵗʰ **T22.00 Burn of unspecified degree of shoulder and upper limb, except wrist and hand, unspecified site**

√6ᵗʰ **T22.01 Burn of unspecified degree of** forearm

√7ᵗʰ **T22.011 Burn of unspecified degree of** right forearm

√7ᵗʰ **T22.012 Burn of unspecified degree of** left forearm

√7ᵗʰ **T22.019 Burn of unspecified degree of unspecified forearm**

√6ᵗʰ **T22.02 Burn of unspecified degree of** elbow

√7ᵗʰ **T22.021 Burn of unspecified degree of** right elbow

√7ᵗʰ **T22.022 Burn of unspecified degree of** left elbow

√7ᵗʰ **T22.029 Burn of unspecified degree of unspecified elbow**

√6ᵗʰ **T22.03 Burn of unspecified degree of** upper arm

√7ᵗʰ **T22.031 Burn of unspecified degree of** right upper arm

√7ᵗʰ **T22.032 Burn of unspecified degree of** left upper arm

√7ᵗʰ **T22.039 Burn of unspecified degree of unspecified upper arm**

√6ᵗʰ **T22.04 Burn of unspecified degree of** axilla

√7ᵗʰ **T22.041 Burn of unspecified degree of** right axilla

√7ᵗʰ **T22.042 Burn of unspecified degree of** left axilla

√7ᵗʰ **T22.049 Burn of unspecified degree of unspecified axilla**

√6ᵗʰ **T22.05 Burn of unspecified degree of** shoulder

√7ᵗʰ **T22.051 Burn of unspecified degree of** right shoulder

√7ᵗʰ **T22.052 Burn of unspecified degree of** left shoulder

√7ᵗʰ **T22.059 Burn of unspecified degree of unspecified shoulder**

√6ᵗʰ **T22.06 Burn of unspecified degree of** scapular region

√7ᵗʰ **T22.061 Burn of unspecified degree of** right scapular region

√7ᵗʰ **T22.062 Burn of unspecified degree of** left scapular region

√7ᵗʰ **T22.069 Burn of unspecified degree of unspecified scapular region**

√6ᵗʰ **T22.09 Burn of unspecified degree of** multiple sites **of shoulder and upper limb, except wrist and hand**

√7ᵗʰ **T22.091 Burn of unspecified degree of multiple sites of** right shoulder and upper limb, except wrist and hand

√7ᵗʰ **T22.092 Burn of unspecified degree of multiple sites of** left shoulder and upper limb, except wrist and hand

√7ᵗʰ **T22.099 Burn of unspecified degree of multiple sites of unspecified shoulder and upper limb, except wrist and hand**

√5ᵗʰ **T22.1 Burn of** first degree **of shoulder and upper limb, except wrist and hand**

Use additional external cause code to identify the source, place and intent of the burn (X00-X19, X75-X77, X96-X98, Y92)

√x7ᵗʰ **T22.10 Burn of first degree of shoulder and upper limb, except wrist and hand, unspecified site**

√6ᵗʰ **T22.11 Burn of first degree of** forearm

√7ᵗʰ **T22.111 Burn of first degree of** right forearm

√7ᵗʰ **T22.112 Burn of first degree of** left forearm

√7ᵗʰ **T22.119 Burn of first degree of unspecified forearm**

√6ᵗʰ **T22.12 Burn of first degree of** elbow

√7ᵗʰ **T22.121 Burn of first degree of** right elbow

√7ᵗʰ **T22.122 Burn of first degree of** left elbow

√7ᵗʰ **T22.129 Burn of first degree of unspecified elbow**

√6ᵗʰ **T22.13 Burn of first degree of** upper arm

√7ᵗʰ **T22.131 Burn of first degree of** right upper arm

√7ᵗʰ **T22.132 Burn of first degree of** left upper arm

√7ᵗʰ **T22.139 Burn of first degree of unspecified upper arm**

√6ᵗʰ **T22.14 Burn of first degree of** axilla

√7ᵗʰ **T22.141 Burn of first degree of** right axilla

√7ᵗʰ **T22.142 Burn of first degree of** left axilla

√7ᵗʰ **T22.149 Burn of first degree of unspecified axilla**

√6ᵗʰ **T22.15 Burn of first degree of** shoulder

√7ᵗʰ **T22.151 Burn of first degree of** right shoulder

√7ᵗʰ **T22.152 Burn of first degree of** left shoulder

√7ᵗʰ **T22.159 Burn of first degree of unspecified shoulder**

√6ᵗʰ **T22.16 Burn of first degree of** scapular region

√7ᵗʰ **T22.161 Burn of first degree of** right scapular region

√7ᵗʰ **T22.162 Burn of first degree of** left scapular region

√7ᵗʰ **T22.169 Burn of first degree of unspecified scapular region**

√6ᵗʰ **T22.19 Burn of first degree of** multiple sites **of shoulder and upper limb, except wrist and hand**

√7ᵗʰ **T22.191 Burn of first degree of multiple sites of** right shoulder and upper limb, except wrist and hand

√7ᵗʰ **T22.192 Burn of first degree of multiple sites of** left shoulder and upper limb, except wrist and hand

√7ᵗʰ **T22.199 Burn of first degree of multiple sites of unspecified shoulder and upper limb, except wrist and hand**

√5ᵗʰ **T22.2 Burn of** second degree **of shoulder and upper limb, except wrist and hand**

Use additional external cause code to identify the source, place and intent of the burn (X00-X19, X75-X77, X96-X98, Y92)

√x7ᵗʰ **T22.20 Burn of second degree of shoulder and upper limb, except wrist and hand, unspecified site**

☑ Additional Character Required   √x7ᵗʰ Placeholder   Questionable PDx   Manifestation   Unspecified Dx   UPD Unacceptable PDx   H1-H14 HAC   HCC CMS-HCC Dx   HIV HIV Dx

ICD-10-CM 2022   1097

√6ᵗʰ **T22.21** Burn of second degree of forearm
- √7ᵗʰ **T22.211** Burn of second degree of right forearm
- √7ᵗʰ **T22.212** Burn of second degree of left forearm
- √7ᵗʰ **T22.219** Burn of second degree of unspecified forearm

√6ᵗʰ **T22.22** Burn of second degree of elbow
- √7ᵗʰ **T22.221** Burn of second degree of right elbow
- √7ᵗʰ **T22.222** Burn of second degree of left elbow
- √7ᵗʰ **T22.229** Burn of second degree of unspecified elbow

√6ᵗʰ **T22.23** Burn of second degree of upper arm
- √7ᵗʰ **T22.231** Burn of second degree of right upper arm
- √7ᵗʰ **T22.232** Burn of second degree of left upper arm
- √7ᵗʰ **T22.239** Burn of second degree of unspecified upper arm

√6ᵗʰ **T22.24** Burn of second degree of axilla
- √7ᵗʰ **T22.241** Burn of second degree of right axilla
- √7ᵗʰ **T22.242** Burn of second degree of left axilla
- √7ᵗʰ **T22.249** Burn of second degree of unspecified axilla

√6ᵗʰ **T22.25** Burn of second degree of shoulder
- √7ᵗʰ **T22.251** Burn of second degree of right shoulder
- √7ᵗʰ **T22.252** Burn of second degree of left shoulder
- √7ᵗʰ **T22.259** Burn of second degree of unspecified shoulder

√6ᵗʰ **T22.26** Burn of second degree of scapular region
- √7ᵗʰ **T22.261** Burn of second degree of right scapular region
- √7ᵗʰ **T22.262** Burn of second degree of left scapular region
- √7ᵗʰ **T22.269** Burn of second degree of unspecified scapular region

√6ᵗʰ **T22.29** Burn of second degree of multiple sites of shoulder and upper limb, except wrist and hand
- √7ᵗʰ **T22.291** Burn of second degree of multiple sites of right shoulder and upper limb, except wrist and hand
- √7ᵗʰ **T22.292** Burn of second degree of multiple sites of left shoulder and upper limb, except wrist and hand
- √7ᵗʰ **T22.299** Burn of second degree of multiple sites of unspecified shoulder and upper limb, except wrist and hand

√5ᵗʰ **T22.3** Burn of third degree of shoulder and upper limb, except wrist and hand

Use additional external cause code to identify the source, place and intent of the burn (X00-X19, X75-X77, X96-X98, Y92)

√x7ᵗʰ **T22.30** Burn of third degree of shoulder and upper limb, except wrist and hand, unspecified site CC H5 SW

√6ᵗʰ **T22.31** Burn of third degree of forearm
- √7ᵗʰ **T22.311** Burn of third degree of right forearm CC H5 SW
- √7ᵗʰ **T22.312** Burn of third degree of left forearm CC H5 SW
- √7ᵗʰ **T22.319** Burn of third degree of unspecified forearm CC H5 SW

√6ᵗʰ **T22.32** Burn of third degree of elbow
- √7ᵗʰ **T22.321** Burn of third degree of right elbow CC H5 SW
- √7ᵗʰ **T22.322** Burn of third degree of left elbow CC H5 SW
- √7ᵗʰ **T22.329** Burn of third degree of unspecified elbow CC H5 SW

√6ᵗʰ **T22.33** Burn of third degree of upper arm
- √7ᵗʰ **T22.331** Burn of third degree of right upper arm CC H5 SW
- √7ᵗʰ **T22.332** Burn of third degree of left upper arm CC H5 SW
- √7ᵗʰ **T22.339** Burn of third degree of unspecified upper arm CC H5 SW

√6ᵗʰ **T22.34** Burn of third degree of axilla
- √7ᵗʰ **T22.341** Burn of third degree of right axilla CC H5 SW
- √7ᵗʰ **T22.342** Burn of third degree of left axilla CC H5 SW
- √7ᵗʰ **T22.349** Burn of third degree of unspecified axilla CC H5 SW

√6ᵗʰ **T22.35** Burn of third degree of shoulder
- √7ᵗʰ **T22.351** Burn of third degree of right shoulder CC H5 SW
- √7ᵗʰ **T22.352** Burn of third degree of left shoulder CC H5 SW
- √7ᵗʰ **T22.359** Burn of third degree of unspecified shoulder CC H5 SW

√6ᵗʰ **T22.36** Burn of third degree of scapular region
- √7ᵗʰ **T22.361** Burn of third degree of right scapular region CC H5 SW
- √7ᵗʰ **T22.362** Burn of third degree of left scapular region CC H5 SW
- √7ᵗʰ **T22.369** Burn of third degree of unspecified scapular region CC H5 SW

√6ᵗʰ **T22.39** Burn of third degree of multiple sites of shoulder and upper limb, except wrist and hand
- √7ᵗʰ **T22.391** Burn of third degree of multiple sites of right shoulder and upper limb, except wrist and hand CC H5 SW
- √7ᵗʰ **T22.392** Burn of third degree of multiple sites of left shoulder and upper limb, except wrist and hand CC H5 SW
- √7ᵗʰ **T22.399** Burn of third degree of multiple sites of unspecified shoulder and upper limb, except wrist and hand CC H5 SW

√5ᵗʰ **T22.4** Corrosion of unspecified degree of shoulder and upper limb, except wrist and hand

Code first (T51-T65) to identify chemical and intent
Use additional external cause code to identify place (Y92)

√x7ᵗʰ **T22.40** Corrosion of unspecified degree of shoulder and upper limb, except wrist and hand, unspecified site

√6ᵗʰ **T22.41** Corrosion of unspecified degree of forearm
- √7ᵗʰ **T22.411** Corrosion of unspecified degree of right forearm
- √7ᵗʰ **T22.412** Corrosion of unspecified degree of left forearm
- √7ᵗʰ **T22.419** Corrosion of unspecified degree of unspecified forearm

√6ᵗʰ **T22.42** Corrosion of unspecified degree of elbow
- √7ᵗʰ **T22.421** Corrosion of unspecified degree of right elbow
- √7ᵗʰ **T22.422** Corrosion of unspecified degree of left elbow
- √7ᵗʰ **T22.429** Corrosion of unspecified degree of unspecified elbow

√6ᵗʰ **T22.43** Corrosion of unspecified degree of upper arm
- √7ᵗʰ **T22.431** Corrosion of unspecified degree of right upper arm
- √7ᵗʰ **T22.432** Corrosion of unspecified degree of left upper arm
- √7ᵗʰ **T22.439** Corrosion of unspecified degree of unspecified upper arm

√6ᵗʰ **T22.44** Corrosion of unspecified degree of axilla
- √7ᵗʰ **T22.441** Corrosion of unspecified degree of right axilla
- √7ᵗʰ **T22.442** Corrosion of unspecified degree of left axilla
- √7ᵗʰ **T22.449** Corrosion of unspecified degree of unspecified axilla

√6ᵗʰ **T22.45** Corrosion of unspecified degree of shoulder
- √7ᵗʰ **T22.451** Corrosion of unspecified degree of right shoulder
- √7ᵗʰ **T22.452** Corrosion of unspecified degree of left shoulder
- √7ᵗʰ **T22.459** Corrosion of unspecified degree of unspecified shoulder

√6ᵗʰ **T22.46** Corrosion of unspecified degree of scapular region
- √7ᵗʰ **T22.461** Corrosion of unspecified degree of right scapular region
- √7ᵗʰ **T22.462** Corrosion of unspecified degree of left scapular region
- √7ᵗʰ **T22.469** Corrosion of unspecified degree of unspecified scapular region

√6ᵗʰ **T22.49** Corrosion of unspecified degree of multiple sites of shoulder and upper limb, except wrist and hand
- √7ᵗʰ **T22.491** Corrosion of unspecified degree of multiple sites of right shoulder and upper limb, except wrist and hand

✓7ᵗʰ **T22.492** Corrosion of unspecified degree of multiple sites of left shoulder and upper limb, except wrist and hand

✓7ᵗʰ **T22.499** Corrosion of unspecified degree of multiple sites of unspecified shoulder and upper limb, except wrist and hand

✓5ᵗʰ **T22.5** Corrosion of first degree of shoulder and upper limb, except wrist and hand
    Code first (T51-T65) to identify chemical and intent
    Use additional external cause code to identify place (Y92)

✓x7ᵗʰ **T22.50** Corrosion of first degree of shoulder and upper limb, except wrist and hand unspecified site

✓6ᵗʰ **T22.51** Corrosion of first degree of forearm

    ✓7ᵗʰ **T22.511** Corrosion of first degree of right forearm

    ✓7ᵗʰ **T22.512** Corrosion of first degree of left forearm

    ✓7ᵗʰ **T22.519** Corrosion of first degree of unspecified forearm

✓6ᵗʰ **T22.52** Corrosion of first degree of elbow

    ✓7ᵗʰ **T22.521** Corrosion of first degree of right elbow

    ✓7ᵗʰ **T22.522** Corrosion of first degree of left elbow

    ✓7ᵗʰ **T22.529** Corrosion of first degree of unspecified elbow

✓6ᵗʰ **T22.53** Corrosion of first degree of upper arm

    ✓7ᵗʰ **T22.531** Corrosion of first degree of right upper arm

    ✓7ᵗʰ **T22.532** Corrosion of first degree of left upper arm

    ✓7ᵗʰ **T22.539** Corrosion of first degree of unspecified upper arm

✓6ᵗʰ **T22.54** Corrosion of first degree of axilla

    ✓7ᵗʰ **T22.541** Corrosion of first degree of right axilla

    ✓7ᵗʰ **T22.542** Corrosion of first degree of left axilla

    ✓7ᵗʰ **T22.549** Corrosion of first degree of unspecified axilla

✓6ᵗʰ **T22.55** Corrosion of first degree of shoulder

    ✓7ᵗʰ **T22.551** Corrosion of first degree of right shoulder

    ✓7ᵗʰ **T22.552** Corrosion of first degree of left shoulder

    ✓7ᵗʰ **T22.559** Corrosion of first degree of unspecified shoulder

✓6ᵗʰ **T22.56** Corrosion of first degree of scapular region

    ✓7ᵗʰ **T22.561** Corrosion of first degree of right scapular region

    ✓7ᵗʰ **T22.562** Corrosion of first degree of left scapular region

    ✓7ᵗʰ **T22.569** Corrosion of first degree of unspecified scapular region

✓6ᵗʰ **T22.59** Corrosion of first degree of multiple sites of shoulder and upper limb, except wrist and hand

    ✓7ᵗʰ **T22.591** Corrosion of first degree of multiple sites of right shoulder and upper limb, except wrist and hand

    ✓7ᵗʰ **T22.592** Corrosion of first degree of multiple sites of left shoulder and upper limb, except wrist and hand

    ✓7ᵗʰ **T22.599** Corrosion of first degree of multiple sites of unspecified shoulder and upper limb, except wrist and hand

✓5ᵗʰ **T22.6** Corrosion of second degree of shoulder and upper limb, except wrist and hand
    Code first (T51-T65) to identify chemical and intent
    Use additional external cause code to identify place (Y92)

✓x7ᵗʰ **T22.60** Corrosion of second degree of shoulder and upper limb, except wrist and hand, unspecified site

✓6ᵗʰ **T22.61** Corrosion of second degree of forearm

    ✓7ᵗʰ **T22.611** Corrosion of second degree of right forearm

    ✓7ᵗʰ **T22.612** Corrosion of second degree of left forearm

    ✓7ᵗʰ **T22.619** Corrosion of second degree of unspecified forearm

✓6ᵗʰ **T22.62** Corrosion of second degree of elbow

    ✓7ᵗʰ **T22.621** Corrosion of second degree of right elbow

    ✓7ᵗʰ **T22.622** Corrosion of second degree of left elbow

    ✓7ᵗʰ **T22.629** Corrosion of second degree of unspecified elbow

✓6ᵗʰ **T22.63** Corrosion of second degree of upper arm

    ✓7ᵗʰ **T22.631** Corrosion of second degree of right upper arm

✓7ᵗʰ **T22.632** Corrosion of second degree of left upper arm

✓7ᵗʰ **T22.639** Corrosion of second degree of unspecified upper arm

✓6ᵗʰ **T22.64** Corrosion of second degree of axilla

    ✓7ᵗʰ **T22.641** Corrosion of second degree of right axilla

    ✓7ᵗʰ **T22.642** Corrosion of second degree of left axilla

    ✓7ᵗʰ **T22.649** Corrosion of second degree of unspecified axilla

✓6ᵗʰ **T22.65** Corrosion of second degree of shoulder

    ✓7ᵗʰ **T22.651** Corrosion of second degree of right shoulder

    ✓7ᵗʰ **T22.652** Corrosion of second degree of left shoulder

    ✓7ᵗʰ **T22.659** Corrosion of second degree of unspecified shoulder

✓6ᵗʰ **T22.66** Corrosion of second degree of scapular region

    ✓7ᵗʰ **T22.661** Corrosion of second degree of right scapular region

    ✓7ᵗʰ **T22.662** Corrosion of second degree of left scapular region

    ✓7ᵗʰ **T22.669** Corrosion of second degree of unspecified scapular region

✓6ᵗʰ **T22.69** Corrosion of second degree of multiple sites of shoulder and upper limb, except wrist and hand

    ✓7ᵗʰ **T22.691** Corrosion of second degree of multiple sites of right shoulder and upper limb, except wrist and hand

    ✓7ᵗʰ **T22.692** Corrosion of second degree of multiple sites of left shoulder and upper limb, except wrist and hand

    ✓7ᵗʰ **T22.699** Corrosion of second degree of multiple sites of unspecified shoulder and upper limb, except wrist and hand

✓5ᵗʰ **T22.7** Corrosion of third degree of shoulder and upper limb, except wrist and hand
    Code first (T51-T65) to identify chemical and intent
    Use additional external cause code to identify place (Y92)

✓x7ᵗʰ **T22.70** Corrosion of third degree of shoulder and upper limb, except wrist and hand, unspecified site   CC H5 SW

✓6ᵗʰ **T22.71** Corrosion of third degree of forearm

    ✓7ᵗʰ **T22.711** Corrosion of third degree of right forearm   CC H5 SW

    ✓7ᵗʰ **T22.712** Corrosion of third degree of left forearm   CC H5 SW

    ✓7ᵗʰ **T22.719** Corrosion of third degree of unspecified forearm   CC H5 SW

✓6ᵗʰ **T22.72** Corrosion of third degree of elbow

    ✓7ᵗʰ **T22.721** Corrosion of third degree of right elbow   CC H5 SW

    ✓7ᵗʰ **T22.722** Corrosion of third degree of left elbow   CC H5 SW

    ✓7ᵗʰ **T22.729** Corrosion of third degree of unspecified elbow   CC H5 SW

✓6ᵗʰ **T22.73** Corrosion of third degree of upper arm

    ✓7ᵗʰ **T22.731** Corrosion of third degree of right upper arm   CC H5 SW

    ✓7ᵗʰ **T22.732** Corrosion of third degree of left upper arm   CC H5 SW

    ✓7ᵗʰ **T22.739** Corrosion of third degree of unspecified upper arm   CC H5 SW

✓6ᵗʰ **T22.74** Corrosion of third degree of axilla

    ✓7ᵗʰ **T22.741** Corrosion of third degree of right axilla   CC H5 SW

    ✓7ᵗʰ **T22.742** Corrosion of third degree of left axilla   CC H5 SW

    ✓7ᵗʰ **T22.749** Corrosion of third degree of unspecified axilla   CC H5 SW

✓6ᵗʰ **T22.75** Corrosion of third degree of shoulder

    ✓7ᵗʰ **T22.751** Corrosion of third degree of right shoulder   CC H5 SW

    ✓7ᵗʰ **T22.752** Corrosion of third degree of left shoulder   CC H5 SW

    ✓7ᵗʰ **T22.759** Corrosion of third degree of unspecified shoulder   CC H5 SW

✓6ᵗʰ **T22.76** Corrosion of third degree of scapular region

    ✓7ᵗʰ **T22.761** Corrosion of third degree of right scapular region   CC H5 SW

√7th **T22.762** Corrosion of third degree of left scapular region `CC` `H5` `SW`

√7th **T22.769** Corrosion of third degree of unspecified scapular region `CC` `H5` `SW`

√6th **T22.79** Corrosion of third degree of multiple sites of shoulder and upper limb, except wrist and hand

√7th **T22.791** Corrosion of third degree of multiple sites of right shoulder and upper limb, except wrist and hand `CC` `H5` `SW`

√7th **T22.792** Corrosion of third degree of multiple sites of left shoulder and upper limb, except wrist and hand `CC` `H5` `SW`

√7th **T22.799** Corrosion of third degree of multiple sites of unspecified shoulder and upper limb, except wrist and hand `CC` `H5` `SW`

√4th **T23** **Burn and corrosion of wrist and hand**

AHA: 2015,1Q,19

The appropriate 7th character is to be added to each code from category T23.
A   initial encounter
D   subsequent encounter
S   sequela

√5th **T23.0** **Burn of unspecified degree of wrist and hand**

Use additional external cause code to identify the source, place and intent of the burn (X00-X19, X75-X77, X96-X98, Y92)

√6th **T23.00** Burn of unspecified degree of hand, unspecified site

√7th **T23.001** Burn of unspecified degree of right hand, unspecified site

√7th **T23.002** Burn of unspecified degree of left hand, unspecified site

√7th **T23.009** Burn of unspecified degree of unspecified hand, unspecified site

√6th **T23.01** Burn of unspecified degree of thumb (nail)

√7th **T23.011** Burn of unspecified degree of right thumb (nail)

√7th **T23.012** Burn of unspecified degree of left thumb (nail)

√7th **T23.019** Burn of unspecified degree of unspecified thumb (nail)

√6th **T23.02** Burn of unspecified degree of single finger (nail) except thumb

√7th **T23.021** Burn of unspecified degree of single right finger (nail) except thumb

√7th **T23.022** Burn of unspecified degree of single left finger (nail) except thumb

√7th **T23.029** Burn of unspecified degree of unspecified single finger (nail) except thumb

√6th **T23.03** Burn of unspecified degree of multiple fingers (nail), not including thumb

√7th **T23.031** Burn of unspecified degree of multiple right fingers (nail), not including thumb

√7th **T23.032** Burn of unspecified degree of multiple left fingers (nail), not including thumb

√7th **T23.039** Burn of unspecified degree of unspecified multiple fingers (nail), not including thumb

√6th **T23.04** Burn of unspecified degree of multiple fingers (nail), including thumb

√7th **T23.041** Burn of unspecified degree of multiple right fingers (nail), including thumb

√7th **T23.042** Burn of unspecified degree of multiple left fingers (nail), including thumb

√7th **T23.049** Burn of unspecified degree of unspecified multiple fingers (nail), including thumb

√6th **T23.05** Burn of unspecified degree of palm

√7th **T23.051** Burn of unspecified degree of right palm

√7th **T23.052** Burn of unspecified degree of left palm

√7th **T23.059** Burn of unspecified degree of unspecified palm

√6th **T23.06** Burn of unspecified degree of back of hand

√7th **T23.061** Burn of unspecified degree of back of right hand

√7th **T23.062** Burn of unspecified degree of back of left hand

√7th **T23.069** Burn of unspecified degree of back of unspecified hand

√6th **T23.07** Burn of unspecified degree of wrist

√7th **T23.071** Burn of unspecified degree of right wrist

√7th **T23.072** Burn of unspecified degree of left wrist

√7th **T23.079** Burn of unspecified degree of unspecified wrist

√6th **T23.09** Burn of unspecified degree of multiple sites of wrist and hand

√7th **T23.091** Burn of unspecified degree of multiple sites of right wrist and hand

√7th **T23.092** Burn of unspecified degree of multiple sites of left wrist and hand

√7th **T23.099** Burn of unspecified degree of multiple sites of unspecified wrist and hand

√5th **T23.1** **Burn of first degree of wrist and hand**

Use additional external cause code to identify the source, place and intent of the burn (X00-X19, X75-X77, X96-X98, Y92)

√6th **T23.10** Burn of first degree of hand, unspecified site

√7th **T23.101** Burn of first degree of right hand, unspecified site

√7th **T23.102** Burn of first degree of left hand, unspecified site

√7th **T23.109** Burn of first degree of unspecified hand, unspecified site

√6th **T23.11** Burn of first degree of thumb (nail)

√7th **T23.111** Burn of first degree of right thumb (nail)

√7th **T23.112** Burn of first degree of left thumb (nail)

√7th **T23.119** Burn of first degree of unspecified thumb (nail)

√6th **T23.12** Burn of first degree of single finger (nail) except thumb

√7th **T23.121** Burn of first degree of single right finger (nail) except thumb

√7th **T23.122** Burn of first degree of single left finger (nail) except thumb

√7th **T23.129** Burn of first degree of unspecified single finger (nail) except thumb

√6th **T23.13** Burn of first degree of multiple fingers (nail), not including thumb

√7th **T23.131** Burn of first degree of multiple right fingers (nail), not including thumb

√7th **T23.132** Burn of first degree of multiple left fingers (nail), not including thumb

√7th **T23.139** Burn of first degree of unspecified multiple fingers (nail), not including thumb

√6th **T23.14** Burn of first degree of multiple fingers (nail), including thumb

√7th **T23.141** Burn of first degree of multiple right fingers (nail), including thumb

√7th **T23.142** Burn of first degree of multiple left fingers (nail), including thumb

√7th **T23.149** Burn of first degree of unspecified multiple fingers (nail), including thumb

√6th **T23.15** Burn of first degree of palm

√7th **T23.151** Burn of first degree of right palm

√7th **T23.152** Burn of first degree of left palm

√7th **T23.159** Burn of first degree of unspecified palm

√6th **T23.16** Burn of first degree of back of hand

√7th **T23.161** Burn of first degree of back of right hand

√7th **T23.162** Burn of first degree of back of left hand

√7th **T23.169** Burn of first degree of back of unspecified hand

√6th **T23.17** Burn of first degree of wrist

√7th **T23.171** Burn of first degree of right wrist

√7th **T23.172** Burn of first degree of left wrist

√7th **T23.179** Burn of first degree of unspecified wrist

√6th **T23.19** Burn of first degree of multiple sites of wrist and hand

√7th **T23.191** Burn of first degree of multiple sites of right wrist and hand

√7th **T23.192** Burn of first degree of multiple sites of left wrist and hand

√7th **T23.199** Burn of first degree of multiple sites of unspecified wrist and hand

√5th **T23.2** **Burn of second degree of wrist and hand**

Use additional external cause code to identify the source, place and intent of the burn (X00-X19, X75-X77, X96-X98, Y92)

√6th **T23.20** Burn of second degree of hand, unspecified site

√7th **T23.201** Burn of second degree of right hand, unspecified site

√7ᵗʰ **T23.202** Burn of second degree of left hand, unspecified site

√7ᵗʰ **T23.209** Burn of second degree of unspecified hand, unspecified site

√6ᵗʰ **T23.21** Burn of second degree of thumb (nail)

    √7ᵗʰ **T23.211** Burn of second degree of right thumb (nail)

    √7ᵗʰ **T23.212** Burn of second degree of left thumb (nail)

    √7ᵗʰ **T23.219** Burn of second degree of unspecified thumb (nail)

√6ᵗʰ **T23.22** Burn of second degree of single finger (nail) except thumb

    √7ᵗʰ **T23.221** Burn of second degree of single right finger (nail) except thumb

    √7ᵗʰ **T23.222** Burn of second degree of single left finger (nail) except thumb

    √7ᵗʰ **T23.229** Burn of second degree of unspecified single finger (nail) except thumb

√6ᵗʰ **T23.23** Burn of second degree of multiple fingers (nail), not including thumb

    √7ᵗʰ **T23.231** Burn of second degree of multiple right fingers (nail), not including thumb

    √7ᵗʰ **T23.232** Burn of second degree of multiple left fingers (nail), not including thumb

    √7ᵗʰ **T23.239** Burn of second degree of unspecified multiple fingers (nail), not including thumb

√6ᵗʰ **T23.24** Burn of second degree of multiple fingers (nail), including thumb

    √7ᵗʰ **T23.241** Burn of second degree of multiple right fingers (nail), including thumb

    √7ᵗʰ **T23.242** Burn of second degree of multiple left fingers (nail), including thumb

    √7ᵗʰ **T23.249** Burn of second degree of unspecified multiple fingers (nail), including thumb

√6ᵗʰ **T23.25** Burn of second degree of palm

    √7ᵗʰ **T23.251** Burn of second degree of right palm

    √7ᵗʰ **T23.252** Burn of second degree of left palm

    √7ᵗʰ **T23.259** Burn of second degree of unspecified palm

√6ᵗʰ **T23.26** Burn of second degree of back of hand

    √7ᵗʰ **T23.261** Burn of second degree of back of right hand

    √7ᵗʰ **T23.262** Burn of second degree of back of left hand

    √7ᵗʰ **T23.269** Burn of second degree of back of unspecified hand

√6ᵗʰ **T23.27** Burn of second degree of wrist

    √7ᵗʰ **T23.271** Burn of second degree of right wrist

    √7ᵗʰ **T23.272** Burn of second degree of left wrist

    √7ᵗʰ **T23.279** Burn of second degree of unspecified wrist

√6ᵗʰ **T23.29** Burn of second degree of multiple sites of wrist and hand

    √7ᵗʰ **T23.291** Burn of second degree of multiple sites of right wrist and hand

    √7ᵗʰ **T23.292** Burn of second degree of multiple sites of left wrist and hand

    √7ᵗʰ **T23.299** Burn of second degree of multiple sites of unspecified wrist and hand

√5ᵗʰ **T23.3** Burn of third degree of wrist and hand

Use additional external cause code to identify the source, place and intent of the burn (X00-X19, X75-X77, X96-X98, Y92)

√6ᵗʰ **T23.30** Burn of third degree of hand, unspecified site

    AHA: 2016,2Q,5

    √7ᵗʰ **T23.301** Burn of third degree of right hand, unspecified site   CC H5 SW

    √7ᵗʰ **T23.302** Burn of third degree of left hand, unspecified site   CC H5 SW

    √7ᵗʰ **T23.309** Burn of third degree of unspecified hand, unspecified site   CC H5 SW

√6ᵗʰ **T23.31** Burn of third degree of thumb (nail)

    √7ᵗʰ **T23.311** Burn of third degree of right thumb (nail)   CC H5 SW

    √7ᵗʰ **T23.312** Burn of third degree of left thumb (nail)   CC H5 SW

    √7ᵗʰ **T23.319** Burn of third degree of unspecified thumb (nail)   CC H5 SW

√6ᵗʰ **T23.32** Burn of third degree of single finger (nail) except thumb

    √7ᵗʰ **T23.321** Burn of third degree of single right finger (nail) except thumb   CC H5 SW

    √7ᵗʰ **T23.322** Burn of third degree of single left finger (nail) except thumb   CC H5 SW

    √7ᵗʰ **T23.329** Burn of third degree of unspecified single finger (nail) except thumb   CC H5 SW

√6ᵗʰ **T23.33** Burn of third degree of multiple fingers (nail), not including thumb

    √7ᵗʰ **T23.331** Burn of third degree of multiple right fingers (nail), not including thumb   CC H5 SW

    √7ᵗʰ **T23.332** Burn of third degree of multiple left fingers (nail), not including thumb   CC H5 SW

    √7ᵗʰ **T23.339** Burn of third degree of unspecified multiple fingers (nail), not including thumb   CC H5 SW

√6ᵗʰ **T23.34** Burn of third degree of multiple fingers (nail), including thumb

    √7ᵗʰ **T23.341** Burn of third degree of multiple right fingers (nail), including thumb   CC H5 SW

    √7ᵗʰ **T23.342** Burn of third degree of multiple left fingers (nail), including thumb   CC H5 SW

    √7ᵗʰ **T23.349** Burn of third degree of unspecified multiple fingers (nail), including thumb   CC H5 SW

√6ᵗʰ **T23.35** Burn of third degree of palm

    √7ᵗʰ **T23.351** Burn of third degree of right palm   CC H5 SW

    √7ᵗʰ **T23.352** Burn of third degree of left palm   CC H5 SW

    √7ᵗʰ **T23.359** Burn of third degree of unspecified palm   CC H5 SW

√6ᵗʰ **T23.36** Burn of third degree of back of hand

    √7ᵗʰ **T23.361** Burn of third degree of back of right hand   CC H5 SW

    √7ᵗʰ **T23.362** Burn of third degree of back of left hand   CC H5 SW

    √7ᵗʰ **T23.369** Burn of third degree of back of unspecified hand   CC H5 SW

√6ᵗʰ **T23.37** Burn of third degree of wrist

    √7ᵗʰ **T23.371** Burn of third degree of right wrist   CC H5 SW

    √7ᵗʰ **T23.372** Burn of third degree of left wrist   CC H5 SW

    √7ᵗʰ **T23.379** Burn of third degree of unspecified wrist   CC H5 SW

√6ᵗʰ **T23.39** Burn of third degree of multiple sites of wrist and hand

    √7ᵗʰ **T23.391** Burn of third degree of multiple sites of right wrist and hand   CC H5 SW

    √7ᵗʰ **T23.392** Burn of third degree of multiple sites of left wrist and hand   CC H5 SW

    √7ᵗʰ **T23.399** Burn of third degree of multiple sites of unspecified wrist and hand   CC H5 SW

√5ᵗʰ **T23.4** Corrosion of unspecified degree of wrist and hand

Code first (T51-T65) to identify chemical and intent
Use additional external cause code to identify place (Y92)

√6ᵗʰ **T23.40** Corrosion of unspecified degree of hand, unspecified site

    √7ᵗʰ **T23.401** Corrosion of unspecified degree of right hand, unspecified site

    √7ᵗʰ **T23.402** Corrosion of unspecified degree of left hand, unspecified site

    √7ᵗʰ **T23.409** Corrosion of unspecified degree of unspecified hand, unspecified site

√6ᵗʰ **T23.41** Corrosion of unspecified degree of thumb (nail)

    √7ᵗʰ **T23.411** Corrosion of unspecified degree of right thumb (nail)

    √7ᵗʰ **T23.412** Corrosion of unspecified degree of left thumb (nail)

    √7ᵗʰ **T23.419** Corrosion of unspecified degree of unspecified thumb (nail)

☑ Additional Character Required   √x7ᵗʰ Placeholder   Questionable PDx   Manifestation   Unspecified Dx   UPD Unacceptable PDx   H1-H14 HAC   HCC CMS-HCC Dx   HIV HIV Dx

ICD-10-CM 2022

1101

T23.202–T23.419

√6ᵗʰ **T23.42** **Corrosion of unspecified degree of** single finger (nail) except thumb
- √7ᵗʰ **T23.421** **Corrosion of unspecified degree of single** right **finger (nail) except thumb**
- √7ᵗʰ **T23.422** **Corrosion of unspecified degree of single** left **finger (nail) except thumb**
- √7ᵗʰ **T23.429** **Corrosion of unspecified degree of unspecified single finger (nail) except thumb**

√6ᵗʰ **T23.43** **Corrosion of unspecified degree of** multiple fingers (nail), not including thumb
- √7ᵗʰ **T23.431** **Corrosion of unspecified degree of multiple** right **fingers (nail), not including thumb**
- √7ᵗʰ **T23.432** **Corrosion of unspecified degree of multiple** left **fingers (nail), not including thumb**
- √7ᵗʰ **T23.439** **Corrosion of unspecified degree of unspecified multiple fingers (nail), not including thumb**

√6ᵗʰ **T23.44** **Corrosion of unspecified degree of** multiple fingers (nail), including thumb
- √7ᵗʰ **T23.441** **Corrosion of unspecified degree of multiple** right **fingers (nail), including thumb**
- √7ᵗʰ **T23.442** **Corrosion of unspecified degree of multiple** left **fingers (nail), including thumb**
- √7ᵗʰ **T23.449** **Corrosion of unspecified degree of unspecified multiple fingers (nail), including thumb**

√6ᵗʰ **T23.45** **Corrosion of unspecified degree of** palm
- √7ᵗʰ **T23.451** **Corrosion of unspecified degree of** right **palm**
- √7ᵗʰ **T23.452** **Corrosion of unspecified degree of** left **palm**
- √7ᵗʰ **T23.459** **Corrosion of unspecified degree of unspecified palm**

√6ᵗʰ **T23.46** **Corrosion of unspecified degree of** back of hand
- √7ᵗʰ **T23.461** **Corrosion of unspecified degree of back of** right **hand**
- √7ᵗʰ **T23.462** **Corrosion of unspecified degree of back of** left **hand**
- √7ᵗʰ **T23.469** **Corrosion of unspecified degree of back of unspecified hand**

√6ᵗʰ **T23.47** **Corrosion of unspecified degree of** wrist
- √7ᵗʰ **T23.471** **Corrosion of unspecified degree of** right **wrist**
- √7ᵗʰ **T23.472** **Corrosion of unspecified degree of** left **wrist**
- √7ᵗʰ **T23.479** **Corrosion of unspecified degree of unspecified wrist**

√6ᵗʰ **T23.49** **Corrosion of unspecified degree of** multiple sites of wrist and hand
- √7ᵗʰ **T23.491** **Corrosion of unspecified degree of multiple sites of** right **wrist and hand**
- √7ᵗʰ **T23.492** **Corrosion of unspecified degree of multiple sites of** left **wrist and hand**
- √7ᵗʰ **T23.499** **Corrosion of unspecified degree of multiple sites of unspecified wrist and hand**

√5ᵗʰ **T23.5** **Corrosion of** first degree **of wrist and hand**
Code first (T51-T65) to identify chemical and intent
Use additional external cause code to identify place (Y92)

√6ᵗʰ **T23.50** **Corrosion of first degree of hand, unspecified site**
- √7ᵗʰ **T23.501** **Corrosion of first degree of** right **hand, unspecified site**
- √7ᵗʰ **T23.502** **Corrosion of first degree of** left **hand, unspecified site**
- √7ᵗʰ **T23.509** **Corrosion of first degree of unspecified hand, unspecified site**

√6ᵗʰ **T23.51** **Corrosion of first degree of** thumb (nail)
- √7ᵗʰ **T23.511** **Corrosion of first degree of** right **thumb (nail)**
- √7ᵗʰ **T23.512** **Corrosion of first degree of** left **thumb (nail)**
- √7ᵗʰ **T23.519** **Corrosion of first degree of unspecified thumb (nail)**

√6ᵗʰ **T23.52** **Corrosion of first degree of** single finger (nail) except thumb
- √7ᵗʰ **T23.521** **Corrosion of first degree of single** right **finger (nail) except thumb**

√7ᵗʰ **T23.522** **Corrosion of first degree of single** left **finger (nail) except thumb**
√7ᵗʰ **T23.529** **Corrosion of first degree of unspecified single finger (nail) except thumb**

√6ᵗʰ **T23.53** **Corrosion of first degree of** multiple fingers (nail), not including thumb
- √7ᵗʰ **T23.531** **Corrosion of first degree of multiple** right **fingers (nail), not including thumb**
- √7ᵗʰ **T23.532** **Corrosion of first degree of multiple** left **fingers (nail), not including thumb**
- √7ᵗʰ **T23.539** **Corrosion of first degree of unspecified multiple fingers (nail), not including thumb**

√6ᵗʰ **T23.54** **Corrosion of first degree of** multiple fingers (nail), including thumb
- √7ᵗʰ **T23.541** **Corrosion of first degree of multiple** right **fingers (nail), including thumb**
- √7ᵗʰ **T23.542** **Corrosion of first degree of multiple** left **fingers (nail), including thumb**
- √7ᵗʰ **T23.549** **Corrosion of first degree of unspecified multiple fingers (nail), including thumb**

√6ᵗʰ **T23.55** **Corrosion of first degree of** palm
- √7ᵗʰ **T23.551** **Corrosion of first degree of** right **palm**
- √7ᵗʰ **T23.552** **Corrosion of first degree of** left **palm**
- √7ᵗʰ **T23.559** **Corrosion of first degree of unspecified palm**

√6ᵗʰ **T23.56** **Corrosion of first degree of** back of hand
- √7ᵗʰ **T23.561** **Corrosion of first degree of back of** right **hand**
- √7ᵗʰ **T23.562** **Corrosion of first degree of back of** left **hand**
- √7ᵗʰ **T23.569** **Corrosion of first degree of back of unspecified hand**

√6ᵗʰ **T23.57** **Corrosion of first degree of** wrist
- √7ᵗʰ **T23.571** **Corrosion of first degree of** right **wrist**
- √7ᵗʰ **T23.572** **Corrosion of first degree of** left **wrist**
- √7ᵗʰ **T23.579** **Corrosion of first degree of unspecified wrist**

√6ᵗʰ **T23.59** **Corrosion of first degree of** multiple sites of wrist and hand
- √7ᵗʰ **T23.591** **Corrosion of first degree of multiple sites of** right **wrist and hand**
- √7ᵗʰ **T23.592** **Corrosion of first degree of multiple sites of** left **wrist and hand**
- √7ᵗʰ **T23.599** **Corrosion of first degree of multiple sites of unspecified wrist and hand**

√5ᵗʰ **T23.6** **Corrosion of** second degree **of wrist and hand**
Code first (T51-T65) to identify chemical and intent
Use additional external cause code to identify place (Y92)

√6ᵗʰ **T23.60** **Corrosion of second degree of hand, unspecified site**
- √7ᵗʰ **T23.601** **Corrosion of second degree of** right **hand, unspecified site**
- √7ᵗʰ **T23.602** **Corrosion of second degree of** left **hand, unspecified site**
- √7ᵗʰ **T23.609** **Corrosion of second degree of unspecified hand, unspecified site**

√6ᵗʰ **T23.61** **Corrosion of second degree of** thumb (nail)
- √7ᵗʰ **T23.611** **Corrosion of second degree of** right **thumb (nail)**
- √7ᵗʰ **T23.612** **Corrosion of second degree of** left **thumb (nail)**
- √7ᵗʰ **T23.619** **Corrosion of second degree of unspecified thumb (nail)**

√6ᵗʰ **T23.62** **Corrosion of second degree of** single finger (nail) except thumb
- √7ᵗʰ **T23.621** **Corrosion of second degree of single** right **finger (nail) except thumb**
- √7ᵗʰ **T23.622** **Corrosion of second degree of single** left **finger (nail) except thumb**
- √7ᵗʰ **T23.629** **Corrosion of second degree of unspecified single finger (nail) except thumb**

√6ᵗʰ **T23.63** **Corrosion of second degree of** multiple fingers (nail), not including thumb
- √7ᵗʰ **T23.631** **Corrosion of second degree of multiple** right **fingers (nail), not including thumb**
- √7ᵗʰ **T23.632** **Corrosion of second degree of multiple** left **fingers (nail), not including thumb**
- √7ᵗʰ **T23.639** **Corrosion of second degree of unspecified multiple fingers (nail), not including thumb**

√6ᵗʰ **T23.64** **Corrosion of second degree of** multiple fingers **(nail),** including thumb

√7ᵗʰ **T23.641** Corrosion of second degree of multiple right fingers (nail), including thumb

√7ᵗʰ **T23.642** Corrosion of second degree of multiple left fingers (nail), including thumb

√7ᵗʰ **T23.649** Corrosion of second degree of unspecified multiple fingers (nail), including thumb

√6ᵗʰ **T23.65** **Corrosion of second degree of** palm

√7ᵗʰ **T23.651** Corrosion of second degree of right palm

√7ᵗʰ **T23.652** Corrosion of second degree of left palm

√7ᵗʰ **T23.659** Corrosion of second degree of unspecified palm

√6ᵗʰ **T23.66** **Corrosion of second degree of** back of hand

√7ᵗʰ **T23.661** Corrosion of second degree back of right hand

√7ᵗʰ **T23.662** Corrosion of second degree back of left hand

√7ᵗʰ **T23.669** Corrosion of second degree back of unspecified hand

√6ᵗʰ **T23.67** **Corrosion of second degree of** wrist

√7ᵗʰ **T23.671** Corrosion of second degree of right wrist

√7ᵗʰ **T23.672** Corrosion of second degree of left wrist

√7ᵗʰ **T23.679** Corrosion of second degree of unspecified wrist

√6ᵗʰ **T23.69** **Corrosion of second degree of** multiple sites **of wrist and hand**

√7ᵗʰ **T23.691** Corrosion of second degree of multiple sites of right wrist and hand

√7ᵗʰ **T23.692** Corrosion of second degree of multiple sites of left wrist and hand

√7ᵗʰ **T23.699** Corrosion of second degree of multiple sites of unspecified wrist and hand

√5ᵗʰ **T23.7** **Corrosion of** third degree **of wrist and hand**

Code first (T51-T65) to identify chemical and intent
Use additional external cause code to identify place (Y92)

√6ᵗʰ **T23.70** **Corrosion of third degree of hand, unspecified site**

√7ᵗʰ **T23.701** Corrosion of third degree of right hand, unspecified site　CC H5 SW

√7ᵗʰ **T23.702** Corrosion of third degree of left hand, unspecified site　CC H5 SW

√7ᵗʰ **T23.709** Corrosion of third degree of unspecified hand, unspecified site　CC H5 SW

√6ᵗʰ **T23.71** **Corrosion of third degree of** thumb **(nail)**

√7ᵗʰ **T23.711** Corrosion of third degree of right thumb (nail)　CC H5 SW

√7ᵗʰ **T23.712** Corrosion of third degree of left thumb (nail)　CC H5 SW

√7ᵗʰ **T23.719** Corrosion of third degree of unspecified thumb (nail)　CC H5 SW

√6ᵗʰ **T23.72** **Corrosion of third degree of** single finger **(nail) except thumb**

√7ᵗʰ **T23.721** Corrosion of third degree of single right finger (nail) except thumb　CC H5 SW

√7ᵗʰ **T23.722** Corrosion of third degree of single left finger (nail) except thumb　CC H5 SW

√7ᵗʰ **T23.729** Corrosion of third degree of unspecified single finger (nail) except thumb　CC H5 SW

√6ᵗʰ **T23.73** **Corrosion of third degree of** multiple fingers (nail), not including thumb

√7ᵗʰ **T23.731** Corrosion of third degree of multiple right fingers (nail), not including thumb　CC H5 SW

√7ᵗʰ **T23.732** Corrosion of third degree of multiple left fingers (nail), not including thumb　CC H5 SW

√7ᵗʰ **T23.739** Corrosion of third degree of unspecified multiple fingers (nail), not including thumb　CC H5 SW

√6ᵗʰ **T23.74** **Corrosion of third degree of** multiple fingers (nail), including thumb

√7ᵗʰ **T23.741** Corrosion of third degree of multiple right fingers (nail), including thumb　CC H5 SW

√7ᵗʰ **T23.742** Corrosion of third degree of multiple left fingers (nail), including thumb　CC H5 SW

√7ᵗʰ **T23.749** Corrosion of third degree of unspecified multiple fingers (nail), including thumb　CC H5 SW

√6ᵗʰ **T23.75** **Corrosion of third degree of** palm

√7ᵗʰ **T23.751** Corrosion of third degree of right palm　CC H5 SW

√7ᵗʰ **T23.752** Corrosion of third degree of left palm　CC H5 SW

√7ᵗʰ **T23.759** Corrosion of third degree of unspecified palm　CC H5 SW

√6ᵗʰ **T23.76** **Corrosion of third degree of** back of hand

√7ᵗʰ **T23.761** Corrosion of third degree of back of right hand　CC H5 SW

√7ᵗʰ **T23.762** Corrosion of third degree of back of left hand　CC H5 SW

√7ᵗʰ **T23.769** Corrosion of third degree back of unspecified hand　CC H5 SW

√6ᵗʰ **T23.77** **Corrosion of third degree of** wrist

√7ᵗʰ **T23.771** Corrosion of third degree of right wrist　CC H5 SW

√7ᵗʰ **T23.772** Corrosion of third degree of left wrist　CC H5 SW

√7ᵗʰ **T23.779** Corrosion of third degree of unspecified wrist　CC H5 SW

√6ᵗʰ **T23.79** **Corrosion of third degree of** multiple sites **of wrist and hand**

√7ᵗʰ **T23.791** Corrosion of third degree of multiple sites of right wrist and hand　CC H5 SW

√7ᵗʰ **T23.792** Corrosion of third degree of multiple sites of left wrist and hand　CC H5 SW

√7ᵗʰ **T23.799** Corrosion of third degree of multiple sites of unspecified wrist and hand　CC H5 SW

√4ᵗʰ **T24** **Burn and corrosion of lower limb, except ankle and foot**

EXCLUDES 2　*burn and corrosion of ankle and foot (T25.-)*
burn and corrosion of hip region (T21.-)

The appropriate 7th character is to be added to each code from category T24.
A　initial encounter
D　subsequent encounter
S　sequela

√5ᵗʰ **T24.0** **Burn of unspecified degree of lower limb, except ankle and foot**

Use additional external cause code to identify the source, place and intent of the burn (X00-X19, X75-X77, X96-X98, Y92)

√6ᵗʰ **T24.00** **Burn of unspecified degree of unspecified site of lower limb, except ankle and foot**

√7ᵗʰ **T24.001** Burn of unspecified degree of unspecified site of right lower limb, except ankle and foot

√7ᵗʰ **T24.002** Burn of unspecified degree of unspecified site of left lower limb, except ankle and foot

√7ᵗʰ **T24.009** Burn of unspecified degree of unspecified site of unspecified lower limb, except ankle and foot

√6ᵗʰ **T24.01** **Burn of unspecified degree of** thigh

√7ᵗʰ **T24.011** Burn of unspecified degree of right thigh

√7ᵗʰ **T24.012** Burn of unspecified degree of left thigh

√7ᵗʰ **T24.019** Burn of unspecified degree of unspecified thigh

√6ᵗʰ **T24.02** **Burn of unspecified degree of** knee

√7ᵗʰ **T24.021** Burn of unspecified degree of right knee

√7ᵗʰ **T24.022** Burn of unspecified degree of left knee

√7ᵗʰ **T24.029** Burn of unspecified degree of unspecified knee

√6ᵗʰ **T24.03** **Burn of unspecified degree of** lower leg

√7ᵗʰ **T24.031** Burn of unspecified degree of right lower leg

√7ᵗʰ **T24.032** Burn of unspecified degree of left lower leg

√7ᵗʰ **T24.039** Burn of unspecified degree of unspecified lower leg

√6ᵗʰ **T24.09** **Burn of unspecified degree of** multiple sites **of lower limb, except ankle and foot**

√7ᵗʰ **T24.091** Burn of unspecified degree of multiple sites of right lower limb, except ankle and foot

✔ Additional Character Required　　√x7ᵗʰ Placeholder　　Questionable PDx　　Manifestation　　Unspecified Dx　　UPD Unacceptable PDx　　H1-H14 HAC　　HCC CMS-HCC Dx　　HIV HIV Dx

ICD-10-CM 2022　　　1103

✓7ᵗʰ **T24.092** Burn of unspecified degree of multiple sites of left lower limb, except ankle and foot

✓7ᵗʰ **T24.099** Burn of unspecified degree of multiple sites of unspecified lower limb, except ankle and foot

✓5ᵗʰ **T24.1** Burn of first degree of lower limb, except ankle and foot

Use additional external cause code to identify the source, place and intent of the burn (X00-X19, X75-X77, X96-X98, Y92)

  ✓6ᵗʰ **T24.10** Burn of first degree of unspecified site of lower limb, except ankle and foot

    ✓7ᵗʰ **T24.101** Burn of first degree of unspecified site of right lower limb, except ankle and foot

    ✓7ᵗʰ **T24.102** Burn of first degree of unspecified site of left lower limb, except ankle and foot

    ✓7ᵗʰ **T24.109** Burn of first degree of unspecified site of unspecified lower limb, except ankle and foot

  ✓6ᵗʰ **T24.11** Burn of first degree of thigh

    ✓7ᵗʰ **T24.111** Burn of first degree of right thigh

    ✓7ᵗʰ **T24.112** Burn of first degree of left thigh

    ✓7ᵗʰ **T24.119** Burn of first degree of unspecified thigh

  ✓6ᵗʰ **T24.12** Burn of first degree of knee

    ✓7ᵗʰ **T24.121** Burn of first degree of right knee

    ✓7ᵗʰ **T24.122** Burn of first degree of left knee

    ✓7ᵗʰ **T24.129** Burn of first degree of unspecified knee

  ✓6ᵗʰ **T24.13** Burn of first degree of lower leg

    ✓7ᵗʰ **T24.131** Burn of first degree of right lower leg

    ✓7ᵗʰ **T24.132** Burn of first degree of left lower leg

    ✓7ᵗʰ **T24.139** Burn of first degree of unspecified lower leg

  ✓6ᵗʰ **T24.19** Burn of first degree of multiple sites of lower limb, except ankle and foot

    ✓7ᵗʰ **T24.191** Burn of first degree of multiple sites of right lower limb, except ankle and foot

    ✓7ᵗʰ **T24.192** Burn of first degree of multiple sites of left lower limb, except ankle and foot

    ✓7ᵗʰ **T24.199** Burn of first degree of multiple sites of unspecified lower limb, except ankle and foot

✓5ᵗʰ **T24.2** Burn of second degree of lower limb, except ankle and foot

Use additional external cause code to identify the source, place and intent of the burn (X00-X19, X75-X77, X96-X98, Y92)

  ✓6ᵗʰ **T24.20** Burn of second degree of unspecified site of lower limb, except ankle and foot

    ✓7ᵗʰ **T24.201** Burn of second degree of unspecified site of right lower limb, except ankle and foot

    ✓7ᵗʰ **T24.202** Burn of second degree of unspecified site of left lower limb, except ankle and foot

    ✓7ᵗʰ **T24.209** Burn of second degree of unspecified site of unspecified lower limb, except ankle and foot

  ✓6ᵗʰ **T24.21** Burn of second degree of thigh

    ✓7ᵗʰ **T24.211** Burn of second degree of right thigh

    ✓7ᵗʰ **T24.212** Burn of second degree of left thigh

    ✓7ᵗʰ **T24.219** Burn of second degree of unspecified thigh

  ✓6ᵗʰ **T24.22** Burn of second degree of knee

    ✓7ᵗʰ **T24.221** Burn of second degree of right knee

    ✓7ᵗʰ **T24.222** Burn of second degree of left knee

    ✓7ᵗʰ **T24.229** Burn of second degree of unspecified knee

  ✓6ᵗʰ **T24.23** Burn of second degree of lower leg

    ✓7ᵗʰ **T24.231** Burn of second degree of right lower leg

    ✓7ᵗʰ **T24.232** Burn of second degree of left lower leg

    ✓7ᵗʰ **T24.239** Burn of second degree of unspecified lower leg

  ✓6ᵗʰ **T24.29** Burn of second degree of multiple sites of lower limb, except ankle and foot

    ✓7ᵗʰ **T24.291** Burn of second degree of multiple sites of right lower limb, except ankle and foot

    ✓7ᵗʰ **T24.292** Burn of second degree of multiple sites of left lower limb, except ankle and foot

    ✓7ᵗʰ **T24.299** Burn of second degree of multiple sites of unspecified lower limb, except ankle and foot

✓5ᵗʰ **T24.3** Burn of third degree of lower limb, except ankle and foot

Use additional external cause code to identify the source, place and intent of the burn (X00-X19, X75-X77, X96-X98, Y92)

  ✓6ᵗʰ **T24.30** Burn of third degree of unspecified site of lower limb, except ankle and foot

    ✓7ᵗʰ **T24.301** Burn of third degree of unspecified site of right lower limb, except ankle and foot `CC` `H5` `SW`

    ✓7ᵗʰ **T24.302** Burn of third degree of unspecified site of left lower limb, except ankle and foot `CC` `H5` `SW`

    ✓7ᵗʰ **T24.309** Burn of third degree of unspecified site of unspecified lower limb, except ankle and foot `CC` `H5` `SW`

  ✓6ᵗʰ **T24.31** Burn of third degree of thigh

    ✓7ᵗʰ **T24.311** Burn of third degree of right thigh `CC` `H5` `SW`

    ✓7ᵗʰ **T24.312** Burn of third degree of left thigh `CC` `H5` `SW`

    ✓7ᵗʰ **T24.319** Burn of third degree of unspecified thigh `CC` `H5` `SW`

  ✓6ᵗʰ **T24.32** Burn of third degree of knee

    ✓7ᵗʰ **T24.321** Burn of third degree of right knee `CC` `H5` `SW`

    ✓7ᵗʰ **T24.322** Burn of third degree of left knee `CC` `H5` `SW`

    ✓7ᵗʰ **T24.329** Burn of third degree of unspecified knee `CC` `H5` `SW`

  ✓6ᵗʰ **T24.33** Burn of third degree of lower leg

    ✓7ᵗʰ **T24.331** Burn of third degree of right lower leg `CC` `H5` `SW`

    ✓7ᵗʰ **T24.332** Burn of third degree of left lower leg `CC` `H5` `SW`

    ✓7ᵗʰ **T24.339** Burn of third degree of unspecified lower leg `CC` `H5` `SW`

  ✓6ᵗʰ **T24.39** Burn of third degree of multiple sites of lower limb, except ankle and foot

    AHA: 2016,2Q,4

    ✓7ᵗʰ **T24.391** Burn of third degree of multiple sites of right lower limb, except ankle and foot `CC` `H5` `SW`

    ✓7ᵗʰ **T24.392** Burn of third degree of multiple sites of left lower limb, except ankle and foot `CC` `H5` `SW`

    ✓7ᵗʰ **T24.399** Burn of third degree of multiple sites of unspecified lower limb, except ankle and foot `CC` `H5` `SW`

✓5ᵗʰ **T24.4** Corrosion of unspecified degree of lower limb, except ankle and foot

Code first (T51-T65) to identify chemical and intent

Use additional external cause code to identify place (Y92)

  ✓6ᵗʰ **T24.40** Corrosion of unspecified degree of unspecified site of lower limb, except ankle and foot

    ✓7ᵗʰ **T24.401** Corrosion of unspecified degree of unspecified site of right lower limb, except ankle and foot

    ✓7ᵗʰ **T24.402** Corrosion of unspecified degree of unspecified site of left lower limb, except ankle and foot

    ✓7ᵗʰ **T24.409** Corrosion of unspecified degree of unspecified site of unspecified lower limb, except ankle and foot

  ✓6ᵗʰ **T24.41** Corrosion of unspecified degree of thigh

    ✓7ᵗʰ **T24.411** Corrosion of unspecified degree of right thigh

    ✓7ᵗʰ **T24.412** Corrosion of unspecified degree of left thigh

    ✓7ᵗʰ **T24.419** Corrosion of unspecified degree of unspecified thigh

  ✓6ᵗʰ **T24.42** Corrosion of unspecified degree of knee

    ✓7ᵗʰ **T24.421** Corrosion of unspecified degree of right knee

    ✓7ᵗʰ **T24.422** Corrosion of unspecified degree of left knee

    ✓7ᵗʰ **T24.429** Corrosion of unspecified degree of unspecified knee

  ✓6ᵗʰ **T24.43** Corrosion of unspecified degree of lower leg

    ✓7ᵗʰ **T24.431** Corrosion of unspecified degree of right lower leg

N Newborn: 0   **P** Pediatric: 0-17   **M** Maternity: 9-64   **A** Adult: 15-124   **MCC** Major Complication/Comorbidity   **CC** Complication/Comorbidity   **SW** Severe Wound Dx

1104   ICD-10-CM 2022

√7ᵗʰ **T24.432** Corrosion of unspecified degree of left lower leg

√7ᵗʰ **T24.439** Corrosion of unspecified degree of unspecified lower leg

√6ᵗʰ **T24.49** Corrosion of unspecified degree of multiple sites of lower limb, except ankle and foot

√7ᵗʰ **T24.491** Corrosion of unspecified degree of multiple sites of right lower limb, except ankle and foot

√7ᵗʰ **T24.492** Corrosion of unspecified degree of multiple sites of left lower limb, except ankle and foot

√7ᵗʰ **T24.499** Corrosion of unspecified degree of multiple sites of unspecified lower limb, except ankle and foot

√5ᵗʰ **T24.5** Corrosion of first degree of lower limb, except ankle and foot

Code first (T51-T65) to identify chemical and intent
Use additional external cause code to identify place (Y92)

√6ᵗʰ **T24.50** Corrosion of first degree of unspecified site of lower limb, except ankle and foot

√7ᵗʰ **T24.501** Corrosion of first degree of unspecified site of right lower limb, except ankle and foot

√7ᵗʰ **T24.502** Corrosion of first degree of unspecified site of left lower limb, except ankle and foot

√7ᵗʰ **T24.509** Corrosion of first degree of unspecified site of unspecified lower limb, except ankle and foot

√6ᵗʰ **T24.51** Corrosion of first degree of thigh

√7ᵗʰ **T24.511** Corrosion of first degree of right thigh

√7ᵗʰ **T24.512** Corrosion of first degree of left thigh

√7ᵗʰ **T24.519** Corrosion of first degree of unspecified thigh

√6ᵗʰ **T24.52** Corrosion of first degree of knee

√7ᵗʰ **T24.521** Corrosion of first degree of right knee

√7ᵗʰ **T24.522** Corrosion of first degree of left knee

√7ᵗʰ **T24.529** Corrosion of first degree of unspecified knee

√6ᵗʰ **T24.53** Corrosion of first degree of lower leg

√7ᵗʰ **T24.531** Corrosion of first degree of right lower leg

√7ᵗʰ **T24.532** Corrosion of first degree of left lower leg

√7ᵗʰ **T24.539** Corrosion of first degree of unspecified lower leg

√6ᵗʰ **T24.59** Corrosion of first degree of multiple sites of lower limb, except ankle and foot

√7ᵗʰ **T24.591** Corrosion of first degree of multiple sites of right lower limb, except ankle and foot

√7ᵗʰ **T24.592** Corrosion of first degree of multiple sites of left lower limb, except ankle and foot

√7ᵗʰ **T24.599** Corrosion of first degree of multiple sites of unspecified lower limb, except ankle and foot

√5ᵗʰ **T24.6** Corrosion of second degree of lower limb, except ankle and foot

Code first (T51-T65) to identify chemical and intent
Use additional external cause code to identify place (Y92)

√6ᵗʰ **T24.60** Corrosion of second degree of unspecified site of lower limb, except ankle and foot

√7ᵗʰ **T24.601** Corrosion of second degree of unspecified site of right lower limb, except ankle and foot

√7ᵗʰ **T24.602** Corrosion of second degree of unspecified site of left lower limb, except ankle and foot

√7ᵗʰ **T24.609** Corrosion of second degree of unspecified site of unspecified lower limb, except ankle and foot

√6ᵗʰ **T24.61** Corrosion of second degree of thigh

√7ᵗʰ **T24.611** Corrosion of second degree of right thigh

√7ᵗʰ **T24.612** Corrosion of second degree of left thigh

√7ᵗʰ **T24.619** Corrosion of second degree of unspecified thigh

√6ᵗʰ **T24.62** Corrosion of second degree of knee

√7ᵗʰ **T24.621** Corrosion of second degree of right knee

√7ᵗʰ **T24.622** Corrosion of second degree of left knee

√7ᵗʰ **T24.629** Corrosion of second degree of unspecified knee

√6ᵗʰ **T24.63** Corrosion of second degree of lower leg

√7ᵗʰ **T24.631** Corrosion of second degree of right lower leg

√7ᵗʰ **T24.632** Corrosion of second degree of left lower leg

√7ᵗʰ **T24.639** Corrosion of second degree of unspecified lower leg

√6ᵗʰ **T24.69** Corrosion of second degree of multiple sites of lower limb, except ankle and foot

√7ᵗʰ **T24.691** Corrosion of second degree of multiple sites of right lower limb, except ankle and foot

√7ᵗʰ **T24.692** Corrosion of second degree of multiple sites of left lower limb, except ankle and foot

√7ᵗʰ **T24.699** Corrosion of second degree of multiple sites of unspecified lower limb, except ankle and foot

√5ᵗʰ **T24.7** Corrosion of third degree of lower limb, except ankle and foot

Code first (T51-T65) to identify chemical and intent
Use additional external cause code to identify place (Y92)

√6ᵗʰ **T24.70** Corrosion of third degree of unspecified site of lower limb, except ankle and foot

√7ᵗʰ **T24.701** Corrosion of third degree of unspecified site of right lower limb, except ankle and foot `CC` `H5` `SW`

√7ᵗʰ **T24.702** Corrosion of third degree of unspecified site of left lower limb, except ankle and foot `CC` `H5` `SW`

√7ᵗʰ **T24.709** Corrosion of third degree of unspecified site of unspecified lower limb, except ankle and foot `CC` `H5` `SW`

√6ᵗʰ **T24.71** Corrosion of third degree of thigh

√7ᵗʰ **T24.711** Corrosion of third degree of right thigh `CC` `H5` `SW`

√7ᵗʰ **T24.712** Corrosion of third degree of left thigh `CC` `H5` `SW`

√7ᵗʰ **T24.719** Corrosion of third degree of unspecified thigh `CC` `H5` `SW`

√6ᵗʰ **T24.72** Corrosion of third degree of knee

√7ᵗʰ **T24.721** Corrosion of third degree of right knee `CC` `H5` `SW`

√7ᵗʰ **T24.722** Corrosion of third degree of left knee `CC` `H5` `SW`

√7ᵗʰ **T24.729** Corrosion of third degree of unspecified knee `CC` `H5` `SW`

√6ᵗʰ **T24.73** Corrosion of third degree of lower leg

√7ᵗʰ **T24.731** Corrosion of third degree of right lower leg `CC` `H5` `SW`

√7ᵗʰ **T24.732** Corrosion of third degree of left lower leg `CC` `H5` `SW`

√7ᵗʰ **T24.739** Corrosion of third degree of unspecified lower leg `CC` `H5` `SW`

√6ᵗʰ **T24.79** Corrosion of third degree of multiple sites of lower limb, except ankle and foot

√7ᵗʰ **T24.791** Corrosion of third degree of multiple sites of right lower limb, except ankle and foot `CC` `H5` `SW`

√7ᵗʰ **T24.792** Corrosion of third degree of multiple sites of left lower limb, except ankle and foot `CC` `H5` `SW`

√7ᵗʰ **T24.799** Corrosion of third degree of multiple sites of unspecified lower limb, except ankle and foot `CC` `H5` `SW`

√4ᵗʰ **T25 Burn and corrosion of ankle and foot**

The appropriate 7th character is to be added to each code from category T25.
A initial encounter
D subsequent encounter
S sequela

√5ᵗʰ **T25.0 Burn of unspecified degree of ankle and foot**

Use additional external cause code to identify the source, place and intent of the burn (X00-X19, X75-X77, X96-X98, Y92)

√6ᵗʰ **T25.01** Burn of unspecified degree of ankle

√7ᵗʰ **T25.011** Burn of unspecified degree of right ankle

√7ᵗʰ **T25.012** Burn of unspecified degree of left ankle

√7ᵗʰ **T25.019** Burn of unspecified degree of unspecified ankle

✔ Additional Character Required   √ˣ⁷ᵗʰ Placeholder   Questionable PDx   Manifestation   Unspecified Dx   `UPD` Unacceptable PDx   `H1`-`H14` HAC   `HCC` CMS-HCC Dx   `HIV` HIV Dx

ICD-10-CM 2022   **1105**

√6ᵗʰ **T25.02** Burn of unspecified degree of foot

> EXCLUDES 2   burn of unspecified degree of toe(s) (nail) (T25.03-)

√7ᵗʰ **T25.021** Burn of unspecified degree of right foot

√7ᵗʰ **T25.022** Burn of unspecified degree of left foot

√7ᵗʰ **T25.029** Burn of unspecified degree of unspecified foot

√6ᵗʰ **T25.03** Burn of unspecified degree of toe(s) (nail)

√7ᵗʰ **T25.031** Burn of unspecified degree of right toe(s) (nail)

√7ᵗʰ **T25.032** Burn of unspecified degree of left toe(s) (nail)

√7ᵗʰ **T25.039** Burn of unspecified degree of unspecified toe(s) (nail)

√6ᵗʰ **T25.09** Burn of unspecified degree of multiple sites of ankle and foot

√7ᵗʰ **T25.091** Burn of unspecified degree of multiple sites of right ankle and foot

√7ᵗʰ **T25.092** Burn of unspecified degree of multiple sites of left ankle and foot

√7ᵗʰ **T25.099** Burn of unspecified degree of multiple sites of unspecified ankle and foot

√5ᵗʰ **T25.1** Burn of first degree of ankle and foot

> Use additional external cause code to identify the source, place and intent of the burn (X00-X19, X75-X77, X96-X98, Y92)

√6ᵗʰ **T25.11** Burn of first degree of ankle

√7ᵗʰ **T25.111** Burn of first degree of right ankle

√7ᵗʰ **T25.112** Burn of first degree of left ankle

√7ᵗʰ **T25.119** Burn of first degree of unspecified ankle

√6ᵗʰ **T25.12** Burn of first degree of foot

> EXCLUDES 2   burn of first degree of toe(s) (nail) (T25.13-)

√7ᵗʰ **T25.121** Burn of first degree of right foot

√7ᵗʰ **T25.122** Burn of first degree of left foot

√7ᵗʰ **T25.129** Burn of first degree of unspecified foot

√6ᵗʰ **T25.13** Burn of first degree of toe(s) (nail)

√7ᵗʰ **T25.131** Burn of first degree of right toe(s) (nail)

√7ᵗʰ **T25.132** Burn of first degree of left toe(s) (nail)

√7ᵗʰ **T25.139** Burn of first degree of unspecified toe(s) (nail)

√6ᵗʰ **T25.19** Burn of first degree of multiple sites of ankle and foot

√7ᵗʰ **T25.191** Burn of first degree of multiple sites of right ankle and foot

√7ᵗʰ **T25.192** Burn of first degree of multiple sites of left ankle and foot

√7ᵗʰ **T25.199** Burn of first degree of multiple sites of unspecified ankle and foot

√5ᵗʰ **T25.2** Burn of second degree of ankle and foot

> Use additional external cause code to identify the source, place and intent of the burn (X00-X19, X75-X77, X96-X98, Y92)

√6ᵗʰ **T25.21** Burn of second degree of ankle

√7ᵗʰ **T25.211** Burn of second degree of right ankle

√7ᵗʰ **T25.212** Burn of second degree of left ankle

√7ᵗʰ **T25.219** Burn of second degree of unspecified ankle

√6ᵗʰ **T25.22** Burn of second degree of foot

> EXCLUDES 2   burn of second degree of toe(s) (nail) (T25.23-)

√7ᵗʰ **T25.221** Burn of second degree of right foot

√7ᵗʰ **T25.222** Burn of second degree of left foot

√7ᵗʰ **T25.229** Burn of second degree of unspecified foot

√6ᵗʰ **T25.23** Burn of second degree of toe(s) (nail)

√7ᵗʰ **T25.231** Burn of second degree of right toe(s) (nail)

√7ᵗʰ **T25.232** Burn of second degree of left toe(s) (nail)

√7ᵗʰ **T25.239** Burn of second degree of unspecified toe(s) (nail)

√6ᵗʰ **T25.29** Burn of second degree of multiple sites of ankle and foot

√7ᵗʰ **T25.291** Burn of second degree of multiple sites of right ankle and foot

√7ᵗʰ **T25.292** Burn of second degree of multiple sites of left ankle and foot

√7ᵗʰ **T25.299** Burn of second degree of multiple sites of unspecified ankle and foot

√5ᵗʰ **T25.3** Burn of third degree of ankle and foot

> Use additional external cause code to identify the source, place and intent of the burn (X00-X19, X75-X77, X96-X98, Y92)

√6ᵗʰ **T25.31** Burn of third degree of ankle

√7ᵗʰ **T25.311** Burn of third degree of right ankle   CC H5 SW

√7ᵗʰ **T25.312** Burn of third degree of left ankle   CC H5 SW

√7ᵗʰ **T25.319** Burn of third degree of unspecified ankle   CC H5 SW

√6ᵗʰ **T25.32** Burn of third degree of foot

> EXCLUDES 2   burn of third degree of toe(s) (nail) (T25.33-)

√7ᵗʰ **T25.321** Burn of third degree of right foot   CC H5 SW

√7ᵗʰ **T25.322** Burn of third degree of left foot   CC H5 SW

√7ᵗʰ **T25.329** Burn of third degree of unspecified foot   CC H5 SW

√6ᵗʰ **T25.33** Burn of third degree of toe(s) (nail)

√7ᵗʰ **T25.331** Burn of third degree of right toe(s) (nail)   CC H5 SW

√7ᵗʰ **T25.332** Burn of third degree of left toe(s) (nail)   CC H5 SW

√7ᵗʰ **T25.339** Burn of third degree of unspecified toe(s) (nail)   CC H5 SW

√6ᵗʰ **T25.39** Burn of third degree of multiple sites of ankle and foot

√7ᵗʰ **T25.391** Burn of third degree of multiple sites of right ankle and foot   CC H5 SW

√7ᵗʰ **T25.392** Burn of third degree of multiple sites of left ankle and foot   CC H5 SW

√7ᵗʰ **T25.399** Burn of third degree of multiple sites of unspecified ankle and foot   CC H5 SW

√5ᵗʰ **T25.4** Corrosion of unspecified degree of ankle and foot

> Code first (T51-T65) to identify chemical and intent
> Use additional external cause code to identify place (Y92)

√6ᵗʰ **T25.41** Corrosion of unspecified degree of ankle

√7ᵗʰ **T25.411** Corrosion of unspecified degree of right ankle

√7ᵗʰ **T25.412** Corrosion of unspecified degree of left ankle

√7ᵗʰ **T25.419** Corrosion of unspecified degree of unspecified ankle

√6ᵗʰ **T25.42** Corrosion of unspecified degree of foot

> EXCLUDES 2   corrosion of unspecified degree of toe(s) (nail) (T25.43-)

√7ᵗʰ **T25.421** Corrosion of unspecified degree of right foot

√7ᵗʰ **T25.422** Corrosion of unspecified degree of left foot

√7ᵗʰ **T25.429** Corrosion of unspecified degree of unspecified foot

√6ᵗʰ **T25.43** Corrosion of unspecified degree of toe(s) (nail)

√7ᵗʰ **T25.431** Corrosion of unspecified degree of right toe(s) (nail)

√7ᵗʰ **T25.432** Corrosion of unspecified degree of left toe(s) (nail)

√7ᵗʰ **T25.439** Corrosion of unspecified degree of unspecified toe(s) (nail)

√6ᵗʰ **T25.49** Corrosion of unspecified degree of multiple sites of ankle and foot

√7ᵗʰ **T25.491** Corrosion of unspecified degree of multiple sites of right ankle and foot

√7ᵗʰ **T25.492** Corrosion of unspecified degree of multiple sites of left ankle and foot

√7ᵗʰ **T25.499** Corrosion of unspecified degree of multiple sites of unspecified ankle and foot

√5ᵗʰ **T25.5** Corrosion of first degree of ankle and foot

> Code first (T51-T65) to identify chemical and intent
> Use additional external cause code to identify place (Y92)

√6ᵗʰ **T25.51** Corrosion of first degree of ankle

√7ᵗʰ **T25.511** Corrosion of first degree of right ankle

√7ᵗʰ **T25.512** Corrosion of first degree of left ankle

√7ᵗʰ **T25.519** Corrosion of first degree of unspecified ankle

---

N Newborn: 0   P Pediatric: 0-17   M Maternity: 9-64   A Adult: 15-124   MCC Major Complication/Comorbidity   CC Complication/Comorbidity   SW Severe Wound Dx

1106   ICD-10-CM 2022

√6ᵗʰ **T25.52 Corrosion of first degree of** foot
    EXCLUDES 2 *corrosion of first degree of toe(s) (nail) (T25.53-)*
    √7ᵗʰ **T25.521 Corrosion of first degree of** right **foot**
    √7ᵗʰ **T25.522 Corrosion of first degree of** left **foot**
    √7ᵗʰ **T25.529 Corrosion of first degree of unspecified foot**

√6ᵗʰ **T25.53 Corrosion of first degree of** toe(s) (nail)
    √7ᵗʰ **T25.531 Corrosion of first degree of** right **toe(s) (nail)**
    √7ᵗʰ **T25.532 Corrosion of first degree of** left **toe(s) (nail)**
    √7ᵗʰ **T25.539 Corrosion of first degree of unspecified toe(s) (nail)**

√6ᵗʰ **T25.59 Corrosion of first degree of** multiple sites **of ankle and foot**
    √7ᵗʰ **T25.591 Corrosion of first degree of multiple sites of** right **ankle and foot**
    √7ᵗʰ **T25.592 Corrosion of first degree of multiple sites of** left **ankle and foot**
    √7ᵗʰ **T25.599 Corrosion of first degree of multiple sites of unspecified ankle and foot**

√5ᵗʰ **T25.6 Corrosion of** second degree **of ankle and foot**
    Code first (T51-T65) to identify chemical and intent
    Use additional external cause code to identify place (Y92)
  √6ᵗʰ **T25.61 Corrosion of second degree of** ankle
    √7ᵗʰ **T25.611 Corrosion of second degree of** right **ankle**
    √7ᵗʰ **T25.612 Corrosion of second degree of** left **ankle**
    √7ᵗʰ **T25.619 Corrosion of second degree of unspecified ankle**

  √6ᵗʰ **T25.62 Corrosion of second degree of** foot
    EXCLUDES 2 *corrosion of second degree of toe(s) (nail) (T25.63-)*
    √7ᵗʰ **T25.621 Corrosion of second degree of** right **foot**
    √7ᵗʰ **T25.622 Corrosion of second degree of** left **foot**
    √7ᵗʰ **T25.629 Corrosion of second degree of unspecified foot**

  √6ᵗʰ **T25.63 Corrosion of second degree of** toe(s) (nail)
    √7ᵗʰ **T25.631 Corrosion of second degree of** right **toe(s) (nail)**
    √7ᵗʰ **T25.632 Corrosion of second degree of** left **toe(s) (nail)**
    √7ᵗʰ **T25.639 Corrosion of second degree of unspecified toe(s) (nail)**

  √6ᵗʰ **T25.69 Corrosion of second degree of** multiple sites **of ankle and foot**
    √7ᵗʰ **T25.691 Corrosion of second degree of** right **ankle and foot**
    √7ᵗʰ **T25.692 Corrosion of second degree of** left **ankle and foot**
    √7ᵗʰ **T25.699 Corrosion of second degree of unspecified ankle and foot**

√5ᵗʰ **T25.7 Corrosion of** third degree **of ankle and foot**
    Code first (T51-T65) to identify chemical and intent
    Use additional external cause code to identify place (Y92)
  √6ᵗʰ **T25.71 Corrosion of third degree of** ankle
    √7ᵗʰ **T25.711 Corrosion of third degree of** right **ankle** CC H5 SW
    √7ᵗʰ **T25.712 Corrosion of third degree of** left **ankle** CC H5 SW
    √7ᵗʰ **T25.719 Corrosion of third degree of unspecified ankle** CC H5 SW

  √6ᵗʰ **T25.72 Corrosion of third degree of** foot
    EXCLUDES 2 *corrosion of third degree of toe(s) (nail) (T25.73-)*
    √7ᵗʰ **T25.721 Corrosion of third degree of** right **foot** CC H5 SW
    √7ᵗʰ **T25.722 Corrosion of third degree of** left **foot** CC H5 SW
    √7ᵗʰ **T25.729 Corrosion of third degree of unspecified foot** CC H5 SW

  √6ᵗʰ **T25.73 Corrosion of third degree of** toe(s) (nail)
    √7ᵗʰ **T25.731 Corrosion of third degree of** right **toe(s) (nail)** CC H5 SW
    √7ᵗʰ **T25.732 Corrosion of third degree of** left **toe(s) (nail)** CC H5 SW

√7ᵗʰ **T25.739 Corrosion of third degree of unspecified toe(s) (nail)** CC H5 SW

√6ᵗʰ **T25.79 Corrosion of third degree of** multiple sites **of ankle and foot**
    √7ᵗʰ **T25.791 Corrosion of third degree of multiple sites of** right **ankle and foot** CC H5 SW
    √7ᵗʰ **T25.792 Corrosion of third degree of multiple sites of** left **ankle and foot** CC H5 SW
    √7ᵗʰ **T25.799 Corrosion of third degree of multiple sites of unspecified ankle and foot** CC H5 SW

Burns and corrosions confined to eye and internal organs (T26-T28)

√4ᵗʰ **T26 Burn and corrosion confined to eye and adnexa**

The appropriate 7th character is to be added to each code from category T26.
A initial encounter
D subsequent encounter
S sequela

√5ᵗʰ **T26.0 Burn of** eyelid and periocular area
    Use additional external cause code to identify the source, place and intent of the burn (X00-X19, X75-X77, X96-X98, Y92)
  √7ᵗʰ **T26.00 Burn of unspecified eyelid and periocular area**
  √7ᵗʰ **T26.01 Burn of** right **eyelid and periocular area**
  √7ᵗʰ **T26.02 Burn of** left **eyelid and periocular area**

√5ᵗʰ **T26.1 Burn of** cornea and conjunctival sac
    Use additional external cause code to identify the source, place and intent of the burn (X00-X19, X75-X77, X96-X98, Y92)
  √7ᵗʰ **T26.10 Burn of cornea and conjunctival sac, unspecified eye**
  √7ᵗʰ **T26.11 Burn of cornea and conjunctival sac,** right **eye**
  √7ᵗʰ **T26.12 Burn of cornea and conjunctival sac,** left **eye**

√5ᵗʰ **T26.2 Burn with resulting** rupture and destruction of eyeball
    Use additional external cause code to identify the source, place and intent of the burn (X00-X19, X75-X77, X96-X98, Y92)
  √7ᵗʰ **T26.20 Burn with resulting rupture and destruction of unspecified eyeball** CC H5
  √7ᵗʰ **T26.21 Burn with resulting rupture and destruction of** right **eyeball** CC H5
  √7ᵗʰ **T26.22 Burn with resulting rupture and destruction of** left **eyeball** CC H5

√5ᵗʰ **T26.3 Burns of other specified parts of eye and adnexa**
    Use additional external cause code to identify the source, place and intent of the burn (X00-X19, X75-X77, X96-X98, Y92)
  √7ᵗʰ **T26.30 Burns of other specified parts of unspecified eye and adnexa**
  √7ᵗʰ **T26.31 Burns of other specified parts of** right **eye and adnexa**
  √7ᵗʰ **T26.32 Burns of other specified parts of** left **eye and adnexa**

√5ᵗʰ **T26.4 Burn of eye and adnexa, part unspecified**
    Use additional external cause code to identify the source, place and intent of the burn (X00-X19, X75-X77, X96-X98, Y92)
  √7ᵗʰ **T26.40 Burn of unspecified eye and adnexa, part unspecified**
  √7ᵗʰ **T26.41 Burn of** right **eye and adnexa, part unspecified**
  √7ᵗʰ **T26.42 Burn of** left **eye and adnexa, part unspecified**

√5ᵗʰ **T26.5 Corrosion of** eyelid and periocular area
    Code first (T51-T65) to identify chemical and intent
    Use additional external cause code to identify place (Y92)
  √7ᵗʰ **T26.50 Corrosion of unspecified eyelid and periocular area**
  √7ᵗʰ **T26.51 Corrosion of** right **eyelid and periocular area**
  √7ᵗʰ **T26.52 Corrosion of** left **eyelid and periocular area**

√5ᵗʰ **T26.6 Corrosion of** cornea and conjunctival sac
    Code first (T51-T65) to identify chemical and intent
    Use additional external cause code to identify place (Y92)
  √7ᵗʰ **T26.60 Corrosion of cornea and conjunctival sac, unspecified eye**
  √7ᵗʰ **T26.61 Corrosion of cornea and conjunctival sac,** right **eye**
  √7ᵗʰ **T26.62 Corrosion of cornea and conjunctival sac,** left **eye**

Chapter 19. Injury, Poisoning and Certain Other Consequences of External Causes *(left margin)*

√5ᵗʰ **T26.7** **Corrosion with resulting rupture and destruction of eyeball**
Code first (T51-T65) to identify chemical and intent
Use additional external cause code to identify place (Y92)

  √x7ᵗʰ **T26.70** **Corrosion with resulting rupture and destruction of unspecified eyeball** `CC` `H5`

  √x7ᵗʰ **T26.71** **Corrosion with resulting rupture and destruction of right eyeball** `CC` `H5`

  √x7ᵗʰ **T26.72** **Corrosion with resulting rupture and destruction of left eyeball** `CC` `H5`

√5ᵗʰ **T26.8** **Corrosions of other specified parts of eye and adnexa**
Code first (T51-T65) to identify chemical and intent
Use additional external cause code to identify place (Y92)

  √x7ᵗʰ **T26.80** **Corrosions of other specified parts of unspecified eye and adnexa**

  √x7ᵗʰ **T26.81** **Corrosions of other specified parts of right eye and adnexa**

  √x7ᵗʰ **T26.82** **Corrosions of other specified parts of left eye and adnexa**

√5ᵗʰ **T26.9** **Corrosion of eye and adnexa, part unspecified**
Code first (T51-T65) to identify chemical and intent
Use additional external cause code to identify place (Y92)

  √x7ᵗʰ **T26.90** **Corrosion of unspecified eye and adnexa, part unspecified**

  √x7ᵗʰ **T26.91** **Corrosion of right eye and adnexa, part unspecified**

  √x7ᵗʰ **T26.92** **Corrosion of left eye and adnexa, part unspecified**

√4ᵗʰ **T27** **Burn and corrosion of respiratory tract**
Use additional external cause code to identify the source and intent of the burn (X00-X19, X75-X77, X96-X98)
Use additional external cause code to identify place (Y92)

> The appropriate 7th character is to be added to each code from category T27.
> A   initial encounter
> D   subsequent encounter
> S   sequela

√x7ᵗʰ **T27.0** **Burn of larynx and trachea** `CC` `H5`

√x7ᵗʰ **T27.1** **Burn involving larynx and trachea with lung** `CC` `H5`

√x7ᵗʰ **T27.2** **Burn of other parts of respiratory tract** `CC` `H5`
    Burn of thoracic cavity

√x7ᵗʰ **T27.3** **Burn of respiratory tract, part unspecified** `CC` `H5`

√x7ᵗʰ **T27.4** **Corrosion of larynx and trachea** `CC` `H5`
    Code first (T51-T65) to identify chemical and intent

√x7ᵗʰ **T27.5** **Corrosion involving larynx and trachea with lung** `CC` `H5`
    Code first (T51-T65) to identify chemical and intent

√x7ᵗʰ **T27.6** **Corrosion of other parts of respiratory tract** `CC` `H5`
    Code first (T51-T65) to identify chemical and intent

√x7ᵗʰ **T27.7** **Corrosion of respiratory tract, part unspecified** `CC` `H5`
    Code first (T51-T65) to identify chemical and intent

√4ᵗʰ **T28** **Burn and corrosion of other internal organs**
Use additional external cause code to identify the source and intent of the burn (X00-X19, X75-X77, X96-X98)
Use additional external cause code to identify place (Y92)

> The appropriate 7th character is to be added to each code from category T28.
> A   initial encounter
> D   subsequent encounter
> S   sequela

√x7ᵗʰ **T28.0** **Burn of mouth and pharynx**

√x7ᵗʰ **T28.1** **Burn of esophagus** `CC` `H5`

√x7ᵗʰ **T28.2** **Burn of other parts of alimentary tract** `CC` `H5`

√x7ᵗʰ **T28.3** **Burn of internal genitourinary organs**

√5ᵗʰ **T28.4** **Burns of other and unspecified internal organs**

  √x7ᵗʰ **T28.40** **Burn of unspecified internal organ**

  √6ᵗʰ **T28.41** **Burn of ear drum**

    √7ᵗʰ **T28.411** **Burn of right ear drum**

    √7ᵗʰ **T28.412** **Burn of left ear drum**

    √7ᵗʰ **T28.419** **Burn of unspecified ear drum**

  √x7ᵗʰ **T28.49** **Burn of other internal organ**

√x7ᵗʰ **T28.5** **Corrosion of mouth and pharynx**
    Code first (T51-T65) to identify chemical and intent

√x7ᵗʰ **T28.6** **Corrosion of esophagus** `CC` `H5`
    Code first (T51-T65) to identify chemical and intent

√x7ᵗʰ **T28.7** **Corrosion of other parts of alimentary tract** `CC` `H5`
    Code first (T51-T65) to identify chemical and intent

√x7ᵗʰ **T28.8** **Corrosion of internal genitourinary organs**
    Code first (T51-T65) to identify chemical and intent

√5ᵗʰ **T28.9** **Corrosions of other and unspecified internal organs**
    Code first (T51-T65) to identify chemical and intent

  √x7ᵗʰ **T28.90** **Corrosions of unspecified internal organs**

  √6ᵗʰ **T28.91** **Corrosions of ear drum**

    √7ᵗʰ **T28.911** **Corrosions of right ear drum**

    √7ᵗʰ **T28.912** **Corrosions of left ear drum**

    √7ᵗʰ **T28.919** **Corrosions of unspecified ear drum**

  √x7ᵗʰ **T28.99** **Corrosions of other internal organs**

Burns and corrosions of multiple and unspecified body regions (T30-T32)

√4ᵗʰ **T30** **Burn and corrosion, body region unspecified**

  T30.0 **Burn of unspecified body region, unspecified degree**
    This code is not for inpatient use. Code to specified site and degree of burns
    Burn NOS
    Multiple burns NOS

  T30.4 **Corrosion of unspecified body region, unspecified degree**
    This code is not for inpatient use. Code to specified site and degree of corrosion
    Corrosion NOS
    Multiple corrosion NOS

√4ᵗʰ **T31** **Burns classified according to extent of body surface involved**

> **NOTE** This category is to be used as the primary code only when the site of the burn is unspecified. It should be used as a supplementary code with categories T20-T25 when the site is specified.

  T31.0 **Burns involving less than 10% of body surface**

√5ᵗʰ **T31.1** **Burns involving 10-19% of body surface**

  T31.10 **Burns involving 10-19% of body surface with 0% to 9% third degree burns** `CC` `H5`
    Burns involving 10-19% of body surface NOS

  T31.11 **Burns involving 10-19% of body surface with 10-19% third degree burns** `CC` `H5` `HCC`

√5ᵗʰ **T31.2** **Burns involving 20-29% of body surface**

  T31.20 **Burns involving 20-29% of body surface with 0% to 9% third degree burns** `CC` `H5`
    Burns involving 20-29% of body surface NOS

  T31.21 **Burns involving 20-29% of body surface with 10-19% third degree burns** `MCC` `H5` `HCC`

  T31.22 **Burns involving 20-29% of body surface with 20-29% third degree burns** `MCC` `H5` `HCC`

√5ᵗʰ **T31.3** **Burns involving 30-39% of body surface**

  T31.30 **Burns involving 30-39% of body surface with 0% to 9% third degree burns** `CC` `H5`
    Burns involving 30-39% of body surface NOS

  T31.31 **Burns involving 30-39% of body surface with 10-19% third degree burns** `MCC` `H5` `HCC`

  T31.32 **Burns involving 30-39% of body surface with 20-29% third degree burns** `MCC` `H5` `HCC`

  T31.33 **Burns involving 30-39% of body surface with 30-39% third degree burns** `MCC` `H5` `HCC`

√5ᵗʰ **T31.4** **Burns involving 40-49% of body surface**

  T31.40 **Burns involving 40-49% of body surface with 0% to 9% third degree burns** `CC` `H5`
    Burns involving 40-49% of body surface NOS

  T31.41 **Burns involving 40-49% of body surface with 10-19% third degree burns** `MCC` `H5` `HCC`

  T31.42 **Burns involving 40-49% of body surface with 20-29% third degree burns** `MCC` `H5` `HCC`

  T31.43 **Burns involving 40-49% of body surface with 30-39% third degree burns** `MCC` `H5` `HCC`

  T31.44 **Burns involving 40-49% of body surface with 40-49% third degree burns** `MCC` `H5` `HCC`

√5ᵗʰ **T31.5**   **Burns involving 50-59% of body surface**

T31.50   **Burns involving 50-59% of body surface with 0% to 9% third degree burns**   `CC` `H5`
Burns involving 50-59% of body surface NOS

T31.51   **Burns involving 50-59% of body surface with 10-19% third degree burns**   `MCC` `H5` `HCC`

T31.52   **Burns involving 50-59% of body surface with 20-29% third degree burns**   `MCC` `H5` `HCC`

T31.53   **Burns involving 50-59% of body surface with 30-39% third degree burns**   `MCC` `H5` `HCC`

T31.54   **Burns involving 50-59% of body surface with 40-49% third degree burns**   `MCC` `H5` `HCC`

T31.55   **Burns involving 50-59% of body surface with 50-59% third degree burns**   `MCC` `H5` `HCC`

√5ᵗʰ **T31.6**   **Burns involving 60-69% of body surface**

T31.60   **Burns involving 60-69% of body surface with 0% to 9% third degree burns**   `CC` `H5`
Burns involving 60-69% of body surface NOS

T31.61   **Burns involving 60-69% of body surface with 10-19% third degree burns**   `MCC` `H5` `HCC`

T31.62   **Burns involving 60-69% of body surface with 20-29% third degree burns**   `MCC` `H5` `HCC`

T31.63   **Burns involving 60-69% of body surface with 30-39% third degree burns**   `MCC` `H5` `HCC`

T31.64   **Burns involving 60-69% of body surface with 40-49% third degree burns**   `MCC` `H5` `HCC`

T31.65   **Burns involving 60-69% of body surface with 50-59% third degree burns**   `MCC` `H5` `HCC`

T31.66   **Burns involving 60-69% of body surface with 60-69% third degree burns**   `MCC` `H5` `HCC`

√5ᵗʰ **T31.7**   **Burns involving 70-79% of body surface**

T31.70   **Burns involving 70-79% of body surface with 0% to 9% third degree burns**   `CC` `H5`
Burns involving 70-79% of body surface NOS

T31.71   **Burns involving 70-79% of body surface with 10-19% third degree burns**   `MCC` `H5` `HCC`

T31.72   **Burns involving 70-79% of body surface with 20-29% third degree burns**   `MCC` `H5` `HCC`

T31.73   **Burns involving 70-79% of body surface with 30-39% third degree burns**   `MCC` `H5` `HCC`

T31.74   **Burns involving 70-79% of body surface with 40-49% third degree burns**   `MCC` `H5` `HCC`

T31.75   **Burns involving 70-79% of body surface with 50-59% third degree burns**   `MCC` `H5` `HCC`

T31.76   **Burns involving 70-79% of body surface with 60-69% third degree burns**   `MCC` `H5` `HCC`

T31.77   **Burns involving 70-79% of body surface with 70-79% third degree burns**   `MCC` `H5` `HCC`

√5ᵗʰ **T31.8**   **Burns involving 80-89% of body surface**

T31.80   **Burns involving 80-89% of body surface with 0% to 9% third degree burns**   `CC` `H5`
Burns involving 80-89% of body surface NOS

T31.81   **Burns involving 80-89% of body surface with 10-19% third degree burns**   `MCC` `H5` `HCC`

T31.82   **Burns involving 80-89% of body surface with 20-29% third degree burns**   `MCC` `H5` `HCC`

T31.83   **Burns involving 80-89% of body surface with 30-39% third degree burns**   `MCC` `H5` `HCC`

T31.84   **Burns involving 80-89% of body surface with 40-49% third degree burns**   `MCC` `H5` `HCC`

T31.85   **Burns involving 80-89% of body surface with 50-59% third degree burns**   `MCC` `H5` `HCC`

T31.86   **Burns involving 80-89% of body surface with 60-69% third degree burns**   `MCC` `H5` `HCC`

T31.87   **Burns involving 80-89% of body surface with 70-79% third degree burns**   `MCC` `H5` `HCC`

T31.88   **Burns involving 80-89% of body surface with 80-89% third degree burns**   `MCC` `H5` `HCC`

√5ᵗʰ **T31.9**   **Burns involving 90% or more of body surface**

T31.90   **Burns involving 90% or more of body surface with 0% to 9% third degree burns**   `CC` `H5`
Burns involving 90% or more of body surface NOS

T31.91   **Burns involving 90% or more of body surface with 10-19% third degree burns**   `MCC` `H5` `HCC`

T31.92   **Burns involving 90% or more of body surface with 20-29% third degree burns**   `MCC` `H5` `HCC`

T31.93   **Burns involving 90% or more of body surface with 30-39% third degree burns**   `MCC` `H5` `HCC`

T31.94   **Burns involving 90% or more of body surface with 40-49% third degree burns**   `MCC` `H5` `HCC`

T31.95   **Burns involving 90% or more of body surface with 50-59% third degree burns**   `MCC` `H5` `HCC`

T31.96   **Burns involving 90% or more of body surface with 60-69% third degree burns**   `MCC` `H5` `HCC`

T31.97   **Burns involving 90% or more of body surface with 70-79% third degree burns**   `MCC` `H5` `HCC`

T31.98   **Burns involving 90% or more of body surface with 80-89% third degree burns**   `MCC` `H5` `HCC`

T31.99   **Burns involving 90% or more of body surface with 90% or more third degree burns**   `MCC` `H5` `HCC`

Rule of Nines Estimation of Total Body Surface Burned

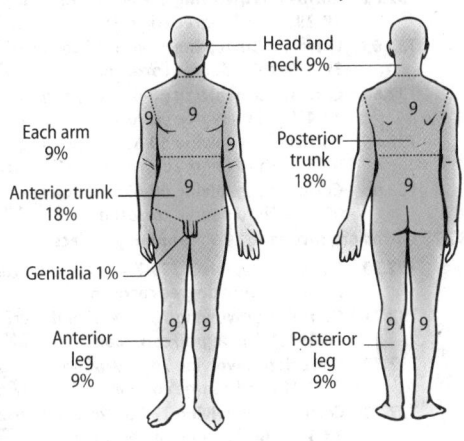

Head and neck 9%
Each arm 9%
Anterior trunk 18%
Posterior trunk 18%
Genitalia 1%
Anterior leg 9%
Posterior leg 9%

√4ᵗʰ **T32**   **Corrosions classified according to extent of body surface involved**

NOTE   This category is to be used as the primary code only when the site of the corrosion is unspecified. It may be used as a supplementary code with categories T20-T25 when the site is specified.

T32.0   **Corrosions involving less than 10% of body surface**

√5ᵗʰ **T32.1**   **Corrosions involving 10-19% of body surface**

T32.10   **Corrosions involving 10-19% of body surface with 0% to 9% third degree corrosion**   `CC` `H5`
Corrosions involving 10-19% of body surface NOS

T32.11   **Corrosions involving 10-19% of body surface with 10-19% third degree corrosion**   `CC` `H5` `HCC`

√5ᵗʰ **T32.2**   **Corrosions involving 20-29% of body surface**

T32.20   **Corrosions involving 20-29% of body surface with 0% to 9% third degree corrosion**   `CC` `H5`

T32.21   **Corrosions involving 20-29% of body surface with 10-19% third degree corrosion**   `MCC` `H5` `HCC`

T32.22   **Corrosions involving 20-29% of body surface with 20-29% third degree corrosion**   `MCC` `H5` `HCC`

√5ᵗʰ **T32.3**   **Corrosions involving 30-39% of body surface**

T32.30   **Corrosions involving 30-39% of body surface with 0% to 9% third degree corrosion**   `CC` `H5`

T32.31   **Corrosions involving 30-39% of body surface with 10-19% third degree corrosion**   `MCC` `H5` `HCC`

T32.32   **Corrosions involving 30-39% of body surface with 20-29% third degree corrosion**   `MCC` `H5` `HCC`

T32.33   **Corrosions involving 30-39% of body surface with 30-39% third degree corrosion**   `MCC` `H5` `HCC`

√5ᵗʰ **T32.4**   **Corrosions involving 40-49% of body surface**

T32.40   **Corrosions involving 40-49% of body surface with 0% to 9% third degree corrosion**   `CC` `H5`

T32.41   **Corrosions involving 40-49% of body surface with 10-19% third degree corrosion**   `MCC` `H5` `HCC`

T32.42   **Corrosions involving 40-49% of body surface with 20-29% third degree corrosion**   `MCC` `H5` `HCC`

T32.43   **Corrosions involving 40-49% of body surface with 30-39% third degree corrosion**   `MCC` `H5` `HCC`

T32.44   **Corrosions involving 40-49% of body surface with 40-49% third degree corrosion**   `MCC` `H5` `HCC`

√5ᵗʰ **T32.5**   **Corrosions involving 50-59% of body surface**

T32.50   **Corrosions involving 50-59% of body surface with 0% to 9% third degree corrosion**   `CC` `H5`

T32.51   **Corrosions involving 50-59% of body surface with 10-19% third degree corrosion**   `MCC` `H5` `HCC`

T32.52   **Corrosions involving 50-59% of body surface with 20-29% third degree corrosion** `MCC` `H5` `HCC`

T32.53   **Corrosions involving 50-59% of body surface with 30-39% third degree corrosion** `MCC` `H5` `HCC`

T32.54   **Corrosions involving 50-59% of body surface with 40-49% third degree corrosion** `MCC` `H5` `HCC`

T32.55   **Corrosions involving 50-59% of body surface with 50-59% third degree corrosion** `MCC` `H5` `HCC`

√5th **T32.6**   **Corrosions involving 60-69% of body surface**

T32.60   **Corrosions involving 60-69% of body surface with 0% to 9% third degree corrosion** `CC` `H5`

T32.61   **Corrosions involving 60-69% of body surface with 10-19% third degree corrosion** `MCC` `H5` `HCC`

T32.62   **Corrosions involving 60-69% of body surface with 20-29% third degree corrosion** `MCC` `H5` `HCC`

T32.63   **Corrosions involving 60-69% of body surface with 30-39% third degree corrosion** `MCC` `H5` `HCC`

T32.64   **Corrosions involving 60-69% of body surface with 40-49% third degree corrosion** `MCC` `H5` `HCC`

T32.65   **Corrosions involving 60-69% of body surface with 50-59% third degree corrosion** `MCC` `H5` `HCC`

T32.66   **Corrosions involving 60-69% of body surface with 60-69% third degree corrosion** `MCC` `H5` `HCC`

√5th **T32.7**   **Corrosions involving 70-79% of body surface**

T32.70   **Corrosions involving 70-79% of body surface with 0% to 9% third degree corrosion** `CC` `H5`

T32.71   **Corrosions involving 70-79% of body surface with 10-19% third degree corrosion** `MCC` `H5` `HCC`

T32.72   **Corrosions involving 70-79% of body surface with 20-29% third degree corrosion** `MCC` `H5` `HCC`

T32.73   **Corrosions involving 70-79% of body surface with 30-39% third degree corrosion** `MCC` `H5` `HCC`

T32.74   **Corrosions involving 70-79% of body surface with 40-49% third degree corrosion** `MCC` `H5` `HCC`

T32.75   **Corrosions involving 70-79% of body surface with 50-59% third degree corrosion** `MCC` `H5` `HCC`

T32.76   **Corrosions involving 70-79% of body surface with 60-69% third degree corrosion** `MCC` `H5` `HCC`

T32.77   **Corrosions involving 70-79% of body surface with 70-79% third degree corrosion** `MCC` `H5` `HCC`

√5th **T32.8**   **Corrosions involving 80-89% of body surface**

T32.80   **Corrosions involving 80-89% of body surface with 0% to 9% third degree corrosion** `CC` `H5`

T32.81   **Corrosions involving 80-89% of body surface with 10-19% third degree corrosion** `MCC` `H5` `HCC`

T32.82   **Corrosions involving 80-89% of body surface with 20-29% third degree corrosion** `MCC` `H5` `HCC`

T32.83   **Corrosions involving 80-89% of body surface with 30-39% third degree corrosion** `MCC` `H5` `HCC`

T32.84   **Corrosions involving 80-89% of body surface with 40-49% third degree corrosion** `MCC` `H5` `HCC`

T32.85   **Corrosions involving 80-89% of body surface with 50-59% third degree corrosion** `MCC` `H5` `HCC`

T32.86   **Corrosions involving 80-89% of body surface with 60-69% third degree corrosion** `MCC` `H5` `HCC`

T32.87   **Corrosions involving 80-89% of body surface with 70-79% third degree corrosion** `MCC` `H5` `HCC`

T32.88   **Corrosions involving 80-89% of body surface with 80-89% third degree corrosion** `MCC` `H5` `HCC`

√5th **T32.9**   **Corrosions involving 90% or more of body surface**

T32.90   **Corrosions involving 90% or more of body surface with 0% to 9% third degree corrosion** `CC` `H5`

T32.91   **Corrosions involving 90% or more of body surface with 10-19% third degree corrosion** `MCC` `H5` `HCC`

T32.92   **Corrosions involving 90% or more of body surface with 20-29% third degree corrosion** `MCC` `H5` `HCC`

T32.93   **Corrosions involving 90% or more of body surface with 30-39% third degree corrosion** `MCC` `H5` `HCC`

T32.94   **Corrosions involving 90% or more of body surface with 40-49% third degree corrosion** `MCC` `H5` `HCC`

T32.95   **Corrosions involving 90% or more of body surface with 50-59% third degree corrosion** `MCC` `H5` `HCC`

T32.96   **Corrosions involving 90% or more of body surface with 60-69% third degree corrosion** `MCC` `H5` `HCC`

T32.97   **Corrosions involving 90% or more of body surface with 70-79% third degree corrosion** `MCC` `H5` `HCC`

T32.98   **Corrosions involving 90% or more of body surface with 80-89% third degree corrosion** `MCC` `H5` `HCC`

T32.99   **Corrosions involving 90% or more of body surface with 90% or more third degree corrosion** `MCC` `H5` `HCC`

Frostbite (T33-T34)

`EXCLUDES 2`   *hypothermia and other effects of reduced temperature (T68, T69.-)*

√4th **T33**   **Superficial frostbite**

> `INCLUDES`   frostbite with partial thickness skin loss
>
> The appropriate 7th character is to be added to each code from category T33.
> A   initial encounter
> D   subsequent encounter
> S   sequela

√5th **T33.0**   **Superficial frostbite of head**

√6th **T33.01**   **Superficial frostbite of ear**

√7th **T33.011**   **Superficial frostbite of right ear** `CC` `H5`

√7th **T33.012**   **Superficial frostbite of left ear** `CC` `H5`

√7th **T33.019**   **Superficial frostbite of unspecified ear** `CC` `H5`

√x7th **T33.02**   **Superficial frostbite of nose** `CC` `H5`

√x7th **T33.09**   **Superficial frostbite of other part of head** `CC` `H5`

√x7th **T33.1**   **Superficial frostbite of neck** `CC` `H5`

√x7th **T33.2**   **Superficial frostbite of thorax** `CC` `H5`

√x7th **T33.3**   **Superficial frostbite of abdominal wall, lower back and pelvis** `CC` `H5`

√5th **T33.4**   **Superficial frostbite of arm**

> `EXCLUDES 2`   *superficial frostbite of wrist and hand (T33.5-)*

√x7th **T33.40**   **Superficial frostbite of unspecified arm** `CC` `H5`

√x7th **T33.41**   **Superficial frostbite of right arm** `CC` `H5`

√x7th **T33.42**   **Superficial frostbite of left arm** `CC` `H5`

√5th **T33.5**   **Superficial frostbite of wrist, hand, and fingers**

√6th **T33.51**   **Superficial frostbite of wrist**

√7th **T33.511**   **Superficial frostbite of right wrist** `CC` `H5`

√7th **T33.512**   **Superficial frostbite of left wrist** `CC` `H5`

√7th **T33.519**   **Superficial frostbite of unspecified wrist** `CC` `H5`

√6th **T33.52**   **Superficial frostbite of hand**

> `EXCLUDES 2`   *superficial frostbite of fingers (T33.53-)*

√7th **T33.521**   **Superficial frostbite of right hand** `CC` `H5`

√7th **T33.522**   **Superficial frostbite of left hand** `CC` `H5`

√7th **T33.529**   **Superficial frostbite of unspecified hand** `CC` `H5`

√6th **T33.53**   **Superficial frostbite of finger(s)**

√7th **T33.531**   **Superficial frostbite of right finger(s)** `CC` `H5`

√7th **T33.532**   **Superficial frostbite of left finger(s)** `CC` `H5`

√7th **T33.539**   **Superficial frostbite of unspecified finger(s)** `CC` `H5`

√5th **T33.6**   **Superficial frostbite of hip and thigh**

√x7th **T33.60**   **Superficial frostbite of unspecified hip and thigh** `CC` `H5`

√x7th **T33.61**   **Superficial frostbite of right hip and thigh** `CC` `H5`

√x7th **T33.62**   **Superficial frostbite of left hip and thigh** `CC` `H5`

√5th **T33.7**   **Superficial frostbite of knee and lower leg**

> `EXCLUDES 2`   *superficial frostbite of ankle and foot (T33.8-)*

√x7th **T33.70**   **Superficial frostbite of unspecified knee and lower leg** `CC` `H5`

√x7th **T33.71**   **Superficial frostbite of right knee and lower leg** `CC` `H5`

√x7th **T33.72**   **Superficial frostbite of left knee and lower leg** `CC` `H5`

√5th **T33.8**   **Superficial frostbite of ankle, foot, and toe(s)**

√6th **T33.81**   **Superficial frostbite of ankle**

√7th **T33.811**   **Superficial frostbite of right ankle** `CC` `H5`

√7th **T33.812**   **Superficial frostbite of left ankle** `CC` `H5`

`N` Newborn: 0   `P` Pediatric: 0-17   `M` Maternity: 9-64   `A` Adult: 15-124   `MCC` Major Complication/Comorbidity   `CC` Complication/Comorbidity   `SW` Severe Wound Dx

1110   ICD-10-CM 2022

√7ᵗʰ **T33.819** Superficial frostbite of unspecified ankle   CC H5

√6ᵗʰ **T33.82** Superficial frostbite of foot

    √7ᵗʰ T33.821 Superficial frostbite of right foot   CC H5

    √7ᵗʰ T33.822 Superficial frostbite of left foot   CC H5

    √7ᵗʰ **T33.829** Superficial frostbite of unspecified foot   CC H5

√6ᵗʰ **T33.83** Superficial frostbite of toe(s)

    √7ᵗʰ T33.831 Superficial frostbite of right toe(s)   CC H5

    √7ᵗʰ T33.832 Superficial frostbite of left toe(s)   CC H5

    √7ᵗʰ **T33.839** Superficial frostbite of unspecified toe(s)   CC H5

√5ᵗʰ **T33.9** Superficial frostbite of other and unspecified sites

    √7ᵗʰ **T33.90** Superficial frostbite of unspecified sites   CC H5
        Superficial frostbite NOS

    √x7ᵗʰ T33.99 Superficial frostbite of other sites   CC H5
        Superficial frostbite of leg NOS
        Superficial frostbite of trunk NOS

√4ᵗʰ **T34** Frostbite with tissue necrosis

> The appropriate 7th character is to be added to each code from category T34.
> A   initial encounter
> D   subsequent encounter
> S   sequela

√5ᵗʰ **T34.0** Frostbite with tissue necrosis of head

    √6ᵗʰ **T34.01** Frostbite with tissue necrosis of ear

       √7ᵗʰ T34.011 Frostbite with tissue necrosis of right ear   CC H5

       √7ᵗʰ T34.012 Frostbite with tissue necrosis of left ear   CC H5

       √7ᵗʰ **T34.019** Frostbite with tissue necrosis of unspecified ear   CC H5

    √x7ᵗʰ **T34.02** Frostbite with tissue necrosis of nose   CC H5

    √x7ᵗʰ **T34.09** Frostbite with tissue necrosis of other part of head   CC H5

√x7ᵗʰ **T34.1** Frostbite with tissue necrosis of neck   CC H5

√x7ᵗʰ **T34.2** Frostbite with tissue necrosis of thorax   CC H5

√x7ᵗʰ **T34.3** Frostbite with tissue necrosis of abdominal wall, lower back and pelvis   CC H5

√5ᵗʰ **T34.4** Frostbite with tissue necrosis of arm

    EXCLUDES 2   *frostbite with tissue necrosis of wrist and hand (T34.5-)*

    √x7ᵗʰ **T34.40** Frostbite with tissue necrosis of unspecified arm   CC H5

    √x7ᵗʰ **T34.41** Frostbite with tissue necrosis of right arm   CC H5

    √x7ᵗʰ **T34.42** Frostbite with tissue necrosis of left arm   CC H5

√5ᵗʰ **T34.5** Frostbite with tissue necrosis of wrist, hand, and finger(s)

    √6ᵗʰ **T34.51** Frostbite with tissue necrosis of wrist

       √7ᵗʰ T34.511 Frostbite with tissue necrosis of right wrist   CC H5

       √7ᵗʰ T34.512 Frostbite with tissue necrosis of left wrist   CC H5

       √7ᵗʰ **T34.519** Frostbite with tissue necrosis of unspecified wrist   CC H5

    √6ᵗʰ **T34.52** Frostbite with tissue necrosis of hand

       EXCLUDES 2   *frostbite with tissue necrosis of finger(s) (T34.53-)*

       √7ᵗʰ T34.521 Frostbite with tissue necrosis of right hand   CC H5

       √7ᵗʰ T34.522 Frostbite with tissue necrosis of left hand   CC H5

       √7ᵗʰ **T34.529** Frostbite with tissue necrosis of unspecified hand   CC H5

    √6ᵗʰ **T34.53** Frostbite with tissue necrosis of finger(s)

       √7ᵗʰ T34.531 Frostbite with tissue necrosis of right finger(s)   CC H5

       √7ᵗʰ T34.532 Frostbite with tissue necrosis of left finger(s)   CC H5

       √7ᵗʰ **T34.539** Frostbite with tissue necrosis of unspecified finger(s)   CC H5

√5ᵗʰ **T34.6** Frostbite with tissue necrosis of hip and thigh

    √x7ᵗʰ **T34.60** Frostbite with tissue necrosis of unspecified hip and thigh   CC H5

    √x7ᵗʰ **T34.61** Frostbite with tissue necrosis of right hip and thigh   CC H5

    √x7ᵗʰ **T34.62** Frostbite with tissue necrosis of left hip and thigh   CC H5

√5ᵗʰ **T34.7** Frostbite with tissue necrosis of knee and lower leg

    EXCLUDES 2   *frostbite with tissue necrosis of ankle and foot (T34.8-)*

    √x7ᵗʰ **T34.70** Frostbite with tissue necrosis of unspecified knee and lower leg   CC H5

    √x7ᵗʰ **T34.71** Frostbite with tissue necrosis of right knee and lower leg   CC H5

    √x7ᵗʰ **T34.72** Frostbite with tissue necrosis of left knee and lower leg   CC H5

√5ᵗʰ **T34.8** Frostbite with tissue necrosis of ankle, foot, and toe(s)

    √6ᵗʰ **T34.81** Frostbite with tissue necrosis of ankle

       √7ᵗʰ T34.811 Frostbite with tissue necrosis of right ankle   CC H5

       √7ᵗʰ T34.812 Frostbite with tissue necrosis of left ankle   CC H5

       √7ᵗʰ **T34.819** Frostbite with tissue necrosis of unspecified ankle   CC H5

    √6ᵗʰ **T34.82** Frostbite with tissue necrosis of foot

       √7ᵗʰ T34.821 Frostbite with tissue necrosis of right foot   CC H5

       √7ᵗʰ T34.822 Frostbite with tissue necrosis of left foot   CC H5

       √7ᵗʰ **T34.829** Frostbite with tissue necrosis of unspecified foot   CC H5

    √6ᵗʰ **T34.83** Frostbite with tissue necrosis of toe(s)

       √7ᵗʰ T34.831 Frostbite with tissue necrosis of right toe(s)   CC H5

       √7ᵗʰ T34.832 Frostbite with tissue necrosis of left toe(s)   CC H5

       √7ᵗʰ **T34.839** Frostbite with tissue necrosis of unspecified toe(s)   CC H5

√5ᵗʰ **T34.9** Frostbite with tissue necrosis of other and unspecified sites

    √x7ᵗʰ **T34.90** Frostbite with tissue necrosis of unspecified sites   CC H5
        Frostbite with tissue necrosis NOS

    √x7ᵗʰ **T34.99** Frostbite with tissue necrosis of other sites   CC H5
        Frostbite with tissue necrosis of leg NOS
        Frostbite with tissue necrosis of trunk NOS

☑ Additional Character Required   √x7ᵗʰ Placeholder   Questionable PDx   Manifestation   Unspecified Dx   UPD Unacceptable PDx   H1–H14 HAC   HCC CMS-HCC Dx   HIV HIV Dx

ICD-10-CM 2022   1111

Chapter 19. Injury, Poisoning and Certain Other Consequences of External Causes

Poisoning by, adverse effects of and underdosing of drugs, medicaments and biological substances (T36-T50)

INCLUDES adverse effect of correct substance properly administered
poisoning by overdose of substance
poisoning by wrong substance given or taken in error
underdosing by (inadvertently) (deliberately) taking less substance than prescribed or instructed

Code first, for adverse effects, the nature of the adverse effect, such as:
adverse effect NOS (T88.7)
aspirin gastritis (K29.-)
blood disorders (D56-D76)
contact dermatitis (L23-L25)
dermatitis due to substances taken internally (L27.-)
nephropathy (N14.0-N14.2)

NOTE The drug giving rise to the adverse effect should be identified by use of codes from categories T36-T50 with fifth or sixth character 5.

Use additional code(s) to specify:
manifestations of poisoning
underdosing or failure in dosage during medical and surgical care (Y63.6, Y63.8-Y63.9)
underdosing of medication regimen (Z91.12-, Z91.13-)

EXCLUDES 1 toxic reaction to local anesthesia in pregnancy (O29.3-)
EXCLUDES 2 abuse and dependence of psychoactive substances (F10-F19)
abuse of non-dependence-producing substances (F55.-)
drug reaction and poisoning affecting newborn (P00-P96)
immunodeficiency due to drugs (D84.821)
pathological drug intoxication (inebriation) (F10-F19)

AHA: 2018,4Q,71; 2016,2Q,8; 2015,3Q,22

√4ᵗʰ **T36 Poisoning by, adverse effect of and underdosing of systemic antibiotics**

EXCLUDES 1 antineoplastic antibiotics (T45.1-)
locally applied antibiotic NEC (T49.0)
topically used antibiotic for ear, nose and throat (T49.6)
topically used antibiotic for eye (T49.5)

> The appropriate 7th character is to be added to each code from category T36.
> A   initial encounter
> D   subsequent encounter
> S   sequela

√5ᵗʰ **T36.0 Poisoning by, adverse effect of and underdosing of penicillins**

√6ᵗʰ   **T36.0X Poisoning by, adverse effect of and underdosing of penicillins**

√7ᵗʰ   **T36.0X1 Poisoning by penicillins, accidental (unintentional)**
Poisoning by penicillins NOS

⁷ √7ᵗʰ **T36.0X2 Poisoning by penicillins, intentional self-harm** HCC

√7ᵗʰ   **T36.0X3 Poisoning by penicillins, assault**

√7ᵗʰ   **T36.0X4 Poisoning by penicillins, undetermined**

√7ᵗʰ   **T36.0X5 Adverse effect of penicillins** UPD

√7ᵗʰ   **T36.0X6 Underdosing of penicillins** UPD

√5ᵗʰ **T36.1 Poisoning by, adverse effect of and underdosing of cephalosporins and other beta-lactam antibiotics**

√6ᵗʰ   **T36.1X Poisoning by, adverse effect of and underdosing of cephalosporins and other beta-lactam antibiotics**

√7ᵗʰ   **T36.1X1 Poisoning by cephalosporins and other beta-lactam antibiotics, accidental (unintentional)**
Poisoning by cephalosporins and other beta-lactam antibiotics NOS

⁷ √7ᵗʰ **T36.1X2 Poisoning by cephalosporins and other beta-lactam antibiotics, intentional self-harm** HCC

√7ᵗʰ   **T36.1X3 Poisoning by cephalosporins and other beta-lactam antibiotics, assault**

√7ᵗʰ   **T36.1X4 Poisoning by cephalosporins and other beta-lactam antibiotics, undetermined**

√7ᵗʰ   **T36.1X5 Adverse effect of cephalosporins and other beta-lactam antibiotics** UPD

√7ᵗʰ   **T36.1X6 Underdosing of cephalosporins and other beta-lactam antibiotics** UPD

√5ᵗʰ **T36.2 Poisoning by, adverse effect of and underdosing of chloramphenicol group**

√6ᵗʰ   **T36.2X Poisoning by, adverse effect of and underdosing of chloramphenicol group**

√7ᵗʰ   **T36.2X1 Poisoning by chloramphenicol group, accidental (unintentional)**
Poisoning by chloramphenicol group NOS

⁷ √7ᵗʰ **T36.2X2 Poisoning by chloramphenicol group, intentional self-harm** HCC

√7ᵗʰ   **T36.2X3 Poisoning by chloramphenicol group, assault**

√7ᵗʰ   **T36.2X4 Poisoning by chloramphenicol group, undetermined**

√7ᵗʰ   **T36.2X5 Adverse effect of chloramphenicol group** UPD

√7ᵗʰ   **T36.2X6 Underdosing of chloramphenicol group** UPD

√5ᵗʰ **T36.3 Poisoning by, adverse effect of and underdosing of macrolides**

√6ᵗʰ   **T36.3X Poisoning by, adverse effect of and underdosing of macrolides**

√7ᵗʰ   **T36.3X1 Poisoning by macrolides, accidental (unintentional)**
Poisoning by macrolides NOS

⁷ √7ᵗʰ **T36.3X2 Poisoning by macrolides, intentional self-harm** HCC

√7ᵗʰ   **T36.3X3 Poisoning by macrolides, assault**

√7ᵗʰ   **T36.3X4 Poisoning by macrolides, undetermined**

√7ᵗʰ   **T36.3X5 Adverse effect of macrolides** UPD

√7ᵗʰ   **T36.3X6 Underdosing of macrolides** UPD

√5ᵗʰ **T36.4 Poisoning by, adverse effect of and underdosing of tetracyclines**

√6ᵗʰ   **T36.4X Poisoning by, adverse effect of and underdosing of tetracyclines**

√7ᵗʰ   **T36.4X1 Poisoning by tetracyclines, accidental (unintentional)**
Poisoning by tetracyclines NOS

⁷ √7ᵗʰ **T36.4X2 Poisoning by tetracyclines, intentional self-harm** HCC

√7ᵗʰ   **T36.4X3 Poisoning by tetracyclines, assault**

√7ᵗʰ   **T36.4X4 Poisoning by tetracyclines, undetermined**

√7ᵗʰ   **T36.4X5 Adverse effect of tetracyclines** UPD

√7ᵗʰ   **T36.4X6 Underdosing of tetracyclines** UPD

√5ᵗʰ **T36.5 Poisoning by, adverse effect of and underdosing of aminoglycosides**
Poisoning by, adverse effect of and underdosing of streptomycin

√6ᵗʰ   **T36.5X Poisoning by, adverse effect of and underdosing of aminoglycosides**

√7ᵗʰ   **T36.5X1 Poisoning by aminoglycosides, accidental (unintentional)**
Poisoning by aminoglycosides NOS

⁷ √7ᵗʰ **T36.5X2 Poisoning by aminoglycosides, intentional self-harm** HCC

√7ᵗʰ   **T36.5X3 Poisoning by aminoglycosides, assault**

√7ᵗʰ   **T36.5X4 Poisoning by aminoglycosides, undetermined**

√7ᵗʰ   **T36.5X5 Adverse effect of aminoglycosides** UPD

√7ᵗʰ   **T36.5X6 Underdosing of aminoglycosides** UPD

√5ᵗʰ **T36.6 Poisoning by, adverse effect of and underdosing of rifampicins**

√6ᵗʰ   **T36.6X Poisoning by, adverse effect of and underdosing of rifampicins**

√7ᵗʰ   **T36.6X1 Poisoning by rifampicins, accidental (unintentional)**
Poisoning by rifampicins NOS

⁷ √7ᵗʰ **T36.6X2 Poisoning by rifampicins, intentional self-harm** HCC

√7ᵗʰ   **T36.6X3 Poisoning by rifampicins, assault**

√7ᵗʰ   **T36.6X4 Poisoning by rifampicins, undetermined**

√7ᵗʰ   **T36.6X5 Adverse effect of rifampicins** UPD

√7ᵗʰ   **T36.6X6 Underdosing of rifampicins** UPD

√5ᵗʰ **T36.7 Poisoning by, adverse effect of and underdosing of antifungal antibiotics, systemically used**

√6ᵗʰ   **T36.7X Poisoning by, adverse effect of and underdosing of antifungal antibiotics, systemically used**

√7ᵗʰ   **T36.7X1 Poisoning by antifungal antibiotics, systemically used, accidental (unintentional)**
Poisoning by antifungal antibiotics, systemically used NOS

⁷ √7ᵗʰ **T36.7X2 Poisoning by antifungal antibiotics, systemically used, intentional self-harm** HCC

√7ᵗʰ   **T36.7X3 Poisoning by antifungal antibiotics, systemically used, assault**

Ⓝ Newborn: 0   Ⓟ Pediatric: 0-17   Ⓜ Maternity: 9-64   Ⓐ Adult: 15-124   **MCC** Major Complication/Comorbidity   **CC** Complication/Comorbidity   **SW** Severe Wound Dx

1112   ICD-10-CM 2022

√7ᵗʰ **T36.7X4** **Poisoning by antifungal antibiotics, systemically used,** undetermined

√7ᵗʰ **T36.7X5** Adverse effect **of antifungal antibiotics, systemically used** `UPD`

√7ᵗʰ **T36.7X6** Underdosing **of antifungal antibiotics, systemically used** `UPD`

√5ᵗʰ **T36.8** **Poisoning by, adverse effect of and underdosing of other systemic antibiotics**

√6ᵗʰ **T36.8X** **Poisoning by, adverse effect of and underdosing of other systemic antibiotics**
AHA: 2017,1Q,39

√7ᵗʰ **T36.8X1** **Poisoning by other systemic antibiotics,** accidental **(unintentional)**
Poisoning by other systemic antibiotics NOS

7 √7ᵗʰ **T36.8X2** **Poisoning by other systemic antibiotics,** intentional self-harm `HCC`

√7ᵗʰ **T36.8X3** **Poisoning by other systemic antibiotics,** assault

√7ᵗʰ **T36.8X4** **Poisoning by other systemic antibiotics,** undetermined

√7ᵗʰ **T36.8X5** Adverse effect **of other systemic antibiotics** `UPD`

√7ᵗʰ **T36.8X6** Underdosing **of other systemic antibiotics** `UPD`

√5ᵗʰ **T36.9** **Poisoning by, adverse effect of and underdosing of unspecified systemic antibiotic**

√x7ᵗʰ **T36.91** **Poisoning by unspecified systemic antibiotic,** accidental **(unintentional)**
Poisoning by systemic antibiotic NOS

7 √x7ᵗʰ **T36.92** **Poisoning by unspecified systemic antibiotic,** intentional self-harm `HCC`

√x7ᵗʰ **T36.93** **Poisoning by unspecified systemic antibiotic,** assault

√x7ᵗʰ **T36.94** **Poisoning by unspecified systemic antibiotic,** undetermined

√x7ᵗʰ **T36.95** Adverse effect **of unspecified systemic antibiotic** `UPD`

√x7ᵗʰ **T36.96** Underdosing **of unspecified systemic antibiotic** `UPD`

√4ᵗʰ **T37** **Poisoning by, adverse effect of and underdosing of other systemic anti-infectives and antiparasitics**

`EXCLUDES 1` *anti-infectives topically used for ear, nose and throat (T49.6-)*
anti-infectives topically used for eye (T49.5-)
locally applied anti-infectives NEC (T49.0-)

The appropriate 7th character is to be added to each code from category T37.
A   initial encounter
D   subsequent encounter
S   sequela

√5ᵗʰ **T37.0** **Poisoning by, adverse effect of and underdosing of sulfonamides**

√6ᵗʰ **T37.0X** **Poisoning by, adverse effect of and underdosing of sulfonamides**

√7ᵗʰ **T37.0X1** **Poisoning by sulfonamides,** accidental **(unintentional)**
Poisoning by sulfonamides NOS

7 √7ᵗʰ **T37.0X2** **Poisoning by sulfonamides,** intentional self-harm `HCC`

√7ᵗʰ **T37.0X3** **Poisoning by sulfonamides,** assault

√7ᵗʰ **T37.0X4** **Poisoning by sulfonamides,** undetermined

√7ᵗʰ **T37.0X5** Adverse effect **of sulfonamides** `UPD`

√7ᵗʰ **T37.0X6** Underdosing **of sulfonamides** `UPD`

√5ᵗʰ **T37.1** **Poisoning by, adverse effect of and underdosing of antimycobacterial drugs**

`EXCLUDES 1` *rifampicins (T36.6-)*
streptomycin (T36.5-)

√6ᵗʰ **T37.1X** **Poisoning by, adverse effect of and underdosing of antimycobacterial drugs**

√7ᵗʰ **T37.1X1** **Poisoning by antimycobacterial drugs,** accidental **(unintentional)**
Poisoning by antimycobacterial drugs NOS

7 √7ᵗʰ **T37.1X2** **Poisoning by antimycobacterial drugs,** intentional self-harm `HCC`

√7ᵗʰ **T37.1X3** **Poisoning by antimycobacterial drugs,** assault

√7ᵗʰ **T37.1X4** **Poisoning by antimycobacterial drugs,** undetermined

√7ᵗʰ **T37.1X5** Adverse effect **of antimycobacterial drugs** `UPD`

√7ᵗʰ **T37.1X6** Underdosing **of antimycobacterial drugs** `UPD`

√5ᵗʰ **T37.2** **Poisoning by, adverse effect of and underdosing of antimalarials and drugs acting on other blood protozoa**

`EXCLUDES 1` *hydroxyquinoline derivatives (T37.8-)*

√6ᵗʰ **T37.2X** **Poisoning by, adverse effect of and underdosing of antimalarials and drugs acting on other blood protozoa**

√7ᵗʰ **T37.2X1** **Poisoning by antimalarials and drugs acting on other blood protozoa,** accidental **(unintentional)**
Poisoning by antimalarials and drugs acting on other blood protozoa NOS

7 √7ᵗʰ **T37.2X2** **Poisoning by antimalarials and drugs acting on other blood protozoa,** intentional self-harm `HCC`

√7ᵗʰ **T37.2X3** **Poisoning by antimalarials and drugs acting on other blood protozoa,** assault

√7ᵗʰ **T37.2X4** **Poisoning by antimalarials and drugs acting on other blood protozoa,** undetermined

√7ᵗʰ **T37.2X5** Adverse effect **of antimalarials and drugs acting on other blood protozoa** `UPD`

√7ᵗʰ **T37.2X6** Underdosing **of antimalarials and drugs acting on other blood protozoa** `UPD`

√5ᵗʰ **T37.3** **Poisoning by, adverse effect of and underdosing of other antiprotozoal drugs**

√6ᵗʰ **T37.3X** **Poisoning by, adverse effect of and underdosing of other antiprotozoal drugs**

√7ᵗʰ **T37.3X1** **Poisoning by other antiprotozoal drugs,** accidental **(unintentional)**
Poisoning by other antiprotozoal drugs NOS

7 √7ᵗʰ **T37.3X2** **Poisoning by other antiprotozoal drugs,** intentional self-harm `HCC`

√7ᵗʰ **T37.3X3** **Poisoning by other antiprotozoal drugs,** assault

√7ᵗʰ **T37.3X4** **Poisoning by other antiprotozoal drugs,** undetermined

√7ᵗʰ **T37.3X5** Adverse effect **of other antiprotozoal drugs** `UPD`

√7ᵗʰ **T37.3X6** Underdosing **of other antiprotozoal drugs** `UPD`

√5ᵗʰ **T37.4** **Poisoning by, adverse effect of and underdosing of anthelminthics**

√6ᵗʰ **T37.4X** **Poisoning by, adverse effect of and underdosing of anthelminthics**

√7ᵗʰ **T37.4X1** **Poisoning by anthelminthics,** accidental **(unintentional)**
Poisoning by anthelminthics NOS

7 √7ᵗʰ **T37.4X2** **Poisoning by anthelminthics,** intentional self-harm `HCC`

√7ᵗʰ **T37.4X3** **Poisoning by anthelminthics,** assault

√7ᵗʰ **T37.4X4** **Poisoning by anthelminthics,** undetermined

√7ᵗʰ **T37.4X5** Adverse effect **of anthelminthics** `UPD`

√7ᵗʰ **T37.4X6** Underdosing **of anthelminthics** `UPD`

√5ᵗʰ **T37.5** **Poisoning by, adverse effect of and underdosing of antiviral drugs**

`EXCLUDES 1` *amantadine (T42.8-)*
cytarabine (T45.1-)

√6ᵗʰ **T37.5X** **Poisoning by, adverse effect of and underdosing of antiviral drugs**

√7ᵗʰ **T37.5X1** **Poisoning by antiviral drugs,** accidental **(unintentional)**
Poisoning by antiviral drugs NOS

7 √7ᵗʰ **T37.5X2** **Poisoning by antiviral drugs,** intentional self-harm `HCC`

√7ᵗʰ **T37.5X3** **Poisoning by antiviral drugs,** assault

√7ᵗʰ **T37.5X4** **Poisoning by antiviral drugs,** undetermined

√7ᵗʰ **T37.5X5** Adverse effect **of antiviral drugs** `UPD`

√7ᵗʰ **T37.5X6** Underdosing **of antiviral drugs** `UPD`

√5ᵗʰ **T37.8** **Poisoning by, adverse effect of and underdosing of other specified systemic anti-infectives and antiparasitics**
Poisoning by, adverse effect of and underdosing of hydroxyquinoline derivatives
EXCLUDES 1   *antimalarial drugs (T37.2-)*

√6ᵗʰ **T37.8X** **Poisoning by, adverse effect of and underdosing of other specified systemic anti-infectives and antiparasitics**

√7ᵗʰ **T37.8X1** **Poisoning by other specified systemic anti-infectives and antiparasitics, accidental (unintentional)**
Poisoning by other specified systemic anti-infectives and antiparasitics NOS

7 √7ᵗʰ **T37.8X2** **Poisoning by other specified systemic anti-infectives and antiparasitics, intentional self-harm**   HCC

√7ᵗʰ **T37.8X3** **Poisoning by other specified systemic anti-infectives and antiparasitics, assault**

√7ᵗʰ **T37.8X4** **Poisoning by other specified systemic anti-infectives and antiparasitics, undetermined**

√7ᵗʰ **T37.8X5** **Adverse effect of other specified systemic anti-infectives and antiparasitics**   UPD

√7ᵗʰ **T37.8X6** **Underdosing of other specified systemic anti-infectives and antiparasitics**   UPD

√5ᵗʰ **T37.9** **Poisoning by, adverse effect of and underdosing of unspecified systemic anti-infective and antiparasitics**

√x7ᵗʰ **T37.91** **Poisoning by unspecified systemic anti-infective and antiparasitics, accidental (unintentional)**
Poisoning by, adverse effect of and underdosing of systemic anti-infective and antiparasitics NOS

7 √x7ᵗʰ **T37.92** **Poisoning by unspecified systemic anti-infective and antiparasitics, intentional self-harm**   HCC

√x7ᵗʰ **T37.93** **Poisoning by unspecified systemic anti-infective and antiparasitics, assault**

√x7ᵗʰ **T37.94** **Poisoning by unspecified systemic anti-infective and antiparasitics, undetermined**

√x7ᵗʰ **T37.95** **Adverse effect of unspecified systemic anti-infective and antiparasitic**   UPD

√x7ᵗʰ **T37.96** **Underdosing of unspecified systemic anti-infectives and antiparasitics**   UPD

√4ᵗʰ **T38** **Poisoning by, adverse effect of and underdosing of hormones and their synthetic substitutes and antagonists, not elsewhere classified**
EXCLUDES 1   *mineralocorticoids and their antagonists (T50.0-)*
oxytocic hormones (T48.0-)
parathyroid hormones and derivatives (T50.9-)

> The appropriate 7th character is to be added to each code from category T38.
> A   initial encounter
> D   subsequent encounter
> S   sequela

√5ᵗʰ **T38.0** **Poisoning by, adverse effect of and underdosing of glucocorticoids and synthetic analogues**
EXCLUDES 1   *glucocorticoids, topically used (T49.-)*

√6ᵗʰ **T38.0X** **Poisoning by, adverse effect of and underdosing of glucocorticoids and synthetic analogues**

√7ᵗʰ **T38.0X1** **Poisoning by glucocorticoids and synthetic analogues, accidental (unintentional)**
Poisoning by glucocorticoids and synthetic analogues NOS

7 √7ᵗʰ **T38.0X2** **Poisoning by glucocorticoids and synthetic analogues, intentional self-harm**   HCC

√7ᵗʰ **T38.0X3** **Poisoning by glucocorticoids and synthetic analogues, assault**

√7ᵗʰ **T38.0X4** **Poisoning by glucocorticoids and synthetic analogues, undetermined**

√7ᵗʰ **T38.0X5** **Adverse effect of glucocorticoids and synthetic analogues**   UPD

√7ᵗʰ **T38.0X6** **Underdosing of glucocorticoids and synthetic analogues**   UPD

√5ᵗʰ **T38.1** **Poisoning by, adverse effect of and underdosing of thyroid hormones and substitutes**

√6ᵗʰ **T38.1X** **Poisoning by, adverse effect of and underdosing of thyroid hormones and substitutes**

√7ᵗʰ **T38.1X1** **Poisoning by thyroid hormones and substitutes, accidental (unintentional)**
Poisoning by thyroid hormones and substitutes NOS

7 √7ᵗʰ **T38.1X2** **Poisoning by thyroid hormones and substitutes, intentional self-harm**   HCC

√7ᵗʰ **T38.1X3** **Poisoning by thyroid hormones and substitutes, assault**

√7ᵗʰ **T38.1X4** **Poisoning by thyroid hormones and substitutes, undetermined**

√7ᵗʰ **T38.1X5** **Adverse effect of thyroid hormones and substitutes**   UPD

√7ᵗʰ **T38.1X6** **Underdosing of thyroid hormones and substitutes**   UPD

√5ᵗʰ **T38.2** **Poisoning by, adverse effect of and underdosing of antithyroid drugs**

√6ᵗʰ **T38.2X** **Poisoning by, adverse effect of and underdosing of antithyroid drugs**

√7ᵗʰ **T38.2X1** **Poisoning by antithyroid drugs, accidental (unintentional)**
Poisoning by antithyroid drugs NOS

7 √7ᵗʰ **T38.2X2** **Poisoning by antithyroid drugs, intentional self-harm**   HCC

√7ᵗʰ **T38.2X3** **Poisoning by antithyroid drugs, assault**

√7ᵗʰ **T38.2X4** **Poisoning by antithyroid drugs, undetermined**

√7ᵗʰ **T38.2X5** **Adverse effect of antithyroid drugs**   UPD

√7ᵗʰ **T38.2X6** **Underdosing of antithyroid drugs**   UPD

√5ᵗʰ **T38.3** **Poisoning by, adverse effect of and underdosing of insulin and oral hypoglycemic [antidiabetic] drugs**

√6ᵗʰ **T38.3X** **Poisoning by, adverse effect of and underdosing of insulin and oral hypoglycemic [antidiabetic] drugs**

√7ᵗʰ **T38.3X1** **Poisoning by insulin and oral hypoglycemic [antidiabetic] drugs, accidental (unintentional)**
Poisoning by insulin and oral hypoglycemic [antidiabetic] drugs NOS

7 √7ᵗʰ **T38.3X2** **Poisoning by insulin and oral hypoglycemic [antidiabetic] drugs, intentional self-harm**   HCC

√7ᵗʰ **T38.3X3** **Poisoning by insulin and oral hypoglycemic [antidiabetic] drugs, assault**

√7ᵗʰ **T38.3X4** **Poisoning by insulin and oral hypoglycemic [antidiabetic] drugs, undetermined**

√7ᵗʰ **T38.3X5** **Adverse effect of insulin and oral hypoglycemic [antidiabetic] drugs**   UPD

√7ᵗʰ **T38.3X6** **Underdosing of insulin and oral hypoglycemic [antidiabetic] drugs**   UPD

√5ᵗʰ **T38.4** **Poisoning by, adverse effect of and underdosing of oral contraceptives**
Poisoning by, adverse effect of and underdosing of multiple- and single-ingredient oral contraceptive preparations

√6ᵗʰ **T38.4X** **Poisoning by, adverse effect of and underdosing of oral contraceptives**

√7ᵗʰ **T38.4X1** **Poisoning by oral contraceptives, accidental (unintentional)**
Poisoning by oral contraceptives NOS

7 √7ᵗʰ **T38.4X2** **Poisoning by oral contraceptives, intentional self-harm**   HCC

√7ᵗʰ **T38.4X3** **Poisoning by oral contraceptives, assault**

√7ᵗʰ **T38.4X4** **Poisoning by oral contraceptives, undetermined**

√7ᵗʰ **T38.4X5** **Adverse effect of oral contraceptives**   UPD

√7ᵗʰ **T38.4X6** **Underdosing of oral contraceptives**   UPD

Ⓝ Newborn: 0   Ⓟ Pediatric: 0-17   Ⓜ Maternity: 9-64   Ⓐ Adult: 15-124   MCC Major Complication/Comorbidity   CC Complication/Comorbidity   SW Severe Wound Dx

1114   ICD-10-CM 2022

T37.8–T38.4X6

√5ᵗʰ **T38.5 Poisoning by, adverse effect of and underdosing of other estrogens and progestogens**
Poisoning by, adverse effect of and underdosing of estrogens and progestogens mixtures and substitutes

√6ᵗʰ **T38.5X Poisoning by, adverse effect of and underdosing of other estrogens and progestogens**

√7ᵗʰ **T38.5X1 Poisoning by other estrogens and progestogens, accidental (unintentional)**
Poisoning by other estrogens and progestogens NOS

7 √7ᵗʰ **T38.5X2 Poisoning by other estrogens and progestogens, intentional self-harm** HCC

√7ᵗʰ **T38.5X3 Poisoning by other estrogens and progestogens, assault**

√7ᵗʰ **T38.5X4 Poisoning by other estrogens and progestogens, undetermined**

√7ᵗʰ **T38.5X5 Adverse effect of other estrogens and progestogens** UPD

√7ᵗʰ **T38.5X6 Underdosing of other estrogens and progestogens** UPD

√5ᵗʰ **T38.6 Poisoning by, adverse effect of and underdosing of antigonadotrophins, antiestrogens, antiandrogens, not elsewhere classified**
Poisoning by, adverse effect of and underdosing of tamoxifen

√6ᵗʰ **T38.6X Poisoning by, adverse effect of and underdosing of antigonadotrophins, antiestrogens, antiandrogens, not elsewhere classified**

√7ᵗʰ **T38.6X1 Poisoning by antigonadotrophins, antiestrogens, antiandrogens, not elsewhere classified, accidental (unintentional)**
Poisoning by antigonadotrophins, antiestrogens, antiandrogens, not elsewhere classified NOS

7 √7ᵗʰ **T38.6X2 Poisoning by antigonadotrophins, antiestrogens, antiandrogens, not elsewhere classified, intentional self-harm** HCC

√7ᵗʰ **T38.6X3 Poisoning by antigonadotrophins, antiestrogens, antiandrogens, not elsewhere classified, assault**

√7ᵗʰ **T38.6X4 Poisoning by antigonadotrophins, antiestrogens, antiandrogens, not elsewhere classified, undetermined**

√7ᵗʰ **T38.6X5 Adverse effect of antigonadotrophins, antiestrogens, antiandrogens, not elsewhere classified** UPD

√7ᵗʰ **T38.6X6 Underdosing of antigonadotrophins, antiestrogens, antiandrogens, not elsewhere classified** UPD

√5ᵗʰ **T38.7 Poisoning by, adverse effect of and underdosing of androgens and anabolic congeners**

√6ᵗʰ **T38.7X Poisoning by, adverse effect of and underdosing of androgens and anabolic congeners**

√7ᵗʰ **T38.7X1 Poisoning by androgens and anabolic congeners, accidental (unintentional)**
Poisoning by androgens and anabolic congeners NOS

7 √7ᵗʰ **T38.7X2 Poisoning by androgens and anabolic congeners, intentional self-harm** HCC

√7ᵗʰ **T38.7X3 Poisoning by androgens and anabolic congeners, assault**

√7ᵗʰ **T38.7X4 Poisoning by androgens and anabolic congeners, undetermined**

√7ᵗʰ **T38.7X5 Adverse effect of androgens and anabolic congeners** UPD

√7ᵗʰ **T38.7X6 Underdosing of androgens and anabolic congeners** UPD

√5ᵗʰ **T38.8 Poisoning by, adverse effect of and underdosing of other and unspecified hormones and synthetic substitutes**

√6ᵗʰ **T38.80 Poisoning by, adverse effect of and underdosing of unspecified hormones and synthetic substitutes**

√7ᵗʰ **T38.801 Poisoning by unspecified hormones and synthetic substitutes, accidental (unintentional)**
Poisoning by unspecified hormones and synthetic substitutes NOS

7 √7ᵗʰ **T38.802 Poisoning by unspecified hormones and synthetic substitutes, intentional self-harm** HCC

√7ᵗʰ **T38.803 Poisoning by unspecified hormones and synthetic substitutes, assault**

√7ᵗʰ **T38.804 Poisoning by unspecified hormones and synthetic substitutes, undetermined**

√7ᵗʰ **T38.805 Adverse effect of unspecified hormones and synthetic substitutes** UPD

√7ᵗʰ **T38.806 Underdosing of unspecified hormones and synthetic substitutes** UPD

√6ᵗʰ **T38.81 Poisoning by, adverse effect of and underdosing of anterior pituitary [adenohypophyseal] hormones**

√7ᵗʰ **T38.811 Poisoning by anterior pituitary [adenohypophyseal] hormones, accidental (unintentional)**
Poisoning by anterior pituitary [adenohypophyseal] hormones NOS

7 √7ᵗʰ **T38.812 Poisoning by anterior pituitary [adenohypophyseal] hormones, intentional self-harm** HCC

√7ᵗʰ **T38.813 Poisoning by anterior pituitary [adenohypophyseal] hormones, assault**

√7ᵗʰ **T38.814 Poisoning by anterior pituitary [adenohypophyseal] hormones, undetermined**

√7ᵗʰ **T38.815 Adverse effect of anterior pituitary [adenohypophyseal] hormones** UPD

√7ᵗʰ **T38.816 Underdosing of anterior pituitary [adenohypophyseal] hormones** UPD

√6ᵗʰ **T38.89 Poisoning by, adverse effect of and underdosing of other hormones and synthetic substitutes**

√7ᵗʰ **T38.891 Poisoning by other hormones and synthetic substitutes, accidental (unintentional)**
Poisoning by other hormones and synthetic substitutes NOS

7 √7ᵗʰ **T38.892 Poisoning by other hormones and synthetic substitutes, intentional self-harm** HCC

√7ᵗʰ **T38.893 Poisoning by other hormones and synthetic substitutes, assault**

√7ᵗʰ **T38.894 Poisoning by other hormones and synthetic substitutes, undetermined**

√7ᵗʰ **T38.895 Adverse effect of other hormones and synthetic substitutes** UPD

√7ᵗʰ **T38.896 Underdosing of other hormones and synthetic substitutes** UPD

√5ᵗʰ **T38.9 Poisoning by, adverse effect of and underdosing of other and unspecified hormone antagonists**

√6ᵗʰ **T38.90 Poisoning by, adverse effect of and underdosing of unspecified hormone antagonists**

√7ᵗʰ **T38.901 Poisoning by unspecified hormone antagonists, accidental (unintentional)**
Poisoning by unspecified hormone antagonists NOS

7 √7ᵗʰ **T38.902 Poisoning by unspecified hormone antagonists, intentional self-harm** HCC

√7ᵗʰ **T38.903 Poisoning by unspecified hormone antagonists, assault**

√7ᵗʰ **T38.904 Poisoning by unspecified hormone antagonists, undetermined**

√7ᵗʰ **T38.905 Adverse effect of unspecified hormone antagonists** UPD

√7ᵗʰ **T38.906 Underdosing of unspecified hormone antagonists** UPD

√6ᵗʰ **T38.99 Poisoning by, adverse effect of and underdosing of other hormone antagonists**

√7ᵗʰ **T38.991 Poisoning by other hormone antagonists, accidental (unintentional)**
Poisoning by other hormone antagonists NOS

7 √7ᵗʰ **T38.992 Poisoning by other hormone antagonists, intentional self-harm** HCC

√7ᵗʰ **T38.993 Poisoning by other hormone antagonists, assault**

√7ᵗʰ **T38.994 Poisoning by other hormone antagonists, undetermined**

√7ᵗʰ **T38.995 Adverse effect of other hormone antagonists** UPD

√7ᵗʰ **T38.996 Underdosing of other hormone antagonists** UPD

Chapter 19. Injury, Poisoning and Certain Other Consequences of External Causes

T38.5–T38.996

✓4th T39 Poisoning by, adverse effect of and underdosing of nonopioid analgesics, antipyretics and antirheumatics

> The appropriate 7th character is to be added to each code from category T39.
> A   initial encounter
> D   subsequent encounter
> S   sequela

✓5th T39.0 Poisoning by, adverse effect of and underdosing of salicylates

     ✓6th T39.01 Poisoning by, adverse effect of and underdosing of aspirin

         Poisoning by, adverse effect of and underdosing of acetylsalicylic acid

         ✓7th T39.011 Poisoning by aspirin, accidental (unintentional)

         ⁷ ✓7th T39.012 Poisoning by aspirin, intentional self-harm `HCC`

         ✓7th T39.013 Poisoning by aspirin, assault

         ✓7th T39.014 Poisoning by aspirin, undetermined

         ✓7th T39.015 Adverse effect of aspirin `UPD`

           AHA: 2016,1Q,15

         ✓7th T39.016 Underdosing of aspirin `UPD`

     ✓6th T39.09 Poisoning by, adverse effect of and underdosing of other salicylates

         ✓7th T39.091 Poisoning by salicylates, accidental (unintentional)

           Poisoning by salicylates NOS

         ⁷ ✓7th T39.092 Poisoning by salicylates, intentional self-harm `HCC`

         ✓7th T39.093 Poisoning by salicylates, assault

         ✓7th T39.094 Poisoning by salicylates, undetermined

         ✓7th T39.095 Adverse effect of salicylates `UPD`

         ✓7th T39.096 Underdosing of salicylates `UPD`

✓5th T39.1 Poisoning by, adverse effect of and underdosing of 4-Aminophenol derivatives

     ✓6th T39.1X Poisoning by, adverse effect of and underdosing of 4-Aminophenol derivatives

         ✓7th T39.1X1 Poisoning by 4-Aminophenol derivatives, accidental (unintentional)

           Poisoning by 4-Aminophenol derivatives NOS

         ⁷ ✓7th T39.1X2 Poisoning by 4-Aminophenol derivatives, intentional self-harm `HCC`

         ✓7th T39.1X3 Poisoning by 4-Aminophenol derivatives, assault

         ✓7th T39.1X4 Poisoning by 4-Aminophenol derivatives, undetermined

         ✓7th T39.1X5 Adverse effect of 4-Aminophenol derivatives `UPD`

         ✓7th T39.1X6 Underdosing of 4-Aminophenol derivatives `UPD`

✓5th T39.2 Poisoning by, adverse effect of and underdosing of pyrazolone derivatives

     ✓6th T39.2X Poisoning by, adverse effect of and underdosing of pyrazolone derivatives

         ✓7th T39.2X1 Poisoning by pyrazolone derivatives, accidental (unintentional)

           Poisoning by pyrazolone derivatives NOS

         ⁷ ✓7th T39.2X2 Poisoning by pyrazolone derivatives, intentional self-harm `HCC`

         ✓7th T39.2X3 Poisoning by pyrazolone derivatives, assault

         ✓7th T39.2X4 Poisoning by pyrazolone derivatives, undetermined

         ✓7th T39.2X5 Adverse effect of pyrazolone derivatives `UPD`

         ✓7th T39.2X6 Underdosing of pyrazolone derivatives `UPD`

✓5th T39.3 Poisoning by, adverse effect of and underdosing of other nonsteroidal anti-inflammatory drugs [NSAID]

     ✓6th T39.31 Poisoning by, adverse effect of and underdosing of propionic acid derivatives

         Poisoning by, adverse effect of and underdosing of fenoprofen

         Poisoning by, adverse effect of and underdosing of flurbiprofen

         Poisoning by, adverse effect of and underdosing of ibuprofen

         Poisoning by, adverse effect of and underdosing of ketoprofen

         Poisoning by, adverse effect of and underdosing of naproxen

         Poisoning by, adverse effect of and underdosing of oxaprozin

         ✓7th T39.311 Poisoning by propionic acid derivatives, accidental (unintentional)

         ⁷ ✓7th T39.312 Poisoning by propionic acid derivatives, intentional self-harm `HCC`

         ✓7th T39.313 Poisoning by propionic acid derivatives, assault

         ✓7th T39.314 Poisoning by propionic acid derivatives, undetermined

         ✓7th T39.315 Adverse effect of propionic acid derivatives `UPD`

         ✓7th T39.316 Underdosing of propionic acid derivatives `UPD`

     ✓6th T39.39 Poisoning by, adverse effect of and underdosing of other nonsteroidal anti-inflammatory drugs [NSAID]

         ✓7th T39.391 Poisoning by other nonsteroidal anti-inflammatory drugs [NSAID], accidental (unintentional)

           Poisoning by other nonsteroidal anti-inflammatory drugs NOS

         ⁷ ✓7th T39.392 Poisoning by other nonsteroidal anti-inflammatory drugs [NSAID], intentional self-harm `HCC`

         ✓7th T39.393 Poisoning by other nonsteroidal anti-inflammatory drugs [NSAID], assault

         ✓7th T39.394 Poisoning by other nonsteroidal anti-inflammatory drugs [NSAID], undetermined

         ✓7th T39.395 Adverse effect of other nonsteroidal anti-inflammatory drugs [NSAID] `UPD`

         ✓7th T39.396 Underdosing of other nonsteroidal anti-inflammatory drugs [NSAID] `UPD`

✓5th T39.4 Poisoning by, adverse effect of and underdosing of antirheumatics, not elsewhere classified

     `EXCLUDES 1` poisoning by, adverse effect of and underdosing of glucocorticoids (T38.0-)

         poisoning by, adverse effect of and underdosing of salicylates (T39.0-)

     ✓6th T39.4X Poisoning by, adverse effect of and underdosing of antirheumatics, not elsewhere classified

         ✓7th T39.4X1 Poisoning by antirheumatics, not elsewhere classified, accidental (unintentional)

           Poisoning by antirheumatics, not elsewhere classified NOS

         ⁷ ✓7th T39.4X2 Poisoning by antirheumatics, not elsewhere classified, intentional self-harm `HCC`

         ✓7th T39.4X3 Poisoning by antirheumatics, not elsewhere classified, assault

         ✓7th T39.4X4 Poisoning by antirheumatics, not elsewhere classified, undetermined

         ✓7th T39.4X5 Adverse effect of antirheumatics, not elsewhere classified `UPD`

         ✓7th T39.4X6 Underdosing of antirheumatics, not elsewhere classified `UPD`

Ⓝ Newborn: 0   Ⓟ Pediatric: 0-17   Ⓜ Maternity: 9-64   Ⓐ Adult: 15-124   `MCC` Major Complication/Comorbidity   `CC` Complication/Comorbidity   `SW` Severe Wound Dx

1116   ICD-10-CM 2022

√5ᵗʰ T39.8 Poisoning by, adverse effect of and underdosing of other nonopioid analgesics and antipyretics, not elsewhere classified
- **√6ᵗʰ T39.8X Poisoning by, adverse effect of and underdosing of other nonopioid analgesics and antipyretics, not elsewhere classified**
  - **√7ᵗʰ T39.8X1 Poisoning by other nonopioid analgesics and antipyretics, not elsewhere classified, accidental (unintentional)**
    Poisoning by other nonopioid analgesics and antipyretics, not elsewhere classified NOS
  - **⁷ √7ᵗʰ T39.8X2 Poisoning by other nonopioid analgesics and antipyretics, not elsewhere classified, intentional self-harm** `HCC`
  - **√7ᵗʰ T39.8X3 Poisoning by other nonopioid analgesics and antipyretics, not elsewhere classified, assault**
  - **√7ᵗʰ T39.8X4 Poisoning by other nonopioid analgesics and antipyretics, not elsewhere classified, undetermined**
  - **√7ᵗʰ T39.8X5 Adverse effect of other nonopioid analgesics and antipyretics, not elsewhere classified** `UPD`
  - **√7ᵗʰ T39.8X6 Underdosing of other nonopioid analgesics and antipyretics, not elsewhere classified** `UPD`

√5ᵗʰ T39.9 Poisoning by, adverse effect of and underdosing of unspecified nonopioid analgesic, antipyretic and antirheumatic
- **√x7ᵗʰ T39.91 Poisoning by unspecified nonopioid analgesic, antipyretic and antirheumatic, accidental (unintentional)**
  Poisoning by nonopioid analgesic, antipyretic and antirheumatic NOS
- **⁷ √x7ᵗʰ T39.92 Poisoning by unspecified nonopioid analgesic, antipyretic and antirheumatic, intentional self-harm** `HCC`
- **√x7ᵗʰ T39.93 Poisoning by unspecified nonopioid analgesic, antipyretic and antirheumatic, assault**
- **√x7ᵗʰ T39.94 Poisoning by unspecified nonopioid analgesic, antipyretic and antirheumatic, undetermined**
- **√x7ᵗʰ T39.95 Adverse effect of unspecified nonopioid analgesic, antipyretic and antirheumatic** `UPD`
- **√x7ᵗʰ T39.96 Underdosing of unspecified nonopioid analgesic, antipyretic and antirheumatic** `UPD`

√4ᵗʰ T40 Poisoning by, adverse effect of and underdosing of narcotics and psychodysleptics [hallucinogens]
> `EXCLUDES 2` drug dependence and related mental and behavioral disorders due to psychoactive substance use (F10.-F19.-)

> The appropriate 7th character is to be added to each code from category T40.
> A   initial encounter
> D   subsequent encounter
> S   sequela

√5ᵗʰ T40.0 Poisoning by, adverse effect of and underdosing of opium
- **√6ᵗʰ T40.0X Poisoning by, adverse effect of and underdosing of opium**
  - **⁶ √7ᵗʰ T40.0X1 Poisoning by opium, accidental (unintentional)** `HCC`
    Poisoning by opium NOS
  - **⁷ √7ᵗʰ T40.0X2 Poisoning by opium, intentional self-harm** `HCC`
  - **√7ᵗʰ T40.0X3 Poisoning by opium, assault**
  - **⁶ √7ᵗʰ T40.0X4 Poisoning by opium, undetermined** `HCC`
  - **√7ᵗʰ T40.0X5 Adverse effect of opium** `UPD`
  - **√7ᵗʰ T40.0X6 Underdosing of opium** `UPD`

√5ᵗʰ T40.1 Poisoning by and adverse effect of heroin
- **√6ᵗʰ T40.1X Poisoning by and adverse effect of heroin**
  - **⁶ √7ᵗʰ T40.1X1 Poisoning by heroin, accidental (unintentional)** `HCC`
    Poisoning by heroin NOS
  - **⁷ √7ᵗʰ T40.1X2 Poisoning by heroin, intentional self-harm** `HCC`
  - **√7ᵗʰ T40.1X3 Poisoning by heroin, assault**
  - **⁶ √7ᵗʰ T40.1X4 Poisoning by heroin, undetermined** `HCC`

√5ᵗʰ T40.2 Poisoning by, adverse effect of and underdosing of other opioids
- **√6ᵗʰ T40.2X Poisoning by, adverse effect of and underdosing of other opioids**
  - **⁶ √7ᵗʰ T40.2X1 Poisoning by other opioids, accidental (unintentional)** `HCC`
    Poisoning by other opioids NOS
  - **⁷ √7ᵗʰ T40.2X2 Poisoning by other opioids, intentional self-harm** `HCC`
  - **√7ᵗʰ T40.2X3 Poisoning by other opioids, assault**
  - **⁶ √7ᵗʰ T40.2X4 Poisoning by other opioids, undetermined** `HCC`
  - **√7ᵗʰ T40.2X5 Adverse effect of other opioids** `UPD`
    AHA: 2020,2Q,24
  - **√7ᵗʰ T40.2X6 Underdosing of other opioids** `UPD`

√5ᵗʰ T40.3 Poisoning by, adverse effect of and underdosing of methadone
- **√6ᵗʰ T40.3X Poisoning by, adverse effect of and underdosing of methadone**
  - **⁶ √7ᵗʰ T40.3X1 Poisoning by methadone, accidental (unintentional)** `HCC`
    Poisoning by methadone NOS
  - **⁷ √7ᵗʰ T40.3X2 Poisoning by methadone, intentional self-harm** `HCC`
  - **√7ᵗʰ T40.3X3 Poisoning by methadone, assault**
  - **⁶ √7ᵗʰ T40.3X4 Poisoning by methadone, undetermined** `HCC`
  - **√7ᵗʰ T40.3X5 Adverse effect of methadone** `UPD`
  - **√7ᵗʰ T40.3X6 Underdosing of methadone** `UPD`

√5ᵗʰ T40.4 Poisoning by, adverse effect of and underdosing of other synthetic narcotics
AHA: 2020,4Q,40
- **√6ᵗʰ T40.41 Poisoning by, adverse effect of and underdosing of fentanyl or fentanyl analogs**
  - **√7ᵗʰ T40.411 Poisoning by fentanyl or fentanyl analogs, accidental (unintentional)** `HCC`
  - **√7ᵗʰ T40.412 Poisoning by fentanyl or fentanyl analogs, intentional self-harm** `HCC`
  - **√7ᵗʰ T40.413 Poisoning by fentanyl or fentanyl analogs, assault**
  - **√7ᵗʰ T40.414 Poisoning by fentanyl or fentanyl analogs, undetermined** `HCC`
  - **√7ᵗʰ T40.415 Adverse effect of fentanyl or fentanyl analogs** `UPD`
  - **√7ᵗʰ T40.416 Underdosing of fentanyl or fentanyl analogs** `UPD`
- **√6ᵗʰ T40.42 Poisoning by, adverse effect of and underdosing of tramadol**
  - **√7ᵗʰ T40.421 Poisoning by tramadol, accidental (unintentional)** `HCC`
  - **√7ᵗʰ T40.422 Poisoning by tramadol, intentional self-harm** `HCC`
  - **√7ᵗʰ T40.423 Poisoning by tramadol, assault**
  - **√7ᵗʰ T40.424 Poisoning by tramadol, undetermined** `HCC`
  - **√7ᵗʰ T40.425 Adverse effect of tramadol** `UPD`
  - **√7ᵗʰ T40.426 Underdosing of tramadol** `UPD`
- **√6ᵗʰ T40.49 Poisoning by, adverse effect of and underdosing of other synthetic narcotics**
  - **√7ᵗʰ T40.491 Poisoning by other synthetic narcotics, accidental (unintentional)** `HCC`
  - **√7ᵗʰ T40.492 Poisoning by other synthetic narcotics, intentional self-harm** `HCC`
  - **√7ᵗʰ T40.493 Poisoning by other synthetic narcotics, assault**
  - **√7ᵗʰ T40.494 Poisoning by other synthetic narcotics, undetermined** `HCC`
  - **√7ᵗʰ T40.495 Adverse effect of other synthetic narcotics** `UPD`
  - **√7ᵗʰ T40.496 Underdosing of other synthetic narcotics** `UPD`

✔ Additional Character Required   √x7ᵗʰ Placeholder   Questionable PDx   Manifestation   Unspecified Dx   `UPD` Unacceptable PDx   H1-H14 HAC   `HCC` CMS-HCC Dx   `HIV` HIV Dx

ICD-10-CM 2022   1117

√5ᵗʰ T40.5 Poisoning by, adverse effect of and underdosing of cocaine

    √6ᵗʰ T40.5X Poisoning by, adverse effect of and underdosing of cocaine

        6 √7ᵗʰ **T40.5X1 Poisoning by cocaine, accidental (unintentional)** HCC
            Poisoning by cocaine NOS
            AHA: 2016,2Q,8

        7 √7ᵗʰ **T40.5X2 Poisoning by cocaine, intentional self-harm** HCC

        √7ᵗʰ **T40.5X3 Poisoning by cocaine, assault**

        6 √7ᵗʰ **T40.5X4 Poisoning by cocaine, undetermined** HCC

        √7ᵗʰ **T40.5X5 Adverse effect of cocaine** UPD

        √7ᵗʰ **T40.5X6 Underdosing of cocaine** UPD

√5ᵗʰ T40.6 Poisoning by, adverse effect of and underdosing of other and unspecified narcotics

    √6ᵗʰ T40.60 Poisoning by, adverse effect of and underdosing of unspecified narcotics

        6 √7ᵗʰ **T40.601 Poisoning by unspecified narcotics, accidental (unintentional)** HCC
            Poisoning by narcotics NOS

        7 √7ᵗʰ **T40.602 Poisoning by unspecified narcotics, intentional self-harm** HCC

        √7ᵗʰ **T40.603 Poisoning by unspecified narcotics, assault**

        6 √7ᵗʰ **T40.604 Poisoning by unspecified narcotics, undetermined** HCC

        √7ᵗʰ **T40.605 Adverse effect of unspecified narcotics** UPD

        √7ᵗʰ **T40.606 Underdosing of unspecified narcotics** UPD

    √6ᵗʰ T40.69 Poisoning by, adverse effect of and underdosing of other narcotics

        6 √7ᵗʰ **T40.691 Poisoning by other narcotics, accidental (unintentional)** HCC
            Poisoning by other narcotics NOS

        7 √7ᵗʰ **T40.692 Poisoning by other narcotics, intentional self-harm** HCC

        √7ᵗʰ **T40.693 Poisoning by other narcotics, assault**

        6 √7ᵗʰ **T40.694 Poisoning by other narcotics, undetermined** HCC

        √7ᵗʰ **T40.695 Adverse effect of other narcotics** UPD

        √7ᵗʰ **T40.696 Underdosing of other narcotics** UPD

√5ᵗʰ T40.7 Poisoning by, adverse effect of and underdosing of cannabis (derivatives)

    ~~T40.7X Poisoning by, adverse effect of and underdosing of cannabis (derivatives)~~

        ~~T40.7X1 Poisoning by cannabis (derivatives), accidental (unintentional)~~

        ~~T40.7X2 Poisoning by cannabis (derivatives), intentional self-harm~~

        ~~T40.7X3 Poisoning by cannabis (derivatives), assault~~

        ~~T40.7X4 Poisoning by cannabis (derivatives), undetermined~~

        ~~T40.7X5 Adverse effect of cannabis (derivatives)~~

        ~~T40.7X6 Underdosing of cannabis (derivatives)~~

    √6ᵗʰ T40.71 Poisoning by, adverse effect of and underdosing of cannabis (derivatives)

        √7ᵗʰ **T40.711 Poisoning by cannabis, accidental (unintentional)**

        √7ᵗʰ **T40.712 Poisoning by cannabis, intentional self-harm**

        √7ᵗʰ **T40.713 Poisoning by cannabis, assault**

        √7ᵗʰ **T40.714 Poisoning by cannabis, undetermined**

        √7ᵗʰ **T40.715 Adverse effect of cannabis**

        √7ᵗʰ **T40.716 Underdosing of cannabis**

    √6ᵗʰ T40.72 Poisoning by, adverse effect of and underdosing of synthetic cannabinoids

        √7ᵗʰ **T40.721 Poisoning by synthetic cannabinoids, accidental (unintentional)**

        √7ᵗʰ **T40.722 Poisoning by synthetic cannabinoids, intentional self-harm**

        √7ᵗʰ **T40.723 Poisoning by synthetic cannabinoids, assault**

        √7ᵗʰ **T40.724 Poisoning by synthetic cannabinoids, undetermined**

        √7ᵗʰ **T40.725 Adverse effect of synthetic cannabinoids**

        √7ᵗʰ **T40.726 Underdosing of synthetic cannabinoids**

√5ᵗʰ T40.8 Poisoning by and adverse effect of lysergide [LSD]

    √6ᵗʰ T40.8X Poisoning by and adverse effect of lysergide [LSD]

        6 √7ᵗʰ **T40.8X1 Poisoning by lysergide [LSD], accidental (unintentional)** HCC
            Poisoning by lysergide [LSD] NOS

        7 √7ᵗʰ **T40.8X2 Poisoning by lysergide [LSD], intentional self-harm** HCC

        √7ᵗʰ **T40.8X3 Poisoning by lysergide [LSD], assault**

        6 √7ᵗʰ **T40.8X4 Poisoning by lysergide [LSD], undetermined** HCC

√5ᵗʰ T40.9 Poisoning by, adverse effect of and underdosing of other and unspecified psychodysleptics [hallucinogens]

    √6ᵗʰ T40.90 Poisoning by, adverse effect of and underdosing of unspecified psychodysleptics [hallucinogens]

        6 √7ᵗʰ **T40.901 Poisoning by unspecified psychodysleptics [hallucinogens], accidental (unintentional)** HCC

        7 √7ᵗʰ **T40.902 Poisoning by unspecified psychodysleptics [hallucinogens], intentional self-harm** HCC

        √7ᵗʰ **T40.903 Poisoning by unspecified psychodysleptics [hallucinogens], assault**

        6 √7ᵗʰ **T40.904 Poisoning by unspecified psychodysleptics [hallucinogens], undetermined** HCC

        √7ᵗʰ **T40.905 Adverse effect of unspecified psychodysleptics [hallucinogens]** UPD

        √7ᵗʰ **T40.906 Underdosing of unspecified psychodysleptics [hallucinogens]** UPD

    √6ᵗʰ T40.99 Poisoning by, adverse effect of and underdosing of other psychodysleptics [hallucinogens]

        6 √7ᵗʰ **T40.991 Poisoning by other psychodysleptics [hallucinogens], accidental (unintentional)** HCC
            Poisoning by other psychodysleptics [hallucinogens] NOS

        7 √7ᵗʰ **T40.992 Poisoning by other psychodysleptics [hallucinogens], intentional self-harm** HCC

        √7ᵗʰ **T40.993 Poisoning by other psychodysleptics [hallucinogens], assault**

        6 √7ᵗʰ **T40.994 Poisoning by other psychodysleptics [hallucinogens], undetermined** HCC

        √7ᵗʰ **T40.995 Adverse effect of other psychodysleptics [hallucinogens]** UPD

        √7ᵗʰ **T40.996 Underdosing of other psychodysleptics [hallucinogens]** UPD

√4ᵗʰ T41 Poisoning by, adverse effect of and underdosing of anesthetics and therapeutic gases

    EXCLUDES 1   *benzodiazepines (T42.4-)*
               cocaine (T40.5-)
               complications of anesthesia during labor and delivery (O74.-)
               complications of anesthesia during pregnancy (O29.-)
               complications of anesthesia during the puerperium (O89.-)
               opioids (T40.0-T40.2-)

> The appropriate 7th character is to be added to each code from category T41.
> A   initial encounter
> D   subsequent encounter
> S   sequela

√5ᵗʰ T41.0 Poisoning by, adverse effect of and underdosing of inhaled anesthetics

    EXCLUDES 1   *oxygen (T41.5-)*

    √6ᵗʰ T41.0X Poisoning by, adverse effect of and underdosing of inhaled anesthetics

        √7ᵗʰ **T41.0X1 Poisoning by inhaled anesthetics, accidental (unintentional)**
            Poisoning by inhaled anesthetics NOS

        7 √7ᵗʰ **T41.0X2 Poisoning by inhaled anesthetics, intentional self-harm** HCC

        √7ᵗʰ **T41.0X3 Poisoning by inhaled anesthetics, assault**

        √7ᵗʰ **T41.0X4 Poisoning by inhaled anesthetics, undetermined**

        √7ᵗʰ **T41.0X5 Adverse effect of inhaled anesthetics** UPD

        √7ᵗʰ **T41.0X6 Underdosing of inhaled anesthetics** UPD

Ⓝ Newborn: 0   Ⓟ Pediatric: 0-17   Ⓜ Maternity: 9-64   Ⓐ Adult: 15-124   **MCC** Major Complication/Comorbidity   **CC** Complication/Comorbidity   **SW** Severe Wound Dx

1118   ICD-10-CM 2022

✓5ᵗʰ **T41.1** **Poisoning by, adverse effect of and underdosing of intravenous anesthetics**
> Poisoning by, adverse effect of and underdosing of thiobarbiturates

  ✓6ᵗʰ **T41.1X** **Poisoning by, adverse effect of and underdosing of intravenous anesthetics**

    ✓7ᵗʰ **T41.1X1** **Poisoning by intravenous anesthetics, accidental (unintentional)**
> Poisoning by intravenous anesthetics NOS

    ⁷ ✓7ᵗʰ **T41.1X2** **Poisoning by intravenous anesthetics, intentional self-harm** `HCC`

    ✓7ᵗʰ **T41.1X3** **Poisoning by intravenous anesthetics, assault**

    ✓7ᵗʰ **T41.1X4** **Poisoning by intravenous anesthetics, undetermined**

    ✓7ᵗʰ **T41.1X5** **Adverse effect of intravenous anesthetics** `UPD`

    ✓7ᵗʰ **T41.1X6** **Underdosing of intravenous anesthetics** `UPD`

✓5ᵗʰ **T41.2** **Poisoning by, adverse effect of and underdosing of other and unspecified general anesthetics**

  ✓6ᵗʰ **T41.20** **Poisoning by, adverse effect of and underdosing of unspecified general anesthetics**

    ✓7ᵗʰ **T41.201** **Poisoning by unspecified general anesthetics, accidental (unintentional)**
> Poisoning by general anesthetics NOS

    ⁷ ✓7ᵗʰ **T41.202** **Poisoning by unspecified general anesthetics, intentional self-harm** `HCC`

    ✓7ᵗʰ **T41.203** **Poisoning by unspecified general anesthetics, assault**

    ✓7ᵗʰ **T41.204** **Poisoning by unspecified general anesthetics, undetermined**

    ✓7ᵗʰ **T41.205** **Adverse effect of unspecified general anesthetics** `UPD`
> **AHA:** 2016,4Q,73

    ✓7ᵗʰ **T41.206** **Underdosing of unspecified general anesthetics** `UPD`

  ✓6ᵗʰ **T41.29** **Poisoning by, adverse effect of and underdosing of other general anesthetics**

    ✓7ᵗʰ **T41.291** **Poisoning by other general anesthetics, accidental (unintentional)**
> Poisoning by other general anesthetics NOS

    ⁷ ✓7ᵗʰ **T41.292** **Poisoning by other general anesthetics, intentional self-harm** `HCC`

    ✓7ᵗʰ **T41.293** **Poisoning by other general anesthetics, assault**

    ✓7ᵗʰ **T41.294** **Poisoning by other general anesthetics, undetermined**

    ✓7ᵗʰ **T41.295** **Adverse effect of other general anesthetics** `UPD`

    ✓7ᵗʰ **T41.296** **Underdosing of other general anesthetics** `UPD`

✓5ᵗʰ **T41.3** **Poisoning by, adverse effect of and underdosing of local anesthetics**
> Cocaine (topical)
> *EXCLUDES 2*   *poisoning by cocaine used as a central nervous system stimulant (T40.5X1-T40.5X4)*

  ✓6ᵗʰ **T41.3X** **Poisoning by, adverse effect of and underdosing of local anesthetics**

    ✓7ᵗʰ **T41.3X1** **Poisoning by local anesthetics, accidental (unintentional)**
> Poisoning by local anesthetics NOS

    ⁷ ✓7ᵗʰ **T41.3X2** **Poisoning by local anesthetics, intentional self-harm** `HCC`

    ✓7ᵗʰ **T41.3X3** **Poisoning by local anesthetics, assault**

    ✓7ᵗʰ **T41.3X4** **Poisoning by local anesthetics, undetermined**

    ✓7ᵗʰ **T41.3X5** **Adverse effect of local anesthetics** `UPD`

    ✓7ᵗʰ **T41.3X6** **Underdosing of local anesthetics** `UPD`

✓5ᵗʰ **T41.4** **Poisoning by, adverse effect of and underdosing of unspecified anesthetic**

  ✓x7ᵗʰ **T41.41** **Poisoning by unspecified anesthetic, accidental (unintentional)**
> Poisoning by anesthetic NOS

  ⁷ ✓x7ᵗʰ **T41.42** **Poisoning by unspecified anesthetic, intentional self-harm** `HCC`

  ✓x7ᵗʰ **T41.43** **Poisoning by unspecified anesthetic, assault**

  ✓x7ᵗʰ **T41.44** **Poisoning by unspecified anesthetic, undetermined**

  ✓x7ᵗʰ **T41.45** **Adverse effect of unspecified anesthetic** `UPD`

  ✓x7ᵗʰ **T41.46** **Underdosing of unspecified anesthetics** `UPD`

✓5ᵗʰ **T41.5** **Poisoning by, adverse effect of and underdosing of therapeutic gases**

  ✓6ᵗʰ **T41.5X** **Poisoning by, adverse effect of and underdosing of therapeutic gases**

    ✓7ᵗʰ **T41.5X1** **Poisoning by therapeutic gases, accidental (unintentional)**
> Poisoning by therapeutic gases NOS

    ⁷ ✓7ᵗʰ **T41.5X2** **Poisoning by therapeutic gases, intentional self-harm** `HCC`

    ✓7ᵗʰ **T41.5X3** **Poisoning by therapeutic gases, assault**

    ✓7ᵗʰ **T41.5X4** **Poisoning by therapeutic gases, undetermined**

    ✓7ᵗʰ **T41.5X5** **Adverse effect of therapeutic gases** `UPD`

    ✓7ᵗʰ **T41.5X6** **Underdosing of therapeutic gases** `UPD`

✓4ᵗʰ **T42** **Poisoning by, adverse effect of and underdosing of antiepileptic, sedative- hypnotic and antiparkinsonism drugs**
> *EXCLUDES 2*   *drug dependence and related mental and behavioral disorders due to psychoactive substance use (F10.- - F19.-)*

> The appropriate 7th character is to be added to each code from category T42.
> A   initial encounter
> D   subsequent encounter
> S   sequela

✓5ᵗʰ **T42.0** **Poisoning by, adverse effect of and underdosing of hydantoin derivatives**

  ✓6ᵗʰ **T42.0X** **Poisoning by, adverse effect of and underdosing of hydantoin derivatives**

    ✓7ᵗʰ **T42.0X1** **Poisoning by hydantoin derivatives, accidental (unintentional)**
> Poisoning by hydantoin derivatives NOS

    ⁷ ✓7ᵗʰ **T42.0X2** **Poisoning by hydantoin derivatives, intentional self-harm** `HCC`

    ✓7ᵗʰ **T42.0X3** **Poisoning by hydantoin derivatives, assault**

    ✓7ᵗʰ **T42.0X4** **Poisoning by hydantoin derivatives, undetermined**

    ✓7ᵗʰ **T42.0X5** **Adverse effect of hydantoin derivatives** `UPD`

    ✓7ᵗʰ **T42.0X6** **Underdosing of hydantoin derivatives** `UPD`

✓5ᵗʰ **T42.1** **Poisoning by, adverse effect of and underdosing of iminostilbenes**
> Poisoning by, adverse effect of and underdosing of carbamazepine

  ✓6ᵗʰ **T42.1X** **Poisoning by, adverse effect of and underdosing of iminostilbenes**

    ✓7ᵗʰ **T42.1X1** **Poisoning by iminostilbenes, accidental (unintentional)**
> Poisoning by iminostilbenes NOS

    ⁷ ✓7ᵗʰ **T42.1X2** **Poisoning by iminostilbenes, intentional self-harm** `HCC`

    ✓7ᵗʰ **T42.1X3** **Poisoning by iminostilbenes, assault**

    ✓7ᵗʰ **T42.1X4** **Poisoning by iminostilbenes, undetermined**

    ✓7ᵗʰ **T42.1X5** **Adverse effect of iminostilbenes** `UPD`

    ✓7ᵗʰ **T42.1X6** **Underdosing of iminostilbenes** `UPD`

✓5ᵗʰ **T42.2** **Poisoning by, adverse effect of and underdosing of succinimides and oxazolidinediones**

  ✓6ᵗʰ **T42.2X** **Poisoning by, adverse effect of and underdosing of succinimides and oxazolidinediones**

    ✓7ᵗʰ **T42.2X1** **Poisoning by succinimides and oxazolidinediones, accidental (unintentional)**
> Poisoning by succinimides and oxazolidinediones NOS

    ⁷ ✓7ᵗʰ **T42.2X2** **Poisoning by succinimides and oxazolidinediones, intentional self-harm** `HCC`

    ✓7ᵗʰ **T42.2X3** **Poisoning by succinimides and oxazolidinediones, assault**

    ✓7ᵗʰ **T42.2X4** **Poisoning by succinimides and oxazolidinediones, undetermined**

    ✓7ᵗʰ **T42.2X5** **Adverse effect of succinimides and oxazolidinediones** `UPD`

    ✓7ᵗʰ **T42.2X6** **Underdosing of succinimides and oxazolidinediones** `UPD`

✓ Additional Character Required   ✓x7ᵗʰ Placeholder   Questionable PDx   Manifestation   Unspecified Dx   `UPD` Unacceptable PDx   `H1`-`H4` HAC   `HCC` CMS-HCC Dx   `HIV` HIV Dx

√5ᵗʰ **T42.3** **Poisoning by, adverse effect of and underdosing of barbiturates**

> EXCLUDES 1   *poisoning by, adverse effect of and underdosing of thiobarbiturates (T41.1-)*

√6ᵗʰ **T42.3X** **Poisoning by, adverse effect of and underdosing of barbiturates**

√7ᵗʰ **T42.3X1** **Poisoning by barbiturates, accidental (unintentional)**
> Poisoning by barbiturates NOS

7 √7ᵗʰ **T42.3X2** **Poisoning by barbiturates, intentional self-harm** HCC

√7ᵗʰ **T42.3X3** **Poisoning by barbiturates, assault**

√7ᵗʰ **T42.3X4** **Poisoning by barbiturates, undetermined**

√7ᵗʰ **T42.3X5** Adverse effect of barbiturates UPD

√7ᵗʰ **T42.3X6** Underdosing of barbiturates UPD

√5ᵗʰ **T42.4** **Poisoning by, adverse effect of and underdosing of benzodiazepines**

√6ᵗʰ **T42.4X** **Poisoning by, adverse effect of and underdosing of benzodiazepines**

√7ᵗʰ **T42.4X1** **Poisoning by benzodiazepines, accidental (unintentional)**
> Poisoning by benzodiazepines NOS

7 √7ᵗʰ **T42.4X2** **Poisoning by benzodiazepines, intentional self-harm** HCC

√7ᵗʰ **T42.4X3** **Poisoning by benzodiazepines, assault**

√7ᵗʰ **T42.4X4** **Poisoning by benzodiazepines, undetermined**

√7ᵗʰ **T42.4X5** Adverse effect of benzodiazepines UPD

√7ᵗʰ **T42.4X6** Underdosing of benzodiazepines UPD

√5ᵗʰ **T42.5** **Poisoning by, adverse effect of and underdosing of mixed antiepileptics**

√6ᵗʰ **T42.5X** **Poisoning by, adverse effect of and underdosing of antiepileptics**

√7ᵗʰ **T42.5X1** **Poisoning by mixed antiepileptics, accidental (unintentional)**
> Poisoning by mixed antiepileptics NOS

7 √7ᵗʰ **T42.5X2** **Poisoning by mixed antiepileptics, intentional self-harm** HCC

√7ᵗʰ **T42.5X3** **Poisoning by mixed antiepileptics, assault**

√7ᵗʰ **T42.5X4** **Poisoning by mixed antiepileptics, undetermined**

√7ᵗʰ **T42.5X5** Adverse effect of mixed antiepileptics UPD

√7ᵗʰ **T42.5X6** Underdosing of mixed antiepileptics UPD

√5ᵗʰ **T42.6** **Poisoning by, adverse effect of and underdosing of other antiepileptic and sedative-hypnotic drugs**

> Poisoning by, adverse effect of and underdosing of methaqualone
> Poisoning by, adverse effect of and underdosing of valproic acid

> EXCLUDES 1   *poisoning by, adverse effect of and underdosing of carbamazepine (T42.1-)*

√6ᵗʰ **T42.6X** **Poisoning by, adverse effect of and underdosing of other antiepileptic and sedative-hypnotic drugs**

√7ᵗʰ **T42.6X1** **Poisoning by other antiepileptic and sedative-hypnotic drugs, accidental (unintentional)**
> Poisoning by other antiepileptic and sedative-hypnotic drugs NOS

7 √7ᵗʰ **T42.6X2** **Poisoning by other antiepileptic and sedative-hypnotic drugs, intentional self-harm** HCC

√7ᵗʰ **T42.6X3** **Poisoning by other antiepileptic and sedative-hypnotic drugs, assault**

√7ᵗʰ **T42.6X4** **Poisoning by other antiepileptic and sedative-hypnotic drugs, undetermined**

√7ᵗʰ **T42.6X5** Adverse effect of other antiepileptic and sedative-hypnotic drugs UPD

√7ᵗʰ **T42.6X6** Underdosing of other antiepileptic and sedative-hypnotic drugs UPD

√5ᵗʰ **T42.7** **Poisoning by, adverse effect of and underdosing of unspecified antiepileptic and sedative-hypnotic drugs**

√x7ᵗʰ **T42.71** **Poisoning by unspecified antiepileptic and sedative-hypnotic drugs, accidental (unintentional)**
> Poisoning by antiepileptic and sedative-hypnotic drugs NOS

7 √x7ᵗʰ **T42.72** **Poisoning by unspecified antiepileptic and sedative-hypnotic drugs, intentional self-harm** HCC

√x7ᵗʰ **T42.73** **Poisoning by unspecified antiepileptic and sedative-hypnotic drugs, assault**

√x7ᵗʰ **T42.74** **Poisoning by unspecified antiepileptic and sedative-hypnotic drugs, undetermined**

√x7ᵗʰ **T42.75** Adverse effect of unspecified antiepileptic and sedative-hypnotic drugs UPD

√x7ᵗʰ **T42.76** Underdosing of unspecified antiepileptic and sedative-hypnotic drugs UPD

√5ᵗʰ **T42.8** **Poisoning by, adverse effect of and underdosing of antiparkinsonism drugs and other central muscle-tone depressants**

> Poisoning by, adverse effect of and underdosing of amantadine

√6ᵗʰ **T42.8X** **Poisoning by, adverse effect of and underdosing of antiparkinsonism drugs and other central muscle-tone depressants**

√7ᵗʰ **T42.8X1** **Poisoning by antiparkinsonism drugs and other central muscle-tone depressants, accidental (unintentional)**
> Poisoning by antiparkinsonism drugs and other central muscle-tone depressants NOS

7 √7ᵗʰ **T42.8X2** **Poisoning by antiparkinsonism drugs and other central muscle-tone depressants, intentional self-harm** HCC

√7ᵗʰ **T42.8X3** **Poisoning by antiparkinsonism drugs and other central muscle-tone depressants, assault**

√7ᵗʰ **T42.8X4** **Poisoning by antiparkinsonism drugs and other central muscle-tone depressants, undetermined**

√7ᵗʰ **T42.8X5** Adverse effect of antiparkinsonism drugs and other central muscle-tone depressants UPD

√7ᵗʰ **T42.8X6** Underdosing of antiparkinsonism drugs and other central muscle-tone depressants UPD

√4ᵗʰ **T43** **Poisoning by, adverse effect of and underdosing of psychotropic drugs, not elsewhere classified**

> EXCLUDES 1   *appetite depressants (T50.5-)*
> *barbiturates (T42.3-)*
> *benzodiazepines (T42.4-)*
> *methaqualone (T42.6-)*
> *psychodysleptics [hallucinogens] (T40.7-T40.9-)*

> EXCLUDES 2   *drug dependence and related mental and behavioral disorders due to psychoactive substance use (F10.- – F19.-)*

The appropriate 7th character is to be added to each code from category T43.
A   initial encounter
D   subsequent encounter
S   sequela

√5ᵗʰ **T43.0** **Poisoning by, adverse effect of and underdosing of tricyclic and tetracyclic antidepressants**

√6ᵗʰ **T43.01** **Poisoning by, adverse effect of and underdosing of tricyclic antidepressants**

√7ᵗʰ **T43.011** **Poisoning by tricyclic antidepressants, accidental (unintentional)**
> Poisoning by tricyclic antidepressants NOS

7 √7ᵗʰ **T43.012** **Poisoning by tricyclic antidepressants, intentional self-harm** HCC

√7ᵗʰ **T43.013** **Poisoning by tricyclic antidepressants, assault**

√7ᵗʰ **T43.014** **Poisoning by tricyclic antidepressants, undetermined**

√7ᵗʰ **T43.015** Adverse effect of tricyclic antidepressants UPD

√7ᵗʰ **T43.016** Underdosing of tricyclic antidepressants UPD

√6ᵗʰ **T43.02** **Poisoning by, adverse effect of and underdosing of tetracyclic antidepressants**

√7ᵗʰ **T43.021** **Poisoning by tetracyclic antidepressants, accidental (unintentional)**
> Poisoning by tetracyclic antidepressants NOS

7 √7ᵗʰ **T43.022** **Poisoning by tetracyclic antidepressants, intentional self-harm** HCC

√7ᵗʰ **T43.023** **Poisoning by tetracyclic antidepressants, assault**

√7ᵗʰ **T43.024 Poisoning by tetracyclic antidepressants, undetermined**

√7ᵗʰ **T43.025** Adverse effect of tetracyclic antidepressants   UPD

√7ᵗʰ **T43.026** Underdosing of tetracyclic antidepressants   UPD

√5ᵗʰ **T43.1 Poisoning by, adverse effect of and underdosing of monoamine-oxidase-inhibitor antidepressants**

√6ᵗʰ **T43.1X Poisoning by, adverse effect of and underdosing of** monoamine-oxidase-inhibitor antidepressants

√7ᵗʰ **T43.1X1 Poisoning by monoamine-oxidase-inhibitor antidepressants, accidental (unintentional)**

Poisoning by monoamine-oxidase-inhibitor antidepressants NOS

7 √7ᵗʰ **T43.1X2 Poisoning by monoamine-oxidase-inhibitor antidepressants, intentional self-harm**   HCC

√7ᵗʰ **T43.1X3 Poisoning by monoamine-oxidase-inhibitor antidepressants, assault**

√7ᵗʰ **T43.1X4 Poisoning by monoamine-oxidase-inhibitor antidepressants, undetermined**

√7ᵗʰ **T43.1X5** Adverse effect of monoamine-oxidase-inhibitor antidepressants   UPD

√7ᵗʰ **T43.1X6** Underdosing of monoamine-oxidase-inhibitor antidepressants   UPD

√5ᵗʰ **T43.2 Poisoning by, adverse effect of and underdosing of other and unspecified antidepressants**

√6ᵗʰ **T43.20 Poisoning by, adverse effect of and underdosing of unspecified antidepressants**

√7ᵗʰ **T43.201 Poisoning by unspecified antidepressants, accidental (unintentional)**

Poisoning by antidepressants NOS

7 √7ᵗʰ **T43.202 Poisoning by unspecified antidepressants, intentional self-harm**   HCC

√7ᵗʰ **T43.203 Poisoning by unspecified antidepressants, assault**

√7ᵗʰ **T43.204 Poisoning by unspecified antidepressants, undetermined**

√7ᵗʰ **T43.205** Adverse effect of unspecified antidepressants   UPD

Antidepressant discontinuation syndrome

√7ᵗʰ **T43.206** Underdosing of unspecified antidepressants   UPD

√6ᵗʰ **T43.21 Poisoning by, adverse effect of and underdosing of** selective serotonin and norepinephrine reuptake inhibitors

Poisoning by, adverse effect of and underdosing of SSNRI antidepressants

√7ᵗʰ **T43.211 Poisoning by selective serotonin and norepinephrine reuptake inhibitors, accidental (unintentional)**

7 √7ᵗʰ **T43.212 Poisoning by selective serotonin and norepinephrine reuptake inhibitors, intentional self-harm**   HCC

√7ᵗʰ **T43.213 Poisoning by selective serotonin and norepinephrine reuptake inhibitors, assault**

√7ᵗʰ **T43.214 Poisoning by selective serotonin and norepinephrine reuptake inhibitors, undetermined**

√7ᵗʰ **T43.215** Adverse effect of selective serotonin and norepinephrine reuptake inhibitors   UPD

√7ᵗʰ **T43.216** Underdosing of selective serotonin and norepinephrine reuptake inhibitors   UPD

√6ᵗʰ **T43.22 Poisoning by, adverse effect of and underdosing of** selective serotonin reuptake inhibitors

Poisoning by, adverse effect of and underdosing of SSRI antidepressants

√7ᵗʰ **T43.221 Poisoning by selective serotonin reuptake inhibitors, accidental (unintentional)**

7 √7ᵗʰ **T43.222 Poisoning by selective serotonin reuptake inhibitors, intentional self-harm**   HCC

√7ᵗʰ **T43.223 Poisoning by selective serotonin reuptake inhibitors, assault**

√7ᵗʰ **T43.224 Poisoning by selective serotonin reuptake inhibitors, undetermined**

√7ᵗʰ **T43.225** Adverse effect of selective serotonin reuptake inhibitors   UPD

√7ᵗʰ **T43.226** Underdosing of selective serotonin reuptake inhibitors   UPD

√6ᵗʰ **T43.29 Poisoning by, adverse effect of and underdosing of other antidepressants**

√7ᵗʰ **T43.291 Poisoning by other antidepressants, accidental (unintentional)**

Poisoning by other antidepressants NOS

7 √7ᵗʰ **T43.292 Poisoning by other antidepressants, intentional self-harm**   HCC

√7ᵗʰ **T43.293 Poisoning by other antidepressants, assault**

√7ᵗʰ **T43.294 Poisoning by other antidepressants, undetermined**

√7ᵗʰ **T43.295** Adverse effect of other antidepressants   UPD

√7ᵗʰ **T43.296** Underdosing of other antidepressants   UPD

√5ᵗʰ **T43.3 Poisoning by, adverse effect of and underdosing of phenothiazine antipsychotics and neuroleptics**

√6ᵗʰ **T43.3X Poisoning by, adverse effect of and underdosing of** phenothiazine antipsychotics and neuroleptics

√7ᵗʰ **T43.3X1 Poisoning by phenothiazine antipsychotics and neuroleptics, accidental (unintentional)**

Poisoning by phenothiazine antipsychotics and neuroleptics NOS

7 √7ᵗʰ **T43.3X2 Poisoning by phenothiazine antipsychotics and neuroleptics, intentional self-harm**   HCC

√7ᵗʰ **T43.3X3 Poisoning by phenothiazine antipsychotics and neuroleptics, assault**

√7ᵗʰ **T43.3X4 Poisoning by phenothiazine antipsychotics and neuroleptics, undetermined**

√7ᵗʰ **T43.3X5** Adverse effect of phenothiazine antipsychotics and neuroleptics   UPD

√7ᵗʰ **T43.3X6** Underdosing of phenothiazine antipsychotics and neuroleptics   UPD

√5ᵗʰ **T43.4 Poisoning by, adverse effect of and underdosing of butyrophenone and thiothixene neuroleptics**

√6ᵗʰ **T43.4X Poisoning by, adverse effect of and underdosing of** butyrophenone and thiothixene neuroleptics

√7ᵗʰ **T43.4X1 Poisoning by butyrophenone and thiothixene neuroleptics, accidental (unintentional)**

Poisoning by butyrophenone and thiothixene neuroleptics NOS

7 √7ᵗʰ **T43.4X2 Poisoning by butyrophenone and thiothixene neuroleptics, intentional self-harm**   HCC

√7ᵗʰ **T43.4X3 Poisoning by butyrophenone and thiothixene neuroleptics, assault**

√7ᵗʰ **T43.4X4 Poisoning by butyrophenone and thiothixene neuroleptics, undetermined**

√7ᵗʰ **T43.4X5** Adverse effect of butyrophenone and thiothixene neuroleptics   UPD

√7ᵗʰ **T43.4X6** Underdosing of butyrophenone and thiothixene neuroleptics   UPD

√5ᵗʰ **T43.5 Poisoning by, adverse effect of and underdosing of other and unspecified antipsychotics and neuroleptics**

EXCLUDES 1   *poisoning by, adverse effect of and underdosing of rauwolfia (T46.5-)*

√6ᵗʰ **T43.50 Poisoning by, adverse effect of and underdosing of unspecified antipsychotics and neuroleptics**

√7ᵗʰ **T43.501 Poisoning by unspecified antipsychotics and neuroleptics, accidental (unintentional)**

Poisoning by antipsychotics and neuroleptics NOS

7 √7ᵗʰ **T43.502 Poisoning by unspecified antipsychotics and neuroleptics, intentional self-harm**   HCC

√7ᵗʰ **T43.503 Poisoning by unspecified antipsychotics and neuroleptics, assault**

√7ᵗʰ **T43.504 Poisoning by unspecified antipsychotics and neuroleptics, undetermined**

✔ Additional Character Required   √x7ᵗʰ Placeholder   Questionable PDx   Manifestation   Unspecified Dx   UPD Unacceptable PDx   H1-H14 HAC   HCC CMS-HCC Dx   HIV HIV Dx

ICD-10-CM 2022   1121

√7ᵗʰ **T43.505** Adverse effect of unspecified antipsychotics and neuroleptics `UPD`

√7ᵗʰ **T43.506** Underdosing of unspecified antipsychotics and neuroleptics `UPD`

√6ᵗʰ **T43.59** Poisoning by, adverse effect of and underdosing of other antipsychotics and neuroleptics
AHA: 2017, 1Q, 40

     √7ᵗʰ **T43.591** Poisoning by other antipsychotics and neuroleptics, accidental (unintentional)
Poisoning by other antipsychotics and neuroleptics NOS

     7 √7ᵗʰ **T43.592** Poisoning by other antipsychotics and neuroleptics, intentional self-harm `HCC`

     √7ᵗʰ **T43.593** Poisoning by other antipsychotics and neuroleptics, assault

     √7ᵗʰ **T43.594** Poisoning by other antipsychotics and neuroleptics, undetermined

     √7ᵗʰ **T43.595** Adverse effect of other antipsychotics and neuroleptics `UPD`

     √7ᵗʰ **T43.596** Underdosing of other antipsychotics and neuroleptics `UPD`

√5ᵗʰ **T43.6** Poisoning by, adverse effect of and underdosing of psychostimulants
   `EXCLUDES 1`   poisoning by, adverse effect of and underdosing of cocaine (T40.5-)

   √6ᵗʰ **T43.60** Poisoning by, adverse effect of and underdosing of unspecified psychostimulant

     6 √7ᵗʰ **T43.601** Poisoning by unspecified psychostimulants, accidental (unintentional) `HCC`
Poisoning by psychostimulants NOS

     7 √7ᵗʰ **T43.602** Poisoning by unspecified psychostimulants, intentional self-harm `HCC`

     √7ᵗʰ **T43.603** Poisoning by unspecified psychostimulants, assault

     6 √7ᵗʰ **T43.604** Poisoning by unspecified psychostimulants, undetermined `HCC`

     √7ᵗʰ **T43.605** Adverse effect of unspecified psychostimulants `UPD`

     √7ᵗʰ **T43.606** Underdosing of unspecified psychostimulants `UPD`

   √6ᵗʰ **T43.61** Poisoning by, adverse effect of and underdosing of caffeine

     6 √7ᵗʰ **T43.611** Poisoning by caffeine, accidental (unintentional) `HCC`
Poisoning by caffeine NOS

     7 √7ᵗʰ **T43.612** Poisoning by caffeine, intentional self-harm `HCC`

     √7ᵗʰ **T43.613** Poisoning by caffeine, assault

     6 √7ᵗʰ **T43.614** Poisoning by caffeine, undetermined `HCC`

     √7ᵗʰ **T43.615** Adverse effect of caffeine `UPD`

     √7ᵗʰ **T43.616** Underdosing of caffeine `UPD`

   √6ᵗʰ **T43.62** Poisoning by, adverse effect of and underdosing of amphetamines
Poisoning by, adverse effect of and underdosing of methamphetamines

     6 √7ᵗʰ **T43.621** Poisoning by amphetamines, accidental (unintentional) `HCC`
Poisoning by amphetamines NOS

     7 √7ᵗʰ **T43.622** Poisoning by amphetamines, intentional self-harm `HCC`

     √7ᵗʰ **T43.623** Poisoning by amphetamines, assault

     6 √7ᵗʰ **T43.624** Poisoning by amphetamines, undetermined `HCC`

     √7ᵗʰ **T43.625** Adverse effect of amphetamines `UPD`

     √7ᵗʰ **T43.626** Underdosing of amphetamines `UPD`

   √6ᵗʰ **T43.63** Poisoning by, adverse effect of and underdosing of methylphenidate

     6 √7ᵗʰ **T43.631** Poisoning by methylphenidate, accidental (unintentional) `HCC`
Poisoning by methylphenidate NOS

     7 √7ᵗʰ **T43.632** Poisoning by methylphenidate, intentional self-harm `HCC`

     √7ᵗʰ **T43.633** Poisoning by methylphenidate, assault

     6 √7ᵗʰ **T43.634** Poisoning by methylphenidate, undetermined `HCC`

√7ᵗʰ **T43.635** Adverse effect of methylphenidate `UPD`

√7ᵗʰ **T43.636** Underdosing of methylphenidate `UPD`

√6ᵗʰ **T43.64** Poisoning by ecstasy
Poisoning by MDMA
Poisoning by 3,4-methylenedioxymethamphetamine
AHA: 2018, 4Q, 30-31

     6 √7ᵗʰ **T43.641** Poisoning by ecstasy, accidental (unintentional) `HCC`
Poisoning by ecstasy NOS

     7 √7ᵗʰ **T43.642** Poisoning by ecstasy, intentional self-harm `HCC`

     √7ᵗʰ **T43.643** Poisoning by ecstasy, assault

     6 √7ᵗʰ **T43.644** Poisoning by ecstasy, undetermined `HCC`

√6ᵗʰ **T43.69** Poisoning by, adverse effect of and underdosing of other psychostimulants

     6 √7ᵗʰ **T43.691** Poisoning by other psychostimulants, accidental (unintentional) `HCC`
Poisoning by other psychostimulants NOS

     7 √7ᵗʰ **T43.692** Poisoning by other psychostimulants, intentional self-harm `HCC`

     √7ᵗʰ **T43.693** Poisoning by other psychostimulants, assault

     6 √7ᵗʰ **T43.694** Poisoning by other psychostimulants, undetermined `HCC`

     √7ᵗʰ **T43.695** Adverse effect of other psychostimulants `UPD`

     √7ᵗʰ **T43.696** Underdosing of other psychostimulants `UPD`

√5ᵗʰ **T43.8** Poisoning by, adverse effect of and underdosing of other psychotropic drugs

   √6ᵗʰ **T43.8X** Poisoning by, adverse effect of and underdosing of other psychotropic drugs

     √7ᵗʰ **T43.8X1** Poisoning by other psychotropic drugs, accidental (unintentional)
Poisoning by other psychotropic drugs NOS

     7 √7ᵗʰ **T43.8X2** Poisoning by other psychotropic drugs, intentional self-harm `HCC`

     √7ᵗʰ **T43.8X3** Poisoning by other psychotropic drugs, assault

     √7ᵗʰ **T43.8X4** Poisoning by other psychotropic drugs, undetermined

     √7ᵗʰ **T43.8X5** Adverse effect of other psychotropic drugs `UPD`

     √7ᵗʰ **T43.8X6** Underdosing of other psychotropic drugs `UPD`

√5ᵗʰ **T43.9** Poisoning by, adverse effect of and underdosing of unspecified psychotropic drug

   √×7ᵗʰ **T43.91** Poisoning by unspecified psychotropic drug, accidental (unintentional)
Poisoning by psychotropic drug NOS

   7 √×7ᵗʰ **T43.92** Poisoning by unspecified psychotropic drug, intentional self-harm `HCC`

   √×7ᵗʰ **T43.93** Poisoning by unspecified psychotropic drug, assault

   √×7ᵗʰ **T43.94** Poisoning by unspecified psychotropic drug, undetermined

   √×7ᵗʰ **T43.95** Adverse effect of unspecified psychotropic drug `UPD`

   √×7ᵗʰ **T43.96** Underdosing of unspecified psychotropic drug `UPD`

√4ᵗʰ **T44** Poisoning by, adverse effect of and underdosing of drugs primarily affecting the autonomic nervous system

> The appropriate 7th character is to be added to each code from category T44.
> A   initial encounter
> D   subsequent encounter
> S   sequela

√5ᵗʰ **T44.0** Poisoning by, adverse effect of and underdosing of anticholinesterase agents

   √6ᵗʰ **T44.0X** Poisoning by, adverse effect of and underdosing of anticholinesterase agents

     √7ᵗʰ **T44.0X1** Poisoning by anticholinesterase agents, accidental (unintentional)
Poisoning by anticholinesterase agents NOS

     7 √7ᵗʰ **T44.0X2** Poisoning by anticholinesterase agents, intentional self-harm `HCC`

☑7ᵗʰ **T44.0X3** Poisoning by anticholinesterase agents, assault

☑7ᵗʰ **T44.0X4** Poisoning by anticholinesterase agents, undetermined

☑7ᵗʰ **T44.0X5** Adverse effect of anticholinesterase agents   UPD

☑7ᵗʰ **T44.0X6** Underdosing of anticholinesterase agents   UPD

☑5ᵗʰ **T44.1** Poisoning by, adverse effect of and underdosing of other parasympathomimetics [cholinergics]

   ☑6ᵗʰ **T44.1X** Poisoning by, adverse effect of and underdosing of other parasympathomimetics [cholinergics]

      ☑7ᵗʰ **T44.1X1** Poisoning by other parasympathomimetics [cholinergics], accidental (unintentional)

         Poisoning by other parasympathomimetics [cholinergics] NOS

   7 ☑7ᵗʰ **T44.1X2** Poisoning by other parasympathomimetics [cholinergics], intentional self-harm   HCC

      ☑7ᵗʰ **T44.1X3** Poisoning by other parasympathomimetics [cholinergics], assault

      ☑7ᵗʰ **T44.1X4** Poisoning by other parasympathomimetics [cholinergics], undetermined

      ☑7ᵗʰ **T44.1X5** Adverse effect of other parasympathomimetics [cholinergics]   UPD

      ☑7ᵗʰ **T44.1X6** Underdosing of other parasympathomimetics [cholinergics]   UPD

☑5ᵗʰ **T44.2** Poisoning by, adverse effect of and underdosing of ganglionic blocking drugs

   ☑6ᵗʰ **T44.2X** Poisoning by, adverse effect of and underdosing of ganglionic blocking drugs

      ☑7ᵗʰ **T44.2X1** Poisoning by ganglionic blocking drugs, accidental (unintentional)

         Poisoning by ganglionic blocking drugs NOS

   7 ☑7ᵗʰ **T44.2X2** Poisoning by ganglionic blocking drugs, intentional self-harm   HCC

      ☑7ᵗʰ **T44.2X3** Poisoning by ganglionic blocking drugs, assault

      ☑7ᵗʰ **T44.2X4** Poisoning by ganglionic blocking drugs, undetermined

      ☑7ᵗʰ **T44.2X5** Adverse effect of ganglionic blocking drugs   UPD

      ☑7ᵗʰ **T44.2X6** Underdosing of ganglionic blocking drugs   UPD

☑5ᵗʰ **T44.3** Poisoning by, adverse effect of and underdosing of other parasympatholytics [anticholinergics and antimuscarinics] and spasmolytics

   Poisoning by, adverse effect of and underdosing of papaverine

   ☑6ᵗʰ **T44.3X** Poisoning by, adverse effect of and underdosing of other parasympatholytics [anticholinergics and antimuscarinics] and spasmolytics

      ☑7ᵗʰ **T44.3X1** Poisoning by other parasympatholytics [anticholinergics and antimuscarinics] and spasmolytics, accidental (unintentional)

         Poisoning by other parasympatholytics [anticholinergics and antimuscarinics] and spasmolytics NOS

   7 ☑7ᵗʰ **T44.3X2** Poisoning by other parasympatholytics [anticholinergics and antimuscarinics] and spasmolytics, intentional self-harm   HCC

      ☑7ᵗʰ **T44.3X3** Poisoning by other parasympatholytics [anticholinergics and antimuscarinics] and spasmolytics, assault

      ☑7ᵗʰ **T44.3X4** Poisoning by other parasympatholytics [anticholinergics and antimuscarinics] and spasmolytics, undetermined

      ☑7ᵗʰ **T44.3X5** Adverse effect of other parasympatholytics [anticholinergics and antimuscarinics] and spasmolytics   UPD

      ☑7ᵗʰ **T44.3X6** Underdosing of other parasympatholytics [anticholinergics and antimuscarinics] and spasmolytics   UPD

☑5ᵗʰ **T44.4** Poisoning by, adverse effect of and underdosing of predominantly alpha-adrenoreceptor agonists

   Poisoning by, adverse effect of and underdosing of metaraminol

   ☑6ᵗʰ **T44.4X** Poisoning by, adverse effect of and underdosing of predominantly alpha-adrenoreceptor agonists

      ☑7ᵗʰ **T44.4X1** Poisoning by predominantly alpha-adrenoreceptor agonists, accidental (unintentional)

         Poisoning by predominantly alpha-adrenoreceptor agonists NOS

   7 ☑7ᵗʰ **T44.4X2** Poisoning by predominantly alpha-adrenoreceptor agonists, intentional self-harm   HCC

      ☑7ᵗʰ **T44.4X3** Poisoning by predominantly alpha-adrenoreceptor agonists, assault

      ☑7ᵗʰ **T44.4X4** Poisoning by predominantly alpha-adrenoreceptor agonists, undetermined

      ☑7ᵗʰ **T44.4X5** Adverse effect of predominantly alpha-adrenoreceptor agonists   UPD

      ☑7ᵗʰ **T44.4X6** Underdosing of predominantly alpha-adrenoreceptor agonists   UPD

☑5ᵗʰ **T44.5** Poisoning by, adverse effect of and underdosing of predominantly beta-adrenoreceptor agonists

   EXCLUDES 1   poisoning by, adverse effect of and underdosing of beta-adrenoreceptor agonists used in asthma therapy (T48.6-)

   ☑6ᵗʰ **T44.5X** Poisoning by, adverse effect of and underdosing of predominantly beta-adrenoreceptor agonists

      ☑7ᵗʰ **T44.5X1** Poisoning by predominantly beta-adrenoreceptor agonists, accidental (unintentional)

         Poisoning by predominantly beta-adrenoreceptor agonists NOS

   7 ☑7ᵗʰ **T44.5X2** Poisoning by predominantly beta-adrenoreceptor agonists, intentional self-harm   HCC

      ☑7ᵗʰ **T44.5X3** Poisoning by predominantly beta-adrenoreceptor agonists, assault

      ☑7ᵗʰ **T44.5X4** Poisoning by predominantly beta-adrenoreceptor agonists, undetermined

      ☑7ᵗʰ **T44.5X5** Adverse effect of predominantly beta-adrenoreceptor agonists   UPD

      ☑7ᵗʰ **T44.5X6** Underdosing of predominantly beta-adrenoreceptor agonists   UPD

☑5ᵗʰ **T44.6** Poisoning by, adverse effect of and underdosing of alpha-adrenoreceptor antagonists

   EXCLUDES 1   poisoning by, adverse effect of and underdosing of ergot alkaloids (T48.0)

   ☑6ᵗʰ **T44.6X** Poisoning by, adverse effect of and underdosing of alpha-adrenoreceptor antagonists

      ☑7ᵗʰ **T44.6X1** Poisoning by alpha-adrenoreceptor antagonists, accidental (unintentional)

         Poisoning by alpha-adrenoreceptor antagonists NOS

   7 ☑7ᵗʰ **T44.6X2** Poisoning by alpha-adrenoreceptor antagonists, intentional self-harm   HCC

      ☑7ᵗʰ **T44.6X3** Poisoning by alpha-adrenoreceptor antagonists, assault

      ☑7ᵗʰ **T44.6X4** Poisoning by alpha-adrenoreceptor antagonists, undetermined

      ☑7ᵗʰ **T44.6X5** Adverse effect of alpha-adrenoreceptor antagonists   UPD

      ☑7ᵗʰ **T44.6X6** Underdosing of alpha-adrenoreceptor antagonists   UPD

☑5ᵗʰ **T44.7** Poisoning by, adverse effect of and underdosing of beta-adrenoreceptor antagonists

   ☑6ᵗʰ **T44.7X** Poisoning by, adverse effect of and underdosing of beta-adrenoreceptor antagonists

      ☑7ᵗʰ **T44.7X1** Poisoning by beta-adrenoreceptor antagonists, accidental (unintentional)

         Poisoning by beta-adrenoreceptor antagonists NOS

   7 ☑7ᵗʰ **T44.7X2** Poisoning by beta-adrenoreceptor antagonists, intentional self-harm   HCC

      ☑7ᵗʰ **T44.7X3** Poisoning by beta-adrenoreceptor antagonists, assault

      ☑7ᵗʰ **T44.7X4** Poisoning by beta-adrenoreceptor antagonists, undetermined

      ☑7ᵗʰ **T44.7X5** Adverse effect of beta-adrenoreceptor antagonists   UPD

☑ Additional Character Required   ☑x7ᵗʰ Placeholder   Questionable PDx   Manifestation   Unspecified Dx   UPD Unacceptable PDx   H1-H14 HAC   HCC CMS-HCC Dx   HIV HIV Dx

ICD-10-CM 2022   1123

Chapter 19. Injury, Poisoning and Certain Other Consequences of External Causes

T44.7X6–T45.2X6

√7ᵗʰ **T44.7X6** Underdosing of beta-adrenoreceptor antagonists UPD

√5ᵗʰ **T44.8** Poisoning by, adverse effect of and underdosing of centrally-acting and adrenergic-neuron- blocking agents

     EXCLUDES 1   *poisoning by, adverse effect of and underdosing of clonidine (T46.5)*

           poisoning by, adverse effect of and underdosing of guanethidine (T46.5)

     EXCLUDES 2   ▶*poisoning by, adverse effect of and underdosing of clonidine (T46.5)*◀

           ▶*poisoning by, adverse effect of and underdosing of guanethidine (T46.5)*◀

√6ᵗʰ **T44.8X** Poisoning by, adverse effect of and underdosing of centrally-acting and adrenergic- neuron-blocking agents

√7ᵗʰ **T44.8X1** Poisoning by centrally-acting and adrenergic-neuron-blocking agents, accidental (unintentional)

     Poisoning by centrally-acting and adrenergic-neuron-blocking agents NOS

⁷ √7ᵗʰ **T44.8X2** Poisoning by centrally-acting and adrenergic-neuron-blocking agents, intentional self-harm HCC

√7ᵗʰ **T44.8X3** Poisoning by centrally-acting and adrenergic-neuron-blocking agents, assault

√7ᵗʰ **T44.8X4** Poisoning by centrally-acting and adrenergic-neuron-blocking agents, undetermined

√7ᵗʰ **T44.8X5** Adverse effect of centrally-acting and adrenergic-neuron-blocking agents UPD

√7ᵗʰ **T44.8X6** Underdosing of centrally-acting and adrenergic-neuron-blocking agents UPD

√5ᵗʰ **T44.9** Poisoning by, adverse effect of and underdosing of other and unspecified drugs primarily affecting the autonomic nervous system

     Poisoning by, adverse effect of and underdosing of drug stimulating both alpha and beta-adrenoreceptors

√6ᵗʰ **T44.90** Poisoning by, adverse effect of and underdosing of unspecified drugs primarily affecting the autonomic nervous system

√7ᵗʰ **T44.901** Poisoning by unspecified drugs primarily affecting the autonomic nervous system, accidental (unintentional)

     Poisoning by unspecified drugs primarily affecting the autonomic nervous system NOS

⁷ √7ᵗʰ **T44.902** Poisoning by unspecified drugs primarily affecting the autonomic nervous system, intentional self-harm HCC

√7ᵗʰ **T44.903** Poisoning by unspecified drugs primarily affecting the autonomic nervous system, assault

√7ᵗʰ **T44.904** Poisoning by unspecified drugs primarily affecting the autonomic nervous system, undetermined

√7ᵗʰ **T44.905** Adverse effect of unspecified drugs primarily affecting the autonomic nervous system UPD

√7ᵗʰ **T44.906** Underdosing of unspecified drugs primarily affecting the autonomic nervous system UPD

√6ᵗʰ **T44.99** Poisoning by, adverse effect of and underdosing of other drugs primarily affecting the autonomic nervous system

√7ᵗʰ **T44.991** Poisoning by other drug primarily affecting the autonomic nervous system, accidental (unintentional)

     Poisoning by other drugs primarily affecting the autonomic nervous system NOS

⁷ √7ᵗʰ **T44.992** Poisoning by other drug primarily affecting the autonomic nervous system, intentional self-harm HCC

√7ᵗʰ **T44.993** Poisoning by other drug primarily affecting the autonomic nervous system, assault

√7ᵗʰ **T44.994** Poisoning by other drug primarily affecting the autonomic nervous system, undetermined

√7ᵗʰ **T44.995** Adverse effect of other drug primarily affecting the autonomic nervous system UPD

√7ᵗʰ **T44.996** Underdosing of other drug primarily affecting the autonomic nervous system UPD

√4ᵗʰ **T45** Poisoning by, adverse effect of and underdosing of primarily systemic and hematological agents, not elsewhere classified

> The appropriate 7th character is to be added to each code from category T45.
> A   initial encounter
> D   subsequent encounter
> S   sequela

√5ᵗʰ **T45.0** Poisoning by, adverse effect of and underdosing of antiallergic and antiemetic drugs

     EXCLUDES 1   *poisoning by, adverse effect of and underdosing of phenothiazine-based neuroleptics (T43.3)*

√6ᵗʰ **T45.0X** Poisoning by, adverse effect of and underdosing of antiallergic and antiemetic drugs

√7ᵗʰ **T45.0X1** Poisoning by antiallergic and antiemetic drugs, accidental (unintentional)

     Poisoning by antiallergic and antiemetic drugs NOS

⁷ √7ᵗʰ **T45.0X2** Poisoning by antiallergic and antiemetic drugs, intentional self-harm HCC

√7ᵗʰ **T45.0X3** Poisoning by antiallergic and antiemetic drugs, assault

√7ᵗʰ **T45.0X4** Poisoning by antiallergic and antiemetic drugs, undetermined

√7ᵗʰ **T45.0X5** Adverse effect of antiallergic and antiemetic drugs UPD

√7ᵗʰ **T45.0X6** Underdosing of antiallergic and antiemetic drugs UPD

√5ᵗʰ **T45.1** Poisoning by, adverse effect of and underdosing of antineoplastic and immunosuppressive drugs

     EXCLUDES 1   *poisoning by, adverse effect of and underdosing of tamoxifen (T38.6)*

     AHA: 2019,1Q,17,20; 2014,4Q,22

√6ᵗʰ **T45.1X** Poisoning by, adverse effect of and underdosing of antineoplastic and immunosuppressive drugs

√7ᵗʰ **T45.1X1** Poisoning by antineoplastic and immunosuppressive drugs, accidental (unintentional)

     Poisoning by antineoplastic and immunosuppressive drugs NOS

⁷ √7ᵗʰ **T45.1X2** Poisoning by antineoplastic and immunosuppressive drugs, intentional self-harm HCC

√7ᵗʰ **T45.1X3** Poisoning by antineoplastic and immunosuppressive drugs, assault

√7ᵗʰ **T45.1X4** Poisoning by antineoplastic and immunosuppressive drugs, undetermined

√7ᵗʰ **T45.1X5** Adverse effect of antineoplastic and immunosuppressive drugs UPD

     AHA: 2020,4Q,11; 2020,3Q,22; 2019,2Q,24,28

√7ᵗʰ **T45.1X6** Underdosing of antineoplastic and immunosuppressive drugs UPD

√5ᵗʰ **T45.2** Poisoning by, adverse effect of and underdosing of vitamins

     EXCLUDES 2   *poisoning by, adverse effect of and underdosing of iron (T45.4)*

           poisoning by, adverse effect of and underdosing of nicotinic acid (derivatives) (T46.7)

           poisoning by, adverse effect of and underdosing of vitamin K (T45.7)

√6ᵗʰ **T45.2X** Poisoning by, adverse effect of and underdosing of vitamins

√7ᵗʰ **T45.2X1** Poisoning by vitamins, accidental (unintentional)

     Poisoning by vitamins NOS

⁷ √7ᵗʰ **T45.2X2** Poisoning by vitamins, intentional self-harm HCC

√7ᵗʰ **T45.2X3** Poisoning by vitamins, assault

√7ᵗʰ **T45.2X4** Poisoning by vitamins, undetermined

√7ᵗʰ **T45.2X5** Adverse effect of vitamins UPD

√7ᵗʰ **T45.2X6** Underdosing of vitamins UPD

     EXCLUDES 1   *vitamin deficiencies (E50-E56)*

Ⓝ Newborn: 0   Ⓟ Pediatric: 0-17   Ⓜ Maternity: 9-64   Ⓐ Adult: 15-124   MCC Major Complication/Comorbidity   CC Complication/Comorbidity   SW Severe Wound Dx

1124   ICD-10-CM 2022

✓5ᵗʰ **T45.3 Poisoning by, adverse effect of and underdosing of enzymes**

    ✓6ᵗʰ **T45.3X Poisoning by, adverse effect of and underdosing of enzymes**

        ✓7ᵗʰ **T45.3X1 Poisoning by enzymes, accidental (unintentional)**
            Poisoning by enzymes NOS

        ⁷ ✓7ᵗʰ **T45.3X2 Poisoning by enzymes, intentional self-harm** `HCC`

        ✓7ᵗʰ **T45.3X3 Poisoning by enzymes, assault**

        ✓7ᵗʰ **T45.3X4 Poisoning by enzymes, undetermined**

        ✓7ᵗʰ **T45.3X5 Adverse effect of enzymes** `UPD`

        ✓7ᵗʰ **T45.3X6 Underdosing of enzymes** `UPD`

✓5ᵗʰ **T45.4 Poisoning by, adverse effect of and underdosing of iron and its compounds**

    ✓6ᵗʰ **T45.4X Poisoning by, adverse effect of and underdosing of iron and its compounds**

        ✓7ᵗʰ **T45.4X1 Poisoning by iron and its compounds, accidental (unintentional)**
            Poisoning by iron and its compounds NOS

        ⁷ ✓7ᵗʰ **T45.4X2 Poisoning by iron and its compounds, intentional self-harm** `HCC`

        ✓7ᵗʰ **T45.4X3 Poisoning by iron and its compounds, assault**

        ✓7ᵗʰ **T45.4X4 Poisoning by iron and its compounds, undetermined**

        ✓7ᵗʰ **T45.4X5 Adverse effect of iron and its compounds** `UPD`

        ✓7ᵗʰ **T45.4X6 Underdosing of iron and its compounds** `UPD`
            EXCLUDES 1   iron deficiency (E61.1)

✓5ᵗʰ **T45.5 Poisoning by, adverse effect of and underdosing of anticoagulants and antithrombotic drugs**

    ✓6ᵗʰ **T45.51 Poisoning by, adverse effect of and underdosing of anticoagulants**

        ✓7ᵗʰ **T45.511 Poisoning by anticoagulants, accidental (unintentional)**
            Poisoning by anticoagulants NOS

        ⁷ ✓7ᵗʰ **T45.512 Poisoning by anticoagulants, intentional self-harm** `HCC`

        ✓7ᵗʰ **T45.513 Poisoning by anticoagulants, assault**

        ✓7ᵗʰ **T45.514 Poisoning by anticoagulants, undetermined**

        ✓7ᵗʰ **T45.515 Adverse effect of anticoagulants** `UPD`
            AHA: 2021,1Q,4; 2016,1Q,14; 2013,2Q,34

        ✓7ᵗʰ **T45.516 Underdosing of anticoagulants** `UPD`

    ✓6ᵗʰ **T45.52 Poisoning by, adverse effect of and underdosing of antithrombotic drugs**
        Poisoning by, adverse effect of and underdosing of antiplatelet drugs
          EXCLUDES 2   poisoning by, adverse effect of and underdosing of aspirin (T39.Ø1-)
                 poisoning by, adverse effect of and underdosing of acetylsalicylic acid (T39.Ø1-)

        ✓7ᵗʰ **T45.521 Poisoning by antithrombotic drugs, accidental (unintentional)**
            Poisoning by antithrombotic drug NOS

        ⁷ ✓7ᵗʰ **T45.522 Poisoning by antithrombotic drugs, intentional self-harm** `HCC`

        ✓7ᵗʰ **T45.523 Poisoning by antithrombotic drugs, assault**

        ✓7ᵗʰ **T45.524 Poisoning by antithrombotic drugs, undetermined**

        ✓7ᵗʰ **T45.525 Adverse effect of antithrombotic drugs** `UPD`
            AHA: 2016,1Q,15

        ✓7ᵗʰ **T45.526 Underdosing of antithrombotic drugs** `UPD`

✓5ᵗʰ **T45.6 Poisoning by, adverse effect of and underdosing of fibrinolysis-affecting drugs**

    ✓6ᵗʰ **T45.6Ø Poisoning by, adverse effect of and underdosing of unspecified fibrinolysis-affecting drugs**

        ✓7ᵗʰ **T45.6Ø1 Poisoning by unspecified fibrinolysis-affecting drugs, accidental (unintentional)**
            Poisoning by fibrinolysis-affecting drug NOS

        ⁷ ✓7ᵗʰ **T45.6Ø2 Poisoning by unspecified fibrinolysis-affecting drugs, intentional self-harm** `HCC`

        ✓7ᵗʰ **T45.6Ø3 Poisoning by unspecified fibrinolysis-affecting drugs, assault**

        ✓7ᵗʰ **T45.6Ø4 Poisoning by unspecified fibrinolysis-affecting drugs, undetermined**

        ✓7ᵗʰ **T45.6Ø5 Adverse effect of unspecified fibrinolysis-affecting drugs** `UPD`

        ✓7ᵗʰ **T45.6Ø6 Underdosing of unspecified fibrinolysis-affecting drugs** `UPD`

    ✓6ᵗʰ **T45.61 Poisoning by, adverse effect of and underdosing of thrombolytic drugs**

        ✓7ᵗʰ **T45.611 Poisoning by thrombolytic drug, accidental (unintentional)**
            Poisoning by thrombolytic drug NOS

        ⁷ ✓7ᵗʰ **T45.612 Poisoning by thrombolytic drug, intentional self-harm** `HCC`

        ✓7ᵗʰ **T45.613 Poisoning by thrombolytic drug, assault**

        ✓7ᵗʰ **T45.614 Poisoning by thrombolytic drug, undetermined**

        ✓7ᵗʰ **T45.615 Adverse effect of thrombolytic drugs** `UPD`
            AHA: 2017,2Q,9

        ✓7ᵗʰ **T45.616 Underdosing of thrombolytic drugs** `UPD`

    ✓6ᵗʰ **T45.62 Poisoning by, adverse effect of and underdosing of hemostatic drugs**

        ✓7ᵗʰ **T45.621 Poisoning by hemostatic drug, accidental (unintentional)**
            Poisoning by hemostatic drug NOS

        ⁷ ✓7ᵗʰ **T45.622 Poisoning by hemostatic drug, intentional self-harm** `HCC`

        ✓7ᵗʰ **T45.623 Poisoning by hemostatic drug, assault**

        ✓7ᵗʰ **T45.624 Poisoning by hemostatic drug, undetermined**

        ✓7ᵗʰ **T45.625 Adverse effect of hemostatic drug** `UPD`

        ✓7ᵗʰ **T45.626 Underdosing of hemostatic drugs** `UPD`

    ✓6ᵗʰ **T45.69 Poisoning by, adverse effect of and underdosing of other fibrinolysis-affecting drugs**

        ✓7ᵗʰ **T45.691 Poisoning by other fibrinolysis-affecting drugs, accidental (unintentional)**
            Poisoning by other fibrinolysis-affecting drug NOS

        ⁷ ✓7ᵗʰ **T45.692 Poisoning by other fibrinolysis-affecting drugs, intentional self-harm** `HCC`

        ✓7ᵗʰ **T45.693 Poisoning by other fibrinolysis-affecting drugs, assault**

        ✓7ᵗʰ **T45.694 Poisoning by other fibrinolysis-affecting drugs, undetermined**

        ✓7ᵗʰ **T45.695 Adverse effect of other fibrinolysis-affecting drugs** `UPD`

        ✓7ᵗʰ **T45.696 Underdosing of other fibrinolysis-affecting drugs** `UPD`

✓5ᵗʰ **T45.7 Poisoning by, adverse effect of and underdosing of anticoagulant antagonists, vitamin K and other coagulants**

    ✓6ᵗʰ **T45.7X Poisoning by, adverse effect of and underdosing of anticoagulant antagonists, vitamin K and other coagulants**

        ✓7ᵗʰ **T45.7X1 Poisoning by anticoagulant antagonists, vitamin K and other coagulants, accidental (unintentional)**
            Poisoning by anticoagulant antagonists, vitamin K and other coagulants NOS

        ⁷ ✓7ᵗʰ **T45.7X2 Poisoning by anticoagulant antagonists, vitamin K and other coagulants, intentional self-harm** `HCC`

        ✓7ᵗʰ **T45.7X3 Poisoning by anticoagulant antagonists, vitamin K and other coagulants, assault**

        ✓7ᵗʰ **T45.7X4 Poisoning by anticoagulant antagonists, vitamin K and other coagulants, undetermined**

        ✓7ᵗʰ **T45.7X5 Adverse effect of anticoagulant antagonists, vitamin K and other coagulants** `UPD`

        ✓7ᵗʰ **T45.7X6 Underdosing of anticoagulant antagonist, vitamin K and other coagulants** `UPD`
          EXCLUDES 1   vitamin K deficiency (E56.1)

✓ Additional Character Required   ✓x7ᵗʰ Placeholder   Questionable PDx   Manifestation   Unspecified Dx   `UPD` Unacceptable PDx   `H1`-`H14` HAC   `HCC` CMS-HCC Dx   `HIV` HIV Dx

ICD-10-CM 2022   1125

√5ᵗʰ **T45.8 Poisoning by, adverse effect of and underdosing of other primarily systemic and hematological agents**

Poisoning by, adverse effect of and underdosing of liver preparations and other antianemic agents

Poisoning by, adverse effect of and underdosing of natural blood and blood products

Poisoning by, adverse effect of and underdosing of plasma substitute

     EXCLUDES 2   *poisoning by, adverse effect of and underdosing of immunoglobulin (T50.Z1)*

         poisoning by, adverse effect of and underdosing of iron (T45.4)

         transfusion reactions (T80.-)

√6ᵗʰ **T45.8X Poisoning by, adverse effect of and underdosing of other primarily systemic and hematological agents**

√7ᵗʰ **T45.8X1 Poisoning by other primarily systemic and hematological agents, accidental (unintentional)**

Poisoning by other primarily systemic and hematological agents NOS

7 √7ᵗʰ **T45.8X2 Poisoning by other primarily systemic and hematological agents, intentional self-harm** HCC

√7ᵗʰ **T45.8X3 Poisoning by other primarily systemic and hematological agents, assault**

√7ᵗʰ **T45.8X4 Poisoning by other primarily systemic and hematological agents, undetermined**

√7ᵗʰ **T45.8X5 Adverse effect of other primarily systemic and hematological agents** UPD

AHA: 2016,4Q,42

√7ᵗʰ **T45.8X6 Underdosing of other primarily systemic and hematological agents** UPD

√5ᵗʰ **T45.9 Poisoning by, adverse effect of and underdosing of unspecified primarily systemic and hematological agent**

√x7ᵗʰ **T45.91 Poisoning by unspecified primarily systemic and hematological agent, accidental (unintentional)**

Poisoning by primarily systemic and hematological agent NOS

7 √x7ᵗʰ **T45.92 Poisoning by unspecified primarily systemic and hematological agent, intentional self-harm** HCC

√x7ᵗʰ **T45.93 Poisoning by unspecified primarily systemic and hematological agent, assault**

√x7ᵗʰ **T45.94 Poisoning by unspecified primarily systemic and hematological agent, undetermined**

√x7ᵗʰ **T45.95 Adverse effect of unspecified primarily systemic and hematological agent** UPD

√x7ᵗʰ **T45.96 Underdosing of unspecified primarily systemic and hematological agent** UPD

√4ᵗʰ **T46 Poisoning by, adverse effect of and underdosing of agents primarily affecting the cardiovascular system**

     EXCLUDES 1   *poisoning by, adverse effect of and underdosing of metaraminol (T44.4)*

The appropriate 7th character is to be added to each code from category T46.

A   initial encounter
D   subsequent encounter
S   sequela

√5ᵗʰ **T46.0 Poisoning by, adverse effect of and underdosing of cardiac-stimulant glycosides and drugs of similar action**

√6ᵗʰ **T46.0X Poisoning by, adverse effect of and underdosing of cardiac-stimulant glycosides and drugs of similar action**

√7ᵗʰ **T46.0X1 Poisoning by cardiac-stimulant glycosides and drugs of similar action, accidental (unintentional)**

Poisoning by cardiac-stimulant glycosides and drugs of similar action NOS

7 √7ᵗʰ **T46.0X2 Poisoning by cardiac-stimulant glycosides and drugs of similar action, intentional self-harm** HCC

√7ᵗʰ **T46.0X3 Poisoning by cardiac-stimulant glycosides and drugs of similar action, assault**

√7ᵗʰ **T46.0X4 Poisoning by cardiac-stimulant glycosides and drugs of similar action, undetermined**

√7ᵗʰ **T46.0X5 Adverse effect of cardiac-stimulant glycosides and drugs of similar action** UPD

√7ᵗʰ **T46.0X6 Underdosing of cardiac-stimulant glycosides and drugs of similar action** UPD

√5ᵗʰ **T46.1 Poisoning by, adverse effect of and underdosing of calcium-channel blockers**

√6ᵗʰ **T46.1X Poisoning by, adverse effect of and underdosing of calcium-channel blockers**

√7ᵗʰ **T46.1X1 Poisoning by calcium-channel blockers, accidental (unintentional)**

Poisoning by calcium-channel blockers NOS

7 √7ᵗʰ **T46.1X2 Poisoning by calcium-channel blockers, intentional self-harm** HCC

√7ᵗʰ **T46.1X3 Poisoning by calcium-channel blockers, assault**

√7ᵗʰ **T46.1X4 Poisoning by calcium-channel blockers, undetermined**

√7ᵗʰ **T46.1X5 Adverse effect of calcium-channel blockers** UPD

√7ᵗʰ **T46.1X6 Underdosing of calcium-channel blockers** UPD

√5ᵗʰ **T46.2 Poisoning by, adverse effect of and underdosing of other antidysrhythmic drugs, not elsewhere classified**

     EXCLUDES 1   *poisoning by, adverse effect of and underdosing of beta-adrenoreceptor antagonists (T44.7-)*

√6ᵗʰ **T46.2X Poisoning by, adverse effect of and underdosing of other antidysrhythmic drugs**

√7ᵗʰ **T46.2X1 Poisoning by other antidysrhythmic drugs, accidental (unintentional)**

Poisoning by other antidysrhythmic drugs NOS

7 √7ᵗʰ **T46.2X2 Poisoning by other antidysrhythmic drugs, intentional self-harm** HCC

√7ᵗʰ **T46.2X3 Poisoning by other antidysrhythmic drugs, assault**

√7ᵗʰ **T46.2X4 Poisoning by other antidysrhythmic drugs, undetermined**

√7ᵗʰ **T46.2X5 Adverse effect of other antidysrhythmic drugs** UPD

√7ᵗʰ **T46.2X6 Underdosing of other antidysrhythmic drugs** UPD

√5ᵗʰ **T46.3 Poisoning by, adverse effect of and underdosing of coronary vasodilators**

Poisoning by, adverse effect of and underdosing of dipyridamole

     EXCLUDES 1   *poisoning by, adverse effect of and underdosing of calcium-channel blockers (T46.1)*

√6ᵗʰ **T46.3X Poisoning by, adverse effect of and underdosing of coronary vasodilators**

√7ᵗʰ **T46.3X1 Poisoning by coronary vasodilators, accidental (unintentional)**

Poisoning by coronary vasodilators NOS

7 √7ᵗʰ **T46.3X2 Poisoning by coronary vasodilators, intentional self-harm** HCC

√7ᵗʰ **T46.3X3 Poisoning by coronary vasodilators, assault**

√7ᵗʰ **T46.3X4 Poisoning by coronary vasodilators, undetermined**

√7ᵗʰ **T46.3X5 Adverse effect of coronary vasodilators** UPD

√7ᵗʰ **T46.3X6 Underdosing of coronary vasodilators** UPD

√5ᵗʰ **T46.4 Poisoning by, adverse effect of and underdosing of angiotensin-converting-enzyme inhibitors**

√6ᵗʰ **T46.4X Poisoning by, adverse effect of and underdosing of angiotensin-converting-enzyme inhibitors**

√7ᵗʰ **T46.4X1 Poisoning by angiotensin-converting-enzyme inhibitors, accidental (unintentional)**

Poisoning by angiotensin-converting-enzyme inhibitors NOS

7 √7ᵗʰ **T46.4X2 Poisoning by angiotensin-converting-enzyme inhibitors, intentional self-harm** HCC

√7ᵗʰ **T46.4X3 Poisoning by angiotensin-converting-enzyme inhibitors, assault**

√7ᵗʰ **T46.4X4 Poisoning by angiotensin-converting-enzyme inhibitors, undetermined**

√7ᵗʰ **T46.4X5** Adverse effect of angiotensin-converting-enzyme inhibitors   UPD

√7ᵗʰ **T46.4X6** Underdosing of angiotensin-converting-enzyme inhibitors   UPD

√5ᵗʰ **T46.5** **Poisoning by, adverse effect of and underdosing of other antihypertensive drugs**

> EXCLUDES 2   poisoning by, adverse effect of and underdosing of beta-adrenoreceptor antagonists (T44.7)
> poisoning by, adverse effect of and underdosing of calcium-channel blockers (T46.1)
> poisoning by, adverse effect of and underdosing of diuretics (T50.0-T50.2)

√6ᵗʰ **T46.5X** **Poisoning by, adverse effect of and underdosing of other antihypertensive drugs**

√7ᵗʰ **T46.5X1** **Poisoning by other antihypertensive drugs,** accidental **(unintentional)**
> Poisoning by other antihypertensive drugs NOS

7 √7ᵗʰ **T46.5X2** **Poisoning by other antihypertensive drugs,** intentional self-harm   HCC

√7ᵗʰ **T46.5X3** **Poisoning by other antihypertensive drugs,** assault

√7ᵗʰ **T46.5X4** **Poisoning by other antihypertensive drugs,** undetermined

√7ᵗʰ **T46.5X5** Adverse effect of other antihypertensive drugs   UPD

√7ᵗʰ **T46.5X6** Underdosing of other antihypertensive drugs   UPD

√5ᵗʰ **T46.6** **Poisoning by, adverse effect of and underdosing of antihyperlipidemic and antiarteriosclerotic drugs**

√6ᵗʰ **T46.6X** **Poisoning by, adverse effect of and underdosing of** antihyperlipidemic and antiarteriosclerotic drugs

√7ᵗʰ **T46.6X1** **Poisoning by antihyperlipidemic and antiarteriosclerotic drugs,** accidental **(unintentional)**
> Poisoning by antihyperlipidemic and antiarteriosclerotic drugs NOS

7 √7ᵗʰ **T46.6X2** **Poisoning by antihyperlipidemic and antiarteriosclerotic drugs,** intentional self-harm   HCC

√7ᵗʰ **T46.6X3** **Poisoning by antihyperlipidemic and antiarteriosclerotic drugs,** assault

√7ᵗʰ **T46.6X4** **Poisoning by antihyperlipidemic and antiarteriosclerotic drugs,** undetermined

√7ᵗʰ **T46.6X5** Adverse effect of antihyperlipidemic and antiarteriosclerotic drugs   UPD

√7ᵗʰ **T46.6X6** Underdosing of antihyperlipidemic and antiarteriosclerotic drugs   UPD

√5ᵗʰ **T46.7** **Poisoning by, adverse effect of and underdosing of peripheral vasodilators**
> Poisoning by, adverse effect of and underdosing of nicotinic acid (derivatives)

> EXCLUDES 1   poisoning by, adverse effect of and underdosing of papaverine (T44.3)

√6ᵗʰ **T46.7X** **Poisoning by, adverse effect of and underdosing of** peripheral vasodilators

√7ᵗʰ **T46.7X1** **Poisoning by peripheral vasodilators,** accidental **(unintentional)**
> Poisoning by peripheral vasodilators NOS

7 √7ᵗʰ **T46.7X2** **Poisoning by peripheral vasodilators,** intentional self-harm   HCC

√7ᵗʰ **T46.7X3** **Poisoning by peripheral vasodilators,** assault

√7ᵗʰ **T46.7X4** **Poisoning by peripheral vasodilators,** undetermined

√7ᵗʰ **T46.7X5** Adverse effect of peripheral vasodilators   UPD

√7ᵗʰ **T46.7X6** Underdosing of peripheral vasodilators   UPD

√5ᵗʰ **T46.8** **Poisoning by, adverse effect of and underdosing of antivaricose drugs, including sclerosing agents**

√6ᵗʰ **T46.8X** **Poisoning by, adverse effect of and underdosing of** antivaricose drugs, including sclerosing agents

√7ᵗʰ **T46.8X1** **Poisoning by antivaricose drugs, including sclerosing agents,** accidental **(unintentional)**
> Poisoning by antivaricose drugs, including sclerosing agents NOS

7 √7ᵗʰ **T46.8X2** **Poisoning by antivaricose drugs, including sclerosing agents,** intentional self-harm   HCC

√7ᵗʰ **T46.8X3** **Poisoning by antivaricose drugs, including sclerosing agents,** assault

√7ᵗʰ **T46.8X4** **Poisoning by antivaricose drugs, including sclerosing agents,** undetermined

√7ᵗʰ **T46.8X5** Adverse effect of antivaricose drugs, including sclerosing agents   UPD

√7ᵗʰ **T46.8X6** Underdosing of antivaricose drugs, including sclerosing agents   UPD

√5ᵗʰ **T46.9** **Poisoning by, adverse effect of and underdosing of other and unspecified agents primarily affecting the cardiovascular system**

√6ᵗʰ **T46.90** **Poisoning by, adverse effect of and underdosing of unspecified agents primarily affecting the cardiovascular system**

√7ᵗʰ **T46.901** **Poisoning by unspecified agents primarily affecting the cardiovascular system,** accidental **(unintentional)**

7 √7ᵗʰ **T46.902** **Poisoning by unspecified agents primarily affecting the cardiovascular system,** intentional self-harm   HCC

√7ᵗʰ **T46.903** **Poisoning by unspecified agents primarily affecting the cardiovascular system,** assault

√7ᵗʰ **T46.904** **Poisoning by unspecified agents primarily affecting the cardiovascular system,** undetermined

√7ᵗʰ **T46.905** Adverse effect of unspecified agents primarily affecting the cardiovascular system   UPD

√7ᵗʰ **T46.906** Underdosing of unspecified agents primarily affecting the cardiovascular system   UPD

√6ᵗʰ **T46.99** **Poisoning by, adverse effect of and underdosing of other agents primarily affecting the cardiovascular system**

√7ᵗʰ **T46.991** **Poisoning by other agents primarily affecting the cardiovascular system,** accidental **(unintentional)**

7 √7ᵗʰ **T46.992** **Poisoning by other agents primarily affecting the cardiovascular system,** intentional self-harm   HCC

√7ᵗʰ **T46.993** **Poisoning by other agents primarily affecting the cardiovascular system,** assault

√7ᵗʰ **T46.994** **Poisoning by other agents primarily affecting the cardiovascular system,** undetermined

√7ᵗʰ **T46.995** Adverse effect of other agents primarily affecting the cardiovascular system   UPD

√7ᵗʰ **T46.996** Underdosing of other agents primarily affecting the cardiovascular system   UPD

√4ᵗʰ **T47** **Poisoning by, adverse effect of and underdosing of agents primarily affecting the gastrointestinal system**

> The appropriate 7th character is to be added to each code from category T47.
> A   initial encounter
> D   subsequent encounter
> S   sequela

√5ᵗʰ **T47.0** **Poisoning by, adverse effect of and underdosing of histamine H2-receptor blockers**

√6ᵗʰ **T47.0X** **Poisoning by, adverse effect of and underdosing of** histamine H2-receptor blockers

√7ᵗʰ **T47.0X1** **Poisoning by histamine H2-receptor blockers,** accidental **(unintentional)**
> Poisoning by histamine H2-receptor blockers NOS

7 √7ᵗʰ **T47.0X2** **Poisoning by histamine H2-receptor blockers,** intentional self-harm   HCC

√7ᵗʰ **T47.0X3** **Poisoning by histamine H2-receptor blockers,** assault

√7ᵗʰ **T47.0X4** **Poisoning by histamine H2-receptor blockers,** undetermined

√7ᵗʰ **T47.0X5** Adverse effect of histamine H2-receptor blockers   UPD

√7ᵗʰ **T47.0X6** Underdosing of histamine H2-receptor blockers   UPD

✔ Additional Character Required   √x7ᵗʰ Placeholder   Questionable PDx   Manifestation   Unspecified Dx   UPD Unacceptable PDx   H1-H14 HAC   HCC CMS-HCC Dx   HIV HIV Dx

ICD-10-CM 2022   1127

✓5th **T47.1** **Poisoning by, adverse effect of and underdosing of other antacids and anti-gastric-secretion drugs**

  ✓6th **T47.1X** **Poisoning by, adverse effect of and underdosing of other antacids and anti-gastric-secretion drugs**

    ✓7th **T47.1X1** **Poisoning by other antacids and anti-gastric-secretion drugs, accidental (unintentional)**
        Poisoning by other antacids and anti-gastric-secretion drugs NOS

    7 ✓7th **T47.1X2** **Poisoning by other antacids and anti-gastric-secretion drugs, intentional self-harm** HCC

    ✓7th **T47.1X3** **Poisoning by other antacids and anti-gastric-secretion drugs, assault**

    ✓7th **T47.1X4** **Poisoning by other antacids and anti-gastric-secretion drugs, undetermined**

    ✓7th **T47.1X5** **Adverse effect of other antacids and anti-gastric-secretion drugs** UPD

    ✓7th **T47.1X6** **Underdosing of other antacids and anti-gastric-secretion drugs** UPD

✓5th **T47.2** **Poisoning by, adverse effect of and underdosing of stimulant laxatives**

  ✓6th **T47.2X** **Poisoning by, adverse effect of and underdosing of stimulant laxatives**

    ✓7th **T47.2X1** **Poisoning by stimulant laxatives, accidental (unintentional)**
        Poisoning by stimulant laxatives NOS

    7 ✓7th **T47.2X2** **Poisoning by stimulant laxatives, intentional self-harm** HCC

    ✓7th **T47.2X3** **Poisoning by stimulant laxatives, assault**

    ✓7th **T47.2X4** **Poisoning by stimulant laxatives, undetermined**

    ✓7th **T47.2X5** **Adverse effect of stimulant laxatives** UPD

    ✓7th **T47.2X6** **Underdosing of stimulant laxatives** UPD

✓5th **T47.3** **Poisoning by, adverse effect of and underdosing of saline and osmotic laxatives**

  ✓6th **T47.3X** **Poisoning by and adverse effect of saline and osmotic laxatives**

    ✓7th **T47.3X1** **Poisoning by saline and osmotic laxatives, accidental (unintentional)**
        Poisoning by saline and osmotic laxatives NOS

    7 ✓7th **T47.3X2** **Poisoning by saline and osmotic laxatives, intentional self-harm** HCC

    ✓7th **T47.3X3** **Poisoning by saline and osmotic laxatives, assault**

    ✓7th **T47.3X4** **Poisoning by saline and osmotic laxatives, undetermined**

    ✓7th **T47.3X5** **Adverse effect of saline and osmotic laxatives** UPD

    ✓7th **T47.3X6** **Underdosing of saline and osmotic laxatives** UPD

✓5th **T47.4** **Poisoning by, adverse effect of and underdosing of other laxatives**

  ✓6th **T47.4X** **Poisoning by, adverse effect of and underdosing of other laxatives**

    ✓7th **T47.4X1** **Poisoning by other laxatives, accidental (unintentional)**
        Poisoning by other laxatives NOS

    7 ✓7th **T47.4X2** **Poisoning by other laxatives, intentional self-harm** HCC

    ✓7th **T47.4X3** **Poisoning by other laxatives, assault**

    ✓7th **T47.4X4** **Poisoning by other laxatives, undetermined**

    ✓7th **T47.4X5** **Adverse effect of other laxatives** UPD

    ✓7th **T47.4X6** **Underdosing of other laxatives** UPD

✓5th **T47.5** **Poisoning by, adverse effect of and underdosing of digestants**

  ✓6th **T47.5X** **Poisoning by, adverse effect of and underdosing of digestants**

    ✓7th **T47.5X1** **Poisoning by digestants, accidental (unintentional)**
        Poisoning by digestants NOS

    7 ✓7th **T47.5X2** **Poisoning by digestants, intentional self-harm** HCC

    ✓7th **T47.5X3** **Poisoning by digestants, assault**

    ✓7th **T47.5X4** **Poisoning by digestants, undetermined**

    ✓7th **T47.5X5** **Adverse effect of digestants** UPD

    ✓7th **T47.5X6** **Underdosing of digestants** UPD

✓5th **T47.6** **Poisoning by, adverse effect of and underdosing of antidiarrheal drugs**

  EXCLUDES 2   *poisoning by, adverse effect of and underdosing of systemic antibiotics and other anti-infectives (T36-T37)*

  ✓6th **T47.6X** **Poisoning by, adverse effect of and underdosing of antidiarrheal drugs**

    ✓7th **T47.6X1** **Poisoning by antidiarrheal drugs, accidental (unintentional)**
        Poisoning by antidiarrheal drugs NOS

    7 ✓7th **T47.6X2** **Poisoning by antidiarrheal drugs, intentional self-harm** HCC

    ✓7th **T47.6X3** **Poisoning by antidiarrheal drugs, assault**

    ✓7th **T47.6X4** **Poisoning by antidiarrheal drugs, undetermined**

    ✓7th **T47.6X5** **Adverse effect of antidiarrheal drugs** UPD

    ✓7th **T47.6X6** **Underdosing of antidiarrheal drugs** UPD

✓5th **T47.7** **Poisoning by, adverse effect of and underdosing of emetics**

  ✓6th **T47.7X** **Poisoning by, adverse effect of and underdosing of emetics**

    ✓7th **T47.7X1** **Poisoning by emetics, accidental (unintentional)**
        Poisoning by emetics NOS

    7 ✓7th **T47.7X2** **Poisoning by emetics, intentional self-harm** HCC

    ✓7th **T47.7X3** **Poisoning by emetics, assault**

    ✓7th **T47.7X4** **Poisoning by emetics, undetermined**

    ✓7th **T47.7X5** **Adverse effect of emetics** UPD

    ✓7th **T47.7X6** **Underdosing of emetics** UPD

✓5th **T47.8** **Poisoning by, adverse effect of and underdosing of other agents primarily affecting gastrointestinal system**

  ✓6th **T47.8X** **Poisoning by, adverse effect of and underdosing of other agents primarily affecting gastrointestinal system**

    ✓7th **T47.8X1** **Poisoning by other agents primarily affecting gastrointestinal system, accidental (unintentional)**
        Poisoning by other agents primarily affecting gastrointestinal system NOS

    7 ✓7th **T47.8X2** **Poisoning by other agents primarily affecting gastrointestinal system, intentional self-harm** HCC

    ✓7th **T47.8X3** **Poisoning by other agents primarily affecting gastrointestinal system, assault**

    ✓7th **T47.8X4** **Poisoning by other agents primarily affecting gastrointestinal system, undetermined**

    ✓7th **T47.8X5** **Adverse effect of other agents primarily affecting gastrointestinal system** UPD

    ✓7th **T47.8X6** **Underdosing of other agents primarily affecting gastrointestinal system** UPD

✓5th **T47.9** **Poisoning by, adverse effect of and underdosing of unspecified agents primarily affecting the gastrointestinal system**

  ✓x7th **T47.91** **Poisoning by unspecified agents primarily affecting the gastrointestinal system, accidental (unintentional)**
    Poisoning by agents primarily affecting the gastrointestinal system NOS

  7 ✓x7th **T47.92** **Poisoning by unspecified agents primarily affecting the gastrointestinal system, intentional self-harm** HCC

  ✓x7th **T47.93** **Poisoning by unspecified agents primarily affecting the gastrointestinal system, assault**

  ✓x7th **T47.94** **Poisoning by unspecified agents primarily affecting the gastrointestinal system, undetermined**

  ✓x7th **T47.95** **Adverse effect of unspecified agents primarily affecting the gastrointestinal system** UPD

  ✓x7th **T47.96** **Underdosing of unspecified agents primarily affecting the gastrointestinal system** UPD

✓4ᵗʰ **T48** **Poisoning by, adverse effect of and underdosing of agents primarily acting on smooth and skeletal muscles and the respiratory system**

> The appropriate 7th character is to be added to each code from category T48.
> A   initial encounter
> D   subsequent encounter
> S   sequela

✓5ᵗʰ **T48.0** **Poisoning by, adverse effect of and underdosing of oxytocic drugs**

> EXCLUDES 1   *poisoning by, adverse effect of and underdosing of estrogens, progestogens and antagonists (T38.4-T38.6)*

   ✓6ᵗʰ **T48.0X** **Poisoning by, adverse effect of and underdosing of oxytocic drugs**

     ✓7ᵗʰ **T48.0X1** **Poisoning by oxytocic drugs, accidental (unintentional)**
       Poisoning by oxytocic drugs NOS

     7 ✓7ᵗʰ **T48.0X2** **Poisoning by oxytocic drugs, intentional self-harm** **HCC**

     ✓7ᵗʰ **T48.0X3** **Poisoning by oxytocic drugs, assault**

     ✓7ᵗʰ **T48.0X4** **Poisoning by oxytocic drugs, undetermined**

     ✓7ᵗʰ **T48.0X5** Adverse effect of oxytocic drugs **UPD**

     ✓7ᵗʰ **T48.0X6** Underdosing of oxytocic drugs **UPD**

✓5ᵗʰ **T48.1** **Poisoning by, adverse effect of and underdosing of skeletal muscle relaxants [neuromuscular blocking agents]**

   ✓6ᵗʰ **T48.1X** **Poisoning by, adverse effect of and underdosing of skeletal muscle relaxants [neuromuscular blocking agents]**

     ✓7ᵗʰ **T48.1X1** **Poisoning by skeletal muscle relaxants [neuromuscular blocking agents], accidental (unintentional)**
       Poisoning by skeletal muscle relaxants [neuromuscular blocking agents] NOS

     7 ✓7ᵗʰ **T48.1X2** **Poisoning by skeletal muscle relaxants [neuromuscular blocking agents], intentional self-harm** **HCC**

     ✓7ᵗʰ **T48.1X3** **Poisoning by skeletal muscle relaxants [neuromuscular blocking agents], assault**

     ✓7ᵗʰ **T48.1X4** **Poisoning by skeletal muscle relaxants [neuromuscular blocking agents], undetermined**

     ✓7ᵗʰ **T48.1X5** Adverse effect of skeletal muscle relaxants [neuromuscular blocking agents] **UPD**

     ✓7ᵗʰ **T48.1X6** Underdosing of skeletal muscle relaxants [neuromuscular blocking agents] **UPD**

✓5ᵗʰ **T48.2** **Poisoning by, adverse effect of and underdosing of other and unspecified drugs acting on muscles**

   ✓6ᵗʰ **T48.20** **Poisoning by, adverse effect of and underdosing of unspecified drugs acting on muscles**

     ✓7ᵗʰ **T48.201** **Poisoning by unspecified drugs acting on muscles, accidental (unintentional)**
       Poisoning by unspecified drugs acting on muscles NOS

     7 ✓7ᵗʰ **T48.202** **Poisoning by unspecified drugs acting on muscles, intentional self-harm** **HCC**

     ✓7ᵗʰ **T48.203** **Poisoning by unspecified drugs acting on muscles, assault**

     ✓7ᵗʰ **T48.204** **Poisoning by unspecified drugs acting on muscles, undetermined**

     ✓7ᵗʰ **T48.205** Adverse effect of unspecified drugs acting on muscles **UPD**

     ✓7ᵗʰ **T48.206** Underdosing of unspecified drugs acting on muscles **UPD**

   ✓6ᵗʰ **T48.29** **Poisoning by, adverse effect of and underdosing of other drugs acting on muscles**

     ✓7ᵗʰ **T48.291** **Poisoning by other drugs acting on muscles, accidental (unintentional)**
       Poisoning by other drugs acting on muscles NOS

     7 ✓7ᵗʰ **T48.292** **Poisoning by other drugs acting on muscles, intentional self-harm** **HCC**

     ✓7ᵗʰ **T48.293** **Poisoning by other drugs acting on muscles, assault**

     ✓7ᵗʰ **T48.294** **Poisoning by other drugs acting on muscles, undetermined**

     ✓7ᵗʰ **T48.295** Adverse effect of other drugs acting on muscles **UPD**

✓7ᵗʰ **T48.296** Underdosing of other drugs acting on muscles **UPD**

✓5ᵗʰ **T48.3** **Poisoning by, adverse effect of and underdosing of antitussives**

   ✓6ᵗʰ **T48.3X** **Poisoning by, adverse effect of and underdosing of antitussives**

     ✓7ᵗʰ **T48.3X1** **Poisoning by antitussives, accidental (unintentional)**
       Poisoning by antitussives NOS

     7 ✓7ᵗʰ **T48.3X2** **Poisoning by antitussives, intentional self-harm** **HCC**

     ✓7ᵗʰ **T48.3X4** **Poisoning by antitussives, assault**

     ✓7ᵗʰ **T48.3X4** **Poisoning by antitussives, undetermined**

     ✓7ᵗʰ **T48.3X5** Adverse effect of antitussives **UPD**

     ✓7ᵗʰ **T48.3X6** Underdosing of antitussives **UPD**

✓5ᵗʰ **T48.4** **Poisoning by, adverse effect of and underdosing of expectorants**

   ✓6ᵗʰ **T48.4X** **Poisoning by, adverse effect of and underdosing of expectorants**

     ✓7ᵗʰ **T48.4X1** **Poisoning by expectorants, accidental (unintentional)**
       Poisoning by expectorants NOS

     7 ✓7ᵗʰ **T48.4X2** **Poisoning by expectorants, intentional self-harm** **HCC**

     ✓7ᵗʰ **T48.4X3** **Poisoning by expectorants, assault**

     ✓7ᵗʰ **T48.4X4** **Poisoning by expectorants, undetermined**

     ✓7ᵗʰ **T48.4X5** Adverse effect of expectorants **UPD**

     ✓7ᵗʰ **T48.4X6** Underdosing of expectorants **UPD**

✓5ᵗʰ **T48.5** **Poisoning by, adverse effect of and underdosing of other anti-common-cold drugs**

> Poisoning by, adverse effect of and underdosing of decongestants
> EXCLUDES 2   *poisoning by, adverse effect of and underdosing of antipyretics, NEC (T39.9-)*
> *poisoning by, adverse effect of and underdosing of non-steroidal antiinflammatory drugs (T39.3-)*
> *poisoning by, adverse effect of and underdosing of salicylates (T39.0-)*

   ✓6ᵗʰ **T48.5X** **Poisoning by, adverse effect of and underdosing of other anti-common-cold drugs**

     ✓7ᵗʰ **T48.5X1** **Poisoning by other anti-common-cold drugs, accidental (unintentional)**
       Poisoning by other anti-common-cold drugs NOS

     7 ✓7ᵗʰ **T48.5X2** **Poisoning by other anti-common-cold drugs, intentional self-harm** **HCC**

     ✓7ᵗʰ **T48.5X3** **Poisoning by other anti-common-cold drugs, assault**

     ✓7ᵗʰ **T48.5X4** **Poisoning by other anti-common-cold drugs, undetermined**

     ✓7ᵗʰ **T48.5X5** Adverse effect of other anti-common-cold drugs **UPD**

     ✓7ᵗʰ **T48.5X6** Underdosing of other anti-common-cold drugs **UPD**

✓5ᵗʰ **T48.6** **Poisoning by, adverse effect of and underdosing of antiasthmatics, not elsewhere classified**

> Poisoning by, adverse effect of and underdosing of beta-adrenoreceptor agonists used in asthma therapy
> EXCLUDES 1   *poisoning by, adverse effect of and underdosing of anterior pituitary [adenohypophyseal] hormones (T38.8)*
> *poisoning by, adverse effect of and underdosing of beta-adrenoreceptor agonists not used in asthma therapy (T44.5)*

   ✓6ᵗʰ **T48.6X** **Poisoning by, adverse effect of and underdosing of antiasthmatics**

     ✓7ᵗʰ **T48.6X1** **Poisoning by antiasthmatics, accidental (unintentional)**
       Poisoning by antiasthmatics NOS

     7 ✓7ᵗʰ **T48.6X2** **Poisoning by antiasthmatics, intentional self-harm** **HCC**

     ✓7ᵗʰ **T48.6X3** **Poisoning by antiasthmatics, assault**

     ✓7ᵗʰ **T48.6X4** **Poisoning by antiasthmatics, undetermined**

     ✓7ᵗʰ **T48.6X5** Adverse effect of antiasthmatics **UPD**

     ✓7ᵗʰ **T48.6X6** Underdosing of antiasthmatics **UPD**

✓ Additional Character Required   ✓x7ᵗʰ Placeholder   Questionable PDx   Manifestation   Unspecified Dx   **UPD** Unacceptable PDx   **H1-H14** HAC   **HCC** CMS-HCC Dx   **HIV** HIV Dx

ICD-10-CM 2022   1129

√5ᵗʰ **T48.9** Poisoning by, adverse effect of and underdosing of other and unspecified agents primarily acting on the respiratory system

√6ᵗʰ **T48.90** Poisoning by, adverse effect of and underdosing of unspecified agents primarily acting on the respiratory system

√7ᵗʰ **T48.901** Poisoning by unspecified agents primarily acting on the respiratory system, accidental (unintentional)

7 √7ᵗʰ **T48.902** Poisoning by unspecified agents primarily acting on the respiratory system, intentional self-harm **HCC**

√7ᵗʰ **T48.903** Poisoning by unspecified agents primarily acting on the respiratory system, assault

√7ᵗʰ **T48.904** Poisoning by unspecified agents primarily acting on the respiratory system, undetermined

√7ᵗʰ **T48.905** Adverse effect of unspecified agents primarily acting on the respiratory system **UPD**

√7ᵗʰ **T48.906** Underdosing of unspecified agents primarily acting on the respiratory system **UPD**

√6ᵗʰ **T48.99** Poisoning by, adverse effect of and underdosing of other agents primarily acting on the respiratory system

√7ᵗʰ **T48.991** Poisoning by other agents primarily acting on the respiratory system, accidental (unintentional)

7 √7ᵗʰ **T48.992** Poisoning by other agents primarily acting on the respiratory system, intentional self-harm **HCC**

√7ᵗʰ **T48.993** Poisoning by other agents primarily acting on the respiratory system, assault

√7ᵗʰ **T48.994** Poisoning by other agents primarily acting on the respiratory system, undetermined

√7ᵗʰ **T48.995** Adverse effect of other agents primarily acting on the respiratory system **UPD**

√7ᵗʰ **T48.996** Underdosing of other agents primarily acting on the respiratory system **UPD**

√4ᵗʰ **T49** Poisoning by, adverse effect of and underdosing of topical agents primarily affecting skin and mucous membrane and by ophthalmological, otorhinolaryngological and dental drugs

INCLUDES poisoning by, adverse effect of and underdosing of glucocorticoids, topically used

The appropriate 7th character is to be added to each code from category T49.
A   initial encounter
D   subsequent encounter
S   sequela

√5ᵗʰ **T49.0** Poisoning by, adverse effect of and underdosing of local antifungal, anti-infective and anti-inflammatory drugs

√6ᵗʰ **T49.0X** Poisoning by, adverse effect of and underdosing of local antifungal, anti-infective and anti-inflammatory drugs

√7ᵗʰ **T49.0X1** Poisoning by local antifungal, anti-infective and anti-inflammatory drugs, accidental (unintentional)
Poisoning by local antifungal, anti-infective and anti-inflammatory drugs NOS

7 √7ᵗʰ **T49.0X2** Poisoning by local antifungal, anti-infective and anti-inflammatory drugs, intentional self-harm **HCC**

√7ᵗʰ **T49.0X3** Poisoning by local antifungal, anti-infective and anti-inflammatory drugs, assault

√7ᵗʰ **T49.0X4** Poisoning by local antifungal, anti-infective and anti-inflammatory drugs, undetermined

√7ᵗʰ **T49.0X5** Adverse effect of local antifungal, anti-infective and anti-inflammatory drugs **UPD**

√7ᵗʰ **T49.0X6** Underdosing of local antifungal, anti-infective and anti-inflammatory drugs **UPD**

√5ᵗʰ **T49.1** Poisoning by, adverse effect of and underdosing of antipruritics

√6ᵗʰ **T49.1X** Poisoning by, adverse effect of and underdosing of antipruritics

√7ᵗʰ **T49.1X1** Poisoning by antipruritics, accidental (unintentional)
Poisoning by antipruritics NOS

7 √7ᵗʰ **T49.1X2** Poisoning by antipruritics, intentional self-harm **HCC**

√7ᵗʰ **T49.1X3** Poisoning by antipruritics, assault

√7ᵗʰ **T49.1X4** Poisoning by antipruritics, undetermined

√7ᵗʰ **T49.1X5** Adverse effect of antipruritics **UPD**

√7ᵗʰ **T49.1X6** Underdosing of antipruritics **UPD**

√5ᵗʰ **T49.2** Poisoning by, adverse effect of and underdosing of local astringents and local detergents

√6ᵗʰ **T49.2X** Poisoning by, adverse effect of and underdosing of local astringents and local detergents

√7ᵗʰ **T49.2X1** Poisoning by local astringents and local detergents, accidental (unintentional)
Poisoning by local astringents and local detergents NOS

7 √7ᵗʰ **T49.2X2** Poisoning by local astringents and local detergents, intentional self-harm **HCC**

√7ᵗʰ **T49.2X3** Poisoning by local astringents and local detergents, assault

√7ᵗʰ **T49.2X4** Poisoning by local astringents and local detergents, undetermined

√7ᵗʰ **T49.2X5** Adverse effect of local astringents and local detergents **UPD**

√7ᵗʰ **T49.2X6** Underdosing of local astringents and local detergents **UPD**

√5ᵗʰ **T49.3** Poisoning by, adverse effect of and underdosing of emollients, demulcents and protectants

√6ᵗʰ **T49.3X** Poisoning by, adverse effect of and underdosing of emollients, demulcents and protectants

√7ᵗʰ **T49.3X1** Poisoning by emollients, demulcents and protectants, accidental (unintentional)
Poisoning by emollients, demulcents and protectants NOS

7 √7ᵗʰ **T49.3X2** Poisoning by emollients, demulcents and protectants, intentional self-harm **HCC**

√7ᵗʰ **T49.3X3** Poisoning by emollients, demulcents and protectants, assault

√7ᵗʰ **T49.3X4** Poisoning by emollients, demulcents and protectants, undetermined

√7ᵗʰ **T49.3X5** Adverse effect of emollients, demulcents and protectants **UPD**

√7ᵗʰ **T49.3X6** Underdosing of emollients, demulcents and protectants **UPD**

√5ᵗʰ **T49.4** Poisoning by, adverse effect of and underdosing of keratolytics, keratoplastics, and other hair treatment drugs and preparations

√6ᵗʰ **T49.4X** Poisoning by, adverse effect of and underdosing of keratolytics, keratoplastics, and other hair treatment drugs and preparations

√7ᵗʰ **T49.4X1** Poisoning by keratolytics, keratoplastics, and other hair treatment drugs and preparations, accidental (unintentional)
Poisoning by keratolytics, keratoplastics, and other hair treatment drugs and preparations NOS

7 √7ᵗʰ **T49.4X2** Poisoning by keratolytics, keratoplastics, and other hair treatment drugs and preparations, intentional self-harm **HCC**

√7ᵗʰ **T49.4X3** Poisoning by keratolytics, keratoplastics, and other hair treatment drugs and preparations, assault

√7ᵗʰ **T49.4X4** Poisoning by keratolytics, keratoplastics, and other hair treatment drugs and preparations, undetermined

√7ᵗʰ **T49.4X5** Adverse effect of keratolytics, keratoplastics, and other hair treatment drugs and preparations **UPD**

√7ᵗʰ **T49.4X6** Underdosing of keratolytics, keratoplastics, and other hair treatment drugs and preparations **UPD**

√5th **T49.5** **Poisoning by, adverse effect of and underdosing of ophthalmological drugs and preparations**
  √6th **T49.5X** **Poisoning by, adverse effect of and underdosing of** ophthalmological drugs and preparations
    √7th **T49.5X1** **Poisoning by ophthalmological drugs and preparations,** accidental (unintentional)
         Poisoning by ophthalmological drugs and preparations NOS
    7 √7th **T49.5X2** **Poisoning by ophthalmological drugs and preparations,** intentional self-harm   HCC
    √7th **T49.5X3** **Poisoning by ophthalmological drugs and preparations,** assault
    √7th **T49.5X4** **Poisoning by ophthalmological drugs and preparations,** undetermined
    √7th **T49.5X5** Adverse effect of ophthalmological drugs and preparations   UPD
    √7th **T49.5X6** Underdosing of ophthalmological drugs and preparations   UPD

√5th **T49.6** **Poisoning by, adverse effect of and underdosing of otorhinolaryngological drugs and preparations**
  √6th **T49.6X** **Poisoning by, adverse effect of and underdosing of** otorhinolaryngological drugs and preparations
    √7th **T49.6X1** **Poisoning by otorhinolaryngological drugs and preparations,** accidental (unintentional)
         Poisoning by otorhinolaryngological drugs and preparations NOS
    7 √7th **T49.6X2** **Poisoning by otorhinolaryngological drugs and preparations,** intentional self-harm   HCC
    √7th **T49.6X3** **Poisoning by otorhinolaryngological drugs and preparations,** assault
    √7th **T49.6X4** **Poisoning by otorhinolaryngological drugs and preparations,** undetermined
    √7th **T49.6X5** Adverse effect of otorhinolaryngological drugs and preparations   UPD
    √7th **T49.6X6** Underdosing of otorhinolaryngological drugs and preparations   UPD

√5th **T49.7** **Poisoning by, adverse effect of and underdosing of dental drugs, topically applied**
  √6th **T49.7X** **Poisoning by, adverse effect of and underdosing of** dental drugs, topically applied
    √7th **T49.7X1** **Poisoning by dental drugs, topically applied,** accidental (unintentional)
         Poisoning by dental drugs, topically applied NOS
    7 √7th **T49.7X2** **Poisoning by dental drugs, topically applied,** intentional self-harm   HCC
    √7th **T49.7X3** **Poisoning by dental drugs, topically applied,** assault
    √7th **T49.7X4** **Poisoning by dental drugs, topically applied,** undetermined
    √7th **T49.7X5** Adverse effect of dental drugs, topically applied   UPD
    √7th **T49.7X6** Underdosing of dental drugs, topically applied   UPD

√5th **T49.8** **Poisoning by, adverse effect of and underdosing of other topical agents**
     Poisoning by, adverse effect of and underdosing of spermicides
  √6th **T49.8X** **Poisoning by, adverse effect of and underdosing of other topical agents**
    √7th **T49.8X1** **Poisoning by other topical agents,** accidental (unintentional)
         Poisoning by other topical agents NOS
    7 √7th **T49.8X2** **Poisoning by other topical agents,** intentional self-harm   HCC
    √7th **T49.8X3** **Poisoning by other topical agents,** assault
    √7th **T49.8X4** **Poisoning by other topical agents,** undetermined
    √7th **T49.8X5** Adverse effect of other topical agents   UPD
    √7th **T49.8X6** Underdosing of other topical agents   UPD

√5th **T49.9** **Poisoning by, adverse effect of and underdosing of unspecified topical agent**
  √x7th **T49.91** **Poisoning by unspecified topical agent,** accidental (unintentional)
  7 √x7th **T49.92** **Poisoning by unspecified topical agent,** intentional self-harm   HCC
  √x7th **T49.93** **Poisoning by unspecified topical agent,** assault

  √x7th **T49.94** **Poisoning by unspecified topical agent,** undetermined
  √7th **T49.95** Adverse effect of unspecified topical agent   UPD
  √7th **T49.96** Underdosing of unspecified topical agent   UPD

√4th **T50** **Poisoning by, adverse effect of and underdosing of diuretics and other and unspecified drugs, medicaments and biological substances**

> The appropriate 7th character is to be added to each code from category T50.
> A   initial encounter
> D   subsequent encounter
> S   sequela

√5th **T50.0** **Poisoning by, adverse effect of and underdosing of mineralocorticoids and their antagonists**
  √6th **T50.0X** **Poisoning by, adverse effect of and underdosing of** mineralocorticoids and their antagonists
    √7th **T50.0X1** **Poisoning by mineralocorticoids and their antagonists,** accidental (unintentional)
         Poisoning by mineralocorticoids and their antagonists NOS
    7 √7th **T50.0X2** **Poisoning by mineralocorticoids and their antagonists,** intentional self-harm   HCC
    √7th **T50.0X3** **Poisoning by mineralocorticoids and their antagonists,** assault
    √7th **T50.0X4** **Poisoning by mineralocorticoids and their antagonists,** undetermined
    √7th **T50.0X5** Adverse effect of mineralocorticoids and their antagonists   UPD
    √7th **T50.0X6** Underdosing of mineralocorticoids and their antagonists   UPD

√5th **T50.1** **Poisoning by, adverse effect of and underdosing of loop [high-ceiling] diuretics**
  √6th **T50.1X** **Poisoning by, adverse effect of and underdosing of** loop [high-ceiling] diuretics
    √7th **T50.1X1** **Poisoning by loop [high-ceiling] diuretics,** accidental (unintentional)
         Poisoning by loop [high-ceiling] diuretics NOS
    7 √7th **T50.1X2** **Poisoning by loop [high-ceiling] diuretics,** intentional self-harm   HCC
    √7th **T50.1X3** **Poisoning by loop [high-ceiling] diuretics,** assault
    √7th **T50.1X4** **Poisoning by loop [high-ceiling] diuretics,** undetermined
    √7th **T50.1X5** Adverse effect of loop [high-ceiling] diuretics   UPD
    √7th **T50.1X6** Underdosing of loop [high-ceiling] diuretics   UPD

√5th **T50.2** **Poisoning by, adverse effect of and underdosing of carbonic-anhydrase inhibitors, benzothiadiazides and other diuretics**
     Poisoning by, adverse effect of and underdosing of acetazolamide
  √6th **T50.2X** **Poisoning by, adverse effect of and underdosing of** carbonic-anhydrase inhibitors, benzothiadiazides and other diuretics
    √7th **T50.2X1** **Poisoning by carbonic-anhydrase inhibitors, benzothiadiazides and other diuretics,** accidental (unintentional)
         Poisoning by carbonic-anhydrase inhibitors, benzothiadiazides and other diuretics NOS
    7 √7th **T50.2X2** **Poisoning by carbonic-anhydrase inhibitors, benzothiadiazides and other diuretics,** intentional self-harm   HCC
    √7th **T50.2X3** **Poisoning by carbonic-anhydrase inhibitors, benzothiadiazides and other diuretics,** assault
    √7th **T50.2X4** **Poisoning by carbonic-anhydrase inhibitors, benzothiadiazides and other diuretics,** undetermined
    √7th **T50.2X5** Adverse effect of carbonic-anhydrase inhibitors, benzothiadiazides and other diuretics   UPD
    √7th **T50.2X6** Underdosing of carbonic-anhydrase inhibitors, benzothiadiazides and other diuretics   UPD

Chapter 19. Injury, Poisoning and Certain Other Consequences of External Causes

T50.3–T50.A92

√5ᵗʰ **T50.3 Poisoning by, adverse effect of and underdosing of electrolytic, caloric and water-balance agents**
Poisoning by, adverse effect of and underdosing of oral rehydration salts

√6ᵗʰ **T50.3X Poisoning by, adverse effect of and underdosing of electrolytic, caloric and water-balance agents**

√7ᵗʰ **T50.3X1 Poisoning by electrolytic, caloric and water-balance agents, accidental (unintentional)**
Poisoning by electrolytic, caloric and water-balance agents NOS

7 √7ᵗʰ **T50.3X2 Poisoning by electrolytic, caloric and water-balance agents, intentional self-harm** HCC

√7ᵗʰ **T50.3X3 Poisoning by electrolytic, caloric and water-balance agents, assault**

√7ᵗʰ **T50.3X4 Poisoning by electrolytic, caloric and water-balance agents, undetermined**

√7ᵗʰ **T50.3X5 Adverse effect of electrolytic, caloric and water-balance agents** UPD

√7ᵗʰ **T50.3X6 Underdosing of electrolytic, caloric and water-balance agents** UPD

√5ᵗʰ **T50.4 Poisoning by, adverse effect of and underdosing of drugs affecting uric acid metabolism**

√6ᵗʰ **T50.4X Poisoning by, adverse effect of and underdosing of drugs affecting uric acid metabolism**

√7ᵗʰ **T50.4X1 Poisoning by drugs affecting uric acid metabolism, accidental (unintentional)**
Poisoning by drugs affecting uric acid metabolism NOS

7 √7ᵗʰ **T50.4X2 Poisoning by drugs affecting uric acid metabolism, intentional self-harm** HCC

√7ᵗʰ **T50.4X3 Poisoning by drugs affecting uric acid metabolism, assault**

√7ᵗʰ **T50.4X4 Poisoning by drugs affecting uric acid metabolism, undetermined**

√7ᵗʰ **T50.4X5 Adverse effect of drugs affecting uric acid metabolism** UPD

√7ᵗʰ **T50.4X6 Underdosing of drugs affecting uric acid metabolism** UPD

√5ᵗʰ **T50.5 Poisoning by, adverse effect of and underdosing of appetite depressants**

√6ᵗʰ **T50.5X Poisoning by, adverse effect of and underdosing of appetite depressants**

√7ᵗʰ **T50.5X1 Poisoning by appetite depressants, accidental (unintentional)**
Poisoning by appetite depressants NOS

7 √7ᵗʰ **T50.5X2 Poisoning by appetite depressants, intentional self-harm** HCC

√7ᵗʰ **T50.5X3 Poisoning by appetite depressants, assault**

√7ᵗʰ **T50.5X4 Poisoning by appetite depressants, undetermined**

√7ᵗʰ **T50.5X5 Adverse effect of appetite depressants** UPD

√7ᵗʰ **T50.5X6 Underdosing of appetite depressants** UPD

√5ᵗʰ **T50.6 Poisoning by, adverse effect of and underdosing of antidotes and chelating agents**
Poisoning by, adverse effect of and underdosing of alcohol deterrents

√6ᵗʰ **T50.6X Poisoning by, adverse effect of and underdosing of antidotes and chelating agents**

√7ᵗʰ **T50.6X1 Poisoning by antidotes and chelating agents, accidental (unintentional)**
Poisoning by antidotes and chelating agents NOS

7 √7ᵗʰ **T50.6X2 Poisoning by antidotes and chelating agents, intentional self-harm** HCC

√7ᵗʰ **T50.6X3 Poisoning by antidotes and chelating agents, assault**

√7ᵗʰ **T50.6X4 Poisoning by antidotes and chelating agents, undetermined**

√7ᵗʰ **T50.6X5 Adverse effect of antidotes and chelating agents** UPD

√7ᵗʰ **T50.6X6 Underdosing of antidotes and chelating agents** UPD

√5ᵗʰ **T50.7 Poisoning by, adverse effect of and underdosing of analeptics and opioid receptor antagonists**

√6ᵗʰ **T50.7X Poisoning by, adverse effect of and underdosing of analeptics and opioid receptor antagonists**

√7ᵗʰ **T50.7X1 Poisoning by analeptics and opioid receptor antagonists, accidental (unintentional)**
Poisoning by analeptics and opioid receptor antagonists NOS

7 √7ᵗʰ **T50.7X2 Poisoning by analeptics and opioid receptor antagonists, intentional self-harm** HCC

√7ᵗʰ **T50.7X3 Poisoning by analeptics and opioid receptor antagonists, assault**

√7ᵗʰ **T50.7X4 Poisoning by analeptics and opioid receptor antagonists, undetermined**

√7ᵗʰ **T50.7X5 Adverse effect of analeptics and opioid receptor antagonists**

√7ᵗʰ **T50.7X6 Underdosing of analeptics and opioid receptor antagonists** UPD

√5ᵗʰ **T50.8 Poisoning by, adverse effect of and underdosing of diagnostic agents**

√6ᵗʰ **T50.8X Poisoning by, adverse effect of and underdosing of diagnostic agents**

√7ᵗʰ **T50.8X1 Poisoning by diagnostic agents, accidental (unintentional)**
Poisoning by diagnostic agents NOS

7 √7ᵗʰ **T50.8X2 Poisoning by diagnostic agents, intentional self-harm** HCC

√7ᵗʰ **T50.8X3 Poisoning by diagnostic agents, assault**

√7ᵗʰ **T50.8X4 Poisoning by diagnostic agents, undetermined**

√7ᵗʰ **T50.8X5 Adverse effect of diagnostic agents** UPD

√7ᵗʰ **T50.8X6 Underdosing of diagnostic agents** UPD

√5ᵗʰ **T50.A Poisoning by, adverse effect of and underdosing of bacterial vaccines**

√6ᵗʰ **T50.A1 Poisoning by, adverse effect of and underdosing of pertussis vaccine, including combinations with a pertussis component**

√7ᵗʰ **T50.A11 Poisoning by pertussis vaccine, including combinations with a pertussis component, accidental (unintentional)**

7 √7ᵗʰ **T50.A12 Poisoning by pertussis vaccine, including combinations with a pertussis component, intentional self-harm** HCC

√7ᵗʰ **T50.A13 Poisoning by pertussis vaccine, including combinations with a pertussis component, assault**

√7ᵗʰ **T50.A14 Poisoning by pertussis vaccine, including combinations with a pertussis component, undetermined**

√7ᵗʰ **T50.A15 Adverse effect of pertussis vaccine, including combinations with a pertussis component** UPD

√7ᵗʰ **T50.A16 Underdosing of pertussis vaccine, including combinations with a pertussis component** UPD

√6ᵗʰ **T50.A2 Poisoning by, adverse effect of and underdosing of mixed bacterial vaccines without a pertussis component**

√7ᵗʰ **T50.A21 Poisoning by mixed bacterial vaccines without a pertussis component, accidental (unintentional)**

7 √7ᵗʰ **T50.A22 Poisoning by mixed bacterial vaccines without a pertussis component, intentional self-harm** HCC

√7ᵗʰ **T50.A23 Poisoning by mixed bacterial vaccines without a pertussis component, assault**

√7ᵗʰ **T50.A24 Poisoning by mixed bacterial vaccines without a pertussis component, undetermined**

√7ᵗʰ **T50.A25 Adverse effect of mixed bacterial vaccines without a pertussis component** UPD

√7ᵗʰ **T50.A26 Underdosing of mixed bacterial vaccines without a pertussis component** UPD

√6ᵗʰ **T50.A9 Poisoning by, adverse effect of and underdosing of other bacterial vaccines**

√7ᵗʰ **T50.A91 Poisoning by other bacterial vaccines, accidental (unintentional)**

7 √7ᵗʰ **T50.A92 Poisoning by other bacterial vaccines, intentional self-harm** HCC

☑7ᵗʰ **T50.A93 Poisoning** by other bacterial vaccines, assault

☑7ᵗʰ **T50.A94 Poisoning** by other bacterial vaccines, undetermined

☑7ᵗʰ **T50.A95 Adverse effect** of other bacterial vaccines   UPD

☑7ᵗʰ **T50.A96 Underdosing** of other bacterial vaccines   UPD

☑5ᵗʰ **T50.B Poisoning** by, adverse effect of and underdosing of viral vaccines

☑6ᵗʰ **T50.B1 Poisoning** by, adverse effect of and underdosing of smallpox vaccines

☑7ᵗʰ **T50.B11 Poisoning** by smallpox vaccines, accidental (unintentional)

7 ☑7ᵗʰ **T50.B12 Poisoning** by smallpox vaccines, intentional self-harm   HCC

☑7ᵗʰ **T50.B13 Poisoning** by smallpox vaccines, assault

☑7ᵗʰ **T50.B14 Poisoning** by smallpox vaccines, undetermined

☑7ᵗʰ **T50.B15 Adverse effect** of smallpox vaccines   UPD

☑7ᵗʰ **T50.B16 Underdosing** of smallpox vaccines   UPD

☑6ᵗʰ **T50.B9 Poisoning** by, adverse effect of and underdosing of other viral vaccines

☑7ᵗʰ **T50.B91 Poisoning** by other viral vaccines, accidental (unintentional)

7 ☑7ᵗʰ **T50.B92 Poisoning** by other viral vaccines, intentional self-harm   HCC

☑7ᵗʰ **T50.B93 Poisoning** by other viral vaccines, assault

☑7ᵗʰ **T50.B94 Poisoning** by other viral vaccines, undetermined

☑7ᵗʰ **T50.B95 Adverse effect** of other viral vaccines   UPD

AHA: 2021,1Q,43

☑7ᵗʰ **T50.B96 Underdosing** of other viral vaccines   UPD

☑5ᵗʰ **T50.Z Poisoning** by, adverse effect of and underdosing of other vaccines and biological substances

☑6ᵗʰ **T50.Z1 Poisoning** by, adverse effect of and underdosing of immunoglobulin

☑7ᵗʰ **T50.Z11 Poisoning** by immunoglobulin, accidental (unintentional)

7 ☑7ᵗʰ **T50.Z12 Poisoning** by immunoglobulin, intentional self-harm   HCC

☑7ᵗʰ **T50.Z13 Poisoning** by immunoglobulin, assault

☑7ᵗʰ **T50.Z14 Poisoning** by immunoglobulin, undetermined

☑7ᵗʰ **T50.Z15 Adverse effect** of immunoglobulin   UPD

☑7ᵗʰ **T50.Z16 Underdosing** of immunoglobulin   UPD

☑6ᵗʰ **T50.Z9 Poisoning** by, adverse effect of and underdosing of other vaccines and biological substances

☑7ᵗʰ **T50.Z91 Poisoning** by other vaccines and biological substances, accidental (unintentional)

7 ☑7ᵗʰ **T50.Z92 Poisoning** by other vaccines and biological substances, intentional self-harm   HCC

☑7ᵗʰ **T50.Z93 Poisoning** by other vaccines and biological substances, assault

☑7ᵗʰ **T50.Z94 Poisoning** by other vaccines and biological substances, undetermined

☑7ᵗʰ **T50.Z95 Adverse effect** of other vaccines and biological substances   UPD

AHA: 2020,1Q,18

☑7ᵗʰ **T50.Z96 Underdosing** of other vaccines and biological substances   UPD

☑5ᵗʰ **T50.9 Poisoning** by, adverse effect of and underdosing of other and unspecified drugs, medicaments and biological substances

☑6ᵗʰ **T50.90 Poisoning** by, adverse effect of and underdosing of unspecified drugs, medicaments and biological substances

☑7ᵗʰ **T50.901 Poisoning** by unspecified drugs, medicaments and biological substances, accidental (unintentional)

7 ☑7ᵗʰ **T50.902 Poisoning** by unspecified drugs, medicaments and biological substances, intentional self-harm   HCC

☑7ᵗʰ **T50.903 Poisoning** by unspecified drugs, medicaments and biological substances, assault

☑7ᵗʰ **T50.904 Poisoning** by unspecified drugs, medicaments and biological substances, undetermined

☑7ᵗʰ **T50.905 Adverse effect** of unspecified drugs, medicaments and biological substances

☑7ᵗʰ **T50.906 Underdosing** of unspecified drugs, medicaments and biological substances

☑6ᵗʰ **T50.91 Poisoning** by, adverse effect of and underdosing of multiple unspecified drugs, medicaments and biological substances

Multiple drug ingestion NOS

Code also any specific drugs, medicaments and biological substances

☑7ᵗʰ **T50.911 Poisoning** by multiple unspecified drugs, medicaments and biological substances, accidental (unintentional)

7 ☑7ᵗʰ **T50.912 Poisoning** by multiple unspecified drugs, medicaments and biological substances, intentional self-harm   HCC

☑7ᵗʰ **T50.913 Poisoning** by multiple unspecified drugs, medicaments and biological substances, assault

☑7ᵗʰ **T50.914 Poisoning** by multiple unspecified drugs, medicaments and biological substances, undetermined

☑7ᵗʰ **T50.915 Adverse effect** of multiple unspecified drugs, medicaments and biological substances   UPD

☑7ᵗʰ **T50.916 Underdosing** of multiple unspecified drugs, medicaments and biological substances   UPD

☑6ᵗʰ **T50.99 Poisoning** by, adverse effect of and underdosing of other drugs, medicaments and biological substances

☑7ᵗʰ **T50.991 Poisoning** by other drugs, medicaments and biological substances, accidental (unintentional)

7 ☑7ᵗʰ **T50.992 Poisoning** by other drugs, medicaments and biological substances, intentional self-harm   HCC

☑7ᵗʰ **T50.993 Poisoning** by other drugs, medicaments and biological substances, assault

☑7ᵗʰ **T50.994 Poisoning** by other drugs, medicaments and biological substances, undetermined

☑7ᵗʰ **T50.995 Adverse effect** of other drugs, medicaments and biological substances

☑7ᵗʰ **T50.996 Underdosing** of other drugs, medicaments and biological substances

Toxic effects of substances chiefly nonmedicinal as to source (T51-T65)

NOTE   When no intent is indicated code to accidental. Undetermined intent is only for use when there is specific documentation in the record that the intent of the toxic effect cannot be determined.

Use additional code(s) for all associated manifestations of toxic effect, such as:
personal history of foreign body fully removed (Z87.821)
respiratory conditions due to external agents (J60-J70)
to identify any retained foreign body, if applicable (Z18.-)

EXCLUDES 1   contact with and (suspected) exposure to toxic substances (Z77.-)

AHA: 2017,1Q,39-40

☑4ᵗʰ **T51 Toxic effect of alcohol**

The appropriate 7th character is to be added to each code from category T51.
A   initial encounter
D   subsequent encounter
S   sequela

☑5ᵗʰ **T51.0 Toxic effect of ethanol**

Toxic effect of ethyl alcohol

EXCLUDES 2   acute alcohol intoxication or "hangover" effects (F10.129, F10.229, F10.929)
drunkenness (F10.129, F10.229, F10.929)
pathological alcohol intoxication (F10.129, F10.229, F10.929)

☑6ᵗʰ **T51.0X Toxic effect of ethanol**

6 ☑7ᵗʰ **T51.0X1 Toxic effect** of ethanol, accidental (unintentional)   HCC

Toxic effect of ethanol NOS

7 ☑7ᵗʰ **T51.0X2 Toxic effect** of ethanol, intentional self-harm   HCC

☑7ᵗʰ **T51.0X3 Toxic effect** of ethanol, assault

☑ Additional Character Required   ☑x7ᵗʰ Placeholder   Questionable PDx   Manifestation   Unspecified Dx   UPD Unacceptable PDx   H1-H4 HAC   HCC CMS-HCC Dx   HIV HIV Dx

ICD-10-CM 2022   **1133**

⁶ √7ᵗʰ **T51.0X4** **Toxic effect of ethanol, undetermined** HCC

√5ᵗʰ **T51.1** **Toxic effect of methanol**
Toxic effect of methyl alcohol

√6ᵗʰ **T51.1X** **Toxic effect of methanol**

√7ᵗʰ **T51.1X1** **Toxic effect of methanol, accidental (unintentional)**
Toxic effect of methanol NOS

⁷ √7ᵗʰ **T51.1X2** **Toxic effect of methanol, intentional self-harm** HCC

√7ᵗʰ **T51.1X3** **Toxic effect of methanol, assault**

√7ᵗʰ **T51.1X4** **Toxic effect of methanol, undetermined**

√5ᵗʰ **T51.2** **Toxic effect of 2-Propanol**
Toxic effect of isopropyl alcohol

√6ᵗʰ **T51.2X** **Toxic effect of 2-Propanol**

√7ᵗʰ **T51.2X1** **Toxic effect of 2-Propanol, accidental (unintentional)**
Toxic effect of 2-Propanol NOS

⁷ √7ᵗʰ **T51.2X2** **Toxic effect of 2-Propanol, intentional self-harm** HCC

√7ᵗʰ **T51.2X3** **Toxic effect of 2-Propanol, assault**

√7ᵗʰ **T51.2X4** **Toxic effect of 2-Propanol, undetermined**

√5ᵗʰ **T51.3** **Toxic effect of fusel oil**
Toxic effect of amyl alcohol
Toxic effect of butyl [1-butanol] alcohol
Toxic effect of propyl [1-propanol] alcohol

√6ᵗʰ **T51.3X** **Toxic effect of fusel oil**

√7ᵗʰ **T51.3X1** **Toxic effect of fusel oil, accidental (unintentional)**
Toxic effect of fusel oil NOS

⁷ √7ᵗʰ **T51.3X2** **Toxic effect of fusel oil, intentional self-harm** HCC

√7ᵗʰ **T51.3X3** **Toxic effect of fusel oil, assault**

√7ᵗʰ **T51.3X4** **Toxic effect of fusel oil, undetermined**

√5ᵗʰ **T51.8** **Toxic effect of other alcohols**

√6ᵗʰ **T51.8X** **Toxic effect of other alcohols**

√7ᵗʰ **T51.8X1** **Toxic effect of other alcohols, accidental (unintentional)**
Toxic effect of other alcohols NOS

⁷ √7ᵗʰ **T51.8X2** **Toxic effect of other alcohols, intentional self-harm** HCC

√7ᵗʰ **T51.8X3** **Toxic effect of other alcohols, assault**

√7ᵗʰ **T51.8X4** **Toxic effect of other alcohols, undetermined**

√5ᵗʰ **T51.9** **Toxic effect of unspecified alcohol**

√x7ᵗʰ **T51.91** **Toxic effect of unspecified alcohol, accidental (unintentional)**

⁷ √x7ᵗʰ **T51.92** **Toxic effect of unspecified alcohol, intentional self-harm** HCC

√x7ᵗʰ **T51.93** **Toxic effect of unspecified alcohol, assault**

√x7ᵗʰ **T51.94** **Toxic effect of unspecified alcohol, undetermined**

√4ᵗʰ **T52** **Toxic effect of organic solvents**

EXCLUDES 1   *halogen derivatives of aliphatic and aromatic hydrocarbons (T53.-)*

The appropriate 7th character is to be added to each code from category T52.
A   initial encounter
D   subsequent encounter
S   sequela

√5ᵗʰ **T52.0** **Toxic effects of petroleum products**
Toxic effects of ether petroleum
Toxic effects of gasoline [petrol]
Toxic effects of kerosene [paraffin oil]
Toxic effects of naphtha petroleum
Toxic effects of paraffin wax
Toxic effects of spirit petroleum

√6ᵗʰ **T52.0X** **Toxic effects of petroleum products**

√7ᵗʰ **T52.0X1** **Toxic effect of petroleum products, accidental (unintentional)**
Toxic effects of petroleum products NOS

⁷ √7ᵗʰ **T52.0X2** **Toxic effect of petroleum products, intentional self-harm** HCC

√7ᵗʰ **T52.0X3** **Toxic effect of petroleum products, assault**

√7ᵗʰ **T52.0X4** **Toxic effect of petroleum products, undetermined**

√5ᵗʰ **T52.1** **Toxic effects of benzene**

EXCLUDES 1   *homologues of benzene (T52.2)*
nitroderivatives and aminoderivatives of benzene and its homologues (T65.3)

√6ᵗʰ **T52.1X** **Toxic effects of benzene**

√7ᵗʰ **T52.1X1** **Toxic effect of benzene, accidental (unintentional)**
Toxic effects of benzene NOS

⁷ √7ᵗʰ **T52.1X2** **Toxic effect of benzene, intentional self-harm** HCC

√7ᵗʰ **T52.1X3** **Toxic effect of benzene, assault**

√7ᵗʰ **T52.1X4** **Toxic effect of benzene, undetermined**

√5ᵗʰ **T52.2** **Toxic effects of homologues of benzene**
Toxic effects of toluene [methylbenzene]
Toxic effects of xylene [dimethylbenzene]

√6ᵗʰ **T52.2X** **Toxic effects of homologues of benzene**

√7ᵗʰ **T52.2X1** **Toxic effect of homologues of benzene, accidental (unintentional)**
Toxic effects of homologues of benzene NOS

⁷ √7ᵗʰ **T52.2X2** **Toxic effect of homologues of benzene, intentional self-harm** HCC

√7ᵗʰ **T52.2X3** **Toxic effect of homologues of benzene, assault**

√7ᵗʰ **T52.2X4** **Toxic effect of homologues of benzene, undetermined**

√5ᵗʰ **T52.3** **Toxic effects of glycols**

√6ᵗʰ **T52.3X** **Toxic effects of glycols**

√7ᵗʰ **T52.3X1** **Toxic effect of glycols, accidental (unintentional)**
Toxic effects of glycols NOS

⁷ √7ᵗʰ **T52.3X2** **Toxic effect of glycols, intentional self-harm** HCC

√7ᵗʰ **T52.3X3** **Toxic effect of glycols, assault**

√7ᵗʰ **T52.3X4** **Toxic effect of glycols, undetermined**

√5ᵗʰ **T52.4** **Toxic effects of ketones**

√6ᵗʰ **T52.4X** **Toxic effects of ketones**

√7ᵗʰ **T52.4X1** **Toxic effect of ketones, accidental (unintentional)**
Toxic effects of ketones NOS

⁷ √7ᵗʰ **T52.4X2** **Toxic effect of ketones, intentional self-harm** HCC

√7ᵗʰ **T52.4X3** **Toxic effect of ketones, assault**

√7ᵗʰ **T52.4X4** **Toxic effect of ketones, undetermined**

√5ᵗʰ **T52.8** **Toxic effects of other organic solvents**

√6ᵗʰ **T52.8X** **Toxic effects of other organic solvents**

√7ᵗʰ **T52.8X1** **Toxic effect of other organic solvents, accidental (unintentional)**
Toxic effects of other organic solvents NOS

⁷ √7ᵗʰ **T52.8X2** **Toxic effect of other organic solvents, intentional self-harm** HCC

√7ᵗʰ **T52.8X3** **Toxic effect of other organic solvents, assault**

√7ᵗʰ **T52.8X4** **Toxic effect of other organic solvents, undetermined**

√5ᵗʰ **T52.9** **Toxic effects of unspecified organic solvent**

√x7ᵗʰ **T52.91** **Toxic effect of unspecified organic solvent, accidental (unintentional)**

⁷ √x7ᵗʰ **T52.92** **Toxic effect of unspecified organic solvent, intentional self-harm** HCC

√x7ᵗʰ **T52.93** **Toxic effect of unspecified organic solvent, assault**

√x7ᵗʰ **T52.94** **Toxic effect of unspecified organic solvent, undetermined**

✓4th **T53** **Toxic effect of halogen derivatives of aliphatic and aromatic hydrocarbons**

The appropriate 7th character is to be added to each code from category T53.
A   initial encounter
D   subsequent encounter
S   sequela

✓5th **T53.0** **Toxic effects of carbon tetrachloride**

Toxic effects of tetrachloromethane

✓6th **T53.0X** **Toxic effects of** carbon tetrachloride

✓7th **T53.0X1** **Toxic effect of carbon tetrachloride,** accidental **(unintentional)**
Toxic effects of carbon tetrachloride NOS

7 ✓7th **T53.0X2** **Toxic effect of carbon tetrachloride,** intentional self-harm   HCC

✓7th **T53.0X3** **Toxic effect of carbon tetrachloride,** assault

✓7th **T53.0X4** **Toxic effect of carbon tetrachloride,** undetermined

✓5th **T53.1** **Toxic effects of chloroform**

Toxic effects of trichloromethane

✓6th **T53.1X** **Toxic effects of** chloroform

✓7th **T53.1X1** **Toxic effect of chloroform,** accidental **(unintentional)**
Toxic effects of chloroform NOS

7 ✓7th **T53.1X2** **Toxic effect of chloroform,** intentional self-harm   HCC

✓7th **T53.1X3** **Toxic effect of chloroform,** assault

✓7th **T53.1X4** **Toxic effect of chloroform,** undetermined

✓5th **T53.2** **Toxic effects of trichloroethylene**

Toxic effects of trichloroethene

✓6th **T53.2X** **Toxic effects of** trichloroethylene

✓7th **T53.2X1** **Toxic effect of trichloroethylene,** accidental **(unintentional)**
Toxic effects of trichloroethylene NOS

7 ✓7th **T53.2X2** **Toxic effect of trichloroethylene,** intentional self-harm   HCC

✓7th **T53.2X3** **Toxic effect of trichloroethylene,** assault

✓7th **T53.2X4** **Toxic effect of trichloroethylene,** undetermined

✓5th **T53.3** **Toxic effects of tetrachloroethylene**

Toxic effects of perchloroethylene
Toxic effect of tetrachloroethene

✓6th **T53.3X** **Toxic effects of** tetrachloroethylene

✓7th **T53.3X1** **Toxic effect of tetrachloroethylene,** accidental **(unintentional)**
Toxic effects of tetrachloroethylene NOS

7 ✓7th **T53.3X2** **Toxic effect of tetrachloroethylene,** intentional self-harm   HCC

✓7th **T53.3X3** **Toxic effect of tetrachloroethylene,** assault

✓7th **T53.3X4** **Toxic effect of tetrachloroethylene,** undetermined

✓5th **T53.4** **Toxic effects of dichloromethane**

Toxic effects of methylene chloride

✓6th **T53.4X** **Toxic effects of** dichloromethane

✓7th **T53.4X1** **Toxic effect of dichloromethane,** accidental **(unintentional)**
Toxic effects of dichloromethane NOS

7 ✓7th **T53.4X2** **Toxic effect of dichloromethane,** intentional self-harm   HCC

✓7th **T53.4X3** **Toxic effect of dichloromethane,** assault

✓7th **T53.4X4** **Toxic effect of dichloromethane,** undetermined

✓5th **T53.5** **Toxic effects of chlorofluorocarbons**

✓6th **T53.5X** **Toxic effects of** chlorofluorocarbons

✓7th **T53.5X1** **Toxic effect of chlorofluorocarbons,** accidental **(unintentional)**
Toxic effects of chlorofluorocarbons NOS

7 ✓7th **T53.5X2** **Toxic effect of chlorofluorocarbons,** intentional self-harm   HCC

✓7th **T53.5X3** **Toxic effect of chlorofluorocarbons,** assault

✓7th **T53.5X4** **Toxic effect of chlorofluorocarbons,** undetermined

✓5th **T53.6** **Toxic effects of other halogen derivatives of aliphatic hydrocarbons**

✓6th **T53.6X** **Toxic effects of** other halogen derivatives of aliphatic hydrocarbons

✓7th **T53.6X1** **Toxic effect of other halogen derivatives of aliphatic hydrocarbons,** accidental **(unintentional)**
Toxic effects of other halogen derivatives of aliphatic hydrocarbons NOS

7 ✓7th **T53.6X2** **Toxic effect of other halogen derivatives of aliphatic hydrocarbons,** intentional self-harm   HCC

✓7th **T53.6X3** **Toxic effect of other halogen derivatives of aliphatic hydrocarbons,** assault

✓7th **T53.6X4** **Toxic effect of other halogen derivatives of aliphatic hydrocarbons,** undetermined

✓5th **T53.7** **Toxic effects of other halogen derivatives of aromatic hydrocarbons**

✓6th **T53.7X** **Toxic effects of** other halogen derivatives of aromatic hydrocarbons

✓7th **T53.7X1** **Toxic effect of other halogen derivatives of aromatic hydrocarbons,** accidental **(unintentional)**
Toxic effects of other halogen derivatives of aromatic hydrocarbons NOS

7 ✓7th **T53.7X2** **Toxic effect of other halogen derivatives of aromatic hydrocarbons,** intentional self-harm   HCC

✓7th **T53.7X3** **Toxic effect of other halogen derivatives of aromatic hydrocarbons,** assault

✓7th **T53.7X4** **Toxic effect of other halogen derivatives of aromatic hydrocarbons,** undetermined

✓6th **T53.9** **Toxic effects of unspecified halogen derivatives of aliphatic and aromatic hydrocarbons**

✓x7th **T53.91** **Toxic effect of unspecified halogen derivatives of aliphatic and aromatic hydrocarbons,** accidental **(unintentional)**

7 ✓x7th **T53.92** **Toxic effect of unspecified halogen derivatives of aliphatic and aromatic hydrocarbons,** intentional self-harm   HCC

✓x7th **T53.93** **Toxic effect of unspecified halogen derivatives of aliphatic and aromatic hydrocarbons,** assault

✓x7th **T53.94** **Toxic effect of unspecified halogen derivatives of aliphatic and aromatic hydrocarbons,** undetermined

✓4th **T54** **Toxic effect of corrosive substances**

The appropriate 7th character is to be added to each code from category T54.
A   initial encounter
D   subsequent encounter
S   sequela

✓5th **T54.0** **Toxic effects of phenol and phenol homologues**

✓6th **T54.0X** **Toxic effects of** phenol and phenol homologues

✓7th **T54.0X1** **Toxic effect of phenol and phenol homologues,** accidental **(unintentional)**
Toxic effects of phenol and phenol homologues NOS

7 ✓7th **T54.0X2** **Toxic effect of phenol and phenol homologues,** intentional self-harm   HCC

✓7th **T54.0X3** **Toxic effect of phenol and phenol homologues,** assault

✓7th **T54.0X4** **Toxic effect of phenol and phenol homologues,** undetermined

✓5th **T54.1** **Toxic effects of other corrosive organic compounds**

✓6th **T54.1X** **Toxic effects of** other corrosive organic compounds

✓7th **T54.1X1** **Toxic effect of other corrosive organic compounds,** accidental **(unintentional)**
Toxic effects of other corrosive organic compounds NOS

7 ✓7th **T54.1X2** **Toxic effect of other corrosive organic compounds,** intentional self-harm   HCC

✓7th **T54.1X3** **Toxic effect of other corrosive organic compounds,** assault

✓7th **T54.1X4** **Toxic effect of other corrosive organic compounds,** undetermined

✓ Additional Character Required   ✓x7th Placeholder   Questionable PDx   Manifestation   Unspecified Dx   UPD Unacceptable PDx   H1 - H14 HAC   HCC CMS-HCC Dx   HIV HIV Dx

ICD-10-CM 2022   1135

Chapter 19. Injury, Poisoning and Certain Other Consequences of External Causes

T53–T54.1X4

✓5ᵗʰ **T54.2** **Toxic effects of corrosive acids and acid-like substances**
Toxic effects of hydrochloric acid
Toxic effects of sulfuric acid

  ✓6ᵗʰ **T54.2X** **Toxic effects of** corrosive acids and acid-like substances

   ✓7ᵗʰ **T54.2X1** **Toxic effect of corrosive acids and acid-like substances,** accidental **(unintentional)**
    Toxic effects of corrosive acids and acid-like substances NOS

   7 ✓7ᵗʰ **T54.2X2** **Toxic effect of corrosive acids and acid-like substances,** intentional self-harm   HCC

   ✓7ᵗʰ **T54.2X3** **Toxic effect of corrosive acids and acid-like substances,** assault

   ✓7ᵗʰ **T54.2X4** **Toxic effect of corrosive acids and acid-like substances,** undetermined

✓5ᵗʰ **T54.3** **Toxic effects of corrosive alkalis and alkali-like substances**
Toxic effects of potassium hydroxide
Toxic effects of sodium hydroxide

  ✓6ᵗʰ **T54.3X** **Toxic effects of** corrosive alkalis and alkali-like substances

   ✓7ᵗʰ **T54.3X1** **Toxic effect of corrosive alkalis and alkali-like substances,** accidental **(unintentional)**
    Toxic effects of corrosive alkalis and alkali-like substances NOS

   7 ✓7ᵗʰ **T54.3X2** **Toxic effect of corrosive alkalis and alkali-like substances,** intentional self-harm   HCC

   ✓7ᵗʰ **T54.3X3** **Toxic effect of corrosive alkalis and alkali-like substances,** assault

   ✓7ᵗʰ **T54.3X4** **Toxic effect of corrosive alkalis and alkali-like substances,** undetermined

✓5ᵗʰ **T54.9** **Toxic effects of unspecified corrosive substance**

  ✓x7ᵗʰ **T54.91** **Toxic effect of unspecified corrosive substance,** accidental **(unintentional)**

  7 ✓x7ᵗʰ **T54.92** **Toxic effect of unspecified corrosive substance,** intentional self-harm   HCC

  ✓x7ᵗʰ **T54.93** **Toxic effect of unspecified corrosive substance,** assault

  ✓x7ᵗʰ **T54.94** **Toxic effect of unspecified corrosive substance,** undetermined

✓4ᵗʰ **T55** **Toxic effect of soaps and detergents**

The appropriate 7th character is to be added to each code from category T55.
A   initial encounter
D   subsequent encounter
S   sequela

  ✓6ᵗʰ **T55.0** **Toxic effect of soaps**

   ✓6ᵗʰ **T55.0X** **Toxic effect of** soaps

    ✓7ᵗʰ **T55.0X1** **Toxic effect of soaps,** accidental **(unintentional)**
     Toxic effect of soaps NOS

    7 ✓7ᵗʰ **T55.0X2** **Toxic effect of soaps,** intentional self-harm   HCC

    ✓7ᵗʰ **T55.0X3** **Toxic effect of soaps,** assault

    ✓7ᵗʰ **T55.0X4** **Toxic effect of soaps,** undetermined

  ✓5ᵗʰ **T55.1** **Toxic effect of detergents**

   ✓6ᵗʰ **T55.1X** **Toxic effect of** detergents

    ✓7ᵗʰ **T55.1X1** **Toxic effect of detergents,** accidental **(unintentional)**
     Toxic effect of detergents NOS

    7 ✓7ᵗʰ **T55.1X2** **Toxic effect of detergents,** intentional self-harm   HCC

    ✓7ᵗʰ **T55.1X3** **Toxic effect of detergents,** assault

    ✓7ᵗʰ **T55.1X4** **Toxic effect of detergents,** undetermined

✓4ᵗʰ **T56** **Toxic effect of metals**

  INCLUDES   toxic effects of fumes and vapors of metals
  toxic effects of metals from all sources, except medicinal substances
  Use additional code to identify any retained metal foreign body, if applicable (Z18.0-, T18.1-)
  EXCLUDES 1   arsenic and its compounds (T57.0)
  manganese and its compounds (T57.2)

The appropriate 7th character is to be added to each code from category T56.
A   initial encounter
D   subsequent encounter
S   sequela

  ✓5ᵗʰ **T56.0** **Toxic effects of lead and its compounds**

   ✓6ᵗʰ **T56.0X** **Toxic effects of** lead and its compounds

    ✓7ᵗʰ **T56.0X1** **Toxic effect of lead and its compounds,** accidental **(unintentional)**
     Toxic effects of lead and its compounds NOS

    7 ✓7ᵗʰ **T56.0X2** **Toxic effect of lead and its compounds,** intentional self-harm   HCC

    ✓7ᵗʰ **T56.0X3** **Toxic effect of lead and its compounds,** assault

    ✓7ᵗʰ **T56.0X4** **Toxic effect of lead and its compounds,** undetermined

  ✓5ᵗʰ **T56.1** **Toxic effects of mercury and its compounds**

   ✓6ᵗʰ **T56.1X** **Toxic effects of** mercury and its compounds

    ✓7ᵗʰ **T56.1X1** **Toxic effect of mercury and its compounds,** accidental **(unintentional)**
     Toxic effects of mercury and its compounds NOS

    7 ✓7ᵗʰ **T56.1X2** **Toxic effect of mercury and its compounds,** intentional self-harm   HCC

    ✓7ᵗʰ **T56.1X3** **Toxic effect of mercury and its compounds,** assault

    ✓7ᵗʰ **T56.1X4** **Toxic effect of mercury and its compounds,** undetermined

  ✓5ᵗʰ **T56.2** **Toxic effects of chromium and its compounds**

   ✓6ᵗʰ **T56.2X** **Toxic effects of** chromium and its compounds

    ✓7ᵗʰ **T56.2X1** **Toxic effect of chromium and its compounds,** accidental **(unintentional)**
     Toxic effects of chromium and its compounds NOS

    7 ✓7ᵗʰ **T56.2X2** **Toxic effect of chromium and its compounds,** intentional self-harm   HCC

    ✓7ᵗʰ **T56.2X3** **Toxic effect of chromium and its compounds,** assault

    ✓7ᵗʰ **T56.2X4** **Toxic effect of chromium and its compounds,** undetermined

  ✓5ᵗʰ **T56.3** **Toxic effects of cadmium and its compounds**

   ✓6ᵗʰ **T56.3X** **Toxic effects of** cadmium and its compounds

    ✓7ᵗʰ **T56.3X1** **Toxic effect of cadmium and its compounds,** accidental **(unintentional)**
     Toxic effects of cadmium and its compounds NOS

    7 ✓7ᵗʰ **T56.3X2** **Toxic effect of cadmium and its compounds,** intentional self-harm   HCC

    ✓7ᵗʰ **T56.3X3** **Toxic effect of cadmium and its compounds,** assault

    ✓7ᵗʰ **T56.3X4** **Toxic effect of cadmium and its compounds,** undetermined

  ✓5ᵗʰ **T56.4** **Toxic effects of copper and its compounds**

   ✓6ᵗʰ **T56.4X** **Toxic effects of** copper and its compounds

    ✓7ᵗʰ **T56.4X1** **Toxic effect of copper and its compounds,** accidental **(unintentional)**
     Toxic effects of copper and its compounds NOS

    7 ✓7ᵗʰ **T56.4X2** **Toxic effect of copper and its compounds,** intentional self-harm   HCC

    ✓7ᵗʰ **T56.4X3** **Toxic effect of copper and its compounds,** assault

    ✓7ᵗʰ **T56.4X4** **Toxic effect of copper and its compounds,** undetermined

√5ᵗʰ **T56.5** **Toxic effects of zinc and its compounds**

  √6ᵗʰ **T56.5X** **Toxic effects of zinc and its compounds**

    √7ᵗʰ **T56.5X1** **Toxic effect of zinc and its compounds, accidental (unintentional)**
           Toxic effects of zinc and its compounds NOS

    ⁷ √7ᵗʰ **T56.5X2** **Toxic effect of zinc and its compounds, intentional self-harm**   HCC

    √7ᵗʰ **T56.5X3** **Toxic effect of zinc and its compounds, assault**

    √7ᵗʰ **T56.5X4** **Toxic effect of zinc and its compounds, undetermined**

√5ᵗʰ **T56.6** **Toxic effects of tin and its compounds**

  √6ᵗʰ **T56.6X** **Toxic effects of tin and its compounds**

    √7ᵗʰ **T56.6X1** **Toxic effect of tin and its compounds, accidental (unintentional)**
           Toxic effects of tin and its compounds NOS

    ⁷ √7ᵗʰ **T56.6X2** **Toxic effect of tin and its compounds, intentional self-harm**   HCC

    √7ᵗʰ **T56.6X3** **Toxic effect of tin and its compounds, assault**

    √7ᵗʰ **T56.6X4** **Toxic effect of tin and its compounds, undetermined**

√5ᵗʰ **T56.7** **Toxic effects of beryllium and its compounds**

  √6ᵗʰ **T56.7X** **Toxic effects of beryllium and its compounds**

    √7ᵗʰ **T56.7X1** **Toxic effect of beryllium and its compounds, accidental (unintentional)**
           Toxic effects of beryllium and its compounds NOS

    ⁷ √7ᵗʰ **T56.7X2** **Toxic effect of beryllium and its compounds, intentional self-harm**   HCC

    √7ᵗʰ **T56.7X3** **Toxic effect of beryllium and its compounds, assault**

    √7ᵗʰ **T56.7X4** **Toxic effect of beryllium and its compounds, undetermined**

√5ᵗʰ **T56.8** **Toxic effects of other metals**

  √6ᵗʰ **T56.81** **Toxic effect of thallium**

    √7ᵗʰ **T56.811** **Toxic effect of thallium, accidental (unintentional)**
           Toxic effect of thallium NOS

    ⁷ √7ᵗʰ **T56.812** **Toxic effect of thallium, intentional self-harm**   HCC

    √7ᵗʰ **T56.813** **Toxic effect of thallium, assault**

    √7ᵗʰ **T56.814** **Toxic effect of thallium, undetermined**

  √6ᵗʰ **T56.89** **Toxic effects of other metals**

    √7ᵗʰ **T56.891** **Toxic effect of other metals, accidental (unintentional)**
           Toxic effects of other metals NOS

    ⁷ √7ᵗʰ **T56.892** **Toxic effect of other metals, intentional self-harm**   HCC

    √7ᵗʰ **T56.893** **Toxic effect of other metals, assault**

    √7ᵗʰ **T56.894** **Toxic effect of other metals, undetermined**

√5ᵗʰ **T56.9** **Toxic effects of unspecified metal**

  √x7ᵗʰ **T56.91** **Toxic effect of unspecified metal, accidental (unintentional)**

  ⁷ √x7ᵗʰ **T56.92** **Toxic effect of unspecified metal, intentional self-harm**   HCC

  √x7ᵗʰ **T56.93** **Toxic effect of unspecified metal, assault**

  √x7ᵗʰ **T56.94** **Toxic effect of unspecified metal, undetermined**

√4ᵗʰ **T57** **Toxic effect of other inorganic substances**

> The appropriate 7th character is to be added to each code from category T57.
> A   initial encounter
> D   subsequent encounter
> S   sequela

√5ᵗʰ **T57.0** **Toxic effect of arsenic and its compounds**

  √6ᵗʰ **T57.0X** **Toxic effect of arsenic and its compounds**

    √7ᵗʰ **T57.0X1** **Toxic effect of arsenic and its compounds, accidental (unintentional)**
           Toxic effect of arsenic and its compounds NOS

    ⁷ √7ᵗʰ **T57.0X2** **Toxic effect of arsenic and its compounds, intentional self-harm**   HCC

    √7ᵗʰ **T57.0X3** **Toxic effect of arsenic and its compounds, assault**

    √7ᵗʰ **T57.0X4** **Toxic effect of arsenic and its compounds, undetermined**

√5ᵗʰ **T57.1** **Toxic effect of phosphorus and its compounds**

   EXCLUDES 1   organophosphate insecticides (T60.0)

  √6ᵗʰ **T57.1X** **Toxic effect of phosphorus and its compounds**

    √7ᵗʰ **T57.1X1** **Toxic effect of phosphorus and its compounds, accidental (unintentional)**
           Toxic effect of phosphorus and its compounds NOS

    ⁷ √7ᵗʰ **T57.1X2** **Toxic effect of phosphorus and its compounds, intentional self-harm**   HCC

    √7ᵗʰ **T57.1X3** **Toxic effect of phosphorus and its compounds, assault**

    √7ᵗʰ **T57.1X4** **Toxic effect of phosphorus and its compounds, undetermined**

√5ᵗʰ **T57.2** **Toxic effect of manganese and its compounds**

  √6ᵗʰ **T57.2X** **Toxic effect of manganese and its compounds**

    √7ᵗʰ **T57.2X1** **Toxic effect of manganese and its compounds, accidental (unintentional)**
           Toxic effect of manganese and its compounds NOS

    ⁷ √7ᵗʰ **T57.2X2** **Toxic effect of manganese and its compounds, intentional self-harm**   HCC

    √7ᵗʰ **T57.2X3** **Toxic effect of manganese and its compounds, assault**

    √7ᵗʰ **T57.2X4** **Toxic effect of manganese and its compounds, undetermined**

√5ᵗʰ **T57.3** **Toxic effect of hydrogen cyanide**

  √6ᵗʰ **T57.3X** **Toxic effect of hydrogen cyanide**

    √7ᵗʰ **T57.3X1** **Toxic effect of hydrogen cyanide, accidental (unintentional)**
           Toxic effect of hydrogen cyanide NOS

    ⁷ √7ᵗʰ **T57.3X2** **Toxic effect of hydrogen cyanide, intentional self-harm**   HCC

    √7ᵗʰ **T57.3X3** **Toxic effect of hydrogen cyanide, assault**

    √7ᵗʰ **T57.3X4** **Toxic effect of hydrogen cyanide, undetermined**

√5ᵗʰ **T57.8** **Toxic effect of other specified inorganic substances**

  √6ᵗʰ **T57.8X** **Toxic effect of other specified inorganic substances**

    √7ᵗʰ **T57.8X1** **Toxic effect of other specified inorganic substances, accidental (unintentional)**
           Toxic effect of other specified inorganic substances NOS

    ⁷ √7ᵗʰ **T57.8X2** **Toxic effect of other specified inorganic substances, intentional self-harm**   HCC

    √7ᵗʰ **T57.8X3** **Toxic effect of other specified inorganic substances, assault**

    √7ᵗʰ **T57.8X4** **Toxic effect of other specified inorganic substances, undetermined**

√5ᵗʰ **T57.9** **Toxic effect of unspecified inorganic substance**

  √x7ᵗʰ **T57.91** **Toxic effect of unspecified inorganic substance, accidental (unintentional)**

  ⁷ √x7ᵗʰ **T57.92** **Toxic effect of unspecified inorganic substance, intentional self-harm**   HCC

  √x7ᵗʰ **T57.93** **Toxic effect of unspecified inorganic substance, assault**

  √x7ᵗʰ **T57.94** **Toxic effect of unspecified inorganic substance, undetermined**

√4ᵗʰ **T58** **Toxic effect of carbon monoxide**

   INCLUDES   asphyxiation from carbon monoxide
             toxic effect of carbon monoxide from all sources

> The appropriate 7th character is to be added to each code from category T58.
> A   initial encounter
> D   subsequent encounter
> S   sequela

√5ᵗʰ **T58.0** **Toxic effect of carbon monoxide from motor vehicle exhaust**
     Toxic effect of exhaust gas from gas engine
     Toxic effect of exhaust gas from motor pump

  √x7ᵗʰ **T58.01** **Toxic effect of carbon monoxide from motor vehicle exhaust, accidental (unintentional)**

  ⁷ √x7ᵗʰ **T58.02** **Toxic effect of carbon monoxide from motor vehicle exhaust, intentional self-harm**   HCC

  √x7ᵗʰ **T58.03** **Toxic effect of carbon monoxide from motor vehicle exhaust, assault**

  √x7ᵗʰ **T58.04** **Toxic effect of carbon monoxide from motor vehicle exhaust, undetermined**

T58.1 Toxic effect of carbon monoxide from utility gas
Toxic effect of acetylene
Toxic effect of gas NOS used for lighting, heating, cooking
Toxic effect of water gas

T58.11 Toxic effect of carbon monoxide from utility gas, accidental (unintentional)

T58.12 Toxic effect of carbon monoxide from utility gas, intentional self-harm   HCC

T58.13 Toxic effect of carbon monoxide from utility gas, assault

T58.14 Toxic effect of carbon monoxide from utility gas, undetermined

T58.2 Toxic effect of carbon monoxide from incomplete combustion of other domestic fuels
Toxic effect of carbon monoxide from incomplete combustion of coal, coke, kerosene, wood

T58.2X Toxic effect of carbon monoxide from incomplete combustion of other domestic fuels

T58.2X1 Toxic effect of carbon monoxide from incomplete combustion of other domestic fuels, accidental (unintentional)

T58.2X2 Toxic effect of carbon monoxide from incomplete combustion of other domestic fuels, intentional self-harm   HCC

T58.2X3 Toxic effect of carbon monoxide from incomplete combustion of other domestic fuels, assault

T58.2X4 Toxic effect of carbon monoxide from incomplete combustion of other domestic fuels, undetermined

T58.8 Toxic effect of carbon monoxide from other source
Toxic effect of carbon monoxide from blast furnace gas
Toxic effect of carbon monoxide from fuels in industrial use
Toxic effect of carbon monoxide from kiln vapor

T58.8X Toxic effect of carbon monoxide from other source

T58.8X1 Toxic effect of carbon monoxide from other source, accidental (unintentional)

T58.8X2 Toxic effect of carbon monoxide from other source, intentional self-harm   HCC

T58.8X3 Toxic effect of carbon monoxide from other source, assault

T58.8X4 Toxic effect of carbon monoxide from other source, undetermined

T58.9 Toxic effect of carbon monoxide from unspecified source

T58.91 Toxic effect of carbon monoxide from unspecified source, accidental (unintentional)

T58.92 Toxic effect of carbon monoxide from unspecified source, intentional self-harm   HCC

T58.93 Toxic effect of carbon monoxide from unspecified source, assault

T58.94 Toxic effect of carbon monoxide from unspecified source, undetermined

T59 Toxic effect of other gases, fumes and vapors

   INCLUDES   aerosol propellants
   EXCLUDES 1   chlorofluorocarbons (T53.5)

The appropriate 7th character is to be added to each code from category T59.
A   initial encounter
D   subsequent encounter
S   sequela

T59.0 Toxic effect of nitrogen oxides

T59.0X Toxic effect of nitrogen oxides

T59.0X1 Toxic effect of nitrogen oxides, accidental (unintentional)
Toxic effect of nitrogen oxides NOS

T59.0X2 Toxic effect of nitrogen oxides, intentional self-harm   HCC

T59.0X3 Toxic effect of nitrogen oxides, assault

T59.0X4 Toxic effect of nitrogen oxides, undetermined

T59.1 Toxic effect of sulfur dioxide

T59.1X Toxic effect of sulfur dioxide

T59.1X1 Toxic effect of sulfur dioxide, accidental (unintentional)
Toxic effect of sulfur dioxide NOS

T59.1X2 Toxic effect of sulfur dioxide, intentional self-harm   HCC

T59.1X3 Toxic effect of sulfur dioxide, assault

T59.1X4 Toxic effect of sulfur dioxide, undetermined

T59.2 Toxic effect of formaldehyde

T59.2X Toxic effect of formaldehyde

T59.2X1 Toxic effect of formaldehyde, accidental (unintentional)
Toxic effect of formaldehyde NOS

T59.2X2 Toxic effect of formaldehyde, intentional self-harm   HCC

T59.2X3 Toxic effect of formaldehyde, assault

T59.2X4 Toxic effect of formaldehyde, undetermined

T59.3 Toxic effect of lacrimogenic gas
Toxic effect of tear gas

T59.3X Toxic effect of lacrimogenic gas

T59.3X1 Toxic effect of lacrimogenic gas, accidental (unintentional)
Toxic effect of lacrimogenic gas NOS

T59.3X2 Toxic effect of lacrimogenic gas, intentional self-harm   HCC

T59.3X3 Toxic effect of lacrimogenic gas, assault

T59.3X4 Toxic effect of lacrimogenic gas, undetermined

T59.4 Toxic effect of chlorine gas

T59.4X Toxic effect of chlorine gas

T59.4X1 Toxic effect of chlorine gas, accidental (unintentional)
Toxic effect of chlorine gas NOS

T59.4X2 Toxic effect of chlorine gas, intentional self-harm   HCC

T59.4X3 Toxic effect of chlorine gas, assault

T59.4X4 Toxic effect of chlorine gas, undetermined

T59.5 Toxic effect of fluorine gas and hydrogen fluoride

T59.5X Toxic effect of fluorine gas and hydrogen fluoride

T59.5X1 Toxic effect of fluorine gas and hydrogen fluoride, accidental (unintentional)
Toxic effect of fluorine gas and hydrogen fluoride NOS

T59.5X2 Toxic effect of fluorine gas and hydrogen fluoride, intentional self-harm   HCC

T59.5X3 Toxic effect of fluorine gas and hydrogen fluoride, assault

T59.5X4 Toxic effect of fluorine gas and hydrogen fluoride, undetermined

T59.6 Toxic effect of hydrogen sulfide

T59.6X Toxic effect of hydrogen sulfide

T59.6X1 Toxic effect of hydrogen sulfide, accidental (unintentional)
Toxic effect of hydrogen sulfide NOS

T59.6X2 Toxic effect of hydrogen sulfide, intentional self-harm   HCC

T59.6X3 Toxic effect of hydrogen sulfide, assault

T59.6X4 Toxic effect of hydrogen sulfide, undetermined

T59.7 Toxic effect of carbon dioxide

T59.7X Toxic effect of carbon dioxide

T59.7X1 Toxic effect of carbon dioxide, accidental (unintentional)
Toxic effect of carbon dioxide NOS

T59.7X2 Toxic effect of carbon dioxide, intentional self-harm   HCC

T59.7X3 Toxic effect of carbon dioxide, assault

T59.7X4 Toxic effect of carbon dioxide, undetermined

T59.8 Toxic effect of other specified gases, fumes and vapors

T59.81 Toxic effect of smoke
Smoke inhalation
   EXCLUDES 2   toxic effect of cigarette (tobacco) smoke (T65.22-)

T59.811 Toxic effect of smoke, accidental (unintentional)
Toxic effect of smoke NOS
AHA: 2013,4Q,121

7 ✓7ᵗʰ **T59.812 Toxic effect of smoke,** intentional self-harm   HCC

✓7ᵗʰ **T59.813 Toxic effect of smoke,** assault

✓7ᵗʰ **T59.814 Toxic effect of smoke,** undetermined

✓6ᵗʰ **T59.89 Toxic effect of other specified gases, fumes and vapors**

✓7ᵗʰ **T59.891 Toxic effect of other specified gases, fumes and vapors,** accidental (unintentional)

7 ✓7ᵗʰ **T59.892 Toxic effect of other specified gases, fumes and vapors,** intentional self-harm   HCC

✓7ᵗʰ **T59.893 Toxic effect of other specified gases, fumes and vapors,** assault

✓7ᵗʰ **T59.894 Toxic effect of other specified gases, fumes and vapors,** undetermined

✓5ᵗʰ **T59.9 Toxic effect of unspecified gases, fumes and vapors**

✓x7ᵗʰ **T59.91 Toxic effect of unspecified gases, fumes and vapors,** accidental (unintentional)

7 ✓x7ᵗʰ **T59.92 Toxic effect of unspecified gases, fumes and vapors,** intentional self-harm   HCC

✓x7ᵗʰ **T59.93 Toxic effect of unspecified gases, fumes and vapors,** assault

✓x7ᵗʰ **T59.94 Toxic effect of unspecified gases, fumes and vapors,** undetermined

✓4ᵗʰ **T60 Toxic effect of pesticides**

INCLUDES   toxic effect of wood preservatives

The appropriate 7th character is to be added to each code from category T60.
A   initial encounter
D   subsequent encounter
S   sequela

✓5ᵗʰ **T60.0 Toxic effect of organophosphate and carbamate insecticides**

✓6ᵗʰ **T60.0X Toxic effect of** organophosphate and carbamate insecticides

✓7ᵗʰ **T60.0X1 Toxic effect of organophosphate and carbamate insecticides,** accidental (unintentional)
Toxic effect of organophosphate and carbamate insecticides NOS

7 ✓7ᵗʰ **T60.0X2 Toxic effect of organophosphate and carbamate insecticides,** intentional self-harm   HCC

✓7ᵗʰ **T60.0X3 Toxic effect of organophosphate and carbamate insecticides,** assault

✓7ᵗʰ **T60.0X4 Toxic effect of organophosphate and carbamate insecticides,** undetermined

✓5ᵗʰ **T60.1 Toxic effect of halogenated insecticides**

EXCLUDES 1   chlorinated hydrocarbon (T53.-)

✓6ᵗʰ **T60.1X Toxic effect of** halogenated insecticides

✓7ᵗʰ **T60.1X1 Toxic effect of halogenated insecticides,** accidental (unintentional)
Toxic effect of halogenated insecticides NOS

7 ✓7ᵗʰ **T60.1X2 Toxic effect of halogenated insecticides,** intentional self-harm   HCC

✓7ᵗʰ **T60.1X3 Toxic effect of halogenated insecticides,** assault

✓7ᵗʰ **T60.1X4 Toxic effect of halogenated insecticides,** undetermined

✓5ᵗʰ **T60.2 Toxic effect of other insecticides**

✓6ᵗʰ **T60.2X Toxic effect of** other insecticides

✓7ᵗʰ **T60.2X1 Toxic effect of other insecticides,** accidental (unintentional)
Toxic effect of other insecticides NOS

7 ✓7ᵗʰ **T60.2X2 Toxic effect of other insecticides,** intentional self-harm   HCC

✓7ᵗʰ **T60.2X3 Toxic effect of other insecticides,** assault

✓7ᵗʰ **T60.2X4 Toxic effect of other insecticides,** undetermined

✓5ᵗʰ **T60.3 Toxic effect of herbicides and fungicides**

✓6ᵗʰ **T60.3X Toxic effect of** herbicides and fungicides

✓7ᵗʰ **T60.3X1 Toxic effect of herbicides and fungicides,** accidental (unintentional)
Toxic effect of herbicides and fungicides NOS

7 ✓7ᵗʰ **T60.3X2 Toxic effect of herbicides and fungicides,** intentional self-harm   HCC

✓7ᵗʰ **T60.3X3 Toxic effect of herbicides and fungicides,** assault

✓7ᵗʰ **T60.3X4 Toxic effect of herbicides and fungicides,** undetermined

✓5ᵗʰ **T60.4 Toxic effect of rodenticides**

EXCLUDES 1   strychnine and its salts (T65.1)
thallium (T56.81-)

✓6ᵗʰ **T60.4X Toxic effect of** rodenticides

✓7ᵗʰ **T60.4X1 Toxic effect of rodenticides,** accidental (unintentional)
Toxic effect of rodenticides NOS

7 ✓7ᵗʰ **T60.4X2 Toxic effect of rodenticides,** intentional self-harm   HCC

✓7ᵗʰ **T60.4X3 Toxic effect of rodenticides,** assault

✓7ᵗʰ **T60.4X4 Toxic effect of rodenticides,** undetermined

✓5ᵗʰ **T60.8 Toxic effect of other pesticides**

✓6ᵗʰ **T60.8X Toxic effect of other pesticides**

✓7ᵗʰ **T60.8X1 Toxic effect of other pesticides,** accidental (unintentional)
Toxic effect of other pesticides NOS

7 ✓7ᵗʰ **T60.8X2 Toxic effect of other pesticides,** intentional self-harm   HCC

✓7ᵗʰ **T60.8X3 Toxic effect of other pesticides,** assault

✓7ᵗʰ **T60.8X4 Toxic effect of other pesticides,** undetermined

✓5ᵗʰ **T60.9 Toxic effect of unspecified pesticide**

✓x7ᵗʰ **T60.91 Toxic effect of unspecified pesticide,** accidental (unintentional)

7 ✓x7ᵗʰ **T60.92 Toxic effect of unspecified pesticide,** intentional self-harm   HCC

✓x7ᵗʰ **T60.93 Toxic effect of unspecified pesticide,** assault

✓x7ᵗʰ **T60.94 Toxic effect of unspecified pesticide,** undetermined

✓4ᵗʰ **T61 Toxic effect of noxious substances eaten as seafood**

EXCLUDES 1   allergic reaction to food, such as:
anaphylactic reaction or shock due to adverse food reaction (T78.0-)
bacterial foodborne intoxications (A05.-)
dermatitis (L23.6, L25.4, L27.2)
food protein-induced enterocolitis syndrome (K52.21)
food protein-induced enteropathy (K52.22)
gastroenteritis (noninfective) (K52.29)
toxic effect of aflatoxin and other mycotoxins (T64)
toxic effect of cyanides (T65.0-)
toxic effect of harmful algae bloom (T65.82-)
toxic effect of hydrogen cyanide (T57.3-)
toxic effect of mercury (T56.1-)
toxic effect of red tide (T65.82-)

The appropriate 7th character is to be added to each code from category T61.
A   initial encounter
D   subsequent encounter
S   sequela

✓5ᵗʰ **T61.0 Ciguatera fish poisoning**

✓x7ᵗʰ **T61.01 Ciguatera fish poisoning,** accidental (unintentional)

7 ✓x7ᵗʰ **T61.02 Ciguatera fish poisoning,** intentional self-harm   HCC

✓x7ᵗʰ **T61.03 Ciguatera fish poisoning,** assault

✓x7ᵗʰ **T61.04 Ciguatera fish poisoning,** undetermined

✓5ᵗʰ **T61.1 Scombroid fish poisoning**
Histamine-like syndrome

✓x7ᵗʰ **T61.11 Scombroid fish poisoning,** accidental (unintentional)

7 ✓x7ᵗʰ **T61.12 Scombroid fish poisoning,** intentional self-harm   HCC

✓x7ᵗʰ **T61.13 Scombroid fish poisoning,** assault

✓x7ᵗʰ **T61.14 Scombroid fish poisoning,** undetermined

✓5ᵗʰ **T61.7 Other fish and shellfish poisoning**

✓6ᵗʰ **T61.77 Other fish poisoning**

✓7ᵗʰ **T61.771 Other fish poisoning,** accidental (unintentional)

7 ✓7ᵗʰ **T61.772 Other fish poisoning,** intentional self-harm   HCC

✓7ᵗʰ **T61.773 Other fish poisoning,** assault

√7ᵗʰ T61.774 **Other fish poisoning,** undetermined

√6ᵗʰ T61.78 **Other** shellfish **poisoning**

√7ᵗʰ T61.781 **Other shellfish poisoning,** accidental **(unintentional)**

7 √7ᵗʰ T61.782 **Other shellfish poisoning,** intentional **self-harm** HCC

√7ᵗʰ T61.783 **Other shellfish poisoning,** assault

√7ᵗʰ T61.784 **Other shellfish poisoning,** undetermined

√5ᵗʰ T61.8 **Toxic effect of other seafood**

√6ᵗʰ T61.8X **Toxic effect of other seafood**

√7ᵗʰ T61.8X1 **Toxic effect of other seafood,** accidental **(unintentional)**

7 √7ᵗʰ T61.8X2 **Toxic effect of other seafood,** intentional **self-harm** HCC

√7ᵗʰ T61.8X3 **Toxic effect of other seafood,** assault

√7ᵗʰ T61.8X4 **Toxic effect of other seafood,** undetermined

√5ᵗʰ T61.9 **Toxic effect of unspecified seafood**

√x7ᵗʰ T61.91 **Toxic effect of unspecified seafood,** accidental **(unintentional)**

7 √x7ᵗʰ T61.92 **Toxic effect of unspecified seafood,** intentional **self-harm** HCC

√x7ᵗʰ T61.93 **Toxic effect of unspecified seafood,** assault

√x7ᵗʰ T61.94 **Toxic effect of unspecified seafood,** undetermined

√4ᵗʰ T62 **Toxic effect of other noxious substances eaten as food**

EXCLUDES 1 *allergic reaction to food, such as:*
anaphylactic shock (reaction) due to adverse food reaction (T78.0-)
bacterial food borne intoxications (A05.-)
dermatitis (L23.6, L25.4, L27.2)
food protein-induced enterocolitis syndrome (K52.21)
food protein-induced enteropathy (K52.22)
gastroenteritis (noninfective) (K52.29)
toxic effect of aflatoxin and other mycotoxins (T64)
toxic effect of cyanides (T65.0-)
toxic effect of hydrogen cyanide (T57.3-)
toxic effect of mercury (T56.1-)

The appropriate 7th character is to be added to each code from category T62.
A initial encounter
D subsequent encounter
S sequela

√5ᵗʰ T62.0 **Toxic effect of ingested mushrooms**

√6ᵗʰ T62.0X **Toxic effect of** ingested mushrooms

√7ᵗʰ T62.0X1 **Toxic effect of ingested mushrooms,** accidental **(unintentional)**
Toxic effect of ingested mushrooms NOS

7 √7ᵗʰ T62.0X2 **Toxic effect of ingested mushrooms,** intentional self-harm HCC

√7ᵗʰ T62.0X3 **Toxic effect of ingested mushrooms,** assault

√7ᵗʰ T62.0X4 **Toxic effect of ingested mushrooms,** undetermined

√5ᵗʰ T62.1 **Toxic effect of ingested berries**

√6ᵗʰ T62.1X **Toxic effect of** ingested berries

√7ᵗʰ T62.1X1 **Toxic effect of ingested berries,** accidental **(unintentional)**
Toxic effect of ingested berries NOS

7 √7ᵗʰ T62.1X2 **Toxic effect of ingested berries,** intentional self-harm HCC

√7ᵗʰ T62.1X3 **Toxic effect of ingested berries,** assault

√7ᵗʰ T62.1X4 **Toxic effect of ingested berries,** undetermined

√5ᵗʰ T62.2 **Toxic effect of other ingested (parts of) plant(s)**

√6ᵗʰ T62.2X **Toxic effect of** other ingested **(parts of)** plant(s)

√7ᵗʰ T62.2X1 **Toxic effect of other ingested (parts of) plant(s),** accidental **(unintentional)**
Toxic effect of other ingested (parts of) plant(s) NOS

7 √7ᵗʰ T62.2X2 **Toxic effect of other ingested (parts of) plant(s),** intentional self-harm HCC

√7ᵗʰ T62.2X3 **Toxic effect of other ingested (parts of) plant(s),** assault

√7ᵗʰ T62.2X4 **Toxic effect of other ingested (parts of) plant(s),** undetermined

√5ᵗʰ T62.8 **Toxic effect of other specified noxious substances eaten as food**

√6ᵗʰ T62.8X **Toxic effect of other specified noxious substances eaten as food**

√7ᵗʰ T62.8X1 **Toxic effect of other specified noxious substances eaten as food,** accidental **(unintentional)**
Toxic effect of other specified noxious substances eaten as food NOS

7 √7ᵗʰ T62.8X2 **Toxic effect of other specified noxious substances eaten as food,** intentional **self-harm** HCC

√7ᵗʰ T62.8X3 **Toxic effect of other specified noxious substances eaten as food,** assault

√7ᵗʰ T62.8X4 **Toxic effect of other specified noxious substances eaten as food,** undetermined

√5ᵗʰ T62.9 **Toxic effect of unspecified noxious substance eaten as food**

√x7ᵗʰ T62.91 **Toxic effect of unspecified noxious substance eaten as food,** accidental **(unintentional)**
Toxic effect of unspecified noxious substance eaten as food NOS

7 √x7ᵗʰ T62.92 **Toxic effect of unspecified noxious substance eaten as food,** intentional self-harm HCC

√x7ᵗʰ T62.93 **Toxic effect of unspecified noxious substance eaten as food,** assault

√x7ᵗʰ T62.94 **Toxic effect of unspecified noxious substance eaten as food,** undetermined

√4ᵗʰ T63 **Toxic effect of contact with venomous animals and plants**

INCLUDES bite or touch of venomous animal
pricked or stuck by thorn or leaf

EXCLUDES 2 *ingestion of toxic animal or plant (T61.-, T62.-)*

The appropriate 7th character is to be added to each code from category T63.
A initial encounter
D subsequent encounter
S sequela

√5ᵗʰ T63.0 **Toxic effect of** snake venom

√6ᵗʰ T63.00 **Toxic effect of unspecified snake venom**

√7ᵗʰ T63.001 **Toxic effect of unspecified snake venom,** accidental **(unintentional)**
Toxic effect of unspecified snake venom NOS

7 √7ᵗʰ T63.002 **Toxic effect of unspecified snake venom,** intentional self-harm HCC

√7ᵗʰ T63.003 **Toxic effect of unspecified snake venom,** assault

√7ᵗʰ T63.004 **Toxic effect of unspecified snake venom,** undetermined

√6ᵗʰ T63.01 **Toxic effect of** rattlesnake **venom**

√7ᵗʰ T63.011 **Toxic effect of rattlesnake venom,** accidental **(unintentional)**
Toxic effect of rattlesnake venom NOS

7 √7ᵗʰ T63.012 **Toxic effect of rattlesnake venom,** intentional self-harm HCC

√7ᵗʰ T63.013 **Toxic effect of rattlesnake venom,** assault

√7ᵗʰ T63.014 **Toxic effect of rattlesnake venom,** undetermined

√6ᵗʰ T63.02 **Toxic effect of** coral snake **venom**

√7ᵗʰ T63.021 **Toxic effect of coral snake venom,** accidental **(unintentional)**
Toxic effect of coral snake venom NOS

7 √7ᵗʰ T63.022 **Toxic effect of coral snake venom,** intentional self-harm HCC

√7ᵗʰ T63.023 **Toxic effect of coral snake venom,** assault

√7ᵗʰ T63.024 **Toxic effect of coral snake venom,** undetermined

√6ᵗʰ T63.03 **Toxic effect of** taipan **venom**

√7ᵗʰ T63.031 **Toxic effect of taipan venom,** accidental **(unintentional)**
Toxic effect of taipan venom NOS

7 √7ᵗʰ T63.032 **Toxic effect of taipan venom,** intentional **self-harm** HCC

√7ᵗʰ T63.033 **Toxic effect of taipan venom,** assault

√7ᵗʰ T63.034 **Toxic effect of taipan venom,** undetermined

N Newborn: 0   P Pediatric: 0-17   M Maternity: 9-64   A Adult: 15-124   MCC Major Complication/Comorbidity   CC Complication/Comorbidity   SW Severe Wound Dx

1140   ICD-10-CM 2022

√6ᵗʰ **T63.04** **Toxic effect of** cobra **venom**

    √7ᵗʰ **T63.041** **Toxic effect of cobra venom,** accidental **(unintentional)**
         Toxic effect of cobra venom NOS

    ⁷ √7ᵗʰ **T63.042** **Toxic effect of cobra venom,** intentional **self-harm**   HCC

    √7ᵗʰ **T63.043** **Toxic effect of cobra venom,** assault

    √7ᵗʰ **T63.044** **Toxic effect of cobra venom,** undetermined

√6ᵗʰ **T63.06** **Toxic effect of venom of** other North and South American snake

    √7ᵗʰ **T63.061** **Toxic effect of venom of other North and South American snake,** accidental **(unintentional)**
         Toxic effect of venom of other North and South American snake NOS

    ⁷ √7ᵗʰ **T63.062** **Toxic effect of venom of other North and South American snake,** intentional self-harm   HCC

    √7ᵗʰ **T63.063** **Toxic effect of venom of other North and South American snake,** assault

    √7ᵗʰ **T63.064** **Toxic effect of venom of other North and South American snake,** undetermined

√6ᵗʰ **T63.07** **Toxic effect of venom of** other Australian snake

    √7ᵗʰ **T63.071** **Toxic effect of venom of other Australian snake,** accidental **(unintentional)**
         Toxic effect of venom of other Australian snake NOS

    ⁷ √7ᵗʰ **T63.072** **Toxic effect of venom of other Australian snake,** intentional self-harm   HCC

    √7ᵗʰ **T63.073** **Toxic effect of venom of other Australian snake,** assault

    √7ᵗʰ **T63.074** **Toxic effect of venom of other Australian snake,** undetermined

√6ᵗʰ **T63.08** **Toxic effect of venom of** other African and Asian snake

    √7ᵗʰ **T63.081** **Toxic effect of venom of other African and Asian snake,** accidental **(unintentional)**
         Toxic effect of venom of other African and Asian snake NOS

    ⁷ √7ᵗʰ **T63.082** **Toxic effect of venom of other African and Asian snake,** intentional self-harm   HCC

    √7ᵗʰ **T63.083** **Toxic effect of venom of other African and Asian snake,** assault

    √7ᵗʰ **T63.084** **Toxic effect of venom of other African and Asian snake,** undetermined

√6ᵗʰ **T63.09** **Toxic effect of venom of** other snake

    √7ᵗʰ **T63.091** **Toxic effect of venom of other snake,** accidental **(unintentional)**
         Toxic effect of venom of other snake NOS

    ⁷ √7ᵗʰ **T63.092** **Toxic effect of venom of other snake,** intentional self-harm   HCC

    √7ᵗʰ **T63.093** **Toxic effect of venom of other snake,** assault

    √7ᵗʰ **T63.094** **Toxic effect of venom of other snake,** undetermined

√5ᵗʰ **T63.1** **Toxic effect of venom of other reptiles**

√6ᵗʰ **T63.11** **Toxic effect of venom of** gila monster

    √7ᵗʰ **T63.111** **Toxic effect of venom of gila monster,** accidental **(unintentional)**
         Toxic effect of venom of gila monster NOS

    ⁷ √7ᵗʰ **T63.112** **Toxic effect of venom of gila monster,** intentional self-harm   HCC

    √7ᵗʰ **T63.113** **Toxic effect of venom of gila monster,** assault

    √7ᵗʰ **T63.114** **Toxic effect of venom of gila monster,** undetermined

√6ᵗʰ **T63.12** **Toxic effect of venom of other venomous lizard**

    √7ᵗʰ **T63.121** **Toxic effect of venom of other venomous lizard,** accidental **(unintentional)**
         Toxic effect of venom of other venomous lizard NOS

    ⁷ √7ᵗʰ **T63.122** **Toxic effect of venom of other venomous lizard,** intentional self-harm   HCC

    √7ᵗʰ **T63.123** **Toxic effect of venom of other venomous lizard,** assault

    √7ᵗʰ **T63.124** **Toxic effect of venom of other venomous lizard,** undetermined

√6ᵗʰ **T63.19** **Toxic effect of venom of other reptiles**

    √7ᵗʰ **T63.191** **Toxic effect of venom of other reptiles,** accidental **(unintentional)**
         Toxic effect of venom of other reptiles NOS

    ⁷ √7ᵗʰ **T63.192** **Toxic effect of venom of other reptiles,** intentional self-harm   HCC

    √7ᵗʰ **T63.193** **Toxic effect of venom of other reptiles,** assault

    √7ᵗʰ **T63.194** **Toxic effect of venom of other reptiles,** undetermined

√5ᵗʰ **T63.2** **Toxic effect of venom of scorpion**

√6ᵗʰ **T63.2X** **Toxic effect of** venom of scorpion

    √7ᵗʰ **T63.2X1** **Toxic effect of venom of scorpion,** accidental **(unintentional)**
         Toxic effect of venom of scorpion NOS

    ⁷ √7ᵗʰ **T63.2X2** **Toxic effect of venom of scorpion,** intentional self-harm   HCC

    √7ᵗʰ **T63.2X3** **Toxic effect of venom of scorpion,** assault

    √7ᵗʰ **T63.2X4** **Toxic effect of venom of scorpion,** undetermined

√5ᵗʰ **T63.3** **Toxic effect of** venom of spider

√6ᵗʰ **T63.30** **Toxic effect of unspecified spider venom**

    √7ᵗʰ **T63.301** **Toxic effect of unspecified spider venom,** accidental **(unintentional)**

    ⁷ √7ᵗʰ **T63.302** **Toxic effect of unspecified spider venom,** intentional self-harm   HCC

    √7ᵗʰ **T63.303** **Toxic effect of unspecified spider venom,** assault

    √7ᵗʰ **T63.304** **Toxic effect of unspecified spider venom,** undetermined

√6ᵗʰ **T63.31** **Toxic effect of venom of** black widow **spider**

    √7ᵗʰ **T63.311** **Toxic effect of venom of black widow spider,** accidental **(unintentional)**

    ⁷ √7ᵗʰ **T63.312** **Toxic effect of venom of black widow spider,** intentional self-harm   HCC

    √7ᵗʰ **T63.313** **Toxic effect of venom of black widow spider,** assault

    √7ᵗʰ **T63.314** **Toxic effect of venom of black widow spider,** undetermined

√6ᵗʰ **T63.32** **Toxic effect of venom of** tarantula

    √7ᵗʰ **T63.321** **Toxic effect of venom of tarantula,** accidental **(unintentional)**

    ⁷ √7ᵗʰ **T63.322** **Toxic effect of venom of tarantula,** intentional self-harm   HCC

    √7ᵗʰ **T63.323** **Toxic effect of venom of tarantula,** assault

    √7ᵗʰ **T63.324** **Toxic effect of venom of tarantula,** undetermined

√6ᵗʰ **T63.33** **Toxic effect of venom of** brown recluse **spider**

    √7ᵗʰ **T63.331** **Toxic effect of venom of brown recluse spider,** accidental **(unintentional)**

    ⁷ √7ᵗʰ **T63.332** **Toxic effect of venom of brown recluse spider,** intentional self-harm   HCC

    √7ᵗʰ **T63.333** **Toxic effect of venom of brown recluse spider,** assault

    √7ᵗʰ **T63.334** **Toxic effect of venom of brown recluse spider,** undetermined

√6ᵗʰ **T63.39** **Toxic effect of venom of** other spider

    √7ᵗʰ **T63.391** **Toxic effect of venom of other spider,** accidental **(unintentional)**

    ⁷ √7ᵗʰ **T63.392** **Toxic effect of venom of other spider,** intentional self-harm   HCC

    √7ᵗʰ **T63.393** **Toxic effect of venom of other spider,** assault

    √7ᵗʰ **T63.394** **Toxic effect of venom of other spider,** undetermined

√5ᵗʰ **T63.4** **Toxic effect of venom of other arthropods**

√6ᵗʰ **T63.41** **Toxic effect of venom of** centipedes and venomous millipedes

    √7ᵗʰ **T63.411** **Toxic effect of venom of centipedes and venomous millipedes,** accidental **(unintentional)**

    ⁷ √7ᵗʰ **T63.412** **Toxic effect of venom of centipedes and venomous millipedes,** intentional self-harm   HCC

    √7ᵗʰ **T63.413** **Toxic effect of venom of centipedes and venomous millipedes,** assault

    √7ᵗʰ **T63.414** **Toxic effect of venom of centipedes and venomous millipedes,** undetermined

✔ Additional Character Required   √x7ᵗʰ Placeholder   Questionable PDx   Manifestation   Unspecified Dx   UPD Unacceptable PDx   H1-H14 HAC   HCC CMS-HCC Dx   HIV HIV Dx

ICD-10-CM 2022   1141

√6ᵗʰ **T63.42** **Toxic effect of venom of** ants

     √7ᵗʰ **T63.421** **Toxic effect of venom of ants,** accidental **(unintentional)**

     7 √7ᵗʰ **T63.422** **Toxic effect of venom of ants,** intentional self-harm   HCC

     √7ᵗʰ **T63.423** **Toxic effect of venom of ants,** assault

     √7ᵗʰ **T63.424** **Toxic effect of venom of ants, undetermined**

√6ᵗʰ **T63.43** **Toxic effect of venom of** caterpillars

     √7ᵗʰ **T63.431** **Toxic effect of venom of caterpillars, accidental (unintentional)**

     7 √7ᵗʰ **T63.432** **Toxic effect of venom of caterpillars, intentional self-harm**   HCC

     √7ᵗʰ **T63.433** **Toxic effect of venom of caterpillars, assault**

     √7ᵗʰ **T63.434** **Toxic effect of venom of caterpillars, undetermined**

√6ᵗʰ **T63.44** **Toxic effect of venom of** bees

     √7ᵗʰ **T63.441** **Toxic effect of venom of bees,** accidental **(unintentional)**

     7 √7ᵗʰ **T63.442** **Toxic effect of venom of bees,** intentional self-harm   HCC

     √7ᵗʰ **T63.443** **Toxic effect of venom of bees,** assault

     √7ᵗʰ **T63.444** **Toxic effect of venom of bees, undetermined**

√6ᵗʰ **T63.45** **Toxic effect of venom of** hornets

     √7ᵗʰ **T63.451** **Toxic effect of venom of hornets, accidental (unintentional)**

     7 √7ᵗʰ **T63.452** **Toxic effect of venom of hornets, intentional self-harm**   HCC

     √7ᵗʰ **T63.453** **Toxic effect of venom of hornets,** assault

     √7ᵗʰ **T63.454** **Toxic effect of venom of hornets, undetermined**

√6ᵗʰ **T63.46** **Toxic effect of venom of** wasps

Toxic effect of yellow jacket

     √7ᵗʰ **T63.461** **Toxic effect of venom of wasps,** accidental **(unintentional)**

     7 √7ᵗʰ **T63.462** **Toxic effect of venom of wasps, intentional self-harm**   HCC

     √7ᵗʰ **T63.463** **Toxic effect of venom of wasps,** assault

     √7ᵗʰ **T63.464** **Toxic effect of venom of wasps, undetermined**

√6ᵗʰ **T63.48** **Toxic effect of venom of other arthropod**

     √7ᵗʰ **T63.481** **Toxic effect of venom of other arthropod, accidental (unintentional)**

     7 √7ᵗʰ **T63.482** **Toxic effect of venom of other arthropod, intentional self-harm**   HCC

     √7ᵗʰ **T63.483** **Toxic effect of venom of other arthropod, assault**

     √7ᵗʰ **T63.484** **Toxic effect of venom of other arthropod, undetermined**

√5ᵗʰ **T63.5** **Toxic effect of contact with** venomous fish

     EXCLUDES 2   *poisoning by ingestion of fish (T61.-)*

√6ᵗʰ **T63.51** **Toxic effect of contact with** stingray

     √7ᵗʰ **T63.511** **Toxic effect of contact with stingray, accidental (unintentional)**

     7 √7ᵗʰ **T63.512** **Toxic effect of contact with stingray, intentional self-harm**   HCC

     √7ᵗʰ **T63.513** **Toxic effect of contact with stingray, assault**

     √7ᵗʰ **T63.514** **Toxic effect of contact with stingray, undetermined**

√6ᵗʰ **T63.59** **Toxic effect of contact with other venomous fish**

     √7ᵗʰ **T63.591** **Toxic effect of contact with other venomous fish,** accidental **(unintentional)**

     7 √7ᵗʰ **T63.592** **Toxic effect of contact with other venomous fish, intentional self-harm**   HCC

     √7ᵗʰ **T63.593** **Toxic effect of contact with other venomous fish, assault**

     √7ᵗʰ **T63.594** **Toxic effect of contact with other venomous fish, undetermined**

√5ᵗʰ **T63.6** **Toxic effect of contact with other** venomous marine animals

     EXCLUDES 1   *sea-snake venom (T63.09)*

     EXCLUDES 2   *poisoning by ingestion of shellfish (T61.78-)*

▲ √6ᵗʰ **T63.61** **Toxic effect of contact with** Portuguese Man-o-war

Toxic effect of contact with bluebottle

▲   √7ᵗʰ **T63.611** **Toxic effect of contact with Portuguese Man-o-war,** accidental **(unintentional)**

▲   7 √7ᵗʰ **T63.612** **Toxic effect of contact with Portuguese Man-o-war, intentional self-harm**   HCC

▲   √7ᵗʰ **T63.613** **Toxic effect of contact with Portuguese Man-o-war, assault**

▲   √7ᵗʰ **T63.614** **Toxic effect of contact with Portuguese Man-o-war, undetermined**

√6ᵗʰ **T63.62** **Toxic effect of contact with other jellyfish**

     √7ᵗʰ **T63.621** **Toxic effect of contact with other jellyfish, accidental (unintentional)**

     7 √7ᵗʰ **T63.622** **Toxic effect of contact with other jellyfish, intentional self-harm**   HCC

     √7ᵗʰ **T63.623** **Toxic effect of contact with other jellyfish, assault**

     √7ᵗʰ **T63.624** **Toxic effect of contact with other jellyfish, undetermined**

√6ᵗʰ **T63.63** **Toxic effect of contact with** sea anemone

     √7ᵗʰ **T63.631** **Toxic effect of contact with sea anemone, accidental (unintentional)**

     7 √7ᵗʰ **T63.632** **Toxic effect of contact with sea anemone, intentional self-harm**   HCC

     √7ᵗʰ **T63.633** **Toxic effect of contact with sea anemone, assault**

     √7ᵗʰ **T63.634** **Toxic effect of contact with sea anemone, undetermined**

√6ᵗʰ **T63.69** **Toxic effect of contact with other venomous marine animals**

     √7ᵗʰ **T63.691** **Toxic effect of contact with other venomous marine animals, accidental (unintentional)**

     7 √7ᵗʰ **T63.692** **Toxic effect of contact with other venomous marine animals, intentional self-harm**   HCC

     √7ᵗʰ **T63.693** **Toxic effect of contact with other venomous marine animals, assault**

     √7ᵗʰ **T63.694** **Toxic effect of contact with other venomous marine animals, undetermined**

√5ᵗʰ **T63.7** **Toxic effect of contact with** venomous plant

√6ᵗʰ **T63.71** **Toxic effect of contact with venomous** marine plant

     √7ᵗʰ **T63.711** **Toxic effect of contact with venomous marine plant,** accidental **(unintentional)**

     7 √7ᵗʰ **T63.712** **Toxic effect of contact with venomous marine plant,** intentional self-harm   HCC

     √7ᵗʰ **T63.713** **Toxic effect of contact with venomous marine plant,** assault

     √7ᵗʰ **T63.714** **Toxic effect of contact with venomous marine plant,** undetermined

√6ᵗʰ **T63.79** **Toxic effect of contact with other venomous plant**

     √7ᵗʰ **T63.791** **Toxic effect of contact with other venomous plant,** accidental **(unintentional)**

     7 √7ᵗʰ **T63.792** **Toxic effect of contact with other venomous plant,** intentional self-harm   HCC

     √7ᵗʰ **T63.793** **Toxic effect of contact with other venomous plant,** assault

     √7ᵗʰ **T63.794** **Toxic effect of contact with other venomous plant,** undetermined

√5ᵗʰ **T63.8** **Toxic effect of contact with other venomous animals**

√6ᵗʰ **T63.81** **Toxic effect of contact with venomous** frog

     EXCLUDES 1   *contact with nonvenomous frog (W62.0)*

     √7ᵗʰ **T63.811** **Toxic effect of contact with venomous frog,** accidental **(unintentional)**

     7 √7ᵗʰ **T63.812** **Toxic effect of contact with venomous frog,** intentional self-harm   HCC

     √7ᵗʰ **T63.813** **Toxic effect of contact with venomous frog,** assault

     √7ᵗʰ **T63.814** **Toxic effect of contact with venomous frog,** undetermined

√6ᵗʰ **T63.82** **Toxic effect of contact with venomous** toad

     EXCLUDES 1   *contact with nonvenomous toad (W62.1)*

     √7ᵗʰ **T63.821** **Toxic effect of contact with venomous toad,** accidental **(unintentional)**

Ⓝ Newborn: 0   Ⓟ Pediatric: 0-17   Ⓜ Maternity: 9-64   Ⓐ Adult: 15-124   MCC Major Complication/Comorbidity   CC Complication/Comorbidity   SW Severe Wound Dx

1142   ICD-10-CM 2022

7 ✓7ᵗʰ **T63.822** **Toxic effect of contact with venomous toad,** intentional self-harm   HCC

✓7ᵗʰ **T63.823** **Toxic effect of contact with venomous toad,** assault

✓7ᵗʰ **T63.824** **Toxic effect of contact with venomous toad,** undetermined

✓6ᵗʰ **T63.83** **Toxic effect of contact with other venomous amphibian**

> EXCLUDES 1   contact with nonvenomous amphibian (W62.9)

✓7ᵗʰ **T63.831** **Toxic effect of contact with other venomous amphibian,** accidental (unintentional)

7 ✓7ᵗʰ **T63.832** **Toxic effect of contact with other venomous amphibian,** intentional self-harm   HCC

✓7ᵗʰ **T63.833** **Toxic effect of contact with other venomous amphibian,** assault

✓7ᵗʰ **T63.834** **Toxic effect of contact with other venomous amphibian,** undetermined

✓6ᵗʰ **T63.89** **Toxic effect of contact with other venomous animals**

✓7ᵗʰ **T63.891** **Toxic effect of contact with other venomous animals,** accidental (unintentional)

7 ✓7ᵗʰ **T63.892** **Toxic effect of contact with other venomous animals,** intentional self-harm   HCC

✓7ᵗʰ **T63.893** **Toxic effect of contact with other venomous animals,** assault

✓7ᵗʰ **T63.894** **Toxic effect of contact with other venomous animals,** undetermined

✓5ᵗʰ **T63.9** **Toxic effect of contact with unspecified venomous animal**

✓x7ᵗʰ **T63.91** **Toxic effect of contact with unspecified venomous animal,** accidental (unintentional)

7 ✓x7ᵗʰ **T63.92** **Toxic effect of contact with unspecified venomous animal,** intentional self-harm   HCC

✓x7ᵗʰ **T63.93** **Toxic effect of contact with unspecified venomous animal,** assault

✓x7ᵗʰ **T63.94** **Toxic effect of contact with unspecified venomous animal,** undetermined

✓4ᵗʰ **T64** **Toxic effect of aflatoxin and other mycotoxin food contaminants**

> The appropriate 7th character is to be added to each code from category T64.
> A   initial encounter
> D   subsequent encounter
> S   sequela

✓5ᵗʰ **T64.0** **Toxic effect of aflatoxin**

✓x7ᵗʰ **T64.01** **Toxic effect of aflatoxin,** accidental (unintentional)

7 ✓x7ᵗʰ **T64.02** **Toxic effect of aflatoxin,** intentional self-harm   HCC

✓x7ᵗʰ **T64.03** **Toxic effect of aflatoxin,** assault

✓x7ᵗʰ **T64.04** **Toxic effect of aflatoxin,** undetermined

✓5ᵗʰ **T64.8** **Toxic effect of other mycotoxin food contaminants**

✓x7ᵗʰ **T64.81** **Toxic effect of other mycotoxin food contaminants,** accidental (unintentional)

7 ✓x7ᵗʰ **T64.82** **Toxic effect of other mycotoxin food contaminants,** intentional self-harm   HCC

✓x7ᵗʰ **T64.83** **Toxic effect of other mycotoxin food contaminants,** assault

✓x7ᵗʰ **T64.84** **Toxic effect of other mycotoxin food contaminants,** undetermined

✓4ᵗʰ **T65** **Toxic effect of other and unspecified substances**

> The appropriate 7th character is to be added to each code from category T65.
> A   initial encounter
> D   subsequent encounter
> S   sequela

✓5ᵗʰ **T65.0** **Toxic effect of cyanides**

> EXCLUDES 1   hydrogen cyanide (T57.3-)

✓6ᵗʰ **T65.0X** **Toxic effect of cyanides**

✓7ᵗʰ **T65.0X1** **Toxic effect of cyanides,** accidental (unintentional)
> Toxic effect of cyanides NOS

7 ✓7ᵗʰ **T65.0X2** **Toxic effect of cyanides,** intentional self-harm   HCC

✓7ᵗʰ **T65.0X3** **Toxic effect of cyanides,** assault

✓7ᵗʰ **T65.0X4** **Toxic effect of cyanides,** undetermined

✓5ᵗʰ **T65.1** **Toxic effect of strychnine and its salts**

✓6ᵗʰ **T65.1X** **Toxic effect of strychnine and its salts**

✓7ᵗʰ **T65.1X1** **Toxic effect of strychnine and its salts,** accidental (unintentional)
> Toxic effect of strychnine and its salts NOS

7 ✓7ᵗʰ **T65.1X2** **Toxic effect of strychnine and its salts,** intentional self-harm   HCC

✓7ᵗʰ **T65.1X3** **Toxic effect of strychnine and its salts,** assault

✓7ᵗʰ **T65.1X4** **Toxic effect of strychnine and its salts,** undetermined

✓5ᵗʰ **T65.2** **Toxic effect of tobacco and nicotine**

> EXCLUDES 2   nicotine dependence (F17.-)

✓6ᵗʰ **T65.21** **Toxic effect of chewing tobacco**

✓7ᵗʰ **T65.211** **Toxic effect of chewing tobacco,** accidental (unintentional)
> Toxic effect of chewing tobacco NOS

7 ✓7ᵗʰ **T65.212** **Toxic effect of chewing tobacco,** intentional self-harm   HCC

✓7ᵗʰ **T65.213** **Toxic effect of chewing tobacco,** assault

✓7ᵗʰ **T65.214** **Toxic effect of chewing tobacco,** undetermined

✓6ᵗʰ **T65.22** **Toxic effect of tobacco cigarettes**
> Toxic effect of tobacco smoke
> Use additional code for exposure to second hand tobacco smoke (Z57.31, Z77.22)

✓7ᵗʰ **T65.221** **Toxic effect of tobacco cigarettes,** accidental (unintentional)
> Toxic effect of tobacco cigarettes NOS

7 ✓7ᵗʰ **T65.222** **Toxic effect of tobacco cigarettes,** intentional self-harm   HCC

✓7ᵗʰ **T65.223** **Toxic effect of tobacco cigarettes,** assault

✓7ᵗʰ **T65.224** **Toxic effect of tobacco cigarettes,** undetermined

✓6ᵗʰ **T65.29** **Toxic effect of other tobacco and nicotine**

✓7ᵗʰ **T65.291** **Toxic effect of other tobacco and nicotine,** accidental (unintentional)
> Toxic effect of other tobacco and nicotine NOS

7 ✓7ᵗʰ **T65.292** **Toxic effect of other tobacco and nicotine,** intentional self-harm   HCC

✓7ᵗʰ **T65.293** **Toxic effect of other tobacco and nicotine,** assault

✓7ᵗʰ **T65.294** **Toxic effect of other tobacco and nicotine,** undetermined

✓5ᵗʰ **T65.3** **Toxic effect of nitroderivatives and aminoderivatives of benzene and its homologues**
> Toxic effect of anilin [benzenamine]
> Toxic effect of nitrobenzene
> Toxic effect of trinitrotoluene

✓6ᵗʰ **T65.3X** **Toxic effect of nitroderivatives and aminoderivatives of benzene and its homologues**

✓7ᵗʰ **T65.3X1** **Toxic effect of nitroderivatives and aminoderivatives of benzene and its homologues,** accidental (unintentional)
> Toxic effect of nitroderivatives and aminoderivatives of benzene and its homologues NOS

7 ✓7ᵗʰ **T65.3X2** **Toxic effect of nitroderivatives and aminoderivatives of benzene and its homologues,** intentional self-harm   HCC

✓7ᵗʰ **T65.3X3** **Toxic effect of nitroderivatives and aminoderivatives of benzene and its homologues,** assault

✓7ᵗʰ **T65.3X4** **Toxic effect of nitroderivatives and aminoderivatives of benzene and its homologues,** undetermined

✓5ᵗʰ **T65.4** **Toxic effect of carbon disulfide**

✓6ᵗʰ **T65.4X** **Toxic effect of carbon disulfide**

✓7ᵗʰ **T65.4X1** **Toxic effect of carbon disulfide,** accidental (unintentional)
> Toxic effect of carbon disulfide NOS

7 ✓7ᵗʰ **T65.4X2** **Toxic effect of carbon disulfide,** intentional self-harm   HCC

✓7ᵗʰ **T65.4X3** **Toxic effect of carbon disulfide,** assault

✓7ᵗʰ **T65.4X4** **Toxic effect of carbon disulfide,** undetermined

✓5ᵗʰ **T65.5 Toxic effect of nitroglycerin and other nitric acids and esters**

Toxic effect of 1,2,3-Propanetriol trinitrate

✓6ᵗʰ **T65.5X Toxic effect of nitroglycerin and other nitric acids and esters**

✓7ᵗʰ **T65.5X1 Toxic effect of nitroglycerin and other nitric acids and esters, accidental (unintentional)**

Toxic effect of nitroglycerin and other nitric acids and esters NOS

7 ✓7ᵗʰ **T65.5X2 Toxic effect of nitroglycerin and other nitric acids and esters, intentional self-harm** HCC

✓7ᵗʰ **T65.5X3 Toxic effect of nitroglycerin and other nitric acids and esters, assault**

✓7ᵗʰ **T65.5X4 Toxic effect of nitroglycerin and other nitric acids and esters, undetermined**

✓5ᵗʰ **T65.6 Toxic effect of paints and dyes, not elsewhere classified**

✓6ᵗʰ **T65.6X Toxic effect of paints and dyes, not elsewhere classified**

✓7ᵗʰ **T65.6X1 Toxic effect of paints and dyes, not elsewhere classified, accidental (unintentional)**

Toxic effect of paints and dyes NOS

7 ✓7ᵗʰ **T65.6X2 Toxic effect of paints and dyes, not elsewhere classified, intentional self-harm** HCC

✓7ᵗʰ **T65.6X3 Toxic effect of paints and dyes, not elsewhere classified, assault**

✓7ᵗʰ **T65.6X4 Toxic effect of paints and dyes, not elsewhere classified, undetermined**

✓5ᵗʰ **T65.8 Toxic effect of other specified substances**

✓6ᵗʰ **T65.81 Toxic effect of latex**

✓7ᵗʰ **T65.811 Toxic effect of latex, accidental (unintentional)**

Toxic effect of latex NOS

7 ✓7ᵗʰ **T65.812 Toxic effect of latex, intentional self-harm** HCC

✓7ᵗʰ **T65.813 Toxic effect of latex, assault**

✓7ᵗʰ **T65.814 Toxic effect of latex, undetermined**

✓6ᵗʰ **T65.82 Toxic effect of harmful algae and algae toxins**

Toxic effect of (harmful) algae bloom NOS
Toxic effect of blue-green algae bloom
Toxic effect of brown tide
Toxic effect of cyanobacteria bloom
Toxic effect of Florida red tide
Toxic effect of pfiesteria piscicida
Toxic effect of red tide

✓7ᵗʰ **T65.821 Toxic effect of harmful algae and algae toxins, accidental (unintentional)**

Toxic effect of harmful algae and algae toxins NOS

7 ✓7ᵗʰ **T65.822 Toxic effect of harmful algae and algae toxins, intentional self-harm** HCC

✓7ᵗʰ **T65.823 Toxic effect of harmful algae and algae toxins, assault**

✓7ᵗʰ **T65.824 Toxic effect of harmful algae and algae toxins, undetermined**

✓6ᵗʰ **T65.83 Toxic effect of fiberglass**

✓7ᵗʰ **T65.831 Toxic effect of fiberglass, accidental (unintentional)**

Toxic effect of fiberglass NOS

7 ✓7ᵗʰ **T65.832 Toxic effect of fiberglass, intentional self-harm** HCC

✓7ᵗʰ **T65.833 Toxic effect of fiberglass, assault**

✓7ᵗʰ **T65.834 Toxic effect of fiberglass, undetermined**

✓6ᵗʰ **T65.89 Toxic effect of other specified substances**

✓7ᵗʰ **T65.891 Toxic effect of other specified substances, accidental (unintentional)**

Toxic effect of other specified substances NOS

AHA: 2018,1Q,5

7 ✓7ᵗʰ **T65.892 Toxic effect of other specified substances, intentional self-harm** HCC

✓7ᵗʰ **T65.893 Toxic effect of other specified substances, assault**

✓7ᵗʰ **T65.894 Toxic effect of other specified substances, undetermined**

✓5ᵗʰ **T65.9 Toxic effect of unspecified substance**

✓x7ᵗʰ **T65.91 Toxic effect of unspecified substance, accidental (unintentional)**

Poisoning NOS

7 ✓x7ᵗʰ **T65.92 Toxic effect of unspecified substance, intentional self-harm** HCC

✓x7ᵗʰ **T65.93 Toxic effect of unspecified substance, assault**

✓x7ᵗʰ **T65.94 Toxic effect of unspecified substance, undetermined**

Other and unspecified effects of external causes (T66-T78)

✓x7ᵗʰ **T66 Radiation sickness, unspecified**

EXCLUDES 1 specified adverse effects of radiation, such as:
burns (T20-T31)
leukemia (C91-C95)
radiation gastroenteritis and colitis (K52.0)
radiation pneumonitis (J70.0)
radiation related disorders of the skin and subcutaneous tissue (L55-L59)
radiation sunburn (L55.-)

The appropriate 7th character is to be added to code T66.
A initial encounter
D subsequent encounter
S sequela

✓4ᵗʰ **T67 Effects of heat and light**

EXCLUDES 1 erythema [dermatitis] ab igne (L59.0)
malignant hyperpyrexia due to anesthesia (T88.3)
radiation-related disorders of the skin and subcutaneous tissue (L55-L59)

EXCLUDES 2 burns (T20-T31)
sunburn (L55.-)
sweat disorder due to heat (L74-L75)

The appropriate 7th character is to be added to each code from category T67.
A initial encounter
D subsequent encounter
S sequela

✓5ᵗʰ **T67.0 Heatstroke and sunstroke**

Use additional code(s) to identify any associated complications of heatstroke, such as:
coma and stupor (R40.-)
rhabdomyolysis (M62.82)
systemic inflammatory response syndrome (R65.1-)
AHA: 2019,4Q,17-18
DEF: Headache, vertigo, cramps, and elevated body temperature due to prolonged exposure to high environmental temperatures that requires emergency intervention.

✓x7ᵗʰ **T67.01 Heatstroke and sunstroke** CC H5

Heat apoplexy
Heat pyrexia
Siriasis
Thermoplegia

✓x7ᵗʰ **T67.02 Exertional heatstroke** CC H5

✓x7ᵗʰ **T67.09 Other heatstroke and sunstroke** CC H5

✓x7ᵗʰ **T67.1 Heat syncope**

Heat collapse

✓x7ᵗʰ **T67.2 Heat cramp**

✓x7ᵗʰ **T67.3 Heat exhaustion, anhydrotic**

Heat prostration due to water depletion

EXCLUDES 1 heat exhaustion due to salt depletion (T67.4)

✓x7ᵗʰ **T67.4 Heat exhaustion due to salt depletion**

Heat prostration due to salt (and water) depletion

✓x7ᵗʰ **T67.5 Heat exhaustion, unspecified**

Heat prostration NOS

✓x7ᵗʰ **T67.6 Heat fatigue, transient**

✓x7ᵗʰ **T67.7 Heat edema**

✓x7ᵗʰ **T67.8 Other effects of heat and light**

✓x7ᵗʰ **T67.9 Effect of heat and light, unspecified**

✓x7ᵗʰ **T68** **Hypothermia**

Accidental hypothermia

Hypothermia NOS

Use additional code to identify source of exposure:

exposure to excessive cold of man-made origin (W93)

exposure to excessive cold of natural origin (X31)

EXCLUDES 1   *hypothermia following anesthesia (T88.51)*

hypothermia not associated with low environmental
temperature (R68.0)

hypothermia of newborn (P80.-)

EXCLUDES 2   *frostbite (T33-T34)*

The appropriate 7th character is to be added to code T68.

A   initial encounter

D   subsequent encounter

S   sequela

✓4ᵗʰ **T69** **Other effects of reduced temperature**

Use additional code to identify source of exposure:

exposure to excessive cold of man-made origin (W93)

exposure to excessive cold of natural origin (X31)

EXCLUDES 2   *frostbite (T33-T34)*

The appropriate 7th character is to be added to each code from
category T69.

A   initial encounter

D   subsequent encounter

S   sequela

✓5ᵗʰ **T69.0** **Immersion hand and foot**

✓6ᵗʰ **T69.01** **Immersion** hand

✓7ᵗʰ **T69.011** **Immersion hand, right hand**

✓7ᵗʰ **T69.012** **Immersion hand, left hand**

✓7ᵗʰ **T69.019** **Immersion hand, unspecified hand**

✓6ᵗʰ **T69.02** **Immersion** foot

Trench foot

✓7ᵗʰ **T69.021** **Immersion foot, right foot** CC H5

✓7ᵗʰ **T69.022** **Immersion foot, left foot** CC H5

✓7ᵗʰ **T69.029** **Immersion foot, unspecified
foot** CC H5

✓x7ᵗʰ **T69.1** **Chilblains**

DEF: Red, swollen, itchy skin primarily affecting the fingers and
toes, nose and ears, and legs. Chilblains follows damp-cold
exposure, and can also be associated with pruritus and a burning
feeling.

✓x7ᵗʰ **T69.8** **Other specified effects of reduced temperature**

✓x7ᵗʰ **T69.9** **Effect of reduced temperature, unspecified**

✓4ᵗʰ **T70** **Effects of air pressure and water pressure**

The appropriate 7th character is to be added to each code from
category T70.

A   initial encounter

D   subsequent encounter

S   sequela

✓x7ᵗʰ **T70.0** **Otitic barotrauma**

Aero-otitis media

Effects of change in ambient atmospheric pressure or water
pressure on ears

✓x7ᵗʰ **T70.1** **Sinus barotrauma**

Aerosinusitis

Effects of change in ambient atmospheric pressure on sinuses

✓5ᵗʰ **T70.2** **Other and unspecified effects of high altitude**

EXCLUDES 2   *polycythemia due to high altitude (D75.1)*

✓x7ᵗʰ **T70.20** **Unspecified effects of high altitude**

✓x7ᵗʰ **T70.29** **Other effects of high altitude**

Alpine sickness

Anoxia due to high altitude

Barotrauma NOS

Hypobaropathy

Mountain sickness

✓x7ᵗʰ **T70.3** **Caisson disease [decompression sickness]** CC H5

Compressed-air disease

Diver's palsy or paralysis

DEF: Rapid reduction in air pressure while breathing compressed
air. Symptoms include skin lesions, joint pains, and respiratory
and neurological problems.

✓x7ᵗʰ **T70.4** **Effects of high-pressure fluids**

Hydraulic jet injection (industrial)

Pneumatic jet injection (industrial)

Traumatic jet injection (industrial)

✓x7ᵗʰ **T70.8** **Other effects of air pressure and water pressure**

✓x7ᵗʰ **T70.9** **Effect of air pressure and water pressure, unspecified**

✓4ᵗʰ **T71** **Asphyxiation**

Mechanical suffocation

Traumatic suffocation

EXCLUDES 1   *acute respiratory distress (syndrome) (J80)*

anoxia due to high altitude (T70.2)

asphyxia NOS (R09.01)

asphyxia from carbon monoxide (T58.-)

asphyxia from inhalation of food or foreign body (T17.-)

asphyxia from other gases, fumes and vapors (T59.-)

respiratory distress (syndrome) in newborn (P22.-)

The appropriate 7th character is to be added to each code from
category T71.

A   initial encounter

D   subsequent encounter

S   sequela

✓5ᵗʰ **T71.1** **Asphyxiation due to** mechanical threat to breathing

Suffocation due to mechanical threat to breathing

✓6ᵗʰ **T71.11** **Asphyxiation due to** smothering under pillow

✓7ᵗʰ **T71.111** **Asphyxiation due to smothering under
pillow, accidental** CC H5

Asphyxiation due to smothering under
pillow NOS

7 ✓7ᵗʰ **T71.112** **Asphyxiation due to smothering under
pillow, intentional
self-harm** CC H5 HCC

✓7ᵗʰ **T71.113** **Asphyxiation due to smothering under
pillow, assault** CC H5

✓7ᵗʰ **T71.114** **Asphyxiation due to smothering under
pillow, undetermined** CC H5

✓6ᵗʰ **T71.12** **Asphyxiation due to** plastic bag

✓7ᵗʰ **T71.121** **Asphyxiation due to plastic bag,
accidental** CC H5

Asphyxiation due to plastic bag NOS

7 ✓7ᵗʰ **T71.122** **Asphyxiation due to plastic bag,
intentional self-harm** CC H5 HCC

✓7ᵗʰ **T71.123** **Asphyxiation due to plastic bag,
assault** CC H5

✓7ᵗʰ **T71.124** **Asphyxiation due to plastic bag,
undetermined** CC H5

✓6ᵗʰ **T71.13** **Asphyxiation due to** being trapped in bed linens

✓7ᵗʰ **T71.131** **Asphyxiation due to being trapped in bed
linens, accidental** CC H5

Asphyxiation due to being trapped in bed
linens NOS

7 ✓7ᵗʰ **T71.132** **Asphyxiation due to being trapped in bed
linens, intentional
self-harm** CC H5 HCC

✓7ᵗʰ **T71.133** **Asphyxiation due to being trapped in bed
linens, assault** CC H5

✓7ᵗʰ **T71.134** **Asphyxiation due to being trapped in bed
linens, undetermined** CC H5

✓6ᵗʰ **T71.14** **Asphyxiation due to** smothering under another
person's body (in bed)

✓7ᵗʰ **T71.141** **Asphyxiation due to smothering under
another person's body (in bed),
accidental** CC H5

Asphyxiation due to smothering under
another person's body (in bed) NOS

✓7ᵗʰ **T71.143** **Asphyxiation due to smothering under
another person's body (in bed),
assault** CC H5

✓7ᵗʰ **T71.144** **Asphyxiation due to smothering under
another person's body (in bed),
undetermined** CC H5

✓6ᵗʰ **T71.15** **Asphyxiation due to** smothering in furniture

✓7ᵗʰ **T71.151** **Asphyxiation due to smothering in
furniture, accidental** CC H5

Asphyxiation due to smothering in
furniture NOS

✓ Additional Character Required   ✓x7ᵗʰ Placeholder   Questionable PDx   Manifestation   Unspecified Dx   UPD Unacceptable PDx   H1 - H1 HAC   HCC CMS-HCC Dx   HIV HIV Dx

7 ✓7ᵗʰ **T71.152** Asphyxiation due to smothering in furniture, intentional self-harm   `CC` `H5` `HCC`

✓7ᵗʰ **T71.153** Asphyxiation due to smothering in furniture, assault   `CC` `H5`

✓7ᵗʰ **T71.154** Asphyxiation due to smothering in furniture, undetermined   `CC` `H5`

✓6ᵗʰ **T71.16** Asphyxiation due to hanging

Hanging by window shade cord
Use additional code for any associated injuries, such as:
crushing injury of neck (S17.-)
fracture of cervical vertebrae (S12.0-S12.2-)
open wound of neck (S11.-)

✓7ᵗʰ **T71.161** Asphyxiation due to hanging, accidental   `CC` `H5`

Asphyxiation due to hanging NOS
Hanging NOS

7 ✓7ᵗʰ **T71.162** Asphyxiation due to hanging, intentional self-harm   `CC` `H5` `HCC`

✓7ᵗʰ **T71.163** Asphyxiation due to hanging, assault   `CC` `H5`

✓7ᵗʰ **T71.164** Asphyxiation due to hanging, undetermined   `CC` `H5`

✓6ᵗʰ **T71.19** Asphyxiation due to mechanical threat to breathing due to other causes

✓7ᵗʰ **T71.191** Asphyxiation due to mechanical threat to breathing due to other causes, accidental   `CC` `H5`

Asphyxiation due to other causes NOS

7 ✓7ᵗʰ **T71.192** Asphyxiation due to mechanical threat to breathing due to other causes, intentional self-harm   `CC` `H5` `HCC`

✓7ᵗʰ **T71.193** Asphyxiation due to mechanical threat to breathing due to other causes, assault   `CC` `H5`

✓7ᵗʰ **T71.194** Asphyxiation due to mechanical threat to breathing due to other causes, undetermined   `CC` `H5`

✓5ᵗʰ **T71.2** Asphyxiation due to systemic oxygen deficiency due to low oxygen content in ambient air

Suffocation due to systemic oxygen deficiency due to low oxygen content in ambient air

✓x7ᵗʰ **T71.20** Asphyxiation due to systemic oxygen deficiency due to low oxygen content in ambient air due to unspecified cause   `CC` `H5`

✓x7ᵗʰ **T71.21** Asphyxiation due to cave-in or falling earth   `CC` `H5`

Use additional code for any associated cataclysm (X34-X38)

✓6ᵗʰ **T71.22** Asphyxiation due to being trapped in a car trunk

✓7ᵗʰ **T71.221** Asphyxiation due to being trapped in a car trunk, accidental   `CC`

7 ✓7ᵗʰ **T71.222** Asphyxiation due to being trapped in a car trunk, intentional self-harm   `CC` `HCC`

✓7ᵗʰ **T71.223** Asphyxiation due to being trapped in a car trunk, assault   `CC`

✓7ᵗʰ **T71.224** Asphyxiation due to being trapped in a car trunk, undetermined   `CC`

✓6ᵗʰ **T71.23** Asphyxiation due to being trapped in a (discarded) refrigerator

✓7ᵗʰ **T71.231** Asphyxiation due to being trapped in a (discarded) refrigerator, accidental   `CC`

7 ✓7ᵗʰ **T71.232** Asphyxiation due to being trapped in a (discarded) refrigerator, intentional self-harm   `CC` `HCC`

✓7ᵗʰ **T71.233** Asphyxiation due to being trapped in a (discarded) refrigerator, assault   `CC`

✓7ᵗʰ **T71.234** Asphyxiation due to being trapped in a (discarded) refrigerator, undetermined   `CC`

✓x7ᵗʰ **T71.29** Asphyxiation due to being trapped in other low oxygen environment   `CC` `H5`

✓x7ᵗʰ **T71.9** Asphyxiation due to unspecified cause   `CC` `H5`

Suffocation (by strangulation) due to unspecified cause
Suffocation NOS
Systemic oxygen deficiency due to low oxygen content in ambient air due to unspecified cause
Systemic oxygen deficiency due to mechanical threat to breathing due to unspecified cause
Traumatic asphyxia NOS

✓4ᵗʰ **T73** Effects of other deprivation.

The appropriate 7th character is to be added to each code from category T73.
A   initial encounter
D   subsequent encounter
S   sequela

✓x7ᵗʰ **T73.0** Starvation

Deprivation of food

✓x7ᵗʰ **T73.1** Deprivation of water

✓x7ᵗʰ **T73.2** Exhaustion due to exposure

✓x7ᵗʰ **T73.3** Exhaustion due to excessive exertion

Exhaustion due to overexertion

✓x7ᵗʰ **T73.8** Other effects of deprivation

✓x7ᵗʰ **T73.9** Effect of deprivation, unspecified

✓4ᵗʰ **T74** Adult and child abuse, neglect and other maltreatment, confirmed

Use additional code, if applicable, to identify any associated current injury
Use additional external cause code to identify perpetrator, if known (Y07.-)

EXCLUDES 1   abuse and maltreatment in pregnancy (O9A.3-, O9A.4-, O9A.5-)

adult and child maltreatment, suspected (T76.-)

The appropriate 7th character is to be added to each code from category T74.
A   initial encounter
D   subsequent encounter
S   sequela

✓5ᵗʰ **T74.0** Neglect or abandonment, confirmed

✓x7ᵗʰ **T74.01** Adult neglect or abandonment, confirmed   `CC` `A`

✓x7ᵗʰ **T74.02** Child neglect or abandonment, confirmed   `CC` `P`

✓5ᵗʰ **T74.1** Physical abuse, confirmed

EXCLUDES 2   sexual abuse (T74.2-)

✓x7ᵗʰ **T74.11** Adult physical abuse, confirmed   `CC` `A`

✓x7ᵗʰ **T74.12** Child physical abuse, confirmed   `CC` `P`

EXCLUDES 2   shaken infant syndrome (T74.4)

✓5ᵗʰ **T74.2** Sexual abuse, confirmed

Rape, confirmed
Sexual assault, confirmed

✓x7ᵗʰ **T74.21** Adult sexual abuse, confirmed   `CC` `A`

✓x7ᵗʰ **T74.22** Child sexual abuse, confirmed   `CC` `P`

✓5ᵗʰ **T74.3** Psychological abuse, confirmed

Bullying and intimidation, confirmed
Intimidation through social media, confirmed

✓x7ᵗʰ **T74.31** Adult psychological abuse, confirmed   `A`

✓x7ᵗʰ **T74.32** Child psychological abuse, confirmed   `CC` `P`

✓x7ᵗʰ **T74.4** Shaken infant syndrome   `CC` `P`

✓5ᵗʰ **T74.5** Forced sexual exploitation, confirmed

AHA: 2018,4Q,32-33,65

✓x7ᵗʰ **T74.51** Adult forced sexual exploitation, confirmed   `CC` `A`

✓x7ᵗʰ **T74.52** Child sexual exploitation, confirmed   `CC` `P`

✓5ᵗʰ **T74.6** Forced labor exploitation, confirmed

AHA: 2018,4Q,32-33,65

✓x7ᵗʰ **T74.61** Adult forced labor exploitation, confirmed   `CC` `A`

✓x7ᵗʰ **T74.62** Child forced labor exploitation, confirmed   `CC` `P`

✓5ᵗʰ **T74.9** Unspecified maltreatment, confirmed

✓x7ᵗʰ **T74.91** Unspecified adult maltreatment, confirmed   `CC` `A`

✓x7ᵗʰ **T74.92** Unspecified child maltreatment, confirmed   `CC` `P`

`N` Newborn: 0   `P` Pediatric: 0-17   `M` Maternity: 9-64   `A` Adult: 15-124   `MCC` Major Complication/Comorbidity   `CC` Complication/Comorbidity   `SW` Severe Wound Dx

1146   ICD-10-CM 2022

✓4ᵗʰ T75 Other and unspecified effects of other external causes

     EXCLUDES 1   adverse effects NEC (T78.-)

     EXCLUDES 2   burns (electric) (T20-T31)

     The appropriate 7th character is to be added to each code from category T75.
     A   initial encounter
     D   subsequent encounter
     S   sequela

  ✓5ᵗʰ T75.0   Effects of lightning

     Struck by lightning

     ✓x7ᵗʰ T75.00   Unspecified effects of lightning

       Struck by lightning NOS

     ✓x7ᵗʰ T75.01   Shock due to being struck by lightning

     ✓x7ᵗʰ T75.09   Other effects of lightning

       Use additional code for other effects of lightning

  ✓x7ᵗʰ T75.1   Unspecified effects of drowning and nonfatal submersion   `CC` `H5`

     Immersion

     EXCLUDES 1   specified effects of drowning - code to effects

  ✓5ᵗʰ T75.2   Effects of vibration

     ✓x7ᵗʰ T75.20   Unspecified effects of vibration

     ✓x7ᵗʰ T75.21   Pneumatic hammer syndrome

     ✓x7ᵗʰ T75.22   Traumatic vasospastic syndrome

     ✓x7ᵗʰ T75.23   Vertigo from infrasound

       EXCLUDES 1   vertigo NOS (R42)

     ✓x7ᵗʰ T75.29   Other effects of vibration

  ✓x7ᵗʰ T75.3   Motion sickness

     Airsickness

     Seasickness

     Travel sickness

     Use additional external cause code to identify vehicle or type of motion (Y92.81-, Y93.5-)

  ✓x7ᵗʰ T75.4   Electrocution

     Shock from electric current

     Shock from electroshock gun (taser)

  ✓5ᵗʰ T75.8   Other specified effects of external causes

     ✓x7ᵗʰ T75.81   Effects of abnormal gravitation [G] forces

     ✓x7ᵗʰ T75.82   Effects of weightlessness

     ✓x7ᵗʰ T75.89   Other specified effects of external causes

✓4ᵗʰ T76 Adult and child abuse, neglect and other maltreatment, suspected

     Use additional code, if applicable, to identify any associated current injury

     EXCLUDES 1   adult and child maltreatment, confirmed (T74.-)

         suspected abuse and maltreatment in pregnancy (O9A.3-, O9A.4-, O9A.5-)

         suspected adult physical abuse, ruled out (Z04.71)

         suspected adult sexual abuse, ruled out (Z04.41)

         suspected child physical abuse, ruled out (Z04.72)

         suspected child sexual abuse, ruled out (Z04.42)

     AHA: 2018,4Q,72

     The appropriate 7th character is to be added to each code from category T76.
     A   initial encounter
     D   subsequent encounter
     S   sequela

  ✓5ᵗʰ T76.0   Neglect or abandonment, suspected

     ✓x7ᵗʰ T76.01   Adult neglect or abandonment, suspected   `CC` `A`

     ✓x7ᵗʰ T76.02   Child neglect or abandonment, suspected   `CC` `P`

  ✓5ᵗʰ T76.1   Physical abuse, suspected

     ✓x7ᵗʰ T76.11   Adult physical abuse, suspected   `CC` `A`

     ✓x7ᵗʰ T76.12   Child physical abuse, suspected   `CC` `P`

       AHA: 2019,2Q,12

  ✓5ᵗʰ T76.2   Sexual abuse, suspected

     Rape, suspected

     EXCLUDES 1   alleged abuse, ruled out (Z04.7)

     ✓x7ᵗʰ T76.21   Adult sexual abuse, suspected   `CC` `A`

     ✓x7ᵗʰ T76.22   Child sexual abuse, suspected   `CC` `P`

  ✓5ᵗʰ T76.3   Psychological abuse, suspected

     Bullying and intimidation, suspected

     Intimidation through social media, suspected

     ✓x7ᵗʰ T76.31   Adult psychological abuse, suspected   `A`

     ✓x7ᵗʰ T76.32   Child psychological abuse, suspected   `CC` `P`

  ✓5ᵗʰ T76.5   Forced sexual exploitation, suspected

     AHA: 2018,4Q,32-33,65

     ✓x7ᵗʰ T76.51   Adult forced sexual exploitation, suspected   `CC` `P`

     ✓x7ᵗʰ T76.52   Child sexual exploitation, suspected   `CC` `P`

  ✓5ᵗʰ T76.6   Forced labor exploitation, suspected

     AHA: 2018,4Q,32-33,65

     ✓x7ᵗʰ T76.61   Adult forced labor exploitation, suspected   `CC` `A`

     ✓x7ᵗʰ T76.62   Child forced labor exploitation, suspected   `CC` `P`

  ✓5ᵗʰ T76.9   Unspecified maltreatment, suspected

     ✓x7ᵗʰ T76.91   Unspecified adult maltreatment, suspected   `CC` `A`

     ✓x7ᵗʰ T76.92   Unspecified child maltreatment, suspected   `CC` `P`

✓4ᵗʰ T78 Adverse effects, not elsewhere classified

     EXCLUDES 2   complications of surgical and medical care NEC (T80-T88)

     The appropriate 7th character is to be added to each code from category T78.
     A   initial encounter
     D   subsequent encounter
     S   sequela

  ✓5ᵗʰ T78.0   Anaphylactic reaction due to food

     Anaphylactic reaction due to adverse food reaction

     Anaphylactic shock or reaction due to nonpoisonous foods

     Anaphylactoid reaction due to food

     ✓x7ᵗʰ T78.00   Anaphylactic reaction due to unspecified food   `CC`

     ✓x7ᵗʰ T78.01   Anaphylactic reaction due to peanuts   `CC`

     ✓x7ᵗʰ T78.02   Anaphylactic reaction due to shellfish (crustaceans)   `CC`

     ✓x7ᵗʰ T78.03   Anaphylactic reaction due to other fish   `CC`

     ✓x7ᵗʰ T78.04   Anaphylactic reaction due to fruits and vegetables   `CC`

     ✓x7ᵗʰ T78.05   Anaphylactic reaction due to tree nuts and seeds   `CC`

       EXCLUDES 2   anaphylactic reaction due to peanuts (T78.01)

     ✓x7ᵗʰ T78.06   Anaphylactic reaction due to food additives   `CC`

     ✓x7ᵗʰ T78.07   Anaphylactic reaction due to milk and dairy products   `CC`

     ✓x7ᵗʰ T78.08   Anaphylactic reaction due to eggs   `CC`

     ✓x7ᵗʰ T78.09   Anaphylactic reaction due to other food products   `CC`

  ✓x7ᵗʰ T78.1   Other adverse food reactions, not elsewhere classified

     Use additional code to identify the type of reaction, if applicable

     EXCLUDES 1   anaphylactic reaction or shock due to adverse food reaction (T78.0-)

         anaphylactic reaction due to food (T78.0-)

         bacterial food borne intoxications (A05.-)

     EXCLUDES 2   allergic and dietetic gastroenteritis and colitis (K52.29)

         allergic rhinitis due to food (J30.5)

         dermatitis due to food in contact with skin (L23.6, L24.6, L25.4)

         dermatitis due to ingested food (L27.2)

         food protein-induced enterocolitis syndrome (K52.21)

         food protein-induced enteropathy (K52.22)

  ✓x7ᵗʰ T78.2   Anaphylactic shock, unspecified   `CC`

     Allergic shock

     Anaphylactic reaction

     Anaphylaxis

     EXCLUDES 1   anaphylactic reaction or shock due to adverse effect of correct medicinal substance properly administered (T88.6)

         anaphylactic reaction or shock due to adverse food reaction (T78.0-)

         anaphylactic reaction or shock due to serum (T80.5-)

☑ Additional Character Required   ✓x7ᵗʰ Placeholder   Questionable PDx   Manifestation   Unspecified Dx   `UPD` Unacceptable PDx   `H1`-`H14` HAC   `HCC` CMS-HCC Dx   `HIV` HIV Dx

ICD-10-CM 2022   1147

Chapter 19. Injury, Poisoning and Certain Other Consequences of External Causes *(left margin)*

T78.3–T79.9 *(left margin bottom)*

√x7ᵗʰ **T78.3** **Angioneurotic edema**
Allergic angioedema
Giant urticaria
Quincke's edema
> *EXCLUDES 1*   serum urticaria (T80.6-)
>   urticaria (L50.-)

√5ᵗʰ **T78.4** **Other and unspecified allergy**
> *EXCLUDES 1*   specified types of allergic reaction such as:
>   allergic diarrhea (K52.29)
>   allergic gastroenteritis and colitis (K52.29)
>   dermatitis (L23-L25, L27.-)
>   food protein-induced enterocolitis syndrome
>   (K52.21)
>   food protein-induced enteropathy (K52.22)
>   hay fever (J30.1)

    √x7ᵗʰ **T78.40** **Allergy, unspecified**
Allergic reaction NOS
Hypersensitivity NOS

    √x7ᵗʰ **T78.41** **Arthus phenomenon**
Arthus reaction

    √x7ᵗʰ **T78.49** **Other allergy**
AHA: 2021,1Q,42

√x7ᵗʰ **T78.8** **Other adverse effects, not elsewhere classified**

Certain early complications of trauma (T79)

√4ᵗʰ **T79** **Certain early complications of trauma, not elsewhere classified**
> *EXCLUDES 2*   acute respiratory distress syndrome (J80)
>   complications occurring during or following medical
>   procedures (T80-T88)
>   complications of surgical and medical care NEC (T80-T88)
>   newborn respiratory distress syndrome (P22.0)

> The appropriate 7th character is to be added to each code from
> category T79.
> A   initial encounter
> D   subsequent encounter
> S   sequela

6 √x7ᵗʰ **T79.0** **Air embolism (traumatic)**   `MCC` `HCC`
>   *EXCLUDES 1*   air embolism complicating abortion or ectopic or
>   molar pregnancy (O00-O07, O08.2)
>   air embolism complicating pregnancy, childbirth and
>   the puerperium (O88.0)
>   air embolism following infusion, transfusion, and
>   therapeutic injection (T80.0)
>   air embolism following procedure NEC (T81.7-)
DEF: Arterial or venous obstruction due to the introduction of air
bubbles into the blood vessels following surgery or trauma.

6 √x7ᵗʰ **T79.1** **Fat embolism (traumatic)**   `MCC` `HCC`
>   *EXCLUDES 1*   fat embolism complicating:
>   abortion or ectopic or molar pregnancy (O00-O07,
>   O08.2)
>   pregnancy, childbirth and the puerperium (O88.8)
DEF: Arterial blockage due to the entrance of fat into the
circulatory system after a fracture of the large bones or
administration of corticosteroids.

6 √x7ᵗʰ **T79.2** **Traumatic secondary and recurrent hemorrhage and seroma**   `CC` `HCC`

6 √x7ᵗʰ **T79.4** **Traumatic shock**   `MCC` `HCC`
Shock (immediate) (delayed) following injury
>   *EXCLUDES 1*   anaphylactic shock due to adverse food reaction
>   (T78.0-)
>   anaphylactic shock due to correct medicinal
>   substance properly administered (T88.6)
>   anaphylactic shock due to serum (T80.5-)
>   anaphylactic shock NOS (T78.2)
>   ~~anesthetic shock (T88.2)~~
>   electric shock (T75.4)
>   nontraumatic shock NEC (R57.-)
>   obstetric shock (O75.1)
>   postprocedural shock (T81.1-)
>   septic shock (R65.21)
>   shock complicating abortion or ectopic or molar
>   pregnancy (O00-O07, O08.3)
>   ►shock due to anesthesia (T88.2)◄
>   shock due to lightning (T75.01)
>   shock NOS (R57.9)

6 √x7ᵗʰ **T79.5** **Traumatic anuria**   `MCC` `HCC`
Crush syndrome
Renal failure following crushing

6 √x7ᵗʰ **T79.6** **Traumatic ischemia of muscle**   `HCC`
Traumatic rhabdomyolysis
Volkmann's ischemic contracture
>   *EXCLUDES 2*   anterior tibial syndrome (M76.8)
>   compartment syndrome (traumatic) (T79.A-)
>   nontraumatic ischemia of muscle (M62.2-)
AHA: 2019,2Q,12

6 √x7ᵗʰ **T79.7** **Traumatic subcutaneous emphysema**   `CC` `HCC`
>   *EXCLUDES 2*   emphysema NOS (J43)
>   emphysema (subcutaneous) resulting from a
>   procedure (T81.82)

√5ᵗʰ **T79.A** **Traumatic compartment syndrome**
>   *EXCLUDES 1*   fibromyalgia (M79.7)
>   nontraumatic compartment syndrome (M79.A-)
>   *EXCLUDES 2*   traumatic ischemic infarction of muscle (T79.6)
DEF: Compression of nerves and blood vessels within an enclosed
muscle space due to previous trauma, which leads to impaired
blood flow and muscle and nerve damage.

   6 √x7ᵗʰ **T79.A0** **Compartment syndrome, unspecified**   `CC` `HCC`
Compartment syndrome NOS

   √6ᵗʰ **T79.A1** **Traumatic compartment syndrome of** upper
extremity
Traumatic compartment syndrome of shoulder, arm,
forearm, wrist, hand, and fingers
    6 √7ᵗʰ **T79.A11** **Traumatic compartment syndrome of**
right upper extremity   `CC` `HCC`
    6 √7ᵗʰ **T79.A12** **Traumatic compartment syndrome of** left
upper extremity   `CC` `HCC`
    6 √7ᵗʰ **T79.A19** **Traumatic compartment syndrome of**
unspecified upper extremity   `CC` `HCC`

   √6ᵗʰ **T79.A2** **Traumatic compartment syndrome of** lower
extremity
Traumatic compartment syndrome of hip, buttock,
thigh, leg, foot, and toes
    6 √7ᵗʰ **T79.A21** **Traumatic compartment syndrome of**
right lower extremity   `CC` `HCC`
    6 √7ᵗʰ **T79.A22** **Traumatic compartment syndrome of** left
lower extremity   `CC` `HCC`
    6 √7ᵗʰ **T79.A29** **Traumatic compartment syndrome of**
unspecified lower extremity   `CC` `HCC`

   6 √x7ᵗʰ **T79.A3** **Traumatic compartment syndrome of**
abdomen   `CC` `HCC`

   6 √x7ᵗʰ **T79.A9** **Traumatic compartment syndrome of other**
sites   `CC` `HCC`

6 √x7ᵗʰ **T79.8** **Other early complications of trauma**   `HCC`

6 √x7ᵗʰ **T79.9** **Unspecified early complication of trauma**   `HCC`

Complications of surgical and medical care, not elsewhere classified (T80-T88)

Use additional code for adverse effect, if applicable, to identify drug (T36-T50 with fifth or sixth character 5)

Use additional code(s) to identify the specified condition resulting from the complication

Use additional code to identify devices involved and details of circumstances (Y62-Y82)

EXCLUDES 2   *any encounters with medical care for postprocedural conditions in which no complications are present, such as:*
     artificial opening status (Z93.-)
     closure of external stoma (Z43.-)
     fitting and adjustment of external prosthetic device (Z44.-)
   burns and corrosions from local applications and irradiation (T20-T32)
   complications of surgical procedures during pregnancy, childbirth and the puerperium (O00-O9A)
   mechanical complication of respirator [ventilator] (J95.850)
   poisoning and toxic effects of drugs and chemicals (T36-T65 with fifth or sixth character 1-4 or 6)
   postprocedural fever (R50.82)
   specified complications classified elsewhere, such as:
     cerebrospinal fluid leak from spinal puncture (G97.0)
     colostomy malfunction (K94.0-)
     disorders of fluid and electrolyte imbalance (E86-E87)
     functional disturbances following cardiac surgery (I97.0-I97.1)
     intraoperative and postprocedural complications of specified body systems (D78.-, E36.-, E89.-, G97.3-, G97.4, H59.3-, H59.-, H95.2-, H95.3, I97.4-, I97.5, J95.6-, J95.7, K91.6-, L76.-, M96.-, N99.-)
     ostomy complications (J95.0-, K94.-, N99.5-)
     postgastric surgery syndromes (K91.1)
     postlaminectomy syndrome NEC (M96.1)
     postmastectomy lymphedema syndrome (I97.2)
     postsurgical blind-loop syndrome (K91.2)
     ventilator associated pneumonia (J95.851)

AHA: 2015,1Q,15

✓4ᵗʰ T80 Complications following infusion, transfusion and therapeutic injection

INCLUDES   complications following perfusion

EXCLUDES 2   *bone marrow transplant rejection (T86.01)*
   febrile nonhemolytic transfusion reaction (R50.84)
   fluid overload due to transfusion (E87.71)
   posttransfusion purpura (D69.51)
   transfusion associated circulatory overload (TACO) (E87.71)
   transfusion (red blood cell) associated hemochromatosis (E83.111)
   transfusion related acute lung injury (TRALI) (J95.84)

> The appropriate 7th character is to be added to each code from category T80.
> A   initial encounter
> D   subsequent encounter
> S   sequela

✓x7ᵗʰ T80.0 Air embolism following infusion, transfusion and therapeutic injection   MCC H2

✓x7ᵗʰ T80.1 Vascular complications following infusion, transfusion and therapeutic injection   CC

Use additional code to identify the vascular complication

EXCLUDES 2   *extravasation of vesicant agent (T80.81-)*
   infiltration of vesicant agent (T80.81-)
   postprocedural vascular complications (T81.7-)
   vascular complications specified as due to prosthetic devices, implants and grafts (T82.8-, T83.8-, T84.8-, T85.8-)

✓5ᵗʰ T80.2 Infections following infusion, transfusion and therapeutic injection

Use additional code to identify the specific infection, such as: sepsis (A41.9)

Use additional code (R65.2-) to identify severe sepsis, if applicable

EXCLUDES 2   *infections specified as due to prosthetic devices, implants and grafts (T82.6-T82.7, T83.5-T83.6, T84.5-T84.7, T85.7)*
   postprocedural infections (T81.4-)

AHA: 2018,4Q,62

✓6ᵗʰ T80.21 Infection due to central venous catheter

Infection due to pulmonary artery catheter (Swan-Ganz catheter)

AHA: 2019,1Q,13-14

DEF: Central venous catheter: Catheter positioned in the superior vena cava or right atrium and introduced through a large vein, such as the jugular or subclavian, and used to measure venous pressure or administer fluids or medication.

TIP: Code assignment is based on the location of the catheter and not how the catheter is being used; for example, for hemodialysis. Infections resulting from catheters that are not central lines should be coded to T82.7-.

✓7ᵗʰ T80.211 Bloodstream infection due to central venous catheter   CC H7

Catheter-related bloodstream infection (CRBSI) NOS

Central line-associated bloodstream infection (CLABSI)

Bloodstream infection due to Hickman catheter

Bloodstream infection due to peripherally inserted central catheter (PICC)

Bloodstream infection due to portacath (port-a-cath)

Bloodstream infection due to pulmonary artery catheter

Bloodstream infection due to triple lumen catheter

Bloodstream infection due to umbilical venous catheter

AHA: 2019,1Q,13,14; 2018,4Q,89

✓7ᵗʰ T80.212 Local infection due to central venous catheter   CC H7

Exit or insertion site infection

Local infection due to Hickman catheter

Local infection due to peripherally inserted central catheter (PICC)

Local infection due to portacath (port-a-cath)

Local infection due to pulmonary artery catheter

Local infection due to triple lumen catheter

Local infection due to umbilical venous catheter

Port or reservoir infection

Tunnel infection

✓7ᵗʰ T80.218 Other infection due to central venous catheter   CC H7

Other central line-associated infection

Other infection due to Hickman catheter

Other infection due to peripherally inserted central catheter (PICC)

Other infection due to portacath (port-a-cath)

Other infection due to pulmonary artery catheter

Other infection due to triple lumen catheter

Other infection due to umbilical venous catheter

☑ Additional Character Required   ✓x7ᵗʰ Placeholder   Questionable PDx   Manifestation   Unspecified Dx   UPD Unacceptable PDx   H1 - H14 HAC   HCC CMS-HCC Dx   HIV HIV Dx

ICD-10-CM 2022   1149

√7ᵗʰ **T80.219 Unspecified infection due to central venous catheter** CC H7

Central line-associated infection NOS

Unspecified infection due to Hickman catheter

Unspecified infection due to peripherally inserted central catheter (PICC)

Unspecified infection due to portacath (port-a-cath)

Unspecified infection due to pulmonary artery catheter

Unspecified infection due to triple lumen catheter

Unspecified infection due to umbilical venous catheter

√x7ᵗʰ **T80.22 Acute infection following transfusion, infusion, or injection of blood and blood products** CC

√x7ᵗʰ **T80.29 Infection following other infusion, transfusion and therapeutic injection** CC

√5ᵗʰ **T80.3 ABO incompatibility reaction due to transfusion of blood or blood products**

> EXCLUDES 1   *minor blood group antigens reactions (Duffy) (E) (K) (Kell) (Kidd) (Lewis) (M) (N) (P) (S) (T80.A-)*

√x7ᵗʰ **T80.30 ABO incompatibility reaction due to transfusion of blood or blood products, unspecified** CC H3

ABO incompatibility blood transfusion NOS

Reaction to ABO incompatibility from transfusion NOS

√6ᵗʰ **T80.31 ABO incompatibility with hemolytic transfusion reaction**

√7ᵗʰ **T80.310 ABO incompatibility with acute hemolytic transfusion reaction** CC H3

ABO incompatibility with hemolytic transfusion reaction less than 24 hours after transfusion

Acute hemolytic transfusion reaction (AHTR) due to ABO incompatibility

√7ᵗʰ **T80.311 ABO incompatibility with delayed hemolytic transfusion reaction** CC H3

ABO incompatibility with hemolytic transfusion reaction 24 hours or more after transfusion

Delayed hemolytic transfusion reaction (DHTR) due to ABO incompatibility

√7ᵗʰ **T80.319 ABO incompatibility with hemolytic transfusion reaction, unspecified** CC H3

ABO incompatibility with hemolytic transfusion reaction at unspecified time after transfusion

Hemolytic transfusion reaction (HTR) due to ABO incompatibility NOS

√x7ᵗʰ **T80.39 Other ABO incompatibility reaction due to transfusion of blood or blood products** CC H3

Delayed serologic transfusion reaction (DSTR) from ABO incompatibility

Other ABO incompatible blood transfusion

Other reaction to ABO incompatible blood transfusion

√5ᵗʰ **T80.4 Rh incompatibility reaction due to transfusion of blood or blood products**

Reaction due to incompatibility of Rh antigens (C) (c) (D) (E) (e)

√x7ᵗʰ **T80.40 Rh incompatibility reaction due to transfusion of blood or blood products, unspecified** CC

Reaction due to Rh factor in transfusion NOS

Rh incompatible blood transfusion NOS

√6ᵗʰ **T80.41 Rh incompatibility with hemolytic transfusion reaction**

√7ᵗʰ **T80.410 Rh incompatibility with acute hemolytic transfusion reaction** CC

Acute hemolytic transfusion reaction (AHTR) due to Rh incompatibility

Rh incompatibility with hemolytic transfusion reaction less than 24 hours after transfusion

√7ᵗʰ **T80.411 Rh incompatibility with delayed hemolytic transfusion reaction** CC

Delayed hemolytic transfusion reaction (DHTR) due to Rh incompatibility

Rh incompatibility with hemolytic transfusion reaction 24 hours or more after transfusion

√7ᵗʰ **T80.419 Rh incompatibility with hemolytic transfusion reaction, unspecified** CC

Rh incompatibility with hemolytic transfusion reaction at unspecified time after transfusion

Hemolytic transfusion reaction (HTR) due to Rh incompatibility NOS

√x7ᵗʰ **T80.49 Other Rh incompatibility reaction due to transfusion of blood or blood products** CC

Delayed serologic transfusion reaction (DSTR) from Rh incompatibility

Other reaction to Rh incompatible blood transfusion

√5ᵗʰ **T80.A Non-ABO incompatibility reaction due to transfusion of blood or blood products**

Reaction due to incompatibility of minor antigens (Duffy) (Kell) (Kidd) (Lewis) (M) (N) (P) (S)

√x7ᵗʰ **T80.A0 Non-ABO incompatibility reaction due to transfusion of blood or blood products, unspecified** CC

Non-ABO antigen incompatibility reaction from transfusion NOS

√6ᵗʰ **T80.A1 Non-ABO incompatibility with hemolytic transfusion reaction**

√7ᵗʰ **T80.A10 Non-ABO incompatibility with acute hemolytic transfusion reaction** CC

Acute hemolytic transfusion reaction (AHTR) due to non-ABO incompatibility

Non-ABO incompatibility with hemolytic transfusion reaction less than 24 hours after transfusion

√7ᵗʰ **T80.A11 Non-ABO incompatibility with delayed hemolytic transfusion reaction** CC

Delayed hemolytic transfusion reaction (DHTR) due to non-ABO incompatibility

Non-ABO incompatibility with hemolytic transfusion reaction 24 or more hours after transfusion

√7ᵗʰ **T80.A19 Non-ABO incompatibility with hemolytic transfusion reaction, unspecified** CC

Hemolytic transfusion reaction (HTR) due to non-ABO incompatibility NOS

Non-ABO incompatibility with hemolytic transfusion reaction at unspecified time after transfusion

√x7ᵗʰ **T80.A9 Other non-ABO incompatibility reaction due to transfusion of blood or blood products** CC

Delayed serologic transfusion reaction (DSTR) from non-ABO incompatibility

Other reaction to non-ABO incompatible blood transfusion

√5ᵗʰ **T80.5 Anaphylactic reaction due to serum**

Allergic shock due to serum

Anaphylactic shock due to serum

Anaphylactoid reaction due to serum

Anaphylaxis due to serum

> EXCLUDES 1   *ABO incompatibility reaction due to transfusion of blood or blood products (T80.3-)*
> *allergic reaction or shock NOS (T78.2)*
> *anaphylactic reaction or shock NOS (T78.2)*
> *anaphylactic reaction or shock due to adverse effect of correct medicinal substance properly administered (T88.6)*
> *other serum reaction (T80.6-)*

DEF: Life-threatening hypersensitivity to a foreign serum causing respiratory distress, vascular collapse, and shock.

√x7ᵗʰ **T80.51 Anaphylactic reaction due to administration of blood and blood products** CC

√x7ᵗʰ **T80.52 Anaphylactic reaction due to vaccination** CC

AHA: 2021,1Q,43

N Newborn: 0   P Pediatric: 0-17   M Maternity: 9-64   A Adult: 15-124   MCC Major Complication/Comorbidity   CC Complication/Comorbidity   SW Severe Wound Dx

     ✓x7ᵗʰ   **T80.59**   **Anaphylactic reaction due to other serum**   `CC`

✓5ᵗʰ   **T80.6**   **Other serum reactions**

     Intoxication by serum

     Protein sickness

     Serum rash

     Serum sickness

     Serum urticaria

     `EXCLUDES 2`   *serum hepatitis (B16–B19)*

     DEF: Serum sickness: Hypersensitivity to a foreign serum that causes fever, hives, swelling, and lymphadenopathy.

     ✓x7ᵗʰ   **T80.61**   **Other serum reaction** due to administration of blood and blood products   `CC`

     ✓x7ᵗʰ   **T80.62**   **Other serum reaction** due to vaccination   `CC`

         AHA: 2021,1Q,42

     ✓x7ᵗʰ   **T80.69**   **Other serum reaction due to other serum**   `CC`

         Code also, if applicable, arthropathy in hypersensitivity reactions classified elsewhere (M36.4)

✓5ᵗʰ   **T80.8**   **Other complications following infusion, transfusion and therapeutic injection**

     ✓6ᵗʰ   **T80.81**   **Extravasation of vesicant agent**

         Infiltration of vesicant agent

         ✓7ᵗʰ   **T80.810**   **Extravasation of vesicant antineoplastic chemotherapy**   `CC`

            Infiltration of vesicant antineoplastic chemotherapy

         ✓7ᵗʰ   **T80.818**   **Extravasation of other vesicant agent**   `CC`

            Infiltration of other vesicant agent

     ●   ✓x7ᵗʰ   **T80.82**   **Complication of immune effector cellular therapy**

         Complication of chimeric antigen receptor (CAR-T) cell therapy

         Complication of IEC therapy

         Use additional code to identify the specific complication, such as:

         cytokine release syndrome (D89.83-)

         immune effector cell-associated neurotoxicity syndrome (G92.0-)

         `EXCLUDES 2`   *complication of bone marrow transplant (T86.0)*

                 complication of stem cell transplant (T86.5)

     ✓x7ᵗʰ   **T80.89**   **Other complications following infusion, transfusion and therapeutic injection**

         Delayed serologic transfusion reaction (DSTR), unspecified incompatibility

         Use additional code to identify graft-versus-host reaction, if applicable, (D89.81-)

         AHA: 2020,4Q,14

✓5ᵗʰ   **T80.9**   **Unspecified complication following infusion, transfusion and therapeutic injection**

     ✓x7ᵗʰ   **T80.90**   **Unspecified complication** following infusion and therapeutic injection

     ✓6ᵗʰ   **T80.91**   **Hemolytic transfusion reaction, unspecified incompatibility**

         `EXCLUDES 1`   *ABO incompatibility with hemolytic transfusion reaction (T80.31-)*

                 non-ABO incompatibility with hemolytic transfusion reaction (T80.A1-)

                 Rh incompatibility with hemolytic transfusion reaction (T80.41-)

         ✓7ᵗʰ   **T80.910**   **Acute hemolytic transfusion reaction, unspecified incompatibility**   `CC`

         ✓7ᵗʰ   **T80.911**   **Delayed hemolytic transfusion reaction, unspecified incompatibility**   `CC`

         ✓7ᵗʰ   **T80.919**   **Hemolytic transfusion reaction, unspecified incompatibility, unspecified as acute or delayed**   `CC`

            Hemolytic transfusion reaction NOS

     ✓x7ᵗʰ   **T80.92**   **Unspecified transfusion reaction**

         Transfusion reaction NOS

✓4ᵗʰ   **T81**   **Complications of procedures, not elsewhere classified**

     Use additional code for adverse effect, if applicable, to identify drug (T36–T50 with fifth or sixth character 5)

     `EXCLUDES 2`   *complications following immunization (T88.0–T88.1)*

         complications following infusion, transfusion and therapeutic injection (T80.-)

         complications of transplanted organs and tissue (T86.-)

         specified complications classified elsewhere, such as:

         complication of prosthetic devices, implants and grafts (T82–T85)

         dermatitis due to drugs and medicaments (L23.3, L24.4, L25.1, L27.0-L27.1)

         endosseous dental implant failure (M27.6-)

         floppy iris syndrome (IFIS) (intraoperative) (H21.81)

         intraoperative and postprocedural complications of specific body system (D78.-, E36.-, E89.-, G97.3-, G97.4, H59.3-, H59.-, H95.2-, H95.3, I97.4-, I97.5, J95, K91.-, L76.-, M96.-, N99.-)

         ostomy complications (J95.0-, K94.-, N99.5-)

         plateau iris syndrome (post-iridectomy) (postprocedural) H21.82

         poisoning and toxic effects of drugs and chemicals (T36–T65 with fifth or sixth character 1-4 or 6)

     AHA: 2019,2Q,21

     The appropriate 7th character is to be added to each code from category T81.

     A   initial encounter

     D   subsequent encounter

     S   sequela

     ✓5ᵗʰ   **T81.1**   **Postprocedural shock**

         Shock during or resulting from a procedure, not elsewhere classified

         `EXCLUDES 1`   *anaphylactic shock due to correct substance properly administered (T88.6)*

            anaphylactic shock due to serum (T80.5-)

            anaphylactic shock NOS (T78.2)

            ~~*anesthetic shock (T88.2)*~~

            electric shock (T75.4)

            obstetric shock (O75.1)

            septic shock (R65.21)

            ▶*shock due to anesthesia (T88.2)*◀

            shock following abortion or ectopic or molar pregnancy (O00–O07, O08.3)

            traumatic shock (T79.4)

         AHA: 2021,1Q,13

         ✓x7ᵗʰ   **T81.10**   **Postprocedural shock unspecified**   `CC`

            Collapse NOS during or resulting from a procedure, not elsewhere classified

            Postprocedural failure of peripheral circulation

            Postprocedural shock NOS

      6   ✓x7ᵗʰ   **T81.11**   **Postprocedural cardiogenic shock**   `MCC` `HCC`

      6   ✓x7ᵗʰ   **T81.12**   **Postprocedural septic shock**   `MCC` `UPD` `HCC`

            Postprocedural endotoxic shock resulting from a procedure, not elsewhere classified

            Postprocedural gram-negative shock resulting from a procedure, not elsewhere classified

            Code first underlying infection

            Use additional code, to identify any associated acute organ dysfunction, if applicable

            AHA: 2018,4Q,63

         ✓x7ᵗʰ   **T81.19**   **Other postprocedural shock**   `MCC`

            Postprocedural hypovolemic shock

     ✓5ᵗʰ   **T81.3**   **Disruption of wound, not elsewhere classified**

         Disruption of any suture materials or other closure methods

         `EXCLUDES 1`   *breakdown (mechanical) of permanent sutures (T85.612)*

            displacement of permanent sutures (T85.622)

            disruption of cesarean delivery wound (O90.0)

            disruption of perineal obstetric wound (O90.1)

            mechanical complication of permanent sutures NEC (T85.692)

         AHA: 2014,1Q,23

         ✓x7ᵗʰ   **T81.30**   **Disruption of wound, unspecified**   `CC` `SW`

            Disruption of wound NOS

☑ Additional Character Required   ✓x7ᵗʰ Placeholder   Questionable PDx   *Manifestation*   Unspecified Dx   `UPD` Unacceptable PDx   `H1`-`H14` HAC   `HCC` CMS-HCC Dx   `HIV` HIV Dx

ICD-10-CM 2022   **1151**

√x 7ᵗʰ **T81.31 Disruption of external operation (surgical) wound, not elsewhere classified** CC SW

Dehiscence of operation wound NOS

Disruption of operation wound NOS

Disruption or dehiscence of closure of cornea

Disruption or dehiscence of closure of mucosa

Disruption or dehiscence of closure of skin and subcutaneous tissue

Full-thickness skin disruption or dehiscence

Superficial disruption or dehiscence of operation wound

EXCLUDES 1 *dehiscence of amputation stump (T87.81)*

√x 7ᵗʰ **T81.32 Disruption of internal operation (surgical) wound, not elsewhere classified** CC SW

Deep disruption or dehiscence of operation wound NOS

Disruption or dehiscence of closure of internal organ or other internal tissue

Disruption or dehiscence of closure of muscle or muscle flap

Disruption or dehiscence of closure of ribs or rib cage

Disruption or dehiscence of closure of skull or craniotomy

Disruption or dehiscence of closure of sternum or sternotomy

Disruption or dehiscence of closure of tendon or ligament

Disruption or dehiscence of closure of superficial or muscular fascia

AHA: 2020,2Q,22; 2017,3Q,4

√x 7ᵗʰ **T81.33 Disruption of traumatic injury wound repair** CC

Disruption or dehiscence of closure of traumatic laceration (external) (internal)

√ 5ᵗʰ **T81.4 Infection following a procedure**

Wound abscess following a procedure

Use additional code to identify infection

Use additional code (R65.2-) to identify severe sepsis, if applicable

EXCLUDES 2 *bleb associated endophthalmitis (H59.4-)*

infection due to infusion, transfusion and therapeutic injection (T80.2-)

infection due to prosthetic devices, implants and grafts (T82.6-T82.7, T83.5-T83.6, T84.5-T84.7, T85.7)

obstetric surgical wound infection (O86.0-)

postprocedural fever NOS (R50.82)

postprocedural retroperitoneal abscess (K68.11)

AHA: 2018,4Q,33-34,62; 2014,1Q,23

√x 7ᵗʰ **T81.40 Infection following a procedure, unspecified** CC H11 H12 H13

√x 7ᵗʰ **T81.41 Infection following a procedure, superficial incisional surgical site** CC H11 H12 H13

Subcutaneous abscess following a procedure

Stitch abscess following a procedure

√x 7ᵗʰ **T81.42 Infection following a procedure, deep incisional surgical site** CC H11 H12 H13

Intra-muscular abscess following a procedure

√x 7ᵗʰ **T81.43 Infection following a procedure, organ and space surgical site** CC H11 H12 H13

Intra-abdominal abscess following a procedure

Subphrenic abscess following a procedure

6 √x 7ᵗʰ **T81.44 Sepsis following a procedure** CC H11 H12 H13 HCC

Use additional code to identify the sepsis

√x 7ᵗʰ **T81.49 Infection following a procedure, other surgical site** CC H11 H12 H13

√ 5ᵗʰ **T81.5 Complications of foreign body accidentally left in body following procedure**

AHA: 2014,4Q,24

√ 6ᵗʰ **T81.50 Unspecified complication of foreign body accidentally left in body following procedure**

√ 7ᵗʰ **T81.500 Unspecified complication of foreign body accidentally left in body following surgical operation** CC H1

√ 7ᵗʰ **T81.501 Unspecified complication of foreign body accidentally left in body following infusion or transfusion** CC H1

√ 7ᵗʰ **T81.502 Unspecified complication of foreign body accidentally left in body following kidney dialysis** CC H1 HCC

√ 7ᵗʰ **T81.503 Unspecified complication of foreign body accidentally left in body following injection or immunization** CC H1

√ 7ᵗʰ **T81.504 Unspecified complication of foreign body accidentally left in body following endoscopic examination** CC H1

√ 7ᵗʰ **T81.505 Unspecified complication of foreign body accidentally left in body following heart catheterization** CC H1

√ 7ᵗʰ **T81.506 Unspecified complication of foreign body accidentally left in body following aspiration, puncture or other catheterization** CC H1

√ 7ᵗʰ **T81.507 Unspecified complication of foreign body accidentally left in body following removal of catheter or packing** CC H1

√ 7ᵗʰ **T81.508 Unspecified complication of foreign body accidentally left in body following other procedure** CC H1

√ 7ᵗʰ **T81.509 Unspecified complication of foreign body accidentally left in body following unspecified procedure** CC H1

√ 6ᵗʰ **T81.51 Adhesions due to foreign body accidentally left in body following procedure**

√ 7ᵗʰ **T81.510 Adhesions due to foreign body accidentally left in body following surgical operation** CC H1

√ 7ᵗʰ **T81.511 Adhesions due to foreign body accidentally left in body following infusion or transfusion** CC H1

√ 7ᵗʰ **T81.512 Adhesions due to foreign body accidentally left in body following kidney dialysis** CC H1 HCC

√ 7ᵗʰ **T81.513 Adhesions due to foreign body accidentally left in body following injection or immunization** CC H1

√ 7ᵗʰ **T81.514 Adhesions due to foreign body accidentally left in body following endoscopic examination** CC H1

√ 7ᵗʰ **T81.515 Adhesions due to foreign body accidentally left in body following heart catheterization** CC H1

√ 7ᵗʰ **T81.516 Adhesions due to foreign body accidentally left in body following aspiration, puncture or other catheterization** CC H1

√ 7ᵗʰ **T81.517 Adhesions due to foreign body accidentally left in body following removal of catheter or packing** CC H1

√ 7ᵗʰ **T81.518 Adhesions due to foreign body accidentally left in body following other procedure** CC H1

√ 7ᵗʰ **T81.519 Adhesions due to foreign body accidentally left in body following unspecified procedure** CC H1

√ 6ᵗʰ **T81.52 Obstruction due to foreign body accidentally left in body following procedure**

√ 7ᵗʰ **T81.520 Obstruction due to foreign body accidentally left in body following surgical operation** CC H1

√ 7ᵗʰ **T81.521 Obstruction due to foreign body accidentally left in body following infusion or transfusion** CC H1

√ 7ᵗʰ **T81.522 Obstruction due to foreign body accidentally left in body following kidney dialysis** CC H1 HCC

√ 7ᵗʰ **T81.523 Obstruction due to foreign body accidentally left in body following injection or immunization** CC H1

√ 7ᵗʰ **T81.524 Obstruction due to foreign body accidentally left in body following endoscopic examination** CC H1

√ 7ᵗʰ **T81.525 Obstruction due to foreign body accidentally left in body following heart catheterization** CC H1

√ 7ᵗʰ **T81.526 Obstruction due to foreign body accidentally left in body following aspiration, puncture or other catheterization** CC H1

N Newborn: 0   P Pediatric: 0-17   M Maternity: 9-64   A Adult: 15-124   MCC Major Complication/Comorbidity   CC Complication/Comorbidity   SW Severe Wound Dx

1152   ICD-10-CM 2022

√7ᵗʰ **T81.527** **Obstruction due to foreign body accidentally left in body following** removal of catheter or packing   `CC` `H1`

√7ᵗʰ **T81.528** **Obstruction due to foreign body accidentally left in body following other procedure**   `CC` `H1`

√7ᵗʰ **T81.529** **Obstruction due to foreign body accidentally left in body following unspecified procedure**   `CC` `H1`

√6ᵗʰ **T81.53** Perforation due to foreign body accidentally left in body following procedure

√7ᵗʰ **T81.530** **Perforation due to foreign body accidentally left in body following** surgical operation   `CC` `H1`

√7ᵗʰ **T81.531** **Perforation due to foreign body accidentally left in body following** infusion or transfusion   `CC` `H1`

√7ᵗʰ **T81.532** **Perforation due to foreign body accidentally left in body following** kidney dialysis   `CC` `H1` `HCC`

√7ᵗʰ **T81.533** **Perforation due to foreign body accidentally left in body following** injection or immunization   `CC` `H1`

√7ᵗʰ **T81.534** **Perforation due to foreign body accidentally left in body following** endoscopic examination   `CC` `H1`

√7ᵗʰ **T81.535** **Perforation due to foreign body accidentally left in body following** heart catheterization   `CC` `H1`

√7ᵗʰ **T81.536** **Perforation due to foreign body accidentally left in body following** aspiration, puncture or other catheterization   `CC` `H1`

√7ᵗʰ **T81.537** **Perforation due to foreign body accidentally left in body following** removal of catheter or packing   `CC` `H1`

√7ᵗʰ **T81.538** **Perforation due to foreign body accidentally left in body following other procedure**   `CC` `H1`

√7ᵗʰ **T81.539** **Perforation due to foreign body accidentally left in body following unspecified procedure**   `CC` `H1`

√6ᵗʰ **T81.59** Other complications of foreign body accidentally left in body following procedure

    EXCLUDES 2   obstruction or perforation due to prosthetic devices and implants intentionally left in body (T82.0-T82.5, T83.0-T83.4, T83.7, T84.0-T84.4, T85.0-T85.6)

√7ᵗʰ **T81.590** **Other complications of foreign body accidentally left in body following** surgical operation   `CC` `H1`

√7ᵗʰ **T81.591** **Other complications of foreign body accidentally left in body following** infusion or transfusion   `CC` `H1`

√7ᵗʰ **T81.592** **Other complications of foreign body accidentally left in body following** kidney dialysis   `CC` `H1` `HCC`

√7ᵗʰ **T81.593** **Other complications of foreign body accidentally left in body following** injection or immunization   `CC` `H1`

√7ᵗʰ **T81.594** **Other complications of foreign body accidentally left in body following** endoscopic examination   `CC` `H1`

√7ᵗʰ **T81.595** **Other complications of foreign body accidentally left in body following** heart catheterization   `CC` `H1`

√7ᵗʰ **T81.596** **Other complications of foreign body accidentally left in body following** aspiration, puncture or other catheterization   `CC` `H1`

√7ᵗʰ **T81.597** **Other complications of foreign body accidentally left in body following** removal of catheter or packing   `CC` `H1`

√7ᵗʰ **T81.598** **Other complications of foreign body accidentally left in body following other procedure**   `CC` `H1`

√7ᵗʰ **T81.599** **Other complications of foreign body accidentally left in body following unspecified procedure**   `CC` `H1`

√5ᵗʰ **T81.6** **Acute reaction to foreign substance accidentally left during a procedure**

    EXCLUDES 2   complications of foreign body accidentally left in body cavity or operation wound following procedure (T81.5-)

√×7ᵗʰ **T81.60** **Unspecified acute reaction to foreign substance accidentally left during a procedure**   `CC` `H1`

√×7ᵗʰ **T81.61** **Aseptic peritonitis due to foreign substance accidentally left during a procedure**   `CC` `H1`
    Chemical peritonitis

√×7ᵗʰ **T81.69** **Other acute reaction to foreign substance accidentally left during a procedure**   `CC` `H1`

√5ᵗʰ **T81.7** **Vascular complications following a procedure, not elsewhere classified**
    Air embolism following procedure NEC
    Phlebitis or thrombophlebitis resulting from a procedure

    EXCLUDES 1   embolism complicating abortion or ectopic or molar pregnancy (O00-O07, O08.2)
        embolism complicating pregnancy, childbirth and the puerperium (O88.-)
        traumatic embolism (T79.0)

    EXCLUDES 2   embolism due to prosthetic devices, implants and grafts (T82.8-, T83.81, T84.8-, T85.81-)
        embolism following infusion, transfusion and therapeutic injection (T80.0)

    AHA: 2019,2Q,22

√6ᵗʰ **T81.71** **Complication of artery following a procedure, not elsewhere classified**

√7ᵗʰ **T81.710** **Complication of** mesenteric **artery following a procedure, not elsewhere classified**   `CC`

√7ᵗʰ **T81.711** **Complication of** renal **artery following a procedure, not elsewhere classified**   `CC`

√7ᵗʰ **T81.718** **Complication of other artery following a procedure, not elsewhere classified**   `CC`
      AHA: 2019,2Q,21-22

√7ᵗʰ **T81.719** **Complication of unspecified artery following a procedure, not elsewhere classified**   `CC`

√×7ᵗʰ **T81.72** **Complication of** vein **following a procedure, not elsewhere classified**   `CC`

√5ᵗʰ **T81.8** **Other complications of procedures, not elsewhere classified**

    EXCLUDES 2   hypothermia following anesthesia (T88.51)
        malignant hyperpyrexia due to anesthesia (T88.3)

√×7ᵗʰ **T81.81** **Complication of inhalation therapy**

√×7ᵗʰ **T81.82** **Emphysema (subcutaneous) resulting from a procedure**

√×7ᵗʰ **T81.83** **Persistent postprocedural fistula**   `CC` `SW`
      AHA: 2017,3Q,3-4

√×7ᵗʰ **T81.89** **Other complications of procedures, not elsewhere classified**   `SW`
      Use additional code to specify complication, such as: postprocedural delirium (F05)
      AHA: 2014,1Q,23

√×7ᵗʰ **T81.9** **Unspecified complication of procedure**

√4ᵗʰ **T82** **Complications of cardiac and vascular prosthetic devices, implants and grafts**

    EXCLUDES 2   failure and rejection of transplanted organs and tissue (T86.-)
    AHA: 2020,3Q,36-37

    The appropriate 7th character is to be added to each code from category T82.
    A   initial encounter
    D   subsequent encounter
    S   sequela

√5ᵗʰ **T82.0** **Mechanical complication of** heart valve prosthesis
    Mechanical complication of artificial heart valve

    EXCLUDES 1   mechanical complication of biological heart valve graft (T82.22-)

√×7ᵗʰ **T82.01** **Breakdown (mechanical) of heart valve prosthesis**   `CC`

√×7ᵗʰ **T82.02** **Displacement of heart valve prosthesis**   `CC`
    Malposition of heart valve prosthesis

√×7ᵗʰ **T82.03** **Leakage of heart valve prosthesis**   `CC`

☑ Additional Character Required   √×7ᵗʰ Placeholder   Questionable PDx   Manifestation   Unspecified Dx   `UPD` Unacceptable PDx   `H1`-`H14` HAC   `HCC` CMS-HCC Dx   `HIV` HIV Dx

ICD-10-CM 2022   **1153**

✓x 7ᵗʰ T82.09 **Other mechanical complication of heart valve prosthesis** `CC`

Obstruction (mechanical) of heart valve prosthesis

Perforation of heart valve prosthesis

Protrusion of heart valve prosthesis

✓5ᵗʰ T82.1 **Mechanical complication of cardiac electronic device**

    ✓6ᵗʰ T82.11 **Breakdown (mechanical) of cardiac electronic device**

        ✓7ᵗʰ T82.110 **Breakdown (mechanical) of cardiac electrode** `CC`

        ✓7ᵗʰ T82.111 **Breakdown (mechanical) of cardiac pulse generator (battery)** `CC`

        ✓7ᵗʰ T82.118 **Breakdown (mechanical) of other cardiac electronic device** `CC`

        ✓7ᵗʰ T82.119 **Breakdown (mechanical) of unspecified cardiac electronic device** `CC`

    ✓6ᵗʰ T82.12 **Displacement of cardiac electronic device**

Malposition of cardiac electronic device

        ✓7ᵗʰ T82.120 **Displacement of cardiac electrode** `CC`

        ✓7ᵗʰ T82.121 **Displacement of cardiac pulse generator (battery)** `CC`

        ✓7ᵗʰ T82.128 **Displacement of other cardiac electronic device** `CC`

        ✓7ᵗʰ T82.129 **Displacement of unspecified cardiac electronic device** `CC`

    ✓6ᵗʰ T82.19 **Other mechanical complication of cardiac electronic device**

Leakage of cardiac electronic device

Obstruction of cardiac electronic device

Perforation of cardiac electronic device

Protrusion of cardiac electronic device

        ✓7ᵗʰ T82.190 **Other mechanical complication of cardiac electrode** `CC`

        ✓7ᵗʰ T82.191 **Other mechanical complication of cardiac pulse generator (battery)** `CC`

        ✓7ᵗʰ T82.198 **Other mechanical complication of other cardiac electronic device** `CC`

        ✓7ᵗʰ T82.199 **Other mechanical complication of unspecified cardiac device** `CC`

✓5ᵗʰ T82.2 **Mechanical complication of coronary artery bypass graft and biological valve heart valve graft**

    `EXCLUDES 1` *mechanical complication of artificial heart valve prosthesis (T82.0-)*

    ✓6ᵗʰ T82.21 **Mechanical complication of coronary artery bypass graft**

        ✓7ᵗʰ T82.211 **Breakdown (mechanical) of coronary artery bypass graft** `CC`

        ✓7ᵗʰ T82.212 **Displacement of coronary artery bypass graft** `CC`

Malposition of coronary artery bypass graft

        ✓7ᵗʰ T82.213 **Leakage of coronary artery bypass graft** `CC`

        ✓7ᵗʰ T82.218 **Other mechanical complication of coronary artery bypass graft** `CC`

Obstruction, mechanical of coronary artery bypass graft

Perforation of coronary artery bypass graft

Protrusion of coronary artery bypass graft

    ✓6ᵗʰ T82.22 **Mechanical complication of biological heart valve graft**

        ✓7ᵗʰ T82.221 **Breakdown (mechanical) of biological heart valve graft** `CC`

        ✓7ᵗʰ T82.222 **Displacement of biological heart valve graft** `CC`

Malposition of biological heart valve graft

        ✓7ᵗʰ T82.223 **Leakage of biological heart valve graft** `CC`

        ✓7ᵗʰ T82.228 **Other mechanical complication of biological heart valve graft** `CC`

Obstruction of biological heart valve graft

Perforation of biological heart valve graft

Protrusion of biological heart valve graft

✓5ᵗʰ T82.3 **Mechanical complication of other vascular grafts**

    ✓6ᵗʰ T82.31 **Breakdown (mechanical) of other vascular grafts**

        6 ✓7ᵗʰ T82.310 **Breakdown (mechanical) of aortic (bifurcation) graft (replacement)** `CC` `HCC`

AHA: 2020,3Q,3-8

        6 ✓7ᵗʰ T82.311 **Breakdown (mechanical) of carotid arterial graft (bypass)** `CC` `HCC`

        6 ✓7ᵗʰ T82.312 **Breakdown (mechanical) of femoral arterial graft (bypass)** `CC` `HCC`

        6 ✓7ᵗʰ T82.318 **Breakdown (mechanical) of other vascular grafts** `CC` `HCC`

        6 ✓7ᵗʰ T82.319 **Breakdown (mechanical) of unspecified vascular grafts** `CC` `HCC`

    ✓6ᵗʰ T82.32 **Displacement of other vascular grafts**

Malposition of other vascular grafts

        6 ✓7ᵗʰ T82.320 **Displacement of aortic (bifurcation) graft (replacement)** `CC` `HCC`

        6 ✓7ᵗʰ T82.321 **Displacement of carotid arterial graft (bypass)** `CC` `HCC`

        6 ✓7ᵗʰ T82.322 **Displacement of femoral arterial graft (bypass)** `CC` `HCC`

        6 ✓7ᵗʰ T82.328 **Displacement of other vascular grafts** `CC` `HCC`

        6 ✓7ᵗʰ T82.329 **Displacement of unspecified vascular grafts** `CC` `HCC`

    ✓6ᵗʰ T82.33 **Leakage of other vascular grafts**

        6 ✓7ᵗʰ T82.330 **Leakage of aortic (bifurcation) graft (replacement)** `CC` `HCC`

AHA: 2020,3Q,3-8

        6 ✓7ᵗʰ T82.331 **Leakage of carotid arterial graft (bypass)** `CC` `HCC`

        6 ✓7ᵗʰ T82.332 **Leakage of femoral arterial graft (bypass)** `CC` `HCC`

        6 ✓7ᵗʰ T82.338 **Leakage of other vascular grafts** `CC` `HCC`

        6 ✓7ᵗʰ T82.339 **Leakage of unspecified vascular graft** `CC` `HCC`

    ✓6ᵗʰ T82.39 **Other mechanical complication of other vascular grafts**

Obstruction (mechanical) of other vascular grafts

Perforation of other vascular grafts

Protrusion of other vascular grafts

        6 ✓7ᵗʰ T82.390 **Other mechanical complication of aortic (bifurcation) graft (replacement)** `CC` `HCC`

AHA: 2020,3Q,3-5

        6 ✓7ᵗʰ T82.391 **Other mechanical complication of carotid arterial graft (bypass)** `CC` `HCC`

        6 ✓7ᵗʰ T82.392 **Other mechanical complication of femoral arterial graft (bypass)** `CC` `HCC`

        6 ✓7ᵗʰ T82.398 **Other mechanical complication of other vascular grafts** `CC` `HCC`

        6 ✓7ᵗʰ T82.399 **Other mechanical complication of unspecified vascular grafts** `CC` `HCC`

✓5ᵗʰ T82.4 **Mechanical complication of vascular dialysis catheter**

Mechanical complication of hemodialysis catheter

    `EXCLUDES 1` *mechanical complication of intraperitoneal dialysis catheter (T85.62)*

    ✓x 7ᵗʰ T82.41 **Breakdown (mechanical) of vascular dialysis catheter** `CC` `HCC`

    ✓x 7ᵗʰ T82.42 **Displacement of vascular dialysis catheter** `CC` `HCC`

Malposition of vascular dialysis catheter

    ✓x 7ᵗʰ T82.43 **Leakage of vascular dialysis catheter** `CC` `HCC`

    ✓x 7ᵗʰ T82.49 **Other complication of vascular dialysis catheter** `CC` `HCC`

Obstruction (mechanical) of vascular dialysis catheter

Perforation of vascular dialysis catheter

Protrusion of vascular dialysis catheter

✓5ᵗʰ T82.5 **Mechanical complication of other cardiac and vascular devices and implants**

    `EXCLUDES 2` *mechanical complication of epidural and subdural infusion catheter (T85.61)*

    ✓6ᵗʰ T82.51 **Breakdown (mechanical) of other cardiac and vascular devices and implants**

        6 ✓7ᵗʰ T82.510 **Breakdown (mechanical) of surgically created arteriovenous fistula** `CC` `HCC`

AHA: 2020,3Q,36

        6 ✓7ᵗʰ T82.511 **Breakdown (mechanical) of surgically created arteriovenous shunt** `CC` `HCC`

AHA: 2020,3Q,37

        ✓7ᵗʰ T82.512 **Breakdown (mechanical) of artificial heart** `CC`

Ⓝ Newborn: 0   Ⓟ Pediatric: 0-17   Ⓜ Maternity: 9-64   Ⓐ Adult: 15-124   `MCC` Major Complication/Comorbidity   `CC` Complication/Comorbidity   `SW` Severe Wound Dx

1154   ICD-10-CM 2022

6 √7ᵗʰ **T82.513** **Breakdown (mechanical) of** balloon (counterpulsation) device CC HCC

6 √7ᵗʰ **T82.514** **Breakdown (mechanical) of** infusion catheter CC HCC

6 √7ᵗʰ **T82.515** **Breakdown (mechanical) of** umbrella device CC HCC

6 √7ᵗʰ **T82.518** **Breakdown (mechanical) of** other cardiac and vascular devices and implants CC HCC

√7ᵗʰ **T82.519** **Breakdown (mechanical) of** unspecified cardiac and vascular devices and implants CC

√6ᵗʰ **T82.52** **Displacement of** other cardiac and vascular devices and implants
  Malposition of other cardiac and vascular devices and implants

6 √7ᵗʰ **T82.520** **Displacement of** surgically created arteriovenous fistula CC HCC
   AHA: 2020,3Q,36

6 √7ᵗʰ **T82.521** **Displacement of** surgically created arteriovenous shunt CC HCC

√7ᵗʰ **T82.522** **Displacement of** artificial heart CC

6 √7ᵗʰ **T82.523** **Displacement of** balloon (counterpulsation) device CC HCC

6 √7ᵗʰ **T82.524** **Displacement of** infusion catheter CC HCC
   AHA: 2020,2Q,21; 2019,3Q,15

6 √7ᵗʰ **T82.525** **Displacement of** umbrella device CC HCC

6 √7ᵗʰ **T82.528** **Displacement of** other cardiac and vascular devices and implants CC HCC

√7ᵗʰ **T82.529** **Displacement of** unspecified cardiac and vascular devices and implants CC

√6ᵗʰ **T82.53** **Leakage of** other cardiac and vascular devices and implants

6 √7ᵗʰ **T82.530** **Leakage of** surgically created arteriovenous fistula CC HCC
   AHA: 2020,3Q,36

6 √7ᵗʰ **T82.531** **Leakage of** surgically created arteriovenous shunt CC HCC

√7ᵗʰ **T82.532** **Leakage of** artificial heart CC

6 √7ᵗʰ **T82.533** **Leakage of** balloon (counterpulsation) device CC HCC

6 √7ᵗʰ **T82.534** **Leakage of** infusion catheter CC HCC

6 √7ᵗʰ **T82.535** **Leakage of** umbrella device CC HCC

6 √7ᵗʰ **T82.538** **Leakage of** other cardiac and vascular devices and implants CC HCC

√7ᵗʰ **T82.539** **Leakage of** unspecified cardiac and vascular devices and implants CC

√6ᵗʰ **T82.59** **Other mechanical complication of** other cardiac and vascular devices and implants
  Obstruction (mechanical) of other cardiac and vascular devices and implants
  Perforation of other cardiac and vascular devices and implants
  Protrusion of other cardiac and vascular devices and implants

6 √7ᵗʰ **T82.590** **Other mechanical complication of** surgically created arteriovenous fistula CC HCC
   AHA: 2020,3Q,36

6 √7ᵗʰ **T82.591** **Other mechanical complication of** surgically created arteriovenous shunt CC HCC

√7ᵗʰ **T82.592** **Other mechanical complication of** artificial heart CC

6 √7ᵗʰ **T82.593** **Other mechanical complication of** balloon (counterpulsation) device CC HCC

6 √7ᵗʰ **T82.594** **Other mechanical complication of** infusion catheter CC HCC

6 √7ᵗʰ **T82.595** **Other mechanical complication of** umbrella device CC HCC

6 √7ᵗʰ **T82.598** **Other mechanical complication of** other cardiac and vascular devices and implants CC HCC

√7ᵗʰ **T82.599** **Other mechanical complication of** unspecified cardiac and vascular devices and implants CC

6 √x7ᵗʰ **T82.6** **Infection and inflammatory reaction due to cardiac valve prosthesis** CC H13 HCC
  Use additional code to identify infection

6 √x7ᵗʰ **T82.7** **Infection and inflammatory reaction due to other cardiac and vascular devices, implants and grafts** CC H13 HCC
  Use additional code to identify infection
  AHA: 2019,1Q,13-14
  DEF: Midline catheter: Long peripheral catheter introduced via the cephalic, basilic, brachial, or median cubital veins in the upper arm and positioned so that the tip is level or near the level of the axilla and distal to the shoulder. Midline catheters are typically used for IV access, fluid replacement, and medication administration.
  TIP: Assign this code for infections and/or cellulitis resulting from catheters that are not centrally placed (e.g., midline catheters).

√5ᵗʰ **T82.8** **Other specified complications of cardiac and vascular prosthetic devices, implants and grafts**
  AHA: 2016,4Q,70

√6ᵗʰ **T82.81** **Embolism** due to cardiac and vascular prosthetic devices, implants and grafts

√7ᵗʰ **T82.817** **Embolism due to** cardiac prosthetic devices, implants and grafts CC

6 √7ᵗʰ **T82.818** **Embolism due to** vascular prosthetic devices, implants and grafts CC HCC

√6ᵗʰ **T82.82** **Fibrosis** due to cardiac and vascular prosthetic devices, implants and grafts

√7ᵗʰ **T82.827** **Fibrosis due to** cardiac prosthetic devices, implants and grafts CC

6 √7ᵗʰ **T82.828** **Fibrosis due** vascular prosthetic devices, implants and grafts CC HCC

√6ᵗʰ **T82.83** **Hemorrhage** due to cardiac and vascular prosthetic devices, implants and grafts

√7ᵗʰ **T82.837** **Hemorrhage due to** cardiac prosthetic devices, implants and grafts CC

6 √7ᵗʰ **T82.838** **Hemorrhage due to** vascular prosthetic devices, implants and grafts CC HCC
   AHA: 2020,3Q,36-37

√6ᵗʰ **T82.84** **Pain** due to cardiac and vascular prosthetic devices, implants and grafts

√7ᵗʰ **T82.847** **Pain due to** cardiac prosthetic devices, implants and grafts CC

6 √7ᵗʰ **T82.848** **Pain due to** vascular prosthetic devices, implants and grafts CC HCC

√6ᵗʰ **T82.85** **Stenosis** due to cardiac and vascular prosthetic devices, implants and grafts

√7ᵗʰ **T82.855** **Stenosis of** coronary artery stent CC
   In-stent stenosis (restenosis) of coronary artery stent
   Restenosis of coronary artery stent

6 √7ᵗʰ **T82.856** **Stenosis of** peripheral vascular stent CC HCC
   In-stent stenosis (restenosis) of peripheral vascular stent
   Restenosis of peripheral vascular stent

√7ᵗʰ **T82.857** **Stenosis of** other cardiac prosthetic devices, implants and grafts CC

6 √7ᵗʰ **T82.858** **Stenosis of** other vascular prosthetic devices, implants and grafts CC HCC

√6ᵗʰ **T82.86** **Thrombosis** of cardiac and vascular prosthetic devices, implants and grafts

√7ᵗʰ **T82.867** **Thrombosis due to** cardiac prosthetic devices, implants and grafts CC

6 √7ᵗʰ **T82.868** **Thrombosis due to** vascular prosthetic devices, implants and grafts CC HCC

√6ᵗʰ **T82.89** **Other specified complication** of cardiac and vascular prosthetic devices, implants and grafts

√7ᵗʰ **T82.897** **Other specified complication of** cardiac prosthetic devices, implants and grafts CC
   AHA: 2019,2Q,33

6 √7ᵗʰ **T82.898** **Other specified complication of** vascular prosthetic devices, implants and grafts CC HCC
   AHA: 2020,3Q,3-5

√x7ᵗʰ **T82.9** **Unspecified complication of cardiac and vascular prosthetic device, implant and graft** CC

☑4ᵗʰ **T83** **Complications of genitourinary prosthetic devices, implants and grafts**

> **EXCLUDES 2** *failure and rejection of transplanted organs and tissue (T86.-)*

AHA: 2016,4Q,70-71

> The appropriate 7th character is to be added to each code from category T83.
> A   initial encounter
> D   subsequent encounter
> S   sequela

☑5ᵗʰ **T83.0** **Mechanical complication of** urinary catheter

> **EXCLUDES 2** *complications of stoma of urinary tract (N99.5-)*

  ☑6ᵗʰ **T83.01** **Breakdown** (mechanical) **of urinary catheter**

    6 ☑7ᵗʰ **T83.010** **Breakdown** (mechanical) **of** cystostomy **catheter** CC HCC

    6 ☑7ᵗʰ **T83.011** **Breakdown** (mechanical) **of** indwelling urethral **catheter** HCC

    6 ☑7ᵗʰ **T83.012** **Breakdown** (mechanical) **of** nephrostomy **catheter** HCC

    6 ☑7ᵗʰ **T83.018** **Breakdown** (mechanical) **of other urinary catheter** HCC
        Breakdown (mechanical) of Hopkins catheter
        Breakdown (mechanical) of ileostomy catheter
        Breakdown (mechanical) urostomy catheter

  ☑6ᵗʰ **T83.02** **Displacement of urinary catheter**
    Malposition of urinary catheter

    6 ☑7ᵗʰ **T83.020** **Displacement of** cystostomy **catheter** CC HCC

    6 ☑7ᵗʰ **T83.021** **Displacement of** indwelling urethral **catheter** HCC

    6 ☑7ᵗʰ **T83.022** **Displacement of** nephrostomy **catheter** HCC

    6 ☑7ᵗʰ **T83.028** **Displacement of other urinary catheter** HCC
        Displacement of Hopkins catheter
        Displacement of ileostomy catheter
        Displacement of urostomy catheter

  ☑6ᵗʰ **T83.03** **Leakage of urinary catheter**

    6 ☑7ᵗʰ **T83.030** **Leakage of** cystostomy **catheter** CC HCC

    6 ☑7ᵗʰ **T83.031** **Leakage of** indwelling urethral **catheter** HCC

    6 ☑7ᵗʰ **T83.032** **Leakage of** nephrostomy **catheter** HCC

    6 ☑7ᵗʰ **T83.038** **Leakage of other urinary catheter** HCC
        Leakage of Hopkins catheter
        Leakage of ileostomy catheter
        Leakage of urostomy catheter

  ☑6ᵗʰ **T83.09** **Other mechanical complication of urinary catheter**
    Obstruction (mechanical) of urinary catheter
    Perforation of urinary catheter
    Protrusion of urinary catheter

    6 ☑7ᵗʰ **T83.090** **Other mechanical complication of** cystostomy **catheter** CC HCC

    6 ☑7ᵗʰ **T83.091** **Other mechanical complication of** indwelling urethral **catheter** HCC

    6 ☑7ᵗʰ **T83.092** **Other mechanical complication of** nephrostomy **catheter** HCC

    6 ☑7ᵗʰ **T83.098** **Other mechanical complication of other urinary catheter** HCC
        Other mechanical complication of Hopkins catheter
        Other mechanical complication of ileostomy catheter
        Other mechanical complication of urostomy catheter

☑5ᵗʰ **T83.1** **Mechanical complication of other urinary devices and implants**

  ☑6ᵗʰ **T83.11** **Breakdown** (mechanical) **of other urinary devices and implants**

    6 ☑7ᵗʰ **T83.110** **Breakdown** (mechanical) **of urinary electronic stimulator device** CC HCC

> **EXCLUDES 2** *breakdown (mechanical) of electrode (lead) for sacral nerve neurostimulator (T85.111)*
> *breakdown (mechanical) of implanted electronic sacral neurostimulator, pulse generator or receiver (T85.113)*

    6 ☑7ᵗʰ **T83.111** **Breakdown** (mechanical) **of** implanted urinary sphincter CC HCC

    6 ☑7ᵗʰ **T83.112** **Breakdown** (mechanical) **of** indwelling ureteral stent CC HCC

    6 ☑7ᵗʰ **T83.113** **Breakdown** (mechanical) **of other urinary stents** CC HCC
        Breakdown (mechanical) of ileal conduit stent
        Breakdown (mechanical) of nephroureteral stent

    6 ☑7ᵗʰ **T83.118** **Breakdown** (mechanical) **of other urinary devices and implants** CC HCC

  ☑6ᵗʰ **T83.12** **Displacement of other urinary devices and implants**
    Malposition of other urinary devices and implants

    6 ☑7ᵗʰ **T83.120** **Displacement of urinary** electronic stimulator device CC HCC

> **EXCLUDES 2** *displacement of electrode (lead) for sacral nerve neurostimulator (T85.121)*
> *displacement of implanted electronic sacral neurostimulator, pulse generator or receiver (T85.123)*

    6 ☑7ᵗʰ **T83.121** **Displacement of** implanted urinary sphincter CC HCC

    6 ☑7ᵗʰ **T83.122** **Displacement of** indwelling ureteral stent CC HCC

    6 ☑7ᵗʰ **T83.123** **Displacement of other urinary stents** CC HCC
        Displacement of ileal conduit stent
        Displacement of nephroureteral stent

    6 ☑7ᵗʰ **T83.128** **Displacement of other urinary devices and implants** CC HCC

  ☑6ᵗʰ **T83.19** **Other mechanical complication of other urinary devices and implants**
    Leakage of other urinary devices and implants
    Obstruction (mechanical) of other urinary devices and implants
    Perforation of other urinary devices and implants
    Protrusion of other urinary devices and implants

    6 ☑7ᵗʰ **T83.190** **Other mechanical complication of urinary electronic stimulator device** CC HCC

> **EXCLUDES 2** *other mechanical complication of electrode (lead) for sacral nerve neurostimulator (T85.191)*
> *other mechanical complication of implanted electronic sacral neurostimulator, pulse generator or receiver (T85.193)*

    6 ☑7ᵗʰ **T83.191** **Other mechanical complication of** implanted urinary sphincter CC HCC

    6 ☑7ᵗʰ **T83.192** **Other mechanical complication of** indwelling ureteral stent CC HCC

    6 ☑7ᵗʰ **T83.193** **Other mechanical complication of other urinary stent** CC HCC
        Other mechanical complication of ileal conduit stent
        Other mechanical complication of nephroureteral stent

    6 ☑7ᵗʰ **T83.198** **Other mechanical complication of other urinary devices and implants** CC HCC

√5ᵗʰ **T83.2** **Mechanical complication of** graft of urinary organ

6 √x7ᵗʰ **T83.21** Breakdown (mechanical) of graft of urinary organ   `CC` `HCC`

6 √x7ᵗʰ **T83.22** Displacement of graft of urinary organ   `CC` `HCC`
Malposition of graft of urinary organ

6 √x7ᵗʰ **T83.23** Leakage of graft of urinary organ   `CC` `HCC`

6 √x7ᵗʰ **T83.24** Erosion of graft of urinary organ   `CC` `HCC`

6 √x7ᵗʰ **T83.25** Exposure of graft of urinary organ   `CC` `HCC`

6 √x7ᵗʰ **T83.29** Other mechanical complication of graft of urinary organ   `CC` `HCC`
Obstruction (mechanical) of graft of urinary organ
Perforation of graft of urinary organ
Protrusion of graft of urinary organ

√5ᵗʰ **T83.3** **Mechanical complication of** intrauterine contraceptive device

√x7ᵗʰ **T83.31** Breakdown (mechanical) of intrauterine contraceptive device   ♀

√x7ᵗʰ **T83.32** Displacement of intrauterine contraceptive device   ♀
Malposition of intrauterine contraceptive device
Missing string of intrauterine contraceptive device
AHA: 2018,1Q,5

√x7ᵗʰ **T83.39** Other mechanical complication of intrauterine contraceptive device   ♀
Leakage of intrauterine contraceptive device
Obstruction (mechanical) of intrauterine contraceptive device
Perforation of intrauterine contraceptive device
Protrusion of intrauterine contraceptive device

√5ᵗʰ **T83.4** **Mechanical complication of other prosthetic devices, implants and grafts of genital tract**

√6ᵗʰ **T83.41** Breakdown (mechanical) of other prosthetic devices, implants and grafts of genital tract

6 √7ᵗʰ **T83.410** Breakdown (mechanical) of implanted penile prosthesis   `CC` `HCC` ♂
Breakdown (mechanical) of penile prosthesis cylinder
Breakdown (mechanical) of penile prosthesis pump
Breakdown (mechanical) of penile prosthesis reservoir

6 √7ᵗʰ **T83.411** Breakdown (mechanical) of implanted testicular prosthesis   `CC` `HCC`

6 √7ᵗʰ **T83.418** Breakdown (mechanical) of other prosthetic devices, implants and grafts of genital tract   `CC` `HCC`

√6ᵗʰ **T83.42** Displacement of other prosthetic devices, implants and grafts of genital tract
Malposition of other prosthetic devices, implants and grafts of genital tract

6 √7ᵗʰ **T83.420** Displacement of implanted penile prosthesis   `CC` `HCC` ♂
Displacement of penile prosthesis cylinder
Displacement of penile prosthesis pump
Displacement of penile prosthesis reservoir

6 √7ᵗʰ **T83.421** Displacement of implanted testicular prosthesis   `CC` `HCC`

6 √7ᵗʰ **T83.428** Displacement of other prosthetic devices, implants and grafts of genital tract   `CC` `HCC`
AHA: 2018,1Q,5

√6ᵗʰ **T83.49** Other mechanical complication of other prosthetic devices, implants and grafts of genital tract
Leakage of other prosthetic devices, implants and grafts of genital tract
Obstruction, mechanical of other prosthetic devices, implants and grafts of genital tract
Perforation of other prosthetic devices, implants and grafts of genital tract
Protrusion of other prosthetic devices, implants and grafts of genital tract

6 √7ᵗʰ **T83.490** Other mechanical complication of implanted penile prosthesis   `CC` `HCC` ♂
Other mechanical complication of penile prosthesis cylinder
Other mechanical complication of penile prosthesis pump
Other mechanical complication of penile prosthesis reservoir

6 √7ᵗʰ **T83.491** Other mechanical complication of implanted testicular prosthesis   `CC` `HCC`

6 √7ᵗʰ **T83.498** Other mechanical complication of other prosthetic devices, implants and grafts of genital tract   `CC` `HCC`

√5ᵗʰ **T83.5** **Infection and inflammatory reaction due to prosthetic device, implant and graft in** urinary system
Use additional code to identify infection

√6ᵗʰ **T83.51** Infection and inflammatory reaction due to urinary catheter
`EXCLUDES 2`   complications of stoma of urinary tract (N99.5-)
AHA: 2019,3Q,17

6 √7ᵗʰ **T83.510** Infection and inflammatory reaction due to cystostomy catheter   `CC` `HCC`

6 √7ᵗʰ **T83.511** Infection and inflammatory reaction due to indwelling urethral catheter   `CC` `H6` `HCC`

6 √7ᵗʰ **T83.512** Infection and inflammatory reaction due to nephrostomy catheter   `CC` `HCC`

6 √7ᵗʰ **T83.518** Infection and inflammatory reaction due to other urinary catheter   `CC` `H6` `HCC`
Infection and inflammatory reaction due to Hopkins catheter
Infection and inflammatory reaction due to ileostomy catheter
Infection and inflammatory reaction due to urostomy catheter

√6ᵗʰ **T83.59** Infection and inflammatory reaction due to prosthetic device, implant and graft in urinary system

6 √7ᵗʰ **T83.590** Infection and inflammatory reaction due to implanted urinary neurostimulation device   `CC` `HCC`
`EXCLUDES 2`   infection and inflammatory reaction due to electrode lead of sacral nerve neurostimulator (T85.732)
infection and inflammatory reaction due to pulse generator or receiver of sacral nerve neurostimulator (T85.734)

6 √7ᵗʰ **T83.591** Infection and inflammatory reaction due to implanted urinary sphincter   `CC` `HCC`

6 √7ᵗʰ **T83.592** Infection and inflammatory reaction due to indwelling ureteral stent   `CC` `HCC`

6 √7ᵗʰ **T83.593** Infection and inflammatory reaction due to other urinary stents   `CC` `HCC`
Infection and inflammatory reaction due to ileal conduit stents
Infection and inflammatory reaction due to nephroureteral stent

6 √7ᵗʰ **T83.598** Infection and inflammatory reaction due to other prosthetic device, implant and graft in urinary system   `CC` `HCC`
AHA: 2020,3Q,25

√5th T83.6 Infection and inflammatory reaction due to prosthetic device, implant and graft in genital tract
Use additional code to identify infection

  6 **√x7th T83.61 Infection and inflammatory reaction due to implanted penile prosthesis** CC HCC
Infection and inflammatory reaction due to penile prosthesis cylinder
Infection and inflammatory reaction due to penile prosthesis pump
Infection and inflammatory reaction due to penile prosthesis reservoir

  6 **√x7th T83.62 Infection and inflammatory reaction due to implanted testicular prosthesis** CC HCC

  6 **√x7th T83.69 Infection and inflammatory reaction due to other prosthetic device, implant and graft in genital tract** CC HCC

√5th T83.7 Complications due to implanted mesh and other prosthetic materials

  √6th T83.71 Erosion of implanted mesh and other prosthetic materials

    6 **√7th T83.711 Erosion of implanted vaginal mesh to surrounding organ or tissue** HCC ♀
Erosion of implanted vaginal mesh into pelvic floor muscles

    6 **√7th T83.712 Erosion of implanted urethral mesh to surrounding organ or tissue** CC HCC
Erosion of implanted female urethral sling
Erosion of implanted male urethral sling
Erosion of implanted urethral mesh into pelvic floor muscles

    6 **√7th T83.713 Erosion of implanted urethral bulking agent to surrounding organ or tissue** CC HCC

    6 **√7th T83.714 Erosion of implanted ureteral bulking agent to surrounding organ or tissue** CC HCC

    6 **√7th T83.718 Erosion of other implanted mesh to organ or tissue** CC HCC

    6 **√7th T83.719 Erosion of other prosthetic materials to surrounding organ or tissue** CC HCC

  √6th T83.72 Exposure of implanted mesh and other prosthetic materials into surrounding organ or tissue
Extrusion of implanted mesh

    6 **√7th T83.721 Exposure of implanted vaginal mesh into vagina** HCC ♀
Exposure of implanted vaginal mesh through vaginal wall

    6 **√7th T83.722 Exposure of implanted urethral mesh into urethra** CC HCC
Exposure of implanted female urethral sling
Exposure of implanted male urethral sling
Exposure of implanted urethral mesh through urethral wall

    6 **√7th T83.723 Exposure of implanted urethral bulking agent into urethra** CC HCC

    6 **√7th T83.724 Exposure of implanted ureteral bulking agent into ureter** CC HCC

    6 **√7th T83.728 Exposure of other implanted mesh into organ or tissue** CC HCC

    6 **√7th T83.729 Exposure of other prosthetic materials into organ or tissue** CC HCC

  6 **√x7th T83.79 Other specified complications due to other genitourinary prosthetic materials** CC HCC

√5th T83.8 Other specified complications of genitourinary prosthetic devices, implants and grafts

  6 **√x7th T83.81 Embolism due to genitourinary prosthetic devices, implants and grafts** CC HCC

  6 **√x7th T83.82 Fibrosis due to genitourinary prosthetic devices, implants and grafts** CC HCC

  6 **√x7th T83.83 Hemorrhage due to genitourinary prosthetic devices, implants and grafts** CC HCC

  6 **√x7th T83.84 Pain due to genitourinary prosthetic devices, implants and grafts** CC HCC

  6 **√x7th T83.85 Stenosis due to genitourinary prosthetic devices, implants and grafts** CC HCC

  6 **√x7th T83.86 Thrombosis due to genitourinary prosthetic devices, implants and grafts** CC HCC

  6 **√x7th T83.89 Other specified complication of genitourinary prosthetic devices, implants and grafts** CC HCC
AHA: 2016,1Q,19

  6 **√x7th T83.9 Unspecified complication of genitourinary prosthetic device, implant and graft** CC HCC

√4th T84 Complications of internal orthopedic prosthetic devices, implants and grafts
  EXCLUDES 2   failure and rejection of transplanted organs and tissues (T86.-)
       fracture of bone following insertion of orthopedic implant, joint prosthesis or bone plate (M96.6)

The appropriate 7th character is to be added to each code from category T84.
A initial encounter
D subsequent encounter
S sequela

√5th T84.0 Mechanical complication of internal joint prosthesis

  √6th T84.01 Broken internal joint prosthesis
Breakage (fracture) of prosthetic joint
Broken prosthetic joint implant
    EXCLUDES 1   periprosthetic joint implant fracture (M97.-)
    AHA: 2016,4Q,42

    6 **√7th T84.010 Broken internal right hip prosthesis** CC HCC

    6 **√7th T84.011 Broken internal left hip prosthesis** CC HCC

    6 **√7th T84.012 Broken internal right knee prosthesis** CC HCC

    6 **√7th T84.013 Broken internal left knee prosthesis** CC HCC

    6 **√7th T84.018 Broken internal joint prosthesis, other site** CC HCC
Use additional code to identify the joint (Z96.6-)

    6 **√7th T84.019 Broken internal joint prosthesis, unspecified site** CC HCC

  √6th T84.02 Dislocation of internal joint prosthesis
Instability of internal joint prosthesis
Subluxation of internal joint prosthesis
    AHA: 2019,2Q,27

    6 **√7th T84.020 Dislocation of internal right hip prosthesis** CC HCC

    6 **√7th T84.021 Dislocation of internal left hip prosthesis** CC HCC

    6 **√7th T84.022 Instability of internal right knee prosthesis** CC HCC

    6 **√7th T84.023 Instability of internal left knee prosthesis** CC HCC

    6 **√7th T84.028 Dislocation of other internal joint prosthesis** CC HCC
Use additional code to identify the joint (Z96.6-)

    6 **√7th T84.029 Dislocation of unspecified internal joint prosthesis** CC HCC

  √6th T84.03 Mechanical loosening of internal prosthetic joint
Aseptic loosening of prosthetic joint

    6 **√7th T84.030 Mechanical loosening of internal right hip prosthetic joint** CC HCC

    6 **√7th T84.031 Mechanical loosening of internal left hip prosthetic joint** CC HCC

    6 **√7th T84.032 Mechanical loosening of internal right knee prosthetic joint** CC HCC

    6 **√7th T84.033 Mechanical loosening of internal left knee prosthetic joint** CC HCC

    6 **√7th T84.038 Mechanical loosening of other internal prosthetic joint** CC HCC
Use additional code to identify the joint (Z96.6-)

    6 **√7th T84.039 Mechanical loosening of unspecified internal prosthetic joint** CC HCC

  √6th T84.05 Periprosthetic osteolysis of internal prosthetic joint
Use additional code to identify major osseous defect, if applicable (M89.7-)

    6 **√7th T84.050 Periprosthetic osteolysis of internal prosthetic right hip joint** CC HCC

    6 **√7th T84.051 Periprosthetic osteolysis of internal prosthetic left hip joint** CC HCC

6 √7ᵗʰ **T84.052** Periprosthetic osteolysis of internal prosthetic **right knee joint** CC HCC

6 √7ᵗʰ **T84.053** Periprosthetic osteolysis of internal prosthetic **left knee joint** CC HCC

6 √7ᵗʰ **T84.058** Periprosthetic osteolysis of other internal prosthetic joint
Use additional code to identify the joint (Z96.6-)

6 √7ᵗʰ **T84.059** Periprosthetic osteolysis of unspecified internal prosthetic joint CC HCC

√6ᵗʰ **T84.06** Wear of articular bearing surface of internal prosthetic joint

6 √7ᵗʰ **T84.060** Wear of articular bearing surface of internal prosthetic **right hip joint** CC HCC

6 √7ᵗʰ **T84.061** Wear of articular bearing surface of internal prosthetic **left hip joint** CC HCC

6 √7ᵗʰ **T84.062** Wear of articular bearing surface of internal prosthetic **right knee joint** CC HCC

6 √7ᵗʰ **T84.063** Wear of articular bearing surface of internal prosthetic **left knee joint** CC HCC

6 √7ᵗʰ **T84.068** Wear of articular bearing surface of other internal prosthetic joint CC HCC
Use additional code to identify the joint (Z96.6-)

6 √7ᵗʰ **T84.069** Wear of articular bearing surface of unspecified internal prosthetic joint CC HCC

√6ᵗʰ **T84.09** Other mechanical complication of internal joint prosthesis
Prosthetic joint implant failure NOS
AHA: 2019,1Q,20

6 √7ᵗʰ **T84.090** Other mechanical complication of internal **right hip prosthesis** CC HCC

6 √7ᵗʰ **T84.091** Other mechanical complication of internal **left hip prosthesis** CC HCC

6 √7ᵗʰ **T84.092** Other mechanical complication of internal **right knee prosthesis** CC HCC

6 √7ᵗʰ **T84.093** Other mechanical complication of internal **left knee prosthesis** CC HCC

6 √7ᵗʰ **T84.098** Other mechanical complication of other internal joint prosthesis CC HCC
Use additional code to identify the joint (Z96.6-)

6 √7ᵗʰ **T84.099** Other mechanical complication of unspecified internal joint prosthesis CC HCC

√5ᵗʰ **T84.1** Mechanical complication of internal fixation device of bones of limb
EXCLUDES 2   *mechanical complication of internal fixation device of bones of feet (T84.2-)*
mechanical complication of internal fixation device of bones of fingers (T84.2-)
mechanical complication of internal fixation device of bones of hands (T84.2-)
mechanical complication of internal fixation device of bones of toes (T84.2-)

√6ᵗʰ **T84.11** Breakdown (mechanical) of internal fixation device of bones of limb

6 √7ᵗʰ **T84.110** Breakdown (mechanical) of internal fixation device of **right humerus** CC HCC

6 √7ᵗʰ **T84.111** Breakdown (mechanical) of internal fixation device of **left humerus** CC HCC

6 √7ᵗʰ **T84.112** Breakdown (mechanical) of internal fixation device of bone of **right forearm** CC HCC

6 √7ᵗʰ **T84.113** Breakdown (mechanical) of internal fixation device of bone of **left forearm** CC HCC

6 √7ᵗʰ **T84.114** Breakdown (mechanical) of internal fixation device of **right femur** CC HCC

6 √7ᵗʰ **T84.115** Breakdown (mechanical) of internal fixation device of **left femur** CC HCC

6 √7ᵗʰ **T84.116** Breakdown (mechanical) of internal fixation device of bone of **right lower leg** CC HCC

6 √7ᵗʰ **T84.117** Breakdown (mechanical) of internal fixation device of bone of **left lower leg** CC HCC

6 √7ᵗʰ **T84.119** Breakdown (mechanical) of internal fixation device of unspecified bone of limb CC HCC

√6ᵗʰ **T84.12** Displacement of internal fixation device of bones of limb
Malposition of internal fixation device of bones of limb

6 √7ᵗʰ **T84.120** Displacement of internal fixation device of **right humerus** CC HCC

6 √7ᵗʰ **T84.121** Displacement of internal fixation device of **left humerus** CC HCC

6 √7ᵗʰ **T84.122** Displacement of internal fixation device of bone of **right forearm** CC HCC

6 √7ᵗʰ **T84.123** Displacement of internal fixation device of bone of **left forearm** CC HCC

6 √7ᵗʰ **T84.124** Displacement of internal fixation device of **right femur** CC HCC

6 √7ᵗʰ **T84.125** Displacement of internal fixation device of **left femur** CC HCC

6 √7ᵗʰ **T84.126** Displacement of internal fixation device of bone of **right lower leg** CC HCC

6 √7ᵗʰ **T84.127** Displacement of internal fixation device of bone of **left lower leg** CC HCC

6 √7ᵗʰ **T84.129** Displacement of internal fixation device of unspecified bone of limb CC HCC

√6ᵗʰ **T84.19** Other mechanical complication of internal fixation device of bones of limb
Obstruction (mechanical) of internal fixation device of bones of limb
Perforation of internal fixation device of bones of limb
Protrusion of internal fixation device of bones of limb

6 √7ᵗʰ **T84.190** Other mechanical complication of internal fixation device of **right humerus** CC HCC

6 √7ᵗʰ **T84.191** Other mechanical complication of internal fixation device of **left humerus** CC HCC

6 √7ᵗʰ **T84.192** Other mechanical complication of internal fixation device of bone of **right forearm** CC HCC

6 √7ᵗʰ **T84.193** Other mechanical complication of internal fixation device of bone of **left forearm** CC HCC

6 √7ᵗʰ **T84.194** Other mechanical complication of internal fixation device of **right femur** CC HCC

6 √7ᵗʰ **T84.195** Other mechanical complication of internal fixation device of **left femur** CC HCC

6 √7ᵗʰ **T84.196** Other mechanical complication of internal fixation device of bone of **right lower leg** CC HCC

6 √7ᵗʰ **T84.197** Other mechanical complication of internal fixation device of bone of **left lower leg** CC HCC

6 √7ᵗʰ **T84.199** Other mechanical complication of internal fixation device of unspecified bone of limb CC HCC

√5ᵗʰ **T84.2** Mechanical complication of internal fixation device of other bones

√6ᵗʰ **T84.21** Breakdown (mechanical) of internal fixation device of other bones

6 √7ᵗʰ **T84.210** Breakdown (mechanical) of internal fixation device of bones of **hand and fingers** CC HCC

6 √7ᵗʰ **T84.213** Breakdown (mechanical) of internal fixation device of bones of **foot and toes** CC HCC

6 √7ᵗʰ **T84.216** Breakdown (mechanical) of internal fixation device of **vertebrae** CC HCC

6 √7ᵗʰ **T84.218** Breakdown (mechanical) of internal fixation device of other bones CC HCC

√6ᵗʰ **T84.22** Displacement of internal fixation device of other bones
Malposition of internal fixation device of other bones

6 √7ᵗʰ **T84.220** Displacement of internal fixation device of bones of **hand and fingers** CC HCC

6 √7ᵗʰ **T84.223** Displacement of internal fixation device of bones of **foot and toes** CC HCC

✓ Additional Character Required   √x7ᵗʰ Placeholder   Questionable PDx   Manifestation   Unspecified Dx   UPD Unacceptable PDx   H1-H4 HAC   HCC CMS-HCC Dx   HIV HIV Dx

6 ✓7ᵗʰ **T84.226** **Displacement of internal fixation device of** vertebrae   cc HCC

6 ✓7ᵗʰ **T84.228** **Displacement of internal fixation device of other bones**   cc HCC

✓6ᵗʰ **T84.29** **Other mechanical complication of internal fixation device of other bones**

Obstruction (mechanical) of internal fixation device of other bones

Perforation of internal fixation device of other bones

Protrusion of internal fixation device of other bones

6 ✓7ᵗʰ **T84.290** **Other mechanical complication of internal fixation device of bones of** hand and fingers   cc HCC

6 ✓7ᵗʰ **T84.293** **Other mechanical complication of internal fixation device of bones of** foot and toes   cc HCC

6 ✓7ᵗʰ **T84.296** **Other mechanical complication of internal fixation device of** vertebrae   cc HCC

6 ✓7ᵗʰ **T84.298** **Other mechanical complication of internal fixation device of other bones**   cc HCC

✓5ᵗʰ **T84.3** **Mechanical complication of other bone devices, implants and grafts**

EXCLUDES 2   other complications of bone graft (T86.83-)

✓6ᵗʰ **T84.31** **Breakdown (mechanical) of other bone devices, implants and grafts**

6 ✓7ᵗʰ **T84.310** **Breakdown (mechanical) of** electronic bone stimulator   cc HCC

6 ✓7ᵗʰ **T84.318** **Breakdown (mechanical) of other bone devices, implants and grafts**   cc HCC

✓6ᵗʰ **T84.32** **Displacement of other bone devices, implants and grafts**

Malposition of other bone devices, implants and grafts

6 ✓7ᵗʰ **T84.320** **Displacement of** electronic bone stimulator   cc HCC

6 ✓7ᵗʰ **T84.328** **Displacement of other bone devices, implants and grafts**   cc HCC

AHA: 2014,4Q,28

✓6ᵗʰ **T84.39** **Other mechanical complication of other bone devices, implants and grafts**

Obstruction (mechanical) of other bone devices, implants and grafts

Perforation of other bone devices, implants and grafts

Protrusion of other bone devices, implants and grafts

6 ✓7ᵗʰ **T84.390** **Other mechanical complication of** electronic bone stimulator   cc HCC

6 ✓7ᵗʰ **T84.398** **Other mechanical complication of other bone devices, implants and grafts**   cc HCC

✓5ᵗʰ **T84.4** **Mechanical complication of other internal orthopedic devices, implants and grafts**

✓6ᵗʰ **T84.41** **Breakdown (mechanical) of other internal orthopedic devices, implants and grafts**

6 ✓7ᵗʰ **T84.410** **Breakdown (mechanical) of** muscle and tendon graft   cc HCC

6 ✓7ᵗʰ **T84.418** **Breakdown (mechanical) of other internal orthopedic devices, implants and grafts**   cc HCC

✓6ᵗʰ **T84.42** **Displacement of other internal orthopedic devices, implants and grafts**

Malposition of other internal orthopedic devices, implants and grafts

6 ✓7ᵗʰ **T84.420** **Displacement of** muscle and tendon graft   cc HCC

6 ✓7ᵗʰ **T84.428** **Displacement of other internal orthopedic devices, implants and grafts**   cc HCC

✓6ᵗʰ **T84.49** **Other mechanical complication of other internal orthopedic devices, implants and grafts**

Mechanical complication of other internal orthopedic devices, implants and grafts NOS

Obstruction (mechanical) of other internal orthopedic devices, implants and grafts

Perforation of other internal orthopedic devices, implants and grafts

Protrusion of other internal orthopedic devices, implants and grafts

6 ✓7ᵗʰ **T84.490** **Other mechanical complication of** muscle and tendon graft   cc HCC

6 ✓7ᵗʰ **T84.498** **Other mechanical complication of other internal orthopedic devices, implants and grafts**   cc HCC

✓5ᵗʰ **T84.5** **Infection and inflammatory reaction due to** internal joint prosthesis

Use additional code to identify infection

AHA: 2019,3Q,16; 2015,1Q,16

6 ✓x7ᵗʰ **T84.50** **Infection and inflammatory reaction due to unspecified internal joint prosthesis**   cc HCC

6 ✓x7ᵗʰ **T84.51** **Infection and inflammatory reaction due to internal** right hip **prosthesis**   cc HCC

6 ✓x7ᵗʰ **T84.52** **Infection and inflammatory reaction due to internal** left hip **prosthesis**   cc HCC

6 ✓x7ᵗʰ **T84.53** **Infection and inflammatory reaction due to internal** right knee **prosthesis**   cc HCC

6 ✓x7ᵗʰ **T84.54** **Infection and inflammatory reaction due to internal** left knee **prosthesis**   cc HCC

6 ✓x7ᵗʰ **T84.59** **Infection and inflammatory reaction due to other internal joint prosthesis**   cc HCC

✓5ᵗʰ **T84.6** **Infection and inflammatory reaction due to** internal fixation device

Use additional code to identify infection

6 ✓x7ᵗʰ **T84.60** **Infection and inflammatory reaction due to internal fixation device of unspecified site**   cc H12 HCC

✓6ᵗʰ **T84.61** **Infection and inflammatory reaction due to internal fixation device of** arm

6 ✓7ᵗʰ **T84.610** **Infection and inflammatory reaction due to internal fixation device of** right humerus   cc H12 HCC

6 ✓7ᵗʰ **T84.611** **Infection and inflammatory reaction due to internal fixation device of** left humerus   cc H12 HCC

6 ✓7ᵗʰ **T84.612** **Infection and inflammatory reaction due to internal fixation device of** right radius   cc H12 HCC

6 ✓7ᵗʰ **T84.613** **Infection and inflammatory reaction due to internal fixation device of** left radius   cc H12 HCC

6 ✓7ᵗʰ **T84.614** **Infection and inflammatory reaction due to internal fixation device of** right ulna   cc H12 HCC

6 ✓7ᵗʰ **T84.615** **Infection and inflammatory reaction due to internal fixation device of** left ulna   cc H12 HCC

6 ✓7ᵗʰ **T84.619** **Infection and inflammatory reaction due to internal fixation device of unspecified bone of arm**   cc H12 HCC

✓6ᵗʰ **T84.62** **Infection and inflammatory reaction due to internal fixation device of** leg

6 ✓7ᵗʰ **T84.620** **Infection and inflammatory reaction due to internal fixation device of** right femur   cc HCC

6 ✓7ᵗʰ **T84.621** **Infection and inflammatory reaction due to internal fixation device of** left femur   cc HCC

6 ✓7ᵗʰ **T84.622** **Infection and inflammatory reaction due to internal fixation device of** right tibia   cc HCC

6 ✓7ᵗʰ **T84.623** **Infection and inflammatory reaction due to internal fixation device of** left tibia   cc HCC

6 ✓7ᵗʰ **T84.624** **Infection and inflammatory reaction due to internal fixation device of** right fibula   cc HCC

6 ✓7ᵗʰ **T84.625** **Infection and inflammatory reaction due to internal fixation device of** left fibula   cc HCC

6 ✓7ᵗʰ **T84.629** **Infection and inflammatory reaction due to internal fixation device of unspecified bone of leg**   cc HCC

6 ✓x7ᵗʰ **T84.63** **Infection and inflammatory reaction due to internal fixation device of** spine   cc H12 HCC

6 ✓x7ᵗʰ **T84.69** **Infection and inflammatory reaction due to internal fixation device of other site**   cc H12 HCC

6 ✓x7ᵗʰ **T84.7** **Infection and inflammatory reaction due to other internal orthopedic prosthetic devices, implants and grafts**   cc H12 HCC

Use additional code to identify infection

✓5ᵗʰ **T84.8** **Other specified complications of internal orthopedic prosthetic devices, implants and grafts**

6 ✓x7ᵗʰ **T84.81** **Embolism due to internal orthopedic prosthetic devices, implants and grafts**   cc HCC

N Newborn: 0   P Pediatric: 0-17   M Maternity: 9-64   A Adult: 15-124   MCC Major Complication/Comorbidity   CC Complication/Comorbidity   SW Severe Wound Dx

1160   ICD-10-CM 2022

6 √x7th **T84.82** Fibrosis due to internal orthopedic prosthetic devices, implants and grafts `CC` `HCC`

6 √x7th **T84.83** Hemorrhage due to internal orthopedic prosthetic devices, implants and grafts `CC` `HCC`

6 √x7th **T84.84** Pain due to internal orthopedic prosthetic devices, implants and grafts `CC` `HCC`

6 √x7th **T84.85** Stenosis due to internal orthopedic prosthetic devices, implants and grafts `CC` `HCC`

6 √x7th **T84.86** Thrombosis due to internal orthopedic prosthetic devices, implants and grafts `CC` `HCC`

6 √x7th **T84.89** Other specified complication of internal orthopedic prosthetic devices, implants and grafts `CC` `HCC`

6 √x7th **T84.9** Unspecified complication of internal orthopedic prosthetic device, implant and graft `CC` `HCC`

√4th **T85 Complications of other internal prosthetic devices, implants and grafts**

> **EXCLUDES 2**   failure and rejection of transplanted organs and tissue (T86.-)

AHA: 2016,4Q,71-72

> The appropriate 7th character is to be added to each code from category T85.
> A   initial encounter
> D   subsequent encounter
> S   sequela

√5th **T85.0 Mechanical complication of** ventricular intracranial (communicating) shunt

6 √x7th **T85.01** Breakdown (mechanical) of ventricular intracranial (communicating) shunt `CC` `HCC`

6 √x7th **T85.02** Displacement of ventricular intracranial (communicating) shunt `CC` `HCC`
Malposition of ventricular intracranial (communicating) shunt

6 √x7th **T85.03** Leakage of ventricular intracranial (communicating) shunt `CC` `HCC`

6 √x7th **T85.09** Other mechanical complication of ventricular intracranial (communicating) shunt `CC` `HCC`
Obstruction (mechanical) of ventricular intracranial (communicating) shunt
Perforation of ventricular intracranial (communicating) shunt
Protrusion of ventricular intracranial (communicating) shunt

√5th **T85.1 Mechanical complication of** implanted electronic stimulator of nervous system

√6th **T85.11** Breakdown (mechanical) of implanted electronic stimulator of nervous system

6 √7th **T85.110** Breakdown (mechanical) of implanted electronic neurostimulator of brain electrode (lead) `CC` `HCC`

6 √7th **T85.111** Breakdown (mechanical) of implanted electronic neurostimulator of peripheral nerve electrode (lead) `CC` `HCC`
Breakdown of electrode (lead) for cranial nerve neurostimulators
Breakdown of electrode (lead) for gastric neurostimulator
Breakdown of electrode (lead) for sacral nerve neurostimulator
Breakdown of electrode (lead) for vagal nerve neurostimulators

6 √7th **T85.112** Breakdown (mechanical) of implanted electronic neurostimulator of spinal cord electrode (lead) `CC` `HCC`

6 √7th **T85.113** Breakdown (mechanical) of implanted electronic neurostimulator, generator `CC` `HCC`
Breakdown (mechanical) of implanted electronic neurostimulator generator, brain, peripheral, gastric, spinal
Breakdown (mechanical) of implanted electronic sacral neurostimulator, pulse generator or receiver

6 √7th **T85.118** Breakdown (mechanical) of other implanted electronic stimulator of nervous system `CC` `HCC`

√6th **T85.12** Displacement of implanted electronic stimulator of nervous system
Malposition of implanted electronic stimulator of nervous system

6 √7th **T85.120** Displacement of implanted electronic neurostimulator of brain electrode (lead) `CC` `HCC`

6 √7th **T85.121** Displacement of implanted electronic neurostimulator of peripheral nerve electrode (lead) `CC` `HCC`
Displacement of electrode (lead) for cranial nerve neurostimulators
Displacement of electrode (lead) for gastric neurostimulator
Displacement of electrode (lead) for sacral nerve neurostimulator
Displacement of electrode (lead) for vagal nerve neurostimulators

6 √7th **T85.122** Displacement of implanted electronic neurostimulator of spinal cord electrode (lead) `CC` `HCC`

6 √7th **T85.123** Displacement of implanted electronic neurostimulator, generator `CC` `HCC`
Displacement of implanted electronic neurostimulator generator, brain, peripheral, gastric, spinal
Displacement of implanted electronic sacral neurostimulator, pulse generator or receiver

6 √7th **T85.128** Displacement of other implanted electronic stimulator of nervous system `CC` `HCC`

√6th **T85.19** Other mechanical complication of implanted electronic stimulator of nervous system
Leakage of implanted electronic stimulator of nervous system
Obstruction (mechanical) of implanted electronic stimulator of nervous system
Perforation of implanted electronic stimulator of nervous system
Protrusion of implanted electronic stimulator of nervous system

6 √7th **T85.190** Other mechanical complication of implanted electronic neurostimulator of brain electrode (lead) `CC` `HCC`

6 √7th **T85.191** Other mechanical complication of implanted electronic neurostimulator of peripheral nerve electrode (lead) `CC` `HCC`
Other mechanical complication of electrode (lead) for cranial nerve neurostimulators
Other mechanical complication of electrode (lead) for gastric neurostimulator
Other mechanical complication of electrode (lead) for sacral nerve neurostimulator
Other mechanical complication of electrode (lead) for vagal nerve neurostimulators

6 √7th **T85.192** Other mechanical complication of implanted electronic neurostimulator of spinal cord electrode (lead) `CC` `HCC`

6 √7th **T85.193** Other mechanical complication of implanted electronic neurostimulator, generator `CC` `HCC`
Other mechanical complication of implanted electronic neurostimulator generator, brain, peripheral, gastric, spinal
Other mechanical complication of implanted electronic sacral neurostimulator, pulse generator or receiver

6 √7th **T85.199** Other mechanical complication of other implanted electronic stimulator of nervous system `CC` `HCC`

√6th **T85.2 Mechanical complication of** intraocular lens

√x7th **T85.21** Breakdown (mechanical) of intraocular lens `CC`

☑ Additional Character Required   √x7th Placeholder   Questionable PDx   Manifestation   Unspecified Dx   `UPD` Unacceptable PDx   `H1`-`H14` HAC   `HCC` CMS-HCC Dx   `HIV` HIV Dx

ICD-10-CM 2022   1161

√x 7ᵗʰ **T85.22** Displacement of intraocular lens   CC
: Malposition of intraocular lens

√x 7ᵗʰ **T85.29** **Other mechanical complication of intraocular lens**   CC
: Obstruction (mechanical) of intraocular lens
: Perforation of intraocular lens
: Protrusion of intraocular lens

√5ᵗʰ **T85.3** **Mechanical complication of other ocular prosthetic devices, implants and grafts**
: EXCLUDES 2   other complications of corneal graft (T86.84-)

√6ᵗʰ **T85.31** Breakdown (mechanical) of other ocular prosthetic devices, implants and grafts

√7ᵗʰ **T85.310** **Breakdown (mechanical) of prosthetic orbit of right eye**   CC

√7ᵗʰ **T85.311** **Breakdown (mechanical) of prosthetic orbit of left eye**   CC

√7ᵗʰ **T85.318** **Breakdown (mechanical) of other ocular prosthetic devices, implants and grafts**

√6ᵗʰ **T85.32** Displacement of other ocular prosthetic devices, implants and grafts
: Malposition of other ocular prosthetic devices, implants and grafts

√7ᵗʰ **T85.320** **Displacement of prosthetic orbit of right eye**   CC

√7ᵗʰ **T85.321** **Displacement of prosthetic orbit of left eye**   CC

√7ᵗʰ **T85.328** **Displacement of other ocular prosthetic devices, implants and grafts**

√6ᵗʰ **T85.39** **Other mechanical complication of other ocular prosthetic devices, implants and grafts**
: Obstruction (mechanical) of other ocular prosthetic devices, implants and grafts
: Perforation of other ocular prosthetic devices, implants and grafts
: Protrusion of other ocular prosthetic devices, implants and grafts

√7ᵗʰ **T85.390** **Other mechanical complication of prosthetic orbit of right eye**   CC

√7ᵗʰ **T85.391** **Other mechanical complication of prosthetic orbit of left eye**   CC

√7ᵗʰ **T85.398** **Other mechanical complication of other ocular prosthetic devices, implants and grafts**

√5ᵗʰ **T85.4** **Mechanical complication of breast prosthesis and implant**

√x 7ᵗʰ **T85.41** Breakdown (mechanical) of breast prosthesis and implant   CC

√x 7ᵗʰ **T85.42** Displacement of breast prosthesis and implant   CC
: Malposition of breast prosthesis and implant

√x 7ᵗʰ **T85.43** Leakage of breast prosthesis and implant   CC

√x 7ᵗʰ **T85.44** Capsular contracture of breast implant   CC

√x 7ᵗʰ **T85.49** **Other mechanical complication of breast prosthesis and implant**   CC
: Obstruction (mechanical) of breast prosthesis and implant
: Perforation of breast prosthesis and implant
: Protrusion of breast prosthesis and implant

√5ᵗʰ **T85.5** **Mechanical complication of gastrointestinal prosthetic devices, implants and grafts**

√6ᵗʰ **T85.51** Breakdown (mechanical) of gastrointestinal prosthetic devices, implants and grafts

√7ᵗʰ **T85.510** **Breakdown (mechanical) of bile duct prosthesis**   CC

√7ᵗʰ **T85.511** **Breakdown (mechanical) of esophageal anti-reflux device**   CC

√7ᵗʰ **T85.518** **Breakdown (mechanical) of other gastrointestinal prosthetic devices, implants and grafts**   CC

√6ᵗʰ **T85.52** Displacement of gastrointestinal prosthetic devices, implants and grafts
: Malposition of gastrointestinal prosthetic devices, implants and grafts

√7ᵗʰ **T85.520** **Displacement of bile duct prosthesis**   CC

√7ᵗʰ **T85.521** **Displacement of esophageal anti-reflux device**   CC

√7ᵗʰ **T85.528** **Displacement of other gastrointestinal prosthetic devices, implants and grafts**   CC

√6ᵗʰ **T85.59** **Other mechanical complication of gastrointestinal prosthetic devices, implants and**
: Obstruction, mechanical of gastrointestinal prosthetic devices, implants and grafts
: Perforation of gastrointestinal prosthetic devices, implants and grafts
: Protrusion of gastrointestinal prosthetic devices, implants and grafts

√7ᵗʰ **T85.590** **Other mechanical complication of bile duct prosthesis**   CC

√7ᵗʰ **T85.591** **Other mechanical complication of esophageal anti-reflux device**   CC

√7ᵗʰ **T85.598** **Other mechanical complication of other gastrointestinal prosthetic devices, implants and grafts**   CC

√5ᵗʰ **T85.6** **Mechanical complication of other specified internal and external prosthetic devices, implants and grafts**

√6ᵗʰ **T85.61** Breakdown (mechanical) of other specified internal prosthetic devices, implants and grafts

√7ᵗʰ **T85.610** **Breakdown (mechanical) of cranial or spinal infusion catheter**   CC
: Breakdown (mechanical) of epidural infusion catheter
: Breakdown (mechanical) of intrathecal infusion catheter
: Breakdown (mechanical) of subarachnoid infusion catheter
: Breakdown (mechanical) of subdural infusion catheter

√7ᵗʰ **T85.611** **Breakdown (mechanical) of intraperitoneal dialysis catheter**   CC HCC
: EXCLUDES 1   mechanical complication of vascular dialysis catheter (T82.4-)

√7ᵗʰ **T85.612** **Breakdown (mechanical) of permanent sutures**   CC
: EXCLUDES 1   mechanical complication of permanent (wire) suture used in bone repair (T84.1-T84.2)

√7ᵗʰ **T85.613** **Breakdown (mechanical) of artificial skin graft and decellularized allodermis**   CC
: Failure of artificial skin graft and decellularized allodermis
: Non-adherence of artificial skin graft and decellularized allodermis
: Poor incorporation of artificial skin graft and decellularized allodermis
: Shearing of artificial skin graft and decellularized allodermis

√7ᵗʰ **T85.614** **Breakdown (mechanical) of insulin pump**   CC

6 √7ᵗʰ **T85.615** **Breakdown (mechanical) of other nervous system device, implant or graft**   CC MCC
: Breakdown (mechanical) of intrathecal infusion pump

√7ᵗʰ **T85.618** **Breakdown (mechanical) of other specified internal prosthetic devices, implants and grafts**   CC

√6ᵗʰ **T85.62** Displacement of other specified internal prosthetic devices, implants and grafts
: Malposition of other specified internal prosthetic devices, implants and grafts

√7ᵗʰ **T85.620** **Displacement of cranial or spinal infusion catheter**   CC
: Displacement of epidural infusion catheter
: Displacement of intrathecal infusion catheter
: Displacement of subarachnoid infusion catheter
: Displacement of subdural infusion catheter

√7ᵗʰ **T85.621** **Displacement of intraperitoneal dialysis catheter**   CC HCC
: EXCLUDES 1   mechanical complication of vascular dialysis catheter (T82.4-)

N Newborn: 0   P Pediatric: 0-17   M Maternity: 9-64   A Adult: 15-124   MCC Major Complication/Comorbidity   CC Complication/Comorbidity   SW Severe Wound Dx

1162   ICD-10-CM 2022

√7ᵗʰ **T85.622 Displacement of** permanent
sutures `CC`
> *EXCLUDES 1* *mechanical complication of permanent (wire) suture used in bone repair (T84.1-T84.2)*

√7ᵗʰ **T85.623 Displacement of** artificial skin graft and
decellularized allodermis `CC`
> Dislodgement of artificial skin graft and decellularized allodermis

√7ᵗʰ **T85.624 Displacement of** insulin pump `CC`

6 √7ᵗʰ **T85.625 Displacement of** other nervous system
device, implant or graft `CC` `HCC`
> Displacement of intrathecal infusion pump

√7ᵗʰ **T85.628 Displacement of other specified internal
prosthetic devices, implants and
grafts** `CC`

√6ᵗʰ **T85.63 Leakage** of other specified internal prosthetic
devices, implants and grafts

√7ᵗʰ **T85.630 Leakage of** cranial or spinal infusion
catheter `CC`
> Leakage of epidural infusion catheter
> Leakage of intrathecal infusion catheter infusion catheter
> Leakage of subdural infusion catheter
> Leakage of subarachnoid infusion catheter

√7ᵗʰ **T85.631 Leakage of** intraperitoneal dialysis
catheter `CC` `HCC`
> *EXCLUDES 1* *mechanical complication of vascular dialysis catheter (T82.4)*

√7ᵗʰ **T85.633 Leakage of** insulin pump `CC`

6 √7ᵗʰ **T85.635 Leakage of other nervous system device,
implant or graft** `CC` `HCC`
> Leakage of intrathecal infusion pump

√7ᵗʰ **T85.638 Leakage of other specified internal
prosthetic devices, implants and
grafts** `CC`

√6ᵗʰ **T85.69 Other mechanical complication of other specified
internal prosthetic devices, implants and grafts**
> Obstruction, mechanical of other specified internal prosthetic devices, implants and grafts
> Perforation of other specified internal prosthetic devices, implants and grafts
> Protrusion of other specified internal prosthetic devices, implants and grafts

√7ᵗʰ **T85.690 Other mechanical complication of** cranial
or spinal infusion catheter `CC`
> Other mechanical complication of epidural infusion catheter
> Other mechanical complication of intrathecal infusion catheter
> Other mechanical complication of subarachnoid infusion catheter
> Other mechanical complication of subdural infusion catheter

√7ᵗʰ **T85.691 Other mechanical complication of**
intraperitoneal dialysis
catheter `CC` `HCC`
> *EXCLUDES 1* *mechanical complication of vascular dialysis catheter (T82.4)*

√7ᵗʰ **T85.692 Other mechanical complication of**
permanent sutures `CC`
> *EXCLUDES 1* *mechanical complication of permanent (wire) suture used in bone repair (T84.1-T84.2)*

√7ᵗʰ **T85.693 Other mechanical complication of**
artificial skin graft and decellularized
allodermis `CC`

√7ᵗʰ **T85.694 Other mechanical complication of** insulin
pump `CC`

6 √7ᵗʰ **T85.695 Other mechanical complication of other
nervous system device, implant or
graft** `CC` `HCC`
> Other mechanical complication of intrathecal infusion pump

√7ᵗʰ **T85.698 Other mechanical complication of other
specified internal prosthetic devices,
implants and grafts** `CC`
> Mechanical complication of nonabsorbable surgical material NOS

√5ᵗʰ **T85.7 Infection and inflammatory reaction** due to other internal
prosthetic devices, implants and grafts
> Use additional code to identify infection

√x7ᵗʰ **T85.71 Infection and inflammatory reaction due to**
peritoneal dialysis catheter `CC` `HCC`

6 √x7ᵗʰ **T85.72 Infection and inflammatory reaction due to** insulin
pump `CC` `HCC`

√6ᵗʰ **T85.73 Infection and inflammatory reaction due to** nervous
system **devices, implants and graft**

6 √7ᵗʰ **T85.730 Infection and inflammatory reaction due
to** ventricular intracranial
(communicating) shunt `CC` `HCC`

6 √7ᵗʰ **T85.731 Infection and inflammatory reaction due
to implanted electronic neurostimulator
of** brain, electrode (lead) `CC` `HCC`

6 √7ᵗʰ **T85.732 Infection and inflammatory reaction due
to implanted electronic neurostimulator
of** peripheral nerve, electrode
(lead) `CC` `HCC`
> Infection and inflammatory reaction due to electrode (lead) for cranial nerve neurostimulators
> Infection and inflammatory reaction due to electrode (lead) for gastric neurostimulator
> Infection and inflammatory reaction due to electrode (lead) for sacral nerve neurostimulator
> Infection and inflammatory reaction due to electrode (lead) for vagal nerve neurostimulators

6 √7ᵗʰ **T85.733 Infection and inflammatory reaction due
to implanted electronic neurostimulator
of** spinal cord, electrode (lead) `CC` `HCC`

6 √7ᵗʰ **T85.734 Infection and inflammatory reaction due
to implanted electronic neurostimulator,
generator** `CC` `HCC`
> Generator pocket infection

6 √7ᵗʰ **T85.735 Infection and inflammatory reaction due
to** cranial or spinal infusion
catheter `CC` `HCC`
> Infection and inflammatory reaction due to epidural catheter
> Infection and inflammatory reaction due to intrathecal infusion catheter
> Infection and inflammatory reaction due to subarachnoid catheter
> Infection and inflammatory reaction due to subdural catheter

6 √7ᵗʰ **T85.738 Infection and inflammatory reaction due
to other nervous system device, implant
or graft** `CC` `HCC`
> Infection and inflammatory reaction due to intrathecal infusion pump

6 √x7ᵗʰ **T85.79 Infection and inflammatory reaction due to other
internal prosthetic devices, implants and
grafts** `CC` `HCC`

√5ᵗʰ **T85.8 Other specified complications of internal prosthetic devices,
implants and grafts, not elsewhere classified**

√6ᵗʰ **T85.81 Embolism** due to internal prosthetic devices,
implants and grafts, not elsewhere classified

5,6 √7ᵗʰ **T85.810 Embolism due to** nervous system
**prosthetic devices, implants and
grafts** `CC` `HCC`

√7ᵗʰ **T85.818 Embolism due to other** internal prosthetic
devices, implants and grafts

√6ᵗʰ **T85.82 Fibrosis** due to internal prosthetic devices, implants
and grafts, not elsewhere classified

5,6 √7ᵗʰ **T85.820 Fibrosis due to** nervous system prosthetic
devices, implants and grafts `CC` `HCC`

√7ᵗʰ **T85.828 Fibrosis due to other** internal prosthetic
devices, implants and grafts

☑ Additional Character Required   √x7ᵗʰ Placeholder   Questionable PDx   *Manifestation*   Unspecified Dx   `UPD` Unacceptable PDx   `H1`-`H14` HAC   `HCC` CMS-HCC Dx   `HIV` HIV Dx

ICD-10-CM 2022   **1163**

Chapter 19. Injury, Poisoning and Certain Other Consequences of External Causes

T85.83–T86.8403

√6ᵗʰ **T85.83 Hemorrhage due to internal prosthetic devices, implants and grafts, not elsewhere classified**

     5,6 √7ᵗʰ **T85.830 Hemorrhage due to nervous system prosthetic devices, implants and grafts** `CC` `HCC`

     √7ᵗʰ **T85.838 Hemorrhage due to other internal prosthetic devices, implants and grafts**

√6ᵗʰ **T85.84 Pain due to internal prosthetic devices, implants and grafts, not elsewhere classified**

     5,6 √7ᵗʰ **T85.840 Pain due to nervous system prosthetic devices, implants and grafts** `CC` `HCC`

     √7ᵗʰ **T85.848 Pain due to other internal prosthetic devices, implants and grafts**

√6ᵗʰ **T85.85 Stenosis due to internal prosthetic devices, implants and grafts, not elsewhere classified**

     5,6 √7ᵗʰ **T85.850 Stenosis due to nervous system prosthetic devices, implants and grafts** `CC` `HCC`

     √7ᵗʰ **T85.858 Stenosis due to other internal prosthetic devices, implants and grafts**

√6ᵗʰ **T85.86 Thrombosis due to internal prosthetic devices, implants and grafts, not elsewhere classified**

     5,6 √7ᵗʰ **T85.860 Thrombosis due to nervous system prosthetic devices, implants and grafts** `CC` `HCC`

     √7ᵗʰ **T85.868 Thrombosis due to other internal prosthetic devices, implants and grafts**

√6ᵗʰ **T85.89 Other specified complication of internal prosthetic devices, implants and grafts, not elsewhere classified**

     Erosion or breakdown of subcutaneous device pocket

     5,6 √7ᵗʰ **T85.890 Other specified complication of nervous system prosthetic devices, implants and grafts** `CC` `HCC`

     √7ᵗʰ **T85.898 Other specified complication of other internal prosthetic devices, implants and grafts**

√x7ᵗʰ **T85.9 Unspecified complication of internal prosthetic device, implant and graft**

     Complication of internal prosthetic device, implant and graft NOS

√4ᵗʰ **T86 Complications of transplanted organs and tissue**

Use additional code to identify other transplant complications, such as:
graft-versus-host disease (D89.81-)
malignancy associated with organ transplant (C80.2)
post-transplant lymphoproliferative disorders (PTLD) (D47.Z1)
AHA: 2020,1Q,18

√5ᵗʰ **T86.0 Complications of bone marrow transplant**

     T86.00 Unspecified complication of bone marrow transplant `CC` `HCC`

     T86.01 Bone marrow transplant rejection `CC` `HCC`

     T86.02 Bone marrow transplant failure `CC` `HCC`

     T86.03 Bone marrow transplant infection `CC` `HCC`

     T86.09 Other complications of bone marrow transplant `CC` `HCC`

√5ᵗʰ **T86.1 Complications of kidney transplant**

     T86.10 Unspecified complication of kidney transplant `CC`

     T86.11 Kidney transplant rejection `CC`

     T86.12 Kidney transplant failure `CC`
         AHA: 2013,1Q,24

     T86.13 Kidney transplant infection `CC`
         Use additional code to specify infection

     T86.19 Other complication of kidney transplant `CC`
         AHA: 2019,2Q,7

√5ᵗʰ **T86.2 Complications of heart transplant**

     EXCLUDES 1   complication of:
         artificial heart device ►(T82.5-)◄
         heart-lung transplant ►(T86.3-)◄

     T86.20 Unspecified complication of heart transplant `CC` `HCC`

     T86.21 Heart transplant rejection `CC` `HCC`

     T86.22 Heart transplant failure `CC` `HCC`

     T86.23 Heart transplant infection `CC` `HCC`
         Use additional code to specify infection

√6ᵗʰ **T86.29 Other complications of heart transplant**

     T86.290 Cardiac allograft vasculopathy `CC` `HCC`
         EXCLUDES 1   atherosclerosis of coronary arteries (I25.75-, I25.76-, I25.81-)

     T86.298 Other complications of heart transplant `CC` `HCC`

√5ᵗʰ **T86.3 Complications of heart-lung transplant**

     T86.30 Unspecified complication of heart-lung transplant `CC` `HCC`

     T86.31 Heart-lung transplant rejection `CC` `HCC`

     T86.32 Heart-lung transplant failure `CC` `HCC`

     T86.33 Heart-lung transplant infection `CC` `HCC`
         Use additional code to specify infection

     T86.39 Other complications of heart-lung transplant `CC` `HCC`

√5ᵗʰ **T86.4 Complications of liver transplant**

     T86.40 Unspecified complication of liver transplant `CC` `HCC`

     T86.41 Liver transplant rejection `CC` `HCC`

     T86.42 Liver transplant failure `CC` `HCC`

     T86.43 Liver transplant infection `CC` `HCC`
         Use additional code to identify infection, such as:
         cytomegalovirus (CMV) infection (B25.-)

     T86.49 Other complications of liver transplant `CC` `HCC`

T86.5 Complications of stem cell transplant `CC` `HCC`
     Complications from stem cells from peripheral blood
     Complications from stem cells from umbilical cord
     AHA: 2020,4Q,14

√5ᵗʰ **T86.8 Complications of other transplanted organs and tissues**

√6ᵗʰ **T86.81 Complications of lung transplant**

     EXCLUDES 1   complication of heart-lung transplant (T86.3-)

     T86.810 Lung transplant rejection `CC` `HCC`

     T86.811 Lung transplant failure `CC` `HCC`

     T86.812 Lung transplant infection `CC` `HCC`
         Use additional code to specify infection

     T86.818 Other complications of lung transplant `CC` `HCC`
         AHA: 2019,2Q,6

     T86.819 Unspecified complication of lung transplant `CC` `HCC`

√6ᵗʰ **T86.82 Complications of skin graft (allograft) (autograft)**

     EXCLUDES 2   complication of artificial skin graft (T85.693)

     T86.820 Skin graft (allograft) rejection `CC`

     T86.821 Skin graft (allograft) (autograft) failure `CC`

     T86.822 Skin graft (allograft) (autograft) infection `CC`
         Use additional code to specify infection

     T86.828 Other complications of skin graft (allograft) (autograft) `CC`

     T86.829 Unspecified complication of skin graft (allograft) (autograft) `CC`

√6ᵗʰ **T86.83 Complications of bone graft**

     EXCLUDES 2   mechanical complications of bone graft (T84.3-)

     T86.830 Bone graft rejection `CC`

     T86.831 Bone graft failure `CC`

     T86.832 Bone graft infection `CC`
         Use additional code to specify infection

     T86.838 Other complications of bone graft `CC`

     T86.839 Unspecified complication of bone graft `CC`

√6ᵗʰ **T86.84 Complications of corneal transplant**

     EXCLUDES 2   mechanical complications of corneal graft (T85.3-)

     AHA: 2020,4Q,40

     √7ᵗʰ **T86.840 Corneal transplant rejection**

         T86.8401 Corneal transplant rejection, right eye `CC`

         T86.8402 Corneal transplant rejection, left eye `CC`

         T86.8403 Corneal transplant rejection, bilateral `CC`

N Newborn: 0   P Pediatric: 0-17   M Maternity: 9-64   A Adult: 15-124   MCC Major Complication/Comorbidity   CC Complication/Comorbidity   SW Severe Wound Dx

1164   ICD-10-CM 2022

T86.8409 Corneal transplant rejection, unspecified eye `cc`

✓7ᵗʰ **T86.841** Corneal transplant failure

T86.8411 Corneal transplant failure, right eye `cc`

T86.8412 Corneal transplant failure, left eye `cc`

T86.8413 Corneal transplant failure, bilateral `cc`

T86.8419 Corneal transplant failure, unspecified eye `cc`

✓7ᵗʰ **T86.842** Corneal transplant infection

Use additional code to specify infection

T86.8421 Corneal transplant infection, right eye `cc` `HCC`

T86.8422 Corneal transplant infection, left eye `cc` `HCC`

T86.8423 Corneal transplant infection, bilateral `cc` `HCC`

T86.8429 Corneal transplant infection, unspecified eye `cc` `HCC`

✓7ᵗʰ **T86.848** Other complications of corneal transplant

T86.8481 Other complications of corneal transplant, right eye `cc`

T86.8482 Other complications of corneal transplant, left eye `cc`

T86.8483 Other complications of corneal transplant, bilateral `cc`

T86.8489 Other complications of corneal transplant, unspecified eye `cc`

✓7ᵗʰ **T86.849** Unspecified complication of corneal transplant

T86.8491 Unspecified complication of corneal transplant, right eye `cc`

T86.8492 Unspecified complication of corneal transplant, left eye `cc`

T86.8493 Unspecified complication of corneal transplant, bilateral `cc`

T86.8499 Unspecified complication of corneal transplant, unspecified eye `cc`

✓6ᵗʰ **T86.85** Complication of intestine transplant

T86.850 Intestine transplant rejection `cc` `HCC`

T86.851 Intestine transplant failure `cc` `HCC`

T86.852 Intestine transplant infection `cc` `HCC`

Use additional code to specify infection

T86.858 Other complications of intestine transplant `cc` `HCC`

T86.859 Unspecified complication of intestine transplant `cc` `HCC`

✓6ᵗʰ **T86.89** Complications of other transplanted tissue

Transplant failure or rejection of pancreas

AHA: 2020,1Q,18

T86.890 Other transplanted tissue rejection `cc`

T86.891 Other transplanted tissue failure `cc`

T86.892 Other transplanted tissue infection `cc`

Use additional code to specify infection

T86.898 Other complications of other transplanted tissue `cc`

T86.899 Unspecified complication of other transplanted tissue `cc`

✓5ᵗʰ **T86.9** Complication of unspecified transplanted organ and tissue

T86.90 Unspecified complication of unspecified transplanted organ and tissue `cc`

T86.91 Unspecified transplanted organ and tissue rejection `cc`

T86.92 Unspecified transplanted organ and tissue failure `cc`

T86.93 Unspecified transplanted organ and tissue infection `cc`

Use additional code to specify infection

T86.99 Other complications of unspecified transplanted organ and tissue `cc`

✓4ᵗʰ **T87** Complications peculiar to reattachment and amputation

✓5ᵗʰ **T87.0** Complications of reattached (part of) upper extremity

✓6ᵗʰ **T87.0X** Complications of reattached (part of) upper extremity

T87.0X1 Complications of reattached (part of) right upper extremity `cc` `HCC`

T87.0X2 Complications of reattached (part of) left upper extremity `cc` `HCC`

T87.0X9 Complications of reattached (part of) unspecified upper extremity `cc` `HCC`

✓5ᵗʰ **T87.1** Complications of reattached (part of) lower extremity

✓6ᵗʰ **T87.1X** Complications of reattached (part of) lower extremity

T87.1X1 Complications of reattached (part of) right lower extremity `cc` `HCC`

T87.1X2 Complications of reattached (part of) left lower extremity `cc` `HCC`

T87.1X9 Complications of reattached (part of) unspecified lower extremity `cc` `HCC`

T87.2 Complications of other reattached body part `cc` `HCC`

✓5ᵗʰ **T87.3** Neuroma of amputation stump

DEF: Non-neoplastic tumor generated at the proximal end of severed, partially transected, or injured nerve following amputation.

T87.30 Neuroma of amputation stump, unspecified extremity `HCC`

T87.31 Neuroma of amputation stump, right upper extremity `HCC`

T87.32 Neuroma of amputation stump, left upper extremity `HCC`

T87.33 Neuroma of amputation stump, right lower extremity `HCC`

T87.34 Neuroma of amputation stump, left lower extremity `HCC`

✓5ᵗʰ **T87.4** Infection of amputation stump

T87.40 Infection of amputation stump, unspecified extremity `cc` `HCC`

T87.41 Infection of amputation stump, right upper extremity `cc` `HCC`

T87.42 Infection of amputation stump, left upper extremity `cc` `HCC`

T87.43 Infection of amputation stump, right lower extremity `cc` `HCC`

T87.44 Infection of amputation stump, left lower extremity `cc` `HCC`

✓5ᵗʰ **T87.5** Necrosis of amputation stump

T87.50 Necrosis of amputation stump, unspecified extremity `HCC`

T87.51 Necrosis of amputation stump, right upper extremity `HCC`

T87.52 Necrosis of amputation stump, left upper extremity `HCC`

T87.53 Necrosis of amputation stump, right lower extremity `HCC`

T87.54 Necrosis of amputation stump, left lower extremity `HCC`

✓5ᵗʰ **T87.8** Other complications of amputation stump

T87.81 Dehiscence of amputation stump `HCC`

T87.89 Other complications of amputation stump `HCC`

Amputation stump contracture

Amputation stump contracture of next proximal joint

Amputation stump flexion

Amputation stump edema

Amputation stump hematoma

EXCLUDES 2 *phantom limb syndrome (G54.6-G54.7)*

T87.9 Unspecified complications of amputation stump `HCC`

☑4ᵗʰ **T88** **Other complications of surgical and medical care, not elsewhere classified**

     EXCLUDES 2   *complication following infusion, transfusion and therapeutic injection (T80.-)*
         complication following procedure NEC (T81.-)
         complications of anesthesia in labor and delivery (O74.-)
         complications of anesthesia in pregnancy (O29.-)
         complications of anesthesia in puerperium (O89.-)
         complications of devices, implants and grafts (T82-T85)
         complications of obstetric surgery and procedure (O75.4)
         dermatitis due to drugs and medicaments (L23.3, L24.4, L25.1, L27.0-L27.1)
         poisoning and toxic effects of drugs and chemicals (T36-T65 with fifth or sixth character 1-4 or 6)
         specified complications classified elsewhere

> The appropriate 7th character is to be added to each code from category T88.
> A   initial encounter
> D   subsequent encounter
> S   sequela

☑x7ᵗʰ **T88.0** **Infection following immunization**   cc
     Sepsis following immunization
     AHA: 2018,4Q,62-63

☑x7ᵗʰ **T88.1** **Other complications following immunization, not elsewhere classified**   cc
     Generalized vaccinia
     Rash following immunization
     EXCLUDES 1   *vaccinia not from vaccine (B08.011)*
     EXCLUDES 2   *anaphylactic shock due to serum (T80.5-)*
         other serum reactions (T80.6-)
         postimmunization arthropathy (M02.2)
         postimmunization encephalitis (G04.02)
         postimmunization fever (R50.83)

☑x7ᵗʰ **T88.2** **Shock due to anesthesia**   cc
     Use additional code for adverse effect, if applicable, to identify drug (T41.- with fifth or sixth character 5)
     EXCLUDES 1   *complications of anesthesia (in):*
         labor and delivery (O74.-)
         postprocedural shock NOS (T81.1-)
         pregnancy (O29.-)
         puerperium (O89.-)

☑x7ᵗʰ **T88.3** **Malignant hyperthermia due to anesthesia**   cc
     Use additional code for adverse effect, if applicable, to identify drug (T41.- with fifth or sixth character 5)

☑x7ᵗʰ **T88.4** **Failed or difficult intubation**

☑5ᵗʰ **T88.5** **Other complications of anesthesia**
     Use additional code for adverse effect, if applicable, to identify drug (T41.- with fifth or sixth character 5)

     ☑x7ᵗʰ **T88.51** **Hypothermia following anesthesia**

     ☑x7ᵗʰ **T88.52** **Failed moderate sedation during procedure**
         Failed conscious sedation during procedure
         EXCLUDES 2   *personal history of failed moderate sedation (Z92.83)*

     ☑x7ᵗʰ **T88.53** **Unintended awareness under general anesthesia during procedure**
         EXCLUDES 2   *personal history of unintended awareness under general anesthesia (Z92.84)*
         AHA: 2016,4Q,72-73

     ☑x7ᵗʰ **T88.59** **Other complications of anesthesia**

☑x7ᵗʰ **T88.6** **Anaphylactic reaction due to adverse effect of correct drug or medicament properly administered**   cc
     Anaphylactic shock due to adverse effect of correct drug or medicament properly administered
     Anaphylactoid reaction NOS
     Use additional code for adverse effect, if applicable, to identify drug (T36-T50 with fifth or sixth character 5)
     EXCLUDES 1   *anaphylactic reaction due to serum (T80.5-)*
         anaphylactic shock or reaction due to adverse food reaction (T78.0-)
     AHA: 2020,1Q,18

☑x7ᵗʰ **T88.7** **Unspecified adverse effect of drug or medicament**
     Drug hypersensitivity NOS
     Drug reaction NOS
     Use additional code for adverse effect, if applicable, to identify drug (T36-T50 with fifth or sixth character 5)
     EXCLUDES 1   *specified adverse effects of drugs and medicaments (A00-R94 and T80-T88.6, T88.8)*

☑x7ᵗʰ **T88.8** **Other specified complications of surgical and medical care, not elsewhere classified**
     Use additional code to identify the complication

☑x7ᵗʰ **T88.9** **Complication of surgical and medical care, unspecified**

N Newborn: 0   P Pediatric: 0-17   M Maternity: 9-64   A Adult: 15-124   MCC Major Complication/Comorbidity   CC Complication/Comorbidity   SW Severe Wound Dx

1166

ICD-10-CM 2022

Chapter 20. External Causes of Morbidity (V00–Y99)

Chapter-specific Guidelines with Coding Examples

The chapter-specific guidelines from the ICD-10-CM Official Guidelines for Coding and Reporting have been provided below. Along with these guidelines are coding examples, contained in the shaded boxes, that have been developed to help illustrate the coding and/or sequencing guidance found in these guidelines.

The external causes of morbidity codes should never be sequenced as the first-listed or principal diagnosis.

External cause codes are intended to provide data for injury research and evaluation of injury prevention strategies. These codes capture how the injury or health condition happened (cause), the intent (unintentional or accidental; or intentional, such as suicide or assault), the place where the event occurred the activity of the patient at the time of the event, and the person's status (e.g., civilian, military).

There is no national requirement for mandatory ICD-10-CM external cause code reporting. Unless a provider is subject to a state-based external cause code reporting mandate or these codes are required by a particular payer, reporting of ICD-10-CM codes in Chapter 20, External Causes of Morbidity, is not required. In the absence of a mandatory reporting requirement, providers are encouraged to voluntarily report external cause codes, as they provide valuable data for injury research and evaluation of injury prevention strategies.

a. General external cause coding guidelines

1) Used with any code in the range of A00.0–T88.9, Z00–Z99

An external cause code may be used with any code in the range of A00.0-T88.9, Z00-Z99, classification that represents a health condition due to an external cause. Though they are most applicable to injuries, they are also valid for use with such things as infections or diseases due to an external source, and other health conditions, such as a heart attack that occurs during strenuous physical activity.

> Actinic reticuloid due to tanning bed use
>
> **L57.1**   **Actinic reticuloid**
>
> **W89.1XXA**   **Exposure to tanning bed, initial encounter**
>
> *Explanation:* An external cause code may be used with any code in the range of A00.0–T88.9, Z00–Z99, classifications that describe health conditions due to an external cause. Code W89.1 Exposure to tanning bed requires a seventh character of A to report this initial encounter, with a placeholder X for the fifth and sixth characters.

2) External cause code used for length of treatment

Assign the external cause code, with the appropriate 7th character (initial encounter, subsequent encounter or sequela) for each encounter for which the injury or condition is being treated.

Most categories in chapter 20 have a 7th character requirement for each applicable code. Most categories in this chapter have three 7th character values: A, initial encounter, D, subsequent encounter and S, sequela. While the patient may be seen by a new or different provider over the course of treatment for an injury or condition, assignment of the 7th character for external cause should match the 7th character of the code assigned for the associated injury or condition for the encounter.

3) Use the full range of external cause codes

Use the full range of external cause codes to completely describe the cause, the intent, the place of occurrence, and if applicable, the activity of the patient at the time of the event, and the patient's status, for all injuries, and other health conditions due to an external cause.

4) Assign as many external cause codes as necessary

Assign as many external cause codes as necessary to fully explain each cause. If only one external code can be recorded, assign the code most related to the principal diagnosis.

5) The selection of the appropriate external cause code

The selection of the appropriate external cause code is guided by the Alphabetic Index of External Causes and by Inclusion and Exclusion notes in the Tabular List.

6) External cause code can never be a principal diagnosis

An external cause code can never be a principal (first-listed) diagnosis.

7) Combination external cause codes

Certain of the external cause codes are combination codes that identify sequential events that result in an injury, such as a fall which results in striking against an object. The injury may be due to either event or both.

The combination external cause code used should correspond to the sequence of events regardless of which caused the most serious injury.

> Toddler tripped and fell while walking and struck his head on an end table, sustaining a scalp contusion
>
> **S00.03XA**   **Contusion of scalp, initial encounter**
>
> **W01.190A**   **Fall on same level from slipping, tripping and stumbling with subsequent striking against furniture, initial encounter**
>
> *Explanation:* Combination external cause codes identify sequential events that result in an injury, such as a fall resulting in striking against an object. The injury may be due to either or both events.

8) No external cause code needed in certain circumstances

No external cause code from Chapter 20 is needed if the external cause and intent are included in a code from another chapter (e.g. T36.0X1-, Poisoning by penicillins, accidental (unintentional)).

b. Place of occurrence guideline

Codes from category Y92, Place of occurrence of the external cause, are secondary codes for use after other external cause codes to identify the location of the patient at the time of injury or other condition.

Generally, a place of occurrence code is assigned only once, at the initial encounter for treatment. However, in the rare instance that a new injury occurs during hospitalization, an additional place of occurrence code may be assigned. No 7th characters are used for Y92.

Do not use place of occurrence code Y92.9 if the place is not stated or is not applicable.

> A farmer was working in his barn and sustained a foot contusion when the horse stepped on his left foot
>
> **S90.32XA**   **Contusion of left foot, initial encounter**
>
> **W55.19XA**   **Other contact with horse, initial encounter**
>
> **Y92.71**   **Barn as the place of occurrence of the external cause**
>
> *Explanation:* A place-of-occurrence code from category Y92 is assigned at the initial encounter to identify the location of the patient at the time the injury occurred.

c. Activity code

Assign a code from category Y93, Activity code, to describe the activity of the patient at the time the injury or other health condition occurred.

An activity code is used only once, at the initial encounter for treatment. Only one code from Y93 should be recorded on a medical record.

The activity codes are not applicable to poisonings, adverse effects, misadventures or sequela.

Do not assign Y93.9, Unspecified activity, if the activity is not stated.

A code from category Y93 is appropriate for use with external cause and intent codes if identifying the activity provides additional information about the event.

> Ranch hand who was grooming a horse sustained a foot contusion when the horse stepped on his left foot
>
> **S90.32XA**   **Contusion of left foot, initial encounter**
>
> **W55.19XA**   **Other contact with horse, initial encounter**
>
> **Y93.K3**   **Activity, grooming and shearing an animal**
>
> *Explanation:* One activity code from category Y93 is assigned at the initial encounter only to describe the activity of the patient at the time the injury occurred.

d. Place of occurrence, activity, and status codes used with other external cause code

When applicable, place of occurrence, activity, and external cause status codes are sequenced after the main external cause code(s). Regardless of the number of external cause codes assigned, generally there should be only one place of occurrence code, one activity code, and one external cause status code assigned to an encounter. However, in the rare instance that a new injury occurs during hospitalization, an additional place of occurrence code may be assigned.

e. If the reporting format limits the number of external cause codes

If the reporting format limits the number of external cause codes that can be used in reporting clinical data, report the code for the cause/intent most related to the principal diagnosis. If the format permits capture of additional external cause codes, the cause/intent, including medical misadventures, of the additional events should be reported rather than the codes for place, activity, or external status.

f. Multiple external cause coding guidelines

More than one external cause code is required to fully describe the external cause of an illness or injury. The assignment of external cause codes should be sequenced in the following priority:

If two or more events cause separate injuries, an external cause code should be assigned for each cause. The first-listed external cause code will be selected in the following order:

External codes for child and adult abuse take priority over all other external cause codes.

See Section I.C.19., Child and Adult abuse guidelines.

External cause codes for terrorism events take priority over all other external cause codes except child and adult abuse.

External cause codes for cataclysmic events take priority over all other external cause codes except child and adult abuse and terrorism.

External cause codes for transport accidents take priority over all other external cause codes except cataclysmic events, child and adult abuse and terrorism.

Activity and external cause status codes are assigned following all causal (intent) external cause codes.

The first-listed external cause code should correspond to the cause of the most serious diagnosis due to an assault, accident, or self-harm, following the order of hierarchy listed above..

30-year-old man accidentally discharged his hunting rifle, sustaining an open gunshot wound to the right thigh, which caused him to fall down the stairs, resulting in closed displaced comminuted fracture of his left radial shaft

S71.131A	**Puncture wound without foreign body, right thigh, initial encounter**
W33.02XA	**Accidental discharge of hunting rifle, initial encounter**
S52.352A	**Displaced comminuted fracture of shaft of radius, left arm, initial encounter for closed fracture**
W10.9XXA	**Fall (on) (from) unspecified stairs and steps, initial encounter**

Explanation: If two or more events cause separate injuries, an external cause code should be assigned for each cause.

---

g. Child and adult abuse guideline

Adult and child abuse, neglect and maltreatment are classified as assault. Any of the assault codes may be used to indicate the external cause of any injury resulting from the confirmed abuse.

For confirmed cases of abuse, neglect and maltreatment, when the perpetrator is known, a code from Y07, Perpetrator of maltreatment and neglect, should accompany any other assault codes.

See Section I.C.19. Adult and child abuse, neglect and other maltreatment

h. Unknown or undetermined intent guideline

If the intent (accident, self-harm, assault) of the cause of an injury or other condition is unknown or unspecified, code the intent as accidental intent. All transport accident categories assume accidental intent.

1) Use of undetermined intent

External cause codes for events of undetermined intent are only for use if the documentation in the record specifies that the intent cannot be determined.

i. Sequelae (late effects) of external cause guidelines

1) Sequelae external cause codes

Sequela are reported using the external cause code with the 7th character "S" for sequela. These codes should be used with any report of a late effect or sequela resulting from a previous injury.

See Section I.B.10 Sequela (Late Effects)

2) Sequela external cause code with a related current injury

A sequela external cause code should never be used with a related current nature of injury code.

3) Use of sequela external cause codes for subsequent visits

Use a late effect external cause code for subsequent visits when a late effect of the initial injury is being treated. Do not use a late effect external cause code for subsequent visits for follow-up care (e.g., to assess healing, to receive rehabilitative therapy) of the injury when no late effect of the injury has been documented.

j. Terrorism guidelines

1) Cause of injury identified by the Federal Government (FBI) as terrorism

When the cause of an injury is identified by the Federal Government (FBI) as terrorism, the first-listed external cause code should be a code from category Y38, Terrorism. The definition of terrorism employed by the FBI is found at the inclusion note at the beginning of category Y38. Use additional code for place of occurrence (Y92.-). More than one Y38 code may be assigned if the injury is the result of more than one mechanism of terrorism.

2) Cause of an injury is suspected to be the result of terrorism

When the cause of an injury is suspected to be the result of terrorism a code from category Y38 should not be assigned. Suspected cases should be classified as assault.

3) Code Y38.9, Terrorism, secondary effects

Assign code Y38.9, Terrorism, secondary effects, for conditions occurring subsequent to the terrorist event. This code should not be assigned for conditions that are due to the initial terrorist act.

It is acceptable to assign code Y38.9 with another code from Y38 if there is an injury due to the initial terrorist event and an injury that is a subsequent result of the terrorist event.

k. External cause status

A code from category Y99, External cause status, should be assigned whenever any other external cause code is assigned for an encounter, including an Activity code, except for the events noted below. Assign a code from category Y99, External cause status, to indicate the work status of the person at the time the event occurred. The status code indicates whether the event occurred during military activity, whether a non-military person was at work, whether an individual including a student or volunteer was involved in a non-work activity at the time of the causal event.

A code from Y99, External cause status, should be assigned, when applicable, with other external cause codes, such as transport accidents and falls. The external cause status codes are not applicable to poisonings, adverse effects, misadventures or late effects.

Do not assign a code from category Y99 if no other external cause codes (cause, activity) are applicable for the encounter.

An external cause status code is used only once, at the initial encounter for treatment. Only one code from Y99 should be recorded on a medical record.

Do not assign code Y99.9, Unspecified external cause status, if the status is not stated.

Chapter 20. External Causes of Morbidity (V00-Y99)

NOTE This chapter permits the classification of environmental events and circumstances as the cause of injury, and other adverse effects. Where a code from this section is applicable, it is intended that it shall be used secondary to a code from another chapter of the Classification indicating the nature of the condition. Most often, the condition will be classifiable to Chapter 19, Injury, poisoning and certain other consequences of external causes (S00-T88). Other conditions that may be stated to be due to external causes are classified in Chapters I to XVIII. For these conditions, codes from Chapter 20 should be used to provide additional information as to the cause of the condition.

AHA: 2018,4Q,58-60

This chapter contains the following blocks:

V00-X58	Accidents
V00-V99	Transport accidents
V00-V09	Pedestrian injured in transport accident
V10-V19	Pedal cycle rider injured in transport accident
V20-V29	Motorcycle rider injured in transport accident
V30-V39	Occupant of three-wheeled motor vehicle injured in transport accident
V40-V49	Car occupant injured in transport accident
V50-V59	Occupant of pick-up truck or van injured in transport accident
V60-V69	Occupant of heavy transport vehicle injured in transport accident
V70-V79	Bus occupant injured in transport accident
V80-V89	Other land transport accidents
V90-V94	Water transport accidents
V95-V97	Air and space transport accidents
V98-V99	Other and unspecified transport accidents
W00-X58	Other external causes of accidental injury
W00-W19	Slipping, tripping, stumbling and falls
W20-W49	Exposure to inanimate mechanical forces
W50-W64	Exposure to animate mechanical forces
W65-W74	Accidental non-transport drowning and submersion
W85-W99	Exposure to electric current, radiation and extreme ambient air temperature and pressure
X00-X08	Exposure to smoke, fire and flames
X10-X19	Contact with heat and hot substances
X30-X39	Exposure to forces of nature
X50	Overexertion and strenuous or repetitive movements
X52-X58	Accidental exposure to other specified factors
X71-X83	Intentional self-harm
X92-Y09	Assault
Y21-Y33	Event of undetermined intent
Y35-Y38	Legal intervention, operations of war, military operations, and terrorism
Y62-Y84	Complications of medical and surgical care
Y62-Y69	Misadventures to patients during surgical and medical care
Y70-Y82	Medical devices associated with adverse incidents in diagnostic and therapeutic use
Y83-Y84	Surgical and other medical procedures as the cause of abnormal reaction of the patient, or of later complication, without mention of misadventure at the time of the procedure
Y90-Y99	Supplementary factors related to causes of morbidity classified elsewhere

ACCIDENTS (V00-X58)

AHA: 2018,2Q,7-8

Transport accidents (V00-V99)

NOTE This section is structured in 12 groups. Those relating to land transport accidents (V00-V89) reflect the victim's mode of transport and are subdivided to identify the victim's 'counterpart' or the type of event. The vehicle of which the injured person is an occupant is identified in the first two characters since it is seen as the most important factor to identify for prevention purposes. A transport accident is one in which the vehicle involved must be moving or running or in use for transport purposes at the time of the accident.

Use additional code to identify:
airbag injury (W22.1)
type of street or road (Y92.4-)
use of cellular telephone and other electronic equipment at the time of the transport accident (Y93.C-)

EXCLUDES 1 agricultural vehicles in stationary use or maintenance (W31.-)
assault by crashing of motor vehicle (Y03.-)
automobile or motor cycle in stationary use or maintenance - code to type of accident
crashing of motor vehicle, undetermined intent (Y32)
intentional self-harm by crashing of motor vehicle (X82)

EXCLUDES 2 transport accidents due to cataclysm (X34-X38)

NOTE Definitions related to transport accidents:

(a) A transport accident (V00-V99) is any accident involving a device designed primarily for, or used at the time primarily for, conveying persons or good from one place to another.

(b) A public highway [trafficway] or street is the entire width between property lines (or other boundary lines) of land open to the public as a matter of right or custom for purposes of moving persons or property from one place to another. A roadway is that part of the public highway designed, improved and customarily used for vehicular traffic.

(c) A traffic accident is any vehicle accident occurring on the public highway [i.e. originating on, terminating on, or involving a vehicle partially on the highway]. A vehicle accident is assumed to have occurred on the public highway unless another place is specified, except in the case of accidents involving only off-road motor vehicles, which are classified as nontraffic accidents unless the contrary is stated.

(d) A nontraffic accident is any vehicle accident that occurs entirely in any place other than a public highway.

(e) A pedestrian is any person involved in an accident who was not at the time of the accident riding in or on a motor vehicle, railway train, streetcar or animal-drawn or other vehicle, or on a pedal cycle or animal. This includes, a person changing a tire, working on a parked car, or a person on foot. It also includes the user of a pedestrian conveyance such as a baby stroller, ice-skates, skis, sled, roller skates, a skateboard, nonmotorized or motorized wheelchair, motorized mobility scooter, or nonmotorized scooter.

(f) A driver is an occupant of a transport vehicle who is operating or intending to operate it.

(g) A passenger is any occupant of a transport vehicle other than the driver, except a person traveling on the outside of the vehicle.

(h) A person on the outside of a vehicle is any person being transported by a vehicle but not occupying the space normally reserved for the driver or passengers, or the space intended for the transport of property. This includes a person travelling on the bodywork, bumper, fender, roof, running board or step of a vehicle, as well as, hanging on the outside of the vehicle.

(i) A pedal cycle is any land transport vehicle operated solely by nonmotorized pedals including a bicycle or tricycle.

(j) A pedal cyclist is any person riding a pedal cycle or in a sidecar or trailer attached to a pedal cycle.

(k) A motorcycle is a two-wheeled motor vehicle with one or two riding saddles and sometimes with a third wheel for the support of a sidecar. The sidecar is considered part of the motorcycle. This includes a moped, motor scooter, or motorized bicycle.

(l) A motorcycle rider is any person riding a motorcycle or in a sidecar or trailer attached to the motorcycle.

(m) A three-wheeled motor vehicle is a motorized tricycle designed primarily for on-road use. This includes a motor-driven tricycle, a motorized rickshaw, or a three-wheeled motor car.

(n) A car [automobile] is a four-wheeled motor vehicle designed primarily for carrying up to 7 persons. A trailer being towed by the car is considered part of the car. It does not include a van or minivan — see definition (o).

(o) A pick-up truck or van is a four or six-wheeled motor vehicle designed for carrying passengers as well as property or cargo weighing less than the local limit for classification as a heavy goods vehicle, and not requiring a special driver's license. This includes a minivan and a sport-utility vehicle (SUV).

(p) A heavy transport vehicle is a motor vehicle designed primarily for carrying property, meeting local criteria for classification as a heavy goods vehicle in terms of weight and requiring a special driver's license.

(q) A bus (coach) is a motor vehicle designed or adapted primarily for carrying more than 10 passengers, and requiring a special driver's license.

(r) A railway train or railway vehicle is any device, with or without freight or passenger cars couple to it, designed for traffic on a railway track. This includes subterranean (subways) or elevated trains.

(s) A streetcar, is a device designed and used primarily for transporting passengers within a municipality, running on rails, usually subject to normal traffic control signals, and operated principally on a right-of-way that forms part of the roadway. This includes a tram or trolley that runs on rails. A trailer being towed by a streetcar is considered part of the streetcar.

(t) A special vehicle mainly used on industrial premises is a motor vehicle designed primarily for use within the buildings and premises of industrial or commercial establishments. This includes battery-powered airport passenger vehicles or baggage/mail trucks, forklifts, coal-cars in a coal mine, logging cars and trucks used in mines or quarries.

(u) A special vehicle mainly used in agriculture is a motor vehicle designed specifically for use in farming and agriculture

(horticulture), to work the land, tend and harvest crops and transport materials on the farm. This includes harvesters, farm machinery and tractor and trailers.

(v) A special construction vehicle is a motor vehicle designed specifically for use on construction and demolition sites. This includes bulldozers, diggers, earth levellers, dump trucks. backhoes, front-end loaders, pavers, and mechanical shovels.

(w) A special all-terrain vehicle is a motor vehicle of special design to enable it to negotiate over rough or soft terrain, snow or sand. Examples of special design are high construction, special wheels and tires, tracks, and support on a cushion of air. This includes snow mobiles, All-terrain vehicles (ATV), and dune buggies. It does not include passenger vehicle designated as Sport Utility Vehicles. (SUV)

(x) A watercraft is any device designed for transporting passengers or goods on water. This includes motor or sailboats, ships, and hovercraft.

(y) An aircraft is any device for transporting passengers or goods in the air. This includes hot-air balloons, gliders, helicopters and airplanes.

(z) A military vehicle is any motorized vehicle operating on a public roadway owned by the military and being operated by a member of the military.

Pedestrian injured in transport accident (V00-V09)

INCLUDES   person changing tire on transport vehicle
person examining engine of vehicle broken down in (on side of) road
EXCLUDES 1   fall due to non-transport collision with other person (W03)
pedestrian on foot falling (slipping) on ice and snow (W00.-)
struck or bumped by another person (W51)

The appropriate 7th character is to be added to each code from categories V00-V09.
A   initial encounter
D   subsequent encounter
S   sequela

✓4ᵗʰ **V00 Pedestrian conveyance accident**

Use additional place of occurrence and activity external cause codes, if known (Y92.-, Y93.-)

EXCLUDES 1   collision with another person without fall (W51)
fall due to person on foot colliding with another person on foot (W03)
fall from non-moving wheelchair, nonmotorized scooter and motorized mobility scooter without collision (W05.-)
pedestrian (conveyance) collision with other land transport vehicle (V01-V09)
pedestrian on foot falling (slipping) on ice and snow (W00.-)

✓5ᵗʰ **V00.0 Pedestrian on foot injured in collision with pedestrian conveyance**

  ✓x7ᵗʰ **V00.01 Pedestrian on foot injured in collision with roller-skater**

  ✓x7ᵗʰ **V00.02 Pedestrian on foot injured in collision with skateboarder**

  ✓6ᵗʰ **V00.03 Pedestrian on foot injured in collision with standing micro-mobility pedestrian conveyance**

    ✓7ᵗʰ **V00.031 Pedestrian on foot injured in collision with rider of** standing electric scooter

    ✓7ᵗʰ **V00.038 Pedestrian on foot injured in collision with rider of other standing micro-mobility pedestrian conveyance**

Pedestrian on foot injured in collision with rider of hoverboard
Pedestrian on foot injured in collision with rider of segway

  ✓x7ᵗʰ **V00.09 Pedestrian on foot injured in collision with other pedestrian conveyance**

✓5ᵗʰ **V00.1 Rolling-type pedestrian conveyance accident**

EXCLUDES 1   accident with baby stroller (V00.82-)
accident with motorized mobility scooter (V00.83-)
accident with wheelchair (powered) (V00.81-)

  ✓6ᵗʰ **V00.11 In-line roller-skate accident**

    ✓7ᵗʰ **V00.111 Fall from in-line roller-skates**

    ✓7ᵗʰ **V00.112 In-line roller-skater colliding with stationary object**

    ✓7ᵗʰ **V00.118 Other in-line roller-skate accident**

EXCLUDES 1   roller-skate collision with other land transport vehicle (V01-V09 with 5th character 1)

  ✓6ᵗʰ **V00.12 Non-in-line roller-skate accident**

    ✓7ᵗʰ **V00.121 Fall from non-in-line roller-skates**

    ✓7ᵗʰ **V00.122 Non-in-line roller-skater colliding with stationary object**

    ✓7ᵗʰ **V00.128 Other non-in-line roller-skating accident**

EXCLUDES 1   roller-skater collision with other land transport vehicle (V01-V09 with 5th character 1)

  ✓6ᵗʰ **V00.13 Skateboard accident**

    ✓7ᵗʰ **V00.131 Fall from skateboard**

    ✓7ᵗʰ **V00.132 Skateboarder colliding with stationary object**

    ✓7ᵗʰ **V00.138 Other skateboard accident**

EXCLUDES 1   skateboarder collision with other land transport vehicle (V01-V09 with 5th character 2)

  ✓6ᵗʰ **V00.14 Scooter (nonmotorized) accident**

EXCLUDES 1   motor scooter accident (V20-V29)

    ✓7ᵗʰ **V00.141 Fall from scooter (nonmotorized)**

    ✓7ᵗʰ **V00.142 Scooter (nonmotorized) colliding with stationary object**

    ✓7ᵗʰ **V00.148 Other scooter (nonmotorized) accident**

EXCLUDES 1   scooter (nonmotorized) collision with other land transport vehicle (V01-V09 with fifth character 9)

  ✓6ᵗʰ **V00.15 Heelies accident**

Rolling shoe
Wheeled shoe
Wheelies accident

    ✓7ᵗʰ **V00.151 Fall from heelies**

    ✓7ᵗʰ **V00.152 Heelies colliding with stationary object**

    ✓7ᵗʰ **V00.158 Other heelies accident**

  ✓6ᵗʰ **V00.18 Accident on other rolling-type pedestrian conveyance**

    ✓7ᵗʰ **V00.181 Fall from other rolling-type pedestrian conveyance**

    ✓7ᵗʰ **V00.182 Pedestrian on other rolling-type pedestrian conveyance colliding with stationary object**

    ✓7ᵗʰ **V00.188 Other accident on other rolling-type pedestrian conveyance**

✓5ᵗʰ **V00.2 Gliding-type pedestrian conveyance accident**

  ✓6ᵗʰ **V00.21 Ice-skates accident**

    ✓7ᵗʰ **V00.211 Fall from ice-skates**

    ✓7ᵗʰ **V00.212 Ice-skater colliding with stationary object**

    ✓7ᵗʰ **V00.218 Other ice-skates accident**

EXCLUDES 1   ice-skater collision with other land transport vehicle (V01-V09 with 5th character 9)

  ✓6ᵗʰ **V00.22 Sled accident**

    ✓7ᵗʰ **V00.221 Fall from sled**

    ✓7ᵗʰ **V00.222 Sledder colliding with stationary object**

    ✓7ᵗʰ **V00.228 Other sled accident**

EXCLUDES 1   sled collision with other land transport vehicle (V01-V09 with 5th character 9)

  ✓6ᵗʰ **V00.28 Other gliding-type pedestrian conveyance accident**

    ✓7ᵗʰ **V00.281 Fall from other gliding-type pedestrian conveyance**

    ✓7ᵗʰ **V00.282 Pedestrian on other gliding-type pedestrian conveyance colliding with stationary object**

√7ᵗʰ **V00.288** **Other accident on other gliding-type pedestrian conveyance**
> EXCLUDES 1   *gliding-type pedestrian conveyance collision with other land transport vehicle (V01-V09 with 5th character 9)*

√5ᵗʰ **V00.3** **Flat-bottomed pedestrian conveyance accident**

√6ᵗʰ **V00.31** Snowboard **accident**

√7ᵗʰ **V00.311** **Fall from** snowboard

√7ᵗʰ **V00.312** **Snowboarder** colliding with stationary object

√7ᵗʰ **V00.318** **Other snowboard accident**
> EXCLUDES 1   *snowboarder collision with other land transport vehicle (V01-V09 with 5th character 9)*

√6ᵗʰ **V00.32** Snow-ski **accident**

√7ᵗʰ **V00.321** **Fall from** snow-skis

√7ᵗʰ **V00.322** **Snow-skier** colliding with stationary object

√7ᵗʰ **V00.328** **Other snow-ski accident**
> EXCLUDES 1   *snow-skier collision with other land transport vehicle (V01-V09 with 5th character 9)*

√6ᵗʰ **V00.38** **Other flat-bottomed pedestrian conveyance accident**

√7ᵗʰ **V00.381** **Fall from** other flat-bottomed pedestrian conveyance

√7ᵗʰ **V00.382** **Pedestrian on other flat-bottomed pedestrian conveyance** colliding with stationary object

√7ᵗʰ **V00.388** **Other accident on other flat-bottomed pedestrian conveyance**

√5ᵗʰ **V00.8** **Accident on other pedestrian conveyance**

√6ᵗʰ **V00.81** **Accident with** wheelchair **(powered)**

√7ᵗʰ **V00.811** **Fall from** moving wheelchair **(powered)**
> EXCLUDES 1   *fall from non-moving wheelchair (W05.0)*

√7ᵗʰ **V00.812** **Wheelchair (powered)** colliding with stationary object

√7ᵗʰ **V00.818** **Other accident with wheelchair (powered)**

√6ᵗʰ **V00.82** **Accident with** baby stroller

√7ᵗʰ **V00.821** **Fall from** baby stroller

√7ᵗʰ **V00.822** **Baby stroller** colliding with stationary object

√7ᵗʰ **V00.828** **Other accident with baby stroller**

√6ᵗʰ **V00.83** **Accident with** motorized mobility scooter

√7ᵗʰ **V00.831** **Fall from** motorized mobility scooter
> EXCLUDES 1   *fall from non-moving motorized mobility scooter (W05.2)*

√7ᵗʰ **V00.832** **Motorized mobility scooter** colliding with stationary object

√7ᵗʰ **V00.838** **Other accident with motorized mobility scooter**

√6ᵗʰ **V00.84** **Accident with** standing micro-mobility pedestrian conveyance

√7ᵗʰ **V00.841** **Fall from** standing electric scooter

√7ᵗʰ **V00.842** **Pedestrian on standing electric scooter** colliding with stationary object

√7ᵗʰ **V00.848** **Other accident with standing micro-mobility pedestrian conveyance**
> Accident with hoverboard
> Accident with segway

√6ᵗʰ **V00.89** **Accident on other pedestrian conveyance**

√7ᵗʰ **V00.891** **Fall from** other pedestrian conveyance

√7ᵗʰ **V00.892** **Pedestrian on other pedestrian conveyance** colliding with stationary object

√7ᵗʰ **V00.898** **Other accident on other pedestrian conveyance**
> EXCLUDES 1   *other pedestrian (conveyance) collision with other land transport vehicle (V01-V09 with 5th character 9)*

√4ᵗʰ **V01** **Pedestrian injured in collision with pedal cycle**

√5ᵗʰ **V01.0** **Pedestrian injured in collision with pedal cycle** in nontraffic accident

√x7ᵗʰ **V01.00** **Pedestrian** on foot **injured in collision with pedal cycle in nontraffic accident**
> Pedestrian NOS injured in collision with pedal cycle in nontraffic accident

√x7ᵗʰ **V01.01** **Pedestrian** on roller-skates **injured in collision with pedal cycle in nontraffic accident**

√x7ᵗʰ **V01.02** **Pedestrian** on skateboard **injured in collision with pedal cycle in nontraffic accident**

√6ᵗʰ **V01.03** **Pedestrian on standing micro-mobility pedestrian conveyance injured in collision with pedal cycle in nontraffic accident**

√7ᵗʰ **V01.031** **Pedestrian** on standing electric scooter **injured in collision with pedal cycle in nontraffic accident**

√7ᵗʰ **V01.038** **Pedestrian on other standing micro-mobility pedestrian conveyance injured in collision with pedal cycle in nontraffic accident**
> Pedestrian on hoverboard injured in collision with pedal cycle in nontraffic accident
> Pedestrian on segway injured in collision with pedal cycle in nontraffic accident

√x7ᵗʰ **V01.09** **Pedestrian with other conveyance injured in collision with pedal cycle in nontraffic accident**
> Pedestrian with baby stroller injured in collision with pedal cycle in nontraffic accident
> Pedestrian on ice-skates injured in collision with pedal cycle in nontraffic accident
> Pedestrian on nonmotorized scooter injured in collision with pedal cycle in nontraffic accident
> Pedestrian on sled injured in collision with pedal cycle in nontraffic accident
> Pedestrian on snowboard injured in collision with pedal cycle in nontraffic accident
> Pedestrian on snow-skis injured in collision with pedal cycle in nontraffic accident
> Pedestrian in wheelchair (powered) injured in collision with pedal cycle in nontraffic accident
> Pedestrian in motorized mobility scooter injured in collision with pedal cycle in nontraffic accident

√5ᵗʰ **V01.1** **Pedestrian injured in collision with pedal cycle** in traffic accident

√x7ᵗʰ **V01.10** **Pedestrian** on foot **injured in collision with pedal cycle in traffic accident**
> Pedestrian NOS injured in collision with pedal cycle in traffic accident

√x7ᵗʰ **V01.11** **Pedestrian** on roller-skates **injured in collision with pedal cycle in traffic accident**

√x7ᵗʰ **V01.12** **Pedestrian** on skateboard **injured in collision with pedal cycle in traffic accident**

√6ᵗʰ **V01.13** **Pedestrian on standing micro-mobility pedestrian conveyance injured in collision with pedal cycle in traffic accident**

√7ᵗʰ **V01.131** **Pedestrian** on standing electric scooter **injured in collision with pedal cycle in traffic accident**

√7ᵗʰ **V01.138** **Pedestrian on other standing micro-mobility pedestrian conveyance injured in collision with pedal cycle in traffic accident**
> Pedestrian on hoverboard injured in collision with pedal cycle in traffic accident
> Pedestrian on segway injured in collision with pedal cycle in traffic accident

✔ Additional Char Req   √x7ᵗʰ Placeholder   Unacceptable PDx   Questionable PDx   Wrong Procedure   Manifestation   Unspecified Dx   H1 - H14 HAC   HCC CMS-HCC Dx   HIV HIV Dx

ICD-10-CM 2022   1171

√x7ᵗʰ V01.19 Pedestrian with other conveyance injured in collision with pedal cycle in traffic accident
Pedestrian with baby stroller injured in collision with pedal cycle in traffic accident
Pedestrian on ice-skates injured in collision with pedal cycle in traffic accident
Pedestrian on nonmotorized scooter injured in collision with pedal cycle in traffic accident
Pedestrian on sled injured in collision with pedal cycle in traffic accident
Pedestrian on snowboard injured in collision with pedal cycle in traffic accident
Pedestrian on snow-skis injured in collision with pedal cycle in traffic accident
Pedestrian in wheelchair (powered) injured in collision with pedal cycle in traffic accident
Pedestrian in motorized mobility scooter injured in collision with pedal cycle in traffic accident

√5ᵗʰ V01.9 Pedestrian injured in collision with pedal cycle, unspecified whether traffic or nontraffic accident

√x7ᵗʰ V01.90 Pedestrian on foot injured in collision with pedal cycle, unspecified whether traffic or nontraffic accident
Pedestrian NOS injured in collision with pedal cycle, unspecified whether traffic or nontraffic accident

√x7ᵗʰ V01.91 Pedestrian on roller-skates injured in collision with pedal cycle, unspecified whether traffic or nontraffic accident

√x7ᵗʰ V01.92 Pedestrian on skateboard injured in collision with pedal cycle, unspecified whether traffic or nontraffic accident

√6ᵗʰ V01.93 Pedestrian on standing micro-mobility pedestrian conveyance injured in collision with pedal cycle, unspecified whether traffic or nontraffic accident

√7ᵗʰ V01.931 Pedestrian on standing electric scooter injured in collision with pedal cycle, unspecified whether traffic or nontraffic accident

√7ᵗʰ V01.938 Pedestrian on other standing micro-mobility pedestrian conveyance injured in collision with pedal cycle, unspecified whether traffic or nontraffic accident
Pedestrian on hoverboard injured in collision with pedal cycle, unspecified whether traffic or nontraffic accident
Pedestrian on segway injured in collision with pedal cycle, unspecified whether traffic or nontraffic accident

√x7ᵗʰ V01.99 Pedestrian with other conveyance injured in collision with pedal cycle, unspecified whether traffic or nontraffic accident
Pedestrian with baby stroller injured in collision with pedal cycle, unspecified whether traffic or nontraffic accident
Pedestrian on ice-skates injured in collision with pedal cycle unspecified, whether traffic or nontraffic accident
Pedestrian on nonmotorized scooter injured in collision with pedal cycle, unspecified whether traffic or nontraffic accident
Pedestrian on sled injured in collision with pedal cycle unspecified, whether traffic or nontraffic accident
Pedestrian on snowboard injured in collision with pedal cycle, unspecified whether traffic or nontraffic accident
Pedestrian on snow-skis injured in collision with pedal cycle, unspecified whether traffic or nontraffic accident
Pedestrian in wheelchair (powered) injured in collision with pedal cycle, unspecified whether traffic or nontraffic accident
Pedestrian in motorized mobility scooter injured in collision with pedal cycle, unspecified whether traffic or nontraffic accident

√4ᵗʰ V02 Pedestrian injured in collision with two- or three-wheeled motor vehicle

√5ᵗʰ V02.0 Pedestrian injured in collision with two- or three-wheeled motor vehicle in nontraffic accident

√x7ᵗʰ V02.00 Pedestrian on foot injured in collision with two- or three-wheeled motor vehicle in nontraffic accident
Pedestrian NOS injured in collision with two- or three-wheeled motor vehicle in nontraffic accident

√x7ᵗʰ V02.01 Pedestrian on roller-skates injured in collision with two- or three-wheeled motor vehicle in nontraffic accident

√x7ᵗʰ V02.02 Pedestrian on skateboard injured in collision with two- or three-wheeled motor vehicle in nontraffic accident

√6ᵗʰ V02.03 Pedestrian on standing micro-mobility pedestrian conveyance injured in collision with two- or three-wheeled motor vehicle in nontraffic accident

√7ᵗʰ V02.031 Pedestrian on standing electric scooter injured in collision with two- or three-wheeled motor vehicle in nontraffic accident

√7ᵗʰ V02.038 Pedestrian on other standing micro-mobility pedestrian conveyance injured in collision with two- or three-wheeled motor vehicle in nontraffic accident
Pedestrian on hoverboard injured in collision with two-or three wheeled motor vehicle in nontraffic accident
Pedestrian on segway injured in collision with two- or three-wheeled motor vehicle in nontraffic accident

√x7ᵗʰ V02.09 Pedestrian with other conveyance injured in collision with two- or three-wheeled motor vehicle in nontraffic accident
Pedestrian with baby stroller injured in collision with two- or three-wheeled motor vehicle in nontraffic accident
Pedestrian on ice-skates injured in collision with two- or three-wheeled motor vehicle in nontraffic accident
Pedestrian on nonmotorized scooter injured in collision with two- or three-wheeled motor vehicle in nontraffic accident
Pedestrian on sled injured in collision with two- or three-wheeled motor vehicle in nontraffic accident
Pedestrian on snowboard injured in collision with two- or three-wheeled motor vehicle in nontraffic accident
Pedestrian on snow-skis injured in collision with two- or three-wheeled motor vehicle in nontraffic accident
Pedestrian in wheelchair (powered) injured in collision with two- or three-wheeled motor vehicle in nontraffic accident
Pedestrian in motorized mobility scooter injured in collision with two- or three-wheeled motor vehicle in nontraffic accident

√5ᵗʰ V02.1 Pedestrian injured in collision with two- or three-wheeled motor vehicle in traffic accident

√x7ᵗʰ V02.10 Pedestrian on foot injured in collision with two- or three-wheeled motor vehicle in traffic accident
Pedestrian NOS injured in collision with two- or three-wheeled motor vehicle in traffic accident

√x7ᵗʰ V02.11 Pedestrian on roller-skates injured in collision with two- or three-wheeled motor vehicle in traffic accident

√x7ᵗʰ V02.12 Pedestrian on skateboard injured in collision with two- or three-wheeled motor vehicle in traffic accident

√6ᵗʰ V02.13 Pedestrian on standing micro-mobility pedestrian conveyance injured in collision with two- or three-wheeled motor vehicle in traffic accident

√7ᵗʰ V02.131 Pedestrian on standing electric scooter injured in collision with two- or three-wheeled motor vehicle in traffic accident

☑7ᵗʰ **V02.138 Pedestrian on other standing micro-mobility pedestrian conveyance injured in collision with two- or three-wheeled motor vehicle in traffic accident**

     Pedestrian on hoverboard injured in collision with two-or three wheeled motor vehicle in traffic accident

     Pedestrian on segway injured in collision with two- or three-wheeled motor vehicle in traffic accident

☑x7ᵗʰ **V02.19 Pedestrian with other conveyance injured in collision with two- or three-wheeled motor vehicle in traffic accident**

     Pedestrian with baby stroller injured in collision with two- or three-wheeled motor vehicle in traffic accident

     Pedestrian on ice-skates injured in collision with two- or three-wheeled motor vehicle in traffic accident

     Pedestrian on nonmotorized scooter injured in collision with two- or three-wheeled motor vehicle in traffic accident

     Pedestrian on sled injured in collision with two- or three-wheeled motor vehicle in traffic accident

     Pedestrian on snowboard injured in collision with two- or three-wheeled motor vehicle in traffic accident

     Pedestrian on snow-skis injured in collision with two- or three-wheeled motor vehicle in traffic accident

     Pedestrian in wheelchair (powered) injured in collision with two- or three-wheeled motor vehicle in traffic accident

     Pedestrian in motorized mobility scooter injured in collision with two- or three-wheeled motor vehicle in traffic accident

☑5ᵗʰ **V02.9 Pedestrian injured in collision with two- or three-wheeled motor vehicle, unspecified whether traffic or nontraffic accident**

☑x7ᵗʰ **V02.90 Pedestrian on foot injured in collision with two- or three-wheeled motor vehicle, unspecified whether traffic or nontraffic accident**

     Pedestrian NOS injured in collision with two- or three-wheeled motor vehicle, unspecified whether traffic or nontraffic accident

☑x7ᵗʰ **V02.91 Pedestrian on roller-skates injured in collision with two- or three-wheeled motor vehicle, unspecified whether traffic or nontraffic accident**

☑x7ᵗʰ **V02.92 Pedestrian on skateboard injured in collision with two- or three-wheeled motor vehicle, unspecified whether traffic or nontraffic accident**

☑6ᵗʰ **V02.93 Pedestrian on standing micro-mobility pedestrian conveyance injured in collision with two- or three-wheeled motor vehicle, unspecified whether traffic or nontraffic accident**

☑7ᵗʰ **V02.931 Pedestrian on standing electric scooter injured in collision with two- or three wheeled motor vehicle, unspecified whether traffic or nontraffic accident**

☑7ᵗʰ **V02.938 Pedestrian on other standing micro-mobility pedestrian conveyance injured in collision with two- or three wheeled motor vehicle, unspecified whether traffic or nontraffic accident**

     Pedestrian on hoverboard injured in collision with two-three-wheeled motor vehicle, unspecified whether traffic or nontraffic accident

     Pedestrian on segway injured in collision with two- or three wheeled motor vehicle, unspecified whether traffic or nontraffic accident

☑x7ᵗʰ **V02.99 Pedestrian with other conveyance injured in collision with two- or three-wheeled motor vehicle, unspecified whether traffic or nontraffic accident**

     Pedestrian with baby stroller injured in collision with two- or three-wheeled motor vehicle, unspecified whether traffic or nontraffic accident

     Pedestrian on ice-skates injured in collision with two- or three-wheeled motor vehicle, unspecified whether traffic or nontraffic accident

     Pedestrian on nonmotorized scooter injured in collision with two- or three-wheeled motor vehicle, unspecified whether traffic or nontraffic accident

     Pedestrian on sled injured in collision with two- or three-wheeled motor vehicle, unspecified whether traffic or nontraffic accident

     Pedestrian on snowboard injured in collision with two- or three-wheeled motor vehicle, unspecified whether traffic or nontraffic accident

     Pedestrian on snow-skis injured in collision with two- or three-wheeled motor vehicle, unspecified whether traffic or nontraffic accident

     Pedestrian in wheelchair (powered) injured in collision with two- or three-wheeled motor vehicle, unspecified whether traffic or nontraffic accident

     Pedestrian in motorized mobility scooter injured in collision with two- or three wheeled motor vehicle, unspecified whether traffic or nontraffic accident

☑4ᵗʰ **V03 Pedestrian injured in collision with car, pick-up truck or van**

☑5ᵗʰ **V03.0 Pedestrian injured in collision with car, pick-up truck or van in nontraffic accident**

☑x7ᵗʰ **V03.00 Pedestrian on foot injured in collision with car, pick-up truck or van in nontraffic accident**

     Pedestrian NOS injured in collision with car, pick-up truck or van in nontraffic accident

☑x7ᵗʰ **V03.01 Pedestrian on roller-skates injured in collision with car, pick-up truck or van in nontraffic accident**

☑x7ᵗʰ **V03.02 Pedestrian on skateboard injured in collision with car, pick-up truck or van in nontraffic accident**

☑6ᵗʰ **V03.03 Pedestrian on standing micro-mobility pedestrian conveyance injured in collision with car, pick-up or van in nontraffic accident**

☑7ᵗʰ **V03.031 Pedestrian on standing electric scooter injured in collision with car, pick-up or van in nontraffic accident**

☑7ᵗʰ **V03.038 Pedestrian on other standing micro-mobility pedestrian conveyance injured in collision with car, pick-up or van in nontraffic accident**

     Pedestrian on hoverboard injured in collision with car, pick-up or van in nontraffic accident

     Pedestrian on segway injured in collision with car, pick-up or van in nontraffic accident

☑x7ᵗʰ **V03.09 Pedestrian with other conveyance injured in collision with car, pick-up truck or van in nontraffic accident**

     Pedestrian with baby stroller injured in collision with car, pick-up truck or van in nontraffic accident

     Pedestrian on ice-skates injured in collision with car, pick-up truck or van in nontraffic accident

     Pedestrian on nonmotorized scooter injured in collision with car, pick-up truck or van in nontraffic accident

     Pedestrian on sled injured in collision with car, pick-up truck or van in nontraffic accident

     Pedestrian on snowboard injured in collision with car, pick-up truck or van in nontraffic accident

     Pedestrian on snow-skis injured in collision with car, pick-up truck or van in nontraffic accident

     Pedestrian in wheelchair (powered) injured in collision with car, pick-up truck or van in nontraffic accident

     Pedestrian in motorized mobility scooter injured in collision with car, pick-up truck or van in nontraffic accident

☑ Additional Char Req   ☑x7ᵗʰ Placeholder   Unacceptable PDx   Questionable PDx   Wrong Procedure   Manifestation   Unspecified Dx   H1-H14 HAC   HCC CMS-HCC Dx   HIV HIV Dx

ICD-10-CM 2022   1173

Chapter 20. External Causes of Morbidity

☑5ᵗʰ **V03.1** **Pedestrian injured in collision with car, pick-up truck or van in traffic accident**

     ☑x7ᵗʰ **V03.10** **Pedestrian on foot injured in collision with car, pick-up truck or van in traffic accident**

         Pedestrian NOS injured in collision with car, pick-up truck or van in traffic accident

     ☑x7ᵗʰ **V03.11** **Pedestrian on roller-skates injured in collision with car, pick-up truck or van in traffic accident**

     ☑x7ᵗʰ **V03.12** **Pedestrian on skateboard injured in collision with car, pick-up truck or van in traffic accident**

     ☑6ᵗʰ **V03.13** **Pedestrian on standing micro-mobility pedestrian conveyance injured in collision with car, pick-up or van in traffic accident**

         ☑7ᵗʰ **V03.131** **Pedestrian on standing electric scooter injured in collision with car, pick-up or van in traffic accident**

         ☑7ᵗʰ **V03.138** **Pedestrian on other standing micro-mobility pedestrian conveyance injured in collision with car, pick-up or van in traffic accident**

             Pedestrian on hoverboard injured in collision with car, pick-up or van in traffic accident

             Pedestrian on segway injured in collision with car, pick-up or van in traffic accident

     ☑x7ᵗʰ **V03.19** **Pedestrian with other conveyance injured in collision with car, pick-up truck or van in traffic accident**

         Pedestrian with baby stroller injured in collision with car, pick-up truck or van in traffic accident

         Pedestrian on ice-skates injured in collision with car, pick-up truck or van in traffic accident

         Pedestrian on nonmotorized scooter injured in collision with car, pick-up truck or van in nontraffic accident

         Pedestrian on sled injured in collision with car, pick-up truck or van in traffic accident

         Pedestrian on snowboard injured in collision with car, pick-up truck or van in traffic accident

         Pedestrian on snow-skis injured in collision with car, pick-up truck or van in traffic accident

         Pedestrian in wheelchair (powered) injured in collision with car, pick-up truck or van in traffic accident

         Pedestrian in motorized mobility scooter injured in collision with car, pick-up truck or van in nontraffic accident

☑5ᵗʰ **V03.9** **Pedestrian injured in collision with car, pick-up truck or van, unspecified whether traffic or nontraffic accident**

     ☑x7ᵗʰ **V03.90** **Pedestrian on foot injured in collision with car, pick-up truck or van, unspecified whether traffic or nontraffic accident**

         Pedestrian NOS injured in collision with car, pick-up truck or van, unspecified whether traffic or nontraffic accident

     ☑x7ᵗʰ **V03.91** **Pedestrian on roller-skates injured in collision with car, pick-up truck or van, unspecified whether traffic or nontraffic accident**

     ☑x7ᵗʰ **V03.92** **Pedestrian on skateboard injured in collision with car, pick-up truck or van, unspecified whether traffic or nontraffic accident**

     ☑6ᵗʰ **V03.93** **Pedestrian on standing micro-mobility pedestrian conveyance injured in collision with car, pick-up or van, unspecified whether traffic or nontraffic accident**

         ☑7ᵗʰ **V03.931** **Pedestrian on standing electric scooter injured in collision with car, pick-up or van, unspecified whether traffic or nontraffic accident**

         ☑7ᵗʰ **V03.938** **Pedestrian on other standing micro-mobility pedestrian conveyance injured in collision with car, pick-up or van, unspecified whether traffic or nontraffic accident**

             Pedestrian on hoverboard injured in collision with car, pick-up or van, unspecified whether traffic or nontraffic accident

             Pedestrian on segway injured in collision with car, pick-up or van, unspecified whether traffic or nontraffic accident

     ☑x7ᵗʰ **V03.99** **Pedestrian with other conveyance injured in collision with car, pick-up truck or van, unspecified whether traffic or nontraffic accident**

         Pedestrian with baby stroller injured in collision with car, pick-up truck or van, unspecified whether traffic or nontraffic accident

         Pedestrian on ice-skates injured in collision with car, pick-up truck or van, unspecified whether traffic or nontraffic accident

         Pedestrian on nonmotorized scooter injured in collision with car, pick-up truck or van, unspecified whether traffic or nontraffic accident

         Pedestrian on sled injured in collision with car, pick-up truck or van in nontraffic accident

         Pedestrian on snowboard injured in collision with car, pick-up truck or van, unspecified whether traffic or nontraffic accident

         Pedestrian on snow-skis injured in collision with car, pick-up truck or van, unspecified whether traffic or nontraffic accident

         Pedestrian in wheelchair (powered) injured in collision with car, pick-up truck or van, unspecified whether traffic or nontraffic accident

         Pedestrian in motorized mobility scooter injured in collision with car, pick-up truck or van, unspecified whether traffic or nontraffic accident

☑4ᵗʰ **V04** **Pedestrian injured in collision with heavy transport vehicle or bus**

     EXCLUDES 1   *pedestrian injured in collision with military vehicle (V09.01, V09.21)*

     ☑5ᵗʰ **V04.0** **Pedestrian injured in collision with heavy transport vehicle or bus in nontraffic accident**

         ☑x7ᵗʰ **V04.00** **Pedestrian on foot injured in collision with heavy transport vehicle or bus in nontraffic accident**

             Pedestrian NOS injured in collision with heavy transport vehicle or bus in nontraffic accident

         ☑x7ᵗʰ **V04.01** **Pedestrian on roller-skates injured in collision with heavy transport vehicle or bus in nontraffic accident**

         ☑x7ᵗʰ **V04.02** **Pedestrian on skateboard injured in collision with heavy transport vehicle or bus in nontraffic accident**

         ☑6ᵗʰ **V04.03** **Pedestrian on standing micro-mobility pedestrian conveyance injured in collision with heavy transport vehicle or bus in nontraffic accident**

             ☑7ᵗʰ **V04.031** **Pedestrian on standing electric scooter injured in collision with heavy transport vehicle or bus in nontraffic accident**

             ☑7ᵗʰ **V04.038** **Pedestrian on other standing micro-mobility pedestrian conveyance injured in collision with heavy transport vehicle or bus in nontraffic accident**

                 Pedestrian on hoverboard injured in collision with heavy transport vehicle or bus in nontraffic accident

                 Pedestrian on segway injured in collision with heavy transport vehicle or bus in nontraffic accident

Ⓝ Newborn: 0   Ⓟ Pediatric: 0-17   Ⓜ Maternity: 9-64   Ⓐ Adult: 15-124   **MCC** Major Complication/Comorbidity   **CC** Complication/Comorbidity   **SW** Severe Wound Dx

1174   ICD-10-CM 2022

✓x 7ᵗʰ **V04.09** **Pedestrian with other conveyance injured in collision with heavy transport vehicle or bus in nontraffic accident**

Pedestrian with baby stroller injured in collision with heavy transport vehicle or bus in nontraffic accident

Pedestrian on ice-skates injured in collision with heavy transport vehicle or bus in nontraffic accident

Pedestrian on nonmotorized scooter injured in collision with heavy transport vehicle or bus in nontraffic accident

Pedestrian on sled injured in collision with heavy transport vehicle or bus in nontraffic accident

Pedestrian on snowboard injured in collision with heavy transport vehicle or bus in nontraffic accident

Pedestrian on snow-skis injured in collision with heavy transport vehicle or bus in nontraffic accident

Pedestrian in wheelchair (powered) injured in collision with heavy transport vehicle or bus in nontraffic accident

Pedestrian in motorized mobility scooter injured in collision with heavy transport vehicle or bus in nontraffic accident

✓5ᵗʰ **V04.1** **Pedestrian injured in collision with heavy transport vehicle or bus in traffic accident**

✓x 7ᵗʰ **V04.10** **Pedestrian on foot injured in collision with heavy transport vehicle or bus in traffic accident**

Pedestrian NOS injured in collision with heavy transport vehicle or bus in traffic accident

✓x 7ᵗʰ **V04.11** **Pedestrian on roller-skates injured in collision with heavy transport vehicle or bus in traffic accident**

✓x 7ᵗʰ **V04.12** **Pedestrian on skateboard injured in collision with heavy transport vehicle or bus in traffic accident**

✓6ᵗʰ **V04.13** **Pedestrian on standing micro-mobility pedestrian conveyance injured in collision with heavy transport vehicle or bus in traffic accident**

✓7ᵗʰ **V04.131** **Pedestrian on standing electric scooter injured in collision with heavy transport vehicle or bus in traffic accident**

✓7ᵗʰ **V04.138** **Pedestrian on other standing micro-mobility pedestrian conveyance injured in collision with heavy transport vehicle or bus in traffic accident**

Pedestrian on hoverboard injured in collision with heavy transport vehicle or bus in traffic accident

Pedestrian on segway injured in collision with heavy transport vehicle or bus in traffic accident

✓x 7ᵗʰ **V04.19** **Pedestrian with other conveyance injured in collision with heavy transport vehicle or bus in traffic accident**

Pedestrian with baby stroller injured in collision with heavy transport vehicle or bus in traffic accident

Pedestrian on ice-skates injured in collision with heavy transport vehicle or bus in traffic accident

Pedestrian on nonmotorized scooter injured in collision with heavy transport vehicle or bus in traffic accident

Pedestrian on sled injured in collision with heavy transport vehicle or bus in traffic accident

Pedestrian on snowboard injured in collision with heavy transport vehicle or bus in traffic accident

Pedestrian on snow-skis injured in collision with heavy transport vehicle or bus in traffic accident

Pedestrian in wheelchair (powered) injured in collision with heavy transport vehicle or bus in traffic accident

Pedestrian in motorized mobility scooter injured in collision with heavy transport vehicle or bus in traffic accident

✓5ᵗʰ **V04.9** **Pedestrian injured in collision with heavy transport vehicle or bus, unspecified whether traffic or nontraffic accident**

✓x 7ᵗʰ **V04.90** **Pedestrian on foot injured in collision with heavy transport vehicle or bus, unspecified whether traffic or nontraffic accident**

Pedestrian NOS injured in collision with heavy transport vehicle or bus, unspecified whether traffic or nontraffic accident

✓x 7ᵗʰ **V04.91** **Pedestrian on roller-skates injured in collision with heavy transport vehicle or bus, unspecified whether traffic or nontraffic accident**

✓x 7ᵗʰ **V04.92** **Pedestrian on skateboard injured in collision with heavy transport vehicle or bus, unspecified whether traffic or nontraffic accident**

✓6ᵗʰ **V04.93** **Pedestrian on standing micro-mobility pedestrian conveyance injured in collision with heavy transport vehicle or bus, unspecified whether traffic or nontraffic accident**

✓7ᵗʰ **V04.931** **Pedestrian on standing electric scooter injured in collision with heavy transport vehicle or bus, unspecified whether traffic or nontraffic accident**

✓7ᵗʰ **V04.938** **Pedestrian on other standing micro-mobility pedestrian conveyance injured in collision with heavy transport vehicle or bus, unspecified whether traffic or nontraffic accident**

Pedestrian on hoverboard injured in collision with heavy transport vehicle or bus, unspecified whether traffic or nontraffic accident

Pedestrian on segway injured in collision with heavy transport vehicle or bus, unspecified whether traffic or nontraffic accident

✓x 7ᵗʰ **V04.99** **Pedestrian with other conveyance injured in collision with heavy transport vehicle or bus, unspecified whether traffic or nontraffic accident**

Pedestrian with baby stroller injured in collision with heavy transport vehicle or bus, unspecified whether traffic or nontraffic accident

Pedestrian on ice-skates injured in collision with heavy transport vehicle or bus, unspecified whether traffic or nontraffic accident

Pedestrian on nonmotorized scooter injured in collision with heavy transport vehicle or bus, unspecified whether traffic or nontraffic accident

Pedestrian on sled injured in collision with heavy transport vehicle or bus, unspecified whether traffic or nontraffic accident

Pedestrian on snowboard injured in collision with heavy transport vehicle or bus, unspecified whether traffic or nontraffic accident

Pedestrian on snow-skis injured in collision with heavy transport vehicle or bus, unspecified whether traffic or nontraffic accident

Pedestrian in wheelchair (powered) injured in collision with heavy transport vehicle or bus, unspecified whether traffic or nontraffic accident

Pedestrian in motorized mobility scooter injured in collision with heavy transport vehicle or bus, unspecified whether traffic or nontraffic accident

✓4ᵗʰ **V05** **Pedestrian injured in collision with railway train or railway vehicle**

✓5ᵗʰ **V05.0** **Pedestrian injured in collision with railway train or railway vehicle in nontraffic accident**

✓x 7ᵗʰ **V05.00** **Pedestrian on foot injured in collision with railway train or railway vehicle in nontraffic accident**

Pedestrian NOS injured in collision with railway train or railway vehicle in nontraffic accident

✓x 7ᵗʰ **V05.01** **Pedestrian on roller-skates injured in collision with railway train or railway vehicle in nontraffic accident**

✓x 7ᵗʰ **V05.02** **Pedestrian on skateboard injured in collision with railway train or railway vehicle in nontraffic accident**

✓6ᵗʰ **V05.03** **Pedestrian on standing micro-mobility pedestrian conveyance injured in collision with railway train or railway vehicle in nontraffic accident**

✓7ᵗʰ **V05.031** **Pedestrian on standing electric scooter injured in collision with railway train or railway vehicle in nontraffic accident**

✓ Additional Char Req   ✓x 7ᵗʰ Placeholder   Unacceptable PDx   Questionable PDx   Wrong Procedure   Manifestation   Unspecified Dx   H1 - H14 HAC   HCC CMS-HCC Dx   HIV HIV Dx

ICD-10-CM 2022   1175

Chapter 20. External Causes of Morbidity

✓7ᵗʰ **V05.038** **Pedestrian on other standing micro-mobility pedestrian conveyance injured in collision with railway train or railway vehicle in nontraffic accident**
> Pedestrian on hoverboard injured in collision with railway train or railway vehicle in nontraffic accident
> Pedestrian on segway injured in collision with railway train or railway vehicle in nontraffic accident

✓×7ᵗʰ **V05.09** **Pedestrian with other conveyance injured in collision with railway train or railway vehicle in nontraffic accident**
> Pedestrian with baby stroller injured in collision with railway train or railway vehicle in nontraffic accident
> Pedestrian on ice-skates injured in collision with railway train or railway vehicle in nontraffic accident
> Pedestrian on nonmotorized scooter injured in collision with railway train or railway vehicle in nontraffic accident
> Pedestrian on sled injured in collision with railway train or railway vehicle in nontraffic accident
> Pedestrian on snowboard injured in collision with railway train or railway vehicle in nontraffic accident
> Pedestrian on snow-skis injured in collision with railway train or railway vehicle in nontraffic accident
> Pedestrian in wheelchair (powered) injured in collision with railway train or railway vehicle in nontraffic accident
> Pedestrian in motorized mobility scooter injured in collision with railway train or railway vehicle in nontraffic accident

✓5ᵗʰ **V05.1** **Pedestrian injured in collision with railway train or railway vehicle in traffic accident**

✓×7ᵗʰ **V05.10** **Pedestrian on foot injured in collision with railway train or railway vehicle in traffic accident**
> Pedestrian NOS injured in collision with railway train or railway vehicle in traffic accident

✓×7ᵗʰ **V05.11** **Pedestrian on roller-skates injured in collision with railway train or railway vehicle in traffic accident**

✓×7ᵗʰ **V05.12** **Pedestrian on skateboard injured in collision with railway train or railway vehicle in traffic accident**

✓6ᵗʰ **V05.13** **Pedestrian on standing micro-mobility pedestrian conveyance injured in collision with railway train or railway vehicle in traffic accident**

    ✓7ᵗʰ **V05.131** **Pedestrian on standing electric scooter injured in collision with railway train or railway vehicle in traffic accident**

    ✓7ᵗʰ **V05.138** **Pedestrian on other standing micro-mobility pedestrian conveyance injured in collision with railway train or railway vehicle in traffic accident**
> Pedestrian on hoverboard injured in collision with railway train or railway vehicle in traffic accident
> Pedestrian on segway injured in collision with railway train or railway vehicle in traffic accident

✓×7ᵗʰ **V05.19** **Pedestrian with other conveyance injured in collision with railway train or railway vehicle in traffic accident**
> Pedestrian with baby stroller injured in collision with railway train or railway vehicle in traffic accident
> Pedestrian on ice-skates injured in collision with railway train or railway vehicle in traffic accident
> Pedestrian on nonmotorized scooter injured in collision with railway train or railway vehicle in traffic accident
> Pedestrian on sled injured in collision with railway train or railway vehicle in traffic accident
> Pedestrian on snowboard injured in collision with railway train or railway vehicle in traffic accident
> Pedestrian on snow-skis injured in collision with railway train or railway vehicle in traffic accident
> Pedestrian in wheelchair (powered) injured in collision with railway train or railway vehicle in traffic accident
> Pedestrian in motorized mobility scooter injured in collision with railway train or railway vehicle in traffic accident

✓5ᵗʰ **V05.9** **Pedestrian injured in collision with railway train or railway vehicle, unspecified whether traffic or nontraffic accident**

✓×7ᵗʰ **V05.90** **Pedestrian on foot injured in collision with railway train or railway vehicle, unspecified whether traffic or nontraffic accident**
> Pedestrian NOS injured in collision with railway train or railway vehicle, unspecified whether traffic or nontraffic accident

✓×7ᵗʰ **V05.91** **Pedestrian on roller-skates injured in collision with railway train or railway vehicle, unspecified whether traffic or nontraffic accident**

✓×7ᵗʰ **V05.92** **Pedestrian on skateboard injured in collision with railway train or railway vehicle, unspecified whether traffic or nontraffic accident**

✓6ᵗʰ **V05.93** **Pedestrian on standing micro-mobility pedestrian conveyance injured in collision with railway train or railway vehicle, unspecified whether traffic or nontraffic accident**

    ✓7ᵗʰ **V05.931** **Pedestrian on standing electric scooter injured in collision with railway train or railway vehicle, unspecified whether traffic or nontraffic accident**

    ✓7ᵗʰ **V05.938** **Pedestrian on other standing micro-mobility pedestrian conveyance injured in collision with railway train or railway vehicle, unspecified whether traffic or nontraffic accident**
> Pedestrian on hoverboard injured in collision with railway train or railway vehicle, unspecified whether traffic or nontraffic accident
> Pedestrian on segway injured in collision with railway train or railway vehicle, unspecified whether traffic or nontraffic accident

Ⓝ Newborn: 0   Ⓟ Pediatric: 0-17   Ⓜ Maternity: 9-64   Ⓐ Adult: 15-124   **MCC** Major Complication/Comorbidity   **CC** Complication/Comorbidity   **SW** Severe Wound Dx

1176   ICD-10-CM 2022

√x7ᵗʰ **V05.99** **Pedestrian with other conveyance injured in collision with railway train or railway vehicle, unspecified whether traffic or nontraffic accident**

Pedestrian with baby stroller injured in collision with railway train or railway vehicle, unspecified whether traffic or nontraffic

Pedestrian on ice-skates injured in collision with railway train or railway vehicle, unspecified whether traffic or nontraffic

Pedestrian on nonmotorized scooter injured in collision with railway train or railway vehicle, unspecified whether traffic or nontraffic

Pedestrian on sled injured in collision with railway train or railway vehicle, unspecified whether traffic or nontraffic

Pedestrian on snowboard injured in collision with railway train or railway vehicle, unspecified whether traffic or nontraffic

Pedestrian on snow-skis injured in collision with railway train or railway vehicle, unspecified whether traffic or nontraffic

Pedestrian in wheelchair (powered) injured in collision with railway train or railway vehicle, unspecified whether traffic or nontraffic

Pedestrian in motorized mobility scooter injured in collision with railway train or railway vehicle, unspecified whether traffic or nontraffic

√4ᵗʰ **V06** **Pedestrian injured in collision with other nonmotor vehicle**

     INCLUDES   collision with animal-drawn vehicle, animal being ridden, nonpowered streetcar

     EXCLUDES 1   *pedestrian injured in collision with pedestrian conveyance (V00.0-)*

√5ᵗʰ **V06.0** **Pedestrian injured in collision with other nonmotor vehicle in nontraffic accident**

√x7ᵗʰ **V06.00** **Pedestrian on foot injured in collision with other nonmotor vehicle in nontraffic accident**

Pedestrian NOS injured in collision with other nonmotor vehicle in nontraffic accident

√x7ᵗʰ **V06.01** **Pedestrian on roller-skates injured in collision with other nonmotor vehicle in nontraffic accident**

√x7ᵗʰ **V06.02** **Pedestrian on skateboard injured in collision with other nonmotor vehicle in nontraffic accident**

√6ᵗʰ **V06.03** **Pedestrian on standing micro-mobility pedestrian conveyance injured in collision with other nonmotor vehicle in nontraffic accident**

√7ᵗʰ **V06.031** **Pedestrian on standing electric scooter injured in collision with other nonmotor vehicle in nontraffic accident**

√7ᵗʰ **V06.038** **Pedestrian on other standing micro-mobility pedestrian conveyance injured in collision with other nonmotor vehicle in nontraffic accident**

Pedestrian on hoverboard injured in collision with other nonmotor vehicle in nontraffic accident

Pedestrian on segway injured in collision with other nonmotor vehicle in nontraffic accident

√x7ᵗʰ **V06.09** **Pedestrian with other conveyance injured in collision with other nonmotor vehicle in nontraffic accident**

Pedestrian with baby stroller injured in collision with other nonmotor vehicle in nontraffic accident

Pedestrian on ice-skates injured in collision with other nonmotor vehicle in nontraffic accident

Pedestrian on nonmotorized scooter injured in collision with other nonmotor vehicle in nontraffic accident

Pedestrian on sled injured in collision with other nonmotor vehicle in nontraffic accident

Pedestrian on snowboard injured in collision with other nonmotor vehicle in nontraffic accident

Pedestrian on snow-skis injured in collision with other nonmotor vehicle in nontraffic accident

Pedestrian in wheelchair (powered) injured in collision with other nonmotor vehicle in nontraffic accident

Pedestrian in motorized mobility scooter injured in collision with other nonmotor vehicle in nontraffic accident

√5ᵗʰ **V06.1** **Pedestrian injured in collision with other nonmotor vehicle in traffic accident**

√x7ᵗʰ **V06.10** **Pedestrian on foot injured in collision with other nonmotor vehicle in traffic accident**

Pedestrian NOS injured in collision with other nonmotor vehicle in traffic accident

√x7ᵗʰ **V06.11** **Pedestrian on roller-skates injured in collision with other nonmotor vehicle in traffic accident**

√x7ᵗʰ **V06.12** **Pedestrian on skateboard injured in collision with other nonmotor vehicle in traffic accident**

√6ᵗʰ **V06.13** **Pedestrian on standing micro-mobility pedestrian conveyance injured in collision with other nonmotor vehicle in traffic accident**

√7ᵗʰ **V06.131** **Pedestrian on standing electric scooter injured in collision with other nonmotor vehicle in traffic accident**

√7ᵗʰ **V06.138** **Pedestrian on other standing micro-mobility pedestrian conveyance injured in collision with other nonmotor vehicle in traffic accident**

Pedestrian on hoverboard injured in collision with other nonmotor vehicle in traffic accident

Pedestrian on segway injured in collision with other nonmotor vehicle in traffic accident

√x7ᵗʰ **V06.19** **Pedestrian with other conveyance injured in collision with other nonmotor vehicle in traffic accident**

Pedestrian with baby stroller injured in collision with other nonmotor vehicle in nontraffic accident

Pedestrian on ice-skates injured in collision with other nonmotor vehicle in traffic accident

Pedestrian on nonmotorized scooter injured in collision with other nonmotor vehicle in traffic accident

Pedestrian on sled injured in collision with other nonmotor vehicle in traffic accident

Pedestrian on snowboard injured in collision with other nonmotor vehicle in traffic accident

Pedestrian on snow-skis injured in collision with other nonmotor vehicle in traffic accident

Pedestrian in wheelchair (powered) injured in collision with other nonmotor vehicle in traffic accident

Pedestrian in motorized mobility scooter injured in collision with other nonmotor vehicle in traffic accident

√5ᵗʰ **V06.9** **Pedestrian injured in collision with other nonmotor vehicle, unspecified whether traffic or nontraffic accident**

√x7ᵗʰ **V06.90** **Pedestrian on foot injured in collision with other nonmotor vehicle, unspecified whether traffic or nontraffic accident**

Pedestrian NOS injured in collision with other nonmotor vehicle, unspecified whether traffic or nontraffic accident

√x7ᵗʰ **V06.91** **Pedestrian on roller-skates injured in collision with other nonmotor vehicle, unspecified whether traffic or nontraffic accident**

✓ Additional Char Req   √x7ᵗʰ Placeholder   Unacceptable PDx   Questionable PDx   Wrong Procedure   Manifestation   Unspecified Dx   H1-H14 HAC   HCC CMS-HCC Dx   HIV HIV Dx

ICD-10-CM 2022   1177

Chapter 20. External Causes of Morbidity

V05.99–V06.91

√x7ᵗʰ **V06.92** **Pedestrian** on skateboard **injured in collision with other nonmotor vehicle, unspecified whether traffic or nontraffic accident**

√6ᵗʰ **V06.93** **Pedestrian on standing micro-mobility pedestrian conveyance injured in collision with other nonmotor vehicle, unspecified whether traffic or nontraffic accident**

√7ᵗʰ **V06.931** **Pedestrian** on standing electric scooter **injured in collision with other nonmotor vehicle, unspecified whether traffic or nontraffic accident**

√7ᵗʰ **V06.938** **Pedestrian on other standing micro-mobility pedestrian conveyance injured in collision with other nonmotor vehicle, unspecified whether traffic or nontraffic accident**

Pedestrian on hoverboard injured in collision with other nonmotor, unspecified whether traffic or nontraffic accident

Pedestrian on segway injured in collision with other nonmotor vehicle, unspecified whether traffic or nontraffic accident

√x7ᵗʰ **V06.99** **Pedestrian with other conveyance injured in collision with other nonmotor vehicle, unspecified whether traffic or nontraffic accident**

Pedestrian with baby stroller injured in collision with other nonmotor vehicle, unspecified whether traffic or nontraffic accident

Pedestrian on ice-skates injured in collision with other nonmotor vehicle, unspecified whether traffic or nontraffic accident

Pedestrian on nonmotorized scooter injured in collision with other nonmotor vehicle, unspecified whether traffic or nontraffic accident

Pedestrian on sled injured in collision with other nonmotor vehicle, unspecified whether traffic or nontraffic accident

Pedestrian on snowboard injured in collision with other nonmotor vehicle, unspecified whether traffic or nontraffic accident

Pedestrian on snow-skis injured in collision with other nonmotor vehicle, unspecified whether traffic or nontraffic accident

Pedestrian in wheelchair (powered) injured in collision with other nonmotor vehicle, unspecified whether traffic or nontraffic accident

Pedestrian in motorized mobility scooter injured in collision with other nonmotorized vehicle, unspecified whether traffic or nontraffic accident

√4ᵗʰ **V09** **Pedestrian injured in other and unspecified transport accidents**

√5ᵗʰ **V09.0** **Pedestrian injured in** nontraffic **accident involving other and unspecified motor vehicles**

√7ᵗʰ **V09.00** **Pedestrian injured in nontraffic accident involving unspecified motor vehicles**

√x7ᵗʰ **V09.01** **Pedestrian injured in nontraffic accident involving** military vehicle

√x7ᵗʰ **V09.09** **Pedestrian injured in nontraffic accident involving other motor vehicles**

Pedestrian injured in nontraffic accident by special vehicle

√x7ᵗʰ **V09.1** **Pedestrian injured in unspecified** nontraffic **accident**

√5ᵗʰ **V09.2** **Pedestrian injured in** traffic accident **involving other and unspecified motor vehicles**

√x7ᵗʰ **V09.20** **Pedestrian injured in traffic accident involving unspecified motor vehicles**

√x7ᵗʰ **V09.21** **Pedestrian injured in traffic accident involving** military vehicle

√x7ᵗʰ **V09.29** **Pedestrian injured in traffic accident involving other motor vehicles**

√x7ᵗʰ **V09.3** **Pedestrian injured in unspecified** traffic **accident**

√x7ᵗʰ **V09.9** **Pedestrian injured in unspecified** transport **accident**

Pedal cycle rider injured in transport accident (V10-V19)

INCLUDES   any non-motorized vehicle, excluding an animal-drawn vehicle, or a sidecar or trailer attached to the pedal cycle

EXCLUDES 2   *rupture of pedal cycle tire (W37.0)*

The appropriate 7th character is to be added to each code from categories V10-V19.
A   initial encounter
D   subsequent encounter
S   sequela

√4ᵗʰ **V10** **Pedal cycle rider injured in collision with pedestrian or animal**

EXCLUDES 1   *pedal cycle rider collision with animal-drawn vehicle or animal being ridden (V16.-)*

√x7ᵗʰ **V10.0** **Pedal cycle** driver **injured in collision with pedestrian or animal** in nontraffic accident

√x7ᵗʰ **V10.1** **Pedal cycle** passenger **injured in collision with pedestrian or animal** in nontraffic accident

√x7ᵗʰ **V10.2** **Unspecified pedal cyclist injured in collision with pedestrian or animal** in nontraffic accident

√x7ᵗʰ **V10.3** Person boarding or alighting **a pedal cycle injured in collision with pedestrian or animal**

√x7ᵗʰ **V10.4** **Pedal cycle** driver **injured in collision with pedestrian or animal** in traffic accident

√x7ᵗʰ **V10.5** **Pedal cycle** passenger **injured in collision with pedestrian or animal** in traffic accident

√x7ᵗʰ **V10.9** **Unspecified pedal cyclist injured in collision with pedestrian or animal** in traffic accident

√4ᵗʰ **V11** **Pedal cycle rider injured in collision with other pedal cycle**

√x7ᵗʰ **V11.0** **Pedal cycle** driver **injured in collision with other pedal cycle** in nontraffic accident

√x7ᵗʰ **V11.1** **Pedal cycle** passenger **injured in collision with other pedal cycle** in nontraffic accident

√x7ᵗʰ **V11.2** **Unspecified pedal cyclist injured in collision with other pedal cycle** in nontraffic accident

√x7ᵗʰ **V11.3** Person boarding or alighting **a pedal cycle injured in collision with other pedal cycle**

√x7ᵗʰ **V11.4** **Pedal cycle** driver **injured in collision with other pedal cycle** in traffic accident

√x7ᵗʰ **V11.5** **Pedal cycle** passenger **injured in collision with other pedal cycle** in traffic accident

√x7ᵗʰ **V11.9** **Unspecified pedal cyclist injured in collision with other pedal cycle** in traffic accident

√4ᵗʰ **V12** **Pedal cycle rider injured in collision with two- or three-wheeled motor vehicle**

√x7ᵗʰ **V12.0** **Pedal cycle** driver **injured in collision with two- or three-wheeled motor vehicle** in nontraffic accident

√x7ᵗʰ **V12.1** **Pedal cycle** passenger **injured in collision with two- or three-wheeled motor vehicle** in nontraffic accident

√x7ᵗʰ **V12.2** **Unspecified pedal cyclist injured in collision with two- or three-wheeled motor vehicle** in nontraffic accident

√x7ᵗʰ **V12.3** Person boarding or alighting **a pedal cycle injured in collision with two- or three-wheeled motor vehicle**

√x7ᵗʰ **V12.4** **Pedal cycle** driver **injured in collision with two- or three-wheeled motor vehicle** in traffic accident

√x7ᵗʰ **V12.5** **Pedal cycle** passenger **injured in collision with two- or three-wheeled motor vehicle** in traffic accident

√x7ᵗʰ **V12.9** **Unspecified pedal cyclist injured in collision with two- or three-wheeled motor vehicle** in traffic accident

√4ᵗʰ **V13** **Pedal cycle rider injured in collision with car, pick-up truck or van**

√x7ᵗʰ **V13.0** **Pedal cycle** driver **injured in collision with car, pick-up truck or van** in nontraffic accident

√x7ᵗʰ **V13.1** **Pedal cycle** passenger **injured in collision with car, pick-up truck or van** in nontraffic accident

√x7ᵗʰ **V13.2** **Unspecified pedal cyclist injured in collision with car, pick-up truck or van** in nontraffic accident

√x7ᵗʰ **V13.3** Person boarding or alighting **a pedal cycle injured in collision with car, pick-up truck or van**

√x7ᵗʰ **V13.4** **Pedal cycle** driver **injured in collision with car, pick-up truck or van** in traffic accident

√x7ᵗʰ **V13.5** **Pedal cycle** passenger **injured in collision with car, pick-up truck or van** in traffic accident

√x7ᵗʰ **V13.9** **Unspecified pedal cyclist injured in collision with car, pick-up truck or van** in traffic accident

√4ᵗʰ **V14** **Pedal cycle rider injured in collision with heavy transport vehicle or bus**

EXCLUDES 1   *pedal cycle rider injured in collision with military vehicle (V19.81)*

√x7ᵗʰ **V14.0** **Pedal cycle** driver **injured in collision with heavy transport vehicle or bus** in nontraffic accident

---

Ⓝ Newborn: 0   Ⓟ Pediatric: 0-17   Ⓜ Maternity: 9-64   Ⓐ Adult: 15-124   **MCC** Major Complication/Comorbidity   **CC** Complication/Comorbidity   **SW** Severe Wound Dx

1178   ICD-10-CM 2022

√x7ᵗʰ **V14.1** Pedal cycle passenger injured in collision with heavy transport vehicle or bus in nontraffic accident

√x7ᵗʰ **V14.2** Unspecified pedal cyclist injured in collision with heavy transport vehicle or bus in nontraffic accident

√x7ᵗʰ **V14.3** Person boarding or alighting a pedal cycle injured in collision with heavy transport vehicle or bus

√x7ᵗʰ **V14.4** Pedal cycle driver injured in collision with heavy transport vehicle or bus in traffic accident

√x7ᵗʰ **V14.5** Pedal cycle passenger injured in collision with heavy transport vehicle or bus in traffic accident

√x7ᵗʰ **V14.9** Unspecified pedal cyclist injured in collision with heavy transport vehicle or bus in traffic accident

√4ᵗʰ **V15** Pedal cycle rider injured in collision with railway train or railway vehicle

√x7ᵗʰ **V15.0** Pedal cycle driver injured in collision with railway train or railway vehicle in nontraffic accident

√x7ᵗʰ **V15.1** Pedal cycle passenger injured in collision with railway train or railway vehicle in nontraffic accident

√x7ᵗʰ **V15.2** Unspecified pedal cyclist injured in collision with railway train or railway vehicle in nontraffic accident

√x7ᵗʰ **V15.3** Person boarding or alighting a pedal cycle injured in collision with railway train or railway vehicle

√x7ᵗʰ **V15.4** Pedal cycle driver injured in collision with railway train or railway vehicle in traffic accident

√x7ᵗʰ **V15.5** Pedal cycle passenger injured in collision with railway train or railway vehicle in traffic accident

√x7ᵗʰ **V15.9** Unspecified pedal cyclist injured in collision with railway train or railway vehicle in traffic accident

√4ᵗʰ **V16** Pedal cycle rider injured in collision with other nonmotor vehicle

     INCLUDES   collision with animal-drawn vehicle, animal being ridden, streetcar

√x7ᵗʰ **V16.0** Pedal cycle driver injured in collision with other nonmotor vehicle in nontraffic accident

√x7ᵗʰ **V16.1** Pedal cycle passenger injured in collision with other nonmotor vehicle in nontraffic accident

√x7ᵗʰ **V16.2** Unspecified pedal cyclist injured in collision with other nonmotor vehicle in nontraffic accident

√x7ᵗʰ **V16.3** Person boarding or alighting a pedal cycle injured in collision with other nonmotor vehicle in nontraffic accident

√x7ᵗʰ **V16.4** Pedal cycle driver injured in collision with other nonmotor vehicle in traffic accident

√x7ᵗʰ **V16.5** Pedal cycle passenger injured in collision with other nonmotor vehicle in traffic accident

√x7ᵗʰ **V16.9** Unspecified pedal cyclist injured in collision with other nonmotor vehicle in traffic accident

√4ᵗʰ **V17** Pedal cycle rider injured in collision with fixed or stationary object

√x7ᵗʰ **V17.0** Pedal cycle driver injured in collision with fixed or stationary object in nontraffic accident

√x7ᵗʰ **V17.1** Pedal cycle passenger injured in collision with fixed or stationary object in nontraffic accident

√x7ᵗʰ **V17.2** Unspecified pedal cyclist injured in collision with fixed or stationary object in nontraffic accident

√x7ᵗʰ **V17.3** Person boarding or alighting a pedal cycle injured in collision with fixed or stationary object

√x7ᵗʰ **V17.4** Pedal cycle driver injured in collision with fixed or stationary object in traffic accident

√x7ᵗʰ **V17.5** Pedal cycle passenger injured in collision with fixed or stationary object in traffic accident

√x7ᵗʰ **V17.9** Unspecified pedal cyclist injured in collision with fixed or stationary object in traffic accident

√4ᵗʰ **V18** Pedal cycle rider injured in noncollision transport accident

     INCLUDES   fall or thrown from pedal cycle (without antecedent collision)
         overturning pedal cycle NOS
         overturning pedal cycle without collision

√x7ᵗʰ **V18.0** Pedal cycle driver injured in noncollision transport accident in nontraffic accident

√x7ᵗʰ **V18.1** Pedal cycle passenger injured in noncollision transport accident in nontraffic accident

√x7ᵗʰ **V18.2** Unspecified pedal cyclist injured in noncollision transport accident in nontraffic accident

√x7ᵗʰ **V18.3** Person boarding or alighting a pedal cycle injured in noncollision transport accident

√x7ᵗʰ **V18.4** Pedal cycle driver injured in noncollision transport accident in traffic accident

√x7ᵗʰ **V18.5** Pedal cycle passenger injured in noncollision transport accident in traffic accident

√x7ᵗʰ **V18.9** Unspecified pedal cyclist injured in noncollision transport accident in traffic accident

√4ᵗʰ **V19** Pedal cycle rider injured in other and unspecified transport accidents

√5ᵗʰ **V19.0** Pedal cycle driver injured in collision with other and unspecified motor vehicles in nontraffic accident

√x7ᵗʰ **V19.00** Pedal cycle driver injured in collision with unspecified motor vehicles in nontraffic accident

√x7ᵗʰ **V19.09** Pedal cycle driver injured in collision with other motor vehicles in nontraffic accident

√5ᵗʰ **V19.1** Pedal cycle passenger injured in collision with other and unspecified motor vehicles in nontraffic accident

√x7ᵗʰ **V19.10** Pedal cycle passenger injured in collision with unspecified motor vehicles in nontraffic accident

√x7ᵗʰ **V19.19** Pedal cycle passenger injured in collision with other motor vehicles in nontraffic accident

√5ᵗʰ **V19.2** Unspecified pedal cyclist injured in collision with other and unspecified motor vehicles in nontraffic accident

√x7ᵗʰ **V19.20** Unspecified pedal cyclist injured in collision with unspecified motor vehicles in nontraffic accident
         Pedal cycle collision NOS, nontraffic

√x7ᵗʰ **V19.29** Unspecified pedal cyclist injured in collision with other motor vehicles in nontraffic accident

√5ᵗʰ **V19.3** Pedal cyclist (driver) (passenger) injured in unspecified nontraffic accident
         Pedal cycle accident NOS, nontraffic
         Pedal cyclist injured in nontraffic accident NOS

√5ᵗʰ **V19.4** Pedal cycle driver injured in collision with other and unspecified motor vehicles in traffic accident

√x7ᵗʰ **V19.40** Pedal cycle driver injured in collision with unspecified motor vehicles in traffic accident

√x7ᵗʰ **V19.49** Pedal cycle driver injured in collision with other motor vehicles in traffic accident

√5ᵗʰ **V19.5** Pedal cycle passenger injured in collision with other and unspecified motor vehicles in traffic accident

√x7ᵗʰ **V19.50** Pedal cycle passenger injured in collision with unspecified motor vehicles in traffic accident

√x7ᵗʰ **V19.59** Pedal cycle passenger injured in collision with other motor vehicles in traffic accident

√5ᵗʰ **V19.6** Unspecified pedal cyclist injured in collision with other and unspecified motor vehicles in traffic accident

√x7ᵗʰ **V19.60** Unspecified pedal cyclist injured in collision with unspecified motor vehicles in traffic accident
         Pedal cycle collision NOS (traffic)

√x7ᵗʰ **V19.69** Unspecified pedal cyclist injured in collision with other motor vehicles in traffic accident

√5ᵗʰ **V19.8** Pedal cyclist (driver) (passenger) injured in other specified transport accidents

√x7ᵗʰ **V19.81** Pedal cyclist (driver) (passenger) injured in transport accident with military vehicle

√x7ᵗʰ **V19.88** Pedal cyclist (driver) (passenger) injured in other specified transport accidents

√x7ᵗʰ **V19.9** Pedal cyclist (driver) (passenger) injured in unspecified traffic accident
         Pedal cycle accident NOS

Motorcycle rider injured in transport accident (V20-V29)

     INCLUDES   moped
         motorcycle with sidecar
         motorized bicycle
         motor scooter
     EXCLUDES 1   *three-wheeled motor vehicle (V30-V39)*

The appropriate 7th character is to be added to each code from categories V20-V29.
A   initial encounter
D   subsequent encounter
S   sequela

√4ᵗʰ **V20** Motorcycle rider injured in collision with pedestrian or animal

     EXCLUDES 1   *motorcycle rider collision with animal-drawn vehicle or animal being ridden (V26.-)*

√x7ᵗʰ **V20.0** Motorcycle driver injured in collision with pedestrian or animal in nontraffic accident

√x7ᵗʰ **V20.1** Motorcycle passenger injured in collision with pedestrian or animal in nontraffic accident

√x7ᵗʰ **V20.2** Unspecified motorcycle rider injured in collision with pedestrian or animal in nontraffic accident

√x7ᵗʰ **V20.3** Person boarding or alighting a motorcycle injured in collision with pedestrian or animal

√x7ᵗʰ **V20.4** Motorcycle driver injured in collision with pedestrian or animal in traffic accident

√x7ᵗʰ **V20.5** Motorcycle passenger injured in collision with pedestrian or animal in traffic accident

√x 7th **V20.9** Unspecified motorcycle rider injured in collision with pedestrian or animal in traffic accident

√4th **V21** Motorcycle rider injured in collision with pedal cycle

√x 7th **V21.0** Motorcycle driver injured in collision with pedal cycle in nontraffic accident

√x 7th **V21.1** Motorcycle passenger injured in collision with pedal cycle in nontraffic accident

√x 7th **V21.2** Unspecified motorcycle rider injured in collision with pedal cycle in nontraffic accident

√x 7th **V21.3** Person boarding or alighting a motorcycle injured in collision with pedal cycle

√x 7th **V21.4** Motorcycle driver injured in collision with pedal cycle in traffic accident

√x 7th **V21.5** Motorcycle passenger injured in collision with pedal cycle in traffic accident

√x 7th **V21.9** Unspecified motorcycle rider injured in collision with pedal cycle in traffic accident

√4th **V22** Motorcycle rider injured in collision with two- or three-wheeled motor vehicle

√x 7th **V22.0** Motorcycle driver injured in collision with two- or three-wheeled motor vehicle in nontraffic accident

√x 7th **V22.1** Motorcycle passenger injured in collision with two- or three-wheeled motor vehicle in nontraffic accident

√x 7th **V22.2** Unspecified motorcycle rider injured in collision with two- or three-wheeled motor vehicle in nontraffic accident

√x 7th **V22.3** Person boarding or alighting a motorcycle injured in collision with two- or three-wheeled motor vehicle

√x 7th **V22.4** Motorcycle driver injured in collision with two- or three-wheeled motor vehicle in traffic accident

√x 7th **V22.5** Motorcycle passenger injured in collision with two- or three-wheeled motor vehicle in traffic accident

√x 7th **V22.9** Unspecified motorcycle rider injured in collision with two- or three-wheeled motor vehicle in traffic accident

√4th **V23** Motorcycle rider injured in collision with car, pick-up truck or van

√x 7th **V23.0** Motorcycle driver injured in collision with car, pick-up truck or van in nontraffic accident

√x 7th **V23.1** Motorcycle passenger injured in collision with car, pick-up truck or van in nontraffic accident

√x 7th **V23.2** Unspecified motorcycle rider injured in collision with car, pick-up truck or van in nontraffic accident

√x 7th **V23.3** Person boarding or alighting a motorcycle injured in collision with car, pick-up truck or van

√x 7th **V23.4** Motorcycle driver injured in collision with car, pick-up truck or van in traffic accident

√x 7th **V23.5** Motorcycle passenger injured in collision with car, pick-up truck or van in traffic accident

√x 7th **V23.9** Unspecified motorcycle rider injured in collision with car, pick-up truck or van in traffic accident

√4th **V24** Motorcycle rider injured in collision with heavy transport vehicle or bus

    EXCLUDES 1   *motorcycle rider injured in collision with military vehicle (V29.81)*

√x 7th **V24.0** Motorcycle driver injured in collision with heavy transport vehicle or bus in nontraffic accident

√x 7th **V24.1** Motorcycle passenger injured in collision with heavy transport vehicle or bus in nontraffic accident

√x 7th **V24.2** Unspecified motorcycle rider injured in collision with heavy transport vehicle or bus in nontraffic accident

√x 7th **V24.3** Person boarding or alighting a motorcycle injured in collision with heavy transport vehicle or bus

√x 7th **V24.4** Motorcycle driver injured in collision with heavy transport vehicle or bus in traffic accident

√x 7th **V24.5** Motorcycle passenger injured in collision with heavy transport vehicle or bus in traffic accident

√x 7th **V24.9** Unspecified motorcycle rider injured in collision with heavy transport vehicle or bus in traffic accident

√4th **V25** Motorcycle rider injured in collision with railway train or railway vehicle

√x 7th **V25.0** Motorcycle driver injured in collision with railway train or railway vehicle in nontraffic accident

√x 7th **V25.1** Motorcycle passenger injured in collision with railway train or railway vehicle in nontraffic accident

√x 7th **V25.2** Unspecified motorcycle rider injured in collision with railway train or railway vehicle in nontraffic accident

√x 7th **V25.3** Person boarding or alighting a motorcycle injured in collision with railway train or railway vehicle

√x 7th **V25.4** Motorcycle driver injured in collision with railway train or railway vehicle in traffic accident

√x 7th **V25.5** Motorcycle passenger injured in collision with railway train or railway vehicle in traffic accident

√x 7th **V25.9** Unspecified motorcycle rider injured in collision with railway train or railway vehicle in traffic accident

√4th **V26** Motorcycle rider injured in collision with other nonmotor vehicle

    INCLUDES   collision with animal-drawn vehicle, animal being ridden, streetcar

√x 7th **V26.0** Motorcycle driver injured in collision with other nonmotor vehicle in nontraffic accident

√x 7th **V26.1** Motorcycle passenger injured in collision with other nonmotor vehicle in nontraffic accident

√x 7th **V26.2** Unspecified motorcycle rider injured in collision with other nonmotor vehicle in nontraffic accident

√x 7th **V26.3** Person boarding or alighting a motorcycle injured in collision with other nonmotor vehicle

√x 7th **V26.4** Motorcycle driver injured in collision with other nonmotor vehicle in traffic accident

√x 7th **V26.5** Motorcycle passenger injured in collision with other nonmotor vehicle in traffic accident

√x 7th **V26.9** Unspecified motorcycle rider injured in collision with other nonmotor vehicle in traffic accident

√4th **V27** Motorcycle rider injured in collision with fixed or stationary object

√x 7th **V27.0** Motorcycle driver injured in collision with fixed or stationary object in nontraffic accident

√x 7th **V27.1** Motorcycle passenger injured in collision with fixed or stationary object in nontraffic accident

√x 7th **V27.2** Unspecified motorcycle rider injured in collision with fixed or stationary object in nontraffic accident

√x 7th **V27.3** Person boarding or alighting a motorcycle injured in collision with fixed or stationary object

√x 7th **V27.4** Motorcycle driver injured in collision with fixed or stationary object in traffic accident

√x 7th **V27.5** Motorcycle passenger injured in collision with fixed or stationary object in traffic accident

√x 7th **V27.9** Unspecified motorcycle rider injured in collision with fixed or stationary object in traffic accident

√4th **V28** Motorcycle rider injured in noncollision transport accident

    INCLUDES   fall or thrown from motorcycle (without antecedent collision)
               overturning motorcycle NOS
               overturning motorcycle without collision

√x 7th **V28.0** Motorcycle driver injured in noncollision transport accident in nontraffic accident

√x 7th **V28.1** Motorcycle passenger injured in noncollision transport accident in nontraffic accident

√x 7th **V28.2** Unspecified motorcycle rider injured in noncollision transport accident in nontraffic accident

√x 7th **V28.3** Person boarding or alighting a motorcycle injured in noncollision transport accident

√x 7th **V28.4** Motorcycle driver injured in noncollision transport accident in traffic accident

√x 7th **V28.5** Motorcycle passenger injured in noncollision transport accident in traffic accident

√x 7th **V28.9** Unspecified motorcycle rider injured in noncollision transport accident in traffic accident

√4th **V29** Motorcycle rider injured in other and unspecified transport accidents

√5th **V29.0** Motorcycle driver injured in collision with other and unspecified motor vehicles in nontraffic accident

√x 7th **V29.00** Motorcycle driver injured in collision with unspecified motor vehicles in nontraffic accident

√x 7th **V29.09** Motorcycle driver injured in collision with other motor vehicles in nontraffic accident

√5th **V29.1** Motorcycle passenger injured in collision with other and unspecified motor vehicles in nontraffic accident

√x 7th **V29.10** Motorcycle passenger injured in collision with unspecified motor vehicles in nontraffic accident

√x 7th **V29.19** Motorcycle passenger injured in collision with other motor vehicles in nontraffic accident

√5th **V29.2** Unspecified motorcycle rider injured in collision with other and unspecified motor vehicles in nontraffic accident

√x 7th **V29.20** Unspecified motorcycle rider injured in collision with unspecified motor vehicles in nontraffic accident

         Motorcycle collision NOS, nontraffic

√x 7th **V29.29** Unspecified motorcycle rider injured in collision with other motor vehicles in nontraffic accident

N Newborn: 0   P Pediatric: 0-17   M Maternity: 9-64   A Adult: 15-124   MCC Major Complication/Comorbidity   CC Complication/Comorbidity   SW Severe Wound Dx

1180   ICD-10-CM 2022

V20.9–V29.29

√7th **V29.3** Motorcycle rider (driver) (passenger) injured in unspecified nontraffic accident
     Motorcycle accident NOS, nontraffic
     Motorcycle rider injured in nontraffic accident NOS

√5th **V29.4** Motorcycle driver injured in collision with other and unspecified motor vehicles in traffic accident

     √7th **V29.40** Motorcycle driver injured in collision with unspecified motor vehicles in traffic accident

     √7th **V29.49** Motorcycle driver injured in collision with other motor vehicles in traffic accident

√5th **V29.5** Motorcycle passenger injured in collision with other and unspecified motor vehicles in traffic accident

     √7th **V29.50** Motorcycle passenger injured in collision with unspecified motor vehicles in traffic accident

     √7th **V29.59** Motorcycle passenger injured in collision with other motor vehicles in traffic accident

√5th **V29.6** Unspecified motorcycle rider injured in collision with other and unspecified motor vehicles in traffic accident

     √7th **V29.60** Unspecified motorcycle rider injured in collision with unspecified motor vehicles in traffic accident
         Motorcycle collision NOS (traffic)

     √7th **V29.69** Unspecified motorcycle rider injured in collision with other motor vehicles in traffic accident

√5th **V29.8** Motorcycle rider (driver) (passenger) injured in other specified transport accidents

     √7th **V29.81** Motorcycle rider (driver) (passenger) injured in transport accident with military vehicle

     √7th **V29.88** Motorcycle rider (driver) (passenger) injured in other specified transport accidents

√7th **V29.9** Motorcycle rider (driver) (passenger) injured in unspecified traffic accident
     Motorcycle accident NOS

Occupant of three-wheeled motor vehicle injured in transport accident (V30-V39)

INCLUDES   motorized tricycle
         motorized rickshaw
         three-wheeled motor car
EXCLUDES 1   all-terrain vehicles (V86.-)
         motorcycle with sidecar (V20-V29)
         vehicle designed primarily for off-road use (V86.-)

The appropriate 7th character is to be added to each code from categories V30-V39.
A   initial encounter
D   subsequent encounter
S   sequela

√4th **V30** Occupant of three-wheeled motor vehicle injured in collision with pedestrian or animal
     EXCLUDES 1   three-wheeled motor vehicle collision with animal-drawn vehicle or animal being ridden (V36.-)

     √7th **V30.0** Driver of three-wheeled motor vehicle injured in collision with pedestrian or animal in nontraffic accident

     √7th **V30.1** Passenger in three-wheeled motor vehicle injured in collision with pedestrian or animal in nontraffic accident

     √7th **V30.2** Person on outside of three-wheeled motor vehicle injured in collision with pedestrian or animal in nontraffic accident

     √7th **V30.3** Unspecified occupant of three-wheeled motor vehicle injured in collision with pedestrian or animal in nontraffic accident

     √7th **V30.4** Person boarding or alighting a three-wheeled motor vehicle injured in collision with pedestrian or animal

     √7th **V30.5** Driver of three-wheeled motor vehicle injured in collision with pedestrian or animal in traffic accident

     √7th **V30.6** Passenger in three-wheeled motor vehicle injured in collision with pedestrian or animal in traffic accident

     √7th **V30.7** Person on outside of three-wheeled motor vehicle injured in collision with pedestrian or animal in traffic accident

     √7th **V30.9** Unspecified occupant of three-wheeled motor vehicle injured in collision with pedestrian or animal in traffic accident

√4th **V31** Occupant of three-wheeled motor vehicle injured in collision with pedal cycle

     √7th **V31.0** Driver of three-wheeled motor vehicle injured in collision with pedal cycle in nontraffic accident

     √7th **V31.1** Passenger in three-wheeled motor vehicle injured in collision with pedal cycle in nontraffic accident

     √7th **V31.2** Person on outside of three-wheeled motor vehicle injured in collision with pedal cycle in nontraffic accident

     √7th **V31.3** Unspecified occupant of three-wheeled motor vehicle injured in collision with pedal cycle in nontraffic accident

     √7th **V31.4** Person boarding or alighting a three-wheeled motor vehicle injured in collision with pedal cycle

     √7th **V31.5** Driver of three-wheeled motor vehicle injured in collision with pedal cycle in traffic accident

     √7th **V31.6** Passenger in three-wheeled motor vehicle injured in collision with pedal cycle in traffic accident

     √7th **V31.7** Person on outside of three-wheeled motor vehicle injured in collision with pedal cycle in traffic accident

     √7th **V31.9** Unspecified occupant of three-wheeled motor vehicle injured in collision with pedal cycle in traffic accident

√4th **V32** Occupant of three-wheeled motor vehicle injured in collision with two- or three-wheeled motor vehicle

     √7th **V32.0** Driver of three-wheeled motor vehicle injured in collision with two- or three-wheeled motor vehicle in nontraffic accident

     √7th **V32.1** Passenger in three-wheeled motor vehicle injured in collision with two- or three-wheeled motor vehicle in nontraffic accident

     √7th **V32.2** Person on outside of three-wheeled motor vehicle injured in collision with two- or three-wheeled motor vehicle in nontraffic accident

     √7th **V32.3** Unspecified occupant of three-wheeled motor vehicle injured in collision with two- or three-wheeled motor vehicle in nontraffic accident

     √7th **V32.4** Person boarding or alighting a three-wheeled motor vehicle injured in collision with two- or three-wheeled motor vehicle

     √7th **V32.5** Driver of three-wheeled motor vehicle injured in collision with two- or three-wheeled motor vehicle in traffic accident

     √7th **V32.6** Passenger in three-wheeled motor vehicle injured in collision with two- or three-wheeled motor vehicle in traffic accident

     √7th **V32.7** Person on outside of three-wheeled motor vehicle injured in collision with two- or three-wheeled motor vehicle in traffic accident

     √7th **V32.9** Unspecified occupant of three-wheeled motor vehicle injured in collision with two- or three-wheeled motor vehicle in traffic accident

√4th **V33** Occupant of three-wheeled motor vehicle injured in collision with car, pick-up truck or van

     √7th **V33.0** Driver of three-wheeled motor vehicle injured in collision with car, pick-up truck or van in nontraffic accident

     √7th **V33.1** Passenger in three-wheeled motor vehicle injured in collision with car, pick-up truck or van in nontraffic accident

     √7th **V33.2** Person on outside of three-wheeled motor vehicle injured in collision with car, pick-up truck or van in nontraffic accident

     √7th **V33.3** Unspecified occupant of three-wheeled motor vehicle injured in collision with car, pick-up truck or van in nontraffic accident

     √7th **V33.4** Person boarding or alighting a three-wheeled motor vehicle injured in collision with car, pick-up truck or van

     √7th **V33.5** Driver of three-wheeled motor vehicle injured in collision with car, pick-up truck or van in traffic accident

     √7th **V33.6** Passenger in three-wheeled motor vehicle injured in collision with car, pick-up truck or van in traffic accident

     √7th **V33.7** Person on outside of three-wheeled motor vehicle injured in collision with car, pick-up truck or van in traffic accident

     √7th **V33.9** Unspecified occupant of three-wheeled motor vehicle injured in collision with car, pick-up truck or van in traffic accident

√4th **V34** Occupant of three-wheeled motor vehicle injured in collision with heavy transport vehicle or bus
     EXCLUDES 1   occupant of three-wheeled motor vehicle injured in collision with military vehicle (V39.81)

     √7th **V34.0** Driver of three-wheeled motor vehicle injured in collision with heavy transport vehicle or bus in nontraffic accident

     √7th **V34.1** Passenger in three-wheeled motor vehicle injured in collision with heavy transport vehicle or bus in nontraffic accident

     √7th **V34.2** Person on outside of three-wheeled motor vehicle injured in collision with heavy transport vehicle or bus in nontraffic accident

     √7th **V34.3** Unspecified occupant of three-wheeled motor vehicle injured in collision with heavy transport vehicle or bus in nontraffic accident

     √7th **V34.4** Person boarding or alighting a three-wheeled motor vehicle injured in collision with heavy transport vehicle or bus

     √7th **V34.5** Driver of three-wheeled motor vehicle injured in collision with heavy transport vehicle or bus in traffic accident

     √7th **V34.6** Passenger in three-wheeled motor vehicle injured in collision with heavy transport vehicle or bus in traffic accident

     √7th **V34.7** Person on outside of three-wheeled motor vehicle injured in collision with heavy transport vehicle or bus in traffic accident

     √7th **V34.9** Unspecified occupant of three-wheeled motor vehicle injured in collision with heavy transport vehicle or bus in traffic accident

Chapter 20. External Causes of Morbidity

V35 Occupant of three-wheeled motor vehicle injured in collision with railway train or railway vehicle

  V35.0 Driver of three-wheeled motor vehicle injured in collision with railway train or railway vehicle in nontraffic accident

  V35.1 Passenger in three-wheeled motor vehicle injured in collision with railway train or railway vehicle in nontraffic accident

  V35.2 Person on outside of three-wheeled motor vehicle injured in collision with railway train or railway vehicle in nontraffic accident

  V35.3 Unspecified occupant of three-wheeled motor vehicle injured in collision with railway train or railway vehicle in nontraffic accident

  V35.4 Person boarding or alighting a three-wheeled motor vehicle injured in collision with railway train or railway vehicle

  V35.5 Driver of three-wheeled motor vehicle injured in collision with railway train or railway vehicle in traffic accident

  V35.6 Passenger in three-wheeled motor vehicle injured in collision with railway train or railway vehicle in traffic accident

  V35.7 Person on outside of three-wheeled motor vehicle injured in collision with railway train or railway vehicle in traffic accident

  V35.9 Unspecified occupant of three-wheeled motor vehicle injured in collision with railway train or railway vehicle in traffic accident

V36 Occupant of three-wheeled motor vehicle injured in collision with other nonmotor vehicle

  INCLUDES collision with animal-drawn vehicle, animal being ridden, streetcar

  V36.0 Driver of three-wheeled motor vehicle injured in collision with other nonmotor vehicle in nontraffic accident

  V36.1 Passenger in three-wheeled motor vehicle injured in collision with other nonmotor vehicle in nontraffic accident

  V36.2 Person on outside of three-wheeled motor vehicle injured in collision with other nonmotor vehicle in nontraffic accident

  V36.3 Unspecified occupant of three-wheeled motor vehicle injured in collision with other nonmotor vehicle in nontraffic accident

  V36.4 Person boarding or alighting a three-wheeled motor vehicle injured in collision with other nonmotor vehicle

  V36.5 Driver of three-wheeled motor vehicle injured in collision with other nonmotor vehicle in traffic accident

  V36.6 Passenger in three-wheeled motor vehicle injured in collision with other nonmotor vehicle in traffic accident

  V36.7 Person on outside of three-wheeled motor vehicle injured in collision with other nonmotor vehicle in traffic accident

  V36.9 Unspecified occupant of three-wheeled motor vehicle injured in collision with other nonmotor vehicle in traffic accident

V37 Occupant of three-wheeled motor vehicle injured in collision with fixed or stationary object

  V37.0 Driver of three-wheeled motor vehicle injured in collision with fixed or stationary object in nontraffic accident

  V37.1 Passenger in three-wheeled motor vehicle injured in collision with fixed or stationary object in nontraffic accident

  V37.2 Person on outside of three-wheeled motor vehicle injured in collision with fixed or stationary object in nontraffic accident

  V37.3 Unspecified occupant of three-wheeled motor vehicle injured in collision with fixed or stationary object in nontraffic accident

  V37.4 Person boarding or alighting a three-wheeled motor vehicle injured in collision with fixed or stationary object

  V37.5 Driver of three-wheeled motor vehicle injured in collision with fixed or stationary object in traffic accident

  V37.6 Passenger in three-wheeled motor vehicle injured in collision with fixed or stationary object in traffic accident

  V37.7 Person on outside of three-wheeled motor vehicle injured in collision with fixed or stationary object in traffic accident

  V37.9 Unspecified occupant of three-wheeled motor vehicle injured in collision with fixed or stationary object in traffic accident

V38 Occupant of three-wheeled motor vehicle injured in noncollision transport accident

  INCLUDES fall or thrown from three-wheeled motor vehicle
    overturning of three-wheeled motor vehicle NOS
    overturning of three-wheeled motor vehicle without collision

  V38.0 Driver of three-wheeled motor vehicle injured in noncollision transport accident in nontraffic accident

  V38.1 Passenger in three-wheeled motor vehicle injured in noncollision transport accident in nontraffic accident

  V38.2 Person on outside of three-wheeled motor vehicle injured in noncollision transport accident in nontraffic accident

  V38.3 Unspecified occupant of three-wheeled motor vehicle injured in noncollision transport accident in nontraffic accident

  V38.4 Person boarding or alighting a three-wheeled motor vehicle injured in noncollision transport accident

  V38.5 Driver of three-wheeled motor vehicle injured in noncollision transport accident in traffic accident

  V38.6 Passenger in three-wheeled motor vehicle injured in noncollision transport accident in traffic accident

  V38.7 Person on outside of three-wheeled motor vehicle injured in noncollision transport accident in traffic accident

  V38.9 Unspecified occupant of three-wheeled motor vehicle injured in noncollision transport accident in traffic accident

V39 Occupant of three-wheeled motor vehicle injured in other and unspecified transport accidents

  V39.0 Driver of three-wheeled motor vehicle injured in collision with other and unspecified motor vehicles in nontraffic accident

    V39.00 Driver of three-wheeled motor vehicle injured in collision with unspecified motor vehicles in nontraffic accident

    V39.09 Driver of three-wheeled motor vehicle injured in collision with other motor vehicles in nontraffic accident

  V39.1 Passenger in three-wheeled motor vehicle injured in collision with other and unspecified motor vehicles in nontraffic accident

    V39.10 Passenger in three-wheeled motor vehicle injured in collision with unspecified motor vehicles in nontraffic accident

    V39.19 Passenger in three-wheeled motor vehicle injured in collision with other motor vehicles in nontraffic accident

  V39.2 Unspecified occupant of three-wheeled motor vehicle injured in collision with other and unspecified motor vehicles in nontraffic accident

    V39.20 Unspecified occupant of three-wheeled motor vehicle injured in collision with unspecified motor vehicles in nontraffic accident

      Collision NOS involving three-wheeled motor vehicle, nontraffic

    V39.29 Unspecified occupant of three-wheeled motor vehicle injured in collision with other motor vehicles in nontraffic accident

  V39.3 Occupant (driver) (passenger) of three-wheeled motor vehicle injured in unspecified nontraffic accident

    Accident NOS involving three-wheeled motor vehicle, nontraffic
    Occupant of three-wheeled motor vehicle injured in nontraffic accident NOS

  V39.4 Driver of three-wheeled motor vehicle injured in collision with other and unspecified motor vehicles in traffic accident

    V39.40 Driver of three-wheeled motor vehicle injured in collision with unspecified motor vehicles in traffic accident

    V39.49 Driver of three-wheeled motor vehicle injured in collision with other motor vehicles in traffic accident

  V39.5 Passenger in three-wheeled motor vehicle injured in collision with other and unspecified motor vehicles in traffic accident

    V39.50 Passenger in three-wheeled motor vehicle injured in collision with unspecified motor vehicles in traffic accident

    V39.59 Passenger in three-wheeled motor vehicle injured in collision with other motor vehicles in traffic accident

  V39.6 Unspecified occupant of three-wheeled motor vehicle injured in collision with other and unspecified motor vehicles in traffic accident

    V39.60 Unspecified occupant of three-wheeled motor vehicle injured in collision with unspecified motor vehicles in traffic accident

      Collision NOS involving three-wheeled motor vehicle (traffic)

    V39.69 Unspecified occupant of three-wheeled motor vehicle injured in collision with other motor vehicles in traffic accident

  V39.8 Occupant (driver) (passenger) of three-wheeled motor vehicle injured in other specified transport accidents

    V39.81 Occupant (driver) (passenger) of three-wheeled motor vehicle injured in transport accident with military vehicle

    V39.89 Occupant (driver) (passenger) of three-wheeled motor vehicle injured in other specified transport accidents

N Newborn: 0　　**P** Pediatric: 0-17　　**M** Maternity: 9-64　　**A** Adult: 15-124　　**MCC** Major Complication/Comorbidity　　**CC** Complication/Comorbidity　　**SW** Severe Wound Dx

1182　　　　　　　　　　　　　　　　　　　　　　　　　　　　　　　　　　　　　ICD-10-CM 2022

✓x7ᵗʰ **V39.9** Occupant (driver) (passenger) of three-wheeled motor vehicle injured in unspecified traffic accident
Accident NOS involving three-wheeled motor vehicle

Car occupant injured in transport accident (V40-V49)

INCLUDES a four-wheeled motor vehicle designed primarily for carrying passengers
automobile (pulling a trailer or camper)

EXCLUDES 1 bus (V50-V59)
minibus (V50-V59)
minivan (V50-V59)
motorcoach (V70-V79)
pick-up truck (V50-V59)
sport utility vehicle (SUV) (V50-V59)

The appropriate 7th character is to be added to each code from categories V40-V49.
A   initial encounter
D   subsequent encounter
S   sequela

✓4ᵗʰ **V40** Car occupant injured in collision with pedestrian or animal
     EXCLUDES 1 car collision with animal-drawn vehicle or animal being ridden (V46.-)
   ✓x7ᵗʰ **V40.0** Car driver injured in collision with pedestrian or animal in nontraffic accident
   ✓x7ᵗʰ **V40.1** Car passenger injured in collision with pedestrian or animal in nontraffic accident
   ✓x7ᵗʰ **V40.2** Person on outside of car injured in collision with pedestrian or animal in nontraffic accident
   ✓x7ᵗʰ **V40.3** Unspecified car occupant injured in collision with pedestrian or animal in nontraffic accident
   ✓x7ᵗʰ **V40.4** Person boarding or alighting a car injured in collision with pedestrian or animal
   ✓x7ᵗʰ **V40.5** Car driver injured in collision with pedestrian or animal in traffic accident
   ✓x7ᵗʰ **V40.6** Car passenger injured in collision with pedestrian or animal in traffic accident
   ✓x7ᵗʰ **V40.7** Person on outside of car injured in collision with pedestrian or animal in traffic accident
   ✓x7ᵗʰ **V40.9** Unspecified car occupant injured in collision with pedestrian or animal in traffic accident

✓4ᵗʰ **V41** Car occupant injured in collision with pedal cycle
   ✓x7ᵗʰ **V41.0** Car driver injured in collision with pedal cycle in nontraffic accident
   ✓x7ᵗʰ **V41.1** Car passenger injured in collision with pedal cycle in nontraffic accident
   ✓x7ᵗʰ **V41.2** Person on outside of car injured in collision with pedal cycle in nontraffic accident
   ✓x7ᵗʰ **V41.3** Unspecified car occupant injured in collision with pedal cycle in nontraffic accident
   ✓x7ᵗʰ **V41.4** Person boarding or alighting a car injured in collision with pedal cycle
   ✓x7ᵗʰ **V41.5** Car driver injured in collision with pedal cycle in traffic accident
   ✓x7ᵗʰ **V41.6** Car passenger injured in collision with pedal cycle in traffic accident
   ✓x7ᵗʰ **V41.7** Person on outside of car injured in collision with pedal cycle in traffic accident
   ✓x7ᵗʰ **V41.9** Unspecified car occupant injured in collision with pedal cycle in traffic accident

✓4ᵗʰ **V42** Car occupant injured in collision with two- or three-wheeled motor vehicle
   ✓x7ᵗʰ **V42.0** Car driver injured in collision with two- or three-wheeled motor vehicle in nontraffic accident
   ✓x7ᵗʰ **V42.1** Car passenger injured in collision with two- or three-wheeled motor vehicle in nontraffic accident
   ✓x7ᵗʰ **V42.2** Person on outside of car injured in collision with two- or three-wheeled motor vehicle in nontraffic accident
   ✓x7ᵗʰ **V42.3** Unspecified car occupant injured in collision with two- or three-wheeled motor vehicle in nontraffic accident
   ✓x7ᵗʰ **V42.4** Person boarding or alighting a car injured in collision with two- or three-wheeled motor vehicle
   ✓x7ᵗʰ **V42.5** Car driver injured in collision with two- or three-wheeled motor vehicle in traffic accident
   ✓x7ᵗʰ **V42.6** Car passenger injured in collision with two- or three-wheeled motor vehicle in traffic accident
   ✓x7ᵗʰ **V42.7** Person on outside of car injured in collision with two- or three-wheeled motor vehicle in traffic accident
   ✓x7ᵗʰ **V42.9** Unspecified car occupant injured in collision with two- or three-wheeled motor vehicle in traffic accident

✓4ᵗʰ **V43** Car occupant injured in collision with car, pick-up truck or van
  ✓5ᵗʰ **V43.0** Car driver injured in collision with car, pick-up truck or van in nontraffic accident
   ✓x7ᵗʰ **V43.01** Car driver injured in collision with sport utility vehicle in nontraffic accident
   ✓x7ᵗʰ **V43.02** Car driver injured in collision with other type car in nontraffic accident
   ✓x7ᵗʰ **V43.03** Car driver injured in collision with pick-up truck in nontraffic accident
   ✓x7ᵗʰ **V43.04** Car driver injured in collision with van in nontraffic accident
  ✓5ᵗʰ **V43.1** Car passenger injured in collision with car, pick-up truck or van in nontraffic accident
   ✓x7ᵗʰ **V43.11** Car passenger injured in collision with sport utility vehicle in nontraffic accident
   ✓x7ᵗʰ **V43.12** Car passenger injured in collision with other type car in nontraffic accident
   ✓x7ᵗʰ **V43.13** Car passenger injured in collision with pick-up truck in nontraffic accident
   ✓x7ᵗʰ **V43.14** Car passenger injured in collision with van in nontraffic accident
  ✓5ᵗʰ **V43.2** Person on outside of car injured in collision with car, pick-up truck or van in nontraffic accident
   ✓x7ᵗʰ **V43.21** Person on outside of car injured in collision with sport utility vehicle in nontraffic accident
   ✓x7ᵗʰ **V43.22** Person on outside of car injured in collision with other type car in nontraffic accident
   ✓x7ᵗʰ **V43.23** Person on outside of car injured in collision with pick-up truck in nontraffic accident
   ✓x7ᵗʰ **V43.24** Person on outside of car injured in collision with van in nontraffic accident
  ✓5ᵗʰ **V43.3** Unspecified car occupant injured in collision with car, pick-up truck or van in nontraffic accident
   ✓x7ᵗʰ **V43.31** Unspecified car occupant injured in collision with sport utility vehicle in nontraffic accident
   ✓x7ᵗʰ **V43.32** Unspecified car occupant injured in collision with other type car in nontraffic accident
   ✓x7ᵗʰ **V43.33** Unspecified car occupant injured in collision with pick-up truck in nontraffic accident
   ✓x7ᵗʰ **V43.34** Unspecified car occupant injured in collision with van in nontraffic accident
  ✓5ᵗʰ **V43.4** Person boarding or alighting a car injured in collision with car, pick-up truck or van
   ✓x7ᵗʰ **V43.41** Person boarding or alighting a car injured in collision with sport utility vehicle
   ✓x7ᵗʰ **V43.42** Person boarding or alighting a car injured in collision with other type car
   ✓x7ᵗʰ **V43.43** Person boarding or alighting a car injured in collision with pick-up truck
   ✓x7ᵗʰ **V43.44** Person boarding or alighting a car injured in collision with van
  ✓5ᵗʰ **V43.5** Car driver injured in collision with car, pick-up truck or van in traffic accident
   ✓x7ᵗʰ **V43.51** Car driver injured in collision with sport utility vehicle in traffic accident
   ✓x7ᵗʰ **V43.52** Car driver injured in collision with other type car in traffic accident
   ✓x7ᵗʰ **V43.53** Car driver injured in collision with pick-up truck in traffic accident
   ✓x7ᵗʰ **V43.54** Car driver injured in collision with van in traffic accident
  ✓5ᵗʰ **V43.6** Car passenger injured in collision with car, pick-up truck or van in traffic accident
   ✓x7ᵗʰ **V43.61** Car passenger injured in collision with sport utility vehicle in traffic accident
   ✓x7ᵗʰ **V43.62** Car passenger injured in collision with other type car in traffic accident
   ✓x7ᵗʰ **V43.63** Car passenger injured in collision with pick-up truck in traffic accident
   ✓x7ᵗʰ **V43.64** Car passenger injured in collision with van in traffic accident
  ✓5ᵗʰ **V43.7** Person on outside of car injured in collision with car, pick-up truck or van in traffic accident
   ✓x7ᵗʰ **V43.71** Person on outside of car injured in collision with sport utility vehicle in traffic accident
   ✓x7ᵗʰ **V43.72** Person on outside of car injured in collision with other type car in traffic accident
   ✓x7ᵗʰ **V43.73** Person on outside of car injured in collision with pick-up truck in traffic accident
   ✓x7ᵗʰ **V43.74** Person on outside of car injured in collision with van in traffic accident

√5ᵗʰ **V43.9** Unspecified car occupant injured in collision with car, pick-up truck or van in traffic accident

√x7ᵗʰ **V43.91** Unspecified car occupant injured in collision with sport utility vehicle in traffic accident

√x7ᵗʰ **V43.92** Unspecified car occupant injured in collision with other type car in traffic accident

√x7ᵗʰ **V43.93** Unspecified car occupant injured in collision with pick-up truck in traffic accident

√x7ᵗʰ **V43.94** Unspecified car occupant injured in collision with van in traffic accident

√4ᵗʰ **V44** Car occupant injured in collision with heavy transport vehicle or bus

> EXCLUDES 1   car occupant injured in collision with military vehicle (V49.81)

√x7ᵗʰ **V44.0** Car driver injured in collision with heavy transport vehicle or bus in nontraffic accident

√x7ᵗʰ **V44.1** Car passenger injured in collision with heavy transport vehicle or bus in nontraffic accident

√x7ᵗʰ **V44.2** Person on outside of car injured in collision with heavy transport vehicle or bus in nontraffic accident

√x7ᵗʰ **V44.3** Unspecified car occupant injured in collision with heavy transport vehicle or bus in nontraffic accident

√x7ᵗʰ **V44.4** Person boarding or alighting a car injured in collision with heavy transport vehicle or bus

√x7ᵗʰ **V44.5** Car driver injured in collision with heavy transport vehicle or bus in traffic accident

√x7ᵗʰ **V44.6** Car passenger injured in collision with heavy transport vehicle or bus in traffic accident

√x7ᵗʰ **V44.7** Person on outside of car injured in collision with heavy transport vehicle or bus in traffic accident

√x7ᵗʰ **V44.9** Unspecified car occupant injured in collision with heavy transport vehicle or bus in traffic accident

√4ᵗʰ **V45** Car occupant injured in collision with railway train or railway vehicle

√x7ᵗʰ **V45.0** Car driver injured in collision with railway train or railway vehicle in nontraffic accident

√x7ᵗʰ **V45.1** Car passenger injured in collision with railway train or railway vehicle in nontraffic accident

√x7ᵗʰ **V45.2** Person on outside of car injured in collision with railway train or railway vehicle in nontraffic accident

√x7ᵗʰ **V45.3** Unspecified car occupant injured in collision with railway train or railway vehicle in nontraffic accident

√x7ᵗʰ **V45.4** Person boarding or alighting a car injured in collision with railway train or railway vehicle

√x7ᵗʰ **V45.5** Car driver injured in collision with railway train or railway vehicle in traffic accident

√x7ᵗʰ **V45.6** Car passenger injured in collision with railway train or railway vehicle in traffic accident

√x7ᵗʰ **V45.7** Person on outside of car injured in collision with railway train or railway vehicle in traffic accident

√x7ᵗʰ **V45.9** Unspecified car occupant injured in collision with railway train or railway vehicle in traffic accident

√4ᵗʰ **V46** Car occupant injured in collision with other nonmotor vehicle

> INCLUDES   collision with animal-drawn vehicle, animal being ridden, streetcar

√x7ᵗʰ **V46.0** Car driver injured in collision with other nonmotor vehicle in nontraffic accident

√x7ᵗʰ **V46.1** Car passenger injured in collision with other nonmotor vehicle in nontraffic accident

√x7ᵗʰ **V46.2** Person on outside of car injured in collision with other nonmotor vehicle in nontraffic accident

√x7ᵗʰ **V46.3** Unspecified car occupant injured in collision with other nonmotor vehicle in nontraffic accident

√x7ᵗʰ **V46.4** Person boarding or alighting a car injured in collision with other nonmotor vehicle

√x7ᵗʰ **V46.5** Car driver injured in collision with other nonmotor vehicle in traffic accident

√x7ᵗʰ **V46.6** Car passenger injured in collision with other nonmotor vehicle in traffic accident

√x7ᵗʰ **V46.7** Person on outside of car injured in collision with other nonmotor vehicle in traffic accident

√x7ᵗʰ **V46.9** Unspecified car occupant injured in collision with other nonmotor vehicle in traffic accident

√4ᵗʰ **V47** Car occupant injured in collision with fixed or stationary object

> AHA: 2016,4Q,73

√x7ᵗʰ **V47.0** Car driver injured in collision with fixed or stationary object in nontraffic accident

√x7ᵗʰ **V47.1** Car passenger injured in collision with fixed or stationary object in nontraffic accident

√x7ᵗʰ **V47.2** Person on outside of car injured in collision with fixed or stationary object in nontraffic accident

√x7ᵗʰ **V47.3** Unspecified car occupant injured in collision with fixed or stationary object in nontraffic accident

√x7ᵗʰ **V47.4** Person boarding or alighting a car injured in collision with fixed or stationary object

√x7ᵗʰ **V47.5** Car driver injured in collision with fixed or stationary object in traffic accident

√x7ᵗʰ **V47.6** Car passenger injured in collision with fixed or stationary object in traffic accident

√x7ᵗʰ **V47.7** Person on outside of car injured in collision with fixed or stationary object in traffic accident

√x7ᵗʰ **V47.9** Unspecified car occupant injured in collision with fixed or stationary object in traffic accident

√4ᵗʰ **V48** Car occupant injured in noncollision transport accident

> INCLUDES   overturning car NOS
> overturning car without collision

√x7ᵗʰ **V48.0** Car driver injured in noncollision transport accident in nontraffic accident

√x7ᵗʰ **V48.1** Car passenger injured in noncollision transport accident in nontraffic accident

√x7ᵗʰ **V48.2** Person on outside of car injured in noncollision transport accident in nontraffic accident

√x7ᵗʰ **V48.3** Unspecified car occupant injured in noncollision transport accident in nontraffic accident

√x7ᵗʰ **V48.4** Person boarding or alighting a car injured in noncollision transport accident

√x7ᵗʰ **V48.5** Car driver injured in noncollision transport accident in traffic accident

√x7ᵗʰ **V48.6** Car passenger injured in noncollision transport accident in traffic accident

√x7ᵗʰ **V48.7** Person on outside of car injured in noncollision transport accident in traffic accident

√x7ᵗʰ **V48.9** Unspecified car occupant injured in noncollision transport accident in traffic accident

√4ᵗʰ **V49** Car occupant injured in other and unspecified transport accidents

√5ᵗʰ **V49.0** Driver injured in collision with other and unspecified motor vehicles in nontraffic accident

√x7ᵗʰ **V49.00** Driver injured in collision with unspecified motor vehicles in nontraffic accident

√x7ᵗʰ **V49.09** Driver injured in collision with other motor vehicles in nontraffic accident

√5ᵗʰ **V49.1** Passenger injured in collision with other and unspecified motor vehicles in nontraffic accident

√x7ᵗʰ **V49.10** Passenger injured in collision with unspecified motor vehicles in nontraffic accident

√x7ᵗʰ **V49.19** Passenger injured in collision with other motor vehicles in nontraffic accident

√5ᵗʰ **V49.2** Unspecified car occupant injured in collision with other and unspecified motor vehicles in nontraffic accident

√x7ᵗʰ **V49.20** Unspecified car occupant injured in collision with unspecified motor vehicles in nontraffic accident

> Car collision NOS, nontraffic

√x7ᵗʰ **V49.29** Unspecified car occupant injured in collision with other motor vehicles in nontraffic accident

√x7ᵗʰ **V49.3** Car occupant (driver) (passenger) injured in unspecified nontraffic accident

> Car accident NOS, nontraffic
> Car occupant injured in nontraffic accident NOS

√5ᵗʰ **V49.4** Driver injured in collision with other and unspecified motor vehicles in traffic accident

√x7ᵗʰ **V49.40** Driver injured in collision with unspecified motor vehicles in traffic accident

√x7ᵗʰ **V49.49** Driver injured in collision with other motor vehicles in traffic accident

√5ᵗʰ **V49.5** Passenger injured in collision with other and unspecified motor vehicles in traffic accident

√x7ᵗʰ **V49.50** Passenger injured in collision with unspecified motor vehicles in traffic accident

√x7ᵗʰ **V49.59** Passenger injured in collision with other motor vehicles in traffic accident

√5ᵗʰ **V49.6** Unspecified car occupant injured in collision with other and unspecified motor vehicles in traffic accident

√x7ᵗʰ **V49.60** Unspecified car occupant injured in collision with unspecified motor vehicles in traffic accident

> Car collision NOS (traffic)

√x7ᵗʰ **V49.69** Unspecified car occupant injured in collision with other motor vehicles in traffic accident

√5ᵗʰ **V49.8** Car occupant (driver) (passenger) injured in other specified transport accidents

√x7ᵗʰ **V49.81** Car occupant (driver) (passenger) injured in transport accident with military vehicle

N Newborn: 0   P Pediatric: 0-17   M Maternity: 9-64   A Adult: 15-124   MCC Major Complication/Comorbidity   CC Complication/Comorbidity   SW Severe Wound Dx

1184   ICD-10-CM 2022

√x7ᵗʰ **V49.88** Car occupant (driver) (passenger) injured in other specified transport accidents

√x7ᵗʰ **V49.9** Car occupant (driver) (passenger) injured in unspecified traffic accident

Car accident NOS

Occupant of pick-up truck or van injured in transport accident (V50-V59)

INCLUDES   a four or six wheel motor vehicle designed primarily for carrying passengers and property but weighing less than the local limit for classification as a heavy goods vehicle

minibus
minivan
sport utility vehicle (SUV)
truck
van

EXCLUDES 1   heavy transport vehicle (V60-V69)

The appropriate 7th character is to be added to each code from categories V50-V59.
A   initial encounter
D   subsequent encounter
S   sequela

✓4ᵗʰ **V50** Occupant of pick-up truck or van injured in collision with pedestrian or animal

EXCLUDES 1   pick-up truck or van collision with animal-drawn vehicle or animal being ridden (V56.-)

√x7ᵗʰ **V50.0** Driver of pick-up truck or van injured in collision with pedestrian or animal in nontraffic accident

√x7ᵗʰ **V50.1** Passenger in pick-up truck or van injured in collision with pedestrian or animal in nontraffic accident

√x7ᵗʰ **V50.2** Person on outside of pick-up truck or van injured in collision with pedestrian or animal in nontraffic accident

√x7ᵗʰ **V50.3** Unspecified occupant of pick-up truck or van injured in collision with pedestrian or animal in nontraffic accident

√x7ᵗʰ **V50.4** Person boarding or alighting a pick-up truck or van injured in collision with pedestrian or animal

√x7ᵗʰ **V50.5** Driver of pick-up truck or van injured in collision with pedestrian or animal in traffic accident

√x7ᵗʰ **V50.6** Passenger in pick-up truck or van injured in collision with pedestrian or animal in traffic accident

√x7ᵗʰ **V50.7** Person on outside of pick-up truck or van injured in collision with pedestrian or animal in traffic accident

√x7ᵗʰ **V50.9** Unspecified occupant of pick-up truck or van injured in collision with pedestrian or animal in traffic accident

✓4ᵗʰ **V51** Occupant of pick-up truck or van injured in collision with pedal cycle

√x7ᵗʰ **V51.0** Driver of pick-up truck or van injured in collision with pedal cycle in nontraffic accident

√x7ᵗʰ **V51.1** Passenger in pick-up truck or van injured in collision with pedal cycle in nontraffic accident

√x7ᵗʰ **V51.2** Person on outside of pick-up truck or van injured in collision with pedal cycle in nontraffic accident

√x7ᵗʰ **V51.3** Unspecified occupant of pick-up truck or van injured in collision with pedal cycle in nontraffic accident

√x7ᵗʰ **V51.4** Person boarding or alighting a pick-up truck or van injured in collision with pedal cycle

√x7ᵗʰ **V51.5** Driver of pick-up truck or van injured in collision with pedal cycle in traffic accident

√x7ᵗʰ **V51.6** Passenger in pick-up truck or van injured in collision with pedal cycle in traffic accident

√x7ᵗʰ **V51.7** Person on outside of pick-up truck or van injured in collision with pedal cycle in traffic accident

√x7ᵗʰ **V51.9** Unspecified occupant of pick-up truck or van injured in collision with pedal cycle in traffic accident

✓4ᵗʰ **V52** Occupant of pick-up truck or van injured in collision with two- or three-wheeled motor vehicle

√x7ᵗʰ **V52.0** Driver of pick-up truck or van injured in collision with two- or three-wheeled motor vehicle in nontraffic accident

√x7ᵗʰ **V52.1** Passenger in pick-up truck or van injured in collision with two- or three-wheeled motor vehicle in nontraffic accident

√x7ᵗʰ **V52.2** Person on outside of pick-up truck or van injured in collision with two- or three-wheeled motor vehicle in nontraffic accident

√x7ᵗʰ **V52.3** Unspecified occupant of pick-up truck or van injured in collision with two- or three-wheeled motor vehicle in nontraffic accident

√x7ᵗʰ **V52.4** Person boarding or alighting a pick-up truck or van injured in collision with two- or three-wheeled motor vehicle

√x7ᵗʰ **V52.5** Driver of pick-up truck or van injured in collision with two- or three-wheeled motor vehicle in traffic accident

√x7ᵗʰ **V52.6** Passenger in pick-up truck or van injured in collision with two- or three-wheeled motor vehicle in traffic accident

√x7ᵗʰ **V52.7** Person on outside of pick-up truck or van injured in collision with two- or three-wheeled motor vehicle in traffic accident

√x7ᵗʰ **V52.9** Unspecified occupant of pick-up truck or van injured in collision with two- or three-wheeled motor vehicle in traffic accident

✓4ᵗʰ **V53** Occupant of pick-up truck or van injured in collision with car, pick-up truck or van

√x7ᵗʰ **V53.0** Driver of pick-up truck or van injured in collision with car, pick-up truck or van in nontraffic accident

√x7ᵗʰ **V53.1** Passenger in pick-up truck or van injured in collision with car, pick-up truck or van in nontraffic accident

√x7ᵗʰ **V53.2** Person on outside of pick-up truck or van injured in collision with car, pick-up truck or van in nontraffic accident

√x7ᵗʰ **V53.3** Unspecified occupant of pick-up truck or van injured in collision with car, pick-up truck or van in nontraffic accident

√x7ᵗʰ **V53.4** Person boarding or alighting a pick-up truck or van injured in collision with car, pick-up truck or van

√x7ᵗʰ **V53.5** Driver of pick-up truck or van injured in collision with car, pick-up truck or van in traffic accident

√x7ᵗʰ **V53.6** Passenger in pick-up truck or van injured in collision with car, pick-up truck or van in traffic accident

√x7ᵗʰ **V53.7** Person on outside of pick-up truck or van injured in collision with car, pick-up truck or van in traffic accident

√x7ᵗʰ **V53.9** Unspecified occupant of pick-up truck or van injured in collision with car, pick-up truck or van in traffic accident

✓4ᵗʰ **V54** Occupant of pick-up truck or van injured in collision with heavy transport vehicle or bus

EXCLUDES 1   occupant of pick-up truck or van injured in collision with military vehicle (V59.81)

√x7ᵗʰ **V54.0** Driver of pick-up truck or van injured in collision with heavy transport vehicle or bus in nontraffic accident

√x7ᵗʰ **V54.1** Passenger in pick-up truck or van injured in collision with heavy transport vehicle or bus in nontraffic accident

√x7ᵗʰ **V54.2** Person on outside of pick-up truck or van injured in collision with heavy transport vehicle or bus in nontraffic accident

√x7ᵗʰ **V54.3** Unspecified occupant of pick-up truck or van injured in collision with heavy transport vehicle or bus in nontraffic accident

√x7ᵗʰ **V54.4** Person boarding or alighting a pick-up truck or van injured in collision with heavy transport vehicle or bus

√x7ᵗʰ **V54.5** Driver of pick-up truck or van injured in collision with heavy transport vehicle or bus in traffic accident

√x7ᵗʰ **V54.6** Passenger in pick-up truck or van injured in collision with heavy transport vehicle or bus in traffic accident

√x7ᵗʰ **V54.7** Person on outside of pick-up truck or van injured in collision with heavy transport vehicle or bus in traffic accident

√x7ᵗʰ **V54.9** Unspecified occupant of pick-up truck or van injured in collision with heavy transport vehicle or bus in traffic accident

✓4ᵗʰ **V55** Occupant of pick-up truck or van injured in collision with railway train or railway vehicle

√x7ᵗʰ **V55.0** Driver of pick-up truck or van injured in collision with railway train or railway vehicle in nontraffic accident

√x7ᵗʰ **V55.1** Passenger in pick-up truck or van injured in collision with railway train or railway vehicle in nontraffic accident

√x7ᵗʰ **V55.2** Person on outside of pick-up truck or van injured in collision with railway train or railway vehicle in nontraffic accident

√x7ᵗʰ **V55.3** Unspecified occupant of pick-up truck or van injured in collision with railway train or railway vehicle in nontraffic accident

√x7ᵗʰ **V55.4** Person boarding or alighting a pick-up truck or van injured in collision with railway train or railway vehicle

√x7ᵗʰ **V55.5** Driver of pick-up truck or van injured in collision with railway train or railway vehicle in traffic accident

√x7ᵗʰ **V55.6** Passenger in pick-up truck or van injured in collision with railway train or railway vehicle in traffic accident

√x7ᵗʰ **V55.7** Person on outside of pick-up truck or van injured in collision with railway train or railway vehicle in traffic accident

√x7ᵗʰ **V55.9** Unspecified occupant of pick-up truck or van injured in collision with railway train or railway vehicle in traffic accident

✓4ᵗʰ **V56** Occupant of pick-up truck or van injured in collision with other nonmotor vehicle

INCLUDES   collision with animal-drawn vehicle, animal being ridden, streetcar

√x7ᵗʰ **V56.0** Driver of pick-up truck or van injured in collision with other nonmotor vehicle in nontraffic accident

√x7ᵗʰ **V56.1** Passenger in pick-up truck or van injured in collision with other nonmotor vehicle in nontraffic accident

✓ Additional Char Req   √x7ᵗʰ Placeholder   Unacceptable PDx   Questionable PDx   Wrong Procedure   Manifestation   Unspecified Dx   H1-H4 HAC   HCC CMS-HCC Dx   HIV HIV Dx

ICD-10-CM 2022   1185

Chapter 20. External Causes of Morbidity   V49.88–V56.1

✓x7ᵗʰ **V56.2** Person on outside of pick-up truck or van injured in collision with other nonmotor vehicle in nontraffic accident

✓x7ᵗʰ **V56.3** Unspecified occupant of pick-up truck or van injured in collision with other nonmotor vehicle in nontraffic accident

✓x7ᵗʰ **V56.4** Person boarding or alighting a pick-up truck or van injured in collision with other nonmotor vehicle

✓x7ᵗʰ **V56.5** Driver of pick-up truck or van injured in collision with other nonmotor vehicle in traffic accident

✓x7ᵗʰ **V56.6** Passenger in pick-up truck or van injured in collision with other nonmotor vehicle in traffic accident

✓x7ᵗʰ **V56.7** Person on outside of pick-up truck or van injured in collision with other nonmotor vehicle in traffic accident

✓x7ᵗʰ **V56.9** Unspecified occupant of pick-up truck or van injured in collision with other nonmotor vehicle in traffic accident

✓4ᵗʰ **V57 Occupant of pick-up truck or van injured in collision with fixed or stationary object**

✓x7ᵗʰ **V57.0** Driver of pick-up truck or van injured in collision with fixed or stationary object in nontraffic accident

✓x7ᵗʰ **V57.1** Passenger in pick-up truck or van injured in collision with fixed or stationary object in nontraffic accident

✓x7ᵗʰ **V57.2** Person on outside of pick-up truck or van injured in collision with fixed or stationary object in nontraffic accident

✓x7ᵗʰ **V57.3** Unspecified occupant of pick-up truck or van injured in collision with fixed or stationary object in nontraffic accident

✓x7ᵗʰ **V57.4** Person boarding or alighting a pick-up truck or van injured in collision with fixed or stationary object

✓x7ᵗʰ **V57.5** Driver of pick-up truck or van injured in collision with fixed or stationary object in traffic accident

✓x7ᵗʰ **V57.6** Passenger in pick-up truck or van injured in collision with fixed or stationary object in traffic accident

✓x7ᵗʰ **V57.7** Person on outside of pick-up truck or van injured in collision with fixed or stationary object in traffic accident

✓x7ᵗʰ **V57.9** Unspecified occupant of pick-up truck or van injured in collision with fixed or stationary object in traffic accident

✓4ᵗʰ **V58 Occupant of pick-up truck or van injured in noncollision transport accident**

> **INCLUDES**   overturning pick-up truck or van NOS
> overturning pick-up truck or van without collision

✓x7ᵗʰ **V58.0** Driver of pick-up truck or van injured in noncollision transport accident in nontraffic accident

✓x7ᵗʰ **V58.1** Passenger in pick-up truck or van injured in noncollision transport accident in nontraffic accident

✓x7ᵗʰ **V58.2** Person on outside of pick-up truck or van injured in noncollision transport accident in nontraffic accident

✓x7ᵗʰ **V58.3** Unspecified occupant of pick-up truck or van injured in noncollision transport accident in nontraffic accident

✓x7ᵗʰ **V58.4** Person boarding or alighting a pick-up truck or van injured in noncollision transport accident

✓x7ᵗʰ **V58.5** Driver of pick-up truck or van injured in noncollision transport accident in traffic accident

✓x7ᵗʰ **V58.6** Passenger in pick-up truck or van injured in noncollision transport accident in traffic accident

✓x7ᵗʰ **V58.7** Person on outside of pick-up truck or van injured in noncollision transport accident in traffic accident

✓x7ᵗʰ **V58.9** Unspecified occupant of pick-up truck or van injured in noncollision transport accident in traffic accident

✓4ᵗʰ **V59 Occupant of pick-up truck or van injured in other and unspecified transport accidents**

✓5ᵗʰ **V59.0** Driver of pick-up truck or van injured in collision with other and unspecified motor vehicles in nontraffic accident

✓x7ᵗʰ **V59.00** Driver of pick-up truck or van injured in collision with unspecified motor vehicles in nontraffic accident

✓x7ᵗʰ **V59.09** Driver of pick-up truck or van injured in collision with other motor vehicles in nontraffic accident

✓5ᵗʰ **V59.1** Passenger in pick-up truck or van injured in collision with other and unspecified motor vehicles in nontraffic accident

✓x7ᵗʰ **V59.10** Passenger in pick-up truck or van injured in collision with unspecified motor vehicles in nontraffic accident

✓x7ᵗʰ **V59.19** Passenger in pick-up truck or van injured in collision with other motor vehicles in nontraffic accident

✓5ᵗʰ **V59.2** Unspecified occupant of pick-up truck or van injured in collision with other and unspecified motor vehicles in nontraffic accident

✓x7ᵗʰ **V59.20** Unspecified occupant of pick-up truck or van injured in collision with unspecified motor vehicles in nontraffic accident

Collision NOS involving pick-up truck or van, nontraffic

✓x7ᵗʰ **V59.29** Unspecified occupant of pick-up truck or van injured in collision with other motor vehicles in nontraffic accident

✓x7ᵗʰ **V59.3** Occupant (driver) (passenger) of pick-up truck or van injured in unspecified nontraffic accident

Accident NOS involving pick-up truck or van, nontraffic
Occupant of pick-up truck or van injured in nontraffic accident NOS

✓5ᵗʰ **V59.4** Driver of pick-up truck or van injured in collision with other and unspecified motor vehicles in traffic accident

✓x7ᵗʰ **V59.40** Driver of pick-up truck or van injured in collision with unspecified motor vehicles in traffic accident

✓x7ᵗʰ **V59.49** Driver of pick-up truck or van injured in collision with other motor vehicles in traffic accident

✓5ᵗʰ **V59.5** Passenger in pick-up truck or van injured in collision with other and unspecified motor vehicles in traffic accident

✓x7ᵗʰ **V59.50** Passenger in pick-up truck or van injured in collision with unspecified motor vehicles in traffic accident

✓x7ᵗʰ **V59.59** Passenger in pick-up truck or van injured in collision with other motor vehicles in traffic accident

✓5ᵗʰ **V59.6** Unspecified occupant of pick-up truck or van injured in collision with other and unspecified motor vehicles in traffic accident

✓x7ᵗʰ **V59.60** Unspecified occupant of pick-up truck or van injured in collision with unspecified motor vehicles in traffic accident

Collision NOS involving pick-up truck or van (traffic)

✓x7ᵗʰ **V59.69** Unspecified occupant of pick-up truck or van injured in collision with other motor vehicles in traffic accident

✓5ᵗʰ **V59.8** Occupant (driver) (passenger) of pick-up truck or van injured in other specified transport accidents

✓x7ᵗʰ **V59.81** Occupant (driver) (passenger) of pick-up truck or van injured in transport accident with military vehicle

✓x7ᵗʰ **V59.88** Occupant (driver) (passenger) of pick-up truck or van injured in other specified transport accidents

✓x7ᵗʰ **V59.9** Occupant (driver) (passenger) of pick-up truck or van injured in unspecified traffic accident

Accident NOS involving pick-up truck or van

Occupant of heavy transport vehicle injured in transport accident (V60-V69)

> **INCLUDES**   18 wheeler
> armored car
> panel truck
> **EXCLUDES 1**   *bus*
> *motorcoach*

The appropriate 7th character is to be added to each code from categories V60-V69.
A   initial encounter
D   subsequent encounter
S   sequela

✓4ᵗʰ **V60 Occupant of heavy transport vehicle injured in collision with pedestrian or animal**

> **EXCLUDES 1**   *heavy transport vehicle collision with animal-drawn vehicle or animal being ridden (V66.-)*

✓x7ᵗʰ **V60.0** Driver of heavy transport vehicle injured in collision with pedestrian or animal in nontraffic accident

✓x7ᵗʰ **V60.1** Passenger in heavy transport vehicle injured in collision with pedestrian or animal in nontraffic accident

✓x7ᵗʰ **V60.2** Person on outside of heavy transport vehicle injured in collision with pedestrian or animal in nontraffic accident

✓x7ᵗʰ **V60.3** Unspecified occupant of heavy transport vehicle injured in collision with pedestrian or animal in nontraffic accident

✓x7ᵗʰ **V60.4** Person boarding or alighting a heavy transport vehicle injured in collision with pedestrian or animal

✓x7ᵗʰ **V60.5** Driver of heavy transport vehicle injured in collision with pedestrian or animal in traffic accident

✓x7ᵗʰ **V60.6** Passenger in heavy transport vehicle injured in collision with pedestrian or animal in traffic accident

✓x7ᵗʰ **V60.7** Person on outside of heavy transport vehicle injured in collision with pedestrian or animal in traffic accident

✓x7ᵗʰ **V60.9** Unspecified occupant of heavy transport vehicle injured in collision with pedestrian or animal in traffic accident

✓4ᵗʰ **V61 Occupant of heavy transport vehicle injured in collision with pedal cycle**

✓x7ᵗʰ **V61.0** Driver of heavy transport vehicle injured in collision with pedal cycle in nontraffic accident

✓x7ᵗʰ **V61.1** Passenger in heavy transport vehicle injured in collision with pedal cycle in nontraffic accident

N Newborn: 0   P Pediatric: 0-17   M Maternity: 9-64   A Adult: 15-124   MCC Major Complication/Comorbidity   CC Complication/Comorbidity   SW Severe Wound Dx

1186   ICD-10-CM 2022

√x7th **V61.2** Person on outside of heavy transport vehicle injured in collision with pedal cycle in nontraffic accident

√x7th **V61.3** Unspecified occupant of heavy transport vehicle injured in collision with pedal cycle in nontraffic accident

√x7th **V61.4** Person boarding or alighting a heavy transport vehicle injured in collision with pedal cycle while boarding or alighting

√x7th **V61.5** Driver of heavy transport vehicle injured in collision with pedal cycle in traffic accident

√x7th **V61.6** Passenger in heavy transport vehicle injured in collision with pedal cycle in traffic accident

√x7th **V61.7** Person on outside of heavy transport vehicle injured in collision with pedal cycle in traffic accident

√x7th **V61.9** Unspecified occupant of heavy transport vehicle injured in collision with pedal cycle in traffic accident

√4th **V62** Occupant of heavy transport vehicle injured in collision with two- or three-wheeled motor vehicle

√x7th **V62.0** Driver of heavy transport vehicle injured in collision with two- or three-wheeled motor vehicle in nontraffic accident

√x7th **V62.1** Passenger in heavy transport vehicle injured in collision with two- or three-wheeled motor vehicle in nontraffic accident

√x7th **V62.2** Person on outside of heavy transport vehicle injured in collision with two- or three-wheeled motor vehicle in nontraffic accident

√x7th **V62.3** Unspecified occupant of heavy transport vehicle injured in collision with two- or three-wheeled motor vehicle in nontraffic accident

√x7th **V62.4** Person boarding or alighting a heavy transport vehicle injured in collision with two- or three-wheeled motor vehicle

√x7th **V62.5** Driver of heavy transport vehicle injured in collision with two- or three-wheeled motor vehicle in traffic accident

√x7th **V62.6** Passenger in heavy transport vehicle injured in collision with two- or three-wheeled motor vehicle in traffic accident

√x7th **V62.7** Person on outside of heavy transport vehicle injured in collision with two- or three-wheeled motor vehicle in traffic accident

√x7th **V62.9** Unspecified occupant of heavy transport vehicle injured in collision with two- or three-wheeled motor vehicle in traffic accident

√4th **V63** Occupant of heavy transport vehicle injured in collision with car, pick-up truck or van

√x7th **V63.0** Driver of heavy transport vehicle injured in collision with car, pick-up truck or van in nontraffic accident

√x7th **V63.1** Passenger in heavy transport vehicle injured in collision with car, pick-up truck or van in nontraffic accident

√x7th **V63.2** Person on outside of heavy transport vehicle injured in collision with car, pick-up truck or van in nontraffic accident

√x7th **V63.3** Unspecified occupant of heavy transport vehicle injured in collision with car, pick-up truck or van in nontraffic accident

√x7th **V63.4** Person boarding or alighting a heavy transport vehicle injured in collision with car, pick-up truck or van

√x7th **V63.5** Driver of heavy transport vehicle injured in collision with car, pick-up truck or van in traffic accident

√x7th **V63.6** Passenger in heavy transport vehicle injured in collision with car, pick-up truck or van in traffic accident

√x7th **V63.7** Person on outside of heavy transport vehicle injured in collision with car, pick-up truck or van in traffic accident

√x7th **V63.9** Unspecified occupant of heavy transport vehicle injured in collision with car, pick-up truck or van in traffic accident

√4th **V64** Occupant of heavy transport vehicle injured in collision with heavy transport vehicle or bus

     EXCLUDES 1   *occupant of heavy transport vehicle injured in collision with military vehicle (V69.81)*

√x7th **V64.0** Driver of heavy transport vehicle injured in collision with heavy transport vehicle or bus in nontraffic accident

√x7th **V64.1** Passenger in heavy transport vehicle injured in collision with heavy transport vehicle or bus in nontraffic accident

√x7th **V64.2** Person on outside of heavy transport vehicle injured in collision with heavy transport vehicle or bus in nontraffic accident

√x7th **V64.3** Unspecified occupant of heavy transport vehicle injured in collision with heavy transport vehicle or bus in nontraffic accident

√x7th **V64.4** Person boarding or alighting a heavy transport vehicle injured in collision with heavy transport vehicle or bus while boarding or alighting

√x7th **V64.5** Driver of heavy transport vehicle injured in collision with heavy transport vehicle or bus in traffic accident

√x7th **V64.6** Passenger in heavy transport vehicle injured in collision with heavy transport vehicle or bus in traffic accident

√x7th **V64.7** Person on outside of heavy transport vehicle injured in collision with heavy transport vehicle or bus in traffic accident

√x7th **V64.9** Unspecified occupant of heavy transport vehicle injured in collision with heavy transport vehicle or bus in traffic accident

√4th **V65** Occupant of heavy transport vehicle injured in collision with railway train or railway vehicle

√x7th **V65.0** Driver of heavy transport vehicle injured in collision with railway train or railway vehicle in nontraffic accident

√x7th **V65.1** Passenger in heavy transport vehicle injured in collision with railway train or railway vehicle in nontraffic accident

√x7th **V65.2** Person on outside of heavy transport vehicle injured in collision with railway train or railway vehicle in nontraffic accident

√x7th **V65.3** Unspecified occupant of heavy transport vehicle injured in collision with railway train or railway vehicle in nontraffic accident

√x7th **V65.4** Person boarding or alighting a heavy transport vehicle injured in collision with railway train or railway vehicle

√x7th **V65.5** Driver of heavy transport vehicle injured in collision with railway train or railway vehicle in traffic accident

√x7th **V65.6** Passenger in heavy transport vehicle injured in collision with railway train or railway vehicle in traffic accident

√x7th **V65.7** Person on outside of heavy transport vehicle injured in collision with railway train or railway vehicle in traffic accident

√x7th **V65.9** Unspecified occupant of heavy transport vehicle injured in collision with railway train or railway vehicle in traffic accident

√4th **V66** Occupant of heavy transport vehicle injured in collision with other nonmotor vehicle

     INCLUDES   collision with animal-drawn vehicle, animal being ridden, streetcar

√x7th **V66.0** Driver of heavy transport vehicle injured in collision with other nonmotor vehicle in nontraffic accident

√x7th **V66.1** Passenger in heavy transport vehicle injured in collision with other nonmotor vehicle in nontraffic accident

√x7th **V66.2** Person on outside of heavy transport vehicle injured in collision with other nonmotor vehicle in nontraffic accident

√x7th **V66.3** Unspecified occupant of heavy transport vehicle injured in collision with other nonmotor vehicle in nontraffic accident

√x7th **V66.4** Person boarding or alighting a heavy transport vehicle injured in collision with other nonmotor vehicle

√x7th **V66.5** Driver of heavy transport vehicle injured in collision with other nonmotor vehicle in traffic accident

√x7th **V66.6** Passenger in heavy transport vehicle injured in collision with other nonmotor vehicle in traffic accident

√x7th **V66.7** Person on outside of heavy transport vehicle injured in collision with other nonmotor vehicle in traffic accident

√x7th **V66.9** Unspecified occupant of heavy transport vehicle injured in collision with other nonmotor vehicle in traffic accident

√4th **V67** Occupant of heavy transport vehicle injured in collision with fixed or stationary object

√x7th **V67.0** Driver of heavy transport vehicle injured in collision with fixed or stationary object in nontraffic accident

√x7th **V67.1** Passenger in heavy transport vehicle injured in collision with fixed or stationary object in nontraffic accident

√x7th **V67.2** Person on outside of heavy transport vehicle injured in collision with fixed or stationary object in nontraffic accident

√x7th **V67.3** Unspecified occupant of heavy transport vehicle injured in collision with fixed or stationary object in nontraffic accident

√x7th **V67.4** Person boarding or alighting a heavy transport vehicle injured in collision with fixed or stationary object

√x7th **V67.5** Driver of heavy transport vehicle injured in collision with fixed or stationary object in traffic accident

√x7th **V67.6** Passenger in heavy transport vehicle injured in collision with fixed or stationary object in traffic accident

√x7th **V67.7** Person on outside of heavy transport vehicle injured in collision with fixed or stationary object in traffic accident

√x7th **V67.9** Unspecified occupant of heavy transport vehicle injured in collision with fixed or stationary object in traffic accident

√4th **V68** Occupant of heavy transport vehicle injured in noncollision transport accident

     INCLUDES   overturning heavy transport vehicle NOS
                overturning heavy transport vehicle without collision

√x7th **V68.0** Driver of heavy transport vehicle injured in noncollision transport accident in nontraffic accident

√x7th **V68.1** Passenger in heavy transport vehicle injured in noncollision transport accident in nontraffic accident

---

✔ Additional Char Req   √x7th Placeholder   Unacceptable PDx   Questionable PDx   Wrong Procedure   Manifestation   Unspecified Dx   H1-H4 HAC   HCC CMS-HCC Dx   HIV HIV Dx

√x7th **V68.2** Person on outside of heavy transport vehicle injured in noncollision transport accident in nontraffic accident

√x7th **V68.3** Unspecified occupant of heavy transport vehicle injured in noncollision transport accident in nontraffic accident

√x7th **V68.4** Person boarding or alighting a heavy transport vehicle injured in noncollision transport accident

√x7th **V68.5** Driver of heavy transport vehicle injured in noncollision transport accident in traffic accident

√x7th **V68.6** Passenger in heavy transport vehicle injured in noncollision transport accident in traffic accident

√x7th **V68.7** Person on outside of heavy transport vehicle injured in noncollision transport accident in traffic accident

√x7th **V68.9** Unspecified occupant of heavy transport vehicle injured in noncollision transport accident in traffic accident

√4th **V69** **Occupant of heavy transport vehicle injured in other and unspecified transport accidents**

√5th **V69.0** Driver of heavy transport vehicle injured in collision with other and unspecified motor vehicles in nontraffic accident

  √x7th **V69.00** Driver of heavy transport vehicle injured in collision with unspecified motor vehicles in nontraffic accident

  √x7th **V69.09** Driver of heavy transport vehicle injured in collision with other motor vehicles in nontraffic accident

√5th **V69.1** Passenger in heavy transport vehicle injured in collision with other and unspecified motor vehicles in nontraffic accident

  √x7th **V69.10** Passenger in heavy transport vehicle injured in collision with unspecified motor vehicles in nontraffic accident

  √x7th **V69.19** Passenger in heavy transport vehicle injured in collision with other motor vehicles in nontraffic accident

√5th **V69.2** Unspecified occupant of heavy transport vehicle injured in collision with other and unspecified motor vehicles in nontraffic accident

  √x7th **V69.20** Unspecified occupant of heavy transport vehicle injured in collision with unspecified motor vehicles in nontraffic accident

    Collision NOS involving heavy transport vehicle, nontraffic

  √x7th **V69.29** Unspecified occupant of heavy transport vehicle injured in collision with other motor vehicles in nontraffic accident

√x7th **V69.3** Occupant (driver) (passenger) of heavy transport vehicle injured in unspecified nontraffic accident

  Accident NOS involving heavy transport vehicle, nontraffic

  Occupant of heavy transport vehicle injured in nontraffic accident NOS

√5th **V69.4** Driver of heavy transport vehicle injured in collision with other and unspecified motor vehicles in traffic accident

  √x7th **V69.40** Driver of heavy transport vehicle injured in collision with unspecified motor vehicles in traffic accident

  √x7th **V69.49** Driver of heavy transport vehicle injured in collision with other motor vehicles in traffic accident

√5th **V69.5** Passenger in heavy transport vehicle injured in collision with other and unspecified motor vehicles in traffic accident

  √x7th **V69.50** Passenger in heavy transport vehicle injured in collision with unspecified motor vehicles in traffic accident

  √x7th **V69.59** Passenger in heavy transport vehicle injured in collision with other motor vehicles in traffic accident

√5th **V69.6** Unspecified occupant of heavy transport vehicle injured in collision with other and unspecified motor vehicles in traffic accident

  √x7th **V69.60** Unspecified occupant of heavy transport vehicle injured in collision with unspecified motor vehicles in traffic accident

    Collision NOS involving heavy transport vehicle (traffic)

  √x7th **V69.69** Unspecified occupant of heavy transport vehicle injured in collision with other motor vehicles in traffic accident

√5th **V69.8** Occupant (driver) (passenger) of heavy transport vehicle injured in other specified transport accidents

  √x7th **V69.81** Occupant (driver) (passenger) of heavy transport vehicle injured in transport accidents with military vehicle

  √x7th **V69.88** Occupant (driver) (passenger) of heavy transport vehicle injured in other specified transport accidents

√x7th **V69.9** Occupant (driver) (passenger) of heavy transport vehicle injured in unspecified traffic accident

  Accident NOS involving heavy transport vehicle

Bus occupant injured in transport accident (V70-V79)

INCLUDES motorcoach
EXCLUDES 1 minibus (V50-V59)

The appropriate 7th character is to be added to each code from categories V70-V79.
A initial encounter
D subsequent encounter
S sequela

√4th **V70** **Bus occupant injured in collision with pedestrian or animal**

EXCLUDES 1 bus collision with animal-drawn vehicle or animal being ridden (V76.-)

√x7th **V70.0** Driver of bus injured in collision with pedestrian or animal in nontraffic accident

√x7th **V70.1** Passenger on bus injured in collision with pedestrian or animal in nontraffic accident

√x7th **V70.2** Person on outside of bus injured in collision with pedestrian or animal in nontraffic accident

√x7th **V70.3** Unspecified occupant of bus injured in collision with pedestrian or animal in nontraffic accident

√x7th **V70.4** Person boarding or alighting from bus injured in collision with pedestrian or animal

√x7th **V70.5** Driver of bus injured in collision with pedestrian or animal in traffic accident

√x7th **V70.6** Passenger on bus injured in collision with pedestrian or animal in traffic accident

√x7th **V70.7** Person on outside of bus injured in collision with pedestrian or animal in traffic accident

√x7th **V70.9** Unspecified occupant of bus injured in collision with pedestrian or animal in traffic accident

√4th **V71** **Bus occupant injured in collision with pedal cycle**

√x7th **V71.0** Driver of bus injured in collision with pedal cycle in nontraffic accident

√x7th **V71.1** Passenger on bus injured in collision with pedal cycle in nontraffic accident

√x7th **V71.2** Person on outside of bus injured in collision with pedal cycle in nontraffic accident

√x7th **V71.3** Unspecified occupant of bus injured in collision with pedal cycle in nontraffic accident

√x7th **V71.4** Person boarding or alighting from bus injured in collision with pedal cycle

√x7th **V71.5** Driver of bus injured in collision with pedal cycle in traffic accident

√x7th **V71.6** Passenger on bus injured in collision with pedal cycle in traffic accident

√x7th **V71.7** Person on outside of bus injured in collision with pedal cycle in traffic accident

√x7th **V71.9** Unspecified occupant of bus injured in collision with pedal cycle in traffic accident

√4th **V72** **Bus occupant injured in collision with two- or three-wheeled motor vehicle**

√x7th **V72.0** Driver of bus injured in collision with two- or three-wheeled motor vehicle in nontraffic accident

√x7th **V72.1** Passenger on bus injured in collision with two- or three-wheeled motor vehicle in nontraffic accident

√x7th **V72.2** Person on outside of bus injured in collision with two- or three-wheeled motor vehicle in nontraffic accident

√x7th **V72.3** Unspecified occupant of bus injured in collision with two- or three-wheeled motor vehicle in nontraffic accident

√x7th **V72.4** Person boarding or alighting from bus injured in collision with two- or three-wheeled motor vehicle

√x7th **V72.5** Driver of bus injured in collision with two- or three-wheeled motor vehicle in traffic accident

√x7th **V72.6** Passenger on bus injured in collision with two- or three-wheeled motor vehicle in traffic accident

√x7th **V72.7** Person on outside of bus injured in collision with two- or three-wheeled motor vehicle in traffic accident

√x7th **V72.9** Unspecified occupant of bus injured in collision with two- or three-wheeled motor vehicle in traffic accident

√4th **V73** **Bus occupant injured in collision with car, pick-up truck or van**

√x7th **V73.0** Driver of bus injured in collision with car, pick-up truck or van in nontraffic accident

√x7th **V73.1** Passenger on bus injured in collision with car, pick-up truck or van in nontraffic accident

√x7th **V73.2** Person on outside of bus injured in collision with car, pick-up truck or van in nontraffic accident

N Newborn: 0   P Pediatric: 0-17   M Maternity: 9-64   A Adult: 15-124   MCC Major Complication/Comorbidity   CC Complication/Comorbidity   SW Severe Wound Dx

1188   ICD-10-CM 2022

√x7ᵗʰ V73.3 Unspecified occupant of bus injured in collision with car, pick-up truck or van in nontraffic accident

√x7ᵗʰ V73.4 Person boarding or alighting from bus injured in collision with car, pick-up truck or van

√x7ᵗʰ V73.5 Driver of bus injured in collision with car, pick-up truck or van in traffic accident

√x7ᵗʰ V73.6 Passenger on bus injured in collision with car, pick-up truck or van in traffic accident

√x7ᵗʰ V73.7 Person on outside of bus injured in collision with car, pick-up truck or van in traffic accident

√x7ᵗʰ V73.9 Unspecified occupant of bus injured in collision with car, pick-up truck or van in traffic accident

√4ᵗʰ V74 Bus occupant injured in collision with heavy transport vehicle or bus

> **EXCLUDES 1**   *bus occupant injured in collision with military vehicle (V79.81)*

√x7ᵗʰ V74.0 Driver of bus injured in collision with heavy transport vehicle or bus in nontraffic accident

√x7ᵗʰ V74.1 Passenger on bus injured in collision with heavy transport vehicle or bus in nontraffic accident

√x7ᵗʰ V74.2 Person on outside of bus injured in collision with heavy transport vehicle or bus in nontraffic accident

√x7ᵗʰ V74.3 Unspecified occupant of bus injured in collision with heavy transport vehicle or bus in nontraffic accident

√x7ᵗʰ V74.4 Person boarding or alighting from bus injured in collision with heavy transport vehicle or bus

√x7ᵗʰ V74.5 Driver of bus injured in collision with heavy transport vehicle or bus in traffic accident

√x7ᵗʰ V74.6 Passenger on bus injured in collision with heavy transport vehicle or bus in traffic accident

√x7ᵗʰ V74.7 Person on outside of bus injured in collision with heavy transport vehicle or bus in traffic accident

√x7ᵗʰ V74.9 Unspecified occupant of bus injured in collision with heavy transport vehicle or bus in traffic accident

√4ᵗʰ V75 Bus occupant injured in collision with railway train or railway vehicle

√x7ᵗʰ V75.0 Driver of bus injured in collision with railway train or railway vehicle in nontraffic accident

√x7ᵗʰ V75.1 Passenger on bus injured in collision with railway train or railway vehicle in nontraffic accident

√x7ᵗʰ V75.2 Person on outside of bus injured in collision with railway train or railway vehicle in nontraffic accident

√x7ᵗʰ V75.3 Unspecified occupant of bus injured in collision with railway train or railway vehicle in nontraffic accident

√x7ᵗʰ V75.4 Person boarding or alighting from bus injured in collision with railway train or railway vehicle

√x7ᵗʰ V75.5 Driver of bus injured in collision with railway train or railway vehicle in traffic accident

√x7ᵗʰ V75.6 Passenger on bus injured in collision with railway train or railway vehicle in traffic accident

√x7ᵗʰ V75.7 Person on outside of bus injured in collision with railway train or railway vehicle in traffic accident

√x7ᵗʰ V75.9 Unspecified occupant of bus injured in collision with railway train or railway vehicle in traffic accident

√4ᵗʰ V76 Bus occupant injured in collision with other nonmotor vehicle

> **INCLUDES**   collision with animal-drawn vehicle, animal being ridden, streetcar

√x7ᵗʰ V76.0 Driver of bus injured in collision with other nonmotor vehicle in nontraffic accident

√x7ᵗʰ V76.1 Passenger on bus injured in collision with other nonmotor vehicle in nontraffic accident

√x7ᵗʰ V76.2 Person on outside of bus injured in collision with other nonmotor vehicle in nontraffic accident

√x7ᵗʰ V76.3 Unspecified occupant of bus injured in collision with other nonmotor vehicle in nontraffic accident

√x7ᵗʰ V76.4 Person boarding or alighting from bus injured in collision with other nonmotor vehicle

√x7ᵗʰ V76.5 Driver of bus injured in collision with other nonmotor vehicle in traffic accident

√x7ᵗʰ V76.6 Passenger on bus injured in collision with other nonmotor vehicle in traffic accident

√x7ᵗʰ V76.7 Person on outside of bus injured in collision with other nonmotor vehicle in traffic accident

√x7ᵗʰ V76.9 Unspecified occupant of bus injured in collision with other nonmotor vehicle in traffic accident

√4ᵗʰ V77 Bus occupant injured in collision with fixed or stationary object

√x7ᵗʰ V77.0 Driver of bus injured in collision with fixed or stationary object in nontraffic accident

√x7ᵗʰ V77.1 Passenger on bus injured in collision with fixed or stationary object in nontraffic accident

√x7ᵗʰ V77.2 Person on outside of bus injured in collision with fixed or stationary object in nontraffic accident

√x7ᵗʰ V77.3 Unspecified occupant of bus injured in collision with fixed or stationary object in nontraffic accident

√x7ᵗʰ V77.4 Person boarding or alighting from bus injured in collision with fixed or stationary object

√x7ᵗʰ V77.5 Driver of bus injured in collision with fixed or stationary object in traffic accident

√x7ᵗʰ V77.6 Passenger on bus injured in collision with fixed or stationary object in traffic accident

√x7ᵗʰ V77.7 Person on outside of bus injured in collision with fixed or stationary object in traffic accident

√x7ᵗʰ V77.9 Unspecified occupant of bus injured in collision with fixed or stationary object in traffic accident

√4ᵗʰ V78 Bus occupant injured in noncollision transport accident

> **INCLUDES**   overturning bus NOS
> overturning bus without collision

√x7ᵗʰ V78.0 Driver of bus injured in noncollision transport accident in nontraffic accident

√x7ᵗʰ V78.1 Passenger on bus injured in noncollision transport accident in nontraffic accident

√x7ᵗʰ V78.2 Person on outside of bus injured in noncollision transport accident in nontraffic accident

√x7ᵗʰ V78.3 Unspecified occupant of bus injured in noncollision transport accident in nontraffic accident

√x7ᵗʰ V78.4 Person boarding or alighting from bus injured in noncollision transport accident

√x7ᵗʰ V78.5 Driver of bus injured in noncollision transport accident in traffic accident

√x7ᵗʰ V78.6 Passenger on bus injured in noncollision transport accident in traffic accident

√x7ᵗʰ V78.7 Person on outside of bus injured in noncollision transport accident in traffic accident

√x7ᵗʰ V78.9 Unspecified occupant of bus injured in noncollision transport accident in traffic accident

√4ᵗʰ V79 Bus occupant injured in other and unspecified transport accidents

√5ᵗʰ V79.0 Driver of bus injured in collision with other and unspecified motor vehicles in nontraffic accident

√x7ᵗʰ V79.00 Driver of bus injured in collision with unspecified motor vehicles in nontraffic accident

√x7ᵗʰ V79.09 Driver of bus injured in collision with other motor vehicles in nontraffic accident

√5ᵗʰ V79.1 Passenger on bus injured in collision with other and unspecified motor vehicles in nontraffic accident

√x7ᵗʰ V79.10 Passenger on bus injured in collision with unspecified motor vehicles in nontraffic accident

√x7ᵗʰ V79.19 Passenger on bus injured in collision with other motor vehicles in nontraffic accident

√5ᵗʰ V79.2 Unspecified bus occupant injured in collision with other and unspecified motor vehicles in nontraffic accident

√x7ᵗʰ V79.20 Unspecified bus occupant injured in collision with unspecified motor vehicles in nontraffic accident
Bus collision NOS, nontraffic

√x7ᵗʰ V79.29 Unspecified bus occupant injured in collision with other motor vehicles in nontraffic accident

√x7ᵗʰ V79.3 Bus occupant (driver) (passenger) injured in unspecified nontraffic accident
Bus accident NOS, nontraffic
Bus occupant injured in nontraffic accident NOS

√5ᵗʰ V79.4 Driver of bus injured in collision with other and unspecified motor vehicles in traffic accident

√x7ᵗʰ V79.40 Driver of bus injured in collision with unspecified motor vehicles in traffic accident

√x7ᵗʰ V79.49 Driver of bus injured in collision with other motor vehicles in traffic accident

√5ᵗʰ V79.5 Passenger on bus injured in collision with other and unspecified motor vehicles in traffic accident

√x7ᵗʰ V79.50 Passenger on bus injured in collision with unspecified motor vehicles in traffic accident

√x7ᵗʰ V79.59 Passenger on bus injured in collision with other motor vehicles in traffic accident

√5ᵗʰ V79.6 Unspecified bus occupant injured in collision with other and unspecified motor vehicles in traffic accident

√x7ᵗʰ V79.60 Unspecified bus occupant injured in collision with unspecified motor vehicles in traffic accident
Bus collision NOS (traffic)

√x7ᵗʰ V79.69 Unspecified bus occupant injured in collision with other motor vehicles in traffic accident

√5ᵗʰ **V79.8 Bus occupant (driver) (passenger) injured in other specified transport accidents**

√x7ᵗʰ **V79.81 Bus occupant (driver) (passenger) injured in transport accidents with** military vehicle

√x7ᵗʰ **V79.88 Bus occupant (driver) (passenger) injured in other specified transport accidents**

√x7ᵗʰ **V79.9 Bus occupant (driver) (passenger) injured in unspecified traffic accident**
Bus accident NOS

Other land transport accidents (V80-V89)

The appropriate 7th character is to be added to each code from categories V80-V89.
A initial encounter
D subsequent encounter
S sequela

√4ᵗʰ **V80 Animal-rider or occupant of animal-drawn vehicle injured in transport accident**

√5ᵗʰ **V80.0 Animal-rider or occupant of animal drawn vehicle injured by fall from or being thrown from animal or animal-drawn vehicle in** noncollision accident

√6ᵗʰ **V80.01 Animal-rider injured by fall from or being thrown from animal in noncollision accident**

√7ᵗʰ **V80.010 Animal-rider injured by fall from or being thrown from horse in noncollision accident**

√7ᵗʰ **V80.018 Animal-rider injured by fall from or being thrown from other animal in noncollision accident**

√x7ᵗʰ **V80.02 Occupant of animal-drawn vehicle injured by fall from or being thrown from animal-drawn vehicle in noncollision accident**
Overturning animal-drawn vehicle NOS
Overturning animal-drawn vehicle without collision

√5ᵗʰ **V80.1 Animal-rider or occupant of animal-drawn vehicle injured in collision with** pedestrian or animal

EXCLUDES 1 animal-rider or animal-drawn vehicle collision with animal-drawn vehicle or animal being ridden (V80.7)

√x7ᵗʰ **V80.11 Animal-rider injured in collision with pedestrian or animal**

√x7ᵗʰ **V80.12 Occupant of animal-drawn vehicle injured in collision with pedestrian or animal**

√5ᵗʰ **V80.2 Animal-rider or occupant of animal-drawn vehicle injured in collision with** pedal cycle

√x7ᵗʰ **V80.21 Animal-rider injured in collision with pedal cycle**

√x7ᵗʰ **V80.22 Occupant of animal-drawn vehicle injured in collision with pedal cycle**

√5ᵗʰ **V80.3 Animal-rider or occupant of animal-drawn vehicle injured in collision with** two- or three-wheeled motor vehicle

√x7ᵗʰ **V80.31 Animal-rider injured in collision with two- or three-wheeled motor vehicle**

√x7ᵗʰ **V80.32 Occupant of animal-drawn vehicle injured in collision with two- or three-wheeled motor vehicle**

√5ᵗʰ **V80.4 Animal-rider or occupant of animal-drawn vehicle injured in collision with** car, pick-up truck, van, heavy transport vehicle or bus

EXCLUDES 1 animal-rider injured in collision with military vehicle (V80.910)
occupant of animal-drawn vehicle injured in collision with military vehicle (V80.920)

√x7ᵗʰ **V80.41 Animal-rider injured in collision with car, pick-up truck, van, heavy transport vehicle or bus**

√x7ᵗʰ **V80.42 Occupant of animal-drawn vehicle injured in collision with car, pick-up truck, van, heavy transport vehicle or bus**

√5ᵗʰ **V80.5 Animal-rider or occupant of animal-drawn vehicle injured in collision with other specified motor vehicle**

√x7ᵗʰ **V80.51 Animal-rider injured in collision with other specified motor vehicle**

√x7ᵗʰ **V80.52 Occupant of animal-drawn vehicle injured in collision with other specified motor vehicle**

√5ᵗʰ **V80.6 Animal-rider or occupant of animal-drawn vehicle injured in collision with** railway train or railway vehicle

√x7ᵗʰ **V80.61 Animal-rider injured in collision with railway train or railway vehicle**

√x7ᵗʰ **V80.62 Occupant of animal-drawn vehicle injured in collision with railway train or railway vehicle**

√5ᵗʰ **V80.7 Animal-rider or occupant of animal-drawn vehicle injured in collision with other nonmotor vehicles**

√6ᵗʰ **V80.71 Animal-rider or occupant of animal-drawn vehicle injured in collision with** animal being ridden

√7ᵗʰ **V80.710 Animal-rider injured in collision with other animal being ridden**

√7ᵗʰ **V80.711 Occupant of animal-drawn vehicle injured in collision with animal being ridden**

√6ᵗʰ **V80.72 Animal-rider or occupant of animal-drawn vehicle injured in collision with** other animal-drawn vehicle

√7ᵗʰ **V80.720 Animal-rider injured in collision with animal-drawn vehicle**

√7ᵗʰ **V80.721 Occupant of animal-drawn vehicle injured in collision with other animal-drawn vehicle**

√6ᵗʰ **V80.73 Animal-rider or occupant of animal-drawn vehicle injured in collision with** streetcar

√7ᵗʰ **V80.730 Animal-rider injured in collision with streetcar**

√7ᵗʰ **V80.731 Occupant of animal-drawn vehicle injured in collision with streetcar**

√6ᵗʰ **V80.79 Animal-rider or occupant of animal-drawn vehicle injured in collision with** other nonmotor vehicles

√7ᵗʰ **V80.790 Animal-rider injured in collision with other nonmotor vehicles**

√7ᵗʰ **V80.791 Occupant of animal-drawn vehicle injured in collision with other nonmotor vehicles**

√5ᵗʰ **V80.8 Animal-rider or occupant of animal-drawn vehicle injured in collision with** fixed or stationary object

√x7ᵗʰ **V80.81 Animal-rider injured in collision with fixed or stationary object**

√x7ᵗʰ **V80.82 Occupant of animal-drawn vehicle injured in collision with fixed or stationary object**

√5ᵗʰ **V80.9 Animal-rider or occupant of animal-drawn vehicle injured in other and unspecified transport accidents**

√6ᵗʰ **V80.91 Animal-rider injured in other and unspecified transport accidents**

√7ᵗʰ **V80.910 Animal-rider injured in transport accident with** military vehicle

√7ᵗʰ **V80.918 Animal-rider injured in other transport accident**

√7ᵗʰ **V80.919 Animal-rider injured in unspecified transport accident**
Animal rider accident NOS

√6ᵗʰ **V80.92 Occupant of animal-drawn vehicle injured in other and unspecified transport accidents**

√7ᵗʰ **V80.920 Occupant of animal-drawn vehicle injured in transport accident with** military vehicle

√7ᵗʰ **V80.928 Occupant of animal-drawn vehicle injured in other transport accident**

√7ᵗʰ **V80.929 Occupant of animal-drawn vehicle injured in unspecified transport accident**
Animal-drawn vehicle accident NOS

√4ᵗʰ **V81 Occupant of railway train or railway vehicle injured in transport accident**

INCLUDES derailment of railway train or railway vehicle
person on outside of train

EXCLUDES 1 streetcar (V82.-)

√x7ᵗʰ **V81.0 Occupant of railway train or railway vehicle injured in collision with motor vehicle in nontraffic accident**

EXCLUDES 1 occupant of railway train or railway vehicle injured due to collision with military vehicle (V81.83)

√x7ᵗʰ **V81.1 Occupant of railway train or railway vehicle injured in collision with motor vehicle in traffic accident**

EXCLUDES 1 occupant of railway train or railway vehicle injured due to collision with military vehicle (V81.83)

√x7ᵗʰ **V81.2 Occupant of railway train or railway vehicle injured in collision with or** hit by rolling stock

√x7ᵗʰ **V81.3 Occupant of railway train or railway vehicle injured in collision with other object**
Railway collision NOS

√x7ᵗʰ **V81.4 Person injured** while boarding or alighting **from railway train or railway vehicle**

√x7ᵗʰ **V81.5 Occupant of railway train or railway vehicle injured by fall in railway train or railway vehicle**

√x7ᵗʰ **V81.6 Occupant of railway train or railway vehicle injured by fall from railway train or railway vehicle**

√x7ᵗʰ **V81.7 Occupant of railway train or railway vehicle injured in derailment without antecedent collision**

√6ᵗʰ **V81.8   Occupant of railway train or railway vehicle injured in other specified railway accidents**

√x7ᵗʰ **V81.81   Occupant of railway train or railway vehicle injured due to explosion or fire on train**

√x7ᵗʰ **V81.82   Occupant of railway train or railway vehicle injured due to object falling onto train**

Occupant of railway train or railway vehicle injured due to falling earth onto train

Occupant of railway train or railway vehicle injured due to falling rocks onto train

Occupant of railway train or railway vehicle injured due to falling snow onto train

Occupant of railway train or railway vehicle injured due to falling trees onto train

√x7ᵗʰ **V81.83   Occupant of railway train or railway vehicle injured due to collision with military vehicle**

√x7ᵗʰ **V81.89   Occupant of railway train or railway vehicle injured due to other specified railway accident**

√x7ᵗʰ **V81.9   Occupant of railway train or railway vehicle injured in unspecified railway accident**

Railway accident NOS

√4ᵗʰ **V82   Occupant of powered streetcar injured in transport accident**

> INCLUDES   interurban electric car
> person on outside of streetcar
> tram (car)
> trolley (car)
>
> EXCLUDES 1   *bus (V70-V79)*
> *motorcoach (V70-V79)*
> *nonpowered streetcar (V76.-)*
> *train (V81.-)*

√x7ᵗʰ **V82.0   Occupant of streetcar injured in collision with motor vehicle in nontraffic accident**

√x7ᵗʰ **V82.1   Occupant of streetcar injured in collision with motor vehicle in traffic accident**

√x7ᵗʰ **V82.2   Occupant of streetcar injured in collision with or hit by rolling stock**

√x7ᵗʰ **V82.3   Occupant of streetcar injured in collision with other object**

> EXCLUDES 1   *collision with animal-drawn vehicle or animal being ridden (V82.8)*

√x7ᵗʰ **V82.4   Person injured while boarding or alighting from streetcar**

√x7ᵗʰ **V82.5   Occupant of streetcar injured by fall in streetcar**

> EXCLUDES 1   *fall in streetcar:*
> *while boarding or alighting (V82.4)*
> *with antecedent collision (V82.0-V82.3)*

√x7ᵗʰ **V82.6   Occupant of streetcar injured by fall from streetcar**

> EXCLUDES 1   *fall from streetcar:*
> *while boarding or alighting (V82.4)*
> *with antecedent collision (V82.0-V82.3)*

√x7ᵗʰ **V82.7   Occupant of streetcar injured in derailment without antecedent collision**

> EXCLUDES 1   *occupant of streetcar injured in derailment with antecedent collision (V82.0-V82.3)*

√x7ᵗʰ **V82.8   Occupant of streetcar injured in other specified transport accidents**

Streetcar collision with military vehicle

Streetcar collision with train or nonmotor vehicles

√x7ᵗʰ **V82.9   Occupant of streetcar injured in unspecified traffic accident**

Streetcar accident NOS

√4ᵗʰ **V83   Occupant of special vehicle mainly used on industrial premises injured in transport accident**

> INCLUDES   battery-powered airport passenger vehicle
> battery-powered truck (baggage) (mail)
> coal-car in mine
> forklift (truck)
> logging car
> self-propelled industrial truck
> station baggage truck (powered)
> tram, truck, or tub (powered) in mine or quarry
>
> EXCLUDES 1   *special construction vehicles (V85.-)*
> *special industrial vehicle in stationary use or maintenance (W31.-)*

√x7ᵗʰ **V83.0   Driver of special industrial vehicle injured in traffic accident**

√x7ᵗʰ **V83.1   Passenger of special industrial vehicle injured in traffic accident**

√x7ᵗʰ **V83.2   Person on outside of special industrial vehicle injured in traffic accident**

√x7ᵗʰ **V83.3   Unspecified occupant of special industrial vehicle injured in traffic accident**

√x7ᵗʰ **V83.4   Person injured while boarding or alighting from special industrial vehicle**

√x7ᵗʰ **V83.5   Driver of special industrial vehicle injured in nontraffic accident**

√x7ᵗʰ **V83.6   Passenger of special industrial vehicle injured in nontraffic accident**

√x7ᵗʰ **V83.7   Person on outside of special industrial vehicle injured in nontraffic accident**

√x7ᵗʰ **V83.9   Unspecified occupant of special industrial vehicle injured in nontraffic accident**

Special-industrial-vehicle accident NOS

√4ᵗʰ **V84   Occupant of special vehicle mainly used in agriculture injured in transport accident**

> INCLUDES   self-propelled farm machinery
> tractor (and trailer)
>
> EXCLUDES 1   *animal-powered farm machinery accident (W30.8-)*
> *contact with combine harvester (W30.0)*
> *special agricultural vehicle in stationary use or maintenance (W30.-)*

√x7ᵗʰ **V84.0   Driver of special agricultural vehicle injured in traffic accident**

√x7ᵗʰ **V84.1   Passenger of special agricultural vehicle injured in traffic accident**

√x7ᵗʰ **V84.2   Person on outside of special agricultural vehicle injured in traffic accident**

√x7ᵗʰ **V84.3   Unspecified occupant of special agricultural vehicle injured in traffic accident**

√x7ᵗʰ **V84.4   Person injured while boarding or alighting from special agricultural vehicle**

√x7ᵗʰ **V84.5   Driver of special agricultural vehicle injured in nontraffic accident**

√x7ᵗʰ **V84.6   Passenger of special agricultural vehicle injured in nontraffic accident**

√x7ᵗʰ **V84.7   Person on outside of special agricultural vehicle injured in nontraffic accident**

√x7ᵗʰ **V84.9   Unspecified occupant of special agricultural vehicle injured in nontraffic accident**

Special-agricultural vehicle accident NOS

√4ᵗʰ **V85   Occupant of special construction vehicle injured in transport accident**

> INCLUDES   bulldozer
> digger
> dump truck
> earth-leveller
> mechanical shovel
> road-roller
>
> EXCLUDES 1   *special industrial vehicle (V83.-)*
> *special construction vehicle in stationary use or maintenance (W31.-)*

√x7ᵗʰ **V85.0   Driver of special construction vehicle injured in traffic accident**

√x7ᵗʰ **V85.1   Passenger of special construction vehicle injured in traffic accident**

√x7ᵗʰ **V85.2   Person on outside of special construction vehicle injured in traffic accident**

√x7ᵗʰ **V85.3   Unspecified occupant of special construction vehicle injured in traffic accident**

√x7ᵗʰ **V85.4   Person injured while boarding or alighting from special construction vehicle**

√x7ᵗʰ **V85.5   Driver of special construction vehicle injured in nontraffic accident**

√x7ᵗʰ **V85.6   Passenger of special construction vehicle injured in nontraffic accident**

√x7ᵗʰ **V85.7   Person on outside of special construction vehicle injured in nontraffic accident**

√x7ᵗʰ **V85.9   Unspecified occupant of special construction vehicle injured in nontraffic accident**

Special-construction-vehicle accident NOS

✓ Additional Char Req   √x7ᵗʰ Placeholder   Unacceptable PDx   Questionable PDx   Wrong Procedure   Manifestation   Unspecified Dx   H1-H14 HAC   HCC CMS-HCC Dx   HIV HIV Dx

ICD-10-CM 2022   1191

✓4th **V86** **Occupant of special all-terrain or other off-road motor vehicle, injured in transport accident**

> EXCLUDES 1 *special all-terrain vehicle in stationary use or maintenance (W31.-)*
> *sport-utility vehicle (V50-V59)*
> *three-wheeled motor vehicle designed for on-road use (V30-V39)*

> AHA: 2017,4Q,26

✓5th **V86.0** **Driver of special all-terrain or other off-road motor vehicle injured in traffic accident**

✓x7th **V86.01** **Driver of ambulance or fire engine injured in traffic accident**

✓x7th **V86.02** **Driver of snowmobile injured in traffic accident**

✓x7th **V86.03** **Driver of dune buggy injured in traffic accident**

✓x7th **V86.04** **Driver of military vehicle injured in traffic accident**

✓x7th **V86.05** **Driver of 3- or 4- wheeled all-terrain vehicle (ATV) injured in traffic accident**

✓x7th **V86.06** **Driver of dirt bike or motor/cross bike injured in traffic accident**

✓x7th **V86.09** **Driver of other special all-terrain or other off-road motor vehicle injured in traffic accident**
> Driver of go cart injured in traffic accident
> Driver of golf cart injured in traffic accident

✓5th **V86.1** **Passenger of special all-terrain or other off-road motor vehicle injured in traffic accident**

✓x7th **V86.11** **Passenger of ambulance or fire engine injured in traffic accident**

✓x7th **V86.12** **Passenger of snowmobile injured in traffic accident**

✓x7th **V86.13** **Passenger of dune buggy injured in traffic accident**

✓x7th **V86.14** **Passenger of military vehicle injured in traffic accident**

✓x7th **V86.15** **Passenger of 3- or 4- wheeled all-terrain vehicle (ATV) injured in traffic accident**

✓x7th **V86.16** **Passenger of dirt bike or motor/cross bike injured in traffic accident**

✓x7th **V86.19** **Passenger of other special all-terrain or other off-road motor vehicle injured in traffic accident**
> Passenger of go cart injured in traffic accident
> Passenger of golf cart injured in traffic accident

✓5th **V86.2** **Person on outside of special all-terrain or other off-road motor vehicle injured in traffic accident**

✓x7th **V86.21** **Person on outside of ambulance or fire engine injured in traffic accident**

✓x7th **V86.22** **Person on outside of snowmobile injured in traffic accident**

✓x7th **V86.23** **Person on outside of dune buggy injured in traffic accident**

✓x7th **V86.24** **Person on outside of military vehicle injured in traffic accident**

✓x7th **V86.25** **Person on outside of 3- or 4- wheeled all-terrain vehicle (ATV) injured in traffic accident**

✓x7th **V86.26** **Person on outside of dirt bike or motor/cross bike injured in traffic accident**

✓x7th **V86.29** **Person on outside of other special all-terrain or other off-road motor vehicle injured in traffic accident**
> Person on outside of go cart in traffic accident
> Person on outside of golf cart injured in traffic accident

✓5th **V86.3** **Unspecified occupant of special all-terrain or other off-road motor vehicle injured in traffic accident**

✓x7th **V86.31** **Unspecified occupant of ambulance or fire engine injured in traffic accident**

✓x7th **V86.32** **Unspecified occupant of snowmobile injured in traffic accident**

✓x7th **V86.33** **Unspecified occupant of dune buggy injured in traffic accident**

✓x7th **V86.34** **Unspecified occupant of military vehicle injured in traffic accident**

✓x7th **V86.35** **Unspecified occupant of 3- or 4- wheeled all-terrain vehicle (ATV) injured in traffic accident**

✓x7th **V86.36** **Unspecified occupant of dirt bike or motor/cross bike injured in traffic accident**

✓x7th **V86.39** **Unspecified occupant of other special all-terrain or other off-road motor vehicle injured in traffic accident**
> Unspecified occupant of go cart injured in traffic accident
> Unspecified occupant of golf cart injured in traffic accident

✓5th **V86.4** **Person injured while boarding or alighting from special all-terrain or other off-road motor vehicle**

✓x7th **V86.41** **Person injured while boarding or alighting from ambulance or fire engine**

✓x7th **V86.42** **Person injured while boarding or alighting from snowmobile**

✓x7th **V86.43** **Person injured while boarding or alighting from dune buggy**

✓x7th **V86.44** **Person injured while boarding or alighting from military vehicle**

✓x7th **V86.45** **Person injured while boarding or alighting from a 3- or 4- wheeled all-terrain vehicle (ATV)**

✓x7th **V86.46** **Person injured while boarding or alighting from a dirt bike or motor/cross bike**

✓x7th **V86.49** **Person injured while boarding or alighting from other special all-terrain or other off-road motor vehicle**
> Person injured while boarding or alighting from go cart
> Person injured while boarding or alighting from golf cart

✓5th **V86.5** **Driver of special all-terrain or other off-road motor vehicle injured in nontraffic accident**

✓x7th **V86.51** **Driver of ambulance or fire engine injured in nontraffic accident**

✓x7th **V86.52** **Driver of snowmobile injured in nontraffic accident**

✓x7th **V86.53** **Driver of dune buggy injured in nontraffic accident**

✓x7th **V86.54** **Driver of military vehicle injured in nontraffic accident**

✓x7th **V86.55** **Driver of 3- or 4- wheeled all-terrain vehicle (ATV) injured in nontraffic accident**

✓x7th **V86.56** **Driver of dirt bike or motor/cross bike injured in nontraffic accident**

✓x7th **V86.59** **Driver of other special all-terrain or other off-road motor vehicle injured in nontraffic accident**
> Driver of go cart injured in nontraffic accident
> Driver of golf cart injured in nontraffic accident

✓5th **V86.6** **Passenger of special all-terrain or other off-road motor vehicle injured in nontraffic accident**

✓x7th **V86.61** **Passenger of ambulance or fire engine injured in nontraffic accident**

✓x7th **V86.62** **Passenger of snowmobile injured in nontraffic accident**

✓x7th **V86.63** **Passenger of dune buggy injured in nontraffic accident**

✓x7th **V86.64** **Passenger of military vehicle injured in nontraffic accident**

✓x7th **V86.65** **Passenger of 3- or 4- wheeled all-terrain vehicle (ATV) injured in nontraffic accident**

✓x7th **V86.66** **Passenger of dirt bike or motor/cross bike injured in nontraffic accident**

✓x7th **V86.69** **Passenger of other special all-terrain or other off-road motor vehicle injured in nontraffic accident**
> Passenger of go cart injured in nontraffic accident
> Passenger of golf cart injured in nontraffic accident

✓5th **V86.7** **Person on outside of special all-terrain or other off-road motor vehicle injured in nontraffic accident**

✓x7th **V86.71** **Person on outside of ambulance or fire engine injured in nontraffic accident**

✓x7th **V86.72** **Person on outside of snowmobile injured in nontraffic accident**

✓x7th **V86.73** **Person on outside of dune buggy injured in nontraffic accident**

✓x7th **V86.74** **Person on outside of military vehicle injured in nontraffic accident**

✓x7th **V86.75** **Person on outside of 3- or 4- wheeled all-terrain vehicle (ATV) injured in nontraffic accident**

✓x7th **V86.76** **Person on outside of dirt bike or motor/cross bike injured in nontraffic accident**

√x7ᵗʰ **V86.79** **Person on outside of other special all-terrain or other off-road motor vehicles injured in nontraffic accident**

Person on outside of go cart injured in nontraffic accident

Person on outside of golf cart injured in nontraffic accident

√5ᵗʰ **V86.9** **Unspecified occupant of special all-terrain or other off-road motor vehicle injured in nontraffic accident**

√x7ᵗʰ **V86.91** **Unspecified occupant of ambulance or fire engine injured in nontraffic accident**

√x7ᵗʰ **V86.92** **Unspecified occupant of snowmobile injured in nontraffic accident**

√x7ᵗʰ **V86.93** **Unspecified occupant of dune buggy injured in nontraffic accident**

√x7ᵗʰ **V86.94** **Unspecified occupant of military vehicle injured in nontraffic accident**

√x7ᵗʰ **V86.95** **Unspecified occupant of 3- or 4- wheeled all-terrain vehicle (ATV) injured in nontraffic accident**

√x7ᵗʰ **V86.96** **Unspecified occupant of dirt bike or motor/cross bike injured in nontraffic accident**

√x7ᵗʰ **V86.99** **Unspecified occupant of other special all-terrain or other off-road motor vehicle injured in nontraffic accident**

Off-road motor-vehicle accident NOS

Other motor-vehicle accident NOS

Unspecified occupant of go cart injured in nontraffic accident

Unspecified occupant of golf cart injured in nontraffic accident

√4ᵗʰ **V87** **Traffic accident of specified type but victim's mode of transport unknown**

EXCLUDES 1   *collision involving:*
pedal cycle (V10-V19)
pedestrian (V01-V09)

√x7ᵗʰ **V87.0** **Person injured in collision between car and two- or three-wheeled powered vehicle (traffic)**

√x7ᵗʰ **V87.1** **Person injured in collision between other motor vehicle and two- or three-wheeled motor vehicle (traffic)**

√x7ᵗʰ **V87.2** **Person injured in collision between car and pick-up truck or van (traffic)**

√x7ᵗʰ **V87.3** **Person injured in collision between car and bus (traffic)**

√x7ᵗʰ **V87.4** **Person injured in collision between car and heavy transport vehicle (traffic)**

√x7ᵗʰ **V87.5** **Person injured in collision between heavy transport vehicle and bus (traffic)**

√x7ᵗʰ **V87.6** **Person injured in collision between railway train or railway vehicle and car (traffic)**

√x7ᵗʰ **V87.7** **Person injured in collision between other specified motor vehicles (traffic)**

√x7ᵗʰ **V87.8** **Person injured in other specified noncollision transport accidents involving motor vehicle (traffic)**

√x7ᵗʰ **V87.9** **Person injured in other specified (collision)(noncollision) transport accidents involving nonmotor vehicle (traffic)**

√4ᵗʰ **V88** **Nontraffic accident of specified type but victim's mode of transport unknown**

EXCLUDES 1   *collision involving:*
pedal cycle (V10-V19)
pedestrian (V01-V09)

√x7ᵗʰ **V88.0** **Person injured in collision between car and two- or three-wheeled motor vehicle, nontraffic**

√x7ᵗʰ **V88.1** **Person injured in collision between other motor vehicle and two- or three-wheeled motor vehicle, nontraffic**

√x7ᵗʰ **V88.2** **Person injured in collision between car and pick-up truck or van, nontraffic**

√x7ᵗʰ **V88.3** **Person injured in collision between car and bus, nontraffic**

√x7ᵗʰ **V88.4** **Person injured in collision between car and heavy transport vehicle, nontraffic**

√x7ᵗʰ **V88.5** **Person injured in collision between heavy transport vehicle and bus, nontraffic**

√x7ᵗʰ **V88.6** **Person injured in collision between railway train or railway vehicle and car, nontraffic**

√x7ᵗʰ **V88.7** **Person injured in collision between other specified motor vehicle, nontraffic**

√x7ᵗʰ **V88.8** **Person injured in other specified noncollision transport accidents involving motor vehicle, nontraffic**

√x7ᵗʰ **V88.9** **Person injured in other specified (collision)(noncollision) transport accidents involving nonmotor vehicle, nontraffic**

√4ᵗʰ **V89** **Motor- or nonmotor-vehicle accident, type of vehicle unspecified**

√x7ᵗʰ **V89.0** **Person injured in unspecified motor-vehicle accident, nontraffic**

Motor-vehicle accident NOS, nontraffic

√x7ᵗʰ **V89.1** **Person injured in unspecified nonmotor-vehicle accident, nontraffic**

Nonmotor-vehicle accident NOS (nontraffic)

√x7ᵗʰ **V89.2** **Person injured in unspecified motor-vehicle accident, traffic**

Motor-vehicle accident [MVA] NOS

Road (traffic) accident [RTA] NOS

√x7ᵗʰ **V89.3** **Person injured in unspecified nonmotor-vehicle accident, traffic**

Nonmotor-vehicle traffic accident NOS

√x7ᵗʰ **V89.9** **Person injured in unspecified vehicle accident**

Collision NOS

Water transport accidents (V90-V94)

The appropriate 7th character is to be added to each code from categories V90-V94.
A   initial encounter
D   subsequent encounter
S   sequela

√4ᵗʰ **V90** **Drowning and submersion due to accident to watercraft**

EXCLUDES 1   *civilian water transport accident involving military watercraft (V94.81-)*
fall into water not from watercraft (W16.-)
military watercraft accident in military or war operations (Y36.0-, Y37.0-)
water-transport-related drowning or submersion without accident to watercraft (V92.-)

√5ᵗʰ **V90.0** **Drowning and submersion due to watercraft overturning**

√x7ᵗʰ **V90.00** **Drowning and submersion due to merchant ship overturning**

√x7ᵗʰ **V90.01** **Drowning and submersion due to passenger ship overturning**

Drowning and submersion due to Ferry-boat overturning

Drowning and submersion due to Liner overturning

√x7ᵗʰ **V90.02** **Drowning and submersion due to fishing boat overturning**

√x7ᵗʰ **V90.03** **Drowning and submersion due to other powered watercraft overturning**

Drowning and submersion due to Hovercraft (on open water) overturning

Drowning and submersion due to Jet ski overturning

√x7ᵗʰ **V90.04** **Drowning and submersion due to sailboat overturning**

√x7ᵗʰ **V90.05** **Drowning and submersion due to canoe or kayak overturning**

√x7ᵗʰ **V90.06** **Drowning and submersion due to (nonpowered) inflatable craft overturning**

√x7ᵗʰ **V90.08** **Drowning and submersion due to other unpowered watercraft overturning**

Drowning and submersion due to windsurfer overturning

√x7ᵗʰ **V90.09** **Drowning and submersion due to unspecified watercraft overturning**

Drowning and submersion due to boat NOS overturning

Drowning and submersion due to ship NOS overturning

Drowning and submersion due to watercraft NOS overturning

√5ᵗʰ **V90.1** **Drowning and submersion due to watercraft sinking**

√x7ᵗʰ **V90.10** **Drowning and submersion due to merchant ship sinking**

√x7ᵗʰ **V90.11** **Drowning and submersion due to passenger ship sinking**

Drowning and submersion due to Ferry-boat sinking

Drowning and submersion due to Liner sinking

√x7ᵗʰ **V90.12** **Drowning and submersion due to fishing boat sinking**

√x7ᵗʰ **V90.13** **Drowning and submersion due to other powered watercraft sinking**

Drowning and submersion due to Hovercraft (on open water) sinking

Drowning and submersion due to Jet ski sinking

√x7ᵗʰ **V90.14** **Drowning and submersion due to sailboat sinking**

✔ Additional Char Req   √x7ᵗʰ Placeholder   Unacceptable PDx   Questionable PDx   Wrong Procedure   Manifestation   Unspecified Dx   HT-H14 HAC   HCC CMS-HCC Dx   HIV HIV Dx

ICD-10-CM 2022   1193

✓x7ᵗʰ **V90.15** **Drowning and submersion due to** canoe or kayak **sinking**

✓x7ᵗʰ **V90.16** **Drowning and submersion due to (nonpowered)** inflatable craft **sinking**

✓x7ᵗʰ **V90.18** **Drowning and submersion due to other** unpowered watercraft sinking

✓x7ᵗʰ **V90.19** **Drowning and submersion due to unspecified watercraft sinking**

Drowning and submersion due to boat NOS sinking

Drowning and submersion due to ship NOS sinking

Drowning and submersion due to watercraft NOS sinking

✓5ᵗʰ **V90.2** **Drowning and submersion due to** falling or jumping from burning watercraft

✓x7ᵗʰ **V90.20** **Drowning and submersion due to falling or jumping from burning** merchant ship

✓x7ᵗʰ **V90.21** **Drowning and submersion due to falling or jumping from burning** passenger ship

Drowning and submersion due to falling or jumping from burning Ferry-boat

Drowning and submersion due to falling or jumping from burning Liner

✓x7ᵗʰ **V90.22** **Drowning and submersion due to falling or jumping from burning** fishing boat

✓x7ᵗʰ **V90.23** **Drowning and submersion due to falling or jumping from other burning** powered **watercraft**

Drowning and submersion due to falling and jumping from burning Hovercraft (on open water)

Drowning and submersion due to falling and jumping from burning Jet ski

✓x7ᵗʰ **V90.24** **Drowning and submersion due to falling or jumping from burning** sailboat

✓x7ᵗʰ **V90.25** **Drowning and submersion due to falling or jumping from burning** canoe or kayak

✓x7ᵗʰ **V90.26** **Drowning and submersion due to falling or jumping from burning (nonpowered)** inflatable craft

✓x7ᵗʰ **V90.27** **Drowning and submersion due to falling or jumping from burning** water-skis

✓x7ᵗʰ **V90.28** **Drowning and submersion due to falling or jumping from other burning** unpowered **watercraft**

Drowning and submersion due to falling and jumping from burning surf-board

Drowning and submersion due to falling and jumping from burning windsurfer

✓x7ᵗʰ **V90.29** **Drowning and submersion due to falling or jumping from unspecified burning watercraft**

Drowning and submersion due to falling or jumping from burning boat NOS

Drowning and submersion due to falling or jumping from burning ship NOS

Drowning and submersion due to falling or jumping from burning watercraft NOS

✓5ᵗʰ **V90.3** **Drowning and submersion due to** falling or jumping from crushed watercraft

✓x7ᵗʰ **V90.30** **Drowning and submersion due to falling or jumping from crushed** merchant ship

✓x7ᵗʰ **V90.31** **Drowning and submersion due to falling or jumping from crushed** passenger ship

Drowning and submersion due to falling and jumping from crushed Ferry boat

Drowning and submersion due to falling and jumping from crushed Liner

✓x7ᵗʰ **V90.32** **Drowning and submersion due to falling or jumping from crushed** fishing boat

✓x7ᵗʰ **V90.33** **Drowning and submersion due to falling or jumping from other crushed** powered **watercraft**

Drowning and submersion due to falling and jumping from crushed Hovercraft

Drowning and submersion due to falling and jumping from crushed Jet ski

✓x7ᵗʰ **V90.34** **Drowning and submersion due to falling or jumping from crushed** sailboat

✓x7ᵗʰ **V90.35** **Drowning and submersion due to falling or jumping from crushed** canoe or kayak

✓x7ᵗʰ **V90.36** **Drowning and submersion due to falling or jumping from crushed (nonpowered)** inflatable craft

✓x7ᵗʰ **V90.37** **Drowning and submersion due to falling or jumping from crushed** water-skis

✓x7ᵗʰ **V90.38** **Drowning and submersion due to falling or jumping from other crushed** unpowered **watercraft**

Drowning and submersion due to falling and jumping from crushed surf-board

Drowning and submersion due to falling and jumping from crushed windsurfer

✓x7ᵗʰ **V90.39** **Drowning and submersion due to falling or jumping from crushed unspecified watercraft**

Drowning and submersion due to falling and jumping from crushed boat NOS

Drowning and submersion due to falling and jumping from crushed ship NOS

Drowning and submersion due to falling and jumping from crushed watercraft NOS

✓5ᵗʰ **V90.8** **Drowning and submersion due to other accident to watercraft**

✓x7ᵗʰ **V90.80** **Drowning and submersion due to other accident to** merchant ship

✓x7ᵗʰ **V90.81** **Drowning and submersion due to other accident to** passenger ship

Drowning and submersion due to other accident to Ferry-boat

Drowning and submersion due to other accident to Liner

✓x7ᵗʰ **V90.82** **Drowning and submersion due to other accident to** fishing boat

✓x7ᵗʰ **V90.83** **Drowning and submersion due to other accident to other** powered **watercraft**

Drowning and submersion due to other accident to Hovercraft (on open water)

Drowning and submersion due to other accident to Jet ski

✓x7ᵗʰ **V90.84** **Drowning and submersion due to other accident to** sailboat

✓x7ᵗʰ **V90.85** **Drowning and submersion due to other accident to** canoe or kayak

✓x7ᵗʰ **V90.86** **Drowning and submersion due to other accident to (nonpowered)** inflatable craft

✓x7ᵗʰ **V90.87** **Drowning and submersion due to other accident to** water-skis

✓x7ᵗʰ **V90.88** **Drowning and submersion due to other accident to other** unpowered **watercraft**

Drowning and submersion due to other accident to surf-board

Drowning and submersion due to other accident to windsurfer

✓x7ᵗʰ **V90.89** **Drowning and submersion due to other accident to unspecified watercraft**

Drowning and submersion due to other accident to boat NOS

Drowning and submersion due to other accident to ship NOS

Drowning and submersion due to other accident to watercraft NOS

✓4ᵗʰ **V91** **Other injury due to accident to watercraft**

INCLUDES any injury except drowning and submersion as a result of an accident to watercraft

EXCLUDES 1 civilian water transport accident involving military watercraft (V94.81-)

military watercraft accident in military or war operations (Y36, Y37.-)

EXCLUDES 2 drowning and submersion due to accident to watercraft (V90.-)

✓5ᵗʰ **V91.0** **Burn due to watercraft on fire**

EXCLUDES 1 burn from localized fire or explosion on board ship without accident to watercraft (V93.-)

✓x7ᵗʰ **V91.00** **Burn due to** merchant ship **on fire**

✓x7ᵗʰ **V91.01** **Burn due to** passenger ship **on fire**

Burn due to Ferry-boat on fire

Burn due to Liner on fire

✓x7ᵗʰ **V91.02** **Burn due to** fishing boat **on fire**

✓x7ᵗʰ **V91.03** **Burn due to other** powered **watercraft on fire**

Burn due to Hovercraft (on open water) on fire

Burn due to Jet ski on fire

✓x7ᵗʰ **V91.04** **Burn due to** sailboat **on fire**

✓x7ᵗʰ **V91.05** **Burn due to** canoe or kayak **on fire**

✓x7ᵗʰ **V91.06** **Burn due to (nonpowered)** inflatable craft **on fire**

Ⓝ Newborn: 0   Ⓟ Pediatric: 0-17   Ⓜ Maternity: 9-64   Ⓐ Adult: 15-124   MCC Major Complication/Comorbidity   CC Complication/Comorbidity   SW Severe Wound Dx

1194

ICD-10-CM 2022

☑x7ᵗʰ **V91.07 Burn due to water-skis on fire**

☑x7ᵗʰ **V91.08 Burn due to other unpowered watercraft on fire**

☑x7ᵗʰ **V91.09 Burn due to unspecified watercraft on fire**
Burn due to boat NOS on fire
Burn due to ship NOS on fire
Burn due to watercraft NOS on fire

☑5ᵗʰ **V91.1 Crushed between watercraft and other watercraft or other object due to collision**
Crushed by lifeboat after abandoning ship in a collision

NOTE   Select the specified type of watercraft that the victim was on at the time of the collision

☑x7ᵗʰ **V91.10 Crushed between merchant ship and other watercraft or other object due to collision**

☑x7ᵗʰ **V91.11 Crushed between passenger ship and other watercraft or other object due to collision**
Crushed between Ferry-boat and other watercraft or other object due to collision
Crushed between Liner and other watercraft or other object due to collision

☑x7ᵗʰ **V91.12 Crushed between fishing boat and other watercraft or other object due to collision**

☑x7ᵗʰ **V91.13 Crushed between other powered watercraft and other watercraft or other object due to collision**
Crushed between Hovercraft (on open water) and other watercraft or other object due to collision
Crushed between Jet ski and other watercraft or other object due to collision

☑x7ᵗʰ **V91.14 Crushed between sailboat and other watercraft or other object due to collision**

☑x7ᵗʰ **V91.15 Crushed between canoe or kayak and other watercraft or other object due to collision**

☑x7ᵗʰ **V91.16 Crushed between (nonpowered) inflatable craft and other watercraft or other object due to collision**

☑x7ᵗʰ **V91.18 Crushed between other unpowered watercraft and other watercraft or other object due to collision**
Crushed between surfboard and other watercraft or other object due to collision
Crushed between windsurfer and other watercraft or other object due to collision

☑x7ᵗʰ **V91.19 Crushed between unspecified watercraft and other watercraft or other object due to collision**
Crushed between boat NOS and other watercraft or other object due to collision
Crushed between ship NOS and other watercraft or other object due to collision
Crushed between watercraft NOS and other watercraft or other object due to collision

☑5ᵗʰ **V91.2 Fall due to collision between watercraft and other watercraft or other object**
Fall while remaining on watercraft after collision

NOTE   Select the specified type of watercraft that the victim was on at the time of the collision

EXCLUDES 1   crushed between watercraft and other watercraft and other object due to collision (V91.1-)
drowning and submersion due to falling from crushed watercraft (V90.3-)

☑x7ᵗʰ **V91.20 Fall due to collision between merchant ship and other watercraft or other object**

☑x7ᵗʰ **V91.21 Fall due to collision between passenger ship and other watercraft or other object**
Fall due to collision between Ferry-boat and other watercraft or other object
Fall due to collision between Liner and other watercraft or other object

☑x7ᵗʰ **V91.22 Fall due to collision between fishing boat and other watercraft or other object**

☑x7ᵗʰ **V91.23 Fall due to collision between other powered watercraft and other watercraft or other object**
Fall due to collision between Hovercraft (on open water) and other watercraft or other object
Fall due to collision between Jet ski and other watercraft or other object

☑x7ᵗʰ **V91.24 Fall due to collision between sailboat and other watercraft or other object**

☑x7ᵗʰ **V91.25 Fall due to collision between canoe or kayak and other watercraft or other object**

☑x7ᵗʰ **V91.26 Fall due to collision between (nonpowered) inflatable craft and other watercraft or other object**

☑x7ᵗʰ **V91.29 Fall due to collision between unspecified watercraft and other watercraft or other object**
Fall due to collision between boat NOS and other watercraft or other object
Fall due to collision between ship NOS and other watercraft or other object
Fall due to collision between watercraft NOS and other watercraft or other object

☑5ᵗʰ **V91.3 Hit or struck by falling object due to accident to watercraft**
Hit or struck by falling object (part of damaged watercraft or other object) after falling or jumping from damaged watercraft

EXCLUDES 2   drowning or submersion due to fall or jumping from damaged watercraft (V90.2-, V90.3-)

☑x7ᵗʰ **V91.30 Hit or struck by falling object due to accident to merchant ship**

☑x7ᵗʰ **V91.31 Hit or struck by falling object due to accident to passenger ship**
Hit or struck by falling object due to accident to Ferry-boat
Hit or struck by falling object due to accident to Liner

☑x7ᵗʰ **V91.32 Hit or struck by falling object due to accident to fishing boat**

☑x7ᵗʰ **V91.33 Hit or struck by falling object due to accident to other powered watercraft**
Hit or struck by falling object due to accident to Hovercraft (on open water)
Hit or struck by falling object due to accident to Jet ski

☑x7ᵗʰ **V91.34 Hit or struck by falling object due to accident to sailboat**

☑x7ᵗʰ **V91.35 Hit or struck by falling object due to accident to canoe or kayak**

☑x7ᵗʰ **V91.36 Hit or struck by falling object due to accident to (nonpowered) inflatable craft**

☑x7ᵗʰ **V91.37 Hit or struck by falling object due to accident to water-skis**
Hit by water-skis after jumping off of waterskis

☑x7ᵗʰ **V91.38 Hit or struck by falling object due to accident to other unpowered watercraft**
Hit or struck by surf-board after falling off damaged surf-board
Hit or struck by object after falling off damaged windsurfer

☑x7ᵗʰ **V91.39 Hit or struck by falling object due to accident to unspecified watercraft**
Hit or struck by falling object due to accident to boat NOS
Hit or struck by falling object due to accident to ship NOS
Hit or struck by falling object due to accident to watercraft NOS

☑5ᵗʰ **V91.8 Other injury due to other accident to watercraft**

☑x7ᵗʰ **V91.80 Other injury due to other accident to merchant ship**

☑x7ᵗʰ **V91.81 Other injury due to other accident to passenger ship**
Other injury due to other accident to Ferry-boat
Other injury due to other accident to Liner

☑x7ᵗʰ **V91.82 Other injury due to other accident to fishing boat**

☑x7ᵗʰ **V91.83 Other injury due to other accident to other powered watercraft**
Other injury due to other accident to Hovercraft (on open water)
Other injury due to other accident to Jet ski

☑x7ᵗʰ **V91.84 Other injury due to other accident to sailboat**

☑x7ᵗʰ **V91.85 Other injury due to other accident to canoe or kayak**

☑x7ᵗʰ **V91.86 Other injury due to other accident to (nonpowered) inflatable craft**

☑x7ᵗʰ **V91.87 Other injury due to other accident to water-skis**

☑x7ᵗʰ **V91.88 Other injury due to other accident to other unpowered watercraft**
Other injury due to other accident to surf-board
Other injury due to other accident to windsurfer

Chapter 20. External Causes of Morbidity

V91.07–V91.88

√x7ᵗʰ **V91.89** **Other injury due to other accident to unspecified watercraft**
Other injury due to other accident to boat NOS
Other injury due to other accident to ship NOS
Other injury due to other accident to watercraft NOS

√4ᵗʰ **V92** **Drowning and submersion due to accident on board watercraft, without accident to watercraft**

EXCLUDES 1 *civilian water transport accident involving military watercraft (V94.81-)*
drowning or submersion due to accident to watercraft (V90-V91)
drowning or submersion of diver who voluntarily jumps from boat not involved in an accident (W16.711, W16.721)
fall into water without watercraft (W16.-)
military watercraft accident in military or war operations (Y36, Y37)

√5ᵗʰ **V92.0** **Drowning and submersion due to fall off watercraft**
Drowning and submersion due to fall from gangplank of watercraft
Drowning and submersion due to fall overboard watercraft

EXCLUDES 2 *hitting head on object or bottom of body of water due to fall from watercraft (V94.0-)*

√x7ᵗʰ **V92.00** **Drowning and submersion due to fall off merchant ship**

√x7ᵗʰ **V92.01** **Drowning and submersion due to fall off passenger ship**
Drowning and submersion due to fall off Ferry-boat
Drowning and submersion due to fall off Liner

√x7ᵗʰ **V92.02** **Drowning and submersion due to fall off fishing boat**

√x7ᵗʰ **V92.03** **Drowning and submersion due to fall off other powered watercraft**
Drowning and submersion due to fall off Hovercraft (on open water)
Drowning and submersion due to fall off Jet ski

√x7ᵗʰ **V92.04** **Drowning and submersion due to fall off sailboat**

√x7ᵗʰ **V92.05** **Drowning and submersion due to fall off canoe or kayak**

√x7ᵗʰ **V92.06** **Drowning and submersion due to fall off (nonpowered) inflatable craft**

√x7ᵗʰ **V92.07** **Drowning and submersion due to fall off water-skis**

EXCLUDES 1 *drowning and submersion due to falling off burning water-skis (V90.27)*
drowning and submersion due to falling off crushed water-skis (V90.37)
hit by boat while water-skiing NOS (V94.X)

√x7ᵗʰ **V92.08** **Drowning and submersion due to fall off other unpowered watercraft**
Drowning and submersion due to fall off surf-board
Drowning and submersion due to fall off windsurfer

EXCLUDES 1 *drowning and submersion due to fall off burning unpowered watercraft (V90.28)*
drowning and submersion due to fall off crushed unpowered watercraft (V90.38)
drowning and submersion due to fall off damaged unpowered watercraft (V90.88)
drowning and submersion due to rider of nonpowered watercraft being hit by other watercraft (V94.-)
other injury due to rider of nonpowered watercraft being hit by other watercraft (V94.-)

√x7ᵗʰ **V92.09** **Drowning and submersion due to fall off unspecified watercraft**
Drowning and submersion due to fall off boat NOS
Drowning and submersion due to fall off ship
Drowning and submersion due to fall off watercraft NOS

√5ᵗʰ **V92.1** **Drowning and submersion due to being thrown overboard by motion of watercraft**

EXCLUDES 1 *drowning and submersion due to fall off surf-board (V92.08)*
drowning and submersion due to fall off water-skis (V92.07)
drowning and submersion due to fall off windsurfer (V92.08)

√x7ᵗʰ **V92.10** **Drowning and submersion due to being thrown overboard by motion of merchant ship**

√x7ᵗʰ **V92.11** **Drowning and submersion due to being thrown overboard by motion of passenger ship**
Drowning and submersion due to being thrown overboard by motion of Ferry-boat
Drowning and submersion due to being thrown overboard by motion of Liner

√x7ᵗʰ **V92.12** **Drowning and submersion due to being thrown overboard by motion of fishing boat**

√x7ᵗʰ **V92.13** **Drowning and submersion due to being thrown overboard by motion of other powered watercraft**
Drowning and submersion due to being thrown overboard by motion of Hovercraft

√x7ᵗʰ **V92.14** **Drowning and submersion due to being thrown overboard by motion of sailboat**

√x7ᵗʰ **V92.15** **Drowning and submersion due to being thrown overboard by motion of canoe or kayak**

√x7ᵗʰ **V92.16** **Drowning and submersion due to being thrown overboard by motion of (nonpowered) inflatable craft**

√x7ᵗʰ **V92.19** **Drowning and submersion due to being thrown overboard by motion of unspecified watercraft**
Drowning and submersion due to being thrown overboard by motion of boat NOS
Drowning and submersion due to being thrown overboard by motion of ship NOS
Drowning and submersion due to being thrown overboard by motion of watercraft NOS

√5ᵗʰ **V92.2** **Drowning and submersion due to being washed overboard from watercraft**
Code first any associated cataclysm (X37.0-)

√x7ᵗʰ **V92.20** **Drowning and submersion due to being washed overboard from merchant ship**

√x7ᵗʰ **V92.21** **Drowning and submersion due to being washed overboard from passenger ship**
Drowning and submersion due to being washed overboard from Ferry-boat
Drowning and submersion due to being washed overboard from Liner

√x7ᵗʰ **V92.22** **Drowning and submersion due to being washed overboard from fishing boat**

√x7ᵗʰ **V92.23** **Drowning and submersion due to being washed overboard from other powered watercraft**
Drowning and submersion due to being washed overboard from Hovercraft (on open water)
Drowning and submersion due to being washed overboard from Jet ski

√x7ᵗʰ **V92.24** **Drowning and submersion due to being washed overboard from sailboat**

√x7ᵗʰ **V92.25** **Drowning and submersion due to being washed overboard from canoe or kayak**

√x7ᵗʰ **V92.26** **Drowning and submersion due to being washed overboard from (nonpowered) inflatable craft**

√x7ᵗʰ **V92.27** **Drowning and submersion due to being washed overboard from water-skis**

EXCLUDES 1 *drowning and submersion due to fall off water-skis (V92.07)*

√x7ᵗʰ **V92.28** **Drowning and submersion due to being washed overboard from other unpowered watercraft**
Drowning and submersion due to being washed overboard from surf-board
Drowning and submersion due to being washed overboard from windsurfer

✓x7ᵗʰ **V92.29 Drowning and submersion due to being washed overboard from unspecified watercraft**

Drowning and submersion due to being washed overboard from boat NOS

Drowning and submersion due to being washed overboard from ship NOS

Drowning and submersion due to being washed overboard from watercraft NOS

✓4ᵗʰ **V93 Other injury due to accident on board watercraft, without accident to watercraft**

> EXCLUDES 1   *civilian water transport accident involving military watercraft (V94.81-)*
>
> *other injury due to accident to watercraft (V91.-)*
>
> *military watercraft accident in military or war operations (Y36, Y37.-)*
>
> EXCLUDES 2   *drowning and submersion due to accident on board watercraft, without accident to watercraft (V92.-)*

✓5ᵗʰ **V93.0 Burn due to localized fire on board watercraft**

> EXCLUDES 1   *burn due to watercraft on fire (V91.0-)*

✓x7ᵗʰ **V93.00 Burn due to localized fire on board merchant vessel**

✓x7ᵗʰ **V93.01 Burn due to localized fire on board passenger vessel**

Burn due to localized fire on board Ferry-boat

Burn due to localized fire on board Liner

✓x7ᵗʰ **V93.02 Burn due to localized fire on board fishing boat**

✓x7ᵗʰ **V93.03 Burn due to localized fire on board other powered watercraft**

Burn due to localized fire on board Hovercraft

Burn due to localized fire on board Jet ski

✓x7ᵗʰ **V93.04 Burn due to localized fire on board sailboat**

✓x7ᵗʰ **V93.09 Burn due to localized fire on board unspecified watercraft**

Burn due to localized fire on board boat NOS

Burn due to localized fire on board ship NOS

Burn due to localized fire on board watercraft NOS

✓5ᵗʰ **V93.1 Other burn on board watercraft**

Burn due to source other than fire on board watercraft

> EXCLUDES 1   *burn due to watercraft on fire (V91.0-)*

✓x7ᵗʰ **V93.10 Other burn on board merchant vessel**

✓x7ᵗʰ **V93.11 Other burn on board passenger vessel**

Other burn on board Ferry-boat

Other burn on board Liner

✓x7ᵗʰ **V93.12 Other burn on board fishing boat**

✓x7ᵗʰ **V93.13 Other burn on board other powered watercraft**

Other burn on board Hovercraft

Other burn on board Jet ski

✓x7ᵗʰ **V93.14 Other burn on board sailboat**

✓x7ᵗʰ **V93.19 Other burn on board unspecified watercraft**

Other burn on board boat NOS

Other burn on board ship NOS

Other burn on board watercraft NOS

✓5ᵗʰ **V93.2 Heat exposure on board watercraft**

> EXCLUDES 1   *exposure to man-made heat not aboard watercraft (W92)*
>
> *exposure to natural heat while on board watercraft (X30)*
>
> *exposure to sunlight while on board watercraft (X32)*
>
> EXCLUDES 2   *burn due to fire on board watercraft (V93.0-)*

✓x7ᵗʰ **V93.20 Heat exposure on board merchant ship**

✓x7ᵗʰ **V93.21 Heat exposure on board passenger ship**

Heat exposure on board Ferry-boat

Heat exposure on board Liner

✓x7ᵗʰ **V93.22 Heat exposure on board fishing boat**

✓x7ᵗʰ **V93.23 Heat exposure on board other powered watercraft**

Heat exposure on board hovercraft

✓x7ᵗʰ **V93.24 Heat exposure on board sailboat**

✓x7ᵗʰ **V93.29 Heat exposure on board unspecified watercraft**

Heat exposure on board boat NOS

Heat exposure on board ship NOS

Heat exposure on board watercraft NOS

✓5ᵗʰ **V93.3 Fall on board watercraft**

> EXCLUDES 1   *fall due to collision of watercraft (V91.2-)*

✓x7ᵗʰ **V93.30 Fall on board merchant ship**

✓x7ᵗʰ **V93.31 Fall on board passenger ship**

Fall on board Ferry-boat

Fall on board Liner

✓x7ᵗʰ **V93.32 Fall on board fishing boat**

✓x7ᵗʰ **V93.33 Fall on board other powered watercraft**

Fall on board Hovercraft (on open water)

Fall on board Jet ski

✓x7ᵗʰ **V93.34 Fall on board sailboat**

✓x7ᵗʰ **V93.35 Fall on board canoe or kayak**

✓x7ᵗʰ **V93.36 Fall on board (nonpowered) inflatable craft**

✓x7ᵗʰ **V93.38 Fall on board other unpowered watercraft**

✓x7ᵗʰ **V93.39 Fall on board unspecified watercraft**

Fall on board boat NOS

Fall on board ship NOS

Fall on board watercraft NOS

✓5ᵗʰ **V93.4 Struck by falling object on board watercraft**

Hit by falling object on board watercraft

> EXCLUDES 1   *struck by falling object due to accident to watercraft (V91.3)*

✓x7ᵗʰ **V93.40 Struck by falling object on merchant ship**

✓x7ᵗʰ **V93.41 Struck by falling object on passenger ship**

Struck by falling object on Ferry-boat

Struck by falling object on Liner

✓x7ᵗʰ **V93.42 Struck by falling object on fishing boat**

✓x7ᵗʰ **V93.43 Struck by falling object on other powered watercraft**

Struck by falling object on Hovercraft

✓x7ᵗʰ **V93.44 Struck by falling object on sailboat**

✓x7ᵗʰ **V93.48 Struck by falling object on other unpowered watercraft**

✓x7ᵗʰ **V93.49 Struck by falling object on unspecified watercraft**

✓5ᵗʰ **V93.5 Explosion on board watercraft**

Boiler explosion on steamship

> EXCLUDES 2   *fire on board watercraft (V93.0-)*

✓x7ᵗʰ **V93.50 Explosion on board merchant ship**

✓x7ᵗʰ **V93.51 Explosion on board passenger ship**

Explosion on board Ferry-boat

Explosion on board Liner

✓x7ᵗʰ **V93.52 Explosion on board fishing boat**

✓x7ᵗʰ **V93.53 Explosion on board other powered watercraft**

Explosion on board Hovercraft

Explosion on board Jet ski

✓x7ᵗʰ **V93.54 Explosion on board sailboat**

✓x7ᵗʰ **V93.59 Explosion on board unspecified watercraft**

Explosion on board boat NOS

Explosion on board ship NOS

Explosion on board watercraft NOS

✓5ᵗʰ **V93.6 Machinery accident on board watercraft**

> EXCLUDES 1   *machinery explosion on board watercraft (V93.4-)*
>
> *machinery fire on board watercraft (V93.0-)*

✓x7ᵗʰ **V93.60 Machinery accident on board merchant ship**

✓x7ᵗʰ **V93.61 Machinery accident on board passenger ship**

Machinery accident on board Ferry-boat

Machinery accident on board Liner

✓x7ᵗʰ **V93.62 Machinery accident on board fishing boat**

✓x7ᵗʰ **V93.63 Machinery accident on board other powered watercraft**

Machinery accident on board Hovercraft

✓x7ᵗʰ **V93.64 Machinery accident on board sailboat**

✓x7ᵗʰ **V93.69 Machinery accident on board unspecified watercraft**

Machinery accident on board boat NOS

Machinery accident on board ship NOS

Machinery accident on board watercraft NOS

✓5ᵗʰ **V93.8 Other injury due to other accident on board watercraft**

Accidental poisoning by gases or fumes on watercraft

✓x7ᵗʰ **V93.80 Other injury due to other accident on board merchant ship**

☑ Additional Char Req ✓x7ᵗʰ Placeholder Unacceptable PDx Questionable PDx Wrong Procedure Manifestation Unspecified Dx H1-H14 HAC HCC CMS-HCC Dx HIV HIV Dx

ICD-10-CM 2022   1197

✓x7ᵗʰ **V93.81** **Other injury due to other accident on board passenger ship**
Other injury due to other accident on board Ferry-boat
Other injury due to other accident on board Liner

✓x7ᵗʰ **V93.82** **Other injury due to other accident on board fishing boat**

✓x7ᵗʰ **V93.83** **Other injury due to other accident on board other powered watercraft**
Other injury due to other accident on board Hovercraft
Other injury due to other accident on board Jet ski

✓x7ᵗʰ **V93.84** **Other injury due to other accident on board sailboat**

✓x7ᵗʰ **V93.85** **Other injury due to other accident on board canoe or kayak**

✓x7ᵗʰ **V93.86** **Other injury due to other accident on board (nonpowered) inflatable craft**

✓x7ᵗʰ **V93.87** **Other injury due to other accident on board water-skis**
Hit or struck by object while waterskiing

✓x7ᵗʰ **V93.88** **Other injury due to other accident on board other unpowered watercraft**
Hit or struck by object while surfing
Hit or struck by object while on board windsurfer

✓x7ᵗʰ **V93.89** **Other injury due to other accident on board unspecified watercraft**
Other injury due to other accident on board boat NOS
Other injury due to other accident on board ship NOS
Other injury due to other accident on board watercraft NOS

✓4ᵗʰ **V94** **Other and unspecified water transport accidents**
> EXCLUDES 1   *military watercraft accidents in military or war operations (Y36, Y37)*

✓x7ᵗʰ **V94.0** **Hitting object or bottom of body of water due to fall from watercraft**
> EXCLUDES 2   *drowning and submersion due to fall from watercraft (V92.0-)*

✓5ᵗʰ **V94.1** **Bather struck by watercraft**
Swimmer hit by watercraft

  ✓x7ᵗʰ **V94.11** **Bather struck by powered watercraft**

  ✓x7ᵗʰ **V94.12** **Bather struck by nonpowered watercraft**

✓6ᵗʰ **V94.2** **Rider of nonpowered watercraft struck by other watercraft**

  ✓x7ᵗʰ **V94.21** **Rider of nonpowered watercraft struck by other nonpowered watercraft**
Canoer hit by other nonpowered watercraft
Surfer hit by other nonpowered watercraft
Windsurfer hit by other nonpowered watercraft

  ✓x7ᵗʰ **V94.22** **Rider of nonpowered watercraft struck by powered watercraft**
Canoer hit by motorboat
Surfer hit by motorboat
Windsurfer hit by motorboat

✓5ᵗʰ **V94.3** **Injury to rider of (inflatable) watercraft being pulled behind other watercraft**

  ✓x7ᵗʰ **V94.31** **Injury to rider of (inflatable) recreational watercraft being pulled behind other watercraft**
Injury to rider of inner-tube pulled behind motor boat

  ✓x7ᵗʰ **V94.32** **Injury to rider of non-recreational watercraft being pulled behind other watercraft**
Injury to occupant of dingy being pulled behind boat or ship
Injury to occupant of life-raft being pulled behind boat or ship

✓x7ᵗʰ **V94.4** **Injury to barefoot water-skier**
Injury to person being pulled behind boat or ship

✓5ᵗʰ **V94.8** **Other water transport accident**

  ✓6ᵗʰ **V94.81** **Water transport accident involving military watercraft**

    ✓7ᵗʰ **V94.810** **Civilian watercraft involved in water transport accident with military watercraft**
Passenger on civilian watercraft injured due to accident with military watercraft

    ✓7ᵗʰ **V94.811** **Civilian in water injured by military watercraft**

    ✓7ᵗʰ **V94.818** **Other water transport accident involving military watercraft**

✓x7ᵗʰ **V94.89** **Other water transport accident**

✓x7ᵗʰ **V94.9** **Unspecified water transport accident**
Water transport accident NOS

Air and space transport accidents (V95-V97)

> EXCLUDES 1   *military aircraft accidents in military or war operations (Y36, Y37)*

The appropriate 7th character is to be added to each code from categories V95-V97.
A   initial encounter
D   subsequent encounter
S   sequela

✓4ᵗʰ **V95** **Accident to powered aircraft causing injury to occupant**

✓5ᵗʰ **V95.0** **Helicopter accident injuring occupant**

  ✓x7ᵗʰ **V95.00** **Unspecified helicopter accident injuring occupant**

  ✓x7ᵗʰ **V95.01** **Helicopter crash injuring occupant**

  ✓x7ᵗʰ **V95.02** **Forced landing of helicopter injuring occupant**

  ✓x7ᵗʰ **V95.03** **Helicopter collision injuring occupant**
Helicopter collision with any object, fixed, movable or moving

  ✓x7ᵗʰ **V95.04** **Helicopter fire injuring occupant**

  ✓x7ᵗʰ **V95.05** **Helicopter explosion injuring occupant**

  ✓x7ᵗʰ **V95.09** **Other helicopter accident injuring occupant**

✓5ᵗʰ **V95.1** **Ultralight, microlight or powered-glider accident injuring occupant**

  ✓x7ᵗʰ **V95.10** **Unspecified ultralight, microlight or powered-glider accident injuring occupant**

  ✓x7ᵗʰ **V95.11** **Ultralight, microlight or powered-glider crash injuring occupant**

  ✓x7ᵗʰ **V95.12** **Forced landing of ultralight, microlight or powered-glider injuring occupant**

  ✓x7ᵗʰ **V95.13** **Ultralight, microlight or powered-glider collision injuring occupant**
Ultralight, microlight or powered-glider collision with any object, fixed, movable or moving

  ✓x7ᵗʰ **V95.14** **Ultralight, microlight or powered-glider fire injuring occupant**

  ✓x7ᵗʰ **V95.15** **Ultralight, microlight or powered-glider explosion injuring occupant**

  ✓x7ᵗʰ **V95.19** **Other ultralight, microlight or powered-glider accident injuring occupant**

✓5ᵗʰ **V95.2** **Other private fixed-wing aircraft accident injuring occupant**

  ✓x7ᵗʰ **V95.20** **Unspecified accident to other private fixed-wing aircraft, injuring occupant**

  ✓x7ᵗʰ **V95.21** **Other private fixed-wing aircraft crash injuring occupant**

  ✓x7ᵗʰ **V95.22** **Forced landing of other private fixed-wing aircraft injuring occupant**

  ✓x7ᵗʰ **V95.23** **Other private fixed-wing aircraft collision injuring occupant**
Other private fixed-wing aircraft collision with any object, fixed, movable or moving

  ✓x7ᵗʰ **V95.24** **Other private fixed-wing aircraft fire injuring occupant**

  ✓x7ᵗʰ **V95.25** **Other private fixed-wing aircraft explosion injuring occupant**

  ✓x7ᵗʰ **V95.29** **Other accident to other private fixed-wing aircraft injuring occupant**

✓5ᵗʰ **V95.3** **Commercial fixed-wing aircraft accident injuring occupant**

  ✓x7ᵗʰ **V95.30** **Unspecified accident to commercial fixed-wing aircraft injuring occupant**

  ✓x7ᵗʰ **V95.31** **Commercial fixed-wing aircraft crash injuring occupant**

  ✓x7ᵗʰ **V95.32** **Forced landing of commercial fixed-wing aircraft injuring occupant**

  ✓x7ᵗʰ **V95.33** **Commercial fixed-wing aircraft collision injuring occupant**
Commercial fixed-wing aircraft collision with any object, fixed, movable or moving

  ✓x7ᵗʰ **V95.34** **Commercial fixed-wing aircraft fire injuring occupant**

  ✓x7ᵗʰ **V95.35** **Commercial fixed-wing aircraft explosion injuring occupant**

  ✓x7ᵗʰ **V95.39** **Other accident to commercial fixed-wing aircraft injuring occupant**

✓5ᵗʰ **V95.4** **Spacecraft accident injuring occupant**

  ✓x7ᵗʰ **V95.40** **Unspecified spacecraft accident injuring occupant**

  ✓x7ᵗʰ **V95.41** **Spacecraft crash injuring occupant**

  ✓x7ᵗʰ **V95.42** Forced landing of spacecraft injuring occupant

  ✓x7ᵗʰ **V95.43** Spacecraft **collision** injuring occupant

       Spacecraft collision with any object, fixed, moveable or moving

  ✓x7ᵗʰ **V95.44** Spacecraft **fire** injuring occupant

  ✓x7ᵗʰ **V95.45** Spacecraft **explosion** injuring occupant

  ✓x7ᵗʰ **V95.49** Other spacecraft accident injuring occupant

✓x7ᵗʰ **V95.8** Other powered aircraft accidents injuring occupant

✓x7ᵗʰ **V95.9** Unspecified aircraft accident injuring occupant

    Aircraft accident NOS

    Air transport accident NOS

✓4ᵗʰ **V96** Accident to nonpowered aircraft causing injury to occupant

  ✓5ᵗʰ **V96.0** **Balloon** accident injuring occupant

    ✓x7ᵗʰ **V96.00** Unspecified balloon accident injuring occupant

    ✓x7ᵗʰ **V96.01** Balloon **crash** injuring occupant

    ✓x7ᵗʰ **V96.02** Forced landing of balloon injuring occupant

    ✓x7ᵗʰ **V96.03** Balloon **collision** injuring occupant

       Balloon collision with any object, fixed, moveable or moving

    ✓x7ᵗʰ **V96.04** Balloon **fire** injuring occupant

    ✓x7ᵗʰ **V96.05** Balloon **explosion** injuring occupant

    ✓x7ᵗʰ **V96.09** Other balloon accident injuring occupant

  ✓5ᵗʰ **V96.1** **Hang-glider** accident injuring occupant

    ✓x7ᵗʰ **V96.10** Unspecified hang-glider accident injuring occupant

    ✓x7ᵗʰ **V96.11** Hang-glider **crash** injuring occupant

    ✓x7ᵗʰ **V96.12** Forced landing of hang-glider injuring occupant

    ✓x7ᵗʰ **V96.13** Hang-glider **collision** injuring occupant

       Hang-glider collision with any object, fixed, moveable or moving

    ✓x7ᵗʰ **V96.14** Hang-glider **fire** injuring occupant

    ✓x7ᵗʰ **V96.15** Hang-glider **explosion** injuring occupant

    ✓x7ᵗʰ **V96.19** Other hang-glider accident injuring occupant

  ✓5ᵗʰ **V96.2** **Glider (nonpowered)** accident injuring occupant

    ✓x7ᵗʰ **V96.20** Unspecified glider (nonpowered) accident injuring occupant

    ✓x7ᵗʰ **V96.21** Glider (nonpowered) **crash** injuring occupant

    ✓x7ᵗʰ **V96.22** Forced landing of glider (nonpowered) injuring occupant

    ✓x7ᵗʰ **V96.23** Glider (nonpowered) **collision** injuring occupant

       Glider (nonpowered) collision with any object, fixed, moveable or moving

    ✓x7ᵗʰ **V96.24** Glider (nonpowered) **fire** injuring occupant

    ✓x7ᵗʰ **V96.25** Glider (nonpowered) **explosion** injuring occupant

    ✓x7ᵗʰ **V96.29** Other glider (nonpowered) accident injuring occupant

  ✓x7ᵗʰ **V96.8** Other nonpowered-aircraft accidents injuring occupant

    Kite carrying a person accident injuring occupant

  ✓x7ᵗʰ **V96.9** Unspecified nonpowered-aircraft accident injuring occupant

    Nonpowered-aircraft accident NOS

✓4ᵗʰ **V97** Other specified air transport accidents

  ✓x7ᵗʰ **V97.0** Occupant of aircraft injured in other specified air transport accidents

    Fall in, on or from aircraft in air transport accident

    EXCLUDES 1 *accident while boarding or alighting aircraft (V97.1)*

  ✓x7ᵗʰ **V97.1** Person injured while boarding or alighting from aircraft

  ✓5ᵗʰ **V97.2** Parachutist accident

    ✓x7ᵗʰ **V97.21** Parachutist entangled in object

       Parachutist landing in tree

    ✓x7ᵗʰ **V97.22** Parachutist injured on landing

    ✓x7ᵗʰ **V97.29** Other parachutist accident

  ✓5ᵗʰ **V97.3** Person on ground injured in air transport accident

    ✓x7ᵗʰ **V97.31** Hit by object falling from aircraft

       Hit by crashing aircraft

       Injured by aircraft hitting house

       Injured by aircraft hitting car

    ✓x7ᵗʰ **V97.32** Injured by rotating propeller

    ✓x7ᵗʰ **V97.33** Sucked into jet engine

    ✓x7ᵗʰ **V97.39** Other injury to person on ground due to air transport accident

  ✓5ᵗʰ **V97.8** Other air transport accidents, not elsewhere classified

    EXCLUDES 1 *aircraft accident NOS (V95.9)*

       exposure to changes in air pressure during ascent or descent (W94.-)

    ✓6ᵗʰ **V97.81** Air transport accident involving military aircraft

      ✓7ᵗʰ **V97.810** Civilian aircraft involved in air transport accident with military aircraft

         Passenger in civilian aircraft injured due to accident with military aircraft

      ✓7ᵗʰ **V97.811** Civilian injured by military aircraft

      ✓7ᵗʰ **V97.818** Other air transport accident involving military aircraft

    ✓x7ᵗʰ **V97.89** Other air transport accidents, not elsewhere classified

       Injury from machinery on aircraft

Other and unspecified transport accidents (V98-V99)

EXCLUDES 1 *vehicle accident, type of vehicle unspecified (V89.-)*

The appropriate 7th character is to be added to each code from categories V98-V99.
A initial encounter
D subsequent encounter
S sequela

✓4ᵗʰ **V98** Other specified transport accidents

  ✓x7ᵗʰ **V98.0** Accident to, on or involving **cable-car, not on rails**

       Caught or dragged by cable-car, not on rails

       Fall or jump from cable-car, not on rails

       Object thrown from or in cable-car, not on rails

  ✓x7ᵗʰ **V98.1** Accident to, on or involving **land-yacht**

  ✓x7ᵗʰ **V98.2** Accident to, on or involving **ice yacht**

  ✓x7ᵗʰ **V98.3** Accident to, on or involving **ski lift**

       Accident to, on or involving ski chair-lift

       Accident to, on or involving ski-lift with gondola

  ✓x7ᵗʰ **V98.8** Other specified transport accidents

✓x7ᵗʰ **V99** Unspecified transport accident

OTHER EXTERNAL CAUSES OF ACCIDENTAL INJURY (W00-X58)

Slipping, tripping, stumbling and falls (W00-W19)

EXCLUDES 1 *assault involving a fall (Y01-Y02)*
    fall from animal (V80.-)
    fall (in) (from) machinery (in operation) (W28-W31)
    fall (in) (from) transport vehicle (V01-V99)
    intentional self-harm involving a fall (X80-X81)

EXCLUDES 2 *at risk for fall (history of fall) Z91.81*
    fall (in) (from) burning building (X00.-)
    fall into fire (X00-X04, X08)

The appropriate 7th character is to be added to each code from categories W00-W19.
A initial encounter
D subsequent encounter
S sequela

✓4ᵗʰ **W00** Fall due to ice and snow

    INCLUDES pedestrian on foot falling (slipping) on ice and snow

    EXCLUDES 1 *fall on (from) ice and snow involving pedestrian conveyance (V00.-)*

       fall from stairs and steps not due to ice and snow (W10.-)

    AHA: 2016,2Q,4

  ✓x7ᵗʰ **W00.0** Fall on **same level** due to ice and snow

  ✓x7ᵗʰ **W00.1** Fall **from stairs** and steps due to ice and snow

  ✓x7ᵗʰ **W00.2** Other fall from one level to another due to ice and snow

  ✓x7ᵗʰ **W00.9** Unspecified fall due to ice and snow

✓ Additional Char Req   ✓x7ᵗʰ Placeholder   Unacceptable PDx   Questionable PDx   Wrong Procedure   Manifestation   Unspecified Dx   H1-H14 HAC   HCC CMS-HCC Dx   HIV HIV Dx

ICD-10-CM 2022   1199

√4ᵗʰ **W01 Fall on same level from slipping, tripping and stumbling**

INCLUDES fall on moving sidewalk

EXCLUDES 1 *fall due to bumping (striking) against object (W18.0-)*
fall in shower or bathtub (W18.2-)
fall on same level NOS (W18.30)
fall on same level from slipping, tripping and stumbling due to ice or snow (W00.0)
fall off or from toilet (W18.1-)
slipping, tripping and stumbling NOS (W18.40)
slipping, tripping and stumbling without falling (W18.4-)

√x7ᵗʰ **W01.0 Fall on same level from slipping, tripping and stumbling without subsequent striking against object**

Falling over animal

√5ᵗʰ **W01.1 Fall on same level from slipping, tripping and stumbling with subsequent striking against object**

√x7ᵗʰ **W01.10 Fall on same level from slipping, tripping and stumbling with subsequent striking against unspecified object**

√6ᵗʰ **W01.11 Fall on same level from slipping, tripping and stumbling with subsequent striking against sharp object**

√7ᵗʰ **W01.110 Fall on same level from slipping, tripping and stumbling with subsequent striking against sharp glass**

√7ᵗʰ **W01.111 Fall on same level from slipping, tripping and stumbling with subsequent striking against power tool or machine**

√7ᵗʰ **W01.118 Fall on same level from slipping, tripping and stumbling with subsequent striking against other sharp object**

√7ᵗʰ **W01.119 Fall on same level from slipping, tripping and stumbling with subsequent striking against unspecified sharp object**

√6ᵗʰ **W01.19 Fall on same level from slipping, tripping and stumbling with subsequent striking against other object**

√7ᵗʰ **W01.190 Fall on same level from slipping, tripping and stumbling with subsequent striking against furniture**

√7ᵗʰ **W01.198 Fall on same level from slipping, tripping and stumbling with subsequent striking against other object**

√x7ᵗʰ **W03 Other fall on same level due to collision with another person**

Fall due to non-transport collision with other person

EXCLUDES 1 *collision with another person without fall (W51)*
crushed or pushed by a crowd or human stampede (W52)
fall involving pedestrian conveyance (V00-V09)
fall due to ice or snow (W00)
fall on same level NOS (W18.30)

AHA: 2012,4Q,108

√x7ᵗʰ **W04 Fall while being carried or supported by other persons**

Accidentally dropped while being carried

√4ᵗʰ **W05 Fall from non-moving wheelchair, nonmotorized scooter and motorized mobility scooter**

EXCLUDES 1 *fall from moving wheelchair (powered) (V00.811)*
fall from moving motorized mobility scooter (V00.831)
fall from nonmotorized scooter (V00.141)

√x7ᵗʰ **W05.0 Fall from non-moving wheelchair**

AHA: 2019,2Q,27

√x7ᵗʰ **W05.1 Fall from non-moving nonmotorized scooter**

√x7ᵗʰ **W05.2 Fall from non-moving motorized mobility scooter**

√x7ᵗʰ **W06 Fall from bed**

√x7ᵗʰ **W07 Fall from chair**

√x7ᵗʰ **W08 Fall from other furniture**

√4ᵗʰ **W09 Fall on and from playground equipment**

EXCLUDES 1 *fall involving recreational machinery (W31)*

√x7ᵗʰ **W09.0 Fall on or from playground slide**

√x7ᵗʰ **W09.1 Fall from playground swing**

√x7ᵗʰ **W09.2 Fall on or from jungle gym**

√x7ᵗʰ **W09.8 Fall on or from other playground equipment**

√4ᵗʰ **W10 Fall on and from stairs and steps**

EXCLUDES 1 *Fall from stairs and steps due to ice and snow (W00.1)*

√x7ᵗʰ **W10.0 Fall (on)(from) escalator**

√x7ᵗʰ **W10.1 Fall (on)(from) sidewalk curb**

√x7ᵗʰ **W10.2 Fall (on)(from) incline**

Fall (on) (from) ramp

√x7ᵗʰ **W10.8 Fall (on) (from) other stairs and steps**

√x7ᵗʰ **W10.9 Fall (on) (from) unspecified stairs and steps**

√x7ᵗʰ **W11 Fall on and from ladder**

√x7ᵗʰ **W12 Fall on and from scaffolding**

√4ᵗʰ **W13 Fall from, out of or through building or structure**

√x7ᵗʰ **W13.0 Fall from, out of or through balcony**

Fall from, out of or through railing

√x7ᵗʰ **W13.1 Fall from, out of or through bridge**

√x7ᵗʰ **W13.2 Fall from, out of or through roof**

√x7ᵗʰ **W13.3 Fall through floor**

√x7ᵗʰ **W13.4 Fall from, out of or through window**

EXCLUDES 2 *fall with subsequent striking against sharp glass ▶(W01.110-)◄*

√x7ᵗʰ **W13.8 Fall from, out of or through other building or structure**

Fall from, out of or through viaduct
Fall from, out of or through wall
Fall from, out of or through flag-pole

√x7ᵗʰ **W13.9 Fall from, out of or through building, not otherwise specified**

EXCLUDES 1 *collapse of a building or structure (W20.-)*
fall or jump from burning building or structure (X00.-)

√x7ᵗʰ **W14 Fall from tree**

√x7ᵗʰ **W15 Fall from cliff**

√4ᵗʰ **W16 Fall, jump or diving into water**

EXCLUDES 1 *accidental non-watercraft drowning and submersion not involving fall (W65-W74)*
effects of air pressure from diving (W94.-)
fall into water from watercraft (V90-V94)
hitting an object or against bottom when falling from watercraft (V94.0)

EXCLUDES 2 *striking or hitting diving board (W21.4)*

√5ᵗʰ **W16.0 Fall into swimming pool**

Fall into swimming pool NOS

EXCLUDES 1 *fall into empty swimming pool (W17.3)*

√6ᵗʰ **W16.01 Fall into swimming pool striking water surface**

√7ᵗʰ **W16.011 Fall into swimming pool striking water surface causing drowning and submersion**

EXCLUDES 1 *drowning and submersion while in swimming pool without fall (W67)*

√7ᵗʰ **W16.012 Fall into swimming pool striking water surface causing other injury**

√6ᵗʰ **W16.02 Fall into swimming pool striking bottom**

√7ᵗʰ **W16.021 Fall into swimming pool striking bottom causing drowning and submersion**

EXCLUDES 1 *drowning and submersion while in swimming pool without fall (W67)*

√7ᵗʰ **W16.022 Fall into swimming pool striking bottom causing other injury**

√6ᵗʰ **W16.03 Fall into swimming pool striking wall**

√7ᵗʰ **W16.031 Fall into swimming pool striking wall causing drowning and submersion**

EXCLUDES 1 *drowning and submersion while in swimming pool without fall (W67)*

√7ᵗʰ **W16.032 Fall into swimming pool striking wall causing other injury**

✓5ᵗʰ **W16.1** **Fall into** natural body of water
Fall into lake
Fall into open sea
Fall into river
Fall into stream

✓6ᵗʰ **W16.11** **Fall into natural body of water** striking water surface

✓7ᵗʰ **W16.111** **Fall into natural body of water striking water surface causing** drowning and submersion
EXCLUDES 1 *drowning and submersion while in natural body of water without fall (W69)*

✓7ᵗʰ **W16.112** **Fall into natural body of water striking water surface causing other injury**

✓6ᵗʰ **W16.12** **Fall into natural body of water** striking bottom

✓7ᵗʰ **W16.121** **Fall into natural body of water striking bottom causing** drowning and submersion
EXCLUDES 1 *drowning and submersion while in natural body of water without fall (W69)*

✓7ᵗʰ **W16.122** **Fall into natural body of water striking bottom causing other injury**

✓6ᵗʰ **W16.13** **Fall into natural body of water** striking side

✓7ᵗʰ **W16.131** **Fall into natural body of water striking side causing** drowning and submersion
EXCLUDES 1 *drowning and submersion while in natural body of water without fall (W69)*

✓7ᵗʰ **W16.132** **Fall into natural body of water striking side causing other injury**

✓5ᵗʰ **W16.2** **Fall in (into) filled** bathtub or bucket of water

✓6ᵗʰ **W16.21** **Fall in (into)** filled bathtub
EXCLUDES 1 *fall into empty bathtub (W18.2)*

✓7ᵗʰ **W16.211** **Fall in (into) filled bathtub causing** drowning and submersion
EXCLUDES 1 *drowning and submersion while in filled bathtub without fall (W65)*

✓7ᵗʰ **W16.212** **Fall in (into) filled bathtub causing other injury**

✓6ᵗʰ **W16.22** **Fall in (into)** bucket of water

✓7ᵗʰ **W16.221** **Fall in (into) bucket of water causing** drowning and submersion

✓7ᵗʰ **W16.222** **Fall in (into) bucket of water causing other injury**

✓5ᵗʰ **W16.3** **Fall into** other water
Fall into fountain
Fall into reservoir

✓6ᵗʰ **W16.31** **Fall into other water** striking water surface

✓7ᵗʰ **W16.311** **Fall into other water striking water surface causing** drowning and submersion
EXCLUDES 1 *drowning and submersion while in other water without fall (W73)*

✓7ᵗʰ **W16.312** **Fall into other water striking water surface causing other injury**

✓6ᵗʰ **W16.32** **Fall into other water** striking bottom

✓7ᵗʰ **W16.321** **Fall into other water striking bottom causing** drowning and submersion
EXCLUDES 1 *drowning and submersion while in other water without fall (W73)*

✓7ᵗʰ **W16.322** **Fall into other water striking bottom causing other injury**

✓6ᵗʰ **W16.33** **Fall into other water** striking wall

✓7ᵗʰ **W16.331** **Fall into other water striking wall causing** drowning and submersion
EXCLUDES 1 *drowning and submersion while in other water without fall (W73)*

✓7ᵗʰ **W16.332** **Fall into other water striking wall causing other injury**

✓5ᵗʰ **W16.4** **Fall into** unspecified water

✓x7ᵗʰ **W16.41** **Fall into unspecified water causing** drowning and submersion

✓x7ᵗʰ **W16.42** **Fall into unspecified water causing other injury**

✓5ᵗʰ **W16.5** **Jumping or diving into** swimming pool

✓6ᵗʰ **W16.51** **Jumping or diving into swimming pool** striking water surface

✓7ᵗʰ **W16.511** **Jumping or diving into swimming pool striking water surface causing** drowning and submersion
EXCLUDES 1 *drowning and submersion while in swimming pool without jumping or diving (W67)*

✓7ᵗʰ **W16.512** **Jumping or diving into swimming pool striking water surface causing other injury**

✓6ᵗʰ **W16.52** **Jumping or diving into swimming pool** striking bottom

✓7ᵗʰ **W16.521** **Jumping or diving into swimming pool striking bottom causing** drowning and submersion
EXCLUDES 1 *drowning and submersion while in swimming pool without jumping or diving (W67)*

✓7ᵗʰ **W16.522** **Jumping or diving into swimming pool striking bottom causing other injury**

✓6ᵗʰ **W16.53** **Jumping or diving into swimming pool** striking wall

✓7ᵗʰ **W16.531** **Jumping or diving into swimming pool striking wall causing** drowning and submersion
EXCLUDES 1 *drowning and submersion while in swimming pool without jumping or diving (W67)*

✓7ᵗʰ **W16.532** **Jumping or diving into swimming pool striking wall causing other injury**

✓5ᵗʰ **W16.6** **Jumping or diving into** natural body of water
Jumping or diving into lake
Jumping or diving into open sea
Jumping or diving into river
Jumping or diving into stream

✓6ᵗʰ **W16.61** **Jumping or diving into natural body of water** striking water surface

✓7ᵗʰ **W16.611** **Jumping or diving into natural body of water striking water surface causing** drowning and submersion
EXCLUDES 1 *drowning and submersion while in natural body of water without jumping or diving (W69)*

✓7ᵗʰ **W16.612** **Jumping or diving into natural body of water striking water surface causing other injury**

✓6ᵗʰ **W16.62** **Jumping or diving into natural body of water** striking bottom

✓7ᵗʰ **W16.621** **Jumping or diving into natural body of water striking bottom causing** drowning and submersion
EXCLUDES 1 *drowning and submersion while in natural body of water without jumping or diving (W69)*

✓7ᵗʰ **W16.622** **Jumping or diving into natural body of water striking bottom causing other injury**

✓5ᵗʰ **W16.7** **Jumping or diving** from boat
EXCLUDES 1 *fall from boat into water - see watercraft accident (V90-V94)*

✓6ᵗʰ **W16.71** **Jumping or diving from boat** striking water surface

✓7ᵗʰ **W16.711** **Jumping or diving from boat striking water surface causing** drowning and submersion

✓7ᵗʰ **W16.712** **Jumping or diving from boat striking water surface causing other injury**

✓6ᵗʰ **W16.72** **Jumping or diving from boat** striking bottom

✓7ᵗʰ **W16.721** **Jumping or diving from boat striking bottom causing** drowning and submersion

✓7ᵗʰ **W16.722** **Jumping or diving from boat striking bottom causing other injury**

Chapter 20. External Causes of Morbidity

W16.8–W21.Ø7

✓5ᵗʰ **W16.8 Jumping or diving into other water**
> Jumping or diving into fountain
> Jumping or diving into reservoir

    ✓6ᵗʰ **W16.81 Jumping or diving into other water striking water surface**

        ✓7ᵗʰ **W16.811 Jumping or diving into other water striking water surface causing drowning and submersion**

            EXCLUDES 1   *drowning and submersion while in other water without jumping or diving (W73)*

        ✓7ᵗʰ **W16.812 Jumping or diving into other water striking water surface causing other injury**

    ✓6ᵗʰ **W16.82 Jumping or diving into other water striking bottom**

        ✓7ᵗʰ **W16.821 Jumping or diving into other water striking bottom causing drowning and submersion**

            EXCLUDES 1   *drowning and submersion while in other water without jumping or diving (W73)*

        ✓7ᵗʰ **W16.822 Jumping or diving into other water striking bottom causing other injury**

    ✓6ᵗʰ **W16.83 Jumping or diving into other water striking wall**

        ✓7ᵗʰ **W16.831 Jumping or diving into other water striking wall causing drowning and submersion**

            EXCLUDES 1   *drowning and submersion while in other water without jumping or diving (W73)*

        ✓7ᵗʰ **W16.832 Jumping or diving into other water striking wall causing other injury**

✓5ᵗʰ **W16.9 Jumping or diving into unspecified water**

    ✓x7ᵗʰ **W16.91 Jumping or diving into unspecified water causing drowning and submersion**

    ✓x7ᵗʰ **W16.92 Jumping or diving into unspecified water causing other injury**

✓4ᵗʰ **W17 Other fall from one level to another**

    ✓x7ᵗʰ **W17.Ø Fall into well**

    ✓x7ᵗʰ **W17.1 Fall into storm drain or manhole**

    ✓x7ᵗʰ **W17.2 Fall into hole**
> Fall into pit

    ✓x7ᵗʰ **W17.3 Fall into empty swimming pool**

        EXCLUDES 1   *fall into filled swimming pool (W16.Ø-)*

    ✓x7ᵗʰ **W17.4 Fall from dock**

    ✓5ᵗʰ **W17.8 Other fall from one level to another**

        ✓x7ᵗʰ **W17.81 Fall down embankment (hill)**

        ✓x7ᵗʰ **W17.82 Fall from (out of) grocery cart**
> Fall due to grocery cart tipping over

        ✓x7ᵗʰ **W17.89 Other fall from one level to another**
> Fall from cherry picker
> Fall from lifting device
> Fall from mobile elevated work platform [MEWP]
> Fall from sky lift
> **AHA:** 2015,2Q,6

✓4ᵗʰ **W18 Other slipping, tripping and stumbling and falls**

    ✓5ᵗʰ **W18.Ø Fall due to bumping against object**
> Striking against object with subsequent fall

        EXCLUDES 1   *fall on same level due to slipping, tripping, or stumbling with subsequent striking against object (WØ1.1-)*

        ✓x7ᵗʰ **W18.ØØ Striking against unspecified object with subsequent fall**

        ✓x7ᵗʰ **W18.Ø1 Striking against sports equipment with subsequent fall**

        ✓x7ᵗʰ **W18.Ø2 Striking against glass with subsequent fall**

        ✓x7ᵗʰ **W18.Ø9 Striking against other object with subsequent fall**

    ✓5ᵗʰ **W18.1 Fall from or off toilet**

        ✓x7ᵗʰ **W18.11 Fall from or off toilet without subsequent striking against object**
> Fall from (off) toilet NOS

        ✓x7ᵗʰ **W18.12 Fall from or off toilet with subsequent striking against object**

    ✓x7ᵗʰ **W18.2 Fall in (into) shower or empty bathtub**

        EXCLUDES 1   *fall in full bathtub causing drowning or submersion (W16.21-)*

    ✓5ᵗʰ **W18.3 Other and unspecified fall on same level**

        ✓7ᵗʰ **W18.3Ø Fall on same level, unspecified**

        ✓7ᵗʰ **W18.31 Fall on same level due to stepping on an object**
> Fall on same level due to stepping on an animal

            EXCLUDES 1   *slipping, tripping and stumbling without fall due to stepping on animal (W18.41)*

        ✓7ᵗʰ **W18.39 Other fall on same level**

    ✓5ᵗʰ **W18.4 Slipping, tripping and stumbling without falling**

        EXCLUDES 1   *collision with another person without fall (W51)*

        ✓7ᵗʰ **W18.4Ø Slipping, tripping and stumbling without falling, unspecified**

        ✓7ᵗʰ **W18.41 Slipping, tripping and stumbling without falling due to stepping on object**
> Slipping, tripping and stumbling without falling due to stepping on animal

            EXCLUDES 1   *slipping, tripping and stumbling with fall due to stepping on animal (W18.31)*

        ✓7ᵗʰ **W18.42 Slipping, tripping and stumbling without falling due to stepping into hole or opening**

        ✓7ᵗʰ **W18.43 Slipping, tripping and stumbling without falling due to stepping from one level to another**

        ✓7ᵗʰ **W18.49 Other slipping, tripping and stumbling without falling**

✓x7ᵗʰ **W19 Unspecified fall**
> Accidental fall NOS
> **AHA:** 2012,4Q,95

Exposure to inanimate mechanical forces (W20-W49)

EXCLUDES 1   *assault (X92-Y09)*
contact or collision with animals or persons (W50-W64)
exposure to inanimate mechanical forces involving military or war operations (Y36.-, Y37.-)
intentional self-harm (X71-X83)

The appropriate 7th character is to be added to each code from categories W20-W49.
A initial encounter
D subsequent encounter
S sequela

✓4ᵗʰ **W20 Struck by thrown, projected or falling object**
> Code first any associated:
> cataclysm (X34-X39)
> lightning strike (T75.ØØ)

    EXCLUDES 1   *falling object in machinery accident (W24, W28-W31)*
falling object in transport accident (VØ1-V99)
object set in motion by explosion (W35-W40)
object set in motion by firearm (W32-W34)
struck by thrown sports equipment (W21.-)

    ✓x7ᵗʰ **W20.Ø Struck by falling object in cave-in**

        EXCLUDES 2   *asphyxiation due to cave-in (T71.21)*

    ✓x7ᵗʰ **W20.1 Struck by object due to collapse of building**

        EXCLUDES 1   *struck by object due to collapse of burning building (XØØ.2, XØ2.2)*

    ✓x7ᵗʰ **W20.8 Other cause of strike by thrown, projected or falling object**

        EXCLUDES 1   *struck by thrown sports equipment (W21.-)*

✓4ᵗʰ **W21 Striking against or struck by sports equipment**

    EXCLUDES 1   *assault with sports equipment (YØ8.Ø-)*
striking against or struck by sports equipment with subsequent fall (W18.Ø1)

    ✓5ᵗʰ **W21.Ø Struck by hit or thrown ball**

        ✓x7ᵗʰ **W21.ØØ Struck by hit or thrown ball, unspecified type**

        ✓x7ᵗʰ **W21.Ø1 Struck by football**

        ✓x7ᵗʰ **W21.Ø2 Struck by soccer ball**

        ✓x7ᵗʰ **W21.Ø3 Struck by baseball**

        ✓x7ᵗʰ **W21.Ø4 Struck by golf ball**

        ✓x7ᵗʰ **W21.Ø5 Struck by basketball**

        ✓x7ᵗʰ **W21.Ø6 Struck by volleyball**

        ✓x7ᵗʰ **W21.Ø7 Struck by softball**

√x7ᵗʰ **W21.Ø9**   **Struck by other hit or thrown ball**

√5ᵗʰ **W21.1**   **Struck by** bat, racquet or club

    √x7ᵗʰ **W21.11**   **Struck by** baseball bat

    √x7ᵗʰ **W21.12**   **Struck by** tennis racquet

    √x7ᵗʰ **W21.13**   **Struck by** golf club

    √x7ᵗʰ **W21.19**   **Struck by other bat, racquet or club**

√5ᵗʰ **W21.2**   **Struck by** hockey stick or puck

    √6ᵗʰ **W21.21**   **Struck by** hockey stick

       √7ᵗʰ **W21.21Ø**   **Struck by** ice **hockey stick**

       √7ᵗʰ **W21.211**   **Struck by** field **hockey stick**

    √6ᵗʰ **W21.22**   **Struck by** hockey puck

       √7ᵗʰ **W21.22Ø**   **Struck by** ice **hockey puck**

       √7ᵗʰ **W21.221**   **Struck by** field **hockey puck**

√5ᵗʰ **W21.3**   **Struck by sports** foot wear

    √x7ᵗʰ **W21.31**   **Struck by shoe** cleats

       Stepped on by shoe cleats

    √x7ᵗʰ **W21.32**   **Struck by skate** blades

       Skated over by skate blades

    √x7ᵗʰ **W21.39**   **Struck by other sports foot wear**

√x7ᵗʰ **W21.4**   **Striking against** diving board

    Use additional code for subsequent falling into water, if applicable (W16.-)

√5ᵗʰ **W21.8**   **Striking against or struck by other sports equipment**

    √x7ᵗʰ **W21.81**   **Striking against or struck by** football helmet

    √x7ᵗʰ **W21.89**   **Striking against or struck by other sports equipment**

√x7ᵗʰ **W21.9**   **Striking against or struck by unspecified sports equipment**

√4ᵗʰ **W22**   **Striking against or struck by other objects**

    EXCLUDES 1   *striking against or struck by object with subsequent fall (W18.Ø9)*

√5ᵗʰ **W22.Ø**   **Striking against** stationary object

    EXCLUDES 1   *striking against stationary sports equipment (W21.8)*

    √x7ᵗʰ **W22.Ø1**   **Walked into** wall

    √x7ᵗʰ **W22.Ø2**   **Walked into** lamppost

    √x7ᵗʰ **W22.Ø3**   **Walked into** furniture

    √6ᵗʰ **W22.Ø4**   **Striking against wall of** swimming pool

       √7ᵗʰ **W22.Ø41**   **Striking against wall of swimming pool causing** drowning and submersion

          EXCLUDES 1   *drowning and submersion while swimming without striking against wall (W67)*

       √7ᵗʰ **W22.Ø42**   **Striking against wall of swimming pool causing other injury**

    √x7ᵗʰ **W22.Ø9**   **Striking against other stationary object**

√5ᵗʰ **W22.1**   **Striking against or struck by** automobile airbag

    √x7ᵗʰ **W22.1Ø**   **Striking against or struck by unspecified automobile airbag**

    √x7ᵗʰ **W22.11**   **Striking against or struck by** driver side **automobile airbag**

    √x7ᵗʰ **W22.12**   **Striking against or struck by** front passenger **side automobile airbag**

    √x7ᵗʰ **W22.19**   **Striking against or struck by other automobile airbag**

√x7ᵗʰ **W22.8**   **Striking against or struck by other objects**

    Striking against or struck by object NOS

    EXCLUDES 1   *struck by thrown, projected or falling object (W2Ø.-)*

√4ᵗʰ **W23**   **Caught, crushed, jammed or pinched in or between objects**

    EXCLUDES 1   *injury caused by cutting or piercing instruments (W25-W27)*
          injury caused by firearms malfunction (W32.1, W33.1-, W34.1-)
          injury caused by lifting and transmission devices (W24.-)
          injury caused by machinery (W28-W31)
          injury caused by nonpowered hand tools (W27.-)
          injury caused by transport vehicle being used as a means of transportation (VØ1-V99)
          injury caused by struck by thrown, projected or falling object (W2Ø.-)

    √x7ᵗʰ **W23.Ø**   **Caught, crushed, jammed, or pinched between** moving objects

√x7ᵗʰ **W23.1**   **Caught, crushed, jammed, or pinched between** stationary objects

√4ᵗʰ **W24**   **Contact with lifting and transmission devices, not elsewhere classified**

    EXCLUDES 1   *transport accidents (VØ1-V99)*

√x7ᵗʰ **W24.Ø**   **Contact with lifting devices, not elsewhere classified**

    Contact with chain hoist
    Contact with drive belt
    Contact with pulley (block)

√x7ᵗʰ **W24.1**   **Contact with transmission devices, not elsewhere classified**

    Contact with transmission belt or cable

√x7ᵗʰ **W25**   **Contact with sharp glass**

    Code first any associated:
       injury due to flying glass from explosion or firearm discharge (W32-W4Ø)
       transport accident (VØØ-V99)

    EXCLUDES 1   *fall on same level due to slipping, tripping and stumbling with subsequent striking against sharp glass ▶(WØ1.11Ø-)◀*
          striking against sharp glass with subsequent fall ▶(W18.Ø2-)◀

    EXCLUDES 2   *glass embedded in skin ▶(W45.-)◀*

√4ᵗʰ **W26**   **Contact with other sharp objects**

    EXCLUDES 2   *sharp object(s) embedded in skin ▶(W45.-)◀*

    AHA: 2016,4Q,73

√x7ᵗʰ **W26.Ø**   **Contact with knife**

    EXCLUDES 1   *contact with electric knife (W29.1)*

√x7ᵗʰ **W26.1**   **Contact with sword or dagger**

√x7ᵗʰ **W26.2**   **Contact with edge of stiff paper**

    Paper cut

√x7ᵗʰ **W26.8**   **Contact with other sharp object(s), not elsewhere classified**

    Contact with tin can lid

√x7ᵗʰ **W26.9**   **Contact with unspecified sharp object(s)**

√4ᵗʰ **W27**   **Contact with nonpowered hand tool**

√x7ᵗʰ **W27.Ø**   **Contact with** workbench tool

    Contact with auger
    Contact with axe
    Contact with chisel
    Contact with handsaw
    Contact with screwdriver

√x7ᵗʰ **W27.1**   **Contact with** garden tool

    Contact with hoe
    Contact with nonpowered lawn mower
    Contact with pitchfork
    Contact with rake

√x7ᵗʰ **W27.2**   **Contact with** scissors

√x7ᵗʰ **W27.3**   **Contact with** needle (sewing)

    EXCLUDES 1   *contact with hypodermic needle (W46.-)*

√x7ᵗʰ **W27.4**   **Contact with** kitchen utensil

    Contact with fork
    Contact with ice-pick
    Contact with can-opener NOS

√x7ᵗʰ **W27.5**   **Contact with** paper-cutter

√x7ᵗʰ **W27.8**   **Contact with other nonpowered hand tool**

    Contact with nonpowered sewing machine
    Contact with shovel

√x7ᵗʰ **W28**   **Contact with powered lawn mower**

    Powered lawn mower (commercial) (residential)

    EXCLUDES 1   *contact with nonpowered lawn mower (W27.1)*

    EXCLUDES 2   *exposure to electric current (W86.-)*

√4ᵗʰ **W29**   **Contact with other powered hand tools and household machinery**

    EXCLUDES 1   *contact with commercial machinery (W31.82)*
          contact with hot household appliance (X15)
          contact with nonpowered hand tool (W27.-)
          exposure to electric current (W86)

√x7ᵗʰ **W29.Ø**   **Contact with powered kitchen appliance**

    Contact with blender
    Contact with can-opener
    Contact with garbage disposal
    Contact with mixer

√x7ᵗʰ **W29.1**   **Contact with electric knife**

☑ Additional Char Req   √x7ᵗʰ Placeholder   Unacceptable PDx   Questionable PDx   Wrong Procedure   Manifestation   Unspecified Dx   H1-H14 HAC   HCC CMS-HCC Dx   HIV HIV Dx

ICD-10-CM 2022   1203

Chapter 20. External Causes of Morbidity

√x7ᵗʰ **W29.2 Contact with other powered household machinery**
    Contact with electric fan
    Contact with powered dryer (clothes) (powered) (spin)
    Contact with washing-machine
    Contact with sewing machine

√x7ᵗʰ **W29.3 Contact with powered garden and outdoor hand tools and machinery**
    Contact with chainsaw
    Contact with edger
    Contact with garden cultivator (tiller)
    Contact with hedge trimmer
    Contact with other powered garden tool
      EXCLUDES 1   *contact with powered lawn mower (W28)*

√x7ᵗʰ **W29.4 Contact with nail gun**

√x7ᵗʰ **W29.8 Contact with other powered hand tools and household machinery**
    Contact with do-it-yourself tool NOS

√4ᵗʰ **W30 Contact with agricultural machinery**
    INCLUDES   animal-powered farm machine
    EXCLUDES 1   *agricultural transport vehicle accident (V01-V99)*
      explosion of grain store (W40.8)
      exposure to electric current (W86.-)

√x7ᵗʰ **W30.0 Contact with combine harvester**
    Contact with reaper
    Contact with thresher

√x7ᵗʰ **W30.1 Contact with power take-off devices (PTO)**

√x7ᵗʰ **W30.2 Contact with hay derrick**

√x7ᵗʰ **W30.3 Contact with grain storage elevator**
      EXCLUDES 1   *explosion of grain store (W40.8)*

√5ᵗʰ **W30.8 Contact with other specified agricultural machinery**

√x7ᵗʰ **W30.81 Contact with agricultural transport vehicle in stationary use**
    Contact with agricultural transport vehicle under repair, not on public roadway
      EXCLUDES 1   *agricultural transport vehicle accident (V01-V99)*

√x7ᵗʰ **W30.89 Contact with other specified agricultural machinery**

√x7ᵗʰ **W30.9 Contact with unspecified agricultural machinery**
    Contact with farm machinery NOS

√4ᵗʰ **W31 Contact with other and unspecified machinery**
    EXCLUDES 1   *contact with agricultural machinery (W30.-)*
      contact with machinery in transport under own power or being towed by a vehicle (V01-V99)
      exposure to electric current (W86)

√x7ᵗʰ **W31.0 Contact with mining and earth-drilling machinery**
    Contact with bore or drill (land) (seabed)
    Contact with shaft hoist
    Contact with shaft lift
    Contact with undercutter

√x7ᵗʰ **W31.1 Contact with metalworking machines**
    Contact with abrasive wheel
    Contact with forging machine
    Contact with lathe
    Contact with mechanical shears
    Contact with metal drilling machine
    Contact with milling machine
    Contact with power press
    Contact with rolling-mill
    Contact with metal sawing machine

√x7ᵗʰ **W31.2 Contact with powered woodworking and forming machines**
    Contact with band saw
    Contact with bench saw
    Contact with circular saw
    Contact with molding machine
    Contact with overhead plane
    Contact with powered saw
    Contact with radial saw
    Contact with sander
      EXCLUDES 1   *nonpowered woodworking tools (W27.0)*

√x7ᵗʰ **W31.3 Contact with prime movers**
    Contact with gas turbine
    Contact with internal combustion engine
    Contact with steam engine
    Contact with water driven turbine

√5ᵗʰ **W31.8 Contact with other specified machinery**

√x7ᵗʰ **W31.81 Contact with recreational machinery**
    Contact with roller coaster

√x7ᵗʰ **W31.82 Contact with other commercial machinery**
    Contact with commercial electric fan
    Contact with commercial kitchen appliances
    Contact with commercial powered dryer (clothes) (powered) (spin)
    Contact with commercial washing-machine
    Contact with commercial sewing machine
      EXCLUDES 1   *contact with household machinery (W29.-)*
      contact with powered lawn mower (W28)

√x7ᵗʰ **W31.83 Contact with special construction vehicle in stationary use**
    Contact with special construction vehicle under repair, not on public roadway
      EXCLUDES 1   *special construction vehicle accident (V01-V99)*

√x7ᵗʰ **W31.89 Contact with other specified machinery**

√x7ᵗʰ **W31.9 Contact with unspecified machinery**
    Contact with machinery NOS

√4ᵗʰ **W32 Accidental handgun discharge and malfunction**
    INCLUDES   accidental discharge and malfunction of gun for single hand use
      accidental discharge and malfunction of pistol
      accidental discharge and malfunction of revolver
      handgun discharge and malfunction NOS
    EXCLUDES 1   *accidental airgun discharge and malfunction (W34.010, W34.110)*
      accidental BB gun discharge and malfunction (W34.010, W34.110)
      accidental pellet gun discharge and malfunction (W34.010, W34.110)
      accidental shotgun discharge and malfunction (W33.01, W33.11)
      assault by handgun discharge (X93)
      handgun discharge involving legal intervention (Y35.0-)
      handgun discharge involving military or war operations (Y36.4-)
      intentional self-harm by handgun discharge (X72)
      Very pistol discharge and malfunction (W34.09, W34.19)

√x7ᵗʰ **W32.0 Accidental handgun discharge**

√x7ᵗʰ **W32.1 Accidental handgun malfunction**
    Injury due to explosion of handgun (parts)
    Injury due to malfunction of mechanism or component of handgun
    Injury due to recoil of handgun
    Powder burn from handgun

√4ᵗʰ **W33 Accidental rifle, shotgun and larger firearm discharge and malfunction**
    INCLUDES   rifle, shotgun and larger firearm discharge and malfunction NOS
    EXCLUDES 1   *accidental airgun discharge and malfunction (W34.010, W34.110)*
      accidental BB gun discharge and malfunction (W34.010, W34.110)
      accidental handgun discharge and malfunction (W32.-)
      accidental pellet gun discharge and malfunction (W34.010, W34.110)
      assault by rifle, shotgun and larger firearm discharge (X94)
      firearm discharge involving legal intervention (Y35.0-)
      firearm discharge involving military or war operations (Y36.4-)
      intentional self-harm by rifle, shotgun and larger firearm discharge (X73)

√5ᵗʰ **W33.0 Accidental rifle, shotgun and larger firearm discharge**

√x7ᵗʰ **W33.00 Accidental discharge of unspecified larger firearm**
    Discharge of unspecified larger firearm NOS

Ⓝ Newborn: 0   Ⓟ Pediatric: 0-17   Ⓜ Maternity: 9-64   Ⓐ Adult: 15-124   MCC Major Complication/Comorbidity   CC Complication/Comorbidity   SW Severe Wound Dx

1204   ICD-10-CM 2022

√x7ᵗʰ **W33.01** **Accidental discharge of** shotgun
Discharge of shotgun NOS

√x7ᵗʰ **W33.02** **Accidental discharge of** hunting rifle
Discharge of hunting rifle NOS

√x7ᵗʰ **W33.03** **Accidental discharge of** machine gun
Discharge of machine gun NOS

√x7ᵗʰ **W33.09** **Accidental discharge of other larger firearm**
Discharge of other larger firearm NOS

√5ᵗʰ **W33.1** **Accidental rifle, shotgun and larger firearm** malfunction
Injury due to explosion of rifle, shotgun and larger firearm (parts)
Injury due to malfunction of mechanism or component of rifle, shotgun and larger firearm
Injury due to piercing, cutting, crushing or pinching due to (by) slide trigger mechanism, scope or other gun part
Injury due to recoil of rifle, shotgun and larger firearm
Powder burn from rifle, shotgun and larger firearm

√x7ᵗʰ **W33.10** **Accidental malfunction of unspecified larger firearm**
Malfunction of unspecified larger firearm NOS

√x7ᵗʰ **W33.11** **Accidental malfunction of** shotgun
Malfunction of shotgun NOS

√x7ᵗʰ **W33.12** **Accidental malfunction of** hunting rifle
Malfunction of hunting rifle NOS

√x7ᵗʰ **W33.13** **Accidental malfunction of** machine gun
Malfunction of machine gun NOS

√x7ᵗʰ **W33.19** **Accidental malfunction of other larger firearm**
Malfunction of other larger firearm NOS

√4ᵗʰ **W34** **Accidental discharge and malfunction from other and unspecified firearms and guns**

√5ᵗʰ **W34.0** **Accidental** discharge **from other and unspecified firearms and guns**

√x7ᵗʰ **W34.00** **Accidental discharge from unspecified firearms or gun**
Discharge from firearm NOS
Gunshot wound NOS
Shot NOS

√6ᵗʰ **W34.01** **Accidental discharge of** gas, air or spring-operated **guns**

√7ᵗʰ **W34.010** **Accidental discharge of** airgun
Accidental discharge of BB gun
Accidental discharge of pellet gun

√7ᵗʰ **W34.011** **Accidental discharge of** paintball gun
Accidental injury due to paintball discharge

√7ᵗʰ **W34.018** **Accidental discharge of other gas, air or spring-operated gun**

√x7ᵗʰ **W34.09** **Accidental discharge from other specified firearms**
Accidental discharge from Very pistol [flare]

√5ᵗʰ **W34.1** **Accidental** malfunction **from other and unspecified firearms and guns**

√x7ᵗʰ **W34.10** **Accidental malfunction from unspecified firearms or gun**
Firearm malfunction NOS

√6ᵗʰ **W34.11** **Accidental malfunction of** gas, air or spring-operated **guns**

√7ᵗʰ **W34.110** **Accidental malfunction of** airgun
Accidental malfunction of BB gun
Accidental malfunction of pellet gun

√7ᵗʰ **W34.111** **Accidental malfunction of** paintball gun
Accidental injury due to paintball gun malfunction

√7ᵗʰ **W34.118** **Accidental malfunction of other gas, air or spring-operated gun**

√x7ᵗʰ **W34.19** **Accidental malfunction from other specified firearms**
Accidental malfunction from Very pistol [flare]

√x7ᵗʰ **W35** **Explosion and rupture of** boiler
> EXCLUDES 1   *explosion and rupture of boiler on watercraft (V93.4)*

√4ᵗʰ **W36** **Explosion and rupture of** gas cylinder

√x7ᵗʰ **W36.1** **Explosion and rupture of** aerosol can

√x7ᵗʰ **W36.2** **Explosion and rupture of** air tank

√x7ᵗʰ **W36.3** **Explosion and rupture of** pressurized-gas tank

√x7ᵗʰ **W36.8** **Explosion and rupture of other gas cylinder**

√x7ᵗʰ **W36.9** **Explosion and rupture of unspecified gas cylinder**

√4ᵗʰ **W37** **Explosion and rupture of** pressurized tire, pipe or hose

√x7ᵗʰ **W37.0** **Explosion of** bicycle tire

√x7ᵗʰ **W37.8** **Explosion and rupture of other pressurized tire, pipe or hose**

√x7ᵗʰ **W38** **Explosion and rupture of other specified** pressurized devices

√x7ᵗʰ **W39** **Discharge of** firework

√4ᵗʰ **W40** **Explosion of other materials**
> EXCLUDES 1   *assault by explosive material (X96)*
> *explosion involving legal intervention (Y35.1-)*
> *explosion involving military or war operations (Y36.0-, Y36.2-)*
> *intentional self-harm by explosive material (X75)*

√x7ᵗʰ **W40.0** **Explosion of** blasting material
Explosion of blasting cap
Explosion of detonator
Explosion of dynamite
Explosion of explosive (any) used in blasting operations

√x7ᵗʰ **W40.1** **Explosion of** explosive gases
Explosion of acetylene
Explosion of butane
Explosion of coal gas
Explosion in mine NOS
Explosion of explosive gas
Explosion of fire damp
Explosion of gasoline fumes
Explosion of methane
Explosion of propane

√x7ᵗʰ **W40.8** **Explosion of other specified explosive materials**
Explosion in dump NOS
Explosion in factory NOS
Explosion in grain store
Explosion in munitions
> EXCLUDES 1   *explosion involving legal intervention (Y35.1-)*
> *explosion involving military or war operations (Y36.0-, Y36.2-)*

√x7ᵗʰ **W40.9** **Explosion of unspecified explosive materials**
Explosion NOS

√4ᵗʰ **W42** **Exposure to noise**

√x7ᵗʰ **W42.0** **Exposure to supersonic waves**

√x7ᵗʰ **W42.9** **Exposure to other noise**
Exposure to sound waves NOS

√4ᵗʰ **W45** **Foreign body or object entering through skin**
> INCLUDES   foreign body or object embedded in skin
> nail embedded in skin
> EXCLUDES 2   *contact with hand tools (nonpowered) (powered) (W27-W29)*
> *contact with other sharp objects (W26.-)*
> *contact with sharp glass (W25.-)*
> *struck by objects (W20-W22)*

√x7ᵗʰ **W45.0** Nail **entering through skin**

√x7ᵗʰ **W45.8** **Other foreign body or object entering through skin**
Splinter in skin NOS

√4ᵗʰ **W46** **Contact with hypodermic needle**

√x7ᵗʰ **W46.0** **Contact with hypodermic needle**
Hypodermic needle stick NOS

√x7ᵗʰ **W46.1** **Contact with** contaminated **hypodermic needle**

√4ᵗʰ **W49** **Exposure to other inanimate mechanical forces**
> INCLUDES   exposure to abnormal gravitational [G] forces
> exposure to inanimate mechanical forces NEC
> EXCLUDES 1   *exposure to inanimate mechanical forces involving military or war operations (Y36.-, Y37.-)*

√5ᵗʰ **W49.0** **Item causing** external constriction

√x7ᵗʰ **W49.01** Hair **causing external constriction**

√x7ᵗʰ **W49.02** String or thread **causing external constriction**

√x7ᵗʰ **W49.03** Rubber band **causing external constriction**

√x7ᵗʰ **W49.04** Ring or other jewelry **causing external constriction**

√x7ᵗʰ **W49.09** **Other specified item causing external constriction**

√x7ᵗʰ **W49.9** **Exposure to other inanimate mechanical forces**

✅ Additional Char Req   √x7ᵗʰ Placeholder   Unacceptable PDx   Questionable PDx   Wrong Procedure   Manifestation   Unspecified Dx   H1-H14 HAC   HCC CMS-HCC Dx   HIV HIV Dx

ICD-10-CM 2022   1205

Chapter 20. External Causes of Morbidity

W50–W58.09

Exposure to animate mechanical forces (W50-W64)

> **EXCLUDES 1**   toxic effect of contact with venomous animals and plants (T63.-)

> The appropriate 7th character is to be added to each code from categories W50-W64.
> A   initial encounter
> D   subsequent encounter
> S   sequela

☑4ᵗʰ W50   Accidental hit, strike, kick, twist, bite or scratch by another person

> **INCLUDES**   hit, strike, kick, twist, bite, or scratch by another person NOS

> **EXCLUDES 1**   assault by bodily force (Y04)
> struck by objects (W20-W22)

   ✓x7ᵗʰ W50.0   Accidental hit or strike by another person
     Hit or strike by another person NOS

   ✓x7ᵗʰ W50.1   Accidental kick by another person
     Kick by another person NOS

   ✓x7ᵗʰ W50.2   Accidental twist by another person
     Twist by another person NOS

   ✓x7ᵗʰ W50.3   Accidental bite by another person
     Human bite
     Bite by another person NOS

   ✓x7ᵗʰ W50.4   Accidental scratch by another person
     Scratch by another person NOS

✓x7ᵗʰ W51   Accidental striking against or bumped into by another person

> **EXCLUDES 1**   assault by striking against or bumping into by another person (Y04.2)
> fall due to collision with another person (W03)

✓x7ᵗʰ W52   Crushed, pushed or stepped on by crowd or human stampede
   Crushed, pushed or stepped on by crowd or human stampede with or without fall

☑4ᵗʰ W53   Contact with rodent

> **INCLUDES**   contact with saliva, feces or urine of rodent

   ☑5ᵗʰ W53.0   Contact with mouse
     ✓x7ᵗʰ W53.01   Bitten by mouse
     ✓x7ᵗʰ W53.09   Other contact with mouse

   ☑5ᵗʰ W53.1   Contact with rat
     ✓x7ᵗʰ W53.11   Bitten by rat
     ✓x7ᵗʰ W53.19   Other contact with rat

   ☑5ᵗʰ W53.2   Contact with squirrel
     ✓x7ᵗʰ W53.21   Bitten by squirrel
     ✓x7ᵗʰ W53.29   Other contact with squirrel

   ☑5ᵗʰ W53.8   Contact with other rodent
     ✓x7ᵗʰ W53.81   Bitten by other rodent
     ✓x7ᵗʰ W53.89   Other contact with other rodent

☑4ᵗʰ W54   Contact with dog

> **INCLUDES**   contact with saliva, feces or urine of dog

   ✓x7ᵗʰ W54.0   Bitten by dog
   ✓x7ᵗʰ W54.1   Struck by dog
     Knocked over by dog
   ✓x7ᵗʰ W54.8   Other contact with dog

☑4ᵗʰ W55   Contact with other mammals

> **INCLUDES**   contact with saliva, feces or urine of mammal

> **EXCLUDES 1**   animal being ridden - see transport accidents
> bitten or struck by dog (W54)
> bitten or struck by rodent (W53.-)
> contact with marine mammals (W56.-)

   ☑5ᵗʰ W55.0   Contact with cat
     ✓x7ᵗʰ W55.01   Bitten by cat
     ✓x7ᵗʰ W55.03   Scratched by cat
     ✓x7ᵗʰ W55.09   Other contact with cat

   ☑5ᵗʰ W55.1   Contact with horse
     ✓x7ᵗʰ W55.11   Bitten by horse
     ✓x7ᵗʰ W55.12   Struck by horse
     ✓x7ᵗʰ W55.19   Other contact with horse

   ☑5ᵗʰ W55.2   Contact with cow
     Contact with bull
     ✓x7ᵗʰ W55.21   Bitten by cow

     ✓x7ᵗʰ W55.22   Struck by cow
     Gored by bull
     ✓x7ᵗʰ W55.29   Other contact with cow

   ☑5ᵗʰ W55.3   Contact with other hoof stock
     Contact with goats
     Contact with sheep
     ✓x7ᵗʰ W55.31   Bitten by other hoof stock
     ✓x7ᵗʰ W55.32   Struck by other hoof stock
     Gored by goat
     Gored by ram
     ✓x7ᵗʰ W55.39   Other contact with other hoof stock

   ☑5ᵗʰ W55.4   Contact with pig
     ✓x7ᵗʰ W55.41   Bitten by pig
     ✓x7ᵗʰ W55.42   Struck by pig
     ✓x7ᵗʰ W55.49   Other contact with pig

   ☑5ᵗʰ W55.5   Contact with raccoon
     ✓x7ᵗʰ W55.51   Bitten by raccoon
     ✓x7ᵗʰ W55.52   Struck by raccoon
     ✓x7ᵗʰ W55.59   Other contact with raccoon

   ☑5ᵗʰ W55.8   Contact with other mammals
     ✓x7ᵗʰ W55.81   Bitten by other mammals
     ✓x7ᵗʰ W55.82   Struck by other mammals
     ✓x7ᵗʰ W55.89   Other contact with other mammals

☑4ᵗʰ W56   Contact with nonvenomous marine animal

> **EXCLUDES 1**   contact with venomous marine animal (T63.-)

   ☑5ᵗʰ W56.0   Contact with dolphin
     ✓x7ᵗʰ W56.01   Bitten by dolphin
     ✓x7ᵗʰ W56.02   Struck by dolphin
     ✓x7ᵗʰ W56.09   Other contact with dolphin

   ☑5ᵗʰ W56.1   Contact with sea lion
     ✓x7ᵗʰ W56.11   Bitten by sea lion
     ✓x7ᵗʰ W56.12   Struck by sea lion
     ✓x7ᵗʰ W56.19   Other contact with sea lion

   ☑5ᵗʰ W56.2   Contact with orca
     Contact with killer whale
     ✓x7ᵗʰ W56.21   Bitten by orca
     ✓x7ᵗʰ W56.22   Struck by orca
     ✓x7ᵗʰ W56.29   Other contact with orca

   ☑5ᵗʰ W56.3   Contact with other marine mammals
     ✓x7ᵗʰ W56.31   Bitten by other marine mammals
     ✓x7ᵗʰ W56.32   Struck by other marine mammals
     ✓x7ᵗʰ W56.39   Other contact with other marine mammals

   ☑5ᵗʰ W56.4   Contact with shark
     ✓x7ᵗʰ W56.41   Bitten by shark
     ✓x7ᵗʰ W56.42   Struck by shark
     ✓x7ᵗʰ W56.49   Other contact with shark

   ☑5ᵗʰ W56.5   Contact with other fish
     ✓x7ᵗʰ W56.51   Bitten by other fish
     ✓x7ᵗʰ W56.52   Struck by other fish
     ✓x7ᵗʰ W56.59   Other contact with other fish

   ☑5ᵗʰ W56.8   Contact with other nonvenomous marine animals
     ✓x7ᵗʰ W56.81   Bitten by other nonvenomous marine animals
     ✓x7ᵗʰ W56.82   Struck by other nonvenomous marine animals
     ✓x7ᵗʰ W56.89   Other contact with other nonvenomous marine animals

✓x7ᵗʰ W57   Bitten or stung by nonvenomous insect and other nonvenomous arthropods

> **EXCLUDES 1**   contact with venomous insects and arthropods (T63.2-, T63.3-, T63.4-)

☑4ᵗʰ W58   Contact with crocodile or alligator

   ☑5ᵗʰ W58.0   Contact with alligator
     ✓x7ᵗʰ W58.01   Bitten by alligator
     ✓x7ᵗʰ W58.02   Struck by alligator
     ✓x7ᵗʰ W58.03   Crushed by alligator
     ✓x7ᵗʰ W58.09   Other contact with alligator

N Newborn: 0   P Pediatric: 0-17   M Maternity: 9-64   A Adult: 15-124   MCC Major Complication/Comorbidity   CC Complication/Comorbidity   SW Severe Wound Dx

1206   ICD-10-CM 2022

☑5ᵗʰ **W58.1** **Contact with** crocodile

  ✓x7ᵗʰ **W58.11** Bitten **by crocodile**

  ✓x7ᵗʰ **W58.12** Struck **by crocodile**

  ✓x7ᵗʰ **W58.13** Crushed **by crocodile**

  ✓x7ᵗʰ **W58.19** **Other contact with crocodile**

☑4ᵗʰ **W59** **Contact with other nonvenomous reptiles**

  EXCLUDES 1 *contact with venomous reptile (T63.0-, T63.1-)*

☑5ᵗʰ **W59.0** **Contact with nonvenomous** lizards

  ✓x7ᵗʰ **W59.01** Bitten **by nonvenomous lizards**

  ✓x7ᵗʰ **W59.02** Struck **by nonvenomous lizards**

  ✓x7ᵗʰ **W59.09** **Other contact with nonvenomous lizards**

    Exposure to nonvenomous lizards

☑5ᵗʰ **W59.1** **Contact with nonvenomous** snakes

  ✓x7ᵗʰ **W59.11** Bitten **by nonvenomous snake**

  ✓x7ᵗʰ **W59.12** Struck **by nonvenomous snake**

  ✓x7ᵗʰ **W59.13** Crushed **by nonvenomous snake**

  ✓x7ᵗʰ **W59.19** **Other contact with nonvenomous snake**

☑5ᵗʰ **W59.2** **Contact with** turtles

  EXCLUDES 1 *contact with tortoises (W59.8-)*

  ✓x7ᵗʰ **W59.21** Bitten **by turtle**

  ✓x7ᵗʰ **W59.22** Struck **by turtle**

  ✓x7ᵗʰ **W59.29** **Other contact with turtle**

    Exposure to turtles

☑5ᵗʰ **W59.8** **Contact with other nonvenomous reptiles**

  ✓x7ᵗʰ **W59.81** Bitten **by other nonvenomous reptiles**

  ✓x7ᵗʰ **W59.82** Struck **by other nonvenomous reptiles**

  ✓x7ᵗʰ **W59.83** Crushed **by other nonvenomous reptiles**

  ✓x7ᵗʰ **W59.89** **Other contact with other nonvenomous reptiles**

✓x7ᵗʰ **W60** **Contact with nonvenomous plant thorns and spines and sharp leaves**

  EXCLUDES 1 *contact with venomous plants (T63.7-)*

☑4ᵗʰ **W61** **Contact with birds (domestic) (wild)**

  INCLUDES contact with excreta of birds

☑5ᵗʰ **W61.0** **Contact with** parrot

  ✓x7ᵗʰ **W61.01** Bitten **by parrot**

  ✓x7ᵗʰ **W61.02** Struck **by parrot**

  ✓x7ᵗʰ **W61.09** **Other contact with parrot**

    Exposure to parrots

☑5ᵗʰ **W61.1** **Contact with** macaw

  ✓x7ᵗʰ **W61.11** Bitten **by macaw**

  ✓x7ᵗʰ **W61.12** Struck **by macaw**

  ✓x7ᵗʰ **W61.19** **Other contact with macaw**

    Exposure to macaws

☑5ᵗʰ **W61.2** **Contact with other** psittacines

  ✓x7ᵗʰ **W61.21** Bitten **by other psittacines**

  ✓x7ᵗʰ **W61.22** Struck **by other psittacines**

  ✓x7ᵗʰ **W61.29** **Other contact with other psittacines**

    Exposure to other psittacines

☑5ᵗʰ **W61.3** **Contact with** chicken

  ✓x7ᵗʰ **W61.32** Struck **by chicken**

  ✓x7ᵗʰ **W61.33** Pecked **by chicken**

  ✓x7ᵗʰ **W61.39** **Other contact with chicken**

    Exposure to chickens

☑5ᵗʰ **W61.4** **Contact with** turkey

  ✓x7ᵗʰ **W61.42** Struck **by turkey**

  ✓x7ᵗʰ **W61.43** Pecked **by turkey**

  ✓x7ᵗʰ **W61.49** **Other contact with turkey**

☑5ᵗʰ **W61.5** **Contact with** goose

  ✓x7ᵗʰ **W61.51** Bitten **by goose**

  ✓x7ᵗʰ **W61.52** Struck **by goose**

  ✓x7ᵗʰ **W61.59** **Other contact with goose**

☑5ᵗʰ **W61.6** **Contact with** duck

  ✓x7ᵗʰ **W61.61** Bitten **by duck**

  ✓x7ᵗʰ **W61.62** Struck **by duck**

  ✓x7ᵗʰ **W61.69** **Other contact with duck**

☑5ᵗʰ **W61.9** **Contact with other birds**

  ✓x7ᵗʰ **W61.91** Bitten **by other birds**

  ✓x7ᵗʰ **W61.92** Struck **by other birds**

  ✓x7ᵗʰ **W61.99** **Other contact with other birds**

    Contact with bird NOS

☑4ᵗʰ **W62** **Contact with nonvenomous amphibians**

  EXCLUDES 1 *contact with venomous amphibians (T63.81-R63.83)*

✓x7ᵗʰ **W62.0** **Contact with nonvenomous** frogs

✓x7ᵗʰ **W62.1** **Contact with nonvenomous** toads

✓x7ᵗʰ **W62.9** **Contact with other nonvenomous amphibians**

✓x7ᵗʰ **W64** **Exposure to other animate mechanical forces**

  INCLUDES exposure to nonvenomous animal NOS

  EXCLUDES 1 *contact with venomous animal (T63.-)*

Accidental non-transport drowning and submersion (W65-W74)

  EXCLUDES 1 *accidental drowning and submersion due to fall into water (W16.-)*
      accidental drowning and submersion due to water transport accident (V90.-, V92.-)

  EXCLUDES 2 *accidental drowning and submersion due to cataclysm (X34-X39)*

The appropriate 7th character is to be added to each code from categories W65-W74.
A initial encounter
D subsequent encounter
S sequela

✓x7ᵗʰ **W65** **Accidental drowning and submersion while in** bath-tub

  EXCLUDES 1 *accidental drowning and submersion due to fall in (into) bathtub (W16.211)*

✓x7ᵗʰ **W67** **Accidental drowning and submersion while in** swimming-pool

  EXCLUDES 1 *accidental drowning and submersion due to fall into swimming pool (W16.011, W16.021, W16.031)*
      accidental drowning and submersion due to striking into wall of swimming pool (W22.041)

✓x7ᵗʰ **W69** **Accidental drowning and submersion while in** natural water

  Accidental drowning and submersion while in lake
  Accidental drowning and submersion while in open sea
  Accidental drowning and submersion while in river
  Accidental drowning and submersion while in stream

  EXCLUDES 1 *accidental drowning and submersion due to fall into natural body of water (W16.111, W16.121, W16.131)*

✓x7ᵗʰ **W73** **Other specified cause of accidental non-transport drowning and submersion**

  Accidental drowning and submersion while in quenching tank
  Accidental drowning and submersion while in reservoir

  EXCLUDES 1 *accidental drowning and submersion due to fall into other water (W16.311, W16.321, W16.331)*

✓x7ᵗʰ **W74** **Unspecified cause of accidental drowning and submersion**

  Drowning NOS

Exposure to electric current, radiation and extreme ambient air temperature and pressure (W85-W99)

  EXCLUDES 1 *exposure to:*
    failure in dosage of radiation or temperature during surgical and medical care (Y63.2-Y63.5)
    lightning (T75.0-)
    natural cold (X31)
    natural heat (X30)
    natural radiation NOS (X39)
    radiological procedure and radiotherapy (Y84.2)
    sunlight (X32)

AHA: 2018,2Q,7-8

The appropriate 7th character is to be added to each code from categories W85-W99.
A initial encounter
D subsequent encounter
S sequela

✓x7ᵗʰ **W85** **Exposure to electric transmission lines**

  Broken power line

☑4ᵗʰ **W86** **Exposure to other specified electric current**

  ✓x7ᵗʰ **W86.0** **Exposure to domestic wiring and appliances**

√x7ᵗʰ **W86.1 Exposure to industrial wiring, appliances and electrical machinery**
Exposure to conductors
Exposure to control apparatus
Exposure to electrical equipment and machinery
Exposure to transformers

√x7ᵗʰ **W86.8 Exposure to other electric current**
Exposure to wiring and appliances in or on farm (not farmhouse)
Exposure to wiring and appliances outdoors
Exposure to wiring and appliances in or on public building
Exposure to wiring and appliances in or on residential institutions
Exposure to wiring and appliances in or on schools

√4ᵗʰ **W88 Exposure to ionizing radiation**
    EXCLUDES 1   exposure to sunlight (X32)

√x7ᵗʰ **W88.0 Exposure to X-rays**

√x7ᵗʰ **W88.1 Exposure to radioactive isotopes**

√x7ᵗʰ **W88.8 Exposure to other ionizing radiation**

√4ᵗʰ **W89 Exposure to man-made visible and ultraviolet light**
    INCLUDES   exposure to welding light (arc)
    EXCLUDES 2   exposure to sunlight (X32)

√x7ᵗʰ **W89.0 Exposure to welding light (arc)**

√x7ᵗʰ **W89.1 Exposure to tanning bed**

√x7ᵗʰ **W89.8 Exposure to other man-made visible and ultraviolet light**

√x7ᵗʰ **W89.9 Exposure to unspecified man-made visible and ultraviolet light**

√4ᵗʰ **W90 Exposure to other nonionizing radiation**
    EXCLUDES 2   exposure to sunlight (X32)
    AHA: 2019,1Q,21

√x7ᵗʰ **W90.0 Exposure to radiofrequency**

√x7ᵗʰ **W90.1 Exposure to infrared radiation**

√x7ᵗʰ **W90.2 Exposure to laser radiation**

√x7ᵗʰ **W90.8 Exposure to other nonionizing radiation**

√x7ᵗʰ **W92 Exposure to excessive heat of man-made origin**

√4ᵗʰ **W93 Exposure to excessive cold of man-made origin**

√5ᵗʰ **W93.0 Contact with or inhalation of dry ice**

√x7ᵗʰ **W93.01 Contact with dry ice**

√x7ᵗʰ **W93.02 Inhalation of dry ice**

√5ᵗʰ **W93.1 Contact with or inhalation of liquid air**

√x7ᵗʰ **W93.11 Contact with liquid air**
Contact with liquid hydrogen
Contact with liquid nitrogen

√x7ᵗʰ **W93.12 Inhalation of liquid air**
Inhalation of liquid hydrogen
Inhalation of liquid nitrogen

√x7ᵗʰ **W93.2 Prolonged exposure in deep freeze unit or refrigerator**

√x7ᵗʰ **W93.8 Exposure to other excessive cold of man-made origin**

√4ᵗʰ **W94 Exposure to high and low air pressure and changes in air pressure**

√x7ᵗʰ **W94.0 Exposure to prolonged high air pressure**

√5ᵗʰ **W94.1 Exposure to prolonged low air pressure**

√x7ᵗʰ **W94.11 Exposure to residence or prolonged visit at high altitude**

√x7ᵗʰ **W94.12 Exposure to other prolonged low air pressure**

√5ᵗʰ **W94.2 Exposure to rapid changes in air pressure during ascent**

√x7ᵗʰ **W94.21 Exposure to reduction in atmospheric pressure while surfacing from deep-water diving**

√x7ᵗʰ **W94.22 Exposure to reduction in atmospheric pressure while surfacing from underground**

√x7ᵗʰ **W94.23 Exposure to sudden change in air pressure in aircraft during ascent**

√x7ᵗʰ **W94.29 Exposure to other rapid changes in air pressure during ascent**

√5ᵗʰ **W94.3 Exposure to rapid changes in air pressure during descent**

√x7ᵗʰ **W94.31 Exposure to sudden change in air pressure in aircraft during descent**

√x7ᵗʰ **W94.32 Exposure to high air pressure from rapid descent in water**

√x7ᵗʰ **W94.39 Exposure to other rapid changes in air pressure during descent**

√x7ᵗʰ **W99 Exposure to other man-made environmental factors**

Exposure to smoke, fire and flames (X00-X08)

    EXCLUDES 1   arson (X97)
    EXCLUDES 2   explosions (W35-W40)
             lightning (T75.0-)
             transport accident (V01-V99)
AHA: 2018,2Q,7-8

The appropriate 7th character is to be added to each code from categories X00-X08.
A   initial encounter
D   subsequent encounter
S   sequela

√4ᵗʰ **X00 Exposure to uncontrolled fire in building or structure**
    INCLUDES   conflagration in building or structure
Code first any associated cataclysm
    EXCLUDES 2   exposure to ignition or melting of nightwear (X05)
             exposure to ignition or melting of other clothing and apparel (X06.-)
             exposure to other specified smoke, fire and flames (X08.-)
    AHA: 2016,2Q,5

√x7ᵗʰ **X00.0 Exposure to flames in uncontrolled fire in building or structure**

√x7ᵗʰ **X00.1 Exposure to smoke in uncontrolled fire in building or structure**

√x7ᵗʰ **X00.2 Injury due to collapse of burning building or structure in uncontrolled fire**
    EXCLUDES 1   injury due to collapse of building not on fire (W20.1)

√x7ᵗʰ **X00.3 Fall from burning building or structure in uncontrolled fire**

√x7ᵗʰ **X00.4 Hit by object from burning building or structure in uncontrolled fire**
    AHA: 2016,2Q,4

√x7ᵗʰ **X00.5 Jump from burning building or structure in uncontrolled fire**

√x7ᵗʰ **X00.8 Other exposure to uncontrolled fire in building or structure**

√4ᵗʰ **X01 Exposure to uncontrolled fire, not in building or structure**
    INCLUDES   exposure to forest fire

√x7ᵗʰ **X01.0 Exposure to flames in uncontrolled fire, not in building or structure**

√x7ᵗʰ **X01.1 Exposure to smoke in uncontrolled fire, not in building or structure**

√x7ᵗʰ **X01.3 Fall due to uncontrolled fire, not in building or structure**

√x7ᵗʰ **X01.4 Hit by object due to uncontrolled fire, not in building or structure**

√x7ᵗʰ **X01.8 Other exposure to uncontrolled fire, not in building or structure**

√4ᵗʰ **X02 Exposure to controlled fire in building or structure**
    INCLUDES   exposure to fire in fireplace
             exposure to fire in stove

√x7ᵗʰ **X02.0 Exposure to flames in controlled fire in building or structure**

√x7ᵗʰ **X02.1 Exposure to smoke in controlled fire in building or structure**

√x7ᵗʰ **X02.2 Injury due to collapse of burning building or structure in controlled fire**
    EXCLUDES 1   injury due to collapse of building not on fire (W20.1)

√x7ᵗʰ **X02.3 Fall from burning building or structure in controlled fire**

√x7ᵗʰ **X02.4 Hit by object from burning building or structure in controlled fire**

√x7ᵗʰ **X02.5 Jump from burning building or structure in controlled fire**

√x7ᵗʰ **X02.8 Other exposure to controlled fire in building or structure**

√4ᵗʰ **X03 Exposure to controlled fire, not in building or structure**
    INCLUDES   exposure to bon fire
             exposure to camp-fire
             exposure to trash fire

√x7ᵗʰ **X03.0 Exposure to flames in controlled fire, not in building or structure**

√x7ᵗʰ **X03.1 Exposure to smoke in controlled fire, not in building or structure**

√x7ᵗʰ **X03.3 Fall due to controlled fire, not in building or structure**

√x7ᵗʰ **X03.4 Hit by object due to controlled fire, not in building or structure**

√x7ᵗʰ **X03.8 Other exposure to controlled fire, not in building or structure**

Ⓝ Newborn: 0   Ⓟ Pediatric: 0-17   Ⓜ Maternity: 9-64   Ⓐ Adult: 15-124   **MCC** Major Complication/Comorbidity   **CC** Complication/Comorbidity   **SW** Severe Wound Dx

1208   ICD-10-CM 2022

☑x7ᵗʰ X04 Exposure to ignition of highly flammable material
Exposure to ignition of gasoline
Exposure to ignition of kerosene
Exposure to ignition of petrol
> **EXCLUDES 2**   exposure to ignition or melting of nightwear (X05)
> exposure to ignition or melting of other clothing and apparel (X06)

AHA: 2016,2Q,4

☑x7ᵗʰ X05 Exposure to ignition or melting of nightwear
> **EXCLUDES 2**   exposure to uncontrolled fire in building or structure (X00.-)
> exposure to uncontrolled fire, not in building or structure (X01.-)
> exposure to controlled fire in building or structure (X02.-)
> exposure to controlled fire, not in building or structure (X03.-)
> exposure to ignition of highly flammable materials (X04.-)

☑4ᵗʰ X06 Exposure to ignition or melting of other clothing and apparel
> **EXCLUDES 2**   exposure to uncontrolled fire in building or structure (X00.-)
> exposure to uncontrolled fire, not in building or structure (X01.-)
> exposure to controlled fire in building or structure (X02.-)
> exposure to controlled fire, not in building or structure (X03.-)
> exposure to ignition of highly flammable materials (X04.-)

   ☑x7ᵗʰ X06.0 Exposure to ignition of plastic jewelry

   ☑x7ᵗʰ X06.1 Exposure to melting of plastic jewelry

   ☑x7ᵗʰ X06.2 Exposure to ignition of other clothing and apparel

   ☑x7ᵗʰ X06.3 Exposure to melting of other clothing and apparel

☑4ᵗʰ X08 Exposure to other specified smoke, fire and flames

   ☑5ᵗʰ X08.0 Exposure to bed fire
     Exposure to mattress fire
     ☑x7ᵗʰ X08.00 Exposure to bed fire due to unspecified burning material
     ☑x7ᵗʰ X08.01 Exposure to bed fire due to burning cigarette
     ☑x7ᵗʰ X08.09 Exposure to bed fire due to other burning material

   ☑5ᵗʰ X08.1 Exposure to sofa fire
     ☑x7ᵗʰ X08.10 Exposure to sofa fire due to unspecified burning material
     ☑x7ᵗʰ X08.11 Exposure to sofa fire due to burning cigarette
     ☑x7ᵗʰ X08.19 Exposure to sofa fire due to other burning material

   ☑5ᵗʰ X08.2 Exposure to other furniture fire
     ☑x7ᵗʰ X08.20 Exposure to other furniture fire due to unspecified burning material
     ☑x7ᵗʰ X08.21 Exposure to other furniture fire due to burning cigarette
     ☑x7ᵗʰ X08.29 Exposure to other furniture fire due to other burning material

   ☑x7ᵗʰ X08.8 Exposure to other specified smoke, fire and flames

Contact with heat and hot substances (X10-X19)

> **EXCLUDES 1**   exposure to excessive natural heat (X30)
> exposure to fire and flames (X00-X08)

AHA: 2018,2Q,7-8

The appropriate 7th character is to be added to each code from categories X10-X19.
A   initial encounter
D   subsequent encounter
S   sequela

☑4ᵗʰ X10 Contact with hot drinks, food, fats and cooking oils

   ☑x7ᵗʰ X10.0 Contact with hot drinks

   ☑x7ᵗʰ X10.1 Contact with hot food

   ☑x7ᵗʰ X10.2 Contact with fats and cooking oils

☑4ᵗʰ X11 Contact with hot tap-water
> **INCLUDES**   contact with boiling tap-water
> contact with boiling water NOS
> **EXCLUDES 1**   contact with water heated on stove (X12)

   ☑x7ᵗʰ X11.0 Contact with hot water in bath or tub
     EXCLUDES 1   contact with running hot water in bath or tub (X11.1)

   ☑x7ᵗʰ X11.1 Contact with running hot water
     Contact with hot water running out of hose
     Contact with hot water running out of tap

   ☑x7ᵗʰ X11.8 Contact with other hot tap-water
     Contact with hot water in bucket
     Contact with hot tap-water NOS

☑x7ᵗʰ X12 Contact with other hot fluids
   Contact with water heated on stove
> **EXCLUDES 1**   hot (liquid) metals (X18)

☑4ᵗʰ X13 Contact with steam and other hot vapors

   ☑x7ᵗʰ X13.0 Inhalation of steam and other hot vapors

   ☑x7ᵗʰ X13.1 Other contact with steam and other hot vapors

☑4ᵗʰ X14 Contact with hot air and other hot gases

   ☑x7ᵗʰ X14.0 Inhalation of hot air and gases

   ☑x7ᵗʰ X14.1 Other contact with hot air and other hot gases

☑4ᵗʰ X15 Contact with hot household appliances
> **EXCLUDES 1**   contact with heating appliances (X16)
> contact with powered household appliances (W29.-)
> exposure to controlled fire in building or structure due to household appliance (X02.8)
> exposure to household appliances electrical current (W86.0)

   ☑x7ᵗʰ X15.0 Contact with hot stove (kitchen)

   ☑x7ᵗʰ X15.1 Contact with hot toaster

   ☑x7ᵗʰ X15.2 Contact with hotplate

   ☑x7ᵗʰ X15.3 Contact with hot saucepan or skillet

   ☑x7ᵗʰ X15.8 Contact with other hot household appliances
     Contact with cooker
     Contact with kettle
     Contact with light bulbs

☑x7ᵗʰ X16 Contact with hot heating appliances, radiators and pipes
> **EXCLUDES 1**   contact with powered appliances (W29.-)
> exposure to controlled fire in building or structure due to appliance (X02.8)
> exposure to industrial appliances electrical current (W86.1)

☑x7ᵗʰ X17 Contact with hot engines, machinery and tools
> **EXCLUDES 1**   contact with hot heating appliances, radiators and pipes (X16)
> contact with hot household appliances (X15)

☑x7ᵗʰ X18 Contact with other hot metals
   Contact with liquid metal

☑x7ᵗʰ X19 Contact with other heat and hot substances
> **EXCLUDES 1**   objects that are not normally hot, e.g., an object made hot by a house fire (X00-X08)

Exposure to forces of nature (X30-X39)

AHA: 2018,2Q,7-8

The appropriate 7th character is to be added to each code from categories X30-X39.
A   initial encounter
D   subsequent encounter
S   sequela

☑x7ᵗʰ X30 Exposure to excessive natural heat
   Exposure to excessive heat as the cause of sunstroke
   Exposure to heat NOS
> **EXCLUDES 1**   excessive heat of man-made origin (W92)
> exposure to man-made radiation (W89)
> exposure to sunlight (X32)
> exposure to tanning bed (W89)

☑x7ᵗʰ X31 Exposure to excessive natural cold
   Excessive cold as the cause of chilblains NOS
   Excessive cold as the cause of immersion foot or hand
   Exposure to cold NOS
   Exposure to weather conditions
> **EXCLUDES 1**   cold of man-made origin (W93.-)
> contact with or inhalation of dry ice (W93.-)
> contact with or inhalation of liquefied gas (W93.-)

☑x7ᵗʰ X32 Exposure to sunlight
> **EXCLUDES 1**   man-made radiation (tanning bed) (W89)
> **EXCLUDES 2**   radiation-related disorders of the skin and subcutaneous tissue (L55-L59)

Chapter 20. External Causes of Morbidity

√x7th **X34 Earthquake**
> EXCLUDES 2   *tidal wave (tsunami) due to earthquake (X37.41)*

√x7th **X35 Volcanic eruption**
> EXCLUDES 2   *tidal wave (tsunami) due to volcanic eruption (X37.41)*

√4th **X36 Avalanche, landslide and other earth movements**
> INCLUDES   victim of mudslide of cataclysmic nature
> EXCLUDES 1   *earthquake (X34)*
> EXCLUDES 2   *transport accident involving collision with avalanche or landslide not in motion (V01-V99)*

√x7th   **X36.0 Collapse of dam or man-made structure causing earth movement**

√x7th   **X36.1 Avalanche, landslide, or mudslide**

√4th **X37 Cataclysmic storm**

√x7th   **X37.0 Hurricane**
> Storm surge
> Typhoon

√x7th   **X37.1 Tornado**
> Cyclone
> Twister

√x7th   **X37.2 Blizzard (snow)(ice)**

√x7th   **X37.3 Dust storm**

√5th   **X37.4 Tidalwave**

√x7th   **X37.41 Tidal wave due to earthquake or volcanic eruption**
> Tidal wave NOS
> Tsunami

√x7th   **X37.42 Tidal wave due to storm**

√x7th   **X37.43 Tidal wave due to landslide**

√x7th   **X37.8 Other cataclysmic storms**
> Cloudburst
> Torrential rain
> EXCLUDES 2   *flood (X38)*

√x7th   **X37.9 Unspecified cataclysmic storm**
> Storm NOS
> EXCLUDES 1   *collapse of dam or man-made structure causing earth movement (X36.0)*

√x7th **X38 Flood**
> Flood arising from remote storm
> Flood of cataclysmic nature arising from melting snow
> Flood resulting directly from storm
> EXCLUDES 1   *collapse of dam or man-made structure causing earth movement (X36.0)*
> *tidal wave NOS (X37.41)*
> *tidal wave caused by storm (X37.42)*

√4th **X39 Exposure to other forces of nature**

√6th   **X39.0 Exposure to natural radiation**
> EXCLUDES 1   *contact with and (suspected) exposure to radon and other naturally occurring radiation (Z77.123)*
> *exposure to man-made radiation (W88-W90)*
> *exposure to sunlight (X32)*

√x7th   **X39.01 Exposure to radon**

√x7th   **X39.08 Exposure to other natural radiation**

√x7th   **X39.8 Other exposure to forces of nature**

Overexertion and strenuous or repetitive movements (X50)

√4th **X50 Overexertion and strenuous or repetitive movements**
> **AHA:** 2018,2Q,7-8; 2016,4Q,73-74

> The appropriate 7th character is to be added to each code from category X50.
> A   initial encounter
> D   subsequent encounter
> S   sequela

√x7th   **X50.0 Overexertion from strenuous movement or load**
> Lifting heavy objects
> Lifting weights

√x7th   **X50.1 Overexertion from prolonged static or awkward postures**
> Prolonged bending
> Prolonged kneeling
> Prolonged reaching
> Prolonged sitting
> Prolonged standing
> Prolonged twisting
> Static bending
> Static kneeling
> Static reaching
> Static sitting
> Static standing
> Static twisting

√x7th   **X50.3 Overexertion from repetitive movements**
> Use of hand as hammer
> EXCLUDES 2   *overuse from prolonged static or awkward postures (X50.1)*

√x7th   **X50.9 Other and unspecified overexertion or strenuous movements or postures**
> Contact pressure
> Contact stress

Accidental exposure to other specified factors (X52-X58)

AHA: 2018,2Q,7-8

> The appropriate 7th character is to be added to each code from categories X52-X58.
> A   initial encounter
> D   subsequent encounter
> S   sequela

√x7th **X52 Prolonged stay in weightless environment**
> Weightlessness in spacecraft (simulator)

√x7th **X58 Exposure to other specified factors**
> Accident NOS
> Exposure NOS

Intentional self-harm (X71-X83)

Purposely self-inflicted injury
Suicide (attempted)

> The appropriate 7th character is to be added to each code from categories X71-X83.
> A   initial encounter
> D   subsequent encounter
> S   sequela

√4th **X71 Intentional self-harm by drowning and submersion**

√x7th   **X71.0 Intentional self-harm by drowning and submersion while in bathtub** HCC

√x7th   **X71.1 Intentional self-harm by drowning and submersion while in swimming pool** HCC

√x7th   **X71.2 Intentional self-harm by drowning and submersion after jump into swimming pool** HCC

√x7th   **X71.3 Intentional self-harm by drowning and submersion in natural water** HCC

√x7th   **X71.8 Other intentional self-harm by drowning and submersion** HCC

√x7th   **X71.9 Intentional self-harm by drowning and submersion, unspecified** HCC

√x7th **X72 Intentional self-harm by handgun discharge** HCC
> Intentional self-harm by gun for single hand use
> Intentional self-harm by pistol
> Intentional self-harm by revolver
> EXCLUDES 1   *Very pistol (X74.8)*

√4th **X73 Intentional self-harm by rifle, shotgun and larger firearm discharge**
> EXCLUDES 1   *airgun (X74.01)*

√x7th   **X73.0 Intentional self-harm by shotgun discharge** HCC

√x7th   **X73.1 Intentional self-harm by hunting rifle discharge** HCC

√x7th   **X73.2 Intentional self-harm by machine gun discharge** HCC

√x7th   **X73.8 Intentional self-harm by other larger firearm discharge** HCC

√x7th   **X73.9 Intentional self-harm by unspecified larger firearm discharge** HCC

✓4ᵗʰ **X74** **Intentional self-harm by other and unspecified firearm and gun discharge**

  ✓5ᵗʰ **X74.0** Intentional self-harm by gas, air or spring-operated guns

    ✓x7ᵗʰ **X74.01** **Intentional self-harm by airgun** `HCC`
      Intentional self-harm by BB gun discharge
      Intentional self-harm by pellet gun discharge

    ✓x7ᵗʰ **X74.02** **Intentional self-harm by paintball gun** `HCC`

    ✓x7ᵗʰ **X74.09** **Intentional self-harm by other gas, air or spring-operated gun** `HCC`

  ✓x7ᵗʰ **X74.8** **Intentional self-harm by other firearm discharge** `HCC`
    Intentional self-harm by Very pistol [flare] discharge

  ✓x7ᵗʰ **X74.9** **Intentional self-harm by unspecified firearm discharge** `HCC`

✓x7ᵗʰ **X75** **Intentional self-harm by explosive material** `HCC`

✓x7ᵗʰ **X76** **Intentional self-harm by smoke, fire and flames** `HCC`

✓4ᵗʰ **X77** **Intentional self-harm by steam, hot vapors and hot objects**

  ✓x7ᵗʰ **X77.0** **Intentional self-harm by steam or hot vapors** `HCC`

  ✓x7ᵗʰ **X77.1** **Intentional self-harm by hot tap water** `HCC`

  ✓x7ᵗʰ **X77.2** **Intentional self-harm by other hot fluids** `HCC`

  ✓x7ᵗʰ **X77.3** **Intentional self-harm by hot household appliances** `HCC`

  ✓x7ᵗʰ **X77.8** **Intentional self-harm by other hot objects** `HCC`

  ✓x7ᵗʰ **X77.9** **Intentional self-harm by unspecified hot objects** `HCC`

✓4ᵗʰ **X78** **Intentional self-harm by sharp object**

  ✓x7ᵗʰ **X78.0** **Intentional self-harm by sharp glass** `HCC`

  ✓x7ᵗʰ **X78.1** **Intentional self-harm by knife** `HCC`

  ✓x7ᵗʰ **X78.2** **Intentional self-harm by sword or dagger** `HCC`

  ✓x7ᵗʰ **X78.8** **Intentional self-harm by other sharp object** `HCC`

  ✓x7ᵗʰ **X78.9** **Intentional self-harm by unspecified sharp object** `HCC`

✓x7ᵗʰ **X79** **Intentional self-harm by blunt object** `HCC`

✓x7ᵗʰ **X80** **Intentional self-harm by jumping from a high place** `HCC`
  Intentional fall from one level to another

✓4ᵗʰ **X81** **Intentional self-harm by jumping or lying in front of moving object**

  ✓x7ᵗʰ **X81.0** **Intentional self-harm by jumping or lying in front of motor vehicle** `HCC`

  ✓x7ᵗʰ **X81.1** **Intentional self-harm by jumping or lying in front of (subway) train** `HCC`

  ✓x7ᵗʰ **X81.8** **Intentional self-harm by jumping or lying in front of other moving object** `HCC`

✓4ᵗʰ **X82** **Intentional self-harm by crashing of motor vehicle**

  ✓x7ᵗʰ **X82.0** **Intentional collision of motor vehicle with other motor vehicle** `HCC`

  ✓x7ᵗʰ **X82.1** **Intentional collision of motor vehicle with train** `HCC`

  ✓x7ᵗʰ **X82.2** **Intentional collision of motor vehicle with tree** `HCC`

  ✓x7ᵗʰ **X82.8** **Other intentional self-harm by crashing of motor vehicle** `HCC`

✓4ᵗʰ **X83** **Intentional self-harm by other specified means**

  EXCLUDES 1 *intentional self-harm by poisoning or contact with toxic substance - see Table of Drugs and Chemicals*

  ✓x7ᵗʰ **X83.0** **Intentional self-harm by crashing of aircraft** `HCC`

  ✓x7ᵗʰ **X83.1** **Intentional self-harm by electrocution** `HCC`

  ✓x7ᵗʰ **X83.2** **Intentional self-harm by exposure to extremes of cold** `HCC`

  ✓x7ᵗʰ **X83.8** **Intentional self-harm by other specified means** `HCC`

Assault (X92-Y09)

INCLUDES homicide
injuries inflicted by another person with intent to injure or kill, by any means

EXCLUDES 1 *injuries due to legal intervention (Y35.-)*
injuries due to operations of war (Y36.-)
injuries due to terrorism (Y38.-)

The appropriate 7th character is to be added to each code from categories X92-Y04 and Y08.
A   initial encounter
D   subsequent encounter
S   sequela

✓4ᵗʰ **X92** **Assault by drowning and submersion**

  ✓x7ᵗʰ **X92.0** **Assault by drowning and submersion while in bathtub**

  ✓x7ᵗʰ **X92.1** **Assault by drowning and submersion while in swimming pool**

  ✓x7ᵗʰ **X92.2** **Assault by drowning and submersion** after push into swimming pool

  ✓x7ᵗʰ **X92.3** **Assault by drowning and submersion** in natural water

  ✓x7ᵗʰ **X92.8** **Other assault by drowning and submersion**

  ✓x7ᵗʰ **X92.9** **Assault by drowning and submersion, unspecified**

✓x7ᵗʰ **X93** **Assault by handgun discharge**
  Assault by discharge of gun for single hand use
  Assault by discharge of pistol
  Assault by discharge of revolver
  EXCLUDES 1 *Very pistol (X95.8)*

✓4ᵗʰ **X94** **Assault by rifle, shotgun and larger firearm discharge**
  EXCLUDES 1 *airgun (X95.01)*

  ✓x7ᵗʰ **X94.0** **Assault by shotgun**

  ✓x7ᵗʰ **X94.1** **Assault by hunting rifle**

  ✓x7ᵗʰ **X94.2** **Assault by machine gun**

  ✓x7ᵗʰ **X94.8** **Assault by other larger firearm discharge**

  ✓x7ᵗʰ **X94.9** **Assault by unspecified larger firearm discharge**

✓4ᵗʰ **X95** **Assault by other and unspecified firearm and gun discharge**

  ✓5ᵗʰ **X95.0** **Assault by gas, air or spring-operated guns**

    ✓x7ᵗʰ **X95.01** **Assault by airgun discharge**
      Assault by BB gun discharge
      Assault by pellet gun discharge

    ✓x7ᵗʰ **X95.02** **Assault by paintball gun discharge**

    ✓x7ᵗʰ **X95.09** **Assault by other gas, air or spring-operated gun**

  ✓x7ᵗʰ **X95.8** **Assault by other firearm discharge**
    Assault by Very pistol [flare] discharge

  ✓x7ᵗʰ **X95.9** **Assault by unspecified firearm discharge**

✓4ᵗʰ **X96** **Assault by explosive material**
  EXCLUDES 1 *incendiary device (X97)*
terrorism involving explosive material (Y38.2-)

  ✓x7ᵗʰ **X96.0** **Assault by antipersonnel bomb**
    EXCLUDES 1 *antipersonnel bomb use in military or war (Y36.2-)*

  ✓x7ᵗʰ **X96.1** **Assault by gasoline bomb**

  ✓x7ᵗʰ **X96.2** **Assault by letter bomb**

  ✓x7ᵗʰ **X96.3** **Assault by fertilizer bomb**

  ✓x7ᵗʰ **X96.4** **Assault by pipe bomb**

  ✓x7ᵗʰ **X96.8** **Assault by other specified explosive**

  ✓x7ᵗʰ **X96.9** **Assault by unspecified explosive**

✓x7ᵗʰ **X97** **Assault by smoke, fire and flames**
  Assault by arson
  Assault by cigarettes
  Assault by incendiary device

✓4ᵗʰ **X98** **Assault by steam, hot vapors and hot objects**

  ✓x7ᵗʰ **X98.0** **Assault by steam or hot vapors**

  ✓x7ᵗʰ **X98.1** **Assault by hot tap water**

  ✓x7ᵗʰ **X98.2** **Assault by hot fluids**

  ✓x7ᵗʰ **X98.3** **Assault by hot household appliances**

  ✓x7ᵗʰ **X98.8** **Assault by other hot objects**

  ✓x7ᵗʰ **X98.9** **Assault by unspecified hot objects**

✓4ᵗʰ **X99** **Assault by sharp object**
  EXCLUDES 1 *assault by strike by sports equipment (Y08.0-)*

  ✓x7ᵗʰ **X99.0** **Assault by sharp glass**

  ✓x7ᵗʰ **X99.1** **Assault by knife**

  ✓x7ᵗʰ **X99.2** **Assault by sword or dagger**

  ✓x7ᵗʰ **X99.8** **Assault by other sharp object**

  ✓x7ᵗʰ **X99.9** **Assault by unspecified sharp object**
    Assault by stabbing NOS

✓x7ᵗʰ **Y00** **Assault by blunt object**
  EXCLUDES 1 *assault by strike by sports equipment (Y08.0-)*

✓x7ᵗʰ **Y01** **Assault by pushing from high place**

✓4ᵗʰ **Y02** **Assault by pushing or placing victim in front of moving object**

  ✓x7ᵗʰ **Y02.0** **Assault by pushing or placing victim in front of motor vehicle**

  ✓x7ᵗʰ **Y02.1** **Assault by pushing or placing victim in front of (subway) train**

✔ Additional Char Req ✓x7ᵗʰ Placeholder Unacceptable PDx Questionable PDx Wrong Procedure Manifestation Unspecified Dx H1-H14 HAC HCC CMS-HCC Dx HIV HIV Dx

ICD-10-CM 2022   1211

✓7th **Y02.8** Assault by pushing or placing victim in front of other moving object

✓4th **Y03** Assault by crashing of motor vehicle

   ✓7th **Y03.0** Assault by being hit or run over by motor vehicle

   ✓7th **Y03.8** Other assault by crashing of motor vehicle

✓4th **Y04** Assault by bodily force

      EXCLUDES 1   assault by:
               submersion (X92.-)
               use of weapon (X93-X95, X99, Y00)

   ✓7th **Y04.0** Assault by unarmed brawl or fight

   ✓7th **Y04.1** Assault by human bite

   ✓7th **Y04.2** Assault by strike against or bumped into by another person

   ✓7th **Y04.8** Assault by other bodily force
          Assault by bodily force NOS

✓4th **Y07** Perpetrator of assault, maltreatment and neglect

    NOTE   Codes from this category are for use only in cases of confirmed abuse (T74.-)

          Selection of the correct perpetrator code is based on the relationship between the perpetrator and the victim

    INCLUDES   perpetrator of abandonment
               perpetrator of emotional neglect
               perpetrator of mental cruelty
               perpetrator of physical abuse
               perpetrator of physical neglect
               perpetrator of sexual abuse
               perpetrator of torture

  ✓5th **Y07.0** Spouse or partner, perpetrator of maltreatment and neglect
          Spouse or partner, perpetrator of maltreatment and neglect against spouse or partner

      Y07.01 Husband, perpetrator of maltreatment and neglect

      Y07.02 Wife, perpetrator of maltreatment and neglect

      Y07.03 Male partner, perpetrator of maltreatment and neglect

      Y07.04 Female partner, perpetrator of maltreatment and neglect

  ✓5th **Y07.1** Parent (adoptive) (biological), perpetrator of maltreatment and neglect

      Y07.11 Biological father, perpetrator of maltreatment and neglect

      Y07.12 Biological mother, perpetrator of maltreatment and neglect

      Y07.13 Adoptive father, perpetrator of maltreatment and neglect

      Y07.14 Adoptive mother, perpetrator of maltreatment and neglect

  ✓6th **Y07.4** Other family member, perpetrator of maltreatment and neglect

    ✓6th **Y07.41** Sibling, perpetrator of maltreatment and neglect

        EXCLUDES 1   stepsibling, perpetrator of maltreatment and neglect (Y07.435, Y07.436)

        Y07.410 Brother, perpetrator of maltreatment and neglect

        Y07.411 Sister, perpetrator of maltreatment and neglect

    ✓6th **Y07.42** Foster parent, perpetrator of maltreatment and neglect

        Y07.420 Foster father, perpetrator of maltreatment and neglect

        Y07.421 Foster mother, perpetrator of maltreatment and neglect

    ✓6th **Y07.43** Stepparent or stepsibling, perpetrator of maltreatment and neglect

        Y07.430 Stepfather, perpetrator of maltreatment and neglect

        Y07.432 Male friend of parent (co-residing in household), perpetrator of maltreatment and neglect

        Y07.433 Stepmother, perpetrator of maltreatment and neglect

        Y07.434 Female friend of parent (co-residing in household), perpetrator of maltreatment and neglect

        Y07.435 Stepbrother, perpetrator or maltreatment and neglect

        Y07.436 Stepsister, perpetrator of maltreatment and neglect

    ✓6th **Y07.49** Other family member, perpetrator of maltreatment and neglect

        Y07.490 Male cousin, perpetrator of maltreatment and neglect

        Y07.491 Female cousin, perpetrator of maltreatment and neglect

        Y07.499 Other family member, perpetrator of maltreatment and neglect

  ✓5th **Y07.5** Non-family member, perpetrator of maltreatment and neglect

      Y07.50 Unspecified non-family member, perpetrator of maltreatment and neglect

    ✓6th **Y07.51** Daycare provider, perpetrator of maltreatment and neglect

        Y07.510 At-home childcare provider, perpetrator of maltreatment and neglect

        Y07.511 Daycare center childcare provider, perpetrator of maltreatment and neglect

        Y07.512 At-home adultcare provider, perpetrator of maltreatment and neglect

        Y07.513 Adultcare center provider, perpetrator of maltreatment and neglect

        Y07.519 Unspecified daycare provider, perpetrator of maltreatment and neglect

    ✓6th **Y07.52** Healthcare provider, perpetrator of maltreatment and neglect

        Y07.521 Mental health provider, perpetrator of maltreatment and neglect

        Y07.528 Other therapist or healthcare provider, perpetrator of maltreatment and neglect
            Nurse perpetrator of maltreatment and neglect
            Occupational therapist perpetrator of maltreatment and neglect
            Physical therapist perpetrator of maltreatment and neglect
            Speech therapist perpetrator of maltreatment and neglect

        Y07.529 Unspecified healthcare provider, perpetrator of maltreatment and neglect

      Y07.53 Teacher or instructor, perpetrator of maltreatment and neglect
          Coach, perpetrator of maltreatment and neglect

      Y07.59 Other non-family member, perpetrator of maltreatment and neglect

     Y07.6 Multiple perpetrators of maltreatment and neglect
          AHA: 2018,4Q,32

     Y07.9 Unspecified perpetrator of maltreatment and neglect

✓4th **Y08** Assault by other specified means

  ✓5th **Y08.0** Assault by strike by sport equipment

    ✓7th **Y08.01** Assault by strike by hockey stick

    ✓7th **Y08.02** Assault by strike by baseball bat

    ✓7th **Y08.09** Assault by strike by other specified type of sport equipment

  ✓5th **Y08.8** Assault by other specified means

    ✓7th **Y08.81** Assault by crashing of aircraft

    ✓7th **Y08.89** Assault by other specified means

Y09 Assault by unspecified means
     Assassination (attempted) NOS
     Homicide (attempted) NOS
     Manslaughter (attempted) NOS
     Murder (attempted) NOS

Event of undetermined intent (Y21-Y33)

Undetermined intent is only for use when there is specific documentation in the record that the intent of the injury cannot be determined. If no such documentation is present, code to accidental (unintentional).

The appropriate 7th character is to be added to each code from categories Y21-Y33.
A   initial encounter
D   subsequent encounter
S   sequela

✓4th **Y21** Drowning and submersion, undetermined intent

  ✓7th **Y21.0** Drowning and submersion while in bathtub, undetermined intent

  ✓7th **Y21.1** Drowning and submersion after fall into bathtub, undetermined intent

---

✓x7th **Y21.2** **Drowning and submersion** while in swimming pool, undetermined intent

✓x7th **Y21.3** **Drowning and submersion** after fall into swimming pool, undetermined intent

✓x7th **Y21.4** **Drowning and submersion** in natural water, **undetermined intent**

✓x7th **Y21.8** **Other drowning and submersion, undetermined intent**

✓x7th **Y21.9** **Unspecified drowning and submersion, undetermined intent**

✓x7th **Y22** **Handgun** **discharge, undetermined intent**

Discharge of gun for single hand use, undetermined intent
Discharge of pistol, undetermined intent
Discharge of revolver, undetermined intent

EXCLUDES 2   Very pistol (Y24.8)

✓4th **Y23** **Rifle, shotgun and larger firearm** **discharge, undetermined intent**

EXCLUDES 2   airgun (Y24.0)

✓x7th **Y23.0** **Shotgun** **discharge, undetermined intent**

✓x7th **Y23.1** **Hunting rifle** **discharge, undetermined intent**

✓x7th **Y23.2** **Military firearm** **discharge, undetermined intent**

✓x7th **Y23.3** **Machine gun** **discharge, undetermined intent**

✓x7th **Y23.8** **Other larger firearm discharge, undetermined intent**

✓x7th **Y23.9** **Unspecified larger firearm discharge, undetermined intent**

✓4th **Y24** **Other and unspecified firearm discharge, undetermined intent**

✓x7th **Y24.0** **Airgun** **discharge, undetermined intent**

BB gun discharge, undetermined intent
Pellet gun discharge, undetermined intent

✓x7th **Y24.8** **Other firearm discharge, undetermined intent**

Paintball gun discharge, undetermined intent
Very pistol [flare] discharge, undetermined intent

✓x7th **Y24.9** **Unspecified firearm discharge, undetermined intent**

✓x7th **Y25** **Contact with explosive material, undetermined intent**

✓x7th **Y26** **Exposure to smoke, fire and flames, undetermined intent**

✓4th **Y27** **Contact with steam, hot vapors and hot objects, undetermined intent**

✓x7th **Y27.0** **Contact with** steam **and hot** vapors, **undetermined intent**

✓x7th **Y27.1** **Contact with hot** tap water, **undetermined intent**

✓x7th **Y27.2** **Contact with hot** fluids, **undetermined intent**

✓x7th **Y27.3** **Contact with hot** household appliance, **undetermined intent**

✓x7th **Y27.8** **Contact with other hot** objects, **undetermined intent**

✓x7th **Y27.9** **Contact with unspecified hot objects, undetermined intent**

✓4th **Y28** **Contact with sharp object, undetermined intent**

✓x7th **Y28.0** **Contact with sharp** glass, **undetermined intent**

✓x7th **Y28.1** **Contact with** knife, **undetermined intent**

✓x7th **Y28.2** **Contact with** sword or dagger, **undetermined intent**

✓x7th **Y28.8** **Contact with other sharp object, undetermined intent**

✓x7th **Y28.9** **Contact with unspecified sharp object, undetermined intent**

✓x7th **Y29** **Contact with blunt object, undetermined intent**

✓x7th **Y30** **Falling, jumping or pushed from a high place, undetermined intent**

Victim falling from one level to another, undetermined intent

✓x7th **Y31** **Falling, lying or running before or into moving object, undetermined intent**

✓x7th **Y32** **Crashing of motor vehicle, undetermined intent**

✓x7th **Y33** **Other specified events, undetermined intent**

Legal intervention, operations of war, military operations, and terrorism (Y35-Y38)

The appropriate 7th character is to be added to each code from categories Y35-Y38.
A   initial encounter
D   subsequent encounter
S   sequela

✓4th **Y35** **Legal intervention**

INCLUDES   any injury sustained as a result of an encounter with any law enforcement official, serving in any capacity at the time of the encounter, whether on-duty or off-duty. Includes injury to law enforcement official, suspect and bystander

AHA: 2019,4Q,18-19

✓5th **Y35.0** **Legal intervention involving** firearm discharge

✓6th **Y35.00** **Legal intervention involving unspecified firearm discharge**

Legal intervention involving gunshot wound
Legal intervention involving shot NOS

✓7th **Y35.001** **Legal intervention involving unspecified firearm discharge,** law enforcement official **injured**

✓7th **Y35.002** **Legal intervention involving unspecified firearm discharge,** bystander **injured**

✓7th **Y35.003** **Legal intervention involving unspecified firearm discharge,** suspect **injured**

✓7th **Y35.009** **Legal intervention involving unspecified firearm discharge, unspecified person injured**

✓6th **Y35.01** **Legal intervention involving injury by** machine gun

✓7th **Y35.011** **Legal intervention involving injury by machine gun,** law enforcement official **injured**

✓7th **Y35.012** **Legal intervention involving injury by machine gun,** bystander **injured**

✓7th **Y35.013** **Legal intervention involving injury by machine gun,** suspect **injured**

✓7th **Y35.019** **Legal intervention involving injury by machine gun, unspecified person injured**

✓6th **Y35.02** **Legal intervention involving injury by** handgun

✓7th **Y35.021** **Legal intervention involving injury by handgun,** law enforcement official **injured**

✓7th **Y35.022** **Legal intervention involving injury by handgun,** bystander **injured**

✓7th **Y35.023** **Legal intervention involving injury by handgun,** suspect **injured**

✓7th **Y35.029** **Legal intervention involving injury by handgun, unspecified person injured**

✓6th **Y35.03** **Legal intervention involving injury by** rifle pellet

✓7th **Y35.031** **Legal intervention involving injury by rifle pellet,** law enforcement official **injured**

✓7th **Y35.032** **Legal intervention involving injury by rifle pellet,** bystander **injured**

✓7th **Y35.033** **Legal intervention involving injury by rifle pellet,** suspect **injured**

✓7th **Y35.039** **Legal intervention involving injury by rifle pellet, unspecified person injured**

✓6th **Y35.04** **Legal intervention involving injury by** rubber bullet

✓7th **Y35.041** **Legal intervention involving injury by rubber bullet,** law enforcement official **injured**

✓7th **Y35.042** **Legal intervention involving injury by rubber bullet,** bystander **injured**

✓7th **Y35.043** **Legal intervention involving injury by rubber bullet,** suspect **injured**

✓7th **Y35.049** **Legal intervention involving injury by rubber bullet, unspecified person injured**

✓6th **Y35.09** **Legal intervention involving other firearm discharge**

✓7th **Y35.091** **Legal intervention involving other firearm discharge,** law enforcement official **injured**

✓7th **Y35.092** **Legal intervention involving other firearm discharge,** bystander **injured**

✓7th **Y35.093** **Legal intervention involving other firearm discharge,** suspect **injured**

✓ Additional Char Req   ✓x7th Placeholder   Unacceptable PDx   Questionable PDx   Wrong Procedure   Manifestation   Unspecified Dx   H1-H1a HAC   HCC CMS-HCC Dx   HIV HIV Dx

ICD-10-CM 2022   **1213**

✓7ᵗʰ **Y35.099** **Legal intervention involving other firearm discharge, unspecified person injured**

✓5ᵗʰ **Y35.1** **Legal intervention involving** explosives

  ✓6ᵗʰ **Y35.10** **Legal intervention involving unspecified explosives**

    ✓7ᵗʰ **Y35.101** **Legal intervention involving unspecified explosives,** law enforcement official **injured**

    ✓7ᵗʰ **Y35.102** **Legal intervention involving unspecified explosives,** bystander **injured**

    ✓7ᵗʰ **Y35.103** **Legal intervention involving unspecified explosives,** suspect **injured**

    ✓7ᵗʰ **Y35.109** **Legal intervention involving unspecified explosives, unspecified person injured**

  ✓6ᵗʰ **Y35.11** **Legal intervention involving injury by** dynamite

    ✓7ᵗʰ **Y35.111** **Legal intervention involving injury by dynamite,** law enforcement official **injured**

    ✓7ᵗʰ **Y35.112** **Legal intervention involving injury by dynamite,** bystander **injured**

    ✓7ᵗʰ **Y35.113** **Legal intervention involving injury by dynamite,** suspect **injured**

    ✓7ᵗʰ **Y35.119** **Legal intervention involving injury by dynamite, unspecified person injured**

  ✓6ᵗʰ **Y35.12** **Legal intervention involving injury by** explosive shell

    ✓7ᵗʰ **Y35.121** **Legal intervention involving injury by explosive shell,** law enforcement official **injured**

    ✓7ᵗʰ **Y35.122** **Legal intervention involving injury by explosive shell,** bystander **injured**

    ✓7ᵗʰ **Y35.123** **Legal intervention involving injury by explosive shell,** suspect **injured**

    ✓7ᵗʰ **Y35.129** **Legal intervention involving injury by explosive shell, unspecified person injured**

  ✓6ᵗʰ **Y35.19** **Legal intervention involving other explosives**

Legal intervention involving injury by grenade

Legal intervention involving injury by mortar bomb

    ✓7ᵗʰ **Y35.191** **Legal intervention involving other explosives,** law enforcement official **injured**

    ✓7ᵗʰ **Y35.192** **Legal intervention involving other explosives,** bystander **injured**

    ✓7ᵗʰ **Y35.193** **Legal intervention involving other explosives,** suspect **injured**

    ✓7ᵗʰ **Y35.199** **Legal intervention involving other explosives, unspecified person injured**

✓5ᵗʰ **Y35.2** **Legal intervention involving** gas

Legal intervention involving asphyxiation by gas

Legal intervention involving poisoning by gas

  ✓6ᵗʰ **Y35.20** **Legal intervention involving unspecified gas**

    ✓7ᵗʰ **Y35.201** **Legal intervention involving unspecified gas,** law enforcement official **injured**

    ✓7ᵗʰ **Y35.202** **Legal intervention involving unspecified gas,** bystander **injured**

    ✓7ᵗʰ **Y35.203** **Legal intervention involving unspecified gas,** suspect **injured**

    ✓7ᵗʰ **Y35.209** **Legal intervention involving unspecified gas, unspecified person injured**

  ✓6ᵗʰ **Y35.21** **Legal intervention involving injury by** tear gas

    ✓7ᵗʰ **Y35.211** **Legal intervention involving injury by tear gas,** law enforcement official **injured**

    ✓7ᵗʰ **Y35.212** **Legal intervention involving injury by tear gas,** bystander **injured**

    ✓7ᵗʰ **Y35.213** **Legal intervention involving injury by tear gas,** suspect **injured**

    ✓7ᵗʰ **Y35.219** **Legal intervention involving injury by tear gas, unspecified person injured**

  ✓6ᵗʰ **Y35.29** **Legal intervention involving other gas**

    ✓7ᵗʰ **Y35.291** **Legal intervention involving other gas,** law enforcement official **injured**

    ✓7ᵗʰ **Y35.292** **Legal intervention involving other gas,** bystander **injured**

    ✓7ᵗʰ **Y35.293** **Legal intervention involving other gas,** suspect **injured**

    ✓7ᵗʰ **Y35.299** **Legal intervention involving other gas, unspecified person injured**

✓5ᵗʰ **Y35.3** **Legal intervention involving** blunt objects

Legal intervention involving being hit or struck by blunt object

  ✓6ᵗʰ **Y35.30** **Legal intervention involving unspecified blunt objects**

    ✓7ᵗʰ **Y35.301** **Legal intervention involving unspecified blunt objects,** law enforcement official **injured**

    ✓7ᵗʰ **Y35.302** **Legal intervention involving unspecified blunt objects,** bystander **injured**

    ✓7ᵗʰ **Y35.303** **Legal intervention involving unspecified blunt objects,** suspect **injured**

    ✓7ᵗʰ **Y35.309** **Legal intervention involving unspecified blunt objects, unspecified person injured**

  ✓6ᵗʰ **Y35.31** **Legal intervention involving** baton

    ✓7ᵗʰ **Y35.311** **Legal intervention involving baton,** law enforcement official **injured**

    ✓7ᵗʰ **Y35.312** **Legal intervention involving baton,** bystander **injured**

    ✓7ᵗʰ **Y35.313** **Legal intervention involving baton,** suspect **injured**

    ✓7ᵗʰ **Y35.319** **Legal intervention involving baton, unspecified person injured**

  ✓6ᵗʰ **Y35.39** **Legal intervention involving other blunt objects**

    ✓7ᵗʰ **Y35.391** **Legal intervention involving other blunt objects,** law enforcement official **injured**

    ✓7ᵗʰ **Y35.392** **Legal intervention involving other blunt objects,** bystander **injured**

    ✓7ᵗʰ **Y35.393** **Legal intervention involving other blunt objects,** suspect **injured**

    ✓7ᵗʰ **Y35.399** **Legal intervention involving other blunt objects, unspecified person injured**

✓5ᵗʰ **Y35.4** **Legal intervention involving** sharp objects

Legal intervention involving being cut by sharp objects

Legal intervention involving being stabbed by sharp objects

  ✓6ᵗʰ **Y35.40** **Legal intervention involving unspecified sharp objects**

    ✓7ᵗʰ **Y35.401** **Legal intervention involving unspecified sharp objects,** law enforcement official **injured**

    ✓7ᵗʰ **Y35.402** **Legal intervention involving unspecified sharp objects,** bystander **injured**

    ✓7ᵗʰ **Y35.403** **Legal intervention involving unspecified sharp objects,** suspect **injured**

    ✓7ᵗʰ **Y35.409** **Legal intervention involving unspecified sharp objects, unspecified person injured**

  ✓6ᵗʰ **Y35.41** **Legal intervention involving** bayonet

    ✓7ᵗʰ **Y35.411** **Legal intervention involving bayonet,** law enforcement official **injured**

    ✓7ᵗʰ **Y35.412** **Legal intervention involving bayonet,** bystander **injured**

    ✓7ᵗʰ **Y35.413** **Legal intervention involving bayonet,** suspect **injured**

    ✓7ᵗʰ **Y35.419** **Legal intervention involving bayonet, unspecified person injured**

  ✓6ᵗʰ **Y35.49** **Legal intervention involving other sharp objects**

    ✓7ᵗʰ **Y35.491** **Legal intervention involving other sharp objects,** law enforcement official **injured**

    ✓7ᵗʰ **Y35.492** **Legal intervention involving other sharp objects,** bystander **injured**

    ✓7ᵗʰ **Y35.493** **Legal intervention involving other sharp objects,** suspect **injured**

    ✓7ᵗʰ **Y35.499** **Legal intervention involving other sharp objects, unspecified person injured**

✓5ᵗʰ **Y35.8** **Legal intervention involving other specified means**

AHA: 2019,4Q,19

  ✓6ᵗʰ **Y35.81** **Legal intervention involving** manhandling

    ✓7ᵗʰ **Y35.811** **Legal intervention involving manhandling,** law enforcement official **injured**

    ✓7ᵗʰ **Y35.812** **Legal intervention involving manhandling,** bystander **injured**

    ✓7ᵗʰ **Y35.813** **Legal intervention involving manhandling,** suspect **injured**

    ✓7ᵗʰ **Y35.819** **Legal intervention involving manhandling, unspecified person injured**

Ⓝ Newborn: 0   Ⓟ Pediatric: 0-17   Ⓜ Maternity: 9-64   Ⓐ Adult: 15-124   **MCC** Major Complication/Comorbidity   **CC** Complication/Comorbidity   **SW** Severe Wound Dx

1214   ICD-10-CM 2022

Chapter 20. External Causes of Morbidity

✓6ᵗʰ **Y35.83** **Legal intervention involving a** conducted energy device
     Electroshock device (taser)
     Stun gun

     ✓7ᵗʰ **Y35.831** **Legal intervention involving a conducted energy device,** law enforcement official **injured**

     ✓7ᵗʰ **Y35.832** **Legal intervention involving a conducted energy device,** bystander **injured**

     ✓7ᵗʰ **Y35.833** **Legal intervention involving a conducted energy device,** suspect **injured**

     ✓7ᵗʰ **Y35.839** **Legal intervention involving a conducted energy device, unspecified person injured**

✓6ᵗʰ **Y35.89** **Legal intervention involving other specified means**

     ✓7ᵗʰ **Y35.891** **Legal intervention involving other specified means,** law enforcement official **injured**

     ✓7ᵗʰ **Y35.892** **Legal intervention involving other specified means,** bystander **injured**

     ✓7ᵗʰ **Y35.893** **Legal intervention involving other specified means,** suspect **injured**
         AHA: 2018,1Q,5

●   ✓7ᵗʰ **Y35.899** **Legal intervention involving other specified means, unspecified person injured**

✓5ᵗʰ **Y35.9** **Legal intervention, means unspecified**

     ✓x7ᵗʰ **Y35.91** **Legal intervention, means unspecified,** law enforcement official **injured**

     ✓x7ᵗʰ **Y35.92** **Legal intervention, means unspecified,** bystander **injured**

     ✓x7ᵗʰ **Y35.93** **Legal intervention, means unspecified,** suspect **injured**

     ✓x7ᵗʰ **Y35.99** **Legal intervention, means unspecified, unspecified person injured**

✓4ᵗʰ **Y36** **Operations of war**

     INCLUDES   injuries to military personnel and civilians caused by war, civil insurrection, and peacekeeping missions

     EXCLUDES 1   injury to military personnel occurring during peacetime military operations (Y37.-)
         military vehicles involved in transport accidents with non-military vehicle during peacetime (V09.01, V09.21, V19.81, V29.81, V39.81, V49.81, V59.81, V69.81, V79.81)

     AHA: 2014,3Q,4

✓5ᵗʰ **Y36.0** **War operations involving** explosion of marine weapons

     ✓6ᵗʰ **Y36.00** **War operations involving explosion of unspecified marine weapon**
         War operations involving underwater blast NOS

         ✓7ᵗʰ **Y36.000** **War operations involving explosion of unspecified marine weapon,** military personnel

         ✓7ᵗʰ **Y36.001** **War operations involving explosion of unspecified marine weapon,** civilian

     ✓6ᵗʰ **Y36.01** **War operations involving explosion of** depth-charge

         ✓7ᵗʰ **Y36.010** **War operations involving explosion of depth-charge,** military personnel

         ✓7ᵗʰ **Y36.011** **War operations involving explosion of depth-charge,** civilian

     ✓6ᵗʰ **Y36.02** **War operations involving explosion of** marine mine
         War operations involving explosion of marine mine, at sea or in harbor

         ✓7ᵗʰ **Y36.020** **War operations involving explosion of marine mine,** military personnel

         ✓7ᵗʰ **Y36.021** **War operations involving explosion of marine mine,** civilian

     ✓6ᵗʰ **Y36.03** **War operations involving explosion of** sea-based artillery shell

         ✓7ᵗʰ **Y36.030** **War operations involving explosion of sea-based artillery shell,** military personnel

         ✓7ᵗʰ **Y36.031** **War operations involving explosion of sea-based artillery shell,** civilian

     ✓6ᵗʰ **Y36.04** **War operations involving explosion of** torpedo

         ✓7ᵗʰ **Y36.040** **War operations involving explosion of torpedo,** military personnel

         ✓7ᵗʰ **Y36.041** **War operations involving explosion of torpedo,** civilian

✓6ᵗʰ **Y36.05** **War operations involving** accidental detonation of onboard marine weapons

     ✓7ᵗʰ **Y36.050** **War operations involving accidental detonation of onboard marine weapons,** military personnel

     ✓7ᵗʰ **Y36.051** **War operations involving accidental detonation of onboard marine weapons,** civilian

✓6ᵗʰ **Y36.09** **War operations involving explosion of other marine weapons**

     ✓7ᵗʰ **Y36.090** **War operations involving explosion of other marine weapons,** military personnel

     ✓7ᵗʰ **Y36.091** **War operations involving explosion of other marine weapons,** civilian

✓5ᵗʰ **Y36.1** **War operations involving** destruction of aircraft

     ✓6ᵗʰ **Y36.10** **War operations involving unspecified destruction of aircraft**

         ✓7ᵗʰ **Y36.100** **War operations involving unspecified destruction of aircraft,** military personnel

         ✓7ᵗʰ **Y36.101** **War operations involving unspecified destruction of aircraft,** civilian

     ✓6ᵗʰ **Y36.11** **War operations involving destruction of aircraft due to** enemy fire or explosives
         War operations involving destruction of aircraft due to air to air missile
         War operations involving destruction of aircraft due to explosive placed on aircraft
         War operations involving destruction of aircraft due to rocket propelled grenade [RPG]
         War operations involving destruction of aircraft due to small arms fire
         War operations involving destruction of aircraft due to surface to air missile

         ✓7ᵗʰ **Y36.110** **War operations involving destruction of aircraft due to enemy fire or explosives,** military personnel

         ✓7ᵗʰ **Y36.111** **War operations involving destruction of aircraft due to enemy fire or explosives,** civilian

     ✓6ᵗʰ **Y36.12** **War operations involving destruction of aircraft due to** collision with other aircraft

         ✓7ᵗʰ **Y36.120** **War operations involving destruction of aircraft due to collision with other aircraft,** military personnel

         ✓7ᵗʰ **Y36.121** **War operations involving destruction of aircraft due to collision with other aircraft,** civilian

     ✓6ᵗʰ **Y36.13** **War operations involving destruction of aircraft due to** onboard fire

         ✓7ᵗʰ **Y36.130** **War operations involving destruction of aircraft due to onboard fire,** military personnel

         ✓7ᵗʰ **Y36.131** **War operations involving destruction of aircraft due to onboard fire,** civilian

     ✓6ᵗʰ **Y36.14** **War operations involving destruction of aircraft due to** accidental detonation of onboard munitions and explosives

         ✓7ᵗʰ **Y36.140** **War operations involving destruction of aircraft due to accidental detonation of onboard munitions and explosives,** military personnel

         ✓7ᵗʰ **Y36.141** **War operations involving destruction of aircraft due to accidental detonation of onboard munitions and explosives,** civilian

     ✓6ᵗʰ **Y36.19** **War operations involving other destruction of aircraft**

         ✓7ᵗʰ **Y36.190** **War operations involving other destruction of aircraft,** military personnel

         ✓7ᵗʰ **Y36.191** **War operations involving other destruction of aircraft,** civilian

✓ Additional Char Req   ✓x7ᵗʰ Placeholder   Unacceptable PDx   Questionable PDx   Wrong Procedure   Manifestation   Unspecified Dx   H1-H14 HAC   HCC CMS-HCC Dx   HIV HIV Dx

ICD-10-CM 2022   1215

✓5ᵗʰ **Y36.2 War operations involving other explosions and fragments**

> EXCLUDES 1   *war operations involving explosion of aircraft (Y36.1-)*
>
> *war operations involving explosion of marine weapons (Y36.0-)*
>
> *war operations involving explosion of nuclear weapons (Y36.5-)*
>
> *war operations involving explosion occurring after cessation of hostilities (Y36.8-)*

✓6ᵗʰ **Y36.20 War operations involving unspecified explosion and fragments**

War operations involving air blast NOS
War operations involving blast NOS
War operations involving blast fragments NOS
War operations involving blast wave NOS
War operations involving blast wind NOS
War operations involving explosion NOS
War operations involving explosion of bomb NOS

✓7ᵗʰ **Y36.200 War operations involving unspecified explosion and fragments, military personnel**

✓7ᵗʰ **Y36.201 War operations involving unspecified explosion and fragments, civilian**

✓6ᵗʰ **Y36.21 War operations involving explosion of aerial bomb**

✓7ᵗʰ **Y36.210 War operations involving explosion of aerial bomb, military personnel**

✓7ᵗʰ **Y36.211 War operations involving explosion of aerial bomb, civilian**

✓6ᵗʰ **Y36.22 War operations involving explosion of guided missile**

✓7ᵗʰ **Y36.220 War operations involving explosion of guided missile, military personnel**

✓7ᵗʰ **Y36.221 War operations involving explosion of guided missile, civilian**

✓6ᵗʰ **Y36.23 War operations involving explosion of improvised explosive device [IED]**

War operations involving explosion of person-borne improvised explosive device [IED]
War operations involving explosion of vehicle-borne improvised explosive device [IED]
War operations involving explosion of roadside improvised explosive device [IED]

✓7ᵗʰ **Y36.230 War operations involving explosion of improvised explosive device [IED], military personnel**

✓7ᵗʰ **Y36.231 War operations involving explosion of improvised explosive device [IED], civilian**

✓6ᵗʰ **Y36.24 War operations involving explosion due to accidental detonation and discharge of own munitions or munitions launch device**

✓7ᵗʰ **Y36.240 War operations involving explosion due to accidental detonation and discharge of own munitions or munitions launch device, military personnel**

✓7ᵗʰ **Y36.241 War operations involving explosion due to accidental detonation and discharge of own munitions or munitions launch device, civilian**

✓6ᵗʰ **Y36.25 War operations involving fragments from munitions**

✓7ᵗʰ **Y36.250 War operations involving fragments from munitions, military personnel**

✓7ᵗʰ **Y36.251 War operations involving fragments from munitions, civilian**

✓6ᵗʰ **Y36.26 War operations involving fragments of improvised explosive device [IED]**

War operations involving fragments of person-borne improvised explosive device [IED]
War operations involving fragments of vehicle-borne improvised explosive device [IED]
War operations involving fragments of roadside improvised explosive device [IED]

✓7ᵗʰ **Y36.260 War operations involving fragments of improvised explosive device [IED], military personnel**

✓7ᵗʰ **Y36.261 War operations involving fragments of improvised explosive device [IED], civilian**

✓6ᵗʰ **Y36.27 War operations involving fragments from weapons**

✓7ᵗʰ **Y36.270 War operations involving fragments from weapons, military personnel**

✓7ᵗʰ **Y36.271 War operations involving fragments from weapons, civilian**

✓6ᵗʰ **Y36.29 War operations involving other explosions and fragments**

War operations involving explosion of grenade
War operations involving explosions of land mine
War operations involving shrapnel NOS

✓7ᵗʰ **Y36.290 War operations involving other explosions and fragments, military personnel**

✓7ᵗʰ **Y36.291 War operations involving other explosions and fragments, civilian**

✓5ᵗʰ **Y36.3 War operations involving fires, conflagrations and hot substances**

War operations involving smoke, fumes, and heat from fires, conflagrations and hot substances

> EXCLUDES 1   *war operations involving fires and conflagrations aboard military aircraft (Y36.1-)*
>
> *war operations involving fires and conflagrations aboard military watercraft (Y36.0-)*
>
> *war operations involving fires and conflagrations caused indirectly by conventional weapons (Y36.2-)*
>
> *war operations involving fires and thermal effects of nuclear weapons (Y36.53-)*

✓6ᵗʰ **Y36.30 War operations involving unspecified fire, conflagration and hot substance**

✓7ᵗʰ **Y36.300 War operations involving unspecified fire, conflagration and hot substance, military personnel**

✓7ᵗʰ **Y36.301 War operations involving unspecified fire, conflagration and hot substance, civilian**

✓6ᵗʰ **Y36.31 War operations involving gasoline bomb**

War operations involving incendiary bomb
War operations involving petrol bomb

✓7ᵗʰ **Y36.310 War operations involving gasoline bomb, military personnel**

✓7ᵗʰ **Y36.311 War operations involving gasoline bomb, civilian**

✓6ᵗʰ **Y36.32 War operations involving incendiary bullet**

✓7ᵗʰ **Y36.320 War operations involving incendiary bullet, military personnel**

✓7ᵗʰ **Y36.321 War operations involving incendiary bullet, civilian**

✓6ᵗʰ **Y36.33 War operations involving flamethrower**

✓7ᵗʰ **Y36.330 War operations involving flamethrower, military personnel**

✓7ᵗʰ **Y36.331 War operations involving flamethrower, civilian**

✓6ᵗʰ **Y36.39 War operations involving other fires, conflagrations and hot substances**

✓7ᵗʰ **Y36.390 War operations involving other fires, conflagrations and hot substances, military personnel**

✓7ᵗʰ **Y36.391 War operations involving other fires, conflagrations and hot substances, civilian**

✓5ᵗʰ **Y36.4 War operations involving firearm discharge and other forms of conventional warfare**

✓6ᵗʰ **Y36.41 War operations involving rubber bullets**

✓7ᵗʰ **Y36.410 War operations involving rubber bullets, military personnel**

✓7ᵗʰ **Y36.411 War operations involving rubber bullets, civilian**

✓6ᵗʰ **Y36.42 War operations involving firearms pellets**

✓7ᵗʰ **Y36.420 War operations involving firearms pellets, military personnel**

✓7ᵗʰ **Y36.421 War operations involving firearms pellets, civilian**

✓6ᵗʰ **Y36.43 War operations involving other firearms discharge**

War operations involving bullets NOS

> EXCLUDES 1   *war operations involving munitions fragments (Y36.25-)*
>
> *war operations involving incendiary bullets (Y36.32-)*

✓7ᵗʰ **Y36.430 War operations involving other firearms discharge, military personnel**

✓7ᵗʰ **Y36.431 War operations involving other firearms discharge, civilian**

Ⓝ Newborn: 0   Ⓟ Pediatric: 0-17   Ⓜ Maternity: 9-64   Ⓐ Adult: 15-124   MCC Major Complication/Comorbidity   CC Complication/Comorbidity   SW Severe Wound Dx

1216

ICD-10-CM 2022

✓6ᵗʰ **Y36.44** **War operations involving** unarmed hand to hand combat

    EXCLUDES 1   *war operations involving combat using blunt or piercing object (Y36.45-)*
        war operations involving intentional restriction of air and airway (Y36.46-)
        war operations involving unintentional restriction of air and airway (Y36.47-)

  ✓7ᵗʰ **Y36.440** **War operations involving unarmed hand to hand combat,** military personnel

  ✓7ᵗʰ **Y36.441** **War operations involving unarmed hand to hand combat,** civilian

✓6ᵗʰ **Y36.45** **War operations involving combat using** blunt or piercing object

  ✓7ᵗʰ **Y36.450** **War operations involving combat using blunt or piercing object,** military personnel

  ✓7ᵗʰ **Y36.451** **War operations involving combat using blunt or piercing object,** civilian

✓6ᵗʰ **Y36.46** **War operations involving** intentional restriction of air and airway

  ✓7ᵗʰ **Y36.460** **War operations involving intentional restriction of air and airway,** military personnel

  ✓7ᵗʰ **Y36.461** **War operations involving intentional restriction of air and airway,** civilian

✓6ᵗʰ **Y36.47** **War operations involving** unintentional restriction of air and airway

  ✓7ᵗʰ **Y36.470** **War operations involving unintentional restriction of air and airway,** military personnel

  ✓7ᵗʰ **Y36.471** **War operations involving unintentional restriction of air and airway,** civilian

✓6ᵗʰ **Y36.49** **War operations involving other forms of conventional warfare**

  ✓7ᵗʰ **Y36.490** **War operations involving other forms of conventional warfare,** military personnel

  ✓7ᵗʰ **Y36.491** **War operations involving other forms of conventional warfare,** civilian

✓5ᵗʰ **Y36.5** **War operations involving** nuclear weapons

  War operations involving dirty bomb NOS

✓6ᵗʰ **Y36.50** **War operations involving unspecified effect of nuclear weapon**

  ✓7ᵗʰ **Y36.500** **War operations involving unspecified effect of nuclear weapon,** military personnel

  ✓7ᵗʰ **Y36.501** **War operations involving unspecified effect of nuclear weapon,** civilian

✓6ᵗʰ **Y36.51** **War operations involving** direct blast **effect of nuclear weapon**

  War operations involving blast pressure of nuclear weapon

  ✓7ᵗʰ **Y36.510** **War operations involving direct blast effect of nuclear weapon,** military personnel

  ✓7ᵗʰ **Y36.511** **War operations involving direct blast effect of nuclear weapon,** civilian

✓6ᵗʰ **Y36.52** **War operations involving** indirect blast **effect of nuclear weapon**

  War operations involving being thrown by blast of nuclear weapon

  War operations involving being struck or crushed by blast debris of nuclear weapon

  ✓7ᵗʰ **Y36.520** **War operations involving indirect blast effect of nuclear weapon,** military personnel

  ✓7ᵗʰ **Y36.521** **War operations involving indirect blast effect of nuclear weapon,** civilian

✓6ᵗʰ **Y36.53** **War operations involving** thermal radiation **effect of nuclear weapon**

  War operations involving direct heat from nuclear weapon

  War operation involving fireball effects from nuclear weapon

  ✓7ᵗʰ **Y36.530** **War operations involving thermal radiation effect of nuclear weapon,** military personnel

  ✓7ᵗʰ **Y36.531** **War operations involving thermal radiation effect of nuclear weapon,** civilian

✓6ᵗʰ **Y36.54** **War operation involving** nuclear radiation **effects of nuclear weapon**

  War operation involving acute radiation exposure from nuclear weapon

  War operation involving exposure to immediate ionizing radiation from nuclear weapon

  War operation involving fallout exposure from nuclear weapon

  War operation involving secondary effects of nuclear weapons

  ✓7ᵗʰ **Y36.540** **War operation involving nuclear radiation effects of nuclear weapon,** military personnel

  ✓7ᵗʰ **Y36.541** **War operation involving nuclear radiation effects of nuclear weapon,** civilian

✓6ᵗʰ **Y36.59** **War operation involving other effects of nuclear weapons**

  ✓7ᵗʰ **Y36.590** **War operation involving other effects of nuclear weapons,** military personnel

  ✓7ᵗʰ **Y36.591** **War operation involving other effects of nuclear weapons,** civilian

✓5ᵗʰ **Y36.6** **War operations involving biological weapons**

✓6ᵗʰ **Y36.6X** **War operations involving** biological weapons

  ✓7ᵗʰ **Y36.6X0** **War operations involving biological weapons,** military personnel

  ✓7ᵗʰ **Y36.6X1** **War operations involving biological weapons,** civilian

✓5ᵗʰ **Y36.7** **War operations involving chemical weapons and other forms of unconventional warfare**

  EXCLUDES 1   *war operations involving incendiary devices (Y36.3-, Y36.5-)*

✓6ᵗʰ **Y36.7X** **War operations involving** chemical weapons and other forms of unconventional warfare

  ✓7ᵗʰ **Y36.7X0** **War operations involving chemical weapons and other forms of unconventional warfare,** military personnel

  ✓7ᵗʰ **Y36.7X1** **War operations involving chemical weapons and other forms of unconventional warfare,** civilian

✓5ᵗʰ **Y36.8** **War operations occurring** after cessation of hostilities

  War operations classifiable to categories Y36.0-Y36.8 but occurring after cessation of hostilities

✓6ᵗʰ **Y36.81** **Explosion of** mine **placed during war operations but exploding after cessation of hostilities**

  ✓7ᵗʰ **Y36.810** **Explosion of mine placed during war operations but exploding after cessation of hostilities,** military personnel

  ✓7ᵗʰ **Y36.811** **Explosion of mine placed during war operations but exploding after cessation of hostilities,** civilian

✓6ᵗʰ **Y36.82** **Explosion of** bomb **placed during war operations but exploding after cessation of hostilities**

  ✓7ᵗʰ **Y36.820** **Explosion of bomb placed during war operations but exploding after cessation of hostilities,** military personnel

  ✓7ᵗʰ **Y36.821** **Explosion of bomb placed during war operations but exploding after cessation of hostilities,** civilian

✓6ᵗʰ **Y36.88** **Other war operations occurring after cessation of hostilities**

  ✓7ᵗʰ **Y36.880** **Other war operations occurring after cessation of hostilities,** military personnel

  ✓7ᵗʰ **Y36.881** **Other war operations occurring after cessation of hostilities,** civilian

✓6ᵗʰ **Y36.89** **Unspecified war operations occurring after cessation of hostilities**

  ✓7ᵗʰ **Y36.890** **Unspecified war operations occurring after cessation of hostilities,** military personnel

  ✓7ᵗʰ **Y36.891** **Unspecified war operations occurring after cessation of hostilities,** civilian

✓6ᵗʰ **Y36.9** **Other and unspecified war operations**

  ✓x7ᵗʰ **Y36.90** **War operations, unspecified**

  ✓x7ᵗʰ **Y36.91** **War operations involving unspecified** weapon of mass destruction [WMD]

  ✓x7ᵗʰ **Y36.92** **War operations involving** friendly fire

---

✓4ᵗʰ **Y37 Military operations**

INCLUDES injuries to military personnel and civilians occurring during peacetime on military property and during routine military exercises and operations

EXCLUDES 1 *military aircraft involved in aircraft accident with civilian aircraft (V97.81-)*

military vehicles involved in transport accident with civilian vehicle (V09.01, V09.21, V19.81, V29.81, V39.81, V49.81, V59.81, V69.81, V79.81)

military watercraft involved in water transport accident with civilian watercraft (V94.81-)

war operations (Y36.-)

✓5ᵗʰ **Y37.0 Military operations involving** explosion of marine weapons

✓6ᵗʰ **Y37.00 Military operations involving explosion of unspecified marine weapon**

Military operations involving underwater blast NOS

✓7ᵗʰ **Y37.000 Military operations involving explosion of unspecified marine weapon, military personnel**

✓7ᵗʰ **Y37.001 Military operations involving explosion of unspecified marine weapon, civilian**

✓6ᵗʰ **Y37.01 Military operations involving explosion of depth-charge**

✓7ᵗʰ **Y37.010 Military operations involving explosion of depth-charge, military personnel**

✓7ᵗʰ **Y37.011 Military operations involving explosion of depth-charge, civilian**

✓6ᵗʰ **Y37.02 Military operations involving explosion of marine mine**

Military operations involving explosion of marine mine, at sea or in harbor

✓7ᵗʰ **Y37.020 Military operations involving explosion of marine mine, military personnel**

✓7ᵗʰ **Y37.021 Military operations involving explosion of marine mine, civilian**

✓6ᵗʰ **Y37.03 Military operations involving explosion of sea-based artillery shell**

✓7ᵗʰ **Y37.030 Military operations involving explosion of sea-based artillery shell, military personnel**

✓7ᵗʰ **Y37.031 Military operations involving explosion of sea-based artillery shell, civilian**

✓6ᵗʰ **Y37.04 Military operations involving explosion of torpedo**

✓7ᵗʰ **Y37.040 Military operations involving explosion of torpedo, military personnel**

✓7ᵗʰ **Y37.041 Military operations involving explosion of torpedo, civilian**

✓6ᵗʰ **Y37.05 Military operations involving accidental detonation of onboard marine weapons**

✓7ᵗʰ **Y37.050 Military operations involving accidental detonation of onboard marine weapons, military personnel**

✓7ᵗʰ **Y37.051 Military operations involving accidental detonation of onboard marine weapons, civilian**

✓6ᵗʰ **Y37.09 Military operations involving explosion of other marine weapons**

✓7ᵗʰ **Y37.090 Military operations involving explosion of other marine weapons, military personnel**

✓7ᵗʰ **Y37.091 Military operations involving explosion of other marine weapons, civilian**

✓5ᵗʰ **Y37.1 Military operations involving** destruction of aircraft

✓6ᵗʰ **Y37.10 Military operations involving unspecified destruction of aircraft**

✓7ᵗʰ **Y37.100 Military operations involving unspecified destruction of aircraft, military personnel**

✓7ᵗʰ **Y37.101 Military operations involving unspecified destruction of aircraft, civilian**

✓6ᵗʰ **Y37.11 Military operations involving destruction of aircraft due to enemy fire or explosives**

Military operations involving destruction of aircraft due to air to air missile

Military operations involving destruction of aircraft due to explosive placed on aircraft

Military operations involving destruction of aircraft due to rocket propelled grenade [RPG]

Military operations involving destruction of aircraft due to small arms fire

Military operations involving destruction of aircraft due to surface to air missile

✓7ᵗʰ **Y37.110 Military operations involving destruction of aircraft due to enemy fire or explosives, military personnel**

✓7ᵗʰ **Y37.111 Military operations involving destruction of aircraft due to enemy fire or explosives, civilian**

✓6ᵗʰ **Y37.12 Military operations involving destruction of aircraft due to collision with other aircraft**

✓7ᵗʰ **Y37.120 Military operations involving destruction of aircraft due to collision with other aircraft, military personnel**

✓7ᵗʰ **Y37.121 Military operations involving destruction of aircraft due to collision with other aircraft, civilian**

✓6ᵗʰ **Y37.13 Military operations involving destruction of aircraft due to onboard fire**

✓7ᵗʰ **Y37.130 Military operations involving destruction of aircraft due to onboard fire, military personnel**

✓7ᵗʰ **Y37.131 Military operations involving destruction of aircraft due to onboard fire, civilian**

✓6ᵗʰ **Y37.14 Military operations involving destruction of aircraft due to** accidental detonation of onboard munitions and explosives

✓7ᵗʰ **Y37.140 Military operations involving destruction of aircraft due to accidental detonation of onboard munitions and explosives, military personnel**

✓7ᵗʰ **Y37.141 Military operations involving destruction of aircraft due to accidental detonation of onboard munitions and explosives, civilian**

✓6ᵗʰ **Y37.19 Military operations involving other destruction of aircraft**

✓7ᵗʰ **Y37.190 Military operations involving other destruction of aircraft, military personnel**

✓7ᵗʰ **Y37.191 Military operations involving other destruction of aircraft, civilian**

✓5ᵗʰ **Y37.2 Military operations involving** other explosions and fragments

EXCLUDES 1 *military operations involving explosion of aircraft (Y37.1-)*

military operations involving explosion of marine weapons (Y37.0-)

military operations involving explosion of nuclear weapons (Y37.5-)

✓6ᵗʰ **Y37.20 Military operations involving unspecified explosion and fragments**

Military operations involving air blast NOS

Military operations involving blast NOS

Military operations involving blast fragments NOS

Military operations involving blast wave NOS

Military operations involving blast wind NOS

Military operations involving explosion NOS

Military operations involving explosion of bomb NOS

✓7ᵗʰ **Y37.200 Military operations involving unspecified explosion and fragments, military personnel**

✓7ᵗʰ **Y37.201 Military operations involving unspecified explosion and fragments, civilian**

✓6ᵗʰ **Y37.21 Military operations involving explosion of aerial bomb**

✓7ᵗʰ **Y37.210 Military operations involving explosion of aerial bomb, military personnel**

✓7ᵗʰ **Y37.211 Military operations involving explosion of aerial bomb, civilian**

✓6ᵗʰ **Y37.22 Military operations involving explosion of guided missile**

✓7ᵗʰ **Y37.220 Military operations involving explosion of guided missile, military personnel**

✓7ᵗʰ **Y37.221** **Military operations involving explosion of guided missile,** civilian

✓6ᵗʰ **Y37.23** **Military operations involving explosion of** improvised explosive device [IED]
Military operations involving explosion of person-borne improvised explosive device [IED]
Military operations involving explosion of vehicle-borne improvised explosive device [IED]
Military operations involving explosion of roadside improvised explosive device [IED]

✓7ᵗʰ **Y37.230** **Military operations involving explosion of improvised explosive device [IED],** military personnel

✓7ᵗʰ **Y37.231** **Military operations involving explosion of improvised explosive device [IED],** civilian

✓6ᵗʰ **Y37.24** **Military operations involving explosion** due to accidental detonation and discharge of own munitions or munitions launch device

✓7ᵗʰ **Y37.240** **Military operations involving explosion due to accidental detonation and discharge of own munitions or munitions launch device,** military personnel

✓7ᵗʰ **Y37.241** **Military operations involving explosion due to accidental detonation and discharge of own munitions or munitions launch device,** civilian

✓6ᵗʰ **Y37.25** **Military operations involving** fragments from munitions

✓7ᵗʰ **Y37.250** **Military operations involving fragments from munitions,** military personnel

✓7ᵗʰ **Y37.251** **Military operations involving fragments from munitions,** civilian

✓6ᵗʰ **Y37.26** **Military operations involving** fragments of improvised explosive device [IED]
Military operations involving fragments of person-borne improvised explosive device [IED]
Military operations involving fragments of vehicle-borne improvised explosive device [IED]
Military operations involving fragments of roadside improvised explosive device [IED]

✓7ᵗʰ **Y37.260** **Military operations involving fragments of improvised explosive device [IED],** military personnel

✓7ᵗʰ **Y37.261** **Military operations involving fragments of improvised explosive device [IED],** civilian

✓6ᵗʰ **Y37.27** **Military operations involving** fragments from weapons

✓7ᵗʰ **Y37.270** **Military operations involving fragments from weapons,** military personnel

✓7ᵗʰ **Y37.271** **Military operations involving fragments from weapons,** civilian

✓6ᵗʰ **Y37.29** **Military operations involving other explosions and fragments**
Military operations involving explosion of grenade
Military operations involving explosions of land mine
Military operations involving shrapnel NOS

✓7ᵗʰ **Y37.290** **Military operations involving other explosions and fragments,** military personnel

✓7ᵗʰ **Y37.291** **Military operations involving other explosions and fragments,** civilian

✓5ᵗʰ **Y37.3** **Military operations involving** fires, conflagrations and hot substances
Military operations involving smoke, fumes, and heat from fires, conflagrations and hot substances

EXCLUDES 1   *military operations involving fires and conflagrations aboard military aircraft (Y37.1-)*
military operations involving fires and conflagrations aboard military watercraft (Y37.0-)
military operations involving fires and conflagrations caused indirectly by conventional weapons (Y37.2-)
military operations involving fires and thermal effects of nuclear weapons (Y36.53-)

✓6ᵗʰ **Y37.30** **Military operations involving unspecified fire, conflagration and hot substance**

✓7ᵗʰ **Y37.300** **Military operations involving unspecified fire, conflagration and hot substance,** military personnel

✓7ᵗʰ **Y37.301** **Military operations involving unspecified fire, conflagration and hot substance,** civilian

✓6ᵗʰ **Y37.31** **Military operations involving** gasoline bomb
Military operations involving incendiary bomb
Military operations involving petrol bomb

✓7ᵗʰ **Y37.310** **Military operations involving gasoline bomb,** military personnel

✓7ᵗʰ **Y37.311** **Military operations involving gasoline bomb,** civilian

✓6ᵗʰ **Y37.32** **Military operations involving** incendiary bullet

✓7ᵗʰ **Y37.320** **Military operations involving incendiary bullet,** military personnel

✓7ᵗʰ **Y37.321** **Military operations involving incendiary bullet,** civilian

✓6ᵗʰ **Y37.33** **Military operations involving** flamethrower

✓7ᵗʰ **Y37.330** **Military operations involving flamethrower,** military personnel

✓7ᵗʰ **Y37.331** **Military operations involving flamethrower,** civilian

✓6ᵗʰ **Y37.39** **Military operations involving other fires, conflagrations and hot substances**

✓7ᵗʰ **Y37.390** **Military operations involving other fires, conflagrations and hot substances,** military personnel

✓7ᵗʰ **Y37.391** **Military operations involving other fires, conflagrations and hot substances,** civilian

✓5ᵗʰ **Y37.4** **Military operations involving firearm discharge and other forms of conventional warfare**

✓6ᵗʰ **Y37.41** **Military operations involving** rubber bullets

✓7ᵗʰ **Y37.410** **Military operations involving rubber bullets,** military personnel

✓7ᵗʰ **Y37.411** **Military operations involving rubber bullets,** civilian

✓6ᵗʰ **Y37.42** **Military operations involving** firearms pellets

✓7ᵗʰ **Y37.420** **Military operations involving firearms pellets,** military personnel

✓7ᵗʰ **Y37.421** **Military operations involving firearms pellets,** civilian

✓6ᵗʰ **Y37.43** **Military operations involving other firearms discharge**
Military operations involving bullets NOS

EXCLUDES 1   *military operations involving munitions fragments (Y37.25-)*
military operations involving incendiary bullets (Y37.32-)

✓7ᵗʰ **Y37.430** **Military operations involving other firearms discharge,** military personnel

✓7ᵗʰ **Y37.431** **Military operations involving other firearms discharge,** civilian

✓6ᵗʰ **Y37.44** **Military operations involving** unarmed hand to hand combat

EXCLUDES 1   *military operations involving combat using blunt or piercing object (Y37.45-)*
military operations involving intentional restriction of air and airway (Y37.46-)
military operations involving unintentional restriction of air and airway (Y37.47-)

✓7ᵗʰ **Y37.440** **Military operations involving unarmed hand to hand combat,** military personnel

✓7ᵗʰ **Y37.441** **Military operations involving unarmed hand to hand combat,** civilian

✓6ᵗʰ **Y37.45** **Military operations involving** combat using blunt or piercing object

✓7ᵗʰ **Y37.450** **Military operations involving combat using blunt or piercing object,** military personnel

✓7ᵗʰ **Y37.451** **Military operations involving combat using blunt or piercing object,** civilian

✓6ᵗʰ **Y37.46** **Military operations involving** intentional restriction of air and airway

✓7ᵗʰ **Y37.460** **Military operations involving intentional restriction of air and airway,** military personnel

✓7ᵗʰ **Y37.461** **Military operations involving intentional restriction of air and airway,** civilian

✓6ᵗʰ **Y37.47** **Military operations involving** unintentional restriction of air and airway

    ✓7ᵗʰ **Y37.470** **Military operations involving unintentional restriction of air and airway,** military personnel

    ✓7ᵗʰ **Y37.471** **Military operations involving unintentional restriction of air and airway,** civilian

✓6ᵗʰ **Y37.49** **Military operations involving other forms of conventional warfare**

    ✓7ᵗʰ **Y37.490** **Military operations involving other forms of conventional warfare,** military personnel

    ✓7ᵗʰ **Y37.491** **Military operations involving other forms of conventional warfare,** civilian

✓5ᵗʰ **Y37.5** **Military operations involving** nuclear weapons

    Military operation involving dirty bomb NOS

    ✓6ᵗʰ **Y37.50** **Military operations involving unspecified effect of nuclear weapon**

        ✓7ᵗʰ **Y37.500** **Military operations involving unspecified effect of nuclear weapon,** military personnel

        ✓7ᵗʰ **Y37.501** **Military operations involving unspecified effect of nuclear weapon,** civilian

    ✓6ᵗʰ **Y37.51** **Military operations involving** direct blast effect of nuclear weapon

        Military operations involving blast pressure of nuclear weapon

        ✓7ᵗʰ **Y37.510** **Military operations involving direct blast effect of nuclear weapon,** military personnel

        ✓7ᵗʰ **Y37.511** **Military operations involving direct blast effect of nuclear weapon,** civilian

    ✓6ᵗʰ **Y37.52** **Military operations involving** indirect blast effect of nuclear weapon

        Military operations involving being thrown by blast of nuclear weapon

        Military operations involving being struck or crushed by blast debris of nuclear weapon

        ✓7ᵗʰ **Y37.520** **Military operations involving indirect blast effect of nuclear weapon,** military personnel

        ✓7ᵗʰ **Y37.521** **Military operations involving indirect blast effect of nuclear weapon,** civilian

    ✓6ᵗʰ **Y37.53** **Military operations involving** thermal radiation effect of nuclear weapon

        Military operations involving direct heat from nuclear weapon

        Military operation involving fireball effects from nuclear weapon

        ✓7ᵗʰ **Y37.530** **Military operations involving thermal radiation effect of nuclear weapon,** military personnel

        ✓7ᵗʰ **Y37.531** **Military operations involving thermal radiation effect of nuclear weapon,** civilian

    ✓6ᵗʰ **Y37.54** **Military operation involving** nuclear radiation effects of nuclear weapon

        Military operation involving acute radiation exposure from nuclear weapon

        Military operation involving exposure to immediate ionizing radiation from nuclear weapon

        Military operation involving fallout exposure from nuclear weapon

        Military operation involving secondary effects of nuclear weapons

        ✓7ᵗʰ **Y37.540** **Military operation involving nuclear radiation effects of nuclear weapon,** military personnel

        ✓7ᵗʰ **Y37.541** **Military operation involving nuclear radiation effects of nuclear weapon,** civilian

    ✓6ᵗʰ **Y37.59** **Military operation involving other effects of nuclear weapons**

        ✓7ᵗʰ **Y37.590** **Military operation involving other effects of nuclear weapons,** military personnel

        ✓7ᵗʰ **Y37.591** **Military operation involving other effects of nuclear weapons,** civilian

✓5ᵗʰ **Y37.6** **Military operations involving** biological weapons

    ✓6ᵗʰ **Y37.6X** **Military operations involving biological weapons**

        ✓7ᵗʰ **Y37.6X0** **Military operations involving biological weapons,** military personnel

        ✓7ᵗʰ **Y37.6X1** **Military operations involving biological weapons,** civilian

✓5ᵗʰ **Y37.7** **Military operations involving chemical weapons and other forms of unconventional warfare**

    EXCLUDES 1   military operations involving incendiary devices (Y36.3-, Y36.5-)

    ✓6ᵗʰ **Y37.7X** **Military operations involving** chemical weapons and other forms of unconventional warfare

        ✓7ᵗʰ **Y37.7X0** **Military operations involving chemical weapons and other forms of unconventional warfare,** military personnel

        ✓7ᵗʰ **Y37.7X1** **Military operations involving chemical weapons and other forms of unconventional warfare,** civilian

✓5ᵗʰ **Y37.9** **Other and unspecified military operations**

    ✓×7ᵗʰ **Y37.90** **Military operations, unspecified**

    ✓×7ᵗʰ **Y37.91** **Military operations unspecified** weapon of mass destruction [WMD]

    ✓×7ᵗʰ **Y37.92** **Military operations involving** friendly fire

✓4ᵗʰ **Y38** **Terrorism**

NOTE   These codes are for use to identify injuries resulting from the unlawful use of force or violence against persons or property to intimidate or coerce a Government, the civilian population, or any segment thereof, in furtherance of political or social objective

Use additional code for place of occurrence (Y92.-)

✓5ᵗʰ **Y38.0** **Terrorism involving explosion of marine weapons**

    Terrorism involving depth-charge

    Terrorism involving marine mine

    Terrorism involving mine NOS, at sea or in harbor

    Terrorism involving sea-based artillery shell

    Terrorism involving torpedo

    Terrorism involving underwater blast

    ✓6ᵗʰ **Y38.0X** **Terrorism involving explosion of** marine weapons

        ✓7ᵗʰ **Y38.0X1** **Terrorism involving explosion of marine weapons,** public safety official **injured**

        ✓7ᵗʰ **Y38.0X2** **Terrorism involving explosion of marine weapons,** civilian **injured**

        ✓7ᵗʰ **Y38.0X3** **Terrorism involving explosion of marine weapons,** terrorist **injured**

✓5ᵗʰ **Y38.1** **Terrorism involving destruction of aircraft**

    Terrorism involving aircraft burned

    Terrorism involving aircraft exploded

    Terrorism involving aircraft being shot down

    Terrorism involving aircraft used as a weapon

    ✓6ᵗʰ **Y38.1X** **Terrorism involving** destruction of aircraft

        ✓7ᵗʰ **Y38.1X1** **Terrorism involving destruction of aircraft,** public safety official **injured**

        ✓7ᵗʰ **Y38.1X2** **Terrorism involving destruction of aircraft,** civilian **injured**

        ✓7ᵗʰ **Y38.1X3** **Terrorism involving destruction of aircraft,** terrorist **injured**

✓5ᵗʰ **Y38.2** **Terrorism involving other explosions and fragments**

    Terrorism involving antipersonnel (fragments) bomb

    Terrorism involving blast NOS

    Terrorism involving explosion NOS

    Terrorism involving explosion of breech block

    Terrorism involving explosion of cannon block

    Terrorism involving explosion (fragments) of artillery shell

    Terrorism involving explosion (fragments) of bomb

    Terrorism involving explosion (fragments) of grenade

    Terrorism involving explosion (fragments) of guided missile

    Terrorism involving explosion (fragments) of land mine

    Terrorism involving explosion of mortar bomb

    Terrorism involving explosion of munitions

    Terrorism involving explosion (fragments) of rocket

    Terrorism involving explosion (fragments) of shell

    Terrorism involving shrapnel

    Terrorism involving mine NOS, on land

    EXCLUDES 1   terrorism involving explosion of nuclear weapon (Y38.5)

        terrorism involving suicide bomber (Y38.81)

    ✓6ᵗʰ **Y38.2X** **Terrorism involving other explosions and fragments**

        ✓7ᵗʰ **Y38.2X1** **Terrorism involving other explosions and fragments,** public safety official **injured**

N Newborn: 0   P Pediatric: 0-17   M Maternity: 9-64   A Adult: 15-124   MCC Major Complication/Comorbidity   CC Complication/Comorbidity   SW Severe Wound Dx

1220   ICD-10-CM 2022

✓7ᵗʰ   **Y38.2X2**   **Terrorism involving other explosions and fragments,** civilian **injured**

✓7ᵗʰ   **Y38.2X3**   **Terrorism involving other explosions and fragments,** terrorist **injured**

✓5ᵗʰ   **Y38.3**   **Terrorism involving fires, conflagration and hot substances**

Terrorism involving conflagration NOS

Terrorism involving fire NOS

Terrorism involving petrol bomb

EXCLUDES 1   terrorism involving fire or heat of nuclear weapon (Y38.5)

✓6ᵗʰ   **Y38.3X**   **Terrorism involving** fires, conflagration and hot substances

✓7ᵗʰ   **Y38.3X1**   **Terrorism involving fires, conflagration and hot substances,** public safety official **injured**

✓7ᵗʰ   **Y38.3X2**   **Terrorism involving fires, conflagration and hot substances,** civilian **injured**

✓7ᵗʰ   **Y38.3X3**   **Terrorism involving fires, conflagration and hot substances,** terrorist **injured**

✓5ᵗʰ   **Y38.4**   **Terrorism involving firearms**

Terrorism involving carbine bullet

Terrorism involving machine gun bullet

Terrorism involving pellets (shotgun)

Terrorism involving pistol bullet

Terrorism involving rifle bullet

Terrorism involving rubber (rifle) bullet

✓6ᵗʰ   **Y38.4X**   **Terrorism involving** firearms

✓7ᵗʰ   **Y38.4X1**   **Terrorism involving firearms,** public safety official **injured**

✓7ᵗʰ   **Y38.4X2**   **Terrorism involving firearms,** civilian **injured**

✓7ᵗʰ   **Y38.4X3**   **Terrorism involving firearms,** terrorist **injured**

✓5ᵗʰ   **Y38.5**   **Terrorism involving nuclear weapons**

Terrorism involving blast effects of nuclear weapon

Terrorism involving exposure to ionizing radiation from nuclear weapon

Terrorism involving fireball effect of nuclear weapon

Terrorism involving heat from nuclear weapon

✓6ᵗʰ   **Y38.5X**   **Terrorism involving** nuclear weapons

✓7ᵗʰ   **Y38.5X1**   **Terrorism involving nuclear weapons,** public safety official **injured**

✓7ᵗʰ   **Y38.5X2**   **Terrorism involving nuclear weapons,** civilian **injured**

✓7ᵗʰ   **Y38.5X3**   **Terrorism involving nuclear weapons,** terrorist **injured**

✓5ᵗʰ   **Y38.6**   **Terrorism involving biological weapons**

Terrorism involving anthrax

Terrorism involving cholera

Terrorism involving smallpox

✓6ᵗʰ   **Y38.6X**   **Terrorism involving** biological weapons

✓7ᵗʰ   **Y38.6X1**   **Terrorism involving biological weapons,** public safety official **injured**

✓7ᵗʰ   **Y38.6X2**   **Terrorism involving biological weapons,** civilian **injured**

✓7ᵗʰ   **Y38.6X3**   **Terrorism involving biological weapons,** terrorist **injured**

✓5ᵗʰ   **Y38.7**   **Terrorism involving chemical weapons**

Terrorism involving gases, fumes, chemicals

Terrorism involving hydrogen cyanide

Terrorism involving phosgene

Terrorism involving sarin

✓6ᵗʰ   **Y38.7X**   **Terrorism involving** chemical weapons

✓7ᵗʰ   **Y38.7X1**   **Terrorism involving chemical weapons,** public safety official **injured**

✓7ᵗʰ   **Y38.7X2**   **Terrorism involving chemical weapons,** civilian **injured**

✓7ᵗʰ   **Y38.7X3**   **Terrorism involving chemical weapons,** terrorist **injured**

✓5ᵗʰ   **Y38.8**   **Terrorism involving other and unspecified means**

✓x7ᵗʰ   **Y38.80**   **Terrorism involving unspecified means**

Terrorism NOS

✓6ᵗʰ   **Y38.81**   **Terrorism involving** suicide bomber

✓7ᵗʰ   **Y38.811**   **Terrorism involving suicide bomber,** public safety official **injured**

✓7ᵗʰ   **Y38.812**   **Terrorism involving suicide bomber,** civilian **injured**

✓6ᵗʰ   **Y38.89**   **Terrorism involving other means**

Terrorism involving drowning and submersion

Terrorism involving lasers

Terrorism involving piercing or stabbing instruments

✓7ᵗʰ   **Y38.891**   **Terrorism involving other means,** public safety official **injured**

✓7ᵗʰ   **Y38.892**   **Terrorism involving other means,** civilian **injured**

✓7ᵗʰ   **Y38.893**   **Terrorism involving other means,** terrorist **injured**

✓5ᵗʰ   **Y38.9**   **Terrorism, secondary effects**

NOTE   This code is for use to identify conditions occurring subsequent to a terrorist attack not those that are due to the initial terrorist attack

✓6ᵗʰ   **Y38.9X**   **Terrorism,** secondary effects

✓7ᵗʰ   **Y38.9X1**   **Terrorism, secondary effects,** public safety official **injured**

✓7ᵗʰ   **Y38.9X2**   **Terrorism, secondary effects,** civilian **injured**

COMPLICATIONS OF MEDICAL AND SURGICAL CARE (Y62-Y84)

INCLUDES   complications of medical devices

surgical and medical procedures as the cause of abnormal reaction of the patient, or of later complication, without mention of misadventure at the time of the procedure

Misadventures to patients during surgical and medical care (Y62-Y69)

EXCLUDES 1   surgical and medical procedures as the cause of abnormal reaction of the patient, without mention of misadventure at the time of the procedure (Y83-Y84)

EXCLUDES 2   breakdown or malfunctioning of medical device (during procedure) (after implantation) (ongoing use) (Y70-Y82)

✓4ᵗʰ   **Y62**   **Failure of** sterile precautions **during surgical and medical care**

Y62.0   **Failure of sterile precautions during** surgical operation

Y62.1   **Failure of sterile precautions during** infusion or transfusion

Y62.2   **Failure of sterile precautions during** kidney dialysis and other perfusion   **HCC**

Y62.3   **Failure of sterile precautions during** injection or immunization

Y62.4   **Failure of sterile precautions during** endoscopic examination

Y62.5   **Failure of sterile precautions during** heart catheterization

Y62.6   **Failure of sterile precautions during** aspiration, puncture and other catheterization

Y62.8   **Failure of sterile precautions during other surgical and medical care**

Y62.9   **Failure of sterile precautions during unspecified surgical and medical care**

✓4ᵗʰ   **Y63**   **Failure in** dosage **during surgical and medical care**

EXCLUDES 2   accidental overdose of drug or wrong drug given in error (T36-T50)

Y63.0   **Excessive amount of blood or other fluid given during transfusion or infusion**

Y63.1   **Incorrect dilution of fluid used during infusion**

Y63.2   **Overdose of radiation given during therapy**

Y63.3   **Inadvertent exposure of patient to radiation during medical care**

Y63.4   **Failure in dosage in electroshock or insulin-shock therapy**

Y63.5   **Inappropriate temperature in local application and packing**

Y63.6   **Underdosing and nonadministration of necessary drug, medicament or biological substance**

AHA: 2018,4Q,72

Y63.8   **Failure in dosage during other surgical and medical care**

AHA: 2018,4Q,72

Y63.9   **Failure in dosage during unspecified surgical and medical care**

AHA: 2018,4Q,72

✓4ᵗʰ   **Y64**   Contaminated **medical or biological** substances

Y64.0   **Contaminated medical or biological substance,** transfused or infused

Y64.1   **Contaminated medical or biological substance,** injected or used for immunization

Y64.8   **Contaminated medical or biological substance administered by other means**

✓ Additional Char Req   ✓x7ᵗʰ Placeholder   Unacceptable PDx   Questionable PDx   Wrong Procedure   Manifestation   Unspecified Dx   ▪️-▪️ HAC   HCC CMS-HCC Dx   HIV HIV Dx

ICD-10-CM 2022   1221

Y64.9   **Contaminated medical or biological substance administered by unspecified means**
Administered contaminated medical or biological substance NOS

✓4ᵗʰ **Y65**   **Other misadventures during surgical and medical care**

     Y65.0   **Mismatched blood in transfusion**

     Y65.1   **Wrong fluid used in infusion**

     Y65.2   **Failure in suture or ligature during surgical operation**

     Y65.3   **Endotracheal tube wrongly placed during anesthetic procedure**

     Y65.4   **Failure to introduce or to remove other tube or instrument**

     ✓5ᵗʰ **Y65.5**   **Performance of** wrong procedure **(operation)**

         Y65.51   **Performance of wrong procedure (operation) on correct patient**
Wrong device implanted into correct surgical site
   EXCLUDES 1   *performance of correct procedure (operation) on wrong side or body part (Y65.53)*

         Y65.52   **Performance of procedure (operation) on patient not scheduled for surgery**
Performance of procedure (operation) intended for another patient
Performance of procedure (operation) on wrong patient

         Y65.53   **Performance of correct procedure (operation) on wrong side or body part**
Performance of correct procedure (operation) on wrong side
Performance of correct procedure (operation) on wrong site

     Y65.8   **Other specified misadventures during surgical and medical care**
AHA: 2019,2Q,23-24

Y66   **Nonadministration of surgical and medical care**
Premature cessation of surgical and medical care
   EXCLUDES 1   *DNR status (Z66)*
           palliative care (Z51.5)

Y69   **Unspecified misadventure during surgical and medical care**

Medical devices associated with adverse incidents in diagnostic and therapeutic use (Y70-Y82)

INCLUDES   breakdown or malfunction of medical devices (during use) (after implantation) (ongoing use)

EXCLUDES 2   *later complications following use of medical devices without breakdown or malfunctioning of device (Y83-Y84)*
misadventure to patients during surgical and medical care, classifiable to (Y62-Y69)
surgical and other medical procedures as the cause of abnormal reaction of the patient, or of later complication, without mention of misadventure at the time of the procedure (Y83-Y84)

✓4ᵗʰ **Y70**   **Anesthesiology** **devices associated with adverse incidents**

     Y70.0   Diagnostic and monitoring **anesthesiology devices associated with adverse incidents**

     Y70.1   Therapeutic (nonsurgical) and rehabilitative **anesthesiology devices associated with adverse incidents**

     Y70.2   Prosthetic and other implants, **materials and accessory anesthesiology devices associated with adverse incidents**

     Y70.3   Surgical instruments, **materials and anesthesiology devices (including sutures) associated with adverse incidents**

     Y70.8   Miscellaneous anesthesiology devices associated with adverse incidents, not elsewhere classified

✓4ᵗʰ **Y71**   **Cardiovascular** **devices associated with adverse incidents**

     Y71.0   Diagnostic and monitoring **cardiovascular devices associated with adverse incidents**

     Y71.1   Therapeutic (nonsurgical) and rehabilitative **cardiovascular devices associated with adverse incidents**

     Y71.2   Prosthetic and other implants, **materials and accessory cardiovascular devices associated with adverse incidents**

     Y71.3   Surgical instruments, **materials and cardiovascular devices (including sutures) associated with adverse incidents**

     Y71.8   Miscellaneous cardiovascular devices associated with adverse incidents, not elsewhere classified

✓4ᵗʰ **Y72**   **Otorhinolaryngological** **devices associated with adverse incidents**

     Y72.0   Diagnostic and monitoring **otorhinolaryngological devices associated with adverse incidents**

     Y72.1   Therapeutic (nonsurgical) and rehabilitative **otorhinolaryngological devices associated with adverse incidents**

     Y72.2   Prosthetic and other implants, **materials and accessory otorhinolaryngological devices associated with adverse incidents**

     Y72.3   Surgical instruments, **materials and otorhinolaryngological devices (including sutures) associated with adverse incidents**

     Y72.8   Miscellaneous otorhinolaryngological devices associated with adverse incidents, not elsewhere classified

✓4ᵗʰ **Y73**   **Gastroenterology and urology** **devices associated with adverse incidents**

     Y73.0   Diagnostic and monitoring **gastroenterology and urology devices associated with adverse incidents**

     Y73.1   Therapeutic (nonsurgical) and rehabilitative **gastroenterology and urology devices associated with adverse incidents**

     Y73.2   Prosthetic and other implants, **materials and accessory gastroenterology and urology devices associated with adverse incidents**

     Y73.3   Surgical instruments, **materials and gastroenterology and urology devices (including sutures) associated with adverse incidents**

     Y73.8   Miscellaneous gastroenterology and urology devices associated with adverse incidents, not elsewhere classified

✓4ᵗʰ **Y74**   **General hospital** **and personal-use devices associated with adverse incidents**

     Y74.0   Diagnostic and monitoring **general hospital and personal-use devices associated with adverse incidents**

     Y74.1   Therapeutic (nonsurgical) and rehabilitative **general hospital and personal-use devices associated with adverse incidents**

     Y74.2   Prosthetic and other implants, **materials and accessory general hospital and personal-use devices associated with adverse incidents**

     Y74.3   Surgical instruments, **materials and general hospital and personal-use devices (including sutures) associated with adverse incidents**

     Y74.8   Miscellaneous general hospital and personal-use devices associated with adverse incidents, not elsewhere classified

✓4ᵗʰ **Y75**   **Neurological** **devices associated with adverse incidents**

     Y75.0   Diagnostic and monitoring **neurological devices associated with adverse incidents**

     Y75.1   Therapeutic (nonsurgical) and rehabilitative **neurological devices associated with adverse incidents**

     Y75.2   Prosthetic and other implants, **materials and neurological devices associated with adverse incidents**

     Y75.3   Surgical instruments, **materials and neurological devices (including sutures) associated with adverse incidents**

     Y75.8   Miscellaneous neurological devices associated with adverse incidents, not elsewhere classified

✓4ᵗʰ **Y76**   **Obstetric and gynecological** **devices associated with adverse incidents**

     Y76.0   Diagnostic and monitoring **obstetric and gynecological devices associated with adverse incidents** ♀

     Y76.1   Therapeutic (nonsurgical) and rehabilitative **obstetric and gynecological devices associated with adverse incidents** ♀

     Y76.2   Prosthetic and other implants, **materials and accessory obstetric and gynecological devices associated with adverse incidents** ♀

     Y76.3   Surgical instruments, **materials and obstetric and gynecological devices (including sutures) associated with adverse incidents** ♀

     Y76.8   Miscellaneous obstetric and gynecological devices associated with adverse incidents, not elsewhere classified ♀

✓4ᵗʰ **Y77**   **Ophthalmic** **devices associated with adverse incidents**

     Y77.0   Diagnostic and monitoring **ophthalmic devices associated with adverse incidents**

     ✓5ᵗʰ **Y77.1**   Therapeutic (nonsurgical) and rehabilitative **ophthalmic devices associated with adverse incidents**
AHA: 2020,4Q,41

         Y77.11   Contact lens **associated with adverse incidents**
Rigid gas permeable contact lens associated with adverse incidents
Soft (hydrophilic) contact lens associated with adverse incidents

         Y77.19   **Other therapeutic (nonsurgical) and rehabilitative ophthalmic devices associated with adverse incidents**

     Y77.2   Prosthetic and other implants, **materials and accessory ophthalmic devices associated with adverse incidents**

     Y77.3   Surgical instruments, **materials and ophthalmic devices (including sutures) associated with adverse incidents**

Y77.8   Miscellaneous ophthalmic devices associated with adverse incidents, not elsewhere classified

☑4ᵗʰ Y78   Radiological devices associated with adverse incidents

Y78.0   Diagnostic and monitoring radiological devices associated with adverse incidents

Y78.1   Therapeutic (nonsurgical) and rehabilitative radiological devices associated with adverse incidents

Y78.2   Prosthetic and other implants, materials and accessory radiological devices associated with adverse incidents

Y78.3   Surgical instruments, materials and radiological devices (including sutures) associated with adverse incidents

Y78.8   Miscellaneous radiological devices associated with adverse incidents, not elsewhere classified

☑4ᵗʰ Y79   Orthopedic devices associated with adverse incidents

Y79.0   Diagnostic and monitoring orthopedic devices associated with adverse incidents

Y79.1   Therapeutic (nonsurgical) and rehabilitative orthopedic devices associated with adverse incidents

Y79.2   Prosthetic and other implants, materials and accessory orthopedic devices associated with adverse incidents

Y79.3   Surgical instruments, materials and orthopedic devices (including sutures) associated with adverse incidents

Y79.8   Miscellaneous orthopedic devices associated with adverse incidents, not elsewhere classified

☑4ᵗʰ Y80   Physical medicine devices associated with adverse incidents

Y80.0   Diagnostic and monitoring physical medicine devices associated with adverse incidents

Y80.1   Therapeutic (nonsurgical) and rehabilitative physical medicine devices associated with adverse incidents

Y80.2   Prosthetic and other implants, materials and accessory physical medicine devices associated with adverse incidents

Y80.3   Surgical instruments, materials and physical medicine devices (including sutures) associated with adverse incidents

Y80.8   Miscellaneous physical medicine devices associated with adverse incidents, not elsewhere classified

☑4ᵗʰ Y81   General- and plastic-surgery devices associated with adverse incidents

Y81.0   Diagnostic and monitoring general- and plastic-surgery devices associated with adverse incidents

Y81.1   Therapeutic (nonsurgical) and rehabilitative general- and plastic-surgery devices associated with adverse incidents

Y81.2   Prosthetic and other implants, materials and accessory general- and plastic-surgery devices associated with adverse incidents

Y81.3   Surgical instruments, materials and general- and plastic-surgery devices (including sutures) associated with adverse incidents

Y81.8   Miscellaneous general- and plastic-surgery devices associated with adverse incidents, not elsewhere classified

☑4ᵗʰ Y82   Other and unspecified medical devices associated with adverse incidents

Y82.8   Other medical devices associated with adverse incidents

Y82.9   Unspecified medical devices associated with adverse incidents

Surgical and other medical procedures as the cause of abnormal reaction of the patient, or of later complication, without mention of misadventure at the time of the procedure (Y83-Y84)

EXCLUDES 1   misadventures to patients during surgical and medical care, classifiable to (Y62-Y69)

EXCLUDES 2   breakdown or malfunctioning of medical device (during procedure) (after implantation) (ongoing use) (Y70-Y82)

☑4ᵗʰ Y83   Surgical operation and other surgical procedures as the cause of abnormal reaction of the patient, or of later complication, without mention of misadventure at the time of the procedure

Y83.0   Surgical operation with transplant of whole organ as the cause of abnormal reaction of the patient, or of later complication, without mention of misadventure at the time of the procedure

Y83.1   Surgical operation with implant of artificial internal device as the cause of abnormal reaction of the patient, or of later complication, without mention of misadventure at the time of the procedure

Y83.2   Surgical operation with anastomosis, bypass or graft as the cause of abnormal reaction of the patient, or of later complication, without mention of misadventure at the time of the procedure

Y83.3   Surgical operation with formation of external stoma as the cause of abnormal reaction of the patient, or of later complication, without mention of misadventure at the time of the procedure

Y83.4   Other reconstructive surgery as the cause of abnormal reaction of the patient, or of later complication, without mention of misadventure at the time of the procedure

Y83.5   Amputation of limb(s) as the cause of abnormal reaction of the patient, or of later complication, without mention of misadventure at the time of the procedure

Y83.6   Removal of other organ (partial) (total) as the cause of abnormal reaction of the patient, or of later complication, without mention of misadventure at the time of the procedure

Y83.8   Other surgical procedures as the cause of abnormal reaction of the patient, or of later complication, without mention of misadventure at the time of the procedure

Y83.9   Surgical procedure, unspecified as the cause of abnormal reaction of the patient, or of later complication, without mention of misadventure at the time of the procedure

☑4ᵗʰ Y84   Other medical procedures as the cause of abnormal reaction of the patient, or of later complication, without mention of misadventure at the time of the procedure

Y84.0   Cardiac catheterization as the cause of abnormal reaction of the patient, or of later complication, without mention of misadventure at the time of the procedure

Y84.1   Kidney dialysis as the cause of abnormal reaction of the patient, or of later complication, without mention of misadventure at the time of the procedure

Y84.2   Radiological procedure and radiotherapy as the cause of abnormal reaction of the patient, or of later complication, without mention of misadventure at the time of the procedure

     AHA: 2019,1Q,21; 2017,1Q,33

Y84.3   Shock therapy as the cause of abnormal reaction of the patient, or of later complication, without mention of misadventure at the time of the procedure

Y84.4   Aspiration of fluid as the cause of abnormal reaction of the patient, or of later complication, without mention of misadventure at the time of the procedure

Y84.5   Insertion of gastric or duodenal sound as the cause of abnormal reaction of the patient, or of later complication, without mention of misadventure at the time of the procedure

Y84.6   Urinary catheterization as the cause of abnormal reaction of the patient, or of later complication, without mention of misadventure at the time of the procedure

Y84.7   Blood-sampling as the cause of abnormal reaction of the patient, or of later complication, without mention of misadventure at the time of the procedure

Y84.8   Other medical procedures as the cause of abnormal reaction of the patient, or of later complication, without mention of misadventure at the time of the procedure

     AHA: 2021,1Q,5; 2014,4Q,24

Y84.9   Medical procedure, unspecified as the cause of abnormal reaction of the patient, or of later complication, without mention of misadventure at the time of the procedure

Supplementary factors related to causes of morbidity classified elsewhere (Y90-Y99)

NOTE   These categories may be used to provide supplementary information concerning causes of morbidity. They are not to be used for single-condition coding.

☑4ᵗʰ Y90   Evidence of alcohol involvement determined by blood alcohol level

Code first any associated alcohol related disorders (F10)

Y90.0   Blood alcohol level of less than 20 mg/100 ml

Y90.1   Blood alcohol level of 20-39 mg/100 ml

Y90.2   Blood alcohol level of 40-59 mg/100 ml

Y90.3   Blood alcohol level of 60-79 mg/100 ml

Y90.4   Blood alcohol level of 80-99 mg/100 ml

Y90.5   Blood alcohol level of 100-119 mg/100 ml

Y90.6   Blood alcohol level of 120-199 mg/100 ml

Y90.7   Blood alcohol level of 200-239 mg/100 ml

Y90.8   Blood alcohol level of 240 mg/100 ml or more

Y90.9   Presence of alcohol in blood, level not specified

☑ Additional Char Req   ✓x7ᵗʰ Placeholder   Unacceptable PDx   Questionable PDx   Wrong Procedure   Manifestation   Unspecified Dx   H1-H4 HAC   HCC CMS-HCC Dx   HIV HIV Dx

ICD-10-CM 2022   1223

☑️⁴ᵗʰ **Y92** **Place of occurrence of the external cause**

The following category is for use, when relevant, to identify the place of occurrence of the external cause. Use in conjunction with an activity code.

Place of occurrence should be recorded only at the initial encounter for treatment

☑️⁵ᵗʰ **Y92.0** **Non-institutional (private) residence** as the place of occurrence of the external cause

> EXCLUDES 1   *abandoned or derelict house (Y92.89)*
> *home under construction but not yet occupied (Y92.6-)*
> *institutional place of residence (Y92.1-)*

☑️⁶ᵗʰ **Y92.00** **Unspecified non-institutional (private) residence** as the place of occurrence of the external cause

Y92.000 **Kitchen** of unspecified non-institutional (private) residence as the place of occurrence of the external cause

Y92.001 **Dining room** of unspecified non-institutional (private) residence as the place of occurrence of the external cause

Y92.002 **Bathroom** of unspecified non-institutional (private) residence as the place of occurrence of the external cause

Y92.003 **Bedroom** of unspecified non-institutional (private) residence as the place of occurrence of the external cause

Y92.007 **Garden or yard** of unspecified non-institutional (private) residence as the place of occurrence of the external cause

Y92.008 **Other place** in unspecified non-institutional (private) residence as the place of occurrence of the external cause

Y92.009 **Unspecified place** in unspecified non-institutional (private) residence as the place of occurrence of the external cause

> Home (NOS) as the place of occurrence of the external cause

☑️⁶ᵗʰ **Y92.01** **Single-family non-institutional (private) house** as the place of occurrence of the external cause

> Farmhouse as the place of occurrence of the external cause

> EXCLUDES 1   *barn (Y92.71)*
> *chicken coop or hen house (Y92.72)*
> *farm field (Y92.73)*
> *orchard (Y92.74)*
> *single family mobile home or trailer (Y92.02-)*
> *slaughter house (Y92.86)*

Y92.010 **Kitchen** of single-family (private) house as the place of occurrence of the external cause

Y92.011 **Dining room** of single-family (private) house as the place of occurrence of the external cause

Y92.012 **Bathroom** of single-family (private) house as the place of occurrence of the external cause

Y92.013 **Bedroom** of single-family (private) house as the place of occurrence of the external cause

Y92.014 **Private driveway** to single-family (private) house as the place of occurrence of the external cause

Y92.015 **Private garage** of single-family (private) house as the place of occurrence of the external cause

Y92.016 **Swimming-pool** in single-family (private) house or garden as the place of occurrence of the external cause

Y92.017 **Garden or yard** in single-family (private) house as the place of occurrence of the external cause

Y92.018 **Other place** in single-family (private) house as the place of occurrence of the external cause

Y92.019 **Unspecified place** in single-family (private) house as the place of occurrence of the external cause

☑️⁶ᵗʰ **Y92.02** **Mobile home** as the place of occurrence of the external cause

Y92.020 **Kitchen** in mobile home as the place of occurrence of the external cause

Y92.021 **Dining room** in mobile home as the place of occurrence of the external cause

Y92.022 **Bathroom** in mobile home as the place of occurrence of the external cause

Y92.023 **Bedroom** in mobile home as the place of occurrence of the external cause

Y92.024 **Driveway** of mobile home as the place of occurrence of the external cause

Y92.025 **Garage** of mobile home as the place of occurrence of the external cause

Y92.026 **Swimming-pool** of mobile home as the place of occurrence of the external cause

Y92.027 **Garden or yard** of mobile home as the place of occurrence of the external cause

Y92.028 **Other place** in mobile home as the place of occurrence of the external cause

Y92.029 **Unspecified place** in mobile home as the place of occurrence of the external cause

☑️⁶ᵗʰ **Y92.03** **Apartment** as the place of occurrence of the external cause

> Condominium as the place of occurrence of the external cause
> Co-op apartment as the place of occurrence of the external cause

Y92.030 **Kitchen** in apartment as the place of occurrence of the external cause

Y92.031 **Bathroom** in apartment as the place of occurrence of the external cause

Y92.032 **Bedroom** in apartment as the place of occurrence of the external cause

Y92.038 **Other place** in apartment as the place of occurrence of the external cause

Y92.039 **Unspecified place** in apartment as the place of occurrence of the external cause

☑️⁶ᵗʰ **Y92.04** **Boarding-house** as the place of occurrence of the external cause

Y92.040 **Kitchen** in boarding-house as the place of occurrence of the external cause

Y92.041 **Bathroom** in boarding-house as the place of occurrence of the external cause

Y92.042 **Bedroom** in boarding-house as the place of occurrence of the external cause

Y92.043 **Driveway** of boarding-house as the place of occurrence of the external cause

Y92.044 **Garage** of boarding-house as the place of occurrence of the external cause

Y92.045 **Swimming-pool** of boarding-house as the place of occurrence of the external cause

Y92.046 **Garden or yard** of boarding-house as the place of occurrence of the external cause

Y92.048 **Other place** in boarding-house as the place of occurrence of the external cause

Y92.049 **Unspecified place** in boarding-house as the place of occurrence of the external cause

☑️⁶ᵗʰ **Y92.09** **Other non-institutional residence** as the place of occurrence of the external cause

> AHA: 2017,2Q,10

Y92.090 **Kitchen** in other non-institutional residence as the place of occurrence of the external cause

Y92.091 **Bathroom** in other non-institutional residence as the place of occurrence of the external cause

Y92.092 **Bedroom** in other non-institutional residence as the place of occurrence of the external cause

Y92.093 **Driveway** of other non-institutional residence as the place of occurrence of the external cause

Y92.094 **Garage** of other non-institutional residence as the place of occurrence of the external cause

Y92.095 **Swimming-pool** of other non-institutional residence as the place of occurrence of the external cause

Y92.096 **Garden or yard** of other non-institutional residence as the place of occurrence of the external cause

Ⓝ Newborn: 0   Ⓟ Pediatric: 0-17   Ⓜ Maternity: 9-64   Ⓐ Adult: 15-124   MCC Major Complication/Comorbidity   CC Complication/Comorbidity   SW Severe Wound Dx

1224   ICD-10-CM 2022

Y92.098 **Other place in other non-institutional residence** as the place of occurrence of the external cause

Y92.099 **Unspecified place in other non-institutional residence** as the place of occurrence of the external cause

√5ᵗʰ Y92.1 **Institutional (nonprivate) residence** as the place of occurrence of the external cause

Y92.10 **Unspecified residential institution** as the place of occurrence of the external cause

√6ᵗʰ Y92.11 **Children's home and orphanage** as the place of occurrence of the external cause

Y92.110 **Kitchen in children's home and orphanage** as the place of occurrence of the external cause

Y92.111 **Bathroom in children's home and orphanage** as the place of occurrence of the external cause

Y92.112 **Bedroom in children's home and orphanage** as the place of occurrence of the external cause

Y92.113 **Driveway of children's home and orphanage** as the place of occurrence of the external cause

Y92.114 **Garage of children's home and orphanage** as the place of occurrence of the external cause

Y92.115 **Swimming-pool of children's home and orphanage** as the place of occurrence of the external cause

Y92.116 **Garden or yard of children's home and orphanage** as the place of occurrence of the external cause

Y92.118 **Other place in children's home and orphanage** as the place of occurrence of the external cause

Y92.119 **Unspecified place in children's home and orphanage** as the place of occurrence of the external cause

√6ᵗʰ Y92.12 **Nursing home** as the place of occurrence of the external cause

Home for the sick as the place of occurrence of the external cause

Hospice as the place of occurrence of the external cause

AHA: 2017,2Q,10

Y92.120 **Kitchen in nursing home** as the place of occurrence of the external cause

Y92.121 **Bathroom in nursing home** as the place of occurrence of the external cause

Y92.122 **Bedroom in nursing home** as the place of occurrence of the external cause

Y92.123 **Driveway of nursing home** as the place of occurrence of the external cause

Y92.124 **Garage of nursing home** as the place of occurrence of the external cause

Y92.125 **Swimming-pool of nursing home** as the place of occurrence of the external cause

Y92.126 **Garden or yard of nursing home** as the place of occurrence of the external cause

Y92.128 **Other place in nursing home** as the place of occurrence of the external cause

Y92.129 **Unspecified place in nursing home** as the place of occurrence of the external cause

√6ᵗʰ Y92.13 **Military base** as the place of occurrence of the external cause

EXCLUDES 1 *military training grounds (Y92.84)*

Y92.130 **Kitchen on military base** as the place of occurrence of the external cause

Y92.131 **Mess hall on military base** as the place of occurrence of the external cause

Y92.133 **Barracks on military base** as the place of occurrence of the external cause

Y92.135 **Garage on military base** as the place of occurrence of the external cause

Y92.136 **Swimming-pool on military base** as the place of occurrence of the external cause

Y92.137 **Garden or yard on military base** as the place of occurrence of the external cause

Y92.138 **Other place on military base** as the place of occurrence of the external cause

Y92.139 **Unspecified place military base** as the place of occurrence of the external cause

√6ᵗʰ Y92.14 **Prison** as the place of occurrence of the external cause

Y92.140 **Kitchen in prison** as the place of occurrence of the external cause

Y92.141 **Dining room in prison** as the place of occurrence of the external cause

Y92.142 **Bathroom in prison** as the place of occurrence of the external cause

Y92.143 **Cell of prison** as the place of occurrence of the external cause

Y92.146 **Swimming-pool of prison** as the place of occurrence of the external cause

Y92.147 **Courtyard of prison** as the place of occurrence of the external cause

Y92.148 **Other place in prison** as the place of occurrence of the external cause

Y92.149 **Unspecified place in prison** as the place of occurrence of the external cause

√6ᵗʰ Y92.15 **Reform school** as the place of occurrence of the external cause

Y92.150 **Kitchen in reform school** as the place of occurrence of the external cause

Y92.151 **Dining room in reform school** as the place of occurrence of the external cause

Y92.152 **Bathroom in reform school** as the place of occurrence of the external cause

Y92.153 **Bedroom in reform school** as the place of occurrence of the external cause

Y92.154 **Driveway of reform school** as the place of occurrence of the external cause

Y92.155 **Garage of reform school** as the place of occurrence of the external cause

Y92.156 **Swimming-pool of reform school** as the place of occurrence of the external cause

Y92.157 **Garden or yard of reform school** as the place of occurrence of the external cause

Y92.158 **Other place in reform school** as the place of occurrence of the external cause

Y92.159 **Unspecified place in reform school** as the place of occurrence of the external cause

√6ᵗʰ Y92.16 **School dormitory** as the place of occurrence of the external cause

EXCLUDES 1 *reform school as the place of occurrence of the external cause (Y92.15-)*
school buildings and grounds as the place of occurrence of the external cause (Y92.2-)
school sports and athletic areas as the place of occurrence of the external cause (Y92.3-)

Y92.160 **Kitchen in school dormitory** as the place of occurrence of the external cause

Y92.161 **Dining room in school dormitory** as the place of occurrence of the external cause

Y92.162 **Bathroom in school dormitory** as the place of occurrence of the external cause

Y92.163 **Bedroom in school dormitory** as the place of occurrence of the external cause

Y92.168 **Other place in school dormitory** as the place of occurrence of the external cause

Y92.169 **Unspecified place in school dormitory** as the place of occurrence of the external cause

√6ᵗʰ Y92.19 **Other specified residential institution** as the place of occurrence of the external cause

AHA: 2017,2Q,10

Y92.190 **Kitchen in other specified residential institution** as the place of occurrence of the external cause

Y92.191 **Dining room in other specified residential institution** as the place of occurrence of the external cause

Y92.192 **Bathroom in other specified residential institution** as the place of occurrence of the external cause

Y92.193 **Bedroom in other specified residential institution** as the place of occurrence of the external cause

Y92.194 **Driveway of other specified residential institution** as the place of occurrence of the external cause

✓ Additional Char Req √x7ᵗʰ Placeholder Unacceptable PDx Questionable PDx Wrong Procedure Manifestation Unspecified Dx H1-H14 HAC HCC CMS-HCC Dx HIV HIV Dx

ICD-10-CM 2022   1225

Y92.195 Garage of other specified residential institution as the place of occurrence of the external cause

Y92.196 Pool of other specified residential institution as the place of occurrence of the external cause

Y92.197 Garden or yard of other specified residential institution as the place of occurrence of the external cause

Y92.198 Other place in other specified residential institution as the place of occurrence of the external cause

Y92.199 Unspecified place in other specified residential institution as the place of occurrence of the external cause

✓5ᵗʰ Y92.2 School, other institution and public administrative area as the place of occurrence of the external cause

Building and adjacent grounds used by the general public or by a particular group of the public

> *EXCLUDES 1* building under construction as the place of occurrence of the external cause (Y92.6)
> residential institution as the place of occurrence of the external cause (Y92.1)
> school dormitory as the place of occurrence of the external cause (Y92.16-)
> sports and athletics area of schools as the place of occurrence of the external cause (Y92.3-)

✓6ᵗʰ Y92.21 School (private) (public) (state) as the place of occurrence of the external cause

Y92.210 Daycare center as the place of occurrence of the external cause

Y92.211 Elementary school as the place of occurrence of the external cause
Kindergarten as the place of occurrence of the external cause

Y92.212 Middle school as the place of occurrence of the external cause

Y92.213 High school as the place of occurrence of the external cause
AHA: 2012,4Q,108

Y92.214 College as the place of occurrence of the external cause
University as the place of occurrence of the external cause

Y92.215 Trade school as the place of occurrence of the external cause

Y92.218 Other school as the place of occurrence of the external cause

Y92.219 Unspecified school as the place of occurrence of the external cause

Y92.22 Religious institution as the place of occurrence of the external cause
Church as the place of occurrence of the external cause
Mosque as the place of occurrence of the external cause
Synagogue as the place of occurrence of the external cause

✓6ᵗʰ Y92.23 Hospital as the place of occurrence of the external cause

> *EXCLUDES 1* ambulatory (outpatient) health services establishments (Y92.53-)
> home for the sick as the place of occurrence of the external cause (Y92.12-)
> hospice as the place of occurrence of the external cause (Y92.12-)
> nursing home as the place of occurrence of the external cause (Y92.12-)

Y92.230 Patient room in hospital as the place of occurrence of the external cause

Y92.231 Patient bathroom in hospital as the place of occurrence of the external cause

Y92.232 Corridor of hospital as the place of occurrence of the external cause

Y92.233 Cafeteria of hospital as the place of occurrence of the external cause

Y92.234 Operating room of hospital as the place of occurrence of the external cause

Y92.238 Other place in hospital as the place of occurrence of the external cause

Y92.239 Unspecified place in hospital as the place of occurrence of the external cause

✓6ᵗʰ Y92.24 Public administrative building as the place of occurrence of the external cause

Y92.240 Courthouse as the place of occurrence of the external cause

Y92.241 Library as the place of occurrence of the external cause

Y92.242 Post office as the place of occurrence of the external cause

Y92.243 City hall as the place of occurrence of the external cause

Y92.248 Other public administrative building as the place of occurrence of the external cause

✓6ᵗʰ Y92.25 Cultural building as the place of occurrence of the external cause

Y92.250 Art Gallery as the place of occurrence of the external cause

Y92.251 Museum as the place of occurrence of the external cause

Y92.252 Music hall as the place of occurrence of the external cause

Y92.253 Opera house as the place of occurrence of the external cause

Y92.254 Theater (live) as the place of occurrence of the external cause

Y92.258 Other cultural public building as the place of occurrence of the external cause

Y92.26 Movie house or cinema as the place of occurrence of the external cause

Y92.29 Other specified public building as the place of occurrence of the external cause
Assembly hall as the place of occurrence of the external cause
Clubhouse as the place of occurrence of the external cause

✓5ᵗʰ Y92.3 Sports and athletics area as the place of occurrence of the external cause

✓6ᵗʰ Y92.31 Athletic court as the place of occurrence of the external cause

> *EXCLUDES 1* tennis court in private home or garden (Y92.09)

Y92.310 Basketball court as the place of occurrence of the external cause

Y92.311 Squash court as the place of occurrence of the external cause

Y92.312 Tennis court as the place of occurrence of the external cause

Y92.318 Other athletic court as the place of occurrence of the external cause

✓6ᵗʰ Y92.32 Athletic field as the place of occurrence of the external cause

Y92.320 Baseball field as the place of occurrence of the external cause

Y92.321 Football field as the place of occurrence of the external cause

Y92.322 Soccer field as the place of occurrence of the external cause

Y92.328 Other athletic field as the place of occurrence of the external cause
Cricket field as the place of occurrence of the external cause
Hockey field as the place of occurrence of the external cause

✓6ᵗʰ Y92.33 Skating rink as the place of occurrence of the external cause

Y92.330 Ice skating rink (indoor) (outdoor) as the place of occurrence of the external cause

Y92.331 Roller skating rink as the place of occurrence of the external cause

Y92.34 Swimming pool (public) as the place of occurrence of the external cause

> *EXCLUDES 1* swimming pool in private home or garden (Y92.016)

Ⓝ Newborn: 0   Ⓟ Pediatric: 0-17   Ⓜ Maternity: 9-64   Ⓐ Adult: 15-124   **MCC** Major Complication/Comorbidity   **CC** Complication/Comorbidity   **SW** Severe Wound Dx

1226

ICD-10-CM 2022

Y92.39   **Other specified sports and athletic area as the place of occurrence of the external cause**

Golf-course as the place of occurrence of the external cause

Gymnasium as the place of occurrence of the external cause

Riding-school as the place of occurrence of the external cause

Stadium as the place of occurrence of the external cause

✓6ᵗʰ **Y92.4**   **Street, highway and other paved roadways as the place of occurrence of the external cause**

EXCLUDES 1   *private driveway of residence (Y92.014, Y92.024, Y92.043, Y92.093, Y92.113, Y92.123, Y92.154, Y92.194)*

   ✓6ᵗʰ **Y92.41**   **Street and highway as the place of occurrence of the external cause**

Y92.410   **Unspecified street and highway as the place of occurrence of the external cause**

Road NOS as the place of occurrence of the external cause

Y92.411   **Interstate highway as the place of occurrence of the external cause**

Freeway as the place of occurrence of the external cause

Motorway as the place of occurrence of the external cause

Y92.412   **Parkway as the place of occurrence of the external cause**

Y92.413   **State road as the place of occurrence of the external cause**

Y92.414   **Local residential or business street as the place of occurrence of the external cause**

Y92.415   **Exit ramp or entrance ramp of street or highway as the place of occurrence of the external cause**

   ✓6ᵗʰ **Y92.48**   **Other paved roadways as the place of occurrence of the external cause**

Y92.480   **Sidewalk as the place of occurrence of the external cause**

Y92.481   **Parking lot as the place of occurrence of the external cause**

Y92.482   **Bike path as the place of occurrence of the external cause**

Y92.488   **Other paved roadways as the place of occurrence of the external cause**

✓5ᵗʰ **Y92.5**   **Trade and service area as the place of occurrence of the external cause**

EXCLUDES 1   *garage in private home (Y92.015)*

schools and other public administration buildings (Y92.2-)

   ✓6ᵗʰ **Y92.51**   **Private commercial establishments as the place of occurrence of the external cause**

Y92.510   **Bank as the place of occurrence of the external cause**

Y92.511   **Restaurant or café as the place of occurrence of the external cause**

Y92.512   **Supermarket, store or market as the place of occurrence of the external cause**

Y92.513   **Shop (commercial) as the place of occurrence of the external cause**

   ✓6ᵗʰ **Y92.52**   **Service areas as the place of occurrence of the external cause**

Y92.520   **Airport as the place of occurrence of the external cause**

Y92.521   **Bus station as the place of occurrence of the external cause**

Y92.522   **Railway station as the place of occurrence of the external cause**

Y92.523   **Highway rest stop as the place of occurrence of the external cause**

Y92.524   **Gas station as the place of occurrence of the external cause**

Petroleum station as the place of occurrence of the external cause

Service station as the place of occurrence of the external cause

   ✓6ᵗʰ **Y92.53**   **Ambulatory health services establishments as the place of occurrence of the external cause**

Y92.530   **Ambulatory surgery center as the place of occurrence of the external cause**

Outpatient surgery center, including that connected with a hospital as the place of occurrence of the external cause

Same day surgery center, including that connected with a hospital as the place of occurrence of the external cause

Y92.531   **Health care provider office as the place of occurrence of the external cause**

Physician office as the place of occurrence of the external cause

Y92.532   **Urgent care center as the place of occurrence of the external cause**

Y92.538   **Other ambulatory health services establishments as the place of occurrence of the external cause**

AHA: 2019,1Q,21

Y92.59   **Other trade areas as the place of occurrence of the external cause**

Office building as the place of occurrence of the external cause

Casino as the place of occurrence of the external cause

Garage (commercial) as the place of occurrence of the external cause

Hotel as the place of occurrence of the external cause

Radio or television station as the place of occurrence of the external cause

Shopping mall as the place of occurrence of the external cause

Warehouse as the place of occurrence of the external cause

✓5ᵗʰ **Y92.6**   **Industrial and construction area as the place of occurrence of the external cause**

Y92.61   **Building [any] under construction as the place of occurrence of the external cause**

Y92.62   **Dock or shipyard as the place of occurrence of the external cause**

Dockyard as the place of occurrence of the external cause

Dry dock as the place of occurrence of the external cause

Shipyard as the place of occurrence of the external cause

Y92.63   **Factory as the place of occurrence of the external cause**

Factory building as the place of occurrence of the external cause

Factory premises as the place of occurrence of the external cause

Industrial yard as the place of occurrence of the external cause

Y92.64   **Mine or pit as the place of occurrence of the external cause**

Mine as the place of occurrence of the external cause

Y92.65   **Oil rig as the place of occurrence of the external cause**

Pit (coal) (gravel) (sand) as the place of occurrence of the external cause

Y92.69   **Other specified industrial and construction area as the place of occurrence of the external cause**

Gasworks as the place of occurrence of the external cause

Power-station (coal) (nuclear) (oil) as the place of occurrence of the external cause

Tunnel under construction as the place of occurrence of the external cause

Workshop as the place of occurrence of the external cause

✓5ᵗʰ **Y92.7**   **Farm as the place of occurrence of the external cause**

Ranch as the place of occurrence of the external cause

EXCLUDES 1   *farmhouse and home premises of farm (Y92.01-)*

Y92.71   **Barn as the place of occurrence of the external cause**

✓ Additional Char Req   ✓x7ᵗʰ Placeholder   Unacceptable PDx   Questionable PDx   Wrong Procedure   Manifestation   Unspecified Dx   H1-H14 HAC   HCC CMS-HCC Dx   HIV HIV Dx

ICD-10-CM 2022   1227

Y92.72 **Chicken coop** as the place of occurrence of the external cause
　Hen house as the place of occurrence of the external cause

Y92.73 **Farm field** as the place of occurrence of the external cause

Y92.74 **Orchard** as the place of occurrence of the external cause

Y92.79 **Other farm location** as the place of occurrence of the external cause

✓6ᵗʰ **Y92.8** **Other places** as the place of occurrence of the external cause

✓6ᵗʰ **Y92.81** **Transport vehicle** as the place of occurrence of the external cause
　EXCLUDES 1　transport accidents (V00-V99)

Y92.810 **Car** as the place of occurrence of the external cause

Y92.811 **Bus** as the place of occurrence of the external cause

Y92.812 **Truck** as the place of occurrence of the external cause

Y92.813 **Airplane** as the place of occurrence of the external cause

Y92.814 **Boat** as the place of occurrence of the external cause

Y92.815 **Train** as the place of occurrence of the external cause

Y92.816 **Subway** car as the place of occurrence of the external cause

Y92.818 **Other transport vehicle** as the place of occurrence of the external cause

✓6ᵗʰ **Y92.82** **Wilderness area**

Y92.820 **Desert** as the place of occurrence of the external cause

Y92.821 **Forest** as the place of occurrence of the external cause

Y92.828 **Other wilderness area** as the place of occurrence of the external cause
　Swamp as the place of occurrence of the external cause
　Mountain as the place of occurrence of the external cause
　Marsh as the place of occurrence of the external cause
　Prairie as the place of occurrence of the external cause

✓6ᵗʰ **Y92.83** **Recreation area** as the place of occurrence of the external cause

Y92.830 **Public park** as the place of occurrence of the external cause

Y92.831 **Amusement park** as the place of occurrence of the external cause

Y92.832 **Beach** as the place of occurrence of the external cause
　Seashore as the place of occurrence of the external cause

Y92.833 **Campsite** as the place of occurrence of the external cause

Y92.834 **Zoological garden (Zoo)** as the place of occurrence of the external cause

Y92.838 **Other recreation area** as the place of occurrence of the external cause

Y92.84 **Military training ground** as the place of occurrence of the external cause

Y92.85 **Railroad track** as the place of occurrence of the external cause

Y92.86 **Slaughter house** as the place of occurrence of the external cause

Y92.89 **Other specified places** as the place of occurrence of the external cause
　Derelict house as the place of occurrence of the external cause

Y92.9 **Unspecified place or not applicable**

✓4ᵗʰ **Y93** **Activity codes**

NOTE　Category Y93 is provided for use to indicate the activity of the person seeking healthcare for an injury or health condition, such as a heart attack while shoveling snow, which resulted from, or was contributed to, by the activity. These codes are appropriate for use for both acute injuries, such as those from chapter 19, and conditions that are due to the long-term, cumulative effects of an activity, such as those from chapter 13. They are also appropriate for use with external cause codes for cause and intent if identifying the activity provides additional information on the event. These codes should be used in conjunction with codes for external cause status (Y99) and place of occurrence (Y92).

This section contains the following broad activity categories:

Y93.0	Activities involving walking and running
Y93.1	Activities involving water and water craft
Y93.2	Activities involving ice and snow
Y93.3	Activities involving climbing, rappelling, and jumping off
Y93.4	Activities involving dancing and other rhythmic movement
Y93.5	Activities involving other sports and athletics played individually
Y93.6	Activities involving other sports and athletics played as a team or group
Y93.7	Activities involving other specified sports and athletics
Y93.A	Activities involving other cardiorespiratory exercise
Y93.B	Activities involving other muscle strengthening exercises
Y93.C	Activities involving computer technology and electronic devices
Y93.D	Activities involving arts and handcrafts
Y93.E	Activities involving personal hygiene and interior property and clothing maintenance
Y93.F	Activities involving caregiving
Y93.G	Activities involving food preparation, cooking and grilling
Y93.H	Activities involving exterior property and land maintenance, building and construction
Y93.I	Activities involving roller coasters and other types of external motion
Y93.J	Activities involving playing musical instrument
Y93.K	Activities involving animal care
Y93.8	Activities, other specified
Y93.9	Activity, unspecified

✓5ᵗʰ **Y93.0** **Activities involving walking and running**
　EXCLUDES 1　activity, walking an animal (Y93.K1)
　　activity, walking or running on a treadmill (Y93.A1)

Y93.01 **Activity, walking, marching and hiking**
　Activity, walking, marching and hiking on level or elevated terrain
　EXCLUDES 1　activity, mountain climbing (Y93.31)

Y93.02 **Activity, running**

✓5ᵗʰ **Y93.1** **Activities involving water and water craft**
　EXCLUDES 1　activities involving ice (Y93.2-)

Y93.11 **Activity, swimming**

Y93.12 **Activity, springboard and platform diving**

Y93.13 **Activity, water polo**

Y93.14 **Activity, water aerobics and water exercise**

Y93.15 **Activity, underwater diving and snorkeling**
　Activity, SCUBA diving

Y93.16 **Activity, rowing, canoeing, kayaking, rafting and tubing**
　Activity, canoeing, kayaking, rafting and tubing in calm and turbulent water

Y93.17 **Activity, water skiing and wake boarding**

Y93.18 **Activity, surfing, windsurfing and boogie boarding**
　Activity, water sliding

Y93.19 **Activity, other involving water and watercraft**
　Activity involving water NOS
　Activity, parasailing
　Activity, water survival training and testing

✓5ᵗʰ Y93.2 Activities involving ice and snow
> EXCLUDES 1   *activity, shoveling ice and snow (Y93.H1)*

Y93.21 Activity, ice skating
Activity, figure skating (singles) (pairs)
Activity, ice dancing
> EXCLUDES 1   *activity, ice hockey (Y93.22)*

Y93.22 Activity, ice hockey

Y93.23 Activity, snow (alpine) (downhill) skiing, snowboarding, sledding, tobogganing and snow tubing
> EXCLUDES 1   *activity, cross country skiing (Y93.24)*

Y93.24 Activity, cross country skiing
Activity, nordic skiing

Y93.29 Activity, other involving ice and snow
Activity involving ice and snow NOS

✓5ᵗʰ Y93.3 Activities involving climbing, rappelling and jumping off
> EXCLUDES 1   *activity, hiking on level or elevated terrain (Y93.01)*
> *activity, jumping rope (Y93.56)*
> *activity, trampoline jumping (Y93.44)*

Y93.31 Activity, mountain climbing, rock climbing and wall climbing

Y93.32 Activity, rappelling

Y93.33 Activity, BASE jumping
Activity, Building, Antenna, Span, Earth jumping

Y93.34 Activity, bungee jumping

Y93.35 Activity, hang gliding

Y93.39 Activity, other involving climbing, rappelling and jumping off

✓5ᵗʰ Y93.4 Activities involving dancing and other rhythmic movement
> EXCLUDES 1   *activity, martial arts (Y93.75)*

Y93.41 Activity, dancing
AHA: 2012,4Q,108

Y93.42 Activity, yoga

Y93.43 Activity, gymnastics
Activity, rhythmic gymnastics
> EXCLUDES 1   *activity, trampolining (Y93.44)*

Y93.44 Activity, trampolining

Y93.45 Activity, cheerleading

Y93.49 Activity, other involving dancing and other rhythmic movements

✓5ᵗʰ Y93.5 Activities involving other sports and athletics played individually
> EXCLUDES 1   *activity, dancing (Y93.41)*
> *activity, gymnastic (Y93.43)*
> *activity, trampolining (Y93.44)*
> *activity, yoga (Y93.42)*

Y93.51 Activity, roller skating (inline) and skateboarding

Y93.52 Activity, horseback riding

Y93.53 Activity, golf

Y93.54 Activity, bowling

Y93.55 Activity, bike riding

Y93.56 Activity, jumping rope

Y93.57 Activity, non-running track and field events
> EXCLUDES 1   *activity, running (any form) (Y93.02)*

Y93.59 Activity, other involving other sports and athletics played individually
> EXCLUDES 1   *activities involving climbing, rappelling, and jumping (Y93.3-)*
> *activities involving ice and snow (Y93.2-)*
> *activities involving walking and running (Y93.0-)*
> *activities involving water and watercraft (Y93.1-)*

✓5ᵗʰ Y93.6 Activities involving other sports and athletics played as a team or group
> EXCLUDES 1   *activity, ice hockey (Y93.22)*
> *activity, water polo (Y93.13)*

Y93.61 Activity, American tackle football
Activity, football NOS

Y93.62 Activity, American flag or touch football

Y93.63 Activity, rugby

Y93.64 Activity, baseball
Activity, softball

Y93.65 Activity, lacrosse and field hockey

Y93.66 Activity, soccer

Y93.67 Activity, basketball

Y93.68 Activity, volleyball (beach) (court)

Y93.6A Activity, physical games generally associated with school recess, summer camp and children
Activity, capture the flag
Activity, dodge ball
Activity, four square
Activity, kickball

Y93.69 Activity, other involving other sports and athletics played as a team or group
Activity, cricket

✓5ᵗʰ Y93.7 Activities involving other specified sports and athletics

Y93.71 Activity, boxing

Y93.72 Activity, wrestling

Y93.73 Activity, racquet and hand sports
Activity, handball
Activity, racquetball
Activity, squash
Activity, tennis

Y93.74 Activity, frisbee
Activity, ultimate frisbee

Y93.75 Activity, martial arts
Activity, combatives

Y93.79 Activity, other specified sports and athletics
> EXCLUDES 1   *sports and athletics activities specified in categories Y93.0-Y93.6*

✓5ᵗʰ Y93.A Activities involving other cardiorespiratory exercise
Activities involving physical training

Y93.A1 Activity, exercise machines primarily for cardiorespiratory conditioning
Activity, elliptical and stepper machines
Activity, stationary bike
Activity, treadmill

Y93.A2 Activity, calisthenics
Activity, jumping jacks
Activity, warm up and cool down

Y93.A3 Activity, aerobic and step exercise

Y93.A4 Activity, circuit training

Y93.A5 Activity, obstacle course
Activity, challenge course
Activity, confidence course

Y93.A6 Activity, grass drills
Activity, guerilla drills

Y93.A9 Activity, other involving cardiorespiratory exercise
> EXCLUDES 1   *activities involving cardiorespiratory exercise specified in categories Y93.0-Y93.7*

✓5ᵗʰ Y93.B Activities involving other muscle strengthening exercises

Y93.B1 Activity, exercise machines primarily for muscle strengthening

Y93.B2 Activity, push-ups, pull-ups, sit-ups

Y93.B3 Activity, free weights
Activity, barbells
Activity, dumbbells

Y93.B4 Activity, pilates

Y93.B9 Activity, other involving muscle strengthening exercises
> EXCLUDES 1   *activities involving muscle strengthening specified in categories Y93.0-Y93.A*

✓5ᵗʰ Y93.C Activities involving computer technology and electronic devices
> EXCLUDES 1   *activity, electronic musical keyboard or instruments (Y93.J-)*

Y93.C1 Activity, computer keyboarding
Activity, electronic game playing using keyboard or other stationary device

Y93.C2 Activity, hand held interactive electronic device
Activity, cellular telephone and communication device
Activity, electronic game playing using interactive device
> EXCLUDES 1   *activity, electronic game playing using keyboard or other stationary device (Y93.C1)*

Y93.C9 Activity, other involving computer technology and electronic devices

✓5ᵗʰ Y93.D Activities involving arts and handcrafts
> EXCLUDES 1   *activities involving playing musical instrument (Y93.J-)*

Y93.D1 Activity, knitting and crocheting

✓ Additional Char Req   ✓x7ᵗʰ Placeholder   <u>Unacceptable PDx</u>   Questionable PDx   Wrong Procedure   Manifestation   Unspecified Dx   H1-H4 HAC   HCC CMS-HCC Dx   HIV HIV Dx

ICD-10-CM 2022   1229

Chapter 20. External Causes of Morbidity

Y93.D2   **Activity,** sewing

Y93.D3   **Activity,** furniture building and finishing
Activity, furniture repair

Y93.D9   **Activity, other involving arts and handcrafts**

✓5ᵗʰ **Y93.E**   **Activities involving personal hygiene and interior property and clothing maintenance**

> *EXCLUDES 1*   *activities involving cooking and grilling (Y93.G-)*
> *activities involving exterior property and land maintenance, building and construction (Y93.H-)*
> *activities involving caregiving (Y93.F-)*
> *activity, dishwashing (Y93.G1)*
> *activity, food preparation (Y93.G1)*
> *activity, gardening (Y93.H2)*

Y93.E1   **Activity,** personal bathing and showering

Y93.E2   **Activity,** laundry

Y93.E3   **Activity,** vacuuming

Y93.E4   **Activity,** ironing

Y93.E5   **Activity,** floor mopping and cleaning

Y93.E6   **Activity,** residential relocation
Activity, packing up and unpacking involved in moving to a new residence

Y93.E8   **Activity, other personal hygiene**

Y93.E9   **Activity, other interior property and clothing maintenance**

✓5ᵗʰ **Y93.F**   **Activities involving** caregiving
Activity involving the provider of caregiving

Y93.F1   **Activity, caregiving,** bathing

Y93.F2   **Activity, caregiving,** lifting

Y93.F9   **Activity, other caregiving**

✓5ᵗʰ **Y93.G**   **Activities involving food preparation, cooking and grilling**

Y93.G1   **Activity,** food preparation and clean up
Activity, dishwashing

Y93.G2   **Activity,** grilling and smoking food

Y93.G3   **Activity,** cooking and baking
Activity, use of stove, oven and microwave oven

Y93.G9   **Activity, other involving cooking and grilling**

✓5ᵗʰ **Y93.H**   **Activities involving exterior property and land maintenance, building and construction**

Y93.H1   **Activity,** digging, shoveling and raking
Activity, dirt digging
Activity, raking leaves
Activity, snow shoveling

Y93.H2   **Activity,** gardening and landscaping
Activity, pruning, trimming shrubs, weeding

Y93.H3   **Activity,** building and construction

Y93.H9   **Activity, other involving exterior property and land maintenance, building and construction**

✓5ᵗʰ **Y93.I**   **Activities involving roller coasters and other types of external motion**

Y93.I1   **Activity,** rollercoaster riding

Y93.I9   **Activity, other involving external motion**

✓5ᵗʰ **Y93.J**   **Activities involving playing musical instrument**
Activity involving playing electric musical instrument

Y93.J1   **Activity,** piano **playing**
Activity, musical keyboard (electronic) playing

Y93.J2   **Activity,** drum and other percussion instrument **playing**

Y93.J3   **Activity,** string instrument **playing**

Y93.J4   **Activity,** winds and brass instrument **playing**

✓5ᵗʰ **Y93.K**   **Activities involving animal care**

> *EXCLUDES 1*   *activity, horseback riding (Y93.52)*

Y93.K1   **Activity,** walking **an animal**

Y93.K2   **Activity,** milking **an animal**

Y93.K3   **Activity,** grooming and shearing **an animal**

Y93.K9   **Activity, other involving animal care**

✓5ᵗʰ **Y93.8**   **Activities, other specified**

Y93.81   **Activity,** refereeing **a sports activity**

Y93.82   **Activity,** spectator **at an event**

Y93.83   **Activity,** rough housing and horseplay

Y93.84   **Activity,** sleeping

Y93.85   **Activity,** choking game
Activity, blackout game
Activity, fainting game
Activity, pass out game
AHA: 2016,4Q,74-76

Y93.89   **Activity, other specified**

Y93.9   **Activity, unspecified**

Y95   **Nosocomial condition**
AHA: 2013,4Q,119

✓4ᵗʰ **Y99**   **External cause status**

> **NOTE**   A single code from category Y99 should be used in conjunction with the external cause code(s) assigned to a record to indicate the status of the person at the time the event occurred.

Y99.0   Civilian **activity done for income or pay**
Civilian activity done for financial or other compensation

> *EXCLUDES 1*   *military activity (Y99.1)*
> *volunteer activity (Y99.2)*

Y99.1   **Military** activity

> *EXCLUDES 1*   *activity of off duty military personnel (Y99.8)*

Y99.2   **Volunteer** activity

> *EXCLUDES 1*   *activity of child or other family member assisting in compensated work of other family member (Y99.8)*

Y99.8   **Other external cause status**
Activity NEC
Activity of child or other family member assisting in compensated work of other family member
Hobby not done for income
Leisure activity
Off-duty activity of military personnel
Recreation or sport not for income or while a student
Student activity

> *EXCLUDES 1*   *civilian activity done for income or compensation (Y99.0)*
> *military activity (Y99.1)*

AHA: 2012,4Q,108

Y99.9   **Unspecified external cause status**

Ⓝ Newborn: 0   Ⓟ Pediatric: 0-17   Ⓜ Maternity: 9-64   Ⓐ Adult: 15-124   **MCC** Major Complication/Comorbidity   **CC** Complication/Comorbidity   **SW** Severe Wound Dx

1230   ICD-10-CM 2022

Chapter 21. Factors Influencing Health Status and Contact with Health Services (Z00–Z99)

Chapter-specific Guidelines with Coding Examples

The chapter-specific guidelines from the ICD-10-CM Official Guidelines for Coding and Reporting have been provided below. Along with these guidelines are coding examples, contained in the shaded boxes, that have been developed to help illustrate the coding and/or sequencing guidance found in these guidelines.

Note: The chapter-specific guidelines provide additional information about the use of Z codes for specified encounters.

a. Use of Z Codes in any healthcare setting

Z codes are for use in any healthcare setting. Z codes may be used as either a first-listed (principal diagnosis code in the inpatient setting) or secondary code, depending on the circumstances of the encounter. Certain Z codes may only be used as first-listed or principal diagnosis.

> Patient with middle lobe lung cancer admitted for initiation of chemotherapy
>
> **Z51.11**   **Encounter for antineoplastic chemotherapy**
>
> **C34.2**   **Malignant neoplasm of middle lobe, bronchus or lung**
>
> *Explanation:* A Z code can be used as first-listed in this situation based on guidelines in this chapter as well as chapter 2, "Neoplasms."

b. Z Codes indicate a reason for an encounter *or provide additional information about a patient encounter*

Z codes are not procedure codes. A corresponding procedure code must accompany a Z code to describe any procedure performed.

c. Categories of Z Codes

1) Contact/exposure

Category Z20 indicates contact with, and suspected exposure to, communicable diseases. These codes are for patients who are suspected to have been exposed to a disease by close personal contact with an infected individual or are in an area where a disease is epidemic.

Category Z77, Other contact with and (suspected) exposures hazardous to health, indicates contact with and suspected exposures hazardous to health.

Contact/exposure codes may be used as a first-listed code to explain an encounter for testing, or, more commonly, as a secondary code to identify a potential risk.

2) Inoculations and vaccinations

Code Z23 is for encounters for inoculations and vaccinations. It indicates that a patient is being seen to receive a prophylactic inoculation against a disease. Procedure codes are required to identify the actual administration of the injection and the type(s) of immunizations given. Code Z23 may be used as a secondary code if the inoculation is given as a routine part of preventive health care, such as a well-baby visit.

3) Status

Status codes indicate that a patient is either a carrier of a disease or has the sequelae or residual of a past disease or condition. This includes such things as the presence of prosthetic or mechanical devices resulting from past treatment. A status code is informative, because the status may affect the course of treatment and its outcome. A status code is distinct from a history code. The history code indicates that the patient no longer has the condition.

A status code should not be used with a diagnosis code from one of the body system chapters, if the diagnosis code includes the information provided by the status code. For example, code Z94.1, Heart transplant status, should not be used with a code from subcategory T86.2, Complications of heart transplant. The status code does not provide additional information. The complication code indicates that the patient is a heart transplant patient.

For encounters for weaning from a mechanical ventilator, assign a code from subcategory J96.1, Chronic respiratory failure, followed by code Z99.11, Dependence on respirator [ventilator] status.

The status Z codes/categories are:

Z14   Genetic carrier

Genetic carrier status indicates that a person carries a gene, associated with a particular disease, which may be passed to offspring who may develop that disease. The person does not have the disease and is not at risk of developing the disease.

Z15   Genetic susceptibility to disease

Genetic susceptibility indicates that a person has a gene that increases the risk of that person developing the disease.

Codes from category Z15 should not be used as principal or first-listed codes. If the patient has the condition to which he/she is susceptible, and that condition is the reason for the encounter, the code for the current condition should be sequenced first. If the patient is being seen for follow-up after completed treatment for this condition, and the condition no longer exists, a follow-up code should be sequenced first, followed by the appropriate personal history and genetic susceptibility codes. If the purpose of the encounter is genetic counseling associated with procreative management, code Z31.5, Encounter for genetic counseling, should be assigned as the first-listed code, followed by a code from category Z15. Additional codes should be assigned for any applicable family or personal history.

Z16   Resistance to antimicrobial drugs

This code indicates that a patient has a condition that is resistant to antimicrobial drug treatment. Sequence the infection code first.

> Penicillin resistant streptococcus pneumoniae meningitis
>
> **G00.1**   **Pneumococcal meningitis**
>
> **Z16.11**   **Resistance to penicillins**
>
> *Explanation:* The status Z code is used to describe the presence of a drug-resistant organism that most likely altered how the meningitis was treated.

Z17   Estrogen receptor status

Z18   Retained foreign body fragments

Z19   Hormone sensitivity malignancy status

Z21   Asymptomatic HIV infection status

This code indicates that a patient has tested positive for HIV but has manifested no signs or symptoms of the disease.

Z22   Carrier of infectious disease

Carrier status indicates that a person harbors the specific organisms of a disease without manifest symptoms and is capable of transmitting the infection.

Z28.3   Underimmunization status

Z33.1   Pregnant state, incidental

This code is a secondary code only for use when the pregnancy is in no way complicating the reason for visit. Otherwise, a code from the obstetric chapter is required.

Z66   Do not resuscitate

This code may be used when it is documented by the provider that a patient is on do not resuscitate status at any time during the stay.

Z67   Blood type

Z68   Body mass index (BMI)

BMI codes should only be assigned when there is an associated, reportable diagnosis (such as obesity). Do not assign BMI codes during pregnancy.

See Section I.B.14 for BMI documentation by clinicians other than the patient's provider.

Z74.01   Bed confinement status

Z76.82   Awaiting organ transplant status

Z78   Other specified health status

Code Z78.1, Physical restraint status, may be used when it is documented by the provider that a patient has been put in restraints during the current encounter. Please note that this code should not be reported when it is documented by the provider that a patient is temporarily restrained during a procedure.

Z79   Long-term (current) drug therapy

Codes from this category indicate a patient's continuous use of a prescribed drug (including such things as aspirin therapy) for the long-term treatment of a condition or for prophylactic use. It is not for use for patients who have addictions to drugs. This subcategory is not for use of medications for detoxification or maintenance programs to prevent withdrawal symptoms (e.g., methadone maintenance for opiate dependence). Assign the appropriate code for the drug use, abuse, or dependence instead.

Assign a code from Z79 if the patient is receiving a medication for an extended period as a prophylactic measure (such as for the prevention of deep vein thrombosis) or as treatment of a chronic condition (such as arthritis) or a disease requiring a lengthy course of treatment (such as cancer). Do not assign a code from category Z79 for medication being administered for a brief period of time to treat an acute illness or injury (such as a course of antibiotics to treat acute bronchitis).

Z88   Allergy status to drugs, medicaments and biological substances

Except: Z88.9, Allergy status to unspecified drugs, medicaments and biological substances status

Z89   Acquired absence of limb

Z90   Acquired absence of organs, not elsewhere classified

Z91.0-   Allergy status, other than to drugs and biological substances

Z92.82   Status post administration of tPA (rtPA) in a different facility within the last 24 hours prior to admission to a current facility

Assign code Z92.82, Status post administration of tPA (rtPA) in a different facility within the last 24 hours prior to admission to current facility, as a secondary diagnosis when a patient is received by transfer into a facility and documentation indicates they were administered tissue plasminogen activator (tPA) within the last 24 hours prior to admission to the current facility.

This guideline applies even if the patient is still receiving the tPA at the time they are received into the current facility.

The appropriate code for the condition for which the tPA was administered (such as cerebrovascular disease or myocardial infarction) should be assigned first.

Code Z92.82 is only applicable to the receiving facility record and not to the transferring facility record.

Z93   Artificial opening status

Z94   Transplanted organ and tissue status

Z95   Presence of cardiac and vascular implants and grafts

Z96   Presence of other functional implants

Z97   Presence of other devices

Z98   Other postprocedural states

Assign code Z98.85, Transplanted organ removal status, to indicate that a transplanted organ has been previously removed. This code should not be assigned for the encounter in which the transplanted organ is removed. The complication necessitating removal of the transplant organ should be assigned for that encounter.

See section I.C19. for information on the coding of organ transplant complications.

Z99   Dependence on enabling machines and devices, not elsewhere classified

Note: Categories Z89-Z90 and Z93-Z99 are for use only if there are no complications or malfunctions of the organ or tissue replaced, the amputation site or the equipment on which the patient is dependent.

4) History (of)

There are two types of history Z codes, personal and family. Personal history codes explain a patient's past medical condition that no longer exists and is not receiving any treatment, but that has the potential for recurrence, and therefore may require continued monitoring.

Family history codes are for use when a patient has a family member(s) who has had a particular disease that causes the patient to be at higher risk of also contracting the disease.

Personal history codes may be used in conjunction with follow-up codes and family history codes may be used in conjunction with screening codes to explain the need for a test or procedure. History codes are also acceptable on any medical record regardless of the reason for visit. A history of an illness, even if no longer present, is important information that may alter the type of treatment ordered.

The reason for the encounter (for example, screening or counseling) should be sequenced first and the appropriate personal and/or family history code(s) should be assigned as additional diagnos(es).

The history Z code categories are:

Z80   Family history of primary malignant neoplasm

Z81   Family history of mental and behavioral disorders

Z82   Family history of certain disabilities and chronic diseases (leading to disablement)

Z83   Family history of other specific disorders

Z84   Family history of other conditions

Z85   Personal history of malignant neoplasm

Z86   Personal history of certain other diseases

Z87   Personal history of other diseases and conditions

Z91.4-   Personal history of psychological trauma, not elsewhere classified

Z91.5-   Personal history of self-harm

Z91.81   History of falling

Z91.82   Personal history of military deployment

Z92   Personal history of medical treatment

Except: Z92.0, Personal history of contraception

Except: Z92.82, Status post administration of tPA (rtPA) in a different facility within the last 24 hours prior to admission to a current facility

Patient has chronic lymphocytic leukemia for which the patient had previous chemotherapy and is now in remission

C91.11   Chronic lymphocytic leukemia of B-cell type in remission

Z92.21   Personal history of antineoplastic chemotherapy

Explanation: The personal history Z code is used to describe a secondary (supplementary) diagnosis to identify that this patient has had chemotherapy in the past.

5) Screening

Screening is the testing for disease or disease precursors in seemingly well individuals so that early detection and treatment can be provided for those who test positive for the disease (e.g., screening mammogram).

The testing of a person to rule out or confirm a suspected diagnosis because the patient has some sign or symptom is a diagnostic examination, not a screening. In these cases, the sign or symptom is used to explain the reason for the test.

A screening code may be a first-listed code if the reason for the visit is specifically the screening exam. It may also be used as an additional code if the screening is done during an office visit for other health problems. A screening code is not necessary if the screening is inherent to a routine examination, such as a pap smear done during a routine pelvic examination.

Should a condition be discovered during the screening then the code for the condition may be assigned as an additional diagnosis.

The Z code indicates that a screening exam is planned. A procedure code is required to confirm that the screening was performed.

The screening Z codes/categories:

Z11   Encounter for screening for infectious and parasitic diseases

Z12   Encounter for screening for malignant neoplasms

Z13   Encounter for screening for other diseases and disorders

Except: Z13.9, Encounter for screening, unspecified

Z36   Encounter for antenatal screening for mother

6) Observation

There are three observation Z code categories. They are for use in very limited circumstances when a person is being observed for a suspected condition that is ruled out. The observation codes are not for use if an injury or illness or any signs or symptoms related to the suspected condition are present. In such cases the diagnosis/symptom code is used with the corresponding external cause code.

The observation codes are primarily to be used as a principal/first-listed diagnosis. An observation code may be assigned as a secondary diagnosis code when the patient is being observed for a condition that is ruled out and is unrelated to the principal/first-listed diagnosis Also, when the principal diagnosis is required to be a code from category Z38, Liveborn infants according to place of birth and type of delivery, then a code from category Z05, Encounter for observation and evaluation of newborn for suspected diseases and conditions ruled out, is sequenced after the Z38

code. Additional codes may be used in addition to the observation code, but only if they are unrelated to the suspected condition being observed.

Codes from subcategory Z03.7, Encounter for suspected maternal and fetal conditions ruled out, may either be used as a first-listed or as an additional code assignment depending on the case. They are for use in very limited circumstances on a maternal record when an encounter is for a suspected maternal or fetal condition that is ruled out during that encounter (for example, a maternal or fetal condition may be suspected due to an abnormal test result). These codes should not be used when the condition is confirmed. In those cases, the confirmed condition should be coded. In addition, these codes are not for use if an illness or any signs or symptoms related to the suspected condition or problem are present. In such cases the diagnosis/symptom code is used.

Additional codes may be used in addition to the code from subcategory Z03.7, but only if they are unrelated to the suspected condition being evaluated.

Codes from subcategory Z03.7 may not be used for encounters for antenatal screening of mother. *See Section I.C.21. Screening.*

For encounters for suspected fetal condition that are inconclusive following testing and evaluation, assign the appropriate code from category O35, O36, O40 or O41.

The observation Z code categories:

Z03	Encounter for medical observation for suspected diseases and conditions ruled out
Z04	Encounter for examination and observation for other reasons
	Except: Z04.9, Encounter for examination and observation for unspecified reason
Z05	Encounter for observation and evaluation of newborn for suspected diseases and conditions ruled out

> Upon initial examination, a heart murmur was heard in a newborn infant delivered vaginally in the hospital; however, after further observation, any serious cardiac conditions were ruled out.
>
> **Z38.00**   **Single liveborn infant, delivered vaginally**
>
> **Z05.0**   **Observation and evaluation of newborn for suspected cardiac condition ruled out**
>
> *Explanation:* Normally an observation code is used as the principal diagnosis except when the patient is a newborn. A code from category Z38 Liveborn infants according to place of birth and type of delivery code would be sequenced first, followed by the encounter for observation and evaluation of newborn for suspected diseases and conditions ruled out.

7) Aftercare

Aftercare visit codes cover situations when the initial treatment of a disease has been performed and the patient requires continued care during the healing or recovery phase, or for the long-term consequences of the disease. The aftercare Z code should not be used if treatment is directed at a current, acute disease. The diagnosis code is to be used in these cases. Exceptions to this rule are codes Z51.0, Encounter for antineoplastic radiation therapy, and codes from subcategory Z51.1, Encounter for antineoplastic chemotherapy and immunotherapy. These codes are to be first listed, followed by the diagnosis code when a patient's encounter is solely to receive radiation therapy, chemotherapy, or immunotherapy for the treatment of a neoplasm. If the reason for the encounter is more than one type of antineoplastic therapy, code Z51.0 and a code from subcategory Z51.1 may be assigned together, in which case one of these codes would be reported as a secondary diagnosis.

The aftercare Z codes should also not be used for aftercare for injuries. For aftercare of an injury, assign the acute injury code with the appropriate 7th character (for subsequent encounter).

The aftercare codes are generally first listed to explain the specific reason for the encounter. An aftercare code may be used as an additional code when some type of aftercare is provided in addition to the reason for admission and no diagnosis code is applicable. An example of this would be the closure of a colostomy during an encounter for treatment of another condition.

Aftercare codes should be used in conjunction with other aftercare codes or diagnosis codes to provide better detail on the specifics of an aftercare encounter visit, unless otherwise directed by the classification. The sequencing of multiple aftercare codes depends on the circumstances of the encounter.

Certain aftercare Z code categories need a secondary diagnosis code to describe the resolving condition or sequelae. For others, the condition is included in the code title.

Additional Z code aftercare category terms include fitting and adjustment, and attention to artificial openings.

Status Z codes may be used with aftercare Z codes to indicate the nature of the aftercare. For example code Z95.1, Presence of aortocoronary bypass graft, may be used with code Z48.812, Encounter for surgical aftercare following surgery on the circulatory system, to indicate the surgery for which the aftercare is being performed. A status code should not be used when the aftercare code indicates the type of status, such as using Z43.0, Encounter for attention to tracheostomy, with Z93.0, Tracheostomy status.

The aftercare Z category/codes:

Z42	Encounter for plastic and reconstructive surgery following medical procedure or healed injury
Z43	Encounter for attention to artificial openings
Z44	Encounter for fitting and adjustment of external prosthetic device
Z45	Encounter for adjustment and management of implanted device
Z46	Encounter for fitting and adjustment of other devices
Z47	Orthopedic aftercare
Z48	Encounter for other postprocedural aftercare
Z49	Encounter for care involving renal dialysis
Z51	Encounter for other aftercare and medical care

8) Follow-up

The follow-up codes are used to explain continuing surveillance following completed treatment of a disease, condition, or injury. They imply that the condition has been fully treated and no longer exists. They should not be confused with aftercare codes, or injury codes with a 7th character for subsequent encounter, that explain ongoing care of a healing condition or its sequelae. Follow-up codes may be used in conjunction with history codes to provide the full picture of the healed condition and its treatment. The follow-up code is sequenced first, followed by the history code.

A follow-up code may be used to explain multiple visits. Should a condition be found to have recurred on the follow-up visit, then the diagnosis code for the condition should be assigned in place of the follow-up code.

The follow-up Z code categories:

Z08	Encounter for follow-up examination after completed treatment for malignant neoplasm
Z09	Encounter for follow-up examination after completed treatment for conditions other than malignant neoplasm
Z39	Encounter for maternal postpartum care and examination

9) Donor

Codes in category Z52, Donors of organs and tissues, are used for living individuals who are donating blood or other body tissue. These codes are for individuals donating for others, **as well as** for self-donations. They are not used to identify cadaveric donations.

10) Counseling

Counseling Z codes are used when a patient or family member receives assistance in the aftermath of an illness or injury, or when support is required in coping with family or social problems.

The counseling Z codes/categories:

Z30.0-	Encounter for general counseling and advice on contraception
Z31.5	Encounter for procreative genetic counseling
Z31.6-	Encounter for general counseling and advice on procreation
Z32.2	Encounter for childbirth instruction
Z32.3	Encounter for childcare instruction
Z69	Encounter for mental health services for victim and perpetrator of abuse
Z70	Counseling related to sexual attitude, behavior and orientation
Z71	Persons encountering health services for other counseling and medical advice, not elsewhere classified
	Note: Code Z71.84, Encounter for health counseling related to travel, is to be used for health risk and safety counseling for future travel purposes.
	Code Z71.85, Encounter for immunization safety counseling, is to be used for counseling of the patient or caregiver regarding the safety of a vaccine. This code should not be used for the provision of general information regarding risks and potential side effects during routine encounters for the administration of vaccines.
Z76.81	Expectant mother prebirth pediatrician visit

11) Encounters for obstetrical and reproductive services

See Section I.C.15. Pregnancy, Childbirth, and the Puerperium, for further instruction on the use of these codes.

Z codes for pregnancy are for use in those circumstances when none of the problems or complications included in the codes from the Obstetrics chapter exist (a routine prenatal visit or postpartum care). Codes in category Z34, Encounter for supervision of normal pregnancy, are always first listed and are not to be used with any other code from the OB chapter.

Codes in category Z3A, Weeks of gestation, may be assigned to provide additional information about the pregnancy. Category Z3A codes should not be assigned for pregnancies with abortive outcomes (categories O00-O08), elective termination of pregnancy (code Z33.2), nor for postpartum conditions, as category Z3A is not applicable to these conditions. The date of the admission should be used to determine weeks of gestation for inpatient admissions that encompass more than one gestational week.

The outcome of delivery, category Z37, should be included on all maternal delivery records. It is always a secondary code.

Codes in category Z37 should not be used on the newborn record.

Z codes for family planning (contraceptive) or procreative management and counseling should be included on an obstetric record either during the pregnancy or the postpartum stage, if applicable.

Z codes/categories for obstetrical and reproductive services:

Z30	Encounter for contraceptive management
Z31	Encounter for procreative management
Z32.2	Encounter for childbirth instruction
Z32.3	Encounter for childcare instruction
Z33	Pregnant state
Z34	Encounter for supervision of normal pregnancy
Z36	Encounter for antenatal screening of mother
Z3A	Weeks of gestation
Z37	Outcome of delivery
Z39	Encounter for maternal postpartum care and examination
Z76.81	Expectant mother prebirth pediatrician visit

12) Newborns and infants

See Section I.C.16. Newborn (Perinatal) Guidelines, for further instruction on the use of these codes.

Newborn Z codes/categories:

Z76.1	Encounter for health supervision and care of foundling
Z00.1-	Encounter for routine child health examination
Z38	Liveborn infants according to place of birth and type of delivery

13) Routine and administrative examinations

The Z codes allow for the description of encounters for routine examinations, such as, a general check-up, or, examinations for administrative purposes, such as, a pre-employment physical. The codes are not to be used if the examination is for diagnosis of a suspected condition or for treatment purposes. In such cases the diagnosis code is used. During a routine exam, should a diagnosis or condition be discovered, it should be coded as an additional code. Pre-existing and chronic conditions and history codes may also be included as additional codes as long as the examination is for administrative purposes and not focused on any particular condition.

Some of the codes for routine health examinations distinguish between "with" and "without" abnormal findings. Code assignment depends on the information that is known at the time the encounter is being coded. For example, if no abnormal findings were found during the examination, but the encounter is being coded before test results are back, it is acceptable to assign the code for "without abnormal findings." When assigning a code for "with abnormal findings," additional code(s) should be assigned to identify the specific abnormal finding(s).

Pre-operative examination and pre-procedural laboratory examination Z codes are for use only in those situations when a patient is being cleared for a procedure or surgery and no treatment is given.

The Z codes/categories for routine and administrative examinations:

Z00	Encounter for general examination without complaint, suspected or reported diagnosis
Z01	Encounter for other special examination without complaint, suspected or reported diagnosis
Z02	Encounter for administrative examination
	Except: Z02.9, Encounter for administrative examinations, unspecified
Z32.0-	Encounter for pregnancy test

14) Miscellaneous Z codes

The miscellaneous Z codes capture a number of other health care encounters that do not fall into one of the other categories. **Some** of these codes identify the reason for the encounter; others are for use as additional codes that provide useful information on circumstances that may affect a patient's care and treatment.

Prophylactic organ removal

For encounters specifically for prophylactic removal of an organ (such as prophylactic removal of breasts due to a genetic susceptibility to cancer or a family history of cancer), the principal or first-listed code should be a code from category Z40, Encounter for prophylactic surgery, followed by the appropriate codes to identify the associated risk factor (such as genetic susceptibility or family history).

If the patient has a malignancy of one site and is having prophylactic removal at another site to prevent either a new primary malignancy or metastatic disease, a code for the malignancy should also be assigned in addition to a code from subcategory Z40.0, Encounter for prophylactic surgery for risk factors related to malignant neoplasms. A Z40.0 code should not be assigned if the patient is having organ removal for treatment of a malignancy, such as the removal of the testes for the treatment of prostate cancer.

Female patient with cancer in lower inner quadrant of right breast and positive BRCA 1 noted on testing is admitted for mastectomy of right breast and prophylactic removal of left breast

C50.311	**Malignant neoplasm of lower-inner quadrant of right female breast**
Z40.01	**Encounter for prophylactic removal of breast**
Z15.01	**Genetic susceptibility to malignant neoplasm of breast**

Explanation: Removal of the current neoplastic disease in the right breast was the focus of treatment for this admission and is sequenced first. The removal of the left breast was not required to treat a current disease process but as a means of prevention. The two Z codes are informational; they capture the reason behind the removal of what is currently a healthy left breast.

Miscellaneous Z codes/categories:

Z28	Immunization not carried out
	Except: Z28.3, Underimmunization status
Z29	Encounter for other prophylactic measures
Z40	Encounter for prophylactic surgery
Z41	Encounter for procedures for purposes other than remedying health state
	Except: Z41.9, Encounter for procedure for purposes other than remedying health state, unspecified
Z53	Persons encountering health services for specific procedures and treatment, not carried out
Z72	Problems related to lifestyle
	Note: These codes should be assigned only when the documentation specifies that the patient has an associated problem
Z73	Problems related to life management difficulty
Z74	Problems related to care provider dependency
	Except: Z74.01, Bed confinement status
Z75	Problems related to medical facilities and other health care
Z76.0	Encounter for issue of repeat prescription
Z76.3	Healthy person accompanying sick person
Z76.4	Other boarder to healthcare facility
Z76.5	Malingerer [conscious simulation]
Z91.1-	Patient's noncompliance with medical treatment and regimen
Z91.83	Wandering in diseases classified elsewhere
Z91.84-	Oral health risk factors
Z91.89	Other specified personal risk factors, not elsewhere classified

See Section I.B.14 for Z55-Z65 Persons with potential health hazards related to socioeconomic and psychosocial circumstances, documentation by clinicians other than the patient's provider

15) Nonspecific Z codes

Certain Z codes are so non-specific, or potentially redundant with other codes in the classification, that there can be little justification for their use in the inpatient setting. Their use in the outpatient setting should be limited to those instances when there is no further documentation to

permit more precise coding. Otherwise, any sign or symptom or any other reason for visit that is captured in another code should be used.

Nonspecific Z codes/categories:

Z02.9	Encounter for administrative examinations, unspecified
Z04.9	Encounter for examination and observation for unspecified reason
Z13.9	Encounter for screening, unspecified
Z41.9	Encounter for procedure for purposes other than remedying health state, unspecified
Z52.9	Donor of unspecified organ or tissue
Z86.59	Personal history of other mental and behavioral disorders
Z88.9	Allergy status to unspecified drugs, medicaments and biological substances status
Z92.0	Personal history of contraception

16) Z codes that may only be principal/first-listed diagnosis

The following Z codes/categories may only be reported as the principal/first-listed diagnosis, except when there are multiple encounters on the same day and the medical records for the encounters are combined:

Z00	Encounter for general examination without complaint, suspected or reported diagnosis
	Except: Z00.6
Z01	Encounter for other special examination without complaint, suspected or reported diagnosis
Z02	Encounter for administrative examination
Z04	Encounter for examination and observation for other reasons
Z33.2	Encounter for elective termination of pregnancy
Z31.81	Encounter for male factor infertility in female patient
Z31.83	Encounter for assisted reproductive fertility procedure cycle
Z31.84	Encounter for fertility preservation procedure
Z34	Encounter for supervision of normal pregnancy
Z39	Encounter for maternal postpartum care and examination
Z38	Liveborn infants according to place of birth and type of delivery
Z40	Encounter for prophylactic surgery
Z42	Encounter for plastic and reconstructive surgery following medical procedure or healed injury
Z51.0	Encounter for antineoplastic radiation therapy
Z51.1-	Encounter for antineoplastic chemotherapy and immunotherapy
Z52	Donors of organs and tissues
	Except: Z52.9, Donor of unspecified organ or tissue
Z76.1	Encounter for health supervision and care of foundling
Z76.2	Encounter for health supervision and care of other healthy infant and child
Z99.12	Encounter for respirator [ventilator] dependence during power failure

17) Social determinants of health

Codes describing social determinants of health (SDOH) should be assigned when this information is documented.

For social determinants of health, such as information found in categories Z55-Z65, Persons with potential health hazards related to socioeconomic and psychosocial circumstances, code assignment may be based on medical record documentation from clinicians involved in the care of the patient who are not the patient's provider since this information represents social information, rather than medical diagnoses.

For example, coding professionals may utilize documentation of social information from social workers, community health workers, case managers, or nurses, if their documentation is included in the official medical record.

Patient self-reported documentation may be used to assign codes for social determinants of health, as long as the patient self-reported information is signed-off by and incorporated into the medical record by either a clinician or provider.

Social determinants of health codes are located primarily in these Z code categories:

Z55	**Problems related to education and literacy**
Z56	**Problems related to employment and unemployment**
Z57	**Occupational exposure to risk factors**
Z58	**Problems related to physical environment**
Z59	**Problems related to housing and economic circumstances**
Z60	**Problems related to social environment**
Z62	**Problems related to upbringing**
Z63	**Other problems related to primary support group, including family circumstances**
Z64	**Problems related to certain psychosocial circumstances**
Z65	**Problems related to other psychosocial circumstances**

See Section I.B.14. Documentation by Clinicians Other than the Patient's Provider.

Chapter 21. Factors Influencing Health Status and Contact With Health Services (Z00-Z99)

NOTE   Z codes represent reasons for encounters. A corresponding procedure code must accompany a Z code if a procedure is performed. Categories Z00-Z99 are provided for occasions when circumstances other than a disease, injury or external cause classifiable to categories A00-Y89 are recorded as "diagnoses" or "problems." This can arise in two main ways:

(a) When a person who may or may not be sick encounters the health services for some specific purpose, such as to receive limited care or service for a current condition, to donate an organ or tissue, to receive prophylactic vaccination (immunization), or to discuss a problem which is in itself not a disease or injury.

(b) When some circumstance or problem is present which influences the person's health status but is not in itself a current illness or injury.

AHA: 2018,4Q,60-61

This chapter contains the following blocks:

Z00-Z13   Persons encountering health services for examinations
Z14-Z15   Genetic carrier and genetic susceptibility to disease
Z16   Resistance to antimicrobial drugs
Z17   Estrogen receptor status
Z18   Retained foreign body fragments
Z19   Hormone sensitivity malignancy status
Z20-Z29   Persons with potential health hazards related to communicable diseases
Z30-Z39   Persons encountering health services in circumstances related to reproduction
Z40-Z53   Encounters for other specific health care
Z55-Z65   Persons with potential health hazards related to socioeconomic and psychosocial circumstances
Z66   Do not resuscitate status
Z67   Blood type
Z68   Body mass index (BMI)
Z69-Z76   Persons encountering health services in other circumstances
Z77-Z99   Persons with potential health hazards related to family and personal history and certain conditions influencing health status

Persons encountering health services for examinations (Z00-Z13)

NOTE   Nonspecific abnormal findings disclosed at the time of these examinations are classified to categories R70-R94.

EXCLUDES 1   examinations related to pregnancy and reproduction (Z30-Z36, Z39.-)

✓4ᵗʰ **Z00**   **Encounter for general examination without complaint, suspected or reported diagnosis**
    EXCLUDES 1   encounter for examination for administrative purposes (Z02.-)
    EXCLUDES 2   encounter for pre-procedural examinations (Z01.81-)
       special screening examinations (Z11-Z13)
    AHA: 2017,4Q,95

   ✓5ᵗʰ **Z00.0**   **Encounter for general adult medical examination**
       Encounter for adult periodic examination (annual) (physical) and any associated laboratory and radiologic examinations
       EXCLUDES 1   encounter for examination of sign or symptom - code to sign or symptom
          general health check-up of infant or child (Z00.12-)

     Z00.00   **Encounter for general adult medical examination without abnormal findings** **UPD** **A**
       Encounter for adult health check-up NOS
       AHA: 2016,1Q,36

     Z00.01   **Encounter for general adult medical examination with abnormal findings** **UPD** **A**
       Use additional code to identify abnormal findings
       AHA: 2016,1Q,35-36

   ✓5ᵗʰ **Z00.1**   **Encounter for newborn, infant and child health examinations**

     ✓6ᵗʰ **Z00.11**   **Newborn health examination**
       Health check for child under 29 days old
       Use additional code to identify any abnormal findings
       EXCLUDES 1   health check for child over 28 days old (Z00.12-)

       Z00.110   **Health examination for newborn under 8 days old** **UPD** **N**
          Health check for newborn under 8 days old

       Z00.111   **Health examination for newborn 8 to 28 days old** **UPD** **N**
          Health check for newborn 8 to 28 days old
          Newborn weight check

     ✓6ᵗʰ **Z00.12**   **Encounter for routine child health examination**
       Health check (routine) for child over 28 days old
       Immunizations appropriate for age
       Routine developmental screening of infant or child
       Routine vison and hearing testing
       EXCLUDES 1   health check for child under 29 days old (Z00.11-)
          health supervision of foundling or other healthy infant or child (Z76.1-Z76.2)
          newborn health examination (Z00.11-)
       AHA: 2018,4Q,36

       Z00.121   **Encounter for routine child health examination with abnormal findings** **UPD** **P**
          Use additional code to identify abnormal findings
          AHA: 2016,1Q,34-35

       Z00.129   **Encounter for routine child health examination without abnormal findings** **UPD** **P**
          Encounter for routine child health examination NOS
          AHA: 2016,1Q,34

   Z00.2   **Encounter for examination for period of rapid growth in childhood** **UPD** **P**

   Z00.3   **Encounter for examination for adolescent development state** **UPD** **P**
       Encounter for puberty development state

   Z00.5   **Encounter for examination of potential donor of organ and tissue** **UPD**

   Z00.6   **Encounter for examination for normal comparison and control in clinical research program**
       Examination of participant or control in clinical research program

   ✓5ᵗʰ **Z00.7**   **Encounter for examination for period of delayed growth in childhood**

     Z00.70   **Encounter for examination for period of delayed growth in childhood without abnormal findings** **UPD** **P**

     Z00.71   **Encounter for examination for period of delayed growth in childhood with abnormal findings** **UPD** **P**
       Use additional code to identify abnormal findings

   Z00.8   **Encounter for other general examination** **UPD**
       Encounter for health examination in population surveys

✓4ᵗʰ **Z01**   **Encounter for other special examination without complaint, suspected or reported diagnosis**
    INCLUDES   routine examination of specific system
    NOTE   Codes from category Z01 represent the reason for the encounter. A separate procedure code is required to identify any examinations or procedures performed
    EXCLUDES 1   encounter for examination for administrative purposes (Z02.-)
       encounter for examination for suspected conditions, proven not to exist (Z03.-)
       encounter for laboratory and radiologic examinations as a component of general medical examinations (Z00.0-)
       encounter for laboratory, radiologic and imaging examinations for sign(s) and symptom(s) - code to the sign(s) or symptom(s)
    EXCLUDES 2   screening examinations (Z11-Z13)

   ✓5ᵗʰ **Z01.0**   **Encounter for examination of eyes and vision**
       EXCLUDES 1   examination for driving license (Z02.4)

     Z01.00   **Encounter for examination of eyes and vision without abnormal findings**
       Encounter for examination of eyes and vision NOS

     Z01.01   **Encounter for examination of eyes and vision with abnormal findings**
       Use additional code to identify abnormal findings
       AHA: 2016,4Q,21

N Newborn: 0   **P** Pediatric: 0-17   **M** Maternity: 9-64   **A** Adult: 15-124   **MCC** Major Complication/Comorbidity   **CC** Complication/Comorbidity   **SW** Severe Wound Dx

1236   ICD-10-CM 2022

√6ᵗʰ **Z01.02 Encounter for examination of eyes and vision following failed vision screening**

> EXCLUDES 1   ▶encounter for examination of eyes and vision with abnormal findings◀ (Z01.01)
> ▶encounter for examination of eyes and vision without abnormal findings◀ (Z01.00)

> AHA: 2019,4Q,20

Z01.020 Encounter for examination of eyes and vision following failed vision screening without abnormal findings

Z01.021 Encounter for examination of eyes and vision following failed vision screening with abnormal findings
> Use additional code to identify abnormal findings

√5ᵗʰ **Z01.1 Encounter for examination of ears and hearing**

Z01.10 Encounter for examination of ears and hearing without abnormal findings UPD
> Encounter for examination of ears and hearing NOS
> AHA: 2016,4Q,24

√6ᵗʰ **Z01.11 Encounter for examination of ears and hearing with abnormal findings**
> AHA: 2016,3Q,17-18

Z01.110 Encounter for hearing examination following failed hearing screening UPD

Z01.118 Encounter for examination of ears and hearing with other abnormal findings
> Use additional code to identify abnormal findings

Z01.12 Encounter for hearing conservation and treatment UPD

√5ᵗʰ **Z01.2 Encounter for dental examination and cleaning**

Z01.20 Encounter for dental examination and cleaning without abnormal findings UPD
> Encounter for dental examination and cleaning NOS

Z01.21 Encounter for dental examination and cleaning with abnormal findings UPD
> Use additional code to identify abnormal findings

√5ᵗʰ **Z01.3 Encounter for examination of blood pressure**

Z01.30 Encounter for examination of blood pressure without abnormal findings UPD
> Encounter for examination of blood pressure NOS

Z01.31 Encounter for examination of blood pressure with abnormal findings UPD
> Use additional code to identify abnormal findings

√5ᵗʰ **Z01.4 Encounter for gynecological examination**

> EXCLUDES 2   pregnancy examination or test (Z32.0-)
> routine examination for contraceptive maintenance (Z30.4-)

√6ᵗʰ **Z01.41 Encounter for routine gynecological examination**
> Encounter for general gynecological examination with or without cervical smear
> Encounter for gynecological examination (general) (routine) NOS
> Encounter for pelvic examination (annual) (periodic)
> Use additional code:
> for screening for human papillomavirus, if applicable, (Z11.51)
> for screening vaginal pap smear, if applicable (Z12.72)
> to identify acquired absence of uterus, if applicable (Z90.71-)

> EXCLUDES 1   gynecologic examination status-post hysterectomy for malignant condition (Z08)
> screening cervical pap smear not a part of a routine gynecological examination (Z12.4)

Z01.411 Encounter for gynecological examination (general) (routine) with abnormal findings ♀
> Use additional code to identify abnormal findings

Z01.419 Encounter for gynecological examination (general) (routine) without abnormal findings ♀

Z01.42 Encounter for cervical smear to confirm findings of recent normal smear following initial abnormal smear ♀

√5ᵗʰ **Z01.8 Encounter for other specified special examinations**

√6ᵗʰ **Z01.81 Encounter for preprocedural examinations**
> Encounter for preoperative examinations
> Encounter for radiological and imaging examinations as part of preprocedural examination

Z01.810 Encounter for preprocedural cardiovascular examination

Z01.811 Encounter for preprocedural respiratory examination

Z01.812 Encounter for preprocedural laboratory examination UPD
> Blood and urine tests prior to treatment or procedure
> AHA: 2020,3Q,14

Z01.818 Encounter for other preprocedural examination UPD
> Encounter for preprocedural examination NOS
> Encounter for examinations prior to antineoplastic chemotherapy

Z01.82 Encounter for allergy testing UPD
> EXCLUDES 1   encounter for antibody response examination (Z01.84)

Z01.83 Encounter for blood typing UPD
> Encounter for Rh typing

Z01.84 Encounter for antibody response examination UPD
> Encounter for immunity status testing
> EXCLUDES 1   encounter for allergy testing (Z01.82)
> AHA: 2020,2Q,11

Z01.89 Encounter for other specified special examinations UPD

√4ᵗʰ **Z02 Encounter for administrative examination**

Z02.0 Encounter for examination for admission to educational institution UPD
> Encounter for examination for admission to preschool (education)
> Encounter for examination for re-admission to school following illness or medical treatment

Z02.1 Encounter for pre-employment examination

Z02.2 Encounter for examination for admission to residential institution UPD
> EXCLUDES 1   examination for admission to prison (Z02.89)

Z02.3 Encounter for examination for recruitment to armed forces

Z02.4 Encounter for examination for driving license UPD

Z02.5 Encounter for examination for participation in sport UPD
> EXCLUDES 1   blood-alcohol and blood-drug test (Z02.83)

Z02.6 Encounter for examination for insurance purposes UPD

√5ᵗʰ **Z02.7 Encounter for issue of medical certificate**
> EXCLUDES 1   encounter for general medical examination (Z00-Z01, Z02.0-Z02.6, Z02.8-Z02.9)

Z02.71 Encounter for disability determination UPD
> Encounter for issue of medical certificate of incapacity
> Encounter for issue of medical certificate of invalidity

Z02.79 Encounter for issue of other medical certificate UPD

√5ᵗʰ **Z02.8 Encounter for other administrative examinations**

Z02.81 Encounter for paternity testing

Z02.82 Encounter for adoption services UPD

Z02.83 Encounter for blood-alcohol and blood-drug test
> Use additional code for findings of alcohol or drugs in blood (R78.-)

Z02.89 Encounter for other administrative examinations UPD
> Encounter for examination for admission to prison
> Encounter for examination for admission to summer camp
> Encounter for immigration examination
> Encounter for naturalization examination
> Encounter for premarital examination
> EXCLUDES 1   health supervision of foundling or other healthy infant or child (Z76.1-Z76.2)

Z02.9 Encounter for administrative examinations, unspecified UPD

☑ Additional Character Required   √x7ᵗʰ Placeholder   Questionable PDx   Manifestation   Unspecified Dx   UPD Unacceptable PDx   H1-H14 HAC   HCC CMS-HCC Dx   HIV HIV Dx

ICD-10-CM 2022   1237

✓4ᵗʰ **Z03 Encounter for** medical observation **for suspected diseases and conditions ruled out**
> This category is to be used when a person without a diagnosis is suspected of having an abnormal condition, without signs or symptoms, which requires study, but after examination and observation, is ruled out. This category is also for use for administrative and legal observation status.
>
> **EXCLUDES 1**   *contact with and (suspected) exposures hazardous to health (Z77.-)*
>> *encounter for observation and evaluation of newborn for suspected diseases and conditions ruled out (Z05.-)*
>> *person with feared complaint in whom no diagnosis is made (Z71.1)*
>> *signs or symptoms under study - code to signs or symptoms*
>
> **AHA:** 2020,2Q,8; 2018,2Q,7-8; 2017,4Q,27

> **Z03.6 Encounter for observation for suspected** toxic effect from ingested substance **ruled out**
>> Encounter for observation for suspected adverse effect from drug
>> Encounter for observation for suspected poisoning

> ✓5ᵗʰ **Z03.7 Encounter for suspected** maternal and fetal conditions **ruled out**
>> Encounter for suspected maternal and fetal conditions not found
>>
>> **EXCLUDES 1**   *known or suspected fetal anomalies affecting management of mother, not ruled out (O26.-, O35.-, O36.-, O40.-, O41.-)*

>> **Z03.71 Encounter for suspected problem with** amniotic cavity and membrane **ruled out**   UPD M ♀
>>> Encounter for suspected oligohydramnios ruled out
>>> Encounter for suspected polyhydramnios ruled out

>> **Z03.72 Encounter for suspected** placental problem **ruled out**   UPD M ♀

>> **Z03.73 Encounter for suspected** fetal anomaly **ruled out**   UPD M ♀

>> **Z03.74 Encounter for suspected** problem with fetal growth **ruled out**   UPD M ♀

>> **Z03.75 Encounter for suspected** cervical shortening **ruled out**   UPD M ♀

>> **Z03.79 Encounter for other suspected maternal and fetal conditions ruled out**   UPD M ♀

> ✓5ᵗʰ **Z03.8 Encounter for** observation **for other suspected diseases and conditions ruled out**

>> ✓6ᵗʰ **Z03.81 Encounter for observation for suspected** exposure to biological agents **ruled out**

>>> **Z03.810 Encounter for observation for suspected exposure to** anthrax **ruled out**

>>> **Z03.818 Encounter for observation for suspected exposure to other biological agents ruled out**
>>>> **AHA:** 2020,2Q,8; 2020,1Q,34-36
>>>> **TIP:** During the COVID-19 pandemic, possible exposure to COVID-19 should be coded using Z20.822 Contact with and (suspected) exposure to COVID-19, even when the COVID-19 infection has been ruled out.

>> ✓6ᵗʰ **Z03.82 Encounter for observation for suspected** foreign body **ruled out**
>>> **EXCLUDES 1**   *retained foreign body (Z18.-)*
>>>> *retained foreign body in eyelid (H02.81)*
>>>> *residual foreign body in soft tissue (M79.5)*
>>> **EXCLUDES 2**   *confirmed foreign body ingestion or aspiration including:*
>>>> *foreign body in alimentary tract (T18)*
>>>> *foreign body in ear (T16)*
>>>> *foreign body on external eye (T15)*
>>>> *foreign body in respiratory tract (T17)*
>>> **AHA:** 2020,4Q,42

>>> **Z03.821 Encounter for observation for suspected** ingested **foreign body ruled out**   UPD

>>> **Z03.822 Encounter for observation for suspected** aspirated (inhaled) **foreign body ruled out**   UPD

>>> **Z03.823 Encounter for observation for suspected** inserted (injected) **foreign body ruled out**   UPD
>>>> Encounter for observation for suspected inserted (injected) foreign body in eye ruled out
>>>> Encounter for observation for suspected inserted (injected) foreign body in orifice ruled out
>>>> Encounter for observation for suspected inserted (injected) foreign body in skin ruled out

>> **Z03.89 Encounter for observation for other suspected diseases and conditions ruled out**

✓4ᵗʰ **Z04 Encounter for examination and observation for other reasons**
> **INCLUDES**   encounter for examination for medicolegal reasons
> This category is to be used when a person without a diagnosis is suspected of having an abnormal condition, without signs or symptoms, which requires study, but after examination and observation, is ruled-out. This category is also for use for administrative and legal observation status.
> **AHA:** 2018,2Q,7-8

> **Z04.1 Encounter for examination and observation following** transport accident
>> **EXCLUDES 1**   *encounter for examination and observation following work accident (Z04.2)*
>> **AHA:** 2019,2Q,11; 2018,2Q,8

> **Z04.2 Encounter for examination and observation following** work accident

> **Z04.3 Encounter for examination and observation following other accident**

> ✓5ᵗʰ **Z04.4 Encounter for examination and observation following** alleged rape
>> Encounter for examination and observation of victim following alleged rape
>> Encounter for examination and observation of victim following alleged sexual abuse

>> **Z04.41 Encounter for examination and observation following alleged** adult rape   A
>>> Suspected adult rape, ruled out
>>> Suspected adult sexual abuse, ruled out

>> **Z04.42 Encounter for examination and observation following alleged** child rape   P
>>> Suspected child rape, ruled out
>>> Suspected child sexual abuse, ruled out

> **Z04.6 Encounter for** general psychiatric examination, requested by authority

> ✓5ᵗʰ **Z04.7 Encounter for examination and observation following** alleged physical abuse

>> **Z04.71 Encounter for examination and observation following alleged** adult physical abuse   A
>>> Suspected adult physical abuse, ruled out
>>> **EXCLUDES 1**   *confirmed case of adult physical abuse (T74.-)*
>>>> *encounter for examination and observation following alleged adult sexual abuse (Z04.41)*
>>>> *suspected case of adult physical abuse, not ruled out (T76.-)*

>> **Z04.72 Encounter for examination and observation following alleged** child physical abuse   P
>>> Suspected child physical abuse, ruled out
>>> **EXCLUDES 1**   *confirmed case of child physical abuse (T74.-)*
>>>> *encounter for examination and observation following alleged child sexual abuse (Z04.42)*
>>>> *suspected case of child physical abuse, not ruled out (T76.-)*

> ✓5ᵗʰ **Z04.8 Encounter for examination and observation for** other specified reasons
>> Encounter for examination and observation for request for expert evidence
>> **AHA:** 2018,4Q,32,35,72

>> **Z04.81 Encounter for examination and observation of** victim following forced sexual exploitation

>> **Z04.82 Encounter for examination and observation of** victim following forced labor exploitation

---

N Newborn: 0   P Pediatric: 0-17   M Maternity: 9-64   A Adult: 15-124   MCC Major Complication/Comorbidity   CC Complication/Comorbidity   SW Severe Wound Dx

1238   ICD-10-CM 2022

Z04.89 Encounter for examination and observation for other specified reasons

Z04.9 Encounter for examination and observation for unspecified reason `UPD`

Encounter for observation NOS

✓4ᵗʰ **Z05** Encounter for observation and evaluation of newborn for suspected diseases and conditions ruled out

This category is to be used for newborns, within the neonatal period (the first 28 days of life), who are suspected of having an abnormal condition, but without signs or symptoms, and which, after examination and observation, is ruled out.

AHA: 2017,4Q,27; 2016,4Q,77

Z05.0 Observation and evaluation of newborn for suspected cardiac condition ruled out `N`

Z05.1 Observation and evaluation of newborn for suspected infectious condition ruled out `N`

AHA: 2019,2Q,10

Z05.2 Observation and evaluation of newborn for suspected neurological condition ruled out `N`

Z05.3 Observation and evaluation of newborn for suspected respiratory condition ruled out `N`

✓5ᵗʰ **Z05.4** Observation and evaluation of newborn for suspected genetic, metabolic or immunologic condition ruled out

Z05.41 Observation and evaluation of newborn for suspected genetic condition ruled out `N`

AHA: 2016,4Q,55

Z05.42 Observation and evaluation of newborn for suspected metabolic condition ruled out `N`

Z05.43 Observation and evaluation of newborn for suspected immunologic condition ruled out `N`

Z05.5 Observation and evaluation of newborn for suspected gastrointestinal condition ruled out `N`

Z05.6 Observation and evaluation of newborn for suspected genitourinary condition ruled out `N`

✓5ᵗʰ **Z05.7** Observation and evaluation of newborn for suspected skin, subcutaneous, musculoskeletal and connective tissue condition ruled out

Z05.71 Observation and evaluation of newborn for suspected skin and subcutaneous tissue condition ruled out `N`

Z05.72 Observation and evaluation of newborn for suspected musculoskeletal condition ruled out `N`

Z05.73 Observation and evaluation of newborn for suspected connective tissue condition ruled out `N`

Z05.8 Observation and evaluation of newborn for other specified suspected condition ruled out `N`

Z05.9 Observation and evaluation of newborn for unspecified suspected condition ruled out `N`

Z08 Encounter for follow-up examination after completed treatment for malignant neoplasm `UPD`

Medical surveillance following completed treatment

Use additional code to identify any acquired absence of organs (Z90.-)

Use additional code to identify the personal history of malignant neoplasm (Z85.-)

EXCLUDES 1 aftercare following medical care (Z43-Z49, Z51)

AHA: 2020,3Q,30

Z09 Encounter for follow-up examination after completed treatment for conditions other than malignant neoplasm `UPD`

Medical surveillance following completed treatment

Use additional code to identify any applicable history of disease code ▶(Z86.-, Z87.-)◀

EXCLUDES 1 aftercare following medical care (Z43-Z49, Z51)
surveillance of contraception (Z30.4-)
surveillance of prosthetic and other medical devices (Z44-Z46)

AHA: 2021,1Q,33; 2020,2Q,10; 2017,1Q,9; 2015,1Q,8

✓4ᵗʰ **Z11** Encounter for screening for infectious and parasitic diseases

Screening is the testing for disease or disease precursors in asymptomatic individuals so that early detection and treatment can be provided for those who test positive for the disease.

EXCLUDES 1 encounter for diagnostic examination - code to sign or symptom

Z11.0 Encounter for screening for intestinal infectious diseases `UPD`

Z11.1 Encounter for screening for respiratory tuberculosis `UPD`

Encounter for screening for active tuberculosis disease

Z11.2 Encounter for screening for other bacterial diseases `UPD`

Z11.3 Encounter for screening for infections with a predominantly sexual mode of transmission `UPD`

EXCLUDES 2 encounter for screening for human immunodeficiency virus [HIV] (Z11.4)
encounter for screening for human papillomavirus (Z11.51)

Z11.4 Encounter for screening for human immunodeficiency virus [HIV] `UPD`

✓5ᵗʰ **Z11.5** Encounter for screening for other viral diseases

EXCLUDES 2 encounter for screening for viral intestinal disease (Z11.0)

Z11.51 Encounter for screening for human papillomavirus (HPV) `UPD`

Z11.52 Encounter for screening for COVID-19 `UPD`

AHA: 2021,1Q,27,37,41

TIP: This code is not appropriate for use during the pandemic phase of COVID-19. Use Z20.822 Contact with or (suspected) exposure to COVID-19, instead.

Z11.59 Encounter for screening for other viral diseases `UPD`

AHA: 2020,3Q,14

Z11.6 Encounter for screening for other protozoal diseases and helminthiases `UPD`

EXCLUDES 2 encounter for screening for protozoal intestinal disease (Z11.0)

Z11.7 Encounter for testing for latent tuberculosis infection `UPD`

AHA: 2019,4Q,20

Z11.8 Encounter for screening for other infectious and parasitic diseases `UPD`

Encounter for screening for chlamydia
Encounter for screening for rickettsial
Encounter for screening for spirochetal
Encounter for screening for mycoses

Z11.9 Encounter for screening for infectious and parasitic diseases, unspecified `UPD`

✓4ᵗʰ **Z12** Encounter for screening for malignant neoplasms

Screening is the testing for disease or disease precursors in asymptomatic individuals so that early detection and treatment can be provided for those who test positive for the disease.

Use additional code to identify any family history of malignant neoplasm (Z80.-)

EXCLUDES 1 encounter for diagnostic examination - code to sign or symptom

Z12.0 Encounter for screening for malignant neoplasm of stomach `UPD`

✓5ᵗʰ **Z12.1** Encounter for screening for malignant neoplasm of intestinal tract

AHA: 2017,1Q,8,9

Z12.10 Encounter for screening for malignant neoplasm of intestinal tract, unspecified `UPD`

Z12.11 Encounter for screening for malignant neoplasm of colon `UPD`

Encounter for screening colonoscopy NOS

AHA: 2019,1Q,32-33; 2018,1Q,6

Z12.12 Encounter for screening for malignant neoplasm of rectum `UPD`

AHA: 2018,1Q,6

Z12.13 Encounter for screening for malignant neoplasm of small intestine

Z12.2 Encounter for screening for malignant neoplasm of respiratory organs `UPD`

✓5ᵗʰ **Z12.3** Encounter for screening for malignant neoplasm of breast

Z12.31 Encounter for screening mammogram for malignant neoplasm of breast `UPD`

EXCLUDES 1 inconclusive mammogram (R92.2)

AHA: 2015,1Q,24

Z12.39 Encounter for other screening for malignant neoplasm of breast `UPD`

Z12.4 Encounter for screening for malignant neoplasm of cervix `UPD` ♀

Encounter for screening pap smear for malignant neoplasm of cervix

EXCLUDES 1 when screening is part of general gynecological examination (Z01.4-)

EXCLUDES 2 encounter for screening for human papillomavirus (Z11.51)

Z12.5 Encounter for screening for malignant neoplasm of prostate ♂

☑ Additional Character Required   ✓x7ᵗʰ Placeholder   Questionable PDx   Manifestation   Unspecified Dx   `UPD` Unacceptable PDx   H1-H14 HAC   HCC CMS-HCC Dx   HIV HIV Dx

ICD-10-CM 2022   1239

Chapter 21. Factors Influencing Health Status and Contact With Health Services

Z12.6   **Encounter for screening for malignant neoplasm of bladder** `UPD`

✓5ᵗʰ **Z12.7**   **Encounter for screening for malignant neoplasm of other genitourinary organs**

    Z12.71   **Encounter for screening for malignant neoplasm of testis** `UPD` ♂

    Z12.72   **Encounter for screening for malignant neoplasm of vagina** `UPD` ♀
       Vaginal pap smear status-post hysterectomy for non-malignant condition
       Use additional code to identify acquired absence of uterus (Z90.71-)
       `EXCLUDES 1`   *vaginal pap smear status-post hysterectomy for malignant conditions (Z08)*

    Z12.73   **Encounter for screening for malignant neoplasm of ovary** `UPD` ♀

    Z12.79   **Encounter for screening for malignant neoplasm of other genitourinary organs** `UPD`

✓5ᵗʰ **Z12.8**   **Encounter for screening for malignant neoplasm of other sites**

    Z12.81   **Encounter for screening for malignant neoplasm of oral cavity** `UPD`

    Z12.82   **Encounter for screening for malignant neoplasm of nervous system** `UPD`

    Z12.83   **Encounter for screening for malignant neoplasm of skin** `UPD`

    Z12.89   **Encounter for screening for malignant neoplasm of other sites** `UPD`
       AHA: 2021,1Q,14

Z12.9   **Encounter for screening for malignant neoplasm, site unspecified** `UPD`

✓4ᵗʰ **Z13**   **Encounter for screening for other diseases and disorders**
    Screening is the testing for disease or disease precursors in asymptomatic individuals so that early detection and treatment can be provided for those who test positive for the disease.
    `EXCLUDES 1`   *encounter for diagnostic examination - code to sign or symptom*

Z13.0   **Encounter for screening for diseases of the blood and blood-forming organs and certain disorders involving the immune mechanism** `UPD`

Z13.1   **Encounter for screening for diabetes mellitus** `UPD`

✓5ᵗʰ **Z13.2**   **Encounter for screening for nutritional, metabolic and other endocrine disorders**

    Z13.21   **Encounter for screening for nutritional disorder** `UPD`

    ✓6ᵗʰ **Z13.22**   **Encounter for screening for metabolic disorder** `UPD`

       Z13.220   **Encounter for screening for lipoid disorders** `UPD`
          Encounter for screening for cholesterol level
          Encounter for screening for hypercholesterolemia
          Encounter for screening for hyperlipidemia

       Z13.228   **Encounter for screening for other metabolic disorders** `UPD`

    Z13.29   **Encounter for screening for other suspected endocrine disorder** `UPD`
       `EXCLUDES 1`   *encounter for screening for diabetes mellitus (Z13.1)*
       `EXCLUDES 2`   ►*encounter for screening for diabetes mellitus (Z13.1)*◄

✓5ᵗʰ **Z13.3**   **Encounter for screening examination for mental health and behavioral disorders**
    AHA: 2018,4Q,35-36

    Z13.30   **Encounter for screening examination for mental health and behavioral disorders, unspecified** `UPD`

    Z13.31   **Encounter for screening for depression** `UPD`
       Encounter for screening for depression, adult
       Encounter for screening for depression for child or adolescent

    Z13.32   **Encounter for screening for maternal depression** `UPD` ♀
       Encounter for screening for perinatal depression

    Z13.39   **Encounter for screening examination for other mental health and behavioral disorders** `UPD`
       Encounter for screening for alcoholism
       Encounter for screening for intellectual disabilities

✓5ᵗʰ **Z13.4**   **Encounter for screening for certain developmental disorders in childhood**
    Encounter for development testing of infant or child
    Encounter for screening for developmental handicaps in early childhood
    `EXCLUDES 2`   *encounter for routine child health examination (Z00.12-)*
    AHA: 2018,4Q,36

    Z13.40   **Encounter for screening for unspecified developmental delays** `UPD`

    Z13.41   **Encounter for autism screening** `UPD`

    Z13.42   **Encounter for screening for global developmental delays (milestones)** `UPD`
       Encounter for screening for developmental handicaps in early childhood

    Z13.49   **Encounter for screening for other developmental delays** `UPD`

Z13.5   **Encounter for screening for eye and ear disorders**
    `EXCLUDES 2`   *encounter for general hearing examination (Z01.1-)*
          encounter for general vision examination (Z01.0-)
    AHA: 2016,3Q,17

Z13.6   **Encounter for screening for cardiovascular disorders** `UPD`

✓5ᵗʰ **Z13.7**   **Encounter for screening for genetic and chromosomal anomalies**
    `EXCLUDES 1`   *genetic testing for procreative management (Z31.4-)*

    Z13.71   **Encounter for nonprocreative screening for genetic disease carrier status** `UPD`

    Z13.79   **Encounter for other screening for genetic and chromosomal anomalies** `UPD`

✓5ᵗʰ **Z13.8**   **Encounter for screening for other specified diseases and disorders**
    `EXCLUDES 2`   *screening for malignant neoplasms (Z12.-)*

    ✓6ᵗʰ **Z13.81**   **Encounter for screening for digestive system disorders**

       Z13.810   **Encounter for screening for upper gastrointestinal disorder** `UPD`

       Z13.811   **Encounter for screening for lower gastrointestinal disorder** `UPD`
          `EXCLUDES 1`   *encounter for screening for intestinal infectious disease (Z11.0)*

       Z13.818   **Encounter for screening for other digestive system disorders** `UPD`

    ✓6ᵗʰ **Z13.82**   **Encounter for screening for musculoskeletal disorder**

       Z13.820   **Encounter for screening for osteoporosis** `UPD`

       Z13.828   **Encounter for screening for other musculoskeletal disorder** `UPD`

    Z13.83   **Encounter for screening for respiratory disorder NEC** `UPD`
       `EXCLUDES 1`   *encounter for screening for respiratory tuberculosis (Z11.1)*

    Z13.84   **Encounter for screening for dental disorders** `UPD`

    ✓6ᵗʰ **Z13.85**   **Encounter for screening for nervous system disorders**

       Z13.850   **Encounter for screening for traumatic brain injury** `UPD`

       Z13.858   **Encounter for screening for other nervous system disorders** `UPD`

    Z13.88   **Encounter for screening for disorder due to exposure to contaminants** `UPD`
       `EXCLUDES 1`   *those exposed to contaminants without suspected disorders (Z57.-, Z77.-)*

    Z13.89   **Encounter for screening for other disorder** `UPD`
       Encounter for screening for genitourinary disorders

Z13.9   **Encounter for screening, unspecified** `UPD`

Genetic carrier and genetic susceptibility to disease (Z14-Z15)

✓4ᵗʰ **Z14 Genetic carrier**

DEF: Individuals carrying a gene mutation associated with a certain disease that typically do not develop the disease but are able to pass the mutated genes to offspring.

✓5ᵗʰ **Z14.Ø Hemophilia A carrier**

  Z14.Ø1 Asymptomatic hemophilia A carrier   UPD

  Z14.Ø2 Symptomatic hemophilia A carrier   UPD

Z14.1 Cystic fibrosis carrier   UPD

Z14.8 Genetic carrier of other disease   UPD

✓4ᵗʰ **Z15 Genetic susceptibility to disease**

  INCLUDES confirmed abnormal gene

  Use additional code, if applicable, for any associated family history of the disease (Z80-Z84)

  EXCLUDES 1 chromosomal anomalies (Q9Ø-Q99)

✓5ᵗʰ **Z15.Ø Genetic susceptibility to malignant neoplasm**

  Code first, if applicable, any current malignant neoplasm (CØØ-C75, C81-C96)

  Use additional code, if applicable, for any personal history of malignant neoplasm (Z85.-)

  Z15.Ø1 Genetic susceptibility to malignant neoplasm of breast   UPD

  Z15.Ø2 Genetic susceptibility to malignant neoplasm of ovary   UPD ♀

  Z15.Ø3 Genetic susceptibility to malignant neoplasm of prostate   UPD ♂

  Z15.Ø4 Genetic susceptibility to malignant neoplasm of endometrium   UPD ♀

  Z15.Ø9 Genetic susceptibility to other malignant neoplasm   UPD

    AHA: 2021,1Q,14

✓5ᵗʰ **Z15.8 Genetic susceptibility to other disease**

  Z15.81 Genetic susceptibility to multiple endocrine neoplasia [MEN]   UPD

    EXCLUDES 1 multiple endocrine neoplasia [MEN] syndromes (E31.2-)

    DEF: Group of conditions in which several endocrine glands grow excessively (such as in adenomatous hyperplasia) and/or develop benign or malignant tumors. Tumors and hyperplasia associated with MEN often produce excess hormones, which impede normal physiology. There is no comprehensive cure known for MEN syndrome. Treatment is directed at the hyperplasia or tumors in each individual gland. Tumors are usually surgically removed and oral medications or hormonal injections are used to correct hormone imbalances.

  Z15.89 Genetic susceptibility to other disease   UPD

Resistance to antimicrobial drugs (Z16)

✓4ᵗʰ **Z16 Resistance to antimicrobial drugs**

  NOTE The codes in this category are provided for use as additional codes to identify the resistance and non-responsiveness of a condition to antimicrobial drugs.

  Code first the infection

  EXCLUDES 1 Methicillin resistant Staphylococcus aureus infection (A49.Ø2)

    Methicillin resistant Staphylococcus aureus pneumonia (J15.212)

    sepsis due to Methicillin resistant Staphylococcus aureus (A41.Ø2)

✓5ᵗʰ **Z16.1 Resistance to beta lactam antibiotics**

  Z16.1Ø Resistance to unspecified beta lactam antibiotics   CC UPD

  Z16.11 Resistance to penicillins   CC UPD

    Resistance to amoxicillin

    Resistance to ampicillin

  Z16.12 Extended spectrum beta lactamase (ESBL) resistance   CC UPD

    EXCLUDES 2 Methicillin resistant Staphylococcus aureus infection in diseases classified elsewhere (B95.62)

  Z16.19 Resistance to other specified beta lactam antibiotics   CC UPD

    Resistance to cephalosporins

✓5ᵗʰ **Z16.2 Resistance to other antibiotics**

  Z16.2Ø Resistance to unspecified antibiotic   CC UPD

    Resistance to antibiotics NOS

  Z16.21 Resistance to vancomycin   CC UPD

  Z16.22 Resistance to vancomycin related antibiotics   CC UPD

  Z16.23 Resistance to quinolones and fluoroquinolones   CC UPD

  Z16.24 Resistance to multiple antibiotics   CC UPD

  Z16.29 Resistance to other single specified antibiotic   CC UPD

    Resistance to aminoglycosides

    Resistance to macrolides

    Resistance to sulfonamides

    Resistance to tetracyclines

✓5ᵗʰ **Z16.3 Resistance to other antimicrobial drugs**

  EXCLUDES 1 resistance to antibiotics (Z16.1-, Z16.2-)

  Z16.3Ø Resistance to unspecified antimicrobial drugs   CC UPD

    Drug resistance NOS

  Z16.31 Resistance to antiparasitic drug(s)   CC UPD

    Resistance to quinine and related compounds

  Z16.32 Resistance to antifungal drug(s)   CC UPD

  Z16.33 Resistance to antiviral drug(s)   CC UPD

✓6ᵗʰ **Z16.34 Resistance to antimycobacterial drug(s)**

    Resistance to tuberculostatics

  Z16.341 Resistance to single antimycobacterial drug   CC UPD

    Resistance to antimycobacterial drug NOS

  Z16.342 Resistance to multiple antimycobacterial drugs   CC UPD

  Z16.35 Resistance to multiple antimicrobial drugs   CC UPD

    EXCLUDES 1 resistance to multiple antibiotics only (Z16.24)

  Z16.39 Resistance to other specified antimicrobial drug   CC UPD

Estrogen receptor status (Z17)

✓4ᵗʰ **Z17 Estrogen receptor status**

  Code first malignant neoplasm of breast (C5Ø.-)

  DEF: Receptor status of breast cancer cells for the hormone estrogen that is used to help determine treatment and evaluate prognosis. ER+ breast cancer responds to hormone therapies while ER- breast cancer does not.

  Z17.Ø Estrogen receptor positive status [ER+]   UPD

  Z17.1 Estrogen receptor negative status [ER-]   UPD

Retained foreign body fragments (Z18)

✓4ᵗʰ **Z18 Retained foreign body fragments**

  INCLUDES embedded fragment (status)

    embedded splinter (status)

    retained foreign body status

  EXCLUDES 1 artificial joint prosthesis status (Z96.6-)

    foreign body accidentally left during a procedure (T81.5-)

    foreign body entering through orifice (T15-T19)

    in situ cardiac device (Z95.-)

    organ or tissue replaced by means other than transplant (Z96.-, Z97.-)

    organ or tissue replaced by transplant (Z94.-)

    personal history of retained foreign body fully removed Z87.821

    superficial foreign body (non-embedded splinter) - code to superficial foreign body, by site

  DEF: Embedded or retained fragment, splinter, or foreign body, natural or synthetic that can cause infection.

✓5ᵗʰ **Z18.Ø Retained radioactive fragments**

  Z18.Ø1 Retained depleted uranium fragments   UPD

  Z18.Ø9 Other retained radioactive fragments   UPD

    Other retained depleted isotope fragments

    Retained nontherapeutic radioactive fragments

✓ Additional Character Required   ✓x7ᵗʰ Placeholder   Questionable PDx   Manifestation   Unspecified Dx   UPD Unacceptable PDx   H1-H14 HAC   HCC CMS-HCC Dx   HIV HIV Dx

ICD-10-CM 2022

1241

Chapter 21. Factors Influencing Health Status and Contact With Health Services

Z18.1–Z22.6

√5ᵗʰ **Z18.1 Retained metal fragments**

     EXCLUDES 1   retained radioactive metal fragments (Z18.01-Z18.09)

     Z18.10 Retained metal fragments, unspecified   UPD
         Retained metal fragment NOS

     Z18.11 Retained magnetic metal fragments   UPD

     Z18.12 Retained nonmagnetic metal fragments   UPD

Z18.2 Retained plastic fragments   UPD
     Acrylics fragments
     Diethylhexyl phthalates fragments
     Isocyanate fragments

√5ᵗʰ **Z18.3 Retained organic fragments**

     Z18.31 Retained animal quills or spines   UPD

     Z18.32 Retained tooth   UPD

     Z18.33 Retained wood fragments   UPD

     Z18.39 Other retained organic fragments   UPD

√5ᵗʰ **Z18.8 Other specified retained foreign body**

     Z18.81 Retained glass fragments   UPD

     Z18.83 Retained stone or crystalline fragments   UPD
         Retained concrete or cement fragments

     Z18.89 Other specified retained foreign body fragments   UPD

Z18.9 Retained foreign body fragments, unspecified material   UPD

Hormone sensitivity malignancy status (Z19)

√4ᵗʰ **Z19 Hormone sensitivity malignancy status**

     Code first malignant neoplasm — see Table of Neoplasms, by site, malignant

     AHA: 2016,4Q,76

Z19.1 Hormone sensitive malignancy status   UPD

Z19.2 Hormone resistant malignancy status   UPD
     Castrate resistant prostate malignancy status

Persons with potential health hazards related to communicable diseases (Z20-Z29)

√4ᵗʰ **Z20 Contact with and (suspected) exposure to communicable diseases**

     EXCLUDES 1   carrier of infectious disease (Z22.-)
           diagnosed current infectious or parasitic disease - see Alphabetic Index
     EXCLUDES 2   personal history of infectious and parasitic diseases (Z86.1-)

√5ᵗʰ **Z20.0 Contact with and (suspected) exposure to intestinal infectious diseases**

     Z20.01 Contact with and (suspected) exposure to intestinal infectious diseases due to Escherichia coli (E. coli)

     Z20.09 Contact with and (suspected) exposure to other intestinal infectious diseases   UPD

Z20.1 Contact with and (suspected) exposure to tuberculosis   UPD

Z20.2 Contact with and (suspected) exposure to infections with a predominantly sexual mode of transmission   UPD

Z20.3 Contact with and (suspected) exposure to rabies   UPD

Z20.4 Contact with and (suspected) exposure to rubella   UPD

Z20.5 Contact with and (suspected) exposure to viral hepatitis

Z20.6 Contact with and (suspected) exposure to human immunodeficiency virus [HIV]

     EXCLUDES 1   asymptomatic human immunodeficiency virus [HIV] HIV infection status (Z21)

Z20.7 Contact with and (suspected) exposure to pediculosis, acariasis and other infestations   UPD

√5ᵗʰ **Z20.8 Contact with and (suspected) exposure to other communicable diseases**

     √6ᵗʰ **Z20.81 Contact with and (suspected) exposure to other bacterial communicable diseases**

         Z20.810 Contact with and (suspected) exposure to anthrax   UPD

         Z20.811 Contact with and (suspected) exposure to meningococcus

         Z20.818 Contact with and (suspected) exposure to other bacterial communicable diseases   UPD
           AHA: 2019,2Q,10

     √6ᵗʰ **Z20.82 Contact with and (suspected) exposure to other viral communicable diseases**

         Z20.820 Contact with and (suspected) exposure to varicella

         Z20.821 Contact with and (suspected) exposure to Zika virus   UPD
           AHA: 2018,4Q,35,64

         Z20.822 Contact with and (suspected) exposure to COVID-19   UPD
           Contact with and (suspected) exposure to SARS-CoV-2
           AHA: 2021,1Q,27-29,37-38,41
           TIP: During the COVID-19 pandemic, this code should be used for any individual being tested due to actual or suspected COVID-19 exposure. This is true regardless of whether the patient is asymptomatic or has symptoms and the infection has been ruled out, is inconclusive, or unknown.

         Z20.828 Contact with and (suspected) exposure to other viral communicable diseases
           AHA: 2021,1Q,37-38; 2020,4Q,99; 2020,3Q,14-15; 2020,2Q,4,8; 2020,1Q,34-36

     Z20.89 Contact with and (suspected) exposure to other communicable diseases   UPD

Z20.9 Contact with and (suspected) exposure to unspecified communicable disease   UPD

Z21 Asymptomatic human immunodeficiency virus [HIV] infection status   HCC

     HIV positive NOS

     Code first human immunodeficiency virus [HIV] disease complicating pregnancy, childbirth and the puerperium, if applicable (O98.7-)

     EXCLUDES 1   acquired immunodeficiency syndrome (B20)
           contact with human immunodeficiency virus [HIV] (Z20.6)
           exposure to human immunodeficiency virus [HIV] (Z20.6)
           human immunodeficiency virus [HIV] disease (B20)
           inconclusive laboratory evidence of human immunodeficiency virus [HIV] (R75)

     AHA: 2019,1Q,8-11

     DEF: Phase of human immunodeficiency virus (HIV) infection with no clinical symptoms. This phase may last for 10 years or more.

√4ᵗʰ **Z22 Carrier of infectious disease**

     INCLUDES   colonization status
           suspected carrier
     EXCLUDES 2   carrier of viral hepatitis (B18.-)

Z22.0 Carrier of typhoid   UPD

Z22.1 Carrier of other intestinal infectious diseases   UPD

Z22.2 Carrier of diphtheria   UPD

√5ᵗʰ **Z22.3 Carrier of other specified bacterial diseases**

     Z22.31 Carrier of bacterial disease due to meningococci   UPD

     √6ᵗʰ **Z22.32 Carrier of bacterial disease due to staphylococci**

         Z22.321 Carrier or suspected carrier of Methicillin susceptible Staphylococcus aureus   UPD
           MSSA colonization

         Z22.322 Carrier or suspected carrier of Methicillin resistant Staphylococcus aureus   UPD
           MRSA colonization
           DEF: Carriers (colonization) of methicillin resistant *Staphylococcus aureus* (MRSA) have MRSA on their skin or in their body but do not exhibit signs of infection. These individuals are able to pass MRSA on to others who may develop an infection.

     √6ᵗʰ **Z22.33 Carrier of bacterial disease due to streptococci**

         Z22.330 Carrier of Group B streptococcus   UPD
           EXCLUDES 1   carrier of streptococcus group B (GBS) complicating pregnancy, childbirth and the puerperium (O99.82-)

         Z22.338 Carrier of other streptococcus   UPD

     Z22.39 Carrier of other specified bacterial diseases   UPD

Z22.4 Carrier of infections with a predominantly sexual mode of transmission   UPD

Z22.6 Carrier of human T-lymphotropic virus type-1 [HTLV-1] infection   UPD

N Newborn: 0   P Pediatric: 0-17   M Maternity: 9-64   A Adult: 15-124   MCC Major Complication/Comorbidity   CC Complication/Comorbidity   SW Severe Wound Dx

1242   ICD-10-CM 2022

Z22.7   **Latent tuberculosis**   `UPD`
    Latent tuberculosis infection (LTBI)
    `EXCLUDES 1`   *nonspecific reaction to cell mediated immunity measurement of gamma interferon antigen response without active tuberculosis (R76.12)*
      nonspecific reaction to tuberculin skin test without active tuberculosis (R76.11)
    AHA: 2019,4Q,19

Z22.8   **Carrier of other infectious diseases**   `UPD`
Z22.9   **Carrier of infectious disease, unspecified**   `UPD`

Z23   **Encounter for immunization**   `UPD`
    `NOTE`   Procedure codes are required to identify the types of immunizations given
    Code first any routine childhood examination
    ▶Code also, if applicable, encounter for immunization safety counseling (Z71.85)◀

`✓4ᵗʰ` **Z28**   **Immunization not carried out and underimmunization status**
    `INCLUDES`   vaccination not carried out
    ▶Code also, if applicable, encounter for immunization safety counseling (Z71.85)◀

`✓5ᵗʰ` **Z28.0**   **Immunization not carried out because of contraindication**
    DEF: Contraindication: Situation where a drug, surgery, or other procedure may negatively affect or cause harm to a patient.

    Z28.01   **Immunization not carried out because of acute illness of patient**   `UPD`
    Z28.02   **Immunization not carried out because of chronic illness or condition of patient**   `UPD`
    Z28.03   **Immunization not carried out because of immune compromised state of patient**   `UPD`
    Z28.04   **Immunization not carried out because of patient allergy to vaccine or component**   `UPD`
    Z28.09   **Immunization not carried out because of other contraindication**   `UPD`

Z28.1   **Immunization not carried out because of patient decision for reasons of belief or group pressure**   `UPD`
    Immunization not carried out because of religious belief

`✓5ᵗʰ` **Z28.2**   **Immunization not carried out because of patient decision for other and unspecified reason**
    Z28.20   **Immunization not carried out because of patient decision for unspecified reason**   `UPD`
    Z28.21   **Immunization not carried out because of patient refusal**   `UPD`
    Z28.29   **Immunization not carried out because of patient decision for other reason**   `UPD`

Z28.3   **Underimmunization status**   `UPD`
    Delinquent immunization status
    Lapsed immunization schedule status

`✓5ᵗʰ` **Z28.8**   **Immunization not carried out for other reason**
    Z28.81   **Immunization not carried out due to patient having had the disease**   `UPD`
    Z28.82   **Immunization not carried out because of caregiver refusal**   `UPD`
      Immunization not carried out because of guardian refusal
      Immunization not carried out because of parent refusal
      `EXCLUDES 1`   *immunization not carried out because of caregiver refusal because of religious belief (Z28.1)*
    Z28.83   **Immunization not carried out due to unavailability of vaccine**   `UPD`
      Delay in delivery of vaccine
      Lack of availability of vaccine
      Manufacturer delay of vaccine
      AHA: 2018,4Q,36
    Z28.89   **Immunization not carried out for other reason**   `UPD`

Z28.9   **Immunization not carried out for unspecified reason**   `UPD`

`✓4ᵗʰ` **Z29**   **Encounter for other prophylactic measures**
    `EXCLUDES 1`   *desensitization to allergens (Z51.6)*
      prophylactic surgery (Z40.-)
    AHA: 2016,4Q,78-79

`✓6ᵗʰ` **Z29.1**   **Encounter for prophylactic immunotherapy**
    Encounter for administration of immunoglobulin
    Z29.11   **Encounter for prophylactic immunotherapy for respiratory syncytial virus (RSV)**   `UPD`

Z29.12   **Encounter for prophylactic antivenin**   `UPD`
Z29.13   **Encounter for prophylactic Rho(D) immune globulin**   `UPD`
    AHA: 2019,3Q,5
Z29.14   **Encounter for prophylactic rabies immune globin**   `UPD`
Z29.3   **Encounter for prophylactic fluoride administration**   `UPD`
Z29.8   **Encounter for other specified prophylactic measures**   `UPD`
Z29.9   **Encounter for prophylactic measures, unspecified**   `UPD`

Persons encountering health services in circumstances related to reproduction (Z30-Z39)

`✓4ᵗʰ` **Z30**   **Encounter for contraceptive management**
    AHA: 2016,4Q,78
    DEF: Contraceptive management to prevent pregnancy. Methods include oral medications, intrauterine devices, and surgical procedures for males and females (sterilization).

`✓5ᵗʰ` **Z30.0**   **Encounter for general counseling and advice on contraception**
    `✓6ᵗʰ` **Z30.01**   **Encounter for initial prescription of contraceptives**
      `EXCLUDES 1`   *encounter for surveillance of contraceptives (Z30.4-)*
      Z30.011   **Encounter for initial prescription of contraceptive pills**   `UPD` ♀
      Z30.012   **Encounter for prescription of emergency contraception**   `UPD` ♀
        Encounter for postcoital contraception
      Z30.013   **Encounter for initial prescription of injectable contraceptive**   `UPD` ♀
      Z30.014   **Encounter for initial prescription of intrauterine contraceptive device**   `UPD` ♀
        `EXCLUDES 1`   *encounter for insertion of intrauterine contraceptive device (Z30.430, Z30.432)*
      Z30.015   **Encounter for initial prescription of vaginal ring hormonal contraceptive**   `UPD` ♀
      Z30.016   **Encounter for initial prescription of transdermal patch hormonal contraceptive device**   `UPD`
      Z30.017   **Encounter for initial prescription of implantable subdermal contraceptive**   `UPD`
      Z30.018   **Encounter for initial prescription of other contraceptives**   `UPD` ♀
        Encounter for initial prescription of barrier contraception
        Encounter for initial prescription of diaphragm
      Z30.019   **Encounter for initial prescription of contraceptives, unspecified**   `UPD` ♀
    Z30.02   **Counseling and instruction in natural family planning to avoid pregnancy**   `UPD`
    Z30.09   **Encounter for other general counseling and advice on contraception**   `UPD`
      Encounter for family planning advice NOS

Z30.2   **Encounter for sterilization**

`✓5ᵗʰ` **Z30.4**   **Encounter for surveillance of contraceptives**
    Z30.40   **Encounter for surveillance of contraceptives, unspecified**   `UPD`
    Z30.41   **Encounter for surveillance of contraceptive pills**   `UPD` ♀
      Encounter for repeat prescription for contraceptive pill
    Z30.42   **Encounter for surveillance of injectable contraceptive**   `UPD` ♀
    `✓6ᵗʰ` **Z30.43**   **Encounter for surveillance of intrauterine contraceptive device**
      Z30.430   **Encounter for insertion of intrauterine contraceptive device**   `UPD` ♀
      Z30.431   **Encounter for routine checking of intrauterine contraceptive device**   `UPD` ♀
      Z30.432   **Encounter for removal of intrauterine contraceptive device**   `UPD` ♀

`✓` Additional Character Required   `✓x7ᵗʰ` Placeholder   Questionable PDx   Manifestation   Unspecified Dx   `UPD` Unacceptable PDx   `H1`-`H14` HAC   `HCC` CMS-HCC Dx   `HIV` HIV Dx

ICD-10-CM 2022   **1243**

Chapter 21. Factors Influencing Health Status and Contact With Health Services

Z30.433–Z34.83

Z30.433 Encounter for removal and reinsertion of intrauterine contraceptive device   UPD ♀
Encounter for replacement of intrauterine contraceptive device

Z30.44 Encounter for surveillance of vaginal ring hormonal contraceptive device   UPD ♀

Z30.45 Encounter for surveillance of transdermal patch hormonal **contraceptive device**   UPD ♀

Z30.46 Encounter for surveillance of implantable subdermal **contraceptive**   UPD ♀
Encounter for checking, reinsertion or removal of implantable subdermal contraceptive

Z30.49 Encounter for surveillance of other contraceptives   UPD ♀
Encounter for surveillance of barrier contraception
Encounter for surveillance of diaphragm

Z30.8 Encounter for other contraceptive management   UPD
Encounter for postvasectomy sperm count
Encounter for routine examination for contraceptive maintenance
EXCLUDES 1   *sperm count following sterilization reversal (Z31.42)*
sperm count for fertility testing (Z31.41)

Z30.9 Encounter for contraceptive management, unspecified   UPD

✓4th **Z31 Encounter for procreative management**
EXCLUDES 1   *complications associated with artificial fertilization (N98.-)*
female infertility (N97.-)
male infertility (N46.-)
EXCLUDES 2   ►*complications associated with artificial fertilization (N98.-)*◄
►*female infertility (N97.-)*◄
►*male infertility (N46.-)*◄

Z31.0 Encounter for reversal of previous sterilization

✓5th **Z31.4 Encounter for** procreative investigation and testing
EXCLUDES 1   *postvasectomy sperm count (Z30.8)*

Z31.41 Encounter for fertility testing   UPD
Encounter for fallopian tube patency testing
Encounter for sperm count for fertility testing

Z31.42 Aftercare following sterilization reversal   UPD
Sperm count following sterilization reversal

✓6th **Z31.43 Encounter for genetic testing of** female **for procreative management**
Use additional code for recurrent pregnancy loss, if applicable (N96, O26.2-)
EXCLUDES 1   *nonprocreative genetic testing (Z13.7-)*

Z31.430 Encounter of female for testing for genetic disease carrier status **for procreative management**   UPD ♀

Z31.438 Encounter for other genetic testing of female for procreative management   UPD ♀

✓6th **Z31.44 Encounter for genetic testing of** male **for procreative management**
EXCLUDES 1   *nonprocreative genetic testing (Z13.7-)*

Z31.440 Encounter of male for testing for genetic disease carrier status **for procreative management**   UPD ♂

Z31.441 Encounter for testing of male partner of patient with recurrent pregnancy loss   UPD A ♂

Z31.448 Encounter for other genetic testing of male for procreative management   UPD A ♂

Z31.49 Encounter for other procreative investigation and testing   UPD

Z31.5 Encounter for procreative genetic counseling   UPD
AHA: 2017,4Q,27

✓5th **Z31.6 Encounter for general counseling and advice on procreation**

Z31.61 Procreative counseling and advice using natural family planning   UPD

Z31.62 Encounter for fertility preservation counseling   UPD
Encounter for fertility preservation counseling prior to cancer therapy
Encounter for fertility preservation counseling prior to surgical removal of gonads

Z31.69 Encounter for other general counseling and advice on procreation   UPD

Z31.7 Encounter for procreative management and counseling for gestational carrier
EXCLUDES 1   *pregnant state, gestational carrier (Z33.3)*
AHA: 2016,4Q,78

✓5th **Z31.8 Encounter for other procreative management**

Z31.81 Encounter for male factor **infertility in female patient**   UPD ♀

Z31.82 Encounter for Rh incompatibility **status**   UPD ♀
AHA: 2015,3Q,40; 2014,4Q,17

Z31.83 Encounter for assisted reproductive fertility procedure cycle   UPD ♀
Patient undergoing in vitro fertilization cycle
Use additional code to identify the type of infertility
EXCLUDES 1   *pre-cycle diagnosis and testing - code to reason for encounter*

Z31.84 Encounter for fertility preservation procedure   UPD
Encounter for fertility preservation procedure prior to cancer therapy
Encounter for fertility preservation procedure prior to surgical removal of gonads

Z31.89 Encounter for other procreative management   UPD

Z31.9 Encounter for procreative management, unspecified   UPD

✓4th **Z32 Encounter for pregnancy test and childbirth and childcare instruction**

✓5th **Z32.0 Encounter for** pregnancy test

Z32.00 Encounter for pregnancy test, result unknown ♀
Encounter for pregnancy test NOS

Z32.01 Encounter for pregnancy test, result positive   M ♀

Z32.02 Encounter for pregnancy test, result negative ♀

Z32.2 Encounter for childbirth instruction   UPD

Z32.3 Encounter for childcare instruction   UPD
Encounter for prenatal or postpartum childcare instruction

✓4th **Z33 Pregnant state**

Z33.1 Pregnant state, incidental   UPD M ♀
Pregnancy NOS
Pregnant state NOS
EXCLUDES 1   *complications of pregnancy (O00-O9A)*
pregnant state, gestational carrier (Z33.3)

Z33.2 Encounter for elective termination of pregnancy   M ♀
EXCLUDES 1   *early fetal death with retention of dead fetus (O02.1)*
late fetal death (O36.4)
spontaneous abortion (O03)
TIP: Do not assign a code from category Z3A with this code.

Z33.3 Pregnant state, gestational carrier   UPD M ♀
EXCLUDES 1   *encounter for procreative management and counseling for gestational carrier (Z31.7)*
AHA: 2016,4Q,78

✓4th **Z34 Encounter for supervision of normal pregnancy**
EXCLUDES 1   *any complication of pregnancy (O00-O9A)*
encounter for pregnancy test (Z32.0-)
encounter for supervision of high risk pregnancy (O09.-)
AHA: 2019,3Q,5; 2014,4Q,17

✓5th **Z34.0 Encounter for supervision of normal** first **pregnancy**

Z34.00 Encounter for supervision of normal first pregnancy, unspecified trimester   UPD M ♀

Z34.01 Encounter for supervision of normal first pregnancy, first trimester   UPD M ♀

Z34.02 Encounter for supervision of normal first pregnancy, second trimester   UPD M ♀

Z34.03 Encounter for supervision of normal first pregnancy, third trimester   UPD M ♀

✓5th **Z34.8 Encounter for supervision of other normal pregnancy**

Z34.80 Encounter for supervision of other normal pregnancy, unspecified trimester   UPD M ♀

Z34.81 Encounter for supervision of other normal pregnancy, first trimester   UPD M ♀

Z34.82 Encounter for supervision of other normal pregnancy, second trimester   UPD M ♀

Z34.83 Encounter for supervision of other normal pregnancy, third trimester   UPD M ♀

✓5ᵗʰ **Z34.9** **Encounter for supervision of normal pregnancy, unspecified**

    Z34.90 **Encounter for supervision of normal pregnancy, unspecified, unspecified trimester** UPD M ♀

    Z34.91 **Encounter for supervision of normal pregnancy, unspecified, first trimester** UPD M ♀

    Z34.92 **Encounter for supervision of normal pregnancy, unspecified, second trimester** UPD M ♀

    Z34.93 **Encounter for supervision of normal pregnancy, unspecified, third trimester** UPD M ♀

✓4ᵗʰ **Z36** **Encounter for antenatal screening of mother**

    INCLUDES   encounter for placental sample (taken vaginally)
         screening is the testing for disease or disease precursors in asymptomatic individuals so that early detection and treatment can be provided for those who test positive for the disease.

    EXCLUDES 1   diagnostic examination - code to sign or symptom
         encounter for suspected maternal and fetal conditions ruled out (Z03.7-)
         suspected fetal condition affecting management of pregnancy - code to condition in Chapter 15

    EXCLUDES 2   abnormal findings on antenatal screening of mother (O28.-)
         genetic counseling and testing (Z31.43-, Z31.5)
         routine prenatal care (Z34)

    AHA: 2017,4Q,28

    Z36.0 **Encounter for antenatal screening for chromosomal anomalies** M ♀

    Z36.1 **Encounter for antenatal screening for raised alphafetoprotein level** M ♀
         Encounter for antenatal screening for elevated maternal serum alphafetoprotein level
         DEF: High levels of alpha-fetoprotein (AFP) that may indicate a possibility of spina bifida and other neural tube defects, anencephaly, or omphalocele in the fetus.

    Z36.2 **Encounter for other antenatal screening follow-up** ♀
         Non-visualized anatomy on a previous scan

    Z36.3 **Encounter for antenatal screening for malformations** M ♀
         Screening for a suspected anomaly

    Z36.4 **Encounter for antenatal screening for fetal growth retardation** M ♀
         Intrauterine growth restriction (IUGR)/small-for-dates

    Z36.5 **Encounter for antenatal screening for isoimmunization** M ♀

✓5ᵗʰ   **Z36.8** **Encounter for other antenatal screening**

       Z36.81 **Encounter for antenatal screening for hydrops fetalis** M ♀
           DEF: Hydrops fetalis: Abnormal accumulation of fluid in two or more parts of the fetus, such as ascites, effusion of the pleural or pericardial tissues, or edema.

       Z36.82 **Encounter for antenatal screening for nuchal translucency** M ♀

       Z36.83 **Encounter for fetal screening for congenital cardiac abnormalities** M ♀

       Z36.84 **Encounter for antenatal screening for fetal lung maturity** M ♀

       Z36.85 **Encounter for antenatal screening for Streptococcus B** ♀

       Z36.86 **Encounter for antenatal screening for cervical length** M ♀
           Screening for risk of pre-term labor

       Z36.87 **Encounter for antenatal screening for uncertain dates** M ♀

       Z36.88 **Encounter for antenatal screening for fetal macrosomia** M ♀
           Screening for large-for-dates

       Z36.89 **Encounter for other specified antenatal screening** M ♀

       Z36.8A **Encounter for antenatal screening for other genetic defects** M ♀

    Z36.9 **Encounter for antenatal screening, unspecified** M ♀

✓4ᵗʰ **Z3A** **Weeks of gestation**

    NOTE   Codes from category Z3A are for use, only on the maternal record, to indicate the weeks of gestation of the pregnancy, if known.

    ▶Code first obstetric condition or encounter for delivery (O09-O6O, O8O-O82)◀
    ~~Code first complications of pregnancy, childbirth and the puerperium (O09-O9A)~~

    AHA: 2019,2Q,11; 2016,2Q,34; 2014,3Q,17; 2014,2Q,9; 2013,2Q,33
    TIP: Do not assign a code from this category with codes from categories O00-O08 or code Z33.2.

✓5ᵗʰ   **Z3A.0** **Weeks of gestation of pregnancy, unspecified or less than 10 weeks**

       Z3A.00 **Weeks of gestation of pregnancy not specified** UPD M ♀

       Z3A.01 **Less than 8 weeks gestation of pregnancy** UPD M ♀

       Z3A.08 **8 weeks gestation of pregnancy** UPD M ♀

       Z3A.09 **9 weeks gestation of pregnancy** UPD M ♀

✓5ᵗʰ   **Z3A.1** **Weeks of gestation of pregnancy, weeks 10-19**

       Z3A.10 **10 weeks gestation of pregnancy** UPD M ♀

       Z3A.11 **11 weeks gestation of pregnancy** UPD M ♀

       Z3A.12 **12 weeks gestation of pregnancy** UPD M ♀

       Z3A.13 **13 weeks gestation of pregnancy** UPD M ♀

       Z3A.14 **14 weeks gestation of pregnancy** UPD M ♀

       Z3A.15 **15 weeks gestation of pregnancy** UPD M ♀

       Z3A.16 **16 weeks gestation of pregnancy** UPD M ♀

       Z3A.17 **17 weeks gestation of pregnancy** UPD M ♀

       Z3A.18 **18 weeks gestation of pregnancy** UPD M ♀

       Z3A.19 **19 weeks gestation of pregnancy** UPD M ♀

✓5ᵗʰ   **Z3A.2** **Weeks of gestation of pregnancy, weeks 20-29**

       Z3A.20 **20 weeks gestation of pregnancy** UPD M ♀

       Z3A.21 **21 weeks gestation of pregnancy** UPD M ♀

       Z3A.22 **22 weeks gestation of pregnancy** UPD M ♀

       Z3A.23 **23 weeks gestation of pregnancy** UPD M ♀

       Z3A.24 **24 weeks gestation of pregnancy** UPD M ♀

       Z3A.25 **25 weeks gestation of pregnancy** UPD M ♀

       Z3A.26 **26 weeks gestation of pregnancy** UPD M ♀

       Z3A.27 **27 weeks gestation of pregnancy** UPD M ♀

       Z3A.28 **28 weeks gestation of pregnancy** UPD M ♀

       Z3A.29 **29 weeks gestation of pregnancy** UPD M ♀

✓5ᵗʰ   **Z3A.3** **Weeks of gestation of pregnancy, weeks 30-39**

       Z3A.30 **30 weeks gestation of pregnancy** UPD M ♀

       Z3A.31 **31 weeks gestation of pregnancy** UPD M ♀

       Z3A.32 **32 weeks gestation of pregnancy** UPD M ♀

       Z3A.33 **33 weeks gestation of pregnancy** UPD M ♀

       Z3A.34 **34 weeks gestation of pregnancy** UPD M ♀

       Z3A.35 **35 weeks gestation of pregnancy** UPD M ♀

       Z3A.36 **36 weeks gestation of pregnancy** UPD M ♀

       Z3A.37 **37 weeks gestation of pregnancy** UPD M ♀

       Z3A.38 **38 weeks gestation of pregnancy** UPD M ♀

       Z3A.39 **39 weeks gestation of pregnancy** UPD M ♀

✓5ᵗʰ   **Z3A.4** **Weeks of gestation of pregnancy, weeks 40 or greater**
       AHA: 2014,4Q,23

       Z3A.40 **40 weeks gestation of pregnancy** UPD M ♀

       Z3A.41 **41 weeks gestation of pregnancy** UPD M ♀

       Z3A.42 **42 weeks gestation of pregnancy** UPD M ♀

       Z3A.49 **Greater than 42 weeks gestation of pregnancy** UPD M ♀

✓4ᵗʰ **Z37** **Outcome of delivery**

    This category is intended for use as an additional code to identify the outcome of delivery on the mother's record. It is not for use on the newborn record.

    EXCLUDES 1   stillbirth (P95)

    Z37.0 **Single live birth** UPD M ♀
         AHA: 2016,2Q,34; 2014,2Q,9

    Z37.1 **Single stillbirth** UPD M ♀

    Z37.2 **Twins, both liveborn** UPD M ♀

    Z37.3 **Twins, one liveborn and one stillborn** UPD M ♀

    Z37.4 **Twins, both stillborn** UPD M ♀

✓5ᵗʰ   **Z37.5** **Other multiple births, all liveborn**

       Z37.50 **Multiple births, unspecified, all liveborn** UPD M ♀

       Z37.51 **Triplets, all liveborn** UPD M ♀

☑ Additional Character Required   ✓×7ᵗʰ Placeholder   Questionable PDx   **Manifestation**   Unspecified Dx   UPD Unacceptable PDx   H1-H14 HAC   HCC CMS-HCC Dx   HIV HIV Dx

Chapter 21. Factors Influencing Health Status and Contact With Health Services

Z37.52–Z43.3

Z37.52	**Quadruplets, all liveborn**	UPD M ♀
Z37.53	**Quintuplets, all liveborn**	UPD M ♀
Z37.54	**Sextuplets, all liveborn**	UPD M ♀
Z37.59	**Other multiple births, all liveborn**	UPD M ♀

✓6ᵗʰ **Z37.6 Other multiple births, some liveborn**

Z37.60	**Multiple births, unspecified, some liveborn**	UPD M ♀
Z37.61	**Triplets, some liveborn**	UPD M ♀
Z37.62	**Quadruplets, some liveborn**	UPD M ♀
Z37.63	**Quintuplets, some liveborn**	UPD M ♀
Z37.64	**Sextuplets, some liveborn**	UPD M ♀
Z37.69	**Other multiple births, some liveborn**	UPD M ♀

Z37.7 Other multiple births, all stillborn   UPD M ♀

Z37.9 Outcome of delivery, unspecified   UPD M ♀
  Multiple birth NOS
  Single birth NOS

✓4ᵗʰ **Z38 Liveborn infants according to place of birth and type of delivery**

This category is for use as the principal code on the initial record of a newborn baby. It is to be used for the initial birth record only. It is not to be used on the mother's record.

AHA: 2020,2Q,13; 2017,2Q,5-7; 2016,3Q,18; 2015,2Q,15

✓5ᵗʰ **Z38.0 Single liveborn infant, born in hospital**

Single liveborn infant, born in birthing center or other health care facility

Z38.00	**Single liveborn infant, delivered vaginally**	N
Z38.01	**Single liveborn infant, delivered by cesarean**	N

Z38.1 Single liveborn infant, born outside hospital   N

Z38.2 Single liveborn infant, unspecified as to place of birth   N
  Single liveborn infant NOS

✓5ᵗʰ **Z38.3 Twin liveborn infant, born in hospital**

Z38.30	**Twin liveborn infant, delivered vaginally**	N
Z38.31	**Twin liveborn infant, delivered by cesarean**	N

Z38.4 Twin liveborn infant, born outside hospital   N

Z38.5 Twin liveborn infant, unspecified as to place of birth   N

✓6ᵗʰ **Z38.6 Other multiple liveborn infant, born in hospital**

Z38.61	**Triplet liveborn infant, delivered vaginally**	N
Z38.62	**Triplet liveborn infant, delivered by cesarean**	N
Z38.63	**Quadruplet liveborn infant, delivered vaginally**	N
Z38.64	**Quadruplet liveborn infant, delivered by cesarean**	N
Z38.65	**Quintuplet liveborn infant, delivered vaginally**	N
Z38.66	**Quintuplet liveborn infant, delivered by cesarean**	N
Z38.68	**Other multiple liveborn infant, delivered vaginally**	N
Z38.69	**Other multiple liveborn infant, delivered by cesarean**	N

Z38.7 Other multiple liveborn infant, born outside hospital   N

Z38.8 Other multiple liveborn infant, unspecified as to place of birth   N

✓4ᵗʰ **Z39 Encounter for maternal postpartum care and examination**

Z39.0 Encounter for care and examination of mother immediately after delivery   M ♀

Care and observation in uncomplicated cases when the delivery occurs outside a healthcare facility

EXCLUDES 1   *care for postpartum complication - see Alphabetic Index*

Z39.1 Encounter for care and examination of lactating mother   UPD M ♀

Encounter for supervision of lactation

EXCLUDES 1   *disorders of lactation (O92.-)*

Z39.2 Encounter for routine postpartum follow-up   UPD M ♀

Encounters for other specific health care (Z40-Z53)

Categories Z40-Z53 are intended for use to indicate a reason for care. They may be used for patients who have already been treated for a disease or injury, but who are receiving aftercare or prophylactic care, or care to consolidate the treatment, or to deal with a residual state

EXCLUDES 2   *follow-up examination for medical surveillance after treatment (Z08-Z09)*

✓4ᵗʰ **Z40 Encounter for prophylactic surgery**

EXCLUDES 1   *organ donations (Z52.-)*

     therapeutic organ removal - code to condition

DEF: Treatment measure intended to prevent or ward off a disease or condition.

✓5ᵗʰ **Z40.0 Encounter for prophylactic surgery for risk factors related to malignant neoplasms**

Admission for prophylactic organ removal
Use additional code to identify risk factor
AHA: 2017,4Q,28-29

Z40.00	**Encounter for prophylactic removal of unspecified organ**
Z40.01	**Encounter for prophylactic removal of breast**
Z40.02	**Encounter for prophylactic removal of ovary(s)** ♀
	Encounter for prophylactic removal of ovary(s) and fallopian tube(s)
Z40.03	**Encounter for prophylactic removal of fallopian tube(s)** ♀
Z40.09	**Encounter for prophylactic removal of other organ**

Z40.8 Encounter for other prophylactic surgery   UPD

Z40.9 Encounter for prophylactic surgery, unspecified   UPD

✓4ᵗʰ **Z41 Encounter for procedures for purposes other than remedying health state**

Z41.1 Encounter for cosmetic surgery

Encounter for cosmetic breast implant
Encounter for cosmetic procedure

EXCLUDES 1   *encounter for plastic and reconstructive surgery following medical procedure or healed injury (Z42.-)*

     encounter for post-mastectomy breast implantation (Z42.1)

Z41.2 Encounter for routine and ritual male circumcision   ♂

AHA: 2018,3Q,15

TIP: Do not report this code when circumcision is performed during the birth admission.

Z41.3 Encounter for ear piercing   UPD

Z41.8 Encounter for other procedures for purposes other than remedying health state

Z41.9 Encounter for procedure for purposes other than remedying health state, unspecified   UPD

✓4ᵗʰ **Z42 Encounter for plastic and reconstructive surgery following medical procedure or healed injury**

EXCLUDES 1   *encounter for cosmetic plastic surgery (Z41.1)*

     encounter for plastic surgery for treatment of current injury - code to relevent injury

Z42.1 Encounter for breast reconstruction following mastectomy   A

EXCLUDES 1   *deformity and disproportion of reconstructed breast (N65.1-)*

Z42.8 Encounter for other plastic and reconstructive surgery following medical procedure or healed injury

AHA: 2017,1Q,42

✓4ᵗʰ **Z43 Encounter for attention to artificial openings**

INCLUDES   closure of artificial openings

     passage of sounds or bougies through artificial openings
     reforming artificial openings
     removal of catheter from artificial openings
     toilet or cleansing of artificial openings

EXCLUDES 1   *complications of external stoma (J95.0-, K94.-, N99.5-)*

EXCLUDES 2   *fitting and adjustment of prosthetic and other devices (Z44-Z46)*

AHA: 2019,2Q,33

Z43.0 Encounter for attention to tracheostomy   HCC

Z43.1 Encounter for attention to gastrostomy   CC HCC

EXCLUDES 2   *artificial opening status only, without need for care (Z93.-)*

Z43.2 Encounter for attention to ileostomy   HCC

Z43.3 Encounter for attention to colostomy   HCC

N Newborn: 0   P Pediatric: 0-17   M Maternity: 9-64   A Adult: 15-124   MCC Major Complication/Comorbidity   CC Complication/Comorbidity   SW Severe Wound Dx

1246   ICD-10-CM 2022

Z43.4 Encounter for attention to other artificial openings of digestive tract `HCC`

Z43.5 Encounter for attention to cystostomy `HCC`

Z43.6 Encounter for attention to other artificial openings of urinary tract `HCC`
- Encounter for attention to nephrostomy
- Encounter for attention to ureterostomy
- Encounter for attention to urethrostomy

Z43.7 Encounter for attention to artificial vagina

Z43.8 Encounter for attention to other artificial openings `HCC`

Z43.9 Encounter for attention to unspecified artificial opening `UPD` `HCC`

☑4ᵗʰ **Z44** Encounter for fitting and adjustment of external prosthetic device
- `INCLUDES` removal or replacement of external prosthetic device
- `EXCLUDES 1` malfunction or other complications of device - see Alphabetical Index
- presence of prosthetic device (Z97.-)

☑5ᵗʰ **Z44.0** Encounter for fitting and adjustment of artificial arm

  ☑6ᵗʰ **Z44.00** Encounter for fitting and adjustment of unspecified artificial arm

    Z44.001 Encounter for fitting and adjustment of unspecified right artificial arm

    Z44.002 Encounter for fitting and adjustment of unspecified left artificial arm

    Z44.009 Encounter for fitting and adjustment of unspecified artificial arm, unspecified arm

  ☑6ᵗʰ **Z44.01** Encounter for fitting and adjustment of complete artificial arm

    Z44.011 Encounter for fitting and adjustment of complete right artificial arm

    Z44.012 Encounter for fitting and adjustment of complete left artificial arm

    Z44.019 Encounter for fitting and adjustment of complete artificial arm, unspecified arm

  ☑6ᵗʰ **Z44.02** Encounter for fitting and adjustment of partial artificial arm

    Z44.021 Encounter for fitting and adjustment of partial artificial right arm

    Z44.022 Encounter for fitting and adjustment of partial artificial left arm

    Z44.029 Encounter for fitting and adjustment of partial artificial arm, unspecified arm

☑5ᵗʰ **Z44.1** Encounter for fitting and adjustment of artificial leg

  ☑6ᵗʰ **Z44.10** Encounter for fitting and adjustment of unspecified artificial leg

    Z44.101 Encounter for fitting and adjustment of unspecified right artificial leg `HCC`

    Z44.102 Encounter for fitting and adjustment of unspecified left artificial leg `HCC`

    Z44.109 Encounter for fitting and adjustment of unspecified artificial leg, unspecified leg `HCC`

  ☑6ᵗʰ **Z44.11** Encounter for fitting and adjustment of complete artificial leg

    Z44.111 Encounter for fitting and adjustment of complete right artificial leg `HCC`

    Z44.112 Encounter for fitting and adjustment of complete left artificial leg `HCC`

    Z44.119 Encounter for fitting and adjustment of complete artificial leg, unspecified leg `HCC`

  ☑6ᵗʰ **Z44.12** Encounter for fitting and adjustment of partial artificial leg

    Z44.121 Encounter for fitting and adjustment of partial artificial right leg `HCC`

    Z44.122 Encounter for fitting and adjustment of partial artificial left leg `HCC`

    Z44.129 Encounter for fitting and adjustment of partial artificial leg, unspecified leg `HCC`

☑5ᵗʰ **Z44.2** Encounter for fitting and adjustment of artificial eye
- `EXCLUDES 1` mechanical complication of ocular prosthesis (T85.3)

  Z44.20 Encounter for fitting and adjustment of artificial eye, unspecified

  Z44.21 Encounter for fitting and adjustment of artificial right eye

  Z44.22 Encounter for fitting and adjustment of artificial left eye

☑5ᵗʰ **Z44.3** Encounter for fitting and adjustment of external breast prosthesis
- `EXCLUDES 1` complications of breast implant (T85.4-)
- encounter for adjustment or removal of breast implant (Z45.81-)
- encounter for initial breast implant insertion for cosmetic breast augmentation (Z41.1)
- encounter for breast reconstruction following mastectomy (Z42.1)

  Z44.30 Encounter for fitting and adjustment of external breast prosthesis, unspecified breast

  Z44.31 Encounter for fitting and adjustment of external right breast prosthesis

  Z44.32 Encounter for fitting and adjustment of external left breast prosthesis

Z44.8 Encounter for fitting and adjustment of other external prosthetic devices

Z44.9 Encounter for fitting and adjustment of unspecified external prosthetic device `UPD`

☑4ᵗʰ **Z45** Encounter for adjustment and management of implanted device
- `INCLUDES` removal or replacement of implanted device
- `EXCLUDES 1` malfunction or other complications of device - see Alphabetical Index
- `EXCLUDES 2` encounter for fitting and adjustment of non-implanted device (Z46.-)

☑5ᵗʰ **Z45.0** Encounter for adjustment and management of cardiac device

  TIP: Assign an additional code for the condition the cardiac device is controlling (e.g., sick sinus syndrome). Even though the cardiac device controls the heart rate, it does not cure the condition and therefore should be reported.

  ☑6ᵗʰ **Z45.01** Encounter for adjustment and management of cardiac pacemaker
- Encounter for adjustment and management of cardiac resynchronization therapy pacemaker (CRT-P)
- `EXCLUDES 1` encounter for adjustment and management of automatic implantable cardiac defibrillator with synchronous cardiac pacemaker (Z45.02)

    Z45.010 Encounter for checking and testing of cardiac pacemaker pulse generator [battery]
- Encounter for replacing cardiac pacemaker pulse generator [battery]

    Z45.018 Encounter for adjustment and management of other part of cardiac pacemaker
- `EXCLUDES 1` presence of other part of cardiac pacemaker (Z95.0)
- `EXCLUDES 2` presence of prosthetic and other devices (Z95.1-Z95.5, Z95.811-Z97)

  Z45.02 Encounter for adjustment and management of automatic implantable cardiac defibrillator
- Encounter for adjustment and management of automatic implantable cardiac defibrillator with synchronous cardiac pacemaker
- Encounter for adjustment and management of cardiac resynchronization therapy defibrillator (CRT-D)

  Z45.09 Encounter for adjustment and management of other cardiac device

Z45.1 Encounter for adjustment and management of infusion pump

Z45.2 Encounter for adjustment and management of vascular access device
- Encounter for adjustment and management of vascular catheters
- `EXCLUDES 1` encounter for adjustment and management of renal dialysis catheter (Z49.01)
- **AHA:** 2020,2Q,21; 2018,3Q,20

☑5ᵗʰ **Z45.3** Encounter for adjustment and management of implanted devices of the special senses

  Z45.31 Encounter for adjustment and management of implanted visual substitution device

☑ Additional Character Required   ☑x7ᵗʰ Placeholder   Questionable PDx   Manifestation   Unspecified Dx   `UPD` Unacceptable PDx   `H1`-`H14` HAC   `HCC` CMS-HCC Dx   `HIV` HIV Dx

ICD-10-CM 2022   1247

Chapter 21. Factors Influencing Health Status and Contact With Health Services

✓6ᵗʰ **Z45.32 Encounter for adjustment and management of implanted hearing device**
> EXCLUDES 1   *encounter for fitting and adjustment of hearing aide (Z46.1)*

Z45.320 Encounter for adjustment and management of bone conduction device

Z45.321 Encounter for adjustment and management of cochlear device

Z45.328 Encounter for adjustment and management of other implanted hearing device

✓5ᵗʰ **Z45.4 Encounter for adjustment and management of implanted nervous system device**

Z45.41 Encounter for adjustment and management of cerebrospinal fluid drainage device
> Encounter for adjustment and management of cerebral ventricular (communicating) shunt

Z45.42 Encounter for adjustment and management of neurostimulator
> Encounter for adjustment and management of brain neurostimulator
> Encounter for adjustment and management of gastric neurostimulator
> Encounter for adjustment and management of peripheral nerve neurostimulator
> Encounter for adjustment and management of sacral nerve neurostimulator
> Encounter for adjustment and management of spinal cord neurostimulator
> Encounter for adjustment and management of vagus nerve neurostimulator

Z45.49 Encounter for adjustment and management of other implanted nervous system device
> AHA: 2014,3Q,19

✓5ᵗʰ **Z45.8 Encounter for adjustment and management of other implanted devices**

✓6ᵗʰ **Z45.81 Encounter for adjustment or removal of breast implant**
> Encounter for elective implant exchange (different material) (different size)
> ▶Encounter for removal of tissue expander with or without synchronous insertion of permanent implant◀
> EXCLUDES 1   *complications of breast implant (T85.4-)*
> *encounter for initial breast implant insertion for cosmetic breast augmentation (Z41.1)*
> *encounter for breast reconstruction following mastectomy (Z42.1)*

Z45.811 Encounter for adjustment or removal of right breast implant

Z45.812 Encounter for adjustment or removal of left breast implant

Z45.819 Encounter for adjustment or removal of unspecified breast implant

Z45.82 Encounter for adjustment or removal of myringotomy device (stent) (tube) UPD

Z45.89 Encounter for adjustment and management of other implanted devices UPD
> AHA: 2014,4Q,26-28

Z45.9 Encounter for adjustment and management of unspecified implanted device UPD

✓4ᵗʰ **Z46 Encounter for fitting and adjustment of other devices**
> INCLUDES   removal or replacement of other device
> EXCLUDES 1   *malfunction or other complications of device - see Alphabetical Index*
> EXCLUDES 2   *encounter for fitting and management of implanted devices (Z45.-)*
> *issue of repeat prescription only (Z76.0)*
> *presence of prosthetic and other devices (Z95-Z97)*

Z46.0 Encounter for fitting and adjustment of spectacles and contact lenses UPD

Z46.1 Encounter for fitting and adjustment of hearing aid UPD
> EXCLUDES 1   *encounter for adjustment and management of implanted hearing device (Z45.32-)*

Z46.2 Encounter for fitting and adjustment of other devices related to nervous system and special senses
> EXCLUDES 2   *encounter for adjustment and management of implanted nervous system device (Z45.4-)*
> *encounter for adjustment and management of implanted visual substitution device (Z45.31)*

Z46.3 Encounter for fitting and adjustment of dental prosthetic device
> Encounter for fitting and adjustment of dentures

Z46.4 Encounter for fitting and adjustment of orthodontic device UPD

✓5ᵗʰ **Z46.5 Encounter for fitting and adjustment of other gastrointestinal appliance and device**
> EXCLUDES 1   *encounter for attention to artificial openings of digestive tract (Z43.1-Z43.4)*

Z46.51 Encounter for fitting and adjustment of gastric lap band UPD

Z46.59 Encounter for fitting and adjustment of other gastrointestinal appliance and device UPD

Z46.6 Encounter for fitting and adjustment of urinary device UPD
> EXCLUDES 2   *attention to artificial openings of urinary tract (Z43.5, Z43.6)*

✓5ᵗʰ **Z46.8 Encounter for fitting and adjustment of other specified devices**

Z46.81 Encounter for fitting and adjustment of insulin pump UPD
> Encounter for insulin pump instruction and training
> Encounter for insulin pump titration

Z46.82 Encounter for fitting and adjustment of non-vascular catheter

Z46.89 Encounter for fitting and adjustment of other specified devices UPD
> Encounter for fitting and adjustment of wheelchair

Z46.9 Encounter for fitting and adjustment of unspecified device UPD

✓4ᵗʰ **Z47 Orthopedic aftercare**
> EXCLUDES 1   *aftercare for healing fracture - code to fracture with 7th character D*

Z47.1 Aftercare following joint replacement surgery
> Use additional code to identify the joint (Z96.6-)
> AHA: 2020,1Q,23

Z47.2 Encounter for removal of internal fixation device
> EXCLUDES 1   *encounter for adjustment of internal fixation device for fracture treatment - code to fracture with appropriate 7th character*
> *encounter for removal of external fixation device - code to fracture with 7th character D*
> *infection or inflammatory reaction to internal fixation device (T84.6-)*
> *mechanical complication of internal fixation device (T84.1-)*

✓5ᵗʰ **Z47.3 Aftercare following explantation of joint prosthesis**
> Aftercare following explantation of joint prosthesis, staged procedure
> Encounter for joint prosthesis insertion following prior explantation of joint prosthesis
> AHA: 2020,1Q,23; 2015,1Q,16
> TIP: For staged removal of elbow joint prosthesis, assign code Z47.1.

Z47.31 Aftercare following explantation of shoulder joint prosthesis
> EXCLUDES 1   *acquired absence of shoulder joint following prior explantation of shoulder joint prosthesis (Z89.23-)*
> *shoulder joint prosthesis explantation status (Z89.23-)*

Z47.32 Aftercare following explantation of hip joint prosthesis
> EXCLUDES 1   *acquired absence of hip joint following prior explantation of hip joint prosthesis (Z89.62-)*
> *hip joint prosthesis explantation status (Z89.62-)*

Ⓝ Newborn: 0   Ⓟ Pediatric: 0-17   Ⓜ Maternity: 9-64   Ⓐ Adult: 15-124   MCC Major Complication/Comorbidity   CC Complication/Comorbidity   SW Severe Wound Dx

1248   ICD-10-CM 2022

Z47.33 **Aftercare following explantation of** knee **joint prosthesis**

> EXCLUDES 1 *acquired absence of knee joint following prior explantation of knee prosthesis (Z89.52-)*
> *knee joint prosthesis explantation status (Z89.52-)*

√5ᵗʰ **Z47.8** **Encounter for other orthopedic aftercare**

Z47.81 **Encounter for orthopedic aftercare** following surgical amputation
> Use additional code to identify the limb amputated (Z89.-)

Z47.82 **Encounter for orthopedic aftercare** following scoliosis surgery

Z47.89 **Encounter for other orthopedic aftercare**
> AHA: 2015,1Q,8

√4ᵗʰ **Z48** **Encounter for other postprocedural aftercare**

> EXCLUDES 1 *encounter for aftercare following injury - code to Injury, by site, with appropriate 7th character for subsequent encounter*
> *encounter for follow-up examination after completed treatment (Z08-Z09)*
> EXCLUDES 2 *encounter for attention to artificial openings (Z43.-)*
> *encounter for fitting and adjustment of prosthetic and other devices (Z44-Z46)*
> AHA: 2015,4Q,38; 2015,1Q,6-7

√5ᵗʰ **Z48.0** **Encounter for** attention to dressings, sutures and drains

> EXCLUDES 1 *encounter for planned postprocedural wound closure (Z48.1)*

Z48.00 **Encounter for change or removal of** nonsurgical wound dressing ⟨UPD⟩
> Encounter for change or removal of wound dressing NOS

Z48.01 **Encounter for change or removal of** surgical wound dressing ⟨UPD⟩
> AHA: 2019,2Q,33

Z48.02 **Encounter for removal of** sutures ⟨UPD⟩
> Encounter for removal of staples

Z48.03 **Encounter for change or removal of** drains
> AHA: 2019,2Q,33

Z48.1 **Encounter for planned** postprocedural **wound closure**
> EXCLUDES 1 *encounter for attention to dressings and sutures (Z48.0-)*

√5ᵗʰ **Z48.2** **Encounter for aftercare following** organ transplant

Z48.21 **Encounter for aftercare following** heart transplant ⟨CC⟩ ⟨HCC⟩

Z48.22 **Encounter for aftercare following** kidney transplant ⟨CC⟩

Z48.23 **Encounter for aftercare following** liver transplant ⟨CC⟩ ⟨HCC⟩

Z48.24 **Encounter for aftercare following** lung transplant ⟨CC⟩ ⟨HCC⟩

√6ᵗʰ **Z48.28** **Encounter for aftercare following** multiple organ transplant

Z48.280 **Encounter for aftercare following** heart-lung transplant ⟨CC⟩ ⟨HCC⟩

Z48.288 **Encounter for aftercare following** multiple organ transplant

√6ᵗʰ **Z48.29** **Encounter for aftercare following other organ transplant**

Z48.290 **Encounter for aftercare following** bone marrow transplant ⟨CC⟩ ⟨HCC⟩

Z48.298 **Encounter for aftercare following other organ transplant**

Z48.3 **Aftercare following** surgery for neoplasm
> Use additional code to identify the neoplasm

√5ᵗʰ **Z48.8** **Encounter for other specified postprocedural aftercare**

√6ᵗʰ **Z48.81** **Encounter for surgical aftercare following** surgery on specified body systems
> These codes identify the body system requiring aftercare. They are for use in conjunction with other aftercare codes to fully explain the aftercare encounter. The condition treated should also be coded if still present.
> EXCLUDES 1 *aftercare for injury - code the injury with 7th character D*
> *aftercare following surgery for neoplasm (Z48.3)*
> EXCLUDES 2 *aftercare following organ transplant (Z48.2-)*
> *orthopedic aftercare (Z47.-)*
> AHA: 2015,4Q,38

Z48.810 **Encounter for surgical aftercare following surgery on the** sense organs

Z48.811 **Encounter for surgical aftercare following surgery on the** nervous system
> EXCLUDES 2 *encounter for surgical aftercare following surgery on the sense organs (Z48.810)*

Z48.812 **Encounter for surgical aftercare following surgery on the** circulatory system
> AHA: 2012,4Q,96

Z48.813 **Encounter for surgical aftercare following surgery on the** respiratory system
> AHA: 2019,2Q,33

Z48.814 **Encounter for surgical aftercare following surgery on the** teeth or oral cavity

Z48.815 **Encounter for surgical aftercare following surgery on the** digestive system

Z48.816 **Encounter for surgical aftercare following surgery on the** genitourinary system
> EXCLUDES 1 *encounter for aftercare following sterilization reversal (Z31.42)*

Z48.817 **Encounter for surgical aftercare following surgery on the** skin and subcutaneous tissue

Z48.89 **Encounter for other specified surgical aftercare**

√4ᵗʰ **Z49** **Encounter for care involving renal dialysis**
> Code also associated end stage renal disease (N18.6)

√5ᵗʰ **Z49.0** Preparatory care **for renal dialysis**
> Encounter for dialysis instruction and training

Z49.01 **Encounter for fitting and adjustment of** extracorporeal dialysis catheter ⟨UPD⟩ ⟨HCC⟩
> Removal or replacement of renal dialysis catheter
> Toilet or cleansing of renal dialysis catheter

Z49.02 **Encounter for fitting and adjustment of** peritoneal dialysis catheter ⟨UPD⟩ ⟨HCC⟩

√5ᵗʰ **Z49.3** **Encounter for** adequacy testing for dialysis

Z49.31 **Encounter for adequacy testing for** hemodialysis ⟨UPD⟩ ⟨HCC⟩

Z49.32 **Encounter for adequacy testing for** peritoneal dialysis ⟨UPD⟩ ⟨HCC⟩
> Encounter for peritoneal equilibration test

√4ᵗʰ **Z51** **Encounter for other aftercare and medical care**
> Code also condition requiring care
> EXCLUDES 1 *follow-up examination after treatment (Z08-Z09)*

Z51.0 **Encounter for antineoplastic** radiation therapy
> AHA: 2017,4Q,103
> TIP: Do not assign when admission is for insertion/implantation of radioactive elements. Assign a code for the malignancy instead. Any complications related to the radioactive elements should be assigned as secondary diagnoses.

√5ᵗʰ **Z51.1** **Encounter for antineoplastic chemotherapy and immunotherapy**
> EXCLUDES 2 *encounter for chemotherapy and immunotherapy for nonneoplastic condition - code to condition*

Z51.11 **Encounter for antineoplastic** chemotherapy
> AHA: 2015,3Q,19

Z51.12 **Encounter for antineoplastic** immunotherapy

Z51.5 **Encounter for** palliative care
> AHA: 2020,4Q,98; 2017,1Q,48

Z51.6   **Encounter for** desensitization to allergens   `UPD`
AHA: 2016,4Q,77

✓5ᵗʰ **Z51.8**   **Encounter for other specified aftercare**
   EXCLUDES 1   holiday relief care (Z75.5)

   Z51.81   **Encounter for** therapeutic drug level **monitoring**
Code also any long-term (current) drug therapy (Z79.-)
     EXCLUDES 1   encounter for blood-drug test for administrative or medicolegal reasons (Z02.83)
     DEF: Drug monitoring: Measurement of the level of a specific drug in the body or measurement of a specific function to assess effectiveness of a drug.

   Z51.89   **Encounter for other specified aftercare**   `UPD`
AHA: 2012,4Q,95-97

✓4ᵗʰ **Z52**   **Donors of organs and tissues**
   INCLUDES   autologous and other living donors
   EXCLUDES 1   cadaveric donor - omit code
           examination of potential donor (Z00.5)
   AHA: 2012,4Q,99

✓5ᵗʰ **Z52.0**   **Blood** donor
   ✓6ᵗʰ **Z52.00**   **Unspecified blood donor**
     Z52.000   **Unspecified donor,** whole **blood**   `UPD`
     Z52.001   **Unspecified donor,** stem cells   `UPD`
     Z52.008   **Unspecified donor, other blood**   `UPD`
   ✓6ᵗʰ **Z52.01**   **Autologous blood donor**
     Z52.010   **Autologous donor,** whole **blood**   `UPD`
     Z52.011   **Autologous donor,** stem cells   `UPD`
     Z52.018   **Autologous donor, other blood**   `UPD`
   ✓6ᵗʰ **Z52.09**   **Other blood donor**
     Volunteer donor
     Z52.090   **Other blood donor,** whole **blood**   `UPD`
     Z52.091   **Other blood donor,** stem cells   `UPD`
     Z52.098   **Other blood donor, other blood**   `UPD`

✓5ᵗʰ **Z52.1**   **Skin** donor
   Z52.10   **Skin donor, unspecified**
   Z52.11   **Skin donor,** autologous
   Z52.19   **Skin donor, other**

✓5ᵗʰ **Z52.2**   **Bone** donor
   Z52.20   **Bone donor, unspecified**
   Z52.21   **Bone donor,** autologous
   Z52.29   **Bone donor, other**

Z52.3   **Bone marrow donor**
Z52.4   **Kidney donor**
Z52.5   **Cornea donor**
Z52.6   **Liver donor**

✓5ᵗʰ **Z52.8**   **Donor of other specified organs or tissues**
   ✓6ᵗʰ **Z52.81**   **Egg (Oocyte) donor**
     Z52.810   **Egg (Oocyte) donor** under age 35, anonymous **recipient**   `UPD` ♀
       Egg donor under age 35 NOS
     Z52.811   **Egg (Oocyte) donor** under age 35, designated **recipient**   `UPD` ♀
     Z52.812   **Egg (Oocyte) donor** age 35 and over, anonymous **recipient**   `UPD` ♀
       Egg donor age 35 and over NOS
     Z52.813   **Egg (Oocyte) donor** age 35 and over, designated **recipient**   `UPD` ♀
     Z52.819   **Egg (Oocyte) donor, unspecified**   `UPD` ♀
   Z52.89   **Donor of other specified organs or tissues**

Z52.9   **Donor of unspecified organ or tissue**
   Donor NOS

✓4ᵗʰ **Z53**   **Persons encountering health services for specific procedures and treatment, not carried out**
   ✓5ᵗʰ **Z53.0**   **Procedure and treatment not carried out because of contraindication**
     Z53.01   **Procedure and treatment not carried out due to** patient smoking   `UPD`
     Z53.09   **Procedure and treatment not carried out because of other contraindication**   `UPD`
   Z53.1   **Procedure and treatment not carried out because of patient's decision for** reasons of belief and group pressure   `UPD`
   ✓5ᵗʰ **Z53.2**   **Procedure and treatment not carried out because of patient's decision for other and unspecified reasons**
     Z53.20   **Procedure and treatment not carried out because of patient's decision for unspecified reasons**   `UPD`

     Z53.21   **Procedure and treatment not carried out due to patient** leaving prior to being seen by health care provider
     Z53.29   **Procedure and treatment not carried out because of patient's decision for other reasons**   `UPD`
   ✓5ᵗʰ **Z53.3**   **Procedure converted to open procedure**
     AHA: 2016,4Q,79
     Z53.31   **Laparoscopic** surgical procedure converted to open **procedure**   `UPD`
     Z53.32   **Thoracoscopic** surgical procedure converted to open procedure   `UPD`
     Z53.33   **Arthroscopic** surgical procedure converted to open **procedure**   `UPD`
     Z53.39   **Other specified procedure converted to open procedure**   `UPD`
   Z53.8   **Procedure and treatment not carried out for other reasons**   `UPD`
   Z53.9   **Procedure and treatment not carried out, unspecified reason**   `UPD`

Persons with potential health hazards related to socioeconomic and psychosocial circumstances (Z55-Z65)

AHA: 2019,4Q,66; 2018,4Q,58,73; 2018,1Q,18
DEF: Social determinants of health: Socioeconomic factors that can affect a person's health, including both environmental and societal conditions such as education and literacy, employment, health behaviors, housing, lack of adequate food or water, occupational exposure to risk factors, social support, transportation, and violence. Tracking social needs that impact patients allows providers to identify population health trends and to promote the personalized care that addresses the medical and social needs of individual patients. *Synonym(s): SDOH.*
TIP: Because codes in these categories represent social information rather than medical diagnoses, they can be assigned based on documentation by nonphysician clinicians involved in the care of these patients as well as self-reported documentation from the patient, as long as the information is approved and incorporated into the medical record by a clinician or provider.

✓4ᵗʰ **Z55**   **Problems related to education and literacy**
   EXCLUDES 1   disorders of psychological development (F80-F89)
   Z55.0   **Illiteracy and low-level literacy**   `UPD`
   Z55.1   **Schooling unavailable and unattainable**   `UPD`
   Z55.2   **Failed school examinations**   `UPD`
   Z55.3   **Underachievement in school**   `UPD`
   Z55.4   **Educational maladjustment and discord with teachers and classmates**   `UPD`
   ● **Z55.5**   **Less than a high school diploma**
     No general equivalence degree (GED)
   Z55.8   **Other problems related to education and literacy**   `UPD`
     Problems related to inadequate teaching
   Z55.9   **Problems related to education and literacy, unspecified**   `UPD`
     Academic problems NOS

✓4ᵗʰ **Z56**   **Problems related to employment and unemployment**
   EXCLUDES 2   occupational exposure to risk factors (Z57.-)
           problems related to housing and economic circumstances (Z59.-)
   Z56.0   **Unemployment, unspecified**   `UPD`
   Z56.1   **Change of job**   `UPD` `A`
   Z56.2   **Threat of job loss**   `UPD`
   Z56.3   **Stressful work schedule**   `UPD`
   Z56.4   **Discord with boss and workmates**   `UPD`
   Z56.5   **Uncongenial work environment**   `UPD`
     Difficult conditions at work
   Z56.6   **Other physical and mental strain related to work**   `UPD`
   ✓5ᵗʰ **Z56.8**   **Other problems related to employment**
     Z56.81   **Sexual harassment on the job**   `UPD`
     Z56.82   **Military deployment status**   `UPD`
       Individual (civilian or military) currently deployed in theater or in support of military war, peacekeeping and humanitarian operations
     Z56.89   **Other problems related to employment**   `UPD`
   Z56.9   **Unspecified problems related to employment**   `UPD`
     Occupational problems NOS

✓4ᵗʰ **Z57**   **Occupational exposure to risk factors**
   Z57.0   **Occupational exposure to** noise   `UPD`
   Z57.1   **Occupational exposure to** radiation   `UPD`
   Z57.2   **Occupational exposure to** dust   `UPD`

√5ᵗʰ **Z57.3** **Occupational exposure to other air contaminants**

     Z57.31 **Occupational exposure to environmental** tobacco smoke `UPD`

        EXCLUDES 2   *exposure to environmental tobacco smoke (Z77.22)*

     Z57.39 **Occupational exposure to other air contaminants** `UPD`

   Z57.4 **Occupational exposure to** toxic agents in agriculture `UPD`

     Occupational exposure to solids, liquids, gases or vapors in agriculture

   Z57.5 **Occupational exposure to** toxic agents in other industries `UPD`

     Occupational exposure to solids, liquids, gases or vapors in other industries

   Z57.6 **Occupational exposure to** extreme temperature `UPD`

   Z57.7 **Occupational exposure to** vibration `UPD`

   Z57.8 **Occupational exposure to other risk factors** `UPD`

   Z57.9 **Occupational exposure to unspecified risk factor** `UPD`

● √4ᵗʰ **Z58** **Problems related to physical environment**

     EXCLUDES 2   *occupational exposure (Z57.-)*

●   **Z58.6** **Inadequate drinking-water supply**

     Lack of safe drinking water

        EXCLUDES 2   *deprivation of water (T73.1)*

√4ᵗʰ **Z59** **Problems related to housing and economic circumstances**

     EXCLUDES 2   *problems related to upbringing (Z62.-)*

▲   √5ᵗʰ **Z59.0** **Homelessness**

●   **Z59.00** **Homelessness unspecified**

●   **Z59.01** **Sheltered homelessness**

       Doubled up

       Living in a shelter such as: motel, scattered site housing, temporary or transitional living situation

●   **Z59.02** **Unsheltered homelessness**

       Residing in place not meant for human habitation such as: abandoned buildings, cars, parks, sidewalk

       Residing on the street

   Z59.1 **Inadequate housing** `UPD`

     Lack of heating

     Restriction of space

     Technical defects in home preventing adequate care

     Unsatisfactory surroundings

       EXCLUDES 1   *problems related to the natural and physical environment (Z77.1-)*

   Z59.2 **Discord with neighbors, lodgers and landlord** `UPD`

   Z59.3 **Problems related to living in residential institution** `UPD`

     Boarding-school resident

       EXCLUDES 1   *institutional upbringing (Z62.2)*

▲   √5ᵗʰ **Z59.4** **Lack of adequate food**

     ~~Inadequate drinking water supply~~

       EXCLUDES 1   ~~*effects of hunger (T73.0)*~~

         ~~*inappropriate diet or eating habits (Z72.4)*~~

         ~~*malnutrition (E40-E46)*~~

       EXCLUDES 2   ▶*deprivation of food (T73.0)*◀

         ▶*effects of hunger (T73.0)*◀

         ▶*inappropriate diet or eating habits (Z72.4)*◀

         ▶*malnutrition (E40-E46)*◀

●   **Z59.41** **Food insecurity**

●   **Z59.48** **Other specified lack of adequate food**

       Inadequate food

       Lack of food

   Z59.5 **Extreme poverty** `UPD`

   Z59.6 **Low income** `UPD`

   Z59.7 **Insufficient social insurance and welfare support** `UPD`

▲ √5ᵗʰ **Z59.8** **Other problems related to housing and economic circumstances**

     ~~Foreclosure on loan~~

     ~~Isolated dwelling~~

     ~~Problems with creditors~~

●   √6ᵗʰ **Z59.81** **Housing instability,** housed

       Foreclosure on home loan

       Past due on rent or mortgage

       Unwanted multiple moves in the last 12 months

●   **Z59.811** **Housing instability, housed,** with risk of homelessness

         Imminent risk of homelessness

●   **Z59.812** **Housing instability, housed,** homelessness in past 12 months

●   **Z59.819** **Housing instability, housed unspecified**

●   **Z59.89** **Other problems related to housing and economic circumstances**

       Foreclosure on loan

       Isolated dwelling

       Problems with creditors

   Z59.9 **Problem related to housing and economic circumstances, unspecified** `UPD`

√4ᵗʰ **Z60** **Problems related to social environment**

   Z60.0 **Problems of adjustment to life-cycle transitions** `UPD`

     Empty nest syndrome

     Phase of life problem

     Problem with adjustment to retirement [pension]

   Z60.2 **Problems related to living alone** `UPD`

   Z60.3 **Acculturation difficulty** `UPD`

     Problem with migration

     Problem with social transplantation

     DEF: Problem adapting to a different culture or environment not based on any coexisting mental disorder.

   Z60.4 **Social exclusion and rejection**

     Exclusion and rejection on the basis of personal characteristics, such as unusual physical appearance, illness or behavior.

       EXCLUDES 1   *target of adverse discrimination such as for racial or religious reasons (Z60.5)*

   Z60.5 **Target of (perceived) adverse discrimination and persecution** `UPD`

       EXCLUDES 1   *social exclusion and rejection (Z60.4)*

   Z60.8 **Other problems related to social environment** `UPD`

   Z60.9 **Problem related to social environment, unspecified** `UPD`

√4ᵗʰ **Z62** **Problems related to upbringing**

     INCLUDES   current and past negative life events in childhood

         current and past problems of a child related to upbringing

     EXCLUDES 2   *maltreatment syndrome (T74.-)*

         problems related to housing and economic circumstances (Z59.-)

   Z62.0 **Inadequate parental supervision and control** `UPD`

   Z62.1 **Parental overprotection** `UPD`

   √5ᵗʰ **Z62.2** **Upbringing away from parents**

       EXCLUDES 1   *problems with boarding school (Z59.3)*

     Z62.21 **Child in welfare custody** `UPD` `P`

       Child in care of non-parental family member

       Child in foster care

         EXCLUDES 2   *problem for parent due to child in welfare custody (Z63.5)*

     Z62.22 **Institutional upbringing** `UPD`

       Child living in orphanage or group home

     Z62.29 **Other upbringing away from parents** `UPD`

   Z62.3 **Hostility towards and scapegoating of child** `UPD` `P`

   Z62.6 **Inappropriate (excessive) parental pressure** `UPD`

   √5ᵗʰ **Z62.8** **Other specified problems related to upbringing**

     √6ᵗʰ **Z62.81** **Personal history of abuse in** childhood

       Z62.810 **Personal history of** physical and sexual abuse in childhood `UPD`

         EXCLUDES 1   *current child physical abuse (T74.12, T76.12)*

           current child sexual abuse (T74.22, T76.22)

☑ Additional Character Required   √x7ᵗʰ Placeholder   Questionable PDx   Manifestation   Unspecified Dx   UPD Unacceptable PDx   H1-H14 HAC   HCC CMS-HCC Dx   HIV HIV Dx

ICD-10-CM 2022   1251

Chapter 21. Factors Influencing Health Status and Contact With Health Services

Z57.3–Z62.810

Z62.811   **Personal history of** psychological abuse **in childhood** `UPD`
> **EXCLUDES 1**   current child psychological abuse (T74.32, T76.32)

Z62.812   **Personal history of** neglect **in childhood** `UPD`
> **EXCLUDES 1**   current child neglect (T74.02, T76.02)

Z62.813   **Personal history of** forced labor **or** sexual exploitation **in childhood** `UPD`
> **AHA:** 2018,4Q,32,35

Z62.819   **Personal history of unspecified abuse in childhood** `UPD`
> **EXCLUDES 1**   current child abuse NOS (T74.92, T76.92)

✓6ᵗʰ **Z62.82**   **Parent-child conflict**

Z62.820   **Parent-**biological **child conflict** `UPD`
> Parent-child problem NOS

Z62.821   **Parent-**adopted **child conflict** `UPD`

Z62.822   **Parent-**foster **child conflict** `UPD`

✓6ᵗʰ **Z62.89**   **Other specified problems related to upbringing**

Z62.890   **Parent-child estrangement NEC** `UPD`

Z62.891   **Sibling rivalry** `UPD`

Z62.898   **Other specified problems related to upbringing** `UPD`

Z62.9   **Problem related to upbringing, unspecified** `UPD`

✓4ᵗʰ **Z63**   **Other problems related to primary support group, including family circumstances**
> **EXCLUDES 2**   maltreatment syndrome (T74.-, T76)
> parent-child problems (Z62.-)
> problems related to negative life events in childhood (Z62.-)
> problems related to upbringing (Z62.-)

Z63.0   **Problems in relationship with** spouse or partner `UPD`
> Relationship distress with spouse or intimate partner
> **EXCLUDES 1**   counseling for spousal or partner abuse problems (Z69.1)
> counseling related to sexual attitude, behavior, and orientation (Z70.-)

Z63.1   **Problems in relationship with** in-laws `UPD`

✓5ᵗʰ **Z63.3**   **Absence of family member**
> **EXCLUDES 1**   absence of family member due to disappearance and death (Z63.4)
> absence of family member due to separation and divorce (Z63.5)

Z63.31   **Absence of family member due to military deployment** `UPD`
> Individual or family affected by other family member being on military deployment
> **EXCLUDES 1**   family disruption due to return of family member from military deployment (Z63.71)

Z63.32   **Other absence of family member** `UPD`

Z63.4   **Disappearance and death of family member** `UPD`
> Assumed death of family member
> Bereavement
> **AHA:** 2014,1Q,25

Z63.5   **Disruption of family by separation and divorce** `UPD`
> Marital estrangement

Z63.6   **Dependent relative needing care at home** `UPD`

✓5ᵗʰ **Z63.7**   **Other stressful life events affecting family and household**

Z63.71   **Stress on family due to return of family member from military deployment** `UPD`
> Individual or family affected by family member having returned from military deployment (current or past conflict)

Z63.72   **Alcoholism and drug addiction in family** `UPD`

Z63.79   **Other stressful life events affecting family and household** `UPD`
> Anxiety (normal) about sick person in family
> Health problems within family
> Ill or disturbed family member
> Isolated family

Z63.8   **Other specified problems related to primary support group** `UPD`
> Family discord NOS
> Family estrangement NOS
> High expressed emotional level within family
> Inadequate family support NOS
> Inadequate or distorted communication within family

Z63.9   **Problem related to primary support group, unspecified** `UPD`
> Relationship disorder NOS

✓4ᵗʰ **Z64**   **Problems related to certain psychosocial circumstances**

Z64.0   **Problems related to unwanted pregnancy** `UPD` ♀

Z64.1   **Problems related to multiparity** `UPD` ♀

Z64.4   **Discord with counselors** `UPD`
> Discord with probation officer
> Discord with social worker

✓4ᵗʰ **Z65**   **Problems related to other psychosocial circumstances**

Z65.0   **Conviction in civil and criminal proceedings without imprisonment** `UPD`

Z65.1   **Imprisonment and other incarceration** `UPD`

Z65.2   **Problems related to release from prison** `UPD`

Z65.3   **Problems related to other legal circumstances** `UPD`
> Arrest
> Child custody or support proceedings
> Litigation
> Prosecution

Z65.4   **Victim of crime and terrorism** `UPD`
> Victim of torture

Z65.5   **Exposure to disaster, war and other hostilities** `UPD`
> **EXCLUDES 1**   target of perceived discrimination or persecution (Z60.5)

Z65.8   **Other specified problems related to psychosocial circumstances** `UPD`
> Religious or spiritual problem

Z65.9   **Problem related to unspecified psychosocial circumstances** `UPD`

Do not resuscitate status (Z66)

Z66   **Do not resuscitate** `UPD`
> DNR status
> **DEF:** Medical order written by a physician that instructs others not to perform cardiopulmonary resuscitation (CPR), intubation, or advanced cardiac life support (ACLS). It prevents unnecessary invasive treatment to prolong life should breathing stop or cardiac arrest occur.

Blood type (Z67)

✓4ᵗʰ **Z67**   **Blood type**
> **AHA:** 2015,3Q,40

Blood Types

Antigen A   Antigen B
Blood Type A
Blood Type B
Anti-B antibody
Anti-A antibody
Blood Type AB
NO ANTIBODIES
NO ANTIGENS
Antigen A
Antigen B
Blood Type O

✓5ᵗʰ **Z67.1**   Type A **blood**

Z67.10   **Type A blood,** Rh positive `UPD`

Z67.11   **Type A blood,** Rh negative `UPD`

✓5ᵗʰ **Z67.2**   Type B **blood**

Z67.20   **Type B blood,** Rh positive `UPD`

N Newborn: 0   P Pediatric: 0-17   M Maternity: 9-64   A Adult: 15-124   MCC Major Complication/Comorbidity   CC Complication/Comorbidity   SW Severe Wound Dx

1252   ICD-10-CM 2022

Z67.21   Type B blood, Rh negative   `UPD`

√5ᵗʰ Z67.3   Type AB blood

     Z67.30   Type AB blood, Rh positive

     Z67.31   Type AB blood, Rh negative   `UPD`

√5ᵗʰ Z67.4   Type O blood

     Z67.40   Type O blood, Rh positive

     Z67.41   Type O blood, Rh negative   `UPD`

√5ᵗʰ Z67.9   Unspecified blood type

     Z67.90   Unspecified blood type, Rh positive   `UPD`

     Z67.91   Unspecified blood type, Rh negative   `UPD`

Body mass index [BMI] (Z68)

√4ᵗʰ Z68   Body mass index [BMI]

     Kilograms per meters squared

     `NOTE`   BMI adult codes are for use for persons 20 years of age or older

          BMI pediatric codes are for use for persons 2-19 years of age.

          These percentiles are based on the growth charts published by the Centers for Disease Control and Prevention (CDC)

     AHA: 2019,4Q,19,57; 2018,4Q,73,77-83; 2017,1Q,39

     DEF: Index used to help determine whether an individual is underweight, a healthy weight, overweight, or obese.

     TIP: A BMI code may be assigned to support an associated condition based on medical record documentation from clinicians who are not the patient's provider.

     TIP: Do not assign when used in association with fluctuations in body fluid during an encounter, such as fluid overload or fluid retention, or during pregnancy.

     TIP: In order to assign a BMI code, the associated condition must meet the definition of a reportable diagnosis for nonoutpatient encounters, per section III of the *ICD-10-CM Official Guidelines for Coding and Reporting.*

     Z68.1   Body mass index [BMI] 19.9 or less, adult   `CC` `UPD` `A`

√5ᵗʰ Z68.2   Body mass index [BMI] 20-29, adult

     Z68.20   Body mass index [BMI] 20.0-20.9, adult   `UPD` `A`

     Z68.21   Body mass index [BMI] 21.0-21.9, adult   `UPD` `A`

     Z68.22   Body mass index [BMI] 22.0-22.9, adult   `UPD` `A`

     Z68.23   Body mass index [BMI] 23.0-23.9, adult   `UPD` `A`

     Z68.24   Body mass index [BMI] 24.0-24.9, adult   `UPD` `A`

     Z68.25   Body mass index [BMI] 25.0-25.9, adult   `UPD` `A`

     Z68.26   Body mass index [BMI] 26.0-26.9, adult   `UPD` `A`

     Z68.27   Body mass index [BMI] 27.0-27.9, adult   `UPD` `A`

     Z68.28   Body mass index [BMI] 28.0-28.9, adult   `UPD` `A`

     Z68.29   Body mass index [BMI] 29.0-29.9, adult   `UPD` `A`

√5ᵗʰ Z68.3   Body mass index [BMI] 30-39, adult

     Z68.30   Body mass index [BMI] 30.0-30.9, adult   `UPD` `A`

     Z68.31   Body mass index [BMI] 31.0-31.9, adult   `UPD` `A`

     Z68.32   Body mass index [BMI] 32.0-32.9, adult   `UPD` `A`

     Z68.33   Body mass index [BMI] 33.0-33.9, adult   `UPD` `A`

     Z68.34   Body mass index [BMI] 34.0-34.9, adult   `UPD` `A`

     Z68.35   Body mass index [BMI] 35.0-35.9, adult   `UPD` `A`

     Z68.36   Body mass index [BMI] 36.0-36.9, adult   `UPD` `A`

     Z68.37   Body mass index [BMI] 37.0-37.9, adult   `UPD` `A`

     Z68.38   Body mass index [BMI] 38.0-38.9, adult   `UPD` `A`

     Z68.39   Body mass index [BMI] 39.0-39.9, adult   `UPD` `A`

√5ᵗʰ Z68.4   Body mass index [BMI] 40 or greater, adult

     Z68.41   Body mass index [BMI] 40.0-44.9, adult   `CC` `UPD` `HCC` `A`

     Z68.42   Body mass index [BMI] 45.0-49.9, adult   `CC` `UPD` `HCC` `A`

     Z68.43   Body mass index [BMI] 50.0-59.9, adult   `CC` `UPD` `HCC` `A`

     Z68.44   Body mass index [BMI] 60.0-69.9, adult   `CC` `UPD` `HCC` `A`

     Z68.45   Body mass index [BMI] 70 or greater, adult   `CC` `UPD` `HCC` `A`

√5ᵗʰ Z68.5   Body mass index [BMI] pediatric

     AHA: 2018,4Q,81-82

     Z68.51   Body mass index [BMI] pediatric, less than 5th percentile for age   `UPD`

     Z68.52   Body mass index [BMI] pediatric, 5th percentile to less than 85th percentile for age   `UPD`

     Z68.53   Body mass index [BMI] pediatric, 85th percentile to less than 95th percentile for age   `UPD`

     Z68.54   Body mass index [BMI] pediatric, greater than or equal to 95th percentile for age   `UPD`

Persons encountering health services in other circumstances (Z69-Z76)

√4ᵗʰ Z69   Encounter for mental health services for victim and perpetrator of abuse

     `INCLUDES`   counseling for victims and perpetrators of abuse

√5ᵗʰ Z69.0   Encounter for mental health services for child abuse problems

     √6ᵗʰ Z69.01   Encounter for mental health services for parental child abuse

         Z69.010   Encounter for mental health services for victim of parental child abuse   `P`

            Encounter for mental health services for victim of child abuse by parent

            Encounter for mental health services for victim of child neglect by parent

            Encounter for mental health services for victim of child psychological abuse by parent

            Encounter for mental health services for victim of child sexual abuse by parent

         Z69.011   Encounter for mental health services for perpetrator of parental child abuse   `UPD`

            Encounter for mental health services for perpetrator of parental child neglect

            Encounter for mental health services for perpetrator of parental child psychological abuse

            Encounter for mental health services for perpetrator of parental child sexual abuse

            `EXCLUDES 1`   *encounter for mental health services for non-parental child abuse (Z69.02-)*

     √6ᵗʰ Z69.02   Encounter for mental health services for non-parental child abuse

         Z69.020   Encounter for mental health services for victim of non-parental child abuse   `P`

            Encounter for mental health services for victim of non-parental child neglect

            Encounter for mental health services for victim of non-parental child psychological abuse

            Encounter for mental health services for victim of non-parental child sexual abuse

         Z69.021   Encounter for mental health services for perpetrator of non-parental child abuse   `UPD`

            Encounter for mental health services for perpetrator of non-parental child neglect

            Encounter for mental health services for perpetrator of non-parental child psychological abuse

            Encounter for mental health services for perpetrator of non-parental child sexual abuse

√5ᵗʰ Z69.1   Encounter for mental health services for spousal or partner abuse problems

     Z69.11   Encounter for mental health services for victim of spousal or partner abuse   `UPD`

         Encounter for mental health services for victim of spouse or partner neglect

         Encounter for mental health services for victim of spouse or partner psychological abuse

         Encounter for mental health services for victim of spouse or partner violence, physical

☑ Additional Character Required   √x7ᵗʰ Placeholder   Questionable PDx   ● Manifestation   Unspecified Dx   `UPD` Unacceptable PDx   `H1`-`H14` HAC   `HCC` CMS-HCC Dx   `HIV` HIV Dx

ICD-10-CM 2022   1253

Chapter 21. Factors Influencing Health Status and Contact With Health Services

Z69.12–Z72.53

Z69.12   **Encounter for mental health services for perpetrator of spousal or partner abuse** [UPD]
> Encounter for mental health services for perpetrator of spouse or partner neglect
> Encounter for mental health services for perpetrator of spouse or partner psychological abuse
> Encounter for mental health services for perpetrator of spouse or partner violence, physical
> Encounter for mental health services for perpetrator of spouse or partner violence, sexual

✓5th **Z69.8**   **Encounter for mental health services for victim or perpetrator of other abuse**

Z69.81   **Encounter for mental health services for victim of other abuse** [UPD]
> Encounter for mental health services for victim of non-spousal adult abuse
> Encounter for mental health services for victim of spouse or partner violence, sexual
> Encounter for rape victim counseling

Z69.82   **Encounter for mental health services for perpetrator of other abuse** [UPD]
> Encounter for mental health services for perpetrator of non-spousal adult abuse

✓4th **Z70**   **Counseling related to sexual attitude, behavior and orientation**
> [INCLUDES] encounter for mental health services for sexual attitude, behavior and orientation
> [EXCLUDES 2] contraceptive or procreative counseling (Z30-Z31)

Z70.0   **Counseling related to sexual attitude** [UPD]

Z70.1   **Counseling related to patient's sexual behavior and orientation** [UPD]
> Patient concerned regarding impotence
> Patient concerned regarding non-responsiveness
> Patient concerned regarding promiscuity
> Patient concerned regarding sexual orientation

Z70.2   **Counseling related to sexual behavior and orientation of third party** [UPD]
> Advice sought regarding sexual behavior and orientation of child
> Advice sought regarding sexual behavior and orientation of partner
> Advice sought regarding sexual behavior and orientation of spouse

Z70.3   **Counseling related to combined concerns regarding sexual attitude, behavior and orientation** [UPD]

Z70.8   **Other sex counseling** [UPD]
> Encounter for sex education

Z70.9   **Sex counseling, unspecified** [UPD]

✓4th **Z71**   **Persons encountering health services for other counseling and medical advice, not elsewhere classified**
> [EXCLUDES 2] contraceptive or procreation counseling (Z30-Z31)
> sex counseling (Z70.-)

Z71.0   **Person encountering health services to consult on behalf of another person** [UPD]
> Person encountering health services to seek advice or treatment for non-attending third party
> [EXCLUDES 2] anxiety (normal) about sick person in family (Z63.7)
> expectant (adoptive) parent(s) pre-birth pediatrician visit (Z76.81)

Z71.1   **Person with feared health complaint in whom no diagnosis is made** [UPD]
> Person encountering health services with feared condition which was not demonstrated
> Person encountering health services in which problem was normal state
> "Worried well"
> [EXCLUDES 1] medical observation for suspected diseases and conditions proven not to exist (Z03.-)

Z71.2   **Person consulting for explanation of examination or test findings** [UPD]

Z71.3   **Dietary counseling and surveillance** [UPD]
> Use additional code for any associated underlying medical condition
> Use additional code to identify body mass index (BMI), if known (Z68.-)

✓5th **Z71.4**   **Alcohol abuse counseling and surveillance**
> Use additional code for alcohol abuse or dependence (F10.-)

Z71.41   **Alcohol abuse counseling and surveillance of alcoholic** [UPD]

Z71.42   **Counseling for family member of alcoholic** [UPD]
> Counseling for significant other, partner, or friend of alcoholic

✓5th **Z71.5**   **Drug abuse counseling and surveillance**
> Use additional code for drug abuse or dependence (F11-F16, F18-F19)

Z71.51   **Drug abuse counseling and surveillance of drug abuser** [UPD]

Z71.52   **Counseling for family member of drug abuser** [UPD]
> Counseling for significant other, partner, or friend of drug abuser

Z71.6   **Tobacco abuse counseling** [UPD]
> Use additional code for nicotine dependence (F17.-)

Z71.7   **Human immunodeficiency virus [HIV] counseling** [UPD]

✓5th **Z71.8**   **Other specified counseling**
> [EXCLUDES 2] counseling for contraception (Z30.0-)
> **AHA:** 2017,4Q,27

Z71.81   **Spiritual or religious counseling** [UPD]

Z71.82   **Exercise counseling** [UPD]

Z71.83   **Encounter for nonprocreative genetic counseling**
> [EXCLUDES 1] counseling for procreative genetics (Z31.5)
> counseling for procreative management (Z31.6)

Z71.84   **Encounter for health counseling related to travel** [UPD]
> Encounter for health risk and safety counseling for (international) travel
> Code also, if applicable, encounter for immunization (Z23)
> [EXCLUDES 2] encounter for administrative examination (Z02.-)
> encounter for other special examination without complaint, suspected or reported diagnosis (Z01.-)
> **AHA:** 2019,4Q,20,57

Z71.85   **Encounter for immunization safety counseling**
> Encounter for vaccine product safety counseling
> Code also, if applicable, encounter for immunization (Z23)
> Code also, if applicable, immunization not carried out (Z28.-)
> [EXCLUDES 1] encounter for health counseling related to travel (Z71.84)

Z71.89   **Other specified counseling** [UPD]

Z71.9   **Counseling, unspecified** [UPD]
> Encounter for medical advice NOS

✓4th **Z72**   **Problems related to lifestyle**
> [EXCLUDES 2] problems related to life-management difficulty (Z73.-)
> problems related to socioeconomic and psychosocial circumstances (Z55-Z65)

Z72.0   **Tobacco use** [UPD]
> Tobacco use NOS
> [EXCLUDES 1] history of tobacco dependence (Z87.891)
> nicotine dependence (F17.2-)
> tobacco dependence (F17.2-)
> tobacco use during pregnancy (O99.33-)

Z72.3   **Lack of physical exercise** [UPD]

Z72.4   **Inappropriate diet and eating habits** [UPD]
> [EXCLUDES 1] behavioral eating disorders of infancy or childhood (F98.2-F98.3)
> eating disorders (F50.-)
> lack of adequate food ▶(Z59.48)◀
> malnutrition and other nutritional deficiencies (E40-E64)

✓5th **Z72.5**   **High risk sexual behavior**
> Promiscuity
> [EXCLUDES 1] paraphilias (F65)

Z72.51   **High risk heterosexual behavior** [UPD]

Z72.52   **High risk homosexual behavior** [UPD]

Z72.53   **High risk bisexual behavior** [UPD]

[N] Newborn: 0   [P] Pediatric: 0-17   [M] Maternity: 9-64   [A] Adult: 15-124   [MCC] Major Complication/Comorbidity   [CC] Complication/Comorbidity   [SW] Severe Wound Dx

1254   ICD-10-CM 2022

Z72.6   **Gambling and betting**   `UPD`
    `EXCLUDES 1`   *compulsive or pathological gambling (F63.0)*

√5ᵗʰ **Z72.8**   **Other problems related to lifestyle**

   √6ᵗʰ **Z72.81**   **Antisocial behavior**
       `EXCLUDES 1`   *conduct disorders (F91.-)*

     Z72.810   **Child and adolescent antisocial behavior**   `P`
       Antisocial behavior (child) (adolescent) without manifest psychiatric disorder
       Delinquency NOS
       Group delinquency
       Offenses in the context of gang membership
       Stealing in company with others
       Truancy from school

     Z72.811   **Adult antisocial behavior**   `A`
       Adult antisocial behavior without manifest psychiatric disorder

   √6ᵗʰ **Z72.82**   **Problems related to sleep**

     Z72.820   **Sleep deprivation**
       Lack of adequate sleep
       `EXCLUDES 1`   *insomnia (G47.0-)*

     Z72.821   **Inadequate sleep hygiene**   `UPD`
       Bad sleep habits
       Irregular sleep habits
       Unhealthy sleep wake schedule
       `EXCLUDES 1`   *insomnia (F51.0-, G47.0-)*

     Z72.89   **Other problems related to lifestyle**   `UPD`
       Self-damaging behavior

   Z72.9   **Problem related to lifestyle, unspecified**   `UPD`

√4ᵗʰ **Z73**   **Problems related to life management difficulty**
    `EXCLUDES 2`   *problems related to socioeconomic and psychosocial circumstances (Z55-Z65)*
    DEF: State of emotional, mental, and physical exhaustion causing difficulties in managing personal, school, or work circumstances. It is usually due to prolonged stress or poor interpersonal relationship skills or parenting skills.

   Z73.0   **Burn-out**   `UPD`
   Z73.1   **Type A behavior pattern**   `UPD`
   Z73.2   **Lack of relaxation and leisure**   `UPD`
   Z73.3   **Stress, not elsewhere classified**   `UPD`
     Physical and mental strain NOS
     `EXCLUDES 1`   *stress related to employment or unemployment (Z56.-)*
   Z73.4   **Inadequate social skills, not elsewhere classified**   `UPD`
   Z73.5   **Social role conflict, not elsewhere classified**   `UPD`
   Z73.6   **Limitation of activities due to disability**   `UPD`
     `EXCLUDES 1`   *care-provider dependency (Z74.-)*

  √5ᵗʰ **Z73.8**   **Other problems related to life management difficulty**

   √6ᵗʰ **Z73.81**   **Behavioral insomnia of childhood**
     DEF: Behaviors on the part of the child or caregivers that cause negative compliance with a child's sleep schedule resulting in lack of adequate sleep.

     Z73.810   **Behavioral insomnia of childhood, sleep-onset association type**   `UPD` `P`
     Z73.811   **Behavioral insomnia of childhood, limit setting type**   `UPD` `P`
     Z73.812   **Behavioral insomnia of childhood, combined type**   `UPD` `P`
     Z73.819   **Behavioral insomnia of childhood, unspecified type**   `UPD` `P`

   Z73.82   **Dual sensory impairment**   `UPD`
   Z73.89   **Other problems related to life management difficulty**   `UPD`

   Z73.9   **Problem related to life management difficulty, unspecified**   `UPD`

√4ᵗʰ **Z74**   **Problems related to care provider dependency**
    `EXCLUDES 2`   *dependence on enabling machines or devices NEC (Z99.-)*

  √5ᵗʰ **Z74.0**   **Reduced mobility**

   Z74.01   **Bed confinement status**   `UPD`
     Bedridden

   Z74.09   **Other reduced mobility**   `UPD`
     Chair ridden
     Reduced mobility NOS
     `EXCLUDES 2`   *wheelchair dependence (Z99.3)*

  Z74.1   **Need for assistance with personal care**   `UPD`
  Z74.2   **Need for assistance at home and no other household member able to render care**   `UPD`
  Z74.3   **Need for continuous supervision**   `UPD`
  Z74.8   **Other problems related to care provider dependency**   `UPD`
  Z74.9   **Problem related to care provider dependency, unspecified**   `UPD`

√4ᵗʰ **Z75**   **Problems related to medical facilities and other health care**

   Z75.0   **Medical services not available in home**   `UPD`
     `EXCLUDES 1`   *no other household member able to render care (Z74.2)*
   Z75.1   **Person awaiting admission to adequate facility elsewhere**   `UPD`
   Z75.2   **Other waiting period for investigation and treatment**   `UPD`
   Z75.3   **Unavailability and inaccessibility of health-care facilities**   `UPD`
     `EXCLUDES 1`   *bed unavailable (Z75.1)*
   Z75.4   **Unavailability and inaccessibility of other helping agencies**   `UPD`
   Z75.5   **Holiday relief care**   `UPD`
   Z75.8   **Other problems related to medical facilities and other health care**   `UPD`
   Z75.9   **Unspecified problem related to medical facilities and other health care**   `UPD`

√4ᵗʰ **Z76**   **Persons encountering health services in other circumstances**

   Z76.0   **Encounter for issue of repeat prescription**   `UPD`
     Encounter for issue of repeat prescription for appliance
     Encounter for issue of repeat prescription for medicaments
     Encounter for issue of repeat prescription for spectacles
     `EXCLUDES 2`   *issue of medical certificate (Z02.7)*
        repeat prescription for contraceptive (Z30.4-)
   Z76.1   **Encounter for health supervision and care of foundling**
   Z76.2   **Encounter for health supervision and care of other healthy infant and child**   `UPD` `P`
     Encounter for medical or nursing care or supervision of healthy infant under circumstances such as adverse socioeconomic conditions at home
     Encounter for medical or nursing care or supervision of healthy infant under circumstances such as awaiting foster or adoptive placement
     Encounter for medical or nursing care or supervision of healthy infant under circumstances such as maternal illness
     Encounter for medical or nursing care or supervision of healthy infant under circumstances such as number of children at home preventing or interfering with normal care
   Z76.3   **Healthy person accompanying sick person**
   Z76.4   **Other boarder to healthcare facility**
     `EXCLUDES 1`   *homelessness ▶(Z59.0-)◀*
   Z76.5   **Malingerer [conscious simulation]**
     Person feigning illness (with obvious motivation)
     `EXCLUDES 1`   *factitious disorder (F68.1-, F68.A)*
        peregrinating patient (F68.1-)
     DEF: Act of intentionally exaggerating an illness or disability in order to receive personal gain or to avoid punishment or responsibility.

  √5ᵗʰ **Z76.8**   **Persons encountering health services in other specified circumstances**

   Z76.81   **Expectant parent(s) prebirth pediatrician visit**   `UPD`
     Pre-adoption pediatrician visit for adoptive parent(s)
   Z76.82   **Awaiting organ transplant status**   `UPD`
     Patient waiting for organ availability
   Z76.89   **Persons encountering health services in other specified circumstances**   `UPD`
     Persons encountering health services NOS
     AHA: 2014,2Q,10

✔ Additional Character Required   √x7ᵗʰ Placeholder   Questionable PDx   Manifestation   Unspecified Dx   `UPD` Unacceptable PDx   `H1`-`H14` HAC   `HCC` CMS-HCC Dx   `HIV` HIV Dx

ICD-10-CM 2022   **1255**

Persons with potential health hazards related to family and personal history and certain conditions influencing health status (Z77-Z99)

Code also any follow-up examination (Z08-Z09)

✓4th **Z77 Other contact with and (suspected) exposures hazardous to health**

INCLUDES   contact with and (suspected) exposures to potential hazards to health

EXCLUDES 2   *contact with and (suspected) exposure to communicable diseases (Z20.-)*

exposure to (parental) (environmental) tobacco smoke in the perinatal period (P96.81)

newborn affected by noxious substances transmitted via placenta or breast milk (P04.-)

occupational exposure to risk factors (Z57.-)

retained foreign body (Z18.-)

retained foreign body fully removed (Z87.821)

toxic effects of substances chiefly nonmedicinal as to source (T51-T65)

✓5th **Z77.0 Contact with and (suspected) exposure to hazardous, chiefly nonmedicinal, chemicals**

   ✓6th **Z77.01 Contact with and (suspected) exposure to hazardous metals**

       Z77.010 Contact with and (suspected) exposure to arsenic UPD

       Z77.011 Contact with and (suspected) exposure to lead UPD

       Z77.012 Contact with and (suspected) exposure to uranium UPD

         EXCLUDES 1   *retained depleted uranium fragments (Z18.01)*

       Z77.018 Contact with and (suspected) exposure to other hazardous metals UPD

         Contact with and (suspected) exposure to chromium compounds

         Contact with and (suspected) exposure to nickel dust

   ✓6th **Z77.02 Contact with and (suspected) exposure to hazardous aromatic compounds**

       Z77.020 Contact with and (suspected) exposure to aromatic amines UPD

       Z77.021 Contact with and (suspected) exposure to benzene UPD

       Z77.028 Contact with and (suspected) exposure to other hazardous aromatic compounds UPD

         Aromatic dyes NOS

         Polycyclic aromatic hydrocarbons

   ✓6th **Z77.09 Contact with and (suspected) exposure to other hazardous, chiefly nonmedicinal, chemicals**

       Z77.090 Contact with and (suspected) exposure to asbestos UPD

       Z77.098 Contact with and (suspected) exposure to other hazardous, chiefly nonmedicinal, chemicals UPD

         Dyes NOS

✓5th **Z77.1 Contact with and (suspected) exposure to environmental pollution and hazards in the physical environment**

   ✓6th **Z77.11 Contact with and (suspected) exposure to environmental pollution**

       Z77.110 Contact with and (suspected) exposure to air pollution UPD

       Z77.111 Contact with and (suspected) exposure to water pollution UPD

       Z77.112 Contact with and (suspected) exposure to soil pollution UPD

       Z77.118 Contact with and (suspected) exposure to other environmental pollution UPD

   ✓6th **Z77.12 Contact with and (suspected) exposure to hazards in the physical environment**

       Z77.120 Contact with and (suspected) exposure to mold (toxic) UPD

       Z77.121 Contact with and (suspected) exposure to harmful algae and algae toxins UPD

         Contact with and (suspected) exposure to (harmful) algae bloom NOS

         Contact with and (suspected) exposure to blue-green algae bloom

         Contact with and (suspected) exposure to brown tide

         Contact with and (suspected) exposure to cyanobacteria bloom

         Contact with and (suspected) exposure to Florida red tide

         Contact with and (suspected) exposure to pfiesteria piscicida

         Contact with and (suspected) exposure to red tide

       Z77.122 Contact with and (suspected) exposure to noise UPD

       Z77.123 Contact with and (suspected) exposure to radon and other naturally occurring radiation

         EXCLUDES 2   *radiation exposure as the cause of a confirmed condition (W88-W90, X39.0-)*

            radiation sickness NOS (T66)

       Z77.128 Contact with and (suspected) exposure to other hazards in the physical environment UPD

✓5th **Z77.2 Contact with and (suspected) exposure to other hazardous substances**

       Z77.21 Contact with and (suspected) exposure to potentially hazardous body fluids UPD

       Z77.22 Contact with and (suspected) exposure to environmental tobacco smoke (acute) (chronic) UPD

         Exposure to second hand tobacco smoke (acute) (chronic)

         Passive smoking (acute) (chronic)

         EXCLUDES 1   *nicotine dependence (F17.-)*

            tobacco use (Z72.0)

         EXCLUDES 2   *occupational exposure to environmental tobacco smoke (Z57.31)*

       Z77.29 Contact with and (suspected) exposure to other hazardous substances UPD

         AHA: 2016,2Q,33

    Z77.9 Other contact with and (suspected) exposures hazardous to health UPD

✓4th **Z78 Other specified health status**

EXCLUDES 2   *asymptomatic human immunodeficiency virus [HIV] infection status (Z21)*

postprocedural status (Z93-Z99)

sex reassignment status (Z87.890)

    Z78.0 Asymptomatic menopausal state UPD A ♀

       Menopausal state NOS

       Postmenopausal status NOS

       EXCLUDES 2   *symptomatic menopausal state (N95.1)*

    Z78.1 Physical restraint status UPD

       EXCLUDES 1   *physical restraint due to a procedure - omit code*

       DEF: Application of mechanical restraining devices or manual restraints to limit physical mobility of a patient.

    Z78.9 Other specified health status UPD

✓4th **Z79 Long term (current) drug therapy**

INCLUDES   long term (current) drug use for prophylactic purposes

Code also any therapeutic drug level monitoring (Z51.81)

EXCLUDES 2   *drug abuse and dependence (F11-F19)*

drug use complicating pregnancy, childbirth, and the puerperium (O99.32-)

AHA: 2021,1Q,12

✓5th **Z79.0 Long term (current) use of anticoagulants and antithrombotics/antiplatelets**

       EXCLUDES 2   *long term (current) use of aspirin (Z79.82)*

    Z79.01 Long term (current) use of anticoagulants

       AHA: 2021,1Q,4; 2020,2Q,20

    Z79.02 Long term (current) use of antithrombotics/antiplatelets UPD

N Newborn: 0   P Pediatric: 0-17   M Maternity: 9-64   A Adult: 15-124   MCC Major Complication/Comorbidity   CC Complication/Comorbidity   SW Severe Wound Dx

1256   ICD-10-CM 2022

Z79.1 Long term (current) use of non-steroidal anti-inflammatories (NSAID) `UPD`
> *EXCLUDES 2*   long term (current) use of aspirin (Z79.82)

Z79.2 Long term (current) use of antibiotics `UPD`

Z79.3 Long term (current) use of hormonal contraceptives
> Long term (current) use of birth control pill or patch

Z79.4 Long term (current) use of insulin `HCC`
> *EXCLUDES 1*   ~~long term (current) use of oral antidiabetic drugs (Z79.84)~~
>
>   ~~long term (current) use of oral hypoglycemic drugs (Z79.84)~~
>
> *EXCLUDES 2*   ►long term (current) use of oral hypoglycemic drugs (Z79.84)◄
>
>   ►long term (current) use of oral antidiabetic drugs (Z79.84)◄

AHA: 2020,3Q,31
TIP: If a patient is being maintained on both insulin and an injectable noninsulin antidiabetic drug, assign this code in addition to code Z79.899.

✓⁵ᵗʰ **Z79.5** Long term (current) use of steroids

     Z79.51 Long term (current) use of inhaled steroids `UPD`

     Z79.52 Long term (current) use of systemic steroids `UPD`

✓⁵ᵗʰ **Z79.8** Other long term (current) drug therapy

     ✓⁶ᵗʰ **Z79.81** Long term (current) use of agents affecting estrogen receptors and estrogen levels
> Code first, if applicable:
> malignant neoplasm of breast (C50.-)
> malignant neoplasm of prostate (C61)
> Use additional code, if applicable, to identify:
> estrogen receptor positive status (Z17.0)
> family history of breast cancer (Z80.3)
> genetic susceptibility to malignant neoplasm (cancer) (Z15.0-)
> personal history of breast cancer (Z85.3)
> personal history of prostate cancer (Z85.46)
> postmenopausal status (Z78.0)
> *EXCLUDES 1*   hormone replacement therapy (Z79.890)

         Z79.810 Long term (current) use of selective estrogen receptor modulators (SERMs) `UPD`
> Long term (current) use of raloxifene (Evista)
> Long term (current) use of tamoxifen (Nolvadex)
> Long term (current) use of toremifene (Fareston)

         Z79.811 Long term (current) use of aromatase inhibitors `UPD`
> Long term (current) use of anastrozole (Arimidex)
> Long term (current) use of exemestane (Aromasin)
> Long term (current) use of letrozole (Femara)

         Z79.818 Long term (current) use of other agents affecting estrogen receptors and estrogen levels `UPD`
> Long term (current) use of estrogen receptor downregulators
> Long term (current) use of fulvestrant (Faslodex)
> Long term (current) use of gonadotropin-releasing hormone (GnRH) agonist
> Long term (current) use of goserelin acetate (Zoladex)
> Long term (current) use of leuprolide acetate (leuprorelin) (Lupron)
> Long term (current) use of megestrol acetate (Megace)

     Z79.82 Long term (current) use of aspirin

     Z79.83 Long term (current) use of bisphosphonates `UPD`
> **AHA:** 2016,4Q,42

Z79.84 Long term (current) use of oral hypoglycemic drugs `UPD`
> Long term (current) use of oral antidiabetic drugs
> *EXCLUDES 2*   long term (current) use of insulin (Z79.4)

AHA: 2020,3Q,31; 2016,4Q,76
TIP: If a patient is being maintained on both oral hypoglycemics and an injectable noninsulin antidiabetic drug, assign this code in addition to code Z79.899.

✓⁶ᵗʰ **Z79.89** Other long term (current) drug therapy

     Z79.890 Hormone replacement therapy `UPD`

     Z79.891 Long term (current) use of opiate analgesic
> Long term (current) use of methadone for pain management
> *EXCLUDES 1*   methodone use NOS (F11.9-)
>   use of methodone for treatment of heroin addiction (F11.2-)

     Z79.899 Other long term (current) drug therapy
> **AHA:** 2020,4Q,11; 2020,3Q,31; 2020,2Q,14; 2015,4Q,34; 2015,3Q,21

✓⁴ᵗʰ **Z80** Family history of primary malignant neoplasm

     Z80.0 Family history of malignant neoplasm of digestive organs `UPD`
> Conditions classifiable to C15-C26
> **AHA:** 2018,1Q,6

     Z80.1 Family history of malignant neoplasm of trachea, bronchus and lung `UPD`
> Conditions classifiable to C33-C34

     Z80.2 Family history of malignant neoplasm of other respiratory and intrathoracic organs `UPD`
> Conditions classifiable to C30-C32, C37-C39

     Z80.3 Family history of malignant neoplasm of breast `UPD`
> Conditions classifiable to C50.-

     ✓⁵ᵗʰ **Z80.4** Family history of malignant neoplasm of genital organs
> Conditions classifiable to C51-C63

         Z80.41 Family history of malignant neoplasm of ovary `UPD`

         Z80.42 Family history of malignant neoplasm of prostate `UPD`

         Z80.43 Family history of malignant neoplasm of testis `UPD`

         Z80.49 Family history of malignant neoplasm of other genital organs `UPD`

     ✓⁵ᵗʰ **Z80.5** Family history of malignant neoplasm of urinary tract
> Conditions classifiable to C64-C68

         Z80.51 Family history of malignant neoplasm of kidney `UPD`

         Z80.52 Family history of malignant neoplasm of bladder `UPD`

         Z80.59 Family history of malignant neoplasm of other urinary tract organ `UPD`

     Z80.6 Family history of leukemia `UPD`
> Conditions classifiable to C91-C95

     Z80.7 Family history of other malignant neoplasms of lymphoid, hematopoietic and related tissues `UPD`
> Conditions classifiable to C81-C90, C96.-

     Z80.8 Family history of malignant neoplasm of other organs or systems `UPD`
> Conditions classifiable to C00-C14, C40-C49, C69-C79

     Z80.9 Family history of malignant neoplasm, unspecified `UPD`
> Conditions classifiable to C80.1

✓⁴ᵗʰ **Z81** Family history of mental and behavioral disorders

     Z81.0 Family history of intellectual disabilities `UPD`
> Conditions classifiable to F70-F79

     Z81.1 Family history of alcohol abuse and dependence `UPD`
> Conditions classifiable to F10.-

     Z81.2 Family history of tobacco abuse and dependence `UPD`
> Conditions classifiable to F17.-

     Z81.3 Family history of other psychoactive substance abuse and dependence `UPD`
> Conditions classifiable to F11-F16, F18-F19

     Z81.4 Family history of other substance abuse and dependence `UPD`
> Conditions classifiable to F55

☑ Additional Character Required   ✓x7ᵗʰ Placeholder   Questionable PDx   Manifestation   Unspecified Dx   `UPD` Unacceptable PDx   H1-H14 HAC   `HCC` CMS-HCC Dx   `HIV` HIV Dx

ICD-10-CM 2022   1257

Z81.8   Family history of other mental and behavioral disorders `UPD`
Conditions classifiable elsewhere in F01-F99

✓4ᵗʰ **Z82   Family history of certain disabilities and chronic diseases (leading to disablement)**

Z82.0   Family history of epilepsy and other diseases of the nervous system `UPD`
Conditions classifiable to G00-G99

Z82.1   Family history of blindness and visual loss `UPD`
Conditions classifiable to H54.-

Z82.2   Family history of deafness and hearing loss `UPD`
Conditions classifiable to H90-H91

Z82.3   Family history of stroke `UPD`
Conditions classifiable to I60-I64

✓5ᵗʰ **Z82.4   Family history of ischemic heart disease and other diseases of the circulatory system**
▶Conditions classifiable to I00-I5A, I65-I99◀

Z82.41   Family history of sudden cardiac death `UPD`

Z82.49   Family history of ischemic heart disease and other diseases of the circulatory system `UPD`

Z82.5   Family history of asthma and other chronic lower respiratory diseases `UPD`
Conditions classifiable to J40-J47
EXCLUDES 2   *family history of other diseases of the respiratory system (Z83.6)*

✓5ᵗʰ **Z82.6   Family history of arthritis and other diseases of the musculoskeletal system and connective tissue**
Conditions classifiable to M00-M99

Z82.61   Family history of arthritis `UPD`

Z82.62   Family history of osteoporosis `UPD`

Z82.69   Family history of other diseases of the musculoskeletal system and connective tissue `UPD`

✓5ᵗʰ **Z82.7   Family history of congenital malformations, deformations and chromosomal abnormalities**
Conditions classifiable to Q00-Q99

Z82.71   Family history of polycystic kidney `UPD`

Z82.79   Family history of other congenital malformations, deformations and chromosomal abnormalities `UPD`

Z82.8   Family history of other disabilities and chronic diseases leading to disablement, not elsewhere classified `UPD`

✓4ᵗʰ **Z83   Family history of other specific disorders**
EXCLUDES 2   *contact with and (suspected) exposure to communicable disease in the family (Z20.-)*

Z83.0   Family history of human immunodeficiency virus [HIV] disease `UPD`
Conditions classifiable to B20

Z83.1   Family history of other infectious and parasitic diseases `UPD`
Conditions classifiable to A00-B19, B25-B94, B99

Z83.2   Family history of diseases of the blood and blood-forming organs and certain disorders involving the immune mechanism `UPD`
Conditions classifiable to D50-D89

Z83.3   Family history of diabetes mellitus `UPD`
Conditions classifiable to E08-E13

✓5ᵗʰ **Z83.4   Family history of other endocrine, nutritional and metabolic diseases**
Conditions classifiable to E00-E07, E15-E88

Z83.41   Family history of multiple endocrine neoplasia [MEN] syndrome `UPD`

Z83.42   Family history of familial hypercholesterolemia `UPD`
AHA: 2016,4Q,77

✓6ᵗʰ **Z83.43   Family history of other disorder of lipoprotein metabolism and other lipidemias**
AHA: 2018,4Q,6,35

Z83.430   Family history of elevated lipoprotein(a) `UPD`
Family history of elevated Lp(a)

Z83.438   Family history of other disorder of lipoprotein metabolism and other lipidemia `UPD`
Family history of familial combined hyperlipidemia

Z83.49   Family history of other endocrine, nutritional and metabolic diseases `UPD`

✓5ᵗʰ **Z83.5   Family history of eye and ear disorders**

✓6ᵗʰ **Z83.51   Family history of eye disorders**
Conditions classifiable to H00-H53, H55-H59
EXCLUDES 2   *family history of blindness and visual loss (Z82.1)*

Z83.511   Family history of glaucoma `UPD`

Z83.518   Family history of other specified eye disorder `UPD`

Z83.52   Family history of ear disorders `UPD`
Conditions classifiable to H60-H83, H92-H95
EXCLUDES 2   *family history of deafness and hearing loss (Z82.2)*

Z83.6   Family history of other diseases of the respiratory system `UPD`
Conditions classifiable to J00-J39, J60-J99
EXCLUDES 2   *family history of asthma and other chronic lower respiratory diseases (Z82.5)*

✓5ᵗʰ **Z83.7   Family history of diseases of the digestive system**
Conditions classifiable to K00-K93

Z83.71   Family history of colonic polyps `UPD`
EXCLUDES 2   *family history of malignant neoplasm of digestive organs (Z80.0)*
AHA: 2021,1Q,14

Z83.79   Family history of other diseases of the digestive system `UPD`

✓4ᵗʰ **Z84   Family history of other conditions**

Z84.0   Family history of diseases of the skin and subcutaneous tissue `UPD`
Conditions classifiable to L00-L99

Z84.1   Family history of disorders of kidney and ureter `UPD`
Conditions classifiable to N00-N29

Z84.2   Family history of other diseases of the genitourinary system `UPD`
Conditions classifiable to N30-N99

Z84.3   Family history of consanguinity `UPD`

✓5ᵗʰ **Z84.8   Family history of other specified conditions**

Z84.81   Family history of carrier of genetic disease `UPD`
AHA: 2021,1Q,14

Z84.82   Family history of sudden infant death syndrome `UPD`
Family history of SIDS
AHA: 2016,4Q,77

Z84.89   Family history of other specified conditions `UPD`

✓4ᵗʰ **Z85   Personal history of malignant neoplasm**
Code first any follow-up examination after treatment of malignant neoplasm (Z08)
Use additional code to identify:
alcohol use and dependence (F10.-)
exposure to environmental tobacco smoke (Z77.22)
history of tobacco dependence (Z87.891)
occupational exposure to environmental tobacco smoke (Z57.31)
tobacco dependence (F17.-)
tobacco use (Z72.0)
EXCLUDES 2   *personal history of benign neoplasm (Z86.01-)*
personal history of carcinoma-in-situ (Z86.00-)
AHA: 2020,3Q,30; 2018,4Q,64

✓5ᵗʰ **Z85.0   Personal history of malignant neoplasm of digestive organs**
AHA: 2017,1Q,9

Z85.00   Personal history of malignant neoplasm of unspecified digestive organ `UPD`

Z85.01   Personal history of malignant neoplasm of esophagus `UPD`
Conditions classifiable to C15

✓6ᵗʰ **Z85.02   Personal history of malignant neoplasm of stomach**

Z85.020   Personal history of malignant carcinoid tumor of stomach `UPD`
Conditions classifiable to C7A.092

Z85.028   Personal history of other malignant neoplasm of stomach `UPD`
Conditions classifiable to C16

☑6ᵗʰ **Z85.03** **Personal history of malignant neoplasm of** large intestine

    Z85.030 **Personal history of malignant** carcinoid tumor of large intestine UPD
        Conditions classifiable to C7A.022-C7A.025, C7A.029

    Z85.038 **Personal history of other malignant neoplasm of large intestine** UPD
        Conditions classifiable to C18

☑6ᵗʰ **Z85.04** **Personal history of malignant neoplasm of** rectum, rectosigmoid junction, and anus

    Z85.040 **Personal history of malignant** carcinoid tumor of rectum UPD
        Conditions classifiable to C7A.026

    Z85.048 **Personal history of other malignant neoplasm of rectum, rectosigmoid junction, and anus** UPD
        Conditions classifiable to C19-C21

Z85.05 **Personal history of malignant neoplasm of liver** UPD
    Conditions classifiable to C22

☑6ᵗʰ **Z85.06** **Personal history of malignant neoplasm of** small intestine

    Z85.060 **Personal history of malignant** carcinoid tumor of small intestine UPD
        Conditions classifiable to C7A.01-

    Z85.068 **Personal history of other malignant neoplasm of small intestine** UPD
        Conditions classifiable to C17

Z85.07 **Personal history of malignant neoplasm of pancreas** UPD
    Conditions classifiable to C25

Z85.09 **Personal history of malignant neoplasm of other digestive organs** UPD

☑5ᵗʰ **Z85.1** **Personal history of malignant neoplasm of** trachea, bronchus and lung

☑6ᵗʰ **Z85.11** **Personal history of malignant neoplasm of** bronchus and lung

    Z85.110 **Personal history of malignant** carcinoid tumor of bronchus and lung UPD
        Conditions classifiable to C7A.090

    Z85.118 **Personal history of other malignant neoplasm of bronchus and lung** UPD
        Conditions classifiable to C34

Z85.12 **Personal history of malignant neoplasm of trachea** UPD
    Conditions classifiable to C33

☑5ᵗʰ **Z85.2** **Personal history of malignant neoplasm of other** respiratory and intrathoracic organs

    Z85.20 **Personal history of malignant neoplasm of unspecified respiratory organ** UPD

Z85.21 **Personal history of malignant neoplasm of larynx** UPD
    Conditions classifiable to C32

Z85.22 **Personal history of malignant neoplasm of** nasal cavities, middle ear, and accessory sinuses UPD
    Conditions classifiable to C30-C31

☑6ᵗʰ **Z85.23** **Personal history of malignant neoplasm of** thymus

    Z85.230 **Personal history of malignant** carcinoid tumor of thymus UPD
        Conditions classifiable to C7A.091

    Z85.238 **Personal history of other malignant neoplasm of thymus** UPD
        Conditions classifiable to C37

Z85.29 **Personal history of malignant neoplasm of other respiratory and intrathoracic organs** UPD

Z85.3 **Personal history of malignant neoplasm of** breast UPD
    Conditions classifiable to C50.-

☑5ᵗʰ **Z85.4** **Personal history of malignant neoplasm of** genital organs
    Conditions classifiable to C51-C63

    Z85.40 **Personal history of malignant neoplasm of unspecified** female genital organ UPD ♀

Z85.41 **Personal history of malignant neoplasm of** cervix uteri UPD ♀

Z85.42 **Personal history of malignant neoplasm of other parts of uterus** UPD ♀

Z85.43 **Personal history of malignant neoplasm of ovary** UPD ♀

Z85.44 **Personal history of malignant neoplasm of other** female genital organs UPD ♀

Z85.45 **Personal history of malignant neoplasm of unspecified** male genital organ UPD ♂

Z85.46 **Personal history of malignant neoplasm of prostate** UPD ♂

Z85.47 **Personal history of malignant neoplasm of testis** UPD ♂

Z85.48 **Personal history of malignant neoplasm of epididymis** UPD ♂

Z85.49 **Personal history of malignant neoplasm of other** male genital organs UPD ♂

☑5ᵗʰ **Z85.5** **Personal history of malignant neoplasm of** urinary tract
    Conditions classifiable to C64-C68

    Z85.50 **Personal history of malignant neoplasm of unspecified urinary tract organ** UPD

Z85.51 **Personal history of malignant neoplasm of bladder** UPD

☑6ᵗʰ **Z85.52** **Personal history of malignant neoplasm of** kidney

    EXCLUDES 1 *personal history of malignant neoplasm of renal pelvis (Z85.53)*

    Z85.520 **Personal history of malignant** carcinoid tumor of kidney
        Conditions classifiable to C7A.093

    Z85.528 **Personal history of other malignant neoplasm of kidney** UPD
        Conditions classifiable to C64

Z85.53 **Personal history of malignant neoplasm of** renal pelvis UPD

Z85.54 **Personal history of malignant neoplasm of ureter** UPD

Z85.59 **Personal history of malignant neoplasm of other urinary tract organ** UPD

Z85.6 **Personal history of** leukemia UPD
    Conditions classifiable to C91-C95
    EXCLUDES 1 *leukemia in remission C91.0-C95.9 with 5th character 1*

☑5ᵗʰ **Z85.7** **Personal history of other malignant neoplasms of lymphoid, hematopoietic and related tissues**

    Z85.71 **Personal history of** Hodgkin lymphoma UPD
        Conditions classifiable to C81

Z85.72 **Personal history of** non-Hodgkin lymphomas UPD
    Conditions classifiable to C82-C85

Z85.79 **Personal history of other malignant neoplasms of lymphoid, hematopoietic and related tissues** UPD
    Conditions classifiable to C88-C90, C96
    EXCLUDES 1 *multiple myeloma in remission (C90.01)*
        plasma cell leukemia in remission (C90.11)
        plasmacytoma in remission (C90.21)

☑5ᵗʰ **Z85.8** **Personal history of malignant neoplasms of other organs and systems**
    Conditions classifiable to C00-C14, C40-C49, C69-C75, C7A.098, C76-C79

☑6ᵗʰ **Z85.81** **Personal history of malignant neoplasm of** lip, oral cavity, and pharynx
    Conditions classifiable to C00-C14

    Z85.810 **Personal history of malignant neoplasm of tongue** UPD

    Z85.818 **Personal history of malignant neoplasm of other sites of lip, oral cavity, and pharynx**

    Z85.819 **Personal history of malignant neoplasm of unspecified site of lip, oral cavity, and pharynx** UPD

☑6ᵗʰ **Z85.82** **Personal history of malignant neoplasm of** skin

    Z85.820 **Personal history of malignant** melanoma of skin UPD
        Conditions classifiable to C43

    Z85.821 **Personal history of** Merkel cell carcinoma UPD
        Conditions classifiable to C4A

    Z85.828 **Personal history of other malignant neoplasm of skin** UPD
        Conditions classifiable to C44

☑6ᵗʰ **Z85.83** **Personal history of malignant neoplasm of** bone and soft tissue
    Conditions classifiable to C40-C41; C45-C49

    Z85.830 **Personal history of malignant neoplasm of bone** UPD

☑ Additional Character Required   ✓x7ᵗʰ Placeholder   Questionable PDx   Manifestation   Unspecified Dx   UPD Unacceptable PDx   H1-H14 HAC   HCC CMS-HCC Dx   HIV HIV Dx

ICD-10-CM 2022   1259

Z85.831 Personal history of malignant neoplasm of soft tissue UPD
> EXCLUDES 2 *personal history of malignant neoplasm of skin (Z85.82-)*

✓6th **Z85.84 Personal history of malignant neoplasm of eye and nervous tissue**
> Conditions classifiable to C69-C72

Z85.840 Personal history of malignant neoplasm of eye UPD

Z85.841 Personal history of malignant neoplasm of brain UPD

Z85.848 Personal history of malignant neoplasm of other parts of nervous tissue UPD

✓6th **Z85.85 Personal history of malignant neoplasm of endocrine glands**
> Conditions classifiable to C73-C75

Z85.850 Personal history of malignant neoplasm of thyroid UPD

Z85.858 Personal history of malignant neoplasm of other endocrine glands UPD

Z85.89 Personal history of malignant neoplasm of other organs and systems UPD
> Conditions classifiable to C7A.098, C76, C77-C79

Z85.9 Personal history of malignant neoplasm, unspecified UPD
> Conditions classifiable to C7A.00, C80.1

✓4th **Z86 Personal history of certain other diseases**
> Code first any follow-up examination after treatment (Z09)

✓5th **Z86.0 Personal history of in-situ and benign neoplasms and neoplasms of uncertain behavior**
> EXCLUDES 2 *personal history of malignant neoplasms (Z85.-)*
>
> **AHA:** 2017,1Q,9

✓6th **Z86.00 Personal history of in-situ neoplasm**
> Conditions classifiable to D00-D09
>
> **AHA:** 2019,4Q,20

Z86.000 Personal history of in-situ neoplasm of breast UPD
> Conditions classifiable to D05

Z86.001 Personal history of in-situ neoplasm of cervix uteri UPD ♀
> Conditions classifiable to D06
>
> Personal history of cervical intraepithelial neoplasia III [CIN III]

Z86.002 Personal history of in-situ neoplasm of other and unspecified genital organs UPD
> Conditions classifiable to D07
>
> Personal history of high-grade prostatic intraepithelial neoplasia III [HGPIN III]
>
> Personal history of vaginal intraepithelial neoplasia III [VAIN III]
>
> Personal history of vulvar intraepithelial neoplasia III [VIN III]

Z86.003 Personal history of in-situ neoplasm of oral cavity, esophagus and stomach UPD
> Conditions classifiable to D00

Z86.004 Personal history of in-situ neoplasm of other and unspecified digestive organs UPD
> Conditions classifiable to D01
>
> Personal history of anal intraepithelial neoplasia (AIN III)

Z86.005 Personal history of in-situ neoplasm of middle ear and respiratory system UPD
> Conditions classifiable to D02

Z86.006 Personal history of melanoma in-situ UPD
> Conditions classifiable to D03
>
> EXCLUDES 2 *sites other than skin - code to personal history of in-situ neoplasm of the site*

Z86.007 Personal history of in-situ neoplasm of skin UPD
> Conditions classifiable to D04
>
> Personal history of carcinoma in situ of skin

Z86.008 Personal history of in-situ neoplasm of other site UPD
> Conditions classifiable to D09

✓6th **Z86.01 Personal history of benign neoplasm**

Z86.010 Personal history of colonic polyps UPD
> **AHA:** 2021,1Q,14; 2017,1Q,14

Z86.011 Personal history of benign neoplasm of the brain UPD

Z86.012 Personal history of benign carcinoid tumor UPD

Z86.018 Personal history of other benign neoplasm UPD
> **AHA:** 2017,1Q,14

Z86.03 Personal history of neoplasm of uncertain behavior UPD

✓5th **Z86.1 Personal history of infectious and parasitic diseases**
> Conditions classifiable to A00-B89, B99
>
> EXCLUDES 1 *personal history of infectious diseases specific to a body system*
>
> *sequelae of infectious and parasitic diseases (B90-B94)*

Z86.11 Personal history of tuberculosis UPD

Z86.12 Personal history of poliomyelitis UPD

Z86.13 Personal history of malaria UPD

Z86.14 Personal history of Methicillin resistant Staphylococcus aureus infection UPD
> Personal history of MRSA infection

Z86.15 Personal history of latent tuberculosis infection UPD

Z86.16 Personal history of COVID-19 UPD
> EXCLUDES 1 ►*post COVID-19 condition (U09.9)*◄
>
> **AHA:** 2021,1Q,28-29,33-35,40-41,44-45

Z86.19 Personal history of other infectious and parasitic diseases UPD
> **AHA:** 2021,1Q,33-34,40; 2020,3Q,13; 2020,2Q,10,12

Z86.2 Personal history of diseases of the blood and blood-forming organs and certain disorders involving the immune mechanism UPD
> Conditions classifiable to D50-D89

✓5th **Z86.3 Personal history of endocrine, nutritional and metabolic diseases**
> Conditions classifiable to E00-E88

Z86.31 Personal history of diabetic foot ulcer UPD
> EXCLUDES 2 *current diabetic foot ulcer (E08.621, E09.621, E10.621, E11.621, E13.621)*

Z86.32 Personal history of gestational diabetes UPD ♀
> Personal history of conditions classifiable to O24.4-
>
> EXCLUDES 1 *gestational diabetes mellitus in current pregnancy (O24.4-)*

Z86.39 Personal history of other endocrine, nutritional and metabolic disease UPD
> **AHA:** 2020,1Q,12

✓5th **Z86.5 Personal history of mental and behavioral disorders**
> Conditions classifiable to F40-F59

Z86.51 Personal history of combat and operational stress reaction UPD A

Z86.59 Personal history of other mental and behavioral disorders UPD

✓5th **Z86.6 Personal history of diseases of the nervous system and sense organs**
> Conditions classifiable to G00-G99, H00-H95

Z86.61 Personal history of infections of the central nervous system UPD
> Personal history of encephalitis
>
> Personal history of meningitis

Z86.69 Personal history of other diseases of the nervous system and sense organs UPD
> **AHA:** 2016,4Q,24

✓5th **Z86.7 Personal history of diseases of the circulatory system**
> Conditions classifiable to I00-I99
>
> EXCLUDES 2 *old myocardial infarction (I25.2)*
>
> *personal history of anaphylactic shock (Z87.892)*
>
> *postmyocardial infarction syndrome (I24.1)*

✓6th **Z86.71 Personal history of venous thrombosis and embolism**

Z86.711 Personal history of pulmonary embolism UPD

N Newborn: 0   P Pediatric: 0-17   M Maternity: 9-64   A Adult: 15-124   MCC Major Complication/Comorbidity   CC Complication/Comorbidity   SW Severe Wound Dx

1260   ICD-10-CM 2022

Z86.718   **Personal history of other venous thrombosis and embolism** `UPD`
> AHA: 2020,2Q,20

Z86.72   **Personal history of** thrombophlebitis `UPD`

Z86.73   **Personal history of** transient ischemic attack **(TIA), and cerebral infarction without residual deficits** `UPD`
> Personal history of prolonged reversible ischemic neurological deficit (PRIND)
> Personal history of stroke NOS without residual deficits
> > EXCLUDES 1   *personal history of traumatic brain injury (Z87.820)*
> > *sequelae of cerebrovascular disease (I69.-)*
> AHA: 2012,4Q,92

Z86.74   **Personal history of** sudden cardiac arrest `UPD`
> Personal history of sudden cardiac death successfully resuscitated

Z86.79   **Personal history of other diseases of the circulatory system** `UPD`
> AHA: 2020,1Q,12

✓4ᵗʰ **Z87**   **Personal history of other diseases and conditions**
> Code first any follow-up examination after treatment (Z09)

✓5ᵗʰ **Z87.0**   **Personal history of diseases of the** respiratory system
> Conditions classifiable to J00-J99

Z87.01   **Personal history of** pneumonia (recurrent) `UPD`

Z87.09   **Personal history of other diseases of the respiratory system** `UPD`

✓5ᵗʰ **Z87.1**   **Personal history of diseases of the** digestive system
> Conditions classifiable to K00-K93

Z87.11   **Personal history of** peptic ulcer **disease** `UPD`

Z87.19   **Personal history of other diseases of the digestive system** `UPD`
> AHA: 2017,1Q,14

Z87.2   **Personal history of diseases of the** skin and subcutaneous **tissue** `UPD`
> Conditions classifiable to L00-L99
> > EXCLUDES 2   *personal history of diabetic foot ulcer (Z86.31)*

✓5ᵗʰ **Z87.3**   **Personal history of diseases of the** musculoskeletal system and connective tissue
> Conditions classifiable to M00-M99
> > EXCLUDES 2   *personal history of (healed) traumatic fracture (Z87.81)*

✓6ᵗʰ **Z87.31**   **Personal history of (healed)** nontraumatic fracture

Z87.310   **Personal history of (healed)** osteoporosis **fracture** `UPD`
> Personal history of (healed) fragility fracture
> Personal history of (healed) collapsed vertebra due to osteoporosis
> **TIP:** Assign for history of osteoporosis fractures that have resolved, even when a code from category M80 indicating current osteoporosis fracture is also reported.

Z87.311   **Personal history of (healed) other pathological fracture** `UPD`
> Personal history of (healed) collapsed vertebra NOS
> > EXCLUDES 2   *personal history of osteoporosis fracture (Z87.310)*

Z87.312   **Personal history of (healed)** stress **fracture** `UPD`
> Personal history of (healed) fatigue fracture

Z87.39   **Personal history of other diseases of the musculoskeletal system and connective tissue** `UPD`

✓5ᵗʰ **Z87.4**   **Personal history of diseases of the** genitourinary system
> Conditions classifiable to N00-N99

✓6ᵗʰ **Z87.41**   **Personal history of** dysplasia of the female genital **tract**
> > EXCLUDES 1   *personal history of intraepithelial neoplasia III of female genital tract (Z86.001, Z86.008)*
> > *personal history of malignant neoplasm of female genital tract (Z85.40-Z85.44)*

Z87.410   **Personal history of** cervical **dysplasia** `UPD` ♀

Z87.411   **Personal history of** vaginal **dysplasia** `UPD` ♀

Z87.412   **Personal history of** vulvar **dysplasia** `UPD` ♀

Z87.42   **Personal history of other diseases of the** female **genital tract** `UPD` ♀

✓6ᵗʰ **Z87.43**   **Personal history of diseases of the** male genital **organs**

Z87.430   **Personal history of** prostatic **dysplasia** `UPD` ♂
> > EXCLUDES 1   *personal history of malignant neoplasm of prostate (Z85.46)*

Z87.438   **Personal history of other diseases of** male **genital organs** `UPD` ♂

✓6ᵗʰ **Z87.44**   **Personal history of diseases of the** urinary system
> > EXCLUDES 1   *personal history of malignant neoplasm of cervix uteri (Z85.41)*

Z87.440   **Personal history of** urinary (tract) **infections** `UPD`

Z87.441   **Personal history of** nephrotic **syndrome** `UPD`

Z87.442   **Personal history of** urinary calculi `UPD`
> Personal history of kidney stones

Z87.448   **Personal history of other diseases of urinary system** `UPD`

✓5ᵗʰ **Z87.5**   **Personal history of complications of** pregnancy, childbirth and the puerperium
> Conditions classifiable to O00-O9A
> > EXCLUDES 2   *recurrent pregnancy loss (N96)*

Z87.51   **Personal history of** pre-term labor `UPD` ♀
> > EXCLUDES 1   *current pregnancy with history of pre-term labor (O09.21-)*

Z87.59   **Personal history of other complications of pregnancy, childbirth and the puerperium** `UPD` ♀
> Personal history of trophoblastic disease

✓5ᵗʰ **Z87.7**   **Personal history of (corrected)** congenital malformations
> Conditions classifiable to Q00-Q89 that have been repaired or corrected
> > EXCLUDES 1   *congenital malformations that have been partially corrected or repair but which still require medical treatment - code to condition*
> > EXCLUDES 2   *other postprocedural states (Z98.-)*
> > *personal history of medical treatment (Z92.-)*
> > *presence of cardiac and vascular implants and grafts (Z95.-)*
> > *presence of other devices (Z97.-)*
> > *presence of other functional implants (Z96.-)*
> > *transplanted organ and tissue status (Z94.-)*

✓6ᵗʰ **Z87.71**   **Personal history of (corrected) congenital malformations of** genitourinary system

Z87.710   **Personal history of (corrected)** hypospadias `UPD` ♂

Z87.718   **Personal history of other specified (corrected) congenital malformations of genitourinary system** `UPD`

✓6ᵗʰ **Z87.72**   **Personal history of (corrected) congenital malformations of** nervous system and sense organs

Z87.720   **Personal history of (corrected) congenital malformations of** eye `UPD`

Z87.721   **Personal history of (corrected) congenital malformations of** ear `UPD`

Z87.728   **Personal history of other specified (corrected) congenital malformations of nervous system and sense organs** `UPD`

✔ Additional Character Required   ✓x7ᵗʰ Placeholder   Questionable PDx   Manifestation   Unspecified Dx   `UPD` Unacceptable PDx   H1-H14 HAC   HCC CMS-HCC Dx   HIV HIV Dx

ICD-10-CM 2022   1261

√6th **Z87.73** **Personal history of (corrected) congenital malformations of** digestive system

Z87.730 **Personal history of (corrected)** cleft lip and palate   UPD

Z87.738 **Personal history of other specified (corrected) congenital malformations of** digestive system   UPD

Z87.74 **Personal history of (corrected) congenital malformations of** heart and circulatory system   UPD

Z87.75 **Personal history of (corrected) congenital malformations of** respiratory system   UPD

Z87.76 **Personal history of (corrected) congenital malformations of** integument, limbs and musculoskeletal system   UPD

√6th **Z87.79** **Personal history of other (corrected) congenital malformations**

Z87.790 **Personal history of (corrected) congenital malformations of** face and neck   UPD

Z87.798 **Personal history of other (corrected) congenital malformations**   UPD

√5th **Z87.8** **Personal history of other specified conditions**

> EXCLUDES 2   personal history of self harm ▶(Z91.5-)◀

Z87.81 **Personal history of (healed)** traumatic fracture   UPD

> EXCLUDES 2   personal history of (healed) nontraumatic fracture (Z87.31-)

√6th **Z87.82** **Personal history of other (healed)** physical injury and trauma

Conditions classifiable to S00-T88, except traumatic fractures

Z87.820 **Personal history of** traumatic brain injury   UPD

> EXCLUDES 1   personal history of transient ischemic attack (TIA), and cerebral infarction without residual deficits (Z86.73)

Z87.821 **Personal history of** retained foreign body fully removed   UPD

Z87.828 **Personal history of other (healed) physical injury and trauma**   UPD

√6th **Z87.89** **Personal history of other specified conditions**

Z87.890 **Personal history of** sex reassignment

Z87.891 **Personal history of** nicotine dependence   UPD

> EXCLUDES 1   current nicotine dependence (F17.2-)

> AHA: 2017, 2Q, 27

Z87.892 **Personal history of** anaphylaxis   UPD

Code also allergy status such as:
allergy status to drugs, medicaments and biological substances (Z88.-)
allergy status, other than to drugs and biological substances (Z91.0-)

Z87.898 **Personal history of other specified conditions**   UPD

> AHA: 2013, 1Q, 21

√4th **Z88** **Allergy status to drugs, medicaments and biological substances**

> EXCLUDES 2   allergy status, other than to drugs and biological substances (Z91.0-)

> AHA: 2015, 3Q, 23

Z88.0 **Allergy status to** penicillin   UPD

Z88.1 **Allergy status to other antibiotic agents**   UPD

Z88.2 **Allergy status to** sulfonamides   UPD

Z88.3 **Allergy status to other anti-infective agents**   UPD

Z88.4 **Allergy status to** anesthetic agent   UPD

Z88.5 **Allergy status to** narcotic agent   UPD

Z88.6 **Allergy status to** analgesic agent   UPD

Z88.7 **Allergy status to** serum and vaccine   UPD

Z88.8 **Allergy status to other drugs, medicaments and biological substances**   UPD

Z88.9 **Allergy status to unspecified drugs, medicaments and biological substances**   UPD

√4th **Z89** **Acquired absence of limb**

> INCLUDES   amputation status
> postprocedural loss of limb
> post-traumatic loss of limb

> EXCLUDES 1   acquired deformities of limbs (M20-M21)
> congenital absence of limbs (Q71-Q73)

√5th **Z89.0** **Acquired absence of** thumb and other finger(s)

√6th **Z89.01** **Acquired absence of** thumb

Z89.011 **Acquired absence of** right thumb   UPD

Z89.012 **Acquired absence of** left thumb   UPD

Z89.019 **Acquired absence of unspecified thumb**   UPD

√6th **Z89.02** **Acquired absence of other** finger(s)

> EXCLUDES 2   acquired absence of thumb (Z89.01-)

Z89.021 **Acquired absence of** right finger(s)   UPD

Z89.022 **Acquired absence of** left finger(s)   UPD

Z89.029 **Acquired absence of unspecified finger(s)**   UPD

√5th **Z89.1** **Acquired absence of** hand and wrist

√6th **Z89.11** **Acquired absence of** hand

Z89.111 **Acquired absence of** right hand   UPD

Z89.112 **Acquired absence of** left hand   UPD

Z89.119 **Acquired absence of unspecified hand**   UPD

√6th **Z89.12** **Acquired absence of** wrist

Disarticulation at wrist

Z89.121 **Acquired absence of** right wrist   UPD

Z89.122 **Acquired absence of** left wrist   UPD

Z89.129 **Acquired absence of unspecified wrist**   UPD

√5th **Z89.2** **Acquired absence of** upper limb above wrist

√6th **Z89.20** **Acquired absence of upper limb, unspecified level**

Z89.201 **Acquired absence of** right upper limb, unspecified level   UPD

Z89.202 **Acquired absence of** left upper limb, unspecified level   UPD

Z89.209 **Acquired absence of unspecified upper limb, unspecified level**   UPD

Acquired absence of arm NOS

√6th **Z89.21** **Acquired absence of** upper limb below elbow

Z89.211 **Acquired absence of** right upper limb below elbow   UPD

Z89.212 **Acquired absence of** left upper limb below elbow   UPD

Z89.219 **Acquired absence of unspecified upper limb below elbow**   UPD

√6th **Z89.22** **Acquired absence of** upper limb above elbow

Disarticulation at elbow

Z89.221 **Acquired absence of** right upper limb above elbow   UPD

Z89.222 **Acquired absence of** left upper limb above elbow   UPD

Z89.229 **Acquired absence of unspecified upper limb above elbow**   UPD

√6th **Z89.23** **Acquired absence of** shoulder

Acquired absence of shoulder joint following explantation of shoulder joint prosthesis, with or without presence of antibiotic-impregnated cement spacer

Z89.231 **Acquired absence of** right shoulder   UPD

Z89.232 **Acquired absence of** left shoulder   UPD

Z89.239 **Acquired absence of unspecified shoulder**   UPD

√5th **Z89.4** **Acquired absence of** toe(s), foot, and ankle

√6th **Z89.41** **Acquired absence of** great toe

Z89.411 **Acquired absence of** right great toe   UPD HCC

Z89.412 **Acquired absence of** left great toe   UPD HCC

Z89.419 **Acquired absence of unspecified great toe**   UPD HCC

N Newborn: 0   P Pediatric: 0-17   M Maternity: 9-64   A Adult: 15-124   MCC Major Complication/Comorbidity   CC Complication/Comorbidity   SW Severe Wound Dx

1262   ICD-10-CM 2022

Chapter 21. Factors Influencing Health Status and Contact With Health Services

√6ᵗʰ **Z89.42** **Acquired absence of** other toe(s)
- EXCLUDES 2   *acquired absence of great toe (Z89.41-)*
- **Z89.421** **Acquired absence of other** right toe(s)   UPD HCC
- **Z89.422** **Acquired absence of other** left toe(s)   UPD HCC
- **Z89.429** **Acquired absence of other** toe(s), unspecified side   UPD HCC

√6ᵗʰ **Z89.43** **Acquired absence of** foot
- **Z89.431** **Acquired absence of** right foot   UPD HCC
- **Z89.432** **Acquired absence of** left foot   UPD HCC
- **Z89.439** **Acquired absence of** unspecified foot   UPD HCC

√6ᵗʰ **Z89.44** **Acquired absence of** ankle
- Disarticulation of ankle
- **Z89.441** **Acquired absence of** right ankle   UPD HCC
- **Z89.442** **Acquired absence of** left ankle   UPD HCC
- **Z89.449** **Acquired absence of** unspecified ankle   UPD HCC

√5ᵗʰ **Z89.5** **Acquired absence of leg below knee**
- √6ᵗʰ **Z89.51** **Acquired absence of** leg below knee
  - **Z89.511** **Acquired absence of** right leg below knee   UPD HCC
  - **Z89.512** **Acquired absence of** left leg below knee   UPD HCC
  - **Z89.519** **Acquired absence of** unspecified leg below knee   UPD HCC
- √6ᵗʰ **Z89.52** **Acquired absence of** knee
  - Acquired absence of knee joint following explantation of knee joint prosthesis, with or without presence of antibiotic-impregnated cement spacer
  - **Z89.521** **Acquired absence of** right knee   UPD
  - **Z89.522** **Acquired absence of** left knee   UPD
  - **Z89.529** **Acquired absence of** unspecified knee   UPD

√5ᵗʰ **Z89.6** **Acquired absence of leg above knee**
- √6ᵗʰ **Z89.61** **Acquired absence of** leg above knee
  - Acquired absence of leg, NOS
  - Disarticulation at knee
  - **Z89.611** **Acquired absence of** right leg above knee   UPD HCC
  - **Z89.612** **Acquired absence of** left leg above knee   UPD HCC
  - **Z89.619** **Acquired absence of** unspecified leg above knee   UPD HCC
- √6ᵗʰ **Z89.62** **Acquired absence of** hip
  - Acquired absence of hip joint following explantation of hip joint prosthesis, with or without presence of antibiotic-impregnated cement spacer
  - Disarticulation at hip
  - **Z89.621** **Acquired absence of** right hip joint   UPD
  - **Z89.622** **Acquired absence of** left hip joint   UPD
  - **Z89.629** **Acquired absence of** unspecified hip joint   UPD

Z89.9 **Acquired absence of limb, unspecified**   UPD

√4ᵗʰ **Z90** **Acquired absence of organs, not elsewhere classified**
- INCLUDES   postprocedural or post-traumatic loss of body part NEC
- EXCLUDES 1   *congenital absence - see Alphabetical Index*
- EXCLUDES 2   *postprocedural absence of endocrine glands (E89.-)*

√5ᵗʰ **Z90.0** **Acquired absence of part of** head and neck
- **Z90.01** **Acquired absence of** eye   UPD
- **Z90.02** **Acquired absence of** larynx   UPD
- **Z90.09** **Acquired absence of** other part of head and neck   UPD
  - Acquired absence of nose
  - EXCLUDES 2   *teeth (K08.1)*

√5ᵗʰ **Z90.1** **Acquired absence of** breast and nipple
- **Z90.10** **Acquired absence of** unspecified breast and nipple
- **Z90.11** **Acquired absence of** right breast and nipple
- **Z90.12** **Acquired absence of** left breast and nipple
- **Z90.13** **Acquired absence of** bilateral breasts and nipples

Z90.2 **Acquired absence of** lung [part of]   UPD
Z90.3 **Acquired absence of** stomach [part of]   UPD

√5ᵗʰ **Z90.4** **Acquired absence of other specified parts of digestive tract**
- √6ᵗʰ **Z90.41** **Acquired absence of** pancreas
  - Code also exocrine pancreatic insufficiency (K86.81)
  - Use additional code to identify any associated:
    - diabetes mellitus, postpancreatectomy (E13.-)
    - insulin use (Z79.4)
  - **Z90.410** **Acquired** total absence **of** pancreas   UPD
    - Acquired absence of pancreas NOS
  - **Z90.411** **Acquired** partial absence **of** pancreas   UPD
  - **Z90.49** **Acquired absence of other specified parts of digestive tract**   UPD

Z90.5 **Acquired absence of** kidney   UPD
Z90.6 **Acquired absence of other parts of urinary tract**   UPD
- Acquired absence of bladder

√5ᵗʰ **Z90.7** **Acquired absence of** genital organ(s)
- EXCLUDES 1   *personal history of sex reassignment (Z87.890)*
- EXCLUDES 2   *female genital mutilation status (N90.81-)*
- √6ᵗʰ **Z90.71** **Acquired absence of** cervix and uterus
  - **Z90.710** **Acquired absence of** both cervix and uterus   UPD ♀
    - Acquired absence of uterus NOS
    - Status post total hysterectomy
  - **Z90.711** **Acquired absence of uterus** with remaining cervical stump   UPD ♀
    - Status post partial hysterectomy with remaining cervical stump
  - **Z90.712** **Acquired absence of cervix** with remaining uterus   UPD ♀
- √6ᵗʰ **Z90.72** **Acquired absence of** ovaries
  - **Z90.721** **Acquired absence of ovaries,** unilateral   UPD ♀
  - **Z90.722** **Acquired absence of ovaries,** bilateral   UPD ♀
- **Z90.79** **Acquired absence of other genital organ(s)**   UPD

√5ᵗʰ **Z90.8** **Acquired absence of other organs**
- **Z90.81** **Acquired absence of** spleen   UPD
- **Z90.89** **Acquired absence of other organs**   UPD

√4ᵗʰ **Z91** **Personal risk factors, not elsewhere classified**
- EXCLUDES 2   *contact with and (suspected) exposures hazardous to health (Z77.-)*
  - *exposure to pollution and other problems related to physical environment (Z77.1-)*
  - *female genital mutilation status (N90.81-)*
  - *personal history of physical injury and trauma (Z87.81, Z87.82-)*
  - *occupational exposure to risk factors (Z57.-)*

√5ᵗʰ **Z91.0** **Allergy status, other than to drugs and biological substances**
- EXCLUDES 2   *allergy status to drugs, medicaments, and biological substances (Z88.-)*
- √6ᵗʰ **Z91.01** **Food allergy status**
  - EXCLUDES 2   *food additives allergy status (Z91.02)*
  - **Z91.010** **Allergy to** peanuts   UPD
  - **Z91.011** **Allergy to** milk products   UPD
    - EXCLUDES 1   *lactose intolerance (E73.-)*
  - **Z91.012** **Allergy to** eggs   UPD
  - **Z91.013** **Allergy to** seafood   UPD
    - Allergy to shellfish
    - Allergy to octopus or squid ink
  - **Z91.014** **Allergy to** mammalian meats
    - Allergy to beef
    - Allergy to lamb
    - Allergy to pork
    - Allergy to red meats
  - **Z91.018** **Allergy to other foods**   UPD
    - Allergy to nuts other than peanuts
- **Z91.02** **Food additives allergy status**   UPD
- √6ᵗʰ **Z91.03** **Insect allergy status**
  - **Z91.030** Bee **allergy status**   UPD
  - **Z91.038** **Other insect allergy status**   UPD
- √6ᵗʰ **Z91.04** **Nonmedicinal substance allergy status**
  - **Z91.040** Latex **allergy status**   UPD
    - Latex sensitivity status

☑ Additional Character Required   √x7ᵗʰ Placeholder   Questionable PDx   Manifestation   Unspecified Dx   UPD Unacceptable PDx   H1-H14 HAC   HCC CMS-HCC Dx   HIV HIV Dx

ICD-10-CM 2022   1263

Z91.041 Radiographic dye **allergy status** `UPD`
     Allergy status to contrast media used for diagnostic X-ray procedure

Z91.048 Other nonmedicinal substance allergy status `UPD`

Z91.09 Other allergy status, other than to drugs and biological substances `UPD`

√5ᵗʰ **Z91.1 Patient's noncompliance with medical treatment and regimen**

Z91.11 Patient's noncompliance with dietary regimen `UPD`

√6ᵗʰ **Z91.12 Patient's** intentional underdosing of medication regimen
     Code first underdosing of medication (T36-T50) with fifth or sixth character 6

     `EXCLUDES 1`   *adverse effect of prescribed drug taken as directed - code to adverse effect*
         poisoning (overdose) - code to poisoning

     AHA: 2018,4Q,72

Z91.120 Patient's intentional underdosing of medication regimen due to financial hardship `UPD`

Z91.128 Patient's intentional underdosing of medication regimen for other reason `UPD`

√6ᵗʰ **Z91.13 Patient's** unintentional underdosing of medication regimen
     Code first underdosing of medication (T36-T50) with fifth or sixth character 6

     `EXCLUDES 1`   *adverse effect of prescribed drug taken as directed - code to adverse effect*
         poisoning (overdose) - code to poisoning

     AHA: 2018,4Q,72

Z91.130 Patient's unintentional underdosing of medication regimen due to age-related debility `UPD`

Z91.138 Patient's unintentional underdosing of medication regimen for other reason `UPD`

Z91.14 Patient's other noncompliance with medication regimen `UPD`
     Patient's underdosing of medication NOS
     AHA: 2018,4Q,72

Z91.15 Patient's noncompliance with renal dialysis `UPD` `HCC`

Z91.19 Patient's noncompliance with other medical treatment and regimen `UPD`
     Nonadherence to medical treatment

√5ᵗʰ **Z91.4 Personal history of psychological trauma, not elsewhere classified**

√6ᵗʰ **Z91.41 Personal history of** adult abuse

     `EXCLUDES 2`   *personal history of abuse in childhood (Z62.81-)*

Z91.410 Personal history of adult physical and sexual abuse `UPD` `A`

     `EXCLUDES 1`   *current adult physical abuse (T74.11, T76.11)*
         current adult sexual abuse (T74.21, T76.11)

Z91.411 Personal history of adult psychological abuse `UPD` `A`

Z91.412 Personal history of adult neglect `UPD` `A`

     `EXCLUDES 1`   *current adult neglect (T74.01, T76.01)*

Z91.419 Personal history of unspecified adult abuse `UPD` `A`

Z91.42 Personal history of forced labor **or** sexual exploitation `UPD`
     AHA: 2018,4Q,32,35

Z91.49 Other personal history of psychological trauma, not elsewhere classified `UPD`

▲ √5ᵗʰ **Z91.5 Personal history of self-harm**
     ~~Personal history of parasuicide~~
     ~~Personal history of self-poisoning~~
     ~~Personal history of suicide attempt~~
     ►Code also mental health disorder, if known◄

● **Z91.51 Personal history of** suicidal behavior
     Personal history of parasuicide
     Personal history of self-poisoning
     Personal history of suicide attempt

● **Z91.52 Personal history of** nonsuicidal self-harm
     Personal history of nonsuicidal self-injury
     Personal history of self-inflicted injury without suicidal intent
     Personal history of self-mutilation

√5ᵗʰ **Z91.8 Other specified personal risk factors, not elsewhere classified**

Z91.81 History of falling `UPD`
     At risk for falling

Z91.82 Personal history of military deployment `UPD` `A`
     Individual (civilian or military) with past history of military war, peacekeeping and humanitarian deployment (current or past conflict)
     Returned from military deployment

Z91.83 *Wandering in diseases classified elsewhere*
     Code first underlying disorder such as:
     Alzheimer's disease (G30.-)
     autism or pervasive developmental disorder (F84.-)
     intellectual disabilities (F70-F79)
     unspecified dementia with behavioral disturbance (F03.9-)

√6ᵗʰ **Z91.84 Oral health risk factors**
     AHA: 2017,4Q,29

Z91.841 Risk for dental caries, low `UPD`

Z91.842 Risk for dental caries, moderate `UPD`

Z91.843 Risk for dental caries, high `UPD`

Z91.849 Unspecified risk for dental caries `UPD`

Z91.89 Other specified personal risk factors, not elsewhere classified `UPD`
     AHA: 2017,1Q,45

√4ᵗʰ **Z92 Personal history of medical treatment**
     `EXCLUDES 2`   *postprocedural states (Z98.-)*

Z92.0 Personal history of contraception `UPD`
     `EXCLUDES 1`   *counseling or management of current contraceptive practices (Z30.-)*
         long term (current) use of contraception (Z79.3)
         presence of (intrauterine) contraceptive device (Z97.5)

√5ᵗʰ **Z92.2 Personal history of** drug therapy
     `EXCLUDES 2`   *long term (current) drug therapy (Z79.-)*

Z92.21 Personal history of antineoplastic chemotherapy `UPD`

Z92.22 Personal history of monoclonal drug therapy `UPD`

Z92.23 Personal history of estrogen therapy `UPD`

√6ᵗʰ **Z92.24 Personal history of** steroid therapy

Z92.240 Personal history of inhaled steroid therapy `UPD`

Z92.241 Personal history of systemic steroid therapy `UPD`
     Personal history of steroid therapy NOS

▲ **Z92.25 Personal history of** immunosuppression therapy `UPD`
     `EXCLUDES 2`   *personal history of steroid therapy (Z92.24)*

Z92.29 Personal history of other drug therapy `UPD`

Z92.3 Personal history of irradiation `UPD`
     Personal history of exposure to therapeutic radiation
     `EXCLUDES 1`   *exposure to radiation in the physical environment (Z77.12)*
         occupational exposure to radiation (Z57.1)

√5ᵗʰ **Z92.8 Personal history of other medical treatment**

Z92.81 Personal history of extracorporeal membrane oxygenation (ECMO) `UPD`

`N` Newborn: 0   `P` Pediatric: 0-17   `M` Maternity: 9-64   `A` Adult: 15-124   `MCC` Major Complication/Comorbidity   `CC` Complication/Comorbidity   `SW` Severe Wound Dx

1264   ICD-10-CM 2022

Z92.82 Status post administration of tPA (rtPA) in a different facility within the last 24 hours prior to admission to current facility `UPD`
Code first condition requiring tPA administration, such as:
acute cerebral infarction (I63.-)
acute myocardial infarction (I21.-, I22.-)
AHA: 2013,4Q,124

Z92.83 Personal history of failed moderate sedation `UPD`
Personal history of failed conscious sedation
> *EXCLUDES 2* *failed moderate sedation during procedure (T88.52)*

Z92.84 Personal history of unintended awareness under general anesthesia `UPD`
> *EXCLUDES 2* *unintended awareness under general anesthesia during procedure (T88.53)*

AHA: 2016,4Q,72-73,77

● ✓6ᵗʰ **Z92.85** Personal history of cellular therapy
●   **Z92.850** Personal history of Chimeric Antigen Receptor T-cell therapy
      Personal history of CAR T-cell therapy
●   **Z92.858** Personal history of other cellular therapy
●   **Z92.859** Personal history of cellular therapy, unspecified
●   **Z92.86** Personal history of gene therapy
    Z92.89 Personal history of other medical treatment `UPD`
      AHA: 2020,1Q,18

✓4ᵗʰ **Z93** Artificial opening status
> *EXCLUDES 1* *artificial openings requiring attention or management (Z43.-)*
> *complications of external stoma (J95.0-, K94.-, N99.5-)*

Z93.0 Tracheostomy status `UPD` `HCC`
  AHA: 2013,4Q,129

Z93.1 Gastrostomy status `UPD` `HCC`

Z93.2 Ileostomy status `UPD` `HCC`

Z93.3 Colostomy status `UPD` `HCC`

Z93.4 Other artificial openings of gastrointestinal tract status `UPD` `HCC`

✓5ᵗʰ **Z93.5** Cystostomy status
  Z93.50 Unspecified cystostomy status `UPD` `HCC`
  Z93.51 Cutaneous-vesicostomy status `UPD` `HCC`
  Z93.52 Appendico-vesicostomy status `UPD` `HCC`
  Z93.59 Other cystostomy status `UPD` `HCC`

Z93.6 Other artificial openings of urinary tract status `UPD` `HCC`
  Nephrostomy status
  Ureterostomy status
  Urethrostomy status

Z93.8 Other artificial opening status `UPD` `HCC`

Z93.9 Artificial opening status, unspecified `UPD` `HCC`

✓4ᵗʰ **Z94** Transplanted organ and tissue status
> *INCLUDES* organ or tissue replaced by heterogenous or homogenous transplant
> *EXCLUDES 1* *complications of transplanted organ or tissue - see Alphabetical Index*
> *EXCLUDES 2* *presence of vascular grafts (Z95.-)*

Z94.0 Kidney transplant status `CC` `UPD`

Z94.1 Heart transplant status `CC` `UPD` `HCC`
> *EXCLUDES 1* *artificial heart status (Z95.812)*
> *heart-valve replacement status (Z95.2-Z95.4)*

Z94.2 Lung transplant status `CC` `UPD` `HCC`

Z94.3 Heart and lungs transplant status `CC` `UPD` `HCC`

Z94.4 Liver transplant status `CC` `UPD` `HCC`

Z94.5 Skin transplant status `UPD`
  Autogenous skin transplant status

Z94.6 Bone transplant status `UPD`

Z94.7 Corneal transplant status `UPD`

✓5ᵗʰ **Z94.8** Other transplanted organ and tissue status
  Z94.81 Bone marrow transplant status `CC` `UPD` `HCC`
  Z94.82 Intestine transplant status `CC` `UPD` `HCC`
  Z94.83 Pancreas transplant status `CC` `UPD` `HCC`
  Z94.84 Stem cells transplant status `CC` `UPD` `HCC`
  Z94.89 Other transplanted organ and tissue status `UPD`
  Z94.9 Transplanted organ and tissue status, unspecified `UPD`

✓4ᵗʰ **Z95** Presence of cardiac and vascular implants and grafts
> *EXCLUDES 2* *complications of cardiac and vascular devices, implants and grafts (T82.-)*

Z95.0 Presence of cardiac pacemaker `UPD`
  Presence of cardiac resynchronization therapy (CRT-P) pacemaker
> *EXCLUDES 1* *adjustment or management of cardiac device (Z45.0-)*
> *adjustment or management of cardiac pacemaker (Z45.0)*
> *presence of automatic (implantable) cardiac defibrillator with synchronous cardiac pacemaker (Z95.810)*

AHA: 2019,1Q,33
TIP: Assign an additional code for the condition the cardiac device is controlling (e.g., sick sinus syndrome). Even though the cardiac device controls the heart rate, it does not cure the condition and therefore should be reported.

Z95.1 Presence of aortocoronary bypass graft `UPD`
  Presence of coronary artery bypass graft

Z95.2 Presence of prosthetic heart valve `UPD`
  Presence of heart valve NOS

Z95.3 Presence of xenogenic heart valve `UPD`

Z95.4 Presence of other heart-valve replacement `UPD`

Z95.5 Presence of coronary angioplasty implant and graft `UPD`
> *EXCLUDES 1* *coronary angioplasty status without implant and graft (Z98.61)*

✓5ᵗʰ **Z95.8** Presence of other cardiac and vascular implants and grafts

✓6ᵗʰ **Z95.81** Presence of other cardiac implants and grafts
  Z95.810 Presence of automatic (implantable) cardiac defibrillator `UPD`
    Presence of automatic (implantable) cardiac defibrillator with synchronous cardiac pacemaker
    Presence of cardiac resynchronization therapy defibrillator (CRT-D)
    Presence of cardioverter-defibrillator (ICD)
    TIP: Assign an additional code for the condition the cardiac device is controlling (e.g., sick sinus syndrome). Even though the cardiac device controls the heart rate, it does not cure the condition and therefore should be reported.
  Z95.811 Presence of heart assist device `CC` `UPD` `HCC`
  Z95.812 Presence of fully implantable artificial heart `CC` `UPD` `HCC`
  Z95.818 Presence of other cardiac implants and grafts `UPD`

✓6ᵗʰ **Z95.82** Presence of other vascular implants and grafts
  Z95.820 Peripheral vascular angioplasty status with implants and grafts `UPD`
> *EXCLUDES 1* *peripheral vascular angioplasty without implant and graft (Z98.62)*
  Z95.828 Presence of other vascular implants and grafts `UPD`
    Presence of intravascular prosthesis NEC

Z95.9 Presence of cardiac and vascular implant and graft, unspecified `UPD`

✓4ᵗʰ **Z96** Presence of other functional implants
> *EXCLUDES 2* *complications of internal prosthetic devices, implants and grafts (T82-T85)*
> *fitting and adjustment of prosthetic and other devices (Z44-Z46)*

Z96.0 Presence of urogenital implants `UPD`

Z96.1 Presence of intraocular lens `UPD`
  Presence of pseudophakia

✓5ᵗʰ **Z96.2** Presence of otological and audiological implants
  Z96.20 Presence of otological and audiological implant, unspecified `UPD`
  Z96.21 Cochlear implant status `UPD`
  Z96.22 Myringotomy tube(s) status `UPD`

Z96.29   **Presence of other otological and audiological implants** `UPD`
Presence of bone-conduction hearing device
Presence of eustachian tube stent
Stapes replacement

Z96.3   **Presence of artificial larynx** `UPD`

✓5ᵗʰ **Z96.4**   **Presence of endocrine implants**

Z96.41   **Presence of insulin pump (external) (internal)** `UPD`

Z96.49   **Presence of other endocrine implants** `UPD`

Z96.5   **Presence of tooth-root and mandibular implants** `UPD`

✓5ᵗʰ **Z96.6**   **Presence of orthopedic joint implants**
AHA: 2019,3Q,16

Z96.60   **Presence of unspecified orthopedic joint implant** `UPD`

✓6ᵗʰ **Z96.61**   **Presence of artificial shoulder joint**

Z96.611   **Presence of right artificial shoulder joint** `UPD`

Z96.612   **Presence of left artificial shoulder joint** `UPD`

Z96.619   **Presence of unspecified artificial shoulder joint** `UPD`

✓6ᵗʰ **Z96.62**   **Presence of artificial elbow joint**

Z96.621   **Presence of right artificial elbow joint** `UPD`

Z96.622   **Presence of left artificial elbow joint** `UPD`

Z96.629   **Presence of unspecified artificial elbow joint** `UPD`

✓6ᵗʰ **Z96.63**   **Presence of artificial wrist joint**

Z96.631   **Presence of right artificial wrist joint** `UPD`

Z96.632   **Presence of left artificial wrist joint** `UPD`

Z96.639   **Presence of unspecified artificial wrist joint** `UPD`

✓6ᵗʰ **Z96.64**   **Presence of artificial hip joint**
Hip-joint replacement (partial) (total)

Z96.641   **Presence of right artificial hip joint** `UPD`

Z96.642   **Presence of left artificial hip joint** `UPD`

Z96.643   **Presence of artificial hip joint, bilateral** `UPD`

Z96.649   **Presence of unspecified artificial hip joint** `UPD`

✓6ᵗʰ **Z96.65**   **Presence of artificial knee joint**

Z96.651   **Presence of right artificial knee joint** `UPD`

Z96.652   **Presence of left artificial knee joint** `UPD`

Z96.653   **Presence of artificial knee joint, bilateral** `UPD`

Z96.659   **Presence of unspecified artificial knee joint** `UPD`

✓6ᵗʰ **Z96.66**   **Presence of artificial ankle joint**

Z96.661   **Presence of right artificial ankle joint** `UPD`

Z96.662   **Presence of left artificial ankle joint** `UPD`

Z96.669   **Presence of unspecified artificial ankle joint** `UPD`

✓6ᵗʰ **Z96.69**   **Presence of other orthopedic joint implants**

Z96.691   **Finger-joint replacement of right hand** `UPD`

Z96.692   **Finger-joint replacement of left hand** `UPD`

Z96.693   **Finger-joint replacement, bilateral** `UPD`

Z96.698   **Presence of other orthopedic joint implants** `UPD`

Z96.7   **Presence of other bone and tendon implants** `UPD`
Presence of skull plate

✓5ᵗʰ **Z96.8**   **Presence of other specified functional implants**

Z96.81   **Presence of artificial skin** `UPD`

Z96.82   **Presence of neurostimulator** `UPD`
Presence of brain neurostimulator
Presence of gastric neurostimulator
Presence of peripheral nerve neurostimulator
Presence of sacral nerve neurostimulator
Presence of spinal cord neurostimulator
Presence of vagus nerve neurostimulator
AHA: 2019,4Q,19

Z96.89   **Presence of other specified functional implants** `UPD`

Z96.9   **Presence of functional implant, unspecified** `UPD`

✓4ᵗʰ **Z97**   **Presence of other devices**
`EXCLUDES 1`   complications of internal prosthetic devices, implants and grafts (T82-T85)
`EXCLUDES 2`   fitting and adjustment of prosthetic and other devices (Z44-Z46)
presence of cerebrospinal fluid drainage device (Z98.2)

Z97.0   **Presence of artificial eye** `UPD`

✓5ᵗʰ **Z97.1**   **Presence of artificial limb (complete) (partial)**

Z97.10   **Presence of artificial limb (complete) (partial), unspecified** `UPD`

Z97.11   **Presence of artificial right arm (complete) (partial)** `UPD`

Z97.12   **Presence of artificial left arm (complete) (partial)** `UPD`

Z97.13   **Presence of artificial right leg (complete) (partial)** `UPD`

Z97.14   **Presence of artificial left leg (complete) (partial)** `UPD`

Z97.15   **Presence of artificial arms, bilateral (complete) (partial)** `UPD`

Z97.16   **Presence of artificial legs, bilateral (complete) (partial)** `UPD`

Z97.2   **Presence of dental prosthetic device (complete) (partial)** `UPD`
Presence of dentures (complete) (partial)

Z97.3   **Presence of spectacles and contact lenses** `UPD`

Z97.4   **Presence of external hearing-aid** `UPD`

Z97.5   **Presence of (intrauterine) contraceptive device** `UPD` ♀
`EXCLUDES 1`   checking, reinsertion or removal of implantable subdermal contraceptive (Z30.46)
checking, reinsertion or removal of intrauterine contraceptive device (Z30.43-)

Z97.8   **Presence of other specified devices** `UPD`

✓4ᵗʰ **Z98**   **Other postprocedural states**
`EXCLUDES 2`   aftercare (Z43-Z49, Z51)
follow-up medical care (Z08-Z09)
postprocedural complication - see Alphabetical Index

Z98.0   **Intestinal bypass and anastomosis status** `UPD`
`EXCLUDES 2`   bariatric surgery status (Z98.84)
gastric bypass status (Z98.84)
obesity surgery status (Z98.84)

Z98.1   **Arthrodesis status** `UPD`

Z98.2   **Presence of cerebrospinal fluid drainage device** `UPD`
Presence of CSF shunt

Z98.3   **Post therapeutic collapse of lung status** `UPD`
Code first underlying disease

✓5ᵗʰ **Z98.4**   **Cataract extraction status**
Use additional code to identify intraocular lens implant status (Z96.1)
`EXCLUDES 1`   aphakia (H27.0)

Z98.41   **Cataract extraction status, right eye** `UPD`

Z98.42   **Cataract extraction status, left eye** `UPD`

Z98.49   **Cataract extraction status, unspecified eye** `UPD`

✓5ᵗʰ **Z98.5**   **Sterilization status**
`EXCLUDES 1`   female infertility (N97.-)
male infertility (N46.-)

Z98.51   **Tubal ligation status** `UPD` ♀

Z98.52   **Vasectomy status** `UPD` `A` ♂

✓5ᵗʰ **Z98.6**   **Angioplasty status**

Z98.61   **Coronary angioplasty status** `UPD`
`EXCLUDES 1`   coronary angioplasty status with implant and graft (Z95.5)

`N` Newborn: 0   `P` Pediatric: 0-17   `M` Maternity: 9-64   `A` Adult: 15-124   `MCC` Major Complication/Comorbidity   `CC` Complication/Comorbidity   `SW` Severe Wound Dx

1266   ICD-10-CM 2022

Z98.62 Peripheral vascular angioplasty status `UPD`
> *EXCLUDES 1*   *peripheral vascular angioplasty status with implant and graft (Z95.820)*

✓5ᵗʰ **Z98.8 Other specified postprocedural states**

✓6ᵗʰ **Z98.81 Dental procedure status**

Z98.810 Dental sealant status `UPD`

Z98.811 Dental restoration status `UPD`
Dental crown status
Dental fillings status

Z98.818 Other dental procedure status `UPD`

Z98.82 Breast implant status `UPD`
> *EXCLUDES 1*   *breast implant removal status (Z98.86)*

Z98.83 Filtering (vitreous) bleb after glaucoma surgery status `UPD`
> *EXCLUDES 1*   *inflammation (infection) of postprocedural bleb (H59.4-)*

AHA: 2020,3Q,29

Z98.84 Bariatric surgery status `UPD`
Gastric banding status
Gastric bypass status for obesity
Obesity surgery status
> *EXCLUDES 1*   *bariatric surgery status complicating pregnancy, childbirth, or the puerperium (O99.84)*
> *EXCLUDES 2*   *intestinal bypass and anastomosis status (Z98.0)*

AHA: 2020,1Q,12

Z98.85 Transplanted organ removal status `UPD`
Transplanted organ previously removed due to complication, failure, rejection or infection
> *EXCLUDES 1*   *encounter for removal of transplanted organ - code to complication of transplanted organ (T86.-)*

Z98.86 Personal history of breast implant removal `UPD`

✓6ᵗʰ **Z98.87 Personal history of in utero procedure**

Z98.870 Personal history of in utero procedure during pregnancy `UPD` ♀
> *EXCLUDES 2*   *complications from in utero procedure for current pregnancy (O35.7)*
> *supervision of current pregnancy with history of in utero procedure during previous pregnancy (O09.82-)*

Z98.871 Personal history of in utero procedure while a fetus `UPD`

✓6ᵗʰ **Z98.89 Other specified postprocedural states**

Z98.890 Other specified postprocedural states `UPD`
Personal history of surgery, not elsewhere classified

Z98.891 History of uterine scar from previous surgery `UPD` ♀
> *EXCLUDES 1*   *maternal care due to uterine scar from previous surgery (O34.2-)*

AHA: 2016,4Q,51-52,76

✓4ᵗʰ **Z99 Dependence on enabling machines and devices, not elsewhere classified**
> *EXCLUDES 1*   ~~*cardiac pacemaker status (Z95.0)*~~

AHA: 2020,1Q,11

Z99.0 Dependence on aspirator `UPD`

✓5ᵗʰ **Z99.1 Dependence on respirator**
Dependence on ventilator

Z99.11 Dependence on respirator [ventilator] status `CC` `HCC`
AHA: 2015,1Q,21

Z99.12 Encounter for respirator [ventilator] dependence during power failure `CC` `HCC`
> *EXCLUDES 1*   *mechanical complication of respirator [ventilator] (J95.850)*

Z99.2 Dependence on renal dialysis `UPD` `HCC`
Hemodialysis status
Peritoneal dialysis status
Presence of arteriovenous shunt for dialysis
Renal dialysis status NOS
> *EXCLUDES 1*   *encounter for fitting and adjustment of dialysis catheter (Z49.0-)*
> *EXCLUDES 2*   *noncompliance with renal dialysis (Z91.15)*

AHA: 2016,1Q,12; 2013,4Q,125

Z99.3 Dependence on wheelchair `UPD`
Wheelchair confinement status
Code first cause of dependence, such as:
muscular dystrophy (G71.0-)
obesity (E66.-)

✓5ᵗʰ **Z99.8 Dependence on other enabling machines and devices**

Z99.81 Dependence on supplemental oxygen `UPD`
Dependence on long-term oxygen
AHA: 2013,4Q,129

Z99.89 Dependence on other enabling machines and devices `UPD`
Dependence on machine or device NOS
AHA: 2020,1Q,11

Chapter 22. Codes for Special Purposes (U00–U85)

Chapter-specific Guidelines

U07.0   Vaping-related disorder (see Section I.C.10.e., Vaping-related disorders)

U07.1   COVID-19 (see Section I.C.1.g.1., COVID-19 infection)

U09.9   **Post COVID-19 condition, unspecified (see Section I.C.1.g.1.m)**

Chapter 22. Codes for Special Purposes (U00-U85)

This chapter contains the following blocks:

U00-U49   Provisional assignment of new diseases of uncertain etiology or emergency use

Provisional assignment of new diseases of uncertain etiology or emergency use (U00-U49)

☑4ᵗʰ **U07   Emergency use of U07**

U07.0   Vaping-related disorder

Dabbing related lung damage

Dabbing related lung injury

E-cigarette, or vaping, product use associated lung injury [EVALI]

Electronic cigarette related lung damage

Electronic cigarette related lung injury

Use additional code, to identify manifestations, such as:

    abdominal pain (R10.84)

    acute respiratory distress syndrome (J80)

    diarrhea (R19.7)

    drug-induced interstitial lung disorder (J70.4)

    lipoid pneumonia (J69.1)

    weight loss (R63.4)

DEF: Respiratory illness or injury caused by harmful aerosolized substances and chemicals produced by electronic cigarettes, vapes, e-pipes, and other battery-powered vaping devices. Symptoms may include shortness of breath and fever, while some patients experience severe, sometimes fatal, lung damage.

Synonym(s): *e-cigarette and vaping product use-associated lung injury, EVALI.*

U07.1   COVID-19   HIV   MCC

Use additional code to identify pneumonia or other manifestations, such as:

    pneumonia due to COVID-19 (J12.82)

EXCLUDES 2   *coronavirus as the cause of diseases classified elsewhere (B97.2-)*

            coronavirus infection, unspecified (B34.2)

            pneumonia due to SARS-associated coronavirus (J12.81)

AHA: 2021,1Q,25-30,31-49; 2020,4Q,14,99; 2020,3Q,9-16; 2020,2Q,3-13

DEF: First diagnosed in December 2019 in China, coronavirus disease 2019 (COVID-19) is a respiratory infection caused by a newly identified (novel) virus not previously seen in humans, known as severe acute respiratory syndrome coronavirus 2 (SARS-CoV-2). Symptoms of this lower respiratory illness include fever, dry cough, and tiredness that may progress to include difficulty breathing. Older patients and those with high blood pressure, heart problems, and diabetes are more likely to develop serious symptoms of the illness. **Synonym(s):** *SARS-CoV-2, coronavirus disease 2019.*

TIP: Only a confirmed diagnosis of COVID-19, either through a positive test result documented in the medical record or documentation by the provider, can be coded to U07.1.

TIP: Assign for asymptomatic individuals who test positive for COVID-19. Even though asymptomatic, the individual is considered to have the COVID-19 infection due to the positive test result.

TIP: Assign appropriate codes for presenting signs/symptoms associated with COVID-19 (cough, fever, shortness of breath), instead of U07.1, if a definitive diagnosis has not been established.

● ☑4ᵗʰ **U09   Post COVID-19 condition**

●   **U09.9   Post COVID-19 condition, unspecified**

    NOTE   This code enables establishment of a link with COVID-19.

           This code is not to be used in cases that are still presenting with active COVID-19. However, an exception is made in cases of re-infection with COVID-19, occurring with a condition related to prior COVID-19.

           Post-acute sequela of COVID-19

Code first the specific condition related to COVID-19 if known, such as:

    chronic respiratory failure (J96.1-)

    loss of smell (R43.8)

    loss of taste (R43.8)

    multisystem inflammatory syndrome (M35.81)

    pulmonary embolism (I26.-)

    pulmonary fibrosis (J84.10)

Ⓝ Newborn: 0   Ⓟ Pediatric: 0-17   Ⓜ Maternity: 9-64   Ⓐ Adult: 15-124   MCC Major Complication/Comorbidity   CC Complication/Comorbidity   SW Severe Wound Dx

1270   ICD-10-CM 2022

Illustrations

Chapter 3. Diseases of the Blood and Blood-forming Organs and Certain Disorders Involving the Immune Mechanism (D50–D89)

Red Blood Cells

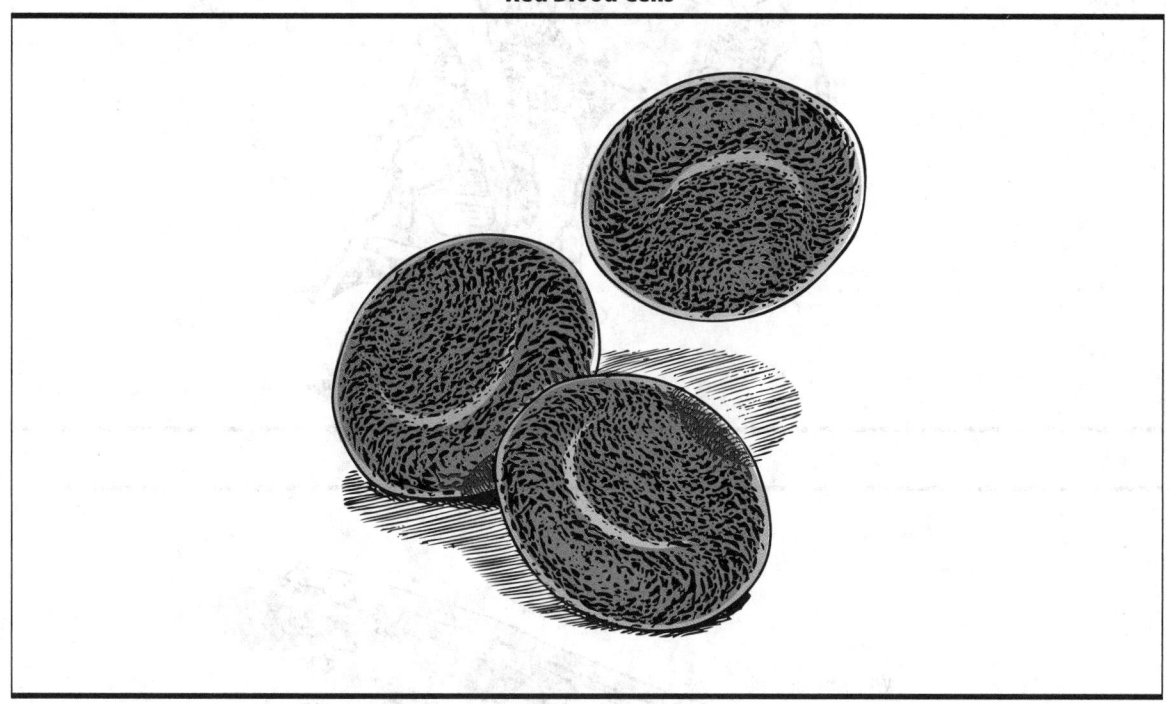

White Blood Cell

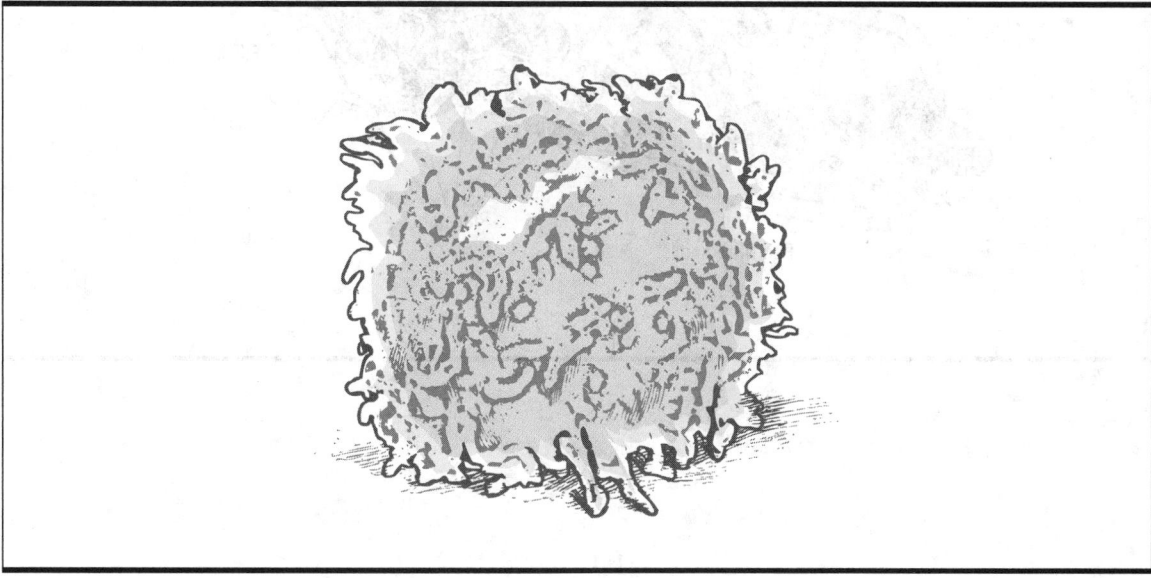

Platelet

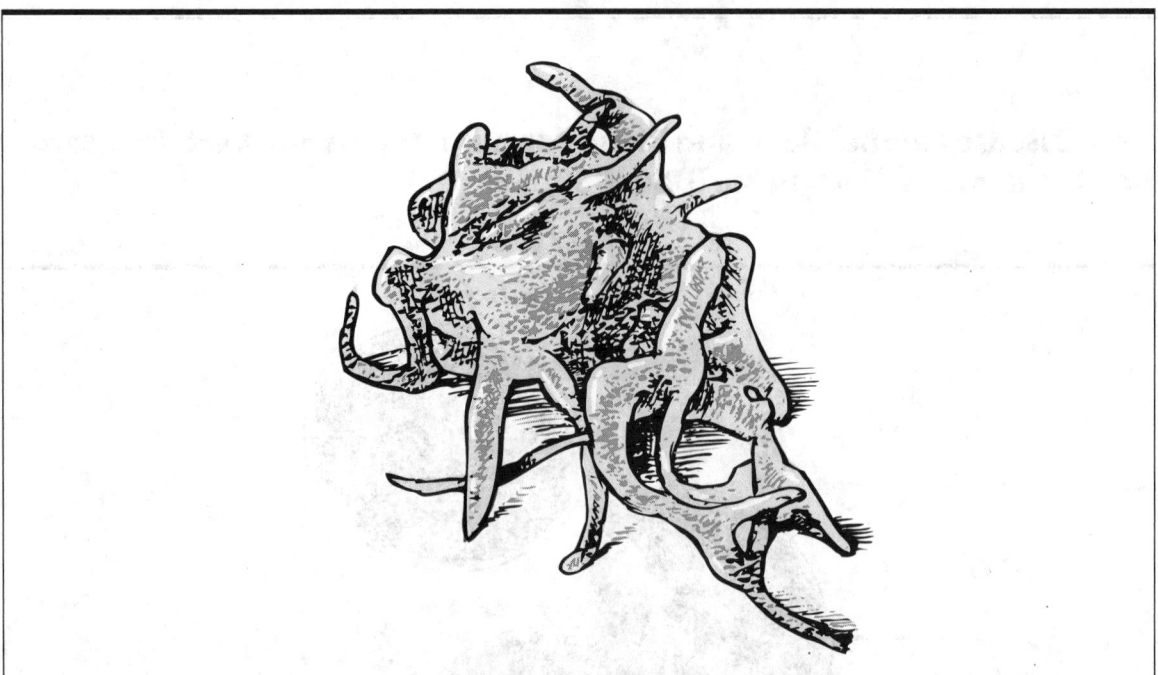

Coagulation

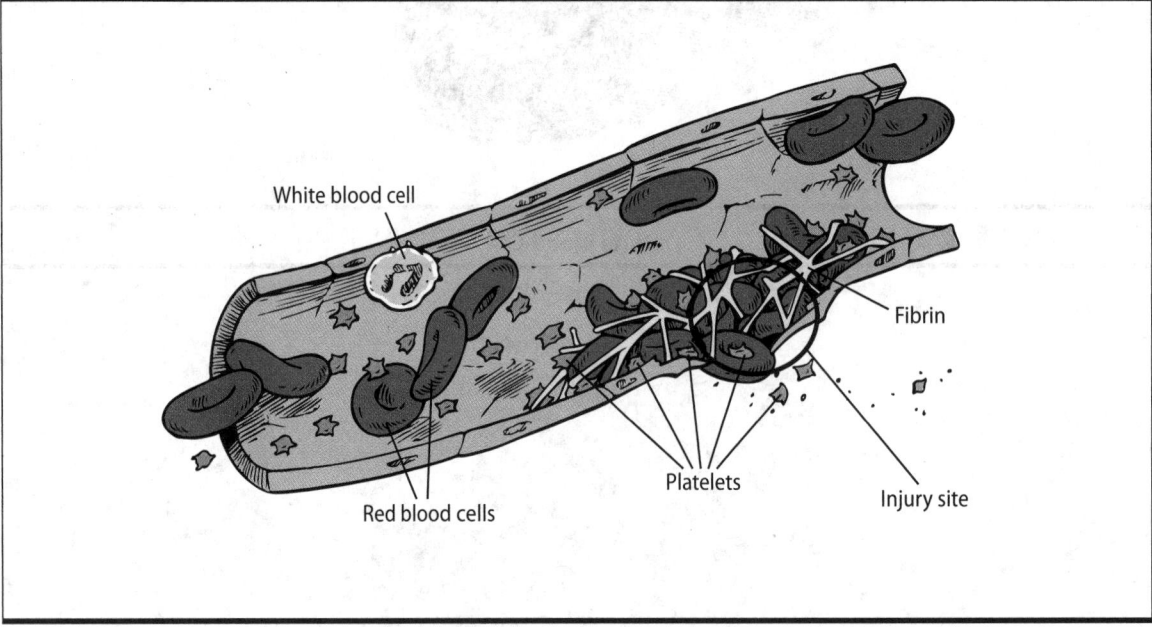

Spleen Anatomical Location and External Structures

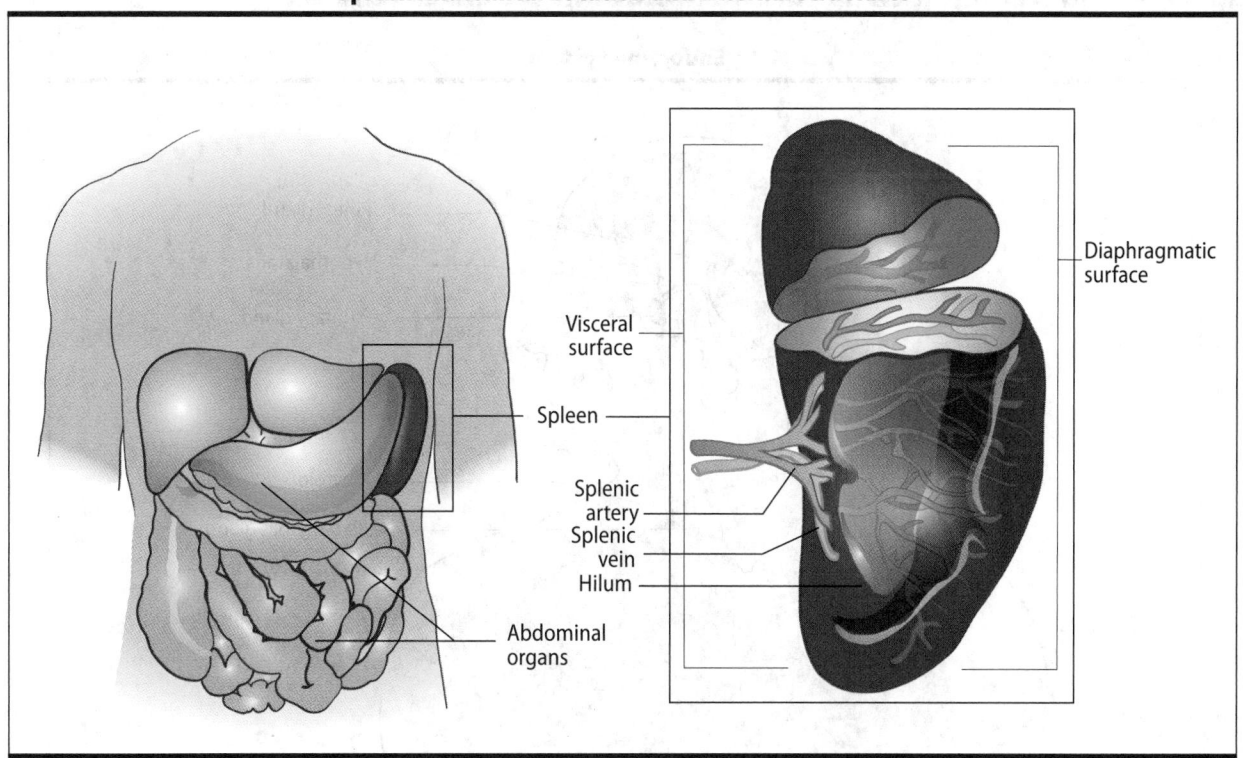

Visceral surface

Spleen

Splenic artery

Splenic vein

Hilum

Abdominal organs

Diaphragmatic surface

Spleen Interior Structures

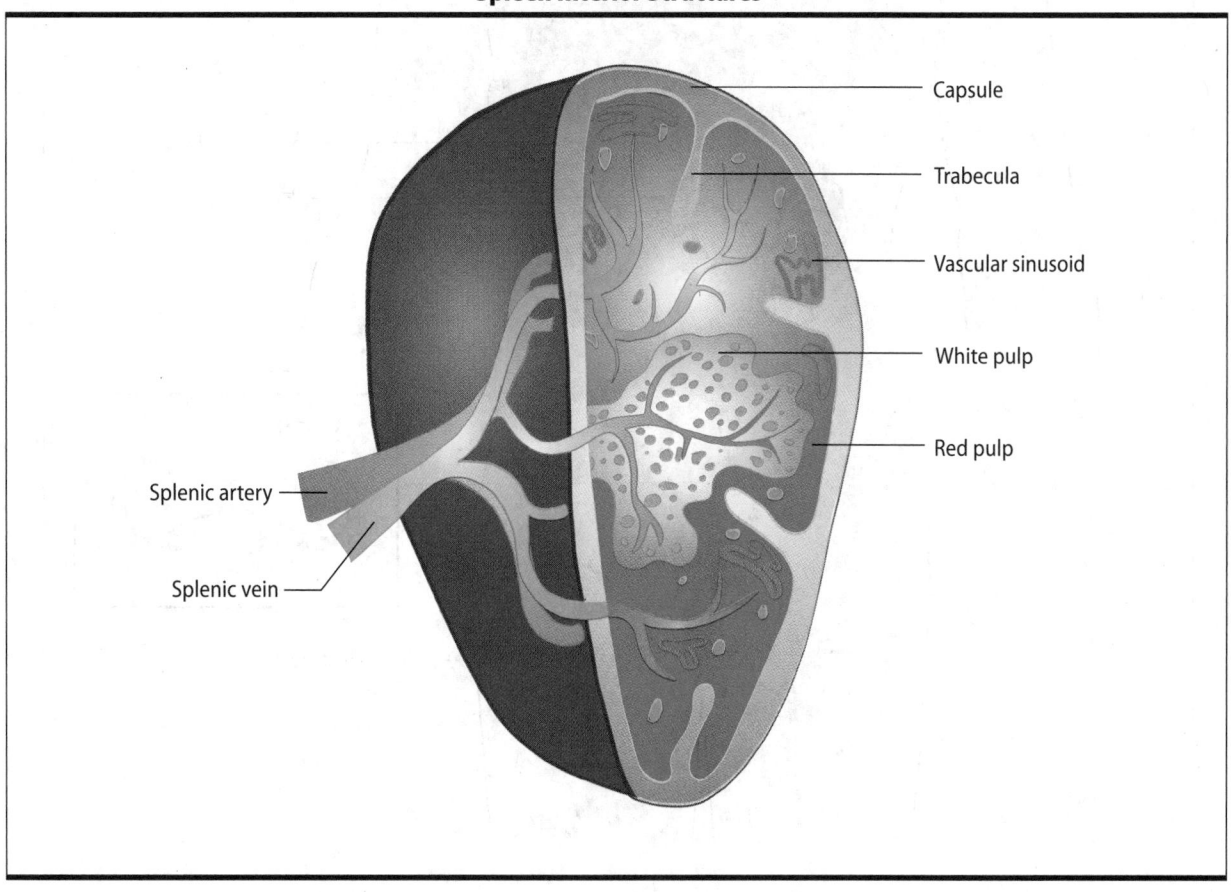

Capsule

Trabecula

Vascular sinusoid

White pulp

Red pulp

Splenic artery

Splenic vein

Chapter 4. Endocrine, Nutritional and Metabolic Diseases (E00–E89)

Endocrine System

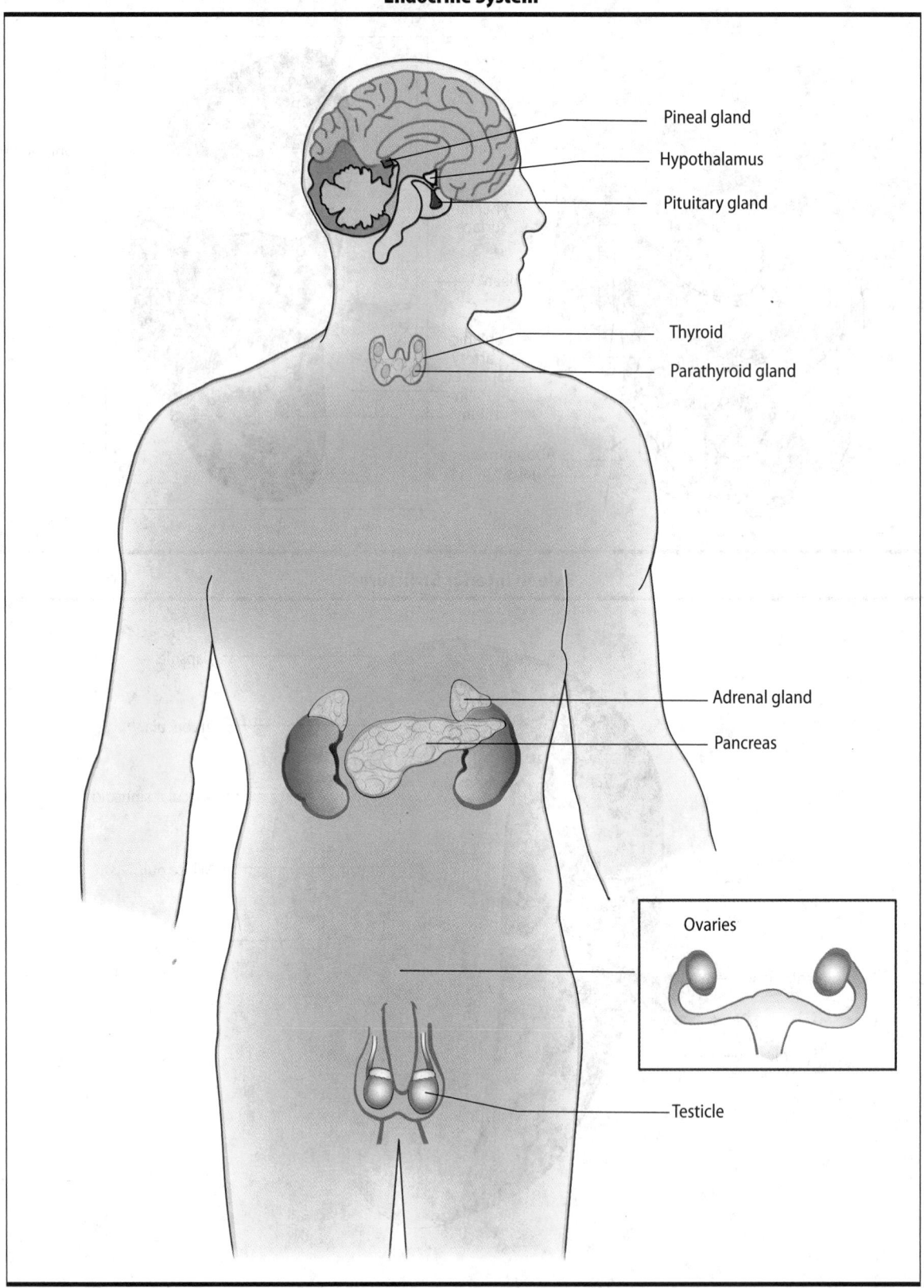

Thyroid

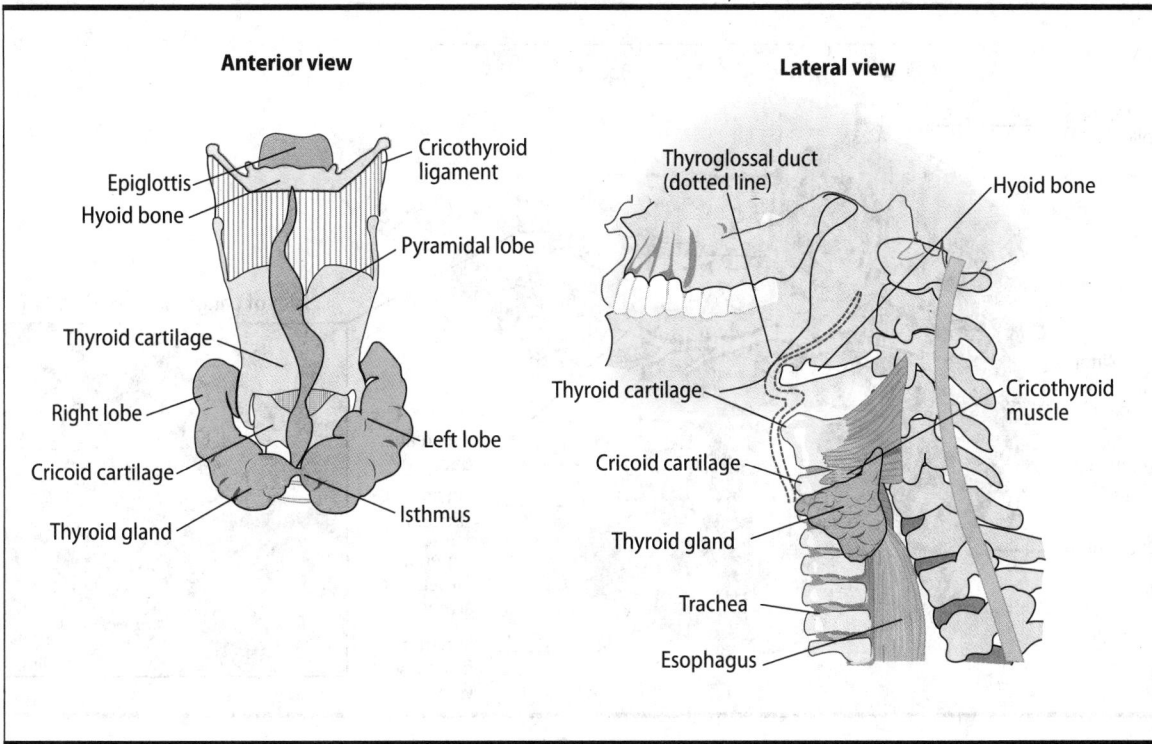

Anterior view

Epiglottis
Hyoid bone
Thyroid cartilage
Right lobe
Cricoid cartilage
Thyroid gland

Cricothyroid ligament
Pyramidal lobe
Left lobe
Isthmus

Lateral view

Thyroglossal duct (dotted line)
Hyoid bone
Thyroid cartilage
Cricothyroid muscle
Cricoid cartilage
Thyroid gland
Trachea
Esophagus

Thyroid and Parathyroid Glands

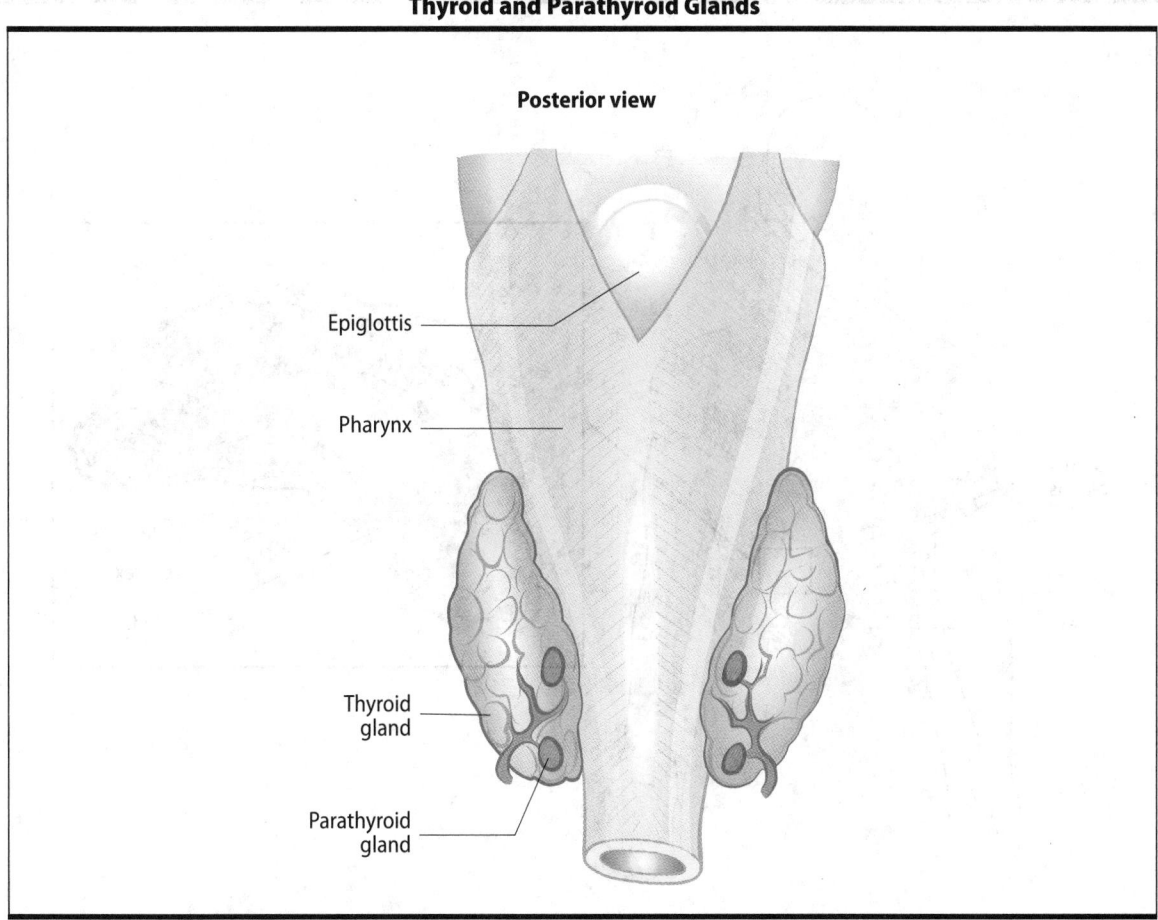

Posterior view

Epiglottis
Pharynx
Thyroid gland
Parathyroid gland

Pancreas

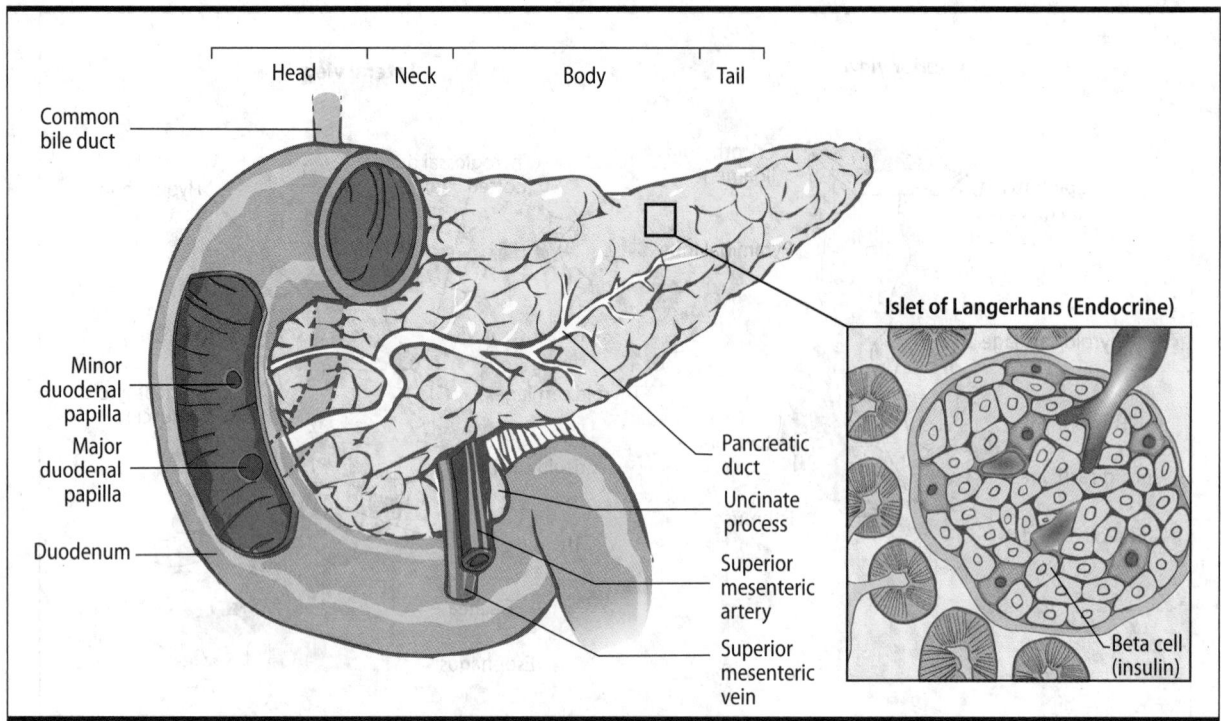

Islet of Langerhans (Endocrine)

Anatomy of the Adrenal Gland

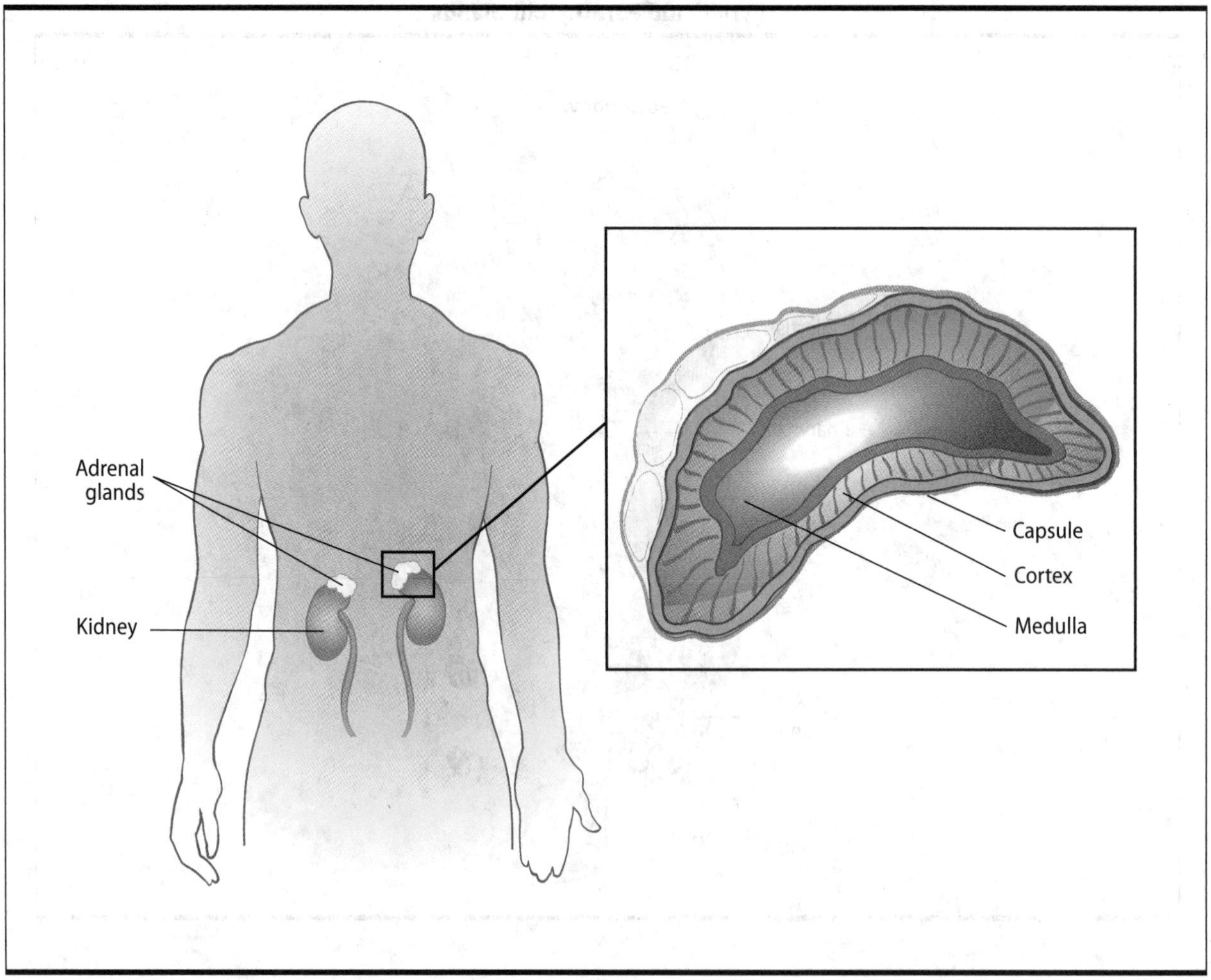

Structure of an Ovary

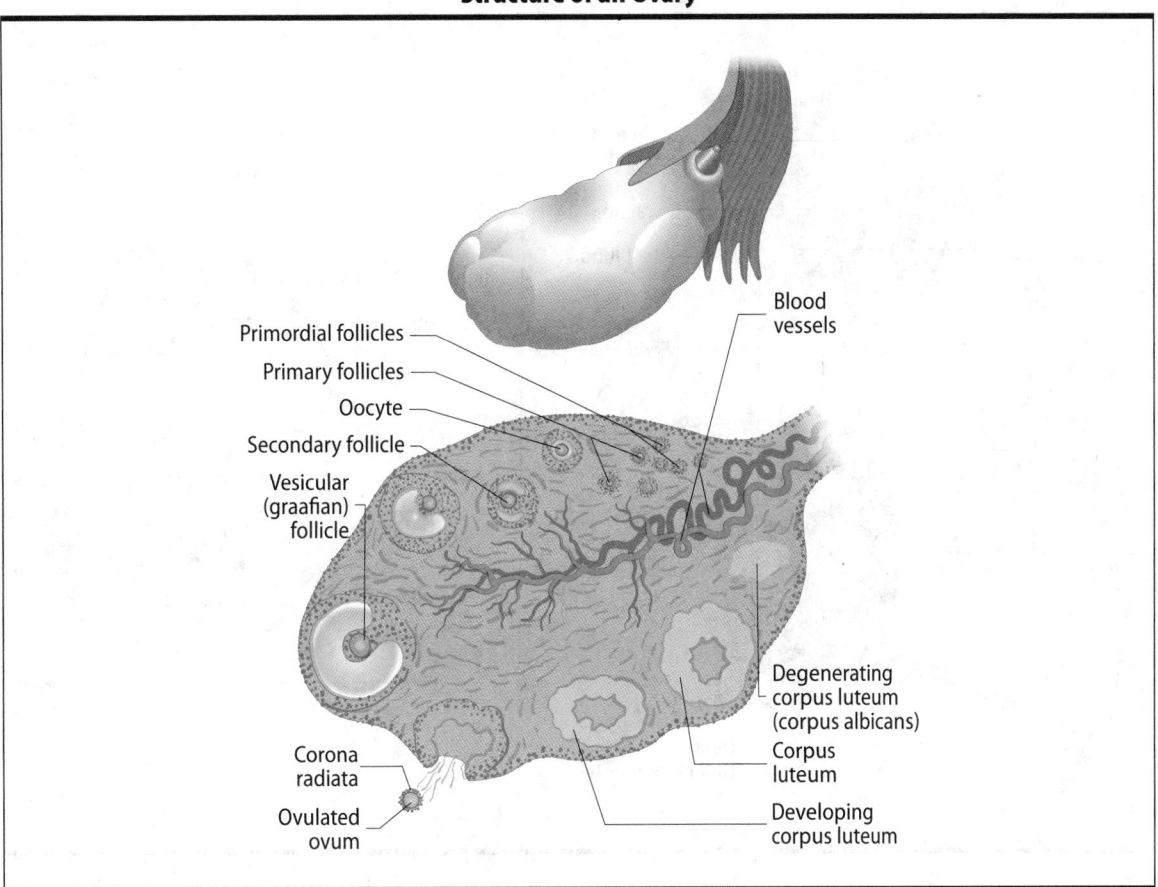

Testis and Associated Structures

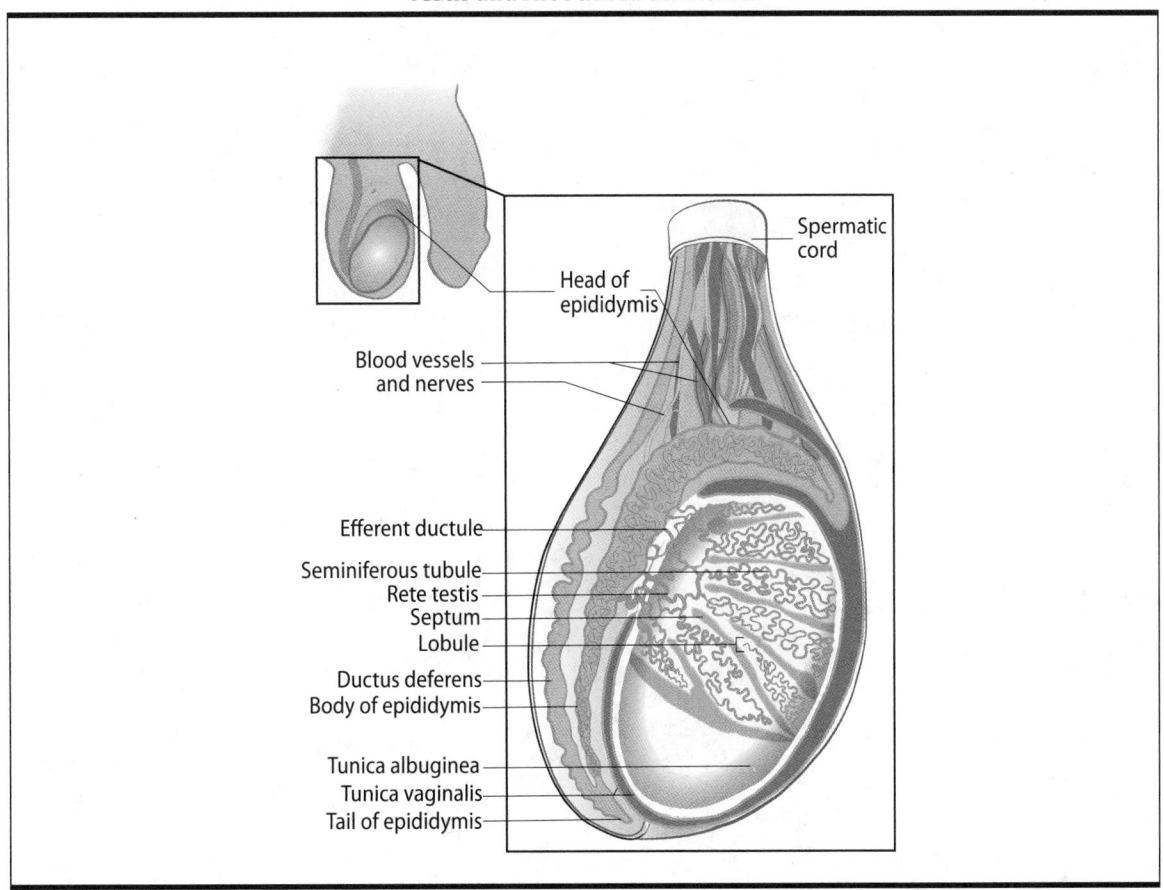

Thymus

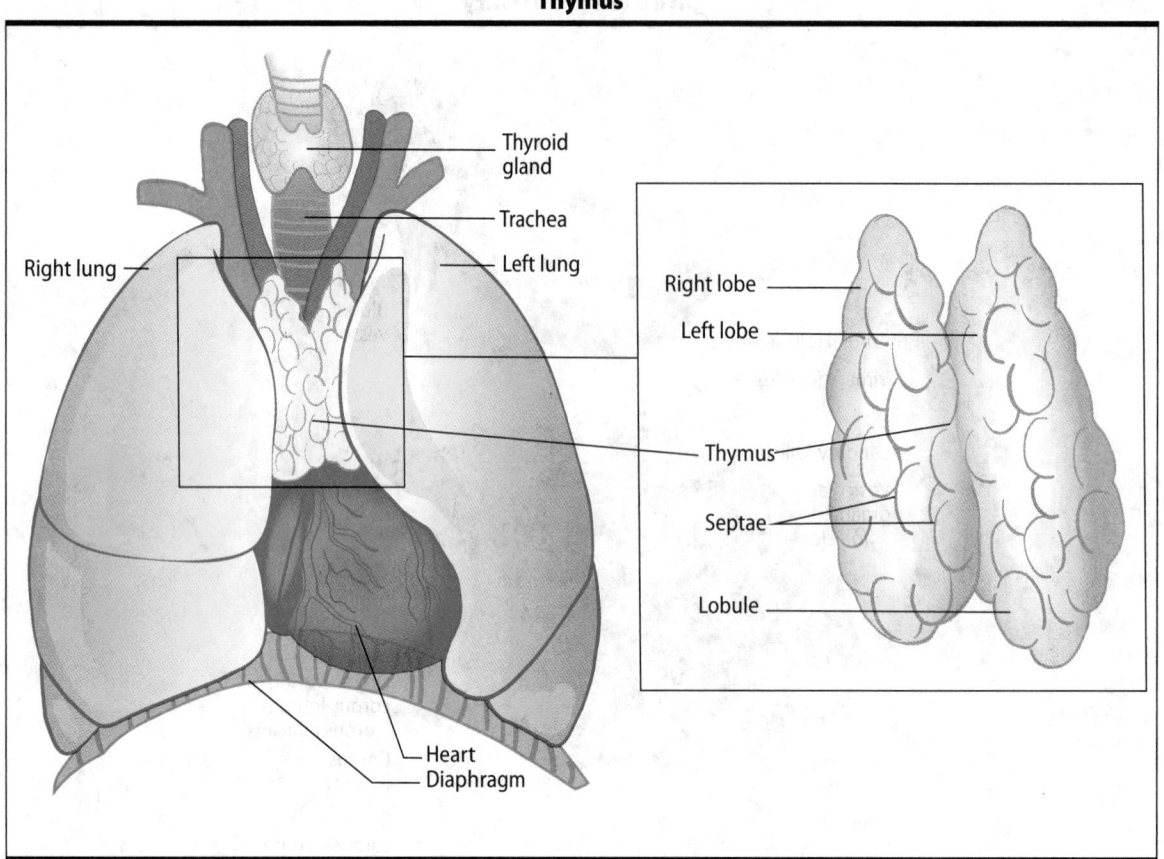

Chapter 6. Diseases of the Nervous System (GØØ–G99)

Brain

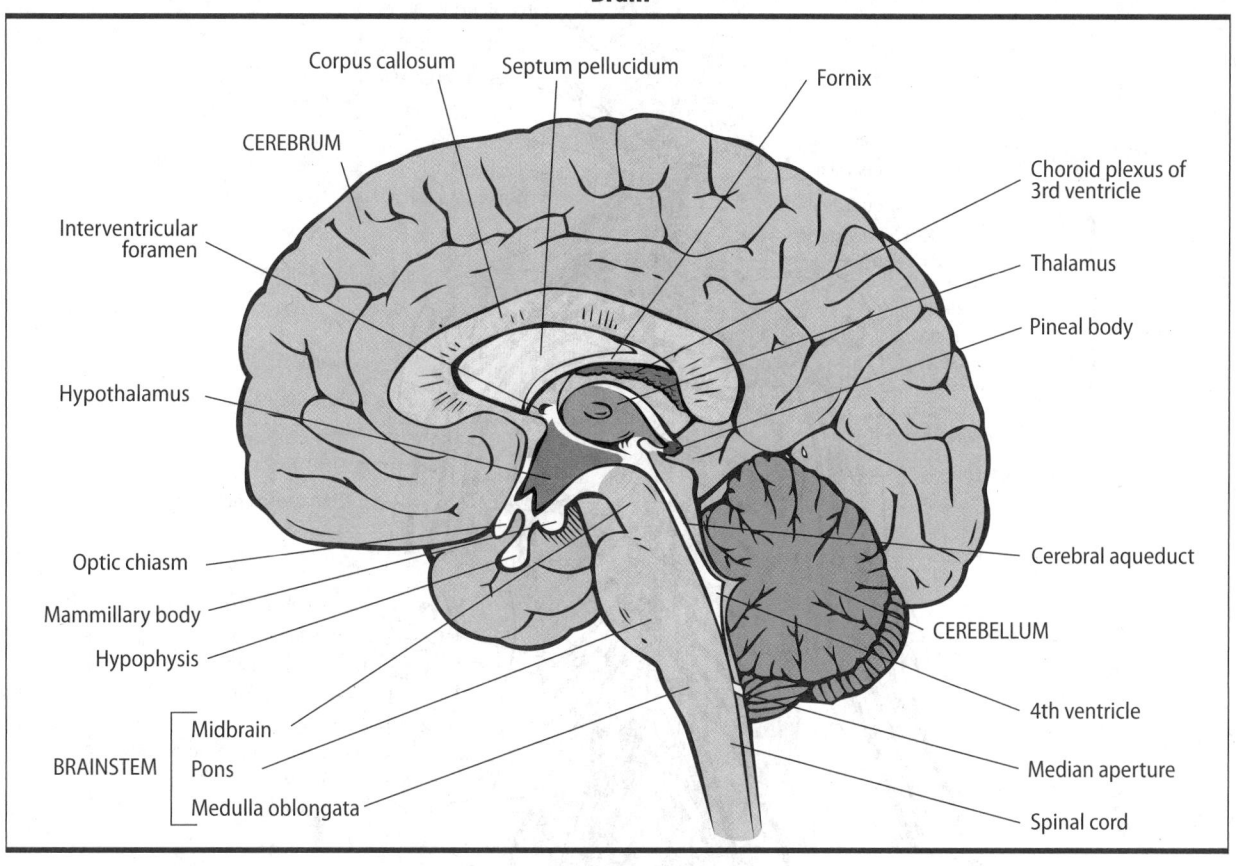

Cranial Nerves

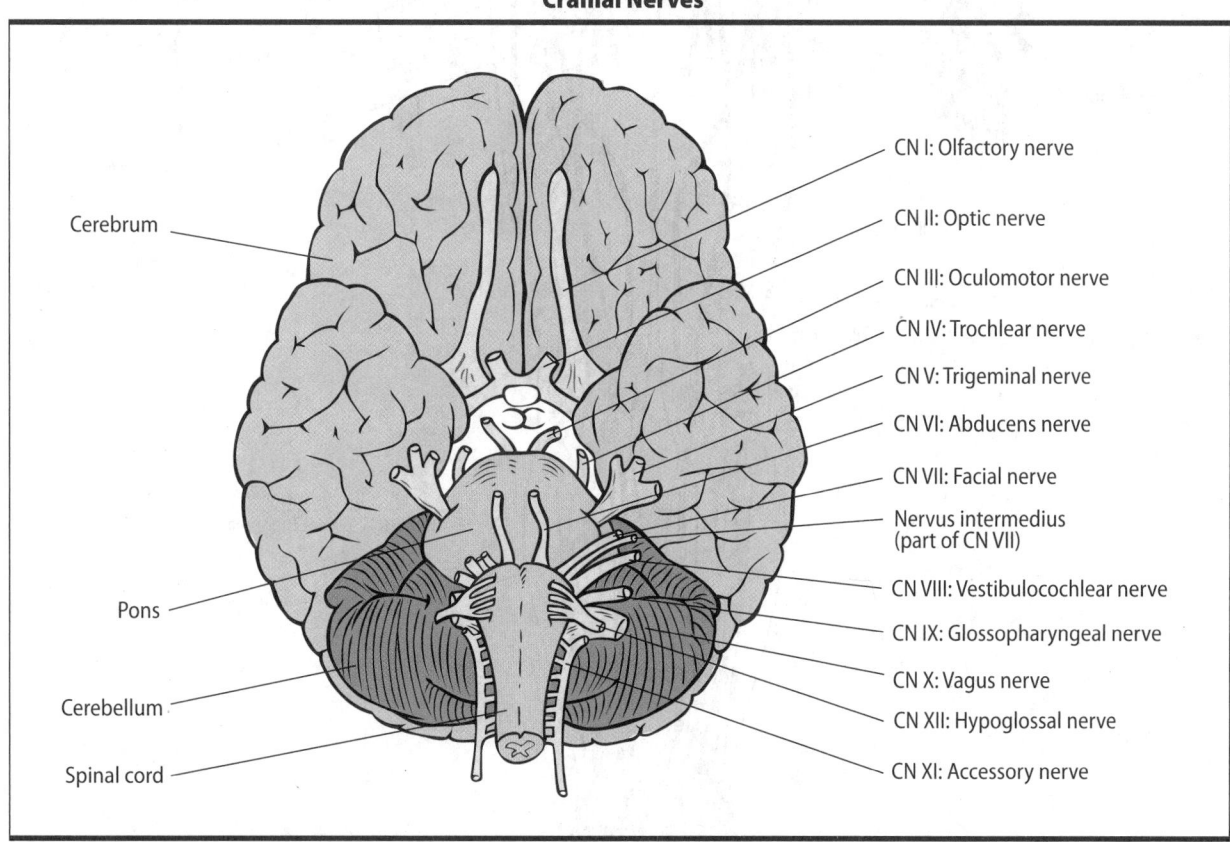

Peripheral Nervous System

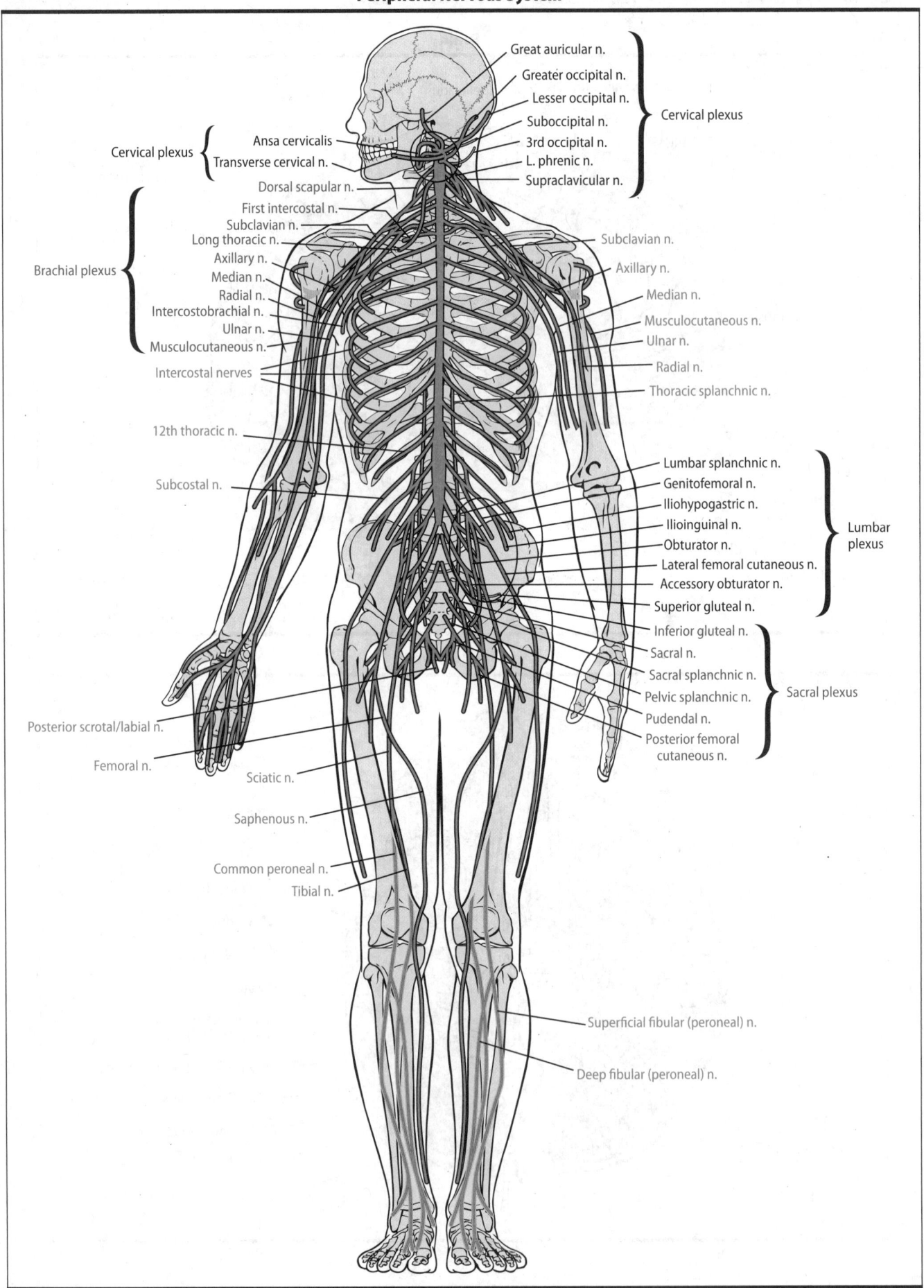

Cervical plexus

Ansa cervicalis
Transverse cervical n.
Dorsal scapular n.
First intercostal n.
Subclavian n.
Long thoracic n.
Axillary n.
Median n.
Radial n.
Intercostobrachial n.
Ulnar n.
Musculocutaneous n.

Brachial plexus

Intercostal nerves

12th thoracic n.

Subcostal n.

Posterior scrotal/labial n.

Femoral n.

Sciatic n.

Saphenous n.

Common peroneal n.

Tibial n.

Great auricular n.
Greater occipital n.
Lesser occipital n.
Suboccipital n.
3rd occipital n.
L. phrenic n.
Supraclavicular n.

Cervical plexus

Subclavian n.
Axillary n.
Median n.
Musculocutaneous n.
Ulnar n.
Radial n.
Thoracic splanchnic n.

Lumbar splanchnic n.
Genitofemoral n.
Iliohypogastric n.
Ilioinguinal n.
Obturator n.
Lateral femoral cutaneous n.
Accessory obturator n.
Superior gluteal n.

Lumbar plexus

Inferior gluteal n.
Sacral n.
Sacral splanchnic n.
Pelvic splanchnic n.
Pudendal n.
Posterior femoral cutaneous n.

Sacral plexus

Superficial fibular (peroneal) n.

Deep fibular (peroneal) n.

Peripheral Nervous System

Spinal Cord and Spinal Nerves

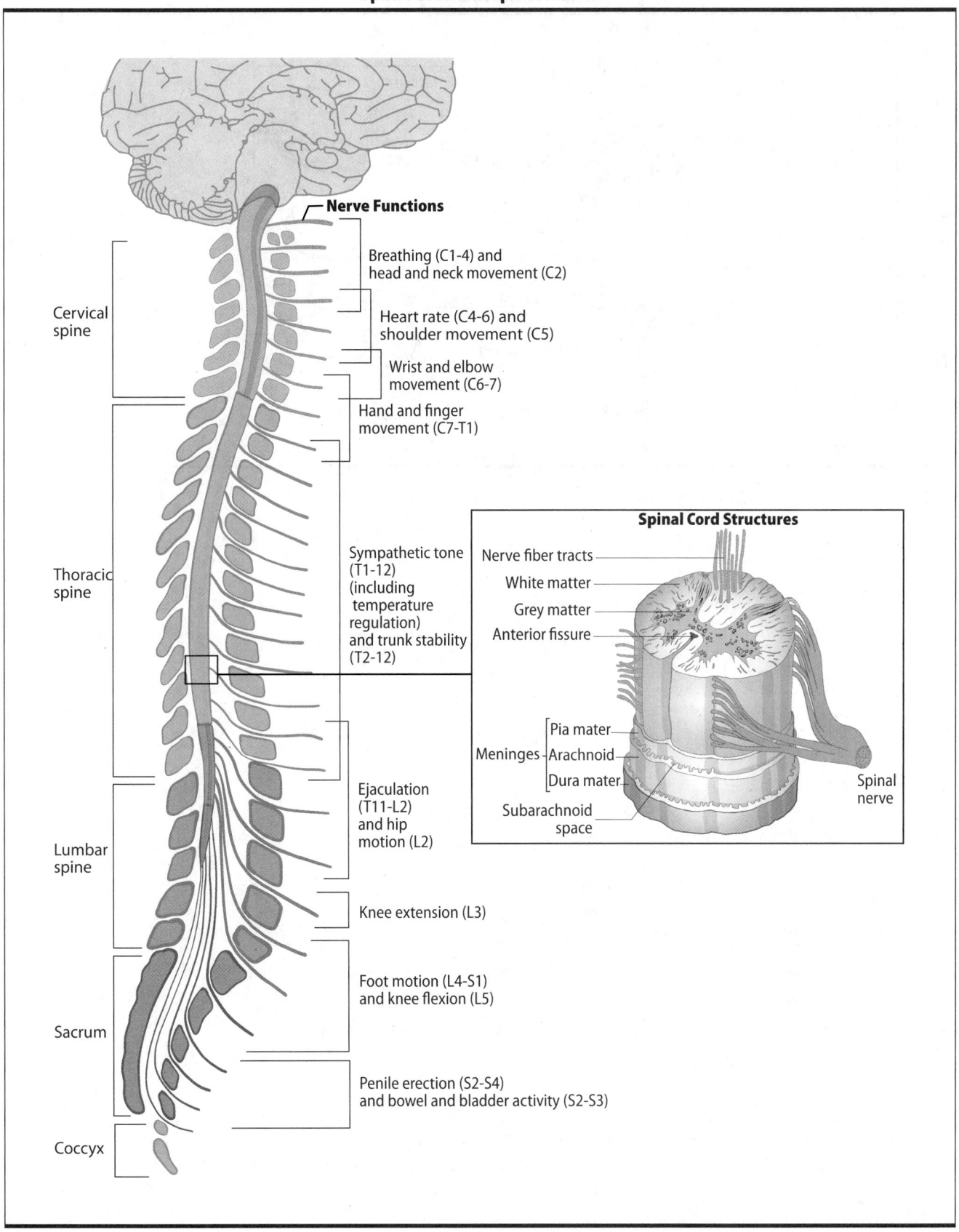

Nerve Functions

Breathing (C1-4) and head and neck movement (C2)

Heart rate (C4-6) and shoulder movement (C5)

Wrist and elbow movement (C6-7)

Hand and finger movement (C7-T1)

Sympathetic tone (T1-12) (including temperature regulation) and trunk stability (T2-12)

Ejaculation (T11-L2) and hip motion (L2)

Knee extension (L3)

Foot motion (L4-S1) and knee flexion (L5)

Penile erection (S2-S4) and bowel and bladder activity (S2-S3)

Cervical spine

Thoracic spine

Lumbar spine

Sacrum

Coccyx

Spinal Cord Structures

Nerve fiber tracts

White matter

Grey matter

Anterior fissure

Meninges — Pia mater, Arachnoid, Dura mater

Subarachnoid space

Spinal nerve

Nerve Cell

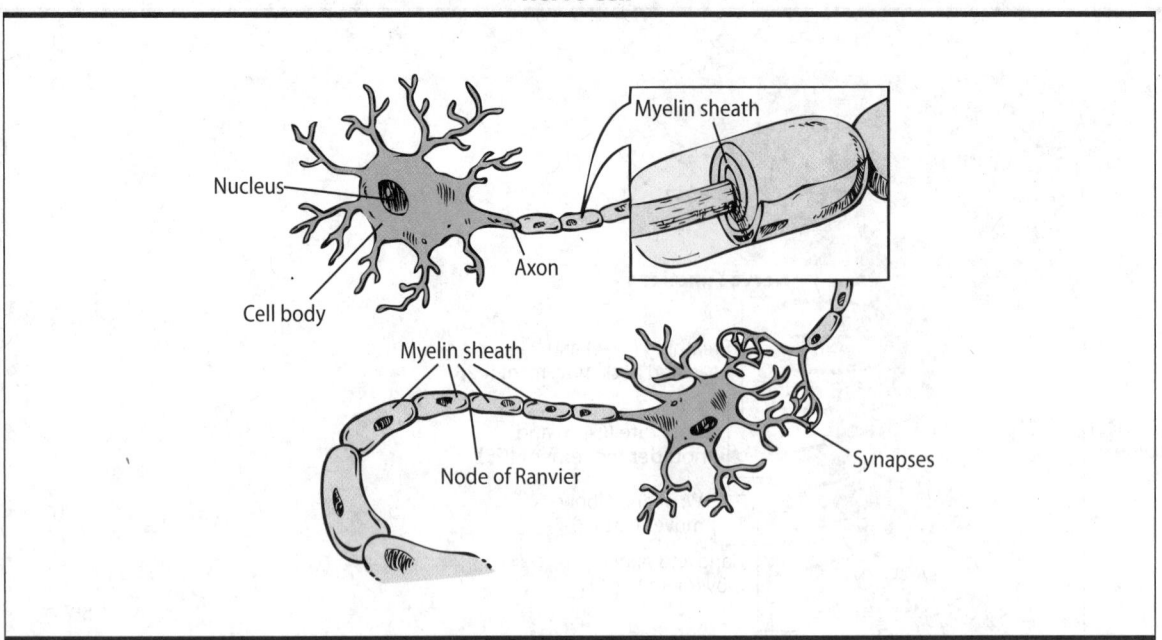

Chapter 7. Diseases of the Eye and Adnexa (H00–H59)

Eye

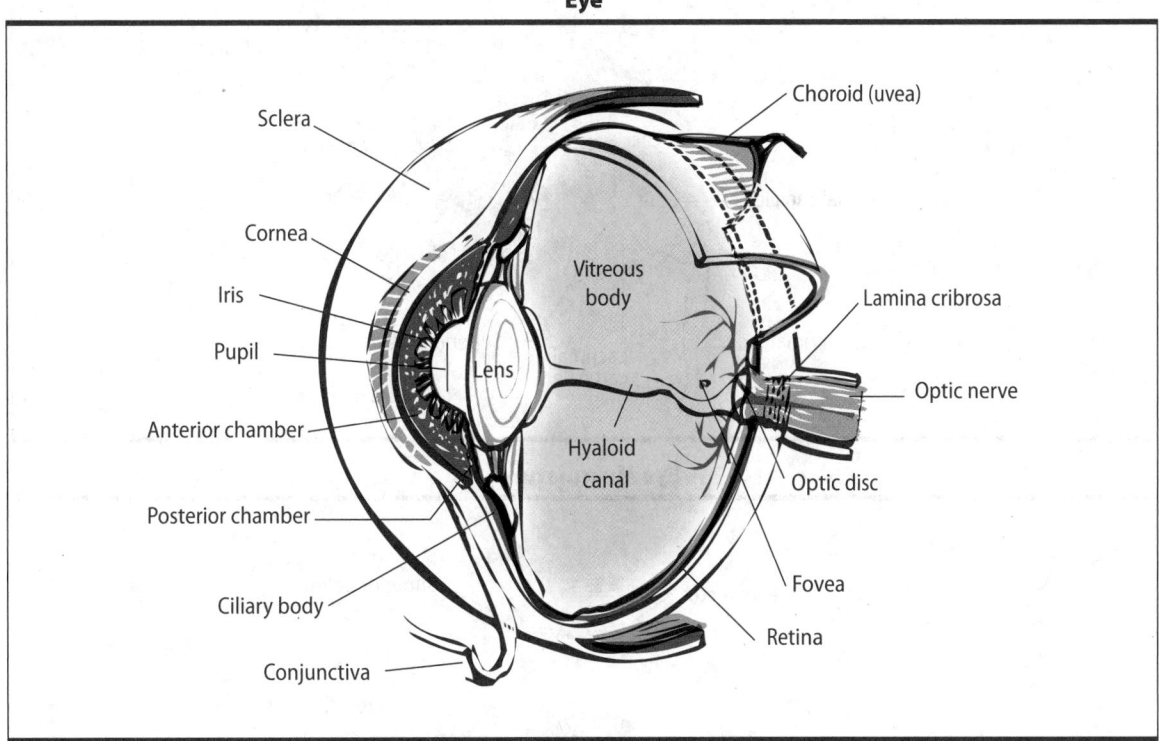

Posterior Pole of Globe/Flow of Aqueous Humor

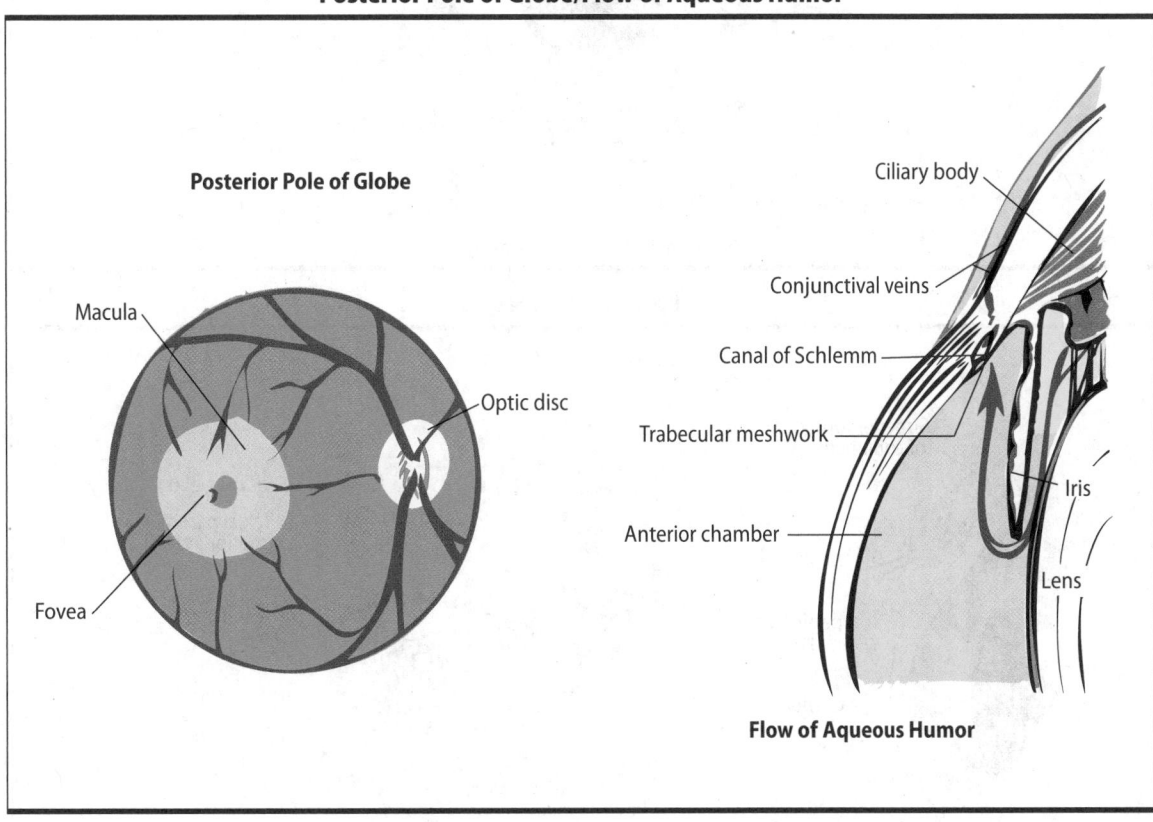

Posterior Pole of Globe

Flow of Aqueous Humor

Lacrimal System

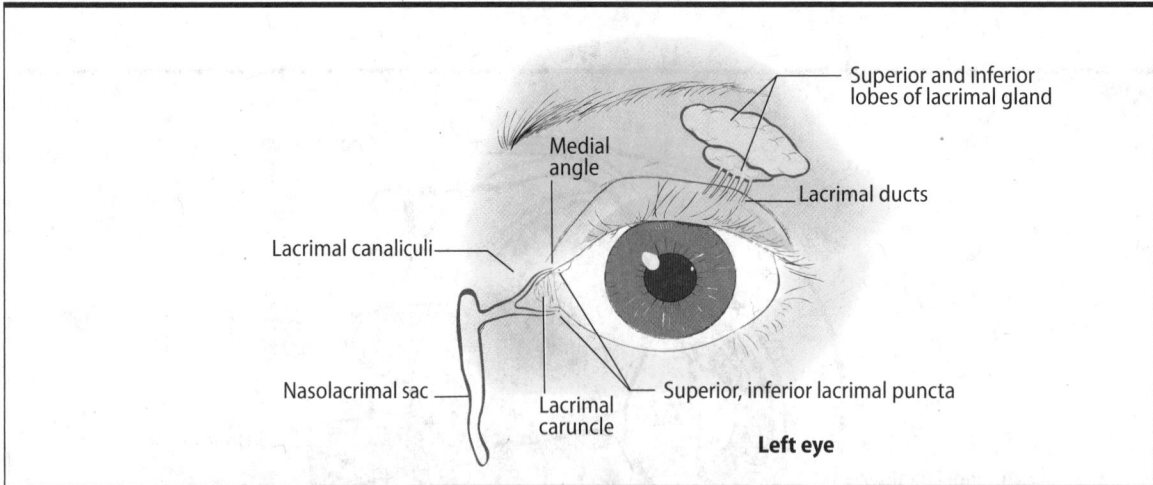

Superior and inferior lobes of lacrimal gland

Medial angle

Lacrimal ducts

Lacrimal canaliculi

Nasolacrimal sac

Lacrimal caruncle

Superior, inferior lacrimal puncta

Left eye

Eye Musculature

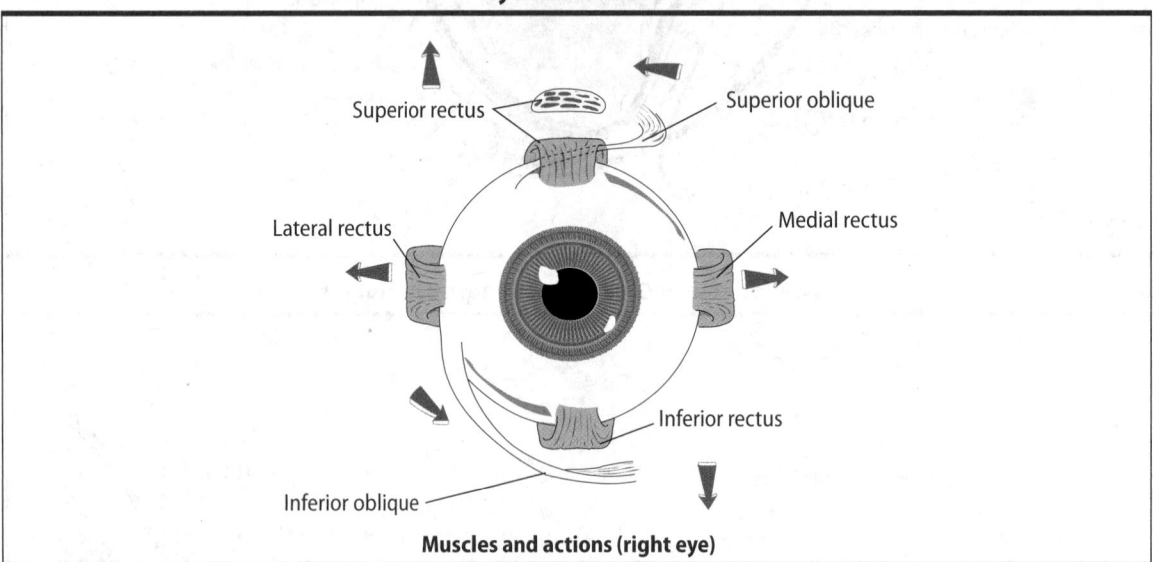

Superior rectus

Superior oblique

Lateral rectus

Medial rectus

Inferior rectus

Inferior oblique

Muscles and actions (right eye)

Eyelid Structures

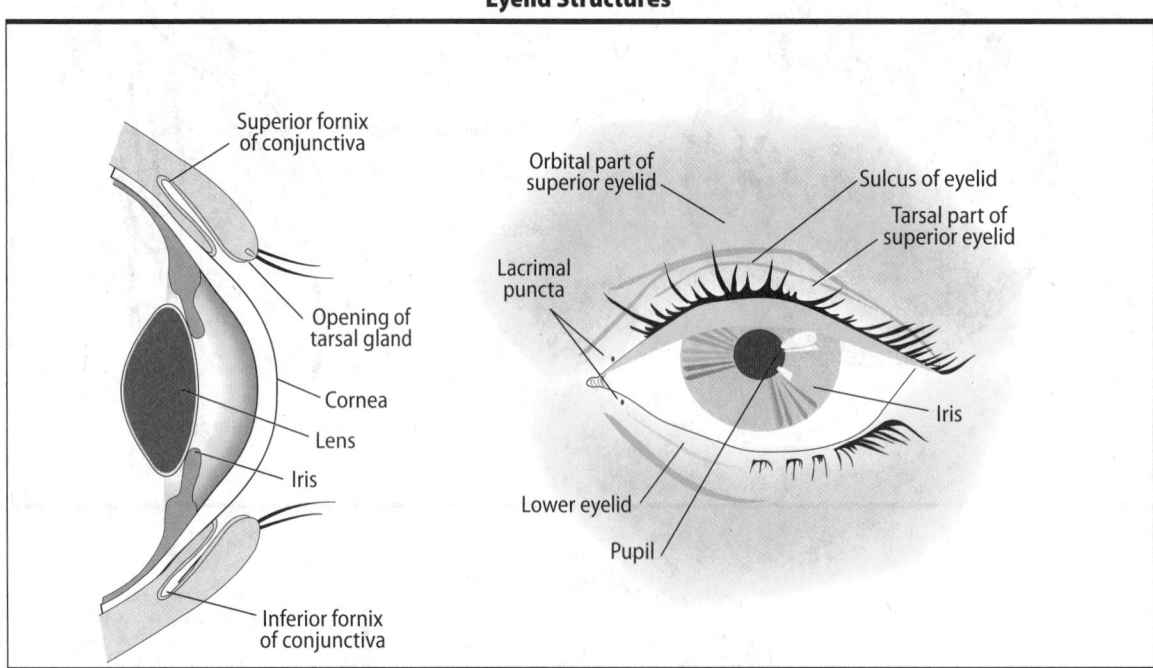

Superior fornix of conjunctiva

Opening of tarsal gland

Cornea

Lens

Iris

Inferior fornix of conjunctiva

Orbital part of superior eyelid

Sulcus of eyelid

Tarsal part of superior eyelid

Lacrimal puncta

Lower eyelid

Pupil

Iris

Chapter 8. Diseases of the Ear and Mastoid Process (H6Ø–H95)

Ear Anatomy

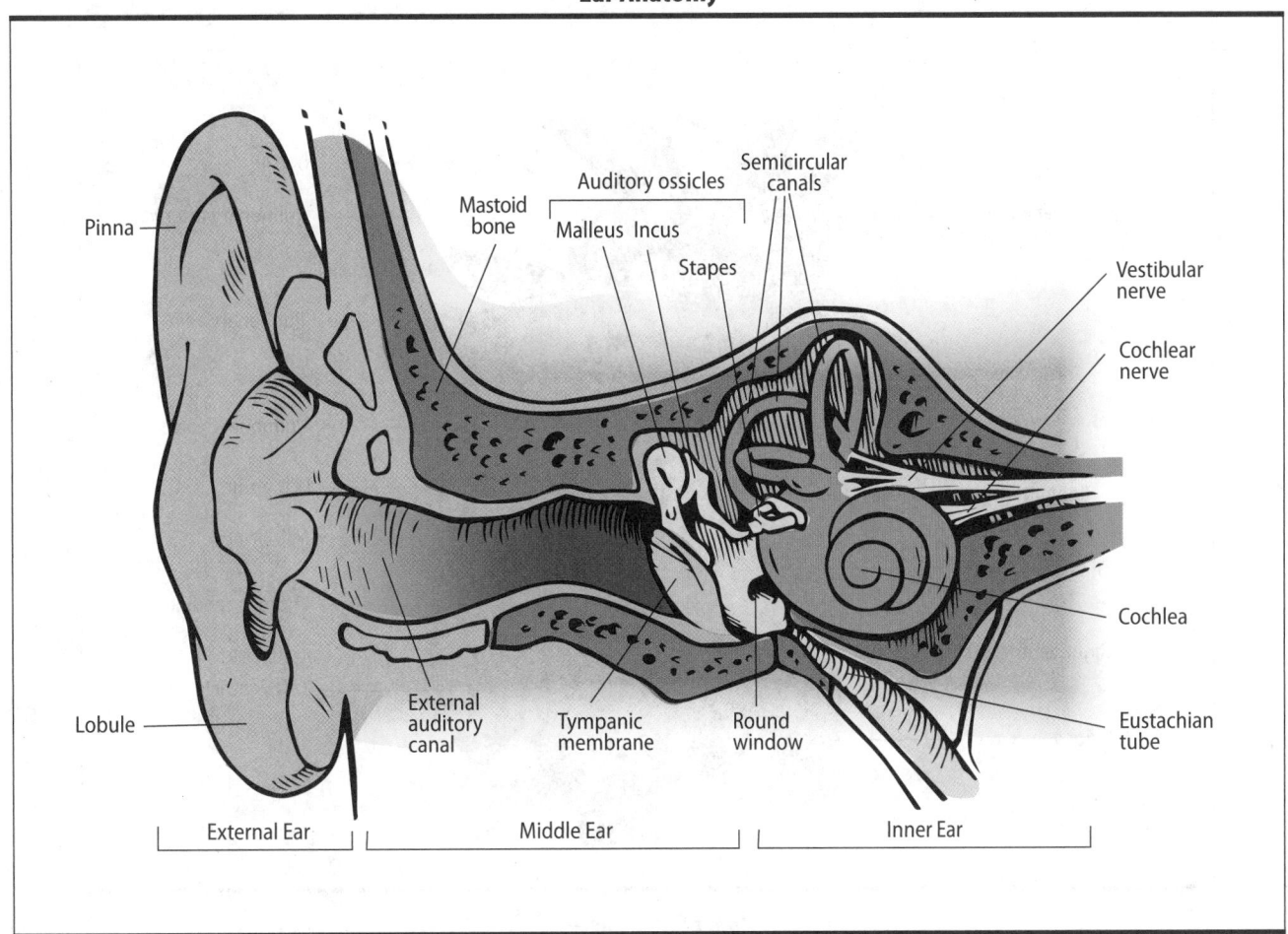

Chapter 9. Diseases of the Circulatory System (I00–I99)

Anatomy of the Heart

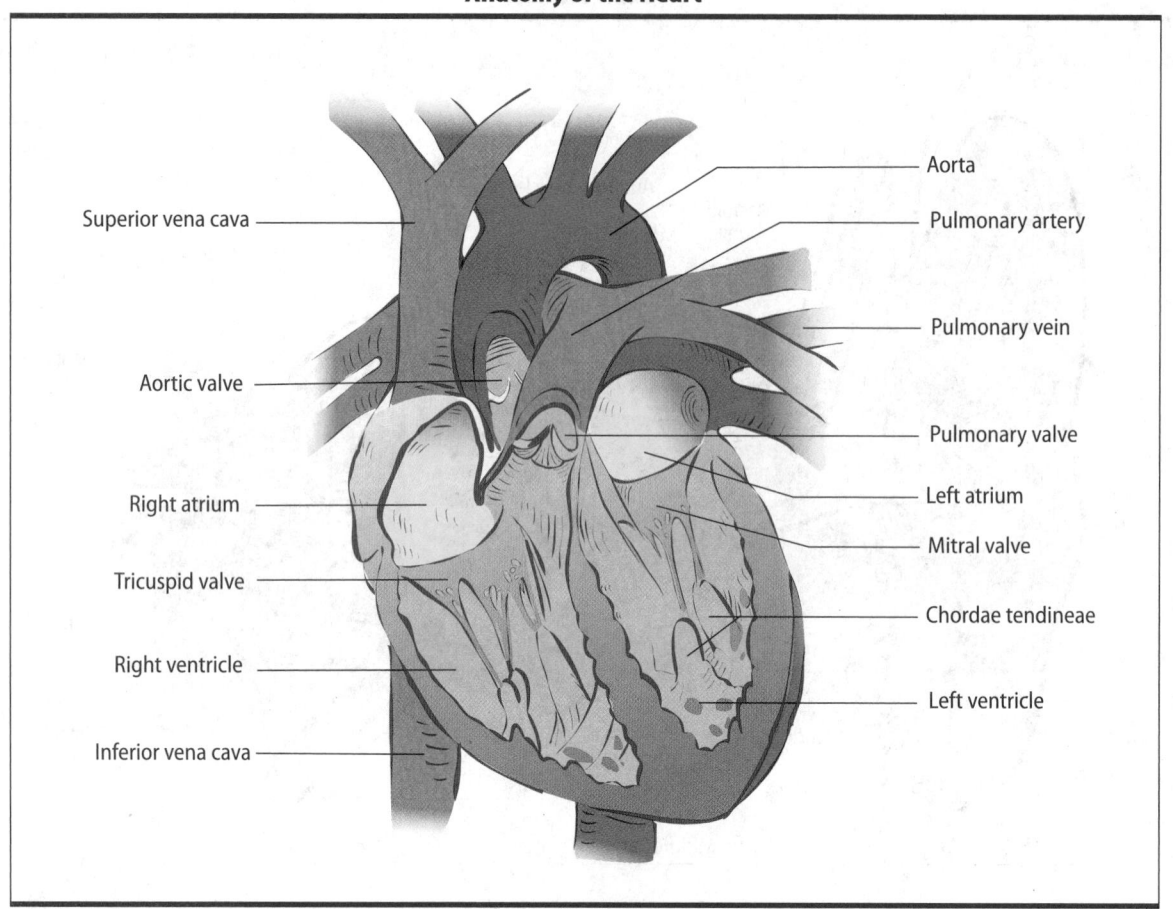

Superior vena cava

Aortic valve

Right atrium

Tricuspid valve

Right ventricle

Inferior vena cava

Aorta

Pulmonary artery

Pulmonary vein

Pulmonary valve

Left atrium

Mitral valve

Chordae tendineae

Left ventricle

Heart Cross Section

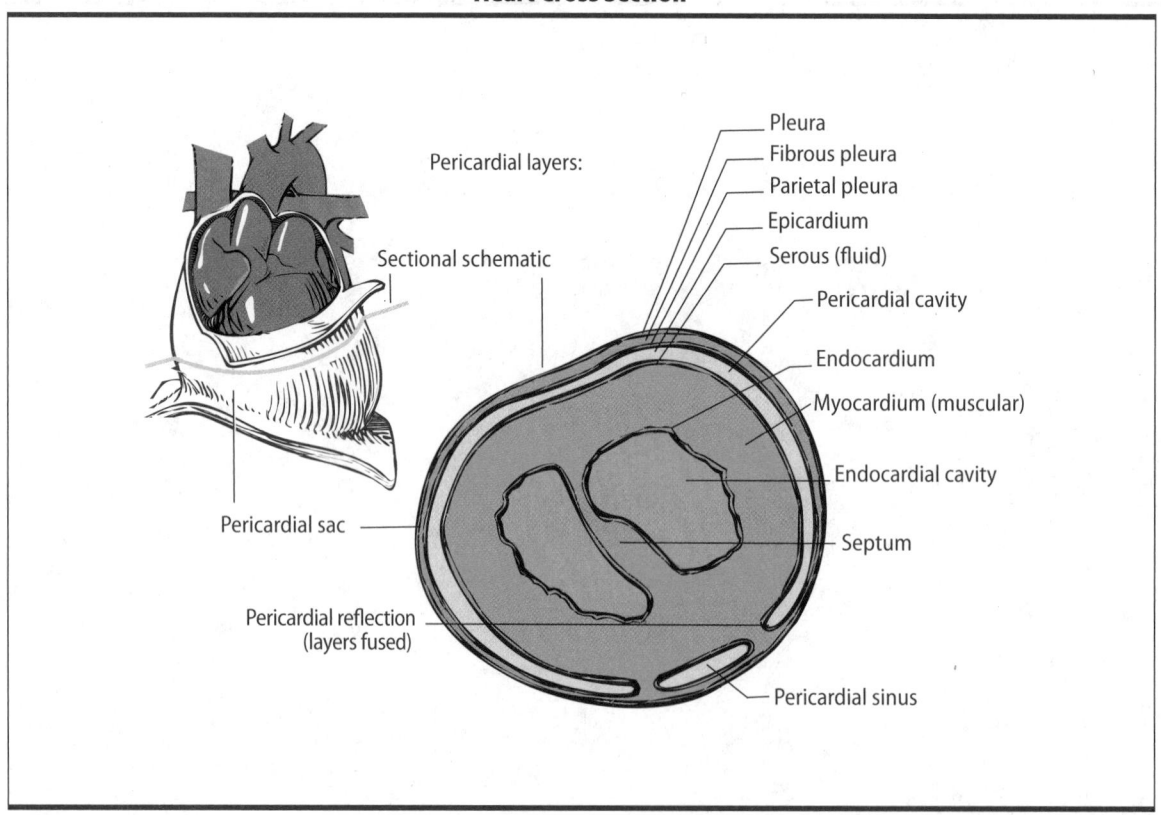

Pericardial layers:

Sectional schematic

Pericardial sac

Pericardial reflection (layers fused)

Pleura

Fibrous pleura

Parietal pleura

Epicardium

Serous (fluid)

Pericardial cavity

Endocardium

Myocardium (muscular)

Endocardial cavity

Septum

Pericardial sinus

Heart Valves

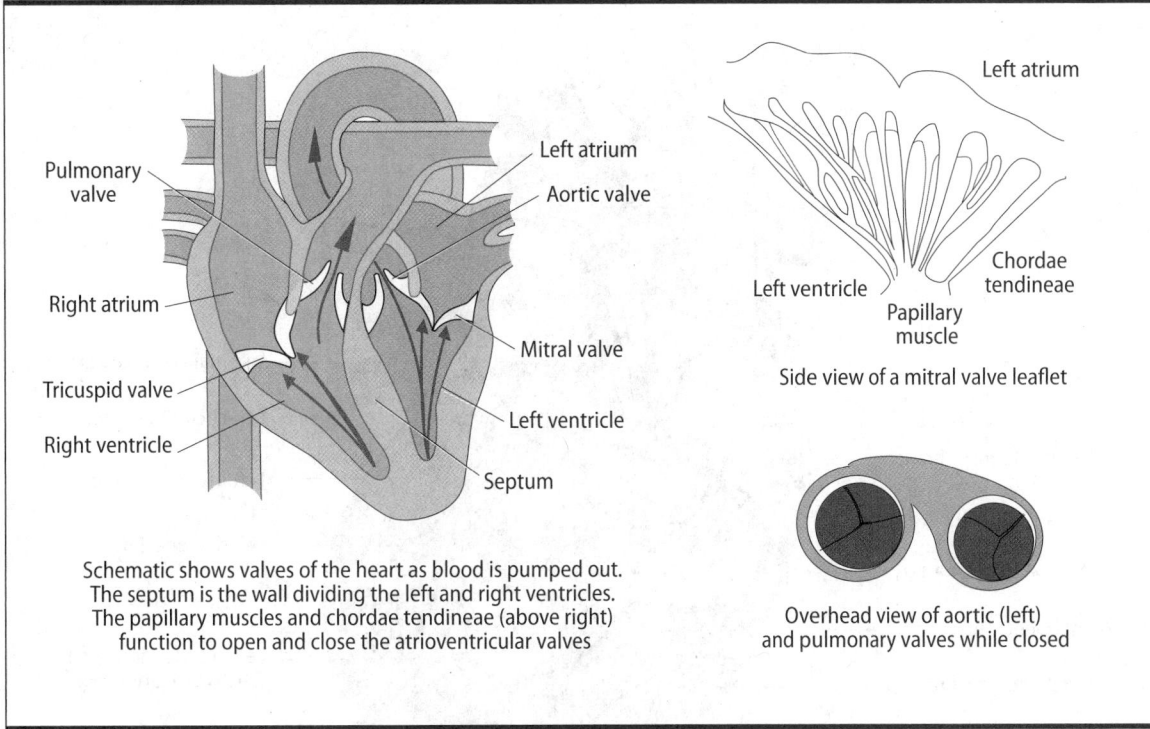

Schematic shows valves of the heart as blood is pumped out.
The septum is the wall dividing the left and right ventricles.
The papillary muscles and chordae tendineae (above right)
function to open and close the atrioventricular valves

Side view of a mitral valve leaflet

Overhead view of aortic (left)
and pulmonary valves while closed

Heart Conduction System

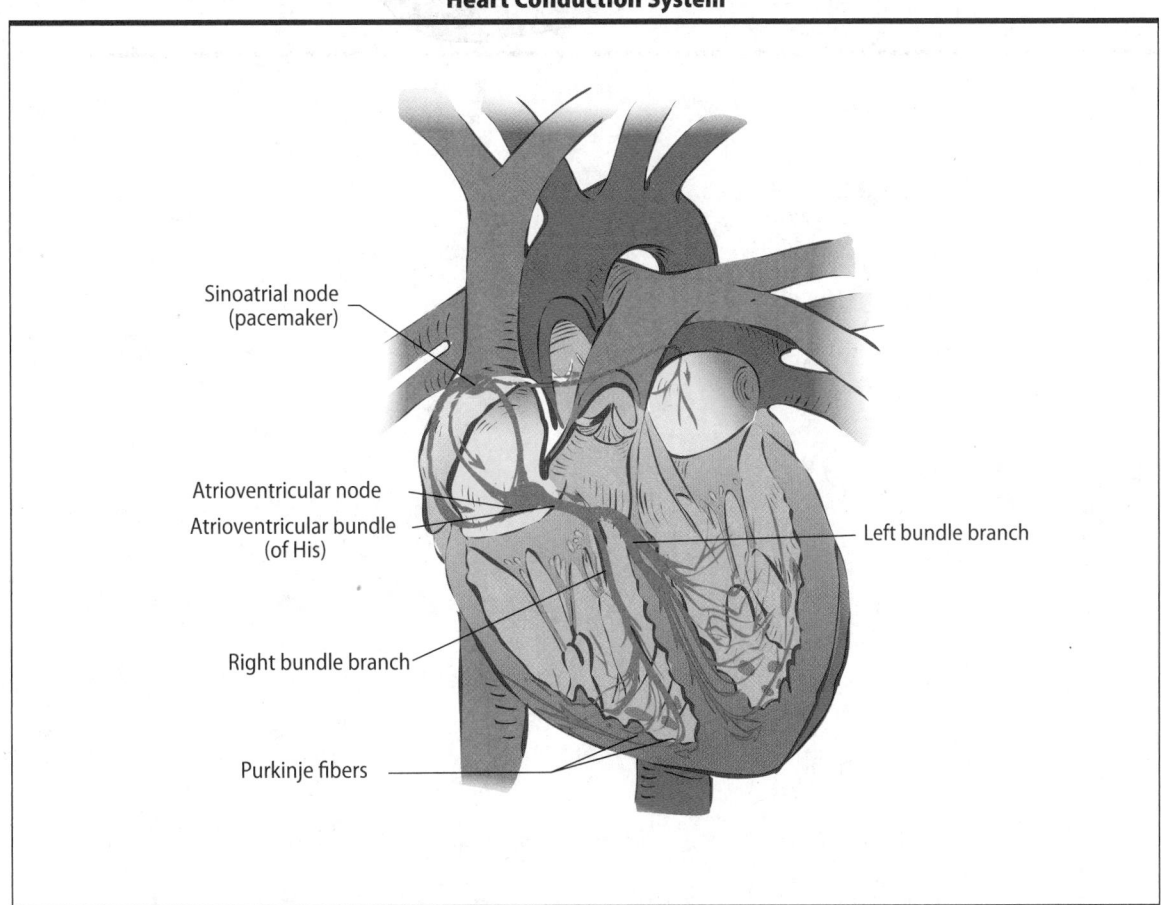

Coronary Arteries

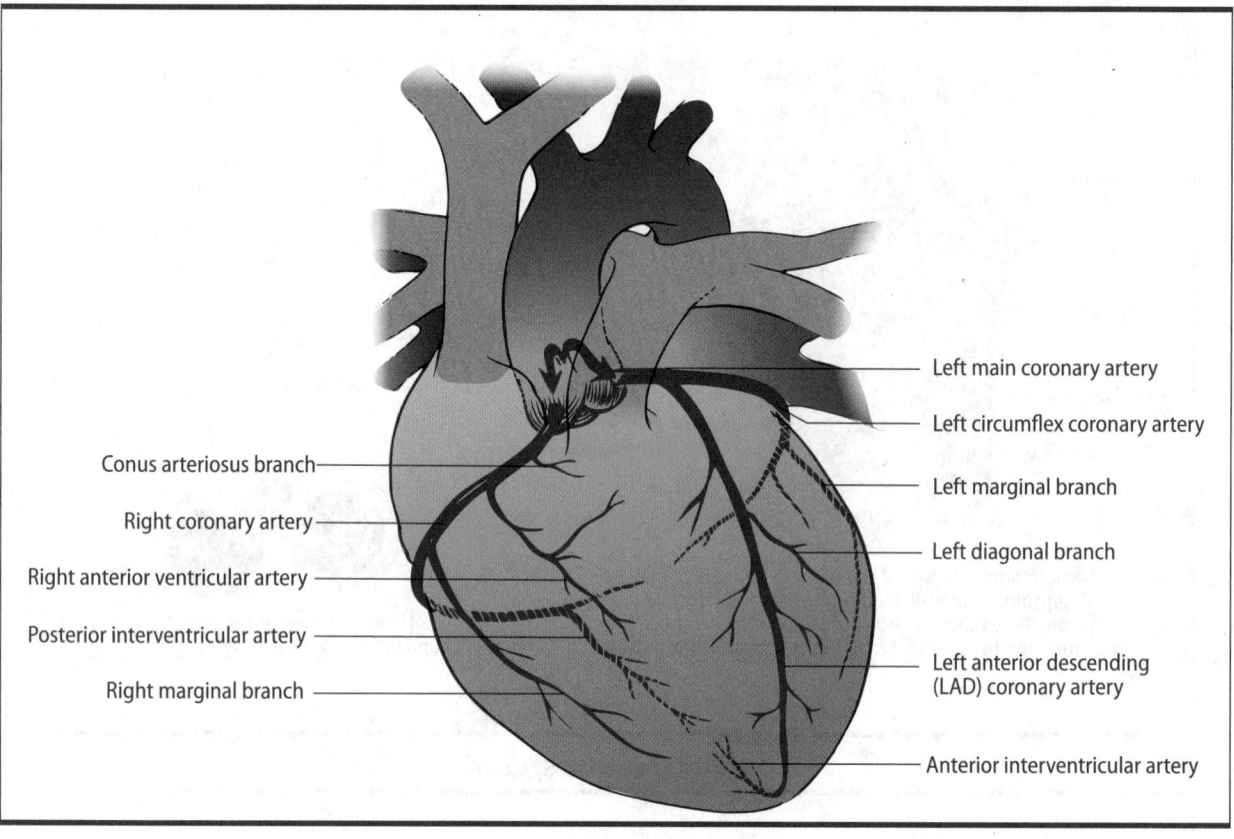

Left main coronary artery

Left circumflex coronary artery

Left marginal branch

Left diagonal branch

Left anterior descending (LAD) coronary artery

Anterior interventricular artery

Conus arteriosus branch

Right coronary artery

Right anterior ventricular artery

Posterior interventricular artery

Right marginal branch

Arteries

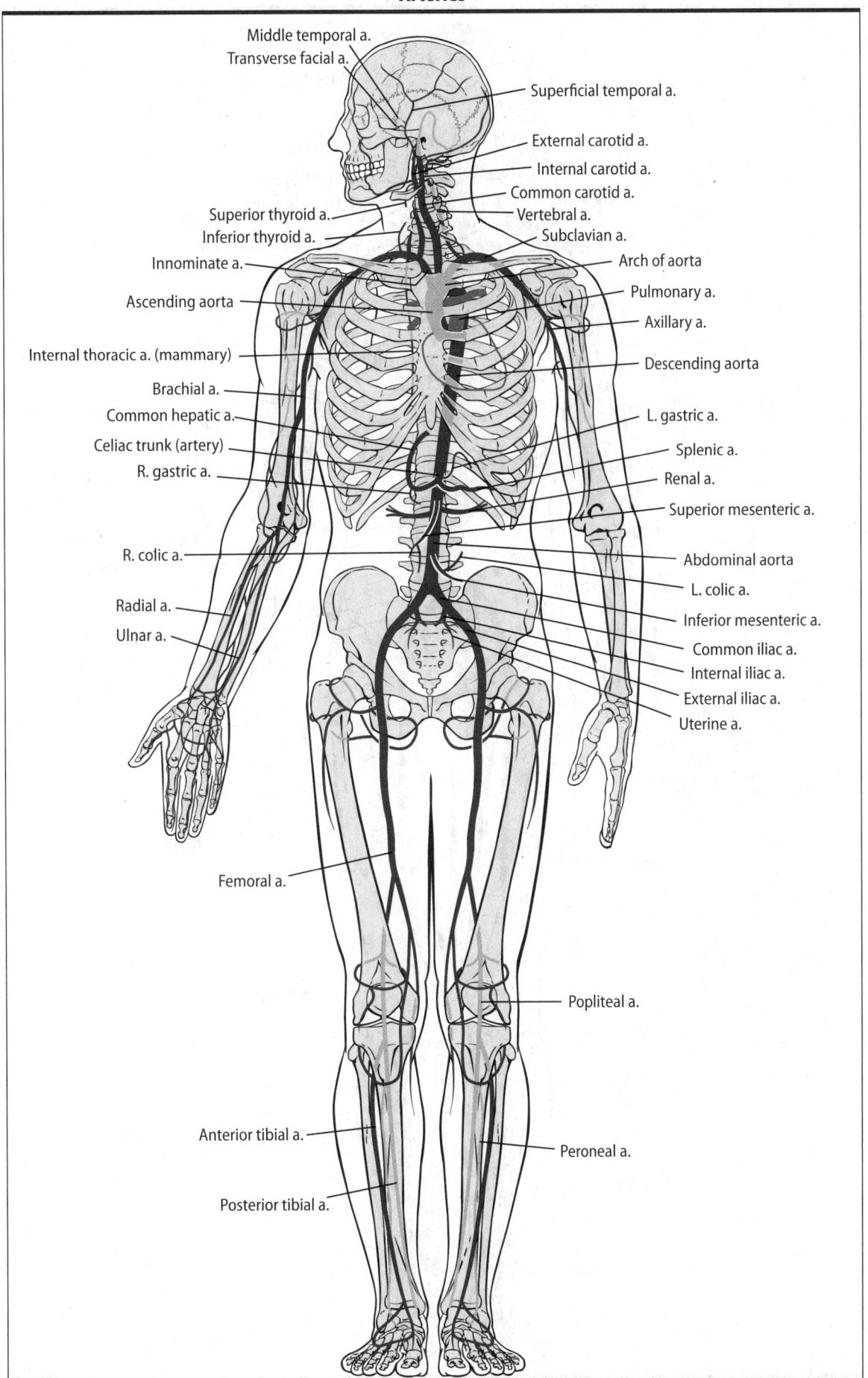

Veins

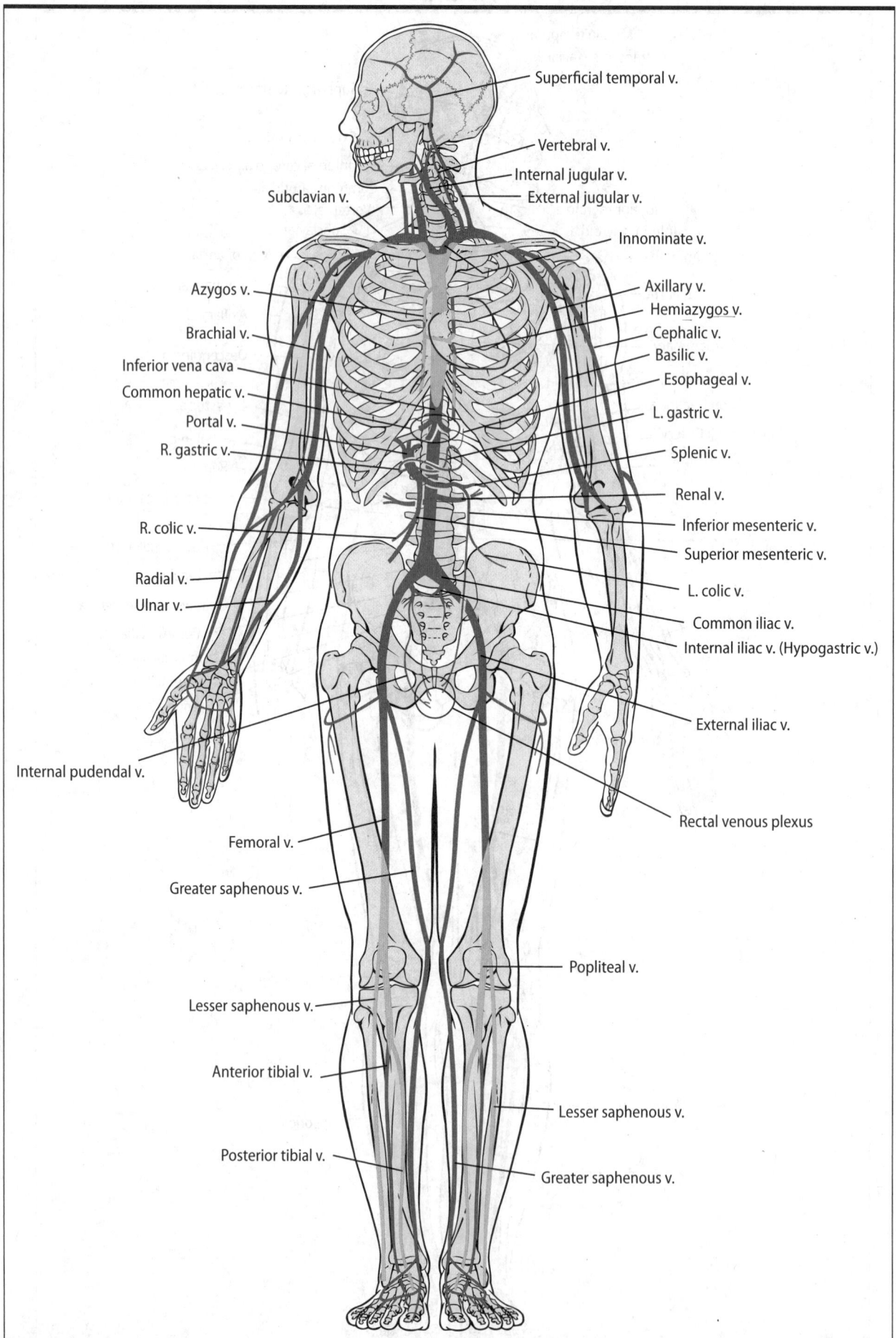

Superficial temporal v.

Vertebral v.

Internal jugular v.

External jugular v.

Subclavian v.

Innominate v.

Azygos v.

Axillary v.

Hemiazygos v.

Brachial v.

Cephalic v.

Basilic v.

Inferior vena cava

Esophageal v.

Common hepatic v.

L. gastric v.

Portal v.

R. gastric v.

Splenic v.

Renal v.

R. colic v.

Inferior mesenteric v.

Superior mesenteric v.

Radial v.

L. colic v.

Ulnar v.

Common iliac v.

Internal iliac v. (Hypogastric v.)

External iliac v.

Internal pudendal v.

Rectal venous plexus

Femoral v.

Greater saphenous v.

Popliteal v.

Lesser saphenous v.

Anterior tibial v.

Lesser saphenous v.

Posterior tibial v.

Greater saphenous v.

Internal Carotid and Vertebral Arteries and Branches

Side View

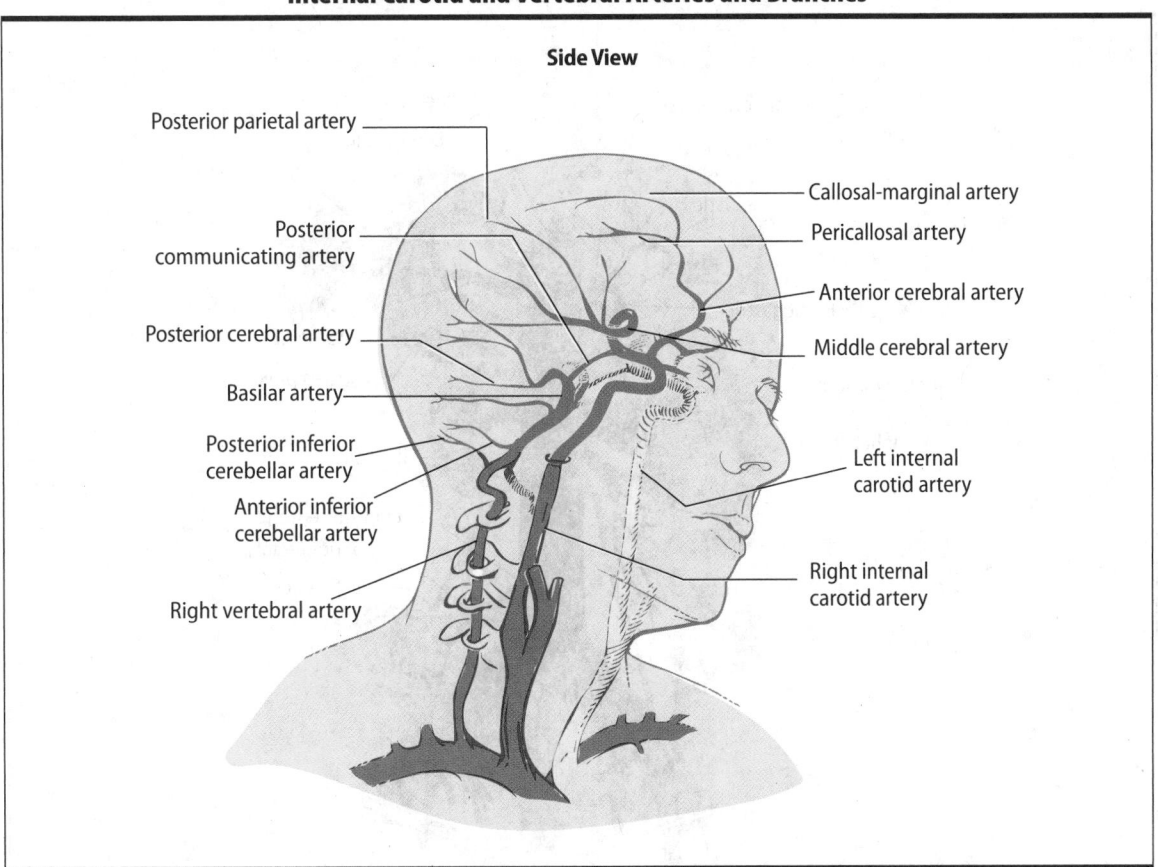

External Carotid Artery and Branches

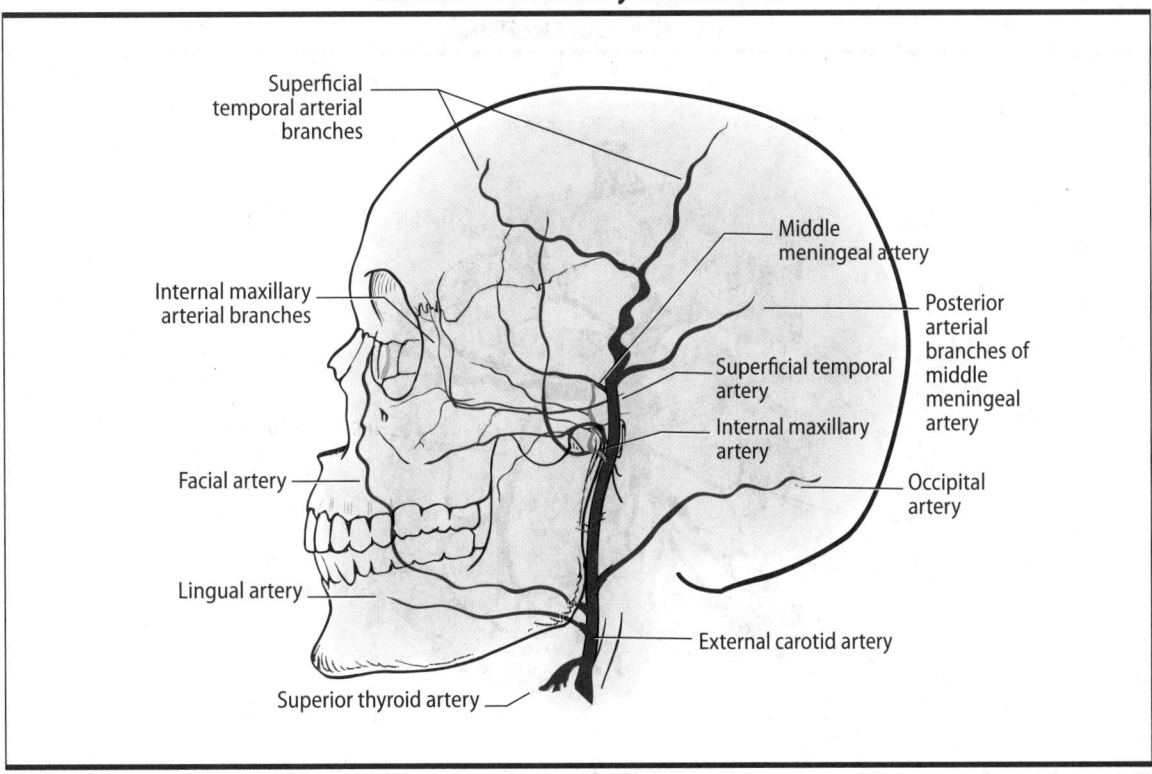

Branches of Abdominal Aorta

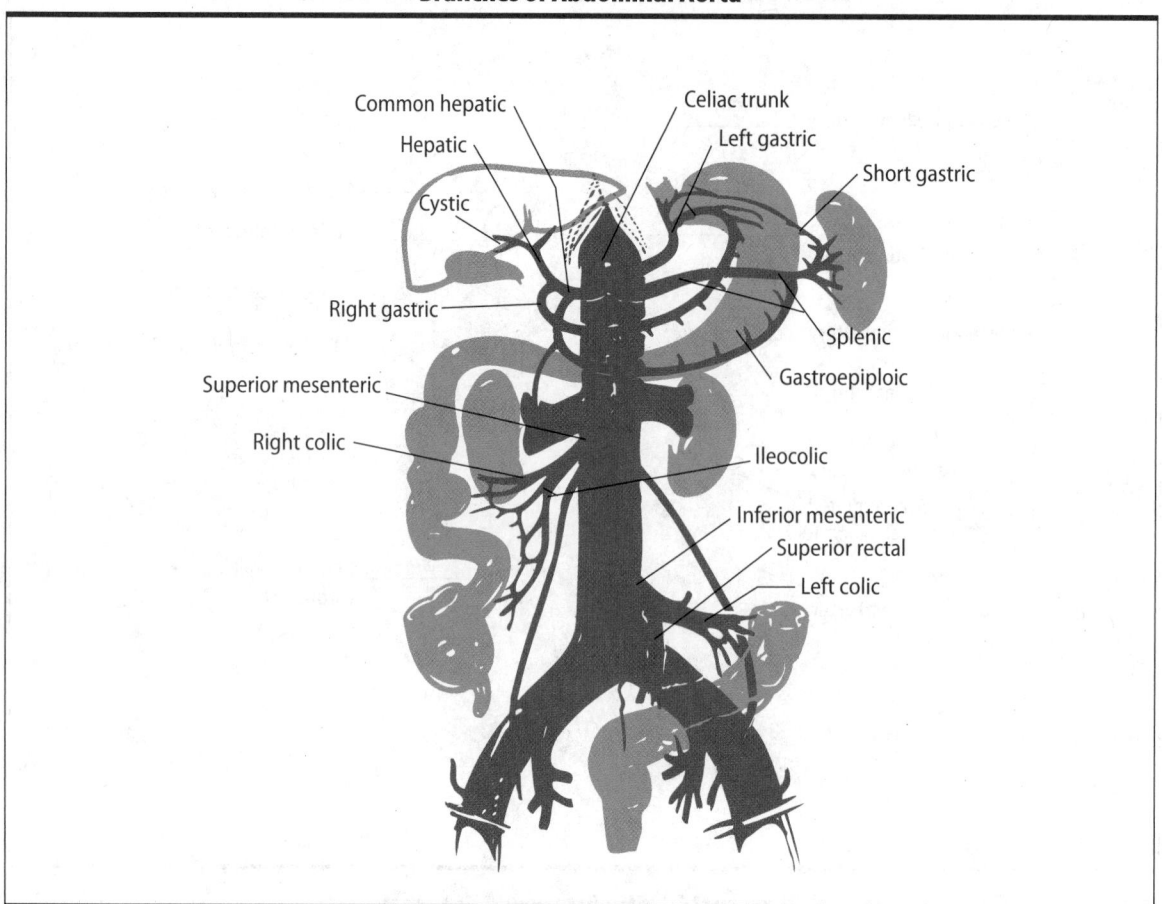

Portal Venous Circulation

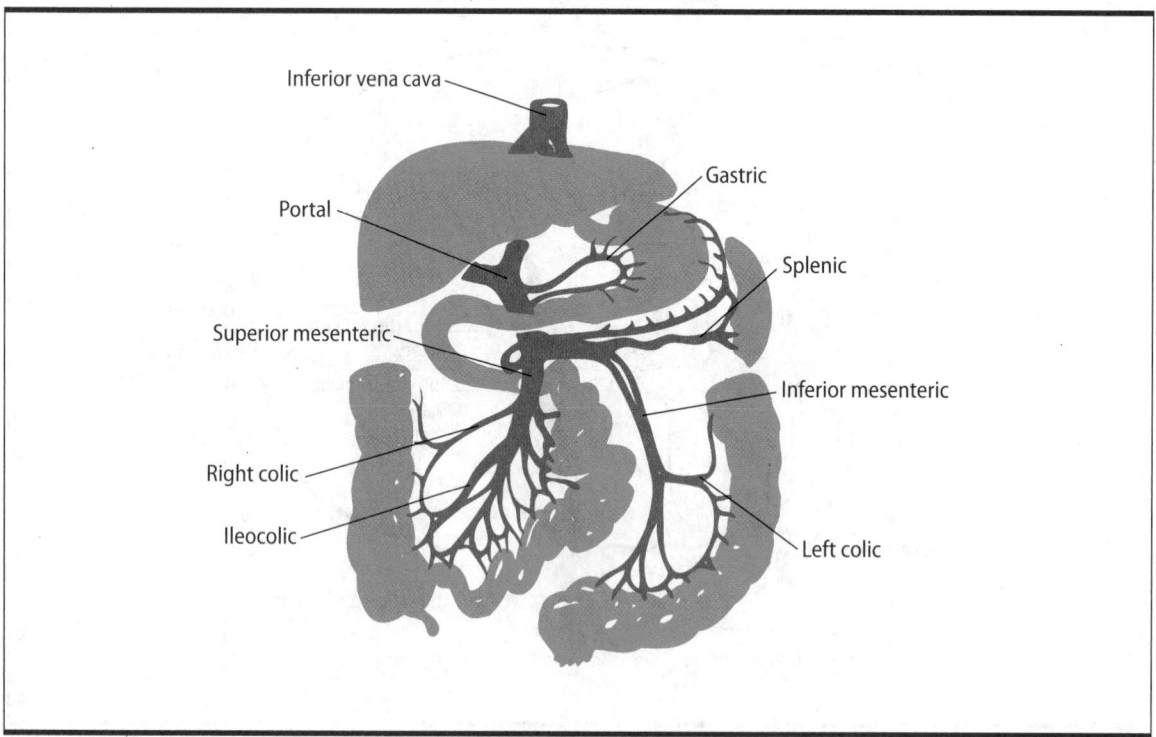

Lymphatic System

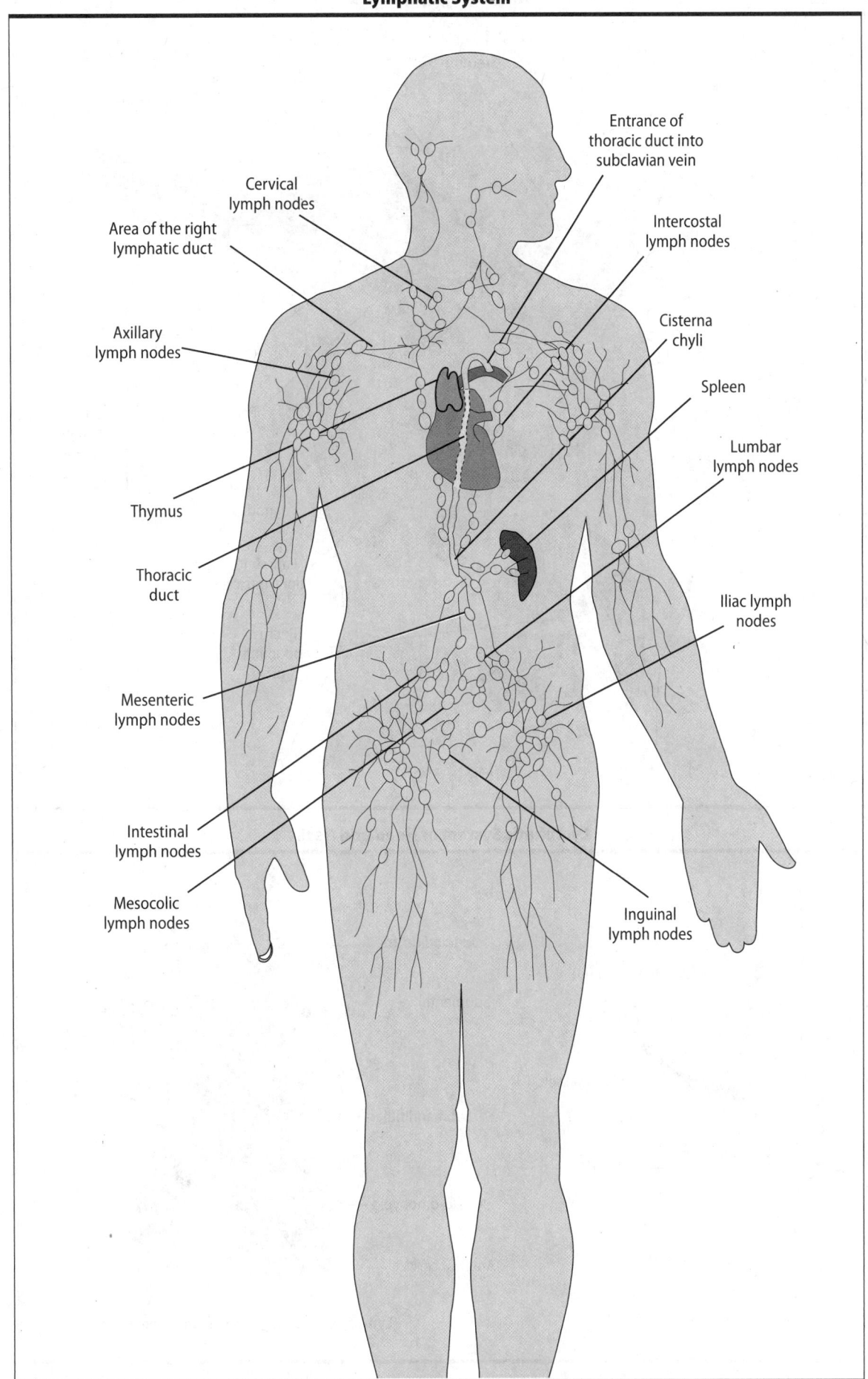

Axillary Lymph Nodes

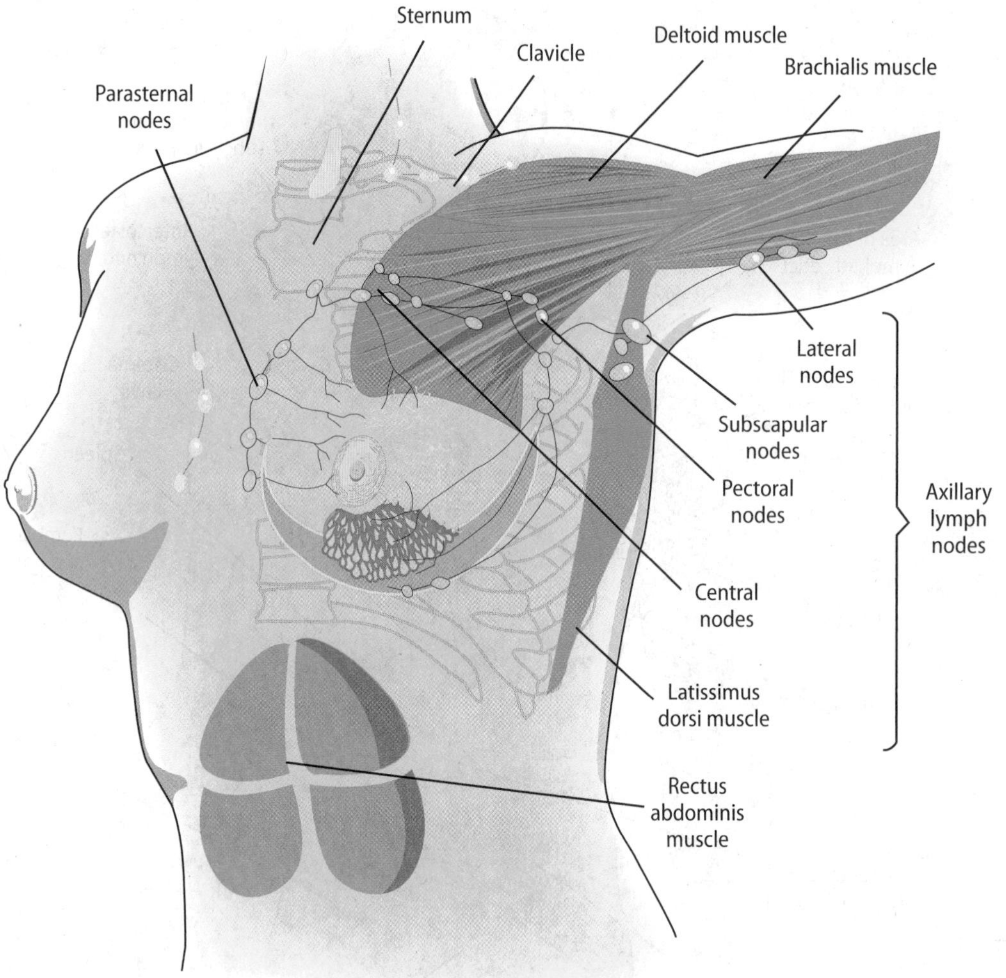

Sternum

Clavicle

Deltoid muscle

Brachialis muscle

Parasternal nodes

Lateral nodes

Subscapular nodes

Pectoral nodes

Axillary lymph nodes

Central nodes

Latissimus dorsi muscle

Rectus abdominis muscle

Lymphatic System of Head and Neck

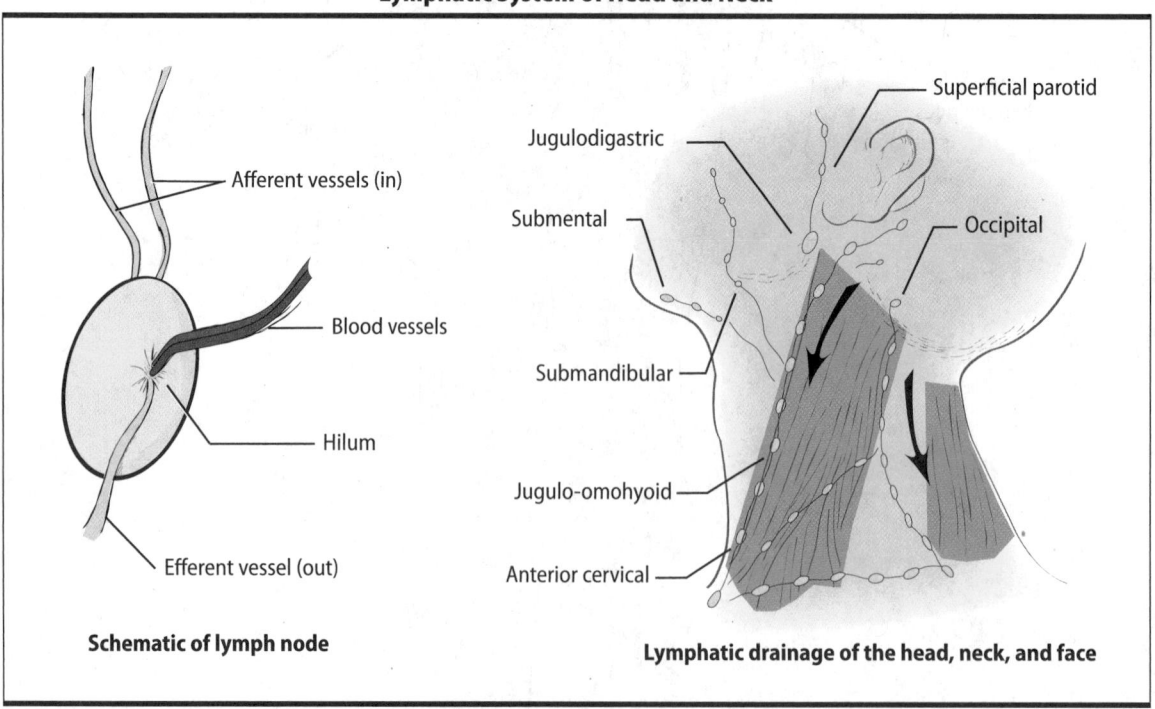

Afferent vessels (in)

Blood vessels

Hilum

Efferent vessel (out)

Schematic of lymph node

Superficial parotid

Jugulodigastric

Submental

Occipital

Submandibular

Jugulo-omohyoid

Anterior cervical

Lymphatic drainage of the head, neck, and face

Lymphatic Capillaries

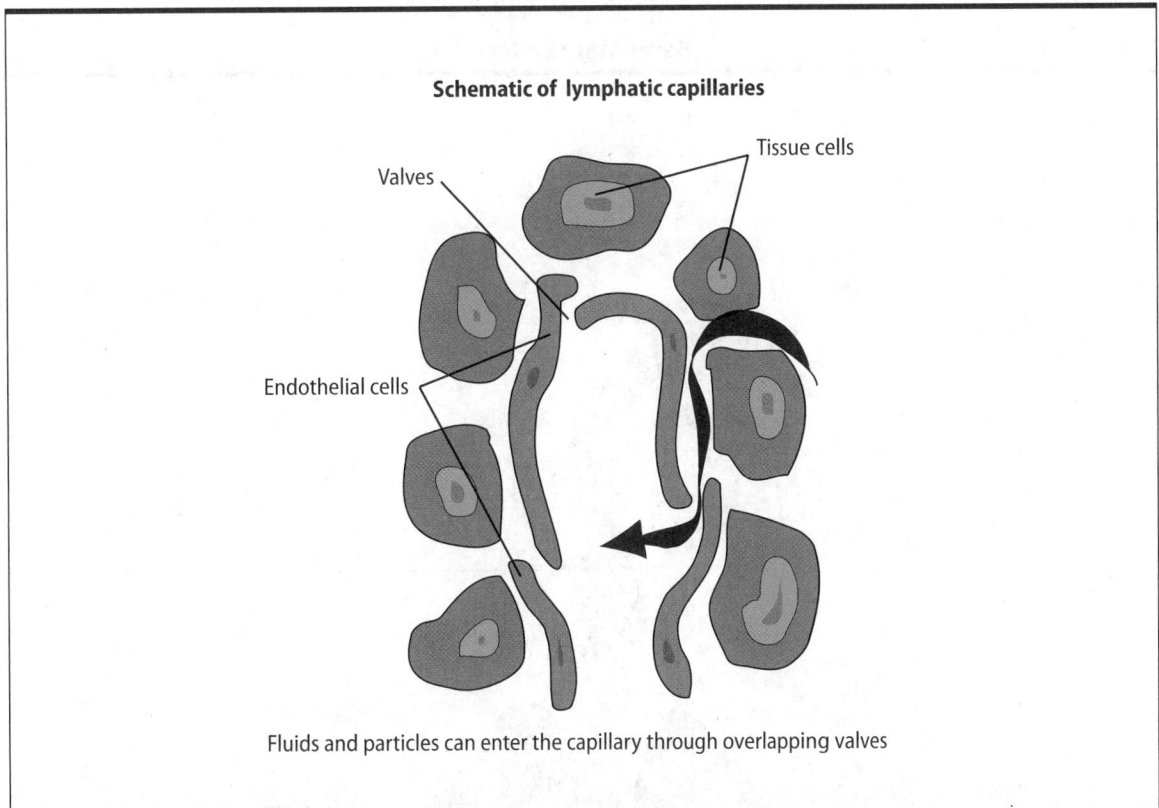

Schematic of lymphatic capillaries
Tissue cells
Valves
Endothelial cells
Fluids and particles can enter the capillary through overlapping valves

Lymphatic Drainage

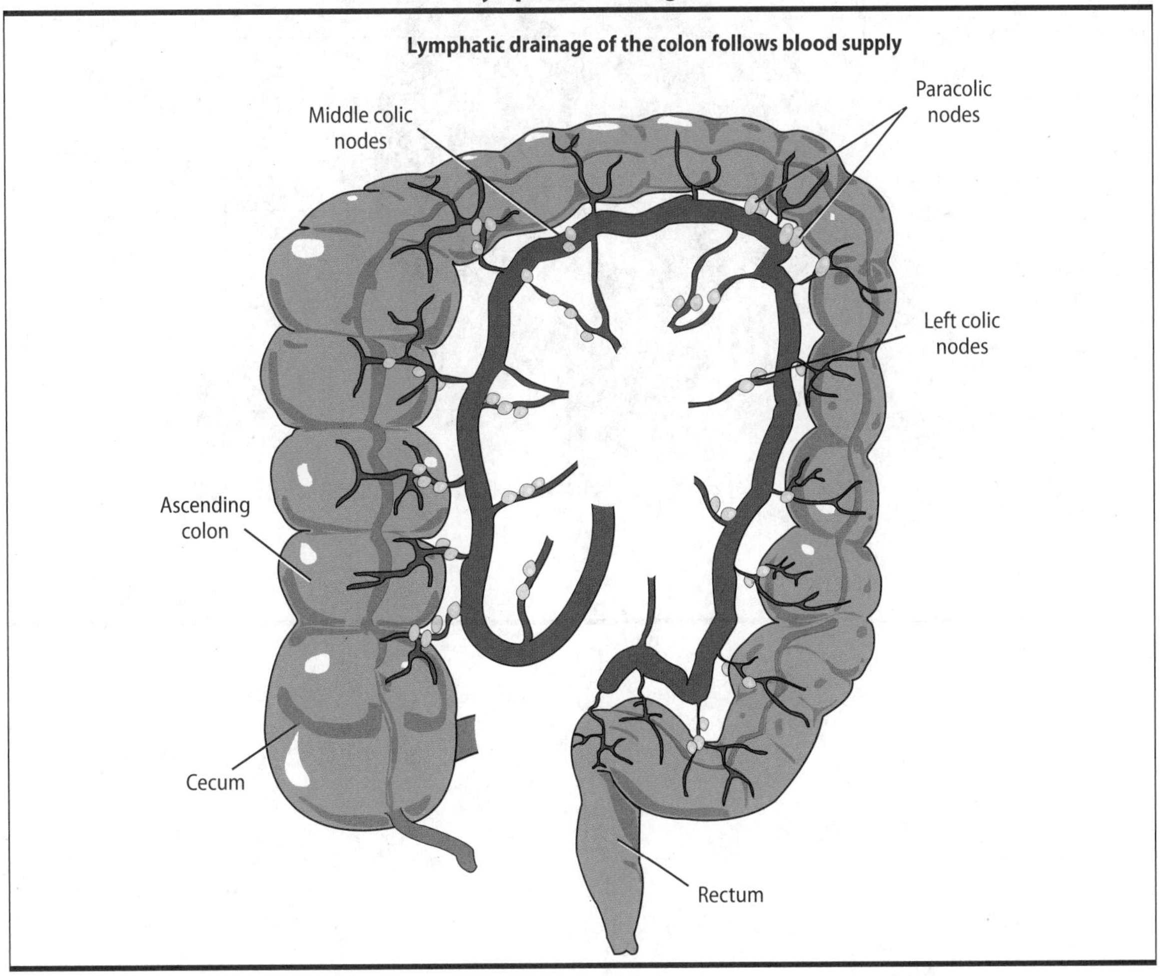

Lymphatic drainage of the colon follows blood supply
Paracolic nodes
Middle colic nodes
Left colic nodes
Ascending colon
Cecum
Rectum

Chapter 10. Diseases of the Respiratory System (J00–J99)

Respiratory System

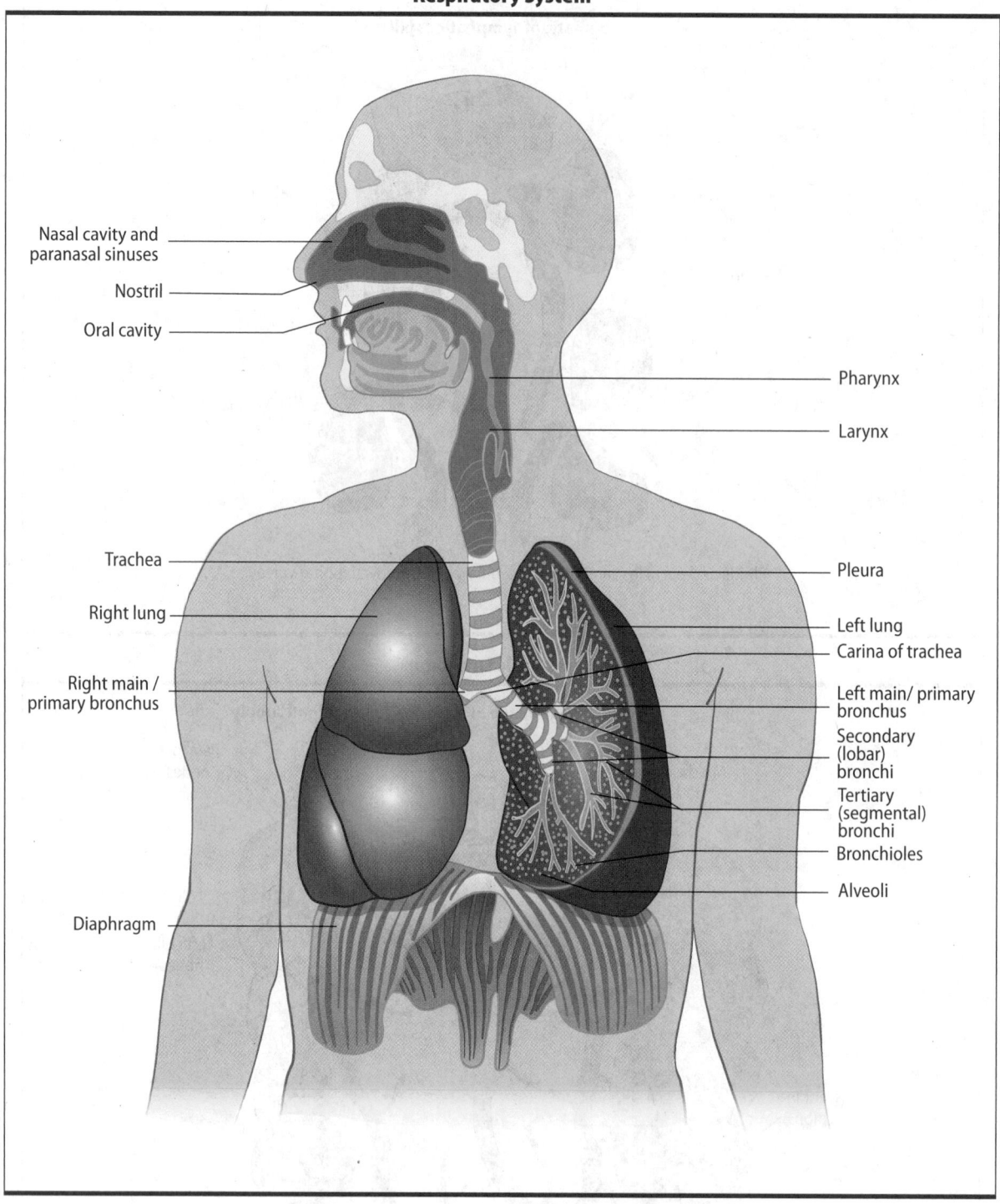

Nasal cavity and paranasal sinuses

Nostril

Oral cavity

Pharynx

Larynx

Trachea

Right lung

Pleura

Left lung

Carina of trachea

Right main / primary bronchus

Left main/ primary bronchus

Secondary (lobar) bronchi

Tertiary (segmental) bronchi

Bronchioles

Alveoli

Diaphragm

Upper Respiratory System

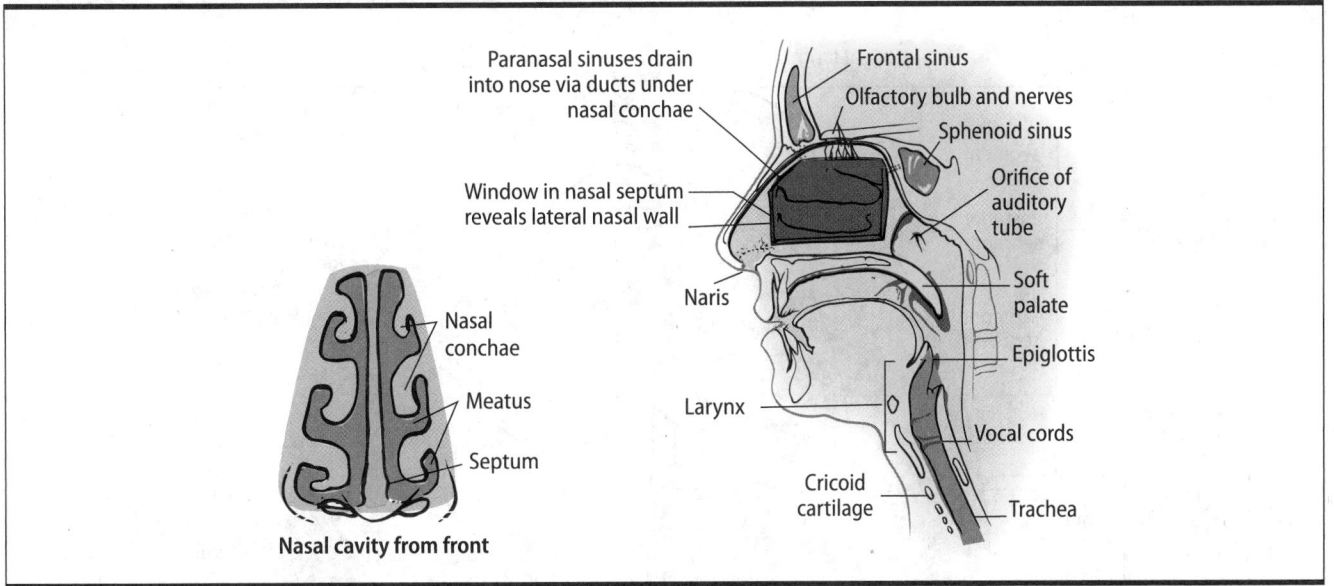

Paranasal sinuses drain into nose via ducts under nasal conchae

Frontal sinus

Olfactory bulb and nerves

Sphenoid sinus

Window in nasal septum reveals lateral nasal wall

Orifice of auditory tube

Naris

Soft palate

Nasal conchae

Meatus

Septum

Larynx

Epiglottis

Vocal cords

Cricoid cartilage

Trachea

Nasal cavity from front

Lower Respiratory System

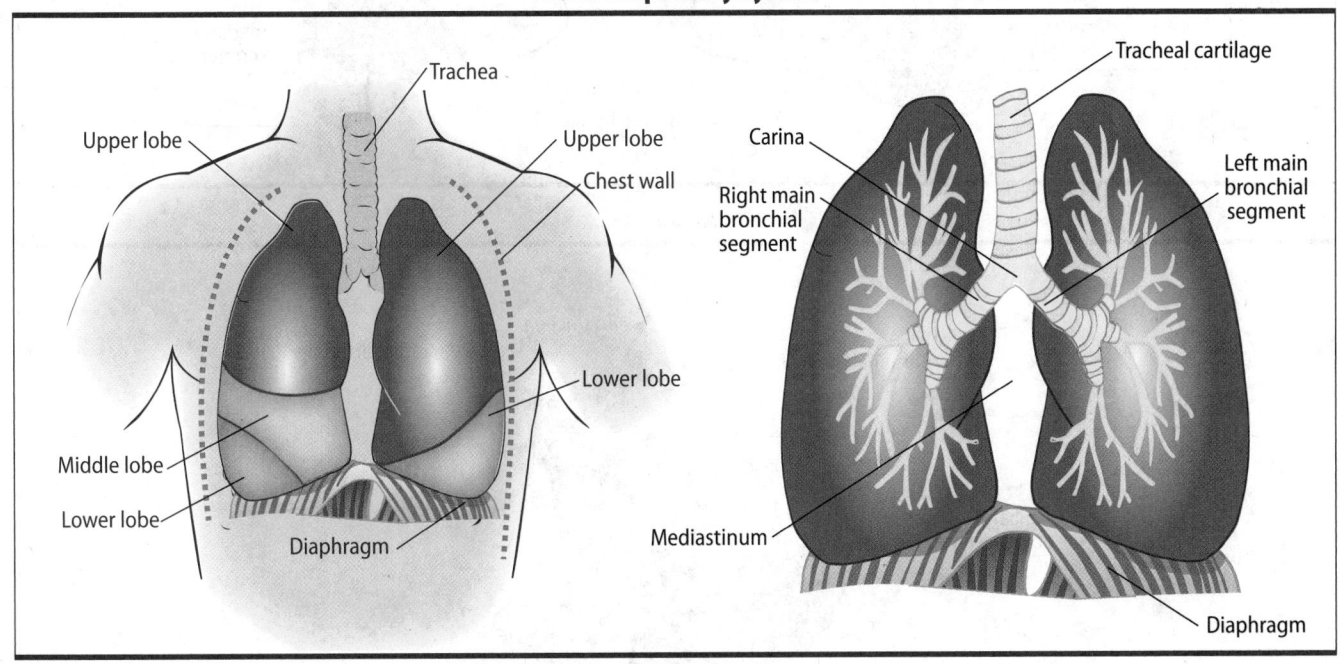

Trachea

Upper lobe

Upper lobe

Chest wall

Tracheal cartilage

Carina

Left main bronchial segment

Right main bronchial segment

Middle lobe

Lower lobe

Lower lobe

Diaphragm

Mediastinum

Diaphragm

Paranasal Sinuses

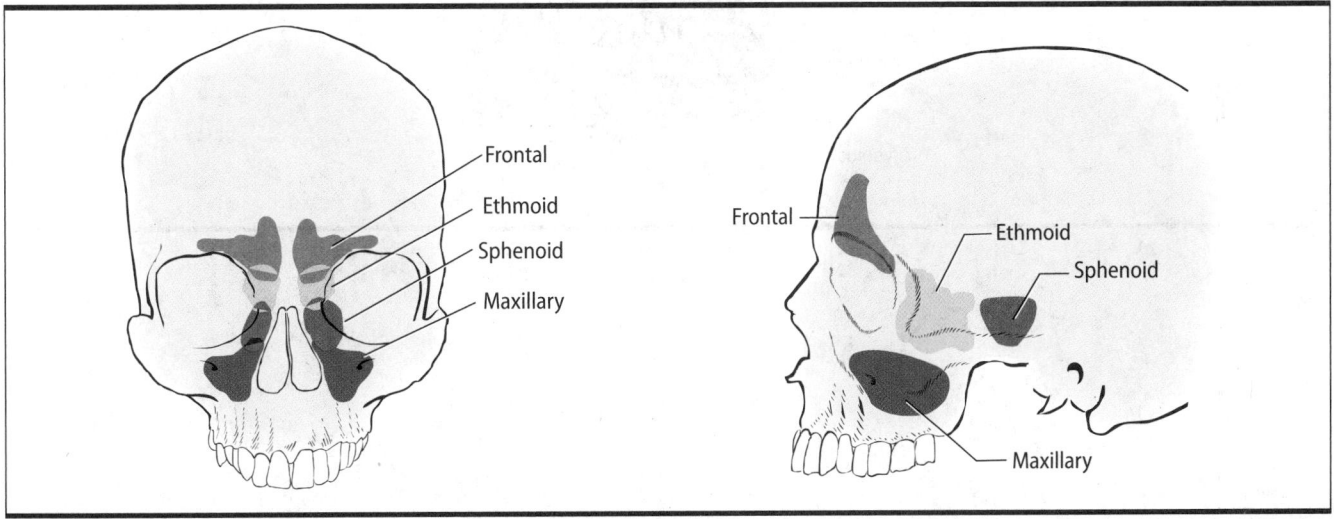

Frontal

Ethmoid

Sphenoid

Maxillary

Frontal

Ethmoid

Sphenoid

Maxillary

Lung Segments

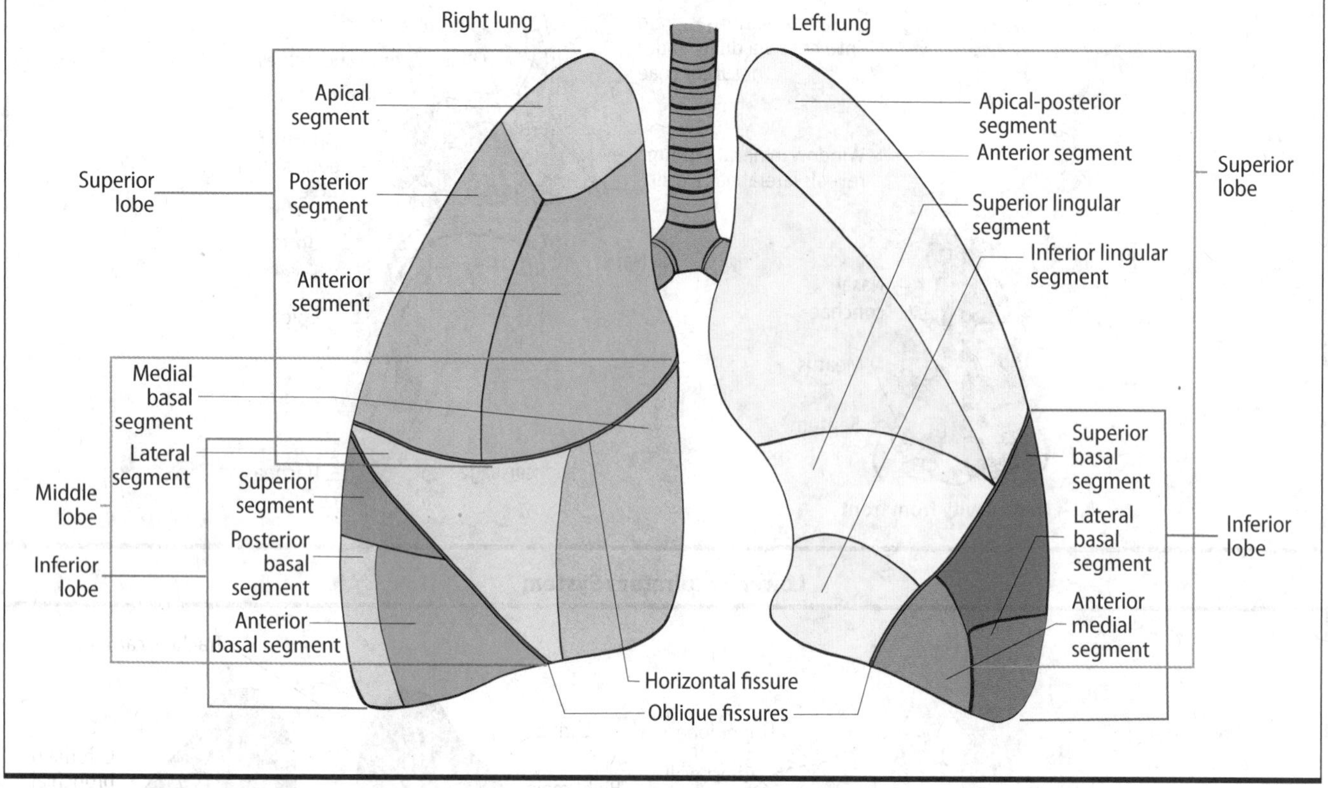

Right lung

Apical segment

Superior lobe

Posterior segment

Anterior segment

Medial basal segment

Lateral segment

Middle lobe

Superior segment

Posterior basal segment

Inferior lobe

Anterior basal segment

Left lung

Apical-posterior segment

Anterior segment

Superior lobe

Superior lingular segment

Inferior lingular segment

Superior basal segment

Lateral basal segment

Inferior lobe

Anterior medial segment

Horizontal fissure

Oblique fissures

Alveoli

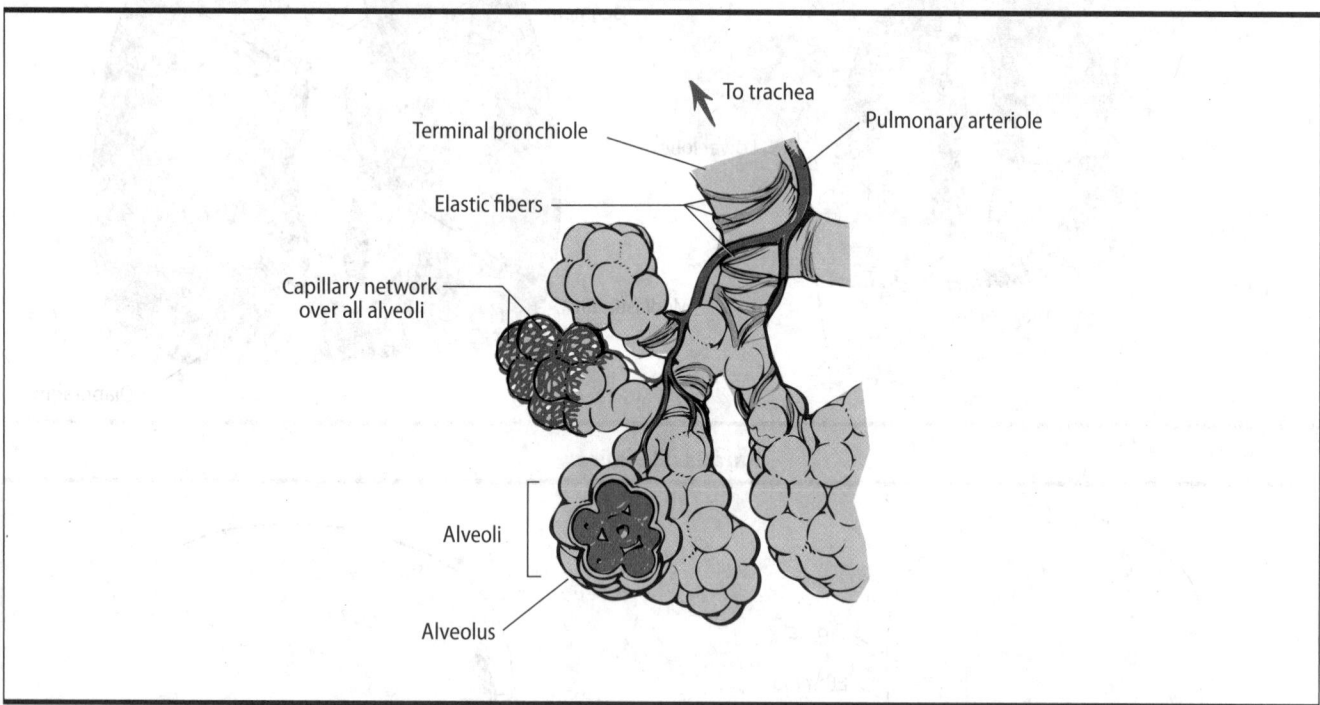

To trachea

Terminal bronchiole

Pulmonary arteriole

Elastic fibers

Capillary network over all alveoli

Alveoli

Alveolus

Chapter 11. Diseases of the Digestive System (K00–K95)

Digestive System

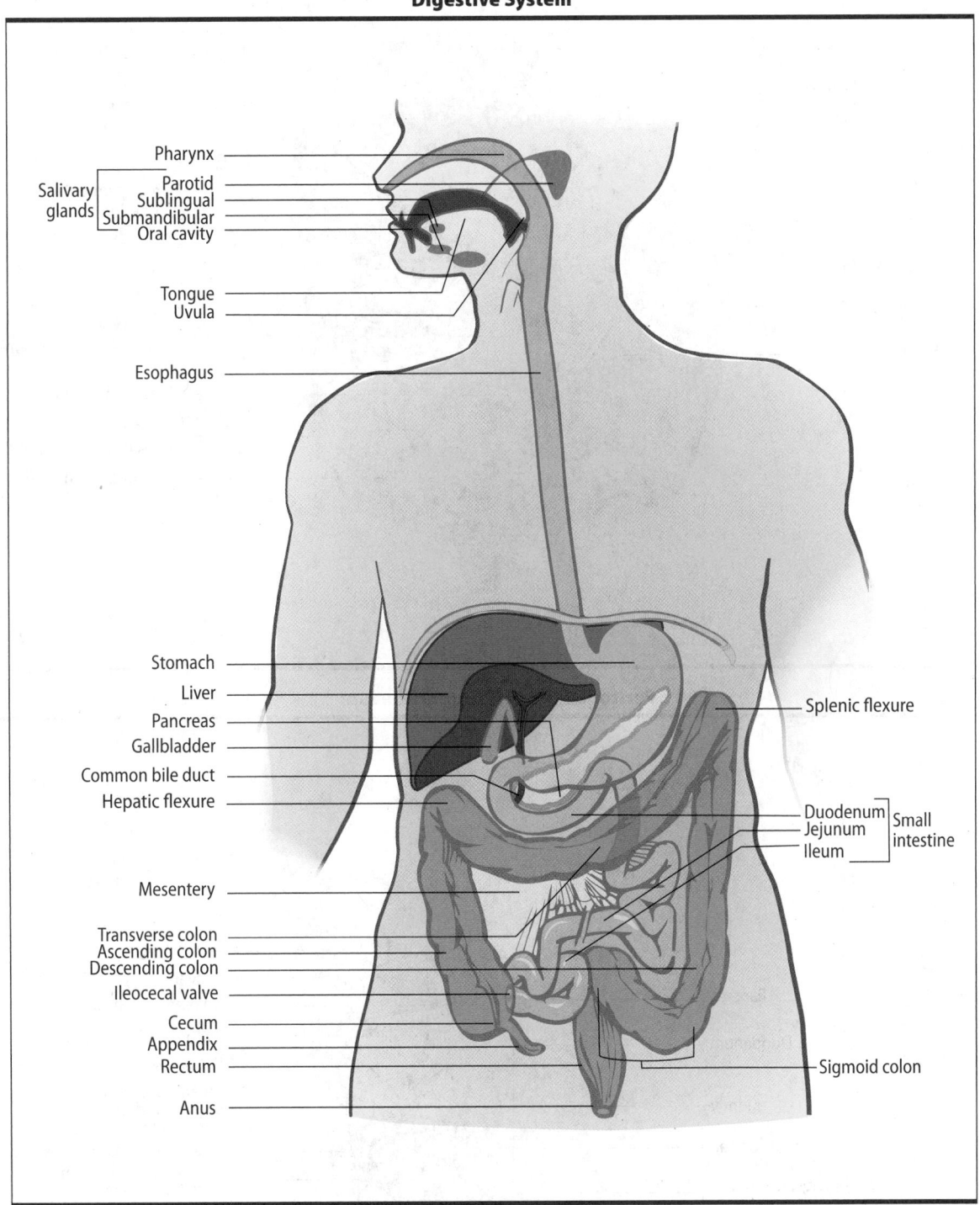

Omentum and Mesentery

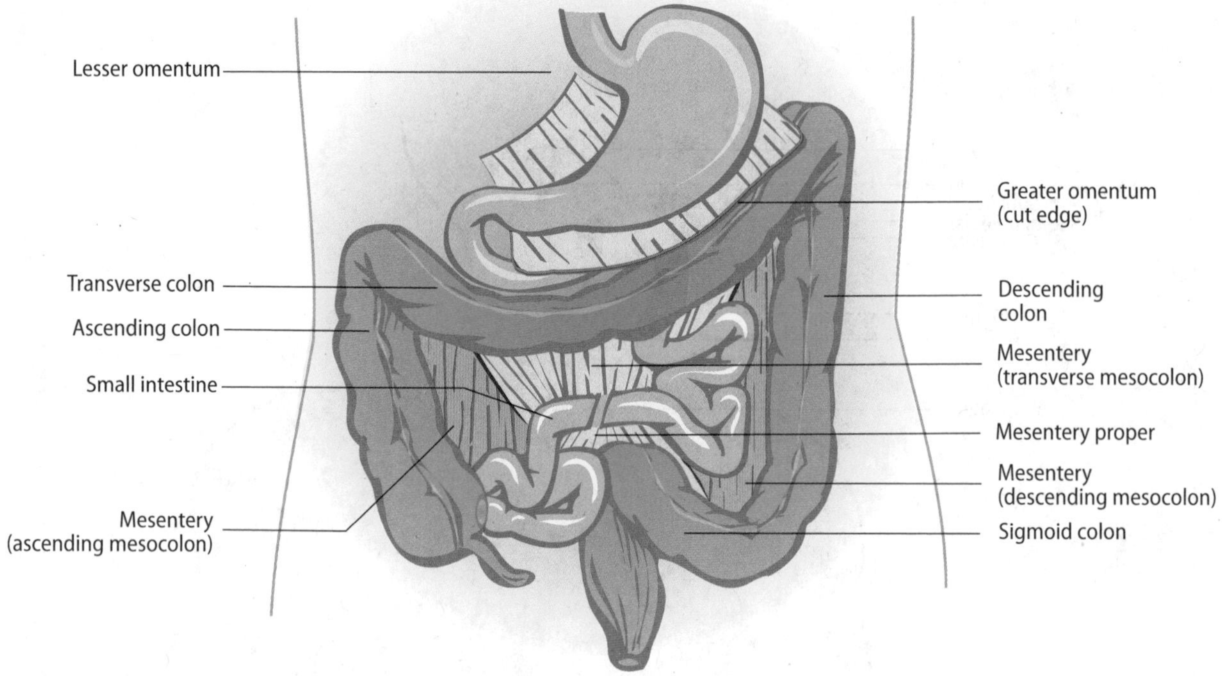

Lesser omentum

Greater omentum (cut edge)

Transverse colon

Descending colon

Ascending colon

Mesentery (transverse mesocolon)

Small intestine

Mesentery proper

Mesentery (descending mesocolon)

Mesentery (ascending mesocolon)

Sigmoid colon

Peritoneum and Retroperitoneum

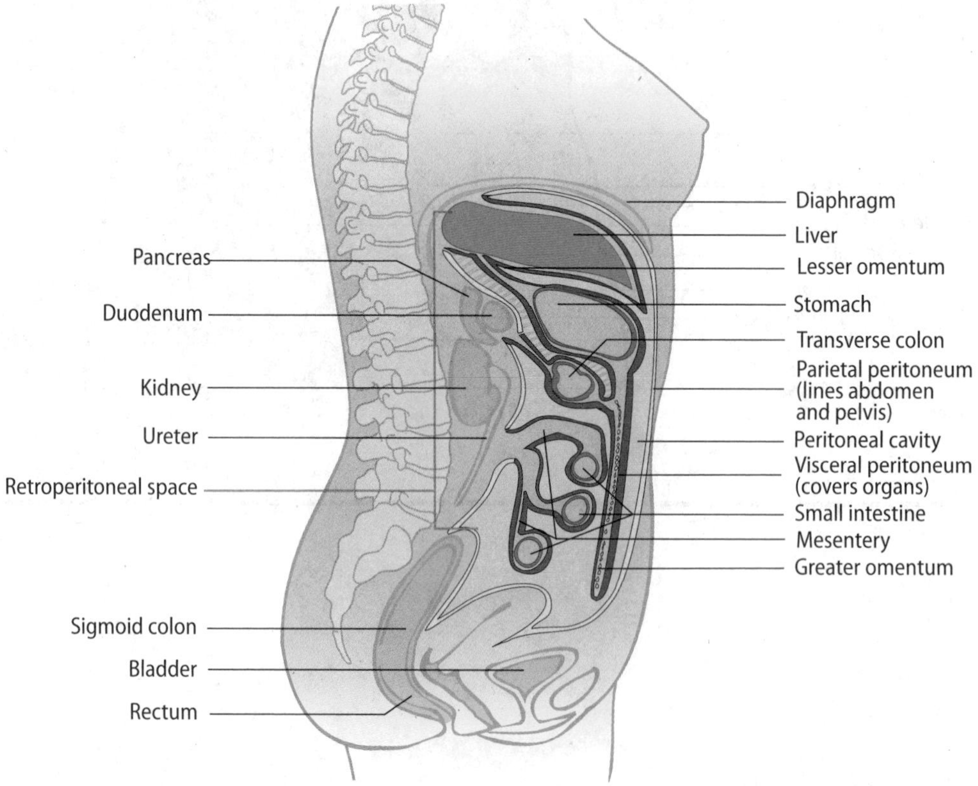

Pancreas

Diaphragm

Liver

Duodenum

Lesser omentum

Stomach

Kidney

Transverse colon

Ureter

Parietal peritoneum (lines abdomen and pelvis)

Retroperitoneal space

Peritoneal cavity

Visceral peritoneum (covers organs)

Small intestine

Mesentery

Greater omentum

Sigmoid colon

Bladder

Rectum

Chapter 12. Diseases of the Skin and Subcutaneous Tissue (LØØ–L99)

Nail Anatomy

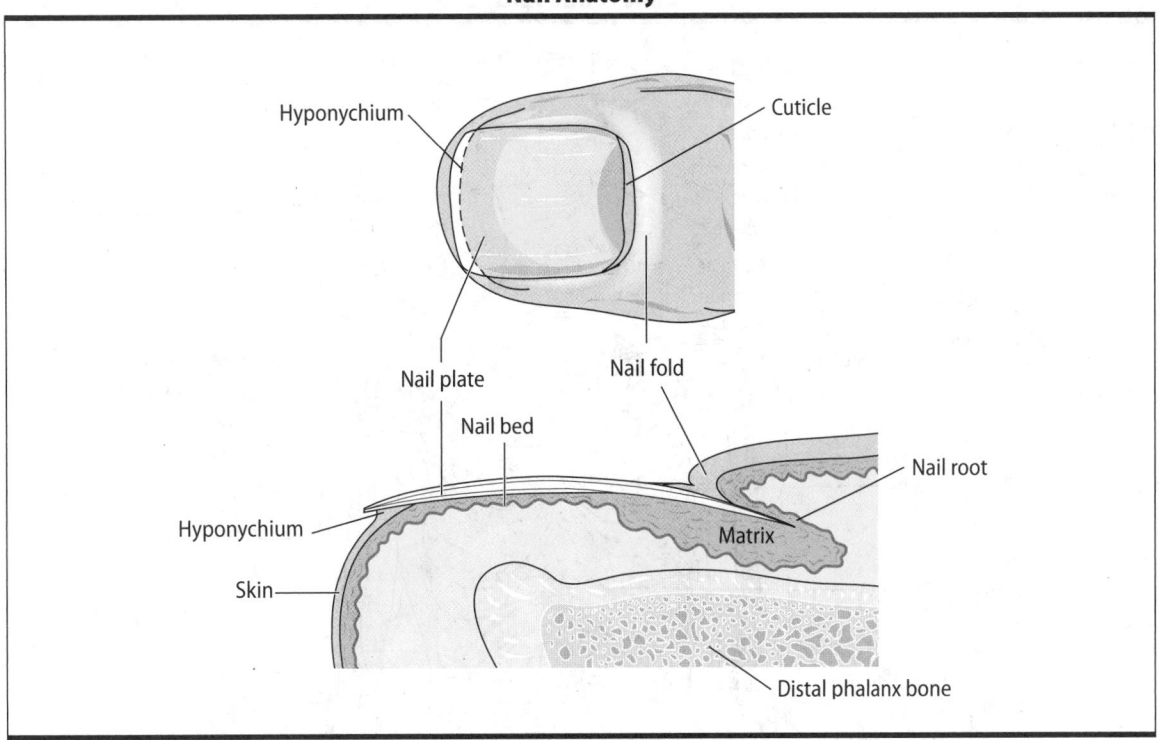

Skin and Subcutaneous Tissue

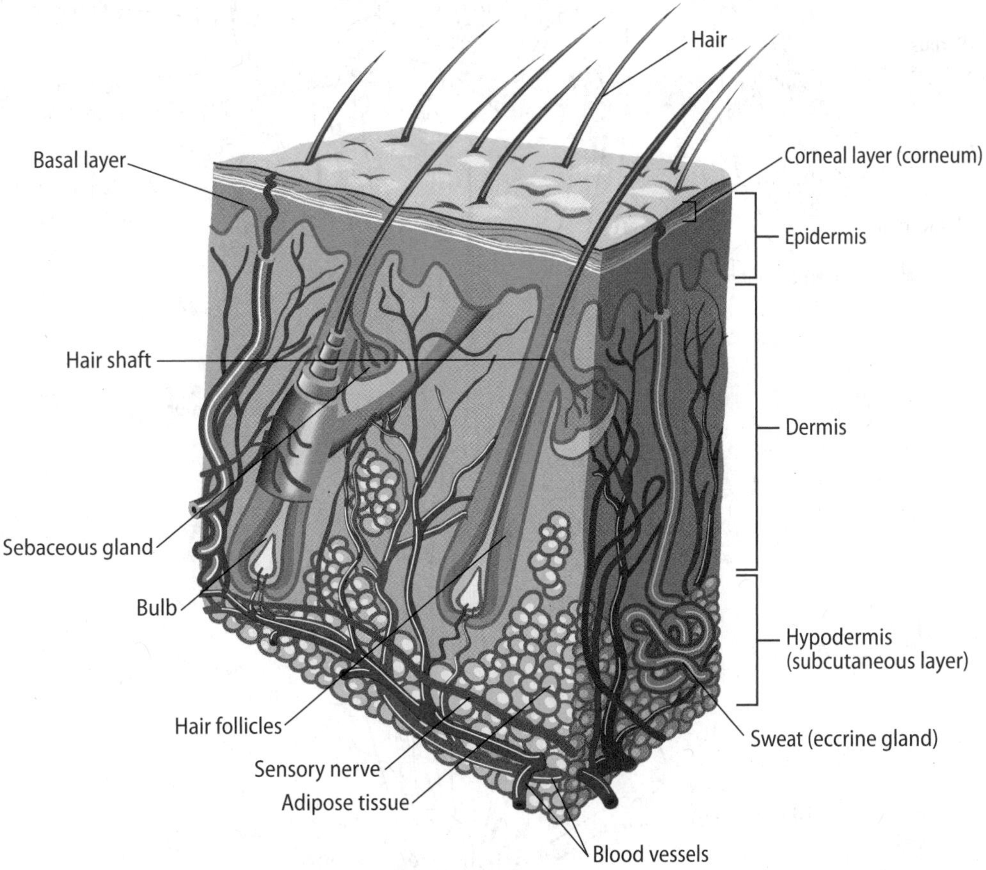

Chapter 13. Diseases of the Musculoskeletal System and Connective Tissue (M00–M99)

Bones and Joints

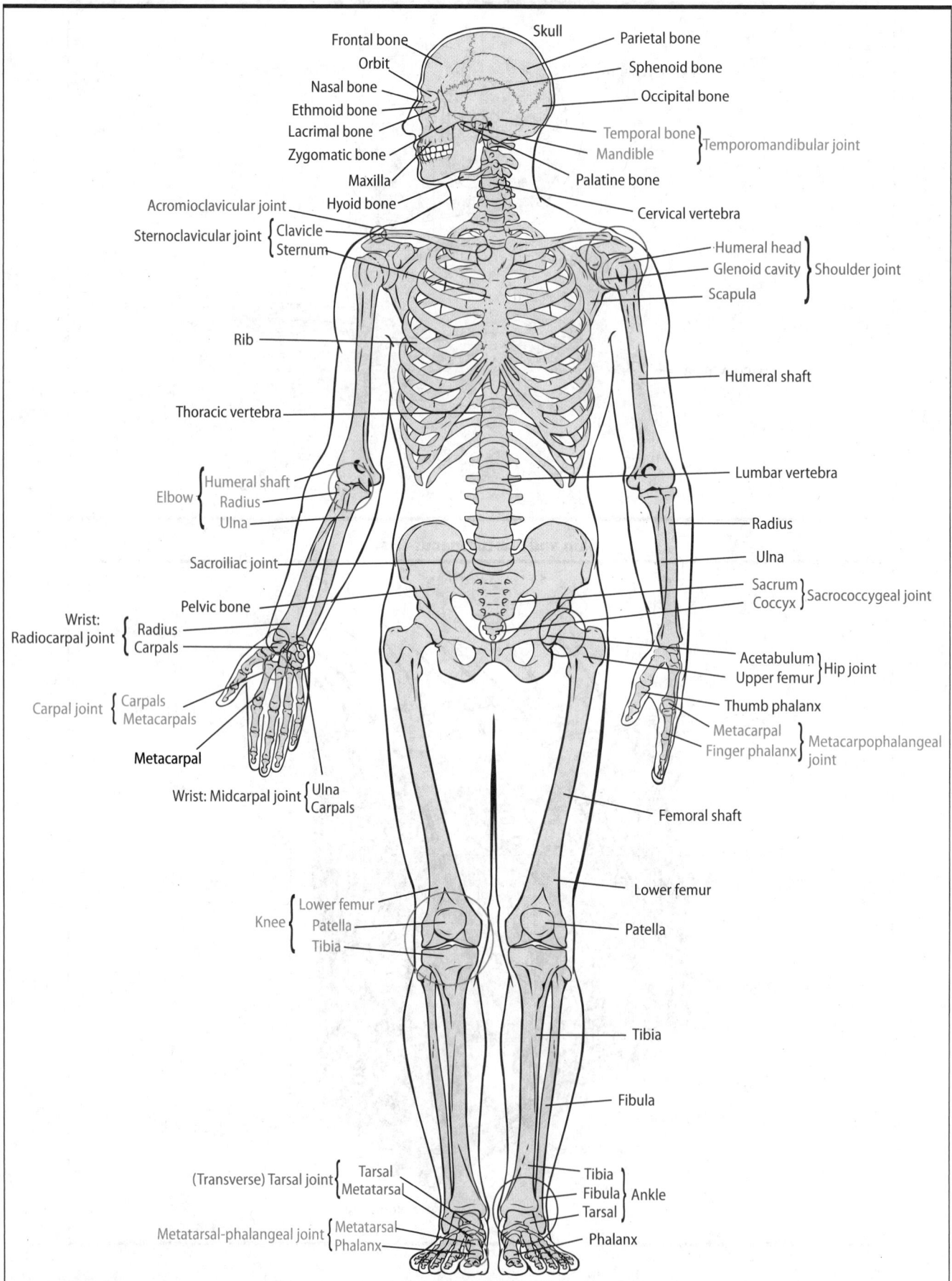

Shoulder Anterior View

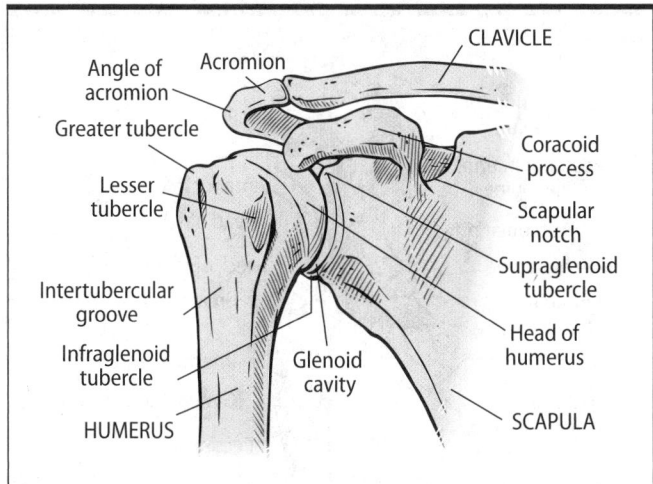

Shoulder Posterior View

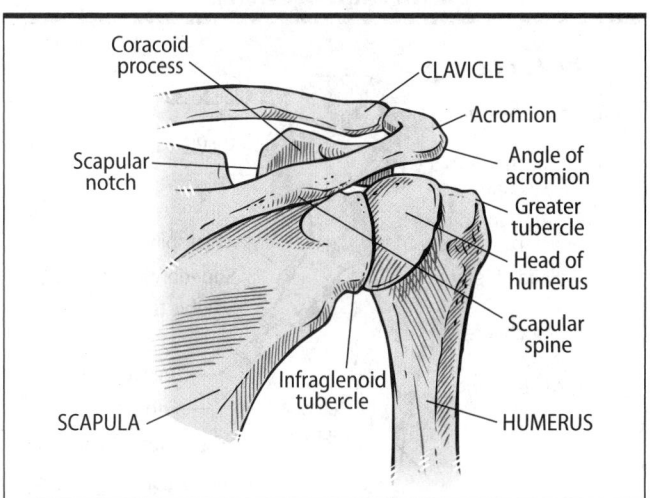

Elbow Anterior View

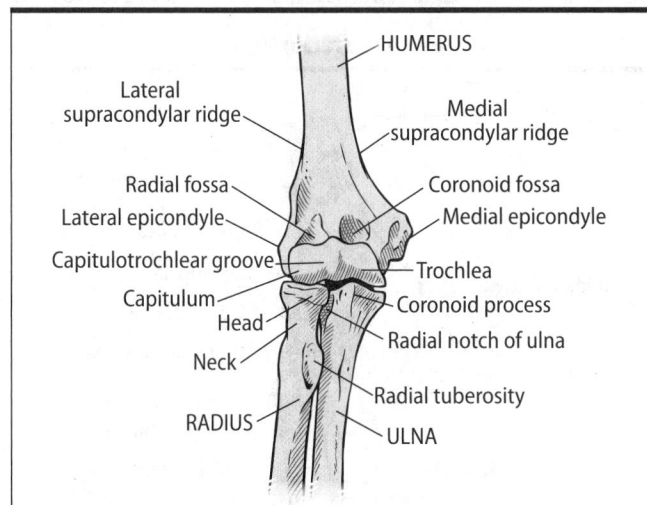

Elbow Posterior View

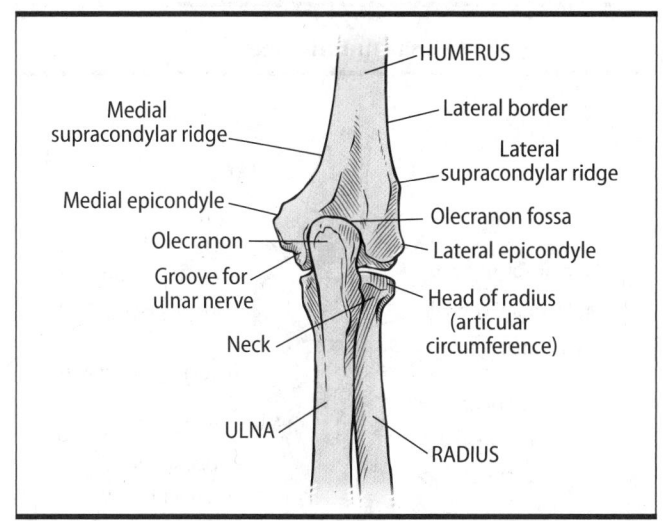

Hand

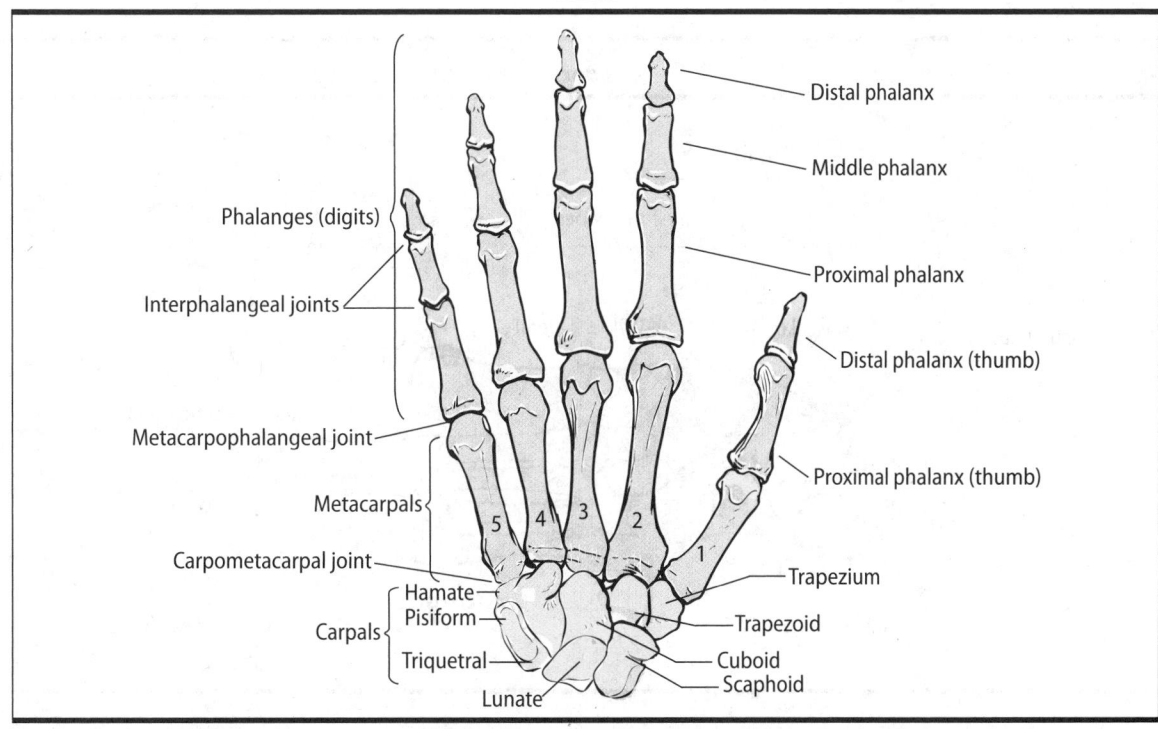

Hip Anterior View

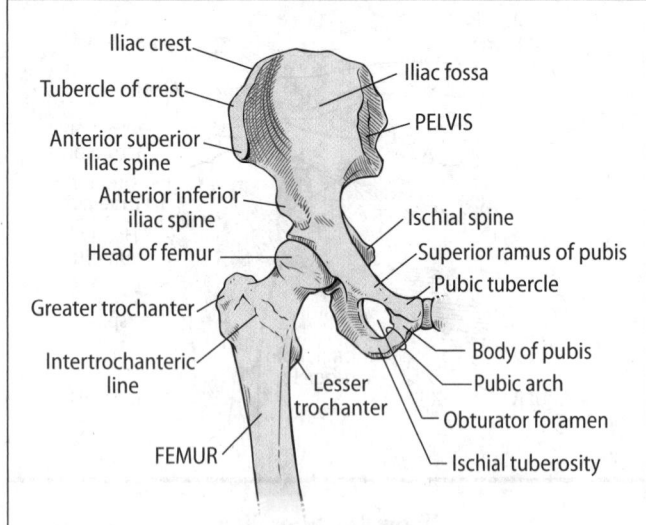

Hip Posterior View

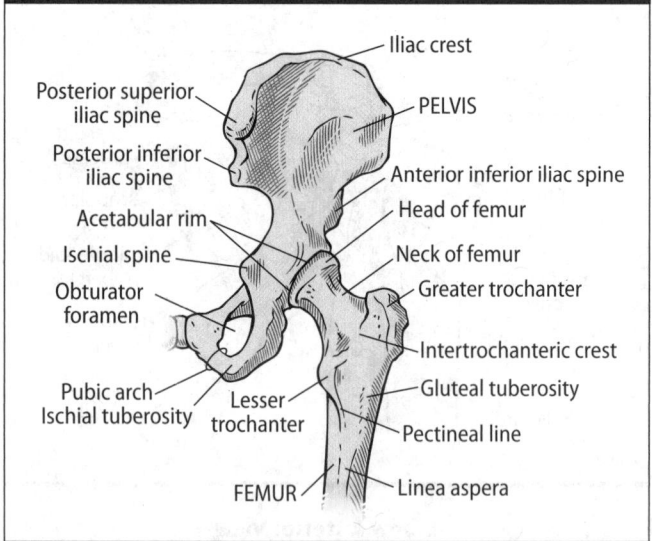

Knee Anterior View

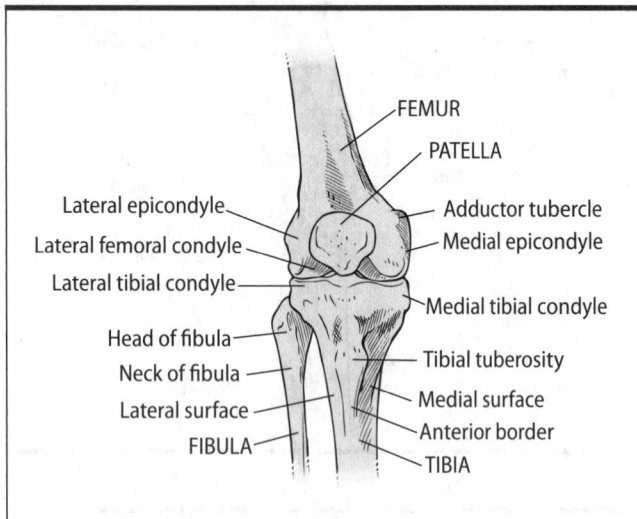

Knee Posterior View

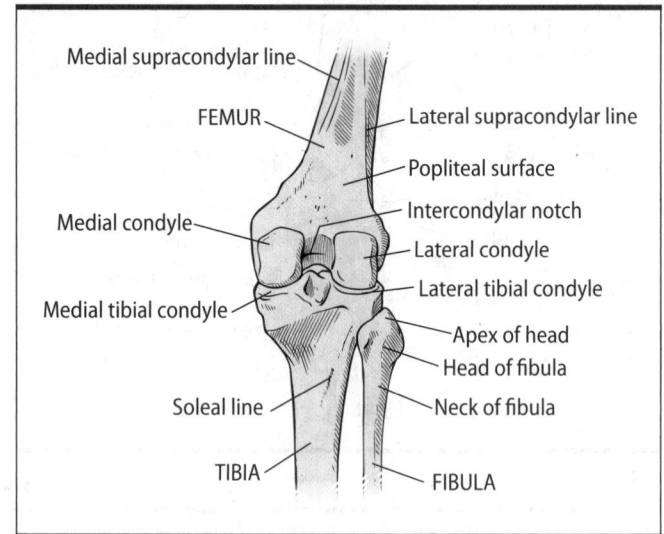

Foot

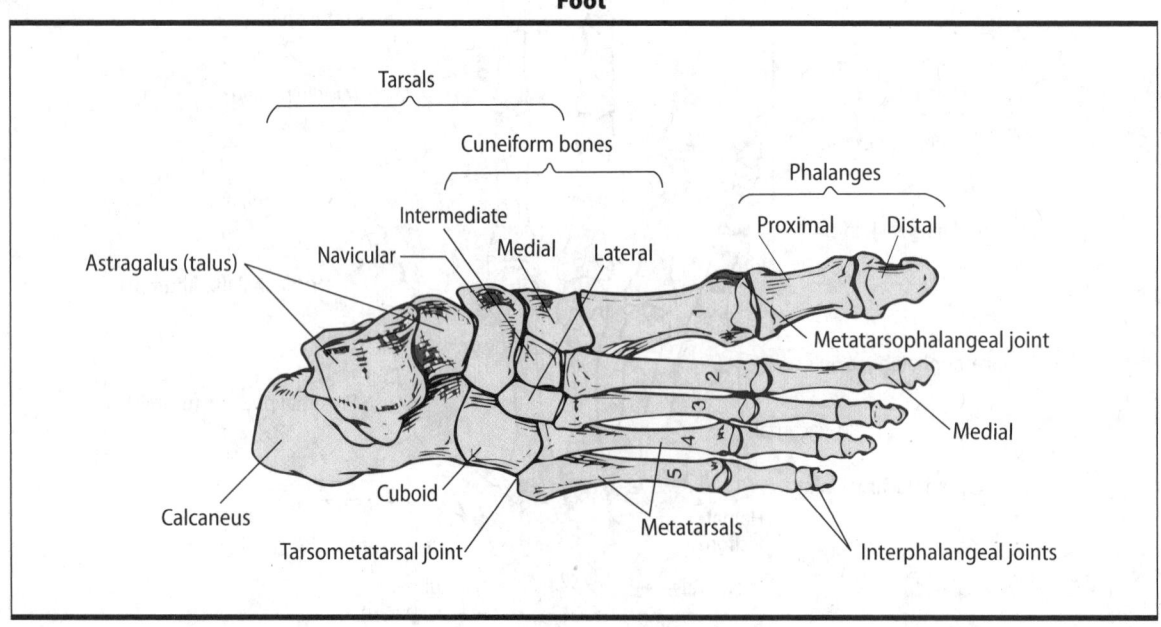

Muscles

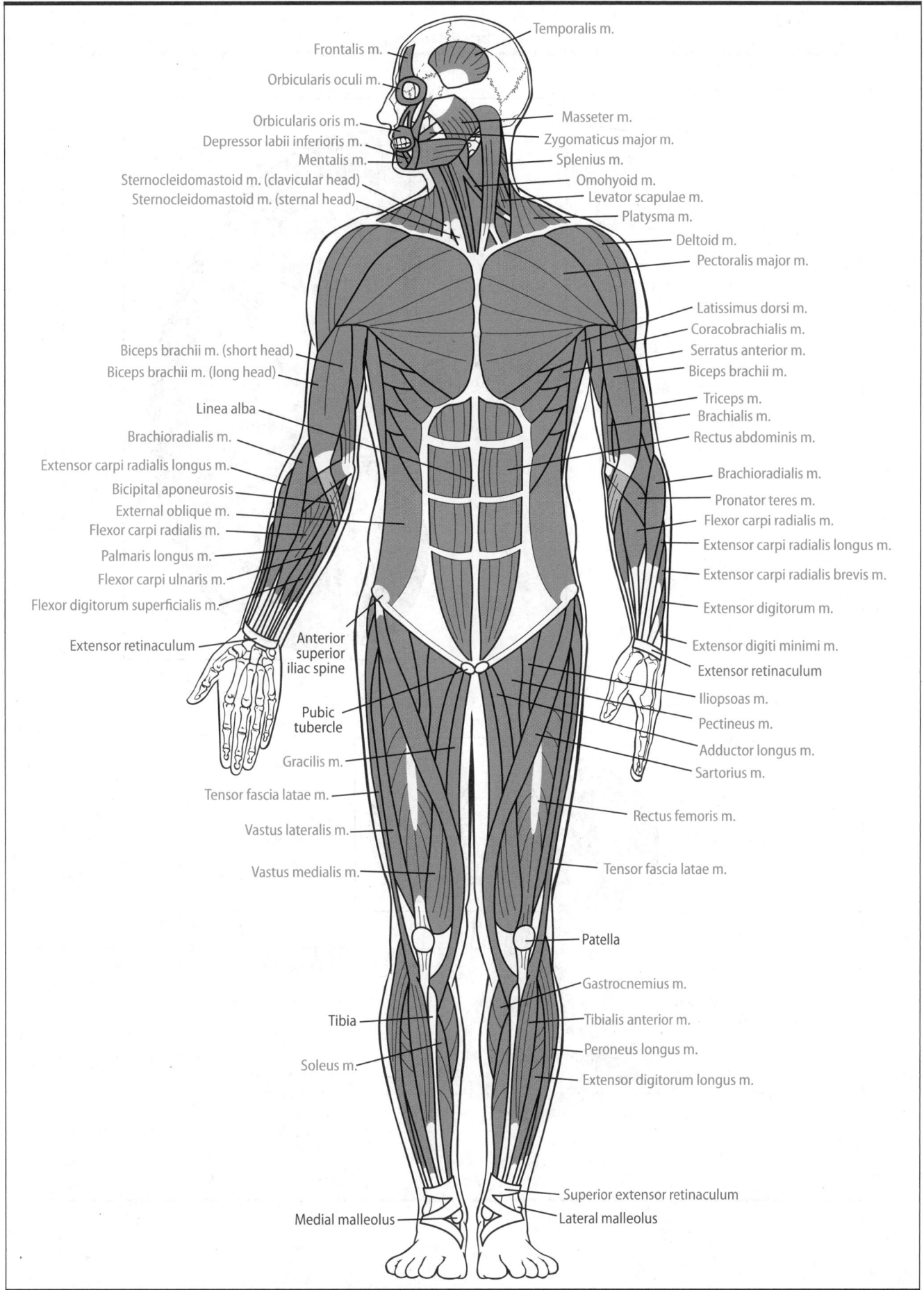

Chapter 14. Diseases of the Genitourinary System (N00–N99)

Urinary System

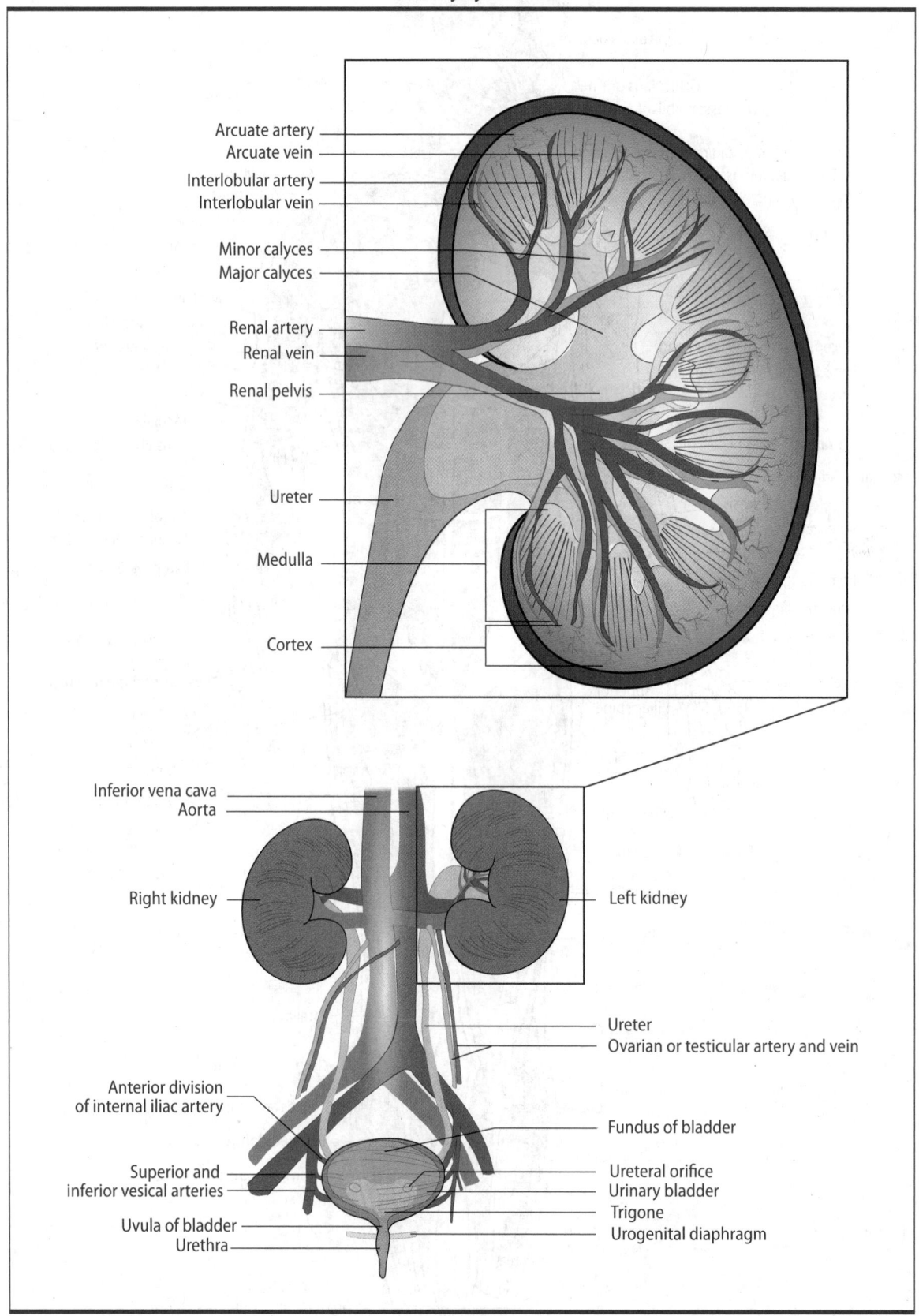

Male Genitourinary System

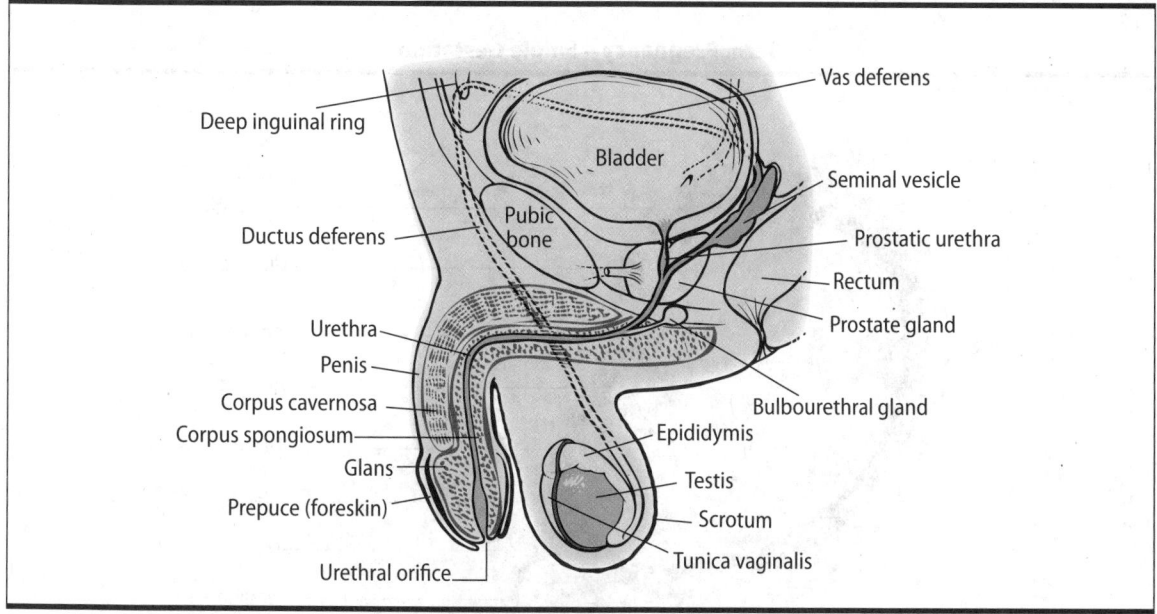

Female Internal Genitalia

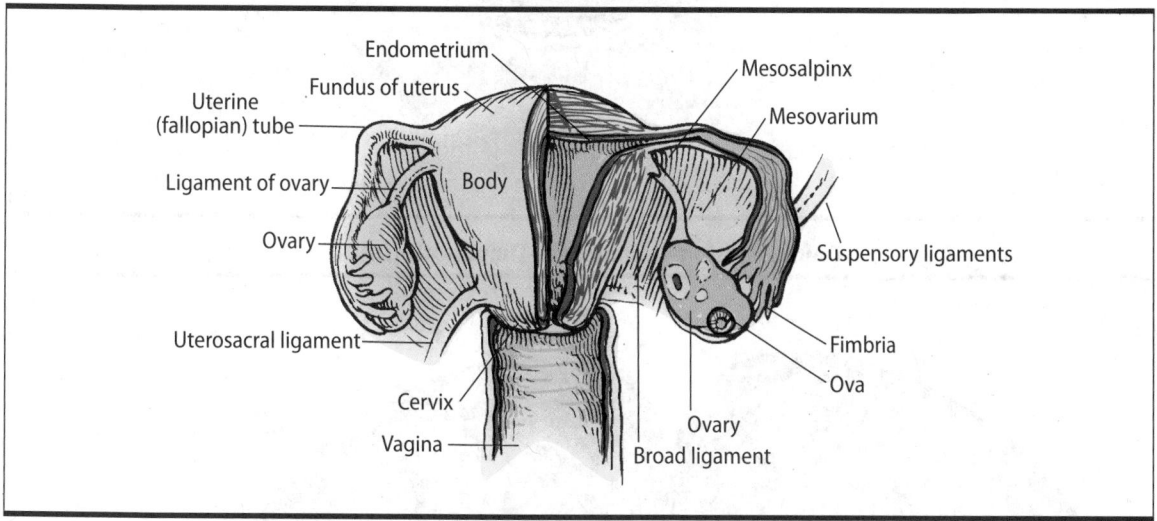

Female Genitourinary Tract Lateral View

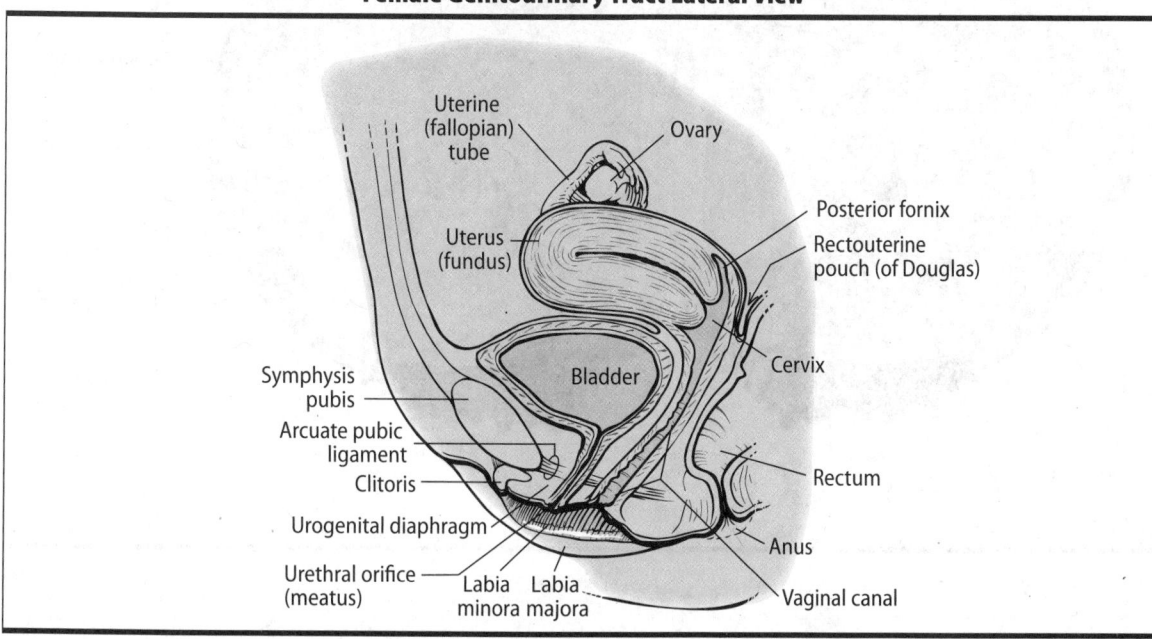

Chapter 15. Pregnancy, Childbirth and the Puerperium (O00–O9A)

Term Pregnancy – Single Gestation

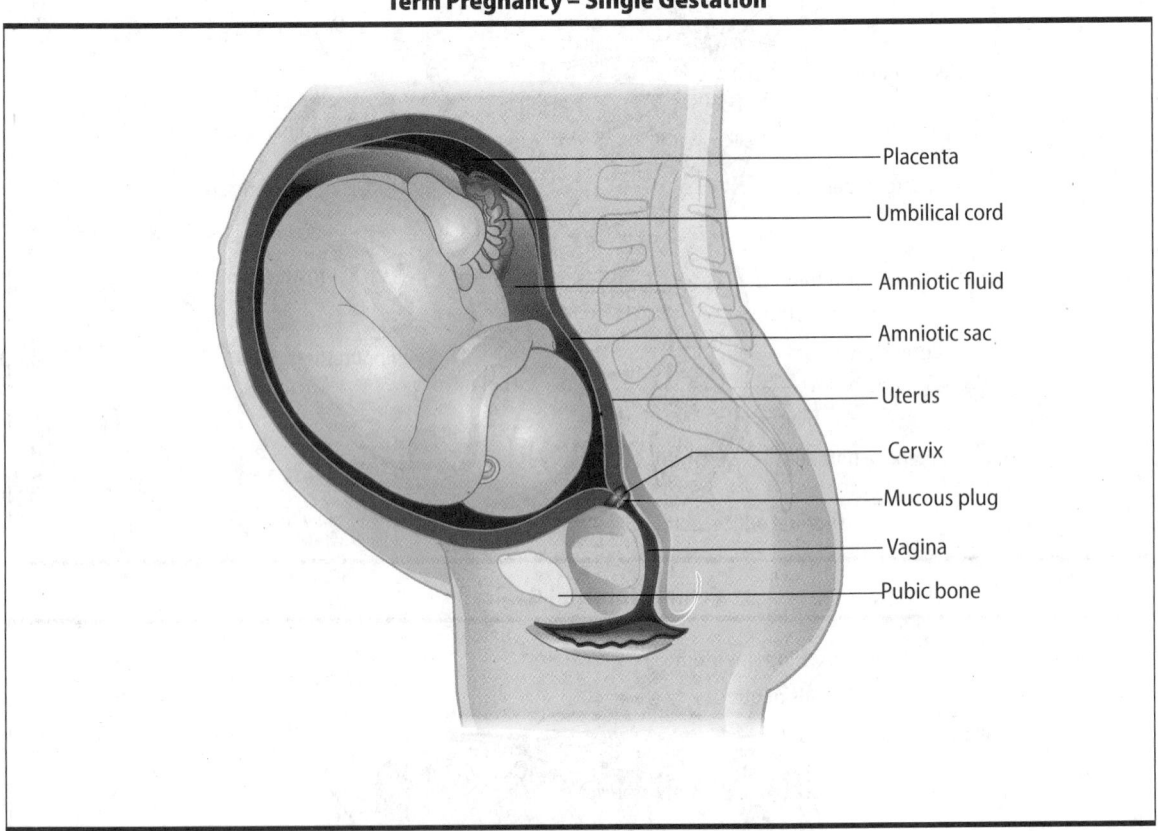

Placenta
Umbilical cord
Amniotic fluid
Amniotic sac
Uterus
Cervix
Mucous plug
Vagina
Pubic bone

Twin Gestation–Dichorionic–Diamniotic (DI-DI)

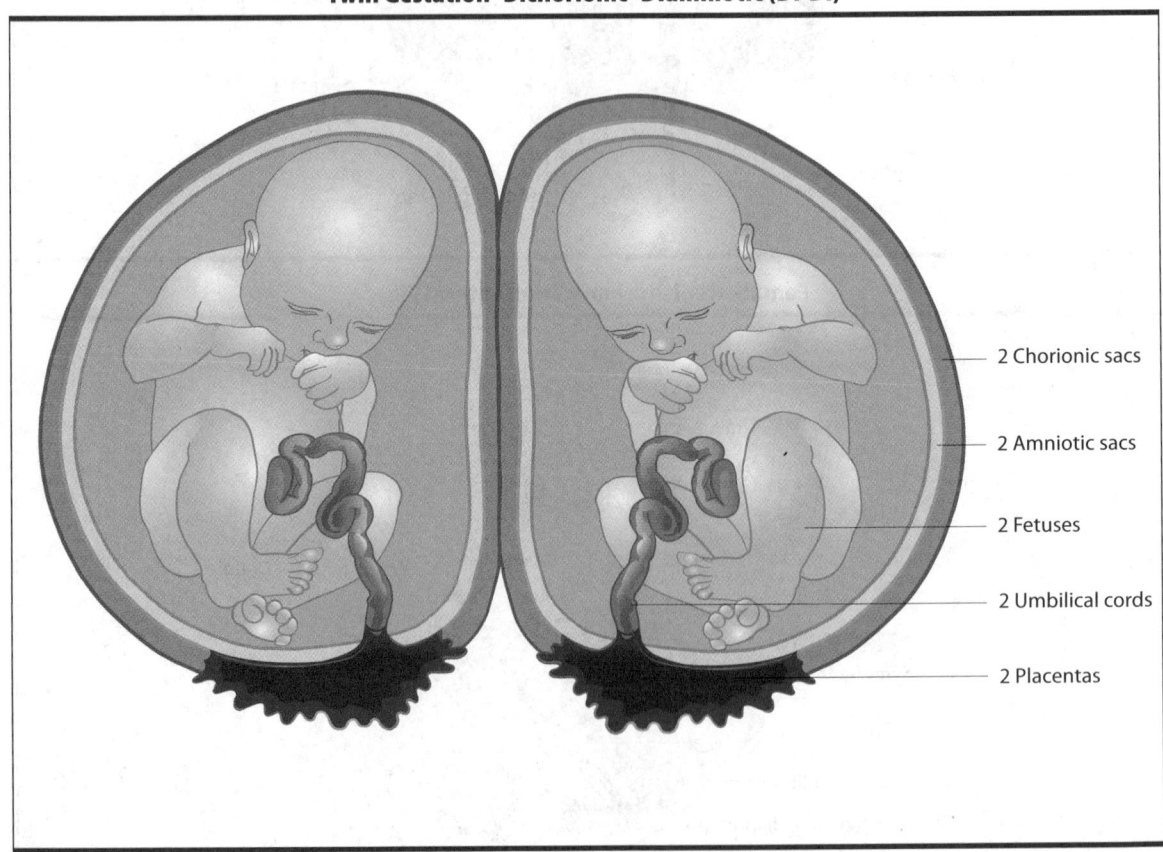

2 Chorionic sacs
2 Amniotic sacs
2 Fetuses
2 Umbilical cords
2 Placentas

Twin Gestation–Monochorionic–Diamniotic (MO-DI)

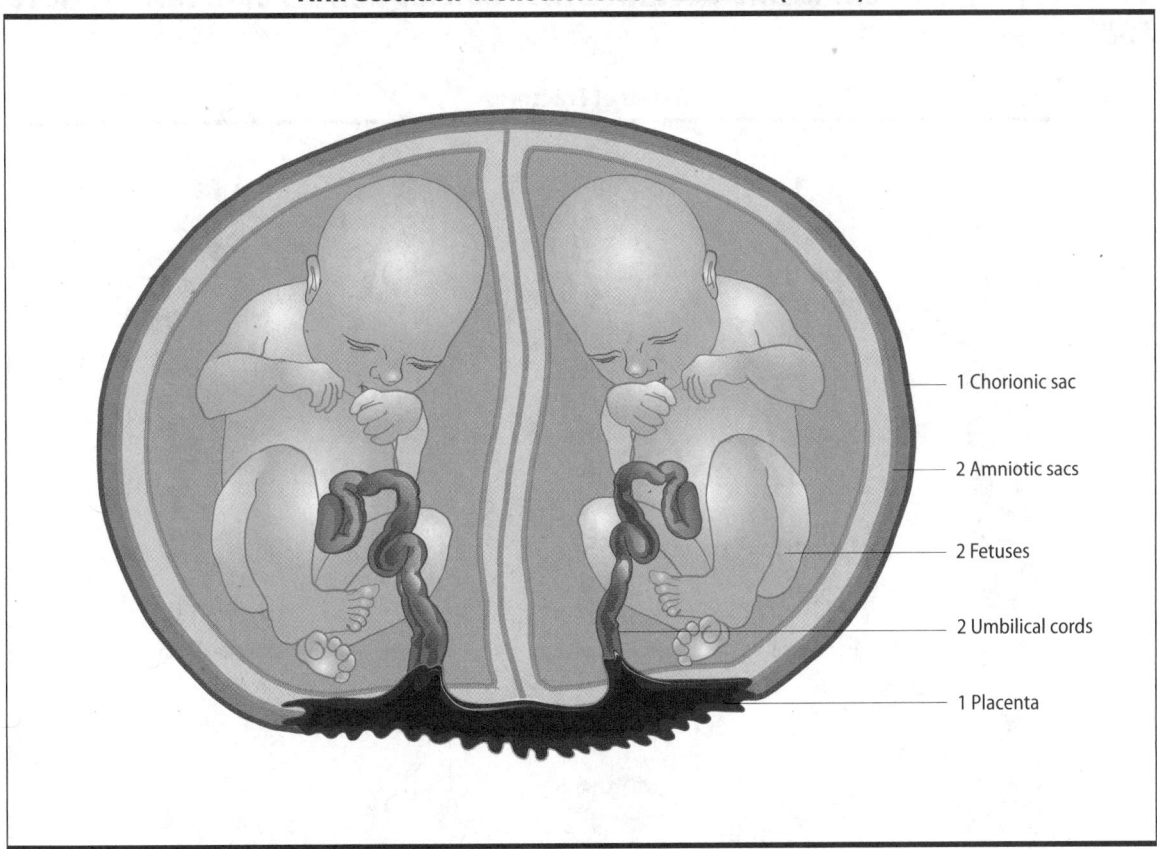

1 Chorionic sac

2 Amniotic sacs

2 Fetuses

2 Umbilical cords

1 Placenta

Twin Gestation–Monochorionic–Monoamniotic (MO-MO)

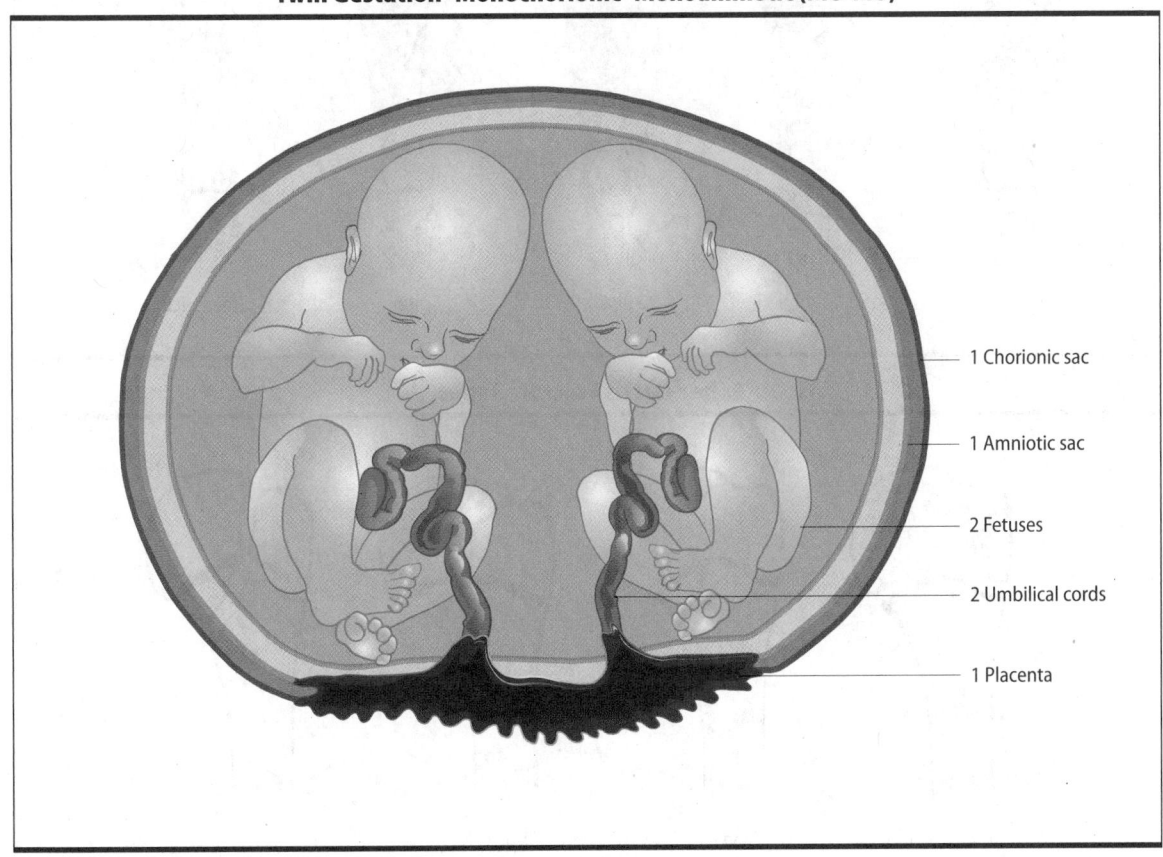

1 Chorionic sac

1 Amniotic sac

2 Fetuses

2 Umbilical cords

1 Placenta

Chapter 19. Injury, Poisoning and Certain Other Consequences of External Causes (SØØ–T88)

Types of Fractures

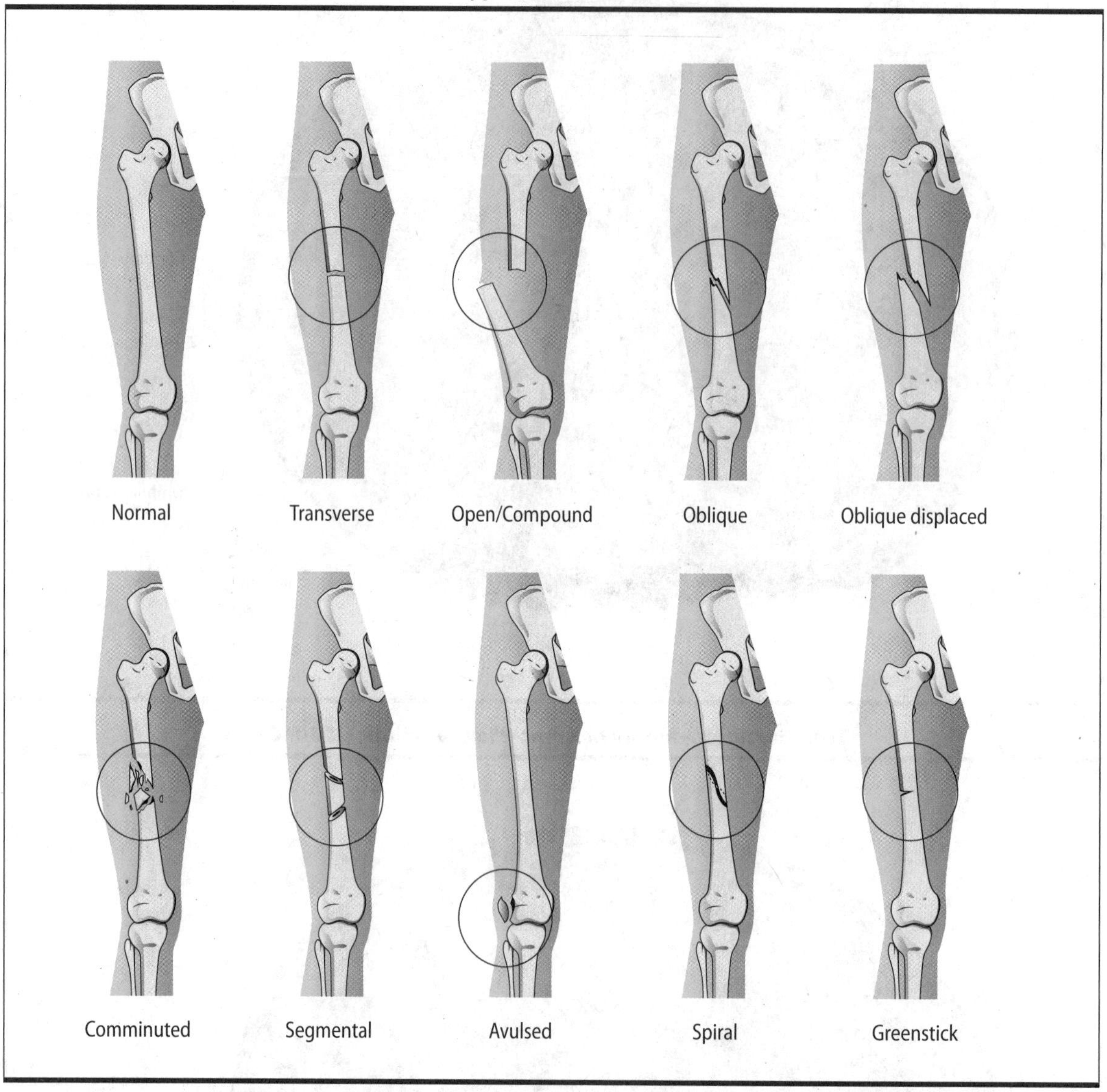

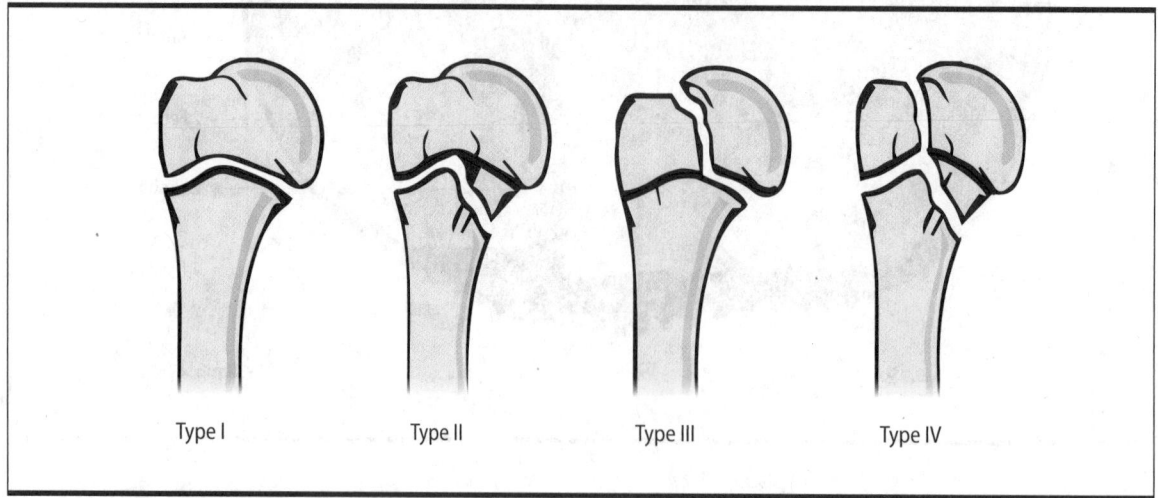

Normal	Transverse	Open/Compound	Oblique	Oblique displaced

Comminuted	Segmental	Avulsed	Spiral	Greenstick

Salter-Harris Fracture Types

Type I	Type II	Type III	Type IV